HUMAN NEEDS OVERVIEW: MOBILITY, SENSATION, AND COGNITION

UNIT X
Problems of Mobility, Sensation, and Cognition: Management of Patients with Problems of the Nervous System

43 Assessment of the Nervous System, 928
44 Care of Patients with Problems of the Central Nervous System: The Brain, 950
45 Care of Patients with Problems of the Central Nervous System: The Spinal Cord, 983
46 Care of Patients with Problems of the Peripheral Nervous System, 1011
47 Care of Critically Ill Patients with Neurologic Problems, 1029

UNIT XI
Problems of Sensation: Management of Patients with Problems of the Sensory System

48 Assessment of the Eye and Vision, 1070
49 Care of Patients with Eye and Vision Problems, 1084
50 Assessment of the Ear and Hearing, 1109
51 Care of Patients with Ear and Hearing Problems, 1120

UNIT XII
Problems of Mobility: Management of Patients with Problems of the Musculoskeletal System

52 Assessment of the Musculoskeletal System, 1140
53 Care of Patients with Musculoskeletal Problems, 1152
54 Care of Patients with Musculoskeletal Trauma, 1178

HUMAN NEEDS OVERVIEW: NUTRITION, METABOLISM, AND BOWEL ELIMINATION

UNIT XIII
Problems of Digestion, Nutrition, and Elimination: Management of Patients with Problems of the Gastrointestinal System

55 Assessment of the Gastrointestinal System, 1216
56 Care of Patients with Oral Cavity Problems, 1231
57 Care of Patients with Esophageal Problems, 1243
58 Care of Patients with Stomach Disorders, 1265
59 Care of Patients with Noninflammatory Intestinal Disorders, 1289
60 Care of Patients with Inflammatory Intestinal Disorders, 1315
61 Care of Patients with Liver Problems, 1344
62 Care of Patients with Problems of the Biliary System and Pancreas, 1366
63 Care of Patients with Malnutrition and Obesity, 1386

UNIT XIV
Problems of Regulation and Metabolism: Management of Patients with Problems of the Endocrine System

64 Assessment of the Endocrine System, 1412
65 Care of Patients with Pituitary and Adrenal Gland Problems, 1425
66 Care of Patients with Problems of the Thyroid and Parathyroid Glands, 1448
67 Care of Patients with Diabetes Mellitus, 1465

HUMAN NEEDS OVERVIEW: URINARY ELIMINATION

UNIT XV
Problems of Excretion: Management of Patients with Problems of the Renal/Urinary System

68 Assessment of the Renal/Urinary System, 1526
69 Care of Patients with Urinary Problems, 1550
70 Care of Patients with Renal Disorders, 1581
71 Care of Patients with Acute Renal Failure and Chronic Kidney Disease, 1600

84
ms,
:ase,

REGISTER TODAY!

evolve
learning system

To access your Student Resources, visit:

http://evolve.elsevier.com/Iggy/

Evolve Student Resources for Ignatavicius & Workman: Medical-Surgical Nursing: Patient-Centered Collaborative Care, *6th edition, include the following:*

- **Self-Assessment Questions for the NCLEX® Examination**
  Interactive NCLEX Examination–style review questions are divided by chapter and address each chapter's Learning Outcomes to help you review important text material and study for the NCLEX Examination.
- **Prioritization and Delegation Questions for the NCLEX® Examination**
  Focusing on the increasingly important NCLEX Examination themes of prioritization and delegation, these interactive questions will help direct your study and reinforce chapter content.
- **Pharmacology Review Questions for the NCLEX® Examination**
  Strengthen your understanding of drug therapy and prepare for safe medication administration—a critical emphasis of the NCLEX Examination. Answers and rationales are provided for each of these interactive questions.
- **Answer Guidelines for Decision-Making Challenges and NCLEX® Examination Challenges**
  The Decision-Making Challenges and NCLEX Examination Challenges that appear throughout the text provide a safe and effective means of simulating the on-the-job decision making that you need to perform in the clinical setting. Suggested Answer Guidelines are provided for these exercises, allowing you to gauge your mastery of essential content and your readiness for clinical practice.
- **Audio Key Points**
  Downloadable MP3 audio files for audio CDs and MP3 players provide an innovative way for auditory learners to review essential chapter content on the go. Reviews include point-by-point highlights from each chapter, along with integrated quizzes.
- **Additional Resources**
  Audio Glossary, Interactive Concept Maps, Concept Map Creator, Fluid and Electrolyte Tutorial, Health Assessment Image Collection, Video Clips, Audio Clips, Animations, and more!

ELSEVIER

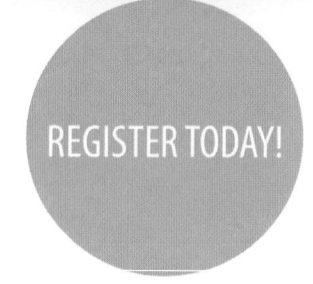

Medical-Surgical Nursing

Patient-Centered Collaborative Care

6
SIXTH EDITION

Medical-Surgical Nursing

Patient-Centered Collaborative Care

Donna D. Ignatavicius, MS, RN, ANEF
Speaker and Curriculum Consultant for Academic Nursing Programs
Founder, Boot Camp for Nurse Educators®
President, DI Associates, Inc.
Placitas, New Mexico

M. Linda Workman, PhD, RN, FAAN
Senior Volunteer Faculty
College of Nursing
University of Cincinnati
Cincinnati, Ohio;
Formerly Gertrude Perkins Oliva Professor of Oncology
Frances Payne Bolton School of Nursing
Case Western Reserve University
Cleveland, Ohio

SAUNDERS
ELSEVIER

SAUNDERS
ELSEVIER

11830 Westline Industrial Drive
St. Louis, Missouri 63146

MEDICAL-SURGICAL NURSING: PATIENT-CENTERED COLLABORATIVE CARE

ISBN (Single volume): 978-1-4160-3762-0
ISBN (2-volume set): 978-1-4160-4903-6

Notice

Knowledge and best practice in this field are constantly changing. As new research and experience broaden our knowledge, changes in practice, treatment and drug therapy may become necessary or appropriate. Readers are advised to check the most current information provided (i) on procedures featured or (ii) by the manufacturer of each product to be administered, to verify the recommended dose or formula, the method and duration of administration, and contraindications. It is the responsibility of the practitioner, relying on their own experience and knowledge of the patient, to make diagnoses, to determine dosages and the best treatment for each individual patient, and to take all appropriate safety precautions. To the fullest extent of the law, neither the Publisher nor the Authors assume any liability for any injury and/or damage to persons or property arising out of or related to any use of the material contained in this book.

The Publisher

Library of Congress Cataloging-in-Publication Data

Medical-surgical nursing : patient-centered collaborative care / [edited by] Donna D. Ignatavicius, M. Linda Workman. -- 6th ed.
p. ; cm.
Includes bibliographical references and index.
ISBN 978-1-4160-3762-0 (single volume, hardcover : alk. paper) -- ISBN 978-1-4160-4903-6 (2 volume set, hardcover : alk. paper) 1. Nursing. 2. Surgical nursing. I. Ignatavicius, Donna D. II. Workman, M. Linda.
[DNLM: 1. Perioperative Nursing. WY 161 M4897 2009]
RT41.I36 2009
617'.0231--dc22
2008045867

Senior Editor: Lee Henderson
Senior Developmental Editor: Rae L. Robertson
Publishing Services Manager: Deborah L. Vogel
Senior Project Manager: Jodi M. Willard
Design Direction: Maggie Reid

Printed in the United States of America
Last digit is the print number: 9 8 7 6 5 4 3 2

To Charles and Stephanie
Thank you for your unending support, love, and understanding during every edition;
I could not do this without you!
To students and faculty
Thank you for your feedback, support, and guidance during my journey as an author.

Donna

To students everywhere, who inspire us to make each edition better.

Linda

About the Authors

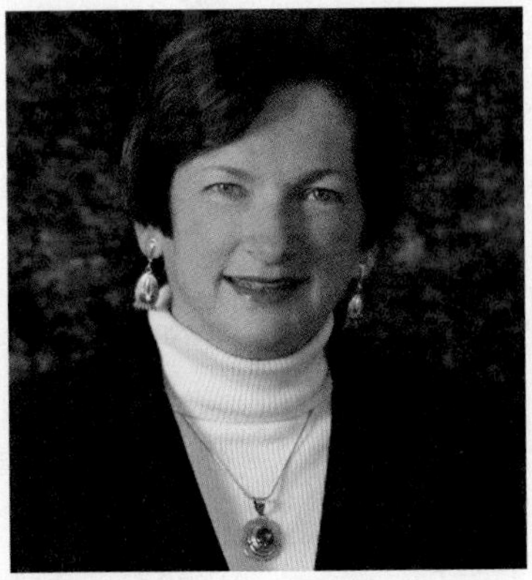

Donna D. Ignatavicius received her diploma in nursing from the Peninsula General School of Nursing in Salisbury, Maryland. After working as a charge nurse in medical-surgical nursing, she became an instructor in staff development at the University of Maryland Medical Center. She then received her BSN from the University of Maryland School of Nursing. For 5 years she taught in several schools of nursing while working toward her MS in Nursing, which she received in 1981. Donna then taught in the BSN program at the University of Maryland, after which she continued to pursue her interest in gerontology and accepted the position of Director of Nursing of a major skilled-nursing facility in her home state of Maryland. She has been a certified gerontologic nurse since 1989 and was certified in nursing case management by the American Nurses Credentialing Center in 1998. Recently she has taught in associate degree nursing programs. Through her consulting and faculty development workshops, Donna has gained national recognition in nursing education. She is currently the President of DI Associates, Inc. (http://www.diassociates.com/), a company dedicated to improving health care through education and consultation for both faculty and clinicians. In recognition of her contributions to the field, she was inducted as a Fellow of the prestigious Academy of Nursing Education in 2007.

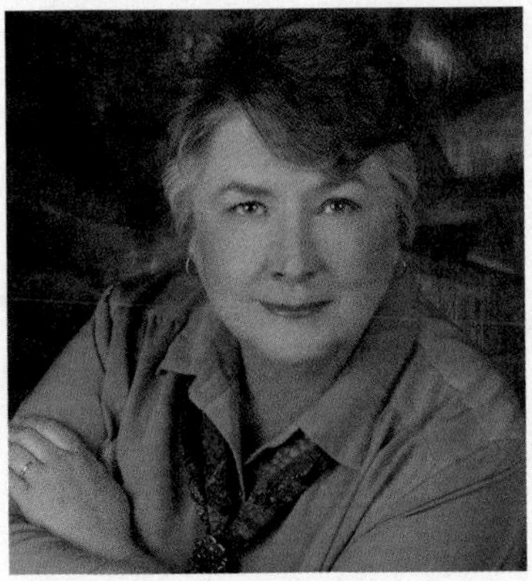

M. Linda Workman, a native of Canada, received her BSN from the University of Cincinnati College of Nursing and Health. After serving in the U.S. Army Nurse Corps and working as an Assistant Head Nurse and Head Nurse in civilian hospitals, Linda earned her MSN from the University of Cincinnati College of Nursing and a PhD in Developmental Biology from the University of Cincinnati College of Arts and Sciences. Linda's 30 years of academic experience include teaching at the diploma, associate degree, baccalaureate, and master's levels. Her areas of teaching expertise include medical-surgical nursing, physiology, pathophysiology, genetics, oncology, and immunology. Linda has been recognized nationally for her teaching expertise and was inducted as a fellow into the American Academy of Nursing in 1992. She received the Excellence in Teaching award at the University of Cincinnati in 2001 and at Case Western Reserve University in 2004, 2005, and 2006. She is a former American Cancer Society Professor of Oncology Nursing and held an endowed chair in oncology for 5 years. Currently, she is Senior Volunteer Faculty at the College of Nursing, University of Cincinnati.

Consultants

Elaine Bishop Kennedy, EdD, RN
Professor, Department of Nursing
Wor-Wic Community College
Salisbury, Maryland
Concept Maps
Plans of Care

Richard Lintner, RT(R), (CV), (MR), (CT), ARRT
Program Director
School of Interventional Radiology;
Manager
Interventional Radiology
Kansas University Medical Center
Kansas City, Kansas
Consultant for interventional radiology

Contributors

Lynne Brophy, RN, MSN, AOCN
Oncology Clinical Nurse Specialist
Bethesda North Hospital
Cincinnati, Ohio

Vicki Brownrigg, PhD, FNP
Associate Professor
Beth-El College of Nursing and Health Sciences
University of Colorado at Colorado Springs
Colorado Springs, Colorado

Katherine L. Byar, MSN, APRN, BC
Hematological Malignancy Nurse Practitioner
University of Nebraska Medical Center
Omaha, Nebraska

Robin Chard, PhD, RN, CNOR
Clinical Assistant Professor
Florida International University
Miami, Florida

John M. Clochesy, PhD, RN, FAAN, FCCM
Independence Foundation Professor of Nursing Education
Frances Payne Bolton School of Nursing
Case Western Reserve University
Cleveland, Ohio

Tammy Coffee, MSN, ACNP, BC
MetroHealth Medical Center
Cleveland, Ohio

Janice Cuzzell, MA, RN
Certified Wound Specialist
Savannah, Georgia

Karrie K. Dietzen, MSN, CGRN
Assistant Professor
Ivy Tech Community College
Muncie, Indiana

Alexandra Falkowski, RN
Nurse Manager, Vascular Access Nursing
Christiana Care Health System
Newark, Delaware

Pat Mahaffee Gingrich, MSN, RN-C, WHNP
Clinical Assistant Professor, School of Nursing
University of North Carolina
Chapel Hill, North Carolina

Kathy A. Hausman, PhD, RN-C
Chair of Nursing and Allied Health
Baltimore City Community College
Baltimore, Maryland

Ronald L. Hickman, Jr., PhD, RN, ACNP-BC
Lecturer and Clinical Research Scholar
Frances Payne Bolton School of Nursing
Case Western Reserve University
Cleveland, Ohio

Mary F. Justice, MSN, RNC, CNE
Associate Professor
University of Cincinnati—Raymond Walters College
Cincinnati, Ohio

Mary K. Kazanowski, PhD, ARNP, BC, CHPN
Professor
Department of Nursing
Saint Anselm College;
Level IV RN, Hospice Department
VNA of Manchester and Southern New Hampshire
Manchester, New Hampshire;
ARNP Wellstone House
Raymond, New Hampshire

Linda A. LaCharity, RN, PhD
Assistant Professor, College of Nursing
University of Cincinnati
Cincinnati, Ohio

Linda Laskowski-Jones, RN, MS, ACNS-BC, CCRN, CEN
Vice President, Emergency, Trauma & Aeromedical Services
Christiana Care Health System
Wilmington, Delaware

Deitra Leonard Lowdermilk, PhD, RNC, FAAN
Adjunct Professor
School of Nursing
University of North Carolina
Chapel Hill, North Carolina

Lora L. McGuire, MS, RN
Professor
Department of Nursing Education and Allied Health
Joliet Junior College
Joliet, Illinois

Margaret Elaine McLeod, MSN, BC-ADM, ACNS-BC, CDE
Clinical Nurse Specialist
Veterans Affairs Medical Center
Tennessee Valley Healthcare System
Nashville, Tennessee

Cathy A. Murray, RN, MSN, CNS, OCNS-C
Clinical Nurse Specialist
Ball Memorial Hospital
Muncie, Indiana

Sarah Pettus, MSN, RN, IBCLC
Assistant Professor
Bellin College of Nursing
Green Way, Wisconsin

Tommie Wright Pniewski, MSN, RN, CNAA, BC
Professor of Nursing
Hopkinsville Community College
Hopkinsville, Kentucky

Harry C. Rees, MSN
Research Intervention Nurse
MetroHealth Medical Center
Cleveland, Ohio

Karen Ruschman, ARNP-C
TriState Gastroenterology Associates
Crestview Hills, Kentucky;
Staff Provider
St. Elizabeth Medical Center
Edgewood, Kentucky;
St. Luke's Hospital
Fort Thomas, Kentucky

Jacquelyn Ann Russek, RN, PhD(c), LTC, AN, USAR
Active Duty
U.S. Army

James G. Sampson, DNP, NP-C
Adult Nurse Practitioner, Internal Medicine
Infectious Disease Clinics
Denver Health Medical Center
Denver, Colorado

Karen L. Toulson, MSN, RN, CEN, NE-BC
Nurse Manager, Emergency Department
Christiana Care Health Services—Christiana Hospital
Newark, Delaware

Shirley E. Van Zandt, MS, MPH, CRNP
Instructor, School of Nursing
Johns Hopkins University
Baltimore, Maryland

Sharon Henry Walicek, MEd, MSN, RN, CCRN, CCNS, CVN, ANP-BC
Professor of Nursing
Elgin Community College;
Cardiac Nurse Practitioner
Elgin Cardiology Associates
Elgin, Illinois

Chris Winkelman, PhD, RN
Assistant Professor
Frances Payne Bolton School of Nursing
Case Western Reserve University;
Staff Nurse, Trauma and Critical Care
MetroHealth Medical Center
Cleveland, Ohio

Pamela C. Zickafoose, EdD, MSN, RN, CAN, BC
Instructor, Department of Nursing
Delaware Technical & Community College—Terry Campus;
ICU Staff Nurse
Bayhealth Medical Center
Dover, Delaware

Reviewers

Michael D. Aldridge, MSN, RN, CCRN, CNS
Instructor in Clinical Nursing
School of Nursing
The University of Texas at Austin
Austin, Texas

Rochelle R. Armola, MSN, RN, CNS
Clinical Nurse Specialist
Division of Critical Care
The Toledo Hospital
Toledo, Ohio

Bridget Bailey, MSN, RN
Associate Professor
Iowa Lakes Community College
Emmetsburg, Iowa

Susan C. Baltrus, MSN, RNC
Director
College of Nursing and Health Professions
Central Maine Medical Center
Lewiston, Maine

Theresa A. Beery, PhD, RN, ACNP
Professor
College of Nursing
University of Cincinnati
Cincinnati, Ohio

Sophia Beydoun, MSN, RN
Nursing Instructor
Henry Ford Community College
Dearborn, Michigan

Jan E. Lawrenz Blasi, MSN, RN
Nursing Instructor
Department of Nursing
Pratt Community College
Pratt, Kansas

Diane C. Bridge, MSN
Nursing Instructor
Maranatha Baptist Bible College
Watertown, Wisconsin

Michele Ruth Bunning, MSN, RN
Associate Professor
Good Samaritan College of Nursing & Health Science
Cincinnati, Ohio

Kathy Burlingame, MSN, CCRN
Associate Dean of Nursing
Minnesota State Community and Technical College;
Intensive Care Unit Nurse
St. Mary's Regional Health Center
Detroit Lakes, Minnesota

Kathryn A. Carney, MSN, APRN, BC
Nursing Instructor
Pennsylvania State University—Worthington-Scranton Campus
Dunmore, Pennsylvania

Gretchen J. Carrougher, MSN, RN
Department of Surgery
University of Washington Burn Center at Harborview Medical Center
Seattle, Washington

Catherine M. Concert, MSN, RN, APRN, BC, FNP, CGRN
Long Island University;
Wyckoff Heights Medical Center
Brooklyn, New York

Patricia B. Conley, MSN, RN
Staff Nurse, Progressive Care Unit
Research Medical Center
Kansas City, Missouri

Angela N. Cornelius, MSN, RN, OCN, CNE
Alumni Nurse, Medical Oncology
Boone Hospital Center
Columbia, Missouri

Patricia A. Cowan, PhD, RN
Associate Professor
College of Nursing
University of Tennessee Health Science Center
Memphis, Tennessee

Shannon M. Donahue, BSN, RN
Assistant Professor of Nursing Education
Santa Fe Community College
Santa Fe, New Mexico

Carrin L. Dvorak, MSN, RN
Assistant Professor
Cuyahoga Community College
Cleveland, Ohio

Pamela J. Ellis, MSN, RN, MS/HCA
Resident Faculty
Mohave Community College
Bullhead City, Kingman, and Lake Havasu City, Arizona

Sherlyn A. Farrish-Barner, MSN
Nursing Educator
Germanna Community College
Locust Grove, Virginia

Linda Fluharty, MSN, RNC
Associate Professor
Ivy Tech Community College
Indianapolis, Indiana

Susan M. Ford, MSN, RN
Nursing Faculty
Tacoma Community College
Tacoma, Washington

Cheryl P. Franklin, MSN, RN, DNS
Assistant Dean
Department of Nursing
Nicholls State University
Thibodaux, Louisiana

Madeline Gervase, PhD(c), MSN, RN, CCRN, FNP
Assistant Professor College of Nursing
Seton Hall University
South Orange, New Jersey

Sherry R. Glover, BSN, RNC
Resident Faculty
Beaufort County Community College
Washington, North Carolina

Linda M. Graham, MSN, RN
Assistant Professor
Thomas More College
Crestview Hills, Kentucky

Audrey Mosley Green, MSN, RN
Nursing Instructor
Gadsden State Community College
Gadsden, Alabama

Annette M. Gunderman, EdD, MSN, RN
Associate Professor of Nursing
Bloomsburg University
Bloomsburg, Pennsylvania

Emily Harder, BScN, RN
Nursing Faculty
Saskatchewan Institute of Applied Science and Technology—Kelsey Campus
Saskatoon, Saskatchewan, Canada

Corinne C. Harmon, EdD, MS, RN, AOCN
Assistant Professor
School of Nursing
Clemson University
Clemson, South Carolina

Susan J. Hart, MSN, RN
Faculty Associate
College of Nursing
Seton Hall University
South Orange, New Jersey

Connie Sue Heflin, MSN, RN, CNE
Professor of Nursing
West Kentucky Community and Technical College
Paducah, Kentucky

Elizabeth A. Hoffman, MS, RN
Assistant Professor of Nursing
Dakota Wesleyan University
Mitchell, South Dakota

Sherrie Nan Holliman, MSN, RN
Resident Faculty, Department of Professional Nursing
School of Health Professions
Baptist Health System
San Antonio, Texas

S. Esther D. Holzbauer, MSN, RN
Assistant Professor of Nursing
Mount Marty College
Yankton, South Dakota

Michelle Hough, MS, RN
Adjunct Professor ADN Evening Option
Massachusetts Bay Community College
Framingham, Massachusetts

Linda K. Houseal, MSN, RN, ACNP, C, CCRN
Clinical Program Manager
Meridian Health Ann May Center for Nursing
Neptune, New Jersey

Donna Walker Hubbard, MSN, RN, CNN
Assistant Professor
College of Nursing
University of Mary Hardin-Baylor
Belton, Texas

Candace Isabell, MSN, RN
RN Educator
St. Anthony's Medical Center;
Adjunct Clinical Faculty
Maryville University
St. Louis, Missouri

Tatiana Isaeff, EdD, RN
Professor of Nursing
College of San Mateo;
Quality Coordinator
Kaiser Home Health and Hospice
San Mateo, California

Kynthia James, MSN, RN
Associate Degree Nursing Instructor
Southwest Georgia Technical College
Thomasville, Georgia

Eileen Kinsella, MS, RN
Associate Professor of Nursing
State University of New York—Morrisville
Morrisville, New York

Beth Knight-Matous, MSN, RN
Instructor
Registered Nursing Program
Sentara School of Health Professions
Chesapeake, Virginia

Barbara A. Konopka, MSN, RN, CCRN, CEN
Nursing Instructor
Pennsylvania State University—Worthington-Scranton Campus
Dunmore, Pennsylvania

Catherine E. Lein, MS, APRN, BC, FNP
Assistant Professor
College of Nursing
Michigan State University
East Lansing, Michigan

Margaret A. Lynch, MSN, FNP, AACRN
Practice Administrator, The Zinberg Clinic
The Cambridge Health Alliance
Cambridge, Massachusetts

Mary Beth Flynn Makic, PhD, RN, CNS, CCNS, CCRN
Clinical Nurse Specialist/Educator
University of Colorado Hospital;
Senior Instructor
School of Nursing
University of Colorado at Denver Health Sciences Center
Denver, Colorado

Kim H. McAlister, MSN, RN
Instructor of Clinical Nursing
San Antonio School of Nursing
University of Texas Health Science Center
San Antonio, Texas

Regina P. McFerren, MSN, RN
Assistant Professor of Nursing
College of Nursing
University of Southern Nevada
Henderson, Nevada

Tara McMillan-Queen, MSN, APRN, BC
Nursing Faculty
Mercy School of Nursing
Carolinas Medical Center—Mercy
Charlotte, North Carolina

Donna T. Mitchell, PhD, RN
Director and Professor
Holzer School of Nursing
University of Rio Grande
Rio Grande, Ohio

Kathleen E. Molden, MSN, RN, CNE
Instructor
School of Nursing
St. Francis Medical Center
Trenton, New Jersey

Sharon E. Moran, MSN, RN, MPH, CS
Associate Professor of Nursing
Hawaii Community College
University of Hawaii
Hilo, Hawaii

Kelly A. Morris, MSN, RN, DNPc
Associate Professor
Nursing Division
Owensboro Community and Technical College
Owensboro, Kentucky

Elizabeth Nix, MSN, APRN-BC, CDE, CPT, ET
Assistant Professor of Nursing
Arkansas State University
Jonesboro, Arkansas

Barbara Penprase, PhD, RN, CNOR
Associate Professor and Director of Accelerated Second Degree Nursing Program
School of Nursing
Oakland University
Rochester, Michigan

Joseph R. Poole Jr., MSN, RN
Nursing Instructor and NLN Ambassador
Central New Mexico Community College
Albuquerque, New Mexico

Bridget A. Porta, MSN, RN, APN
Instructor
Seton Hall University
South Orange, New Jersey;
Educator
Visiting Nurse Association of Central Jersey
Red Bank, New Jersey

Betty Ann Powers-Luhn, MSN, RN
Assistant Professor of Nursing
University of Southern Nevada
Henderson, Nevada

Sharon R. Redding, MSN, RN, CNE
Associate Professor of Nursing
College of Saint Mary;
Staff Nurse
Alegent Bergan Mercy Medical Center
Omaha, Nebraska

Charlene M. Romer, PhD, RN
Associate Professor
Clayton State University
Morrow, Georgia

Erin Rosfeld, MSN, RN
Nursing Faculty
Pueblo Community College
Pueblo, Colorado

Nancy Jo Ross, MSN, RN
Instructor
College of Nursing and Health Professions
Central Maine Medical Center
Lewiston, Maine

Connie J. Schroeder, MSN, RN
Director of Nursing Education
Danville Area Community College
Danville, Illinois

Tamara Sadie Seavey, MSN, RN, BC
Nursing Professor
Central Arizona College
Coolidge, Arizona

Jaime Michelle Sinutko, BSN, RN
RN Project Manager
Oakland University
Rochester, Michigan;
Emergency Room Nurse
William Beaumont Hospital
Troy, Michigan

Sharon Souter, PhD, RN, CNE
Dean and Associate Professor
University of Mary Hardin-Baylor
Belton, Texas

Susan Spooner-Holland, MSN, APRN, BC, GNP
Assistant Professor
College of Nursing
Northwestern State University
Shreveport, Louisiana

Ann D. Sprengel, EdD, MSN, RN
Professor
Southeast Missouri State University
Cape Girardeau, Missouri

Barbara Kim Cundiff Stevens, MSN
Assistant Professor
Holzer School of Nursing
University of Rio Grande
Rio Grande, Ohio

Wendy B. Stewart, MSN, RN
Professor of Nursing
San Jacinto College—Central
Pasadena, Texas

Rebeca M. Tacy, MSN, RN, CFN
Assistant Professor
Thomas More College
Crestview Hills, Kentucky;
St. Elizabeth Medical Center
Edgewood, Kentucky

Jean M. Truman, MSN, RN, CMSRN
ASN Program Coordinator and Assistant Professor of Nursing
Division of Biological and Health Sciences
University of Pittsburgh at Bradford
Bradford, Pennsylvania

Samantha J. Venable, MSN, RN, FNP
Nursing Instructor
Department of Health Sciences
Saddleback College
Mission Viejo, California

Wendi Walcer, MSN, RNC, NP
Obstetrics Nurse Practitioner
Foothills Primary Care Network
Calgary, Alberta, Canada

Coleen M. Weil, MSN, RN
Assistant Professor of Nursing
Wor-Wic Community College
Salisbury, Maryland

Cecilia Elaine Wilson, MSN, RN, CPN
Associate Clinical Professor
College of Nursing
Texas Woman's University
Dallas, Texas

Rebecca Lee Zumbo, BSN, RN
Adjunct Faculty
Okaloosa-Walton College
Niceville, Florida;
Registered Nurse
Fort Walton Beach Medical Center
Fort Walton Beach, Florida

Preface

The first edition of this text, entitled *Medical-Surgical Nursing: A Nursing Process Approach,* received widespread acclaim in the early 1990s. The following four editions built on that achievement and further solidified the book's position as a major trendsetter for the practice of adult health nursing. Now in its sixth edition, "Iggy" charts an essential course for the future of adult nursing practice—a course reflected in its current title: *Medical-Surgical Nursing: Patient-Centered Collaborative Care.* The focus of this new edition is to help students learn how to provide safe, quality care that is both patient-centered and collaborative.

The new title for this edition was carefully chosen to emphasize the nurse's role in providing patient care in collaboration with members of the interdisciplinary team in both acute care and community-based settings. The Institute of Medicine, The Joint Commission, and other health care organizations have called for all health professionals to coordinate and deliver patient care as a collaborative care team.

Patient safety is also emphasized in this edition. A new icon highlights important content that reflects The Joint Commission's National Patient Safety Goals initiative. The National Patient Safety Goals themselves are included in the back of the book, and safety points are highlighted in the chapter-ending Key Points.

KEY THEMES FOR THE SIXTH EDITION

Throughout the sixth edition, the term "client" has been replaced with "patient." Although the use of these terms remains a subject of discussion among nursing educators, we have not defined the patient as a dependent person. Rather, the patient can be an individual, a family, or a group who has rights that are respected in a mutually trusting nurse-patient relationship. Health care agencies and professional organizations use "patient" in their practice and publications, and many nursing organizations also support the term.

As in the extraordinarily successful fifth edition, a key theme of this edition is critical thinking, and the sixth edition sharpens that focus to an emphasis on clinical decision making. To help achieve that new focus, case-based Decision-Making Challenges have been inserted throughout the text. These exercises provide clinical situations in which students can practice on-the-spot decision making to help prepare them for the fast-paced world of medical-surgical nursing. Suggested answer guidelines for these Decision-Making Challenges are provided on the book's Evolve website (http://evolve.elsevier.com/Iggy/).

In addition to this key theme of clinical decision making, the sixth edition emphasizes "readiness"—readiness for the NCLEX® Examination, readiness for major emergencies such as we saw in the aftermath of 9/11, readiness for safe drug administration, and readiness for the new world of genetics that is unfolding before us.

As the nursing shortage becomes more acute, it is more critical than ever that students be ready to pass the licensure exam on the first try. To help both students and faculty reach that outcome, the sixth edition continues to include an innovative end-of-chapter feature called "Get Ready for the NCLEX Examination!" This unique and popular learning aid consists of a list of Key Points *organized by NCLEX Client Needs Category* as found in the NCLEX Test Plan. Also included in these sections are highlighted reminders to go to the Companion CD or Evolve website for Self-Assessment Questions for the NCLEX Examination and to the Evolve website for Prioritization and Delegation Questions for the NCLEX Examination. The Self-Assessment Questions for the NCLEX Examination are keyed to the Learning Outcomes at the start of each chapter. These Learning Outcomes are now congruent with the objectives listed in the detailed NCLEX Test Plan and are organized by NCLEX Client Needs Categories.

The Prioritization and Delegation Questions for the NCLEX Examination focus on delegation and supervision, assignment, and prioritization/decision making. These questions are aimed at stimulating and validating decision making to help students apply the material covered in the text and integrate it with material they have learned elsewhere in the curriculum.

To further help students connect previously learned concepts with new information in the text, six Human Needs Overviews have been added to introduce groups of content units. These new and unique features review basic concepts learned in nursing fundamentals courses—such as oxygenation and protection—to help students make connections between these fundamental concepts and patient care for medical-surgical conditions. At the end of each body system chapter, these same concepts are applied (in a bulleted format) to the health problems presented in the chapter. Tanner's clinical judgment framework is used to help students apply these concepts (Tanner, 2006).* The components of this model include that clinical nurses:

- Notice
- Interpret
- Respond
- Reflect

This sixth edition includes a new chapter (Chapter 12: Concepts of Emergency and Disaster Preparedness) that introduces the principles of emergency nursing and disaster preparedness, including common triage systems. At the end of this chapter, we walk the reader through a case scenario related to bioterrorism and the response of the interdisciplinary health care team. Chapter 25 (Infection) has been expanded to increase attention to emerging infections and the rapid rise of multidrug-resistant organisms.

To promote readiness for safe drug administration, the sixth edition provides Pharmacology Review Questions for the NCLEX Examination on the Evolve website. These questions, which are keyed to the text with distinctive Evolve Online Pharm Review icons, give students practice in the concepts of safe drug and parenteral therapy administration—a major theme of the NCLEX Examination.

Additional themes carried over from the previous edition are an emphasis on women's health issues, genetic consider-

*Tanner, C.A. (2006). Thinking like a nurse: A research-based model of clinical judgement in nursing. *Journal of Nursing Education, 45*(6), 204-211.

ations, cultural awareness, complementary and alternative therapies, and the special needs of older adults. In addition, the concepts of case management and community-based care are interwoven throughout to help students identify the role of the nurse in providing continuing patient care.

CLINICAL CURRENCY AND ACCURACY

To ensure the book's currency and accuracy, we listened to students and faculty who have used the previous editions, focusing on their impressions of and experiences with the book. We reviewed documents crafted by a variety of health care organizations, including the Institute of Medicine (IOM), The Joint Commission (TJC), and the Institute for Healthcare Improvement (IHI). We also examined recent nursing education publications, such as those authored by the National League for Nursing (NLN) and the American Association of Colleges of Nursing (AACN). A thorough nursing education literature search helped us validate best practices and national health care trends to help shape the focus of the sixth edition.

We also commissioned in-depth reviews of every chapter by clinicians and instructors from across the United States and Canada and used their reviews to guide us in revising the chapters into their final form. A well-respected interventional radiologist ensured the accuracy of selected diagnostic testing procedures and associated patient care.

The results of these efforts are reflected in the sixth edition's:

- Strong, consistent focus on clinical decision making, patient-centered collaborative care, pathophysiology, drug therapy, evidence-based clinical practice, and community-based care.
- Foundation of relevant research and best practice guidelines.
- Emphasis on the critical "need to know" information that nurses must master to provide safe patient care.

Best Practice for Patient Safety & Quality Care charts help highlight the most important nursing care. In addition, our Evidence-Based Practice boxes now include a Commentary section, as well as a rating of the level of evidence based on a scale outlined in Chapter 1.

With today's knowledge explosion, it is easy for a book to become larger with each new edition. However, today's nursing students have limited time to absorb and begin to apply the information essential for safe patient care. Therefore for the sixth edition we redesigned the first unit to eliminate some of the content found in previous foundational courses. We limited our discussions to how these concepts are used in adult nursing, and we expanded Chapter 3 (Common Health Problems of Older Adults) and Chapter 4 (Cultural Aspects of Health and Illness). We also omitted content that was trivial and not "need to know" for nursing practice. Examples include excessive incidence and prevalence statistics and detailed surgical techniques. Content on fluids and electrolytes and acid-base balance has been reduced from six chapters to three to emphasize nursing care related to these needs.

OUTSTANDING READABILITY

The sixth edition has been carefully revised from cover to cover for improved readability. Today's students need to be able to read information once and understand it. They do not have time to repeatedly read the same information. To achieve this level of readability, we took two steps: (1) wherever appropriate, we revised the text into a more direct-address style that speaks directly to the reader; and (2) we kept sentences as short as possible without sacrificing essential content.

Reading level is highly influenced by the length of sentences and words. Although we can control sentence length, medical terms often consist of four or five syllables and tend to skew a chapter's reading level. Nevertheless, the result of our efforts for this edition is a med-surg text of consistently outstanding readability. The average reading level is 10th to 11th grade.

It is important to note that reducing the reading level of this edition did not reduce the quality or depth of content that students need to know. Instead the content is clear, focused, and accessible.

EASE OF ACCESS

To make the text as easy to use as possible, we have maintained the fifth edition's approach of smaller chapters of more uniform length. We also have maintained the last edition's unit structure, with vital body systems (cardiovascular, respiratory, and neurologic) appearing earlier in the book. In these three units, we have continued to provide complex care content in separate chapters that discuss managing critically ill patients with coronary artery disease, respiratory problems, and neurologic problems.

To help break up long blocks of text and also to highlight key information, we have included numerous headings, bulleted lists, tables, charts, and in-text highlights. We end each chapter with a Selected Bibliography (with classic sources before 2005 noted with an asterisk [*]). Key Terms are in boldface type and are defined in the text to foster the learning of need-to-know vocabulary. A glossary is now located in the back of the book.

A PATIENT-CENTERED COLLABORATIVE CARE APPROACH

As in all previous editions, we take a collaborative care approach to patient care. We believe that in the real world of health care, nurses, patients, and other health care providers (including physicians, advanced practice nurses, and physician's assistants) *share* responsibility for the management of patient problems. Thus we present patient care in a collaborative care framework. In this framework we make no *artificial* distinctions between medical treatment and nursing care. Instead, under each Patient-Centered Collaborative Care heading we discuss how the nurse coordinates care and interacts with members of the health care team as appropriate for the patient's health problems.

As in the fifth edition, this edition includes patient-centered Concept Maps that underscore this collaborative care approach. Each Concept Map contains a case scenario and shows how a selected complex health problem is addressed. Each one spells out the steps of the nursing process and related concepts to illustrate the relationships among disease processes, medical treatments, nursing interventions, and more.

Although our approach is collaborative, the text is first and foremost a *nursing* text. We therefore use a nursing process approach to organize discussions of patient health problems and their management. Discussions of major health problems follow a full nursing process format using this structure:

[Health problem]
    Pathophysiology
        Etiology (and Genetic Risk when appropriate)
        Incidence/Prevalence

Patient-Centered Collaborative Care
Assessment
Analysis
Common Nursing Diagnoses and Collaborative Problems
Additional Nursing Diagnoses and Collaborative Problems
Planning and Implementation
Nursing Diagnosis/Collaborative Problem
Planning: Expected Outcomes
Interventions
Community-Based Care
Health Teaching
Home Care Management
Health Care Resources
Evaluation: Outcomes

Health Promotion and Maintenance sections are found in selected discussions. The nursing diagnoses used in this edition are the 2007-2008 NANDA-I diagnoses—the most recently approved diagnoses at the time of this revision.

Discussions of less common or less complex disorders do not have this complete subhead structure but do follow the same basic format: a discussion of the problem itself (including pertinent information on pathophysiology) followed by a section on the collaborative care of patients with the disorder. Common nursing diagnoses/collaborative problems are often identified.

Integral to this collaborative care approach is a clear delineation of just who is responsible for what. When a responsibility is primarily the nurse's, the text says so. When a decision must be made jointly by, for example, the patient, nurse, physician, and physical therapist, this is clearly stated. When different health care practitioners in different care settings might be involved in the patient's care, this is stated.

To further emphasize the nurse's role, we include pertinent components of the Nursing Interventions Classification (NIC) system and the Nursing Outcomes Classification (NOC) system. These systems were developed by the Center for Nursing Classification to standardize nursing interventions and outcomes and the terminology used to describe them. Where appropriate for health problems that receive full nursing process coverage, NIC interventions are clearly identified with a NIC symbol. Selected activities associated with each identified intervention are listed in NIC Intervention Activities charts.

The expected outcomes for patient care in this edition are consistent with the NOC system. However, NOC continues to be developed and refined to ensure that outcomes are evidence based. Therefore, when appropriate, we have included NOC outcomes and specified indicators as well as other outcome statements validated empirically by clinical practice. Statements that are particularly consistent with NOC language are identified with a NOC symbol.

ORGANIZATION

The 76 chapters of *Medical-Surgical Nursing: Patient-Centered Collaborative Care* are grouped into 16 units. Unit I, Foundations for Medical-Surgical Nursing, lays the foundation for the health care concepts incorporated throughout the text. Unit II consists of three chapters on concepts of emergency care and disaster preparedness.

Unit III consists of three chapters on the management of patients with fluid, electrolyte, and acid-base imbalances. These three chapters have been condensed from six in the previous edition. Chapters 13 and 14 review key assessments and related patient care in a clear, concise discussion. The expanded chapter on infusion therapy (Chapter 15) is supplemented with an online fluid and electrolyte tutorial on the companion Evolve website.

Unit IV presents the perioperative nursing content that medical-surgical nurses need to know. This content provides a solid foundation to help the student better understand the collaborative care required by the surgical patient.

The remaining 12 units, subdivided and introduced by the six new Human Needs Overviews, cover medical-surgical content by body system. Each of these units begins with an Assessment chapter and continues with one or more collaborative care chapters for patients with selected health problems in that body system.

MULTINATIONAL, MULTICULTURAL, MULTIGENERATIONAL FOCUS

To reflect the increasing diversity of our society, *Medical-Surgical Nursing: Patient-Centered Collaborative Care* takes a multinational, multicultural, and multigenerational focus. Addressing the needs of both U.S. and Canadian readers, we have included examples of trade names of drugs available in the United States and those available in Canada. Drug brands that are available only in Canada are designated with a 🍁 symbol. When appropriate, we identify specific Canadian health care resources, including websites.

To help nurses provide quality care for patients whose cultural background may differ from their own, numerous Cultural Awareness in-text boxes highlight important aspects of culturally competent care. A revised and expanded cultural health chapter (Chapter 4) now includes specific information about lesbian, gay, bisexual, and transgender (LGBT) health and health care. Located in an appendix is an innovative Communication Quick Reference for Spanish-Speaking Patients. This Quick Reference helps ensure clear communication between native English speakers and the rapidly growing population that speaks Spanish as a first language.

Increases in life expectancy and the "graying" of the baby-boom generation add up to a steadily increasing older adult population. To help equip nurses for this challenge, the sixth edition continues to provide thorough coverage of the care of older adults. Chapter 3 expands coverage of the role of the nurse and the health care team in promoting health for older adults in the community. It also provides expanded coverage of the common health problems that older adults may have in the health care setting. The text includes a greater number of Nursing Focus on the Older Adult charts. Laboratory values and drug dosages typical for older patients are also included throughout the book. Charts specifying the normal physiologic changes to expect in the older population are found in each Assessment chapter. In addition, Considerations for Older Adults in-text boxes are included throughout the text to emphasize key points to remember when caring for these patients.

Also appearing throughout the text is an increased number of Women's Health Considerations boxes, which address topics of concern to women and their health care providers. These in-text highlights alert the reader to gender-related differences in assessment parameters and in the incidence, severity, and treatment of common health problems.

ADDITIONAL LEARNING AIDS

As in previous editions, the sixth edition includes a rich array of learning aids geared toward adult learners to help them quickly identify and understand key information and to serve as study aids. Several of these features are new to this edition:

- Written in "patient-friendly" language, Patient and Family Education Guide charts provide the types of instructions that nurses must learn to provide to patients and their families to help them cope with the life changes caused by illness.
- Laboratory Profile charts summarize important information on laboratory tests commonly ordered to evaluate health problems. Information typically includes normal ranges of laboratory values (including differences for older adults, when appropriate) and the possible significance of abnormal findings.
- Common Examples of Drug Therapy charts summarize important information about commonly used drugs. Most charts include both U.S. and Canadian trade names for typically used drugs, usual dosages (including dosages for older patients, as appropriate), and nursing interventions with rationales. In addition, "Med Error Alerts" are included where common mistakes could be made in medication administration. Drug errors are a major health problem in health care today, and our goal with this feature is to help students administer drugs safely.
- Key Features charts highlight the clinical manifestations of important health problems.
- Evidence-Based Practice boxes, provided in nearly every chapter, give synopses of recent nursing research articles and other scientific articles applicable to nursing. Each box provides a summary of the research, its level of evidence, and a brief commentary with implications for nursing practice and future research. The purpose of this feature is to help students identify the strengths and weaknesses of the research and see how research can help guide nursing practice.
- Plans of Care are sometimes used to help students learn the nursing process. The sixth edition therefore includes selected examples of these care-planning tools. Our Plans of Care continue to include a distinctive icon (**D**) to designate interventions that can be delegated to assistive nursing personnel.
- As in the fifth edition, Home Care Assessment charts serve as a convenient summary of essential assessment points for patients who need follow-up home health nursing care.
- Assessment Using Gordon's Functional Health Patterns charts provide a convenient one-stop list of questions to ask patients regarding the impact of health conditions on their everyday function.
- Legal/Ethical issues are discussed in the text and are also examined in one subtype of our new Decision-Making Challenges. These Decision-Making Challenges introduce students to some of the dilemmas they will face in the increasingly high-tech world of medical-surgical nursing.
- Additional subtypes of Decision-Making Challenges emphasize three other aspects of care: Critical Rescue, Delegation/Supervision, and Coordination of Care. Each Critical Rescue Decision-Making Challenge presents an emergent or urgent patient care situation and asks students to explain their priority actions in each case. Each Coordination of Care Decision-Making Challenge presents a patient care scenario that requires students to identify the appropriate health care team members needed and to explain how they would coordinate interdisciplinary care. Each Delegation/Supervision Decision-Making Challenge presents a scenario that challenges students to explain how and why they would assign and delegate specific patient care.

AN INTEGRATED MULTIMEDIA RESOURCE BASED ON PROVEN LEARNING STRATEGIES

Medical-Surgical Nursing: Patient-Centered Collaborative Care, sixth edition, is the centerpiece of a comprehensive package of electronic and print learning resources that break new ground in the application of proven learning strategies and evidence-based educational practice. This integrated multimedia resource actively engages the student in problem solving and clinical decision making.

Resources for Instructors

For the convenience of faculty, all primary Instructor Resources are available on both a streamlined, secure instructor area of the **Evolve website** (http://evolve.elsevier.com/Iggy/) and on an **Instructor's Electronic Resource CD-ROM.**

Included among these Instructor Resources is an exciting new **Integrated Lesson Plan Manual** (ILPM). The ILPM incorporates the best content from the former Instructor's Resource Manual and builds on that excellent resource to provide ready-made lesson plans for each chapter. Each ILPM chapter (corresponding to the equivalent textbook chapter) includes four parts:

Part One: Chapter Resources for Instructors Only
Part Two: Chapter Resources for Students and Instructors
Part Three: Supplemental Resources for Students and Instructors
Part Four: Adoptable Resources for Students and Instructors

At the heart of Part One in each ILPM chapter are lesson plans with four columns: Chapter Outline, Teaching Strategies, Collaborative/Active Learning, and Putting It All Together. The Putting It All Together column integrates all major learning resources to make preparing for teaching easier than ever. Also provided in the ILPM are four introductory chapters that cover facilitating learning in today's diverse educational settings, incorporating technology into the medical-surgical nursing course, promoting critical thinking, and test construction.

Additional Instructor Resources provided on the Evolve website and on the Instructor's Electronic Resource CD-ROM include:

- A high-quality, 2350-item **Test Bank**—includes both traditional multiple-choice and NCLEX "alternate" item types of questions. Each question is coded for correct answer, rationale, cognitive level, NCLEX Integrated Process, NCLEX Client Needs Category, and Learning Outcome. Page references are provided for Knowledge- and Comprehension-level questions. (Questions at the Application level and above require the student to draw on their understanding of broader concepts not limited to a single textbook page; therefore page cross references are not provided for these higher-level questions.) The

Test Bank is provided in ExamView, ParTest, and rich-text formats.
- An electronic **Image Collection**—contains virtually all images in the book (approximately 650 images) delivered in a format that makes incorporation into lectures and presentations easier than ever.
- **Bonus Animations**—100 three-dimensional animations that faculty can use to enhance classroom or online presentations.
- **PowerPoint Presentations**—a collection of 1800 slides corresponding to each chapter in the text and highlighting key content, *now with integrated images and animations.*
- **Audience Response System Questions**—a collection of five discussion-oriented questions per chapter delivered in PowerPoint format for use with iClicker and other audience response systems.

In addition, the following resources are provided on the Evolve website:
- **Guest Lectures**—Seven ready-to-use narrated PowerPoint presentations by Dr. Workman covering topics with which both students and faculty tend to struggle.
- **Faculty Development Videos**—two videos (one completely new) by Donna Ignatavicius that address (1) the implications of changes in the NCLEX Examination for faculty, and (2) curriculum transformation.

Also available for adoption and separate purchase, new **Clinical Simulation Scenarios** help faculty make the best use of high-fidelity patient simulators.

Resources for Students

Resources for students include a free Companion CD, a thoroughly revised and updated Clinical Decision-Making Study Guide, a Clinical Companion, a Virtual Clinical Excursions workbook/CD-ROM, and Evolve Learning Resources.

The **Companion CD** features Self-Assessment Questions for the NCLEX Examination—one for each Learning Outcome at the beginning of each chapter. Also included on the Companion CD are animations and video clips (each keyed to the text by a distinctive icon), as well as a revised Audio Glossary. The Audio Glossary includes the definitions of all Key Terms from the text along with audio pronunciations for each term.

The Clinical Decision-Making Study Guide has been carefully revised and updated for an increased emphasis on clinical decision making. The Study Guide now features an increased number of multiple-choice questions that are written in NCLEX Examination format and emphasize the NCLEX priorities of delegation, management of care, and pharmacology. The use of Case Studies is expanded in this edition.

The pocket-sized Clinical Companion has undergone its most thorough revision ever for this edition. This handy clinical resource retains its popular alphabetical organization and streamlined format and now includes new "Critical Rescue" and "Clinical Landmine" highlights throughout. New National Patient Safety Goals highlights underscore the importance of observing vital patient safety standards. This "pocket-sized Iggy" has been tailored to the special needs of students preparing for clinicals and clinical practice.

The Virtual Clinical Excursions workbook/CD-ROM package, featuring an updated and easy-to-navigate "virtual" clinical setting, will once again be available for the sixth edition. This unique learning tool guides students through a virtual clinical environment and helps them "learn by doing" in the safety of a "virtual" hospital. The clinical simulations and workbook represent the next generation of research-based learning tools to promote critical thinking and meaningful learning.

Also available for students is a dynamic collection of Evolve Student Resources, available at http://evolve.elsevier.com/Iggy/. The Evolve Student Resources—*now organized by student learning needs*—include the following:
- Pharmacology Review Questions for the NCLEX Examination (keyed to icons in the textbook evolve ONLINE PHARM REVIEW)
- Self-Assessment Questions for the NCLEX Examination (also on the Companion CD)
- Prioritization and Delegation Questions for the NCLEX Examination
- Answer Key for Decision-Making Challenges
- Answer Key for NCLEX Examination Challenges
- Interactive Concept Maps ("building" versions of the 12 Concept Maps from the text)
- Concept Map Creator (a handy tool for creating customized Concept Maps)
- Fluid & Electrolyte Tutorial (a complete self-paced tutorial on this perennially difficult content)
- Audio Clips (keyed to the text by an icon) for key sounds in health assessment.
- Audio Key Points (new downloadable chapter reviews with integrated quizzing)
- Study Tips chapter (formerly in the Study Guide)
- Health Assessment Image Collection (supplemental images of common assessment findings)
- Complete listings of the Nursing Interventions Classification (NIC) and Nursing Outcomes Classification (NOC)
- The Audio Glossary, Animations, and Video Clips from the Companion CD
- Content Updates

For more information on any of these innovative companion publications, contact your Elsevier sales representative, visit http://www.us.elsevierhealth.com/, or contact Elsevier Faculty Support at 1-800-222-9570 or sales.inquiry@elsevier.com.

In summary, *Medical-Surgical Nursing: Patient-Centered Collaborative Care,* sixth edition, together with its fully integrated multimedia ancillary package, provides the tools you will need to meet the challenge of nursing in the 21st century. The only elements that remain to be added to this package are those that you alone can provide—your diligence, your commitment, your innovation, *your nursing expertise.*

Donna D. Ignatavicius
M. Linda Workman

Acknowledgments

Publishing a textbook and ancillary package of this depth and breadth would not be possible without the combined efforts of many people. Irene Owens, Instructor at Lake Sumter Community College, provided helpful feedback on Chapter 73 (Care of Patients with Breast Disorders). Paul W. Elliott, Jr. helped develop the Human Needs Overview feature for Mobility, Sensation, and Cognition.

Our contributing authors once again provided consistently excellent manuscripts in a timely fashion. Special thanks to Elaine Kennedy, who developed our Concept Maps and Plans of Care. Our reviewers—expert clinicians and instructors from around the United States and Canada—provided invaluable suggestions and encouragement throughout the book's development.

The staff of Saunders/Elsevier once again provided us with crucial guidance and support throughout the planning, writing, revision, and production of the sixth edition. In particular, Senior Editor Lee Henderson worked closely with us from the early stages of this edition to help us hone and focus our revision plan, and he coordinated the project from start to finish. Senior Developmental Editor Rae Robertson then worked with us step-by-step to bring the sixth edition from vision to publication. Rae, Jacqueline Twomey, and Mary Ann Zimmerman held the reins of our complex ancillary package and worked with a gifted group of writers and content experts to provide an outstanding library of resources to complement and enhance the text. Special thanks to Editorial Assistant Julie Eisen, who not only managed the *Clinical Companion* but handled the countless administrative details associated with a project of this size.

Senior Project Manager Jodi Willard was once again a joy to work with. If, as is said, the mark of a good copy editor is that her work is invisible to the reader, then Jodi is the consummate copy editor. Her unwavering attention to detail, flexibility, and conscientiousness not only helped to make this edition the most consistently readable ever but also made the entire production process incredibly smooth and headache-free.

Special thanks also to Publishing Services Manager Debbie Vogel. For three editions now, Debbie has worked quietly behind the scenes to help bring the book to publication precisely on schedule and with a very high level of quality.

Designer Margaret Reid is responsible for the beautiful cover and the completely new interior design for the sixth edition. The praise of a book designer's work is often unsung, but Maggie's work on this edition has cast important features in exactly the right light, with neither too much nor too little emphasis, making this edition not only practical and easy to read but also beautiful.

Our acknowledgments would not be complete without recognizing our dedicated team of sales representatives and other key members of the Sales and Marketing staff who helped to put this book into your hands.

Finally, we wish to thank Executive Vice President, Nursing and Health Professions, Sally Schrefer. Sally's personal leadership style continues to create a unique publishing environment in which authors and editors have the freedom to interact creatively to produce the best books in the field.

Donna D. Ignatavicius
M. Linda Workman

Contents

UNIT I
Foundations for Medical-Surgical Nursing

CHAPTER 1
Introduction to Medical-Surgical Nursing, 2
Donna D. Ignatavicius

National Patient Safety Goals, *2*
Protecting Five Million Lives from Harm, *3*
Institute of Medicine Core Competencies for Health Professionals, *3*
Providing Patient-Centered Care, *3*
Collaborating with the Interdisciplinary Health Care Team, *5*
Implementing Evidence-Based Practice, *5*
Using Quality Improvement in Patient Care, *6*
Using Informatics for Patient Care, *6*

CHAPTER 2
Introduction to Complementary and Alternative Therapies, 8
Donna D. Ignatavicius

Overview, *8*
National Center for Complementary and Alternative Medicine, *8*
CAM Domains, *9*
Systems of Health Care, *9*
Mind-Body Therapies, *9*
Manipulative and Body-Based Therapies, *11*
Biologically-Based Therapies, *11*
Energy Therapies, *12*
Summary of Implications for Nursing, *13*

CHAPTER 3
Common Health Problems of Older Adults, 15
Donna D. Ignatavicius

Overview, *15*
Health Issues for Older Adults in the Community, *16*
Nutrition, *16*
Mobility, *17*
Stress and Loss, *17*
Accidents, *18*
Drug Use and Misuse, *18*
Mental Health/Behavioral Health, *20*
Elder Neglect and Abuse, *22*
Health Care Issues in Hospitals, *23*
Sleep, Nutrition, and Incontinence, *23*
Confusion, Falls, and Skin Breakdown, *23*

CHAPTER 4
Cultural Aspects of Health and Illness, 27
Donna D. Ignatavicius

Culture and Cultural Competence, *27*
Health and Health Care Disparities, *28*
Purnell's Domains of Culture, *29*
Culture Overview and Communication, *29*
Family and Workplace Issues, *29*
Biologic Ecology, *31*
Nutrition, *31*
Spirituality, *31*
Health Care Practices and Practitioners, *32*

CHAPTER 5
Pain: The Fifth Vital Sign, 35
Lora L. McGuire

Overview, *36*
Definitions of Pain, *36*
Scope of the Problem, *36*
Categorizing Pain, *36*
Theoretical Bases for Pain, *38*
Patient-Centered Collaborative Care, *41*

CHAPTER 6
Genetic Concepts for Medical-Surgical Nursing, 62
M. Linda Workman

Genetic Biology, *62*
Deoxyribonucleic Acid, *63*
Gene Structure and Function, *68*
Gene Expression, *69*
Protein Synthesis, *70*
Mutations, *70*
Patterns of Inheritance, *71*
Pedigree, *71*
Autosomal Dominant Pattern of Inheritance, *73*
Autosomal Recessive Pattern of Inheritance, *73*
Sex-Linked Recessive Pattern of Inheritance, *74*
Complex Inheritance and Familial Clustering, *74*
Genetic Testing, *74*
Purpose of Testing, *74*
Benefits and Risks of Testing, *74*
Genetic Counseling, *75*
Ethical Issues, *75*
The Role of the Medical-Surgical Nurse in Genetic Counseling, *77*
Communication, *77*
Privacy and Confidentiality, *77*
Information Accuracy, *78*
Patient Advocacy and Support, *78*

CHAPTER 7
Substance Abuse and Medical-Surgical Nursing, 80
Tommie Wright Pniewski

Overview of Substance Abuse and Misuse, *80*
Substance Abuse, Stress, and Addiction, *81*
Substance Abuse or Misuse and the Hospitalized Patient, *81*
Substance Use and Abuse Among Nurses, *82*
Substances That Are Abused or Misused, *82*
Alcohol, *82*
Nicotine, *84*
Stimulants, *85*
Hallucinogens and Related Compounds, *86*
Depressants, *88*
Barbiturates, *89*

Opioids, *90*
Inhalants, *91*
Steroids, *91*

CHAPTER 8
Rehabilitation Concepts for Chronic and Disabling Health Problems, 94
Donna D. Ignatavicius

Overview, *94*
Concepts Related to Rehabilitation, *95*
The Rehabilitation Team, *95*
Patient-Centered Collaborative Care, *97*

CHAPTER 9
End-of-Life Care, 111
Mary K. Kazanowski

Overview of Death and Dying, *111*
Perception of Death in the United States, *111*
Pathophysiology of Dying, *112*
Incidence of Death, *113*
Planning for End of Life, *113*
Hospice and Palliative Care, *113*
Symptoms at End of Life, *115*
Overview, *115*
Patient-Centered Collaborative Care, *115*
Postmortem Care, *121*
Euthanasia, *121*

UNIT II
Concepts of Emergency Care and Disaster Preparedness

CHAPTER 10
Concepts of Emergency and Trauma Nursing, 126
Linda Laskowski-Jones
Karen L. Toulson

The Emergency Department Environment of Care, *126*
Demographic Data, *126*
Special Populations, *127*
Special Nursing Teams, *127*
Interdisciplinary Team Collaboration, *127*
Staff and Patient Safety Considerations, *128*
Scope of Emergency Nursing Practice, *130*
Core Competencies, *130*
Training and Certification, *131*
Emergency Nursing Principles, *131*
Triage, *131*
Care of the Emergency Department Patient, *132*
Trauma Nursing Principles, *134*
Trauma Centers and Trauma Systems, *135*
Mechanism of Injury, *136*
The Primary Survey and Resuscitation Interventions, *136*
The Secondary Survey and Resuscitation Interventions, *138*
Disposition, *138*

CHAPTER 11
Care of Patients with Common Environmental Emergencies, 141
Linda Laskowski-Jones

Heat-Related Illnesses, *141*
Health Promotion and Maintenance, *141*
Heat Exhaustion, *142*
Heat Stroke, *142*
Snakebite, *143*
Health Promotion and Maintenance, *144*
North American Pit Vipers, *144*
Coral Snakes, *145*
Arthropod Bites and Stings, *146*
Brown Recluse Spider, *147*
Black Widow Spider, *147*
Tarantulas, *148*
Scorpions, *148*
Bees and Wasps, *149*
Lightning Injuries, *150*
Cold Injuries, *152*
Health Promotion and Maintenance, *152*
Hypothermia, *152*
Frostbite, *154*
Altitude-Related Illnesses, *154*
Drowning, *156*

CHAPTER 12
Concepts of Emergency and Disaster Preparedness, 159
Linda Laskowski-Jones

Impact of Recent Disasters, *159*
Emergency Preparedness and Response, *160*
Mass Casualty Triage, *160*
Notification and Activation of Emergency Preparedness Plans, *161*
Hospital Emergency Preparedness: Personnel Roles and Responsibilities, *162*
Event Resolution, *164*
Debriefing, *164*
Psychosocial Response of Survivors to Mass Casualty Events, *165*
Emergency Room Case Scenario: Possible Anthrax Exposure, *166*
Case Presentation, *166*
Case Discussion, *166*

UNIT III
Management of Patients with Fluid, Electrolyte and Acid-Base Imbalances

CHAPTER 13
Assessment and Care of Patients with Fluid and Electrolyte Imbalances, 170
M. Linda Workman

Homeostasis, *170*
Anatomy and Physiology Review, *171*
Physiologic Influences on Fluid and Electrolyte Balance, *171*

Fluid Balance, *174*
Body Fluids, *174*
Hormonal Regulation of Fluid Balance, *175*
Fluid Imbalances, *176*
Dehydration, *176*
Fluid Overload, *181*
Electrolyte Balance and Imbalances, *183*
Sodium, *183*
Potassium, *187*
Calcium, *191*
Phosphorus, *194*
Magnesium, *195*
Chloride, *197*

CHAPTER 14
Assessment and Care of Patients with Acid-Base Imbalances, 199
M. Linda Workman

Acid-Base Balance, *199*
Acid-Base Chemistry, *200*
Body Fluid Chemistry, *201*
Acid-Base Regulatory Mechanisms, *202*
Acid-Base Imbalances, *204*
Acidosis, *204*
Alkalosis, *210*

CHAPTER 15
Infusion Therapy, 213
Linda Laskowski-Jones
Alexandra Falkowski

Overview, *213*
Types of Infusion Therapy Fluids, *214*
Prescribing Infusion Therapy, *215*
Vascular Access Devices, *215*
Peripheral Intravenous Therapy, *215*
Short Peripheral Catheters, *215*
Midline Catheters, *217*
Central Intravenous Therapy, *217*
Peripherally Inserted Central Catheters, *217*
Nontunneled Percutaneous Central Catheters, *218*
Tunneled Central Catheters, *218*
Implanted Ports, *218*
Dialysis Catheters, *219*
Infusion Systems, *219*
Containers, *219*
Administration Sets, *220*
Rate-Controlling Devices, *221*
Nursing Care for Patients Receiving Intravenous Therapy, *222*
Educating the Patient, *222*
Confirming Tip Location, *222*
Performing the Nursing Assessment, *222*
Securing and Dressing the Catheter, *223*
Changing Administration Sets and Needleless Connectors, *224*
Controlling Infusion Pressure, *224*
Flushing the Catheter, *224*
Obtaining Blood Samples from the Catheter, *225*
Removing the Catheter, *225*
Documenting Intravenous Therapy, *225*
Complications of Infusion Therapy, *225*
Older Adult Care, *235*
Skin Care, *235*
Vein and Catheter Selection, *235*
Cardiac and Renal Changes, *235*
Alternative Sites for Infusion, *236*
Arterial Therapy, *236*
Intraperitoneal Infusion, *236*
Subcutaneous Infusion, *237*
Intraspinal Infusion, *237*
Intraosseous Therapy, *238*

UNIT IV
Management of Perioperative Patients

CHAPTER 16
Care of Preoperative Patients, 242
Robin Chard

Overview, *243*
Categories and Purposes of Surgery, *243*
Surgical Settings, *244*
Patient-Centered Collaborative Care, *244*

CHAPTER 17
Care of Intraoperative Patients, 264
Robin Chard

Overview, *264*
Members of the Surgical Team, *264*
Preparation of the Surgical Suite and Team Safety, *267*
Anesthesia, *270*
Patient-Centered Collaborative Care, *277*

CHAPTER 18
Care of Postoperative Patients, 285
Robin Chard

Overview, *285*
Patient-Centered Collaborative Care, *286*

HUMAN NEEDS OVERVIEW:
Protection, 304

UNIT V
Problems of Protection: Management of Patients with Problems of the Immune System

CHAPTER 19
Inflammation and the Immune Response, 306
M. Linda Workman

Overview, *306*
Purpose of Inflammation and Immunity, *307*
Self Versus Non-Self, *307*
Organization of the Immune System, *308*
Inflammation, *309*
Purpose, *309*
Infection, *309*
Cell Types Involved in Inflammation, *310*
Phagocytosis, *311*
Sequence of Inflammatory Responses, *312*
Antibody-Mediated Immunity, *313*
Purpose, *313*
Antigen-Antibody Interactions, *313*

Antibody Classification, *316*
Acquiring Antibody-Mediated Immunity, *316*
Cell-Mediated Immunity, *317*
Cell Types Involved in Cell-Mediated Immunity, *317*
Cytokines, *317*
Protection Provided by Cell-Mediated Immunity, *319*
Transplant Rejection, *319*

CHAPTER 20
Care of Patients with Arthritis and Other Connective Tissue Diseases, 322
Donna D. Ignatavicius
Cathy A. Murray

Osteoarthritis, *323*
Pathophysiology, *323*
Health Promotion and Maintenance, *324*
Patient-Centered Collaborative Care, *324*
Rheumatoid Arthritis, *337*
Pathophysiology, *337*
Patient-Centered Collaborative Care, *337*
Lupus Erythematosus, *347*
Pathophysiology, *347*
Patient-Centered Collaborative Care, *348*
Scleroderma, *351*
Pathophysiology, *351*
Patient-Centered Collaborative Care, *351*
Gout, *353*
Pathophysiology, *353*
Patient-Centered Collaborative Care, *353*
Other Connective Tissue Diseases, *354*
Polymyositis/Dermatomyositis, *354*
Systemic Necrotizing Vasculitis, *354*
Polymyalgia Rheumatica and Temporal Arteritis, *355*
Anklyosing Spondylitis, *355*
Reiter's Syndrome, *355*
Marfan Syndrome, *355*
Infectious Arthritis, *356*
Lyme Disease, *356*
Pseudogout, *356*
Psoriatic Arthritis, *357*
Other Disease-Associated Arthritis, *357*
Fibromyalgia Syndrome, *357*
Chronic Fatigue Syndrome, *358*
Mixed Connective Tissue Disease, *358*

CHAPTER 21
Care of Patients with HIV Disease and Other Immune Deficiencies, 362
James G. Sampson
M. Linda Workman

Acquired (Secondary) Immune Deficiencies, *363*
HIV Disease and Acquired Immune Deficiency Syndrome (AIDS), *363*
Therapy-Induced Immune Deficiencies, *384*
Congenital (Primary) Immune Deficiencies, *385*
Bruton's Agammaglobulinemia, *385*
Common Variable Immune Deficiency, *385*
Selective Immunoglobulin A Deficiency, *385*

CHAPTER 22
Care of Patients with Immune Function Excess: Hypersensitivity (Allergy) and Autoimmunity, 387
M. Linda Workman

Hypersensitivities/Allergies, *387*
Type I: Rapid Hypersensitivity Reactions, *387*
Type II: Cytotoxic Reactions, *394*
Type III: Immune Complex Reactions, *394*
Type IV: Delayed Hypersensitivity Reactions, *395*
Type V: Stimulatory Reactions, *395*
Autoimmunity, *395*
Sjögren's Syndrome, *396*
Goodpasture's Syndrome, *397*

CHAPTER 23
Cancer Development, 399
M. Linda Workman

Pathophysiology, *399*
Biology of Normal Cells, *400*
Biology of Abnormal Cells, *402*
Cancer Development, *403*
Carcinogenesis/Oncogenesis, *403*
Cancer Classification, *405*
Cancer Grading, Ploidy, and Staging, *406*
Cancer Etiology and Genetic Risk, *407*
Cancer Prevention, *411*
Primary Prevention, *411*
Secondary Prevention, *412*

CHAPTER 24
Care of Patients with Cancer, 414
M. Linda Workman

General Disease-Related Consequences of Cancer, *415*
Reduced Immunity and Blood-Producing Functions, *415*
Altered GI Structure and Function, *415*
Motor and Sensory Deficits, *415*
Decreased Respiratory Function, *417*
Cancer Management, *417*
Surgery, *417*
Radiation Therapy, *418*
Chemotherapy, *421*
Hormonal Manipulation, *431*
Photodynamic Therapy, *432*
Immunotherapy: Biological Response Modifiers, *433*
Gene Therapy, *434*
Targeted Therapy, *434*
Oncologic Emergencies, *434*
Sepsis and Disseminated Intravascular Coagulation, *435*
Syndrome of Inappropriate Antidiuretic Hormone, *435*
Spinal Cord Compression, *436*
Hypercalcemia, *436*
Superior Vena Cava Syndrome, *436*
Tumor Lysis Syndrome, *437*

CHAPTER 25
Care of Patients with Infection, 440
Donna D. Ignatavicius
Overview of the Infectious Process, *440*
Health Promotion and Maintenance, *443*
Centers for Disease Control and Prevention Transmission-Based Guidelines, *446*
Multidrug-Resistant Organism Infections and Colonizations, *448*
Occupational Exposure to Sources of Infection, *449*
Problems from Inadequate Antimicrobial Therapy, *449*
Patient-Centered Collaborative Care, *449*
Critical Issues for the Next Decade: Bioterrorism and Emerging Infections, *453*

UNIT VI
Problems of Protection: Management of Patients with Problems of the Skin, Hair, and Nails

CHAPTER 26
Assessment of the Skin, Hair, and Nails, 460
Janice Cuzzell
M. Linda Workman
Anatomy and Physiology Review, *461*
Structure of the Skin, *461*
Structure of the Skin Appendages, *462*
Functions of the Skin, *462*
Skin Changes Associated with Aging, *462*
Assessment Methods, *466*
Patient History, *466*
Skin Assessment, *467*
Hair Assessment, *473*
Nail Assessment, *473*
Skin Assessment Methods for Patients with Dark Skin, *475*
Psychosocial Assessment, *476*
Diagnostic Assessment, *476*

CHAPTER 27
Care of Patients with Skin Problems, 479
Janice Cuzzell
M. Linda Workman
Minor Skin Irritations, *480*
Dryness, *480*
Pruritus, *480*
Sunburn, *481*
Urticaria, *481*
Trauma, *481*
Pressure Ulcers, *484*
Common Infections, *499*
Cutaneous Anthrax, *503*
Parasitic Disorders, *504*
Pediculosis, *504*
Scabies, *504*
Common Inflammations, *504*
Psoriasis, *506*
Benign Tumors, *508*
Cysts, *508*
Seborrheic Keratoses, *508*
Keloids, *509*
Nevi, *509*
Skin Cancer, *509*
Plastic or Reconstructive Surgery, *513*
Other Skin Disorders, *515*
Acne, *515*
Lichen Planus, *516*
Pemphigus Vulgaris, *516*
Toxic Epidermal Necrolysis, *516*
Stevens-Johnson Syndrome, *516*
Leprosy, *516*

CHAPTER 28
Care of Patients with Burns, 519
Tammy Coffee
Introduction to the Burn Problem, *520*
Health Promotion and Maintenance, *527*
Resuscitation/Emergent Phase of Burn Injury, *528*
Acute Phase of Burn Injury, *537*
Rehabilitative Phase of Burn Injury, *545*

HUMAN NEEDS OVERVIEW: OXYGENATION AND TISSUE PERFUSION, 548

UNIT VII
Problems of Oxygenation: Management of Patients with Problems of the Respiratory Tract

CHAPTER 29
Assessment of the Respiratory System, 552
Harry C. Rees
Anatomy and Physiology Review, *553*
Upper Respiratory Tract, *553*
Lower Respiratory Tract, *554*
Accessory Muscles of Respiration, *556*
Respiratory Changes Associated with Aging, *556*
Assessment Methods, *556*
Patient History, *556*
Physical Assessment, *559*
Psychosocial Assessment, *564*
Diagnostic Assessment, *564*

CHAPTER 30
Care of Patients Requiring Oxygen Therapy or Tracheostomy, 571
Harry C. Rees
Oxygen Therapy, *571*
Tracheostomy, *580*

CHAPTER 31
Care of Patients with Noninfectious Upper Respiratory Problems, 590
M. Linda Workman
Noninfectious Disorders of the Nose and Sinuses, *590*
Fracture of the Nose, *590*
Epistaxis, *591*
Nasal Polyps, *592*
Cancer of the Nose and Sinuses, *592*
Facial Trauma, *593*
Noninfectious Disorders of the Oral Pharynx and Tonsils, *594*
Obstructive Sleep Apnea, *594*

Noninfectious Disorders of the Larynx, *594*
Vocal Cord Paralysis, *594*
Vocal Cord Nodules and Polyps, *595*
Laryngeal Trauma, *596*
Other Upper Airway Disorders, *596*
Upper Airway Obstruction, *596*
Neck Trauma, *596*
Head and Neck Cancer, *597*

CHAPTER 32
Care of Patients with Noninfectious Lower Respiratory Problems, 609
M. Linda Workman
Chronic Airflow Limitation, *610*
Asthma, *610*
Chronic Obstructive Pulmonary Disease, *621*
Cystic Fibrosis, *635*
Primary Pulmonary Hypertension, *637*
Interstitial Pulmonary Diseases, *638*
Sarcoidosis, *638*
Idiopathic Pulmonary Fibrosis, *639*
Occupational Pulmonary Disease, *639*
Bronchiolitis Obliterans Organizing Pneumonia (BOOP), *641*
Lung Cancer, *641*

CHAPTER 33
Care of Patients with Infectious Respiratory Problems, 653
M. Linda Workman
Disorders of the Nose and Sinuses, *654*
Rhinitis, *654*
Sinusitis, *654*
Disorders of the Oral Pharynx and Tonsils, *655*
Pharyngitis, *655*
Tonsillitis, *657*
Peritonsillar Abscess, *657*
Disorders of the Larynx and Lungs, *658*
Laryngitis, *658*
Influenza, *658*
Pneumonia, *659*
Severe Acute Respiratory Syndrome (SARS), *666*
Avian Influenza—"Bird Flu," *667*
Pulmonary Tuberculosis, *668*
Lung Abscess, *672*
Inhalation Anthrax, *672*
Pulmonary Empyema, *673*

CHAPTER 34
Care of Critically Ill Patients with Respiratory Problems, 677
John M. Clochesy
Ronald L. Hickman
Pulmonary Embolism, *677*
Acute Respiratory Failure, *685*
Acute Respiratory Distress Syndrome, *686*
The Patient Requiring Intubation and Ventilation, *689*
Chest Trauma, *697*
Pulmonary Contusion, *697*
Rib Fracture, *698*
Flail Chest, *698*
Pneumothorax, *698*
Tension Pneumothorax, *699*
Hemothorax, *699*
Tracheobronchial Trauma, *699*

UNIT VIII
Problems of Cardiac Output and Tissue Perfusion: Management of Patients with Problems of the Cardiovascular System

CHAPTER 35
Assessment of the Cardiovascular System, 704
Donna D. Ignatavicius
Sharon Henry Walicek
Anatomy and Physiology Review, *704*
Heart, *704*
Vascular System, *708*
Cardiovascular Changes Associated with Aging, *709*
Assessment Methods, *709*
Patient History, *709*
Functional History, *714*
Physical Assessment, *714*
Psychosocial Assessment, *719*
Diagnostic Assessment, *719*

CHAPTER 36
Care of Patients with Dysrhythmias, 730
Pamela C. Zickafoose
Review of Cardiac Electrophysiology, *730*
Electrophysiologic Properties, *730*
Cardiac Conduction System, *731*
Electrocardiography, *731*
Lead Systems, *732*
Continuous Electrocardiographic Monitoring, *732*
Electrocardiographic Complexes, Segments, and Intervals, *733*
Determination of Heart Rate, *736*
Electrocardiographic Rhythm Analysis, *736*
Normal Rhythms, *737*
Dysrhythmias, *738*

CHAPTER 37
Care of Patients with Cardiac Problems, 764
Donna D. Ignatavicius
Sharon Henry Walicek
Heart Failure, *765*
Valvular Heart Disease, *779*
Inflammations and Infections, *783*
Infective Endocarditis, *783*
Pericarditis, *785*
Rheumatic Carditis, *787*
Cardiomyopathy, *787*

CHAPTER 38
Care of Patients with Vascular Problems, 793
Donna D. Ignatavicius
Sharon Henry Walicek
Arteriosclerosis and Atherosclerosis, *793*
Hypertension, *796*
Peripheral Arterial Disease, *804*

Acute Peripheral Arterial Occlusion, *810*
Aneurysms of Central Arteries, *810*
Aneurysms of the Peripheral Arteries, *814*
Aortic Dissection, *814*
Buerger's Disease, *815*
Subclavian Steal, *815*
Thoracic Outlet Syndrome, *815*
Raynaud's Phenomenon, *815*
Popliteal Entrapment, *816*
Peripheral Venous Disease, *816*
Venous Thromboembolism, *816*
Venous Insufficiency, *821*
Varicose Veins, *822*
Phlebitis, *823*
Vascular Trauma, *823*

CHAPTER 39
Care of Patients with Shock, 826
M. Linda Workman
Overview, *826*
Review of Oxygenation and Tissue Perfusion, *827*
Types of Shock, *828*
Hypovolemic Shock, *830*
Sepsis and Septic Shock, *838*

CHAPTER 40
Care of Patients with Acute Coronary Syndromes, 847
Vicki Brownrigg
Sharon Henry Walicek
Donna D. Ignatavicius
Pathophysiology, *847*
Chronic Stable Angina Pectoris, *847*
Acute Coronary Syndromes, *848*
Etiology and Genetic Risk, *850*
Incidence/Prevalence, *850*
Health Promotion and Maintenance, *850*
Elevated Serum Lipid Levels, *850*
Tobacco Use, *851*
Physical Activity, *852*
Other Factors, *852*
Patient-Centered Collaborative Care, *853*

UNIT IX
Problems of Tissue Perfusion: Management of Patients with Problems of the Hematologic System

CHAPTER 41
Assessment of the Hematologic System, 876
M. Linda Workman
Anatomy and Physiology Review, *876*
Bone Marrow, *876*
Blood Components, *877*
Accessory Organs of Blood Formation, *879*
Hemostasis/Blood Clotting, *879*
Anti-Clotting Forces, *881*
Hematologic Changes Associated with Aging, *881*
Assessment Methods, *882*
Patient History, *882*
Physical Assessment, *885*
Psychosocial Assessment, *886*
Diagnostic Assessment, *886*

CHAPTER 42
Care of Patients with Hematologic Problems, 892
Katherine L. Byar
Red Blood Cell Disorders, *893*
Anemia, *893*
Polycythemia, *901*
Myelodysplastic Syndromes, *901*
White Blood Cell Disorders, *902*
Leukemia, *902*
Malignant Lymphomas, *913*
Coagulation Disorders, *915*
Platelet Disorders, *916*
Clotting Factor Disorders, *916*
Transfusion Therapy, *917*
Pretransfusion Responsibilities, *917*
Transfusion Responsibilities, *919*
Types of Transfusions, *919*
Transfusion Reactions, *920*
Autologous Blood Transfusions, *921*

HUMAN NEEDS OVERVIEW: MOBILITY, SENSATION, AND COGNITION, 924

UNIT X
Problems of Mobility, Sensation, and Cognition: Management of Patients with Problems of the Nervous System

CHAPTER 43
Assessment of the Nervous System, 928
Kathy A. Hausman
Anatomy and Physiology Review, *928*
Nervous System Cells: Structure and Function, *928*
Central Nervous System: Structure and Function, *929*
Peripheral Nervous System: Structure and Function, *933*
Autonomic Nervous System: Structure and Function, *933*
Neurologic Changes Associated with Aging, *933*
Assessment Methods, *935*
Patient History, *935*
Physical Assessment, *936*
Psychosocial Assessment, *942*
Diagnostic Assessment, *943*

CHAPTER 44
Care of Patients with Problems of the Central Nervous System: The Brain, 950
Kathy A. Hausman
Donna D. Ignatavicius
Headaches, *951*
Migraine Headache, *951*
Cluster Headache, *954*
Tension Headache, *955*
Seizures and Epilepsy, *955*
Infections, *961*
Meningitis, *961*
Encephalitis, *963*

Parkinson Disease, *965*
Alzheimer's Disease, *969*
Huntington Disease, *979*

CHAPTER 45
Care of Patients with Problems of the Central Nervous System: The Spinal Cord, 983
Kathy A. Hausman
Donna D. Ignatavicius

Back Pain, *983*
Lumbosacral Back Pain (Low Back Pain), *984*
Cervical Neck Pain, *989*
Spinal Cord Injury, *990*
Spinal Cord Tumors, *1000*
Multiple Sclerosis, *1002*
Amyotrophic Lateral Sclerosis, *1007*

CHAPTER 46
Care of Patients with Problems of the Peripheral Nervous System, 1011
Kathy A. Hausman
Donna D. Ignatavicius

Guillain-Barré Syndrome, *1011*
Myasthenia Gravis, *1016*
Peripheral Nerve Trauma, *1022*
Restless Legs Syndrome, *1024*
Diseases of the Cranial Nerves, *1025*
Trigeminal Neuralgia, *1025*
Facial Paralysis, *1026*

CHAPTER 47
Care of Critically Ill Patients with Neurologic Problems, 1029
Donna D. Ignatavicius
Kathy A. Hausman

Transient Ischemic Attack and Reversible Ischemic Neurologic Deficit, *1030*
Stroke (Brain Attack), *1030*
Traumatic Brain Injury, *1049*
Brain Tumors, *1060*
Brain Abscess, *1065*

UNIT XI
Problems of Sensation: Management of Patients with Problems of the Sensory System

CHAPTER 48
Assessment of the Eye and Vision, 1070
M. Linda Workman

Anatomy and Physiology Review, *1070*
Structure, *1070*
Function, *1073*
Eye Changes Associated with Aging, *1074*
Health Promotion and Maintenance, *1074*
Assessment Methods, *1075*
Patient History, *1075*
Physical Assessment, *1077*
Psychosocial Assessment, *1079*
Diagnostic Assessment, *1079*

CHAPTER 49
Care of Patients with Eye and Vision Problems, 1084
M. Linda Workman

Eyelid Disorders, *1084*
Blepharitis, *1084*
Entropion, *1085*
Ectropion, *1085*
Hordeolum, *1085*
Chalazion, *1087*
Keratoconjunctivitis Sicca, *1087*
Conjunctival Disorders, *1087*
Hemorrhage, *1087*
Conjunctivitis, *1087*
Trachoma, *1088*
Corneal Disorders, *1088*
Corneal Abrasion, Ulceration, and Infection, *1089*
Keratoconus and Corneal Opacities, *1089*
Cataract, *1091*
Glaucoma, *1095*
Vitreous Hemorrhage, *1098*
Uveitis, *1100*
Retinal Disorders, *1100*
Macular Degeneration, *1100*
Retinal Holes, Tears, and Detachments, *1101*
Retinitis Pigmentosa, *1102*
Refractive Errors, *1102*
Trauma, *1103*
Hyphema, *1103*
Contusion, *1103*
Foreign Bodies, *1103*
Lacerations, *1104*
Penetrating Injuries, *1104*
Ocular Melanoma, *1104*
Reduced Vision, *1106*

CHAPTER 50
Assessment of the Ear and Hearing, 1109
Jacquelyn Ann Russek

Anatomy and Physiology Review, *1109*
Structure, *1109*
Function, *1111*
Ear and Hearing Changes Associated with Aging, *1111*
Assessment Methods, *1111*
Patient History, *1111*
Physical Assessment, *1114*
Auditory Assessment, *1115*
Psychosocial Assessment, *1116*
Diagnostic Assessment, *1116*

CHAPTER 51
Care of Patients with Ear and Hearing Problems, 1120
Jacquelyn Ann Russek

Conditions Affecting the External Ear, *1120*
External Otitis, *1121*
Furuncle, *1122*
Perichondritis, *1122*
Cerumen or Foreign Bodies, *1122*
Conditions Affecting the Middle Ear, *1123*
Otitis Media, *1123*

Mastoiditis, *1125*
Trauma, *1126*
Neoplasms, *1126*
Conditions Affecting the Inner Ear, *1126*
Tinnitus, *1126*
Vertigo and Dizziness, *1126*
Labyrinthitis, *1127*
Ménière's Disease, *1127*
Acoustic Neuroma, *1129*
Hearing Loss, *1129*

UNIT XII
Problems of Mobility: Management of Patients with Problems of the Musculoskeletal System

CHAPTER 52
Assessment of the Musculoskeletal System, 1140
Cathy A. Murray

Anatomy and Physiology Review, *1140*
Skeletal System, *1140*
Muscular System, *1143*
Musculoskeletal Changes Associated with Aging, *1143*
Assessment Methods, *1143*
Patient History, *1143*
Assessment of the Skeletal System, *1145*
Assessment of the Muscular System, *1147*
Psychosocial Assessment, *1147*
Diagnostic Assessment, *1147*

CHAPTER 53
Care of Patients with Musculoskeletal Problems, 1152
Cathy A. Murray

Metabolic Bone Diseases, *1153*
Osteoporosis, *1153*
Osteomalacia, *1160*
Paget's Disease of the Bone, *1162*
Osteomyelitis, *1164*
Benign Bone Tumors, *1167*
Bone Cancer, *1168*
Disorders of the Hand, *1172*
Dupuytren's Contracture, *1172*
Ganglion, *1172*
Disorders of the Foot, *1172*
Foot Deformities, *1172*
Morton's Neuroma, *1173*
Plantar Fasciitis, *1173*
Other Problems of the Foot, *1173*
Scoliosis, *1173*
Progressive Muscular Dystrophies, *1174*

CHAPTER 54
Care of Patients with Musculoskeletal Trauma, 1178
Cathy A. Murray

Fractures, *1179*
Fractures of Specific Sites, *1195*
Upper Extremity Fractures, *1195*
Lower Extremity Fractures, *1195*
Fractures of the Chest and Pelvis, *1198*
Compression Fractures of the Spine, *1198*
Fractures at Other Sites, *1199*
Amputations, *1199*
Complex Regional Pain Syndrome, *1204*
Sports-Related Injuries, *1204*
Knee Injuries: Patellofemoral Pain Syndrome, *1205*
Knee Injuries: Meniscus, *1205*
Knee Injuries: Ligaments, *1206*
Other Injuries, *1206*
Carpal Tunnel Syndrome, *1206*
Tendon Rupture and Joint Dislocation, *1208*
Strains and Sprains, *1208*
Rotator Cuff Injuries, *1208*

HUMAN NEEDS OVERVIEW:
NUTRITION, METABOLISM, AND BOWEL ELIMINATION, 1212

UNIT XIII
Problems of Digestion, Nutrition, and Elimination: Management of Patients with Problems of the Gastrointestinal System

CHAPTER 55
Assessment of the Gastrointestinal System, 1216
Karrie K. Dietzen

Anatomy and Physiology Review, *1216*
Overview of the Gastrointestinal System, *1216*
Oral Cavity, *1217*
Esophagus, *1217*
Stomach, *1217*
Pancreas, *1218*
Liver and Gallbladder, *1218*
Small Intestine, *1219*
Large Intestine, *1219*
Gastrointestinal Changes Associated with Aging, *1219*
Assessment Methods, *1219*
Patient History, *1219*
Physical Assessment, *1221*
Psychosocial Assessment, *1223*
Diagnostic Assessment, *1223*

CHAPTER 56
Care of Patients with Oral Cavity Problems, 1231
Karrie K. Dietzen

Stomatitis, *1231*
Oral Tumors, *1234*
Premalignant Lesions, *1234*
Oral Cancer, *1234*
Disorders of the Salivary Glands, *1239*
Acute Sialadenitis, *1239*
Postirradiation Sialadenitis, *1240*
Salivary Gland Tumors, *1240*

CHAPTER 57
Care of Patients with Esophageal Problems, 1243
Donna D. Ignatavicius

Gastroesophageal Reflux Disease, *1243*
Hiatal Hernia, *1249*
Achalasia, *1254*
Esophageal Tumors, *1255*
Esophageal Diverticula, *1261*
Esophageal Trauma, *1262*

CHAPTER 58
Care of Patients with Stomach Disorders, 1265
Donna D. Ignatavicius

Gastritis, *1265*
Peptic Ulcer Disease, *1270*
Zollinger-Ellison Syndrome, *1279*
Gastric Cancer, *1279*

CHAPTER 59
Care of Patients with Noninflammatory Intestinal Disorders, 1289
Lynne Brophy
Donna D. Ignatavicius

Irritable Bowel Syndrome, *1289*
Herniation, *1291*
Colorectal Cancer, *1293*
Intestinal Obstruction, *1302*
Abdominal Trauma, *1307*
Polyps, *1308*
Hemorrhoids, *1309*
Malabsorption Syndrome, *1310*

CHAPTER 60
Care of Patients with Inflammatory Intestinal Disorders, 1315
Karen Ruschman

Acute Inflammatory Bowel Disorders, *1316*
Appendicitis, *1316*
Peritonitis, *1317*
Gastroenteritis, *1319*
Inflammatory Bowel Disease, *1321*
Ulcerative Colitis, *1321*
Crohn's Disease, *1330*
Diverticular Disease, *1334*
Anal Disorders, *1337*
Anorectal Abscess, *1337*
Anal Fissure, *1337*
Anal Fistula, *1338*
Parasitic Infection, *1338*
Helminthic Infestation, *1339*
Roundworms, *1339*
Tapeworms, *1340*
Food Poisoning, *1340*
Salmonellosis, *1340*
Staphylococcal Infection, *1341*
Escherichia coli Infection, *1341*
Botulism, *1341*

CHAPTER 61
Care of Patients with Liver Problems, 1344
Donna D. Ignatavicius

Cirrhosis, *1344*
Hepatitis, *1356*
Fatty Liver (Steatosis), *1360*
Hepatic Abscess, *1361*
Liver Trauma, *1361*
Cancer of the Liver, *1362*
Liver Transplantation, *1362*

CHAPTER 62
Care of Patients with Problems of the Biliary System and Pancreas, 1366
Donna D. Ignatavicius
Sarah Pettus

Gallbladder Disorders, *1366*
Cholecystitis, *1366*
Cancer of the Gallbladder, *1371*
Pancreatic Disorders, *1371*
Acute Pancreatitis, *1371*
Chronic Pancreatitis, *1377*
Pancreatic Abscess, *1379*
Pancreatic Pseudocyst, *1380*
Insulinoma, *1380*
Pancreatic Cancer, *1380*

CHAPTER 63
Care of Patients with Malnutrition and Obesity, 1386
Donna D. Ignatavicius

Nutrition Standards for Health Promotion and Maintenance, *1386*
Nutritional Assessment, *1387*
Initial Nutritional Screening, *1389*
Anthropometric Measurements, *1389*
Malnutrition, *1392*
Obesity, *1402*

UNIT XIV
Problems of Regulation and Metabolism: Management of Patients with Problems of the Endocrine System

CHAPTER 64
Assessment of the Endocrine System, 1412
M. Linda Workman

Anatomy and Physiology Review, *1413*
Hypothalamus and Pituitary Glands, *1414*
Gonads, *1415*
Adrenal Glands, *1415*
Thyroid Gland, *1417*
Parathyroid Glands, *1417*
Pancreas, *1418*
Endocrine Changes Associated with Aging, *1418*
Assessment Methods, *1419*
Patient History, *1419*
Physical Assessment, *1421*
Psychosocial Assessment, *1422*
Diagnostic Assessment, *1423*

CHAPTER 65
Care of Patients with Pituitary and Adrenal Gland Problems, 1425
M. Linda Workman

Disorders of the Anterior Pituitary Gland, *1426*
Hypopituitarism, *1426*
Hyperpituitarism, *1428*

Disorders of the Posterior Pituitary Gland, *1432*
Diabetes Insipidus, *1432*
Syndrome of Inappropriate Antidiuretic Hormone, *1433*
Disorders of the Adrenal Gland, *1436*
Adrenal Gland Hypofunction, *1436*
Adrenal Gland Hyperfunction, *1439*

CHAPTER 66
Care of Patients with Problems of the Thyroid and Parathyroid Glands, 1448
M. Linda Workman

Thyroid Disorders, *1448*
Hyperthyroidism, *1448*
Hypothyroidism, *1455*
Thyroiditis, *1460*
Thyroid Cancer, *1460*
Parathyroid Disorders, *1461*
Hyperparathyroidism, *1461*
Hypoparathyroidism, *1463*

CHAPTER 67
Care of Patients with Diabetes Mellitus, 1465
Margaret Elaine McLeod

Pathophysiology, *1466*
Classification of Diabetes, *1466*
The Endocrine Pancreas, *1466*
Insulin Physiology, *1466*
Glucose Homeostasis, *1467*
Absence of Insulin, *1467*
Acute Complications of Diabetes, *1468*
Chronic Complications of Diabetes, *1468*
Etiology and Genetic Risk, *1471*
Incidence/Prevalence, *1472*
Health Promotion and Maintenance, *1472*
Patient-Centered Collaborative Care, *1473*

HUMAN NEEDS OVERVIEW: URINARY ELIMINATION, 1522

UNIT XV
Problems of Excretion: Management of Patients with Problems of the Renal/Urinary System

CHAPTER 68
Assessment of the Renal/Urinary System, 1526
Chris Winkelman

Anatomy and Physiology Review, *1526*
Kidneys, *1526*
Ureters, *1532*
Urinary Bladder, *1532*
Urethra, *1533*
Renal/Urinary Changes Associated with Aging, *1533*
Renal Changes, *1533*
Urinary Changes, *1533*
Assessment Methods, *1533*
Patient History, *1533*
Physical Assessment, *1536*
Psychosocial Assessment, *1537*
Diagnostic Assessment, *1537*

CHAPTER 69
Care of Patients with Urinary Problems, 1550
Chris Winkelman

Infectious Disorders, *1550*
Cystitis, *1551*
Urethritis, *1559*
Noninfectious Disorders, *1559*
Urethral Strictures, *1559*
Urinary Incontinence, *1559*
Urolithiasis, *1570*
Urothelial Cancer, *1575*
Bladder Trauma, *1578*

CHAPTER 70
Care of Patients with Renal Disorders, 1581
Chris Winkelman

Congenital Disorders, *1581*
Polycystic Kidney Disease, *1581*
Obstructive Disorders, *1585*
Hydronephrosis, Hydroureter, and Urethral Stricture, *1585*
Infectious Disorders: Pyelonephritis, *1586*
Immunologic Renal Disorders, *1589*
Acute Glomerulonephritis, *1590*
Rapidly Progressive Glomerulonephritis, *1591*
Chronic Glomerulonephritis, *1592*
Nephrotic Syndrome, *1592*
Immunologic Interstitial and Tubulointerstitial Disorders, *1593*
Degenerative Disorders, *1593*
Nephrosclerosis, *1593*
Renovascular Disease, *1593*
Diabetic Nephropathy, *1594*
Renal Cell Carcinoma, *1595*
Renal Trauma, *1596*

CHAPTER 71
Care of Patients with Acute Renal Failure and Chronic Kidney Disease, 1600
Linda A. LaCharity

Acute Renal Failure, *1601*
Chronic Kidney Disease, *1609*
Renal Replacement Therapies, *1620*

HUMAN NEEDS OVERVIEW: SEXUALITY, 1638

UNIT XVI
Problems of Reproduction: Management of Patients with Problems of the Reproductive System

CHAPTER 72
Assessment of the Reproductive System, 1642
Deitra Leonard Lowdermilk

Anatomy and Physiology Review, *1642*
Structure and Function of the Female Reproductive System, *1642*
Structure and Function of the Male Reproductive System, *1645*

Reproductive Changes Associated with Aging, *1646*
Assessment Methods, *1647*
Patient History, *1647*
Physical Assessment, *1649*
Psychosocial Assessment, *1651*
Diagnostic Assessment, *1652*

CHAPTER 73
Care of Patients with Breast Disorders, 1660
Mary F. Justice

Benign Breast Disorders, *1660*
Fibroadenoma, *1660*
Fibrocystic Breast Condition, *1661*
Ductal Ectasia, *1661*
Intraductal Papilloma, *1662*
Issues of Large-Breasted Women, *1662*
Issues of Smaller-Breasted Women, *1662*
Gynecomastia, *1662*
Breast Cancer, *1663*

CHAPTER 74
Care of Patients with Gynecologic Problems, 1684
Pat Mahaffee Gingrich

Menstrual Cycle Disorders, *1684*
Primary Dysmenorrhea, *1684*
Premenstrual Syndrome, *1685*
Endometriosis, *1687*
Dysfunctional Uterine Bleeding, *1688*
Menopause, *1689*
Vulvovaginitis, *1690*
Toxic Shock Syndrome, *1691*
Uterine Prolapse, *1691*
Fistulas, *1694*
Benign Neoplasms, *1694*
Ovarian Cyst, *1694*
Uterine Leiomyoma, *1694*
Bartholin Cyst, *1699*
Cervical Polyp, *1699*
Gynecologic Cancers, *1699*
Endometrial (Uterine) Cancer, *1699*
Cervical Cancer, *1702*
Ovarian Cancer, *1705*
Vulvar Cancer, *1707*
Vaginal Cancer, *1708*
Fallopian Tube Cancer, *1709*

CHAPTER 75
Care of Male Patients with Reproductive Problems, 1712
Donna D. Ignatavicius

Benign Prostatic Hypertrophy, *1712*
Prostate Cancer, *1719*
Erectile Dysfunction, *1725*
Testicular Cancer, *1726*
Other Problems Affecting the Testes and Adjacent Structures, *1730*
Hydrocele, *1730*
Spermatocele, *1731*
Varicocele, *1731*
Cancer of the Penis, *1732*
Phimosis and Paraphimosis, *1732*
Priapism, *1733*
Prostatitis, *1733*
Epididymitis, *1734*
Orchitis, *1734*

CHAPTER 76
Care of Patients with Sexually Transmitted Disease, 1737
Shirley E. Van Zandt

Infections Associated with Ulcers, *1738*
Syphilis, *1738*
Genital Herpes, *1742*
Infections of the Epithelial Structures, *1743*
Condylomata Acuminata (Genital Warts), *1743*
Gonorrhea, *1744*
Chlamydia Infection, *1746*
Other Gynecologic Conditions, *1747*
Pelvic Inflammatory Disease, *1747*
Vaginal Infections, *1753*
Other Sexually Transmitted Diseases, *1753*
Lymphogranuloma Venereum, *1753*
Chancroid, *1753*
Granuloma Inguinale, *1753*

APPENDIXES
A Do-Not-Use Abbreviations and Symbols, 1757
B Communication Quick Reference for Spanish-Speaking Patients, 1760

GLOSSARY, 1765

Guide to Special Features

Assessment Using Gordon's Functional Health Patterns

Acid-Base Assessment, 207
Cardiovascular Assessment, 711
Ear and Hearing Assessment, 1112
Endocrine Assessment, 1420
Eye and Vision Assessment, 1076
Fluid and Electrolyte Assessment, 178
Gastrointestinal Assessment, 1220
Hematologic Assessment, 882
Musculoskeletal Assessment, 1144
Neurologic Assessment, 937
Renal/Urinary Assessment, 1534
Reproductive Assessment, 1648
Respiratory Assessment, 558

Best Practice for Emergency Care

Adrenal Insufficiency, Acute, 1436
Anaphylaxis, 392
Autonomic Dysreflexia, 998
Benzodiazepine Overdose, 300
Burns, 528
Chest Discomfort, 856
Extremity Fracture, 1186
Heatstroke, 143
Hypertensive Crisis, 803
Malignant Hyperthermia, 275
Myxedema Coma, 1459
Nosebleed, Anterior, 592
Opioid Overdose, 299
Sports-Related Injuries, 1205
Surgical Wound Evisceration, 296
Thyroid Storm, 1455

Best Practice for Patient Safety & Quality Care

AIDS, Infection Control for Home Care, 384
Altitude-Related Illnesses, Preventing, Recognizing, and Treating, 156
Alzheimer's Disease, Promoting Communication, 976
Anterior Cervical Diskectomy and Fusion, 990
Anticoagulant or Fibrinolytic Therapy, Prevention of Injury, 683
Anticoagulant Therapy, 819
Arteriovenous Fistula, Arteriovenous Graft, or Arteriovenous Shunt, 1624
Artificial Airway, Suctioning, 584
Aspiration Prevention During Swallowing, 586, 603
Autologous Blood Salvage and Transfusion, 279
Breast Mass Assessment, 1670
Breast Reconstruction, Postoperative Care, 1677
Cancer, Colorectal, Screening Recommendations, 1295
Caregiver Stress Reduction, 978
Carpal Tunnel Syndrome Prevention in Health Care Organizations, 1207
Catheter-Related Infection Prevention, 1553
Chest Tube Drainage Systems, 648
Colonoscopy, 1229
Communicating with LGBT Patients, 30
Communicating with Non–English-Speaking Patients, 29
Continuous Passive Motion Machine, 334
Contracture Prevention, 544
Contrast Agent Precautions, 943
Contrast Media, Assessing the Patient, 1545
Dark Skin, Assessing Changes, 476
Diarrhea, Skin Care, 1312
Driver Safety Improvement, Older Adults, 19
Dying Patient and the Family, Psychosocial Interventions, 120
Ear Irrigation, 1123
Eardrops Instillation, 1121
Electroencephalogram, 947
Emergency Department, Maintaining Patient and Staff Safety, 129
Endocrine Testing, 1423
Endotracheal Tube Securement, 691
Extravasation Documentation, 424
Eye Patch Application, 1088
Eyedrop Instillation, 1081
Fall Prevention in Older Adults, 24
Falls Precautions, 180
Feeding Tube Maintenance, 1398
Fundoplication, Assessment of Postoperative Complications, 1254
Gait Training, 101
Genetic Testing and Counseling, 76
Genital Herpes, 1742
Hand Hygiene, 444
Hearing Impairment and Communication, 1135
Heart Transplant Rejection, Assessment, 790
Hemodialysis, 1626
HIV Postexposure Prophylaxis, 369
HIV, Recommendations for Preventing Transmission by Health Care Workers, 369
Home Hospice, Symptom Relief, 121
Hypophysectomy, 1432
Hypovolemic Shock, 836
Immunosuppressed Patient, 376
Inflammatory Bowel Disease, Pain Control and Skin Care, 1328
Infusing an Intermittent Drug, Backpriming Method, 220
Intraoperative Positioning, Prevention of Complications, 281
IV Administration of rtPA, 1037
Lumbar Spinal Surgery, Assessment and Management of Complications, 987
Magnetic Resonance Imaging, 1149
Mechanical Ventilation, 692
Meningitis, 963

Best Practice for Patient Safety & Quality Care—*cont'd*

Mental Status Assessment, 937
Mucositis, Mouth Care, 429
Musculoskeletal Injury, Assessment of Neurovascular Status, 1184
Myasthenia Gravis, Improving Nutrition, 1020
Nasogastric Tube After Esophageal Surgery, 1260
Nasogastric Tubes, 1277
Neutropenia, 426
Nursing Database, 937
Nutrition Screening Assessment, 1390
Ocular Irrigation, 1104
Ocular Prosthesis, Insertion and Removal, 1105
Ophthalmic Ointment Instillation, 1085
Oral Cavity Problems, 1233
Osteoporosis and Assessment of Risk Factors, 1153
Oxygen Therapy, 574
Pain, Reducing Postoperatively with Nonpharmacologic Interventions, 299
Paracentesis, 1352
Parkinson Disease, 967
Pericarditis, 786
Perineal Comfort Promotion, 1337
Perineal Wound Care, 1300
Peripheral Venous Catheters, Placement, 216
Peritoneal Dialysis Catheter, 1629
Phlebostatic Axis Identification, 727
Piggybacking an Intermittent Drug, 220
Plasmapheresis Complications, 1014
Pleurodesis, 650
Postmortem Care, 122
Postoperative Hand-off Report, 286
Post-Traumatic Stress Disorder Prevention in Staff During a Mass Casualty Event, 164
Pressure Ulcer Prevention, 485
Prostatectomy, 1722
Pulmonary Embolism Prevention, 678
Radioactive Sealed Implants, 420
Relocation Stress in Older Adults, Minimizing Effects, 18
Reproductive Health Problems, 1649
Restraint Alternatives, 24
Sealed Implants of Radioactive Sources, 1701
Sickle Cell Crisis, 897
Sinus Surgery, 655
Skin Problems, Nursing History, 466
Spinal Cord Injury and Motor Function Assessment, 994
Systemic Sclerosis and Esophagitis, 352
Thrombocytopenia, 910
Thrombocytopenia, Prevention of Injury, 427
Tonic-Clonic or Complete Partial Seizure, 959
Total Parenteral Nutrition, 1401
Tracheostomy Care, 585
Transfer Techniques, 100
Transfusion Therapy, 918
Transfusion, Older Adult, 919
Transurethral Resection of the Prostate, 1718
T-Tube, 1370
Tube Feeding Care and Maintenance, 1398
Ventilator-Associated Pneumonia Prevention, 660
Vertebroplasty or Kyphoplasty, Nursing Care, 1198
Viral Hepatitis Prevention in Health Care Workers, 1358
Wound Monitoring, 497
Z-Track Injection Method, 899

Common Examples of Drug Therapy

Adrenal Gland Hypofunction, 1439
Anaphylaxis, 393
Anthrax, Prophylaxis and Treatment, 673
Antiepileptic Drugs, 957
Arthritis and Connective Tissue Disease, 341
Asthma, 616
Burns, 542
Cardiac Arrest, 752
Coronary Artery Disease, 857
Diabetes Insipidus, 1434
Diabetes Mellitus, 1477
Dysrhythmias, 741
Eye Inflammation and Infection, 1086
Gastroesophageal Reflux Disease, 1246
Glaucoma, 1099
HIV Infection, 376
Hyperthyroidism, 1453
Hypovolemic Shock, 837
Methicillin-Resistant *Staphylococcus aureus*, 503
Nausea and Vomiting, Chemotherapy-Induced, 429
Osteoporosis, 1158
Pain, Postoperative, 297
Pelvic Inflammatory Disease, Acute, 1750
Peptic Ulcer Disease, 1268
Pulmonary Embolism, 681
Renal Failure, 1606
Tuberculosis, 671
Urinary Incontinence, 1565
Urinary Tract Infections, 1556
Vasodilators and Inotropes, Intravenous, 863

Concept Map

Bacterial Pneumonia, 662
Benign Prostatic Hypertrophy, 1716
Chronic Cancer Pain, 416
Cirrhosis, 1351
Diabetes Mellitus–Type 2, 1476
End-Stage Kidney Disease, 1616
Glaucoma, 1096
Hypertension, 800
Hypovolemic Shock, 834
Multiple Sclerosis, 1005
Pressure Ulcer, 492
Respiratory Acidosis (COPD Related), 625

Evidence-Based Practice

Blood Pressure Telemonitoring Program and Blood Pressure Lowering, 803
Breast Cancer and Chemotherapy Side Effects, 1678
Cardiovascular Risks and Ankle-Brachial Index Values, 717
Cataract Surgery Delays and Increased Risk for Negative Events, 1093
Catheters and Urinary Tract Infections, 1554
Coronary Artery Disease and Dietary Supplements for Prevention, 851
Dementia and Oral Hygiene in Long-Term Care Residents, 1232
Dentures and Surgery, 278
Distraction During Chemotherapy, 425
Fluid Intake and Acute Lung Injury, 688
Heart Failure and Home Care Management, 777
Hip Surgery and Functional Status, 1197
Implanted Cardiac Devices, 758
Insulin Therapy, 1500
Kidney Transplantation and Adherence to Immunosuppressive Therapy, 1634
Lung Cancer, Early Diagnosis, 643
Needle Sticks, 888
Oral Care to Prevent Ventilator-Associated Pneumonia, 661
Osteoarthritis, Daily Stressors and Coping Strategies, 326
Osteoporosis and Strategies for Prevention, 1155
Ostomies and Sexuality Challenges, 1302
Pain and Anxiety, 249
Pain Assessment in Older Adults with Cognitive or Communication Impairments, 44
Pain, Anxiety, and Patient Satisfaction, Effect of Music Therapy, 10
Pin Site Care and Improved Patient Outcomes, 1191
Prostate Cancer Stages, 1724
Skin Examination with Partners, 511
Stem Cell Donation, 908
Stool Collection and Patient Compliance, 1225
Stroke Patients and Community-Based Rehabilitation, 1048
Vertigo and Effectiveness of Self-Administered Treatment, 1128

Focused Assessment

AIDS, 383
Cancer, Oral, Older Adults, 1238
Diabetic Foot, 1503
Diabetic Patient, Home or Clinic Visit, 1516
Hearing Loss, 1131
Hysterectomy, Total Abdominal, 1697
Infection Risk in Hospitalized or Home Care Patients, 905
Kidney Disease, Chronic, 1634
Pneumonia, 665
Postanesthesia Care Unit Discharge to Medical-Surgical Unit, 289
Preoperative Patient, 251
Seizures, Nursing Observations and Documentation, 960
Sexually Transmitted Disease, 1740
Testicular Lump, 1728
Tracheostomy, 585
Urinary Incontinence, 1562

Home Care Assessment

Amputation, Lower Extremity, 1204
Breast Cancer Surgery, 1680
Cataract Surgery, 1095
Chronic Obstructive Pulmonary Disease, 634
Colostomy, 1301
Heart Failure, 776
Hyperpituitarism, Transsphenoidal Hypophysectomy, 1432
Inflammatory Bowel Disease, 1329
Laryngectomy, 605
Myocardial Infarction, 870
Peripheral Vascular Disease, 809
Pressure Ulcers, 499
Pulmonary Embolism, 684
Sepsis, 844
Thyroid Dysfunction, 1460
Ulcer Disease, 1279

Key Features

Acidosis, 207
Adrenal Insufficiency, 1437
AIDS, 371
Alkalosis, 211
Alzheimer's Disease, 972
Amyotrophic Lateral Sclerosis, 1007
Anemia, 894
Angina and Myocardial Infarction, 854
Anthrax, 673
Asthma, 613
Autonomic Dysreflexia, 998
Benign Prostatic Hyperplasia, 1714
Bowel Obstructions, Small and Large, 1304
Brain Tumors, 1061
Cancer, Gastric, Early Versus Advanced, 1280
Cancer, Pancreatic, 1381
Cervical Diskectomy and Fusion, 990
Cholecystitis, 1368
Compartment Syndrome, 1181
Cor Pulmonale, 623
Diabetes Insipidus, 1433
Endocarditis, Infective, 784
Fluid Overload, 182
Gastritis, 1267
Gastroesophageal Reflux Disease, 1244
GI Bleeding, 1271
Giant Cell (Temporal) Arteritis, 355
Guillain-Barré Syndrome, 1012

Key Features—*cont'd*

Heart Disease, Valvular, 779
Heart Failure, Left-Sided, 768
Heart Failure, Right-Sided, 768
Hernias, Hiatal, 1250
Hypercortisolism (Cushing's Disease/Syndrome), 1441
Hyperthyroidism, 1449
Hypothyroidism, 1456
Intracranial Pressure, Increased, 1037
Kidney Disease, Severe, Chronic, 1613
Leukemia, 903
Liver Trauma, 1361
Meningitis, 962
Migraine Headaches, 952
Multiple Sclerosis, 1003
Myasthenia Gravis, 1017
Nephrotic Syndrome, 1593
Occupational Pulmonary Diseases, 640
Opiate Use, Manifestations That Require Emergency Interventions, 91
Osteomyelitis, Acute and Chronic, 1166
Paget's Disease of the Bone, 1163
Pancreatitis, Chronic, 1378
Parkinson Disease, 966
Peripheral Arterial Disease, Chronic, 805
Peritonitis, 1317
Pharyngitis, Acute Viral and Bacterial, 656
Pituitary Hyperfunction, 1430
Pituitary Hypofunction, 1427
Polycystic Kidney Disease, 1583
Premenstrual Syndrome, 1686
Pressure Ulcers, 489
Pulmonary Edema, 775
Pulmonary Emboli: Fat Embolism Versus Blood Clot Embolism, 1182
Pulmonary Embolism, 679
Pyelonephritis, Acute, 1587
Pyelonephritis, Chronic, 1587
Renal Failure, Acute, 1604
Renovascular Disease, 1594
Rheumatoid Arthritis, 337
Shock, 829
Skin Conditions, Inflammatory, 505
Skin Infections, 500
Spinal Cord Tumors, 1001
Stroke Syndromes, 1033
Strokes, Left and Right Hemisphere, 1034
Systemic Lupus Erythematosus and Systemic Sclerosis, 348
Tachydysrhythmias and Bradydysrhythmias, Sustained, 738
Tonsillitis, Acute, 657
Toxic Shock Syndrome, 1692
Transient Ischemic Attack, 1030
Traumatic Brain Injury, 1049
Tumors, Esophageal, 1256
Ulcers, Lower Extremity, 806
Uremia, 1609
Urinary Tract Infection, 1555

Laboratory Profile

Acid-Base Assessment, 202
Acid-Base Imbalances, 208
Adrenal Gland Assessment, 1438
Anticoagulation Therapy, Blood Tests, 682
Blood Glucose Values, 1473
Burn Assessment During the Resuscitation/Emergent Phase, 532
Cardiovascular Assessment, 720
Connective Tissue Disease, 339
Gastrointestinal Assessment, 1224
Hematologic Assessment, 887
Hypovolemic Shock, 836
Musculoskeletal Assessment, 1148
Parathyroid Function, 1462
Perioperative Assessment, 250
Renal Failure, 1605
Renal Function Blood Studies, 1538
Reproductive Assessment, 1653
Respiratory Assessment, 565
Thyroid Function, 1451
Urinalysis, 1539
Urine Collections, 24-Hour, 1542

NIC Intervention Activities

Adrenal Insufficiency, 1439
Alcohol Withdrawal, 84
Alzheimer's Disease, 974
Burns, Resuscitation/Emergent Phase, 533
Cancer, Bone (Psychosocial Care), 1171
Caregiver Support, 22
Chronic Obstructive Pulmonary Disease, 629
Cirrhosis, 1353
Coronary Artery Disease and Acute Coronary Syndrome, 861
Diabetic Patient, Hypoglycemia, 1508
Diabetic Patient, Pain, 1505
Diabetic Patient, Physical Activity, 1497
Diabetic Patient, Reduced Sensation in the Lower Extremities, 1502
Dysrhythmias, 751
Esophageal Problems, 1258
Fluid Volume, Deficient, 180
Genetic Problem Risk, 77
Guillain-Barré Syndrome, 1015
Heart Failure, 771
Hypersensitivity/Allergy, 390
Hypokalemia, 189
Infection, 452
Infection, Risk, 443
Inflammatory Bowel Disease, 1324
Intestinal Disorders, Noninflammatory, 1297
Kidney Disease, Chronic, 1617
Leukemia, Bone Marrow/Stem Cell Transplantation, 911
Malnutrition, 1395
Metabolic Acidosis, 209
Oral Cancer, 1236
Osteoarthritis, 327

NIC Intervention Activities—*cont'd*

Pelvic Floor Muscles, Weak, 1693
Peptic Ulcer Disease, 1276
Peripheral Neurovascular Dysfunction, 1186
Pneumonia, 664
Pressure Ulcers, 493
Pulmonary Embolism, 680
Rehabilitation, 103
Renal Problems, 1584
Respiratory Problems, 572
Shock Progression, 833
Spinal Cord Injury, 995
Stroke, 1037
Urinary Incontinence, 1567
Vision, Reduced, 1106
Vocalization Problems, 595

Nursing Focus on the Older Adult

Acid-Base Imbalance, 205
Burn Injury Complications, 529
Cardiovascular System Changes, 710
Cerumen Impaction, 1123
Coronary Artery Bypass Graft Surgery, 871
Coronary Artery Disease, 861
Diverticulitis, 1335
Dysrhythmias, 760
Ear and Hearing Changes, 1112
Electrolyte Values, 184
Endocrine System Changes, 1419
Eye and Vision Changes, 1075
Fecal Impaction Prevention, 1306
Fluid Balance, 174
Gastrointestinal System Changes, 1220
Head Injury, 1054
Hematologic Assessment, 409, 882
Immune Function Changes, 308
Impaired Vision, Promoting Independent Living, 1098
Infection, Risk Factors, 442
Intraoperative Nursing Interventions, 279
Integumentary System Changes, 463
Low Back Pain, 984
Malnutrition, Risk Assessment, 1393
Musculoskeletal System Changes, 1143
Nervous System Changes, 936
Nutritional Intake, 1396
Pain, 40
Preoperative Considerations for Care Planning, 247
Rehabilitation Considerations, 104
Renal/Urinary System Changes, 1534
Reproductive System Changes, 1646
Respiratory Disorder, Chronic, 610
Respiratory System Changes, 557
Shock, Risk Factors, 841
Skin Care, Postoperative, 295
Spinal Cord Injury, 999
Surgical Risk Factors, 245
Teaching Older Adults, 4
Thyroid Problems, 1458
Total Hip Arthroplasty, 330
Urinary Incontinence, 1562

Patient and Family Education Guide

Arthritis and Energy Conservation, 346
Arthropod Bite/Sting Prevention, 150
Asthma Management, 615
Back Injury Prevention Through Proper Body Mechanics, 988
Bariatric Surgery, Discharge Teaching, 1408
Beta Blocker/Digoxin Therapy, 778
Bleeding and Injury Prevention with Anticoagulants, 684
Bleeding or Injury Prevention, 428
Bleeding Risk, 912
Blood Glucose Testing, 1474
Breast Cancer Surgery, Recovery, 1679
Breathing Exercises, 631
Cancer, Dietary Habits to Reduce Risk, 408
Cast Removal, Extremity Care, 1194
Catheter Care at Home, 1725
Central Venous Catheter, Home Care, 911
Cerumen Removal, Self–Ear Irrigation, 1113
Cervical Ablation Therapy, 1704
Cervical Biopsy, 1657
Chest Pain, Home Management, 872
Cirrhosis, 1355
Condoms, 1743
Coronary Artery Disease and Activity, 871
Coronary Artery Disease Prevention, 854
Cortisol Replacement Therapy, 1445
Death, Emotional Signs of Approaching, 116
Death, Physical Signs and Symptoms of Approaching, 115
Death, Signs That It Has Occurred, 121
Diabetes, Sick-Day Rules, 1512
Diabetes, Travel Tips, 1517
Dry Powder Inhaler, 619
Dry Skin Prevention, 480
Dysrhythmias, Preventing and Decreasing, 759
Ear Infection or Trauma, Prevention, 1134
Ear Surgery Recovery, 1125
Epilepsy Instructions, 959
Estrogen Replacement Therapy, 1690
Excretory Urogram, 1545
Eyedrops, 1076
Foot Care Instructions, 1504
Gastroenteritis, Transmission Prevention, 1321
Gastroesophageal Reflux Disease, Postoperative Instructions, 1248
Gastritis Prevention, 1266
Glucosamine Supplements, 328
Halo Device, 1000
Head Injury, Minor, 1056

Patient and Family Education Guide—*cont'd*

Hearing Aid Care, 1133
Heart Disease, Valvular, 783
Heat-Related Illness Prevention, 142
HIV Testing Recommendations, 370
HIV, Nonoccupational Postexposure Prophylaxis, 368
Hyperkalemia, Dietary Management, 191
Hypoglycemia, Home Treatment, 1508
Hypophosphatemia, Dietary Management, 195
Hysterectomy, Total Abdominal, 1698
Ileostomy Care, 1329
Implantable Cardioverter-Defibrillator, 761
Infection Precautions, 844
Infection Prevention, 375, 427, 912
Inhaler Use, 619
Insulin Administration, Subcutaneous, 1488
Insulin Mixing, 1488
Joint Protection Instructions, 336
Laparoscopic Nissen Fundoplication, Postoperative Instructions, 1253
Laryngectomy, Home Care, 605
Leg Exercises, Postoperative, 257
Lightning Strike Prevention, 151
Low Back Pain and Injury Prevention, 984
Low Back Pain Exercises, 986
Lupus Erythematosus and Skin Protection, 350
Lyme Disease, Prevention and Early Dectection, 356
Migraine Attack, Triggers, 954
MRSA, Prevention of Spread, 502
Myasthenia Gravis, Drug Therapy Instruction, 1022
Ocular Compress Application, 1087
Oral Cavity Maintenance, 1232
Osteoarthritis and Rheumatoid Arthritis Exercises, 336
Pacemakers, Permanent, 760
Pancreatitis, Chronic, Enzyme Replacement, 1378
Pancreatitis, Chronic, Prevention of Exacerbations, 1379
Pelvic Muscle Exercises, 1564
Peripheral Neuropathy, Chemotherapy-Induced, 431
Peripheral Vascular Disease and Foot Care, 810
Photodynamic Therapy, 432
Pneumonia Prevention, 660
Polycystic Kidney Disease, 1585
Polycythemia Vera, 901
Postmastectomy Exercises, 1675
Prostate Screening and Detection Guidelines (2008), 1719
Radiation Therapy and Skin Protection, 420
Reflux Control, 1245
Renal and Genitourinary Trauma Prevention, 1597
Renal and Urinary Problems Prevention, 1612
Respiratory Care, Perioperative, 257
Sexually Transmitted Diseases, Condom Use for Prevention, 368
Sexually Transmitted Diseases, Oral Antibiotic Therapy, 1752
Sickle Cell Crisis Prevention, 898
Skin Cancer Prevention, 511
Smoking Cessation, 614
Snakebite Prevention, 144
Sperm Banking, 1729
STEC *(E. coli)* Infection Prevention, 1341
Stroke, Risk Factors, 1033
Supraglottic Method of Swallowing, 604
Testicular Self-Examination, 1726
Total Hip Arthroplasty, 332
Toxic Shock Syndrome, Prevention, 1692
Urinary Calculi, 1575
Urinary Incontinence, 1570
Urinary Tract Infection Prevention, 1554
Vaginal Infections, 1691
Venous Insufficiency, 822
Viral Hepatitis, 1361
Viral Hepatitis Prevention, 1358
Vulvar Self-Examination, 1650
Vulvovaginitis, Prevention, 1691
Warfarin (Coumadin), Interference of Food and Drugs, 821
Wellness Promotion Through Lifestyles and Practices, 16
West Nile Virus Prevention, 964

Plan of Care

Critically Ill Neurologic Problem Affecting the Brain/Postoperative Craniotomy, 1038
Gastrectomy, 1282
Open Conventional Esophageal Surgery, 1250

Electronic Resources
Companion CD and Evolve

The following electronic resources are available to supplement and reinforce the content discussed in this textbook.

- Animations
- Answer Key for Decision-Making Challenges
- Answer Key for NCLEX® Examination Challenges
- Audio Key Points
- Audio and Video Clips
- Audio Glossary
- Interactive Concept Maps
- Concept Map Creator
- Fluid and Electrolyte Tutorial
- Health Assessment Image Collection
- Health Assessment Video Clips
- Pharmacology Review Questions for the NCLEX® Examination
- Prioritization and Delegation Questions for the NCLEX® Examination
- Self-Assessment Questions for the NCLEX® Examination
- Additional Reference Information

Each of the following resources is available for *every chapter* in the book:

(CD) Audio Glossary

(evolve) Answer Key for Decision-Making Challenges

(evolve) Answer Key for NCLEX® Examination Challenges

(evolve) Audio Key Points

(evolve) Nursing Interventions Classification and Nursing Outcomes Classification Listings

(evolve) Prioritization and Delegation Questions for the NCLEX® Examination

(CD) Self-Assessment Questions for the NCLEX® Examination

Following is a complete listing of specific resources available for select chapters in the book.

UNIT I
Foundations for Medical-Surgical Nursing

Chapter 6
Genetic Concepts for Medical-Surgical Nursing

(CD) Animation: Hereditary Traits

UNIT III
Management of Patients with Fluid, Electrolyte, and Acid-Base Imbalances

Chapter 15
Infusion Therapy

(evolve) Fluid and Electrolyte Tutorial

UNIT IV
Management of Perioperative Patients

Chapter 16
Care of Preoperative Patients

(evolve) Pharmacology Review Questions for the NCLEX® Examination

Chapter 17
Care of Intraoperative Patients

(evolve) Pharmacology Review Questions for the NCLEX® Examination

Chapter 18
Care of Postoperative Patients

(evolve) Audio Clip: Stridor

(evolve) Pharmacology Review Questions for the NCLEX® Examination

UNIT V
Problems of Protection: Management of Patients with Problems of the Immune System

Chapter 19
Inflammation and the Immune Response

(CD) Animation: Inflammatory Response

Chapter 20
Care of Patients with Arthritis and Other Connective Tissue Diseases

(evolve) Pharmacology Review Questions for the NCLEX® Examination

Chapter 21
Care of Patients with HIV Disease and Other Immune Deficiencies

(evolve) Pharmacology Review Questions for the NCLEX® Examination

Chapter 22
Care of Patients with Immune Function Excess: Hypersensitivity (Allergy) and Autoimmunity

(CD) Animation: Allergy

(evolve) Audio Clip: High- and Low-Pitched Crackles

(evolve) Audio Clip: High- and Low-Pitched Wheezes

(CD) available on Companion CD and Evolve website

(evolve) available on Evolve website at http://evolve.elsevier.com/Iggy/

Chapter 23
Cancer Development

- Animation: Metastatic Spread of Breast Cancer

Chapter 24
Care of Patients with Cancer

- evolve Interactive Concept Map: Chronic Cancer Pain

Chapter 25
Care of Patients with Infection

- evolve Pharmacology Review Questions for the NCLEX® Examination

UNIT VI
Problems of Protection: Management of Patients with Problems of the Skin, Hair, and Nails

Chapter 27
Care of Patients with Skin Problems

- evolve Interactive Concept Map: Pressure Ulcer
- evolve Pharmacology Review Questions for the NCLEX® Examination

Chapter 28
Care of Patients with Burns

- evolve Audio Clip: High- and Low-Pitched Crackles
- evolve Audio Clip: High- and Low-Pitched Wheezes
- evolve Pharmacology Review Questions for the NCLEX® Examination

UNIT VII
Problems of Oxygenation: Management of Patients with Problems of the Respiratory Tract

Chapter 29
Assessment of the Respiratory System

- Animation: Pulmonary Circulation
- evolve Audio Clip: Bronchial Breath Sounds
- evolve Audio Clip: Bronchovesicular Breath Sounds
- evolve Audio Clip: High- and Low-Pitched Crackles
- evolve Audio Clip: High- and Low-Pitched Wheezes
- evolve Audio Clip: Pleural Friction Rub
- evolve Audio Clip: Vesicular Breath Sounds
- Video Clip: Diaphragmatic Excursion
- Video Clip: Inspection of the Nose
- Video Clip: Percussion: Anterior Thorax
- Video Clip: Respiratory Excursion
- Video Clip: Tactile Fremitus

Chapter 30
Care of Patients Requiring Oxygen Therapy or Tracheostomy

- Animation: Pulse Oximeter
- Animation: Suctioning

Chapter 31
Care of Patients with Noninfectious Upper Respiratory Problems

- evolve Audio Clip: Stridor
- evolve Pharmacology Review Questions for the NCLEX® Examination

Chapter 32
Care of Patients with Noninfectious Lower Respiratory Problems

- evolve Animation: Asthma
- evolve Audio Clip: High- and Low-Pitched Wheezes
- evolve Audio Clip: Pleural Friction Rub
- evolve Interactive Concept Map: Respiratory Acidosis (COPD Related)
- evolve Pharmacology Review Questions for the NCLEX® Examination

Chapter 33
Care of Patients with Infectious Respiratory Problems

- Animation: Tuberculosis
- evolve Audio Clip: High- and Low-Pitched Crackles
- evolve Audio Clip: High- and Low-Pitched Wheezes
- evolve Audio Clip: Stridor
- evolve Interactive Concept Map: Bacterial Pneumonia
- evolve Pharmacology Review Questions for the NCLEX® Examination

Chapter 34
Care of Critically Ill Patients with Respiratory Problems

- Animation: Endotracheal Intubation
- Animation: Pulmonary Embolism
- evolve Audio Clip: Stridor
- evolve Pharmacology Review Questions for the NCLEX® Examination

UNIT VIII
Problems of Cardiac Output and Tissue Perfusion: Management of Patients with Problems of the Cardiovascular System

Chapter 35
Assessment of the Cardiovascular System

- Animation: Heart Valves and Sounds
- evolve Audio Clip: Single S_1
- evolve Audio Clip: S_1 at Various Locations
- evolve Audio Clip: Single S_2
- evolve Audio Clip: S_2 at Various Locations
- evolve Audio Clip: S_4
- evolve Audio Clip: S_3

- Audio Clip: Murmurs: High, Medium, and Low
- Audio Clip: Murmurs: Blowing, Harsh or Rough, and Rumble
- Audio Clip: Systolic Murmur
- Audio Clip: Diastolic Murmur
- Audio Clip: Pericardial Friction Rub
- Video Clip: Anterior Chest
- Video Clip: Auscultation with Diaphragm and Bell
- Video Clip: Auscultatory Landmarks
- Video Clip: Carotid Artery
- Video Clip: Pulses, Lower Extremities

Chapter 36
Care of Patients with Dysrhythmias

- Animation: Conduction of Heart Impulses
- Animation: Events Represented by the ECG
- Pharmacology Review Questions for the NCLEX® Examination

Chapter 37
Care of Patients with Cardiac Problems

- Animation: Congestive Heart Failure
- Animation: Pericardial Tamponade
- Pharmacology Review Questions for the NCLEX® Examination

Chapter 38
Care of Patients with Vascular Problems

- Animation: Abdominal Aortic Aneurysm
- Animation: Physiology of Blood Pressure
- Interactive Concept Map: Hypertension
- Pharmacology Review Questions for the NCLEX® Examination

Chapter 39
Care of Patients with Shock

- Interactive Concept Map: Hypovolemic Shock
- Pharmacology Review Questions for the NCLEX® Examination

Chapter 40
Care of Patients with Acute Coronary Syndromes

- Animation: Acute Coronary Syndrome
- Animation: Coronary Artery Bypass Graft
- Pharmacology Review Questions for the NCLEX® Examination

UNIT IX
Problems of Tissue Perfusion: Management of Patients with Problems of the Hematologic System

Chapter 42
Care of Patients with Hematologic Problems

- Pharmacology Review Questions for the NCLEX® Examination

UNIT X
Problems of Mobility, Sensation, and Cognition: Management of Patients with Problems of the Nervous System

Chapter 43
Assessment of the Nervous System

- Animation: Cranial Nerves
- Animation: Physiology of the Brain
- Video Clip: Central Vision
- Video Clip: Deep Tendon Reflex
- Video Clip: Fine Motor Coordination
- Video Clip: Light Touch
- Video Clip: Pupil Responses
- Video Clip: Sensory Evaluation
- Video Clip: Smell

Chapter 44
Care of Patients with Problems of the Central Nervous System: The Brain

- Animation: Meningitis
- Animation: Parkinson's Disease
- Pharmacology Review Questions for the NCLEX® Examination

Chapter 45
Care of Patients with Problems of the Central Nervous System: The Spinal Cord

- Animation: Spinal Cord Structure
- Interactive Concept Map: Multiple Sclerosis
- Pharmacology Review Questions for the NCLEX® Examination

Chapter 46
Care of Patients with Problems of the Peripheral Nervous System

- Animation: Guillain-Barré Syndrome
- Pharmacology Review Questions for the NCLEX® Examination

Chapter 47
Care of Critically Ill Patients with Neurologic Problems

- Animation: Subarachnoid Hemorrhage
- Pharmacology Review Questions for the NCLEX® Examination

UNIT XI
Problems of Sensation: Management of Patients with Problems of the Sensory System

Chapter 48
Assessment of the Eye and Vision

- Video Clip: Central Vision
- Video Clip: External Eye
- Video Clip: Pupil Responses

Chapter 49
Care of Patients with Eye and Vision Problems

- evolve Interactive Concept Map: Glaucoma
- evolve Pharmacology Review Questions for the NCLEX® Examination

Chapter 50
Assessment of the Ear and Hearing

- Video Clip: Ear Canal
- Video Clip: External Ear

Chapter 51
Care of Patients with Ear and Hearing Problems

- evolve Pharmacology Review Questions for the NCLEX® Examination

UNIT XII
Problems of Mobility: Management of Patients with Problems of the Musculoskeletal System

Chapter 52
Assessment of the Musculoskeletal System

- Video Clip: Gait
- Video Clip: Muscular Development and Strength

Chapter 53
Care of Patients with Musculoskeletal Problems

- evolve Pharmacology Review Questions for the NCLEX® Examination

Chapter 54
Care of Patients with Musculoskeletal Trauma

- evolve Pharmacology Review Questions for the NCLEX® Examination

UNIT XIII
Problems of Digestion, Nutrition, and Elimination: Management of Patients with Problems of the Gastrointestinal System

Chapter 55
Assessment of the Gastrointestinal System

- Animation: Digestion
- Video Clip: Abdomen, Bowel Sounds
- Video Clip: Palpation of Abdomen
- Video Clip: Percussion, Abdomen
- Video Clip: Percussion, Liver, Spleen

Chapter 56
Care of Patients with Oral Cavity Problems

- evolve Pharmacology Review Questions for the NCLEX® Examination

Chapter 57
Care of Patients with Esophageal Problems

- evolve Pharmacology Review Questions for the NCLEX® Examination

Chapter 58
Care of Patients with Stomach Disorders

- Animation: Bleeding Ulcer, Pathophysiology
- evolve Pharmacology Review Questions for the NCLEX® Examination

Chapter 59
Care of Patients with Noninflammatory Intestinal Disorders

- Animation: Nasogastric Tube Placement
- evolve Pharmacology Review Questions for the NCLEX® Examination

Chapter 60
Care of Patients with Inflammatory Intestinal Disorders

- evolve Pharmacology Review Questions for the NCLEX® Examination

Chapter 61
Care of Patients with Liver Problems

- evolve Interactive Concept Map: Cirrhosis
- evolve Pharmacology Review Questions for the NCLEX® Examination

Chapter 62
Care of Patients with Problems of the Biliary System and Pancreas

- Animation: Laparoscopic Cholecystectomy; Gallbladder Removal
- evolve Pharmacology Review Questions for the NCLEX® Examination

Chapter 63
Care of Patients with Malnutrition and Obesity

- evolve Pharmacology Review Questions for the NCLEX® Examination

UNIT XIV
Problems of Regulation and Metabolism: Management of Patients with Problems of the Endocrine System

Chapter 65
Care of Patients with Pituitary and Adrenal Gland Problems

- evolve Pharmacology Review Questions for the NCLEX® Examination

Chapter 66
Care of Patients with Problems of the Thyroid and Parathyroid Glands

- evolve Pharmacology Review Questions for the NCLEX® Examination

Chapter 67
Care of Patients with Diabetes Mellitus

- Animation: Insulin Function
- evolve Interactive Concept Map: Diabetes Mellitus—Type 2
- evolve Pharmacology Review Questions for the NCLEX® Examination

UNIT XV
Problems of Excretion: Management of Patients with Problems of the Renal/Urinary System

Chapter 68
Assessment of the Renal/Urinary System

- Animation: Filtration
- Animation: Nephrons

Chapter 69
Care of Patients with Urinary Problems

- Animation: Renal Stone; Kidney Stone; Nephrolithiasis
- Animation: Insertion of Foley Catheter
- evolve Pharmacology Review Questions for the NCLEX® Examination

Chapter 70
Care of Patients with Renal Disorders

- evolve Pharmacology Review Questions for the NCLEX® Examination

Chapter 71
Care of Patients with Acute Renal Failure and Chronic Kidney Disease

- Animation: Renal and Urinary Disorders
- evolve Interactive Concept Map: End-Stage Kidney Disease (ESKD)
- evolve Pharmacology Review Questions for the NCLEX® Examination

UNIT XVI
Problems of Reproduction: Management of Patients with Problems of the Reproductive System

Chapter 72
Assessment of the Reproductive System

- Video Clip: Bimanual Examination
- Video Clip: External Genitalia
- Video Clip: Inguinal Hernia Evaluation
- Video Clip: Inspection (Standing)
- Video Clip: Speculum Examination

Chapter 73
Care of Patients with Breast Disorders

- evolve Pharmacology Review Questions for the NCLEX® Examination
- Video Clip: Inspection (Sitting)
- Video Clip: Inspection (Supine)

Chapter 74
Care of Patients with Gynecologic Problems

- evolve Pharmacology Review Questions for the NCLEX® Examination

Chapter 75
Care of Male Patients with Reproductive Problems

- evolve Interactive Concept Map: Benign Prostatic Hypertrophy
- evolve Pharmacology Review Questions for the NCLEX® Examination

Chapter 76
Care of Patients with Sexually Transmitted Disease

- evolve Pharmacology Review Questions for the NCLEX® Examination

Medical-Surgical Nursing

Patient-Centered Collaborative Care

I

UNIT

Foundations for Medical-Surgical Nursing

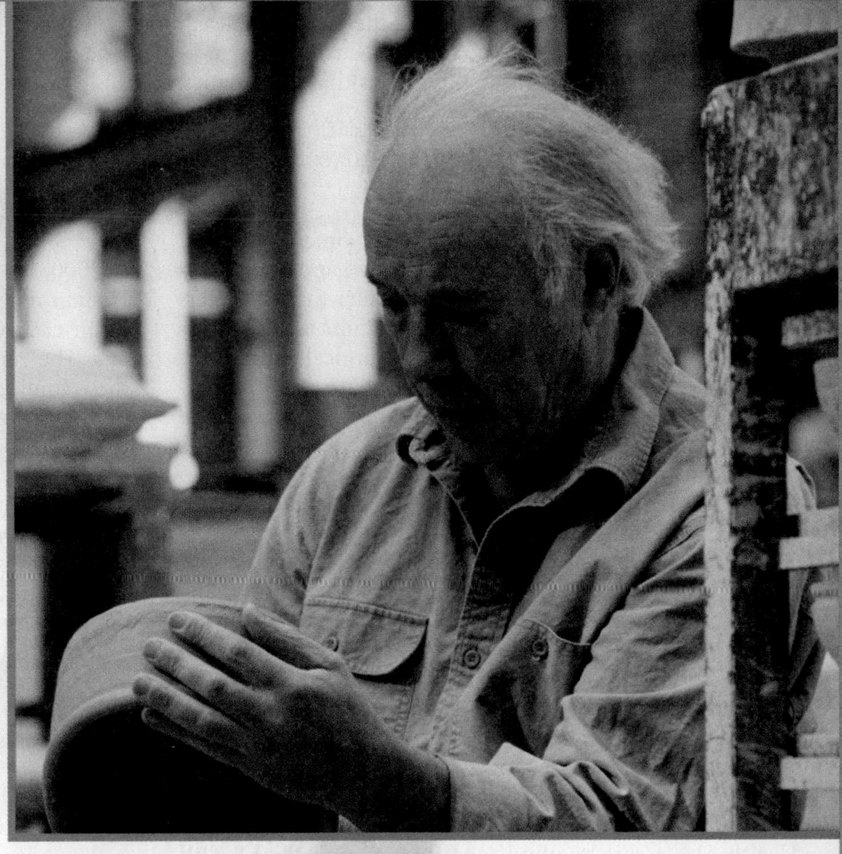

CHAPTER 1

Introduction to Medical-Surgical Nursing

Donna D. Ignatavicius

LEARNING OUTCOMES

For clinical competence and success on the NCLEX Examination, study this chapter with these Learning Outcomes in mind:

1. Describe the scope of medical-surgical nursing.
2. Explain the recent increased focus on patient safety and quality of care.
3. Identify the purpose of the Rapid Response Team (RRT).
4. Explain when to call the RRT.
5. Explain the primary roles of the medical-surgical nurse.
6. Identify three ethical principles that help guide clinical decision making.
7. Explain the importance of communication when collaborating with the interdisciplinary team.
8. Identify best practice interventions when teaching older adults.
9. List the steps of the evidence-based practice process.
10. Describe the nurse's role in the systematic quality improvement process.
11. Identify three ways that informatics is used in health care.

evolve Go to your Companion CD or Evolve at http://evolve.elsevier.com/Iggy/ for *Self-Assessment Questions for the NCLEX Examination* keyed to these Learning Outcomes.

The scope of medical-surgical nursing, sometimes called *adult health nursing,* is to promote health and prevent illness or injury in patients from 18 to older than 100 years of age. A separate chapter on care of older adults is part of this textbook because the majority of medical-surgical patients are over 65 years of age (see Chapter 3). To be consistent with current health care literature, the authors use the term *patient* rather than *client* (except in *NCLEX Examination Challenge* questions). In this textbook, **patients** are recipients of care in mutually trusting relationships with nurses and other members of the health care team.

Although medical-surgical nursing is considered a specialty practice, nurses who practice medical-surgical nursing must have a broad knowledge base to meet the needs of patients in a variety of health care settings across the continuum (Academy of Medical-Surgical Nursing [AMSN], 2007). The most common area of practice, though, is the acute care hospital. Rapid advances in technology, massive increases in knowledge, and dramatic changes in the health care delivery system require that medical-surgical nurses use expert clinical judgment *to ensure patient safety as the priority in practice.*

Health care errors by physicians, nurses, and other health care professionals have been widely publicized for the past 10 years. Many of these errors have resulted in patient deaths and injuries. As a result of these findings, a number of national and international organizations have implemented new programs and standards to combat this growing problem.

NATIONAL PATIENT SAFETY GOALS

In 2000, the Institute of Medicine (IOM) stated in its *To Err is Human* report that between 44,000 and 98,000 patient *deaths* result each year from preventable errors in acute care hospitals. The report identified several factors that contribute to these findings and motivated other national bodies to examine ways they could improve patient safety and quality care. One of these groups, The Joint Commission (TJC), requires that health care organizations create a *culture of safety*.

The Joint Commission (formerly the Joint Commission for the Accreditation of Healthcare Organizations [JCAHO]) offers peer evaluation for accreditation every 3 years for all types of health care agencies that meet their standards. Although acute care hospitals are accredited more often than other types of settings, many home care agencies, nursing homes, and ambulatory care centers are also TJC-accredited.

In 2002, TJC published its first annual **National Patient Safety Goals (NPSGs).** These Goals require health care organizations to focus on specific priority safety practices, many of which involve nursing care. Since that time, TJC continues to add new Goals each year. NPSGs address high-risk issues such as drug administration, fall reduction, pressure ulcer prevention, and communication among health care team members. When appropriate, this textbook discusses related NPSGs and highlights them with a special icon. A complete list of these goals can be found on TJC website at www.jointcommission.org.

PROTECTING FIVE MILLION LIVES FROM HARM

As a result of the IOM report and other data from national studies, the Institute for Healthcare Improvement (IHI) estimates that there are nearly 15 million *health care errors* in U.S. hospitals each year, or 40,000 per day (www.ihi.org). In 2004, the IHI and its partner health care organizations launched the *100,000 Lives Campaign*—an effort to save patient lives over an 18-month targeted time frame. Six interventions for quality improvement changes in care were implemented by partnering health care agencies (Table 1-1). As a result of this project, an estimated 122,000 patient lives were saved!

The next IHI objective was to *protect patients from five million incidents of medical harm* over a 2-year period (December, 2006–December, 2008) (www.ihi.org). **Medical harm** refers not just to physician incidents but to errors caused by *all* members of the health care team that lead to patient injury or death. To meet this IHI objective, six interventions for changes in care were added to the original list. As seen in Table 1-1, many of these interventions are within the scope of nursing practice and are therefore emphasized throughout this textbook. Some interventions, such as pressure ulcer prevention and adverse drug event reduction, are also part of TJC's National Patient Safety Goals.

One of the most successful IHI initiatives was the creation of the Rapid Response Team (RRT), also called the *Medical Emergency Team (MET).* **Rapid Response Teams** save lives and decrease the risk for harm by providing care to patients *before* a respiratory or cardiac arrest occurs. Although the RRT does not replace the Code Team who responds to patient arrests, it intervenes rapidly for those who are beginning to clinically decline. Clinical changes in condition occur in most patients for up to 48 hours before a "Code Blue." *Observe for and report common clinical manifestations of patient decline, including hypotension, tachycardia, and mental status changes* (Morse et al., 2007).

Members of an RRT are critical care experts who are on-site and available at any time. Although membership varies among facilities, the team may consist of an ICU nurse, respiratory therapist, and **intensivist** (physician who specializes in critical care). In other hospitals, acute care nurse practitioners or medical residents may be part of the team. The team responds to emergency calls, usually from nurses, according to established agency protocols and policies. Outcome data demonstrate that using this approach to emergency care reduces medical complications and decreases the number of cardiac and respiratory arrests (Durkin, 2006). *Therefore call the RRT whenever a patient has a slow or sudden deterioration in clinical condition.* This textbook presents *Decision-Making Challenges: Critical Rescue* exercises to help you decide what to do as patient conditions change.

The Joint Commission's 2008 National Patient Safety Goals also include the need for early intervention for patients who are clinically changing. They require each health care organization to establish criteria for patients, families, or staff to call for additional assistance in response to an actual or perceived change in the patient's condition.

TABLE 1-1 Institute for Healthcare Improvement (IHI) Interventions to Save Patient Lives and Prevent Patient Harm

Interventions to Save Patient Lives	Interventions to Prevent Patient Harm
Deploy Rapid Response Teams.	Prevent harm from High-Alert Drugs (e.g., anticoagulants, insulin, opioids).
Provide reliable, evidence-based care for acute myocardial infarction.	Reduce surgical complications.
Prevent central line infections.	Prevent pressure ulcers.
Prevent adverse drug events (ADEs).	Reduce methicillin-resistant *Staphylococcus aureus* (MRSA) infections.
Prevent surgical site infections.	Provide reliable, evidence-based care for congestive heart failure.
Prevent ventilator-associated pneumonia.	Get boards of health care organizations to support measures to promote safe patient care.

INSTITUTE OF MEDICINE CORE COMPETENCIES FOR HEALTH PROFESSIONALS

The Institute of Medicine (IOM) has published many reports suggesting ways to improve patient safety and quality care. One of its reports, *Health Professions Education: A Bridge to Quality,* identified five broad core competencies for today's practice reality to ensure patient safety and quality care (IOM, 2003). All of these competencies are interrelated and include:

- Provide patient-centered care.
- Collaborate with the interdisciplinary health care team.
- Implement evidence-based practice.
- Use quality improvement in patient care.
- Use informatics in patient care.

The nursing profession has taken these recommendations very seriously and is continuing to study how to best apply them to nursing education and practice. One major project is the Quality and Safety Education for Nurses (QSEN) initiative, funded by the Robert Wood Johnson Foundation. The project leaders support the IOM competencies and have added *providing patient safety* as a separate competency to emphasize its importance to nursing.

Providing Patient-Centered Care

The primary concern of medical-surgical nursing care is to meet the biologic, psychosocial, cultural, and spiritual needs of the adult patient in a mutually trusting, respectful, and caring relationship. These basic human needs, also referred to as *concepts,* were introduced in your Fundamentals of Nursing course. This textbook builds on those concepts but focuses most on the role of nurses in meeting biologic (physiologic) human needs for selected medical-surgical patients. Discussions of psychosocial (emotional), cultural, and spiritual needs are presented when appropriate to describe a holistic approach to patient care. In addition, a separate chapter (Chapter 4) discusses cultural aspects. Chapter 2 presents an introduction to complementary and alternative therapies.

To further build a bridge between your basic fundamentals course and medical-surgical nursing care, several special features at the beginning of each textbook section visually review these selected human needs:

- Protection
- Oxygenation and Tissue Perfusion
- Mobility, Sensation, and Cognition
- Nutrition, Bowel Elimination, and Metabolism
- Urinary Elimination
- Human Sexuality

To meet these human needs for patient-centered care, the medical-surgical nurse functions in a variety of roles, including caregiver, educator, and advocate.

In the *caregiver* role, medical-surgical nurses assess patients, analyze collected information to determine their needs, develop nursing diagnoses and collaborative problems, plan care and carry out the plan with the health care team, and evaluate the care given. This process, which is referred to as the *nursing process*, is used throughout this text as an organizational tool.

As a caregiver, you will provide physical care through skills such as administering medications and performing comprehensive assessments. Some nursing tasks and activities may be delegated to unlicensed assistive personnel (UAP)—nursing staff members such as patient care technicians (PCTs) or patient care assistants (PCAs). Examples are turning and positioning, vital signs, and recording intake and output. Other activities may be assigned to licensed practical or vocational nurses (LPNs or LVNs), depending on the state in which practice occurs. Interventions that you can usually delegate or assign are indicated throughout this text and in the Plans of Care. *Decision-Making Challenge: Delegation and Supervision* questions provide the opportunity for you to make decisions about what and when to delegate and supervise UAP and LPNs/LVNs.

The RN or LPN/LVN also implements emotional and spiritual interventions, such as encouraging the patient to discuss concerns with a clergyperson or offering measures to reduce anxiety. Nursing interventions to help patients meet their spiritual needs are discussed in Chapter 4.

Activities that you will perform are often categorized as *collaborative* (interdependent) or *independent*. **Collaborative nursing functions** include:

- Those that are mutually determined by the nurse and the physician or other health care team member, such as setting activity limitations or providing a special diet
- Those that are directed or prescribed by the health care provider (physician, nurse practitioner, or physician assistant) but require nursing judgment to perform (e.g., administering medications)

Independent nursing functions are initiated and carried out without direction from the health care provider. Examples are:

- Weighing a patient
- Listening to breath sounds
- Elevating the head of the bed to facilitate breathing

This text discusses both types of nursing functions—collaborative and independent—in an interrelated framework under the heading *Patient-Centered Collaborative Care.* Charts entitled *Best Practice for Patient Safety and Quality Care* identify the most important collaborative care for patients with selected health problems. The roles for each member of the health care team are clearly identified.

Patient education is a major component of medical-surgical nursing care. In collaboration with the interdisciplinary team, the nurse strives to improve health by facilitating patient learning regarding health promotion, disease and illness, and specific treatment. As *educators,* you will teach individual patients and family members or other caregivers. The role of education has become increasingly important because patients are discharged "quicker and sicker" from the hospital, transitional care, or skilled nursing home unit.

Assess the patient's learning needs and barriers to learning. A patient with a disease for 25 years may need as much teaching as one with a newly diagnosed condition. Make no assumptions. Instead, assess each patient individually. Determine the patient's goals and willingness to learn. If he or she has no interest in learning, wait for another time or setting before beginning health teaching. Consider the special needs of older adults when providing patient teaching (Chart 1-1).

Health teaching may occur in a spontaneous, informal manner, or it may follow a more structured, formal approach based on written teaching plans. Most facilities provide written teaching plans and tools for the interdisciplinary team to ensure that every patient receives the same accurate information.

Chart 1-1 NURSING FOCUS ON THE OLDER ADULT

Best Practices Interventions for Teaching Older Adults

- Ensure that the patient wears glasses, contact lenses, or hearing aids if needed.
- Be sure that the area for teaching has ample lighting and minimal distraction.
- Speak slowly (but not loudly unless the patient has a hearing problem), and provide small amounts of new information at a time.
- Ask the patient to repeat the information to make sure that he or she has learned it.
- Provide written information so the patient can refer to it later if needed.
- Provide as much privacy as possible.
- Ask the patient whether family or significant others should be present during the interview.
- Refer to the patient by his or her last name (e.g., Mrs. Brown) unless he or she prefers another name.
- Provide health teaching when the patient is not experiencing pain and after basic comfort needs have been met.
- Sit at the patient's eye level during the interview.
- Be aware that the patient may not be able to distinguish soft consonant blends such as "sh" or "ch."
- Teach the patient in the morning, after breakfast, or in the early afternoon, after the patient has rested.
- Whenever possible, use open-ended questions to gather more information; avoid questions that can be answered "yes" or "no."
- Consider the patient's education, culture, and age when teaching, especially about sensitive or controversial issues.
- Observe the patient's nonverbal behavior as well as what he or she says.

Document what was taught and what the patient learned using the appropriate paper or electronic record. A signed copy of the information that was taught becomes a part of the medical record. Give a copy to the patient or family member or significant other at discharge. Some Community-Based Care sections within this text include a subsection entitled Health Teaching. *Patient and Family Education Guides* for health teaching are also included as appropriate throughout the text.

As an *advocate*, the medical-surgical nurse assists the patient and family through caring interventions. **Caring** is a process, set of actions, and attitude that show genuine physical and emotional concern for others. Examples of caring behaviors are:

- Protecting the patient from harm and providing a safe environment
- Responding promptly to patients' call lights or questions
- Being physically present for emotional support
- Interpreting information for patients and families
- Clarifying misunderstandings with patients and families
- Making eye contact with patients and families, if culturally appropriate
- Providing privacy and maintaining patient dignity
- Being culturally sensitive to patients and their families
- Taking time to listen to patients and their families
- Being respectful to patients and their families

Respect for people is one of three basic *ethical principles* that nurses and other health care professionals should use as a basis for clinical decision making. Respect implies that patients are treated as autonomous individuals capable of making informed decisions about their care. This patient autonomy is referred to as **self-determination** *or* **self-management.** When the patient is not capable of self-determination, you are ethically obligated to protect him or her as an advocate within the professional scope of practice, according to the American Nurses Association (ANA) Code of Ethics for Nurses.

The second ethical principle is **beneficence,** which emphasizes the importance of preventing harm and ensuring the patient's well-being. Harm can be avoided only if its causes or possible causes are identified. As described earlier in this chapter, patient safety is currently a major national focus to prevent deaths and injuries.

Justice, the third principle, refers to equality; that is, all patients should be treated equally and fairly. For example, a patient who cannot afford health care should receive the same quality and level of care as one who has extensive insurance coverage. An older patient with dementia should be shown the same respect as a younger patient who can communicate. *Decision-Making Challenge: Legal/Ethical* features are found throughout this textbook to help you think about this important concept for nursing practice.

Collaborating with the Interdisciplinary Health Care Team

Patient-centered care requires that all members of the interdisciplinary (ID) team collaborate to achieve optimal clinical outcomes. The nurse functions as the *coordinator of patient care* through effective communication with the nursing and health care team—for example, by conducting ID clinical rounds and developing ID plans of care.

One of the most important members of the ID team is the case manager (CM), who is usually a nurse or social worker in acute care hospitals. The goal of the **case management** process is to provide quality and cost-effective services and resources to achieve positive patient outcomes. In collaboration with the nurse, the CM coordinates inpatient and community-based care before discharge from a hospital or other facility. Part of that process may involve communicating with other CMs who are employed by third-party health care payers (e.g., Medicare).

Poor communication between professional caregivers and health care agencies has caused many medical errors and patient safety risks. In 2006, The Joint Commission began to require systematic strategies for improving communication. Two years later, another National Patient Safety Goal mandated that nurses communicate continuing patient care needs, such as pain management or respiratory support, to post-discharge caregivers.

Health care organizations must also establish procedures for "hand-off" communication between shifts and between departments. A popular procedure used in many agencies today is called *SBAR* (pronounced S-Bar). **SBAR** is a formal method of communication between two or more members of the health care team. It is used most often when there is an unmet patient need or problem. It can also be used to communicate continuing care issues when a patient is transferred from one agency to another. You will most likely be using this method of communication in the hospital setting. The SBAR process includes these four steps:

- **S**ituation: Describe what is happening at the time to require this communication.
- **B**ackground: Explain any relevant background information that relates to the situation.
- **A**ssessment: Provide an analysis of the problem or patient need based on assessment data.
- **R**ecommendation: State what is needed or what the desired outcome is.

Other agency-specific "hand-off" methods may be used to share information between nursing shifts in an inpatient facility or from one nurse to another in any setting. For example, Schroeder (2006) described a method for patient reporting called *PACE.* PACE stands for Patient Problem, Assessment/Actions, Continuing/Changes, and Evaluation. This type of focused information helps the receiving nurse maintain continuity of care and address any new patient problems that may have occurred. Be sure to follow the established documentation and reporting protocols in your agency to prevent miscommunication.

Implementing Evidence-Based Practice

Evidence-based practice (EBP) is the deliberate use of current best evidence to make decisions about patient care; it considers the patient's preferences and values, as well as one's own clinical expertise (Melnyk & Fineout-Overholt, 2005). All health care professions should use the EBP process to maintain patient safety and quality care. The steps of this process include:

1. Critically think about nursing or interdisciplinary practice to formulate important clinical questions.
2. Access resources to retrieve the most relevant and best evidence that may answer the clinical question (e.g., www.cochrane.org; www.nlm.nih.gov).
3. Critically analyze the evidence for validity, reliability, and utility to answer the clinical question.
4. Integrate the evidence findings with one's own expertise and patient preferences and values to make clinical decisions to answer the question.
5. Implement the evidence-based practice change or seek appropriate channels for making the change in practice.

6. Evaluate the practice change for its effectiveness in promoting patient safety and quality care.

As stated in the first step, critical thinking is an essential tool for the EBP process to provide quality, cost-effective, and safe patient care. Alfaro-LeFevre (2008) describes **critical thinking** as purposeful, outcome-directed thinking that is used to make clinical judgments based on scientific evidence, rather than on tradition or conjecture (guesswork). Clinical judgment is used to make timely and appropriate clinical decisions about patient care. This textbook includes many *Decision-Making Challenges* and *NCLEX Examination Challenges* that require critical thinking to answer.

The best source of scientific evidence is research. However, available nursing research is limited and often does not represent the highest or best level of evidence. As seen in Table 1-2, the highest level of evidence, or LOE-1, is based on a systematic review or meta-analysis of all relevant randomized controlled trials (RCTs), or evidence-based clinical practice guidelines based on systematic reviews of RCTs (Melynk & Fineout-Overholt, 2005). However, most nursing research consists of small descriptive studies at LOE-6. The findings of these studies cannot be generalized, but they provide a basis for future larger and better-controlled research. Each study in this text's *Evidence-Based Practice* feature is rated by level of evidence using the scale in Table 1-2. "Commentary and Nursing Implications" discussions are also presented to help you consider these findings for daily practice.

Using Quality Improvement in Patient Care

Ensuring patient safety requires individual and systematic evaluation. You should not only continuously reflect and examine your own practice but also assess potential systematic problems that impact the quality of nursing care—a more global approach. One of the ways to evaluate care is to be part of the quality improvement (QI) process in your setting. As a medical-surgical nurse, you will be expected to:

- Identify indicators to monitor quality and effectiveness of nursing care.
- Collect data to monitor the quality and effectiveness of nursing care.
- Recommend ways to improve nursing care.
- Implement activities to improve the quality of nursing care.

More information about your role in the QI process can be found in books that focus on the leadership role of nurses.

Using Informatics for Patient Care

Informatics is a specialized computer science that is used to manage information and technology (Yoder-Wise, 2007). Although most health care settings have information technology (IT) departments, nurses need to retrieve and use valuable information for patient care. The largest application of health care informatics is the growing trend of electronic medical records, or EMRs, for documenting interdisciplinary care. Computers may be centrally located or at the patient's bedside or treatment room (Fig. 1-1).

Another major purpose of informatics is for retrieval of data for the evidence-based practice process described earlier in this chapter. The Internet provides ways to search for multiple sources of information very efficiently. However, all electronic sources must be evaluated for their credibility and reliability.

The other main use of the Internet is to send and receive electronic mail. This method allows for quick communication among health care professionals to enhance collaboration and coordination of care. *However, it should not replace face-to-face and phone communication.*

TABLE 1-2 Level of Evidence (LOE) Rating Scale and Hierarchy of Evidence

LOE	Origin of Evidence
HIGHEST	
LOE-1	Systematic review or meta-analysis of all randomized controlled trials (RCTs) or evidence-based clinical practice guidelines based on systematic reviews of RCTs
LOE-2	At least one properly designed RCT
LOE-3	Well-designed controlled trials without randomization
MODERATE	
LOE-4	Well-designed case control and cohort studies
LOE-5	Systematic reviews of descriptive and qualitative studies
LOE-6	Single descriptive or qualitative study
LOWEST	
LOE-7	Opinion of authorities and/or reports of expert committees

Modified from Melnyk, B.M., & Fineout-Overholt, E. (2005). *Evidence-based practice in nursing and healthcare.* Philadelphia: Lippincott Williams & Wilkins.

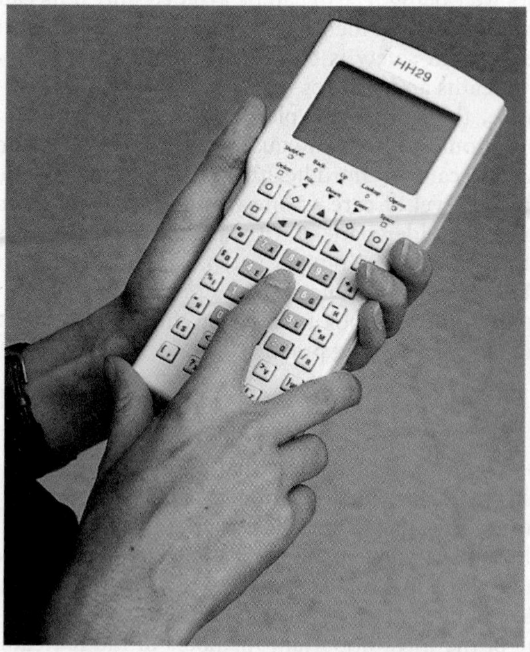
HH29

Fig. 1-1 • A handheld electronic documentation system that is used at the bedside.

GET READY FOR THE NCLEX EXAMINATION!

Key Points

Review these Key Points.

- Medical-surgical nursing requires a broad knowledge base to meet the needs of adult patients in a variety of settings across the continuum.
- The Joint Commission requires that health care organizations create a *culture of safety* by following the National Patient Safety Goals (NPSGs).
- The Institute of Healthcare Improvement (IHI) interventions to save lives and prevent patient harm are listed in Table 1-1.
- Rapid Response Teams (RRTs) save lives and decrease the risk for patient harm before a respiratory or cardiac arrest occurs.
- Remember to always observe for slow and sudden changes in patient condition, especially changes in vital signs and mental status.
- Nurses help meet human needs of adult patients, such as mobility and oxygenation, in a caring, mutually respectful relationship.
- The primary roles of medical-surgical nurses include patient caregiver, educator, and advocate.
- Special considerations for teaching older adults are found in Chart 1-1.
- The three ethical principles to consider when making clinical decisions are self-determination, beneficence, and justice.
- Nurses function as coordinators of care by communicating and collaborating with members of the health care team.
- Nurses use critical thinking and the nursing process to make timely and appropriate clinical decisions. Critical thinking is purposeful, outcome-directed thinking involving judgment based on sound, scientific evidence, when available.
- Evidence-based practice (EBP) is the deliberate use of current best evidence to make decisions about patient care. It considers the patient's preferences and values, as well as one's own clinical expertise.
- The levels of evidence are listed in Table 1-2.
- Nurses are active participants in the systematic quality improvement process in their health care agency.
- Informatics is used for patient documentation, Internet searches, and e-mail communication in health care.

Additional Study Resources

Go to your Companion CD or Evolve at http://evolve.elsevier.com/Iggy/ for *Self-Assessment Questions for the NCLEX Examination.*

Go to Evolve at http://evolve.elsevier.com/Iggy/ for *Prioritization and Delegation Questions for the NCLEX Examination.*

SELECTED BIBLIOGRAPHY

Asterisk indicates a classic or definitive work on this subject.

Academy of Medical-Surgical Nursing (AMSN). (2007). *Scope and standards of medical-surgical nursing practice* (4th ed.). Pitman, NJ: Anthony J. Janetti, Inc.

Alfaro-LeFevre, R. (2006). *Applying the nursing process: A tool for critical thinking* (6th ed.). Philadelphia: Lippincott Williams & Wilkins.

Alfaro-LeFevre, R. (2008). *Critical thinking and clinical judgment: A practical approach to outcome-focused thinking* (4th ed.). Philadelphia: Saunders.

Durkin, S.E. (2006). Implementing a rapid response team. *AJN, 106*(10), 50-53.

Gordon, M. (2007). *Manual of nursing diagnosis* (11th ed.). Boston: Jones & Bartlett.

Halvorsen, L., Garolis, S., Wallace-Scroggs, A., Stenstrom, J., & Maunder, R. (2007). Building a rapid response team. *AACN Advanced Critical Care, 18*(2), 129-140.

*Institute of Medicine (IOM). (2001). *To err is human.* Washington, DC: National Academies Press.

*Institute of Medicine (IOM). (2003). *Health professions education: A bridge to quality.* Washington, DC: National Academies Press.

Jarvis, C. (2008). *Physical examination and health assessment* (5th ed.). Philadelphia: Saunders.

Melnyk, B.M., & Fineout-Overholt, E. (2005). *Evidence-based practice in nursing and healthcare.* Philadelphia: Lippincott Williams & Wilkins.

*Mohide, E.A., & King, B. (2003). Building a foundation for evidence-based practice: Experiences in a tertiary hospital. *Evidence-Based Nursing, 6*(4), 100-103.

Morse, K.J., Warshawsky, D., Moore, J.M., & Pecora, D.C. (2007). Rapid response teams: Reducers of death. *Nursing2007, Spring* (Suppl.), 2-8.

Schroeder, S.J. (2006). Picking up the PACE: A new template for shift report. *Nursing2006, 36*(10), 22-23.

Yoder-Wise, P.S. (2007). *Leading and managing in nursing* (4th ed.). St. Louis: Mosby.

2

CHAPTER

Introduction to Complementary and Alternative Therapies

Donna D. Ignatavicius

LEARNING OUTCOMES

For clinical competence and success on the NCLEX Examination, study this chapter with these Learning Outcomes in mind:

Health Promotion and Maintenance

1. Teach patients about the risks and precautions when using herbal preparations.
2. Evaluate patient and family use of complementary and alternative medicine (CAM) practices to determine the need for patient and family education.

Physiological Integrity

3. Describe the purposes of the National Center for Complementary and Alternative Medicine (NCCAM).
4. Differentiate five domains of CAM therapies.
5. Provide examples of each domain and their purpose.
6. Assess the patient's need or desire for CAM therapies.
7. Incorporate CAM therapies into the patient's plan of care.
8. Explain the purposes of commonly used therapies in nursing practice.
9. Evaluate patient outcomes of CAM therapies.

Go to your Companion CD or Evolve at http://evolve.elsevier.com/Iggy/ for *Self-Assessment Questions for the NCLEX Examination* keyed to these Learning Outcomes.

OVERVIEW

Western biomedicine has been the predominant health care system in the United States and other Western countries for the past 100 years. However, during the past 25 years, a growing interest in **complementary** (together with traditional treatment) and **alternative** (in place of traditional treatment) medicine has rapidly evolved. **Complementary and alternative medicine (CAM)** is a diverse group of practices, products, and systems that are not an official part of today's U.S. traditional biomedical health care system. However, there is growing scientific evidence that some CAM therapies can be effective as conventional therapies. **Integrative medicine** combines therapies from traditional Western medicine and CAM. A number of health care systems have an integrated medicine department.

Most people who seek complementary and alternative therapies pay for them out-of-pocket, because most third-party payers reimburse for only selected therapies such as chiropractic treatment and acupuncture. More women than men and people with high formal educational levels are most likely to use CAM (www.nncam.nih.gov).

The advantage of CAM therapies is the focus on holistic care. Biomedicine is based on the philosophy in which the body, mind, and spirit are treated as separate entities. Nurses and other health care providers believe in a holistic, caring approach to care. In most cases, no special or advanced training is needed to use these modalities. Some therapies, such as acupuncture, require specialized education and, in some states, licensure or certification. This chapter briefly *introduces* some of the CAM therapies used by nurses in a variety of settings.

NATIONAL CENTER FOR COMPLEMENTARY AND ALTERNATIVE MEDICINE

The National Institutes of Health established the Office of Alternative Medicine in 1992. This office has since been renamed the *National Center for Complementary and Alternative Medicine* (NCCAM). The purposes of the center are to:

- Fund studies examining the effectiveness of various complementary therapies
- Advance the knowledge about complementary therapies of health professionals
- Serve as a clearinghouse for information about these therapies

NCCAM has identified five complementary and alternative medicine domains, or categories, as listed in Table 2-1.

TABLE 2-1 **NCCAM Domains of Complementary and Alternative Medicine with Examples**

Domain	Examples
Systems of health care	Traditional Chinese medicine, Ayurvedic, Native American/American Indian medicine, homeopathy
Mind-body therapies	Imagery, meditation, music, journaling, humor, biofeedback, yoga, prayer
Manipulative and body-based therapies	Chiropractic treatment, massage, rolfing, light and color therapies, hydrotherapy
Biologically based therapies	Herbs, aromatherapy, special diets (Ornish, Atkins), nutritional and food supplements
Energy therapies	Healing Touch, Therapeutic Touch, Reiki, external Qigong, magnets

NCCAM, National Center for Complementary and Alternative Medicine.

CAM DOMAINS

Systems of Health Care

As indicated in Table 2-1, many systems of health care exist in the world. Each of these systems is based on a philosophy that guides practitioners in their assessments and the therapies to use. Most people living in the world use therapies other than ones in the traditional U.S. biomedical system. With the growing immigrant (newcomer) population in the United States, it is vital that nurses increase their knowledge about other large systems of health care.

Nontraditional health care systems incorporate many specific practices that nurses and others use to treat patients. For example, meditation and massage are part of India's Ayurveda medicine. **Homeopathic medicine** uses small doses of specially prepared plant extracts and minerals to promote healing. **Naturopathic medicine** employs herbs and nutrition into its health care practice. Traditional Chinese medicine (TCM), especially acupressure and acupuncture, has gained popularity in the United States and other Western countries. Although these therapies require additional intensive training, they are commonly used by consumers for a variety of health problems.

Acupressure, a TCM therapy, is used in health care for a number of conditions, particularly in the treatment of pain, nausea, and vomiting. **Acupressure** is an ancient healing art that uses the fingers to press certain points on the body to stimulate the body's self-healing ability. According to the philosophy of traditional Chinese medicine, *qi* or energy flows along 12 major meridians. Illness or pain occurs when the flow of *qi* is blocked or diminished. The philosophy of acupressure is similar to acupuncture. For **acupuncture,** needles are used on one of the 365 to 700 **acupoints** that are located on meridians throughout the body. Although most research has been done on acupuncture, studies on the effectiveness of acupressure are increasing (www.nccam.nih.gov).

In the United States, many American Indian tribes have maintained their ancient healing ways. Herbs, prayer, and massage are just a few of the many therapies that are practiced on many pueblos and reservations throughout the country. Chapter 4 describes this culture in more detail.

Mind-Body Therapies

Mind-body therapies are the most commonly used CAM. Because these therapies are used to enhance the mind's ability to affect body function, they fit with the holistic, caring philosophy of nursing. Nurses have traditionally used a number of mind-body therapies such as journaling, imagery, meditation, music, and animal-assisted therapy. *Prayer is the most commonly used mind-body therapy by health care professionals and patients with a number of health care problems.* Chapter 4 discusses this practice as part of spirituality.

Journaling

Journaling is a reflective therapy; it is a tool for recording the process of one's life. Writing provides a vehicle for a person to express feelings, to gain new perspectives, and to pay attention to what is in the unconscious. A number of techniques for journaling can be used.

Although journal writing has been done for centuries, little formal research exists to support its use. Free-flowing journaling is the technique most often used. The person writes whatever comes to mind without censoring any thoughts or feelings or correcting grammar or punctuation. The writing done is for oneself and need not be shared. The expectation to share what is written usually places constraints on what is being recorded. Entries are made in a book dedicated to journaling. This may be a loose-leaf notebook, a special journal entry book, or a computer.

Imagery

Imagery has been used for many years in nursing. **Imagery** is the formation of a mental representation of an object, place, event, or situation that is perceived through the patient's senses. Visualization is sometimes used interchangeably with imagery, but in reality, all senses can be used in imagery. For example, while changing dressings or doing other procedures that may produce pain, ask the patient to think about a pleasant event or a beautiful scene.

Imagery has been used in a wide variety of conditions, including:

- Reducing pain
- Reducing nausea and vomiting
- Decreasing anxiety
- Promoting comfort during treatment for cancer

Many techniques can be used to help people use their senses to create images. Guided imagery in which the patient is provided with images or prompts by a nurse, a family member, or a friend or via a tape is the technique frequently used by nurses. Before suggestions for imagery are presented, provide the patient with instructions that will help produce relaxation. These may include tensing and relaxing muscle groups and focusing attention on one's breathing.

When the person seems relaxed (slower respirations and relaxed muscles), give specific suggestions for imagery. The patient may be asked to choose a place he or she enjoys and to think about the sights, smells, tastes, and feelings associated with the place. Time allowed for imagery varies, but it is usually between 15 and 20 minutes. Opportunities are provided for the person to enjoy being in this place; the patient is informed that he or she can return to this "place" at anytime. Some patients like to create their own imagery tape to listen to, whereas others prefer listening to commercial tapes or having the nurse or family member guide them through the session. Use of guided imagery has few risks. However, be attentive to any adverse effects such as heightened anxiety or difficulty in breathing.

Meditation

Meditation has been a part of many religions and cultures for thousands of years. Although often thought of in terms of religion, meditation, or focusing on the moment, can be used in a nonreligious context. Meditation has been used to reduce anxiety, reduce pain, relieve symptoms of psoriasis, lower blood pressure, and promote health (Fig. 2-1).

Kreitzer (2002) defined **meditation** as "a self-directed practice for relaxing the body and calming the mind" (p. 101). Some of the most common types of meditation are:

- Mental repetition such as using a mantra
- Physical repetition such as focusing on breathing or walking
- Problem contemplation such as solving a riddle
- Visual concentration that is similar to imagery

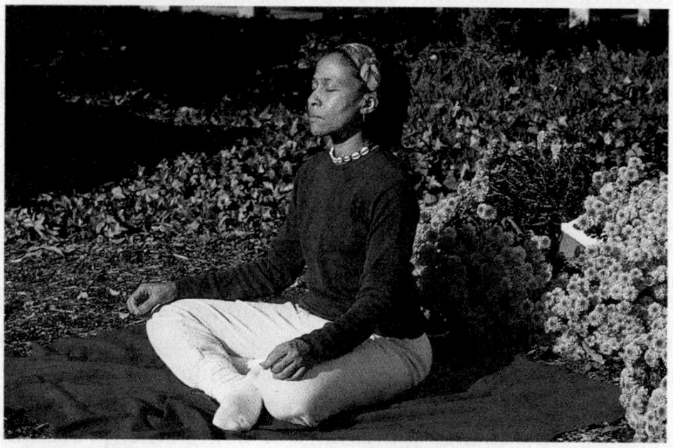

Fig. 2-1 • Meditation can be used to relax the body and calm the mind.

Walking meditation, a commonly used type, contains both active and meditative elements. While walking, the person focuses attention on the sound of the foot hitting the ground, the feelings in the muscles and joints, or the movements of the body. This type of meditation may be appealing to persons who are more active and have difficulty concentrating while sitting. The walking meditation should be done for about 20 minutes.

The labyrinth is an ancient form of walking meditation that has attracted renewed attention. Labyrinths are found in many cultures such as Hindu, Hopi Indians, Crete, and medieval European religions. The labyrinth is not a maze. The person walks the circles meditatively. Walkers may ask themselves a question and search for answers, they may pray, or they might focus on feelings they are experiencing.

Music Therapy

Music therapy has been part of CAM for many years. Nursing homes and other long-term care settings have used music as an important part of their activity program for many years. Music often calms agitated patients and provides reminiscence for older adults, particularly when familiar music is played.

Several universities offer training to certify musicians to play therapeutic music for patients in a variety of settings. A systematic review of the literature conducted by Richards et al. (2007) found that music therapy decreased pain and anxiety. It also showed that patients were more satisfied with their hospital care when music therapy was provided (see the Evidence-Based Practice box below). Results were best when an individual patient listened to calming live music such as that provided by a harp, when compared with listening to recorded music and other instruments.

Animal-Assisted Therapy

It is not unusual to see dogs, cats, or other animals when visiting a hospital or nursing home. Since the 1970s, studies have sought to validate the link between animal companionship

EVIDENCE-BASED PRACTICE

What is the effect of music therapy on pain, anxiety, and patient satisfaction?

Richards, T., Johnson, J., Sparks, A., & Emerson, H. (2007). The effect of music therapy on patients' perception and manifestation of pain, anxiety, and patient satisfaction. *MEDSURG Nursing, 16*(1), 7-15.

The researchers conducted an extensive systematic review of over 20 descriptive and quasi-experimental studies on how hospital patients perceive the effects of listening to music on their pain, anxiety, or patient satisfaction. Although the study findings did not show consensus or no statistical significance was found, the results did indicate that some patients did benefit from music therapy in the hospital setting.

As a result of this review, the authors established a music therapy program in their large, mid-Atlantic hospital. Live harp music was provided at the patient's or family's request. No physician's request was needed. The most significant results were related to patient satisfaction with their care.

Level of Evidence—5. Systematic review of descriptive studies.

Commentary: Implications for Practice and Research. The authors reviewed the literature before making a decision about whether to begin a new intervention for patients in a hospital setting. They asked a question, reviewed and analyzed the literature, and used the findings to make decisions to improve patient care, using patient preferences and their own clinical expertise—the evidence-based practice process.

This study also indicates the need for further research in the use of music therapy for patients in hospitals and other settings. Although the authors did not show consistency in the effect of music to decrease pain and/or anxiety, some patients did experience improvement in their pain and anxiety levels.

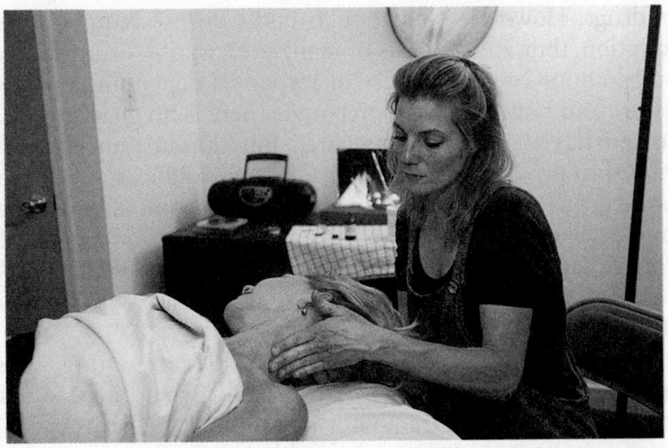

Fig. 2-2 • Massage therapy can be effectively used to relieve tension.

and positive health outcomes. Jorgenson (2002) differentiates between animal-assisted therapy (AAT) and pet visitation. In AAT, the animal, often a dog, is an integral part of the treatment plan. For example, a dog may be used to assist a patient to improve motor skills or increase ability to concentrate. In contrast, the goal of pet visitation is aimed more at increasing socialization or keeping the person in touch with reality.

Animal-assisted therapy has been used with many different patient groups including hospice, behavioral health, and dementia. Jorgenson (2002) recommends that any facility planning to implement AAT should first develop guidelines that specify the inclusion and exclusion criteria for patients who might receive AAT, the procedure to be used during the visitation, and the responsibilities of the nursing staff. Some institutions do not allow dogs to be on site for more than 1 hour because the animal becomes exhausted.

Manipulative and Body-Based Therapies

Three large groups of therapies make up the manipulative and body-based NCCAM category: chiropractic, osteopathy, and massage. Chiropractic and osteopathic medicine require years of specialized training. Massage and tai chi are common manipulative and body-based therapies that nurses can learn and teach to their patients. Other movement therapies such as dance and yoga also are sometimes placed in this category.

Massage

Massage has a long history within nursing. Until recently, back rubs were a standard nursing procedure provided for all hospitalized patients on a daily basis. **Massage** involves using various strokes and pressure to manipulate soft tissues for therapeutic purposes. Many types of massage exist: Swedish (rather vigorous massage with long, flowing strokes), Esalen (light touch), neuromuscular (deep tissue), Shiatsu (Japanese pressure-point), and reflexology (massage of various points on the foot). Many different strokes are used in massage. Massage can be of the entire body or of selected areas such as foot, hand, shoulder/neck, or back (Fig. 2-2). Specialized licensed therapists use various types of massage in both health care and non–health care settings.

Hand massage can be readily used with any patient group. Table 2-2 details one technique that can be used. Massage can be used to produce relaxation and help lessen aggressive behaviors in patients with dementia. It can also reduce pain in some patients (see Chapter 5).

TABLE 2-2 Directions for Giving Hand Massage

Do not massage the hand if it is injured, reddened, swollen, or infected. Each hand is massaged for about $2\frac{1}{2}$ minutes.

BACK OF HAND
- Use medium pressure strokes from the wrist to the fingertips.
- Make large half-circle stretching strokes from the center to the side of the hand using moderate pressure.
- Make small circular strokes (like an O) over the entire back of the hand.
- Use light pressure strokes from the wrist to the fingertips.

PALM OF HAND
- Make medium pressure strokes from the wrist to the fingertips.
- Use gentle strokes to lift the muscle tissue of the palms.
- Use small circular strokes, applying moderate pressure over the palm.
- Use large stretching strokes from the center of the palm to the sides (like opening up the palm).

FINGERS
- Gently squeeze each finger from the base to the tip on both sides using the thumb and index finger.
- Do gentle range of motion.
- Apply gentle pressure on the nail bed.

COMPLETION
- Place the patient's hand on yours and cover it with your other hand.
- Gently draw your top hand toward you several times.
- Turn the hand over and gently draw your other hand toward you several times.

Modified from Snyder, M., & Lindquist, R. (Eds.). (2002). *Complementary/alternative therapies in nursing* (4th ed.). New York: Springer.

Because of cultural differences related to touch and personal preferences related to touch, the nurse needs to obtain the person's permission before using massage. Massage should not be used over reddened, bruised, or infected areas of skin.

Tai Chi

Tai chi is a holistic movement therapy that has wide popularity in China, Taiwan, and Japan. It is a traditional Chinese martial art that has been adapted to be a mind-body exercise. The goal is to integrate body movements, mind concentration, muscle relaxation, and breathing to achieve the desired outcome. Several styles of tai chi exist: *chen* (quick and slow large movements), *yang* (slow large movements), *sun* (quick compact), and tai chi *chih* (simple repetitive movements). The latter is a style that is popular in the United States and Canada and originated in the West. Tai chi is closely tied to the philosophy of traditional Chinese medicine (TCM); the movements promote the flow of *qi* or energy throughout the body.

Biologically Based Therapies

Biologically based therapies (BBT) use natural substances for healing, including herbs, foods, vitamins, and minerals. The regulations governing herbal preparations and food additives are less strict than those for drug therapy, which has raised concern about their safety. The most common BBTs used in the United States are aromatherapy and herbal preparations.

Aromatherapy

Aromatherapy is one of the fastest growing areas in complementary therapies. Clinical **aromatherapy** uses essential oils from various parts of plants to promote comfort or healing. Essential oils may be applied in compresses, used in baths, or applied topically to the skin.

Numerous oils can be used. For example, lavender and rose are two common oils that promote relaxation and sleep. Peppermint has been used for stimulation and to promote concentration. Sandalwood and lavender may improve mood in patients with depression.

Before using aromatherapy, assess the patient for any allergies and any negative associations with particular smells. Essential oils are potent and need to be diluted before being applied topically.

Herbal Preparations

Herbal preparations are plants used for medicinal purposes in many societies for years. Today they are regularly used in the United States. Herbs have become increasingly popular as a means to promote health, to prevent diseases, or to cure a variety of ailments. For example, they may be used to control high blood pressure, control high serum glucose levels, or manage painful chronic conditions. The list of available herbal preparations is extensive. Several common herbs, their intended purposes, and precautions are listed in Table 2-3.

Herbal preparations are attractive alternatives or supplements to conventional health care because they are "natural." However, they have pharmacoactive effects that may be serious or deadly, as in cases of overuse, inappropriate use, herbal toxicities, and herb-drug and herb-herb interactions. Increased popularity of herbs has increased concern about their safety.

There are other drawbacks to herbal therapies. Herbs may be self-administered to treat a serious health problem that could more effectively be treated by conventional medicine, potentially resulting in a delay of diagnosis and treatment. In some cases, patients may neglect or choose not to tell their health care providers about their use of herbs.

In the United States, herbal preparations are regulated as food and nutritional supplements by the Food and Drug Administration (FDA). However, these regulations are less strict than for drugs. Because herbs are not classified as drugs, they do not receive the same oversight in their preparation and use as drugs. However, even though herbs do not require a prescription, they are the basis of many prescription drugs. Herbal preparations cause a variety of responses depending on their nature and how they were prepared. There is no guarantee that an herb has been properly prepared, thus there are uncertainties related to product quality. Herbs that are sold as standardized extracts are more likely to contain accurate amounts of herbs and less likely to contain other inactive elements or contamination. *Because an herb is natural, it does not mean that it is safe.* Because a given herb is considered "safe," it does not mean it is effective.

When caring for patients in any health care setting, question them about the use of herbs and for what purpose. Ask the patient about the frequency and dose of the herbs used. If appropriate, remind the patient about the importance of informing future care providers about herbal therapy use. For example, to avoid increased risks of bleeding, one should not use ginkgo, ginseng, or garlic before surgery.

Caution patients about unreliable sources of health information, and refer them to credible resources for herbal remedies. Examples are the National Library of Medicine's PubMed website: www.ncbi.nlm.nih.gov/PubMed/; the American Botanical Council's website: http://herbalgram.org; and the Herb Research Foundation's website: www.herbs.org.

Energy Therapies

Energy therapies include both biofield therapies and bioelectromagnetics. They are based on the belief that the body has a subtle energy that extends beyond it (Pierce, 2007). In nursing, biofield therapies are most commonly used. Examples include Therapeutic Touch (TT), Healing Touch (HT), and Reiki. Two of these modalities were developed by nurses—TT by Dolores Krieger in the 1970s and HT by Janet Mentgen in the 1980s. *The most well-known energy therapy is Therapeutic Touch.*

Therapeutic Touch is based on the assumption that illness is an imbalance in the flow of energy or the energy pattern within the body. Using TT, the practitioner intervenes in the patient's energy field to stimulate healing potential. This therapy has been used to achieve numerous health outcomes: reduced anxiety, decreased pain, improved immune system, and improved functional ability.

TT consists of five steps: centering, assessing the energy field, clearing and mobilizing the patient's energy field, di-

TABLE 2-3 Commonly Used Herbal Preparations

Herb	Intended Effects/Uses	Cautions/Adverse Effects
Ginkgo biloba	Reduce memory problems, dementia, peripheral vascular disease; has antioxidant and vasodilator properties.	Use with anticoagulants may cause bleeding; rarely dizziness, headache, GI upset.
Garlic	Lower cholesterol or blood pressure; act as a natural antibiotic; act as an antiplatelet agent.	Bleeding when used with other antiplatelet agents; potentiates antidiabetic drugs; avoid before surgery.
Echinacea	Build immunity; help wound healing.	Not recommended for people with immune diseases. May suppress immune function if used for more than 8 weeks.
Ginseng	Promote general well-being; anti-aging.	Observe INR with warfarin. Side effects may depend on type of ginseng used.
St. John's wort	Ease mild to moderate depression.	Photosensitivity; avoid use in major depression or with other antidepressants.

INR, International Normalized Ratio.

recting energy for healing, and balancing the energy field. In centering, the practitioner is quiet and focuses attention on the patient with the intention to heal. The practitioner uses his or her hands to assess the flow of energy. They are then moved from head to foot, noting any blockages in the flow of energy or absences or excesses in energy in a particular spot. In the clearing and mobilizing step, the practitioner holds his or her hands 2 to 4 inches from the patient's body and moves them with the palms facing the patient, from head to foot in a sweeping motion (Fig. 2-3). This process may be repeated. Based on the assessment, the practitioner directs energy so that imbalances are resolved. The practitioner's hands are placed on the patient, and energy is directed toward him or her. Finally, the practitioner seeks to balance the patient's energy by using head-to-toe clearing motions with the intention of smoothing the energy. *Caution should be used in administering TT to the very young and very old.*

SUMMARY OF IMPLICATIONS FOR NURSING

Complementary and alternative therapies are being used increasingly to promote health, prevent disease, or address illness and symptoms. Increased nursing research is essential to evaluate the usefulness of therapies and their role in medical-surgical nursing practice. Throughout this text, discussions of specific complementary and alternative therapies are included as part of the collaborative management of various diseases and illnesses. These descriptions are labeled with a separate heading and an icon ( ) to help locate this information.

Nurses have an important role in assessing the patients' use of therapies in order to discuss safety, perceived effectiveness, and satisfaction. Furthermore, the knowledge of patients' use of complementary and alternative therapies is important in the planning of care. A better understanding of therapies enhances your ability to educate patients about specific therapies and their effects, to discuss therapies with potential benefits, and to make referrals to appropriate providers of the desired CAM therapies.

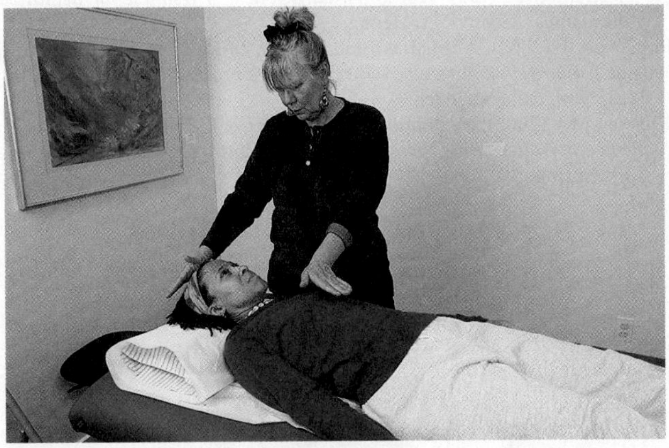

Fig. 2-3 • In Therapeutic Touch, the practitioner directs the practitioner's own interpersonal energy to help or heal another.

GET READY FOR THE NCLEX EXAMINATION!

Key Points

Review these Key Points for each NCLEX Examination Client Needs Category.

Health Promotion and Maintenance

- Evaluate patient and family use of CAM practices to determine the need for patient education.
- Teach patients taking herbal preparations about overuse, toxicities, herb-herb interactions, and herb-drug interactions.

Physiological Integrity

- Complementary and alternative therapies include a broad range of healing approaches and therapies that are not commonly used as part of Western medicine. Many of these therapies are derived from Eastern medicine, such as traditional Chinese medicine (e.g., acupressure).
- As part of the National Institutes of Health, the National Center for Complementary and Alternative Medicine is funding research to determine the usefulness of selected therapies.
- The five domains of CAM are listed with examples on Table 2-1.
- Assess the patient's need or desire for CAM therapies.
- Include CAM therapies in the patient's plan of care as needed.
- Examples of mind-body therapies are journaling, imagery, meditation, music therapy, and animal-assisted therapy.
- Journaling allows an opportunity for reflection as the person records thoughts and feelings.
- Imagery is often used for reducing pain, nausea and vomiting, and anxiety.
- Massage is a commonly used manipulative and body-based therapy in nursing (e.g., giving a back rub).
- Aromatherapy and herbal preparations are commonly used biologic therapies; these interventions are used for an assortment of problems (see Table 2-3).
- Therapeutic Touch promotes healing by balancing a person's energy field.
- Evaluate whether CAM therapies are effective for patients in a variety of settings.

Additional Study Resources

Go to your Companion CD or Evolve at http://evolve.elsevier.com/Iggy/ for *Self-Assessment Questions for the NCLEX Examination.*

Go to Evolve at http://evolve.elsevier.com/Iggy/ for *Prioritization and Delegation Questions for the NCLEX Examination.*

SELECTED BIBLIOGRAPHY

Asterisk indicates a classic or definitive work on this subject.

American Polarity Therapy Association. (2007). Retrieved November 15, 2007, from www.polaritytherapy.org.

*Bodeker, G. (2002). Lessons on integration from the developing world's experience. *British Medical Journal, 322,* 154-167.

*Chen, K.M., Snyder, M., & Kirchbaum, K. (2001). Clinical use of tai chi in elderly populations. *Geriatric Nursing, 22,* 198-200.

*Eliopoulos, C. (1999). Using complementary and alternative therapies wisely. *Geriatric Nursing, 20,* 139-143.

Facente, A. (2006). Humor in health care: Irreverent or invaluable? *Nursing2006, 36*(4), 64hn6-7.

Healing Touch International, Inc. (2007). Retrieved November 15, 2007, from www.healingtouchinternational.org.

*Hover-Kramer, D. (Ed.). (2001). *Healing Touch: A resource for health care professionals.* Albany, NY: Delmar.

*Jorgenson, J. (2002). Animal-assisted therapy. In M. Snyder & R. Lindquist (Eds.), *Complementary/alternative therapies in nursing* (4th ed., pp. 152-162). New York: Springer.

*Kreitzer, M.J. (2002). Meditation. In M. Snyder & R. Lindquist (Eds.), *Complementary/alternative therapies in nursing* (4th ed., pp. 101-113). New York: Springer.

*Krieger, D. (1976). Healing by laying on of hands as facilitators of bioenergetic change: The response of in-vivo hemoglobin. *Psychoenergetic Systems, 1,* 121-129.

*Lu, Y. (2003). Herb use in critical care: What to watch for. *Critical Care Nursing Clinics of North America, 15*(3), 313-319.

*McNamara, M.E., Burnham, D.C., Smith, C., & Carroll, D.L. (2003). The effects of back massage before diagnostic cardiac catheterization. *Alternative Therapies in Health and Medicine, 9,* 50-57.

National Center for Complementary and Alternative Medicine. (2007). Retrieved November 15, 2007, from www.nccam.nih.gov.

Pierce, B. (2007). The use of biofield therapies in cancer care. *Clinical Journal of Oncology Nursing, 11*(2), 253-258.

Richards, T., Johnson, J., Sparks, A., & Emerson, H. (2007). The effect of music therapy on patients' perception and manifestation of pain, anxiety, and patient satisfaction. *MEDSURG Nursing, 16*(1), 7-15.

Snyder, M., & Lindquist, R. (Eds.). (2006). *Complementary/alternative therapies in nursing* (5th ed.). New York: Springer.

*Wardell, D.W., & Weymouth, K.F. (2004). Review of studies of Healing Touch. *Journal of Nursing Scholarship, 36,* 147-154.

Common Health Problems of Older Adults

3

CHAPTER

Donna D. Ignatavicius

LEARNING OUTCOMES

For clinical competence and success on the NCLEX Examination, study this chapter with these Learning Outcomes in mind:

Safe and Effective Care Environment

1. Collaborate with members of the interdisciplinary health care team when providing care to older adults.
2. Identify risk factors for falls and driving ability in older adults who live in the community or are hospitalized.
3. Report suspected neglect and abuse to appropriate health care team members or agencies.
4. Follow The Joint Commission and federal/state standards when using patient restraints.

Health Promotion and Maintenance

5. Teach selected lifestyle practices to promote health in the older adult.
6. Provide special needs care for patients over 65 years of age.

Psychosocial Integrity

7. Assess the older patient's risk for neglect and abuse.
8. Explain the results of undiagnosed depression in the older adult.
9. Assist the older adult to cope with stress and loss.

Physiological Integrity

10. Identify four subgroups of older adults.
11. Describe nursing interventions for relocation stress syndrome.
12. Explain the effects of drugs on the older adult.
13. Compare and contrast delirium and dementia.
14. Assess the older adult's risk for sleep disturbance, and implement interventions to promote rest.

Go to your Companion CD or Evolve at http://evolve.elsevier.com/Iggy/ for *Self-Assessment Questions for the NCLEX Examination* keyed to these Learning Outcomes.

About 13% of the people in the United States are older than 65 years. Women live longer than men, although the exact reason for this difference is not known. The older population is expected to grow as "baby boomers" approach late adulthood in the next 5 to 10 years. Most patients on adult acute care units are over 65 years of age. Many of these patients are discharged for home health services. Over 90% of patients in long-term care (LTC) facilities are older than 65 years. Therefore health care professionals need to know about the special needs of older adults to care for them in a variety of settings.

This chapter describes the major health issues associated with late adulthood in community and inpatient settings. The care of older adults (sometimes referred to as *elders*) with acute and chronic health problems is discussed in appropriate chapters throughout this text. The specialized care for older adults with these problems is emphasized throughout this book. In addition, Nursing Focus on the Older Adult charts and Considerations for Older Adults headings highlight the most important information. A brief review of major physiologic changes of aging are listed in each body system unit.

OVERVIEW

Late adulthood can be divided into four subgroups:

- 65 to 74 years of age: the young old
- 75 to 84 years of age: the middle old
- 85 to 99 years of age: the old old
- 100 years of age or more: the elite old

The fastest growing subgroup is the old old, sometimes referred to as the advanced older adult population. The members of this subgroup are sometimes referred to as the "frail elderly," although a number of 85 to 95 year olds are very healthy. In general, the needs and problems of this subgroup are different from those of adults between 65 and 74 years of age. The incidence of chronic disease like cancer increases with advanced age.

Most older adults are relatively healthy and live in the community at home, in assisted-living facilities, or in retirement complexes. Men over 65 years of age are less likely to live in a single-person household than women of that age. Of all older adults, 5% reside in long-term care facilities (mostly nursing homes) and another 10% to 15% are ill but are cared for at home. Older adults from any setting usually experience one or more hospitalizations in their lifetime. About half of all older adults are admitted for short-term stays in a nursing home, usually for rehabilitation services (see Chapter 8).

HEALTH ISSUES FOR OLDER ADULTS IN THE COMMUNITY

Health is a major concern for many older adults. Health status can affect the ability to perform ADLs and to participate in social roles. A failure to perform these activities may increase dependence on others and may have a negative effect on morale and life satisfaction. When older adults lose the ability to function independently, they often feel empty and worthless. Loss of autonomy is a painful event related to the physical and mental changes of aging.

Older adults may also experience a number of losses that can affect their sense of control over their lives, such as the death of a spouse and friends or the loss of social and work roles. Support their self-esteem and feelings of independence by encouraging them to maintain as much control as possible over their lives, to participate in decision making, and to perform as many tasks as possible.

Like younger and middle-aged adults, older adults need to practice health promotion and illness prevention to maintain or achieve a high level of wellness. Teach them the importance of promoting wellness and strategies for accomplishing this goal (Chart 3-1).

Common health issues and problems that can affect older adults in the community include:

- Nutrition
- Mobility
- Stress and loss
- Accidents
- Drug use and misuse
- Mental health/behavioral health
- Elder neglect and abuse

Chart 3-1 PATIENT AND FAMILY EDUCATION GUIDE

Lifestyles and Practices to Promote Wellness

HEALTH-PROTECTING BEHAVIORS

- Have yearly influenza vaccinations (after October 1).
- Obtain a pneumococcal vaccination. (A routine revaccination may be necessary.)
- Have a tetanus immunization, and get a booster every 10 years.
- Wear seat belts when you are in an automobile.
- Use alcohol in moderation or not at all.
- Avoid smoking.
- If you smoke at home, do not smoke in bed.
- Install and maintain working smoke detectors.
- Create a hazard-free environment to prevent falls; eliminate hazards such as scatter rugs and waxed floors.
- Use medications according to your physician's prescription.
- Avoid over-the-counter medications unless your physician directs you to use them.
- Take one aspirin every day (any dose between 81 and 325 mg) to decrease the risk of myocardial infarction and colon cancer (if not contraindicated for another reason).

HEALTH-ENHANCING BEHAVIORS

- Have a yearly physical examination; see your health care provider more often if health problems occur.
- Reduce dietary fat to not more than 30% of calories; saturated fat should provide less than 10% of your calories.
- Increase your dietary intake of complex carbohydrate and fiber-containing food to five or more servings of fruits and vegetables and six or more servings of grain products daily.
- Increase calcium intake to between 1000 and 1500 mg daily.
- Allow at least 10 to 15 minutes of sun exposure two to three times weekly for vitamin D intake; avoid prolonged sun exposure.
- Exercise regularly three to five times a week for 30 minutes per session.
- Manage stress through coping mechanisms that have been successful in the past.
- Get together with people in different settings.
- Reminisce about your life.

Nutrition

A person's need for adequate nutrition remains constant throughout the life span, yet many older adults are at risk for undernutrition—usually protein-calorie malnutrition, also known as protein energy malnutrition (Chapman, 2006). Inflation, reduced income, and a lack of transportation are factors that contribute to inadequate nutrition among older adults. Those whose diets consist of the wrong types of foods or the wrong amounts of some types of foods may also be poorly nourished. Some older adults reduce their intake of food to near-starvation levels, even with the availability of programs such as food stamps, food banks, and Meals on Wheels. Many senior centers offer meals, as well as group social activities. The lack of transportation, the necessity of traveling to obtain such services, and the inability to carry large or heavy groceries prevent some older adults from taking advantage of food programs. Others are too proud to accept free services.

Poor nutrition may also be related to loneliness. Older adults may respond to loneliness, depression, and boredom by not eating, which can lead to undernutrition. Many who live alone lose the incentive to prepare or eat balanced diets, especially if they do not "feel well." Still others respond to stress by overeating, which leads to obesity.

The minimum nutritional requirements of the human body remain consistent from youth through old age, with a few exceptions. Older adults need an increased dietary intake of calcium, vitamin D, vitamin C, and vitamin A because aging changes disrupt the ability to store, use, and absorb these substances. A sedentary lifestyle and reduced metabolic rate require a reduction in total caloric intake to maintain an ideal body weight.

Other physical aging changes influence nutritional status or the ability to consume needed nutrients. Diminished senses of taste and smell often result in a loss of desire for food. Older adults have less ability to taste sweet and salt than to taste bitter

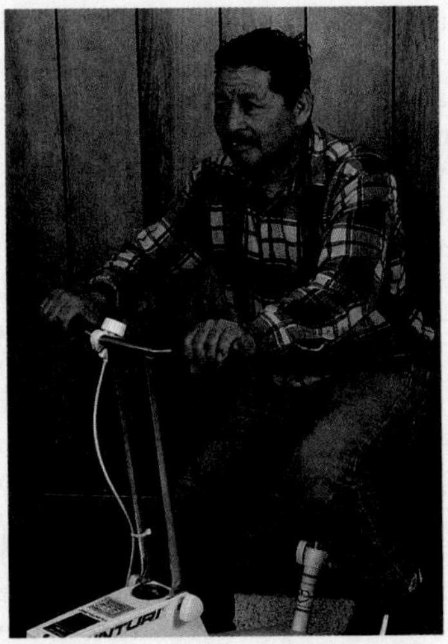

Fig. 3-1 • Exercise is important to older adults for health promotion and maintenance.

and sour. This aging change may result in an overuse of table sugar and salt to compensate. Teach the patient to substitute herbs and spices to season food or to vary the textures of food substances to feel satisfied.

Tooth loss and poorly fitting dentures from inadequate dental care or calcium loss can also cause the older adult to avoid important foods. Unlike today, dental preventive programs were not readily available or stressed as being important when older adults were younger. Older people with dentition problems may resort to eating soft, high-calorie foods such as ice cream and mashed potatoes, which lack roughage and fiber. Unless the person carefully chooses more nutritious soft foods, vitamin deficiencies, constipation, and other problems can result. The extensive use of prescribed and over-the-counter (OTC) drugs, including herbal supplements, may affect appetite, food tolerances, and food absorption and use.

Older adults sometimes respond to problems associated with mobility, prescribed diuretics, and limited bladder capacity by limiting fluid intake, especially in the evening. *Teach older adults that fluid restrictions make them susceptible to dehydration and electrolyte imbalances that can cause serious illness or death.* Incontinence may actually increase because the urine becomes more concentrated and irritating to the bladder and urinary sphincter.

Mobility

Exercise and activity are important for older adults as a means of promoting and maintaining health (Fig. 3-1). Physical activity can help keep the body in shape and maintain an optimal level of functioning. Regular exercise has many benefits, including:

- Decreased risk for falls
- Increased muscle strength and balance
- Increased mobility
- Increased sleep
- Reduced or maintained weight
- Improved sense of well-being and self-esteem
- Decreased depression symptoms
- Improved longevity
- Reduced risks for diabetes and coronary artery disease

Teach older adults about the value of physical activity. For people who are homebound, focus on functional fitness, such as performing ADLs. For those who are not homebound, teach the importance of other types of exercise. Resistance exercise, for example, maintains muscle mass. Aerobic exercise, like walking, improves strength and endurance. One of the best exercises is walking at least 30 minutes, three to five times a week (Struck & Ross, 2006). The person may walk for 30 continuous minutes or walk 3 times a day for 10 minutes. During the winter, indoor shopping centers and other public places can be used. In addition, many senior centers and community centers offer exercise programs for older adults.

Swimming is also recommended but does not offer the weight-bearing advantage of walking. Weight bearing helps build bone, an especially important advantage for older women to prevent osteoporosis (see Chapter 53). Older adults who have been sedentary should start their exercise programs slowly and gradually increase the frequency and duration of activity over time, under the direction of their health care provider.

Stress and Loss

Stress can speed up the aging process over time, or it can lead to diseases that increase the rate of degeneration. It can also impair the reserve capacity of older adults and lessen their ability to respond and adapt to changes in their environment.

Although no period of the life cycle is free from stress, the later years can be a time of especially high risk. Frequent sources of stress for the older population include:

- Rapid environmental changes that require immediate reaction
- Changes in lifestyle resulting from retirement or physical incapacity
- Acute or chronic illness
- Loss of significant others
- Financial hardships
- Relocation

How people react to these stresses depends on their personal coping skills and support networks. The loss of roles experienced by older adults often limits the availability of external support networks. For instance, losses leave many older adults without friends for support and help. As a result, many must rely solely on their personal resources to maintain their mental health/behavioral health. A combination of poor physical health and social problems leaves older adults susceptible to stress overload, which can result in illness and premature death.

The ways in which people adapt to old age depend largely on the personality traits and coping strategies that have characterized them throughout their lives. Establishing and maintaining relationships with others throughout life is especially important to the older person's happiness. Even more important than having friends is the nature of the friendships. People who have close, intimate, stable relationships with others in whom they confide are more likely to cope with crisis.

Most older adults are relatively healthy and live in and own their own homes. Physical health problems may force some to relocate to a retirement center or an assisted-living facility, although these facilities can be very expensive. Others move in with family members or apartment buildings funded and designated for seniors. Older adults usually have more difficulty adjusting to major change when compared with younger and middle-aged adults. Being admitted to a hospital or nursing home is a particularly traumatic experience. Older adults often suffer from relocation stress syndrome, also known as *relocation trauma.* **Relocation stress syndrome** is the physical and emotional distress that occurs after the person moves from one setting to another. Examples of physiologic behaviors are sleep disturbance and increased physical symptoms, such as GI distress. Examples of emotional manifestations are withdrawal, anxiety, anger, and depression. Chart 3-2 lists nursing interventions that may help decrease the effects of relocation.

Family members and facility staff need to be aware that older adults need personal space in their new surroundings. Older adults need to participate in deciding how the space will be arranged and what they can keep in their new home to help offset the feelings of powerlessness. Suggest that the patient or family bring in personal items, such as pictures of relatives and friends, favorite clothing, and valued knickknacks, to assist in making the new setting seem more familiar and comfortable. This same intervention can be carried out in a hospital setting.

Accidents

Fall Prevention

Most accidents occur at home. Teach older adults about the need to be aware of safety precautions to prevent accidents, such as falls. Incapacitating accidents are a primary cause of decreased mobility in old age. Some people develop **fallophobia** (fear of falling) and avoid leaving their homes.

Home modifications may be helpful to prevent falls. Involve family and significant others when recommending useful changes to prevent patient injury. Safeguards such as handrails, slip-proof underpads for rugs, and adequate lighting are essential in the home. Avoiding scatter rugs, slippery floors, and clutter is also important to prevent falls. Installing grab bars and using non-slip bathmats can help prevent falls in the bathroom. Raised toilet seats are also important. Remind older adults to avoid going out on days when steps are wet or icy and to ask for help when ambulating. To minimize sensory overload, advise the older adult to concentrate on one activity at a time.

Changes in vision, touch, and motor ability can create challenges for older adults in any environment. For example, **presbyopia** (farsightedness that worsens with aging) may make walking more difficult; the person is less aware of the location of each step. In addition, the older adult may have disorders that affect visual acuity, such as macular degeneration, cataracts, glaucoma, or diabetic retinopathy.

A reduced sense of touch decreases the awareness of body orientation (e.g., whether the foot is squarely on the step). The decreased reaction time that commonly results from age-related changes in the neurologic system may also impair the ability to recognize or move from a dangerous setting. Chronic diseases can affect mobility and sensation in the older adult as well, such as peripheral neuropathy and arthritis. If needed, encourage the use of visual, hearing, or ambulatory assistive devices. High costs and a fear of appearing old sometimes prevent older adults from obtaining or using hearing aids, eyeglasses, walkers, or canes.

Once an older person has been identified as being at high risk for falls, choose interventions that help prevent falls and possible serious injury. For those in the community, tai chi exercise is very helpful to improve balance and functional mobility, as well as to decrease the fear of falling, especially among older women.

Chart 3-2 BEST PRACTICE FOR PATIENT SAFETY & QUALITY CARE

Minimizing the Effects of Relocation Stress in Older Adults

- Provide opportunities for the patient to assist in decision making.
- Carefully explain all procedures and routines to the patient before they occur.
- Ask the family or significant other to provide familiar or special keepsakes to keep at the patient's bedside (e.g., family picture, favorite hairbrush).
- Reorient the patient frequently to his or her location.
- Ask the patient about his or her expectations during hospitalization or nursing home placement.
- Encourage the patient's family and friends to visit often.
- Establish a trusting relationship with the patient as early as possible.
- Assess the patient's usual lifestyle and daily activities, including food likes and dislikes and preferred time for bathing.
- Avoid unnecessary room changes.
- If possible, have a family member, significant other, staff member, or volunteer accompany the patient when leaving the unit for special procedures or therapies.

Driving Safety

Motor vehicle accidents are the most common cause of injury-related death in the young-old population, those between 65 and 74 years of age (Odenheimer, 2006). Increased national concerns about this growing problem have prompted many states to require more frequent testing for older drivers. As one ages, reaction time and the ability to multi-task decrease. Sleep disturbances, especially insomnia, are also common in older adults but are not part of normal aging. Some accidents occur because the person falls asleep while driving.

The older the person, the more likely he or she will have chronic diseases and the drugs needed to manage them. These health problems and treatments can contribute to vehicle accidents. For instance, drugs used for hypertension can cause orthostatic hypotension (low blood pressure when changing body position).

Physicians and other health care professionals play a major role in identifying driver safety issues. Yet, many are reluctant to intervene because older patients feel they will lose their independence if they cannot drive. They may also be angry and resistant to the idea of giving up perhaps their only means of transportation (Odenheimer, 2006). As an alternative, health care professionals can recommend driving refresher courses and suggest that high-risk driving conditions, like wet roads, be avoided. Newer vehicles on the market have some safety features to help older adults, such as large-print digital readouts for speed and other data. Chart 3-3 lists additional ways to improve older adult driver safety.

Drug Use and Misuse

Drug therapy for the older population is another major health issue. Because of the multiple chronic and acute health problems that occur in this age-group, drugs for older adults account for about one third of all prescription drug costs. The term **polypharmacy** has been used to describe the use of multiple drugs by older adults.

Older adults also commonly use nonprescription drugs, such as analgesics, antacids, cold and cough preparations, laxatives, and herbal/vitamin supplements, often without consulting a health care provider. The occurrence of adverse drug events (ADEs) is directly related to the number of drugs taken and the frequency with which they are taken. Therefore older adults are at high risk for ADEs or interactions, either drug-drug or food-drug, often leading to hospital admission.

Effects of Drugs on Older Adults

Older adults may not tolerate the standard dosage of drugs traditionally prescribed for younger adults. The physiologic changes related to aging make drug therapy more complex and challenging. These changes affect the absorption, distribution, metabolism, and excretion of drugs from the body. Even common antibiotics can lead to temporary memory loss or confusion.

Age-related changes that can potentially affect drug absorption from an oral route include an increase in gastric pH, a decrease in gastric blood flow, and a decrease in GI motility. Despite these changes, most older adults do not have major absorption difficulties because of age-related changes alone.

Age-related changes that affect drug distribution include smaller amounts of total body water, an increased ratio of adipose tissue to lean body mass, a decreased albumin level, and a decreased cardiac output. Increased adipose tissue in proportion to lean body mass can cause increased storage of lipid-soluble drugs. This leads to a decreased concentration of the drug in plasma but an increased concentration in tissue.

Drug metabolism usually occurs in the liver. Age-related changes affecting metabolism include a decrease in liver size, a decrease in liver blood flow, and a decrease in liver enzyme activity. These changes can result in increased plasma concentrations of a drug. Monitor liver function studies, and teach older adults to have regular physical examinations.

Changes in the kidneys can also result in high plasma concentrations of drugs. The excretion of drugs usually involves the renal system. Age-related changes of the renal system include decreased renal blood flow and reduced glomerular filtration rate. These changes result in a decreased creatinine clearance and thus a slower excretion time for medications. Consequently, serum drug levels can become toxic and the patient can become extremely ill or die. Monitor renal studies, especially creatinine, when giving drugs to older adults. Teach patients to have regular physical examinations and renal evaluations.

When chronic disease is added to the physiologic changes of aging, drug reactions have a more dramatic effect and take a longer time to correct. Often a lower dose of a drug is necessary to prevent ADEs. *The policy of "start low, go slow" is essential when health care providers prescribe drugs for older adults.* The physiologic changes of aging are highly individual. Alterations in drug therapy should always be individualized according to the actual physiologic changes present and the occurrence and severity of chronic disease. Common ADEs are listed in Table 3-1.

Chart 3-3 BEST PRACTICE FOR PATIENT SAFETY & QUALITY CARE

Recommendations for Improving Older Driver Safety

- Discuss driving ability with the patient to assess his or her perception.
- Assess physical and mental deficits that could affect driving ability.
- Consult with appropriate health care providers to treat health problems that could interfere with driving.
- Suggest community-based transportation options instead of driving.
- Discuss driving concerns with patients and their families.
- Remind the patient to wear glasses and hearing aids, if prescribed.
- Encourage driver refresher classes, often offered by AAA and AARP.
- Consult a certified driving specialist for an on-road driving assessment.
- Encourage avoiding high-risk driving locations or conditions, such as busy urban interstates and wet or icy weather conditions.
- Report unsafe drivers to the state department of motor vehicles if they continue to drive.

Self-Administration of Drugs

Most people older than 65 years take their own medications. Because the risk of drug toxicity is considerably increased in the older population, assist patients in assuming this task responsibly. Teach patients and their caregivers, providing clear and concise directions and developing ways to assist them in overcoming difficulties with self-administration.

Older adults may make errors in self-administration or do not adhere to the drug regimen for several reasons. First, they may simply forget. In the rush of daily activities, they may not take their drugs or may take them too often because they cannot remember when or whether the medications have been taken. It is often helpful if they associate pill taking with daily events (e.g., meals) or keep a simple chart or calendar. Pill boxes are available for a daily, weekly, or monthly supply of medicine that can be placed in small compartments (Fig. 3-2). Egg cartons can be very cost-effective pill boxes. Large print on the drug label assists patients who have poor vision. Writing the drug regimen on the top of the bottle with large letters and numbers is helpful for some older adults. Colored labels or dots can also be applied. Easy-open bottle caps help older adults with limited hand mobility or strength.

A second reason for drug errors is poor communication with health care professionals. These problems result from poor explanations that are not understood because of educational limitations, language barriers, or difficulty with hearing

TABLE 3-1 **Common Adverse Drug Events (ADEs) in Older Adults**

Edema	Dizziness
Severe nausea and vomiting	Syncope
Anorexia	Urinary retention
Dehydration	Diarrhea
Dysrhythmias	Constipation/Impaction
Fatigue	Hypotension
Weakness	Acute confusion

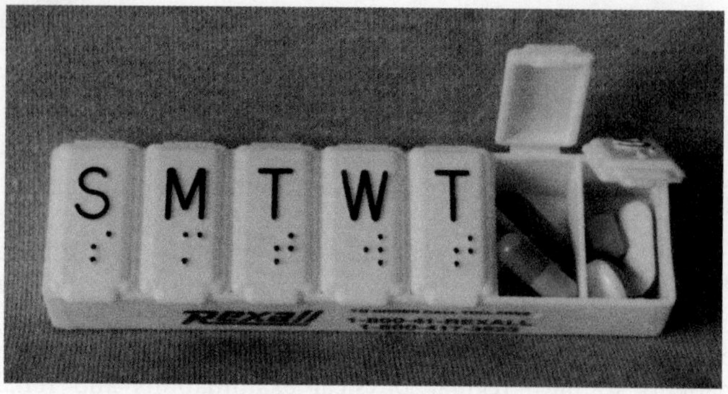
S
M
T
W
T
Rexall

Fig. 3-2 • A medication system for safe self-administration.

and vision. Health care professionals often presume that their patients have learned the information if they have taught them about the drugs. Assist older adults plan their drug therapy schedules.

A third reason for errors is the varying ways that patients take their medications. Some add to their drug regimen by taking over-the-counter (OTC) drugs, which can interact with prescription drugs and cause serious problems. For example, a patient receiving warfarin (Coumadin, Warfilone ♣) for anticoagulation may take ibuprofen (Motrin) regularly for arthritis. Because ibuprofen has anticoagulant ability, this combination can cause serious bleeding. When obtaining a drug history, ask patients about all OTC drugs, including herbal and food supplements.

Some other older adults avoid taking drugs. The fear of dependency or the cost of the drugs may cause many to discontinue their drug therapy too soon. In addition, the actions or side effects of some drugs may not be desirable. For example, diuretics may cause incontinence when patients cannot get to the bathroom quickly enough. Others may think that two pills are twice as effective as one. Some older adults take a drug that is leftover from a previous illness or one that has been prescribed for someone else.

Health care providers can influence the beliefs and practices of older adults about drug therapy and its effects. One method being tried in some hospitals and nursing homes is supervised drug self-administration, in which patients are allowed to take their own medications under supervision. In this way, the nurse can be sure of the patient's understanding and ability to self-administer medications at home or in another health care setting.

Mental Health/Behavioral Health

Most older adults are mentally sound and competent. A few changes in cognition have been identified as age related and are linked to specific cognitive functions rather than intellectual capacity. These changes include a decreased reaction time to stimuli and an impairment of memory for recent events. *However, severe cognitive impairment, depression, hallucinations, and delusions are not part of the normal aging process.*

Two forms of competence exist: legal competence and clinical competence. A person is **legally competent** if he or she is:

- 18 years of age or older
- Pregnant or a married minor
- A legally emancipated (free) minor who is self-supporting
- Not declared incompetent by a court of law

If a court determines that a person is not legally competent, a **guardian** is appointed to make financial and health care decisions. Guardians may be family members or a person who is not related to the patient.

A person is **clinically competent** if he or she is legally competent and can make clinical decisions. Decisional capacity is determined by a person's ability to identify problems, recognize options, make decisions, and provide the rationale supporting the decisions. Behavioral/mental illnesses often affect both legal and clinical competence and are briefly discussed here. Complete discussion of these problems can be found in behavioral/mental health textbooks. Depression, delirium, and dementia are often referred to as the *3Ds* of cognitive problems in older adults. None of these disorders are a result of normal aging changes. Diagnosis of the 3Ds is often difficult because they have some cognitive manifestations in common (Milisen et al., 2006).

Depression

Depression is the most common mental health/behavioral health problem among older adults in the community. It increases in incidence when older adults are admitted to the hospital or nursing home. **Depression** is broadly defined as a mood disorder that can have cognitive, affective, and physical manifestations. It can be primary or secondary and can range from mild to severe, or major. As a *primary* problem, depression is thought to result from a lack of the neurotransmitters norepinephrine and serotonin in the brain. *Secondary* depression, sometimes called *situational* depression, can result when there is a sudden change in the person's life, such as an illness or loss. Common illnesses that can cause secondary depression include stroke, arthritis, and cardiac disease. It is often underdiagnosed by physicians and is therefore undertreated (Greenberg, 2007).

Families and nurses are in the best position to suspect depression in an older adult. Several screening tools are available to help determine if the patient has clinical depression. The **Geriatric Depression Scale—Short Form (GDS-SF)** is a valid and reliable screening tool and is available in multiple languages. The patient selects "yes" or "no" to 15 questions, or a nurse or other health care professional can ask the questions to the patient. A score of 10 or greater is consistent with a possible diagnosis of clinical depression (Fig. 3-3). These patients are then evaluated more thoroughly by the health care provider for treatment.

Without diagnosis and treatment, depression can result in:

- Worsening of medical conditions
- Risk of physical illness
- Alcoholism
- Increased pain and disability
- Delayed recovery from illness
- Suicide

Older adults have the highest suicide rate of any age-group. Non-Hispanic white men who are older than 85 years are the most likely to die from suicide than any other older subgroup. Many of these patients visited their health care provider the week before the suicide (Greenberg, 2007).

Older adults with depression may have early morning insomnia, excessive daytime sleeping, poor appetite, a lack of energy, and an unwillingness to participate in social and recreational activities. The primary treatment for depression usually includes drug therapy and psychotherapy. In some parts

Geriatric Depression Scale: Short Form

Choose the best answer for how you have felt over the past week:

1. Are you basically satisfied with your life? YES / **NO**
2. Have you dropped many of your activities and interests? **YES** / NO
3. Do you feel that your life is empty? **YES** / NO
4. Do you often get bored? **YES** / NO
5. Are you in good spirits most of the time? YES / **NO**
6. Are you afraid that something bad is going to happen to you? **YES** / NO
7. Do you feel happy most of the time? YES / **NO**
8. Do you often feel helpless? **YES** / NO
9. Do you prefer to stay at home, rather than going out and doing new things? **YES** / NO
10. Do you feel you have more problems with memory than most? **YES** / NO
11. Do you think it is wonderful to be alive now? YES / **NO**
12. Do you feel pretty worthless the way you are now? **YES** / NO
13. Do you feel full of energy? YES / **NO**
14. Do you feel that your situation is hopeless? **YES** / NO
15. Do you think that most people are better off than you are? **YES** / NO

Answers in bold indicate depression. Score 1 point for each bolded answer.

A score > 5 points is suggestive of depression.
A score ≥ 10 points is almost always indicative of depression.
A score > 5 points should warrant a follow-up comprehensive assessment.

Fig. 3-3 • The Geriatric Depression Scale—Short Form.

of the country, electroconvulsive therapy (ECT) may be used either as a last resort or when drugs are not effective.

Selective serotonin reuptake inhibitors (SSRIs) are the first choice for drug therapy but take 2 to 3 weeks to work. They act by increasing the amount of serotonin and norepinephrine at nerve synapses in the brain. More information about depression, including strategies for preventing depression, is available in mental health/behavioral health nursing textbooks.

Dementia

Dementia is a broad term used for a syndrome that involves a slowly progressive cognitive decline, sometimes referred to as *chronic confusion*. Formerly called *organic brain syndrome* (OBS) and *chronic brain syndrome* (CBS), dementia represents a global impairment of intellectual function and is generally chronic and progressive. There are many types of dementia, the most common being Alzheimer's disease. Multi-infarct dementia, the second most common dementia, is a vascular disorder and accounts for 20% to 25% of all dementias. Chapter 44 discusses dementias in detail, with a focus on Alzheimer's disease.

Delirium

Whereas dementia is a chronic, progressive disorder, **delirium** is an *acute* state of confusion. Delirium also differs from dementia in that it is usually short-term and reversible within 3 weeks or less. It is often seen among older adults in a setting with which they are unfamiliar. It occurs in up to 50% of older adults who are in hospitals (Rigney, 2006). In addition to cognitive changes, some patients have physical manifestations and are *hyperactive*. Hyperactive patients may try to climb out of bed or become agitated and combative. *Hypoactive* patients are quiet, apathetic, and withdrawn.

Some of the multiple factors that can cause delirium are:

- Drug therapy (especially anticholinergic drugs)
- Electrolyte imbalances
- Infections, especially urinary tract or pneumonia
- Surgery
- Metabolic problems, such as hypoglycemia
- Neurologic disorders, such as tumors
- Circulatory, renal, and pulmonary disorders
- Nutritional deficiencies
- Hypoxia
- Relocation
- Major loss

Acutely confused patients who are discharged from the hospital are at an increased risk for functional decline, falls, and incontinence at home. Therefore assess older patients in any setting for acute confusion. A number of assessment tools have been developed, including the Confusion Assessment Method (CAM), Delirium Rating Scale (DRS), and NEECHAM Confusion Scale. Although the CAM is easy to use (Table 3-2), the nurse-developed NEECHAM Confusion Scale is also popular.

TABLE 3-2 **The Confusion Assessment Method (CAM)**

1. Acute onset and fluctuating course (e.g., Is there evidence of an acute change in mental status from the patient's baseline?)
2. Inattention (e.g., Does the patient have difficulty focusing attention or keeping track of what is being said?)
3. Disorganized thinking (e.g., Is the patient's thinking and conversation disorganized or incoherent?)
4. Altered level of consciousness (e.g., Is the patient lethargic, hyperalert, or difficult to arouse?)

The diagnosis of delirium by the CAM is the presence of features 1 *and* 2 and either 3 *or* 4.

TABLE 3-3 **Differences in the Characteristics of Delirium and Dementia**

Variable	Dementia	Delirium
Description	A chronic, progressive cognitive decline	An acute confusional state
Onset	Slow	Fast
Duration	Months to years	Hours to less than 1 month
Cause	Unknown, possibly familial, chemical	Multiple, such as surgery, infection, drugs
Reversibility	None	Usually
Management	Treat signs and symptoms	Remove or treat the cause
Nursing interventions	Reorientation not effective in the late stages; use validation therapy (acknowledge the patient's feelings, and do not argue); provide a safe environment; observe for associated behaviors, such as delusions and hallucinations	Reorient the patient to reality; provide a safe environment

To help manage delirium, use a calm voice to reorient the patient. A number of other nursing interventions have been used with some success. For example, playing tapes of soothing music may have a calming effect. Providing a doll or stuffed animal to "fidget" with may prevent the patient from removing important medical tubes or equipment. Some nurses believe that providing dolls and stuffed animals is treating the adult like a child, but this intervention can sometimes be very effective when used for therapeutic purposes. If the patient has a favorite item, such as an afghan blanket or a picture, ask the family or significant others to provide it for the same purpose.

Table 3-3 briefly differentiates delirium and dementia and lists the major nursing considerations for each. The most difficult challenge is caring for a patient who is experiencing both problems at the same time.

Chart 3-4 **NIC INTERVENTION ACTIVITIES**
Caregiver Support

Caregiver Support: *Provision of the necessary information, advocacy, and support to facilitate primary patient care by someone other than a health care professional*

- Determine caregiver's level of knowledge.
- Determine caregiver's acceptance of role.
- Teach caregiver stress management techniques.
- Monitor for indicators of stress.
- Identify sources of respite care.
- Teach the caregiver health care maintenance strategies to sustain own physical and mental health.
- Encourage caregiver participation in support groups.
- Educate caregiver about the grieving process.
- Teach caregiver strategies to access and maximize health care and community resources.
- Foster caregiver social networking.

NIC intervention activities selected from Bulechek, G.M., Butcher, H.K., & McCloskey Dochterman, J. (Eds). (2008). *Nursing interventions classification (NIC)* (5th ed.). St. Louis: Mosby. No part of this work is to be altered without prior written permission from the Publisher.

Elder Neglect and Abuse

Another problem for some older adults is neglect and abuse, both verbal and physical. Some older adults are more vulnerable to these problems than others, especially widows who may have difficulty being assertive. Older persons who are neglected or abused are often physically dependent. The abuser is often a family member who becomes frustrated or distraught over the burden of caring for the older adult.

Prolonged caregiving by a family member is a new and unexpected role for adult children, usually women. This new role may result in role fatigue and role conflict. Caregiver Role Strain and Risk for Caregiver Role Strain are nursing diagnoses approved by North American Nursing Diagnosis Association International (NANDA-I). From their research, Bulechek, Butcher, and Dochterman (2008) identified Caregiver Support as a major nursing intervention (Chart 3-4).

Neglect occurs when a caregiver fails to provide for an older adult's basic needs, such as food, clothing, medications, or assistance with ADLs. The caregiver refuses to let other people, like nursing assistants or home care nurses, into the home. Whether intentional or unintentional, neglect accounts for almost half of all cases of actual elder abuse.

Physical abuse is the use of physical force that results in bodily injury, especially in the "bathing suit" zone (abdomen, buttocks, genital area, upper thighs). Examples of physical abuse are hitting, burning, pushing, and molesting the patient. Sedating the older adult is also abusive. **Financial abuse** occurs when the older adult's property or resources are mismanaged or misused; this is more common than physical abuse. **Emotional abuse** is the intentional use of threats, humiliation, intimidation, and isolation toward older adults.

Carefully assess the patient for signs of abuse, such as bruises in clusters or regular patterns; burns, commonly to the buttocks or the soles of the feet; unusual hair loss; or multiple injuries, especially fractures. If the older adult is too weak or has no other resources or support systems, he or she may not admit that abuse is occurring. Neglect may be manifested by pressure ulcers, contractures, dehydration or undernutrition, urine burns, excessive body odor, and listlessness. Depression and dementia are common in community older adults who are abused or neglected.

All states in the United States and other Western countries have laws requiring health care professionals to report suspected elder abuse. In the community, if physical abuse or neglect is suspected, notify the local Adult Protective Services agency. In a hospital or nursing home, notify the social worker or case manager, who then will report the problem to the appropriate agency.

HEALTH CARE ISSUES IN HOSPITALS

Older adults who are admitted to hospitals and nursing homes have special needs and potential problems. Whereas nursing homes have multiple federal and state laws to prevent negative patient outcomes, hospitals are not required to follow these protective laws. However, The Joint Commission and other agencies have recently addressed some of the most common problems seen in older adults. In addition, since 1996, the Hartford Institute for Gerontological Nursing has worked to ensure that all hospitalized patients 65 years of age and older be given quality care.

Many nurses are not aware that the needs of older adults differ from those for younger adults (Fulmer, 2007). Some health care systems have designated Acute Care of the Elderly (ACE) units with geriatric resources nurses and geriatric clinical nurse specialists. The patients are cared for by geriatricians who specialize in the care of older adults.

Other hospitals have developed interdisciplinary programs system-wide to meet the special needs of older patients. The incentive for these new programs is the Nurses Improving Care for Health System Elders (NICHE) project, which continues to generate evidence-based practice guidelines for older adult care.

The purpose of all of these programs and units is to focus on the special health care issues seen in the older population. The **Fulmer SPICES** framework was developed as part of the NICHE project and identifies six serious "marker conditions" that can lead to longer hospital stays, higher medical costs, and even deaths. These conditions are:

- Sleep disorders
- Problems with eating or feeding
- Incontinence
- Confusion
- Evidence of falls
- Skin breakdown

Each of these problems is briefly described here and also is discussed in more detail in other parts of this chapter and the textbook. Other problems, such as depression and constipation, are also common in older hospitalized patients. Rather than being fully comprehensive, the SPICES framework is intended to be an easy tool that has been called "geriatric vital signs" (Fulmer, 2007).

Sleep, Nutrition, and Incontinence

Sleep disorders are common in hospitalized patients, especially older adults. Adequate rest is important for healing, as well as for physical and mental functioning. Pain, chronic disease, environmental noise and lighting, and staff conversations are a few of the many contributing factors to insomnia in the acute care setting. Assess the patient, and ask how he or she is sleeping. If the patient is not able to answer, observe for restlessness and other behaviors that could indicate lack of adequate rest. Manage the patient's pain by giving pain medication before bedtime. Attempt to keep patients awake during the day to prevent insomnia. Keep staff conversations as quiet as possible and away from patients' rooms. Dim the lights to make the patient area as dark as possible. Postpone treatments until waking hours or early morning if they can be delayed safely. If possible, place a "Do not Disturb" sign on the patient's door to avoid unnecessary interruptions in sleep (Cole & Richards, 2007).

Problems with eating and feeding prevent the older patient from receiving adequate nutrition. Some older patients become undernourished during prolonged hospital stays. Malnutrition has been linked to increased death rates in this population. Collaborate with the nutritionist about the patient's diet. Consider cultural preferences, and determine what foods the patient likes. Manage symptoms such as pain, nausea, and vomiting. If the patient has difficulty chewing or swallowing, coordinate a plan of care with the speech-language pathologist and nutritionist. If there are no dietary restrictions, encourage family members or friends to bring in food that the patient might enjoy. Additional interventions to prevent undernutrition are discussed in Chapter 63.

Incontinence varies in type and severity and may be caused by many factors, including acute or chronic disease, ADL ability, and available staff. Assess the patient to identify causes for incontinence. *Incontinence is not a physiologic change of aging, but it is very common in both the hospital and long-term care setting.* Place the patient on a toileting schedule or a bowel or bladder training program, if appropriate. Delegate and supervise this activity to unlicensed assistive personnel. Chapters 8 and 69 discuss bladder training in detail; Chapter 8 describes bowel training as well.

Confusion, Falls, and Skin Breakdown

Confusion affects many older patients in both the hospital and nursing home. Whereas chronic confusion states such as dementia are not reversible, acute confusion, or delirium, may be avoidable and is often reversible when the cause is resolved or removed. For example, avoiding multiple drugs and promoting adequate sleep can help prevent acute confusion. Help the patient by reorienting him or her to reality as much as needed. Keep the patient as comfortable as possible; for example, provide interventions to control pain. Chapter 44 describes acute and chronic confusion in detail.

The most common accident among older patients in a hospital or nursing home setting is falling. A ***fall*** is an unintentional change in body position that results in the patient's body coming to rest on the floor or ground. Some falls result in serious injuries such as fractures and head trauma. The Joint Commission's **National Patient Safety Goals (NPSG)** requires that all inpatient health care settings have admission and daily fall risk assessment tools and a fall reduction program for patients who are at high risk.

Assess the older adult for risk of falls. Many assessment tools have been developed to help the nurse focus on factors that increase an older person's risk of falling. Chart 3-5 lists some of the common risk factors that should be assessed and evidence-based, collaborative interventions for preventing falls. *A recent history of falling is the single most important predictor for falls.*

Older patients often have **nocturia** (urination at night) and get out of bed to go to the bathroom. They may forget to ask for assistance and may subsequently fall as a result of disorientation in the darkness in an unfamiliar environment. In some cases, they may crawl over the siderail, which can make the fall more serious. Because of this, full or split siderails are used far less often in both hospitals and nursing homes. In both settings, siderails are classified as restraints unless the use of rails helps patients increase mobility.

A **restraint** is any device or drug that prevents the patient from moving freely and must be prescribed by a health care provider. In 1990, the federal government enforced a law that gives nursing home residents the right to be restraint free. Removing physical restraints from nursing home residents has reduced serious injuries, although falls and minor injuries have increased in some cases. Mattresses placed on floors next to patient beds or "low beds" have helped reduce injury. The Joint Commission requires hospitals to reduce the risk of patient harm resulting from falls.

Hospitals have also reduced the use of physical restraints. The Joint Commission has specific standards that limit the use of physical restraints in hospitals and nursing homes. Chemical restraints (psychoactive drugs) such as haloperidol (Haldol) have sometimes been used in place of physical restraints.

Experts agree that older adults should not be placed in a physical restraint or sedated just because they are old. Use alternatives before applying any type of restraint (Chart 3-6). However, if all other interventions (e.g., reminding patients to call for assistance when needed; asking a family member to stay with patients) are not effective in fall prevention, a physical restraint may be required for a limited period. Applying a restraint is a serious intervention and should be analyzed for its risk versus its benefit. Check the patient in a restraint every 30 to 60 minutes, and release the restraint at least every 2 hours for turning, repositioning, and toileting. Physical restraints such as vests have caused serious injury and even death. If

Chart 3-5 BEST PRACTICE FOR PATIENT SAFETY & QUALITY CARE

Assessing Risk Factors and Preventing Falls in Older Adults

Assess for the presence of these risk factors:
- History of falls
- Advanced age (>80 years)
- Multiple illnesses
- Generalized weakness or decreased mobility
- Disorientation or confusion
- Use of drugs that can cause increased confusion, mobility limitations, or orthostatic hypotension
- Urinary incontinence
- Communication impairments
- Major visual impairment or visual impairment without correction
- Substance abuse
- Location of patient's room away from the nurses' station (in the hospital or nursing home)
- Change of shift or mealtime (in the hospital or nursing home)

Implement these nursing interventions for all patients, regardless of risk:
- Monitor the patient's activities and behavior as often as possible, preferably every 30 to 60 minutes.
- Remind the patient to call for help before getting out of bed or a chair.
- Help the patient to get out of bed or a chair if needed.
- Provide or remind the patient to use a walker or cane for ambulating if needed.
- Remind the patient to wear eyeglasses or a hearing aid if needed.
- Help the incontinent patient to toilet every 1 to 2 hours.
- Clean up spills immediately.
- Arrange the furniture in the patient's room or hallway to eliminate clutter or obstacles that could contribute to a fall.
- Provide adequate lighting at all times, especially at night.
- Observe for side effects and toxic effects of drug therapy.
- Orient the patient to the environment.
- Keep the call light within reach, and ensure that the patient can use it.
- Place the bed in the lowest position with the brakes locked.
- Place objects that the patient needs within reach.
- Ensure that adequate handrails are present in the patient's room, bathroom, and hall.
- Have the physical therapist assess the patient for mobility and safety.

For patients at a high risk for falls:
- Implement all interventions listed above.
- Relocate the patient for best visibility and supervision.
- Use bed and chair alarms.
- Encourage family members or significant other to stay with the patient.

Chart 3-6 BEST PRACTICE FOR PATIENT SAFETY & QUALITY CARE

Using Restraint Alternatives

- If the patient is acutely confused, reorient him or her to reality as often as possible.
- If the patient has dementia, use validation to reaffirm his or her feelings and concerns.
- Check the patient often, at least every hour.
- If the patient pulls tubes and lines, cover them with roller gauze or another protective device.
- Provide activities that keep the patient busy, such as an activity, pillow or apron, puzzle, or art activity.
- Provide soft, calming music.
- Place the patient in an area where he or she can be supervised. (If the patient is agitated, do not place him or her in a noisy area.)
- Turn off the television if the patient is agitated.
- Ask a family member or friend to stay with the patient at night.
- Help the patient to toilet every 2 to 3 hours, including during the night.
- Be sure that the patient's needs for food, fluids, and comfort are met.
- If agency policy allows, provide the patient with a pet visit.
- Provide familiar objects or cherished items that the patient can touch.
- Document the use of all alternative interventions.
- If a restraint is applied, use the least restrictive device (e.g., mitts rather than wrist restraints, a roller belt rather than a vest).

restraint is needed, the least restrictive device should be used. Be sure to follow your facility's policy and procedure for using restraints.

Chemical restraints are often overused in hospital settings. Patients who are noisy, agitated, abusive, or combative may have an "as needed" prescription for a psychoactive drug. Such medications include:

- Antipsychotic drugs
- Antianxiety drugs
- Antidepressant drugs
- Sedative-hypnotic drugs

These drugs produce serious adverse drug events and therefore should be reserved for patients with a documented mental health or behavioral health problem, such as severe anxiety or psychosis. Those receiving these medications must be closely monitored for therapeutic and adverse effects.

The most potent group of psychoactive drugs is the antipsychotics. These drugs may be appropriate for the control of certain behavioral symptoms, such as hallucinations, delusions, and violent episodes. However, fewer than half of patients respond to these drugs. *If a psychoactive drug is used as a last resort to control behavior, the lowest dose should be given.*

Skin breakdown, especially pressure ulcers, is a major problem among older adults in hospitals and nursing homes. In some cases, these wounds cause death from infection. Therefore prevention is the best approach. The Joint Commission's 2007 NPSGs require that all health care agencies have a program to prevent agency-associated pressure ulcers. The program should include these evidence-based interventions:

- Nutritional support
- Avoidance of skin injury from friction or shearing forces
- Repositioning and support surfaces
- A plan to increase mobility and activity level, when appropriate
- Skin cleansing and use of moisture barriers

Assess older adults for their risk for pressure ulcers, using an assessment tool such as the Braden Scale for Predicting Pressure Sore Risk (see Chapter 27). Implement evidence-based interventions to prevent agency-acquired pressure ulcers. Coordinate these interventions with members of the health care team, including the nutritionist and wound care specialist. Supervise unlicensed assistive personnel (UAP) for frequent turning and repositioning for the patient who is immobile. Assess the skin every 8 hours for reddened areas that do not blanch. Remind UAP to keep the skin clean and dry. Use pressure-relieving mattresses, and avoid briefs or absorbent pads that can cause skin irritation and excess moisture. Chapter 27 describes additional interventions for prevention and management of pressure ulcers in detail.

Skin tears are also common in older adults, especially the old-old group and those who are on chronic steroid therapy. Teach UAP to use extreme caution when handling these patients. Use a gentle touch, and report any open areas. Avoid bruising because older adults have increased capillary fragility.

GET READY FOR THE NCLEX EXAMINATION!

Key Points

Review these Key Points for each NCLEX Examination Client Needs Category.

Safe and Effective Care Environment

- Coordinate care by collaborating with members of the health care team when providing care to older adults in the community or inpatient setting.
- Assess all older adults for risk for falls and driving ability (see Charts 3-3 and 3-5).
- Assess for signs of elder neglect and abuse; if suspected, it should be reported.
- Physical and chemical restraints should not be used for older adults until all other alternatives have been tried.
- Follow The Joint Commission's National Patient Safety Goals and federal/state standards when using patient restraints.

Health Promotion and Maintenance

- Relocation stress syndrome is the reaction of an older adult when transferred to a different environment; ways to minimize this problem are listed in Chart 3-2.
- Nutrition and mobility are two health problems experienced by older adults.
- Teach older adults about the benefits of regular physical exercise.
- Provide information regarding community resources for older adults to help them meet their basic needs.
- Teach health promotion practices as listed in Chart 3-1.

Psychosocial Integrity

- Depression is the most common yet most underdiagnosed and undertreated mental health/behavioral health disorder among older adults.
- Elder neglect and abuse are serious problems; family caregivers are usually the abusers.
- Use interventions listed in Chart 3-4 to support caregivers for older adults.
- Many older adults are not prepared for retirement in view of increased expenses and income that is not adequate to meet basic needs, health care treatments, and medications.

Physiological Integrity

- The four subgroups of the older adult population are the young old, middle old, old old, and elite old.
- The biggest concern regarding accidents among older adults in both the community and inpatient setting is falls.
- Physiologic changes of aging predispose older adults to toxic effects of medication; drugs are absorbed, metabolized, and distributed more slowly than in younger people. They are also excreted more slowly by the kidneys.
- Medication use in older adults is often a problem when they commit errors when self-medicating, avoid needed medications, or have problems understanding their medication regimen.
- Delirium is acute confusion that is short-lived; dementia is chronic confusion that progresses slowly and worsens. Table

3-3 compares these two health problems commonly seen in older adults.

- Follow The Joint Commission's National Patient Safety Goals and best practice guidelines to prevent agency-acquired pressure ulcers.
- Promote sleep and rest for older adults to decrease the incidence of delirium and prevent falls.
- Use alternatives for physical or chemical restraints to provide patient safety, as listed in Chart 3-6.
- Use the SPICES assessment tool for identifying serious health problems that can be prevented or managed early.

Additional Study Resources

Go to your Companion CD or Evolve at http://evolve.elsevier.com/Iggy/ for Self-Assessment Questions for the NCLEX Examination.

Go to Evolve at http://evolve.elsevier.com/Iggy/ for Prioritization and Delegation Questions for the NCLEX Examination.

SELECTED BIBLIOGRAPHY

Asterisk indicates a classic or definitive work on this subject.

Bulechek, G.M., Butcher, H.K., & McCloskey Dochterman, J. (Eds.). (2008). *Nursing interventions classification (NIC)* (5th ed.). St. Louis: Mosby.

Chapman, I.M. (2006). Nutritional disorders in the elderly. *Medical Clinics of North America, 90*(5), 887-907.

Cole, C., & Richards, K. (2007). Sleep disruption in older adults. *AJN, 107*(5), 40-48.

*Davidhizar, R., Eshleman, J., & Moody, M. (2002). Health promotion in aging adults. *Geriatric Nursing, 23*(1), 28-35.

DiMaria-Ghalili, R.A., & Amella, E. (2005). Nutrition in older adults. *AJN, 105*(3), 40-50.

Forrest, J., Willis, L., Holm, K., Kwon, M.S., Anderson, M.A., & Foreman, M.D. (2007). Recognizing quiet delirium. *AJN, 107*(4), 35-39.

Fulmer, T. (2007). How to try this: Fulmer SPICES. *AJN, 107*(10), 40-48.

*Gray-Vickery, P. (2000). Protecting the older adult. *Nursing2000, 30*(7), 34-37.

Greenberg, S.A. (2007). How to try this: The Geriatric Depression Scale—Short Form. *AJN, 107*(10), 60-69.

Gustafson, S.E. (2007). Assess for fall risk, intervene, and bump up patient safety. *Nursing2007, 37*(12), 24-25.

Hendrich, A. (2007). Predicting patient falls: Using the Hendrich II Fall Risk Model in clinical practice. *AJN, 107*(11), 50-59.

Hook, M.L., & Winchel, S. (2006). Fall-related injuries in acute care: Reducing the risk of harm. *MEDSURG Nursing, 15*(6), 370-377.

*Ignatavicius, D. (2000). Do you help staff rise to the fall-prevention challenge? *Nursing Management, 31*(1), 27-30.

Jasniewski, J. (2006). Take steps to protect your patient from falls. *Nursing2006, 36*(4), 24-25.

King, B.D. (2006). Functional decline in hospitalized elders. *MEDSURG Nursing, 15*(5), 265-270.

Mauk, K.L. (2005). Keeping an older adult on her toes with exercise. *Nursing2005, 35*(1), 24.

Milisen, K., Braes, T., Fick, T.M., & Foreman, M.D. (2006). Cognitive assessment and differentiating the 3 Ds (dementia, depression, delirium). *Nursing Clinics of North America, 41*(1), 1-22.

NANDA International. (2007). *Nursing diagnoses: Definitions and classification 2007-2008.* Philadelphia: Author.

O'Connell, B., Gardner, A., Takase, M., Hawkins, M.T., Ostaszkiewicz, J., Ski, C., et al. (2007). Clinical usefulness and feasibility of using Reality Orientation with patients who have dementia in acute care settings. *International Journal of Nursing Practice, 13*(3), 182-192.

Odenheimer, G.L. (2006). Driver safety in older adults: The physician's role in assessing driving skills in older patients. *Geriatrics, 61*(10), 14-21.

Pountney, D. (2007). Dementia, delirium, or depression? *Nursing Older People, 19*(5), 12-16.

Rigney, T.S. (2006). Delirium in the hospitalized elder and recommendations for practice. *Geriatric Nursing, 27*(3), 151-157.

Struck, B.D., & Ross, K.M. (2006). Health promotion in older adults: Prescribing exercise for the frail and home bound. *Geriatrics, 61*(5), 22-27.

Sweeny, S.J., Bridges, E.J., Wild, L.M., & Sayre, C.A. (2008). Care of the patient with delirium. *AJN, 108*(5), 72CC-72GG.

*Taggart, H.M. (2002). Effects of tai chi exercise on balance, functional mobility, and fear of falling among older women. *Applied Nursing Research, 15*(4), 235-242.

*Theodus, P. (2003). Fall prevention in frail elderly nursing home residents: A challenge to case management. Part I. *Lippincott's Case Management, 8*(6), 246-251.

Cultural Aspects of Health and Illness

CHAPTER 4

Donna D. Ignatavicius*

LEARNING OUTCOMES

For clinical competence and success on the NCLEX Examination, study this chapter with these Learning Outcomes in mind:

Health Promotion and Maintenance

1. Explain the purpose of *Healthy People 2010* as related to culture.
2. Incorporate cultural practices and beliefs into the patient's plan of care.

Psychosocial Integrity

3. Define culture, cultural diversity, cultural competence, and cultural sensitivity.
4. Discuss specific cultural practices, such as family roles and nutrition, which should be part of a cultural assessment.
5. Identify two major health issues related to the lesbian, gay, bisexual, and transgender (LGBT) population.
6. Identify two influences of culture on drug therapy.
7. Collaborate with the professional chaplain to manage a patient's spiritual distress.
8. Describe two examples of generic and folk medicine that are used in the United States today.
9. Explain ways that nurses can communicate sensitively with patients from various cultural groups.

Go to your Companion CD or Evolve at http://evolve.elsevier.com/Iggy/ for *Self-Assessment*

evolve *Questions for the NCLEX Examination* keyed to these Learning Outcomes.

In the 1950s, Madeline Leininger, a nurse anthropologist and theorist, provided a large body of knowledge called *transcultural nursing*. She defined **transcultural** nursing as an area of study and practice that focuses on the care, health, and illness patterns of people with similarities and differences in their cultural beliefs, values, and practices. Since that time, other researchers have continued her work as the United States has become more culturally diverse.

It is still the case that the majority of people in the United States are white and of European descent (Euro-American). However, the population is increasing by more than 2.5 million people *each year,* and 1 million of them are newcomers (also called immigrants) from other countries. In 2000, the number of minority populations in the United States accounted for 28% of the total population; Hispanic/Latinos are the largest minority group (Giger et al., 2007). Asian Americans are currently the fastest growing group.

In addition to racial and ethnic diversity, people differ in gender, age (generation), education, occupation, geographic location, and religion. Each of these differences represents varying cultures. As a nurse, you will care for many diverse patients and work with diverse staff. Therefore you will need to learn about cultural diversity and become culturally competent.

CULTURE AND CULTURAL COMPETENCE

When considering cultural aspects of health, nurses and other health care staff need to understand the differences in commonly used terms: culture, cultural diversity, cultural competency, and cultural sensitivity. Culture is not restricted to race or ethnicity. Instead, **culture** is a broad term that refers to integrated patterns of behavior acquired over time, including beliefs, values, customs, norms, habits, language, thoughts, and ways of life (Wilson-Stronks & Galvez, 2007). It is learned and transmitted primarily within the family unit, generation, and/or other social organizations and is shared by most of the members of the group. A person's culture provides his or her worldview, which helps guide decision making and enhances self-worth (Fig. 4-1) (Giger et al., 2007).

Cultural diversity refers to differences among people, which may or may not be visible, For example, a person's *race* describes his or her visible physical characteristics, such as skin tone, head shape, and hair texture. *Ethnicity* describes common social customs, values, and beliefs of a group. *A person's race does not determine his or her ethnicity.* For instance, a woman

*Special thanks to Stephanie M. Ignatavicius for her contributions to this chapter in the areas of LGBT issues and cultural bias.

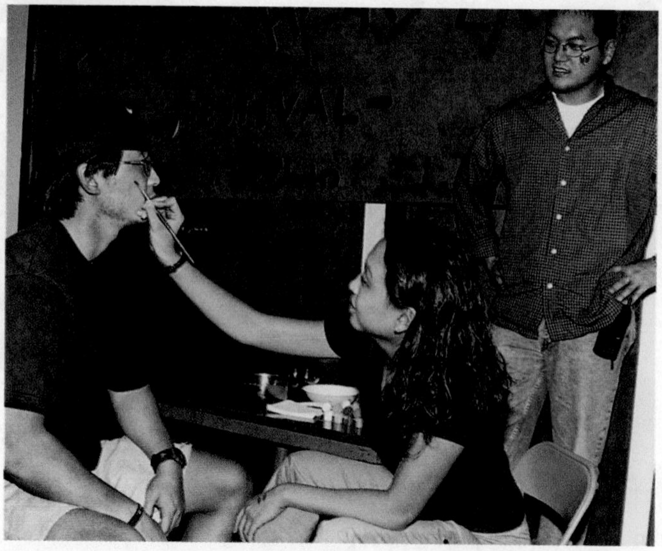

Fig. 4-1 • Healthy self-esteem in young adulthood is tied to appreciation of one's cultural heritage. These Korean Americans demonstrate pride in their cultural heritage through participation in a cultural celebration.

TABLE 4-1 Campinha-Bacote's ASKED Model of Cultural Competence

Awareness: Are you aware of your personal biases and prejudices towards cultures different than yours?
Skill: Do you have the skill to conduct a cultural assessment and perform a culturally based physical assessment?
Knowledge: Do you have knowledge of the patient's **worldview** (the way that a person looks at the universe to form values in their lives and the world)?
Encounters: How many face-to-face encounters have you had with patients from diverse cultural backgrounds?
Desire: What is your desire to want to be culturally competent?

Courtesy Dr. Josie Campinha-Bacote, expert in cultural nursing.

may be white and of Russian descent. Therefore her customs and beliefs about health care or family roles may be different from those of a white woman from Italian ancestry. Another example is the use of the U.S. census category "African American," which implies that all black people come from an African background. There are a number of problems with that assumption. First, all African countries do not have the same customs and values. Second, although many black people are of African heritage, some are from Haiti, Jamaica, and other countries. Therefore to refer to all black people as African American is not culturally correct.

Cultural competence is a process that involves respecting all differences and not letting one's own biases influence others. It requires having the knowledge, skills, and understanding about diverse groups (Giger et al., 2007). In health care, cultural competence refers to the *ability of health care providers and organizations to understand and respond effectively to the cultural and linguistic needs that patients bring to the health care setting.* The Joint Commission standards and National Patient Safety Goals require that cultural differences be respected and incorporated into the plan of care for patient safety and quality care.

Becoming culturally competent first requires you to examine your feelings and experiences regarding diversity, starting with an understanding of your own heritage. Then, you will need to learn more about specific cultural differences so you can develop an appreciation for the values and beliefs of both patients and staff co-workers.

Campinha-Bacote's (2003) **ASKED** Model of Cultural Competence provides a beginning self-assessment tool. Ask yourself the questions listed in Table 4-1.

Cultural sensitivity occurs when a person is aware of and appreciates cultural differences and thus avoids biased, negative, impolite, and offensive language and actions when interacting with people of diverse cultures. Sensitivity also means avoiding stereotyping. **Stereotyping** occurs when you assume that all people in a particular culture have the group's values and beliefs or practice the group's customs. Everyone in a particular group is a unique person.

Some groups continually strive to preserve their heritage. The most common example is the American-Indian population, which consists of many subgroups, also called *councils* or *nations,* across the United States. This multi-cultural group teaches the importance of maintaining traditions from generation to generation. However, specific beliefs and rituals vary among its subgroups. For instance, the Lakota Council is made up of several tribes that have specific customs. These customs differ from those of other American Indians like the Cherokee or Navajo nations. However, some generalizations apply to all American Indians, such as their value for respect, spirituality, and nature.

According to U.S. government treaties in the 1800s, the Lakotas and other like subgroups are American Indians, not Native Americans. For that reason, they refer to themselves as American Indian because that is their legal designated name (Personal communication, Ogala Lakota College, Pine Ridge, SD, August 6, 2003). This textbook uses *American Indian* rather than *Native American* to refer to this large cultural group.

HEALTH AND HEALTH CARE DISPARITIES

Health disparities are the differences in the incidence of health care problems among minority racial and ethnic groups when compared with the white majority. To date, no research has definitely supported either a genetic or environmental cause for these disparities, but both may contribute to the problem. Disparities in health care quality may also help explain the differences in health status among minority groups. Possible factors that may contribute to this problem include socioeconomic status, individual discrimination, access to care, and language barriers (Giger et al., 2007).

Healthy People 2010 is a health promotion program created by the U.S. Department of Health and Human Services (USDHHS) to decrease disparities in health and health care (2001). The goal by 2010 is to eliminate the differences in the health status of racial and ethnic minorities while trying to continually improve the overall health of all American individuals. A few of the main target areas are:

- Infant mortality
- Cancer screening and management
- Diabetes mellitus
- Cardiovascular disease

PURNELL'S DOMAINS OF CULTURE

No one is expected to know the specific traits of every type of culture, including racial and ethnic groups. But you will need to continue learning as you interact with more and more diverse groups to develop cultural competence. Purnell & Paulanka (2008) have suggested 12 essential areas, or domains, to assess and understand any culture (Table 4-2). The most relevant of these cultural practices for nursing care are briefly reviewed here.

Culture Overview and Communication

The first domain is *overview and localities.* This area refers to a person's residence, heritage, education, and occupation. The ancestors of a large portion of the U.S. population left their native countries many decades or centuries ago. One of the biggest movements of newcomers was in the early 1990s. Many of these people were European, fleeing persecution or war-torn countries. More recent immigrants come to the United States for better opportunities for education, jobs, religious freedom, and democracy (Purnell & Paulanka, 2008).

Although ethnic minorities can be found anywhere throughout the United States, some have chosen to live in specific geographic areas with members of their group for support and practice of traditional customs. For example, the Chinese are concentrated in New York and California. Mexicans tend to live in the Southwestern United States, Florida, and California (Purnell & Paulanka, 2008).

Other cultural groups also tend to congregate in specific locations. For instance, older adults tend to retire to warmer climates like Florida and Arizona. Many younger people are attracted to large urban areas for access to multiple social activities and job opportunities. When you are caring for patients, assess where they live and whether they have a support system within their culture.

The second area to assess is the ability of your patient to *communicate.* Language continues to be the largest barrier for people who do not speak English or cannot communicate in English effectively. If your patient is not fluent in English, determine his or her primary language. The Joint Commission National Patient Safety Goals require that professional *interpreters* (also called *trained medical interpreters* or *medical language interpreters*) be available in health care facilities to prevent errors in communication that could lead to patient harm. In addition, telephone interviews with patients who cannot communicate in English should involve the use of telephonic interpretation services, such as Language Line Services (www.languageline.com) or Language Services Associates (www.lsaweb.com) (Galanti, 2006). Chart 4-1 lists guidelines to help you communicate with non–English-speaking patients. Remember that many groups (e.g., Japanese Americans, Appalachians, and Mexican Americans) are not as open with expressing their feelings to strangers as most Euro-Americans.

Communication also includes nonverbal forms, such as body language, eye contact, facial expression, and touch. *Be sure to find out which forms are acceptable for your patient.* For instance, eye contact can be interpreted differently depending on the patient's cultural background. American Indians may find it offensive to make direct eye contact. Many Middle-Eastern cultures are not likely to accept touch by strangers, for example, Egyptian Americans.

Family and Workplace Issues

Ask about *family roles, organization,* and *lifestyle,* as well as *workforce issues.* Information about family and gender roles will influence your plan of care. For example, an Arab Muslim woman cannot be exposed and only a female is allowed to care for her. If you are preparing the patient for a procedure, keep her entire body including her head covered and provide additional draping. Make sure that all staff caring for her is female (Galanti, 2006).

Assess who makes the decisions in the family; do not assume that the patient will want to make them. Autonomy and independence are core American values but may not be valued by some of your patients. The family as a unit may make decisions—not the individual patient. In cultures in which men dominate, the husband makes all decisions for the woman. If the woman works outside the home, she may have difficulty being assertive or making workplace decisions. This is especially true among Nigerian, Chinese, and Iranian women (Purnell & Paulanka, 2008).

TABLE 4-2 Purnell's Domains for Assessing Cultural Groups or Persons

- Nutrition
- Communication
- Family roles and organization
- Workforce issues
- Biocultural ecology
- High-risk behaviors
- Overview (e.g., heritage)
- Pregnancy and childbirth practices
- Death rituals
- Spirituality
- Health care practices
- Health care practitioners

Data from Purnell L. (2000). A description of the Purnell model for cultural competence. *Journal of Transcultural Nursing, 11*(1), 40-46.

Chart 4-1 BEST PRACTICE FOR PATIENT SAFETY & QUALITY CARE

Guidelines for Communicating with Non–English-Speaking Patients

- Use dialect-specific interpreters who are the same gender and about the same age as the patient if possible.
- Use interpreters who are familiar with health and health care.
- Avoid the use of relatives to prevent bias and misinterpretation.
- Speak slowly, and allow the patient time to translate and process what is being discussed.
- Use common words in the patient's language if known; become familiar with Spanish terms that are frequently used in health care.
- Maintain eye contact with the patient and family while communicating, *unless it is not culturally acceptable.*
- Remember that most patients can understand English better than they can speak it.
- Be careful with nonverbal facial expressions and body language.

In some cultures, entire families insist on staying with patients while they are hospitalized to show their love and support. On the other hand, some patients may not want family members present. Hospitals and other health care facilities are not designed to meet these special needs. A "culture clash" may result, causing conflict and patient dissatisfaction. Work to meet the needs of your patients and negotiate with both families and administration. For example, request extra cots or recliners for family sleeping arrangements if possible.

Another aspect of family roles and organization is how members view and treat their older adult relatives. Some groups, such as Asian subcultures, highly value and respect older adults. Euro-Americans tend to value children and their immediate nuclear families rather than their extended families, including grandparents, cousins, and uncles.

The makeup of a family in the United States varies greatly. For example, some families have single parents; others have grandparents who rear their grandchildren. Domestic partnerships with the opposite or same gender are also very common and acceptable in most societies. However, the health status and the quality of health care may differ depending on a person's sexual identity. Do not assume that every patient is heterosexual or clearly gendered. *Include questions about sexual identity and sexual activity as part of your patient's health assessment* (Neville & Henrickson, 2006).

Lesbian, Gay, Bisexual, and Transgender Health

The health care system, like other facets of society, often overlooks genders and sexualities that are alternative to the "norm." To best characterize these identities, this textbook uses **"LGBT"** to refer to the lesbian, gay, bisexual, and transgender culture. This terminology is widely accepted by the LGBT community and is commonly seen in the literature. Members within this population vary by race, ethnicity, and age. The exact size of the group is not known.

LGBT health has not been widely studied because the group is very diverse. Selecting an accurate sample is difficult and therefore may not represent the entire group. As a result, any research findings may be less reliable than desired and more difficult to generalize for the entire culture.

In 1999, the Institute of Medicine (IOM) drafted a document to summarize its findings of lesbian health and recommendations for improvement. In 2001, the USDHHS published a companion document for the *Healthy People 2010* program on LGBT health. However, the research findings may have limitations because of inaccuracies in sample identity.

Using the best scientific findings available, the report outlined major health disparities when the LGBT population was compared with other groups. For example, women who identify as lesbians have a higher incidence of alcohol abuse, smoking, and obesity than non-lesbian women. As a result, lesbians may have more gynecologic cancers, especially breast and ovarian; lung cancer; and cardiovascular disease. Nulliparity (not giving birth to a child) or low parity is also a risk factor for gynecologic cancer. Depression and suicide are also higher among lesbians. These mental health problems may be caused by substance abuse and poor self-esteem, possibly related to their lack of acceptance in society (USDHHS, 2001). Some health problems occur less often in women who identify as lesbians when compared with other groups. For example, sexually transmitted diseases are not as common among lesbians.

Gay men or men having sex with men have a higher incidence of anal and colon cancer than other men. Like lesbians, they experience substance abuse, depression, and suicide. Kaposi's sarcoma associated with acquired immune deficiency syndrome (AIDS) is much more common in gay men when compared with other men (USDHHS, 2001). More research on health disparities for the LGBT population is needed to validate the beginning work that has been done in this area.

Quality of LGBT Health Care

The *Healthy People 2010* companion document also reported differences in health care access and quality between the LGBT population and other groups. Additional studies have confirmed these findings. For example, women who identify as lesbians report experiencing health care provider discrimination and may therefore avoid routine preventive care like Papanicolaou (Pap) smears and mammograms. In addition, some physicians assure them that they are at low risk for cervical cancer, assuming they do not have sex with men. Patients are also told that they cannot transmit the human papillomavirus (HPV). However, a number of lesbians have had sexual contact with men and HPV can be transmitted from one woman to another (O'Hanlan et al., 2004).

Because of health care discrimination, people who are LGBT may not disclose their sexual identity to health care professionals. First, many health care team members assume that anyone seeking health care is heterosexual. Second, these patients have special health needs that are often not understood by the health care community. Neville and Henrickson (2006) found that the attitudes of health professionals are important to the LGBT population, but they know that the health care community is not culturally competent about their group. The researchers referred to the need to provide "culturally safe care" for all patients. Chart 4-2 provides guidelines to increase communication and trust between LGBT patients and health care professionals.

Chart 4-2 **BEST PRACTICE FOR PATIENT SAFETY & QUALITY CARE**

Guidelines for Communicating with LGBT Patients

- Create a culturally safe, trusting environment to help the patient feel more comfortable.
- Ask open-ended questions about sexual identity and sexual activity (see Table 4-3).
- Do not be judgmental or offensive in your interactions with the patient.
- If the patient does not feel comfortable with disclosing his or her sexual identity, provide additional opportunities for disclosure.
- Listen to your patient, and show respect.
- Teach LGBT patients the need for preventive health interventions, such as the importance of regular mammograms and screening colonoscopies.
- Be sure that the patient has access to a primary health care provider and payer source; if not, collaborate with the case manager or social worker.
- Respect the patient's right to have his or her partner present.
- Recognize that the patient's partner and friends are the major support system for most patients; biologic family members may not be accepting of the patient's lifestyle.

LGBT, Lesbian, gay, bisexual, transgender.

Part of culturally safe care requires that nurses and other providers know their patient's sexual identity. Some health care team members are uncomfortable with interviewing or providing services to the LGBT population. Assessment forms traditionally ask questions such as "Are you married, divorced, widowed, or single?" This question has no options for LGBT patients to answer. This type of barrier interferes with communication between the patient and the nurse. Better questions to ask about sexual identity during a patient interview are recommended in Table 4-3.

Biologic Ecology

Biologic ecology includes biologic variations, health disparities, and drug metabolism differences. Race and health disparities have already been discussed. A new field related to culture is ethnopharmacology. **Ethnopharmacology** is the study of the effect of ethnicity on how drugs work in the body, including drug absorption, distribution, metabolism, and excretion. For example, some angiotensin-converting enzyme (ACE) inhibitors for hypertension typically work better for Euro-American patients than for African Americans and other blacks. On the other hand, the thiazide diuretics are more effective for lowering blood pressure in African-American and other blacks when compared with Euro-Americans. The exact causes for these differences are being studied. Although nurse generalists do not prescribe drug therapy, they need to understand why selected drugs are given to certain groups.

The lifestyle and values of patients can also affect drug response. For instance, excess tobacco and alcohol use can increase or decrease the rate at which a drug is metabolized and excreted, depending on the specific drug. Another concern about drug therapy is whether the patient adheres to the drug regimen. For example, older adults may be less likely than younger adults to follow the prescribed therapy because of drug costs. Some groups, such as Hispanics, are less likely than Euro-Americans or African Americans and other blacks to continue taking their medication as prescribed (Muñoz & Hilgenberg, 2005). Again, the reasons for the differences among cultural groups are unknown but may include language or transportation barriers. Consider these cultural factors when teaching patients about their drug therapy.

TABLE 4-3 Recommended Patient Interview Questions About Sexual Identity and Health Care

- Do you have sex with men, women, with both or neither?
- Does anyone live with you in your household?
- Are you in a relationship with someone who does not live with you?
- If you have a sexual partner, have you or your partner been evaluated about the possibility of transmitting infections to each other?
- If you have more than one sexual partner, how are you protecting both of you from infections, such as Hepatitis B or C or HIV?
- Have you disclosed your sexual identity and sexual activity to your health care provider?
- If you have not, could I have your permission to provide that information to members of the health care team who are involved in your care?
- Who do you consider as your closest family members?

HIV, Human immune deficiency virus.

Nutrition

Nutritional assessment is part of the comprehensive health assessment (see Chapter 63). Determine what food means to your patient and which foods are preferred. For example, Korean and Chinese foods tend to be high in salt; other Asian cultures prepare very spicy food that can contribute to GI cancers. Also assess the patient's eating patterns, which may be different from your own.

Rituals and customs surrounding food are also important to assess. American-Indian subgroups may celebrate Feast Days. Muslims may observe Ramadan by fasting during the day; Catholics may give up a certain food during Lent. The British have tea in the afternoon, and many people in the United States have coffee during their morning breaks. Hot dogs and sports events seem to go together, and turkey is traditionally served at Thanksgiving. Assess how your patient connects food with customs or rituals, especially if the patient is being cared for during one of these special times.

Some ethnic groups have food intolerances. For example, many Vietnamese Americans and African Americans and other blacks are lactose intolerant. Some Greek Americans have glucose-6-phosphate dehydrogenase deficiency, an enzyme problem (Purnell & Paulanka, 2008). Coordinate the diet with the nutritionist to ensure that patients receive foods that they can tolerate and are culturally appropriate. For new immigrants who may not know where to obtain ethnic foods, collaborate with the nutritionist to provide a list of specialty stores in the community.

Spirituality

Spirituality is a broad concept that involves the behaviors that give purpose to life and provide individual strength; it may or may not include religious practices. Religion is a more narrow term and refers to a formal belief system that is expressed in public (McClung et al., 2006).

Only some of your patients will reveal they are religious, but everyone is spiritual. Therefore many of your patients will have spiritual needs or experience spiritual distress. Since 1998, patients have rated emotional and spiritual needs as the second most important aspect of their hospital care (Clark et al., 2003). Spiritual issues, in particular, influence patient healing (McClung et al., 2006). Helping patients meet their spiritual needs improves satisfaction and helps them cope with their health problems or crisis.

The Joint Commission requires all health care facilities and agencies to address the spiritual needs of their patients. Yet nurses may not know how to help them or may not feel they have time for this aspect of care. Today professional chaplains are specifically trained and certified to help patients meet their spiritual needs.

Since 2000, The Joint Commission has required hospitals to have a qualified chaplain as part of the health care team. Chaplains may come from any religious affiliation, but all must know about health problems, health care, and interpersonal skills. Although they may perform religious ceremonies or rituals, their role is much broader. Chaplains have the time and expertise to manage spiritual distress. They are uniquely qualified to help patients cope with their responses to health crises, which is typically guilt and anger at first. They can also assist families to allay fear and anxiety and help them cope with their loved one's illness or end of life. Collaborate with your facility's chaplain if patients or families have any of these needs.

In addition to providing direct services to patients and their families, chaplains can provide a liaison between patients and families and clinical staff. They can also support staff when difficult situations occur, such as a serious illness or death of a staff member. Do not hesitate to ask a chaplain to help you or your health care team.

Health Care Practices and Practitioners

Assess your patient's health promotion and maintenance practices, such as exercise and a healthy diet. Ask about preventive screening tests, such as mammograms and prostate examinations, and current immunizations, such as the influenza vaccine. Recent newcomers may not have been tested or immunized if they came from less affluent countries where the technology and resources are not available. Other patients may have access to resources but may chose or not be able to not follow recommended testing or other health promotion practices.

Determine if your patient is able to afford health care and what type of insurance coverage he or she has. Most people have health insurance through their employer, but if the patient is not employed or is working part-time, he or she may not have that benefit. Collaborate with the case manager or social worker to help find resources to pay for health care.

Another aspect of health care practices that is important to ask about is the use of alternative health care systems and healers. Although many people in the United States use the traditional medical and nursing system for health care, some do not seek professional care for many reasons, such as:

- Transportation difficulties
- High cost of care
- Fear and distrust of health care workers
- Poor communication between patients and professionals

Therefore cultural ways of healing might be sought before or while seeking care from the traditional health care system. Although considered unscientific and strange to many health care professionals, it is essential to assess and support patients in their cultural practices when appropriate.

Many cultures work to preserve both their heritage and their health. Folk health beliefs, practices, and values are learned from experience and observations. They are passed down from generation to generation and have been found to be valuable. For example, acupressure and acupuncture are ancient Chinese therapies and are widely used today. Information about these treatments and other common complementary and alternative therapies is found in Chapter 2. In addition, they are discussed in many interventions chapters as they relate to specific health problems.

Generic and folk systems of caring for and curing people have been around for thousands of years. For example, early ancestors found they could prevent or cure disease with plants. Digitalis (which comes from the foxglove plant) and belladonna have been used for many generations to treat heart failure and tuberculosis. Methods other than plants are also used. There are also numerous hot/cold beliefs related to healing. These beliefs may not necessarily be based on a nurse's definition of temperature. Hot/cold theories of healing are found among Hispanic, Arab, Asian, Southeast Indian, Southern Anglo-American, African-American, and other black cultures. For example, some Hispanic women believe that partaking of "cold" foods and medicines after pregnancy will cause bleeding to stop. They believe this blood is reabsorbed into the body to cause nervousness or insanity later in life. A similar belief is that cold can get into the open vagina after childbirth and stay in the body to cause arthritis in adult life. Health care providers must realize that the patient's view of the cause of the problem may be quite different from the scientific explanation.

The "evil eye" is a prominent belief in some cultures, including Hispanic and Arab cultures. The Spanish term for this belief is *mal de ojo.* Some people believe that "the gods" give the evil eye when they become envious or jealous when a person is excessively praised or admired. Another belief is that a person who is angry with another person can "put the evil eye" on him or her. Various amulets are worn to reflect the evil eye back onto the person who caused it (Fig. 4-2).

A very important point to consider with folk medicine is the use of particular phrases to describe health problems. Some African Americans and others refer to blood in various ways. For example, "high blood" can mean hypertension, or too much blood in the body, or it can mean the movement of blood to a higher part of the body such as the brain or head. The movement of blood into the head is commonly believed to cause strokes or nervousness or to make the person "fall out" (faint). A similar situation is "low blood," which can mean low blood pressure or anemia. These different terms can cause communication problems. When taking care of your patients, ask questions to determine the intended meaning of certain phrases.

Some patients may not seek traditional health care providers, such as physicians and nurse practitioners, as their first

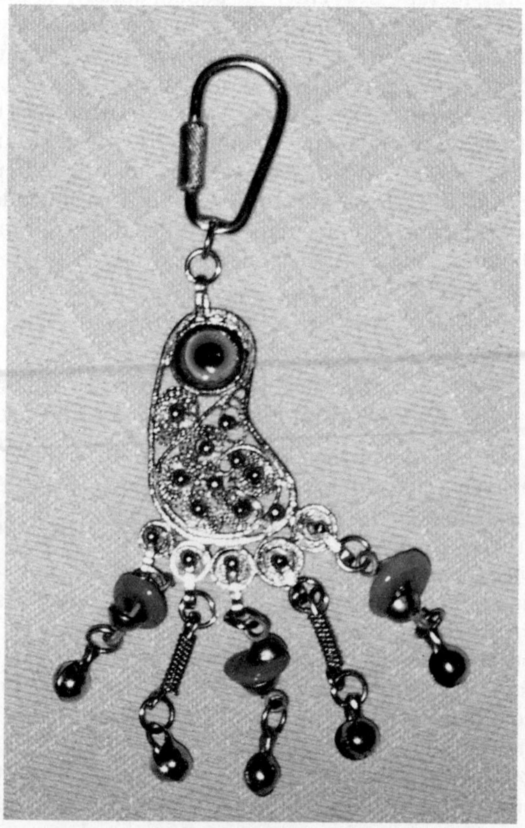

Fig. 4-2 • "Hand of God" amulet to protect the wearer from the "evil eye."

source for treatment. Instead, they go to cultural healers, especially in American-Indian and some Hispanic cultures. For instance, in the Mexican-American medicine system, the folk healer is called a **curandero** (male) or **curandera** (female). He or she considers health and health care from a holistic, spiritual perspective rather than the traditional scientific viewpoint (Fig. 4-3).

When performing a cultural assessment, be sure to ask your patients whom they consider as their primary source of treatment or healing and what methods they use. Do not be judgmental, and show respect for their values and beliefs at all times. Use an interpreter if you cannot understand their responses.

Culture is a very broad area but an essential aspect of nursing care. Be sure to document your cultural assessment findings for communication with other members of the health care team. For additional information about cultural assessment, review the culture chapter in your fundamentals textbook. For more information about specific cultures, refer to the bibliography resources.

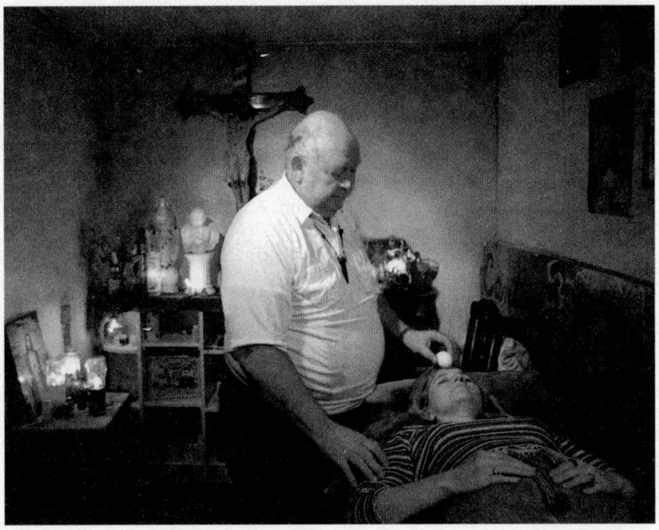

Fig. 4-3 • Within the Mexican-American folk medicine system, the *curandero* is the folk healer.

GET READY FOR THE NCLEX EXAMINATION!

Key Points

Review these Key Points.

- Culture refers to integrated patterns of behavior acquired over time that includes thought, language, beliefs, customs, norms, and ways of life.
- Cultural competence is the ability of health care providers and organizations to understand and respond effectively to the cultural and linguistic needs of patients.
- To assess your cultural competence, answer the questions in Table 4-1.
- One of the major purposes of *Healthy People 2010* is to eliminate differences in health and health care access for various ethnic and racial groups in the United States.
- Nurses need to be educated in and assess specific cultural practices that affect assessment and planning of patient care, including spirituality, nutrition, and communication (see Table 4-2).
- Communication techniques vary among cultural groups and may be misinterpreted; nurses need to learn how groups communicate (verbal and nonverbal) to avoid misperceptions (see Chart 4-1).
- The Joint Commission requires that professional interpreters be available to prevent communication errors with patients and their families.
- Two major issues related to the very diverse LGBT culture are health disparities and the quality of LGBT health care.
- Use the recommendations in Chart 4-2 and Table 4-3 when communicating about sexual identity.
- Patients may avoid the traditional health care system because of transportation problems, high cost of care, fear and distrust of health care staff, or poor communication between patients and health care providers; generic or folk medicine may be used as an alternative.
- Examples of generic and folk medicine are the use of the curandero by some members of the Mexican-American culture and the use of clay for healing in some Southeastern and Appalachian people.

Additional Study Resources

Go to your Companion CD or Evolve at http://evolve.elsevier.com/lggy/ for *Self-Assessment Questions for the NCLEX Examination.*

evolve Go to Evolve at http://evolve.elsevier.com/lggy/ for *Prioritization and Delegation Questions for the NCLEX Examination.*

SELECTED BIBLIOGRAPHY

Asterisk indicates a classic or definitive work on this subject.

*Anderson, L.M., Scrimshaw, S.C., Fullilove, M.T., Fielding, J.E., Normand, J.; Task Force on Community Preventive Services. (2003). Culturally competent healthcare systems: A systematic review. *American Journal of Preventive Medicine, 24*(Suppl. 3), 68-79.

*Campinha-Bacote, J. (2003). Many faces: Addressing diversity in health care. *Online Journal of Issues in Nursing, 8*(1). Retrieved January 15, 2008, from www.nursingworld.com.

*Clark, P.A., Drain, M., & Malone, M.P. (2003). Addressing patients' emotional and spiritual needs. *Joint Commission Journal on Quality and Safety, 29*(12), 659-670.

Galanti, G. (2006). Applying cultural competence to perianesthesia nursing. *Journal of Perianesthesia Nursing, 21*(3), 97-102.

Giger, J., Davidhizar, R.E., Purnell, L., Harden, J.T., Phillips, J., Strickland, O.; American Academy of Nursing. (2007). American Academy of Nursing

Expert Panel Report: Developing cultural competence to eliminate health disparities in ethnic minorities and other vulnerable populations. *Journal of Transcultural Nursing, 18*(2), 95-102.

Katz, A. (2005). Do ask, do tell. Why do so many nurses avoid the topic of sexuality? *AJN, 105*(7), 66-68.

*Leininger, M. (2002). Culture care theory: A major contribution to advance transcultural nursing knowledge and practices. *Journal of Transcultural Nursing, 13*(3), 189-192.

McClung, E., Grossoehme, D.H., & Jacobson, A.F. (2006). Collaborating with chaplains to meet spiritual needs. *MEDSURG Nursing, 15*(3), 147-156.

Muñoz, C., & Hilgenberg, C. (2005). Ethnopharmacology. *AJN, 105*(8), 41-48.

*Narayanasamy, A. (2003). Transcultural nursing: How do nurses respond to cultural needs? *British Journal of Nursing, 12*(3), 185-194.

Neville, S., & Henrickson, M. (2006). Perceptions of lesbian, gay, and bisexual people of primary healthcare services. *Journal of Advanced Nursing, 55*(4), 407-415.

*O'Hanlan, K.A., Dibble, S.L., Hagan, H.J.J., & Davids, R. (2004). Advocacy for women's health includes lesbian health. *Journal of Women's Health, 13*(2), 1-8.

Pullen, R.L. (2007). Tips for communicating with a patient from another culture. *Nursing2007, 37*(10), 48.

Purnell, L.D., & Paulanka, B.J. (2005). *Guide to culturally competent care.* Philadelphia: Davis.

Purnell, L.D., & Paulanka, B.J. (2008). *Transcultural healthcare: A culturally competent approach* (3rd ed.). Philadelphia: Davis.

Smith, L.S. (2007). Speaking up for medical language interpreters. *Nursing2007, 37*(12), 48-49.

*Spector, R.E. (2004). *Cultural diversity in health and illness* (6th ed.). Upper Saddle River, NJ: Prentice-Hall Health.

*U.S. Department of Health and Human Services (U.S. DHHS), Office of Disease Prevention and Health Promotion. (2001). *Tracking Healthy People 2010* (2nd ed.). Pittsburgh: U.S. Government Printing Office.

Wells, J.N., Cagle, C.S., & Bradley, P.J. (2006). Building on Mexican-American cultural values. *Nursing2006, 36*(7), 20-21.

Wilson-Stronks, A., & Galvez, E. (2007). *Hospitals, language, and culture: A snapshot of the nation.* Chicago: The Joint Commission. Retrieved January 15, 2008, from www.jointcommission.com.

5

CHAPTER

Pain: The Fifth Vital Sign

Lora L. McGuire

LEARNING OUTCOMES

For clinical competence and success on the NCLEX Examination, study this chapter with these Learning Outcomes in mind:

Safe and Effective Care Environment

1. Act as an advocate for patients in acute and chronic pain.
2. Develop a teaching/learning plan for managing pain as part of community-based care.

Health Promotion and Maintenance

3. Teach patients in pain about complementary and alternative therapies as additions to their established plan of care.
4. Perform a complete pain assessment, and document per agency policy.

Psychosocial Integrity

5. Discuss the attitudes and knowledge of nurses, physicians, and patients regarding pain assessment and management.

Physiological Integrity

6. Differentiate between addiction, pseudoaddiction, tolerance, and physical dependence.
7. Compare and contrast the characteristics of the major types of pain and examples of each.
8. Explain the role of non-opioid analgesics in pain management.
9. Compare common opioid analgesics, using an equianalgesic chart.
10. Develop a plan of care to prevent common side effects of opioid analgesics.
11. Compare the advantages and disadvantages of drug administration routes.
12. Determine the patient's need for pain medication, including PRN and adjuvant therapy.
13. Prioritize care for the patient receiving patient-controlled analgesia.
14. Provide care for a patient receiving epidural analgesia.
15. Identify special considerations for older adults related to pain assessment and management.
16. Incorporate complementary and alternative therapies into the patient's plan of care as needed to control pain.

Go to your Companion CD or Evolve at http://evolve.elsevier.com/Iggy/ for *Self-Assessment Questions for the NCLEX Examination* keyed to these Learning Outcomes.

Pain is a universal, complex, subjective experience. It is the most common reason for a patient to seek medical care and the number-one reason for a person to take medication. It alters or diminishes quality of life more than any other single health-related problem. Despite more than 30 years of work by clinicians and professional and lay organizations, unrelieved and undertreated pain remains a major yet often avoidable public health problem in the United States.

The nurse's primary role in pain management is to advocate for the patient by *believing* reports of pain. Because many practitioners have difficulty with this concept, it must be emphasized repeatedly that there is no diagnostic test for pain. Even though some nurses with many years of experience think that they can identify patients in pain, it is impossible. To assist in advocating for adequate pain relief, the American Pain Foundation has developed a "Pain Care Bill of Rights" (Table 5-1).

Many hospitals and other health care agencies have **multidisciplinary pain teams**, also known as **analgesia teams**, who consult with staff and prescribers on how best to control the patient's pain. The team typically consists of one or more nurses, pharmacists, case managers, and physicians. In larger facilities, pain teams may specialize by type of pain (e.g., orthopedic pain team, postoperative pain team, cancer pain team). Although a large part of the team's plan may center on drug therapy, this group also recommends nonpharmacologic measures for individual patients upon request.

Overview

Everyone experiences pain at some point in life. Because pain is such a private and personal experience, it may be difficult to describe or explain to others. The amount of pain and responses to it vary from person to person; therefore interpreting pain solely on actions or behaviors can be misleading.

Pain is generally related to some type of tissue damage and serves as a warning signal (e.g., pain signals a person to immediately remove a hand from a hot stove). Although pain is familiar to everyone, it is so complex that there is no single, universal treatment.

Definitions of Pain

Pain is an unpleasant sensory and emotional experience associated with actual or potential tissue damage. McCaffery (McCaffery & Pasero, 1999) offered a more personal explanation of pain when she stated that pain is whatever the experiencing person says it is and exists whenever he or she says it does. This understanding of pain requires that the patient be seen as the authority on the pain and as the only one who can define the experience. *In other words, self-report is always the most reliable indication of pain.* Nurses who approach pain from this perspective can help the patient achieve effective pain management by advocating for proper control. If the patient cannot communicate, self-report is not possible. In this case, a variety of methods and observation of nonverbal indicators are used to assess the pain.

Scope of the Problem

Pain is a major economic problem and a major cause of disability that hampers the lives of many people. About 9 in 10 Americans regularly suffer pain. Chronic pain is the most common cause of long-term disability, affecting millions of Americans and others throughout the world.

Pain is not adequately treated in all areas of health care. Populations at the highest risk are older adults, minorities, and addicts. Older adults in nursing homes are especially at risk. In patients who are substance abusers, unrelieved pain can contribute to relapses or increased substance use.

Inadequate pain management can lead to many consequences affecting the patient and family members. These consequences often affect the patient's and family's quality of life (Table 5-2). Therefore, as a nurse, you have a legal and ethical responsibility to ensure that patients receive adequate pain control. In 2000, The Joint Commission published pain standards that were approved by the American Pain Society. This document states that patients in all health care settings, including home care, have a right to effective pain management.

Patients rely on nurses to adequately assess and manage their pain. As the coordinator of patient care, advocate for proper treatment of pain and always document your actions, including patient teaching.

Categorizing Pain

Pain can be categorized in two ways: by type related to the characteristics of the pain (Table 5-3) or by the physiologic source of the pain. The two major types of pain are acute and chronic. *Acute pain* results from acute injury, disease, or surgery. *Chronic pain* or *persistent pain* is further divided into two subtypes. **Chronic cancer pain** is pain associated with cancer or another progressive disease such as acquired immune deficiency syn-

TABLE 5-1 Pain Care Bill of Rights

As a person with pain, you have the right to:

- Have your report of pain taken seriously and to be treated with dignity and respect by doctors, nurses, pharmacists, and other health care professionals.
- Have your pain thoroughly assessed and promptly treated.
- Be informed by your health care provider about what may be causing your pain, possible treatments, and the benefits, risks, and costs of each.
- Participate actively in decisions about how to manage your pain.
- Have your pain reassessed regularly and your treatment adjusted if your pain has not been eased.
- Be referred to a pain specialist if your pain persists.
- Get clear and prompt answers to your questions, take time to make decisions, and refuse a particular type of treatment if you choose.

Although not always required by law, these are the rights you should expect for your pain care.

From American Pain Foundation, Baltimore, MD.

TABLE 5-2 Impact of Unrelieved Pain

PHYSIOLOGIC IMPACT
- Prolongs stress response
- Increases heart rate, blood pressure, and oxygen demand
- Decreases GI motility
- Causes immobility
- Decreases immune response
- Delays healing
- Increases risk for chronic pain

QUALITY-OF-LIFE IMPACT
- Interferes with ADLs
- Causes anxiety, depression, fear, anger, and sleeplessness
- Impairs family, work, and social relationships

FINANCIAL IMPACT
- Costs Americans $100 billion per year
- Increases hospital lengths of stay
- Leads to lost income and productivity

Modified from McCaffery, M., & Pasero, C. (1999). *Pain: Clinical manual* (2nd ed.). St. Louis: Mosby.

TABLE 5-3 Characteristics of Acute and Chronic Pain

Acute	Chronic* (*or Persistent*)
Has short duration	Lasts longer than several months (usually longer than 3)
Usually has a well-defined cause	May or may not have well-defined cause
Decreases with healing	Begins gradually and persists
Is reversible	Is exhausting and useless
Ranges from mild to severe intensity	Ranges from mild to severe intensity
May be accompanied by anxiety and restlessness	May be accompanied by depression and fatigue, as well as decreased functional ability

*Includes chronic cancer pain and chronic non-cancer pain.

drome (AIDS). The cause of pain is usually life threatening. **Chronic non-cancer pain** is associated with tissue injury that has healed or is not associated with cancer, such as arthritis or chronic back pain. This type of pain is the most common.

Acute Pain

Almost everyone experiences acute pain at some time. Certain characteristics distinguish this type of pain from the more chronic (long-term) pain often associated with chronic illness. A major distinction between acute and chronic pain is the effect on biologic responses. **Acute pain** serves a biologic purpose. It acts as a warning signal because it can activate the sympathetic nervous system, causing various physiologic responses. These responses are similar to those found in "fight-or-flight" reactions and include:

- Increased heart rate
- Increased blood pressure
- Increased respiratory rate
- Dilated pupils
- Sweating

Behavioral signs of acute pain may include restlessness, an inability to concentrate, apprehension, and overall distress.

Acute pain is usually temporary, of sudden onset, and easily localized. The patient can often describe the pain, which may subside with or without treatment. Acute pain often results from sudden, accidental trauma (e.g., fractures, burns, lacerations) or from surgery, ischemia, or acute inflammation. The pain is usually confined to the affected area. As this area heals, the quality of sensation of the pain changes. Although possibly severe, acute pain is limited over time and generally can be managed successfully. Both the caregiver and the patient can see an end to the pain, which makes coping somewhat easier.

Pain that accompanies surgery is one of the most common examples of acute pain, but it is not always well managed. Usually poorly managed postoperative pain is a result of inadequate drug therapy.

The severity of postoperative pain may be a predictor of long-term pain. The use of **preemptive analgesia** is a technique designed to decrease pain in the postoperative period, decrease the requirements for a postoperative analgesic, prevent morbidity, and decrease hospital stay. Preemptive analgesia includes administering local anesthetics, opioids, and nonsteroidal anti-inflammatory drugs (NSAIDs) in the preoperative, intraoperative, and/or postoperative period. This intervention may inhibit changes in the spinal cord—changes that can lead to a central sensitization that results in chronic pain.

In general, intrathoracic and upper intra-abdominal surgical approaches are associated with more severe, steady wound pain and with pain on movement after surgery. Many patients who undergo superficial surgery of the head and neck, chest wall, or limbs report minimal postoperative pain. Muscle-splitting procedures, like thoracotomy, are generally far more painful than muscle-stretching procedures, such as open hysterectomy.

Chronic Pain

Chronic pain or **persistent pain** is defined as pain that persists or recurs for indefinite periods, usually for more than 3 months. The onset is gradual, and the character and quality of the pain change over time. Because chronic pain often involves deep body structures, it is usually poorly localized (hard to pinpoint) and often difficult to describe. If the underlying cause cannot be treated, controlling the long-term effects of chronic pain may be a difficult clinical challenge.

Because chronic pain persists for extended periods, it can interfere with personal relationships and activities of daily living. It can also result in emotional and financial burdens. Thus the efforts of an interdisciplinary health care team are needed to manage the situation effectively. Inadequately managed pain is an overwhelming, frustrating experience for both the sufferer and the caregiver. Over half of patients with chronic pain become clinically depressed. *Although many characteristics of chronic pain are similar in different patients, be aware that each situation is unique and requires a highly specialized plan of care.*

Chronic Cancer Pain. About two thirds of patients with advanced cancer have moderate to severe pain. What is frustrating is that we have known for over 30 years that 90% of cancer pain can be treated simply by giving adequate amounts of oral opioids around the clock. Yet patients with terminal cancer are often inadequately treated for their excruciating pain.

Most cancer pain is caused by the disease itself. The sources of pain include nerve compression, invasion of tissue, and/or bone metastasis. Cancer treatments also can cause pain (e.g., from surgery and toxicities from chemotherapy and radiation therapy).

Patients with cancer pain generally have pain in two or more areas but usually talk about only the primary area of pain. Be sure to perform a complete pain assessment to locate all areas of pain.

Chronic Non-Cancer Pain. Chronic non-cancer pain is a major health problem, usually occurring in patients older than 65 years. *Unlike acute pain, chronic pain serves no biologic purpose.* After the initial warning signal of pain, the body must learn to adapt to the persistent pain impulses by blocking or adjusting to sympathetic nervous system response (which causes the fight-or-flight reaction in acute pain). Because of this adaptation, the symptoms often associated with acute pain, such as increased pulse, are *absent* with chronic pain.

Chronic non-cancer pain was formerly called *chronic nonmalignant pain.* However, most pain experts, and certainly patients who suffer with daily pain, believe that all pain is malignant—thus the newer term. Chronic non-cancer pain may be caused by chronic diseases such as rheumatoid arthritis and osteoporosis (Table 5-4).

TABLE 5-4 Examples of Acute and Chronic Pain

ACUTE PAIN
• Postoperative
• Trauma
• Burns
• Procedural
• Obstetric
CHRONIC CANCER PAIN
• Tumor invasion
• Nerve compression
• Bone metastasis
• HIV-related pain
• Treatment-related pain (radiation, surgery, chemotherapy)
CHRONIC NON-CANCER PAIN
• Arthritis
• Low back pain
• Neuropathic (diabetic neuropathy, phantom limb, postherpetic neuralgia)

HIV, Human immune deficiency virus.

TABLE 5-5 Physiologic Sources of Pain

Physiologic Structure	Characteristics of Pain	Sources of Acute Postoperative Pain	Sources of Chronic Pain Syndromes
NOCICEPTIVE PAIN			
SOMATIC PAIN			
Cutaneous or superficial: skin and subcutaneous tissues	Sharp, burning	Incisional pain, pain at insertion sites of tubes and drains, wound complications, orthopedic procedures, skeletal muscle spasms	Bony metastases, osteoarthritis and rheumatoid arthritis, low back pain, peripheral vascular diseases
Deep somatic: bone, muscle, blood vessels, connective tissues	Dull, aching, cramping		
VISCERAL PAIN			
Organs and the linings of the body cavities	Poorly localized Diffuse, deep cramping or splitting, sharp, stabbing	Chest tubes, abdominal tubes and drains, bladder distention or spasms, intestinal distention	Pancreatitis, liver metastases, colitis, appendicitis
NEUROPATHIC PAIN			
Nerve fibers, spinal cord, and central nervous system	Poorly localized Shooting, burning, fiery, shocklike, sharp, painful numbness	Phantom limb pain, postmastectomy pain, nerve compression	HIV-related pain, diabetic neuropathy, postherpetic neuralgia, chemotherapy-induced neuropathies, cancer-related nerve injury, radiculopathies

HIV, Human immune deficiency virus.

Pain is also categorized as either nociceptive (normal processing of pain) or neuropathic (abnormal pain processing). **Nociceptive pain** is either visceral or somatic (Table 5-5). *Somatic* pain arises from the skin and musculoskeletal structures and *visceral* pain arises from organs. **Neuropathic pain** is one of the most challenging types of chronic non-cancer pains; it results from some type of nerve injury. Neuropathic pain is still not completely understood. It is divided into centrally or peripherally generated pain. Regardless of the cause, neuropathic pain is described as burning, shooting, stabbing, and feeling "pins and needles."

Theoretical Bases for Pain

Pain Transmission

Painful stimuli often originate in the periphery (extremities) of the body. To be perceived, the stimuli must be transmitted first to the spinal cord and then to the central areas of the brain. If the pain impulse is not transmitted to the brain, the person feels no pain. In the periphery, two specific fibers can transmit stimuli: (1) A delta fibers, which are found primarily in the skin and muscle; and (2) C fibers, which are distributed in muscle, periosteum, and viscera. Both of these nerve fibers are capable of accepting nociceptive stimuli.

A delta fibers are myelinated fibers that carry rapid, sharp, pricking, or piercing sensations. A person feeling these sensations can generally localize them readily to a fairly well-defined area. Because these fibers respond mainly to mechanical rather than chemical or thermal stimuli, they are called *mechanical nociceptors.*

C fibers are unmyelinated or poorly myelinated fibers that conduct thermal, chemical, and strong mechanical impulses. Pain conduction from C fibers is slow, more diffuse (widespread) and dull, burning, or achy—quite different from the sensations of A delta fibers. In contrast to the intermittent nature of A delta sensations, C fibers usually produce persistent pain.

Although many theories of pain have been proposed, the **gate control theory** by Melzack and Wall (1982) still forms the basis of what is believed by pain researchers today. According to this theory, a gating mechanism occurs in the spinal cord. Nerve fibers (A delta and C fibers) transmit pain impulses from the periphery of the body. These impulses travel to the dorsal horn of the spinal cord, specifically to the *substantia gelatinosa,* where the gating mechanism occurs. When the gate is opened, pain impulses ascend to the brain; when the gate is closed, the impulses do not get through and pain is not perceived (Fig. 5-1).

Morphine-like substances called **endorphins** are released when the large-diameter nerve fibers are stimulated. These fibers close the gate and decrease pain transmission. This helps explain why many noninvasive pain management techniques work to relieve pain. Endorphins are thought to be a gene product, and producing them requires a stimulus to the brain.

Similar gating mechanisms exist in the nerve fibers descending from the thalamus and cerebral cortex. These areas of the brain regulate thoughts and emotions, including beliefs and values. When pain occurs, a person's thoughts and emotions can modify perceptual phenomena as they reach the level of conscious awareness.

The gate control theory has helped nurses and other health care professionals recognize the *holistic* nature of pain. As a result, many cognitive-behavioral therapies (e.g., imagery and distraction described on p. 56) are used to help relieve pain.

Attitudes and Practices Related to Pain

The attitudes of health care professionals toward pain influence the way they perceive and interact with patients in pain. Without adequate assessment skills or knowledge of pain and analgesic therapy, they may not be able to understand their patients' pain.

Nurses who have little personal experience with pain may not appreciate the magnitude of painful conditions associated with diseases and medical and surgical interventions. They may expect patients with chronic pain to react similarly to those

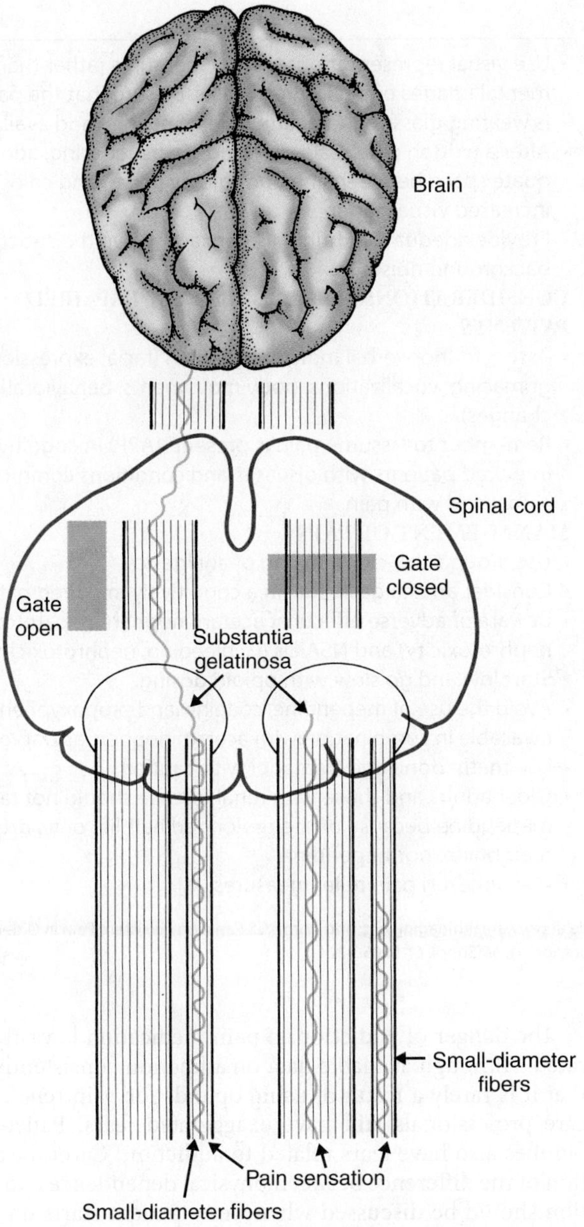
Brain
Spinal cord
Gate closed
Gate open
Substantia gelatinosa
Small-diameter fibers
Pain sensation
Small-diameter fibers

Fig. 5-1 • The gate control theory of pain.

with acute pain. Nurses may assume that reactions to pain fall within a certain norm on the basis of their own cultural values. The more that a patient's response varies from these expected norms, the more likely it is that a nurse's attitude toward the patient will be positively or negatively biased.

Not only do the health care professionals need continued education about pain management—the public needs education as well. Nurses can help patients and their families achieve and maintain successful pain management through education.

Many patients are reluctant to report pain. When they do, they may underreport its severity. Patients may not state their pain because they want to be "good" patients or do not want to bother or distract their caregivers from other issues in their care. In patients with a history of cancer, pain can be an unwanted reminder of the disease and its progression.

Some patients are also reluctant to take pain medications, especially opioid analgesics, because they fear becoming addicted to or used to the drug, especially older adults. Address these exaggerated fears of addiction so that the patient will adhere to the drug regimen.

Pain Perception and Disparities in Care

Many variables affect the perception of and response to pain. Factors such as age, gender, sociocultural background, and genetics influence the patient's ability to process and react to pain. These factors also put patients at risk for undertreatment.

CONSIDERATIONS FOR OLDER ADULTS

Age can influence how pain is perceived, assessed, and treated. It has been well documented that the incidence of pain in older adults is high, as is risk for undertreatment. Chart 5-1 addresses key components in assessment and management of pain in older adults.

Certain painful conditions are more common in either men or women. Most chronic pain sufferers are women. Women have more migraine headaches, tension headaches, rheumatoid arthritis and osteoarthritis, fibromyalgia, and multiple sclerosis. Men have more cluster headaches, back pain, gout, peripheral vascular disease, and postherpetic neuralgia.

Women are at a higher risk for undertreatment of pain than men. A classic study by Cleeland et al. (1994) found that female cancer patients were more likely to be undertreated than male patients. Follow-up of chest pain is more extensive in men than women. Researchers are currently exploring gender and cultural differences in response to pain and opioids.

Addiction, Pseudoaddiction, Tolerance, and Physical Dependence

It is crucial that nurses and other health care professionals not refer to patients as "addict," "clock-watcher," or "drug seeker." These labels have caused biases and have an impact on patient care.

Addiction is as "a primary, chronic neurobiologic disease with genetic, psychosocial, and environmental factors influencing its development and manifestations. It is characterized by behaviors that include one or more of the following: impaired control over drug use, compulsive use, continued use despite harm, and craving" (American Society for Pain Management Nursing [ASPMN], 2002, p. 1). Addiction occurs over time—not as a result of one hospital stay. The stress of unrelieved pain could cause a relapse in a recovering patient or an increase in drug use in the person who is actively using drugs.

Pseudoaddiction is "an iatrogenic syndrome created by the undertreatment of pain. It is characterized by patient behaviors such as anger and escalating demands for more or different medications, and results in suspicion and avoidance by staff"(ASPMN, 2002, p. 1). Pseudoaddiction can be distinguished from true addiction in that the behaviors resolve when pain is effectively treated.

Tolerance is "a state of adaptation in which exposure to a drug induces changes that result in a decrease in one or more of the drug's effects over time" (ASPMN, 2002, p. 1). Some of these changes include increasing drug excretion and reducing the number of receptors to bind the drug.

Chart 5-1 **NURSING FOCUS ON THE OLDER ADULT**

Pain

PREVALENCE OF PAIN

- Recognize that older adults are at great risk for undertreated pain.
- Consider the older adult at risk for the undertreatment of cancer pain because of inappropriate beliefs about pain sensitivity, tolerance, and ability to take opioids.

BELIEFS ABOUT PAIN

- In addition to receiving less analgesia, older adults tend to report pain less often than do younger adults. These findings may be related to beliefs and concerns about pain and the reporting of pain. Many older people hold these beliefs and concerns about pain:
  - Pain is something that must be lived with.
  - Expressing pain is unacceptable or is a sign of weakness.
  - Reporting pain will result in being labeled as a "bad" patient.
  - Nurses are too busy to listen to reports of pain.
  - Pain signifies a serious illness or impending death.
- Nurses should be aware of the beliefs of older patients regarding pain management. Nurses and other caregivers often undermedicate these patients and are sometimes reluctant to administer the prescribed analgesics.

ASSESSMENT

- Ask about present pain only.
- Use a standard scale, such as the numerical FACES rating scales.
- Explain the scale each time it is used.
- Use verbal descriptions such as "ache," "sore," and "hurt," *rather than the word "pain."*
- Use visual representations of pain measures rather than mental images of pain rating scales. Be sure that the patient is wearing glasses and hearing aids if needed and available.
- Alter a written pain scale to include large lettering, adequate space between lines, nonglossy paper, and color for increased visualization.
- Provide adequate lighting and privacy to avoid distracting background noise.

CONSIDERATIONS FOR COGNITIVELY IMPAIRED PATIENTS

- Assess for nonverbal indicators of pain (facial expressions, grimacing, vocalizations, body movements, behavioral changes).
- Remember to "assume pain is present" (APP) in cognitively impaired patients with diseases and conditions commonly associated with pain.

MANAGEMENT OF PAIN

- Use around-the-clock dosing of analgesics.
- Consider an analgesic trial in a cognitively impaired patient.
- Beware of adverse effects of acetaminophen (hepatotoxicity, nephrotoxicity) and NSAIDs (GI bleeding, nephrotoxicity).
- Start low and go slow with opioid dosing.
- Avoid the use of meperidine, codeine, and propoxyphene (available in combination with acetaminophen, as Darvocet).
- Use methadone and tramadol with caution.
- Older adults and those with renal disease should not take meperidine because of the prolonged half-life of its drug metabolite, normeperidine.
- Use nondrug pain relief measures.

Data is, in part, from The American Geriatrics Society Foundation for Health in Aging. Available at www.healthinaging.org; and from AGS Panel on Persistent Pain in Older Persons. (2002). The management of persistent pain in older persons. *Journal of the American Geriatrics Society, 50*(Suppl. 6), S205-S224.

Physical dependence is the "adaptation manifested by a drug-class–specific withdrawal syndrome that can be produced by abrupt cessation, rapid dose reduction, decreasing blood level of the drug, and/or administration of an antagonist" (ASPMN, 2002, p. 1). A person who is drug tolerant does not experience withdrawal, even when the drug is stopped suddenly.

Physical dependence occurs in *everyone* who takes opioids over a period of time. *It is important to prevent physical withdrawal.* So-called **withdrawal** or **abstinence syndrome** results when a patient who is physically dependent on opioids abruptly ceases using them. *Abstinence syndrome may also occur if a patient on opioids receives a reversal agent, such as naloxone (Narcan).* These symptoms result from autonomic nervous system responses and include nausea and vomiting, abdominal cramping, muscle twitching, profuse perspiration, delirium, and convulsions. When it is necessary to discontinue opioid analgesia for a patient who is opioid dependent, a slow tapering (weaning) of the drug dosage lessens or alleviates the physical withdrawal symptoms. Doses of opioids should be tapered by 10% to 20% daily for patients on chronic opioid therapy. Clonidine (Catapres, Dixarit♣) may be used to help alleviate the distressing symptoms of withdrawal.

Tolerance, physical dependence, and addiction are separate conditions, but they may coexist. However, it is important to distinguish tolerance and physical dependence from addiction.

The danger of addiction to pain medication is vastly overrated. Although available data on addiction consistently show that it is rarely a result of using opioids for pain relief, health care professionals still have exaggerated fears. Patients and families also have fears related to addiction. Careful explanation of the difference between physical dependence and addiction should be discussed whenever a patient starts on opioid therapy.

Patients who are substance abusers often have traumatic injuries and other health problems that cause pain. It is important for the nurse to recognize that substance abusers, typically those abusing opioids, are often tolerant to the pain-relieving effects of opioid analgesics and generally require increased doses. Abrupt physiologic withdrawal is always a danger when recreational users of opioid agonists are given mixed agonist-antagonists and partial agonists.

The clinical use of placebos in non–research-based therapies has not been shown to have a sustained effect on pain relief. A **placebo** is any medical treatment or nursing care that produces an effect in a patient because of its therapeutic intent and not because of its actual physical or chemical properties. When a patient responds favorably to a placebo, it is known as the **placebo effect.** Placebos do not indicate whether or not a patient has real pain. *Because of the deception involved and the need for informed consent, never administer a placebo to your patient.*

Most health care agencies have developed educational programs to inform professionals about pain management, including the inappropriate use of placebos. Ethics committees should be consulted for assistance in formulating policies and procedures regarding the use of placebos. Because of The Joint Commission's commitment to effective pain control, a policy against the use of placebos is recommended to be in place in all accredited institutions and agencies. The American Society for Pain Management Nurses has a position statement available on the website against the use of placebos for the management of pain (see www.aspmn.org).

Patient-Centered Collaborative Care

Assessment

History

The American Pain Society refers to pain as the *fifth vital sign.* Like for vital signs, health care agencies require initial and ongoing pain assessments. Begin by asking the patient about the pain experience, including the sequence of events (precipitating and relieving factors); the nature of adjustments, if any, in life or in the family; and beliefs about the cause of the pain and what should be done about it (patient's expectations). Personal characteristics (e.g., age, culture) influence attitudes about reporting a pain history. Families and significant others are included in this information-gathering process.

Patients may report pain in the absence of any observable or documented physiologic changes. Respect the patient's verbal and nonverbal expressions of pain without making judgments or inferences about the reality of the pain. If patients perceive that health care professionals doubt the existence of their pain, mistrust and other negative feelings can arise and interfere with a therapeutic nurse-patient relationship.

Assess the length of time the patient has experienced pain. Patients may welcome an opportunity to discuss acute pain with the nurse because it is a relatively short-term experience and is easily described. However, those with chronic pain can become frustrated when they are unable to adequately describe their vague, diffuse pain experience. Structured interviews using assessment aids (e.g., pain scales, descriptors) often help patients express their pain.

Information about a person's pain can be helpful in understanding the factors associated with the present pain or previous episodes of pain. If the patient is in pain when you are obtaining the history, keep the session reasonably short or continue at a later time. Essential data include:

- *Precipitating factors.* Does the person associate any activities, food, or other environmental factors with the onset of pain? What does the patient think causes the present pain? Was the onset of pain sudden or slow? Has the patient done anything or taken anything to relieve the pain? What were the results of the intervention?
- *Aggravating factors.* What factors make the pain worse? What influence has this pain had on the patient's activity? What lifestyle changes have been affected (e.g., diet, job, sleep)?
- *Localization of pain.* Can the person localize the pain or describe where it travels or radiates?
- *Character and quality of pain.* What words does the patient use to describe the pain and its character, quality, or intensity?
- *Duration of pain.* How long has the patient experienced this pain?

Physical Assessment/Clinical Manifestations

Although physiologic changes occur in response to acute noxious stimuli, these changes are usually *not* reliable indicators of pain. Acute pain, with its property of warning a person about harm, *may,* but not always, cause several physiologic manifestations, which are largely a function of sympathetic nervous system stimulation. People with acute pain may have changes in vital signs, such as tachycardia and blood pressure changes. Blood pressure is usually increased initially and then decreased. However, not all patients with acute pain have these signs, *so the patient's statement of pain is the only reliable indicator.*

A person usually adapts to physiologic changes in response to chronic pain as the body attempts to compensate for and adapt to noxious stimuli. The pain no longer serves as a necessary warning. Chronic pain patients, then, frequently have developed coping skills and may appear to look quite well.

Certain motor or body movements may be associated with either acute or chronic pain. Some may be more exaggerated or obvious than others. Patients in pain may support or shield ("splint"), holding painful body parts while moving, or they may lie listlessly because they are afraid to move. Assess the functional status and degree of impairment in the patient with pain.

Location of Pain. Assess the level and location of pain. Most patients can usually describe the severity of acute pain or chronic pain. The actual area or location of the pain, however, may not be as easily identified. Ask the patient whether the pain is superficial or deep. In general, those with pain involving superficial or cutaneous (skin) structures describe their pain as superficial and can often localize the pain to a specific area.

Pain may be described as belonging to one of four categories related to its location:

- **Localized pain** is pain confined to the site of origin.
- **Projected pain** is pain along a specific nerve or nerves.
- **Radiating pain** is diffuse pain around the site of origin that is not well localized.
- **Referred pain** is pain perceived in an area distant from the site of painful stimuli.

A patient who has difficulty specifying the exact location of pain can be asked to point to the painful areas on his or her own body or on another person. If able to communicate, have the patient point to or shade in the painful areas on a diagram of the front and back of the human body (Fig. 5-2). Those who cannot identify the painful areas and state that they just "hurt all over" are encouraged to focus on parts of the body that are not painful. Ask the patient to concentrate on different body parts, beginning with the hand and fingers of one extremity, and identify the presence or absence of pain. By focusing attention on selected areas of the body, the patient is assisted in localizing painful areas. People who state that they hurt everywhere often begin to realize that some parts of the body are not painful.

Patients may present with more than one discrete painful site. In fact, about one half of persons with advanced cancer report having pain in more than one location. Identifying painful areas helps the patient understand the origin of the pain. This understanding is particularly important for those with cancer, because every new pain often raises the suspicion of metastasis (spread of disease). The pain may be caused by other reasons, such as immobility or constipation.

Intensity and Quality of Pain. After asking the patient to locate the pain, ask him or her to describe it. He or she may use

McGill-Melzack PAIN QUESTIONNAIRE

Patient's name ______________ Age ______

File No. ______________ Date ______________

Clinical category (e.g., cardiac, neurologic)

Diagnosis: ______________

____

Analgesic (if already administered):

1. Type ______________
2. Dosage ______________
3. Time given in relation to this test ______________

Patient's intelligence: circle number that represents best estimate.

1 (low) 2 3 4 5 (high)

****

This questionnaire has been designed to tell us more about your pain. Four major questions we ask are

1. Where is your pain?
2. What does it feel like?
3. How does it change with time?
4. How strong is it?

It is important that you tell us how your pain feels now. Please follow the instructions at the beginning of each part.

Part 1. Where Is Your Pain?

Please mark, on the drawings below, the areas where you feel pain. Put E if external, or I if internal, near the areas you mark. Put EI if both external and internal.

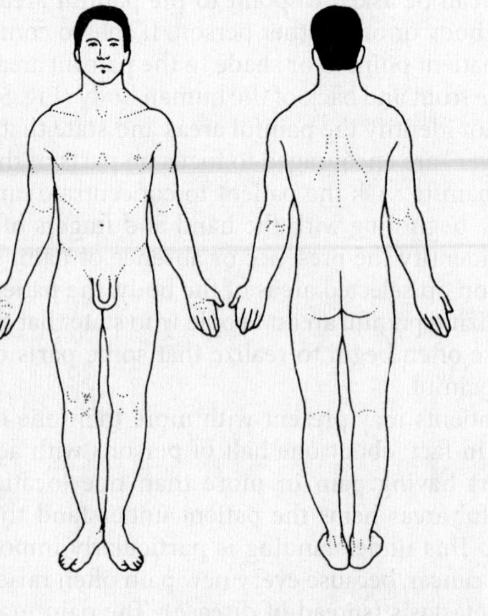

Part 2. What Does Your Pain Feel Like?

Some of the words below describe your *present* pain. Circle *ONLY* those words that best describe it. Leave out any category that is not suitable. Use only a single word in each appropriate category—the one that applies best.

1
Flickering
Quivering
Pulsing
Throbbing
Beating
Pounding

2
Jumping
Flashing
Shooting

3
Pricking
Boring
Drilling
Stabbing
Lancinating

4
Sharp
Cutting
Lacerating

5
Pinching
Pressing
Gnawing
Cramping
Crushing

6
Tugging
Pulling
Wrenching

7
Hot
Burning
Scalding
Searing

8
Tingling
Itchy
Smarting
Stinging

9
Dull
Sore
Hurting
Aching
Heavy

10
Tender
Taut
Rasping
Splitting

11
Tiring
Exhausting

12
Sickening
Suffocating

13
Fearful
Frightful
Terrifying

14
Punishing
Grueling
Cruel
Vicious
Killing

15
Wretched
Blinding

16
Annoying
Troublesome
Miserable
Intense
Unbearable

17
Spreading
Radiating
Penetrating
Piercing

18
Tight
Numb
Drawing
Squeezing
Tearing

19
Cool
Cold
Freezing

20
Nagging
Nauseating
Agonizing
Dreadful
Torturing

Part 3. How Does Your Pain Change With Time?

1. Which word or words would you use to describe the *pattern* of your pain?

1	2	3
Continuous	Rhythmic	Brief
Steady	Periodic	Momentary
Constant	Intermittent	Transient

2. What kind of things *relieve* your pain?

3. What kind of things *increase* your pain?

Part 4. How Strong Is Your Pain?

People agree that the following 5 words represent pain of increasing intensity. They are:

1	2	3	4	5
Mild	Discomforting	Distressing	Horrible	Excruciating

To answer each question below, write the number of the most appropriate word in the space beside the question.

1. Which word describes your pain right now? ___
2. Which word describes it at its worst? ___
3. Which word describes it when it is least? ___
4. Which word describes the worst toothache you ever had? ___
5. Which word describes the worst headache you ever had? ___
6. Which word describes the worst stomachache you ever had? ___

Fig. 5-2 • The McGill-Melzack Pain Questionnaire.

one word or a group of words to convey the sensations or feelings of the pain. *Avoid suggesting descriptive words for the pain.*

Subjective measurements of pain intensity are more reliable and accurate than observable qualities of pain. Only the patient can determine the amount or severity of pain being experienced. Various visual analog scales (VASs), number rating scales (NRSs), descriptive word scales, and other measures have been designed to help patients communicate the magnitude or severity of pain and to help nurses quantify the pain (Fig. 5-3).

Use pain intensity scales to measure pain in the clinical or home setting and to assess and determine the effectiveness of pain relief interventions. For most pain scales, the patient is asked to rate the amount of painful stimuli. Patients with more than one discrete painful site may wish to specify their pain levels by location. Some scales also assess the emotional aspect of pain. Be sure to use the *same* scale over time for the patient, and assess pain intensity both with and without activity.

Verbal descriptive scales typically group words such as "none," "moderate," or "severe" and permit an intensity rating of pain. However, the 0-to-10 NRS is used most commonly in clinical practice for adult patients who can communicate in English (see Fig. 5-3). For culturally diverse patients with language barriers, the Wong-Baker FACES Pain Rating Scale (pain rating scale of smile to frown) may be helpful. This scale is also used for children, older adults, and developmentally disabled populations (Flaherty, 2008).

Assessing Pain in Cognitively Impaired or Critically Ill Nonverbal Patients. *Although it seems obvious, nonverbal, intubated, and cognitively impaired patients do feel pain! It is important to be proactive and assume pain is present, or "APP."*

In 2006, the American Society for Pain Management Nursing published its position statement on evidence-based recommendations when performing pain assessments for nonverbal patients (Herr et al., 2006). Five general recommendations for pain assessment were presented:

- Self-report (when possible)
- Search for potential causes of pain
- Observe patient behaviors

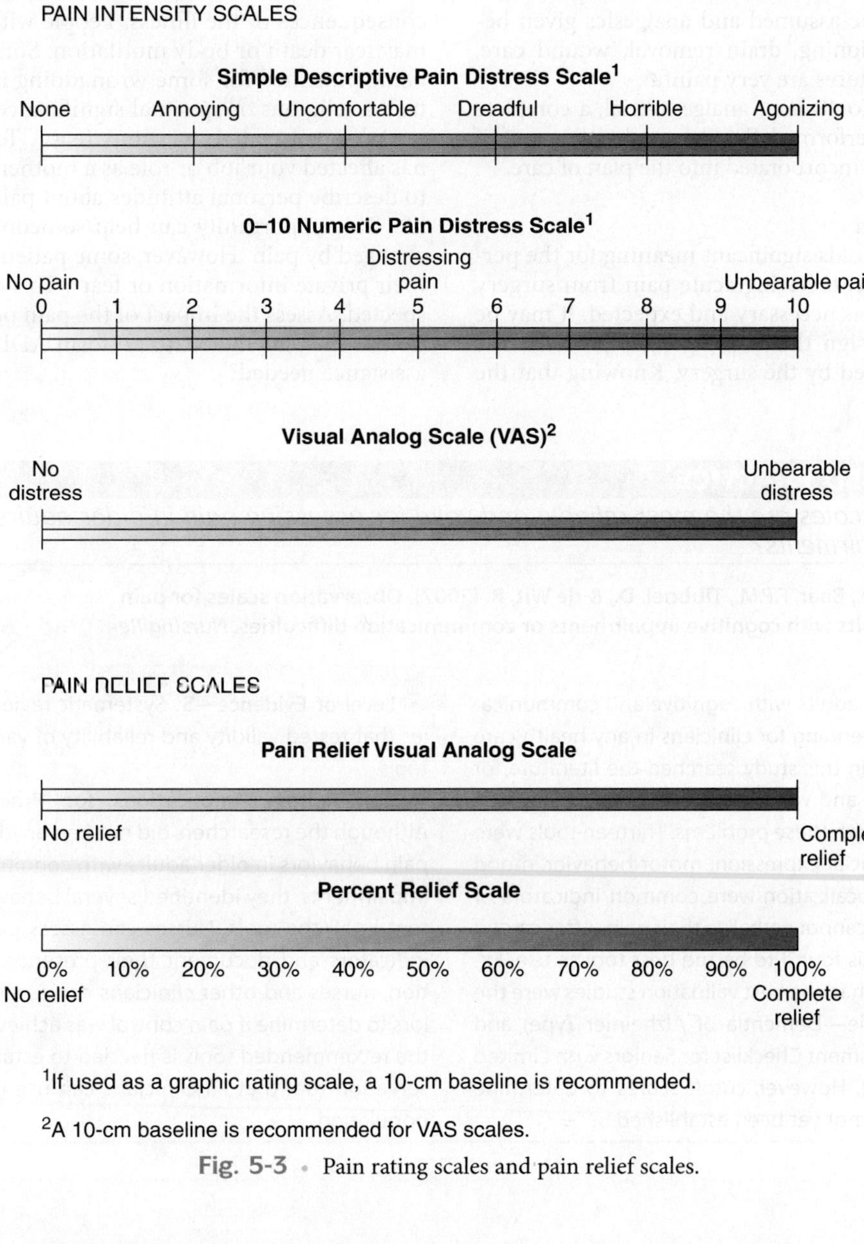
PAIN INTENSITY SCALES
Simple Descriptive Pain Distress Scale[1]
None
Annoying
Uncomfortable
Dreadful
Horrible
Agonizing
0–10 Numeric Pain Distress Scale[1]
No pain
Distressing pain
Unbearable pain
0
1
2
3
4
5
6
7
8
9
10
Visual Analog Scale (VAS)[2]
No distress
Unbearable distress
PAIN RELIEF SCALES
Pain Relief Visual Analog Scale
No relief
Complete relief
Percent Relief Scale
0%
10%
20%
30%
40%
50%
60%
70%
80%
90%
100%
No relief
Complete relief
[1]If used as a graphic rating scale, a 10-cm baseline is recommended.
[2]A 10-cm baseline is recommended for VAS scales.

Fig. 5-3 • Pain rating scales and pain relief scales.

- Surrogate reporting (e.g., family member)
- Attempt an analgesic trial

Nurses and other clinicians have recently been researching assessment tools to measure observable nonverbal behaviors that indicate the patient is in pain (see the Evidence-Based Practice box below). A variety of valid and reliable tools are published in the literature. Most of them are designed to be used for patients with severe dementia. Fewer tools have been developed for intubated patients.

The American Geriatrics Society Panel on Persistent Pain in Older Persons found six common pain indicators that you can observe and document (2002):

- Facial expression (e.g., grimacing, crying)
- Verbalizations or vocalizations (e.g., screaming)
- Body movements (e.g., restlessness)
- Changes in interpersonal interactions
- Changes in activity patterns or routines
- Mental status changes (e.g., confusion, increased confusion)

Patients with painful chronic conditions such as arthritis, osteoporosis, cancer, pressure ulcers, and contractures should receive an analgesic trial of around-the-clock drugs. Procedural pain should also be assumed and analgesics given beforehand. Turning, suctioning, drain removal, wound care, and other routine procedures are very painful.

After receiving a 24- to 48-hour analgesic trial, a complete reassessment should be performed. Family members' reports of a patient's pain should be incorporated into the plan of care.

Psychosocial Assessment

Acute Pain. All pain holds significant meaning for the person experiencing it. Patients having acute pain from surgery may interpret their pain as necessary and expected. It may be viewed with relief as a sign that some greater problem has been resolved or alleviated by the surgery. Knowing that the duration of the pain is limited may allow the patient to deal with unpleasant sensations without too much difficulty. In contrast, acute chest pain associated with angina may mark the beginning of a life of fear and uncertainty.

Chronic Pain. Various psychosocial factors influence chronic pain. Some factors are similar to those found in the acute pain experience, such as anxiety or fear related to the meaning of the pain. Because chronic pain persists or is perhaps only partially relieved, the patient may feel powerless, angry, hostile, or desperate. He or she is also vulnerable to labels such as "chronic complainer" or "fake." *Remain objective, and advocate for proper pain control for all patients.*

Assess the status of family and other close relationships, along with the range of social resources available to the chronic pain patient. The existence of a pain-specific conflict with a spouse or significant other may affect or limit pain coping strategies. Other people may react to chronic pain with depression, social withdrawal, and preoccupation with physical symptoms.

If the chronic pain is associated with a progressive disease such as cancer, rheumatoid arthritis, or peripheral vascular disease, the patient may have worries and concerns about the consequences of the illness. People with cancer-related pain may fear death or body mutilation. Some may think they are being punished for some wrongdoing in life. Others may attach a religious or spiritual significance to lingering pain.

Ask open-ended questions (e.g., "Tell me how your pain has affected your job or role as a mother") to allow the patient to describe personal attitudes about pain and its influence on life. This opportunity can help someone whose life has been changed by pain. However, some patients choose not to share their private information or fears. This decision should be respected. Assess the impact of the pain on their ability to function. Is the patient able to perform ADLs independently, or is assistance needed?

EVIDENCE-BASED PRACTICE

Which observation scales are the most reliable and valid for assessing pain in older adults with cognitive or communication impairments?

van Herk, R., van Dijk, M., Baar, F.P.M., Tibboel, D., & de Wit, R. (2007). Observation scales for pain assessment in older adults with cognitive impairments or communication difficulties. *Nursing Research, 56*(1), 34-43.

Pain assessment in older adults with cognitive and communication impairments is challenging for clinicians in any health care setting. The researchers in this study searched the literature for the most useful, reliable, and valid observation tools for assessing pain in older adults with these problems. Thirteen tools were included in the study. Facial expression, motor behavior, mood and socialization, and vocalization were common indicators of pain in older adults who cannot verbalize their pain. After careful analysis, no one scale was found to be the best tool to use. Examples of the scales that had the best validation studies were the DS-DAT (Discomfort Scale—Dementia of Alzheimer Type) and the PACSLAC (Pain Assessment Checklist for Seniors with Limited Ability to Communicate). However, cutoff scores to determine the severity of pain have not yet been established.

Level of Evidence—5. Systematic review of descriptive studies that tested validity and reliability of various pain assessment tools.

Commentary: Implications for Practice and Research. Although the researchers did not find an ideal tool for observing pain behaviors in older adults with cognitive or communication impairments, they identified several behaviors that were consistent in all the tools. Nurses can assess patients for these pain indicators and document their presence. After pain intervention, nurses and other clinicians can assess these same behaviors to determine if pain control was achieved. More research on the recommended tools is needed to establish a consistent observation tool that all clinicians can use with their older adult population.

DECISION-MAKING CHALLENGE
Critical Rescue

A 76-year-old patient was admitted yesterday to your skilled nursing unit for physical therapy after a hip replacement 2 days ago. On admission, she was alert and oriented. However, today she seems very confused and refuses to attend physical therapy. She is receiving acetaminophen 650 mg three times daily as needed for pain, but she has received only two doses since admission.

1. What are possible reasons for this patient's change in mental status? (Hint: Think of all the possibilities.)
2. Why do you think the patient refused to go to physical therapy?
3. Is acetaminophen the best medication for a patient who had a total hip replacement 2 days ago? Why or why not?
4. What action should you take at this time and why?

evolve For suggested answer guidelines, go to http://evolve.elsevier.com/Iggy/.

▪ *Interventions*
Pharmacologic Therapy

Drug therapy is commonly used for pain control if nonpharmacologic methods are not helpful. Three groups of drugs are used to manage pain: non-opioids, opioids, and adjuvants. To advocate for your patient, a thorough understanding of the drugs used to treat pain is necessary (Table 5-6).

Non-Opioid Analgesics. The non-opioid analgesics are the first-line therapy for mild to moderate pain. The two most common non-opioids are acetylsalicylic acid (aspirin) and acetaminophen (Tylenol). The analgesic effects are the same in equal doses. The single optimal dose of aspirin or acetaminophen is between 650 and 1000 mg.

There is a ceiling to the analgesic effect of these non-opioids. In other words, if the dose of the non-opioid analgesic is greater than 1000 mg, there will be no additional analgesic effect—only more side effects. Many people underestimate the effectiveness of non-opioid analgesics, also referred to as *peripheral-acting analgesics.* For mild pain, the non-opioids aspirin 650 mg and acetaminophen (Tylenol) 650 mg produce pain relief comparable to that of the opioids codeine 32 mg orally and meperidine (Demerol) 50 mg orally. Most non-opioids (other than acetaminophen) are potent anti-inflammatory agents called **nonsteroidal anti-inflammatory drugs (NSAIDs).**

Nonsteroidal Anti-Inflammatory Drugs. Aspirin and other NSAIDs are very effective for inflammatory-type pain, such as rheumatoid arthritis, postoperative pain, dental pain, menstrual pain, migraines, and muscle pain. These agents inhibit the synthesis of prostaglandins, which are fatty-acid substances found throughout the body. The release of prostaglandins in inflamed tissues causes pain, edema, and inflammation. By inhibiting the synthesis of these prostaglandins, anti-inflammatory drugs decrease inflammation and pain. NSAIDs are particularly useful in the management of acute inflammation such as that which causes postoperative pain. **Ketorolac (Toradol)** is one of the most popular NSAIDs prescribed for short-term use in cases of acute pain because it can be given orally or by IV push.

Aspirin and other NSAIDs can cause GI disturbances and can prevent platelet aggregation, which results in GI bleeding. Therefore observe the patient for gastric discomfort or vomiting and for bleeding or bruising. Report these problems to the health care provider immediately.

TABLE 5-6 Examples of Analgesics by Classification

Non-Opioids	Opioids	Adjuvants
Acetaminophen (Tylenol)	Pure agonists:	Tricyclic antidepressants:
NSAIDs (nonselective):	Morphine (MS Contin, Kadian, Avinza)	Amitriptyline (Elavil)
Aspirin	Fentanyl (Duragesic, Actiq, Fentora)	Desipramine (Norpramin)
Ibuprofen (Motrin)	Hydrocodone (Vicoden)	Nortriptyline (Pamelor)
Naproxen (Naprosyn)	Oxycodone (OxyContin, Percodan [also contains aspirin])	Doxepin (Sinequan)
Etodolac (Lodine)	Hydromorphone (Dilaudid)	Anticonvulsants:
Ketoprofen (Toradol, Orudis)	Meperidine (Demerol) (outdated drug)	Gabapentin (Neurontin)
Piroxicam (Feldene)	Methadone	Pregabalin (Lyrica)
Salsalate (Disalcid)	Codeine	Valproic acid (Depakene)
NSAIDs (selective):	Agonist/antagonists (not commonly used):	Topiramate (Topamax)
Celecoxib (Celebrex)	Pentazocine (Talwin)	Clonazepam (Klonopin)
	Butorphanol (Stadol)	Baclofen (Lioresal)
	Nalbuphine (Nubain)	Alpha-2 adrenergics:
	Buprenorphine (Buprenex)	Clonidine (Catapres)
		Tizanidine (Zanaflex)
		Local anesthetics:
		Mexiletine (Mexitil)
		Topical lidocaine (Lidoderm)
		NMDA antagonists:
		Ketamine
		Dextromethorphan

Modified from McCaffery, M., & Pasero, C., (1999). *Pain: Clinical manual* (2nd ed.) St. Louis: Mosby.
NMDA, N-methyl-D-aspartate.

When taking a patient history, ask about the use of NSAIDs, keeping in mind that store brand names may not be considered as NSAIDs. For example, Walprofen is Wal-Mart's brand name for ibuprofen; Walproxen is Wal-Mart's brand name for naproxen. Orudis contains ketoprofen, and Aleve contains naproxen. Ask the patient or patient's family to provide the name of each drug that the patient is taking, as well as the daily dosage. Some patients may unknowingly take several types of NSAIDs at the same time, putting them at a high risk for adverse drug effects.

The side effects of individual NSAIDs differ. For example, ibuprofen (Motrin) and naproxen (Naprosyn) appear to cause fewer GI problems than ketoprofen (Orudis). By adding a GI protective drug such as misoprostol (Cytotec), GI side effects may be reduced.

Because of the high incidence of GI bleeding caused by NSAID use, particularly in older adults, selective cyclooxygenase-2 (COX-2) inhibitors, such as celecoxib (Celebrex), are recommended for long-term use. This newer class of NSAIDs, COX-2 inhibitors, selectively block the COX-2 enzyme responsible for inflammation and the production of substances associated with pain (e.g., prostaglandins). However, all COX-2 inhibitors have recently been associated with increased cardiovascular disease and may have limited use or be unavailable in the future. Most older NSAIDs block both COX-1 and COX-2 enzymes. The COX-1 enzyme is responsible for the gastric and renal side effects associated with older NSAID use. Patients with dental pain, osteoarthritis, and rheumatoid arthritis treated with COX-2 inhibitors often demonstrate effective analgesia without GI side effects. There is no difference in the COX-2 analgesic efficacy or in renal side effects, but the decreased risk of GI bleeding makes these drugs more beneficial.

Acetaminophen. Unlike the rest of the non-opioid analgesics, acetaminophen (Tylenol) has few anti-inflammatory properties. Acetaminophen has some advantages over aspirin in that it is available in a liquid form (which is the best way to take oral analgesics) and it can be taken on an empty stomach. Acetaminophen causes no adverse GI effects. Therefore it is preferred for any patient who has a history of ulcer disease. Acetaminophen also has no effect on platelet aggregation as most of the other non-opioids do. This drug is preferred, then, for people in whom bleeding is likely, such as preoperative or postoperative patients. Acetaminophen does have several serious side effects, however, especially hepatotoxicity (liver toxicity) and **nephrotoxicity** (renal toxicity) with long-term use.

Health care providers commonly prescribe acetaminophen for pain. The drug exerts its analgesic action by blocking peripheral pain receptors, thus increasing the threshold of these receptors to painful stimuli. Reports of liver toxicity have been associated with higher doses of the drug (1000 mg) taken more frequently than every 4 hours for long-term use. Current recommendations restrict the total daily amount of acetaminophen to no more than 4000 mg (4 g). For long-term use, no more than 3600 mg daily should be taken. Less than 2400 mg daily should be used in older adults. Teach patients to be aware of the amount of acetaminophen in combination products such as hydrocodone (e.g., Vicodin) and propoxyphene (e.g., Darvocet). The acetaminophen in these products limits their use for chronic pain.

Opioid Analgesics. Opioid analgesics are the mainstay in the management of all types of pain. They work centrally by blocking the release of neurotransmitters in the spinal cord. Opioids are classified as full or mu agonists (morphine-like), partial agonists, or mixed agonists/antagonists. There are no advantages to the partial or mixed agonists, and they could precipitate a withdrawal if given to someone taking a full agonist.

The opioid **full agonists** bind to mu receptors and block the release of substance P, preventing the transmission of pain. The full agonists are the most potent of all analgesics.

Most opioid agonists are similar in pharmacologic effects, so a patient does not need more than one. Response varies widely from one person to another. Although the oral route is generally the preferred route, most opioids can be administered in many different routes. For patients on very large doses of opioids in end-of-life care, "opioid rotation" is another choice when ineffective analgesia or intolerable side effects occur.

There is no ceiling in the dose of a pure opioid agonist. The use of an equianalgesic chart when changing opioids is necessary, though, because these drugs vary in their oral to parenteral dosages (Table 5-7). The term **equianalgesic** refers to the dose and route of administration of one drug that produces about the same degree of analgesia as the given dose and route of another drug. This chart is useful when switching opioids or routes of administration of opioids because it helps you learn the dosage of the drugs being administered for pain.

Most commonly, 10 mg IM of morphine is the standard dose against which other opioids are measured. Equianalgesic opioid drug guides provide only the comparative analgesic potencies among these drugs. Dose modifications may be necessary according to each patient's response, and as always, with older adults, the guideline is to "start low and go slow" with drug dosing.

Commonly Used Opioids. A number of opioids can be used for pain control. Some are not as strong as others in their ability to control pain. For instance, *codeine* is a short-acting weak opioid. It is considered a pro-drug, and is converted to morphine after ingestion. An enzyme, CYP2D, is necessary to convert codeine to morphine to be effective. An estimated 5% to 10% of the population lack this enzyme, which could account for codeine's ineffectiveness in certain patients. For these patients, the conversion of codeine is so slow the drug is excreted before pain is relieved. This drug also has limited value for severe pain and should not be used in older adults because of the possible accumulation of a toxic metabolite, as well as constipation.

Hydrocodone is available as a combination product with acetaminophen (Lortab, Vicodin) and ibuprofen (Vicoprofen). Because of this, the dose cannot be escalated because of the toxicities from the non-opioids. Therefore hydrocodone has limited usefulness for chronic, long-term pain.

More potent opioids are available when weaker drugs are not appropriate for the level of pain or if they are ineffective in controlling pain. *Oxycodone*, for example, is available as a single-agent, both in short- and long-acting preparations (OxyContin). It is also available in combination with aspirin (Percodan, Oxycodan🍁) or acetaminophen (Percocet, Tylox, Roxicet, Oxycocet🍁). Oxycodone is recommended for acute and chronic pain. *The long-acting form, OxyContin, is given every 12 hours and should never be crushed, chewed, or broken.* These actions destroy the "time release." An advantage of Oxycodone is that, unlike other mu agonists, it has no active metabolites.

TABLE 5-7 Dose Equivalents for Opioid Analgesics in Opioid-Naive Adults[a]

	APPROXIMATE EQUIANALGESIC DOSE		USUAL STARTING DOSE FOR MODERATE TO SEVERE PAIN	
Drug	**Oral**	**Parenteral**	**Oral**	**Parenteral**
OPIOID AGONIST[b]				
Morphine[c]	30 mg every 3-4 hr (repeat around-the-clock dosing) 60 mg every 3-4 hr (single dose or intermittent dosing)	10 mg every 3-4 hr	30 mg every 3-4 hr	10 mg every 3-4 hr
Morphine, controlled-release[b,d] (MS Contin, Oramorph)	90-120 mg every 12 hr	N/A	90-120 mg every 12 hr	N/A
Hydromorphone[c] (Dilaudid)	7.5 mg every 3-4 hr	1.5 mg every 3-4 hr	6 mg every 3-4 hr	1.5 mg every 3-4 hr
Levorphanol (Levo-Dromoran)	4 mg every 6-8 hr	2 mg every 6-8 hr	4 mg every 6-8 hr	2 mg every 6-8 hr
Meperidine (Demerol)	300 mg every 2-3 hr	100 mg every 3 hr	N/R	100 mg every 3 hr
Methadone (Dolophine, other)	20 mg every 6-8 hr	10 mg every 6-8 hr	20 mg every 6-8 hr	10 mg every 6-8 hr
Oxymorphone[c] (Opana, Opana ER)	5, 10 mg or ER 5, 10, 20, 40 mg	New formulation of oxymorphone so unsure of equivalents		
COMBINATION OPIOID/NSAID PREPARATIONS[e]				
Codeine[f] (with aspirin or acetaminophen)	180-200 mg every 3-4 hr	120 mg every 3-4 hr	60 mg every 3-4 hr	60 mg every 2 hr (IM/subcutaneous)
Hydrocodone (in Lorcet, Lortab, Vicodin, others)	30 mg every 3-4 hr	N/A	10 mg every 3-4 hr	N/A
Oxycodone (Roxicodone, also in Percocet, Percodan, Tylox, others)	30 mg every 3-4 hr	N/A	10 mg every 3-4 hr	N/A

From Management of Cancer Pain Guideline Panel. (1994). *Management of cancer pain: Clinical practice guidelines.* AHCPR Publication No. 94-0592. Rockville, MD: Agency for Health Care Policy and Research, Public Health Service, U.S. Department of Health and Human Services.

N/A, Not available; *N/R*, not recommended.

Note: Published tables vary in the suggested doses that are equianalgesic to morphine. Clinical response is the criterion that must be applied for each patient; titration to clinical responses is necessary. Because there is not complete cross tolerance among these drugs, it is usually necessary to use a lower-than-equianalgesic dose when changing drugs and to retitrate to response.

[a]**Caution:** Recommended doses do not apply for adult patients with body weight less than 50 kg.

[b]**Caution:** Recommended doses do not apply to patients with renal or hepatic insufficiency or other conditions affecting drug metabolism and kinetics.

[c]**Caution:** For morphine, hydromorphone, and oxymorphone, rectal administration is an alternate route for patients unable to take oral medications. Equianalgesic doses may differ from oral and parenteral doses because of pharmacokinetic differences.

[d]Transdermal fentanyl (Duragesic) is an alternative option. Transdermal fentanyl dosage is not calculated as equianalgesic to a single morphine dosage. See the package insert for dosing calculations. Doses above 25 mcg/hr should not be used in opioid-naive patients.

[e]**Caution:** Doses of aspirin and acetaminophen in combination opioid-NSAID preparations must also be adjusted to the patient's body weight. Aspirin is contraindicated in children in the presence of fever or other viral disease because of its association with Reye's syndrome.

[f]**Caution:** Codeine doses above 65 mg often are not appropriate because of diminishing incremental analgesia with increasing doses, as well as a higher incidence of nausea, constipation, and other side effects.

Morphine (Roxanol, Avinza, Kadian♣) is the gold standard opioid for both acute and chronic pain. It is available in many dosage strengths (both short- and long-acting) and can be given in virtually any route, including rectally. MS Contin, Avinza, and Kadian are examples of long-acting or slow-release forms of the drug. Morphine 10 mg intramuscularly equals 30 mg orally. All other pain drugs are compared with morphine for effectiveness.

Hydromorphone (Dilaudid) is eight times more potent than morphine. It is currently available only in the short-acting form. Like morphine, hydromorphone is useful for all types of moderate to severe pain. Hydromorphone is being used more frequently for patients on IV patient-controlled analgesia (PCA) pumps.

Fentanyl (Sublimaze) is a potent opioid available in several forms for *chronic* pain:

- 72-hour transdermal patch (Duragesic)
- Oral transmucosal lozenge (Actiq)
- Effervescent buccal oralets (Fentora)

Duragesic is used on a continuous basis to maintain pain control, especially in terminal cancer patients. Actiq lozenges and Fentora tablets are indicated for breakthrough cancer pain and should not be given to opioid-naive patients (i.e., those who are not on opioids) (D'Arcy, 2007b). Breakthrough pain occurs primarily in patients with severe terminal cancer pain. The patient with breakthrough pain experiences pain between scheduled doses of the drug regimen. Other drugs may also be used for this purpose, but lozenges and buccal tablets are less invasive. Actiq is also being used "off-label" (not FDA approved) for procedural-type pain.

For acute pain, fentanyl can be administered either IV, usually with a PCA pump, or as an iontophoretic transdermal system (IONSYS). IONSYS is a needle-free, patient-activated transdermal system that forces medication deep into the skin using a weak electrical current powered by a battery-operated device. The most common use for this system is for patients with acute postoperative pain.

Methadone (Dolophine) is the only full opioid agonist with a dual mechanism of action. It works on both the mu receptors and the *N*-methyl-D-aspartate (NMDA) receptors. Methadone is inexpensive and very effective for chronic pain but very complex and potentially unsafe to use. Practitioners need to be educated on the many drug/drug interactions, potential cardiac toxicity, and long half-life (24 to 36 hours). The FDA has recently come out with a black box warning because of several fatal overdoses. Analgesia lasts only 4 hours, but because of the long half-life, sedation and respiratory depression can occur more frequently than with other opioids. Patients must be monitored for sedation (especially days 2 to 3), and it should be used cautiously in older adults. When managing pain in a patient in a methadone maintenance program for substance abuse, be sure to increase the methadone dose for pain relief or add a second opioid.

Tramadol (Ultram) is classified as an atypical opioid. It binds weakly to the mu receptors in the central nervous system and inhibits the reuptake of norepinephrine and serotonin. Tramadol can be used for *either* acute pain or chronic pain. It should not be given in doses greater than 400 mg daily because it can cause seizures. It should be used cautiously in patients who are taking antidepressant medications.

Meperidine (Demerol) used to be routinely prescribed in acute care settings. Most health care agencies now have policies in place restricting its use to less than 48 hours or no more than 600 mg in 24 hours. Many agencies have discontinued its use altogether for older adults because of the resulting toxicities. Because of the accumulation of the toxic metabolite normeperidine, central nervous system toxicities may occur. Repetitive doses of meperidine, particularly in older adults or in people with decreased renal clearance, may cause numbness, twitching, confusion, and seizures. It is never a good idea to give meperidine orally because of its poor oral absorption—75 mg IM equals 300 mg orally. *Meperidine use is considered to be outdated pain management. In fact, it is not recommended for use in PCA, since morphine, hydromorphone, and fentanyl are more commonly used.* The only benefit to the use of meperidine is for postoperative rigors (shivering) in postanesthesia recovery.

Numorphan is now available as Opana. This is a new, oral form of an old opioid that was available only rectally in the past. Opana is twice as strong as morphine milligram per milliliter. It is available in strengths of 5 and 10 milligrams or Opana ER (extended-release) 5-, 10-, 20-, and 40-mg doses. The drug is indicated for moderate to severe pain and should be administered around the clock. Teach the patient to take Opana on an empty stomach or 2 hours after meals.

World Health Organization Analgesic Ladder. Although you will not prescribe drug therapy for your patients as a nurse generalist, you will evaluate its effectiveness in achieving pain control. The World Health Organization (WHO) recommends guidelines to help prescribers select the most appropriate medications based on the patient's level of pain. The patient does not need to begin with the weakest drugs and then progress to stronger, more potent opioids. Rather, the level of pain determines the type of drug required based on a 1-to-10 (10 being the worse pain) pain intensity scale:

- Level 1 pain (1-3 rating): Use non-opioids, such as acetaminophen or NSAIDs.
- Level 2 pain (4-6 rating): Use weak opioids alone or in combination with an adjuvant drug, such as Ultram or Vicodin.
- Level 3 pain (7-10 rating): Use strong opioids, such as morphine, hydromorphone (Dilaudid), or fentanyl (Duragesic patch or Fentanyl Oralets).

Side Effects of Opioids. The most important type of opioid receptor is the mu receptor. **Mu opioids** cause side effects that include constipation, nausea and vomiting, urinary retention, pruritus (itching), sedation, and respiratory depression. These side effects are often mistakenly viewed as allergies, but it is rare to be allergic to morphine-type medications. The side effects (other than constipation) are time limited and easily managed (Table 5-8).

Nausea and vomiting may occur initially as a side effect in patients taking opioids for pain relief. Treating the nausea and vomiting with an appropriate antiemetic usually helps. In addition, if the patient needs to continue the opioid therapy longer than 1 week, the problem usually resolves on its own.

Opioids inhibit peristalsis in the GI tract. Patients who take regular doses of opioids almost always become *constipated.* Also, many patients in pain lack proper exercise and have an inadequate diet, both making the problem of constipation worse. Although constipation may seem like a minor side effect, it is not to the patient, especially the older adult. Often the discomfort of constipation is more distressing to the older adult than the pain itself.

Whenever a patient is started on regular doses of opioids at home, teach him or her how to prevent constipation (see Table 5-8). If the patient is unable to provide self-care, provide these interventions in the inpatient facility.

Because opioids have a depressant effect on the central nervous system, some drowsiness can be anticipated. However, *sedation* is not always caused by opioids. If the patient is still in pain, other causes of sedation should be ruled out before decreasing the opioid dosage or changing drugs. For example, drugs such as hypnotics or tranquilizers (diazepam [Valium], alprazolam [Xanax], or promethazine [Phenergan]) can cause the sedation. Often the elimination of other central nervous system–depressant medications resolves the sedation problem.

Sedation occurs before opioid-induced respiratory depression, so nurse-monitored sedation levels are recommended by use of a sedation scale for opioid-naive (not currently on an opioid) patients or those receiving opioids IV or epidurally. An example of a sedation scale is shown in Table 5-9. The key to assessing sedation is determining how easily the patient is aroused. *Stop the medication if the patient is difficult to arouse.*

TABLE 5-8 Nursing Interventions to Prevent Side Effects of Opioids

CONSTIPATION
- Assess previous bowel habits.
- Use measures to *prevent* this problem because constipation is the most common side effect (push fluids, encourage activity, give foods high in bulk and roughage).
- Keep a record of bowel movements.
- Administer stool softeners and stimulant laxatives.
- If ineffective, try suppository or Fleet's enema.

NAUSEA AND VOMITING (N/V)
- Assess actual cause of nausea.
- Recognize that N/V may be only an initial, temporary side effect for the first 24 to 48 hours because tolerance seems to develop quickly to this side effect.
- Try an antiemetic prophylactically before administration, as prescribed.
- Treat with prochlorperazine (Compazine) 5 mg orally every 4 hours, as prescribed.
- Give metoclopramide (Reglan) 10 mg before meals and at bedtime, or ondansetron (Zofran) 4 mg IV.

SEDATION AND CONFUSION
- Assess actual cause of sedation because the patient may also be on hypnotics and antianxiety agents; eliminate unnecessary sedating medications.
- Recall that tolerance to this side effect generally occurs after 2 to 3 days.
- Be aware that stimulants such as caffeine may counteract opioid-induced sedation.
- Consider opioid rotation using an equianalgesic chart.

RESPIRATORY DEPRESSION
- Be aware that clinically significant respiratory depression is rarely seen in patients with severe pain caused by cancer, even when large doses of opioids are given.
- Recognize that pain and stress seem to counteract the respiratory depression effects of opioids.
- Recall that respiratory depression is usually preceded by sedation.
- Monitor sedation level and respiratory status frequently for the first 24 to 48 hours, especially in opioid-naive patients.
- If increased sedation occurs, decrease opioid dose and attempt to stimulate patient.
- Be aware that respiratory rate alone is not indicative of respiratory status.
- If absolutely necessary in an unresponsive patient, administer naloxone (Narcan) 0.4 mg diluted in 10 mL of normal saline; push 0.5 mL IV slowly for 2 minutes and observe the patient.

TABLE 5-9 Example of a Sedation Scale*

Score	Meaning
1	Awake and alert
2	Slightly drowsy, but easy to arouse
3	Always drowsy, but arousable
4	Somnolent, little or no response to stimuli

*For scores of 3 or 4, stop the medication and notify the health care provider.

Assess each person's response to the first dose of an opioid. Be sure to assess the patient's level of consciousness. Monitor respiratory rate and depth, especially while sleeping.

A main reason for inadequate pain control is the exaggerated fear of respiratory depression. However, this problem rarely occurs, especially in patients taking opioids for chronic, long-term pain.

The pain, stress, and anxiety experienced by the patient are potent respiratory stimulants that may override or negate the respiratory depression resulting from the drugs. Consider that the effect of all opioid analgesics may be greater in a person who is older, has reduced blood volume or renal disease, or has received anesthetic agents or other central nervous system depressants.

McCaffery (McCaffery & Pasero, 1999) states that patients develop tolerance to respiratory depression at the same time that they become tolerant to the analgesic effect of an opioid. Pain appears to be nature's antidote to the respiratory depressant effects of opioids.

Opioid-induced respiratory depression can be treated. Respiratory depression is generally more apt to occur in an opioid-naive patient than in an opioid-tolerant (currently on an opioid) one. Also, it probably occurs at the onset and peak effect of the opioid. Naloxone (Narcan) is a fast-acting medication given IV to reverse the opioid effect. It should be administered only when absolutely necessary because it removes all of the pain-relieving effects of the opioid and leads to withdrawal symptoms. When giving naloxone, be sure to dilute with normal saline and administer slowly until respirations increase to eight or more per minute. The respiratory depressant effect of the opioid is usually longer-acting than naloxone. Continue to monitor the patient after giving the drug because respiratory depression can recur.

Pain Management at End of Life. Nurses caring for patients at the end of life should continue the same opioid regimen that was followed before the last weeks of life. Even though a patient may be unconscious, it is generally believed that he or she still feels pain. Because patients become tolerant to the respiratory depressant effects of an opioid, it does not hasten death unless the dose was not properly and gradually titrated. Chapter 9 discusses end-of-life issues in further detail.

Routes of Opioid Administration. Opioids can be administered by every route used. Table 5-10 lists the routes with advantages and disadvantages. Effective management of pain requires the knowledge that the oral route is always the preferred route for most types of pain. The IV route is the most efficient route because of its rapid titration. The IM route is no longer acceptable for pain management because of its ineffectiveness in controlling pain.

TABLE 5-10 Routes of Analgesic Administration

ORAL

ADVANTAGES

- Preferred route of analgesic
- Allows greater mobility and convenience
- Drug levels peak in 1 to 2 hours
- Greater patient satisfaction
- If patient is NPO or has a nasogastric or gastrostomy tube, medications can still be given enterally
- Cost efficient
- Relatively steady blood levels produced

DISADVANTAGES

- Slow onset
- Long-acting opioids cannot be crushed, broken, or chewed
- Some patients are unable to swallow or are NPO
- Requires functional GI system

RECTAL

ADVANTAGES

- Good for patients who are NPO, nauseated, or at home
- Easy for patients to self-administer, especially older adults
- Duration of action 4 to 6 hours
- Any opioid can be compounded by a pharmacist for rectal route
- Clinical practice suggests oral and rectal doses of analgesics fairly equal

DISADVANTAGES

- May be more expensive than oral route and difficult to obtain
- Contraindicated in thrombocytopenic patients

INTRAMUSCULAR

ADVANTAGES

- Should be used for acute short-term pain

DISADVANTAGES

- Rapid peak effect but short duration of action and rapid fall-off
- Problems with absorption lead to inconsistent blood levels
- Painful administration
- Not recommended for chronic long-term pain, especially cancer pain
- Patient depends on others to administer injection
- Not recommended for use with emaciated patients or patients with decreased muscle mass
- Long-term use can cause fibrosis and sterile abscesses

TRANSDERMAL

ADVANTAGES

- Available as fentanyl (Duragesic)
- Doses of 25, 50, 75, and 100 mcg/hr patches applied every 72 hours
- Noninvasive, easy to use, well accepted by patients

DISADVANTAGES

- Because of gradual increases in plasma concentration, may need to supplement with short-acting analgesics for first 12 to 24 hours after initial application
- Costly
- Difficult to adjust dose
- Febrile patients absorb medication quickly
- Concerns over disposal

ORAL TRANSMUCOSAL FENTANYL CITRATE (OTFC)

ADVANTAGES

- Good bioavailability, rapid peak effect
- FDA-approved for breakthrough cancer pain
- May be useful off-label for procedural pain

DISADVANTAGES

- Sweetened matrix contains 2 g sugar
- Short-acting, short half-life
- Must be swabbed inside mouth for at least 10 minutes to dissolve completely

TOPICAL

ADVANTAGES

- Easy to use
- Little systemic absorption
- Lidoderm patch, EMLA topical cream, and capsaicin cream are examples

DISADVANTAGES

- May cause skin reactions
- Capsaicin causes burning initially

SUBLINGUAL

ADVANTAGES

- Most opioids can be absorbed sublingually
- Good for patients with no IV access and/or impaired swallowing

DISADVANTAGES

- May not be absorbed or may cause mucosal irritation

INTRANASAL

ADVANTAGES

- Butorphanol (Stadol NS) opioid agonist-antagonist and sumatriptan for migraines are examples
- Convenient delivery form
- Good for outpatient use

DISADVANTAGES

- Butorphanol is not to be given to patient on pure opioid; can precipitate a withdrawal

SUBCUTANEOUS

ADVANTAGES

- Available as bolus, continuous infusion, or continuous infusion with patient-controlled analgesia (PCA)
- Avoids need for IV access and cheaper than IV
- Readily managed at home
- Recommended for cancer patients who cannot take anything by mouth and in whom IV access is not desirable
- Avoids repetitive injections and is less painful
- Continuous infusion
- Avoids peaks and valleys in bloodstream; maintains steady blood level
- Provides prolonged parenteral administration of opioid
- No delay in drug administration

DISADVANTAGES

- Subcutaneous boluses have slower onset and a lower peak effect than IV boluses
- Requires use of ambulatory infusion pump, which is not always patient acceptable

FDA, Food and Drug Administration.

TABLE 5-10 Routes of Analgesic Administration—cont'd

INTRAVENOUS • Available as bolus, continuous infusion, or continuous infusion with PCA IV bolus *ADVANTAGES* • Good for acute pain or procedures • Immediate pain relief • Provides fastest onset but shortest duration • Peaks in 5 to 15 minutes • Eliminates anxiety and prevents pain • Recommended when unable to achieve pain control through oral or rectal routes with high dosages of opioid or unable to use oral/rectal route • Continuous IV administration provides steady blood level *DISADVANTAGES* • Not recommended for constant pain because of peaks and valleys in bloodstream • Requires use of infusion pump with an alarm **PATIENT-CONTROLLED ANALGESIA (PCA)** *ADVANTAGES* • Allows patient to receive a predetermined intravenous bolus of an opioid by hitting a syringe pump mechanism • Gives patient sense of control, less anxiety • Provides quick and consistent pain relief • Maintains a constant level of pain relief • Eliminates the need for repeated injections	• Saves time • Especially recommended for acute pain such as postoperative pain *DISADVANTAGES* • Requires use of a pump • Requires reinforced patient teaching for maximum effectiveness • Requires two nurses to program to prevent errors (in hospitals) • Requires designated person to hit button if patient cannot **SPINAL (EPIDURAL AND INTRATHECAL) ADMINISTRATION** *ADVANTAGES* • Opioid (usually morphine or fentanyl) administered through catheter into epidural or intrathecal space • Preservative-free morphine or fentanyl used • Useful for postoperative pain (abdominal, thoracic, orthopedic) or chronic pain • May be intermittent bolus or by continuous infusion pump *DISADVANTAGES* • Careful patient selection is necessary because procedure is expensive and may be risky • Side effects include nausea, vomiting, pruritus, sedation, urinary retention, and respiratory depression • Possible complication of hematoma and infection and/or meningitis

PRN Range Orders. Nurses have administered PRN range orders for opioid analgesia for many years. Although this approach is meant to manage the pain of individual patients based on accurate assessments, obvious safety issues are involved. Because of The Joint Commission's and the Institute of Medicine's recent concerns regarding safety of drug range orders, the American Society for Pain Management Nurses recently developed a consensus statement, "Use of As-Needed Range Orders for Opioid Analgesics in the Management of Acute Pain." The intent was to promote quality pain management through safe drug practices (ASPMN, 2004). Nurses are required to follow institutional guidelines when administering range order analgesics. These policies should contain prescribing guidelines and appropriate monitoring guidelines.

Patient-Controlled Analgesia. **Patient-controlled analgesia (PCA)** is a common way to combat the problem of inadequate analgesia by allowing the patient to control the dosage of opioid received. This approach to pain control can improve pain relief and increase patient satisfaction. It can also decrease the amount of opioid consumption per day when compared with nurse-administered intermittent dosing methods.

Patients who have ready access to an analgesic are more likely to medicate themselves before the pain becomes severe, and thus they may require a reduced amount. Having such control over drug administration also reduces anxiety, which helps relieve pain.

PCA is achieved through the use of a PCA infusion pump (Fig. 5-4). Both stationary pole pumps (for hospital use) and ambulatory pumps (for nursing home or home use) are available. The infusion pump delivers the desired amount of drug through an IV access for pain. Morphine, fentanyl, and hydromorphone are the most commonly used drugs for PCA. Standing or preprinted orders from the health care provider are commonly used for PCA administration.

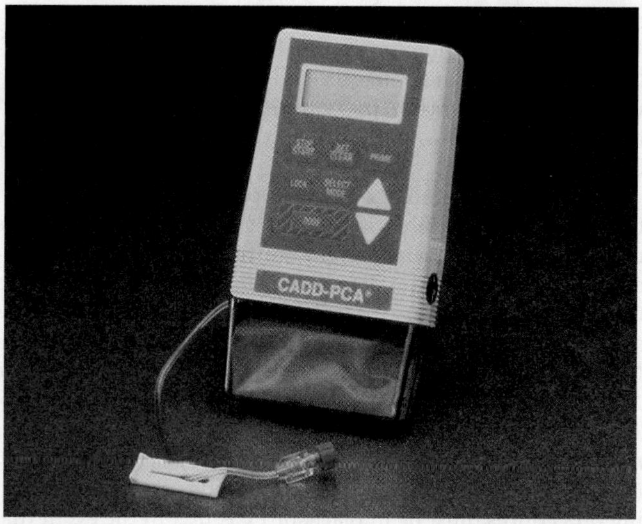
CADD-PCA
Fig. 5-4 • An ambulatory patient-controlled analgesia (PCA) infusion pump.

Drug security to avoid overdosing is achieved through a locked syringe pump system or locked drug reservoir system.

The device is programmed to deliver a certain amount of drug **(demand dose)** within a specific interval known as a **lockout interval.** The health care provider specifies the amount of the demand dose. Morphine doses are typically 1 mg/mL, hydromorphone 0.2 mg/mL, and fentanyl 10 mcg/mL. Doses vary according to the patient's degree of pain. The lockout interval is typically 5 to 15 minutes.

To prevent drug errors, it is recommended that two nurses program the dosing parameters into the PCA delivery device. When the patient presses the button or pendant (on ambulatory pumps), the appropriate bolus or demand dose is delivered. No drug is administered if the patient attempts to access the drug before the programmed time interval between doses. With this technique, there is little chance that patients will overmedicate themselves. *It is also recommended that all pumps have warning labels with large print that read "Patient only to push button" to prevent other people or staff from administering the medication, unless otherwise designated.*

The PCA regimen may consist of a demand-dosing-only schedule or a continuous infusion or **basal rate** and demand dosing. With demand or self-administered dosing only, the patient relies solely on a push of the pendant or bolus feature to seek pain relief. Continuous infusion of the opioid in addition to demand dosing provides more consistent analgesia and allows the patient to sleep without fear of missing any pain medication. However, when a continuous infusion is added to the regimen, some patients may be at greater risk for opioid-induced side effects (e.g., nausea and vomiting, sedation, respiratory depression), especially if the hourly dose is too much.

Teach patients how to use the PCA and to report side effects, such as dizziness, nausea and vomiting, and inability to void. As with all opioids, monitor the patient's vital signs, particularly respirations, and check sedation level at least every 2 hours or per agency protocol.

When a patient is cognitively impaired or unable to push the PCA button, another method of administration should be considered. PCA means **patient-controlled,** so having someone else push the button defeats the purpose. More important, this practice can cause oversedation and possible serious safety issues. The American Society for Pain Management Nursing recently developed a position statement on the Authorized and Unauthorized ("PCA by Proxy") Dosing of Analgesic Infusion Pumps. *Because of serious sentinel events related to PCA overdoses, PCA by Proxy is not recommended but may be used in special cases.* Clear guidelines and monitoring procedures must be in place for PCA use. In the event that a patient is unable to push the button, *one authorized agent,* such as a close family member, for controlled analgesia may be clearly designated.

Epidural Analgesia. **Epidural analgesia** (also known as *peridural* or *extradural analgesia*) refers to the instillation of a pain-blocking agent, usually an opioid analgesic alone or in combination with a local anesthetic, such as bupivacaine, into the epidural space. Epidural analgesia is more commonly used for the management of acute pain, such as postoperative pain. It has been used since the 1950s but has become more popular as newer and more innovative approaches to acute pain control are explored. Epidural analgesia is used primarily in patients who are predisposed to respiratory complications, including those undergoing thoracic, orthopedic, and abdominal surgery), those with pre-existing respiratory disease, and those who are obese. In some states, the nurse practice act allows registered nurses to remove epidural catheters. All practitioners who care for patients with epidural catheters must be properly educated. If given, low-molecular-weight heparin is withheld on the day the epidural is to be discontinued. This intervention reduces the chance of bleeding complications.

Intrathecal (subarachnoid) analgesia, in which a pain-blocking agent is introduced into the space between the arachnoid mater and pia mater of the spinal cord (where cerebrospinal fluid is located), may be considered for long-term management of **intractable pain** (chronic pain that cannot be managed using standard therapies). However, it is not used as commonly as epidural analgesia because of increased central nervous system risks.

Morphine (preservative free), hydromorphone (Dilaudid), and fentanyl (Sublimaze) are the most commonly used opioids for epidural administration and are often given by a patient-controlled epidural analgesia (PCEA) pump. Sufentanil (Sufenta), a derivative of fentanyl but more potent, may also be used. A local anesthetic such as bupivacaine (Marcaine), which affects both sensory and motor nerves, may be given alone or in combination with an opioid. *Low* concentrations of local anesthetics are used to prevent significant sensory and motor deficits. Lower motor weakness is far less common with ropivacaine (Naropin) when compared with bupivacaine because it is more selective for sensory nerves.

Using a combination of opioids, non-opioids, and local anesthetics for postoperative pain (as described above) is sometimes referred to as **multimodal analgesia** or **balanced analgesia.** The advantage of these drug combinations is to provide better pain control at lower doses than any single drug does. Another advantage is that these drugs *decrease* the surgical stress response, which is typically mediated by multiple endocrine and metabolic changes. These changes contribute to increased pain, GI distress, confusion (especially in older adults), and cardiopulmonary complications. Balanced analgesia, then, not only decreases pain but also helps decrease other problems that result from the stress of surgery. It is especially appropriate for patients having complex surgeries, such as those undergoing abdominal or thoracic procedures.

A temporary, externalized epidural catheter is used for acute pain control. This device is not sutured to the skin and is easily dislodged. Be sure to tape the catheter in two places to anchor it properly. Some clinicians do not recommend transparent dressings because the catheter may be dislodged when the dressing is removed. The catheter is generally placed in either the lumbar or the thoracic region. Rarely is the catheter placed above the level of the sixth thoracic vertebra, because the diaphragmatic muscle may be affected by the analgesic.

Complications that occur with epidural analgesia are directly related to catheter placement, catheter maintenance, and type of analgesic. Infection, *although rare,* results from a failure to maintain aseptic technique during catheter placement, direct drug instillation, and infusion solution and tubing changes. Infection also results from a failure to maintain aseptic conditions for indwelling catheters at the site of insertion or at the site of tube junctions. To prevent infections, ensure that all catheter line connections are secure and that an occlusive sterile dressing is maintained over the site.

For some surgical patients, a single injection of a morphine sulfate extended-release liposome (DepoDur) may be administered. This procedure does not require an indwelling epidural catheter and can be given before or after surgery. Most typically this drug is used for patients having total joint replacements or abdominal surgery. The drug often lasts up to 48 hours, which reduces the patient's need for usual postoperative medications.

Pruritus (itching) and nausea and vomiting are common side effects of epidural opioids. Pruritus is first treated with a small amount of naloxone (Narcan). Because epidural-induced pruritus does not appear to be caused by histamine release, diphenhydramine (Benadryl, Allerdryl🍁) may not be effective in relieving itching and may work only via its sedating effects. The health care provider usually prescribes an antiemetic as needed for nausea and vomiting.

Patients who receive epidural opioids are also at risk for respiratory depression resulting from high plasma or cerebrospinal fluid concentrations of the instilled drug. Those receiving epidural therapy with only a local anesthetic are not at risk for respiratory depression. Because of its potential for greater spread up the spinal cord, morphine is more likely than fentanyl to cause respiratory depression. Morphine is preferred to fentanyl when a larger distribution of analgesia is required (e.g., pain relief from extensive abdominal wounds).

Monitor the patient's respirations and sedation level at frequent intervals during and after the administration of epidural opioids, and immediately report any concerns to the health care provider (see Table 5-9). Opioid-induced respiratory depression usually occurs within the first few hours of administering fentanyl but may not be seen for 12 hours or more when morphine is given. This complication is managed by administering low doses (0.2 mg) of IV naloxone (Narcan).

Urinary retention is another common problem associated with epidural analgesia, but it occurs no more frequently than urinary retention after surgery in patients not receiving epidural analgesia. Although the cause is not clear, this problem usually occurs during the first or second day of analgesic administration and may be treated with bethanechol chloride (Urecholine) or intermittent urinary catheterization. The incidence of this complication is less than 25% and is more likely to occur in men than in woman.

Lower motor weakness is common when an epidural local anesthetic is used in combination with the opioid. Assist patients who get out of bed for the first time to determine the degree of leg weakness. *Do not delegate this activity and assessment to unlicensed assistive personnel!*

Epidural analgesia may also be used for *long-term* chronic pain relief. Such pain is usually the result of cancer or central sensitization. A permanent epidural catheter may be inserted, and several catheter devices are available for this purpose. The DuPen Silastic catheter (Davol) is a commonly used **external catheter.** A portion of the catheter exits the skin. Drugs can be intermittently injected into this portion, or the catheter can be attached to an infusion device for continuous drug administration.

Implantable devices are also used to treat chronic pain. The epidural Port-A-Cath (SIMS Deltec, Inc.) is implanted under the skin, and the catheter portion is inserted into the epidural space. As with the DuPen catheter, this device can be injected with drugs intermittently or can be connected to an infusion device for continuous opioid delivery. Injectable ports have been shown to reduce the incidence of catheter dislodgement and early infection. Systems consisting of either an externalized catheter or a drug delivery device are rarely used for intrathecal drug administration. The SynchroMed pump (Medtronic, Inc.) is a totally implantable system that contains a drug reservoir. The drug reservoir is filled on a routine basis and is capable of continuously administering a certain volume of drug each day (Fig. 5-5).

The side effects of long-term epidural opioids are common in patients who have had little exposure to opioids. Those who receive this therapy are usually more tolerant of the effects of opioids and may not require the rigorous monitoring needed for postoperative analgesia. Male patients receiving long-term epidural opioids may have sexual dysfunction, decreased li-

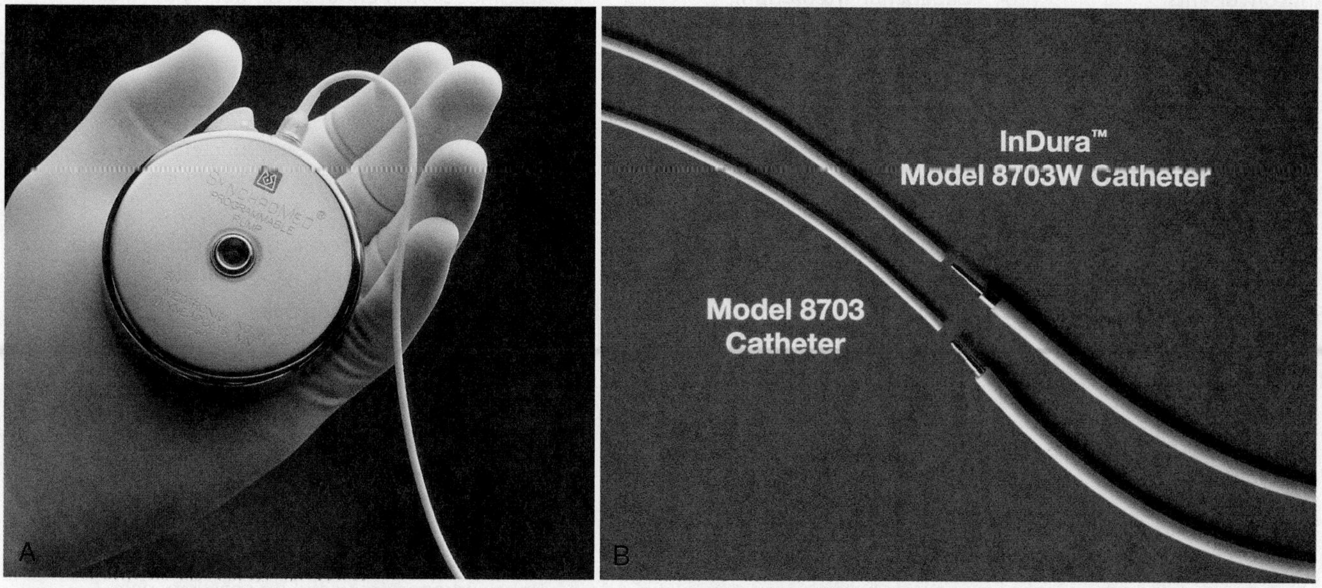
A
B
InDura™
Model 8703W Catheter
Model 8703
Catheter

Fig. 5-5 • A SynchroMed implantable pump (**A**) and spinal catheters (**B**) for delivery of a precise volume of long-term intraspinal analgesic each day.

bido, and difficulty maintaining an erection; female patients may experience amenorrhea. Testosterone injections seem to help improve sexual function in males.

NCLEX EXAMINATION CHALLENGE

The nurse assesses the sedation level of a client receiving epidural morphine analgesia after a knee replacement. When assessing the client for side effects of the drug, the nurse notes that the client is slightly drowsy but can be easily aroused. What is the nurse's best action at this time?

A. Stop the morphine infusion immediately.
B. Document the assessment on the sedation scale.
C. Notify the charge nurse on the unit.
D. Ask another nurse to assess the client.

evolve For the correct answer, go to http://evolve.elsevier.com/Iggy/.

Adjuvant Analgesics. Always consider the use of adjuvant analgesics, especially for patients with chronic pain or complex pain syndromes. Although not true analgesics, the **adjuvant drugs** relieve pain either alone or in combination with analgesics. These drugs can potentiate or enhance the effectiveness of the analgesic.

Some nurses and other health care professionals confuse potentiators with additives. **Additives** are drugs that add an effect, either harmful or beneficial. A common example of this is the drug promethazine (Phenergan). Phenergan is a phenothiazine that has been given for years with opioids such as meperidine (Demerol) to enhance the opioid effects. However, it does just the opposite. Phenergan does not have any analgesic or analgesia-potentiating properties. In fact, it is thought to actually have anti-analgesic properties.

The use of adjuvant analgesics not only can provide additional pain relief in some cases but also can help control other discomforts associated with pain (anxiety, depression, nausea, insomnia). Table 5-11 gives examples of adjuvant medications.

Some *antiepileptic drugs* (AEDs or anticonvulsants), such as gabapentin (Neurontin) and pregabalin (Lyrica), are effective in treating postherpetic neuralgia and the painful neuropathy associated with diabetes mellitus and cancer. They have been useful in many patients with neuropathic pain from back injuries as well. Doses of gabapentin can be escalated up to 3600 mg daily with few side effects compared with other anticonvulsants. Topiramate (Topamax) is another AED with promise for neuropathic pain, and it causes weight loss, rather than gain like most of the tricyclic antidepressants. Because most AEDs can cause hyponatremia, monitor electrolyte values carefully, especially in older adults.

The older **tricyclic antidepressants,** such as amitriptyline (Elavil), nortriptyline (Pamelor), and imipramine (Tofranil), may also be beneficial in treating chronic neuropathic pain. Both tricyclic antidepressants and other antidepressants such as trazodone (Desyrel), paroxetine (Paxil), and sertraline (Zoloft) help treat the depression that can accompany chronic pain. They also stimulate the activity of endogenous opiates (endorphins and enkephalins) by increasing levels of the neurotransmitter *serotonin.* Perhaps the greatest advantage of this group of drugs is the sedative effect. This effect can be helpful in promoting sleep when administered at bedtime.

TABLE 5-11 Examples of Adjuvant Analgesics

Drug Class	Example	Indications
Tricyclic antidepressants	Amitriptyline (Elavil) Nortriptyline (Pamelor) Desipramine (Norpramin)	Multipurpose; any chronic pain; pain associated with depression
Anticonvulsants	Gabapentin (Neurontin) Pregabalin (Lyrica) Carbamazepine (Tegretol) Valproic acid (Depakene) Clonazepam (Klonopin)	First-line recommendation for neuropathic pain Any lancinating, burning, neuropathic pain
Stimulants	Methylphenidate (Ritalin) Dextroamphetamine (Dexedrine) Dronabinol (Marinol)	Lethargy: counteract opioid-induced sedation; used for anorexia with associated weight loss in HIV and cancer patients
Steroids	Dexamethasone (Decadron) Prednisone	Severe bone pain; nerve compression; increased intracranial pressure; soft tissue infiltration
Systemic local anesthetics	Lidocaine (Xylocaine) Mexiletine (Mexitil)	Any lancinating, burning pain
Topical anesthetics	EMLA, Numby Stuff Capsaicin Lidoderm patch	Procedural, invasive pain Postherpetic neuralgia; diabetic neuropathy; postmastectomy pain
Miscellaneous	Clonidine Baclofen Calcitonin Tizanidine (Zanaflex)	Nonspecific analgesic; may be helpful for select group of chronic pain patients Trigeminal neuralgia; other neuropathic pains Sympathetically maintained pain; phantom limb pain Alpha$_2$-adrenergics useful for spasticity pain

HIV, Human immune deficiency virus.

The tricyclics are contraindicated in people with a history of seizures or cardiac disease. They should also be used with caution in older adults because they have long half-lives and can cause toxicities.

In some cases, antianxiety agents help relax the patient and thus help relieve pain. However, many of these drugs cause confusion, drowsiness, and hypotension; the health care provider selects the drugs with the fewest side effects. Examples of antianxiety agents are alprazolam (Xanax), lorazepam (Ativan), and oxazepam (Serax, Zapex♣). Clonazepam (Klonopin), also used for anxiety, has been shown to be particularly helpful for certain types of nerve injury pain.

Oral local anesthetics, such as mexiletine (Mexitil), act by suppressing the electrical activity of both peripheral nerves and neurons in the central nervous system. They are useful for electric shock–like pain and continuous pain. Mexiletine is contraindicated for patients who have cardiac conduction defects or dysrhythmias or are currently taking cardiac antidysrhythmia drugs.

Other agents known to have some effect in relieving mild to moderate chronic pain include dextromethorphan (the active ingredient in many cough syrups) and ketamine. Both of these agents are *N*-methyl-D-aspartate (NMDA) antagonists. NMDA receptors are involved in the development of tolerance to opioids. The administration of NMDA antagonists is thought to potentiate the action of opioids and prevent the development of opioid tolerance.

A new technique used for postoperative pain management is *local anesthesia infusion pumps.* Several brands are on the market: ON-Q, I-Flow, and Stryker. These pumps are filled with a local anesthetic, such as bupivacaine, and slowly release the drug over several days. They are inserted by the surgeon and used mainly for spinal fusions, total hip repair, and other orthopedic surgeries. Most patients are taught to remove the pump themselves when they return home. Health professionals need to be aware that some of these pumps may contain latex, so people with allergies must be made aware. The principle of combination treatment is very useful with these pumps because patients use less systemic drugs and therefore experience fewer side effects.

Topical drugs can be useful, particularly for localized neuropathic pain. For example, the *Lidoderm patch* is approved for postherpetic neuralgia. Up to three patches can be applied at once, or they can be fitted to the painful area. The patch should be put on for 12 hours and removed for 12 hours. There is virtually no systemic absorption of lidocaine.

EMLA and *ELA-Max* creams are combinations of topical lidocaine and prilocaine. These must be applied to intact skin at least 45 minutes before needle sticks. The topical medications for pain relief have rare side effects, including local skin reactions.

Local, short-acting gels and creams may provide *cryotherapy* to decrease pain, especially for muscle aches and pains. Bio-Freeze is an example of a commonly used gel that is often used by physical therapists to "cool down" an area after it has been manipulated. Other products can be bought over the counter (OTC) (e.g., Bengay). The effects of this type of application last about 1 to 2 hours, depending upon the patient.

Nonpharmacologic Interventions

A number of effective interventions for pain are nonpharmacologic. These may be used alone, for mild to moderate pain, or in combination with drug therapy for more severe pain. Nonpharmacologic therapies are classified as either physical measures or cognitive-behavioral measures. Some may be referred to as part of complementary and alternative medicine (CAM), such as imagery, therapeutic touch, and hypnosis. CAM is not considered part of conventional medicine. Many patients pay a great deal of money out of pocket because these techniques are rarely covered by insurance. These therapies often enhance, not replace, drugs for pain management. Chapter 2 discusses CAM in more detail.

Physical Measures. Physical measures may be used instead of or in addition to drug therapy to relieve pain. Most of these measures are categorized in the literature as complementary and alternative therapies. *Cutaneous (skin) stimulation* strategies to relieve pain have been in use for many years. Various types of stimulation to the skin and subcutaneous tissue produce pain relief. Nurses play an important role in educating patients about these techniques. Methods of cutaneous stimulation include these techniques:

- Application of heat, cold, and pressure
- Therapeutic touch
- Massage
- Vibration

Whichever method is used, several issues must be considered:

- The benefits of these techniques are highly unpredictable and may vary from application to application.
- Pain relief is generally sustained only as long as the stimulation continues.
- Multiple trials may be necessary to establish the desired effects.
- Stimulation itself may aggravate pre-existing pain or may produce new pain.

Despite the drawbacks to cutaneous stimulation, it is effective in the management of both acute pain and chronic pain. These techniques have both physiologic and psychological effects on the patient. Cutaneous stimulation techniques also give patients an opportunity to participate actively in the management of their pain.

Physical therapy and occupational therapy are used for patients having pain to increase function, decrease pain, compensate for decreased function, and prevent further deterioration. Exercises and physical modalities such as heat, cold, or massage may be used. Measures of patient progress include an increase in the range of motion, strength, and function of the affected area, as well as impact of pain on quality of life. Collaborate with the physical therapist to evaluate these treatments.

The occupational therapist may also help decrease pain by making one or more splints to rest severely inflamed joints. These devices are most often used short-term and intermittently for patients with osteoarthritis or rheumatoid arthritis.

Transcutaneous electrical nerve stimulation (TENS), also referred to as **percutaneous electrical nerve stimulation (PENS),** involves the use of a battery-operated device capable of delivering small electrical currents to the skin and underlying tissues. This technique is not as widely used today as when it first was developed. However, for older adults, it may be safer and just as effective as medications. Electrodes connected to a small box are placed over the painful sites. The voltage or current is regulated by adjusting a dial to the point at which the patient perceives a prickly, "pins-and-needles" sensation. The current is adjusted on the basis of the degree of pain relief and level of comfort.

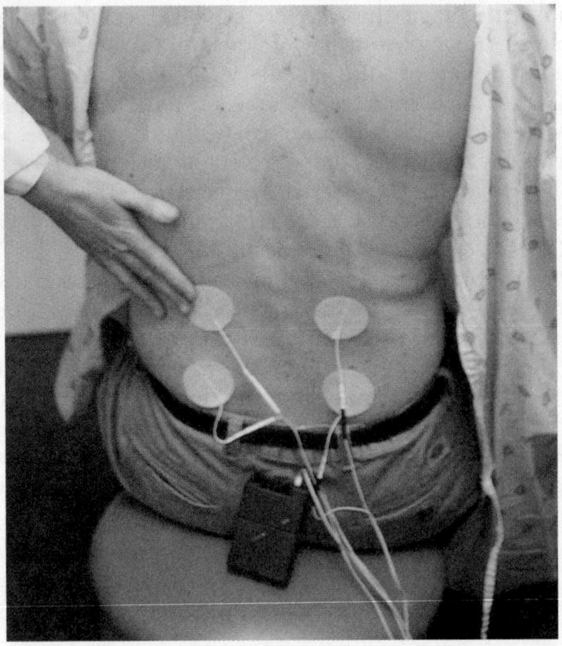

Fig. 5-6 • Application of a transcutaneous electrical nerve stimulation (TENS) unit.

The health care provider, nurse, or physical therapist (depending on the health care setting) assists the person in applying the electrodes either on the painful area or above or below it (Fig. 5-6). A conducting substance (usually a gel) is placed between the electrode and the patient's skin.

Other cutaneous techniques, such as touch, pressure, massage, vibration, and heat and cold application, stimulate the skin and somehow interrupt the pain pathway. These interventions are relatively easy to learn and are fairly economical. Cold applications are especially helpful for inflamed areas. Heat is appropriate when an increased blood flow is desired, such as for patients with chronic arthritis. Paraffin dips for the hands are particularly helpful for those patients to increase movement. Warm showers and compresses that can be done at home are also useful in reducing stiffness and promoting movement in patients with arthritis, especially after awakening.

Cognitive-Behavioral Measures. Cognitive-behavioral strategies to relieve pain (e.g., distraction) have been popular for years, mainly as adjuncts to drug therapy. Theoretic explanations for the effectiveness of these measures reflect the premises of the gate control theory. Examples of cognitive-behavioral measures are distraction, imagery, relaxation, hypnosis, music therapy, aromatherapy, prayer and meditation, and other coping skills (see Chapter 2).

Distraction can be an effective method of acute pain relief. Simple measures such as holding a patient's hand, taking him or her for a walk, or encouraging deep-breathing exercises can divert attention from the pain. Nurses often observe that patients request less pain medication when family members are present and when talking on the phone. After visiting hours, many patients request something for pain because they are no longer distracted.

Instead of viewing distraction as a therapeutic pain relief measure, as they should, some nurses may question the presence or severity of the pain if a patient is easily distracted from it. Distraction alters the perception of pain but does not influence the cause or peripheral mechanism of pain. It is a transient method of pain relief and is probably best used with other pain control measures.

The nurse can provide several methods of distraction. For example, visual distractors (e.g., pictures, television) can divert the attention to something pleasant or interesting. Auditory distractors, including music or relaxation tapes, can have a calming effect. Changing the environment can remove unpleasant stressors or reminders that may enhance pain. Physical distractions (e.g., deep-breathing exercises) help the patient concentrate on other physiologic sensations.

Distraction can be particularly useful in these situations:
- Exacerbations of pain
- Painful procedures (e.g., dressing changes, invasive procedures)
- Interrupting the patient's constant perception of pain

Imagery is a form of distraction in which the patient is encouraged to visualize or think about some pleasant or desirable feeling, sensation, or event. Guided imagery occurs when a person, often a nurse, assists the patient in sustaining a sequence of thoughts aimed at diverting attention away from the pain. Intense concentration is required to visualize images. Those who are extremely anxious, agitated, or unable to concentrate may first benefit from mild distraction.

Imagery is particularly useful for chronic pain. Patients who practice this technique can mentally and vividly experience sights, sounds, smells, events, or other sensations. The nurse first assesses the patient's level of concentration to determine whether he or she can sustain a particular thought or thoughts for a desired time. The time interval for mental imagery can vary from 5 to 60 minutes. Behaviors that are helpful in assessing the capacity for imagery include:
- Reading and comprehending the newspaper
- Listening to music or other auditory stimuli
- Having the ability to follow and participate in sustained conversation
- Having an interest in environmental surroundings

When the patient has demonstrated some ability to concentrate, assist him or her in identifying a pleasant or favorable thought. Encourage the patient to focus on this thought to divert attention away from painful stimuli. Audiotapes or CDs may help in forming and maintaining images. The nurse, patient, or family may wish to create these, or commercially available tapes and CDs may be used. This is an example of guided imagery instructions: "Imagine yourself on the beach on some deserted island. You can hear the sound of waves rushing onto the shore, the cry of seagulls flying high above, and the rustling of trees as they are brushed gently by the wind. You can feel the warmth of the sun over your body and the cooling breeze."

Imagery works for some patients but not for others. The capacity to become engaged in the reality of the image may be important for the successful use of this therapy.

Patients may use *relaxation techniques* to reduce anxiety, tension, and emotional stress, all of which may exacerbate pain. Techniques to promote relaxation can be both physical and psychological. Physical relaxation techniques include:
- Receiving a body massage, back rub, or warm or hot bath
- Modifying the environment to reduce distractions
- Moving into a comfortable position

Psychological relaxation techniques include:

- Pleasant conversation
- Music
- Relaxation tapes

Some relaxation tapes assist the patient with progressive relaxation of the muscles. Relaxation exercises can be effectively coupled with guided imagery, distraction, and hypnosis.

Hypnosis is an altered state of consciousness in which a person enters a trance and loses an overall sense of reality. Although the person is in a trance, he or she has some sense of awareness and contact with reality and has an understanding of what is actually happening. Hypnosis can be used to treat a variety of pain syndromes, particularly chronic pain. It is used to help patients overcome the emotional consequences of pain and can promote a positive state of mind. Although nurses do not usually teach hypnosis, they are in a key position to help clarify misconceptions, instruct patients about relaxation and distraction, and encourage them to practice self-hypnosis.

Other Complementary and Alternative Therapies. The data are scarce regarding the usefulness of other pain management techniques, such as magnet therapy, acupuncture, and herbal supplements. Although not supported by research, some patients believe that magnets applied to the skin or worn in shoes can reduce pain. This is a noninvasive therapy, and there is no harm to those who use this modality.

The practice of **acupuncture** originated in China. According to ancient beliefs, the body is divided into sections by lines, or meridians. Specific acupuncture points are located within these meridians. The acupuncturist inserts tiny needles into the skin and subcutaneous tissues at these points, and manual vibration or electrical stimulation is delivered. This technique is used to relieve pain and is thought to cure certain diseases.

Acupuncture is still widely acclaimed in China but is less popular in the West because the physiologic basis for this technique is unclear. Many Western health care professionals are skeptical about its usefulness. Nonetheless, acupuncture is practiced for the treatment of pain and for anesthetic purposes during diagnostic procedures, labor and delivery, and surgery. It is also used to help patients change their behavior (e.g., smoking cessation). Certain parts of the United States (e.g., the Southwest) and other countries are expanding the use of this therapy for various purposes.

Glucosamine is a commonly used supplement for patients who have arthritis. It is believed to restore joint health and thus relieve pain and inflammation. Ask the patient about the use of herbal supplements, because some can cause serious interactions with other pharmacologic agents. This drug can also increase blood glucose in diabetic patients.

Invasive Techniques for Chronic Pain

Invasive techniques are used to interrupt the pain pathways when pain is intractable (not able to be relieved) or severely debilitating. Depending on the technique, some degree of neurologic deficit and nerve destruction is expected. Various invasive techniques are used when chronic or persistent pain can no longer be adequately controlled with drugs or other pain-reducing methods. *Because of high failure rates and serious neurologic complications, these procedures are rarely used.*

Nerve blocks can be used for both diagnostic and treatment purposes. These procedures are usually indicated for pain confined to a specific area or nerve distribution. This technique involves localizing a nerve root (or roots) and injecting it with either a local anesthetic for temporary relief or diagnostic evaluations or with a chemical agent (e.g., phenol or alcohol) to achieve permanent **neurolysis** or nerve destruction. Temporary blocks or permanent destruction (neuroablation) might be considered in areas such as the intercostal nerves, celiac plexus, superior hypogastric plexus, or craniofacial nerves.

The complications associated with nerve block vary. In general, injecting a local anesthetic or chemical agent into a peripheral nerve root leads to decreased sensation in the area; motor function is not affected. Injecting a local anesthetic into the lumbosacral area of the spinal cord area may cause transient motor and bowel and bladder dysfunction. Neurolysis of the lumbosacral nerves can damage motor nerve roots, resulting in lost or impaired bowel, bladder, or sexual function. This procedure is reserved for patients with intractable cancer-related pain.

Before permanent neurolysis is considered, a temporary nerve block may be given to determine the degree of relief obtained from disrupting the nerve impulses. Although the intent of neurolysis is to permanently destroy nerve transmission, patients may experience only short-term pain relief because of nerve cell regeneration or the development of alternative pathways capable of transmitting pain. Permanent ablation of nerve roots can be performed with thermal techniques such as **radiofrequency ablation** (uses heat) or **cryoanalgesia** (uses cold).

Because a nerve block is an invasive procedure performed by anesthesiologists, neurosurgeons, surgeons, and neurologists, the health care provider is responsible for informing the patient about the procedure and its risks and alternative treatments. The nurse reinforces this information with the patient and family.

Spinal cord stimulation offers a more invasive method of nerve stimulation and is becoming more popular as a method of chronic pain control when other methods fail. This technique involves the use of electrodes implanted under the skin and into the area of the nerve responsible for the pain. At first, a trial of spinal cord stimulation is attempted through the use of temporary externalized electrodes that are implanted and connected to a stimulator device. The amount of electrical current is adjusted to provide pain relief without additional discomfort. If this trial is successful, the patient undergoes surgery for placement of a permanent implantable stimulator.

The *surgical techniques* aimed at interrupting the transmission of pain include rhizotomy and cordotomy. These two procedures are not performed as commonly today because of newer, improved pain management measures available (Fig. 5-7).

In **rhizotomy,** sensory nerve roots are destroyed where they enter the spinal cord. In a *closed* rhizotomy, a percutaneous catheter is inserted into the area and the sensory nerve roots are destroyed by chemicals, coagulation, or cryodestruction (extreme cold). A laminectomy is necessary for an *open* rhizotomy. During this surgery, the health care provider isolates and destroys the nerve roots.

In a **cordotomy,** the surgeon cuts the pain pathways at the midline portion of the spinal cord before nerve impulses ascend to the spinothalamic tract. As with the other surgical procedures, patients may experience impaired bowel, bladder, or sexual function. Because of the complexity of the pain

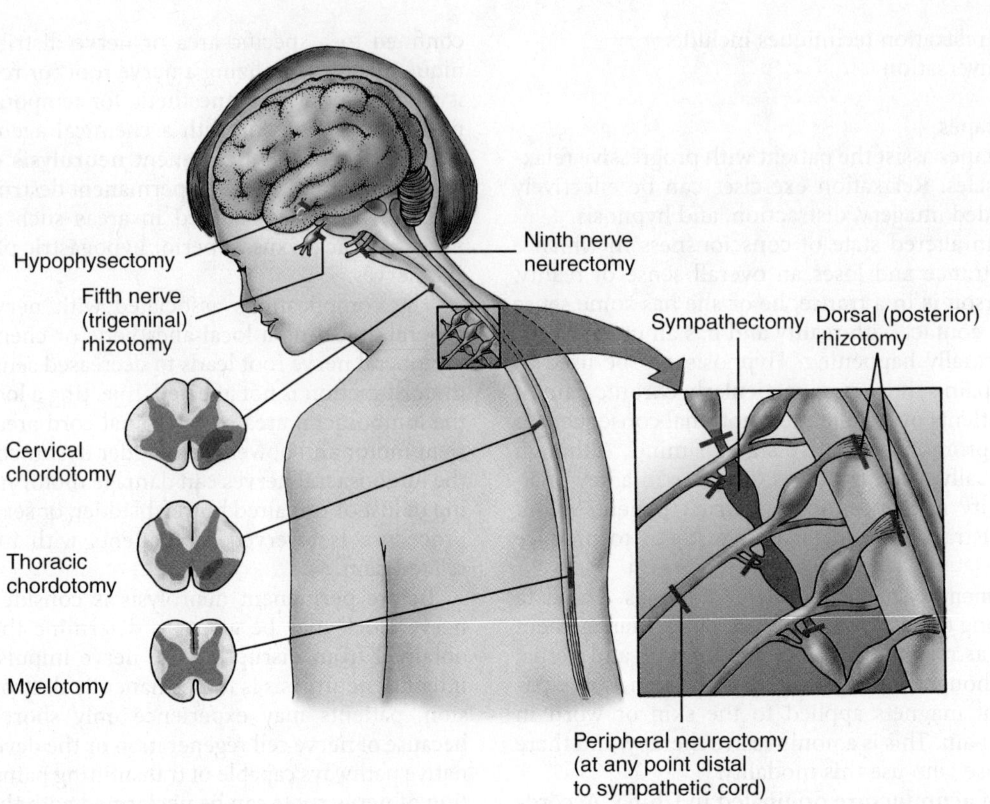
Hypophysectomy
Fifth nerve (trigeminal) rhizotomy
Cervical chordotomy
Thoracic chordotomy
Myelotomy
Ninth nerve neurectomy
Sympathectomy
Dorsal (posterior) rhizotomy
Peripheral neurectomy (at any point distal to sympathetic cord)

Fig. 5-7 • Surgical procedures designed to alleviate pain.

experience, the interruption of nerve conduction and pain pathways may not completely interrupt the sensation of pain.

After surgical intervention, assess the nature of the neurologic deficits, if any, and teach the patient how to adapt to them. If the patient has lost sensation in a body area, he or she will need to learn how to protect that area from harm. Assess expectations in relation to the surgery, and help the patient express realistic expectations.

Community-Based Care

The pain experience extends beyond hospitalization. Many patients have chronic pain but are not hospitalized. Others are in nursing homes or assisted-living facilities and have chronic pain, often not well managed. Effective analgesic regimens or pain relieving strategies should be coordinated before discharge if patients are to leave the hospital still having pain. Ensure that the patient, especially one who is on opioids, has enough pain medication to last at least until the first follow-up visit.

Home Care Management

Together with the patient and family, the nurse, case manager, discharge planner, or occupational therapist determines whether modifications are necessary for maintaining a reasonably pain-free regimen after discharge. Fatigue heightens the awareness of pain. If physical modifications (e.g., installing a downstairs bathroom) are unrealistic, suggest schedule changes, role responsibilities, and daily routines to help avoid fatigue.

At home, patients may require a referral for physical therapy, especially to start or continue treatment with cutaneous stimulation, TENS, or heat or cold techniques. Patients may need a clinical nurse specialist in pain management or social worker to assist them in developing coping strategies or maintaining adequate family dynamics. A hospice referral (hospital- or community-based) can help maintain continuity of care in the management of terminally ill patients. Those with cancer may be at risk for developing uncontrolled pain that results in hospitalization if it cannot be managed at home. It is important that nurses be knowledgeable about palliative care and end-of-life issues so they are better able to manage pain crises (see Chapter 9).

The growing number of home infusion therapy programs provides a wide variety of services to patients who require technology-supported pain care at home. Many of these services depend on approval by the insurance carrier, usually before analgesic options are considered and therapy is started. Well-defined home agency practices and professional support at home are required if patients leave the hospital with infusion therapy for pain management.

Health Teaching

Teach the patient and family about analgesic regimens, including any technical skills needed to administer or deliver the analgesic, the purpose and action of various drugs, their side effects or adverse reactions, and the importance of dosage intervals. Explain how to prevent or treat the constipation commonly associated with taking opioid analgesics and other pain medications.

In addition, explain that, ideally, the analgesic regimen should not interfere with the patient's sleep, rest, appetite, level of physical mobility, or driving ability. If such interference occurs, encourage the family or significant other to consult with the health care provider or home care nurse.

In patients with pain from advanced cancer, all efforts should be directed toward maximizing pain relief and symptom control at home to eliminate unnecessary readmissions. This may mean that the health care provider prescribes a flexible analgesic schedule that allows the patient to adjust analgesics according to the amount of pain. Teach the patient and family how to safely increase the drug within the prescribed dosing guidelines.

Evaluate family support systems to assist the patient in adhering to and continuing the proposed medical treatment and nursing plans. Inform and include family members in activities during and after hospitalization.

To achieve a reasonable level of expectation for the patient, suggest ways to continue participation in household, social, sexual, and work-oriented activities after discharge. Help identify important activities, and plan them around adequate rest schedules.

The patient with chronic pain needs continued support to cope with the anxiety, fear, and powerlessness that often accompany this pain. Help the patient and family or significant others identify coping strategies that have worked in the past. Outside support systems are also identified, such as self-help organizations.

Health Care Resources

A home care nurse referral is made when it is anticipated that patients will require assistance or supervision with their pain relief regimen at home. This referral should include specific information from the hospital-based staff nurse about the patient's overall physical condition, general level of sedation, weakness or fatigue, possible constipation or nutritional problems, sleep patterns, and functional status.

In addition to explaining the patient's physical status to the home care nurse, the staff nurse or case manager also describes the patient's level of anxiety and general expectations about pain status after discharge. Close relationships and available support network are important factors in providing ongoing support for effective pain intervention strategies.

Referral to an advanced practice nurse pain specialist, social worker, or psychologist is an appropriate way to continue providing support to the patient and family, reinforce instructions for cognitive-behavioral strategies to deal with pain, and evaluate overall physical and emotional adaptation after discharge. When severe chronic or intractable pain exists, health care professionals should direct the patient and family to appropriate resources such as pain centers or health care providers who specialize in pain management.

Patients with chronic pain often require treatment and support beyond that available in the traditional health care system. For this reason, pain clinics or programs have evolved over the past 25 years. The underlying premise of these resources is to foster independence and self-care behaviors while promoting pain control and maximizing quality of life. These programs use analgesics, adjuvant drug therapy, physical measures, cognitive-behavioral strategies, surgical interventions, and individual and group counseling for patients and family.

GET READY FOR THE NCLEX EXAMINATION!

Key Points

Review these Key Points for each NCLEX Examination Client Needs Category.

Safe and Effective Care Environment

- The nurse is legally and ethically responsible for acting as an advocate for patients experiencing pain.
- Coordinate the patient's plan of care as he or she transfers between health care agencies; be sure that the plan of care is communicated clearly.

Health Promotion and Maintenance

- Provide information to the patient and family about complementary and alternative therapies as needed; these modalities are additions to, not replacements for, the established plan of care.
- Perform a complete pain assessment, including duration, location, intensity, and quality of pain.

Psychosocial Integrity

- Be aware that some nurses and physicians have biases about pain assessment and management; be objective when caring for any patient in pain.
- Provide information to patients who have misperceptions about pain and pain management.

Physiological Integrity

- Pain is what the patient says it is; self-report is always the most reliable indication of pain.
- Three major types of pain have been identified—acute, chronic cancer, and chronic non-cancer.
- Acute pain serves as a warning to the body, causing sympathetic responses such as increased heart rate, increased blood pressure and pulse, dilated pupils, and sweating.
- Both types of chronic pain do not cause sympathetic reactions; therefore some patients do not appear to be in pain, even when they are.
- The gate control theory has helped explain the mechanism of pain and its management.
- Factors that affect pain and its management include age, gender, genetics, and culture.
- Tolerance implies that the patient has adapted to a drug and that, over time, its effects decline; physical dependence is manifested by a withdrawal reaction; addiction is a primary, chronic disease that occurs over a long period. Behaviors in addiction include craving, compulsive drug use, and continued use despite harm.
- Never use placebos for any patient; their use in non–research-based practice is unethical.
- Special considerations for older adults experiencing pain are summarized in Chart 5-1.
- Non-opioid drugs are the first-line therapy for mild to moderate pain; NSAIDs and acetaminophen (Tylenol) are commonly used drugs in this category.
- NSAIDs should be used with caution in older adults because of adverse effects, such as GI disturbances, bleeding, and sodium and water retention.

- Acetaminophen can cause hepatotoxicity and nephrotoxicity with long-term use.
- The opioid full agonists are most effective for both acute and chronic pain management; they bind to mu receptors and block pain transmission.
- Equianalgesic charts are useful when changing from one opioid to another; morphine 10 mg is the standard dose against which other opioids are measured.
- Morphine and *similar mu agonists* are the gold standard drugs for both acute and chronic pain and are available in many forms, both short acting and long acting.
- Other commonly used mu agonists include oxycodone, hydromorphone, and fentanyl.
- Meperidine is an outdated drug and is rarely used. Its toxic metabolite (normeperidine) can accumulate, especially in the older adult or someone with decreased renal clearance, and can cause seizures and confusion.
- Observe for and prevent common side effects of opioids including nausea and vomiting, constipation, sedation, and respiratory depression (see Table 5-8).
- Table 5-10 summarizes the advantages and disadvantages of drug therapy by route of administration.
- Multimodal (balanced) analgesia for epidural pain management is a combination of opioids, non-opioids, and/or local anesthetics to relieve acute pain, usually postoperative pain.
- Assess for sedation in patients receiving PCA or epidural medication.
- Common adjuvant analgesics, as an addition to other drug regimens, are listed in Table 5-11.
- Nonpharmacologic therapies for pain management may be used in place of or in combination with drug therapy; these therapies are classified as physical measures or cognitive-behavioral therapies.
- Examples of physical measures to manage pain are transcutaneous electrical nerve stimulation (TENS), heat, cold, and massage.
- Distraction, imagery, relaxation techniques, and hypnosis are examples of cognitive-behavioral therapies.
- Acupuncture, magnet therapy, and herbal supplements are examples of other complementary and alternative therapies used for chronic pain management.
- Nerve blocks and surgical techniques are uncommon, invasive techniques performed by health care specialists to treat chronic pain; rhizotomy and cordotomy are examples of surgeries.
- Pain can be managed in any setting, including the home; some patients require parenteral pain medications at home; therefore provide health teaching to ensure continuity of care.
- Refer patients whose pain is difficult to manage to pain specialists and/or pain centers.

Additional Study Resources

Go to your Companion CD or Evolve at http://evolve.elsevier.com/Iggy/ for *Self-Assessment Questions for the NCLEX Examination.*

evolve Go to Evolve at http://evolve.elsevier.com/Iggy/ for *Prioritization and Delegation Questions for the NCLEX Examination.*

SELECTED BIBLIOGRAPHY

Asterisk indicates a classic or definitive work on this subject.

*Acute Pain Management Guideline Panel. (1992). *Acute pain management: Operative or medical procedures and trauma. Clinical Practice Guidelines.* AHCPR Publication No. 92-0032. Rockville, MD: Agency for Health Care Policy and Research, Public Health Services, U.S. Department of Health and Human Services.

*American Geriatric Society. (2002). The management of persistent pain in older persons. *Journal of the American Geriatric Society, 50*(56), 205-224.

*American Pain Society. (2003). *Principles of analgesic use in the treatment of acute pain and cancer pain* (5th ed.). Glenview, IL: Author.

American Pain Society and the American Academy of Pain Medicine. *The use of opioids for the treatment of chronic pain* (consensus statement). Retrieved November 10, 2007, from www.painmed.org/productpub/statements/pdfs/opioids.pdf.

*American Society of Pain Management Nurses and the American Pain Society. (2004). *A position statement on the use of "as-needed" range orders for opioid analgesics in the management of acute pain.* Retrieved February 8, 2008, from www.aspmn.org.

*American Society for Pain Management Nursing (ASPMN). (2002). *ASPMN position statement: Pain management in patients with addictive disease* (pp. 1-4). Retrieved January 15, 2008, from www.aspmn.org.

*Cleeland, C.S., Gonin, R., Hatfield, A.K., Edmonson, J.H., Blum, R.H., Stewart, J.A., et al. (1994). Pain and its treatment in outpatients with metastatic cancer. *The New England Journal of Medicine, 330*(9), 592-596.

Cranwell-Bruce, L. (2007). Update on pain management: New methods of opiate delivery. *MEDSURG Nursing, 16*(5), 333-335.

D'Arcy, Y. (2005a). Pain management standards, the law, and you. *Nursing2005, 35*(4), 17.

D'Arcy, Y. (2005b). Patching together transdermal pain control options. *Nursing2005, 35*(9), 17.

D'Arcy, T. (2005c). What you need to know about fentanyl patches. *Nursing2005, 35*(8), 73.

D'Arcy, Y. (2006d). Which analgesic is right for my patient? *Nursing2006, 36*(7), 50-55.

D'Arcy, Y. (2007a). Managing pain in a patient who's drug dependent. *Nursing2007, 37*(3), 37-40.

D'Arcy, Y. (2007b). New pain management options: Delivery systems and techniques. *Nursing2007, 372,* 26-27.

Eshkevari, L., & Heath, J. (2005). Use of acupuncture for chronic pain: Optimizing clinical practice. *Holistic Nursing Practice, 19*(5), 217-221.

Flaherty, E. (2008). Using pain-rating scales with older adults. *AJN, 108*(6), 40-48.

Foley, K.M. (2006). Appraising the WHO Analgesic Ladder on its 20th anniversary. *Cancer Pain Release, 19*(1), 1-4.

Gelinas, C., Fillion, L., Puntillo, K.A., Viens, C., & Fortier, M. (2006). Validation of the critical-care pain observation tool in adult patients. *American Journal of Critical Care, 15*(4), 420-427.

Gevirtz, C. (2007). Treating sleep disturbances in patients with chronic pain. *Nursing2007, 37*(4), 26-27.

*Gordon, D.B., Dahl, J., Phillips, P., Frandsen, J., Cowley, C., Foster R.L., et al., American Society for Pain Management Nursing; American Pain Society. (2004). The use of "as needed" range orders for opioid analgesics in the management of acute pain: a consensus statement of the American Society for Pain Management Nursing and the American Pain Society. *Pain Management Nursing, 5*(2), 53-58.

Herr, K., Coyne, P.J., Key, T., Manworren, R., McCaffery, M., Merkel, S., et al.; American Society for Pain Management Nursing. (2006). Pain assessment in the nonverbal patient: Position statement with clinical practice recommendations. *Pain Management Nursing, 7*(2), 44-52.

Kirk, T.W. (2007). Managing pain, managing ethics. *Pain Management Nursing, 8*(1), 25-34.

Laurenson, M. (2006). Working complementary therapies into mainstream health care. *British Journal of Nursing, 15*(7), 356-358.

LeFort, S.M. (2005). Intravenous and oral opioids reduce chronic non-cancer pain but are associated with high rates of constipation, nausea, and sleepiness. *Evidence-Based Nursing, 8*(3), 88.

Manias, E., Bucknall, T., & Botti, M. (2005). Nurses' strategies for managing pain in the postoperative setting. *Pain Management Nursing, 6*(1), 18-29.

Manworren, R. (2007). A call to action to protect range orders. *AJN,* 106(7), 65-58.

*McCaffery, M., & Pasero, C. (1999). Harmful effects of unrelieved pain. In M. McCaffery & C. Pasero, *Pain: Clinical manual* (2nd ed., pp. 15-34). St. Louis: Mosby.

*Melzack, R., & Wall, P.D., (1982). *The challenge of pain.* New York: Basic Books.

Miaskowski, C. (2005). The next step to improving cancer pain management. *Pain Management Nursing, 6*(1), 1-2.

Pasero, C., Manworren, R., & McCaffery, M. (2007). IV opioid range orders for acute pain management. *AJN, 107*(2), 52-59.

Pasero, C., & McCaffery, M. (2004). Comfort-function goals: A way to establish accountability for pain relief. *AJN, 104*(9), 77-78, 81.

Pasero, C., & McCaffery, M. (2005a). Authorized and unauthorized use of PCA pumps. *AJN, 105*(7), 30-33.

Pasero, C., & McCaffery, M. (2005b). Ketamine. *AJN, 105*(4), 60-64.

Sopalski, M.A. (2007). Pain control with fentanyl patch. *Journal of Hospice and Palliative Nursing, 9*(1), 13-14.

Stewart, M.W. (2005). Evidence-based assessment of acute pain in older adults: Current nursing practices and perceived barriers. *Journal of Peri-Anesthesia Nursing, 20*(1), 59-63.

Valente, S.M. (2006). Hypnosis for pain management: Focusing on pleasant sensations—like being on a beach, lake, or mountaintop—can relieve pain, tension, and anxiety. *Journal of Psychosocial Nursing and Mental Health Services, 44*(2), 22-30, 48-49.

van Herk, R., van Dijk, M., Baar, F.P.M., Tibboel, D., & de Wit, R. (2007). Observation scales for pain assessment in older adults with cognitive impairments or communication difficulties. *Nursing Research, 56*(1), 34-43.

Vaughn, F., Wichowski, H., & Bosworth, G. (2007). Does preoperative anxiety level predict postoperative pain? *AORN Journal, 85*(3), 589-594, 597-604.

Wuhrman, E., Cooney, M.F., Dunwoody, C.J., Eksterowicz, N., Merkel, S., Oakes, L.L.; American Society for Pain Management Nursing. (2007). Authorized and unauthorized ("PCA by Proxy") dosing of analgesic infusion pumps: Position statement with clinical practice recommendations. *Pain Management Nursing, 8*(1), 4-11.

6

CHAPTER

Genetic Concepts for Medical-Surgical Nursing

M. Linda Workman

LEARNING OUTCOMES

For clinical competence and success on the NCLEX Examination, study this chapter with these Learning Outcomes in mind:

Safe and Effective Care Environment

1. Coordinate with health care team members and genetics professionals when providing genetic testing information to patients and families.
2. Advocate for the patient with regard to whether or not to have genetic testing, informed consent before testing, and sharing of test results.
3. Ensure that confidentiality of genetic test results is maintained by all health care team members.

Health Promotion and Maintenance

4. Teach the patient and family who are at increased genetic risk for a disease or disorder to participate in an appropriate screening plan.

Psychosocial Integrity

5. Assess patient and family responses to the findings of genetic testing.
6. Support the decision of the patient and family to have or not to have genetic counseling or testing.

Physiological Integrity

7. Describe the structure and forms of DNA.
8. Describe the relationship between genes and proteins.
9. Compare the concept of phenotype with that of genotype.
10. Compare the patterns of inheritance for single gene traits.
11. Explain how genetic variations can induce or affect adult health problems.
12. Analyze a three-generation pedigree.
13. Identify patients at increased genetic risk for health problems.
14. Explain how genetic testing is different from other laboratory tests.
15. Describe the role of the medical-surgical nurse in genetic counseling.

Go to your Companion CD or Evolve at http://evolve.elsevier.com/Iggy/ for *Self-Assessment*
evolve *Questions for the NCLEX Examination* keyed to these Learning Outcomes.

One of the most important areas of health advancement this century is in the understanding of the influence of genetic factors on adult health and adult illness. The use of these advances, called *genomic medicine* or "*genomics,*" will lead to disease prevention strategies and therapies that take into account each person's genetic differences.

Organizations such as the American Nurses Association, the American Association of Colleges of Nursing, and the American Academy of Nursing support the need for all nurses to have a basic understanding of genetics to provide the best possible care for patients and families. Many common adult health problems (e.g., hypertension, diabetes, heart disease, cancer, arthritis, and many others) have a genetic basis.

The purpose of this chapter is to help present the essentials about basic genetics and how this information relates to adult health care. Although nurses are not expected to be genetics experts, they need to know enough about basic genetics to recognize when a patient or family has a possible genetic risk for a health problem and to coordinate the attention of health care team members to ensure appropriate care.

GENETIC BIOLOGY

All living things, including people, have genes. Genes are the instructions for the making of all the different substances any organism produces. Think of all the hormones, enzymes, and other proteins the human body makes. It is the specific genes

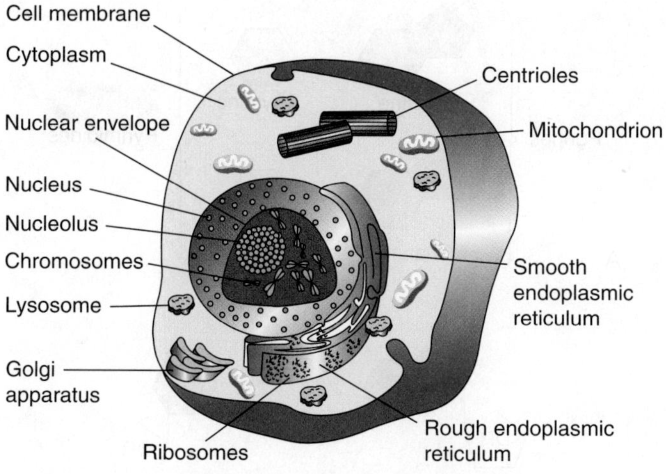
Cell membrane
Cytoplasm
Centrioles
Nuclear envelope
Mitochondrion
Nucleus
Nucleolus
Chromosomes
Smooth endoplasmic reticulum
Lysosome
Golgi apparatus
Rough endoplasmic reticulum
Ribosomes

Fig. 6-1 • Anatomy of a cell.

that tell each cell what protein to make, how to make it, when to make it, and how much to make. Think of each gene as a specific "recipe" for making proteins.

So where are these genes? The genes are located in the nucleus of most body cells. As shown in Fig. 6-1, the cell nucleus contains DNA in the form of chromosomes. All cells with a nucleus contain all the genes. (Mature red blood cells do not have a nucleus and thus contain no genes; the germ cells [sperm and ova] have only half of the chromosomes that regular body cells have.) For example, all cells have the gene for insulin. However, even though all cells have the gene for insulin, the only cell type that allows the insulin gene to be active and make insulin is the beta cell of the pancreas. So, although the insulin gene is present in skin cells, heart cells, brain cells, and other cells, only in the beta cells is this gene selectively "turned on" **(expressed)** when you need to make insulin.

An important fact to remember is that every human cell with a nucleus contains the entire set of human genes. This complete set of genes is called the **genome.** The human genome contains about 25,000 individual genes.

One area that is somewhat confusing about genetics is how DNA is different from the genes and from the chromosomes. DNA, chromosomes, and genes are all the same basic thing; only the structures differ. Fig. 6-2 shows that if any one chromosome is pulled out from the nucleus and "unwound," its framework is the DNA. Each chromosome has many genes within it. Humans have 23 pairs of chromosomes—46 individual chromosomes. The Y chromosome, a small chromosome, has fewer than 100 genes. Larger chromosomes, such as the number 1 chromosome, contain thousands of genes.

One way to think of it is to consider all the DNA in any cell's nucleus to be a giant "cookbook" containing all the recipes needed to make all the proteins, hormones, enzymes, and other substances your body needs. The chromosome pairs are the different book chapters (so the human genome cookbook has 23 chapters), and the genes are the individual recipes contained within the chapters.

There is a specific chromosome location **(locus)** for every gene. For example, the locus for the gene for blood type is on chromosome 9. The locus for the gene for part of hemoglobin is on chromosome 6. We now know the location and the exact DNA sequence for many, but not all, genes. Fig. 6-2 shows that each chromosome is made up of a large chunk of DNA that

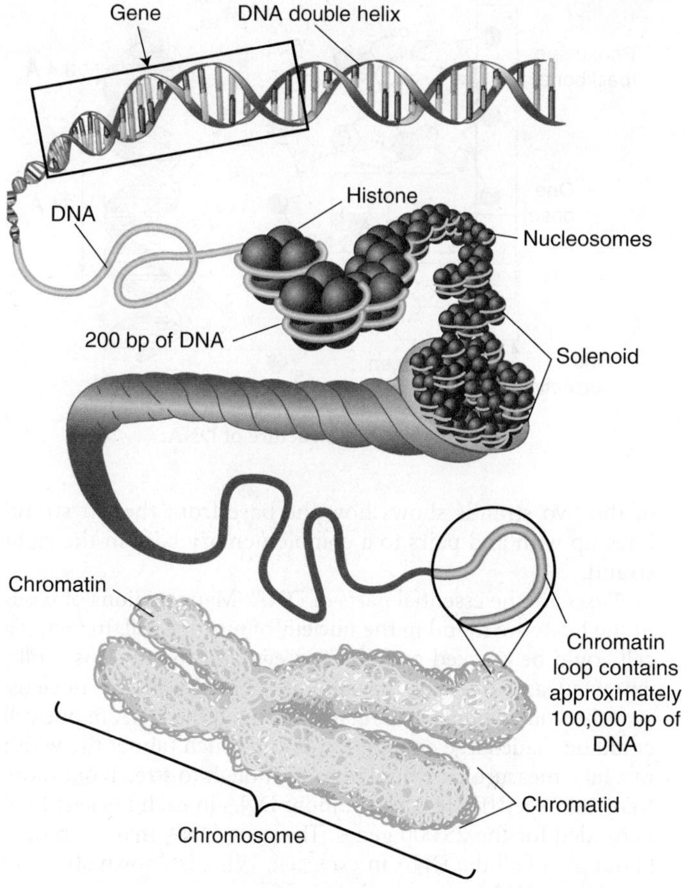
Gene
DNA double helix
DNA
Histone
Nucleosomes
200 bp of DNA
Solenoid
Chromatin
Chromatin loop contains approximately 100,000 bp of DNA
Chromatid
Chromosome

Fig. 6-2 • Coiling loose DNA tightly into a chromosome.

has been twisted (like a length of rope) until it coils up tightly into a very dense structure. Thus in each cell the DNA is divided into 46 separate chunks.

Deoxyribonucleic Acid

DNA is short for **deoxyribonucleic acid,** which is the basic genetic material of a cell. Most DNA (about 99.99%) is in the nucleus, although other cell parts also contain very small amounts of DNA. This chapter focuses on the nuclear DNA.

DNA Structure

In humans, DNA is a linear, double-stranded structure composed of multiple units of four different nitrogenous bases, each attached to a sugar molecule. The bases in each strand are connected together by phosphate groups. These two individual strands are held together loosely. This double-stranded DNA is arranged like a long set of railroad tracks. The "backbones" of the track are the two long steel rails. For DNA, these backbones are the phosphate groups that hold the bases in place. The bases are the individual railroad ties. Think of each tie as having two pieces—one piece attached to the right-hand rail and one piece attached to the left-hand rail.

Fig. 6-3 shows a very small piece of double-stranded DNA on the left (containing only four base pairs) taken from the larger piece of DNA on the right. The phosphate groups that hold the nucleotides together as a strand are in the red box. The green box in the lower left-hand section shows a whole nucleotide (a base with the sugar and the phosphate group) in place in the left-hand DNA strand. The blue box in the middle

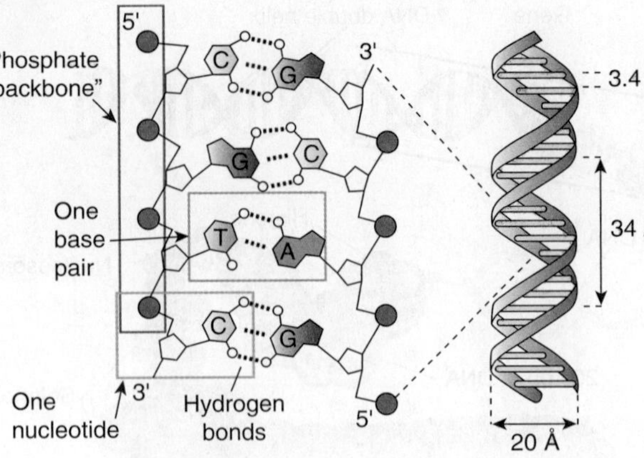
5'
Phosphate "backbone"
3'
3.4 Å
One base pair
34 Å
One nucleotide
3'
Hydrogen bonds
5'
20 Å
C
G
T
A

Fig. 6-3 • The structure of DNA.

of the two strands shows how the base from the left strand lines up with and pairs to a complementary base in the right strand.

Bases are the essential parts of DNA. Many trillions of bases in the DNA are found in the nucleus of just one cell. In fact, if a cell could be cracked open like an egg and the nucleus (yolk) extracted and opened, the amount of DNA in the nucleus, stretched out, would be about 6 feet long. If the DNA in one cell could be made large enough to see and touch (about the width of a tape measure), it would be long enough to stretch out more than 1000 feet! There is much more DNA in each nucleus than is needed for the 25,000 genes. The gene DNA makes up only about 5% of all the DNA in each cell. What is known about all that other DNA is discussed on p. 66.

The four bases in DNA are adenine (A), guanine (G), cytosine (C), and thymine (T). These four bases are made from vitamins and the nitrogen atoms from amino acids. For example, thymine is made from folic acid and nitrogen. Two of the bases (thymine and cytosine) are *pyrimidines,* and the other two bases (adenine and guanine) are *purines* (Fig. 6-4, *A*).

Each base becomes a **nucleoside** when a five-sided sugar (known as a *deoxyribose sugar*) is attached to it. Fig. 6-4, *B*, shows how the four bases become four nucleosides. Each nucleoside becomes a complete **nucleotide** when phosphate groups are attached (Fig. 6-4, *C*). The final form of a base that actually gets put into the DNA strand is a nucleotide. The phosphate groups hold each base in place in a strand of DNA.

Base pairs are the linked bases in the two opposite strands of DNA. The bases always link together across from each other in a very specific way. First, the two DNA strands need to remain perfectly parallel to each other so that the strands remain the same distance apart down the total length of DNA. So a pyrimidine must always pair up with a purine to maintain the proper distance (Fig. 6-4, *D*). The two DNA strands are held together by loose bonds that form between the base pairs. Cytosine and guanine connect with three bonds, whereas adenine and thymine connect with only two bonds (Fig. 6-4, *D*). Adenine can pair only with thymine, and cytosine can pair only with guanine.

These complementary base pairs in DNA are specific. Thus, if the base sequence of one strand of DNA is known, the opposite strand's sequence could be accurately predicted. For example, if the left-hand section of DNA (strand 1 in Fig. 6-5) had the sequence A-G-G-C-T-C-A-A-C-C-T-G, the corresponding (complementary) right-hand section (strand 2 in Fig. 6-5) of

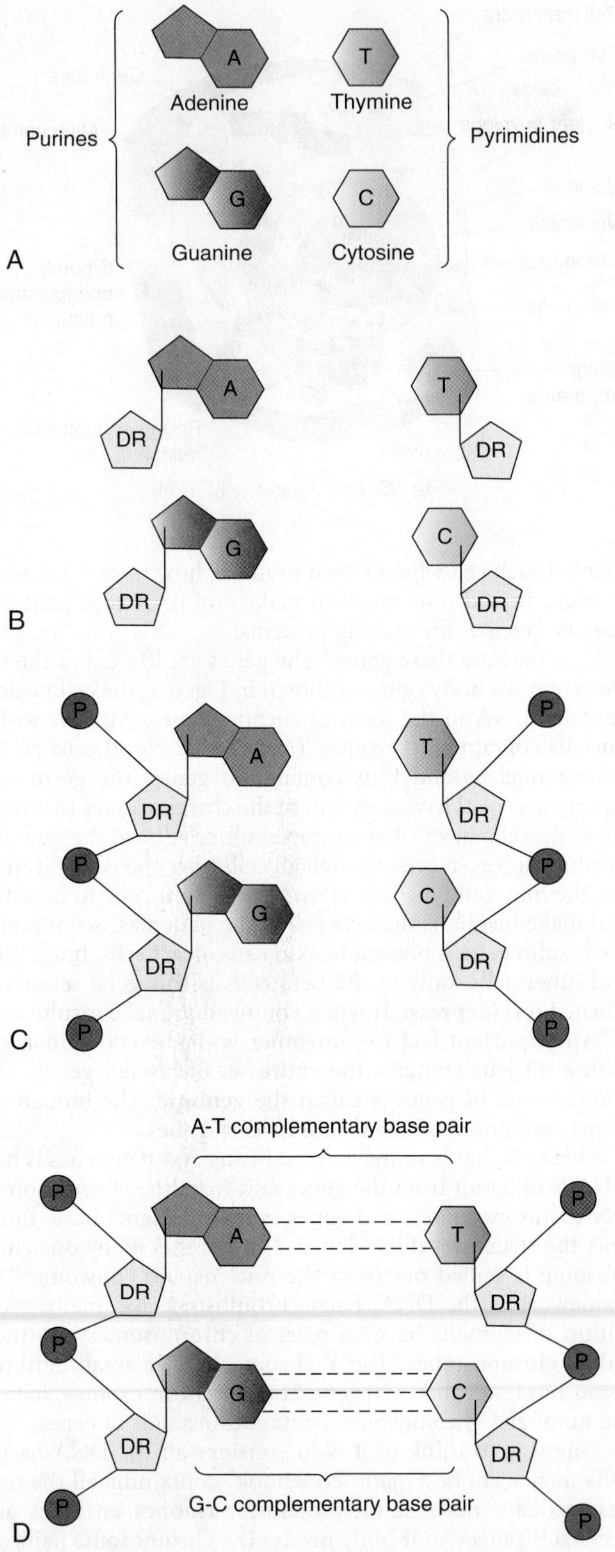
A
Adenine
T
Thymine
Purines
Pyrimidines
G
Guanine
C
Cytosine
A
DR
B
P
C
A-T complementary base pair
G-C complementary base pair
D

Fig. 6-4 • Close view of DNA. **A,** The four nitrogenous bases of DNA. **B,** Nitrogenous bases converted into nucleosides by attaching a deoxyribose sugar (DR). **C,** The four nucleosides converted into nucleotides by attaching phosphate groups (P). **D,** Two short strands of DNA held loosely together by hydrogen bonds forming complementary base pairs. ——— = weak hydrogen bonds.

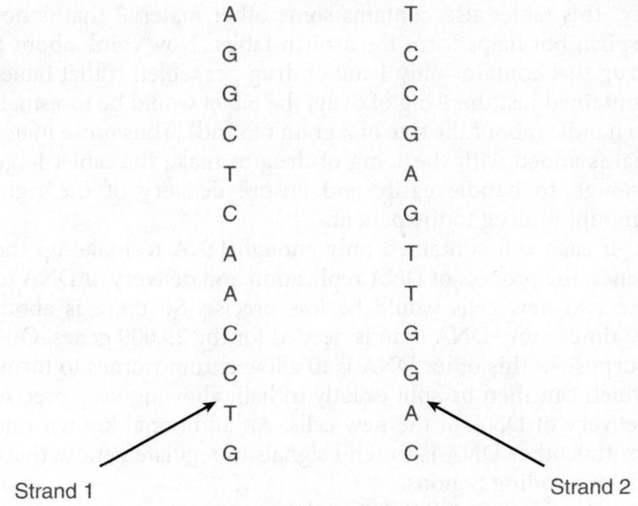
A T
G C
G C
C G
T A
C G
A T
A T
C G
C G
T A
G C
Strand 1
Strand 2

Fig. 6-5 • Complementary strands of DNA.

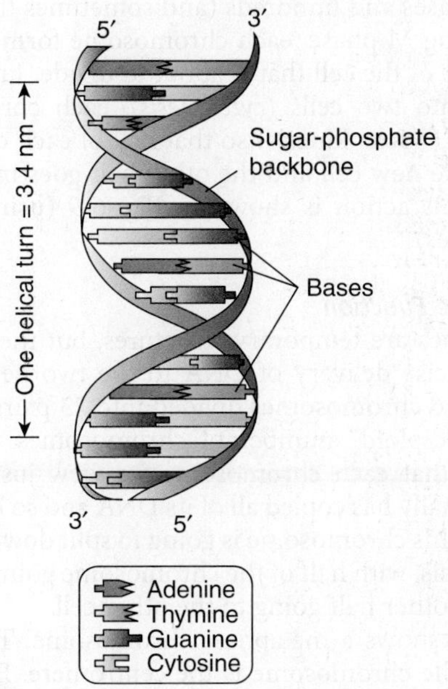
5′
3′
One helical turn = 3.4 nm
Sugar-phosphate backbone
Bases
3′
5′
Adenine
Thymine
Guanine
Cytosine

Fig. 6-6 • Complementary strands of DNA twisted into a loose helical shape.

DNA would have the sequence T-C-C-G-A-G-T-T-G-G-A-C. When the two strands of DNA are lined up properly, they twist in a loose helical shape (Fig. 6-6; see also Fig. 6-2). DNA keeps this shape most of the time. In this shape, the DNA is so fine that it can be seen only with electron microscopes. Only when a cell begins to divide (i.e., undergoes mitosis) does the DNA super-coil tightly into dense pieces called *chromosomes* (see Fig. 6-2), which can be seen with standard microscopes.

These two strands separate completely during the DNA synthesis phase of cell division. The weak bonds allow this separation to occur easily.

DNA Replication

Cell Division

DNA must reproduce itself (replicate) every time a cell divides (undergoes mitosis). Cell division (mitosis) occurs in a regulated pattern known as the *cell cycle.* The purpose of mitosis is for one cell to reproduce into two new cells, each of which is identical to the cell that started mitosis. For each new cell to

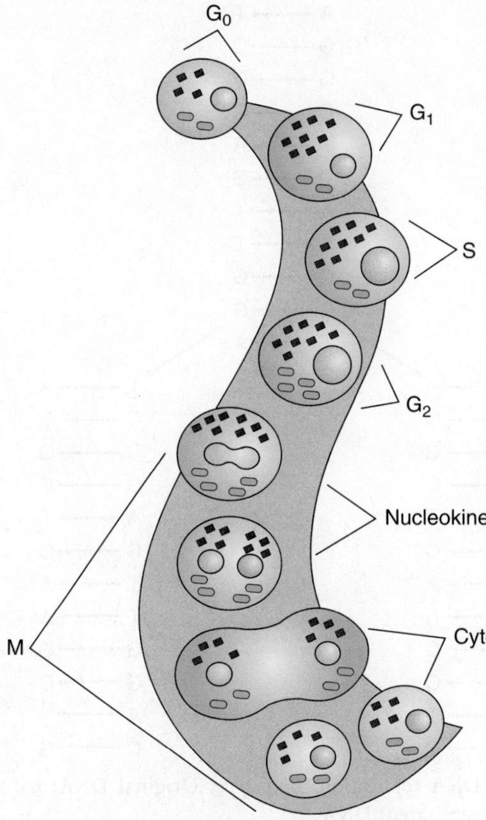
G0
G1
S
G2
Nucleokinesis
M
Cytokinesis

Fig. 6-7 • The cell cycle.

have exactly the right amount of DNA and genes, the DNA in the dividing cell must exactly replicate. Fig. 6-7 shows the phases of the cell cycle.

Living cells that are not actively reproducing are in a "resting state" called G_0. During the G_0 period, cells carry out their normal functions but do not divide. Normal cells spend most of their lives in the G_0 state, just as most humans spend more time not pregnant than pregnant.

Mitosis makes one cell divide into two identical cells. Cells go through four phases of the cell cycle to divide:

1. ***G_1:*** The cell is getting ready for division by taking on extra nutrients, making more energy, and growing extra membrane. The amount of cell fluid (cytoplasm) also increases.
2. ***S:*** Because making one cell into two cells requires twice as much DNA, the cell doubles its DNA content through DNA synthesis. This process occurs in S phase. First the double strands of DNA separate, and then enzymes read the sequence of the original strands and build two new strands complementary to the original strands (Fig. 6-8). The process of making a new copy of an entire strand of DNA is called **DNA replication.**

Many enzymes are involved in DNA synthesis. Some of the enzymes "relax" and then "unwind" the double-stranded DNA. Other enzymes separate the two strands and keep them separate. Different enzymes "read" the original DNA strands and determine the order of the bases for the new strands. Special enzymes actually build the new strands by placing and linking nucleotides together. Finally, other enzymes actually "spell check" the new strands of DNA to ensure that each

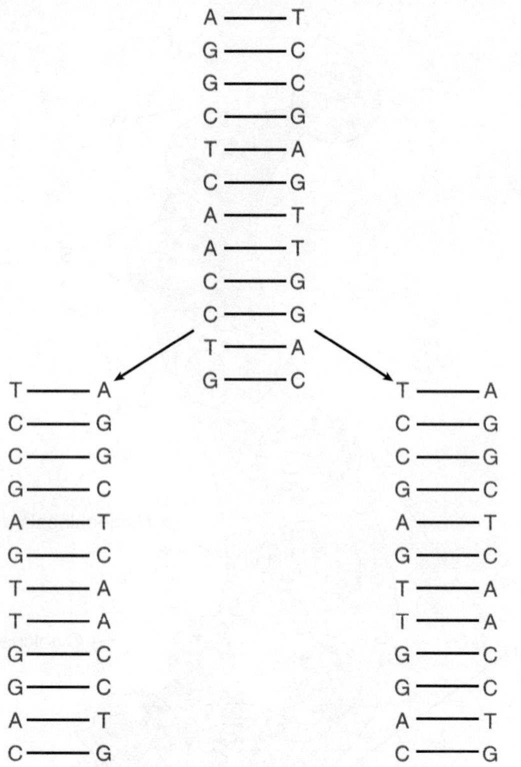
A—T
G—C
G—C
C—G
T—A
C—G
A—T
A—T
C—G
C—G
T—A
G—C
T—A
C—G
C—G
G—C
A—T
G—C
T—A
T—A
G—C
G—C
A—T
C—G
T—A
C—G
C—G
G—C
A—T
G—C
T—A
T—A
G—C
G—C
A—T
C—G

Fig. 6-8 • DNA replication. *Blue type,* Original DNA; *red type,* newly made (replicated) DNA.

base in the new strand is complementary to its base pair on the original strand.

When DNA synthesis is complete, the result is two sets of double-stranded DNA. Each of the two sets has one old strand and one new strand. Notice in Fig. 6-7 that the nucleus during S phase is twice as large as it was during G_1 because it now has twice as much DNA.

During M phase of the cell cycle, one set of DNA will move into one of the two new cells made during mitosis and the second set will move into the other new cell. In this way, every new cell ends up with exactly the right amount of DNA with all the genes.

3. ***G_2:*** The cell makes important proteins that will be used in actual cell division and in normal physiologic function after cell division is complete.
4. ***M:*** The single cell splits apart into two cells (actual mitosis). It is in this phase, after the DNA has completely replicated itself, that the 46 separate chunks of DNA twist very tightly and form dense "chromosomes" that can be seen using a standard microscope.

Chromosome Formation

During M phase, the fact that there is much more DNA in each cell than just the genes is helpful. The delivery of genes to each new cell during mitosis is critical for the new cells to be able to function. Thus this DNA delivery must be precise and perfect. Having the DNA pack down into chromosomes makes for precise DNA delivery. This works in much the same way that oral drugs do. For example, think about the size of a single aspirin tablet that contains 325 mg of the drug *aspirin.* This tablet is not very large—only a little over 1 cm in diameter. This tablet also contains some other material that is not aspirin but helps form the aspirin tablet. Now think about a drug that contains only 1 mg of drug per tablet. If that tablet contained just the 1 mg of drug, the tablet would be too small to handle (about the size of a grain of sand). Thus more material is added with the 1 mg of drug to make the tablet large enough to handle easily and ensure delivery of the right amount of drug to the patient.

If each cell contained only enough DNA to make up the genes, the process of DNA replication and delivery of DNA to the two new cells would be less precise. So there is about 20 times more DNA than is needed for the 25,000 genes. One purpose of this other DNA is to allow chromosomes to form, which can then be split exactly in half, allowing very precise delivery of DNA to the new cells. An additional known role for this other DNA is to send signals to regulate gene activity in gene coding regions.

So, as shown in Fig. 6-2, a chromosome is a specific large chunk of double-stranded DNA, with each chunk containing billions of bases and hundreds (and sometimes thousands) of genes. During M phase, each chromosome forms and moves to the center of the cell that is about to divide. Just before the cell splits into two cells *(cytokinesis),* each chromosome is pulled apart (nucleokinesis) so that half of each chromosome goes into one new cell and the other half goes into the other new cell. This action is shown in Fig. 6-9 (using just three chromosomes).

Chromosome Function

Chromosomes are temporary structures, but their job is important: precise delivery of DNA to the two new cells. Humans have 46 chromosomes divided into 23 pairs. This number is the "diploid" number of chromosomes for humans. Remember that each chromosome we view just before cell division actually has copied all of its DNA and so has twice the DNA in it. This chromosome is going to split down the middle during mitosis, with half of the chromosome going to one new cell and the other half going to the other cell.

Fig. 6-10 shows a metaphase chromosome. The "pinched in" area of the chromosome is the centromere. Each left and right half of the chromosome is a chromatid. The "arms" above the centromere are the short arms, or the "p" arms. The longer arms (not legs) below the centromere are the "q" arms. A particular gene may be listed as located on 9q, meaning that the gene has its location **(locus)** on the long arm of the number 9 chromosome.

The very "tips" of the chromosomes are the **telomeres,** or the telomeric DNA (deep pink area of Fig. 6-10 and Fig. 6-11). This DNA actually caps each chromosome in the same way that a plastic tip caps shoestrings. The purpose is the same—to keep the strands from unraveling. Fig. 6-11 shows a chromosome lying on its side. The deep pink areas at each end are the telomeres. The inset figure below the chromosome is the enlarged end region and telomere of the chromosome. This region contained many thousands of bases at birth. With every cell division, the telomeres of the chromosomes in the cell that just divided are shortened by 50 to 100 bases. Telomeres are not replaced by the cell. As a person ages, the telomeres become shorter. Eventually, the telomere DNA is gone and the chromosomes unravel, which is a signal for the cell to commit "cellular suicide" **(apoptosis)** and die.

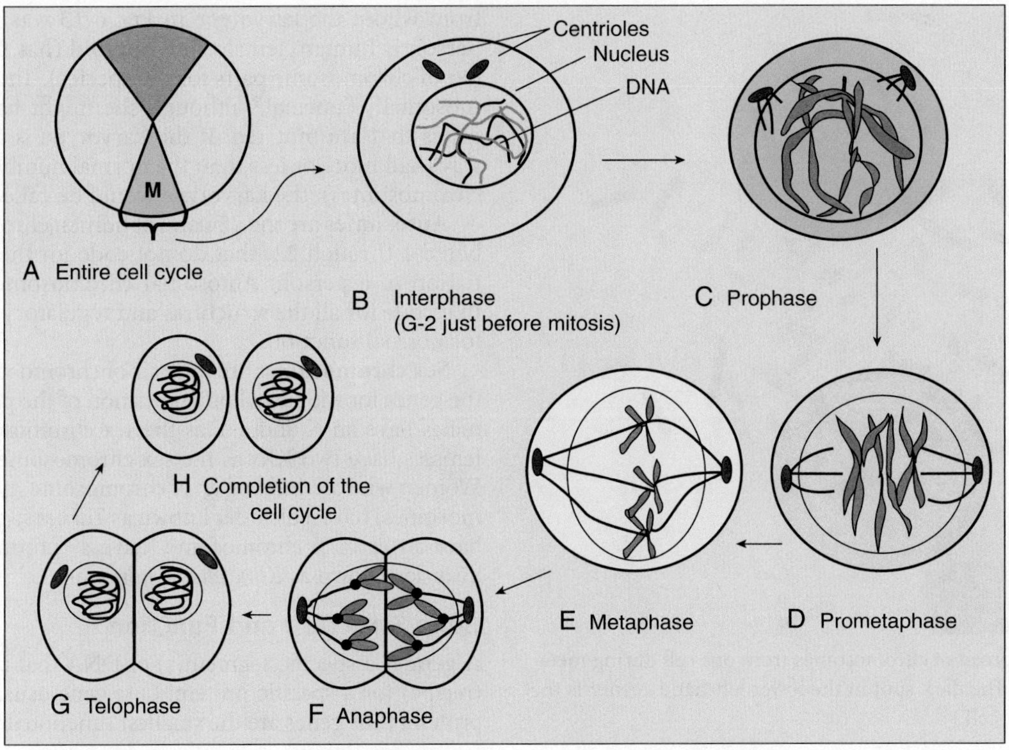
Centrioles
Nucleus
DNA
M
A Entire cell cycle
B Interphase
(G-2 just before mitosis)
C Prophase
D Prometaphase
E Metaphase
F Anaphase
G Telophase
H Completion of the
cell cycle

Fig. 6-9 • The activities of M phase of the cell cycle.

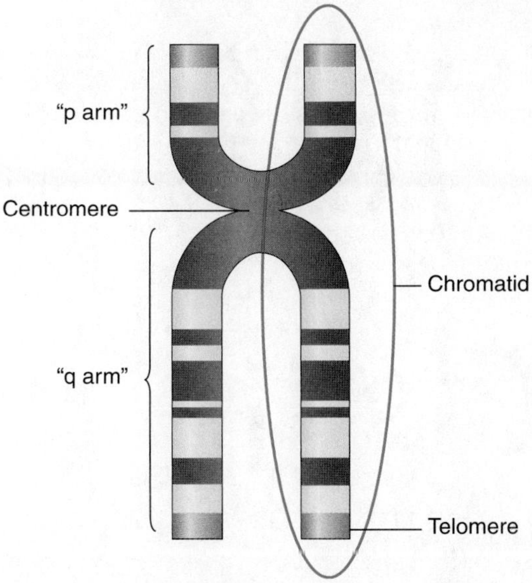
"p arm"
Centromere
Chromatid
"q arm"
Telomere

Fig. 6-10 • A single metaphase chromosome.

Telomeres are related to aging and other important events that happen in the life of the cell. With normal aging, these telomeres shorten until they are gone and the cell then dies. When the cell death rate in any one organ occurs faster than cells can be replaced, the organ cannot function and the person dies. The normal loss of telomeric DNA with each cell division gives each of our normal cells a finite life span. The rate at which a person ages is related to the rate of telomere loss. Faster cellular aging occurs among people who have faster rates of telomere loss. Slower cellular aging occurs among people who have slower rates of telomere loss.

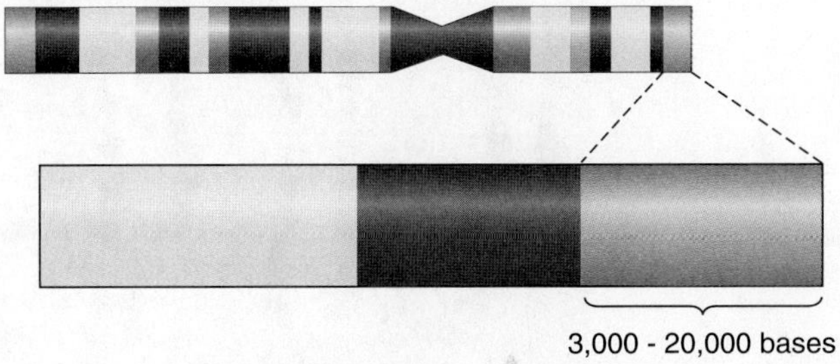
3,000 - 20,000 bases

Fig. 6-11 • Telomeric DNA.

Chromosomal Analysis

Some things about a person can be known by examining his or her chromosomes. It is important to remember that the information that can be obtained by chromosomal analysis is limited because each chromosome is composed of a large chunk of DNA. Only very large deletions, additions, or rearrangements of DNA show up at the level of the chromosome. Losses or gains of just a few bases (or even tens of thousands) cannot be detected by chromosome analysis. Fig. 6-12 shows how the chromosomes of one cell look just before cell division. To analyze chromosomes, they must first be organized into a karyotype.

A **karyotype** is an organized arrangement of all of the chromosomes within one cell during the metaphase section of mitosis (Fig. 6-13). A technician first collects pictures of the chromosomes into pairs and then lines them up according to size (largest first) and centromere position. This gross organization of DNA can be used to determine missing or extra whole chromosomes and some large structural rearrangements. *A missing gene or a mutated gene would not show up at this level of analysis.* What can be learned about the person

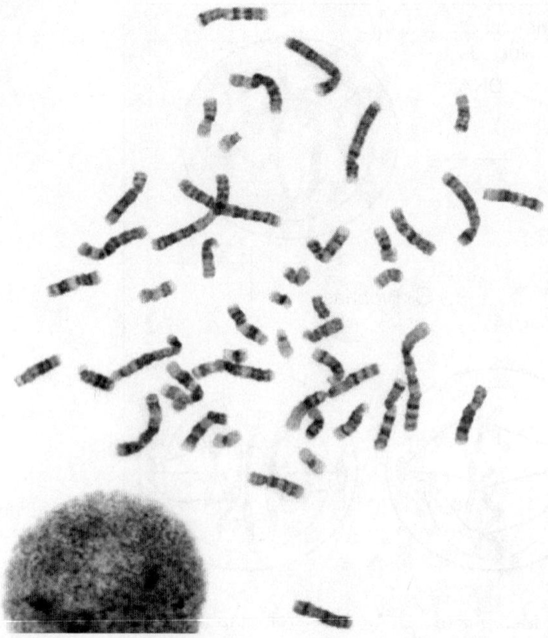

Fig. 6-12 • A spread of chromosomes from one cell during metaphase of mitosis. (The dark spot in the lower left-hand corner is the nucleus of another cell.)

from whom the karyotype in Fig. 6-13 was made is that the person is human, female, and **euploid** (has the correct number of chromosome pairs for the species). This person is chromosomally "normal," although she might have one or more genes that are mutated. If the karyotype is abnormal in any way (had more or less than the normal number or had broken chromosomes), the karyotype would be called **aneuploid.**

Autosomes are the 22 pairs of human chromosomes (numbered 1 through 22) that do not code for the sexual differentiation of a person. Autosomal chromosomes contain genes that code for all the structures and regulatory proteins needed for normal function.

Sex chromosomes are the pair of chromosomes that contain the genes for the sexual differentiation of the person. Almost all males have an X and a Y as the sex chromosomes. Almost all females have two XXs as the sex chromosomes (see Fig. 6-13). Women who are missing an X chromosome (have only 45 chromosomes) have a disorder known as *Turner syndrome.* Men who have an extra X chromosome (have 47 chromosomes) have a disorder known as *Klinefelter syndrome.*

Gene Structure and Function

A **gene** is a specific segment(s) of DNA that contains the code (recipe) for a specific protein. One gene usually codes for one protein; thus genes are the smallest functional unit of the DNA.

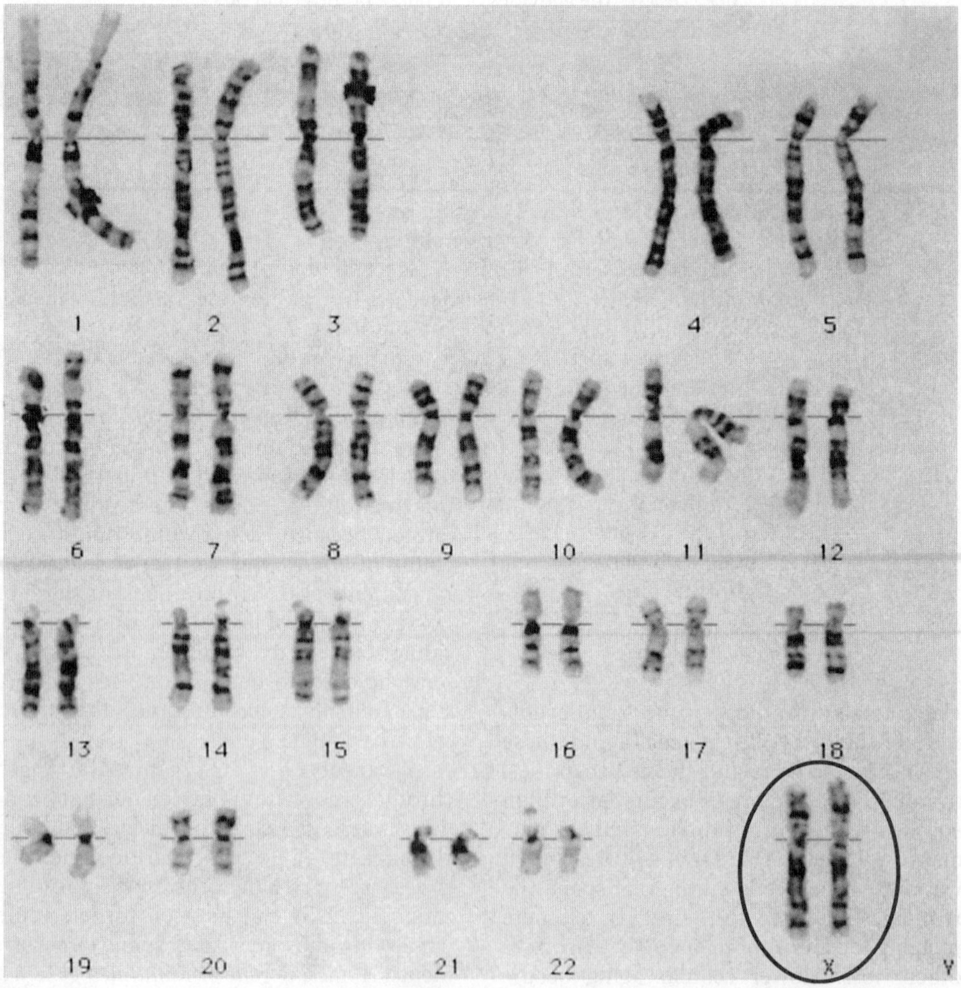
1
2
3
4
5
6
7
8
9
10
11
12
13
14
15
16
17
18
19
20
21
22
X
Y

Fig. 6-13 • A karyotype of a chromosomally normal female. (The sex chromosomes are circled in red.)

Each chromosome contains hundreds of genes (and remember that each chromosome is made up of a large segment of DNA). Thus an individual gene is a very small segment of DNA.

For many human traits, one gene controls the expression of that trait in any person. Such traits are known as "single gene traits." For each single gene, we have two alleles. An **allele** (pronounced "ah-**lee**-el") is an alternate form (or variation) of a gene. For example, there is one gene for blood type but there are three possible gene alleles (A, B, and O). Each person has only two of the three specific gene alleles for blood type. One of these alleles is on one chromosome 9 of the pair; the other allele is located on the other number 9 chromosome. Because each person only has two number 9 chromosomes, he or she can have only two alleles for blood type. One gene allele was inherited from the person's mother, and the other gene allele was inherited from the person's father. *Some traits have even more than three possible alleles, but each person has only two.* Which blood type gene alleles are inherited from a person's parents determines his or her blood type.

If a person has inherited a blood type A allele from his or her mother and a blood type B allele from his or her father, he or she has the A and B alleles; the blood type expressed when the blood bank determines type is type AB. Fig. 6-14 shows this concept. In Fig. 6-14, two people are about to become pregnant. What are the possibilities for this baby to have a specific type of ear shape (pointy, rounded, square, triangular)? The gene for ear shape is trait 1, and it (for the purposes of this explanation) is on chromosome number 6.

Each of the father's sperm contains only one number 6 chromosome, and each of the mother's eggs contains only one number 6 chromosome (so that when the sperm fertilizes the egg, the resulting person conceived will have only one pair of chromosome number 6 instead of two pairs of chromosome number 6).

Half the father's sperm have the 1a allele for ear shape, and the other half have allele 1b for ear shape. Half the mother's eggs have 1c for ear shape, and the other half have 1d. The resulting baby can inherit only a 1a or a 1b from the father, not both; and this same baby can inherit only a 1c or a 1d from the mother—again, not both. The lower portion of Fig. 6-14 shows all the combinations possible for each ear shape gene alleles for any child these two people have.

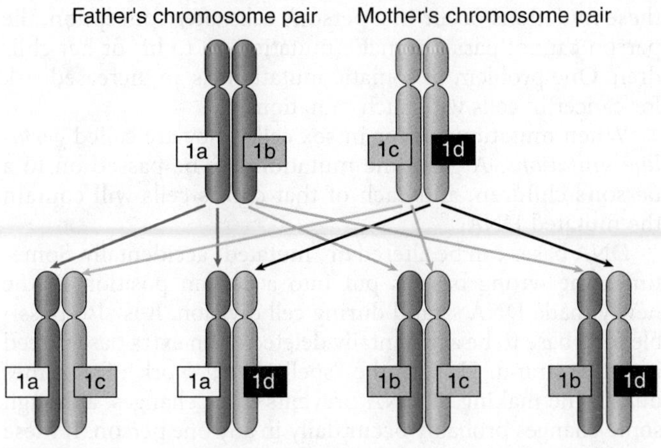
Father's chromosome pair
Mother's chromosome pair
1a
1b
1c
1d
1a
1c
1a
1d
1b
1c
1b
1d

Fig. 6-14 • Inheritance of four possible alleles for the single gene trait 1. (Any one person can have only two alleles for a single gene trait.)

If a person has two identical alleles for a single gene trait, that person is said to be *homozygous* for that trait. So if a person has an A blood-type gene allele on one number 9 chromosome and an A blood-type gene allele on the other number 9 chromosome, he or she is homozygous for that trait and will express the A blood type.

If a person has two different alleles for a single gene trait, he or she is *heterozygous* for that trait. So if a person has an A blood-type gene allele on one number 9 chromosome and a B blood-type gene allele on the other number 9 chromosome, that person is heterozygous for that trait and will express the AB blood type. Because the A and B alleles are equally dominant *(co-dominant),* they will both be expressed in the actual blood type.

There are differences in expression of the alleles for a trait depending on whether an allele is dominant or is recessive. If a person has an A blood-type gene allele on one number 9 chromosome and an O blood-type gene allele on the other number 9 chromosome, that person is heterozygous for that trait and expresses only the A blood type. Because the A allele is dominant and the O allele is recessive, they will not both be expressed in the actual blood type. Only the dominant allele is expressed, and the recessive allele is "silent." More information about dominant, recessive, and co-dominant expression is presented later on p. 73.

Phenotype

The **phenotype** of any gene for a person is what characteristic can actually be observed or, in some cases, determined by a laboratory test. For example, the person who has the AO gene alleles for blood type has the phenotype of type A blood. A person with curly hair has a curly hair phenotype regardless of whether he or she has two alleles for curly hair or one allele for curly hair and one allele for straight hair.

Genotype

The **genotype** for a person's single gene trait is what the actual alleles are for that trait—not just what can be observed. A person with a phenotype of type A blood could have either an AA genotype or an AO genotype. The person who has type O blood would have an OO genotype. When a person has homozygous alleles for a trait, we would expect the genotype and phenotype to be the same. When a person has heterozygous alleles for a trait, the phenotype and the genotype are not always the same. Recessive traits are expressed only when the person is homozygous for the alleles. Thus for recessive traits, phenotype and genotype are the same. Dominant traits are expressed whether the person is homozygous for the gene alleles or heterozygous for the gene alleles. Thus for dominant traits, phenotype and genotype can be the same but do not have to be the same.

Gene Expression

The purpose of a gene is to code for the making of a specific protein used by a cell, tissue, or organ within a person. For example, the hormone *insulin* is a protein. When a person's blood glucose level starts to rise, the beta cells of the pancreas rapidly make insulin to meet the immediate needs of the person for blood glucose homeostasis.

To continue the cookbook analogy, each gene is the recipe needed to make a specific protein. All the "stuff" that a human body makes—every hormone, every enzyme, every growth factor, every chemical needed to keep the person functioning—is a protein. These proteins are *gene products* because they are produced when the right gene is "turned on" or *expressed.* Just a few examples of gene products are insulin, hemoglobin, erythropoietin, angiotensin, and estrogen.

Protein Synthesis

Protein synthesis is the process by which genes are used to make the proteins needed for physiologic function. Remember from the science class, proteins are made up of individual amino acids hooked together like beads on a string. There are 22 different amino acids. Every protein has a specific amount of the amino acids and a specific order in which they are put together. If even one amino acid is out of order or completely deleted from the sequence, the protein will be incorrect and unable to do its job in the body.

For example, the hormone *insulin* is a protein that contains 51 amino acids in a specific sequence. If some of the amino acids are missing or are in the wrong position, the protein made would be different from real insulin and could not reduce blood glucose levels. So the actual order of the amino acids is critical for the final function of any protein.

Within the DNA there is a code for each amino acid (Table 6-1). Each amino acid code is three bases (nucleotides) long. A gene is the recipe for making a specific protein. It contains all the amino acid codes in exactly the right order for that protein. For example, the final active form of the protein *insulin* has 51 amino acids. Thus the minimum number of bases needed in the gene for insulin would be 153 (3 bases per amino acid × 51 amino acids). Fig. 6-15 shows an example of short protein made up of only seven amino acids.

Fig. 6-16 shows the model of using DNA to make proteins. To think of this process in terms of the cookbook, the entire genome in each cell is the giant cookbook in the library. When a specific protein needs to be made, the chapter for that protein is opened (the chromosome) and the right recipe is found (the gene). The recipe is copied (transcribed) onto a note card (messenger ribonucleic acid, or mRNA) and taken to the kitchen (endoplasmic reticulum). In the kitchen, all the ingredients (amino acids) are put together (translated) in the right order with the help of bowls, ovens, pans, potholders, and other kitchen tools (adapter and transfer molecules).

TABLE 6-1 Examples of DNA Codes and RNA Codons for Selected Amino Acids

Amino Acid	DNA Code(s)	RNA Codons
Alanine	CGA, CGG, CGT, CGC	GCU, GCC, GCA, GCG
Glycine	CCA, CCG, CCT, CCC	GGU, GGC, GGA, GGG
Isoleucine	TAA, TAG, TAT	AUU, AUC, AUA
Lysine	TTT, TTC	AAA, AAG
Tryptophan	ACC	UGG
Tyrosine	ATA, ATG	UAU, UAC
Start		AUG
Stop		UAA, UAG, UGA

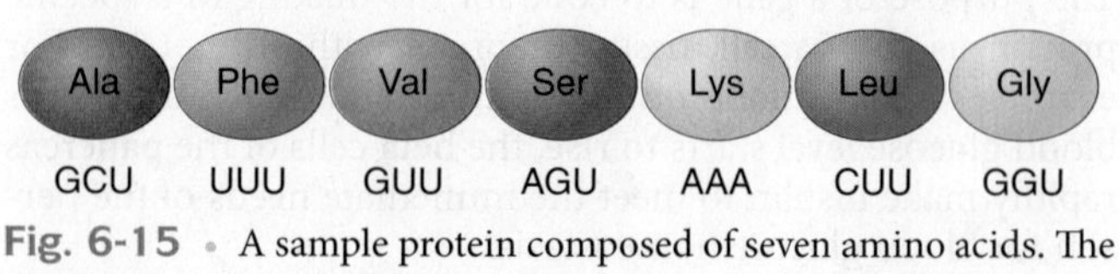
Ala
Phe
Val
Ser
Lys
Leu
Gly
GCU
UUU
GUU
AGU
AAA
CUU
GGU

Fig. 6-15 • A sample protein composed of seven amino acids. The RNA codons for the individual amino acids are listed below each amino acid.

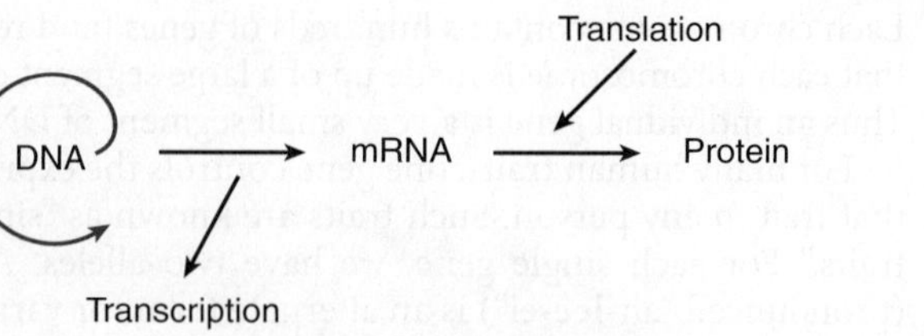
Translation
DNA
mRNA
Protein
Transcription

Fig. 6-16 • The genetic model for protein synthesis.

Many of the steps of protein synthesis use the same enzymes and similar processes as in DNA synthesis, although there are a few differences. During DNA synthesis, the entire DNA strand is replicated into a new DNA strand. For protein synthesis, only the area of the DNA that contains the gene for the specific protein needed is transcribed into RNA.

RNA itself is similar to DNA with a few differences. First, the sugar attached to the base is a ribose sugar (hence the name "ribo"nucleic acid). In addition, thymine does not exist in RNA. Instead, a similar base called *uracil* is placed in RNA instead of thymine. This means there is a specific three-base RNA code (called a *codon*) for each amino acid (see Table 6-1). These RNA codes are complementary to the DNA amino acid codes, with uracil in place of thymine. In addition to the amino acid codes, RNA contains some "stop" codes that tell the process when the protein is finished. Last, RNA is single-stranded instead of double-stranded (Fig. 6-17).

Mutations

Mutations are DNA changes that are passed from one generation to another and thus are *inherited.* An inherited mutation does not have to mean that the mutation is passed from one human generation to another. It can mean that the mutation is passed from one *cell* generation to another and may affect only certain tissues within a person rather than be a problem within a family. These mutations occur in general body cells (somatic cells) and are known as *somatic mutations.* Because these mutations occur in a person's cells after conception, the person cannot pass a somatic mutation on to his or her children. One problem of somatic mutations is an increased risk for cancer in cells with such mutations.

When mutations occur in sex cells, they are called *germline mutations.* A germline mutation *can* be passed on to a person's children, and each of that child's cells will contain the mutated DNA.

DNA bases can be altered or "mutated" accidentally. Sometimes the wrong base is put into a certain position in the newly made DNA strand during cell division. It is also possible for a base to be accidentally deleted or an extra base placed into the strand. Usually the "spell check" work of enzymes during the making of DNA prevents these changes, although some changes probably occur daily in any one person. If these changes occur in a gene area of the DNA, the change can alter the expression of that gene and an incorrect gene product

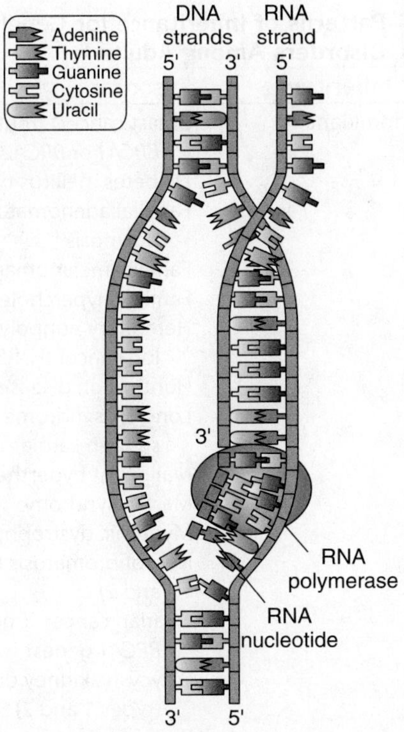
Adenine
Thymine
Guanine
Cytosine
Uracil
DNA strands
RNA strand
5'
3'
5'
3'
RNA polymerase
RNA nucleotide
3'
5'

Fig. 6-17 • RNA transcription for protein synthesis.

(protein) might result. So mutations can have serious results, although some mutations may actually be beneficial. Gene mutations or variations that increase the risk for a disorder are known as *susceptibility* genes. Gene mutations or variations that decrease the risk for a disorder are known as *protective* or *resistance* genes.

The genes for most proteins are generally the same in all people. Sometimes a base in one person's gene for a specific protein is not the same as that in most people. This difference can be either a variation known as a *single nucleotide polymorphism,* or *SNP* ("snip"), or it can be a mutation. When a base difference allows the protein to be made but there are differences in how well the protein works, the difference is called a variation or a **polymorphism.** When a base difference causes a loss of protein function, it is called a **mutation.** The two types of mutations are point mutations and frameshift mutations.

Point mutations are the substitution of one base for another. A change has been made at a single point of DNA, and the type of change is a base substitution, not a deletion or addition. So the triplets, or three-base codes, remain intact, although one may be incorrect. This change may or may not alter amino acid position or protein synthesis.

Below is an analogy to a point mutation. The top sentence represents the "reading sequence" for a specific gene:

THE BIG DOG ATE THE CAT

THE BIG DOG ATE THE CAP

A point mutation, as seen in the bottom sentence, has changed the *t* in cat to a *p*. The coded message is similar but not exactly the same.

Sometimes a point mutation can change the protein (gene product) a little, but it can still function. Sometimes, however, a point mutation changes the protein just enough that it does not work at all. It all depends on how critical the amino acid that changed was to the function of the protein.

Frameshift mutations occur when a whole base or group of bases is added or deleted. This type of mutation always alters amino acid position, disrupts the reading frame, and stops protein synthesis. These changes ruin the reading sequence of the gene from the mutation on down. *These changes are very serious because a normal product cannot be made from a gene with such a mutation.*

Below is an analogy to a frameshift mutation. The top sentence represents the correct "reading sequence" for a specific gene.

THE BIG DOG ATE THE CAT

THB IGD OGA TET HEC AT

THE PBI GDO GAT ETH ECA T

A base deletion mutation, as seen in the middle sentence, has removed the *E* in "THE," shifting the rest of the bases to the left (for the three-base codes) and disrupting the reading frame. A base addition mutation, as seen in the bottom sentence, has added a *P* to "BIG," shifting the three-base reading codes to the right and disrupting the reading frame. The coded message (recipe) has been lost completely.

Changes in genes, even small changes, can have serious results. Some changes would inactivate a protein. Other changes may alter how often or how well a group of cells divides. Gene variations may cause one person to have a greater-than-normal risk for developing a disease. A different variation in the same gene may cause another person to have a smaller-than-normal risk for developing the same disease.

PATTERNS OF INHERITANCE

For every single gene trait, a person inherits one allele for that gene from his or her mother and one allele from his or her father. How these traits are expressed depend on whether one or both alleles are "dominant" or whether one or both alleles are "recessive." Expression also depends on whether the gene for the trait is located on an autosome or on a sex chromosome.

◄ ANIMATION: Hereditary Traits

It is possible to determine how the gene for a specific trait is passed from one human generation to the next **(transmitted).** By looking at how that trait is expressed through several generations of a family, patterns emerge that indicate whether that gene is dominant or recessive and whether it is located on an autosomal chromosome or on one of the sex chromosomes. This information can be determined through pedigree analysis. Determining inheritance patterns for a specific trait makes it possible to predict the risk for any one person to have a trait or transmit that trait to his or her children.

Pedigree

A **pedigree** is a graph of a family history for a specific trait or health problem over several generations. Fig. 6-18 shows a typical three-generation pedigree. Fig. 6-19 shows the most common symbols used when creating a pedigree. Although the term *pedigree* is the correct genetic term, some patients are offended by this term. Use the term *family tree* in place of pedigree when

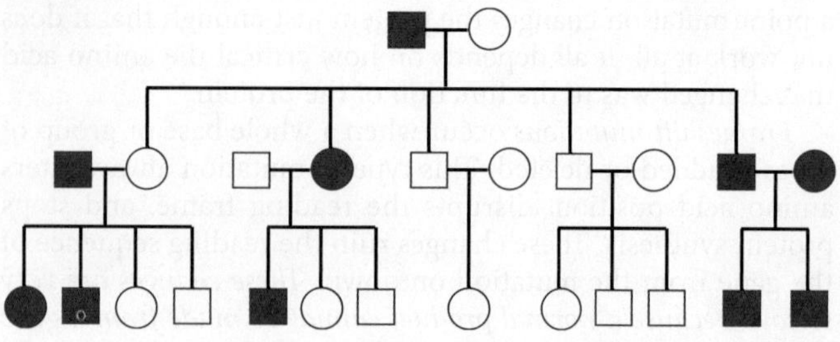

Fig. 6-18 • A three-generation pedigree showing an autosomal dominant pattern of inheritance.

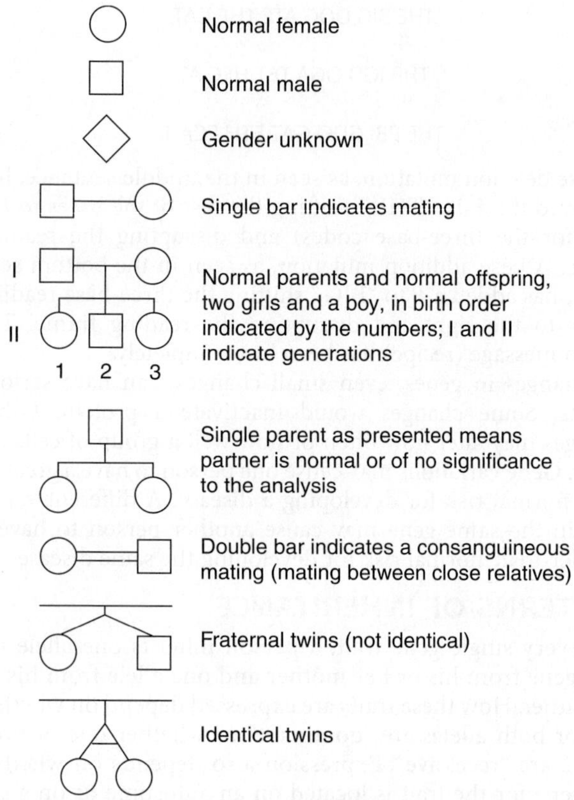
Normal female
Normal male
Gender unknown
Single bar indicates mating
I
II
1 2 3
Normal parents and normal offspring, two girls and a boy, in birth order indicated by the numbers; I and II indicate generations
Single parent as presented means partner is normal or of no significance to the analysis
Double bar indicates a consanguineous mating (mating between close relatives)
Fraternal twins (not identical)
Identical twins

Fig. 6-19 • Standard pedigree symbols.

TABLE 6-2 Patterns of Inheritance for Genetic Disorders Among Adults

Pattern of Inheritance	Disorder
Autosomal dominant	Breast cancer* (mutation of *BRCA1* or *BRCA2* genes)
	Diabetes mellitus type 2*
	Familial adenomatous polyposis
	Familial melanoma
	Familial hypercholesterolemia
	Hereditary nonpolyposis colon cancer (HNCC)
	Huntington disease
	Long QT syndrome and sudden cardiac death
	Malignant hyperthermia (MH)
	Marfan syndrome
	Myotonic dystrophy
	Neurofibromatosis (types 1 and 2)
	Ovarian cancer* (mutation of *BRCA1* genes)
	Polycystic kidney disease† (types 1 and 2)
	Retinitis pigmentosa†
	von Willebrand's disease
Autosomal recessive	Albinism
	Alpha$_1$-antitrypsin deficiency
	Beta thalassemia
	Bloom syndrome
	Cystic fibrosis
	Hereditary hemochromatosis
	Sickle cell disease
	Xeroderma pigmentosum
Sex-linked recessive	Glucose-6-phosphate dehydrogenase deficiency
	Hemophilia
	Red-green color blindness
Complex disorders/ Familial clustering	Alzheimer's disease
	Autoimmune disorders
	Bipolar disorder
	Parkinson disease
	Schizophrenia
	Hypertension
	Rheumatoid arthritis

*Some disorders have both a genetic and nongenetic form.
†Some disorders have more than one genetic form and can also be autosomal recessive.

talking with patients. Construct a pedigree that includes at least three generations when taking the family history. When analyzing a pedigree, note the answers to these questions:

- Is any pattern of inheritance recognized, or does the trait appear sporadic?
- Is the trait expressed equally among male and female family members or unequally?
- Is the trait present in every generation, or does it skip one or more generations?
- Do only affected people have children affected with the trait, or do unaffected people also have children who express the trait?

The four types of inheritance patterns associated with single gene-controlled traits are autosomal dominant, autosomal recessive, sex-linked dominant, and sex-linked recessive. Each inheritance pattern has specific defining criteria. Table 6-2 lists the patterns of inheritance for some disorders that either are identified in adults or may be identified in children who live to adulthood.

Some traits and disorders cluster within a family but do not follow any known pattern of inheritance. Although no specific gene has yet been found for some of these disorders, the clustering suggests a genetic basis. It is thought that for some of the disorders that show familial clustering, environmental factors may modify a genetic predisposition. Continued genetic research may solve the familial clustering gene puzzle.

Autosomal Dominant Pattern of Inheritance

Autosomal dominant (AD) single gene traits require that the gene alleles controlling the trait be located on an autosomal chromosome. A dominant gene allele is expressed even when only one allele of the pair is dominant. Other criteria for AD patterns of inheritance include:

- The trait appears in every generation with no skipping.
- The risk for an affected person to pass the trait to a child is 50% with each pregnancy.
- Unaffected people do not have affected children; therefore their risk is essentially 0%.
- The trait is found about equally in males and females.

An example of an AD trait is blood type A. If a person is homozygous for the blood type A allele, he or she will express type A blood (with genotype being identical to the phenotype). If a person is heterozygous for the blood type A allele, with the other allele being type O (which is a recessive trait), he or she will also express type A blood. In this case, however, the phenotype is not identical to the genotype. *When a dominant allele is paired with a recessive allele, only the dominant allele is expressed.* The blood type B allele is a dominant allele. When a B allele is paired with an O allele, B blood type is expressed. When a person has one blood type A allele and a blood type B allele, however, both alleles are expressed (because they are equally dominant) and the person has type AB blood.

When a person actually has a specific gene allele, he or she is said to "carry" that gene allele. This issue is different from being a "carrier" of a recessive allele. Carrier status is discussed later under Autosomal Recessive Pattern of Inheritance.

Some health problems inherited as autosomal dominant (AD) single gene traits are not apparent at birth but develop as the person ages (see Table 6-2). Two factors that affect the expression of some AD single gene traits are penetrance and expressivity.

Penetrance

Penetrance is how often or how well, within a population, a gene is expressed when it is present. Some genes are more penetrant than others. For example, the gene for Huntington disease (HD) has an autosomal dominant pattern of transmission. Therefore a person who has one HD allele is at risk for developing HD. This gene is "highly penetrant" (sometimes called "fully penetrant"). This means that if a person has the HD gene allele, his or her risk of expressing the gene and developing the disease is about 99.99%.

Some dominant gene alleles have "reduced" penetrance. This means that a person who has the gene mutation has a lower risk for this gene being expressed and actually developing the disorder.

Penetrance is calculated by examining a population of people known to have the gene mutation and assessing the percentage that go on to express the gene by developing the disorder. For example, the *BRCA2* gene mutation increases a person's risk for breast cancer. This gene is not fully penetrant, so some women (and men) who have the gene do not develop breast cancer. The penetrance rate for this gene mutation is calculated to be between 60% and 80%, meaning that a person who has the gene mutation has a 60% to 80% risk for developing breast cancer. Although this risk is far higher than among people who do not have this mutant gene, the risk is not 100%. Having the gene mutation does not absolutely predict that the person will develop breast cancer—just that the risk is high.

Expressivity

Expressivity is the degree of expression a person has when a dominant gene is present. So it is a personal issue, not a population issue. The gene is *always* expressed, but some people have more severe problems than do other people. For example, the gene mutation for one form of neurofibromatosis (NF1) is dominant. Some people with this gene have only a few light brown skin tone areas known as *café au lait spots.* These skin lesions can be so minor that the person may not even be aware that they are present. Other people with the same gene mutation develop hundreds of tumors (neurofibromas) that protrude through the skin. Expressivity accounts for some variation in genetic disease severity.

Autosomal Recessive Pattern of Inheritance

Autosomal recessive (AR) single gene traits require that the gene controlling the trait be located on an autosomal chromosome. The trait can be expressed *only* when both alleles are present. Table 6-2 lists some AR adult disorders. Fig. 6-20 shows a typical pedigree for an AR disorder. Criteria for AR patterns of inheritance include:

- The trait may not appear in all generations of any one branch of a family.
- The trait or characteristic often first appears only in siblings rather than in the parents themselves.
- About 25% of a family will be affected and express the trait.
- The children of two affected parents will *always* be affected (risk is 100%).
- Unaffected people who are carriers (heterozygous for the trait) and do not express the trait themselves *can* transmit the trait to their children if their partner is either also a carrier or is affected.
- The trait is found about equally in male and female members of the same family.

An example of an AR trait is type O blood. The blood-type O allele is recessive, and both alleles must be type O (homozygous) for the person to express type O blood. If only one allele is a type O allele and the other allele is either type A or type B, the dominant allele will be expressed and the O allele, although present, is not expressed. For AR single gene traits, phenotype and genotype are always the same

A person who has one mutated allele for a recessive genetic disorder is a **carrier.** A carrier, even though he or she may have one mutated allele, does not usually have any manifesta-

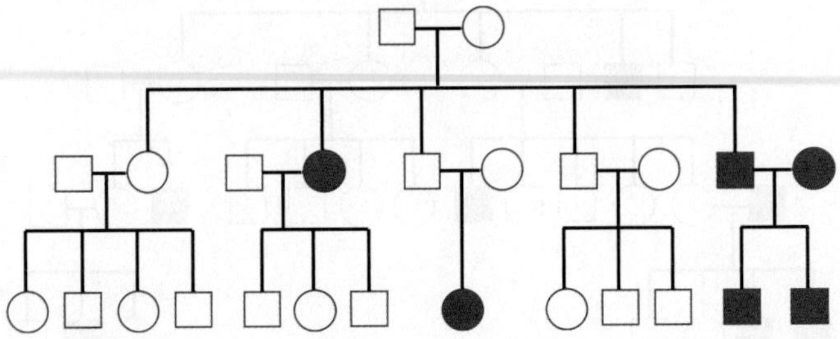

Fig. 6-20 • A typical pedigree showing an autosomal recessive pattern of inheritance.

tions of the disorder but can pass this mutated allele on to his or her children. For some autosomal recessive disorders, a carrier may have very mild manifestations. One example is sickle cell trait. A person with two sickle cell alleles has the disease and has many associated health problems. A carrier with one sickle cell allele (and is said to have the "sickle cell trait") may be healthy most of the time and have manifestations only under conditions of severe hypoxia.

Sex-Linked Recessive Pattern of Inheritance

Some genes are present only on the sex chromosomes. The Y chromosome has only a few genes that are not also present on the X chromosome. These few genes are important for male sexual development. The X chromosome, however, has many single genes that are not present on the Y or elsewhere in the human genome. Some of these genes are specific for female sexual development, but there are also several hundred genes on the X chromosome that code for other functions. Few traits or disorders have an X-linked dominant pattern of expression, and they are not discussed in this chapter.

Because the number of X chromosomes in males and females is not the same (1:2), the number of X-linked chromosome genes in the two genders is also unequal. Males have only one X chromosome. As a result, X-linked recessive genes have dominant expression in males and recessive expression in females. This difference in expression is because males do not have a second X chromosome to balance the presence of a recessive gene on the first X chromosome.

Sex-linked (X-linked) recessive single gene traits require that the gene allele be present on both of the X chromosomes for the trait to be expressed in females (homozygous) and on only one X chromosome for the trait to be expressed in males. Fig. 6-21 shows a typical pedigree for a sex-linked recessive disorder. Features of a sex-linked recessive pattern of inheritance include:

- The incidence of the trait is much higher among males in a family than among females.
- The trait cannot be passed down (transmitted) from father to son.
- Transmission of the trait is from father to all daughters (who will be carriers).
- Female carriers have a 50% risk (with each pregnancy) of passing the gene to their children.

Complex Inheritance and Familial Clustering

Some health problems appear in families at a rate higher than normal and greater than can be accounted for by chance alone; however, no specific pattern occurs within a family.

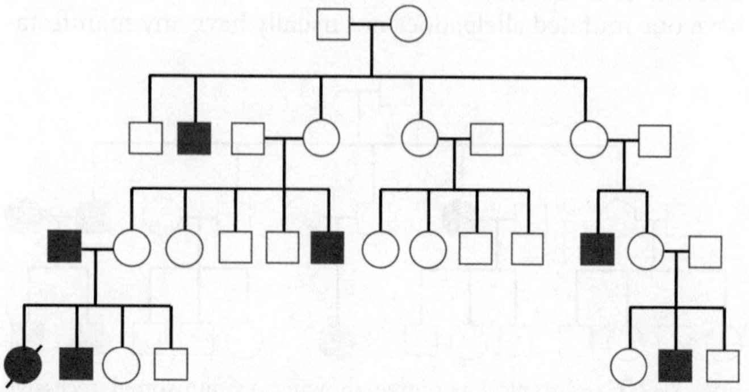

Fig. 6-21 • A typical pedigree showing a sex-linked (X-linked) recessive pattern of inheritance.

Although clusters suggest a genetic influence, it is likely that additional factors, such as gender and the environment, also influence disease development or disease severity. Such disorders include Alzheimer's disease, type 1 diabetes, and many others. These disorders are often called *complex* and *multifactorial,* because although an increased genetic risk may be present, the risk is changed by diet, lifestyle, exposure to toxins, infectious agents, and other factors. For example, the risk for developing type 2 diabetes mellitus appears to be inherited as an autosomal dominant pattern. However, whether the person who has inherited the genetic risk ever actually develops the disease depends on other factors, such as obesity and a sedentary lifestyle.

GENETIC TESTING

Purpose of Testing

Many people are eager to have genetic testing but also are fearful of genetic testing. The lay public often believe that a single genetic test can "tell everything about a person." Although genetic testing has the potential to be that informative, this is not currently the case. *It is important to remember that no single person is genetically perfect.*

Genetic testing can be performed with many different techniques. Some genetic tests are specific for a disorder. Others may show a gene variation but the significance of the variation may not be known. Unexpected information can be found during genetic testing. Some ordinary tests, such as blood typing and tissue typing, provide genetic information. Tests that measure the amount of an enzyme or protein also provide genetic information.

Actual genetic testing can be performed at many levels. Cellular or biochemical tests provide information about gene products made by a cell, tissue, or organ. Chromosomes can be assessed for missing, extra, or broken chromosomes. Chromosome segments can be analyzed for abnormalities or changes from normal positions. The sequence of a gene can be examined to determine variation or mutation. At present, not all genes can be analyzed and the analysis of even one gene is limited by expense and availability. Specific base pairs can be evaluated for mutations. These tests are currently expensive, and the results may not be conclusive. Table 6-3 lists purposes of genetic testing for adults.

Benefits and Risks of Testing

Genetic testing is different from any other type of testing for many reasons. *It is important to remember that just because the technology exists does not mean it should be used in all cases.* Informed consent is required before genetic testing is undertaken. The person tested is the one who gives consent, even though genetic testing *always* gives information about a family and family members—not just the patient.

Benefits of genetic testing include the ability to confirm a diagnosis or to test people who are at risk for a health problem but do not as yet have any symptoms (presymptomatic testing). The information can help a person, family, and their health care provider develop a specific plan of care or early detection. For example, in the case of a strong genetic predisposition for colon cancer, identifying a patient before symptoms appear allows interventions to prevent the disease or to diagnosis it earlier, when cure is more likely.

Risks are associated with genetic testing that are not associated with other types of tests. Genetic testing results do not

TABLE 6-3 Purposes of Genetic Testing for Adults

Purpose/Type	Definition
Carrier testing	Determining whether a patient without symptoms has an allele for a recessive disorder that could be transmitted to his or her children. Disorders for which carrier testing is common include sickle cell disease, hemophilia, hereditary hemochromatosis, cystic fibrosis, beta thalassemia, and Tay-Sachs disease.
Diagnostic testing	Determining whether a patient has or does not have a mutation that increases the risk for a specific disorder.
Symptomatic	Patient has clinical manifestations; test results confirm a diagnosis.
Presymptomatic	Patient has no clinical manifestations but is at high risk for inheriting a specific genetic disorder for which there is no known prevention or treatment. A disorder for which presymptomatic testing is commonly performed is Huntington disease.
Predisposition	Family history or genetic testing indicates risk is high for a known genetic disorder. The patient does not have any manifestations but wants to know whether he or she has the specific mutation and what the chances are that it will be expressed. Disorders for which predisposition testing is often performed include hereditary breast/ovarian cancer and hereditary colorectal cancers. The advantage of predisposition testing is that the patient can then engage in heightened screening activities or medical and surgical interventions that reduce risk.

change. This means that a positive test result cannot be "taken back." The risks of genetic testing may include psychological or social risks, as well as a risk for family disruption. Often genetic tests are expensive and may not be covered by insurance. Some genetic tests have limited value for predicting future risk. Testing may identify a patient at great risk for the future development of a serious health problem that cannot be prevented. Such a disorder is Huntington disease (HD), which currently has no treatment. Knowing positive test results in this case can lead to depression, blame, and guilt.

Another risk of genetic testing is that positive results may be used to discriminate against a person or a family. Some protection is in place to prevent health insurance companies from failing to insure a person or dropping the coverage of a person who is at high risk for developing a serious illness (e.g., breast or ovarian cancer). However, there are no protections against rate hikes or exclusions of specific treatments. Patients often fear workplace discrimination and personal discrimination if positive test results become known.

Genetic Counseling

Genetic testing is not a standard test that any person should have performed without knowing the advantages and disadvantages. Counseling patients before, during, and after testing is critical. Entire families may be a part of the genetic evaluation and follow-up. For example, a 45-year-old woman has breast cancer. In her family, her mother, grandmother, brother, and one sister have all had breast cancer. This woman's older daughter wonders whether she has a gene mutation for breast cancer and asks to be tested. When she and her younger sister are tested, the older daughter does not have the mutation but the younger sister does.

Genetic counseling is a process—not a single session or a single recommendation. This process should begin when the patient or family is first identified as potentially having a genetic problem. The process continues through actual testing if the decision to test is made, and it continues through interpretation of results and follow-up. Steps in the process are listed in Chart 6-1.

As a nurse and patient advocate, determine whether the patient understands the consequences of testing. Often a patient may request genetic testing even when there is no indication of an increased risk for a genetic disorder. Counseling and evaluation can help patients understand whether any useful information could be obtained from testing.

Counseling is performed by a professional or a team who have defined expertise in interpretation of genetic testing results. Such professionals include advanced practice nurses with specialization in genetics, certified genetic counselors, clinical geneticists, and medical geneticists. Each profession has a different level of preparation in genetics and different skills or roles in the counseling process. For example, an advanced practice nurse may counsel a patient about the Huntington disease gene mutation because this test is not ambiguous and the gene is highly penetrant. When the test shows a variation or mutation in an unusual gene region or when penetrance is reduced, the patient may best be served by counseling from a clinical or medical geneticist.

No matter which professional is involved in genetic counseling, a key feature of this counseling is to be "nondirective." The counselor provides as much information as possible about the risks and benefits but does not in any way influence the patient's decision to test or not to test. Once the patient has made the decision, the counselor supports the patient and the decision. Chart 6-2 lists NIC intervention activities for adult patients considering or having genetic testing.

Ethical Issues

Many ethical issues are considered with genetic testing. Some of the most important issues focus on the patient's right to know versus the right not to know his or her gene status, confidentiality, coercion, and sharing of information.

The right to know genetic risk versus the right to not know is the individual patient's choice. Sometimes a patient's right to know has an impact on the right of another family member not to know. For example, if a patient's maternal grandfather had Huntington disease (HD) and the patient wants to know whether he or she has that gene, he or she is tested. This person's mother does not want to know whether she has the gene. If the patient is tested and found to have the gene, because HD is autosomal dominant, the only way he or she could have the gene is if this person's mother also has it. Thus when the patient finds out he or she is positive and tells the mother, the mother will learn that she is also positive, even if she did not want to know.

Confidentiality is crucial to the genetic counseling process. The results of a genetic test must remain confidential to the pa-

Chart 6-1 BEST PRACTICE FOR PATIENT SAFETY & QUALITY CARE

Steps for Genetic Testing and Counseling

PRE-TESTING ASSESSMENT AND PATIENT EDUCATION (MAY TAKE MULTIPLE SESSIONS)

- Determining patient understanding and why testing or counseling is being sought
- Determining whether testing is reasonable (considering cost of the test, specificity, probable risk, accuracy of testing)
- Establishing a trusting professional relationship
- Ensuring privacy and confidentiality
- Reviewing informed consent procedures
- Assessing the patient's ability to communicate accurately (including language issues, cognitive function, sensory perception)
- Assessing the patient's psychosocial status and availability of social support
- Taking a detailed patient health history (including drugs, diet, exercise, hormonal history, lifestyle issues)
- Obtaining physical assessment data relevant to the at-risk disorder
- Taking a detailed family history and constructing a three-generation pedigree (minimum)
- Obtaining and verifying information obtained from:
  - Patient
  - Family members
  - Medical records
  - Pathology reports
  - Death certificates
- Interpreting the family history
- Discussing the consequences of testing
- Discussing patient rights and obligations regarding disclosure of information
- Discussing testing options
- Assessing to determine whether coercion is occurring
- Obtaining material to be tested (usually blood)

TEST RESULT PRESENTATION

- Re-assessing the patient's wish to know or not know the test results
- Respecting the patient's decision not to know the test results
- Ensuring privacy and confidentiality
- Presenting the test results
- Interpreting the test results
- Assessing the patient's perception of the test results

FOLLOW-UP

- Supporting the patient's decision to disclose or not disclose the information to other family members
- Discussing the potential risks for other family members
- Ensuring privacy and confidentiality
- Addressing the patient's concerns
- Discussing prevention, early detection, and treatment options
- Discussing family concerns
- Addressing psychosocial issues
- Discussing available resources for information, support, and further counseling
- Providing summary of results and consultation to the patient

tient. The results cannot be given to a family member, other health care provider, or insurance carrier without the patient's permission.

Coercion is possible by other family members and even by health care professionals.

The final decision to have genetic testing or to not have testing rests with the patient. Other people may believe it is important for the patient to have the test; however, the patient must make the decision without such pressures. As a patient advocate, assess whether the patient is freely making the decision to have genetic testing or if someone else is urging the patient to test. This important issue can be difficult to assess. Ask the patient who else in his or her family wants to know the results of testing. An important question to ask is "Will you do anything differently for screening or treatment if the test is positive versus if the test is negative?"

Sharing of test result information, negative or positive, can induce stress. The patient makes the final decision to share the information with family members. Some patients choose not to share this information even when other family members may also be at risk. This can be difficult for the health care provider who knows the patient has a positive test result for a serious inherited condition and the patient chooses not tell other family members who may be at risk. For example, hereditary non-polyposis colon cancer (HNPCC) has an autosomal dominant inheritance pattern and each child of the patient has a 50% risk for having the gene. If the patient chooses not to tell his or her grown children, they then do not have the opportunity for increased screening to find the cancer at an early stage when cure is possible. An ethical dilemma arises when the health care provider wants to inform the children of their risk.

Chart 6-2 **NIC INTERVENTION ACTIVITIES**

The Adult Patient with or at Risk for a Genetic Problem

Genetic Counseling: *Use of an interactive helping process focusing on assisting an individual, family, or group, manifesting or at risk for developing or transmitting a birth defect or genetic condition, to cope*

- Provide privacy and ensure confidentiality.
- Establish a therapeutic relationship based on trust and respect.
- Determine the patient's purpose, goals, and agenda for the genetic counseling session.
- Determine knowledge base, myths, perceptions, and misperceptions related to a birth defect or genetic condition.
- Determine presence and quality of family support, other support systems, and previous coping skills.
- Provide estimates of patient's risk based upon phenotype (patient characteristics), family history (pedigree analysis), calculated risk information, or genotype (genetic testing results).
- Provide estimates of occurrence or recurrence risks for patient and at-risk family members.
- Provide information on the natural history of the disease or condition, treatment and/or management strategies, and preventions strategies, if known.
- Provide information about the risks, benefits, and limitations of treatment/management options, as well as options for dealing with recurrence risk in a nondirective manner.
- Provide decision-making support as patients consider their options.
- Prioritize areas of risk reduction in collaboration with the individual, family, or group.
- Monitor response when patient learns about own genetic risk factors.
- Allow expression of feelings.
- Support patient's coping process.
- Institute crisis support measures as needed.
- Provide referral to genetic health care specialists, as necessary.
- Provide referral to community resources, including genetic support groups, as needed.
- Provide patient a written summary of genetic counseling session, as indicated.

NIC intervention activities selected from Bulechek, G.M., Butcher, H.K., & McCloskey Dochterman, J. (Eds.). (2008). *Nursing interventions classification (NIC)* (5th ed.). St. Louis: Mosby. No part of this work is to be altered without prior written permission from the Publisher.

THE ROLE OF THE MEDICAL-SURGICAL NURSE IN GENETIC COUNSELING

Medical-surgical nurses help patients during the assessing, testing, and counseling processes in many areas, although they do not provide in-depth genetic counseling. Patients often feel most comfortable sharing information with nurses and asking nurses to clarify information.

Nurses may be the first health care professionals to identify a patient at specific genetic risk. Some of the "red flags" that a patient may have an increased genetic risk for a disease or disorder are:

- The disease or disorder occurs at a higher incidence within the family compared with the general population.
- The patient or close family members have another identified genetic problem.
- The incidence of a specific disease or disorder occurs in the patient or in family members at an unusually early age.
- A rare disease is present in two or more family members.
- More than one type of cancer is present in any one person.
- The specific manifestation is associated with one or more genetic disorders (e.g., unusual freckling or skin pigmentation, bicuspid aortic valve, deafness).

The nurse may be the health care professional who first verifies information to bring a genetic problem to light. For example, during an assessment, the patient reveals that her mother died of bone cancer when she was 40 years old. Bone cancer is quite rare among adults; thus the nurse might then ask, "Did your mother ever have any other type of cancer?" Often the patient may then reveal that her mother had breast cancer some years before that ("bone cancer" was actually breast cancer that had spread to the bones). Breast cancer at an early age can indicate a genetic predisposition.

Patients may ask questions that indicate they have an interest in genetic testing. These are examples of questions that may be cues that the patient has genetic concerns:

- Will my children get this disease?
- Because my sister has this problem, what are the chances I might also develop it?
- Is there a way to test and see whether my chances of getting this disease or problem are high or low?

Areas of responsibility for any medical-surgical nurse in working with a patient who is considering or having genetic testing include communication, privacy and confidentiality, information accuracy, patient advocacy, and support.

Communication

Act as a patient advocate by ensuring that communication between the patient and whoever is providing the genetic information is clear. First assess the patient's ability to receive and process information. Can the patient see and hear clearly, or are assistive devices needed? Does the patient understand English, or will an interpreter be needed? Does the patient have adequate cognition at the time of meeting with the genetic professional, or is it impaired by medication, disease, anxiety, or fear?

If the patient appears not to understand terms or jargon during a discussion between him or her and a genetic professional, ask the professional to use common terms and examples for the patient. Verify with the patient that he or she understands or does not understand.

After any discussion about genetic risk or genetic testing, assess the patient's understanding of what was said. Ask the patient to explain, in his or her own words, what the issue means and what his or her expectations are.

Privacy and Confidentiality

All conversations regarding potential diagnoses or genetic testing need to occur in a private environment. The patient has the right to determine who may be a part of the discussion. The patient can decide to exclude his or her primary physician and any family member from the discussion with a genetic professional. It is important that health care professionals who may be present during such discussion do not disclose information, formally or informally, without the patient's permission. It is the nurse's responsibility to protect this information from improper disclosure to family members, other health care professionals, other patients, insurance providers, or anyone not specified by the patient.

Information Accuracy

Correct myths about genetic disorders, and teach patients about the nature of genetic testing. In addition, help patients find accurate and helpful resource materials or websites. Medical-surgical nurses are not genetics experts and would not be expected to be the final source of definitive information; however, they can help ensure that the patient is referred to the correct level of genetic counseling. If you are present during the patient's discussions with a genetics professional, assess whether the patient understands the issues regarding his or her health problem.

Patient Advocacy and Support

Ensure that the patient's rights are not neglected or ignored. Ask the patient privately what his or her wishes are regarding genetic testing. Ask whether another person or agency is insisting on the testing. Remind the patient that he or she does not have to agree to be tested. Verify that he or she has signed an informed consent statement for the test.

Considering or having genetic testing is a stressful experience. The patient and family require strong support and may need help to find the best way to cope. Genetic testing should be performed only after genetic counseling has occurred and should be followed with an opportunity for more counseling.

Patients may feel anger, depression, guilt, or hopelessness. Patients who have positive results from genetic testing may have issues of role changes, risk for early death or disability, and the possibility of having passed the risk for a health problem on to their children. Patients who have an ambiguous test result or one of unknown significance may feel that they have agonized over a decision, spent money, and still have no clear answer or direction. Even patients who have negative genetic test results need counseling and support. Some patients may have an unrealistic view of what a negative result means for their general health. Others may feel guilty that they were "spared" when other family members were not.

Assess the patient's response to genetic test results. Ask about how he or she may have used coping mechanisms in the past. If the patient has disclosed information to family members, assess whether they can help provide patient support or need support themselves. Assess whether the information about positive test results has strained family relationships. Refer the patient to appropriate support groups and general counseling services.

For some positive genetic test results, such as having a *BRCA1* gene mutation, the risk for developing breast cancer is high but is not a certainty. Because the risk is high, the patient should have a plan for prevention and risk reduction. One form of prevention is early detection. Thus a patient who tests positive for a *BRCA1* mutation should have at least yearly mammograms and ovarian ultrasounds to detect cancer at an early stage when it is more easily cured. Teach the patient who has positive test results that indicate an increased risk for a specific health problem about the types of screening procedures that are available and how often screening should occur. For example, some patients at known high genetic risk for breast cancer and ovarian cancer choose the primary prevention methods of bilateral prophylactic mastectomies (surgical removal of the breasts) and oophorectomies (surgical removal of the ovaries). Although these strategies are severe, they are effective and the patient should be informed about their availability.

GET READY FOR THE NCLEX EXAMINATION!

Key Points

Review these Key Points for each NCLEX Examination Client Needs Category.

Safe and Effective Care Environment

- Determine whether an informed consent statement was obtained before any genetic test is performed.
- Keep all patient and family information regarding genetic testing confidential.

Health Promotion and Maintenance

- Identify patients and families at increased genetic risk for disease or disorder.
- Teach patients and families at known increased risk for disease or disorder what types of screening procedures and schedules are most appropriate (check specific disorder chapters for the appropriate screening guidelines).

Psychosocial Integrity

- Assess patients who have received results of genetic testing for responses such as anger, guilt, or depression.
- Allow the patient and family who have been identified as being at increased genetic risk for serious health problems to express concerns and feelings.
- Ensure that the patient who undergoes genetic testing is appropriately counseled before testing, while waiting for test results, and after test results are obtained.

Physiological Integrity

- DNA, genes, and chromosomes are different forms of the same substance.
- All human cells with a nucleus contain all the genes.
- Every time a cell divides, it must replicate its DNA.
- The normal human chromosome number is 46.
- The purpose of a gene is to serve as the instructions for making a specific protein.
- Mutations can change the activity of a protein and have adverse effects on health.
- Many common adult diseases or disorders have a genetic basis (hypertension, diabetes, cancer) although some of these diseases also may occur among people with no genetic risk.
- Having a gene for a disorder does not necessarily mean that the disorder will ever develop.
- Genetic testing reveals information about the patient and his or her family members.

Additional Study Resources

Go to your Companion CD or Evolve at http://evolve.elsevier.com/Iggy/ for *Self-Assessment Questions for the NCLEX Examination.*

evolve Go to Evolve at http://evolve.elsevier.com/Iggy/ for *Prioritization and Delegation Questions for the NCLEX Examination.*

SELECTED BIBLIOGRAPHY

Asterisk indicates a classic or definitive work on this subject.

American Association of Colleges of Nursing. (2006). *Essential nursing competencies and curricula guidelines for genetics and genomics* (endorsed by the AACN, January 2006).

Ashcraft, P.F., Coleman, E.A., Lange, U., Enderlin, C., & Stewart, C.B. (2007). Obtaining family histories from patients with cancer. *Clinical Journal of Oncology Nursing, 11*(1), 119-124, 130-134.

Frazier, L., Johnson, R., & Sparks, E. (2005). Genomics and cardiovascular disease. *Journal of Nursing Scholarship, 37*(4), 315-321.

Hamilton, R., & Bowers, B. (2007). The theory of genetic vulnerability: A Roy model exemplar. *Nursing Science Quarterly, 20*(3), 254-265.

*Jenkins, J. (2002). Genetics competency: New directions for nursing. *AACN Clinical Issues: in Advanced Practice in Acute and Critical Care, 13*(4), 486-491.

Jenkins, J., & Calzone, K. (2007). Establishing the essential nursing competencies for genetics and genomics. *Journal of Nursing Scholarship, 39*(1), 10-16.

Jenkins, J., & Lea, D. (2005). Nursing care in the genomic era: A case-based approach. Boston: Jones & Bartlett.

Kelly, P. (2008). Understanding genomics: No longer an option for gastroenterology nurses. *Gastroenterology Nursing, 31*(1), 45-54.

Kirk, M., Tonkin, E., & Patch, C. (2006). Genetics: Is it part of your role? *Nursing Older People, 18*(8), 22-26.

*Lea, D. (2002). Position statement: Integrating genetics competencies into baccalaureate and advanced nursing education. *Nursing Outlook, 50*(4), 167-168.

Lea, D., Feero, G. & Jenkins, J. (2008). Warfarin therapy and pharmacogenomics: A step toward personalized medicine. *American Nurse Today, 3*(5), 12-13.

Loescher, L., & Merkle, C. (2005). The interface of genomic technology and nursing. *The Journal of Nursing Scholarship, 37*(2), 111-119.

Nussbaum, R., McInnes, R., & Willard, H. (2007). *Thompson & Thompson: Genetics in medicine* (7th ed.). Philadelphia: Saunders.

Nyrhinen, T., Hietala, M., Puukka, P., & Leino-Kilpi, H. (2007). Privacy and equality in diagnostic genetic testing. *Nursing Ethics, 14*(3), 295-308.

*Prows, C., & Prows, D. (2004). Medication selection by genotype. *AJN, 104*(5), 60-70.

Schutte, D. (2006). Alzheimer disease and genetics: Anticipating the questions. *AJN, 106*(12), 40-48.

*Spahis, J. (2002). Human genetics: Constructing a family pedigree. *AJN, 102*(7), 44-50.

Trossman, S. (2006). It's in the genes. *AJN, 106*(2), 74-75.

Warren, B., & Alley, S. (2005). Culture and genetics: Critical aspects within nursing education. *Journal of Nursing Education, 44*(6), 291.

*Winkelman, C. (2004). What every critical care nurse needs to know about the genetic contribution to critical illness. *Critical Care Nurse, 24*(3), 34-45.

7 CHAPTER

Substance Abuse and Medical-Surgical Nursing

Tommie Wright Pniewski

LEARNING OUTCOMES

For clinical competence and success on the NCLEX Examination, study this chapter with these Learning Outcomes in mind:

Safe and Effective Care Environment

1. Prioritize nursing care to keep patients safe when they are in alcohol withdrawal.

Psychosocial Integrity

2. Explain the effects of substance abuse or misuse on the psychological and physical health of individuals and society.
3. Describe the relationship between stress and substance abuse or misuse.

Physiological Integrity

4. Discuss substance abuse or misuse as a major health issue in the United States.
5. Discuss recent biologic and genetic research in the etiology of substance abuse or misuse.
6. Identify assessment findings associated with use of alcohol, nicotine, stimulants, hallucinogens, depressants, opioids, inhalants, and steroids.
7. Identify symptoms that indicate emergency situations associated with the use of alcohol, nicotine, stimulants, hallucinogens, depressants, opioids, inhalants, and steroids.
8. Explain the responsibilities of the nurse when a peer or other health care worker is suspected of abusing or misusing substances.
9. Identify common medication regimens that are used in the emergency treatment of drug withdrawal and adverse reactions to drugs and alcohol.

evolve Go to your Companion CD or Evolve at http://evolve.elsevier.com/Iggy/ for *Self-Assessment Questions for the NCLEX Examination* keyed to these Learning Outcomes.

OVERVIEW OF SUBSTANCE ABUSE AND MISUSE

This chapter provides an introduction to substance abuse and misuse and their importance in caring for medical-surgical patients. Refer to your mental health textbook for more detailed information.

Substance abuse is the excessive use of a chemical substance, such as drugs and alcohol, and the resulting physical and psychological dependence that interferes with life's activities. **Dependence** is a condition that causes a habitual, compulsive, and uncontrollable urge to use a substance. Without the substance, the body experiences severe physiological, psychological, and emotional disturbances.

By contrast, **substance use** is taking chemicals for pleasure without dependence. **Substance misuse** occurs when people use chemicals for reasons other than their intended action. **Addiction** causes negative outcomes after abusers stop using the substance(s). It is a disease caused by changes in the brain that affect human behavior and is manifested by substance craving, seeking, and subsequent use. Symptoms of **withdrawal syndrome** may result if the drug is eliminated suddenly, such as hallucinations, severe irritability, and hyperactivity.

When a patient is addicted, life-threatening health risks increase, especially if he or she already has a health problem. For example, liver, lung, and cardiovascular diseases can occur or worsen as a result of drug abuse. The spread of human immune deficiency virus/acquired immune deficiency syndrome (HIV/AIDS) and sexually transmitted diseases is also linked to substance use and abuse.

Abuse substances may be legal, as in the case of alcohol, or illegal, such as the non-medical use of prescription drugs or methamphetamines. Each year there are alarming increases in the use and abuse of mind- and mood-altering substances, such as alcohol, marijuana, and cocaine and in the use of nontherapeutic prescription drugs. Productivity is drastically reduced, and the cost of drug abuse to society is enormous.

TABLE 7-1 Commonly Abused Substances

STIMULANTS
• Amphetamines
• Methamphetamines
• Cocaine
HALLUCINOGENS AND RELATED COMPOUNDS
• Lysergic acid (LSD)
• Phencyclidine (PCP)
• Ketamine
• 3,4-Methylenedioxymethamphetamine
• Marijuana
DEPRESSANTS
• Benzodiazepines
• Rohypnol
• Gamma hydroxybutyrate (GHB)
• Barbiturates
• Alcohol
INHALANTS
• Solvents
• Gases
• Nitrites
STEROIDS (ANABOLIC)
NARCOTICS: OPIOIDS AND MORPHINE DERIVATIVES

In addition to alcohol and nicotine, categories of substances commonly abused or have the potential for misuse include (Table 7-1):

- Stimulants
- Hallucinogens
- Depressants
- Opioids (narcotics)
- Inhalants
- Steroids

Stimulants are abused because Western society seeks a "faster, better, and longer" way of life. *Hallucinogens* continue to be popular in various forms but are most commonly mind-altering drugs, such as phencyclidine (PCP) and lysergic acid (LSD). *Depressants*, including the anxiolytics, are used as a way to respond to the ever-increasing demands of today's busy lifestyles. *Opioids*, although important for therapeutic uses for pain relief, continue to be misused or abused in the drug community. The incidence and prevalence of substance abuse vary among the drug categories.

WOMEN'S HEALTH CONSIDERATIONS

Women of all races, ages, educational backgrounds, cultures, and community types are among the drug users in the United States. Data about the misuse or abuse of drugs among women are becoming increasingly more available as the nursing profession seeks to improve women's health. Women usually abuse more than one drug. Research also shows that women are less likely to enter treatment for substance abuse than men. However, once in treatment, success rates are the same as those of men. Factors that affect successful outcomes for women are correlated with education level and a history of victimization (National Institute of Drug Abuse [NIDA], 2006).

CULTURAL AWARENESS

Culture influences every aspect of a person's life. The nurse needs to demonstrate competence in understanding the cultural influences that are related to drug abuse to plan care that will be effective. In addition, an understanding of the patient's culture helps avoid making assumptions about substance abuse. Some behaviors that are interpreted within the Western culture as negative responses are considered normal, even reverent, in some cultures, as in the case of avoiding eye contact. Chapter 4 discusses culture in detail.

SUBSTANCE ABUSE, STRESS, AND ADDICTION

Many people abuse substances for stress relief. Stress results in stimulation of the hypothalamus, the center for emotional responses. Responses to external stress (situational or ingested chemicals) or internal stress (disease or withdrawal of drugs) trigger chemical and hormonal responses in the body that are controlled by the hypothalamus. For example, corticotropin-releasing hormone (CRH) increases to stimulate adrenocorticotropic hormone (ACTH) in the pituitary gland, resulting in more cortisol secretion by the adrenal cortex. Cortisol travels throughout the body enabling the body to cope with the stress. It influences the continued response to the stress or reduction depending on the severity of the stressor.

Frequently triggered stress responses can result in a more sensitive response. Continued abuse of the substance creates a cycle of ever-increasing amounts of the drug needed to sustain the desired level of response to the drug. The body also responds with "withdrawal" responses when deprived of the substance. The cyclic ingestion-withdrawal response creates the environment for addiction.

GENETIC CONSIDERATIONS

Efforts continue to identify links between substance abuse and genetics. Current National Institute of Drug Abuse (NIDA) research is directed toward assessment of cognitive deficits associated with illicit drug use. A relationship between patients with antisocial personalities, environmental risk factors, and illicit drug abuse seems to exist. There is evidence that cognitive deficits due to antisocial behavioral tendencies may have a biologic component in association with substance abuse.

A study by the Virginia Commonwealth University identified evidence that suggests that genetic factors contribute to misuse, abuse, or dependence from illicit drug use (Nauert, 2006). Another study suggests that the genes associated with illegal drug abuse are not the same as those associated with legal substances like alcohol and nicotine. Studies of twins also found a strong influence of genetics associated with susceptibility to drug abuse and dependence (Nauert, 2007).

SUBSTANCE ABUSE OR MISUSE AND THE HOSPITALIZED PATIENT

Substance abuse occurs when these criteria are met:

- Losing control in use of the drug
- Ingesting the drug even though the drug has caused adverse conditions in the body

- Demonstrating cognitive, behavioral, and physiologic disturbances with the abuse of drugs or inhalants

The patient who has coexisting problems with substance use or abuse and medical problems presents a complex challenge for the health care team. As part of the comprehensive health assessment, they carefully assess for signs, symptoms, and/or history of substance abuse.

Alcohol, tobacco, prescription, over-the-counter (OTC), and illicit drug use must be determined. As a complementary therapy, herbal use is important to identify to be alert for interactions or symptomatic withdrawal from natural substances. The patient who habitually uses any substance requires closer observation for withdrawal symptoms than the occasional user. The health care team needs to anticipate complications associated with specific substances of abuse to adequately address the health and safety needs of the patient.

Effective pain management may present special problems if the patient has received long-term treatment for chronic pain. When opioids are used for chronic pain, effective pain management is often more difficult to achieve. Assessment and subsequent relief of pain are altered with the patient who currently abuses or misuses substances. Interference with the administration of the patient's daily use of routine opioids or other substances can result in withdrawal symptoms. Undertreatment of patient-reported pain when he or she has a history of nontherapeutic substance use is common. Refer to Chapter 5 for interventions for pain management.

Understanding the influence of abusive substances is an important aspect of patient education. Some chemicals affect therapeutic medications and can increase the severity of life-threatening risks. Room assignment, delegation to personnel, staffing assignments, and other nursing decisions are important when caring for the patient with a substance abuse diagnosis. The length and course of hospitalization and recovery may be altered as a result of complications related to the abuse.

Caring for the patient with coexisting substance abuse and medical problems includes determining the discharge destination. If he or she desires treatment and recovery from the substance, discharge to a residential treatment center may be the setting of choice. If the patient intends to continue using substances, returning to the home may be the choice for discharge. Regardless of the planned interventions, the patient may choose to handle the substance abuse problem without help.

SUBSTANCE USE AND ABUSE AMONG NURSES

Nurses and other heath care professionals tend to be susceptible to substance abuse because of the availability of drugs and stress at work. Drug diversion by nurses can occur in facilities that have drugs with a high potential for abuse. The best safeguard to discourage diversion is to have effective policies and procedures that account for these drugs. *Safeguard your own practice by demonstrating responsible and accountable professional behaviors when giving medication.* For example, open drug packages in front of the patient before giving them. Ask another nurse to witness disposal of substances that are not needed, and document as such to account for missing drugs that were not administered. Be aware of the facility drug administration policies and those policies for reporting suspected diversion. *Report any colleague to the board whom you suspect of substance use or abuse, even though it may be difficult. Public safety is your primary responsibility as a nurse.*

In supporting safe and competent nursing care, state boards of nursing have peer-assistance programs to assist in identifying and effectively managing substance abuse by nurses. All nurses need to be knowledgeable about their state board of nursing laws and the consequences for drug use or abuse. Alternative programs for impaired health care workers can be identified by contacting the National Organization of Alternative Programs (www.alternativeprograms.org). Returning to the workforce after treatment has challenges, but through professional support, nurses can return to their careers. Support and encouragement are important for the nurse who returns after treatment because of the availability of drugs in the workplace.

CONSIDERATIONS FOR OLDER ADULTS

Substance abuse should not be overlooked in the older adult population. The potential is high because of the number of different drugs taken by this age-group. Alcohol may also be consumed in large quantities. As part the aging process, older adults have more difficulty metabolizing and excreting drugs and alcohol; therefore toxicity is a common complication. A thorough history is necessary for identifying patterns of substance use that could be harmful to the patient. Misuse of prescription medications, OTC medications, and herbal preparations may result from impaired memory. Regular drug administration times are difficult to remember, resulting in either overdosing or underdosing.

DECISION-MAKING CHALLENGE
Legal/Ethical

You are working the night shift with three other nurses. When you walk into the break room, you find one of the nurses self-injecting an IV opioid that he obtained from the Emergency Department. He pleads with you not to report this incident to anyone in order to protect his reputation and RN license. He tells you that he plans to move to another state next month.

1. Are you legally required to do anything with this information? If so, what?
2. Do you have any professional or ethical obligations? Why or why not?
3. Does the nurse's rationale for not reporting the incident have any legal or ethical basis? Why or why not?

evolve For suggested answer guidelines, go to http://evolve.elsevier.com/lggy/.

SUBSTANCES THAT ARE ABUSED OR MISUSED

The following sections describe the most common groups of addictive and abused substances and the effects on the body. Many drugs can cause coma or death. When nontherapeutic drug use is suspected, blood and urine testing may be indicated to determine the type(s) of substance present in the body.

ALCOHOL
Overview

A substantial number of people in the United States and other countries drink alcoholic beverages. For most people, alcohol is used for a pleasurable experience. It acts as a depressant on the central nervous system (CNS) and the respiratory system.

Therefore the signs and symptoms of the effects of alcohol use are primarily neurologic. Many visits to emergency departments each year are related to alcohol use. Increased binge-drinking among young adults in colleges and universities has resulted in major complications and death. Nearly one third of all adults in the United States engage in "at-risk drinking" behaviors according to the National Institute of Alcohol Abuse and Alcoholism (NIAAA) (2005b).

At-risk drinking is described as five or more of these beverages for men, or four or more for women:

- 12 ounces of beer
- 5 ounces of wine
- 1½ ounces of 80-proof spirits

Alcoholism (alcohol dependence) is a disease in which the patient:

- Has a strong need (craving) or compulsion to consume alcohol
- Is unable to limit alcohol consumption once drinking has begun (loss of control)
- Experiences physical dependence
- Has a need to increase the amount of alcohol to get the desired effect **(tolerance)**

Physical dependence is present when the person experiences alcohol withdrawal symptoms after habitual use is suddenly stopped, resulting in nausea, sweating, shakiness, and disorientation. The brain becomes hyper-excitable. As alcohol is ingested, it enters the bloodstream, affecting the CNS as a depressant. It then causes relaxation and a calming effect manifested by euphoria and a loss of inhibitions or self-control. Once these effects subside, sedation occurs. *When drinking alcohol relieves the symptoms of withdrawal, the person has developed a true physical dependence on alcohol and is considered an alcoholic.*

Alcohol abuse exists when a person *does not* have a strong craving for alcohol, loss of control, or physical dependence but has problems resulting from alcohol use. Examples include when the person fails to fulfill responsibilities at home, work, or school; drinks in unsafe situations; and/or continues to drink when problems have been caused or worsened by use of alcohol. When one or more of these events occur within a 12-month period, the person is abusing alcohol (NIAAA, 2005d).

CONSIDERATIONS FOR OLDER ADULTS

The older adult also faces risks for alcohol-related problems. Using even a small amount of alcohol in combination with other drugs increases the risk for intoxication and serious drug-alcohol interactions. Older adults may have a long history of alcohol use and are therefore at greater risk for severe withdrawal.

Because of the normal aging process, it is sometimes difficult to distinguish alcohol withdrawal from expected changes of aging. Disorientation may be interpreted as a sign of aging rather than a more serious alcohol problem. The change in function of the aging body needs to be considered in the treatment of the older person in withdrawal. He or she may need close monitoring and adjusted dosages of medications to avoid oversedation.

Patient-Centered Collaborative Care

Nursing care of the patient with alcohol problems or alcoholism depends on the patient's desire to reduce or stop alcohol consumption. The nurse in the medical-surgical setting must be knowledgeable about the signs, symptoms, and complications of alcohol use because the influence of alcohol can interfere with treatment of the medical-surgical health problem.

Assessment

The most objective assessment of alcohol intoxication is a blood alcohol level (BAL). If measured by a breathalyzer, a BAL of 0.08% is the legal limit. In health care settings, a blood sample is used to test for the ethanol (ETOH or alcohol) level (Table 7-2).

Additional assessment tools used by nurses and other health care professionals are the CAGE and T-ACE. The CAGE questionnaire is a popular, simple tool used in primary care settings. This tool identifies alcohol problems over the patient's lifetime. Another four-item assessment tool is the T-ACE adapted from the CAGE (Table 7-3). It is particularly useful in identifying the range of alcohol use. Additional in-depth screening is usually

TABLE 7-2 Alcohol Toxicity: Blood Alcohol Level, Classification, and Assessment Findings

80-200 mg/dL *(mild to moderate intoxication).* Behaviors include mood and behavior changes, impaired judgment, and poor motor coordination. Hypotension may occur in patients with levels greater than 100 mg/dL.

250-400 mg/dL *(marked intoxication).* This level of intoxication results in staggering ataxia and emotional lability. Symptoms may progress to confusion and stupor or coma.

Greater than 500 mg/dL *(severe intoxication).* Death is due to respiratory depression.

TABLE 7-3 Two Typical Tools for Alcohol Use Assessment

CAGE*	T-ACE*†
C Have you ever felt you should *cut* down on your drinking?	T *Tolerance*: How many drinks does it take to make you feel high?
A Have people *annoyed* you by criticizing your drinking?	A Have people *annoyed* you by criticizing your drinking?
G Have you ever felt bad or *guilty* about your drinking?	C Have you ever felt you ought to *cut* down your drinking?
E *Eye opener*: Have you ever had a drink first thing in the morning to steady your nerves or to get rid of a hangover?	E *Eye Opener*: Have you ever had a drink first thing in the morning to steady your nerves or to get rid of a hangover?

*For both CAGE and T-ACE, two or more positive responses indicate a need for further assessment.

†NOTE: The T-ACE is valuable in determining range and lifetime of use.

TABLE 7-4 Typical Signs and Symptoms of Alcohol Withdrawal Syndrome

Mild Symptoms of Alcohol Withdrawal (6-24 hours after last drink)	More Severe Symptoms (24-72 hours after last drink)
Restlessness, anxiety	In addition to mild symptoms, also includes delirium tremens (DTs), as manifested by:
Low-grade fever	Alcohol withdrawal delirium (can last up to a week)
Tremors	Hallucinations (visual/auditory)
Headache	Disorientation
Palpitations	Tachycardia (heart rate more than 100 beats/min)
Mild hypertension	Hypertension (diastolic more than 100 mm Hg)
GI discomfort	Low-grade fever
Insomnia	Agitation
Diaphoresis	Pronounced diaphoresis
	Vomiting

reserved for other disciplines or specialty health care workers who work with substance addictions.

The most threatening result of alcohol abuse or alcoholism is withdrawal from the substance. Symptoms of withdrawal range from mild to severe and can progress to death (Table 7-4). *The life-threatening stage of alcohol withdrawal requires emergency medical interventions. Alcohol seizures may occur 12 to 48 hours after the last drink.*

Interventions

When the patient is experiencing withdrawal from alcohol or another depressant, the priority is to prevent him or her from self-harm or potential harm to others! Reorient him or her frequently. The health care provider often prescribes medications to calm or sedate the patient according to agency protocol or physician preference. For example, benzodiazepines, such as chlordiazepoxide (Librium) and diazepam (Valium), are given to prevent seizures and **delirium tremens (DTs),** the most severe symptom of alcohol withdrawal. DTs are manifested by hallucinations, acute confusion, restlessness, and hyperactivity of the autonomic nervous system (e.g., tachycardia, hypertension, fever).

Other commonly used drugs include beta blockers to reduce cravings and decrease pulse and blood pressure and alpha-adrenergic blockers to decrease withdrawal symptoms. IV fluids and vitamins, such as thiamine, are also prescribed. In collaboration with the nutritionist, plan ways to increase protein and calories to address the patient's nutritional needs.

Nursing care for the patient with alcohol use or abuse includes thorough assessment to identify dependence and frequency of use. Chart 7-1 lists nursing activities that should be implemented when caring for a patient experiencing alcohol withdrawal.

Patients with alcoholism and their families require extensive rehabilitation and support. Collaborate with the case manager, social worker, and/or discharge planner to ensure patient and family awareness of community resources such as Alcoholics Anonymous for patients and Al-Anon for family members and friends. If supportive group work is not effective, aversion therapy with disulfiram (Antabuse) may be an option for treatment. Mental health/behavioral health texts discuss psychosocial support and alcohol abuse treatment in more detail.

Chart 7-1 NIC INTERVENTION ACTIVITIES

The Patient in Alcohol Withdrawal

Substance Use Treatment: Alcohol Withdrawal: *Care of the patient experiencing sudden cessation of alcohol consumption*

- Create a low-stimulation environment.
- Monitor vital signs during withdrawal.
- Monitor for delirium tremens (DTs).
- Administer anticonvulsants or sedatives, as appropriate.
- Medicate to relieve physical discomfort, as needed.
- Address hallucinations in a therapeutic manner.
- Maintain adequate nutrition and fluid intake.
- Administer vitamin therapy as appropriate.
- Provide emotional support to patient/family, as appropriate.
- Provide reality orientation, as appropriate.

NIC intervention activities selected from Bulechek, G.M., Butcher, H.K., & McCloskey Dochterman, J. (Eds.). (2008). *Nursing interventions classification (NIC)* (5th ed.). St. Louis: Mosby. No part of this work is to be altered without prior written permission from the Publisher.

NICOTINE

Overview

Nicotine is one of the most addictive substances in the United States and is the addictive component of tobacco. Although the U.S. Surgeon General issued a report in 1989 about the health hazards of tobacco and cigarette smoking, tobacco products continue to be used. Tobacco use remains the leading cause of *preventable* death in the United States. Nicotine continues to be a major contributing factor to the occurrence of cardiovascular disease. A number of nicotine products are available: cigarettes, pipe tobacco, chewing tobacco, and "spit tobacco" (Fig. 7-1).

The smoker is not the only person affected by tobacco use. *Secondhand smoke has become a public health issue in contributing to the development of cardiovascular disease and lung cancer in nonsmokers.* The presence of carbon monoxide, formaldehyde, cyanide, ammonia, and nicotine from secondhand smoke continues to present environmental hazards to people and the environment.

Physiologically, nicotine has both stimulant and sedative properties that affect the central nervous system (CNS). It stimulates the discharge of epinephrine from the adrenal glands, causing a sudden release of glucose. After recovery from the stimulant effects of the nicotine, depressant effects are manifested as feelings of depression and fatigue. When used daily, nicotine accumulates in the body and lasts up to 24 hours. Because of the cyclic properties of nicotine, the body begins to require more usage to maintain the stimulant effects of the drug.

The addictive power of nicotine has been compared to that of cocaine. Withdrawal symptoms occur when nicotine is discontinued. Lack of nicotine use in a 24-hour period can result in aggression, hostility, anger, and inappropriate social interactions.

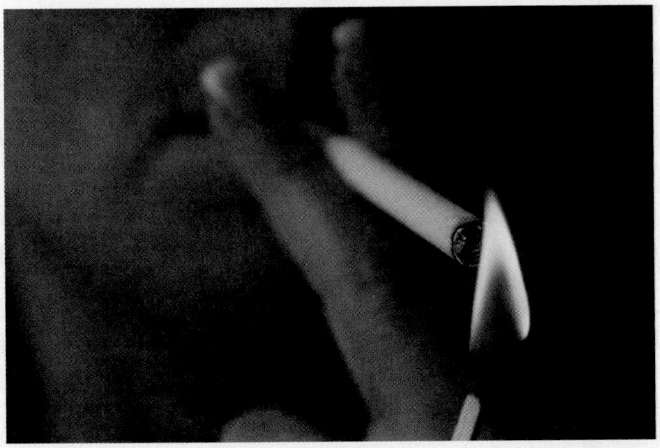

Fig. 7-1 • The incidence of smoking is increasing among women.

Patient-Centered Collaborative Care

As advocates of good health practices, nurses should help motivate the patient to quit using nicotine through education. The negative effects of smoking, including chronic cardiovascular and respiratory diseases, as well as the risks to others from secondhand smoke, should be stressed. When teaching the value of smoking cessation, it is especially necessary to exhibit sensitivity to the actual addiction present with tobacco use. A number of community-based support groups and smoking cessation programs are available using behavioral models, hypnosis, acupressure, or other modalities tailored to the person. Success has been found when behavioral interventions are used with bupropion (Zyban or Wellbutrin) to help diminish nicotine craving. Nicotine patches or gums are helpful with withdrawal in a titrated reduction of nicotine ingestion. Coping strategies are essential to overcome the person's desire to smoke. Many people gain weight as they wean from nicotine and therefore return to tobacco. The smoking cessation rate is increased for some patients by combining low-dose naltrexone (Revia, Depade), an opiate blocker, and the nicotine patch. Naltrexone helps prevent weight gain, especially in women. Smoking cessation is discussed further in the cardiovascular unit (Unit VIII) of this text and in Chart 32-3 in Chapter 32.

STIMULANTS

Stimulants are drugs that excite the cerebral cortex of the brain, producing a variety of behavioral responses. Any substance that is introduced into the body that excites or stimulates an increase in body activity is referred to as a *stimulant.* Examples are caffeine, nicotine, amphetamines, and methamphetamines. Although amphetamines and methamphetamines can be used for therapeutic purposes, their use is limited. Agents that are considered to be illicit and abused stimulants are crack (a potent form of cocaine), cocaine, and illegally produced methamphetamines.

The therapeutic effects of stimulants are:

- Improved sense of well-being
- Increased mental alertness
- Increased capacity to work
- Improved performance of motor skills
- Stimulation of general metabolism by increasing respiratory and cardiac function

When a large amount of stimulant is introduced into the body, the effects can cause insomnia, tremor, and restlessness, with resulting loss of motor function. The prolonged and sustained use of a stimulant can result in toxicity. An overdose can cause hallucinations, seizures, and cardiac dysrhythmias.

AMPHETAMINES AND METHAMPHETAMINES

Overview

Prescribed therapeutically as psychomotor stimulants, amphetamines and methamphetamines are effective in the treatment of attention deficit hyperactivity disorder (ADHD), obesity, and narcolepsy. When *amphetamines* are used for recreation, the desired effect is to achieve a state of euphoria and grandiosity. Street names for amphetamines in the drug culture include *black beauties, cross,* and *hearts.* These can be taken by a variety of methods including orally or by injection, smoking, or sniffing. Amphetamines have a very high potential for addiction both physically and psychologically. Use of stimulants results in energy, excitement, relief of fatigue, decreased appetite, insomnia, and aggression.

Although similar to amphetamines, *methamphetamine* is more powerful because its effects last longer and it is more harmful to the CNS. High levels of the neurotransmitter *dopamine* are released as a result of taking this drug. It has neurotoxic effects on the brain, damaging cells that contain other transmitters such as serotonin. Symptoms of parkinsonism can be found in the long-term user. Even small amounts can result in severe damage. This drug can be taken orally, intranasally, by injection, or by inhalation.

Recreational methamphetamine is used to obtain a rush or flash. Commonly known as *biker dope, chalk, speed, crank, crystal, glass,* and *hillbilly crack,* methamphetamine is produced illegally in "meth" labs across the United States. It can produce life-threatening conditions, such as myocardial infarction, liver damage, hyperthermia, and acute renal failure (McGuinness, 2006). Irreversible damage to the vessels in the brain can cause strokes. Methamphetamine users often die from cardiovascular collapse.

Not only is "meth" harmful to the person who is using the drug, but also it is an extreme safety hazard to those who make the drug or live in the building in which it is made. Home production of methamphetamines is increasingly common, creating an environmental hazard. Produced from combinations of OTC pseudoephedrine, drain cleaner, fertilizer, and starter fluid, the environment becomes toxic, requiring decontamination of exposed people as well as the lab structure. As a result of home methamphetamine production, the Combat Methamphetamine Epidemic Act of 2005 now requires that products containing pseudoephedrine be kept behind counters in the retail market.

Patient-Centered Collaborative Care

Clinical manifestations of amphetamine and methamphetamine use range from increased wakefulness and physical activity with appetite suppression to increased respirations, rapid irregular heart rate, increased blood pressure, and hyperthermia. Additional symptoms include irritability, anxiety, insomnia, confusion, tremors, convulsions, cardiovascular collapse, and death. Long-term effects are noted by severe dental problems, paranoia, aggressiveness, memory loss, anorexia, and hallucination or delusions.

Dental problems are significant manifestations of methamphetamine use because the user craves carbonated sweet beverages. Dental care is usually neglected during use; therefore repetitive use results in tooth decay. The acidic nature of the methamphetamine components gives rise to tooth decay as does the lack of saliva production created by the drug. Methamphetamine users also have a tendency to grind their teeth. See Fig. 7-2 for an example of "meth mouth."

For both overdose and withdrawal, the priority for care is to maintain a safe environment both physically and psychologically for the patient. Emergency care is briefly outlined in Table 7-5. Vital sign monitoring is essential. Hypertension and hyperthermia are difficult complications that must be managed. Because hyperthermia can lead to death, evaporation temperature-reducing methods may be necessary to keep the core temperature within limits compatible with optimal function.

Psychiatric symptoms may alert the caregiver to a history of methamphetamine use. Hallucinations, rage, paranoia, and depression are common (McGuinness, 2006).

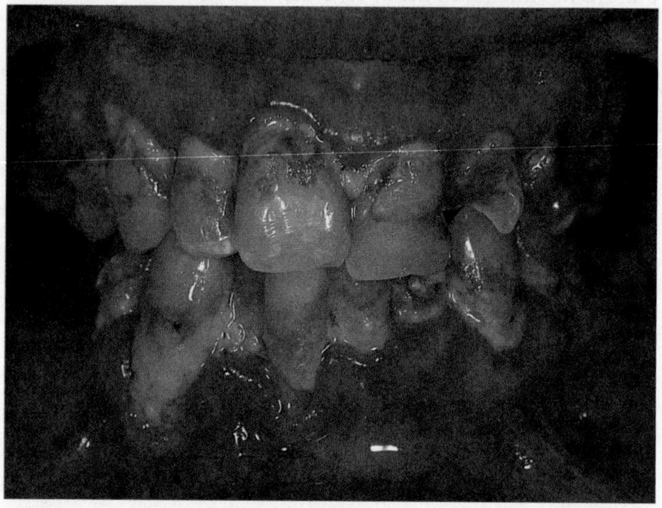

Fig. 7-2 • "Meth mouth" is caused by the caustic ingredients in methamphetamines, including battery acid, drain cleaner, and lye. A craving for sugary carbonated beverages and dryness of mouth lead to further decay.

TABLE 7-5 Clinical Manifestations and Emergency Care for Patients Who Abuse Stimulants

	Clinical Manifestations	Emergency Care
Stimulant Overdose	Respiratory distress Ataxia Fever Convulsions Coma Myocardial infarction Stroke Death	Respiratory support Cooling blanket Anticonvulsants Antipsychotics Ammonium chloride (to acidify urine for excretion of amphetamines [bases])
Stimulant Withdrawal	Fatigue Depression Agitation Apathy Anxiety Insomnia Disorientation Craving	Antianxiety medications Antidepressants Dopamine agonists (to reduce tremors)

COCAINE

Cocaine, commonly known as *coke, crack, flake, rocks,* and *snow,* is also a stimulant. This drug interferes with the reabsorption process of dopamine. As a chemical messenger related to pleasure and movement, dopamine is released as part of the brain's reward system and is associated with the euphoria achieved with cocaine use. Processing cocaine using ammonia or sodium bicarbonate transforms the cocaine into "crack cocaine," a preparation that can be inhaled. Inhalation of cocaine is referred to as *freebasing.* Smoking cocaine is a more direct method of getting the drug to the brain.

Physical dependence can occur, but psychological dependence is more common. Cocaine use is severely addicting, and withdrawal can be a life-threatening situation. When caring for the patient using cocaine, observe for symptoms that are associated with crack cocaine use. With *moderate* amounts of this drug, the patient may exhibit increased alertness, euphoria, anorexia, high blood pressure, increased heart rate, and dilated pupils. In *high* doses or an overdose, agitation, confusion, hallucinations, panic attacks, paranoia, or convulsions may occur. Withdrawal symptoms include irritability, sluggishness, and depression. The drug is detectable in the urine 1 to 4 hours after ingestion and may remain up to 3 days after use.

Nursing care of the patient with an overdose or withdrawal from cocaine includes critical observations for cardiac symptoms, including frequent vital signs. Assess for signs of depression and potential suicide gestures during the withdrawal period. Help reduce nausea by ensuring that the environmental temperature is comfortable and that odors are eliminated. Nutritional and hydration assessment is pertinent because the persons tends to omit eating or drinking fluids while using.

During the initial and ongoing physical assessment, pay careful attention to the mucous membranes of the nose because prolonged snorting can deteriorate the membranes and the nasal septum. Nosebleeds are common with "snorting" (sniffing) the drug and can be a valuable tool in assessment of use. Cardiopulmonary arrest can also occur with the first use of cocaine. Generally the medical treatment for cocaine withdrawal or overdose is the same as that for other stimulants.

HALLUCINOGENS AND RELATED COMPOUNDS

Chemical substances that possess mind-altering or mental perception–altering properties are known as **hallucinogens.** Examples of these substances are lysergic acid (LSD), phencyclidine (PCP), 3,4-methylenedioxymethamphetamine (MDMA), and marijuana. LSD has no known therapeutic purpose for humans at present. Marijuana is being used for cancer pain relief and as an appetite enhancer for patients with AIDS in some states in the United States.

Hallucinogenic compounds are desirable to the user because of their thrill-seeking effects caused by an alteration in perception. Action of these drugs produces changes in the neurotransmitters of the brain. Alterations in mood, sensory distortions, delusions, and depersonalization are some of the resulting behaviors. Physical changes are elevated vital signs and dilated pupils. A psychological dependence may occur, or the patient may experience suicidal or psychotic states. Flashbacks are a common problem when psychedelic drugs are used and can occur at any time. The user is returned to the initial drug experience without warning, which can be very disturbing and create a threat to safety. Observe for objective signs of use, as well as paranoia and suspicious behavior.

LYSERGIC ACID

Overview

Lysergic acid (LSD) is the prototype and major hallucinogenic drug, commonly known as "acid." LSD exerts its hallucinogen effects by interrupting the interaction of nerve cells and the neurotransmitter *serotonin.* Normally, serotonin is distributed throughout the brain and the spinal cord and is involved in regulation of behavioral, perceptual, and regulatory systems. These systems affect mood, hunger, body temperature, sexual behavior, muscle control, and sensory perception. Usually taken orally, LSD is distributed on absorbent, decorative paper, making it very attractive to adolescents and children. The health hazards of LSD are very unpredictable and are affected by dose, personality or mood of the user, anticipated outcome, and the environment at the time of use. The effects of the drug can last up to 12 hours and can result in either a pleasant experience (good trip) or an unpleasant experience (bad trip).

Introspective thinking may occur with the person experiencing personal revelations about himself or herself, the truth of the universe, or other bizarre thoughts. Sensory experiences are powerful in LSD use because of the perception of surroundings. Colors seem more vivid and tangible. Thoughts and feelings can be so bizarre that a "trip" can result in suicide. LSD use can also result in severe and chronic mental illness, such as schizophrenia. Because the drug does not result in compulsive drug-seeking behaviors, it is not considered addictive, but a strong tolerance can develop. An increased amount is needed to attain the same level of stimulation as earlier experiences. LSD stimulates the sympathetic nervous system causing tremors and hyperreflexia.

Patient-Centered Collaborative Care

Observe for intoxication from LSD, such as:
- Dilated pupils
- Tachycardia
- Palpitations
- Diaphoresis
- Tremors
- Poor coordination
- Elevated body temperature
- Increased pulse and respiration

Many psychological symptoms also occur as paranoid ideas, anxiety, and depression, transforming sounds and sights into sensation (hearing colors). Overdose can result in brain damage, psychosis, or death.

Treatment for the patient in an LSD crisis includes (1) one-to-one observation to keep him or her safe, and (2) helping him or her sort reality as the effects subside. Fears can be comforted to prevent the person from acting on psychotic thoughts. Because there is such a sensory influence on him or her, the environment should be calming with a comfortable temperature and few disturbances. Reducing the stimuli can significantly limit the response to the drug's effects. In an emergency situation, the person is exposed to varied and powerful stimuli that contribute to intense behavioral responses to the powerful stimulus created by the LSD. Antianxiety drugs (benzodiazepines) or drugs to control or eliminate the symptoms of mental illness may be prescribed. Haloperidol (Haldol) has been found to be effective in the treatment of LSD symptoms. Effects created by other hallucinogens such as mescaline and psilocybin (derived from peyote cactus and mushrooms) respond to the same treatment regimen as used with LSD.

DISSOCIATIVE DRUGS

Dissociative drugs are anesthetics that create distortions of the perception of sight and sound (hallucinations). The clinical manifestations of toxicity in these drugs are increased heart rate and blood pressure, nausea and vomiting, impaired motor responses, and memory loss. Drugs in this category are phencyclidine (PCP) and ketamine. They can be smoked, injected, or used intranasally. These drugs act in the body by altering the distribution of the neurotransmitter *glutamate* throughout the brain. The action of glutamate involves the perception of pain, responses to the environment, and memory.

Phencyclidine

Phencyclidine, commonly known as *PCP,* is an animal anesthetic that causes a feeling of detachment in humans. Patients using PCP (also known as *angel dust, ozone, wack, rocket fuel*) are unaware of their surroundings, creating feelings of detachment. It affects primarily the CNS, and the patient exhibits flushing, increased perspiration, aggression, and incoherence. The user may experience feelings of superior strength and physical power. Some users report that their use is related to the numbing effects on the mind. However, the results may progress to a comatose state. With the sophistication of newer drugs, PCP is not as prevalent as in the past.

There is no evidence of physical addiction; however, psychological addiction is common. Low to moderate ingestion produces a slight increase in shallow respirations and a significant rise in the heart rate and blood pressure with flushing and profuse diaphoresis. High doses of PCP are manifested by decreased blood pressure, pulse, and respiratory rates. Other manifestations with high amounts of ingestion may include nausea/vomiting, blurred vision, drooling, eye flickers (up and down motion of the eyes), loss of balance, and dizziness. Seizures, coma, and death may also occur with high does of PCP. The patient's symptoms may mimic those of schizophrenia, such as hallucinations or catatonia. With long-term use, these symptoms may persist for a year or cause permanent disabilities.

Ketamine

Closely associated with PCP, ketamine is sometimes known as "businessman's LSD." *Moderate* doses produce euphoria, loss of inhibition, confusion, ringing in the ears, a quick burst of energy, and drunken feeling. Tolerance can occur as well as physical and psychological dependence. Street names for ketamine are *Special K, K,* and *Kat.* Ketamine is also referred to as a "techno" drug because of its attractiveness to the "rave" culture.

Complications associated with ketamine *overdose* include:
- Tunnel vision
- Shortness of breath
- Loss of balance
- Numbness of the body

- Clinical depression
- No sense of time
- Seizures
- Coma

A calm and stimulus-free environment is very important for the patient recovering from a ketamine overdose, as well as availability of supportive therapies. Respiratory support is a priority because of the anesthetic effects of the drug.

DECISION-MAKING CHALLENGE
Critical Rescue

A young adult was admitted yesterday to the medical unit with chest pain and atrial fibrillation. He has a history of congenital heart disease and type 1 diabetes mellitus. This morning he reports nausea; he also has diaphoresis and is trembling. He states that he saw spiders on the wall in the middle of the night and wants to be in a different room.

1. What further assessment should you conduct at this time?
2. What might explain his physical complaints?
3. How do you explain the spiders he saw on the wall?
4. What is your current priority in caring for this patient?

evolve For suggested answer guidelines, go to http://evolve.elsevier.com/Iggy/.

3,4-Methylenedioxymethamphetamine

Amphetamines can be altered to become hallucinogens, as in the case of 3,4-methylenedioxymethamphetamine (MDMA), also called *Adam.* Other names for the drug are *ecstasy, XTC, hug, beans,* and the *"date rape" drug.* MDMA is a synthetic, psychoactive drug chemically similar to methamphetamine. It can be taken orally, smoked, snorted, or injected. Desired effects by the user include development of trust in others, which eases inhibitions between people, and an increased level of confidence, euphoria, and physical energy.

Part of the popularity of MDMA is the relaxation of voluntary muscles and the amnesiac effect for the period in which the drug is most active in the body; hence the name "date rape" drug. The physiological effects of MDMA occur at the serotonin receptor sites, which create the inhibition of behaviors. Action of MDMA at the serotonin site accounts for the report of heightened sexual experiences and tranquility. Demonstrating a structural relationship to methamphetamine, MDMA causes a degeneration of neurons containing dopamine, a neurotransmitter, resulting in parkinsonism. It is neurotoxic and can cause brain damage. Its interference with the temperature control mechanism of the body can result in hyperthermia. Though rare, physiological manifestations of MDMA use are multiorgan failure and death.

Assess the patient for psychological symptoms including confusion, depression, sleep disturbances, drug craving, severe anxiety, and paranoia. With *moderate* doses, other effects are euphoria, nervousness, hyperexcitability, and a rapid heart rate. Physical symptoms of *high* dose ingestion are muscle tension, involuntary teeth clenching, nausea, visual disturbances, faintness, and chills or sweating. Increased heart rate and blood pressure are also observed. Nursing care of the patient is based on the symptoms at the time of assessment.

If acute symptoms are present, the *priority for care is safety* and symptomatic relief of the psychological manifestations. Treatment regimens are focused on reduction or elimination of the adverse effects of the drug.

Marijuana

Marijuana is commonly called *weed, smoke, pot, grass, Mary Jane,* and *herb.* Widely used and distributed, this drug is illegal in most states and does not have any evidence-based therapeutic uses. For some patients, it helps control chronic pain. Synthetic derivatives of marijuana are available for treatment of complications associated with cancer therapy such as nausea and vomiting, as well as an appetite stimulant for patients with AIDS. Debate continues about the uses and need for legalization of marijuana in the United States.

Though physical dependence for marijuana is seemingly nonexistent, it has a high risk for psychological dependence if it is used over long periods. The desired effects of marijuana are sensations of euphoria, sexual arousal, and relaxation. The "high" experience that users feel is a result of the action of tetrahydrocannabinol (THC), the main active substance in marijuana. THC changes the method by which sensory information enters and is processed in the hippocampus. As a component of the brain's limbic system, the hippocampus is necessary for the integration of sensory experiences and emotion, as well as learning and memory. Frequent and long-term use of marijuana can create the same respiratory changes seen in long-term tobacco smokers. Studies of young adults who use marijuana demonstrate that learning and social behaviors are affected by heavy marijuana use. Evidence suggests that marijuana use affects critical skills related to attention, memory, and learning. Heavy marijuana users make more mistakes in their work and have more difficulty maintaining attention.

Research comparing marijuana use with tobacco smoking suggests that marijuana creates precarcinogenic effects in the respiratory tract. Marijuana smokers hold their breath longer than the tobacco smoker, thereby increasing lung exposure to carcinogens within the tar. Epithelial cells become injured, which can predispose the user to abnormal cell replication in the airway and lungs (Tashkin, 2005).

Whether marijuana is smoked or taken orally, the physical and psychological effects in moderate doses include relaxation, happiness, euphoria, increased heart rate, and impaired short-term memory. High doses produce more pronounced effects such paranoia, restlessness, anxiety attacks, panic attacks, increased appetite, impaired coordination, and altered perceptions. Withdrawal symptoms include insomnia, decreased appetite, nausea, irritability, and anxiety.

Nursing interventions for the person who is under the influence of marijuana are based on the severity of symptoms presented. Frequent vital sign assessment and a complete physical assessment are needed to determine stability of the person's physical condition. Pain control may be more difficult in the patient with a history of marijuana use. Impaired judgment and loss of memory are significant long-term effects of marijuana use.

DEPRESSANTS

Drugs that reduce the activity of the central nervous system (CNS) are referred to as **depressants.** Benzodiazepines and barbiturates are discussed as depressants because of their activity in the ascending reticular activating system in the CNS. Both classes have valuable therapeutic properties in treating anxiety and emotional disorders. CNS depressants are therapeutically used as adjuncts to sleep and can be used as needed for situational tension. The route of ingestion may be oral or by injection. On the illicit drug market, barbiturates are called *barbs* or *ludes,* depending on the chemical makeup. A commonly abused benzodiazepine, Rohypnol, is referred to as *rophies, ruffies, R2s, Mexican Valium, Rib, roach,* or *Roches.* Sometimes Rohypnol (flunitrazepam) is referred to as "forget me pill" or "forget pill." These are Schedule IV drugs because of the high potential for abuse.

Depressants are used to produce decreased feelings of anxiety and improve one's sense of well-being. Use of depressants can lower inhibitions. Physiological manifestations of depressants include lowered heart rate, blood pressure, and respirations; poor concentration; fatigue; confusion; and impaired coordination, memory, and judgment. Long-term depressant use can cause addiction, respiratory depression, cardiac arrest, and death. Treatment and nursing interventions are symptomatic relief and comfort measures.

Benzodiazepines

The desired results for the use of prescribed benzodiazepines include relaxation, sleep, seizure control, withdrawal from alcohol, and relief of anxiety. Abuse is present when the patient continues to use the drug after the clinical signs have subsided. The street value of benzodiazepines and the drug effects make these drugs popular. Physical and psychological dependence on benzodiazepines are prevalent. Users can develop a high tolerance for these drugs, causing the need for increasing amounts to achieve the desired feeling. Benzodiazepines act to depress the CNS; therefore combination with other CNS substances has a potentiating effect.

Commonly used street terms for benzodiazepines are *candy, downers, sleeping beauties,* and *tranks* (short for tranquilizers). Physiological effects include sedation, drowsiness/depression, unusual excitement, fever, irritability, poor judgment, slurred speech, dizziness, and life-threatening withdrawal. The drugs can be injected or swallowed. Treatment for overdose is symptomatic relief of symptoms and being alert to cardiovascular and respiratory symptoms of sedation.

Rohypnol

Flunitrazepam (Rohypnol) is a highly potent benzodiazepine (10 times more potent than diazepam [Valium]) available through a provider prescription. This drug is not available in the United States; however, it is used legally in other countries. Use of Rohypnol is for treatment of severe sleep disorders and inpatient psychiatric care. Combined with alcohol, this drug is also referred to as a *date rape drug,* or a *club drug.* Being colorless and tasteless, Rohypnol can be dissolved in beverages without being detected. This drug can be swallowed, inhaled, injected, smoked, or dissolved in a drink. Effects of Rohypnol are:

- Relief from tension
- Anticonvulsant action
- Sedation
- Amnesia
- Muscle relaxation
- Sleep
- Slowing of motor performance (greatly increased when combined with alcohol)

Young adults use this drug to engage in violent or destructive activities without feelings of guilt. Rohypnol has physical and psychological dependence properties. *Moderate* doses create a loss of inhibition, drunken state, dizziness, tranquility, and slurred speech. Signs and symptoms associated with *withdrawal or overdosing* from Rohypnol are more severe, including delirium, seizures, respiratory depression, and shock.

Nursing care should focus on the severity of the symptoms and astute assessment for deterioration in the patient's physical condition. Treatment of Rohypnol abuse is aimed at a medical model of detoxification using titrating doses.

Gamma Hydroxybutyrate

Gamma hydroxybutyrate (GHB) is also considered a club drug. When taken in small amounts, GHB, referred to as "liquid ecstasy," reduces one's social inhibitions and increases libido. It is produced illegally in the United States and was referred to as the *date rape drug of the 90s.* GBH may be inhaled, injected, or swallowed. In small doses, it produces euphoria, anxiety, increased sexual pleasure, impaired judgment, a loss of coordination, and nausea, along with the loss of inhibition.

Effects of high doses of GHB can range from dizziness to death. Common symptoms of overdose include respiratory depression, memory loss, bradycardia, muscular fatigue, and coma. The adverse effects of the drug can be devastating. When it is combined with alcohol, deaths are more prevalent. Anyone presenting at the emergency department in a coma of unknown origin should be evaluated for GHB use.

BARBITURATES

Barbiturates are drugs that depress the CNS through action in the cerebral cortex and the reticular formation (helps regulate the sleep-wake cycle). Effects of barbiturates include sedation, drowsiness, and a decrease in motor activity of the body similar to that seen with alcohol. Common barbiturates are Amytal, Nembutal, and Phenobarbital, also known on the street as *barbs, reds, red birds, phennies, tooies, yellows,* and *yellow jackets.* Therapeutic uses of barbiturates are treatment of short-term insomnia or preanesthesia and anticonvulsant therapy. Because of the aging process, older adults can tolerate only small doses of the barbiturate group.

Dependence and addiction to barbiturates can occur in a very short time and can lead to withdrawal symptoms if the drug is discontinued abruptly. Initial withdrawal symptoms are anxiety, restlessness, insomnia, irritability, and impaired attention, with more severe symptoms if the person has a chronic pattern of use. Physical illness may accompany the withdrawal of barbiturates with nausea, vomiting, abdominal cramping, seizures, and varied behavioral responses. *With severe dependence, the effects of withdrawal can be life threatening. Toxic or overdose symptoms include respiratory depression, coma, and pinpoint pupils.* Laboratory testing for barbiturates can be done by direct immunoassay from blood, urine, or gastric contents.

Nursing interventions for the patient in crisis due to overdose or withdrawal of barbiturates are to ensure safety through frequent vital signs, neurological checks, and emotional support. Symptomatic treatment such as drug tapering is needed to avoid the more severe response to drug elimination. Food, fluids, and a calm environment are necessary to achieve the initial outcomes for the patient. Because barbiturates are constipating, monitor for elimination patterns, being sure to provide high fiber in the diet. Immediate and long-term care of the person with physical addiction requires various members of the health care team to plan and implement holistic care.

TABLE 7-6 Commonly Abused Opioid Prescription Drugs: Trade (Street) Names

Generic Name	Trade Name (Street Name)	Generic Name	Trade Name (Street Name)
Codeine	Empirin w/codeine, Fiorinal w/codeine, Robitussin A-C, Tylenol w/codeine (Captain Cody, Cody, schoolboy) Preparations with glutethimide (doors & fours, loads, pancakes & syrup)	Opium	laudanum, paregoric (big O, black stuff, block, gum, hop)
Fentanyl	Actiq, Duragesic, Sublimaze (Apache, China girl, China white, dance fever, friend goodfella, jackpot, murder B, TNT, tango & cash)	Oxycodone	Tylox, OxyContin, Percodan, Percocet (oxy 80s, oxycet, hillbilly heroin, percs)
Morphine	Roxanol, Duramorph (M, Miss Emma, monkey, white stuff)	Meperidine	Demerol, meperidine hydrochloride (demmies, pain killer)
		Hydromorphone	Dilaudid (juice)
		Hydrocodone	Vicodin, Lortab, Lorcet
		Propoxyphene	Darvon, Darvocet

OPIOIDS

Overview

Opioids is a broad term encompassing all drugs that are made from the Asian poppy or produced as a synthetic drug that produces the same effects of the opium plant. The street term for opioids is *narcotics, or "narcs."* A desired (therapeutic) action of opioids is to reduce the patient's perception of pain. Drugs included in this category are codeine, morphine, heroin, methadone, hydromorphone (Dilaudid), meperidine (Demerol), and oxycodone (OxyContin). Opium and morphine derivatives have become drugs of dependence because of their analgesic and euphoric effects.

Common street names are *horse, junk, H,* and *smack* for heroin. *Dover's powder* refers to opium. The sites of action of these drugs are in the brain, binding in the receptor sites of the CNS (causing CNS depression) and in the GI system (producing the antidiarrheal effects of opium [e.g., Lomotil]). Desired effects of substance abuse with these drugs are the escape effect in the mind and analgesia. Aggression and sexual drives are usually minimized with use of the opioids and morphine-like drugs (Table 7-6).

A high potential for addiction, tolerance, and dependence occurs with this class of drugs. The withdrawal effects can range from mild withdrawal symptoms to death. According to the National Institute on Drug Abuse, there are four categories of opiate withdrawal manifestations (NIDA, 2008c):

- Grade 0—drug craving, anxiety, and drug-seeking behaviors
- Grade 1—yawning, sweating, lacrimation, and rhinorrhea ("runny nose")
- Grade 2—mydriasis (pupillary dilation), gooseflesh, muscle twitching, and anorexia
- Grade 3—increased pulse, respiratory rate, and blood pressure; abdominal cramps; diarrhea; vomiting; and weakness; considered as the most dangerous of the grades in opiate withdrawal

These drugs may be taken orally, injected, or inhaled. *Heroin,* a highly addictive drug, is an opiate derivative. Unlike other opiate drugs, heroin has no medical use. The health hazards of heroin are very serious and include fatal overdoses and spontaneous abortions. IV use of heroin or other abused substances increases the risk of acquiring infectious diseases such as HIV infection or AIDS and hepatitis. Short-term effects of heroin are felt immediately and continue for a few hours after a single dose. Users report an immediate "rush" when using. The person experiences a dry mouth, heavy extremities, and a warm, flushed feeling. There may be alternate sensations of wakefulness and sleep. Chronic use of heroin results in many physical problems, such as emaciation, frequent infections, cellulitis, and liver disease. Morphine, heroin, and codeine use can be identified in the urine from 2 hours to up to 3 days after use.

Patient-Centered Collaborative Care

When possible, determine the patient's history of drug use, drug of choice, and the last dose taken. A small percentage of people become addicted to opioids while being treated for severe, chronic pain. An example is the pain associated with sickle cell anemia. These patients have episodes of extreme pain during an exacerbation of their disease and require large amounts of pain medication.

Three major problems that require emergency intervention may occur when opiates are used: intoxication, overdose, and withdrawal. Assessment findings for each of these conditions are listed in Chart 7-2.

Care of the patient with an opiate or heroin addiction becomes complex because of the physical condition, the addictive behaviors, and safety concerns both physically and psychologically. Anticonvulsant drugs are commonly prescribed to prevent seizures. Other drugs, such as naloxone (Narcan) and naltrexone (Revia), work as opioid antagonists, competing with opioids at the receptor sites. Midazolam (Versed) may also be given to induce amnesic effects. Anxiety-reducing medications (anxiolytics) help relieve anxiety. In some cases of severe dependence, methadone is prescribed to relieve pain. Other drugs may be given to treat symptoms such as nausea.

Provide supportive measures for the patient, including nonpharmacologic measures to relieve pain, reduction of stimuli, and basic comfort measures. Monitor vital signs frequently, and assess for major changes, both physiologic and

Chart 7-2 KEY FEATURES

Manifestations of Opiate Use That Require Emergency Interventions

OPIATE INTOXICATION
- Constricted pupils
- Decreased blood pressure
- Decreased respirations
- Drowsiness
- Slurred speech
- Initial euphoria followed by dysphoria (depression)
- Cognitive impairments resulting in judgment and memory losses

OPIATE OVERDOSE
- Dilated pupils
- Respiratory depression
- Coma
- Shock
- Convulsions
- Respiratory arrest
- Death

OPIATE WITHDRAWAL
- Yawning
- Insomnia
- Irritability
- Rhinorrhea
- Diaphoresis
- Abdominal cramps
- Nausea and vomiting
- Muscle aches
- Chills, cold flashes with goose bumps (referred to as "cold turkey")

psychological. Alterations in respiratory rate and quality are of special concern.

INHALANTS

Breathable chemical vapors that produce psychoactive effects are called **inhalants.** These substances are popular with children, adolescents, and young adults because of their accessibility and price. Three categories of inhalants are common household items. *Solvents* produce an exhilarating high when inhaled. Examples of solvents are paint thinners, gasoline, glues, paper correction fluid, felt-tip markers, and electronic contact cleaners. *Gases* are another source of inhalants and include products such as butane lighters, propane tanks, whipping cream aerosols, spray paints, hair and deodorant sprays, chloroform, ether, and nitrous oxide (laughing gas). *Nitrites* are the third source of inhalants, which include cyclohexyl nitrite, amyl nitrite, and butyl nitrite. Slang terms that readily identify inhalant use are *glue, kick, bang, sniff, huffing, poppers, whippets,* and *Texas shoe-shine.*

Inhalants produce anesthetic results, consequently slowing body functions. Persons who use inhalants feel intoxicated, less inhibited, and less in control with repeated use. They may inhale to the point of causing unconsciousness. Sniffing highly concentrated chemicals can result in death from cardiac failure. Suffocation can also occur because the inhalant takes the place of oxygen in the lungs and respirations cease. Irreversible effects, including hearing losses, limb spasms, brain damage, and/or bone marrow suppression, can occur from inhalants. Reversible effects that can occur with inhalants include liver and kidney damage and blood oxygen depletion. Pouring the inhalant into a paper bag increases the concentration of the substance, inducing a quicker, more pronounced effect.

Signs of inhalant use are:
- Slurred speech
- Drunk, dizzy, or dazed appearance
- Chemical smell on the person
- Paint stains on body or face
- Red eyes
- Rhinorrhea

Users may require hospitalization for complications of inhalant use or for medical conditions complicated by substance use. Management and treatment of inhaled chemicals is primarily supportive and using antidotes for inhalant overdose or toxicity. Once the patient is stabilized, try to explore potential underlying reasons for substance use.

STEROIDS

Anabolic-androgenic steroids are growing in popularity among young athletes. The term *anabolic* indicates muscle building, and the term *androgenic* refers to increased masculinity. **Anabolic steroids** are synthetic substances that mimic the actions of testosterone. They are legally available through prescription use for people with hormonal difficulties such as delayed puberty or impotence. Known as *roids, juice, hype,* or *pump,* steroids can boost athletic performance—but not without complications for the user. Athletes have been known to use steroids to increase strength and performance even when they are known to be unhealthy, life threatening, and illegal for use in amateur, professional, and international events. The pressure to become stronger, achieve, and succeed often tempts the person to use steroids to "bulk up" for mastery in select sports.

Misuse of steroids can lead to serious medical problems, some of which are irreversible. Possible effects of steroids include:
- For men: shrinking testicles, reduced sperm count, infertility, baldness, development of breasts, and an increased risk for cancer
- For women: growth of facial hair, male pattern baldness, changes or cessation of menses, enlargement of the clitoris, and deepened voice

When using steroids, negative emotional effects are characterized by "roid rage," which is manifested by severe, aggressive behavior with the potential for violence. Severe mood swings are also common. Other clinical symptoms may include hallucinations, paranoia, anxiety or panic attacks, depression, or thoughts of suicide.

For both genders, these side effects may occur with steroid use:
- High blood pressure and heart disease
- Liver damage
- Stroke and blood clots
- Urinary and bowel problems such as diarrhea
- Headaches, muscle cramps, aching joints
- Sleep problems

- Increased risk of ligament and tendon injuries
- Severe acne
- Baldness

Steroid use has been banned by the International Olympic Committee, the National Football League (NFL), the National Collegiate Athletic Association (NCAA), and other public and private intuitions. Vigilant oversight for steroid use in sports continues to be difficult to implement. Public education is important to reduce the use of steroids for performance enhancement.

GET READY FOR THE NCLEX EXAMINATION!

Key Points

Review these Key Points.

- Substance abuse interferes with life's activities, which can endanger the patient when hospitalized. Therefore a complete drug history is essential in identification of substance abuse in the hospitalized patient.
- Substance use/misuse/abuse, treatment, and recovery are affected by the cultural background of the patient.
- Pain threshold is altered in the patient with a history of substance abuse or misuse.
- Nursing assessment of the older adult includes information about substance abuse or misuse, including alcohol or prescription and OTC drugs.
- Common drugs of abuse are alcohol, stimulants, hallucinogens, depressants, opioids, inhalants, and steroids.
- Research findings indicate a linkage between genetics and substance use.
- Stimulants increase mental alertness, improve a person's sense of well-being, increase the capacity to work, improve performance of motor skills, and increase metabolism through increased respiratory and cardiac function. Common stimulants of abuse are amphetamines, methamphetamines, cocaine, and nicotine.
- Common slang terms for illicit substance use are:
  - Amphetamines: crosses, hearts, black beauties
  - Methamphetamines: crank, crystal, ice, glass, speed, chalk
  - Cocaine: coke, snow, flake, rocks, crack
- Symptoms of stimulant abuse requiring emergency interventions are elevated vital signs, dehydration, and neurological changes, including convulsions or coma.
- Drug therapy common in the treatment of overdose or withdrawal of stimulants includes antipsychotics, antiparkinsonism agents, antidepressants, antianxiety medications, and IV therapy.
- Hallucinogenic substances, which create an alteration in perception and a subsequent euphoria, include LSD, PCP, ketamine, MDMA (ecstasy), and marijuana.
- Effects of hallucinogenic substances, such as enhanced sexual arousal, create the environment for risk behaviors of the euphoria and false sense of abilities experienced when using these drugs.
- PCP creates a feeling of detachment and is referred to as "angel dust" because it exerts numbing effects on the mind.
- Depressants, including benzodiazepines, gamma hydroxybutyrate (GHB), barbiturates, alcohol, and opioids, are among some of the most popular abused substances.
- Barbiturates, commonly referred to as "barbs" and "ludes," are addictive and can result in physical withdrawal symptoms if stopped abruptly.
- Alcohol withdrawal (syndrome) is classified as minor, major, and life threatening.
- Life-threatening symptoms of alcohol withdrawal are delirium tremens (DTs), disorientation, confusion, and inability to recognize familiar objects or persons.
- Interventions for acute alcohol withdrawal are administration of sedatives, vitamins, magnesium sulfate, anticonvulsants, and folic acid.
- Minor to moderate symptoms of opiate or narcotic withdrawal are yawning, insomnia, irritability, rhinorrhea, diaphoresis, chills, and "goose bumps."
- The most dangerous grade of opiate withdrawal is characterized by increased blood pressure and pulse and respiratory rates; abdominal cramps; diarrhea; vomiting; and weakness requiring emergency interventions to prevent death.
- Interventions for symptoms associated with narcotic withdrawal range from supportive care to use of IV fluids, anticonvulsants, opioid antagonists, methadone substitution, clonidine, and midazolam hydrochloride (Versed).
- Inhalants are used by children and adolescents because of availability, inducing slurred speech; drunk, dizzy, or dazed appearance; red eyes; and rhinorrhea.
- Inhalants create anesthetic results and slow body functions, resulting in feelings of intoxication.
- Continuous steroid use is found primarily in athletes to build strength and muscle mass for success.

Additional Study Resources

Go to your Companion CD or Evolve at http://evolve.elsevier.com/Iggy/ for *Self-Assessment Questions for the NCLEX Examination.*

Go to Evolve at http://evolve.elsevier.com/Iggy/ for *Prioritization and Delegation Questions for the NCLEX Examination.*

SELECTED BIBLIOGRAPHY

Asterisk indicates a classic or definitive work on this subject.

D'arcy, Y. (2007). Managing pain in a patient who's drug-dependent. *Nursing 2007, 37*(3), 36-40.

Harkreader, M. (2006). Differentiating between substance use, abuse and addiction. *Nursing Perspectives: A Publication of the Tennessee Board of Nursing in collaboration with the Tennessee Center for Nursing, 1*(3), 12-13.

Leeuwen, A., Dranpitz, T., & Smith, L. (2006). *Laboratory and diagnostic tests with nursing implications* (2nd ed.). Philadelphia: Davis.

Lussier-Cushing, M., Repper-DeLisi, J., Mitchell, M.T., Latatos, B.E., Mahmoud, F., & Lipkis-Orlando, R. (2007). Is your medical/surgical patient withdrawing from alcohol? *Nursing2007, 37*(10), 50-55.

*McCloskey, J. (2003). *Unifying nursing languages: The harmonization of NANDA, NIC, and NOC.* Washington, DC: American Nurses Association.

McGuinness, T. (2006). Methamphetamine abuse. *AJN, 106*(12), 54-59.

Mosby's dictionary of medicine, nursing & health professions (7th ed.). (2006). St. Louis: Mosby.

National Institute on Alcohol Abuse and Alcoholism (NIAAA). (2005a). *Alcohol alert: Screening for alcohol use and alcohol related problems.* Retrieved January 29, 2008, from http://pubs.niaaa.nih.gov/publications/aa65/AA65.htm.

National Institute on Alcohol Abuse and Alcoholism (NIAAA). (2005b). *Alcoholism: Getting the facts last.* Retrieved January 15, 2008, from www.collegedrinkingprevention.gov.

National Institute on Alcohol Abuse and Alcoholism (NIAAA). (2005c). *Alcoholism: Facts about alcohol poisoning.* Retrieved January 15, 2008, from www.collegedrinkingprevention.gov.

National Institute on Alcohol Abuse and Alcoholism (NIAAA). (2005d). *Helping patients who drink too much: A clinician's guide.* Retrieved January 24, 2008, from http://pubs.niaaa.nih.gov/publications/Practitioner/CliniciansGuide2005/clinicians.guide.htm.

National Institute on Drug Abuse (NIDA). (2006). *News Scan: NIDA Addiction Research News. Women and Substance Abuse Issue.* Retrieved January 27, 2007, from www.drugabuse.gov/newsroom/06/NS-10.html.

National Institute of Drug Abuse (NIDA). (2007). Naltrexone-nicotine patch combination shows promise. *NIDA Notes, 21*(3), 3.

National Institute of Drug Abuse (NIDA). (2008a). *Commonly abused drugs.* Retrieved January 15, 2008, from www.drugabuse.gov/DrugPages/DrugsofAbuse.html.

National Institute of Drug Abuse (NIDA). (2008b). *InfoFacts: Science-based facts on drug abuse and addiction.* Retrieved January 8, 2008, from www.drugabuse.gov/infoFacts/.

National Institute on Drug Abuse (NIDA). (2008c). *Medical consequences of drug abuse.* Retrieved January 15, 2008, from www.nida.nih.gov/consequences/.

Nauert, R. (2006). *Genetic link to substance abuse confirmed. PsychCentral.* Retrieved January 6, 2008, from http://psychcentral.com/news/2006/07/06/genetic-link-to-substance-abuse-confirmed/72.html.

Nauert, R. (2007). *Genetic basis for drug abuse. PsychCentral.* Retrieved January 6, 2008, from http://psychcentral.com/news/2007/11/09/genetic-basis-for-drug-abuse/1512.html.

Piano, M.R. (2005). The cardiovascular effects of alcohol: The good and the bad. *AJN, 105*(7), 87-91.

Salladay, S. (2006). Ethical problems: Suspected drug diversion. *Nursing2006, 36*(12), 28.

Tashkin, D.P. (2005). Smoked marijuana as a cause of lung injury. *Monaldi Archives for Chest Disease, 63*(2), 93-100.

Tobacco Information and Prevention Source (TIPS). Retrieved February 8, 2007, from www.cdc.gov/tobacco/.

Varcarolis, E., Carson, V., & Shoemaker, N. (2006). *Foundations of psychiatric mental health nursing: A clinical approach* (5th ed.). Philadelphia: Saunders.

Volkow, N. (2007). *Fentanyl use in combination with street drugs leading to death in some cases.* NIDA. Retrieved January 5, 2008, from www.nida.nih.gov/about/.

Volkow, N. (2007). Steroid abuse is a high-risk route to the finish line. *NIDA Notes, 21*(1), 2.

Weiss, B. (2005). Winning the battle with addiction. *RN, 68*(7), 63-66.

Whitten, L. (2006). Studies identify factors surrounding rise in abuse of prescription drugs by college students. *NIDA Notes, 20*(4), 1, 6-10.

Zickler, P. (2006a). Buprenorphine plus a behavioral therapy is effective for adolescents with opioid addiction. *NIDA Notes, 21*(1), 7-8.

Zickler, P. (2006b). Marijuana smoking is associated with a spectrum of respiratory disorders. *NIDA NOTES, 21*(1), 12-13.

8

CHAPTER

Rehabilitation Concepts for Chronic and Disabling Health Problems

Donna D. Ignatavicius

LEARNING OUTCOMES

For clinical competence and success on the NCLEX Examination, study this chapter with these Learning Outcomes in mind:

Safe and Effective Care Environment

1. Identify the roles of each member of the interdisciplinary rehabilitation team.
2. Collaborate with members of the rehabilitation team when providing patient care.
3. Delegate and supervise selected nursing tasks as part of care for the rehabilitation patient.
4. Coordinate recommendations for home modifications with the patient, family, occupational therapist, and case manager.
5. Transfer and ambulate patients safely, avoiding lifting and possible self-injury.

Health Promotion and Maintenance

6. Assess the patient's ability to perform ADLs.
7. Interpret physical and psychosocial assessment findings for the patient in a rehabilitation program.
8. Develop a teaching plan for the rehabilitation patient who has impaired physical mobility.

Psychosocial Integrity

9. Assess the patient's response to chronic or disabling health problems.
10. Assess the family's response to the patient's chronic or disabling health problems.
11. Promote independence for the rehabilitation patient and family.

Physiological Integrity

12. Assess the ability of patients to use assistive/adaptive devices to promote independence.
13. Differentiate training techniques for a patient with a spastic versus flaccid bladder and bowel.
14. Evaluate patient outcomes of the interdisciplinary rehabilitation program.
15. Explain the primary concerns for patients being discharged to home after rehabilitation.

Go to your Companion CD or Evolve at http://evolve.elsevier.com/Iggy/ for *Self-Assessment Questions for the NCLEX Examination* keyed to these Learning Outcomes.

A **chronic health problem** is one that has existed for at least 3 months. A **disabling health problem** is any physical or mental health/behavioral health problem that can cause disability. This text focuses on physical health problems; mental health/behavioral health problems are discussed in textbooks on mental health/behavioral health nursing.

Patients with chronic and disabling health problems often participate in rehabilitation programs to prevent further disability, maintain functional ability, and restore as much function as possible. The nurse is a vital member of the rehabilitation team and the coordinator of the patient's care.

Overview

Chronic and disabling illnesses are a major health problem in the United States, with almost half of the population having one or more chronic health problems. Chronic disease accounts for the majority of all deaths, and associated medical costs account for over two thirds of the nation's health care cost. The rate of chronic and disabling conditions is expected to increase as more "baby boomers" approach late adulthood. Some people with chronic and disabling problems are in residential settings like rehabilitation centers and skilled nursing facilities, whereas others are managed at home.

Stroke is the leading cause of disability. Coronary artery disease, cancer, chronic obstructive pulmonary disease (COPD), asthma, and arthritis are other common chronic conditions that may result in varying degrees of disability. Most occur in people older than 65 years. These health problems are discussed throughout this text.

Chronic and disabling conditions are not always illnesses such as heart disease; they may also result from accidents. Accidents are a leading cause of death among young and middle-aged adults. Increasing numbers of people survive accidents because of advances in medical technology and safety equipment such as car air bags. These survivors are often faced with chronic or disabling conditions, such as traumatic brain injuries (TBIs) and spinal cord injuries (SCIs). Many of them require months to years of follow-up health care after returning to the community. As a result, the need for rehabilitation is on the rise.

Concepts Related to Rehabilitation

Rehabilitation is the continuous process of learning to live with chronic and disabling conditions, often those resulting from trauma. The main outcome of rehabilitation is that the patient will return to the best possible physical, mental, social, vocational, and economic capacity. Rehabilitation is not limited to the return of function in post-traumatic situations. It also includes education and therapy for any chronic illness characterized by a change in a body system function or body structure. Rehabilitation programs related to respiratory, cardiac, and musculoskeletal health problems are common examples that do not involve trauma.

The terms *impairment, disability,* and *handicap* were defined by the World Health Organization (WHO) in 1980 and are still sometimes used interchangeably. However, in 2001, WHO updated its definitions in *International Classification of Functioning, Disability, and Health.* This resolution states that every person can experience a decline in health resulting in some degree of disability, including both physical and social dysfunction (WHO, 2001).

After the acute condition or injury has been stabilized in a hospital, the patient may be discharged to continue the healing process at home, generally under the follow-up care of a nonhospital health care provider (e.g., a family physician). The nurse provides home care preparation, health teaching, psychosocial preparation, and information about various health care resources to help the patient resume his or her usual roles in society.

Some health problems require the intermediate step of rehabilitation ("rehab"), which can occur in a number of settings. Rehabilitation starts in the acute care hospital (sometimes called *acute rehabilitation*) and continues after discharge from the hospital. The nurse's coordination of care from acute care through community-based care is critical to the success of rehabilitation.

For continuing rehabilitation services, the most common settings are freestanding rehabilitation hospitals, rehabilitation units within hospitals, and skilled nursing facilities (SNFs) to which the patient is typically admitted for 1 to 3 weeks (Fig. 8-1). Ambulatory care rehabilitation departments and home rehabilitation programs may be needed for continuing less intensive rehabilitative services.

Some hospitals and nursing homes have converted one or more inpatient units into transitional care units (TCUs) or skilled nursing units. In this way, the patient can stay in the same health care system for both acute and continuing rehabilitative care.

After disabled patients become more confident and independent in the inpatient setting, they may choose to live at home or in a group home. Group homes are facilities in which patients live independently together with other disabled adults. Each patient or group of patients has a care provider, such as a personal care aide, to assist with ADLs and decisions requiring accurate judgments. The patients may or may not be employed. The goal of these centers is to provide independent living arrangements outside an institution, especially for younger patients with traumatic brain injury (TBI).

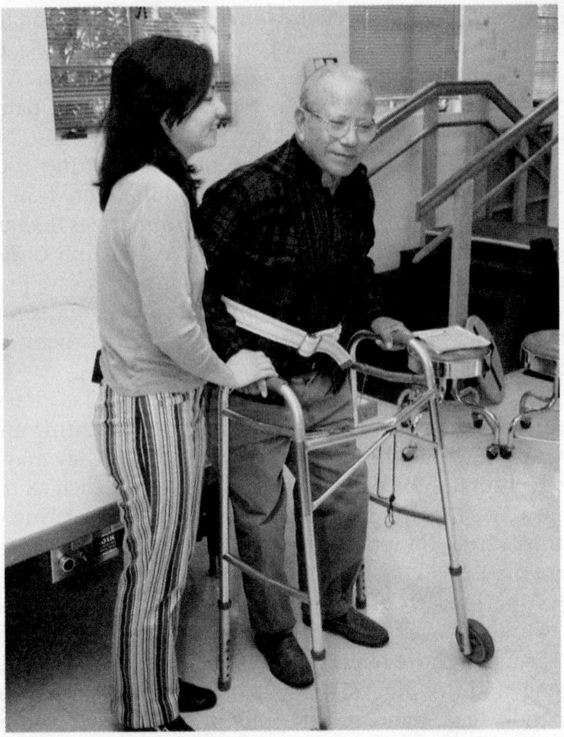

Fig. 8-1 • A physical therapist helping a patient ambulate with a walker.

The Rehabilitation Team

Successful rehabilitation depends on the coordinated effort of a group of health care professionals, the interdisciplinary rehabilitation team, and the involvement of the patient, family, and other support systems in planning and implementing care. The focus of the rehabilitation team is to restore and maintain the patient's function.

In addition to the patient, family, and/or significant others, members of the interdisciplinary health care team in the rehabilitation setting may include (Association of Rehabilitation Nurses, 2007):

- Physicians
- Nurses and nursing assistants
- Physical therapists and assistants
- Occupational therapists and assistants
- Speech-language pathologists and assistants
- Rehabilitation assistants/restorative aides
- Recreational or activity therapists
- Cognitive therapists or neuropsychologists
- Social workers
- Psychologists
- Vocational counselors
- Spiritual care counselors
- Nutritionists (formerly called *dietitians*)

Not all settings that offer rehabilitation services have all of these members on their team. All patients do not require the services of all health care team members.

A physician who specializes in rehabilitative medicine is called a **physiatrist.** Except for community-based SNFs, most inpatient rehabilitation settings employ physiatrists. A primary care physician may also oversee care for the patient's medical problems.

The **rehabilitation nurse** in the inpatient setting coordinates the efforts of the team members and therefore functions as the patient's case manager. Table 8-1 summarizes the nurse's role as part of the rehabilitation team (Association of Rehabilitation Nurses, 2007). Nurses and other health care professionals may be designated as **rehabilitation case managers** in the home or in acute care settings. Case management is described in Chapter 1.

Physical therapists (RPTs), usually called PTs, intervene to help the patient achieve mobility (e.g., by facilitating ambulation and teaching the patient to use a walker). They may also teach techniques for performing certain ADLs, such as transferring (e.g., moving into and out of bed), ambulating, and toileting. Physical therapy assistants (PTAs) may be employed to help the PT.

Occupational therapists (OTRs), usually referred to as OTs, work to develop the patient's fine motor skills used for ADLs, such as those required for eating, maintaining hygiene, dressing, and driving. OTs may also teach skills related to coordination (e.g., hand movements) and cognitive retraining (Fig. 8-2). Occupational therapy assistants (OTAs) may be available to help the OT.

Speech-language pathologists (SLPs) evaluate and retrain patients with speech, language, or swallowing problems. *Speech* is the ability to say words, and *language* is the ability to understand and put words together in a meaningful way. Some patients, especially those who have experienced a head injury or stroke, have difficulty with both speech and language. Those who have had a stroke also may have dysphagia (difficulty with swallowing). SLPs provide screening and testing for dysphagia. If the patient has this problem, the SLP recommends appropriate foods and feeding techniques. Speech-language pathology assistants (SLPAs) may be employed to help the SLP.

In the United Kingdom and Canada, assistants to PTs, OTs, and SLPs are called *rehabilitation assistants* (Stanmore et al., 2006). In the United States, **restorative aides,** often within the nursing department, assist the therapists, especially in the long-term care setting.

TABLE 8-1 Nurse's Role in the Rehabilitation Team

- Advocates for the patient and family
- Provides and coordinates holistic patient care in a variety of health care settings, including the home
- Collaborates with the rehabilitation team to establish expected patient outcomes to develop a plan of care
- Coordinates rehabilitation team activities to ensure implementation of the plan of care
- Acts as a resource to the rehabilitation team having specialized knowledge and clinical skills needed to care for patient with chronic and disabling health problems
- Communicates effectively with all members of the rehabilitation team, including the patient and family
- Plans continuity of care when the patient is discharged from the health care facility
- Evaluates the effectiveness of the interdisciplinary plan of care for the patient and family

Adapted from the Association of Rehabilitation Nurses, 2007.

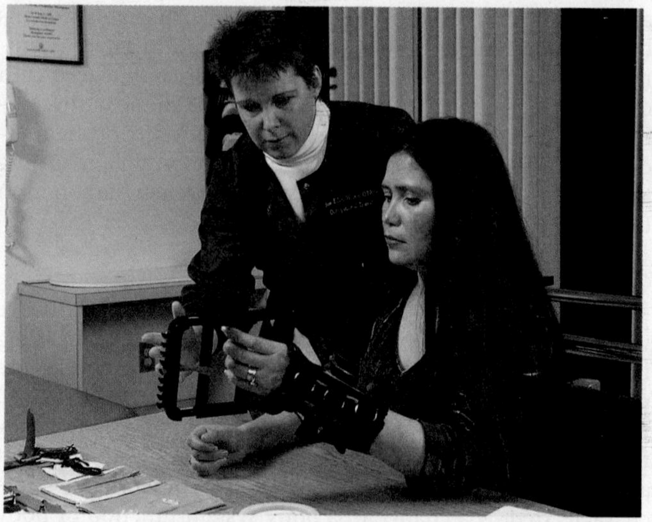

Fig. 8-2 • A registered occupational therapist working with a patient on improving hand strength.

Recreational or **activity therapists** work to help patients continue or develop hobbies or interests. These therapists often coordinate their efforts with those of the OT.

Cognitive therapists, usually neuropsychologists, work primarily with patients who have experienced head injuries with cognitive impairments. These therapists often use computers to assist with cognitive retraining.

Nutritionists, formerly called *dietitians,* ensure that patients meet their nutritional needs. For example, to prevent the constipation that often results form impaired mobility, the nutritionist can help patients select foods high in fiber content. For patients who need weight reduction, a restricted calorie diet can be planned. For patients who need additional calories or other nutrients, including vitamins, nutritionists can plan a patient-specific diet.

Nursing assistants work in the nursing departments to assist in the care of patients. These members of the rehabilitation team are under the direct supervision of the registered nurse.

Various counselors are helpful in promoting community reintegration of the patient and acceptance of the disability or chronic illness. **Social workers** help patients identify support services and resources, including financial assistance, and coordinate transfers to or discharges from the rehabilitation setting. Psychologists also counsel patients and families on their psychological problems and on strategies to cope with disability. Spiritual counselors specialize in spiritual assessments and care.

Vocational counselors assist with job placement, training, or further education. Work-related skills are taught if the patient needs to change careers because of the disability. If the patient has not yet completed high school, tutors may help with completion of the requirements for graduation.

Depending on the patient's health care needs, additional team members may be included in the rehabilitation program, such as respiratory therapists and audiologists.

Interdisciplinary team conferences for the exchange of ideas are held regularly with the patient, family members and significant others, and health care providers. Chart documentation is shared and read by all team members.

Patient-Centered Collaborative Care

evolve ONLINE PHARM REVIEW

Assessment

History

Collect the history of the patient's present condition, any current drug therapy, and any treatment programs in progress. Begin by obtaining general background data about the patient and family. This information includes cultural practices and the patient's home situation. In collaboration with the occupational therapist, the nurse or case manager addresses the layout of the home. Together they discuss whether the physical layout at home, such as stairs or the width of doorways, will present a problem to the patient after discharge.

Assess the patient's usual daily schedule and habits of everyday living. These include hygiene practices, eating, elimination, sexual activity, and sleep. Ask about the patient's preferred method and time of bathing and hygiene activity. In assessing dietary patterns, note food likes and dislikes. Also obtain information about bowel and bladder function and the normal pattern of elimination.

In assessing sexuality patterns, ask about changes in sexual function since the onset of the disability. The patient's current and previous sleep habits, patterns, usual number of hours of sleep, and use of hypnotics are also assessed. Question whether the patient feels well rested after sleep. Sleep patterns have a significant impact on activity patterns. The assessment of activity patterns focuses on work, exercise, and recreational activities.

Physical Assessment/Clinical Manifestations

Collect the physical assessment data systematically according to major body systems on admission for baseline and every day, according to agency policy and type of setting (Table 8-2). The focus of the assessment related to rehabilitation and chronic disease is on the functional abilities of the patient.

Cardiovascular and Respiratory Assessment. An alteration in cardiac status may affect the patient's cardiac output or cause activity intolerance. Assess associated signs and symptoms of decreased cardiac output (e.g., chest pain, fatigue). If present, determine when the patient experiences these symptoms and what relieves them. The physician may prescribe a change in drug therapy or may prescribe a prophylactic dose of nitroglycerin to be taken before the patient resumes activities. Collaborate with the physician and appropriate therapists to determine whether activities need to be modified.

For the patient showing fatigue, the nurse and patient plan methods for using limited energy resources. For instance, frequent rest periods can be taken throughout the day, especially before performing activities. Major tasks could be performed in the morning because most people have the most energy at that time.

A hindrance to rehabilitation for patients with cardiac disorders is fear. These patients may have survived a life-threatening experience (e.g., myocardial infarction) and are now so afraid of recurrence or death that they are unable or unwilling to resume any activity. They usually benefit from participation in a structured cardiac rehabilitation program. (See Chapter 40 for a complete description of cardiac rehabilitation.)

Ask the patient whether he or she has shortness of breath during or after activity. *Determine the level of activity that can be accomplished without experiencing shortness of breath.* For example, can the patient climb one flight of stairs without shortness of breath or does shortness of breath occur after climbing only two steps?

The fear associated with any inability to breathe normally can make a person dependent in many aspects of life. Some problems related to disorders of the respiratory system can be resolved or diminished, but some chronic diseases, such as emphysema, often continue to worsen.

Gastrointestinal and Nutritional Assessment. Monitor the patient's oral intake and pattern of eating. Also assess for the presence of anorexia, dysphagia (difficulty swallowing), nausea, vomiting, or discomfort that may interfere with oral intake. Review the patient's height, weight, hemoglobin and hematocrit levels, serum prealbumin, and blood glucose levels (see Chapter 63 for discussion of how to perform a nutritional assessment). Weight loss or weight gain is particularly significant and may be related to an associated disease or to the illness that caused the disability.

Bowel elimination habits vary from person to person. They are often related to daily job or activity schedules, dietary patterns, and family or cultural background. Elimination habits may be difficult to assess, because many nurses are hesitant to request (and many patients are afraid to volunteer) information pertaining to elimination. Ask about usual bowel patterns before the injury or the illness.

TABLE 8-2 Assessment of Patients in Rehabilitation

Body System	Relevant Data
Cardiovascular system	Chest pain Fatigue Fear of cardiac failure
Respiratory system	Shortness of breath or dyspnea Activity tolerance Fear of inability to breathe
Gastrointestinal system and nutrition	Oral intake, eating pattern Anorexia, nausea, and vomiting Dysphagia Laboratory data (e.g., serum prealbumin level) Weight loss or gain Bowel elimination pattern or habits Change in stool Ability to get to toilet
Renal-urinary system	Urinary pattern Fluid intake Urinary incontinence or retention Urine culture or urinalysis
Neurologic system	Motor function Sensation Cognitive abilities
Musculoskeletal system	Functional ability Range of motion Endurance Muscle strength
Integumentary system	Risk of skin breakdown Presence of skin lesions

Note any changes in the patient's bowel routine or stool consistency. If the patient reports any change in elimination pattern, try to determine whether it is due to a change in diet, activity pattern, or medication use. Bowel habits are evaluated on the basis of what is normal for that person.

The nurse also asks whether the patient can manage bowel functions independently. Independence in bowel elimination requires cognition, manual dexterity, sensation, muscle control, and mobility. If the patient requires help, determine whether someone is available at home to provide the assistance. The patient's and family's ability to cope with any dependency in bowel elimination should also be assessed.

Renal and Urinary Assessment. Ask about the patient's baseline urinary patterns, including the number of times the patient usually voids. Determine whether he or she routinely awakens during the night to empty the bladder or has uninterrupted sleep. Record fluid intake patterns and volume, including the type of fluids ingested and the time they were consumed.

Question whether the patient has ever had any problems with urinary incontinence or retention. Also monitor laboratory reports, especially the results of the urinalysis.

Neurologic and Musculoskeletal Assessment. In rehabilitation, the neurologic assessment includes motor function, sensation, and cognition. Assess the patient's pre-existing problems, general physical condition, and communication abilities.

Determine if the patient has **paresis** (weakness) or **paralysis** (absence of movement). Observe the patient's gait. Identify sensory-perceptual changes that could contribute to the patient's risk for injury. Assess his or her response to light touch, hot or cold temperature, and position change in each extremity and on the trunk. Identify levels of decreased sensation. For a perceptual assessment, the nurse evaluates the patient's ability to receive and understand what is heard and seen and the ability to express appropriate motor and verbal responses. During this portion of the assessment, begin to assess short-term and long-term memory.

Ascertain the patient's cognitive abilities, especially if there is a head injury or stroke. Several tools are available to evaluate cognition. One of the most common is the Mini-Mental State Examination, which is described in detail in Chapter 44.

As with other body systems, the rehabilitation nursing assessment of the musculoskeletal system focuses on function. Assess the patient's musculoskeletal status, response to the impairment, and demands of the home, work, or school environment. Determine the patient's endurance level, and measure active and passive joint range of motion (ROM). Review the results of manual muscle testing by physical therapy, which identifies the patient's ROM and resistance against gravity. In this procedure, the therapist determines the degree of muscle strength present in each body segment. The grading system usually ranges from 0 (no evidence of muscle contractility) to 5 (normal muscle contractility) (see Chapter 52).

Skin Assessment. Identify actual or potential interruptions in skin integrity. To maintain healthy skin, the body must have adequate food, water, and oxygen intake; intact waste removal mechanisms; sensation; and functional mobility. Changes in any of these variables can lead to rapid and extensive skin breakdown. If the patient cannot protect or maintain the skin, assess and plan for his or her needs. *Monitor the patient to determine the risk of skin breakdown before it occurs.*

Most rehabilitation settings use special skin assessment tools to identify patients at risk for skin breakdown. For example, the classic Braden Scale for Predicting Pressure Ulcer Risk (see Chapter 27) assesses several areas: sensory perception, skin moisture, activity level, nutritional status, and potential for friction and shear.

Other skin risk assessment tools are available. Some tools also include additional indicators of nutritional status, such as the serum prealbumin. When these levels are low, the patient is at high risk for pressure ulcers. Some tools include incontinence and altered mental state as risk factors.

If a pressure ulcer or other change in skin integrity develops, accurately assess the problem and its possible causes. Inspect the skin every 2 hours until the patient learns to inspect his or her own skin several times a day. Measure the depth and diameter of any open skin areas in centimeters or inches, depending on the policy of the facility. Assess the area around the open lesion. Determine the presence of cellulitis or other tissue damage. Chapter 27 includes several widely used classification systems for assessing skin breakdown. Determine the patient's knowledge about the cause and treatment of skin breakdown, as well as his or her ability to inspect the skin and participate in maintaining skin integrity.

In many health care agencies, a skin assessment and documentation tool ("skin sheet") is used to keep track of each area of skin breakdown. A baseline assessment is conducted on admission to the agency, and the form is updated periodically depending on the agency's policy and the nurse's judgment. In most long-term care, acute care, and rehabilitation settings, and with the patient's (or family's if the patient cannot communicate) permission, photographs of the skin are taken on admission and at various intervals for documentation.

Functional Assessment

Functional ability refers to the ability to perform **activities of daily living (ADLs),** such as bathing, dressing, feeding, and ambulating. **Independent living skills** include activities such as using the telephone, shopping, preparing food, and housekeeping. These skills are sometimes referred to as **instrumental activities of daily living (IADLs).** Functional assessment tools are used to assess a patient's abilities. Rehabilitation nurses, physiatrists, or therapists complete one or more of these assessment tools on the basis of the patient's abilities and the policy of the health care setting. The most commonly used tool is the Functional Independence Measure, although many other tools are available.

A uniform data system used for outcome data collection across the United States is the Functional Independence Measure (FIM) developed by Granger & Gresham (1984). As a basic indicator of the severity of a disability, the FIM attempts to quantify what the person actually does, whatever the diagnosis or impairment. It does not measure what a person should do or how the person would perform under a different set of circumstances. To eliminate the bias of a particular discipline, the assessment may be performed by trained clinicians. The entire assessment may be performed by one person, or certain categories may be completed by professionals from various disciplines.

Categories for assessment are self-care, sphincter control, mobility and locomotion, communication, and cognition. Scoring is done with numbers that use predetermined criteria for measurement. The patient is evaluated when he or she is admitted to and discharged from a rehabilitation institution and at other specified times to determine progress. The FIM system has also been adapted for use in other health care settings, including acute care and home care, and is available in multiple languages.

In U.S. long-term care settings, the interdisciplinary Minimum Data Set (MDS) is used to assess patients (residents) in nursing homes. The resident's motor ability, sensation, and cognition are evaluated, as well as the overall health status. Similar to the FIM, all health care team members involved in the resident's care record their assessments on the MDS.

Psychosocial Assessment

Theories of body image and self-esteem are important to assess the patient's psychosocial needs adequately. These concepts serve as a basis for understanding psychological responses to chronic illness and the resulting disability. The patient's self-esteem and body image are assessed through verbal indicators and descriptions of self-care. Encourage the family to allow the patient to perform as many functions as possible independently to promote feelings of self-worth.

Assess the patient's use of defense mechanisms and manifestations of anxiety. To assess the patient's response to loss, ask the patient to describe feelings concerning the loss of a body part or function. Assess for the presence of any stress-related physical problem. The patient may have symptoms of depression, such as fatigue, a change in appetite, or feelings of powerlessness. See Chapter 9 for a more thorough discussion of loss and grieving.

Determine the availability of support systems for the patient. The major support system is typically the family or significant others. Assess the patient's spiritual and religious needs, and refer to a counselor as needed.

Vocational Assessment

To assist patients in maximizing functional status, allow them to resume many usual activities. Vocational counselors can help patients find meaningful training, education, or employment after discharge from the rehabilitation setting.

Patients in the United States should be informed about the Americans with Disabilities Act, which was passed by Congress in 1991 to prevent employer discrimination against disabled people. The employer must offer reasonable assistance to a disabled employee to allow him or her to perform the job. For example, if an employee has a severe hearing loss, the employer may need to hire an interpreter for sign language. Workers have a right to ask for special adaptations based on their disabilities.

The rehabilitation team assesses the cognitive and physical demands of the patient's job to determine whether he or she can return to the former job or whether retraining in another field is necessary. The physical demands of jobs range from light in sedentary occupations (0-10 lb often lifted) to heavy (more than 100 lb often lifted). The nurse must also consider other aspects of the job, such as strength, mobility, or senses required (e.g., hearing).

Job analysis also involves assessing the work environment of the patient's former job. Collaborate with the vocational counselor to determine whether the environment is conducive to the patient's return. Job modifications may be needed to accommodate the patient at work. If an injured worker requires vocational rehabilitation, refer him or her to vocational rehabilitation personnel to evaluate present skills and learn new skills for employment if needed. In most states, Workers' Compensation insurance helps support vocational rehabilitation.

▪ *Analysis*

Common Nursing Diagnoses and Collaborative Problems

Regardless of age or specific disability, these nursing diagnoses are commonly applicable to the patient with chronic illness or disability:

1. Impaired Physical Mobility related to neuromuscular impairment, sensory-perceptual impairment, and/or pain
2. Self-Care Deficit (specify deficits) related to neuromuscular impairment and/or perceptual or cognitive impairment
3. Risk for Impaired Skin Integrity related to altered sensation and/or altered nutritional state
4. Impaired Urinary Elimination related to neurologic dysfunction and/or trauma or disease affecting spinal cord nerves
5. Constipation related to neurologic impairment
6. Ineffective Coping related to situational crisis and/or inadequate time to prepare for stressor

Additional Nursing Diagnoses and Collaborative Problems

Additional nursing diagnoses may apply depending on the patient's specific disability. For example, a person with rheumatoid arthritis also experiences Chronic Pain related to chronic physical disability. The patient with a spinal cord injury may also have Sexual Dysfunction related to altered body function.

▪ *Planning and Implementation*

Impaired Physical Mobility

NOC **Planning: Expected Outcomes.** Most patients with chronic illness or disability are expected to move purposefully in their environment with or without assistive device. Not all patients are able to achieve all indicators for this outcome because of physical limitations. Indicators include that the patient has normal or baseline:

- Balance
- Coordination
- Gait
- Muscle movement
- Body positioning performance
- Transfer performance

Interventions. Most problems requiring rehabilitation relate to impaired physical mobility. Patients with neurologic disease or injury, amputations, arthritis, severe burns, and cardiopulmonary disease experience some degree of impaired mobility. Coordinate care with physical and occupational therapists who are the key rehabilitation team members in helping patients meet their mobility goals. Depending on the setting, patients spend 2 to 6 hours every day working in the physical/occupational therapy department to regain function and skills.

Transfer Techniques. Patients with decreased mobility may require assistance with transfers, such as from a bed to a chair, commode, or wheelchair. Because the degree of assistance required varies with the patient and the specific disability, carefully assess mobility status before attempting a transfer. The physical or occupational therapist usually specifies the type of transfer. For example, a quadriplegic patient may use a sliding board for transfer, whereas a patient with an above-knee amputation may need a wheelchair with removable arms. In any case, for safety, always plan the transfer technique before ini-

Chart 8-1 **BEST PRACTICE FOR PATIENT SAFETY & QUALITY CARE**

Transfer Techniques

BED TO WHEELCHAIR OR CHAIR
- Place the chair at an angle to the bed on the patient's strong side.
- Lock the wheelchair brakes, or secure the chair position.
- Assist the patient to stand, and move his or her strong hand to the armrest.
- Keep the patient's body weight forward, and pivot.
- When the patient's legs touch the chair edge, assist the patient in sitting.

WHEELCHAIR OR CHAIR TO BED
- Place the chair with the patient's strong side next to the bed.
- Lock the wheelchair brakes, or secure the chair position.
- Assist the patient to stand, and move his or her strong hand to the armrest.
- Keep the patient's body weight forward, and pivot.
- When the patient's legs touch the bed edge, assist the patient in sitting and then reclining.

USE OF A SLIDING BOARD
- Place the chair or wheelchair as close to the bed as possible.
- Remove the armrest from the chair or (if removable) wheelchair.
- Powder the sliding board.
- Place the sliding board under the patient's buttocks.
- Instruct the patient to reach toward his or her side.
- Assist the patient in sliding gently to the bed.

tiating it. The desired outcome is that the patient will eventually be able to transfer independently and safely.

Basic techniques for assisting patient transfer from a bed to a chair or wheelchair (and vice versa) are identified in Chart 8-1. These techniques are also taught to the family member or other caregiver who will be caring for the patient at home. Additional information about transfers can be found in basic nursing textbooks.

Some patients cannot bear weight or are very obese. For example, a spinal cord injury resulting in quadriplegia often involves using a **sliding board** (which requires balance skills). In the past, if the patient did not have sufficient balance, nurses and therapists used a "bear hug" technique to lift the patient from bed to chair or back again. Obese patients were also lifted with multiple staff assistance. Heavy lifting has resulted in a high incidence of back injuries, which are often preventable. For that reason, some health care facilities have adopted a "no lift" or limited lift policy as part of creating an ergonomically designed and safe work environment (Waters, 2007).

The Department of Veterans' Affairs and other systems have a no-lift policy in place for all of their facilities. That means that nurses and therapists either rely on the patient to independently transfer or use a mechanical patient lift. **Mechanical patient lifts** are electrically operated devices used to lift, transfer, move, and reposition patients. Most of them use slings that are comfortable, safe, and easy to apply. They may be portable, ceiling-mounted, or wall-mounted. In 2002, the U.S. government requested that nursing homes voluntarily use mechanical lifts rather than manual transfers. Instead of a no-lift policy, though, most acute and long-term care facilities limit lifting to 35 pounds (15.9 kg). These changes involve intensive staff training and compliance to prevent staff injury. Mechanical lifts are also available for home use.

Before any transfer, carefully observe for potential problems. Orthostatic, or postural, hypotension is a common problem in rehabilitation and contributes to falls, which are common in any patient with impaired mobility. If the patient moves from a lying to a sitting or standing position too quickly, his or her blood pressure drops; as a result, he or she becomes dizzy or faints. This problem is worsened by antihypertensive drugs, especially in older adults. To prevent this situation, help the patient change positions slowly, with frequent rest periods to allow the blood pressure to stabilize. If needed, measure blood pressure with the patient in the lying, sitting, and standing positions to examine the differences. Orthostatic hypotension is indicated by a drop of more than 20 mm Hg in systolic pressure or 10 mm Hg in diastolic pressure between positions. Notify the health care provider and the therapists about this change.

If the patient has problems in maintaining blood pressure while out of bed, the physical therapist starts the patient on a tilt table to gradually increase tolerance. A low blood pressure is a particularly common problem for patients who are quadriplegic because they have a delayed blood flow to the brain and upper part of the body.

Weight gain is another potential problem. Because the patient undergoing rehabilitation has impaired mobility, he or she tends to gain weight. Excessive weight hinders transfers both for the nurse or the therapist who is assisting and for the patient who is learning to transfer independently. Weight is usually checked every week to monitor gains or losses.

Gait Training. The physical therapist works with patients for gait training if they are able to ambulate. While regaining the ability to ambulate, patients may need to use canes or walkers (Fig. 8-3). When working with patients who are using such assistive devices, also known as **ambulatory aids,** the physical therapist ensures that there is a level surface on which to walk. The patient wears a gait belt for safety so that the therapist can hold onto him or her during ambulation if needed. Falls are common when patients have mobility problems.

Reinforce the physical therapist's instructions and encourage practice, with the outcome being to walk independently with or without an assistive device. Older patients typically use a walker, with or without rollers, for a broader base of support. Younger or minimally impaired patients often progress to the use of a hemi-cane or straight cane. Chart 8-2 outlines best practices for patient safety when using assistive devices for ambulation.

Some patients never regain the ability to walk because of their impairment, such as advanced multiple sclerosis or complete high spinal cord injury. They may become wheelchair dependent and need to learn wheelchair mobility skills. With the help of physical and occupational therapy, most patients can learn to move anywhere in a wheelchair. For example, quadriplegic patients often use motorized wheelchairs that can be directed and propelled by moving their head or blowing into a device.

During the rehabilitation phase, patients are at risk for complications of immobility. Table 8-3 lists the common complications and the major strategies the nurse can use to help prevent each complication. Implementing range-of-motion (ROM) routines, adhering to schedules for turning and repositioning, and maintaining skin care are constant components

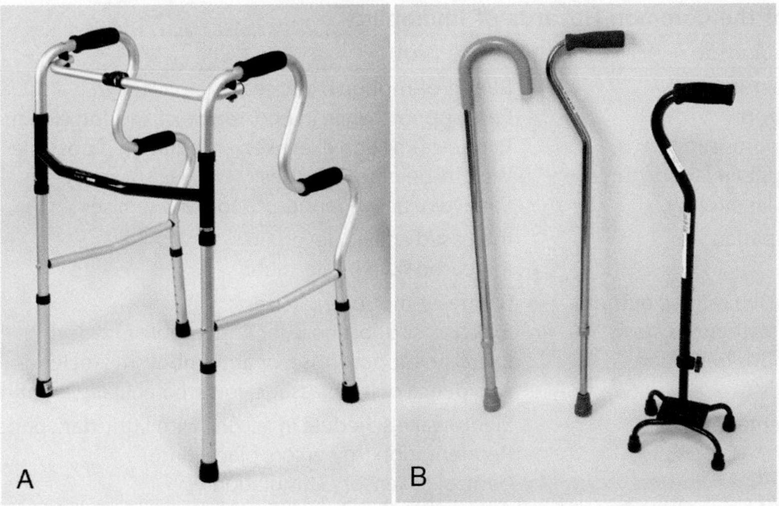

Fig. 8-3 • Assistive devices for ambulation. Assistive devices vary in the amount of support they provide. A straight cane provides less support than a walker (**A**) or quadripod cane (**B**).

Chart 8-2 **BEST PRACTICE FOR PATIENT SAFETY & QUALITY CARE**

Gait Training

WALKER ASSISTED

- Apply a gait belt around the patient's waist.
- Assist the patient to a standing position.
- Assist the patient in placing both hands on the walker.
- Ensure that the patient is well balanced.
- Assist the patient repeatedly to perform this sequence:
  - Lift the walker.
  - Move the walker 2 feet forward, and set it down on all legs.
  - While resting on the walker, take small steps.
  - Check balance.

CANE ASSISTED

- Apply a gait belt around the patient's waist.
- Assist the patient to a standing position.
- Assist the patient in placing his or her strong hand on the cane.
- Ensure that the patient is well balanced.
- Assist the patient to perform this sequence repeatedly:
  - Move the cane forward.
  - Move the weaker leg one step forward.
  - Move the stronger leg one step forward.
  - Check balance.

of rehabilitation nursing care to prevent complications of immobility. The key is to increase mobility.

One way to increase mobility, even with patients who are bedridden, is through ROM exercises. ROM techniques are beneficial for any patient with decreased mobility (Table 8-4). Although simple ROM techniques are presented in basic nursing textbooks, a few key principles are pertinent to rehabilitation nursing care:

- The human body contains more joints than simply the knees, hips, elbows, and shoulders. For ROM techniques to be effective in preventing musculoskeletal contractures, the patient must exercise all joints, including each joint of the fingers, hands, toes, and so forth.
- In performing ROM activities, the nurse or patient performs full-range movement of each joint at least five times and completes the entire process at least three times daily.
- *The nurse does not move the joints beyond the point at which the patient expresses pain or beyond the point at which resistance occurs.*

Patients with decreased mobility who are able to follow directions are taught by the nurse and the physical therapist to perform active or active-assisted ROM exercises.

NCLEX EXAMINATION CHALLENGE

The nurse observes that a nursing assistant is preparing to transfer a newly admitted 250-lb client with severe arthritis and recent left hip surgery from the bed to the chair. What is the nurse's best response to the assistant at this time?

A. "I'll help you with the client's transfer as soon as I've finished giving my meds."
B. "Does the client need any help to transfer from the bed to the chair?"
C. "Be sure to get some help when you transfer the client to the chair."
D. "Let me check with PT to make sure that he can transfer by himself."

evolve For the correct answer, go to http://evolve.elsevier.com/Iggy/.

Self-Care Deficit

NOC **Planning: Expected Outcomes.** Most patients with chronic illness or disability are expected to perform basic physical tasks and personal care activities independently with or without assistive devices. Indicators include that the patient demonstrates the ability to perform these activities independently or with minimal assistance:

- Eating
- Dressing
- Toileting
- Bathing
- Grooming
- Hygiene
- Oral hygiene
- Walking or wheelchair mobility
- Transfer performance
- Positioning of self

TABLE 8-3 Prevention of the Common Hazards of Immobility

Body System	Complication	Prevention
Musculoskeletal	Contractures	Range-of-motion exercises
	Foot drop	Foot support while in bed, range-of-motion exercises, high-top tennis shoes
	Osteoporosis	Range-of-motion exercises, ambulation if possible (walking)
	Susceptibility to fractures	Weight-bearing exercises
	Muscular atrophy	Passive or active range-of-motion exercises
Gastrointestinal	Constipation	Increased activity level Increased fluid intake, fiber
Cardiovascular	Decreased cardiac output	Range-of-motion exercises
	Increased venous stasis	Exercise, support hose, or antiembolism stockings
	Thrombus formation	Exercise, support hose, or antiembolism stockings
	Embolism	Avoidance of leg massage, low–molecular weight heparin
Neurologic	Disorientation	Sleep-wake schedule in accord with light-dark pattern Reorientation (to person, place, time) Control of sensory stimulation
	Postural hypotension	Avoidance of sudden position changes, tilt table
Renal/urinary	Calculi	Decreased dietary calcium level, if needed Increased fluid intake Maintenance of acidic urine
	Infection	Use intermittent catheterization instead of indwelling if possible
Respiratory	Pneumonia	Frequent repositioning in wheelchair or bed Respiratory exercises
Integumentary (Skin)	Pressure ulcers	Frequent repositioning in wheelchair or bed Pressure relief devices (bed and wheelchair) Skin care Adequate nutrition Skin monitoring

TABLE 8-4 Types of Range-of-Motion Exercises

Type	Description	Indications
Passive	Exercises are performed by the nurse for the patient.	The patient is too weak to participate actively.
Active	Exercises are performed by the patient.	The patient is able to complete range-of-motion movements.
Assisted, or active assisted	Exercises are performed by the patient but are guided by the nurse or therapist.	The patient is weak and needs assistance.
Resistive	The actions of the patient are in opposition to those performed by the nurse or therapist.	The patient has full range of motion, and an increase in strength is desired.

Interventions. ADLs, or self-care activities, include eating, bathing, dressing, grooming, and toileting. Encourage the patient to perform as much self-care as possible. Be patient because he or she often takes more time to complete a task than healthy adults do. Collaborate with the occupational therapist (OTR) to identify ways in which self-care activities can be modified so the patient can perform them independently and with minimal frustration if possible. For example, the OTR teaches a hemiplegic patient to put on a shirt by first placing the affected arm in the sleeve and then putting the unaffected arm in the appropriate sleeve. Reinforce this dressing technique, and encourage the patient to practice.

In long-term care (LTC) settings (e.g., nursing homes), federal regulations require that residents not lose their functional skills while they are in the facility. Therefore most facilities have developed *restorative nursing* programs and have coordinated these programs with rehabilitation therapy and activity therapy. The focus of this coordinated effort includes:

- Bed mobility
- Walking
- Transfers
- Dressing
- Grooming
- Active range of motion
- Communication

A variety of devices are available for patients with chronic illness and disability for *assisting with self-care*. An **assistive/adaptive device,** or self-care support device, is any item that enables the patient to perform all or part of an activity independently and safely. Table 8-5 identifies common devices and describes their use.

Many department stores and large pharmacies carry clothing and assistive/adaptive devices designed for patients with disabilities. The occupational therapist determines specific patient needs for this equipment. Collaborate with the occupational therapist to look for creative and inexpensive alternatives to meeting these needs. For example, barbecue tongs may be used as "reachers" for pulling up pants or obtaining items on high shelves. A foam curler with the plastic insert

TABLE 8-5 Examples and Uses of Common Assistive/Adaptive Devices

Device	Use
Buttonhook	Threaded through the buttonhole to enable patients with weak finger mobility to button shirts Alternative uses include serving as pencil holder or cigarette holder
Extended shoehorn	Assists in the application of shoes for patients with decreased mobility Alternative uses include turning light switches off or on while patient is in a wheelchair
Plate guard and spork (spoon and fork in one utensil)	Applied to a plate to assist patients with weak hand and arm mobility to feed themselves; spork allows one utensil to serve two purposes
Gel pad	Placed under a plate or a glass to prevent dishes from slipping and moving Alternative uses include placement under bathing and grooming items to prevent them from moving
Foam buildups	Applied to eating utensils to assist patients with weak hand grasps to feed themselves Alternative uses include application to pens and pencils to assist with writing or over a buttonhook to assist with grasping the device
Hook and loop fastener (Velcro) straps	Applied to utensils, a buttonhook, or a pencil to slip over the hand and provide a method of stabilizing the device when the patient's hand grasp is weak
Long-handled reacher	Assists in obtaining items located on high shelves or at ground level for patients who are unable to change positions easily
Elastic shoelaces or Velcro shoe closure	Prevents the need for tying shoes

removed may be placed over a pencil or eating utensil to make a built-up device. The patient might use an extended shoehorn to operate light switches from wheelchair height. Hook-and-loop fasteners (Velcro) sewn on clothes can prevent the frustrations caused by buttons and zippers. Chart 8-3 lists nursing interventions for patients who need self-care assistance.

Assistive technology has further increased the ability for disabled patients to care for themselves through the use of electronic equipment. For example, telephones can be dialed using a voice-activated dialing device. Computer keyboards can also be operated by voice-activation devices.

Fatigue often occurs with chronic and disabling conditions. Therefore collaborate with the occupational therapist to assess the patient's self-care abilities and to determine possible ways of *conserving energy*. Coordinate with the therapist to develop strategies for energy conservation after evaluating the patient's self-care routines. Preparation for ADLs can help reduce effort and energy expenditure (e.g., gathering all necessary equipment before starting grooming routines). If a patient has high energy levels in the morning, he or she can be taught to schedule energy-intensive activities in the morning rather than later in the day or evening. Spacing activities is also helpful for conserving energy. In addition, allowing time to rest before and after eating and toileting decreases the strain on energy level.

Chart 8-3 NIC INTERVENTION ACTIVITIES

The Patient in Rehabilitation

Self-Care Assistance: *Assisting another to perform activities of daily living*

- Monitor patient's ability for independent self-care.
- Monitor patient's need for adaptive devices for personal hygiene, dressing, grooming, toileting, and eating.
- Provide assistance until the patient is fully able to assume self-care.
- Use consistent repetition of health routines as a means of establishing them.
- Encourage patient to perform normal activities of daily living to level of ability.
- Teach family to encourage independence, to intervene only when the patient is unable to perform.
- Establish a routine for self-care activities.

NIC intervention activities selected from Bulechek, G.M., Butcher, H.K., & McCloskey Dochterman, J. (Eds.). (2008). *Nursing interventions classification (NIC).* (5th ed.). St. Louis: Mosby. No part of this work is to be altered without prior written permission from the Publisher.

Risk for Impaired Skin Integrity

NOC Planning: Expected Outcomes The patient with chronic illness or disability is expected to have structural intactness and physiologic function of the skin as indicated by having none of these:

- Skin lesions
- Erythema
- Blanching
- Necrosis
- Induration
- Skin flaking

Interventions. *The best intervention to prevent skin impairment is frequent position changes in combination with adequate skin care and sufficient nutritional intake.* Teach staff to *turn and reposition all patients every 2 hours* if they are unable to perform this activity. This time frame may not be sufficient for people who are frail and have thin skin, especially older adults (Chart 8-4). To determine the best turning schedule, assess the patient's skin condition during each turning and repositioning. For example, if the patient has been sleeping for 2 hours and the nursing assistant decides to postpone turning for 1 hour, reddened areas over the bony prominences may be present. If reddened areas do not fade within 30 minutes after pressure relief or do not blanch, they may be classified as pre-ulcer areas, or stage I pressure areas (see Chapter 27).

Patients who sit for prolonged periods in a wheelchair need to be repositioned at least every 1 to 2 hours. Each patient is evaluated by the physical or occupational therapist for the best seating pad or cushion that is comfortable yet reduces pressure on bony prominences. Patients who are able are taught to perform "wheelchair push-ups" by using their arms to lift their buttocks off the wheelchair seat for 10 seconds or longer every hour, or more often if needed. The physical therapist helps them strengthen their arm muscles in preparation for performing wheelchair push-ups.

If the patient wears tennis shoes for foot positioning to prevent footdrop, remove the shoes and assess for pressure areas every 2 hours. Many patients with neurologic problems have decreased or absent sensation and may not be able to feel the discomfort of increased pressure. Also check patients who are sitting in wheelchairs for signs of pressure, especially on the lower legs where the leg of the wheelchair could rub against the skin.

Adequate skin care is an essential component of prevention. Perform or assist patients in completing skin care each time they are turned, repositioned, or bathed. Delegate and supervise skin care to unlicensed assistive personnel (UAP), including cleaning soiled areas, drying carefully, and applying body lotion. If a patient is incontinent, topical barrier creams or ointments can help protect the skin from moisture, which facilitates skin breakdown. *Teach UAP to avoiding rubbing reddened areas to prevent damage to the already fragile capillary system.* Instead, carefully observe the areas for further breakdown and relieve pressure on the areas as much as possible. Bed pillows are often good pressure-relieving devices. (See Chapter 27 for a complete discussion of skin care interventions.)

Sufficient nutrition is needed both to repair wounds and to prevent pressure ulcers. Collaborate with the nutritionist to assess the patient's food selection and ensure that it contains adequate protein and carbohydrates. Both the nurse and the nutritionist closely monitor the patient's weight and serum prealbumin levels. If either of these indices decreases significantly, the patient may be given high-protein, high-carbohydrate food supplements (e.g., milkshakes) or commercial preparations (also see Chapter 63).

Pressure-relieving devices include waterbeds, gel mattresses or pads, air mattresses, low–air loss overlays or beds, and air-fluidized beds. Mattress overlays, such as air and gel types, and replacement mattresses are often effective in reducing pressure. The use of any mechanical device (except air-fluidized beds) does not eliminate the need for turning and repositioning.

Specialty beds are categorized as either "low air loss" or "air fluidized." Air-fluidized therapy (e.g., Clinitron or FluidAir bed) provides the most effective pressure relief by distributing the patient's weight to prevent pressure in any one area (Fig. 8-4). These beds are not used to *prevent* skin breakdown because most insurers will not reimburse the agency for the use of the bed. Therefore these special beds are usually reserved for *severe skin problems* that have not healed with the use of a conventional bed or other mechanical device. The primary disadvantage of this therapy is its expense, which may exceed several hundred dollars for each day of use. Patients also report the heat generated by the bed. Although air-fluidized beds are heavy to move, lighter and more portable versions are available for home use. The cost of air-fluidized therapy is re-

Chart 8-4 NURSING FOCUS ON THE OLDER ADULT

Special Considerations in Rehabilitation

- When getting the patient out of bed, move him or her (or instruct him or her to move or sit up) slowly to prevent orthostatic hypotension. This problem is most common in older adults who take antihypertensive medications.
- Turn the patient *more* often than every 2 hours, even if it is just a minor position change. Skin becomes thinner and more fragile with age, and subcutaneous tissue thins.
- Determine whether the patient had any problem with urinary patterns before the illness or rehabilitation. A patient with a previous problem may not have a successful bladder training program.
- Be aware that intestinal motility decreases with age, which leads to constipation.
- Assess the patient's support system of family and significant others. Many older adults have no spouse or close friends, who would usually serve as a support network.

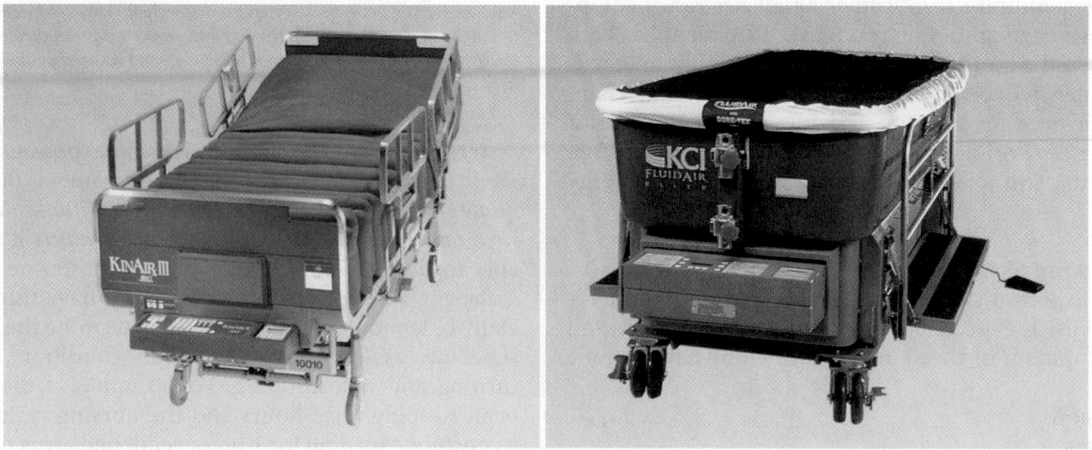
KinAir III
KCI
FLUIDAIR

Fig. 8-4 • Pressure relief devices. *Left,* KinAir III beds provide controlled air suspension to redistribute body weight away from bony prominences. *Right,* FluidAir Elite beds use airflow and bead fluidizations. Both of these beds are covered with GORE-TEX fabric, which resists tearing. This fabric is also waterproof and acts as a barrier against bacteria.

imbursed by some health insurance providers if the bed is deemed medically necessary for the patient's skin problem.

Impaired Urinary Elimination

NOC **Planning: Expected Outcomes.** Most patients with chronic illness or disability are expected to have a normal collection and discharge of urine. Not all patients are able to meet the following indicators because of physiologic impairment. Indicators include that the patient has normal or baseline:

- Elimination pattern
- Adequacy of fluid intake
- Emptying of bladder

In addition, the patient is expected to have none of these:

- Hesitancy with urination
- Urinary retention (which can lead to urinary tract infection)
- Urinary incontinence

Interventions. Neurologic disabilities may interfere with successful bladder control in a patient undergoing rehabilitation. These disabilities result in three basic functional types of neurogenic bladder: reflex (spastic) bladder, flaccid bladder, and uninhibited bladder.

A **spastic** or **reflex** (upper motor neuron) **bladder** causes incontinence with sudden, gushing voids. The bladder does not usually empty completely. A reflex bladder is also sometimes referred to as a *spastic bladder.* Neurologic problems affecting the upper motor neuron typically occur with high-level or mid-level spinal cord injuries above the twelfth thoracic vertebra (T12). These injuries result in a failure of impulse transmission from the lower spinal cord areas to the cortex of the brain. When the bladder fills and transmits impulses to the spinal cord, the patient is not conscious of the filling sensation. However, because there is no injury to the lower spinal cord and the voiding reflex arc is intact, the efferent (motor) impulse is relayed and the bladder contracts.

A **flaccid** or **areflexic** (lower motor neuron) **bladder** results in urinary retention and overflow (dribbling). Injuries that cause damage to the lower motor neuron at the spinal cord level of S2-4 (e.g., multiple sclerosis, spinal cord injury below T12) may directly interfere with the reflex arc or may result in improper interpretation of impulses to the brain. The bladder fills, and afferent (sensory) impulses conduct the message via the spinal cord to the brain cortex. Because of the injury, the impulse is not interpreted correctly by the brain's bladder center and there is a failure to respond with a message for the bladder to contract.

An **uninhibited bladder** is similar to a reflex bladder in that it is the result of damage to upper motor neurons. It frequently occurs when the patient has a neurologic problem that affects the brain's bladder center in the frontal lobe, such as stroke or brain injury. When the bladder needs to empty, the patient has little sensorimotor control and cannot wait until he or she is on the commode or bedpan before voiding. The patient is incontinent, but the bladder may not completely empty.

Post-Void Residual Assessment. Patients who cannot completely empty their bladder are at risk for post-void residual. **Post-void residual (PVR)** is the amount of urine remaining in the bladder within 20 minutes after voiding (Newman, 2007). PVR assessments using a noninvasive ultrasound device called the *BladderScan* are performed by nurses at the bedside. The residual amount measured is accurate if the device is used correctly. It is not accurate when used for patients who are morbidly obese. The outcome of bladder ultrasonography is to prevent an indwelling urinary catheter. Long-term urinary catheters cause urinary tract infections that are often chronic. A picture of the BladderScan device is in Chapter 68 (see Fig. 68-10).

Bladder Training. The nurse can teach a variety of techniques to assist the patient in "repatterning" voiding, also called *bladder training:*

- Facilitating, or triggering, techniques
- Intermittent catheterization
- Consistent scheduling of toileting routines; "timed void"

These techniques may not be as effective in patients with physiologic changes associated with aging.

Facilitating (triggering) techniques are used to stimulate voiding (Table 8-6). If there is an upper motor neuron problem but the reflex arc is intact (reflex bladder pattern), the voiding response can be initiated by any stimulus that sends the message to the spinal cord level S2-4 that the bladder might be full. Such techniques include stroking the medial aspect of the thigh, pinching the area above the groin, massaging the penoscrotal area, pinching the posterior aspect of the glans penis, and providing digital anal stimulation.

When the patient has a lower motor neuron problem, the voiding reflex arc is not intact (flaccid bladder pattern) and additional stimulation may be needed to initiate voiding. Two techniques used to facilitate voiding are the Valsalva maneuver and the Credé maneuver. In teaching the Valsalva maneu-

TABLE 8-6 Management of Impaired Urinary Elimination

Functional Type	Neurologic Disability	Clinical Manifestations	Re-establishing Voiding Patterns
Reflex (spastic)	Upper motor neuron spinal cord injury above T12	Urinary frequency, incontinence	Triggering or facilitating techniques Medications Bedside bladder ultrasound Intermittent catheterization Consistent toileting schedule
Flaccid	Lower motor neuron spinal cord injury below T12 (affects S2-4 reflex arc)	Urinary retention, overflow	Valsalva and Credé maneuvers Medications
Uninhibited	Brain damage from injury or stroke	Frequency, urgency, incontinence, voiding in small amounts	Intermittent catheterization Consistent toileting schedule Regulation of fluid intake

ver, teach the patient to hold his or her breath and bear down as if trying to defecate. Assist the patient in performing the Credé maneuver by placing the patient's hand in a cupped position directly over the bladder area and instructing him or her to push inward and downward as if massaging the bladder to empty.

Intermittent catheterization may be used for disorders that involve a flaccid or spastic bladder. A urinary catheter is inserted to drain urine every 2 to 3 hours—after the patient has attempted voiding and has used the Valsalva and Credé maneuvers. If less than 150 mL of post-void residual is obtained, the nurse typically increases the interval between catheterizations. This interval may be up to 3 to 4 hours according to the health care provider's prescription or health care agency protocol. *The patient should not go beyond 8 hours between catheterizations.* If the patient will be performing intermittent self-catheterization at home after discharge from the rehabilitation facility, teach the patient about clean (not sterile) technique. In some cases, a specialized appliance may be used to help patients perform self-catheterization, especially for those who have problems with manual dexterity. For patients who cannot catheterize themselves, a family member or significant other may need to be taught how to perform the procedure.

Consistent toileting routines may be the best way to re-establish voiding continence when the patient displays an *uninhibited bladder* pattern (associated with stroke or head injury). Assess the patient's previous voiding pattern, and determine his or her daily routine. At a minimum, the nurse assists the patient with voiding after awakening in the morning, before and after meals, before and after physical activity, and at bedtime. *Remind the staff to toilet the patient every 2 hours during the day and every 3 to 4 hours at night.*

Consider the patient's bladder capacity, which may range from 100 to 500 mL, as well as mobility limitations and restrictive clothing. Bladder capacity is determined by measuring urine output. Ensure that the patient is aware of nearby bathrooms at all times or has a call system to contact the nurse or unlicensed assistive personnel for assistance. Chapter 69 also describes methods of achieving bladder control.

Drug Therapy. Drugs that may be used for urinary elimination problems include cholinergics (to promote bladder emptying), antispasmodics (to prevent incontinence), and skeletal muscle relaxants (to decrease spasticity, which promotes self-care). Drug therapy is not usually prescribed by the health care provider in the initial management of bladder problems but may be used to assist with the initial bladder training program. Report the patient's progress in bladder training to the rehabilitation team so that the best decision regarding drug therapy can be made. In general, cholinergics, antispasmodics, and skeletal muscle relaxants help promote continence in patients with a reflex (upper motor neuron) bladder. Cholinergics, such as bethanechol chloride (Urecholine), may decrease urinary retention problems resulting from a flaccid bladder. They may also facilitate complete bladder emptying in a patient with a large residual volume, which occurs with reflex bladder problems. An uninhibited bladder does not routinely require medications for bladder training programs unless urinary function is affected by additional pathologic changes.

Fluid Intake. Instruct the patient to maintain an adequate intake of fluids—at least 2000 to 2500 mL/day. An acidic urine may minimize the risk of urinary tract infection and calculus (stone) formation, although this belief is controversial. Some microorganisms, such as *Escherichia coli,* grow best in acidic environments. Encourage the patient to drink fluids, including large amounts of cranberry juice, prune juice, bouillon, tomato juice, and water. Discourage fluids that promote an alkaline urine, including citrus juices, excessive amounts of milk and milk products, and carbonated beverages. Remind patients that water is the preferred liquid to help prevent urinary infection. Teach them to avoid excessive caffeinated beverages because they tend to contribute to dehydration, especially in older adults.

In addition, discourage high-calorie fluids for overweight patients. Disabled patients have more difficulty with mobility and self-care if their weight is not controlled.

Constipation

NOC **Planning: Expected Outcomes.** The patient with chronic illness or disability is expected to have a normal formation and evacuation of stool. Indicators include that the patient has:

- Return of usual elimination pattern
- Control of bowel movements
- Ease of stool passage
- Comfort of stool passage
- Muscle tone to evacuate stool

Interventions. Neurologic problems often affect the patient's bowel pattern by causing a reflex (spastic) bowel, a flaccid bowel, or an uninhibited bowel.

Upper motor neuron diseases and injuries, such as a cervical or mid-level spinal cord injury, may result in a reflex (spastic) bowel pattern, with defecation occurring suddenly and without warning. With a reflex pattern, any facilitating or triggering mechanism may lead to defecation if the lower colon contains stool. An example of facilitating or triggering techniques is digital stimulation. For this technique, use a lubricated glove or finger cot and massage the anus in a circular motion for no less than 1 full minute. *Digital stimulation should not be used for patients with cardiac disease because of the risk of inducing a vagal response (a rapid decrease in heart rate).*

Lower motor neuron diseases and injuries interfere with transmission of the nervous impulse across the reflex arc and may result in a flaccid bowel pattern, with defecation occurring infrequently and in small amounts. The use of facilitating and triggering mechanisms in combination with a toileting schedule, suppository use, and disimpaction may get the best results. Patients may be able to self-administer the suppository or disimpact if necessary.

Neurologic injuries that affect the brain may cause an uninhibited bowel pattern, with frequent defecation, urgency, and reports of hard stool. Patients may manage uninhibited bowel patterns through a consistent toileting schedule, a high-fiber diet, and the use of stool softeners.

An overview of management techniques for bowel dysfunction is presented in Table 8-7. In many cases, patients are not able to regain their previous level of control over their bowel function. The rehabilitation team assists in designing a bowel elimination program that accommodates the disability.

Work with patients to schedule bowel elimination as close as possible to their previous routine. For example, a patient who had stools at noon every other day before the illness or injury should have the bowel program scheduled in the same way. An exception is the patient who prefers another time that best fits into his or her daily routine. If the patient is employed

TABLE 8-7 Management of Bowel Dysfunction

Functional Type	Neurologic Disability	Dysfunction	Re-establishing Defecation Patterns
Reflex (spastic)	Upper motor neuron spinal cord injury above T12	Defecation without warning	Triggering mechanisms Facilitation techniques High-fiber diet Suppository use Consistent toileting schedule
Flaccid	Lower motor neuron spinal cord injury below T12 (affects S2-4 reflex arc)	Infrequent, small stools	Triggering or facilitating techniques High-fiber diet Suppository use Consistent toileting schedule Manual disimpaction
Uninhibited	Brain damage from injury or stroke	Frequency, urgency, constipation	Consistent toileting schedule High-fiber diet Stool softener use

during the day, a time-consuming bowel elimination program in the morning may not be reasonable. It may be preferable to change the bowel protocol to the evening, when there is more time.

Bowel training programs for patients with neurologic problems are often designed to include a combination of suppository use and a consistent toileting schedule. Although drug therapy should not be a first choice when formulating a bowel training program, consider the need for a suppository if the patient does not re-establish defecation habits through a consistent toileting schedule, dietary modification, anal stimulation, and disimpaction.

Bisacodyl (Dulcolax) and glycerin are common agents prescribed by health care providers as suppositories in bowel training programs. Suppositories must be placed against the bowel wall to stimulate the sacral reflex arc and promote rectal emptying. Both agents are equivalent in effect, with results occurring in 15 to 30 minutes. Administer the suppository when the patient expects to defecate, for example, after a meal to coincide with the gastrocolic reflex. Using the suppository every second or third day is usually effective in re-establishing defecation patterns. Depending on each patient's need, other drugs (e.g., laxatives) may be indicated for bowel training programs.

For patients at risk for constipation, encourage fluids and plenty of fiber in the diet. Whole grains, fruits, and nuts are good sources of fiber. Do not offer a bedpan when toileting. Instead, be sure that the patient sits upright on a bedside commode or bathroom toilet to facilitate defecation. Stool softeners and bulk-forming laxatives, such as psyllium hydrophilic mucilloid (Metamucil), may be needed to promote bowel elimination. Remember that Metamucil may bind with some drugs, such as anticoagulants, thyroid replacements, and digoxin, and prevent their absorption. Timing of this drug is best when it is separated from other prescribed drugs by at least 3 hours.

DECISION-MAKING CHALLENGE
Coordination of Care

You are a nurse working in a facility that specializes in rehabilitation of stroke patients. One of your recently admitted patients reports that she dribbles urine and does not want to "wet" herself. She also says that she hasn't had a bowel movement in at least 3 days. The patient walks with a walker but remains unsteady at times when ambulating. Your unit on the night shift has been short-handed, and you are concerned that patients are not being toileted as often as they should be.

1. With what members of the interdisciplinary team should you collaborate to manage the patient's current concerns?
2. What should you report to your nursing assistant related to this patient's care?
3. What will you report to the physiatrist, and why?

evolve For suggested answer guidelines, go to http://evolve.elsevier.com/Iggy/.

Ineffective Coping

NOC **Planning: Expected Outcomes.** The patient with chronic illness or disability is expected to take personal actions to manage stressors that impact the patient's resources. Indicators include that the patient consistently:

- Identifies ineffective and effective coping patterns
- Verbalizes a sense of control
- Reports decrease in stress
- Seeks information concerning illness and treatment
- Modifies lifestyle as needed
- Adapts to life changes
- Uses available social support

Interventions. The patient with a disability often has a poor self-concept because of changes in body image from structural or functional changes. The use of an assistive device, such as a wheelchair, also makes the patient different from other people, and he or she may not want to accept the need for the device. Encourage patients to discuss their feelings, and ask questions to obtain information that can help in assessing acceptance of and ability to cope with the disability.

A disability also affects a person's role in society. For instance, a young medical student may fall from a ladder and become a quadriplegic; as a result, plans for a career as a surgeon are altered. A middle-aged farmer may be burned severely when his tractor catches on fire. He can no longer care for his farm, and his wife takes over during his rehabilitation process. An older adult who cares for her grandchildren is crippled with rheumatoid arthritis and can no longer provide childcare. Disability requires role changes and always involves losses in the lives of those affected.

In addition to role changes, relationships with people change. Socializing with friends and family may be a strain when a person feels different. Intimate relationships may be affected because sexual dysfunction may result from disability. Be sensitive to these issues, and do not avoid discussing them.

Assess the patient's previous coping strategies and support systems so they can be used during rehabilitation if needed. Ask the patient what strategies have been used to cope successfully with previous life crises, if any. Spiritual and religious beliefs are important for some people and should not be overlooked when helping identify sources of support.

Some patients use complementary and alternative medicine (CAM) to cope with chronic disease and disability, especially if chronic pain is a problem. Examples of these therapies are acupuncture, acupressure, imagery, and music. Chapter 2 discusses CAM in detail.

Community-Based Care

Discharge planning begins at the time of the patient's admission. If the patient is transferred from a hospital to a rehabilitation unit or long-term care facility, orient him or her to the change in routine and emphasize the importance of self-care. When the patient is admitted, a case manager or OTR assesses his or her current living situation at home. Together with the patient and family members or significant others, they determine the adequacy of the current situation and the potential needs after discharge to home. The patient with chronic illness and disability may require home care, assistance with ADLs, nursing care, or physical or occupational therapy after discharge.

Other health care professionals may be necessary to meet the unique needs of special populations. For example, patients with brain injury may benefit from life planning—a process that examines and plans to meet lifelong needs. Case managers specializing in life planning may be part of the interdisciplinary rehabilitation team.

Home Care Management

Before the patient returns home, the nurse assesses his or her readiness for discharge from the rehabilitation facility or hospital. The home may be assessed in multiple ways.

Predischarge Assessment. Before discharge, the case manager or OT may visit the home to assess its layout and accessibility. These professionals may be employed by the health care agency or by a third-party payer, such as a health maintenance organization. Because of the stress of hospitalization, a patient with a fractured hip who is ambulating well with a walker may neglect to explain to the nurse that the bathroom in the home is accessible by stairway only. The patient may not consider it important to mention that throw rugs, which can cause falls, are scattered throughout the apartment. Other fall prevention strategies in the home environment are discussed in Chapter 3.

During a predischarge visit to the home, the accessibility of bathrooms, bedrooms, and kitchen is assessed. If the patient will be wheelchair dependent after discharge from the facility, home modifications may be needed, such as ramps to replace steps. Doorways should be checked for adequate width. A doorway width of 36 to 38 inches (slightly less than 1 m) is usually sufficient for a standard-size wheelchair. Any room that the patient needs to use is checked. The bedroom should have sufficient space for the patient to maneuver transfers to and from the wheelchair and the bed. The bathroom may need a raised toilet seat to at least 17 inches (43 cm).

Space requirements depend on the patient's need to use a wheelchair, walker, or cane. In the bathroom, grab bars may need to be installed before the patient comes home. Bathtub benches can provide support for the patient who has difficulty with mobility and, when used in combination with a handheld shower head, can provide easily accessible bathing facilities. Assessment of the kitchen may or may not be critical, depending on whether the patient has help with cooking and preparing meals. If the patient will be cooking after discharge, the kitchen is assessed for wheelchair or walker accessibility, appliance accessibility, and the need for adaptive equipment.

Leave-of-Absence Visit. A second method of assessing the patient's home is through a brief home visit, also called a *leave-of-absence (LOA)* visit, before discharge. Explain the need for the trial home visit, and assess the patient's comfort level with this idea. The patient who has been hospitalized for a lengthy period may feel intense anxiety about returning home. The nurse may allay such anxieties with careful preparation. Before the visit, the rehabilitation nurse meets with the patient and family members or significant others to set goals for the visit and to identify specific tasks to be attempted while at home. After the home visit, interview the patient to determine the success of the visit and to assess additional education or training needs before final discharge.

Going home may not be an option for everyone. Some patients may not have a support network of family members or significant others. For example, many older adults have no spouse or close friends living nearby. Children may live far away, which can make home care difficult. If no caregiver is available, the family must decide whether care can be provided in the home by an outside resource. The patient may need to be admitted to a 24-hour supervised health care setting, such as a nursing home. Continued rehabilitation services are available in most long-term care settings (skilled nursing facilities) at least 5 days a week if it is medically necessary.

Health Teaching

The OTR and RPT teach the patient to perform ADLs independently. The patient's learning potential and cognitive capacity are assessed. The patient is asked to perform or direct each skill or technique independently to verify understanding. Written material explaining the steps in the procedure is provided to the patient and family members to reinforce learning and to provide support with the technique after discharge. Before distributing written material, the rehabilitation team assesses the reading level of the material and determines whether it is appropriate for the patient's reading ability and language skills.

Any chronic illness or disability necessitates changes in lifestyle and body image. Assist the patient in dealing with such changes by encouraging verbalization of feelings and emotions. A focus on existing capabilities instead of disabilities is emphasized.

The patient may fail to relate psychologically to the disability during hospitalization. For example, he or she may display anger or frustration in attempting to perform self-care routines before discharge from the rehabilitation facility. Encourage the patient to be open about such feelings and to talk about ways to prevent worries from becoming realities after discharge. If needed, refer the patient to a mental health professional to help with adjustment and coping strategies.

The leave-of-absence home visit assists the patient and family members or significant others in psychosocial preparation for discharge. It allows the experience of the home situation while being able to return to the hospital environment after a few hours. Often the patient finds new problems in the home that must be addressed before discharge. Review this information with the patient in preparation for discharge to the home.

Health Care Resources

After discharge to the home, various health care resources (e.g., physical therapy, home care nursing, vocational counseling) are available to the patient with chronic illness and disability. Assess the need for additional care and support throughout the hospitalization, and coordinate with the case manager and physician in arranging for home services. A new technology, home-telehealth, allows for care coordination in the home setting. Through the use of various electronic devices, a health care team member can monitor the patient's vital signs, weight, and other assessment data through the use of wireless Internet (Lutz et al., 2007).

Evaluation: Outcomes

The patient and rehabilitation team evaluate the effectiveness of interdisciplinary interventions on the basis of the identified nursing diagnoses and collaborative problems. Expected outcomes may include that the patient will:

- Move purposefully in his or her environment with or without assistive devices.
- Perform the most basic physical tasks and personal care activities independently with or without assistive devices.
- Have structural intactness and physiologic function of the skin.
- Have normal collection and discharge of urine.
- Have normal formation and evacuation of stool.
- Take personal actions to manage stressors that tax the patient's resources.

GET READY FOR THE NCLEX EXAMINATION!

Key Points

Review these Key Points for each NCLEX Examination Client Needs Category.

Safe and Effective Care Environment

- Rehabilitation is the process of learning to live with chronic and disabling conditions.
- Patients in a rehabilitation setting are managed by an interdisciplinary team of health care professionals; the patient is also a member of the team.
- Collaborate with the rehabilitation health care team when planning and providing patient care.
- Assessment of the patient in rehabilitation includes the components that are listed in Table 8-2.
- The Functional Independence Measure (FIM) system is used to assess functional ability of the patient in rehabilitation.
- After assessing the home environment, the case manager, OTR, and rehabilitation nurse make recommendations to the patient and family about home modifications.
- The members of the interdisciplinary team teach patients transfer, bed mobility, and gait training techniques (see Charts 8-1 and 8-2)
- The patient is taught how to perform ADLs with or without using adaptive devices; encourage the patient to be as independent as possible.

Health Promotion and Maintenance

- In coordination with the RPT and OTR, assess the patient's ability to perform ADLs using a functional assessment process.
- Assess rehabilitation patients as outlined in Table 8-2.
- Prevent complications of immobility for patients, and teach patients how to prevent complications by using interventions listed in Table 8-3.

Psychosocial Integrity

- Assess the patient's self-esteem and changes in body image caused by chronic or disabling health problems.
- Assess the patient's and family's response to chronic and disabling conditions, including feelings of loss and grief.
- Assist patients in coping with their loss, and assess the availability of patient support systems.

Physiological Integrity

- Assess patients in rehabilitation for risk factors that make them likely to develop skin breakdown; interventions to prevent skin problems include repositioning and adequate nutrition.
- Patients with bladder and bowel problems are managed by training programs; spastic, flaccid, and uninhibited elimination are managed differently (see Tables 8-6 and 8-7).
- Evaluate the ability of patients to use assistive/adaptive devices to promote independence.

Additional Study Resources

Go to your Companion CD or Evolve at http://evolve.elsevier.com/Iggy/ for *Self-Assessment Questions for the NCLEX Examination.*

evolve Go to Evolve at http://evolve.elsevier.com/Iggy/ for *Prioritization and Delegation Questions for the NCLEX Examination.*

SELECTED BIBLIOGRAPHY

Asterisk indicates a classic or definitive work on this subject.

*Association of Rehabilitation Nurses. (2000a). *Standards and scope of rehabilitation nursing practice.* Glenview, IL: Author.

*Association of Rehabilitation Nurses. (2000b). *The specialty practice of rehabilitation nursing: A core curriculum* (4th ed.). Skokie, IL: Author.

Association of Rehabilitation Nurses. (2007). *ARN position statement on role of the nurse in the rehabilitation team.* Retrieved September 9, 2007, from www.rehabnurse.org/profresources/roleofnurse.html.

*Braden, B.J., & Bergstrom, N. (1992). Pressure reduction. In G.M. Bulechek & J.C. McCloskey (Eds.), *Nursing interventions: Essential nursing treatments* (2nd ed., pp. 94-108). Philadelphia: Saunders.

Bulechek, G.M., Butcher, H.K., & McCloskey Dochterman, J. (Eds.). (2008). *Nursing interventions classification (NIC)* (5th ed.). St. Louis: Mosby.

*Gallagner, R.M. (2000). How long-term care is changing. *AJN, 100*(2), 65-67.

*Gibson, K.L. (2003). Caring for a patient who lives with a spinal cord injury. *Nursing, 33*(7), 36-41.

*Glenn, J. (2003). Restorative Nursing Bladder Training Program: Recommending a strategy. *Rehabilitation Nursing, 28*(1), 15-22.

*Granger, C.V., & Gresham, G.E. (1984). *Functional assessment in rehabilitation medicine.* Baltimore: Williams & Wilkins.

*Granger, C.V., Hamilton, B.B., Linacre, J.M., Heinemann, A.W., & Wright, B.D. (1993). Performance profiles of the Functional Independence Measure. *Journal of Physical Medicine and Rehabilitation, 72,* 84-89.

*Ignatavicius, D.D. (1998). *Introduction to long term care nursing.* Philadelphia: Davis.

Lutz, B.J., Chumbler, N.R., & Roland, K. (2007). Care coordination/home telehealth for veterans with stroke and their caregivers: Addressing an unmet need. *Topics in Stroke Rehabilitation, 14*(2), 32-42.

Moorhead, S., Johnson, M., & Maas, M. (2008). *Nursing outcomes classification (NOC)* (4th ed.). St. Louis: Mosby.

Newman, D.K. (2007). *Managing and treating urinary incontinence* (2nd ed.). Baltimore: Health Professions Press.

Pullen, R.L. (2008). Transferring a patient from bed to wheelchair. *Nursing2008, 38*(2), 46-48.

Quigley, P.A., Bulat, T., & Hart-Hughes, S. (2007). Strategies to reduce risk of fall-related injuries in rehabilitation nursing. *Rehabilitation Nursing, 32*(3), 120-125.

Rieg, L.S., Mason, C.H., & Preston, K. (2006). Spiritual care: Practical guidelines for rehabilitation nurses. *Rehabilitation Nursing, 31*(6), 249-256.

Robinson, J. (2006). Intermittent self-catheterisation appliances for disabled patients. *British Journal of Community Nursing, 11*(2), 520-523.

*Sorensen, B., & Luken, K. (1999). Improving functional outcomes with recreational therapy. *The Case Manager, 10*(5), 48-53.

Stanmore, E., Ormrod, S., & Waterman, H. (2006). New roles in rehabilitation—The implications for nurses and other professionals. *Journal of Evaluation of Clinical Practice, 12*(6), 656-664.

Waters, T.R. (2007). When is it safe to manually lift a patient? *AJN, 107*(8), 53-58.

Whipple, K. (2007). Therapeutic use of assistive technology: A clinical perspective. *Rehabilitation Nursing, 32*(2), 48-50.

*World Health Organization (WHO). (1980). *International classification of impairments, disabilities, and handicaps.* Geneva: Author.

*World Health Organization (WHO). (2001). *International classification of functioning, disability, and health.* Geneva: Author.

End-of-Life Care

Mary K. Kazanowski

CHAPTER 9

LEARNING OUTCOMES

For clinical competence and success on the NCLEX Examination, study this chapter with these Learning Outcomes in mind:

Safe and Effective Care Environment

1. Assess the patient's and family's knowledge about advance directives.
2. Explain the purpose and value of advance directives to patients and their families.
3. Collaborate with members of the interdisciplinary team when caring for the dying patient and family or other caregivers.

Psychosocial Integrity

4. Assess the patient's and family's ability to cope with the dying process.
5. Assess and plan interventions to meet the dying patient's spiritual needs.
6. Incorporate the patient's cultural practices and beliefs when providing care during the dying process.
7. Provide psychosocial support to the family or other caregivers during the patient's dying process.

Physiological Integrity

8. Apply knowledge of the pathophysiology of death to palliative care interventions.
9. Assess patients for signs and symptoms related to the end of life.
10. Provide evidence-based end-of-life care to the dying patient.
11. Assess the need for complementary and alternative therapies to manage symptoms associated with the dying process.
12. Incorporate appropriate complementary and alternative therapies into the plan of care for the dying patient.
13. Evaluate outcomes of palliative care interdisciplinary interventions.
14. Explain best practice guidelines for performing postmortem care.
15. Discuss the ethical and legal obligations of the nurse with regard to end-of-life care.

Go to your Companion CD or Evolve at http://evolve.elsevier.com/Iggy/ for *Self-Assessment Questions for the NCLEX Examination* keyed to these Learning Outcomes.

OVERVIEW OF DEATH AND DYING

Although dying is part of the normal life cycle, it is often feared as a time of pain and suffering. For the family, death of a member is a life-altering loss that can cause significant and prolonged suffering. As sad and difficult as the death may be, the experience of dying need not be physically painful for the patient or emotionally agonizing for the family. The dying process is an opportunity to change a potentially difficult situation into one that is tolerable, peaceful, and meaningful for the patient and the family left behind.

Because nurses spend more time with patients than do any other health care providers, it is the nurse who often has the greatest impact on a person's experience with death. It is the nurse who can impact the dying process to prevent a death without dignity ("bad" death) from occurring, while striving to promote a peaceful and meaningful death ("good death"). To accomplish this, the nurse needs to have knowledge of end-of-life care, compassion, advocacy, and competent communication skills.

Perception of Death in the United States

The U.S. health care system is based on the acute care model, which is focused on prevention, early detection, and cure of disease. This focus and the advances in survival rates for once deadly diseases have made it difficult for many patients and health care providers to accept death as an outcome of many health problems. Many view death as a failure.

These views have led to a major deficiency in the care and quality of life for many Americans at the end of life. In 1995, a landmark study highlighted the poor quality of dying that hospitalized patients experienced at the end of their lives. The Study to Understand Prognoses and Preferences for Outcomes and Risks of Treatment (SUPPORT) showed that more than 50% of a sample of 9105 hospitalized patients with a life-threatening disease had moderate to severe pain during the last days of their lives. In addition, they did not have their wishes met, even when their wishes had been made known.

As a result of the SUPPORT study, the Institute of Medicine (IOM) studied death in America. The Institute recommended that a major initiative be undertaken to improve care at the end of life, with the outcome of facilitating good death. A **good death** is one that is free from avoidable distress and suffering for patients, families, and caregivers; in agreement with patients' and families' wishes; and consistent with clinical practice standards. Pain, not having one's wishes followed at the end of one's life, isolation, abandonment, and constant agonizing about losses associated with death are characteristics of a **bad death**.

In response to this initiative, core curricula on end-of-life care were developed and implemented to educate medical and nursing students, physicians, and nurses on how to provide quality end-of-life care. In 1998, the American Association of Colleges of Nursing (AACN) published "Peaceful Death," which outlined 15 undergraduate nursing competencies for providing quality end-of-life care (Table 9-1).

Pathophysiology of Dying

Death is defined as the cessation of integrated tissue and organ function, manifested by cessation of heartbeat, absence of spontaneous respirations, or irreversible brain dysfunction. It generally occurs as a result of an illness or trauma that overwhelms the compensatory mechanisms of the body, eventually leading to cardiopulmonary failure/arrest. Direct causes of death include:

- Heart failure secondary to cardiac dysrhythmias, myocardial infarction, or cardiogenic shock
- Respiratory failure secondary to pulmonary embolism, heart failure, pneumonia, lung disease, or respiratory arrest caused by increased intracranial pressure
- Shock secondary to infection, blood loss, or organ dysfunction, which leads to lack of blood flow (i.e., perfusion) to vital organs

Inadequate perfusion to body tissues deprives cells of their source of oxygen, which leads to anaerobic metabolism with acidosis, hyperkalemia, and tissue ischemia. Dramatic changes in vital organs lead to the release of toxic metabolites and destructive enzymes, referred to as *multiple organ dysfunction syndrome (MODS)*. As illness or organ damage progresses, the syndrome occurs with renal and liver failure. Renal or liver failure can also begin the dying process.

When the body is hypoxic and acidotic, a lethal dysrhythmia such as ventricular fibrillation or asystole can occur, which ultimately leads to the cessation of cardiac output. Shortly after cardiac arrest, respiratory arrest occurs. When respiratory arrest occurs first, cardiac arrest follows within minutes.

Cardiopulmonary resuscitation (CPR) is a procedure that involves forcing air into the lungs of the patient who has stopped breathing and giving chest compressions in the absence of a carotid pulse. By law, health care providers must initiate CPR for a person who is not breathing or is pulseless unless that person has a Do Not Resuscitate (DNR) order. Although CPR may be effective in patients with reversible illness or single organ dysfunction, patients with terminal cancer, multisystem organ failure, and renal failure rarely survive after a cardiac arrest (Weil & Fries, 2005).

TABLE 9-1 Peaceful Death AACN Undergraduate Nursing Competencies

1. Recognize dynamic changes in population demographics, health care economics, and service delivery that necessitate improved professional preparation for end-of-life care.
2. Promote the provision of comfort care to the dying as an active, desirable, and important skill, and an integral component of nursing care.
3. Communicate effectively and compassionately with the patient, family, and health care team members about end-of-life issues.
4. Recognize one's own attitudes, feelings, values, and expectations about death and the individual, cultural, and spiritual diversity existing in these beliefs and customs.
5. Demonstrate respect for the patient's views and wishes during end-of-life care.
6. Collaborate with interdisciplinary team members while implementing the nursing role in end-of-life care.
7. Use scientifically based standardized tools to assess symptoms experienced by patients at the end of life.
8. Use data from symptom assessment to plan and intervene in symptom management using state-of-the-art traditional approaches.
9. Evaluate the impact of traditional, complementary, and technologic therapies on patient-centered outcomes.
10. Assess and treat multiple dimensions, including physical, psychological, social, and spiritual needs, to improve quality of care at the end of life.
11. Assist the patient, family, colleagues, and one's self to cope with suffering, grief, loss, and bereavement in end-of-life care.
12. Apply legal and ethical principles in the analysis of complex issues in end-of-life care, recognizing the influence of personal values, professional codes, and patient preferences.
13. Identify barriers and facilitators to patients' and caregivers' effective use of resources.
14. Demonstrate skill at implementing a plan for improved end-of-life care within a dynamic and complex health care delivery system.
15. Apply knowledge gained from palliative care research to end-of-life education and care.

AACN, American Association of Colleges of Nursing.

Incidence of Death

In 2004, over 2 million deaths occurred in the United States. The most common causes of death in the United States are diseases of the heart, followed by cancer.

Of all people who die, only a few die suddenly and unexpectedly. Most people die after a long period of illness (e.g., cardiac, renal, respiratory disease), with gradual deterioration until an active dying phase before the death. Most people who die are older than 65 years.

About 25% of all deaths in the United States take place at home, but this figure varies among states. About 75% of deaths in the United States occur in hospitals or nursing homes (Hooyman & Kiyak, 2005). In a review of published research, Carlson (2007) found that deaths occurring in nursing homes were problematic for the residents, family members, and nursing home staff. For example, many residents needlessly suffered from pain and other symptoms associated with dying. This problem is probably because of inadequate understanding of how to ensure a peaceful death.

Planning for End of Life

Advance Directives

An **advance directive** is a written document prepared by a competent person that specifies what, if any, extraordinary actions a person would want when he or she can no longer make decisions about personal health care. Advance directives such as the durable power of attorney (DPOA) for health care and the living will ideally are completed long before a medical crisis. A **DPOA for Health Care** is a legal document in which a person appoints someone else to make his or her health care decisions in the event he or she becomes incapable of making decisions (Fig. 9-1). A **living will** is also a legal document that instructs physicians and family members about what life-sustaining treatment a person does or does not want at some future time if he or she becomes unable to make decisions.

The Patient Self-Determination Act of 1990 requires that all patients admitted to any health care agency be asked if they have written advance directives. Those who do not have advance directives should be given information about the process and the implications of having (or not having) these in place and should be assisted in drafting them. Each agency has its own policies and procedures to direct this process. Advance directives vary from state to state but are readily available through Caring Connections, an online program of the National Hospice and Palliative Care Organization (2005).

Advance directives guide physicians in planning care for seriously ill people. If the patient has advanced or terminal disease and has indicated that he or she does not want cardiopulmonary resuscitation (CPR) performed, then the physician can initiate a Do Not Resuscitate (DNR) order with confidence that this is the person's wish. However, most Americans do not have advance directives in place and many physicians do not talk to patients about their wishes for end-of-life care. Nurses are often in the position of initiating discussions with patients about their wishes regarding end-of-life care, especially when their condition declines quickly. Be sure to communicate and document any discussion regarding a person's wishes for end-of-life care.

Desired Outcomes for End-of-Life Care

The desired outcomes for a patient near the end of life are:

- Identification of patient needs
- Control of symptoms of distress
- Promotion of meaningful interactions between the patient and family
- Facilitation of a peaceful death

Interventions that attend to the physical, psychological, social, and spiritual needs of patients require an interdisciplinary approach. The coordinated, interdisciplinary care of hospice is the most successful approach to end-of-life care to date. *Although the perception of hospice is that it provides care for the dying, the emphasis of hospice care is on its provision of quality of life.*

Hospice and Palliative Care

The concept of hospice in the United States came about as a grassroots effort in response to the unmet needs of terminally ill people. As both a philosophy and a system of care, **hospice care** uses an interdisciplinary approach to assess and address the holistic needs of patients and families to facilitate quality of life and a peaceful death. This holistic approach neither hastens nor postpones death but provides relief of symptoms experienced by the dying patient. Hospice systems of care are provided in a variety of settings. They are often affiliated with home care agencies, providing services to patients at home or in a long-term care facility. Some communities also have hospice houses, which admit patients in the terminal phase of their lives and provide a comfortable place and care. In other cases, some hospitals have hospice units or dedicated hospice beds.

The Medicare Hospice Benefit serves as a guide for hospice care in the United States. This benefit pays for hospice services for Medicare recipients who have a prognosis of 6 months or less to live and who agree to forgo curative treatment for their terminal illness. Historically, those with terminal cancer have been the most common recipients of hospice care. However, those with other life-limiting conditions and life expectancies of 6 months or less are also appropriate for hospice. Examples of those conditions are end-stage heart failure and end-stage cirrhosis. Guidelines are available to assist health care providers and families in identifying who is entitled to hospice care under Medicare. Patients who are hospice-appropriate but do not qualify for Medicare may use benefits through private insurance or managed care. In some states, Medical Assistance (Medicaid) pays for hospice care.

Because hospice benefits and care generally require a prognosis of 6 months or less, its use is limited. Unfortunately, the many people with chronic, serious illness whose prognosis may be longer than 6 months often do not have access to the support services that work so well within the hospice model. In an attempt to address this need, the concept of palliative care is being used to address the holistic needs of chronically/seriously ill patients who may not be hospice-appropriate. **Palliative care** is both a philosophy of care and an organized, structured system for delivering care for people with a life-threatening illness. The goal of palliative care is to prevent and relieve suffering and to support the best possible quality of life for patients and their families, regardless of the stage of the disease or the need for other therapies.

NEW HAMPSHIRE DURABLE POWER OF ATTORNEY FOR HEALTH CARE

INSTRUCTIONS

PRINT YOUR NAME

I, ______________________ (name), hereby appoint ______________________ (name of agent)

PRINT THE NAME AND ADDRESS OF YOUR AGENT

of ______________________ (address)

as my agent to make any and all health care decisions for me, except to the extent I state otherwise in this document or as prohibited by law. This durable power of attorney for health care shall take effect in the event I become unable to make my own health care decisions.

INSTRUCTION STATEMENTS

STATEMENT OF DESIRES, SPECIAL PROVISIONS, AND LIMITATIONS REGARDING HEALTH CARE DECISIONS.

CIRCLE AND INITIAL THE RESPONSES THAT REFLECT YOUR WISHES

For your convenience in expressing your wishes, some general statements concerning the withholding or removal of life-sustaining treatment are set forth below. (Life-sustaining treatment is defined as procedures without which a person would die, such as but not limited to the following: cardiopulmonary resuscitation, mechanical respiration, kidney dialysis or the use of other external mechanical and technological devices, drugs to maintain blood pressure, blood transfusions, and antibiotics.) There is also a section that allows you to set forth specific directions for these or other matters. If you wish, you may indicate your agreement or disagreement with any of the following statements and give your agent power to act in those specific circumstances.

TERMINAL ILLNESS

1. If I become permanently incompetent to make health care decisions, and if I am also suffering from a terminal illness, I authorize my agent to direct that life-sustaining treatment be discontinued.
   YES NO (Circle your choice and initial beneath it.)

PERMANENTLY UNCONSCIOUS

2. Whether terminally ill or not, if I become permanently unconscious I authorize my agent to direct that life-sustaining treatment be discontinued.
   YES NO (Circle your choice and initial beneath it.)

ARTIFICIAL NUTRITION AND HYDRATION

3. I realize that situations could arise in which the only way to allow me to die would be to discontinue artificial feeding (artificial nutrition and hydration). In carrying out any instructions I have given above in #1 or #2 or any instructions I may write in #4 below, I authorize my agent to direct that (circle your choice of [a] or [b] and initial beside it):

   (a) artificial nutrition and hydration not be started or, if started, be discontinued,

   —OR—

   (b) although all other forms of life-sustaining treatment be withdrawn, artificial nutrition and hydration continue to be given to me.

If you do not complete item 3, your agent will not have the power to direct the withdrawal of artificial nutrition and hydration.

ADD PERSONAL INSTRUCTIONS (IF ANY)

4. Here you may include any specific desires or limitations you deem appropriate, such as when or what life-sustaining treatment you would want used or withheld, or instructions about refusing any specific types of treatment that are inconsistent with your religious beliefs or unacceptable to you for any other reason. You may leave this question blank if you desire.

(attach additional pages as necessary)

ALTERNATE AGENT

In the event the person I appoint above is unable, unwilling or unavailable, or ineligible to act as my health care agent, I hereby appoint

PRINT THE NAME AND ADDRESS OF YOUR ALTERNATE AGENT

______________________ (name of alternate agent) of ______________________ (address of alternate agent)

as alternate agent.

I hereby acknowledge that I have been provided with a disclosure statement explaining the effect of this document. I have read and understand the information contained in the disclosure statement.

LOCATION OF THE ORIGINAL AND COPIES

The original of this document will be kept at ____________ and the following persons and institutions will have signed copies:

DATE AND SIGN THE DOCUMENT HERE

In witness, whereof, I have hereunto signed my name this ________ (day) day of ____________ (month), 20 ____ (year).

______________________ (signature)

WITNESSING PROCEDURE

WITNESSES MUST SIGN AND PRINT THEIR ADDRESSES

I declare that the principal appears to be of sound mind and free from duress at the time the durable power of attorney for health care is signed and that the principal has affirmed that he or she is aware of the nature of the document and is signing it freely and voluntarily.

Witness: ______________ Address: ______________

Witness: ______________ Address: ______________

AND A NOTARY PUBLIC OR JUSTICE OF THE PEACE MUST COMPLETE THIS SECTION

STATE OF NEW HAMPSHIRE, COUNTY OF ______________

The foregoing instrument was acknowledged before me this ______ day of _____, 20 ___, by __________.

____

Notary Public/Justice of the Peace

My commission expires:

Fig. 9-1 • An example of a Durable Power of Attorney (DPOA) for Health Care.

SYMPTOMS AT END OF LIFE

Overview

As death nears, patients often have signs and symptoms of decline in physical function, manifested as weakness, anorexia, and changes in cardiovascular function, breathing patterns, and GI and genitourinary function. As death nears, peripheral circulation decreases and the patient's skin often becomes cold, mottled, and cyanotic. Blood pressure decreases and often is only palpable. The dying person's pulse may increase in rate, become irregular in rhythm, gradually decrease, and stop. Changes in breathing pattern are common, with breaths becoming very shallow and rapid. Periods of apnea and **Cheyne-Stokes respirations** (apnea alternating with periods of rapid breathing) are also common. Death has taken place when respirations and heartbeat cease.

Although these symptoms of physical decline are often disturbing to patients and families, they generally do not cause physical discomfort to the patient. *However, symptoms of distress such as pain, dyspnea, agitation, nausea, and vomiting can also occur, and these should be treated with medication.* When patients have access to health care providers knowledgeable in palliative care, symptoms of distress are effectively controlled in most cases.

Patient-Centered Collaborative Care

Assessment

Obtain information about the patient's diagnosis, past medical history, and recent state of health to identify the risks for symptoms of distress at end of life. For example, people with lung cancer, cardiac failure, or chronic respiratory disease are at high risk for respiratory distress and dyspnea near death. Those with brain tumors are at risk for seizure activity. Patients with tumors near major arteries (e.g., head and neck cancer) are at risk for hemorrhage. Those who have been experiencing pain often continue to have pain at the end of life, which may increase, decrease, or remain at the same level of intensity.

Physical Assessment/Clinical Manifestations

Near the end of life, the patient may become weak and drowsy, often sleeping most of the time. Eventually the person can become unresponsive. As the patient's ability to talk diminishes, it is difficult to assess his or her perception of symptoms. When caring for those who are unable to communicate their distress or needs, it is essential that health care providers identify alternative ways to assess symptoms of distress. Teach family caregivers to watch closely for objective signs of discomfort (e.g., restlessness, grimacing, moaning) and identify when these symptoms occur in relation to positioning, movement, medication, or other external stimuli (Chart 9-1).

Although the patient's point of view is the most valid indicator of comfort or distress, the family's perception of symptoms is also important. Family caregivers, health care providers, and dying patients may differ in their perceptions of symptoms in terms of intensity, significance, and meaning. Whereas health care providers are often more able to identify symptoms of distress, families are often more knowledgeable about the patient's habits and preferences. Incorporate all pertinent information into the plan for symptom management, and work with patients and families toward a common outcome.

Chart 9-1 PATIENT AND FAMILY EDUCATION GUIDE

Common Physical Signs and Symptoms of Approaching Death

COOLNESS OF EXTREMITIES

Circulation to the extremities is decreased; the skin may become mottled or discolored.

- Cover the person with a blanket.
- Do not use an electric blanket, hot water bottle, electric heating pad, or hair dryer to warm the person.

INCREASED SLEEPING

Metabolism is decreased.

- Spend time sitting quietly with the person.
- Do not force the person to stay awake.
- Talk to the person as you normally would, even if he or she does not respond.

FLUID AND FOOD DECREASE

Metabolic needs have decreased.

- Do not force the person to eat or drink.
- Offer small sips of liquids or ice chips at frequent intervals if the person is alert and able to swallow.
- Use moist swabs to keep the mouth and lips moist and comfortable.
- Coat the lips with lip balm.

INCONTINENCE

The perineal muscles relax.

- Keep the perineal area clean and dry. Use disposable underpads (Chux) and disposable undergarments.
- If the person would be more comfortable, consider a Foley catheter.

CONGESTION AND GURGLING

The person is unable to cough up secretions effectively.

- Position the patient on his or her side.
- Administer medications to decrease the production of secretions.

BREATHING PATTERN CHANGE

Slowed circulation to the brain may cause the breathing pattern to become irregular, with brief periods of no breathing or shallow breathing.

- Elevate the person's head.
- Position the person on his or her side.

DISORIENTATION

Decreased metabolism and slowed circulation to the brain may occur.

- Identify yourself whenever you communicate with the person.
- Reorient the patient as needed.
- Speak softly, clearly, and truthfully.

RESTLESSNESS

Decreased metabolism and slowed circulation to the brain may occur.

- Play soothing music, and use aromatherapy.
- Do not restrain the person.
- Massage the person's forehead.
- Reduce the number of people in the room.
- Talk quietly.
- Keep the room dimly lit.
- Keep the noise level to a minimum.
- Consider sedation if other methods do not work.

Modified from the Hospice of North Central Florida, Inc.

Assess any symptom of distress in terms of intensity, frequency, duration, quality, exacerbating (worsening) and relieving factors, and effect on the patient's comfort when awake or asleep. A method for rating the intensity of symptoms should be used to facilitate ongoing assessments and evaluate treatment response. A rating scale of 0 to 10 is commonly used, with 0 indicating no distress and 10 indicating the worst possible distress. The intensity of the symptom before and after an intervention (e.g., medication) is documented by the nurse or the family caregiver and is used daily to evaluate the patient's overall comfort. (See Chapter 5 for a complete discussion of pain assessment.)

Psychosocial Assessment

People facing death may have coping difficulties, fear, and anxiety with regard to their decline and/or impending death. Cultural considerations, values, and religious beliefs of the patient and family should be assessed for their influence on the dying experience, control of symptoms, and family bereavement. Families of people near death are also likely to manifest fear, anxiety, and knowledge deficits regarding the process of death and their role in providing care.

Assess the patient and family members for their expectations regarding death and for fear and anxiety. Families may have a preconceived notion about the dying process that may or may not be realistic. Chart 9-2 describes the common emotional signs of approaching death that the nurse should explain to the patient, family, or significant others.

▪ *Interventions*

Disturbing symptoms reported by patients and their families as death nears include weakness, pain, dyspnea, nausea and vomiting, restlessness, and agitation. Interventions are aimed at promoting comfort and controlling symptoms. With the exception of weakness, these symptoms usually require drug therapy to provide relief and/or prevent reoccurrence. A variety of complementary and alternative therapies may also relieve these symptoms.

Weakness Management

Patients commonly experience weakness and fatigue as death nears. Weakness combined with decreased neurologic function may impair the ability to swallow. Once the patient is unable to swallow, oral intake should stop. Warn families of the risk for aspiration, and reassure them that anorexia is normal at this stage. Giving fluid or food can actually lead to discomfort. Families may have great difficulty accepting that their loved ones are not being fed and may request that IV fluids be started. With great sensitivity, reinforce that the cessation of food and liquids and dehydration are natural processes. Inform families that giving fluids can actually increase discomfort in a person with multisystem slowdown. Discomfort from fluid replacement could lead to respiratory secretions (and distress), increased GI secretions, nausea, vomiting, edema, and ascites. Most experts believe that dehydration in the last hours of life (i.e., terminal dehydration) does not cause distress and may stimulate endorphin release that promotes a patient's sense of well-being. One side effect of dehydration that may be uncomfortable is dry lips and mouth. Apply emollient to the lips, and moisten the mouth and lips with applicators to help prevent and/or relieve this symptom.

Impaired swallowing near death presents a problem for drug therapy. Although some pills may be crushed, drugs such as sustained-release capsules should not be taken apart. Reassess the need for each medication. Collaborate with the prescriber about discontinuing drugs that are not needed to control pain, dyspnea, agitation, nausea, vomiting, cardiac workload, or seizures. In collaboration with a pharmacist experienced in palliative care, identify alternative routes and/or alternative medications to maintain control of symptoms. Choose the least invasive route such as oral, buccal mucosa, transdermal, or rectal. Many oral drugs can be given rectally. The subcutaneous or IV routes are used only if necessary, and the IM route is almost never used at the end of life. These methods are invasive and painful and can cause infection.

Pain Management

Pain is the symptom that dying patients fear the most. Although it is not universal, this fear is common and has many possible causes. Diseases such as cancer often cause tumor pain as a result of the infiltration of cancer cells into organs, nerves, and bones. Other causes of pain in dying patients include osteoarthritis, muscle spasms, and stiff joints secondary to immobility.

Patients who have had their pain controlled with long-acting opioids should continue their scheduled doses of opioids to prevent pain reoccurrence. Depending on the brand of long-acting opioid, oral capsules may be given rectally (same dose and same capsule) when swallowing is impaired. Increases in pain require immediate-relief analgesics (e.g., morphine sulfate immediate-release). Morphine sulfate elixir can be given sublingually, rectally, or via the buccal mucosa. It is quick-acting, effective, and safe to administer, even to comatose patients.

Some experts in palliative care recommend discontinuing routine doses of opioids as patients become oliguric or anuric. The rationale for this measure is to decrease the risk for delirium that may occur as a result of an increase in serum me-

Chart 9-2 PATIENT AND FAMILY EDUCATION GUIDE

Common Emotional Signs of Approaching Death

WITHDRAWAL

The person is preparing to "let go" from surroundings and relationships.

VISION-LIKE EXPERIENCES

The person may talk to people you cannot see or hear and see objects and places not visible to you. These are not hallucinations or drug reactions.

- Do not deny or argue with what the person claims.
- Affirm the experience.

LETTING GO

The person may become agitated or continue to perform repetitive tasks. Often this indicates that something is unresolved or is preventing the person from letting go. As difficult as it may be to do or say, the dying person takes on a more peaceful demeanor when loved ones are able to say things such as "It's okay to go. We'll be all right."

SAYING GOODBYE

When the person is ready to die and you are ready to let go, saying "goodbye" is important for both of you. Touching, hugging, crying, and saying "I love you," "Thank you," "I'm sorry," or "I'll miss you so much" are all natural expressions of sadness and loss. Verbalizing these sentiments can bring comfort both to the dying person and to those left behind.

Modified from the Hospice of North Central Florida, Inc.

tabolite levels when renal excretion is reduced (Emanuel et al., 2006). Chapter 5 describes in detail the management of chronic malignant and nonmalignant pain.

Complementary and Alternative Therapies. In addition to drug therapy to manage chronic pain, nonpharmacologic interventions are often integrated into the pain management plan. Some common approaches are presented here, and Chapters 2 and 5 provide additional information and detail.

Massage has been shown to decrease pain in people with cancer (Cassileth & Vickers, 2004), and it is one of the most popular complementary services being offered to patients at end of life (Demmer, 2004). This technique involves the manipulation of a person's muscles and soft tissue, which improves circulation and promotes relaxation. Patients who are frail may not tolerate an extensive treatment but may benefit from a short treatment to sites of their choice. In working with patients with cancer, light pressure is best and deep or intense pressure should be avoided (Berenson, 2005; Deng et al., 2004). Massage is contraindicated over the site of tissue damage (e.g., open wounds, tissue undergoing radiation therapy), in patients with bleeding disorders, and in those who are uncomfortable with touch (Layman-Goldstein & Coyle, 2006).

Music therapy is another complementary therapy used by people near end of life that has been shown to decrease pain (Layman-Goldstein & Coyle, 2006). The nurse arranges for music to meet the patient's preferences. Music promotes relaxation and therefore may reduce discomfort.

Therapeutic Touch, which involves moving one's hands through the patient's energy field, has also been shown to relieve pain (Newshan & Schuller-Citella, 2003). This approach requires specialized training in the method. Reiki therapy is another type of energy therapy being evaluated for its role in pain and symptom management. Use of Reiki requires access to a Reiki practitioner who is trained in the method.

Aromatherapy can be used in conjunction with other treatments to relieve pain near end of life. Lavender, capsicum, bergamot, chamomile, rose, ginger, rosemary, lemongrass, sage, and camphor have been recommended for use in palliative care (Mariano, 2006). Aromatherapy promotes relaxation and reduces anxiety, a contributing factor to pain.

Dyspnea Management

Dyspnea is a subjective experience in which the patient has an uncomfortable feeling of breathlessness, which is often described as terrifying. It can manifest itself as air hunger, copious secretions, cough, chest pain, or fatigue. Dyspnea is a common symptom of distress near the end of life. Many patients, families, and health care providers consider this to be the worst symptom of distress near death. Dyspnea can be:

- Directly related to the primary diagnosis (e.g., lung cancer, breast cancer, coronary artery disease)
- Secondary to the primary diagnosis (e.g., pleural effusion, metastasis to the lung or pleura)
- Related to treatment of the primary disease (e.g., heart failure caused by chemotherapy, constrictive pericarditis caused by radiation therapy, anemia related to chemotherapy)
- Unrelated to the primary disease (e.g., pneumonia)

Depending on the cause, the pathophysiology of dyspnea can involve:

- Obstructive, restrictive, or vascular disturbances in the airways with tumor or nodal involvement
- Pulmonary congestion secondary to fluid overload and/or cardiac dysfunction
- Bronchoconstriction and bronchospasm as seen with respiratory infection, chronic obstructive pulmonary disease (COPD), or airway blockage by a tumor
- Decreased hemoglobin-carrying capacity, as with anemia
- Hyperventilation secondary to neuromuscular disease, with limited movement of the diaphragm

Diagnostic testing to identify the cause of dyspnea is usually inappropriate at end of life. Treatment is determined based on physical assessment and knowledge of the underlying condition.

Pharmacologic interventions should begin early in the course of dyspnea near death. Nonpharmacologic interventions can be used in conjunction with, but not in place of, drug therapy.

Opioids such as morphine elixir are the standard treatment for dyspnea near death. They work by (1) altering the perception of air hunger, reducing anxiety and associated oxygen consumption; and (2) reducing pulmonary congestion by dilating pulmonary blood vessels. Patients who have not been receiving opioids are given starting doses of 5 to 6 mg orally. Those who have taken morphine or other opioids for pain may need much higher doses of morphine (up to 50% more than their usual dose) for relief of dyspnea. If IV access is available, health care providers may prescribe 1 to 2 mg of morphine to be given every 5 to 10 minutes until relief is obtained. However, IV access for dying patients is not started unless it is absolutely necessary.

Bronchodilators, such as albuterol or ipratropium bromide via a metered dose inhaler (MDI) or nebulizer, may be given for symptoms of bronchospasm (heard as wheezes). *Corticosteroids*, such as prednisone or dexamethasone, may also be given for bronchospasm and inflammatory problems within and exterior to the lung. Superior vena cava syndrome and lymphangitis carcinomatosis causing dyspnea may also respond to corticosteroids.

People who have fluid overload with dyspnea, crackles on auscultation, peripheral edema, and other signs of heart failure may be given a *diuretic* such as furosemide (Lasix) to decrease blood volume, reduce vascular congestion, and reduce the workload of the heart. Furosemide can be administered by mouth, intravenously, subcutaneously, or intramuscularly. IV administration, which is effective within minutes, may be preferred for heart failure and pulmonary edema to promote comfortable breathing.

Antibiotics may be indicated for dyspnea from a respiratory infection. A thorough workup for a respiratory infection is not appropriate when death is imminent. However, if signs or symptoms of a respiratory infection are present (i.e., fever, adventitious breath sounds, congested cough) along with the dyspnea, a trial of an appropriate antibiotic may be considered to make the patient comfortable.

Secretions in the respiratory tract and oral cavity may contribute to dyspnea near death. Loud, wet respirations (referred to as **death rattle**) are disturbing to family and caregivers even when they do not seem to cause dyspnea or respiratory distress. Reposition the patient onto one side to reduce gurgling, and place a towel under his or her mouth to collect secretions. *Anticholinergics*, such as transdermal or subcutaneous scopolamine, reduce the production of secretions. Oropharyngeal suctioning is not recommended for loud secretions in the bronchi or oropharynx because it is not effective and may only agitate the patient.

Sedatives such as benzodiazepines are used when morphine does not fully control the patient's dyspnea. Lorazepam (Ativan) 0.5 mg is given orally or sublingually every 4 hours as needed or around the clock.

Oxygen therapy for dyspnea near death has not been established as a standard of care for all patients. However, those who do not respond promptly to morphine or other drugs should be tried on oxygen (2 to 6 L by nasal cannula) to assess its effect. If it provides relief, oxygen should be continued.

Nonpharmacologic interventions include:

- Altering the environment to facilitate the circulation of cool air (e.g., via air conditioner and fan)
- Applying wet cloths on the patient's face
- Positioning the patient to facilitate chest expansion
- Intervening to conserve the patient's energy through frequent rest periods
- Encouraging imagery and deep breathing

Positioning the person with the head of the bed elevated and the upper body supported to facilitate diaphragmatic movement can be accomplished with a hospital bed or pillows or with the patient in a chair. Insertion of a Foley catheter to avoid the need for exertion with voiding may be a comfort measure if the patient or family agrees.

Nausea and Vomiting Management

Although not as common a problem as pain or dyspnea, nausea and vomiting are thought to occur in almost half of terminally ill patients during the last week of life. It is particularly prevalent in patients with acquired immune deficiency syndrome (AIDS) or breast, stomach, or gynecologic cancers.

Common causes of nausea and vomiting at the end of life include:

- Uremia
- Hypercalcemia
- Increased intracranial pressure from brain tumors
- Vagal stimulation secondary to oral candida
- Stretching of the hepatic capsule
- Constipation or impaction
- Bowel obstruction

If constipation is identified as the cause, a biphosphate enema is administered to release stool quickly. If stool in the rectum cannot be evacuated, a mineral oil enema followed by gentle disimpaction may relieve the patient's distress.

Nausea and vomiting related to other causes can be controlled by one or more antiemetic agents. Combinations of antiemetics as rectal suppositories, gels, or oral troches can be tried and individualized for maximum relief and control. In addition to medications, be sure to remove sources of odors and keep the room temperature at a level that the patient desires. Dietary changes may also be needed to decrease nausea and vomiting. Coordinate the diet with the nutritionist.

Complementary and Alternative Therapies. Aromatherapy using peppermint and rosewood has been found to be helpful in relieving nausea. Aromatherapy using chamomile, camphor, fennel, lavender, peppermint, and rose may reduce or relieve vomiting.

Restlessness and Agitation Management

Agitation at the end of life first requires assessing for pain or urinary retention, constipation, or another reversible cause. If constipation is ruled out as the cause and if analgesia and catheterization do not relieve the restlessness, sedatives should be administered.

Benzodiazepines such as lorazepam (Ativan) elixir or a tablet (1-2 mg) dissolved in 0.5 mL of water can be placed against the buccal mucosa. Most patients become more relaxed with 2 to 10 mg in 24 hours. To prevent agitation, Ativan should be given every 3 to 4 hours around the clock. If paradoxical agitation occurs, the lorazepam is discontinued and a neuroleptic such as haloperidol (0.5-2 mg IV, subcutaneously, or rectally) is usually given.

Complementary and Alternative Therapies. Music therapy may produce relaxation by quieting the mind and removing a patient's inner restlessness (Guzzetta, 2005). Aromatherapy with chamomile has been used to overcome anxiety, anger, tension, stress, and insomnia in dying patients (Mariano, 2006).

Seizure Management

Seizures are uncommon at end of life but may occur with brain tumors, advanced AIDS, and pre-existing seizure disorders. If patients have been taking antiepileptic drugs (AEDs) and can no longer swallow them or if they are at risk for seizures, around-the-clock medication to maintain a high seizure threshold should be given. Benzodiazepines, such as diazepam (Valium) and lorazepam (Ativan), are the drugs of choice. For home use, rectal diazepam gel or sublingual lorazepam oral solution (2 mg/mL) is preferred. Barbiturates such as phenobarbital 60 to 120 mg rectally, intravenously, or intramuscularly are alternatives if necessary.

Management of the Refractory Symptoms of Distress

A small percentage of patients experience symptoms of distress that are refractory (resistant to treatment) near the end of life. They may require such high doses of analgesics that sedation occurs as a side effect, or they may actually need to be sedated to control symptoms of distress. Although sedation is not ideal, its occurrence as a side effect of treatment for symptoms of distress at the end of life may be acceptable if there is no alternative for comfort. It is important that health care providers and the public understand that adequate symptom management may at times result in sedation. The sedation that occurs is a side effect of treatment—it is not a treatment goal or an effect meant to hasten death.

Drug therapy for symptoms of distress at the end of life is guided by protocols using doses of medications that are considered safe. These guidelines and protocols are used with the intention of alleviating suffering, not hastening death. Although it is true that patients are more likely to receive higher doses of both opioids and sedatives as they get closer to death, there is no evidence that increases in dose of opioids or sedatives hasten death (Sykes & Thorns, 2003). Despite this fact, some health care providers may continue to express concern that opioids or benzodiazepines cause death. Health care providers with this concern should be reminded that an increased risk of earlier death counts little against the benefit of pain relief and painless death in a person who faces imminent death from progression of a primary disease. *The ethical responsibility of the nurse in caring for patients near death is to follow guidelines for drug use to manage symptoms and to facilitate prompt and effective symptom management.*

Psychosocial Management

The personal experience of dying or of losing a loved one through death can be extremely difficult. But unexpected deaths, particularly in young people, tend to be most traumatic for families. When a person has a chronic life-threatening disease, he or she and the family often have some knowledge of the expected outcome. This knowledge and the gift of time may provide patients and families the opportunity to make their wishes known and develop plans of care consistent with their values and needs.

Whereas death is the termination of life, dying is a process. People facing death may demonstrate emotional signs and symptoms of their response to the dying process through behaviors that equate to saying goodbye or through actual withdrawal. Families need to be educated that such behaviors are normal to the process of dying (see Chart 9-2).

Grief is the emotional feeling related to the perception of the loss. **Mourning** is the outward social expression of the loss. Interventions to assist patients and families in grieving and mourning are based on their cultural beliefs, values, and practices. Table 9-2 lists basic beliefs regarding death, dying, and afterlife for some of the major subcultures and religions.

Interventions are aimed at providing appropriate emotional support to allow patients and their families to verbalize their fears and concerns. Support includes keeping the patient and family involved in health care decisions and emphasizing that the patient will remain as comfortable as possible until death. Interventions for providing psychosocial support are summarized in Chart 9-3.

Intervene with those grieving an impending death by "being with" as opposed to "being there." "Being with" implies that you are physically and psychologically with the grieving patient, empathizing to provide emotional support. Listening and acknowledging the legitimacy of the patient's and/or family's pain are often more therapeutic than speaking; this concept is often referred to as **presence.** Nurses facilitate the expression of grief by giving the person who is mourning permission to express himself or herself. Your manner and words show that these expressions of grief are acceptable and

TABLE 9-2 Basic Beliefs Regarding Death, Dying, and Afterlife for Selected Cultures and Religions

AFRICAN AMERICAN
- Primarily Protestant or Muslim but there is diversity among different communities.
- Belief in afterlife and judgment.
- Funerals tend to be highly involved ceremonies with defined rituals; family, friends, and acquaintances of the deceased make an effort to attend.

ASIAN—ENCOMPASSES SEVERAL COUNTRIES AND RELIGIONS (E.G., CHINESE, FILIPINO, JAPANESE, LAOTIAN, CAMBODIAN, KOREAN, VIETNAMESE)
- There is a traditional strong family and extended family with male dominance.
- Herbal medicine plays an important role.
- Direct eye contact is considered impolite.
- For Southeast Asians, discussing dying brings bad luck and hospitals and treatments are alien. Some Southeast Asians, especially if uneducated, are likely to avoid visiting terminally ill family members for fear of contracting the disease.
- The number or character "4" is avoided because it symbolizes death.
- Funeral and burial customs vary greatly depending on culture, religion, and generation involved.

LATINO/HISPANIC
- Many subcultures within this population with diverse cultural variations exist (e.g., Mexico, Central America, the Caribbean, South America).
- Catholicism is the predominant religion, but many people depend on folk healers for treatment of ailments.
- Death is viewed as a direct result of life; one naturally follows the other.
- There is an acceptance of death based on religious and cultural beliefs.
- Family and family life are important, especially regarding deaths and funerals.
- Expression of grief is open, especially among women.

NATIVE AMERICANS/AMERICAN INDIANS
- Over 350 distinct tribes in the United States exist with variation in cultural practices.
- The focus of identity is on the tribe or council rather than on ancestry; each tribe has its own belief system.
- Most tribes have the belief that spirits are attached to living things.
- Indian healers (Shamans) are common.
- Family is usually a large, extended unit, often including as many as a hundred or more.
- Family may not want the patient to die at home, but to allow a family member to die alone is also not appropriate.
- Material possessions often are dispersed before or after death to friends and family members.
- Bereavement follow-up may not be appropriate because some tribes have a taboo against speaking of the dead.

JUDAISM
- This religion encompasses Orthodox, Conservative, and Reformed Jews.
- There is a strong belief in the sacredness of life and one, indivisible God.
- Funerals have two common themes: honor the dead and comfort the mourners.
- The body must not be left unattended until burial, which should take place as soon as possible (preferably within 24 hours).
- Autopsies and cremation are opposed.
- The deceased is often dressed in a white shroud and buried in a plain pine box.
- A 7-day mourning period, called *Shiva,* follows the person's death for the immediate next of kin.
- Because of acculturation to American society, funeral and mourning traditions may vary.

Modified from Antelope, T., Eighmy, J., & Nahman, E. (2002). Care of the patient and family. In Hospice and Palliative Nurses Association (Ed.), *Core curriculum for the generalist hospice and palliative care nurse* (pp. 155-180). Dubuque, IA: Kendall/Hunt.

Chart 9-3 **BEST PRACTICE FOR PATIENT SAFETY & QUALITY CARE**

Psychosocial Interventions for Care of the Dying Patient and the Family

- Offer physical and emotional support by "being with" the patient.
- Be realistic.
- Encourage reminiscence.
- Promote spirituality.
- Foster hope.
- Avoid explanations of the loss.
- Communicate with the patient.
- Provide referrals to bereavement specialists.
- Teach about the physical signs of death (see Chart 9-1).
- Ensure that the patient is receiving palliative care, with an emphasis on symptom management.

expected. An example of therapeutic communication might be "This must be very difficult for you" or "I'm sorry this is happening."

A patient's or family member's pain of loss should not be minimized. Avoid trite assurances such as "Things will be fine. Don't cry," "Don't be upset. She wouldn't want it that way," or "In a year you will have forgotten." Such comments can actually be barriers to demonstrating care and concern. Accept whatever the grieving person says about the situation, and remain present, be ready to listen attentively, and guide gently. In this way, you can help the bereaved prepare for the necessary reminiscence and integration of the loss.

Storytelling through reminiscence and life review can be an important activity for patients who are dying. **Life review** is a structured process of reflecting on one's life, which is often facilitated by an interviewer. **Reminiscence** is the process of randomly reflecting on memories of events in one's life. The benefits of storytelling through either method include catharsis, the ability to attain perspective, and enhancement of meaning. Suggest that the patient and family tape autobiographic stories, record memories in a journal, or develop a scrapbook. If the patient does not have enough energy for these activities, familiar objects such as photographs and favorite jewelry pieces can be used to spark ideas for stories.

Spirituality is the connection to self, others, the environment, and a "higher power" (e.g., God, Allah, spirit). **Religion** is the formal expression of one's spirituality. Spirituality helps people cope with death and contributes to quality of life during the dying process. *Therefore perform an assessment to identify the patient's spiritual needs and to facilitate open expression of his or her beliefs and needs.* Although a number of spiritual assessment tools are available, few of them are specific to end of life.

People who have been alienated from their religious or spiritual community and have difficulty finding meaning in their suffering or approaching death may have spiritual distress. Possible causes include guilt, regrets, lack of meaning, poor relationships, and fear of the unknown. Acknowledge the patient's spiritual pain, and encourage verbalization. Use a family tree to discuss relationships, fears, hopes, and unfinished business. Explore issues related to forgiveness for possible resolution.

Hope involves picturing a reality that is not yet present and imagining what a situation might be like. This image sets the direction for patients and their families to provide purpose in life and to help them find the strength to go forward, even in the darkest times. *Foster hope for patients and their families by listening and caring, but remain realistic.*

Do not try to explain the loss in philosophic or religious terms. Statements such as "Everything happens for the best" or "God sends us only as much as we can bear" are not helpful when the bereaved person has yet to express feelings of anguish or anger. Telling someone too soon that he or she has other children to rely on or that other family members need them does not diminish the intensity of the grief. In fact, doing so can create feelings of anger and resentment toward the nurse because it reflects insensitivity to the patient's emotional pain. "Being with" remains important as the weeks or months pass and the funeral crisis supports dissipate. The out-of-town relatives leave, and friends and local relatives resume their own lives. Consider contacting family members after the death to allow them the opportunity to voice their perceptions of the experience. Family caregivers who assumed the role of symptom manager in the home often welcome the opportunity to discuss their experience.

Patients near death are often obtunded or withdrawn from the external environment. However, it is believed that their sense of hearing remains intact until death. *Conversation in the room and near the patient should occur as if he or she is alert.* Caregivers are encouraged to talk softly to the patient and to touch and gently stroke the skin, if culturally acceptable. Although the dying person may not respond, these actions foster a sense of communication between the patient and the caregiver.

Bereavement includes grief and mourning—the inner feelings and outward reactions of the survivor. *Inform the patient and family about bereavement counselors who can assist them to cope both before and after the death.* Bereavement counselors are extremely knowledgeable about the grieving process and can be accessed through hospice agencies. Any nurse caring for people who are dying or have died should know how to access this resource.

Participation in bereavement support groups by people who are grieving a person's pending or past death has been shown to facilitate the grieving process. Being a part of a support group can help people discover that others have suffered through an experience just as devastating as their own. This discovery makes them more likely to share their feelings with others and work toward some resolution of the experience.

Although emotionally challenging, witnessing the death of a loved one may actually facilitate the family's acceptance of death. Witnessing how ill a person is makes the event real and enhances an understanding of how disease affects bodily function and decline. If death is anticipated, use nontechnical language to give the patient and family information about the signs of death. The physical signs are described in detail—realistic enough to be unmistakable yet not so graphic as to alarm the listeners. Chart 9-1 describes the common signs and symptoms of approaching death, and Chart 9-2 describes the common emotional signs of impending death.

Family and friends who are anticipating the death of a loved one often fear that the death will be characterized by pain and suffering. *Reassure families that patients in health care settings*

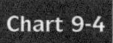

Chart 9-4 BEST PRACTICE FOR PATIENT SAFETY & QUALITY CARE

Symptom Relief Kit for Patients in Home Hospice

- For unrelieved pain: Morphine solution (20 mg/1 mL solution) 0.25 to 0.5 mL orally or sublingually every 2 to 3 hours as needed.
- For unrelieved dyspnea: Morphine solution (20 mg/1 mL solution) 0.25 to 0.5 mL orally or sublingually every 2 hours as needed.
- For nausea or vomiting: Prochlorperazine, 25-mg suppository rectally or 25 mg/0.5 mL transdermal gel to inner wrist every 8 hours as needed.
- For severe agitation and restlessness:
  - Determine if patient is in pain; treat accordingly.
  - Determine if patient is experiencing urinary retention; insert straight or Foley catheter.
  - Lorazepam, 1 to 2 mg elixir or tablet dissolved in 0.5 mL water, administered against buccal mucosa. Give 0.5 to 1 mg every 4 hours to keep patient comfortable. If patient becomes excited after lorazepam, discontinue and contact hospice.
- For oral secretions or loud, wet respirations: Scopolamine 1 to 3 transdermal patches every 72 hours.
- For unrelieved pain, dyspnea, nausea, vomiting, agitation, or secretions, call hospice.

will be monitored closely for any sign or symptom of distress and that appropriate drugs will be administered as needed. Families providing direct care in the home (including medication administration) are contacted daily to offer assistance with symptom management. The home care or hospice nurse also emphasizes that he or she is available by phone or pager 24 hours a day.

Most people who choose hospice care prefer the home to other environments during the final episodes of illness. Although there are exceptions, being surrounded by familiar people and things, having ready access to friends and relatives, and being free from institutional restrictions make the home setting more comfortable and give the person and family more control. If patients are not able to stay at home until death, they should be offered information about the nearest inpatient hospice unit or facility. In these settings, families are allowed to remain with patients. Interdisciplinary hospice team meetings are routinely conducted in both home hospice and inpatient hospice agencies to review the patient's plan of care.

It is not always possible to predict the final phase of the terminal process or the development of symptoms of distress. To address this problem, some hospices have arranged for pharmacies to supply patients with "symptom relief kits by prescription." These kits provide a limited amount of commonly used drugs that are effective in treating symptoms near death (Chart 9-4).

POSTMORTEM CARE

Nurses or family members usually discover cessation of breathing when the patient dies. Chart 9-5 lists other physical manifestations of death. If the death was in the home, and expected, there is no need to call for emergency assistance. If the person was a patient in a hospice program, the family calls hospice. If a death is unexpected or malice is suspected, the medical examiner is notified. Otherwise the nurse or physician performs the pronouncement and completes a death certificate.

Chart 9-5 PATIENT AND FAMILY EDUCATION GUIDE

Signs That Death Has Occurred

- Breathing stops.
- Heart stops beating.
- Pupils become fixed and dilated.
- Body color becomes pale and waxen.
- Body temperature drops.
- Muscles and sphincters relax.
- Urine and stool may be released.
- Eyes may remain open, and there is no blinking.
- The jaw may fall open.
- Observers may hear trickling of fluids internally.

Ask the family or other caregivers if they would like to spend time with the body to come to terms with what has happened and say their good-byes. Even if the death has been anticipated, no one knows how he or she will feel until it occurs. It may take hours to days to weeks or months for each person to realize the full effect of the event. Some family members may find it therapeutic to bathe and prepare the person's body for transfer to the funeral home or the hospital morgue. Offer families this opportunity if it is culturally acceptable.

Before preparing the body for transfer, ask the physician whether an autopsy will be ordered. When the death is expected, an autopsy is not likely. But when the physician or family members do not know the cause of death, an autopsy may be performed.

After the family or significant others view the body, follow agency procedure for preparing the patient for transfer to either the morgue or a funeral home. In the hospital, a postmortem kit is generally used with a shroud and identification tags. Chart 9-6 describes best practice guidelines for postmortem care.

EUTHANASIA

Nurses are usually in the best and most immediate position to discuss end-of-life issues. This includes assisting in the decision-making process regarding immediate or future needs. To do this, nurses must be knowledgeable about terminology and ethical issues related to death and dying (Table 9-3).

Much confusion exists regarding the concept of euthanasia. **Withdrawing or withholding life-sustaining therapy (WWLST)**, formerly called **passive euthanasia,** involves discontinuing one or more therapies that might prolong the life of a person who cannot be cured by the therapy. Another term that is sometimes used instead of WWLST is "letting die." *In this situation, the withdrawal of the intervention does not directly cause the patient's death.* The progression of the patient's disease or poor health status is the cause of death. Professional organizations (e.g., American Nurses Association, American Medical Association) and religious communities (e.g., the Catholic church) support the right of patients and their surrogate decision makers to refuse or stop treatment (e.g., mechanical ventilation, antibiotics, IV fluids) when patients are close to death and interventions are considered medically futile and/or capable of causing harm. The U.S. court system also supports WWLST (Ersek, 2005).

Active euthanasia involves a health care provider taking action that purposefully and directly causes the patient's death. Active euthanasia is not supported by most professional organizations, including the American Nurses Association. In

Chart 9-6 BEST PRACTICE FOR PATIENT SAFETY & QUALITY CARE

Postmortem Care

- Ensure that the nurse or physician has completed and signed the death certificate.
- Ask the family or significant others if they wish to help wash the patient.
- If no autopsy is planned, remove or cut all tubes and lines according to health care agency policy.
- Close the patient's eyes.
- Insert dentures if the patient wore them.
- Straighten the patient, and lower the bed to a flat position.
- Place a pillow under the patient's head.
- Wash the patient as needed; comb and arrange the patient's hair.
- Place pads under the patient's hips and around the perineum to absorb feces and urine.
- Clean the patient's room or unit.
- Allow the family or significant others to see the patient in private and to perform any religious or cultural customs they wish.
- Notify the hospital chaplain or appropriate community religious leader if requested by the family or significant others.
- Prepare the patient for transfer to either a morgue or funeral home; wrap the patient in a shroud and attach identification tags per agency policy (if the patient is to be transferred to the morgue).

TABLE 9-3 **Definitions of Ethical Concepts Related to Issues at End of Life**

Withdrawing or withholding life-sustaining therapy (WWLST) (formerly called **passive euthanasia**) An act of omission (e.g., withholding or withdrawing treatment) that might prolong the life of a person who cannot be cured by the treatment. In this situation, the withdrawal of the intervention does not directly cause the patient's death.

Principle of double effect Involves taking an action (e.g., administering an opioid) intended to have a good effect, which also has a known harmful effect. This is not active euthanasia.

Voluntary active euthanasia An act by which the causative agent in the death of a patient is administered directly by another.

Involuntary active euthanasia The action to end the patient's life is taken without the patient's consent.

Physician-assisted suicide Refers to a practice whereby a physician provides a means (e.g., medication) to a patient with the knowledge that the patient will use the means to commit suicide.

the state of Oregon, physician-assisted suicide is legal in certain situations.

Nurses should not be involved in active euthanasia or physician-assisted euthanasia. They do, however, play a major role in end-of-life care by advocating for patients' wishes and ensuring quality symptom management and support at the end of life.

GET READY FOR THE NCLEX EXAMINATION!

Key Points

Review these Key Points for each NCLEX Examination Client Needs Category.

Safe and Effective Care Environment

- Assess the patient and family regarding whether they have written advance directives, such as a Durable Power of Attorney (DPOA) for Health Care or Living Will.
- If necessary, teach the patient and family that an advance directive is a written document that specifies what, if any, extraordinary actions that person would want if he or she could no longer make decisions about care.
- Be aware that hospice care uses an interdisciplinary approach to assess and address the holistic needs of patients who are dying. Current criteria for Medicare Hospice require a prognosis of 6 months or less.

Psychosocial Integrity

- Assess the patient's emotional signs of impending death; assess coping ability of the patient and family or other caregiver.
- Assess the patient's spiritual needs in order to assist in planning appropriate interventions such as obtaining clergy.
- Incorporate the patient's personal cultural practices and beliefs regarding death and dying (see Table 9-2).
- Provide psychosocial interventions to support the patient and family during the dying process, as listed in Chart 9-3.

Physiological Integrity

- Death is defined as the cessation of integrated tissue and organ function, manifested by cessation of heartbeat, absence of spontaneous respirations, or irreversible brain dysfunction.
- Assess the patient for pain, dyspnea, agitation, nausea, and vomiting, which are common problems at the end of life.
- Assess for the common physical signs of approaching death, as listed in Chart 9-1.
- Medications are frequently given to control dyspnea, pain, agitation, and nausea and vomiting in patients near death (see Chart 9-4).
- Common complementary and alternative therapies used for symptom management at end of life include aromatherapy, music therapy, and energy therapies, such as Therapeutic Touch.
- Best practice guidelines for postmortem care are described in Chart 9-6.

- Withdrawing or withholding life-sustaining therapy (WWLST) involves withholding treatment that might prolong a patient's life; active euthanasia involves giving a patient a treatment or agent that causes death (see Table 9-3).

Additional Study Resources

Go to your Companion CD or Evolve at http://evolve.elsevier.com/Iggy/ for *Self-Assessment Questions for the NCLEX Examination.*

Go to Evolve at http://evolve.elsevier.com/Iggy/ for *Prioritization and Delegation Questions for the NCLEX Examination.*

SELECTED BIBLIOGRAPHY

Asterisk indicates a classic or definitive work on this subject.

*American Association of Colleges of Nursing. (1998). *Peaceful death: Recommended competencies and curricular guidelines for end-of-life nursing care.* Washington, DC: Author.

*American Nurses Association. (1994a). *Position statement on active euthanasia.* Washington, DC: Author.

*American Nurses Association. (1994b). *Position statement on assisted suicide.* Washington, DC: Author.

Berenson, S. (2005). Complementary and alternative therapies in palliative care. In B.R. Ferrell & N. Coyle (Eds.), *Textbook of palliative care nursing.* St. Louis: Mosby.

Burkhardt, M.A., & Nagai-Jacobson, M.G. (2005). Spirituality and health. In B.M. Dossey, L. Keegan, & C.E. Guzzetta (Eds.), *Holistic nursing: A handbook for practice* (4th ed., pp. 137-172). Sudbury, MA: Jones & Bartlett.

Carlson, A.L. (2007). Death in the nursing home: Resident, family, and staff perspectives. *Journal of Gerontological Nursing, 33*(4), 32-41.

*Cassileth, B.R., & Vickers, A.J. (2004). Massage therapy for symptom control: Outcome study at a major cancer center. *Journal of Pain and Symptoms Management, 28,* 244-249.

*Demmer, C. (2004). A survey of complementary therapy services provided by hospices. *Journal of Palliative Medicine, 7,* 510-516.

*Deng, G., Cassileth, B.R., & Simon Yeung, K. (2004). Complementary therapies for cancer-related symptoms. *Supportive Oncology, 2,* 419-429.

*Doyle, D., & Woodruff, R. (2004). *The IAHPC manual of palliative care* (2nd ed.). Houston: International Association for Hospice and Palliative Care Press.

Emanuel, L., Ferris, F.D., von Gunten, C.F., & von Roenn, J.H. (August 28, 2006). *The last hours of living: Practical advice for clinicians.* Medscape. Retrieved November 28, 2007, from www.medscape.com.

*End-of-Life Nursing Education Consortium (ELNEC). (2000). *ELNEC faculty guide.* Washington, DC: American Association of Colleges of Nursing and City of Hope National Medical Center.

Ersek, M. (2005). Assisted suicide: Unraveling a complex issue. *Nursing2005, 35*(4), 48-52.

*Escalante, C.P., Martin, C.G., Elting, L.S., Cantor, S.B., Harle, T.S., Price, K.J., et al. (1996). Dyspnea in cancer patients: Etiology, resource utilization, and survival implications in a managed care world. *Cancer, 78*(6), 1314-1319.

*Ferrell, B., & Coyle, N. (2002). An overview of palliative nursing care. *AJN, 102*(5), 26-31.

*Field, M.J., & Cassel, C.K.; Committee on Care at the End of Life, Institute of Medicine. (1997). *Approaching death: Improving care at the end of life.* Washington, DC: National Academies Press.

Granda-Cameron, C., Viola, S.R., Lynch, M.P., & Polomano, R.C. (2008). Measuring patient-oriented outcomes in palliative care: Functionality and quality of life. *Clinical Journal of Oncology Nursing, 12*(1), 65-77.

Guzzetta, C. (2005). Music therapy: Healing the melody of the soul. In B. Dossey, L. Keegan, & C. Guzzetta (Eds.), *Holistic nursing: A handbook for practice* (4th ed., pp. 617-640). Sudbury, MA: Jones & Bartlett.

Halpern, L.M. (2006). Reflections: Tahara. *AJN, 106*(4), 39.

Hermann, C.P. (2006). Development and testing of the spiritual needs inventory for patients near the end of life. *Oncology Nursing Forum, 33*(4), 737-744.

Hooyman, N., & Kiyak, H. (2005). *Social gerontology* (7th ed.). Boston: Pearson.

*Hospice and Palliative Nurses Association. (1996). *Clinical practice protocol: Dyspnea.* Pittsburgh, PA: Author.

*Hospice and Palliative Nurses Association. (1997). *Clinical practice protocol: Terminal restlessness.* Pittsburgh, PA: Author.

Kehl, K. (2006). Moving toward peace: An analysis of the concept of a good death. *American Journal of Hospice & Palliative Medicine, 23*(4), 277-286.

*Kübler-Ross, E. (1969). *On death and dying.* New York: Macmillan.

Layman-Goldstein, M., & Coyle, N. (2006). Nondrug pain interventions. In M.L. Matzo & D.W. Sherman (Eds.), *Palliative care nursing* (2nd ed., pp. 407-442). New York: Springer.

*MacDonald, G. (2000). *Medicine hands: Massage therapy for people with cancer.* Tallahassee, FL: Findhorn.

*Management of Cancer Pain Guideline Panel. (1994). *Management of cancer pain: Clinical practice guidelines.* AHCPR Publication No. 94-0592. Rockville, MD: Agency for Health Care Policy and Research, Public Health Service, U.S. Department of Health and Human Services.

*March, P.A. (1998). Terminal restlessness. *American Journal of Hospice & Palliative Care, 15*(1), 51-53.

Mariano, C. (2006). Holistic integrative therapies in palliative care. In M.L. Matzo & D.W. Sherman (Eds.), *Palliative care nursing: Quality care to the end of life* (pp. 51-86). New York: Springer.

Matzo, M.L., & Sherman, D.W. (Eds.). (2006). *Palliative care nursing: Quality care to the end of life.* New York: Springer.

National Center for Health Statistics. (2006). *Deaths: Final data for 2004. National vital statistics reports.* Hyattsville, MD: Author.

National Hospice and Palliative Care Organization. (2005). *Caring connections.* Retrieved November 15, 2007, from www.caringinfo.org.

Newshan, G., & Schuller-Citella, D. (2003). Large clinical study shows value of Therapeutic Touch program. *Holistic Nursing Practice, 17*(4), 189-192.

Oregon Hospice Association. (2005). *Hospice FAQ.* Retrieved November 15, 2007, from www.oregonhospice.org.

Patient Education Series. (2006). Advance directives. *Nursing2006, 36*(9), 43.

Perrin, K.Q. (in press). Ethical issues at the end of life. In K. Perrin & J. McGee (Eds.), *Ethics and conflict.* Sudbury, MA: Jones & Bartlett

Sherman, D.W. (2006). Spirituality and culture as domains of quality palliative care. In M.L. Matzo & D.W. Sherman (Eds.), *Palliative care nursing* (2nd ed., pp. 3-49). New York: Springer.

*Support Study Principal Investigators. (1995). A controlled trial to improve care for seriously ill hospitalized patients: The Study to Understand Prognoses and Preferences for Outcomes and Risks for Treatments (SUPPORT). *Journal of the American Medical Association, 274,* 1591-1598.

*Sykes, N., & Thorns, A. (2003). Sedative use in the last week of life and the implications for end-of-life decision making. *Archives of Internal Medicine, 163*(3), 341-344.

*Taylor, E.J. (2003). Nurses caring for the spirit: Patients with cancer and family caregiver expectations. *Oncology Nursing Forum, 30,* 585-590.

*Taylor, E.J. (2003). Prayer's clinical issues and implications. *Holistic Nursing Practice, 17*(4), 179-188.

Weil, M.H., & Fries, M. (2005). In-hospital cardiac arrest. *Critical Care Medicine, 33*(12), 2825-2830.

*Wilkie, D.J. (2001). *Toolkit for nursing excellence at end-of-life transition for nurse educators (TNEEL-NE).* Seattle, WA: University of Washington.

Zerwekh, J.V. (2006). *Nursing care at the end of life.* Philadelphia: Davis.

II

UNIT

Concepts of Emergency Care and Disaster Preparedness

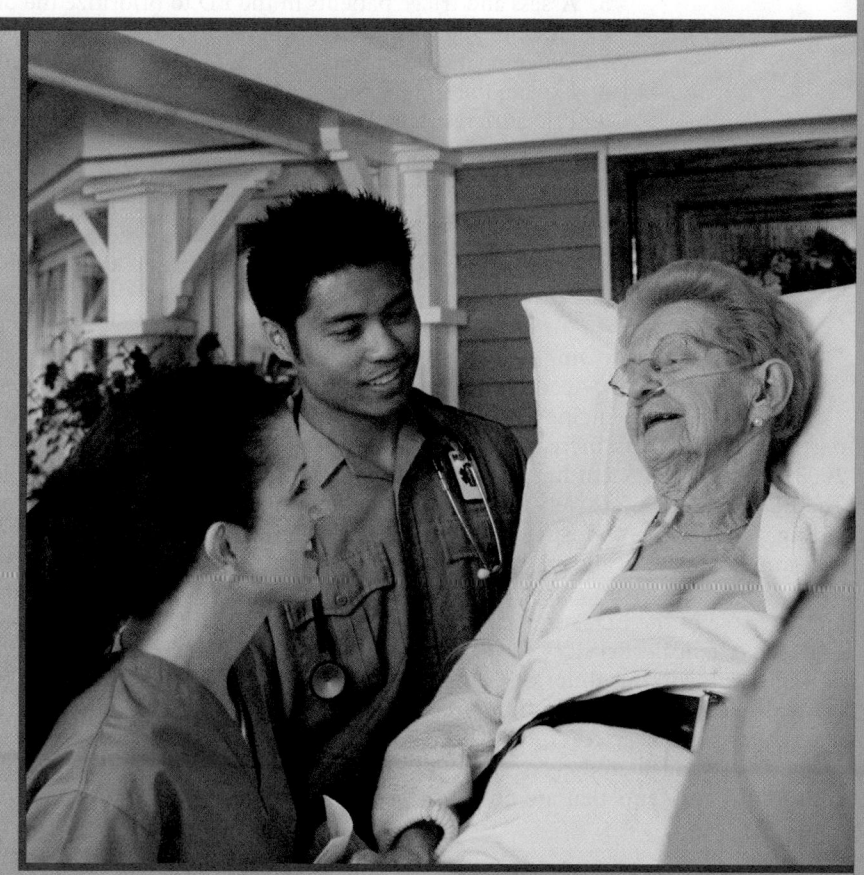

10 CHAPTER

Concepts of Emergency and Trauma Nursing

Linda Laskowski-Jones • Karen L. Toulson

LEARNING OUTCOMES

For clinical competence and success on the NCLEX Examination, study this chapter with these Learning Outcomes in mind:

Safe and Effective Care Environment

1. Describe the emergency department (ED) environment, including vulnerable populations and interdisciplinary team members.
2. Identify the roles and responsibilities of the health care team members in the ED.
3. Plan and implement best practices to prevent staff and patient injury in the ED.
4. Explain the core competencies that nurses need to function in the ED.
5. Assess and triage patients in the ED to prioritize the order of care delivery.
6. Describe the general process of admission through disposition of a patient in the ED.
7. Differentiate the various levels of trauma centers based on clinical capabilities.
8. Explain the significance of knowing the patient's mechanism of injury.
9. Prioritize resuscitation interventions based on the primary survey of the injured patient.

Psychosocial Integrity

10. Incorporate behavioral management techniques when caring for patients with mental illness in the ED.

Go to your Companion CD or Evolve at http://evolve.elsevier.com/Iggy/ for *Self-Assessment Questions for the NCLEX Examination* keyed to these Learning Outcomes.

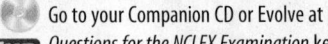

There is a fast-growing demand for emergency care in the United States. According to a report released by the Institute of Medicine (IOM) (2006), emergency department (ED) visits increased by 26% between 1993 and 2003, yet the number of hospitals and EDs nationwide fell. The ED functions as a safety net for the community by providing services to both insured and uninsured patients seeking immediate medical care. It is also responsible for public health surveillance and emergency disaster preparedness. In fact, the role of the ED is so vital that the Centers for Medicare and Medicaid Services (2006) has a process for designating small, rural facilities of 15 inpatient beds or fewer as **critical access hospitals** if they provide around-the-clock emergency care services 7 days per week. Critical access hospitals are considered *necessary providers of health care* to community residents that are not close to other hospitals in a given region.

THE EMERGENCY DEPARTMENT ENVIRONMENT OF CARE

In the emergency care environment, rapid change is the rule. The typical ED is fast paced and, at the height of activity, might even appear chaotic. Patients seek treatment for a number of physical, psychological, spiritual, and social reasons. In general, nurses are drawn to this environment because they dislike routines and thrive in challenging, stimulating work settings. Although most EDs have treatment areas that are designated for certain populations such as patients with trauma or cardiac, psychiatric, or gynecologic problems, care can actually take place almost anywhere. In an overcrowded ED, many patients receive initial treatment outside of the usual treatment rooms, including the waiting room and hallways.

Patient care areas are typically alive with activity and noise, although the pace can slow at times. Emergency nurses can expect background sounds that include ringing telephones, monitor alarms, vocal patients, crying children, and radio transmissions between staff and incoming ambulance or helicopter personnel. Interruptions are the norm.

Demographic Data

Staff members in the ED provide care for people across the life span with a broad spectrum of issues, illnesses, and injuries—as well as various cultural and religious values. During a given shift, for example, the emergency nurse may function as a cardiac nurse, a pediatric nurse, a psychiatric nurse, and a trauma nurse. Patient acuity runs the range from life-threatening emergencies to minor maladies that could be addressed in a primary care office or community clinic. Some of the most common reasons that people seek ED care are chest pain, abdominal pain, headache, and fever.

Because of the multispecialty nature of the environment, EDs play a unique role within the U.S. health care system. More than 113.9 million people visit the ED each year (Institute of Medicine [IOM], 2006). The demand for emergency care has greatly increased over the past 15 years, and the health care consumer has higher expectations—but the capacity to provide necessary resources has not kept pace in most systems. When ED patient census and acuity exceed available resources, inpatient bed capacity is limited (Laskowski-Jones, 2005b).

Emergency department overcrowding has become a national problem, with frequent boarding or holding of admitted patients in the ED because of lack of beds in the hospital. In February 2006, the Emergency Nurses Association published a position statement on crowding in the ED. This statement called for action to resolve the causes of overcrowding, promote collaborative problem-solving efforts, and ensure access, quality, and safety for patients in need of emergency services. Shortly thereafter, the IOM released a comprehensive report in June of 2006 that outlined the crisis in emergency care and trauma centers in the United States.

Special Populations

The ED serves as an important safety net for patients who are ill or injured but lack access to health care. Especially vulnerable populations include the underinsured and uninsured. Because the current health care system is complex, expensive, and difficult to navigate, some patients view the ED as an easy access route to basic health care services. The ED may become a temporary bridge to establishing a relationship with a primary care provider or a clinic.

Special Nursing Teams

Many EDs have specialized teams that deal with high-risk populations of patients. One example is the forensic nurse examiner team. **Forensic nurse examiners (RN-FNEs)** are educated to obtain patient histories, collect forensic evidence, and offer counseling and follow-up care for victims of rape, child abuse, and domestic violence—also known as *intimate partner violence (IPV)* (Markowitz et al., 2005). They are trained to recognize evidence of abuse and to intervene on the patient's behalf. Forensic nurses who specialize in helping victims of sexual assault are called *sexual assault nurse examiners (SANE)* or *sexual assault forensic nurses (SAFE)*.

Interventions performed by forensic nurses may include providing information about developing a safety plan or how to escape a violent relationship. Forensic nurse examiners document injuries and collect physical and photographic evidence. They may also provide testimony in court as to what was observed during the examination and information about the type of care provided.

The **psychiatric crisis nurse team** is another example of an ED specialty team. These nurses interact with patients and families in crisis. The sudden illness, serious injury, or death of a loved one may have precipitated the crisis. This team also evaluates people with psychiatric complaints or mental illness and facilitates follow-up or admission to an appropriate psychiatric facility. The presence of psychiatric nurses can improve the quality of care delivered to patients who require mental health intervention in the ED, and it can offer valuable expertise to the emergency health care team.

Interdisciplinary Team Collaboration

The emergency nurse is one member of the large interdisciplinary team who provides care for patients in the ED. A collaborative team approach to emergency care is considered a standard of practice. In this setting, the nurse coordinates care with all levels of health care team providers, from prehospital emergency medical services (EMS) personnel to physicians, hospital technicians, and professional and ancillary staff.

Prehospital Care Providers

Prehospital care providers are typically the first caregivers encountered by the patient before transport to the ED by an ambulance or helicopter (Fig. 10-1). Local protocols define the skill level of the EMS responders dispatched to provide assistance. **Emergency medical technicians (EMTs)** offer basic life support (BLS) interventions such as oxygen, basic wound care, splinting, spinal immobilization, and monitoring of vital signs. Some units carry automatic external defibrillators (AEDs) and may be authorized to administer selected drugs such as an EpiPen or nitroglycerin based on established medical command protocols. For patients who require care that exceeds BLS resources, paramedics are usually dispatched. **Paramedics** are advanced life support (ALS) providers who can perform advanced techniques, which may include cardiac monitoring, advanced airway management and intubation, establishing IV access, and administering drugs en route to the ED (Fig. 10-2).

The prehospital provider is a key source for valuable patient data. Emergency nurses rely on these providers to be the "eyes and ears" of the health care team in the prehospital set-

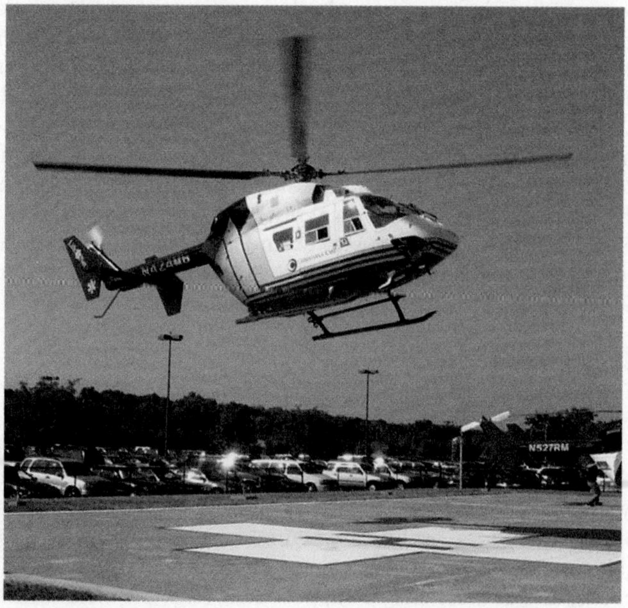

Fig. 10-1 • Advanced life support helicopter arriving at emergency department landing zone. Helicopters are used to rapidly transport critically ill and injured patients to the hospital for emergent care.

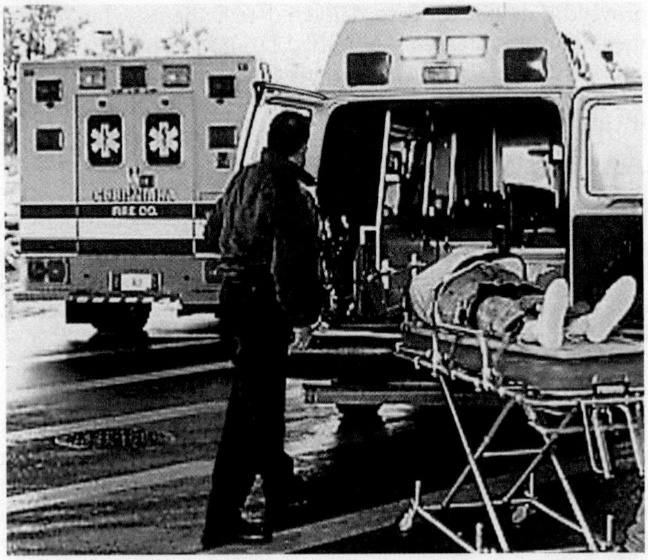

Fig. 10-2 • Prehospital providers take a patient from the ambulance to be brought into the emergency department.

ting and to communicate this information to other staff members for continuity of care.

Physicians

Another integral member of the emergency health care team is the **emergency medicine physician.** These medical professionals receive specialized education and training in emergency patient management. In the past, physicians of all types of skills rotated through the ED. As emergency care became increasingly complex and specialized, emergency medicine became a recognized physician specialty practice, complete with board certification requirements.

The emergency nurse interacts with a number of staff and community physicians involved in patient care but works most closely with emergency medicine physicians. Even though other physician specialists may be involved in ED patient treatment, the emergency medicine physician typically directs the overall care in the department. Many EDs also employ nurse practitioners and physician assistants to assume designated roles in patient assessment and treatment. Teaching hospitals also have medical residents who train in the ED. They act in collaboration with or under the supervision of the emergency medicine physician to expedite emergency care delivery.

Support Staff

The emergency nurse also interacts on a regular basis with professional and ancillary staff who function in support roles. These personnel include radiology and ultrasound technicians, respiratory therapists, laboratory technicians, and social workers. Each support staff member is essential to the success of the emergency health care team. The ED nurse is accountable for communicating pertinent staff considerations, patient needs, and restrictions to support staff (e.g., physical limitations, isolation precautions) to ensure that ongoing patient and staff safety issues are addressed. For example, the respiratory therapist can assist the nurse to troubleshoot mechanical ventilator issues. Laboratory technicians can offer advice regarding best practice techniques for specimen collection. During the discharge planning process, social workers or case managers can be tremendous patient advocates in locating community resources, including temporary housing, durable medical equipment (DME), drug and alcohol counseling, health insurance information, and prescription services.

Inpatient Unit Staff

The emergency nurse's interactions extend beyond the walls of the ED. Communication with staff nurses from the inpatient units is necessary to ensure continuity of patient care. Providing a concise but comprehensive report of the patient's ED experience is essential for the *hand-off communication* process and patient safety. Information should include the patient's:

- Situation (reason for being in the ED)
- Brief medical history
- Assessment and diagnostic findings
- Transmission-based precautions needed
- Interventions
- Response to those interventions

The 2009 Joint Commission National Patient Safety Goals require hospitals and other health care agencies to use a standardized approach to hand-off communications to prevent errors that are caused by poor or inadequate communication.

Both emergency nurses and nurses on inpatient units should strive to understand the unique aspects of their two practice environments to prevent conflicts. For example, nurses on inpatient units can be critical of the push to move patients out of the ED setting quickly, particularly when the unit activity is high. Similarly, the emergency nurse may be critical of the inpatient unit's lack of understanding or enthusiasm for accepting admissions rapidly. Effective interpersonal communication skills and respectful negotiation can optimize teamwork between the emergency nurse and the inpatient unit nurse. For instance, when ED patient volume or acuity is overwhelming, the unit nurse can volunteer to assist the ED nurse by moving a monitored patient to the hospital bed. By the same token, the emergency nurse may elect to delay sending admitted patients to inpatient units during change of shift or crisis periods such as a cardiac arrest on the unit whenever possible.

STAFF AND PATIENT SAFETY CONSIDERATIONS

In the emergency department (ED) setting, staff and patient safety is an ever-present concern (Chart 10-1). *Staff safety* concerns center on the potential for transmission of disease and on personal safety when dealing with aggressive, agitated, or violent patients and visitors.

The emergency nurse uses Standard Precautions at all times when a potential for contamination by blood or other body fluids exists. Patients with tuberculosis or other airborne pathogens are preferentially placed in a negative pressure room if available. The nurse wears a positive air-purifying respirator (PAPR) or a specially fitted facemask before engaging in any close interaction with these patients.

Hostile patient and visitor behavior also poses an injury risk to ED staff members. Recognizing volatile situations or people who show evidence of violent tendencies through verbal abuse or acting out is critical to planning an escape route or attempting de-escalation strategies before harm can occur. Emergency visits stemming from gang violence produce particularly hazardous conditions. Many EDs have at least one

Chart 10-1 **BEST PRACTICE FOR PATIENT SAFETY & QUALITY CARE**

Maintaining Patient and Staff Safety in the Emergency Department

Safety Consideration	Interventions to Minimize Risk
Patient identification	Provide an identification (ID) bracelet for each patient. Use two unique identifiers (e.g., name, date of birth). If patient identity is unknown, use a special identification system.
Injury prevention for patients	Keep rails up on stretcher. Keep stretcher in lowest position. Remind the patient to use call light/bell for assistance. Reorient confused patient frequently. If patient is confused, ask a family member or significant other to remain with him or her. Implement skin prevention measures for patient at risk for skin breakdown.
Risk for errors and adverse events	Obtain a thorough patient and family history. Check the patient for a medical alert bracelet or necklace. Search the patient's belongings when he or she has altered mental status.
Injury prevention for staff	Use Standard Precautions at all times. Anticipate hostile, violent patient, family, and/or visitor behavior. Plan options if violence occurs, including assistance from the security department.

security guard present at all times for immediate assistance with these situations. Metal detectors may be used as a screening device for patients and visitors who are suspected of having weapons. Strategically located panic buttons and remote door access controls allow staff to summon help and secure major ED or hospital entrances. The triage reception area—a particularly vulnerable access point into the ED—is often designed to serve as a security barrier with bullet-proof glass (Laskowski-Jones et al., 2005a). Hospitals may even employ canine units made up of specially trained officers and dogs to patrol high-risk areas and respond to handle threatening situations (Johnson et al., 2005).

In addition to concerns about staff safety, some of the most common *patient safety* issues are:

- Patient identification
- Fall risk
- Skin breakdown in vulnerable populations
- High risk for medical errors or adverse events

Hospital emergency departments have unique factors that can impact patient safety. These factors include the provision of complex emergency care, constant interruptions, and the need to interact with the many providers involved in caring for one patient.

Correct *patient identification* is critical in any health care setting. All patients are issued an identification bracelet at their point of entry of the ED—generally at the triage registration desk or at the bedside if emergent needs exist. For patients with an unknown identity and those with emergent conditions that prevent the proper identification process (e.g., unconscious patient without identification, emergent trauma patient), hospitals commonly use a "Jane/John Doe" or another identification system. Whatever method is used, the emergency nurse must verify the patient's identity using two unique identifiers before each intervention and before medication administration per The Joint Commission's 2008 National Patient Safety Goals. The fast pace of the ED often complicates ensuring proper identification. However, the nurse must adhere to patient identification standards to optimize safety and to reduce personal liability risk.

The nurse also ensures that the patient is safe at all times in the ED. Two primary safety considerations are to protect patients from falls and to prevent skin breakdown.

Fall prevention starts with identifying people at risk for falls and then applying appropriate fall precautions. Patients can enter the ED without apparent fall risk factors, but because of interventions such as pain medication, sedation, or even lower extremity cast application, for example, they can become vulnerable. Many medical conditions can also induce syncope ("blackouts"), especially with postural blood pressure changes. Ensure that patients are assisted when moving from a supine to an upright position and when ambulating, if needed. Also confirm that siderails are up and locked on stretchers, that the call bell or light is within reach, and that a patient's fall risk is communicated clearly to visitors and staff members who may assume responsibility for care. Additional strategies are listed in Chart 10-1.

CONSIDERATIONS FOR OLDER ADULTS

Older adults who are on beds or stretchers should always have all siderails up and the bed or stretcher in the lowest position. Access to a call light or bell is especially important; the patient is instructed to call for the nurse if assistance is needed rather than attempt independent ambulation. Older patients may become confused and need reorientation. In some cases, the nurse should ask a family member, significant other, or sitter to stay with the patient to prevent falls.

Some patients spend a lengthy time on stretchers while awaiting unit bed availability—possibly as long as 1 to 2 days. During that time, basic health needs require attention, including providing nutrition, hygiene, and privacy for all ED patients. *Protecting skin integrity* also begins in the ED. Emergency nurses assess the skin frequently and implement preventive interventions into the ED plan of care, especially when caring for older adults or those of any age who are immobilized. Interventions that promote clean, dry skin for incontinent patients, mobility techniques that decrease shearing forces when moving the immobile patient, and routine turning to help prevent skin breakdown. Chapter 27 describes additional nursing interventions for preventing skin breakdown.

A significant risk for all patients who enter the emergency care environment is the *potential for medical errors or adverse events,* especially those associated with medication administration. The episodic and often chaotic nature of emergency management can easily lead to errors.

To reduce error potential, the emergency nurse makes every attempt to obtain essential medical history information from the patient, family, or reliable significant others as necessary. When dealing with patients who arrive with an altered mental status, a quick survey to determine whether the person is wearing a medical alert bracelet or necklace is important to gain medical information. In addition, a two-person search of patient belongings may yield medication containers; the name of a physician, pharmacy, or family contact person; or a medication list. In this case, the nurse serves as a detective to find clues, which may not only promote safety but also help determine the diagnosis and influence the overall emergency treatment plan. Automated electronic tracking systems are also available in some EDs to assist staff in identifying the location of patients at any given time and in monitoring the progress of care delivery during the visit. These valuable safety measures are especially important in large or busy EDs (Laskowski-Jones, 2005a).

SCOPE OF EMERGENCY NURSING PRACTICE

The scope of emergency nursing practice encompasses management of patients across the life span—from birth through death—and all health conditions that prompt a person of any age to seek emergency care.

Core Competencies

Emergency nursing practice requires that nurses be skilled in patient assessment, priority setting and clinical decision making, multitasking, and communication. A sound knowledge base is essential. Flexibility and adaptability are vital traits because situations within the ED, as well as individual patients, can change rapidly.

Like that of any nurse in practice, the foundation of the emergency nurse's skill base is *assessment.* He or she must be able to rapidly and accurately discern normal from abnormal and interpret assessment findings according to acuity and age. For example, mottling of the extremities may be a normal finding in a newborn but it may indicate poor peripheral perfusion and a shock state in an adult. The significance of preexisting disease states **(comorbidities)** must also be factored into the assessment in regard to how the condition might adversely affect or complicate a seemingly unrelated health problem. For example, a patient who has rib fractures and chronic obstructive pulmonary disease (COPD) may not be able to maintain adequate oxygenation without endotracheal intubation and mechanical ventilatory support in the ED. Another common assessment scenario involves the type I diabetic patient who presents to the ED with an altered mental status after a fall: Is the altered mental status caused by hypoglycemia or by intracranial injury? The nurse must quickly assess blood glucose in this case, as well as follow trauma protocols for managing a potential head injury.

Another essential skill for the emergency nurse is *priority setting,* which is essential in the triage process and is described on p. 131. Priority setting depends on accurate assessment, as well as good clinical decision-making skills. These skills are generally gained through hands-on clinical experience in the ED. However, discussion of case studies and the use of simulation software can help prepare nurses to acquire this skill base in a nonthreatening environment and then apply it in the actual clinical situation.

The knowledge base for emergency nurses is broad and ranges from critical care emergencies to less common problems, such as snake bites and hazardous materials contamination (see Chapters 11 and 12). ED nurses also learn to recognize and manage the legal implications of societal problems such as child abuse, domestic violence, elder abuse, and sexual assault.

Although most EDs have physicians available around the clock who are physically located within the ED, the nurse often initiates interdisciplinary protocols for life-saving interventions such as cardiac monitoring, oxygen therapy, insertion of IV catheters, and infusion of appropriate parenteral solutions. In many EDs, nurses function under medical protocols that allow them to initiate drug therapy for emergent conditions such as anaphylactic shock and cardiac arrest. Emergency care principles extend to knowing what essential laboratory and diagnostic tests may be needed and, when necessary, obtaining them.

The emergency nurse must also be proficient in performing a variety of technical skills (multitasking), sometimes in a stressful, high-pressure environment such as a cardiac or trauma resuscitation. In addition to basic skills, he or she may also need to be proficient with critical care equipment, such as invasive pressure monitoring devices and mechanical ventilators. This type of equipment is found in EDs that are part of a Level I trauma center.

The nurse also assists the physician with a number of procedures. Knowledge and skills related to procedural setup, patient preparation, teaching, and post-procedural care are also key aspects of emergency nursing practice. Common ED procedures include:

- Simple and complex suturing for wound closure
- Foreign body removal
- Central line insertion
- Endotracheal intubation
- Transvenous pacemaker insertion
- Lumbar puncture
- Pelvic examination
- Chest tube insertion
- Peritoneal lavage
- Paracentesis
- Fracture management

More than one nurse may be necessary to assist with some procedures. For example, if moderate sedation is used to produce amnesia and relaxation during fracture reduction, one nurse assists the physician with the actual procedure while the other nurse monitors the patient before, during, and after the moderate sedation medications are administered.

Finally, an essential aspect of the emergency nurse's skill base is *communication.* The ED environment is complex—barriers to effective communication exist at all levels of interaction. Overcrowding and insufficient nursing personnel to meet the demand for services create difficulties with communication of pertinent patient information and quality of written documentation. The high-stress ED environment can negatively impact effective interpersonal behaviors, particularly when nurses must deal with angry, violent, or demanding patients as well as co-workers with challenging attitudes. Despite the obstacles, the nurse upholds professional standards of communication to the best of his or her ability when confronted with adversity and seeks administrative support when barriers cannot seem to be overcome. Sometimes practice modifications need to be made based on overwhelming patient volume or acuity, but the nurse should strive to maintain patient safety, quality, and dignity.

Training and Certification

Two general types of certification are referred to in emergency nursing practice: the "certification" that marks successful completion of a particular course of study; and emergency nursing specialty certification (Table 10-1). As part of the orientation and employment requirements for staff nurses in most U.S. EDs, successful completion of the Health Care Provider Basic Cardiac Life Support (BCLS) and Advanced Cardiac Life Support (ACLS) provider courses through the American Heart Association is necessary (Cummins, 2005). These courses provide instruction in fundamental, evidence-based management theory and techniques for cardiopulmonary resuscitation (CPR). Course participants include physicians, nurses, and prehospital personnel. BCLS emphasizes hands-on, noninvasive assessment and management skills to restore an effective airway, breathing, and circulation. The participant performs basic airway maneuvers and CPR. The ACLS course builds on the BCLS content to include advanced concepts in cardiac monitoring, invasive airway management skills, pharmacologic and electrical therapies, intravascular access techniques, special resuscitation situations, and post-resuscitation management considerations.

EMERGENCY NURSING PRINCIPLES

Triage

The concept of ED **triage** is based on sorting or classifying patients into priority levels depending on illness or injury severity. The organization of emergency care and even the ED is structured through triage principles. The key concept is that patients who present to the ED with the highest acuity needs receive the quickest evaluation, treatment, and prioritized resource utilization such as x-ray studies, laboratory work, and computed tomography (CT) scans. These patients also have priority for hospital service areas, such as the operating room or cardiac catheterization laboratory. A person with a lower acuity problem may wait longer in the ED, because the higher acuity patient is moved to the "head of the line." The staff may need to explain this system to the patient and family who may not understand why other patients are treated first.

The triage nurse is the gatekeeper in the emergency care system. When patients present to the ED, regulatory standards dictate that a registered nurse (RN), physician, or physician assistant perform a rapid assessment to determine triage priority. The RN is typically the person assigned to perform the triage function in most hospitals, however. The triage nurse should have appropriate training and experience in both emergency nursing and triage decision-making concepts. Typically, the RN determines the patient's triage priority independently. In rare instances, the triage nurse may seek the input of an emergency physician, advanced practice nurse, or physician assistant to help establish the acuity level if the patient's presentation is highly unusual.

Based on the triage priority, patients may be rushed into a treatment room, directed to a lower acuity area within the ED, or asked to sit in the waiting room. Variations on this theme include:

- Triage nurse–initiated protocols for laboratory work or diagnostic studies that may be performed before the patient is actually evaluated by a physician
- Initiation of care while the patient is on a stretcher in the hallway of an overcrowded ED.

These protocols are especially beneficial for certain populations, such as those with a clinical presentation suspicious for pneumonia, who require rapid diagnosis and treatment with antibiotics within 4 hours of ED arrival to meet established standards of care (VanHoy & Laskowski-Jones, 2006).

Emergent, Urgent, and Nonurgent Categories

Many triage schemes can be used by a hospital ED. Whatever scheme is used, it must be applied consistently by all triage nursing staff and endorsed by the emergency medicine physician staff. Based on the severity of the patient's condition, a typical triage scheme used in the United States is the three-tiered model of "emergent, urgent, and nonurgent" (Table 10-2). In this system, for example, a patient experiencing crushing substernal chest pain, shortness of breath, and diaphoresis would be classified as emergent and triaged immediately to a treatment room within the ED. Similarly, a critically injured trauma patient or a person with an active hemorrhage would also be prioritized as emergent. The **emergent triage** category implies that a condition exists that poses an immediate threat to life or limb.

The **urgent triage** category indicates that the patient should be treated quickly but that an immediate threat to life does not exist at the moment. Reassessment must occur if a physician cannot evaluate the patient in a timely manner. In people with evidence of clinical deterioration, triage priority may be upgraded from urgent to emergent. Examples of patients who typically fall into the urgent category are those with a new

TABLE 10-1 Descriptions of Training and Certifications for Emergency Nursing

Certification	Description
Basic Cardiac Life Support (BCLS) (required)	Noninvasive assessment and management skills for airway maintenance and cardiopulmonary resuscitation (CPR)
Advanced Cardiac Life Support (ACLS) (usually required)	Invasive airway management skills, pharmacology, and electrical therapies, special resuscitation
Pediatric Advanced Life Support (PALS) (may be required)	Neonatal and pediatric resuscitation
Certified Emergency Nurse (CEN) (optional)	Validates core emergency nursing knowledge base

TABLE 10-2 Three-Tiered Triage System and Examples of Patients Triaged in Each Tier

Tier Level	Examples of Patients Triaged in Each Tier
Emergent (life-threatening)	Respiratory distress Chest pain with diaphoresis Active hemorrhage Unstable vital signs
Urgent (needs quick treatment, but not immediately life threatening)	Severe abdominal pain Renal colic Displaced or multiple fractures Complex or multiple soft tissue injuries New-onset respiratory infection, especially pneumonia in older adults
Nonurgent (could wait several hours if needed without fear of deterioration)	Skin rash Strains and sprains "Colds" Simple fracture

onset of pneumonia (as long as respiratory failure does not appear imminent), renal colic, complex lacerations not associated with major hemorrhage, displaced fractures or dislocations, and temperature greater than 101° F (38.3° C).

Those categorized as **nonurgent** can generally tolerate waiting several hours for health care services without a significant risk of clinical deterioration. Conditions within this classification include patients with sprains and strains, simple fractures, "cold" symptoms, and skin rashes.

Other Multitiered Models

To further sort patient conditions within an acuity classification or triage priority system, four- and five-tier triage models also exist. Such models are based either on comprehensive lists of conditions that indicate the particular triage priority to which a patient should be assigned or on the nature of resources that a patient will use in the ED setting. A patient situation may generate various triage classifications in different hospitals depending on the triage priority system used at that particular institution. Some schemes may even take into account the presence of pre-existing conditions such as a history of warfarin (Coumadin) use, diabetes, heart disease, and organ transplantation.

Surprisingly, there is no universally accepted triage system recognized in the United States. Thus there is no standardization of triage acuity data to compare patient acuity among hospitals. The Emergency Nurses Association in collaboration with the American College of Emergency Physicians studied the available research literature on acuity scales and concluded that two standardized five-level systems, the **Emergency Severity Index (ESI)** and the **Canadian Triage Acuity Scale (CTAS),** are the most reliable (Fernandes et al., 2005). The ESI model uses an algorithm that fosters rapid, reliable, and clinically pertinent categorization of patients into five groups, from level 1 (emergent) to level 5 (nonurgent). The CTAS model differs from ESI in that lists of descriptors are used to establish the triage level.

Williams and Crouch (2006) also conducted a systematic review in search of the most valid and reliable ED triage system. They found that the Jones Dependency Tool, developed and used primarily in the United Kingdom, was deemed the most simple, easy to use, valid, and reliable when compared with 12 other systems, including the ESI and CTAS.

Whatever triage model is used, McNair (2005) asserts that "education, experience, and empathy are still the most important factors at triage…" (p. 600). Triage nurses are educated to use a systematic approach, apply solid clinical-decision making skills, and maintain a caring ethic (McNair, 2005). Compassion fatigue, or burn-out, can hinder objectivity in dealing with patients who present to the ED. A biased approach threatens the ED nurse's ability to triage patients accurately. Mistriage is another patient safety risk that can be the "root cause" of delayed or inadequate treatment—with potentially deadly consequences.

Care of the Emergency Department Patient

Perhaps the hallmark public image of emergency nursing is the resuscitation scene as viewed on television in which the emergency team acts rapidly and competently to save a human life. This drama is actually played out daily in EDs. Although only a small percentage of patients who seek emergency services actually require this level of care, emergency nurses often define their roles in terms of their resuscitation skills and experience. The opportunity to participate in resuscitation on a regular basis is a primary reason many nurses choose to work in the ED setting. There is much pride in the frequently heard emergency nurse's statement that "we save lives." Even for the experienced nurse, however, resuscitation can be challenging because of the critical nature of the patient's illness or injuries and the impact of other issues in the emergency environment, such as overcrowding and competing needs for limited resources. Updating resuscitation skills as new techniques and devices become available and regularly seeking continuing education opportunities are essential for maintaining competency.

The vast majority of those who come to the ED do not need resuscitation; they come for a variety of reasons. For instance, they are afraid that symptoms they are experiencing may indicate a very serious condition such as a stroke or heart attack. They have an acute illness, an exacerbation of a chronic illness, or an injury that requires urgent intervention. Patients may have nagging problems that they just cannot tolerate, like a urinary tract infection, until they get an appointment with a primary care provider.

Because patients have a variety of health care needs in the ED setting, nursing care needs are highly variable as well. However, certain commonalties for the care of all emergency patients exist. After triage, the nurse assigned to the patient reviews or completes a nursing assessment. Based on established treatment protocols in some emergency departments (EDs), the nurse may take action when necessary. These interventions may include application of oxygen, cardiac monitoring, IV access, and collection of blood or urine specimens, even before the patient is seen by a physician.

The patient is asked to undress to allow for an appropriate examination. Maintaining privacy and dignity and maintaining confidentiality of information are essential to the ethical provision of nursing care as well as patient satisfaction. In a busy ED environment with overcrowding issues, maintaining dignity, privacy, and confidentiality can be challenging, especially when care may sometimes take place on stretchers in the hallway. Keeping voices low when discussing confidential information; employing alternative areas for undressing when no treatment room is available (e.g., a bathroom or an office with a locking door); and providing two patient gowns (one to wear as a robe over the first gown) and a sheet or blanket as a cover are appropriate strategies.

After the physician has evaluated the patient, the nurse is responsible for providing follow-up care, such as medication administration, specimen collection, and assistance with bedside procedures. The nurse's role is to reassess and reprioritize needs whenever necessary, because the patient's condition can improve or deteriorate.

CULTURAL AWARENESS

The emergency nurse needs to be aware of the various cultural and religious values of patients that may impact care. Many people have distinct beliefs that must be respected in the health care setting. For example, some Mexican Americans are modest and do not like to have their bodies exposed. They tend to be very family-oriented and affectionate toward each other.

Patients with language barriers can present a challenge. The Spanish-speaking population in the United States, for instance, is rapidly increasing. When a bilingual staff member is not available to interpret, the emergency nurse employs resources such as telephone language lines and dedicated interpreters contracted by the hospital.

A religious belief system can also affect the delivery of care. For example, Jehovah's Witness patients do not accept blood transfusions.

Care of Patients with Mental Illness

The care and management of patients with mental illness pose a particular challenge for the emergency nurse. Patients exhibit mental health problems that range from anxiety and depression to suicidal and homicidal ideation. Their behaviors can be highly unpredictable and problematic and include agitation, combativeness, and a tendency to harm themselves or others. When substance abuse coexists with mental illness, assessment and treatment are further complicated. Some EDs have established psychiatric rooms or areas within the emergency care environment by design. However, many EDs do not have such facilities, necessitating that emergency nurses use flexibility and creativity to care for these patients within the general ED treatment setting.

Wherever care is delivered, the top priority is to provide a safe environment for patients, families, and staff. Therefore patients with mental illness undergo a thorough search upon entry into the ED. The patient is typically brought to a designated private area accompanied by two staff members. In some EDs, a metal-detecting hand wand may be used before the search to rule out the presence of any weapons or other contraband such as a hypodermic needle. Belongings are searched, and personal effects are secured. The goal is to prevent the patient from gaining access to any items that could harm self or others.

Similarly, the treatment area used for the patient with mental illness also must be safe. Equipment, supplies, extra linen, plastic trashcan liners, and nonessential furniture are removed. The environment is carefully scanned to identify objects that are in a treatment room but could pose a safety hazard in this instance. Examples are the call light cord, oxygen flowmeter and tubing, telephone, and sharps containers. Emergency equipment such as the bag-valve-mask, suction tubing, and canisters should be placed outside the treatment room, if the patient's condition permits, for ready access if needed.

Until the person with mental illness can be admitted or transferred to an appropriate psychiatric facility, the emergency nurse strives to create a therapeutic environment using a variety of assessment skills and interventions—both pharmacologic and nonpharmacologic. Some nonpharmacologic interventions include observation, de-escalation techniques, and behavioral contracts. Direct observation requires that an appropriately trained staff member is assigned to stay close to the patient at all times. De-escalation techniques involve decreasing stimulation in the environment by reducing noise and harsh light. Once the patient is made comfortable, the nurse can also establish behavioral expectations and set firm limits. Frequent reinforcement may be necessary. Social workers, case managers, and behavioral intake coordinators may assist the nurse in caring for the psychiatric patient.

Disposition

At the conclusion of the workup, the physician must make a decision regarding patient disposition. Should the patient be admitted to the hospital, transferred to a specialty care center, or be discharged to home with instructions for continued care and follow-up? Usually, the answer is straightforward. A patient who has an evolving myocardial infarction, stroke, or acute surgical need is admitted. Sometimes, though, the ED disposition decision is less clear. Often the emergency nurse and physician discuss this decision collaboratively. The nurse may have a greater sense of how well a patient will fare in a home setting depending on whether other family members or friends are available to assist and are reliable. For example, in the event a patient with a minor head injury has suffered a loss of consciousness, someone is typically expected to remain with that person for the first 12 to 24 hours to be sure that he or she does not show any evidence of neurologic deterioration. Another common scenario involves the potential risk to the patient in cases of actual or suspected domestic violence. If discharge to home is not deemed safe, the patient may be admitted to the hospital until resources can be organized to provide for a safe environment. Social workers or case managers are consulted to investigate resource needs and to plan accordingly.

Case Management

Some EDs employ registered nurse case managers who screen ED patients and intervene when necessary to arrange appropriate referral and follow-up. This is a new and evolving role in the ED setting that can be beneficial in the provision of comprehensive care and as a strategy to avoid inappropriate use of resources in an era of ED overcrowding.

ED case managers, supported by electronic information systems, can review the ED census on both a "real-time" and a retrospective basis to determine which patients have visited the ED frequently in a given period. The case manager can then determine the reasons they sought emergency services, such as lack of a primary health care provider, exacerbation ("flare-up") of a chronic condition, or lack of health education.

Case management interventions include facilitating referrals to primary care providers who are accepting new patients or to subsidized community-based health clinics for patients or families in need of routine services.

For those with needs related to chronic conditions, the case manager can arrange referral into appropriate disease management programs in the community if available (see Chapter 1). Disease management programs are specific to a particular condition such as asthma, COPD, diabetes, hypertension, heart failure, and renal failure. They help patients learn how to manage their condition on a day-to-day basis to prevent exacerbations or clinical deterioration. The main goal is to keep the person out of the hospital as long as possible. Health teaching is a key component of these programs. For other health teaching needs, the ED case manager directs the patient to the appropriate educational resources such as a health educator, nutritionist, or organization (e.g., the American Cancer Society, the American Heart Association).

Other functions of the ED case manager might include working with staff to plan disposition for homeless people, locating a safe environment for victims of domestic violence or elder abuse, providing information on community resources for low-cost prescription plans and health insurance, and referral to a home health agency.

Patient and Family Education

A key role of the emergency nurse is health teaching. At the most basic level, nurses review discharge instructions with the patient and family before signing them out of the department.

> **CULTURAL AWARENESS**
>
> Most discharge instructions are either preprinted or computer generated and can be customized to address the patient's needs. His or her reading level, primary language, and visual acuity must be considered. Educational materials and instructions should be available no higher than the 6th-grade reading level. For patients who have English as a second language, many hospitals have educational materials available in Spanish and other regional languages. However, interpreters may be necessary to assist the health care provider customize the information appropriately. The nurse may need to demonstrate how to care for a wound, for example, or how to measure the correct drug dosage. When follow-up is necessary, specific information regarding the timing and type of follow-up must be communicated. For older adults and others with vision deficits, large-print materials are helpful.

In addition to discharge instructions, the ED environment and community-at-large present many opportunities for health education. Emergency nurses are in an ideal position to educate the public about wellness and injury prevention strategies. If the patient presented after a motor vehicle crash, for instance, the nurse can reinforce the need to wear seat belts or use child safety seats correctly. ED visits that result from mishaps in the home provide an excellent circumstance to discuss home safety issues (e.g., the need for smoke detectors and carbon monoxide detectors) and fall prevention tips (e.g., the need for proper lighting, removal of throw rugs). Injury is not the only topic that affords a teaching opportunity. A new onset or an exacerbation of a medical condition also allows for education, such as how to measure blood glucose and ways to control blood pressure or reduce the risk of heart disease.

Death in the Emergency Department

Not all patients who come to the ED can be saved. Sometimes a patient's death is expected by family members, typically when they have dealt with a loved one's terminal condition or age-related decline. Usually, however, a death in the ED is a sudden and unexpected event that produces a state of crisis and chaos for family and significant others. Emergency department staff must turn their attention to addressing the needs of the family members in this overwhelming time.

If resuscitation efforts are still underway when the family arrives, one or two family members may be given the opportunity to be present during life-saving procedures. Family presence during resuscitation is gaining wider acceptance in the health care community. Resources are available to help nurses offer this option when appropriate (Laskowski-Jones, 2007).

If the patient has died by the time family members arrive, ED staff make every effort to prepare the body and the room for viewing by the family. However, certain types of ED deaths may require forensic investigation or become medical examiner's cases. Therefore ED staff may not be able to remove IV lines and indwelling tubes or clean the patient's skin if these actions could potentially damage evidence. Trauma deaths, suspected homicide, or abuse cases always fall into this category. In these situations, covering the body with a sheet or blanket while leaving the patient's face exposed and dimming the lights may be all that can be done in the ED before family viewing.

When dealing with family members in crisis, communication that is simple and concrete is best. Words such as *death* or *died,* although seemingly harsh, create less confusion than terms such as *expired* or *passed away.* Demonstrate caring, compassion, and empathy during all interactions, even in periods of heightened emotions. Intense grief can provoke a range of family reactions from silence to violence. Many EDs have crisis staff (social workers or psychiatric nurses) to assist families. Offer the family the option of speaking with clergy or calling someone of their choice for additional support. A family member may need to be admitted to the ED to be treated for anxiety or physical manifestations of stress such as chest pain, difficulty breathing, or headache.

Dealing with death is often difficult for ED personnel, especially during busy periods when the ability to console family members may be limited. In response, some emergency departments have developed bereavement committees that focus on meeting the needs of grieving families. Activities such as sending sympathy cards, attending funerals, making follow-up phone calls, and creating memory boxes are common. These actions help communicate caring and compassion after the moment of crisis.

TRAUMA NURSING PRINCIPLES

The general public tends to use the term *trauma* to mean any type of crisis ranging from a heart attack to psychological stress. Among health care professionals, though, **trauma** refers to bodily injury. More than 160,000 people in the United States die each year as a result of injuries, and nearly 2 million are hospitalized, often with permanent and disabling consequences (National Center for Health Statistics, 2006). Injuries can be categorized as either intentional (i.e., assault, homicide, suicide) or unintentional (i.e., accidents). *Unintentional injury* is the leading cause of death for Americans younger than 35 years and is one of today's most significant public health problems (National Center for Health Statistics, 2006).

Injury management is a key component of emergency department services. About 30 million people in the United States visit the ED each year to receive treatment for injuries (National Center for Health Statistics, 2006). Therefore an important part of emergency nursing practice is a core competency in general trauma care. For emergency nurses who work in accredited trauma centers, opportunities typically exist to further develop expertise in trauma nursing through ongoing clinical practice, specialty training programs, and continuing education. But **trauma nursing** as a specialty does not begin and end solely in the ED. It is actually a field that encompasses the continuum of care from injury prevention and prehospital services, to acute care, rehabilitation, and, ultimately, community reintegration. Nurses who provide trauma care in any setting along this continuum are considered to be trauma nurses.

Trauma Centers and Trauma Systems

The trauma center concept has its roots in military medicine. Injured soldiers who received rapid transport from the battlefield and treatment from skilled health care personnel had a survival advantage in the mobile army surgical hospital (MASH) units first deployed in the Korean and Vietnam wars. Consequently, the MASH unit became the original model for the development of civilian trauma centers. Today's **trauma center** in the United States is a specialty care facility that provides competent and timely trauma services to patients, depending on its designated level of capability.

Trauma Centers

It is important to realize that not all EDs that offer around-the-clock emergency services are trauma centers. The American College of Surgeons Committee on Trauma (2006) has set forth national standards for trauma center accreditation in its publication *Resources for Optimal Care of the Injured Patient* and categorizes the resource requirements necessary for the highest capability trauma center (Level I) to the lowest (Level IV) (Table 10-3). Although this document is typically viewed as the "gold standard" for trauma center accreditation across the United States, the process varies from state to state. Some states—and even some individual hospitals—define their own criteria for accreditation. Accordingly, there are "self-designated" trauma centers that may deviate from national standards in their processes and operations.

TABLE 10-3 Levels and Functions of Trauma Centers

Levels of Trauma Center	Functions of Trauma Center
Level I	Usually located in large teaching hospital systems in densely populated areas. Provides full continuum of care for all patient care.
Levels II and III	Both located in community hospitals. Level II provides care to most injured patients; Level III stabilizes major injuries. Both levels often transport patients to higher trauma center levels.
Level IV	Located in rural and remote areas. Provides advanced life support. Transports to higher trauma center levels when able.

The American College of Surgeons (2006) defines a **Level I trauma center** as a regional resource facility that is capable of "providing leadership and total care for every aspect of injury, from prevention through rehabilitation" (p. 2). Level I centers also have a responsibility to offer professional and community education programs, conduct research, and participate in system planning. Because a significant resource and experience commitment is required to maintain strict accreditation standards, Level I trauma centers are usually located in large teaching hospitals and serve dense population areas.

Level II trauma centers generally reside in community hospitals and are capable of providing care to the vast majority of injured patients. However, a Level II trauma center may not be able to meet the resource needs of patients who require very complex injury management, such as those in need of advanced surgical care. These people are generally transferred to a Level I trauma center for specialty care. In communities without a Level I trauma center, Level II centers play a significant leadership role in injury management, education, prevention, and emergency preparedness planning.

A **Level III trauma center** is a critical link to higher capability trauma centers in communities that do not have ready access to Level I or Level II centers. The primary focus is injury stabilization and patient transfer. Level III trauma centers are usually found in smaller, rural hospitals and serve areas with less population density. Because Level III trauma centers have general surgeons and orthopedic surgeons immediately available, patients with lower severity injuries may be admitted to a Level III trauma center for care. However, if the injuries are major, transfer to a Level I or II trauma center will happen after ED assessment, resuscitation, and stabilization—sometimes after emergent, life-saving surgery. Patients are typically transported out in either an advanced life support ambulance or helicopter with critical care transport personnel in attendance.

The function of a **Level IV trauma center** is to offer advanced life support care in rural or remote settings that do not have ready access to a higher level trauma center, such as a ski area. Patients are stabilized to the best degree possible before transfer, using available personnel such as advanced practice nurses, physician assistants, nurses, and paramedics. Resources, including the consistent availability of a physician, may be extremely limited. Transport time to the definitive care center can be prolonged because of both distance and inclement weather conditions that may prevent transfer by air.

Level III and Level IV trauma centers must establish close working relationships with Level I and Level II trauma centers. Based on accreditation standards, care providers at Levels I and II trauma centers have a responsibility to readily accept injured patients in transfer. They provide timely feedback to trauma personnel at referring hospitals and share expertise by offering educational opportunities to advance trauma care delivery in the region. In addition, personnel from all levels of trauma centers are required to participate in focused performance improvement and patient safety initiatives that enhance quality of care and solve identified problems.

Trauma Systems

Trauma centers save lives—but a trauma center is only as good as the overall trauma system that supports it. A **trauma system** is an organized and integrated approach to trauma care designed to ensure that all critical elements of trauma care delivery are aligned to meet the injured patient's needs. These elements include (Cooper & Laskowski-Jones, 2006):

- Access to care through communication technology (e.g., an enhanced 911 service)
- Timely availability of prehospital emergency medical care
- Rapid transport to a qualified trauma center
- Early provision of rehabilitation services
- System-wide injury prevention, research, and education initiatives

The overall goal of an organized trauma system is to enable an injured patient not only to recover from trauma but also to return to a productive role in society.

A well-functioning trauma system is also essential to general public health and safety. It provides the structure necessary for disaster readiness and community emergency preparedness (see Chapter 12). Although most states now have at least some basic elements of a trauma system in place, significant gaps still exist in many regions.

Mechanism of Injury

The **mechanism of injury (MOI)** describes the manner in which the patient's traumatic event occurred, such as a high-speed motor vehicle crash, a fall from a standing height, or a gunshot wound to the torso. Knowing key details about the MOI can provide insight into the energy forces involved and may enable trauma care providers to predict injury types and, in some cases, patient outcomes. Prehospital care providers report the MOI as a communication standard when handing off care to ED and trauma personnel. Similarly, patients who present to the ED for medical care will often relate the MOI by describing the particular chain of events that caused their injuries.

Two of the most common injury-producing mechanisms are blunt trauma and penetrating trauma. **Blunt trauma** results from impact forces like those sustained in a motor vehicle crash, a fall, and an assault with fists, kicks, or a baseball bat. **Blast effect** from an exploding bomb also causes blunt trauma. The energy transmitted from a blunt trauma mechanism, particularly the rapid **acceleration-deceleration** forces involved in high-speed crashes or falls from a great height, produces injury by tearing, shearing, and compressing anatomic structures. Trauma to bones, blood vessels, and soft tissues occurs. **Penetrating trauma** is caused by injury from sharp objects and projectiles. Examples are wounds from knives, ice picks, and other comparable implements, as well as bullets or pellets. Fragments of metal, glass, or other materials that become airborne in an explosion (shrapnel) can also produce penetrating trauma. Each mechanism has the risk for specific injury patterns and severity that the trauma team considers when planning diagnostic evaluation and management strategies. Certain injury mechanisms, such as a gunshot wound to the torso or a stab wound to the neck, are so highly associated with life-threatening consequences that they also serve as criteria for summoning the trauma team (**trauma activation criteria**) for a rapid and coordinated resuscitation response.

The Primary Survey and Resuscitation Interventions

A basic tenet of emergency care in any environment is scene safety. In the prehospital setting, emergency care providers must ensure that they are aware of any hazards that might pose a threat to rescuers and take actions to decrease or eliminate the risk. This same concept applies to the hospital ED setting. Before engaging in trauma resuscitation as a nurse member of the trauma team, keep in mind that there is a high risk of contamination with blood and body fluids. For this reason, Standard Precautions attire must be worn in *all* resuscitation situations—and at other times when exposure to blood and body fluids is likely. Proper attire consists of an impervious cover gown, gloves, eye protection, a facemask, and even a surgical cap and shoe covers if *significant* blood loss is anticipated (e.g., during performance of an ED thoracotomy).

To remain focused on priorities and keep the situation under control, an organized approach is essential. This approach is applicable for *every* resuscitation situation and promotes rapid identification and intervention techniques to address the most immediate life threats. Although both medical and trauma resuscitation scenes may appear chaotic and complex to the lay person, if performed according to widely accepted protocols and standards, they are actually highly planned events that are based on established priorities of care.

These priorities of care are addressed in order as part of the initial assessment termed the **"primary survey."** The primary survey organizes the approach to the patient so that immediate threats to life are rapidly identified and effectively managed. The primary survey is based on a standard "ABC" mnemonic with a "D" and "E" added for trauma patients: airway/cervical spine **(A)**; breathing **(B)**; circulation **(C)**; disability **(D)**; and exposure **(E)**. Resuscitation efforts occur simultaneously with each element of the primary survey (American College of Surgeons, 2004; Cummins, 2005; Laskowski-Jones, 2006a). Even though the resuscitation team may encounter multiple clinical problems or injuries, issues identified in the primary survey must be managed before the team engages in interventions of lower priority, such as splinting fractures and dressing wounds.

A: Airway/Cervical Spine

The highest priority intervention is to establish a patent airway. Even minutes without an adequate oxygen supply in humans can lead to cerebral injury that can progress to anoxic brain death. The airway is cleared of any secretions or debris either with a suction catheter or manually if necessary. The cervical spine is protected in any trauma patient with the potential for spinal injury by manually aligning the neck in a neutral, in-line position and using a jaw-thrust maneuver when establishing an airway. Supplemental oxygen is required for all patients who require resuscitation. In general, a non-rebreather mask is best for the spontaneously breathing patient. Bag-valve-mask (BVM) ventilation with the appropriate airway adjunct and a 100% oxygen source is indicated for the person who needs ventilatory assistance during resuscitation. A patient with significantly impaired consciousness requires a definitive airway such as an endotracheal tube (American College of Surgeons, 2004) (Fig. 10-3). After endotracheal intubation, a mechanical ventilator is employed. Initially, oxygen in high concentration (FIO_2 100%) is administered; lower concentrations may be requested after the patient's condition has improved.

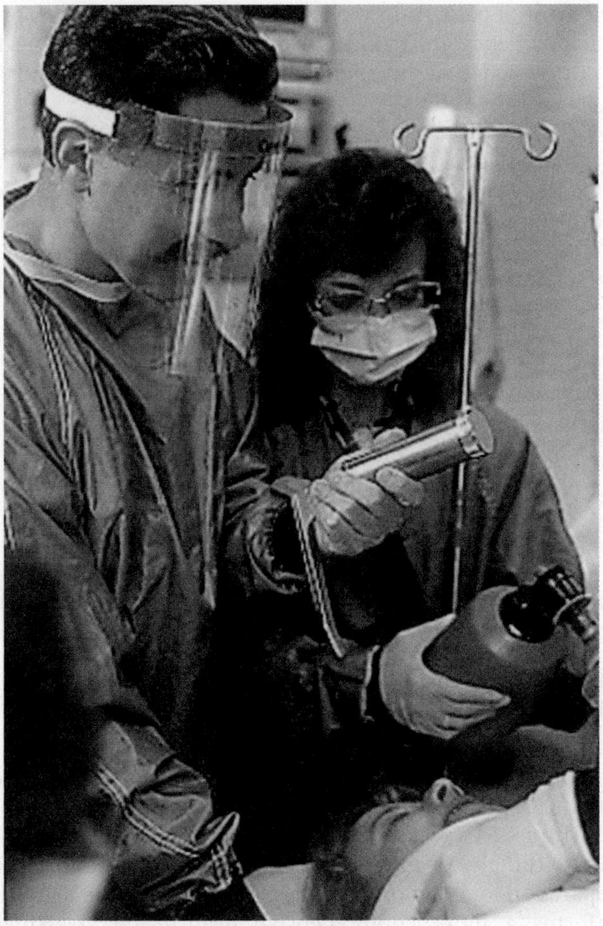

Fig. 10-3 • Emergency department trauma resuscitation room. Wearing Standard Precautions attire, trauma team members prepare to intubate the injured patient.

B: Breathing

After the airway is successfully secured, breathing becomes the next priority in the primary survey. *This assessment determines whether or not ventilatory efforts are effective—not only whether or not the patient is breathing.* The focus is on auscultation of breath sounds and evaluation of chest expansion, respiratory effort, and any evidence of chest wall trauma or physical abnormalities. Both apneic patients and those with poor ventilatory effort need BVM ventilation for support until endotracheal intubation is performed and a mechanical ventilator is used. If cardiopulmonary resuscitation (CPR) becomes necessary, the mechanical ventilator must be disconnected and the patient manually ventilated with a BVM device. Lung compliance can be assessed through sensing the degree of difficulty in ventilating the patient with the BVM.

Another lifesaving intervention that may be performed in this phase is chest decompression, either with a needle or chest tube to vent trapped air. The main indication for chest decompression is clinical evidence of a tension pneumothorax, which can pose a critical threat to both breathing and circulation. Symptoms include decreased to absent breath sounds over the affected side, respiratory distress, hypotension, jugular vein distention, and tracheal deviation (late). If unrelieved, a tension pneumothorax causes mediastinal shift, cardiovascular collapse, and death. Causes of tension pneumothorax include barotrauma from BVM ventilation or other positive-pressure ventilation, blunt or penetrating chest trauma, and expansion of a simple pneumothorax.

Chest decompression is performed in two ways: needle thoracostomy and tube thoracostomy. **Needle thoracostomy** is a quick, temporary maneuver used in an emergency to vent trapped air before chest tube insertion. A large-bore needle (14- or 16-gauge IV catheter, 3 to 6 cm in length) is inserted into the second intercostal space in the midclavicular line; a "rush of air" is expected as the trapped air is expelled from the pleural space under pressure (American College of Surgeons, 2004). Documentation of the air rush out of the catheter confirms the presence of a tension pneumothorax. After needle thoracostomy, a chest tube is inserted **(tube thoracostomy)** into the fifth intercostal space, just anterior to the midaxillary line. Chest tube placement in this anatomic position promotes air and fluid drainage. If a hemothorax is anticipated, prepare a chest tube drainage system with autotransfusion capabilities so that the pleural blood collected can be transfused into the patient as needed. An anticoagulant-preservative solution must be added according to the manufacturer's recommendations to prevent the pleural blood from clotting.

C: Circulation

When effective ventilation is ensured, the priority shifts to circulation. The adequacy of heart rate, blood pressure, and overall perfusion becomes the focus of the assessment. Common threats to circulation include cardiac arrest, myocardial dysfunction, and hemorrhage leading to a shock state. Interventions are targeted at restoring effective circulation through cardiopulmonary resuscitation, hemorrhage control, IV vascular access with fluid and blood administration as necessary, and drug therapy. *External* hemorrhage is usually quite obvious and best controlled with firm, direct pressure on the bleeding site with thick, dry dressing material (Laskowski-Jones, 2006c). This method is effective in decreasing blood flow for the majority of wounds—even those caused by amputations (Laskowski-Jones, 2006b). *Thus tourniquets that occlude arterial blood flow distal to the injury should not be used to control bleeding unless hemorrhage is so severe that the risk to limb viability is justified to save a life. Internal* hemorrhage is a more hidden complication that must be suspected in injured patients or those who present in a shock state.

In a resuscitation situation, blood pressure can be quickly and easily estimated before a manual cuff pressure can be obtained by palpating for the presence or absence of peripheral and central pulses:

- Presence of a radial pulse: BP at least 80 mm Hg systolic
- Presence of a femoral pulse: BP at least 70 mm Hg systolic
- Presence of a carotid pulse: BP at least 60 mm Hg systolic

By the time hypotension occurs, compensatory mechanisms used by the body in an attempt to maintain vital signs in a shock state have been exhausted. Timely, effective intervention is critical to preserve life and vital organ function.

IV access is best achieved initially with insertion of large-bore (16-gauge) peripheral IV lines in the antecubital area (inside bend of the elbow). Additional access can be obtained via central veins in the femoral, subclavian, or jugular sites using large-bore (≥8.5 Fr) central venous catheters. In some cases, intraosseous access may be used for critically ill patients if veins cannot be accessed by prehospital health care providers (see Chapter 15 for discussion of intraosseous infusion therapy). Resuscitation solutions of choice are Ringer's lactate and 0.9% normal saline (NS). Fluids and blood products should be warmed before administration to prevent hypothermia. A good rule of thumb is to consider the need for blood product administration in a hemorrhagic shock state when significant hypotension persists after infusion of 2 L of solution.

D: Disability

The disability examination provides a rapid baseline assessment of neurologic status. A simple method to evaluate level of consciousness is the "AVPU" mnemonic:

- A: Alert
- V: Responsive to voice
- P: Responsive to pain
- U: Unresponsive

Another common way of assessing and documenting level of consciousness is the **Glasgow Coma Scale (GCS),** which scores eye opening, verbal response, and motor response. The lowest score is 3, which indicates a totally unresponsive patient; a normal GCS score is 15. Metabolic abnormalities, hypoxia, neurologic injury, and intoxicants can impair level of consciousness. Frequent reassessment is needed for rapid intervention in the event of neurologic compromise or deterioration.

E: Exposure

The final component of the primary survey is **exposure.** All clothing is removed to allow for thorough assessment. Always *cut away* clothing with scissors in these situations (Laskowski-Jones, 2006d):

- During resuscitation when rapid access to the patient's body is critical
- When manipulating a patient's limbs to remove clothing could cause further injury
- When thermal or chemical burns have caused fabrics to melt into the patient's skin

If evidence preservation is an issue, items should be handled per institutional policy. Evidence may include articles of clothing, impaled objects, weapons, drugs, and bullets. Emergency nurses are often called upon to provide testimony in court regarding their recollections of the presentation and treatment of patients in the ED. Examples of types of cases in which evidence collection is vital are rape, elder abuse, domestic violence, homicide, suicide, drug overdose, and assault.

Once clothing is removed, hypothermia (body temperature less than or equal to 97° F [36° C]) poses a risk to injured patients, especially those with burns (Laskowski-Jones, 2006d). Specifically, hypothermia complicates management of the injured patient by causing:

- Vasoconstriction
- Difficulty with venous access and arterial assessment
- Coagulopathy
- Increased bleeding
- Slowed drug metabolism

Interventions to prevent hypothermia are basic:

- Remove wet sheets or clothing.
- Cover the patient with blankets.
- Infuse only warm solutions and blood products.
- Set the room temperature at 75° to 80° F.
- Use devices such as heat lamps and warming blankets.

Table 10-4 highlights the primary survey and associated resuscitation interventions.

The Secondary Survey and Resuscitation Interventions

After the ED resuscitation team addresses the immediate life threats, other activities that the emergency nurse can anticipate include insertion of a gastric tube for decompression of the GI tract to prevent vomiting and aspiration, insertion of a urinary catheter to allow careful measure of urine output, and preparation for diagnostic studies. The resuscitation team also performs a more comprehensive head-to-toe assessment, known as the **secondary survey,** to identify other injuries or medical issues that need to be managed or that might impact the course of treatment.

Disposition

The patient may be transported immediately to the operating room or interventional radiology suite directly from the ED, depending on the nature of the injury. When no immediate procedural intervention is indicated, patients are admitted to

TABLE 10-4 The Primary Survey and Resuscitation Interventions

Priorities of the Primary Survey	Examples of Specific Interventions
A: Airway/cervical spine	Establish a patent airway by positioning, suctioning, and oxygen, as needed. Protect the cervical spine by maintaining alignment. If the Glasgow Coma Scale (GCS) score is 8 or less or the patient is at risk for airway compromise, prepare for endotracheal intubation and mechanical ventilation.
B: Breathing	Assess breath sounds and respiratory effort. Observe for chest wall trauma or other physical abnormality. Prepare for chest decompression, if needed.
C: Circulation	Monitor vital signs, especially blood pressure and pulse. Maintain vascular access using a large-bore catheter. Use direct pressure for external bleeding.
D: Disability	Evaluate the patient's level of consciousness (LOC) using the AVPU system and the GCS. Re-evaluate the patient's LOC frequently.
E: Exposure	Remove all clothing for a complete physical assessment. Prevent hypothermia (e.g., cover the patient with blankets, use heat lamps, infuse warm solutions).

the trauma critical care unit, step-down unit, or surgical floor for continued medical management and nursing care based on the nature and severity of their injuries, as well as any other pre-existing medical conditions (e.g., coagulopathy from liver disease, heart disease, cancer) that could complicate trauma care. However, if the facility does not have the resource capabilities to manage the injured patient, the physician will arrange for transfer to a higher level of care at this point.

An interdisciplinary team approach is essential to address the trauma patient's complex health care needs, including early consultation of social services and the rehabilitation team. Other support services may be called upon as necessary and can involve pastoral care, nutrition support, psychiatry, behavioral health specialists, and substance abuse counselors. The needs of family members in crisis are considered and are addressed when planning nursing care. A trauma nurse case manager, if available, can help coordinate trauma care by offering clinical expertise, facilitating communication among caregivers, and serving as an educator for the patient, staff, and family (Umbrell, 2006).

GET READY FOR THE NCLEX EXAMINATION!

Key Points

Review these Key Points for each NCLEX Examination Client Needs Category.

Safe and Effective Care Environment

- Emergency departments (EDs) are fast-paced and overcrowded environments that care for patients across the life span with a variety of health problems.
- Vulnerable populations who present to the ED include patients who are uninsured, underinsured, mentally ill, and abused.
- Anticipate that the most common reasons that patients seek ED care are chest pain, abdominal pain, headache, and fever.
- The interdisciplinary ED team includes prehospital providers, physicians, nurses, specialty teams, and support staff.
- Use the best practices listed in Chart 10-1 to maintain safety in the ED.
- Core competencies for the ED nurse include assessment, priority setting/critical thinking, knowledge of the ED, technical skills, and communication.
- The triage system most commonly used under usual conditions is the three-level model: emergent, urgent, and nonurgent (see Table 10-2). The Emergency Severity Index is a five-tier triage system that uses both acuity and the prediction of resources to rapidly categorize the priority of patients.
- Trauma centers are categorized as Levels I through IV, based on their resource capabilities as listed in Table 10-3.
- The mechanism of injury describes the manner in which the traumatic event occurred.
- Two of the most common injury-producing mechanisms are blunt trauma and penetrating trauma.
- Implement the steps of the primary survey and trauma resuscitation interventions outlined in Table 10-4.
- Patient education as part of the discharge plan is an important part of ED nursing practice.

Psychosocial Integrity

- Use behavioral management strategies for patients with mental illness in the ED, including de-escalation techniques, behavioral contracts, direct observation, and creating a safe environment to prevent the patient from harming himself or herself or others. If needed, consult with the psychiatric crisis team.

Additional Study Resources

Go to your Companion CD or Evolve at http://evolve.elsevier.com/Iggy/ for *Self-Assessment Questions for the NCLEX Examination.*

Go to Evolve at http://evolve.elsevier.com/Iggy/ for *Prioritization and Delegation Questions for the NCLEX Examination.*

SELECTED BIBLIOGRAPHY

Asterisk indicates a classic or definitive work on this subject.

American Academy of Pediatrics, & American Heart Association. (2005). *PALS provider manual.* Dallas: American Heart Association.

*American College of Surgeons Committee on Trauma. (2004). *Advanced trauma life support course for doctors student manual* (7th ed.). Chicago, IL: Author.

American College of Surgeons Committee on Trauma. (2006). *Resources for optimal care of the injured patient 2006.* Chicago, IL: Author.

Beachley, M. (2005). The evolution of trauma nursing and the Society of Trauma Nurses: A noble history. *Journal of Trauma Nursing, 12*(4), 105-115.

Centers for Medicare and Medicaid Services. (May 31, 2006). *Critical access hospitals.* Retrieved April 4, 2007, from www.cms.hhs.gov/Certification andComplianc/04_CAHs.asp.

Clarke, D.E., Hughes, L., Brown, A.M., & Motluk, L. (2005). Psychiatric emergency nurses in the emergency department: The success of the Winnipeg, Canada, experience. *Journal of Emergency Nursing, 31*(4), 351-356.

Cooper, G., & Laskowski-Jones, L. (2006). Development of trauma care systems. *Prehospital Emergency Care, 10*(3), 328-331.

Cummins, R.O. (Ed.). (2005). *ACLS: Principles and practice.* Dallas: American Heart Association.

*Emergency Medical Treatment and Active Labor Act, 42 U.S.C.SS 1395dd. (1986).

Emergency Nurses Association. (2006). Emergency Nurses Association position statements: Crowding in the emergency department. *Journal of Emergency Nursing, 32*(1), 12-17.

Fernandes, C.M., Tanabe, P.L., Gilboy, N., Johnson, L.A., McNair, R.S., Rosenau, A.M., Sawchuk, P., et al. (2005). Five-level triage: A report from the ACEP/ENA five-level triage task force. *Journal of Emergency Nursing, 31*(1), 39-50.

*Hawkins, H. (Ed.). (2004). *ENPC provider manual* (3rd ed.). Park Ridge, IL: Emergency Nurses Association.

Howard, M.S., Davis, B.A., Anderson, C., Cherry, D., Koller, P., & Shelton, D. (2005). Patients' perspective on choosing the emergency department for nonurgent medical care: A qualitative study exploring one reason for overcrowding. *Journal of Emergency Nursing, 31*(5), 429-435.

Institute of Medicine (IOM) Committee on the Future of Emergency Care in the U.S. Health System. (2006). *Hospital-based emergency care: At the breaking point.* Washington, DC: National Academies Press.

Johnson, D., Laskowski-Jones, L., Vickers, S., Parker, D., Marine, M., & Workman R. (2005). Canine units: The softer side of security. *Nursing2005, 35*(7), 54-55.

*Joint Commission Resources. (2003). *Accreditation issues for emergency departments.* Oakbrook Terrace, IL: Joint Commission on Accreditation of Health Care Organizations.

Laskowski-Jones L. (2005a). Rx for busy EDs: Patient-tracking technology. *Nursing2005, 35*(11), 32cc1-32cc2.

Laskowski-Jones, L. (2005b). Starling's curve: A way to conceptualize emergency department overcrowding. *Journal of Emergency Nursing, 31*(3), 229-230.

Laskowski-Jones, L. (2006a). Emergency! Responding to trauma—Your priorities in the first hour. *Nursing2006, 36*(9), 52-59.

Laskowski-Jones, L. (2006b). First aid for amputations. *Nursing2006, 36*(4), 50-52.

Laskowski-Jones, L. (2006c). First aid for bleeding wounds. *Nursing2006, 36*(9), 50-51.

Laskowski-Jones, L. (2006d). First aid for burns. *Nursing2006, 36*(1), 41-43.

Laskowski-Jones, L. (2007). Should families be present during resuscitation? *Nursing2007, 37*(5), 44-47.

Laskowski-Jones, L., Toulson, K., & McConnell, L. (2005). Assessing and planning for triage redesign. *Journal of Emergency Nursing, 31*(3), 315-318.

Markowitz, J.R., Steer, S., & Garland, M. (2005). Hospital-based intervention for intimate partner violence victims: A forensic nursing model. *Journal of Emergency Nursing, 31*(2), 166-170.

McNair, R.S. (2005). It takes more than string to fly a kite: 5-Level acuity scales are effective, but education, clinical expertise, and compassion are still essential. *Journal of Emergency Nursing, 31*(6), 600-603.

National Center for Health Statistics. (June 30, 2006). *NCHS data on injuries*, Retrieved April 9, 2007, from www.cdc.gov/nchs.injury.htm.

Scalise, D. (August 10, 2006). Patient safety in the ED. *Hospitals and health networks*, Retrieved August 10, 2006, from www.hhnmag.com.

The Joint Commission. (2008). *National Patient Safety Goals.* Retrieved July 29, 2007, from www.thejointcommission.com.

Toulson, K., Laskowski-Jones, L., & McConnell, L. (2005). Implementation of the five-level Emergency Severity Index in a Level I trauma center emergency department with a three-tiered triage scheme. *Journal of Emergency Nursing, 31*(3), 259-264.

Umbrell, C.E. (2006). Trauma case management: A role for the advanced practice nurse. *Journal of Trauma Nursing, 13*(2), 70-73.

VanHoy, S., & Laskowski-Jones, L. (2006). Early intervention for the pneumonia patient: An emergency department triage protocol. *Journal of Emergency Nursing, 32*(2), 154-158.

Williams, S., & Crouch, R. (2006). Emergency department patient classification systems: A systematic review. *Accident and Emergency Nursing, 14*(3), 160-170.

Care of Patients with Common Environmental Emergencies

11 CHAPTER

Linda Laskowski-Jones

LEARNING OUTCOMES

For clinical competence and success on the NCLEX Examination, study this chapter with these Learning Outcomes in mind:

Safe and Effective Care Environment

1. Determine patient knowledge of safety procedures to prevent heat-related and cold injuries.
2. Determine patient knowledge of safety procedures to prevent drowning or submersion accidents.

Health Promotion and Maintenance

3. Assess people for lifestyle practice risks that may impact health, including excessive sun and cold exposures.
4. Teach people how to prevent heat-related and cold injuries.
5. Teach people how to prevent arthropod bites, stings, and snakebites.

Physiological Integrity

6. Prioritize first aid interventions for patients who have heat-related or cold injuries.
7. Prioritize first aid interventions for patients who have arthropod bites.
8. Prioritize first aid interventions for patients experiencing snakebites.
9. Apply knowledge of best practices for care of patients with environmental emergencies.
10. Develop a plan of care for a patient who is allergic to bees and experiences a bee sting.
11. Prioritize care for patients who have been struck by lightning.
12. Employ best practices for patients who are at risk for or experience altitude-related illnesses.
13. Determine priorities for managing patients who are victims of drowning or submersion incidents.

Go to your Companion CD or Evolve at http://evolve.elsevier.com/Iggy/ for *Self-Assessment Questions for the NCLEX Examination* keyed to these Learning Outcomes.

Recreational activities, as well as home and work responsibilities, make people of all ages leave the shelter of their homes for the great outdoors. Seemingly harmless outside activities can have associated environmental risks. Some of these hazards, such as insect bites or stings, reptile bites, and environmental conditions, may also pose threats indoors. This chapter gives an overview of selected environmental emergencies and their management for immediate emergency care needs. Acute care interventions for these hazards are also presented. Illness and injury prevention strategies for nurses to incorporate into their own lifestyle and health teaching opportunities are also discussed.

HEAT-RELATED ILLNESSES

High environmental temperature (above 95° F) and high humidity (above 80%) are the most common environmental factors for heat-related illnesses. Physical factors range from extremes of age to a patient's health status. For example, dehydration, fatigue, lack of sleep, obesity, heart disease, fever, strenuous exercise, seizures, and all degrees of burns (even sunburn) cause people to become more susceptible to heat stress. In addition, the use of drugs such as alcohol, beta-adrenergic blockers, angiotensin-converting enzyme (ACE) inhibitors, diuretics, thyroid medications, and illegal drugs increases the risk of heat-related illness (Glazer, 2005). Before participating in any hot weather activity, all people should be taught to consider their risk factors and take steps to eliminate or minimize them whenever possible.

HEALTH PROMOTION AND MAINTENANCE

Chart 11-1 lists heat-related illness prevention strategies. Include this important information into health teaching opportunities with people who participate in warm weather activities, as well as those with health risk factors that predispose them to heat-related illness. *Older adults and the homeless are particu-*

Chart 11-1 PATIENT AND FAMILY EDUCATION GUIDE
Heat-Related Illness Prevention

- Ensure adequate intake of nutritious foods and fluids before, during, and after exercise (e.g., commercially available sports bars; drinks that contain carbohydrates, sodium, and other essential electrolytes). Avoid alcohol and caffeine.
- Prevent overexposure to the sun; use a sunscreen with an SPF of at least 30.
- Take time to get used to the heat by gradually increasing time spent working or playing in a hot environment.
- Rest frequently when working in a hot environment. Plan to limit activity at the hottest time of day.
- Wear clothing suited to the environment. Lightweight, light-colored, and loose-fitting clothing is best.
- Pay attention to your personal physical limitations; modify activities accordingly.
- Take cool baths or showers to help reduce body temperature.
- Stay indoors in air-conditioned buildings, if possible.
- Check on neighbors and family members (especially older adults) at least twice a day during a heat wave (Lewis, 2007).

larly at risk for heat-related illnesses as a result of decreased body fluid volume or overexposure to the sun (Lewis, 2007).

HEAT EXHAUSTION

Pathophysiology

Heat exhaustion is a syndrome resulting primarily from dehydration. It is caused by heavy perspiration, as well as inadequate fluid and electrolyte intake during heat exposure over hours to days. Patients feel ill, and their clinical manifestations resemble the flu. Although not a true emergency condition, if untreated, heat exhaustion can lead to heat stroke, a more serious problem.

Patient-Centered Collaborative Care

In heat exhaustion, patients have a normal mental status and a flu-like syndrome with headache, weakness, fatigue, anorexia, nausea, and vomiting. Assess the patient for orthostatic hypotension and tachycardia, especially the older adult. Keep in mind that body temperature is not significantly elevated in this condition. The patient may continue to perspire despite dehydration.

Treat the patient by immediately stopping physical activity, moving him or her to a cool place, and using cooling measures. Effective cooling measures include placing cold packs on the neck, chest, abdomen, and groin; soaking the person in cool water; or fanning him or her while spraying water on the skin (Glazer, 2005; Smith, 2005). Remove any constrictive clothing. Provide an oral rehydrating solution such as a sports drink. Do not give salt tablets—they can cause stomach irritation, nausea, and vomiting. If these signs and symptoms persist, call an ambulance to transport the patient to the hospital.

In the clinical setting, vital sign assessment and temperature monitoring are necessary. The patient is rehydrated with IV 0.9% saline solution if nausea or vomiting is present. Blood is drawn for serum electrolyte analysis. Hospital admission is indicated for patients who have other health problems that are worsened by the heat-related illness or for those with manifestations that do not improve.

HEAT STROKE

Pathophysiology

Heat stroke is a true medical emergency in which body temperature may exceed 104° F (40° C). It has a high mortality rate if not treated in a timely manner. The victim's heat regulatory mechanisms fail and cannot adjust for a critical elevation in body temperature (Glazer, 2005). If it is uncorrected, organ dysfunction and death result.

The two major types of heat stroke are exertional and classic. **Exertional heat stroke** has a sudden onset and is often the result of strenuous physical activity in hot, humid conditions. Not being used to hot weather and wearing clothing too heavy for the environment are common contributing factors. **Classic heat stroke** occurs over a period of time as a result of chronic exposure to a hot, humid environment, such as a home without air-conditioning in the high heat of the summer. It generally affects ill and older adults. The body's ability to handle heat effectively is significantly impaired in this disorder. The risk factors for heat stroke are the same as for heat exhaustion.

Patient-Centered Collaborative Care

evolve ONLINE PHARM REVIEW

Assessment

Victims of heat stroke have a profoundly elevated body temperature (above 104° F [40° C]). Mental status changes occur as a result of thermal injury to the brain. Common changes are evidenced by the appearance of anxiety, confusion, bizarre behavior, loss of coordination, hallucinations, agitation, seizures, and coma. Vital sign abnormalities may include hypotension, tachycardia, and tachypnea (increased respiratory rate). *Although the patient's skin is described as hot and dry, the presence of sweating does not rule out heat stroke—persons may continue to perspire in this state.*

Complications of classic heat stroke include multiple organ dysfunction syndrome, renal impairment, electrolyte and acid-base disturbances, coagulopathy (abnormal clotting), pulmonary edema, and cerebral edema (Glazer, 2005). Any of these problems can lead to death.

Interventions

Heat stroke must be recognized and treated immediately and aggressively for optimal patient outcomes (Chart 11-2).

First Aid

In the prehospital setting, rapid cooling is the first priority of care after ensuring the patient has a patent airway, effective breathing, and circulation. Methods for rapidly cooling include:

- Stripping away clothing
- Placing ice packs on the neck, axillae, chest, and groin
- Immersing the victim in cold water
- Wetting the patient's body with tepid water and then fanning rapidly to aid in cooling by evaporation

Recent evidence suggests that ice immersion is the fastest, most effective means to reduce core body temperature (Glazer, 2005; Smith, 2005). Do not give food or liquid by mouth because vomiting and aspiration are risks in patients experiencing neurologic impairment. Immediate medical care is essential. Call an ambulance with advanced life support capabilities as soon as possible.

Chart 11-2 BEST PRACTICE FOR PATIENT SAFETY & QUALITY CARE

Emergency Care of the Patient with Heatstroke

EMERGENCY CARE

AT THE SCENE
- Ensure a patent airway.
- Remove the patient from the hot environment (into air-conditioning or into the shade).
- Remove the patient's clothing.
- Pour or spray water on the patient's body and scalp.
- Fan the patient (not only the person providing care, but all surrounding people should fan the patient with newspapers or whatever is available).
- If ice is available, place ice in cloth or bags and position the packs on the patient's scalp, in the groin area, behind the neck, and in the armpits.
- Get the patient to the nearest emergency department.

AT THE HOSPITAL
- Give oxygen by mask or nasal cannula.
- Start at least one IV with a large-bore needle or cannula.
- Administer normal saline (0.9% sodium chloride) as rapidly as possible, using cooled solutions if available.
- Use a cooling blanket.
- *Do not give aspirin or any other antipyretics.*
- Insert a rectal probe to measure core body temperature continuously, or use a rectal thermometer and assess temperature every 15 minutes.
- Insert a Foley catheter.
- Monitor vital signs at least every 15 minutes.
- Obtain these laboratory tests as quickly as possible: serum electrolytes, cardiac enzymes, liver enzymes, and complete blood count (CBC).
- Assess arterial blood gases.
- Administer muscle relaxants (benzodiazepines) if the patient begins to shiver.
- Measure urine output and specific gravity to determine fluid needs.
- Slow cooling interventions when core body temperature is reduced to 102° F (39° C).
- Obtain urinalysis, and monitor urine output.

Hospital Care

Once in a clinical setting, monitor and support the patient's airway, breathing, and circulatory status. Initiation of high-concentration oxygen therapy, IV lines with 0.9% saline solution, and a urinary catheter are indicated. Do not use Ringer's lactate solution because the liver cannot metabolize lactate effectively during hyperthermia, worsening lactic acidosis (Yeo, 2004). Continue aggressive interventions to cool the patient until the rectal temperature is 100.4° F (38° C) (Glazer, 2005). External methods include using cooling blankets and applying ice packs in the axilla and groin and on the neck and head. Internal cooling methods consist of iced gastric and bladder lavage. In severe cases, iced peritoneal and thoracic lavage may be used (Glazer, 2005). Use a continuous core temperature monitoring device (e.g., rectal or esophageal probe) or a temperature-monitoring urinary bladder catheter to prevent hypothermia. If shivering occurs during the cooling process, chlorpromazine (Thorazine) 25 to 50 mg IM or IV may be prescribed.

Seizure activity is a serious problem because it can further elevate body temperature. Be sure that a benzodiazepine such as diazepam (Valium) is immediately available for IV administration. Admission to a critical care unit for continued support and hemodynamic monitoring is usually indicated because complication and mortality rates for heatstroke are very high.

SNAKEBITE

Many people fear snakes. Although most snake species are nonvenomous (nonpoisonous) and harmless, there are two families of poisonous snakes in North America: the Crotalidae and the Elapidae.

The *Crotalidae* are the "pit vipers," named for the characteristic depression between each eye and nostril that serves as a heat-sensitive organ for locating warm-blooded prey. They include various species of rattlesnakes, copperheads, and cottonmouths and account for the majority of the poisonous snakebites in the United States (Figs. 11-1 and 11-2).

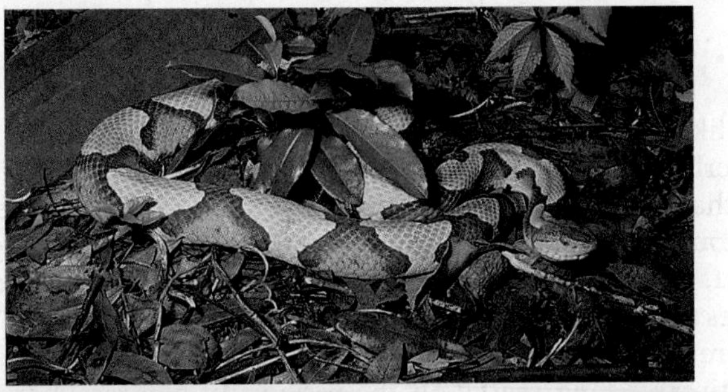

Fig. 11-1 • Southern copperhead *(Agkistrodon contortrix)* has markings that make it almost invisible when lying in leaf litter.

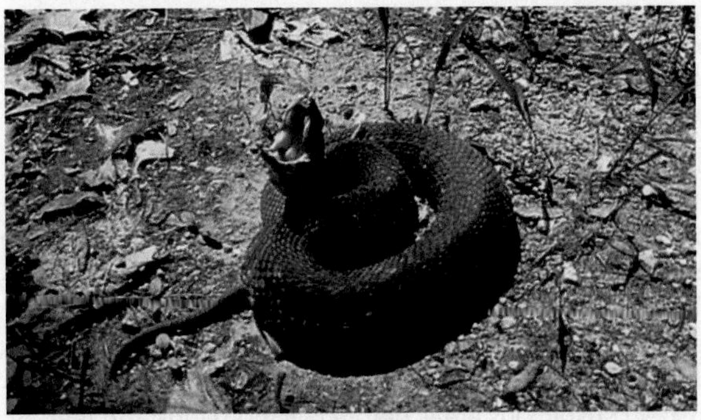

Fig. 11-2 • Cottonmouth water moccasin *(Agkistrodon piscivorus)*. The open-mouthed threat gesture is characteristic of this semiaquatic pit viper.

The *Elapidae* include the coral snakes, which are found from North Carolina to Florida and in the Gulf states through Texas and the southwestern United States. Coral snakes have broad bands of red and black rings, separated by yellow or cream rings. These nonaggressive snakes have short, fixed fangs and inject highly neurotoxic venom into prey.

Of the venomous snakebites that occur each year in the United States, fatalities are few but tend to occur in children, older adults, and people who are inadequately treated (Gold et al., 2004). Most bites occur between April and October, with a peak incidence in July and August (Gold et al., 2004). This time frame corresponds to an increase in both human and reptile activity in the outdoor environment during the warm weather months. Most snakes fear humans and attempt to avoid contact with them. Sudden, unexpected confrontations at close range often lead to defensive strikes. Awareness is the key to snakebite prevention.

HEALTH PROMOTION AND MAINTENANCE

Chart 11-3 provides common sense actions to avoid being bitten by a poisonous snake.

NORTH AMERICAN PIT VIPERS

North American pit vipers can be differentiated from harmless snakes by noting these key anatomic features:

- A heat-sensing "pit"
- A triangular head that indicates the presence of venom glands and elliptical pupils
- Two retractable, curved fangs that have canals for venom flow
- Up to three sets of developing "replacement" fangs behind the primary fangs

Unlike copperheads and cottonmouths, rattlesnakes also have interlocking horny rings in their tails that vibrate and serve as a characteristic warning signal. Pit vipers can regulate the amount of venom flow through their fangs, depending, in part, on the size of the prey. The amount of venom injected in bites to humans varies. A bite might actually be "dry," meaning there is no **envenomation** (venom injection), yet there are distinctive fang marks on the patient. In contrast, harmless snakes do not have venom glands or fangs but can bite and leave skin marks.

Chart 11-3 PATIENT AND FAMILY EDUCATION GUIDE

Snakebite Prevention

- Do not keep venomous snakes as pets.
- Be extremely careful in locations that may harbor snakes such as tall grass, rock piles, ledges and crevices, woodpiles, brush, swamps, and caves. Snakes are most active on warm nights.
- Don protective attire such as boots, heavy pants, and leather gloves. When walking or hiking, use a walking stick or trekking poles.
- Inspect suspicious areas before placing hands and feet in them.
- Do not harass any snakes you may encounter. Striking distance is at least the length of the snake. Even young snakes pose a threat; they are capable of envenomation from birth.
- Be aware that newly dead or decapitated snakes can inflict a bite for 20 to 60 minutes after death because of persistence of the bite reflex.
- Use extreme caution if attempting to transport the snake with the victim to the medical facility for identification purposes. Ensure that the snake is placed in a sealed container.

Pathophysiology

When providing emergency care to a victim of snakebite, the key question is whether the venom has been injected into the skin. Understanding venom's purpose and function is essential to recognizing the manifestations of venom injection and planning appropriate interventions. The primary functions of venom are to immobilize, kill, and aid in digestion of prey. Therefore venom causes local and systemic toxic effects. The enzymes in venom break down human tissue proteins, alter membrane integrity, and impair blood clotting. The pathophysiologic effects of pit viper envenomation can lead to local tissue necrosis, massive tissue swelling, intravascular fluid shifts and hypovolemic shock, pulmonary edema, renal failure, and hemorrhagic complications from disseminated intravascular coagulation (DIC). Any of these complications can lead to death.

Patient-Centered Collaborative Care

Assessment

The clinical manifestations of venom release are based on the type and amount of venom injected, the bite location, and the age, size, and health status of the victim. Puncture wounds in the skin are a key local sign of pit viper envenomation. One or more puncture wounds may be present, depending on how many fangs the snake has and how many times the snake struck the patient. Severe pain, swelling, and redness or ecchymosis (bruising) in the area around the bite are common. Hours later, vesicles or hemorrhagic bullae may form. Systemic responses to venom must be distinguished from the effects of anxiety and panic related to being bitten by a snake. Commonly reported complaints include a minty, rubbery, or metallic taste in the mouth and tingling or paresthesias of the scalp, face, and lips. Other effects include muscle **fasciculations** (twitching) and weakness, nausea, vomiting, hypotension, seizures, and coagulopathy (clotting abnormalities) or DIC. If the bite site does not show evidence of local tissue swelling or redness within 8 hours, systemic effects are less likely to develop.

Interventions

First Aid

First aid interventions for snakebite should begin in the field and can improve the victim's outcome. *The first priority is to move the person to a safe area away from the snake and encourage rest to decrease venom circulation.* Next, remove jewelry and constricting clothing before swelling becomes significant. Immobilizing the affected extremity in a position of function with a splint helps limit the spread of the venom. Maintain the extremity below the level of the heart. Keep the person warm, and provide calm reassurance. Do not offer any alcohol or stimulants such as caffeinated beverages because these may speed the absorption of venom (Gold et al., 2004).

If transportation and treatment are delayed, a 2- to 4-cm constricting band may be applied proximal to an extremity wound to slow venom circulation via lymphatic flow, but it should not be tight enough to impair venous drainage or arterial flow. *This band should not be used as a tourniquet.* Placement of the band may worsen the local tissue necrosis by retaining venom in the tissues—the risk of increased limb damage must be weighed against the consequences of systemic venom effects (Auerbach et al., 2003). Assess distal circulation every hour. Loosen the band if edema occurs. *Do not incise or suck the wound or apply ice to it.* However, a commercially available device called the *Sawyer extractor* has been found to remove significant amounts of venom if used within 3 minutes of the bite and left in place for at least 30 minutes (Auerbach et al., 2003).

Hospital Care

Acute care in a hospital is required as soon as possible because envenomation is a medical emergency. Acute care management in the hospital provides supportive care, including supplemental oxygen, two large-bore IV lines, and infusion of crystalloid fluids such as normal saline solution or Ringer's lactate solution. Apply continuous cardiac and blood pressure monitoring equipment to quickly detect clinical deterioration. Because venom can cause severe pain at the bite site, opioids are indicated. Snakebite also poses tetanus and wound infection risks. Tetanus prophylaxis, attention to wound care, and broad-spectrum antibiotics are incorporated into the management plan.

Severe pit viper bites cause coagulopathy and promote hemorrhage and tissue destruction. Along with typical baseline laboratory studies, anticipate obtaining specimens for a coagulation profile, complete blood count, creatinine kinase, type and crossmatch, and urinalysis. An electrocardiogram (ECG) is necessary to detect evidence of myocardial ischemia or other cardiac abnormalities. Pertinent patient history related to the event includes a full account of the snake's appearance, the time the bite was inflicted, prehospital interventions, and any past incidence of snakebite or antivenom use. To accurately assess the development of tissue edema at the bite site, measure and record the circumference of the bitten extremity every 15 to 30 minutes.

Venom potency varies. Not all snakebite victims need antivenom administration. The decision whether or not to give antivenom is based on the severity of the snakebite. Table 11-1 classifies envenomation severity. *Contact the regional poison control center so that toxicologists can provide advice in antivenom dosing and medical management.*

Two types of antivenom are available and approved by the Food and Drug Administration (FDA) for the treatment of North American crotalids bites (e.g., rattlesnakes, copperheads, cottonmouths) (U.S. Food and Drug Administration, 2007; Wozniak et al., 2006). The older drug, Antivenin (Crotalidae) Polyvalent (ACP), is made from hyperimmune horse (equine) serum that contains antibodies against the venom. This drug is associated with an adverse drug event (ADE) known as *serum sickness.* **Serum sickness** is a type III hypersensitivity reaction that develops first as a skin rash that occurs within 3 to 21 days of ACP administration. This allergic response is often accompanied by other manifestations, such as fever, arthralgias (joint pains), and pruritus (itching) (see Chapter 22). *Be sure to perform skin testing before giving equine antivenom.*

TABLE 11-1 Grades of Pit Viper Envenomation

ENVENOMATION CHARACTERISTICS
• None. Fang marks, but no local or systemic reactions
• Minimal. Fang marks, local swelling and pain, but no systemic reactions
• Moderate. Fang marks and swelling progressing beyond the site of the bite; systemic signs and symptoms, such as nausea, vomiting, paresthesias, and hypotension
• Severe. Fang marks present with marked swelling of the extremity, subcutaneous ecchymosis, severe symptoms, including manifestations of coagulopathy

From Auerbach, P.S., Donner, H.J., & Weiss, E.A. (2003). *Field guide to wilderness medicine* (2nd ed.). St. Louis: Mosby.

The newest, safest, and most preferred antivenom is Crotalidae Polyvalent Immune Fab (CroFab), which is derived from sheep (ovine). This drug consists of specific antibody fragments of immunoglobulin G (IgG) that bind, neutralize, and redistribute toxins in crotalid venom so that they may be removed from the patient's body (Protherics, Inc., 2006). Serum sickness rarely occurs from CroFab administration, and less drug is needed to neutralize the toxins from the snakebite. Mild to moderate allergic reactions such as pruritus and urticaria can occur, but anaphylaxis is rare. Skin testing before administration is not necessary.

If the patient has a known hypersensitivity to papain or papaya, which is used during the manufacturing process, CroFab is contraindicated unless the benefits are believed to outweigh the risks (Protherics, Inc., 2006). Give CroFab cautiously to patients who have:

- A previous allergic reaction to antivenom therapy
- A hypersensitivity to bromelain (a pineapple-derived enzyme) or sheep protein
- Prior CroFab therapy for a past envenomation (patients can become sensitized to the foreign sheep protein)
- Pregnancy
- Sensitivity to mercury-containing products (the antivenin contains mercury)

CroFab should be given to patients as soon as possible, with the optimal timing within 6 hours of the bite (Protherics, Inc., 2006). The recommended initial IV dose is 4 to 6 vials infused over 60 minutes. During the first 10 minutes, the infusion should be slow (25-50 mL/hr). Monitor the patient closely for an allergic reaction (e.g., hives, rash, difficulty breathing). If symptoms are not effectively controlled with the first dose, an additional four to six vials are recommended. Once the symptoms are under control, two vials of CroFab are administered every 6 hours for a total of 18 hours of administration (Protherics, Inc., 2006).

CORAL SNAKES

Pathophysiology

North American coral snakes are found in the southeastern and southwestern United States (Fig. 11-3). These snakes burrow into the ground and are nonaggressive. Their ability to inject venom is less efficient than that of the pit vipers. Their maxillary fangs are small and fixed in an upright position. The coral snake must use a chewing motion to inject venom from glands through its maxillary fangs. Most bites occur when people attempt to handle the snake. Coral snake venom is less complex than pit viper venom but can be extremely potent. It has only two toxins: a nerve toxin and a muscle toxin. The amount of venom in an adult coral snake is enough to kill an adult.

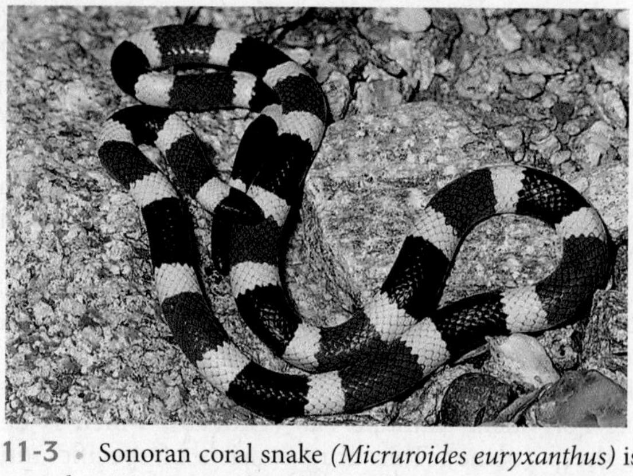

Fig. 11-3 • Sonoran coral snake *(Micruroides euryxanthus)* is also known as the *Arizona coral snake.* No documented fatality has followed a bite by this species.

Coral snakes can be recognized by bands of black, red, and yellow that completely encircle the body of the snake. If a black band lies between the red and yellow bands, the snake is often nonvenomous. Several harmless species closely resemble the coral snake. A helpful memory aid for identifying coral snakes is "red on yellow can kill a fellow" and "red and black, venom lack." *Be aware that this saying applies only to coral snakes found in the United States!*

Patient-Centered Collaborative Care

Assessment

Manifestations of coral snake envenomation are the result of its neurotoxic properties. The physiologic effect is to block neurotransmission, which produces ascending paralysis, reduced perception of pain, and, ultimately, respiratory paralysis (Wozniak et al., 2006). Unlike the pain from pit viper bites, pain at the coral snakebite site may be only mild and transient. The venom is spread via the lymphatic system, but swelling is unlikely. Fang marks may be difficult to find because of the coral snake's small teeth. Clotting changes do not occur. The toxic effects of coral snake venom also may be delayed up to 12 to 18 hours after a bite but then produce rapid clinical deterioration. Early signs and symptoms are nausea, vomiting, headache, pallor, and abdominal pain. Assess for neurologic manifestations, such as paresthesias (painful tingling), numbness, and mental status changes, as well as cranial nerve and peripheral nerve deficits. Total flaccid paralysis may occur later, and the patient may have difficulty speaking, swallowing, and breathing.

Respiratory problems and cardiovascular collapse can occur in severe cases (Norris, 2007). Arterial blood gas analysis reveals respiratory insufficiency. The muscle toxin in the venom can cause an elevation in creatinine kinase (CK) levels from muscle breakdown and produce **myoglobinuria** (release of muscle myoglobulin into the urine). Despite these clinical effects, death is rare if the patient receives timely management.

Interventions

First Aid

Because several varieties of harmless snakes resemble the coral snake, the first priority, if possible, is to identify the snake as a coral snake. Identification is easier if the snake is captured and brought to the health care facility with the victim. *However, if the snake cannot be safely caught or positively identified, the victim should be treated as if venom has been injected.* The field care is the same as for that of a pit viper bite without the added concern over tissue necrosis if a constricting band is used; coral snake venom does not destroy tissue. The affected extremity is encircled snugly with an elastic bandage or roller gauze dressing to impede lymphatic flow and then splinted to slow the spread of venom in coral snakebites (Wozniak et al., 2006). *This compression bandage must not be so tight that it impairs arterial flow. It should not be removed until the victim is managed at an acute care facility* (Norris, 2007).

Hospital Care

Once in an acute care setting, patients who have had an actual or potential coral snake envenomation should have continuous cardiac, blood pressure, and pulse oximetry monitoring and should be admitted to a critical care unit. Prepare to provide aggressive airway management via endotracheal intubation if respiratory insufficiency or severe neurologic impairment occurs. Aspiration of secretions is a significant risk for this patient.

The regional poison control center should be contacted immediately for advice on antivenom administration and patient management. Antivenom administration is recommended even when clinical evidence of envenomation is not present, because a delay can lead to rapid neurotoxicity once it develops (Gold et al., 2004). The onset of symptoms after coral snakebites can be delayed but can persist for a week in spite of treatment (Norris, 2007). The antivenom indicated for the North American coral snake is Antivenin *Micrurus fulvius* (Wyeth-Ayerst) made from horse serum. Although this drug is no longer in active production, limited supplies are still available (Gold et al., 2004; Wozniak et al., 2006).

The same precautions are applied when administering coral snake antivenom as with Crotalidae (pit viper) antivenom. The most significant risk to the victim is an anaphylactic response to the antivenom. *Therefore ensure that the patient's IV lines are patent and that emergency drugs (e.g., epinephrine, antihistamines, steroids) and resuscitation equipment are immediately available.* Anticipate premedication with H_2-blocking antihistamines when steroids are given.

The adult dose of Antivenin *Micrurus fulvius* is three to six vials (Norris, 2007). Begin the infusion slowly, and then increase to complete the entire infusion within about 2 hours. *If an allergic reaction occurs, stop the infusion while the patient is treated with epinephrine and/or antihistamines.* Then restart the infusion at a slower rate. For severe reactions, the physician determines whether to continue antivenom administration. The initial dose of coral snake antivenom may need to be repeated if neurotoxicity continues to progress.

ARTHROPOD BITES AND STINGS

Several North American insects are members of the phylum *Arthropoda.* These insects include spiders, scorpions, bees, and wasps. Unlike snakes, almost all species of spiders are venomous to some degree—most are not harmful to humans either because their mouthparts are too small to pierce human skin or the quantity or quality of their venom is inadequate to produce significant health problems. However, the venom of some spiders indigenous to the United States does produce major pathologic effects. These spiders include the brown recluse, black widow, and tarantula. Scorpions, bees, and wasps are other venomous arthropods that produce toxic reactions in humans.

BROWN RECLUSE SPIDER

Pathophysiology

The brown spiders of the *Loxosceles* genus are known for producing bites that result in ulcerative lesions. In the United States, the brown recluse spider *(L. reclusa)* is the best known of this spider type. Brown recluse spiders, also known as "fiddlebacks" or "violin spiders," are medium-sized spiders (body length 8-15 mm) that are light brown in color and have a dark brown, fiddle-shaped mark that extends from their eyes down their back (Fig. 11-4). Like their name implies, brown recluse spiders are shy and hide in areas that are dark and secluded, such as boxes, closets, basements, sheds, garages, luggage, shoes, clothing, and even bed sheets. Most indoor bites occur when people are sleeping, reaching into boxes or closets, or donning clothing that contains the spider. Few people ever see the spider that bit them. The only evidence may be a simple skin lesion; a necrotic wound **(necrotic arachnidism)**; or, less often, systemic effects from the injected toxin, commonly referred to as **loxoscelism** (Zeglin, 2005).

Patient-Centered Collaborative Care

Assessment

Brown recluse spider venom causes cell damage. The bite may be described as painless or stinging to sharp and painful. Some victims are unaware that they were bitten until intense local aching and pruritus develop over minutes to hours. The central bite site may appear as a bleb or vesicle surrounded by edema and erythema, which may expand over the course of hours as the toxin spreads to surrounding tissues. The center of the bite becomes bluish purple at the site of the bite. Over the next 1 to 3 days, the central lesion becomes dark and necrotic (Fig. 11-5). Eschar eventually forms. The combination of these tissue changes is often referred to as the classic "red, white, and blue sign" that is associated with severe brown recluse spider bites. Some people have few or no tissue changes and therefore do not require medical attention.

When the eschar sloughs, an open wound or ulcer can remain for weeks to months. In rare cases, some patients may also have manifestations of systemic toxicity to brown recluse spider bites. These can include a rash, fever, chills, nausea, vomiting, malaise, and joint pain (Furbee et al., 2006). At the extreme end, massive hemolytic reactions, renal failure, cardiovascular collapse, and death have been reported (Furbee et al., 2006).

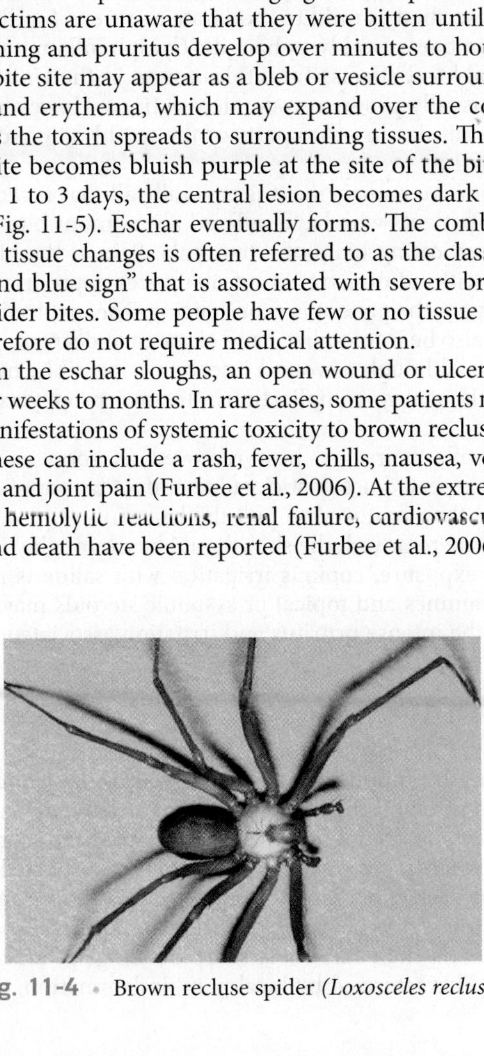

Fig. 11-4 • Brown recluse spider *(Loxosceles reclusa)*.

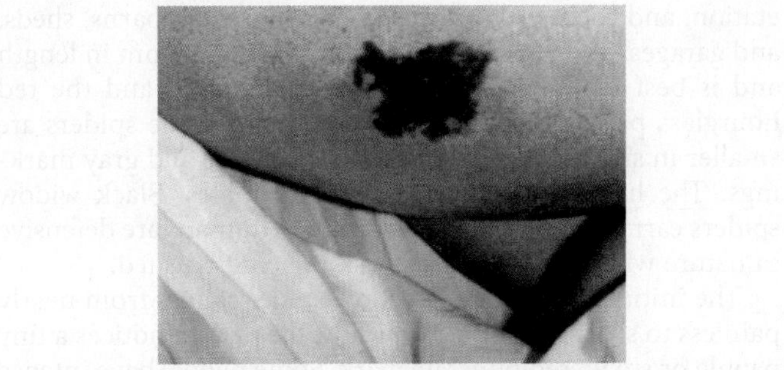

Fig. 11-5 • Brown recluse spider bite after 24 hours, with central ischemia and rapidly advancing cellulitis.

Interventions

First Aid

The basic first aid for a brown recluse spider bite is to apply ice intermittently during the first 4 days after the bite (Auerbach et al., 2003; Swanson & Vetter, 2005). Ice helps decrease the enzyme activity of the venom and may limit tissue necrosis. *Do not use heat because it increases the enzyme activity and potentially worsens the wound.* Recommended actions include elevation of the affected extremity and local wound care and rest (Swanson & Vetter, 2005).

Hospital Care

For patients with wounds that appear infected, a topical antiseptic and sterile dressing are necessary; antibiotics are also indicated. For severe wounds, therapy with dapsone (Avlosulfon) may be considered (Swanson & Vetter, 2005). Dapsone, administered in doses of 50 mg orally twice daily, is a neutrophil inhibitor that prevents extension of crater lesions. Because this drug increases the risk of blood dyscrasias in persons with glucose-6-phosphate dehydrogenase (G6PD) deficiency, G6PD screening and careful monitoring of blood studies are important to detect abnormalities (see Chapter 42). Agranulocytosis (decreased granulocytic white blood cells, such as neutrophils) and aplastic anemia (anemia caused by deficient red blood cell production from the bone marrow) are other potential adverse drug events (ADEs) of dapsone.

A surgeon should evaluate patients whose wounds require interventions beyond conservative management. Debridement and skin grafting may be required to promote healing in severe wounds. In all cases, tetanus prophylaxis is indicated. Where available, referral to a wound specialist nurse should be made.

About 10% of patients experience severe systemic complications, or loxoscelism. Manifestations include renal failure, leukopenia (decreased white blood cell count), seizures, hemolytic anemia (anemia caused by destruction of red blood cells), thrombocytopenia (decreased platelets), and coma, any of which can cause death (Zeglin, 2005). Critical care management, including aggressive hydration, blood transfusions, systemic steroids, and supportive therapies, is required to prevent further deterioration and promote recovery.

BLACK WIDOW SPIDER

Pathophysiology

Black widow spiders can be found in every state in the United States except Alaska. They can inflict deadly bites and are found in cool, damp environments like outdoor log piles, vegetation, and rocks. They also commonly inhabit barns, sheds, and garages. The female spider is about 12 to 16 mm in length and is best identified by her shiny black color and the red hourglass pattern on her ventral abdomen. Male spiders are smaller in size and lighter in color with white and gray markings. The hourglass pattern is faint in males. Black widow spiders carry neurotoxic venom. Bites to humans are defensive in nature when the spider is at risk of being crushed.

The initial bite of a black widow spider ranges from nearly painless to sharply painful. Typically, the person notices a tiny papule or small, red punctate mark. Some people have intense pain, which seems out of proportion to the lesion. In many cases, the symptoms do not progress beyond a local reaction in the area of the bite site. If systemic signs and symptoms do occur, they generally develop within 1 hour and involve the neuromuscular system.

Patient-Centered Collaborative Care

Assessment

Black widow spider venom produces a syndrome known as **latrodectism,** in which the venom causes neurotransmitter release from nerve terminals. Severe abdominal pain, muscle rigidity and spasm, hypertension, and nausea and vomiting are common. The problem may be incorrectly diagnosed as an acute abdomen, and surgical consultation may be considered because of the clinical features similar to peritonitis. The muscle spasms involve the large muscles of the abdomen, back, and limbs. Other problems include facial edema (*Latrodectus* facies), ptosis (eyelid drooping), diaphoresis, weakness, increased salivation, priapism (sustained erection), respiratory difficulty, increased respiratory secretions, fasciculations (twitching), and paresthesias (painful tingling or numbness). The effects of the bite are self-limited and generally resolve in a few days. *However, older adults with other health problems (comorbid conditions), such as cardiovascular disease, are at much higher risk for complications.*

Interventions

First Aid

The primary first aid intervention for a black widow spider bite in the prehospital setting is to apply an ice pack. Ice inhibits the action of the neurotoxin. Monitor the person for evidence of systemic toxicity as described above. If this problem occurs, support the patient's airway, breathing, and circulation. Patients should be transported to a medical facility as soon as possible for advanced life support care.

Hospital Care

In the emergency department, closely monitor vital signs, with special attention to blood pressure and respiratory function. Supportive therapy in the hospital includes administration of opioid pain medication and muscle relaxants such as diazepam (Valium). Calcium gluconate (10 mL of a 10% solution) also may be given for muscle spasms, rigidity, and pain. Tetanus prophylaxis is necessary. Observe the patient for seizures related to a rapidly rising blood pressure (Auerbach et al., 2003). Antihypertensive agents may be needed. Although relapses may occur, recovery usually occurs within a week.

Less often, pulmonary edema, uncontrollable hypertension, and shock occur. These patients require critical care management. Antivenom is available for black widow spider bites. However, this agent is rarely used because it carries a risk for anaphylaxis and serum sickness, both of which are potentially fatal. It is generally administered to treat only severe reactions in which respiratory arrest, seizures, or uncontrolled hypertension occurs. Because pregnant women may have uterine contractions from a black widow spider bite that can cause a premature delivery, antivenom is also indicated for them. The typical dose is one to three ampules. A poison control center can assist in antivenom dosing and patient management under these circumstances.

TARANTULAS

Pathophysiology

Tarantulas are the largest spiders in the arachnid class. They are found mainly in the tropical and subtropical areas of the United States and on all continents of the world. However, a number of species are also found in dry, arid states, such as New Mexico and Arizona. Tarantulas can grow to 10 cm in length and live as long as 25 years. These spiders possess venom that paralyzes prey and causes muscle necrosis. However, most bites to humans result in only local effects. A more serious issue is that several types of tarantulas have hairs in their dorsal abdominal area that can be launched into the air as a defensive maneuver and onto a victim. Thousands of these barbed hairs may land on a victim, penetrate skin and eyes, and cause a severe inflammatory reaction.

Patient-Centered Collaborative Care

Tarantula bites typically produce pain at the bite site, variously described as mild to moderate to severe. Swelling, redness, numbness, and lymphangitis (lymph inflammation) are the usual local effects. Tarantulas found in the United States do not usually produce systemic reactions. However, venom from tarantulas in other parts of the world may induce systemic illness.

Supportive management is generally all that is required to manage patients who have suffered a venomous bite or exposure to urticating hairs of a tarantula. Pain at the bite site is treated with administration of analgesics appropriate to the level of pain the patient is experiencing. The involved extremity may also be immobilized and elevated to decrease pain and swelling. Although a wound infection is possible, most bites heal without any complications. Tetanus prophylaxis is required.

Tarantula hairs are best removed as soon as possible through repeated use of sticky tape or duct tape applied to the skin and then removed to pull the hairs from the skin. After all hairs are removed, the skin should be thoroughly irrigated. For eye exposure, copious irrigation with saline is required. Antihistamines and topical or systemic steroids may be used to treat the intense pruritus and irritation associated with the spider's hairs.

SCORPIONS

Pathophysiology

Scorpions are found in many states within the United States although not typically in the Midwest or New England. However, stings are always possible when people keep scorpions as pets or when scorpions are accidentally transported in baggage and packaging. Unlike spiders that envenom their prey by inflicting a bite, scorpions inject venom through a stinging apparatus on their tail. Most scorpion stings produce a mild reaction characterized by local pain, inflammation, and mild

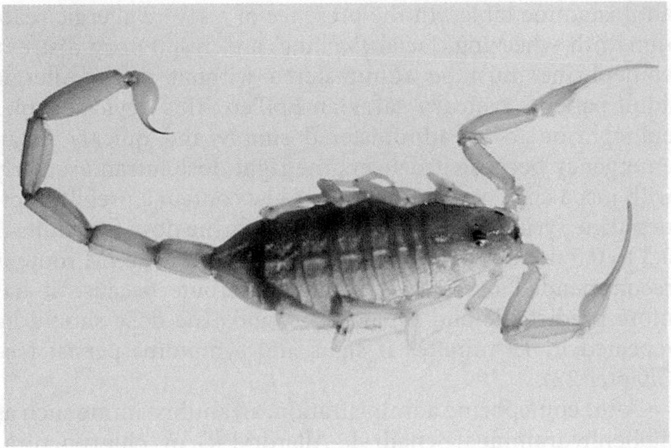

Fig. 11-6 • *Centruroides exilicauda (C. sculpturatus),* the bark scorpion of Arizona.

systemic symptoms. These effects are usually self-limiting and best treated by analgesics, supportive management, and basic wound care.

One species of scorpion found in the United States that can inflict a sting associated with a severe, potentially fatal systemic response is the bark scorpion (Fig. 11-6). It is often found in trees and woodpiles and around debris. Humans are usually stung when the scorpion gets into clothing, shoes, blankets, and personal items left on the ground. The small bark scorpion is about 5 cm (2 inches) in length and may be solid yellow, brown, or tan in color. There are also some striped varieties though not as common. Whereas many scorpions have thick claws and thick tails, distinctive features of the bark scorpion include thin pincers and a thin tail, as well as a tubercle (enlarged round area) at the base of the stinger. This scorpion is found throughout Arizona and in some areas of New Mexico, Texas, Nevada, and California. The venom of the bark scorpion is neurotoxic.

Patient-Centered Collaborative Care

Assessment

Because bark scorpion venom is neurotoxic, manifestations involve the cranial nerves and/or the musculoskeletal system. The sting site may or may not show evidence of the venom release. There may be no redness or other obvious sign of inflammation. Gentle tapping at the potential sting site that greatly increases pain is confirmation of a bark scorpion sting (Saucier, 2004). The severity of the reaction varies, from local pain to severe systemic manifestations such as high fever, hypertension, GI disorders, tachycardia, cardiac dysfunction, pulmonary edema, paresthesias, and central nervous system involvement. In rare cases, death can occur.

Symptoms usually begin immediately after the sting and can reach a crisis level within 12 hours. Recovery occurs gradually. Pain, tachycardia, and paresthesias can remain for up to 2 weeks (Saucier, 2004).

Interventions

The first priority of patient management is vital sign assessment and continuous monitoring for several hours in a hospital emergency department or critical care unit to enable rapid intervention if symptoms progress. The patient may require intubation and mechanical ventilation for respiratory failure. Supplemental oxygen and IV fluid replacement are instituted immediately. Apply an ice pack to the sting site to control pain. Give analgesic and sedative agents with caution in the non-intubated, spontaneously breathing patient. Potent opioids, benzodiazepines, and barbiturates can cause loss of airway reflexes and precipitate respiratory failure. Fever is treated with acetaminophen (Tylenol) and application of a cooling blanket as needed. Because scorpion stings produce a puncture wound, tetanus prophylaxis and basic wound care with an antiseptic agent are indicated.

Contact the poison control center as soon as possible to assist with patient management, particularly in regard to use of pharmacologic agents. Supportive care to address symptoms constitutes the typical course of treatment. For hypersalivation (excessive saliva) that may compromise the patient's airway after a bark scorpion sting, a dose of atropine may be recommended to decrease secretions.

An antivenom derived from goat serum is available for bark scorpion stings (*Centruroides exilicauda* Antivenin), but its use is controversial and its availability is limited to Arizona. It is generally not administered unless the patient had a severe envenomation. Hypersensitivity reactions are possible, especially if patients have a history of asthma, a prior hypersensitivity response to the scorpion antivenin, or allergies to goats or goat products. *Consult the poison control center for preparation and dosing of the antivenom if it is both available and indicated for the patient.* Be sure that advanced life support equipment is available to treat an anaphylactic response to the antivenom if it should occur. Serum sickness often develops days to weeks after antivenom administration and is treated with antihistamines and a tapering regimen of corticosteroids.

BEES AND WASPS

Pathophysiology

Bees and wasps are venomous arthropods. Stings can produce a wide range of reactions from discomfort at the sting site to severe pain and life-threatening anaphylaxis in allergic people. Bees and wasps are capable of stinging repeatedly when disturbed. Only the honeybee does not have this tendency. "Africanized" bees, also called "killer bees," are a very aggressive bee species found in the southwestern states that are known to attack in groups and can remain agitated for several hours. People under attack should attempt to outrun the bees, if possible, and keep their mouth and eyes protected from the swarm. When a person sustains multiple stings, reactions are more severe and may be fatal because multiple venom doses have cumulative toxic effects.

Health Promotion and Maintenance

Chart 11-4 lists actions that may help prevent arthropod bites and stings.

Patient-Centered Collaborative Care

Assessment

The person who is stung by a bee or wasp first has a local reaction of immediate pain and a wheal-and-flare reaction. Swelling can be extensive and involve an entire limb or body area. Systemic effects can then develop based on the venom load and the person's sensitivity to the venom. These effects may include generalized edema, nausea, vomiting, and diarrhea and are a reaction to the toxic effects of the venom itself, not necessarily an allergic reaction (Mitchell, 2006). Other toxic venom effects

Chart 11-4 PATIENT AND FAMILY EDUCATION GUIDE
Arthropod Bite/Sting Prevention

- Wear appropriate protective clothing, including gloves and shoes, when working in areas known to harbor venomous arthropods, such as spiders, scorpions, bees, and wasps.
- Cover garbage cans. Bees and wasps are attracted to uncovered garbage.
- Use screens in windows and doors to prevent flying insects from entering buildings.
- Inspect clothing, shoes, and gear for insects before putting on these items.
- Shake out clothing and gear that have been on the ground to prevent arthropod "stowaways" and inadvertent bites and stings.
- Consult an exterminator to control arthropod populations in and around the home. Eliminating insects that are part of the arthropod's food source may also limit their presence.
- Identify nesting areas such as yard debris and rock piles; remove them whenever possible.
- Do not place unprotected hands where the eyes cannot see.
- Avoid handling insects or keeping them as "pets."
- Do not swat insects, wasps, and Africanized bees because they can send chemical signals that alert others to attack.
- Carry prescription epinephrine preparations and antihistamines if known to be allergic to bee and wasp stings.

include destruction of red and white blood cells and platelets, damage to the blood vessel walls, acute renal failure, liver injury, and cardiac dysrhythmias (Mitchell, 2006).

If the patient has an allergy to the venom, then **urticaria** (hives), pruritus, and swelling of the lips and tongue may ensue. An allergic response can progress to an anaphylactic reaction rapidly in highly sensitive patients. **Anaphylaxis** is evidenced by respiratory distress with bronchospasm and laryngeal edema, hypotension, deterioration in mental status, and cardiac dysrhythmias. *This type of reaction constitutes a true medical emergency that is imminently life threatening and may lead to cardiac arrest.* Realize that initially it may be impossible to distinguish an allergic reaction from a toxic venom reaction because they can both cause the same types of early signs and symptoms.

Interventions

First Aid

Basic emergency care for bee and wasp stings includes quick removal of the stinger and application of an ice pack (Laskowski-Jones, 2006). Tweezers are not used to remove a stinger to avoid pinching the venom sac in the stinger and causing additional venom to be injected during removal. The commonly preferred method is to remove the stinger by gently scraping or brushing it off with the edge of a knife blade, credit card, or needle. However, it is important to realize that the method used to remove the stinger is not as relevant as the speed of removal (Mitchell, 2006).

Emergency Care

Advanced emergency care interventions are prioritized to ensure that airway, breathing, and circulation are maintained. First, it is essential to determine whether the patient has a history of allergic reactions to bee stings and whether he or she has an epinephrine kit. These kits sometimes also contain an antihistamine tablet. In the presence of a severe allergic reaction with wheezing, facial swelling, and respiratory distress, epinephrine must be administered without delay. Allergic adult patients typically carry an EpiPen. This device enables epinephrine to be administered simply and quickly in an emergency because it delivers the right dose intramuscularly with just a click of a button. Other kits contain a prefilled epinephrine syringe. The standard epinephrine dose for adults is 0.3 to 0.5 mg of a 1:1000 solution given IM. `The IM route is recommended over the subcutaneous route because it has more predictable and rapid absorption. The dose should be repeated in 15 minutes if signs and symptoms persist (see Chapter 22).

After epinephrine administration, an antihistamine such as diphenhydramine (Benadryl, Allerdryl🍁) or chlorpheniramine (Chlor-Trimeton, Novopheniram🍁) should also be given immediately. In the field setting, oral liquid diphenhydramine (available over the counter) may be easier for the victim to swallow than the tablet form if there is tongue or pharyngeal edema. For reactions that cause just pruritus and urticaria, only an antihistamine may be indicated initially. *It is critical to call 911 to transport the patient to a medical facility as soon as possible.*

Hospital Care

Once in a clinical setting, patients who sustain serious reactions to bee or wasp stings need oxygen and continuous cardiac and blood pressure monitoring. Establish an IV infusion with normal saline solution to support blood pressure. Advanced life support drugs and equipment should be made immediately available. If epinephrine IM fails to relieve the life-threatening reaction, epinephrine 0.1 mg to 0.25 mg of a 1:10,000 solution may be requested as a very slow IV bolus. IV epinephrine administration has much greater risk of adverse cardiovascular effects than IM epinephrine. Use the IV form of epinephrine with extreme caution, especially in older adults with cardiovascular disease, because it can increase pulse rate and blood pressure. Bronchospasm can be treated with albuterol via inhalation or a similar bronchodilating agent.

Parenteral antihistamines and corticosteroids are also prescribed to decrease the immune response. The toxin in the bee and wasp venom may outlast the effects of the initial doses of epinephrine and antihistamines and cause a recurrence of the allergic reaction over time. Therefore doses may need to be repeated for hours or days. Corticosteroids prescribed in tapered doses are usually given to manage or prevent delayed allergic effects, as well as serum sickness.

All patients who have sustained multiple stings (particularly more than 50) should be observed in an emergency care setting for several hours to monitor for the development of toxic venom effects. A critical care admission may be needed. Anyone who develops an allergic reaction to bee or wasp stings also should be urged to always carry a prescription epinephrine emergency kit and wear a medical alert tag or bracelet.

LIGHTNING INJURIES

Pathophysiology

Lightning is a year-round force of nature responsible for multiple injuries and deaths each year. It is caused by an electric charge generated within thunderclouds that may become cloud-to-ground lightning—the most dangerous form to people and structures. Young adult males account for the majority of lightning-related deaths. Most lightning-related injuries occur in the summer months during the afternoon and early evening because of increased thunderstorm activity and greater numbers of people spending time outside. Anyone without adequate shelter, including golfers, hikers, campers, beach-goers, and swimmers, is at risk.

Lightning has an enormous magnitude of energy and a much shorter duration of contact and a different current flow than a typical high-voltage electric shock. *High-voltage* electricity is considered to exceed 1000 volts. The energy in a single lightning stroke can exceed millions of volts (Spies & Trohman, 2006). The duration of contact, however, is nearly instantaneous, resulting in a flashover phenomenon—an effect that may account for the relatively low overall mortality rate. Because water is a conductor of electricity and current takes the path of least resistance to the ground, any wetness on the body increases the flashover effect of a lightning strike. Lightning flashover produces an explosive force that can injure victims directly, as well as cause them to fall or to be thrown. The clothing and shoes of victims may be damaged or blown off in the process.

Lightning produces injury by directly striking a victim, by splashing off a nearby object, or by traveling through the ground—also called *step voltage.* Although few people die after a lightning strike, many survivors are left with permanent disabilities.

Health Promotion and Maintenance

Perhaps the best remedy for lightning injuries is avoidance. Injuries caused by lightning strike are highly preventable. Chart 11-5 lists common prevention strategies.

Chart 11-5 PATIENT AND FAMILY EDUCATION GUIDE

Lightning Strike Prevention

- Observe weather forecasts when planning to be outside.
- Seek shelter when you hear thunder. Safe areas include the nearest building or an enclosed vehicle. Isolated sheds and the entrances to caves are dangerous, however. Do not stand under an isolated tall tree or structure (e.g., ski lift, flag pole, boat mast, power line) in an open area such as a field, ridge, or hilltop; lightning seeks the highest point. A stand of dense trees offers better protection.
- Leave the water immediately (including an indoor shower or bathtub), and move away from any open bodies of water.
- Avoid metal objects: put down tools, fishing rods, garden equipment, golf clubs, and umbrellas; stand clear of fences, exposed pipes, motorcycles, bicycles, tractors, and golf carts.
- If camping in a tent, stay away from the metal tent poles and wet walls.
- Once inside a building, stay away from open doors, windows, fireplaces, metal fixtures, and plumbing.
- Turn off electrical equipment including computers, televisions, and stereos.
- Stay off the telephone. Lightning can enter through the telephone line and produce head and neck trauma, including cataracts and tympanic membrane disruption. Death can result.
- If you are caught out in the open and cannot seek shelter, attempt to move to lower ground such as a ravine or valley; stay away from any tall trees or objects that could result in a lightning strike splashing over to you; place insulating material between you and the ground (e.g., sleeping pad, rain parka, life jacket), and bend down on your knees, bend forward, and place your hands on your knees. A lightning strike is imminent if your hair stands on end, you see blue halos around objects, and hear high-pitched or crackling noises. If you cannot move away from the area immediately, crouch on the balls of your feet and tuck your head down to minimize the target size; do not lie down on the ground or have hand contact with the ground.

Data from Auerbach, P.S., Donner, H.J., & Weiss, E.A. (2003). *Field guide to wilderness medicine* (2nd ed.). St. Louis: Mosby.

Patient-Centered Collaborative Care

Assessment

Both the cardiopulmonary and the central nervous systems are profoundly affected by lightning injuries. The most lethal initial effect of the massive current discharge on the cardiopulmonary system is asystole. Apnea results in hypoxia-induced ventricular fibrillation (Spies & Trohman, 2006). Because cardiac cells are autorhythmic, an effective cardiac rhythm may return spontaneously. However, prolonged respiratory arrest from impairment of the medullary respiratory center produces hypoxia and, subsequently, a second cardiac arrest. Therefore the principle of "reverse triage" is the rule when attempting to manage multiple victims of a lightning strike: provide care to those who are in cardiopulmonary arrest first. Initiate resuscitation measures with immediate airway and ventilatory management, chest compressions, and other appropriate life support interventions. People who exhibit signs of life immediately after a lightning strike have the best chance of survival and may be treated in a less emergent fashion. Keep in mind, however, that victims of lightning strike can suffer serious myocardial injury, which may be manifested by ECG and myocardial perfusion abnormalities. The initial appearance of mottled skin and decreased to absent peripheral pulses usually arises from arterial vasospasm and typically resolves spontaneously in several hours.

Central nervous system (CNS) injury is common in lightning strike victims. A classic finding is an immediate but temporary paralysis that affects the lower limbs to a greater extent than the upper limbs (Cherington, 2005). This condition usually resolves within hours. Other effects include loss of consciousness, amnesia, confusion or disorientation, photophobia, and seizures. Intracranial hemorrhage, cerebral infarction, post-hypoxic encephalopathy, cerebellar dysfunction, and spinal cord injury may also occur (Cherington, 2005). Chronic fatigue, depression, headache, chronic pain syndromes, cognitive impairments, and post-traumatic stress disorder are all long-term consequences that have been reported in many lightning strike survivors (Cherington, 2005; Yarnell, 2005). Other complications include ruptured tympanic membranes, blindness, cataracts, fractures, and retinal detachment, which may be due to both blast effect and intense heat production and can occur with lightning-mediated telephone injury (Gatewood & Zane, 2004).

Lightning strike also causes skin burns. Most burns are superficial and heal without incident. Patients may have full-thickness burns, charring, and contact burns from overlying metal objects. An uncommon but characteristic skin manifestation of lightning is the appearance of branching or ferning marks on the skin called **Lichtenberg figures.**

Interventions

First Aid

Because of lightning's powerful impact to the body, patients are at great risk for multisystem trauma. The full extent of injury may not be known until thorough monitoring and diagnostic evaluation can be performed in the hospital. Initial care includes spinal immobilization with attention to stabilization of airway, breathing, and circulation through standard basic and advanced life support measures. CPR is performed immediately when a person is in cardiac arrest. In the presence of cardiopulmonary or CNS injury, skin burns are *not* an initial priority. However, if time and resources permit, a sterile dressing may be applied to cover the sites. *Victims of lightning strike are not electrically charged; the rescuer is in no danger from physical contact.* Nonetheless, the storm can present a continued threat to everyone in the vicinity who lacks adequate shelter. Contrary to popular belief, lightning can and does strike in the same place more than once.

Hospital Care

Once in the acute care hospital setting, the patient requires advanced life support management, including cardiac monitoring to detect cardiac dysrhythmias and a 12-lead ECG. Airway, breathing, and circulatory support are performed as needed. The patient may require mechanical ventilation until spontaneous breathing returns. A thorough physical and diagnostic evaluation to identify obvious and occult traumatic injuries is important because the patient may have suffered a fall or blast effect during the strike. A creatinine kinase (CK) measurement may be requested to detect skeletal muscle damage resulting from the lightning strike. In severe cases, rhabdomyolysis (by-products of skeletal muscle destruction) can occur and can lead to renal failure. Burn wounds should be assessed and treated according to standard burn care protocols. Tetanus prophylaxis is necessary for burns or any break in skin integrity. Care of the patient is supportive as recovery begins. Some institutions transfer these victims to a burn center for follow-up management.

COLD INJURIES

Two common cold injuries are hypothermia and frostbite. Both types of injuries can be prevented by implementing protection from the cold. Teach patients at risk ways to prevent these injuries, which can range from mild discomfort to major systemic complications.

HEALTH PROMOTION AND MAINTENANCE

When participating in cold weather activities, clothing choices are critical to the prevention of hypothermia and frostbite. Synthetic clothing is best because it wicks away moisture from the body and dries fast. Cotton clothing, especially as an undergarment, holds moisture, becomes wet, and contributes to the development of hypothermia. Cotton clothing should be strictly avoided in a cold outdoor environment; this rule applies to gloves and socks as well. The classic mountaineering adage that "cotton kills" is important to remember. Wet socks and gloves promote frostbite in the toes and fingers. Wearing too many pairs of socks can impair circulation and predispose to frostbite.

Clothing should be layered so that it can be easily added or removed as the temperature changes. The inner layers should provide warmth and insulation. Polyester fleece is a good choice. The outer layer's purpose is to block the wind and provide moisture protection. This layer is best made of a windproof, waterproof, breathable fabric such as GORE-TEX. A hat is an essential clothing item that significantly decreases body heat loss through the head. Face protection with a facemask should be used on particularly cold days when wind chill poses a risk. Sunscreen (at least SPF 30) and sunglasses are also important to protect skin and eyes from the sun's harmful rays.

When driving in winter cannot be avoided, water, extra clothing, and food should be kept in the car in case the vehicle becomes stranded. Maintaining personal fitness and conditioning are also important considerations to prevent hypothermia and frostbite. People should not diet or restrict food or fluid intake when participating in winter outdoor activities. Malnutrition and dehydration contribute to cold-related illnesses and injuries. Finally, it is important for people to know their physical limits and to come in out of the cold when these limits have been reached.

HYPOTHERMIA

Pathophysiology

Hypothermia is a core body temperature below 95° F (35° C). An understanding of the causes and risk factors involved in the development of hypothermia is the key to both recognition and prevention. Predisposing conditions that promote hypothermia include:

- Cold water immersion
- Illness
- Traumatic injury
- Shock states
- Immobilization
- Weather (especially for homeless)
- Extremes of age
- Select medications (e.g., phenothiazines, barbiturates)
- Alcohol intoxication
- Malnutrition
- Hypothyroidism
- Inadequate clothing or shelter

An important point, however, is that an environmental temperature below 82° F can produce hypothermia in any susceptible person. Therefore people, especially older adults, are actually at risk on a *year-round* basis in most areas of the world. Wind chill is a significant factor: heat loss increases as wind speed rises. Wet conditions further increase heat loss through evaporation. Weather is the most common cause of hypothermia for outdoor sports enthusiasts and for those with inadequate clothing or shelter. It is also a problem for the older adult, homeless, and poor who cannot afford heating.

Patient-Centered Collaborative Care

Assessment

Hypothermia is commonly divided into the categories of *mild* (32° to 35° C), *moderate* (28° to 32° C), and *severe* (below 28° C). Treatment decisions are based on the degree of hypothermia present. *Mild* hypothermia is manifested by shivering, dysarthria, muscular incoordination, impaired cognitive abilities (i.e., mental slowness), and "cold diuresis." Cold diuresis results from peripheral vasoconstriction and shunting of blood to the core of the body. With core hypervolemia, blood flow to the kidneys increases, causing an increase in urine output. Dehydration results and worsens the hypothermic condition because of impaired circulation. Shivering and an increased metabolic rate are the body's compensatory mechanisms to stimulate heat production. Early cardiopulmonary manifestations include tachycardia and increased respiratory rate.

Patients with *moderate* (28° to 32° C) to *severe* hypothermia (below 28° C) have obvious motor impairment and weakness. They become uncoordinated and may stumble or fall. Cognitive abilities and mental processes deteriorate. Confusion and apathy progress to irrationality and incoherence, stupor, and unconsciousness. Shivering stops in severe hypothermia. Victims may even mistakenly perceive warmth and engage in "paradoxical undressing" in which they undress, an action that worsens their already hypothermic condition (Auerbach et al., 2003). Vital signs become depressed; bradycardia and hypotension are typical. Respiratory rate and effort and cardiac output decline. Prolongation of the P-R, QRS, and Q-Tc intervals occurs; J waves or Osborn waves may appear on the ECG (Aslam et al., 2006). A cold heart is an irritable heart; atrial and ventricular dysrhythmias are common. The ventricular fibrillation threshold is decreased. Deterioration to ventricular fibrillation and asystole is easily precipitated by rough handling or jolting of the patient's body, as well as procedures like central line insertion. In severe hypothermia (below 28° C), neurologic reflexes and responsiveness to pain are absent. Profound hypotension, acid-base abnormalities, ventricular fibrillation, and asystole are characteristic.

In moderate to severe hypothermia, laboratory values may reveal blood clotting abnormalities, including platelet dysfunction. Clotting factor function is temperature dependent and is reduced in hypothermia. Platelet aggregation is impaired; thrombocytopenia develops because of destruction of platelets in the liver and spleen (Watts, 1998). Prolonged bleeding times result. *An important concept is that hypothermia causes clotting problems over a range of temperatures—the greater the degree of hypothermia, the more likely the patient will hemorrhage from injury or invasive procedures.* This problem is especially critical for the injured patient in shock who requires resuscitation: hypothermia must be identified and treated effectively to prevent further blood loss.

Interventions

First Aid

Treatment of mild hypothermia is straightforward: the person needs to be sheltered from the cold environment, have all wet clothing removed, and undergo passive or active external rewarming. Passive methods involve applying warm clothing or blankets. Active methods incorporate heating blankets, warm packs, and convective air heaters or warmers to speed rewarming. If a heating blanket is used, monitor the patient's skin at least every 15 to 30 minutes to reduce the risk of burn injury.

In a camping or wilderness setting, a rescuer can share the same sleeping bag with a hypothermic victim to promote transfer of body heat as an effective means of active external rewarming. Both the rescuer and the victim should be only minimally clothed to facilitate heat transfer. In the case of mild, uncomplicated hypothermia as the only health problem, having the victim drink warm high-carbohydrate liquids that do not contain alcohol or caffeine can aid in rewarming. Alcohol is a peripheral vasodilator; both alcohol and caffeine are diuretics. These effects can potentially worsen dehydration and hypothermia.

Hospital Care

General management principles apply to both *moderate* and *severe* hypothermia. The patient should be protected from further heat loss and handled gently to prevent ventricular fibrillation. The horizontal position prevents orthostatic changes in blood pressure from cardiovascular instability. Standard resuscitation efforts are indicated with special attention to maintenance of airway, breathing, and circulation as recommended by the American Heart Association (2005b):

- Administer drugs with caution and/or spaced at longer intervals because metabolism is unpredictable in hypothermic conditions.
- Remember that drugs can accumulate without obvious therapeutic effect while the patient is cold but may become active and potentially lead to drug toxicity as effective rewarming is underway.
- Consider withholding IV drugs until the core temperature is above 86° F (30° C).
- Initiate CPR for patients without spontaneous circulation.
- Be aware that defibrillation attempts may be ineffective until the core temperature is above 86° F (30° C).

Treatment of *moderate* hypothermia may involve active external and core rewarming methods. Applying external heat with heating blankets can promote core temperature "after-drop" by producing peripheral vasodilation. **After-drop** is the continued decrease in core body temperature after the victim is removed from the cold environment caused by the return of cold blood from the periphery to the central circulation. Therefore the patient's trunk should be actively rewarmed before the extremities (Aslam et al., 2006). Core rewarming methods for moderate hypothermia include administration of warm IV fluids, heated oxygen or inspired gas to prevent further heat loss via the respiratory tract, and heated peritoneal, pleural, gastric, or bladder lavage.

The patient who is *severely* hypothermic is at high risk of cardiac arrest. Active external rewarming with heating devices is dangerous and is contraindicated in this population because it produces vasodilation in the extremities with core temperature after-drop. The treatment of choice is to employ extracorporeal (outside of the body) rewarming methods such as cardiopulmonary bypass, hemodialysis, or continuous arteriovenous rewarming (CAVR). The advantage of CAVR for the trauma patient with hemorrhage is that heparin is not required. A limitation is that the patient's systolic blood pressure must be greater than 60 mm Hg for blood to flow through the circuit. Cardiopulmonary bypass is the fastest core rewarming technique. It supports the circulation and allows for timely correction of fluid, electrolyte, and metabolic abnormalities. However, this device is not available in all hospitals. It also requires specialized personnel and resources to operate it properly. Complications can occur after weaning from cardiopulmonary bypass, such as acute respiratory distress syndrome (ARDS), acute renal failure, and pneumonia.

A long-standing principle in the treatment of patients with hypothermic cardiac arrest is that "no one is dead until they are warm and dead." There is a factual basis to this statement when considering the number of survivors who have suffered a prolonged hypothermic cardiac arrest. Prolonged resuscitation efforts may not be reasonable in cases in which survival appears highly unlikely, such as in an anoxic event followed by a hypothermic cardiac arrest. Clinical judgment must always be used in each situation, however.

FROSTBITE

Pathophysiology

Another significant cold-related injury that may or may not be associated with hypothermia is frostbite. The main risk factor is inadequate insulation against cold weather; that is, either the skin is exposed to the cold or the person's clothing offers insufficient protection. Wet clothing, in particular, is a poor insulator and facilitates the development of frostbite. Fatigue, dehydration, and poor nutrition are other contributing factors. People who smoke, consume alcohol, or have impaired peripheral circulation have a higher incidence of frostbite. These factors aggravate cold injuries. Any previous history of frostbite further increases a person's susceptibility.

Patient-Centered Collaborative Care

Assessment

Frostbite is characterized by the degree of tissue freezing and the resultant damage it produces. Like burns, frostbite injuries can be superficial, partial, or full thickness. **Frostnip** is a type of superficial cold injury that may produce initial pain, numbness, and pallor of the affected area but is easily remedied with application of warmth and does not induce tissue damage. Frostnip typically develops on skin areas such as the face, nose, finger, or toes. Untreated, frostnip is a precursor to more severe forms of frostbite. *First-degree frostbite*, the least severe type of frostbite, involves hyperemia (increased blood flow) of the involved area and edema formation. In *second-degree frostbite*, large fluid-filled blisters develop with partial-thickness skin necrosis (Fig. 11-7). *Third-degree frostbite* appears as small blisters that contain dark fluid and an affected body part that is cool, numb, blue, or red and does not blanch. Full-thickness and subcutaneous tissue necrosis occur and require débridement. In *fourth-degree frostbite*, the most severe form, there are no blisters or edema; the part is numb, cold, and bloodless. The full-thickness necrosis extends into the muscle and bone. At this stage, gangrene develops, which may necessitate amputation of the affected part.

Interventions

First Aid

Recognition of frostbite is essential to early, effective intervention and prevention of further tissue damage. Asking a partner to frequently observe for early signs of frostbite such as a white, waxy appearance to exposed skin, especially on the nose, cheeks, and ears, is an effective strategy to identify the problem before it worsens. In this case, the best remedy is to have the person seek shelter from the wind and cold and to attend to the affected body part. Superficial frostbite is easily managed in the prehospital setting using body heat to warm the affected area. Teach patients to place their warm hands over the affected areas on their face or to place cold hands under the arms in the axillary region.

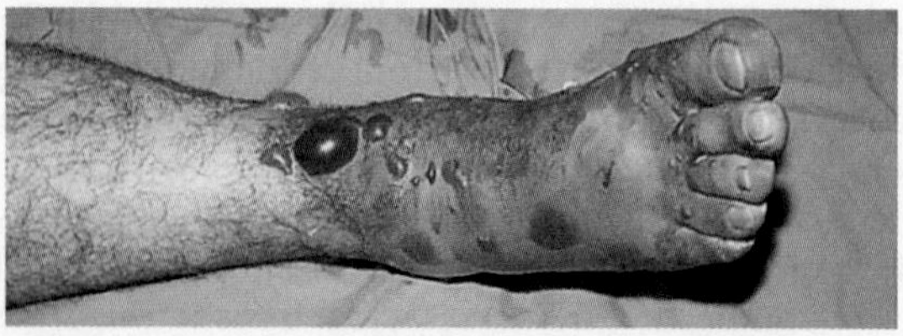

Fig. 11-7 • Edema and blister formation 24 hours after frostbite injury occurring in an area covered by a tightly fitted boot.

Hospital Care

Patients with more severe and deeper forms of frostbite need aggressive management. For all degrees of partial to full-thickness frostbite, rapid rewarming in a water bath at a temperature range of 104° to 108° F (40°-42° C) is indicated to thaw the frozen part (Ulrich & Rathlev, 2004). If a warming tub is not available, use hot towels instead. Because patients experience severe pain during the rewarming process, this intervention is best accomplished in a medical facility; however, it may be done in another setting if no other options exist for prompt transport or rescue. Analgesic agents, especially IV opiates, and IV rehydration are essential aspects of the plan of care. *Dry heat should never be applied, nor should the frostbitten areas be rubbed or massaged as part of the warming process. These actions produce further tissue injury.*

When the rewarming process is complete, handle the injured areas gently and elevate them above heart level if possible to decrease tissue edema. Sometimes splints are used to immobilize extremities during the healing process. Assess the person at least hourly for the development of compartment syndrome—a limb-threatening complication of frostbite that requires surgical intervention. Frostbite destroys tissue and produces a deep tetanus-prone wound; the patient should be immunized for tetanus prophylaxis. Apply only loose, nonadherent sterile dressings to the damaged areas. Avoid compression of the injured tissues. Both topical and systemic antibiotics may be used. Once a patient's frozen part has been thawed, do not allow it to refreeze, which worsens the injury.

In cases of severe, deep frostbite, surgical intervention is needed to evaluate tissue viability and provide wound management. Débridement of necrotic tissue is necessary. Amputation may be indicated for patients with severe injuries or for those who develop gangrene.

ALTITUDE-RELATED ILLNESSES

Pathophysiology

High altitude is an elevation above 5000 feet that can produce a range of physiologic responses in the body and can be fatal. Because many people visit mountainous areas for sport and recreation, such as skiing and hiking, it is important to understand altitude physiology and how to recognize the most common emergency situations that may be caused by its effect on the human body.

As altitude increases, atmospheric pressure decreases. Oxygen makes up 21% of the pressure. Therefore as this pressure falls, the partial pressure of oxygen in the air decreases, resulting in less available oxygen to humans. The physiologic consequence is hypoxia. Hypoxia is more pronounced as elevation increases. High altitude is considered to be about 5,000 to 11,500 feet—the same elevation as most Western ski areas in the United States. Very high altitude is an elevation between about 11,500 feet and 18,000 feet. The peaks of some Western ski areas are in the 12,000- to 13,000-foot range. Elevations higher than 18,000 feet are extreme altitudes. Supplemental oxygen is necessary at these altitudes to prevent altitude-related illness, including death, from occurring during abrupt ascent.

The process of adapting to high altitude is called *acclimatization.* **Acclimatization** involves physiologic changes that help the body adapt to less available oxygen in the atmosphere. As the carotid bodies sense a decline in Pao_2 at about 5000 feet, the respiratory rate increases to improve oxygen delivery. This mechanism is called the "hypoxic ventilatory response." Increased respiratory rate causes **hypocapnia** (decreased carbon dioxide) and respiratory alkalosis, which limit further increases in respiratory rate. At this point, sleep disturbances characterized by periodic respirations are common. Rapid eye movement (REM) sleep is impaired. Hypoxia can occur from periods of apnea. Within 24 to 48 hours of being at high altitude, the kidneys excrete the excess bicarbonate and enable the pH to return to normal and ventilatory rate to again increase as an important compensatory response. Greater sympathetic nervous system activity increases heart rate, blood pressure, and cardiac output. Pulmonary artery pressure rises as an effect of generalized hypoxia-induced pulmonary vasoconstriction. Cerebral blood flow increases to maintain cerebral oxygen delivery. Hypoxia also induces red blood cell production by stimulating the release of erythropoietin. The result is an increase in red blood cells and hemoglobin concentration. Over time, polycythemia can develop in people who remain in a high-altitude environment.

People who plan to ascend to high altitudes are advised to ascend slowly, over the course of days or even weeks, depending on the degree of elevation. Ascending too rapidly is the primary cause of altitude-related illness. This illness is more common in people who sleep at elevations above 8000 feet. Dehydration and central nervous system (CNS) depressants, such as alcohol, increase the risk of altitude-related illness.

The three most common clinical conditions that pose a risk to people at high altitude are acute mountain sickness (AMS), high altitude cerebral edema (HACE), and high altitude pulmonary edema (HAPE). These conditions may overlap in the same person; the underlying pathophysiology is hypoxia. Although each syndrome has some unique manifestations, the basic assessment and management approach are the same.

Patient-Centered Collaborative Care

Assessment

Acute mountain sickness (AMS) usually occurs before high altitude cerebral edema (HACE) and/or high altitude pulmonary edema (HAPE). People who make a rapid ascent without acclimatization to altitudes above 8000 feet from altitudes below 5000 feet are most often affected (Hackett & Roach, 2007). Findings from the assessment of the typical patient with AMS include reports of throbbing headache, anorexia, nausea, and vomiting. Feeling chilled, irritable, and apathetic are also associated with AMS. The syndrome produces effects similar to an alcohol-induced hangover. The patient may relate a feeling of extreme illness. Vital signs are variable: the patient can be tachycardic or bradycardic, have normal blood pressure, or have postural hypotension. He or she may experience dyspnea both on exertion and at rest. Exertional dyspnea is expected as a person adjusts to high altitude. However, dyspnea at rest is abnormal and may signal the onset of HAPE.

If AMS progresses to *high altitude cerebral edema (HACE),* the extreme form of this disorder, the patient cannot perform ADLs and exhibits extreme apathy. A key sign of HACE is the development of ataxia (defective muscular coordination) (Hackett & Roach, 2007). The patient has a change in mental status with confusion and impaired judgment. Cranial nerve dysfunction and seizures may occur. If untreated, a further decline in the patient's level of consciousness results. Stupor, coma, and death can result from brain swelling and the subsequent damage caused by increased intracranial pressure over the course of 1 to 3 days.

High altitude pulmonary edema (HAPE) often appears in conjunction with HACE but may occur during the progression of AMS within the first 2 to 4 days of a rapid ascent to high altitude, commonly on the second night. It is the most common cause of death associated with high altitude (Hackett & Roach, 2007). Patients notice poor exercise tolerance and a prolonged recovery time after exertion. Fatigue and weakness, as well as other signs and symptoms of AMS, are present. Important clinical indicators of HAPE include a persistent, dry cough and cyanosis of the lips and nail beds. Tachycardia and tachypnea occur at rest. Crackles may be auscultated in one or both lungs. Pink, frothy sputum is a late sign of HAPE. A chest x-ray demonstrates pulmonary infiltrates and pulmonary edema. Arterial blood gas analysis shows respiratory alkalosis and hypoxemia (decreased oxygen). Pneumonia also may be present. When a pulmonary artery catheter is inserted for hemodynamic monitoring, pulmonary artery pressure is very elevated. The patient may also have an elevated body temperature.

Interventions

First Aid

The most important intervention to manage serious altitude-related illnesses is descent to a lower altitude. Patients must be monitored carefully for any evidence of symptom progression. With mild AMS, the victim should be allowed to rest and acclimate at the current altitude. The person is instructed not to ascend to a higher altitude, especially for sleep, until symptoms dissipate. If symptoms persist or worsen, he or she should be moved to a lower altitude as soon as possible. Even a descent of about 1600 feet to 3300 feet may improve the patient's condition and reverse altitude-related pathologic effects. Oxygen should also be administered if available to effectively treat symptoms of AMS.

Hospital Care

The oral drug *acetazolamide* (Diamox, Apo-Acetazolamide♣) is used to both prevent and treat AMS (Wagner et al., 2006). Acetazolamide is a carbonic anhydrase inhibitor. It acts by causing a bicarbonate diuresis, which rids the body of excess fluid, and induces metabolic acidosis. The acidotic state increases respiratory rate and decreases the occurrence of periodic respiration during sleep at night. In this way it helps patients acclimate faster to a high altitude. For best results, acetazolamide should be taken 24 hours before ascent and be continued for the first 2 days of the trip. Dosing regimens vary. The most common regimens are in the range of 125 mg to 250 mg orally once or twice daily. Because acetazolamide is a sulfa drug, it may cause hypersensitivity reactions in allergic people. An herbal remedy that may have benefit in reducing the severity of acute mountain sickness symptoms, but not as a substitute for acetazolamide, is *Ginkgo biloba* (Gertsch et al., 2002; Wagner et al., 2006).

The other drug that may be helpful in the treatment of moderate to severe AMS is dexamethasone (Decadron, Deronil♣) 4 mg to 8 mg either orally or IM as an initial dose, and then 4 mg every 6 hours while the patient is undergoing descent to a lower altitude. This drug's mechanism of action is unclear for AMS treatment, but it reduces cerebral edema by dehydrating the CNS. It does not speed acclimatization like acetazolamide does, but it does relieve the symptoms of AMS. Symptoms may recur when the drug is stopped.

For the treatment of HACE, early recognition of ataxia or a change in level of consciousness should prompt a rapid descent by rescuers or companions to a lower altitude. While undergoing descent, the patient can be given supplemental oxygen and dexamethasone 4 mg to 8 mg initially as an oral, IM, or IV dose, followed by 4 mg every 6 hours if available. If mental status is severely impaired and the patient's airway is at risk, all drugs should be given parenterally. Loop diuretics such as furosemide (Lasix) may be prescribed to decrease brain swelling. Ultimately, the patient with HACE must be admitted to the hospital. Critical care management may be necessary.

Like HACE, early recognition of HAPE is essential to improve the patient's chance for survival. This is a serious condition that requires prompt evacuation to a lower altitude, oxygen administration, and bedrest to save the patient's life. If descent must be delayed because of weather conditions or other factors, oxygen administration is essential as soon as possible. Cold stress must be avoided because it can increase pulmonary artery pressure. Keep the patient warm at all times. Drugs are not substitutes for descent and oxygen. However, the treatment of HAPE may include diuretics such as furosemide to reduce pulmonary edema, morphine, and vasodilators to decrease pulmonary vascular resistance. Hospital admission is warranted. In uncomplicated cases of HAPE, recovery occurs quickly but effects such as weakness and fatigue may persist for 2 weeks.

Chart 11-6 provides best practice strategies for preventing, recognizing, and treating altitude-related illnesses.

Chart 11-6 BEST PRACTICE FOR PATIENT SAFETY & QUALITY CARE

Preventing, Recognizing, and Treating Altitude-Related Illnesses

- Plan a slow ascent to allow for acclimatization.
- Learn to recognize clinical manifestations of altitude-related illnesses.
- Avoid overexertion and overexposure to cold; rest at present altitude.
- Ensure adequate hydration and nutrition.
- Avoid alcohol and sleeping pills when at high altitude.
- For progressive or advanced acute mountain sickness (AMS), recognize symptoms and implement an immediate descent; provide oxygen at high concentration.
- To prevent the occurrence of AMS, discuss the use of acetazolamide (Diamox) with your health care provider.
- Protect skin and eyes from the sun's harmful ultraviolet rays at high altitude. Wear sunscreen (at least SPF 30) and high-quality wraparound sunglasses or goggles.

DROWNING

Pathophysiology

Drowning is a leading cause of accidental death in the United States. The victim dies by suffocation from submersion in a liquid medium (usually water). Although suffocation usually results from aspiration of fresh or salt water into the lungs, about 10% to 20% of victims experience laryngospasm with subsequent glottic closure followed by asphyxiation. **Near-drowning** was previously defined as recovery after submersion; however, this term is not commonly used today (American Heart Association, 2005a; Idris et al., 2003). Males—more often engaged in risk-taking behavior like diving—have a significantly greater incidence of drowning than females.

Health Promotion and Maintenance

Prevention is the key to avoiding drowning events. Health teaching should include these points:

- Maintain constant surveillance of people who cannot swim and are in or around water.
- Do not swim alone.
- Test the water depth before diving in head first; never dive into shallow water.
- Avoid alcoholic beverages when swimming and boating and while in proximity to water.
- Ensure that water rescue equipment, such as life jackets, floatation devices, and rope, is immediately available when around water.

Patient-Centered Collaborative Care

Assessment

When water is aspirated into the lungs, the composition of the water is a factor in the pathophysiology of the drowning event. Aspiration of fresh water causes surfactant to wash out of the lungs. Surfactant reduces surface tension within the alveoli, increases lung compliance and alveolar radius, and decreases the work of breathing. Loss of surfactant from fresh water aspiration destabilizes the alveoli and leads to increased airway resistance. Conversely, salt water—a hypertonic fluid—creates an osmotic gradient that draws protein-rich fluid from the vascular space into the alveoli. Another concern is water quality during the submersion event. The victim's outcome may be negatively affected by contaminants in the water such as chemicals, algae, microbes, sand, and mud. These substances can worsen lung injury and cause a lung infection.

The duration and severity of hypoxia are the two most important factors that determine outcomes for victims of drowning (American Heart Association, 2005a). Very cold water seems to have a protective effect. Successful resuscitations have been reported even after prolonged arrest intervals. Hypothermia might offer some protection to the hypoxic brain by reducing cerebral metabolic rate. The diving reflex is a physiologic response to asphyxia, which produces bradycardia, a reduction in cardiac output, and vasoconstriction of vessels in the intestine, skeletal muscles, and kidneys. These physiologic effects are thought to reduce myocardial oxygen use and enhance blood flow to the heart and cerebral tissues. Survival may be linked to some combination of the effects of hypothermia and the diving reflex.

The cause of the submersion should also be discerned if possible. The patient may have suffered a medical condition or injury that precipitated the drowning event such as a seizure, myocardial infarction, stroke, or spinal cord injury while in the water. Injuries sustained from diving into shallow water or body surfing, such as cervical spine trauma, can also increase the difficulty of rescue and resuscitation efforts.

Interventions

First Aid

Immediate emergency care focuses on a safe rescue of the victim. Potential rescuers must consider their own swimming abilities and limitations, as well as any natural or human-made hazards, before attempting to save the victim; failure to do so could place additional lives in jeopardy. *Once rescuers gain access to the victim, the priority is safe removal from the water.* Spine stabilization with a board or floatation device should be considered only for those victims who are at high risk for spine trauma (e.g., history of diving, use of a water slide, signs of injury or alcohol intoxication), as opposed to all drowning victims (American Heart Association, 2005a; Watson et al., 2001). Time is of the essence; efforts directed toward a rapid rescue have the most potential benefit. Initiate airway clearance and ventilatory support measures as soon as possible—usually once the person is in shallow water or out of the water altogether, because effective airway and ventilation measures are very difficult to perform in deep water. If hypothermia is a concern, handle the victim gently to prevent ventricular fibrillation. *Do not attempt to get the water out of the victim's lungs; deliver abdominal or chest thrusts only if airway obstruction is suspected.*

Hospital Care

Once the person is safely removed from the water, airway and cardiopulmonary support interventions should begin, including oxygen administration, endotracheal intubation, and CPR if necessary. In the clinical setting, gastric decompression with a nasogastric or orogastric tube is indicated to prevent aspiration of gastric contents and improve ventilatory function. After a period of artificial ventilation by mask, the victim typically has a distended abdomen, which impairs movement of the diaphragm and inhibits lung ventilation if it is not decompressed as described. Patients who experience drowning require complex care to support their body systems. The full spectrum of critical care technology may be needed to manage the physiologic complications of drowning, including pulmonary infection, acute respiratory distress syndrome (ARDS), and CNS impairment. These complications are discussed elsewhere in this text.

GET READY FOR THE NCLEX EXAMINATION!

Key Points

Review these Key Points for each NCLEX Examination Client Needs Category.

Safe and Effective Care Environment

- Assess high-risk patients, especially older adults, for their knowledge of safety precautions to prevent heat-related and cold injuries.
- Assess high-risk patients, including those who do not know how to swim, for their knowledge of safety precautions to avoid drowning or submersion accidents.

Health Promotion and Maintenance

- Teach people how to prevent heat-related illnesses as outlined in Chart 11-1.
- Teach people how to prepare for cold environments, including proper clothing (no cotton) and avoidance of wind and wet weather.
- Teach people how to prevent arthropod bites and stings as described in Chart 11-4.
- Teach people how to avoid getting bitten by a snake as listed in Chart 11-3.

Physiological Integrity

- Heat-related injuries can be mild (heat exhaustion) to severe (heat stroke).
- The priority for first aid for heat stroke, after a patent airway is established, is to cool the patient as quickly as possible (see Chart 11-2).
- North American pit vipers can be identified by the triangular-shaped head and retractable fangs; nonpoisonous snakes do not have these features.
- The management of a patient who has a snakebite depends on the severity of envenomation (venom injection) (see Table 11-1); both local and systemic manifestations can occur.
- The priority for first aid when a patient has a snakebite is to decrease the venom circulation; do not use a tourniquet.
- Antivenom drugs are available for most types of poisonous snakebites; monitor for an allergic response when these medications are given.
- The bite of a brown recluse spider can cause tissue necrosis; in rare cases, systemic manifestations can occur, including death.
- Cold applications, such as ice, should be used as first aid for poisonous spider bites.
- The venom of a bark scorpion is neurotoxic; monitor the patient for signs of respiratory failure that may require mechanical ventilation.
- Single bee and wasp stings cause local reactions unless the person is allergic to them.
- Epinephrine is the drug of choice for bee and wasp sting allergic reactions, followed by an antihistamine drug.
- The best way to prevent lightning injuries is to avoid places where lightning is likely to strike (see Chart 11-5).
- Lightning causes central nervous system and cardiovascular complications, as well as skin burns.
- Two common cold injuries are hypothermia and frostbite; both can be prevented by selecting appropriate layered clothing; cotton should not be worn.
- In moderate to severe cases of hypothermia, coagulopathy (abnormal clotting) or cardiac failure can occur.
- The priority for care of a patient with a cold injury is warming; alcohol should be avoided.
- Frostbite can be mild (frostnip) to serious (fourth degree); severe frostbite can result in amputation due to tissue necrosis and gangrene.
- High altitude can cause a range of physiologic consequences in the body, primarily due to hypoxia.

- The priority for care of the patient with illness related to high altitude is descent to a lower altitude.
- Acetazolamide (Diamox, Apo-Acetazolamide 🍁) is the drug of choice for prevention and treatment of mild altitude-related illness.
- Chart 11-6 outlines best practice strategies for preventing, recognizing, and treating altitude-related illnesses.
- Drowning victims often require cardiopulmonary support, including CPR.
- The patient who has been submersed in water is at risk for pulmonary infection, ARDS, and central nervous system impairment.

Additional Study Resources

Go to your Companion CD or Evolve at http://evolve.elsevier.com/Iggy/ for *Self-Assessment Questions for the NCLEX Examination.*

Go to Evolve at http://evolve.elsevier.com/Iggy/ for *Prioritization and Delegation Questions for the NCLEX Examination.*

SELECTED BIBLIOGRAPHY

Asterisk indicates a classic or definitive work on this subject.

American Heart Association. (2005a). Part 10.3: Drowning. *Supplement to Circulation: Journal of the American Heart Association, 112*(24), IV-133-IV-135.

American Heart Association. (2005b). Part 10.4: Hypothermia. *Supplement to Circulation: Journal of the American Heart Association, 112*(24), IV-136-IV-137.

Aslam, A.F., Aslam, A.K., Vasavada, B.C., & Khan, I.A. (2006). Hypothermia: Evaluation, electrocardiographic manifestations, and management. *The American Journal of Medicine, 119,* 297-301.

Auerbach, P.S. (2007). *Wilderness medicine* (5th ed.). St. Louis: Mosby.

*Auerbach, P.S., Donner, H.J., & Weiss, E.A. (2003). *Field guide to wilderness medicine* (2nd ed.). St. Louis: Mosby.

Beattie, S. (2006). In from the cold. *RN, 69*(11), 22-28.

Bernardo, L.M., Crane, P.A., & Veenema, T.G. (2006). Treatment and prevention of pediatric heat-related illnesses at mass gatherings and special events. *Dimensions of Critical Care Nursing, 25*(4), 165-171.

Cherington, M. (2005). Spectrum of neurologic complications of lightning injuries. *NeuroRehabilitation, 20,* 3-8.

*Dinakaran, S., Desai, S.P., & Elsom, D.M. (1998). Telephone-mediated lightning injury causing cataract. *Injury, 29*(8), 645-646.

*Espaillat, A., Janigian, R., & To, K. (1999). Cataracts, bilateral macular holes, and rhegmatogenous retinal detachment induced by lightning. *American Journal of Ophthalmology, 127*(2), 216-217.

Furbee, R.B., Kao, L.W., & Ibrahim, D. (2006). Brown recluse spider envenomation. *Clinics in Laboratory Medicine, 26,* 211-226.

*Gatewood, M.O., & Zane, R.D. (2004). Lightning injuries. *Emergency Medical Clinics of North America, 22,* 369-403.

*Gertsch, J.H., Seto, T.B., Mor, J., & Onopa, J. (2002). Gingko biloba for the prevention of severe acute mountain sickness (AMS) starting one day before rapid ascent. *High Altitude Medicine & Biology, 3,* 29-37.

Glazer, J.L. (2005). Management of heatstroke and heat exhaustion. *American Family Physician, 71*(11), 2133-2140.

*Gold, B.S., Barish, R.A., & Dart, R.C. (2004). North American snake envenomation: Diagnosis, treatment, and management. *Emergency Medical Clinics of North America, 22,* 423-443.

Hackett, P.H., & Roach, R.C. (2007). High-altitude medicine. In P.S. Auerbach (Ed.), *Wilderness medicine* (5th ed., pp. 2-36). St. Louis: Mosby.

*Idris, A.H., Berg, R.A., Bierens, J., Bossaert, L., Branche, C.M., Gabrielli, A., et al. (2003). Recommended guidelines for uniform reporting of data from drowning: The "Utstein style." *Resuscitation, 59,* 45-57.

Laskowski-Jones, L. (2006). First aid for bee, wasp & hornet stings. *Nursing2006, 36*(7), 58-59.

Lewis, A.M. (2007). Heatstroke in older adults. *AJN, 107*(6), 52-56.

Mitchell, A. (2006). Africanized killer bees: A case study. *Critical Care Nurse, 26*(3), 23-32.

Norris, R. (Last updated January 4, 2007). *Snake envenomation, Coral.* e-Medicine. Retrieved March 10, 2007, from WebMD, www.emedicine.com/EMERG/topic542.htm.

*Project Team of the Resuscitation Council (UK). (1999). Consensus guidelines: Emergency medical treatment of anaphylactic reactions. *Resuscitation, 41,* 93-99.

Protherics, Inc. (2006). *CroFab: Crotalidae Polyvalent Immune Fab (Ovine).* (Product brochure). Melville, NY: Savage Laboratories.

*Saucier, J.R. (2004). Arachnid envenomation. *Emergency Medicine Clinics of North America, 22,* 405-422.

Smith, J.E. (2005). Cooling methods used in the treatment of exertional heat illness. *British Journal of Sports Medicine, 39,* 503-507.

Spies, C., & Trohman, R.G. (2006). Narrative review: Electrocution and life-threatening electrical injuries. *Annals of Internal Medicine, 145,* 531-537.

Swanson, D.L., & Vetter, R.S. (2005). Bites of brown recluse spiders and suspected necrotic arachnidism. *The New England Journal of Medicine, 352,* 700-707.

*Ulrich, A.S., & Rathlev, N.K. (2004). Hypothermia and localized cold injuries. *Emergency Medical Clinics of North America, 22,* 281-298.

U.S. Food and Drug Administration, Department of Health & Human Services, Center for Biologics Evaluation and Research. (2007). Product Approval Information—Licensing Action: *Crotalidae Polyvalent Immune Fab (Ovine) (CroFab).* Retrieved March 4, 2007, from www.fda.gov/cber/products/cropro100200.htm.

*Visscher, P.K., Vetter, R.S., & Camazine, S. (1996). Removing bee stings. *Lancet, 348*(9023), 301-302.

Wagner, D.R., Fargo, J.D., Parker, D., Tatsugawa, K., & Young, T.A. (2006). Variables contributing to acute mountain sickness on the summit of Mt. Whitney. *Wilderness and Environmental Medicine, 17*(4), 221-228.

*Watson, R.S., Cummings, P., Quan, L., Bratton, S., & Weiss, N.S. (2001). Cervical spine injuries among submersion victims. *Journal of Trauma, 51,* 658-662.

*Watts, D.D. (1998). Hypothermic coagulopathy in trauma: Effect of varying levels of hypothermia on enzyme speed, platelet function, and fibrinolytic activity. *Journal of Trauma, 44,* 846-854.

Wozniak, E.J., Wisser, J., & Schwartz, M. (2006). Venomous adversaries: A reference to snake identification, field safety, and bite-victim first aid for disaster-response personnel deploying into the hurricane-prone regions of North America. *Wilderness and Environmental Medicine, 17*(4), 246-266.

Yarnell, P.R. (2005). Neurorehabilitation of cerebral disorders following lightning and electrical trauma. *NeuroRehabilitation, 20,* 15-18.

*Yeo, T.P. (2004). Heat stroke: A comprehensive review. *AACN Clinical Issues, 15*(2), 280-293.

Zeglin, D. (2005). Emergency: Brown recluse spider bites. *AJN, 105*(2), 64-68.

Concepts of Emergency and Disaster Preparedness

12
CHAPTER

Linda Laskowski-Jones

LEARNING OUTCOMES

For clinical competence and success on the NCLEX Examination, study this chapter with these Learning Outcomes in mind:

Safe and Effective Care Environment

1. Triage patients to prioritize care delivery in a disaster situation.
2. Compare the key personnel roles in an Emergency Preparedness and Response Plan.
3. Implement an Emergency Preparedness and Response Plan.
4. Develop a personal emergency preparedness plan.
5. Differentiate two types of debriefing that occur after a disaster.
6. Identify the role of the nurse when a bioterrorism agent is suspected.

Psychosocial Integrity

7. Assess the person/family/significant others affected by a disaster for ability to adapt to temporary/permanent role changes.
8. Provide support to the person and/or family in coping with life changes due to a disaster.

Go to your Companion CD or Evolve at http://evolve.elsevier.com/Iggy/ for *Self-Assessment Questions for the NCLEX Examination* keyed to these Learning Outcomes.

A **disaster** is commonly defined as an event in which illness or injuries exceed resource capabilities of a community or medical facility. Disasters strike around the world because of acts of violence, illness outbreaks, severe weather, earthquakes, avalanches, fire, catastrophic building collapse, and transportation calamities. The American College of Surgeons (2006) distinguishes between multi-casualty and mass casualty (disaster) events. The main difference is based on the scope and scale of the incident, considering the number and severity of victims or casualties involved. Both require specific response plans to activate necessary resources. In general, a **multi-casualty event** can be managed by a hospital using local resources. A **mass casualty event** overwhelms local medical capabilities and may require the collaboration of multiple agencies and health care facilities to handle the crisis. State, regional, and/or national resources may be needed to support the areas impacted by the event. Trauma centers have a special role in all emergency preparedness activities because they provide a critical level of expertise in complex injury management.

To maintain ongoing disaster preparedness, hospital personnel participate in emergency training and drills regularly. In the United States, The Joint Commission mandates that hospitals have an emergency preparedness plan that is tested through drills or actual participation in a real event at least twice yearly. One of the drills or events must involve community-wide resources and an influx of actual or simulated patients to assess the ability of collaborative efforts and command structures (The Joint Commission, 2007). In addition, accredited health care organizations are required to take an "all-hazards approach" to disaster planning. Using this approach, preparedness activities must address *all credible threats* to the community that could result in a disaster situation. Disaster drills, then, are ideally planned based on a risk assessment that identifies the events most likely to occur in a particular community. For example, a flood is more likely in the Gulf of Mexico and an avalanche is more likely in ski areas of the Rocky Mountains.

Hospitals are not the only health care agencies that are required to practice disaster drills. Nursing homes and other long-term care (LTC) facilities are also mandated to have annual drills to prepare for mass casualty events. Part of the response plan must include a method for evacuation of residents from the facility in a timely and safe manner.

IMPACT OF RECENT DISASTERS

The events of September 11, 2001, changed hospital and community disaster planning efforts. With the shocking terrorist attacks on the Twin Towers of the World Trade Center and the Pentagon and the actual and perceived threat of domestic terrorism including anthrax exposure that followed, hospital emergency preparedness concepts became much more fully integrated into the daily operations of emergency departments (ED) by necessity. Weapons of mass destruction (WMD) rapidly became the focus of public health risk.

The term "NBC" was coined to describe nuclear, biologic, and chemical threats. In response, emergency medical services (EMS) agencies and hospitals upgraded their decontamination facilities, equipment, and all levels of personal protective gear to better protect staff. ED physician and nursing staff underwent hazardous materials (HAZMAT) training and learned how to recognize patterns of illness in patients who present for treatment that potentially indicate biologic terrorism agents, such as anthrax or smallpox. Protocols for the pharmacologic treatment of infectious disease agents, as well as stockpiles of antibiotics and nerve agent antidotes, were made readily available.

The most immediate outcome of enhancing emergency preparedness after September 11 is that the ability to competently handle the more typical multi-casualty or mass casualty incident such as a bus crash, tornado, or building collapse has been greatly improved in many communities. However, disaster situations can still exceed the scope of usual day-to-day crisis operations, pointing to the necessity of well-defined regional and national emergency preparedness plans.

In 2005, Hurricane Katrina made landfall in Louisiana and other Gulf states as a category-4 storm and caused more than 1000 deaths and devastating environmental and property damage (Fig. 12-1). Volunteers from all over the United States, as well as local, regional, and federal agencies, took part in the large-scale disaster evacuation, rescue, and relief effort that severely challenged available resources and established disaster plans. Critical systems failed and were eventually re-established through coordination with multiple agencies and people to ensure that the most basic human needs were met (Fig. 12-2). Hurricane Katrina overwhelmed the existing emergency care system and caused the mobilization of a national mutual aid response on a level that had not been experienced in recent U.S. history.

Lessons learned from Hurricane Katrina, as well as recent worldwide incidents such as tsunamis, earthquakes, and terrorist attacks, enable improved preparation and coordination of efforts that are beneficial for future disasters. For example, these insights can be applied to health care facility and community agency plans for pandemic infections. Pandemics are

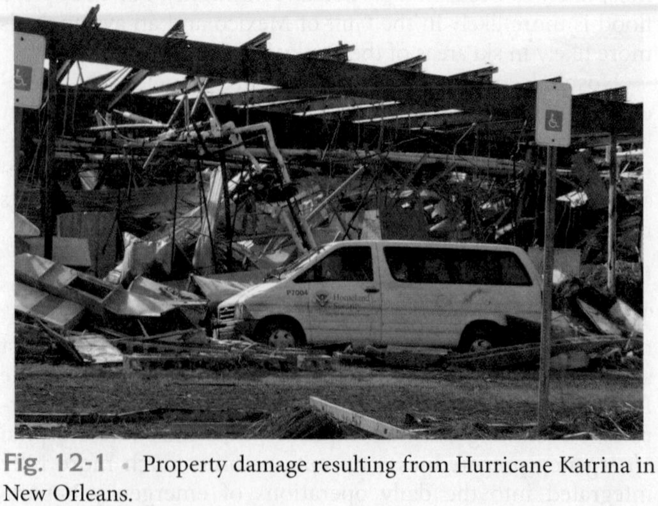

Fig. 12-1 • Property damage resulting from Hurricane Katrina in New Orleans.

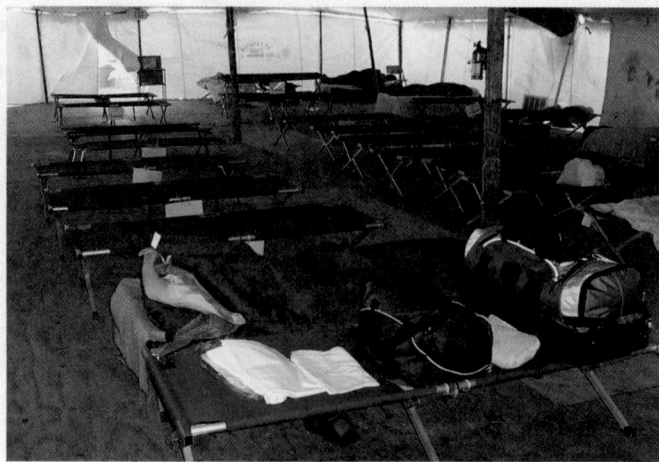

Fig. 12-2 • Temporary shelter set up for homeless victims of Hurricane Katrina in New Orleans.

a future threat that would lead a vast number of people to seek medical care. In addition to those patients needing care, the health care system would encounter many "worried well." Those people are not yet ill but want evaluation, preventive treatment, or reassurance from a health care provider. A pandemic influenza outbreak, such as avian influenza caused by the H5N1 virus ("bird flu"), would not only overwhelm the resource capabilities of the entire health care system but also could severely damage community systems and critical supply chains. Worker illness, absenteeism, and personal choices to remain quarantined to avoid being exposed to the illness would negatively affect the number of health care staff available to care for patients.

Because of the mass casualty nature of pandemic influenza, emergency preparedness planners must incorporate strategies to handle an influx of ill patients into the system as part of ongoing disaster readiness (Russo, 2006). Quarantine of certain nursing units or the entire hospital could become necessary, prompting closure until the risk has passed.

Common to all mass casualty events, the goal of **emergency preparedness** is to define ways to meet the extraordinary need for hospital beds, staff, drugs, personal protective equipment (PPE), supplies, and medical devices, such as mechanical ventilators (Casani & Romanosky, 2006). The U.S. government is currently stockpiling critical equipment and supplies in case they are needed for a pandemic influenza outbreak. In addition, the Food and Drug Administration (FDA) approved the first vaccine to protect humans against H5N1 avian influenza virus (see Chapter 25 for more information on emerging infections). Each state has its own specific emergency preparedness plan for pandemic influenza, including who would receive vaccines in a mass casualty event. Most of these plans are posted on the Internet.

EMERGENCY PREPAREDNESS AND RESPONSE

Mass Casualty Triage

Triage Process

A key process in any multi-casualty or mass casualty response is effective **triage** to rapidly sort ill or injured patients into priority categories based on their acuity and survival potential. In mass casualty or disaster situations, a military form of triage is implemented with the overall goal of doing the greatest good for the greatest number of people (Reisner, 2006). This means that patients who are critically ill or injured and might otherwise receive attempted resuscitation during usual operations could be triaged into an "expectant" or "black-tagged" category and allowed to die or not be treated until others received care. Typical examples of black-tagged patients are those with massive head trauma, extensive full-thickness body burns, and high cervical spinal cord injury requiring mechanical ventilation. The rationale for this seemingly heartless decision is that the limited resources must be dedicated to saving the most lives rather than expending valuable resources to save one life at the possible expense of many others.

Triage functions may be performed by EMS providers in the field, such as:

- Emergency medical technicians (EMTs) and paramedics
- Nurse and physician field teams who are called from the hospital to a disaster scene to assist EMS providers
- Nurse and physician hospital teams to assess and reassess incoming patients

Before going to the incident in the field, nurses, physicians, and support staff must have adequate training to prepare them to recognize the risks in an unstable environment. Such risks can include the potential for structural collapse, becoming the secondary target of a terrorist attack, and working in an environment in which natural hazards are common (e.g., poisonous snake bites). Disaster workers must take measures to protect themselves so that they do not become victims as well.

The National Disaster Life Support Foundation offers Basic and Advanced Disaster Life Support training courses to health care professionals that cover all essential aspects of disaster response and management. In addition, the Federal Emergency Management Agency (FEMA) provides Community Emergency Response Team (CERT) training to citizens so that they are better prepared for disasters and are able to respond more self-sufficiently to incidents and hazard situations in their own communities. These courses include mass casualty triage education.

Triage Method

An important point to recognize is that triage concepts in a mass casualty incident differ from the "civilian triage" methods covered in Chapter 10 that are practiced during usual ED operations (Table 12-1). Although disaster triage practices can vary widely based on local EMS protocols, some concepts are fairly universal. Most mass casualty response teams both in the field and in the hospital setting use a **disaster triage tag system** that categorizes triage priority by color and number (Reisner, 2006):

- Emergent (class I) patients are identified with a red tag.
- Patients who can wait a short time for care (class II) are marked with a yellow tag.
- Nonurgent or "walking wounded" (class III) patients are given a green tag.
- Patients who are expected to die or are dead are issued a black tag (class IV).

In general, *red-tagged* patients have immediate threats to life, such as airway obstruction or shock, and require immediate attention. *Yellow-tagged* patients have major injuries, such as open fractures with a distal pulse and large wounds that need treatment within 30 minutes to 2 hours. *Green-tagged* patients have minor injuries that can be managed in a delayed fashion, generally more than 2 hours. Examples of green-tag injuries include closed fractures, sprains, strains, abrasions, and contusions.

TABLE 12-1 Comparison of Triage Under Usual Versus Mass Casualty Conditions

Triage Under Usual Conditions	Triage Under Mass Casualty Conditions
Emergent (immediate threat to life)	Emergent or Class I (red tag) (immediate threat to life)
Urgent (major injuries that require immediate treatment)	Urgent or Class II (yellow tag) (major injuries that require treatment)
Nonurgent (minor injuries that do not require immediate treatment)	Nonurgent or Class III (green tag) (minor injuries that do not require immediate treatment)
	Expectant or Class IV (black tag) (expected and allowed to die)

The green-tagged patients are often referred to as the "walking wounded"; they may actually evacuate themselves from the mass casualty scene and go to the hospital in a private vehicle. Green-tagged patients usually make up the greatest number in most large-scale multi-casualty situations. Therefore they can overwhelm the system if provisions are not made to handle them as part of the disaster plan. Also, because they often come to the hospital on their own, the hospital may not be able to determine how many actual casualties will arrive. A related concern is that green-tagged patients who self-transport may unknowingly carry contaminants from a nuclear, biologic, or chemical incident into the hospital environment with potentially disastrous consequences. ED staff must anticipate these issues and devise emergency response plans accordingly.

Once patients are in the triage area of the hospital, they typically receive a special bracelet with a disaster number. Preprinted labels with this number can be applied to the patients' chart forms and personal belongings. Digital photos may also be incorporated into the identification process in some systems. The standard hospital identification band can be applied after the patient's identity is confirmed.

Automated tracking systems using infrared and radiofrequency technology are available in some emergency departments; these systems may be used to track a patient's triage priority upon arrival, location, and process of care. The interactions the patient has with caregivers can also be tracked, an important safety strategy if the patient is later found to have contaminants or a disease that could pose a risk to staff members who had close contact and require decontamination or prophylaxis (Laskowski-Jones, 2005). These newer systems are valuable components of the hospital's emergency preparedness infrastructure because they can rapidly portray the overall census and acuity of patients. They also enable ED leaders to determine how many casualties of a particular acuity level a hospital can safely accept from the incident scene in a disaster situation.

Notification and Activation of Emergency Preparedness Plans

When the number of casualties exceeds the usual resource capabilities, a disaster situation is recognized to exist. What may be a routine day in the emergency department (ED) of a large urban trauma center could be defined as a disaster for a small rural community hospital if the same number of patients were to arrive. Each facility, then, defines its own parameters to identify when a disaster situation is present. Flexibility is needed because resources may change by time of day and by day of the week. For instance, hospitals typically have the fewest human resources available after midnight on the weekend. An incident that occurs in this time frame may require activation of the emergency preparedness plan to bring extra resources into the hospital. The same incident during weekday business hours might be handled with on-site personnel alone without the need for activation of the plan.

Notification that a multi-casualty or mass casualty situation exists usually occurs by radio or cellular communication between the ED and EMS providers at the scene. A state or regional emergency management agency may also notify the ED of the event. Each hospital has its own policy that specifies *who* has the authority to activate and *how* to activate the disaster or emergency preparedness plan. Group paging systems, telephone trees, and instant computer-based alert messages are the most common means of notifying essential personnel of a mass casualty incident or disaster.

A catastrophic event, such as a major earthquake or tornado, or a terrorist incident involving weapons of mass destruction (WMD) also requires volunteer assistance from all levels of health care providers in the region. In this case, the media may be contacted to broadcast messages to the health care community-at-large via television, radio, and electronic announcements. For such incidents, the National Guard, the American Red Cross, the Public Health Department, various military units, a Medical Reserve Corps (MRC) or a Disaster Medical Assistance Team (DMAT) can be activated by state and federal government authorities.

An MRC is made up of a group of volunteer medical and public health care professionals, including physicians and nurses. They offer their services to health care facilities or to the community in a supportive or supplemental capacity during times of need such as a disaster or pandemic disease outbreak. This group may help staff hospitals or community health settings that face personnel shortages and establish first aid stations or special needs shelters (Hoard & Tosatto, 2005). The MRC may also set up an acute care center (ACC) in the community for patients who need acute care (but not intensive care) for days to weeks as a means to alleviate emergency department and hospital overcrowding (Casani & Romanosky, 2006).

A DMAT is a medical relief team made up of about 35 medical, paraprofessional, and support personnel that is deployed to a disaster area with enough medical equipment and supplies to sustain operations for 72 hours (Stopford, 2005). DMATs are part of the National Disaster Medical System (NDMS), a component of FEMA, under the Department of Homeland Security in the United States. They provide relief services ranging from primary health care and triage to evacuation and staffing to assist health care facilities that have become overwhelmed with casualties (Stopford, 2005). *Because licensed health care providers such as nurses act as federal employees when they are deployed, their professional licenses are recognized and valid in all states.*

Examples of what the NDMS provides are (Stopford, 2005):

- Disaster Mortuary Teams (DMORTs) to manage mass fatalities
- Veterinary Medical Assistance Teams (VMATs) for emergency animal care
- International Medical Surgical Response Teams (MSRTs) to establish fully functional field surgical facilities wherever they are needed in the world
- National Nurse and National Pharmacist Response Teams (NNRTs and NPRTs) to assist with large-scale public health crises
- National Medical Response Teams—Weapons of Mass Destruction (NMRTs) to decontaminate and manage victims of hazardous materials incidents

Nurses can join these teams, complete the required training, and offer their expertise as part of a coordinated federal response team in times of critical need.

Hospital Emergency Preparedness: Personnel Roles and Responsibilities

Hospital Incident Command System

A common organizational model for disaster management is the **Hospital Incident Command System (HICS).** In this system, roles are formally structured under the hospital or long-term care facility incident commander with clear lines of authority and accountability for specific resources. Officers are named to oversee essential emergency preparedness functions such as public information, safety and security, and medical command. Chiefs are appointed to manage logistics, planning, finance, and operations as appropriate to the type and scale of the event. In turn, chiefs delegate specific duties to other departmental officers and unit leaders. The idea is to achieve a manageable span of control over the personnel or resources allocated to achieve efficiency (Sutingco, 2006).

Because mass casualty events typically involve large numbers of people and can create a chaotic work environment, many EMS agencies and health care facilities use brightly colored vests with large lettering to help identify key leadership positions. Specific job action sheets are distributed to all personnel with leadership roles in HICS that pre-define reporting relationships and list prioritized tasks and responsibilities. The HICS personnel also establish an **emergency operations center (EOC)** or **command center** in a designated location with accessible communication technology. They then use their collective expertise to manage the overall incident (Sutingco, 2006). All internal requests for additional personnel and resources, as well as communication with field teams and external agencies, should be coordinated through the EOC to maintain unity of command.

The roles and responsibilities of health care personnel in a mass casualty event or disaster are defined within the institution's emergency response or preparedness plan (Table 12-2). Each plan can be as individual as the particular facility's operations. However, virtually all plans identify certain key functions. For example, one of the primary roles in a hospital to be established at the onset of an incident is the role of a **hospital incident commander** who assumes overall leadership for implementing the institutional plan. This person is usually either a physician in the ED or a hospital administrator who has the authority to activate resources. The hospital incident commander's role is to take a global view of the entire situation and facilitate patient movement through the system. The commander brings in both human and supply resources to meet patient needs. For example, a hospital incident commander might dictate that all patients due to be discharged

TABLE 12-2 Summary of Key Personnel Roles and Functions for Emergency Preparedness and Response Plan

Personnel Role	Personnel Function
Hospital incident commander	Physician or administrator who assumes overall leadership for implementing the emergency plan
Medical command physician	Physician who decides the number, acuity, and resource needs of patients
Triage officer	Physician or nurse who rapidly evaluates each patient to determine priorities for treatment
Community relations or public information officer	Person who serves as a liaison between the health care facility and the media

from an inpatient unit be moved to a lounge area immediately to free up hospital beds for mass casualty victims. He or she could also direct departments such as physical therapy or a surgical clinic to cancel their usual operations to convert the space into a minor treatment area. The incident commander assists in the organization of hospital-wide services to rapidly expand hospital capacity, recruit paid or volunteer staff, and ensure the availability of medical supplies.

Another typical role defined in hospital or other health care emergency preparedness plans is that of the **medical command physician.** This person focuses on determining the number, acuity, and medical resource needs of victims arriving from the incident scene to the hospital and organizing the emergency health care team response to the injured or ill patients. Responsibilities include identifying the need for and calling in specialty-trained providers such as:

- Trauma surgeons
- Neurosurgeons
- Orthopedic surgeons
- Pulmonologists
- Plastic surgeons
- Burn surgeons
- Infectious disease physicians
- Industrial hygienists
- Radiation safety personnel

In smaller hospitals with limited specialty resources, the medical command physician would also help determine which patients should be transported out of the facility to a higher level of care.

Closely affiliated with the medical command physician is the **triage officer.** Again, this person is generally a physician in a large hospital who is assisted by triage nurses. When physician resources are limited, an experienced nurse may assume this role. The triage officer rapidly evaluates each person who presents to the hospital, even those who come in with triage tags in place. Patient acuity is re-evaluated for appropriate disposition to the area within the ED or hospital best suited to meet the patient's medical needs.

Many other roles and responsibilities can be defined within the institutional emergency response plan and may include the supply officer, the communications officer, the infection control officer, and the community relations/public information officer, to name a few. The community relations or public information officer is an especially important role to delineate in advance. Mass casualty incidents tend to attract a large amount of media attention. This staff member can draw media away from the clinical areas so that essential hospital operations are not hindered. He or she can also serve as the liaison between hospital administration and the media to release only appropriate and accurate information.

Role of Nursing

The ED charge nurse, trauma program manager, and other ED nursing leadership personnel act in collaboration with the medical command physician and triage officer to organize nursing and ancillary services to meet patient needs. Telephone trees can be activated to call in off-duty emergency nurses. Nurses from medical-surgical nursing units can be recruited to provide care for stable ED patients, thus freeing up emergency nurses to aid mass casualty victims. Critical care unit nurses can supplement emergency nurses in the resuscitation setting or assist in monitored care and transport to critical care units. Emergency nurse leaders also typically direct the ancillary departments to deliver supplies, instrument trays, medications, food, and personnel to meet service demands.

Hospital staff of all levels may be required to alter their routine operations to accommodate a high volume of patients. Emergency plans dictate specific actions by staff members, such as who should be called when the plan is activated, who should report, where to report, what supplies or equipment carts should be brought to a pre-designated location, and what type of paperwork or system should be implemented for patient identification in a large-scale event. Some staff may even have their roles changed completely. For example, nurses from the performance improvement department or case management may be reassigned to fulfill a clinical responsibility for a nursing unit. The key concept is that staff members are expected to remain flexible in a mass casualty situation and perform at their highest level to address both the needs of the health care system and those of the patients. The greatest good for the greatest number of people is still the organizing principle when considering roles and responsibilities in mass casualty events—not necessarily individual staff preferences. However, the safety of all patients is vital.

Creativity and flexibility of nursing leaders and nursing staff are essential to provide the staffing coverage necessary for a large-scale or extended incident. A **personal emergency preparedness plan** for each nurse can help in such situations. It should outline the preplanned specific arrangements that are to be made for childcare, pet care, and older adult care if the need arises, especially if the event prevents returning home for an extended period. Emergency contact names, addresses, and telephone numbers should be included for optimal usefulness in a crisis. In addition, pre-assembling **personal readiness supplies** or **"go bag"** (disaster supply kit) for the home and automobile with clothing and basic survival supplies aids allows for a rapid response for disaster staffing coverage (Table 12-3). "Go bags" are essential for all members of the family, including pets, in the event the disaster requires evacuation of the community or people are required to take shelter in their own homes.

When called to respond to work during a mass casualty event, some nurses may experience ethical and moral conflict

TABLE 12-3 Basic Supplies for Personal Preparedness (3-Day Supply)

Backpack	Emergency blanket and/or sleeping bag and pillow
Clean clothing, sturdy footwear	Work gloves
Potable water—1 gallon per person per day	Personal first aid kit with over-the-counter (OTC) and prescription medications/vitamins
Food—non-perishable, no cooking required	Rain gear
Flashlight—battery powered; extra batteries and/or chemical light sticks	Roll of duct tape and plastic sheeting
Pocket knife or multi-tool	Radio—battery powered or hand-crank generator
Personal ID with emergency contacts and phone numbers, allergies, and medical information; lists of credit card numbers and bank accounts (keep in watertight container)	Toiletries (toothbrush and toothpaste, comb, brush, razor, shaving cream, mirror, feminine supplies, deodorant, shampoo, lip balm, sunscreen, insect repellent, toilet paper)
Towel and washcloth; towelettes, soap, hand sanitizer	Plastic garbage bags and ties, re-sealable plastic bags
Paper, pens, and pencils; regional maps	Matches in a waterproof container
Cell phone	Whistle
Sunglasses/eyewear	Household liquid bleach for disinfection

between their family obligations and professional responsibilities (Chaffee, 2006). The American Nurses Association's (ANA's) *Code of Ethics for Nurses with Interpretive Statements* (2001) does not offer clear guidance in this situation. Each person has to make a choice about whether to be involved in helping during the emergency or when to become involved.

EVENT RESOLUTION

When the last major casualties have been treated and no more are expected to arrive in numbers that could overwhelm the health care system, the incident commander considers "standing down" or deactivating the emergency response plan. However, although the casualties may have left the ED, other areas in the hospital may still be under stress and need the support of the supplemental resources provided by emergency plan activation. Before terminating the response, it is essential to ensure that the needs of the other hospital departments have been met and all are in agreement to resume normal operations.

A vital consideration in event resolution is staff and supply availability to meet ongoing operational needs. If nursing staff and other personnel were called in from home during their off hours or if they worked well beyond their scheduled shifts to meet patient and departmental needs, provision for adequate rest periods should be made. Exhaustion poses a risk not only to patient safety but also to the nurse when he or she must drive home. Sleeping quarters at the hospital might be necessary in this case, especially if the disaster event contributed to treacherous travel conditions.

Severe shortages of supplies also pose a threat to normal operations at the conclusion of a mass casualty incident. Taking inventory and restocking the ED are high priority assignments. Collaboration between the ED and the central supply department is essential to resolving stock availability problems. Instrument trays must be washed, packaged, and resterilized. Critical supplies that have been depleted from hospital stores must be reordered and delivered to the hospital quickly. Contracts with key vendors outlining emergency resupply expectations and arrangements should be a part of the hospital's overall emergency preparedness plan.

Debriefing

Two general types of **debriefing,** or formal systematic review and analysis, occur after a mass casualty incident or disaster. The first type entails bringing in critical incident stress debriefing (CISD) teams to provide sessions for small groups of staff to promote effective coping strategies. The second type of debriefing involves an administrative review of staff and system performance during the event to determine whether opportunities for improvement in the emergency management plan exist.

Critical Incident Stress Debriefing

CISD is only one component of a much broader critical incident stress management (CISM) program. CISM programming addresses pre-crisis through post-crisis interventions for small to large groups, including communities. After working through the turmoil and the emotional impact of the incident as well as the aftermath, the staff may find it difficult to "get back to normal." Without intervention during *and* after the emergency, they may develop post-traumatic stress disorder (PTSD). PTSD can lead to multiple characteristic psychological and physical effects, including flashbacks, avoidance, less interest in previously enjoyable events, and detachment, as well as rapid heart rate and insomnia. People suffering from PTSD can have great difficulty relating in their usual way to family and friends. Ultimately, professional "burnout" can stem from the inability to cope with the stress effectively. Chart 12-1 lists recommendations proposed by several national organizations to help prevent PTSD during the emergency situation.

A CISD team comprises two or three specially trained people who come together quickly when called to deal with the emotional needs of health care team members after a par-

Chart 12-1 BEST PRACTICE FOR PATIENT SAFETY & QUALITY CARE

Preventing Staff Post-Traumatic Stress Disorder (PTSD) During a Mass Casualty Event

- Use available counseling.
- Encourage and support co-workers.
- Monitor each other's stress level and performance.
- Take breaks when needed.
- Talk about feelings with staff and managers.
- Drink plenty of water, and eat healthy snacks for energy.
- Keep in touch with family, friends, and significant others.
- Do not work for more than 12 hours per day.

Adapted from Papp, E. (2005). Preparing for disasters. *AJN, 105*(5), 112.

ticularly devastating or disturbing incident. The team leader typically has background in a mental health/behavioral health field. The co-leader is ideally a peer of the group being debriefed. Thus if nurses are debriefed, then a nurse member of the CISD team is generally assigned to the session. CISD-trained physicians, police, firefighters, EMTs, and paramedics may also be used, depending on the needs of the group. The third member of the team is known as the "doorkeeper." This person is responsible for keeping inappropriate people out (e.g., media, spectators) and talking with anyone who leaves the session early in an effort to have him or her return or accept follow-up (Mitchell et al., 2003b). Staff involved in the incident need protected time to undergo stress debriefing, which generally lasts from 1 to 3 hours per session.

Typical "ground rules" for stress debriefing include strict confidentiality of information shared during the session and unconditional acceptance of the thoughts and feelings expressed by people within the group. The usual arrangement for the most effective group interaction is a circular configuration of chairs in a private setting. Food should be available so that hunger is not a distraction. CISD group leaders encourage group discussion through asking a series of questions designed to make everyone involved tell his or her own story about the incident and explain the personal impact. The group leaders enable participants to place the incident into perspective and dispel any feelings of blame or guilt. They also educate participants about self-care concepts and coping strategies to use immediately. People who require more than a CISD session may need referral for mental health/behavioral health counseling. Research efforts using meta-analysis techniques have produced mixed results regarding the efficacy of CISD. However, the technique is thought to be clinically effective (Mitchell et al., 2003b).

Administrative Review

The second type of debriefing is an administrative function directed at analyzing the hospital or agency response to an event while it is still in the forefront of the minds of everyone who participated in it. The goal of this type of debriefing is to discern what went right and what went wrong during activation and implementation of the emergency preparedness plan so that changes can be made. Typically, representatives from all groups that were involved in the incident come together soon after plan activation has been discontinued. They each are given an opportunity to hear and express both positive and negative comments related to their experiences with the event. Then, in the days after the plan activation, written critique forms are also solicited to gain additional information after participants have had time to consider their overall impressions of the response as well as the impact it had on their respective departments or clinical areas.

Although drills are important, implementing the emergency preparedness plan during an actual mass casualty event is the most effective means of "reality testing" the plan's utility. Feedback provided by participants can be used to modify or revise the plan and create new processes in preparation for future events.

Psychosocial Response of Survivors to Mass Casualty Events

Experiencing a disaster can produce both immediate and long-lasting psychosocial effects in people personally affected by the event. Depending on the nature and magnitude of the incident, survivors can be confronted with the tragic loss of loved ones, property, and valued possessions. They and their family members may have suffered injuries or illnesses brought about by the catastrophe. Lifestyles, roles, and routines are drastically altered, preventing people from achieving any sense of normalcy in the hours, the days, and perhaps even the weeks and months that follow a disaster. Coping abilities in survivors are severely stressed, leading to many individual responses that can range from functional and adaptive behaviors to maladaptive coping.

Survivors have to confront feelings of vulnerability resulting from the devastating event, knowing that it could occur again—a particularly relevant issue for people who live in areas prone to acts of terrorism or to natural disasters. The decision—be it voluntary or involuntary—to abandon a family home or geographic region and then relocate to a "safe" area either temporarily or permanently results in a further sense of loss and grief. Some people may feel guilty about living through an event that caused so many others to die. The range of intense emotions can appear as physical illness, as well as psychological and social dysfunction (Mitchell et al., 2005).

The disaster serves as the catalyst for some survivors to experience PTSD. This condition, which can potentially last for a lifetime, is characterized by recurrent intrusive memories, hyperarousal, and avoidance of any triggers that cause PTSD symptoms (Olszewski & Varrasse, 2005). Such triggers include sounds, scents, weather, and images that produce flashbacks, severe anxiety, and agitation in affected people. Real or imagined threats stimulate the body to release a surge of norepinephrine and subsequently enter into a state of alarm or a conditioned fear response (Olszewski & Varrasse, 2005). Patients with PTSD are at a higher risk for stress-related illnesses and maladaptive coping. Sleep disturbances and nightmares are common. Cognitive abilities, as well as relationships with significant others and co-workers, may become significantly impaired.

Consider strategies that promote effective coping in survivors. Weiss et al. (2006) found that victims of a devastating hurricane collectively felt "paralyzed" after the storm. They exhibited powerlessness related to fear, loss, hopelessness, and uncertainty. The researchers concluded that people needed to engage in a process they termed "returning to life" to successfully overcome this paralysis. Steps included "moving forward to survive," accessing both internal and external resources to rebuild their lives, and recognizing benefits such as the realization that things could have been worse or that some good came out of the pain.

Becker (2006) studied techniques for training disaster field workers in mental health interventions after the India tsunami in 2004. General emotional support principles included:

- Allowing patients to ventilate their feelings so that they could be normalized
- Listening and encouraging relaxation
- Using culturally appropriate proverbs or storytelling to help restore coping mechanisms
- Facilitating community cohesion through recreational activities and support groups

These practices were incorporated into the overall tsunami relief and rehabilitation efforts. An integral aspect of the program was to "restore normalcy" by providing a sense of security and predictability through structured routines in the refugee camps.

When working with people in crisis after a mass casualty event, use calm reassurance while offering choices whenever feasible to enhance a sense of personal control. Actively listen, and communicate honest information. Help survivors adapt to their new surroundings and routines through simple, concrete explanations. Convey caring behaviors, and provide a sense of safety and security to the best extent possible. If needed to combat the detrimental and recurrent effects of PTSD, refer victims for ongoing peer support, group therapy, or psychotherapy. Some survivors may need medication to manage PTSD (Olszewski & Varrasse, 2005).

EMERGENCY ROOM CASE SCENARIO: POSSIBLE ANTHRAX EXPOSURE

Case Presentation

M.C., a 34-year-old woman, presents to the triage desk of a large suburban emergency department (ED) with a box with a dusting of white powder on it. M.C. quickly explains to the triage nurse that she is afraid an employee at her office has contaminated the box with anthrax. The patient exhibits signs of severe anxiety while she relates that this employee was born in an Arab country and obviously "hates America." Nearly sobbing now, she expresses her fears that she has been deliberately exposed to anthrax by a terrorist and needs treatment.

The triage nurse immediately notifies security and escorts the patient outside of the building. The patient is confused and angry as to why she cannot be placed in a treatment room. She wants the substance on the box tested to determine if it is indeed anthrax. The emergency nurse instructs M.C. to place the box on the ground in a grassy area outside of the ED. She then asks that the security guard place a sheet over the box to prevent spread of the powder, establish a safe perimeter around the suspicious item, and place calls to both the local police agency and the Department of Public Health. These agencies will collaborate on removal of the box, investigation of the woman's claim, and appropriate testing of the white powder.

In the meantime, the emergency nurse also activates the ED's hazardous materials decontamination plan. Nursing staff don appropriate protective attire, which includes an impervious gown, gloves, facemask, and eye protection, and prepare the decontamination facility (Fig. 12-3). When ready to begin decontamination, M.C. is directed to enter the decontamination room through the outside door from the parking lot to avoid the potential for contamination of the ED. Staff assist M.C. to remove all of her clothing. She is directed into a shower stall and washed thoroughly with soap and water. When decontamination is complete, she is given a hospital gown, robe, and slippers and is placed in a wheelchair for transport to an ED treatment room in the "fast track" area for low-acuity patients.

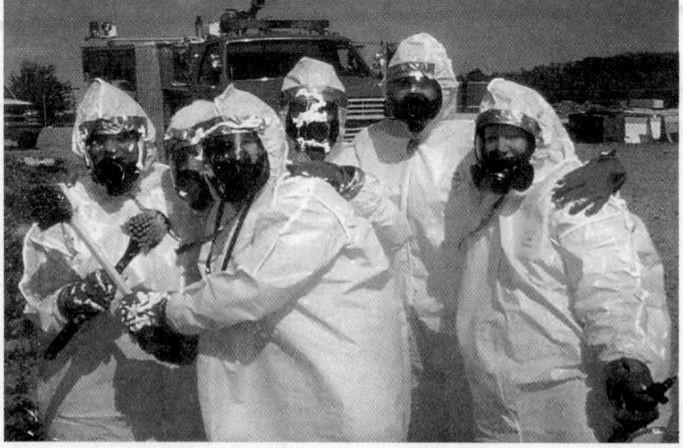

Fig. 12-3 • Hazardous materials team members wearing protective clothing and respirators prepare to decontaminate people exposed to toxic chemicals in an outdoor decontamination area.

Upon arrival to the treatment room, M.C. appears much less anxious. A physician examines her and determines that she has no clinical evidence of infectious disease. For this reason and because an actual exposure to anthrax has not yet been confirmed by the Public Health Department, the physician elects *not* to prescribe the typical 60-day course of an oral prophylactic antibiotic for *Bacillus anthracis*—either ciprofloxacin (Cipro) 500 mg twice daily or doxycycline 100 mg twice daily. The emergency physician explains that her plan is to discharge the patient to home with referral for outpatient follow-up at the Public Health Department. M.C. again becomes tearful and demands that she be given a prescription for an antibiotic because she is afraid she will die. She contends that she will sue the hospital if anything should happen to her.

The emergency physician and nurse actively engage M.C. in discharge teaching about anthrax. With compassion and empathy, they explain that taking antibiotics unnecessarily will promote the growth of resistant bacteria and may cause serious drug-related side effects. They tell M.C. that the Department of Public Health will analyze the substance on the box, and if it is found to be *B. anthracis*, she will be notified right away. She will then be re-evaluated by the Public Health Department and started on post-exposure prophylactic antibiotics. M.C. is reassured and offered the services of a community mental health/behavioral health clinic if she desires counseling to address her anxiety about this situation as well as her perceived threat from the Arab employee at her work site. After this teaching episode, she appears to have her anxiety and anger under control. Because M.C.'s own clothing was confiscated and placed in a hazardous materials container for disposal during the decontamination process, the emergency nurse contacts the social worker to request that female apparel be made available from the hospital's supply of donated clothing so that she can get dressed. The patient is given written discharge instructions.

Case Discussion

Although it may seem odd that the emergency nurse escorted M.C. outside of the building, this action prevented the potential spread of *B. anthracis* into the ED and potentially the hospital environment. Contamination of innocent bystanders, as well as the hospital, with a hazardous material can force the closure of key areas within the facility and can require evacuation of patients and staff. Because M.C. was a "walk-in" patient, she accessed the triage area before undergoing decontamination. Had M.C. been a known potentially contaminated patient before arrival (e.g., if she was treated by an ambulance crew), she would have been taken to the decontamination facility upon arrival. Decontamination should precede triage; only the most basic life-sustaining interventions should be performed before or during decontamination. M.C. also brought a potentially contaminated item into the ED. It is important to realize that the ED has no ability to conduct "point of care" testing to determine whether the unknown white powder substance was actually *B. anthracis*, the bacterium responsible for causing anthrax infection. This testing is the domain of the Public Health Department.

Local, state, and federal law enforcement agencies also must become involved in the overall investigation of an actual or potential bioterrorism event so that the suspected perpetrators can be apprehended, even in the event of a hoax or practical joke. Hoaxes are not taken lightly by law enforcement in this era of heightened terrorist awareness. The practical jokers may find themselves prosecuted as criminals and serving prison time for their actions. More common, however, are the panicked reactions from innocent people like M.C. who come to the ED believing that they have suffered an exposure to a bioterrorism agent.

M.C. was sent into the decontamination room through an outside door. Most ED decontamination facilities have both outside and inside doors. The patient enters from the outside, is decontaminated, and is then transported into the ED. Containment tanks to collect wastewater run-off from the decontamination process and separate air-handling systems are typical components of new facility designs. Potentially contaminated clothing is removed from the victim and destroyed.

According to Centers for Disease Control and Prevention guidelines, unless the person exhibits clinical evidence of disease or the substance under question tests positive for *B. anthracis*, antibiotics are *not* indicated. Anthrax can occur in three forms: cutaneous, gastrointestinal, and inhalational or pulmonary. Cutaneous anthrax is caused by direct contact with *B. anthracis*. It presents as a pruritic papular lesion that turns into a vesicle, which, in 2 to 6 days, becomes a lesion with depressed black eschar; this form of anthrax is generally nonfatal if treated with antibiotics. Gastrointestinal anthrax is caused by ingestion of contaminated food and is characterized by abdominal pain, nausea, vomiting (hematemesis), fever, bloody diarrhea, and sepsis in late stages. Mortality rate is high, especially after the patient exhibits sepsis. Pulmonary or inhalational anthrax stems from inhalation of anthrax spores. This illness begins as a flu-like syndrome with fever and drenching sweats that progresses rapidly to respiratory failure. Classic x-ray findings reveal a widened mediastinum and pleural effusions. These findings may not appear until later in the course of illness. Unless treatment is instituted very early in the disease process, mortality rates are exceptionally high. See Chapter 33 for further discussion of anthrax management.

Once in the fast-track setting in this case scenario, attention was directed at reducing the anxiety level of the patient and providing effective health teaching. The psychosocial harm that occurs with actual or potential victims of bioterrorism events cannot be overestimated. When large groups of people are involved in a potential exposure, there is great potential for hysteria. Effective interventions include calmly providing factual information about the potential threat and offering follow-up with public health and mental health/behavioral health care professionals as needed to address both physical and mental health/behavioral health issues.

GET READY FOR THE NCLEX EXAMINATION!

Key Points

Review these Key Points for each NCLEX Examination Client Needs Category.

Safe and Effective Care Environment

- All medical centers must have an emergency preparedness and response team in case of mass casualty (disaster).
- The typical triage system for a mass casualty situation includes an additional category for those patients allowed to die (black-tagged) (see Table 12-1).
- Special roles are assigned in a mass casualty incident as identified in Table 12-2.
- In the emergency department, assist in determining the need for initiating the emergency preparedness plan based on available resources, including staffing.
- Be prepared for an emergency, including a plan for child, pet, and older adult care; have a "to go" bag, or disaster supply kit, packed for both the automobile and home (see Table 12-3).
- Two types of debriefing occur after a mass casualty event or period—critical incident stress debriefing and an administrative review.
- In a situation wherein exposure to a biologic agent is suspected, the decontamination team wears special protective gear to decontaminate the patients who were exposed. Those patients are separated from others in the ED.

Psychosocial Integrity

- Assess families and other survivors for their reaction to temporary or permanent loss as a result of a mass casualty event.
- Provide emotional support through encouraging relaxation, listening to survivor feelings, and referring to support groups.
- Be honest with victims and their families, and help them adapt to their changed or new surroundings.
- Take precautions to prevent staff from developing post-traumatic stress disorder (PTSD) as outlined in Chart 12-1.

Additional Study Resources

Go to your Companion CD or Evolve at http://evolve.elsevier.com/Iggy/ for *Self-Assessment Questions for the NCLEX Examination.*

evolve Go to Evolve at http://evolve.elsevier.com/Iggy/ for *Prioritization and Delegation Questions for the NCLEX Examination.*

SELECTED BIBLIOGRAPHY

Asterisk indicates a classic or definitive work on this subject.

American College of Surgeons. (2006). *Resources for optimal care of the injured patient.* Chicago: Author.

*American Nurses Association. (2001). *Code of ethics for nurses with interpretive statements.* Washington, DC: Author.

Becker, S.M. (2006). Psychosocial care for adult and child survivors of the 2004 tsunami disaster in India. *American Journal of Public Health, 96*(8), 1397-1398.

Casini, J.A.P., & Romanosky, A.J. (2006). Surge capacity. In G.R. Ciottone (Ed.), *Disaster medicine* (pp. 193-202). St. Louis: Mosby.

Centers for Disease Control and Prevention. (2006). *Fact Sheet: Anthrax information for health care providers.* Retrieved March 25, 2007, from www.bt.cdc.gov/agent/anthrax/anthrax-hcp-factsheet.asp.

Chaffee, M. (2006). Making the decision to report to work in a disaster. *AJN, 106*(9), 54-57.

*Everly, G.S., & Mitchell, J.T. (1999). *Critical incident stress management (CISM): A new era and standard of care in crisis intervention.* Ellicott City, MD: Chevron.

*Federal Emergency Management Agency (FEMA). (2004). *Are you ready? An in-depth guide to citizen preparedness.* Jessup, MD: Author.

Frank, I.C. (2005). Emergency response to the Gulf Coast devastation by hurricanes Katrina and Rita: Experiences and impressions. *Journal of Emergency Nursing, 31*(6), 526-547.

Hoard, M.L., & Tosatto, R.J. (2005). Medical reserve corps: Strengthening public health and improving preparedness. *Disaster Management & Response, 3*(2), 48-52.

Laskowski-Jones L. (2005). Rx for busy EDs: Patient-tracking technology. *Nursing2005, 35*(11), 32cc1-2.

*Mitchell, A.M., Kameg, K., & Sakraida, T.J. (2003a). Post-traumatic stress: Clinical implications. *Disaster Management & Response, 1*(1), 14-18.

*Mitchell, A.M., Sakraida, T.J., & Kameg, K. (2003b). Critical incident stress debriefing: Implications for best practice. *Disaster Management & Response, 1*(2), 46-51.

Mitchell, A.M., Sakraida, T.J., & Zalice, K.K. (2005). Disaster care: Psychological considerations. *Nursing Clinics of North America, 40*(3), 535-550.

Olszewski, T.M., & Varrasse, J.F. (2005). The neurobiology of PTSD: Implications for nurses. *Journal of Psychosocial Nursing, 43*(6), 40-47.

Papp, E. (2005). Preparing for disasters: Helping yourself as well as others. *AJN, 105*(5), 112.

Reisner, A. (2006). Triage. In G.R. Ciottone (Ed.), *Disaster medicine* (pp. 283-290). St. Louis: Mosby.

Rice, K.L., Colletti, L.S., Hartmann, S., Schaubhut, R., & Davis, N.L. (2006). Learning from Katrina. *Nursing2006, 36*(4), 44-47.

Russo, T. (2006). Pandemic planning. *Emergency Medical Services, 35*(10), 51-61.

Stopford, B.M. (2005). The National Disaster Medical System—America's medical readiness force. *Disaster Management & Response, 3*(2), 53-56.

Sutingco, N. (2006). The incident command system. In G.R. Ciottone (Ed.), *Disaster medicine* (pp. 208-214). St. Louis: Mosby.

The Joint Commission. (2007). Standards FAQs—Disaster drills: Planning and implementation activities. Retrieved March 25, 2007, from www.jointcommission.org/AccreditationPrograms/CriticalAccessHospitals/Standards/FAQs/Management+of+Env+of+Care/Planning+and+Implementation+Activities/Disaster_Drills.htm.

Weiss, J.A., Holcomb, L., & Crigger, N.J. (2006). Lessons learned from Hurricane Mitch: A guide for holistic practice. *Holistic Nursing Practice, 20*(6), 282-287.

Wielawski, I.M. (2006). The health legacy of September 11. *AJN, 106*(9), 27-28.

III

UNIT

Management of Patients with Fluid, Electrolyte, and Acid-Base Imbalances

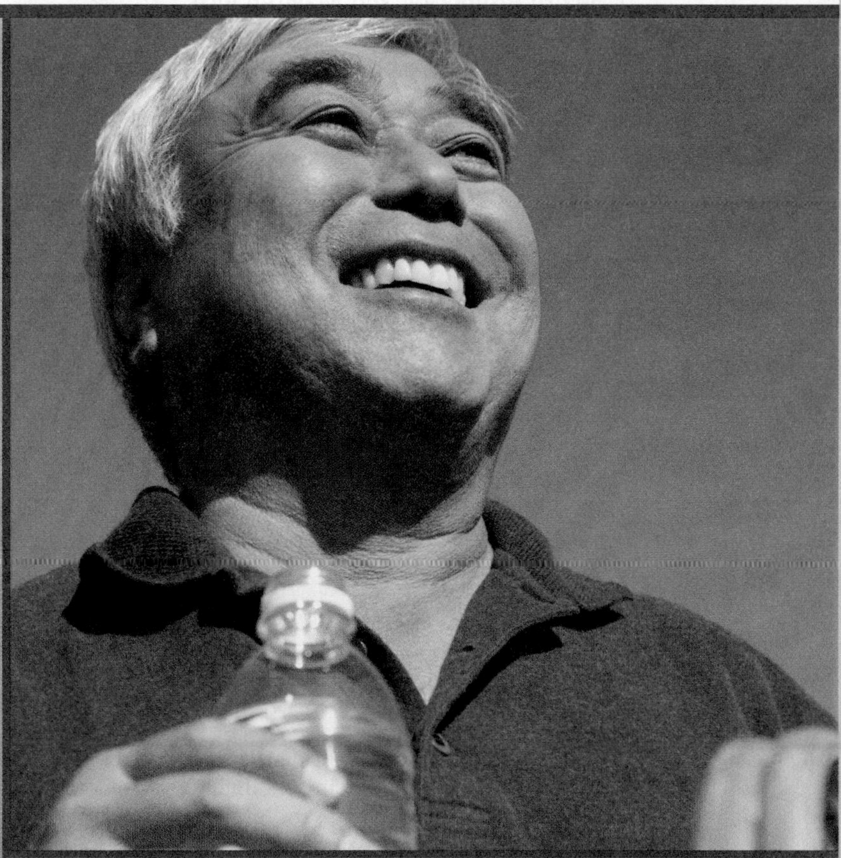

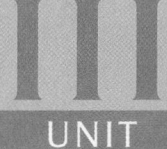

13
CHAPTER

Assessment and Care of Patients with Fluid and Electrolyte Imbalances

M. Linda Workman

LEARNING OUTCOMES

For clinical competence and success on the NCLEX Examination, study this chapter with these Learning Outcomes in mind:

Safe and Effective Care Environment

1. Assess the patient with a fluid or electrolyte imbalance for falls.
2. Use appropriate safety techniques to prevent injury or death when administering parenteral potassium-containing solutions.
3. Supervise the oral fluid therapy and intake and output measurements aspects of care delegated to unlicensed assistive personnel.

Health Promotion and Maintenance

4. Teach healthy adults and patients how to prevent dehydration.
5. Assess patients for lifestyle practices and drug therapies that increase the risk for fluid and electrolyte imbalances.
6. Teach patients at risk for fluid or electrolyte imbalances as a result of drug therapy about the manifestations of the imbalance.

Physiological Integrity

7. Explain the relationship between weight gain or loss and fluid imbalances.
8. Identify patients at risk for fluid or electrolyte imbalances.
9. Apply knowledge of the anatomic and physiologic responses to aging when assessing hydration status of an older adult.
10. Use laboratory data and clinical manifestations to determine the presence of fluid or electrolyte imbalances.
11. Correctly interpret blood chemistry laboratory results to determine whether the patient has a fluid or electrolyte imbalance and to determine effectiveness of interventions.
12. Assess the breathing effectiveness of any patient with skeletal muscle weakness from an electrolyte imbalance.
13. Prioritize interventions for patients who have dehydration or fluid overload.
14. Prioritize interventions for patients who have specific electrolyte imbalances.

Go to your Companion CD or Evolve at http://evolve.elsevier.com/Iggy/ for *Self-Assessment Questions for the NCLEX Examination* keyed to these Learning Outcomes.

HOMEOSTASIS

The human body works best when conditions inside the body are kept within a narrow range of normal. Examples include body temperature, blood electrolyte values (e.g., sodium, potassium, calcium), blood pH, and blood volume. No body system works well if 2 liters of blood volume are gained or lost. To keep conditions as close to normal as possible (a situation called **homeostasis**), the body has many control mechanisms **(homeostatic mechanisms)** to prevent dangerous changes.

An important area for homeostasis is maintaining the body's normal fluid volume and composition. Water is the most common substance in the body, making up about 55% to 60% of total body weight for healthy younger adults and 50% to 55% of total body weight for healthy older adults. This water (fluid) is divided into two main spaces or compartments—the fluid outside the cells, which is the **extracellular fluid (ECF);** and the fluid inside the cells, which is the **intracellular fluid (ICF).** The ECF space contains about one third (about 15 L) of the total body water. The ECF includes **interstitial fluid** (fluid between cells, sometimes called the "third space"); blood, lymph, bone, and connective tissue water; and the transcellular fluids. **Transcellular fluids** are the fluids in special body spaces and include cerebrospinal fluid, synovial fluid, peritoneal fluid, and pleural fluid. ICF contains the remaining two thirds (about 25 L) of total body water. Fig. 13-1 shows the normal distribution of total body water.

Water is needed to deliver dissolved nutrients, electrolytes, and other substances to all organs, tissues, and cells. In the healthy adult, the volume of water in the fluid compartments remains within the normal range although the water moves constantly between compartments. Changes in either the amount of water or the amount of electrolytes in body fluids can affect the functioning of all cells, tissues, and organs. *For proper function, the volume of all body fluids and the types and amount of dissolved substances must be carefully controlled.*

ANATOMY AND PHYSIOLOGY REVIEW

PHYSIOLOGIC INFLUENCES ON FLUID AND ELECTROLYTE BALANCE

Body fluids are composed of water and particles dissolved or suspended in water. The **solvent** is the water portion of fluids. **Solutes** are the particles dissolved or suspended in the water. Solutes vary in type and amount from one fluid space to another. Body function depends on keeping the correct balance of fluid and electrolytes within each body fluid space.

Three processes are important to control normal fluid and electrolyte balance and work together to maintain balance so the internal environment remains stable even when the external environment changes. These processes are filtration, diffusion, and osmosis. They determine how, when, and where fluids and particles move across cell membranes.

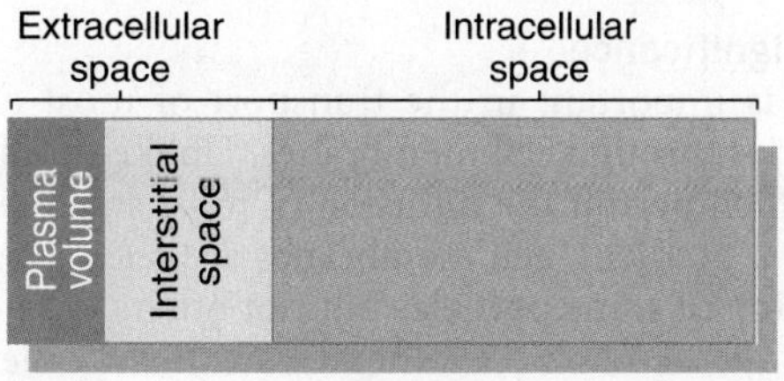
Extracellular space
Intracellular space
Plasma volume
Interstitial space

Fig. 13-1 • Normal distribution of total body water.

Filtration

Physiologic Action

Filtration is the movement of fluid through a cell or blood vessel membrane because of hydrostatic pressure differences on both sides of the membrane. Filtration occurs because of differences in water volume pressing against the confining walls of the space.

Fluid weight in a confined space is related to the amount of fluid present in that area. Water molecules in a confined space constantly press outward against the confining walls. This pressing of water molecules is **hydrostatic pressure.** It is a "water-pushing" pressure, because it is the force that pushes water outward from a confined space through a membrane.

The amount of water in any body fluid space determines the hydrostatic pressure of that space. Blood, a fluid that is "thicker" than water (more **viscous**), is confined within the blood vessels. Blood has hydrostatic pressure because of its weight and volume and also because the heart is pumping blood into the arteries, creating more pressure.

The hydrostatic pressures of two fluid spaces can be compared whenever a porous **(permeable)** membrane separates the two spaces. If the hydrostatic pressure is the same in both fluid spaces, there is no pressure difference between the two spaces and the hydrostatic pressure is now at **equilibrium.** If the hydrostatic pressure is not the same in both spaces, **disequilibrium** exists. This means that the two spaces have a graded difference **(gradient)** for hydrostatic pressure: one space has a higher hydrostatic pressure than the other. The human body constantly seeks equilibrium. When a gradient exists, water movement (filtration) occurs until the hydrostatic pressure is the same in both spaces (Fig. 13-2).

When nothing stops it, water moves **(filters)** through the membrane from the space with higher hydrostatic pressure to the space with lower pressure. This filtration continues only as long as the hydrostatic pressure gradient exists. Equilibrium is

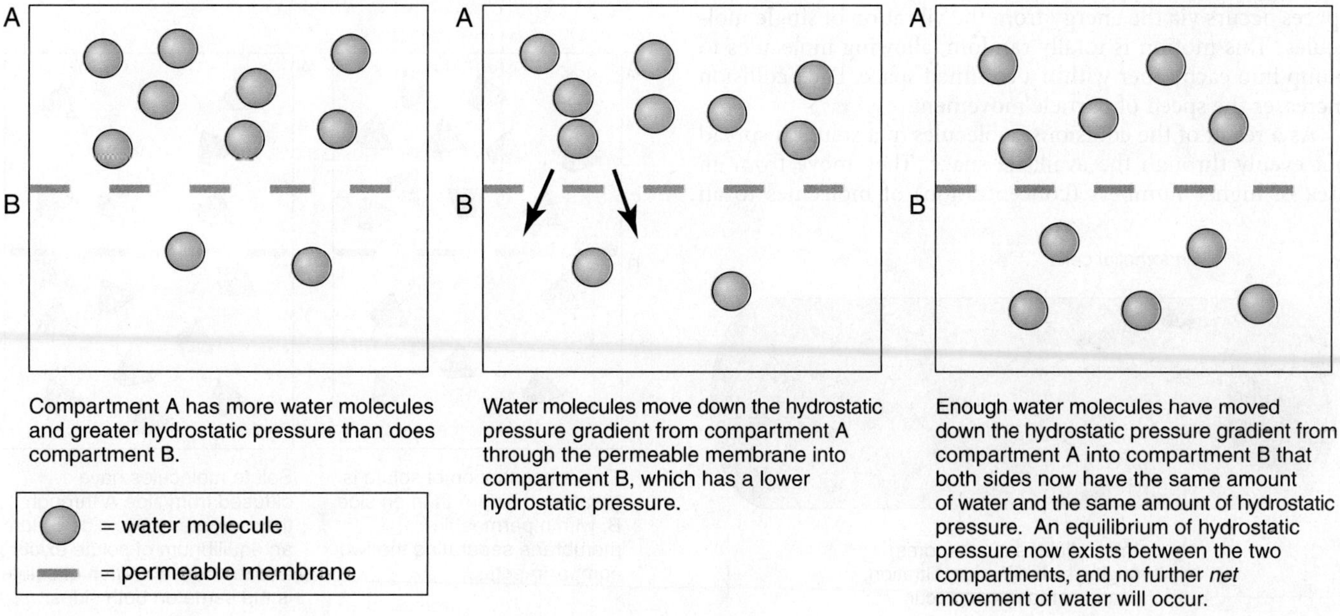
A
B
A
B
A
B
Compartment A has more water molecules and greater hydrostatic pressure than does compartment B.
Water molecules move down the hydrostatic pressure gradient from compartment A through the permeable membrane into compartment B, which has a lower hydrostatic pressure.
Enough water molecules have moved down the hydrostatic pressure gradient from compartment A into compartment B that both sides now have the same amount of water and the same amount of hydrostatic pressure. An equilibrium of hydrostatic pressure now exists between the two compartments, and no further *net* movement of water will occur.
= water molecule
= permeable membrane

Fig. 13-2 • The process of filtration.

reached when enough fluid leaves one space and enters the other space to make the hydrostatic pressure in both spaces equal. At this point, water molecules may be exchanged evenly between two spaces in equilibrium, but no net further filtration of fluid occurs. Neither space gains or loses water molecules, and the hydrostatic pressure in both spaces remains the same.

Clinical Significance

Blood pressure is an example of a hydrostatic filtering force. It moves whole blood from the heart to capillaries where filtration can occur to exchange water, nutrients, and waste products between the blood and the tissues. One factor that determines whether fluid leaves the blood vessels and enters the tissue spaces (interstitial fluid) is the difference between the hydrostatic pressure of capillary blood and that of the interstitial fluid.

Capillaries are only one cell layer thick, making a thin "wall" to hold blood in the capillaries. Large spaces **(pores)** in the capillary membrane help water filter freely when a hydrostatic pressure gradient is present (Fig. 13-3).

Edema (tissue swelling with fluid collection) develops with changes in normal hydrostatic pressure differences, such as in patients with right-sided heart failure. In this condition, the volume of blood in the right side of the heart increases greatly because the right ventricle is too weak to pump blood efficiently into the pulmonary blood vessels. As blood backs up into the venous system, venous hydrostatic pressure rises, which causes capillary hydrostatic pressure to rise until it is higher than the hydrostatic pressure in the interstitial space. Then excess filtration of fluid from the capillaries into the interstitial tissue space occurs, forming visible edema.

Diffusion

Physiologic Action

Diffusion is the free movement of particles (solute) across a permeable membrane from an area of higher concentration to an area of lower concentration (down a *concentration gradient*). This action controls the movement of solute particles in solution across various body membranes.

The diffusion of particles into and out from cells and fluid spaces occurs via the energy from the vibration of single molecules. This motion is totally random, allowing molecules to bump into each other within a confined space. Each collision increases the speed of particle movement.

As a result of the collisions, molecules in a solution spread out evenly through the available space. They move from an area of higher numbers (concentration) of molecules to an area of lower numbers until an equal number is present in all areas. The number of collisions is related to the number of molecules in a confined space. Fluid spaces with many particles have more collisions and faster particle movement than spaces with fewer particles.

A concentration gradient exists when two fluid spaces have different numbers of the same type of particles. Particle collisions cause them to move down the concentration gradient. Any membrane that separates two spaces is struck repeatedly by particles. When the particle strikes a pore in the membrane that is large enough for it to pass through, diffusion occurs (Fig. 13-4). The chance of any single particle hitting the membrane and going through a pore is much greater on the side of the membrane with a higher particle concentration.

The speed of diffusion is related to the difference in number of particles (concentration gradient) between the two sides of the membrane. The degree of difference is the *steepness* of the gradient: the larger the concentration difference between the two sides, the steeper the gradient. Diffusion is more rapid when the gradient is steeper (just as a ball rolls downhill more rapidly when the hill is steep than when the hill is nearly flat). Particles move from the fluid space with a higher concentration to the fluid space with a lower concentration.

Diffusion of particles continues as long as a concentration gradient exists between the two sides of the membrane. *When the concentration of particles is the same on both sides of the membrane, the particles are in equilibrium and only an equal exchange of particles continues.*

Clinical Significance

Diffusion is important in the transport of most electrolytes and particles through cell membranes. Unlike capillary membranes, which permit the diffusion of most small-sized particles down a gradient, cell membranes are *selective.* They permit diffusion of some particles but not others. Some particles cannot move across a cell membrane, even when a steep "downhill" gradient exists, because the membrane is not open **(impermeable)** to that particle. Then the concentration gradient is maintained across the membrane.

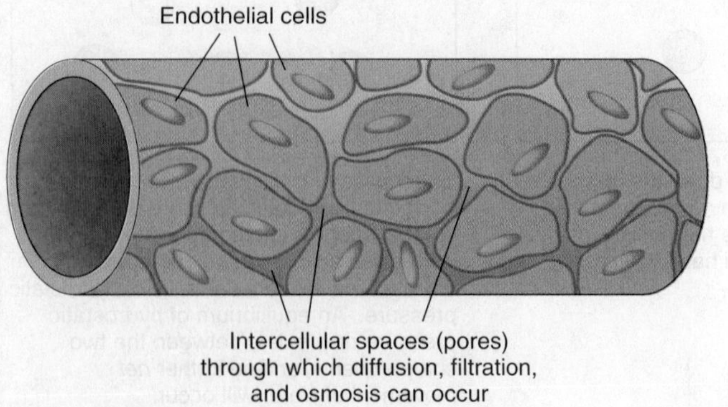
Endothelial cells
Intercellular spaces (pores) through which diffusion, filtration, and osmosis can occur

Fig. 13-3 • The basic structure of a capillary.

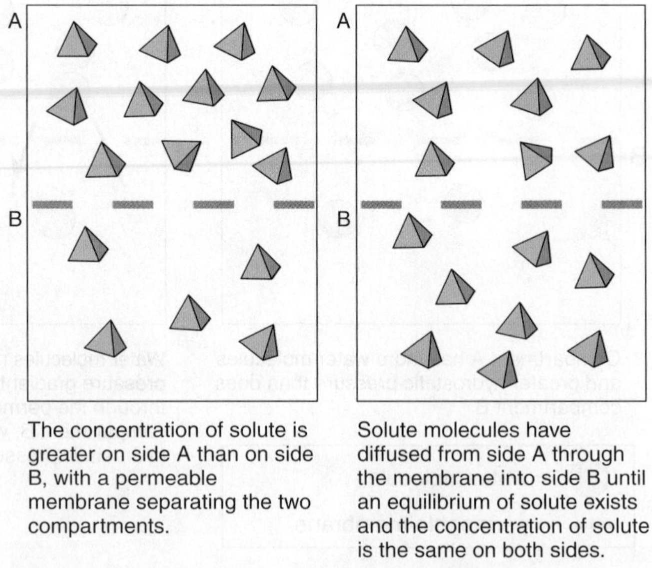
A
B
The concentration of solute is greater on side A than on side B, with a permeable membrane separating the two compartments.
A
B
Solute molecules have diffused from side A through the membrane into side B until an equilibrium of solute exists and the concentration of solute is the same on both sides.

Fig. 13-4 • Diffusion of a solute.

Impermeability and special transport systems cause differences in the numbers of specific particles from one fluid space to another. For example, usually the fluid outside of the cells, the extracellular fluid (ECF), has ten times more sodium ions than the fluid inside the cell, the intracellular fluid (ICF). This extreme difference is caused by cell membrane impermeability to sodium and by special "sodium pumps" that move any extra sodium out of the cell "uphill" against its concentration gradient and back into the ECF.

In some instances, diffusion cannot occur without help, even down steep concentration gradients, because of membrane selectivity. One example is glucose. Even though the amount of glucose may be much higher in the ECF than in the ICF (creating a steep gradient for glucose), glucose cannot cross most cell membranes without the help of insulin. When insulin is present, it binds to insulin receptor sites on cell membranes, which makes the membranes much more permeable to glucose. Glucose can then cross the cell membrane down its concentration gradient until equilibrium of glucose concentration is created.

Diffusion across a cell membrane that requires the assistance of a membrane-altering system (e.g., insulin) is called **facilitated diffusion** or **facilitated transport.** This type of movement is still a form of diffusion.

Osmosis

Physiologic Action

Osmosis is the movement of water only through a selectively permeable (semipermeable) membrane. For osmosis to occur, a membrane must separate two fluid spaces and one space must have particles that cannot move through the membrane. (The membrane is impermeable to this particle.) A concentration gradient of this particle must also exist. Because the membrane is impermeable to these particles, they cannot cross the membrane but water molecules can.

For the fluid spaces to have equal concentrations of the particle, the water molecules move down their concentration gradient from the side with the higher concentration of water molecules (and thus a lower concentration of particles) to the side with the lower concentration of water molecules (and a higher concentration of particles). This movement continues until both spaces contain the same proportions of particles to water. Dilute (less concentrated) fluid has fewer particles and more water molecules than the more concentrated fluid. Thus water moves by osmosis down its pressure gradient from the dilute fluid to the more concentrated fluid until equilibrium occurs (Fig. 13-5).

At this point, the concentrations of particles in the fluid spaces on both sides of the membrane are equal even though the total numbers of particles and volumes of water are different. Equilibrium occurs by the movement of water molecules rather than the movement of particles.

Factors that determine whether and how fast osmosis occurs include the overall concentration of particles in solution, how easily the solute dissolves in water (solubility), and the amount of membrane available for osmosis.

Particle concentration in body fluids is expressed in milliequivalents per liter (mEq/L), millimoles per liter (mmol/L), and milliosmoles per liter (mOsm/L). **Osmolarity** is the number of milliosmoles in a *liter* of solution; **osmolality** is the number of milliosmoles in a *kilogram* of solution. The normal osmolarity value for plasma and other body fluids ranges from 270 to

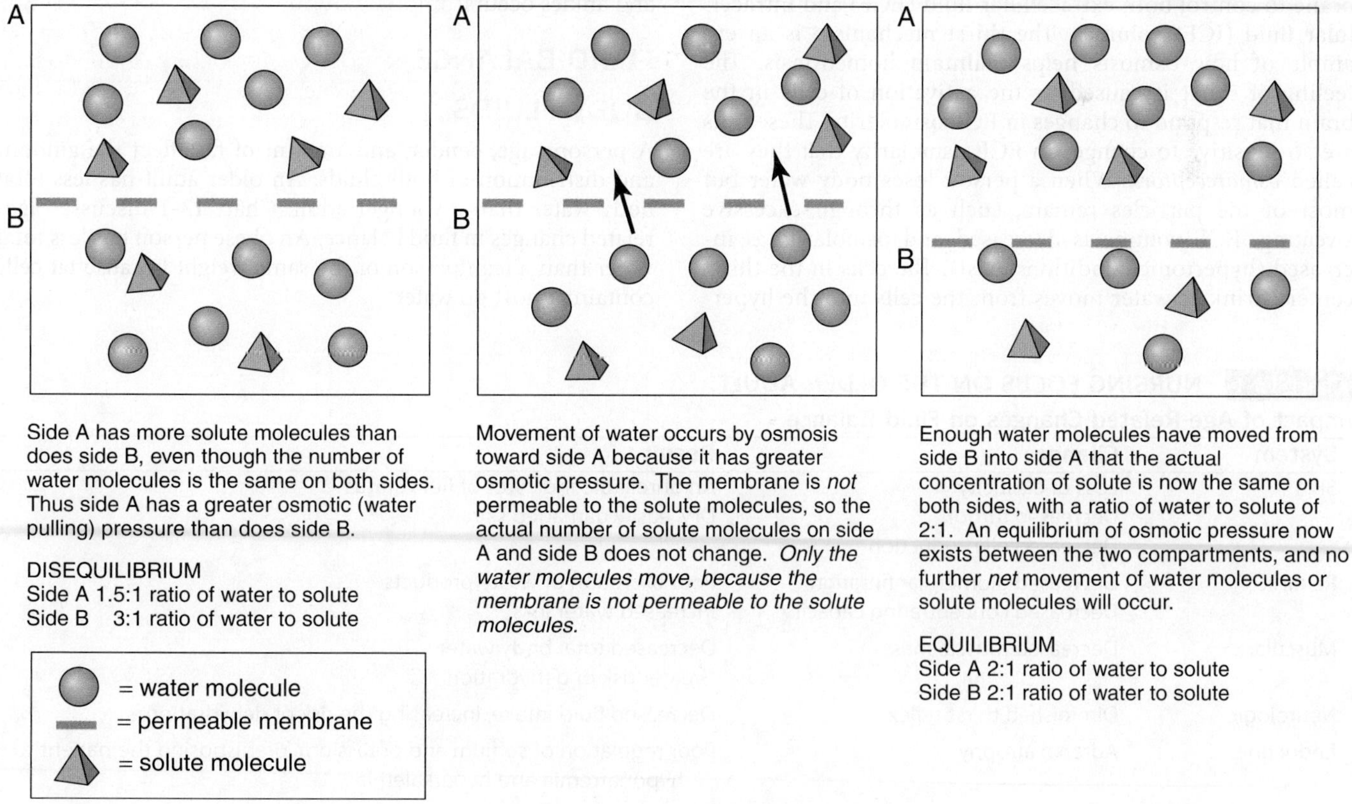
A
B
A
B
A
B
Side A has more solute molecules than does side B, even though the number of water molecules is the same on both sides. Thus side A has a greater osmotic (water pulling) pressure than does side B.
DISEQUILIBRIUM
Side A 1.5:1 ratio of water to solute
Side B 3:1 ratio of water to solute
Movement of water occurs by osmosis toward side A because it has greater osmotic pressure. The membrane is not permeable to the solute molecules, so the actual number of solute molecules on side A and side B does not change. Only the water molecules move, because the membrane is not permeable to the solute molecules.
Enough water molecules have moved from side B into side A that the actual concentration of solute is now the same on both sides, with a ratio of water to solute of 2:1. An equilibrium of osmotic pressure now exists between the two compartments, and no further net movement of water molecules or solute molecules will occur.
EQUILIBRIUM
Side A 2:1 ratio of water to solute
Side B 2:1 ratio of water to solute
= water molecule
= permeable membrane
= solute molecule

Fig. 13-5 • The process of osmosis.

about 300 mOsm/L. The body functions best when the osmolarity of the fluids in all body fluid spaces is close to 300 mOsm/L. When all body fluids have this particle concentration, the body fluids are **isosmotic** to each other. Another term with the same meaning is **isotonic** (also called **normotonic**).

Fluids with osmolarities greater than 300 mOsm/L are **hyperosmotic,** or **hypertonic,** compared with isosmotic fluids. These fluids have a *greater* osmotic pressure than do isosmotic fluids and tend to pull water from the isosmotic fluid space into the hyperosmotic fluid space until an osmotic balance occurs. If a hyperosmotic IV solution (e.g., 2% saline) were infused into a patient with normal ECF osmolarity, the infusing fluid would make the person's blood hyperosmotic. To balance this situation, the interstitial fluid would be pulled into the circulation in an attempt to dilute the blood osmolarity back to normal. As a result, the interstitial volume would shrink and the plasma volume would expand.

Fluids with osmolarities of less than 270 mOsm/L are **hypo-osmotic,** or **hypotonic,** compared with isosmotic fluids. Hypo-osmolar fluids have a *lower* osmotic pressure than isosmotic fluids, and water is pulled from the hypo-osmotic fluid space into the isosmotic fluid space.

Solubility is how well a particle type dissolves in water. Fluids that have particles with greater solubility have higher osmotic pressures than fluids with insoluble particles.

Amount of membrane available for osmosis affects the speed of osmosis. More membrane increases the chances that water molecules will hit the membrane at a point where penetration is possible and thus increases the speed of osmosis.

Clinical Significance

Osmosis and filtration act together at the capillary membrane to control both extracellular fluid (ECF) and intracellular fluid (ICF) volumes. The thirst mechanism is an example of how osmosis helps maintain homeostasis. The feeling of thirst is caused by the activation of cells in the brain that respond to changes in ECF osmolarity. These cells are so sensitive to changes in ECF osmolarity that they are called *osmoreceptors.* When a person loses body water but most of the particles remain, such as through excessive sweating, ECF volume is decreased and osmolarity is increased (hypertonic conditions exist). The cells in the thirst center shrink as water moves from the cells into the hypertonic ECF. The shrinking of these cells triggers a person's awareness of thirst and increases the urge to drink. Drinking replaces the amount of water lost through sweating and restores the ECF osmolarity to normal. *It is important to remember that the thirst mechanism is less sensitive in older adults, making them more at risk for dehydration.*

Lymph

At the capillary level, fluid moves out from the capillary at its arterial end (because hydrostatic pressure is greater there) into the interstitial space and moves from the interstitial space back into the capillary at the venous end. In most cases, not all of the fluid that leaves the capillary at the arterial end and enters the interstitial space is returned to the capillary at the venous end. A small amount remains in the tissues. If this situation is not balanced by another mechanism to return the fluid to the systemic circulation, blood volume would become depleted and the interstitial areas would constantly be edematous. Instead, this extra fluid leaking out from the capillaries is returned to the systemic circulation as lymph.

Lymph fluid is similar to blood plasma (from which it is formed) but contains far less protein. It is returned to the circulation by lymph vessels, or lymphatics. These vessels drain lymph back into the circulatory system at the left and right subclavian veins. Lymph nodes are situated along the lymphatic paths and filter the lymph fluid. Lymph flow is slower than blood flow because lymph has no pump. Flow is enhanced by skeletal muscle contractions, breathing, and a peristalsis-like motion in the lymph vessels. When skeletal muscle contractions are reduced, like when a person is sitting for hours during a long airplane trip, lymph moves very slowly in the dependent areas (lower legs and feet) and swelling of the feet and ankles occurs.

FLUID BALANCE

BODY FLUIDS

A person's age, gender, and amount of fat affect the amount and distribution of body fluids. An older adult has less total body water than a younger adult. Chart 13-1 discusses age-related changes in fluid balance. An obese person has less total water than a lean person of the same weight because fat cells contain almost no water.

Chart 13-1 NURSING FOCUS ON THE OLDER ADULT

Impact of Age-Related Changes on Fluid Balance

System	Change	Result
Skin	Loss of elasticity Decreased turgor Decreased oil production	An unreliable indicator of fluid status Dry, easily damaged skin
Renal	Decreased glomerular filtration Decreased concentrating capacity	Poor excretion of waste products Increased water loss
Muscular	Decreased muscle mass	Decreased total body water Greater risk of dehydration
Neurologic	Diminished thirst reflex	Decreased fluid intake, increasing the risk of dehydration
Endocrine	Adrenal atrophy	Poor regulation of sodium and potassium, predisposing the patient to hyponatremia and hyperkalemia

WOMEN'S HEALTH CONSIDERATIONS

Women of any age have less total body water than men of similar sizes and ages. This difference is because men have more muscle mass than women and because women have more body fat. (Muscle cells contain mostly water, and fat cells have little water.) Differences in muscle mass and body fat are partly a result of sex hormones. This difference in water distribution may be responsible for some differences seen in women's and men's responses to drugs.

Body fluids are constantly filtered and replaced as fluid balance is maintained through intake and output. The total amount of water within each fluid space is stable, but water moves continually among all spaces. Water in all spaces is exchanged continually while maintaining constant fluid volume.

Fluid intake is regulated through the thirst drive. Fluids enter the body mainly as liquids (Table 13-1). Solid foods also contain up to 85% water, and some fluid also enters the body with ingested solid foods.

A rising blood osmolarity or a decreasing blood volume triggers the sensation of thirst. Sensations such as mouth dryness or the thought that a person has not had a drink recently also trigger the thirst drive. An adult drinks an average of 1500 mL of fluid per day and ingests an additional 800 mL of fluid from food.

Fluid loss occurs through several routes (see Table 13-1). Of all the water loss pathways, the kidney is the most important and the most sensitive. Water loss by the kidney is regulated and is adjustable. The volume of urine excreted daily varies depending on the amount of fluid intake and the body's need to conserve fluids.

The minimum amount of urine per day needed to excrete toxic waste products is 400 to 600 mL. This minimum volume is called the **obligatory urine output.** If the 24-hour urine output falls below the obligatory output amount, wastes are retained and can cause lethal electrolyte imbalances, acidosis, and a toxic buildup of nitrogen.

The ability of the kidneys to make either concentrated or very dilute urine helps maintain fluid balance. The kidney works with various hormones to maintain fluid balance when extracellular fluid concentrations, volumes, or pressures change.

Other normal water loss occurs through the skin, the lungs, and the intestinal tract. Water losses can occur via salivation, drainage from fistulas and drains, and GI suction.

TABLE 13-1 Routes of Fluid Ingestion and Excretion

Intake	Output
MEASURABLE	
Oral fluids	Urine
Parenteral fluids	Emesis†
Enemas*	Feces†
Irrigation fluids*	Drainage from body cavities
NOT MEASURABLE	
Solid foods	Perspiration
Metabolism	Vaporization through the lungs

*Measured by subtracting the amount returned from the amount instilled.
†Measurement is accurate only when these substances are excreted in liquid form.

Water loss from the skin, lungs, and stool is called **insensible water loss,** because it cannot be controlled. The amount lost can be significant. In a healthy adult, insensible water loss is about 500 to 1000 mL/day. This loss increases greatly during thyroid crisis, trauma, burns, states of extreme stress, and fever. For every degree increase in body temperature, insensible water loss increases by about 10%. Insensible water loss also increases when the environment is hot and dry. Patients at risk for increased insensible water loss include those being mechanically ventilated and those with rapid respirations (tachypnea). Insensible water loss, if not balanced by intake, can lead to severe dehydration and electrolyte imbalances.

Loss by sweating is variable and can reach a maximum rate of about 2 L/hr. The amount of sweating is controlled by the autonomic nervous system, body temperature, and blood flow in the skin.

Water loss through stool is normally minimal. However, this loss can increase greatly with severe diarrhea or excessive fistula drainage.

HORMONAL REGULATION OF FLUID BALANCE

The endocrine system helps control fluid and electrolyte balance. Three hormones that help control these critical balances are aldosterone, antidiuretic hormone (ADH), and natriuretic peptide (NP).

Aldosterone is a hormone secreted by the adrenal cortex whenever sodium level in the extracellular fluid (ECF) is decreased (Fig. 13-6). Aldosterone prevents both water and sodium loss.

When aldosterone is secreted, it acts on the kidney nephrons, triggering them to reabsorb sodium and water from the urine back into the blood. This action increases blood osmolarity and blood volume. Aldosterone prevents excessive kidney excretion of sodium. It also helps prevent blood potassium levels from becoming too high.

Antidiuretic hormone (ADH), or vasopressin, is produced in the brain and stored in the posterior pituitary gland. ADH release from the posterior pituitary gland is controlled by the hypothalamus in response to changes in blood osmolarity. The hypothalamus contains specialized cells (osmoreceptors) that are sensitive to changes in blood osmolarity. Increased blood osmolarity, especially an increase in the level of plasma sodium, results in a slight shrinkage of these cells and triggers ADH release from the posterior pituitary gland.

ADH acts directly on kidney tubules and collecting ducts, making them more permeable to water. As a result, more water is *reabsorbed* by these tubules and returned to the blood, decreasing blood osmolarity by making it more dilute. When blood osmolarity decreases, especially when the plasma sodium level is below normal, the osmoreceptors swell slightly and inhibit ADH release. Less water is then reabsorbed, and more is lost from the body in the urine. As a result, the amount of water in the extracellular fluid (ECF) decreases, bringing osmolarity to normal.

Natriuretic peptides (NPs) are hormones secreted by special cells that line the atria of the heart (atrial natriuretic peptide [ANP]) and the ventricles of the heart (brain natriuretic peptide [BNP]). They are secreted in response to increased blood volume and blood pressure, which stretch the heart tissue. NP

TABLE 13-2 Common Causes of Fluid Imbalances

Dehydration	Fluid Overload
Hemorrhage	Excessive fluid replacement
Vomiting	Renal failure (late phase)
Diarrhea	Heart failure
Profuse salivation	Long-term corticosteroid therapy
Fistulas	Syndrome of inappropriate antidiuretic hormone (SIADH)
Ileostomy	Psychiatric disorders with polydipsia
Profuse diaphoresis	Water intoxication
Burns	
Severe wounds	
Long-term nothing-by-mouth (NPO) status	
Diuretic therapy	
GI suction	
Hyperventilation	
Renal failure (early phase)	
Diabetes insipidus	
Difficulty swallowing	
Impaired thirst	
Unconsciousness	
Fever	
Impaired motor function	

binds to receptor sites in the nephrons, creating effects that are opposite of aldosterone. Kidney reabsorption of sodium is inhibited at the same time that glomerular filtration is increased, causing increased urine output. The outcome is decreased circulating blood volume and decreased blood osmolarity.

FLUID IMBALANCES

All patients are at risk for some degree of fluid imbalance because many health problems can disrupt fluid intake or output. Fluid imbalances can occur in any setting.

DEHYDRATION

Pathophysiology

In **dehydration,** fluid intake is less than what is needed to meet the body's fluid needs, resulting in a fluid volume deficit. It is a condition rather than a disease and can be caused by many factors (Table 13-2). Dehydration may be an *actual* decrease in total body water caused by either too little intake of fluid or too great a loss of fluid. It also can occur without an actual loss of total body water, such as when water shifts from the plasma into the interstitial space. This condition is called *relative* dehydration.

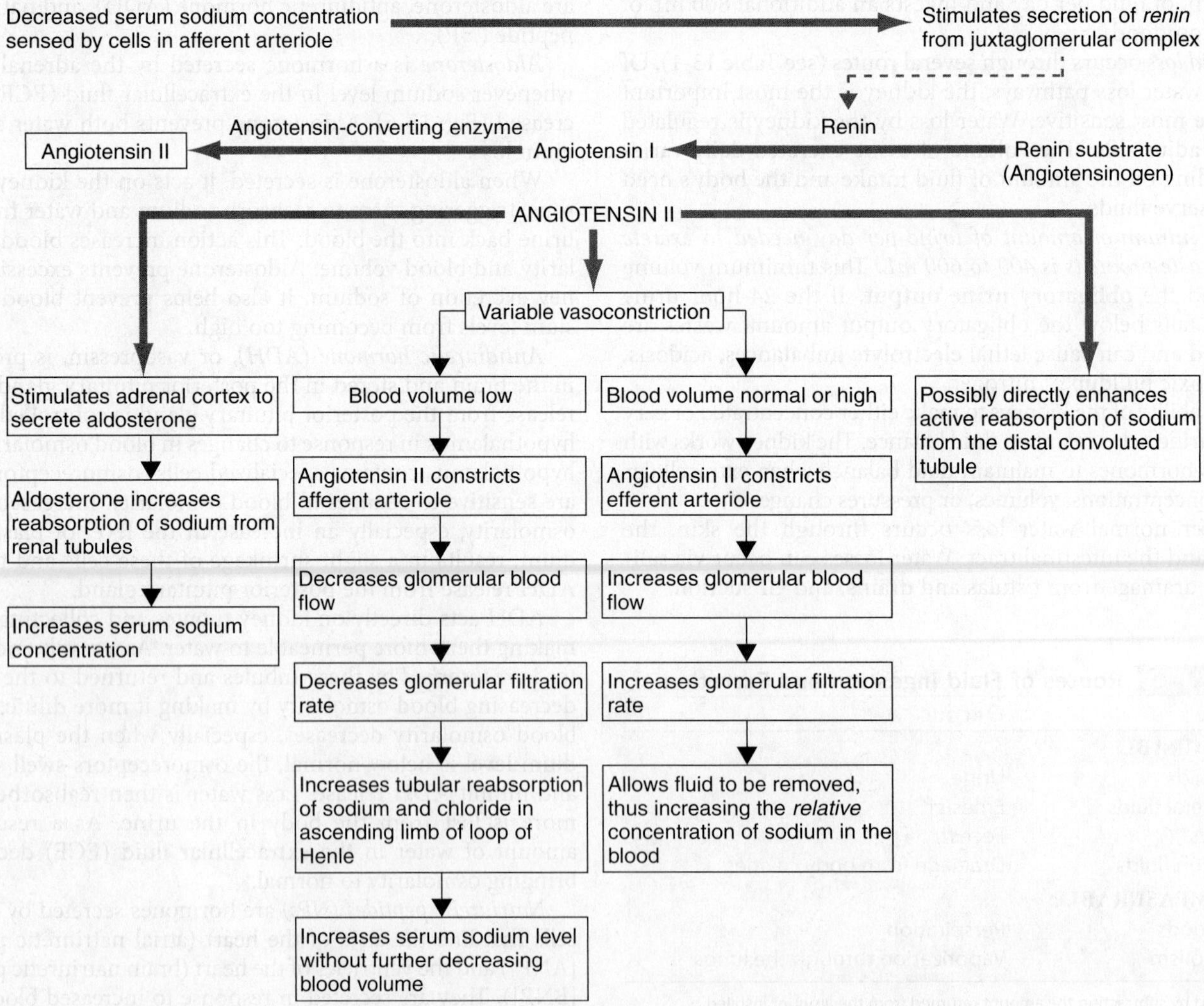
Decreased serum sodium concentration sensed by cells in afferent arteriole
Stimulates secretion of renin from juxtaglomerular complex
Renin
Renin substrate (Angiotensinogen)
Angiotensin I
Angiotensin-converting enzyme
Angiotensin II
ANGIOTENSIN II
Variable vasoconstriction
Stimulates adrenal cortex to secrete aldosterone
Aldosterone increases reabsorption of sodium from renal tubules
Increases serum sodium concentration
Blood volume low
Angiotensin II constricts afferent arteriole
Decreases glomerular blood flow
Decreases glomerular filtration rate
Increases tubular reabsorption of sodium and chloride in ascending limb of loop of Henle
Increases serum sodium level without further decreasing blood volume
Blood volume normal or high
Angiotensin II constricts efferent arteriole
Increases glomerular blood flow
Increases glomerular filtration rate
Allows fluid to be removed, thus increasing the relative concentration of sodium in the blood
Possibly directly enhances active reabsorption of sodium from the distal convoluted tubule

Fig. 13-6 • The role of aldosterone, angiotensinogen, angiotensin I, and angiotensin II in the renal regulation of water and sodium.

CONSIDERATIONS FOR OLDER ADULTS

Older patients are at high risk for dehydration because they have less total body water than younger adults. In addition, many older adults have decreased thirst sensation and may have difficulty with walking or other motor skills needed for ingesting fluids. They also may take drugs such as diuretics, antihypertensives, and laxatives that increase fluid excretion.

Dehydration may occur with just water loss or with water and electrolyte loss (isotonic dehydration). *Isotonic dehydration is the most common type of fluid volume deficit.* Fluid is lost only from the extracellular fluid (ECF) space, including both the plasma and the interstitial spaces. There is no shift of fluids between spaces, so the intracellular fluid (ICF) volume remains normal (Fig. 13-7). Circulating blood volume is decreased **(hypovolemia)** and leads to inadequate tissue perfusion. The body's defenses adapt (compensate) during dehydration to maintain adequate blood flow to vital organs in spite of hypovolemia (Fig. 13-8).

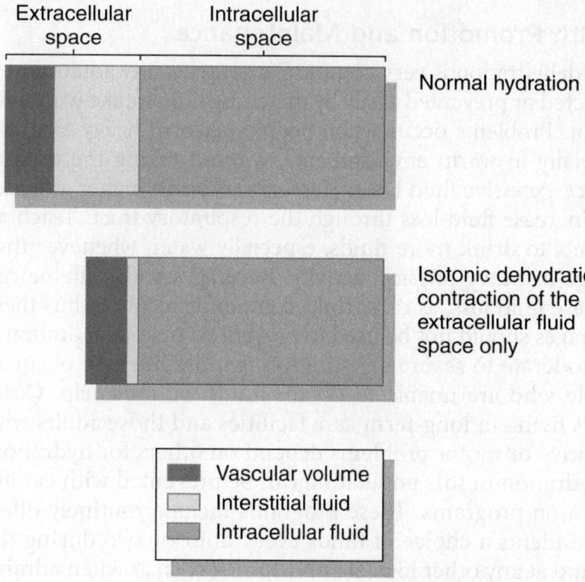
Extracellular space
Intracellular space
Normal hydration
Isotonic dehydration: contraction of the extracellular fluid space only
Vascular volume
Interstitial fluid
Intracellular fluid

Fig. 13-7 • Fluid changes with dehydration.

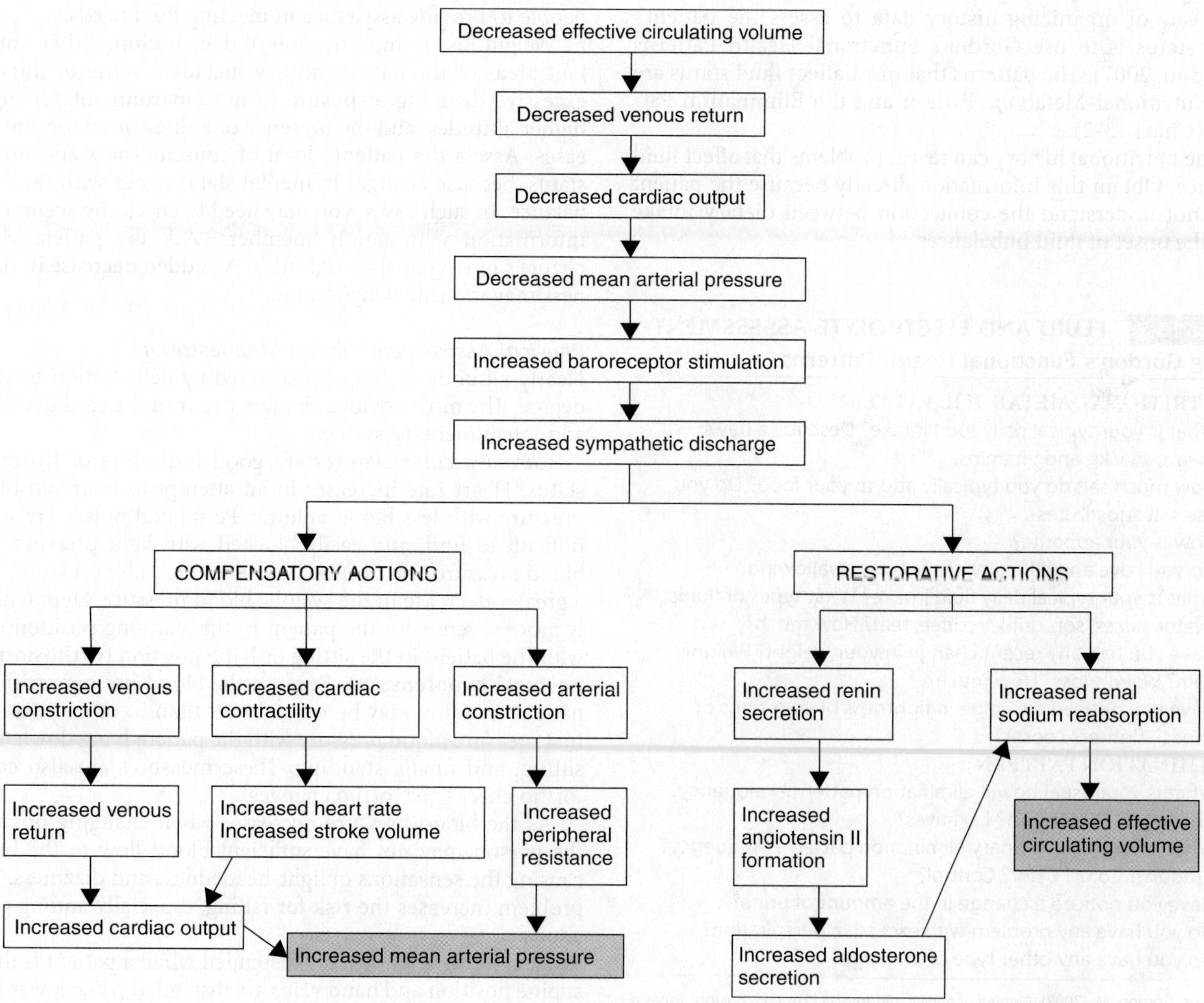
Decreased effective circulating volume
Decreased venous return
Decreased cardiac output
Decreased mean arterial pressure
Increased baroreceptor stimulation
Increased sympathetic discharge
COMPENSATORY ACTIONS
RESTORATIVE ACTIONS
Increased venous constriction
Increased cardiac contractility
Increased arterial constriction
Increased renin secretion
Increased renal sodium reabsorption
Increased venous return
Increased heart rate
Increased stroke volume
Increased peripheral resistance
Increased angiotensin II formation
Increased effective circulating volume
Increased cardiac output
Increased mean arterial pressure
Increased aldosterone secretion

Fig. 13-8 • Adaptive mechanisms during dehydration.

Health Promotion and Maintenance

Mild dehydration is very common among healthy adults and is corrected or prevented easily by matching fluid intake with fluid output. Problems occur when people perform heavy exercise, especially in warm environments, without taking the time to replace excessive fluid losses. Dry climates and higher altitudes also increase fluid loss through the respiratory tract. Teach all patients to drink more fluids, especially water, whenever they engage in heavy physical activity. Beverages with caffeine can increase fluid loss, as can drinks containing alcohol; thus these beverages should not be used to prevent or treat dehydration.

Moderate to severe dehydration is more likely to occur in people who are unable to obtain fluids without help. Older adults living in long-term care facilities and those adults with cognitive or motor problems depend on others for hydration. Dehydration in this population can be prevented with careful hydration programs. These programs include routinely offering residents a choice of fluids every hour or two during the day and at any other logical opportunity, such as when administering medications.

Patient-Centered Collaborative Care

evolve ONLINE PHARM REVIEW

Assessment

History

One way of organizing history data to assess the patient's fluid status is to use Gordon's Functional Health Patterns (Gordon, 2007). The patterns that most affect fluid status are the Nutritional-Metabolic Pattern and the Elimination Pattern (Chart 13-2).

The nutritional history can reveal problems that affect fluid balance. Obtain this information directly because the patient may not understand the connection between dietary intake and the onset of fluid imbalances.

Chart 13-2 FLUID AND ELECTROLYTE ASSESSMENT

Using Gordon's Functional Health Patterns

NUTRITIONAL-METABOLIC PATTERN

- What is your typical daily food intake? Describe a day's meals, snacks, and vitamins.
- How much salt do you typically add to your food? Do you use salt substitutes?
- How is your appetite?
- Do you have any difficulty chewing or swallowing?
- What is your typical daily fluid intake? What types of fluids (water, juices, soft drinks, coffee, tea)? How much?
- Have you had any recent change in your weight? Weight gain? Weight loss? How much?
- Have you noticed a change in tightness of your rings or shoes? Tighter? Looser?

ELIMINATION PATTERN

- What is your usual bowel elimination pattern? Frequency? Character? Discomfort? Laxatives?
- What is your usual urinary elimination pattern? Frequency? Amount? Color? Odor? Control?
- Have you noticed a change in the amount of urine?
- Do you have any problem with excessive perspiration?
- Do you have any other type of drainage?

Based on Gordon, M. (2007). *Manual of nursing diagnosis* (11th ed.). Boston: Jones & Bartlett.

The guidelines for obtaining a thorough fluid history do not differ from those for assessing any other system; however, the information collected is more specific. For example, exact intake and output volumes are important, as are serial daily weight measurements. If possible, weigh the patient directly. Because 1 L of water weighs 2.2 pounds (1 kg), changes in daily weights are the best indicators of fluid losses or gains. A weight change of 1 pound corresponds to a fluid volume change of about 500 mL.

Guide the patient in reporting accurately the amount of fluid ingested and changes in urine patterns. Also assess the types of fluids and foods ingested to determine amount and osmolarity. Many patients do not know that solid foods contain liquid. Solid foods such as ice cream, gelatin, and ices are liquids at body temperature, and these must be included when calculating fluid intake.

Output includes losses not only as urine but also as sweat, diarrhea, and insensible loss during fevers. Ask specific questions about prescribed and over-the-counter drugs, and check the dosage, the length of time taken, and the patient's adherence with the drug regimen.

Older adults often use diuretics and laxatives, which can disturb fluid balance. Misuse and overuse of these drugs can lead to dehydration and electrolyte imbalances. An important issue for many older adults is that they may depend on other people to provide assistance in meeting fluid needs.

Weight loss is an indication of dehydration. Other important areas of the patient history include a sense of thirst or excessive drinking, exposure to hot environments, living at higher altitudes, and the presence of kidney or endocrine diseases. Assess the patient's level of consciousness and mental status, because changes in mental status occur with fluid imbalance. In such cases, you may need to check the accuracy of information with family members. Ask the patient about changes in ring or shoe tightness. A sudden decrease in tightness may indicate dehydration.

Physical Assessment/Clinical Manifestations

Nearly all body systems are affected by dehydration to some degree. The most obvious changes occur in the cardiovascular and integumentary systems.

Cardiovascular changes are good indicators of hydration status. Heart rate increases in an attempt to maintain blood pressure with less blood volume. Peripheral pulses are weak, difficult to find, and easily blocked with light pressure. The blood pressure also decreases, as does the pulse pressure, with a greater decrease in the systolic blood pressure. Hypotension is more severe with the patient in the standing position than with the patient in the sitting or lying position (**orthostatic** or **postural hypotension**). Because the blood pressure with the patient standing may be much lower than in other positions, first measure blood pressure with the patient lying down, then sitting, and finally standing. These measures are also called "ortho checks" or "ortho changes."

As the blood pressure decreases when changing position, the person may not have sufficient blood flow to the brain, causing the sensations of light-headedness and dizziness. This problem increases the risk for falling, especially among older adults.

Neck veins are normally distended when a patient is in the supine position and hand veins are distended when lower than the level of the heart. Neck veins normally flatten when the patient moves to a sitting position. With dehydration, neck and hand veins are flat, even when the neck and hands are not raised above the level of the heart.

Respiratory changes include an increased rate because the decreased blood volume is perceived by the body as decreased oxygen levels **(hypoxia).** The increased respiratory rate is an attempt to maintain oxygen delivery.

Skin changes can indicate dehydration. Assess the skin and mucous membranes for color, moisture, and turgor. In older patients this information is less reliable because of poor skin turgor resulting from the loss of elastic tissue and increased skin dryness from the loss of tissue fluids with aging. Assess skin turgor by checking:

- How easily the skin over the back of the hand and arm can be gently pinched between the thumb and the forefinger to form a "tent"
- How soon the pinched skin resumes its normal position after release

In generalized dehydration, skin turgor is poor, with the tenting remaining for minutes after pinching the skin, and no skin depressions occur with gentle pressure. The skin is dry and scaly.

CONSIDERATIONS FOR OLDER ADULTS

Assess skin turgor in an older adult by pinching the skin over the sternum or on the forehead, rather than the back of the hand, because these areas more reliably indicate hydration (Fig. 13-9). As a person ages, the skin loses elasticity and tents on hands and arms even when the person is well hydrated.

In dehydration, oral mucous membranes are not moist. They may be covered with a thick, sticky, pastelike coating and may have cracks and fissures. The surface of the tongue may have deep furrows. This manifestation may not be accurate for dehydration in patients taking drugs that have the side effect of dry mouth.

Neurologic changes with dehydration include alterations of mental status and body temperature status because blood flow in the brain is reduced. Mental status changes, especially confusion, are more common among older adults and may be the first indication of a fluid balance problem. Check to determine whether the patient is alert and oriented. Chapter 43 provides more information about assessment of mental status.

The patient with dehydration often has a low-grade fever, and fever can also cause dehydration. A patient with a temperature higher than 102° F (39° C) for longer than 6 hours is

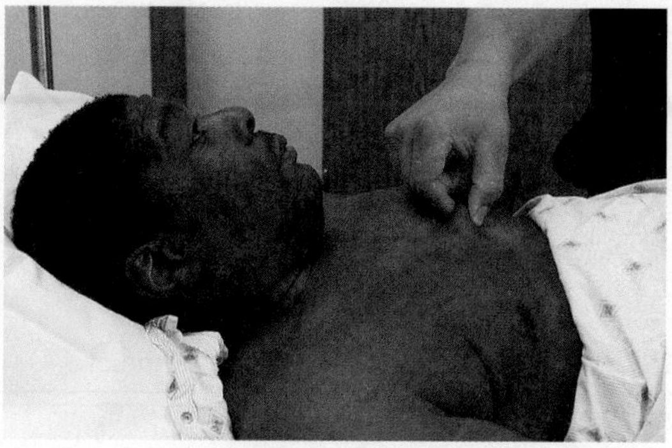

Fig. 13-9 • Examining the skin turgor of an older patient.

especially at risk because the increased body temperature increases the rate at which fluids are lost. For every degree (Celsius) increase in body temperature above normal, a minimum of an additional 500 mL of body fluid is lost. The older adult begins to lose more body water at lower levels of fever.

Renal changes in dehydration affect urine volume and composition. Monitor urine output, comparing total output with total fluid intake and daily weights. The urine may be concentrated, with a specific gravity greater than 1.030. The color is dark amber and has a strong odor. *Urine output below 500 mL/day for any patient without renal disease is cause for concern. Weigh the patient each day at the same time and on the same scale.* When possible, have the patient wear the same amount and type of clothing for each weigh-in. Any weight loss over a half pound per day is fluid loss.

Laboratory Assessment

No single laboratory test result confirms or rules out dehydration. Instead, dehydration is determined by laboratory findings along with clinical manifestations. Usually, laboratory findings with dehydration show elevated levels of hemoglobin, hematocrit, serum osmolarity, glucose, protein, blood urea nitrogen, and various electrolytes because more water is lost and other substances remain, increasing the osmolarity or concentration of the blood **(hemoconcentration).** Hemoconcentration is not present when dehydration is caused by hemorrhage, because loss of all blood and plasma products occurs together.

▪ Common Nursing Diagnoses and Collaborative Problems

Nursing diagnoses and collaborative problems that may apply to patients with dehydration include:

- Deficient Fluid Volume related to excessive fluid loss or inadequate fluid intake
- Decreased Cardiac Output related to decreased plasma volume
- Impaired Oral Mucous Membrane related to inadequate oral secretions
- Confusion (Acute or Chronic) related to neurologic changes
- Risk for Falls related to orthostatic (postural) hypotension
- Risk for Impaired Skin Integrity related to changes in fluid status and skin turgor
- Potential for Dysrhythmias
- Potential for Electrolyte Imbalances

▪ Interventions

Management of dehydration aims to prevent injury, prevent further fluid losses, and increase fluid compartment volumes to normal ranges. Main strategies include patient safety, fluid replacement, and drug therapy.

Patient safety issues and strategies are priorities of care before and during other therapies for dehydration. Monitor vital signs, especially heart rate and blood pressure. The patient with dehydration is at risk for falls because of the accompanying orthostatic hypotension, dysrhythmia, muscle weakness, and possible confusion. Assess his or her muscle strength, gait stability, and level of alertness. Instruct the patient to get up slowly from a lying or sitting position and to immediately sit down if he or she feels light-headed. Implement the falls precautions listed in Chart 13-3.

Chart 13-3 **BEST PRACTICE FOR PATIENT SAFETY & QUALITY CARE**

Falls Precautions

- Assess for orthostatic hypotension.
- Assess muscle strength in legs.
- Orient the patient to the environment.
- Remind the patient to call for help before getting out of bed or a chair.
- Help the patient get out of bed or a chair.
- Provide, or remind the patient to use, a walker or cane for ambulating.
- Help the incontinent patient toilet every 1 to 2 hours.
- Clean up spills immediately.
- Provide adequate lighting at all times, especially at night.
- Keep the call light within reach, and ensure that the patient can use it.
- Place the bed in the lowest position with the brakes locked.
- Place objects that the patient needs within reach.
- Ensure that adequate handrails are present in the patient's room, bathroom, and hall.
- Encourage family members or significant other to stay with the patient.

Chart 13-4 **NIC INTERVENTION ACTIVITIES**

The Patient with Deficient Fluid Volume

Fluid Management: *Promotion of fluid balance and prevention of complications resulting from abnormal or undesired fluid levels*

- Administer IV therapy, as prescribed.
- Give fluids, as appropriate.
- Promote oral intake (e.g., provide a drinking straw, offer fluids between meals, change ice water routinely), as appropriate.
- Distribute the fluid intake over 24 hours, as appropriate.
- Encourage significant other to assist patient with feedings, as appropriate.
- Offer snacks (e.g., frequent drinks and fresh fruits/fruit juice), as appropriate.

NIC intervention activities selected from Bulechek, G.M., Butcher, H.K., & McCloskey Dochterman, J. (Eds.). (2008). *Nursing interventions classification (NIC)* (5th ed.). St. Louis: Mosby. No part of this work is to be altered without prior written permission from the Publisher.

Fluid replacement is key to correcting dehydration. Chart 13-4 lists NIC intervention activities for fluid management. Mild to moderate dehydration is corrected with oral fluid replacement if the patient is alert enough to swallow and can tolerate oral fluids. Verify that he or she does not have a health problem that requires restriction of fluid volume or fluid types. Encourage and measure fluid intake.

Determine whether the patient has any special fluid needs (e.g., sugar-free fluids, thickened fluids). Provide fluids the patient enjoys, and carefully time the intake schedule. Dividing the total amount of fluids needed by nursing shifts helps meet fluid needs more evenly over 24 hours with less danger of overload. Offer the conscious patient small volumes of fluids every hour to increase intake.

Coordinate with unlicensed assistive personnel (UAP) to meet patients' specific fluid needs. Teach UAP to offer 2 to 4 ounces of fluid every hour to patients who are dehydrated or who are at risk for dehydration. If incontinence is a concern, ensure that UAP understand that withholding fluids is not an appropriate means to prevent the problem. Instruct them to take the time to stay with patients while they drink the fluid and to note the exact amounts ingested. Ask UAP to report any difficulties patients may have in swallowing or managing fluids.

Oral rehydration therapy (ORT) is a cost-effective way to replace fluids for the patient with dehydration. Specifically formulated solutions containing glucose and electrolytes are absorbed even when the patient is vomiting or has diarrhea. These are more often used in the home setting, in long-term care, and for patients who have poor veins, making IV therapy difficult. Available ORT solutions for adults include EQUALYTE, Oralyte, and Rehydralyte.

Drug therapy for dehydration is directed at restoring fluid balance and controlling the causes of dehydration. Whenever possible, fluids are replaced orally. When dehydration is severe or life threatening or the patient cannot tolerate oral fluids, IV fluid replacement is needed. Calculation of how much fluid to replace is based on the patient's weight loss and clinical manifestations. The rate of fluid replacement depends on the degree of dehydration and the presence of other cardiac, pulmonary, or renal problems.

The type of fluid prescribed by the health care provider varies with the patient's cardiovascular status and the osmolarity of the blood. Table 13-3 lists the composition of common IV fluids. *The two most important areas to monitor during rehydration are pulse rate and quality and urine output.*

TABLE 13-3 **Characteristics of Common Intravenous Therapy Solutions**

Solution	Osmolarity (mOsm/L)	pH	Calories* (kcal)	Tonicity
0.9% saline	308	5	0	Isotonic
0.45% saline	154	5	0	Hypotonic
5% dextrose in water (D_5W)	272	3.5-6.5	170	Isotonic†
10% dextrose in water ($D_{10}W$)	500	3.5-6.5	340	Hypertonic†
5% dextrose in 0.9% saline	560	3.5-6.5	170	Hypertonic†
5% dextrose in 0.45% saline	406	4	170	Hypertonic†
5% dextrose in 0.225% saline	321	4	170	Isotonic†
Ringer's lactate	273	6.5	9	Isotonic
5% dextrose in Ringer's lactate	525	4-6.5	179	Hypertonic†

Data from Trissel, L. (2007). *Handbook on injectable drugs* (14th ed.). Bethesda, MD: American Society of Hospital-System Pharmacists.

*Calories are calculated on the basis of a volume of 1000 mL.

†*Solution tonicity at the time of administration.* Within a short time after administration, the dextrose is metabolized and the tonicity of the infused solution decreases in proportion to the osmolarity or tonicity of the non-dextrose components (electrolytes) within the water.

Drug therapy may correct some causes of the dehydration. For example, antidiarrheal drugs are prescribed when diarrhea causes dehydration. Antimicrobial therapy may be used in patients with bacterial diarrhea. Antiemetics to control vomiting may be needed when vomiting causes dehydration. Antipyretics to reduce fever are helpful when fever makes dehydration worse.

FLUID OVERLOAD

Pathophysiology

Fluid overload, also called **overhydration,** is an excess of body fluid. It is not a disease but, rather, a clinical sign of a problem in which fluid intake or retention is greater than the body's fluid needs. Fluid overload may be either an actual excess of total body fluid or a relative fluid excess. The most common type of fluid overload is hypervolemia (Fig. 13-10) because the problems result from excessive fluid in the extracellular fluid (ECF) space. Most problems caused by fluid overload are related to fluid volume excess in the vascular space or to dilution of specific electrolytes and blood components. The conditions leading to overhydration (fluid overload) are related to excessive intake or inadequate excretion of fluid. See Table 13-2 for causes of fluid overload. Fig. 13-11 outlines the adaptive changes the body makes in response to mild or moderate fluid overload. When overload is severe or when it occurs in a person with poor cardiac function, fluid overload can lead to heart failure and pulmonary edema.

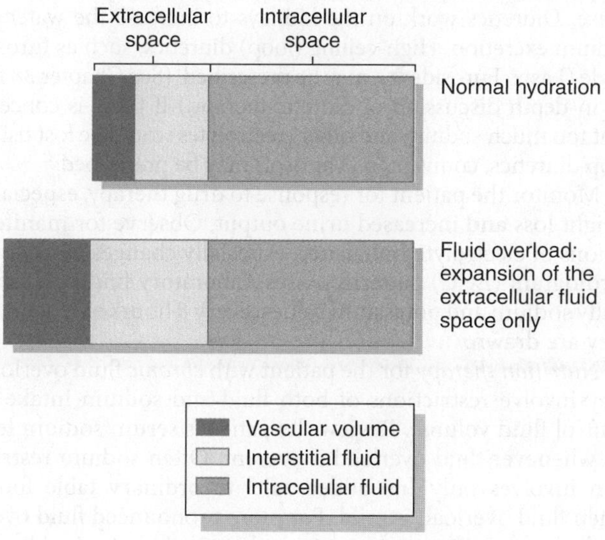
Extracellular space
Intracellular space
Normal hydration
Fluid overload: expansion of the extracellular fluid space only
Vascular volume
Interstitial fluid
Intracellular fluid

Fig. 13-10 • Fluid overload.

Patient-Centered Collaborative Care

Assessment

Patients with fluid overload often have pitting edema (Fig. 13-12). Other manifestations are usually seen in the cardiovascular, respiratory, neuromuscular, integumentary, and gastrointestinal systems (Chart 13-5).

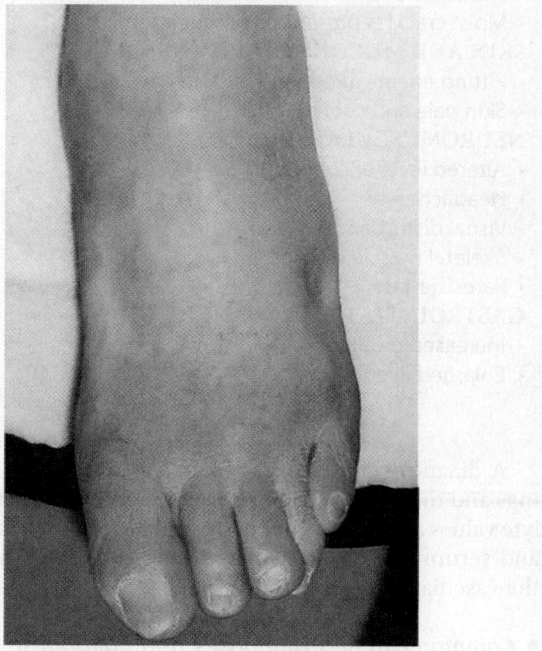

Fig. 13-12 • Pitting edema.

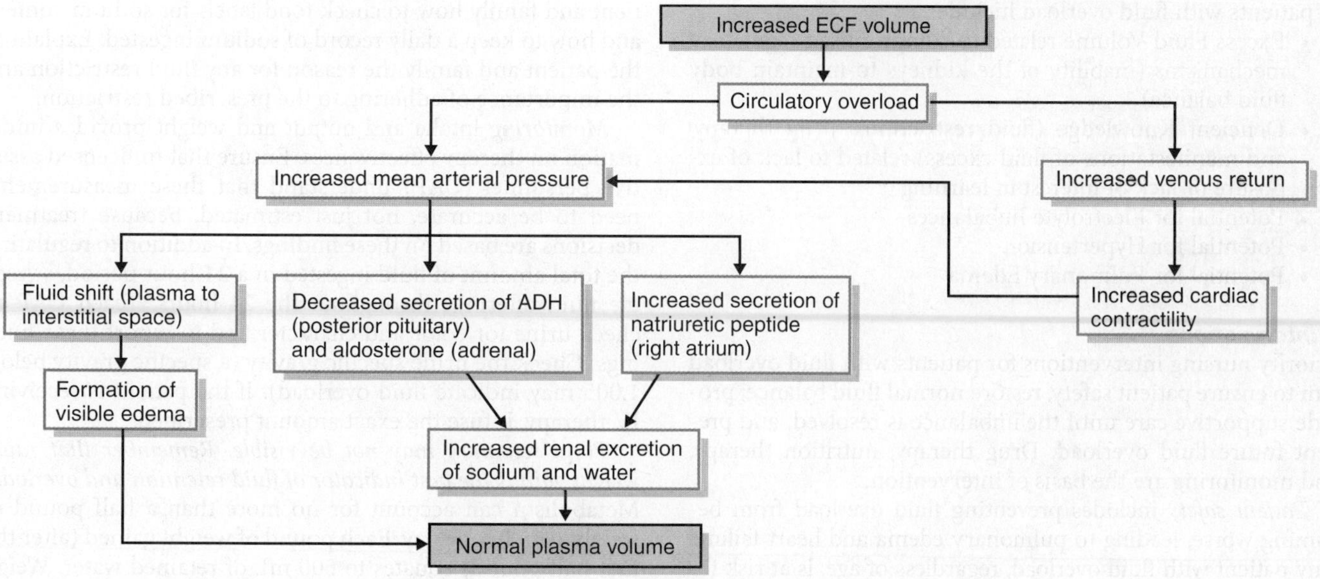
Increased ECF volume
Circulatory overload
Increased mean arterial pressure
Increased venous return
Fluid shift (plasma to interstitial space)
Decreased secretion of ADH (posterior pituitary) and aldosterone (adrenal)
Increased secretion of natriuretic peptide (right atrium)
Increased cardiac contractility
Formation of visible edema
Increased renal excretion of sodium and water
Normal plasma volume

Fig. 13-11 • Adaptive mechanisms associated with fluid overload. (*ADH,* Antidiuretic hormone; *ECF,* extracellular fluid.)

Chart 13-5 KEY FEATURES

Fluid Overload

CARDIOVASCULAR CHANGES
- Increased pulse rate
- Bounding pulse quality
- Full peripheral pulses
- Elevated blood pressure
- Decreased pulse pressure
- Elevated central venous pressure
- Distended neck and hand veins
- Engorged varicose veins
- Weight gain

RESPIRATORY CHANGES
- Increased respiratory rate
- Shallow respirations
- Increased dyspnea with exertion or in the supine position
- Moist crackles present on auscultation

SKIN AND MUCOUS MEMBRANE CHANGES
- Pitting edema in dependent areas
- Skin pale and cool to touch

NEUROMUSCULAR CHANGES
- Altered level of consciousness
- Headache
- Visual disturbances
- Skeletal muscle weakness
- Paresthesias

GASTROINTESTINAL CHANGES
- Increased motility
- Enlarged liver

A diagnosis of fluid overload is based on assessment findings and the results of laboratory tests. Usually, serum electrolyte values are normal, but decreased hemoglobin, hematocrit, and serum protein levels may result from excessive water in the vascular space **(hemodilution).**

Common Nursing Diagnoses and Collaborative Problems

Nursing diagnoses and collaborative problems that may apply to patients with fluid overload include:

- Excess Fluid Volume related to compromised regulatory mechanisms (inability of the kidneys to maintain body fluid balance)
- Deficient Knowledge (fluid restrictions, drug therapy, and manifestations of fluid excess) related to lack of exposure or lack of interest in learning
- Potential for Electrolyte Imbalances
- Potential for Hypertension
- Potential for Pulmonary Edema

Interventions

Priority nursing interventions for patients with fluid overload aim to ensure patient safety, restore normal fluid balance, provide supportive care until the imbalance is resolved, and prevent future fluid overload. Drug therapy, nutrition therapy, and monitoring are the basis of intervention.

Patient safety includes preventing fluid overload from becoming worse, leading to pulmonary edema and heart failure. Any patient with fluid overload, regardless of age, is at risk for these complications. The older adult or one who has co-existing cardiac problems, kidney problems, pulmonary problems, or liver problems is at greater risk.

Monitor for indicators of increased fluid overload (bounding pulse, increasing neck vein distention, presence of crackles in lungs, increasing peripheral edema, reduced urine output) at least every 2 hours. *Pulmonary edema can occur very quickly and can lead to death.* Notify the health care provider of any change that indicates the fluid overload either is not responding to therapy or is becoming worse.

The patient with fluid overload and dependent edema is at risk for skin breakdown. Use a pressure-reducing or pressure-relieving overlay on the mattress. Assess skin pressure areas daily for signs of redness or open areas, especially the coccyx, elbows, hips, and heels. Because many patients with fluid overload may be receiving oxygen by mask or nasal cannula, check the skin around the mask, nares, and ears and under the elastic band for loss of integrity. Assist the patient to change positions every 2 hours, or ensure that others delegated to perform this intervention are diligent in this action.

Drug therapy focuses on removing the excess fluid. Diuretics are prescribed for patients with overload if renal failure is not the cause. Diuretics work on the kidneys to increase the water or sodium excretion. High-ceiling (loop) diuretics, such as furosemide (Lasix, Furoside♣), may be prescribed. (See Chapter 38 for an in-depth discussion of diuretic therapy.) If there is concern that too much sodium and other electrolytes would be lost using loop diuretics, conivaptan (Vaprisol) may be prescribed.

Monitor the patient for response to drug therapy, especially weight loss and increased urine output. Observe for manifestations of electrolyte imbalance, especially changes in electrocardiogram (ECG) patterns. Assess laboratory findings, especially sodium and potassium values, every 8 hours or whenever they are drawn.

Nutrition therapy for the patient with *chronic* fluid overload may involve restrictions of both fluid and sodium intake to control fluid volume. Review the patient's serum sodium levels whenever fluid overload is present. Often sodium restriction involves only "no added salt" to ordinary table foods when fluid overload is mild. For more pronounced fluid overload, the patient may be restricted to 2 g/day to 4 g/day of sodium. When sodium restriction is ongoing, teach the patient and family how to check food labels for sodium content and how to keep a daily record of sodium ingested. Explain to the patient and family the reason for any fluid restriction and the importance of adhering to the prescribed restriction.

Monitoring intake and output and weight provides information on therapy effectiveness. Ensure that unlicensed assistive personnel (UAP) understand that these measurements need to be accurate, not just estimated, because treatment decisions are based on these findings. In addition to regulating the total amount of fluid ingested in a 24-hour period, schedule fluid offerings throughout the 24 hours. Teach UAP to check urine for color and character and to report these findings. Check the urine specific gravity (a specific gravity below 1.005 may indicate fluid overload). If the patient is receiving IV therapy, infuse the exact amount prescribed.

Fluid retention may not be visible. Remember that rapid weight gain is the best indicator of fluid retention and overload. Metabolism can account for no more than a half pound of weight gain in one day. Each pound of weight gained (after the first half pound) equates to 500 mL of retained water. Weigh the patient at the same time every day (before breakfast), using the same scale. Whenever possible, have the patient wear the same type of clothing for each weigh-in.

If the patient either is discharged to home before the fluid overload has completely resolved or has continuing risk for fluid overload, teach him or her and the family to monitor weight at home. Verify that the patient understands the relationship between body weight and fluid balance. Suggest that a record of these daily weights be kept to show the health care provider at checkups. Also, instruct the patient to call his or her health care provider for more than a 3-pound gain in a week or more than a 1- to 2-pound gain in 24 hours.

DECISION-MAKING CHALLENGE
Delegation/Supervision

The nurse is the only RN working the day shift at a large extended-care facility. The unlicensed nursing assistant tells the nurse that Mrs. Fletcher has gained 3 pounds since she was weighed 4 days ago. The patient is 82 years old and has had mild heart failure for 4 years, after an MI. She takes digoxin 0.125 mg daily, furosemide (Lasix) 40 mg daily, and an ACE inhibitor.

1. What other questions should the nurse ask the nursing assistant?
2. What risk factors does this patient have for fluid overload?
3. Should the nurse check this patient's vital signs, or can this action be delegated to the nursing assistant? (Provide a rationale for your decision.)
4. What other assessment findings would support the existence of fluid overload?
5. What should the nurse teach this nursing assistant about this patient's care to ensure the patient's safety?

evolve For suggested answer guidelines, go to http://evolve.elsevier.com/Iggy/.

ELECTROLYTE BALANCE AND IMBALANCES

Electrolytes, or **ions,** are substances in body fluids that carry an electrical charge. **Cations** have positive charges; **anions** have negative charges. Body fluids are electrochemically neutral, which means that the number of positive ions is balanced by an equal number of negative ions. However, the distribution of ions differs in the extracellular fluid (ECF) and the intracellular fluid (ICF) (Fig. 13-13).

Most electrolytes have different concentrations in the ICF and ECF. This concentration difference helps maintain membrane excitability and allows nerve impulse transmission. The normal ranges of electrolyte concentration are very narrow. So, even small changes in these levels can cause major problems.

Electrolyte imbalances can occur in healthy people as a result of changes in fluid intake and output. These imbalances are usually mild and are easily corrected. Severe electrolyte imbalances are life threatening and can occur in any setting. *People at greatest risk for severe imbalances are older patients, patients with chronic renal or endocrine disorders, patients who are mentally impaired, and patients who are taking drugs that alter fluid and electrolyte levels. All ill people are at some risk for electrolyte imbalances.*

Table 13-4 lists major electrolytes, their normal serum levels, and main functions. Most electrolytes enter the body in ingested food. The normal concentration of blood electrolytes changes slightly with the aging process. Chart 13-6 lists the normal electrolyte values for people older than 60 years.

Electrolyte homeostasis is controlled by balancing the dietary intake of electrolytes with the renal excretion or reabsorption of electrolytes. For example, the plasma level of potassium is maintained between 3.5 and 5.0 mmol/L. The high potassium level in common foods could increase the ECF potassium level and lead to major problems. This does not occur because kidney excretion of potassium keeps pace with potassium intake and prevents major changes in the blood potassium level.

CONSIDERATIONS FOR OLDER ADULTS

Older adults are at risk for most electrolyte imbalances as a result of age-related organ changes. For example, older adults have less total body water than younger adults and therefore are more at risk for fluid imbalances. They also are more likely to be taking drugs that affect fluid or electrolyte balance.

SODIUM

Sodium (Na^+), a mineral, is the major cation (positively charged particle) in the extracellular fluid (ECF) and maintains ECF osmolarity. Sodium levels of the ECF are high (135 to

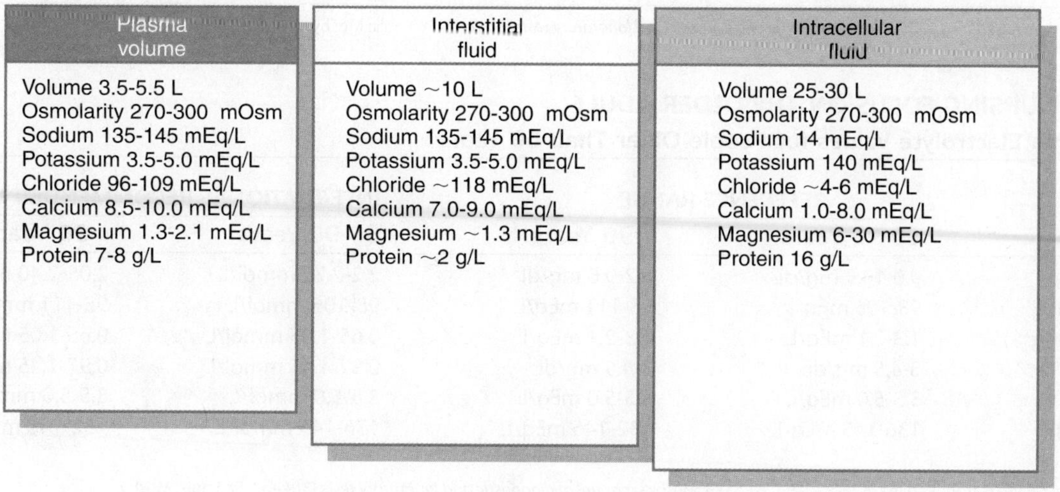
Plasma volume
Volume 3.5-5.5 L
Osmolarity 270-300 mOsm
Sodium 135-145 mEq/L
Potassium 3.5-5.0 mEq/L
Chloride 96-109 mEq/L
Calcium 8.5-10.0 mEq/L
Magnesium 1.3-2.1 mEq/L
Protein 7-8 g/L
Interstitial fluid
Volume ~10 L
Osmolarity 270-300 mOsm
Sodium 135-145 mEq/L
Potassium 3.5-5.0 mEq/L
Chloride ~118 mEq/L
Calcium 7.0-9.0 mEq/L
Magnesium ~1.3 mEq/L
Protein ~2 g/L
Intracellular fluid
Volume 25-30 L
Osmolarity 270-300 mOsm
Sodium 14 mEq/L
Potassium 140 mEq/L
Chloride ~4-6 mEq/L
Calcium 1.0-8.0 mEq/L
Magnesium 6-30 mEq/L
Protein 16 g/L

Fig. 13-13 • The composition of various body fluids.

145 mmol/L), and the intracellular fluid (ICF) sodium levels are low (about 14 mmol/L). Keeping this difference in sodium levels is vital for skeletal muscle contraction, cardiac contraction, nerve impulse transmission, and normal osmolarity and volume of the ECF. Sodium levels and movement influence water balance because "where sodium goes, water follows." The ECF sodium level determines whether water is retained, excreted, or moved from one fluid space to another.

To maintain electrical balance, the sodium (a cation) level within a body fluid must be matched by an equal number of anions (negatively charged substances). Each positive charge in the ECF is balanced by a negative charge so the fluid does not carry either an overall positive or an overall negative charge. When this balance is present, the fluid is electrically neutral. Changes in the plasma sodium level seriously change fluid volume and the distribution of other electrolytes.

Sodium enters the body through the ingestion of many foods and fluids. Foods with the highest sodium levels are those that are processed or preserved, such as ham and smoked or pickled meats. Snack foods are often very high in sodium. Condiments, such as salt, soy sauce, and relishes, are also high in sodium. Foods lowest in sodium include fresh fish and poultry and most fresh vegetables and fruit. The average dietary intake of sodium among North Americans is about 6 to 13 g/day. Sodium is also stored deep within the kidney tissues and can be released to the ECF as needed.

TABLE 13-4 Major Serum Electrolyte Concentrations and Functions

Electrolyte	Reference Range	International Recommended Units	Functions
Sodium (Na^+)	136-145 mEq/L	136-145 mmol/L	Maintenance of plasma and interstitial osmolarity Generation and transmission of action potentials Maintenance of acid-base balance Maintenance of electroneutrality
Potassium (K^+)	3.5-5.0 mEq/L	3.5-5.0 mmol/L	Regulation of intracellular osmolarity Maintenance of electrical membrane excitability Maintenance of plasma acid-base balance
Calcium (Ca^{2+})	9.0-10.5 mg/dL	2.25-2.75 mmol/L	Cofactor in blood-clotting cascade Excitable membrane stabilizer Adds strength/density to bones and teeth Essential element in cardiac, skeletal, and smooth muscle contraction
Chloride (Cl^-)	98-106 mEq/L	98-106 mmol/L	Maintenance of plasma acid-base balance Maintenance of plasma electroneutrality Formation of hydrochloric acid
Magnesium (Mg^{2+})	1.3-2.1 mEq/L	0.65-1.05 mmol/L	Excitable membrane stabilizer Essential element in cardiac, skeletal, and smooth muscle contraction Cofactor in blood-clotting cascade Cofactor in carbohydrate metabolism Cofactor in DNA and protein synthesis
Phosphorus (P)	3.0-4.5 mg/dL	0.97-1.45 mmol/L	Activation of B-complex vitamins Formation of adenosine triphosphate and other high-energy substances Cofactor in carbohydrate, protein, and lipid metabolism

Data from Pagana, K., & Pagana, T. (2006). *Mosby's manual of diagnostic and laboratory tests* (3rd ed.). St. Louis: Mosby.

Chart 13-6 NURSING FOCUS ON THE OLDER ADULT

Normal Plasma Electrolyte Values for People Older Than 60 Years

	REFERENCE RANGE		INTERNATIONAL RECOMMENDED UNITS	
Electrolyte	60-90 Years	>90 Years	60-90 Years	>90 Years
Calcium (Ca^{2+})	9.0-10.5 mg/dL	8.2-9.6 mg/dL	2.2-2.75 mmol/L	2.05-2.40 mmol/L
Chloride (Cl^-)	98-106 mEq/L	98-111 mEq/L	98-106 mmol/L	98-111 mmol/L
Magnesium (Mg^{2+})	1.3-2.1 mEq/L	1.3-2.1 mEq/L	0.65-1.05 mmol/L	0.65-1.05 mmol/L
Phosphorus (P)	3-4.5 mg/dL	3-4.5 mg/dL	0.97-1.45 mmol/L	0.97-1.45 mmol/L
Potassium (K^+)	3.5-5.0 mEq/L	3.5-5.0 mEq/L	3.5-5.0 mmol/L	3.5-5.0 mmol/L
Sodium (Na^+)	136-145 mEq/L	132-146 mEq/L	136-145 mmol/L	132-146 mmol/L

Data for adults 60 to 90 years from Pagana, K., & Pagana, T. (2006). *Mosby's manual of diagnostic and laboratory tests* (3rd ed.). St. Louis: Mosby.
Data for adults >90 years from Tietz, N.W. (Ed.). (1995). *Clinical guide to laboratory tests* (3rd ed.). Philadelphia: Saunders.

Despite variation in sodium intake from one day to the next, the blood sodium level usually remains within the normal range. Serum sodium balance is regulated by the kidney under the influences of aldosterone, antidiuretic hormone (ADH), and natriuretic peptide (NP), as described on p. 175.

Low serum sodium levels inhibit the secretion of ADH and NP and trigger aldosterone secretion. Together these actions increase serum sodium levels by increasing kidney reabsorption of sodium and enhancing kidney loss of water.

High serum sodium levels inhibit aldosterone secretion and directly stimulate secretion of ADH and NP. Together these hormones increase kidney excretion of sodium and kidney reabsorption of water.

HYPONATREMIA

Pathophysiology

Hyponatremia is a serum sodium (Na^+) level below 136 mEq/L (mmol/L). Sodium imbalances often occur with fluid volume imbalances because the same hormones regulate both sodium and water balance. The problems caused by hyponatremia involve two mechanisms—reduced excitable depolarization and cellular swelling.

Excitable cell membrane depolarization depends on high extracellular fluid (ECF) levels of sodium being available to cross cell membranes and move into cells in response to a stimulus. Hyponatremia makes depolarization slower so that excitable membranes are less excitable.

With hyponatremia, the osmolarity of the ECF is lower than that of the intracellular fluid (ICF). As a result, water moves into the cell, causing swelling. Even a small amount of swelling can reduce cell function. Larger amounts of swelling can make the cell burst and die (lysis).

Many conditions and drugs can lead to hyponatremia (Table 13-5). One of the most common causes of low sodium levels is the prolonged use and overuse of diuretics, especially in older adults or in anyone who is also restricting sodium intake. When these drugs are used to manage fluid overload, sodium is lost along with the extra water. Hyponatremia can result from the loss of total body sodium, the movement of sodium from the blood to other fluid spaces, or the dilution of serum sodium from excessive water in the plasma.

TABLE 13-5 Common Causes of Hyponatremia

ACTUAL SODIUM DEFICITS
- Excessive diaphoresis
- Diuretics (high-ceiling diuretics)
- Wound drainage (especially gastrointestinal)
- Decreased secretion of aldosterone
- Hyperlipidemia
- Renal disease (scarred distal convoluted tubule)
- Nothing by mouth
- Low-salt diet

RELATIVE SODIUM DEFICITS (DILUTION)
- Excessive ingestion of hypotonic fluids
- Psychogenic polydipsia
- Freshwater submersion accident
- Renal failure (nephrotic syndrome)
- Irrigation with hypotonic fluids
- Syndrome of inappropriate antidiuretic hormone secretion
- Hyperglycemia
- Heart failure

Patient-Centered Collaborative Care

Assessment

The manifestations of hyponatremia are caused by its effects on excitable cellular activity. The cells especially affected are those involved in cerebral, neuromuscular, and intestinal smooth muscle functions.

Cerebral changes are the most obvious problems of hyponatremia. First establishing the patient's usual cognitive and behavioral patterns is essential because either depressed activity or excessive activity (and sometimes both) may occur. Behavioral changes result from cerebral edema and increased intracranial pressure. Closely observe and document the patient's behavior, level of consciousness, and mental status. A sudden onset of acute confusion or increased confusion is often seen in older adults who have low serum sodium levels.

Neuromuscular changes are seen as general muscle weakness. Assess the patient's neuromuscular status during each nursing shift for changes from baseline. Deep tendon reflexes diminish, and muscle weakness is worse in the legs and arms. Assess muscle strength in several ways, including arm muscle strength and leg muscle strength. Test arm muscle strength first by having the patient squeeze your hand. Another way to test arm muscle strength is to have the patient flex his or her arms against the chest and keep them flexed while you attempt to pull them away from the chest. Test leg muscle strength by having the patient push both feet against a flat surface (like a box or a board) while you apply resistance to the opposite side of the flat surface. *If muscle weakness is present, immediately check respiratory effectiveness because ventilation depends on adequate strength of respiratory muscles.*

Intestinal changes include increased motility, causing nausea, diarrhea, and abdominal cramping. Assess the GI system by listening to bowel sounds and observing stools. Bowel sounds are hyperactive, with rushes and gurgles over the splenic flexure and in the lower left quadrant. Bowel movements are frequent and watery.

Cardiovascular changes are seen as changes in cardiac output. The cardiac responses to hyponatremia with **hypovolemia** (decreased plasma volume) are a rapid, weak, thready pulse. Peripheral pulses are difficult to palpate and are easily blocked with light pressure. Blood pressure is decreased, and the patient may have severe hypotension when moving from a lying or sitting position to a standing position (orthostatic hypotension), leading to light-headedness or dizziness. The central venous pressure is low.

When hyponatremia occurs with **hypervolemia** (fluid overload), cardiac changes include a bounding pulse with normal or high blood pressure. Peripheral pulses are full and difficult to block; however, they may not be palpable if edema is present.

Interventions

The health care provider determines the specific cause of the low sodium level to plan the most appropriate medical treatment. Interventions with drug therapy and nutrition therapy are used to restore serum sodium levels to normal and prevent complications from fluid overload or a too-rapid change in serum sodium level. *The priority for nursing care of the patient with hyponatremia is monitoring the patient's response to therapy to prevent hypernatremia and fluid overload.*

Drug therapy first involves reducing the doses of any drugs that increase sodium loss, such as loop diuretics and thiazide diuretics. Other regimens vary depending on whether fluid imbalance occurs with hyponatremia. When hyponatremia occurs with a fluid deficit, IV saline infusions are prescribed to restore both sodium and fluid volume. Severe hyponatremia may be treated with small-volume infusions of hypertonic (2%-3%) saline. These infusions are delivered through a controller to prevent accidental increases in infusion rate. Monitor the infusion rate and the patient's response.

When hyponatremia occurs with fluid excess, drug therapy includes giving osmotic diuretics that promote the excretion of water rather than sodium, such as mannitol (Osmitrol), or conivaptan (Vaprisol). Assess hourly for signs of excessive fluid loss, potassium loss, and increased sodium levels.

Drug therapy for hyponatremia caused by inappropriate secretion of antidiuretic hormone (ADH) includes agents that antagonize ADH, such as lithium and demeclocycline (Declomycin).

Nutrition therapy can help restore normal sodium balance in mild hyponatremia. Collaborate with the nutritionist to teach the patient about which foods to increase in the diet. Therapy involves increasing oral sodium intake and restricting oral fluid intake. Fluid restriction may be needed long-term when fluid overload is the cause of the hyponatremia or when renal fluid excretion is impaired. Nursing actions for patient safety, skin protection, measurement of fluid intake and output, and patient and family teaching are the same as those for fluid overload on pp. 181-183.

HYPERNATREMIA

Pathophysiology

Hypernatremia is a serum sodium level over 145 mEq/L (mmol/L). High serum sodium levels can be caused by or can cause changes in fluid volumes. Table 13-6 lists common causes of hypernatremia.

As serum sodium level rises, a larger difference in sodium levels occurs between the extracellular fluid (ECF) and the intracellular fluid (ICF). More sodium is present to move rapidly across cell membranes during depolarization, making excitable tissues more easily excited. This condition is called **irritability,** and excitable tissues over-respond to stimuli. In addition, water moves from the cells into the ECF to dilute the hyperosmolar ECF. So, when serum sodium levels are high, severe cellular dehydration occurs. The dehydrated excitable tissues may no longer be able to respond to stimuli.

TABLE 13-6 Common Causes of Hypernatremia

ACTUAL SODIUM EXCESSES
- Hyperaldosteronism
- Renal failure
- Corticosteroids
- Cushing's syndrome or disease
- Excessive oral sodium ingestion
- Excessive administration of sodium-containing IV fluids

RELATIVE SODIUM EXCESSES
- Nothing by mouth
- Increased rate of metabolism
- Fever
- Hyperventilation
- Infection
- Excessive diaphoresis
- Watery diarrhea
- Dehydration

Patient-Centered Collaborative Care

Assessment

The manifestations of hypernatremia vary with the severity of sodium imbalance and whether a fluid imbalance is also present. Changes are first seen in excitable membrane activity, especially cerebral, neuromuscular, and cardiac function.

Nervous system changes start with altered cerebral function. Assess the patient's mental status for attention span, recall of recent events, and cognitive function. In hypernatremia with normal or decreased fluid volumes, the patient may have a short attention span and be agitated or confused about recent events. Manic episodes or seizures may occur if serum sodium continues to rise. When hypernatremia occurs with fluid overload, the patient may be lethargic, drowsy, stuporous, and even comatose.

Skeletal muscle changes vary with the degree of sodium increases. Mild rises cause muscle twitching and irregular muscle contractions. As hypernatremia worsens, the muscles and nerves are less able to respond to a stimulus and muscles become progressively weaker. Deep tendon reflexes are reduced or absent. Muscle weakness occurs bilaterally and has no specific pattern. Observe for twitching in muscle groups. Assess muscle strength by having the patient perform handgrip and arm flexion against resistance as described on p. 185. The advanced practice nurse may check reflexes by lightly tapping the patellar (knee) tendons and Achilles (heel) tendons with a reflex hammer and measuring the movement.

Cardiovascular changes include decreased contractility because high sodium levels slow the movement of calcium into the heart cells. Measure blood pressure and the rate and quality of the apical and peripheral pulses. Pulse rate and blood pressure may be normal, above normal, or below normal, depending on the fluid volume and how rapidly the imbalance occurred.

Pulse rate is increased in patients with hypernatremia and hypovolemia. Peripheral pulses are difficult to palpate and are easily blocked. Hypotension and severe orthostatic (postural) hypotension are present, and pulse pressure is reduced.

Patients with hypernatremia and hypervolemia have slow to normal bounding pulses. Peripheral pulses are full and difficult to block. Neck veins are distended, even with the patient in the upright position. Blood pressure, especially diastolic blood pressure, is increased.

Common Nursing Diagnoses and Collaborative Problems

Nursing diagnoses and collaborative problems that may apply to patients with hypernatremia include:
- Excess Fluid Volume related to excess sodium intake
- Decreased Cardiac Output related to poor cardiac contractility
- Risk for Falls related to skeletal muscle weakness
- Impaired Memory related to fluid and electrolyte imbalances
- Potential for Pulmonary Edema

Interventions

Drug and nutrition therapies aim to prevent further increases in serum sodium and decrease high serum sodium levels. Other medical interventions used when sodium levels become life threatening include hemodialysis and blood ultrafiltration. *Priorities for nursing care of the patient with hypernatremia include monitoring the patient's response to therapy and preventing hyponatremia and dehydration.*

Drug therapy is used to restore fluid balance when hypernatremia is caused by fluid loss. Hypotonic IV infusions, usually 0.225% or 0.45% sodium chloride, are prescribed. Hypernatremia caused by poor renal excretion of sodium requires drug therapy with diuretics that promote sodium loss, such as furosemide (Lasix, Furoside♣) or bumetanide (Bumex). Assess the patient hourly for symptoms of excessive losses of fluid, sodium or potassium.

Nutrition therapy can prevent or correct mild hypernatremia by ensuring adequate water intake, especially among older adults or those who may not have self-access to water. Dietary sodium restriction may be needed to prevent sodium excess when renal problems are present. In addition, fluids must often be restricted. Collaborate with the nutritionist to teach the patient how to determine the sodium content of foods, beverages, and drugs. Nursing actions for patient safety, skin protection, measurement of fluid intake and output, and patient and family teaching are similar to those for fluid overload on pp. 181-183.

POTASSIUM

Potassium (K^+) is the major cation of the intracellular fluid (ICF). The normal plasma potassium level ranges from 3.5 to 5.0 mEq/L or mmol/L (see Table 13-4). The normal ICF potassium level is about 140 mEq/L (mmol/L). Because of its high levels inside cells, potassium has some control over intracellular osmolarity and volume. Keeping this large difference in potassium concentration between the ICF and the extracellular fluid (ECF) is critical for excitable tissues to depolarize and generate action potentials. Other functions of potassium include regulating protein synthesis and regulating glucose use and storage.

Because potassium levels in the blood and interstitial fluid are so low, any change seriously affects physiologic activities. For example, a decrease in blood potassium of only 1 mEq/L (from 4 mEq/L to 3 mEq/L) is a 25% difference in total ECF potassium concentration. In contrast, a 1 mEq/L decrease in blood sodium level (from 130 mEq/L to 139 mEq/L) is, overall, a much smaller change (less than 1%) in total ECF sodium concentration.

Almost all foods contain potassium. It is highest in meat, fish, and many (but not all) vegetables and fruits. It is lowest in eggs, bread, and cereal grains. Potassium intake is about 2 to 20 g/day. Despite heavy potassium intake, the healthy adult keeps plasma potassium levels within the narrow range of normal values needed for physiologic function.

The main controller of ECF potassium level is the sodium-potassium pump within the membranes of all body cells. This pump moves extra sodium ions from the ICF and moves extra potassium ions from the ECF back into the cell. In this way, the serum potassium level remains low and the cellular potassium remains high. At the same time, this action also helps the serum sodium level remain high and the cellular sodium level remain low.

Potassium control also occurs through kidney function, because about 80% of potassium removed from the body occurs via the kidney. Kidney excretion of potassium is enhanced by aldosterone. No hormone has been identified that enhances kidney reabsorption of potassium.

HYPOKALEMIA

Pathophysiology

Because 98% of total body potassium (K^+) is inside cells, minor changes in extracellular potassium levels cause major changes in cell membrane excitability and in other cellular processes. **Hypokalemia** is a serum potassium level below 3.5 mEq/L (mmol/L). *It can be life threatening because every body system is affected.*

Low serum potassium levels increase the difference in the amount of potassium between the fluid inside the cells (ICF) and the fluid outside the cells (ECF). This increased difference reduces the excitability of cells. As a result, the cell membranes of all excitable tissues, such as nerve and muscle, are less responsive to normal stimuli.

When the loss of ECF potassium is gradual, cells adjust and cellular potassium decreases in proportion to the ECF potassium level. The potassium difference between the two fluid spaces remains unchanged, and symptoms of hypokalemia may not appear until the potassium loss is extreme. Rapid reduction of serum potassium levels causes dramatic changes in function.

Hypokalemia may result either from an *actual* total body potassium loss or from the movement of potassium from the ECF to the ICF, causing a *relative* decrease in extracellular potassium level. Table 13-7 lists the common causes of hypokalemia.

Actual potassium depletion occurs when potassium loss is excessive or when potassium intake is not adequate to match normal potassium loss. Relative hypokalemia occurs when total body potassium levels are normal but the potassium distribution between fluid spaces is abnormal.

Patient-Centered Collaborative Care

Assessment

Age is important because renal urine concentration decreases with aging, which increases potassium loss. Older adults are more likely to use drugs that lead to potassium loss.

TABLE 13-7 Common Causes of Hypokalemia

ACTUAL POTASSIUM DEFICITS
- Inappropriate or excessive use of drugs
  - Diuretics
  - Digitalis
  - Corticosteroids
- Increased secretion of aldosterone
- Cushing's syndrome
- Diarrhea
- Vomiting
- Wound drainage (especially gastrointestinal)
- Prolonged nasogastric suction
- Heat-induced excessive diaphoresis
- Renal disease impairing reabsorption of potassium
- Nothing by mouth

RELATIVE POTASSIUM DEFICITS
- Alkalosis
- Hyperinsulinism
- Hyperalimentation
- Total parenteral nutrition
- Water intoxication
- IV therapy with potassium-poor solutions

Drugs, especially diuretics, corticosteroids, and beta-adrenergic agonists or antagonists, can increase potassium loss through the kidneys. Ask about prescription and over-the-counter drug use. A common cause of hypokalemia is the prolonged use and misuse of diuretics. In patients taking digoxin (Lanoxin, Novodigoxin♣), hypokalemia increases the sensitivity of the cardiac muscle to the drug and may result in digoxin toxicity, even when the digoxin level is within the therapeutic range. Ask whether the patient takes a potassium supplement, such as potassium chloride (KCl), or eats foods that have high concentrations of potassium, such as bananas, citrus fruits or juices, raisins, and meat. The patient may not be taking the supplement as prescribed because of its unpleasant taste.

Any acute or chronic disease may lead to potassium loss. Ask the patient about recent illnesses and medical or surgical interventions. A thorough diet history, including a typical day's food and beverage intake, helps identify patients at risk for hypokalemia.

Respiratory changes are likely because of weakness of the muscles needed for breathing. Skeletal muscle weakness results in shallow respirations. *Thus respiratory status should be assessed first in any patient who might have hypokalemia.* Assess the patient's breath sounds, ease of respiratory effort, color of nail beds and mucous membranes, and rate and depth of respiration. Assess respiratory status at least every 2 hours because respiratory insufficiency is a major cause of death.

Musculoskeletal changes include skeletal muscle weakness in response to hypokalemia. A stronger stimulus is needed to begin muscle contraction. A patient may be so weak that he or she is unable to stand. Hand grasps are weak, and a decreased response to deep tendon reflex stimulation **(hyporeflexia)** may be seen. Severe hypokalemia causes flaccid paralysis. Assess for muscle weakness, and determine the patient's ability to perform ADLs.

Cardiovascular changes are assessed by first palpating the peripheral pulses. In the patient with hypokalemia, the pulse is usually thready and weak. Palpation is difficult, and the pulse is easily blocked with light pressure. The pulse rate can range from very slow to very rapid, and an irregular heartbeat (dysrhythmia) may be present. Measure blood pressure with the patient in the lying, sitting, and standing positions, because orthostatic (postural) hypotension occurs with hypokalemia.

Neurologic changes from hypokalemia include altered mental status. The patient may have short-term irritability and anxiety followed by lethargy that progresses to acute confusion and coma as hypokalemia worsens.

Behavioral changes caused by hypokalemia can occur quickly. If needed, obtain information about the patient's behavior from close family members or friends if the patient is confused. The patient may be lethargic and unable to perform simple problem-solving tasks such as counting by threes. As hypokalemia progresses, the patient may become more confused, especially to time and place. In severe hypokalemia, coma may develop.

Intestinal changes occur with hypokalemia because smooth muscle contractions in the intestinal tract are decreased, which leads to decreased peristalsis. The patient has hypoactive bowel sounds and may have nausea, vomiting, constipation, and abdominal distention. Assess distention by measuring abdominal girth. Auscultate for bowel sounds in all four abdominal quadrants to assess the extent of decreased peristalsis. *Severe hypokalemia can cause the absence of peristalsis* **(paralytic ileus).**

Laboratory data confirm hypokalemia (serum potassium value below 3.5 mEq/L (mmol/L). Hypokalemia causes ECG changes in the heart, including ST-segment depression, flat or inverted T waves, and increased U waves. *Dysrhythmias can lead to death, particularly in older adults who are taking digoxin.*

DECISION-MAKING CHALLENGE
Coordination of Care

The patient is a 75-year-old woman who fell when she attempted to get up during intermission while attending a concert with a friend. When asked if she takes any drugs, she tells the nurse that she has been taking Diuril for 20 years to manage her high blood pressure. The only other drugs she takes are an aspirin each day and a multivitamin. She is alert and just a little anxious. Her vital signs are:

T = 98.4° F; P = 102, thready, slightly irregular; R = 30, shallow; BP = 98/50; Spo_2 = 95%

1. What other assessment data should the nurse obtain?
2. What question should the nurse ask about her drug regimen?
3. Should oxygen be applied? Why or why not?
4. Should she be monitored by ECG? Why or why not?

evolve For suggested answer guidelines, go to http://evolve.elsevier.com/Iggy/.

Common Nursing Diagnoses and Collaborative Problems

Nursing diagnoses and collaborative problems that may apply to patients with hypokalemia include:

- Impaired Physical Mobility related to skeletal muscle weakness
- Decreased Cardiac Output related to dysrhythmia
- Risk for Falls related to skeletal muscle weakness
- Constipation related to smooth muscle atony
- Potential for Respiratory Insufficiency

Interventions

Interventions for hypokalemia aim to prevent potassium loss, increase serum potassium levels, and provide a safe environment for the patient. (See Chart 13-7 for NIC interventions for hypokalemia.) Drug and nutrition therapies help restore normal serum potassium levels. *The priorities for nursing care of the patient with hypokalemia are ensuring adequate oxygenation, patient safety for falls prevention, and prevention of injury from potassium administration and monitoring the patient's response to therapy.*

Drug therapy for the treatment and prevention of hypokalemia includes additional potassium and drugs to prevent potassium loss. Most potassium supplements are potassium chloride, potassium gluconate, potassium citrate, and a combination of these salts. The amount and the route of potassium replacement depend on the degree of potassium loss.

Potassium is given IV for severe hypokalemia. The drug is available in different concentrations, and this drug carries a high alert warning as a concentrated electrolyte solution. Although the drug is usually added to the IV solution in the pharmacy, it may be added on the nursing unit. *Check and recheck the concentration of the drug in the vial with another registered nurse, a pharmacist, or a physician, and carefully calculate the required dilution before adding it to the IV solution. A dilution of no more than 1 mEq/10 mL of solution is*

Chart 13-7 NIC INTERVENTION ACTIVITIES

The Patient with Hypokalemia

Electrolyte Management: Hypokalemia: *Promotion of potassium balance and prevention of complications resulting from serum potassium levels lower than desired*

- Monitor lab values associated with hypokalemia (e.g., elevated glucose, metabolic alkalosis, reduced urine osmolality, urine potassium, hypochloremia, and hypocalcemia).
- Administer prescribed supplemental potassium (PO, NG, or IV), per policy.
- Prevent/reduce irritation from potassium supplement (e.g., administer PO or NG potassium supplements during or after meals to minimize GI irritation, dilute IV potassium adequately, administer IV supplement slowly, and apply topical anesthetic to IV site), as appropriate.
- Administer potassium-sparing diuretics (e.g., spironolactone [Aldactone] or triamterene [Dyrenium]), as appropriate.
- Avoid administration of alkaline substances (e.g., IV sodium bicarbonate and PO or NG antacids), as appropriate.
- Monitor neurologic manifestations of hypokalemia (e.g., muscle weakness, altered level of consciousness, drowsiness, apathy, lethargy, confusion, and depression).
- Monitor cardiac manifestations of hypokalemia (e.g., hypotension, broad T wave, U wave, ectopy, tachycardia, and weak pulse).
- Monitor renal manifestations of hypokalemia (e.g., acidic urine, reduced urine osmolality, nocturia, polyuria, and polydipsia).
- Monitor GI manifestations of hypokalemia (e.g., anorexia, nausea, cramps, constipation, distention, and paralytic ileus).
- Monitor pulmonary manifestations of hypokalemia (e.g., hypoventilation and respiratory muscle weakness).
- Monitor for symptoms of respiratory failure (e.g., low Pao_2 and elevated $Paco_2$ levels and respiratory muscle fatigue).
- Monitor for rebound hyperkalemia.

NIC intervention activities selected from Bulechek, G.M., Butcher, H.K., & McCloskey Dochterman, J. (Eds.). (2008). *Nursing interventions classification (NIC)* (5th ed.). St. Louis: Mosby. No part of this work is to be altered without prior written permission from the Publisher.
$Paco_2$, Partial pressure of arterial carbon dioxide; *Pao_2*, partial pressure of arterial oxygen.

recommended. The maximum recommended infusion rate is 5 to 10 mEq/hr; this rate is never to exceed 20 mEq/hr under any circumstances. Older patients may not be able to handle this rate. Because rapid infusion of potassium can cause cardiac arrest, potassium is not given by IV push.

Potassium is a severe tissue irritant and is never given by IM or subcutaneous injection. Tissues damaged by potassium can become necrotic and slough, causing loss of function and requiring reconstructive surgery. IV potassium solutions irritate veins and can cause phlebitis. Check the prescription carefully to ensure that the patient receives the correct amount of potassium. Assess the IV site every 2 hours, and ask the patient whether he or she feels burning or pain at the site. *Stop the IV solution immediately if infiltration occurs, remove the venous access, and notify the health care provider or Rapid Response Team.* Document these actions along with a complete description of the IV site.

Oral potassium preparations may be taken as liquids or solids. Potassium has a strong, unpleasant taste that is difficult to mask, although it can be mixed with many liquids. Some preparations are already flavored. Because potassium chloride can cause nausea and vomiting, give the drug during or after a meal and advise patients using the drug at home not to take it on an empty stomach.

Diuretics that increase the renal excretion of potassium can cause hypokalemia. These classes of diuretics include high-ceiling (loop) diuretics (e.g., furosemide [Lasix, Furoside♣] and bumetanide [Bumex]) and the thiazide diuretics. Avoid these drugs in patients with hypokalemia. A potassium-sparing diuretic may be prescribed for patients with hypokalemia who need diuretic therapy. Potassium-sparing diuretics increase urine output without increasing potassium loss. Potassium-sparing diuretics include spironolactone (Aldactone, Novo-Spiroton♣), triamterene (Dyrenium), and amiloride (Midamor).

Nutrition therapy involves coordination with a nutritionist to teach the patient how to increase dietary potassium intake. Eating foods that are naturally rich in potassium helps prevent further loss, but supplementation is needed to restore normal potassium levels when hypokalemia is present.

Implement safety measures with a patient who has muscle weakness from hypokalemia, including the falls precautions listed in Chart 13-3. Measures include eliminating hazards and assisting with ambulation. Instruct UAP to remove obstacles or slippery areas from the ambulation path, and make certain the patient wears nonslip footgear. Be sure to have the patient wear a gait belt when ambulating with assistance.

Respiratory monitoring is performed at least hourly for severe hypokalemia and includes rate and depth, especially checking for increasing rate and decreasing depth. Also check oxygen saturation by pulse oximetry to determine breathing effectiveness. Assess respiratory muscle effectiveness by checking the patient's ability to cough. Examine the face, oral mucosa, and nail beds for pallor or cyanosis. Evaluate arterial blood gas values (when available) for decreased blood oxygen levels **(hypoxemia)** and increased arterial carbon dioxide levels **(hypercapnia)**, which indicate inadequate breathing effectiveness.

DECISION-MAKING CHALLENGE

Coordination of Care

The 75-year-old patient with hypokalemia described earlier tells the nurse that she took two doses of Diuril today because she and her friend were going to a Chinese restaurant after the concert and she was afraid the salty food would make her hypertension worse. She has not eaten in the past 7 hours and has had only one cup of coffee in the past 4 hours. She says she last saw her doctor 6 months ago and that the blood work done at that time was "okay."

1. Is she at risk for any other fluid or electrolyte imbalance?
2. If so, what specific imbalance(s) and why?
3. What should the nurse teach this patient to prevent future problems with potassium balance?

evolve For suggested answer guidelines, go to http://evolve.elsevier.com/Iggy/.

HYPERKALEMIA

Pathophysiology

Hyperkalemia is a serum potassium level higher than 5.0 mEq/L (mmol/L). The normal range for serum potassium values is narrow, so even slight increases above normal values can affect excitable tissues, especially the heart.

A high serum potassium level decreases the potassium difference between the intracellular fluid (ICF) and the extracellular fluid (ECF). This decreased difference increases cell excitability; as a result, excitable tissues respond to less intense stimuli and may even discharge spontaneously. The heart is very sensitive to serum potassium increases, and the most serious complication of hyperkalemia is altered cardiac function.

The problems that occur with hyperkalemia are related to how rapidly ECF potassium levels increase. Sudden rises in serum potassium cause severe problems at potassium levels between 6 and 7 mEq/L. When serum potassium rises slowly, problems may not occur until potassium levels reach 8 mEq/L or higher.

Hyperkalemia may result from an actual increase in total body potassium or from the movement of potassium from the cells into the blood. Hyperkalemia is rare in people with normal kidney function. Most cases of hyperkalemia occur in hospitalized patients and in those undergoing medical treatment. Those at greatest risk for hyperkalemia are chronically ill patients, debilitated patients, and older adults. Table 13-8 lists common causes of hyperkalemia.

Patient-Centered Collaborative Care

Assessment

Age is important because renal function decreases with aging. Ask about chronic illnesses (particularly renal disease and diabetes mellitus), recent medical or surgical treatment, and urine output, including frequency and amount of voidings. Ask about drug use, particularly potassium-sparing diuretics and angiotensin-converting enzyme (ACE) inhibitors. Obtain a diet history to determine the intake of potassium-rich foods and the use of salt substitutes (which contain potassium).

Collect data regarding symptoms related to hyperkalemia. Ask whether the patient has had palpitations, skipped heartbeats, other cardiac irregularities, muscle twitching, weakness in the leg muscles, or unusual tingling or numbness in the hands, feet, or face. Ask about recent changes in bowel habits, especially diarrhea.

Cardiovascular changes are the most severe problems from hyperkalemia and are the most common cause of death in patients with hyperkalemia. Cardiac manifestations of hyperkalemia include bradycardia, hypotension, and ECG changes of tall, peaked T waves, prolonged PR intervals, flat or absent P waves, and wide QRS complexes. As serum potassium levels rise, heartbeats generated outside the normal conduction system in the ventricles **(ectopic beats)** may appear. Complete heart block, asystole, and ventricular fibrillation are life-threatening complications of severe hyperkalemia.

Neuromuscular changes with hyperkalemia have two phases. Skeletal muscles twitch in the early stages of hyperkalemia, and the patient may be aware of tingling and burning sensations followed by numbness in the hands and feet and around the mouth **(paresthesia).** As hyperkalemia worsens, muscle twitching changes to weakness followed by flaccid paralysis. The weakness moves up from the hands and feet and first affects the muscles of the arms and legs. Respiratory muscles are not affected until serum potassium levels reach lethal levels.

Intestinal changes include increased motility. The patient may have diarrhea and spastic colonic activity. Bowel sounds are hyperactive, with audible rushes and gurgles. Bowel movements are frequent and watery.

Laboratory data confirm hyperkalemia (potassium level over 5.0 mEq/L). If it is caused by dehydration, levels of other electrolytes, hematocrit, and hemoglobin also are elevated. Hyperkalemia caused by renal failure occurs with elevated serum creatinine and blood urea nitrogen, decreased blood pH, and normal or low hematocrit and hemoglobin levels.

Interventions

Interventions for hyperkalemia are aimed at rapidly reducing the serum potassium level, preventing recurrences, and ensuring patient safety during the electrolyte imbalance. Drug therapy is the main medical intervention. *The priorities for nursing care of the patient with hyperkalemia are monitoring to prevent cardiac complications, patient safety for falls prevention, monitoring the patient's response to therapy, and health teaching.*

Drug therapy can restore normal potassium balance by enhancing potassium excretion and promoting the movement of potassium from the extracellular fluid (ECF) into the cells.

Eliminate extra potassium by stopping potassium-containing infusions. Keeping the IV catheter open is useful in managing hyperkalemia. Withhold oral potassium supplements, and provide a potassium-restricted diet.

Increasing potassium excretion helps reduce hyperkalemia if renal function is normal. Potassium-excreting diuretics, such as furosemide, are prescribed. For a patient with renal problems, drug therapy to increase potassium excretion includes cation exchange resins that promote intestinal sodium absorption and potassium excretion, such as sodium polystyrene sulfonate (Kayexalate). However, this therapy may take many hours to reduce potassium levels. If potassium levels are dangerously high, additional measures, such as dialysis, are needed.

Movement of potassium from the extracellular fluid (ECF) to the intracellular fluid (ICF) can help reduce serum potassium levels temporarily. Potassium movement into the cells is enhanced by insulin. Insulin increases the activity of the sodium-

TABLE 13-8 Common Causes of Hyperkalemia

ACTUAL POTASSIUM EXCESSES
- Overingestion of potassium-containing foods or medications
  - Salt substitutes
  - Potassium chloride
  - Rapid infusion of potassium-containing IV solution
  - Bolus IV potassium injections
- Transfusions of whole blood or packed cells
- Adrenal insufficiency (Addison's disease, adrenalectomy)
- Renal failure
- Potassium-sparing diuretics

RELATIVE POTASSIUM EXCESSES
- Tissue damage
- Acidosis
- Hyperuricemia
- Uncontrolled diabetes mellitus

potassium pumps, which move potassium from the ECF into the cell. IV fluids containing glucose and insulin are prescribed to help decrease serum potassium levels (usually 100 mL of 10% to 20% glucose with 10 to 20 units of regular insulin). These IV solutions are hypertonic and are infused through a central line or in a vein with a high blood flow to avoid local vein inflammation. Observe the patient for manifestations of hypokalemia and hypoglycemia during this therapy.

Cardiac monitoring allows for the early recognition of dysrhythmias and other manifestations of hyperkalemia on cardiac muscle. Compare recent ECG tracings with the patient's baseline tracings or with tracings obtained when the patient's serum potassium level was close to normal. *Notify the health care provider or Rapid Response Team if the patient's heart rate falls below 60 beats per minute or if the T waves become spiked.*

Health teaching is key to the prevention of hyperkalemia and the early detection of complications. The teaching plan for the patient at risk for hyperkalemia includes diet, drugs, and recognition of the manifestations of hyperkalemia. Collaborate with the nutritionist to teach the patient and family about which foods to avoid (those high in potassium). Foods that contain little potassium and are allowed are listed in Chart 13-8. Instruct the patient and family to read the labels on drug and food packages to determine the potassium content. Warn them to avoid salt substitutes, which contain potassium.

Chart 13-8 PATIENT AND FAMILY EDUCATION GUIDE

Dietary Management of Hyperkalemia

YOU SHOULD AVOID

- Meats, especially organ meat and preserved meat
- Dairy products
- Dried fruit
- Fruits high in potassium
  - Bananas
  - Cantaloupe
  - Kiwi
  - Oranges
- Vegetables high in potassium
  - Avocados
  - Broccoli
  - Dried beans or peas
  - Lima beans
  - Mushrooms
  - Potatoes (white or sweet)
  - Seaweed
  - Soybeans
  - Spinach

YOU MAY EAT

- Eggs
- Breads
- Butter
- Cereals
- Sugar
- Fruits low in potassium (fresh, frozen, or canned)
  - Apples
  - Apricots
  - Berries
  - Cherries
  - Grapefruit
  - Peaches
  - Pineapple
  - Cranberries
- Vegetables low in potassium
  - Alfalfa sprouts
  - Cabbage
  - Carrots
  - Cauliflower
  - Celery
  - Eggplant
  - Green beans
  - Lettuce
  - Onions
  - Peas
  - Peppers
  - Squash

Data from Pennington, J. (2004). *Bowe's and Church's food values of portions commonly used* (18th ed.). Philadelphia: Lippincott-Raven.

CALCIUM

Calcium (Ca^{2+}) is a mineral with functions closely related to those of phosphorus and magnesium. Calcium is an ion having two positive charges **(divalent cation)** that exists in the body in a bound form and an ionized (unbound or free) form.

Bound calcium is usually attached to serum proteins, especially albumin. Ionized calcium is present in the blood and other extracellular fluid (ECF) as free calcium. Free calcium is the active form and must be kept within a narrow range in the ECF. The body functions best when blood calcium levels are maintained between 9.0 and 10.5 mg/dL, or between 2.25 and 2.75 mmol/L (see Table 13-4). Calcium has a steep gradient between ECF and intracellular fluid (ICF) because the amount of calcium in the ICF is very low. This mineral is important for maintaining bone strength and density, activating enzymes, allowing skeletal and cardiac muscle contraction, controlling nerve impulse transmission, and allowing blood clotting.

Calcium enters the body by dietary intake and absorption through the intestinal tract. Dairy products are common foods high in calcium. Absorption of dietary calcium requires the active form of vitamin D. Calcium is stored in the bones. When both plasma calcium levels and stored calcium levels are adequate, intestinal absorption of dietary calcium is reduced and urine excretion of excess calcium increases. When more calcium is needed, *parathyroid hormone (PTH)* is released from the parathyroid glands. PTH increases serum calcium levels by releasing free calcium from bone storage sites (bone resorption of calcium), stimulating vitamin D activation to help increase intestinal absorption of dietary calcium, inhibiting kidney calcium excretion, and stimulating kidney calcium reabsorption.

When excess calcium is present in plasma, PTH secretion is inhibited and the secretion of *thyrocalcitonin (TCT)*, a hormone secreted by the thyroid gland, is increased. TCT causes the plasma calcium level to decrease by inhibiting bone resorption of calcium, inhibiting vitamin D–associated intestinal uptake of calcium, and increasing kidney excretion of calcium in the urine.

HYPOCALCEMIA

Pathophysiology

Hypocalcemia is a total serum calcium (Ca^{2+}) level below 9.0 mg/dL or 2.25 mmol/L. Calcium is stored in bone, with only a small amount of total body calcium present in extracellular fluid

TABLE 13-9 Common Causes of Hypocalcemia

ACTUAL CALCIUM DEFICITS
- Inadequate oral intake of calcium
- Lactose intolerance
- Malabsorption syndromes
  - Celiac sprue
  - Crohn's disease
- Inadequate intake of vitamin D
- End-stage kidney disease
- Renal failure—polyuric phase
- Diarrhea
- Steatorrhea
- Wound drainage (especially gastrointestinal)

RELATIVE CALCIUM DEFICITS
- Hyperproteinemia
- Alkalosis
- Calcium chelators or binders
- Citrate
- Mithramycin
- Penicillamine
- Sodium cellulose phosphate (Calcibind)
- Aredia
- Acute pancreatitis
- Hyperphosphatemia
- Immobility
- Removal or destruction of parathyroid glands

(ECF). Because the normal blood level of calcium is so low, any change in calcium levels has major effects on function.

Calcium is an excitable membrane stabilizer, regulating depolarization and the generation of action potentials. It decreases sodium movement across excitable membranes, slowing the rate of depolarization. Low serum calcium levels increase sodium movement across excitable membranes, allowing depolarization to occur more easily and at inappropriate times.

Hypocalcemia is caused by many chronic and acute conditions, as well as medical or surgical treatments. Table 13-9 lists the common causes of hypocalcemia. Acute hypocalcemia results in the rapid onset of life-threatening manifestations, even when the serum calcium level is not very low. Chronic hypocalcemia occurs slowly over time, and excitable membrane manifestations may not be severe because the body has adjusted to the gradual reduction of serum calcium levels.

Actual calcium loss (a reduction in total body calcium) occurs when the absorption of calcium from the GI tract slows or when calcium is lost from the body. Relative calcium loss causes total body calcium amounts to remain normal while serum calcium levels are low. This problem occurs when the unbound calcium in the body is reduced or when parathyroid gland function is decreased.

CULTURAL AWARENESS

Lactose intolerance caused by a deficiency of the enzyme *lactase* occurs in 75% to 90% of all Asians, African Americans, and American Indians (McCance & Huether, 2006). Although this problem also does occur in Caucasians, the incidence is much higher in nonwhites. People with lactose intolerance cannot use the nutrients in milk and have cramping, diarrhea, and abdominal pain after ingesting dairy products. Dairy products, especially milk, are common and rich sources of both calcium and vitamin D. People with lactose intolerance may, therefore, have difficulty obtaining enough calcium and vitamin D from other sources to maintain normal calcium levels in the blood and bones.

WOMEN'S HEALTH CONSIDERATIONS

Postmenopausal women are at risk for chronic calcium loss. This problem is related to reduced weight-bearing activities and a decrease in estrogen levels. In general, women have smaller frames than men and the female skeleton does not bear as much weight as the male skeleton. As they age, many women decrease weight-bearing activities such as running and walking. Osteoporosis occurs when weight-bearing activity decreases or is limited. In addition, the estrogen secretion that protects against osteoporosis diminishes. All of these factors increase the risk for calcium loss in postmenopausal women (see Chapter 53 for a complete discussion of osteoporosis).

Patient-Centered Collaborative Care

Assessment

The diet history is important to assess for the risk of hypocalcemia. Ask the patient about his or her intake of dairy products and whether a calcium supplement is taken regularly.

One indicator of hypocalcemia is a report of frequent, painful muscle spasms ("charley horses") in the calf or foot during rest or sleep. Other information that indicates possible hypocalcemia is a history of recent orthopedic surgery or bone healing. Endocrine disturbances and treatments are risk factors for hypocalcemia. A history of thyroid surgery, therapeutic irradiation of the upper middle chest and neck area, or a recent anterior neck injury increase the risk for hypocalcemia. Most manifestations of acute hypocalcemia are caused by overstimulation of the nerves and muscles.

Neuromuscular changes often occur first in the hands and feet. Paresthesias occur at first, with sensations of tingling and numbness. If hypocalcemia continues or worsens, actual muscle twitching or painful cramps and spasms occur. Tingling may also affect the lips, nose, and ears. These problems may signal the onset of neuromuscular overstimulation and tetany.

Assess for hypocalcemia by testing for Trousseau's and Chvostek's signs. To test for Trousseau's sign, place a blood pressure cuff around the upper arm, inflate the cuff to greater than the patient's systolic pressure, and keep the cuff inflated for 1 to 4 minutes. Under these hypoxic conditions, a positive Trousseau's sign occurs when the hand and fingers go into spasm in palmar flexion (Fig. 13-14). To test for Chvostek's sign, tap the face just below and in front of the ear (over the facial nerve) to trigger facial twitching of one side of the mouth, nose, and cheek (Fig. 13-15).

Cardiovascular changes involve heart rate and ECG changes. The heart rate may be slower or slightly faster than normal, with a weak, thready pulse. Severe hypocalcemia causes severe hypotension and ECG changes of a prolonged ST interval and a prolonged QT interval.

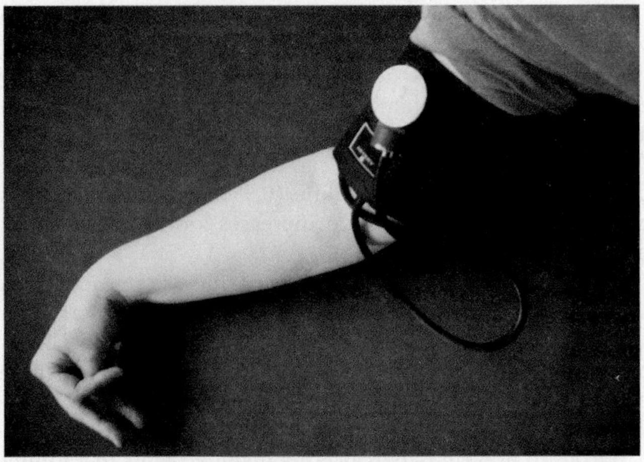

Fig. 13-14 • Palmar flexion–positive Trousseau's sign in hypocalcemia.

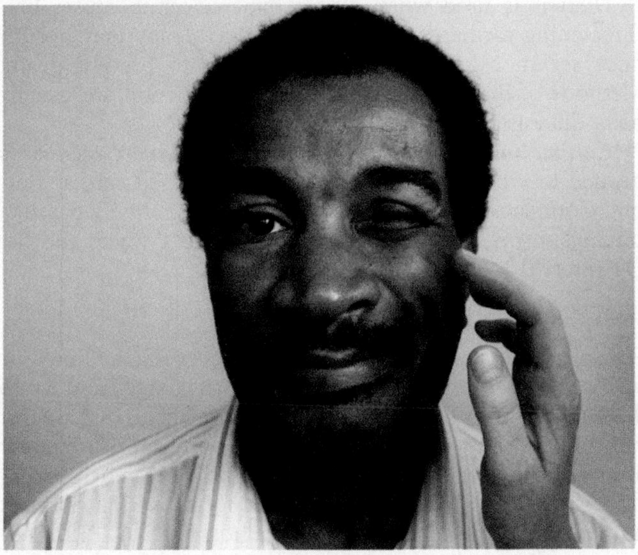

Fig. 13-15 • Facial muscle response–positive Chvostek's sign in hypocalcemia.

Intestinal changes include increased peristaltic activity. Auscultate the abdomen for hyperactive bowel sounds. The patient may report painful abdominal cramping and diarrhea.

Skeletal changes are most common with chronic hypocalcemia. Calcium is moved from bone storage sites, causing a loss of bone density (osteoporosis). The bones are thinner, more brittle, and fragile. These bones break easily with even slight trauma. Vertebrae become more compact and may bend forward, leading to an overall loss of height. See Chapter 53 for more discussion about osteoporosis.

Ask about changes in height and any unexplained bone pain. Observe for spinal curvatures and any unusual bumps or protrusions in bone areas that may indicate old fractures.

Common Nursing Diagnoses and Collaborative Problems

Nursing diagnoses that may apply to patients with hypocalcemia include:

- Acute Pain related to hypocalcemia-induced muscle spasms and hyperactive gastric motility
- Decreased Cardiac Output related to hypocalcemia-induced dysrhythmias or reduced myocardial contractility
- Deficient Knowledge (dietary calcium) related to lack of exposure
- Risk for Injury related to bone density loss

Interventions

Interventions aim to restore normal calcium levels and prevent complications. These include drug therapy, nutrition therapy, reducing environmental stimuli, and preventing injury.

Drug therapy for hypocalcemia includes direct calcium replacement (oral and IV) and drugs that enhance the absorption of calcium, such as aluminum hydroxide and vitamin D. When neuromuscular manifestations are troublesome, drugs that decrease nerve and muscle responses may be used also. These drugs may include magnesium sulfate and various muscle relaxants.

Nutrition therapy involves a high-calcium diet for patients with mild hypocalcemia and for those with chronic conditions that cause them to be at continuous risk for hypocalcemia. Coordinate with the nutritionist to assist the patient in selecting calcium-rich foods.

Environmental management is needed because the excitable membranes of the nervous system and the skeletal system are overstimulated in hypocalcemia. Interventions to reduce stimulation include keeping the room quiet, limiting visitors, adjusting the lighting, and using a soft but reassuring voice.

Use seizure precautions for the patient with hypocalcemia. Such precautions include padding the siderails of the bed and keeping emergency equipment (e.g., oxygen, suction) at the bedside. Keep an emergency cart equipped with emergency drugs and an endotracheal tray just outside the patient's room.

Injury prevention strategies are needed because the patient with long-standing calcium loss may have brittle, fragile bones that fracture easily and cause little pain. When lifting or moving a patient with fragile bones, use a lift sheet rather than pulling the patient. Observe for normal range of joint motion and for any unusual surface bumps or depressions over bony areas.

HYPERCALCEMIA

Pathophysiology

Hypercalcemia is a total serum calcium level above 10.5 mg/dL or 2.75 mmol/L. Because the normal range for serum calcium is so narrow, even small increases have severe effects. Although the effects of hypercalcemia occur first in excitable tissues, all systems are affected.

Hypercalcemia means either that the amount of serum calcium is so great that the normal calcium-controlling mechanisms cannot keep pace or that at least one control mechanism is not functioning properly (Table 13-10). Hypercalcemia causes excitable tissues to be less sensitive to normal stimuli, thus requiring a stronger stimulus to function. The excitable tissues affected most by hypercalcemia are the heart, muscles, nerves, and intestinal smooth muscles.

Calcium is needed by many of the enzymes involved in blood clotting. Hypercalcemia causes faster clotting times. Clots may form when they are not needed to control bleeding. Excessive clotting from hypercalcemia occurs more easily in vessels with slow blood flow.

TABLE 13-10 Common Causes of Hypercalcemia

ACTUAL CALCIUM EXCESSES
• Excessive oral intake of calcium
• Excessive oral intake of vitamin D
• Renal failure
• Use of thiazide diuretics
RELATIVE CALCIUM EXCESSES
• Hyperparathyroidism
• Malignancy
• Direct invasion (cancers of breast, lung, prostate, and osteoclastic bone and multiple myeloma)
• Indirect resorption (liver cancer, small cell lung cancer, and cancer of the adrenal gland)
• Hyperthyroidism
• Immobility
• Use of glucocorticoids
• Dehydration

Patient-Centered Collaborative Care

Assessment

The manifestations of hypercalcemia are related to its severity and how quickly the imbalance occurred. The patient with a mild but rapidly occurring calcium excess usually has more severe problems than the patient whose imbalance is severe but has developed slowly.

Cardiovascular changes are the most serious and life-threatening problems of hypercalcemia. Mild hypercalcemia at first causes increased heart rate and blood pressure. Severe or prolonged calcium imbalance depresses electrical conduction, slowing heart rate.

Measure pulse rate and blood pressure, and observe for indications of poor tissue blood flow, such as cyanosis and pallor. Examine ECG tracings for dysrhythmias, especially a shortened QT interval.

Hypercalcemia allows blood clots to form more easily whenever blood flow is poor. Blood clotting is more likely in the lower legs, the pelvic region, areas where blood flow is blocked by internal or external constrictions, and areas where venous obstruction occurs.

Assess for slowed or impaired blood flow. Measure and record calf circumferences with a soft tape measure. Assess the feet for temperature, color, and capillary refill to determine the blood flow to and from the area.

Neuromuscular changes include severe muscle weakness and decreased deep tendon reflexes without paresthesia. The patient may have an altered level of consciousness that can range from confusion and lethargy to coma. Psychiatric problems also can occur.

Intestinal changes are first reflected as decreased peristalsis. Constipation, anorexia, nausea, vomiting, and abdominal pain are common. Bowel sounds are hypoactive or absent. The abdomen increases in size because the intestinal contents remain in the tract instead of being moved forward. Assess abdominal size by measuring abdominal girth with a soft tape measure in a line circling the abdomen at the umbilicus.

Interventions

Interventions for hypercalcemia aim to reduce serum calcium levels through drug therapy and dialysis. Rehydration and cardiac monitoring are also important.

Drug therapy involves preventing increases in calcium, as well as drugs to lower calcium levels. IV solutions containing calcium (e.g., Ringer's lactate) are stopped. Oral drugs containing calcium or vitamin D (e.g., calcium-based antacids) are discontinued.

Fluid volume replacement can help restore normal serum calcium levels. IV normal saline (0.9% sodium chloride) is usually given because sodium increases kidney excretion of calcium.

Thiazide diuretics are discontinued and are replaced with diuretics that enhance the excretion of calcium, such as furosemide (Lasix, Furoside♣). Calcium chelators (calcium binders) help lower serum calcium levels. Such drugs include plicamycin (Mithracin) and penicillamine (Cuprimine, Pendramine♣).

Drugs to prevent hypercalcemia include agents that inhibit calcium resorption from bone, such as phosphorus, calcitonin (Calcimar), bisphosphonates (etidronate), and prostaglandin synthesis inhibitors (aspirin, NSAIDs).

Dialysis is used when severe hypercalcemia causes life-threatening cardiac problems and drug therapy may not reduce serum calcium levels fast enough to prevent death. Methods of dialysis for rapid calcium reduction are usually hemodialysis or blood ultrafiltration.

Cardiac monitoring of patients with hypercalcemia is needed to identify dysrhythmias and decreased cardiac output. Compare recent ECG tracings with the patient's baseline tracings. Especially look for changes in the T waves and the QT interval and changes in rate and rhythm.

PHOSPHORUS

Phosphorus (P) is in the body in both inorganic and organic forms. Normal serum levels of phosphorus range from 3.0 to 4.5 mg/dL, or 0.97 to 1.45 mmol/L (see Table 13-4). Most phosphorus (80%) can be found in the bones. It is the major anion in the ICF, and its levels inside cells are much higher than in the ECF. Phosphorus is needed for activating vitamins and enzymes, forming adenosine triphosphate (ATP) for energy supplies, and assisting in cell growth and metabolism. It also functions in acid-base balance and calcium homeostasis.

The average North American diet is high in phosphorus (1 to 2 g/day). Food sources of phosphorus include meats, fish, dairy products, and nuts.

Phosphorus balance and calcium balance are intertwined. Plasma levels of calcium and phosphorus exist in a balanced, reciprocal relationship, which means that when you multiply the two values, the product remains constant. Therefore a change in the amount of plasma phosphorus results in an equal and opposite change in the amount of plasma calcium (and vice versa).

The regulation of ECF phosphorus occurs through the activity of parathyroid hormone (PTH). Increased PTH levels cause a net loss of phosphorus. Reduced PTH levels enhance kidney reabsorption of phosphorus, resulting in increased plasma levels of phosphorus.

HYPOPHOSPHATEMIA

Pathophysiology

Hypophosphatemia is a serum phosphorus level below 3.0 mEq/L. Even though the serum level has a narrow range of normal (3.0 to 4.5 mEq/L), body functions are not usually impaired with rapid, wide changes in serum phosphorus lev-

TABLE 13-11 Common Causes of Phosphorus Imbalance

HYPOPHOSPHATEMIA
- Malnutrition
- Starvation
- Use of aluminum hydroxide–based antacids
- Use of magnesium-based antacids
- Hyperparathyroidism
- Hypercalcemia
- Renal failure
- Malignancy
- Hyperglycemia
- Hyperalimentation
- Respiratory alkalosis
- Uncontrolled diabetes mellitus
- Alcohol abuse

HYPERPHOSPHATEMIA
- Decreased renal excretion resulting from renal insufficiency
- Tumor lysis syndrome
- Increased intake of phosphorus
- Hypoparathyroidism

els. Reduced function occurs more often with chronic hypophosphatemia.

Most of the effects of hypophosphatemia are related to decreased energy metabolism and imbalances of other electrolytes and body fluids. Because of the relationship between phosphorus and calcium, *decreases* in serum phosphorus levels cause *increases* in serum calcium levels.

Three main processes lead to decreased serum phosphorus levels: decreased absorption of phosphorus, increased excretion of phosphorus, and intracellular phosphorus shift (Table 13-11).

Patient-Centered Collaborative Care

Assessment

Manifestations occur when low serum phosphorus levels are severe or prolonged. They are related to the decreased amounts of high-energy compounds (e.g., adenosine triphosphate [ATP]) needed for normal metabolism. Manifestations are most apparent in the cardiac, musculoskeletal, hematologic, and central nervous systems.

Cardiac changes include decreased stroke volume and decreased cardiac output. Peripheral pulses are slow, difficult to find, and easy to block. Cardiac depression is caused by low stores of intracellular energy. Without sufficient energy in myocardial cells, contractions are weak and ineffective. Prolonged hypophosphatemia causes progressive but reversible cardiac muscle damage.

Musculoskeletal changes include weak skeletal muscles that may progress to acute muscle breakdown **(rhabdomyolysis).** The weakness is generalized, and paresthesias usually are not present. When muscle weakness becomes profound, respiratory movements are ineffective, leading to respiratory failure. Assess for muscle strength, and observe respiratory effort.

The manifestations of *chronic* hypophosphatemia are most evident in the skeletal system. Bone density is decreased, which leads to fractures and changes in bone shape. These changes are caused by the bone calcium loss that occurs with hypophosphatemia. Assess the patient for unusual lumps or depressions over bony areas that indicate bone fractures.

Chart 13-9 PATIENT AND FAMILY EDUCATION GUIDE
Dietary Management of Hypophosphatemia

YOU SHOULD AVOID	YOU MAY EAT
Milk	Fish
Cheese	Beef
Yogurt	Chicken
Collard greens	Pork
Rhubarb	Organ meats
	Nuts
	Whole-grain breads and cereals

Central nervous system changes are not apparent until hypophosphatemia is severe. These first appear as irritability and may progress to seizure activity followed by coma.

Interventions

Drugs that promote phosphorus loss (e.g., antacids, osmotic diuretics, calcium supplements) are discontinued. Oral replacement of phosphorus along with a vitamin D supplement may correct moderate hypophosphatemia. IV phosphorus is given only when serum phosphorus levels fall below 1 mg/dL and the patient has serious manifestations. Infuse IV phosphorus slowly because the problems caused by hyperphosphatemia are equally serious.

Nutrition therapy involves increasing the intake of phosphorus-rich foods while decreasing the intake of calcium-rich foods (Chart 13-9). Collaborate with the nutritionist to teach the patient and family which foods to eat and which to avoid.

HYPERPHOSPHATEMIA

Hyperphosphatemia is a serum phosphorus level above 4.5 mEq/L. High levels are well tolerated by most body systems.

The problems caused by hyperphosphatemia center on the hypocalcemia that results when serum phosphorus levels increase. These problems include increased membrane excitability (see pp. 192-193).

Causes of increased serum phosphorus levels include renal insufficiency, certain cancer treatments, increased phosphorus intake, and hypoparathyroidism. Table 13-11 lists common causes of hyperphosphatemia.

Hyperphosphatemia causes few direct problems with body function. However, hypocalcemia is usually present because calcium and phosphorus exist in the blood in a balanced reciprocal relationship: when one increases, the other decreases. The hypocalcemia greatly alters many body system functions and can cause life-threatening side effects. Thus the management of hyperphosphatemia entails the management of hypocalcemia (see p. 193).

MAGNESIUM

Magnesium (Mg^{2+}) is a mineral that forms a cation when dissolved in water. Adults have an average total body level of 25 g of magnesium, most of which (60%) is stored in bones and cartilage. Little magnesium is present in the extracellular fluid (ECF). Plasma levels of free magnesium range from 1.3 to 2.1 mg/dL, or 0.65 to 1.05 mmol/L (see Table 13-4). Much more magnesium is present in the intracellular fluid (ICF), and it has more functions inside the cells than in the blood. Magnesium is critical for skeletal muscle contraction, carbohydrate metabolism, adenosine triphosphate (ATP) formation, vitamin activation, and cell growth. Extracellular magnesium regulates blood coagulation and skeletal muscle contractility.

The daily magnesium requirement for adults is about 300 mg. Magnesium is present in most foods only in low levels.

Magnesium regulation occurs through the kidney and the intestinal tract although the exact mechanisms are not known. When blood magnesium levels are low, ingested magnesium is rapidly absorbed and kidney excretion of magnesium stops. When blood magnesium levels are high, little magnesium is absorbed from food and kidney magnesium excretion increases.

HYPOMAGNESEMIA

Pathophysiology

Hypomagnesemia is a serum magnesium (Mg^{2+}) level below 1.3 mEq/L. Most problems leading to hypomagnesemia are caused by decreased magnesium intake or increased magnesium loss. As a result, hypomagnesemia reflects a decrease in the total body magnesium content.

The effects of hypomagnesemia are caused by increased membrane excitability and the accompanying serum calcium and potassium imbalances. Excitable membranes, especially nerve cell membranes, may depolarize spontaneously.

Hypomagnesemia is caused by decreased absorption of dietary magnesium or increased renal magnesium excretion. Table 13-12 lists the specific causes of hypomagnesemia.

Patient-Centered Collaborative Care

Common clinical manifestations of hypomagnesemia are seen in the neuromuscular, central nervous, and intestinal systems.

Neuromuscular changes are caused by increased nerve impulse transmission. Normally, magnesium inhibits nerve impulse transmission at synapse areas. Decreased levels increase impulse transmission from nerve to nerve or from nerve to skeletal muscle. The patient has hyperactive deep tendon reflexes, numbness and tingling, and painful muscle contractions. Positive Chvostek's and Trousseau's signs may be present because hypomagnesemia may occur with hypocalcemia (see the earlier discussion of these assessment signs of neuromuscular changes on pp. 192-193 in the Hypocalcemia section). Skeletal muscle weakness occurs when intracellular magnesium levels are also decreased. The patient may have tetany and seizures as hypomagnesemia worsens.

Central nervous system (CNS) changes are caused by increased nerve impulse transmission. These changes may present as psychological depression, psychosis, and confusion.

Intestinal changes are from decreased intestinal smooth muscle contraction. Reduced motility, anorexia, nausea, constipation, and abdominal distention are common. A paralytic ileus may occur when hypomagnesemia is severe.

Interventions for hypomagnesemia aim to correct the imbalance and manage the specific problem that caused it. In addition, because hypocalcemia often occurs with hypomagnesemia, interventions also aim to restore normal serum calcium levels.

Drugs that promote magnesium loss, such as high-ceiling (loop) diuretics, osmotic diuretics, aminoglycoside antibiotics, and drugs containing phosphorus, are discontinued. Magnesium is replaced intravenously with magnesium sulfate ($MgSO_4$) when hypomagnesemia is severe. *The IV route is used because $MgSO_4$ causes pain and tissue damage when injected IM.* Assess deep tendon reflexes at least hourly in the patient receiving IV magnesium to monitor effectiveness and prevent hypermagnesemia. Oral magnesium often causes diarrhea and can increase magnesium loss. If hypocalcemia is also present, drug therapy to increase serum calcium levels is prescribed.

TABLE 13-12 Common Causes of Magnesium Imbalance

HYPOMAGNESEMIA

- Malnutrition
- Starvation
- Diarrhea
- Steatorrhea
- Celiac disease
- Crohn's disease
- Drugs (diuretics, aminoglycoside antibiotics, cisplatin, amphotericin B, cyclosporine)
- Citrate (blood products)
- Ethanol ingestion

HYPERMAGNESEMIA

- Increased magnesium intake
  - Magnesium-containing antacids and laxatives
  - IV magnesium replacement
- Decreased renal excretion of magnesium resulting from renal insufficiency

HYPERMAGNESEMIA

Pathophysiology

Hypermagnesemia is a serum magnesium level above 2.1 mEq/L. Magnesium is a membrane stabilizer. When magnesium excess occurs, excitable membranes are less excitable and need a stronger-than-normal stimulus to respond. With severe hypermagnesemia, excitable membranes may not respond to any stimulus.

The imbalance results from increased intake of magnesium coupled with decreased renal excretion of magnesium. Table 13-12 lists the specific causes of hypermagnesemia.

Patient-Centered Collaborative Care

Most manifestations of hypermagnesemia occur as a result of reduced membrane excitability. They usually are not apparent until serum magnesium levels exceed 4 mEq/L. The most common problems are seen in the cardiac, central nervous, and neuromuscular systems.

Cardiac changes include bradycardia, peripheral vasodilation, and hypotension. These problems become more severe as serum magnesium levels increase. ECG changes show a prolonged PR interval with a widened QRS complex. Bradycardia can be severe, and cardiac arrest is possible. Hypotension is also severe, with a diastolic pressure lower than normal. *Patients with severe hypermagnesemia are in grave danger of cardiac arrest.*

Central nervous system changes result from depressed nerve impulse transmission. Patients may be drowsy or lethargic. Coma may occur if the imbalance is prolonged or severe.

Neuromuscular changes result from decreased nerve impulse transmission to the skeletal muscles. Deep tendon reflexes are reduced or even absent. Voluntary skeletal muscle contractions become progressively weaker and finally stop.

Hypermagnesemia has no direct effect on the lungs; however, when the respiratory muscles are weak, respiratory insufficiency can lead to respiratory failure and death.

Interventions for hypermagnesemia aim to reduce the serum level and correct the underlying problem that caused the imbalance.

All oral and parenteral magnesium is discontinued. When renal failure is not present, giving magnesium-free IV fluids can reduce serum magnesium levels. High-ceiling (loop) diuretics such as furosemide (Lasix, Furoside🍁) can further reduce serum magnesium levels. When cardiac problems are severe, giving calcium may reverse the cardiac effects of hypermagnesemia.

CHLORIDE

Chloride (Cl^-) is the major anion of the extracellular fluid (ECF) and works with sodium to maintain ECF osmotic pressure. Chloride is important in the formation of hydrochloric acid in the stomach. The normal plasma concentration of chloride ranges from 98 to 106 mEq/L or mmol/L (see Table 13-4).

Only a small amount of chloride is present inside the cells because negative charges on the cell membrane repel chloride and prevent it from crossing the membrane. However, extracellular chloride can enter cells when exchanged for another anion that is leaving the cell. This situation, called a *chloride shift,* decreases plasma chloride without a net body loss of chloride. Bicarbonate (HCO_3^-) is the anion most commonly exchanged for chloride.

Chloride enters the body through dietary intake. Because chloride (along with sodium, potassium, and many other minerals) is a part of a salt, most diets contain enough chloride to meet the normal needs of the body.

Imbalances of chloride usually occur as a result of other electrolyte imbalances. An exception is chloride loss from excessive vomiting or prolonged gastric suction. Imbalances of chloride are usually corrected by interventions for correcting other electrolyte or acid-base problems.

GET READY FOR THE NCLEX EXAMINATION!

Key Points

Review these Key Points for each NCLEX Examination Client Needs Category.

Safe and Effective Care Environment

- Assess any patient with a fluid or electrolyte imbalance for falls risk.
- Ensure access to adequate fluids for patients who are unable to talk or who have limited mobility.
- Use a pump or controller to deliver IV fluids to patients with fluid overload.
- Do not give IV potassium at a rate greater than 20 mEq/hr.
- Never give potassium supplements by the IM, subcutaneous, or IV push routes.
- Use a pump or controller when giving IV potassium-containing solutions.
- Use a gait belt when assisting a patient with muscle weakness to walk or transfer.
- Collaborate with the nutritionist to teach patients about diets that are restricted in potassium, sodium, or calcium.
- Use a lift sheet to move or reposition a patient with chronic hypocalcemia.

Health Promotion and Maintenance

- Encourage all patients to maintain an adequate fluid intake (minimum of 3 L/day) unless another condition requires fluid restriction.
- Teach all people to increase fluid intake when exercising, when in hot or dry environments, or during conditions that increase metabolism (e.g., fever).
- Instruct patients at risk for fluid imbalance to weigh themselves on the same scale daily, close to the same time each day, and with about the same amount of clothing on each time and to monitor these daily weights for changes or trends.
- Instruct patients who exercise heavily (athletes) to take scheduled fluid replacement breaks.
- Instruct caregivers of older adults who have cognitive impairments or mobility problems to schedule offerings of fluids at regular intervals throughout the day.
- Teach patients how to determine electrolyte content of processed foods by reading labels.
- Teach patients who are prescribed to take diuretics to take the drugs as prescribed.
- Teach patients who are taking digoxin to measure their pulse for rate, rhythm, and quality.
- Teach patients who are taking diuretics to measure their pulse for rate, rhythm, and quality.
- Include the person who prepares the patient's meals when teaching about dietary electrolyte restrictions.

Psychosocial Integrity

- Explain the purpose of fluid restriction to the patient and the family to ensure cooperation and prevent any misunderstandings.
- Assess patients who have a sudden change in cognition for fluid and electrolyte imbalances.
- Determine the patient's food preferences when planning an electrolyte restricted diet.

Physiological Integrity

- Assess skin turgor on the forehead or the sternum of older patients.
- Use daily weights to determine fluid gains or losses.
- Ask patients about the use of drugs such as diuretics, laxatives, salt substitutes, and antihypertensives that may alter fluid and electrolyte status.
- Correctly interpret laboratory electrolyte values.
- Do not give oral fluids to an unconscious patient.
- Monitor the cardiac and pulmonary status at least every hour when patients with dehydration are receiving IV fluid replacement therapy.
- Offer or perform oral care at least every 4 hours for patients with dehydration.

- Assess the IV site of a person receiving IV solutions containing potassium hourly, and document its condition.
- Immediately stop the infusion of potassium-containing solutions if infiltration is suspected.
- Avoid administering magnesium sulfate by the IM route.
- Assess all patients with hyperkalemia for cardiac dysrhythmias and ECG abnormalities, especially tall T waves, conduction delays, and heart block.
- Assess the respiratory status of all patients with hypokalemia.
- Assess the bowel sounds; heart rate, rhythm, and quality; and muscle strength to evaluate the patient's responses to therapy for an electrolyte imbalance.

Additional Study Resources

Go to your Companion CD or Evolve at http://evolve.elsevier.com/Iggy/ for Self-Assessment Questions for the NCLEX Examination.

Go to Evolve at http://evolve.elsevier.com/Iggy/ for Prioritization and Delegation Questions for the NCLEX Examination.

SELECTED BIBLIOGRAPHY

Atassi, K. (2008). Action STAT: Water intoxication. *Nursing2008, 38*(2), 72.

Astle, S. (2005). Restoring electrolyte balance. *RN, 68*(5), 34-40.

David, K. (2007). IV fluids: Do you know what's hanging and why? *RN, 70*(10), 35-40.

Edwards, N. (2005). Interpreting laboratory values in older adults. *MEDSURG Nursing, 14*(4), 220-229.

Edwards, S. (2005). Maintaining calcium balance: Physiology and implications. *Nursing Times, 101*(19), 58-61.

Fox, T. (2005). About hypercalcemia. *Nursing2005, 35*(7), 74.

Goertz, S. (2006). Gauging fluid balance with osmolarity. *Nursing2006, 36*(10), 70-71.

Gordon, M. (2007). *Manual of nursing diagnosis* (11th ed.). Boston: Jones & Bartlett.

Hankins, J. (2006). The role of albumin in fluid and electrolyte balance. *Journal of Infusion Nursing, 29*(5), 260-265.

Hayes, D. (2007). How to respond to abnormal serum sodium levels. *Nursing2007, 37*(12), 56hn1-56hn4.

Hayes, D. (2007). When potassium takes dangerous detours. *Nursing2007, 37*(11), 56hn1-56hn4.

Holcomb, S. (2008). Third-spacing: When body fluid shifts. *Nursing2008, 38*(7), 51-53.

Lecko, C. (2008). Improving hydration: An issue of safety. *Nursing & Residential Care, 10*(3), 149-150.

Legg, V. (2005). Complications of chronic kidney disease. *AJN, 105*(6), 40-49.

Lien, Y., & Shapiro, J. (2007). Hyponatremia: Clinical diagnosis and management. *American Journal of Medicine, 120*(8), 653-658.

Lin, M., Liu, S., & Lim, I. (2005). Disorders of water balance. *Emergency Medicine Clinics of North America, 23*(3), 749-770.

McCance, K., & Huether, S. (2006). *Pathophysiology: The biologic basis for disease in adults and children* (5th ed.). St. Louis: Mosby.

Meiner, S., & Lueckenotte, A. (Eds.). (2006). *Gerontologic nursing* (3rd ed.). St. Louis: Mosby.

Mentes, J. (2006). Oral hydration in older adults. *AJN, 106*(6), 40-49.

Miller, W., & Graham, M. (2006). Life-threatening electrolyte abnormalities. *Patient Care, 40*(12), 19-27.

Moe, S. (2005). Disorders of calcium, phosphorus, and magnesium. *American Journal of Kidney Diseases, 45*(1), 213-218.

Munger, M. (2007). New agents for managing hyponatremia in hospitalized patients. *American Journal of Health-System Pharmacy, 64*(3), 253-265.

O'Neill, P. (2007). Helping your patient to restrict potassium. *Nursing2007, 37*(4), 64hn6, 64hn8.

Pagana, K., & Pagana, T. (2006). *Mosby's manual of diagnostic and laboratory tests* (3rd ed.). St. Louis: Mosby.

Reynolds, G. (2007). Discovering and stopping hyperkalemia. *American Nurse Today, 2*(11), 52.

Reynolds, R., Padfield, P., & Secki, J. (2006). Disorders of sodium balance. *British Medical Journal, 332*(7543), 702-705.

Schaefer, T., & Wolford, R. (2005). Disorders of potassium. *Emergency Medicine Clinics of North America, 23*(3), 723-747.

Sweeney, J. (2005a). What causes hyponatremia? *Nursing2005, 35*(6), 18.

Sweeney, J. (2005b). What causes sudden hypokalemia? *Nursing2005, 35*(4), 12.

Vacca, V. (2008). Hyperkalemia. *Nursing2008, 38*(7), 72.

Assessment and Care of Patients with Acid-Base Imbalances

14
CHAPTER

M. Linda Workman

LEARNING OUTCOMES

For clinical competence and success on the NCLEX Examination, study this chapter with these Learning Outcomes in mind:

Physiological Integrity

1. Describe the relationship between free hydrogen ion level and pH.
2. Explain the role of bicarbonate in the blood.
3. Explain the concept of compensation.
4. Compare the roles of the respiratory system and the renal system in maintaining acid-base balance.
5. Describe the role of oxygen in maintaining acid-base balance.
6. Identify patients at risk for acid-base imbalances.
7. Use laboratory data and clinical manifestations to determine the presence of acid-base imbalances.
8. Correctly interpret arterial blood gases to determine whether acidosis is respiratory or metabolic in origin.
9. Coordinate nursing care for the patient with an acid-base imbalance.

Go to your Companion CD or Evolve at http://evolve.elsevier.com/Iggy/ *for Self-Assessment Questions for the NCLEX Examination* keyed to these Learning Outcomes.

Acid-base balance occurs through control of hydrogen ion (H^+) production and elimination. Body fluid **pH** is a measure of the body fluid's free hydrogen ion level. *This value has the narrowest range of normal and the tightest control mechanisms of all electrolytes.* The level of free hydrogen ions, formed from acids, must be rigidly controlled for proper function. Even small changes in the free hydrogen ion level, or pH, of body fluids can cause major problems in function. Keeping the pH within the normal range involves balancing acids and bases in body fluids. Normal pH ranges from 7.35 to 7.45 for arterial blood and from 7.31 to 7.41 for venous blood.

The normal free hydrogen ion level of blood and other body fluids is quite low (<0.0001 mEq/L) compared with the levels of other electrolytes (see Chapter 13). Because it is so low, it is not measured directly but, instead, is a calculated value. The pH value is calculated as the negative logarithm of the concentration in milliequivalents per liter. Because it is calculated in negative logarithm units, the value of pH is inversely related (negatively related) to the level of free hydrogen ions. In other words, the *lower* the pH value of a fluid, the *higher* the level of free hydrogen ions in that fluid. The pH of a solution may range from 1 (as acidic as possible) to 14 (as alkaline as possible), with 7 being neutral. *A change of 1 pH unit actually represents a tenfold change in free hydrogen ion level.* Therefore any pH unit change (e.g., a change from 7.4 to 7.3) represents a large increase in the free hydrogen ion level.

Keeping the pH of the blood within the normal range is important because changes from normal interfere with many normal physiologic functions. These changes include:

- Changing the shape and reducing the function of hormones and enzymes
- Changing the distribution of other electrolytes, causing fluid and electrolyte imbalances
- Changing excitable membranes, making the heart, nerves, muscles, and GI tract either less or more active than normal
- Decreasing the effectiveness of many drugs

Fortunately, the body has many mechanisms to ensure minimal changes in free hydrogen ion level.

ACID-BASE BALANCE

As discussed in Chapter 13, body fluids are electrically neutral even though they contain ions with overall positive charges and ions with overall negative charges. When fluids contain an equal number of positive and negative charges, the electrical charge of the fluid remains neutral. The body keeps blood pH between 7.35 and 7.45 in a similar manner; however, this value is not strictly neutral (7.0 is neutral) but, rather, is slightly alkaline. Normal body fluid pH remains at a near-neutral value when the acids and bases are nearly balanced, limiting the total number of free or unbalanced hydrogen

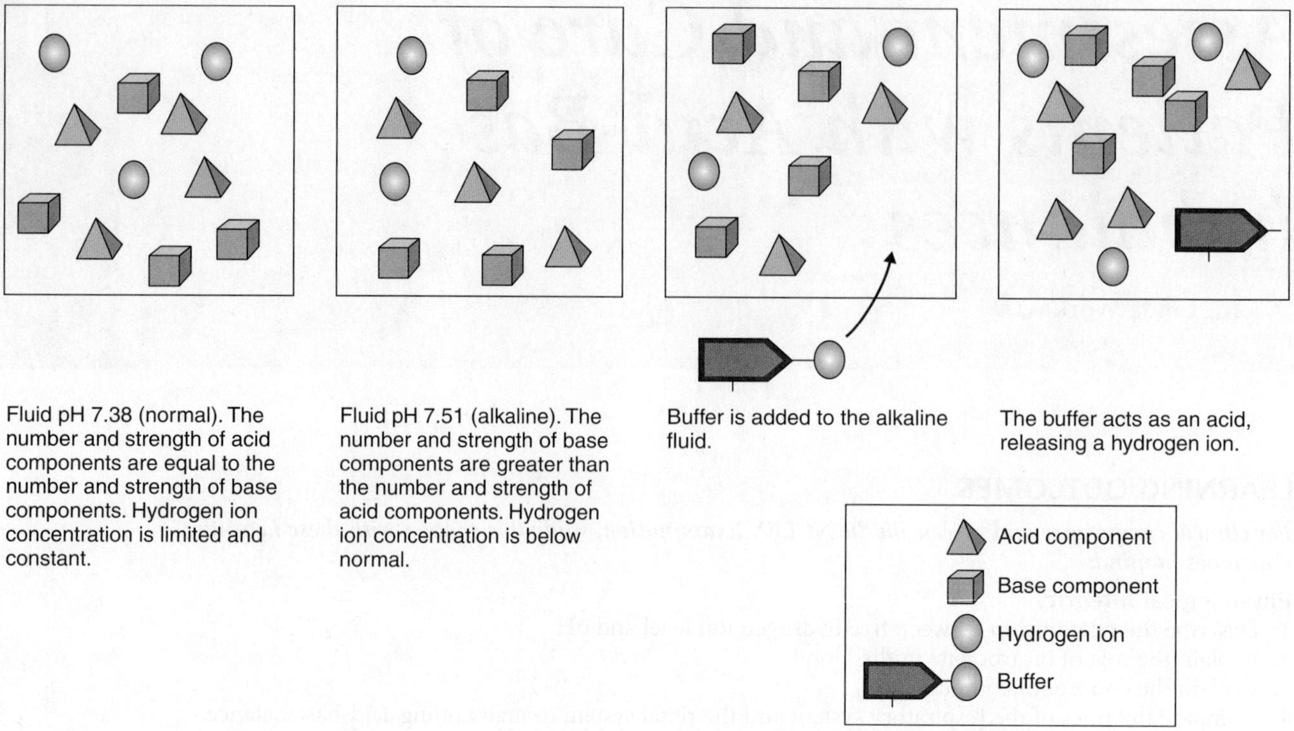
Fluid pH 7.38 (normal). The number and strength of acid components are equal to the number and strength of base components. Hydrogen ion concentration is limited and constant.
Fluid pH 7.51 (alkaline). The number and strength of base components are greater than the number and strength of acid components. Hydrogen ion concentration is below normal.
Buffer is added to the alkaline fluid.
The buffer acts as an acid, releasing a hydrogen ion.
Acid component
Base component
Hydrogen ion
Buffer

Fig. 14-1 • Action of buffer in solution.

ions. Acid-base balance occurs by matching the rate of hydrogen ion production with hydrogen ion loss.

ACID-BASE CHEMISTRY

Acids

Acids are substances that release hydrogen ions when dissolved in water (H_2O). An acid in solution *increases* the amount of free hydrogen ions in that solution. The strength of an acid is measured by how easily it releases a hydrogen ion in solution. A strong acid, such as hydrochloric acid (HCl), separates **(dissociates)** completely in water and readily releases all of its hydrogen ions:

HCl	+	H_2O	→	H^+	+	Cl^-	+	H_2O
Hydrochloric acid		Water		Hydrogen ion		Chloride ion		Water

A weak acid does not completely separate in water; it releases only some of its hydrogen ions. In the following example, each molecule of acetic acid (CH_3COOH), a weak acid, contains a total of four hydrogen molecules. When acetic acid combines with water, it releases only one of its four hydrogen molecules. The other three hydrogen molecules remain bound to the acetic acid molecule (CH_3COO^-).

Bases

A **base** is a substance that binds free hydrogen ions in solution. Thus bases are "hydrogen acceptors" that reduce the amount of free hydrogen ions in solution. Strong bases bind hydrogen ions easily. Examples of strong bases include sodium hydroxide (NaOH) and ammonia (NH_3).

Weak bases bind hydrogen ions less readily. Examples of weak bases are aluminum hydroxide ($AlOH_3$) and bicarbonate (HCO_3^-). Although bicarbonate is a weak base, bicarbonate ions in the body prevent major changes in body fluid pH.

AAABBB	AAAABBB	AAABB
AAABBB	AAAABBB	AAABB
AAABBB	AAAABBB	AAABB
Neutral or acid-base balance	Acidic (acid excess) (actual acidosis)	Acidic (base deficit) (relative acidosis)

Fig. 14-2 • Concept of acidic versus normal pH. (A = acid; B = base.)

Buffers

Buffers can either release a hydrogen ion into a fluid or bind a hydrogen ion from a fluid. Buffers dissolved in water can react in two ways: either as an acid (releasing a hydrogen ion) or as a base (binding a hydrogen ion). How a buffer reacts when dissolved in water depends on the existing acid-base balance of that fluid. Buffers always try to bring the fluid as close as possible to the normal body fluid pH of 7.35 to 7.45. If the fluid is basic (with few free hydrogen ions), the buffer releases hydrogen ions into the fluid (Fig. 14-1). If the fluid is acidic (with many free hydrogen ions), the buffer acts as a base, binding some hydrogen ions. In this way, buffers act like hydrogen ion "sponges," soaking up hydrogen ions when too many are present and squeezing out hydrogen ions when too few are present. Because of this flexibility, buffers are important in keeping body fluid pH in the normal range.

Liquids with a pH of 7.0 are neutral; they have a free hydrogen ion level in which the amount and strength of acids and bases are equal. Fig. 14-2 shows the concept of neutral pH. This figure shows that the combined *strength* and *amount* of all acids are equal to the combined *strength* and *amount* of all bases in a given solution. This is not the actual case in human physiology. However, in acid-base homeostasis, the relative

Neutral	Alkaline (base excess)	Alkaline (acid deficit)
AAABBB	AAABBBB	AABBB
AAABBB	AAABBBB	AABBB
AAABBB	AAABBBB	AABBB

Fig. 14-3 • Concept of alkaline versus normal pH. (A = acid; B = base.)

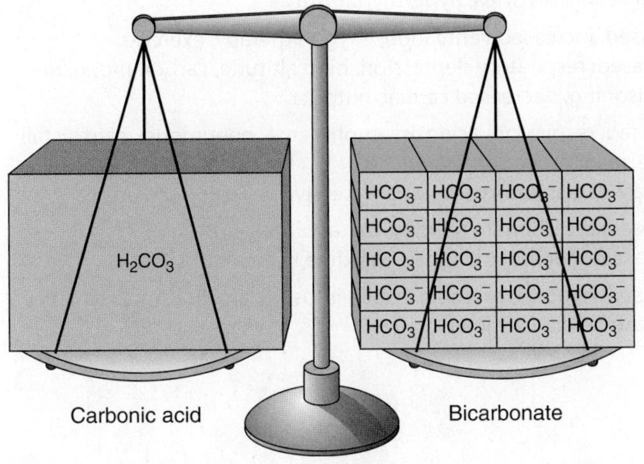

H_2CO_3
HCO_3^-
Carbonic acid
Bicarbonate

Fig. 14-4 • Normal ratio of carbonic acid to bicarbonate is 1:20.

amounts and strengths of acids and bases are nearly equal, so the overall free hydrogen ion levels remain constant.

Liquids with a pH ranging from 1.0 to 6.99 have more or stronger (or both) acids compared with the amount or strength (or both) of bases. These liquids are *acidic* (see Fig. 14-2), which means that more free hydrogen ions are being released than bound, increasing the amount of free hydrogen ions.

Liquids with a pH ranging from 7.01 to 14.0 have more or stronger (or both) bases compared with the amount or strength (or both) of acids. These liquids are *basic,* which means that more hydrogen ions are being bound than released, decreasing the amount of free hydrogen ions (Fig. 14-3).

BODY FLUID CHEMISTRY

Bicarbonate Ions

Body fluids contain many different types of acids and a few types of bases. The most common base in human body fluid is bicarbonate (HCO_3^-); the most common acid is carbonic acid (H_2CO_3). In health, the body keeps these substances at a constant ratio of one molecule of carbonic acid to 20 free bicarbonate ions (1:20) (Fig. 14-4). To maintain this ratio, both carbonic acid and bicarbonate must be carefully controlled. This constant ratio is related to balancing the production and elimination of carbon dioxide (CO_2) and hydrogen ions (H^+).

A key concept in understanding acid-base balance is the *carbonic anhydrase equation.* This equation, driven by the enzyme *carbonic anhydrase,* shows how hydrogen ion levels and carbon dioxide levels are directly related to one another, so that an increase in one causes an equal increase in the other:

$$\underset{\text{Carbon dioxide}}{CO_2} + \underset{\text{Water}}{H_2O} \Leftrightarrow \underset{\text{Carbonic acid}}{H_2CO_3} \Leftrightarrow \underset{\text{Hydrogen ion}}{H^+} + \underset{\text{Bicarbonate ion}}{HCO_3^-}$$

Carbon dioxide is a gas that forms carbonic acid when combined with water. Carbon dioxide is a changeable part of carbonic acid. Carbonic acid is not stable, and the body needs to keep a 1:20 ratio of carbonic acid to bicarbonate. As soon as carbonic acid is formed from water and carbon dioxide, it immediately separates into free hydrogen ions and bicarbonate ions. *Therefore the carbon dioxide content of a fluid is directly related to the amount of hydrogen ions in that fluid. Whenever conditions cause carbon dioxide to increase, more free hydrogen ions are created. Likewise, whenever free hydrogen ion production increases, more carbon dioxide is produced.*

Relationship Between Carbon Dioxide and Hydrogen Ions

When excess carbon dioxide is produced, the amount of carbon dioxide increases and the equation shifts to the right, causing an increase in hydrogen ions (and a decrease in pH):

$$\mathbf{CO_2} + H_2O \Longrightarrow H_2CO_3 \Longrightarrow H^+ + HCO_3^-$$

When very little carbon dioxide is produced, no free hydrogen ions are created by this equation.

When excess hydrogen ions are produced or brought into the body, the carbonic anhydrase equation shifts to the left, causing the creation of more carbon dioxide:

$$CO_2 + H_2O \Longleftarrow H_2CO_3 \Longleftarrow \mathbf{H^+} + HCO_3^-$$

When the amount of free hydrogen ions in body fluids is low, no extra carbon dioxide is produced.

Calculation of Free Hydrogen Ion Level

The pH is a calculation of the free hydrogen ion level in body fluids. A formula is used because the actual number of free hydrogen ions is not easily measured. The pH calculations come from an equation that shows how three factors are related: the level of free hydrogen ions, the amount of bases, and the strength of acids in a solution. In the body, if two of these three factors are known, the third factor can then be calculated.

Because the normal ratio of carbonic acid and bicarbonate level in ECF is 1:20, the only factor that changes is the carbon dioxide (CO_2) level. Whenever the CO_2 level changes, the pH changes to the same degree, in the opposite direction. Thus when the CO_2 level of a liquid increases, the pH drops, indicating more free hydrogen ions (more acidic). On the other hand, when the CO_2 level of a liquid decreases, the pH rises, indicating fewer free hydrogen ions (more alkaline).

An increase in bicarbonate causes the amount of hydrogen ions to decrease and the pH to increase, or become more alkaline (basic). On the other hand, an increase in the CO_2 level causes the free hydrogen ion level to increase and the pH to decrease, or become more acidic.

Because the kidneys control bicarbonate levels and the lungs control CO_2 levels in the healthy person, pH is also described as the function of the kidneys divided by the function of the lungs:

$$\text{pH} = \frac{\text{Kidneys (bicarbonate)}}{\text{Lungs (carbon dioxide)}}$$

Sources of Acids and Bicarbonate

Normal metabolism of carbohydrate, protein, and fat creates natural waste products. Carbohydrate metabolism forms carbon dioxide (CO_2). Carbon dioxide is exhaled by the lungs during breathing. One factor that determines blood pH is how

Chart 14-1 LABORATORY PROFILE

Acid-Base Assessment

Test	NORMAL RANGE FOR ADULTS Arterial	Venous	Significance of Abnormal Findings
pH		7.31-7.41	Increased: metabolic alkalosis, loss of gastric fluids, decreased potassium intake, diuretic therapy, fever, salicylate toxicity
Adult <90 yr	7.35-7.45		Decreased: metabolic or respiratory acidosis, ketosis, renal failure, starvation, diarrhea, hyperthyroidism
>90 yr	7.25-7.45		
Pao_2			Increased: increased ventilation, oxygen therapy, exercise
Adult <90 yr	80-100 mm Hg		Decreased: respiratory depression, high altitude, carbon monoxide poisoning, decreased cardiac output
>90 yr	>70-90 mm Hg		
$Paco_2$	35-45 mm Hg	40-50 mm Hg	Increased: respiratory acidosis, emphysema, pneumonia, cardiac failure, respiratory depression Decreased: respiratory alkalosis, excessive ventilation, diarrhea
Bicarbonate	21-28 mEq/L	24-29 mEq/L	Increased: bicarbonate therapy, metabolic alkalosis Decreased: metabolic acidosis, diarrhea, pancreatitis
Lactate	3-7 mg/dL 0.3-0.8 mmol/L	5-20 mg/dL 0.6-2.2 mmol/L	Increased: hypoxia, exercise, insulin infusion, alcoholism, pregnancy Decreased: fluid overload

$Paco_2$, Partial pressure of arterial carbon dioxide; *Pao_2*, partial pressure of arterial oxygen.

much CO_2 is produced by body cells during metabolism versus how rapidly that CO_2 is removed by breathing. Protein breakdown forms sulfuric acid. Fat breakdown forms fatty acids and ketoacids.

Incomplete breakdown of glucose, which occurs whenever cells metabolize under **anaerobic** (no oxygen) conditions, forms lactic acid. Anaerobic conditions occur with hypoxia, sepsis, and shock. Incomplete breakdown of fatty acids, occurring when large amounts of fatty acids are being metabolized, forms ketoacids.

Destruction of cells allows cell contents to be released. Some cell structures contain acids. When these acids are released into the extracellular fluid (ECF), free hydrogen ions are dissociated.

Bicarbonate is the main buffer of the ECF. It comes from the breakdown of carbonic acid, intestinal absorption of ingested bicarbonate, pancreatic production of bicarbonate, movement of cellular bicarbonate into the ECF, and kidney reabsorption of filtered bicarbonate. Once bicarbonate is in the ECF, it is kept at a level 20 times greater than that of carbonic acid.

ACID-BASE REGULATORY MECHANISMS

As long as body cells are healthy, they continually produce acids, carbon dioxide, and hydrogen ions. Despite this production, hydrogen ions, bicarbonate, oxygen, and carbon dioxide levels are kept within normal limits when physiologic function is normal. Chart 14-1 lists normal values for these substances in arterial and venous blood. This homeostasis depends on three factors:

- Hydrogen ion production is consistent and not excessive.
- CO_2 loss from the body through breathing keeps pace with hydrogen ion production.
- The ratio between carbonic acid and bicarbonate remains at 1:20.

To keep the free hydrogen ion level (pH) of the ECF within the narrow range of normal, the body has chemical, respiratory, and renal mechanisms for acid-base balance (Table 14-1).

Chemical Acid-Base Control Mechanisms

Buffers are the first line of defense against changes in the amount of free hydrogen ions. Because they are always present in body fluids, buffers act fast to reduce or raise the amount of free hydrogen ions to normal. By acting as hydrogen ion "sponges," buffers can bind hydrogen ions when too many are present or release hydrogen ions when not enough are present. Buffers are composed of chemicals or proteins.

Chemical buffers are paired mixtures—usually a weak base and an acid salt. The two most common chemical buffers are bicarbonate (which is active in both the extracellular fluid [ECF] and intracellular fluid [ICF]) and phosphate (which is active in the ICF).

Protein buffers are the most common buffers. Proteins in body fluids can either bind or release free hydrogen ions as needed. Both ICF and ECF proteins serve as buffers. Extracellular protein buffers are albumin and globulins. A major cell protein buffer is hemoglobin. Hemoglobin buffers hydrogen ions directly and also buffers acids formed during the production of carbon dioxide. When the amount of free hydrogen ions in the blood increases, some of the excess hydrogen ions cross the membranes of red blood cells and bind to the large numbers of hemoglobin molecules in each red blood cell. This binding of hydrogen ions to hemoglobin results in fewer hydrogen ions remaining in the blood, bringing blood pH back up toward normal.

Respiratory Acid-Base Control Mechanisms

When chemical buffers alone cannot prevent changes in blood pH, the respiratory system is the second line of defense against changes. Breathing controls the amount of free

TABLE 14-1 Acid-Base Regulatory Mechanisms

Mechanism Type	Key Characteristics
CHEMICAL	
Protein buffers (albumin, globulins, hemoglobin) Chemical buffers (bicarbonate, phosphate)	Very rapid response Provide immediate response to changing conditions Can handle relatively small fluctuations in hydrogen ion production and elimination encountered under normal metabolic and health conditions
RESPIRATORY	
Increased hydrogen ions or increased carbon dioxide Stimulates central respiratory neurons, leading to increased rate and depth of breathing, causing more carbon dioxide to be lost and decreasing the hydrogen ion concentration Decreased hydrogen ions or decreased carbon dioxide Inhibits central respiratory neurons, leading to decreased rate and depth of breathing, causing normally produced carbon dioxide to be retained, increasing the hydrogen ion concentration	Primarily assist buffering systems when the fluctuation of hydrogen ion concentration is acute
RENAL	
Mechanisms to decrease pH Increased renal excretion of bicarbonate Increased renal reabsorption of hydrogen ions Mechanisms to increase pH Decreased renal excretion of bicarbonate Decreased renal reabsorption of hydrogen ions	The most powerful regulator of acid-base balance Respond to large or chronic fluctuations in hydrogen ion production or elimination Slowest response (hours to days) Longest duration

hydrogen ions by controlling the amount of carbon dioxide (CO_2) in arterial blood. Remember, because CO_2 is converted into hydrogen ions through the carbonic anhydrase reaction, the CO_2 level is *directly* related to the hydrogen ion level. Breathing rids the body of the excess CO_2 created through metabolism.

The amount of CO_2 in venous blood increases during normal metabolism. This CO_2 is moved in the blood to the lung capillaries. Because the amount (pressure) of CO_2 is far higher in capillary blood than in the air in the alveoli, CO_2 diffuses freely from the blood into the alveolar air. Once in the alveoli, CO_2 is exhaled during breathing and is lost from the body. Because the amount (pressure) of CO_2 in atmospheric air is nearly zero, CO_2 usually continues to be exhaled even when breathing is impaired.

Respiratory regulation of acid-base balance is under the control of the central nervous system (Fig. 14-5). Special receptors in the respiratory areas of the brain are sensitive to changes in the amount of CO_2 in brain tissues. As the amount of CO_2 begins to rise above normal in brain blood and tissues, these central receptors trigger the neurons to increase the rate and depth of breathing **(hyperventilation)**. As a result, more CO_2 is exhaled ("blown off") from the lungs and the amount of CO_2 in the ECF decreases. When the amount of arterial CO_2 returns to normal, the rate and depth of breathing return to levels that are normal for the person.

If the amount of ECF free hydrogen ions is too low, then the amount of CO_2 also is too low. Central receptors sense these low CO_2 levels and stop or slow the neuron activity in the respiratory centers, decreasing the rate and depth of breathing **(hypoventilation)**. As a result, less CO_2 is lost through the lungs and more CO_2 is retained in arterial blood. This retention of already-formed CO_2, together with the normal production of CO_2 from metabolism, results in a rapid return of the arterial CO_2 levels (and hydrogen ion levels) to normal. When these levels are normal, the rate and depth of breathing also return to normal levels.

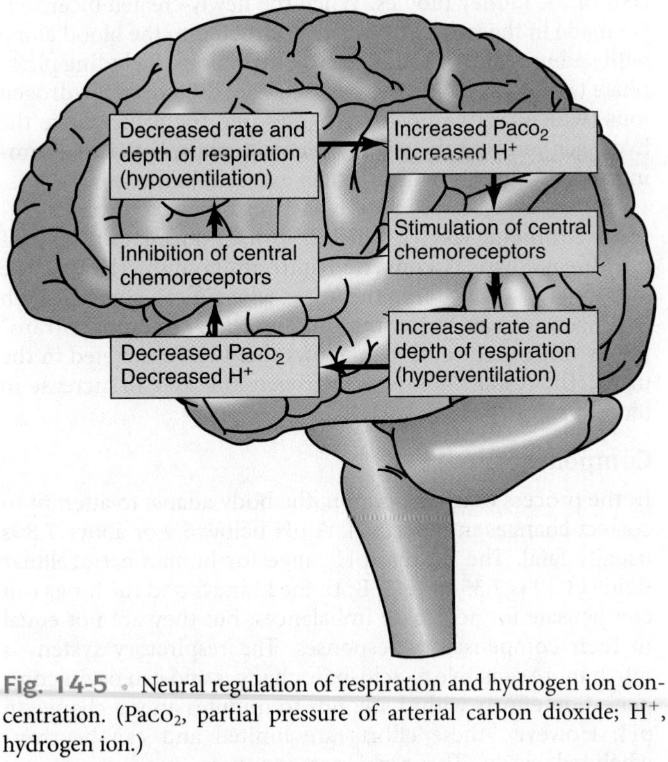

Decreased rate and depth of respiration (hypoventilation)
Increased Pa_{CO_2}
Increased H^+
Stimulation of central chemoreceptors
Inhibition of central chemoreceptors
Increased rate and depth of respiration (hyperventilation)
Decreased Pa_{CO_2}
Decreased H^+

Fig. 14-5 • Neural regulation of respiration and hydrogen ion concentration. (Pa_{CO_2}, partial pressure of arterial carbon dioxide; H^+, hydrogen ion.)

The respiratory system's response in acid-base balance is rapid. Changes in the rate and depth of breathing occur within minutes after changes in the hydrogen ion level or CO_2 level of the ECF occur.

Renal Acid-Base Control Mechanisms

The kidneys are the third line of defense against wide changes in body fluid pH. Renal mechanisms are stronger for regulating acid-base balance but take longer than chemical and respiratory mechanisms to completely respond. (They take 24 to 48 hours to respond.) When blood pH changes are persistent, renal mechanisms that increase excretion and reabsorption rates of acids or bases (depending on the direction of the pH changes) begin to operate. These mechanisms are kidney movement of bicarbonate, formation of acids, and formation of ammonium.

Kidney movement of bicarbonate is the first renal control mechanism. It occurs in the kidney tubules in two ways: (1) kidney movement of bicarbonate produced elsewhere in the body and (2) kidney movement of bicarbonate produced in the kidneys. Much of the bicarbonate made in other body areas is excreted in the urine. When blood hydrogen ion levels are high, this bicarbonate is reabsorbed from the kidneys back into circulation, where it can help buffer excess hydrogen ions. When blood hydrogen ion levels are low, the bicarbonate remains in the urine and is excreted. When hydrogen ion excess occurs, the kidney tubules also can make additional bicarbonate that will be reabsorbed.

Formation of acids is the second renal control mechanism. It occurs through the phosphate-buffering system inside the cells of the kidney tubules. When the newly created bicarbonate made in the kidney cells is reabsorbed into the blood along with sodium, the urine has an excess of anions, including phosphate (HPO_4^{2-}). This negatively charged fluid draws hydrogen ions (which carry a positive charge) into the urine. Once the hydrogen ion is in the urine, it binds to phosphate ions, forming an acid, H_2PO_4, which is then excreted in the urine.

Formation of ammonium is the third renal control mechanism. Ammonia (NH_3), which is formed during normal protein breakdown, is converted into ammonium (NH_4^+). The ammonia is secreted into the urine, where it can combine with hydrogen ions to form ammonium. The ammonium "traps" the hydrogen ions and then allows them to be excreted in the urine. The result is a loss of hydrogen ions and an increase in blood pH.

Compensation

In the process of *compensation,* the body adapts to attempt to correct changes in blood pH. A pH below 6.9 or above 7.8 is usually fatal. The normal pH range for human extracellular fluid (ECF) is 7.35 to 7.45. Both the kidneys and the lungs can compensate for acid-base imbalances, but they are not equal in their compensatory responses. The respiratory system is much more sensitive to acid-base changes and can begin compensation efforts within seconds to minutes after a change in pH. However, these efforts are limited and can be overwhelmed easily. The renal compensatory mechanisms are much more powerful and result in rapid changes in ECF composition. However, these more powerful mechanisms are not fully triggered unless the acid-base imbalance continues for several hours to several days.

Respiratory compensation occurs through the lungs, usually to correct for acid-base imbalances from metabolic problems. For example, when prolonged running causes buildup of lactic acid, hydrogen ion levels in the ECF increase and the pH drops. To bring the pH back to normal, breathing is triggered in response to increased carbon dioxide levels. Both the rate and depth of respiration increase. These respiratory efforts cause the blood to lose carbon dioxide with each exhalation, so ECF levels of carbon dioxide and free hydrogen ions gradually decrease. When the lungs can *fully compensate*, the pH returns to normal.

Renal compensation results when a healthy kidney works to correct for changes in blood pH that occur when the respiratory system either is overwhelmed or is not healthy. For example, in a person with chronic obstructive pulmonary disease (COPD), the respiratory system cannot exchange gases adequately. Carbon dioxide is retained continually, and the blood pH falls (becomes more acidic). To oppose this process, the kidney excretes more hydrogen ions and increases the reabsorption of bicarbonate back into the blood. As a result, the blood pH remains either within or closer to the normal range. When these backup mechanisms are completely effective, acid-base problems are *fully compensated* and the pH of the blood returns to normal even though the levels of oxygen and bicarbonate may be abnormal.

Sometimes, however, the respiratory problem causing the acid-base imbalance is so severe that kidney actions can only *partially compensate* and the pH is not quite normal. Partial compensation is helpful because it prevents the acid-base imbalance from becoming severe or life threatening.

ACID-BASE IMBALANCES

Acid-base imbalances are changes in the blood hydrogen ion level or pH. These changes are caused by problems with the acid-base regulatory mechanisms of the body or by exposure to dangerous conditions. Imbalances in which blood pH is below normal reflect **acidosis,** and imbalances in which blood pH is above normal reflect **alkalosis.** Acid-base imbalances impair the function of many organs and can be life threatening.

ACIDOSIS

Pathophysiology

In acidosis, the acid-base balance of the blood and other extracellular fluid (ECF) is upset by an excess of hydrogen ions (H^+). This problem is reflected as an arterial blood pH below 7.35. The amount or strength (or both) of acids is greater than normal compared with the amount or strength of bases.

Acidosis is not a disease; it is a condition caused by a disorder or pathologic process. Acidosis can be caused by metabolic problems, respiratory problems, or both. Patients at greatest risk for acute acidosis are those with problems that impair breathing. Older adults with chronic health problems are at greater risk for developing acidosis (Chart 14-2).

Acidosis can result from an actual or relative increase in the amount or strength of acids. An *actual acid excess* results in acidosis by either overproducing acids (and release of hydrogen ions) or undereliminating normally produced acids (retention of hydrogen ions). Examples of problems that actually increase acid production are diabetic ketoacidosis and seizures. Examples of problems that actually decrease acid elimination are respiratory impairment and renal impairment.

Chart 14-2 NURSING FOCUS ON THE OLDER ADULT

The Older Patient Experiencing Acid-Base Imbalance

WHEN OBTAINING A PATIENT'S HISTORY

- Assess risk factors for acid-base imbalance, including medications, chronic health problems (especially renal disease, pulmonary disease), and acute health problems.
- Obtain the history when the patient is awake and more familiar with his or her surroundings.
- Ask the patient to list all prescribed and over-the-counter drugs (especially diuretics and antacids). If he or she cannot recall this information or seems confused, ask the significant other to bring drugs from home to show the nurse.
- Ask the patient to recall what liquids he or she has taken in the past 24 hours and whether he or she has urinated as much as usual.

WHEN ASSESSING THE PATIENT

- Compare the patient's mental status with what the family, significant other, or health record states is the patient's baseline.
- Observe the rate and depth of respiration.
  Can the patient complete a sentence without stopping to take a breath?
- Examine the color of the patient's nail beds and mucous membranes.
- Obtain a urine specimen, and observe for color and character. Test for specific gravity and pH.
- Examine skin turgor for dehydration. Attempt to pinch the skin to form a tent over the sternum and on the forehead. If a tent forms, record how long it remains.
- Measure the rate and quality of the pulse.
- Observe the patient's clinical responses and laboratory values carefully while the acid-base imbalance is being corrected.
- Administer IV therapy by pump or controller.

In *relative* acidosis, the amount or strength of acids does not increase. Instead, the amount or strength (or both) of the bases decreases (to create a *base deficit*), which makes the fluid relatively more acidic than basic. A relative acidosis *(base deficit)* is caused by either overeliminating bases (bicarbonate ions [HCO_3^-]) or underproducing bases (see Fig. 14-2). Examples of problems that underproduce bases are pancreatitis and dehydration. A condition that overeliminates bases is diarrhea.

Regardless of its origin, acidosis causes major changes in body function. The main problems are related to the fact that hydrogen ions are positively charged ions. An increase in hydrogen ions creates imbalances of other positively charged electrolytes, especially potassium. The changes in potassium levels because of excess hydrogen ions is described on p. 208 in the Laboratory Assessment section. These electrolyte imbalances then disrupt the functions of nerves, cardiac muscle, and skeletal muscle. The early manifestations of acidosis first appear in the musculoskeletal, cardiac, respiratory, and central nervous systems. Even slight increases in blood hydrogen ion levels reduce the activity of many hormones and enzymes, leading to death. Many drugs are less effective during acidosis.

Acidosis can be caused by metabolic problems, respiratory problems, or combined metabolic and respiratory problems. Specific causes of acidosis are listed in Table 14-2.

Metabolic Acidosis

Four processes can result in metabolic acidosis: overproduction of hydrogen ions, underelimination of hydrogen ions, underproduction of bicarbonate ions, and overelimination of bicarbonate ions.

Overproduction of hydrogen ions can occur with excessive breakdown of fatty acids, anaerobic glucose breakdown (lactic acidosis), and excessive intake of acids. Excessive breakdown of fatty acids occurs with diabetic ketoacidosis or starvation. When glucose is not available for fuel, the body breaks down

TABLE 14-2 Common Causes of Acidosis

Pathology	Condition
METABOLIC ACIDOSIS	
Overproduction of hydrogen ions	Excessive oxidation of fatty acids
	Diabetic ketoacidosis
	Starvation
	Hypermetabolism
	Heavy exercise
	Seizure activity
	Fever
	Hypoxia, ischemia
	Excessive ingestion of acids
	Ethanol intoxication
	Methanol ingestion
	Salicylate intoxication
Underelimination of hydrogen ions	Renal failure
Underproduction of bicarbonate	Renal failure
	Pancreatitis
	Liver failure
	Dehydration
Overelimination of bicarbonate	Diarrhea
	Buffering of organic acids
RESPIRATORY ACIDOSIS	
Underelimination of hydrogen ions	Respiratory depression
	Anesthetics
	Drugs (especially opioids)
	Electrolyte imbalance
	Head or neck trauma
	Inadequate chest expansion
	Skeletal deformities
	Muscle weakness
	Nonpulmonary restriction
	Obesity, casts, eschar
	Airway obstruction
	Alveolar-capillary block

fats (lipids). The products of excessive fatty acid breakdown are strong acids *(ketoacids),* which release large amounts of hydrogen ions.

Lactic acidosis occurs when cells are forced to use glucose without adequate oxygen (anaerobic metabolism); as a result, glucose is incompletely broken down and forms lactic acid. Lactic acid leaves the cell, enters the blood, and releases hydrogen ions, causing acidosis. Lactic acidosis occurs whenever the body has too little oxygen, such as during heavy exercise, seizure activity, fever, and reduced oxygen intake.

Excessive intake of acids floods the body with hydrogen ions. Agents that cause acidosis when ingested in excess include alcoholic beverages, methyl alcohol, and acetylsalicylic acid (aspirin).

Underelimination of hydrogen ions leads to acidosis when hydrogen ions are produced at the normal rate but are not removed at the same rate they are produced. Most hydrogen ion loss occurs through the lungs and the kidneys. Kidney failure causes acidosis when the kidney tubules cannot secrete hydrogen ions into the urine. As a result, too many hydrogen ions are retained.

Underproduction of bicarbonate ions (base deficit) leads to acidosis when hydrogen ion production and removal are normal but too few bicarbonate ions are present to balance the hydrogen ions. Such base deficits occur when bicarbonate ions are not produced at the normal rate. Because bicarbonate is made in the kidneys and in the pancreas, renal failure and impaired liver or pancreatic function can cause a base-deficit acidosis.

Overelimination of bicarbonate ions (base-deficit) leads to acidosis when hydrogen ion production and removal are normal but too many bicarbonate ions have been lost. One cause of base-deficit acidosis is diarrhea.

Respiratory Acidosis

Respiratory acidosis results when any area of respiratory function is impaired, reducing the exchange of oxygen (O_2) and carbon dioxide (CO_2). This problem causes CO_2 retention. Because any increase in CO_2 levels causes the same increase in hydrogen ion levels, CO_2 retention leads to acidosis. (See the carbonic anhydrase equation on p. 201.)

Unlike metabolic acidosis, respiratory acidosis results from only one mechanism—retention of CO_2, causing increased production of free hydrogen ions. Respiratory acidosis is caused by four types of problems: respiratory depression, inadequate chest expansion, airway obstruction, and reduced alveolar-capillary diffusion (see Table 14-2).

Respiratory depression is caused by reduced function of the brainstem neurons that trigger breathing movements. The result is a reduced rate and depth of breathing, which leads to poor gas exchange and retention of carbon dioxide. Respiration can be depressed by anesthetic agents, drugs (especially opioids), and poisons such as methyl alcohol, pesticides, and botulinus toxin. Specific electrolyte imbalances also inhibit these neurons (see Chapter 13 for electrolyte imbalances).

Physical depression of respiration occurs when neurons are damaged or destroyed by trauma or when problems in other areas of the brain increase the intracranial pressure. This increase causes edema, which presses on the respiratory centers located in the brainstem. Problems causing cerebral edema and respiratory depression include brain tumors, cerebral aneurysm, stroke, and overhydration.

Inadequate chest expansion reduces gas exchange and leads to acidosis. Chest expansion can be restricted by skeletal trauma or deformities, respiratory muscle weakness, or external constriction. Skeletal problems restrict chest wall movement when broken or malformed bones distort the shape of the chest or when the rigidity of the rib cage is lost (flail chest). Respiratory muscle weakness, caused by electrolyte imbalances, fatigue, muscular dystrophy, muscle damage or breakdown, reduces chest movement. External conditions also can restrict chest movement and gas exchange. Such conditions include body casts, tight scar tissue around the chest, obesity, and ascites.

Airway obstruction prevents air movement into and out from the lungs and leads to poor gas exchange, CO_2 retention, and acidosis. The upper airway can be obstructed externally by clothing, neck edema, and local lymph node enlargement. Internal obstruction of the upper airway can be caused by aspiration of foreign objects, bronchoconstriction, mucus, and edema.

Reduced alveolar-capillary diffusion causes poor gas exchange and leads to CO_2 retention and acidosis. Disorders that reduce diffusion include pneumonia, pneumonitis, tuberculosis, emphysema, acute respiratory distress syndrome, chest trauma, pulmonary emboli, pulmonary edema, and drowning.

Combined Metabolic and Respiratory Acidosis

Metabolic and respiratory acidosis can occur at the same time. Uncorrected acute respiratory acidosis always leads to poor oxygenation and lactic acidosis (McCance & Huether, 2006). Combined acidosis is more severe than either metabolic acidosis or respiratory acidosis alone. Cardiac arrest is an example of a problem leading to combined metabolic and respiratory acidosis.

Patient-Centered Collaborative Care

Assessment

History

When taking the history from any patient, collect data about risk factors related to the development of acidosis, specifically age, nutrition, and presenting symptoms. One way of organizing data to assess acid-base status is to use Gordon's Functional Health Patterns, especially Activity-Exercise, Elimination, and the Cognitive-Perceptual patterns (Chart 14-3).

Older adults are more at risk for problems leading to acid-base imbalance, including cardiac, renal, or pulmonary impairment. In addition, older adults are more likely to be taking drugs that disrupt acid-base, fluid, and electrolyte balance, especially diuretics and aspirin. Ask about specific risk factors, such as any type of breathing problem, kidney failure, diabetes mellitus, diarrhea, pancreatitis, and fever.

Obtain a detailed nutrition history to determine total caloric intake and the proportions of carbohydrates, fats, and proteins ingested. Ask the patient specifically whether he or she has fasted or followed a strict diet within the past week.

Ask about headaches, behavior changes, increased drowsiness, reduced alertness, reduced attention span, lethargy, anorexia, abdominal distention, nausea or vomiting, muscle weakness, or increased fatigue. Having the patient relate activities of the previous 24 hours may help identify activity intolerance, behavior changes, and unexplained fatigue. Because the central nervous system is often depressed in acidosis, you may need to obtain this information from the patient's family.

Chart 14-3 ACID-BASE ASSESSMENT
Using Gordon's Functional Health Patterns

ACTIVITY-EXERCISE PATTERN
- Have you had any shortness of breath or difficulty breathing at rest or during activity?
- Have you noticed any changes in your breathing rate or depth?
- Do you have a hard time "catching" your breath?
- Do you have any difficulty clearing excretions?
- Do you feel the need for additional energy to accomplish routine tasks?
- Do you have any difficulty concentrating?
- Have you noticed any changes in your interest in normal daily activities?
- Have you noticed any changes in your leisure activities?

ELIMINATION PATTERN
- What is your usual urinary elimination pattern? Frequency? Amount? Color? Odor? Control?
- Have you noticed any changes in the amount of urine?
- Has your urine changed color or odor?
- What is your usual bowel elimination pattern? Frequency? Amount? Control?
- Have you noticed any changes in the number or consistency of your stools?

COGNITIVE-PERCEPTUAL PATTERN
- Have you noticed any changes in memory lately?
- Have you noticed an increase in anxiety or feelings of apprehension?
- Are you sleeping more or sleeping less than usual for you?
- Have you noticed any changes in your attention span?
- Have your muscles seemed weak or "twitchy" lately?

Based on Gordon, M. (2007). *Manual of nursing diagnosis* (11th ed.). Boston: Jones & Bartlett.

Physical Assessment/Clinical Manifestations

Manifestations of acidosis are similar whether the cause is metabolic or respiratory (Chart 14-4). These are changes in the excitable membranes of neurons, skeletal muscle, and gastric smooth muscle.

Central nervous system (CNS) changes include depression of CNS function. Problems may range from lethargy to confusion, especially in older patients. As acidosis worsens, the patient may become stuporous and unresponsive. Assess the patient's mental status (see Chapter 43).

Neuromuscular changes with acidosis include reduced muscle tone and deep tendon reflexes. The cause of these changes is high blood levels of potassium (hyperkalemia) along with acidosis. Assess muscle strength in several ways, including arm muscle strength and leg muscle strength. Test arm muscle strength first by having the patient squeeze your hand. Another way to test arm muscle strength is to have the patient flex his or her arms against the chest and keep them flexed while you attempt to pull the arms away from the chest. Test leg muscle strength by having the patient push both feet against a flat surface (like a box or a board) while you apply resistance to the opposite side of the flat surface. The muscle weakness from acidosis is bilateral and can progress to flaccid paralysis.

Chart 14-4 KEY FEATURES
Acidosis

CENTRAL NERVOUS SYSTEM MANIFESTATIONS
- Depressed activity (lethargy, confusion, stupor, coma)

NEUROMUSCULAR MANIFESTATIONS
- Hyporeflexia
- Skeletal muscle weakness
- Flaccid paralysis

CARDIOVASCULAR MANIFESTATIONS
- Delayed electrical conduction
  - Ranges from bradycardia to heart block
  - Tall T waves
  - Widened QRS complex
  - Prolonged PR interval
- Hypotension
- Thready peripheral pulses

RESPIRATORY MANIFESTATIONS
- Kussmaul respirations (in metabolic acidosis with respiratory compensation)
- Variable respirations (generally ineffective in respiratory acidosis)

INTEGUMENTARY MANIFESTATIONS
- Warm, flushed, dry skin in metabolic acidosis
- Pale to cyanotic and dry skin in respiratory acidosis

Cardiovascular changes are first seen with mild acidosis and are more severe as the condition worsens. Early changes include increased heart rate and cardiac output. With worsening acidosis or with acidosis and hyperkalemia, heart rate decreases, T waves become tall and peaked, and QRS complexes are widened. Peripheral pulses may be hard to find and are easily blocked. Hypotension may occur as a result of vasodilation.

Respiratory changes may cause the acidosis and can be caused by the acidosis. Assess the patient's rate, depth, and ease of breathing. Use pulse oximetry to determine how well oxygen is delivered to the peripheral tissues.

If acidosis is metabolic in origin, the rate and depth of breathing increase as the hydrogen ion level rises. Breaths are deep and rapid and not under voluntary control. This pattern is called **Kussmaul respiration.**

If acidosis is caused by respiratory problems, breathing efforts are reduced. Respirations are usually shallow and rapid. Muscle weakness makes this problem worse.

Skin changes occur with metabolic or respiratory acidosis. With metabolic acidosis, breathing is unimpaired and the rate is increased and CO_2 is lost. This causes vasodilation and makes the skin and mucous membranes warm, dry, and pink. With respiratory acidosis, breathing is ineffective and skin and mucous membranes are pale to cyanotic.

Psychosocial Assessment

It is vital to complete a psychosocial assessment, because behavioral changes may be the first manifestations of acidosis. Observe and document the patient's behavior by description (objectively) rather than by interpretation (subjectively). For example, you should state that "the patient does not recognize close family members" rather than "the patient is confused" or state that "the patient spit out the oral drugs" rather than "the patient is uncooperative." Ask family members if the patient's behavior is typical for him or her, and establish a baseline for comparison with later assessment findings.

Laboratory Assessment

Arterial blood pH is the laboratory value used to confirm acidosis. Acidosis is present when arterial blood pH is less than 7.35. However, this test alone does not indicate what is causing the acidosis or its origin. Manifestations of metabolic acidosis and respiratory acidosis are similar, but their treatments are different. Therefore it is critical to obtain and interpret other laboratory data, such as arterial blood gas (ABG) values and blood levels of electrolytes (Chart 14-5).

Metabolic acidosis is reflected by several changes in ABG values. The pH is low (<7.35). It is low because buffering and respiratory compensation are not adequate to keep the amount of free hydrogen ions at a normal level. The bicarbonate level is low (<21 mEq/L). It is low because (1) bicarbonate has been lost, causing a base-deficit acidosis; (2) bicarbonate production is inadequate, causing a base-deficit acidosis; or (3) bicarbonate may be bound to other substances. The partial pressure of arterial oxygen (Pa_{O_2}) is normal because gas exchange is adequate. The partial pressure of arterial carbon dioxide (Pa_{CO_2}) is normal or even slightly decreased because gas exchange is adequate and carbon dioxide retention is not a factor.

The serum potassium level is often high in acidosis as the body attempts to maintain electroneutrality during buffering. Fig. 14-6 shows the movement of potassium ions as serum pH changes. As the blood hydrogen ion level rises, some of the excess hydrogen ions enter red blood cells for intracellular buffering. The movement of hydrogen ions into the cells creates an excess of positive ions inside the cells. To balance these extra positive charges, an equal number of potassium ions move from the cells into the blood. This increases the blood potassium level, causing hyperkalemia.

Respiratory acidosis is reflected by several changes in ABG values. The pH is low (<7.35). It is lowered by the increased

Chart 14-5 LABORATORY PROFILE

Acid-Base Imbalances (Uncompensated)

Imbalance	pH	HCO_3^-	Pa_{O_2}	Pa_{CO_2}	K^+	Ca^{2+}	Cl^-
Metabolic acidosis	↓	↓	Ø	Ø and ↓	↑	Ø	Ø and ↑
Respiratory acidosis	↓	Ø	↓	↑	↑	Ø	↑↓
Combined acidosis	↓	↓↑	↓	↑	↑	Ø	↑
Metabolic alkalosis	↑	↑	Ø	Ø and ↑	↓	↓	↓
Respiratory alkalosis	↑	Ø	Ø	↓↓	↓	↓	↑
Combined alkalosis	↑	↑	Ø	↓	↓	↓	↓

(Columns pH through Cl^-: LABORATORY VALUE CHANGES)

↑, Above normal; ↓, below normal; ↑↓, value can increase or decrease depending on other factors; Ø, normal; Ca^{2+}, calcium ions; Cl^-, chloride ions; Pa_{CO_2}, partial pressure of arterial carbon dioxide; Pa_{O_2}, partial pressure of arterial oxygen; HCO_3^-, bicarbonate ions; K^+, potassium ions.

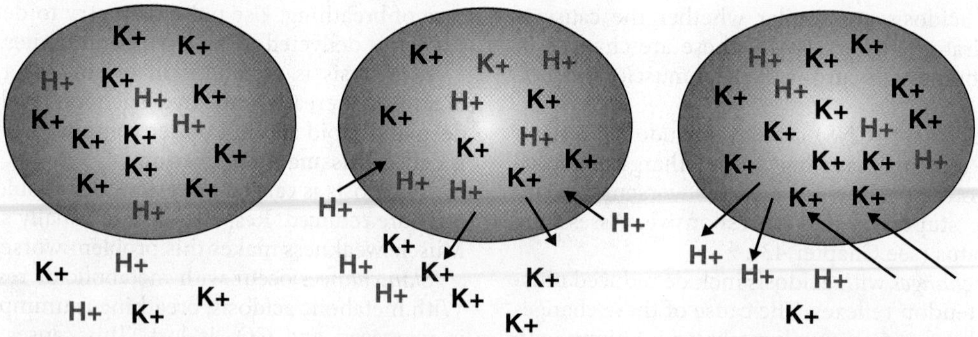

Under normal conditions, the intracellular potassium content is much greater than that of the extracellular fluid. The concentration of hydrogen ions is low in both compartments.

In acidosis, the extracellular hydrogen ion content increases, and the hydrogen ions move into the intracellular fluid. To keep the intracellular fluid electrically neutral, an equal number of potassium ions leave the cell, creating a relative hyperkalemia.

In alkalosis, more hydrogen ions are present in the intracellular fluid than in the extracellular fluid. Hydrogen ions move from the intracellular fluid into the extracellular fluid. To keep the intracellular fluid electrically neutral, potassium ions move from the extracellular fluid into the intracellular fluid, creating a relative hypokalemia.

Fig. 14-6 • Movement of potassium in response to changes in the extracellular fluid hydrogen ion concentration.

amount of free hydrogen ions in the blood. Buffering and renal compensation are not adequate to keep the amount of free hydrogen ions at a normal level. If the kidneys partially compensate for this acidosis, pH is low but not as abnormal as could be expected with the degree of CO_2 retention.

The partial pressure of arterial oxygen (Pao_2) is low and the partial pressure of arterial carbon dioxide ($Paco_2$) is high because the pulmonary problem impairs gas exchange, causing poor oxygenation and CO_2 retention. Carbon dioxide is 20 times more able than oxygen to diffuse across the alveolar membrane. Therefore a decreased Pao_2 usually occurs before an increased $Paco_2$.

The serum bicarbonate level is variable. A patient with rapid onset of respiratory acidosis often has a normal bicarbonate level because kidney compensation has not started. When respiratory acidosis persists for 24 hours or longer, kidney compensation increases the levels of bicarbonate. Chronic respiratory acidosis is indicated by an elevated bicarbonate level and increased $Paco_2$.

Serum potassium levels are elevated in acute respiratory acidosis. They are normal or low in chronic respiratory acidosis when renal compensation is present.

Common Nursing Diagnoses and Collaborative Problems

Nursing diagnoses that may apply to patients with acidosis include:

- Deficient Fluid Volume related to dehydration
- Decreased Cardiac Output related to poor cardiac contractility and decreased vascular volume
- Risk for Falls related to skeletal muscle weakness
- Impaired Memory related to fluid and electrolyte imbalances
- Ineffective Breathing Pattern related to reduced gas exchange
- Fatigue related to inadequate tissue oxygenation

Interventions

Interventions for acidosis focus on correcting the underlying problem and monitoring for changes. To ensure appropriate interventions, the specific type of acidosis must first be identified.

Metabolic Acidosis

Interventions for metabolic acidosis include hydration and drugs or treatments to control the problem causing the acidosis. For example, if the acidosis is a result of diabetic ketoacidosis, insulin is given to correct the hyperglycemia and halt the production of ketone bodies. Rehydration and antidiarrheal drugs are given if the acidosis is a result of prolonged diarrhea. *Bicarbonate is administered only if serum bicarbonate levels are low.* Chart 14-6 lists NIC interventions for patients with metabolic acidosis.

Chart 14-6 NIC INTERVENTION ACTIVITIES

The Patient with Metabolic Acidosis

Acid-Base Management: Metabolic Acidosis: *Promotion of acid-base balance and prevention of complications resulting from serum bicarbonate levels lower than desired*

- Monitor ABG levels for decreasing pH level, as appropriate.
- Maintain patent IV access.
- Monitor intake and output.
- Monitor determinants of tissue oxygen delivery (e.g., Pao_2, Sao_2, and hemoglobin levels and cardiac output), if available.
- Monitor loss of bicarbonate through the GI tract (e.g., diarrhea, pancreatic fistula, small bowel fistula, and ileal conduit), as appropriate.
- Administer fluids as prescribed.
- Administer insulin and fluid hydration (isotonic and hypotonic) for diabetic ketoacidosis, causing metabolic acidosis, as appropriate.
- Prepare patient for dialysis (e.g., assist with catheter placement for dialysis), as appropriate.
- Institute seizure precautions.

NIC intervention activities selected from Bulechek, G.M., Butcher, H.K., & McCloskey Dochterman, J. (Eds.). (2008). *Nursing interventions classification (NIC)* (5th ed.). St. Louis: Mosby. No part of this work is to be altered without prior written permission from the Publisher.

ABG, Arterial blood gas; *GI,* gastrointestinal; *$Paco_2$,* partial pressure of arterial carbon dioxide; *Pao_2,* partial pressure of arterial oxygen; *Sao_2,* arterial oxygen saturation.

Respiratory Acidosis

Interventions aim to maintain a patent airway and enhance gas exchange. These include drug therapy, oxygen therapy, pulmonary hygiene (positioning and breathing techniques), ventilatory support, and prevention of complications. (See Chapter 32 for disorders causing respiratory acidosis.)

Drug therapy includes agents to increase the diameter of upper and lower airways and to thin pulmonary secretions. Drug therapy is not aimed directly at altering arterial pH. The major categories of drugs useful for respiratory problems that lead to acidosis include bronchodilators, anti-inflammatories, and mucolytics.

Oxygen therapy helps promote gas exchange for patients with respiratory acidosis. However, use caution when giving oxygen to patients with chronic obstructive pulmonary disease (COPD) and CO_2 retention as evidenced by a high $Paco_2$ level. The only breathing trigger for these patients is a decreased arterial oxygen level. *Giving too much oxygen to these patients decreases their respiratory drive and may lead to respiratory arrest.*

Pulmonary hygiene promotes gas exchange with the use of positioning techniques to enhance the removal of lung secretions and specific breathing techniques to keep alveoli inflated. Help the patient assume an upright position (mid- to high-Fowler's position) to increase lung expansion. Increasing fluid intake may reduce the thickness of lung secretions and assist in their removal.

Ventilation support with mechanical ventilation may be needed for patients who cannot keep their oxygen saturation at 90% or who have respiratory muscle fatigue. Chapter 34 discusses the nursing care needs of patients who are being mechanically ventilated.

Preventing complications is a major nursing responsibility. Monitoring breathing status and intervening when changes occur are critical in preventing complications. For patients who have chronic respiratory acidosis, assess breathing status at least every 2 hours. Listen to breath sounds, and assess how easily air moves into and out of the lungs. Check for any muscle retractions, the use of accessory muscles (especially the neck muscles [sternocleidomastoids]), and whether breathing produces a sound (like a grunt or a wheeze) that can be heard without a stethoscope. Assess the color of the nail beds and oral membranes for cyanosis (a late finding).

ALKALOSIS

Pathophysiology

In patients with alkalosis, the acid-base balance of the blood is disturbed and has an excess of bases, especially bicarbonate (HCO_3^-). The amount or strength (or both) of the bases is greater than normal compared with the amount or strength of the acids. Alkalosis is a decrease in the free hydrogen ion level of the blood and is reflected by an arterial blood pH above 7.45. Like acidosis, alkalosis is not a disease but, rather, a manifestation of a problem. Alkalosis can be caused by metabolic problems, respiratory problems, or both (Table 14-3).

Alkalosis can result from an actual or relative increase in the amount or strength (or both) of bases. In an actual base excess, alkalosis occurs when base (usually bicarbonate) is either overproduced or undereliminated.

In *relative* alkalosis, the actual amount or strength of bases does not increase. Instead, the amount or strength (or both) of the acids decrease, creating an *acid deficit* and making the blood more basic than acidic. A relative base-excess alkalosis (acid deficit) results from an overelimination or underproduction of acids (Fig. 14-7).

TABLE 14-3 Common Causes of Alkalosis

Pathology	Condition
METABOLIC ALKALOSIS	
Increase of base components	Oral ingestion of bases
	Antacids
	Milk-alkali syndrome
	Parenteral base administration
	Blood transfusion
	Sodium bicarbonate
	Total parenteral nutrition
Decrease of acid components	Prolonged vomiting
	Nasogastric suctioning
	Hypercortisolism
	Hyperaldosteronism
	Thiazide diuretics
RESPIRATORY ALKALOSIS	
Excessive loss of carbon dioxide	Hyperventilation
	Fear, anxiety
	Mechanical ventilation
	Salicylate toxicity
	Hypoxemia-stimulated hyperventilation
	High altitudes
	Shock
	Early-stage acute pulmonary problems

AAABBB	AAABBBB	AABBB
AAABBB	AAABBBB	AABBB
AAABBB	AAABBBB	AABBB
Acid-base balance	Actual alkalosis (base excess)	Relative alkalosis (acid deficit)

Fig. 14-7 • Concepts of actual and relative alkalosis. (A = acid; B = base.)

The problems of alkalosis are serious and potentially life threatening. Treatment is aimed at correcting the cause of alkalosis after identifying whether it is respiratory or metabolic in origin.

Whether metabolic, respiratory, or both, alkalosis affects specific functions. The pathologic effects are caused by the electrolyte imbalances that occur in response to decreased blood cation levels. Most problems of alkalosis are related to increased stimulation of the nervous, neuromuscular, and cardiac systems.

Metabolic alkalosis is caused by conditions that create the acid-base imbalance through either an increase of bases (base excess) or a decrease of acids (acid deficit). Base excesses are caused by excessive intake of bicarbonates, carbonates, acetates, and citrates. Excessive use of oral antacids containing sodium bicarbonate or calcium carbonate can also cause a metabolic alkalosis. Other base excesses can occur during medical treatments, such as citrate excesses during massive blood transfusions and IV sodium bicarbonate given to correct acidosis.

Acid deficits can be caused by disease processes or medical treatment. Disorders include prolonged vomiting, excess cortisol, and hyperaldosteronism. Medical treatments that promote acid loss causing metabolic alkalosis include thiazide diuretics and prolonged nasogastric suctioning.

Respiratory alkalosis is usually caused by an excessive loss of CO_2 through hyperventilation (rapid respirations). Patients may hyperventilate in response to anxiety, fear, or improper settings on mechanical ventilators. Hyperventilation can also result from direct stimulation of central respiratory centers because of fever, central nervous system lesions, and salicylates.

Patient-Centered Collaborative Care

Assessment

Manifestations are the same for metabolic and respiratory alkalosis. Many symptoms are the result of the low calcium levels (hypocalcemia) and low potassium levels (hypokalemia) that usually occur with alkalosis (see Fig. 14-6). These problems change the function of the nervous, neuromuscular, cardiac, and respiratory systems (Chart 14-7).

Central nervous system (CNS) changes are caused by overexcitement of the nervous systems. Patients have dizziness, agitation, confusion, and hyperreflexia, which may progress to seizure activity. Tingling or numbness around the mouth and in the toes may be present. Other indicators of alkalosis with hypocalcemia are positive Chvostek's and Trousseau's signs (see Chapter 13).

Neuromuscular changes are related to the hypocalcemia and hypokalemia that occur with alkalosis. Hypocalcemia increases nervous system activity, causing muscle cramps, twitches, and "charley horses." Deep tendon reflexes are hyperactive. **Tetany** (continuous contractions) of muscle groups also may be present. Tetany is painful and indicates a rapidly worsening condition.

Skeletal muscles may contract as a result of nerve overstimulation, but they become weaker because of the hypokalemia. Handgrip strength decreases, and the patient may be unable to stand or walk. Respiratory efforts become less effective as the skeletal muscles of respiration weaken.

Cardiovascular changes occur because alkalosis increases myocardial irritability, especially when accompanied by hypokalemia. Heart rate increases, and the pulse is thready. When hypovolemia (decreased blood volume) is also present, the patient may have severe hypotension. The hypokalemia increases myocardial sensitivity to digoxin, which increases the risk for digoxin toxicity.

Chart 14-7 KEY FEATURES

Alkalosis

CENTRAL NERVOUS SYSTEM MANIFESTATIONS
- Increased activity
- Anxiety, irritability, tetany, seizures
- Positive Chvostek's sign
- Positive Trousseau's sign
- Paresthesias

NEUROMUSCULAR MANIFESTATIONS
- Hyperreflexia
- Muscle cramping and twitching
- Skeletal muscle weakness

CARDIOVASCULAR MANIFESTATIONS
- Increased heart rate
- Normal or low blood pressure
- Increased digitalis toxicity

RESPIRATORY MANIFESTATIONS
- Increased rate and depth of ventilation in respiratory alkalosis
- Decreased respiratory effort associated with skeletal muscle weakness in metabolic alkalosis

Respiratory changes, especially increases in the rate of breathing, are the main causes of respiratory alkalosis. Although the volume of air inhaled and exhaled with each breath is nearly normal, the total volume of air inhaled and exhaled each minute rises with the increased respiratory rate. The increased minute volume may be caused by anxiety or physiologic changes.

Arterial blood pH greater than 7.45 confirms alkalosis, but this test alone does not identify its cause. Because the manifestations of metabolic alkalosis and respiratory alkalosis are similar, it is critical to obtain additional laboratory data, especially arterial blood gas (ABG) values and specific serum electrolyte levels (see Chart 14-5).

Interventions

Interventions are planned to prevent further losses of hydrogen, potassium, calcium, and chloride ions; to restore fluid balance; and to monitor changes. Drug therapy is used for alkalosis. Drugs are prescribed to resolve the causes of alkalosis and to restore normal fluid, electrolyte, and acid-base balance. For example, the patient with metabolic alkalosis caused by diuretic therapy receives fluid and electrolyte replacement. Fluids and electrolytes are replaced orally or parenterally. Antiemetic drugs are prescribed if the patient is vomiting. Carefully monitor the patient's progress, and adjust fluid and electrolyte therapy. Serum electrolyte values are monitored daily until they return to normal or near normal.

GET READY FOR THE NCLEX EXAMINATION!

Key Points

Review these Key Points for each NCLEX Examination Client Needs Category.

Safe and Effective Care Environment
- Use caution in giving oxygen to people who have COPD.

Health Promotion and Maintenance
- Teach all patients to take drugs as prescribed, especially diuretics, antihypertensives, and cardiac drugs.
- Instruct all patients at continuing risk for respiratory acidosis to stop smoking.

Psychosocial Integrity
- Assess the oxygenation status of any patient with acute confusion.
- Monitor the neurologic status at least every 2 hours in patients being treated for an acid-base imbalance.
- Assist patients who have anxiety-induced respiratory alkalosis to identify causes of anxiety.
- Teach patients who have anxiety-induced respiratory alkalosis to use stress management techniques.

Physiological Integrity
- The normal pH of the body's extracellular fluids (including blood) is 7.35 to 7.45.
- The normal pH of arterial blood is slightly higher (less acidic) than venous blood.
- The more hydrogen ions present, the more acidic the fluid.
- The fewer hydrogen ions present, the more alkaline the fluid.
- Lower pH values (below 7.35) mean acidosis is present.
- Higher pH values (above 7.45) mean alkalosis is present.
- The pH in the body can be described as the relationship of bicarbonate to carbonic acid, or a 20:1 ratio.
- Carbon dioxide (CO_2) is the most changeable component of carbonic acid.
- The concentration of CO_2 is directly related to the concentration of hydrogen ions.
- Anything that increases the CO_2 level in the blood increases the hydrogen ion content and lowers the pH.
- An acid gives up hydrogen ions in solution; a base binds hydrogen ions in solution.
- Acids are normally formed in the body as a result of metabolism and incomplete breakdown of glucose and fats.
- Acid-base balance is regulated by chemical, respiratory, and renal mechanisms.
- Chemical buffers are the immediate way that acid-base imbalances are corrected.
- The lungs control the amount of CO_2 that is retained or exhaled.
- The kidneys regulate the amount of hydrogen and bicarbonate ions that are retained or excreted by the body.
- Compensation is the process in which the body uses its three regulatory mechanisms to correct for changes in the pH of body fluids.
- If a lung problem causes retention of carbon dioxide, the healthy kidney compensates by increasing the amount of bicarbonate that is produced and retained.

- The best way to determine acid-base balance is to analyze arterial blood gases (ABGs).
- Check the serum potassium level for any patient who has acidosis.
- Assess heart rate and rhythm at least every 2 hours for any patient with an acid-base imbalance.
- Assess the airway of any patient who has acute respiratory acidosis.
- Monitor arterial blood gas values to evaluate the effectiveness of therapy for acid-base imbalances.
- Assess the oxygenation status of any patient with acidosis.

Additional Study Resources

Go to your Companion CD or Evolve at http://evolve.elsevier.com/Iggy/ for *Self-Assessment Questions for the NCLEX Examination.*

evolve Go to Evolve at http://evolve.elsevier.com/Iggy/ for *Prioritization and Delegation Questions for the NCLEX Examination.*

SELECTED BIBLIOGRAPHY

Astle, S. (2005). Restoring electrolyte balance. *RN, 68*(5), 34-40.

Casaletto, J. (2005). Differential diagnosis of metabolic acidosis. *Emergency Medicine Clinics of North America, 23*(3), 771-787.

Charles, J., & Heilman, R. (2005). Metabolic acidosis. *Hospital Physician, 41*(3), 37-42.

Gordon, M. (2007). *Manual of nursing diagnosis* (11th ed.). Boston: Jones & Bartlett.

Jarvis, C. (2008). *Physical examination and health assessment* (5th ed.). Philadelphia: Saunders.

McCance, K., & Huether, S. (2006). *Pathophysiology: The biologic basis for disease in adults and children* (5th ed.). St. Louis: Mosby.

Meiner, S., & Lueckenotte, A. (Eds.). (2006). *Gerontologic nursing* (3rd ed.). St. Louis: Mosby.

Pagana, K., & Pagana, T. (2006). *Mosby's manual of diagnostic and laboratory tests* (3rd ed.). St. Louis: Mosby.

Ruholl, L. (2006). Arterial blood gases: Analysis and nursing responses. *MEDSURG Nursing, 15*(6), 343-351.

Swiderski, D., & Byrum, D. (2007). Are you an ABG ace? *American Nurse Today, 2*(4), 18-21.

Vacca, V. (2008). Hyperkalemia. *Nursing2008, 38*(7), 72.

Infusion Therapy

Linda Laskowski-Jones • Alexandra Falkowski

15
CHAPTER

LEARNING OUTCOMES

For clinical competence and success on the NCLEX Examination, study this chapter with these Learning Outcomes in mind:

Safe and Effective Care Environment

1. Check the accuracy of requests for intravenous (IV) fluids and medications.
2. Prevent IV administration errors by following agency policies and using systems that ensure patient safety.
3. Prevent staff injury by using appropriate needleless connection devices.
4. Document care for the patient receiving any type of infusion therapy.

Health Promotion and Maintenance

5. Teach the patient and family about care of the patient receiving infusion therapy.

Physiological Integrity

6. Identify the appropriate veins for peripheral IV catheter insertion.
7. Differentiate types of vascular access devices (VADs) used for peripheral and central IV therapy.
8. Use best practice for inserting peripheral VADs.
9. Use best practice for administering an intermittent IV medication.
10. Assess the patient's infusion site frequently for local complications such as phlebitis and infiltration.
11. Prioritize nursing interventions for maintaining an infusion system.
12. Assess, prevent, and manage systemic complications related to infusion therapy and VADs.
13. Determine special needs of older adults receiving IV therapy.
14. Identify nursing considerations for intra-arterial, intraperitoneal, subcutaneous, intraosseous, epidural, and intrathecal infusion therapy.

Go to your Companion CD or Evolve at *http://evolve.elsevier.com/Iggy/* for Self-Assessment *Questions for the NCLEX Examination* keyed to these Learning Outcomes.

Infusion therapy is the delivery of parenteral medications and fluids through a wide variety of catheter types and locations using multiple procedures. IV therapy is the most common route for infusion therapy. It delivers solutions directly into the veins of the vascular system. This chapter focuses on access for and administration of all types of infusion therapy.

OVERVIEW

Infusion therapy is delivered in all health care settings, including hospitals, home care, ambulatory clinics, physicians' offices, and long-term care facilities (Fig. 15-1). The most common reasons for using infusion therapy are to:

- Maintain fluid balance or correct fluid balance
- Maintain electrolyte or acid-base balance or correct electrolyte or acid-base imbalance
- Administer medications
- Replace blood or blood products

Having a specialized team of infusion nurses to initiate and maintain infusion therapy is recommended by the Centers for Disease Control and Prevention to reduce complications of infusion therapy (O'Grady et al., 2002). Infusion nurses may perform these activities:

- Develop evidence-based policies and procedures
- Insert several types of peripheral and central venous catheters
- Monitor patient outcomes
- Educate staff, patients, and families
- Consult on product selection and purchasing decisions

Rapid advances in technology for infusion therapy have driven the need for nurses specializing in vascular access and infusion therapy. Yet not all health care agencies have an infusion

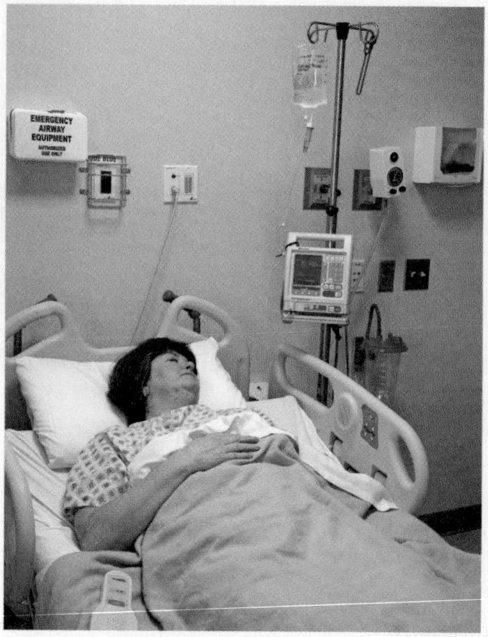
EMERGENCY
AIRWAY
EQUIPMENT

Fig. 15-1 • A patient receiving IV therapy using an infusion pump.

therapy team. All nurses who provide direct patient care are expected to perform basic infusion therapy procedures, although responsibilities vary widely among facilities. Most agencies require that nurses complete an in-house certification course before they are allowed to start IV therapy.

In many states, licensed practical/vocational nurses (LPNs/LVNs) are limited in their scope of practice related to IV therapy. For example, most states do not allow LPNs/LVNs to hang hyperosmolar solutions. Others do not allow them to change central line dressings or draw blood from a central line. The RN can delegate and supervise selected nursing tasks to the LPN/LVN as designated by the health care agency and/or state nurse practice act. The RN is accountable for comprehensive patient care and outcomes of that care.

Several professional organizations strive to improve patient outcomes with infusion therapy and vascular access through education and publications. The Infusion Nurses Society (INS), formerly the Intravenous Nurses Society, publishes guidelines and standards of practice for policy and procedure development in all health care settings. These standards establish the criteria for all nurses delivering infusion therapy (Infusion Nurses Society [INS], 2006). The Infusion Nurses Certification Corporation (INCC) offers a written certifying examination. Nurses who successfully complete this examination have mastered an advanced body of knowledge in this specialty and may use the initials *CRNI*, which stand for *certified registered nurse infusion*. The Association for Vascular Access (AVA) is a multidisciplinary organization focusing on advanced practices with vascular access. The Oncology Nursing Society (ONS) develops guidelines about chemotherapy and biotherapy administration. The American Society of Parenteral and Enteral Nutrition (ASPEN) publishes standards for all types of nutrition.

Types of Infusion Therapy Fluids

Many types of parenteral fluids are used for infusion therapy. These fluids include:

- IV solutions, including parenteral nutrition
- Blood and blood components
- Drugs

Intravenous Solutions

More than 200 IV fluids (solutions) are available that meet the requirements established by the United States Pharmacopeia (USP). Each solution is classified by its tonicity (concentration) and pH. Tonicity is typically categorized by comparison with normal blood plasma as osmolarity (mOsm/L). As discussed in Chapter 13, normal serum osmolarity for adults is between 270 and 300 mOsm/L. Parenteral solutions within that normal range are **isotonic;** those fluids greater than 300 mOsm/L are **hypertonic;** and those fluids less than 270 mOsm/L are **hypotonic.** Table 13-3 in Chapter 13 lists common IV solutions according to their tonicity.

When an *isotonic* **infusate** (solution that is infused into the body) is used, water does not move into or out of the body's cells. Therefore patients receiving isotonic solutions are at risk for fluid overload, especially older adults. This complication is discussed in Chapter 13. *Hypertonic* fluids are used to correct fluid, electrolyte, and acid-base imbalances by moving water out of the body's cells and into the bloodstream. Parenteral nutrition solutions are also hypertonic (see Chapter 63). Instead of moving water out of cells, *hypotonic* infusates move water into cells to expand them. Patients receiving either hypertonic or hypotonic fluids are at risk for phlebitis and infiltration, discussed in Tables 15-2 and 15-6.

The pH of IV solutions measures the acidity or alkalinity and usually ranges from 3.5 to 6.2. Extremes of both osmolarity and pH can cause vein damage leading to phlebitis and thrombosis. Thus fluids and medications with a pH value less than 5 and more than 9 and with an osmolarity more than 500 mOsm/L should not be infused through a peripheral vein (INS, 2006).

Blood and Blood Components

Blood transfusion is accomplished using packed red blood cells, created by removing a large portion of the plasma from whole blood. Other blood components include platelets, fresh frozen plasma, albumin, and several specific clotting factors. Each component has detailed requirements for blood-type compatibility and infusion techniques. Facilities that are accredited by The Joint Commission (TJC) (formerly the Joint Commission on Accreditation of Healthcare Organizations [JCAHO]) are required to ensure that blood components are properly ordered, handled and dispensed, and administered, along with appropriate patient monitoring. Positive patient identification is essential before any blood or blood component is administered. An acute hemolytic transfusion reaction due to an incompatible blood transfusion is a "sentinel event" requiring an intense analysis of the contributing factors and corrective action. Established policies and procedures must be rigidly followed to ensure a safe transfusion and reduce the risk of complications. (See Chapter 42 for a complete discussion of blood transfusions.)

Drug Therapy

IV drugs provide a rapid therapeutic effect but can lead to immediate serious reactions, called **adverse drug events (ADE).** Hundreds of drugs are available for infusion by a variety of techniques. As with all drug administration, nurses must be knowledgeable about drug indications, proper dosage, contraindications, and precautions. IV administration also requires knowledge of appropriate dilution, rate of infusion, pH and osmolarity, compatibility with other IV medications, and specific aspects of patient monitoring because of its immediate effect. *Regardless of familiarity with the drug, never assume that*

IV administration is the same as giving that drug by other routes. New information is continuously being published, and new drugs are rapidly being introduced.

Medication safety is extremely important in all health care settings today. The Joint Commission publishes new and updated National Patient Safety Goals every year. One major goal is improving the safety of high-alert drugs. An example of these drugs is concentrated electrolyte solutions (e.g., potassium chloride), which require restricted access, prominent warnings about the concentration, and storage in a secured location. Other strategies to reduce errors include limiting available concentrations of drugs and dispensing all drugs, including catheter flush solutions, in single-dose containers. Smart pumps, in combination with computer physician order entry (CPOE) and bar code medication administration (BCMA) systems, use recent technology to help reduce adverse drug events (ADEs). Electronic medication administration records (MARs) and multiple checks by pharmacists also help reduce errors.

Prescribing Infusion Therapy

A prescription for infusion therapy written by a physician or other authorized health care provider is necessary before IV therapy begins. To be complete, the prescription for infusion fluids should include:

- Specific type of fluid
- Rate of administration written in milliliters per hour, or the total amount of fluid and the total number of hours for infusion (e.g., 125 mL/hr or 1000 mL/8 hr)
- Drugs and the specific dose to be added to the solution, such as electrolytes or vitamins

A drug prescription should include:

- Drug name, preferably by generic name
- Specific dose and route
- Frequency of administration
- Time of administration
- Length of time for infusion
- Purpose (required in some health care agencies, especially nursing homes)

Some continuously infused drugs, such as those for pain management, are prescribed as milligrams per hour. The type and volume of dilution for infusion medications may be included in the prescription or calculated by the infusion pharmacist.

The nurse is responsible for determining that the prescription is appropriate for the patient and clarifying any questions before administration. Be sure to check for the accuracy and completeness of the treatment prescription. An example of an incomplete one is "5% dextrose in water to keep the vein open (TKO or KVO). This statement does not specify the rate of infusion and is not considered complete (INS, 2006).

Vascular Access Devices

An infusion catheter, also known as a **vascular access device (VAD),** is a plastic tube placed in a blood vessel to deliver fluids and medications. The specific type and purpose of the therapy determine whether the infusion can be given safely through peripheral veins or if the large central veins of the chest are needed. Advances in catheter materials and insertion techniques have radically expanded the types of VAD currently used. This discussion includes the description of each type of catheter used for peripheral and central IV therapy. Seven major types are described:

- Short peripheral catheters
- Midline catheters
- Peripherally inserted central catheters (PICC)
- Nontunneled percutaneous central catheters
- Tunneled catheters
- Implanted ports
- Hemodialysis catheters

Assess the patient's needs for vascular access, and choose the device that has the best chance of infusing the prescribed therapy for the required length of time. Be sure to use a topical anesthetic agent before inserting a VAD to decrease patient discomfort.

PERIPHERAL INTRAVENOUS THERAPY

Short infusion catheters and midline catheters are the most commonly used vascular access devices (VADs) for **peripheral IV therapy.** They are usually placed in the veins of the arm.

Short Peripheral Catheters

Short peripheral catheters are composed of a plastic cannula built around a sharp stylet extending slightly beyond the cannula (Fig. 15-2). The stylet (sharp) allows for the venipuncture, and the cannula is advanced into the vein. These catheters are designed with a safety mechanism to cover the sharp end of the stylet after it is removed from the patient. These stylets are hollow-bore, blood-filled needles that carry a high risk of exposure to bloodborne pathogens if needle stick injury occurs. A federal law enacted in 2000 amended the Bloodborne Pathogen Standards from the Occupational Safety and Health Administration (OSHA) requiring the use of catheters with an engineered safety mechanism to prevent needle sticks.

Insertion

Short peripheral catheters are usually inserted into superficial veins of the forearm using sterile technique. In emergent situations, these catheters can be used also in the external jugular vein of the neck. *The use of veins in the hands or feet of adults should be avoided if possible because of an increased risk of deep vein thrombosis and infiltration.*

Short catheters range in length from $\frac{3}{4}$ inch to $1\frac{1}{4}$ inch with gauge sizes from 26 gauge (the smallest) to 14 gauge (large bore). *Choose the smallest gauge catheter capable of delivering the prescribed therapy.* Current design allows for a thin-wall construction, providing a larger lumen (opening) without increasing the outer diameter. This design improves the fluid flow through the catheter while using a smaller gauge and thereby decreases the possibility of vein irritation from a large catheter. For example, a thin-walled 24-gauge Insyte (BD Medical) catheter has about the same flow-rate ability as a 22-gauge non–thin-walled Angiocath (BD Medical). Larger gauge sizes allow for faster flow rates but also cause phlebitis more often. Table 15-1 lists each gauge size and its common uses.

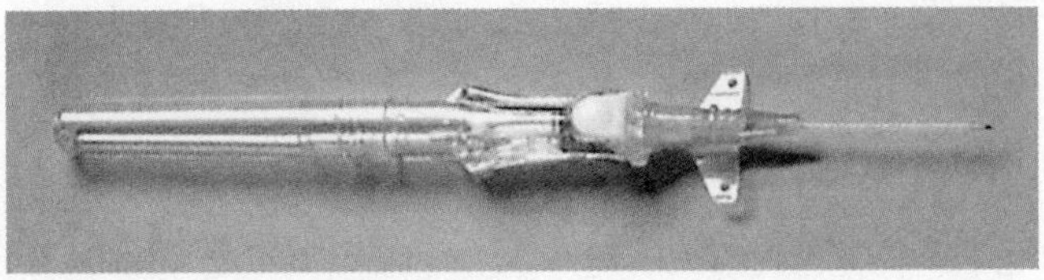

Fig. 15-2 • Insyte AutoGuard IV catheters. With the push of a button, the needle instantly retracts, reducing the risk of accidental needle stick injuries.

TABLE 15-1 Choosing the Gauge Size for Peripheral Catheters

24- and 26-gauge	Used for neonates and pediatric and older patients Recommended when extremely small-diameter veins are the only choice Blood return in the flash chamber may be slower Suitable for most infusions, but flow rates are slower May be used for blood transfusion without an infusion pump; a unit of packed red blood cells should be divided into two bags to accommodate the extended infusion time
22-gauge	Used for all infusions including blood and blood products Infusion rates will be slightly slower Recommended for most adults, especially those with small or fragile veins Not appropriate when rapid flow rates are required such as trauma or surgery
20-gauge	Used for all infusions including blood and blood products; suitable for minor surgical procedures Most commonly used size
18-gauge	Used for trauma and surgery Rapid flow rates Requires a large vein to allow room for blood to flow in the vein around the catheter Irritation to the vein wall and phlebitis result when the catheter is too large for the chosen vein
16- and 14-gauge	Used for high-risk surgical procedures and trauma Large volumes and rapid flow Requires a large vein Mechanical irritation and phlebitis are likely

Chart 15-1 BEST PRACTICE FOR PATIENT SAFETY & QUALITY CARE

Placement of Short Peripheral Venous Catheters

- Verify that the prescription for infusion therapy is complete and appropriate for infusion through a short peripheral catheter.
- For adults, choose a site for placement in the upper extremity.
- Choose the patient's nondominant arm when possible.
- Choose a distal site, and make all subsequent venipunctures proximal to previous sites.
- Do not use the arm on the side of a mastectomy, lymph node dissection, arteriovenous shunt or fistula, or paralysis.
- Avoid choosing a site in an area of joint flexion.
- Avoid choosing a site in a vein that feels hard or cordlike.
- Avoid choosing a site close to areas of cellulitis, dermatitis, or complications from previous catheter sites.

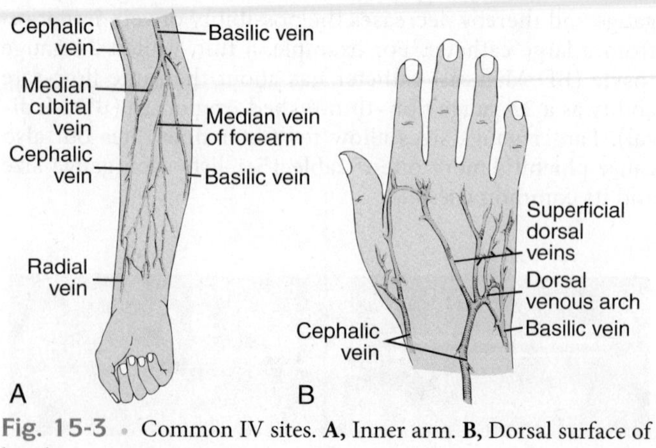
Cephalic vein
Basilic vein
Median cubital vein
Median vein of forearm
Cephalic vein
Basilic vein
Radial vein
A
Superficial dorsal veins
Dorsal venous arch
Basilic vein
Cephalic vein
B

Fig. 15-3 • Common IV sites. **A,** Inner arm. **B,** Dorsal surface of hand.

Short peripheral catheters are allowed to dwell (stay in) for 72 to 96 hours but then require removal and insertion at another venous site. If the length of the patient's therapy is expected to be longer than 6 days, a midline catheter or PICC should be chosen (O'Grady et al., 2002). When selecting the site for insertion of a peripheral catheter, consider the patient's age, history, and diagnosis; the type and duration of the prescribed therapy; and, whenever possible, the patient's preference (Rosenthal, 2005b). Chart 15-1 lists the major criteria for the placement of peripheral VADs.

Placement

Though not yet widely used in most clinical settings, vein transilluminators and ultrasound devices are now available as tools to assist in IV line placement. One of the most popular tools, VeinViewer, is a mobile infrared device that locates the vein. Veinlite LED is also mobile but uses transillumination to find the vein (Krueger, 2007). Training and practice are required to develop the skills needed to use these devices properly. If these devices are not used, nurses must rely on sight and touch to insert an IV catheter.

The most appropriate veins for peripheral catheter placement include the dorsal venous network, basilic, cephalic, and median veins, as well as their branches (Fig. 15-3). *Veins on the hand are not appropriate, especially for older patients with a loss of skin turgor and poor vein condition and for active patients receiving infusion therapy in an ambulatory clinic or home care.* Mastectomy, axillary lymph node dissection, lymphedema, paralysis of the upper extremity, and the presence of dialysis grafts or fistulas alter the normal pattern of blood flow through the arm. Using veins in the extremity affected by these conditions requires a physician's request. Short peripheral catheters are not recommended for obtaining routine blood samples (INS, 2006).

Veins on the palm side of the wrist should be avoided because the median nerve is located close to veins in this area, making the venipuncture more painful and difficult to stabilize (Rosenthal,

2005b). The cephalic vein begins above the thumb and extends up the entire length of the arm. This vein is usually large and prominent, appearing as a prime site for catheter insertion. However, the sensory branch of the median nerve can intersect with the cephalic vein up to three times from its origin to about 4 to 5 inches up the lateral aspect of the arm. Transection of the nerve can result in permanent loss of function, and local nerve damage can become a chronic systemic pain syndrome. *Reports of tingling, feeling "pins and needles" in the extremity, or numbness during the venipuncture procedure can indicate nerve puncture. The procedure should be stopped immediately, the catheter removed, and a new site chosen.*

Winged needles are easy to insert but are associated with a high frequency of infiltration. They are most commonly used for injection of single-dose drugs or for drawing blood samples. Like a short peripheral catheter, winged needles should also have an engineered safety mechanism to house the needle when removed.

Midline Catheters

Midline catheters are 6 to 8 inches long and are inserted through the veins of the antecubital fossa. The basilic vein is preferred over the cephalic vein because of its larger diameter and straighter path. It also allows greater hemodilution of the fluids and medications being infused. The catheter tip is located in the upper-arm level below the axilla. These catheters are used for therapies lasting from 1 to 4 weeks; however, there are no recommendations for the optimal dwell time. Because of the extended dwell time, strict sterile technique is used for insertion of a midline catheter. Additional education and skill assessment are required for the nurse to be considered qualified to insert midline catheters.

A midline catheter can be used when skin integrity or limited peripheral veins make it difficult to maintain a short peripheral catheter. Other indications include:

- Fluids for hydration
- Five to 10 days of antibiotics to treat urosepsis or pneumonia
- Heparin infusions for deep vein thrombosis
- Bronchodilators, such as aminophylline
- Steroids

Limiting venipunctures in patients who have received anticoagulation agents is desirable to avoid excessive bruising and hematoma formation. Steroid-dependent patients experience changes in their skin and vein fragility, making repeated venipuncture difficult. Therefore midline catheters are preferred in these instances.

The fluids and medications infused through a midline catheter should have a pH between 5 and 9 and a final osmolarity of less than 500 mOsm/L (INS, 2006). The pH and osmolarity outside these parameters increase the risk of complications like phlebitis and thrombosis. Midline catheters should not be used for infusion of **vesicant medications**—drugs that cause severe tissue damage if they escape into the subcutaneous tissue **(extravasation).** At a midline tip location, larger amounts of the drug can extravasate before the problem is detected. All parenteral nutrition formulas, including those with low concentrations of dextrose, have an osmolarity greater than 500 mOsm/L and should not be infused through a midline catheter. Blood sampling from them should not be routinely performed (INS, 2006). Midline catheters should not be placed in extremities affected by mastectomy with lymphedema, paralysis, or dialysis grafts and fistulas.

Midline catheters may be designed with pressure-sensitive valves located near the internal catheter tip (e.g., Groshong, made by Bard Access Systems) or in the external catheter hub (e.g., PASV, made by Boston Scientific). These valves open when pressure is applied, allowing for infusion and aspiration. However, when no pressure is applied, they are closed to prevent blood refluxing (backing) into the lumen or air entering the bloodstream. The manufacturers of both catheters state that saline only can be used to flush these lines.

CENTRAL INTRAVENOUS THERAPY

In **central IV therapy,** the vascular access device (VAD) is placed in the central blood vessels, such as the superior vena cava (SVC). A number of types of central venous catheters (CVC) are available, depending on the purpose, duration, and insertion site availability.

Peripherally Inserted Central Catheters

Placement

A peripherally inserted central catheter (PICC) is a long catheter inserted through a vein of the antecubital fossa (inner aspect of the bend of the arm) or the middle of the upper arm. In adults, the catheter length ranges from 18 to 29 inches (45 to 72 cm), with the tip residing in the SVC. Placement of the catheter tip in veins distal to the SVC should be avoided. This inappropriate tip location, often called a *mid-clavicular catheter,* is associated with much higher rates of thrombosis than when the tip is located in the SVC (INS, 2006). Mid-clavicular tip locations should be used only when anatomic or pathophysiologic changes prohibit placing the catheter into the SVC.

PICCs should be inserted early in the course of therapy before veins of the extremity have been damaged from multiple venipunctures and infusions. Insertion methods using guidewires and ultrasound greatly improve insertion success. The basilic vein is the preferred site for insertion; the cephalic vein can be used if necessary. *Sterile technique is used for insertion to reduce the risk of catheter-related bloodstream infections (CR-BSIs). A chest x-ray indicating that the tip resides in the lower SVC is required before the catheter can be used for infusion.* PICCs are available in single-, dual-, or triple-lumen configurations and are available with both the Groshong valve and the pressure-activated safety valve (PASV).

PICCs have low complication rates because of the insertion site in the upper extremity. The dry skin of the arm has fewer types and numbers of microorganisms, leading to lower rates of infection. Inadvertent arterial puncture or excessive bleeding can be controlled by direct pressure. Insertion complications such as pneumothorax associated with other central venous catheters do not occur with PICCs. In addition, PICC lines are less expensive than central catheters (Moureau, 2006).

Indications

PICCs can accommodate the infusion of all types of therapy because the tip resides in the SVC where the rapid blood flow will quickly dilute the fluids being infused. Therefore there are no limitations on the pH or osmolality of fluids that can be infused through a PICC. Patients requiring lengthy courses of antibiotics, chemotherapy agents, parenteral nutrition formulas, vasopressor agents, and numerous other fluids can benefit from a PICC. These catheters have been reported to dwell successfully for months or even years; however, the optimal dwell time is not known (O'Grady et al., 2002).

PICCs can be used for blood sampling; however, lumen sizes of 4 Fr or larger are recommended. Using lumens with small diameters may not yield a sample capable of producing the needed test results. Transfusion of blood through a PICC usually requires the use of an infusion pump. Packed red blood cells are cold and viscous. The length of the PICC adds resistance and may prevent the blood from infusing within the 4-hour limit.

Teach patients with a PICC to perform normal ADLs; however, they should avoid excessive physical activity. Muscle contractions in the arm from physical activity like heavy lifting can lead to catheter dislodgment and possible lumen occlusion.

PICC insertion is commonly performed in the patient's hospital room, an outpatient treatment facility, or the imaging department. Nurses placing these catheters require a high level of skill with venipuncture and central venous catheter management. Additional education, along with documented competency assessment, is required.

Nontunneled Percutaneous Central Catheters

Nontunneled percutaneous central catheters are inserted by a physician through the subclavian vein in the upper chest or the jugular veins in the neck using sterile technique. They are usually 7 to 10 inches (15 to 25 cm) long and have dual or triple lumens. The tip resides in the SVC, confirmed by a chest x-ray. Nontunneled percutaneous central catheters are most commonly used for emergent or trauma situations, critical care, and surgery. There is no recommendation for optimal dwell time. However, these catheters are commonly used for short-term situations and are not the catheter of choice for home care or ambulatory clinic settings.

Insertion of these central catheters requires the patient to be placed in the Trendelenburg position, usually with a rolled towel between the shoulder blades. This position may be difficult or contraindicated for patients with respiratory conditions, spinal curvatures, and increased intracranial pressure. Trauma, surgery, or radiation in the neck or chest prohibits the use of these devices as well. The presence of a tracheotomy increases the risk of cross-contamination of the insertion site. The oily skin of the neck and upper chest has more types and higher numbers of microorganisms, resulting in more bloodstream infections (BSI) with this type of catheter.

Tunneled Central Catheters

Tunneled central venous catheters have a portion of the catheter lying in a subcutaneous tunnel, separating the points where the catheter enters the vein from where it exits the skin. This separation is intended to prevent the organisms on the skin from reaching the bloodstream (Fig. 15-4). The catheter has a cuff made of a rough material that is positioned inside the subcutaneous tunnel. The tissue granulates into this cuff, providing a mechanical barrier to microorganisms and anchoring the catheter in place. This design requires surgical techniques for insertion. Single, dual, and triple lumens are available. These catheters were originally named for the physicians who designed them, including Broviac, Hickman, and Leonard catheters. These names are trade names and should be used when referring to those particular catheters.

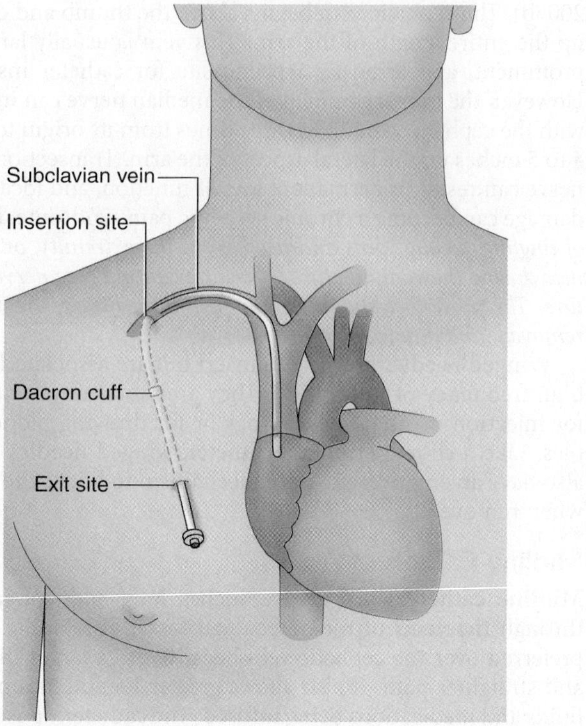
Subclavian vein
Insertion site
Dacron cuff
Exit site

Fig. 15-4 • Tunneled catheter. A portion of this catheter lies in a subcutaneous tunnel, separating the point where the catheter enters the vein from where it exits the skin.

Tunneled catheters are used primarily when the need for infusion therapy is frequent and long-term. Patients needing parenteral nutrition for months, years, or the remainder of their life commonly choose a tunneled catheter. Tunneled catheters are also chosen when several weeks or months of infusion therapy are needed and a PICC is not a good choice. For example, paraplegic patients needing 6 to 8 weeks of antibiotics are not good candidates for a PICC because of the excessive use of the upper extremities for mobility. Some oncology patients may prefer a tunneled catheter instead of an implanted port because they cannot tolerate the needle sticks required for accessing those devices.

Implanted Ports

Implanted ports consist of a portal body, a dense septum over a reservoir, and a catheter (Fig. 15-5). A subcutaneous pocket is surgically created to house the port body. The catheter is inserted into the vein and attached to the portal body. The septum is made of self-sealing silicone and is located in the center of the port body over the reservoir. The catheter extends from the side of the port body. The incision is closed, and no part of the catheter is visible externally; therefore this device has the least impact on body image.

Placement

Venous ports may be placed on the upper chest or the upper extremity. The venous catheter may enter either the subclavian or internal jugular vein and is available as a single- or double-lumen device. Although an implanted port is most commonly

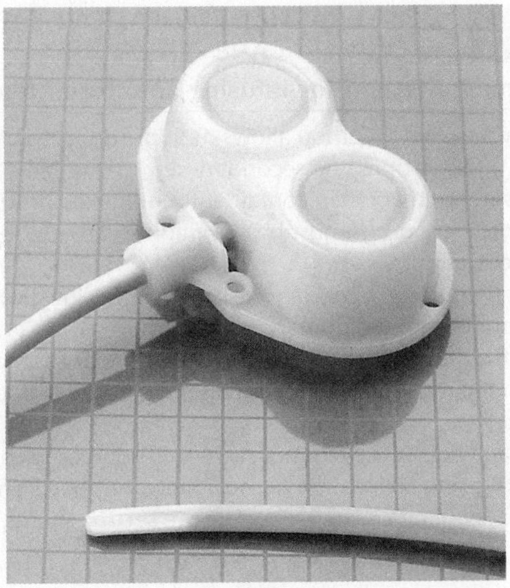

Fig. 15-5 • A dual-lumen implanted port for venous access.

used in the venous system, the catheter may be placed in arteries, the epidural space, or the peritoneal cavity, with the port pocket located over a bony prominence.

Maintenance

Implanted ports are accessed by using a noncoring needle specially designed with a deflected tip. This design slices through the dense septum without coring out a small piece of it, thus preserving the integrity of the septum. Port bodies placed in the chest have a larger septum and will usually tolerate about 2000 punctures. Port bodies placed in the upper extremity are smaller and are rated to tolerate about 750 punctures. Before puncture, palpate the port to locate the septum. Carefully palpate to feel the shape and depth of the port body to ensure puncture of the septum, not the attached catheter. Noncoring port access needles, also called **Huber needles,** may have a straight shaft or may be bent at a right angle. Some have attached extension sets and wings to stabilize the needle. One important feature is an engineered safety mechanism to contain the needle when it is removed from the septum. Because the dense septum holds tightly to the needle, there can be a rebound when it is pulled from the septum, often resulting in needle stick injury to the nurse (see Fig. 15-5).

An implanted port needs to be flushed after each use and at least once a month between courses of therapy. When the port is not accessed, there is no external catheter requiring a dressing. Puncture of the skin over the port is required to gain access to the port body, causing pain for some patients. Topical anesthetic creams can be used to make the access procedure more tolerable.

Dialysis Catheters

Dialysis catheters have very large lumens to accommodate the hemodialysis procedure or a pheresis procedure that harvests specific blood cells. They may be tunneled for long-term needs or nontunneled for short-term needs. A dialysis catheter is critical to the management of renal failure and must function well. CR-BSI and vein thrombosis are common problems; therefore this catheter should not be used for administration of other fluids or medications except in an emergency.

INFUSION SYSTEMS

Nurses administering infusion therapies need to understand how infusion systems work. This knowledge ensures that the patient can benefit from a particular system's advantages while minimizing any potential complications.

Containers

Infusion containers are made of glass or plastic. *Glass* bottles were the original fluid container to be mass produced. They are easily sterilized, and it is easy to read the amount of fluid remaining in the bottle. Also, they do not have the problems of compatibility with some drugs like plastic does. However, glass bottles are heavy and cannot easily be used in many situations, such as patient transport during emergencies. These containers require an air vent for fluids to flow freely from them. The most common method is to use an administration set with a special filtered vent. Some bottles may have a straw tube open to the room air through the rubber stopper in the bottle and extending to above the level of the fluid. Bottles with a venting straw do not have a barrier to prevent contaminants in the air from entering the fluid.

Plastic containers are considered *closed systems* because they do not rely on outside air to allow the fluid to infuse. Instead, atmospheric pressure pushes against the flexible sides of the container, allowing the fluid to flow by gravity. For this reason, plastic containers do not require vented administration sets. These containers are lightweight, unbreakable, and easy to use in emergency conditions. Therefore they are used more frequently than glass containers.

Plastic containers are commonly made of polyvinyl chloride (PVC). To increase flexibility and strength, PVC requires the addition of plasticizers. The most common chemical used as a plasticizer is di-2-ethylhexyl-phthalate or DEHP. Concern has been growing in the past few years over the exposure of patients to this chemical. DEHP does not chemically bind to the PVC and can leach from the plastic fluid container or tubing and can be infused to the patient with the IV fluid or medication.

Plastic containers are incompatible with insulin, nitroglycerin, lorazepam (Ativan), fat emulsions, and lipid-based drugs. Nitroglycerin and insulin adhere to the walls of the PVC container, making it impossible to know exactly how much medication the patient is receiving.

Another concern with plastic bags is the accuracy of reading the amount of fluid remaining in the container. The middle graduations have been shown to be 10% above or below the actual amount of fluid, but the first and last markings could be inaccurate by as much as 40% (Perucca, 2001).

Semirigid containers are made of plastic but offer some of the benefits of glass, such as the absence of plasticizers and drug incompatibility. These containers are lightweight and unbreakable but are more bulky and less flexible. They also require an air vent to allow the fluid to flow freely. Recent changes have led to a traditional flexible plastic bag made from materials other than PVC and do not require DEHP.

Regardless of the type of fluid container being used, it should be checked for cracks or pinholes before use. Always check the fluid for **turbidity** (cloudiness) or any unusual color that could indicate contamination.

Chart 15-2 BEST PRACTICE FOR PATIENT SAFETY & QUALITY CARE

Piggybacking an Intermittent Drug

1. Verify the prescription from the health care provider.
2. Check the compatibility between the drug and the large-volume parenteral (LVP) infusion and its additives.
3. Spike the medication mini-bag with the secondary set.
4. Prime the secondary set, close the roller clamp, and hang the mini-bag on the other arm of the IV pole.
5. Place the hanger that comes with the secondary set on the IV pole with the LVP.
6. Cleanse the Y-site injection port on the LVP administration set.
7. Attach the secondary set to the Y-site.
8. Lower the level of the LVP by hanging it from the hanger. Do not adjust the LVP roller clamp. (The rate will decrease and then stop when the secondary set is opened.)
9. Open the roller clamp on the secondary set, and regulate the flow to the desired rate.
10. When the intermittent infusion completes, the LVP will automatically begin again. Hang the LVP from the IV pole, and adjust the roller clamp to deliver the prescribed rate.

Chart 15-3 BEST PRACTICE FOR PATIENT SAFETY & QUALITY CARE

Backpriming Method for Infusing an Intermittent Drug

- The backpriming method allows multiple drugs to be infused through the same secondary set.
- Assess the primary fluid container for premixed drugs. If present, these drugs must be compatible with the secondary medication.
- Lower the empty secondary container, and allow fluid to flow into it from the primary container.
- Close the clamp, and disconnect the secondary container.
- Attach the new secondary container with the next dose of medication.
- Hang and adjust the rate or set the infusion pump as indicated. If using an infusion pump, follow the specific manufacturer's guidelines to backprime the secondary set.

Administration Sets

The administration set is the connection between the catheter and the fluid container. Numerous sets are available in many different configurations. The type and purpose of the infusion determine the type of administration set needed. Some sets are *generic,* meaning that they are appropriate for most infusions. Other sets are used for specific types of infusions, such as blood transfusion. Still others are *dedicated,* meaning that they must be used with a specific manufacturer's infusion controlling device. Information that describes their proper use is usually provided on the packaging of administration sets.

Secondary Administration Sets

A primary continuous administration set is used to infuse the primary IV fluid by either a gravity infusion or an electronic infusion pump. A short **secondary administration set,** also known as a **piggyback set,** is attached to the primary set at a Y–injection site and is used to deliver intermittent medications. Chart 15-2 describes the procedure for piggybacking. Once attached, these sets should remain connected together as an infusion system. If multiple intermittent medications are required, it may be possible to use only one secondary set rather than a secondary set for each medication. This depends on the compatibility of the drugs. Chart 15-3 explains how to infuse multiple medications using the backpriming method. This process eliminates the costs of using multiple secondary sets and follows the INS standards of practice. These sets are changed every 72 to 96 hours (INS, 2006; O'Grady et al., 2002).

Intermittent Administration Sets

When no primary continuous fluid is being infused, an intermittent administration set is used to infuse multiple doses of medications through a catheter that has been capped with a needleless connection device. The medication container from the previous dose is removed and the new one attached. The sterile cap covering the distal end of the set is removed, and the set is attached to the catheter. Because both ends of the set are being manipulated with each dose, the INS standards of practice state that this set should be changed every 24 hours. If a secondary administration set is detached from the primary set, it should be considered an intermittent set and changed every 24 hours (INS, 2006).

Administration sets are sterile in the fluid pathway and under the sterile caps on each end of the set. The set is not packaged as a completely sterile product and cannot be added to a sterile field. Careful attention is required to maintain the sterility of the spike and the connection end of the tubing to prevent introduction of microorganisms into the catheter and bloodstream.

Add-on Devices

Several other types of add-on devices include short extension sets, injection caps, and filters. Extension sets may be packaged as a sterile product for adding to a sterile field; however, always check the product label to ascertain this information.

Administration sets have two ways to connect to the catheter hub: a slip lock or a Luer-Lok. The *slip lock* is a male end that slips into the female catheter hub. A *Luer-Lok* connection has the same male end with a threaded collar that requires twisting onto the corresponding threads of the catheter hub. All connections, including *extension sets,* should have a Luer-Lok design to ensure that the set remains firmly connected. Loose connections lead to fluid leakage and increase the risk of contamination and subsequent bloodstream infection. When using a central venous catheter, a Luer-Lok connection is critical to reduce the risk of air embolism. Tape is not considered an adequate mechanism for securing set connections.

Luer-Lok devices may be purposefully or accidentally disconnected. Patients or visitors may disconnect the system to allow the patient to get out of bed or the chair. Or, the device may become accidentally disconnected when the patient turns or moves. In either case, be sure to reconnect the device by following the proper sequence to reassemble the IV system components. Reports of fatalities have resulted when nurses have reconnected IV tubing to a tracheostomy or blood pressure cuff (Eackle et al., 2005; Paparella, 2005).

Filters may be part of the administration set or may be separate add-on pieces. Their purpose is to remove particulate matter, microorganisms, and air from the infusion system. Filter sizes depend on the pore size, with common sizes being 5 microns intended to remove gross particles, 1.2 microns used to filter lipid-containing parenteral nutrition, and 0.22 microns intended to remove all particles and microorganisms. Filters should be placed as close to the catheter hub as possible.

Particulate matter in the IV fluid, a primary reason to use filters, comprises undissolved, unintended substances and may include rubber pieces, glass particles, cotton fibers, drug particles, paper, and metal fibers. These particles become trapped in the small circulation of the lungs. A red blood cell is about 5 microns in diameter and is the largest size that can pass through the pulmonary capillary bed, and yet IV fluids may contain particles larger than this. For patients receiving infusion therapy for long periods, a significant number of particles could block the blood flow through the pulmonary circulation. Microcirculation in the spleen, kidneys, and liver could also be affected. Particulate matter has also been implicated in the development of phlebitis in peripheral veins.

Other concerns with using filters include the possibility for their rupture, their use with certain drugs that bind to the filter surface, using the correct size of filter for drugs with large molecules, and choosing a filter that will tolerate the pressure exerted by infusion pumps. Rupture is most commonly associated with the exertion of high pressure exceeding the limit tolerated by the specific filter. Some drugs cannot be filtered because they are retained inside the filter because of their chemical nature or molecule size. For these reasons, medication filtration during the process of admixing is now used as an alternative to final filtration at the bedside. Drugs of a very small quantity should be administered below the filter.

Filters used on blood administration sets have much larger pore size and are not interchangeable with filters used for fluids and medications. A standard blood filter ranges from 170 to 220 microns and removes microclots and other debris caused by blood collection and storage. Microaggregate filters have a pore size of 20, 40, or 80 microns and are used to remove degenerating platelets, white blood cells, and fibrin strands. Leukocyte-removal filters are used to remove white blood cells that cause febrile and allergic blood transfusion reactions, cytomegalovirus, and some herpes viruses.

Needleless Connection Devices

In July 1992, the Occupational Safety and Health Administration (OSHA) published guidelines entitled *Occupational Exposure to Bloodborne Pathogens, Final Rule*. This document requires health care organizations to initiate engineering controls "that isolate or remove the bloodborne pathogen hazard from the workplace." This standard was amended in 2001 with the passage of the Needlestick Safety and Prevention Act. This regulation requires the use of devices engineered with safety mechanisms and mandates that staff who perform these tasks be directly involved with selecting products. It also requires each employer to maintain a sharps injury log with details of each incident. Many products are designed to minimize health care workers' exposure to contaminated needles. Luer-activated devices are the most common design for needleless systems today (Fig. 15-6).

Although these devices have reduced the incidence of accidental needle sticks for health care professionals, concern remains about a possible increase in the risk of catheter-related bloodstream infections (CR-BSIs) (Rosenthal, 2006a). However, well-designed conclusive studies need to be conducted to determine the best design for needleless systems. Until then, implement these interventions to reduce infection risk:

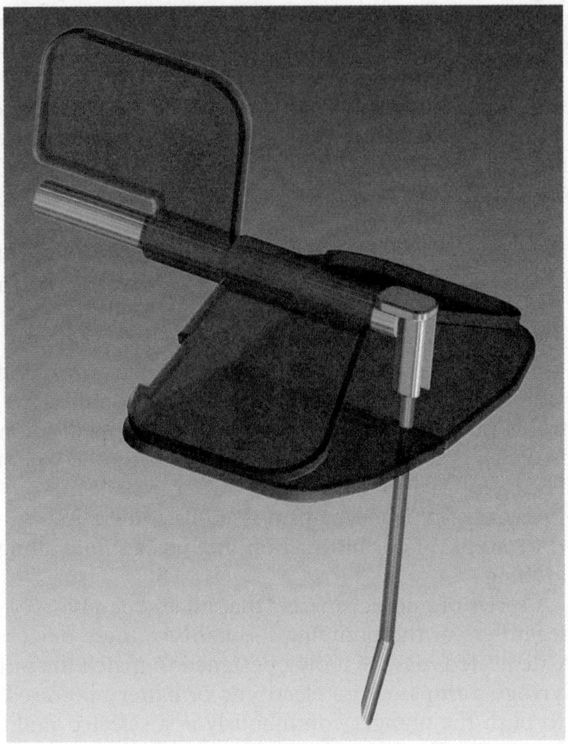

Fig. 15-6 • Huber Plus noncoring needle. The safety mechanism traps the needle to prevent needle stick injury.

- Clean all needleless system connections vigorously with antimicrobial (usually chlorhexidine) swabs before connecting infusion sets or syringes.
- Do not tape connections between tubing sets.
- Use evidence-based hand hygiene guidelines from the CDC and OSHA.
- Attend educational offerings about new products or guidelines to prevent or minimize CR-BSIs.

Rate-Controlling Devices

The ability to regulate the rate and volume of infusions is critical to the safe and accurate administration of medications and fluids to patients. Nurses have a choice of numerous devices that can be mechanically or electronically regulated.

Mechanically regulated systems include elastomeric balloons, spring-coiled syringes and containers, and a multichambered fluid container placed in a mechanical roller. These devices are commonly used to deliver intermittent medications such as antibiotics in community-based health care settings. They are powered by positive pressure from the collapsing balloon or roller returning to its coiled position. Fluid volume is determined by the size of the fluid container; however, most hold 50 to 100 mL. They deliver a preset infusion rate determined by the size of the opening in the tubing connected to the fluid container; therefore additional tubing is not required. These small, portable devices do not require power sources such as batteries or electricity.

Electronic infusion devices fall into two categories—controllers and pumps—based on the mechanism of operation. Both nurses and patients reap the benefits of some of the latest infusion computer technology. Electronic infusion devices can save nursing time, prevent patients from receiving too much infusion solution, and keep infusion access devices patent. However, remember that the use of these devices does not decrease your responsibility to carefully monitor the patient's infusion site and the infusion rate.

A **controller** is a stationary, pole-mounted electronic device that uses a sensor to monitor fluid flow and to detect when flow has been interrupted. Controllers rely completely on gravity to create fluid flow and do not create pressure. Because controllers rely on counting drops, which vary in size and therefore volume, controllers are not as accurate as pumps.

Pumps may be either large and pole-mounted or ambulatory and portable (see Fig. 15-1). As their name indicates, these electronic devices with battery backup pump medications or fluids under pressure. They accurately measure the volume of fluid being infused by using one of three mechanisms:

- A syringe-type mechanism that fills and empties
- A wavelike, peristaltic action that pushes fluid along the tubing
- A series of microchambers that fill and empty

Regardless of the pumping mechanism, these devices require dedicated cassette tubing designed to match the pump.

Syringe pumps use an electronic or battery-powered piston to push the plunger continuously at a selected milliliter-per-hour rate. The use of syringe pumps is limited to small-volume continuous or intermittent infusions and depends on the syringe size. Antibiotics and patient-controlled analgesia are frequently delivered with syringe pumps. Patients requiring fluid restrictions can also benefit from using a syringe pump because smaller yet accurate volumes can be used to dilute medications. Syringe pumps are generally not appropriate for continuous administration of larger volumes because they require frequent syringe changes.

Ambulatory pumps are generally used for home care patients and allow them to return to their usual activities while receiving infusion therapy. These pumps have a wide range of sizes, with some requiring a backpack, but they usually weigh less than 6 pounds. They are typically used to accurately deliver continuous infusions, such as parenteral nutrition and many programmable medication schedules. Frequent battery recharging or replacement is usually necessary.

Electronic infusion devices can be programmed in many different ways and require a thorough knowledge of the specific brand being used. Infusion rate and the volume to be infused are usually entered in single milliliter increments, but some can be programmed as fractions of a milliliter. Some pumps allow the rate to be programmed to taper or ramp up and down at the beginning and ending of the infusion. Secondary syringe infusion, secondary infusion rate, remote site programming, adjustable infusion pressure, and integration into the nurse call system also are possible.

Electronic infusion devices have a variety of alarms, such as air-in-line, upstream and downstream occlusion, infusion complete, and low-battery or power warnings. All devices must have some mechanism to prevent free flow of the infusing fluid or medication. When the cassette or tubing is removed from the pump, this mechanism automatically stops fluid flow until it is properly replaced in the pump. This safety measure prevents accidental rapid infusion of large amounts of fluid or medication, which could lead to serious clinical problems.

In the past few years, **smart pumps** (infusion pumps with dosage calculation software) have been promoted to reduce adverse drug events (ADEs). Incorrect programming of pumps without this feature is one of the most common types of medication errors, especially in hospitals. Multiple libraries of drug information are stored in the pump manufacturer's medical management system. This software allows the facility to pre-program dosing limits, especially for high-alert drugs. For example, Hospira's MedNet works with its Plum A+ smart pump. In addition to preventing drug errors, smart pump systems record potential errors that would have occurred without these safety mechanisms (Jacobs, 2006).

NCLEX EXAMINATION CHALLENGE

A client receiving morphine delivered by continuous infusion on an electronic pump returns from the PACU screaming "Do something now nurse; I can't stand this pain any more!" What is the nurse's best action at this time?

A. Tell the client that the pain is expected but it takes a while for morphine to work.
B. Ask the client to describe the quality of pain being experienced at this time
C. Check the infusion pump to be sure that it is working properly.
D. Report the client's pain experience to the surgeon immediately.

evolve For the correct answer, go to http://evolve.elsevier.com/Iggy/.

NURSING CARE FOR PATIENTS RECEIVING INTRAVENOUS THERAPY

Educating the Patient

Before catheter insertion, educate the patient and family about:

- The type of catheter to be used
- The therapy required
- Alternatives to the catheter and therapy
- Activity limitations
- Any signs or symptoms of complications that should be reported to a health care professional

Although written information should be provided before placement of a long-term catheter, continue to assess the patient's understanding and provide more information or answers as needed. Most manufacturers of PICCs, tunneled catheters, and implanted ports provide patient information booklets. However, specific information about the chosen procedures and supplies may be required. The booklets may be useless to those patients who cannot read or have difficulty with reading.

Confirming Tip Location

All central venous catheters require a post-insertion chest x-ray to document the tip location. The initial verbal and subsequent written report should contain specific information about the catheter tip location in relation to anatomic structures. The nurse's knowledge of accurate tip location is required before beginning infusion through the catheter. Repeating the x-ray during catheter use may be necessary if the patient reports unusual pain or sensation.

Performing the Nursing Assessment

Nursing assessment of all infusion systems should be systematic. Begin with the insertion site and work upward, following the tubing. Know the type of catheter your patient has in place. Be sure to find out the length of catheter, the insertion site, and tip location to do a complete assessment. Assess the insertion site by looking for redness, swelling, hardness, or drainage. Lightly palpate the area over the dressing. When a midline catheter or PICC is used, assess the entire extremity and upper chest for signs of phlebitis and thrombosis. When a tunneled catheter is used, assess the exit site, the entire length of the tunnel, and the point where the catheter enters the vein. For a well-healed catheter, it may not be possible to detect the vein entrance site. On newly inserted catheters, there could be a small puncture site with a suture or securement device. For implanted ports, assess the incision and surgically created subcutaneous pocket.

Assess the integrity of the dressing, making sure it is clean, dry, and adherent to the skin on all sides. Check all connections on the administration set, and ensure that they are secure. Be sure they are not taped. Check the rate of infusion for all fluids by either counting drops or checking the infusion pump. Assess the amount of fluid that has infused from the container. Is it accurate, or is it infusing too fast or too slow? Adjust the rate to the prescribed flow rate. Check all labels on fluid containers for the patient's name and fluid or medication. Be sure that the correct solution is being infused.

Avoid taking blood pressures in an extremity with any type of catheter in place. If a short peripheral catheter is being used for continuous infusion, the compression while taking the blood pressure can increase venous pressure, causing fluid to overflow from the puncture site and infiltration. When a midline catheter or PICC is being used, compression from the blood pressure cuff could increase vein irritation and lead to phlebitis.

Venipuncture for blood sampling should be performed in the extremity opposite from all catheters. Blood samples should not be drawn from a venipuncture site proximal to an infusing peripheral catheter because the infusing fluid could alter the results of the test to be performed. Venipuncture at or near the insertion site of a midline catheter or PICC could inadvertently damage the catheter and add to areas of venous inflammation.

Securing and Dressing the Catheter

Adequate catheter securement is vital to prevent many complications. Tape, sutures, and specially designed securement devices can be used for this purpose. For a short peripheral catheter, tape strips are most common; however, the tape should be *clean*. Tape strips from a peripheral IV start kit are preferred. Strips of tape should not be taken from rolls of tape moved between patient's rooms, from other procedures, or from uniform pockets. Precutting tape and placing it on the patient's bedrails or other object should also be avoided to prevent infection.

Newer *securement devices* are designed for all catheter types and provide an evidence-based method to prevent IV catheter movement (INS, 2006) (Fig. 15-7). Recent studies have shown that these devices, such as the StatLock IV Stabilization Device, prevent peripheral and central catheters from becoming dislodged. In addition, they prevent catheter complications, like phlebitis and infiltration (Schears, 2006; Smith, 2006). Use of securement devices, rather than tape, also provides significant cost savings by decreasing the number of IV restarts.

PICCs and nontunneled percutaneous central catheters may be sutured in place; however, this creates additional breaks in the skin that could become infected. If these sutures are loose or broken, the physician must be notified to replace them. Therefore IV catheter sutures are being replaced with securement devices in some facilities.

Tunneled catheters usually have sutures placed near the skin exit site that are removed after the tunnel has healed. The incision over a port pocket will have sutures until it has healed.

Sterile dressings used over the insertion site protect the skin and puncture site. For a short peripheral catheter, the transparent membrane dressings do not require routine changes. Tape and sterile gauze or a transparent membrane dressing can be used for midline catheters and all types of central venous dressings. Tape and gauze dressings should be changed every 48 hours; transparent membrane dressings are changed at least every 7 days (Gorski, 2007). The initial dressing on a midline catheter or PICC is usually tape and gauze, changed within 24 hours after insertion because some bleeding is likely. Transparent membrane dressings can be used for subsequent dressing. Document all sterile dressing changes and site assessments in the appropriate medical record.

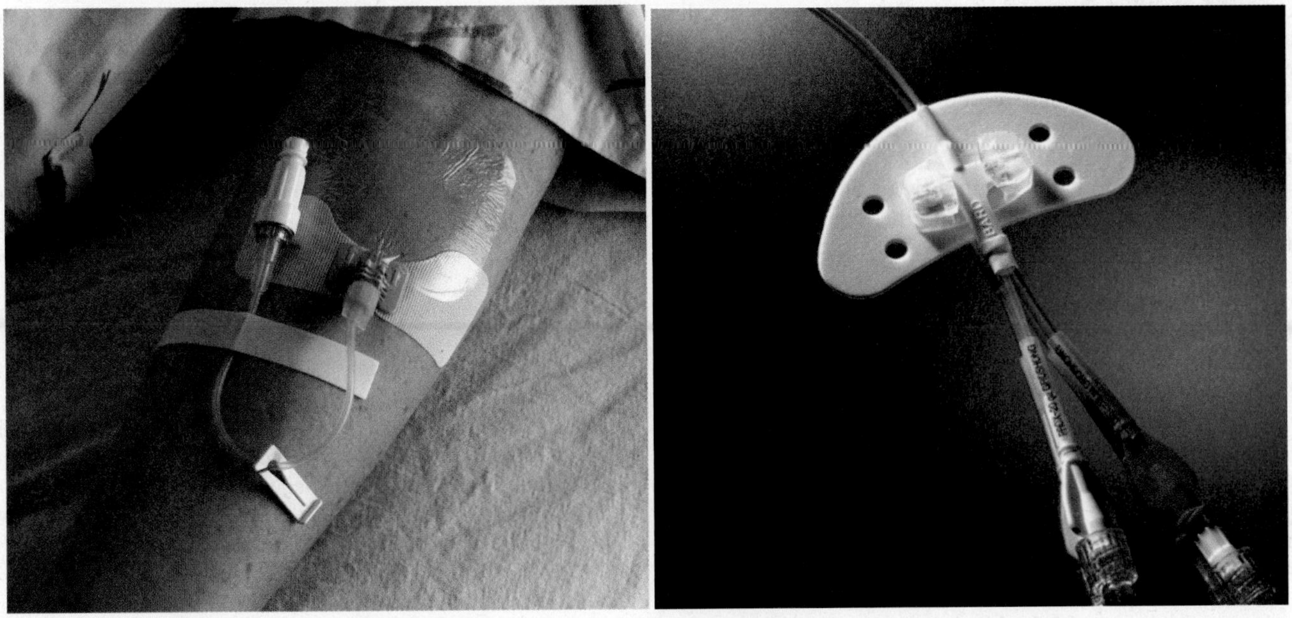

Fig. 15-7 • The Statlock provides a standardized method to prevent catheter movement.

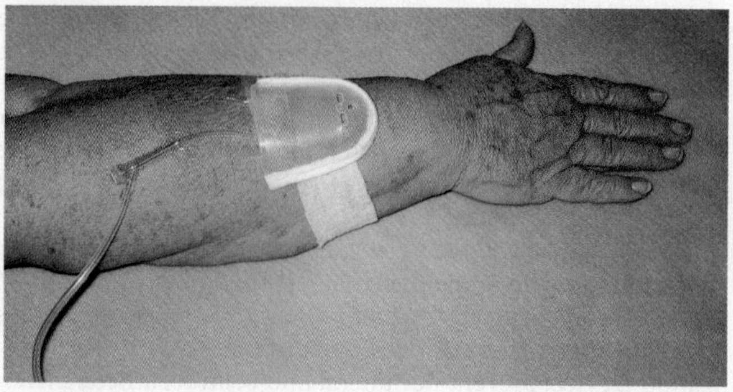

Fig. 15-8 • I.V. House, a commercially available safety device used for IV site protection, guards the integrity of the older adult's skin while helping secure the site.

Site protection may be needed for short peripheral catheters or for port access needles. Plastic shields can be placed over the site to prevent accidental bumping or pressure from clothing (Fig. 15-8).

When changing the dressing, remove it by pulling laterally from side to side. It can also be removed by holding the external catheter and pulling it off toward the insertion site. Never pull it off by pulling away from the insertion site because this could dislodge the catheter.

After removing the dressing from a midline catheter or any central venous catheter, take note of the external catheter length. Compare this length with the original length at insertion. If this length has changed, the catheter tip location has also changed and may no longer be in a vein appropriate for infusion. This situation may require a repeat chest x-ray and careful assessment of the type of therapy and remaining length of therapy required.

The external catheter, dressing, and all attached tubing must be protected from water because water is a source of contamination. While bathing, the extremity should be covered. Plastic trash bags can be taped over the extremity; however, devices specially designed for this purpose are usually more convenient for your patient to use.

Changing Administration Sets and Needleless Connectors

Primary and secondary administration sets are usually changed using sterile technique every 72 or 96 hours; however, certain types of fluids require more frequent change. These include lipid emulsion, blood products, and drugs such as propofol. Identify when the tubing was changed according to agency protocol, and document.

All connections must be secured by using a Luer-Lok device. Do not rely on tape to secure connections. Tape residue attracts organisms and increases the risk of infection.

Plan the change of administration sets and fluid containers to occur at the same time, if possible, to minimize the number of times the system is opened. For short peripheral catheters, the administration set and catheter should also be changed at the same time to avoid excessive manipulation of the catheter. Identify and document these changes.

Needleless connector devices can be changed when the administration set is changed. If it is being used for intermittent infusions, the device should be changed at least once per week. Fluid leakage from the device indicates the integrity has been compromised, and it should be changed immediately.

Precautions to prevent *air emboli* are required when changing the set or connectors attached to any catheter; however, central venous catheters require special attention. The patient should be lying flat to ensure that the catheter exit site is at or below the level of the heart. Some catheters may have a pinch clamp that can be closed during this procedure. Ask the patient to perform a Valsalva maneuver by holding his or her breath and bearing down while you disconnect the old set and reconnect the new. This action prevents air from entering the lumen, the heart, and pulmonary circulation.

Controlling Infusion Pressure

Fluid flow through the infusion system requires that the pressure on the external side be greater than the pressure at the catheter tip. Fluid flow can be slowed or obstructed by many causes. At or above the catheter hub, kinked tubing, tubing or syringe diameter, and fluid temperature or viscosity could create resistance to flow. Inside the catheter lumen, resistance is created by the catheter length and diameter or by deposits of fibrin, thrombus, or drug precipitate. Near the catheter tip, resistance to flow comes from the catheter tip impinging on the vein wall, thrombus, or venous spasm.

All catheter manufacturers have warnings about the use of excessive pressure. Gravity and infusion pumps do not exert pressure too high for the catheter to handle; however, excessive pressure from syringes can lead to catheter damage. For this reason, use of 10-mL syringes is often recommended for use with central venous catheters. Although these larger syringes generate less pressure, it is still possible to reach excessive pressure levels if great force is applied against a syringe attached to a catheter that is partially occluded. Catheter patency must be carefully assessed before each use. Attach a 10-mL syringe filled with saline, and attempt to flush the catheter without excessive force. *If resistance is felt, always stop the flush! Never forcefully flush any catheter with any size of syringe.* Catheter rupture or forcing a blood clot into circulation could result.

Flushing the Catheter

Catheter flushing prevents contact between incompatible drugs and maintains patency of the lumens (Hadaway, 2006b). Normal saline alone or normal saline followed by heparinized saline (less commonly) may be used. When using valved catheters and certain positive fluid-displacement needleless devices, normal saline alone is acceptable because these devices have mechanisms that prevent the backflow of blood into the catheter lumen.

Before using any catheter, use sterile technique to flush with normal saline to determine lumen patency. Apply slow, gentle pressure to the syringe plunger. *If you feel any resistance, stop the procedure immediately.* During the flushing procedure, always aspirate for a brisk blood return from the catheter lumen. If the catheter will not yield a blood return, further diagnostic studies may be needed to determine the cause of the problems.

For short peripheral catheters, usually 3 mL normal saline is adequate to flush the catheter. For all other catheters, 5 to 10 mL of preservative-free normal saline is needed. Bacteriostatic normal saline is limited to no more than 30 mL in a 24-hour period in adults. By using 10 mL before and after each dose of medication, it is easy to exceed this limitation. Check your agency's policy and procedure about specific flushing amounts.

Catheters should be flushed immediately after each use. Delay in disconnecting the intermittent administration set and flushing the catheter could cause lumen occlusion from blood that backflows into the lumen when the infusion pressure is lower than venous pressure.

All fluids used to flush catheters should be obtained from single-dose containers or prefilled syringes. Vials used for multiple doses contribute to medication errors and increase the risk of contamination.

Obtaining Blood Samples from the Catheter

Short peripheral and midline catheters should not be routinely used for obtaining blood samples. This additional manipulation could lead to vein irritation that requires removal of the catheter. Central venous catheters can be used for obtaining blood samples after a careful assessment of the risks versus the benefits. If your patient has no peripheral venipuncture sites or is fearful of needles, using the central venous catheter may be appropriate. The risks associated with obtaining blood samples from a central venous catheter are numerous. This procedure requires additional hub manipulation, which is a major cause of catheter-related bloodstream infection (CR-BSI). Consider the laboratory tests needed and the types of fluids that have recently been infused. Heparin interferes with coagulation studies. Electrolytes in the fluid may alter the results of serum electrolytes. Antibiotics such as vancomycin may interfere with measuring the peak serum levels of the drug.

If blood sampling from a central venous catheter is the best alternative, use methods that do not require the use of needles. Vacuum tubes attached directly to the catheter hub eliminate the need to transfer the blood from a syringe into the tubes. For small-diameter catheters, the vacuum in the tube may cause the catheter to temporarily collapse, preventing the backflow of blood into the tube. In this situation, small syringes should be used because they create less pressure on aspiration, the opposite of what small syringes do on injection. Transfer of the blood from the syringe to the vacuum tube requires the use of a special transfer device to avoid the use of needles.

Removing the Catheter

Short peripheral catheters are usually removed 72 or 96 hours after insertion. If a complication develops, they should be removed immediately. Lift opposite sides of the transparent dressing and pull laterally to remove the dressing from the site while stabilizing the catheter. Slowly withdraw the catheter from the skin, and immediately cover the puncture site with dry gauze. Do not use an alcohol pad because this will interfere with coagulation. Hold pressure on the site until hemostasis is achieved. Assess the catheter tip to make sure it is intact and completely removed. Document catheter removal and the appearance of the IV site.

Removal of midline catheters and PICCs must be performed with the same slow, gentle techniques used to insert the catheter. Veins can develop venospasms when rapid or forceful techniques are used. After explaining to the patient that this procedure will not be painful, remove the dressing and withdraw the catheter in short segments by pulling from the insertion site. *If you feel resistance, always stop and never apply force to the catheter. Extreme traction or force could cause the catheter to break and embolize to the heart or pulmonary circulation.*

Simple distraction techniques and deep breathing may be sufficient to relax the patient and remove the catheter. If these fail, replace the dressing and apply heat; allow time for the vein wall to relax. Keeping the extremity warm and dry and asking the patient to drink warm liquids could facilitate removal. Use of medications to relax the vein wall may be required if the catheter cannot be removed after several hours. Imaging studies may also be needed to determine whether the cause is a thrombosis instead of venospasm.

Nontunneled percutaneous central catheters are removed by clipping any sutures and withdrawing the catheter in short segments. Venospasm does not commonly occur when removing these catheters because the vein diameter is large.

For all catheters, immediately after the catheter comes out of the skin, apply digital pressure with a dry gauze dressing to stop any bleeding. Apply a sterile occlusive gauze dressing with an antiseptic ointment as per agency protocol or procedure. When a central venous catheter is removed, a tract between the skin and vein creates a conduit for air to be pulled into the vein. The ointment seals off the tract. After removal, measure the catheter length and compare it with the length documented on insertion. If the entire catheter length was not removed, contact the physician immediately.

Removal of tunneled catheters and implanted ports requires surgical techniques and is usually performed by nurse practitioners or physicians.

Documenting Intravenous Therapy

Nurses often are sued for malpractice related to infusion therapy, especially IV therapy. Therefore document after insertion of a VAD and throughout the course of the therapy. When inserting a venous catheter, remember to document the:

- Date and time of the VAD insertion
- Name of the nurse (you) who inserted the VAD
- Vein that was used for insertion
- Type of VAD used
- Number of insertion attempts and locations of attempts before successful insertion
- Response of the patient to the VAD insertion process
- Type of dressing applied
- Type of securement device, if used
- Special barrier precautions used, if any
- Patient and family education provided related to IV therapy

During the course of the patient's infusion therapy, be sure to continue documenting your assessments and any interventions needed as a result of complications. Follow your agency's policies and procedures for additional requirements.

COMPLICATIONS OF INFUSION THERAPY

Complications from infusion therapy can be minor and limited or life threatening. Serious life-altering or life-threatening complications are dramatically increasing in frequency and severity and present a tremendous financial burden to the U.S. health care system. Catheter-related bloodstream infections (CR-BSIs) are one of the most serious problems, often resulting in patient death. They are more common in patients with central venous catheters than with peripheral catheters.

Local complications of IV therapy occur at or near the catheter. A priority for care for patients with IV therapy is to prevent, assess, and detect these complications. In some cases, nurses also manage these problems. Definitions, causes, signs and symptoms, treatment, and prevention of local complications are summarized in Table 15-2. *Systemic complications* of IV therapy involve the entire vascular system or multiple systems. Information on common systemic complications can be found in Table 15-3. For central venous catheters (CVCs), complications can occur during the insertion procedure or during the dwell time; these problems are described in Tables 15-4 and 15-5.

Text continued on p. 235.

TABLE 15-2 Local Complications of Intravenous Therapy

Complication	Definition	Cause	Signs and Symptoms	Treatment	Prevention
Infiltration	Leakage of a nonvesicant IV solution or medication into the extravascular tissue	Peripheral catheter has punctured the vein in a second location Obstruction of blood flow causing increased pressure and fluid overflow from peripheral puncture site Inflammatory process causing fluid leakage at the capillary level Fibrin sheath fully encasing a central venous catheter leading to retrograde flow and leakage from venipuncture site Damaged septum of implanted port Dislodged port access needle	IV rate slows; increasing edema at or above the insertion site; patient may report skin tightness; blanching or coolness of skin; burning, tenderness or general discomfort at the insertion site; fluid leaking from puncture site; presence or absence of a blood return is not reliable diagnostic tool on a short peripheral catheter	Stop infusion and remove short peripheral catheter immediately after identification of problem. Apply sterile dressing if weeping from tissue occurs. Apply cold compresses. Elevate extremity if it increases patient comfort. Insert a new catheter in the opposite extremity. For all central venous catheters, obtain a study to determine the cause of the problem. For implanted port, remove and insert a new port access needle.	Stabilize short peripheral catheter well; use smallest catheter that will accomplish the infusion; avoid placement over area of flexion; use armboard if sites in an area of flexion must be used. Avoid placing restraints in the area of an IV site; make successive venipunctures proximal to the previous site. Monitor site frequently; educate patient about activities and signs and symptoms. For all central venous catheters, always obtain a brisk blood return before using the catheter for infusion. Frequently assess proper positioning of port access needle. Stabilize it well, and protect from clothing.
Extravasation	Leakage of a vesicant IV solution or medication into the extravascular tissue	Same as infiltration	Same as infiltration Tissue sloughing appears in 1-4 wk	Stop infusion, and disconnect administration set. Aspirate drug from short peripheral catheter or port access needle. Leave short peripheral catheter or port access needle in place to deliver antidote, if indicated by established policy. If possible, aspirate residual drug from the exit site of a central venous catheter. Administer antidote according to established policy. Apply cold compresses for all drugs EXCEPT vinca alkaloids and epipodophyllotoxins. Photograph site. Monitor at 24 hr, 1 wk, 2 wk, and as needed. Surgical interventions may be required. Provide written instructions to patient and family.	Same as infiltration. Know the vesicant potential before giving any IV medication.

Phlebitis and post-infusion phlebitis	Inflammation of the vein Post-infusion phlebitis presents within 48-96 hr after the catheter has been removed	Mechanical cause from insertion technique, catheter size, and lack of catheter securement Chemical cause from extremes of pH and/or osmolarity of the fluid or medication Bacterial cause from a break in aseptic technique, poor securement, and extended dwell time	Patient may report pain at the IV site; nurse may observe that vein appears red and inflamed along the length; vein may become hard and cordlike (Table 15-6)	Remove short peripheral catheter at the first sign of phlebitis; use warm compresses to relieve pain. Monitor frequently. Document using Phlebitis Scale. Insert a new catheter using the opposite extremity. Mechanical phlebitis occurring in the first week after PICC insertion may be treated without catheter removal. Apply continuous heat; rest and elevate the extremity. Significant improvement is seen in 24 hr, and complete resolution is seen within 72 hr. Remove catheter if treatment is unsuccessful.	Choose the smallest gauge catheter for the required therapy. Avoid sites of joint flexion or stabilize with an armboard. Avoid infusing fluids or medications with a pH below 5 or above 9 through a peripheral vein. Avoid infusing fluids or medications with a final osmolarity above 500 mOsm/L through a peripheral vein. Rotate sites every 72-96 hr according to established policy. Adequately secure the catheter. Use aseptic technique. For PICCs, teach patient to avoid excessive physical activity with the extremity.
Thrombosis	Blood clot inside the vein	Traumatic venipuncture Multiple venipuncture attempts Use of catheters too large for the chosen vein Contact between the catheter and the vein wall, especially at or near the central venous catheter tip Fluid volume deficits in patients with a central venous catheter	Slowed or stopped infusion rate Swollen extremity Tenderness and redness Engorged peripheral veins of the ipsilateral chest and extremity Difficulty moving the neck or jaw	Stop infusion and remove short peripheral catheter immediately. Apply cold compresses to decrease blood flow and stabilize the clot. Elevate extremity. Surgical intervention may be required. For central venous catheters, notify the physician and obtain requests for a diagnostic study. Low-dose thrombolytic agents can be used to lyse the clot.	Use good venipuncture technique. Make only two attempts to perform venipuncture. Choose the smallest-gauge catheter in the largest vein possible. Secure catheter adequately. Use armboards if short peripheral catheters are placed in areas of joint flexion. Ensure adequate hydration to avoid changes in blood composition and flexion. Prophylactic low-dose warfarin (Coumadin, Warfilone🍁) may be prescribed for patients with a central venous catheter.
Thrombophlebitis	The presence of a blood clot and vein inflammation	Same as phlebitis and thrombosis	Same as phlebitis and thrombosis	Same as phlebitis and thrombosis. Apply cold compresses initially, followed by warm.	Same as phlebitis and thrombosis.

PICC, Peripherally inserted central catheter.

Continued

TABLE 15-2 Local Complications of Intravenous Therapy—cont'd

Ecchymosis and hematoma	Ecchymosis from infiltration of blood into the surrounding tissue Hematoma is the uncontrolled bleeding from a venipuncture site creating a painful lump	Venipuncture by unskilled person Venipuncture attempts into veins that cannot be seen or palpated Anticoagulated and steroid-dependent patients are at the greatest risk Using fragile veins or areas of poor skin turgor Excessive pressure or failure to apply direct pressure for the required time when removing a catheter	Swelling usually seen first Bruising at the insertion site Pain or tenderness	Remove IV device, and apply light pressure; excessive pressure could cause other fragile veins in the area to rupture. For hematoma, apply direct pressure until bleeding has stopped. See treatment for infiltration.	Avoid veins that cannot be easily seen or palpated. Know your patient's history. Use good venipuncture technique. Apply direct pressure long enough to control bleeding.
Site infection	Localized redness and hardness at the IV site caused by invasion of microorganisms in the absence of simultaneous bloodstream infection	Break in aseptic technique during insertion or the handling of sterile equipment Lack of proper hand hygiene and skin antisepsis	Site appears red, swollen, and warm; patient may report tenderness at the site; may observe purulent or malodorous exudate	Clean exit site with alcohol, expressing drainage if present. For short peripheral, midline catheter or PICC, remove using sterile technique and avoid contact between skin and catheter. Amputate catheter tip into a sterile container. Send catheter tip for culture, if requested. Clean site with alcohol, and cover with dry sterile dressing; physician to evaluate for septic phlebitis and need for antimicrobial therapy or surgical intervention.	Use strict aseptic technique when inserting, maintaining, or removing catheters. Practice good hand hygiene. Ensure dressing remains clean, dry, and adherent to skin at all times.

Venous spasm	A sudden contraction of the vein or artery	Catheter advancement immediately after tourniquet removal Infusion of cold fluids such as blood Sudden changes in the infusion pressure Removal of a midline catheter or PICC	Cramping or pain at or above the insertion site Numbness in the area Slowing of the infusion rate Inability to withdraw midline catheter or PICC	Temporarily slow infusion rate. Apply warm compress. Do not immediately remove short peripheral catheter. If occurring during midline catheter or PICC removal, do not apply tension or attempt forceful removal. Reapply a dressing, apply heat, encourage patient to drink warm liquids, and keep extremity covered and dry. 12-24 hr may be required before catheter can be removed.	Allow time for vein diameter to return to normal after tourniquet removal and before advancing catheter. Infuse fluids at room temperature, if possible. For a midline catheter or PICC, gently withdraw the catheter in short segments.
Nerve damage	Inadvertent piercing or complete transection of a nerve	Venipuncture near known nerve locations Unanticipated nerve locations	Reports of tingling or feeling pins and needles at or below the insertion site Numbness at or near the insertion site	Immediately stop the insertion procedure if the patient reports extreme pain. Remove the catheter if reports of discomfort do not improve when the catheter is secured.	Avoid using the cephalic vein near the wrist. Avoid using veins on the palm side of the wrist. Adequately secure the catheter, but avoid tape that is too tight. Support areas of joint flexion with an armboard.

PICC, Peripherally inserted central catheter.

TABLE 15-3 Systemic Complications of Intravenous Therapy

Complication	Definition	Cause	Signs and Symptoms	Treatment	Prevention
Circulatory overload	Disruption of fluid homeostasis with excess fluid in the circulatory system	Infusion of fluids at a rate greater than the patient's system can accommodate	Patient may report shortness of breath and cough; patient's blood pressure is elevated, and there is puffiness around the eyes and edema in dependent areas; patient's neck veins may be engorged, and nurse may hear moist breath sounds.	Slow the IV rate, and notify physician; raise patient to an upright position; monitor vital signs, and administer oxygen as prescribed; administer diuretics as prescribed.	Monitor intake and output carefully and notify physician as soon as an imbalance is noticed between the patient's intake and output.
Speed shock	Systemic reaction to the rapid infusion of a substance unfamiliar to the patient's circulatory system	Rapid infusion of drugs or bolus infusion, which causes the drug to reach toxic levels quickly	Patient may report lightheadedness or dizziness and chest tightness; nurse may note that patient has a flushed face and an irregular pulse; without intervention, patient may lose consciousness and go into shock and cardiac arrest.	Immediately discontinue the drug infusion and hang isotonic solution to keep the vein open; monitor vital signs carefully, and notify physician for further treatments.	Be aware of the appropriate infusion rate of medications and adhere to them; use of infusion control devices assists in prevention of speed shock.
Allergic reaction	Local or general response to an allergen	May be a response to tape, cleansing agent, drug, solution, or IV device	A patient having a local reaction may exhibit a wheal, redness, or itching at the IV site; in the case of a general reaction, patient may report itching, running nose, and tearing; nurse may note bronchospasm, wheezing, and a truncal rash; without treatment, patient may experience anaphylaxis.	For a local reaction, use a nonallergenic type or other securement device. For a general reaction, remove the offending agent (tape) or stop the IV infusion immediately.	Check patient's medical record for drug or other allergies
Catheter embolism	A shaving or piece of catheter breaks off and floats freely in the vessel	May occur if the needle of an over-the-needle catheter is reinserted into the catheter or if the needle of a through-the-needle catheter is inadvertently pulled back through the catheter	Patient will experience a decrease in blood pressure and report pain along the vein; pulse becomes weak, rapid, and thready, and nurse may note circumoral and nail bed cyanosis; patient may lapse into unconsciousness.	Remove the catheter, and apply a tourniquet high on the limb of the catheter site; inspect catheter for any rough edges; an x-ray is taken to determine the presence of any catheter piece; surgical intervention may be necessary.	When inserting over-the-needle catheters, never reinsert the needle into the catheter; avoid pulling a through-the-needle catheter back through the needle during insertion.

TABLE 15-4 **Insertion-Related Complications of Central Venous Catheters**

Problem	Definition	Possible Causes	Signs and Symptoms	Treatment	Prevention
Pneumothorax	Collection of air in the pleural space (space between the lung and chest wall)	Puncture of the pleural covering of the lung by the introducer on insertion of a direct subclavian approach	Chest pain Dyspnea Apprehension Cyanosis Decreased breath sounds on the affected side Abnormal chest x-ray findings	Remove catheter, or assist with removal. Assess patient by monitoring vital signs, and assess breath sounds. Notify physician immediately if suspected after insertion. Administer oxygen as prescribed. Assist with insertion of a chest tube.	Use jugular or upper extremity insertion sites instead of subclavian sites. Use ultrasound to locate veins.
Hemothorax	Collection of blood in the pleural cavity	Result of puncture or transection of the subclavian vein or artery	Similar to pneumothorax; usually see dyspnea first and then tachycardia Decreased hemoglobin because of blood pooling	Same as for pneumothorax. Apply pressure on insertion site after introducer needle and catheter are removed.	Use jugular or upper extremity insertion sites instead of subclavian sites. Use ultrasound to locate veins.
Chylothorax	Lymph (chyle) enters the pleural cavity	Transection of the thoracic duct on the left side	Same as in hemothorax Usually noted on insertion with withdrawal of a milklike substance	Same as for pneumothorax.	Use right side for subclavian insertion. Use jugular or upper extremity insertion sites. Use ultrasound to locate veins.
Hydrothorax	Infusion of IV fluids directly into the thoracic cavity	Transection of the subclavian vein and placement of the catheter into the thoracic cavity	Same as in pneumothorax with absence of vesicular breath sounds and a murmur with a flat sound over the location	Same as for pneumothorax with removal of the catheter and aspiration of fluid.	Use jugular or upper extremity insertion sites instead of subclavian sites. Use ultrasound to locate veins.
Air embolism	Air enters the central venous system	Air is introduced into the central venous system during catheter insertion, tubing changes, catheter rupture, and catheter removal	Chest pain, dyspnea, hypoxia Anxiety, tachycardia, hypotension Nausea Light-headed, dizzy Loud churning heard over the pericardium on auscultation is possible but not always heard	Clamp catheter immediately. Place patient in left lateral Trendelenburg position. Notify physician immediately. Oxygen therapy. Arterial blood gases. Electrocardiogram.	Have patient lie flat when changing administration sets or needleless connectors. Close slide clamp on catheter extension, if present. Ask patient to perform a Valsalva maneuver, if possible. Use Luer-Lok connections on all catheters. Apply occlusive dressing with antiseptic ointment when removing a central venous catheter; allow to remain in place for at least 24 hr.

Continued

TABLE 15-4 Insertion-Related Complications of Central Venous Catheters—cont'd

Problem	Definition	Possible Causes	Signs and Symptoms	Treatment	Prevention
Arterial puncture	Cannulation of an artery	Accessed the artery instead of the vein	Pulsating of bright red blood from the introducer needle	Remove needle immediately, and apply pressure to the site. Secure a pressure dressing for 5-10 min.	Use ultrasound to locate veins during insertion procedure.
Nerve injury	Damage to one of the ulnar, median, or radial cords	Ineffective cannulation of the vein	Tingling to sensory motor deficit to complete paralysis	Immediately remove catheter.	Use ultrasound during cannulation.
Malpositioned catheters	Catheter has passed into the jugular vein, the right atrium, the azygos vein, or several other tributary veins	Improper patient positioning during insertion Insertion of catheter length that is too short or too long for patient	No signs or symptoms may be experienced before detection on initial chest radiograph to confirm tip location Ear, neck, or back pain Palpitations or dysrhythmias Inability to irrigate	Place patient in semi-Fowler's position, and flush catheter with 20-50 mL of saline. Notify physician to reposition catheter by guidewire exchange. Refer to radiology for repositioning under fluoroscopy.	Insert under fluoroscopy. Ensure proper patient measurement for catheter length. Position patient properly.

PICC, Peripherally inserted central catheter; *SVC*, superior vena cava.

TABLE 15-5 Complications During the Dwell of Central Venous Catheters

Complication	Definition	Possible Causes	Signs and Symptoms	Treatment	Prevention
Catheter migration	Movement of a properly placed catheter tip to another vein No change in the external catheter length	Changes in intrathoracic pressure caused by coughing, vomiting, sneezing, heavy lifting, and congestive heart failure	For migration to the jugular vein: reports of hearing a running stream or gurgling sound on the side of catheter insertion For migration to the azygos vein: back pain between the shoulder blades Neurologic complications if medications are infused	Stop all infusions, and flush catheter. Notify physician. Obtain a chest radiograph to assess tip location. Spontaneous repositioning back to the SVC is possible. Repositioning by radiology may be required.	Place catheter tip properly in the lower third of the SVC near the junction with the right atrium. Instruct patient to perform usual ADLs but to avoid excessive physical activity.
Catheter dislodgment	Movement of catheter into or out of the insertion site	Inadequate catheter securement Excessive physical activity with a PICC	External catheter length has changed, also changing the internal tip location No other signs or symptoms may be immediately noticed	Stop all infusions, and flush catheter. NEVER re-advance the catheter into the insertion site. Determine the amount of external catheter length, and compare with the length documented on insertion. Notify the physician or nurse inserting the catheter for further assessment.	Proper catheter securement. Instruct patient to perform normal ADLs but to avoid excessive physical activity.

TABLE 15-5 Complications During the Dwell of Central Venous Catheters—cont'd

Complication	Definition	Possible Causes	Signs and Symptoms	Treatment	Prevention
Catheter rupture	Catheter is broken, damaged, or separated from hub or port body	Forcefully flushing a catheter with any size syringe against resistance Using scissors to remove a dressing Catheter compression of a subclavian inserted catheter between the clavicle and first rib (also known as pinch-off syndrome)	Fluid leaking from insertion site Pain or swelling during infusion Reflux of blood into the catheter extension Inability to aspirate blood from catheter	Repair the damaged segment; depends on the availability of a repair kit designed for the specific brand of catheter being used; repair may be considered a temporary measure instead of a permanent treatment. Remove catheter.	NEVER use excessive force when flushing a catheter, regardless of syringe size. On injection, small syringes generate more pressure than larger syringes. Use of a 10-mL syringe is generally recommended for flushing procedures. Insert catheter through jugular or upper extremity sites instead of subclavian site.
Lumen occlusion	Catheter lumen is partially or totally blocked	Drug or mineral precipitate (calcium, diazepam, and phenytoin are common) Lipid sludge from long-term infusion of fat emulsion Blood clots and fibrin sheath caused by blood reflux into lumen Allowing administration sets to remain connected for extended periods after medication has infused	Infusion stops or pump alarm sounds Inability or difficulty administering fluids Inability or difficulty drawing blood Increased resistance to flushing of the catheter	Assess history of catheter use. A suddenly developing problem may indicate contact between incompatible medications. A problem that develops over an extended period may indicate a gradual clot formation. For drug precipitate, determine the pH of the precipitated drug. Use hydrochloric acid for acidic drug. Use sodium bicarbonate for alkaline drugs. For blood clot, use thrombolytic enzymes such as alteplase.	Always flush with normal saline between, before, and after each medication given through the catheter. Use positive-pressure flushing techniques when a negative fluid displacement needleless connector is being used. Use a positive fluid displacement needleless connector. Flush catheters immediately when medication infusion is complete.
Phlebitis	Inflammation of the vein wall	Mechanical phlebitis is common with PICC lines and will appear within 7 days after insertion Chemical phlebitis may be seen with catheter rupture	Pain, redness, slight swelling May progress to cellulitis and palpable cord or collateral circulation	For mechanical phlebitis: use conservative measures, warm compresses applied for 20 min four times daily for about 48-72 hr.	

Continued

TABLE 15-5 Complications During the Dwell of Central Venous Catheters—cont'd

Complication	Definition	Possible Causes	Signs and Symptoms	Treatment	Prevention
Thrombosis	Formation of a blood clot in a vessel within the neck, chest, or arms that occurs in the presence of a central venous catheter	Stasis, vessel wall injury, or hypercoagulability	Chest pain, earache, or jaw pain Edema of neck, supraclavicular area, or extremities Edema at puncture site Jugular distention Collateral circulation on the affected side	Provide anticoagulant therapy. Consider possible catheter removal.	
Exit, port pocket, or tunnel infection	Infection may be localized at the insertion site or in the catheter or may progress to systemic infection	Failure to maintain sterile technique during catheter insertion or care Wet or soiled dressing remaining on site Immunosuppression Contaminated catheter or solution	Redness, warmth, tenderness, swelling at the insertion site Cellulitis Possible exudate of purulent material Local rash or pustules Fever, chills, malaise Leukocytosis Nausea and vomiting Elevated urine glucose level	Monitor vital signs closely. Monitor culture site. Redress with sterile technique. Treat systemically with antibiotics or antifungals, depending on culture results. Blood cultures. Remove catheter.	Maintain sterile technique.
Bloodstream infection	Pathogenic organisms invade the patient's circulation	Inadequate skin antiseptic agents and application techniques Manipulation of the catheter hub leading to intraluminal contamination Inadequate hand hygiene	Early symptoms include fever, chills, headache, and general malaise If left, patient may experience severe infection, which may lead to vascular collapse and death	Change the entire infusion system from solution to IV device; notify physician, obtain cultures, and administer antibiotics as prescribed. If the infusate is the suspected cause, send a specimen to the laboratory for evaluation.	Maintain sterile technique.

PICC, Peripherally inserted central catheter; *SVC*, superior vena cava.

DECISION-MAKING CHALLENGE

Critical Rescue

You are caring for a patient who is admitted with diabetes and cellulitis of his left upper arm secondary to a large mole extraction. He has been receiving IV antibiotics through a short peripheral venous access device (VAD) in his right forearm for the past 24 hours. When you perform his shift assessment, you note that the insertion site has minimal swelling. He tells you that he told the night nurse that the area around the VAD feels "a little funny" and that his arm has been tingling and quite painful since the catheter was inserted. He is alert and oriented.

1. What do you think is a possible cause for this patient's reports and your observation and why?
2. What action should you take now and why?
3. What should you document on the medical record?
4. What follow-up interventions should be implemented?
5. Should you approach the night nurse about what the patient told you? Why or why not?

evolve For suggested answer guidelines, go to http://evolve.elsevier.com/Iggy/.

TABLE 15-6 Phlebitis Scale from INS Standards of Practice

Grade	Criteria
0	No symptoms
1	Erythema with or without pain
2	Pain at access site with erythema and/or edema
3	Pain at access site with erythema and/or edema Streak formation Palpable cord
4	Pain at access site with erythema and/or edema Streak formation Palpable venous cord more than 1 inch long Purulent drainage

Data from Infusion Nurses Society (INS). (2006). Infusion nursing standards of practice. *Journal of Infusion Nursing, 29*(1, Suppl. 6S), S1-S92.

OLDER ADULT CARE

The aging process causes numerous changes in all body functions, and yet aging occurs differently in each person. Nutrition, environment, genetics, social factors, and education are just a few of the factors that influence the older adult's needs. Because all body functions are affected, infusion therapy can be affected by these changes.

Skin Care

Aging skin becomes thinner and loses subcutaneous fat, decreasing the skin's ability for thermal regulation. Fewer nerve endings mean the decreased ability to feel pain. Your patient *may* not perceive pain from traumatic venipuncture requiring excessive probing or multiple attempts. However, this action increases the risk of fluid leakage and subsequent infiltration or extravasation injury. Inserting and removing a catheter and dressing could tear the skin layers.

Skin antisepsis is extremely important because of the possible compromised immune status of the older patient. Lipids are normally found in skin as a protective agent, and alcohol easily dissolves lipids. Although greater numbers of organisms may be killed, the skin can also become excessively dry and cracked. Current recommendations call for using friction when cleaning the skin to penetrate the layers of the epidermis. However, excessive friction may damage fragile skin. Chlorhexidine is now the preferred agent, and the product currently available contains alcohol. Check for allergies to iodine before using iodine or iodophors. Iodophors such as povidone-iodine require contact with the skin for a minimum of 2 minutes to be effective. All antiseptic solutions must be thoroughly dry before applying the dressing or tape.

Skin should never be shaved before venipuncture, but excessive amounts of hair should be clipped. Shaving causes micro-abrasions that can lead to infection. The skin of an older adult may be more delicate and therefore more easily nicked while shaving.

Skin integrity can easily be compromised by the application of tape or dressings. Use of skin protectant solutions puts a protective barrier between the skin and dressing and improves the adherence of the dressing to the skin. Removal of tape and dressings may require adhesive remover solutions, or an alcohol pad may accomplish the same purpose. Newer securement devices (e.g., the Statlock) require the use of a skin protectant (e.g., Skin-Prep) before applying the device. The protectant prevents skin tearing when the device is removed.

Vein and Catheter Selection

Vein and catheter selection are of highest importance in older adults. Choose insertion sites carefully after consideration of skin integrity, vein condition, and ADLs. The general principle of starting with the most distal sites usually indicates use of hand veins. However, avoid fragile skin and small, tortuous veins on the back of the hand (dorsum); select the initial IV site higher on the arm.

Venous distention must be accomplished with a flat tourniquet; however, the veins may require longer to distend. Allowing a tourniquet to remain in place for extended periods causes an overfilling of the vein and can result in a hematoma when the vein is punctured. On extremely fragile skin, the tourniquet application can lead to ecchymotic areas or skin tears. A tourniquet may not be required in veins that are already distended; however, carefully palpate these veins to determine their condition. Avoid hard, cordlike veins. Blood pressure cuffs can also be used for venous distention. Inflate the cuff and release until the pressure is slightly less than diastolic pressure. Other methods to distend veins include:

- Tapping lightly, but avoiding forceful slapping
- Asking the patient to open and close the fist so the muscles can force blood into the veins, making sure the hand is relaxed when the venipuncture is attempted
- Placing the extremity lower than the heart
- Applying heat to the entire extremity for 10 to 20 minutes and removing just before making the venipuncture

As with all patients, venipuncture technique requires adequate skin and vein stabilization during the puncture and complete catheter advancement. Veins of an older adult are more likely to roll away from the needle. Low angles of 10 to 15 degrees between the skin and catheter will improve your success with venipuncture.

As soon as the catheter enters the vein, it may be necessary to release the tourniquet. Release of venous pressure from the puncture can lead to ecchymosis. Allowing the tourniquet to remain in place during the complete catheter advancement could increase this problem.

Catheter securement may mean that the administration sets are placed out of easy reach of a confused patient. Using flexible netting over the extremity may prevent the patient from pulling at the dressing or tubing while allowing easy assess to the site. A device such as the I.V. House shown in Fig. 15-8 can also protect the site. Rolled bandages should not be used to cover the extremity because they will prevent easy visualization of the site, allowing complications to progress to an advanced state before recognition.

Choosing a midline catheter or PICC may be best in older patients with poor skin turgor, limited venous sites, or veins that are fragile, tortuous, or hard. These catheters are placed in the upper extremity where venous distention techniques can be used. Inserting nontunneled percutaneous central catheters in older adults may be a great challenge. Venous distention for insertion requires the Trendelenburg position and a well-hydrated patient. Fluid volume deficit prevents adequate distention of the subclavian or jugular veins. Respiratory conditions like chronic obstructive pulmonary disease, spinal curvatures, and increased intracranial pressure may contraindicate this position. Tunneled catheters and implanted ports may be appropriate after consideration of the surgical techniques required to insert these catheters.

Cardiac and Renal Changes

Because of changes in cardiac and renal status, the accuracy of infusion volume and flow rate measurements is very important in the older adult. The health care provider's prescription for infusion therapy should be assessed for appropriateness for the patient's condition. Older adults are very prone to fluid overload and resulting congestive heart failure. Electronic controlling devices may be required to ensure the necessary accuracy. Clinical manifestations of fluid overload are described in Chapter 13.

When fluid restrictions are required, medications could be diluted in small quantities and delivered using a syringe pump or a manual IV push. For instance, 1 g of an antibiotic could be diluted in 10 mL normal saline instead of the more common 50 mL. This alternative allows the patient to have more fluid to drink. Serum sodium levels should be considered when normal saline is routinely used for dilution in patients with hypertension or cardiac problems.

For a poorly controlled diabetic patient, dextrose solutions for dilution may not be preferred, although well-controlled diabetic patients may not have a problem with the small amount of dextrose in the solution. Consult with the pharmacist and prescriber to answer these questions.

ALTERNATIVE SITES FOR INFUSION

Many reasons drive the need for infusion through sites other than the venous circulation. Through numerous technologic advances, we are now capable of infusion into arteries, peritoneum, bone marrow, epidural and intrathecal space, and subcutaneous tissue.

Arterial Therapy

Description

Catheters are placed into arteries to obtain repeated arterial blood samples, to monitor various hemodynamic pressures continuously, and to infuse chemotherapy agents. Catheters placed in the radial, brachial, or femoral arteries are used for obtaining blood samples or arterial pressure monitoring. Pulmonary artery pressure measures the function of the left heart and is accomplished by advancing a catheter through the central venous system, through the right heart chambers, and into the pulmonary artery.

Arterial waveforms and pressures are converted to digital values displayed on attached monitors. Between the catheter and the monitor is a special administration set capable of handling high infusion pressure, a pressurized fluid container, a continuous flush attachment, a three-way stopcock, and a transducer. In the past, it was common to use a heparinized saline flush solution in the pressurized fluid container. Studies have shown that this solution increases the risk of heparin-induced thrombocytopenia, and the use of heparin is now generally avoided (Kaur, 2006; Swanson, 2007). The transducer is positioned at the level of the patient's atrium and secured to an IV pole to enable correct arterial pressure measurements.

Catheters used for pressure monitoring are inserted percutaneously through veins of the upper extremity or the subclavian or jugular sites. Insertion procedures are similar to the procedures used for venous cannulation. Removal requires deflating arterial balloons, if used, and applying digital pressure for longer than when removing a venous catheter to prevent a significant hematoma from forming.

Chemotherapy agents administered arterially allow infusion of a high concentration of drug directly to the tumor site before it is diluted in the circulatory system or metabolized by the liver or kidneys. Drug infusion through the same blood supply feeding the tumor optimizes cell kill at the tumor site while minimizing systemic side effects. The most common arterial sites include the hepatic and celiac arteries for liver tumors, although the carotid artery for tumors of the head, neck, or brain and pelvic arteries for cervical tumors have been used.

Arterial catheter insertion can be performed percutaneously, via a surgical procedure or through an interventional radiologic procedure. Implanted ports are commonly used for extended therapies. For short-term therapy, an external catheter may be used for 3 to 7 days, although longer periods result in high complication rates.

One other device used for arterial infusion of chemotherapy agents is an implanted pump with an attached catheter. This small device holds 50 mL of fluid in an upper chamber. The lower chamber exerts pressure when the upper chamber is filled, causing the drug to flow at 1 to 2 mL/day. Changes in blood pressure, body temperature, and altitudes alter the flow rate. The patient must return for refilling the fluid chamber every 14 days.

Nursing Care

All arterial catheters require close attention to securing all junctions on the administration sets with Luer-Lok devices. Life-threatening hemorrhage can occur if an accidental disconnection occurs. When an infusion pump is used, it should have a pumping pressure high enough to overcome arterial pressure. Observe the insertion site and involved extremity closely. Assess for warmth, sensation, capillary refill, and pulse. When the carotid artery is involved, perform neurologic assessments. When a femoral catheter is used, antiembolic stockings or other measures are indicated.

Complications from arterial catheters are similar to those from venous catheters, including infection, bleeding from the insertion site, hemorrhage from a catheter disconnection, catheter migration, infiltration, and catheter lumen or arterial occlusion.

Intraperitoneal Infusion

Description

Intraperitoneal (IP) therapy is the administration of chemotherapy agents into the peritoneal cavity. IP therapy is used to treat intra-abdominal malignancies such as ovarian and gastrointestinal tumors that have moved into the peritoneum after surgery (Almadrones, 2007).

Catheters used for IP therapy may be an implanted port for long-term treatment or an external catheter for temporary use. These catheters, including those attached to an implanted port, have large internal lumens with multiple side-holes along the catheter length to allow for delivery of large quantities of fluid. Administration of IP therapy includes three phases: the instillation phase; the dwell phase, usually 1 to 4 hours; and the drain phase. Because this treatment involves the delivery of biohazardous agents, additional competency is required to handle the infusion properly.

Nursing Care

The patient should be in the semi-Fowler's position for the infusion. He or she may experience nausea and vomiting caused by increasing pressure on the internal organs from the infusing fluid. Pressure on the diaphragm may cause respiratory distress. Reducing the flow rate and treatment with antiemetic drugs are indicated. Severe pain may indicate that the catheter has migrated, and an abdominal radiograph is needed to determine its location.

During the dwell and drainage phases, the patient may need assistance in frequently moving from side to side to distribute the fluid evenly around the abdominal cavity. After the fluid has drained, the catheter is flushed with normal saline, although heparinized saline may be used in implanted ports. Catheter lumen occlusion is caused by the formation of fibrous sheaths or fibrin clots or plugs inside the catheter or around the tip.

Exit site infection, indicated by redness, tenderness, and warmth of the tissue around the catheter, can occur. Microbial peritonitis and inflammation of the peritoneal membranes from the invasion of microorganisms are other complications. If peritonitis occurs, the patient may experience a fever and report abdominal pain. Abdominal rigidity and rebound tenderness may be present. This condition is preventable by using strict aseptic technique in the handling of all equipment and infusion supplies. Management includes antimicrobial therapy administered either intravenously or intraperitoneally.

Subcutaneous Infusion

Description

Subcutaneous therapy has rapidly expanded in the past few years, with many drugs being infused to treat numerous conditions (Table 15-7). Subcutaneous therapy may be used in palliative care patients who cannot tolerate oral medications, when IM injections are too painful, or when vascular access is not available or is too difficult to obtain. Most often, subcutaneous infusion is used in hospices in the United States for pain management.

Hypodermoclysis involves the slow infusion of isotonic fluids into the patient's subcutaneous tissue. Although common in the early twentieth to mid-twentieth century, this method had not been widely used again until the 1990s. The growth of geriatric and palliative health care has helped spur the use of this method of infusion therapy for select patients (Khan & Younger, 2007).

Hypodermoclysis can be used for short-term fluid volume replacement. The patient must have sufficient sites of intact skin without infection, inflammation, bruising, scarring, or edema. The most common sites are the front and sides of the thighs and hips, the upper abdomen, and the area under the clavicle. Unlike IV therapy, the upper extremity should not be used because fluid is absorbed more readily from sites on the torso with larger stores of adipose tissue. Hypodermoclysis should not be used if the fluid replacement needs exceed 2000 to 3000 mL/day, in emergency situations, or if there are bleeding or coagulation problems (Brown & Worobec, 2000; Khan & Younger, 2007).

Hyaluronidase 150 units may be mixed with each liter of infusion fluid. This is an enzyme that improves the absorption of the infusing fluids from the subcutaneous tissue. An intradermal test dose is required because of the possibility of an allergic reaction. If the enzyme is not used, the infusion may not be well absorbed and redness at the insertion site is more likely (Brown & Worobec, 2000; Khan & Younger, 2007).

A small-gauge, winged infusion or "butterfly" needle, a small-gauge, short peripheral catheter, or an infusion set specially designed for subcutaneous infusion can be chosen. The subcutaneous infusion sets have a small needle extending at a right angle from a flat disk that helps stabilize the needle.

TABLE 15-7 Examples of Subcutaneous Infusion Therapy

Disease or Condition	Drug or Therapy
Chronic iron overload	Deferoxamine mesylate (Desferal)
Chronic pain management	Morphine (Morphitec♣) Hydromorphone (Dilaudid) Fentanyl Haloperidol (Haldol, Peridol♣) Midazolam (Versed)
Diabetes, type 1	Insulin
Rheumatoid arthritis	Etanercept (Enbrel)
Head and neck malignant tumors	Amifostine (Ethyol)
Pulmonary arterial hypertension	Treprostinil (Remodulin)
Chronic asthma	Terbutaline (Brethine)

Nursing Care

When choosing the infusion site, consider the patient's level of activity. The area under the clavicle or the abdomen may interfere the least with ambulation. Clip excess hair in the area, and clean the chosen site with the antiseptic solution, preferably chlorhexidine gluconate. Prime the infusion tubing and the attached subcutaneous infusion set or winged needle. Gently pinch an area of about 2 inches (1 cm), and insert the needle using sterile technique. After securing the needle, cover the site with a transparent dressing. Hydrocortisone cream can be applied to the skin to prevent irritation.

Flow rates for hydration fluids begin at 30 mL/hr. After 1 hour, the rate can be increased if the patient has experienced no discomfort. The maximum rate is usually 75 to 80 mL/hr. For pain medication infusion, the flow rate is usually 2 or 3 mL/hr. If required for adequate pain control, two subcutaneous sites may be needed (Pasero, 2002).

Assess the site at least twice daily. Redness, heat, leakage, bruising, swelling, and reports of pain indicate tissue irritation, and the infusion needle should be removed. Rotate the subcutaneous site at least once per week.

Other complications include pooling of the fluid at the insertion site and an uneven fluid drip rate. Both of these problems may be resolved by restarting the infusion in another location. An infusion pump may also be used. Small ambulatory infusion pumps can be used to allow for greater mobility.

Intraspinal Infusion

The spinal column is covered by three layers: the dura mater, or outermost covering; the arachnoid, or middle layer; and the pia mater, which is closest to the spinal cord. Two spaces used for infusion are the **epidural** space between the dura mater and vertebrae and the **subarachnoid** space. The epidural space consists of fat, connective tissue, and blood vessels that protect the spinal cord. Medications infused into the epidural space must diffuse through the dura mater, and there is the possibility that some drug will be absorbed systemically. **Intrathecal** medications are infused into the subarachnoid space closer to the spinal cord, allowing reduced doses.

Description

Postoperative and chronic pain management are the primary indications for epidural infusion. Opioids administered epidurally slowly diffuse across the dura mater to the dorsal horn of the spinal cord. They lock onto receptors and block pain impulses from ascending to the brain. The patient receives pain relief from the level of the injection caudally (toward the toes). Local anesthetics administered epidurally work on the sensory nerve roots in the epidural space to block pain impulses. The physician administers the first dose of medication; then, depending on state law, the type of medication, and facility policies, nurses trained in epidural therapy may administer subsequent doses.

Intrathecal infusion is used for treating cancers that cross the blood-brain barrier and involve the central nervous system (CNS). Some medications used to treat CNS neoplasms, such as methotrexate and cytarabine, are not effective IV because they cannot cross the blood-brain barrier. Others must be administered in large doses to cross this natural protective mechanism. It may not be possible to administer large doses of chemotherapeutic agents IV because of the severe systemic side effects associated with them. Administration of medications via the intrathecal route eliminates this problem because they are administered directly into the cerebrospinal fluid (CSF). Intrathecal infusion is also used to treat spasticity of neurologic diseases such as cerebral palsy, multiple sclerosis, reflex sympathetic dystrophy, and traumatic and anoxic acquired brain injuries.

A temporary catheter used for epidural therapy can be a percutaneous catheter that is secured at the site and extends up the back toward the shoulder. These catheters are used for postoperative pain management and usually dwell for only several hours or a few days. Infection and subsequent meningitis and catheter migration are the possible complications.

Epidural catheters used for longer periods include a tunneled catheter and implanted port. Tunneled catheters are tunneled toward the abdomen and have a subcutaneous cuff to act as a barrier to infection. The external catheter exits the skin on the abdomen, so it can be easily reached for use by the patient or caregiver. An epidural implanted port is the same design as an IV implanted port and is accessed with the same noncoring needle. The catheter extends from the lumbar puncture site to the port pocket and is located over a bony prominence on the abdomen through a subcutaneous tunnel. Surgically implanted pumps, described on p. 236 for intra-arterial infusion, can also be used to deliver epidural and intrathecal infusion.

Nursing Care

Intraspinal catheters are usually inserted using sterile technique in the lumbar region. The external portion of a temporary epidural catheter is laid along the back toward the head and usually extends over the shoulder. The entire catheter length is taped for added security. Dressings are usually not routinely changed because they are only used for short periods. If bleeding or fluid leakage requires dressing removal, extreme care is required to prevent dislodging the catheter.

For a tunneled catheter or implanted port, the entire subcutaneous tunnel and port pocket should be frequently assessed. Measurement of an external catheter segment could help identify catheter migration.

An in-line filter is used on all intraspinal infusions to block the infusion of particulate matter. Medications commonly contain preservatives such as alcohol, phenols, or sulfites; however, these are toxic to the CNS. All medications used for intraspinal infusion must be free of preservatives. Alcohol and products containing alcohol should not be applied to the insertion site because the solution could track along the catheter and cause nerve damage. Povidone-iodine solutions are preferred for skin antisepsis before insertion and during catheter dwell, including tunneled catheter exit sites and implanted port pockets.

Complications from epidural and intrathecal infusion can be caused by the type of medication being infused or can be related to the catheter. It is important to know the specific location of the intraspinal catheter because the doses of medications are quite different. When used for pain management, doses are usually 10 times greater for epidural than for intrathecal infusion. Assess the patient for response to the drugs being given, level of alertness, respiratory status, and itching.

Catheter-related complications include infection, bleeding or leakage of CSF, occlusion of the catheter lumen, and catheter migration. Infection in the patient receiving either epidural or intrathecal therapy could be the result of a lack of asepsis when handling the medication or during the administration. Evidence of local infection, such as redness or swelling at the catheter exit site, may be present. The patient may also exhibit neurologic and systemic signs of infection, such as headache, stiff neck, or temperature higher than 101° F (38.3° C).

Intraosseous Therapy

Description

Intraosseous (IO) therapy allows access to the rich vascular network located in the long bones. This vascular network is more prominent in children younger than 6 years. Though IO was typically regarded as a pediatric procedure, it is now considered acceptable for use in adults. Victims of trauma, burns, cardiac arrest, and other life-threatening conditions benefit from this therapy because often clinicians cannot access these patients' vascular systems for traditional IV therapy (American Heart Association, 2005). Intraosseous catheters may be established in the prehospital setting when IV access cannot be readily obtained in an emergency (Fowler et al., 2007). Research indicates that absorption rates of large-volume parenteral (LVP) infusions and medications administered via the IO route are similar to those achieved with peripheral or central venous administration. The IO route should be used only during the immediate period of resuscitation and should not be used longer than 24 hours. After establishing IO access, efforts should continue to obtain IV access as well.

Theoretically, any needle can be used to provide therapy and access the medullary space. Adults require a 15- or 16-gauge needle. Needles specifically designed for IO are preferred because they have:

- A needle with a removable stylet that screws into the cannula to keep the needle from retracting during insertion
- A short shaft to eliminate accidental dislodgment after placement
- An adjustable guard to stabilize the needle at skin level
- Graduations along the needle to guide the practitioner during insertion

Kits to facilitate rapid IO needle insertion are now available commercially and are very helpful in the emergency resuscitation setting (Curran, 2005). Sites chosen include the distal or proximal tibia and the distal femur. As a general rule, the sternum is not typically recommended because it is too thin to accommodate a needle. It could lead to pneumothorax and may interfere with other resuscitation efforts.

Nursing Care

If IV access cannot be obtained within the first few minutes of resuscitation procedures, IO may be attempted. The leg is restrained, and the site is cleaned with an antiseptic agent. After successful insertion, the needle must be secured to prevent movement out of the bone. The same doses of fluids and medications can be infused IO as IV. An infusion pump may be used for rapid flow rates.

Improper needle placement is the most common complication of IO therapy. An accumulation of fluid under the skin at either the insertion site or on the other side of the limb indicates that the needle is either not far enough in to penetrate the bone marrow or is too far into the limb and has protruded through the other side of the shaft. Needle obstruction occurs when the puncture has been accomplished but flushing has been delayed. This delay may cause the needle to become clotted with bone marrow.

Osteomyelitis is an unusual but serious complication of IO therapy. This bone infection is generally caused by allowing the IO needle to remain in place for a lengthy period.

Compartment syndrome is a condition in which increased tissue pressure in a confined anatomic space causes decreased blood flow to the area. The decreased circulation to the area leads to hypoxia and pain in the area. Although the complication is rare in IO therapy, the nurse should monitor the site carefully and alert the physician promptly if the patient exhibits any signs of decreased circulation to the limb, such as coolness, swelling, mottling, or discoloration. Without improvement in perfusion to the limb, the patient could ultimately require amputation of the limb.

GET READY FOR THE NCLEX EXAMINATION!

Key Points

Review these Key Points for each NCLEX Examination Client Needs Category.

Safe and Effective Care Environment

- Check intravenous (IV) administration orders for accuracy and completeness before implementing them.
- Prevent IV administration errors by using smart pumps and other safety infusion systems.
- Devices engineered with safety mechanisms are required by the Occupational Safety and Health Administration (OSHA) to prevent staff injuries from needles, thus preventing bloodborne pathogen hazards.
- Document care for the patient receiving IV therapy, including the type of vascular access device (VAD) inserted.

Health Promotion and Maintenance

- Teach the patient and family about care of the patient receiving infusion therapy, including purpose and safety precautions.

Physiological Integrity

- Infusion therapy is the delivery of parenteral medications and fluids through a wide variety of catheters and locations.
- Infusion therapy is used for establishing fluid and electrolyte balance, achieving optimum nutrition, maintaining hemostasis, and treating or preventing illnesses with medications.
- VADs are catheters that are used to deliver fluids, electrolytes, and medications into the intravascular space.
- Common types of VADs include short peripheral catheters, midline catheters, peripherally inserted central catheters (PICCs), nontunneled percutaneous and tunneled central catheters, implanted ports, and hemodialysis catheters.
- Use best practice for placement of short peripheral VADs, including avoiding the small veins of the hands (see Chart 15-1).
- The type of VAD that is used depends on the reason for infusion therapy, the patient's condition, and the length of therapy.
- Choose the appropriate peripheral catheter gauge size of the VAD depending on its purpose (see Table 15-1).
- PICCs, tunneled central catheters, and implanted ports are commonly used for long-term infusion therapy.
- Infusion controllers and pumps are electronic devices used to regulate the flow of infusion fluids and medications, but be sure to monitor the infusion rate.
- Use best practice for administering intermittent IV medications by either of two methods: piggybacking or backpriming (see Charts 15-2 and 15-3).
- Nursing care for patients receiving IV therapy includes using sterile technique when starting the therapy and when changing components of the infusion system, changing and securing the site dressing, and assessing the site for local complications (see Table 15-2).
- Document the presence of phlebitis using the INS Phlebitis Scale (see Table 15-6).
- Use normal saline to flush IV catheters on a periodic basis per agency policy.
- Assess, prevent, and manage systemic complications related to IV therapy as outlined in Table 15-3.
- Assess for common complications associated with CVAD insertion as described in Table 15-4.
- Assess, prevent, and manage complications during the course of central IV therapy as listed in Table 15-5.
- Older adults present special challenges when infusion therapy is used; physiologic changes of the skin and cardiac/renal systems must be considered.
- Use small IV catheters for older adults, and insert using a 10- to 15-degree angle to prevent rolling of the vein.
- Arterial therapy is used primarily for the administration of chemotherapy agents directly into a tumor site; the liver is the most common arterial site for this purpose.
- Intraperitoneal therapy is used for chemotherapy agent administration into the peritoneal cavity, especially for ovarian and gastrointestinal tumors that have metastasized into the peritoneum.
- Subcutaneous therapy of fluids (hypodermoclysis) involves a slow infusion for a short time; the thighs, hips, and abdomen are commonly used sites (see Table 15-7).
- Epidural and intrathecal administration of medications is the common use for intraspinal infusion. Epidural infusions are usually for pain management; intrathecal infusions are usually chemotherapy agents used for cancers that cross the blood-brain barrier into the central nervous system.
- Intraosseous therapy allows fluids and medications to be absorbed by the rich vascular network of the long bones; it is used for both children and adults, particularly in emergency situations.

Additional Study Resources

Go to your Companion CD or Evolve at http://evolve.elsevier.com/Iggy/ for *Self-Assessment Questions for the NCLEX Examination.*

evolve

Go to Evolve at http://evolve.elsevier.com/Iggy/ for *Prioritization and Delegation Questions for the NCLEX Examination.*

SELECTED BIBLIOGRAPHY

Asterisk indicates a classic or definitive work on this subject.

Almadrones, L. (2007). Evidence-based research for intraperitoneal chemotherapy in epithelial ovarian cancer. *Clinical Journal of Oncology Nursing, 11*(2), 211-216.

American Heart Association. (2005). 2005 American Heart Association guidelines for cardiopulmonary resuscitation and emergency cardiovascular care. *Supplement to Circulation, 112*(Suppl. 24), IV58-IV66.

*Brown, M., & Worobec, F. (2000). Hypodermoclysis: Another way to replace fluids. *Nursing2000, 30*(5), 58-59.

*CDRH. (2001). *Safety assessment of di(2ethylhexyl)phthalate (DEHP) released from PVC medical devices.* Rockville, MD: Center for Devices and Radiological Health, Food and Drug Administration.

Curran, A. (2005). Bone injection gun placement of intraosseous needles. *Emergency Medicine Journal, 22*(5), 366.

Eackle, M., Gallauresi, B.A., & Morrison, A. (2005). Luer-lock misconnects can be deadly. *Nursing2005, 35*(9), 73.

Earhart, A., & Kaminski, D. (2007). Evidence-based practice in infusion nursing: 2007 NACNS National Conference abstracts. *Clinical Nurse Specialist, 21*(2), 107.

Forauer, A.R. (2007). Pericardial tamponade in patients with central venous catheters. *Journal of Infusion Nursing, 30*(3), 161-167.

Fowler, R., Gallagher, J.V., Isaacs, S.M., Ossman, E., Pepe, P., & Wayne, M. (2007). The role of intraosseous vascular access in the out-of-hospital environment. *Prehospital Emergency Care, 11*(1), 63-66.

Francis, J.L., & Drexler, A.J. (2005). Striking back at heparin-induced thrombocytopenia. *Nursing2005, 35*(9), 48-51.

Gillies, D., O'Riordan, L., Wallen, M., Morrison, A., Rankin, K., & Nagy, S. (2007). Optimal timing for intravenous administration set replacement. *Cochrane Database of Systematic Reviews,* 2005, Issue 4.

Gorski, L. (2007). Standard 44: Dressings. *Journal of Infusion Nursing, 30*(2), 87-88.

Guthrie, D., Dreher, D., & Munson, M. (2007). What you need to know about PICCs, Part 1. *Nursing2007, 37*(8), 18.

Hadaway, L. (2007). Emergency: Infiltration and extravasation. *AJN, 107*(8), 62-72.

Hadaway, L.C. (2005a). Reopen the pipeline for I.V. therapy. *Nursing2005, 35*(8), 54-61.

Hadaway, L.C. (2005b). Caring for a nontunneled CVC site. *Nursing2005, 35*(12), 54-56.

Hadaway, L.C. (2006a). Keeping central line infection at bay. *Nursing2006, 36*(4), 58-63.

Hadaway, L.C. (2006b). Technology of flushing vascular access devices. *Journal of Infusion Nursing, 29*(3), 137-145.

Hawes, M. (2007). A proactive approach to combating venous depletion in the hospital setting. *Journal of Infusion Nursing, 30*(1), 33-44.

*Herndon, C., & Fike, D. (2001). Continuous subcutaneous infusion practices of United States hospices. *Journal of Pain Symptom Management, 22*(6), 1027-1034.

Higuchi, K.A., Edwards, N., Danseco, E., Davies, B., & McConnell, H. (2007). Development of an evaluation tool for a clinical practice guideline on nursing assessment and device selection for vascular access. *Journal of Infusion Nursing, 30*(1), 45-54.

Infusion Nurses Society (INS). (2006). Infusion nursing standards of practice. *Journal of Infusion Nursing, 29*(1, Suppl. 6S), S1-S92.

Jacobs, B. (2006). Using an infusion pump safely. *Nursing2006, 36*(10), 24.

Kaur, A. (2006). Caring for a patient with an arterial line. *Nursing2006, 36*(4), 64cc1-64cc4.

Khan, M., & Younger, G. (2007). Promoting safe administration of subcutaneous infusions. *Nursing Standard, 21*(31), 50-56.

Krueger, A. (2007). Need help finding a vein? *Nursing2007, 37*(6), 39-41.

Moureau, N. (2006). Vascular safety: It's all about PICCs. *Nursing Management, 37*(5), 22-27.

*National Association of Vascular Access Networks (NAVAN). (1998). Position paper: Tip location of peripherally inserted central catheters. *Journal of Vascular Access Devices, 3*(2), 8-10.

*O'Grady, N.P., Alexander, M., Dellinger, E.P., Gerberding, J.L., Heard, S.O., Maki, D.G., et al. (2002). Guidelines for the prevention of intravascular catheter-related infections. *Centers for Disease Control and Prevention, Morbidity and Mortality Weekly Report, 51*(RR-10), 1-29.

Paparella, S. (2005). Inadvertent attachment of a blood pressure device to a needleless IV "Y-site": Surprising, fatal connections. *Journal of Emergency Nursing, 31*(2), 180-182.

*Pasero, C. (2002). Subcutaneous opioid infusion. *AJN, 102*(7), 61-62.

*Perucca, R. (2001). Infusion therapy equipment: Types of infusion therapy equipment. In J. Hankins, R.A. Lonsway, C. Hedrick, & M. Perdue (Eds.), *Infusion therapy in clinical practice* (2nd ed.). Philadelphia: Saunders.

Rosenthal, K. (2005a). Documenting peripheral I.V. therapy. *Nursing2005, 35*(7), 28.

Rosenthal, K. (2005b). Tailor your I.V. insertion techniques for special populations. *Nursing2005, 35*(5), 37-41.

Rosenthal, K. (2006a). Do needleless connectors increase bloodstream infection risk? *Nursing Management, 37*(4), 78-80.

Rosenthal, K. (2006b). Guarding against vascular site infection. *Nursing Management, 37*(4), 54-66.

Rosenthal, K. (2006c). Intravenous fluids: The whys and wherefores. *Nursing2006, 36*(7), 26-27.

Schears, G.J. (2006). Summary of product trials for 10,164 patients: Comparing an intravenous stabilizing device to tape. *Journal of Infusion Nursing, 29*(4), 225-231.

*Slesak, G. Schnürle, J.W., Kinzel, E., Jakob, J., & Dietz, P.K. (2003). Comparison of subcutaneous and intravenous rehydration in geriatric patients: A randomized trial. *Journal of the American Geriatric Society, 51*(2), 155-160.

Smith, B. (2006). Peripheral intravenous catheter dwell times: A comparison of 3 securement methods for implementation of a 96-hour scheduled change protocol. *Journal of Infusion Nursing, 29*(1), 14-17.

Swanson, J.M. (2007). Heparin-induced thrombocytopenia: A general review. *Journal of Infusion Nursing, 30*(4), 232-240.

Tilton, D. (2006). PICC care. *RN, 69*(9), 30-36.

Vialle, R., Pietin Vialle, C., Cronier, P., Brillu, C., Villapadnierna, F., & Mercier, P. (2001). Anatomic relations between the cephalic vein and the sensory branches of the radial nerve: How can nerve lesions during vein puncture be prevented? *Anesthesia and Analgesia, 93,* 1058-1061.

Walsh, G. (2005). Hypodermoclysis: An alternate method for rehydration in long-term care. *Journal of Infusion Nursing, 28*(2), 123-129.

Weinstein, S. (2006). *Plumer's principles and practice of intravenous therapy* (8th ed.). Philadelphia: Lippincott Williams & Wilkins.

*West, V. (1998). Alternative routes of administration. *Journal of Intravenous Nursing, 21*(4), 221-231.

Winfield. C., Davis, S., Schwaner, S., Conaway, M., et al. (2007). Evidence: The first word in safe I.V. practice. *American Nurse Today, 2*(5), 31-33.

*Zwicker, C.D. (2003). The elderly patient at risk. *Journal of Infusion Nursing, 26*(3), 137-143.

IV

UNIT

Management of Perioperative Patients

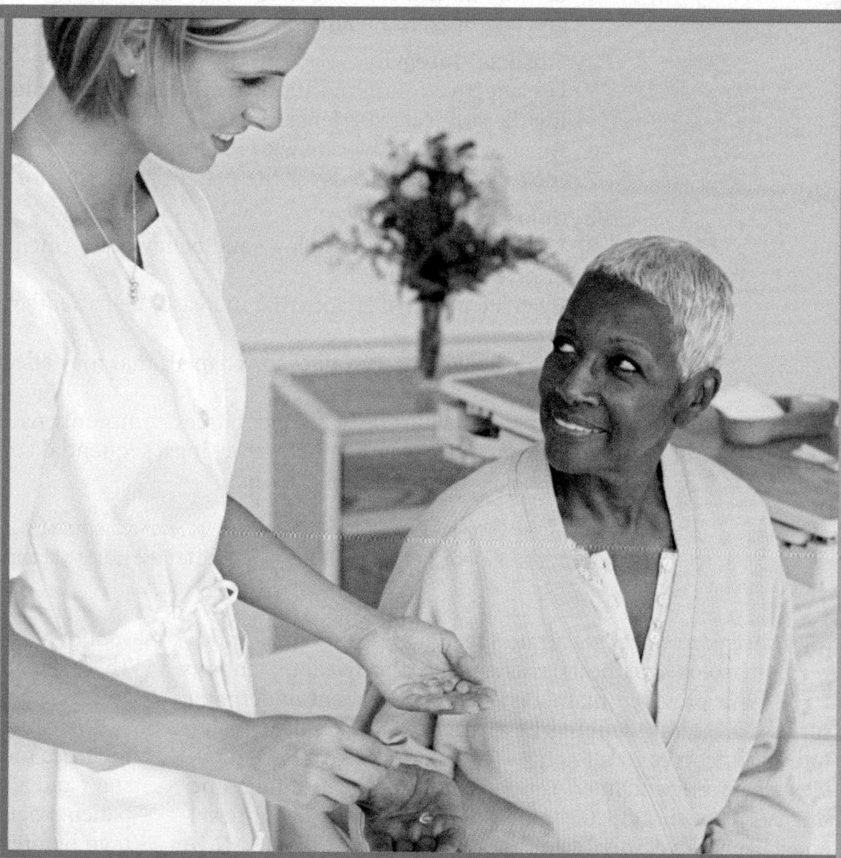

16

CHAPTER

Care of Preoperative Patients

Robin Chard

LEARNING OUTCOMES

For clinical competence and success on the NCLEX Examination, study this chapter with these Learning Outcomes in mind:

Safe and Effective Care Environment

1. Differentiate among the various types and purposes of surgery.
2. Use appropriate patient identifiers when providing instruction, administering drugs, marking surgical sites, and performing any procedure.
3. Verify that the patient has given informed consent for the surgical procedure and that the presurgical checklist is complete and accurate.
4. Identify patient conditions or issues that need to be communicated to other members of the surgical and postoperative teams.

Psychosocial Integrity

5. Use effective communication when teaching patients and family members about what to expect during the surgical experience.
6. Act as a patient advocate with regard to patients' rights, informed consent, and advance directives.
7. Identify learning needs for the patient preparing for surgery.

Physiological Integrity

8. Use knowledge of physiology and behavioral principles to describe an accurate and complete preoperative assessment.
9. Evaluate personal factors that increase the patient's risk for complications during and immediately after surgery.
10. Evaluate laboratory values for changes that may affect the patient's response to drugs, anesthesia, and surgery.
11. Explain the purposes and techniques commonly used for patient preoperative preparation.
12. Correctly apply antiembolic stockings, sequential compression boots, or other devices to reduce or prevent vascular complications.

Go to your Companion CD or Evolve at http://evolve.elsevier.com/Iggy/ for *Self-Assessment Questions for the NCLEX Examination* keyed to these Learning Outcomes.

Recent advances in surgical techniques, anesthesia, pharmacology, medical devices, and supportive interventions have provided many benefits to the patient undergoing surgery. Research defining best practices has resulted in improved outcomes in all areas of the perioperative experience. New diagnostic and intervention devices for the use and refinement of new surgical techniques are continually being developed. Examples of such technical advances include the GAMMA knife for brain tumor resections, robotics, and other types of minimally invasive surgeries (MISs). Advances in anesthetic agents and techniques improve the ways that a surgical patient is treated and has made anesthesia safer than ever before. Many procedures that used to be performed only in the operating room are now being done in other departments such as interventional radiology, cardiac catheterization, and endoscopy. These advancements affect the role of the perioperative nurse and have an impact on how patient teaching is performed.

Cost-reduction policies by third-party payers are also a driving force for the management of the surgical patient. Shortened stays and ambulatory surgical services are common, with more patients being admitted as inpatients *after* a procedure, rather than before. Some patients may only be observed after surgery and may not be admitted as an inpatient. In response to the ongoing health care delivery changes and the use of multiple settings, nurses have modified their interventions, remaining focused on patient care before **(preoperative)**, during **(intraoperative)**, and after **(postoperative)** surgery. Together, these time periods are known as the **perioperative** experience.

Overview

The preoperative period begins when the patient is scheduled for surgery and ends at the time of transfer to the surgical suite. As a nurse, you will function as an educator, an advocate, and a promoter of health. The surgical environment demands the use of knowledge, judgment, and skills based on the principles of nursing science. Perioperative nursing places special emphasis on safety, advocacy, and patient education, although ensuring a "culture of safety" is the responsibility of all health care team members (Scherer & Fitzpatrick, 2008).

The patient's readiness for surgery is critical to the outcome. Preoperative care focuses on preparing the patient for the surgery and patient safety. This care includes education and any intervention needed before surgery to reduce anxiety and complications and to promote patient cooperation in procedures after surgery. Use adult teaching and learning principles in teaching patients and families before surgery. Validate and clarify information the patient has received from the surgeon or other members of the surgical team. In addition, during the nursing assessment before surgery, it is not uncommon to identify problems that warrant further patient assessment or intervention before the procedure. Communication and collaboration with the surgical team are essential so that correct actions are taken to achieve the desired outcome.

Categories and Purposes of Surgery

Surgical procedures are categorized by the purpose, body location, extent, and degree of urgency. Table 16-1 explains the categories and gives examples of surgical procedures.

TABLE 16-1 Selected Categories of Surgical Procedures

Category	Description	Condition or Surgical Procedure
REASONS FOR SURGERY		
Diagnostic	Performed to determine the origin and cause of a disorder or the cell type for cancer	Breast biopsy Exploratory laparotomy Arthroscopy
Curative	Performed to resolve a health problem by repairing or removing the cause	Cholecystectomy Appendectomy Hysterectomy
Restorative	Performed to improve a patient's functional ability	Total knee replacement Finger reimplantation
Palliative	Performed to relieve symptoms of a disease process, but does not cure	Colostomy Nerve root resection Tumor debulking Ileostomy
Cosmetic	Performed primarily to alter or enhance personal appearance	Liposuction Revision of scars Rhinoplasty Blepharoplasty
URGENCY OF SURGERY		
Elective	Planned for correction of a nonacute problem	Cataract removal Hernia repair Hemorrhoidectomy Total joint replacement
Urgent	Requires prompt intervention; may be life threatening if treatment is delayed more than 24-48 hr	Intestinal obstruction Bladder obstruction Kidney or ureteral stones Bone fracture Eye injury Acute cholecystitis
Emergent	Requires immediate intervention because of life-threatening consequences	Gunshot or stab wound Severe bleeding Abdominal aortic aneurysm Compound fracture Appendectomy
DEGREE OF RISK OF SURGERY		
Minor	Procedure without significant risk; often done with local anesthesia	Incision and drainage (I&D) Implantation of a venous access device (VAD) Muscle biopsy
Major	Procedure of greater risk; usually longer and more extensive than a minor procedure	Mitral valve replacement Pancreas transplant Lymph node dissection

Continued

TABLE 16-1 Selected Categories of Surgical Procedures—cont'd

Category	Description	Condition or Surgical Procedure
EXTENT OF SURGERY		
Simple	Only the most overtly affected areas involved in the surgery	Simple/partial mastectomy
Radical	Extensive surgery beyond the area obviously involved; is directed at finding a root cause	Radical prostatectomy Radical hysterectomy
Minimally invasive surgery (MIS)	Surgery performed in a body cavity or body area through one or more endoscopes; can correct problems, remove organs, take tissue for biopsy, re-route blood vessels and drainage systems; is a fast-growing and ever-changing type of surgery	Arthroscopy Tubal ligation Hysterectomy Lung lobectomy Coronary artery bypass Cholecystectomy

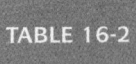

TABLE 16-2 Selected Factors That Increase Surgical Risk or Increase the Risk of Postoperative Complications

AGE
- Older than 65 years

MEDICATIONS
- Antihypertensives
- Tricyclic antidepressants
- Anticoagulants
- Nonsteroidal anti-inflammatory drugs (NSAIDs)

MEDICAL HISTORY
- Decreased immunity
- Diabetes
- Pulmonary disease
- Cardiac disease
- Hemodynamic instability
- Multisystem disease
- Coagulation defect or disorder
- Anemia
- Dehydration
- Infection
- Hypertension
- Hypotension
- Any chronic disease

PRIOR SURGICAL EXPERIENCES
- Less-than-optimal emotional reaction
- Anesthesia reactions or complications
- Postoperative complications

HEALTH HISTORY
- Malnutrition or obesity
- Drug, tobacco, alcohol, or illicit substance use or abuse
- Altered coping ability

FAMILY HISTORY
- Malignant hyperthermia
- Cancer
- Bleeding disorder

TYPE OF SURGICAL PROCEDURE PLANNED
- Neck, oral, or facial procedures (airway complications)
- Chest or high abdominal procedures (pulmonary complications)
- Abdominal surgery (paralytic ileus, deep vein thrombosis)

Surgical Settings

The term **inpatient** refers to a patient who is admitted to a hospital. The patient may be admitted the day before or, more often, the day of surgery (often termed *same-day admission [SDA]*), or the patient may already be an inpatient when surgery is needed. The terms **outpatient** and **ambulatory** refer to a patient who goes to the surgical area the day of the surgery and returns home on the same day (i.e., *same-day surgery [SDS]*). Hospital-based ambulatory surgical centers, freestanding surgical centers, physicians' offices, and ambulatory care centers are common. About 70% to 90% of all surgical procedures in North America are performed in ambulatory centers (data retrieved September 2007, from www.cdc.gov/nchs/nsas.htm).

One advantage of outpatient surgery is that patients are not separated from the comfort and security of their home and family. With improvements in surgical techniques and anesthesia, more procedures are performed safely on an outpatient basis. Same-day surgery, however, presents new challenges for the patient who does not have an adequate or available support system. An older spouse may be unable to assist in care before or after surgery. Patients who are responsible for others may be unable to perform their usual tasks within the family. They may try to continue their family role but jeopardize their own health by doing so. As a result, their stress, fears, and anxieties about the surgical experience and about returning home immediately after surgery may increase. In these circumstances, a case manager may be assigned to coordinate post-discharge care for the patient.

Patient-Centered Collaborative Care

evolve ONLINE PHARM REVIEW

Assessment

History

Data collection about the patient before surgery begins in various settings (e.g., the surgeon's office, the preadmission or admission office, the inpatient unit, the telephone). Use privacy to increase the patient's comfort with the interview process. Anesthesia and surgery are both physical and emotional stressors. Collect these data:

- Age
- Use of tobacco, alcohol, or illicit substances, including marijuana
- Current drugs
- Use of complementary or alternative practices, such as herbal therapies, folk remedies, or acupuncture
- Medical history
- Prior surgical procedures and how these were tolerated

Chart 16-1 NURSING FOCUS ON THE OLDER ADULT

Changes of Aging as Surgical Risk Factors

Physiologic Change	Nursing Interventions	Rationales
CARDIOVASCULAR SYSTEM		
Decreased cardiac output Increased blood pressure	Determine normal activity levels, and note when the patient tires.	Knowing limits helps prevent fatigue.
Decreased peripheral circulation	Monitor vital signs, peripheral pulses, and capillary refill.	Having baseline data helps detect deviations.
RESPIRATORY SYSTEM		
Reduced vital capacity Loss of lung elasticity	Teach coughing and deep-breathing exercises.	Pulmonary exercises help prevent pulmonary complications.
Decreased oxygenation of blood	Monitor respirations and breathing effort.	Having baseline data helps detect deviations.
RENAL/URINARY SYSTEM		
Decreased blood flow to kidneys Reduced ability to excrete waste products Decline in glomerular filtration rate	Monitor intake and output. Assess overall hydration. Monitor electrolyte status.	Ongoing assessment helps detect fluid and electrolyte imbalances and decreased renal function.
Nocturia common	Assist frequently with toileting needs, especially at night.	Frequent toileting helps prevent incontinence and falls.
NEUROLOGIC SYSTEM		
Sensory deficits Slower reaction time Decreased ability to adjust to changes in the surroundings	Orient the patient to the surroundings. Allow extra time for teaching the patient.	An individualized preoperative teaching plan is developed on the basis of the patient's orientation and any neurologic deficits.
	Provide for the patient's safety.	Safety measures help prevent falls and injury.
MUSCULOSKELETAL SYSTEM		
Increased incidence of deformities related to osteoporosis or arthritis	Assess the patient's mobility. Teach turning and positioning. Encourage ambulation.	Interventions help prevent complications of immobility.
	Place on falls precautions, if indicated.	Safety measures help prevent injury.
SKIN		
Dry with less subcutaneous fat makes the skin at greater risk for damage; slower skin healing increases risk for infection	Assess the patient's skin before surgery for lesions, bruises, and areas of decreased circulation.	Having baseline data helps detect changes and evaluate interventions.
	Pad bony prominences.	Padding can protect at-risk areas.
	Use pressure-avoiding or pressure-reducing overlays.	Overlays can prevent pressure ulcer formation by redistributing body weight.
	Avoid applying tape to skin.	Tape removal damages thin skin.
	Teach the patient to change position at least every 2 hours.	Changing position frequently helps prevent reduced blood flow to an area and changes external pressure patterns.

- Prior experience with anesthesia, pain control, and management of nausea or vomiting
- Autologous or directed blood donations
- Allergies, including sensitivity to latex products
- General health
- Family history
- Type of surgery planned
- Knowledge about and understanding of events during the perioperative period
- Adequacy of the patient's support system

When taking a history, screen the patient for problems that increase the risk for complications during and after surgery. Some problems that increase the surgical risk or increase the risk for complications after surgery are listed in Table 16-2.

Older patients are at increased risk for complications (Dunn, 2004). The normal aging process decreases immune system functioning and delays wound healing. The frequency of chronic illness increases in older patients. In addition, the reduced muscle mass and body water increase the risk for dehydration. See Chart 16-1 for other changes in older adults that may alter the operative response or risk.

Drugs and substance use may affect patient responses to surgery. The use of tobacco increases the risk for pulmonary complications because of changes it causes to the lungs and chest cavity. Excessive alcohol and illicit substance use can alter the patient's responses to anesthesia and pain medication. Withdrawal of alcohol before surgery may lead to delirium tremens. Prescription and over-the-counter drugs may

TABLE 16-3 Potential Effects of Herbs

Herb	Potential Effect
Black cohosh	Bradycardia, hypotension, joint pains
Bloodroot	Bradycardia, dysrhythmia, dizziness, impaired vision, intense thirst
Boneset	Liver toxicity, mental changes, respiratory problems
Coltsfoot	Fever, liver toxicity
Dandelion	Interactions with diuretics, increased concentration of lithium or potassium
Ephedra	Headache, dizziness, insomnia, tachycardia, hypertension, anxiety, irritability, dry mouth
Feverfew	Interference with blood-clotting mechanisms
Garlic	Hypotension, blood-clotting inhibition, potentiation of diabetes drugs
Ginseng	Headache, anxiety, insomnia, hypertension, tachycardia, asthma attacks, postmenopausal bleeding
Goldenseal	Vasoconstriction
Hawthorn	Hypotension
Kava	Damage to the eyes, skin, liver, and spinal cord from long-term use
Licorice	Hyperkalemia, hypernatremia
Lobelia	Hearing and vision problems
Motherwort	Increased anticoagulation
Nettle	Hypokalemia
Senna	Potentiation of digoxin
St. John's wort	Antidepressant, photosensitivity
Valerian root	Mild sedative or tranquilizer effect, hepatotoxicity

also affect how the patient reacts to the operative experience. Adverse effects can occur with the use of some herbs, such as those listed in Table 16-3.

Medical history is important to obtain because many chronic illnesses increase surgical risks and need to be considered when planning care. For example, a patient with systemic lupus erythematosus may need additional drugs to offset the stress of the surgery. A diabetic patient may need a more extensive bowel preparation because of decreased intestinal motility. An infection may need to be treated before surgery.

Ask the patient specifically about cardiac disease because complications from anesthesia occur more often in patients with cardiac problems. A patient with a history of rheumatic heart disease may be prescribed antibiotics before surgery. Cardiac problems that increase surgical risks include coronary artery disease, angina, myocardial infarction (MI) within 6 months before surgery, heart failure, hypertension, and dysrhythmias. These problems impair the patient's ability to withstand hemodynamic changes and alter the response to anesthesia. The risk for an MI during surgery is higher in patients who have heart problems.

Pulmonary complications during or after surgery are more likely to occur in older patients, those with chronic respiratory problems, and smokers because of smoking- or age-related lung changes (Gazarian, 2006). Increased chest rigidity and loss of lung elasticity reduce anesthetic excretion. Smoking increases the blood level of **carboxyhemoglobin** (carbon monoxide on oxygen-binding sites of the hemoglobin molecule), which decreases oxygen delivery to organs. Action of cilia in pulmonary mucous membranes decreases, which leads to retained secretions and predisposes the patient to infection (pneumonia) and **atelectasis** (collapse of alveoli). Atelectasis reduces gas exchange and causes intolerance of anesthesia. It is also a common problem after general anesthesia.

Chronic lung problems such as asthma, emphysema, and chronic bronchitis also reduce the elasticity of the lungs, which reduces gas exchange. As a result, patients with these problems have reduced tissue oxygenation.

Previous surgical procedures and anesthesia affect the patient's readiness for surgery. Previous experiences, especially with complications, may increase anxiety about the scheduled surgery. Ask about the patient's experience with anesthesia and all allergies. These data provide information about tolerance of and possible fears about the use of anesthesia. The family medical history and problems with anesthetics may indicate possible reactions to anesthesia, such as malignant hyperthermia (see Chapter 17).

A sensitivity or allergy to certain substances alerts you to a possible reaction to anesthetic agents or to substances that are used before or during surgery. For example, povidone-iodine (e.g., Betadine) used for skin cleansing contains the same allergens found in shellfish. Patients who are allergic to shellfish may have an adverse reaction to povidone-iodine. The patient with an allergy to bananas and other fruits often also has a latex allergy.

Blood donation for surgery can be made by the patient **(autologous donations)** a few weeks just before the scheduled surgery date. Then, if blood is needed during or after surgery, an autologous blood transfusion can be given. This practice eliminates transfusion reactions and reduces the risk of acquiring bloodborne disease.

Patients can donate their own blood up to 5 weeks before surgery if they are infection free, have a hemoglobin level greater than 11 g/dL (110 g/L), and have a physician's recommendation. Patients with cardiac disease may need additional clearance from their cardiologist before making an autologous donation. The physician may prescribe supplemental iron before the first donation. Autologous donations can be made as often as every 3 days if other criteria are met. Usually a total of 2 to 4 units are donated. The last donation cannot be made within 72 hours before surgery.

A special tag is placed on the blood bag when an autologous blood donation has been made. The blood donor center gives the patient a matching tag that he or she wears or brings to the surgical area before surgery. This procedure helps ensure that patients receive only their own blood. If the blood is not used, some agencies discard it. In other agencies, the blood goes to the blood bank where it is processed into various blood components (e.g., plasma, packed cells, platelets).

Patients may wish to have family and friends donate blood exclusively for their use, if needed. This practice (called *directed blood donation*) is possible only if the blood types are compatible and the donor's blood is acceptable. Patients may fear disease transmission from unknown blood and feel more comfortable knowing who gave the blood. Many centers do not accept directed blood, stating that it gives a false sense of security. As with autologous blood donations, a special tag is attached to the blood bag. This tag notes the names of the patient and the donor and bears the patient's signature.

Ask whether autologous or directed blood donations have been made, and document this information in the chart. It is important to know the specific blood collection center where the donation was made and whether the blood has arrived before the patient goes into surgery. The hospital receives and stores the blood units until they are used or are no longer needed. Unused blood is returned to the collection center.

Increased use of "bloodless surgery" and minimally invasive surgery provides alternatives for patients with religious or medical restrictions to blood transfusions. These programs reduce the need for transfusion during and after surgery. Some techniques used include limiting blood samples (the number of samples, as well as the volume of blood drawn per sample) before surgery and stimulating the patient's own red blood cell production with epoetin alpha (Epogen, Procrit) before, during, and after surgery. Supplemental iron, folic acid, vitamin B_{12}, and vitamin C may be prescribed before surgery to help red blood cell formation. Newer equipment and surgical techniques cause less blood loss than older techniques. Such advances include recycling blood suctioned during surgery and immediately transfusing it back into the patient. Assess, monitor, teach, and support the patient during the bloodless surgery process.

Discharge planning is started before surgery (Tappen et al., 2001). Assess the patient's home environment, self-care capabilities, and support systems, and anticipate postoperative needs before surgery. *All patients, regardless of how minor the procedure or how often they have had surgery, should have discharge planning.* Older patients and dependent adults may need transportation referrals to and from the physician's office or the surgical setting. A home care nurse may be needed to monitor recovery and to provide instructions. All patients with few support systems may need follow-up care at home. Some patients need a planned direct admission to a rehabilitation hospital or center for physical therapy after surgery (e.g., a total hip replacement). Shortened hospital stays require adequate discharge planning to achieve the desired outcomes after surgery.

Physical Assessment/Clinical Manifestations

The preoperative patient may be any age, with a health status that varies from well to debilitated. Perform a complete assessment before surgery to obtain baseline data. During assessment, identify current health problems, potential complications related to anesthesia, and possible complications that may occur after surgery.

When beginning the assessment, obtain a complete set of vital signs. You may need to obtain vital signs several times at different time intervals for accurate baseline values. Previous vital signs from another admission (if available) are helpful to compare with current vital signs. Abnormal vital signs may require postponement of surgery until the problem is treated and the patient's condition is stable. Also assess for anxiety, which could increase blood pressure, pulse, and respiratory rate. Document these findings as part of the overall assessment.

Throughout the physical assessment, focus on problem areas identified from the patient's history and on all body systems affected by the surgical procedure. The older adult (Chart 16-2; see also Chapter 3) or chronically ill patient is at increased risk for complications during and after surgery. The number of serious problems (**morbidity**) and deaths (**mortality**) during or after surgery is higher in older and chronically ill patients.

Chart 16-2 NURSING FOCUS ON THE OLDER ADULT

Specific Considerations When Planning Care for the Older Preoperative Patient

- Greater incidence of chronic illness
- Greater incidence of malnutrition
- More allergies
- Increased incidence of impaired self-care abilities
- Inadequate support systems
- Decreased ability to withstand the stress of surgery and anesthesia
- Increased risk for cardiopulmonary complications after surgery
- Risk of a change in mental status when admitted (e.g., related to unfamiliar surroundings, change in routine, drugs)
- Increased risk of a fall and resultant injury

Report any abnormal assessment findings to the surgeon and to anesthesia personnel. In this way, you are a proactive patient advocate exercising professional legal responsibility. Often, established protocols or care maps identify what interventions are to be performed before surgery.

Cardiovascular status is critical to assess because cardiac problems may cause as many as 30% of surgery-related deaths. Check the patient for hypertension, which is common, is often undiagnosed, and can affect the response to surgery. Cardiac assessment includes listening to heart sounds for rate, regularity, and abnormalities. Examine the patient's hands and feet for temperature, color, peripheral pulses, capillary refill, and edema. Report any problems (e.g., absent peripheral pulses, pitting edema, cardiac symptoms such as chest pain, shortness of breath, and dyspnea) to the physician for further assessment and evaluation. (Cardiac assessment is discussed further in Chapter 35.)

Respiratory status considers age, smoking history (including exposure to secondhand smoke), and any chronic illness (Gazarian, 2006). Observe the patient's posture; respiratory rate, rhythm, and depth; overall respiratory effort; and lung expansion. Document any clubbing of the fingertips (swelling at the base of the nail beds caused by a chronic lack of oxygen) or cyanosis. Auscultate the lungs to assess for any abnormal breath sounds (crackles, wheezes, rubs). (More information on respiratory assessment is found in Chapter 29.)

Renal status and function affect the excretion of drugs and waste products, including anesthetic and analgesic agents. If renal function is reduced, fluid and electrolyte balance can be altered, especially in older patients. Ask about problems such as urinary frequency, **dysuria** (painful urination), **nocturia** (awakening during nighttime sleep because of a need to void), difficulty starting urine flow, and **oliguria** (scant amount of urine). Ask the patient about the appearance and odor of the urine. Equally important is an assessment of usual fluid intake and degree of continence. If the patient has renal or urinary problems, consult with the physician about further workup. (Renal/urinary assessment is discussed further in Chapter 68.)

Kidney impairment decreases the excretion of drugs and anesthetic agents. As a result, drug effectiveness may be altered. Scopolamine (Buscopan), morphine, meperidine

(Demerol), and barbiturates often cause confusion, disorientation, apprehension, and restlessness when given to patients with decreased kidney function.

Neurologic status includes the patient's overall mental status, level of consciousness, orientation, and ability to follow commands. This information is needed before planning preoperative teaching and care after surgery. A problem in any of these areas affects the type of care needed during the surgical experience. Determine the patient's baseline neurologic status to be able to identify changes that may occur later. Also assess for any motor or sensory deficits. (See Chapter 43 for complete nervous system assessment.)

The usual neurologic status of a mentally impaired patient may be difficult to assess. The patient who has been independent and oriented at home may become disoriented in the hospital setting. Family members can often provide information about what the patient was like at home.

Ensure patient safety by assessing the patient's risk for falling, especially the older patient. Evaluate factors such as mental status, muscle strength, steadiness of gait, and sense of independence to determine the patient's risk. Document the patient's ability to ambulate and the steadiness of gait as baseline data (Metules & Bauer, 2006).

Musculoskeletal status problems may interfere with positioning during and after surgery. For example, patients with arthritis may be able to assume surgical positions but have discomfort after surgery from prolonged joint immobilization. Other anatomic features, such as the shape and length of the neck and the shape of the chest cavity, may interfere with respiratory and cardiac function or require special positioning during surgery.

Ask about a history of joint replacements, and document the exact location of any prostheses. *During surgery, ensure that electrocautery pads, which could cause an electrical burn, are not placed on or near the area of the prosthesis.*

Nutritional status, especially malnutrition and obesity, can increase surgical risk (Baugh et al., 2007). Surgery increases metabolic rate and depletes potassium, vitamin C, and B vitamins, all of which are needed for wound healing and blood clotting. In malnourished patients, decreased serum protein levels slow recovery. Negative nitrogen balance may result from depleted protein stores. This problem increases the risk for skin breakdown, delayed wound healing, possible dehiscence or evisceration (see Chapter 18), dehydration, and sepsis.

Some older patients may have poor nutrition because of chronic illness, diuretic or laxative use, poor dietary planning or habits, anorexia, and lack of motivation or financial limitations (Meiner & Lueckenotte, 2006). Indications of poor fluid or nutritional status include:

- Brittle nails
- Muscle wasting
- Dry or flaky skin, decreased skin turgor, and hair changes (e.g., dull, sparse, dry)
- Orthostatic (postural) hypotension
- Decreased serum protein levels and abnormal serum electrolyte values

The obese patient is often malnourished because of an imbalanced diet. Obesity increases the risk for poor wound healing because of excessive **adipose** (fatty) tissue. Fatty tissue has few blood vessels, little collagen, and decreased nutrients, all of which are needed for wound healing. Obesity stresses the heart and reduces the lung volumes, which can affect the surgery and recovery. In addition, obese patients may need larger doses of drugs and may retain them longer after surgery.

Psychosocial Assessment

Perform a psychosocial assessment to determine the patient's level of anxiety, coping ability, and support systems. Provide information and offer support as needed.

Most patients have some degree of anxiety before surgery; other may be fearful. The extent of these reactions varies according to the type of surgery, the perceived effects of the surgery and its potential outcome, and the patient's personality. Surgery may be seen as a threat to life, body image, self-esteem, self-concept, or lifestyle. Patients may fear death, pain, helplessness, a change in role or work status, a diagnosis of life-threatening conditions, possible disabling or crippling effects, or the unknown.

Anxiety or fear affects the patient's ability to learn, cope, and cooperate with teaching and operative procedures. Anxiety may also influence the amount and type of anesthetic needed and may slow recovery (Vaughn et al., 2007). In addition, severe preoperative anxiety appears to increase the degree of pain some patients have after surgery (see the Evidence-Based Practice box on p. 249). Be aware of potential anxiety when interviewing the patient and planning teaching.

Assess coping mechanisms used by the patient under similar situations or in the past when confronted with a stressful situation. Ask open-ended questions about the patient's feelings about the entire surgical experience. Factors that influence coping include age; previous surgical or sick-role experiences; and emotional and physical signs of fear, anxiety, or discomfort. Signs of anxiety include anger, crying, restlessness, profuse sweating, increased pulse rate, palpitations, sleeplessness, diarrhea, and urinary frequency.

Laboratory Assessment

Laboratory tests before surgery provide baseline data about the patient's health and help predict potential complications. The patient scheduled for surgery in an ambulatory surgical center or admitted to the hospital on the morning of or day before surgery may have preadmission testing (PAT) performed from 24 hours to 28 days before the scheduled surgery. These test results are usually valid unless there has been a change in the patient's condition that warrants repeated testing or the patient is taking drugs that can alter laboratory values (e.g., warfarin [Coumadin], aspirin, diuretics). Some facilities have time limits for tests, especially pregnancy testing or any other test results that would require altering the surgical plan.

The choice of laboratory testing before surgery varies among facilities and depends on the patient's age, medical history, and type of anesthesia planned (Rothrock & McEwen, 2007). The most common tests include:

- Urinalysis
- Blood type and screen
- Complete blood count or hemoglobin level and hematocrit
- Clotting studies (prothrombin time [PT], international normalized ratio [INR], activated partial thromboplastin time [aPTT], platelet count)
- Electrolyte levels
- Serum creatinine and blood urea nitrogen levels
- Depending on a female patient's age and the nature of the planned procedure, a pregnancy test may also be needed

EVIDENCE-BASED PRACTICE

Relationship between anxiety and postoperative pain is controversial

Vaughn, F., Wichowski, H., & Bosworth, G. (2007). Does preoperative anxiety level predict postoperative pain? *AORN Journal, 85*(3), 589-604.

Nurses have been taught that anxiety can have an impact on a patient's perception of pain. The first study exploring the influence of anxiety on surgical recovery was conducted in 1958. This concept has provided the rationale for preoperative teaching, relaxation techniques, and medications. However, the evidence linking high levels of preoperative anxiety to increased pain levels after surgery has shown conflicting results. The authors of this article attempted to analyze appropriate previous research in this area to determine possible sources of the different results.

A variety of research reports and previous meta-analyses regarding preoperative anxiety and postoperative factors were examined for study design, numbers of subjects, methodology, and control variables. These studies employed different designs and often used different instruments to measure anxiety and pain. Few studies also examined the level of pain in the preoperative period. Some studies using an experimental design compared the anxiety levels and postoperative pain levels in patients who received anti-anxiety drugs in the preoperative period with patients who did not receive such drugs. For those studies that did not use anti-anxiety drugs, a statistical difference was seen with patients having higher levels of preoperative anxiety, especially state anxiety, also having higher levels of pain or using higher amounts of analgesics in the postoperative period than those patients with lower preoperative anxiety.

Level of Evidence—3. The study is a report of a meta-analysis of previous research on the topic of preoperative anxiety and postoperative pain.

Commentary: Implications for Practice and Research. Although anxiety reduction techniques can include drug therapy, there are many nonpharmacologic ways to help reduce anxiety. Many of these are considered nursing interventions, which can be low risk to the patient. Therefore, although the authors of this meta-analysis identify the need for large, prospective, unified design, intervention studies examining the influence of preoperative anxiety on the level of postoperative pain among surgical patients, they also advocate the continued use of nursing strategies to lower anxiety among patients during the perioperative experience.

Urinalysis is performed to assess abnormal substances in the urine such as protein, glucose, blood, and bacteria. If kidney disease is suspected or if the patient is older, the physician may request other tests to determine the type and degree of disease present.

Report electrolyte imbalances or other abnormal results to the anesthesia team and the surgeon before surgery. **Hypokalemia** (decreased serum potassium level) increases the risk for toxicity if the patient is taking digoxin, slows recovery from anesthesia, and increases cardiac irritability. **Hyperkalemia** (increased serum potassium level) increases the risk for dysrhythmias, especially with the use of anesthesia. *Potassium problems must be corrected before the surgery.*

Other studies may be needed, depending on the patient's medical history. For example, baseline arterial blood gas (ABG) values are assessed before surgery for patients with chronic pulmonary problems. Chart 16-3 lists abnormal laboratory findings and their possible causes.

Imaging Assessment

A chest x-ray may be requested before surgery. Often, young healthy adults are not required to have a chest x-ray. A chest x-ray determines the size and shape of the heart, lungs, and major vessels and determines the presence of pneumonia or tuberculosis. It also provides baseline data in case of complications. Abnormal x-ray findings alert the surgeon to potential cardiac or pulmonary complications. Heart failure, cardiomyopathy, pneumonia, or infiltrates may cause cancellation or delay of elective surgery. For emergency surgery, x-ray results assist the anesthesia provider in selecting anesthesia.

Other imaging studies are based on patient need, medical history, and the nature of the surgical procedure. For example, a patient with back pain may have computed tomography (CT) or magnetic resonance imaging (MRI) examinations before spinal surgery to identify the exact location of the problem.

Other Diagnostic Assessment

An electrocardiogram (ECG) may be required for all patients older than a specific age who are to have general anesthesia. The age varies among facilities but is often 40 to 45 years. An ECG may also be ordered for patients with a history of cardiac disease or those at risk for cardiac complications. It provides baseline information on new or existing cardiac problems, such as an old myocardial infarction (MI). A patient with a known cardiac problem may need a cardiology consultation before surgery. Drugs for problem prevention, such as nitroglycerin and antibiotics, may be needed throughout the surgical period to reduce or prevent stress on the heart. Abnormal or potentially life-threatening ECG results may cause the cancellation of surgery until the patient's cardiac status is stable.

A focused assessment of the preoperative patient is shown in Chart 16-4.

NCLEX EXAMINATION CHALLENGE

While the nurse is taking the client's history before elective cosmetic surgery, the client reports all the following facts. Which one should be reported to the surgeon and may result in a cancellation of this surgery?

A. She delivered a baby 8 weeks ago and still has some vaginal discharge.
B. She has three large "boils" (furuncles) on the skin of her left shoulder.
C. She has been taking oral contraceptives for the last 2 weeks.
D. She is allergic to aspirin, dust, peanuts, and fall pollens.

evolve For the correct answer, go to http://evolve.elsevier.com/Iggy/.

Chart 16-3 LABORATORY PROFILE

Perioperative Assessment

Test	Normal Range for Adults	Significance of Abnormal Findings: Increased in	Significance of Abnormal Findings: Decreased in
Potassium (K^+)	3.5-5.0 mEq/L, or 3.5-5.0 mmol/L	Dehydration Renal failure Acidosis Cellular/tissue damage Hemolysis of the specimen	NPO status when potassium replacement is inadequate Excessive use of non–potassium-sparing diuretics Vomiting Malnutrition Diarrhea Alkalosis
Sodium (Na^+)	90 yr old or younger: 136-145 mEq/L, or 136-145 mmol/L Older than 90 yr: 132-146 mEq/L, or 132-146 mmol/L	Cardiac or renal failure Hypertension Excessive amounts of IV fluids containing normal saline Edema Dehydration (hemoconcentration)	Nasogastric drainage Vomiting or diarrhea Excessive use of laxatives or diuretics Excessive amounts of IV fluids containing water Syndrome of inappropriate antidiuretic hormone (SIADH)
Chloride (Cl^-)	90 yr old or younger: 98-106 mEq/L, or 98-106 mmol/L Older than 90 yr: 98-111 mEq/L, or 98-111 mmol/L	Respiratory alkalosis Dehydration Renal failure Excessive amounts of IV fluids containing sodium chloride (NaCl)	Excessive nasogastric drainage Vomiting Excessive use of diuretics Diarrhea
Carbon dioxide (CO_2)	60 yr or younger: 23-30 mEq/L, or 23-30 mmol/L 60-90 yr: 23-31 mEq/L, or 23-31 mmol/L Older than 90 yr: 20-29 mEq/L, or 20-29 mmol/L	Chronic pulmonary disease Intestinal obstruction Vomiting or nasogastric suctioning Metabolic alkalosis	Hyperventilation Diabetic ketoacidosis Diarrhea Lactic acidosis Renal failure Salicylate toxicity
Glucose (fasting)	60 yr or younger: 70-110 mg/dL, or 4.1-5.9 mmol/L 60-90 yr: 82-115 mg/dL, or 4.6-6.4 mmol/L Older than 90 yr: 75-121 mg/dL, or 4.2-6.7 mmol/L	Hyperglycemia Excessive amounts of IV fluids containing glucose Stress Steroid use Pancreatic or hepatic disease	Hypoglycemia Excess insulin
Creatinine	*Females:* 60 yr or younger: 0.5-1.1 mg/dL, or 44-97 μmol/L 60-90 yr: 0.6-1.2 mg/dL, or 53-106 μmol/L Older than 90 yr: 0.6-1.3 mg/dL, or 53-115 μmol/L *Males:* 60 yr or younger: 0.6-1.2 mg/dL, or 53-106 μmol/L 60-90 yr: 0.8-1.3 mg/dL, or 71-115 μmol/L Older than 90 yr: 1.0-1.7 mg/dL, or 88-150 μmol/L	Renal damage with destruction of large number of nephrons Renal insufficiency Acute renal failure Chronic kidney disease End-stage kidney disease (ESKD)	Atrophy of muscle tissue
Blood urea nitrogen (BUN)	Younger than 60 yr: 10-20 mg/dL, or 2.1-7.1 mmol/L 60-90 yr: 8-23 mg/dL, or 2.9-8.2 mmol/L Older than 90 yr: 10-31 mg/dL, or 3.6-11.1 mmol/L	Dehydration Renal failure Excessive protein in diet Liver failure	Overhydration Malnutrition

IRU, International recommended unit; *NPO*, nothing by mouth.

Chart 16-3 LABORATORY PROFILE

Perioperative Assessment—cont'd

Test	Normal Range for Adults	SIGNIFICANCE OF ABNORMAL FINDINGS: Increased in	SIGNIFICANCE OF ABNORMAL FINDINGS: Decreased in
Prothrombin time (pro time, PT)	11-12.5 sec, 85%-100%, or 1:1.1 patient-control ratio	Coagulation defect (bleeding disorder)	Coagulation (clotting) disorder, such as thrombophlebitis or pulmonary embolus
International normalized ratio (INR)	0.7-1.8	Anticoagulant therapy (aspirin, warfarin)	Extensive cancer
Partial thromboplastin time, activated (aPTT)	30-40 sec	Coagulation defect (bleeding disorder) Anticoagulant therapy (heparin) Liver disease	Coagulation (clotting) disorder, such as thrombophlebitis or pulmonary embolus Extensive cancer
White blood cell (WBC) count (leukocyte count)	Total: 5,000-10,000/mm^3	Infection Inflammation Stress Tissue necrosis	Immune disorder Immunosuppressant therapy
Hemoglobin, total	*Females:* 18-44 yr: 12-16 g/dL, or 117-155 g/L 45-64 yr: 11.7-16.0 g/dL, or 117-160 g/L 65-74 yr: 11.7-16.1 g/dL, or 117-161 g/L *Males:* 18-44 yr: 14-18 g/dL, or 132-173 g/L 45-64 yr: 13.1-17.2 g/dL, or 131-172 g/L 65-74 yr: 12.6-17.4 g/dL, or 126-174 g/L	Dehydration Polycythemia Chronic pulmonary disease Congestive heart failure	Blood loss Anemia Renal failure
Hematocrit	*Females:* 18-44 yr: 35%-45% 45-74 yr: 37%-47% *Males:* 18-44 yr: 42%-52% 45-64 yr: 39%-50% 65-74 yr: 37%-51%	Dehydration Polycythemia High altitude	Blood loss Anemia Renal failure

Chart 16-4 FOCUSED ASSESSMENT

The Preoperative Patient

As part of the cardiopulmonary assessment, take and record vital signs; report:
- Hypotension or hypertension
- Heart rate less than 60 or more than 120 beats/min
- Irregular heart rate
- Chest pain
- Shortness of breath or dyspnea
- Tachypnea
- Pulse oximetry reading of less than 94%

Assess for and report any signs or symptoms of infection, including:
- Fever
- Purulent sputum
- Dysuria or cloudy, foul-smelling urine
- Any red, swollen, draining IV or wound site
- Increased white blood cell count

Assess for and report signs or symptoms that could contraindicate surgery, including:
- Increased prothrombin time (PT), international normalized ratio (INR), or activated partial thromboplastin time (aPTT)
- Hypokalemia or hyperkalemia
- Patient report of possible pregnancy or positive pregnancy test

Assess for and report other clinical conditions that may need to be evaluated by a physician or advanced nurse practitioner before proceeding with the surgical plans, including:
- Change in mental status
- Vomiting
- Rash
- Recent administration of an anticoagulant drug

Analysis

Common Nursing Diagnoses and Collaborative Problems

Priority nursing diagnoses for preoperative patients are:

1. Deficient Knowledge (specific experiences before, during, and after surgery) related to unfamiliarity with available resources
2. Anxiety related to the threat of a change in health status or fear of the unknown

Additional Nursing Diagnoses and Collaborative Problems

In addition to the common nursing diagnoses, preoperative patients may have one or more of these:

- Sleep Deprivation related to internal sensory alterations (e.g., illness, anxiety)
- Ineffective Coping related to the impending surgery
- Grieving related to the effects of surgery
- Disturbed Body Image related to anticipated changes in the body's appearance or function
- Compromised Family Coping related to temporary family disorganization and role changes
- Powerlessness related to the health care environment, loss of independence, and loss of control of one's body

Planning and Implementation

As the nurse, your role is to ensure coordination of care for the patient before surgery. This responsibility continues until the patient is transferred to the OR.

Deficient Knowledge

NOC **Planning: Expected Outcomes.** The patient needs to know what to expect during and after surgery and participate in his or her recovery as indicated by consistently demonstrating these behaviors:

- Explaining the purpose and expected results of the planned surgery
- Asking questions when a term or procedure is not known
- Adhering to the NPO requirements
- Stating an understanding of preoperative preparations (e.g., skin preparation, bowel preparation)
- Demonstrating correct use of exercises and techniques to be used after surgery for the prevention of complications (e.g., splinting the incision, coughing/deep breathing, performing leg exercises, ambulating as early as permitted)

Interventions. Because the surgical experience is foreign to many people, focus on teaching the patient and family members. Teaching may begin in the surgeon's office for planned or elective surgery. Pamphlets, written instructions, and videotapes and DVDs may be given or sent to the patient. More teaching may occur when the patient has preadmission testing. Some facilities hold classes before surgery for groups of patients or show videos for those who are having the same or similar surgical procedures. A tour of the operating suite and the postanesthesia care unit (PACU) may be included.

Explore the patient's level of knowledge and understanding. Increased access to information via the Internet may be helpful but is also a concern. Some Internet information may not be accurate or may not apply to a specific patient's plan of care.

Information about informed consent, dietary restrictions, specific preparation for surgery (bowel and skin preparations), exercises after surgery, and plans for pain management promote patients' participation and help achieve the desired outcome. A sample educational checklist is shown in Table 16-4. Because education occurs in a variety of settings, coordination of patient teaching efforts is challenging. When you care for the patient just before surgery (same-day, ambulatory surgery [outpatient] unit, inpatient hospital unit), assess the patient's and family members' knowledge and provide additional information as needed. Document in the patient record information about who was involved in teaching, what specifically was taught, and what education materials were given to the patient and family (Pearce, 2006).

Ensuring Informed Consent. Surgery of any type involves invasion of the body and requires informed consent from the patient or legal guardian (Fig. 16-1). Patients deserve, and rightly demand, to be informed and involved in decisions affecting their health care. Consent implies that the patient has sufficient information to understand:

- The nature of and reason for surgery
- Who will be performing the surgery and whether others will be present during the procedure (e.g., students)
- All available options and the risks associated with each option
- The risks associated with the surgical procedure and its potential outcomes
- The risks associated with the use of anesthesia

Informed consent is one way to help ensure patient safety. It helps protect the patient from any unwanted procedures and protects the surgeon and the facility from lawsuit claims related to unauthorized surgery or uninformed patients. Written record of informed consent is documented on a "consent form" but can also be documented in the surgeon's notes. The consent form documents the patient's consent and signature for the procedure listed.

As a competent adult, it is the patient's right to refuse treatment for any reason, even when refusal might lead to death. For example, in the case of Jehovah's Witnesses, some patients will not accept blood transfusions because of their religious convictions.

The surgeon is responsible for having the consent form signed before sedation is given and before surgery is performed. *You, as a nurse, are not responsible for providing detailed information about the surgical procedure. Rather, your*

TABLE 16-4 Preoperative Teaching Checklist

Consider these items when planning individualized preoperative teaching for patients and families:

- Fears and anxieties
- Surgical procedure
- Preoperative routines (e.g., NPO, blood samples, showering)
- Invasive procedures (e.g., lines, catheters)
- Coughing, turning, deep breathing
- Incentive spirometer
  - How to use
  - How to tell when used correctly
- Lower extremity exercises
- Stockings and pneumatic compression devices
- Early ambulation
- Splinting
- Pain management

NPO, Nothing by mouth.

GENERAL REQUEST AND CONSENT

FOR OFFICE USE ONLY:
Patient Name: ______
Date of Birth: ______
Date of Procedure: ______

I ____________________ request and give consent to ____________________
(Type or print patient name) (Type or print Doctor or Practitioner Name(s))

to perform the following procedure(s) ____________________
(Please list site and side if appropriate)

____

____

The benefits, risks, complications, and alternatives to the above procedure(s) have been explained to me.

I understand that the procedure(s) will be performed at Christiana Care by and under supervision of my doctor or practitioner. My doctor or practitioner may use the services of other doctors or practitioners, or members of the resident staff as he or she deems necessary or advisable.

I authorize my doctor or practitioner and his or her associates and assistants to perform such additional procedures, which in their judgment are necessary and appropriate to carry out my diagnosis or treatment.

I authorize the hospital to retain, preserve and use for scientific, teaching or transplant purposes, or to make other dispositions of, at their convenience, any specimens, tissues, or parts taken from my body during the course of this operation.

I consent to observers in the operating room in accordance with hospital policy. I consent to photography or video taping of my surgical procedure for educational purposes, provided my identity remains anonymous and confidential.

I agree to being given blood or blood products as deemed advisable during the course of my procedure. The risks, benefits, and alternatives to receiving blood or blood products have been explained to me.

I consent to the administration of sedation or analgesia during my procedure. The risks, benefits, and alternatives to receiving sedation or analgesia have been explained to me.

If anesthesia is required, I consent to the administration of anesthesia by members of the Department of Anesthesiology. I also consent to the use of non-invasive and invasive monitoring techniques as deemed necessary. I understand that anesthesia involves risks that are in addition to those resulting from the operation itself including, but not limited to, dental injury, hoarseness, vocal cord injury, infection, nerve injury, corneal abrasion, seizures, heart attack, stroke and even death.

Please initial one of the following statements (females only):

______ To the best of my knowledge I am not pregnant. ______ I believe I am pregnant.

I certify that I have read and understand the above consent statements. In addition, I have been offered the opportunity to ask my doctor or practitioner any questions I have regarding the procedure(s) to be performed and they have been answered to my satisfaction. I acknowledge that I have been given no guarantee or assurance as to the results that may be obtained from the procedure(s).

Signature of Patient or Decision Maker — Date and Time	Doctor or Practitioner Signature — Date and Time
Relationship to Patient if Decision Maker	Doctor ID # or Print Name
Witness Signature — Date and Time	Practitioner Print Name/Title
Witness Print Name	

Telephone Consent: ____________________
Name of person obtained from/Relationship to Patient

Witness's (es') Signature(s) — Date and Time	Witness's (es') Signature(s) — Date and Time
Witness's (es') Print Name(s)	Witness's (es') Print Name(s)

Fig. 16-1 • A surgical consent form.

role is to clarify facts that have been presented by the physician and dispel myths that the patient or family may have about the surgical experience. You verify that the consent form is signed, and you serve as a witness to the signature, not to the fact that the patient is informed. If you believe that the patient has not been adequately informed, contact the surgeon and request that he or she see the patient for further clarification. Document this action in the chart.

Patients who cannot write may sign with an X, which must be witnessed by two persons. In an emergency, telephone or telegram authorization is acceptable and should be followed up with written consent as soon as possible. The number of witnesses (usually two) and the type of documentation vary according to the facility's policy. In a life-threatening situation in which every effort has been made to contact the person with medical power of attorney, consent is desired but not essential. In place of written or oral consent, written consultation by at least two physicians who are not associated with the case may be requested by the physician. This formal consultation legally supports the decision for surgery until the appropriate person can sign a consent form. If the patient is not capable of giving consent and has no family, the court can appoint a legal guardian to represent the patient's best interests.

A blind patient may sign his or her own consent form, which usually needs to be witnessed by two persons. Patients who have English as a second language (ESL), who do not speak the general language of the facility, or who are hearing impaired may require a qualified translator and a second witness. Many facilities have consent forms written in more than one language and also have health care professionals who are proficient with American Sign Language. Qualified translators may be health care professionals, other types of hospital employee, or family members (Smith, 2007). They are required to keep patient information confidential.

Some surgical procedures, such as intraocular lens implants, sterilization, and experimental procedures, may require a special permit in addition to the standard consent. National and local governing bodies and the individual facility determine which procedures require a separate permit. Separate consents for anesthesia and blood products may be required.

Surgical procedures that are site-specific, such as left, right, or bilateral, require patient identification before surgery. The patient is asked to mark the site with a marker to ensure the correct site is used and the wrong site is avoided. The nurse is an important part of this safety measure. Before starting the operative procedure, several facilities are adopting a "time-out" procedure. *At a minimum, the patient's identity, correct side and site, correct patient position, agreement on the proposed procedure, and availability of correct implants and equipment must be verified by all members of the surgical team.* The perioperative nurse is in a position of ensuring these safety measures are again implemented immediately before the procedure is started (Association of periOperative Registered Nurses [AORN], 2007a; Beyea, 2007; Metules & Bauer, 2006).

Patient Self-Determination. Patients receiving medical care have the right to have or to initiate advance directives, such as a living will or durable power of attorney, as mandated by the Patient Self-Determination Act. Advance directives provide legal instructions to the health care providers about the patient's wishes and are to be followed. *Surgery does not provide an exception to a patient's advance directives or living will* (AORN, 2007c). Chapter 9 discusses advance directives in more detail.

Implementing Dietary Restrictions. Regardless of the type of surgery and anesthesia planned, the patient is restricted to NPO status before surgery. **NPO** means no eating, drinking (including water), or smoking (nicotine stimulates gastric secretions). The exact amount of time a patient must be NPO before surgery is controversial. Patients, especially older adults, who fast for 8 or more hours may have imbalances of fluids, electrolytes, and blood glucose levels. The American Society of Anesthesiologists (ASA) recommends a reduced NPO time—6 or more hours for easily digested solid food and 2 hours for clear liquids (American Society of Anesthesiologists Task Force, 1999).

NPO status ensures that the stomach contains a limited volume of gastric secretions, which decreases the risk for aspiration. Outpatients and patients who are scheduled for admission to the hospital on the same day that surgery is performed must receive written and oral instructions about when to begin NPO status. *Emphasize the importance of adherence. Failure to adhere can result in cancellation of surgery or increase the risk for aspiration during or after surgery.*

Administering Regularly Scheduled Drugs. On the day of surgery, the patient's usual drug schedule may need to be altered. Consult the medical physician and the anesthesia provider for instructions about drugs such as those taken for diabetes, cardiac disease, or glaucoma, as well as regularly scheduled anticonvulsants, antihypertensives, anticoagulants, antidepressants, and corticosteroids. The physician may prescribe some drugs, including over-the-counter drugs such as aspirin, and herbal supplements to be stopped until after surgery. Other drugs may be given IV to maintain the drug level in the blood. *Drugs for cardiac disease, respiratory disease, seizures, and hypertension are commonly allowed with a sip of water before surgery.* Some antihypertensive or antidepressant drugs are withheld on the day of surgery to reduce adverse effects on blood pressure during surgery.

The diabetic patient who takes insulin may be given a reduced dose of intermediate- or long-acting insulin based on the blood glucose level or may be given regular (fast-acting) insulin in divided doses on the day of surgery. As an alternative, an IV infusion of 5% dextrose in water may be given with the insulin to prevent low blood sugar during surgery. Because of the many treatment approaches to diabetes, clarify drug and IV prescriptions with the physician. (See Chapter 67 for more information about diabetes.)

Intestinal Preparation. Bowel or intestinal preparations are performed to prevent injury to the colon and to reduce the number of intestinal bacteria. Evacuation of the bowel is needed when a patient is having major abdominal, pelvic, perineal, or perianal surgery. The surgeon's preference and the type of surgical procedure determine the type of bowel preparation. An enema ordered to be given until return flow is clear is a stressful procedure, especially for the older patient. Repeated enemas can cause electrolyte imbalance, fluid volume imbalances, vagal stimulation, and postural (orthostatic) hypotension. Enemas also cause severe anorectal discomfort in patients with hemorrhoids. Some physicians prescribe potent laxatives (e.g., polyethylene glycol electrolyte solution [GoLYTELY]) instead of enemas, especially for older patients. Bowel preparations can be exhausting, and you must take safety precautions to prevent falls.

Skin Preparation. The skin preparation may be embarrassing or uncomfortable for the patient, especially if the surgical site is in a sensitive or private body area. Provide a warm, comfortable, and private environment during the procedure. The skin is the body's first line of defense against infection. A break in this barrier increases the risk for infection, especially for older patients. Skin preparation before surgery is the first step in the prevention of surgical wound infection (AORN, 2007d).

One or two days before the scheduled surgery, the surgeon may ask the patient to shower using an antiseptic solution. Instruct the patient to be especially careful to clean around the proposed surgical site. If the patient is hospitalized before surgery, showering and cleaning are repeated the night before surgery or in the morning before transfer to the surgical suite. This cleaning reduces contamination of the surgical field and reduces the number of organisms at the site. Remove any soil or debris from the surgical site and surrounding areas.

Factors that predispose to wound contamination include bacteria found in hair follicles, disruption of the normal protective mechanisms of the skin, and nicks in the skin. Shaving of hair creates the potential for infection. Hair clipping with electrical clippers is often used to decrease the problems caused by traditional razors. The Centers for Disease Control and Prevention (CDC) recommends that if shaving is necessary, the hair should be removed using disposable sterile supplies and aseptic principles *immediately* before the start of the surgical procedure. If needed, shaving is performed in the treatment room, the holding area of the operating suite, or the operating room (OR). Fig. 16-2 shows areas shaved for various surgical procedures. Shaving is considered an inappropriate hair removal method. Beginning in 2010, only clippers or depilatories are to be used for hair removal.

Preparing the Patient for Tubes, Drains, and Vascular Access. Prepare the patient for possible placement of tubes, drains, and vascular access devices. Preparation reduces the patient's anxiety and fear and the family's negative reaction. Be careful not to scare the patient while providing information about the purpose of each tube.

Tubes of all sorts are common after surgery. The patient may need an indwelling urinary (Foley) catheter before, during, or after surgery to keep the bladder empty and to monitor kidney function. The patient having abdominal or genitourinary surgery usually has a Foley catheter.

A nasogastric (NG) tube may be inserted before abdominal surgery to decompress or empty the stomach and the upper bowel. More often, however, the tube is placed after the induction of anesthesia, when insertion is less disturbing to the patient and is easier to perform.

Drains are often placed during surgery to help remove fluid from the surgical site. Some drains are under the dressing; others are visible and require emptying. Drains come in various shapes and sizes (see Chapter 18). Inform the patient that drains are often used routinely and that generally they are not painful but may cause some discomfort. Discuss the reasons drains should not be kinked or pulled.

Vascular access is placed for patients receiving a general anesthetic and most patients receiving other types of anesthetics. Access is needed to give drugs and fluids before, during, and after surgery. Patients who are dehydrated or are at risk for dehydration may receive fluids before surgery.

CONSIDERATIONS FOR OLDER ADULTS

Older adult patients are at greater risk for dehydration because their fluid reserves are lower than those of young or middle-aged adults. Carefully monitor older adult patients and patients with cardiac disease receiving IV fluids. (See Chapter 15 for more information on IV therapy.)

The IV access is usually placed in the arm using a large, short catheter (e.g., 18-gauge, 1-inch catheter) or placed in the back of the hand using a smaller (20-gauge) catheter. A larger vein provides the least resistance to fluid or blood infusion, especially in an emergency when rapid infusions may be needed. Depending on the patient's needs and the facility's policies, the IV access can be placed before surgery when the patient is in the hospital room, in the holding or admission area of the surgical suite, or in the OR.

Postoperative Procedures and Exercises. Teach the patient and family members about exercises and procedures (e.g., checking dressings, obtaining vital signs frequently) to be performed after surgery. Family members can be helpful in reminding patients to perform these exercises. Teaching before surgery reduces apprehension and fear, increases cooperation and participation in care after surgery, and decreases respiratory and vascular complications. When the fear or anxiety level is high, explore the patient's feelings before discussing procedures.

Discussion, demonstration with return demonstration, and practice by the patient aid in the ability to perform various breathing (Chart 16-5) and leg (Chart 16-6) exercises after surgery. Stress the need to begin exercises early in the recovery phase and to continue them, with 5 to 10 repetitions each, every 1 to 2 hours after surgery for at least the first 48 hours. Explain that the patient may need to be awakened for these activities.

Procedures and exercises to prevent respiratory complications. *Breathing exercises* include deep, or diaphragmatic, breathing to enlarge the chest cavity and expand the lungs. After you demonstrate and explain the technique, urge the patient to practice the five steps of deep breathing.

For patients with chronic lung disease or limited chest expansion, as seen in older patients because of the aging process, expansion breathing exercises are useful. For the patient having chest surgery, expansion breathing exercises strengthen accessory muscles and are started before surgery. Expansion breathing may be used after surgery during chest physiotherapy (percussion, vibration, postural drainage) to help loosen secretions and maintain an adequate air exchange.

Incentive spirometry is another way to encourage the patient to take deep breaths. Its purpose is to promote complete lung expansion and to prevent pulmonary problems. Various types of incentive spirometers are available; Fig. 16-3 shows a patient using one type. With all types, the patient must be able to seal the lips tightly around the mouthpiece, inhale spontaneously, and hold his or her breath for 3 to 5 seconds for effective lung expansion. Goals (e.g., attaining specific volumes) can be set according to the patient's ability and the type of incentive spirometer. Seeing a light move up a column or a bellows expanding reinforces and motivates the patient to continue performance.

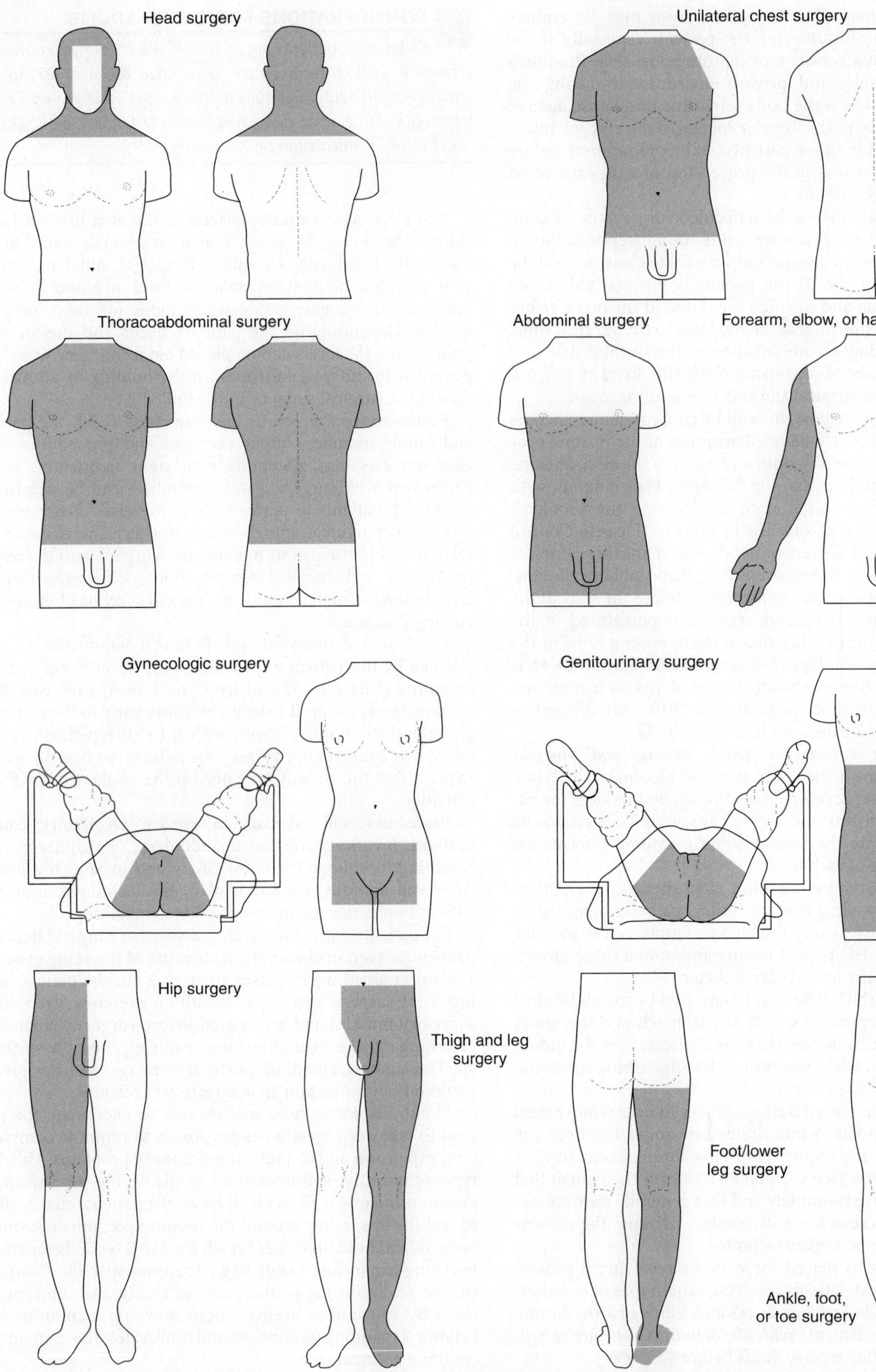
Head surgery
Unilateral chest surgery
Thoracoabdominal surgery
Abdominal surgery
Forearm, elbow, or hand surgery
Gynecologic surgery
Genitourinary surgery
Hip surgery
Thigh and leg surgery
Foot/lower leg surgery
Ankle, foot, or toe surgery

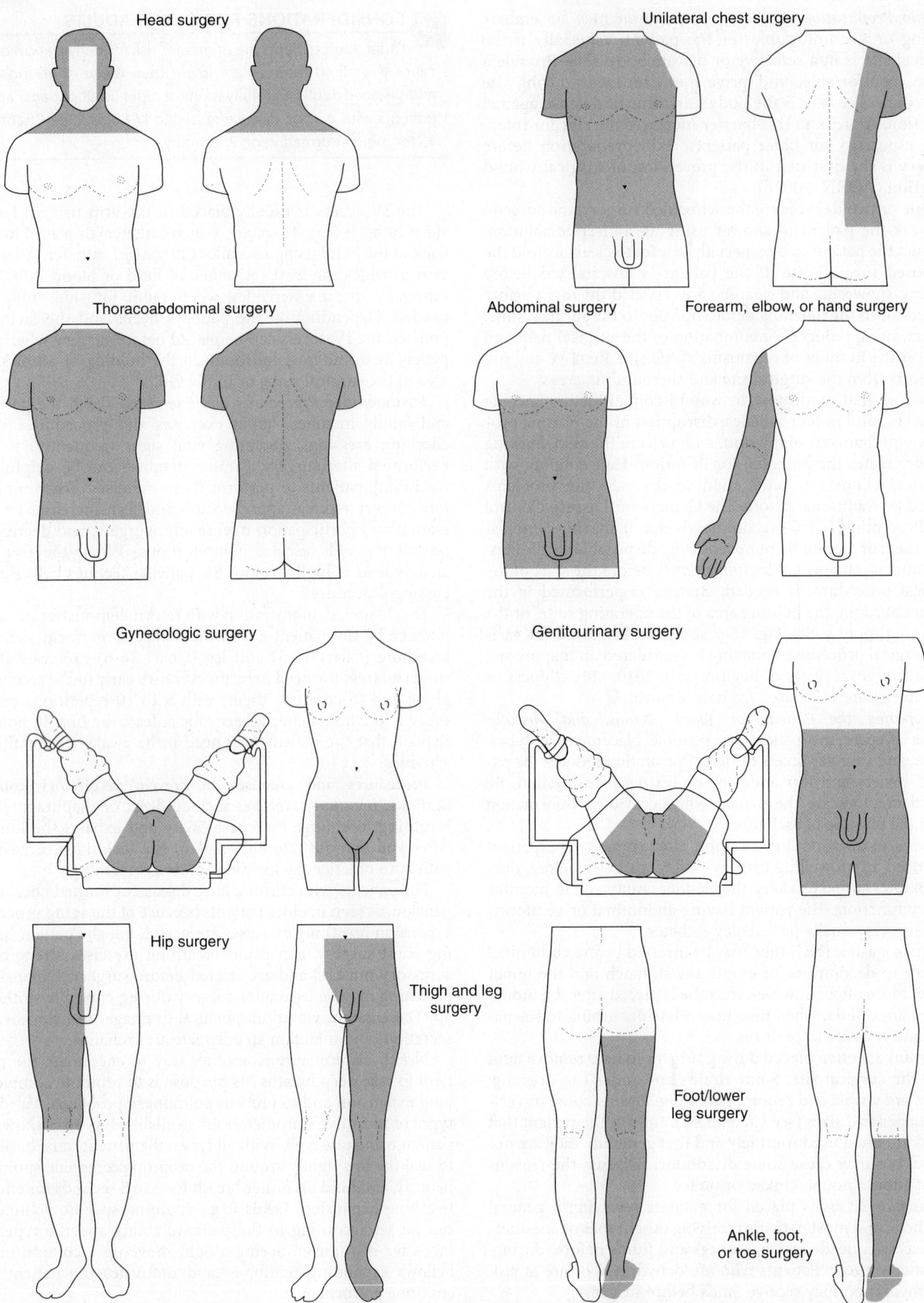

Fig. 16-2 • Skin preparation of common surgical sites. *Shaded areas* indicate preparation areas.

Chart 16-5 PATIENT AND FAMILY EDUCATION GUIDE

Perioperative Respiratory Care

DEEP (DIAPHRAGMATIC) BREATHING

1. Sit upright on the edge of the bed or in a chair, being sure that your feet are placed firmly on the floor or a stool. (After surgery, deep breathing is done with the patient in Fowler's position or in semi-Fowler's position.)
2. Take a gentle breath through your mouth.
3. Breathe out gently and completely.
4. Then take a deep breath through your nose and mouth, and hold this breath to the count of five.
5. Exhale through your nose and mouth.

EXPANSION BREATHING

1. Find a comfortable upright position, with your knees slightly bent. (Bending the knees decreases tension on the abdominal muscles and decreases respiratory resistance and discomfort.)
2. Place your hands on each side of your lower rib cage, just above your waist.
3. Take a deep breath through your nose, using your shoulder muscles to expand your lower rib cage outward during inhalation.
4. Exhale, concentrating first on moving your chest, then on moving your lower ribs inward, while gently squeezing the rib cage and forcing air out of the base of your lungs.

SPLINTING OF THE SURGICAL INCISION

1. Unless coughing is contraindicated, place a pillow, towel, or folded blanket over your surgical incision and hold the item firmly in place.
2. Take three slow, deep breaths to stimulate your cough reflex.
3. Inhale through your nose, and then exhale through your mouth.
4. On your third deep breath, cough to clear secretions from your lungs while firmly holding the pillow, towel, or folded blanket against your incision.

Chart 16-6 PATIENT AND FAMILY EDUCATION GUIDE

Postoperative Leg Exercises

EXERCISE NO. 1

1. Lie in bed with the head of your bed elevated to about 45 degrees.
2. Beginning with your right leg, bend your knee, raise your foot off the bed, and hold this position for a few seconds.
3. Extend your leg by unbending your knee, and lower the leg to the bed.
4. Repeat this sequence four more times with your right leg; then perform this same exercise five times with your left leg.

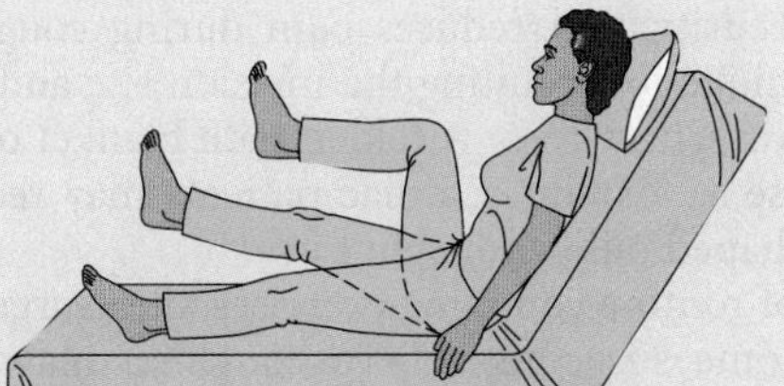

EXERCISE NO. 2

1. Beginning with your right leg, point your toes toward the bottom of the bed.
2. With the same leg, point your toes up toward your face.
3. Repeat this exercise several times with your right leg; then perform this same exercise with your left leg.

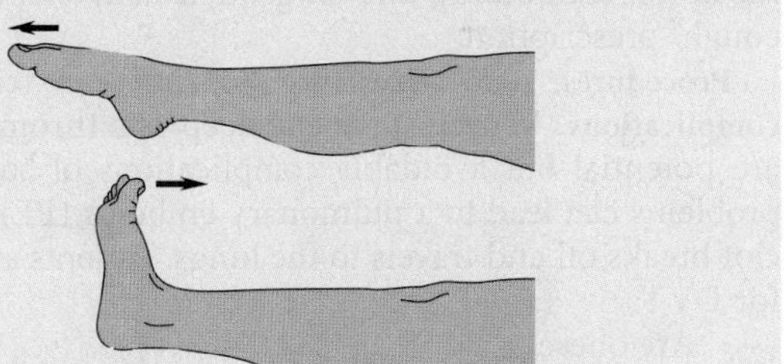

EXERCISE NO. 3

1. Beginning with your right leg, make circles with your ankles, first to the left and then to the right.
2. Repeat this exercise several times with your right leg; then perform this same exercise with your left leg.

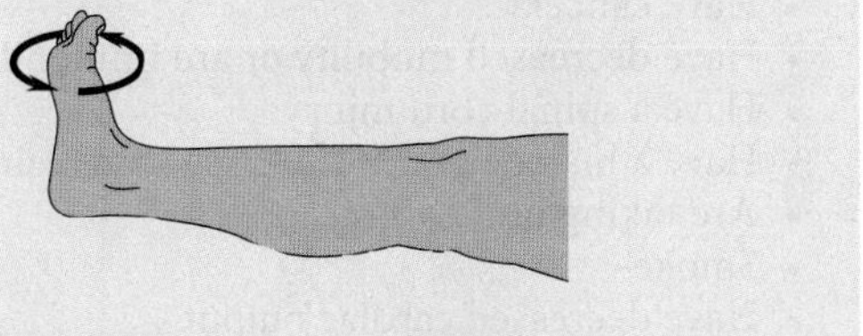

EXERCISE NO. 4

1. Beginning with your right leg, bend your knee and *push* the ball of your foot into the bed or floor until you feel your calf and thigh muscles contracting.
2. Repeat this exercise several times with your right leg; then perform this same exercise with your left leg.

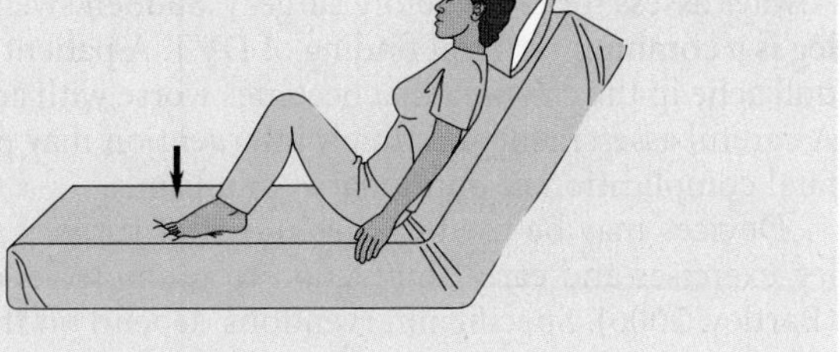

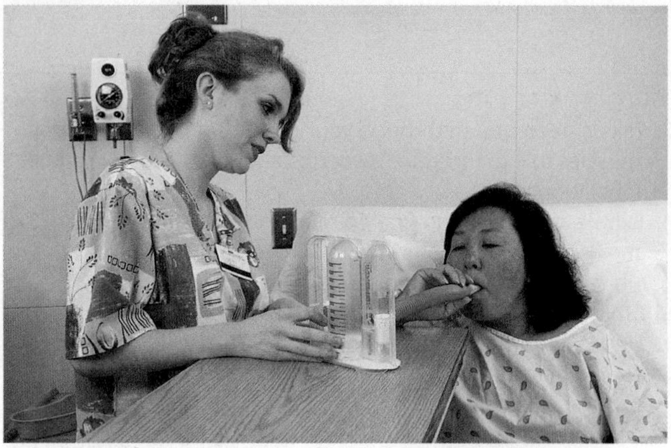

Fig. 16-3 • A patient using an incentive spirometer.

Coughing and splinting may be performed along with deep breathing every 1 to 2 hours after surgery. The purposes of coughing are to expel secretions, keep the lungs clear, allow full aeration, and prevent pneumonia and atelectasis. Coughing may be uncomfortable for the patient, but when performed correctly, it should not harm the incision. Splinting (i.e., holding) the incision area provides support, promotes a feeling of security, and reduces pain during coughing. The proper technique for splinting the incision site and coughing is described in Chart 16-5. A folded bath blanket or pillow is helpful to use as a splint. Cardiac patients may receive their own heart-shaped pillow for splint use.

The use of routine coughing exercises after surgery is controversial. Some surgeons believe coughing may harm the surgical wound and that it would be better to use other, safer measures for lung hygiene, such as deep breathing and incentive spirometer exercises. When routine coughing exercises should be avoided for a specific patient, such as after a hernia repair or craniotomy, the surgeon usually writes a "do not cough" prescription.

Procedures and exercises to prevent cardiovascular complications. Venous stasis and deep vein thrombosis (DVT) are potential but avoidable complications of surgery. These problems can lead to a pulmonary embolus (PE) if the blood clot breaks off and travels to the lungs. Patients at greater risk for DVT:

- Are obese
- Are older than 40 years
- Have cancer
- Have decreased mobility or are immobile
- Have a spinal cord injury
- Have a history of DVT, PE, varicose veins, or edema
- Are taking oral contraceptives
- Smoke
- Have decreased cardiac output
- Have hip fracture or total hip or total knee surgery

Always assess for DVT before surgery. Sudden swelling in one leg is a common physical finding of DVT. A patient may feel a dull ache in the calf area that becomes worse with ambulation. A careful assessment and timely intervention may prevent the fatal complication of pulmonary embolism.

Devices may be used during and after surgery along with leg exercises and early ambulation to promote venous return (Bartley, 2006). Specific interventions depend on the patient's risk factors.

Antiembolism stockings (TED or Jobst stockings) and elastic (Ace) wraps provide graduated compression of the legs, starting at the end of the foot and ankle. Measure the patient's leg length and circumference before ordering the stocking size. Elastic wraps are used when the legs are too large or too small for the stockings. Assist the patient in applying the devices, and ensure that they are neither too loose (are ineffective) nor too tight (inhibit blood flow). The devices need to be worn properly and should be removed one to three times per day for 30 minutes for skin care and inspection.

Pneumatic compression devices enhance venous blood flow by providing intermittent periods of compression on the legs. Measure the patient's legs, and order the correct size. Place the boots on the patient's legs, and then set and check the compression pressures (usually 35-55 mm Hg). Fig. 16-4 shows various types of sequential devices. Antiembolism stockings may be worn in addition to the boots and may reduce some of the uncomfortable sensations of the boots (e.g., itching, sweating, heat).

Leg exercises also promote venous return. Teach the leg exercises outlined in Chart 16-6, and then urge the patient to practice these exercises before surgery. The exercises are important, even when other devices are used.

Mobility soon after surgery (early ambulation) has many cardiovascular and other benefits. It stimulates intestinal motility, enhances lung expansion, mobilizes secretions, promotes venous return, prevents joint rigidity, and relieves pressure. For most types of surgery, teach the patient to turn at least every 2 hours after surgery while confined to bed. Teach patients how to use the bed siderails safely for turning and how to protect the surgical wound (splinting) when turning. Assure patients that assistance and pain drugs will be given as needed to reduce any anxiety and pain they may have with this activity.

For certain surgical procedures, such as some brain, spinal, and orthopedic procedures, the surgeon may prescribe turning restrictions. Ask the surgeon about other interventions to prevent complications of immobility in patients with turning restrictions. Inform the patient of anticipated turning restrictions during teaching before surgery.

Most patients are allowed and encouraged to get out of bed the day of or the day after surgery. Assist the patient into a chair or with ambulation after the surgery, the next day, or when the surgeon specifies. If a patient must remain in bed, help him or her turn, deep breathe, and perform leg exercises at least every 2 hours to prevent complications from immobility.

Anxiety

NOC **Planning: Expected Outcomes.** Before surgery, the patient is expected to have manageable anxiety as indicated by consistently demonstrating these behaviors:

- Expressing a reduced level of anxiety
- Showing an absence of body language indicators of anxiety (e.g., hand wringing, facial tension, restlessness, dilated pupils, sweating, elevated blood pressure, elevated pulse rate)

Interventions. Anxiety often causes restlessness and sleeplessness. The patient may perceive the surgical experience as a threat to life and function. Assess the patient's level of anxiety, as discussed on p. 248 in the Psychosocial Assessment section. Interventions such as teaching and communicating with the patient before surgery, enabling the patient to use previously successful coping mechanisms, and giving antianxiety drugs

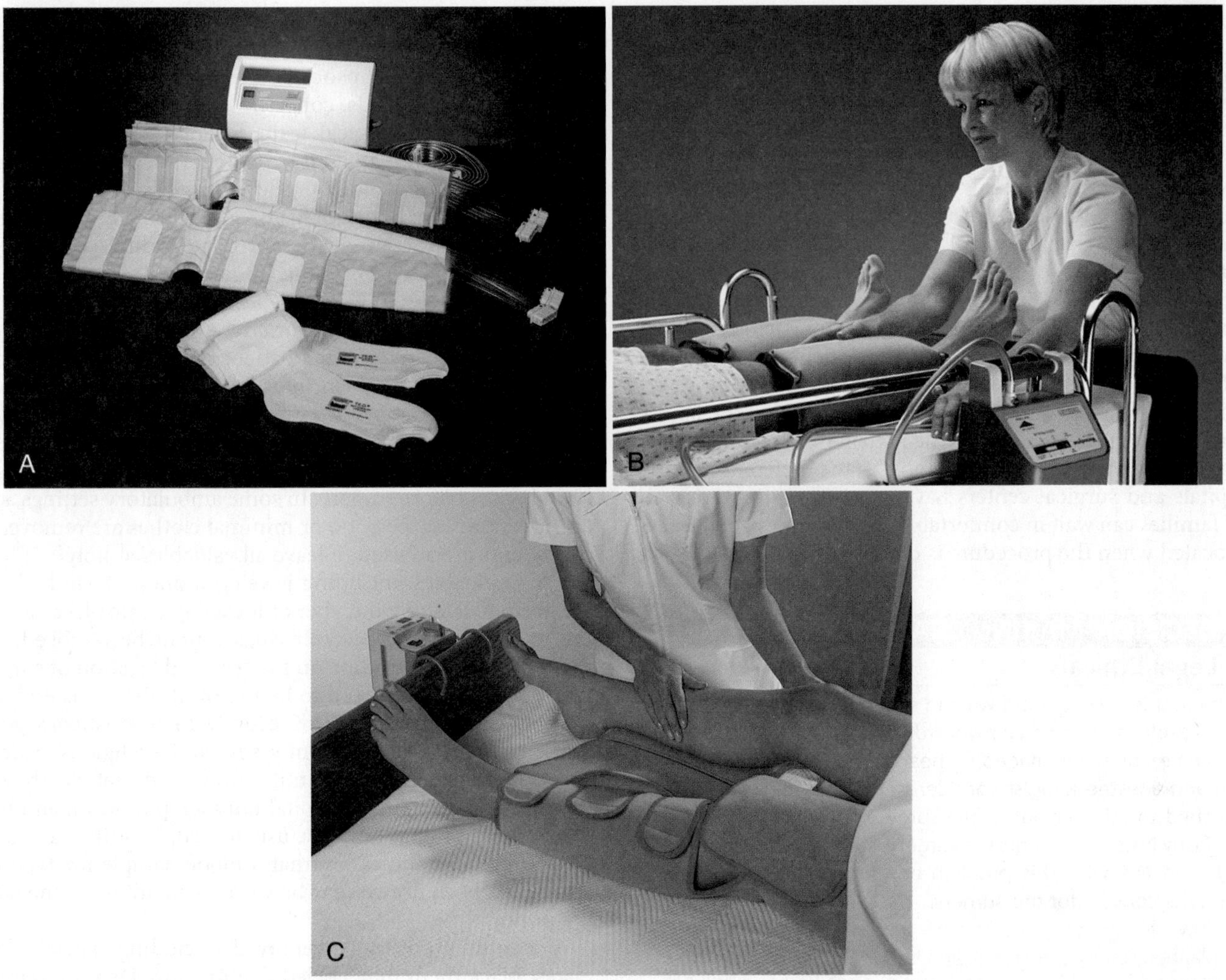
A
B
C

Fig. 16-4 • Examples of external pneumatic compression devices used to promote venous return and prevent deep vein thrombosis (DVT). **A,** Kendall SCD machine, sleeves, and TED stockings. **B,** Venodyne pneumatic compression system. **C,** Flowtron DVT calf garments.

help reduce the anxiety. Incorporate available support systems into the plan of care.

Preoperative teaching involves first assessing the patient's knowledge about the surgical experience (see p. 252 in the Deficient Knowledge section) and then providing factual information to promote the patient's understanding. Allow ample time for questions. Respond to the questions accurately, and refer unanswered questions to the proper person. During the discussion, continually assess the patient's responses and anxiety level. Be careful not to provide information that might increase anxiety. Patients have ranked psychosocial support as the most important part of preoperative teaching. The informed, educated patient is better able to anticipate events and maintain self-control and is thus less anxious.

Encouraging communication by having the patient state feelings, fears, and concerns can help reduce anxiety. Use an honest and open approach so that the patient can express feelings freely without fear of ridicule or judgment. Keep the patient informed by clarifying information, answering questions, and allaying fears about the surgery.

Promoting rest is helpful because the stress and anxiety of impending surgery often interfere with the patient's ability to sleep and rest the night before surgery. The period before surgery is physically and emotionally stressful. To help the patient relax, determine what the patient usually does to relax and fall asleep. If the patient is able, urge him or her to continue these methods of relaxation. A back rub is relaxing and can be performed by a nurse or family member. The surgeon may prescribe a sedative or hypnotic drug to help the patient be well rested for surgery.

Distraction may be used as an intervention for anxiety, especially in the 24 hours immediately before surgery. Listening to music may decrease anxiety, as may watching television, reading, or visiting with family members.

Teaching family members helps reduce anxiety by increasing the likelihood of support and involvement in the patient's care. Assess the readiness and desire of the family to take an active part in the patient's care. A positive sign of family interest is that of members asking questions about the surgical experience. After family readiness is determined, keep family members informed and encourage their involvement in all aspects of education. Emphasize the important role of the family before surgery, but guide discussions and practice sessions so that family members do not dominate the sessions. Family members can encourage and help the patient practice exercises to be performed after surgery.

Inform the family of the time for surgery, if known, and of any schedule changes. If the patient is an outpatient, provide clear directions to the patient and family regarding any specific night-before procedures, what time and where to report, and what to bring with them. Encourage the family to stay with the patient before surgery for support.

Most families are anxious about the surgery planned for their loved one. To reduce their anxiety, explain the routines expected before, during, and after surgery. Tell the family that after the patient leaves the hospital room or admission area, there is usually a 30- to 60-minute preparation period in the operating area (holding room, treatment area) before the surgery actually begins. After surgery, the patient is taken to the postanesthesia care unit (PACU) for 1 to 2 hours before returning to the hospital room or discharge area. Tell the family about the best place to wait for the patient or surgeon according to the facility's policy and the physician's preference. Many hospitals and surgical centers have surgical waiting areas so that families can wait in comfortable surroundings and be easily located when the procedure is completed.

DECISION-MAKING CHALLENGE
Legal/Ethical

The patient is a 92-year-old woman scheduled to have a repair of a rectal prolapse. She had a myocardial infarction 4 years ago and has been medically managed for heart failure ever since. Her surgeon and anesthesiologist consider her a poor surgical risk and have tried to talk her out of the surgery, as has her family. She steadfastly insists she wants the surgery, stating "I would rather be dead than live with this problem any longer." She has already signed the consent for this surgery.

1. How will you determine whether this patient understands the planned surgical procedure and its risks?
2. Given her age, should consent also be obtained from the family? Why or why not?
3. What ethical conviction is most endangered for this patient in this situation?
4. How can you best act as an advocate for this patient?

evolve For suggested answer guidelines, go to http://evolve.elsevier.com/Iggy/.

Preoperative Chart Review

Review the patient's chart to ensure that all documentation, preoperative procedures, and orders are completed. Check the surgical informed consent form and, if indicated, any other special consent forms to see that they are signed and dated and that they contain the witnesses' signatures. Confirm that the scheduled procedure, including the identification of left versus right when necessary, is what is listed on the consent form. Even though it might be obvious, have the patient mark the correct area for surgery. If the patient cannot reach the area, coordinate with the surgeon to mark the area before the patient is transferred to the OR. Document allergies according to facility policy. Accurate measuring and recording of height and weight are important for proper dosage of the anesthetic agents. Ensure that the results of all laboratory, radiographic, and diagnostic tests are on the chart. Document any abnormal results, and report them to the surgeon and the anesthesia provider. If the patient is an autologous blood donor or has had directed blood donations made, those special slips must be included in the chart. Record a current set of vital signs (within 1 to 2 hours of the scheduled surgery time), and document any significant physical or psychosocial observations.

Report special needs, concerns, and instructions (advance directives) to the surgical team. For example, advise the surgical team if the patient is a member of Jehovah's Witnesses and does not accept blood products or if the patient is hard of hearing and does not have his or her hearing aid. This information assists the surgical team in providing continuity of care while the patient is in the surgical area.

Preoperative Patient Preparation

Facilities usually require the patient to remove most clothing and wear a hospital gown into the OR; however, underwear may be worn in above-the-waist surgery and socks may be worn, except in foot or leg surgery. If prescribed by the surgeon, apply antiembolism stockings or pneumatic compression devices before surgery. In some ambulatory settings, such as for cataract surgery, no or minimal clothes are removed.

Patients are advised to leave all valuables at home. If he or she has valuables, including jewelry, money, or clothes, they are given to a family member or locked in a safe place, according to the facility's policy. If rings cannot be removed, tape them in place. Depending on the type and location of surgery, pierced jewelry may need to be removed. Religious emblems may be pinned or fastened securely to the patient's gown. Some facilities have paper emblems from a religious leader.

The patient wears an identification band that clearly gives the first and last name, hospital number, physician, and birth date. An additional bracelet, usually red, identifies any allergies. A bracelet indicating that a blood sample for type and screen has been drawn may be worn, depending on the facility's policy.

If dentures are to be removed, including partial dental plates, place them in a labeled denture cup. Denture removal is a safety measure to prevent aspiration and obstruction of the airway. If a patient has any capped teeth, document this finding on the checklist.

All prosthetic devices, such as artificial eyes and limbs, are removed and given to a family member or safely stored, as are contact lenses, glasses, wigs, and toupees. Check and remove hairpins and clips, which can conduct electrical current used during surgery and cause scalp burns.

Some facilities allow hearing aids in the surgical suite to help communication before and after surgery. If the patient is sent to surgery with a hearing aid, communicate this to the surgical nurse to prevent accidental loss of or damage to the device. Some facilities allow dentures, wigs, and glasses to be worn into the operating suite to prevent embarrassment to the patient. These items are removed when absolutely necessary.

The removal of fingernail polish or artificial nails is controversial. Polish and artificial nails have been thought to affect the accuracy of pulse oximetry readings. Recent studies have indicated that pulse oximetry readings taken on fingers is affected by brown or blue polish but not by red or lighter color polish (Rodden et al., 2007). In addition, pulse oximetry does not have to be measured on fingers only. Some facilities still require that at least one artificial nail must be removed to monitor oxygen saturation by pulse oximetry.

After the patient is prepared for surgery and the operating suite is ready to receive him or her, ask him or her to empty the bladder. This action prevents incontinence or overdistention and is a starting point for intake and output measurement. A full bladder may hinder access to the surgical site. Answer questions, offer reassurance as needed, and give prescribed drugs.

Preoperative Drugs

Preoperative drugs may be prescribed regardless of the type of planned anesthesia. Various drugs reduce anxiety, promote relaxation, reduce nasal and oral secretions, prevent laryngospasm, reduce vagal-induced bradycardia, inhibit gastric secretions, and decrease the amount of anesthetic needed for the induction and maintenance of anesthesia. Drug selection is based on the patient's age, physical and psychological condition, medical history, and height and weight; other drugs the patient takes routinely; test results; and the type and extent of the planned surgical procedure. If more than one response is required, combination therapy may be prescribed.

Drug types for preoperative preparation may include sedatives (hydroxyzine [Atarax, Vistaril]); hypnotics (e.g., lorazepam [Ativan]); anxiolytics (e.g., midazolam [Versed]); opioid analgesics (e.g., morphine, hydromorphone, meperidine); and an anticholinergic agent (e.g., atropine). Other specific-purpose drugs also may be added. For example, if rapid emptying of the stomach is needed, metoclopramide (Reglan) may be prescribed. When procedures are long or stress ulcers are likely, an H_2 histamine blocker (e.g., cimetidine [Tagamet]; ranitidine [Zantac]) is used (DeLamar, 2007).

Preoperative drugs may be given when the patient is "on call" to the surgical suite. After positively identifying the patient (using the armband and asking the patient to state his or her name) and making sure the operative permit is signed, give the correct drugs in the correct doses. Then raise the siderails, place the call light within easy reach of the patient, and remind him or her not to try to get out of bed. Place the bed in a low position. Tell the patient that he or she may become drowsy and have a dry mouth as a result of the drugs.

A more common practice is for the preoperative drugs to be given *after* the patient is transferred to the operating area (DeLamar, 2007). This practice permits the surgical team and anesthesia personnel to make more accurate assessments and have last-minute discussions with a patient not yet affected by drugs. In addition, after the patient is in the preoperative area, drugs can be given by the IV route. Monitoring equipment such as continuous pulse oximetry and ECG are more readily available in this area. The oral or IM route is used less often because of variable absorption rates. The surgeon may prescribe a prophylactic antibiotic to be given right before or during surgery to reduce the risk for a surgical site infection. The antibiotic is usually given within 60 minutes before the incision is made.

Patient Transfer to the Surgical Suite

In the immediate preoperative period, review and update the patient's chart, reinforce teaching, ensure that the patient is correctly dressed for surgery, and give prescribed preoperative drugs. Use a preoperative checklist for a smooth, efficient transfer to the surgical suite (Fig. 16-5). The patient, along with the signed consent form, the completed preoperative checklist, the chart, and the patient identification card, is transported to the surgical suite.

Most patients in the hospital setting are transferred to the surgical suite on a stretcher with the siderails up. In special circumstances (e.g., patients requiring traction, those having orthopedic surgery, those who should be moved as little as possible), the patient is transferred in the hospital bed. Other factors that influence the decision to transfer in a bed are the patient's age, size, and physical condition. In ambulatory settings, patients either walk or are transferred to the surgical suite on a stretcher or in a wheelchair.

DECISION-MAKING CHALLENGE
Legal/Ethical

You are about to send the patient, described earlier in the Decision-Making Challenge on p. 260, to the surgical suite. After her competency was established, she signed her consent form but refused to sign a Do Not Resuscitate (DNR) order. As you are giving her the prescribed preoperative drugs, she asks you just what the DNR means and says she did not sign it because she was afraid that if she was "choking" no one would do anything to help her.

1. How would you explain a DNR order to this patient?
2. Should you have her sign such a document at this time? Why or why not?
3. What risk factors does this patient have for specific intraoperative or postoperative complications? Why?

evolve For suggested answer guidelines, go to http://evolve.elsevier.com/Iggy/.

▪ *Evaluation: Outcomes*

Evaluate the care of the preoperative patient on the basis of the identified nursing diagnoses. The expected outcomes include that the patient:

- States understanding of the informed consent and preoperative procedures
- Demonstrates postoperative exercises and techniques for prevention of complications
- Has reduced anxiety

Specific indicators for these outcomes are listed for each nursing diagnosis in the Planning and Implementation section (see earlier).

GET READY FOR THE NCLEX EXAMINATION!

Key Points

Review these Key Points for each NCLEX Examination Client Needs Category.

Safe and Effective Care Environment

- Ask the patient if an advance directive has been completed.
- Ask the patient to explain in his or her own words what surgical procedure is being done and why.
- If the patient's explanation of the scheduled surgery is not consistent with the documentation, notify the surgeon and request that he or she speak to the patient.
- Use appropriate identifiers (e.g., hospital number, the identification band, asking the patient to state his or her name) to identify the patient. *Do not use room number or bed number to identify the patient.*
- Ensure that the patient is wearing proper identification.

PRESURGICAL CHECKLIST

Date: ______________

Side 1

	INITIALS: UNIT	INITIALS: Prep & Holding	COMMENTS
1. Allergies: ☐ Latex ☐ Environmental ☐ Medications			Green allergy band intact if allergies are present
2. Isolation/Precautions: ☐ MRSA ☐ VRE ☐ C-diff Other: ______			☐ Operating Room notified (OR) ☐ Post-Anesthesia Care Unit notified (PACU)
3. Side/Site identification form completed			
4. Pre-Surgical Testing (RESULTS ON CHART) ☐ CBC ☐ SMA6 ☐ Glucose ______ ☐ Chest X-ray ☐ UA ☐ ECG ☐ Hemoglobin & Hematocrit ☐ Other: ______			Pending Results:
5. Vital Signs: Time performed: ______ Temperature: ______ Blood Pressure: ______ Pulse: ______ SpO₂: ______ % Respiratory Rate: ______			
6. NPO since: ______ Solids: ______ Liquids: ______			
7. Weight (last 24 hours): ______kg Height: ______ cm			
8. Last Menstrual Period: ______			
9. Patient's belongings including valuables secured/removed: ☐ wedding band taped ☐ dentures ☐ contact lenses ☐ glasses Drawer number (Surgicenter only): ______			Secure all valuables.
10. ☐ Type & Cross-Match ☐ Blood consent on chart # of autologous units available: ______			
11. Voiding or catheter: ______ (Time)			
12. Preoperative surgical antimicrobial prophylaxis guideline checklist instituted and faxed to pharmacy.			Call placed to physician if not ordered ______ (time) ______ initials
13. Intravenous antimicrobials should be administered within 0-60 minutes prior to surgical incision.			
14. Surgical site prep: ☐ Prep ordered by physician ☐ If no prep ordered, call placed to physician for Surgical Site prep order			☐ Clip Only ☐ Scrub Only Location: ______ ☐ Site prep location: ______ ☐ Clip & Scrub-Betadine ☐ Clip & Scrub-Hibiclens Signature: ______ Time: ______
15. Equipment to go to OR with patient ☐ X-ray films ☐ Old records ☐ Chart volumes			
Signature/Initials	Signature/Initials		
Print Name	Print Name		

Fig. 16-5 • A preoperative checklist.

- Ensure that the patient is not asked to sign an operative permit or any other legal document after the preoperative drugs have been given.
- After the patient has received preoperative drugs, keep the siderails up and the bed in the low position.
- Communicate to the surgeon and anesthesia personnel any physical or laboratory change that may alter the patient's response to drugs, anesthesia, or surgery.

Health Promotion and Maintenance

- Teach patients about dietary restrictions and preoperative preparations.
- Teach the patient specific interventions to perform after surgery to prevent complications (incision splinting, deep-breathing exercises, range-of-motion exercises—as described in Charts 16-5 and 16-6).

Psychosocial Integrity

- Pace your interview to match the learning needs and style of the individual patient.
- Encourage the patient to express his or her feelings regarding the surgical procedure or its possible outcome.
- Explain and provide written information for all diagnostic procedures, restrictions, and follow-up care to the patient and his or her family.
- Communicate any concerns or fears the patient has to the surgeon and anesthesia personnel.

Physiological Integrity

- Check that documentation for any procedure to be performed on one of a paired organ or extremity clearly indicates which organ or extremity is involved.
- If required, ensure that dentures and any other personal items are removed from the patient before the patient is transferred to the surgical suite.

Additional Study Resources

Go to your Companion CD or Evolve at http://evolve.elsevier.com/Iggy/ for *Self-Assessment Questions for the NCLEX Examination.*

evolve Go to Evolve at http://evolve.elsevier.com/Iggy/ for *Prioritization and Delegation Questions for the NCLEX Examination.*

SELECTED BIBLIOGRAPHY

Asterisk indicates a classic or definitive work on this subject.

Adams, A. (2008). Is hair removal necessary before the surgical incision? *Perioperative Nursing Clinics, 3*(2), 107-113.

*American Society of Anesthesiologists Task Force. (1999). Practice guidelines for preoperative fasting and the use of pharmacologic agents to reduce the risk of pulmonary aspiration: Application to healthy patients undergoing elective procedures. *Anesthesiology, 90*(3), 896-905.

American Society of PeriAnesthesia Nurses (ASPAN). (2004). *Standards, recommended practices, and guidelines.* Denver: Author.

Association of periOperative Registered Nurses (AORN). (2006). AORN clinical path template. In *Standards, recommended practices and guidelines* (pp. 157-165). Denver: Author.

Association of periOperative Registered Nurses (AORN). (2007a). Statement on correct site surgery. In *Standards, recommended practices and guidelines* (pp. 371-374). Denver: Author.

Association of periOperative Registered Nurses (AORN). (2007b). ANA code for nurses with interpretive statements: Explications perioperative nursing. In *Standards, recommended practices and guidelines* (pp. 171-201). Denver: Author.

Association of periOperative Registered Nurses (AORN). (2007c). Perioperative care of patients with do-not-resuscitate (DNR) orders. In *Standards, recommended practices and guidelines* (pp. 377-388). Denver: Author.

Association of periOperative Registered Nurses (AORN). (2007d). Recommended practices for skin preparation of patients. In *Standards, recommended practices and guidelines* (pp. 653-656). Denver: Author.

Bartley, M. (2006). Preventing venous thromboembolism. *Nursing2006, 36*(1), 64cc1-64cc4.

Baugh, N., Zuelzer, H., Meador, J., & Blankenship, J. (2007). Wounds in surgical patients who are obese. *AJN, 107*(6), 40-50.

*Beyea, S. (2002). Accident prevention in surgical settings: Keeping patients safe. *AORN Journal, 75*(2), 361-363.

*Beyea, S. (2004). Evidence-based practice in perioperative nursing. *American Journal of Infection Control, 32*(2), 97-100.

Beyea, S. (2007). Update on correct site surgery. *AORN Journal, 85*(2), 415-417.

Bulechek, G.M., Butcher, H.K., & McCloskey Dochterman, J. (Eds.). (2008). *Nursing interventions classification (NIC)* (5th ed.). St. Louis: Mosby.

Carney, B.L. (2006). Evolution of wrong site surgery prevention strategies. *AORN Journal, 83*(5), 1115-1118, 1121-1122.

Daniels, S. (2007). Protecting patients from harm: Improving hospital care for surgical patients. *Nursing2007, 37*(8), 36-41.

DeLamar, L. (2007). Anesthesia. In J.C. Rothrock & D. McEwen (Eds.), *Alexander's care of the patient in surgery* (13th ed., Chapter 4). St. Louis: Mosby.

*Dunn, D. (2004). Preventing perioperative complications in an older adult. *Nursing2004, 34*(11), 36-41.

Dunn, D. (2005). Preventing perioperative complications in special populations. *Nursing2005, 35*(11), 36-43.

Gazarian, P.K. (2006). Identifying risk factors for postoperative pulmonary complications. *AORN Journal, 84*(4), 616-625.

McEwen, D. (2007). Ambulatory surgery. In J.C. Rothrock & D. McEwen (Eds.), *Alexander's care of the patient in surgery* (13th ed.). St. Louis: Mosby.

Meiner, S., & Lueckenotte, A. (Eds.). (2006). *Gerontologic nursing* (3rd ed.). St. Louis: Mosby.

Metules, T., & Bauer, J. (2006). JCAHO's patient safety goals: A practical guide, Part 1. *RN, 69*(12), 21-26.

Metules, T., & Bauer, J. (2007). JCAHO's patient safety goals: Preventing med errors, Part 2. *RN, 70*(1), 39-43.

Moorhead, S., Johnson, M., & Maas, M. (Eds.). (2004). *Nursing outcomes classification (NOC)* (3rd ed.). St. Louis: Mosby.

Neil, J.A. (2007). Perioperative care of the immunocompromised patient. *AORN Journal, 85*(3), 544-560.

Odom-Forren, J. (2006). Preventing surgical site infections. *Nursing2006, 36*(6), 59-63.

Pagana, K., & Pagana, T. (2006). *Mosby's manual of diagnostic and laboratory tests* (3rd ed.). St. Louis: Mosby.

Pearce, J. (2006). Documenting preoperative teaching. *Nursing2006, 36*(8), 71.

Ridge, R. (2008). Patient safety: Doing right to prevent wrong-site surgery. *Nursing2008, 38*(3), 24-25.

Rodden, A., Spicer, L., Diaz, V., & Steyer, T.E. (2007). Does fingernail polish affect pulse oximeter readings? *Intensive and Critical Care Nursing, 23*(1), 51-55.

Rothrock, J.C., & McEwen, D. (2007). *Alexander's care of the patient in surgery* (13th ed.). St. Louis: Mosby.

Scherer, D., & Fitzpatrick, J. (2008). Perceptions of patient safety culture among physicians and RNs in the perioperative area. *AORN Journal, 87*(1), 163-164, 166, 168-174.

Schweon, S. (2006) Stamping out surgical site infections. *RN, 69*(8), 36-40.

Smith, L. (2007). Speaking up for medical language interpreters. *Nursing2007, 37*(12), 48-49.

*Tappen, R., Muzic, J., & Kennedy, P. (2001). Preoperative assessment and discharge planning for older adults undergoing ambulatory surgery. *AORN Journal, 73*(2), 464-474.

Vaughn, F., Wichowski, H., & Bosworth, G. (2007). Does preoperative anxiety level predict postoperative pain? *AORN Journal, 85*(3), 589-604.

White, A., & Schneider, T. (2007). Improving compliance with prophylactic antibiotic administration guidelines. *AORN Journal, 85*(1), 173-180.

17 CHAPTER

Care of Intraoperative Patients

Robin Chard

LEARNING OUTCOMES

For clinical competence and success on the NCLEX Examination, study this chapter with these Learning Outcomes in mind:

Safe and Effective Care Environment

1. Use appropriate patient identifiers when administering drugs or marking surgical sites.
2. Verify that the patient has given informed consent for the surgical procedure.
3. Differentiate the roles and responsibilities of intraoperative personnel.
4. Understand the principles of infection prevention as they apply to aseptic technique in setting up a sterile field.
5. Explain correct technique to apply and remove surgical attire.
6. Understand the nurse's role in monitoring all OR personnel for possible breaks in sterile technique.

Psychosocial Integrity

7. Apply nursing interventions to reduce patient and family anxiety.
8. Explain procedures to ensure the identity of the patient and the accuracy of the planned surgical procedure.
9. Act as a patient advocate with regard to patients' rights, informed consent, and advance directives.
10. Apply interventions to ensure the patient's safety and dignity during an operative procedure.

Physiological Integrity

11. Assess patients for specific problems related to positioning during surgical procedures.
12. Understand anatomic principles for modifying patient positioning and OR bed padding to prevent skin breakdown, promote comfort, and prevent positioning injury during surgical procedures.
13. Coordinate appropriate care for the patient with malignant hyperthermia.

Go to your Companion CD or Evolve at http://evolve.elsevier.com/Iggy/ for *Self-Assessment Questions for the NCLEX Examination* keyed to these Learning Outcomes.

The intraoperative period begins when the patient enters the surgical suite and ends at the time of transfer to the postanesthesia recovery area, same-day surgery unit, or the intensive care unit. The main concerns of perioperative nurses are the safety and advocacy for the patient during surgery. Nursing observations and actions can prevent, reduce, control, and manage many hazards. Once in the operating room (OR), the patient is at risk for infection, impaired skin integrity, increased anxiety, altered body temperature, and injury related to positioning and other hazards. The surgical phase is filled with unfamiliar experiences and uncertain outcomes. Nursing care during this period is critical because the patient's physical needs, spiritual needs, comfort, safety, dignity, and psychological status depend on the perioperative nurse. Specific procedures and policies may differ among agencies but should all reflect the standards and recommended practices for perioperative nursing, as published by the Association of periOperative Registered Nurses (AORN) (2007a). Perioperative nurses practice within a specific, patient-focused model that incorporates professional practice with attainable, measurable outcomes.

Overview

Members of the Surgical Team

The surgical team consists of the surgeon, one or more surgical assistants, the anesthesia provider, and the OR nursing staff. Perioperative, or OR, nurses include the holding area nurse, circulating nurse, scrub nurse, and specialty nurse. The number of assistants, circulating nurses, and scrub nurses depends on the complexity and projected length of the surgical procedure. For some minor procedures, only a circulating nurse and scrub person may be needed in addition to the surgeon. More complex procedures may require additional nursing staff to either circulate or scrub.

Surgeon and Surgical Assistant

The *surgeon* is a physician who assumes responsibility for the surgical procedure and any surgical judgments about the patient. The *surgical assistant* might be another surgeon (or physician, such as a resident or intern) or a physician assistant, certified registered nurse first assistant (CRNFA), or surgical technologist. Under the direction of the surgeon and within the legal scope of practice for each state, the assistant may hold retractors, suction the wound (to improve viewing of the operative site), cut tissue, suture, and dress wounds.

Anesthesia Providers

The *anesthesiologist* is a physician who specializes in giving anesthetic agents. A *certified registered nurse anesthetist (CRNA)* is a registered nurse with additional education and credentials who delivers anesthetic agents under the supervision of an anesthesiologist, surgeon, dentist, or podiatrist. The anesthesia provider gives anesthetic drugs to induce and maintain anesthesia and delivers other drugs as needed to support the patient during surgery.

The anesthesia provider monitors the patient during surgery by assessing and monitoring:

- The level of anesthesia (i.e., by using a peripheral nerve stimulator or electroencephalogram [EEG] bispectral analysis)
- Cardiopulmonary function (using electrocardiographic [ECG] monitoring, pulse oximetry, end-tidal carbon dioxide monitoring, arterial blood gases [ABGs], and hemodynamic monitoring via arterial lines and/or pulmonary artery catheters)
- Vital signs
- Intake and output

Depending on the patient's needs, anesthesia personnel give IV fluids, including blood and blood products.

Perioperative Nursing Staff

Perioperative, or OR, staff have several roles during surgery, depending on their education, experience, skill, and job responsibilities. Regardless of their role, the OR nurse uses clinical decision-making skills, develops a plan of nursing care, and coordinates care delivery to patients and their family members.

Holding area nurses work in those operating suites that have a presurgical holding area next to the main ORs. The patient waits in this area until the OR is ready. The holding area nurse coordinates and manages the care while the patient is in this area. Responsibilities include greeting the patient on arrival, reviewing the medical record and preoperative checklist, verifying that the operative consent forms are signed, and documenting the risk assessment (Fig. 17-1). This nurse also assesses the patient's physical and emotional status, gives emotional support, answers questions, and provides additional education as needed.

The holding area is busy, with many staff members performing different procedures before surgery (e.g., starting IV lines, inserting epidural catheters). The holding area nurse promotes an atmosphere of comfort, privacy, and confidentiality. Depending on the facility's policy, family members may wait with the patient.

Circulating nurses or "circulators" are registered nurses who coordinate, oversee, and are involved in the patient's nursing care in the OR. The circulating nurse's actions are vital to the smooth flow of events before, during, and after surgery. He or she is responsible for coordinating all activities within that particular OR. The circulator sets up the OR and ensures that supplies, including blood products and diagnostic support, are available as needed. All anticipated equipment is gathered and inspected by the circulator to make certain that it is safe and functional before the surgery. Depending on the procedure and position required, the circulator makes up the operating bed (OR table) with gel pads (to prevent pressure ulcers), safety straps and armboards (for patient positioning), and either heating pads under the sheets or disposable warming blankets placed over the patient as indicated (to prevent hypothermia) (Weirich, 2008).

If there is no holding area nurse, the circulator assumes the responsibilities of that nursing role as well. Even when there is a holding area nurse, the circulator also greets the patient and reviews findings with the holding area nurse.

Once the patient is ready to be moved into the OR, the circulating nurse assists the OR team in the transfer to the operating bed. The nurse positions the patient, protecting bony areas with extra padding while providing comfort and reassurance. While observing the patient, the circulating nurse also assists the anesthesia provider with the induction of anesthesia. The circulator then may assist with additional positioning, insert a Foley catheter if needed, and "prep" (scrub) the surgical site before the patient is draped with sterile drapes.

Throughout the surgery, the circulating nurse:

- Monitors traffic in the room
- Assesses the amount of urine and blood loss
- Reports findings to the surgeon and anesthesia provider
- Ensures that the surgical team maintain sterile technique and a sterile field
- Anticipates the patient's and surgical team's needs, providing supplies and equipment
- Communicates information about the patient's status to family members during long or unique procedures
- Documents care, events, interventions, and findings

Depending on facility policy, the circulating nurse may record drugs, blood, and blood components given. (This also may be a function of the anesthesia provider.)

Before the procedure is over, the circulating nurse completes documentation in the OR and nursing records, including the presence of drains or catheters, the length of the surgery, and a count of all sponges, "sharps" (needles, blades), and instruments. He or she notifies the postanesthesia care unit (PACU) of the patient's estimated time of arrival and any special needs.

Scrub nurses set up the sterile field (Fig. 17-2), drape the patient, and hand sterile supplies, sterile equipment, and instruments to the surgeon and the assistant. Knowledge of the surgical procedure allows the scrub person to anticipate which instruments and types of sutures the surgeon will need. Anticipating these needs reduces the duration of anesthesia for the patient. In addition, the surgeon's anxiety and tension are reduced when the nurse is familiar with the procedure and can anticipate and respond accordingly. Throughout the surgical procedure, the scrub person (with the circulating nurse) maintains an accurate count of sponges, sharps, instruments, and amounts of irrigation fluid and drugs used.

A specially trained person who is not a nurse may perform the scrub role. Such people are called *operating room technicians (ORTs)* or *surgical technologists*. Often certified surgical technologists (CSTs) are used in the OR.

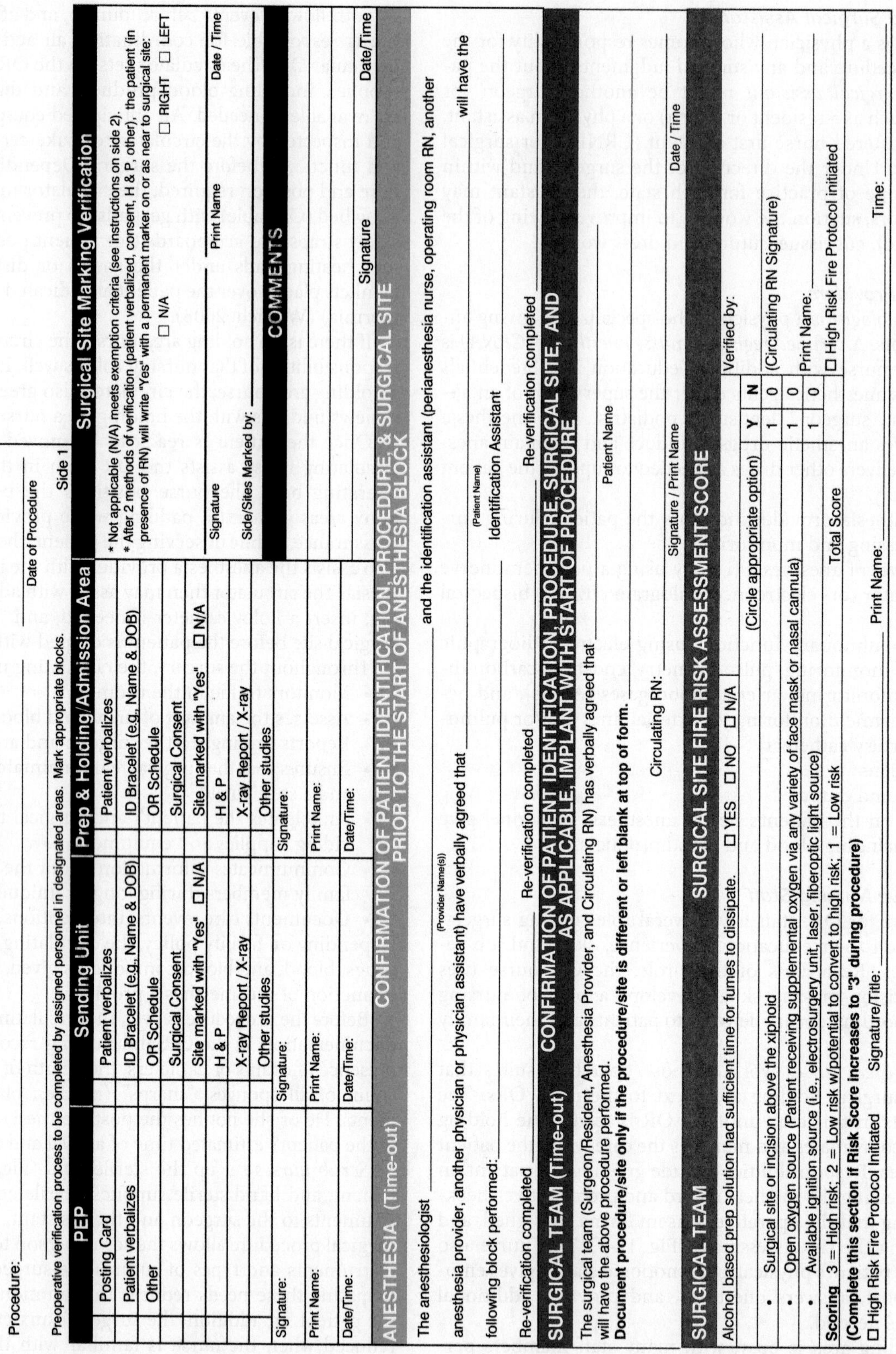

Identification of Patient, Procedure, and Surgical Side/Sites, and Fire Risk Assessment

Procedure: ______ Date of Procedure ______

Preoperative verification process to be completed by assigned personnel in designated areas. Mark appropriate blocks.

Side 1

PEP	Sending Unit	Prep & Holding/Admission Area
Posting Card	Patient verbalizes	Patient verbalizes
Patient verbalizes	ID Bracelet (e.g., Name & DOB)	ID Bracelet (e.g., Name & DOB)
Other	OR Schedule	OR Schedule
	Surgical Consent	Surgical Consent
	Site marked with "Yes" ☐ N/A	Site marked with "Yes" ☐ N/A
	H & P	H & P
	X-ray Report / X-ray	X-ray Report / X-ray
	Other studies	Other studies
Signature:	Signature:	Signature:
Print Name:	Print Name:	Print Name:
Date/Time:	Date/Time:	Date/Time:

Surgical Site Marking Verification

* Not applicable (N/A) meets exemption criteria (see instructions on side 2).
* After 2 methods of verification (patient verbalized, consent, H & P, other), the patient (in presence of RN) will write "Yes" with a permanent marker on or as near to surgical site:

☐ N/A ☐ RIGHT ☐ LEFT

Signature ______ Print Name ______ Date / Time

Side/Sites Marked by: ______

COMMENTS

Signature ______ Date/Time

ANESTHESIA (Time-out) CONFIRMATION OF PATIENT IDENTIFICATION, PROCEDURE, & SURGICAL SITE PRIOR TO THE START OF ANESTHESIA BLOCK

The anesthesiologist ______ (Provider Name(s)) and the identification assistant (perianesthesia nurse, operating room RN, another anesthesia provider, another physician or physician assistant) have verbally agreed that ______ (Patient Name) will have the following block performed: ______ Identification Assistant ______

Re-verification completed ______ Re-verification completed ______ Re-verification completed ______

SURGICAL TEAM (Time-out) CONFIRMATION OF PATIENT IDENTIFICATION, PROCEDURE, SURGICAL SITE, AND AS APPLICABLE, IMPLANT WITH START OF PROCEDURE

The surgical team (Surgeon/Resident, Anesthesia Provider, and Circulating RN) has verbally agreed that ______ (Patient Name) will have the above procedure performed.
Document procedure/site only if the procedure/site is different or left blank at top of form. ______

Circulating RN: ______ Signature / Print Name ______ Date / Time

SURGICAL TEAM SURGICAL SITE FIRE RISK ASSESSMENT SCORE

Alcohol based prep solution had sufficient time for fumes to dissipate. ☐ YES ☐ NO ☐ N/A

(Circle appropriate option)	Y	N
• Surgical site or incision above the xiphoid	1	0
• Open oxygen source (Patient receiving supplemental oxygen via any variety of face mask or nasal cannula)	1	0
• Available ignition source (i.e., electrosurgery unit, laser, fiberoptic light source)	1	0
Scoring 3 = High risk; 2 = Low risk w/potential to convert to high risk; 1 = Low risk — Total Score		

Verified by: ______ (Circulating RN Signature)
Print Name: ______
☐ High Risk Fire Protocol initiated

(Complete this section if Risk Score increases to "3" during procedure)
☐ High Risk Fire Protocol Initiated Signature/Title: ______ Print Name: ______ Time: ______

Fig. 17-1 • Identification of patient, procedures, and surgical side/site and fire risk assessment.

Specialty nurses may be in charge of a particular type of surgical specialty (e.g., orthopedic, cardiac, ophthalmologic) and are responsible for nursing care specific to patients needing that type of surgery. The specialty nurse assesses, maintains, and recommends equipment, instruments, and supplies used in that specialty.

If the facility uses laser technology, a nurse specially trained in the use, care, and maintenance of the laser is needed. He or she may be called a *laser specialty nurse* or a *laser nurse coordinator.* (**Laser** is an acronym for **l**ight **a**mplification by the **s**timulated **e**mission of **r**adiation.) A laser gives off a high-powered beam of light that cuts tissue more cleanly than do

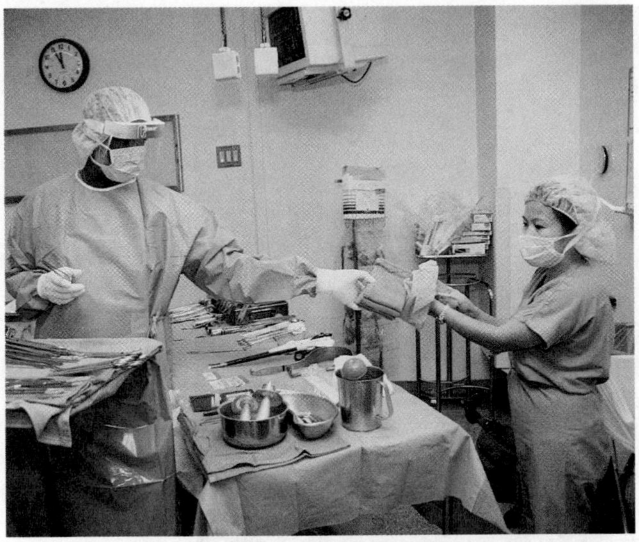

Fig. 17-2 • Setting up the sterile table.

scalpel blades. This process creates intense heat, rapidly clots blood vessels or tissue, and turns target tissue (e.g., a tumor) into vapor. All personnel must observe safety measures (e.g., wear eye shields, read door signs) during laser procedures to prevent injury to the patient and staff (AORN, 2007h).

Preparation of the Surgical Suite and Team Safety

The patient is unable to protect himself or herself during surgery; protection is provided by all members of the surgical team. The OR layout helps prevent infection by reducing contaminants through air exchanges in the room, maintaining recommended temperature and humidity levels, and limiting the traffic and activities in the OR. Safety straps are used for the patient, and the operating bed is locked in place. Blankets or warming units are used to prevent hypothermia, and interventions are used to prevent skin breakdown.

The nurse ensures electrical safety through proper placement of grounding pads and use of electrical equipment that meets safety standards. All equipment used during surgery must be functional and in proper working condition as determined by the safety procedure of that facility. Equipment is cleaned and, when required, sterilized so that it can be used as a part of the procedure. The scrub and circulating nurses together ensure a correct count of surgical instruments, sharps, and sponges. Counts are performed before the procedure, during the procedure as items are added or at the time personnel are relieved from that assignment, at closure of the first layer of the surgical wound, and immediately before complete skin closure (AORN, 2007l; Jackson & Brady, 2008).

Fire prevention and prevention of complications from the use of hazardous or toxic substances are concerns of all OR personnel. Ignition sources, oxidizers, and fuels are present in the OR and increase the risk for fires. Such events are rare but can occur during any kind of procedure. A cool room temperature (between 68° and 73° F [20° and 23° C]) with low humidity (30% to 60%) is optimal. The nurse is aware of emergency measures to take in the event of a fire or spill.

Layout

The surgical suite is located out of the mainstream of the hospital and near the PACU and support services (e.g., blood bank, pathology, and laboratory departments). Traffic flow is patterned to reduce contamination from outside the suite. Within the suite, clean and contaminated areas are separate. The surgical area is divided into three zones—unrestricted, semirestricted, and restricted—to ensure proper movement of patients and personnel.

The size of a surgical suite depends on the size and surgical capabilities of the facility. Most suites contain staff areas as well as areas related to patient care, surgery, and surgical support. Staff areas include locker rooms and staff lounges. Patient care areas include an admission or preoperative holding area and operating rooms. Surgical support areas include a number of ORs, cabinets for sterile supplies, separate utility rooms for clean and soiled equipment, and a clean linen room.

Fig. 17-3 shows a typical OR. The exact number of tables and equipment used in a room is based on the needs of each patient. A communication system links the OR and the main desk of the surgical suite. The system includes an intercom with separate systems for routine and emergency calls.

New OR designs use computers with the surgical equipment, lights, OR bed, and communications. These "hi-tech" rooms are similar to traditional ORs with the addition of computer equipment and panels. They are larger and more efficient for the surgical team with voice-activated commands operating some equipment that used to require manual operation.

Minimally Invasive and Robotic Surgery

Minimally invasive surgery (MIS) is now a common practice. Once used only for minor procedures and joint surgery, MIS is the preferred technique for many types of surgery, including cholecystectomy, cardiac surgery, splenectomy, and spinal surgery. It is even being used for cancer surgeries, such as the removal of a lung lobe (lobectomy) or even the entire lung (pneumonectomy), and colectomy. Research has verified many benefits of MIS, including reduced surgery time for some surgeries, smaller incisions, reduced blood loss, faster recovery time, and less pain and other discomfort after surgery (Bragg et al., 2005; Harrell & Heniford, 2005).

MIS involves making one or more small incisions in the area of the surgery and placing an endoscope through the opening. An **endoscope** is a tube that allows viewing and manipulation of internal body areas (Fig. 17-4). Some endoscopes also magnify the view. These instruments may be rigid, semirigid, or flexible. Some have light sources, whereas others require that a separate light source be inserted into the surgical area. Endoscopes have different names and shapes for different surgical purposes. For example, laparoscopes are used for abdominal surgery, arthroscopes are used for joint surgery, and ureteroscopes are used for urinary tract surgery.

At one time, endoscopes were used only for examination and obtaining small specimens for biopsy. Now, these instruments can be used by surgeons for organ removal, reconstruction, blood vessel grafting, and many other procedures. Cutting, suturing, stapling, cautery, and laser surgery can all be performed through or with endoscopes. An important part of MIS for abdominal surgery, pelvic surgery, and surgery in some other body cavity areas is injecting gas or air into the cavity before the surgery to separate organs and improve visualization. This injection is known as **insufflation** and may contribute to complications and patient discomfort. It is one factor that is considered when deciding to perform a procedure by traditional "open" surgery or by endoscopy.

Patient preparation for endoscopic surgery is much the same as the preparation for the same procedure when per-

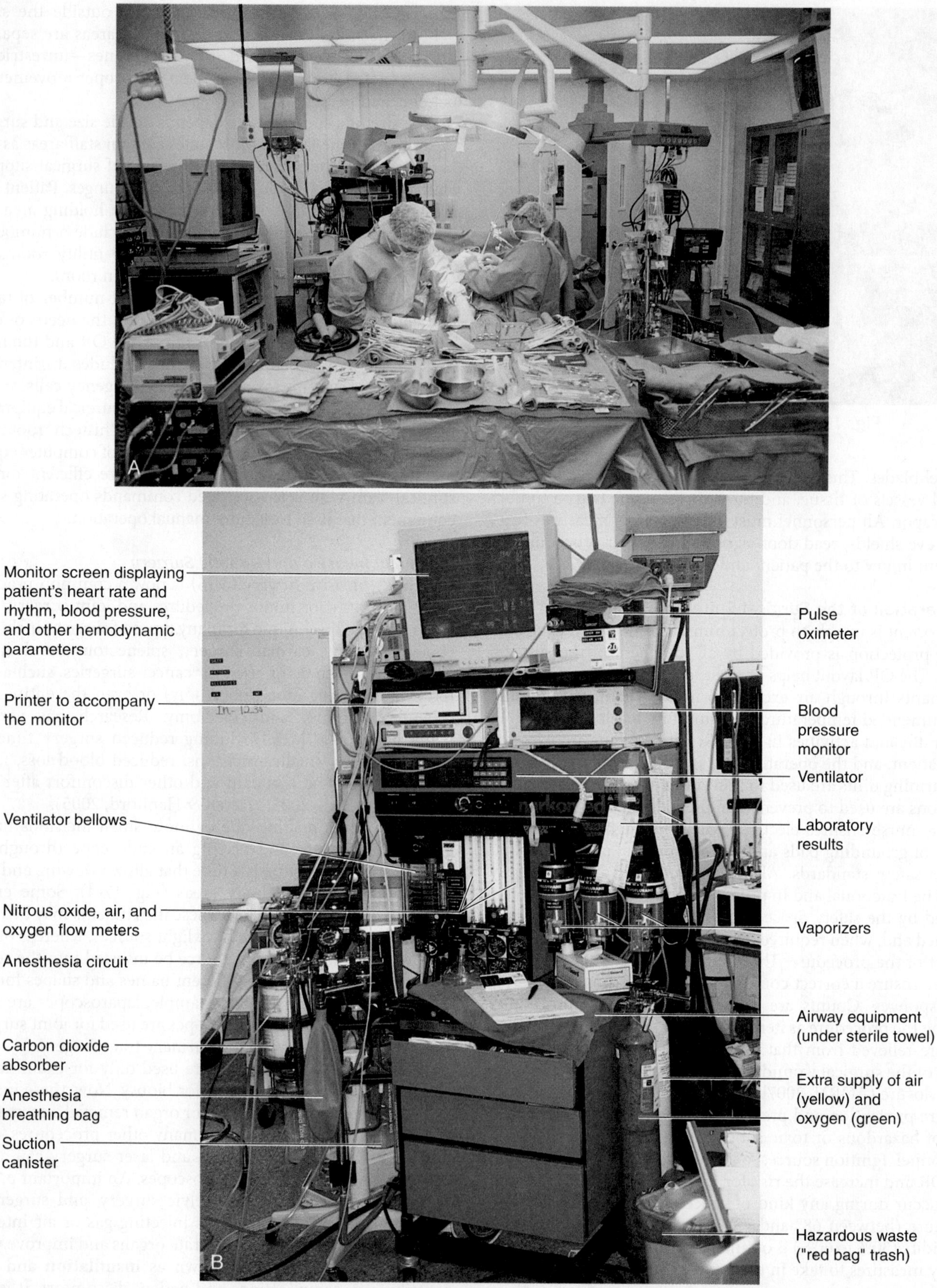
A
B
Monitor screen displaying patient's heart rate and rhythm, blood pressure, and other hemodynamic parameters
Printer to accompany the monitor
Ventilator bellows
Nitrous oxide, air, and oxygen flow meters
Anesthesia circuit
Carbon dioxide absorber
Anesthesia breathing bag
Suction canister
Pulse oximeter
Blood pressure monitor
Ventilator
Laboratory results
Vaporizers
Airway equipment (under sterile towel)
Extra supply of air (yellow) and oxygen (green)
Hazardous waste ("red bag" trash)

Fig. 17-3 • **A,** A typical operating room. **B,** A typical anesthesia station with an anesthesia machine.

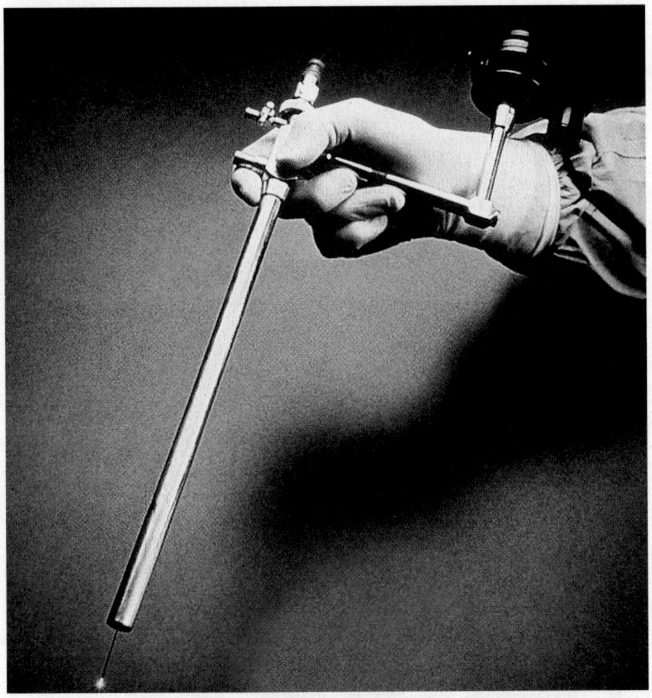

Fig. 17-4 • An operative laparoscope.

formed by open surgical methods, especially for abdominal surgery. An endoscopic surgical procedure has a chance for becoming an open surgical procedure depending on what patient-related or procedure-related variables are discovered or develop during the surgery.

Robotic technology is drastically changing how surgery is performed and how the OR is organized. Robotic surgery takes minimally invasive surgery to a new level. Many gynecologic, urologic, and cardiovascular procedures are being performed by using robotics. The robotic system consists of several components (Fig. 17-5). These include a console, surgical arm cart, and video cart. Initially, the surgeon inserts the required instruments and positions the articulating arms and then breaks scrub and performs the surgery while sitting at the console. A three dimensional (3-D) view of the patient's anatomy provides the surgeon with precise control and dexterity. The vision cart holds the monitors, cameras, and recorder equipment. This new technology requires a perioperative robotics nurse specialist who provides education for patients and family and training for members of the surgical team.

One limitation for both minimally invasive surgery and robotic surgery is the cost of special equipment and OR setting. In addition, surgeons require lengthy training and prac-

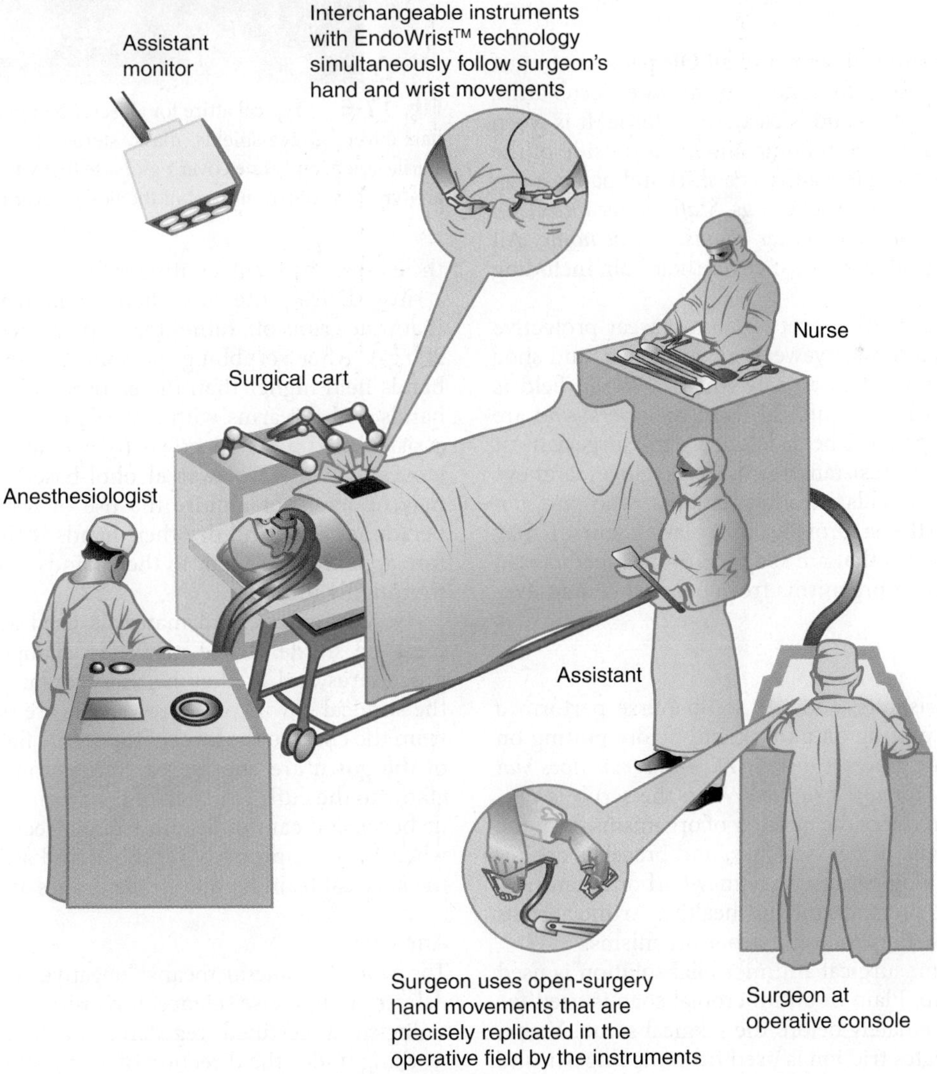
Interchangeable instruments with EndoWrist™ technology simultaneously follow surgeon's hand and wrist movements
Assistant monitor
Nurse
Surgical cart
Anesthesiologist
Assistant
Surgeon uses open-surgery hand movements that are precisely replicated in the operative field by the instruments
Surgeon at operative console

Fig. 17-5 • The operating room layout when the da Vinci Robotic Surgery System is used.

tice periods to become proficient in even one procedure performed using these endoscopic methods (Birch et al., 2007).

Health and Hygiene of the Surgical Team

People are a source of bacteria in the surgical setting. Everyone has bacteria on the skin and the hair and in the airways. Because these organisms can be transmitted to the patient, special health standards and dress are needed. Every surgical setting has policies and procedures for personnel and attire. Health standards require that all members of the surgical team and other support personnel in the surgical suite be free of communicable diseases. Anyone who has an open wound, cold, or any infection should not participate in surgery.

Good personal hygiene helps prevent and control infection, as does frequent handwashing. Jewelry carries many organisms and should be minimal. All personnel must wash their hands between touching patients and performing procedures and more often when indicated. Hands of surgical personnel may be cultured on a regular basis to determine the potential for **nosocomial** (hospital-acquired) **infections** and to identify sources of pathogens. Further interventions or cultures are needed if quality reports (e.g., through the facility's quality improvement program) indicate a problem. Routine cultures are usually obtained every 3 to 6 months. Surgical attire and the surgical scrub help prevent contaminations.

Surgical Attire

All members of the surgical team and all OR personnel must wear scrub attire for use within the surgical suite. Scrub attire is provided by the hospital and is clean, not sterile. It is worn to reduce contamination from home and areas outside of the surgical setting. Basic surgical attire is a shirt and pants, a cap or hood (Fig. 17-6), and shoe coverings. *Staff change into clean surgical attire in the OR suite locker rooms, not at home.* All members of the surgical team must cover their hair, including any facial hair.

In addition to basic attire, everyone must wear protective attire. This includes a mask, eyewear, gloves, gown, and shoe covers. Everyone who enters an OR where a sterile field is present must wear a mask. Surgical team members who are scrubbed and at the patient's bedside during the surgery must also wear a sterile fluid-resistant gown, sterile gloves, and eye protectors, or face shields. Team members who are *not* scrubbed (e.g., anesthesia provider, circulating nurse) may wear cover scrub jackets that are snapped or buttoned closed (to prevent shedding of organisms from bare arms) and eyewear, as warranted.

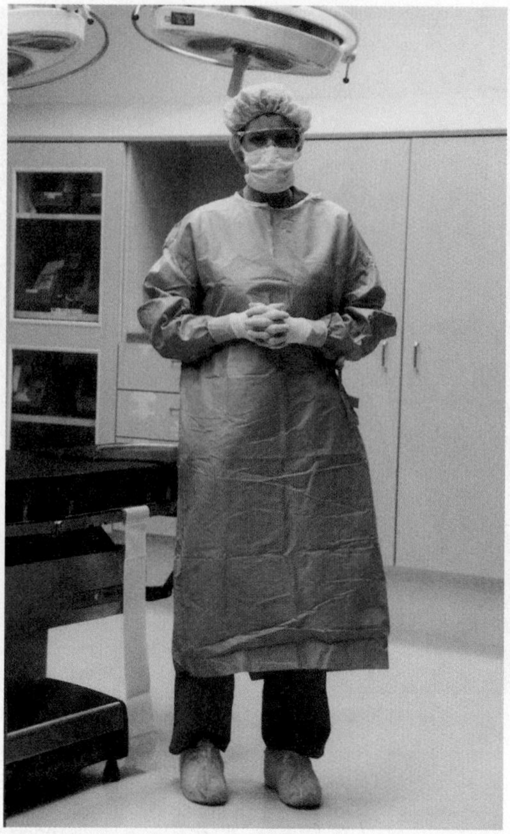

Fig. 17-6 • Typical attire for all scrubbed personnel. Note complete hair covering, eye shields, mask, sterile gloves over the cuffs of the sterile gown, and shoe coverings. Note that when not in use, the hands are typically folded in front of the body, never below the waist.

Surgical Scrub

The surgeon, all assistants, and the scrub nurse perform a surgical scrub after putting on a mask and before putting on the sterile gown and gloves (Fig. 17-7). *The scrub does not make the hands and forearms sterile.* When the scrub is performed correctly, it reduces the number of organisms from the hands, arms, and nails. Rings, watches, and bracelets are removed before scrubbing because they may harbor organisms. Fingernails are kept short, clean, and healthy. Artificial nails are not worn because they too can harbor organisms.

A broad-spectrum, surgical antimicrobial solution is used for the surgical scrub. Plain or antimicrobial soap is used for washing hands immediately before the surgical scrub. Vigorous rubbing that creates friction is used from the fingertips to the elbow. The scrub continues for 3 to 5 minutes, followed by a rinse. During the rinse, hands and arms are positioned so that water runs off, rather than up or down, the arms (AORN, 2007p). After scrubbing, personnel enter the OR with their hands held higher than the elbows and thoroughly dry their hands and forearms with a sterile towel. This person is then assisted into a sterile gown *("gowning")* and puts on sterile gloves *("gloving")*. Newer, alcohol-based surgical scrub agents may or may not require the use of water. Operating room personnel wash and dry their hands with soap and water before applying the agent to their hands and forearms, rubbing thoroughly until dry.

Gowns, gloves, and materials used at the operative field must be sterile. These items are changed between surgical procedures and as they become contaminated. The areas of the surgical gown considered sterile are the front of the gown from the chest to the level of the sterile field. The entire sleeves of the gown are considered sterile from 2 inches above the elbow to the cuff. The back of the gown is not considered sterile because it cannot be consistently seen by the wearer. Only when they are properly scrubbed and attired do members of the surgical team handle sterile drapes and equipment.

Anesthesia

The word *anesthesia* means "negative sensation." Anesthesia delivery is a precise science. It requires the skill of an anesthesiologist, a certified registered nurse anesthetist (CRNA) working under the direction of an anesthesiologist or another

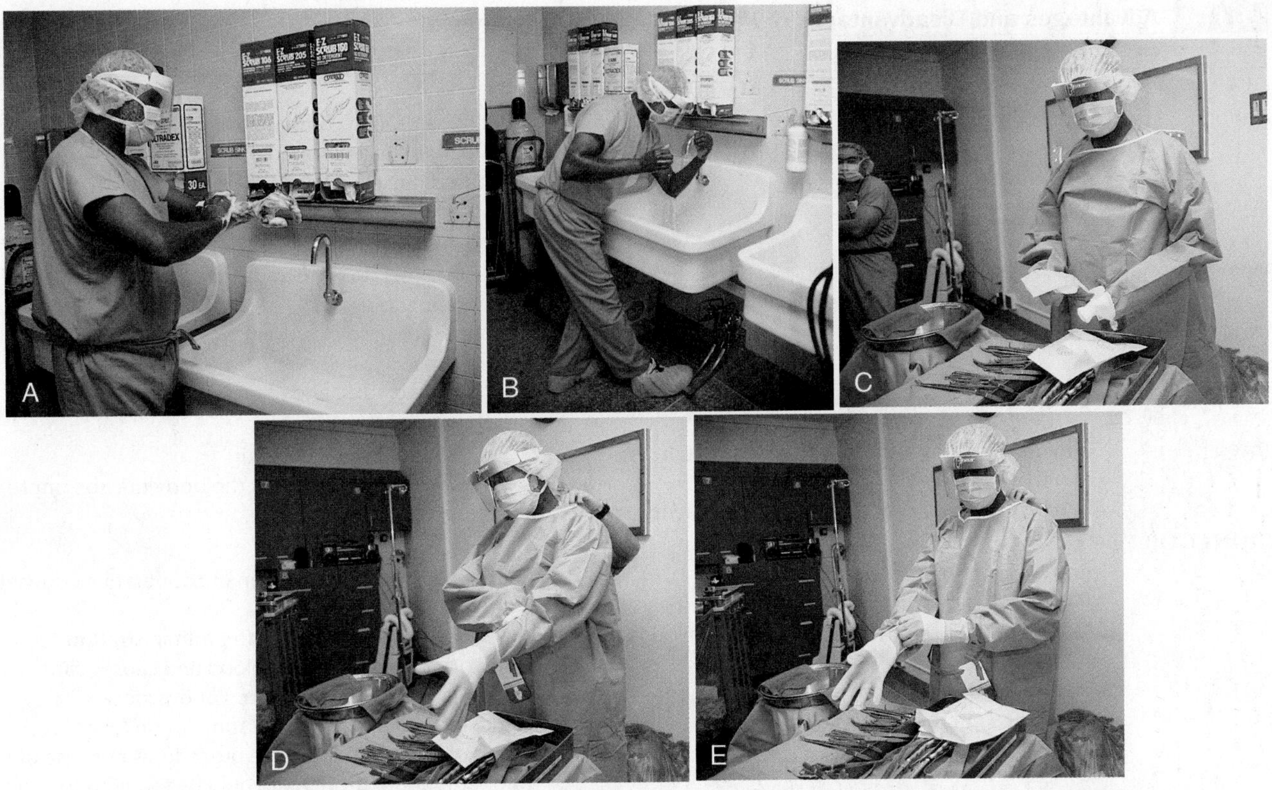

Fig. 17-7 • The scrubbing, gowning, and gloving process. **A,** The surgical scrub. **B,** Rinsing. Note the water falling off the hands and arms. Also note the foot-operated handle that controls the water flow. (After scrubbing and rinsing, the scrub nurse dries his hands and arms with a sterile towel inside the operating room and then is assisted into a sterile gown.) **C,** The scrub nurse prepares sterile gloves. Note that the scrub nurse's hands are *inside* the sleeve of the gown and that he is touching the sterile gloves only with the sterile sleeve. **D,** The scrub nurse puts on his first sterile glove while the sterile gown is being tied in the back. Note again that his hand never emerges from under the sterile sleeve. **E,** The scrub nurse puts on his second sterile glove.

physician, or an anesthesiologist assistant (AA—similar to a physician assistant) working under the direction of an anesthesiologist.

Anesthesia is an induced state of partial or total loss of sensation, occurring with or without loss of consciousness. The purpose of anesthesia is to block nerve impulse transmission, suppress reflexes, promote muscle relaxation, and, in some cases, achieve a controlled level of unconsciousness. Anesthesia providers use a separate anesthesia record for documentation.

Usually the anesthesia provider selects the anesthesia after consulting with the patient and surgeon and after considering specific patient-related factors. The nurse and patient communicate patient preferences and fears about anesthesia to the anesthesia provider. Patient health problems are major factors in the selection and dose of anesthesia. Selection is also influenced by:

- Type and duration of the procedure
- Area of the body having surgery
- Safety issues to reduce injury, such as airway management
- Whether the procedure is an emergency
- Options for management of pain after surgery
- How long it has been since the patient ate, had any liquids, or had any drugs
- Patient position needed for the surgical procedure
- Whether the patient must be alert enough to follow instructions during surgery
- The patient's previous responses and reactions to anesthesia

The physical status of a patient is ranked according to a classification system developed by the American Society of Anesthesiologists (ASA). The anesthesiologist assesses the patient and assigns him or her to one of six categories based on current health and the presence of diseases and disorders. The categories rank patients in a range from a totally healthy patient (P1 ranking) to a patient who is brain dead (P6 ranking) (DeLamar, 2007). This system is used to estimate potential risks during surgery and patient outcomes.

Anesthesia delivery begins with selecting and giving preoperative drugs (see Chapter 16). The nurse must know the actions of commonly used drugs and their effects during and after surgery. Anesthesia affects many systems and can worsen other health problems, increasing the patient's need for care. For example, most anesthetics are metabolized by the liver and excreted by the kidneys. Liver or kidney impairment increases anesthetic effects and the risk for toxicity. In addition, interactions may occur between the anesthetics and other drugs the patient has received.

Anesthesia can be induced in many ways (Table 17-1). The most common forms of anesthesia used in North America in-

TABLE 17-1 Advantages and Disadvantages of Various Types of Anesthesia

Type	Advantages	Disadvantages
GENERAL		
Inhalation	Most controllable method Induction and reversal accomplished with pulmonary ventilation Few side effects	Must be used in combination with other agents for painful or prolonged procedures Limited muscle relaxant effects Postoperative nausea and shivering common Explosive
Intravenous	Rapid and pleasant induction Low incidence of postoperative nausea and vomiting Requires little equipment	Must be metabolized and excreted from the body for complete reversal Contraindicated in presence of hepatic or renal disease Increased cardiac and respiratory depression Retained by fat cells
Balanced	Minimal disturbance to physiologic function Minimal side effects Can be used with older and high-risk patients	Drug interactions can occur Pharmacologic effects on the body may be unpredictable
REGIONAL OR LOCAL		
	Gag and cough reflexes stay intact Allows participation and cooperation by the patient Less disruption of physical and emotional body functions Decreased chance of sensitivity to the agent Decreased intraoperative stress	Difficult to administer to an uncooperative or upset patient No way to control agent after administration Absorbs rapidly into the blood and causes cardiac depression (hypotension) or overdose Increased nervous system stimulation (overdose) Not practical for extensive procedures because of the amount of drug that would be required to maintain anesthesia
CRYOTHERMIA		
	Reflexes remain intact Decreases chance of adverse reactions Decreased intraoperative stress	No way to control depth of anesthesia Not used in long or extensive procedures May not be appropriate for an anxious patient
HYPNOSIS/HYPNOANESTHESIA		
	Reflexes remain intact	Requires patient cooperation Requires special training

clude general, regional, or local anesthesia. Hypnosis or hypnoanesthesia (which induces a passive, trancelike state), cryothermia (use of cold [e.g., ice] reduces the surface temperature of the surgical site), and acupuncture are used less often.

General Anesthesia

General anesthesia is a reversible loss of consciousness induced by inhibiting neuronal impulses in several areas of the central nervous system (CNS). This state can be achieved with a single agent or a combination of agents. General anesthesia depresses the CNS, resulting in **analgesia** (pain relief or pain suppression), **amnesia** (memory loss of the surgery), and unconsciousness, with loss of muscle tone and reflexes. The patient is unconscious and unaware. This type of anesthesia is used most often in surgery of the head, neck, upper torso, and abdomen. It may also be used when patients cannot cooperate.

Stages of General Anesthesia. Induction of general anesthesia involves four stages. Table 17-2 lists the expected patient responses and nursing care for each stage. The speed of **emergence** (recovery from the anesthesia) depends on the type of anesthetic agent, the length of time the patient is anesthetized, and whether a reversal agent is used. Retching, vomiting, and restlessness may occur during emergence, although not all patients have these responses. Suction equipment must be available to prevent aspiration. During recovery, shivering, rigidity, and slight cyanosis may occur. These responses are caused by a temporary change in the body's temperature control. The nurse provides warm blankets, radiant light, and oxygen to decrease the effects of emergence.

Administration of General Anesthesia. General anesthesia agents are administered by inhalation and IV injection. Table 17-3 lists common agents for general anesthesia along with their advantages and disadvantages. At times, both inhalation and IV agents are used together as "balanced anesthesia" to obtain specific effects. A combination is used to provide hypnosis, amnesia, analgesia, muscle relaxation, and reduced reflexes with minimal disturbance of physiologic function. This method provides safe and controlled anesthetic delivery, especially for older and high-risk patients. An example of balanced anesthesia is the use of thiopental for induction, nitrous oxide for amnesia, morphine for analgesia, and pancuronium for muscle relaxation. Many combinations are possible, and selection is based on the individual patient and the specific surgical procedure.

Other drugs, such as hypnotics, opioid analgesics, and neuromuscular blocking agents, may be used as part of the anesthesia regimen (see Table 17-3). Hypnotics and opioid analgesics can be used for sedation before surgery, IV moderate sedation for short procedures, and as an adjunct to general anesthesia during surgery. The neuromuscular blocking agents are used to relax the jaw and vocal cords immediately after induction so that the

TABLE 17-2 The Four Stages of General Anesthesia and Related Nursing Interventions

Description	Nursing Interventions	Rationales
STAGE 1 (ANALGESIA AND SEDATION, RELAXATION)		
Begins with induction and ends with loss of consciousness.	Close operating room doors, dim the lights, and control traffic in the operating room.	Avoiding external stimuli in the environment promotes relaxation.
Patient feels drowsy and dizzy, has a reduced sensation to pain, and is amnesic.	Position patient securely with safety belts.	Using safety measures in stage 1 prepares for stage 2.
Hearing is exaggerated.	Keep discussions about the patient to a minimum.	Being sensitive to the patient maintains his or her dignity.
STAGE 2 (EXCITEMENT, DELIRIUM)		
Begins with loss of consciousness and ends with relaxation, regular breathing, and loss of the eyelid reflex.	Avoid auditory and physical stimuli.	Sensory stimuli can contribute to the patient's response.
Patient may have irregular breathing, increased muscle tone, and involuntary movement of the extremities during this stage.	Protect the extremities.	Safety measures help prevent injury.
Laryngospasm or vomiting may occur.	Assist the anesthesiologist or CRNA with suctioning as needed.	
Patient is susceptible to external stimuli.	Stay with patient.	Staying with the patient is emotionally supportive.
STAGE 3 (OPERATIVE ANESTHESIA, SURGICAL ANESTHESIA)		
Begins with generalized muscle relaxation and ends with loss of reflexes and depression of vital functions.	Assist the anesthesiologist or CRNA with intubation.	Providing assistance helps promote smooth intubation and prevent injury.
The jaw is relaxed, and breathing is quiet and regular.	Place patient into operative position.	Performing procedures as soon as possible promotes time management to minimize total anesthesia time for the patient.
The patient cannot hear.	Prep (scrub) the patient's skin over the operative site as directed.	
Sensations (i.e., to pain) are lost.		
STAGE 4 (DANGER)		
Begins with depression of vital functions and ends with respiratory failure, cardiac arrest, and possible death.	Prepare for and assist in treatment of cardiac and/or pulmonary arrest.	Teamwork and preparedness help decrease injuries and complications and promote the possibility of a desired outcome for the patient.
Respiratory muscles are paralyzed; apnea occurs.	Document occurrence in the patient's chart.	
Pupils are fixed and dilated.		

CRNA, Certified registered nurse anesthetist.

endotracheal tube can be placed. These drugs also may be used during surgery to provide continued muscle relaxation.

Complications from General Anesthesia. Complications can range from minor and annoying (sore throat) to death. Improvement in anesthesia delivery and surgical techniques has resulted in a decline in anesthesia-related deaths, even among higher-risk patients. Although the anesthesia provider has the main responsibility for monitoring patient responses during surgery, the circulating nurse also remains alert for changes in the patient's condition.

Malignant hyperthermia (MH) is an acute, life-threatening complication of certain drugs used for general anesthesia. The reaction begins in skeletal muscle exposed to specific agents, causing increased calcium levels in muscle cells and increased muscle metabolism. Serum calcium and potassium levels are increased, as is the metabolic rate, leading to acidosis, cardiac dysrhythmias, and a high body temperature.

Onset of MH may occur immediately after induction of anesthesia, several hours into the procedure, or, rarely, even after the anesthetic has been terminated. Clinical features reflect the increased muscle calcium level and the greatly increased body metabolism. Manifestations include tachycardia, dysrhythmias, muscle rigidity (especially of the jaw and upper chest), hypotension, tachypnea, skin mottling, cyanosis, and **myoglobinuria** (presence of muscle proteins in the urine). The most sensitive indication is an unexpected rise in the end-tidal carbon dioxide level with a decrease in oxygen saturation. Another early indication is sinus tachycardia. *Extremely elevated temperature, as high as 111.2° F (44° C), is a late sign of MH.* Survival depends on early diagnosis and the actions of the entire surgical team. Time is crucial when MH is diagnosed. Dantrolene sodium, a skeletal muscle relaxant, is the drug of choice along with other interventions (Hommertzheim & Steinke, 2006).

For a known history or risk, the patient can be treated before, during, and after surgery with dantrolene to prevent this problem. Chart 17-1 lists best practices for care of the patient with MH. The AORN recommends that all operating rooms have a dedicated MH cart containing drugs for management (normal saline, dantrolene, sodium bicarbonate, insulin, 50% dextrose, and calcium chloride), a protocol card listing interventions, and the MH hotline number. Additional nursing support is needed during this true perioperative emergency.

TABLE 17-3 Advantages and Disadvantages of Common Agents for General Anesthesia

Agent	Advantages	Disadvantages
INHALATION ANESTHETICS		
Desflurane (Suprane)	Rapid induction and recovery	May increase heart rate and lower BP during induction Can induce malignant hyperthermia*
Enflurane (Ethrane)	Rapid induction and recovery Less likely to induce dysrhythmias	Respiratory depression may occur Hypotension may occur Can induce malignant hyperthermia* Lowers seizure threshold
Halothane (Fluothane)	Rapid and smooth induction Low incidence of postoperative nausea and vomiting Less irritating to the respiratory tract than other inhalation agents	Shivering common postoperatively Can induce malignant hyperthermia* Hypotension and bradycardia may occur Can increase dysrhythmias Can cause permanent liver damage (rare)
Isoflurane (Forane)	Rapid induction and recovery Induces additional muscle relaxation	Respiratory depression possible Irritating odor
Sevoflurane (Ultane)	Rapid induction and recovery Induces additional muscle relaxation	Can induce renal impairment (rare)
Nitrous oxide (N_2O)	Rapid induction and recovery Useful for short procedures When used with other agents, reduces the required concentration of the other agents Minimal cardiovascular and respiratory depression	Relatively weak anesthetic agent May produce hypoxia if the concentration is high Needs addition of other agents for longer procedures
INTRAVENOUS ANESTHETICS		
Etomidate (Amidate)	Rapid induction and recovery Useful for short procedures Little "hang-over" effect	Can cause pain at injection site Laryngospasms (rare)
Ketamine (Ketalar)	Rapid induction and recovery Protective reflexes remain intact	Stimulates cardiovascular responses Dissociative emergence reactions Can induce nausea and vomiting
Midazolam (Versed)	Induces amnesia around the event	Slower induction than other IV agents
Propofol (Diprivan)	Rapid induction and recovery	Can cause pain at injection site May induce propofol infusion syndrome (PrIS): Severe metabolic acidosis, rhabdomyolysis, hyperkalemia, renal failure, cardiovascular collapse
Methohexital sodium (Brevital)	Acts directly on the central nervous system	Can induce bradycardia and hypotension
Thiopental sodium (Pentothal)	Rapid induction and recovery	Can depress respiratory and cardiac functions
NEUROMUSCULAR BLOCKERS		
Succinylcholine (SUX, Anectine)	Rapid induction and recovery	Causes fasciculations on induction
Atracurium (Tracrium)	Rapid induction and recovery	Temporarily paralyzes muscles but does not block sensation
Cisatracurium (Nimbex)	Same as for atracurium	Same as for atracurium
Mivacurium (Mivacron)	Same as for atracurium	Same as for atracurium
Vecuronium (Norcuron)	Same as for atracurium	Same as for atracurium
Pancuronium (Pavulon)	Slower onset and longer duration than atracurium	Same as for atracurium
OPIOIDS		
Alfentanil (Alfenta)	Rapid induction and recovery	
Fentanyl (Sublimaze)	Outstanding analgesia, anesthesia (epidural)	
Remifentanil (Ultiva)	Effective at very low doses	
Sufentanil (Sufenta)	Rapid induction and recovery	Can induce prolonged respiratory depression

*May induce malignant hyperthermia only in susceptible people.

GENETIC CONSIDERATIONS

MH is a genetic disorder with an autosomal dominant pattern of inheritance. The patient with a genetic predisposition for MH is at risk for this complication from halothane, enflurane, isoflurane, desflurane, sevoflurane, and succinylcholine (Hommertzheim & Steinke, 2006). This rare syndrome is most common in young adults. Males are affected more often than females (despite the autosomal dominant pattern of inheritance) because of gender differences in muscle mass. Once a patient or family history of MH is known, family members can have a muscle biopsy to determine whether they are at risk. When a patient is determined to be at risk for MH, he or she can still have anesthesia and surgery; however, more precautions are needed and different anesthetic agents are used.

Chart 17-1 BEST PRACTICE FOR PATIENT SAFETY & QUALITY CARE

Emergency Care of the Patient with Malignant Hyperthermia

EMERGENCY CARE

- Stop all inhalation anesthetic agents and succinylcholine.
- If an endotracheal (ET) tube is not already in place, intubate immediately.
- Ventilate the patient with 100% oxygen, using the highest possible flow rate.
- Administer dantrolene sodium (Dantrium) IV at a dose of 2 to 3 mg/kg.
- Change the anesthesia machine or disconnect breathing circuit and flush carbon dioxide absorbent with 100% oxygen.
- If possible, terminate surgery. If termination is not possible, continue surgery using anesthetic agents that do not trigger malignant hyperthermia (MH).
- Assess arterial blood gases (ABGs) and serum chemistries for metabolic acidosis and hyperkalemia.
- If metabolic acidosis is evident by ABG analysis, administer sodium bicarbonate IV.
- If hyperkalemia is present, administer 0.15 units/kg regular insulin in 1 mL/kg 50% dextrose IV.
- Use active cooling techniques:
  - Administer iced saline (0.9% NaCl) IV at a rate of 15 mL/kg every 15 minutes as needed.
  - Apply a cooling blanket over the torso.
  - Wrap or rub extremities with cold, wet towels or ice wrapped in towels.
  - Lavage the stomach, bladder, rectum, and open body cavities with sterile iced normal saline.
- Insert a nasogastric tube and a rectal tube.
- Monitor core body temperature to assess effectiveness of interventions and avoid hypothermia.
- Monitor cardiac rhythm by electrocardiography (ECG) to assess for dysrhythmias.
- Insert a Foley catheter to monitor urine output.
- Treat any dysrhythmias that do not resolve on correction of hyperthermia and hyperkalemia with antidysrhythmic agents *other than calcium channel blockers*.
- Administer IV fluids at a rate and volume sufficient to maintain urine output above 2 mL/kg/hr.
- Monitor urine for presence of blood or myoglobin.
- If urine output falls below 2 mL/kg/hr, consider using osmotic or loop diuretics, depending on the patient's cardiac and renal status.
- Contact the Malignant Hyperthermia Association of the United States (MHAUS) hotline for more information regarding treatment: (800) 644-9737.
- Transfer the patient to the intensive care unit (ICU) when stable.
- Continue to monitor the patient's temperature, ECG, ABGs, electrolytes, creatine kinase, coagulation studies, and serum and urine myoglobin levels until they have remained normal for 24 hours.
- Instruct the patient and family about testing for MH risk.
- Refer the patient and family to the Malignant Hyperthermia Association of the United States at (800) 986-4287 or www.mhaus.org.
- Report the incident to the North American Malignant Hyperthermia Registry at the University of Pittsburgh: (412) 692-5464.

Data from Malignant Hyperthermia Association of the United States; and Hommertzheim, R., & Steinke, E.E. (2006). Malignant hyperthermia: The perioperative nurse's role. *AORN, 83*(1), 149-164.

Overdose of anesthesia can occur if the patient's metabolism and drug elimination are slower than expected. This is more likely to occur in patients who are older or who have liver or kidney problems. Other drugs (e.g., antihypertensives) also alter metabolism, and interactions can occur between the anesthetic and the patient's regular drugs. Accurate information about the patient's height, weight, and medical history, especially liver and kidney function, is vital in determining the anesthetic type and dosage. Death during surgery is more often related to pre-existing health problems than to anesthesia overdose.

Unrecognized hypoventilation occurs as an anesthesia-induced complication. Failure to exchange gases adequately can lead to cardiac arrest, permanent brain damage, and death. Monitoring standards include the use of an end-tidal carbon dioxide monitor to confirm carbon dioxide in the patient's expired gas and a breathing system disconnect monitor to detect any break in the breathing circuit equipment.

Intubation complications can include many problems (e.g., broken or injured teeth and caps, swollen lip, vocal cord trauma). Intubation may be difficult because of anatomic variance or disease presence (e.g., small oral cavity, tight jaw joint, presence of tumor). Improper neck extension during intubation also may cause injury. The surgeon should be in the operating room (OR) during the intubation process in case a tracheostomy is needed when the endotracheal (ET) tube is placed. ET placement causes tracheal irritation and edema. Often the patient has a sore throat after surgery.

Local or Regional Anesthesia

Local or regional anesthesia briefly disrupts sensory nerve impulse transmission from a specific body area or region. Motor function may or may not be affected. The patient remains conscious and can follow instructions. Because the gag and cough reflexes remain intact, the risk for aspiration is low. Local or regional anesthesia is often supplemented with sedatives, opioid analgesics, or hypnotics to reduce anxiety and increase comfort. The OR nurse provides the patient with information, directions, and emotional support before, during, and after the procedure.

Local anesthesia is delivered topically (applied to the skin or mucous membranes of the area to be anesthetized) and by local infiltration (injected directly *into* the tissue around an incision, wound, or lesion). Sometimes when the term *local* is used, it means *any* form of anesthesia that is not general anesthesia.

Regional anesthesia is a type of local anesthesia that blocks multiple peripheral nerves in a specific body region. It may be used when general anesthesia cannot be used because of medical problems, when the patient has had adverse reactions to general anesthesia, when the patient has a preference and a choice is possible, and when pain management after surgery is enhanced by regional anesthesia. If the patient has eaten and the surgery is an emergency, it may be possible to perform surgery with the patient under regional anesthesia (depending on the procedure) to decrease the risk for aspiration. Types of regional anesthesia include field block, nerve block, spinal, and epidural. Table 17-4 defines the types of regional anesthesia. Figs. 17-8 and 17-9 show common sites of nerve blocks, spinal anesthesia, and epidural anesthesia.

TABLE 17-4 Types of Regional Anesthesia

Anesthesia Type	Definition and Common Use
Field block	A series of injections *around* the operative field Most commonly used for chest procedures, hernia repair, dental surgery, and some plastic surgeries
Nerve block	Injection of the local anesthetic agent *into or around* one nerve or group of nerves in the involved area Most commonly used for limb surgery or to relieve chronic pain
Spinal anesthesia	Injection of an anesthetic agent into the cerebrospinal fluid in the subarachnoid space (see Fig. 17-9) Most commonly used for lower abdominal, pelvic, hip, and knee surgery
Epidural anesthesia	Injection of an agent into the epidural space (see Fig. 17-9) Most commonly used for anorectal, vaginal, perineal, hip, and lower extremity surgeries

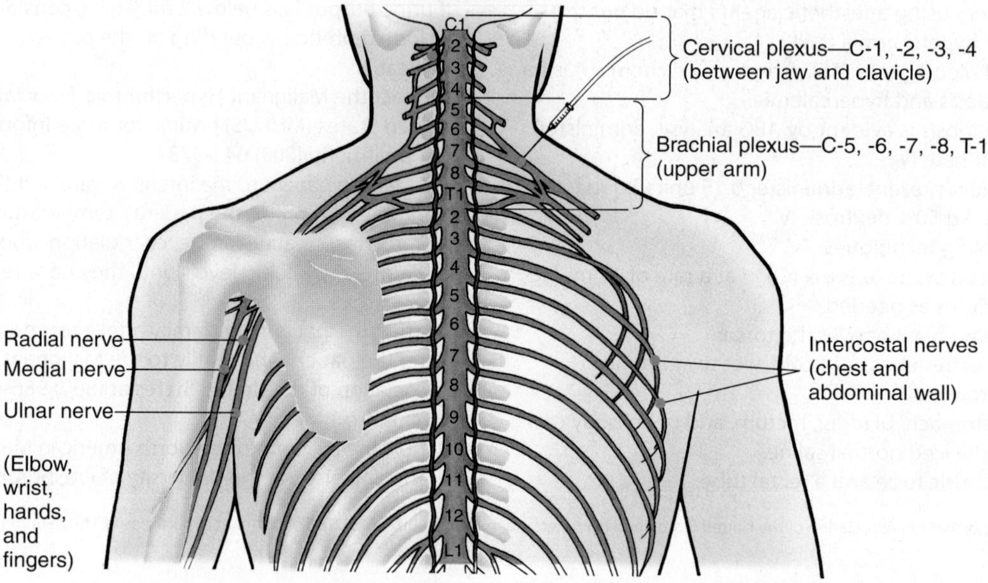

Cervical plexus—C-1, -2, -3, -4
(between jaw and clavicle)
Brachial plexus—C-5, -6, -7, -8, T-1
(upper arm)
Radial nerve
Medial nerve
Ulnar nerve
(Elbow, wrist, hands, and fingers)
Intercostal nerves
(chest and abdominal wall)
C1
2
3
4
5
6
7
8
T1
2
3
4
5
6
7
8
9
10
11
12
L1

Fig. 17-8 • Nerve block sites.

The nurse's role in the delivery of regional anesthesia consists of:

- Assisting the anesthesia provider
- Observing for breaks in sterile technique
- Providing emotional support for the patient
- Staying with the patient
- Offering information and reassurance
- Positioning the patient comfortably and safely

Complications of local or regional anesthesia are related to patient sensitivity to the anesthetic agent (anaphylaxis), incorrect delivery technique, systemic absorption, and overdose. The nurse observes for central nervous system (CNS) stimulation followed by CNS and cardiac depression, which are signs of a systemic toxic reaction. The nurse also assesses for restlessness, excitement, incoherent speech, headache, blurred vision, metallic taste, nausea, vomiting, tremors, seizures, and increased pulse, respirations, and blood pressure. Interventions include establishing an open airway, giving oxygen, and notifying the surgeon. Usually a fast-acting barbiturate is needed for treatment. If the toxic reaction is untreated, unconsciousness, hypotension, apnea, cardiac arrest, and death may result.

Cardiac arrest may occur as a rare complication of spinal anesthesia. Epinephrine is given to prevent cardiac arrest in patients who develop sudden, unexplained bradycardia.

Local complications include edema and inflammation as early problems. Abscess formation, tissue necrosis, and/or gangrene may occur later. Abscesses result from contamination during injection of the agent. Necrosis and gangrene are rare but may occur as a result of prolonged blood vessel constriction in the injected area.

Moderate (Conscious) Sedation

Moderate sedation, still commonly called *conscious* sedation, is the IV delivery of sedative, hypnotic, and opioid drugs to reduce the level of consciousness but allow the patient to maintain a patent airway and to respond to verbal commands. The amnesia action is short, and the patient usually has a rapid return to ADLs. Etomidate (Amidate), diazepam (Valium, Vivol♣, Novo-Dipam♣), midazolam (Versed), meperidine (Demerol), fentanyl (Sublimaze), alfentanil (Alfenta), and morphine sulfate are the most commonly used drugs. Moderate sedation is used for endoscopy, cardiac catheterization, closed fracture reduction, cardioversion, and other special but short procedures.

Selection of patients for moderate sedation is based on specific criteria. The physician determines whether the patient is a candidate. In most states, a credentialed registered nurse may deliver moderate sedation under physician supervision and within the state-defined scope of nursing practice. Credentialing includes advanced training in IV drug delivery, airway management, and advanced cardiac life support (ACLS).

The nurse monitors the patient during and after the procedure for response to the procedure and the drugs. The airway,

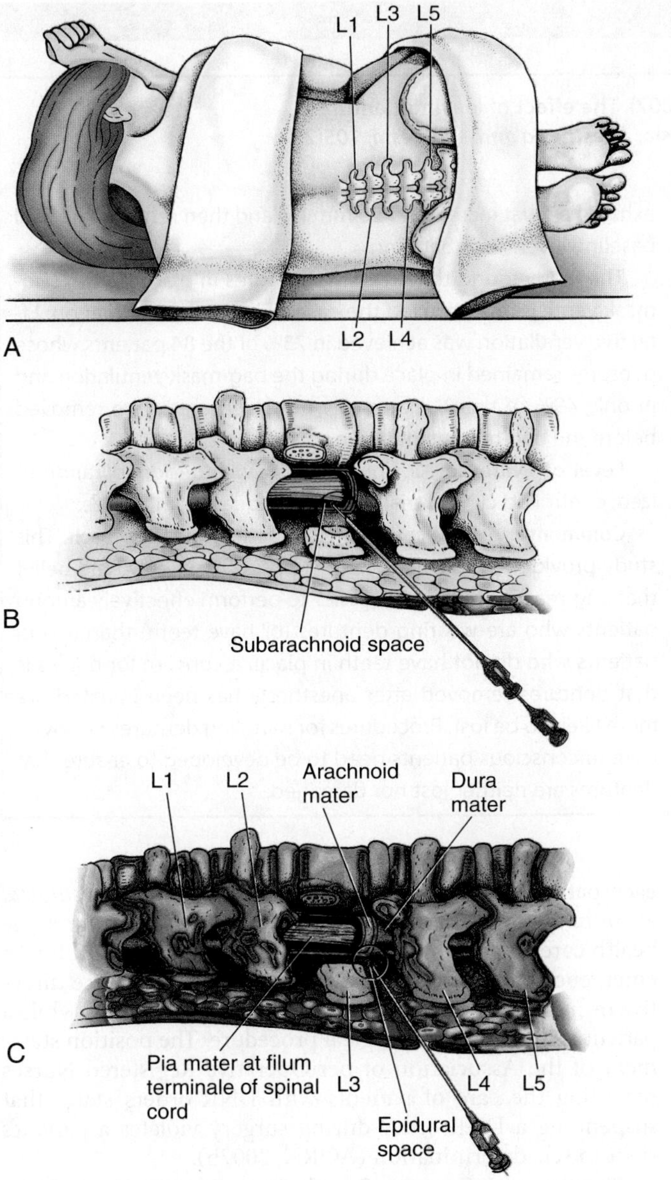
L1
L3
L5
L2
L4
A
B
Subarachnoid space
L1
L2
Arachnoid mater
Dura mater
C
Pia mater at filum terminale of spinal cord
L3
L4
L5
Epidural space

Fig. 17-9 • Administration of spinal and epidural anesthesia. **A,** Spinal or epidural anesthesia is administered by inserting a spinal needle between the second and third or the third and fourth lumbar vertebrae (L2-3 or L3-4). The patient is placed in the flexed lateral (fetal) position *(shown here)* or seated on the edge of the operating bed with the back arched and the chin tucked to the chest. **B,** Spinal anesthesia *(viewed from the side).* A large needle is inserted to the surface of the dura mater, and a second, smaller needle is passed through the first to penetrate the dura mater and arachnoid mater. An anesthetic is injected, sometimes through an indwelling catheter, directly into the cerebrospinal fluid in the subarachnoid space. **C,** Epidural anesthesia *(viewed from the side).* The needle is inserted to the surface of the dura mater, and the anesthetic is injected, usually through an indwelling catheter, into the epidural space.

level of consciousness, oxygen saturation, ECG status, and vital signs are monitored every 15 to 30 minutes until the patient is awake and oriented and vital signs have returned to baseline levels (AORN, 2007i).

The patient receiving IV moderate sedation can be discharged to go home with a responsible adult. If the patient returns to the general medical-surgical nursing unit, the unit staff nurses continue monitoring. The patient is expected to be sleepy but arousable for several hours after the procedure. Oral intake is not permitted until 30 minutes after the patient has received the sedation or according to the physician's prescription. When fluids are permitted, the nurse makes sure that the patient is awake and positioned to avoid aspiration.

Patient-Centered Collaborative Care

evolve ONLINE PHARM REVIEW

Assessment

History

On arrival in the surgical suite, the patient is taken to the holding area or directly into the operating suite. The holding area nurse or the circulating nurse greets the patient on arrival. *Correct identification of the patient is the responsibility of every member of the health care team.* The nurse verifies the patient's identity with *two types of identifiers* (name, birth date, medical record number, or social security number). For example, the nurse checks the patient's identification bracelet and asks, "What is your name and when were you born?" This practice prevents errors by drowsy or confused patients. For example, if a patient is asked, "Are you Mr. Gates?," he may respond inappropriately if he is anxious or sedated. The nurse always validates identification using the medical record and identification bracelet and by asking the patient or family.

After completing the identification process, the nurse validates that the surgical consent form has been signed and witnessed. The nurse asks, "What kind of operation are you having today?" to ascertain that the patient's perception of the procedure, the operative permit, and the operative schedule are the same. *When the procedure involves a specific site, validating the side on which a procedure is to be performed (e.g., for amputation, cataract removal, hernia repair) is the responsibility of each health care professional before and at the time of surgery. Facilities usually have the patient and/or nurse initial the correct surgical site* (Ridge, 2008). Before proceeding, each health care professional thoroughly investigates *any* discrepancy and notifies the surgeon and anesthesia provider. The Joint Commission (TJC) has developed a Universal Protocol for Preventing Wrong Site, Wrong Procedure, Wrong Person Surgery and the Association of periOperative Registered Nurses has developed recommendations based on this protocol (AORN, 2007t). The nurse asks the patient about any allergies and determines whether autologous blood was donated. A red allergy bracelet on the patient's wrist and the medical record must be verified with what has been communicated.

The nurse checks the patient's attire to ensure adherence with facility policy. Dentures and dental prostheses (e.g., bridges, retainers), jewelry (including body piercing), eyeglasses, contact lenses, hearing aids, wigs, and other prostheses are removed. Denture removal before anesthesia is controversial (Conlon et al., 2007). Although the denture plate could become loose and obstruct the airway during surgery, the anesthesia provider may request that dentures be left in place to ensure a snug fit of the bag-mask. Research indicates that leaving the dentures in place during induction of general anesthesia does allow a better fit of the bag-mask (see the Evidence-Based Practice box on p. 278). In some facilities, patients may wear eyeglasses and hearing aids until after anesthesia induction.

EVIDENCE-BASED PRACTICE

The "dentures-in or dentures-out" dilemma!

Conlon, N., Sullivan, R., Herbison, P., Zacharias, M., & Buggy, D. (2007). The effect of leaving dentures in place on bag-mask ventilation at induction of general anesthesia. *Anesthesia and Analgesia, 105*(2), 370-373.

For decades patients undergoing general anesthesia have been required to remove their dentures before surgery. This practice is embarrassing to patients; it often interferes with their ability to speak clearly and increases anxiety. The rationale for denture removal is to prevent denture damage and dislodgement, which leads to airway obstruction. However, anesthesia providers have said that establishing effective ventilation by bag-mask is more difficult because of the shape of the patient's mouth when dentures are not in place. (Effective ventilation using the bag-mask requires a seal of the mask around the mouth.)

This prospective study sought to evaluate the ease and effectiveness of bag-mask ventilation among patients with and without dentures in place after induction of anesthesia. The subjects were 166 patients with dentures. These patients were then randomly assigned to have either the dentures removed immediately after induction of general anesthesia (and before bag-mask ventilation) or left in place after the induction of general anesthesia and during bag-mask ventilation. Effective ventilation was determined by having the end-tidal carbon dioxide level of exhaled air first increase to 20 mm Hg and then return to normal baseline levels with bagging.

The study found that keeping dentures in place during bag-mask ventilation improved the ease of bag-mask ventilation. Effective ventilation was achieved in 73% of the 84 patients whose dentures remained in place during the bag-mask ventilation and in only 49% of the 81 patients whose dentures were removed before the bag-mask ventilation.

Level of Evidence—2. The study is a well-designed, randomized, controlled clinical trial with an adequate sample size.

Commentary: Implications for Practice and Research. This study provided solid evidence to support the largely held belief that bag-mask ventilation is easier to perform effectively among patients who are wearing dentures (or have teeth) than it is in patients who do not have teeth in place. A concern for nurses is that dentures removed after anesthesia has been initiated are more likely to be lost. Procedures for handling dentures removed from unconscious patients need to be developed to ensure that dentures are neither lost nor damaged.

NCLEX EXAMINATION CHALLENGE

The client has entered the surgical suite about 30 minutes after she has received atropine and midazolam as preoperative drugs. The OR schedule lists that she is to have a vaginal hysterectomy. When the nurse asks her what kind of surgery she is having today, her response is "I am going to have a hemorrhoidectomy." What is the nurse's next best action?

A. Notify the surgeon that the client is uninformed and that consent must be obtained again.
B. Ask the client to describe what the surgery is supposed to be in her own words.
C. Ask the client her name and compare it with the name on the chart.
D. Delay further preparations until the preoperative drugs have worn off.

evolve For the correct answer, go to http://evolve.elsevier.com/Iggy/.

Medical Record Review

The circulating nurse and anesthesia provider review the patient's medical record in the holding area or the operating room (OR). The medical record provides information needed to identify patient needs during surgery and allows the circulating nurse to assess and plan specific care during and after surgery. The medical record is the main source of information on the type and location of the planned surgery. The nurse checks the medical record to ensure required data are present before surgery is started.

Advance Directives and Do-Not-Resuscitate Orders. Ethical dilemmas may occur during or after surgery. As a patient advocate, the nurse may have to intervene on behalf of the patient's rights and wishes. The nurse must be familiar with the advance directives and do-not-resuscitate (DNR) orders for each patient. *These directives are to be honored in the surgical environment regardless of the situation.* It is difficult for some health care providers not to treat the patient in the OR for an emergency situation, and they may ignore an advance directive or living will. Some agencies suspend DNR orders while a patient is undergoing a surgical procedure. The position statement of the Association of periOperative Registered Nurses regarding the care of patients with DNR orders states that suspending a DNR order during surgery violates a patient's right to self-determination (AORN, 2007b).

Allergies and Previous Reactions to Anesthesia or Transfusions. The nurse asks about allergies and previous reactions to anesthesia or blood transfusions. Allergies to iodine products or shellfish indicate a risk for a reaction to the agents used to clean the surgical area. Latex allergies are assessed with all patients. Latex-induced anaphylaxis accounts for about 10% of the anaphylactic reactions that occur during surgery (see Chapters 19 and 22). Latex-free equipment and supplies are used when there is a latex allergy (Wadlund, 2006). The nurse documents the allergy in the medical record and notifies the OR team.

The patient's previous experience with anesthesia helps the nurse and anesthesia provider anticipate needs and plan interventions. For example, if a patient is restless or agitated as a reaction to anesthesia, the nurse can have padding for the siderails and protective restraints available. The use of blood and blood products during surgery may be influenced by the patient's history, religious beliefs, preferences, and past transfusion reactions.

Autologous Blood Transfusion. Autologous blood transfusion (reinfusing the patient's own blood) may be used for surgery. Chapters 16 and 42 discuss autologous transfusion in more detail. Chart 17-2 outlines best practices for autologous blood transfusion during surgery.

Laboratory and Diagnostic Test Results. The OR nurse reviews the most recent laboratory findings and test results to inform the surgical team about the patient's health and to alert them for potential problems. These results are usually obtained within 24 to 48 hours before surgery for hospitalized patients and within 4 weeks for ambulatory surgery patients. The nurse reports all abnormal findings or results to the surgeon and anesthesia provider. Laboratory values greater than or less than the normal range are potentially life threatening for patient having surgery (see Chapter 16). For example, if the hemoglobin level is less than 10 g/dL, oxygen transport capacity is reduced, affecting the amount and type of anesthesia used as well as the impact of blood loss during surgery.

Medical History and Physical Examination Findings. The OR nurse checks that the medical history and examination findings, including usual pulse and blood pressure, are recorded. This information provides the circulating nurse, surgeon, anesthesia provider, and PACU nurse with baseline data to assess the patient's reaction to the surgery and anesthesia. Drugs taken before surgery may affect the patient's reaction to surgery and wound healing. For example, aspirin reduces platelet action, increasing clotting time and the risk for hemorrhage.

Knowing the patient's medical history and age allows the nurse to plan interventions for the care and safety of high-risk patients (Chart 17-3). The nurse carefully monitors older patients and those with cardiac disease for potential fluid overload.

Chart 17-2 BEST PRACTICE FOR PATIENT SAFETY & QUALITY CARE

Intraoperative Autologous Blood Salvage and Transfusion

- Be aware of the cell-processing method to be used.
- Make sure that collection containers are labeled for the patient.
- Assist with sterile setup as necessary.
- Assist with processing and reinfusing procedures as needed.
- Document the transfusion process.
- Monitor the patient's vital signs during the transfusion procedure.

Chart 17-3 NURSING FOCUS ON THE OLDER ADULT

Intraoperative Nursing Interventions

- Allow patients to retain eyeglasses and hearing aids until anesthesia has been administered.
- Use a small pillow under the patient's head if his or her head and neck are normally bent slightly forward.
- Lift patients into position to prevent shearing forces on fragile skin.
- Position arthritic and artificial joints carefully to prevent postoperative pain and discomfort from strain on those joints.
- Pad bony prominences to prevent pressure sores.
- Provide extra padding for those patients with decreased peripheral circulation.
- Use head caps to prevent heat loss through the scalp.
- Place stockinette on extremities to conserve body heat.
- Warm prepping solutions and IV and irrigation fluids as indicated.
- Follow strict aseptic technique.
- Carefully monitor intake and output, including blood loss.

After completing the medical record review, the nurse may insert an IV catheter and perform a surgical shave. The circulating nurse provides emotional support and explains procedures to the patient. *The patient is never left unattended.* If the patient is in the holding area, he or she is moved to the OR after the preoperative routine is completed.

DECISION-MAKING CHALLENGE

Legal/Ethical

The patient, a 48-year-old secretary, has entered the surgical suite about 30 minutes after she has received the preoperative drugs *atropine* and *midazolam.* The OR schedule lists that she is scheduled to have a left mastectomy as treatment for breast cancer. When you ask her what kind of surgery she is having today, her response is "I am going to have the size of my breast reduced." You ask her if she means breast removal, and she responds, "No, that's for people with cancer, I am just reducing the size of my breast." When you check the informed consent page, the consent states *mastectomy* and the patient's signature is present, as is the surgeon's signature. The witness signature is a name that you do not know and does not indicate professional status. When you ask the patient who was in the room with her when the surgeon told her about her surgery and she signed the paper, she tells you no one was in the room other than she and the surgeon.

1. Is there any question about whether the consent form is complete?
2. What does a witness's signature mean?
3. What additional questions should you ask this patient?

When you ask the surgeon whether he believes this patient understands her surgery, he says that she knows she needs surgery and trusts that he knows what he is doing. As you continue to determine whether this patient understands the proposed surgery, you are convinced that she does not clearly understand what will be done during this surgery.

4. Should you explain this surgery to the patient? Why or why not?
5. To whom should you report your concerns?
6. Can this patient now sign a new consent form? Why or why not?
7. The surgeon is insisting that the patient now be brought into the OR. What should you do? What is the rationale for your choice of action?

evolve For suggested answer guidelines, go to http://evolve.elsevier.com/Iggy/.

Analysis

Common Nursing Diagnoses and Collaborative Problems

Priority nursing diagnoses for patients during surgery are:

1. Risk for Perioperative Positioning Injury related to immobilization and effects of anesthesia
2. Risk for Infection related to a break in skin integrity (e.g., incision, invasive lines)

A primary collaborative problem is Potential for Hypoventilation.

Additional Nursing Diagnoses and Collaborative Problems

In addition to the common nursing diagnoses and collaborative problems, patients during surgery may have one or more of these:

- Risk for Injury related to the surgical environment, extraneous objects, and equipment (laser, electrical, use of x-rays/radiation)
- Risk for Disuse Syndrome related to a decreased level of consciousness or to immobilization

- Hypothermia related to evaporation from skin and exposed tissue in a cool environment, body heat loss, changes in the hypothalamus from anesthetic agents, or inadequate body covering
- Fear related to the threat of death, actual or perceived, or anticipation of events posing a threat to self-esteem
- Anxiety related to loss of control or the threat of death
- Deficient Fluid Volume related to decreased intake, evaporative fluid loss through the skin and exposed tissue, or blood loss
- Potential for Peripheral Neurovascular Dysfunction related to intraoperative positioning

Planning and Implementation

Risk for Perioperative Positioning Injury

NOC **Planning: Expected Outcomes.** The patient is expected to be free of injury as indicated by:

- Adequate capillary refill and peripheral pulses in all extremities
- Sensory perception and motor function after surgery at the same level as before surgery
- Absence of skin redness or open skin areas
- Absence of bruising

Interventions. Interventions are used to prevent injury from positioning during surgery. Because of anesthesia and the narrow OR bed, the patient's normal defense mechanisms cannot guard against nerve or joint damage and muscle stretch or strain. In addition, pressure ulcers often start to develop during surgery (Schoohoven et al., 2002). Thus proper positioning is important. The circulating nurse pads the operating bed with foam and/or silicone gel pads and properly places the grounding pads. He or she coordinates the transfer to the operating bed and helps the patient to a comfortable position. The skin is assessed, especially of older patients, for bruising or injury, and extra padding is placed as indicated.

The patient is usually in a supine position after transfer to the operating bed. Anesthesia may be given with the patient supine, and he or she may then be repositioned for surgery (Fig. 17-10).

The circulating nurse coordinates positioning of the patient for surgery and modifies the position according to the patient's safety and special needs. Factors influencing the *timing* of repositioning include:

- The surgical site
- The age and size of the patient
- The anesthetic delivery technique
- Pain on movement (conscious patient)

Factors influencing the actual *position* include:

- The specific procedure being performed
- The surgeon's request
- The patient's age, size, and weight
- Any pulmonary, skeletal, or muscular limitations, such as arthritis, joint replacements, emphysema, or implanted devices

Chart 17-4 lists best practices to prevent complications related to prolonged immobility during surgery.

The dorsal recumbent, prone, lithotomy, and lateral positions are most often used for surgery. Fig. 17-10 shows many surgical positions and the use of protective padding. When general anesthesia is used, the nurse positions the patient

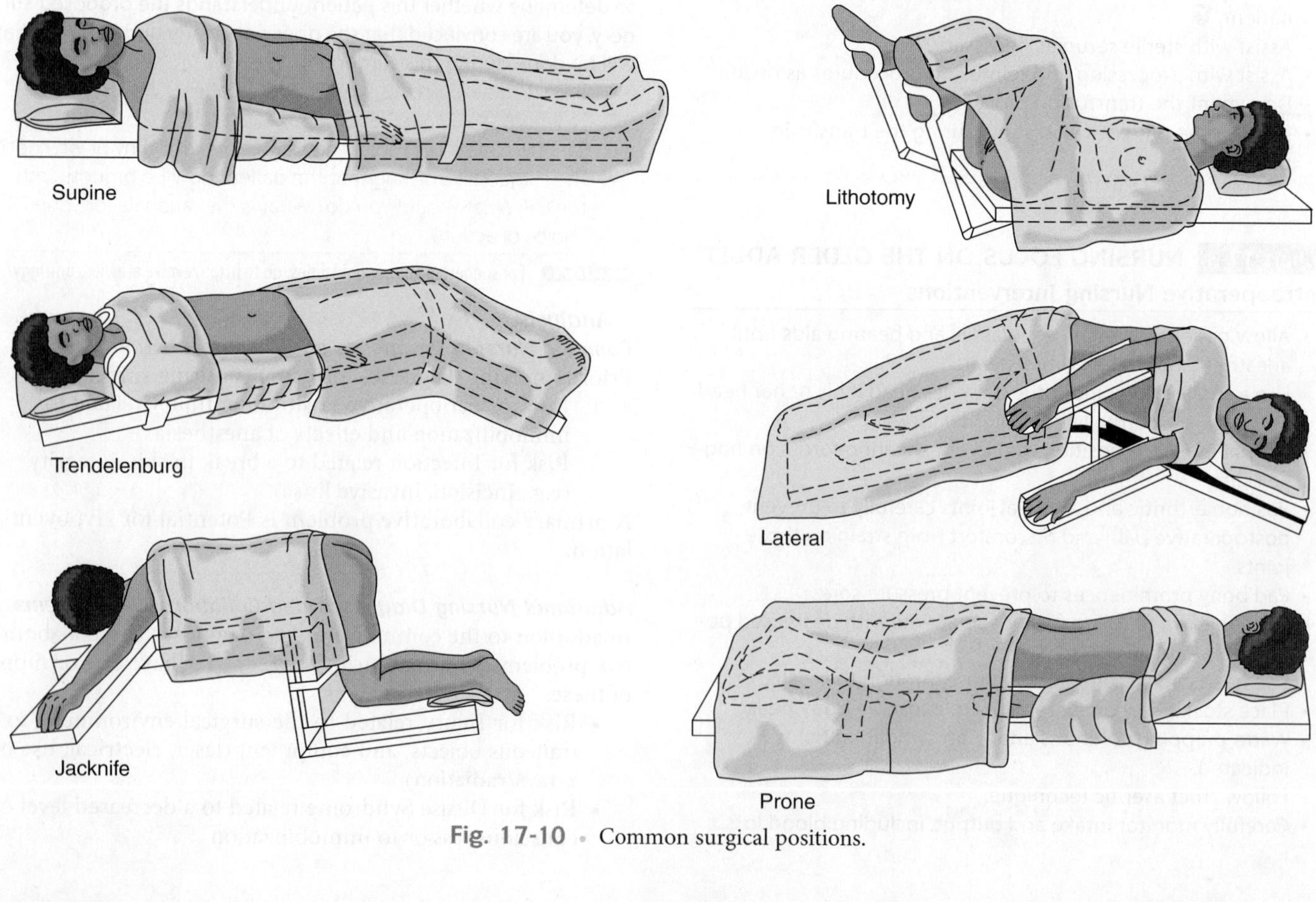
Supine
Lithotomy
Trendelenburg
Lateral
Jacknife
Prone

Fig. 17-10 • Common surgical positions.

Chart 17-4 BEST PRACTICE FOR PATIENT SAFETY & QUALITY CARE

Prevention of Complications Related to Intraoperative Positioning

PREVENTION OF BRACHIAL PLEXUS COMPLICATIONS (PARALYSIS, LOSS OF SENSATION IN ARM AND SHOULDER)
- Pad the elbow.
- Avoid excessive abduction.
- Secure the arm firmly on an armboard, positioned at shoulder level.

PREVENTION OF RADIAL NERVE COMPLICATIONS (WRIST DROP)
- Support the wrist with padding.
- Be careful not to overtighten wrist straps.

PREVENTION OF MEDIAL OR ULNAR NERVE COMPLICATIONS (HAND WEAKNESS, CLAW HAND)
- Place the safety strap above or below the nerve locations.

PREVENTION OF PERONEAL NERVE COMPLICATIONS (FOOT DROP)
- Pad knees and ankles.
- Maintain minimal external rotation of the hips.
- Support the lower extremities.
- Be careful not to overtighten leg straps.

PREVENTION OF TIBIAL NERVE COMPLICATIONS (LOSS OF SENSATION ON THE PLANTAR SURFACE OF THE FOOT)
- Place the safety strap above the ankle.
- Do not place equipment on lower extremities.
- Urge OR personnel to avoid leaning on the patient's lower extremities.

PREVENTION OF JOINT COMPLICATIONS (STIFFNESS, PAIN, INFLAMMATION, LIMITED MOTION)
- Place a pillow or foam padding under bony prominences.
- Maintain the patient's extremities in good anatomical alignment.
- Slightly flex joints and support with pillows, trochanter rolls, or pads.

slowly to prevent hypotension from blood vessel dilation. Proper positioning is ensured by assessing for:
- Anatomic alignment
- Interference with circulation and breathing
- Protection of skeletal and neuromuscular structures
- Optimal exposure of the operative site and IV line
- Adequate access to the patient for the anesthesia provider
- The patient's comfort and safety
- Preservation of the patient's dignity

Care is modified to reduce the potential complications related to specific positions. For example, patients in the lithotomy position may develop leg swelling, pain in the legs or back, reduced foot pulses, or reduced sensation from compression of the peroneal nerve. The nurse ensures proper padding and position changes at regular intervals. Throughout the surgery, the nurse prevents obstruction of circulation, respiration, or nerve conduction caused by tight straps, poorly placed pads and pillows, or the position of the bed (Wadlund, 2006).

DECISION-MAKING CHALLENGE
Coordination of Care

The patient is an 82-year-old thin woman (100 lbs) who has a pacemaker in place in the upper left side of her chest, just under the skin. She will be placed in the prone position for repair of a rectal prolapse. She also has arthritis in both shoulders.

1. What special interventions should be made for her weight and pacemaker?
2. What areas on this patient are most likely to be injured as a result of poor positioning or inadequate padding?
3. How will you determine safe arm positioning for this patient during her surgery?

evolve For suggested answer guidelines, go to http://evolve.elsevier.com/Iggy/.

Risk for Infection

NOC **Planning: Expected Outcomes.** The patient is expected to have an uninfected surgical wound or wounds. Indicators include:
- Wound edges are closed and not excessively red or swollen
- Wound is free from purulent drainage
- White blood cell counts remain at expected levels after surgery
- Patient is afebrile

Interventions. Surgical wound infections interfere with the patient's recovery, delay wound healing, contribute to rising health care costs, and are a major source of hospital-acquired infections. The Centers for Disease Control and Prevention (CDC) defines surgical site infections as occurring 30 days post-surgery and up to 1 year for transplant surgery (National Center for Health Care Statistics, 2007). Aseptic technique must be strictly practiced by all OR personnel to ensure that the patient is free from infection.

Assess the risk for infection, including identifying patients with pre-existing health problems such as diabetes mellitus, immune deficiency, obesity, and renal failure. The nurse performs the prescribed skin preparation, protects the patient's exposure to cross-contamination, keeps traffic control to a minimum, and administers prescribed antimicrobial prophylaxis. Surgery places the patient at risk for wound complications (e.g., incisional tears, lacerations), infection, and loss of body fluids. Sterile surgical technique and the use of protective drapes, skin closures, and dressings reduce complications and promote wound healing. When a wound is already infected or is at high risk for infection, antibiotics may be used directly in the wound by irrigation or by placing drug-impregnated beads into the surgical site before wound closure.

Skin and tissue closures include sutures, staples, and special tape. Fig. 17-11 shows commonly used wound closures. They are used to:
- Hold wound edges in place until wound healing is complete
- Occlude blood vessels, preventing hemorrhage and fluid loss
- Prevent wound contamination

Sutures are absorbable or nonabsorbable. **Absorbable sutures** are digested over time by body enzymes. **Nonabsorbable sutures** become encapsulated in the tissue during the healing process and remain in the tissue unless they are removed. Body enzymes do not affect nonabsorbable sutures. Retention

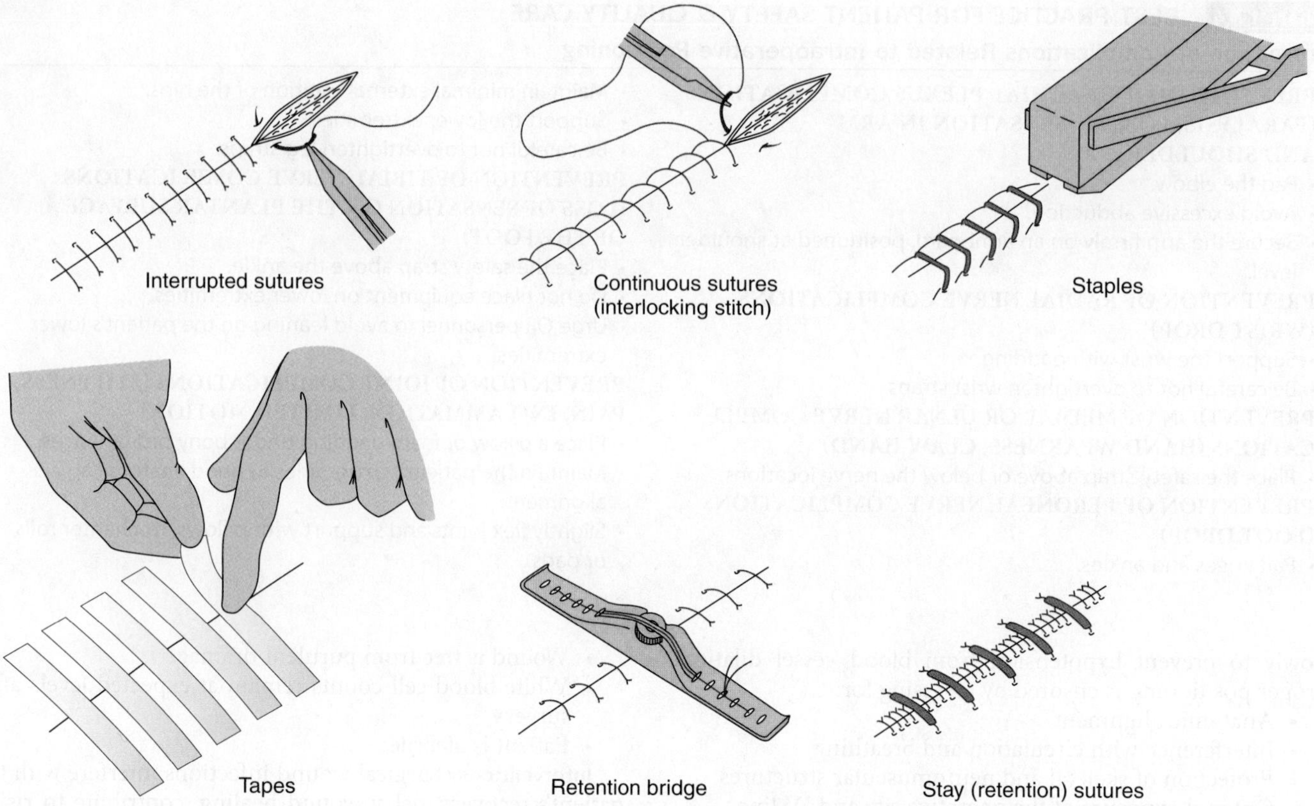

Interrupted sutures
Continuous sutures
(interlocking stitch)
Staples
Tapes
Retention bridge
Stay (retention) sutures

Fig. 17-11 • Common skin closures.

(stay) sutures (see Fig. 17-11) may be used in addition to standard sutures for patients at high risk for impaired wound healing (those having major abdominal surgery, obese patients, patients with diabetes, and those taking steroids).

After the incision is closed, the surgeon may inject a local anesthetic or instill an antibiotic into the wound. A gauze or spray dressing may be applied to protect the incision from contamination. A variety of dressings may also be used to absorb drainage and support the incision. A pressure dressing may be applied to prevent bleeding. One or more drains (see Chapter 18) may be inserted to remove secretions and fluids from within tissues around the surgical area. These secretions, if not drained, slow healing and promote bacterial growth, which could result in wound infection.

After the dressing is secure, the nurse coordinates the surgical team in positioning and transferring the patient. A roller board or a lift sheet is used to move the patient from the operating bed to a stretcher or bed. Some patients are able to move themselves over to the stretcher. The circulating nurse and anesthesia provider go with the patient to the PACU and report the patient's surgical experience to the PACU nurse (see Chapter 18).

Potential for Hypoventilation

NOC **Planning: Expected Outcomes.** The patient is expected to be free of damaging events related to hypoventilation as indicated by:

- Maintenance of Sao_2, Pao_2, and blood pH within normal limits
- Vital signs within normal limits
- Return to presurgical level of cognitive function

Interventions. Interventions aim to prevent injury resulting from anesthesia (see discussion on pp. 273-275). The nurse, surgeon, and anesthesia provider monitor the patient according to official standards. These standards, adopted by both the American Society of Anesthesiologists and the American Association of Nurse Anesthetists, include continuous monitoring of breathing, circulation, and cardiac rhythms; blood pressure and heart rate recordings every 5 minutes; and the continuous presence of an anesthesia provider during the case.

Evaluation: Outcomes

The nurse evaluates the care of the patient during surgery on the basis of the identified nursing diagnoses and collaborative problems. The expected outcomes are that the patient:

- Is safely anesthetized without complications
- Does not experience any injury related to surgical positioning or equipment
- Is free of skin or tissue contamination during surgery
- Is free of skin tears, bruises, redness, abrasion, or maceration over pressure points and elsewhere

Specific indicators for these outcomes are listed for each nursing diagnosis and collaborative problem under the Planning and Implementation section (see earlier).

GET READY FOR THE NCLEX EXAMINATION!

Key Points

Review these Key Points for each NCLEX Examination Client Needs Category.

Safe and Effective Care Environment

- Ensure that all personnel entering the OR are wearing proper OR attire for their role.
- Observe for and inform OR personnel of any break in sterile field or sterile technique.
- Use two identifiers to check the identity of the patient.
- Report to the surgeon any discrepancy between what type of surgery the patient says is going to be performed and what the informed consent form indicates.
- Review preoperative checklist and informed consent forms.
- Highlight any known allergies.
- Apply grounding pads as needed.
- Complete any needed skin preparation.
- Perform an accurate "sharps" and sponge count with the scrub nurse or surgical technologist.

Health Promotion and Maintenance

- Apply padding to the OR bed to maintain the patient's skin integrity.
- Position the patient comfortably and safely.

Psychosocial Integrity

- Encourage the patient to express his or her feelings about the surgical procedure or its possible outcome.
- Communicate patient preferences or fears about anesthesia to the anesthesia provider.
- Preserve the patient's privacy and dignity by keeping body exposure to a minimum.
- Stay with the patient during induction of anesthesia.
- Communicate information about the patient's status to waiting family members.
- Ensure that the patient's wishes, as expressed in the advance directives statement, are honored in the surgical setting.

Physiological Integrity

- Ask the patient when was the last time he or she had anything to eat or drink.
- Assess the patient for tachycardia, increased end-tidal carbon dioxide level, and increased body temperature as indicators of malignant hyperthermia.
- Maintain the malignant hyperthermia cart.
- Monitor the patient's airway, level of consciousness, oxygen saturation, ECG, and vital signs during and immediately after moderate sedation.
- Assess all skin areas and document findings before transferring the patient to the postanesthesia care unit.

Additional Study Resources

Go to your Companion CD or Evolve at http://evolve.elsevier.com/Iggy/ for *Self-Assessment Questions for the NCLEX Examination.*

Go to Evolve at http://evolve.elsevier.com/Iggy/ for *Prioritization and Delegation Questions for the NCLEX Examination.*

SELECTED BIBLIOGRAPHY

Asterisk indicates a classic or definitive work on this subject.

*American Society of PeriAnesthesia Nurses (ASPAN). (2000). *Standards of perianesthesia nursing practice.* New Jersey: Author.

Association of periOperative Registered Nurses (AORN). (2007a). Position statement: AORN official statement on RN first assistants. In *Standards, recommended practices and guidelines* (pp. 404-405). Denver: Author.

Association of periOperative Registered Nurses (AORN). (2007b). Position statement: Perioperative care of patients with do not resuscitate (DNR) orders. In *Standards, recommended practices and guidelines* (pp. 377-378). Denver: Author.

Association of periOperative Registered Nurses (AORN). (2007c). Recommended practices for the care and cleaning of surgical instruments and powered equipment. In *Standards, recommended practices and guidelines* (pp. 583-591). Denver: Author.

Association of periOperative Registered Nurses (AORN). (2007d). Recommended practices for high-level disinfection. In *Standards, recommended practices and guidelines* (pp. 503-509). Denver: Author.

Association of periOperative Registered Nurses (AORN). (2007e). Recommended practices for documentation of perioperative nursing care. In *Standards, recommended practices and guidelines* (pp. 511-513). Denver: Author.

Association of periOperative Registered Nurses (AORN). (2007f). Recommended practices for environmental cleaning in the surgical practice setting. In *Standards, recommended practices and guidelines* (pp. 551-557). Denver: Author.

Association of periOperative Registered Nurses (AORN). (2007g). Recommended practices for safe care through identification of potential hazards in the surgical environment. In *Standards, recommended practices and guidelines* (pp. 575-581). Denver: Author.

Association of periOperative Registered Nurses (AORN). (2007h). Recommended practices for laser safety in the practice settings. In *Standards, recommended practices and guidelines* (pp. 593-598). Denver: Author.

Association of periOperative Registered Nurses (AORN). (2007i). Recommended practices for managing the patient receiving moderate sedation/analgesia. In *Standards, recommended practices and guidelines* (pp. 467-474). Denver: Author.

Association of periOperative Registered Nurses (AORN). (2007j). Recommended practices for positioning the patient in the perioperative practice setting. In *Standards, recommended practices and guidelines* (pp. 631-636). Denver: Author.

Association of periOperative Registered Nurses (AORN). (2007k). Recommended practices for skin preparation of patients. In *Standards, recommended practices and guidelines* (pp. 653-656). Denver: Author.

Association of periOperative Registered Nurses (AORN). (2007l). Recommended practices for sponge, sharp, and instrument counts. In *Standards, recommended practices and guidelines* (pp. 493-502). Denver: Author.

Association of periOperative Registered Nurses (AORN). (2007m). Recommended practices for maintaining a sterile field. In *Standards, recommended practices and guidelines* (pp. 665-672). Denver: Author.

Association of periOperative Registered Nurses (AORN). (2007n). Recommended practices for sterilization in the perioperative practice setting. In *Standards, recommended practices and guidelines* (pp. 673-687). Denver: Author.

Association of periOperative Registered Nurses (AORN). (2007o). Recommended practices for surgical attire. In *Standards, recommended practices and guidelines* (pp. 485-491). Denver: Author.

Association of periOperative Registered Nurses (AORN). (2007p). Recommended practices for surgical hand antisepsis/hand scrubs. In *Standards, recommended practices and guidelines* (pp. 565-573). Denver: Author.

Association of periOperative Registered Nurses (AORN). (2007q). Recommended practices for traffic patterns in the perioperative practice setting. In *Standards, recommended practices and guidelines* (pp. 703-706). Denver: Author.

Association of periOperative Registered Nurses (AORN). (2007r). Recommended practices for selection and use of surgical gowns and drapes. In *Standards, recommended practices and guidelines* (pp. 559-563). Denver: Author.

Association of periOperative Registered Nurses (AORN). (2007s). Recommended practices for skin preparation of patients. In *Standards, recommended practices and guidelines* (pp. 653-656). Denver: Author.

Association of periOperative Registered Nurses (AORN). (2007t). Statement on correct site surgery. In *Standards, recommended practices and guidelines* (p. 371). Denver: Author.

Bartely, M. (2006). Preventing venous thromboembolism. *Nursing2006, 36*(1), 64cc1-64cc4.

Birch, D., Asiri, A., & de Gara, C. (2007). The impact of a formal mentoring program for minimally invasive surgery on surgeon practice and patient outcomes. *American Journal of Surgery, 193*(5), 589-591.

Bragg, K., VanBalen, N., & Cook, N. (2005). Future trends in minimally invasive surgery. *AORN Journal, 82*(6), 1006-1018.

Bulechek, G.M., Butcher, H.K., & McCloskey Dochterman, J. (Eds.). (2008). *Nursing interventions classification (NIC)* (5th ed.). St. Louis: Mosby.

Conlon, N., Sullivan, R., Herbison, P., Zacharias, M., & Buggy, D. (2007). The effect of leaving dentures in place on bag-mask ventilation at induction of general anesthesia. *Anesthesia and Analgesia, 105*(2), 370-373.

DeLamar, L. (2007). Anesthesia. In J.C. Rothrock & D. McEwen (Eds.), *Alexander's care of the patient in surgery* (13th ed., Chapter 4). St. Louis: Mosby.

Dixon, B. (2006). Is your patient susceptible to malignant hyperthermia? *Nursing2006, 36*(12), 26-27.

Dunn, D. (2005). Preventing perioperative complications in special populations. *Nursing2005, 35*(11), 36-43.

Harrell, A., & Heniford, B.T. (2005). Minimally invasive surgery: Lux et veritas past, present, and future. *American Journal of Surgery, 190*(2), 239-243.

Hommertzheim, R., & Steinke, E.E. (2006). Malignant hyperthermia: The perioperative nurse's role. *AORN, 83*(1), 149-164.

Jackson, S., & Brady, S. (2008). Counting difficulties: Retained instruments, sponges, and needles. *AORN Journal, 87*(2), 315-321.

McCance, K., & Huether, S. (2006). *Pathophysiology: The biologic basis for disease in adults and children* (5th ed.). St. Louis: Mosby.

McEwen, D. (2007). Ambulatory surgery. In J.C. Rothrock & D. McEwen (Eds.), *Alexander's care of the patient in surgery* (13th ed.). St. Louis: Mosby.

Meiner, S., & Lueckenotte, A. (Eds.). (2006). *Gerontologic nursing* (3rd ed.). St. Louis: Mosby.

Metules, T., & Bauer, J. (2006). JCAHO's patient safety goals: A practical guide, Part 1. *RN, 69*(12), 21-26.

Millsaps, C. (2006). Pay attention to patient positioning! *RN, 69*(1), 59-63.

Moorhead, S., Johnson, M., & Maas, M. (Eds.). (2004). *Nursing outcomes classification (NOC)* (3rd ed.). St. Louis: Mosby.

National Center for Health Care Statistics. (2007). *National survey of ambulatory surgery.* Retrieved March 15, 2008, from www.cdc.gov/nchs/nsas.htm.

Nussbaum, R., McInnes, R., & Willard, H. (2007). *Thompson & Thompson: Genetics in medicine* (7th ed.). Philadelphia: Saunders.

Odom-Forren, J. (2006). Preventing surgical site infections. *Nursing2006, 36*(6), 59-63.

Ridge, R. (2008). Patient safety: Doing right to prevent wrong-site surgery. *Nursing2008, 38*(3), 24-25.

Rothrock, J.C., & McEwen, D. (2007). *Alexander's care of the patient in surgery* (13th ed.). St. Louis: Mosby.

*Schoonhoven, L., Defloor, T., & Grypdonck, M. (2002). Incidence of pressure ulcers due to surgery. *Journal of Clinical Nursing, 11*(4), 479-487.

Schwoen, S. (2006). Stamping out surgical site infections. *RN, 69*(8), 36-40.

Wadlund, D. (2006). Prevention, recognition, and management of nursing complications in the intraoperative and postoperative surgical patient. *Nursing Clinics of North America, 41*(2), 151-171.

Weirich, T. (2008). Hypothermia/warming protocols: Why are they not widely used in the OR? *AORN Journal, 87*(2), 333-344.

Care of Postoperative Patients

Robin Chard

18 CHAPTER

LEARNING OUTCOMES

For clinical competence and success on the NCLEX Examination, study this chapter with these Learning Outcomes in mind:

Safe and Effective Care Environment

1. Apply concepts of sterile technique, asepsis, and Standard Precautions during wound assessment and dressing changes.
2. Use specific agency criteria for determining readiness of the patient to be discharged from the postanesthesia care unit.

Health Promotion and Maintenance

3. Evaluate patient risk for complications of wound healing.
4. Provide postoperative education for patients and family members after surgery.

Physiological Integrity

5. Perform an ongoing head-to-toe assessment of the postoperative patient.
6. Prioritize nursing interventions for the patient recovering from surgery and anesthesia during the first 24 hours.
7. Apply knowledge of pathophysiology to monitor the patient for the complications of shock, respiratory depression, or impaired wound healing after surgery.
8. Assess the patient's level of postoperative pain, and evaluate his or her responses to coordinated pain management strategies and interventions.
9. Explain the actions, dosages, side effects, and nursing implications for different types of drug therapy for pain management after surgery.
10. Evaluate surgical incisions and wounds for complications.
11. Collaborate with health care team members to perform emergency care procedures for surgical wound dehiscence or wound evisceration.

Go to your Companion CD or Evolve at http://evolve.elsevier.com/Iggy/ for *Self-Assessment Questions for the NCLEX Examination* keyed to these Learning Outcomes.

The postoperative period starts at the completion of surgery and transfer of the patient to either the postanesthesia care unit (PACU), the same-day surgery (SDS) unit (ambulatory care unit), or the intensive care unit (ICU). Discharge from these areas is based on the stability of the patient and the meeting of specific discharge criteria. Many patients can be discharged to home shortly after the surgery is completed. They are observed and monitored until discharge criteria are met and are then discharged. Some patients move from the specialized nursing care in the PACU to a hospital inpatient floor or ICU for additional nursing care.

The postoperative period continues after the patient's condition is stabilized, as well as after the patient is discharged from the ambulatory surgery facility or hospital. The actual time spent away from home after surgery varies according to age, physical health, self-care ability, support systems, type and length of surgical procedure, anesthesia, any complications, and community resources.

Overview

The purpose of a **postanesthesia care unit (PACU)** (recovery room) is the ongoing evaluation and stabilization of patients to anticipate, prevent, and treat complications after surgery. The PACU is usually located close to the surgical suite for ease of access and patient transfer. The unit is usually a large and open room to provide best observation of all patients and easy access to supplies and emergency equipment. Adults are usually separated from children. The patient area may be divided into individual cubicles. So that each patient can be observed continuously, privacy curtains or screens are closed only during bedside procedures. Each cubicle has equipment to monitor and care for the patient, such as oxygen, suction equipment, cardiac monitors, pulse oximetry, airway equipment, and emergency drugs.

After the surgery is completed, the circulating nurse and the anesthesia provider accompany the patient to the PACU. When the patient is in critical condition, transfer may be directly from the operating room (OR) to the ICU. On arrival, the anesthesia provider and the circulating nurse give the PACU nurse a verbal "hand-off" report to communicate the patient's condition and care needs.

A hand-off report that meets National Patient Safety Goal 2 requires effective communication between health care professionals. It is at least a two-way verbal interaction between the professional giving the report and the nurse receiving it. The language used by the person or persons giving the report is clear and cannot be interpreted in more than one way. The nurse receiving the report focuses on the report and is not distracted by the environment or other responsibilities. Standardizing the information reported helps prevent omission of critical patient-centered information and helps avoid irrelevant details. The receiving nurse takes the time to restate (report back) the information to verify what was said and to make certain both the reporting professional and the receiving nurse have the same understanding. The receiving nurse takes the time to ask questions and the reporting professional must respond to the questions until a common understanding is established. Chart 18-1 gives an example of critical information to include in a standard hand-off report.

The PACU nurse is skilled in the care of patients with multiple medical and surgical problems immediately after a surgical procedure. This area requires in-depth knowledge of anatomy and physiology, anesthetic agents, pharmacology, pain management, extubation, and surgical procedures. The PACU nurse is skilled in assessment and can make quick decisions if emergencies or complications occur. The patient is monitored closely. The anesthesia provider and surgeon are consulted as needed.

Patient-Centered Collaborative Care

evolve ONLINE PHARM REVIEW

Assessment

History

Use the surgical team's report to plan the care for an individual patient. After receiving the report and assessing the patient, review the medical record for information about the patient's history, presurgical physical condition, and emotional status. If the patient remains as an inpatient, the surgical and anesthesia information is incorporated into the postoperative plan of care. Chapter 16 identifies situations that increase a patient's risk for the potential complications listed in Table 18-1.

Physical Assessment/Clinical Manifestations

Assess the patient, and record data on a PACU flow chart record (Fig. 18-1). Assessment data include level of consciousness, temperature, pulse, respiration, oxygen saturation, and blood pressure. *The most important assessment is respiratory* (Pruitt, 2006; Wadlund, 2006). Examine the surgical area for bleeding. Monitor vital signs as often as your facility's policy states, the patient's condition warrants, and the surgeon prescribes. Once the patient is discharged from the PACU, vital signs are often measured every 15 minutes for four times, every 30 minutes for four times, every 2 hours for four times, and then every 4 hours for 24 to 48 hours if the patient's condition is stable. Thereafter, if the patient is admitted, vital signs are assessed according to the facility's policy, the patient's condition, and the nurse's judgment.

The health care team determines the patient's readiness for discharge from the PACU by the presence of a recovery score rating of at least 10 on the recovery scale (see Fig. 18-1). Other criteria for discharge (e.g., stable vital signs; normal body temperature; no overt bleeding; return of gag, cough, and swallow reflexes; and the ability to take liquids) may be specific to the facility. After you determine that all criteria have been met, the patient is discharged by the anesthesia provider to the hospital unit or to home. If an anesthesia provider has not been involved, which may be the case with local anesthesia or moderate sedation, the surgeon or nurse discharges the patient once the discharge criteria have been met.

Chart 18-1 BEST PRACTICE FOR PATIENT SAFETY & QUALITY CARE

Postoperative Hand-off Report

- Type and extent of the surgical procedure
- Type of anesthesia and length of time the patient was under anesthesia
- Tolerance of anesthesia and the surgical procedure
- Allergies (especially to latex or drugs)
- Pathologic condition
- Oxygen saturation
- Status of vital signs
- Core body temperature
- Type and amount of IV fluids and drugs administered
- Estimated blood loss (EBL)
- Any intraoperative complications, such as a traumatic intubation
- Preoperative drugs and patient responses
- Primary language, any sensory impairments, any communication difficulties
- Anxiety level before receiving anesthesia
- Special requests that were verbalized by the patient preoperatively
- Preoperative and intraoperative respiratory function and dysfunction
- Pertinent medical history, including substance abuse
- Location and type of incisions, dressings, catheters, tubes, drains, or packing
- Intake and output, including current IV fluid administration and estimated blood loss
- Prosthetic devices
- Joint or limb immobility while in the operating room, especially in the older patient
- Other intraoperative positioning that may be relevant in the postoperative phase
- Intraoperative complications, how managed, patient responses
- Any other important intraoperative occurrences

Assessment continues from the PACU to the intensive care or medical-surgical nursing unit. If the patient is to be discharged from the PACU to home, assessment is continued by home care nurses or by the patient or family members after health teaching. When the patient is transferred to an inpatient unit, complete an initial assessment on arrival (Chart 18-2).

During the postoperative period, all patients remain at risk for pneumonia, shock, cardiac arrest, respiratory arrest, deep vein thrombosis, and GI bleeding. These serious complications can be prevented or the consequences reduced with coordinated care (Pruitt, 2006; Wadlund, 2006). Nursing observations and interventions are part of critical rescue management for patient safety and quality care to reduce the risk for an adverse patient outcome after surgery.

Respiratory System. *When the patient is admitted to the PACU, immediately assess for a patent airway and adequate gas exchange. Although some patients may be awake and able to speak, talking is not a good indicator of adequate gas exchange.*

TABLE 18-1 General Potential Complications of Surgery

RESPIRATORY SYSTEM COMPLICATIONS
• Atelectasis
• Pneumonia
• Pulmonary embolism (PE)
• Laryngeal edema
• Ventilator dependence
• Pulmonary edema
CARDIOVASCULAR COMPLICATIONS
• Hypertension
• Hypotension
• Hypovolemic shock
• Dysrhythmias
• Deep vein thrombosis (DVT)
• Heart failure
• Sepsis
• Disseminated intravascular coagulation (DIC)
• Anemia
• Anaphylaxis
SKIN COMPLICATIONS
• Pressure ulcers
• Wound infection
• Wound dehiscence
• Wound evisceration
• Skin rashes
• Contact allergies
GASTROINTESTINAL COMPLICATIONS
• Paralytic ileus
• Gastrointestinal ulcers and bleeding
NEUROMUSCULAR COMPLICATIONS
• Hypothermia
• Hyperthermia
• Nerve damage and paralysis
• Joint contractures
RENAL URINARY COMPLICATIONS
• Urinary tract infection
• Acute urinary retention
• Electrolyte imbalances
• Renal failure

An artificial airway, such as an endotracheal (ET) tube, a nasal trumpet, or an oral airway, may be in place. If the patient is receiving oxygen, document the type of delivery device and the concentration or liter flow of the oxygen. Continuously monitor pulse oximetry for oxygen saturation (Spo_2) while the patient is in the PACU. The Spo_2 should be above 95% (or at the patient's presurgery baseline). If it drops below this level, notify the surgeon or anesthesia provider. If it drops by 10 percentage points and you are certain it is an accurate measure, call the Rapid Response Team.

Assess the rate, pattern, and depth of breathing to determine adequacy of air exchange. A respiratory rate of less than 10 breaths per minute may indicate anesthetic- or opioid analgesic–induced depression. Rapid, shallow respirations may signal shock, cardiac problems, increased metabolic rate, or pain.

Listen to the lungs over all lung fields to assess breath sounds. Also check symmetry of breath sounds and chest movement. If, for example, the patient has an ET tube, it could move down into the right mainstem bronchus and prevent left lung expansion. In this case, lung sounds on the left are absent or decreased and only the right chest wall rises and falls with breathing.

Perform ongoing inspection of the chest wall for accessory muscle use, sternal retraction, and diaphragmatic breathing. These signs could indicate an excessive anesthetic effect, airway obstruction, or paralysis, which could result in hypoxia. Listen for snoring and **stridor** (a high-pitched crowing sound). Snoring and stridor occur with airway obstruction resulting from tracheal or laryngeal spasm or edema, mucus in the airway, or blockage of the airway from edema or tongue relaxation. When neuromuscular blocking agents are retained, the patient has muscle weakness, which could affect gas exchange. Indicators of muscle weakness include the inability to maintain a head lift, weak hand grasps, and an abdominal breathing pattern.

◄ AUDIO CLIP: Stridor

If the patient returns to an inpatient unit, complete an initial assessment on arrival (see Chart 18-2) and then continue to assess for respiratory depression or hypoxemia. Listen to the lungs to check for effective expansion and for abnormal breath sounds. Check the lungs at least every 4 hours during the first 24 hours after surgery and then every 8 hours, or more often, as indicated. Older patients, smokers, and patients with a history of lung disease are at greater risk for respiratory complications after surgery and need more frequent assessment (Litwack, 2006). Obese patients are also at high risk for respiratory complications (Wadlund, 2006).

Cardiovascular System. *Vital signs* and heart sounds are assessed on admission to the PACU and then at least every 15 minutes until the patient's condition is stable. Automated blood pressure cuffs and cardiac monitoring assist in continuous assessment.

Review vital signs after surgery for trends, and compare them with those taken before surgery. Report blood pressure changes that are 25% higher or lower than values obtained before surgery (15- to 20-point difference, systolic or diastolic) to the anesthesia provider or the surgeon. Decreased blood pressure and pulse pressure and abnormal heart sounds indicate possible cardiac depression, fluid volume deficit, shock, hemorrhage, or the effects of drugs (see Chapters 13 and 39). Bradycardia could indicate an anesthesia effect or

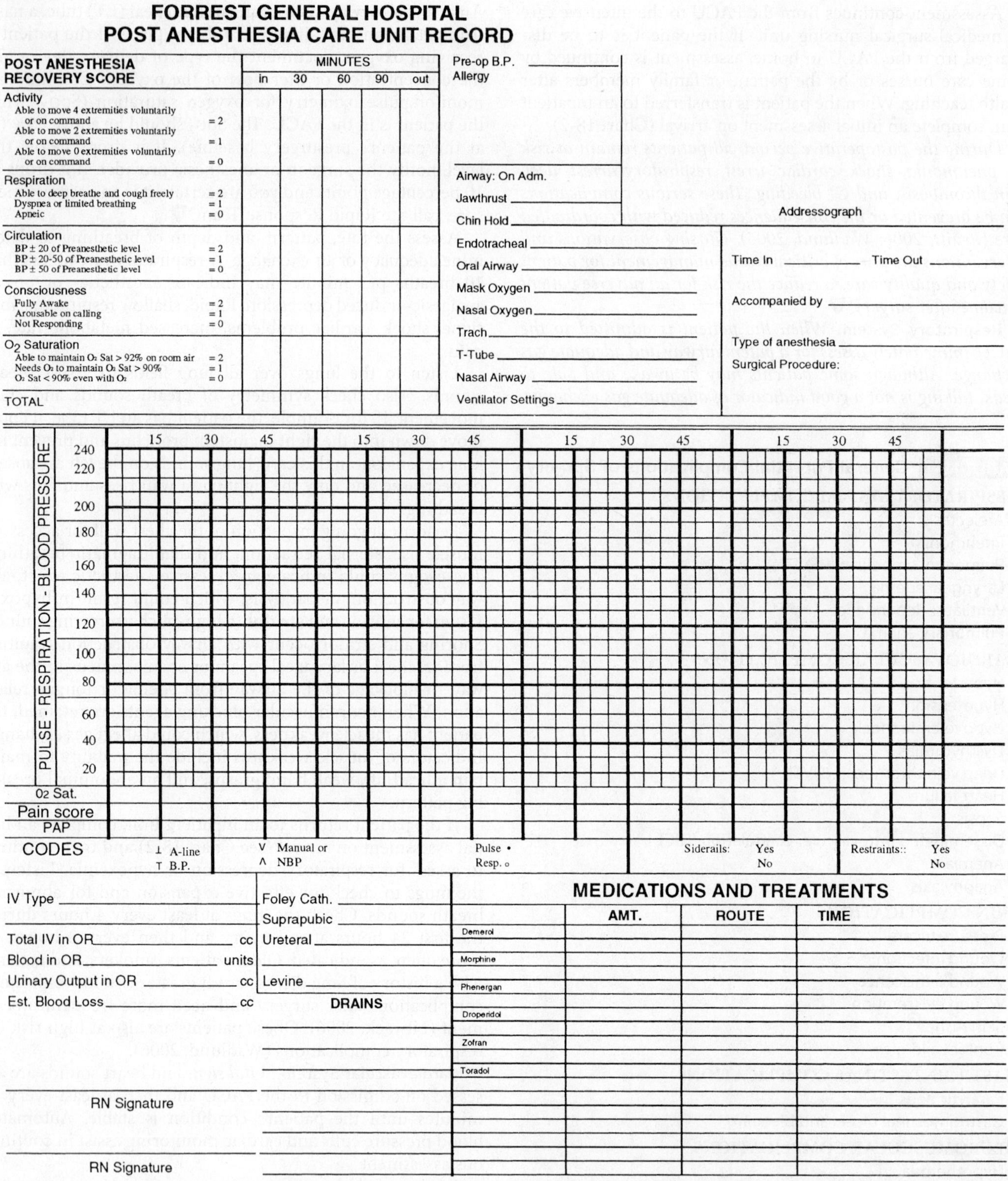

FORREST GENERAL HOSPITAL
POST ANESTHESIA CARE UNIT RECORD

POST ANESTHESIA RECOVERY SCORE		MINUTES in	30	60	90	out
Activity						
Able to move 4 extremities voluntarily or on command	= 2					
Able to move 2 extremities voluntarily or on command	= 1					
Able to move 0 extremities voluntarily or on command	= 0					
Respiration						
Able to deep breathe and cough freely	= 2					
Dyspnea or limited breathing	= 1					
Apneic	= 0					
Circulation						
BP ± 20 of Preanesthetic level	= 2					
BP ± 20-50 of Preanesthetic level	= 1					
BP ± 50 of Preanesthetic level	= 0					
Consciousness						
Fully Awake	= 2					
Arousable on calling	= 1					
Not Responding	= 0					
O_2 Saturation						
Able to maintain O_2 Sat > 92% on room air	= 2					
Needs O_2 to maintain O_2 Sat > 90%	= 1					
O_2 Sat < 90% even with O_2	= 0					
TOTAL						

Pre-op B.P. ______
Allergy
Airway: On Adm.
Jawthrust ______
Chin Hold ______
Endotracheal ______
Oral Airway ______
Mask Oxygen ______
Nasal Oxygen ______
Trach ______
T-Tube ______
Nasal Airway ______
Ventilator Settings ______

Addressograph
Time In ______ Time Out ______
Accompanied by ______
Type of anesthesia ______
Surgical Procedure:

PULSE - RESPIRATION - BLOOD PRESSURE
15 30 45 15 30 45 15 30 45 15 30 45
240
220
200
180
160
140
120
100
80
60
40
20
O_2 Sat.
Pain score
PAP
CODES ⊥ A-line T B.P. V Manual or Λ NBP Pulse • Resp. ○ Siderails: Yes No Restraints:: Yes No

IV Type ______
Total IV in OR ______ cc
Blood in OR ______ units
Urinary Output in OR ______ cc
Est. Blood Loss ______ cc

Foley Cath.
Suprapubic
Ureteral
Levine
DRAINS

MEDICATIONS AND TREATMENTS

	AMT.	ROUTE	TIME
Demerol			
Morphine			
Phenergan			
Droperidol			
Zofran			
Toradol			

RN Signature ______
RN Signature ______

Fig. 18-1 • Example of a postanesthesia care unit record.

hypothermia. Older patients are at risk for hypothermia because of age-related changes in the hypothalamus (the temperature regulation center), low levels of body fat, and coolness of the OR suite (Meiner & Lueckenotte, 2006). An increased pulse rate could indicate hemorrhage, shock, or pain.

Cardiac monitoring is maintained until the patient is discharged from the PACU. For patients at risk for dysrhythmias, monitoring may continue either on telemetry units or on general medical-surgical units. In assessing the vital signs of a patient who is not being monitored continuously, compare the rate, rhythm, and quality of the apical pulse with the rate,

Chart 18-2 FOCUSED ASSESSMENT

The Patient on Arrival at the Medical-Surgical Unit After Discharge from the Postanesthesia Care Unit

AIRWAY
- Is it patent?
- Is the neck in proper alignment?

BREATHING
- What is the quality and pattern of the breathing?
- What is the respiratory rate and depth?
- Is the patient receiving oxygen? At what setting? What is the pulse oximetry result?

MENTAL STATUS
- Is the patient awake, able to be aroused, oriented, and aware?
- Does the patient respond to verbal stimuli?

SURGICAL INCISION SITE
- How is it dressed?
- Mark the amount of drainage on the dressing immediately.
- Is there any bleeding or drainage under the patient?
- Are any drains present?
- Are the drains set properly (e.g., compressed if they should be compressed, not kinked, patient not lying on them)?
- How much drainage is present in the drainage container?

TEMPERATURE, PULSE, AND BLOOD PRESSURE
- Are these values within the patient's baseline range?
- Are these values significantly different from when the patient was in the postanesthesia care unit (PACU)?

INTRAVENOUS FLUIDS
- What type of solution is infusing and with what additives?
- How much solution was remaining on arrival?
- How much solution infused in the transport time from PACU?
- At what rate is the infusion supposed to be set? Is it?

OTHER TUBES
- Is there a nasogastric or other intestinal tube?
- What is the color, consistency, and amount of drainage?
- Is suction applied to the tube if ordered? Is the suction setting correct?
- Is there a Foley catheter?
- Is the Foley draining properly?
- What is the color, clarity, and volume of urine output?

TABLE 18-2 Immediate Postoperative Neurologic Assessment: Return to Preoperative Level

ORDER OF RETURN TO CONSCIOUSNESS AFTER GENERAL ANESTHESIA
1. Muscular irritability
2. Restlessness and delirium
3. Recognition of pain
4. Ability to reason and control behavior

ORDER OF RETURN OF MOTOR AND SENSORY FUNCTIONING AFTER LOCAL OR REGIONAL ANESTHESIA
1. Sense of touch
2. Sense of pain
3. Sense of warmth
4. Sense of cold
5. Ability to move

rhythm, and quality of a peripheral pulse, such as the radial pulse. A **pulse deficit** (a difference between the apical and peripheral pulses) could indicate a dysrhythmia.

Peripheral vascular assessment needs to be performed because anesthesia and positioning during surgery (e.g., the lithotomy position for genitourinary procedures) may impair the peripheral circulation and contribute to deep vein thrombosis (DVT) (Owens, 2008; Wadlund, 2006). Compare distal pulses on both feet for the quality of pulsation, observe the color and temperature of extremities, evaluate sensation, and determine the speed of capillary refill. Palpable pedal pulses indicate adequate circulation and perfusion of the legs.

Assess the feet and legs for redness, pain, warmth, and swelling, which may occur with DVT. Foot and leg assessment may be performed once during a nursing shift, once daily, or once per visit, depending on the patient's risk for complications and the facility's or agency's policy. (See Chapters 16 and 38 for more information on DVT.)

Neurologic System. *Cerebral functioning* and the level of consciousness or awareness must be assessed in *all* patients who have received general anesthesia (Table 18-2) or any type of sedation. Observe for lethargy, restlessness, or irritability, and test coherence and orientation. Determine awareness by observing responses to calling the patient's name, touching the patient, and giving simple commands such as "Open your eyes" and "Take a deep breath." Eye opening in response to a command indicates wakefulness or arousability but not necessarily awareness. Determine the degree of orientation to person, place, and time by asking the conscious patient to answer questions such as "What is your name?" (person), "Where are you?" (place), and "What day is it?" (time).

CONSIDERATIONS FOR OLDER ADULTS

For an older adult, a rapid return to his or her level of orientation before surgery may not be realistic. Preoperative drugs and anesthetics often delay the older patient's return of orientation (see Chapters 16 and 17).

Compare the patient's baseline neurologic status (obtained before surgery) with the findings after surgery. Patients who had altered cerebral functioning before surgery as a result of another condition usually continue to have that alteration after surgery. After the patient is alert (and all other criteria have been met), he or she is discharged from the PACU. On the medical-surgical nursing unit, assess the level of consciousness every 4 to 8 hours or as indicated by the patient's condition and the facility's policy.

Motor function and sensory function are assessed for all patients who received general or regional anesthesia. General anesthesia depresses all voluntary motor function. Regional anesthesia alters the motor and sensory function of only part of the body. (See Chapter 17 for more information on anesthesia.) *Motor and sensory assessments are very important after epidural or spinal anesthesia.* Evaluate motor function by asking the patient to move each extremity. The patient who had epidural or spinal anesthesia remains in the PACU until sensory function (feeling) and voluntary motor movement of the legs have returned (see Table 18-2). Also assess the strength of each limb, and compare the results on both sides.

Test for the return of sympathetic nervous system tone by gradually elevating the patient's head and monitoring for hypotension. Begin this evaluation after the patient's sensation has returned to at least the spinal dermatome level of T10. (See Chapter 43 for further neurologic assessment.) After the patient is transferred to the nursing unit, continue neurologic assessment as indicated.

Fluid, Electrolyte, and Acid-Base Balance. Fasting before and during surgery, the loss of fluid during the procedure, and the type and amount of blood or fluid given affect the patient's fluid and electrolyte balance after surgery. Fluid volume deficit or fluid volume overload may occur after surgery. Sodium, potassium, chloride, and calcium imbalances also may result, as may changes in other electrolyte levels. Fluid and electrolyte imbalances occur more often in older or debilitated patients and in those with health problems such as diabetes mellitus, Crohn's disease, or heart failure.

Intake and output measurement is part of the operative record and is reported by the circulating nurse to the PACU nurse. Record any intake or output, including IV fluid intake, vomitus, urine, wound drainage, and nasogastric (NG) tube drainage. You must know the total intake and output from both the OR and the PACU to assess fluid balance accurately and to complete the 24-hour intake and output record.

Hydration status is assessed in the PACU and the medical-surgical unit. To determine hydration status, inspect the color and moisture of mucous membranes; the turgor, texture, and "tenting" of the skin (test over the sternum or forehead of an older patient); the amount of drainage on dressings; and the presence of axillary sweat. Measure and compare total output (e.g., NG tube drainage, urine output, wound drainage) with total intake to identify a possible fluid imbalance. Consider insensible fluid loss, such as sweat, when reviewing total output. Continue to assess intake and output as long as the patient is at risk for fluid imbalances. Some facilities require intake and output to be measured if the patient receives IV fluids or has a catheter, drains, or an NG tube. In addition, patients who have heart disease or kidney disease may need a longer period of intake and output measurement.

IV fluids are closely monitored to promote fluid and electrolyte balance. Isotonic solutions such as lactated Ringer's (LR), 0.9% saline, and 5% dextrose with lactated Ringer's (D_5/LR) are used for IV fluid replacement in the PACU. After the patient returns to the medical-surgical unit, the type and rate of IV infusions are based on need. A typical IV solution for the patient being admitted to the nursing unit is 5% dextrose with 0.45% normal saline (D_5 0.45% NS). (See Chapters 13 and 15 for further discussion of IV fluids, electrolyte balance, and hydration assessment.)

Acid-base balance is affected by the patient's respiratory status before and during surgery; metabolic changes during surgery; and losses of acids or bases in drainage. For example, NG tube drainage or vomitus causes a loss of hydrochloric acid and leads to metabolic alkalosis. Examine arterial blood gas values and other laboratory values. (See Chapter 14 for more detailed information on acid-base imbalances.)

Renal/Urinary System. Control of urination may return immediately after surgery or may not return for hours after general or regional anesthesia. The effects of preoperative drugs (especially atropine), anesthetic agents, or manipulation during surgery can cause urine retention. Assess for urine retention by inspection, palpation, and percussion of the lower abdomen for bladder distention or by the use of a bladder scanner (see Chapter 68). Assessment may be difficult to perform after lower abdominal surgery. Urine retention is common early after surgery and requires intervention, such as intermittent (straight) catheterization, to empty the bladder.

When the patient has an indwelling urinary (Foley) catheter, assess the urine for color, clarity, and amount. If the patient is voiding, assess the frequency, amount per void, and any symptoms. Urine output should be close to the total intake for a 24-hour period. Consider other sources of output, such as sweat, vomitus, or diarrhea stools. Report a urine output of less than 30 mL/hr (240 mL per 8-hour nursing shift) to the physician. Decreased urine output may indicate hypovolemia or renal complications. (See Chapter 68 for renal/urinary assessment.)

Gastrointestinal System. *Nausea and vomiting* are among the most common reactions after surgery. About 30% of patients who receive general anesthesia have some form of GI upset within the first 24 hours after surgery. Preventive drug therapy is effective in reducing the incidence. A drug often used is ondansetron (Zofran), a serotonin antagonist. Patients with a history of motion sickness are more likely to develop nausea and vomiting after surgery. Obese patients may be at risk because many anesthetics are retained by fat cells and remain in the body longer. Abdominal surgery and the use of opioid analgesics reduce intestinal peristalsis after surgery. These problems increase the risk for prolonged nausea and vomiting after surgery.

Nausea and vomiting can stress and irritate abdominal and GI wounds, increase intracranial pressure in patients who had head and neck surgery, elevate intraocular pressure in patients who had eye surgery, and increase the risk for aspiration. Assess the patient continuously for nausea and vomiting. Often patients have nausea as the head of the bed is raised early after surgery. This symptom may occur with or without dizziness. You can help reduce this distressing symptom by having the patient in a side-lying position before raising the head slowly.

Intestinal peristalsis may be delayed because of long anesthesia time, the amount of bowel handling during surgery, and opioid analgesic use. In the PACU and later on the medical-surgical unit, assess for the return of peristalsis. Patients who have abdominal surgery often have decreased or no peristalsis for at least 24 hours. This problem may persist for several days for those who have GI surgery.

Listen for bowel sounds in all four abdominal quadrants and at the umbilicus. If NG suction is being used, turn off the suction before listening to prevent mistaking the sound of the suction for bowel sounds. *The presence of active bowel sounds usually indicates return of peristalsis; however, the absence of bowel sounds does not confirm a lack of peristalsis. The best indicator of intestinal activity is the passage of flatus or stool.* Abdominal cramping along with distention denotes trapped, nonmoving gas—not peristalsis.

Decreased peristalsis occurs in patients who have a paralytic ileus. The abdominal wall is distended, and there is no movement of the intestinal wall. Assess for the manifestations of paralytic ileus (few or absent bowel sounds, a distended abdomen, abdominal discomfort, vomiting, no passage of flatus or stool).

A nasogastric (NG) tube may be inserted during surgery to decompress and drain the stomach, to promote GI rest, to allow the lower GI tract to heal, and to provide an enteral feeding route. It may also be used to monitor any gastric bleeding and to prevent intestinal obstruction. One of the most common tubes used is the Salem sump. The Salem sump is a double-lumen tube with an air vent to keep the tube from grabbing the gastric mucosa. This feature allows easy drainage of the stomach and prevents mucosal damage. Less commonly used is the Levin tube, which is a single-lumen tube with no air vent. To promote drainage, suction (usually low) is applied to the NG tube. Suction is either continuous (recommended for the Salem sump) or intermittent.

Record the color, consistency, and amount of the drainage every 8 hours (Table 18-3). In some instances, an occult blood test (Gastroccult) may be performed. Normal NG drainage fluid is greenish yellow. Red drainage fluid indicates active bleeding, and brown liquid or drainage with a "coffee-ground" appearance indicates old bleeding. Assess that the NG tube is securely taped to the nose, and note any skin irritation.

Assess the patient for complications related to NG tube use, such as fluid and electrolyte imbalances, aspiration, and nares discomfort. To prevent aspiration, check the tube placement every 4 to 8 hours and before instilling any liquid into the tube. (See Chapter 58 for information on tube placement and care.) *After gastric surgery, do not move or irrigate the tube without an order from the surgeon.* Fluid and electrolyte imbalances can result from NG drainage and tube irrigation with water instead of saline. Imbalances include fluid volume deficit, hypokalemia and hyponatremia (see Chapter 13), hypochloremia, and metabolic alkalosis (see Chapter 14).

Constipation may occur after surgery as a result of anesthesia, analgesia (especially opioid analgesics), decreased activity, and decreased oral intake. Assess the abdomen by inspection, auscultation, palpation, and percussion, and record the elimination pattern to determine whether interventions are needed. For abdominal assessment, auscultate before palpation or percussion because these two maneuvers can affect peristalsis. Increased dietary fiber intake, the use of mild laxatives or bulk-forming agents, or the use of enemas may be needed.

Skin Assessment. The clean surgical wound heals at skin level in about 2 weeks in the absence of trauma, connective tissue disease, malnutrition, or the use of some drugs, such as steroids. Smokers and patients who are older, obese, or diabetic or whose immunity is reduced have delayed wound healing. Complete healing of all tissue layers within the surgical wound may take 6 months to 2 years. The physical health and age of the patient, size and location of the wound, and stress on the wound all affect healing time. Head and facial wounds heal more quickly than abdominal and leg wounds because of the better blood flow to the head and neck.

Normal Wound Healing. During the first few days of normal wound healing, the incised tissue regains blood supply and begins to bind together. Fibrin and a thin layer of epithelial cells seal the incision. After 1 to 4 days, epithelial cells continue growing in the fibrin and strands of collagen begin to fill in the wound gaps. This process continues for 2 to 3 weeks. *At that time, the wound appears to be healed; however, healing is not complete for up to 2 years, until the scar is strengthened* (Greenhalgh, 2005; McEwen, 2007). (See Chapter 26 for discussion of wound healing and wound infection.)

When the patient is an inpatient, the surgeon usually removes the original dressing on the first or second day after surgery. Assess the incision on a regular basis, at least every 8 hours, for redness, increased warmth, swelling, tenderness or pain, and the type and amount of drainage. Some drainage, changing from **sanguineous** (bloody) to serosanguineous to **serous** (serum-like, or yellow), is normal during the first few days. Serosanguineous drainage continuing beyond the fifth day after surgery or increasing in amount instead of decreasing alerts you to the possibility of dehiscence (discussed below), and the surgeon should be notified. Crusting on the incision line is normal, as is a pink color to the line itself, which is caused by inflammation from the surgical procedure. Slight swelling under the sutures or staples is also normal. Redness or swelling of or around the incision line, excessive tenderness or pain on palpation, and purulent or odorous drainage indicates wound infection and must be reported to the surgeon.

Ineffective Wound Healing. Ineffective wound healing may be caused by infection, distention from edema or paralytic ileus, stress at the surgical site, and health problems that cause delayed wound healing (e.g., diabetes). Wound **dehiscence** is a partial or complete separation of the outer wound layers, sometimes described as a "splitting open of the wound." **Evisceration** is the total separation of all wound layers and protrusion of internal organs through the open wound (Fig. 18-2). Both of these problems occur most often between the fifth and tenth days after surgery (Beattie, 2007; Hahler, 2006). Wound separation occurs more often in obese patients and those with diabetes, immune deficiency, or malnutrition or who are using

TABLE 18-3 Calculating Nasogastric Tube Drainage

FORMULA

Drainage in collection device − Amount of irrigant = True (actual) amount of drainage

EXAMPLE

A patient's drainage container was marked at 150 mL at 7 AM. At 3 PM, there was 525 mL in the container. During the nursing shift, the nurse instilled 30 mL of saline as an irrigant into the tube four times, as prescribed by the physician.

525 mL − 150 mL = 375 mL of drainage

30 mL × 4 = 120 mL of irrigant

375 mL − 120 mL = 255 mL of actual drainage

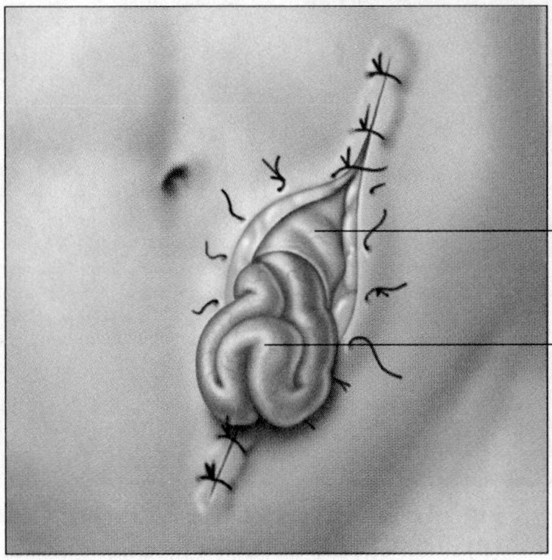
Dehiscence
Evisceration

Fig. 18-2 • Complications of wound healing.

steroids (Baugh et al., 2007). Dehiscence or evisceration may follow forceful coughing, vomiting, or straining and when not splinting the surgical site during movement. The patient may state, "Something gave way" or "I feel as if I just split open."

Dressings and Drains. Assess all dressings, including casts and elastic (Ace) bandages, for bleeding or other drainage on admission to the PACU and then hourly thereafter. When the patient is on the nursing unit, assess the dressing each time vital signs are taken (at least every 8 hours). During dressing inspection, check for drainage and record its amount, color, consistency, and odor. If drainage is present on a dressing or cast, monitor its progression by outlining it with a pen and indicating the date and time. Check the area underneath the patient also, because drainage or blood may leak from the side of the dressing and not appear on the dressing itself.

Ensure that the dressing does not restrict circulation or sensation. This problem is most likely to occur when dressings are tight or completely surround an arm or a leg. Chest dressings that are too tight or that encircle the chest can restrict breathing.

The surgeon inserts a drain into or close to the wound if more than a minimal amount of drainage is expected. A Penrose drain (a single-lumen, soft, open, latex tube) is a gravity-type drain under the dressing. Drainage on the dressing is expected with open tube drains but is not expected with closed drainage systems. Assess closed-suction drains, such as Hemovac, Vacu-Drain, and Jackson-Pratt drains, for maintenance of suction. Specialty drains, such as a T-tube, may be placed for specific drainage purposes. For example, a T-tube drains bile after a cholecystectomy. Fig. 18-3 shows commonly used drains.

Assess all drains for patency when the patient is admitted to the PACU and every time vital signs are taken. Monitor the amount, color, and type of drainage while the patient is in the PACU and at least every 8 hours after he or she is transferred to the medical-surgical nursing unit. Large amounts of sanguineous drainage may indicate internal bleeding.

Discomfort/Pain Assessment. The patient almost always has pain or discomfort after surgery. Pain is a subjective experience and may be more intense than the health care professional can appreciate. Pain after surgery is related to the surgical wound, tissue manipulation, drains, positioning during surgery, presence of an endotracheal (ET) tube, and the patient's experience with pain. In assessing his or her discomfort and need for medication, consider the type, extent, and length of the surgical procedure. Assess for physical and emotional signs of acute pain, such as increased pulse and blood pressure, increased respiratory rate, profuse sweating, restlessness, confusion (in the older adult), wincing, moaning, and crying. When possible, ask the patient to rate the pain before and after drugs are given (e.g., on a scale of 1 to 10, with 1 being no pain and 10 being extreme pain). Plan the patient's activities around the timing of analgesia to improve mobility. Observe for a return of normal (baseline) physical behaviors. (See Chapter 5 for further discussion of pain assessment.)

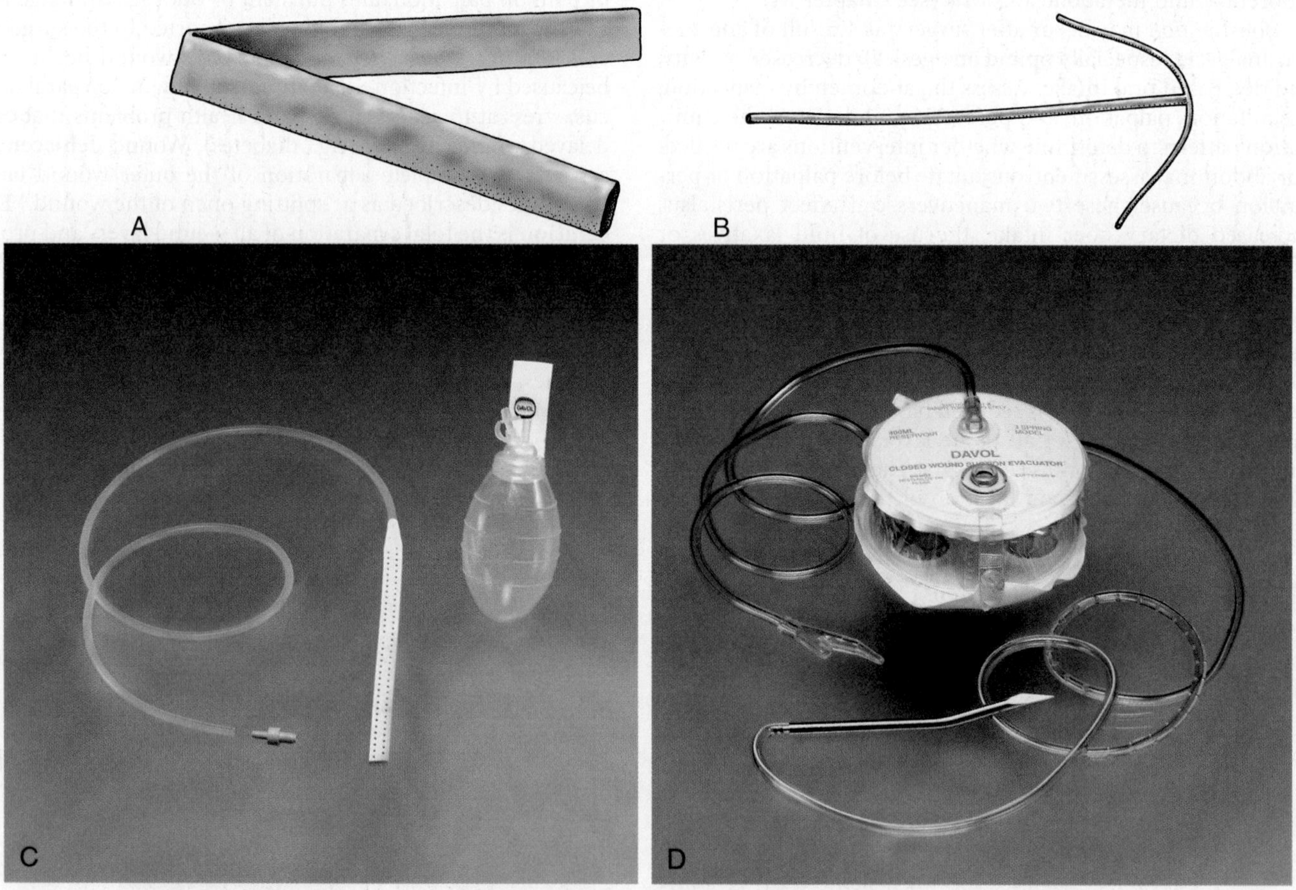
A
B
C
D
DAVOL

Fig. 18-3 • Types of surgical drains. Gravity drains, such as the Penrose (**A**) and the T-tube (**B**) drain directly through a tube from the surgical area. In closed wound drainage systems, such as the Jackson-Pratt (**C**) and Hemovac (**D**), drainage collects in a collecting vessel by means of compression and re-expansion of the system.

Pain assessment is started by the PACU nurse. After the patient is transferred from the PACU, the medical-surgical nurse continues to assess the patient's comfort level. Pain usually reaches its peak on the second day after surgery, when the patient is more awake and more active and the anesthetic agents and drugs given during surgery have been excreted.

Psychosocial Assessment

Consider the psychological, social, and cultural issues of the patient after surgery as you provide physical care. This assessment may be delayed or difficult to perform in the PACU when the patient is drowsy or confused. Consider the patient's age and medical history, the surgical procedure, and the impact of surgery on recovery, body image, roles, and lifestyle.

Physical signs of anxiety include restlessness; increased pulse, blood pressure, and respiratory rate; and crying. The patient may be anxious and ask questions about the results or findings of the surgical procedure. Reassure the patient that the surgeon will speak with him or her after he or she is fully awake. If the surgeon has already spoken with the patient, reinforce what was said.

After the patient returns to the medical-surgical unit, continue the psychosocial assessment and also assess significant others for psychological discomfort.

NCLEX EXAMINATION CHALLENGE

The client who had abdominal surgery for colon cancer is transferred to the medical-surgical unit after 4 hours in the PACU. The nurse notes all the following assessment findings. For which one should the nurse notify the surgeon, anesthesia provider, or Rapid Response Team?

A. There is a large amount of serosanguineous drainage on the dressing around the ostomy stoma.
B. SpO_2 is 80% when measured by pulse oximetry on the fingers, nose, and ear.
C. The client is confused and trying to pull out the nasogastric tube.
D. Bowel sounds are absent in all four abdominal quadrants.

evolve For the correct answer, go to http://evolve.elsevier.com/Iggy/.

Laboratory Assessment

Laboratory tests are performed after surgery to monitor for complications. Tests are based on the surgical procedure, the patient's medical history, and clinical manifestations after surgery. Common tests include analysis of electrolytes and a complete blood count (see Chart 16-3 in Chapter 16). A change in laboratory test results (e.g., electrolyte, hematocrit, hemoglobin levels) often occurs during the first 24 to 48 hours after surgery because of blood and fluid loss and the body's reaction to the surgical process. Fluid loss with minimal blood loss may cause hemoconcentration of laboratory values. Such test results are reported as increased but actually represent a concentrated normal value.

An indication of infection is an increase in the band cells (immature neutrophils) in the white blood cell differential count. This increase is termed a "left shift" (sometimes called *bandemia*). The source of infection may be the respiratory system, urinary tract, wound, or IV site. Obtain specimens for culture and sensitivity testing, and monitor the culture reports at 24, 48, and 72 hours. Notify the surgeon of positive culture results. (See Chapters 19 and 25 for information on infection and assessment of immune function.)

Arterial blood gas (ABG) tests may be needed for patients who have respiratory or cardiac disease, those undergoing mechanical ventilation after surgery, and those who had chest surgery. Review ABG results, and notify the surgeon of any acid-base imbalance or hypoxemia. (For more discussion on arterial blood gases and acidosis, see Chapter 14.)

Urine and renal laboratory tests also may be obtained (e.g., urinalysis, urine electrolyte levels, serum creatinine levels). Other laboratory tests depend on the diagnosis, type of surgical procedure, and other health problems. Examples are a serum amylase level for a patient who had pancreatic surgery and a blood glucose level for a patient with diabetes.

DECISION-MAKING CHALLENGE
Critical Rescue

The patient is a 32-year-old woman who is returned to the day-surgery area after a tubal ligation performed by laparoscopic surgery. While you are assessing her, she tells you that her left shoulder really hurts and that she is nauseated. Her vital signs are as follows: HR = 110 bpm; BP = 90/68; R = 24. Her last vital signs recorded before leaving the OR were HR = 90 bpm; BP = 128/82; R = 14. She received morphine sulfate 4 mg IV 20 minutes ago.

1. What additional assessment data should you obtain?
2. Where should you assess for hemorrhage?
3. What are the possible causes for her left shoulder pain?
4. What is the most likely cause for her change in vital signs?
5. Should the surgeon be notified? Why or why not?

evolve For suggested answer guidelines, go to http://evolve.elsevier.com/Iggy/.

Analysis

Common Nursing Diagnoses and Collaborative Problems

Priority nursing diagnoses for the patient after surgery are:

1. Impaired Gas Exchange related to the effects of anesthesia, pain, opioid analgesics, and immobility
2. Impaired Skin Integrity related to surgical wounds, decreased mobility, drains and drainage, and tubes
3. Acute Pain related to the surgical incision, positioning during surgery, and endotracheal (ET) tube irritation

A common collaborative problem is Potential for Hypoxemia.

Additional Nursing Diagnoses and Collaborative Problems

In addition to the common nursing diagnoses and collaborative problems, patients may have one or more of these problems after surgery:

- Risk for Aspiration related to decreased mobility, anesthesia, and opioid analgesic use
- Ineffective Airway Clearance related to ineffective or absent cough
- Constipation related to decreased mobility, anesthesia, and opioid analgesic use
- Risk for Infection related to surgery and invasive lines, catheters, and tubes
- Urinary Retention related to anesthesia, surgical procedures, and decreased mobility
- Delayed Surgical Recovery related to presence of other health problems (diabetes, obesity) or complications of surgery
- Bathing/hygiene Self-Care Deficit related to surgical procedures, pain, and decreased mobility

- Disturbed Body Image related to surgical procedures, loss of a body part or function, and pain
- Interrupted Family Processes related to the impact of surgery and illness on the family system
- Potential for Hypovolemic Shock
- Potential for Deep Vein Thrombosis and Pulmonary Embolism

Planning and Implementation

Impaired Gas Exchange

NOC **Planning: Expected Outcomes.** The patient is expected to attain or maintain optimal lung expansion and breathing patterns after surgery as indicated by:

- Partial pressure of arterial oxygen ($Pa{O_2}$) within normal range
- Partial pressure of arterial carbon dioxide ($Pa{CO_2}$) within normal range
- Oxygen saturation values within normal range

Interventions

Airway Maintenance. After assessing the airway, you may need to insert an oral airway if the patient does not already have one. The oral airway pulls the tongue forward and holds it down to prevent obstruction. If the patient had oral surgery or has clenched teeth, a large tongue, or upper airway obstruction, insert a nasal airway (nasal trumpet) to keep the airway open. Keep the manual resuscitation bag and emergency equipment for intubation or tracheostomy nearby. For patients whose only airway is a tracheostomy or laryngectomy stoma, alert other staff members by posting signs in the room and notes on the chart.

Positioning. *In the PACU, immediately position the patient in a side-lying position or turn his or her head to the side to prevent aspiration.* Suction the mouth, nose, and throat to keep the airway clear of mucus or vomitus as needed.

Keep the patient's head flat to prevent hypotension and possible shock unless this position is contraindicated by the condition or surgical procedure. (For example, after intracranial surgery, the head of the bed or stretcher is elevated to promote ventilation and prevent cerebral edema.) Apply oxygen by face tent, nasal cannula, or mask to eliminate inhaled anesthetic agents, increase oxygen levels, raise the level of consciousness, and reduce confusion (Pruitt, 2006). After the patient is fully reactive and stable, raise the head of the bed to promote respiratory function.

Breathing Exercises. After the patient regains the gag and cough reflexes and meets the agency's criteria for extubation (if intubated), remove the airway or ET tube. Usual extubation criteria are the ability to raise and hold the head up and evidence of thoracic breathing. Help the patient cough (with the incision splinted) and deep breathe to expand the lungs, promote gas exchange, and eliminate inhalation anesthetic agents. Chart 16-5 (in Chapter 16) reviews breathing exercises and splinting of the surgical area. As soon as the patient is awake enough to follow commands, urge him or her to cough, use the incentive spirometer, and take deep breaths (Wadlund, 2006). Remind him or her to continue these activities throughout the postoperative period. The patient who is unable to remove mucus or sputum requires oral or nasal suctioning. Perform mouth care after removing secretions.

Movement. Assist the patient out of bed and to ambulate as soon as possible to help remove secretions and promote lung expansion. Even when the patient has had extensive surgery, the goal may be to get out of bed the day of or the first day after surgery. If this is not possible, assist him or her to turn at least every 2 hours (side to side) and ensure that breathing exercises and leg exercises are performed (see Charts 16-5 and 16-6 in Chapter 16). Early ambulation reduces the risk for pulmonary complications, especially after abdominal, pelvic, or spinal surgery. The patient may report pain and resist getting up, but you should stress the importance of activity to prevent complications. When indicated, offer pain medication 30 to 45 minutes before he or she gets out of bed.

Impaired Skin Integrity

NOC **Planning: Expected Outcomes.** The patient is expected to have incision healing without wound complications as indicated by:

- Wound edges remaining together
- Absence of purulent drainage, induration, or redness in, from, or around the incision

Interventions. Nursing assessment of the surgical area is critical (see the discussion of skin assessment on p. 291). Although most wound complications do not require additional surgical intervention, emergency surgical procedures may be needed.

Nonsurgical Management. Wound care includes reinforcing the dressing, changing the dressing, assessing the wound for healing and infection, and caring for drains, including emptying drainage containers/reservoirs and measuring and documenting drainage. Emphasize the importance of early deep-breathing exercises to prevent forceful coughing. Encourage hip flexion when the patient is in the supine position to reduce tension on a chest or abdominal wound. Remind the patient to always splint the incision when coughing. Promote wound healing and protection of the skin in general, especially for the older patient (Litwack, 2006). Chart 18-3 lists best practices for skin care of the older patient after surgery.

Dressings. The surgeon usually performs the first dressing change to assess the wound, remove any packing, and advance (pull partially out) or remove drains. Before the first dressing change, reinforce the dressing (add more dressing material to the existing dressing) if it becomes wet from drainage. Document the added material, as well as the color, type, amount, and odor of drainage fluid and time of observation. Assess the surgical site at least every shift, and report any unexpected findings to the surgeon.

After removal of the dressing, the surgeon may leave the suture or staple line open to the air, which allows easy assessment of the wound and early detection of poor wound edge adherence, drainage, swelling, or redness. Some surgeons believe that air-drying promotes healing. A draining wound, however, is always covered with a dressing.

Dressing changes are prescribed by the surgeon; however, the facility or unit may have standards or policies that dictate specific protocols for dressing changes and incision care. An unchanged wet or damp dressing is a source of infection. Change dressings using aseptic technique until the sutures or staples are removed (Wright, 2005).

Dressings vary with the surgical procedure and the surgeon's preference. Common dressings for large incisions consist of gauze or nonadherent pads covered with a larger absorbent pad held in place by tape, a tubular stretchy net, or Montgomery straps (Fig. 18-4). Some incisions may be covered with a transparent plastic surgical dressing (e.g., OpSite) or a spray in the operating room. This type of dressing stays intact for 3 to 6 days and allows direct observation of the

Chart 18-3 NURSING FOCUS ON THE OLDER ADULT

Best Practice in Postoperative Skin Care

Improve perfusion to the wound to promote wound healing:
- Keep the patient adequately hydrated to maintain cardiac output.
- Keep the airway patent, and provide adequate oxygenation.
- Keep the patient's oxygen saturation on pulse oximetry at greater than 93%.

Conserve the patient's energy:
- Allow the patient to sleep in a darkened, quiet room.
- Administer drugs to combat pain and sleeplessness, as prescribed.
- Provide rest periods throughout the day.
- Control the patient's room temperature.
- Assist in ADLs.

Place the patient on a safety program to prevent falls, if indicated.

Use strict aseptic technique in caring for breaks in the integument (e.g., IV or other catheters, indwelling urethral catheter, wound).

Maintain the patient's psychosocial health:
- Prevent unnecessary stressors.
- Allow the patient liberal visitation of supportive others.
- Enable the patient to use individual successful coping mechanisms.
- Keep the patient well groomed and bathed.

Protect fragile skin:
- Minimize the use of tape on the skin.
- Use hypoallergenic tape or Montgomery straps.
- Change dressings as soon as they become wet.
- Lift the patient during transfer or repositioning.

Data from Jones, P.L., & Millman, A. (1990). Wound healing and the aged patient. *Nursing Clinics of North America, 25*(1), 263-277.

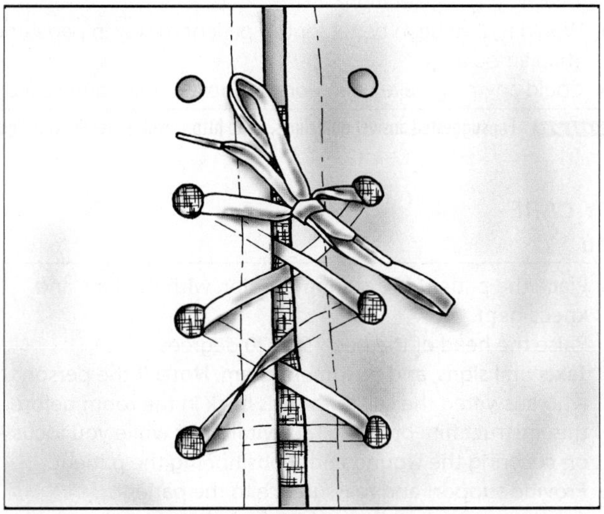

Fig. 18-4 • Montgomery straps may be used when frequent dressing changes are anticipated. They help prevent skin irritation from frequent tape removal.

wound. It also prevents contamination and eliminates the need for dressing changes (Wright, 2005).

Wound or suture line care consists of changing gauze dressings at least once during a nursing shift or daily and may include cleaning the area with sterile saline or some other solution. Some suture lines are left open to air without any dressing to cover the incision. The hospital's policy, the unit's standards, and the surgeon's preference determine what solution, if any, is used to clean the wound and how often dressings are changed (McEwen, 2007). For large dressing changes or drain removal, offer the patient a prescribed analgesic before the procedure. Always assess the skin for redness, rash, or blisters in areas where tape has been used. Tape can cause a skin reaction after surgery even among patients who are not known to be tape sensitive (Glenn, 2006).

Skin sutures or staples are usually removed 6 to 8 days after surgery, and the incision is secured with Steri-Strips. The surgeon or the nurse removes the sutures or staples, depending on the agency's policy. Clean the incision before removing sutures or staples. Before removing sutures, examine the condition and healing stage of the wound. First remove every other suture or staple and re-assess the wound for integrity. If wound healing is progressing normally, the rest of the sutures or staples may then be removed or may be removed the next day. If the wound does not appear to be healing well, notify the surgeon before removing any sutures.

Drains. Drains (see Fig. 18-3) may be placed in the wound or through a separate small incision (known as a "stab" wound) close to the incision during surgery. Drains provide an exit route for air, blood, and bile. Drains also help prevent deep infections and abscess formation during healing.

The Penrose drain is placed into the external aspect of the incision and drains directly onto the dressing and skin around the incision. Change a damp or soiled dressing, and carefully clean under and around the Penrose drain. Then place absorbent pads under and around the exposed drain to prevent skin irritation and wound contamination. Whether sutured in place or not, the drain can be dislodged or pulled out accidentally during a dressing change. It is also possible for the drain to slip back through the wound into the patient. Usually this complication is prevented when the drain is first placed in the OR. The surgeon pins a sterile safety pin through the drain at an angle perpendicular to the drain and the wound. The safety pin acts as a barrier to prevent the drain from slipping. As the wound heals, the surgeon or nurse shortens (advances) the drain by pulling it out a short distance and trimming off the excess external portion so that only 2 to 3 inches of drain protrudes through the incision. The stabilizing safety pin must be repositioned each time the drain is advanced. The drain remains in place until drainage stops.

Jackson-Pratt and Hemovac drains are two self-contained drainage systems that drain wounds directly through a tube via gravity and vacuum. These drains are sutured in place with a suture that seals the area when the drain is removed. Use sterile technique to empty the reservoir. Record the amount and color of drainage during every nursing shift or more often if prescribed. After emptying and compressing the reservoir to restore suction, secure the drain to the patient's gown (never to the sheet or mattress) to prevent pulling and stress on the surgical wound.

Drug therapy. Wound infection is a major complication after surgery. It usually results from contamination during surgery, preoperative infection, debilitation, or immunosuppression (Odom-Forren, 2006; Sarvis, 2006; Schwoen, 2006). A patient at risk for wound infection may receive antibiotic therapy with drugs that are effective against organisms common to the specific surgical site. These antibiotics are usually continued for at least 24 hours after surgery. The first dose may be given IV before or during surgery.

Wounds that become infected and open are treated with dressing changes and systemic antibiotic therapy. Depending on the surgeon's prescription, irrigate the wound (e.g., with sterile saline, hydrogen peroxide, povidone-iodine, or acetic acid), loosely pack it with solution-soaked gauze (e.g., neomycin, gentamicin, iodoform, povidone-iodine, saline, or acetic acid), and cover the wound with dry, sterile dressings. This procedure (wet-to-damp dressings) may be done one to three times daily. The packing promotes healing from within the wound and **débridement** (removal of the infected or dead tissue) as the wound heals (Schwoen, 2006).

Surgical Management. Poorly healing wounds, infected wounds, or complicated wounds may require surgical intervention.

Management of dehiscence. *If dehiscence (wound opening) occurs, apply a sterile nonadherent (e.g., Telfa) or saline dressing to the wound and notify the surgeon* (Beattie, 2007). Instruct the patient to bend the knees and to avoid coughing. A wound that becomes infected dehisces by itself, or it may be opened by the surgeon through an incision and drainage (I&D) procedure. In either case, the wound is left open rather than resutured and is treated as described previously.

Management of evisceration. *An* ***evisceration*** *(a wound opening with protrusion of internal organs) is a surgical emergency.* One nurse tends to the patient while another nurse immediately notifies the surgeon (Beattie, 2007). Chart 18-4 lists best practices for emergency care of the patient with surgical wound evisceration. Provide emotional support by explaining what happened and reassuring the patient that the emergency will be handled competently.

The surgeon may prescribe a nasogastric (NG) tube to decompress the stomach and relieve internal pressure or to remove the stomach's contents if the patient has been eating and general anesthesia is needed. Prepare the patient for surgery (see Chapter 16) to close the wound. Regional or local anesthesia may be used, depending on the location and type of wound. Nausea and vomiting, which stress the already fragile incision, are reduced when regional or local anesthesia is used. To increase the incision's integrity, stay or retention sutures of wire or nylon are used along with standard sutures or staples (see Fig. 17-11).

Prevention. Patients also are at risk for developing pressure ulcers from positioning during surgery, prolonged contact with damp surgical linens, and contact with unpadded surfaces. Pressure ulcers acquired during the surgical period increase lengths of stay and the risk for complications. Addressing early-stage pressure ulcers can prevent progression and limit complications.

Examine the patient's skin for areas of redness or open areas. Document and report any abnormalities. Use padding and positioning to relieve pressure. Treat any open areas according to facility guidelines and the surgeon's prescription. Ensure that information about the patient's skin condition in the PACU is communicated to the medical-surgical nurse.

DECISION-MAKING CHALLENGE
Coordination of Care

The patient is a 52-year-old obese woman who had abdominal surgery 4 days ago for an ovarian abscess. She takes Avandia for type 2 diabetes and prednisone 10 mg daily for rheumatoid arthritis. She is still on IV antibiotics and has been very adherent to her postoperative prevention regimen. She walks unassisted several times a day in the hallway, drinks 4 liters of water each day, and uses her incentive spirometer every 2 hours while she is awake. When you make your rounds at midnight, she is awake and tells you that she has felt incision pressure all day but when she climbed back into bed a few minutes ago, she felt something "pop" and now the pressure is gone. When you look under her loose dressing, you see loops of bowel protruding. You are the only registered nurse on this small (12-bed) unit, and you have one LPN/LVN and one unlicensed nursing assistant working with you.

1. What is your first action?
2. Who should stay with the patient—you, the LPN/LVN, or the nursing assistant? Why?
3. Who should be notified first—the surgeon or the Rapid Response Team? Provide a rationale for your answer.
4. What risk factors does this patient have for impaired wound healing and evisceration?
5. Would it have been better for this patient to stay in bed rather than ambulate?
6. Could anything have been done to prevent this complication?

evolve For suggested answer guidelines, go to http://evolve.elsevier.com/Iggy/.

Chart 18-4 BEST PRACTICE FOR PATIENT SAFETY & QUALITY CARE
Emergency Care of the Patient with Surgical Wound Evisceration

EMERGENCY CARE

1. Call for help! Instruct the person who responds to notify the surgeon or Rapid Response Team immediately and to bring any needed supplies into the patient's room.
2. Stay with the patient.
3. Cover the wound with a nonadherent dressing premoistened with warmed sterile normal saline. **Note:** The supplies needed for this emergency should be in the patient's room, especially if the patient is at high risk.
4. If premoistened dressings are not available, moisten sterile gauze or sterile towels in a sterile irrigation tray with sterile saline and then cover the wound.
5. If saline is not immediately available, cover the wound with gauze and then moisten with sterile saline using a sterile irrigation tray as soon as someone brings saline.
6. Do not attempt to reinsert the protruding organ or viscera.
7. While covering the wound, note the patient's response and assess for manifestations of shock.
8. Place the patient in a supine position with the hips and knees bent.
9. Raise the head of the bed 15 to 20 degrees.
10. Take vital signs, and document them. **Note:** If the person who answered the call for help is back in the room before this, instruct him or her to take vital signs while you focus on covering the wound and repositioning the patient.
11. Provide support and reassurance to the patient.
12. Continue assessing the patient, including vital signs assessment, every 5 to 10 minutes until the surgeon arrives.
13. Keep dressings continuously moist by adding warmed sterile saline to the dressing as often as necessary. Do not let the dressing become dry.
14. When the surgeon arrives, report your finding and your interventions. Then follow the surgeon's directions.
15. Document the incident, the activity the patient was engaged in at the time of the incident, your actions, and your assessments.

Acute Pain

NOC **Planning: Expected Outcomes.** The postoperative patient is expected to attain or maintain optimal comfort levels. Indicators include:

- Reporting that pain is controlled
- Absence of physiologic indicators of acute pain (increased heart rate and blood pressure)
- Absence of facial grimacing, teeth clenching
- Willingness to move and participate in self-care

Interventions. Pain management after surgery includes drug therapy and other methods of management, such as positioning, massage, relaxation techniques, and diversion. Often the patient has better pain relief from a combination of approaches. Assess the patient's comfort level and the effectiveness of the therapies. See Chapter 5 for discussion of pain assessment and management. The patient who has optimal pain control is better able to cooperate with the therapies and exercises to prevent complications and promote rehabilitation.

Drug Therapy. *The use of opioids or other analgesics for pain management may mask or increase the severity of symptoms of an anesthesia reaction. Therefore give these drugs with caution, especially in the PACU when the patient's condition is not stable.* When pain drugs are used in the PACU, they are usually given IV in small doses. After receiving any drug for pain, the patient remains in the PACU for a defined period (often 45 to 60 minutes). Assess for hypotension, respiratory depression, and other side effects. Within 5 to 10 minutes after an IV injection, assess the effectiveness of the drug (i.e., on a rating scale) in relieving pain.

Opioid analgesics are given during the first 24 to 48 hours after surgery to control acute pain. Around-the-clock scheduling is more effective than "on demand" scheduling because more constant blood levels are achieved. Drugs commonly used include morphine (Statex♣), hydromorphone (Dilaudid), ketorolac (Toradol), meperidine (Demerol), codeine, butorphanol (Stadol), and oxycodone with aspirin (Percodan) or oxycodone with acetaminophen (Tylox, Percocet).

Assess the type, location, and intensity of the pain before and after giving medication (see also pp. 292-293 in the Discomfort/Pain Assessment section). Monitor the patient's vital signs for hypotension and hypoventilation after giving opioid drugs. Chart 18-5 lists more information about analgesics used after surgery.

Patient-controlled analgesia (PCA) by IV infusion or internal pump (the catheter is sutured into or near the surgical area) and epidural analgesia are often used for better pain control. In PCA, the patient adjusts the dosage of the analgesic on the basis of the pain level and response to the drug. This method allows more consistent pain relief and more control by the patient. The maximum dose per hour is "locked in" to the pump so that the patient cannot accidentally overdose. Drugs given by the PCA method include morphine, meperidine, and hydromorphone.

Epidural analgesia can be given intermittently by the anesthesia provider or by continuous drip through an epidural catheter left in place after epidural anesthesia. Drugs given by epidural catheter include the opioids *fentanyl* (Sublimaze), *preservative-free morphine* (Duramorph), and *bupivacaine* (Marcaine).

Take care not to overmedicate or undermedicate, especially with older patients. In assessing for overmedication, monitor vital signs, especially blood pressure and respiratory rate, and level of consciousness. Complications from the use of opioid analgesics include respiratory depression, hypotension, nausea, vomiting, and constipation. An opioid antagonist, such as naloxone (Narcan), may be needed to reverse the acute effects of opioid depression. Because of the short effect of the opioid antagonist, monitor the patient's blood pressure and respirations every 15 to 30 minutes until the full effect of the opioid analgesic has passed. You may need to give more doses of the antagonist during this time because it is eliminated from the body more quickly than is the opioid. (See Chart 18-6 for more information on using opioid antagonists to reverse opioid overdose.) In addition, the patient has breakthrough pain after the opioid antagonist is given, so other interventions to promote comfort are needed.

Chart 18-5 COMMON EXAMPLES OF DRUG THERAPY
Management of Postoperative Pain

Drug	Usual Dosage	Nursing Interventions	Rationales
Morphine sulfate (Epimorph♣, Statex♣) **Med Error Alert!** Watch dosage; the dosage of morphine is only one-tenth that of meperidine.	2-15 mg IM or IV incrementally 10-30 mg orally every 4 hr Maximum 6 doses	Monitor respiratory status. Monitor blood pressure. Assess for GI motility and urine output.	Respiratory depression can be severe and require medical intervention. Hypotension, constipation, and urinary retention can occur.
Hydromorphone hydrochloride (Dilaudid) **Med Error Alert!** Watch dosage; the dosage of hydromorphone is only one-tenth that of morphine.	1-4 mg IV or IM every 3-4 hr 2-4 mg orally every 3-4 hr	Monitor respirations. Monitor blood pressure. Monitor for food intolerance. Monitor fluid and electrolyte balance. Assess GI motility.	Respiratory depression, hypotension, anorexia, nausea, vomiting, and constipation can occur.

Continued

Chart 18-5 COMMON EXAMPLES OF DRUG THERAPY
Management of Postoperative Pain—cont'd

Drug	Usual Dosage	Nursing Interventions	Rationales
Meperidine hydrochloride (Demerol)	50-150 mg orally or IM every 3-4 hr 12.5-25 mg IV Maximum 6-8 doses	Monitor blood pressure. Move and ambulate the patient slowly. Monitor pulse rate. Assess for decreased GI motility or GI upset.	Common side effects include decreased blood pressure, orthostatic (postural) hypotension, and bradycardia. Constipation, nausea, and vomiting can occur.
Codeine sulfate, codeine phosphate (Paveral🍁)	15-60 mg IM or orally every 4 hr Maximum 6 doses	Monitor respiratory status. Monitor for food intolerance. Monitor fluid and electrolyte balance. Assess GI motility.	Respiratory depression, nausea, and vomiting can occur. Constipation is common; prophylactic interventions may be indicated.
Butorphanol tartrate (Stadol)	1-4 mg IM every 3-4 hr 0.5-2 mg IV Maximum 6-8 doses	Monitor neurologic status and changes in level of consciousness. Monitor respiratory status.	Butorphanol can cause increased intracranial pressure and respiratory depression.
Oxycodone hydrochloride and aspirin (Percodan, Endodan🍁, Oxycodan🍁)	1-2 tablets (5-10 mg) orally every 3-4 hr Maximum 80 mg	Assess GI tolerance of medication. Assess for GI bleeding. Monitor GI motility. Monitor coagulation studies (PT, aPTT). Monitor respiratory status.	The aspirin component can irritate the stomach and could cause GI bleeding. Bleeding times and other coagulation study results may be increased because of the aspirin component. Respiratory depression and constipation can be caused by the oxycodone component.
Oxycodone hydrochloride and acetaminophen (Tylox, Percocet, Endocet🍁, Oxycocet🍁)	1-2 tablets (5-10 mg) orally every 3-4 hr Maximum 12 tablets	Monitor blood pressure and respiratory status. Assess for GI motility.	Respiratory depression, hypotension, and constipation can occur.
Ketorolac tromethamine (Toradol) **Med Error Alert!** Do not confuse Toradol with Tramadol, a drug used for central analgesia.	15-60 mg IM or IV every 6 hr Maximum 120 mg 5-day administration maximum	Monitor for GI bleeding. Monitor for renal effects, especially in older adults.	GI bleeding, ulceration, and perforation can occur. Decreased urine output, increased serum creatinine, hematuria, and proteinuria can occur. Ketorolac is cleared more slowly in older adults. Older persons are more sensitive to the renal effects of NSAIDs.
Ibuprofen (Motrin, Amersol🍁, Novo-profen🍁)	300-800 mg orally every 4-6 hr Maximum 2400 mg daily	Monitor upper GI tolerance of medication. Give with food or milk. Monitor coagulation studies (PT, aPTT). Assess for signs of bleeding or delayed clotting.	Food or milk helps decrease irritation of the stomach. Bleeding times and other coagulation study results may be increased. Monitoring leads to early detection of complications.

aPTT, Activated partial thromboplastin time; *GI*, gastrointestinal; *NSAID*, nonsteroidal anti-inflammatory drug; *PT*, prothrombin time.

Assess for undermedication by asking the patient about the effects of the drug and observing for nonverbal cues of pain or discomfort (e.g., restlessness, increased confusion, "picking" at bedcovers, aggressive behaviors). Offer prescribed pain drug(s) after checking for hypotension and respiratory depression.

As recovery progresses, reduce the doses and frequency of pain drugs. Drugs are changed from injectable or PCA to oral as soon as the patient can tolerate oral agents. Non-opioid analgesics, such as acetaminophen (Tylenol, Atasol🍁), and nonsteroidal anti-inflammatory drugs (NSAIDs), such as ibuprofen (Motrin, Novo-Profen🍁, Amersol🍁) and ketorolac (Toradol),

Chart 18-6 **BEST PRACTICE FOR PATIENT SAFETY & QUALITY CARE**

Emergency Care of the Patient Experiencing an Opioid Overdose

EMERGENCY CARE

- Prepare to administer naloxone hydrochloride (Narcan)* in a dose of 1 to 2 mg IV.
- Repeat drug every 2 to 3 minutes up to 10 mg, as needed, depending on the patient's response.
- Maintain an open airway.
- Give oxygen if hypoxia is present or if respirations are below 10 breaths per minute.
- Have suction equipment available because naloxone can trigger vomiting and a drowsy patient is at risk for aspiration.
- Continuously monitor vital signs and level of consciousness for reversal of overdose.
- Do not leave the patient until he or she is fully responsive.
- Assess the patient for pain because reversal of the opioid overdose also reverses the analgesic effects.
- Continue to monitor the patient's vital signs and level of consciousness every 10 to 15 minutes for the first hour because naloxone is eliminated from the body more quickly than is the opioid and because the antagonist may induce side effects, including blood pressure changes, tachycardia, and dysrhythmias.
- Determine the need for additional antagonist therapy 1 hour after the patient initially becomes fully responsive.

*There are other opioid antagonists; however, naloxone hydrochloride is used most often to manage adult opioid overdose in the postoperative period.

are used alone or with an opioid analgesic. Antianxiety drugs, such as hydroxyzine (Vistaril, Novo-Hydroxyzin♣), may be given with an opioid analgesic. This combination decreases pain-related anxiety, reduces muscle tension, and controls nausea.

Complementary and Alternative Therapies. Provide other comfort measures that may lower the amount of pain drugs needed (Good et al., 2005). These measures, such as positioning, massage, relaxation, and diversion, reduce anxiety and allow the patient to relax and rest.

In positioning the patient, consider the position during surgery, the location of the surgical incision and drains, and problems such as arthritis and chronic lung disease. Assist the patient to a position of comfort. Support the extremities with pillows. *Unless the surgeon prescribes pillow support, place no pillows under the knees, and do not raise the knee gatch, because this position could restrict circulation and increase the risk for thrombophlebitis.* Turn or help the patient turn at least every 2 hours while he or she is bedridden to prevent complications caused by immobility.

On the basis of the surgeon's prescription and your assessment of the patient's tolerance, urge the patient to increase activity progressively. Activity decreases stiffness, helps lung expansion, and promotes venous blood return. When he or she is first allowed out of bed, assist the patient to the side of the bed and into a chair. Teach him or her to splint the surgical wound for support and comfort during the transfer.

Use gentle massage on stiff joints or a sore back to decrease discomfort. Assist the patient to a side-lying position, and apply lotion with smooth, gentle strokes to increase blood flow to the area and promote relaxation. *Do not massage the calves because of the risk of loosening a clot and causing a life-threatening pulmonary embolus.*

Chart 18-7 **BEST PRACTICE FOR PATIENT SAFETY & QUALITY CARE**

Nonpharmacologic Interventions to Reduce Postoperative Pain and Promote Comfort

- Control or remove noxious stimuli.
- Cushion and elevate painful areas; avoid tension or pressure on those areas.
- Provide adequate rest to increase pain tolerance.
- Encourage the patient's participation in diversional activities.
- Instruct the patient in relaxation techniques; use audiotapes or CDs and breathing exercises.
- Provide opportunities for meditation.
- Help the patient stimulate sensory nerve endings near the painful areas to inhibit ascending pain impulses.
- Use ice to reduce and prevent swelling, as indicated.
- Find a general position of comfort for the patient.
- Help the patient stimulate the area contralateral (opposite) to the painful area.

Relaxation and diversion are also used to control acute episodes of pain that may occur during dressing changes and injections. Chapters 2 and 5 discuss how to instruct and guide the patient through these pain control methods. Music and noise reduction have also been shown to decrease awareness of discomfort (Good et al., 2005). Chart 18-7 lists other interventions that may help reduce pain and promote comfort.

Potential for Hypoxemia

NOC **Planning: Expected Outcomes.** The patient is expected to attain or maintain preoperative baseline partial pressure of arterial oxygen (Pao_2) values.

Interventions. The key to preventing hypoxemia is to follow the interventions for the nursing diagnoses of Impaired Gas Exchange (p. 294), Ineffective Airway Clearance, and Ineffective Breathing Pattern. After surgery, monitor the patient's oxygen saturation (Spo_2) with pulse oximetry. An older adult is often prescribed to receive low-dose oxygen therapy for the first 12 to 24 hours after surgery to reduce confusion from anesthesia and sedation. A patient who received moderate sedation with a benzodiazepine such as midazolam (Versed) or lorazepam (Ativan, Nu-Loraz♣) may be overly sedated or have pulmonary depression sufficient to need reversal with flumazenil (Romazicon) (Chart 18-8). Hypothermia after surgery causes shivering that increases oxygen demand and can induce hypoxemia. Many rewarming methods can be used, although prevention is more important. The highest incidence of hypoxemia after surgery occurs on the second postoperative day. Patients who normally have a low Pao_2, such as those with lung disease or older adults, are at higher risk for hypoxemia.

Hypoxemia is treated with oxygen therapy. Depending on the surgeon's preference and established guidelines, oxygen therapy may continue through the second day after surgery. When hypoxemia occurs despite preventive care, interventions to manage the cause of the hypoxemia are prescribed (Pruitt, 2006). These may include respiratory treatments and mechanical ventilation (if needed).

Community-Based Care

Many patients are discharged after a brief hospital stay or directly from the PACU to home. Because of the shortened length of hospital stays, discharge planning, teaching, and referral begin before surgery and continue after surgery.

Chart 18-8 **BEST PRACTICE FOR PATIENT SAFETY & QUALITY CARE**

Emergency Care of the Patient Experiencing a Benzodiazepine Overdose

EMERGENCY CARE

- Secure the airway and IV access before starting benzodiazepine antagonist therapy.
- Prepare to administer flumazenil (Romazicon)* in a dose of 0.2 mg to 1 mg IV.
- Repeat drug every 2 to 3 minutes up to 3 mg, as needed, depending on the patient's response.
- Give oxygen if hypoxia is present or if respirations are below 10 breaths per minute.
- Have suction equipment available because flumazenil can trigger vomiting and a drowsy patient is at risk for aspiration.
- Continuously monitor vital signs and level of consciousness for reversal of overdose.
- Do not leave the patient until he or she is fully responsive.
- Continue to monitor the patient's vital signs and level of consciousness every 10 to 15 minutes for the first 2 hours because flumazenil is eliminated from the body more quickly than is the benzodiazepine.
- Determine the need for additional flumazenil therapy 1 to 2 hours after the patient initially becomes fully responsive.
- Observe the patient for tremors or convulsions because flumazenil can lower the seizure threshold in patients who have seizure disorders.
- Assess the IV site every shift because flumazenil can cause thrombophlebitis at the injection site.
- Observe the patient for side effects of flumazenil, including skin rash, hot flushes, dizziness, headache, sweating, dry mouth, and blurred vision. The incidence of these side effects increases with higher total doses of flumazenil.

*There are other benzodiazepine antagonists; however, flumazenil is used most often to manage adult benzodiazepine overdose in the postoperative period.

Home Care Management

If the patient is discharged directly to home, assess information about the home environment for safety, cleanliness, and availability of caregivers. Use the database obtained on admission before surgery to determine the patient's needs. For example, if the patient is unable or not allowed to climb stairs and lives in a two-story house with only one bathroom, advise the patient to rent a bedside commode. Collaborate with the social worker or discharge planner to identify needs related to care after surgery, including meal preparation, dressing changes, drain management, drug administration, physical therapy, and personal hygiene. A referral to a home care nursing agency may be indicated.

The patient is usually concerned about complications, pain, changes in the usual activity level, or payment of the hospital bill. The more extensive the surgical procedure is, the more fearful the patient is of assuming self-care. Support the patient and family members as they make discharge plans. The patient with visible scars after surgery may need more emotional support from and acceptance of his or her family. The patient may be angry about the surgical outcome or about role changes. He or she may be concerned about financial matters and work. The surgical outcome may not have met the patient's expectations, and further interventions may be needed to assist in resolving his or her feelings. Ensure that referrals are made for additional counseling as indicated.

Health Teaching

The teaching plan for the patient and family after surgery includes:

- Prevention of infection
- Care and assessment of the surgical wound
- Management of drains or catheters
- Nutrition therapy
- Pain management
- Drug therapy
- Progressive increase in activity

If dressing changes and drain or catheter care are needed, instruct the patient and family members on the importance of proper handwashing to prevent infection. Explain and demonstrate wound care to the patient and family, who then perform a return demonstration. During teaching sessions, evaluate learning and promote adherence after discharge. At the same time, teach about the manifestations of complications such as wound infection. Also instruct the patient and family about what to do if complications occur.

A diet high in protein, calories, and vitamin C promotes wound healing. Supplemental vitamin C, iron, zinc, and other vitamins are often prescribed after surgery to aid in wound healing and red blood cell formation. Instruct the patient who needs dietary restrictions about the importance of following the prescribed diet while recovering from surgery. Encourage the older adult or debilitated patient to continue using dietary supplements, if prescribed, between meals until the wound is completely healed and the energy levels are restored.

Teach the patient about drugs for pain, especially about the proper dosage and frequency. Instruct the patient to notify the surgeon if pain is not controlled or if the pain suddenly increases. If antibiotics or other drugs are prescribed, stress the importance of completing the entire prescription.

Surgery stresses the body, and time and rest are needed for healing. Teach the patient to increase activity level slowly, rest often, and avoid straining the wound or the surrounding area. The surgeon decides when the patient may climb stairs, return to work, drive, and resume other usual activities, such as sexual intercourse. The amount of weight that the patient can lift safely after surgery is specifically defined by the surgeon (i.e., in pounds or kilograms). Remind patients of the weights of grocery bags, women's handbags, laundry baskets, children, and books.

Instruct the patient in the use of proper body mechanics. A patient whose work involves a moderate amount of physical labor may return to work about 6 weeks after abdominal surgery. However, he or she may be eager to return to normal activities and may not follow restrictions. Stress the importance of adherence to prevent complications or disability. *The patient must receive written discharge instructions to follow at home.* A referral for a home care nurse may be needed for follow-up.

Health Care Resources

After returning home, the patient may need equipment and assistance with dressing changes, ADLs, and meal preparation. Referral to a home care agency is made, if needed. Home care may be paid for by third-party insurance payers, including Medicare, if the patient is homebound and requires skilled care such as dressing changes or physical therapy. The home care nurse provides skilled nursing assessments, dressing supplies, education in self-care, and referrals for services as needed. Such referrals include Meals on Wheels, support groups, and homemaker services (e.g., for housekeeping, food shopping).

Evaluation: Outcomes

Evaluate the care of the patient after surgery on the basis of the identified nursing diagnoses and collaborative problems. The expected outcomes include that the patient:

- Attains and maintains adequate lung expansion and respiratory function
- Has complete wound healing without complications
- Has acceptable comfort levels after surgery

Specific indicators for these outcomes are listed for each nursing diagnosis and collaborative problem in the Planning and Implementation sections (see earlier).

GET READY FOR THE NCLEX EXAMINATION!

Key Points

Review these Key Points for each NCLEX Examination Client Needs Category.

Safe and Effective Care Environment

- Use aseptic technique during all dressing changes.
- Use established criteria to determine when a patient is ready to leave the postanesthesia care unit (PACU) for discharge to home or a medical-surgical nursing unit.
- Keep suction equipment, oxygen, and artificial breathing equipment near the patient in the PACU.

Health Promotion and Maintenance

- Reinforce to the patient after surgery the specific interventions to use to prevent complications (incision splinting, deep-breathing exercises, range-of-motion exercises—as described in Chart 16-6 in Chapter 16).
- Encourage early ambulation.
- Stress the need for following the activity restrictions prescribed by the surgeon.

Psychosocial Integrity

- Explain all procedures, restrictions, drugs, and follow-up care to the patient and family.
- Allow the patient to verbalize feelings about any change in physical appearance or lifestyle as a result of surgery.
- Reassure patients that taking pain medication when needed, even opioids, does not make them drug abusers.
- Remain with the patient if wound dehiscence or evisceration occurs.
- Offer alternative therapies for relaxation, pain reduction, and distraction, such as massage, music therapy, and guided imagery.

Physiological Integrity

- Begin every assessment of the patient after surgery by checking the airway and breathing effectiveness.
- Assess the incision site each shift (on the medical-surgical nursing unit).
- In the event of wound dehiscence or evisceration, have the patient lie flat (supine) with knees bent to reduce intra-abdominal pressure; apply sterile, nonadherent dressing materials to the wound; and follow the steps outlined in Chart 18-4.
- Teach the patient about any drugs to be continued after discharge from the facility.
- Instruct the patient and family about the clinical manifestations of complications and when to seek assistance.

Additional Study Resources

Go to your Companion CD or Evolve at http://evolve.elsevier.com/Iggy/ for *Self-Assessment Questions for the NCLEX Examination.*

evolve Go to Evolve at http://evolve.elsevier.com/Iggy/ for *Prioritization and Delegation Questions for the NCLEX Examination.*

SELECTED BIBLIOGRAPHY

Asterisk indicates a classic or definitive work on this subject.

*Acute Pain Management Guideline Panel. (1992). *Acute pain management in adults: Operative procedures.* AHCPR Publication No. 92-0022. Rockville, MD: Agency for Health Care Policy and Research, Public Health Service, U.S. Department of Health and Human Services.

*American Society of PeriAnesthesia Nurses (ASPAN). (2000). *Standards of perianesthesia nursing practice.* Cherry Hill, NJ: Author.

Baugh, N., Zuelzer, H., Meador, J., & Blankenship, J. (2007). Wounds in surgical patients who are obese. *AJN, 107*(6), 40-50.

Beattie, S. (2007). Wound dehiscence. *RN, 70*(6), 34-37.

Blaney-Koen, L. (2007). Safe surgery: A patient's guide. *Journal of Patient Safety, 3*(1), 56.

Bulechek, G.M., Butcher, H.K., & McCloskey Dochterman, J. (Eds.). (2008). *Nursing interventions classification (NIC)* (5th ed.). St. Louis: Mosby.

Dunn, D. (2005). Preventing perioperative complications in special populations. *Nursing2005, 35*(11), 36-43.

Glenn, Y. (2006). When your patient is sensitive to tape. *Nursing2006, 36*(1), 17.

Good, M., Anderson, G., Ahn, S., Cong, X., & Stanton-Hicks, M. (2005). Relaxation and music reduce pain after intestinal surgery. *Research in Nursing and Health, 28*(3), 240-251.

Greenhalgh, D. (2005). Models of wound healing. *Journal of Burn Care and Rehabilitation, 26*(4), 293-305.

Hahler, B. (2006). Surgical wound dehiscence. *MEDSURG Nursing, 15*(5), 296-300.

Halliday, A. (2006). Shades of sedation: Learning about moderate sedation and analgesia. *Nursing2006, 36*(4), 36-41.

Litwack, K. (2006). Adjusting postsurgical care for older patients. *Nursing2006, 26*(1), 66-67.

McCance, K., & Huether, S. (2006). *Pathophysiology: The biologic basis for disease in adults and children* (5th ed.). St. Louis: Mosby.

McEwen, D. (2007). Wound healing, dressings, and drains. In J.C. Rothrock & D. McEwen (Eds.), *Alexander's care of the patient in surgery* (13th ed.). St. Louis: Mosby.

Meiner, S., & Lueckenotte, A. (Eds.). (2006). *Gerontologic nursing* (3rd ed.). St. Louis: Mosby.

Metules, T., & Bauer, J. (2006). JCAHO's patient safety goals: A practical guide, Part 1. *RN, 69*(12), 21-26.

Moorhead, S., Johnson, M., & Maas, M. (Eds.). (2004). *Nursing outcomes classification (NOC)* (3rd ed.). St. Louis: Mosby.

Odom-Forren, J. (2006). Preventing surgical site infections. *Nursing2006, 36*(6), 59-63.

Owens, R. (2008). Teaming up to improve the quality of surgical care. *American Nurse Today, 3*(5), 25-26.

Pruitt, B. (2006). Help your patient combat postoperative atelectasis. *Nursing2006, 36*(5), 64hn1-64hn6.

Rothrock, J.C., & McEwen, D. (2007). *Alexander's care of the patient in surgery* (13th ed.). St. Louis: Mosby.

Sarvis, C. (2006). Postoperative wound care. *Nursing2006, 36*(12), 56-57.

Schwoen, S. (2006). Stamping out surgical site infections. *RN, 69*(8), 36-40.

Wadlund, D. (2006). Prevention, recognition, and management of nursing complications in the intraoperative and postoperative surgical patient. *Nursing Clinics of North America, 41*(2), 151-171.

Walker, C., Hogstel, M., & Curry, L. (2007). Hospital discharge of older adults. *AJN, 107*(6), 60-70.

Wright, K. (2005). Ensure your patient's wounds are best dressed. *Nursing Management, 36*(11), 49-50.

HUMAN NEEDS OVERVIEW

Protection

The human body works best when the internal environment is kept separate from the external environment. This is especially important for substances and organisms that could harm body cells, tissues, and organs. Normal protection is provided by three types of defenses—similar to how people living in a castle are protected against invaders (Fig. 1).

The first line of defense is the moat surrounding the castle walls. Although the moat seldom kills invaders directly, it slows them down and sometimes repels them. The human "moat" consists of the normal flora on the surface of the skin and mucous membranes. This normal flora is made up of bacteria and other organisms that belong on the skin, live peacefully with the human host, and help repel more harmful microorganisms. When the normal flora is changed as a result of some types of drug therapy, procedures, diseases, excessive dryness, and normal aging, this small protection is damaged or lost.

The second line of defense is the castle wall and the "watchers" and alarm systems embedded within it. When the wall is tall, thick, and intact, and when the watchers and alarms are working, penetration of the castle by invaders is greatly reduced. In humans, this type of protection is provided by intact skin and mucous membranes. These structures are a major barrier to invaders and help prevent dangerous changes in the internal environment. However, the castle walls do suffer some damage over time and must be repaired and maintained in order to provide continuing protection.

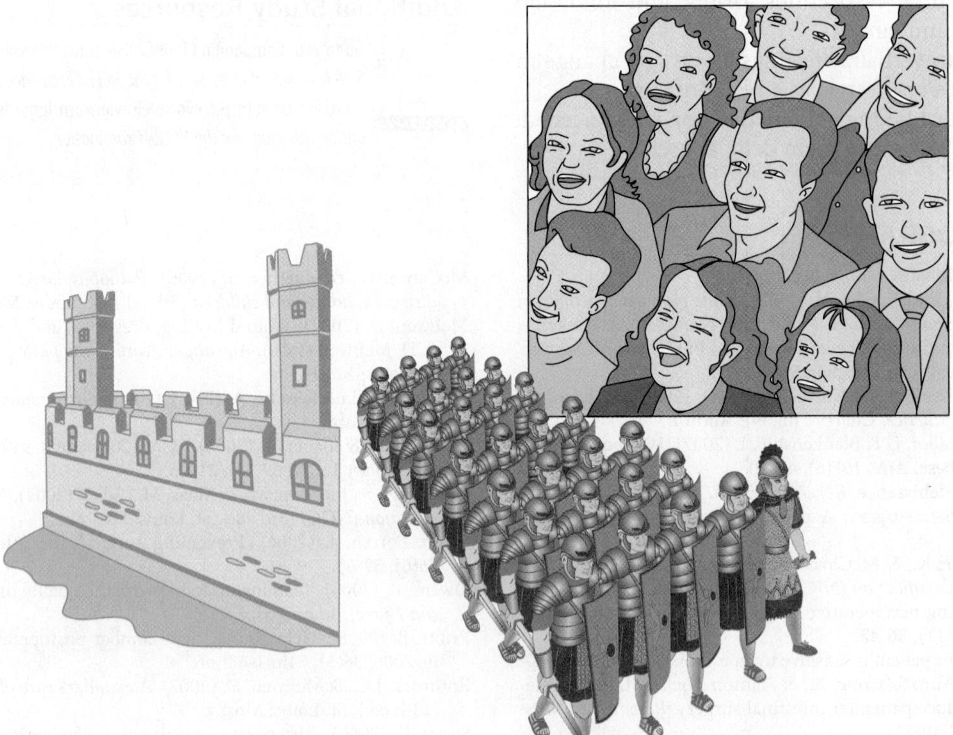

Three levels of protection (moat, castle wall, knights and soldiers) for humans

Fig. 1

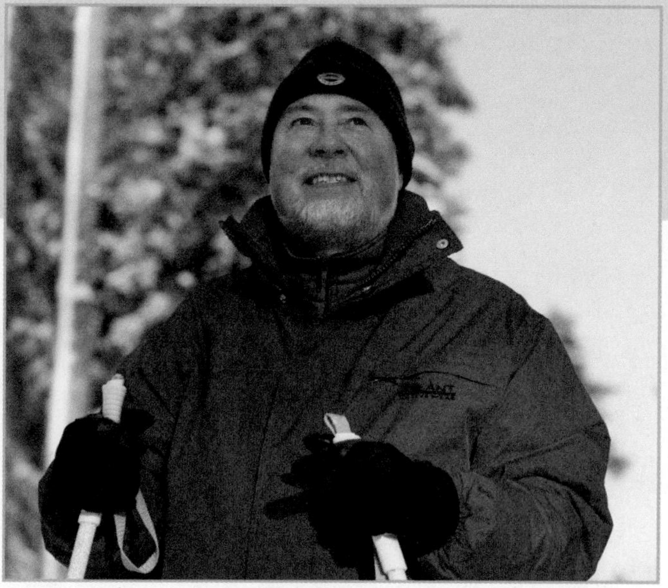

The last and strongest line of defense consists of the knights and soldiers within the castle. These individuals have the skills to kill or capture invaders. Some of these skills are common to all knights and soldiers, and others are unique to different groups. In humans, the white blood cells (leukocytes) and the substances they produce serve as the knights and soldiers. In addition to the work related directly to the invaders, this defense helps repair and maintain the castle walls. It is important to remember that this level of protection relies on both the alarms of the castle wall and its physical barrier to recognize invaders and trigger the protective responses of the knights and soldiers.

The human need for protection is best met when all three defenses are intact and are working at their highest functional levels. These defenses begin at birth and reach their maximum function in early to middle adulthood. The defenses decline slowly over time, making an older adult at greater risk for illnesses related to invasion and a decreased ability to repair damage. External factors and health status can reduce the ability of these defenses to provide complete protection. Specific nursing strategies can help reduce risk and protect the person whose defenses are less than perfect.

V

UNIT

Problems of Protection

Management of Patients with Problems of the Immune System

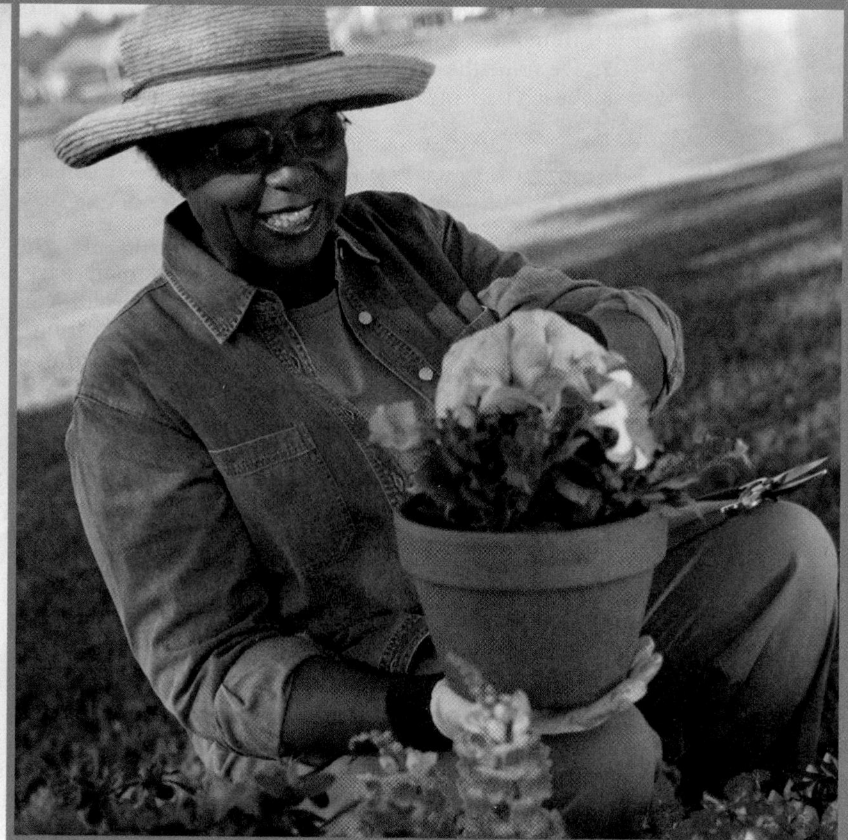

19

CHAPTER

Inflammation and the Immune Response

M. Linda Workman

LEARNING OUTCOMES

For clinical competence and success on the NCLEX Examination, study this chapter with these Learning Outcomes in mind:

Physiological Integrity

1. Describe the concept of self-tolerance.
2. Explain the differences between inflammation and infection.
3. Compare the cells, purposes, and features of inflammation and immunity.
4. Use knowledge of physiology to describe the basis for the five cardinal manifestations of inflammation.
5. Interpret correctly a white blood cell count with differential to indicate no immune problems, immunosuppression, infection, or an allergic reaction.
6. Compare the cells, function, and protective actions of antibody-mediated immunity and cell-mediated immunity.
7. Describe the expected immune system responses to the presence of transplanted organs.
8. Teach patients the need for and actions of drug therapy to prevent transplant rejection.

Go to your Companion CD or Evolve at http://evolve.elsevier.com/Iggy/ for *Self-Assessment Questions for the NCLEX Examination* keyed to these Learning Outcomes.

The human body's internal environment works best when invaders from the external world are destroyed, inactivated, or confined. Inflammation and the immune system work with other defenses to provide *protection* from harmful microorganisms and cells.

As indicated in the section opener defining the *human need for protection,* the cells and cell products of inflammation and immunity are represented mostly by the knights and soldiers behind the castle walls. The products made by cells, such as cytokines, growth factors, and antibodies, are the weapons of the knights and soldiers. In addition, some of these cells serve as watchers and alarm systems actually within the castle walls (skin and mucous membranes). They also help maintain and repair these walls when damage occurs.

Injury and infectious diseases are common. Most people, however, are healthy more often than they are ill. Inflammation and immunity are the two major defenses that protect a person against diseases and other problems when the body is invaded by organisms. These same defenses also help the body recover after injury or tissue damage. For these reasons, inflammation and immunity are critical to maintaining health and preventing disease. When all the different parts and functions of inflammation and immunity are working well, the person is **immunocompetent.**

Immune function is reduced by many diseases, injuries, and medical therapies. Reduction of immune function may be temporary or permanent, but it always endangers the patient's health. Chapter 21 discusses issues related to loss of protection from poor function of any or all parts of inflammation and immunity. Other problems occur when immunity overfunctions or functions at inappropriate times. Then this normally protective response becomes an enemy (Stephensen & Kelley, 2006). Chapters 20 and 22 discuss issues related to damage from excessive or inappropriate inflammation and immune responses.

OVERVIEW

Immunity is composed of many cell functions that protect people against the effects of injury or microscopic invasion. People interact with many other living organisms in the environment. The size of these organisms varies from large (other humans and animals) to microscopic (bacteria, viruses, molds, spores, pollens, protozoa, and cells from other people or animals). As long as organisms do not enter the body's internal environment, they pose no threat to health. The body has some defenses to prevent organisms from gaining access to the internal environment, such as intact skin and mucous membranes, skin surface normal flora, and natural chemicals that inhibit bacterial growth. These defenses are not perfect, and invasion of the body's internal environment by organisms occurs often. Invasion occurs much more often than does an actual disease or illness because of proper immune functioning.

Purpose of Inflammation and Immunity

The purpose of inflammation and immunity is to meet the *human need for protection* by neutralizing, eliminating, or destroying organisms that invade the internal environment. To meet protection needs without harming the body, immune system cells use protective actions only against non-self proteins and cells. Immune system cells can distinguish between the body's own healthy self cells and other, non-self proteins and cells.

Self Versus Non-Self

Non-self proteins and cells include infected body cells, cancer cells, and all invading cells and organisms. This ability to recognize self versus non-self, which is necessary to prevent healthy body cells from being destroyed along with the invaders, is called **self-tolerance.** The immune system cells are the only body cells capable of determining self from non-self. Self-tolerance is possible because of the different kinds of proteins present on cell membranes.

All organisms are made up of cells. Each cell is surrounded by a plasma membrane with different proteins protruding through the membrane (Fig. 19-1). For example, in liver cells, many different protein types are present on the cell membrane surface. The amino acid sequence of each protein type differs from that of all other protein types. Some of these proteins are found on the liver cells of all animals (including humans) that have livers, because these protein types are specific to the liver and serve as a marker for liver tissues. Other protein types are found only on the liver cells of humans, because these protein types are specific markers for human tissues. Still other protein types are found only on the liver cells of humans with a specific blood type. In addition, each person's liver cells have surface proteins that are specific to that person. These proteins are unique to the person and would be identical only to the proteins of an identical sibling. These unique proteins, found on the surface of all body cells of that person, serve as a "universal product code" or a "cellular fingerprint" for that person. The proteins that make up the universal product code for one person are recognized as "foreign," or non-self, by the immune system of another person. Because the cell-surface proteins are non-self to another person's immune system, they are **antigens,** which are proteins capable of stimulating an immune response.

Human leukocyte antigens (HLAs) are this unique universal product code for each person. These antigens are also present on the surfaces of nearly all body cells—not just on leukocytes. HLAs are a normal part of the person and act as antigens only if they enter another person's body. These antigens determine the *tissue type* of a person. Other names for these cellular fingerprints are *human transplantation antigens, human histocompatibility antigens, major histocompatibility antigens,* and *class I antigens.*

Humans have about 40 major HLAs that are determined by a set of genes called the *major histocompatibility complex (MHC).* The exact number of *minor* HLAs that any person has is not known. The specific antigens that any person has (of a large number of possible antigens) are determined by which MHC gene alleles were inherited from his or her parents.

The HLA is key for recognition and self-tolerance. The immune system cells constantly come into contact with other body cells and with any invader that enters the body. At each encounter, the immune system cells compare the surface protein HLAs to determine whether the encountered cell belongs in the body (Fig. 19-2). If the encountered cell's HLA perfectly matches the HLA of the immune system cell, the encountered cell is "self" and is not attacked by the immune system cell. If the encountered cell's HLA does not perfectly match the HLA of the immune system cell, the encountered cell is non-self, or foreign. The immune system cell then takes action to neutralize, destroy, or eliminate this foreign invader.

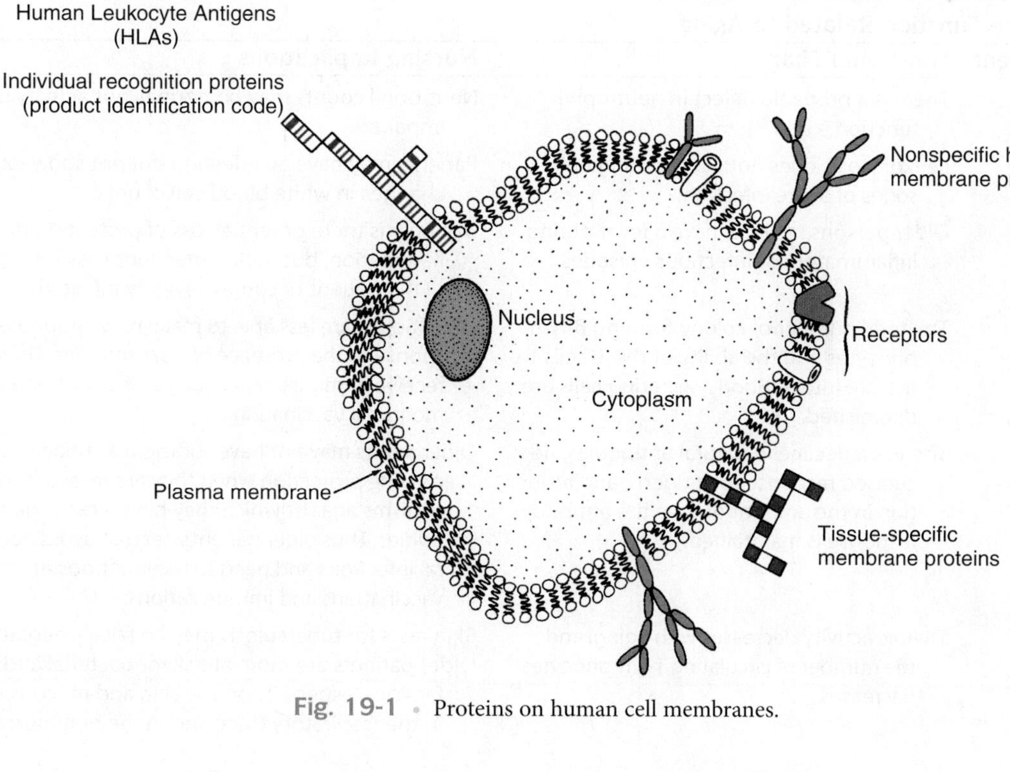
Human Leukocyte Antigens (HLAs)
Individual recognition proteins (product identification code)
Nonspecific human membrane proteins
Nucleus
Receptors
Cytoplasm
Plasma membrane
Tissue-specific membrane proteins

Fig. 19-1 • Proteins on human cell membranes.

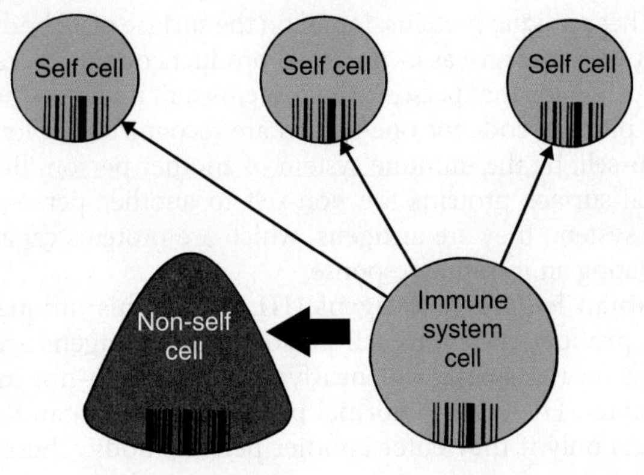

Self cell
Self cell
Self cell
Non-self cell
Immune system cell

Fig. 19-2 • Determination of self versus non-self cells.

Immune function changes during a person's life, according to nutritional status, environmental conditions, drugs, disease, and age. Immune function is most efficient when people are in their 20s and 30s and slowly declines with increasing age (Graham et al., 2006). Older adults have decreased immune function, increasing their risk for many health problems (Chart 19-1).

Organization of the Immune System

The immune system is not located in any one organ or body area but is influenced by many body systems, especially the nervous system, the endocrine system, and the GI system (Blalocke, 2005). Most immune system cells come from the bone marrow. Some cells mature in the bone marrow; others leave the bone marrow and mature in different body sites. When mature, many immune system cells are released into the blood, where they circulate to most body areas and have specific effects.

The bone marrow is the source of all blood cells, including immune system cells. The bone marrow produces immature, undifferentiated cells called **stem cells** (Abbas et al., 2007). Stem cells are **pluripotent,** meaning that each cell has more than one potential outcome. When the stem cell is first created in the bone marrow, it is undifferentiated. The cell is not yet committed to maturing into a specific blood cell type. At this stage, the stem cell is flexible (pluripotent) and could become any one of many mature blood cells. Fig. 19-3 shows the possible outcomes for maturation of the pluripotent stem cell. The type of mature cell that the stem cell becomes depends on which pathway it follows.

The maturational pathway of any stem cell depends on body needs at the time and on the presence of specific chemicals that direct growth (growth factors). For example, erythropoietin is a growth factor for red blood cells that is made in the kidney. When immature stem cells are exposed to erythropoietin, they commit to the erythrocyte pathway and eventually become mature red blood cells.

White blood cells **(leukocytes or WBCs)** protect the body from the effects of invasion by organisms. These cells are the immune system cells, the knight and soldiers protecting the castle inhabitants after invaders get through the castle wall. Table 19-1 lists the functions of different immune system cells. The leukocytes provide protection through many defensive actions (Abbas et al., 2007). These actions include:

- Recognition of self versus non-self
- Destruction of foreign invaders, cellular debris, and unhealthy or abnormal self cells
- Production of antibodies directed against invaders
- Complement activation
- Production of cytokines that stimulate increased formation of leukocytes in bone marrow and increase specific leukocyte activity

Chart 19-1 NURSING FOCUS ON THE OLDER ADULT

Changes in Immune Function Related to Aging

Immune Component	Functional Change	Nursing Implications
Inflammation	There is a probable defect in neutrophil function.	Neutrophil counts may be normal, but activity is reduced or impaired.
	Leukocytosis does not occur during episodes of acute infection.	Patients may have an infection but not show expected changes in white blood cell counts.
	Older persons may not have a fever during inflammatory or infectious episodes.	Not only is there potential loss of protection through inflammation, but minor infections may be overlooked until the patient becomes severely infected or septic.
Antibody-mediated immunity	The total number of colony-forming B-lymphocytes and the ability of these cells to mature into antibody-secreting cells are diminished.	Older adults are less able to make new antibodies in response to the presence of new antigens. Thus they should receive immunizations, such as "flu shots" and the pneumococcal vaccination.
	There is a decline in natural antibodies, decreased response to antigens, and reduction in the amount of time the antibody response is maintained.	Older adults may not have sufficient antibodies present to provide protection when they are re-exposed to microorganisms against which they have already generated antibodies. Thus older patients need to avoid people with viral infections and need to receive "booster" shots for old vaccinations and immunizations.
Cell-mediated immunity	Thymic activity decreases with aging, and the number of circulating T-lymphocytes decreases.	Skin tests for tuberculosis may be falsely negative. Older patients are more at risk for bacterial and fungal infections, especially on the skin and mucous membranes, in the respiratory tract, and in the genitourinary tract.

The three processes needed for human protection through immunity are (1) inflammation; (2) antibody-mediated immunity (AMI), also known as *humoral immunity;* and (3) cell-mediated immunity (CMI). Each process uses different defensive actions, and each influences or requires assistance from the other two processes (Fig. 19-4). *Therefore full immunity* ***(immunocompetence)*** *requires the function and interaction of all three processes.*

INFLAMMATION

Inflammation, also called *natural immunity,* provides immediate protection against the effects of tissue injury and invading foreign proteins. The ability to produce an inflammatory response is critical to health and well-being. Inflammation differs from AMI and CMI in two important ways (O'Neill, 2005):

- Inflammatory protection is immediate but short-term against injury or invading organism. It does not provide true immunity on repeated exposure to the same organisms.
- Inflammation is a *nonspecific* body defense to invasion or injury and can be started quickly by almost any event, regardless of where it occurs or what causes it.

So, inflammation triggered by a scald burn to the hand is the same as inflammation triggered by excess stomach acid or by bacteria in the middle ear. How widespread the symptoms of inflammation are depends on the intensity, severity, and duration of exposure to the initiating injury or invasion. For example, a splinter in the finger triggers inflammation only at the splinter site, whereas a burn injuring 50% of the skin leads to an inflammatory response involving the entire body.

Purpose

Inflammatory responses start tissue actions that cause visible and uncomfortable symptoms. Despite the discomfort, these actions are important in ridding the body of harmful organisms. However, if the inflammatory response is excessive, tissue damage may result. Inflammatory responses also help start both antibody-mediated and cell-mediated actions to activate a full immune response (O'Neill, 2005).

Infection

A confusing issue about inflammation is that this process occurs in response to tissue injury, as well as to invasion by organisms. *Infection is usually accompanied by inflammation;*

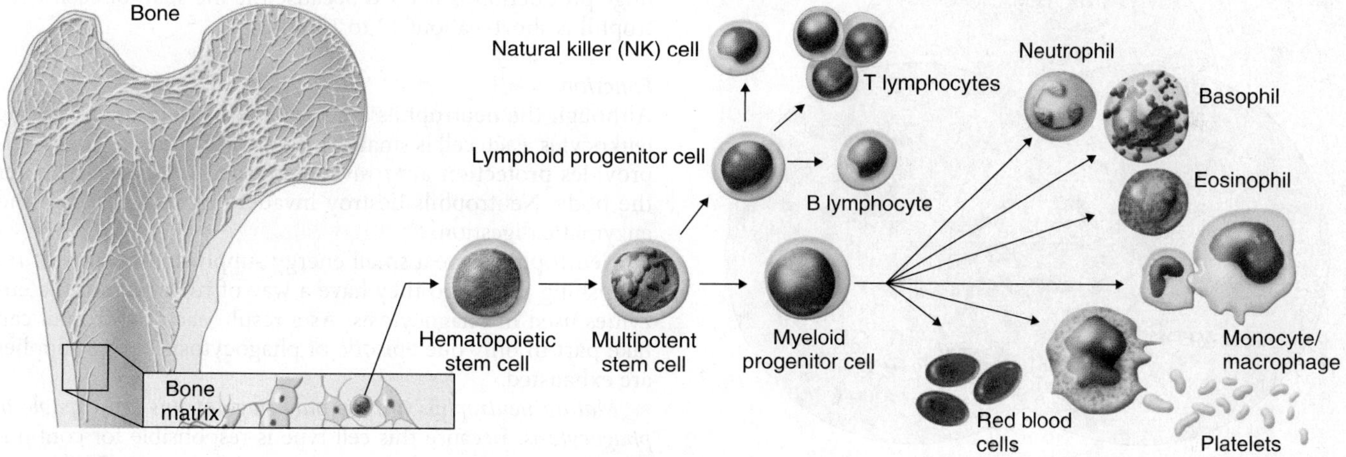
Bone
Bone matrix
Hematopoietic stem cell
Multipotent stem cell
Lymphoid progenitor cell
Natural killer (NK) cell
T lymphocytes
B lymphocyte
Myeloid progenitor cell
Neutrophil
Basophil
Eosinophil
Monocyte/ macrophage
Red blood cells
Platelets

Fig. 19-3 • Stem cell differentiation and maturation.

TABLE 19-1 Immune Functions of Specific Leukocytes

Variable	Leukocyte	Function
Inflammation	Neutrophil	Nonspecific ingestion and phagocytosis of microorganisms and foreign protein
	Macrophage	Nonspecific recognition of foreign proteins and microorganisms; ingestion and phagocytosis
	Monocyte	Destruction of bacteria and cellular debris; matures into macrophage
	Eosinophil	Weak phagocytic action; releases vasoactive amines during allergic reactions
	Basophil	Releases histamine and heparin in areas of tissue damage
Antibody-mediated immunity	B-lymphocyte	Becomes sensitized to foreign cells and proteins
	Plasma cell	Secretes immunoglobulins in response to the presence of a specific antigen
	Memory cell	Remains sensitized to a specific antigen and can secrete increased amounts of immunoglobulins specific to the antigen on re-exposure
Cell-mediated immunity	T-lymphocyte helper/ inducer T-cell	Enhances immune activity through secretion of various factors, cytokines, and lymphokines
	Cytotoxic/cytolytic T-cell	Selectively attacks and destroys non-self cells, including virally infected cells, grafts, and transplanted organs
	Natural killer cell	Nonselectively attacks non-self cells, especially body cells that have undergone mutation and become malignant; also attacks grafts and transplanted organs

however, inflammation can occur without infection. Examples of inflammation without infection include sprain injuries to joints, myocardial infarction, sterile surgical incisions, blister formation, and thrombophlebitis. Examples of inflammation caused by noninfectious invasion by foreign proteins include allergic rhinitis, contact dermatitis, and other allergic reactions. Inflammations caused by infection include otitis media, appendicitis, peritonitis, and viral hepatitis, among many others. *Inflammation does not always mean that an infection is present.*

Cell Types Involved in Inflammation

The leukocytes involved in inflammation are neutrophils, macrophages, eosinophils, and basophils. Neutrophils and macrophages use phagocytosis to destroy and eliminate foreign invaders. Basophils and eosinophils release chemicals that act on blood vessels to cause tissue-level responses.

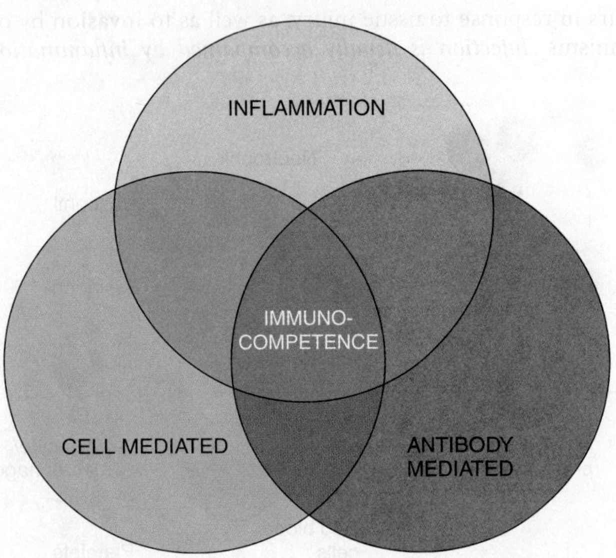
INFLAMMATION
IMMUNO-
COMPETENCE
CELL MEDIATED
ANTIBODY
MEDIATED

Fig. 19-4 • The three divisions of immunity. Each division (inflammation, antibody-mediated immunity, and cell-mediated immunity) has an important independent function. In addition, the function of each division of immunity is profoundly influenced by the other two divisions. Most important, optimal function of all three divisions is necessary for complete immunity.

Neutrophils

Description and Origin

Mature neutrophils make up between 55% and 70% of the normal total white blood cell (WBC) count. Neutrophils come from the stem cells and complete the maturation process in the bone marrow (Fig. 19-5). They are also called **granulocytes** because of the large number of granules present inside each cell. Other names for neutrophils are based on their appearance and maturity. Mature neutrophils are also called *segmented neutrophils* ("segs") or *polymorphonuclear cells* ("polys," PMNs,) because of their segmented nucleus. Less mature neutrophils are called *band neutrophils* ("bands" or "stabs") because of their nuclear shape.

Usually, growth of a stem cell into a mature neutrophil requires 12 to 14 days. This time is shortened by conditions that trigger the body to produce specific growth factors (cytokines), such as granulocyte-macrophage colony-stimulating factor (GM-CSF) and granulocyte colony-stimulating factor (G-CSF). The purpose and action of cytokines are described on pp. 317-318 in the Cytokines section.

In the immunocompetent healthy person, more than 100 billion fresh, mature neutrophils are released from the bone marrow into the circulation daily (Abbas et al., 2007). This huge production is needed because the life span of each neutrophil is short—about 12 to 18 hours.

Function

Although the neutrophils are the largest group of circulating leukocytes, each cell is small. This powerful army of small cells provides protection after invaders (especially bacteria) enter the body. Neutrophils destroy invaders by phagocytosis and enzymatic digestion.

Neutrophils have a small energy supply and no way of replenishing it; nor do they have a way of replenishing the enzymes used in phagocytosis. As a result, each neutrophil can take part in only one episode of phagocytosis before supplies are exhausted.

Mature neutrophils are the only stage of this cell capable of phagocytosis. Because this cell type is responsible for continuous, instant, nonspecific protection against organisms, the percentage and actual number of mature circulating neutrophils are used to measure a patient's risk for infection: the higher the numbers, the greater the resistance to infection. This measurement is the **absolute neutrophil count (ANC),** also called the *absolute granulocyte count* or *total granulocyte count.*

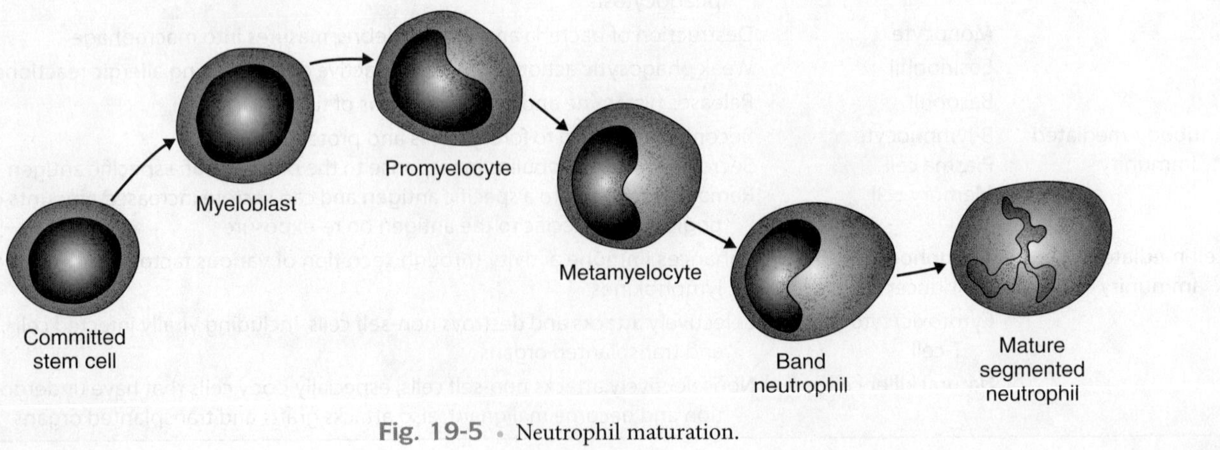
Committed
stem cell
Myeloblast
Promyelocyte
Metamyelocyte
Band
neutrophil
Mature
segmented
neutrophil

Fig. 19-5 • Neutrophil maturation.

The differential of a normal white blood cell count shows the number and percent of many different types of circulating leukocytes (Table 19-2). The values in this table indicate that most of the neutrophils released into the blood from the bone marrow are segmented neutrophils; only a small percentage are band neutrophils. The less mature neutrophil forms should not be in the blood. Some problems, such as sepsis, cause the neutrophils in the blood to change from being mostly segmented neutrophils to being less mature forms. This situation is termed a **left shift** or *bandemia* because the segmented neutrophil, which is seen at the far right of the neutrophil pathway (see Fig. 19-5), is no longer the most numerous type of circulating neutrophils. Instead, more of the circulating cells are bands—the less mature cell type found farther left on the neutrophil pathway.

A left shift indicates that the patient's bone marrow cannot produce enough mature neutrophils to keep pace with the continuing infection and is releasing immature neutrophils into the blood. Unfortunately, most of these immature cells are of no benefit because they are not capable of phagocytosis.

Macrophages

Description and Origin

Macrophages come from the committed myeloid stem cells in the bone marrow and form the mononuclear-phagocyte system. The stem cells first form monocytes, which are released into the blood at this stage. Until they mature, monocytes have limited activity. Most monocytes move from the blood into body tissues, where they mature into macrophages. Some macrophages become "fixed" in position within the tissues, whereas others can move within and between tissues. Macrophages in various tissues have slightly different appearances and names (Table 19-3). The liver, spleen, and intestinal tract contain large numbers of these cells.

TABLE 19-2 Values of a White Blood Cell Differential for Peripheral Blood Representing a Normal Count

WBC Type	%	/mm³
Total WBC	**100.5**	**10,000**
Segs	62	6,200
Bands	5	500
Monos	3	300
Lymphs	28	2,800
Eosin	1.5	150
Baso	0.5	50

TABLE 19-3 Tissue Macrophages

Tissue	Macrophage
Lung	Alveolar macrophage
Connective tissue	Histiocyte
Brain	Microglial cell
Liver	Kupffer cell
Peritoneum	Peritoneal macrophage
Bone	Osteoclast
Joint	Synovial type A cell
Kidney	Mesangial cell

Function

Macrophages play more than one role in *protection.* These cells are important in immediate inflammatory responses and also stimulate the longer-lasting immune responses of antibody-mediated immunity (AMI) and cell-mediated immunity (CMI). Specific macrophage functions include phagocytosis, repair, antigen presenting/processing, and secretion of cytokines that help control the immune system.

The inflammatory function of macrophages is phagocytosis. Macrophages can easily distinguish between self and nonself, and their large size makes them very effective at trapping invading cells. Unlike neutrophils, macrophages have long life spans and can renew the energy supplies and enzymes needed to degrade foreign protein. Therefore each macrophage can take part in many phagocytic events.

Basophils

Description and Origin

Basophils come from myeloid stem cells and make up only about 1% of the total circulating WBC count. These cells cause the manifestations of inflammation.

Function

Basophils have granules containing many chemicals (vasoactive amines) that act on blood vessels. These chemicals include heparin, histamine, serotonin, kinins, and leukotrienes. When released into the blood, most of these chemicals act on smooth muscle and blood vessel walls. Heparin inhibits blood and protein clotting. Histamine constricts small veins and respiratory smooth muscles. Constriction of respiratory smooth muscle narrows airways and restricts breathing. Constriction of veins inhibits blood flow and decreases venous return. This effect causes blood to collect in capillaries and arterioles. Kinins dilate arterioles and increase capillary permeability. These actions cause blood plasma to leak into the interstitial space *(vascular leak syndrome).*

Eosinophils

Description and Origin

Eosinophils come from the myeloid line and contain many vasoactive chemicals. Usually, only 1% to 2% of the total white blood cell (WBC) count is composed of eosinophils.

Function

Eosinophils act against infestations of parasitic larvae. Their granules contain many different substances. Some substances induce inflammation when released. In addition, enzymes from eosinophils degrade the vasoactive chemicals released by other leukocytes and can limit inflammatory reactions. This is why the number of circulating eosinophils increases during an allergic response.

Phagocytosis

A key process of inflammation is phagocytosis. **Phagocytosis** is the engulfing and destruction of invaders. This action also rids the body of debris after tissue injury. Neutrophils and macrophages are most efficient at phagocytosis. Phagocytosis involves the seven steps shown in Fig. 19-6.

Exposure and invasion occur as the first step. Leukocytes that engage in phagocytosis and stimulate inflammation are present in the blood and other extracellular fluids. For phagocytosis to start, leukocytes must first be exposed to organisms,

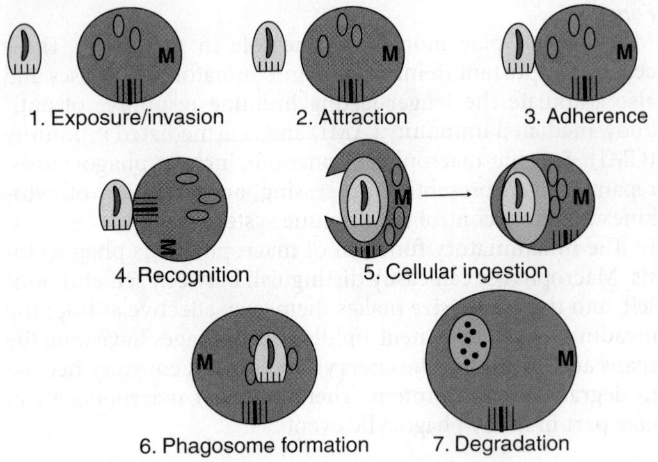
M
1. Exposure/invasion
2. Attraction
3. Adherence
4. Recognition
5. Cellular ingestion
6. Phagosome formation
7. Degradation

Fig. 19-6 • Steps of phagocytosis.

foreign proteins, or debris from damaged tissues. Phagocytosis is triggered by injury or invasion.

Attraction is needed as the second step because phagocytosis can occur only when the WBC comes into direct contact with the target (antigen, invader, or foreign protein). Some substances attract neutrophils and macrophages. These substances are called **chemotaxins.** Damaged tissues and blood vessels secrete chemotaxins and release debris that can combine with the surface of invading foreign proteins.

Adherence is important because phagocytosis requires that the phagocytic cell first bind to the surface of the target. Opsonins are substances that increase contact of the cell with its target by coating the target cell (antigen or organism). During inflammation, coating the target makes it easier for phagocytic cells to stick to it. Many substances can act as opsonins. Some are particles from dead neutrophils, antibodies, and activated (fixated) complement components.

Complement activation and fixation are part of opsonization and help with adherence. Twenty different types of inactive complement proteins are present in the blood. When stimulated, each complement protein is activated, joins other activated complement proteins, surrounds an antigen, and "fixes" or sticks to the antigen. Complement fixation occurs quickly as a cascade or chain reaction.

Recognition occurs when the phagocytic cell sticks to the surface of the target cell and "recognizes" it as non-self. The phagocytic cells examine the universal product codes (human leukocyte antigens [HLAs]) of whatever they encounter. Recognition of non-self is made easier by opsonins on the target cell surface. Phagocytic cells start phagocytosis only when the target cell is recognized either as non-self or as debris from damaged self cells.

Cellular ingestion is needed because phagocytic destruction occurs inside the cell. The target cell is brought inside the phagocytic cell by phagocytosis (engulfment). The phagocytic cell bends its membrane around to enclose (engulf) the target cell and form a vacuole.

Phagosome formation occurs when the phagocyte's granules are inside the vacuole. These granules break and release enzymes that attack the ingested target.

Degradation is the final step. The enzymes in the phagosome digest the engulfed target. The target is broken into smaller pieces until only small particles of debris remain.

Sequence of Inflammatory Responses

Inflammatory responses occur in a predictable sequence of three stages. The sequence is the same regardless of the triggering event. Responses at the tissue level cause the **five cardinal manifestations of inflammation:** warmth, redness, swelling, pain, and decreased function. The timing of the stages may overlap.

◀ ANIMATION: Inflammatory Response

Stage I is the vascular part of the inflammatory response. In this stage, the early effects involve changes in blood vessels. Injured tissues and the leukocytes in this area secrete histamine, serotonin, and kinins that constrict the small veins and dilate the arterioles in the area of injury. These blood vessel changes cause redness and warmth of the tissues. This increased blood flow increases delivery of nutrients to injured tissues.

Blood flow to the area increases **(hyperemia)** and **edema** (swelling) forms at the site of injury or invasion. Capillary leak also occurs, allowing blood plasma to leak into the tissues. This response causes swelling and pain. Edema at the site of injury or invasion protects the area from further injury by creating a cushion of fluid. The extra fluid also can dilute any toxins or organisms that have entered the area. The duration of these responses depends on the severity of the initiating event, but usually they subside within 24 to 72 hours.

The macrophage is the major cell involved in stage I of inflammation. The action is rapid because macrophages are already in place at the site of injury or invasion. This action is limited because the number of macrophages is so small. To enhance the inflammatory response, the tissue macrophages secrete several cytokines. One cytokine is colony-stimulating factor (CSF), which triggers the bone marrow to shorten the length of time to produce white blood cells (WBCs) from 14 days to a matter of hours. Some of the cytokines also increase the release of neutrophils from the bone marrow and attract them to the site of injury or invasion, which leads to the next stage of inflammation.

Stage II is the cellular exudate part of the response. In this stage, **neutrophilia** (an increased number of circulating neutrophils) occurs. Exudate in the form of pus occurs, containing dead WBCs, necrotic tissue, and fluids that escape from damaged cells.

The most active cell in this stage is the neutrophil. Under the influence of cytokines, the neutrophil count can increase up to five times within 12 hours after the onset of inflammation. At the site of inflammation, neutrophils attack and destroy organisms and remove dead tissue through phagocytosis.

In acute inflammation, the healthy person produces enough mature neutrophils to keep pace with invasion and prevent the organisms from growing. At the same time, the WBCs and inflamed tissues secrete cytokines, which allow tissue macrophages to increase and trigger bone marrow production of monocytes. This reaction begins slowly, but its effects are long lasting.

During this phase, the arachidonic acid cascade starts to increase the inflammatory response. This action begins by the conversion of fatty acids in plasma membranes into arachidonic acid (AA). Then, enzymes (including cyclooxygenase) convert AA into many chemicals that are further processed into the substances that continue the inflammatory response in the tissues. Some of these substances include histamine, leukotrienes, prostaglandins, serotonin, and kinins. Many anti-inflammatory drugs stop this cascade by preventing cyclooxygenase from converting AA into inflammatory substances.

When an infection stimulating inflammation lasts longer than just a few days, the bone marrow cannot produce and release enough mature neutrophils into the blood to keep pace with the growth of organisms. In this situation, the bone marrow begins to release immature neutrophils, reducing the number of circulating mature neutrophils. This reduction of mature neutrophils limits the helpful effects of inflammation and increases the risk for sepsis.

Stage III features tissue repair and replacement. Although this stage is completed last, it begins at the time of injury and is critical to the final function of the inflamed area.

Some of the WBCs involved in inflammation start the replacement of lost tissues or repair of damaged tissues by inducing the remaining healthy cells to divide. In tissues that cannot divide, WBCs trigger new blood vessel growth (angiogenesis) and scar tissue formation. Because scar tissue does not behave like normal tissue, function is lost wherever damaged tissues are replaced with scar tissue. The degree of function lost is determined by how much tissue is replaced by scar tissue. For example, when heart muscles are destroyed because of a myocardial infarction (heart attack), scar tissue forms in the area to prevent a hole from forming in the muscle wall as the ischemic cells die. (Remember that heart muscle is non-dividing tissue and the heart cannot replace these muscle cells.) The scar tissue serves only as a patch; it does not contract or act in any way like heart muscle. So, if 20% of the left ventricle is replaced with scar tissue, the effectiveness of left ventricular contraction is reduced by at least 20%.

Inflammation alone cannot provide immunity. Inflammatory cells must interact with lymphocytes to provide long-lasting immunity (O'Neill, 2005). Long-lasting immune actions develop through antibody-mediated immunity (AMI) and cell-mediated immunity (CMI).

ANTIBODY-MEDIATED IMMUNITY

Antibody-mediated immunity (AMI), also known as *humoral immunity,* involves antigen-antibody interactions to neutralize, eliminate, or destroy foreign proteins. Antibodies are produced by B-lymphocytes (B-cells).

Purpose

The main purposes of B-cells are to become sensitized to a specific foreign protein (antigen) and to produce antibodies directed specifically against that protein. The antibody (rather than the actual B-cell) causes one of several actions to neutralize, eliminate, or destroy that antigen.

B-cells have the most direct role in AMI. Macrophages and T-lymphocytes (discussed on p. 317 in the Cell-Mediated Immunity section) work with B-cells to start and complete antigen-antibody interactions. For optimal AMI, the entire immune system must function adequately.

B-cells start as stem cells in the bone marrow, the primary lymphoid tissue. Those stem cells that become B-cells commit early to the lymphocyte pathway (see Fig. 19-3) and are then restricted in development. The lymphocyte stem cells are released from the bone marrow into the blood. They then migrate into many secondary lymphoid tissues, where maturation is completed. The secondary lymphoid tissues for B-cell maturation are the spleen, parts of lymph nodes, tonsils, and the mucosa of the intestinal tract.

Antigen-Antibody Interactions

The body learns to make enough of any specific antibody to provide long-lasting immunity and protection against specific organisms or toxins. Seven steps are needed to produce a specific antibody directed against a specific antigen whenever the person is exposed to that antigen. These steps are exposure (invasion), antigen recognition, lymphocyte sensitization, antibody production and release, antigen-antibody binding, antibody-binding reactions, and sustained immunity, or memory (Fig. 19-7).

Exposure or invasion is needed because antibody actions occur inside the body or on a few body surfaces. For a person to make an antibody that can exert its effects on a specific antigen, the antigen must first enter the person. Not all exposures or invasions result in antibody production. Invasion by the antigen must occur in such large numbers that some of the antigen evades detection by the body's natural nonspecific defenses or overwhelms the ability of the inflammatory response to get rid of the invader.

Take, for example, a person who has never been exposed to the childhood viral disease *chickenpox.* This person baby-sits for three children who develop chickenpox lesions within the next 10 hours. These children, in the pre-eruption stage, shed many millions of live chickenpox virus particles via droplets from the upper respiratory tract. Because small children are often unconcerned about the finer points of infection control, they drink out of the baby-sitter's cup, kiss him or her directly on the lips, and sneeze and cough directly into his or her face. During the 5 hours spent with the children, the baby-sitter is heavily invaded by the chickenpox virus (varicella-zoster) and will become sick with this disease within 14 to 21 days. While the virus is growing and the disease is developing, the baby-sitter's white blood cells are taking part in antibody-antigen actions to prevent him or her from having chickenpox more than once.

Antigen recognition is the next step to begin making antibodies against an antigen. The "naive," or "virgin," unsensitized B-cell must first recognize the antigen as non-self. B-cells need the help of macrophages and helper/inducer T-cells to recognize an antigen.

Recognition is started by the macrophages. After the antigen surface has been altered by opsonization (see discussion of "Adherence" on p. 312), the macrophage recognizes the invading antigen as non-self and physically attaches itself to the antigen. This attachment does not result in phagocytosis or in antigen destruction. Instead, the macrophage presents the attached antigen to the helper/inducer T-cell. Then, the helper/inducer T-cell and the macrophage together process the antigen to expose the antigen's recognition sites (universal product code). After processing the antigen, the helper/inducer T-cell brings the antigen into contact with the B-cell so that the B-cell can recognize the antigen as non-self.

Lymphocyte sensitization occurs when the B-cell recognizes the antigen as non-self and is now "sensitized" to this antigen. A single naive B-cell can become sensitized only once. *So, each B-cell can be sensitized to only one type of antigen.*

Sensitizing allows this B-cell to respond to any substance that carries the same antigens (codes) as the original antigen. The sensitized B-cell always remains sensitized to that specific antigen. In addition, all cells produced by that sensitized B-cell also are sensitized to that same specific antigen.

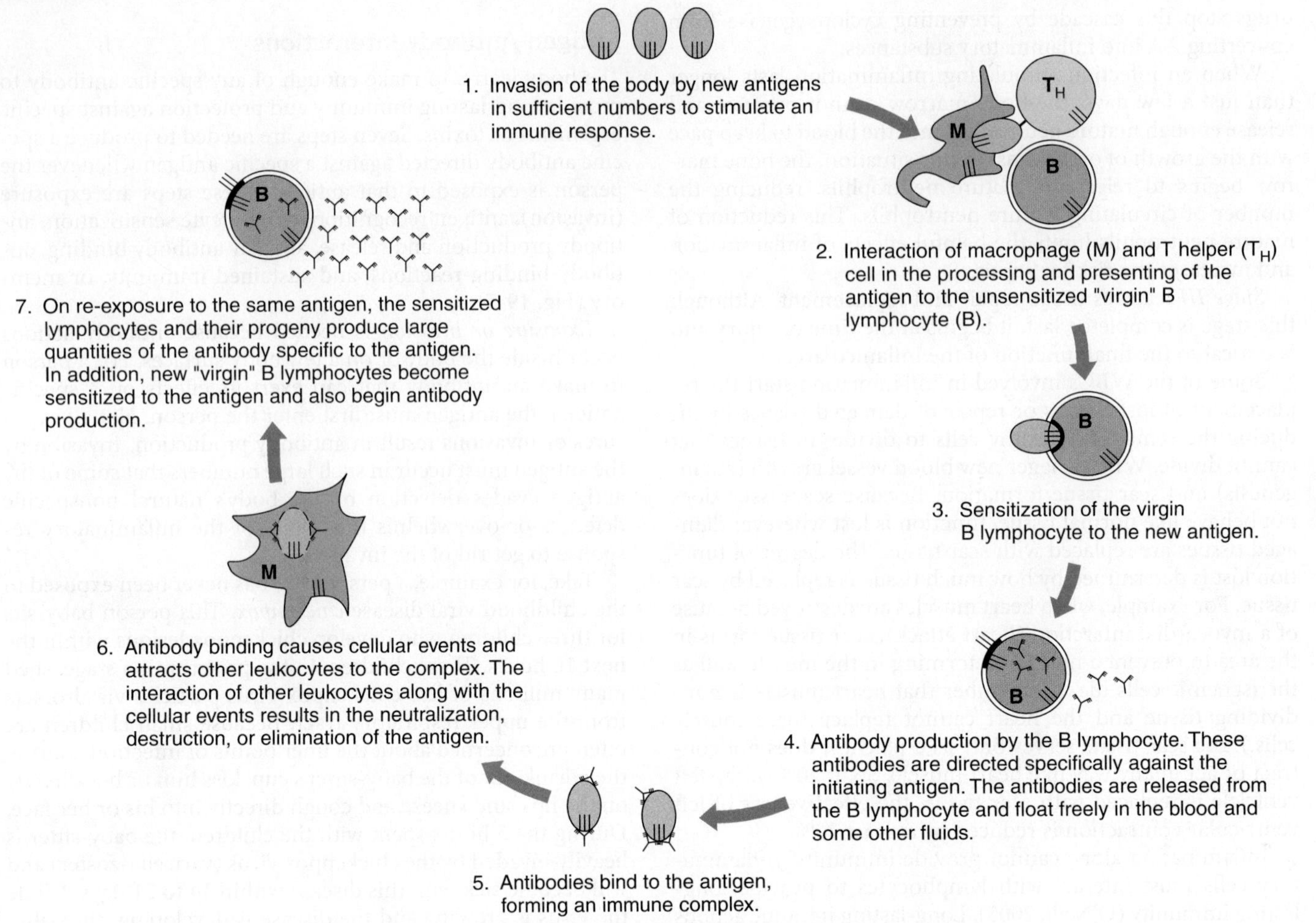
1. Invasion of the body by new antigens in sufficient numbers to stimulate an immune response.
TH
M
B
2. Interaction of macrophage (M) and T helper (TH) cell in the processing and presenting of the antigen to the unsensitized "virgin" B lymphocyte (B).
B
3. Sensitization of the virgin B lymphocyte to the new antigen.
B
4. Antibody production by the B lymphocyte. These antibodies are directed specifically against the initiating antigen. The antibodies are released from the B lymphocyte and float freely in the blood and some other fluids.
5. Antibodies bind to the antigen, forming an immune complex.
6. Antibody binding causes cellular events and attracts other leukocytes to the complex. The interaction of other leukocytes along with the cellular events results in the neutralization, destruction, or elimination of the antigen.
M
7. On re-exposure to the same antigen, the sensitized lymphocytes and their progeny produce large quantities of the antibody specific to the antigen. In addition, new "virgin" B lymphocytes become sensitized to the antigen and also begin antibody production.
B

Fig. 19-7 • Sequence of events stimulating antibody-mediated immunity.

Immediately after it is sensitized, the B-cell divides and forms two types of B-lymphocytes, each one remaining sensitized to that specific antigen (Fig. 19-8). One new cell becomes a **plasma cell,** which can start immediately to produce antibodies against the sensitizing antigen. This new plasma cell functions immediately but has a short life span. The other new cell becomes a memory cell. The **memory cell** is a sensitized B-cell but does not start to function until the next exposure to the same antigen (see discussion of "Sustained immunity (memory)" on p. 316).

Antibody production and release allow the antibodies to search out specific antigens. Antibodies are produced by plasma cells. When fully stimulated, each plasma cell can make as many as 300 molecules of antibody per second. Each plasma cell produces antibody specific only to the antigen that originally sensitized the parent B-cell. For example, in the case of the baby-sitter who was exposed to and invaded by the chickenpox virus, the plasma cells from those B-cells sensitized to the chickenpox virus can make only anti-chickenpox antibodies. The antibody class (e.g., immunoglobulin G [IgG] or immunoglobulin M [IgM]) that the plasma cell produces may vary, but the antibody can be forever directed only against the chickenpox virus.

Antibody molecules made by plasma cells are released into the blood and other body fluids as free antibody. Each free antibody molecule remains in the blood for 3 to 30 days. Because the antibody is in body fluids (or body "humors") and is separate from the B-cells, this type of immunity is sometimes called **humoral immunity.** *Circulating antibodies can be transferred from one person to another to provide the receiving person with immediate immunity of short duration.*

Antibody-antigen binding is needed for anti-antigen actions. Antibodies are Y-shaped molecules (Fig. 19-9). The tips of the short arms of the Y recognize the specific antigen and bind to it. Because each antibody molecule has two tips (Fab fragments, or arms), each antibody can bind either to two separate antigens or to two areas of the same antigen.

The stem of the Y is the "Fc fragment." This area can bind to Fc receptor sites on white blood cells (WBCs). The WBC then not only has its own means of attacking antigens but also has the added power of having surface antibodies that can stick to antigens (see Fig. 19-9).

The binding of antibody to antigen may not be lethal to the antigen. Instead, antibody-antigen binding starts other actions that neutralize, eliminate, or destroy the antigen.

Antibody-binding actions are triggered by binding of antibody to antigen. The resulting reactions neutralize, eliminate, or destroy the bound antigen. These actions include agglutination, lysis, complement fixation, precipitation, and inactivation or neutralization.

Agglutination is a clumping action that results from the antibody linking antigens together, forming large and small im-

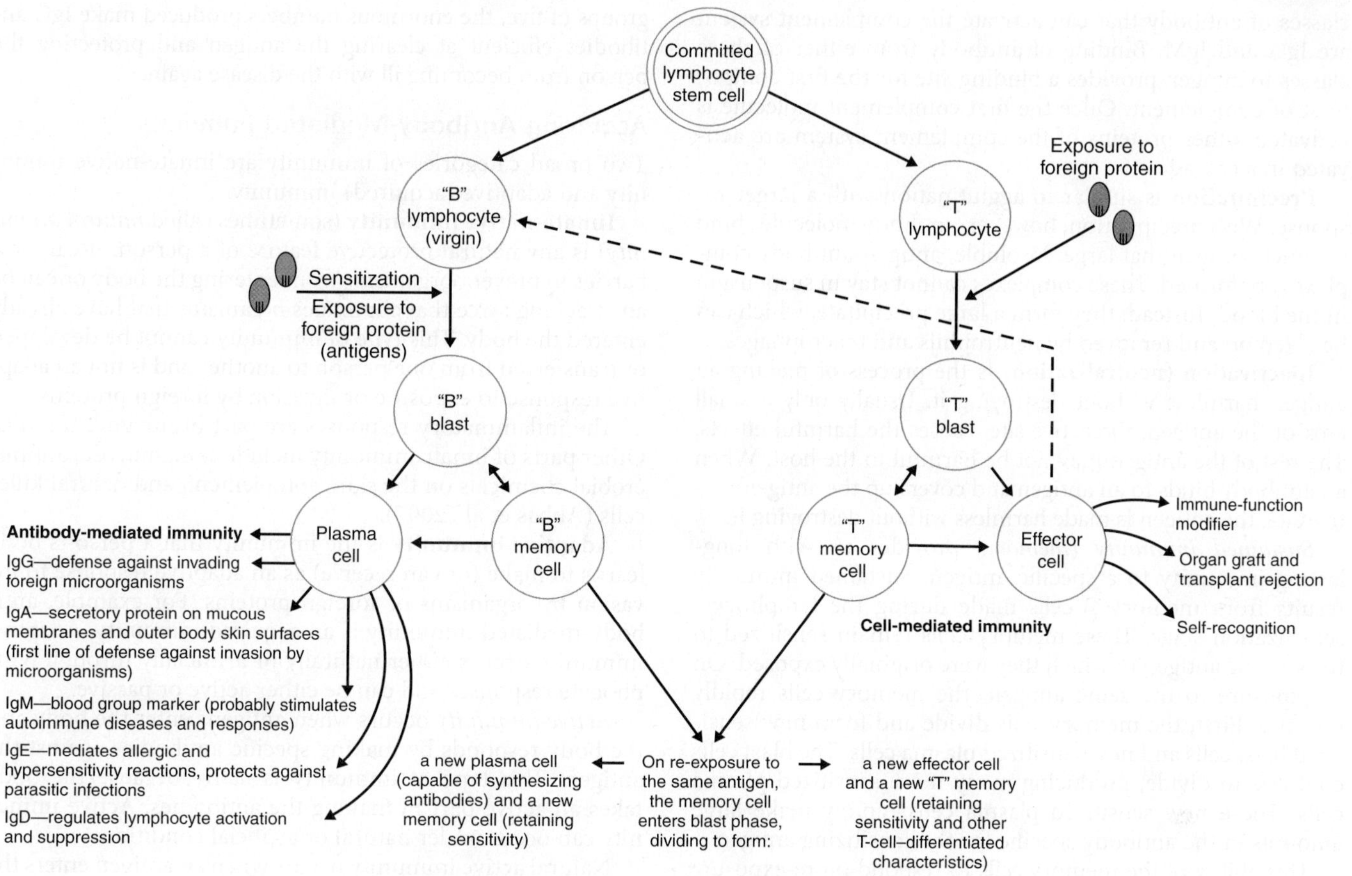
Committed lymphocyte stem cell
"B" lymphocyte (virgin)
Sensitization
Exposure to foreign protein (antigens)
"B" blast
Plasma cell
"B" memory cell
Antibody-mediated immunity
IgG—defense against invading foreign microorganisms
IgA—secretory protein on mucous membranes and outer body skin surfaces (first line of defense against invasion by microorganisms)
IgM—blood group marker (probably stimulates autoimmune diseases and responses)
IgE—mediates allergic and hypersensitivity reactions, protects against parasitic infections
IgD—regulates lymphocyte activation and suppression
a new plasma cell (capable of synthesizing antibodies) and a new memory cell (retaining sensitivity)
On re-exposure to the same antigen, the memory cell enters blast phase, dividing to form:
a new effector cell and a new "T" memory cell (retaining sensitivity and other T-cell–differentiated characteristics)
Exposure to foreign protein
"T" lymphocyte
"T" blast
"T" memory cell
Effector cell
Immune-function modifier
Organ graft and transplant rejection
Self-recognition
Cell-mediated immunity

Fig. 19-8 • Differentiated functions of lymphocytes.

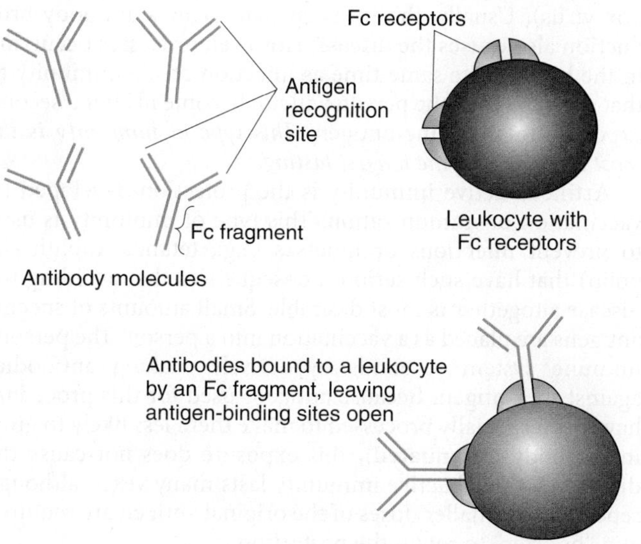
Fc receptors
Antigen recognition site
Fc fragment
Antibody molecules
Leukocyte with Fc receptors
Antibodies bound to a leukocyte by an Fc fragment, leaving antigen-binding sites open

Fig. 19-9 • Antibody structure and the Fc receptors on leukocytes.

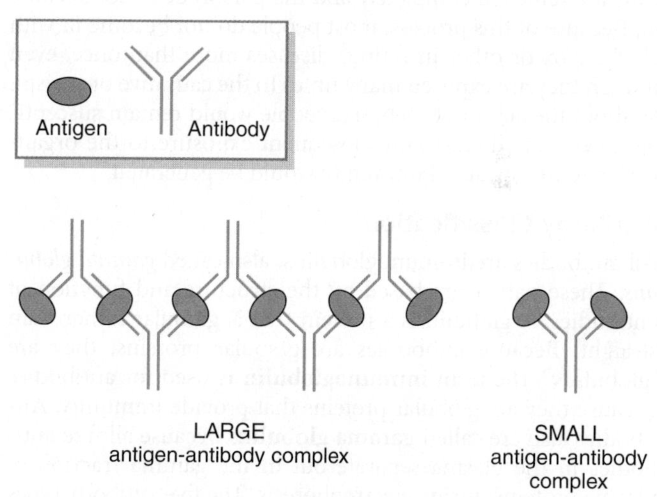
Antigen
Antibody
LARGE antigen-antibody complex
SMALL antigen-antibody complex

Fig. 19-10 • Antibody-antigen complexes.

mune complexes (Fig. 19-10). Agglutination alone does not directly destroy the antigen. This action starts other defensive effects. First, it slows the movement of the antigen through body fluids. Second, the irregular shape of the antigen-antibody complex (see Fig. 19-10) increases the chances of the complex being attacked by other WBCs (e.g., macrophages, neutrophils).

Lysis is cell membrane destruction, and it occurs now because of antibody binding to membrane-bound antigens of some invaders. The actual binding makes holes in the invader's membrane, weakening the invader. This response usually requires that complement be activated and "fixed" to the immune complex. Bacteria and viruses are the non-self cells that are damaged most through lysis caused by the binding of antibody to antigens.

Complement activation and fixation are actions triggered by some classes of antibodies that can remove or destroy antigen. (See "Adherence" on p. 312 for a discussion of the mechanism by which complement assists in immunity.) The two classes of antibody that can activate the complement system are IgG and IgM. Binding of antibody from either of these classes to antigen provides a binding site for the first component of complement. Once the first complement molecule is activated, other proteins of the complement system are activated in a cascade.

Precipitation is similar to agglutination with a larger response. With precipitation, however, antibody molecules bind so much antigen that large, insoluble, antigen-antibody complexes are formed. These complexes cannot stay in suspension in the blood. Instead, they form a large precipitate, which can be acted on and removed by neutrophils and macrophages.

Inactivation (neutralization) is the process of making an antigen harmless without destroying it. Usually only a small area of the antigen, the active site, causes the harmful effects. The rest of the antigen may not be harmful to the host. When an antibody binds to an antigen and covers up the antigen's active site, the antigen is made harmless without destroying it.

Sustained immunity (memory) provides us with long-lasting immunity to a specific antigen. Sustained immunity results from memory B-cells made during the lymphocyte sensitization stage. These memory cells remain sensitized to the specific antigen to which they were originally exposed. On re-exposure to the same antigen, the memory cells rapidly respond. First, the memory cells divide and form new sensitized blast cells and new sensitized plasma cells. The blast cells continue to divide, producing many more sensitized plasma cells. These new sensitized plasma cells rapidly make large amounts of the antibody specific for the sensitizing antigen.

This ability of the memory cells to respond on re-exposure to the same antigen that originally sensitized the B-cell allows a rapid and large immune (anamnestic) response to the antigen. Because so much antibody is made, usually the invading organisms are removed completely and the person does not become ill. Because of this process, most people do not become ill with chickenpox or other infectious diseases more than once, even though they are exposed many times to the causative organism. Without the action of memory, people would remain susceptible to specific diseases on subsequent exposure to the organisms and no sustained immunity would be generated.

Antibody Classification

All antibodies are immunoglobulins, also called *gamma globulins.* These names are based on the structure and function of antibodies. A globulin is a protein that is globular rather than straight. Because antibodies are globular proteins, they are "globulins." The term **immunoglobulin** is used for antibodies because they are globular proteins that provide immunity. Antibodies also are called **gamma globulins** because all free antibodies in the plasma separate out in the gamma fraction of plasma proteins during electrophoresis. The five antibody types are classified by differences in size and timing (see Fig. 19-8).

On first exposure to an antigen, the newly sensitized B-cell produces the IgM antibody type against the antigen. IgM is special because it forms itself into a five-member group. Each IgM group, then, has ten antigen binding sites. So, even though antibody production is slow on first exposure, the antibody type produced forms groups that are very efficient at antigen binding. This process ensures that the initial illness, like chickenpox, lasts only 5 to 10 days. On re-exposure to the same antigen, the already sensitized B-cell makes large amounts of the IgG type of antibody against that antigen. Although IgG does not form groups of five, the enormous numbers produced make IgG antibodies efficient at clearing the antigen and protecting the person from becoming ill with the disease again.

Acquiring Antibody-Mediated Immunity

Two broad categories of immunity are innate-native immunity and adaptive (acquired) immunity.

Innate-native immunity (sometimes called *natural immunity*) is any natural protective feature of a person. It can be a barrier to prevent organisms from entering the body or can be an attacking force that eliminates organisms that have already entered the body. This type of immunity cannot be developed or transferred from one person to another and is not an adaptive response to exposure or invasion by foreign proteins.

The inflammatory responses are part of innate immunity. Other parts of innate immunity include skin, mucosa, antimicrobial chemicals on the skin, complement, and natural killer cells (Abbas et al., 2007).

Adaptive immunity is the immunity that a person's body learns to make (or can receive) as an adaptive response to invasion by organisms or foreign proteins. For example, antibody-mediated immunity is an acquired immunity. Adaptive immunity occurs either naturally or artificially through lymphocyte responses and can be either active or passive.

Active immunity occurs when antigens enter the body and the body responds by making specific antibodies against the antigen. This type of immunity is *active* because the body takes an active part in making the antibodies. Active immunity can occur under natural or artificial conditions.

Natural active immunity occurs when an antigen enters the body without human assistance and the body responds by actively making antibodies against that antigen (e.g., chickenpox virus). Usually, the invasion that triggers antibody production also causes the disease. However, processes occurring in the body at the same time as infection create immunity to that antigen. Thus the person will not become ill after a second exposure to the same antigen. *This type of immunity is the most effective and the longest lasting.*

Artificial active immunity is the protection developed by vaccination or immunization. This type of immunity is used to prevent infections or illnesses (e.g., tetanus, diphtheria, polio) that have such serious consequences that avoiding the disease altogether is most desirable. Small amounts of specific antigens are placed as a vaccination into a person. The person's immune system responds by actively making antibodies against the antigen. Because antigens used for this procedure have been specially processed to make them less likely to grow in the body **(attenuated)**, this exposure does not cause the disease. Artificial active immunity lasts many years, although repeated but smaller doses of the original antigen are required as a "booster" to retain the protection.

Passive immunity occurs when antibodies against an antigen are in a person's body but were not created there. Rather, these antibodies are transferred to the person's body after being made in the body of another person or animal. Because these antibodies are foreign to the receiving person, the antibodies are recognized as non-self and eliminated quickly. For this reason, passive immunity provides only immediate, short-term protection against a specific antigen.

Natural passive immunity occurs when antibodies are passed from the mother to the fetus via the placenta or to the infant through colostrum and breast milk.

Artificial passive immunity involves injecting a person with antibodies that were produced in another person or animal. This type of immunity is used when a person is exposed to a serious disease for which he or she has little or no actively acquired immunity. Instead, the injected antibodies are expected to inactivate the antigen. This type of immune protection is temporary, lasting only days to a few weeks. Artificial passive immunity may be used to prevent disease or death for patients exposed to rabies, tetanus, and poisonous snake bites.

AMI works with inflammation to protect against infection. However, AMI can provide the most effective, long-lasting immunity only when its actions are combined with those of cell-mediated immunity (CMI).

CELL-MEDIATED IMMUNITY

Cell-mediated immunity (CMI), or cellular immunity, involves many white blood cell (WBC) actions and interactions. This type of immunity is provided by lymphocyte stem cells that mature in the secondary lymphoid tissues of the thymus and pericortical areas of lymph nodes. Certain CMI responses influence and regulate the activities of antibody-mediated immunity (AMI) and inflammation by producing and releasing cytokines. For total immunocompetence, then, CMI must function optimally.

Cell Types Involved in Cell-Mediated Immunity

The WBCs with the most important roles in CMI include several specific T-lymphocytes (T-cells) along with a special population of cells known as *natural killer (NK) cells.* T-cells have a variety of subsets, each of which has a specific function.

One way of identifying different T-cell subsets is to examine certain "marker proteins" (antigens) on the cell membrane's surface. More than 200 different T-cell proteins have been identified on the cell membrane, and 11 of these (named *T1* through *T11*) are commonly used clinically to identify specific cells. Antibodies have been made against each of these 11 proteins. Thus each T-cell subset can be identified by its reaction to the commercial antibodies. Most T-cells have more than one antigen on their cell membrane. For example, all mature T-cells contain T1, T3, T10, and T11 proteins. Certain T-cells also contain other specific T-cell membrane antigens.

The names used to identify specific T-cell subsets include the specific membrane antigen and the overall actions of the cells in a subset. The three T-lymphocyte subsets that are critically important for the development and continuation of CMI are helper/inducer T-cells, suppressor T-cells, and cytotoxic/cytolytic T-cells. An additional cell, the natural killer cell, although not a true T-cell, also contributes to CMI.

Helper/inducer T-cells have the T4 protein on their membranes. These cells are usually called *T4+ cells* or T_H cells. The most correct name for helper/inducer T-cells is CD4+ (cluster of differentiation 4). The T4 cells may also be referred to as cells that are *OKT4 positive* or *Leu-3 positive* because of the specific antigens on the membrane surface.

Helper/inducer T-cells easily recognize self cells versus non-self cells. In response to the recognition of non-self (antigen), helper/inducer T-cells secrete lymphokines that can enhance the activity of other WBCs.

Most lymphokines secreted by the helper/inducer T-cells increase immune function. These lymphokines increase bone marrow production of stem cells and speed up their maturation. Thus helper/inducer T-cells act as organizers in "calling to arms" various squads of WBCs involved in inflammatory, antibody, and cellular protective actions to destroy or neutralize antigens.

Suppressor T-cells have the T8-lymphocyte antigen on their membrane surfaces. These cells are commonly called *T8+ cells, CD8+ cells,* or T_S cells. Suppressor T-cells help regulate CMI.

Suppressor T-cells prevent **hypersensitivity** (continuous overreactions) when a person is exposed to non-self cells or proteins. This function is important in preventing the formation of antibodies directed against normal, healthy self cells, which is the basis for many autoimmune diseases.

The suppressor T-cells secrete lymphokines that have an overall *inhibitory* action on most cells of the immune system. These lymphokines inhibit both the growth and activation of immune system cells.

Suppressor T-cells have the opposite action of helper/inducer T-cells. For optimal function of CMI, then, a balance between helper/inducer T-cell activity and suppressor T-cell activity must be maintained. This balance occurs when the helper/inducer T-cells outnumber the suppressor T-cells by a ratio of 2:1. When this ratio increases, indicating that helper/inducer T-cells vastly outnumber the suppressor cells, overreactions can occur, some of which are tissue damaging as well as unpleasant. When the helper-suppressor ratio decreases, indicating fewer-than-normal helper/inducer T-cells, immune function is suppressed and the person's risk for infections increases.

Cytotoxic/cytolytic T-cells are also called T_C cells. Because they have the T8 protein present on their surfaces, they are a subset of suppressor cells. Cytotoxic/cytolytic T-cells destroy cells that contain a processed antigen's major histocompatibility complex (MHC). This activity is most effective against self cells infected by parasites, such as viruses or protozoa.

Parasite-infected self cells have both self MHC proteins (universal product code) and the parasite's antigens on the cell surface. This allows the person's immune system cells to recognize the infected self cell as abnormal, and the cytotoxic/cytolytic T-cell can bind to it.

When the cytotoxic/cytolytic T-cell binds to the infected cell's MHC complex, the cytotoxic/cytolytic T-cell makes holes in the membrane of the infected cell and delivers a "lethal hit" of enzymes to the infected cell, causing it to lyse and die. Once the lethal hit has been delivered to the infected cell, the cytotoxic/cytolytic T-cell releases the dying infected cell and can then attack and destroy other infected cells that carry the same antigen MHC complex.

Natural killer (NK) cells are also known as *CD16+ cells* and are very important in providing CMI. The actual site of NK cell differentiation and maturation is unknown. Although this cell type has some T-cell features, it is not a true T-cell subset (Abbas et al., 2007).

NK cells have direct cytotoxic effects on some non-self cells without first being sensitized. The cell killing actions of NK cells are independent of the interactions of other white blood cells. NK cells conduct "seek and destroy" missions in the body to eliminate non-self cells.

NK cells are most effective in destroying unhealthy or abnormal self cells. The non-self cells most often harmed by NK cells are cancer cells and virally infected body cells.

Cytokines

CMI regulates the immune system by the production and activity of cytokines. **Cytokines** are small protein hormones produced by the many WBCs (and some other tissues). Cytokines

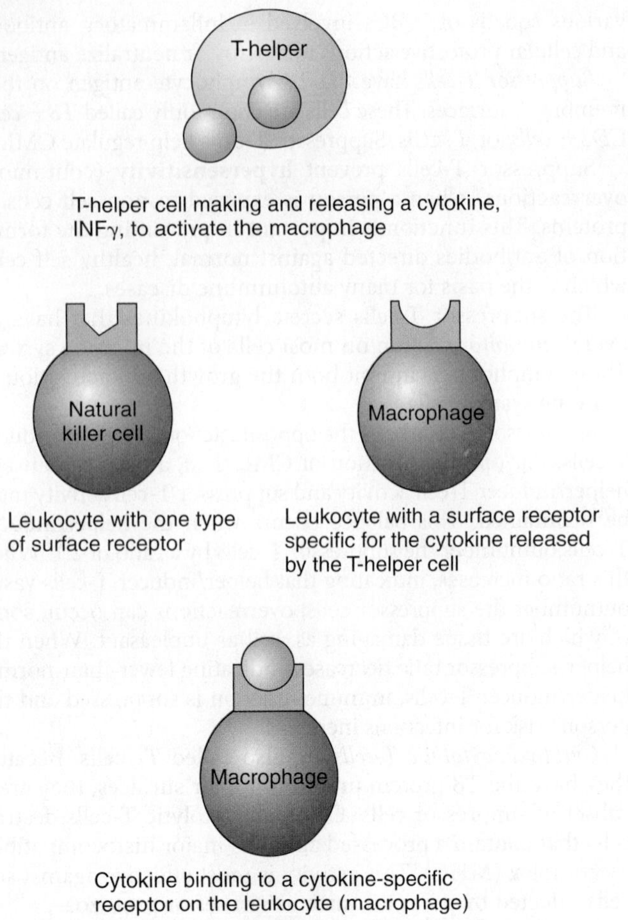
T-helper
T-helper cell making and releasing a cytokine, INFγ, to activate the macrophage
Natural killer cell
Macrophage
Leukocyte with one type of surface receptor
Leukocyte with a surface receptor specific for the cytokine released by the T-helper cell
Macrophage
Cytokine binding to a cytokine-specific receptor on the leukocyte (macrophage)

Fig. 19-11 • Cytokine receptors on leukocytes.

made by the macrophages, neutrophils, eosinophils, and monocytes are called **monokines.** Cytokines produced by T-cells are called **lymphokines.**

Cytokines work like other types of hormone: one cell produces a cytokine, which in turn exerts its effects on other cells of the immune system and on other body cells. The cells responding to the cytokine may be located close to or remote from the cytokine-secreting cell. Thus cytokines act like "messengers" that tell specific cells how and when to respond. The cells that change their activity when a cytokine is present are "responder" cells. For a responder cell to respond to the presence of a cytokine, the responder cell must have a specific receptor to which the cytokine can bind. Once the cytokine binds to its receptor, the responder cell changes its activity (Fig. 19-11).

Cytokines control many inflammatory and immune responses and are controlled by interactions with other systems, especially the nervous system (Blalocke, 2005). Some cytokines are **pleiotropic** (their effects are widespread within the immune system) and set into motion many different immune actions. Other cytokines have specific actions limited to only one type of cell. Cytokines include the interleukins, interferons, colony-stimulating factors, and tumor necrosis factor. The interleukins are the largest group of cytokines, with interleukin-27 (IL-27) being the most recently defined. Although there are many cytokines, not all are clinically useful at this time; however, this is an area of continuing research and discovery. Table 19-4 lists the cytokines that have current clinical importance. Chapters discussing specific diseases (e.g., lymphoma, rheumatoid arthritis) caused by or treated with certain cytokines have more information about the role of cytokines in the disease and its treatment.

TABLE 19-4 Activity of Selected Cytokines

Cytokine	Actions
PRO-INFLAMMATORY CYTOKINES	
Interleukin-1 (IL-1)	Induces fever Stimulates production of prostaglandins Increases growth of CD4+ T-cells
Interleukin-2 (IL-2)	Increases growth and differentiation of T-lymphocytes Enhances natural killer cell activity against cancer cells
Interleukin-6 (IL-6)	Stimulates liver to produce fibrinogen and protein C Increases rate of bone marrow production of stem cells Increases numbers of sensitized B-lymphocytes
Tumor necrosis factor (TNF)	Induces fever Major cytokine involved in rheumatoid arthritis damage Increases leukocyte adhesion Participates in graft rejection Induces cachexia and muscle breakdown Induces cell death Stimulates delayed hypersensitivity reactions and allergy
GROWTH FACTORS	
Granulocyte Colony-Stimulating Factor (G-CSF)	Increases numbers and maturity of neutrophils
Granulocyte-Macrophage Colony-Stimulating Factor (GM-CSF)	Increases growth and maturation of myeloid stem cells
Erythropoietin	Increases growth and differentiation of erythrocytes
Thrombopoietin	Increases growth and differentiation of platelets

Protection Provided by Cell-Mediated Immunity

Cell-mediated immunity (CMI) helps protect the body through the ability to differentiate self from non-self. The non-self cells most easily recognized by CMI are cancer cells and those self cells infected by organisms that live within host cells. CMI watches for and rids the body of self cells that might potentially harm the body. *CMI is important in preventing the development of cancer and metastasis after exposure to carcinogens.*

Transplant Rejection

Natural killer (NK) cells and cytotoxic/cytolytic T-cells also destroy cells from other people or animals. Although this action is usually helpful, it is also responsible for rejection of tissue grafts and transplanted organs (also termed *grafts*). Because the solid organ transplanted into the host is seldom a perfectly identical match of human leukocyte antigens (unless the organ is obtained from an identical sibling) between the donated organ and the recipient host, the patient's immune system cells recognize a newly transplanted organ as non-self. Without intervention, the host's immune system starts inflammatory and immunologic actions to destroy or eliminate these non-self cells. This activity causes rejection of the transplanted organ. Rejection of transplanted solid organs and other grafts is a result of a complex series of responses that change over time and involve different components of the immune system. Rejection can be hyperacute, acute, or chronic.

Hyperacute Rejection

Hyperacute rejection begins immediately on transplantation and is an antibody-mediated response. Antigen-antibody complexes form in the blood vessels of the transplanted organ. The host's blood has pre-existing antibodies to one or more of the antigens (including blood group antigens) present in the donated organ. The antigen-antibody complexes adhere to the lining of blood vessels and activate complement. The activated complement in the blood vessel linings triggers the blood clotting cascade, causing small clots to form throughout the new organ. Widespread clotting occludes blood vessels and leads to ischemic necrosis, inflammation with phagocytosis of the necrotic blood vessels, and release of lytic enzymes into the new organ. These enzymes cause massive cellular destruction and graft loss.

Hyperacute rejection occurs mostly in transplanted kidneys but is less common now as a result of greater efforts in HLA matching. The patients at greatest risk for hyperacute rejection are those who have received donated organs of an ABO blood type different from their own, have received multiple blood transfusions at any time in life before transplantation, have a history of multiple pregnancies, or have received a previous transplant.

The manifestations of hyperacute rejection are apparent within minutes of attachment of the donated organ to the host's blood supply. The process cannot be stopped once it has started, and the rejected organ is removed as soon as hyperacute rejection is diagnosed.

Acute Rejection

Acute rejection occurs within 1 week to 3 months after transplantation. Two mechanisms are responsible. The first mechanism is antibody mediated and results in vasculitis within the transplanted organ. This reaction differs from that of hyperacute rejection in that blood vessel necrosis (rather than occlusion) leads to the organ's destruction.

The second mechanism is cellular. Host cytotoxic/cytolytic T-cells and NK cells enter the transplanted organ through the blood, penetrate the organ cells, start an inflammatory response, and cause lysis of the organ cells (Abbas et al., 2007).

Diagnosis of acute rejection is made by laboratory tests that show impaired function of the donated organ and by biopsy of the donated organ. Symptoms of acute rejection vary with each patient and with the specific organ transplanted. For example, when acute rejection occurs in a transplanted kidney, the patient usually has some tenderness in the kidney area and may have other general symptoms of inflammation.

An episode of acute rejection after solid organ transplantation does not automatically mean that the patient will lose the new organ. Drug management of host immune responses at this time may limit the damage to the organ and allow the graft to be maintained.

Chronic Rejection

The origin of *chronic rejection* is not clear, but it is similar to chronic inflammation and scarring. The smooth muscles of blood vessels overgrow and occlude the vessels. The donated organ tissues are replaced with fibrotic, scarlike tissue. Because this fibrotic tissue is not organ tissue, the transplanted organ's function is reduced in proportion to the amount of normal tissue that is replaced by fibrotic tissue. This type of reaction is long-standing and occurs continuously as a response to chronic ischemia caused by blood vessel injury. The results of chronic rejection are unique to different transplanted organs. For example, in transplanted lungs, chronic rejection thickens small airways. In transplanted livers, chronic rejection destroys bile ducts. In transplanted hearts, this process is called *accelerated graft atherosclerosis (AGA)* and is the major cause of death in patients who have survived 1 or more years after heart transplantation.

Although good control over host immune function can delay this type of rejection, the process probably occurs to some degree with all transplanted solid organs obtained from donors who are not identical siblings of the recipient. Because the fibrotic changes are permanent, there is no cure for chronic graft rejection. When the fibrosis increases to the extent that the transplanted organ can no longer function, the only recourse is retransplantation.

Treatment of Transplant Rejection

Rejection of transplanted solid organs involves all three components of immunity, although cell-mediated immune (CMI) responses contribute the most to the rejection process.

Maintenance therapy is the continuous immune suppression used after a solid organ transplant. The drugs used for routine therapy after solid organ transplantation are combinations of specific immunosuppressants (cyclosporine [Sandimmune, Neoral, Gengraf]); less specific immunosuppressants (azathioprine [Imuran] or mycophenolate [CellCept, Myfortic]); and one of the corticosteroids, such as prednisone (Apo-Prednisone🍁, Deltasone🍁) or prednisolone (Delta-Cortef). Cyclosporine induces the specific and effective suppression of rejection. This drug, however, induces major long-term adverse actions and is expensive. A new similar drug under investigation is gusperimus (Spandin). The dosage of all immunosuppressive agents is adjusted to the immune response of each patient. Treatment with these agents increases the risk for bacterial and fungal infections and for cancer development.

Tacrolimus (Prograf) is similar to erythromycin and specifically suppresses T-cell actions, including production of interleukin-2 (IL-2). These effects occur through several mechanisms. Without continuous stimulation by IL-2, helper/inducer T-cells and cytotoxic/cytolytic T-cells are slow to reproduce and do not perform their usual functions. Suppression of these two cell populations allows the donated organ to remain free from immunologic destruction. The general immunosuppression is not as profound, and the host's risk for infection is not greatly increased. Tacrolimus also prevents activation of unsensitized cytotoxic/cytolytic T-cells. Other drugs with similar actions include sirolimus (Rapamune) and the investigational drug everolimus (Certican).

Another approach to prevent transplant rejection for patients undergoing kidney transplantation is the use of monoclonal antibodies directed against the IL-2 receptor site on activated T-cells (especially helper/inducer T-cells). These antibodies, basiliximab (Simulect) or daclizumab (Zenapax), are given IV within 2 hours before the transplant surgery and within the first few days after the surgery. By binding the antibodies to the IL-2 receptor site, T-cell growth and activation are reduced for several months.

Rescue therapy is used to treat acute rejection episodes. These agents may be used in addition to or in place of the maintenance drugs in the host's normal treatment regimen.

Antilymphocyte globulin (ALG) is an antibody (or group of antibodies) produced in an animal after the animal has been exposed to human lymphocytes. The globulin can be made more specific by exposing the animal to human T-cells instead of mixed lymphocytes. When these antihuman lymphocyte antibodies are given to humans, the antibodies selectively attack and clear lymphocytes from body fluids, blood, and the transplanted organ. These agents are given only for a short time to combat the acute rejection episode because of the immunologic side effects, ranging from low-grade fever and malaise to serum sickness and anaphylaxis. The side effects usually increase in intensity on repeated exposure to ALG.

Muromonab-CD3 (OKT3) is an antibody directed specifically against the human T-cell cell-surface antigen CD3. This antibody is generated in mice rather than in horses. Because the agent is generated in mice, the patients receiving it rapidly develop antimouse antibodies. These antimouse antibodies attack the CD3 and prevent its anti–T-cell activities. This antibody is most effective against rejection during the first episode in which it is used. Its effect in combating graft rejection decreases with each use. Like ALG, this drug is given only for a short time to combat the acute rejection episode because of the immunologic side effects, which increase in intensity on repeated exposure.

Antibodies made in other animals, especially mice, cause side effects in humans because the animal proteins in the antibodies are recognized as foreign by the human immune system. The incidence of side effects is decreasing because newer antibodies have been "humanized." This process removes most of the mouse-specific proteins from the antibody and replaces them with human specific proteins. The humanized antibodies made by mice now contain up to 95% human proteins rather than mouse proteins.

GET READY FOR THE NCLEX EXAMINATION!

Key Points

Review these Key Points for each NCLEX Examination Client Needs Category.

Physiological Integrity

- Inflammation and immunity are provided through the actions and products of white blood cells (WBCs), also called *leukocytes.*
- Different types of WBCs provide different types of immune or inflammatory protection.
- The differential of the WBC count can be used to determine the patient's risk for infection, the presence or absence of infection, the presence or absence of an allergic reaction, and whether an infection is bacterial or viral.
- WBCs are the only body cells able to recognize non-self cells and to attack them.
- Self-tolerance is the special ability of WBCs to recognize healthy self cells and not attempt to attack or destroy them.
- Human leukocyte antigens (HLAs) are a person's tissue type and are inherited from parents.
- Immunocompetence requires that all three parts of inflammation and immunity have optimal functioning.
- Inflammation is a general, nonspecific protective response.
- The five cardinal manifestations of inflammation are redness, warmth, swelling, pain, and loss of function.
- Inflammation and infection are not the same thing. Infection almost always is accompanied by inflammation, but inflammation often occurs without infection.
- The tissue responses to inflammation are helpful if confined to the area of invasion or infection and do not extend beyond the acute phase.
- Chronic inflammation can damage tissues and reduce function.
- The cells and actions of cell-mediated immunity control and coordinate the entire inflammatory and immune responses.
- Inflammation cannot be transferred from one person to another.
- Immune function declines with age, making the older adult at increased risk for infection and cancer development.
- Antibody-mediated immunity (also known as *humoral immunity*) can be transferred from one person or animal to another.
- Antibodies transferred from one person into another person have a short-term effect.
- Natural, active immunity is the most beneficial and long-lasting type of immunity.

- Vaccinations cause artificial active immunity and require "boosting" for best long-term effects.
- A person's normal membrane proteins would be antigens in another person.
- Transplant rejection is a normal response of the immune system that can damage or destroy the transplanted organ.
- Patients who receive transplanted organs (unless from an identical sibling) need to take immunosuppressive drugs daily to prevent transplant rejection.
- Patients who take immunosuppressive drugs have an increased risk for infection and cancer development.

Additional Study Resources

Go to your Companion CD or Evolve at http://evolve.elsevier.com/Iggy/ for *Self-Assessment Questions for the NCLEX Examination.*

evolve Go to Evolve at http://evolve.elsevier.com/Iggy/ for *Prioritization and Delegation Questions for the NCLEX Examination.*

SELECTED BIBLIOGRAPHY

Asterisk indicates a classic or definitive work on this subject.

Abbas, A., Lichtman, A., & Pillai, S. (2007). *Cellular and molecular immunology* (6th ed.). Philadelphia: Saunders.

Blalocke, J. (2005). The immune system as the sixth sense. *Journal of Internal Medicine, 257*(2), 126-138.

Edwards, N., & Baird, C. (2005). Interpreting laboratory values in older adults. *MEDSURG Nursing, 14*(4), 220-229.

Graham, J., Christian, L., & Kiecolt-Glaser, J. (2006). Stress, age, and immune function: Toward a lifespan approach. *Journal of Behavioral Medicine, 29*(4), 389-400.

McCance, K., & Huether, S. (2006). *Pathophysiology: The biologic basis for disease in adults and children* (5th ed.). St. Louis: Mosby.

Nussbaum, R., McInnes, R., & Willard, H. (2007). *Thompson & Thompson: Genetics in medicine* (7th ed.). Philadelphia: Saunders.

O'Neill, L. (2005). Immunity's early-warning system. *Scientific American, 292*(1), 38-45.

*Otto, S. (2003). Understanding the immune system. *Journal of Infusion Nursing, 26*(2), 79-85.

Stephensen, C., & Kelley, D. (2006). The innate immune system: Friend and foe. *American Journal of Clinical Nutrition, 83*(2), 187-188.

*Workman, M.L. (2003). The cellular basis of bacterial infection. *Critical Care Clinics of North America, 15*(1), 1-11.

20
CHAPTER

Care of Patients with Arthritis and Other Connective Tissue Diseases

Donna D. Ignatavicius • Cathy A. Murray

LEARNING OUTCOMES

For clinical competence and success on the NCLEX Examination, study this chapter with these Learning Outcomes in mind:

Safe and Effective Care Environment

1. Collaborate with members of the health care team when providing care to patients with arthritis or other connective tissue disease (CTD).
2. Prioritize collaborative interventions for patients with osteoarthritis (OA) and rheumatoid arthritis (RA).
3. Identify community resources to help patients achieve or maintain independence in ADLs.

Health Promotion and Maintenance

4. Identify risk factors for the development of arthritis and other CTDs.
5. Provide information for patients and families about the use and side effects of drug therapy for arthritis or other CTD.
6. Teach patients about how to protect and exercise their joints and conserve their energy.
7. Teach patients how to prevent Lyme disease and detect it early if it occurs.
8. Teach patients and their families about the postoperative care required after a total joint arthroplasty.

Psychosocial Integrity

9. Assess the patient's and family's response to arthritis or other CTD, their support systems, and available resources.
10. Assess the patient's and family's sources of stress and coping mechanisms when living with arthritis or other CTD.

Physiological Integrity

11. Compare and contrast the pathophysiology and clinical manifestations of OA and RA.
12. Interpret laboratory findings for patients with RA and other autoimmune CTDs.
13. Apply knowledge of pathophysiology to monitor for and prevent complications of total hip and knee arthroplasty.
14. Identify the nursing implications associated with drug therapy for patients with rheumatoid arthritis.
15. Evaluate and document patient response to drug therapy.
16. Differentiate between discoid lupus erythematosus and systemic lupus erythematosus.
17. Prioritize nursing interventions for patients who have systemic sclerosis.
18. Discuss the treatment of gout based on knowledge of pathophysiology.
19. Explain the differences between polymyositis, systemic necrotizing vasculitis, polymyalgia rheumatica, ankylosing spondylitis, Reiter's syndrome, and Sjögren's syndrome.
20. Describe current treatment strategies for patients with fibromyalgia.

Go to your Companion CD or Evolve at http://evolve.elsevier.com/Iggy/ for *Self-Assessment Questions for the NCLEX Examination* keyed to these Learning Outcomes.

Connective tissue disease (CTD) is the major focus of *rheumatology,* the study of rheumatic disease. A **rheumatic disease** is any disease or condition involving the musculoskeletal system. In this text, CTDs are discussed separately from other musculoskeletal conditions because most CTDs are classified as autoimmune disorders. In autoimmune disease, antibodies attack healthy normal cells and tissues. For reasons that are unclear, the immune system does not recognize body cells as self and therefore triggers an immune response. The usual *protective* nature of the immune system does not function properly in patients with autoimmune CTDs.

Most common CTDs are characterized by chronic pain and progressive joint deterioration, which results in decreased function. Some of these disorders have additional localized clinical manifestations, whereas others are systemic. The economic and social costs of these diseases are staggering and will increase steadily as "baby boomers" continue to age. Patient care management requires an interdisciplinary approach, including medicine, surgery, nursing, and physical and occupational therapy.

More than 46 million people in the United States (nearly 1 in 4) have at least one of more than 100 types of CTDs, or "arthritis" (www.cdc.gov/arthritis/data_statistics/index.htm). **Arthritis** means inflammation of one or more joints. In clinical practice, however, arthritis is categorized as either noninflammatory or inflammatory. Noninflammatory arthritis such as osteoarthritis (OA) is not systemic; OA is not an autoimmune disease. Systemic autoimmune diseases, such as RA and systemic lupus erythematosus, are connective tissue diseases that are inflammatory.

OSTEOARTHRITIS

Pathophysiology

Osteoarthritis is the most common arthritis and a major cause of disability among adults in the United States and the world. It is sometimes called *degenerative joint disease (DJD);* however, this term is no longer current. Joint pain and loss of function are common problems with OA.

Osteoarthritis is characterized by the progressive deterioration and loss of cartilage in one or more joints (articular cartilage). Primarily weight-bearing joints (hips and knees), the vertebral column, and the hands are affected, possibly because they are used most often or bear the mechanical stress of body weight. Most patients have the *primary (idiopathic)* form of the disease; *secondary* OA can result from other musculoskeletal conditions or from trauma. The disease can also be classified as *nodal* (with hand involvement) or *non-nodal* (without hand involvement).

Joint cartilage consists of a matrix of proteoglycans and collagen. Enzymes, such as stromelysin, break down this matrix in patients with OA. Proteoglycans then can no longer manage the amount of fluid in the joint space, and cartilage loses some of its strength. In early disease, the cartilage changes from its normal bluish white, translucent color to an opaque and yellowish brown appearance. As cartilage and the bone beneath the cartilage begin to erode, the joint space narrows and **osteophytes** (bone spurs) form (Fig. 20-1). As the disease progresses, fissures, pitting, and ulcerations develop and the cartilage thins. Inflammatory cytokines (enzymes) such as interleukin-1 (IL-1) enhance this deterioration. The body's normal repair process then cannot overcome the rapid process of degeneration (McCance & Huether, 2006). Bone cysts and secondary **synovitis** (synovial inflammation) are common in advanced disease. **Subluxation** (partial joint dislocation) and joint deformities eventually lead to immobility, pain, muscle spasm, and localized inflammation.

Etiology and Genetic Risk

Although the exact etiology of *primary* OA has not been identified, the disease may be triggered by aging, genetic changes, obesity, smoking, and/or trauma.

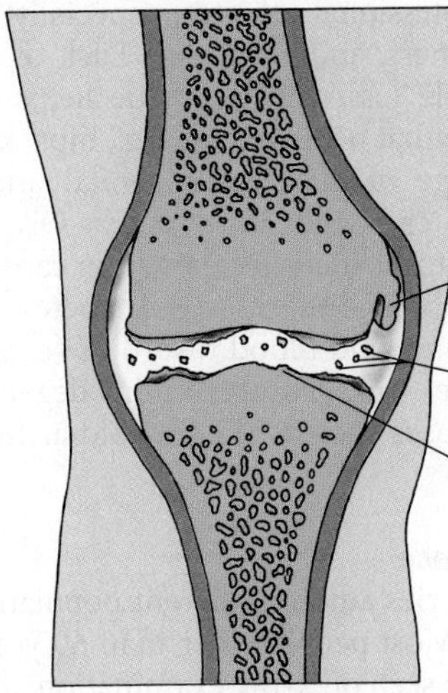
Bone hypertrophy (bone spur)
Cartilage particles
Loss of cartilage

Fig. 20-1 • Joint changes in degenerative joint disease.

CONSIDERATIONS FOR OLDER ADULTS

Age is the biggest risk factor for OA. As a person ages, the proteoglycans in the joint cartilage decrease, which affects cartilage strength. Prolonged weight bearing also contributes to joint changes, especially in the knees, sometimes referred to as "wear and tear."

GENETIC CONSIDERATIONS

Some patients report a family history of OA, which supports a possible genetic cause, especially for women who have the nodal type. Genetic changes may contribute to cartilage destruction, osteophyte formation, or the inability of the cartilage to repair itself. For instance, Interleukin-1 (IL-1), a cytokine, may increase cartilage breakdown by releasing and activating destructive enzymes. Variations in the IL-1 gene family have been shown to increase the risk of other bone diseases and thus may also be a factor in the pathophysiology of OA (McCance & Huether, 2006).

A study reported by Sunk et al. (2007) found a genetic link in OA of the knee. They reported that an increase in discoidin domain receptor 2 (DDR-2) expression in diseased joint cartilage was correlated with the degree of tissue damage. The authors concluded that this change occurs after the decrease in proteoglycans from aging. Studies are being conducted to further explore the genetic factors related to OA.

Other factors that can lead to OA are obesity and smoking. Obesity causes joint degeneration, particularly in the knees. Smoking leads to knee cartilage loss, especially in patients with a family history of knee OA. This finding shows a gene-environment interaction in the cause of knee OA (Ding et al., 2007).

Trauma to the joints from excessive use or abuse predisposes a person to OA. Certain heavy manual occupations (e.g., carpet laying, construction, farming) cause high-intensity or repetitive stress to the joints. The risk of hip and knee OA is also increased in professional athletes, especially football and soccer players, runners, and gymnasts. Lack of exercise can contribute to muscle loss. Muscle tissue helps support joints, particularly those that bear weight (e.g., hips, knees).

In a small percentage of people, congenital anomalies, trauma, and joint sepsis can result in *secondary* OA. For example, injuries from motor vehicle accidents can cause OA in later years. Certain metabolic diseases (e.g., diabetes mellitus, Paget's disease of the bone) and blood disorders (e.g., hemophilia, sickle cell disease) can also cause joint degeneration. Inflammatory joint diseases such as rheumatoid arthritis can lead to secondary OA.

Incidence and Prevalence

The prevalence of OA varies among different populations but is a universal problem. Most people older than 60 years have joint changes that can be seen on x-ray examination, although not all of those people actually develop the disease. More women older than 50 years have OA than men.

Health Promotion and Maintenance

Several lifestyle changes can help prevent or slow joint degeneration. These practices include:

- Keep body weight within normal limits; obesity causes excess wear on joints, especially hips and knees.
- Stop or do not start smoking.
- Avoid or limit activities that promote stress on joints, such as jogging.
- Limit participation in recreational sports that can damage joints, such as football.
- Wear supportive shoes to prevent damage to foot joints, especially metatarsal joints.
- Do not perform repetitive stress activities, such as knitting or typing, for prolonged periods.
- Avoid risk-seeking activities to prevent trauma that can result in OA later in life.

Patient-Centered Collaborative Care

evolve ONLINE PHARM REVIEW

Assessment

Patient History

Patients with OA usually seek medical attention in ambulatory care settings for their joint pain. However, you will also care for those who have OA as a secondary diagnosis in acute and chronic care facilities. Ask the patient about the course of the disease. Collect information specifically related to OA, such as the nature and location of joint pain and how much pain he or she is experiencing. *Remember that older patients may underreport pain, resulting in inadequate pain management.* Use a 0-to-10 scale or other assessment tool to assess pain intensity. Chapter 5 discusses pain assessment in detail.

Other questions to ask include:

- If joint stiffness has occurred, where and for how long?
- When and where has any joint swelling occurred?
- What do you do to control the pain or stiffness?
- Is there any loss of function or difficulty in performing ADLs?

Because this disease occurs more often in older women, age and gender are important factors for the nursing history. Ask patients about their occupation, nature of work, history of trauma, weight history, smoking history, and current or previous involvement in sports, because these are all risk factors for the disease. A history of obesity is significant, even for those currently within the ideal range for body weight. Document any family history of arthritis. Determine whether the patient has a current or previous medical condition that may cause joint manifestations.

Physical Assessment/Clinical Manifestations

In the early stage of the disease, the clinical manifestations of OA may appear similar to those of rheumatoid arthritis (RA). The distinction between OA and RA becomes more evident as the disease progresses. Table 20-1 differentiates the major characteristics of both diseases and their general treatments.

The typical patient with OA is a middle-aged or older woman who reports *chronic joint pain and stiffness.* Early in the course of the disease, the pain diminishes after rest and worsens after activity. Later the pain occurs with slight motion or even when at rest. Because cartilage has no nerve supply, the pain is probably due to joint and soft-tissue involvement and to spasms of the surrounding muscles. During the joint examination, the patient may have pain or tenderness by palpation or by putting the joint through range of motion. **Crepitus,** a continuous grating sensation caused by irregular cartilage, may be felt or heard as the joint goes through range of motion. One or more joints may be affected. The patient may also report joint stiffness that usually lasts less than 30 minutes after a period of inactivity.

On inspection, the joint is often enlarged because of bony hypertrophy; rarely does a joint appear to be hot and inflamed. The presence of inflammation in patients with OA indicates a secondary synovitis. About half of patients with hand involvement have **Heberden's nodes** (at the distal interphalangeal [DIP] joints) and **Bouchard's nodes** (at the proximal interphalangeal [PIP] joints). Although OA is not a bilateral, symmetric disease, these large bony nodes appear on both hands, especially in women. The nodes may be painful and red. Some patients experience pain in developing nodes or when nodes are palpated. These deformities tend to be familial and are often a cosmetic concern to patients.

Joint effusions (excess joint fluid) are common when the knees are involved. When trying to differentiate the presence of fluid from subcutaneous tissue, you may be able to move fluid from the **infrapatellar notch** (the area directly below the knee) into the **suprapatellar area** (directly above the knee). Other ways to detect fluid in the knee involve grasping the medial and lateral aspect of the knee between the thumb and third finger and pushing down on the top surface of the patella with the forefinger **(ballottement).** If fluid is present, the patella will be able to be pressed down a distance and then rise back up when the forefinger is removed. Subcutaneous tissue cannot be relocated.

Observe any *atrophy of skeletal muscle* from disuse. The vicious pain cycle of the disease discourages the movement of painful joints, which may result in contractures, muscle atrophy, and further pain. *Loss of function* may result, depending on which joints are involved. Hip or knee pain may cause the patient to limp and restrict walking distance.

Osteoarthritis (OA) can affect the spine, especially the lumbar region at the L3-4 level or the cervical region at C4-6 (neck). Compression of spinal nerve roots may occur as a result of vertebral facet bone spurs. The patient typically reports radiating pain, stiffness, and muscle spasms in one or both extremities.

Severe pain and deformity interfere with ambulation and self-care. In addition to performing a musculoskeletal assessment, collaborate with the physical and occupational thera-

TABLE 20-1 **Differential Features of Rheumatoid Arthritis and Osteoarthritis**

Characteristic	Rheumatoid Arthritis	Osteoarthritis
Typical onset (age)	35-45 yr	Older than 60 yr
Gender affected	Female (3:1)	Female (2:1)
Risk factors or cause	Autoimmune (genetic basis) Emotional stress (triggers exacerbation) Environmental factors	Aging Genetic factor (possible) Obesity Trauma Occupation
Disease process	Inflammatory	Degenerative
Disease pattern	Bilateral, symmetric, multiple joints Usually affects upper extremities first Distal interphalangeal joints of hands spared Systemic	May be unilateral, single joint Affects weight-bearing joints and hands, spine Metacarpophalangeal joints spared Nonsystemic
Laboratory findings	Elevated rheumatoid factor, antinuclear antibody, ESR	Normal or slightly elevated ESR
Common drug therapy	NSAIDs (short-term use) Methotrexate Leflunomide (Arava) Corticosteroids Biological response modifiers Other immunosuppressive agents	NSAIDs (short-term use) Acetaminophen Other analgesics

ESR, Erythrocyte sedimentation rate; *NSAIDs*, nonsteroidal anti-inflammatory drugs.

pists to conduct a functional assessment. Assess the patient's mobility and ability to perform ADLs. Chapter 8 describes functional assessment in depth.

Psychosocial Assessment

OA is a chronic condition that may cause permanent changes in lifestyle. An inability to care for oneself in advanced disease prevents socialization and results in role changes and other losses. Constant pain interferes with quality of life. Chronic pain can also affect sexuality. Patients may not have the energy for sexual intercourse or may find positioning uncomfortable (Gevirtz, 2008).

Patients with arthritis experience daily stress from health problems and other causes that can lead to mental health problems such as depression (Tak, 2006). Assess the specific causes of your patient's stress to plan how to best minimize it (see the Evidence-Based Practice box on p. 326).

The patient may also have a role change in the family, workplace, or both. To identify changes that have been or need to be made, ask his or her roles before the disease developed. Identify coping strategies to help live with the disease. Ask the patient about his or her goals and expectations regarding treatment for OA.

In addition to role changes, joint deformities and bony nodules often alter body image and self-esteem. Observe the patient's response to body changes. Does he or she ignore them or seem overly occupied with them? Ask the patients directly how they perceive their body image? Document your assessment findings in the interdisciplinary record.

Laboratory Assessment

The health care provider uses the history and physical examination to make the diagnosis of OA. The results of routine laboratory tests are usually normal but can be helpful in screening for associated conditions. The erythrocyte sedimentation rate (ESR) and high-sensitivity C-reactive protein (hsCRP) may be slightly elevated when secondary synovitis (synovial inflammation) occurs. The ESR also tends to rise with age and infection.

Imaging Assessment

Routine x-rays are useful in determining structural joint changes. Specialized views are obtained when the disease cannot be visualized on standard x-ray film but is suspected. Magnetic resonance imaging (MRI) may be used to determine vertebral or knee involvement.

▪ *Analysis*

Common Nursing Diagnoses and Collaborative Problems

The priority nursing diagnoses for patients with osteoarthritis (OA) are:

1. Chronic Pain related to muscle spasm, cartilage deterioration, or joint inflammation
2. Impaired Physical Mobility related to pain and muscle atrophy

Additional Nursing Diagnoses and Collaborative Problems

In addition to the common nursing diagnoses, patients may have secondary problems caused by the pain and immobility common in OA, including one or more of these:

- Activity Intolerance related to pain and fatigue
- Self-Care Deficit (Partial) related to pain, fatigue, and immobility
- Disturbed Body Image related to the effects of loss of body function
- Impaired Walking related to joint pain
- Ineffective Coping related to chronic pain and decreased function
- Imbalanced Nutrition: More Than Body Requirements related to decreased activity and mobility

EVIDENCE-BASED PRACTICE

What are the daily stressors and coping strategies for patients who have osteoarthritis?

Tak, S.H. (2006). An insider perspective of daily stress and coping in elders with arthritis. *Orthopaedic Nursing, 25*(2), 127-132.

This qualitative study examined the daily stress and coping strategies of 13 older adults with osteoarthritis using semistructured, individual interviews. Content analysis of the interview transcriptions was performed. Results indicated that there were six sources of stress in the daily lives of the sample subjects: health, routine tasks, family issues, financial management, social relationships, and living conditions. Although coping strategies for dealing with these sources varied, they could be classified as (1) participating in diversional activities, (2) using cognitive efforts, such as problem-solving techniques, and (3) assertive actions, such as finding resources to help them.

Level of Evidence—8. Small qualitative study.

Commentary: Implications for Practice and Research. The participants represented a very small convenience sample. However, qualitative research in nursing often has small samples to allow for in-depth interview and analysis of psychosocial aspects of care. Nurses and other health care professionals should assess their patients for sources of stress and assist them in coping, such as locating community resources or teaching them cognitive-mind therapies that can help them cope (see Chapter 2).

Planning and Implementation

Chronic Pain

NOC **Planning: Expected Outcomes.** The major concern of the patient with OA is pain control. Therefore he or she is expected to take personal actions to control pain. When pain is not well controlled, the interdisciplinary health care team assists with pain management. Indicators include that the patient will:

- Recognize pain onset
- Use previous measures that were effective
- Use analgesics appropriately
- Use nonanalgesic relief measures
- Report changes in pain symptoms or sites to health care professional
- Report that pain is controlled

Interventions. Pain control may involve drug and nonpharmacologic measures. If these measures become ineffective, surgery may be performed to reduce pain as a last resort. Perform a pain assessment before and after implementing interventions (Chart 20-1).

Nonsurgical Management. Management of chronic joint pain is difficult for both the patient and the health care professional. A combination of modalities is often used, including analgesics, rest, positioning, thermal modalities, weight control, and integrative therapies. Chapter 5 elaborates on methods of pain control for chronic pain.

NIC **Analgesic administration.** The purpose of drug therapy is to reduce pain and secondary joint inflammation if present. The American Pain Society recommends regular *acetaminophen* (Tylenol, Atasol♣) as the primary drug of choice although it is not an anti-inflammatory medication. *Patients are at risk for liver damage if they take more than 4000 mg daily, have alcoholism, or have liver disease. Older adults are particularly at risk due to normal changes of aging, such as slowed excretion of drug metabolites.* Remind patients to read the labels of over-the-counter (OTC) drugs that could contain acetaminophen before taking them. Teach them that their liver enzyme levels will be monitored while taking this drug.

Topical drug applications may help with temporary relief of pain. Lidocaine 5% patches have been used for neuralgia but may also relieve joint pain. Teach the patient to apply the patch on clean, intact skin for 12 hours each day. Up to three patches may be applied to painful joints at one time. Remind him or her that topical lidocaine can cause skin irritation. Topical salicylates, such as OTC Aspercreme and prescription 1% diclofenac sodium (Voltaren), are also useful for some patients as a temporary pain reliever, especially for knee pain.

If acetaminophen or topical agents do not relieve pain, the analgesic drug class of choice may be *nonsteroidal anti-inflammatory drugs (NSAIDs)* if the patient can tolerate them (see Chart 20-10 later in this chapter). Before beginning NSAID therapy, baseline laboratory information is obtained, including a complete blood count (CBC) and kidney and liver function tests. Celecoxib (Celebrex), a COX-2 inhibitor, is usually the first choice unless the patient has hypertension, renal disease, or cardiovascular disease. All of the COX-2 inhibiting drugs are thought to cause cardiovascular disease, such as myocardial infarction, and may be unavailable on the market at some time in the future. Older NSAIDs, such as ibuprofen, can cause severe GI side effects, bleeding, and acute renal failure. *Teach your patient about adverse effects from NSAIDs and the need to report them to his or her health care provider. Examples include having dark, tarry stools; shortness of breath; and frequent dyspepsia (indigestion).*

Opioids may be needed when all other drug therapy does not control pain. *Dosages should be as low as possible, especially for older adults. Teach the patient and family to monitor for adverse drug effects in older adults, including confusion, sedation, respiratory depression, and hallucinations.* Teach the patient to take a mild stimulant laxative or stool softener as needed, especially if codeine products are taken.

For temporary relief of pain in a single joint, the health care provider may inject an individual joint with cortisone. Frequently injected joints include the knee, base of the thumb, shoulder, and trochanteric bursa, which people often call the *hip*.

Other agents, such as hyaluronate (Hyalgan) and hylan GF 20 (Synvisc), are joint injections for OA of the knee. These synthetic joint fluid implants replace or supplement the body's natural hyaluronic acid, which is broken down by inflammation. Muscle relaxants, such as cyclobenzaprine hydrochloride (Flexeril), are sometimes given for painful muscle spasms, especially those occurring in the back. *Remind the patient not to drive or operate dangerous machinery when taking muscle relaxants.*

Chart 20-1 NIC INTERVENTION ACTIVITIES
The Patient with Osteoarthritis

Analgesic Administration: *Use of pharmacologic agents to reduce or eliminate pain*

- Determine pain location, characteristics, quality, and severity before medicating patient.
- Check medical order for drug, dose, and frequency of analgesic prescribed.
- Attend to comfort needs and other activities that assist in relaxation to facilitate response to analgesia.
- Administer analgesics around-the-clock to prevent peaks and troughs of analgesia, especially with severe pain.
- Set positive expectations regarding the effectiveness of analgesics to optimize patient response.
- Document response to analgesic and any untoward effects.

Pain Management: *Alleviation of pain or a reduction in pain to a level of comfort that is acceptable to the patient*

- Observe for nonverbal cues of discomfort, especially in those unable to communicate effectively.
- Consider cultural influences on pain response.
- Determine the impact of the pain experience on quality of life (e.g., sleep, appetite, activity, cognition, mood, relationships, performance of job, and role responsibilities).
- Evaluate, with the patient and the health care team, the effectiveness of past pain control measures that have been used.
- Consider the patient's willingness to participate, ability to participate, preference, support of significant others for method, and contraindications when selecting a pain relief strategy.
- Teach the use of nonpharmacologic techniques (e.g., biofeedback, hypnosis, relaxation, guided imagery, music therapy, distraction, activity therapy, acupressure, hot/cold application, and massage) before, after and, if possible, during painful activities; before pain occurs or increases; and along with other pain relief measures.
- Promote adequate rest/sleep to facilitate pain relief.
- Utilize an interdisciplinary approach to pain management, when appropriate.
- Consider referrals for patient, family, and significant others to support groups, and other resources, as appropriate.
- Monitor patient satisfaction with pain management at specified intervals.

NIC intervention activities selected from Bulechek, G.M., Butcher, H.K., & McCloskey Dochterman, J. (Eds.). (2008). *Nursing interventions classification (NIC)* (5th ed.). St. Louis: Mosby. No part of this work is to be altered without prior written permission from the Publisher.

NIC **Pain management.** In addition to analgesics, many nonpharmacologic measures can be used for patients with OA, such as rest, joint positioning, heat or cold applications, weight control, or a variety of complementary and alternative therapies. Several types of *rest* are used to treat patients with OA:

- *Local* rest involves immobilizing a joint with a splint or brace. If a joint becomes acutely inflamed, the joint is rested until inflammation subsides. Rest the joint when painful, but exercise it to maintain mobility and tone. Balance rest and activity. Consult the physical therapist or occupational therapist (PT/OT), who fits the patient for the appropriate device and explains its use.
- *Systemic* rest refers to immobilizing the entire body, such as during a nap. Teach the patient about the importance of sleeping about 8 to 10 hours and, if possible, resting an additional 1 to 2 hours each day.
- *Psychological* rest is equally important because it allows relief from the daily stresses that can enhance pain.

Teach the patient to *position joints in their functional position*. For example, when in a supine position (recumbent), he or she should use a small pillow under the head or neck but avoid the use of other pillows. The use of large pillows under the knees or head may result in flexion contractures. If needed, the legs may be elevated 8 to 12 inches (20 to 30 cm) to reduce back discomfort. Remind him or her to use proper posture when standing and sitting to reduce undue strain on the vertebral column.

Most patients apply *heat* or *cold* for temporary relief of pain. Heat may help decrease the muscle tension around the tender joint and thereby decreases pain. Suggest hot showers and baths, hot packs or compresses, and moist heating pads. *Regardless of treatment, teach him or her to check that the heat source is not too heavy or so hot that it causes burns.* A temperature just above body temperature is adequate to promote comfort.

A physical therapist may provide special heat treatments, such as paraffin dips, diathermy (electrical current), and ultrasonography (sound waves). A 15- to 20-minute application usually is sufficient to temporarily reduce pain, spasm, and stiffness. Cold packs or gels that feel hot and cold at the same time may also be used.

Cold therapy may also be used to control pain. Cold works by numbing nerve endings and decreasing secondary joint inflammation. *Teach the patient to use ice packs that are not too heavy. Be sure they are not placed directly on skin by wrapping them in a towel or soft cloth.*

There is no one food that causes or cures arthritis. Instead, a well-balanced diet is recommended. Gradual *weight loss* for obese patients may lessen the stress on weight-bearing joints, decrease pain, and perhaps slow joint degeneration. If needed, collaborate with the nutritionist to provide more in-depth teaching and meal planning.

Complementary and alternative therapies. Many patients use a variety of complementary and alternative therapies (CAMs), such as acupuncture, acupressure, tai chi, music therapy, and cognitive-behavioral therapies like imagery, prayer, and meditation, for pain relief (see Chapters 2 and 5). Topical capsaicin products may also be used. This expensive OTC drug may work by blocking substance P, a neurotransmitter for pain. Tell the patient to expect a burning sensation for a short time after applying capsaicin. Recommend the use of plastic gloves for application. To prevent burning of eyes or other body areas, wash hands immediately after applying the substance.

Other dietary supplements, such as gamma-linolenic acid (GLA, Efamol), glucosamine, and chondroitin, complement traditional drug therapies. GLA can be found in evening primrose oil, borage seed oil, and black currant seed oil. GLA is an omega-6 fatty acid, one of the body's essential fatty acids, and is used for both OA and rheumatoid arthritis (RA).

Omega-3 fatty acids are found in certain types of fish (e.g., salmon) or may be taken in fish oil capsules.

Glucosamine and chondroitin are the most widely used nonprescription supplements taken to decrease pain and improve functional ability (Clegg et al., 2006). These natural products are found in and around bone cartilage for repair and maintenance. Glucosamine may decrease inflammation, and chondroitin may play a role in strengthening cartilage. These drugs may be used topically or taken in oral form. In 2006, the results of the Glucosamine/Chondroitin Arthritis Intervention Trial (GAIT) found that these substances did not significantly reduce joint pain in patients with OA (Clegg et al., 2006). Chart 20-2 summarizes what you should teach your patients about glucosamine, with or without chondroitin.

NCLEX EXAMINATION CHALLENGE

A diabetic client has been taking a glucosamine and chondroitin OTC combination drug for several years. Which of these statements by the client indicates a need for further teaching?

A. "I should take the drug based on my weight and not on the amount of pain I have."
B. "I should tell my doctor if I have stomach problems or loose stools."
C. "It's OK if I take this drug along with my Lisinopril and Norvasc."
D. "I have to be careful and not hurt myself to cause bruises or bleeding."

evolve For the correct answer, go to http://evolve.elsevier.com/Iggy/.

Chart 20-2 PATIENT AND FAMILY EDUCATION GUIDE

Considerations for Taking Glucosamine Supplements

- Tell your health care provider if you decide to take glucosamine.
- Do not take glucosamine if you have hypertension.
- Do not take glucosamine is you are pregnant or breast-feeding.
- Monitor for bleeding if you take chondroitin with glucosamine or chondroitin alone if you are on anticoagulant therapy.
- If diabetic, monitor your blood glucose levels carefully because taking glucosamine for a prolonged time can increase them.
- Be aware that glucosamine can cause adverse effects such as a rash; GI disturbances, especially diarrhea; drowsiness; and headache.
- Be sure to take the recommended dosage based on your weight.
- Read drug labels to ensure that you do not take too much glucosamine for your weight; some drug names may not indicate they contain glucosamine (e.g., Bioflex, Arth-X Plus, Nutri-Joint).

As stated earlier, IL-1 may be an important factor in the pathophysiology of OA. Evans et al. (2005) reported that the anti-inflammatory and cartilage-protective IL-1 Ra gene therapy may be helpful in treating the disease, especially knee OA. This experimental treatment has the potential to stimulate regeneration of cartilage and inhibit joint destruction if the disease is diagnosed early.

Surgical Management. Surgery may be indicated when conservative measures no longer provide pain control, when mobility becomes so restricted that the patient cannot participate in activities he or she enjoys, and when he or she cannot maintain the desired quality of life. The most common surgical procedure performed is **total joint arthroplasty (TJA)** (surgical creation of a joint), also known as **total joint replacement (TJR).** Almost any synovial joint of the body can be replaced with a prosthetic system that consists of at least two parts, one for each joint surface.

A less invasive procedure using arthroscopy may be used to remove damaged cartilage (see Chapter 52). An **osteotomy** (bone resection) may be performed to correct joint deformity, but this procedure is less common because of the success rate of TJR.

Indications. Total joint arthroplasty is a procedure used most often to manage the pain of OA and to improve mobility, although other conditions causing cartilage destruction may require the surgery. These disorders include RA, congenital anomalies, trauma, and osteonecrosis. **Osteonecrosis** is bony necrosis secondary to lack of blood flow, usually from trauma or chronic steroid therapy. Hip and knee joints are most commonly replaced, but replacement of finger and wrist joints, elbows, shoulders, toe joints, and ankles have become more popular in the past 20 years.

Contraindications. The contraindications for TJA are active infection anywhere in the body, advanced osteoporosis, and rapidly progressive inflammation. An infection elsewhere in the body or from the joint being replaced can result in an infected TJA and subsequent prosthetic failure. Therefore if a patient has a urinary tract infection, for example, the physician treats the infection before surgery. Advanced osteoporosis can cause bone shattering during insertion of the prosthetic device. Severe medical problems, such as uncontrolled diabetes or hypertension, put the patient at risk for major postoperative complications and possible death.

As a group, TJAs are very successful. Many patients who have lived with chronic, unbearable pain for years and could not function independently at home or in the workplace no longer experience pain in the diseased joint. The pain relief and psychological benefit often outweigh the perioperative risks and costs, but the surgeon and patient must make that decision. When the patient is older than 85 years, this decision may become an ethical issue in addition to a physical risk and cost-versus-benefit decision.

Total hip arthroplasty. The number of total hip arthroplasty (THA) procedures (also known as total hip replacement [THR]) has steadily increased over the past 30 years. The first time a patient receives THA, it is referred to as **primary arthroplasty.** If the implant loosens, **revision arthroplasty** may be performed. Availability of joint implants with better custom design features allows longer life of a replaced hip. Although patients of any age can undergo THR, the procedure is performed most often in those older than 60 years. The special needs and normal physiologic changes of older adults often complicate the perioperative period and may result in additional postoperative complications. The preferred criteria for those planning to have a THR include (Hohler, 2005):

- The pain interrupts the patient's sleep.
- The pain limits ADLs.
- Drug therapy no longer controls pain.
- The patient is able to participate in physical therapy after surgery.

Preoperative care. As with any procedure, preoperative care begins with assessing the patient's level of understanding about the surgery. The surgeon explains the procedure and postoperative expectations during the office visit, but this education may have occurred weeks or months before the scheduled surgery. Some patients may not know what questions to ask or may forget the important information that was taught. Orthopedic surgeons often hire nurses who follow up and address patient concerns. Information may be provided in a notebook or DVD format that the patient can take home to review and share with family. This is particularly useful to patients with poor reading skills or poor memory. Written materials or other media provided in the patient's language are essential. An interdisciplinary plan of care that outlines expectations during preadmission, hospitalization, and posthospitalization phases of care should be reviewed with the patient and family or significant other.

In some hospitals or orthopedic office practices, the physical therapist (PT) may meet the patient before surgery to explain transfers, positioning, ambulation, and postoperative exercises. An occupational therapist (OT) may be available to demonstrate assistive/adaptive devices that facilitate independent ADLs. For patients having *minimally invasive surgery* (MIS), the PT teaches how to perform muscle-strengthening exercises at home before the procedure.

Patients are also told to have any necessary dental procedures done before surgery. After surgery, he or she must take extreme care not to acquire an infection that could migrate to the surgical area and cause prosthetic failure. *Remind the patient to tell any future health care provider that he or she has had a THA.*

In addition to usual preoperative laboratory tests, the surgeon may require that the patient with RA have a cervical spine x-ray if he or she is having general anesthesia. Those with RA often have cervical spine disease that can lead to subluxation during intubation. Hip x-rays, computed tomography (CT) scan, and/or MRI may be done to assess the operative joint and surrounding soft tissues.

Because venous thromboembolism (VTE) is a serious postoperative complication, especially for hip surgery, the patient's risk factors for clotting problems are assessed, including history of previous clotting, obesity, smoking, and advanced age. *Drugs that increase the risk of clotting, such as NSAIDs and hormone replacement therapy (HRT), are discontinued about a week before surgery.* Some patients begin taking a low-molecular-weight heparin (LMWH) or other anticoagulant before surgery, whereas others take it after surgery.

Because THAs are elective procedures, autologous blood transfusions are appropriate. The patient may donate blood before surgery to be used as needed during and after surgery. This pre-deposit autologous blood donation is a safe and cost-effective blood replacement alternative for those who are undergoing elective surgeries. It also decreases the risk of blood transfusion reaction.

Many surgeons prescribe several weeks of epoetin alfa (Epogen, Procrit, Eprex♣) with or without iron to prevent anemia that often occurs after hip or knee surgery. Epoetin alfa is recombinant human erythropoietin, a cytokine that is essential for developing red blood cells. This drug is particularly useful for older adults, who frequently have mild anemia before surgery.

Remind patients that they will be asked to take a shower with antiseptic soap before surgery. Review which drugs are safe to take or necessary the morning of the operation, such as antihypertensives, and which ones should be avoided. Medication should be taken with a very small amount of water.

Operative procedures. For total hip arthroplasty, the patient receives an IV antibiotic, usually a cephalosporin such as cefazolin (Ancef), at least 1 hour before the initial surgical incision is made or during surgery. Other drugs may be used for those who are allergic to cephalosporins.

The anesthesiologist or nurse anesthetist places the patient under general or **neuroaxial** (epidural/spinal) anesthesia for lower extremity surgery. Neuroaxial induction reduces blood loss and the incidence of deep vein thrombosis. Intraoperative blood loss with hypotensive neuroaxial anesthesia is usually less than that with general anesthesia, thereby decreasing the need for postoperative blood transfusions.

Several types of incisions for hip replacement may be used. The more *traditional* 8- to 10-inch (20 to 24 cm) incision is usually longitudinal on the anterolateral thigh. The anterolateral approach results in more damage to muscle but less risk for dislocation. A posterior incision, posterolateral on the thigh and into the buttock, may be used to preserve muscle but with increased risk for dislocation and sciatic nerve injury.

Some patients are candidates for *minimally invasive surgery* (MIS) using one or two smaller (2- to 4-inch [5- to 10-cm) incisions with special instruments to reduce muscle cutting. This newer technique cannot be used for patients who are obese or those with osteoporosis. It is done only for primary THAs, not for revision surgeries. The benefits of MIS are decreased soft tissue damage and postoperative pain and often a shorter hospital stay and quicker recovery (Hohler, 2005). Postoperative complications are not as common in patients having MIS when compared with those having the traditional technique.

Regardless of procedure type, two components are used in the THA—the acetabular component and the femoral component. A non-cemented prosthesis is most often used in THA. Bone surfaces are smoothed as they are prepared to receive the artificial components. The non-cemented components are press-fitted into the prepared bone. The acetabular cup may be placed using computer assistance. If the prosthesis is cemented, polymethyl methacrylate (an acrylic fixating substance) is used. A closed wound drainage system may be placed in the wound before the surgeon closes the incision.

Considerations of a non-cemented prosthesis include protection of weight-bearing status to allow bone to ingrow into the prosthesis and decreased problems with loosening of the prosthesis. With a cemented prosthesis, cement can fracture or deteriorate over time, leading to loosening of the prosthesis, which causes pain and can lead to the need for a revision arthroplasty. In revision arthroplasty, the old prosthesis is removed and new components are replaced. Bone graft may be placed if bone loss is significant. Outcomes from revision arthroplasty may not be as good as with primary arthroplasty.

Postoperative care. In addition to providing the routine postoperative care discussed in Chapter 18, assess for and assist in the prevention of possible postoperative complications. Table 20-2 summarizes these common complications, including nursing measures for prevention, assessment, and intervention. Chart 20-3 highlights special concerns for the care of older adults in the postoperative period.

PREVENTION OF DISLOCATION. A common complication of THA is **subluxation** (partial dislocation) or total dislocation. *Therefore correct positioning is maintained at all times. When the patient returns from the postanesthesia care unit (PACU), place him or her in a supine position with the head slightly*

TABLE 20-2 Nursing Interventions to Prevent Complications of Total Joint Arthroplasty

Complication	Prevention/Intervention
Dislocation	Position correctly. For hip, keep leg slightly abducted. For hip, prevent hip flexion beyond 90 degrees. Assess for pain, rotation, and extremity shortening. Report immediately to physician.
Infection	Use aseptic technique for wound care and emptying of drains. Wash hands thoroughly when caring for patient. Culture drainage fluid, if change. Monitor temperature. Report excessive inflammation or drainage to physician.
Venous thromboembolism	Have patient wear elastic stockings and/or sequential compression device. Teach leg exercises to patient. Encourage fluid intake. Observe for signs of thrombosis (redness, swelling, or pain). Observe patient for changes in mental status. Administer anticoagulant as prescribed. Do not massage legs. Do not use knee gatch on bed.
Hypotension, bleeding, or infection	Take vital signs at least every 4 hours. Observe patient for bleeding. Report excessively low blood pressure or bleeding to physician.

Chart 20-3 NURSING FOCUS ON THE OLDER ADULT

Postoperative Care of the Older Adult with a Total Hip Arthroplasty

- Use an abduction pillow or splint to prevent adduction after surgery if the patient is very restless or has an altered mental state.
- Keep the patient's heels off the bed to prevent pressure ulcers.
- Do not rely on fever as a sign of infection; older patients often have infection without fever. Decreasing mental status typically occurs when the patient has an infection.
- When assisting the patient out of bed, move him or her slowly to prevent orthostatic (postural) hypotension.
- Encourage the patient to deep breathe and cough, and use the incentive spirometer every 2 hours to prevent atelectasis and pneumonia.
- As soon as permitted, get the patient out of bed to prevent complications of immobility.
- Anticipate the patient's need for pain medication, especially if he or she cannot verbalize the need for pain control.
- Expect a temporary change in mental state immediately after surgery as a result of the anesthetic and unfamiliar sensory stimuli. Reorient the patient frequently.

elevated. Place a trapezoid-shaped abduction pillow, wedge, sling, or splint (with or without straps) between the patient's legs to prevent adduction beyond the midline of the body. In some hospitals, this device is no longer used because it is uncomfortable and unnecessary in most cases. Abduction devices are usually reserved for patients who are restless or cannot follow instructions, especially older adults with delirium or dementia. One or two regular bed pillows are used in most cases. For devices with straps, be sure to loosen the straps every 2 hours and check the patient's skin for irritation or breakdown.

Place and support the affected leg in neutral rotation. *Keep the patient's heels off the bed to prevent skin breakdown, particularly for older adults.* The procedure for postoperative turning is controversial and specified by agency policy or surgeon preference. In most cases, you are safe to turn the patient toward either side as long as the abduction device or other pillow is in place. Some surgeons allow only turning directly onto one side or the other.

Observe for possible signs of hip dislocation, which include increased hip pain, shortening of the affected leg, and leg rotation. If any of these clinical manifestations occur, keep the patient in bed and notify the surgeon immediately. The surgeon manipulates and relocates the affected hip after the patient receives an analgesic or is anesthetized. The hip is then immobilized by an abduction splint or other device until healing occurs—usually in about 6 weeks.

PREVENTION OF THROMBOEMBOLIC COMPLICATIONS. *The most potentially life-threatening complication after THA is venous thromboembolism (VTE), which includes deep venous thrombosis (DVT) and pulmonary embolism (PE). Older patients are especially at increased risk for VTE because of age and compromised circulation before surgery.* Obese patients and those with a history of VTE are also at high risk for thrombi. The most common sites for DVT are the anterior and posterior tibial veins, the peroneal vein, the popliteal vein, the saphenous vein, and the femoral vein. Nonpharmacologic or mechanical prophylaxis includes the use of graduated antiembolism stockings and sequential compression devices (see Chapter 18 for more information about these measures).

Anticoagulants, such as warfarin (Coumadin, Warfilone♣), subcutaneous LMWH, or factor Xa inhibitors, help prevent VTE. During the past 15 years, the use of LMWHs has markedly increased for patients with total hip and knee replacements. Examples include enoxaparin (Lovenox), dalteparin (Fragmin), and tinzaparin (Innohep). These drugs work to inhibit factor Xa, which is a key component in the clotting process. Given in a low prophylactic dose based on the patient's weight, they do not significantly affect prothrombin time (PT) or activated partial thromboplastin time (aPTT). Although not as commonly seen with these drugs when compared with unfractionated heparin (UFH), **thrombocytopenia** (decreased platelets) can occur. Therefore monitor the patient's complete blood count and platelet count per agency policy. Assess for bleeding, including occult blood in stool and bruising. Protamine sulfate can be given as an antidote for all heparins; however, it is not as effective for LMWH when compared with UFH. Be especially alert for signs and symptoms of neurologic dysfunction because spinal and epidural hematomas can occur in patients who received neuroaxial anesthesia. Patients typically receive LMWH for at least 5 days and start on oral anticoagulant therapy for at least 72 hours before it is discontinued.

Fondaparinux (Arixtra), a factor Xa inhibiting agent, may also be prescribed for patients undergoing hip and knee arthroplasty. Its action is similar to that of LMWHs and has no effect on coagulation tests. Like other drugs, however, the patient is at risk for bleeding. No antidote exists at this time for fondaparinux. Like LMWHs, Arixtra is given for at least 5 days with an overlap while anticoagulants begin to work. A complete discussion of nursing care associated with patients taking anticoagulants and VTE is found in Chapter 38.

Early ambulation and exercise help prevent VTE. Collaborate with the physical therapist (PT) in teaching leg exercises, which are begun in the immediate postoperative period and continue through the rehabilitation period. These exercises include plantar flexion and dorsiflexion (heel pumping), circumduction (circles) of the feet, gluteal and quadriceps muscle setting, and straight-leg raises (SLRs). Teach the patient to perform gluteal exercises by pushing the heels into the bed and achieve **quadriceps-setting exercises** ("quad sets") by straightening the legs and pushing the back of the knees into the bed. In addition to preventing clots, these exercises improve muscle tone, which aids restoring the function of the extremity.

Prevention of infection. Another common potential complication of hip replacement is infection. Infection can occur during hospitalization or for months or years later. Most infections are caused by contamination during surgery.

Monitor the surgical incision and vital signs carefully—every 4 hours for the first 24 hours and every 8 hours thereafter. Observe for signs of infection, such as an elevated temperature and excessive or foul-smelling drainage from the incision. *An older patient may not have a fever with infection but instead may experience an altered mental state.* Obtain a sample of the drainage for culture and sensitivity to determine the offending organisms and the antibiotics that may be needed for treatment.

Assessment of bleeding and management of anemia. Observe the surgical hip dressing for bleeding or other type of drainage at least every 4 hours or when vital signs are taken. Empty and measure the bloody fluid in the surgical drain(s) every shift. The total amount of drainage is usually less than 50 mL/8 hr. Patients who have the minimally invasive procedure may not have a drain. The surgeon usually removes the drains and operative dressing 24 to 48 hours after surgery. *Take special care when removing tape from the skin to prevent tape burns as the surgical dressing is changed, especially for older adults.*

The surgeon also requests periodic hemoglobin and hematocrit (H&H) tests to assess for anemia. Patients who took LMWH before surgery but not epoetin alfa are most at risk for postoperative anemia. Although some patients receive several units of blood during surgery, the H&H levels may continue to fall below the normal level, in which case additional blood is needed 1 to 2 days after surgery. Blood pressure may be lower than usual because of blood loss during surgery or because cement was used during surgery. Cement can dilate blood vessels and cause hypotension.

If the patient did not donate his or her own blood, another method for blood replacement is intraoperative or postoperative blood salvage. The shed blood is collected intraoperatively via aspiration from the surgical site. Using a cell saver, about 50% of the red blood cells are saved for reinfusion. This procedure is used most commonly for bilateral joint replacements or revision surgeries. Blood can be replaced postoperatively by collecting shed blood via suction into a reservoir, filtering the blood, and reinfusing it within a few hours.

Assessment for neurovascular compromise. As with other musculoskeletal surgery, frequent neurovascular assessments are necessary to monitor for a possible compromise in circulation to the distal extremity. *Check and document color, temperature, distal pulses, capillary refill, movement, and sensation.* Remember to compare the operative leg with the nonoperative leg. These assessments are performed at the same time the vital signs are checked. Any changes in neurovascular assessment should be reported to the surgeon and carefully monitored. Early detection of changes in neurovascular status can prevent permanent tissue damage.

Management of pain. Although hip arthroplasty is performed to relieve joint pain, the patient does experience pain related to the surgical procedure. Many state that they have pain after surgery but that it is of a different type and is less excruciating than the pain before surgery. Pain control is typically achieved by epidural analgesia, intraspinal analgesia, patient-controlled analgesia (PCA), IV opioid analgesia, or a combination of techniques. Chapter 5 contains information on commonly used opioid analgesics used for acute pain and related nursing interventions. *Keep in mind that the patient may also receive other analgesics or anti-inflammatory drugs for chronic arthritic pain in other joints.*

Regardless of the pain management method used, most patients do not require parenteral analgesics after the first day. Oral opioids, such as oxycodone plus acetaminophen (Percocet, Tylox), are then commonly prescribed until the pain can be controlled by NSAIDs such as ketorolac (Toradol, Acular) or ibuprofen (Motrin, Apo-Ibuprofen🍁). Patients who have orthopedic surgery should take NSAIDs only on a short-term basis, up to 14 days. Nonpharmacologic methods for acute and chronic pain control should also be used to decrease the amount of drug therapy used (see Chapter 5).

Progression of activity. The patient with a THA gets out of bed the day after surgery with help and physical therapy is initiated. Permitted activities differ among surgeons and hospitals, but prolonged bedrest can cause numerous complications (e.g., atelectasis, pneumonia), especially in older adults. When getting the patient out of bed, stand on the same side of the bed as the affected leg. After achieving a sitting position, the patient stands on the unaffected leg and pivots to the chair with assistance. To prevent hip dislocation, ensure that he or she does not flex the hips beyond 90 degrees (Fig. 20-2). Raised toilet seats, straight-back chairs, and reclining wheelchairs help prevent hyperflexion of the replaced hip joint.

The surgeon, type of prosthesis, and surgical procedure determine the amount of weight bearing that can be applied to

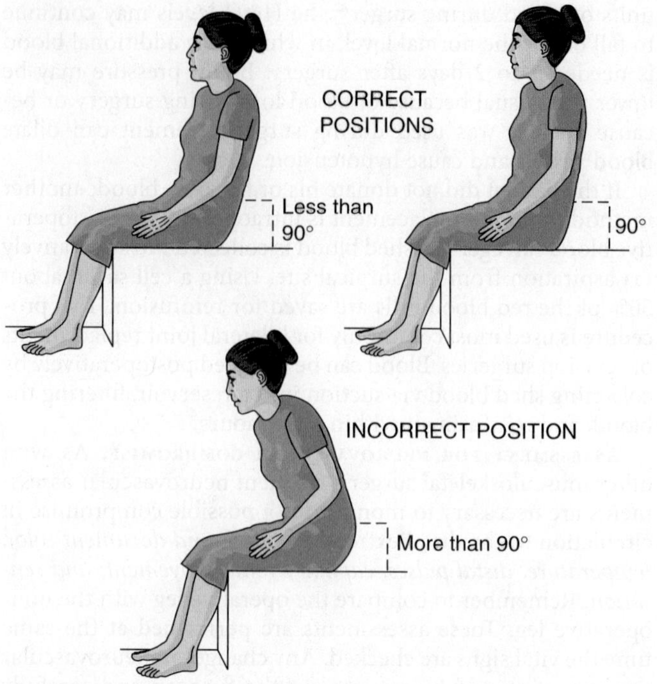
CORRECT
POSITIONS
Less than
90°
90°
INCORRECT POSITION
More than 90°

Fig. 20-2 • Correct and incorrect hip flexion after a total hip replacement.

the affected leg. A patient with a cemented implant is usually allowed immediate partial weight bearing (PWB) or full weight bearing (FWB) to tolerance. One with an uncemented prosthesis cannot tolerate FWB until bony ingrowth occurs. Typically, only PWB is permitted for the first few weeks or until there is x-ray evidence of bony ingrowth.

In collaboration with the physical therapist (PT), teach the patient how to follow weight-bearing restrictions and progress to FWB status, when possible. Most patients use a walker, but younger adults may use crutches. They are usually advanced to a single cane or crutch if they can walk without a severe limp 4 to 6 weeks after surgery. When the limp disappears, they no longer need an ambulatory/assistive device and may be permitted to sit in chairs of normal height, use regular toilets, and drive a car.

Promotion of self-care. The hospital's occupational therapy department often supplies assistive/adaptive devices to help with ADLs, especially for those having traditional surgery. Particularly important are devices designed for reaching to prevent patients from bending or stooping and flexing the hips more than 90 degrees. Extended handles on shoehorns and dressing sticks are particularly useful to achieve ADL independence.

For those who have *traditional surgery,* the length of stay in the acute care hospital is typically 3 days, but older adults or those experiencing postoperative complications may stay longer. Those who have *MIS procedures* may be discharged on the second postoperative day or, in a few cases, the day of surgery. Those patients are discharged to home on crutches to do their own rehabilitative exercises. Most of them are able to return to work in 2 weeks. For that reason, some hospitals have started Rapid Recovery Hip Replacement programs for patients who are candidates for MIS.

Discharge for patients having *traditional surgery* may be to the home, a rehabilitation unit, transitional care unit, or skilled long-term care facility. The interdisciplinary team provides written instructions for posthospital care and reviews them with patients and their family members (Chart 20-4). Be sure to provide a copy of these instructions for the patient.

Acute rehabilitation usually takes 1 to 2 weeks or longer, depending on the patient's age and tolerance as well as the type of prosthesis used. However, it often takes 6 weeks or longer for complete recovery. Some patients who are discharged to their home are able to attend PT sessions in an office or ambulatory care setting. Others have no means or cannot use community resources and need PT in the home, depending on their health insurance coverage. *Collaborate with the case manager to determine which option is best for your patient.*

Total knee arthroplasty. Although many older adults require total knee arthroplasty (TKA, also known as total knee

Chart 20-4 PATIENT AND FAMILY EDUCATION GUIDE

Care of Patients with Total Hip Arthroplasty After Hospital Discharge

HIP PRECAUTIONS
- Do not sit or stand for prolonged periods.
- Do not cross your legs beyond the midline of your body.
- Do not bend your hips more than 90 degrees.
- Use an ambulatory aid, such as a walker, when walking.
- Use assistive/adaptive devices for dressing, such as for putting on shoes and socks.
- Resume sexual intercourse as usual on the advice of your surgeon.

PAIN MANAGEMENT
- Report increased hip pain to the physician immediately.
- Take oral analgesics as prescribed and only as needed.
- Do not overexert yourself; take frequent rests.

INCISIONAL CARE
- Inspect your hip incision every day for redness, heat, or drainage; if any of these are present, call your physician immediately.
- Cleanse your hip incision with a mild soap and water every day; be sure to dry it thoroughly.

OTHER CARE
- Continue walking and performing the leg exercises as you learned in the hospital.
- Report pain, redness, or swelling in your legs to your physician immediately.
- Report chest pain or shortness of breath to your physician immediately.
- If you are taking an anticoagulant, follow the precautions learned in the hospital to prevent bleeding; avoid using a straight razor, avoid injuries, and report bleeding or excessive bruising to your surgeon immediately.

replacement [TKR]), those who have a knee replaced may be younger than those who have a hip replaced. Continued improvements in total knee implants in the past 15 years have increased the expected life of a TKA to 15 years or more, depending on the age and activity level of the patient. An increasing number of patients who have TKAs are overweight or obese. Obesity can increase wear and tear on weight-bearing joints, which can lead to revision surgeries.

Preoperative care. TKA, like hip replacement, is performed when joint paint cannot be managed by conservative measures. When activity and mobility severely prevent patients from participating in work or activities they enjoy, this procedure can restore a high quality of life. The preoperative care and teaching for patients undergoing a TKA are similar to that for total hip replacement. Differences in patient and family teaching depend on the procedure used by the orthopedic surgeon.

Like the minimally invasive surgery (MIS) for the hip, the knee can also be replaced using MIS. Candidates for this newer surgery should not have severe bone loss or previous knee surgery. They should be in good health, including normal weight for their height. Patients having MIS usually have less blood loss during surgery, less pain, more joint range of motion (less stiffness from scarring), and a faster recovery, leading to a shorter hospital stay. Rapid Recovery Knee Replacement programs for patients having MIS total knee arthroplasty are becoming popular in a number of hospitals.

All patients are given verbal and either written or video preoperative instructions, which include the activity protocol to follow after surgery. The PT and OT provide information about transfers, ambulation, and postoperative exercises. Some surgeons prescribe a continuous passive motion (CPM) machine after knee surgery to increase joint mobility. Others have found that the range of motion for the surgical knee is not improved by using this device. If the patient will have a CPM machine after surgery, be sure to explain what it is and how it is used.

Routine diagnostic testing is requested, as well as any additional tests, such as cervical spine x-rays for patients with rheumatoid arthritis (RA). Knee x-rays, CT scan, and/or MRI may be done to assess the joint and surrounding soft tissues.

Patients having a TKA are at risk for many of the same postoperative complications as those who have a hip replacement. The most common problems include venous thromboembolism (VTE), anemia, and infection. The Preoperative Care section in the Total Hip Arthroplasty section explains the care needed to prevent these same problems in patients having knee surgery (see pp. 328-329).

Operative procedures. As with the hip, the knee can be replaced with the patient under general or neuroaxial (epidural or spinal) anesthesia. Antibiotics are given before surgical opening. In the *traditional surgery,* the surgeon makes a central longitudinal incision about 8 inches (20 cm) or more long. Osteotomies of the femoral and tibial condyles and of the posterior patella are performed, and the surfaces are prepared for the prosthesis. The femoral component is often non-cemented (using a press-fit) with the tibial component being cemented. The surgeon may insert a surgical drain, and a pressure dressing is applied to decrease edema and bleeding. Some patients have bilateral knee replacements as part of one surgery.

Minimally invasive procedures for TKA may be performed using a 2- to 4-inch incision and special instruments to spare muscle and other soft tissue. Computer-guided equipment is being studied to address concerns about accurate positioning of the knee implants.

Complementary and alternative therapies. An experimental treatment to reduce the severe pain that occurs after knee arthroplasty is the intraoperative insertion of Adlea, a refined capsaicin product, directly into the surgical joint. Capsaicin binds to and opens C fiber receptors, especially TRPV1, which causes extra calcium to enter the nerve cells. The cells become overloaded and shut down, causing numbness. Preliminary results from several studies show that patients who were given Adlea during knee surgery had less acute postoperative pain when compared with others who did not receive the treatment (www.anesiva.com/wt/page/postsurgical_pain). Additional studies for patients having total hip replacements and bunionectomies are currently being conducted. Adlea could help decrease the need for opioid analgesia for many patients having surgery.

Postoperative care. Postoperative nursing care of the patient with a TKA is similar to that for the patient with a total hip arthroplasty; however, maintaining hip abduction is not necessary. The surgeon may prescribe a continuous passive motion (CPM) machine, which can be applied in the postanesthesia care unit (PACU) or soon after the patient is admitted to the postoperative unit (Fig. 20-3). The CPM machine keeps the prosthetic knee in motion and may prevent the formation of scar tissue, which could decrease knee mobility and increase postoperative pain. In the immediate postoperative period, the surgeon may also prescribe ice packs or other cold therapy to decrease swelling at the surgical site. Swelling and bruising are more common with this type of surgery than with hip surgery.

The surgeon, PT, or technician presets the CPM machine for the appropriate range of motion and cycles per minute. A typical initial setting is 20 to 30 degrees of flexion and full extension (0 degrees) at two cycles per minute, but this setting varies according to surgeon preference. The machine is generally used on an intermittent schedule of a designated number of hours several times a day, with the range of motion increased gradually. Observe and document the patient's response to the device, and follow the surgeon's protocol for

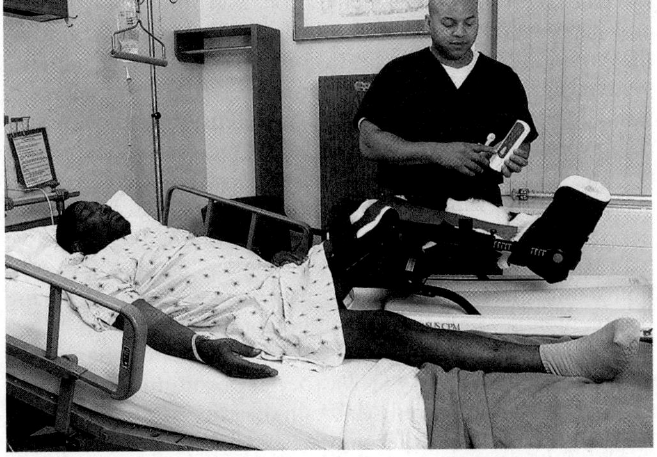

Fig. 20-3 • A continuous passive motion (CPM) machine in use.

Chart 20-5 **BEST PRACTICE FOR PATIENT SAFETY & QUALITY CARE**

The Patient Using a Continuous Passive Motion (CPM) Machine

- Ensure that the machine is well padded.
- Check the cycle and range-of-motion settings at least once every 8 hours.
- Ensure that the joint being moved is properly positioned on the machine.
- If the patient is confused, place the controls to the machine out of his or her reach.
- Assess the patient's response to the machine.
- Turn off the machine while the patient is having a meal in bed.
- When the machine is not in use, do not store it on the floor.

settings. Chart 20-5 outlines your responsibility when caring for a patient using the CPM machine.

In general, pain-control measures for patients with TKA are similar to those with total hip arthroplasty. Many patients report higher ratings on the pain scale and require IV opioid medications longer than patients with THA, particularly if they have had bilateral surgery. *Be sure to manage your patient's pain to provide comfort, increase their participation in physical therapy, and improve joint mobility.*

One of the most recent advances in postoperative pain management for lower extremity total joint arthroplasty is *continuous peripheral nerve blockade (CPNB).* In this procedure, the anesthesiologist injects the femoral or sciatic nerve with local anesthetic and the patient receives a continuous infusion by portable pump. This method of pain management not only decreases pain but also allows patients to participate in rehabilitation earlier than when using opioid analgesia alone. Duarte et al. (2006) reported that patients having a continuous femoral nerve blockade (CFNB) after TKA required less opioids and antiemetics when compared with patients receiving no CFNB and those who had a single shot FNB. The authors concluded that FNB was an effective way to control postoperative pain after TKA.

When caring for a patient receiving a CPNB, perform neurovascular assessments every 2 to 4 hours or according to hospital protocol. The patient should be able to plantar flex and dorsiflex the affected foot but not feel pain in the extremity. Check for movement, sensation, warmth, color, pulses, and capillary refill. Also monitor the patient for symptoms that could indicate that the infusion is getting into the patient's system, such as a metallic taste, tinnitus, restlessness, nervousness, slurred speech, bradycardia, hypotension, and decreased respirations. In some cases, the patient may have one or more seizures (Turjanica, 2007).

Nonpharmacologic interventions, such as music therapy, have also been used with success in controlling postoperative pain (Giaquinto et al., 2006). See Chapters 2 and 5 for additional information about acute pain management, including complementary and alternative therapies.

Because dislocation is a rare problem for a patient with total knee replacement (TKR), special positioning to prevent adduction is not required. Maintain the knee in a neutral position and not rotated internally or externally. Some surgeons recommend that the knee should rest flat on the bed or with one pillow under the lower calf and foot to encourage slight extension of the knee joint. Be sure that the surgical knee does not hyperextend.

Other complications that affect patients with THA may also affect those having TKA, such as venous thromboembolism, infection, and bleeding. *Monitor neurovascular status frequently to check for compromise to the distal operative leg.* The preventive postoperative measures for total hip arthroplasty are also used for TKA (see Postoperative Care section in the Total Hip Arthroplasty section on pp. 329-331).

The ideal goal for discharge from the acute hospital unit is that the patient can walk independently with crutches, walker, or cane and has close to 90 degrees of flexion in the operative knee. Patients who had the *MIS procedure* are discharged to home in 1 to 2 days with instructions for postoperative exercises and activity progression. During the home rehabilitation phase, the use of a stationary bicycle or CPM machine may help gain flexion. These patients can return to work and other usual activities in 2 weeks.

Acute rehabilitation for *traditional* surgery usually takes about 1 to 2 weeks or longer, depending on the age and tolerance of the patient. These patients may be discharged to their home or to an acute rehabilitation unit, transitional care unit, or skilled long-term care facility for therapy. If able, they may attend PT sessions in an office or ambulatory care setting. If not, home care services can provide PT in their home, depending on the insurance available. *Collaborate with the case manager to determine which option is best for your patient.* Total recovery takes 6 weeks or longer, especially for those older than 75 years.

Other joint arthroplasties. After the hip and knee, the shoulder and hand are the most common joints replaced for severe OA, RA, or trauma. Elbow, wrist, ankle, and foot replacements are not performed as often as other types of arthroplasties. The shoulder and other upper extremity joints do not bear weight and therefore tend to have less degeneration and subsequent pain. Preoperative teaching for patients having any of these surgeries depends on the surgeon's technique and postoperative protocols. For example, the continuous passive motion (CPM) machine may be prescribed postoperatively in the hospital and in the posthospital setting (home or other facility). These devices are available for almost any joint surgery in the body. Some surgeons find that the CPM machine is not helpful in promoting joint mobility and may be uncomfortable for patients.

Total shoulder arthroplasty (TSA) has gained popularity as newer prostheses and technology have been developed. This procedure usually decreases arthritic pain and increases the patient's ability to perform ADLs. Because the shoulder joint is complex and has many **articulations** (joint surfaces), **subluxation** (partial dislocation) or complete dislocation is a major complication. Usually the glenohumeral joint, created by the glenoid cavity of the shoulder blade (scapula) and the head of the humerus, is replaced because it moves the most and is therefore most affected by arthritis. A **hemiarthroplasty** (replacement of part of the joint), typically the humeral component, may be performed as an alternative to TSA.

The surgeon makes a 3- to 4-inch (8- to 10-cm) incision to replace the joint while the patient is under general anesthesia. The implant may be cemented or press-fitted without cement. A few surgeons are beginning to perform *minimally invasive shoulder arthroplasty,* which should decrease postoperative complications like infection and nerve damage. A sling is applied to immobilize the joint until therapy begins.

In addition to dislocation, postoperative complications are similar to those for other THAs and include infection, loosening, and nerve and blood vessel damage. Active and passive exercises are needed to begin shoulder movement. *As for any other total joint arthroplasty, perform frequent neurovascular assessments, at least every 4 to 8 hours.* The hospital stay for TSA is shorter than for a total hip or knee replacement—usually 1 to 2 days until pain is controlled. Rehabilitation with an occupational therapist generally takes 2 to 3 months.

Total elbow arthroplasty (TEA) is performed most often for patients with rheumatoid arthritis (RA), but it is done for anyone whose severe arthritis limits movement and causes uncontrolled pain. TEA may be successful in increasing range of motion, but infection and loosening may occur because of extensive tissue cutting during surgery. Active and passive exercises are used postoperatively. In general, elbow motion is allowed as tolerated. Occupational therapy may not be necessary, but the need depends on the individual patient. Lifting is usually restricted on a long-term basis after TEA. Generalized swelling usually resolves in 3 to 6 months.

Any joint of the hand or foot can be replaced *(phalangeal joint, metacarpal or metatarsal arthroplasties),* often for patients with RA. Hand prostheses are implanted without the use of cement because they stay in place and do not bear weight.

For the hand, a bulky dressing is used temporarily after surgery and is then replaced with a dynamic splint. Edema is controlled by having the patient elevate the arm as much as possible. The rehabilitation program for phalangeal joint arthroplasties may last for many weeks until normal function and strength return. These procedures are typically performed in specialized hand centers. Joint replacements in the toe usually require less rehabilitation.

Any bone of the *wrist* can also be replaced, including the heads of the radius and ulna. The postoperative pressure dressing is removed in 1 to 2 days, and a splint is applied. The patient usually regains full function within 6 to 12 weeks, but lifting may be restricted for a longer period. Special hand therapists work with these patients for the extensive rehabilitation that is required for phalangeal and wrist replacements.

Because the ankles support about 25% of the body's weight and are complex joints, developing an implant that is both small enough and strong enough has been difficult. Although total ankle arthroplasties (TAAs) have been problematic for more than three decades, newer non-cemented prosthetic systems have renewed interest in ankle replacements.

Postoperative complications include infection, delayed wound healing, nerve injuries, and loosening. Therefore TAA is not as successful as total hip or knee replacements. Noncemented prostheses seem to be preferred over cemented ones to prevent loosening. The patient is allowed to begin weight bearing at about 6 weeks, and rehabilitation continues for about 3 months.

DECISION-MAKING CHALLENGE

Critical Rescue

An 82-year-old active man had a left total knee arthroplasty 2 days ago and has been progressing well in physical therapy. Plans are being made for him to be discharged to home to live with his daughter for several weeks. While you are busy administering 10 AM meds, the nursing assistant tells you that the patient's surgical leg is swollen and looks "angry." When you asked her what she means, she explains that his leg is very "red-looking and hot."

1. What response should you give the nursing assistant at this time?
2. What might explain the nursing assistant's observations? Think of all the possibilities.
3. When you check on the patient, you find that he is having shortness of breath and reports that he thinks he has indigestion. What should your action be at this time and why?

evolve For suggested answer guidelines, go to http://evolve.elsevier.com/Iggy/.

Impaired Physical Mobility

NOC **Planning: Expected Outcomes.** The patient with osteoarthritis (OA) is expected to move in his or her own environment independently, with or without an assistive device. Indicators include that he or she will have no problems with:

- Balance and coordination
- Gait
- Joint movement
- Transfer performance
- Walking

Interventions. *Management of the patient with OA is an interdisciplinary effort. Collaborate with the physical therapist (PT) and occupational therapist (OT) to meet the goal of independent function.* Major interventions include therapeutic exercise and the promotion of ADLs and ambulation by teaching about health and the use of assistive devices.

Two types of *exercise* are recommended for the patient with OA: recreational and therapeutic. **Recreational exercise** includes hobbies and sports, with no planned purpose other than relaxation. **Therapeutic exercise** includes carefully planned activities that are designed to improve muscle strength, muscle tone, and joint range of motion. Therapeutic exercise can also reduce pain and improve the patient's psychological health.

Certain recreational activities may also be therapeutic, such as swimming to enhance chest and arm muscles. Aerobic exercises (e.g., walking, biking, swimming, aerobic dance) are recommended. Usually the PT prescribes exercises for the patient with OA, but you will need to reinforce their techniques and principles. The ideal time for exercise is immediately after the application of heat. To prevent further joint damage, teach patients to carefully follow the instructions for exercise outlined in Chart 20-6.

Collaborate with the PT to evaluate the patient's need for ambulatory aids such as canes, walkers, or platform crutches. Although many patients do not like to use these aids or may forget how to use them, they do help prevent further joint deterioration and pain. Collaborate with the OT to assess the patient's ability to perform ADLs and to provide ideas and devices for assistance.

Community-Based Care

The patient with OA is not usually hospitalized for the disease itself but for surgical management. Expect that any patient older than 60 years will have some degree of arthritis and possibly chronic pain that need to be managed.

Home Care Management

If weight-bearing joints are severely involved, the patient may have difficulty going up or down stairs. Making arrangements to live on one floor with accessibility to all rooms is often the

Chart 20-6 PATIENT AND FAMILY EDUCATION GUIDE

Exercises for Patients with Osteoarthritis or Rheumatoid Arthritis

- Follow the exercise instructions that have been prescribed specifically for you. There are no universal exercises; your exercises have been specifically tailored to your needs.
- Do your exercises on both "good" and "bad" days. Consistency is important.
- Respect pain. If pain increases as you exercise, stop and report this to your health care provider.
- Use active rather than active-assist or passive exercise whenever possible.
- Reduce the number of repetitions when the inflammation is severe and you have more pain.
- Do not substitute your normal activities or household tasks for the prescribed exercises.
- Avoid resistive exercises when your joints are severely inflamed.

best solution. A home care nurse, PT, and OT collaborate to assess the need for structural alterations to the home to accommodate ambulatory aids and enable the patient to perform ADLs. For example, a kitchen counter may need to be lowered or a seat and handrails may need to be installed in the shower. If the patient has undergone a total hip replacement, an elevated toilet seat is necessary for several weeks postoperatively to prevent excessive hip flexion.

Health Teaching

Learning how to protect joints is the most important part of patient and family education. Preventing further damage to joints slows the progression of OA and minimizes pain. Explain the general principles of joint protection, and give practical examples (Chart 20-7).

As with other diseases in which drugs and nutritional therapy are used, teach the patient and family the medication protocol, desired and potential side effects, and toxic effects. Emphasize the importance of reducing weight and eating a well-balanced diet to promote tissue healing.

Many patients with arthritis look for a cure after becoming frustrated and desperate about the course of the disease and treatment. Better control of arthritis is possible, but cure is not yet available. Unfortunately tabloids, books, media, and the Internet often report "curative" remedies. People spend billions of dollars each year on quackery, including liniments, special diets, and copper bracelets. More hazardous substances, such as snake venom and industrial cleaners, are also advertised as remedies. Refer the patient to the Arthritis Foundation for up-to-date information about these "cures." The practice of wearing a copper bracelet will not cure arthritis, but it will not cause harm. If the patient is using a potentially harmful substance or method, however, reinforce the need to avoid the unproven remedy and explain why it should not be used.

With most types of arthritis and connective tissue disease (CTD), patients must live with a chronic, unpredictable, and painful disorder. Their roles, self-esteem, and body image may be affected by these diseases. Body image is often not as devastating in OA as in the inflammatory arthritic diseases, such as RA. The psychosocial component is discussed in more detail in the Psychosocial Assessment section on p. 339 of the Rheumatoid Arthritis section.

Chart 20-7 PATIENT AND FAMILY EDUCATION GUIDE

Evidence-Based Instructions for Joint Protection

- Use large joints instead of small ones; for example, place your purse strap over your shoulder instead of grasping the purse with your hand.
- Do not turn a doorknob clockwise. Turn it counterclockwise to avoid twisting your arm and promoting ulnar deviation.
- Use two hands instead of one to hold objects.
- Sit in a chair that has a high, straight back.
- When getting out of bed, do not push off with your fingers; use the entire palm of both hands.
- Do not bend at your waist; instead, bend your knees while keeping your back straight.
- Use long-handled devices, such as a hairbrush with an extended handle.
- Use assistive/adaptive devices, such as Velcro closures and built-up utensil handles, to protect your joints.
- Do not use pillows in bed except a small one under your head.
- Avoid twisting or wringing your hands.

Health Care Resources

The patient who has undergone surgery probably will need help from community resources. After an arthroplasty, he or she needs extensive assistance with mobility. The patient may be discharged to home, a long-term care facility, a transitional care unit, or a rehabilitation unit. Collaborate with the case manager and physician to find the best placement. If the patient is discharged to home, home care nurses may be approved for several visits, depending on the concurrent systemic diseases. A nursing assistant may visit the home to help with hygiene-related needs, and a physical therapist may work with ambulatory and mobility skills. For older patients, a family member, significant other, or other caregiver should be in the home for at least the first 4 to 6 weeks when the patient needs the most assistance.

Provide written instructions about the required care, regardless of whether the patient goes home or to another inpatient facility. Hand-off communication with the new care provider is essential for seamless continuity of care.

The Arthritis Foundation (www.arthritis.org) is an important community resource for all patients with arthritis and CTD. This organization provides information to lay people and health care professionals and refers patients and their families to other resources as needed. Local support groups can help them cope with these diseases.

▪ *Evaluation: Outcomes*

Evaluate the care of the patient with OA on the basis of the identified nursing diagnoses. The expected outcomes are that he or she:

- Takes personal actions to control pain, if possible
- Moves in his or her own environment independently with or without an assistive device

Specific indicators for these outcomes are listed for each nursing diagnosis under the Planning and Implementation section (see earlier).

RHEUMATOID ARTHRITIS

Pathophysiology

Rheumatoid arthritis (RA) is one of the most common connective tissue diseases and is the most destructive to the joints. It is a chronic, progressive, systemic inflammatory autoimmune disease process that affects primarily the synovial joints. **Systemic** means this disease affects the body system, affecting many joints and other tissues. RA affects over 2 million people, and European Americans have the disease more often than other groups (www.arthritis.org).

In RA, autoantibodies (rheumatoid factors [RFs]) are formed that attack healthy tissue, especially synovium, causing inflammation. RFs consist mainly of immunoglobulins M and G, and they bind with antigens forming immune complexes. Phagocytes attempt to engulf these complexes and, as a result, release powerful enzymes, such as cytokines. The B- and T-lymphocytes of the immune system are also stimulated and increase the inflammatory response.

Inflammation occurs first in the synovial membrane, which lines the joint cavity. It then begins to involve the articular cartilage, joint capsule, and surrounding ligaments and tendons. Several processes cause cartilage damage in patients with RA (McCance & Huether, 2006):

- Neutrophils and other cells in synovial fluid are activated and break down the joint cartilage.
- Synovium digests cartilage, releasing inflammatory substances, such as IL-1 and TNFA. (See Chapter 19 for a complete discussion of the inflammatory response.)
- Cytokines, especially interleukin-1 (IL-1) and tumor necrosis factor–alpha (TNFA), cause chondrocytes to attack cartilage. TNF has effects on lipid metabolism, coagulation, insulin resistance, and endothelial function.

The synovium then thickens and becomes hyperemic, fluid accumulates in the joint space, and a pannus forms. The **pannus** is vascular granulation tissue composed of inflammatory cells; it erodes articular cartilage and eventually destroys bone. As a result, in late disease, fibrous adhesions, bony ankylosis, and calcifications occur; bone loses density, and secondary osteoporosis occurs.

Permanent joint changes may be avoided if RA is diagnosed early. Early, aggressive treatment to suppress synovitis may lead to a remission. RA is a disease characterized by natural remissions and exacerbations. Interdisciplinary management helps control the disease to decrease the intensity and number of exacerbations. Preventing flares helps prevent joint erosion and permanent joint damage.

Because rheumatoid arthritis is a systemic disease, areas of the body besides the synovial joints can be affected. Inflammatory responses similar to those occurring in synovial tissue may be seen in any organ or body system in which connective tissue is prevalent. If blood vessel involvement **(vasculitis)** occurs, the organ supplied by that vessel can be affected. The result is malfunction and eventual failure of the organ or system. These pathologic changes may occur late in the disease process and cause life-threatening problems.

The etiology of RA remains unclear, but research suggests a *combination of environmental and genetic factors*. Some researchers suspect that female reproductive hormones influence the development of RA because it affects women more often than men—usually young- to middle-aged women. Others suspect that infectious organisms may play a role, particularly the Epstein-Barr virus (McCance & Huether, 2006). Physical and emotional stresses have been linked to exacerbations of the disorder and may be contributing factors or "triggers" to its development.

GENETIC CONSIDERATIONS

Research has shown that there is a strong association between RA and several human leukocyte antigen (HLA)-DR alleles. The cause of this association is not clear, but most HLA diseases are autoimmune (Nussbaum et al., 2007). DR alleles, especially DR4 and DRB1, are the primary genetic factors contributing to the development of RA. DR4 is associated with more severe forms of the disease (Klippel, 2007). Other contributing factors are being researched.

Patient-Centered Collaborative Care

Assessment

The onset of rheumatoid arthritis (RA) may be acute and severe or slow and progressive; patients may have vague symptoms that last for several months before diagnosis. The onset of the disease is more common in the winter months than in the warmer months. The manifestations of RA can be categorized as early or late disease and as articular (joint) or extra-articular (Chart 20-8).

Physical Assessment/Clinical Manifestations

Early Disease Manifestations. *The patient with RA typically reports joint stiffness, swelling, pain, and fatigue. He or she may report generalized weakness and morning stiffness.* Anorexia

Chart 20-8 KEY FEATURES

The Patient with Rheumatoid Arthritis

EARLY MANIFESTATIONS

JOINT

- Inflammation

SYSTEMIC

- Low-grade fever
- Fatigue
- Weakness
- Anorexia
- Paresthesias

LATE MANIFESTATIONS

JOINT

- Deformities (e.g., swan neck or ulnar deviation)
- Moderate to severe pain and morning stiffness

SYSTEMIC

- Osteoporosis
- Severe fatigue
- Anemia
- Weight loss
- Subcutaneous nodules
- Peripheral neuropathy
- Vasculitis
- Pericarditis
- Fibrotic lung disease
- Sjögren's syndrome
- Renal disease

and a weight loss of about 2 or 3 pounds (1 kg) usually occur early in the disease process. Persistent low-grade fever may accompany these manifestations. In patients with early disease, the upper-extremity joints are involved initially—often the proximal interphalangeal (PIP) and metacarpophalangeal (MCP) joints of the hands. These joints may be slightly reddened, warm, stiff, swollen, and tender or painful, particularly on palpation (caused by synovitis). The typical pattern of joint involvement in RA is bilateral and symmetric (e.g., both wrists), and the number of joints involved usually increases as the disease progresses. In early disease, the patient may report migrating symptoms known as **migratory arthritis.**

The presence of only *one* hot, swollen, painful joint (out of proportion to the other joints) may mean the joint is infected. *Refer the patient to the health care provider (generally the rheumatologist) immediately if this is the case.* Single hot, swollen joints are considered infected until proven otherwise and require immediate long-term antibiotic treatment.

Late Disease Manifestations. As the disease worsens, the joints become progressively inflamed and very painful. The patient usually has frequent morning stiffness (also called the **gel phenomenon**), which lasts for 45 minutes to several hours after awakening. On palpation, the joints feel soft and look puffy because of synovitis and **effusions** (joint swelling with fluid, especially the knees). The fingers often appear spindle-like. Note any muscle atrophy (which can result from disuse secondary to joint pain) and a decreased range of motion in the affected joints.

Most or all synovial joints are eventually affected. The temporomandibular joint (TMJ) may be involved in severe disease, but such involvement is uncommon. When the TMJ is affected, the patient may have pain when chewing or opening the mouth.

When the spinal column is involved, the cervical joints are most likely to be affected. During clinical examination, gently palpate the posterior cervical spine and identify it as cervical pain, tenderness, or loss of motion. *Cervical disease may result in subluxation, especially with the first and second vertebrae. This complication may be life threatening because branches of the phrenic nerve that supply the diaphragm are restricted and respiratory function may be compromised. The patient is also in danger of becoming quadriparetic (weak in all extremities) or quadriplegic (paralyzed in all extremities). If you identify cervical pain or loss of range of motion in the cervical spine of a person with RA, report this information to the physician, generally the rheumatologist.*

Joint Involvement. *Joint deformity* occurs as a late, articular manifestation, and secondary osteoporosis can cause bone fractures. Observe common deformities, especially in the hands and feet (Fig. 20-4). Extensive wrist involvement can result in carpal tunnel syndrome (see Chapter 54 for assessment and management of carpal tunnel syndrome).

Gently palpate the tissues around the joints to elicit pain or tenderness associated with other rheumatoid complications, unless the patient is having severe joint pain. For example, **Baker's cysts** (enlarged popliteal bursae behind the knee) may occur and cause tissue compression and pain. Tendon rupture is also possible, particularly rupture of the Achilles tendon.

Systemic Complications. Numerous extra-articular clinical manifestations are associated with advanced disease. Assess other body systems to ascertain systemic involvement. In addition to increased joint swelling and tenderness, moderate to severe *weight loss, fever, and extreme fatigue* are common in

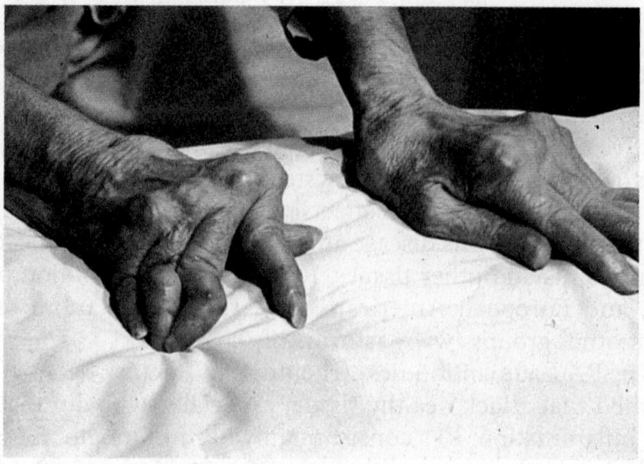

Fig. 20-4 • Common joint deformities seen in rheumatoid arthritis.

late disease **exacerbations,** often called "flare-ups." Some patients have the characteristic round, movable, nontender **subcutaneous nodules,** which usually appear on the ulnar surface of the arm, on the fingers, or along the Achilles tendon. These nodules can disappear and reappear at any time and are associated with severe, destructive disease. Rheumatoid nodules usually are not a problem themselves; however, they occasionally open and become infected and may interfere with ADLs. Bumping nodules may cause discomfort or pain. Occasionally, nodules are identified within the lungs.

Inflammation of the blood vessels results in *vasculitis,* particularly of small- to medium-sized vessels. When arterial involvement occurs, major organs and body systems become ischemic and malfunction. Assess for ischemic skin lesions that appear in groups as small, brownish spots, most commonly around the nail bed **(periungual lesions).** Monitor the number of lesions, note their location each day, and report vascular changes to the health care provider. Increased lesions indicate increased vasculitis, and a decreased number indicates decreased vasculitis. Also carefully assess any larger lesions that appear on the lower extremities. These lesions can lead to ulcerations, which heal slowly as a result of decreased circulation. Peripheral neuropathy associated with decreased circulation can cause foot drop and **paresthesias** (burning and tingling sensations), usually in older adults.

Respiratory complications may manifest as *pleurisy, pneumonitis, diffuse interstitial fibrosis, and pulmonary hypertension.* Cardiac complications include *pericarditis and myocarditis.* Assess for eye involvement, which typically manifests as *iritis and scleritis.* If either of these complications is present, the sclera of one or both eyes is reddened and the pupils have an irregular shape. Clinical manifestations of each of these health problems can be found elsewhere in this text under the specific body system affected.

Associated Syndromes. Several syndromes are seen in patients with advanced RA. The most common is **Sjögren's syndrome,** which includes a triad of:

- Dry eyes (keratoconjunctivitis sicca [KCS], or the sicca syndrome)
- Dry mouth **(xerostomia)**
- Dry vagina (in some cases)

Note the patient's report of dry mouth or dry eyes. Some patients state that their eyes feel "gritty," as if sand is in their eyes. Inspect the mouth for dry, sticky membranes and the eyes for redness and lack of tearing.

Less commonly observed is **Felty's syndrome,** which is characterized by RA, hepatosplenomegaly (enlarged liver and spleen), and leukopenia. **Caplan's syndrome** is characterized by the presence of rheumatoid nodules in the lungs and pneumoconiosis, which is noted primarily in coal miners and asbestos removal workers.

Psychosocial Assessment

Rheumatoid arthritis (RA) and other inflammatory types of arthritis are chronic diseases that can be crippling if not well controlled. Fear of becoming disabled and dependent, uncertainty about the disease process, altered body image, devaluation of self, frustration, and depression are common psychosocial problems. Physical limitations caused by disease may limit ADLs. These limitations result in role changes in the family and society. For example, the person may not be able to cook for the family or be an active sexual partner. In addition, extreme fatigue often causes patients to desire an early bedtime and may result in a reluctance to socialize.

Body changes caused by joint changes and steroid therapy (if used) may also cause poor self-esteem and body image. Because many societies value people with physically fit, attractive bodies, the patient with RA may be embarrassed to be seen in public places. The patient may grieve or experience degrees of depression. He or she may have feelings of helplessness caused by a loss of control over a disease that can "consume" the body. Fortunately, newer drugs have improved the treatment of RA and provide the patient with hope and better disease control.

Living with a chronic disease and its pain is difficult for the patient and family. Patients may experience a loss of control and independence, especially if they are older than 65 years. Chronic suffering affects quality of life. Assess their emotional and mental status in relation to the disease and its problems. Evaluate their support systems and resources. Patients who are knowledgeable about their disease and treatment options feel emotionally stronger to cope with their disease and better able to discuss treatment options with their physician.

Laboratory Assessment

Laboratory tests help support a diagnosis of RA, but no single test or group of tests can confirm it. Chart 20-9 summarizes the most common laboratory tests that the health care provider uses for diagnosing connective tissue diseases.

The test for *rheumatoid factor (RF)* measures the presence of unusual antibodies of the immunoglobulins G (IgG) and M (IgM) types that develop in a number of connective tissue diseases. Many patients with RA have a positive titer, but not all positive results indicate the disease, *especially in older adults* (Pagana & Pagana, 2006).

The *antinuclear antibody (ANA)* test measures the titer of unusual antibodies that destroy the nuclei of cells and cause tissue death in patients with autoimmune disease. The fluorescent method is sometimes referred to as *FANA*. If this test result is positive (a value higher than 1:40), various subtypes of this antibody are identified and measured. ANA is often

Chart 20-9 LABORATORY PROFILE

Connective Tissue Disease

Test	Normal Range for Adults	Significance of Abnormal Findings
Rheumatoid factor	Negative	Positive or increase indicative of possible RA or other CTD; may also be elevated in leukemia, liver disease, and renal disease
ANA (total)	Negative (if positive, types of ANA identified [e.g., anti-ENA, anti-Smith, anti-ss-A (Ro)] to indicate what part of cells are involved)	Elevations common in SLE, SSc, RA, and other inflammatory CTDs (5% of healthy adults have positive ANA results)
Serum complement	*Total*: 75-160 units/mL (*C3*: 55-120 mg/dL; *C4*: 20-50 mg/dL)	Decreased values indicative of active autoimmune disease such as SLE, and other problems like anemia, infection, and malnutrition
Erythrocyte sedimentation rate (ESR)	*Male:* up to 15 mm/hr *Female:* up to 20 mm/hr	Increased in inflammatory diseases, like RA, SLE, PMR, temporal arteritis; also elevated in patients with bacterial infections or severe anemias
SPEP	*Total:* 6.4-8.3 g/dL	
Albumin	3.5-5.0 g/dL	Decreased level occurs with chronic inflammation or infection; also decreased in malnutrition and advanced cirrhosis
Globulin		
$Alpha_1$ globulin	0.1-0.3 g/dL	Increased level possible in RA
$Alpha_2$ globulin	0.6-1.0 g/dL	
Beta globulin	0.7-1.1 g/dL	
Gamma globulin	0.8-1.6 g/dL	Increased levels indicative of CTD (inflammatory type)
HLA testing (HLA-B27)	None	Presence of HLA-B27 indicative of Reiter's syndrome or ankylosing spondylitis

ANA, Antinuclear antibody; *CTD,* connective tissue disease; *HLA,* human leukocyte antigen; *PMR,* polymyalgia rheumatica; *RA,* rheumatoid arthritis; *SLE,* systemic lupus erythematosus; *SPEP,* serum protein electrophoresis; *SSc,* systemic sclerosis.

negative until later in the disease process and is positive in only 30% of patients with RA (Pagana & Pagana, 2006). It is more commonly positive in other rheumatic diseases, such as systemic lupus erythematosus and scleroderma.

When RA patients also have Sjögren's syndrome or if the syndrome occurs as a separate disease, several unusual anti-SS antibody types may be present. In particular, *anti-SS-A (Ro)* is positive in about 75% of those with RA or those with secondary Sjögren's with RA. The higher the titer of anti-SS antibodies, the more likely that Sjögren's syndrome is present (Pagana & Pagana, 2006).

Serum *complement,* especially C3 and C4, are usually decreased in autoimmune diseases, including RA and lupus. An elevated *erythrocyte sedimentation rate (ESR),* or "sed rate," can confirm inflammation or infection anywhere in the body. An elevated ESR helps confirm a diagnosis of an unspecified inflammatory disease. The test is most useful to monitor the course of a disease, especially for inflammatory autoimmune diseases. In general, the more severe the disease gets, the higher the ESR rises; as the disease improves or goes into remission, the ESR level decreases.

The *high-sensitivity C-reactive protein,* or *hsCRP,* is another useful test to measure inflammation and may be done with or instead of the ESR. As the name implies, it is more sensitive to inflammatory changes than the ESR. It is also very useful for detecting infection anywhere in the body.

The presence of most chronic diseases usually causes mild to moderate anemia, which contributes to the patient's fatigue. Therefore monitor the patient's complete blood count (CBC) for a low hemoglobin, hematocrit, and red blood cell (RBC) count. An increase in white blood cell (WBC) count is consistent with an inflammatory response. A decrease in the WBC count may indicate Felty's syndrome. Thrombocytosis (increased platelets) is common in patients with RA. Additional laboratory tests may be performed depending on the body systems and organs that may be affected by the disease. For example, if heart involvement is suspected, the health care provider may request cardiac enzymes.

Other Diagnostic Assessment

A standard x-ray is used to visualize the joint changes and deformities typical of RA. A CT scan may help determine the presence and degree of cervical spine involvement.

An *arthrocentesis* is an invasive procedure that may be used for patients with joint swelling caused by excess synovial fluid (effusion). It may be performed at the bedside or in a physician's office or clinic. After administering a local anesthetic, the physician inserts a large-gauge needle into the joint (usually the knee) to aspirate a sample of synovial fluid to relieve pressure. The fluid is analyzed for inflammatory cells and immune complexes, including RF. Fluid from patients with RA shows increased WBCs, cloudiness, and volume. *After the procedure, monitor the insertion site for bleeding or leakage of synovial fluid. Notify the physician if either of these problems occurs.* Teach the patient to use ice and rest the affected joint for 24 hours. Often the health care provider will recommend acetaminophen as needed for pain. If increased pain or swelling occurs, teach the patient or family to notify the health care provider.

A bone scan or joint scan can also assess the extent of joint involvement. MRI may be performed to assess spinal column disease or other joint involvement.

Because RA can affect multiple body systems, tests to diagnose specific systemic manifestations are performed as necessary. For example, electromyography helps confirm peripheral neuropathy. Pulmonary function tests help determine the presence of lung involvement.

Interventions

As in other types of arthritis, the interdisciplinary health care team manages pain by using a combination of pharmacologic and nonpharmacologic measures. A **synovectomy** to remove inflamed synovium may be needed for joints like the knee or elbow. Total joint arthroplasty may be indicated when other measures fail to relieve pain. These surgeries are discussed under Osteoarthritis.

Drug Therapy

Some drugs prescribed for RA have analgesic, antipyretic, and anti-inflammatory actions. Other drugs are immunosuppressive and disease modifying, which may cause remission of the illness and prevent erosive joint changes. Biological response modifiers make up the newest class of disease-modifying drugs that help reduce signals for the immune system to cause inflammation (Chart 20-10). Patients with inflammatory diseases other than RA are also using various biological response modifying medications successfully. Future genetic research will further advance these medications to give even better control of autoimmune diseases. Although RA is a chronic disease and no cure is yet available, drugs now used can better control the disease and prevent further deterioration.

The health care provider, usually a rheumatologist, makes decisions about appropriate drug therapy for patients with rheumatoid disease based on the severity of the disease. Initially, most patients are managed with **disease-modifying antirheumatic drugs (DMARDs)**. As the name implies, these drugs are given to slow the progression of the disease.

Disease-Modifying Antirheumatic Drugs. *Methotrexate (Rheumatrex), an immunosuppressive medication, in a low, once-a-week dose (generally 25 mg or less per week) has become the mainstay of therapy for RA because it is effective and relatively inexpensive.* It is a slow-acting drug, taking 4 to 6 weeks to begin to control inflammatory joint symptoms. Observe for desired drug effects, such as a decrease in joint pain and swelling.

Monitor patients for potential adverse effects, such as decreasing WBCs and platelets (as a result of bone marrow suppression) or elevations in liver enzymes or serum creatinine. *Remind patients to avoid alcoholic beverages while taking methotrexate to prevent liver toxicity. Teach them to observe and report other side and toxic effects, which include mouth sores and acute dyspnea from pneumonitis.* Rarely, lymph node tumor (lymphoma) has been associated in those who have RA and are taking methotrexate. Folic acid, one of the B vitamins, is often given to those who are taking methotrexate to help decrease some of the drug's side effects.

Pregnancy is not recommended while taking methotrexate because birth defects are possible. *Strict birth control is recommended for childbearing women who are in need of methotrexate to control their RA.* If pregnancy is ever desired, instruct the patient to consult the rheumatologist as well as an obstetric/gynecologic (OB/GYN) health care provider. Generally, the health care provider will discontinue the drug at least 3 months before planned pregnancy. Methotrexate may be restarted after birth if the patient does not breast-feed.

Chart 20-10 COMMON EXAMPLES OF DRUG THERAPY

Arthritis and Connective Tissue Disease*

Drug and Usual Dosage	Purpose of Drug	Nursing Interventions	Rationales
NSAIDs Dosage varies depending on which drug is being used	Relieves chronic pain by inhibiting prostaglandin synthesis	Observe for fluid retention, increased blood pressure, and changes in renal function.	Most NSAIDs cause sodium retention, which can lead to edema, hypertension, renal damage, and heart failure. Drugs should be used with caution in older adults.
		Monitor electrolyte and CBC values.	Most NSAIDs cause increased sodium levels and can cause bone marrow suppression.
		Observe for CNS changes (e.g., dizziness or confusion).	Most NSAIDs can cause CNS effects, *especially in older adults.*
Hydroxychloroquine sulfate (Plaquenil) 200 mg orally daily	An antimalarial agent that helps decrease inflammation and slow disease process	Instruct patient to have frequent (every 6-12 mo) ophthalmologic examination.	Drug can cause retinal damage.
Immunosuppressive agents (e.g., methotrexate [Rheumatrex] [most commonly used], azathioprine [Imuran], cyclophosphamide [Cytoxan]) Usual dose of oral methotrexate (MTX) is 7.5 to 20 mg/wk. Dosage of other drugs varies depending on disease activity and route of drug administration	Suppresses bone marrow to reduce immune response	Monitor for side effects and toxic effects, including but not limited to nausea/vomiting, bone marrow suppression, and increased liver enzymes.	The side effects and toxic effects of these drugs can be devastating.
		Instruct patient to avoid crowds and people with infections such as influenza. If ill, seek medical attention.	Immune suppression increases the risk of infection.
Prednisone (Deltasone, Apo-Prednisone♣) 10-150 mg orally daily; for maintenance, attempt to give dose every other day (to allow patient's adrenal glands to function)	Decreases inflammatory and immune response by decreasing WBC count	Observe for cushingoid changes, such as moon face, buffalo hump, striae, acne, thin skin, bruising, fluid retention, and increased blood pressure.	These changes are expected and tend to be dose related. Changes diminish as dose decreases.
		Monitor electrolyte and glucose levels. Monitor weight.	Chronic steroid therapy can cause sodium or fluid retention, potassium depletion, and elevated glucose level.
		Observe for long-term effects of chronic steroid therapy, such as osteoporosis, cataracts, hypertension, diabetes, and impaired healing.	These complications may need to be treated with other drugs or modalities.
		Teach patient to increase dietary calcium and vitamin D and to take a supplement.	
		Instruct patient to avoid crowds and persons with infections such as influenza.	Drug suppresses immune system (lymphocytes) and increases risk of infection or decreased healing.

CBC, Complete blood count; *CNS*, central nervous system; *IL*, interleukin; *MS*, multiple sclerosis; *MTX*, methotrexate; *NSAIDs*, nonsteroidal anti-inflammatory drugs; *TB*, tuberculosis; *TNF*, tumor necrosis factor; *WBC*, white blood cell.

*This is not a comprehensive list; this chart lists only the common drugs used for arthritis and connective tissue disease.

Continued

Chart 20-10 COMMON EXAMPLES OF DRUG THERAPY

Arthritis and Connective Tissue Disease*—cont'd

Drug and Usual Dosage	Purpose of Drug	Nursing Interventions	Rationales
Sulfasalazine (Azulfidine) 500 to 3000 mg orally daily in 2 to 4 doses	Decreases inflammation and slows disease process	Check for sulfa allergy or kidney or liver disease.	Drug is a sulfa medication that has potential renal/liver toxicities.
		Teach patient to drink adequate fluids.	Failure to drink fluids may cause formation of urine crystals.
		Teach men that the drug can lower sperm count.	Low sperm count may interfere with ability to conceive.
Leflunomide (Arava) 10 to 20 mg orally daily	Decreases inflammation by inhibiting an enzyme	Teach patient to have prescribed laboratory tests, usually every 6 to 8 weeks.	Increased liver enzymes and decreased blood count have been reported.
		Avoid alcohol while taking drug.	Alcohol can increase liver enzymes.
		Remind patient to use strict birth control.	Drug can cause birth defects.
Biological response modifiers (BRMs):	Neutralize biological activity of either TNF or IL to decrease immune response	Do not give BRMs if patient has a serious infection, TB, or MS.	Drugs may exacerbate infections, MS, or lupus.
Etanercept (Enbrel): Usually 25 mg subcutaneously weekly		Teach patient to report site reaction.	Site reactions can be painful.
Infliximab (Remicade): Varies from 200 to 400 mg IV every 2 mo		Refrigerate all BRMs except Remicade.	Refrigeration prevents drug decomposition.
		Teach patient to report chest pain or difficulty breathing during infusion; monitor blood pressure.	These are potentially life-threatening adverse drug events.
Adalimumab (Humira): 40 mg subcutaneously every 2 wk with MTX or every week with no MTX		Teach patients to report site reaction.	Site reactions may occur.
Anakinra (Kineret): Typically 100 mg subcutaneously daily		Teach patient to monitor site for reaction.	Site reactions may occur.
		Monitor WBC count.	Drug can cause a severe decrease in WBC count and make patient very susceptible to infection.
Abatacept (Orencia): Based on body weight from 500 to 1000 mg IV each week for 3 wks; then every 2 wks		Report cough, dizziness, and sore throat.	Serious infections can occur.
		Monitor for dyspnea, wheezing, flushing, itching.	This drug can cause a mild to moderate allergic reaction.
Rituximab (Rituxan): Two 1000-mg IV doses given 2 weeks apart		Observe for infusion reaction as above.	

CBC, Complete blood count; *CNS*, central nervous system; *IL*, interleukin; *MS*, multiple sclerosis; *MTX*, methotrexate; *NSAIDs*, nonsteroidal anti-inflammatory drugs; *TB*, tuberculosis; *TNF*, tumor necrosis factor; *WBC*, white blood cell.

*This is not a comprehensive list; this chart lists only the common drugs used for arthritis and connective tissue disease.

Leflunomide (Arava) may be prescribed instead of methotrexate for some patients. It is a slow-acting immune-modulating medication that helps diminish inflammatory arthritis symptoms of joint swelling and stiffness and improves mobility. The drug is generally prescribed as follows: a loading dose of 100 mg daily for 3 days followed by 20 mg daily thereafter. Inform the patient that Arava takes 4 to 6 weeks and sometimes up to 3 months before maximum benefit is realized.

Arava is a potent medication that is generally tolerated, but side effects of hair loss, diarrhea, decreased WBCs and platelets, or increased liver enzymes have been reported. *Teach patients to report these changes and monitor laboratory results carefully. Remind them to avoid alcohol. Inform them that Arava can cause birth defects, and therefore recommend strict birth control to women of childbearing age. Tell patients to contact the health care provider immediately if pregnancy occurs while taking the drug.* Cholestyramine (Questran) is available to help block the drug's action.

Other DMARDs include hydroxychloroquine (Plaquenil) and sulfasalazine. These drugs slow the progression of mild rheumatoid disease before it worsens (see Chart 20-10). *Hydroxychloroquine (Plaquenil)* is an antimalarial drug that helps decrease joint and muscle pain and often helps patients with early RA or other inflammatory autoimmune diseases such as systemic lupus erythematosus (SLE), described later in this chapter. Some health care providers may use Plaquenil as one of the initial treatments for mild disease. The patient usually takes 400 mg each evening with a light snack. Occasionally the dose is divided into 200 mg twice daily with food.

Patients generally tolerate Plaquenil quite well. In a few cases, mild stomach discomfort, light-headedness, or headache has been reported. The most serious adverse effect of the drug is retinal damage. Teach patients to report blurred vision or headache. Remind them to have an eye examination every 6 to 12 months to detect changes in the cornea, lens, or retina. If this complication occurs, the health care provider discontinues the drug. Eye complications are rare, but prevention safety is the reason for the recommendation.

Sulfasalazine (Azulfidine) is a medication that may be prescribed for mild to moderate inflammatory arthritis conditions such as RA or psoriatic arthritis (an inflammatory arthritis variant described on p. 357). The usual dosage is 1000 mg twice daily taken with breakfast and supper. Starting doses may be less, such as 500 mg once or twice daily, gradually building up to the standard adult dose. Minimization of such GI side effects as sulfa taste, bloating, stomach discomfort, and gas occurs by gradually increasing drug dosing. Monitor the complete blood count (CBC), paying special attention for a decrease in white blood cells (WBCs) or platelet count. Changes in blood counts are rare but severe potential side effects for which the medication must be discontinued. Patients with an allergy to sulfa drugs or aspirin should not take sulfasalazine.

Nonsteroidal Anti-inflammatory Drugs. *NSAIDs are sometimes used on a short-term basis for inflammatory arthritis to relieve pain and inflammation* (see Chart 20-10). The choice of which one to prescribe depends on the patient's needs and tolerance, as well as the scientific evidence supporting the drug therapy. To decrease GI problems, the NSAID may be given with an H2-blocking agent, such as ranitidine (Zantac) or misoprostol (Cytotec). If there is no clinical change after 6 to 8 weeks, the health care provider may discontinue the current NSAID and try another one or change to a different drug class.

It was once thought that Celecoxib (Celebrex), a COX-2 inhibiting NSAID, should be given rather than the older NSAIDs like ibuprofen. However, all COX-2 inhibiting drugs have recently been associated with cardiovascular disease, such as myocardial infarction, and some have been taken off the market. The risk of GI bleeding is also high in patients taking Celebrex, and the drug cannot be given to those who have recent open heart surgery.

Salicylates are an older type of NSAID and were previously the drug of choice for pain and inflammation. They remain excellent anti-inflammatory drugs and relatively inexpensive, and therefore they are still used within some countries or when a patient has specific needs or restrictions. Salicylates must be taken with food and are sometimes given with GI acid–lowering agents providing GI protection such as proton pump inhibitors. *Monitor the patient for heartburn, indigestion, stomach discomfort, or black, tarry bowel movements (signs and symptoms of ulceration or GI bleeding).* Report such symptoms to the health care provider.

Biological Response Modifiers. As a group, **biological response modifiers (BRMs)** are classified as the newest antiarthritic drugs. Most BRMs neutralize the biological activity of tumor necrosis factor (TNF) by inhibiting its binding with TNF receptors. Any one of the BRMs may be tried. If one drug is not effective, the health care provider prescribes another drug in the same class. All these medications are extremely expensive at this time, and insurance companies may not completely pay for their use. Some patients receive one of these drugs in addition to the drugs in this Drug Therapy section.

Patients with multiple sclerosis or tuberculosis are not given TNF inhibitors. Determine whether the patient has had a recent negative purified protein derivative (PPD) test. If not, a PPD skin test is typically administered and the selected BRM is not started until the results are known to be negative. Collaborate with the health care provider to ensure that this process is complete.

Etanercept (Enbrel) is given subcutaneously by injection either as 50 mg once weekly or as 25 mg twice weekly. Immunosuppression with medications such as methotrexate is generally tried before using Enbrel or other biological response modifiers. Methotrexate may also be continued in combination with biological therapies because the combination may be more effective than either drug alone. Most patients tolerate Enbrel or Enbrel and methotrexate together; however, laboratory monitoring is important. Combination therapy requires CBC, serum creatinine, and a liver panel to be drawn regularly, generally every 4 to 8 weeks. In general, clinical outcomes with Enbrel have been excellent.

Teach the patient or family member how to self-administer Enbrel injections. Injection site reactions and infections (especially respiratory) are possible adverse effects. Ice and hydrocortisone 1% cream can be used if a red, itchy rash at the injection site develops. The drug manufacturer cannot yet predict long-term potential side effects regarding severity of infection or cancer risk. To date, what has been seen is mild increase in upper respiratory infections with occasional serious infections. Teach the patient to notify the health care provider if infection or a delay in wound healing occurs.

Infliximab (Remicade), first approved to treat Crohn's disease, is given in a single IV infusion over several hours. The initial dose generally used for RA is 3 mg/kg of body weight. After the first few weeks of therapy, the drug is repeated at intervals between 2 and 8 weeks, depending on the response of the patient. Patients typically take methotrexate before starting Remicade and continue on combination therapy.

Teach the patient to report and observe for symptoms of infusion reaction: chest discomfort, tachycardia, shortness of breath, or lightheadedness. If any of these symptoms are reported, decrease the IV rate or discontinue it! These symptoms generally subside, but the physician must be notified in case medical assistance is needed. Dose, rate, and interval changes may be needed. Acetaminophen and Benadryl are medications often given before the start of Remicade and are often used at the time of reported infusion reaction. Those who experience serious adverse effects, such as hypertension or anaphylaxis, require permanent discontinuation of the drug.

Adalimumab (Humira) is the first fully human TNF inhibitor. It is a 40-mg once every 2 weeks subcutaneous injection. Symptoms of inflammatory arthritis tend to decrease with the use of Humira, including less joint swelling, less stiffness, and better movement.

Injection site reactions and adverse effects similar to the other TNF inhibitors have been reported. Careful monitoring, especially with combination therapy of Humira and methotrexate or other immunosuppressive medication, is important and similar to combination therapy with other BRMs.

Anakinra (Kineret) is another biological response modifier. Instead of affecting tumor necrosis factor (TNF), however, it works to inhibit a different protein signal of the immune system called *interleukin-1 (IL-1).* IL-1 is also a pro-inflammatory protein that signals the immune system to increase inflammation. It is thought that IL-1 is a weaker protein than TNF, but having an alternative drug that targets a different receptor site is helpful when a patient cannot take other biologicals. Those who have multiple sclerosis or tuberculosis cannot take TNF inhibitors, but Kineret can be used with this population.

Injection site reactions occur more often with Kineret compared with other BRMs. Ice and hydrocortisone 1% cream are recommended. Remind patients to rotate injection sites. Kineret is administered with a simple jet for self-administration. The patient has the option to use the simple jet or administer the subcutaneous injection traditionally.

Abatacept (Orencia) and *rituximab (Rituxan)* require IV infusions every 2 weeks to start and then may be more spread out, depending on the drug. Like the results of the other BRMs, patients usually report feeling a benefit from these drugs in 2 weeks, but it may take months for the maximum benefit to be seen.

The newest BRM that has been approved in several countries but is awaiting U.S. approval is *tocilizumab (Actemra).* Tocilizumab is different from other drugs in this class because it is the first humanized interleukin-6 (IL-6) receptor-inhibiting monoclonal antibody that is available for patients with RA. It can be used alone or in combination with other DMARDs.

Other Drugs. A few drugs may be given as adjuncts to or instead of the previously described drugs. It is not unusual for a patient to be taking several disease-modifying drugs, such as methotrexate, a BRM, and an adjunct medication. Each drug works differently to relieve symptoms and slow the progression of the disease.

Glucocorticoids (steroids)—usually prednisone (Deltasone)—are given for their fast-acting anti-inflammatory and immunosuppressive effects. Prednisone may be given in high dose for short duration **(pulse therapy)** or as a low chronic dose. Moderate-dose, short-term tapering bridge therapy may be used when inflammation is symptomatic and other RA medications are insufficient or have not yet had an effect.

Chronic steroid therapy can result in numerous complications, such as diabetes mellitus, infection, fluid and electrolyte imbalances, hypertension, osteoporosis, and glaucoma. Some drug effects are dose related, whereas others are not. Observe the patient for complications associated with chronic steroid therapy, and report them to the health care provider. For example, if blood pressure becomes elevated or significant laboratory values change, notify the health care provider.

Instruct patients taking chronic steroids to take calcium 1200 to 1500 mg daily plus vitamin D 400 mg daily to help prevent osteoporosis. Bisphosphonate drugs such as Fosamax or Actonel are often prescribed as well. Bone density measurements are recommended.

Patients with RA may experience one or a few joints that have more pain and inflammation than the others. Cortisone injections in single joints may be used to relieve local pain and inflammation. Have the patient ice and rest the joint for 24 hours after the procedure. Oral analgesics also are sometimes needed during that time.

Other immunosuppressive agents that may be used are *azathioprine (Imuran)* and *cyclophosphamide (Cytoxan).* Cyclophosphamide is sometimes given specifically to control RA vasculitis. Such immunosuppressive drugs may cause bone marrow suppression and occasionally leukemia or lymphoma. White blood cell counts are expected to decrease 7 to 14 days after the administration of IV cyclophosphamide; therefore laboratory results are closely monitored to ensure safe limits. Hemorrhagic cystitis is a concern more with oral cyclophosphamide. Instruct the patient to drink water and void frequently (about every 2 hours while awake), which dilutes the urine and empties the bladder, thus decreasing opportunity for bladder irritation from residual drug. Hair thinning or loss can be seen with immunosuppressive medications. Cyclophosphamide may also cause sterility; strict birth control is recommended.

Although rarely prescribed today in the United States, some patients from other countries may have been on *gold therapy* for their RA. The oral and injectable forms of gold have caused many toxicities and therefore has been replaced by DMARDs and BRMs in the United States.

Analgesic drugs may be prescribed to supplement the pain relief property in anti-inflammatory drugs specific for RA. Some analgesics include acetaminophen (Tylenol) and propoxyphene napsylate (Darvocet-N). Propoxyphene and its associated products can cause headache, dizziness, and drowsiness. *In older adults and others with decreased metabolic rates, this slowly excreted drug may accumulate in the body over a long period and can cause death. Teach about the side effects and toxic effects of these drugs, and advise the patient to report any unusual symptoms to the health care provider.*

Nonpharmacologic Interventions

Adequate rest, proper positioning, and ice and heat applications are important in pain management. If acute inflammation is present, the physical therapist (PT) or assistive nursing personnel under the supervision of a licensed professional applies ice to the "hot" joints for pain relief until the inflammation lessens. The ice pack should not be too heavy. Heated paraffin (wax) dips may help decrease pain and increase comfort of arthritic hands. Finger and hand exercises are often done more easily after paraffin treatment.

To relieve morning stiffness or the pain of late-stage disease, recommend a hot shower rather than a sponge bath or a tub bath. It is often difficult for the patient with RA to get into and out of a bathtub, although special hydraulic lifts and tub chairs may be available. Grab bars and nonskid tread in the tub or shower floor are important safety features to discuss with all patients. Some older adults prefer using shower chairs and a walk-in shower that does not have a ledge that could cause falls.

Hot packs applied directly to involved joints may be beneficial. Most physical therapy departments have machines that keep hot packs ready anytime they are needed (Fig. 20-5). Teach patients to use the microwave or stovetop heating instructions to warm the heat pack at home. Remind them to follow the instructions given with each heating device used.

Plasmapheresis (sometimes called *plasma exchange*) is an in-hospital procedure prescribed by a health care provider in which the patient's plasma is treated to remove the antibodies causing the disease. This procedure may be combined with pulse therapy for patients with severe, life-threatening disease.

Gene Therapy

A small number of patients with severe RA have received injections of the IL-1 receptor antagonist (IL-1Ra) or other transgene into MCP joints. This experimental approach holds promise for synovial healing and could replace traditional synovectomy in the future (Evans et al., 2005).

Complementary and Alternative Therapies

Some patients may have pain relief from hypnosis, acupuncture, imagery, music therapy, or other technique. Stress management is also popular as a pain relief intervention. Chapters 2 and 5 discuss these therapies in detail.

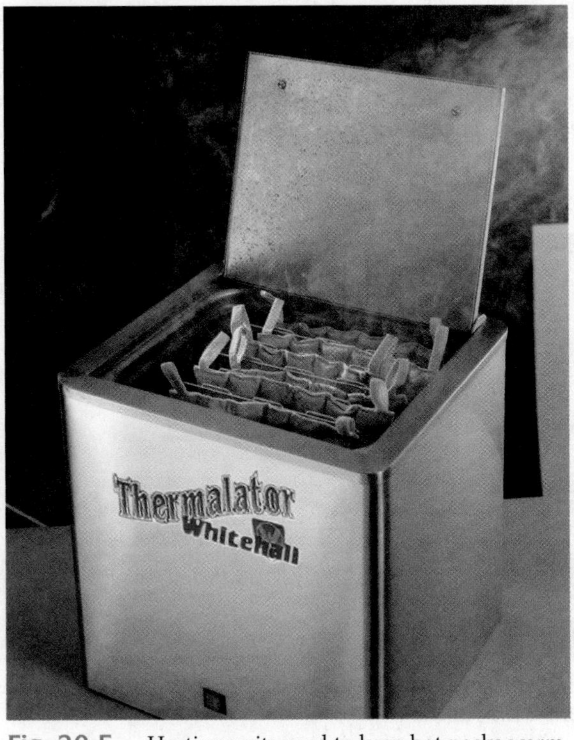
Thermalator
Whitehall

Fig. 20-5 • Heating units used to keep hot packs warm.

Adequate nutrition is an important part of the management of RA. Obesity should be avoided. The inflammatory state may place a greater burden on the metabolism of some essential nutrients. This catabolic state may be related to increased cytokine production, specifically tumor necrosis factor. Some attention has been given to specific foods and supplements that can be helpful (National Center for Complementary and Alternative Medicine [NCCAM], 2005):

- Foods high in calcium or calcium supplements to prevent bone loss (should not be taken in excess to prevent kidney stones)
- Cold-water fish or fish oil capsules containing omega-3 fatty acids at 2.5 to 5 g daily to reduce inflammation (should not be taken if the patient is taking anticoagulant therapy)
- Foods high in antioxidant vitamins (e.g., C and E) or vitamin supplements to help maintain the normal function of the immune system
- Herbs, such as valerian to promote sleep; and ginger, curcumin, and boswellia to decrease inflammation

According to the Arthritis Foundation, no one food causes or cures RA; however, healthy nutrition in general is supported. Refer the patient to the Arthritis Foundation's pamphlet regarding diet and arthritis. Refer him or her to the nutritionist for vitamin- and nutrition-specific questions or recommendations. Any herbal or nutrition supplement should be taken under the supervision of a qualified health care provider to prevent adverse events and drug-food or drug-drug interactions.

Other complementary and alternative medicine (CAM) therapies are safe but have not been scientifically proven to be effective for most people. Examples include magnets (static magnets and electromagnets), hydrotherapy, and homeopathy. Mind-body therapies, such as meditation, relaxation techniques, and spirituality, and acupuncture have been proven to be safe and effective for arthritic pain (NCCAM, 2005). For information about these techniques, see Chapter 2.

Promotion of Self-Care

Although the physical appearance of a patient with severe RA may create the image that independence in ADLs is not possible, a number of alternative methods can be used to perform these activities. *Do not automatically perform these activities for the patient. Those with RA do not want to be dependent.* For example, hand deformities often prevent a patient from opening packages of food, such as a box of crackers; however, he or she may prefer to use the teeth to open the crackers rather than depend on someone else.

In the hospital or long-term care facility, a patient may not eat because of the barriers of heavy plate covers, milk cartons, small packages of condiments, and heavy containers. Styrofoam or paper cups may bend and collapse as he or she attempts to hold them. A china or heavy plastic cup with handles may be easier to manipulate. Collaborate with the nutritionist to assist with access to food and total independence in eating.

When fine motor activities (e.g., squeezing a tube of toothpaste) become impossible, larger joints or body surfaces can substitute for smaller ones. For example, teach how to use the palm of the hand to press the paste onto the brush. Devices such as long-handled brushes can help patients brush their hair; dressing sticks can assist with putting on pants. These examples illustrate the need to assess the problem area, suggest alternative methods, and refer the patient to an occupational or physical therapist for special assistive and adaptive devices if necessary.

Management of Fatigue

Nursing interventions depend in part on identifying the factors contributing to fatigue. For example, increases in pain, sleep disturbances, and weakness are positively associated with increased fatigue. Anemia may also be a contributing factor and may be treated with iron (if an iron deficiency anemia is present), folic acid, or vitamin supplements prescribed by the health care provider. Chronic normochromic or chronic hypochromic anemia often occurs in most chronic, systemic diseases. Assess for drug-related blood loss, such as that caused by NSAIDs, by checking the stool for gross or occult blood. *Older white women are the most likely to experience GI bleeding as a result of taking these medications.*

When fatigue results from muscle atrophy, the health care provider prescribes an aggressive physical therapy program to strengthen muscles and prevent further atrophy. Patients experience increased fatigue when pain prevents them from getting adequate rest and sleep. Measures to facilitate sleep include promoting a quiet environment, giving warm beverages, and administering hypnotics or relaxants as prescribed, if necessary.

In addition to identifying and managing specific reasons for fatigue, determine the patient's usual daily activities and teach principles of **energy conservation,** including:

- Pacing activities
- Allowing rest periods
- Setting priorities
- Obtaining assistance when needed

Chart 20-11 lists specific suggestions for conserving energy and thus increasing activity tolerance.

Enhancement of Body Image

Body image may be affected by both the disease process and drug therapy. Steroids can cause a moonfaced appearance, acne, striae, "buffalo humps," and weight gain. Determine the patient's perception of these changes and the impact of the reactions of family and significant others. The most important intervention is communicating acceptance of the patient. When a trusting relationship is established, encourage him or her to express personal feelings.

Another way to improve body image while in the hospital or nursing home is to use personal items. A hospital gown reinforces the sick role. Encourage patients to wear their own clothes, to brush their hair, and to use makeup if desired. Assist or teach the family to assist the patient as needed. The use of colored hair accessories, nail polish, and perfume may improve a female's image and self-concept.

As a reaction to body image disturbance and the presence of a chronic, painful disease, some patients display behaviors indicative of loss. They may use coping strategies that range from denial or fear to anger or depression. In an attempt to regain control over the effects of the disease process, they may appear to be "manipulative and demanding" and sometimes may be referred to as having an "arthritis personality." *This personality, which represents a negative label, is a myth; using these terms should be avoided.* Patients are trying to cope with the effects of their illness and should be treated with patience and understanding. Continually assess and accept these behaviors, but remain realistic in discussing goals to improve self-esteem. Emphasize their strengths, and help them identify previously successful coping strategies.

Chart 20-11 PATIENT AND FAMILY EDUCATION GUIDE

Energy Conservation for the Patient with Arthritis

- Balance activity with rest. Take one or two naps each day.
- Pace yourself; do not plan too much for one day.
- Set priorities. Determine which activities are most important, and do them first.
- Delegate responsibilities and tasks to your family and friends.
- Plan ahead to prevent last-minute rushing and stress.
- Learn your own activity tolerance, and do not exceed it.

Community-Based Care

Patients with rheumatoid arthritis (RA) are usually managed at home but, in a few cases, may be institutionalized in a long-term care facility if they become restricted to bed or a wheelchair. Some patients may be transferred to a rehabilitation facility for several weeks to aid in developing strategies, techniques, and skills for independent living at home.

Home Care Management

The amount of home care preparation depends on the severity of the disease. Structural changes may be necessary if there are deficits in ADLs or mobility. Doors must be wide enough to accommodate a wheelchair or walker if one is used. Ramps are needed to prevent the patient in a wheelchair from becoming homebound. If the person cannot use stairs, he or she must have access to facilities for all ADLs on one floor. Handrails should be available in the bathroom and halls.

To promote continued homemaking functions, countertops and appliances may require structural changes. The patient may also require handrails and elevated chairs and toilet seats, which facilitate transfers (Fig. 20-6). *These devices are especially important for older adults with arthritis.*

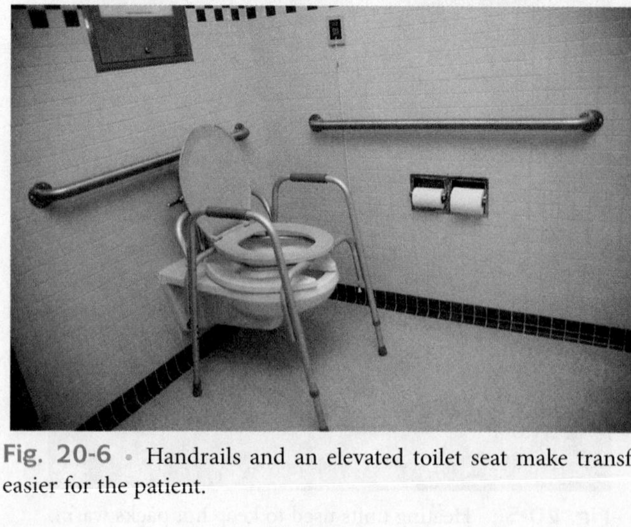

Fig. 20-6 • Handrails and an elevated toilet seat make transfers easier for the patient.

Health Teaching

Health teaching is a vital role for nurses in the diagnosis and management of arthritis. Many people have signs and symptoms of joint inflammation but do not seek medical attention. Teach them to seek professional health care to reduce pain and disability.

Health teaching is also important for promoting adherence with a treatment plan. A patient who understands the disease process and the treatment rationale can better follow and ask questions about the treatment plan.

Teach patients to discuss any questions with their health care provider before trying any over-the-counter or home remedies. Some remedies may be harmful. Check with the Arthritis Foundation for the latest information on arthritis myths and quackery (www.arthritis.org).

Information about drug therapy, joint protection, energy conservation, rest, and exercise should be taught to the patient, family, and significant others. This information is summarized in Charts 20-6, 20-7, 20-10, and 20-11.

The patient with RA often reports being on an "emotional roller coaster" from coping with a chronic illness every day. Control over one's life is an important human need. The patient with an unpredictable chronic disease may lose this control, and this lowers self-esteem. Health care providers must allow him or her to make decisions about care. Families and significant others must also include him or her in decision making. Although the patient's behavior may be perceived as demanding or manipulative, his or her self-esteem cannot be improved without this important aspect of interpersonal relationships.

Increased dependency also affects a sense of control and self-esteem. Some people ignore their health needs and portray a tough image for others by insisting that they need no assistance. Emphasize to the patient and family that asking for help may be the best decision at times to prevent further joint damage and disease progression.

Rheumatoid arthritis (RA) may also affect work and social roles. The patient may have physical difficulty doing tasks that require lifting, climbing, grasp, or gross or fine motor activities. The severity of RA disease may cause difficulty with total number of hours worked. Some people with RA can do their jobs well without problem; others may have varying degrees of difficulty. Those who can no longer do their job at work may need to discuss with their employer having a lighter workload, but some may need to file for disability with their company and Social Security.

Arthritis support groups and self-help courses provide the education and the support that patients, families, and friends need. Refer the patient to a psychological counselor or religious or spiritual leader for emotional support and guidance during times of crisis or as needed. Identify and recommend other support systems within the family and community when necessary.

Health Care Resources

The need for health care resources for the patient with RA is similar to that for the patient with osteoarthritis. A home care nurse or aide, physical therapist, or occupational therapist may be needed. In collaboration with the case manager, identify these resources and make sure they are available before transfer or discharge. The Arthritis Foundation (www.arthritis.org) is an excellent source of information and support.

NCLEX EXAMINATION CHALLENGE

A client with rheumatoid arthritis has been receiving infliximab for the past 2 months. She states that her joint pain is much better but that she has been having terrible headaches and a "runny nose" for the past 2 days. What is the nurse's best action?

A. Perform a comprehensive pain assessment.
B. Take her vital signs and compare with her baseline.
C. Call her physician immediately.
D. Teach her meditation and relaxation techniques.

evolve For the correct answer, go to http://evolve.elsevier.com/Iggy/.

LUPUS ERYTHEMATOSUS

Pathophysiology

In the mid-nineteenth century, the facial rash accompanying this disease was thought to look like the facial markings of a wolf. The rash was usually red, and thus the term *erythematosus,* a Latin word meaning "reddened," was added to describe the disease.

The two main classifications of lupus are discoid lupus erythematosus (DLE) and systemic lupus erythematosus (SLE). A small percentage of patients with lupus have the DLE type, which affects only the skin.

Unlike DLE, **systemic lupus erythematosus** is a chronic, progressive, inflammatory connective tissue disorder that can cause major body organs and systems to fail. It is characterized by spontaneous remissions and **exacerbations** ("flare-ups"), and the onset may be acute or insidious (slow). The condition is potentially fatal, but the survival rate has improved dramatically in countries where SLE is diagnosed early and treated adequately. Today most patients with SLE are living many years after diagnosis and can lead normal lives. Improvements in determining the cause, diagnosis, and treatment of lupus account for the prolonged survival.

Lupus is thought to be an autoimmune process. Antinuclear antibodies (ANAs) primarily affect the DNA within the cell nuclei. As a result, immune complexes form in the serum and organ tissues, which cause inflammation and damage (McCance & Huether, 2006). These complexes invade organs directly or cause **vasculitis** (vessel inflammation), which deprives the organs of arterial blood and oxygen.

Autoimmune complexes tend to be attracted to the glomeruli of the kidneys. Therefore many patients with SLE have some degree of kidney involvement—the leading cause of death. Other causes of death from the disease are cardiac and central nervous system involvement.

In kidney disease, renal biopsies show these progressive changes within the glomeruli:

- In minimal lupus nephritis, the glomeruli are slightly irregular; immunoglobulins and complement are seen by electron microscopy.
- Focal, or mild, lupus nephritis is characterized by further glomerular changes, and immune complex deposits are common. In this type of lupus, the patient begins to show clinical signs of renal impairment.
- In diffuse, severe proliferative nephritis, more than 50% of the glomeruli are affected and the patient is in renal failure.

CULTURAL AWARENESS

Lupus affects women more than men. About 1 in 700 European-American women between the ages of 15 and 64 years have the disease compared with 1 in 245 African-American women. The reason for this difference is unknown. Lupus is therefore one of the most common chronic diseases among African-American women. The disease is also more common among Native Americans, Asian Americans, and Hispanics than among Euro-Americans (www.lupus.org).

The onset of the disease occurs most often during the childbearing years, but it has been reported in young children and older adults. A genetic predisposition is based on the trend to develop the disease in some twins and the occurrence of autoimmune disease in some families of patients who have lupus. However, it is not the only basis of the disease. Like RA, lupus is probably caused by a *combination of genetic and environmental factors.*

GENETIC CONSIDERATIONS

Over the past several decades, more than 100 genetic risk factors have been identified as possible causes of lupus. The research challenge is that patients with lupus differ from each other in their genetic risk and makeup. To complicate this situation, environmental factors can trigger an autoimmune response in some people and not in others with the same risk. For example, SLE may be triggered by a virus, such as Epstein-Barr, in some people who have a genetic risk for the disease (Sestak et al., 2007).

The genetic basis of SLE is very complex and somewhat conflicting in research findings. The major factors associated with the inflammatory process of SLE include:

- Complement , especially C2, C4d, and CR1q
- HLA alleles, such as DR3 and DR2
- Interferon-related genes, such as IRF5
- Interleukin (IL)-10, a cytokine

Information on these factors can be found in Chapter 19.

A transient lupus-like syndrome can occur in some patients taking select medications, especially procainamide (Pronestyl) and hydralazine (McCance & Huether, 2006). When these drugs are discontinued, the syndrome usually resolves. Neither of these drugs is commonly used as much today. Long-term use of newer biological response modifiers (BRMs) like infliximab, which is used to treat RA and other autoimmune diseases, may also cause a lupus-like syndrome.

Patient-Centered Collaborative Care

Assessment

It is impossible to describe a typical textbook picture of a patient with lupus because of the extreme range of symptoms. There is no classic presentation of this disease. When lupus is in remission, the patient may appear healthy and have no activity limitations. When the disease flares, some patients may be so ill that admission to a critical care unit is needed. Chart 20-12 highlights the clinical manifestations that occur with systemic lupus.

Chart 20-12 KEY FEATURES

Systemic Lupus Erythematosus (SLE) and Systemic Sclerosis (SSc)

Systemic Lupus Erythematosus	Systemic Sclerosis
SKIN MANIFESTATIONS	
Inflamed, red rash	Inflamed
Discoid lesions	Fibrotic
	Sclerotic
	Edematous
RENAL MANIFESTATIONS	
Nephritis	Renal failure
CARDIOVASCULAR MANIFESTATIONS	
Pericarditis	Myocardial fibrosis
Raynaud's phenomenon	Raynaud's phenomenon
PULMONARY MANIFESTATIONS	
Pleural effusions	Interstitial fibrosis
	Pulmonary hypertension
NEUROLOGIC MANIFESTATIONS	
CNS lupus	Not common
GASTROINTESTINAL MANIFESTATIONS	
Abdominal pain	Esophagitis
	Ulcers
MUSCULOSKELETAL MANIFESTATIONS	
Joint inflammation	Joint inflammation
Myositis	Myositis
OTHER MANIFESTATIONS	
Fever	Fever
Fatigue	Fatigue
Anorexia	Anorexia
Vasculitis	Vasculitis

CNS, Central nervous system.

Physical Assessment/Clinical Manifestations

Skin Involvement. *The major skin manifestation of DLE and SLE is a dry, scaly, raised rash on the face **("butterfly" rash)*** (Fig. 20-7). This rash may also appear on other sun-exposed areas. The rash is generally nonscarring and may increase in a lupus flare and disappear when the disease is in remission.

Individual round **discoid** (coinlike) **lesions** are the scarring lesions of discoid lupus. The lesions are especially evident when the patient is exposed to sunlight or ultraviolet light. Alopecia is also common in lupus. Observe and document all skin changes, and monitor them daily while the patient is in an acute care setting or during an ambulatory care or home visit. Mouth ulcers are not uncommon.

Other Manifestations. In addition to skin changes, *polyarthritis* occurs in most patients with SLE. The early joint changes are similar to those seen in rheumatoid arthritis (RA), but severe deformities are not common even in late disease. Small joints and the knees are most commonly involved. **Osteonecrosis** (bone necrosis from lack of oxygen) is often seen in those who have been treated for at least 5 years with steroids like prednisone. Chronic steroid therapy may cause the constriction of small blood vessels supplying the joint, which causes the tissue to die. The hip is most commonly affected, and reports of pain and decreased mobility result. As a result, a total hip arthroplasty may be done.

Observe for *muscle atrophy,* which can result from disuse, from skeletal muscle invasion by the immune complexes

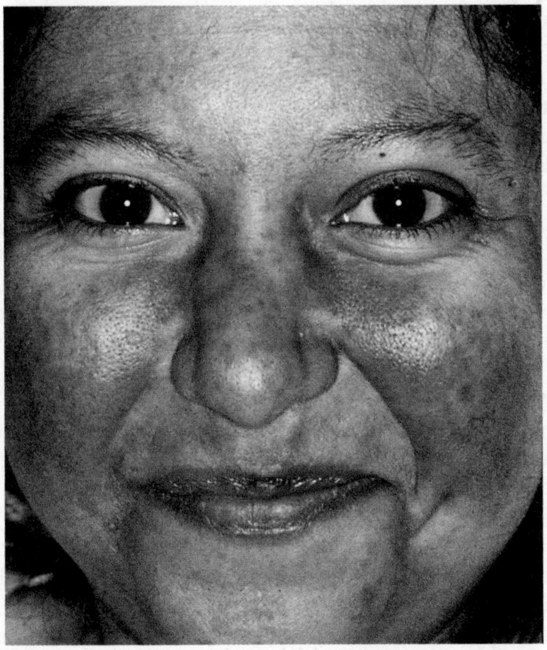

Fig. 20-7 • The characteristic "butterfly" rash of systemic lupus erythematosus.

(myositis), or from chronic steroid therapy. Myalgia (muscle pain) may also occur. Inspect and palpate the major muscles, especially those in the extremities.

Because SLE is an inflammatory condition, *fever* and *fatigue* are common findings. *Fever is the classic sign of a flare, or exacerbation.* Various degrees of generalized weakness, fatigue, anorexia, and weight loss may occur. These signs may be the only evidence of disease, which makes diagnosis by the health care provider difficult. Therefore some patients have a diagnosis of "probable SLE."

Any or all body systems may be affected by SLE. Because lupus nephritis is the leading cause of death, carefully assess for signs of renal involvement (e.g., changes in urine output, proteinuria, hematuria, fluid retention).

Pleural effusions or *pneumonia* is found in almost half of all cases of SLE, but this complication is usually not life threatening. Pulmonary restrictive or obstructive changes may not result in overt clinical signs; however, progressive involvement can lead to dyspnea and arterial blood gas abnormalities. Perform a complete respiratory assessment to determine any abnormalities in respiratory pattern or breath sounds.

Pericarditis is the most common cardiovascular manifestation and causes tachycardia, chest pain, and myocardial ischemia. Monitor the vital signs at least every 4 hours while the patient is in the hospital, and report chest pain immediately to the physician. *Anemia, leukopenia, and thrombocytopenia* are also common in patients with SLE.

Raynaud's phenomenon occurs in a small portion of lupus patients. On exposure to cold or extreme stress, the patient reports the characteristic red, white, and blue color changes and severe pain in the digits; these changes are caused by arteriolar vasospasm. Ask patients whether color changes occur when their hands or feet are exposed to cold or when they are extremely stressed.

Neurologic manifestations are varied. Central nervous system effects include psychoses, paresis, seizures, migraine headaches, and cranial nerve palsies. Peripheral neuropathies are also common. Perform a neurologic assessment as described in Chapter 43.

Monitor *abdominal pain,* which usually results from **serositis** (peritoneal involvement). Mesenteric arteritis, pancreatitis from arteritis of the pancreatic artery, and colonic ulcers also can cause abdominal pain with lupus. Jaundice is rare. Many patients have lymph enlargement, and a few have splenomegaly (enlarged spleen). Palpate the lymph nodes, and document findings. Vasculitis affecting any major or small vessels can lead to organ failure.

Psychosocial Assessment

The psychosocial results of lupus can be devastating. With either DLE or SLE, the rash can be disfiguring and embarrassing. Young adult women who never had a blemish are confronted with a rash that cannot be completely covered with makeup. If chronic steroid therapy is used, side effects such as acne, striae, fat pads, and weight gain intensify the problem of an already altered body image.

Chronic fatigue and generalized weakness may prevent the patient from being as active as in the past. He or she may avoid social gatherings and may withdraw from family activities. The unpredictability and chronicity of SLE can cause fear and anxiety. Fear may increase if the patient knows another person with the disease, particularly if the other person has more advanced severe disease. Unfortunately, the myth that lupus is fatal is still common. Inform the patient and family that control of lupus is generally possible with regular medical monitoring, medications, and healthy practices, such as limiting sun exposure to prevent exacerbation of the disease.

Assess the patient's and family's feelings about the illness to identify areas requiring intervention. Determine their usual coping mechanisms and support systems before developing a plan of care. See p. 339 in the Psychosocial Assessment section of the Rheumatoid Arthritis section for additional information.

Laboratory Assessment

Because discoid lupus erythematosus (DLE) is not a systemic condition, the only significant test is a *skin biopsy.* The physician gently scrapes skin cells from the rash for microscopic evaluation. The characteristic lupus cell and a number of inflammatory cells confirm the diagnosis.

Some of the immunologic-based laboratory tests used to diagnose SLE are the same as those performed for rheumatoid arthritis (RA): rheumatoid factor, antinuclear antibody, erythrocyte sedimentation rate, serum protein electrophoresis, serum complement (especially C3 and C4), and immunoglobulins (see Chart 20-9). A false-positive Venereal Disease Research Laboratory (VDRL) syphilis test is common with lupus.

Newer and more specific immunologic tests, such as anti-SS-a (Ro), anti-SS-b (La), anti-Smith (anti-Sm), anti-DNA, and extractable nuclear antigens (ENA), are also performed. High titers of some of these antibodies are associated with lupus, but some of these antibodies can be found in people without the disease. Some patients with lupus do not have high titers of these antibodies (Rooney, 2005).

A complete blood count (CBC) commonly shows **pancytopenia** (a decrease of all cell types), probably caused by direct attack of the blood cells or bone marrow by immune complexes. Serum electrolyte levels, renal function, cardiac and liver enzymes, and clotting factors are also routinely assessed to determine other body system functioning.

Interventions

The health care provider often prescribes potent drugs that are used topically and systemically. In addition, precautions are taken to prevent further skin impairment and exacerbations. Many of the skin lesions do not disappear, even with treatment, but they usually fade when the disease is in remission.

Drug Therapy

With DLE, the patient's major concern is the rash or discoid lesions. Patients with SLE also may be concerned about skin changes. Topical cortisone preparations help reduce inflammation and promote fading of the skin lesions. In addition, the health care provider may prescribe the anti-malarial agent *hydroxychloroquine* (Plaquenil) for some patients to decrease the inflammatory response; other systemic medications are usually not used (see Chart 20-10). *Teach patients to have frequent eye examinations if they are receiving Plaquenil.* Acetaminophen (Tylenol) or NSAIDs may be used to treat musculoskeletal problems like arthritis and myalgias.

The aim of management of SLE is to treat the disease aggressively until remission. In addition to medications for skin lesions, the health care provider often prescribes chronic steroid therapy to treat the systemic disease process. For renal or central nervous system lupus, the health care provider may also prescribe immunosuppressive agents, such as methotrexate (Rheumatrex) or azathioprine (Imuran) (see Chart 20-10). Although clinical manifestations improve during remission, maintenance doses of these drugs are usually continued to prevent further exacerbations of the disease. These drugs make patients susceptible to infections. *Stress the importance of avoiding large crowds and people who are ill. Teach them to report any early sign of infection to their health care provider.* Observe for side effects and toxic effects of these drugs, and report their occurrence immediately.

For severe renal involvement, immunosuppressants may be given in combination with steroids. For patients who do not respond to this regimen, a high-dose IV bolus of glucocorticoids, cyclophosphamide, and plasmapheresis may be tried for 3 consecutive days. Renal transplantation has been successful for some patients.

Skin Protection

Teach patients to avoid prolonged exposure to sunlight and other forms of ultraviolet lighting, including certain types of fluorescent light. Remind them to wear long sleeves and a large-brimmed hat when outdoors. They should use sun-blocking agents with a sun protection factor (SPF) of 30 or higher on exposed skin surfaces.

In addition, teach the patient to clean the skin with mild soap (e.g., Ivory) and to avoid harsh, perfumed substances. The skin should be rinsed and dried well and lotion applied. Excess powder and other drying substances should be avoided. Cosmetics must be carefully selected and should include moisturizers and sun protectors. Refer the patient to a medical cosmetologist who specializes in applying makeup for skin lesions of all types, if requested.

The patient's hair should receive special attention because alopecia (hair loss) is common. Recommend the use of mild protein shampoos and the avoidance of harsh treatments (e.g., permanents or highlights) until the hair regrows during remission.

Community-Based Care

Community-based care for the patient with lupus is similar to that for RA. In general, the patient is home but may need repeated hospitalizations during exacerbations of disease. He or she usually does not need rehabilitation unless having surgery, because severe joint deformity and prolonged immobility are not common in lupus.

Two major differences exist between SLE and RA in terms of education of the patient and family or significant others. First, instruct patients how to protect the skin (Chart 20-13). Second, teach them to monitor body temperature. Fever is the major sign of an exacerbation, during which they can become seriously ill. Teach the importance of reporting any other unusual or new clinical manifestations to the health care provider immediately.

Many patients become frustrated that family members, significant others, and lay people do not have a thorough understanding of lupus. When lupus is in complete remission, patients appear to be healthy; however, an exacerbation can lead to a critical care admission. This unpredictability disrupts the patient's life and can cause fear and anxiety. Help him or her identify coping strategies and support systems that can help with functioning in the community.

Teach the possible effects of the disease on lifestyle, including fatigue. Women of childbearing age need to know that pregnancy can be a stressor and can cause an exacerbation of the disease, either during pregnancy or after delivery. The pregnant woman also has an increased risk of miscarriage, stillbirth, or premature birth. Pregnancy is not recommended for those with cardiac, renal, or central nervous system involvement. Sexual counseling regarding contraception options may be necessary.

The Arthritis Foundation (www.arthritis.org) is a general resource for all patients with connective tissue disease. The Lupus Foundation (www.lupus.org) is a resource specific for patients with lupus. It is a national organization and has chapters in every state to provide information and assistance for patients with lupus and their families. Local support groups and services are offered free of charge.

Chart 20-13 PATIENT AND FAMILY EDUCATION GUIDE

Evidence-Based Practice for Skin Protection in Patients with Lupus Erythematosus

- Cleanse your skin with a mild soap, such as Ivory.
- Dry your skin thoroughly by patting rather than rubbing.
- Apply lotion liberally to dry skin areas.
- Avoid powder and other drying agents, such as rubbing alcohol.
- Use cosmetics that contain moisturizers.
- Avoid direct sunlight and any other type of ultraviolet lighting, including tanning beds.
- Wear a large-brimmed hat, long sleeves, and long pants when in the sun.
- Use a sun-blocking agent with a sun protection factor (SPF) of at least 30.
- Inspect your skin daily for open areas and rashes.

SCLERODERMA

Pathophysiology

Scleroderma, also called **systemic sclerosis (SSc),** is a chronic, inflammatory, autoimmune connective tissue disease. Formerly called *progressive systemic disease,* or *PSS,* this illness is not always progressive. *Scleroderma* means hardening of the skin, which is only one clinical manifestation of the problem. Some patients have only skin involvement, or localized scleroderma (also called *linear scleroderma*). However, most have skin and other body system involvement. SSc is less common than systemic lupus erythematosus (SLE) but is associated with a higher mortality rate. See Chart 20-12 for a comparison of the clinical manifestations of these two diseases. The manifestations for both diseases vary widely from person to person.

The early inflammatory process of SSc is so similar to that of lupus that patients may first be diagnosed as having probable SLE until the disease progresses or until antibody testing supports the diagnosis. The inflamed tissue in patients with SSc becomes fibrotic and then **sclerotic** (hard). Renal involvement is the leading cause of death. Respiratory involvement and hypertension are also common. Patients with SSc do not respond well to the steroids and immunosuppressants used for lupus, and therefore the mortality rate is higher.

The classification for systemic sclerosis is:

- **Diffuse scleroderma**—skin thickening on the trunk, face, and proximal and distal extremities
- **Limited scleroderma**—thick skin limited to sites distal to the elbows and knees but also involves the face and neck.

Patients often have the **CREST syndrome:**

Calcinosis (calcium deposits)
Raynaud's phenomenon
Esophageal dysmotility
Sclerodactyly (scleroderma of the digits)
Telangiectasia (spider-like hemangiomas)

Little is known about the cause of SSc, but autoimmunity is suspected. The occurrence of more than one case per family is uncommon, but other connective tissue diseases may be noted in the family history.

Systemic sclerosis has been described in people of all races and in all geographic areas and affects over 300,000 people. Women are affected four times more often than men. The onset of the disease is usually between 25 and 65 years of age, with most women getting it in their 40s (www.scleroderma.org). The incidence is higher in coal miners, who have a high incidence of silicosis, a possible predisposing or contributing factor to SSc. Prolonged exposure to other toxins, such as industrial solvents and epoxy resins, may also predispose a person to the disease. The Choctaw American Indians from Oklahoma have the highest incidence of SSc (www.scleroderma.org).

GENETIC CONSIDERATIONS

Like lupus erythematosus, systemic sclerosis is a complex disease that is probably caused by a combination of genetic and environmental factors. Research findings are conflicting but seem to imply that certain gene variants are associated with the disease. These genetic factors include HLA alleles, such as HLA-DRB1; cytokines, such as interleukin (IL); endothelin; fibrillin; and tumor necrosis factor (TNF)-alpha (Fonseca & Denton, 2007).

Patient-Centered Collaborative Care

Assessment

Physical Assessment/Clinical Manifestations

Arthralgia (joint pain) and stiffness are common manifestations that you can elicit during the musculoskeletal examination. The acute inflammation that occurs with rheumatoid arthritis (RA) is not common, and deformities are rare.

Findings on inspection of the skin depend on the stage of the scleroderma. Typically, a painless, symmetric, pitting edema of the hands and fingers is present. The edema may progress to include the entire upper and lower extremities and face. In this phase, the fingers are described as *sausage-like.* The skin is taut, shiny, and free of wrinkles. If diffuse scleroderma occurs, swelling is replaced by tightening, hardening, and thickening of skin tissue; this phase is sometimes called the *indurative phase* (Fig. 20-8). The skin loses its elasticity, and range of motion is markedly decreased; ulcerations may occur. Joint contractures may develop, and the patient may be unable to perform ADLs independently.

Major organ damage is likely to develop with diffuse scleroderma, specifically affecting the:

- GI tract
- Cardiovascular system

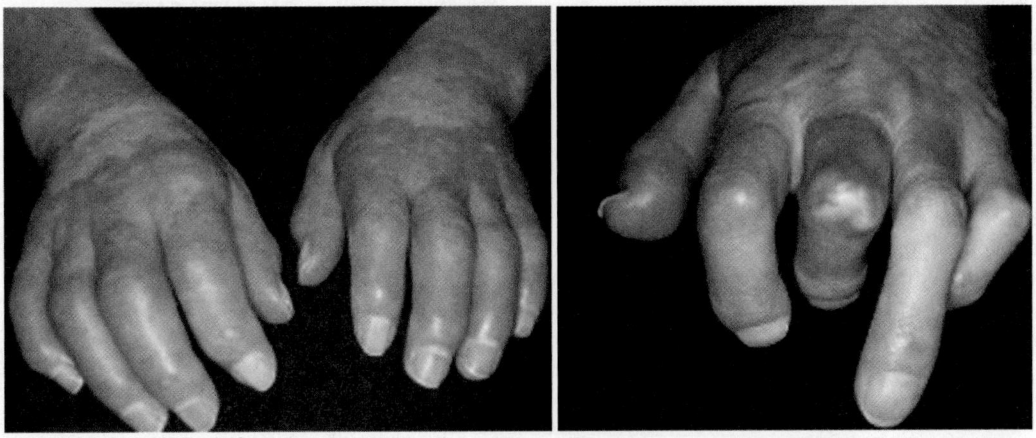

Fig. 20-8 • Late-stage skin changes seen in patients with systemic sclerosis.

- Pulmonary system
- Renal system

Involvement of the *GI tract,* particularly the esophagus, is very common. The esophagus loses its motility, resulting in *dysphagia* and *esophageal reflux.* Assess for the ability of the patient to swallow before allowing him or her to drink or eat food. A small, sliding hiatal hernia may be present, and swallowing may be difficult. Reflux of the gastric contents can cause esophagitis and subsequent ulceration, particularly in the lower two thirds of the esophagus. Intestinal changes are similar to those of the esophagus. Peristalsis is diminished, which causes clinical manifestations similar to a partial bowel obstruction. Malabsorption is a common complication, causing malodorous *diarrheal stools.*

In addition to assessing problems of the digestive tract, observe for *cardiovascular manifestations. Raynaud's phenomenon* occurs in various degrees in most patients with SSc. On exposure to cold or emotional stress, the small arterioles in the digits of both hands and feet rapidly constrict, which causes decreased blood flow. In severe cases, the patient experiences digit necrosis, excruciating pain, and **autoamputation of the distal digits** (the tips of the digits fall off spontaneously). In many patients, vasculitic lesions, often around the nail beds **(periungual lesions),** are evident. *Myocardial fibrosis,* another common problem, is evidenced by electrocardiographic (ECG) changes, cardiac dysrhythmias, and chest pain.

Lung involvement in the patient with SSc may go undetected until late in the disease or sometimes until autopsy. *Fibrosis of the alveoli and interstitial tissues* is present in almost all cases of the disease, but clinical manifestations may not be present. Patients with scleroderma and *pulmonary arterial hypertension* have a more serious prognosis. Recently, bosentan (Tracleer), the first of a new class of drugs called *endothelin receptor antagonists,* demonstrated (in clinical trials) improved walk tests for patients with class III-IV pulmonary arterial hypertension. Various doses improved patients' breathing during exercise, but the potential for liver injury at the highest dose caused recommended doses to be lowered. Teach the patient the desired and potential adverse effects, including liver toxicity and birth defects.

Renal involvement is an important aspect of the overall disease process and often causes malignant hypertension and death. Assess for signs of impending organ failure, such as changes in urine output and increased blood pressure.

Laboratory Assessment

The laboratory findings for SSc are similar to those for SLE. Clinical findings and the patient's response to drug therapy help the health care provider differentiate between the two diseases. Additional tests depend on which organs seem to be affected. Upper and lower GI series are commonly performed because of the frequency of GI clinical manifestations.

Interventions

The medical management of SSc aims to force the disease into remission and thus slow disease progression. The health care provider uses drug therapy primarily for this purpose, but it is often unsuccessful. Systemic steroids and immunosuppressants are used in large doses and often in combination (see Chart 20-10). Another desired outcome of disease management is to identify early organ involvement and treat it before it becomes severe and irreversible. For example, a patient who has lung involvement receives aggressive respiratory therapy and other treatments as the condition requires.

Local skin protective measures can help maintain skin integrity. Teach the patient to use mild soap and lotions and gentle cleaning techniques. Inspect the skin for further changes or open lesions. Skin ulcers are treated according to their type and location.

In addition to drug therapy to control the overall disease process, specific measures can provide comfort. The patient with SSc not only experiences chronic joint pain but also has severe, acute pain during episodes of Raynaud's phenomenon. Remind unlicensed nursing personnel to use a bed cradle and foot board to keep bed covers away from the skin in severe cases. Adjust the room temperature to prevent chilling, which can precipitate digit vasospasm. The patient who can tolerate touching of the affected areas can wear gloves and socks to increase warmth. Because cigarette smoking and extreme emotional stress can also cause symptoms to recur, teach the patient to avoid or minimize these factors as much as possible.

If the patient has esophageal involvement, collaborate with the speech and language pathologist to schedule a swallowing study. The patient may need small, frequent meals rather than the traditional three meals daily. He or she should minimize the intake of foods and liquids that stimulate gastric secretion (e.g., spicy foods, caffeine, alcohol). Teach the patient to keep his or her head elevated for 1 to 2 hours after meals. He or she may need to be in this position continuously. Histamine antagonists and antacids help reduce and neutralize gastric acid. To help prevent choking, collaborate with the nutritionist for dietary changes (Chart 20-14).

Nursing care for the patient with joint pain and decreased mobility is very similar to that for rheumatoid arthritis (see the Interventions section of the Rheumatoid Arthritis section). NSAIDs are given for inflammation and pain. Joint protection and energy conservation are also important for these patients.

Community-Based Care

Community-based care for the person with SSc is similar to that for lupus. The patient is treated at home but may need frequent hospitalizations if major organ involvement occurs during exacerbations. The Arthritis Foundation (www.arthritis.org) and Scleroderma Foundation (www.scleroderma.org)

Chart 20-14 BEST PRACTICE FOR PATIENT SAFETY & QUALITY CARE

The Patient with Systemic Sclerosis and Esophagitis

- Keep the patient's head elevated at least 60 degrees during meals and for at least 1 hour after each meal.
- Provide small, frequent meals rather than three large meals each day.
- Give the patient small amounts of food for each bite, and explain the importance of chewing each bite carefully before swallowing.
- Provide semisoft foods, such as mashed potatoes and pudding or custard; liquids are most likely to cause choking.
- Collaborate with the nutritionist about the patient's diet.
- Teach the patient to avoid foods that increase gastric secretion, such as caffeine, pepper, and other spices.
- Give antacids or histamine antagonists as needed.

are excellent resources for more information about the disease and how to manage it.

DECISION-MAKING CHALLENGE
Delegation/Supervision

A 38-year-old female patient with late-stage scleroderma has been admitted to your skilled unit with pneumonia on IV antibiotic therapy. She has esophageal involvement, kidney disease, and cardiac complications. Her skin is hardened and dry, and her hands are severely contracted. She cannot perform ADLs without assistance. She is allowed out of bed twice a day into a chair with maximum assistance.

1. What part of the patient's care can you safely delegate to unlicensed nursing personnel?
2. What is the safest way to get her out of bed?
3. Should you ask the nursing assistant to feed her? Why or why not?
4. With what members of the health care team should you collaborate and why?

evolve For suggested answer guidelines, go to http://evolve.elsevier.com/Iggy/.

GOUT
Pathophysiology

Gout, or gouty arthritis, is a systemic disease in which urate crystals deposit in the joints and other body tissues, causing inflammation. It is the most common inflammatory arthritis in older adults. The cause and treatment of gout have been firmly established. The classic case of well-advanced disease is seldom seen today unless the patient does not adhere to the therapeutic regimen. The two major types of gout are primary and secondary.

Primary gout is the most common type and results from one of several inborn errors of purine metabolism. An end product of purine metabolism is uric acid, which is usually excreted by the kidneys. In primary gout, the production of uric acid exceeds the excretion capability of the kidneys. Sodium urate is deposited in synovium and other tissues, resulting in inflammation. For some patients, primary gout is inherited as an X-linked trait; males are affected through female carriers. A number of patients have a family history of gout. Primary gout affects middle-aged and older men and postmenopausal women. The peak time of onset in men is between 40 and 50 years of age (McCance & Huether, 2006).

Secondary gout involves **hyperuricemia** (excessive uric acid in the blood) caused by another disease or factor Secondary gout affects people of all ages. Renal insufficiency, diuretic therapy, "crash" diets, and certain chemotherapeutic agents decrease the normal excretion of uric acid and other waste products. Disorders such as multiple myeloma and certain carcinomas result in increased production of uric acid because of a greater turnover of cellular nucleic acids. Treatment involves management of the underlying disorder.

Hyperuricemia and gout are often seen in older patients with cardiovascular health problems. There is some debate as to whether gout actually contributes to the development of coronary artery disease (CAD). The exact cause of this relationship needs further study (Ene-Stroescu & Gorbien, 2005).

The three clinical stages of the primary disease process are asymptomatic hyperuricemic, acute gouty arthritis, and chronic or tophaceous gout (McCance & Huether, 2006). The patient is usually unaware of the *asymptomatic hyperuricemic stage* unless he or she has had a serum uric acid level determination. The serum level is elevated, but no obvious signs of the disease are present. No treatment is needed in this stage.

The first "attack" of gouty arthritis begins the *acute stage.* The patient experiences excruciating pain and inflammation in one or more small joints, usually the metatarsophalangeal joint of the great toe, called **podagra.** The erythrocyte sedimentation rate (ESR) is usually increased as a result of the inflammatory process.

Months or years may pass before additional attacks occur. The patient is asymptomatic, and no abnormalities are found during examination of the joints.

After repeated episodes of acute gout, deposits of urate crystals develop under the skin and within the major organs, particularly in the renal system. The patient is then classified as having *chronic tophaceous gout.* In chronic gout, urate kidney stone formation is more common than renal insufficiency. Chronic gout can begin anywhere between 3 and 40 years after the initial gout symptoms occur (McCance & Huether, 2006).

Patient-Centered Collaborative Care

Assessment

Note the patient's age, gender, and family history of gout. A complete history is needed to determine whether gout has been caused by another problem. Some women overuse diuretics, which can lead to secondary gout.

Acute Gout

Overt manifestations are present in the acute and chronic phases of gout. You probably will encounter a patient with acute gout; chronic gout is not common in the United States today. *Joint inflammation is the most common finding and is usually so painful that the patient seeks medical care immediately.* Inspect the inflamed area. It is usually too painful and swollen to be touched or moved.

The health care provider requests a serum uric acid level to check for hyperuricemia. Because the level can be altered by food intake, several measurements may be obtained. A consistent level of more than 8.5 mg/dL is generally considered abnormal. Urinary uric acid levels are also measured; an overproduction of uric acid is confirmed by an excretion of more than 750 mg/24 hr (Pagana & Pagana, 2006).

The health care provider may requests renal function tests, such as blood urea nitrogen (BUN) and serum creatinine levels, to monitor possible kidney involvement. A definitive diagnostic test for the disease is synovial fluid aspiration (arthrocentesis) to detect the needle-like crystals in the affected joint that are characteristic of the disorder.

Chronic Gout

With chronic gout, inspect the skin for **tophi,** or deposits of sodium urate crystals (Fig. 20-9). Although tophi may occur anywhere, they commonly appear on the outer ear. Other common sites for tophi are the arms and fingers near the joints. The tophi are hard on palpation and are irregular in shape. When the skin over the tophi is irritated, it may break open and a yellow, gritty substance is discharged. Infection may result.

Other manifestations of chronic gout include signs of renal calculi (stones) or renal dysfunction, such as severe pain or changes in urinary output. In some cases, urate kidney stones occur before the arthritis is present.

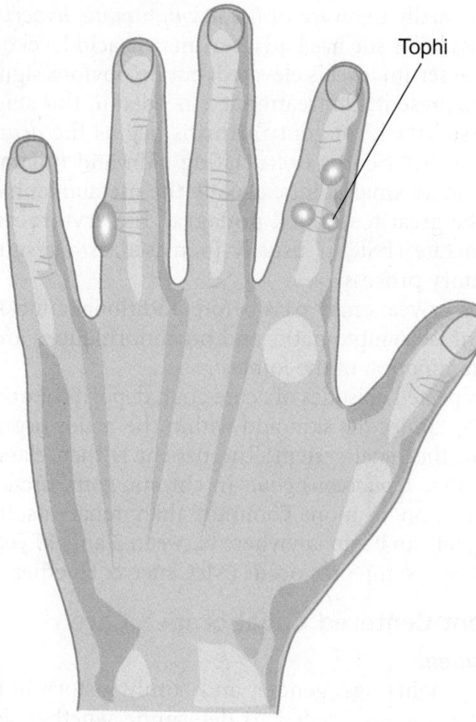
Tophi

Fig. 20-9 • Typical appearance of tophi, which may occur in chronic gout, on an index finger.

Interventions

Gout is one of the easiest diseases for the health care provider to diagnose and treat in its early phases. If the patient receives treatment and adheres to drug therapy, he or she should experience no further symptoms and no change in body image or lifestyle. The patient with gout is treated on an ambulatory basis, but hospitalized patients may have a secondary diagnosis of the disease.

Drug Therapy

Drug therapy is the key to managing patients with gout. In acute gouty "attacks," the inflammation subsides spontaneously within 3 to 5 days; however, most patients cannot tolerate the pain for that long. The drugs used for acute gout are different from those used for chronic gout. The health care provider typically prescribes a combination of colchicine (Colsalide) and an NSAID, such as indomethacin (Indocin, Novomethacin♣) or ibuprofen (Motrin, Amersol♣) for acute gout. IV colchicine works within 12 hours. The patient takes oral medications until the inflammation subsides, usually for 4 to 7 days.

For patients with repeated acute episodes or with chronic gout, the health care provider prescribes drugs to promote uric acid excretion or to reduce its production on a continuous, maintenance basis. Allopurinol (Zyloprim) is the drug of choice. As a xanthine oxidase inhibitor, it prevents the conversion of xanthine to uric acid. Probenecid (Benemid, Benuryl♣) is also effective as a uricosuric drug in gout because it promotes the excretion of excess uric acid. Combination drugs that contain probenecid and colchicine (e.g., ColBENEMID) are also available. The health care provider and nurse monitor serum uric acid levels to determine the effectiveness of these medications. Aspirin should be avoided because it inactivates the effects of the drug.

Nutrition Therapy

Whether or not to recommend special nutritional restrictions for patients with gout is controversial. Some physicians advocate a strict low-purine diet and advise patients to avoid foods such as organ meats, shellfish, and oily fish with bones (e.g., sardines). Some health care providers and nutritionists believe that limiting protein foods, especially red and organ meats, is sufficient. Still others do not believe that diet restrictions affect treatment. It is well known, however, that excessive alcohol intake and fad "starvation" diets can cause a gouty attack. *Teach patients to determine which foods precipitate acute attacks and try to avoid them.*

In addition to food and beverage restrictions, patients with gout should avoid all forms of aspirin and diuretics because they may precipitate an attack. Likewise, excessive physical or emotional stress can exacerbate the disease. Surgery or acute illness, like a myocardial infarction, can also trigger an attack. Stress-management techniques may be helpful for the patient with gout.

Teach the patient to drink plenty of fluids to prevent the formation of urinary stones. Increasing fluid intake helps dilute urine and prevent sediment formation. Uric acid is more soluble in urine with a high pH and therefore is less likely to form urinary stones in that environment. The patient's urinary pH can be increased with an intake of alkaline ash foods, such as citrus fruits and juices, milk, and certain other dairy products. The value of adhering to a strict diet rich in these foods is questionable, however.

OTHER CONNECTIVE TISSUE DISEASES

The care of patients with connective tissue diseases (CTDs) is often similar regardless of the specific diagnosis. This section describes other fairly common diseases that are classified as CTDs.

Polymyositis/Dermatomyositis

Polymyositis is a diffuse inflammatory disease of skeletal (striated) muscle that causes symmetric weakness and atrophy. When a rash accompanies polymyositis, the disease is called **dermatomyositis.** Both diseases vary in their mode of onset and progression and are characterized by spontaneous remissions and exacerbations. Women are affected twice as often as men, and men and women between 30 and 60 years of age are most susceptible to either disease.

In addition to proximal muscle and possible skin involvement, patients typically have polyarthritis, **polyarthralgia** (aching around multiple joints), and Raynaud's phenomenon (see Chapter 38). Patients with dermatomyositis have the characteristic heliotrope (lilac) rash and periorbital (around the eyes) edema. Malignant neoplasms are more common in these patients than in the rest of the population; some patients older than 55 years have malignancies. Most patients develop difficulty swallowing or talking because of severe muscle weakness.

These conditions are treated with high-dose steroids, immunosuppressive agents, and supportive care. Particular attention is given to nutrition due to swallowing problems.

Systemic Necrotizing Vasculitis

Necrotizing vasculitis is a term for a group of diseases whose primary manifestation is **arteritis** (inflammation of arterial walls), which causes ischemia in the tissues usually supplied by the involved vessels. The drug of choice for most types of vasculitis is chronic steroid therapy (prednisone), although immunosuppressive drugs may be used also.

Polyarteritis nodosa affects middle-aged men most often and involves every body system. Treatment is similar to that for systemic lupus, but the prognosis is not as promising. Renal disorders and cardiac involvement are the most common causes of death. *Hypersensitivity vasculitis* is the most common form of vasculitis and primarily causes skin lesions as an allergic response to drugs, infections, or tumors. *Takayasu's arteritis,* or the *aortic arch syndrome,* is also called the "pulseless" disease. Women in their 20s, particularly those of Japanese descent, are affected most often. Cerebral ischemia is manifested by visual changes, syncope, and vertigo.

Polymyalgia Rheumatica and Temporal Arteritis

Polymyalgia rheumatica (PMR) is a clinical syndrome characterized by stiffness, weakness, and aching of the proximal musculature (i.e., the shoulder and pelvic girdles). Systemic manifestations such as low-grade fever, arthralgias (aching around joints) and stiffness, fatigue, and weight loss occur in most cases. The most common joints affected are the neck, shoulder, and hip joints. Stiffness is worse in the morning.

Most patients have an increased erythrocyte sedimentation rate (ESR) and a normochromic, normocytic anemia (see Chart 20-9). The disease commonly occurs in women older than 50 years and typically responds to low-dose steroid therapy in several days.

Giant cell arteritis (GCA), or *temporal arteritis (TA),* occurs in as many as 20% of people with PMR. GCA is a systemic vasculitis that affects large and midsized arteries. Clinical manifestations may be classified as systemic, myalgic, and arteritic (Chart 20-15).

The cause of both PMR and GCA is unknown, but a genetic predisposition related to HLA-DRB1 is likely. The disorder is easy to miss because most patients are older women who report declining vision (also an age-related change). GCA is treated *urgently* with high doses of corticosteroids, often as high as 40 to 80 mg daily. Taking calcium and vitamin D is important for preventing osteoporosis that can result from steroid therapy, especially in middle-aged women.

Chart 20-15 KEY FEATURES
Giant Cell (Temporal) Arteritis

SYSTEMIC MANIFESTATIONS
- Fatigue, malaise
- Fever
- Weight loss
- Night sweats

MYALGIC MANIFESTATIONS (IF PATIENT HAS POLYMYALGIA RHEUMATICA [PMR])
- Proximal, symmetric muscle pain
- Stiffness

ARTERITIC MANIFESTATIONS
- Erythema
- Pain (especially localized temporal headache)
- Swelling
- Tenderness (especially scalp)
- Amaurosis fugax (temporary vision loss in one eye)
- Diplopia or any vision change (requires urgent management)

Ankylosing Spondylitis

Ankylosing spondylitis (AS) is also known as *Marie-Strümpell disease* or *rheumatoid spondylitis.* The disease affects the vertebral column and causes spinal deformities. Although this disorder is present in both men and women at any age in adulthood, white men younger than 40 years are most commonly affected. Other features include **iritis** (inflammation of the iris), arthritis or **arthralgia** (joint aching), and nonspecific systemic manifestations such as malaise and weight loss.

GENETIC CONSIDERATIONS

Although the exact cause is unknown, ankylosing spondylitis is associated with the HLA-B27 alleles. The risk of developing AS is 150 times greater for people with HLA-B27 than for those without it. However, only a small percentage of people who have it actually develop the disease. One explanation is that there are many subtypes of HLA-B27 that need further research for predicting who is most at risk for AS (Nussbaum et al., 2007).

Compromised respiratory function caused by a rigid chest wall is the major threat to health. Most patients function normally but live with chronic discomfort. As in other types of inflammatory arthritis, anti-inflammatory drugs, heat applications, and physical therapy are the key components of management (see earlier discussion of pain management for rheumatoid arthritis, p. 344).

Disease-modifying antirheumatic drugs (DMARDs), such as methotrexate (Rheumatrex), have been successful in slowing disease progress. Biological response modifiers (TNF inhibitors), such as infliximab (Remicade), have also been approved for managing ankylosing spondylitis (see Chart 20-10).

Reiter's Syndrome

As with ankylosing spondylitis, Reiter's syndrome is associated with the HLA-B27 antigen. This disease usually affects young white men. The complete syndrome is a triad of arthritis, conjunctivitis, and **urethritis** (inflammation of the urethra) resulting from exposure to sexually transmitted disease or dysentery (infectious diarrhea). Urethritis is often the first clinical manifestation.

Although the disease is characterized by this triad of manifestations, other conditions such as **balanitis circinata** (ringlike inflammation of the glans penis) and skin lesions are equally significant for confirmation of the diagnosis.

Management is symptomatic and may be complex if there is organ involvement. NSAIDs and physical therapy are generally prescribed.

Marfan Syndrome

Marfan syndrome is an autosomal dominant, connective tissue disease in which abnormalities of the skeletal, ocular, cardiopulmonary, and central nervous systems result from a basic defect in extracellular microfibrils. Microfibrils are very small fibers within cells.

GENETIC CONSIDERATIONS

Marfan syndrome results from mutations in the fibrillin 1 gene (FBN1). This gene encodes fibrillin 1, which forms microfibrils in both elastic and nonelastic tissues (e.g., the skin, the outer layer of the aorta). Patients with Marfan syndrome have a 50% chance of having a child with the disease (Nussbaum et al., 2007). Genetic counseling should also be part of the interdisciplinary plan of care, especially for women of childbearing age.

Patients with the classic form of Marfan syndrome tend to be excessively *tall* and have *elongated hands and feet.* The diagnosis of milder forms of Marfan syndrome is often missed in young men, especially athletes involved in sports such as basketball.

Other skeletal abnormalities include *scoliosis,* a funnel-shaped chest, loss of the normal cervical curve, and hyperextensibility of the joints. Subluxation of the lens is usually bilateral and occurs by the age of 5 years, causing decreased visual acuity or glaucoma.

Cardiovascular problems are responsible for most deaths resulting from Marfan syndrome. The average life span is shortened, often with death in the 30s. Mitral valve prolapse with regurgitation and aortic aneurysm with regurgitation and rupture are common. The patient is closely monitored by echocardiography.

Management is both palliative and preventive and includes careful monitoring, cardiovascular medications, and orthopedic surgery if needed.

Infectious Arthritis

Any infectious agent can invade the joint space and cause inflammation and tissue destruction. Certain pathogens, such as *Staphylococcus aureus,* destroy tissue rapidly; others, especially viruses, do not cause irreversible damage. The cornerstone of management is local or systemic antibiotic therapy for 6 to 8 weeks.

Lyme Disease

Lyme disease is a reportable systemic infectious disease caused by the spirochete *Borrelia burgdorferi* and results from the bite of an infected deer tick, also known as the *black-legged tick.* It is the most common vector-borne disease in the United States and Europe. Most cases of the disease in the United States are seen in New England; the mid-Atlantic states, including Maryland and Virginia; the upper Midwest, including Wisconsin and Minnesota; and northern California, especially during the summer months.

In the early and *localized stage I,* the patient appears with *flu-like symptoms,* **erythema migrans** (round or oval, flat or slightly raised rash), and *pain and stiffness in the muscles and joints.* Most patients in the United States tend to have only one lesion, sometimes referred to as a *"bull's-eye lesion."* Symptoms begin within 3 to 30 days of the tick bite, but most present in 7 to 14 days. Antibiotic therapy using doxycycline, amoxicillin, or cefuroxime (Ceftin) should be prescribed during this uncomplicated stage for 14 to 21 days. Erythromycin can be used for patients who are allergic to penicillin. Without treatment, these symptoms tend to disappear in about 4 to 5 weeks (Wormser, 2006).

If not treated or if treatment is not successful, the patient progresses to the more serious complications of Lyme disease. *Stage II (early disseminated stage)* occurs 2 to 12 weeks after the tick bite. The patient may develop *carditis* with *dysrhythmias, dyspnea, dizziness, or palpitations,* as well as central nervous system disorders such as *meningitis, facial paralysis* (often misdiagnosed as Bell's palsy), and *peripheral neuritis.* For severe disease, IV antibiotics (e.g., ceftriaxone or cefotaxime) are given for at least 30 days (Bratton & Corey, 2005).

If Lyme disease is not diagnosed and treated in the earlier stages, later chronic complications (e.g., *arthritis, chronic fatigue, memory/thinking problems*) can result. This *late stage III (chronic persistent stage)* occurs months to years after the tick bite. *For some patients, the first and only sign of Lyme disease is arthritis.* In some cases, the disease may not respond to antibiotics in any stage and the patient develops permanent damage to joints and the nervous system. *Prevention is the best strategy for Lyme disease.* Teach patients to follow the measures outlined in Chart 20-16 to prevent Lyme and other tick-borne diseases. Tell them about community resources such as the Lyme Disease Foundation (www.lyme.org) for more information.

Pseudogout

Pseudogout is a disease that mimics the clinical manifestations of gout. In this disease, however, the crystals deposited in the joints are calcium pyrophosphate, not sodium urate. These crystals usually migrate to cartilage, but they can also deposit in tendons, ligaments, and synovium.

The patient most susceptible to pseudogout is an older hospitalized male. Although the cause is not certain, the incidence is highest in men with metastatic cancer or endocrine imbalances such as hypothyroidism. NSAIDs usually control manifestations of the disease.

Chart 20-16 PATIENT AND FAMILY EDUCATION GUIDE

Prevention and Early Detection of Lyme Disease

- Avoid heavily wooded areas or areas with thick underbrush, especially in the spring and summer months.
- Walk in the center of the trail.
- Avoid dark clothing. Lighter-colored clothing makes spotting ticks easier.
- Use an insect repellent (DEET) on your skin and clothes when in an area where ticks are likely to be found.
- Wear long-sleeved tops and long pants; tuck your shirt into your pants and your pants into your socks or boots.
- Wear closed shoes or boots and a hat or cap.
- Bathe immediately after being in an infested area, and inspect your body for ticks (about the size of a pinhead); pay special attention to your arms, legs, and scalp.
- Check your pets for ticks.
- Gently remove with tweezers or fingers covered with tissue or gloves any tick that you find (do not squeeze). Dispose of the tick by flushing it down the toilet (burning a tick could spread infection).
- After removal, clean the tick area with an antiseptic such as rubbing alcohol.
- Wait 4 to 6 weeks after being bitten by a tick before being tested for Lyme disease (testing before this time is not reliable).
- Report symptoms, such as a rash or influenza-like illness, to your physician immediately.

Psoriatic Arthritis

Psoriatic arthritis (PsA) affects about 5% to 10% of people who have psoriasis, a skin condition characterized by a scaly, itchy rash, usually on the elbows, knees, and scalp. Fingernail and toenail lifting and pitting may also occur (see Chapter 27 for discussion of this disease). The joint pain associated with psoriasis is often associated with stiffness, especially in the morning. Neck and back pain are particularly common, but various forms of the disease can cause small joint arthritis or involvement of the sacroiliac joints of the spine.

PsA occurs most often in people between 20 and 50 years of age in men and women of all races. Nail symptoms are common in patients who have the associated arthritis. Causes may include genetic and environmental factors, infectious agents, and immune system dysfunction.

TABLE 20-3 Common Disorders Associated with Arthritis

- Crohn's disease
- Ulcerative colitis
- Tuberculosis
- Hemophilia
- Whipple's disease
- Intestinal bypass surgery
- Hyperparathyroidism
- Hyperthyroidism
- Diabetes mellitus
- Sickle cell anemia crisis
- Psoriasis
- Infection

Most patients do not experience destructive and deforming arthritis, but those who do have a major impact on their quality of life. Treatment is focused on managing joint pain and inflammation, controlling skin lesions, and slowing the progression of the disease. Health teaching for skin care is similar to that for lupus. Management of joint inflammation is similar to that for rheumatoid arthritis. Methotrexate (Rheumatrex), sulfasalazine (Azulfidine), and biological response modifiers have been used with success. Further discussion regarding management of psoriasis can be found in Chapter 27.

Other Disease-Associated Arthritis

A number of other diseases can cause secondary arthritis. Tuberculosis, Crohn's disease, ulcerative colitis, hemophilia, and sickle cell anemia are typical examples. To manage joint involvement, the primary disease is treated. For example, when a patient with Crohn's disease is in remission, joint manifestations also subside. Conditions in which joint involvement can occur are presented in Table 20-3.

Fibromyalgia Syndrome

Fibromyalgia syndrome (FMS), also referred to as simply *fibromyalgia,* was previously known as *fibrositis.* The name was changed because FMS is now understood to be a chronic pain syndrome, not an inflammatory disease. Pain and tenderness are located at specific sites in the back of the neck, upper chest, trunk, low back, and extremities. These tender points are also known as **trigger points** and can typically be palpated to elicit pain in a predictable, reproducible pattern. The pain is typically described as burning and gnawing. As seen in the theoretic pathophysiologic model in Fig. 20-10, increased muscle tenderness may be due to the inability to tolerate pain, possibly related to dysfunction in the brain, especially the thalamus and hypothalamus (McCance & Huether, 2006).

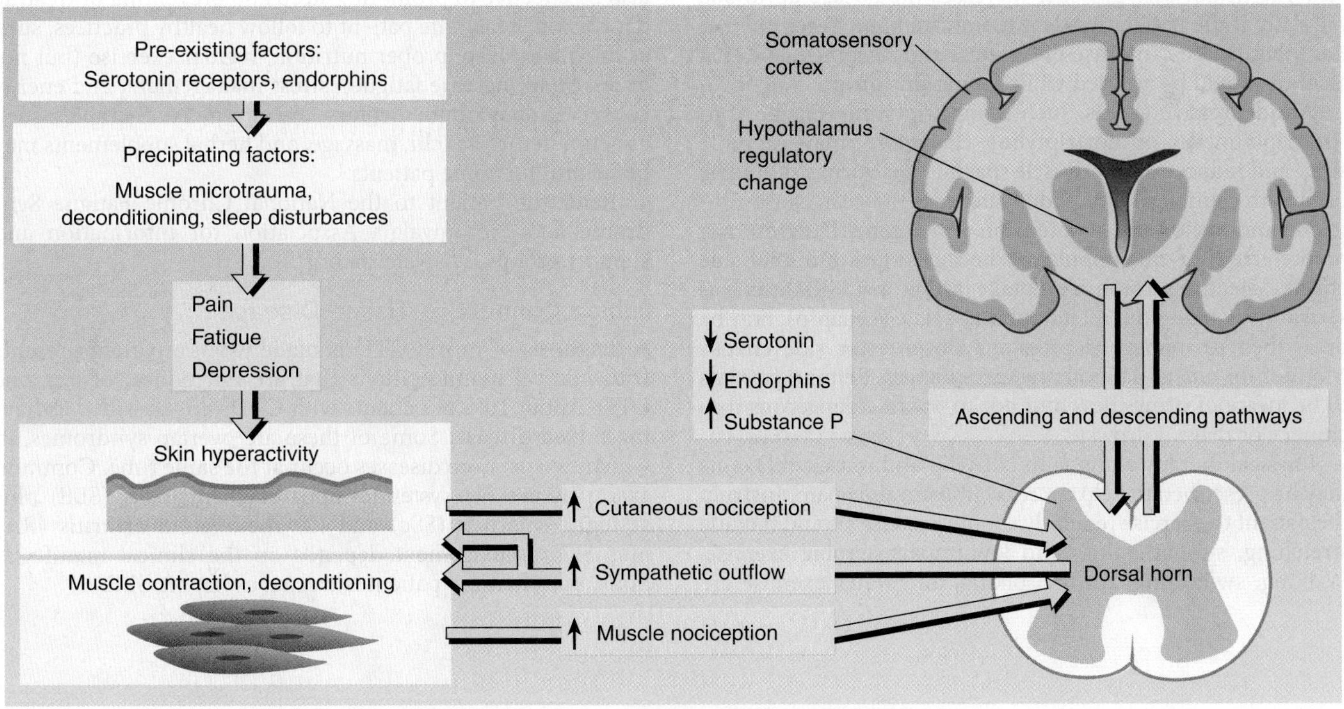

Pre-existing factors:
Serotonin receptors, endorphins
Precipitating factors:
Muscle microtrauma, deconditioning, sleep disturbances
Pain
Fatigue
Depression
Skin hyperactivity
Muscle contraction, deconditioning
Somatosensory cortex
Hypothalamus regulatory change
↓ Serotonin
↓ Endorphins
↑ Substance P
Ascending and descending pathways
↑ Cutaneous nociception
↑ Sympathetic outflow
↑ Muscle nociception
Dorsal horn

Fig. 20-10 • Theoretic pathophysiologic model of fibromyalgia.

The pain and tenderness tend to come and go but typically worsen in response to stress, increased activity, and weather conditions. The patient reports mild to severe fatigue, and sleep disturbances are common. Some people report numbness or tingling in their extremities, and others are sensitive to noxious odors, loud noises, and bright lights. Headaches and jaw pain are also common.

Other symptoms include:

- Gastrointestinal (GI), including abdominal pain, diarrhea and constipation, and heartburn
- Genitourinary, including dysuria, urinary frequency, urgency, and pelvic pain
- Cardiovascular, including dyspnea, chest pain, and dysrhythmias
- Visual, including blurred vision and dry eyes

Many with these symptoms become frustrated because they are not properly diagnosed and are in constant pain and discomfort.

Some patients are diagnosed as having chronic fatigue syndrome (CFS). CFS, migraine headache, irritable bowel syndrome (IBS), and myofascial pain are often present in those with FMS. As a result, patients can become depressed and anxious.

Most patients are women between 30 and 50 years of age. It is unlikely that the disease is caused by one factor. Possible precipitating factors include CFS, Lyme disease, trauma, medications, and flu-like illness (McCance & Huether, 2006). FMS may also be aggravated by deep-sleep deprivation. Teach patients to limit caffeine, alcohol, or other unnecessary substances that could interfere with deep sleep. Establish a regular sleep pattern.

Secondary FMS can accompany any connective tissue disease (CTD), particularly lupus and rheumatoid disease, and may not necessarily be related to sleep patterns. Pregabalin (Lyrica) is the first drug approved for fibromyalgia nerve pain. The starting dose is 150 mg daily divided into three times a day. The health care provider increases the dosage up to 300 mg daily if the patient needs it to control pain. Teach the patient that Lyrica can cause drowsiness and sleepiness and that alcohol should be avoided while taking this drug.

Antidepressive agents, such as amitriptyline (Elavil, Apo-Amitriptyline🍁) or nortriptyline (Pamelor), may promote sleep and reduce pain or muscle spasm. These drugs should be used with caution in older adults because they can cause confusion and orthostatic hypotension. Trazodone (Desyrel) may be preferred for this population because of its minimal side effects. Selective serotonin reuptake inhibitors (SSRIs), such as sertraline (Zoloft) and escitalopram oxalate (Lexapro), may be prescribed to manage depression. Observe for side effects. Monitor for postural blood pressure changes. Remind patients to be aware of drowsiness and not to operate dangerous machinery or drive if drowsy.

Physical therapy along with NSAIDs and muscle relaxants may be prescribed to help decrease fibromyalgia pain. Instruct the patient to exercise regularly. Home exercise should include stretching, strengthening, and low-impact aerobic exercise. Walking, swimming, rowing, biking, and water exercise are good examples of low-impact exercise. Complementary and alternative therapies, such as tai chi, acupuncture, hypnosis, and stress management, may help some patients with symptom relief (Taggart et al., 2003). Refer patients to the land, water, and walking exercise pamphlets produced by the Arthritis Foundation (www.arthritis.org). Inform them about the National Fibromyalgia Association for additional information (www.fmaware.org).

Chronic Fatigue Syndrome

Chronic fatigue syndrome (CFS), also known as *chronic fatigue and immune dysfunction syndrome (CFIDS),* is a chronic illness in which patients have severe fatigue for 6 months or longer, usually following flu-like symptoms. In addition, four or more of these criteria must be met for a diagnosis of CFS:

- Sore throat
- Substantial impairment in short-term memory or concentration
- Tender lymph nodes
- Muscle pain
- Multiple joint pain with redness or swelling
- Headaches of a new type, pattern, or severity (not familiar to the patient)
- Unrefreshing sleep
- Postexertional malaise lasting more than 24 hours

Chronic fatigue syndrome is most common in women and is not limited to any socioeconomic group or age. There is no laboratory test to confirm the diagnosis, and therefore many people with the disease probably have not been diagnosed. The cause is unknown, although immune, endocrine, neurologic, and environmental factors are being studied.

Management of the patient is challenging in that there is no cure for FMS. Treatment is supportive and focuses on alleviation or reduction of symptoms. For example, NSAIDs may help with body aches and pain. Low-dose antidepressants may also be effective in promoting sleep and preventing or treating depression. Teach the patient to follow healthy practices, such as adequate sleep, proper nutrition, regular exercise (but not excessive to increase fatigue), stress management, and energy conservation. Complementary and alternative therapies, such as acupuncture, tai chi, massage, and herbal supplements may be helpful for some patients.

Refer the patient to the National Chronic Fatigue Syndrome and Fibromyalgia Association for information and support groups (www.ncfsfa.org).

Mixed Connective Tissue Disease

A diagnosis of mixed CTD is made when a patient presents with clinical manifestations that are not typical of any one CTD. About 10% of patients with CTDs are classified as having mixed disease. Some of these are overlap syndromes, in which two or more diseases occur at the same time. Common examples are (1) systemic lupus erythematosus (SLE) plus systemic sclerosis (SSc) and (2) rheumatoid arthritis (RA) plus SLE. Management depends on the clinical manifestations, but often the patient is treated as having SLE.

HUMAN NEEDS NURSING CARE REVIEW

What might you NOTICE if the patient has impaired protection as a result of arthritis or other connective tissue disease (CTD)?

- Joint inflammation (redness, swelling, pain)
- Impaired joint mobility
- Joint deformity
- Difficulty ambulating
- Fever
- Rash
- Report of weight loss and fatigue
- Other manifestations that indicate organ involvement, such as dysrhythmias (heart) and decreased urinary output (kidneys)

What should you INTERPRET and how should you RESPOND to a patient with impaired protection as a result of arthritis or other CTD?

Perform and interpret focused physical assessment findings, including:

- Joint assessment, including range of motion
- ADL ability
- Pain intensity and quality
- Body weight
- Ability to cope with disease
- Vital signs
- Other assessments related to specific organ involvement (e.g., cardiac assessment)

Respond:

- Provide pain control interventions, including drug therapy and nonpharmacologic measures (e.g., music, diversional therapy).
- Collaborate with members of the health care team to improve mobility and ambulation, if needed.
- Teach about drug therapy, including the expected and adverse effects.
- Teach about nonpharmacologic measures to control pain, including ice and heat, and CAM therapies, such as glucosamine.
- Report manifestations of organ involvement to the health care provider for possible immediate intervention (e.g., drug therapy for severe dysrhythmias).
- Monitor laboratory test results to determine progress of treatment.
- Continue to assess for changes in the patient's condition, including new or additional manifestations of organ involvement.
- Encourage patients and their families to discuss their feelings about chronic illness and possible body image changes.
- Help identify coping strategies, and provide information about community and professional resources and support groups.

On what should you REFLECT?

- Monitor the patient's response to pain control interventions.
- Evaluate the patient's and family's knowledge of the disease and its management.
- Evaluate the patient's and family's stress levels and coping strategies.
- Think about what else you might do to promote mobility.
- Decide whether you need to provide alternative interventions or additional health teaching.

GET READY FOR THE NCLEX EXAMINATION!

Key Points

Review these Key Points for each NCLEX Examination Client Needs Category.

Safe and Effective Care Environment

- Provide information about community resources for patients, especially professional organizations such as the Arthritis Foundation.
- Collaborate with the health care team to manage chronic pain and increase mobility for patients with arthritis and other CTDs.
- Prioritize care for patients with systemic lupus erythematosus (SLE) by monitoring for life-threatening complications, such as renal failure.

Health Promotion and Maintenance

- Teach patients who have osteoarthritis (OA) or are prone to the disease to lose weight (if obese), avoid trauma, and limit strenuous weight-bearing activities.
- Instruct patients with arthritic pain to use multiple modalities for pain relief, including ice/heat, rest, positioning, complementary and alternative therapies, and medications as prescribed.
- Teach patients to monitor and report side and adverse effects of drugs used to treat OA and connective tissue diseases.
- Teach patients who are taking hydroxychloroquine (Plaquenil) to have frequent (every 6 months) eye examinations to monitor for retinal changes.
- Remind patients to avoid crowds and other possible sources of infection when they are taking immunosuppressant drugs.
- Reinforce the importance of good health practices, such as adequate sleep, proper nutrition, regular exercise, and stress-management techniques.
- Teach patients with arthritis what exercises to do (Chart 20-6), joint protection techniques (Chart 20-7), and energy conservation guidelines (Chart 20-11).
- Teach patients with SLE to avoid sunlight; exacerbations of the disease may be triggered.
- Remind patients with gout to avoid factors that trigger an attack, such as aspirin, organ meats, and alcohol.
- Teach people ways to prevent or detect early Lyme disease as listed in Chart 20-16.

Psychosocial Integrity

- Recognize that patients with rheumatoid arthritis (RA) may have body image disturbance as a result of potentially deforming joint involvement and nodules.
- Encourage patients with arthritis and connective tissue diseases to discuss their chronic illness and identify coping strategies that have previously been successful.

- Be aware that chronic, painful diseases affect the patient's quality of life and role performance.
- Recognize that patients with fibromyalgia syndrome (FMS) and chronic fatigue syndrome (CFS) are often frustrated because they have not been diagnosed or have been misdiagnosed.
- Teach patients with FMS and CFS that antidepressant drugs can promote sleep and decrease pain, as well as prevent or treat the depression that is common with these illnesses.

Physiological Integrity

- Be aware that most of the connective tissue diseases and arthritic disorders have a genetic basis as part of their etiology; most are also classified as autoimmune diseases and have remissions and exacerbations.
- Differentiate OA as primarily a degenerative joint problem and RA as a systemic disease.
- Realize that older patients have OA more than younger patients; younger patients have RA more than older adults; other differences between the two diseases are summarized in Table 20-1.
- Implement interventions to prevent venous thromboembolitic complications (e.g., anticoagulants, exercises, sequential compression devices); observe the patient for bleeding when he or she is taking anticoagulants.
- Be careful when positioning a patient after a total hip arthroplasty (THA) to prevent dislocation; do not hyperflex the hips or adduct the legs.
- Administer biological response modifiers (BRMs) and other disease-modifying agents with caution.
- Monitor and interpret laboratory test results for patients with autoimmune connective tissue diseases as highlighted in Chart 20-9.
- Assess for therapeutic and adverse effects of drugs used for arthritis and connective tissue diseases as specified in Chart 20-10.
- Be aware that disease-modifying antirheumatic drugs (DMARDs) and BRMs slow the progression of connective tissue diseases, especially RA and SLE.
- Assess patients with rheumatoid arthritis for early or late clinical manifestations as listed in Chart 20-8.
- Differentiate clinical manifestations and prognosis for patients with SLE versus systemic sclerosis (SSc) as listed in Chart 20-12.
- Prioritize care by assessing for swallowing ability in patients who have SSc; collaborate with the nutritionist for food modifications if needed.
- Monitor for acute joint inflammation in patients with a history of gout; the great toe and other small joints are most typically affected.
- Assess for visual symptoms (indicating possible giant cell arteritis) in patients with polymyalgia rheumatica; report changes immediately to the health care provider.
- Be aware that arthritis often accompanies other diseases, such as psoriasis, Crohn's disease, and hemophilia.

Additional Study Resources

Go to your Companion CD or Evolve at http://evolve.elsevier.com/Iggy/ for *Self-Assessment Questions for the NCLEX Examination.*

evolve Go to Evolve at http://evolve.elsevier.com/Iggy/ for *Prioritization and Delegation Questions for the NCLEX Examination.*

SELECTED BIBLIOGRAPHY

Asterisk indicates a classic or definitive work on this subject.

*Barry, F.P. (2003). Mesenchymal stem cell therapy in joint disease. *Novartis Foundation Symposium, 249,* 86-96.

Bratton, R.L., & Corey, G.R. (2005). Tick-borne disease. *American Family Physician, 71*(12), 2323-2330.

Bruce, M.L.O., & Peck, B. (2005). New rheumatoid arthritis treatments. *Holistic Nursing Practice, 19*(5), 197-206.

Bulechek, G.M., Butcher, H.K., & McCloskey Dochterman, J. (Eds.). (2008). *Nursing interventions classification (NIC)* (5th ed.). St. Louis: Mosby.

Chen, S.Y., & Wang, H.H. (2007). The relationship between physical function, knowledge of disease, social support and self-care behavior in patients with rheumatoid arthritis. *Journal of Nursing Research, 15*(3), 183-192.

Clegg, D.O., Reda, D.J., Harris, C.L., Klein, M.A., O'Dell, J.R., Hooper, M.M., et al. (2006). Glucosamine, chondroitin sulfate, and the two in combination for painful knee osteoarthritis. *New England Journal of Medicine, 354*(8), 795-808.

*Cohen, M., Wolfe, R., Mai, T., & Lewis, D. (2003). A randomized, double blind, placebo controlled trial of a topical cream containing glucosamine sulfate, chondroitin sulfate, and camphor for osteoarthritis of the knee. *Journal of Rheumatology, 30*(3), 523-528.

Dahlen, L., Zimmerman, L., & Barron, C. (2006). Pain perception and its relation to functional status post total knee arthroplasty: A pilot study. *Orthopaedic Nursing, 25*(4), 264-270.

*D'Arcy, Y. (2002). How to treat arthritis pain. *Nursing2002, 32*(7), 30-31.

D'Arcy, Y. (2006). Treating pain after a total joint replacement. *Nursing2006, 36*(5), 26, 28.

Ding, C., Cicuttini, F., Blizzard, L., & Jones, G. (2007). Smoking interacts with family history with regard to change in knee cartilage volume and cartilage defect development. *Arthritis and Rheumatology, 56*(5), 1521-1528.

Duarte, V.M., Fallis, W.M., Slonowsky, D., Kwarteng, K., & Yeung, C.K. (2006). Effectiveness of femoral nerve blockade for pain control after knee arthroplasty. *Journal of Perianesthesia Nursing, 21*(1), 311-316.

Ene-Stroescu, D., & Gorbien, M.J. (2005). Gouty arthritis: A primer on late-onset gout. *Geriatrics, 60*(7), 24-31.

Evans, C.H., Ghivizzani, S.C., Herndon, J.H., & Robbins, P.D. (2005). Gene therapy for the treatment of musculoskeletal diseases. *Journal of the American Academy of Orthopaedic Surgeons, 13*(4), 230-242.

Fonesca, C., & Denton, C.P. (2007). Genetic association studies in systemic sclerosis: More evidence of a complex disease. *The Journal of Rheumatology, 34*(5), 903-905.

Gevirtz, C. (2008). How chronic pain affects sexuality. *Nursing2008, 38*(1), 17.

Giaquinto, S., Cacciato, A., Minasi, S., Sostero, E., & Amanda, S. (2006). Effects of music-based therapy on distress following knee arthroplasty. *British Journal of Nursing, 15*(10), 576-579.

Hathaway, L. (2005). Lyme disease. *Nursing2005, 35*(4), 44-45.

Hohler, S.E. (2005). Looking into minimally invasive total hip arthroplasty. *Nursing2005, 35*(6), 54-57.

Jakonsson, U., & Hallberg, I.R. (2006). Quality of life among older adults with osteoarthritis: An explorative study. *Journal of Gerontological Nursing, 32*(8), 51-60.

Klippel, J.H. (2007). *Primer on the rheumatic diseases* (13th ed.). Atlanta: The Arthritis Foundation.

*Kuper, B.C., & Failla, S. (2000). Systemic lupus erythematosus: A multisystem autoimmune disorder. *Nursing Clinics of North America, 35*(1), 253-266.

*McCaffrey, R., & Freeman, E. (2003). Effect of music on chronic osteoarthritis pain in older people. *Journal of Advanced Nursing, 44*(5), 517-524.

McCance, K.L., & Huether, S.E. (2006). *Pathophysiology: The biologic basis for disease in adults and children* (5th ed.). St. Louis: Mosby.
*Morris, N.S. (2004). Complications associated with orthopaedic surgery. In C.M. Mosher (Ed.), *An introduction to orthopaedic nursing* (3rd ed.). Chicago: National Association of Orthopaedic Nurses.
National Center for Complementary and Alternative Medicine (NCCAM). (2005). *Research report on rheumatoid arthritis and complementary and alternative medicine.* Retrieved January 5, 2008, from *www.nccam.nih.gov/health/RA/.*
Nussbaum, R.L., McInnes, R., & Willard, H. (2007). *Thompson & Thompson genetics in medicine* (7th ed.). Philadelphia: Saunders.
Pagana, K.D., & Pagana, T.J. (2006). *Mosby's manual of diagnostic and laboratory tests.* St. Louis: Mosby.
Pellino, T.A., Gordon, D.B., Engelke, Z.K., Busse, K.L., Collins, M.A., Silver, C.E., et al. (2005). Use of nonpharmacologic interventions for pain and anxiety after total hip and knee arthroplasty. *Orthopaedic Nursing, 24*(3), 182-192.
Rooney, J. (2005). Systemic lupus erythematosus. *Nursing2005, 35*(11), 54-60.
Sestak, A.L., Nath, S.K., Sawalha, A.H., & Harley, J.B. (2007). Current status of lupus genetics. *Arthritis Research and Therapy, 9*(3), 210-219.
*Siebold, J.R. (2001). Scleroderma and mixed connective tissue diseases In S. Ruddy, E.D. Harris, & C.B. Sledge (Eds.), *Kelley's textbook of rheumatology* (6th ed., pp. 1211-1239). Philadelphia: Saunders.
Sunk, I.G., Bobacz, K., Hofstaetter, J.G., Amoyo, L., Soleiman, A., Smolen, J., et al. (2007). Increased expression of discoidin domain receptor 2 is linked to the degree of cartilage damage in human knee joints: A potential role in osteoarthritis pathogenesis. *Arthritis and Rheumatology, 56*(11), 3685-3692.
*Taggert, H.M., Arslanian, C.L., Bae, S., & Singh, K. (2003). Effects of T'ai Chi exercise on fibromyalgia symptoms and health-related quality of life. *Orthopaedic Nursing, 22*(5), 353-360.
Tak, S.H. (2006). An insider perspective of daily stress and coping in elders with arthritis. *Orthopeadic Nursing, 25*(2), 127-132.
Theis, L.M., & Kahn, B. (2006). The hip, femur, and pelvis. In H.M. Taggart (Ed.), *Core curriculum for orthopaedic nursing* (5th ed.). Boston: National Association of Orthopaedic Nurses.
Turjanica, M.A. (2007). Postoperative continuous peripheral nerve blockade in the lower extremity total joint arthroplasty population. *MEDSURG Nursing, 16*(3), 151-154.
Wormser, G.P. (2006). Early Lyme disease. *New England Journal of Medicine, 354*(26), 2794-2801.

21
CHAPTER

Care of Patients with HIV Disease and Other Immune Deficiencies

James G. Sampson • M. Linda Workman

LEARNING OUTCOMES

For clinical competence and success on the NCLEX Examination, study this chapter with these Learning Outcomes in mind:

Safe and Effective Care Environment

1. Use appropriate techniques to reduce the risk for infection in an immunocompromised patient.
2. Use Standard Precautions to prevent human immune deficiency virus (HIV) transmission to you, patients, and other members of the health care team.
3. Ensure that confidentiality of HIV status is maintained by all health care team members.

Health Promotion and Maintenance

4. Teach all sexually active people to use safer sex practices.
5. Assess all patients for high-risk behaviors for HIV disease.

Psychosocial Integrity

6. Teach family members reorientation techniques when the patient is confused.
7. Respect the patient's right to inform or not to inform family members about his or her HIV status.
8. Use a nonjudgmental approach when discussing sexual practices and sexual behaviors that are different from your own.

Physiological Integrity

9. Compare primary and secondary immune deficiencies for cause and onset of problems.
10. Explain the differences in nursing care required for a patient with a pathogenic infection versus a patient with an opportunistic infection.
11. Distinguish between the conditions of HIV infection and acquired immune deficiency syndrome (AIDS) for clinical manifestations and risks for complications.
12. Describe the ways in which HIV is transmitted.
13. Coordinate nursing care for the patient with AIDS who has impaired gas exchange.
14. Identify teaching priorities for the HIV-positive patient receiving highly active antiretroviral therapy.

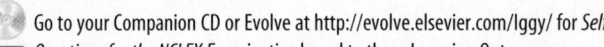

evolve Go to your Companion CD or Evolve at http://evolve.elsevier.com/Iggy/ for *Self-Assessment Questions for the NCLEX Examination* keyed to these Learning Outcomes.

Immune system function is concerned with helping the body stay healthy by preventing the growth of infectious organisms. It assists the body to monitor and maintain those cells and substances that are considered "self," belonging to the body. For example, newly made cells and compatible blood transfusions are deemed self and safe by the immune system. However, when the immune system detects the presence of a protein or cell that does not belong to the body and represents a potential threat, its job is then to attack and destroy the "non-self" or "foreign" substance. Infection is a major threat. We are exposed to many organisms every day. The efficiency of the immune system prevents disease despite this exposure.

When the immune system fails to recognize infectious agents, severe local and systemic infections are not suppressed or controlled. Immune system failure can be the result of a primary (congenital) immune deficiency in which one or more parts of the system are not functioning properly from birth. These problems are usually genetic mutations that are discovered in the infant or child who is repeatedly sick. Immune system failure can also be secondary (acquired after birth) as the result of viral infection, contact with a toxin, or medical therapy. These problems can cause a normal immune system to stop functioning or to function less efficiently. In either case, the immune system can no longer distinguish what should be in the body from a foreign invader. The consequences for the immune-deficient patient can range from mild, localized health problems to total immune system failure, leaving the body open to attack from any foreign pathogen.

ACQUIRED (SECONDARY) IMMUNE DEFICIENCIES

HIV DISEASE AND ACQUIRED IMMUNE DEFICIENCY SYNDROME (AIDS)

Pathophysiology

Acquired immune deficiency syndrome (AIDS) is the most common secondary immune deficiency disease in the world. First identified in 1981, HIV/AIDS is now a serious worldwide epidemic.

Etiology and Genetic Risk

The cause of HIV infection is a virus—the human immune deficiency virus. Like most viruses, HIV is a parasite looking for a way into a cell, to take over the cell, and to force the cell into making more copies of the virus. These new virus particles then look for additional cells to infect, repeating the cycle as long as there are new host cells to infect.

The HIV Infectious Process

Viral particle features include an outer envelope with special "docking proteins," known as *gp41* and *gp120,* that assist in finding a host (Fig. 21-1). Inside, the virus has two protein coatings and the genetic material along with the enzymes *reverse transcriptase (RT)* and *integrase.* The first challenge is for the HIV particle to get inside a host cell. HIV accomplishes this task by first finding a way into the host's bloodstream. Once in the blood, HIV "hijacks" certain cells. One of the cells that it hijacks is the CD4+ T-cell, also known as the *CD4+ cell, helper/inducer T-cell,* or *T4-cell* (see Chapter 19). This cell directs immune system defenses and regulates the activity of all immune system cells. If HIV successfully enters a CD4+ T-cell, it can then create more virus particles.

Virus-host interactions are needed for disease development. When a person is infected with HIV, the virus randomly "bumps" into many cells. The docking proteins on the outside of the virus try to find special receptors on a host cell that will allow the virus to bind and then enter the cell. The CD4+ T-cell has receptors on its surface known as *CD4, CCR5,* and *CXCR4* (Fig. 21-2). Proteins on the HIV particle surface, known as *gp120* and *gp41,* recognize these receptors on the CD4+ T-cell. For the virus to enter this cell, *both* the gp120 and the gp41 must bind to the receptors. The gp120 first binds to the primary CD4 receptor, which changes its shape and allows the gp41 to bind to one of the co-receptors (either the CCR5 receptor or the CXCR4 receptor). This attachment allows the virus to then enter the CD4+ T-cell (Fig. 21-3). *Viral binding to the CD4 receptor and to either of the co-receptors is needed to enter the cell.* (The new drug class known as *entry inhibitors* work here to prevent gp41 from binding to the CCR5 receptor and entering the CD4+ T-cell.)

Viruses, like human cells, have genetic material. After entering a host cell, HIV must get its genetic material into the host cell's DNA. HIV belongs to a family of viruses called **retroviruses.** Viruses, like human cells, have genetic material. The genetic material of the human cell is double-stranded DNA (ds-DNA). The genetic material of HIV is single-stranded ribonucleic acid (ss-RNA). To infect and take over a human cell, the genetic material must be the same. HIV overcomes this problem by bringing along an enzyme at the time of infection, *reverse transcriptase (RT).* RT takes HIV's ss-RNA and converts it into ds-DNA, which makes the viral genetic material the same as human DNA. (The drug classes known as *nucleoside analog reverse transcriptase inhibitors [NARTIs]* and *non-nucleoside reverse transcriptase inhibitors [NNRTIs]* work here to inhibit HIV reverse transcriptase.) Then HIV must get its DNA into the nucleus of the CD4+ T-cell and place it within the human DNA. HIV also makes an enzyme called *integrase.* This enzyme allows the viral ds-DNA to be inserted into the host ds-DNA, which completes the infection of the CD4+ T-cell. (The new drug class known as *integrase inhibi-*

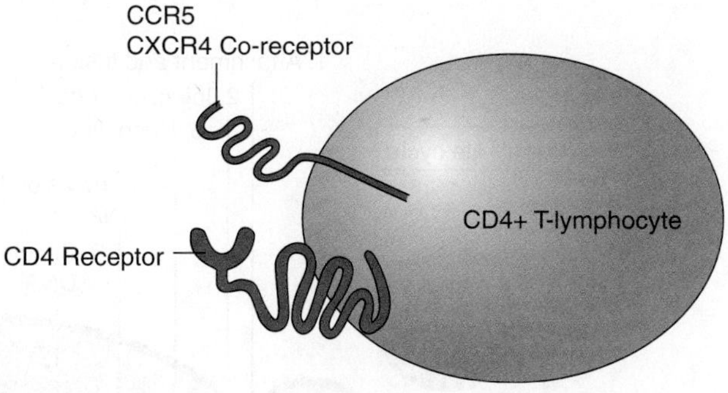
CCR5
CXCR4 Co-receptor
CD4+ T-lymphocyte
CD4 Receptor

Fig. 21-2 • The CD4+ T-lymphocyte receptors for the HIV "docking" proteins.

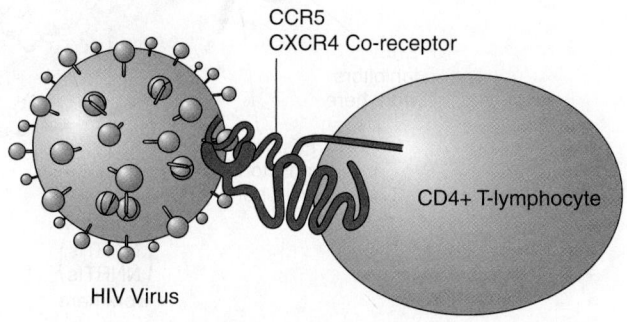

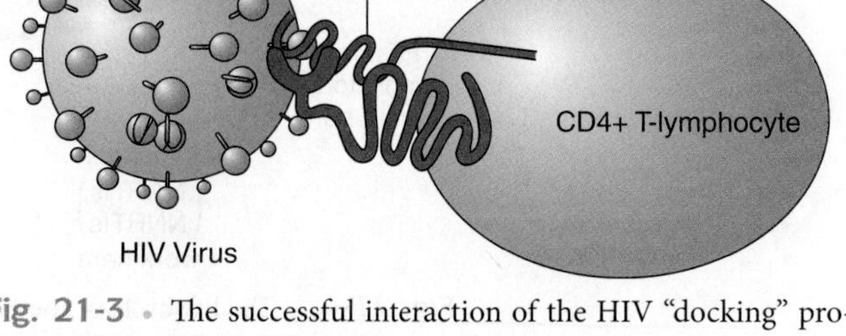
CCR5
CXCR4 Co-receptor
CD4+ T-lymphocyte
HIV Virus

Fig. 21-3 • The successful interaction of the HIV "docking" proteins with the CD4+ T-lymphocyte receptors.

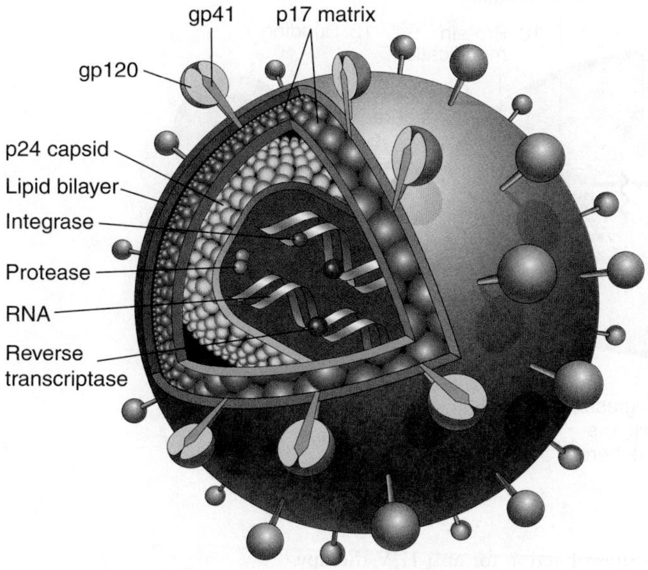
gp41
p17 matrix
gp120
p24 capsid
Lipid bilayer
Integrase
Protease
RNA
Reverse transcriptase

Fig. 21-1 • The human immune deficiency virus (HIV).

tors works here to prevent viral DNA from integrating into the cell's normal human DNA.)

HIV particles are made within the infected CD4+ T-cell, using all the metabolic machinery of the host. The new virus particle is made in the form of one long protein strand. The strand is clipped, using chemical scissors called *HIV protease,* into several small functional pieces. These pieces are formed into a new finished viral particle. (The drug class known as *protease inhibitors* works here to inhibit HIV protease.) Once the new virus particle is finished, it fuses with the infected cell's membrane and then buds off in search of another CD4+ T-cell to infect (Fig. 21-4).

Effects of HIV infection are related to the new genetic instructions that now direct CD4+ T-cells to change their role in immune system defenses. The new role is to be an "HIV factory." Not only is the immune system made weaker by removing some CD4+ T-cells from circulation, but also the most important cell in the immune system becomes an HIV factory. Up to 10 billion virus particles are made daily. In early HIV infection, the immune system can still attack and destroy most of the newly created virus particles. With time, however, the number of HIV particles overwhelms the immune system. Gradually, CD4+ T-cell counts fall, viral numbers (viral load) rise, and without treatment the patient eventually dies of opportunistic infections or cancer.

Everyone who has AIDS has HIV infection; however, not everyone who has HIV infection has AIDS. The distinction rests with the number of CD4+ T-cells the patient has and whether any opportunistic infections have occurred. A healthy adult usually has at least 800 to 1000 of these cells/mm^3 of blood. The number of CD4+ T-cells is reduced in the person with HIV disease.

When a person is infected with HIV, the first manifestations are fever, night sweats, chills, headache, and muscle aches. All of these problems can be caused by exposure to almost any virus, such as influenza—not just to HIV. Many people with this acute HIV infection also have a rash and a sore throat, which is often confused with mononucleosis and viral meningitis. With time, these symptoms cease and the person feels well again. Actually, a "war is going on" in the body between HIV and the immune system.

As time passes, with more CD4+ T-cells infected and taken out of service, this cell count drops to below normal levels and those that remain may not function normally. Poor CD4+ T-cell function as a result of HIV infection leads to these immune system abnormalities:

- Lymphocytopenia (decreased numbers of lymphocytes)
- Increased production of incomplete and nonfunctional antibodies
- Abnormally functioning macrophages

As the CD4+ T-cell level drops, the patient is at risk for bacterial, fungal, and viral infections, as well as some opportunistic cancers. **Opportunistic infections** are those caused by organisms that are present as part of the normal environment and are kept in check by normal immune function. They occur because of the profound immune suppression of the person with AIDS. These infections may result from a newly acquired infection or reactivation of an old infection.

A diagnosis of AIDS requires that the person be HIV positive and have either a CD4+ T-cell count of less than 200 cells/mm^3 or an opportunistic infection. Once AIDS is diagnosed, even if the patient's cell count goes higher than 200 cells/mm^3 or if the infection is successfully treated, the AIDS diagnosis remains and the patient never reverts to being just HIV positive.

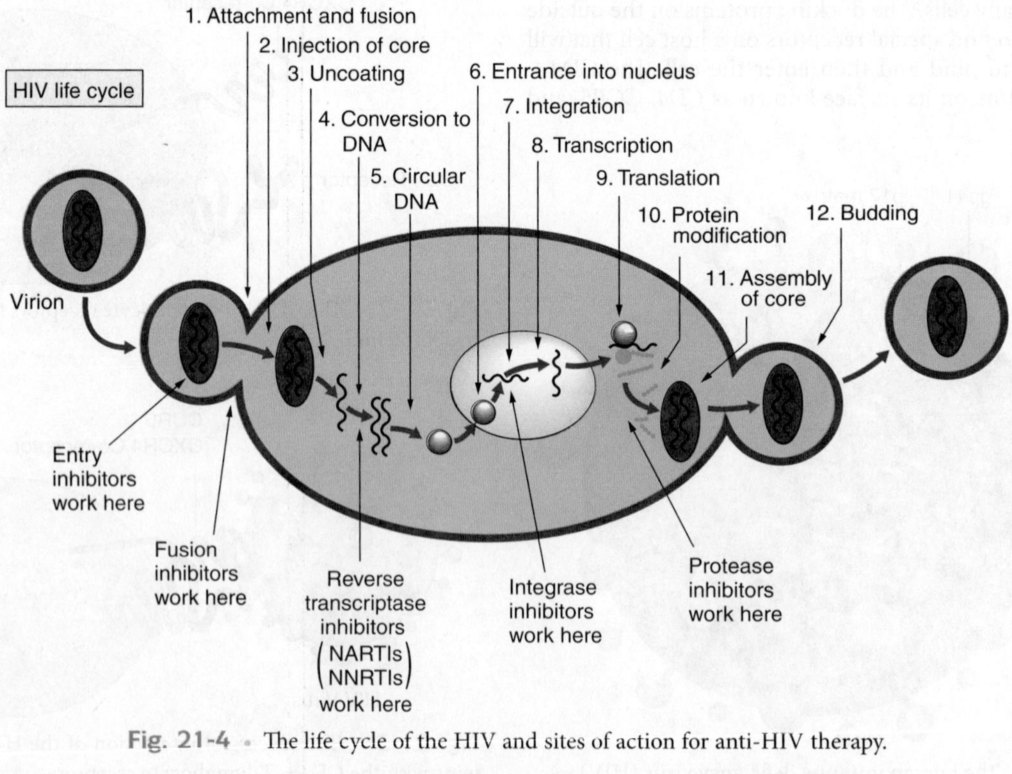
HIV life cycle
1. Attachment and fusion
2. Injection of core
3. Uncoating
4. Conversion to DNA
5. Circular DNA
6. Entrance into nucleus
7. Integration
8. Transcription
9. Translation
10. Protein modification
11. Assembly of core
12. Budding
Virion
Entry inhibitors work here
Fusion inhibitors work here
Reverse transcriptase inhibitors (NARTIs NNRTIs) work here
Integrase inhibitors work here
Protease inhibitors work here

Fig. 21-4 • The life cycle of the HIV and sites of action for anti-HIV therapy.

HIV Classification

The Centers for Disease Control and Prevention (CDC) classifies HIV infection by combining clinical conditions that occur with HIV infection and three ranges of CD4+ T-cell counts (Table 21-1). The classification begins with acute HIV infection (clinical category A) and spans a continuum that ends with AIDS (clinical category C). The classifications are further divided into 1, 2, and 3 based on the CD4+ T-cell count. *The person with HIV infection can transmit the virus to others at all stages of disease, but the recently infected person with a high viral load can be particularly infectious.*

Clinical category A is used to describe a person who is HIV positive. Manifestations may not be present at this stage, or the person may have persistently enlarged lymph nodes **(lymphadenopathy).** He or she may have acute but temporary "flu-like" symptoms as the only disease manifestations. Patients have the additional classification of A1, A2, or A3, depending on their CD4+ T-cell counts. When the count is at least 500/μL, the disease is classified as *A1.* When the count is between 200 and 499/μL, the disease is classified as *A2.* When the count is less than 200/μL, the disease is classified as *A3.*

Clinical category B is used to describe a patient with HIV infection who *also* has one or more of the problems listed in column B of Table 21-1 that are (1) caused by HIV infection or indicate a deficiency in cell-mediated immunity or (2) are complicated by HIV infection. The list gives examples of category B clinical conditions but is not comprehensive. The additional classification 1, 2, or 3 depends on the CD4+ T-cell count and is the same as for category A as just described.

Clinical category C is used to describe an HIV-positive patient who has AIDS if any one of the health problems listed on Table 21-1, column C, is present. These problems meet the CDC case definition for AIDS. The additional classification 1, 2, or 3 depends on the CD4+ T-cell count and is the same as for category A as just described.

TABLE 21-1 Centers for Disease Control and Prevention Classification System for HIV Infection and AIDS Case Definition

CD4+ Cell Categories	CLINICAL CATEGORIES A	B	C*
	HIV positive, asymptomatic *OR* Persistent generalized lymphadenopathy *OR* Acute (primary) HIV infection with accompanying illness or history of acute infection as the only manifestations	Bacterial endocarditis, meningitis, pneumonia, or sepsis Vulvovaginal candidiasis that is persistent for more than 1 month or is poorly responsive to therapy Oropharyngeal candidiasis (thrush) Severe cervical dysplasia or carcinoma Constitutional symptoms, such as fever or diarrhea lasting longer than 1 month Oral hairy leukoplakia Herpes zoster (shingles), involving at least two distinct episodes or more than one dermatome Idiopathic thrombocytopenic purpura Listeriosis Pulmonary *Mycobacterium tuberculosis* infection Nocardiosis Pelvic inflammatory disease Peripheral neuropathy	Bronchial, tracheal, pulmonary, or esophageal candidiasis Invasive cervical cancer Disseminated or extrapulmonary coccidioidomycosis Chronic intestinal cryptosporidiosis Cytomegalovirus disease other than that of the liver, spleen, or lymph nodes Cytomegalovirus retinitis with vision loss HIV-related encephalopathy Herpes simplex (chronic; bronchitis, pneumonitis; or esophagitis) Disseminated or extrapulmonary histoplasmosis Chronic intestinal isosporiasis Kaposi's sarcoma Lymphoma (Burkitt's, immunoblastic, or primary brain) Disseminated or extrapulmonary *M. avium* complex or *M. kansasii* Extrapulmonary *M. tuberculosis* *Pneumocystis jiroveci* pneumonia Recurrent infectious pneumonia Progressive multifocal leukoencephalopathy Salmonella septicemia Toxoplasmosis (brain) Wasting syndrome
1 ≥500/μL	A1	B1	C1
2 200-499/μL	A2	B2	C2
3 <200/μL*	A3	B3	C3

Data from Centers for Disease Control and Prevention, 1992.
*AIDS indicator conditions or counts.

HIV Progression

The time from the beginning of HIV infection to development of AIDS ranges from months to years. The range depends on how HIV was acquired, personal factors, and interventions. For people who have been transfused with HIV-contaminated blood, for example, AIDS develops quickly. For those who become HIV positive as a result of a single sexual encounter, the period is much longer before progression to AIDS. Other personal factors that may influence progression to AIDS include frequency of re-exposure to HIV, presence of other sexually transmitted diseases (STDs), nutritional status, and stress.

GENETIC CONSIDERATIONS

About 1% of people with HIV infection are **long-term nonprogressors (LTNPs).** These people have been infected with HIV for at least 10 years and have remained asymptomatic, with CD4+ T-cell counts within a normal range.

A genetic difference for this population is that their CCR5/CXCR4 co-receptors on the CD4+ T-cells are abnormal and nonfunctional. Most LTNPs have mutations in both pairs of the co-receptors' gene alleles. The mutation creates a defective receptor called *delta32.* This defective receptor does not bind to the HIV docking proteins. Cells with this defective receptor successfully resist the entrance of the HIV. People who have only one mutated co-receptor gene allele have fewer normal co-receptors. Although these people can be infected with HIV, disease progression is slow compared with that in people who have normal co-receptor gene alleles.

Incidence/Prevalence

Currently in the United States, almost 1 million cases of HIV/AIDS have been diagnosed, and more than 550,000 people have died of AIDS (Centers for Disease Control and Prevention [CDC], 2007). This number is less than the total number of people in the United States estimated to be infected with HIV (1.1 million to 1.8 million). Worldwide, AIDS has caused more than 30 million deaths and an estimated 40 to 60 million people are currently infected with HIV (CDC, 2007).

AIDS hits hardest among people between 21 and 44 years of age. The loss of productivity and wage-earning power among this group devastates the patient and strains the insurance and health care industry.

Most AIDS cases in North America occur among men who have had sex with other men (MSM) (46%) or persons of either gender who have used injection drugs (20%) (CDC, 2007). *The changing demographics of the infection indicate that the perception that HIV/AIDS is only a problem for homosexual white men is false.*

CULTURAL AWARENESS

More than 72% of new HIV infections reported in the United States occur in racial and ethnic minority groups, particularly among African Americans and Hispanics (CDC, 2007) (Fig. 21-5). These two groups show an increasing trend in HIV infection compared with a leveling off among white people.

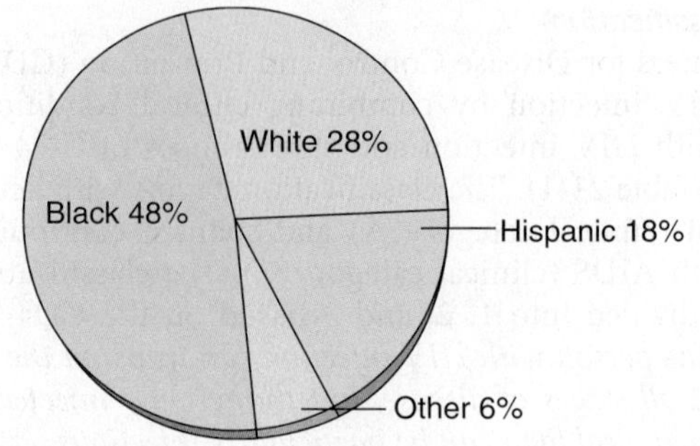
White 28%
Black 48%
Hispanic 18%
Other 6%

Fig. 21-5 • Estimates of annual new HIV infections in the United States by ethnicity and race.

Factors that may increase the incidence of HIV infection and progression to AIDS among minority groups include:
- Fear of or lack of faith in the U.S. health care system
- Poverty and limited access to high-cost drugs
- Homophobia leading to increased bisexual activity among men of color
- Health beliefs about HIV treatment

CONSIDERATIONS FOR OLDER ADULTS

Infection with HIV can occur at any age. Assess the older patient for risk behaviors, including a sexual and drug use history (Tangredi et al., 2008). Age-related decline in immune function increases the likelihood that the older adult will develop the infection after an HIV exposure. In the older woman, thinning of vaginal tissue as a result of decreased estrogen may increase susceptibility to all sexually transmitted diseases, including HIV infection.

WOMEN'S HEALTH CONSIDERATIONS

Women are the fastest growing group with HIV infection and AIDS. In North America, about 16% of people with HIV infection are women. Twenty-six percent of newly diagnosed cases are women (Fig. 21-6). In less affluent countries, 50% of cases occur in women. Risk factors are sexual exposure (75%) and IV drug use (25%). Strategies specifically targeted to reducing sexual exposures of HIV to women may help prevent an increase in HIV infection in that group. Women with HIV infection have a poorer outcome with shorter mean survival time than that of men. This outcome may be the result of late diagnosis and social or economic factors that reduce access to medical care.

Gynecologic problems, especially persistent or recurrent vaginal candidiasis, may be the first signs of HIV infection in women. Other common problems include genital herpes, pelvic inflammatory disease, and cervical dysplasia or cancer.

Most women with HIV are of childbearing age. The effect of HIV on pregnancy outcomes includes higher incidence of premature delivery, low-birth-weight infants, and transmission of the disease to the infant.

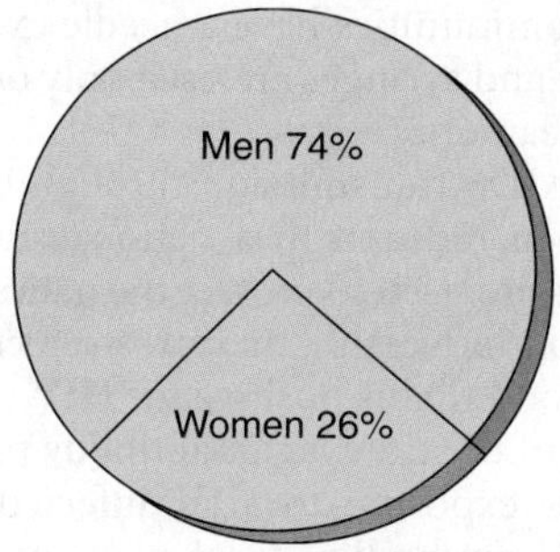
Men 74%
Women 26%

Fig. 21-6 • Estimates of annual new HIV infections in the United States by gender.

AIDS is a disease with a high mortality rate. The fatality rate is at least 60% for adults and, to date, there is no cure, just like other viral diseases have no cure. Thus a major focus for health care in North America and worldwide is prevention of HIV infection. For those infected with HIV, drug therapy slows disease progression and, to be effective, it must be taken as prescribed for the rest of the patient's life.

Health Promotion and Maintenance

The most important aspect for prevention of HIV transmission is education. Teach all people, regardless of age, gender, ethnicity, or sexual orientation, that they are susceptible to HIV infection. HIV infection is preventable because of the modes of viral transmission and the fragile nature of the virus.

HIV has been found in most body fluids of infected patients, including blood, semen, vaginal secretions, breast milk, amniotic fluid, urine, feces, saliva, tears, cerebrospinal fluid, lymph nodes, cervical cells, corneal tissue, and brain tissue. The fluids with the highest concentrations of HIV are the semen and the blood, causing HIV to be transmitted most often in these three ways:

- Sexual: genital, anal, or oral sexual contact with exposure of mucous membranes to infected semen or vaginal secretions
- Parenteral: sharing of needles or equipment contaminated with infected blood or receiving contaminated blood products
- Perinatal: from the placenta, from contact with maternal blood and body fluids during birth, or from breast milk from an infected mother to child

Teach everyone about the transmission routes and ways to reduce their exposure (discussed below). Also stress that HIV is not transmitted by casual contact in the home, school, or workplace. Sharing household utensils, towels and linens, and toilet facilities does not transmit HIV. In addition, HIV is not spread by mosquitoes or other insects.

Sexual Transmission

The CDC describes the ABC safer sex methods as A, abstinence; B, be faithful; and C, condoms (CDC, 2007). *Abstinence and mutually monogamous sex with a noninfected partner are the only absolutely safe methods of preventing HIV infection from sexual contact.* Many forms of sexual expression can spread HIV infection if one partner is infected. *The risk for becoming infected from a partner who is HIV positive is always present,* although some sexual practices are more risky than others. The virus concentrates most heavily in blood and seminal fluid, although it is also present in vaginal secretions. Thus risk differs by gender, sexual act, and the viral load of the infected partner.

Gender affects HIV transmission. HIV is most easily transmitted when infected body fluids come into contact with mucous membranes or nonintact skin. The vagina has much more mucous membrane than does the penis. Thus HIV, like all other sexually transmitted diseases (STDs), is more easily transmitted from infected male to uninfected female than vice versa. Teach women the importance of always either using a vaginal or dental dam or having their male partners use a condom.

Sexual acts or practices that permit infected seminal fluid to come into contact with mucous membranes or nonintact skin are the most risky for sexual transmission of HIV. The practice with the highest risk is anal intercourse. In anal intercourse, the risk increases when the penis and seminal fluid of an infected person come into contact with the mucous membranes of the uninfected partner's rectum. *Anal intercourse in which the semen depositor is infected is a very risky sexual practice regardless of whether the semen receiver is male or female.* Anal intercourse not only allows seminal fluid to make contact with the mucous membranes of the rectum but also tears the mucous membranes, making infection more likely. Teach patients who engage in anal intercourse that the safer sex practice is for the semen depositor to wear a condom during this act.

Viral load, or the amount of virus present in blood and other body fluids, affects transmission. The higher the blood level of HIV **(viremia),** the greater the risk for sexual and perinatal transmission. Current highly active antiretroviral therapy (HAART) has caused the viral load of some infected patients to drop below detectable levels. *Although there is less virus in seminal or vaginal fluids of people receiving HAART, the risk for disease transmission still exists.*

Safer sex practices are those that reduce the risk of nonintact skin or mucous membranes coming in contact with infected body fluids and blood. Teach everyone the importance of consistently using these safer sex practices:

- A latex condom for genital and anal intercourse (Chart 21-1)
- A condom or latex barrier (dental dam) over the genitals or anus during oral-genital or oral-anal sexual contact
- Latex gloves for finger or hand contact with the vagina or rectum

For those who believe they have been exposed to HIV as a result of sexual relations or other types of non-occupational exposure, the CDC has guidelines for post-exposure prophylaxis. The length and type of prophylaxis therapy depend on the nature of the exposure (Chart 21-2).

Parenteral Transmission

Preventive practices to reduce transmission among injection drug users include the use of proper cleaning of "works" (needles, syringes, other drug paraphernalia). Instruct patients to clean a used needle and syringe by first filling and flushing them with clear water. Next, the syringe should be filled with ordinary household bleach. The bleach-filled syringe should be shaken for 30 to 60 seconds. Advise drug users to carry a small container with this solution whenever sharing

Chart 21-1 PATIENT AND FAMILY EDUCATION GUIDE

Condom Use to Prevent Sexually Transmitted Diseases

- Use latex condoms rather than natural membrane condoms.
- Store condoms in a cool, dry place.
- Do not use condoms that were in damaged packages or those that show signs of age, such as those that are brittle, sticky, or discolored.
- Handle condoms carefully to avoid puncturing them.
- Put a condom on before making any genital contact.
- Hold the tip of the condom and unroll it onto the erect penis, making sure that no air is trapped in the tip. Leave space at the tip to collect semen.
- Use adequate lubrication. Use water-based lubricants only. Petroleum or oil-based lubricants such as petroleum jelly, cooking oil, shortening, and lotions can damage the condom.
- Replace a broken condom immediately. If ejaculation occurs after the condom breaks, there may be some protection in the immediate use of a spermicide.
- After ejaculation, the condom must remain on until the penis is withdrawn. While the penis is still erect, hold the condom against the base of the penis while withdrawing.
- Never reuse condoms.

From Centers for Disease Control. (1988). Condoms for prevention of sexually transmitted diseases. *Morbidity and Mortality Weekly Report, 37*(9), 133-137.

Chart 21-2 PATIENT AND FAMILY EDUCATION GUIDE

Nonoccupational Postexposure Prophylaxis (nPEP) to HIV

Recommendations for nPEP with a *substantial risk* for HIV exposure is a 28-day course of the preferred regimen of HAART* †

NNRTI-based	Efavirenz plus either lamivudine or emtricitabine plus either zidovudine or tenofovir
or	
PI-based	Lopinavir/ritonavir plus either lamivudine or emtricitabine plus zidovudine

A substantial risk is exposure of any of these:

- Vagina
- Rectum
- Eye
- Mouth
- Other intact mucous membrane
- Nonintact skin or mucous membrane

With:

- Blood
- Semen
- Vaginal secretions
- Rectal secretions
- Breast milk
- Any body fluid visibly contaminated with blood

When:

- The source person is known to be HIV-infected

Data from Centers for Disease Control and Prevention. (2005). Antiretroviral postexposure prophylaxis after sexual, injection-drug use, or other nonoccupational exposure to HIV in the United States. *Morbidity and Mortality Weekly Report, 54*(RR-2), 1-27.

*Either when a substantial risk has occurred and more than 72 hours has passed since the exposure or when the exposure is considered to be a negligible risk, nPEP is not recommended.

†When a substantial risk has occurred and less than 72 hours has passed since the exposure but the HIV-infection status of the source person is not known, nPEP is determined on a case-by-case basis.

HAART, Highly active antiretroviral therapy; *NNRTI,* non-nucleoside reverse transcriptase inhibitor; *PI,* protease inhibitor.

needles. Some communities have a needle exchange program in which needles and syringes are used only once and are then exchanged for clean ones.

The risk for AIDS transmission through blood and blood products has been reduced to a national average of 0.02%. Several measures are used to protect the nation's blood supply. All donated blood in North America is screened for the HIV antibody, and blood that is positive for HIV antibodies is discarded. Because of the time lag in antibody production (seroconversion) after exposure to HIV, infected blood can test negative for HIV antibodies. False-negative results also can occur for other reasons. Inform patients that there is a small but real possibility of HIV transmission through blood and blood products. As a result, methods for reducing transfusion-related infections have included less reliance on standard transfusion therapy through more stringent criteria for transfusion, the use of growth factors to promote more rapid blood production in the patient, and an increase in autologous transfusion in which the patient donates his or her own blood to be transfused back at a later time.

Perinatal Transmission

The risk for perinatal transmission to infants in pregnant patients with HIV infection is about 25% in woman who are not using drug therapy for the disease compared with about 8% for women who are using drug therapy for HIV. Therefore encourage HIV-positive women who are pregnant to continue the therapy, or if they are not on antiviral therapy, to start the therapy as soon as possible.

HIV transmission can occur across the placenta during pregnancy, with infant exposure to blood and vaginal secretions during birth, or with exposure after birth through breast milk. Inform women of childbearing age with HIV infection about the risks for perinatal transmission. Consult a maternal-child textbook for more information about reducing perinatal transmission of HIV.

Transmission and Health Care Workers

Needle stick or "sharps" injuries are the main means of occupation-related HIV infection for health care workers. In addition, health care workers can be infected through exposure of nonintact skin and mucous membranes to blood and body fluids. Because of the time lag between the time of infection with HIV and the production of serum antibodies (seroconversion), infected people can test negative for HIV and still transmit the virus. *The best prevention for health care providers is the consistent use of Standard Precautions for all patients as recommended by the CDC and required by The Joint Commission (TJC)* (see Chapter 25). Chart 21-3 lists the recommended actions for prevention of HIV infection after a needle stick or other occupational exposure (postexposure prophylaxis [PEP]). When the source patient is known to be HIV negative, PEP is not recommended.

The public may be alarmed about HIV transmission by health care workers. It is recommended that HIV-infected health care workers wear gloves when in contact with patients' mucous membranes or nonintact skin. Infected workers with weeping dermatitis or open lesions should not perform direct care. The CDC guidelines for preventing HIV transmission by health care workers during exposure-prone invasive procedures are listed in Chart 21-4. These include any procedure in which there is a risk for broken

Chart 21-3 BEST PRACTICE FOR PATIENT SAFETY & QUALITY CARE

Postexposure Prophylaxis (PEP) for Occupational HIV Exposure

Basic PEP	Expanded PEP
Small volume (few drops) exposure to mucous membranes or nonintact skin • Source patient is HIV positive, asymptomatic with known low viral load • Source patient is HIV positive, symptomatic or AIDS with high viral load	Large volume (major splash) exposure to mucous membranes or nonintact skin • Source patient is HIV positive, symptomatic or AIDS with high viral load
Large volume (major splash) exposure to mucous membranes or nonintact skin • Source patient is HIV positive, asymptomatic with known low viral load • Optional when source patient is unknown or known with HIV risk factors	Less severe percutaneous injury (solid needle or superficial injury) • Source patient is HIV positive, symptomatic or AIDS with high viral load
Less severe percutaneous injury (solid needle or superficial injury) • Source patient is HIV positive, asymptomatic with known low viral load • Optional when source patient is unknown or known with HIV risk factors	More severe percutaneous injury (large-bore hollow needle, deep punctures, visible blood on the device, needle was in the patient's artery or vein) • Source patient is HIV positive, asymptomatic with known low viral load • Source patient is HIV positive, symptomatic or AIDS with high viral load

Data from Centers for Disease Control and Prevention. (2005). Updated Public Health Service guidelines for the management of health-care worker exposure to HIV and recommendations for postexposure prophylaxis. *Morbidity and Mortality Weekly Report, 54*(RR-9), 1-22.

Basic PEP = Two drugs: (zidovudine plus lamivudine or emtricitabine); or (stavudine plus lamivudine or emtricitabine); or (tenofovir plus lamivudine or emtricitabine).

Expanded PEP = Three or more drugs: (zidovudine plus lamivudine or emtricitabine plus lopinavir/ritonavir); or (stavudine plus lamivudine or emtricitabine plus lopinavir/ritonavir); or (tenofovir plus lamivudine or emtricitabine plus lopinavir/ritonavir).

When PEP therapy is instituted, the recommended course is 28 days.

Chart 21-4 BEST PRACTICE FOR PATIENT SAFETY & QUALITY CARE

Recommendations for Preventing HIV Transmission by Health Care Workers

- Workers should adhere to Standard Precautions.
- Workers with exudative lesions or weeping dermatitis should not perform direct patient care or handle patient care equipment and devices used in invasive procedures.
- Workers must follow guidelines for disinfection and sterilization of reusable equipment used in invasive procedures.
- Workers infected with HIV are not restricted from practice of non–exposure-prone procedures, as long as they comply with Standard Precautions and sterilization and disinfection recommendations.
- Workers should identify exposure-prone procedures by institutions where they are performed.
- Workers who perform exposure-prone procedures should know their HIV antibody status.
- Workers who are infected with HIV should seek advice from an expert review panel before performing exposure-prone procedures to determine under what circumstances they may continue to practice these procedures. These circumstances would include notification of prospective patients of HIV positivity.

Modified from Centers for Disease Control. (1991). Recommendations for preventing transmission of human immunodeficiency virus and hepatitis B virus to patients during exposure-prone invasive procedures. *Morbidity and Mortality Weekly Report, 40*(RR-8), 1-9.

skin injury to the health care worker and the worker's blood is likely to make contact with the patient's body cavity, subcutaneous tissues, or mucous membranes. These recommendations aim to reduce the risk of HIV transmission to patients.

DECISION-MAKING CHALLENGE

Delegation/Supervision

One of the UAP on your unit is assigned to care for a 36-year-old man who has bone fractures and extensive open wounds as a result of a car crash. You find that she is reluctant to enter the patient's room and note that she is trying to exchange patient assignments with another one of the UAP. When you question her about this behavior, she tells you that although she does not know this man personally, he lives in her neighborhood and is known to be HIV positive. (This information is not documented anywhere in his inpatient medical record.) She says she does not want to touch anyone who may have AIDS.

1. What are the main issues with this situation?
2. Should this person continue to be assigned to this patient? Why or why not?
3. What should you teach this person about protecting herself while providing care for this patient?
4. What are your responsibilities in this situation?

evolve For suggested answer guidelines, go to http://evolve.elsevier.com/Iggy/.

Testing

Testing for HIV antibodies or other features of the virus is complex, requiring interpretation, counseling, and confidentiality. Testing plays a role in prevention because tests are a way of diagnosing HIV infection before immune changes or symptoms develop. A primary health care focus for testing is to teach those who test positive to modify their behaviors to prevent transmission to others. *Therefore all sexually active people should know their HIV status.* Chart 21-5 lists additional conditions for which HIV antibody testing is advised.

Pretest and post-test counseling must be performed by personnel trained in HIV issues. These counselors may be

Chart 21-5 PATIENT AND FAMILY EDUCATION GUIDE

CDC Recommendations for HIV Testing

You should be tested for AIDS if you fall within one or more of these groups:

- People with sexually transmitted disease
- Injection drug users
- People who consider themselves at risk
- Women of childbearing age with identifiable risks, including:
  - Used injection drugs
  - Engaged in prostitution
  - Had sexual partners who were infected or at risk
  - Had contact with men from countries with high HIV prevalence
  - Received a transfusion between 1978 and 1985
- People planning to get married
- People undergoing medical evaluation or treatment for manifestations that may be HIV related
- People admitted to hospitals
- People in correctional institutions such as jails and prisons
- Prostitutes and their customers

Modified from Centers for Disease Control. (1987). Public Health Service guidelines for counseling and antibody testing to prevent HIV infection and AIDS. *Morbidity and Mortality Weekly Report, 36*(31), 509-515.
CDC, Centers for Disease Control and Prevention.

nurses, physicians, social workers, health educators, or even lay educators who have specialized training. Counseling helps the patient make an informed decision about testing and provides an opportunity to teach risk reduction behaviors. Post-test counseling is needed to interpret the results, discuss risk reduction, and provide psychological support and health promotion information for the patient with a positive test result. People who test positive should also be counseled on how to inform sexual partners and those with whom they have shared needles. Testing methods, their accuracy, and indications are presented on pp. 373-374 in the Laboratory Assessment section.

Patient-Centered Collaborative Care

evolve ONLINE PHARM REVIEW

Assessment

The person who has HIV disease is monitored on a regular basis for changes in immune function or health status that indicate disease progression and warrant prophylaxis or intervention. Early in the course of HIV disease, yearly monitoring may be sufficient; however, as the disease progresses, routine monitoring and re-assessment are needed more frequently. This comprehensive and continuing assessment of the patient with HIV infection is crucial, because he or she may have problems related to disease in many organ systems. Assess subtle changes so that infections and other problems can be found early and treated.

History

Ask specifically about age, gender, occupation, and where the person lives. Thoroughly assess the current illness, including its nature, when it started, the severity of symptoms, associated problems, and any interventions to date. Ask the patient about when HIV infection was diagnosed and what clinical symptoms led to that diagnosis. Ask him or her to give a chronologic history of infections and clinical problems since the diagnosis. Assess his or her health history, including whether he or she received a blood transfusion between 1978 and 1985 in the United States (before routine blood testing for HIV contamination). Blood testing for HIV contamination is not consistently performed in all parts of the world and is a source of infection for immigrants. Ask the immigrant patient about his or her history of transfusion therapy before coming to the United States.

Ask the patient about sexual practices, sexually transmitted diseases (STDs), and any major infectious diseases, including tuberculosis and hepatitis. If the patient has hemophilia, ask about treatment with clotting factors. Determine whether the patient has engaged in past or present injection drug use, including needle exposure and needle sharing. Assess the patient's level of knowledge regarding the diagnosis, symptom management, diagnostic tests, treatments, community resources, and modes of HIV transmission. Also assess his or her understanding and use of safer sex practices. If knowledge deficits are found, provide the appropriate patient teaching.

Physical Assessment/Clinical Manifestations

HIV disease and AIDS are a progression continuum. The patient with HIV disease may either have few manifestations and problems or may have problems that are acute rather than chronically present. As the disease progresses, however, more health problems of long duration and greater severity occur. He or she may not realize that the disease is progressing. Assess for manifestations that cluster as symptoms of disease progression and may indicate that the treatment regimen needs to be modified (Chart 21-6).

Opportunistic Infections. The patient with HIV/AIDS often develops pathogenic infections and opportunistic infections. *Pathogenic infections* are caused by virulent organisms and occur even among people whose immune systems are functioning normally. *Opportunistic infections* are those caused by organisms that are present as part of the normal environment and are kept in check by normal immune function. Only when immune function is depressed are such organisms capable of causing infection.

Opportunistic infections occur because of the profound immune suppression of the person with HIV infection. They may result from primary infection or reactivation of a latent infection. Opportunistic infections account for many of the clinical symptoms observed in HIV infection and can be protozoan, fungal, bacterial, or viral. More than one infection may be present at the same time. The presence of opportunistic infections may represent disease progression or a temporary further reduction of immune status. *In either case, these infections can result in death if appropriate treatment is not started quickly.* Priority nursing actions when caring for a patient who is HIV positive are continually assessing for the presence of an opportunistic infection and monitoring the patient's response to therapy. Document all assessment findings in the patient's medical record, and report to the health care provider those manifestations that may indicate an infection.

Opportunistic infections do not pose a threat to the immunocompetent health care worker caring for a patient with HIV infection or AIDS. When the patient with HIV infection or AIDS has a pathogenic infection, however, health care personnel must use precautions appropriate to the specific disease to prevent disease spread. For example, when the person with HIV/AIDS also has tuberculosis at a transmissible stage, Airborne Precautions are needed in addition to Standard Precautions. See Chapter 25 for a more complete discussion on transmission precautions for specific infectious diseases.

Chart 21-6 KEY FEATURES
AIDS

IMMUNOLOGIC MANIFESTATIONS
- Low white blood cell counts:
  - CD4+/CD8+ ratio <2
  - CD4+ count <200/mm^3
- Hypergammaglobulinemia
- Opportunistic infections
- Lymphadenopathy
- Fatigue

INTEGUMENTARY MANIFESTATIONS
- Dry skin
- Poor wound healing
- Skin lesions
- Night sweats

RESPIRATORY MANIFESTATIONS
- Cough
- Shortness of breath

GASTROINTESTINAL MANIFESTATIONS
- Diarrhea
- Weight loss
- Nausea and vomiting

CENTRAL NERVOUS SYSTEM MANIFESTATIONS
- Confusion
- Dementia
- Headache
- Fever
- Visual changes
- Memory loss
- Personality changes
- Pain
- Seizures

OPPORTUNISTIC INFECTIONS
- Protozoal infections
  - *Pneumocystis jiroveci* pneumonia
  - Toxoplasmosis
  - Cryptosporidiosis
  - Isosporiasis
  - Microsporidiosis
  - Strongyloidiasis
  - Giardiasis
- Fungal infections
  - Candidiasis
  - Cryptococcosis
  - Histoplasmosis
  - Coccidioidomycosis
- Bacterial infections
  - Mycobacterium avium complex infection
  - Tuberculosis
  - Nocardiosis
- Viral infections
  - Cytomegalovirus infection
  - Herpes simplex virus infection
  - Varicella-zoster virus infection

MALIGNANCIES
- Kaposi's sarcoma
- Non-Hodgkin's lymphoma
- Hodgkin's lymphoma
- Invasive cervical carcinoma

Protozoal infections are common among patients with AIDS. *Pneumocystis jiroveci* pneumonia (PCP) is the most common opportunistic infection in persons infected with HIV. Assess for dyspnea on exertion, tachypnea, a persistent dry cough, and fever. The patient with PCP may report fatigue and weight loss. Listen to breath sounds for crackles that may be present on lung auscultation.

Toxoplasmosis encephalitis, caused by *Toxoplasma gondii,* is acquired through contact with contaminated cat feces or by ingesting infected, undercooked meat. Assess the patient for subtle changes in mental status, neurologic deficits, headaches, and fever. Other symptoms to assess include difficulties with speech, gait, and vision; seizures; lethargy; and confusion. Perform a comprehensive baseline mental status examination and monitor the patient to detect subtle changes.

Cryptosporidiosis is an intestinal infection caused by *Cryptosporidium* organisms. In AIDS, this illness ranges from a mild diarrhea to a severe wasting with electrolyte imbalance. Diarrhea may result in fluid loss of up to 15 to 20 L/day. Ask the patient about the presence of diarrhea and whether he or she has had an unplanned weight loss of 5 pounds or more.

Fungal infections occur by overgrowth of normal body flora. *Candida albicans* is part of the natural flora of the intestinal tract. In the person with AIDS, candidiasis (overgrowth of the *Candida* fungus) occurs because the weakened immune system can no longer control fungal growth. *Candida* stomatitis or esophagitis is a frequent finding in AIDS. Patients may report food tasting "funny," mouth pain, difficulty in swallowing, and retrosternal pain (pain behind the ribs). On examination of the mouth and the back of the throat, you may see cottage cheese–like, yellowish white plaques and inflammation. Esophagitis is diagnosed by endoscopic biopsy and culture. Women with HIV disease or AIDS may have persistent vaginal candidiasis with severe pruritus (itching), perineal irritation, and a thick, white vaginal discharge.

Cryptococcosis is a debilitating meningitis and is sometimes a widely spread infection in AIDS. It is caused by *Cryptococcus neoformans.* Ask about fever, headache, blurred vision, nausea and vomiting, nuchal rigidity (stiff neck), mild confusion, and other mental status changes. Some patients have seizures and other focal neurologic problems, or they may have mild symptoms of malaise and fever with or without headaches.

Histoplasmosis, caused by *Histoplasma capsulatum,* begins as a respiratory infection and progresses to widespread infection in the person with AIDS. Assess whether dyspnea, fever, cough, and weight loss are present. Check for enlargement of lymph nodes, the spleen, or the liver.

Bacterial infections are acquired from other people or sources and as overgrowth of skin flora. *Mycobacterium avium* complex (MAC) is the most common bacterial infection associated with AIDS. This problem is caused by *M. intracellulare* or *M. avium,* which infects the respiratory or GI tract. MAC is a systemic infection. Positive cultures may be obtained from lymph nodes, bone marrow, and blood. Assess for fever, debility, weight loss, malaise, and sometimes swollen lymph glands or organ disease.

Tuberculosis (TB), caused by *Mycobacterium tuberculosis,* occurs in 2% to 10% of persons with AIDS (CDC, 2007). More than 50% of all patients with AIDS and TB have extrapulmonary disease sites, including the central nervous system, bones, liver, spleen, skin, and intestinal tract. Ask about the presence of cough, dyspnea, chest pain, fever, chills, night sweats, weight loss, and anorexia. Symptoms of extrapulmonary infection vary with the site. *The person with TB and a CD4+ T-cell count below 200/mm³ may not have a positive TB skin test (purified protein derivative [PPD]) because of an inability to mount an immune response to the antigen, a condition known as* ***anergy.*** Other diagnostic tests include a chest x-ray, acid-fast sputum smear, and sputum culture.

The tuberculosis bacillus is spread by airborne routes. When particles from the patient's respiratory tract are aerosolized, anyone near the patient is at risk for inhaling the particles and the bacillus. Therefore the nurse or respiratory therapist who gives cough-inducing aerosol treatments, such as pentamidine isethionate, to patients with AIDS should be screened with a PPD skin test every 6 months to determine whether he or she has been infected with TB.

Recurrent pneumonia from bacterial infections occurs often among patients with AIDS. In the current CDC classification system for AIDS, two or more episodes of pneumonia in a 12-month period are an AIDS case definition. Assess for chest pain, productive cough, fever, and dyspnea.

Viral infection from a virus other than HIV is common among people with HIV disease and AIDS. Cytomegalovirus (CMV) can infect many sites in persons with AIDS, including the eye (CMV retinitis), respiratory and GI tracts, and the central nervous system. CMV infection can also cause many nonspecific problems such as fever, malaise, weight loss, fatigue, and swollen lymph nodes. CMV retinitis impairs vision, ranging from slight impairment to total blindness. It can also cause diarrhea, abdominal bloating and discomfort, and weight loss. Ask the patient whether he or she has any of these manifestations. In addition, CMV can cause encephalitis, pneumonitis, adrenalitis, hepatitis, and disseminated infection.

Herpes simplex virus (HSV) infections in people with HIV disease or AIDS occur in the perirectal, oral, and genital areas. The manifestations are more widespread and of longer duration among patients with HIV/AIDS than among those who are immunocompetent. Numbness or tingling at the site of infection occurs up to 24 hours before blisters form. Lesions are painful, with chronic open areas after blisters rupture. Assess for fever, pain, bleeding, and lymph node enlargement in the affected area. Other manifestations include headache, myalgia, and malaise.

Varicella-zoster virus (VZV) infection (shingles) is usually not a new infection for people with AIDS. This virus, present in the nerve ganglia of many people, causes chickenpox. When people who have had chickenpox previously are immunocompromised, VZV leaves the nerve ganglia and enters body fluids and other tissue areas, causing shingles. Ask whether the patient has pain and burning along sensory nerve tracts (see Chapter 43 for the dermatomes of sensory nerve locations). Examine the skin for fluid-filled blisters with or without crusts. Other problems include headache and low-grade fever.

Malignancies. The weakened immune response increases the risk for cancer. Cancers occurring with AIDS include Kaposi's sarcoma, Hodgkin's lymphoma, non-Hodgkin's lymphoma, and invasive cervical cancer (CDC, 2007).

Kaposi's sarcoma (KS) is the most common AIDS-related malignancy, occurring in 1% to 21% of patients with AIDS. The risk for KS appears to be related to co-infection with some types of herpes virus.

KS develops as small, purplish brown, raised lesions that are usually not painful or itchy. The lesions can occur anywhere on the body. Most patients with KS have skin or mucous membrane lesions. In some patients, lesions develop in the lymph nodes, intestinal tract, or lungs. KS is diagnosed by biopsy and histologic examination of the lesion. Assess KS lesions for number, size, location, and whether they are intact, and monitor their progression.

Malignant lymphomas occurring with AIDS are non-Hodgkin's B-cell lymphomas, such as Burkitt's lymphoma, immunoblastic lymphoma, and primary brain lymphoma. Manifestations include weight loss, fever, and night sweats.

Endocrine Changes. Patients with HIV disease may have disease-related endocrine problems, such as gonadal dysfunction, body shape changes, adrenal insufficiency, diabetes mellitus, and elevated triglycerides and cholesterol (Table 21-2).

Many HIV-positive men have low testosterone levels, and HIV-positive women often have irregular menstrual cycles. With this gonadal dysfunction comes a decrease in body muscle mass for both genders and a change in libido.

Body shape changes from fat redistribution or lipodystrophy are common in patients receiving antiretroviral therapies, especially protease inhibitors. Manifestations include "buffalo humps" or cervical (neck) fat development and large abdominal fat accumulations. Other body areas, such as the face, arms, and legs, have a wasted appearance.

TABLE 21-2 Endocrine Complications of HIV Infection or Treatment

Endocrine Gland	Problems/Dysfunction
Gonads	Decreased testosterone Reduced libido Reduced fertility Decreased muscle mass Decreased estrogen Reduced libido Premature menopause Decreased muscle mass
Adrenal cortex	Increased cortisol Fat redistribution Decreased muscle mass Decreased cortisol Adrenal insufficiency Hypoglycemia Hyperkalemia Hypotension Fatigue Weight loss
Pancreas	Reduced exocrine function Fatty food intolerance Cholelithiasis Pancreatitis Reduced endocrine function Diabetes mellitus Hyperlipidemia

Adrenal dysfunction can result from the glands being infected by opportunistic infections (cytomegalovirus, *M. avium*, or tuberculosis), resulting in adrenal insufficiency. This problem manifests as fatigue, weight loss, nausea, vomiting, low blood pressure, and electrolyte disturbances and can be life threatening.

Patients taking protease inhibitors have a higher-than-expected incidence of type 1 diabetes and hyperlipidemia. These problems are seen even among patients who have no other risks for these problems or the associated heart disease.

Other Clinical Manifestations. All body systems are affected to some degree in AIDS. *AIDS dementia complex (ADC),* also called *HIV-associated dementia complex,* refers to the manifestations of central nervous system involvement. ADC occurs in about 70% of people with AIDS. It is a result of infection of cells within the central nervous system by HIV. ADC causes cognitive, motor, and behavioral impairments. Manifestations range from barely noticeable to severe dementia. (See Chapter 44 for more discussion on dementia.)

Some neurologic problems may be a result of HIV infection or drug side effects, including peripheral neuropathies and myopathies. Assess for symptoms of peripheral neuropathies, which include paresthesias and burning sensations, pain, and gait changes. Myopathies are accompanied by leg weakness, ataxia, and muscle pain.

AIDS wasting syndrome is not due to any single factor. It may be a result of altered metabolism from cancer or infection. Diarrhea, malabsorption, anorexia, and oral and esophageal lesions can all contribute to persistent and sometimes extreme weight loss, and the patient may appear quite emaciated.

Skin changes include dry, itchy, irritated skin and many types of rashes. Folliculitis, eczema, or psoriasis may occur. Ask the patient about skin sensation changes, and examine any rash or irritation. When the platelet count is low, petechiae or bleeding gums may be present.

Psychosocial Assessment

Psychosocial data collection for a patient with AIDS is very important. Ask about the patient's social support system, including family, significant others, and friends. To protect confidentiality, learn who in this support system is aware of the patient's diagnosis so that it is not inadvertently mentioned. Some patients, because of fear of discrimination, are quite selective about whom they tell. Health care professionals must respect the patient's choices as much as possible without compromising care. Offer resources to help with disclosure to sexual partners or significant others.

The patient may be closest to a lover or a friend who is not legally recognized as next of kin. Obtain the name and telephone number of that person, and learn whether a health care proxy or durable power-of-attorney document has been signed.

Ask about the patient's ADLs, as well as any changes that may have occurred since the diagnosis. Also assess his or her employment status and occupation, immigration status, social activities and hobbies, living arrangements, and financial resources, including health insurance. Also ask whether he or she uses drugs, including alcohol, supplements, opioids, benzodiazepines, or crystal methamphetamine.

To plan care and monitor changes, assess the patient's anxiety level, mood, cognitive ability, and level of energy. Ask about any experiences with discrimination and how they were handled. After assessing the patient's level of self-esteem and changes in body image, work with him or her to identify strengths and coping strategies. Gather information about any suicidal ideation, depression, or other psychological problems. Also ask about the use of support groups or other community resources.

The patient with HIV infection has less energy as the disease progresses. Many factors contribute to this energy loss, and many cannot be treated. Pace interviews, assessments, and intervention activities to match his or her energy level. When he or she is greatly fatigued, postpone or eliminate nonurgent tests or care activities.

Laboratory Assessment

Lymphocyte Counts. Lymphocyte counts are performed as part of a complete blood count (CBC) with differential (see Chapter 19). The normal white blood cell (WBC) count is between 4500 and 11,000 cells/mm^3, with a differential of about 30% to 40% lymphocytes (an absolute number of 1500 to 4500). Patients with AIDS are often leukopenic, with a WBC count of less than 3500 cells/mm^3, and lymphopenic (<1500 lymphocytes/mm^3).

CD4+ T-cell and CD8+ T-cell counts and percentages are an important part of an immune profile. People with HIV disease usually have a lower-than-normal number of CD4+ T-cells. Some patients with AIDS have fewer than 100 cells/mm^3 (normal: 500 to 1600 cells/mm^3), whereas the number of CD8+ T-cells remains normal. The normal ratio of CD4+ to CD8+ T-cells is 2:1. In HIV disease and AIDS, because of the low number of CD4+ T-cells, this ratio is low. Low CD4+ T-cell counts and a low ratio are associated with increased manifestations of disease.

Antibody Tests. These tests are used to measure the patient's response to the virus (the antigen) rather than to measure parts of the virus. When the body is infected with HIV, the normal response is to make an antibody to the infecting agent. This antibody is usually made 3 weeks to 3 months after the infection first occurs, although in some people antibodies are not made until 36 months after initial infection.

Thus antibody tests for HIV antibody can be measured by enzyme-linked immunosorbent assay (ELISA) and Western blot analysis. False-negative results (incorrectly indicating the absence of HIV infection) have been reported early in the infection, in people with cancer, and in people receiving long-term immunosuppressive therapy.

ELISA is an inexpensive and accurate test. The patient's serum is mixed with HIV grown in culture. If the patient has antibodies to HIV, they bind to the HIV antigens and can be detected (a positive test). However, this test can be negative even when the person has HIV infection if the test is performed before antibodies are made in sufficient amounts. The period between when a person is first infected with the virus and when viral replication is occurring but the immune system has not yet started making antibodies is called the "window period." *This means that if the patient has an episode of unprotected sex with an HIV-positive person one night and comes in for testing a week later, the ELISA will be negative even though the patient may have active HIV. Thus testing during the window does not provide useful information.*

False-positive test results (incorrectly indicating HIV infection) occur in about 0.1% (1 of 1000) of those tested with ELISA. False-positive results sometimes occur in pregnant women and women who have had children, injection drug users, people who have had malaria, patients with lymphomas, and other conditions. Therefore anyone who has a positive ELISA needs to have additional testing to confirm or rule out infection.

Western blot is used to confirm the diagnosis when the results of an ELISA are positive. This test is more sophisticated and expensive than the ELISA. The Western blot detects serum antibodies to four specific major HIV antigens. A positive Western blot result is based on the presence of antibodies to at least two of the major HIV antigens.

The result is considered inconclusive if two of the major antibodies are not detected but other antibodies to HIV are. The person should then be retested. *If a person has a positive test result for HIV antibodies, it does not mean that he or she has AIDS—only that he or she has been infected with the virus.*

Both the ELISA and Western blot are blood-based tests. This requires special equipment and trained personnel to test for HIV infection. Some HIV testing is simpler, using techniques that are not blood-based so that testing can be done anywhere, even at home. One test involves oral testing for HIV antibody. This test uses a device that is placed against the gum and cheek for 2 minutes. Fluid (not saliva) is drawn into an absorbable pad, which, in an HIV-positive person, contains HIV-specific antibodies. The pad is placed in a solution; a positive result shows a change similar to a positive result in a urine pregnancy test. Total testing time is about 20 minutes. This test has the same accuracy as blood testing and can provide results quickly. If results are positive for HIV, a blood test is needed to confirm the result.

Home test kits require that a drop of blood be placed on a test card with a special code number. The card is mailed to a laboratory where the blood is tested for HIV antibodies. A special telephone number is called and the code entered. Test results are then given.

Viral Load Testing. **Viral load testing** (also called *viral burden testing*) measures the presence of HIV viral genetic material (RNA) or other viral proteins in the patient's blood rather than the body's response to the virus. These tests are quantitative and indicate the level of viral burden or viral load. Such tests are useful in monitoring disease progression and treatment effectiveness.

Quantitative RNA assays are used for quantitative viral load testing. These assays include the reverse transcriptase–polymerase chain reaction (RT-PCR), the branched DNA (bDNA) method, and the nucleic acid sequence–based assay (NASBA). All three assays use gene amplification to determine the amount of HIV RNA present in a patient's serum, and all have a specificity of 100%. Even if only a few infected cells are present in a serum sample, tiny amounts of the HIV RNA are amplified by these methods to allow detection and diagnosis in people who have no indication of infection. These tests are used to monitor therapy effectiveness and as indicators of the need to change drug regimens.

Other Laboratory Tests. Other laboratory tests monitor the overall health of the patient and detect or diagnose any infections or other problems related to HIV disease. These tests include blood chemistries, a CBC with differential and platelets, toxoplasmosis antibody titer, liver function tests, a serologic test for syphilis (STS), and antigens to hepatitis A, hepatitis B, and hepatitis C. Tests to further evaluate the immune profile of a patient may include bone marrow aspiration with biopsy and cultures.

Other Diagnostic Assessment

Other diagnostic tests are performed on the basis of the patient's manifestations. Such tests may include testing stool for ova and parasites; biopsies of the skin, lymph nodes, lungs, liver, GI tract, or brain; a chest x-ray; gallium scans; bronchoscopy, endoscopy, or colonoscopy; liver and spleen scans; computed tomography scans; pulmonary function tests; and arterial blood gas analysis.

DECISION-MAKING CHALLENGE

Coordination of Care

The patient is a 32-year-old Hispanic nurse from your unit who is admitted for surgery to repair a fractured wrist sustained in a fall while she was working at the hospital. She divorced her first husband, who was unfaithful to her, after 5 years. She recently remarried and is hoping to start a family in the near future. She tells you she has symptoms of a vaginal yeast infection and reports that this is her sixth yeast infection in 7 months even though she has treated herself each time with an over-the-counter antifungal product. Her preoperative blood work indicates a lower-than-normal total white blood count and a low lymphocyte count.

1. In view of the laboratory results and her yeast infections, what other assessment information should you obtain?
2. Should you inform this patient at this time about her laboratory results? Why or why not?
3. Should you inform the surgeon about these results? Why or why not?
4. What should you change with regard to providing care to this patient until you know her HIV status?
5. What questions should you ask about this patient's sexual activity?
6. How should you approach this patient about her HIV status?

evolve For suggested answer guidelines, go to http://evolve.elsevier.com/Iggy/.

▪ *Analysis*

Common Nursing Diagnoses and Collaborative Problems

The most common nursing diagnoses for patients with AIDS are:

1. Risk for Infection related to immune deficiency
2. Impaired Gas Exchange related to anemia, respiratory infection (*P. jiroveci* pneumonia [PCP], cytomegalovirus [CMV] pneumonitis), pulmonary Kaposi's sarcoma (KS), anemia, fatigue, or pain
3. Acute Pain or Chronic Pain related to neuropathy, myelopathy, cancer, or infection
4. Imbalanced Nutrition: Less Than Body Requirements related to high metabolic need, nausea and vomiting, diarrhea, difficulty chewing or swallowing, or anorexia
5. Diarrhea related to infection, food intolerance, or drugs
6. Impaired Skin Integrity related to KS, infection, altered nutritional state, incontinence, immobility, hyperthermia, or cancer
7. Disturbed Thought Processes related to AIDS dementia complex (ADC), central nervous system infection, or cancer
8. Chronic Low Self-Esteem related to changes in body image, decreased self-esteem, or helplessness
9. Social Isolation related to stigma, virus transmissibility, infection control practices, or fear

The primary collaborative problem is Potential for Infection (processed in the Risk for Infection section).

Additional Nursing Diagnoses and Collaborative Problems

In addition to the common nursing diagnoses and collaborative problems, patients with AIDS may have one or more of these:

- Activity Intolerance related to fatigue, discomfort, central nervous system defect, weakness, or anemia
- Risk for Injury related to central nervous system defect, mental status changes, depression, or thrombocytopenia
- Disturbed Sensory Perception (Visual) related to CMV retinitis or blindness
- Sleep Deprivation related to pain, discomfort, anxiety, or depression
- Ineffective Coping related to the diagnosis of AIDS
- Disabled Family Coping related to the diagnosis of AIDS
- Grieving related to anticipated loss of role and function or impending death

Planning and Implementation

Risk for Infection

The patient with AIDS is susceptible to opportunistic infections and other infections because of immune deficiency secondary to HIV infection.

NOC **Planning: Expected Outcomes.** The patient is expected to remain free of opportunistic diseases and other infections. Indicators include:

- Absence of chills, fever, or temperature instability
- Absence of purulent drainage or sputum
- Absence of diarrhea
- Absence of chest x-ray infiltration
- Maintenance of white blood cell (WBC) count within the patient's normal range

Interventions. The person who has HIV infection and is immunocompromised is at greater risk for any type of infection. Teach him or her to avoid exposure to infection (Chart 21-7). Chart 21-8 outlines best practices for prevention of infection in a hospitalized immunocompromised patient. Some strategies are investigational, including drug therapy and immune function enhancement.

Drug Therapy. Some drugs have demonstrated antiretroviral effects; however, *it is important to remember that antiretroviral therapy only inhibits viral replication and does not kill the virus.* Treatment with only one antiretroviral agent, known as *monotherapy,* promotes drug resistance and does not improve the duration or quality of life for the patient with HIV/AIDS. Instead, multiple drugs are used together in regimens popularly called "cocktails." These regimens consist of combinations of different types of antiretroviral agents. This approach is termed *highly active antiretroviral therapy (HAART)* and is showing good results as measured by reduced viral load and improved CD4+ T-cell counts.

An important issue with HAART is the development of drug-resistant mutations in the HIV organism. When resistance develops, viral replication is no longer suppressed by the drugs. Several factors contribute to the development of drug resistance to HAART, with the most important being missed doses of drugs. When doses are missed, the blood drug concentrations become lower than what are needed for inhibition of viral replication (often called *the inhibitory concentration*). When this concentration is too low, the organism can replicate and produce new organisms that are resistant to the drugs being used. *Therefore it is critical to ensure that HAART drugs are not missed, delayed, or administered in lower-than-prescribed doses in the inpatient setting. Teach patients the importance of taking their drugs exactly as prescribed to maintain the effectiveness of HAART drugs. Even a few missed doses per month can promote drug resistance.*

The main actions of each drug category are explained in the following pages. Representative drugs in each category are presented in Chart 21-9. Drawbacks to HIV/AIDS drug

Chart 21-7 PATIENT AND FAMILY EDUCATION GUIDE

Prevention of Infection

During the times when your white blood cell counts are low:

- Avoid crowds and other large gatherings of people who might be ill.
- Do not share personal toilet articles, such as toothbrushes, toothpaste, washcloths, or deodorant sticks, with others.
- If possible, bathe daily, using an antimicrobial soap. If total bathing is not possible, wash the armpits, groin, genitals, and anal area twice a day with an antimicrobial soap.
- Clean your toothbrush daily by either running it through the dishwasher or rinsing it in liquid laundry bleach.
- Wash your hands thoroughly with an antimicrobial soap before you eat or drink, after touching a pet, after shaking hands with anyone, as soon as you come home from any outing, and after using the toilet.
- Eat a low-bacteria diet, and avoid salads; raw fruit and vegetables; undercooked meat, fish, and eggs; and pepper and paprika.
- Wash dishes between use with hot, sudsy water, or use a dishwasher.
- Do not drink water, milk, juice, or other cold liquids that have been standing for longer than an hour.
- Do not reuse cups and glasses without washing.
- Do not change pet litter boxes. If unavoidable, use gloves and wash hands immediately.
- Avoid turtles and reptiles as pets.
- Do not feed pets raw or undercooked meat.
- Take your temperature at least once a day and whenever you do not feel well.
- Report any of the following signs or symptoms of infection to your physician immediately:
  - Temperature greater than 100° F (38° C)
  - Persistent cough (with or without sputum)
  - Pus or foul-smelling drainage from any open skin area or normal body opening
  - Presence of a boil or abscess
  - Urine that is cloudy or foul smelling or that causes burning on urination
- Take all prescribed drugs.
- Do not dig in the garden or work with houseplants.
- Wear a condom (if you are a man) when having sex. If you are a woman having sex with a male partner, ensure that he wears a condom.
- Avoid travel to areas of the world with poor sanitation or less-than-adequate health care facilities.

Chart 21-8 BEST PRACTICE FOR PATIENT SAFETY & QUALITY CARE

Care of the Hospitalized Immunosuppressed Patient

- Place the patient in a private room whenever possible.
- Use good handwashing technique or use alcohol-based hand rubs before touching the patient or any of his or her belongings.
- Ensure that the patient's room and bathroom are cleaned at least once each day.
- Do not use supplies from common areas for neutropenic patients. For example, keep a sleeve or box of paper cups in his or her room and do not share this box with any other patient. Other articles include drinking straws, plastic knives and forks, dressing materials, gloves, and bandages.
- Limit the number of health care personnel entering the patient's room.
- Monitor vital signs every 4 hours, including temperature.
- Inspect the patient's mouth at least every 8 hours.
- Inspect the patient's skin and mucous membranes (especially the anal area) for the presence of fissures and abscesses at least every 8 hours.
- Inspect open areas, such as IV sites, every 4 hours for manifestations of infection.
- Change wound dressings daily.
- Obtain specimens of all suspicious areas for culture (as specified by the agency), and promptly notify the physician.
- Assist the patient in performing coughing and deep-breathing exercises.
- Encourage activity at a level appropriate for the patient's current health status.
- Change IV tubing daily.
- Keep frequently used equipment in the room for use with this patient only (e.g., blood pressure cuff, stethoscope, thermometer).
- Limit visitors to healthy adults.
- Use strict aseptic technique for all invasive procedures.
- Avoid the use of indwelling urinary catheters.
- Keep fresh flowers and potted plants out of the patient's room.
- Teach the patient to eat a low-bacteria diet (e.g., avoiding raw fruits and vegetables; undercooked meat, eggs, and fish; pepper and paprika as seasonings sprinkled on food right before eating).

Chart 21-9 COMMON EXAMPLES OF DRUG THERAPY

HIV Infection

Drug/Usual Dosage	Physiologic Purpose	Nursing Interventions	Rationale
NUCLEOSIDE ANALOG REVERSE TRANSCRIPTASE INHIBITORS (NARTIs)			
Abacavir (Ziagen) 300 mg orally twice daily	Suppress viral replication in infected cells by inhibiting the activity of reverse transcriptase.	Assess for flu-like symptoms (fever, rash, headache, nausea, sore throat, fatigue, shortness of breath).	These are manifestations of a hypersensitivity reaction to this drug.
Combivir (zidovudine 300 mg + lamivudine 150 mg) 1 tab orally twice daily		Same as with zidovudine and lamivudine individually.	This combination agent contains both drugs.
Didanosine (ddl, Videx 125-300 mg orally twice daily; Videx EC 400 mg orally once daily)		Teach the patient to take this drug on an empty stomach.	Food inhibits the absorption of this drug.
Emtricitabine (Emtriva) 200 mg orally daily		Teach the patient to avoid eating fatty foods while on this drug.	The drug in combination with a high-fat diet can cause pancreatitis.
Epzicom (*abacavir* 600 mg + lamivudine 300 mg) 1 tab daily		Same as with abacavir and lamivudine individually.	This combination agent contains both drugs.
Lamivudine (Epivir, 3TC🍁)		Teach the patient to avoid eating fatty foods while on this drug.	The drug in combination with a high-fat diet can cause pancreatitis.
Stavudine (d4T, Zerit) 40 mg orally twice daily		Assess vision, hearing, touch, and balance. Teach the patient to change positions slowly and watch the floor or ground when walking.	The drug induces peripheral neuropathy, causing orthostatic hypotension, reduced touch sensation, and decreased balance.
Tenofovir (Viread) 250 mg orally daily		Teach the patient who is also prescribed didanosine to separate these drugs by at least 2 hours.	This drug can boost the blood levels of didanosine to toxic levels in some people.

CBC, Complete blood count; *CNS,* central nervous system.

Chart 21-9 COMMON EXAMPLES OF DRUG THERAPY

HIV Infection—cont'd

Drug/Usual Dosage	Physiologic Purpose	Nursing Interventions	Rationale
NUCLEOSIDE ANALOG REVERSE TRANSCRIPTASE INHIBITORS (NARTIs)—cont'd			
Trizivir (three drugs in one) (zidovudine 300 mg + lamivudine 150 mg + abacavir 300 mg) 1 tab orally twice daily		Same as with zidovudine, lamivudine, and abacavir individually.	This combination agent contains all three drugs.
Truvada (tenofovir 300 mg + emtricitabine 200 mg) 1 tab orally daily		Same as with tenofovir and emtricitabine individually.	This combination agent contains both drugs.
Zidovudine (Retrovir) 300 mg orally twice daily		Teach the patient to take care when driving and avoid operating heavy machinery.	Drug crosses the blood-brain barrier, causing dizziness.
		Monitor CBC, hepatic and renal function.	The drug suppresses bone marrow function and can be both renal and liver toxic.
NON-NUCLEOSIDE REVERSE TRANSCRIPTASE INHIBITORS (NNRTIs)			
Delavirdine (Rescriptor) 400 mg orally three times daily	Suppress viral replication in infected cells by inhibiting the activity of reverse transcriptase.	Teach the patient who also takes antacids to take this drug either 1 hour before the antacid or 2 hours after the antacid.	Antacids inhibit the absorption of this drug from the stomach.
Etravirine 200 mg orally twice daily		Teach the patient who is also taking a protease inhibitor to watch for more side effects.	This new drug appears to have some interactions with the protease inhibitors.
Efavirenz (Sustiva) 600 mg orally daily		Warn the patient about dizziness, insomnia, and nightmares while taking this drug.	Drug crosses blood-brain barrier and can induce CNS manifestations.
Nevirapine (Viramune) 200 mg orally twice daily		Instruct the patient to stop the drug if a rash develops.	Allergic reactions to this drug are common.
		Instruct the patient to report persistent abdominal pain.	This drug can induce liver problems.
PROTEASE INHIBITORS			
Atazanavir (Reyataz) 300 mg orally daily	Prevents viral replication and release of viral particles by inhibiting viral protease.	Teach the patient to take this drug with food.	Food reduces GI side effects and enhances absorption of this drug.
		Teach the patient to check his or her skin and sclera weekly for a yellowish tint and report its presence.	The drug can increase blood bilirubin levels, which tint the skin and sclera with a yellow color.
Darunavir (Prezista) 600 mg orally twice daily		Monitor the patient's blood glucose levels.	The drug can increase blood glucose levels and make diabetes worse.
		Ask whether the patient is allergic to any drugs containing sulfa.	There is some cross-reactivity and allergic reactions to this drug in people who have sulfa allergies.
Fosamprenavir (Lexiva) 1400 mg orally twice daily		Monitor serum lipid levels and blood pressure.	This drug can induce hyperlipidemia and atherosclerosis.
Indinavir (Crixivan) 800 mg orally every 8 hours		Teach the patient to take this drug on an empty stomach.	Food inhibits the absorption of this drug.
		Teach the patient to check his or her skin and sclera weekly for a yellowish tint and report its presence.	The drug can increase blood bilirubin levels, which tint the skin and sclera with a yellow color.
		Teach the patient to report flank pain or bloody urine.	The drug can induce kidney stones.

Continued

Chart 21-9 COMMON EXAMPLES OF DRUG THERAPY

HIV Infection—cont'd

Drug/Usual Dosage	Physiologic Purpose	Nursing Interventions	Rationale
PROTEASE INHIBITORS—cont'd			
Kaletra (lopinavir 133 mg + ritonavir 33 mg) 2 capsules orally twice daily		Teach the patient to take this drug with food.	Food reduces GI side effects and enhances absorption of this drug.
		Ask whether the patient is allergic to any drugs containing sulfa.	There is some cross-reactivity and allergic reactions to this drug in people who have sulfa allergies.
Nelfinavir (Viracept) 625 mg orally every 12 hours		Teach the patient to take this drug with food.	This drug causes diarrhea, which is lessened when taken with food.
		Monitor the patient's blood glucose levels.	The drug can increase blood glucose levels and make diabetes worse.
Ritonavir (Norvir) 600 mg orally every 12 hours		Teach the patient to take this drug with food.	Food reduces GI side effects and enhances absorption of this drug.
Saquinavir (Invirase) 600 mg orally every 12 hours		Teach the patient to take this drug with or just after a high-fat, high-calorie meal.	This drug is best absorbed with a fatty meal.
		Warn the patient to avoid direct sunlight, wear protective clothing when out of doors, and use sunscreen.	This drug increases skin sun sensitivity and increases the risk for severe sunburn even for patients with dark skin.
FUSION INHIBITORS			
Enfuvirtide (Fuzeon) 90 mg subcutaneously twice daily	Prevents HIV infection by blocking the ability of gp41 to fuse with the host cell.	Teach the patient how to self-administer subcutaneous injections.	This drug is available only as a parenteral agent.
		Teach the patient to rotate injection sites.	The risk for infection and lipodystrophy are increased when the site is not rotated.
ENTRY INHIBITORS			
Maraviroc (Selzentry) 300 mg orally twice daily	This new type drug prevents HIV infection by blocking the CCR5 receptor on CD4+ T-lymphocytes.	Teach patients who are also taking an antihypertensive drug that severe hypotension is possible.	This drug lowers blood pressure.
		Monitor liver function tests.	Some liver toxicities are possible while taking this drug.
INTEGRASE INHIBITORS			
Raltegravir (Isentress) 400 mg orally twice daily	Prevents viral protein synthesis and viral replication by inhibiting the enzyme *integrase,* which is needed to insert the viral DNA into the host cell's human DNA.	Warn the patient about diarrhea.	Common side effect for this drug.

therapy include the expense of the drugs, side effects, food and timing requirements, and the number of daily drugs. The daily regimen is lifelong and burdensome.

Nucleoside analog reverse transcriptase inhibitors (NARTIs) have a similar structure to the four nucleoside bases of DNA. These drugs are converted in the virally infected cell into a "counterfeit" form of a nucleotide base and compete with the actual nucleotide for placement in DNA. Thus they suppress production of reverse transcriptase (RT) and inhibit viral DNA synthesis and replication. This class of anti-HIV agents includes zidovudine (Retrovir), didanosine (ddI, Videx), zalcitabine (ddC, HIVID), lamivudine (Epivir, 3TC♣), stavudine (d4T, Zerit), tenofovir (Viread), emtricitabine (Emtriva), and abacavir (Ziagen).

Non-nucleoside reverse transcriptase inhibitors (NNRTIs) also inhibit synthesis of reverse transcriptase. These drugs suppress viral replication but do not kill the virus. These drugs include nevirapine (Viramune), delavirdine (Rescriptor), efavirenz (Sustiva), and etravirine.

Protease inhibitors block the HIV protease enzyme, preventing viral replication and release of viral particles. The HIV initially produces all of its proteins, including the ones needed to move viral particles out of a cell, in one long strand. For the proteins to be active, this large protein must be broken down into separate smaller proteins through the action of the viral enzyme *HIV protease.* The protease inhibitor drugs, when taken into an HIV-infected cell, make the protease enzyme work on the drug rather than on the initial large protein. Thus active proteins are not produced and the viral particles cannot leave the cell to infect other cells. Drugs include ritonavir (Norvir), indinavir (Crixivan), saquinavir (Invirase), nelfinavir (Viracept), lopinavir (Kaletra), atazanavir (Reyataz), fosamprenavir (Lexiva), and darunavir (Prezista).

Fusion inhibitors work by blocking the fusion of HIV with a host cell by blocking the ability of gp41 to fuse with the host cell. Remember, after gp120 and the CD4+ T-cell interact, the next step is for gp41 to fuse HIV and the host cell together for transfer of genetic information. Without fusion, infection of new cells does not occur. The major drug in this category is enfuvirtide (Fuzeon).

Entry inhibitors are a new type of anti-HIV drug. They work to prevent infection by blocking the CCR5 receptor on CD4+ T-cells. Remember, for HIV to enter the cell, the virus' gp120 must bind to the CD4 receptor and its gp41 must bind to the CCR5 receptor or to the CXCR4 receptor (see Fig. 21-3). Viral binding to both receptors is needed to enter the cell. So, this class of drug prevents cellular infection with HIV. The major drug in this category is maraviroc (Selzentry).

Integrase inhibitors are the newest type of anti-HIV drug. They work to prevent infection by inhibiting the enzyme *integrase,* which is needed to insert the viral DNA into the host cell's human DNA. Without this action, viral proteins are not made and viral replication is inhibited. The major drug in this category is raltegravir (Isentress).

Immune Enhancement. Research is being conducted to evaluate treatments that may enhance or replenish the immune system of patients with AIDS. Some of these methods include bone marrow transplantation, lymphocyte transfusion, and infusions of lymphokines, particularly interleukin-2, and other biological response modifiers.

Complementary and Alternative Therapies. Complementary therapies are often used by people with HIV/AIDS. Such therapies include vitamins, shark cartilage, and botanical products available at health food stores. The usefulness of these products has yet to be established through well-controlled clinical trials. In addition, some botanicals alter the effects of prescription drugs. Ask the patient which botanicals are being used, and check with the pharmacist to determine known drug interactions with HAART therapy.

Impaired Gas Exchange

NOC **Planning: Expected Outcomes.** The patient is expected to maintain adequate oxygenation and perfusion and to have minimal dyspnea. Indicators include:

- Rate and depth of respiration within the normal range
- Pulse oximetry within the normal range
- Absence of cyanosis or pallor

Interventions. The nurse or respiratory therapist uses drug therapy, respiratory support and maintenance, comfort, and rest.

Drug therapy is a mainstay for gas exchange problems resulting from infection. Appropriate drug therapy is started after an infectious or other cause for respiratory difficulty is identified. A common respiratory infection among people with HIV disease or AIDS is *P. jiroveci* pneumonia (PCP). The treatment of choice for PCP is trimethoprim/sulfamethoxazole (Apo-Sulfatrim♣, Bactrim, Cotrim, Septra). Many patients with AIDS have adverse reactions to this drug, including nausea, vomiting, hyponatremia, rashes, fever, leukopenia, thrombocytopenia, and hepatitis.

Pentamidine isethionate (Pentacarinat♣, Pentam), usually given IV or IM, is also used to treat PCP. Aerosolized pentamidine isethionate is used for patients with CD4+ T-cell counts below 200 and for those who have already had PCP.

Other drug therapies include dapsone (Avlosulfon) and atovaquone (Mepron), which can be used as therapy for existing PCP or as prophylaxis. For moderate to severe PCP, steroids may be used to reduce the inflammation.

Respiratory support and maintenance are important to maintain respiratory function and avoid complications. Assess the respiratory rate, rhythm, and depth; breath sounds; and vital signs and monitor for cyanosis at least every 8 hours. Apply oxygen and humidify the room as prescribed. Also monitor mechanical ventilation, perform suctioning and chest physical therapy as needed, and evaluate blood gas results.

Comfort can help improve gas exchange. Assess the patient's comfort. The patient with difficulty breathing may be more comfortable with the head of the bed elevated. Pace activities to reduce shortness of breath and fatigue. Provide psychological support during periods of breathing difficulty.

Rest and activity changes are needed when gas exchange is impaired. Most patients with HIV/AIDS have fatigue, especially when respiratory problems also are present. Certain treatments worsen fatigue. Consult with the patient to pace activities to conserve energy. Guide the patient in active and passive range-of-motion (ROM) exercises. Schedule non–time-critical activities, such as bathing, so that he or she is not fatigued at mealtime.

Pain

The patient with severe HIV disease or AIDS often has pain from many causes. Pain can result from enlarged organs stretching the viscera or compressing nerves. Tumor invasion of bone and other tissues can cause pain. Many patients with

AIDS have peripheral neuropathy–induced pain from the disease or drug therapies. Many have generalized joint and muscle pain.

NOC **Planning: Expected Outcomes.** The patient is expected to achieve an acceptable level of comfort and pain reduction. Indicators include:

- Reporting that pain is controlled
- Absence of indicators of acute pain (increased heart rate and blood pressure)
- Absence of facial grimacing, teeth clenching
- Willingness to move and participate in self-care

Interventions. Drug therapy and other approaches are used together to manage pain in the patient with HIV/AIDS, depending on the cause of the pain.

Comfort measures include the use of pressure-relieving mattress pads, warm baths or other forms of hydrotherapy, massage, and applying heat or cold to painful areas to help reduce pain levels, with or without drug therapy. Take care when moving or assisting the patient. Use lift sheets to avoid pulling or grasping the patient with joint pain. The patient may be thin and have poor circulation, contributing to pain and discomfort. Help the patient change positions often.

Drug therapy with different classes of drugs is used to manage pain from different causes. For arthralgia and myalgia, NSAIDs may reduce inflammation and increase comfort without inducing drowsiness. The neuropathic pain of peripheral neuropathy may respond best to tricyclic antidepressants such as amitriptyline (Elavil) or to anticonvulsant drugs such as phenytoin (Dilantin) or carbamazepine (Tegretol). Drugs for neuropathic pain may take from several days to weeks before a full effect is seen. During this time, opioids may be needed to control pain.

When opioids are used, assess the patient for pain intensity and quality. Mild to moderate pain is treated with weaker opioids such as oxycodone or codeine. More intense pain is treated with stronger opioids such as morphine, hydromorphone (Dilaudid), or fentanyl transdermal (Duragesic). Combinations of weak and strong opioids along with non-opioid drugs may be used to provide the best sustained pain relief and allow the patient to participate in activities to the extent that he or she wishes.

Complementary and alternative therapies are used by many patients with pain from HIV/AIDS. These include such therapies as guided imagery, distraction, progressive relaxation, body-talk, and biofeedback to help control pain. Such therapies can be used with more traditional and pharmacologic measures to improve comfort.

Imbalanced Nutrition: Less Than Body Requirements

Many patients with AIDS have difficulty maintaining their weight and nutritional status. This problem may be caused by fatigue, anorexia, nausea and vomiting, difficult or painful swallowing, diarrhea, or wasting syndrome.

Planning: Expected Outcomes. The patient is expected to maintain optimal weight through adequate nutrition and hydration. Indicators include:

- Selecting foods high in calories and protein
- Maintaining current weight or gaining weight
- Drinking at least 3 L of oral fluids per day
- Maintaining blood levels of albumin, prealbumin, and hemoglobin within normal ranges

Interventions. Because there are many factors for poor nutrition in AIDS, diagnostic procedures are needed to determine the cause. Once the cause is determined, appropriate therapy is initiated. For example, in the patient who has candidal esophagitis, nutrition is affected because of swallowing difficulties.

Drug therapy can include ketoconazole (Nizoral) or fluconazole (Diflucan) orally, or IV amphotericin B (Fungizone). Administer the drug as prescribed, and monitor for side effects such as nausea and vomiting, which also affect nutrition. Provide mouth care and ice chips, and keep unpleasant odors out of the patient's environment. Antiemetics are used as needed.

Nutrition therapy includes monitoring weight, intake and output, and calorie count. Assess food preferences and any dietary cultural or religious practices. Teach the patient about a high-calorie, high-protein, nutritionally sound diet. Encourage him or her to avoid dietary fat, because fat intolerance often occurs as a result of the disease and as a side effect of some antiretroviral medications. Collaborate with the nutritionist to provide an appropriate diet, including small, frequent meals (better tolerated than large meals). Supplemental vitamins and fluids are indicated in some cases. For the patient who cannot achieve adequate nutrition through food, tube feedings or total parenteral nutrition may be needed.

Mouth care performed frequently can improve appetite. When this nursing action is delegated to unlicensed assistive personnel (UAP), instruct them to offer the patient rinses of sodium bicarbonate with normal saline every 2 hours or several times a day. Explain to UAP why the patient should use a soft toothbrush and the need to drink plenty of fluids. For oral pain, analgesics or viscous lidocaine may be needed.

Diarrhea

Patients with AIDS often suffer from diarrhea. Sometimes an infectious cause (e.g., *Giardia* or amoeba) can be determined and treated, or the cause is determined but no effective therapy is available. Many patients are lactose intolerant, and HIV disease worsens the condition. Diarrhea may occur as a side effect of therapy with protease inhibitors. In some cases, patients with AIDS have diarrhea and no cause can be identified.

NOC **Planning: Expected Outcomes.** The patient is expected to have decreased diarrhea; to maintain fluid, electrolyte, and nutritional status; and to reduce incontinence. Indicators include:

- Has a stool amount that is appropriate for the diet
- Expels stools that are formed and soft
- Recognizes urge to defecate
- Maintains control of stool passage

Interventions. For most patients with AIDS and diarrhea, symptom management is all that is available. Antidiarrheals, such as diphenoxylate hydrochloride (Diarsed♣, Lomotil) or loperamide (Imodium), given on a regular schedule, provide some relief. Consult with the nutritionist and offer dietary counseling about appropriate foods. Recommended dietary changes include less roughage; less fatty, spicy, and sweet food; and no alcohol or caffeine. Some patients obtain relief when they eliminate dairy products from the diet or eat smaller amounts of food more often and drink plenty of fluids, especially between meals.

Assess the perineal skin of the patient with diarrhea every 8 to 12 hours for a change in skin integrity. Provide him or her with a bedside commode or a bedpan if needed. Some patients cannot reach the bathroom in time because of immobility or anal sphincter weakness and others because of the urgency to defecate. Teach UAP performing this care to provide the patient with privacy, support, and understanding. Explain the need to keep the patient's perineal area clean and dry. Instruct UAP to report any skin changes in the perineal area, including persistent redness, rashes, blisters, or open areas.

Impaired Skin Integrity

The most common skin lesion in AIDS is Kaposi's sarcoma (KS). Lesions may be localized or widespread. Large lesions can cause pain and restrict movement. They can impede circulation, causing open, weeping, painful lesions. Another cause of impaired skin integrity is herpes simplex virus (HSV) infection.

NOC **Planning: Expected Outcomes.** The patient is expected to have healing of any existing lesions and avoid increased skin breakdown or secondary infection. Indicators include:

- Absence of new lesions or open skin areas
- Existing lesions become smaller in diameter
- Absence of pus, induration, or redness in, from, or around skin lesions

Interventions. KS can be treated with local radiation, intralesional chemotherapy, or cryotherapy. Systemic therapy is used in patients with rapidly progressive disease or with major involvement of the intestinal tract, lungs, or other organs. Therapies include chemotherapy (single agent or combination), interferon-alpha, and interferon-alpha plus zidovudine.

Treatment of painful KS lesions includes analgesics and comfort measures. Keep open, weeping KS lesions clean and dressed to reduce the risk for secondary infection. Many patients with skin KS are concerned about their appearance and the risk of being identified as HIV positive. Makeup (if lesions are not open), long-sleeved shirts, and hats may help maintain a normal appearance.

For the patient with an HSV abscess, provide good skin care directly or delegate this care to UAP. Stress the importance of keeping the area clean and dry. Teach UAP to clean abscesses at least once per shift with normal saline and allow them to air-dry. This infection is painful and requires analgesics, assistance with position, and other comfort measures. Modified Burow's solution (Domeboro) soaks promote healing for some patients. HSV infection is treated with acyclovir (Zovirax) or valacyclovir (Valtrex).

Disturbed Thought Processes

Neurologic changes with disturbed thought processes are major areas of concern for patients with HIV infection or AIDS. These changes may be due to psychological stressors accompanying the disease or to organic disorders caused by opportunistic infections, cancer, or HIV encephalitis.

NOC **Planning: Expected Outcomes.** The patient is expected to show improved mental status. Indicators include that the patient demonstrates these behaviors:

- Identifies self and significant others
- Identifies correct month and year
- Recalls immediate, recent, and remote information accurately

Interventions. Patients with AIDS suffer from enormous loss and psychological stress, which complicates the assessment of any changes in behavior or affect. Assess baseline neurologic and mental status by using neurologic assessment tools (see Chapter 43) to compare any changes. Evaluate the patient for subtle changes in memory, ability to concentrate, affect, and behavior. It is important to determine whether the cause of the neurologic changes is treatable.

Reorient the confused patient to person, time, and place as needed. Coordinate with all members of the health care team to ensure that reorientation methods are performed by everyone who interacts with the patient. Remind the patient of your identity and explain what is to be done at any given time. Give simple directions; use short, uncomplicated sentences; explain activities in simple language; and involve him or her in planning the daily schedule. Ask relatives or significant others to bring in familiar items from home. Arrange all items in the patient's environment in the same location as at home. Using calendars, clocks, and radios and putting the bed close to a window also may help keep the patient oriented.

Drug therapy is used for different conditions that can alter thought processes in the person with AIDS. Psychotropic drugs are used to treat ongoing behavioral problems or emotional disorders. Antidepressants and anxiolytics may be prescribed.

Safety measures are crucial to the well-being of the neurologically impaired patient with AIDS. He or she may not be aware of activities or surroundings and may need help with bathing, dressing, eating, ambulating, and other ADLs. Make the environment, whether a hospital room or long-term care facility, safe and comfortable.

Some patients with AIDS have seizures. Institute seizure precautions, including using padded siderails and having an artificial oral airway available. Anticonvulsants may be added to the drug therapy.

Assess the patient with neurologic manifestations for increased intracranial pressure. Document and report immediately any changes in level of consciousness (one of the earliest signs of increased intracranial pressure), vital signs, pupil size or reactivity, or limb strength to the physician for appropriate intervention. Corticosteroids may be given to reduce intracranial pressure.

Support the family and friends of the patient who has neurological impairment. There is great trauma in seeing a loved one unable to care for himself or herself or showing childlike behavior. Answer questions honestly and sensitively. Teach UAP, the family, and significant others how to reorient the patient. Encourage them to continue to provide the patient with news of family happenings or current events. Coordinate with the social worker to identify community resources for the patient and family.

Chronic Low Self-Esteem

The patient with AIDS may have changes in self-esteem and self-concept. Contributing to this are dramatic changes in appearance that alter the person's body image. Many patients also have abrupt, significant changes in their relationships with others and in day-to-day activities, including a job or other productive activities. All changes can disrupt the self-concept.

NOC **Planning: Expected Outcomes.** The patient is expected to identify his or her positive aspects and accept himself or herself. Indicators include that he or she often or consistently demonstrates these behaviors:

- Maintaining eye contact
- Accepting compliments from others
- Expressing feelings of self-worth

Interventions. Provide a climate of acceptance for patients with AIDS by promoting a trusting relationship. Help them express feelings and identify positive aspects of themselves. Allow for privacy, but do not avoid or isolate the patient. Encourage self-care, independence, control, and decision making by helping him or her set short-term, attainable goals and offering praise when goals are achieved.

Guided imagery is a form of complementary therapy used by many patients to increase their sense of control and enhance self-esteem. Imagery can focus on helping them cope with distressing side effects or painful procedures. Other uses include picturing battle scenes in which the virus is killed by immune system cells.

Social Isolation

Many patients with AIDS face discrimination, rejection, and isolation. Friends or health care workers sometimes avoid or refuse to have anything to do with them. Misunderstanding and fear lead to misuse of proper infection control procedures, and patients are inappropriately isolated.

NOC **Planning: Expected Outcomes.** The patient is expected to identify behaviors that cause social isolation and demonstrate behaviors that reduce social isolation. Indicators include that the patient often or consistently demonstrates these behaviors:

- Interacting with close friends and family members
- Cooperating with others
- Using assertive behaviors as appropriate

Interventions. Interventions for social isolation focus on promoting interactions and on education to reduce fear of AIDS transmission.

Promote patient interaction first by establishing a therapeutic nurse-patient relationship, and do not isolate the patient. Spend time with him or her, even when not performing a procedure or assessment, just to be present. Model this behavior for UAP, and encourage them to spend extra time with the patient. Show understanding and concern while helping the patient find ways to reduce feelings of rejection and isolation. Reduce barriers to social contact. Assess his or her social support resources. Teach family and significant others about HIV transmission and the use of Standard Precautions to reduce anxiety and increase contact with the patient (see Chapter 25).

Encourage the patient to state feelings about self, coping skills, and a sense of control over the situation. Help him or her identify support systems, including those already in place and those that need to be arranged.

Teaching about HIV transmission is the most important aspect for prevention of HIV. All people, regardless of age, gender, ethnicity, or sexual orientation, are susceptible to HIV infection. HIV infection is preventable because of the mode of viral transmission and the fragile nature of the virus. (See discussion on pp. 367-368 in the Health Promotion and Maintenance section.)

DECISION-MAKING CHALLENGE

Legal/Ethical

The patient described on p. 374 had the same CBC results on a repeat blood test. After outpatient surgery, the surgeon tells her the results of the test and suggests she be tested for HIV. She agrees, and her test comes back positive. She is completely devastated and is worried about losing both her new husband and her job. She begs you not to tell your (and her) co-workers. In addition, she says she needs time before telling her husband.

1. Are her fears about her job realistic? Why or why not?
2. How should you handle her request not to tell her husband about her HIV status?
3. What specifically can you do to support her at this time?

evolve For suggested answer guidelines, go to http://evolve.elsevier.com/Iggy/.

Community-Based Care

Many health care providers are beginning to regard HIV infection as a manageable chronic disease. The usual course of illness is one of intermittent acute infections and periods of relative wellness over months or years. This period is often followed by chronic, progressive debilitation. Because of the cyclic nature of HIV disease and AIDS, the patient often spends long periods at home between hospital admissions or clinic visits. In some instances, especially as the illness becomes more severe, he or she may need referral to a long-term care facility, home care agency, or hospice. In collaboration with the social worker, nutritionist, and other available resources, work with patients to plan what will be needed and how they will manage at home with self-care and ADLs.

Home Care Management

Before the patient is discharged to home, assess his or her status and ability to perform self-care activities. Some patients do not need home care but do need to maintain a link with primary care providers. Home care can range from help with ADLs for those with weakness, debility, or limited function to around-the-clock nursing care, drugs, and nutritional support for severely or terminally ill patients. Assess available resources, including family members and significant others willing and able to be caregivers. Help the family make arrangements for outside caregivers or respite care, if needed. Patients may need referrals or help in planning housing, finances, insurance, legal services, funeral arrangements, and spiritual counseling. Coordinate with the case manager to ensure these issues are addressed.

Home care aides may be involved in daily or weekly care of the patient with AIDS in the home. Usually a home care nurse makes an initial visit for assessment purposes, and care is followed up by home care aides. If the patient becomes increasingly debilitated, a nurse re-assesses his or her status. Chart 21-10 lists focused assessment areas for the patient with AIDS at home.

NCLEX EXAMINATION CHALLENGE

The home care nurse is making a regularly scheduled visit to a client with AIDS for assessment purposes. The client's overall personal care is being performed by his significant other and many friends in the local "buddy system" care community. At this visit, the client, who has PCP, is confused and is incontinent with diarrhea. What precautions should the home care nurse make (in addition to Standard Precautions) while performing a respiratory and skin assessment?

A. A mask to reduce the risk for PCP.
B. Gown and glove Contact Precautions.
C. Eye protection to reduce the risk for HIV transmission.
D. No additional protection beyond Standard Precautions is needed.

evolve For the correct answer, go to http://evolve.elsevier.com/Iggy/.

Chart 21-10 FOCUSED ASSESSMENT

The Person with AIDS

Assess cardiovascular and respiratory status:
- Vital signs
- Presence of acute chest pain or dyspnea
- Presence of cough
- Presence of fever
- Activity tolerance

Assess nutritional status:
- Food intake
- Weight loss or gain
- General condition of skin
- Financial resources

Assess neurologic status:
- Cognitive changes
- Motor changes
- Sensory disturbances

Assess gastrointestinal status:
- Mouth and oropharynx
- Presence of dysphagia
- Presence of abdominal pain
- Presence of nausea, vomiting, diarrhea

Assess psychological status:
- Presence of anxiety
- Presence of depression

Assess activity and rest:
- Activities of daily living (ADLs)
- Mobility and ambulation
- Fatigue
- Sleep pattern
- Presence of pain

Assess home environment:
- Safety hazards
- Structural barriers affecting functional ability

Assess patient's and caregiver's adherence and understanding of illness and treatment, including:
- Manifestations to report to nurse
- Medication schedule and side or toxic effects

Assess patient's and caregiver's coping skills.

Health Teaching

Teaching the patient, family, and friends is a high priority when preparing for discharge. Instruct about modes of transmission and preventive behaviors (guidelines for safer sex; not sharing toothbrushes, razors, and other potentially blood-contaminated articles). Caregivers also need instruction about best practices for infection control precautions to prevent transmission while caring for the patient in the home (Chart 21-11), nursing techniques to use in the home, and coping or support strategies.

Teach the patient, family, and friends how to protect the patient from infection, how to identify the presence of infections, and what to do if these appear. Teach about the use of self-care strategies, such as good hygiene, balanced rest and exercise, skin care, mouth care, and safe administration and potential side effects of all prescribed drugs. During diet teaching, stress good nutrition; the need to avoid raw or rare fish, fowl, or meat; thorough washing of fruits and vegetables; and proper food refrigeration.

Teach the patient to avoid large crowds, especially in enclosed areas, not to travel to countries with poor sanitation, and to avoid cleaning pet litter boxes. Chart 21-7 lists more strategies to teach the patient and family how to avoid infections.

Psychosocial Preparation

Patients with AIDS often fear social stigma and rejection. Be aware that this fear is realistic, and help identify ways to avoid problems, as well as identify coping strategies for difficult situations. Support family members and friends in efforts to help the patient and provide protection from discrimination.

Encourage patients to continue as many usual activities as possible. Except when too ill or too weak, they can continue to work and participate in most social activities. Support them in their selection of friends and relatives with whom to discuss the diagnosis. Stress that sexual partners and care providers should be informed; beyond that, it is up to the patient. Some patients have severe depression or anxiety about the future. Almost all feel the burden of having a fatal disease widely considered unacceptable and feel compelled to maintain some secrecy about the illness. Referrals to community resources, mental health/behavioral health professionals, and support groups can help the patient verbalize fears and frustrations and cope with the illness.

Health Care Resources

In many cities, community groups exist to assist people with AIDS. Often composed of volunteers, they offer excellent services to the community. The types and number of services vary by agency and city, but many include HIV testing and counseling, clinic services, buddy systems, support groups, respite care, education and outreach, referral services, and even housing. Patients may also need referrals to other local resources, such as home care agencies, companies that provide home IV therapy, community mental health/behavioral health agencies, Meals on Wheels, and others. In addition, educational materials and support groups are available through Internet access.

Evaluation: Outcomes

The overall goals for care of patients with AIDS are to maintain the highest possible level of function for as long as possible, reduce infections, and maintain quality of life and dignity during the course of progressive illness. Evaluate the care of the patient with AIDS on the basis of the identified nursing diagnoses and collaborative problems. Expected outcomes include that he or she should:
- Adhere to the prescribed drug therapy regimen more than 95% of the time
- Practice safer sex techniques all of the time
- Remain free from opportunistic infections
- Have adequate respiratory function
- Achieve an acceptable level of physical comfort
- Attain adequate weight and nutritional and fluid status
- Maintain skin integrity
- Remain oriented
- Maintain self-esteem
- Maintain a support system and involvement with others

Specific indicators for these outcomes are listed for each nursing diagnosis and collaborative problem in the Planning and Implementation section (see earlier).

Chart 21-11 BEST PRACTICE FOR PATIENT SAFETY & QUALITY CARE

Infection Control for Home Care of the Person with AIDS

DIRECT CARE
- Follow Standard Precautions and good handwashing techniques.
- Do not share razors or toothbrushes.

HOUSEKEEPING
- Wipe up feces, vomitus, sputum, urine, or blood or other body fluids and the area with soap and water. Dispose of solid wastes and solutions used for cleaning by flushing them down the toilet. Disinfect the area by wiping with a 1:10 solution of household bleach (1 part bleach to 10 parts water). Wear gloves during cleaning.
- Soak rags, mops, and sponges used for cleaning in a 1:10 bleach solution for 5 minutes to disinfect them.
- Wash dishes and eating utensils in hot water and dishwashing soap or detergent.
- Clean bathroom surfaces with regular household cleaners, and then disinfect them with a 1:10 solution of household bleach.

LAUNDRY
- Rinse clothes, towels, and bedclothes if they become soiled with feces, vomitus, sputum, urine, or blood. Then dispose of the soiled water by flushing it down the toilet. Launder these clothes with hot water and detergent with 1 cup of bleach added per load of laundry.
- Keep soiled clothes in a plastic bag.

WASTE DISPOSAL
- Dispose of needles and other "sharps" in a labeled puncture-proof container such as a coffee can with a lid, using Standard Precautions, to avoid needle stick injuries. Decontaminate full containers by adding a 1:10 bleach solution. Then seal the container with tape and place it in a paper bag. Dispose of the container in the regular trash.
- Remove solid waste from contaminated trash (e.g., paper towels or tissues, dressings, disposable incontinence pads, disposable gloves); then flush the solid waste down the toilet. Place the contaminated trash items in tied plastic bags, and dispose of them in the regular trash.

THERAPY-INDUCED IMMUNE DEFICIENCIES

Some acquired secondary immune deficiencies may be related to other conditions that cause the loss of immunoglobulins or destruction of lymphocytes. The most common cause of secondary immune deficiency is the use of drugs and other treatment modalities for various diseases. Sometimes immunosuppression is a desired effect, as in organ transplantation or for the treatment of autoimmune disorders. Often immunosuppression is an undesirable, complicating side effect of therapy that is used for another intent, such as cancer chemotherapy, and may even require changing the therapeutic regimen. Various therapies cause different types and degrees of immunosuppression. The challenge is to have maximum therapeutic effect without leaving the patient overly immunosuppressed and susceptible to serious complications.

Drug-Induced Immune Deficiencies

Several drug classes have major immunosuppressive effects. Some induce general immunosuppression; others are more specific and target one part of the immune system more than another.

Cytotoxic drugs are mostly those used in the treatment of cancer and autoimmune disorders. Most of these drugs interfere with all rapidly dividing cells. White blood cells (WBCs), including lymphocytes and phagocytes, rapidly divide and are susceptible to this type of destruction. The result is a decrease in the number of lymphocytes and phagocytes. Cytotoxic drugs interfere with the ability of lymphocytes to produce and release products such as lymphokines and antibodies, causing general immunosuppression. Most cytotoxic drugs are used for cancer and autoimmune disorders.

Corticosteroids are hormones used to treat many autoimmune diseases, neoplasms, and endocrine disorders. Corticosteroids have both anti-inflammatory and immunosuppressive effects. They inhibit inflammation by stabilizing blood vessel membranes and decreasing permeability, blocking the movement of neutrophils and monocytes. These drugs disrupt the synthesis of arachidonic acid, the main precursor for a variety of inflammatory chemicals.

Corticosteroids keep T-cells in the bone marrow, reducing the number of circulating T-cells and resulting in lymphopenia and suppressed cell-mediated immunity. They also interfere with immunoglobulin G (IgG) production and reduce antibody-antigen binding. These drugs have many effects that alter disease activity, and numerous side effects, including:

- Central nervous system changes, such as euphoria, insomnia, or psychosis
- Cardiovascular changes, such as edema and hypertension
- GI effects, such as gastric irritation, ulcers, and increased appetite (with weight gain)
- Other changes (e.g., hyperglycemia, muscle weakness, delayed wound healing, bone density loss, body fat redistribution)

Cyclosporine (Sandimmune, Neoral) is a specific immunosuppressant that selectively suppresses the helper-inducer T-cells by blocking their growth and development. Cyclosporine is used to prevent organ transplant rejection and graft-versus-host disease. This drug is occasionally used for disorders such as uveitis, rheumatoid arthritis, and other autoimmune disorders.

Radiation-Induced Immune Deficiencies

Radiation is toxic to dividing and resting cells. Because most lymphocytes are sensitive to radiation, exposure can induce profound lymphopenia, causing general immunosuppression. Whether immune deficiency occurs after radiation therapy depends on the location and dose of radiation. Exposure to the ilium and femur in adults can cause generalized immunosuppression because these bone areas are the primary blood cell–producing sites.

Management of the patient with treatment-induced immune deficiency aims to improve immune function and protect him or her from infection. The most severe immunosuppression occurs while he or she is receiving the immunosuppressive drugs or during radiation treatment. The severity and duration of the immunosuppression are related to the dosage of specific drugs. Although this impairment is usually temporary, with good recovery of immune and inflammatory responses within weeks or months of therapy completion, the potential for severe infections makes this problem a major treatment concern. Common infections occurring during this period include those of fungal origin, yeast, residual viral breakthrough, and a variety of bacteria.

Coordinate with patients and other health care professionals to provide safe care to those at risk for infection. Chart 21-8 lists specific nursing actions to prevent infection among patients with drug-induced or any type of immunosuppression. Good handwashing by all health care personnel before contact with the patient is essential for infection prevention. Health care professionals must use aseptic technique with any invasive procedure.

In some instances, drug-induced immunosuppression can be reduced or avoided by giving biological response modifiers (BRMs) to stimulate bone marrow production of immune system cells. Although not appropriate for all types of disorders, this treatment can reduce the patient's risk for infection during drug therapy. BRMs are expensive, however, and not consistently covered by insurance. See Chapters 24 and 42 for further discussion about this treatment.

Many patients remain at home during periods of immunosuppression. Teach the patient and family best practices to reduce the patient's risk for infection (see Chart 21-7).

For patients receiving long-term therapy with immunosuppressive drugs, drug dosages are altered according to their responses. The lowest dose that achieves the desired effect is given.

CONGENITAL (PRIMARY) IMMUNE DEFICIENCIES

Congenital, or primary, immune deficiencies are disorders in which the person is born with a defect in the development or function of one or more immune components. As a result, the immune response does not adequately protect him or her from infection, cancer, or other disease. Most congenital immune deficiencies are rare.

Some congenital immune deficiencies are inherited as an X-linked trait (e.g., Bruton's agammaglobulinemia or Wiskott-Aldrich syndrome), and some are recessive (e.g., ataxia-telangiectasia). For many congenital immune deficiencies, however, the genetic defect and inheritance pattern have not been clearly identified.

Congenital immune deficiencies are classified according to the type of immune function that is impaired: antibody mediated, cell mediated, or combined. Because cell-mediated and combined immune deficiencies are so severe that the affected person usually does not survive childhood, only antibody-mediated problems (seen in adults) are discussed in this chapter.

BRUTON'S AGAMMAGLOBULINEMIA

A classic congenital antibody-mediated immune deficiency is Bruton's disease or Bruton's agammaglobulinemia. Boys born with this disease usually start to have problems at about 6 months of age, after maternal antibodies, transferred through the placenta, have been lost. The first manifestations are recurrent otitis, sinusitis, pneumonia, furunculosis, meningitis, and septicemia with organisms such as *Pneumococcus, Streptococcus,* and *Haemophilus.* Laboratory assessment shows an absence of circulating immunoglobulin (antibodies).

Except for patients with poliomyelitis, chronic echovirus infection, or a lymphoreticular cancer, the prognosis for Bruton's disease is good if antibody replacement is started early. Immune serum globulin is regularly given to these patients, usually about 100 to 400 mg/kg IV every 3 to 4 weeks (Scherf & White-Reid, 2008). The dosage and schedule are individualized. Antibiotics are used for specific infections. Long-term prophylactic antibiotic therapy may also be used. Often, severe sinus and pulmonary problems later develop in some patients.

COMMON VARIABLE IMMUNE DEFICIENCY

The patient with common variable immune deficiency, or hypogammaglobulinemia, has recurrent bacterial infections similar to those seen with Bruton's disease. The patient has low levels of circulating antibodies (immunoglobulins) of all classes.

Hypogammaglobulinemia differs from Bruton's disease in that it usually first appears later (in adolescence or young adulthood), it occurs almost equally in men and women, and the infections are less severe. Common problems include giardiasis (intestinal infection with *Giardia lamblia*), pneumonia, sinusitis, gastric cancer, bronchiectasis, and gallstones).

Treatment is similar to that for Bruton's disease. Regular infusions of immune serum globulin and regular or intermittent use of antibiotics protect the affected person against infection.

SELECTIVE IMMUNOGLOBULIN A DEFICIENCY

Selective immunoglobulin A (IgA) deficiency is the most common congenital immune deficiency seen in adults, occurring in 1 per 600 to 800 people (McCance & Huether, 2006). The patient may be asymptomatic or have chronic recurrent upper respiratory tract infections, skin infections, urinary tract infections, vaginal infections, and diarrhea. Selective IgA deficiency does not reduce life span. Because IgA is the major antibody in secretions, bacterial infections are seen mostly in the respiratory, GI, and urogenital tracts. Some patients with IgA deficiency also have malabsorption syndrome.

Treatment for IgA deficiency is limited to vigorous treatment of infections. *Unlike other immunoglobulin deficiencies, IgA deficiency should never be treated with exogenous immune globulin for two reasons. First, exogenous immune globulin contains very little IgA and would not help boost IgA levels. Second, because patients with IgA deficiency make normal amounts of all other antibodies, they are at high risk for severe allergic reactions to exogenous immune globulin.* If malabsorption syndrome occurs with IgA deficiency, the patient needs nutritional supplements (e.g., partial or total enteral or parenteral nutrition).

GET READY FOR THE NCLEX EXAMINATION!

Key Points

Review these Key Points for each NCLEX Examination Client Needs Category.

Safe and Effective Care Environment

- Use Standard Precautions for all patients regardless of age, gender, race or ethnicity, sexual orientation, education level, and profession.
- Ask patients about advance directives, and document the status.
- Use good handwashing techniques before providing any care to a patient who is immune deficient.
- Ensure the confidentiality of the patient's HIV status.

Health Promotion and Maintenance

- Identify patients at high risk for infection as a result of work environment or leisure activities.
- Urge all patients who are HIV positive to use condoms and other precautions during sexual intimacy even if the partner is also HIV positive.
- Teach patients with protein-calorie malnutrition what foods to include in the diet.
- Teach the patient and family about the manifestations of infection and when to seek medical advice.

Psychosocial Integrity

- Treat all patients, regardless of diagnosis, with dignity.
- Do not assume that any visitor or family member knows the patient's diagnosis.
- Pace your interview to match the learning needs and energy level of each patient.
- Encourage the patient the opportunity to express his or her feelings about a change in health status or the diagnosis of an "incurable" disease.
- Refer patients newly diagnosed with HIV infection to local resources and support groups.
- Urge all patients who are HIV positive to inform their sexual partners of their HIV status.
- Explain all diagnostic procedures, restrictions, and follow-up care to the patient scheduled for tests.
- Allow patients who have a change in physical appearance to mourn this change.

Physiological Integrity

- Urge patients to adhere to their antiviral drug regimen.
- Pace nonurgent health care activities to reduce the risk for fatigue among patients with AIDS.
- Teach patients the expected side effects and possible adverse reactions to prescribed drugs.
- Assess the immune deficient patient every shift for manifestations of infection; document the assessment findings, and report any manifestation of infection immediately to the health care provider.
- Assess the skin integrity of the perianal region of a patient with AIDS-related diarrhea after every bowel movement.

Additional Study Resources

Go to your Companion CD or Evolve at http://evolve.elsevier.com/Iggy/ for *Self-Assessment Questions for the NCLEX Examination.*

evolve Go to Evolve at http://evolve.elsevier.com/Iggy/ for *Prioritization and Delegation Questions for the NCLEX Examination.*

SELECTED BIBLIOGRAPHY

Asterisk indicates a classic or definitive work on this subject.

Abbas, A., Lichtman, A., & Pillai, S. (2007). *Cellular and molecular immunology* (6th ed.). Philadelphia: Saunders.

Bulechek, G.M., Butcher, H.K., & McCloskey Dochterman, J. (Eds.). (2008). *Nursing interventions classification (NIC)* (5th ed.). St. Louis: Mosby.

Buseh, A.G., Stevens, P.E., McManus, P., Addison, R.J., Morgan, S., & Millon-Underwood, S. (2006). Challenges and opportunities for HIV prevention and care: Insights from focus groups of HIV-infected African American men. *Journal of the Association of Nurses in AIDS Care, 17*(4), 3-15.

Capili, B., & Anastasi, J. (2006). HIV and hyperlipidemia: Current recommendations and treatment. *MEDSURG Nursing, 15*(1), 14-19.

*Centers for Disease Control (CDC). (1987). Public Health Service guidelines for counseling and antibody testing to prevent HIV infection and AIDS. *Morbidity and Mortality Weekly Report, 36*(31), 509-515.

*Centers for Disease Control (CDC). (1991). Recommendations for preventing transmission of human immunodeficiency virus and hepatitis B virus to clients during exposure-prone invasive procedures. *Morbidity and Mortality Weekly Report, 40*(RR-8), 1-9.

Centers for Disease Control and Prevention (CDC). (2005a). Antiretroviral postexposure prophylaxis after sexual, injection-drug use, or other non-occupational exposure to HIV in the United States. *Morbidity and Mortality Weekly Report, 54*(RR-2), 1-27.

Centers for Disease Control and Prevention (CDC). (2005b). Updated Public Health Service guidelines for the management of health-care worker exposure to HIV and recommendations for postexposure prophylaxis. *Morbidity and Mortality Weekly Report, 54*(RR-9), 1-22.

Centers for Disease Control and Prevention (CDC). (2007, revised report). *HIV/AIDS surveillance report 2005*, Author. Retrieved November 2007, from www.cdc.gov/hiv/stats/.

Cohen, B. (2007). Caring for a patient with HIV/AIDS. *MEDSURG Nursing, 16*(1), 53-54.

Cosby, C. (2007). Hematologic disorders associated with human immunodeficiency virus and AIDS. *Journal of Infusion Nursing, 30*(1), 22-32.

Dulak, S. (2006). Stop the assault in skin in HIV. *RN, 69*(6), 25-29.

Holzemer, W., & Marefat, S. (2007). Poverty, development, and PEPFAR: A U.S. strategy for combating the global HIV/AIDS epidemic. *Nursing Outlook, 55*(5), 215-217.

Jones, S. (2006). A step-by-step approach to HIV/AIDS. *The Nurse Practitioner, 31*(6), 26-39.

Levine, A. (2006). AIDS-related lymphoma. *Seminars in Oncology Nursing, 22*(2), 80-89.

McCance, K., & Huether, S. (2006). *Pathophysiology: The biologic basis for disease in adults and children* (5th ed.). St. Louis: Mosby.

Nussbaum, R., McInnes, R., & Willard, H. (2007). *Thompson & Thompson: Genetics in medicine* (7th ed.). Philadelphia: Saunders.

Pagana, K., & Pagana, T. (2006). *Mosby's manual of diagnostic and laboratory tests* (3rd ed.). St. Louis: Mosby.

*Sande, M.A., & Volberding, P.A. (2002). *The medical management of AIDS* (6th ed.). Philadelphia: Saunders.

Scherf, R., & White-Reid, K. (2008). Giving intravenous immunoglobulin. *RN, 71*(1), 29-34.

Stark, S. (2007). The aging face of HIV/AIDS. *American Nurse Today, 2*(6), 30-34.

Swan, A., Daley, A., & Crowley, A. (2007). Contraceptive counseling for adolescents with HIV. *The Nurse Practitioner, 32*(5), 38-44.

Tangredi, L.A., Danvers, K., Molony, S.L., & Williams, A. (2008). New CDC recommendations for HIV testing in older adults. *The Nurse Practitioner, 33*(6), 37-44.

Villarreal, H., & Fogg, C. (2006). Syringe-exchange programs and HIV prevention. *AJN, 106*(5), 58-63.

Care of Patients with Immune Function Excess: Hypersensitivity (Allergy) and Autoimmunity

22
CHAPTER

M. Linda Workman

LEARNING OUTCOMES

For clinical competence and success on the NCLEX Examination, study this chapter with these Learning Outcomes in mind:

Safe and Effective Care Environment

1. Verify that known hypersensitivities of each patient are documented in the medical record and communicated to all members of the health care team.
2. Coordinate with other members of the health care team to ensure a safe environment for the patient with a latex allergy.
3. Implement measures to prevent anaphylaxis.

Health Promotion and Maintenance

4. Encourage all patients with a severe allergy or history of anaphylaxis to wear a medical alert bracelet or other identification.
5. Teach patients with allergies how to avoid known allergens.

Physiological Integrity

6. Describe allergy testing techniques.
7. Compare the characteristics of type I, type II, type III, type IV, and type V hypersensitivity reactions.
8. Explain the rationale for types of drug therapy for autoimmune disorders.
9. Identify the manifestations of hypersensitivity reactions.
10. Prioritize care for the patient experiencing anaphylaxis.

Go to your Companion CD or Evolve at http://evolve.elsevier.com/Iggy/ for *Self-Assessment Questions for the NCLEX Examination* keyed to these Learning Outcomes.

The inflammatory and immune responses are normally helpful in meeting the *human need for protection* against infection and cancer development. These responses also stimulate tissue growth and repair after injury. When inflammation or immune responses are prolonged or excessive or occur at an inappropriate time, however, normal tissues are damaged. These responses are "overreactions" to invaders and foreign antigens and are known as *hypersensitivity* or *allergic responses.* When these responses fail to recognize and protect self cells, normal body tissues are attacked and harmed. This type of reaction is known as an *autoimmune response.* Hypersensitivity and autoimmune responses can severely damage cells, tissues, and organs (Abbas et al., 2007).

HYPERSENSITIVITIES/ALLERGIES

Hypersensitivity or **allergy** is an increased or excessive response to the presence of an **antigen** (foreign protein or allergen) to which the patient has been previously exposed. These responses cause problems that range from uncomfortable (e.g., itchy, watery eyes or sneezing) to life threatening (e.g., allergic asthma, anaphylaxis, bronchoconstriction, or circulatory collapse). The terms *hypersensitivity* and *allergy* are used interchangeably. Hypersensitivity reactions are classified into five basic types, determined by differences in timing, pathophysiology, and clinical manifestations (Table 22-1). Each type may occur alone or along with one or more other types (McCance & Huether, 2006).

TYPE I: RAPID HYPERSENSITIVITY REACTIONS

Type I, or rapid, hypersensitivity, also called *atopic allergy,* is the most common type of hypersensitivity. This type results from the increased production of the immunoglobulin E (IgE) antibody class. Acute inflammation occurs when IgE responds to an antigen, such as pollen, and causes the release of histamine and other vasoactive amines from basophils, eosinophils, and mast cells. Examples of type I reactions include anaphylaxis and allergic asthma (discussed in Chapter 32); atopic allergies such as hay fever and allergic rhinitis; and al-

TABLE 22-1 Mechanisms and Examples of Types of Hypersensitivities

Mechanism	Clinical Examples
TYPE I: IMMEDIATE	
Reaction of IgE antibody on mast cells with antigen, which results in release of mediators, especially histamine	Hay fever Allergic asthma Anaphylaxis
TYPE II: CYTOTOXIC	
Reaction of IgG with host cell membrane or antigen adsorbed by host cell membrane	Autoimmune hemolytic anemia Goodpasture's syndrome Myasthenia gravis
TYPE III: IMMUNE COMPLEX–MEDIATED	
Formation of immune complex of antigen and antibody, which deposits in walls of blood vessels and results in complement release and inflammation	Serum sickness Vasculitis Systemic lupus erythematosus Rheumatoid arthritis
TYPE IV: DELAYED	
Reaction of sensitized T-cells with antigen and release of lymphokines, which activates macrophages and induce inflammation	Poison ivy Graft rejection Positive TB skin tests Sarcoidosis
TYPE V: STIMULATED	
Reaction of autoantibodies with normal cell-surface receptors, which stimulates a continual overreaction of the target cell	Graves' disease B-cell gammopathies

IgE, Immunoglobulin E; *IgG,* immunoglobulin G; *TB,* tuberculosis.

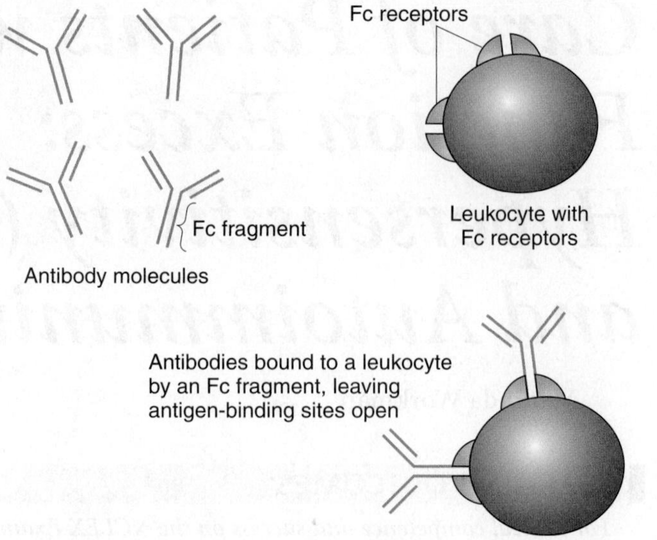
Fc receptors
Leukocyte with
Fc receptors
Fc fragment
Antibody molecules
Antibodies bound to a leukocyte
by an Fc fragment, leaving
antigen-binding sites open

Fig. 22-1 • Antibody Fc receptors on basophils and mast cells.

lergies to specific allergens such as latex, bee venom, peanut, iodine, shellfish, drugs, and thousands of other environmental antigens. Allergens can be contacted in these ways:

- Inhaled (plant pollens, fungal spores, animal dander, house dust, grass, ragweed)
- Ingested (foods, food additives, drugs)
- Injected (bee venom, drugs, biologic substances such as contrast dyes)
- Contacted (latex, pollens, foods, environmental proteins)

Some reactions occur just in the areas exposed to the antigen, such as the mucous membranes of the nose and eyes, causing symptoms of rhinorrhea, sneezing, and itchy, red, watery eyes. Other reactions may involve all blood vessels and bronchiolar smooth muscle causing widespread blood vessel dilation, decreased cardiac output, and bronchoconstriction. This condition is known as **anaphylaxis.**

ANIMATION: Allergy ▶

ALLERGIC RHINITIS

Pathophysiology

Allergic rhinitis, also called *hay fever,* is triggered by reactions to airborne allergens, especially plant pollens, molds, dust, animal dander, wool, food, and air pollutants. Some acute episodes are "seasonal," tending to recur at the same time each year. They often coincide with the timing of large environmental exposure and last only a few weeks. Chronic rhinitis, or perennial rhinitis, tends to occur intermittently (with no predictable seasonal pattern) or continuously when a person is exposed to certain allergens. In "nonallergic rhinitis," the same manifestations are present although no allergic cause is identified and the immune system does not appear to be involved.

On first exposure to an **allergen** (an antigen that provokes allergic sensitization), the person responds by making antigen-specific IgE. This antigen-specific IgE binds to the surface of basophils and mast cells (Fig. 22-1). These cells have many granules containing vasoactive amines (including histamine) that are released when stimulated. Once the antigen-specific IgE is formed, the person is sensitized to that allergen.

In a type I allergic reaction, the already sensitized person is re-exposed to the provoking allergen. The resulting response has a primary phase and a secondary phase. In the primary phase, the allergen binds to two adjacent IgE molecules on the surface of a basophil or mast cell, which breaks or distorts the cell membrane. These changes cause the cell membrane to open and release the vasoactive amines within the granules into the tissue fluids (Fig. 22-2).

The most common vasoactive amine is *histamine,* a short-acting biochemical. Histamine causes capillary leak, nasal and conjunctival mucus secretion, and itching (pruritus), often occurring with erythema (redness). These symptoms last for about 10 minutes after histamine is first released. When the allergen is continuously present, mast cells continuously release histamine and other proteins, prolonging the response.

The secondary phase results from the release of other proteins. These other proteins draw more white blood cells to the area and stimulate a more general inflammatory reaction through actions of leukotriene and prostaglandins (other mediators of inflammation; see Chapter 19). This reaction occurs in addition to the allergic reaction stimulated in the primary phase. The resulting inflammation increases the clinical manifestations and is probably responsible for continuing the response.

The tendency to produce IgE in response to antigen exposure is based on genetic inheritance, but no single gene has been found to be responsible. Although allergic tendencies are inherited, specific allergies are *not* inherited (Nussbaum et al., 2007). For example, a mother who has an allergy to penicillin

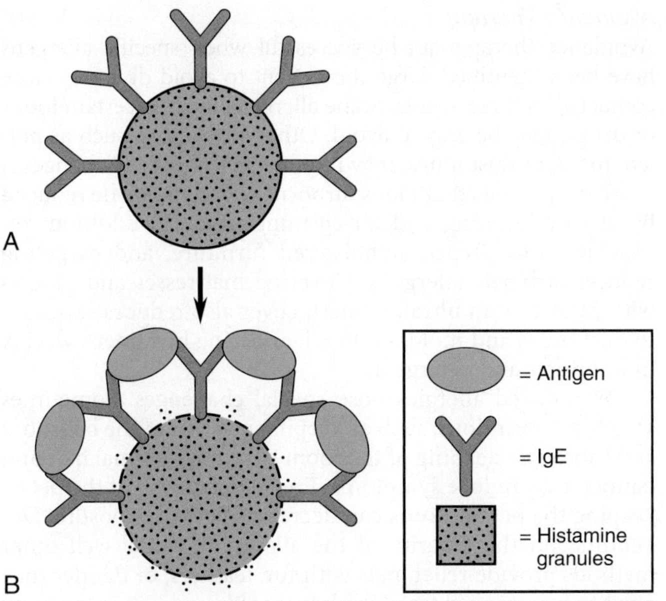
A
B
= Antigen
= IgE
= Histamine granules

Fig. 22-2 • Degranulation and histamine release. **A,** Mast cell with IgE. **B,** Mast cell degranulation and histamine release when allergen binds to IgE.

but not to peanuts may have a child with an allergy to peanuts but not to penicillin. About 50% of patients with allergic rhinitis have one parent with type I allergies. Atopic allergies, including allergic rhinitis, affect about 10% of the population in North America (McCance & Huether, 2006).

Patient-Centered Collaborative Care

evolve ONLINE PHARM REVIEW

Assessment

History

An accurate and detailed history may provide insight into the possibility of allergic rhinitis. Ask the patient to describe the onset and duration of problems in relation to possible allergen exposure. Ask about work, school, and home environments and about possible exposures through hobbies, leisure time, or sports activities. Because a tendency toward type I allergic responses can be inherited, ask about the presence of allergies among close relatives.

Physical Assessment/Clinical Manifestations

The patient with allergic rhinitis usually has **rhinorrhea** (a "runny" nose), a "stuffy" nose, and itchy, watery eyes. He or she may breathe through the mouth, and the voice has a nasal sound. Drainage from the nose is usually clear or white. The nasal mucosa appears swollen and pink. The patient may have a headache or feel pressure over the frontal and maxillary sinuses. Placing a penlight directly on the skin over the sinuses and observing for a glow (transillumination) usually shows reduced glow when rhinitis is present. If nasal secretions drip posteriorly, he or she may have a dry, scratchy throat and pharyngitis. The patient often feels as though he or she has a cold that has lasted longer than a week. Fever is rare unless an infection occurs with the rhinitis.

Laboratory Assessment

A complete blood count (CBC) and differential indicate the presence of an allergic response by an increase in eosinophils. A patient with severe seasonal allergic rhinitis may have an eosinophil count as high as 12% (normal being 1% to 2%). Some patients have an increased total white blood cell (WBC) count, but the percentage of neutrophils remains normal (55% to 70%). If an acute infection occurs with allergic rhinitis, both the total WBC count and the number of neutrophils increase.

Other laboratory tests that indicate the presence of an allergic reaction include serum immunoglobulin E (IgE) levels and the radioallergosorbent test (RAST). A normal level of IgE for adults is about 39 IU/mL (or $<$100 IU/mL). This level can increase greatly with allergies. The usual IgE test does not indicate the specific allergen—only the tendency to have allergic responses. The RAST shows the blood level of IgE directed against a specific antigen and thus can determine specific allergies. However, the expense of this study limits its use in allergy testing.

Allergy Testing

Skin testing can show which specific allergens are the cause of most type I reactions. Skin testing can be performed as scratch testing and intradermal testing. Patch testing is often reserved for contact dermatitis and other manifestations of type IV hypersensitivities.

A scratch or prick test can show an *immediate* hypersensitivity reaction to an allergen. Scratch tests are used in routine allergy testing to determine the cause of allergic rhinitis, asthma, urticaria (hives), or any other type I reactions. Allergens introduced through a scratch or prick cause a localized reaction (wheal) when the test result is positive. Results are usually determined after 15 to 20 minutes.

Patient Preparation. For best results, systemic glucocorticoids and antihistamines are discontinued for 5 days before the test to avoid suppressing an allergic response during the test. Nasal sprays to reduce mucous membrane swelling are permitted, except for sprays that contain an antihistamine. Some allergists recommend that aspirin and other NSAIDs also be withheld before allergy testing.

Procedure. The best site for scratch testing is the inside of the forearm or on the back. Other sites are used if a rash or skin problem is present on the arms or back. Gently clean the skin with soap and water, and remove surface oils with alcohol.

Small drops of sera containing different known allergens are placed on the skin. The skin is scratched or pricked through the drop with a bifurcated skin testing needle. Control drops are also applied to determine how a person reacts to substances that do not normally stimulate a reaction (negative control) and to substances that normally should stimulate a reaction (positive control). Normal saline drops are negative controls, and histamine drops are positive controls. The allergen-tested areas are examined for the presence and size of positive reactions. These areas are then compared with the control areas. Areas showing erythema and wheal formation are considered positive for that antigen. Degree of sensitivity is estimated by the size of the response.

Serious reactions in response to scratch testing are rare. Ensure that emergency equipment, including manual resuscitation bag, oxygen, suction equipment, IV infusion set, and drugs for anaphylaxis (epinephrine and diphenhydramine), is readily available during a scratch test.

Follow-up Care. After testing is completed for the day, wash the solution from the skin. Topical steroids and oral antihistamines may be given to reduce itching and increase patient comfort. If an antihistamine that causes sedation is given, another person must drive the patient home.

Intradermal testing is reserved for substances that are strongly suspected of causing allergy but did not test positive with scratch testing. Intradermal testing increases the risk for an adverse reaction, including anaphylaxis, but it is usually a safe procedure. Ensure that emergency equipment is in the room with the patient. Small amounts of testing sera (0.1 mL) are injected intradermally on the patient's upper arm, and the area is observed for erythema and wheal formation. The degree of allergy is estimated by the size of the response. Patient preparation and follow-up care are the same as for scratch testing.

Oral food challenges are used for patients who have allergic rhinitis when the allergen is eaten and does not come into direct contact with the nasal mucosa. This type of testing is used to identify specific allergens if skin testing is not conclusive and if keeping a food diary has failed to determine the offending food items. The test requires the patient to eliminate suspected foods for 7 to 14 days before testing. After this time, the patient is directed to eat specific suspected food for at least 1 day and to monitor for manifestations of allergy. When many food allergies are present, the patient may have to eat only one food type per day of testing.

Interventions

Chart 22-1 lists NIC interventions for allergy management. Common interventions include avoidance therapy, drug therapy, complementary and alternative therapies, and desensitization therapy. Many patients use a combination of these types of therapy for management of allergic rhinitis and other manifestations of type I allergy.

Chart 22-1 NIC INTERVENTION ACTIVITIES

The Patient with Hypersensitivity/Allergy

Allergy Management: *Identification, treatment, and prevention of allergic responses to food, medications, insect bites, contrast material, blood, and other substances*

- Identify known allergies (e.g., medication, food, insect, environmental) and usual reaction.
- Notify caregivers and health care providers of known allergies.
- Document all allergies in clinical record, according to protocol.
- Place an allergy band on patient, as appropriate.
- Monitor patient for allergic reactions to new medications, formulas, foods, latex, and/or test dyes.
- Encourage patient to wear a medical alert tab, as appropriate.
- Provide medication to reduce or minimize an allergic response.
- Assist with allergy testing, as appropriate.
- Administer allergy injections, as needed.
- Instruct patient to avoid allergic substances, as appropriate.
- Instruct patient to avoid further use of substances causing allergic responses.
- Discuss methods to control environmental allergens (e.g., dust, mold, and pollen).
- Instruct patient and caregiver(s) on how to avoid situations that put them at risk and how to respond if an anaphylactic reaction should occur.
- Instruct patient and caregiver on use of epinephrine pen.

NIC interventions selected from Bulechek, G.M., Butcher, H.K., & McCloskey Dochterman J. (Eds.). (2008). *Nursing interventions classification (NIC)* (5th ed.). St. Louis: Mosby. No part of this work is to be altered without prior written permission from the Publisher.

Avoidance Therapy

Avoidance therapy can be successful when specific allergens have been identified. Urge the patient to avoid direct or close contact with these agents. Some allergens, such as certain foods or drugs, may be easy to avoid. Other substances, such as pollen, mold, or dust mites, may require environmental changes.

Teach patients that many airborne allergens can be reduced by air-conditioning and air-cleaning units. In addition, removing cloth drapes, upholstered furniture, and carpeting reduces airborne allergens. Covering mattresses and pillows with plastic or an ultrafine mesh cover also reduces exposure to dust mites and mold, as does laundering bed linens weekly in hot water and detergent.

Pet-induced allergies pose special challenges. Sometimes simple interventions, such as keeping pets out of the bedroom and thorough cleaning of the room to remove animal hair and dander, may reduce symptoms. Frequent bathing of the pet or keeping the pet outdoors can decrease allergen exposure. Depending on the severity of the allergy and how well other methods provide relief, pets with fur, feathers, or dander may need to be removed from the household.

Drug Therapy

Drug therapy for symptom relief may be tried when avoidance therapy is impractical. It can be effective in reducing the allergic response and making the patient more comfortable. Drug therapy involves the use of steroidal and nonsteroidal agents (to reduce inflammation), vasoconstrictors, antihistamines, mast cell stabilizers, and drugs that inhibit the release or action of leukotrienes. Some drugs reduce the response, and other drugs prevent the response.

Decongestants are available as systemic oral drugs or nasal sprays. These drugs do not clear the allergen or prevent the release of mediators such as histamine. They have actions similar to adrenergic drugs and work by causing vasoconstriction in the inflamed tissue, thereby reducing the edema. Decongestants often contain ephedrine, phenylephrine, or pseudoephedrine. Secretions are reduced when vasoconstricting drugs are combined with an anticholinergic drug, such as scopolamine or atropine. Many combination decongestants are available by prescription and as over-the-counter cold and allergy drugs. Side effects include dry mouth, increased blood pressure, and sleep difficulties. *Because effects are systemic, instruct patients with high blood pressure, glaucoma, or urinary retention to consult with a health care professional before taking any decongestant.*

Antihistamines compete with histamine at its receptor site and block histamine from binding to the receptor. This action prevents vasodilation and capillary leak. Many antihistamines also decrease secretions. Older antihistamines, such as diphenhydramine (Benadryl, Allerdryl🍁) and chlorpheniramine (Allergy, Aller-Chlor, Chlor-Trimeton), often induce sedation. Newer antihistamines, such as desloratadine (Clarinex), cetirizine (Zyrtec), and fexofenadine (Allegra), are less sedating. Not every patient responds to each drug in the same way.

Corticosteroids decrease inflammatory and immune responses in many ways, one of which is by preventing the synthesis of mediators. Corticosteroid nasal sprays can prevent the symptoms of rhinitis. Systemic corticosteroids can produce severe side effects. These drugs are avoided for rhinitis and are used only on a short-term basis for other problems associated with type I reactions.

Mast cell stabilizing drugs include nasal sprays, such as cromolyn sodium (Nasalcrom), that prevent mast cell membranes from opening when an allergen binds to IgE. Thus these drugs prevent the symptoms of allergic rhinitis but are not useful during an acute episode.

Leukotriene antagonists may be used to treat allergic rhinitis. Zileuton (Zyflo) prevents leukotriene synthesis. (See Chapter 19 for a discussion of the role of leukotriene in inflammatory and allergic responses.) Zafirlukast (Accolate) blocks the leukotriene receptor. Both are oral agents and work best in the prevention of allergic rhinitis.

Complementary and Alternative Therapy

Complementary and alternative therapies have helped some patients with rhinitis obtain relief, especially through the use of aromatherapy. Possible mechanisms of action include competition and desensitization. Patients with pollen allergies report decreased problems after eating unprocessed honey.

Desensitization Therapy

Desensitization therapy, commonly called "allergy shots," may be needed when allergens are identified and cannot be avoided easily. It involves subcutaneous injections of small amounts of the allergen. After the allergen has been identified, a very dilute injection solution (1:100,000 or 1:1,000,000) of the allergen is compounded. A 0.05-mL dose of this solution is injected subcutaneously. Usually an increasing dose is given weekly (or more often) until the patient is receiving a 0.5-mL dose. The patient is then started on the lowest dose of the next higher concentration of allergen solution. The process is repeated with increasing concentrations of allergen solutions until the patient is receiving the maximum dose of the greatest concentration (usually 1:100), depending on his or her response. Injections are usually given at weekly intervals during the first year, every other week for the second year, and then every 3 to 4 weeks for the third year. The recommended course of treatment is about 5 years.

Desensitization appears to reduce allergic responses by competition. In theory, the very small amounts of allergen first injected are too low to bind to the IgE already present but are enough to induce immunoglobulin G (IgG) production against that allergen. Because IgG is not associated with either mast cells or basal cells, allergens that bind to IgG do not trigger allergic responses. IgG removes the allergen from the body by precipitation (see Chapter 19). By gradually increasing the allergen injection, large amounts of IgG are produced against the allergen. When the patient is then exposed to the allergen in the environment, the IgG binds to it and clears it from the body before IgE can bind to it and trigger an allergic reaction. Because so much more IgG can be produced compared with IgE, IgG is successful in the competition to bind the allergen.

NCLEX EXAMINATION CHALLENGE

What precaution is most important for the nurse to teach a client with allergic rhinitis who also has hypertension?

A. "Change positions slowly when rising from sitting or lying to prevent falls from a sudden drop in blood pressure."
B. "If you experience dry mouth or an increase in heart rate, be sure to contact your health care provider as soon as possible."
C. "Read the labels of over-the-counter allergy drugs and avoid those containing pseudoephedrine or phenylephrine."
D. "Be sure to reduce the amount of water or other fluids you drink whenever you take an over-the-counter antihistamine or decongestant to prevent water retention."

evolve For the correct answer, go to http://evolve.elsevier.com/Iggy/.

ANAPHYLAXIS

Pathophysiology

Anaphylaxis, the most dramatic and life-threatening example of a type I hypersensitivity reaction, occurs rapidly and systemically. It affects many organs within seconds to minutes after allergen exposure. Anaphylaxis is not common, and the episodes can vary in severity. *It can be fatal.* Many substances can trigger anaphylaxis in a susceptible person (Table 22-2).

Health Promotion and Maintenance

Anaphylaxis has a rapid onset and a potentially fatal outcome (even with appropriate medical intervention); thus prevention is critical. *Teach the patient with a history of allergic reactions to avoid allergens whenever possible, to wear a medical alert bracelet, and to alert health care personnel about specific allergies.* Some patients must carry an emergency anaphylaxis kit (e.g., a bee sting kit with injectable epinephrine) or an epinephrine injector, such as the EpiPen automatic injector. The EpiPen device is a spring-loaded injector that delivers 0.3 mg of epinephrine per 2-mL dose (Fig. 22-3). Although the device is relatively easy to use, it requires some assembly first. Practice devices containing no drug are available from the manufacturer. When a patient is prescribed to carry the device, teach him or her how to assemble and use it. Obtain a return demonstration.

TABLE 22-2 Common Agents That Cause Anaphylaxis

DRUGS/FOREIGN PROTEINS	
Antibiotics (penicillin, cephalosporins, tetracycline, sulfonamides, streptomycin, vancomycin, chloramphenicol, amphotericin B, others)	
Adrenocorticotropic hormone, insulin, vasopressin, protamine*	
Allergen extracts, muscle relaxants, hydrocortisone, vaccines, local anesthetics (lidocaine, procaine)*	
Whole blood, cryoprecipitate, immune serum globulin*	
Radiocontrast media*	
Opiates	
FOODS	**OTHER AGENTS**
Shellfish	Pollens
Eggs	Exercise
Legumes, nuts	Heat/cold
Grains	Latex
Berries	Other
Preservatives	
Bananas	
Peanuts	
INSECTS/ANIMALS	
Hymenoptera: bees, wasps, hornets	
Fire ants	
Snake venom	

*Anaphylaxis caused by these substances is probably a result of direct mast cell degranulation rather than an IgE-mediated hypersensitivity event.

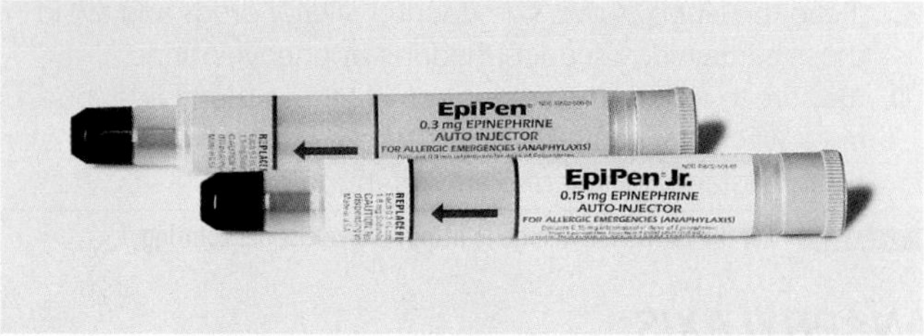
EpiPen
0.3 mg EPINEPHRINE
AUTO INJECTOR
FOR ALLERGIC EMERGENCIES (ANAPHYLAXIS)
EpiPen Jr.
0.15 mg EPINEPHRINE
AUTO-INJECTOR
FOR ALLERGIC EMERGENCIES (ANAPHYLAXIS)

Fig. 22-3 • EpiPen and EpiPen Jr. self-injectors for epinephrine.

The medical records of patients with a history of anaphylaxis should prominently display the list of specific allergens. Ask the patient about drug allergies before giving any drug or therapeutic agent. If he or she has a known allergy, be sure to document this response in the medical record and communicate the allergy to other members of the health care team. Skin tests should be performed before giving any substance that has a high incidence of causing anaphylactic reactions, such as iodine-containing dyes. Be aware of common cross-reacting agents. For example, a patient who is allergic to penicillin is also likely to react to cephalosporins because both have a similar chemical structure. People who have an allergy to bananas, avocados, nuts, or any plant-based food are likely to have a latex allergy.

Take precautionary measures if an agent must be used despite a history of allergic reactions. Start an IV solution, and place intubation equipment and a tracheostomy set at the bedside. The patient is often premedicated with diphenhydramine (Benadryl, Allerdryl♣) or a corticosteroid. The substance is given first intradermally, then subcutaneously, and then intramuscularly in increasing doses at 20- to 30-minute intervals so the initial dose by the next route does not exceed the final dose by the previous route.

Patient-Centered Collaborative Care

Assessment

A patient having an anaphylactic reaction first has feelings of uneasiness, apprehension, weakness, and impending doom. Often the patient is anxious and frightened. These feelings are followed, often quickly, by generalized itching and urticaria (hives). Erythema and sometimes **angioedema** (diffuse swelling) of the eyes, lips, or tongue occur next (Fig. 22-4). Intensely itchy skin wheals or hives may appear and sometimes merge to form large, red blotches.

Histamine and other biochemicals cause bronchoconstriction, mucosal edema, and excess mucus production. Respiratory symptoms include congestion, rhinorrhea, dyspnea, and increasing respiratory distress with audible wheezing.

AUDIO CLIPS: High- and Low-Pitched Crackles; High- and Low-Pitched Wheezes

On auscultation, crackles, wheezing, and reduced breath sounds are heard. Patients may have laryngeal edema as a "lump in the throat," hoarseness, and stridor (a crowing sound). Distress increases as the tongue and larynx swell and more mucus is produced. Stridor and anxiety increase as the airway begins to close. Respiratory failure may follow from laryngeal edema, suffocation, or lower airway constriction causing hypoxemia (poor blood oxygenation).

The patient is usually hypotensive and has a rapid, weak, irregular pulse. These findings are due to vasodilation and extensive capillary leak. He or she is faint and diaphoretic with increasing anxiety and confusion. *If the patient is not treated immediately, he or she may lose consciousness. Dysrhythmias, shock, and cardiac arrest may occur within minutes as intravascular volume is lost and the heart becomes hypoxic. Most anaphylactic deaths are caused by respiratory failure or by shock and cardiac dysrhythmias.*

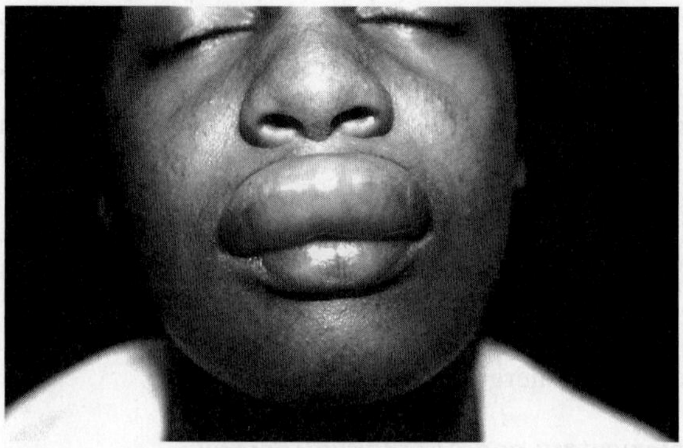

Fig. 22-4 • Angioedema of the lips and mouth.

Chart 22-2 BEST PRACTICE FOR PATIENT SAFETY & QUALITY CARE

Emergency Care of the Patient with Anaphylaxis

EMERGENCY CARE

- Immediately assess the respiratory status, airway, and oxygen saturation of patients who show any symptom of an allergic reaction.
- Call the Rapid Response Team.
- Ensure that intubation and tracheotomy equipment is ready.
- Apply oxygen using a high-flow, non-rebreather mask at 40% to 60%.
- Immediately discontinue the IV drug of a patient having an anaphylactic reaction to that drug. **Do not** discontinue the IV, but change the IV tubing and hang normal saline.
- If the patient does not have an IV, start one immediately and run normal saline.
- Be prepared to administer diphenhydramine (Benadryl) and epinephrine IV.
  - Diphenhydramine 25 mg to 50 mg IV push
  - Epinephrine 1:1000 concentration, 0.3 to 0.5 mL IV push
  - Repeat as needed every 10 to 15 minutes until the patient responds
- Keep the head of the bed elevated about 10 degrees if hypotension is present; if blood pressure is normal, elevate the head of the bed to 45 degrees or higher to improve ventilation.
- Raise the feet and legs.
- Stay with the patient.
- Reassure the patient that the appropriate interventions are being instituted.

Interventions

Assess respiratory function first. Emergency respiratory management is critical during an anaphylactic reaction, because the severity of the reaction increases with time. Call the Rapid Response Team immediately to establish or stabilize the airway. If an IV drug is suspected to be causing the anaphylaxis, stop the drug immediately but do not remove the venous access because restarting an IV may be very difficult if the patient experiences a rapid decline in blood pressure. Instead, change the IV tubing and hang normal saline. More emergency interventions for patients with anaphylaxis are listed in Chart 22-2.

Chart 22-3 COMMON EXAMPLES OF DRUG THERAPY
Anaphylaxis

Drug	Mechanism	Side Effects
SYMPATHOMIMETICS		
Epinephrine (Adrenalin)	Rapidly stimulates alpha- and beta-adrenergic receptors of autonomic nervous system (alpha: vasoconstriction; beta: bronchodilation).	Pallor, tachycardia and palpitations, nervousness, muscle twitching, sweating, anxiety, insomnia, hypertension, headache, hyperglycemia.
Isoproterenol (Isuprel)	Stimulates beta-adrenergic receptors, relaxing bronchial smooth muscles and dilating vessels.	Same as for epinephrine.
Ephedrine sulfate (Vatronol)	Similar to isoproterenol, but with longer duration of action.	Same as for epinephrine.
ANTIHISTAMINES		
Diphenhydramine HCl (Allerdryl🍁, Benadryl)	Competes with histamine for H_1 receptors on effector cells, thus blocking effects of histamine on bronchioles, gastrointestinal tract, and blood vessels.	Drowsiness, confusion, insomnia, headache, vertigo, photosensitivity, diplopia, nausea, vomiting, dry mouth.
CORTICOSTEROIDS		
Prednisone (orally) Hydrocortisone sodium succinate (Solu-Cortef) (IV/IM) Methylprednisolone sodium succinate (Solu-Medrol) (IV/IM) Beclomethasone (inhalant)	Anti-inflammatory; inhibits mast cell degranulation.	Fluid and sodium retention, hypertension, cushingoid state, gastric distress, adrenal suppression, psychosis, osteoporosis, susceptibility to infection.
METHYLXANTHINES		
Aminophylline (Truphylline)	Relaxes bronchial smooth muscle.	Restlessness, dizziness, palpitations, tachycardia, nausea, vomiting, epigastric distress, headache, convulsions.
VASOPRESSORS		
Norepinephrine (Levophed)	Raises blood pressure and cardiac output in severely decompensated states.	Headache, tachycardia, fibrillation, decreased urine output, hypertension, metabolic acidosis.
Dopamine (Intropin)	Raises blood pressure and cardiac output in severely decompensated states.	Dysrhythmias, tachycardia, hypertension, dyspnea, nausea and vomiting, azotemia, headache.
INHALED BETA-ADRENERGIC AGONISTS		
Metaproterenol (Alupent, Metaprel)	Rapidly stimulates $beta_2$-receptor sites in pulmonary smooth muscle, causing bronchodilation.	Palpitations, tachycardia, dysrhythmias, hypokalemia.
Albuterol (Proventil, Ventolin)	Same as for metaproterenol.	Same as for metaproterenol, plus painful urination, flushing of the face.

The patient with anaphylaxis is usually anxious or frightened. Stay with the patient, and reassure him or her that the appropriate interventions are being instituted.

Cardiopulmonary resuscitation may be needed. Epinephrine (1:1000) 0.3 to 0.5 mL is given subcutaneously as soon as symptoms of systemic anaphylaxis appear. This drug constricts blood vessels, improves cardiac contraction, and dilates the bronchioles. The same dose may be repeated every 10 to 15 minutes if needed. Other drugs used to treat anaphylaxis are listed in Chart 22-3.

Antihistamines, such as diphenhydramine (Benadryl, Allerdryl🍁) 25 to 100 mg are usually given IV, IM, or orally to treat angioedema and urticaria. If needed, an endotracheal tube may be inserted or an emergency tracheostomy may be performed.

If the patient can breathe independently, give oxygen to reduce hypoxemia. Start oxygen therapy via a high-flow nonrebreather facemask at 40% to 60% before arterial blood gas results are obtained. Monitor pulse oximetry to determine oxygenation adequacy, with the goal of maintaining oxygen saturation greater than 90%. Arterial blood gases may be ordered to determine therapy effectiveness. Use suction to remove excess mucus and other secretions, if indicated. Continually assess the patient's respiratory rate and depth. Assess breath sounds continually for bronchospasm, wheezing, crackles, and stridor. Elevate the bed to 45 degrees unless severe hypotension is also present.

For severe bronchospasm, the patient is given theophylline 6 mg/kg IV over 20 to 30 minutes. If he or she is taking aminophylline regularly, no more than 3 mg/kg is given. Maintenance aminophylline (0.3 to 0.5 mg/kg/hr) is initiated. The patient may be given an inhaled beta-adrenergic agonist such as metaproterenol (Alupent) or albuterol (Proventil) via high-flow nebulizer every 2 to 4 hours. Corticosteroids are added to emergency interventions but are not effective immediately. Oral steroids are continued (at lower doses) after the anaphylaxis is under control to prevent the late recurrence of symptoms.

Continually assess for changes in any body system or for adverse effects of drug therapy. For severe anaphylaxis, the patient is admitted to a critical care unit for cardiac, pulmonary arterial, and capillary wedge pressure monitoring. Observe the patient for fluid overload from the rapid drug and IV fluid infusions, and report changes to the physician immediately. The patient is discharged from the hospital when respiratory and cardiovascular systems have returned to baseline.

DECISION-MAKING CHALLENGE

Critical Rescue

The patient is a 42-year-old first-grade teacher who is diabetic and has an ulcer on her right foot seriously infected with staphylococcus. She had a débriding procedure earlier today and is prescribed to receive clindamycin 1 g IV as soon as possible. She is 5 feet tall and weighs 202 pounds.

Her medical record indicates an allergy to cortisone. When you ask her whether she has any other drug allergies, she replies, "No, only to cortisone." The drug comes up from the pharmacy about 7 PM, 3 hours after she returned to your unit after the débridement.

About 5 minutes after the infusion is started, the patient says she is having a hard time catching her breath and feels dizzy and scared. You find her pulse to be too rapid to count and thready. Her lips are dusky, and she begins to wheeze.

1. Should you continue the clindamycin? Why or why not?
2. How should you manage her current IV access?
3. Should you call her surgeon or the Rapid Response Team (provide a rationale for your choice)?
4. Why should you or should you not start oxygen on this patient?
5. Would epinephrine be helpful in this situation? Why or why not? Where, how much, and by what route would you expect to administer it?
6. Would diphenhydramine (Benadryl) be helpful in this situation? Why or why not?
7. How likely is an allergy to cortisone?

evolve For suggested answer guidelines, go to http://evolve.elsevier.com/Iggy/.

LATEX ALLERGY

Latex allergy is a type I hypersensitivity reaction in which the specific allergen is a protein found in processed natural latex rubber products. When the allergen enters the body through inhalation or direct contact with blood vessels (e.g., as might occur during surgery), interaction with IgE occurs, leading to a type I reaction. For some people, latex allergen contact is limited to the skin or mucous membranes, causing contact dermatitis, a type IV delayed hypersensitivity reaction (see p. 395). Others may have a "mixed" allergic response to latex, with symptoms of both type I and type IV hypersensitivities. Others may have only one or the other type of reaction.

The incidence of latex hypersensitivity is increasing. People at greatest risk are those with a high exposure to natural latex products, such as patients with spina bifida, people who routinely use latex condoms, and health care workers who use latex gloves. The incidence of latex allergy among health care workers is falling, largely as a response to changes in latex exposure in the workplace.

Ask all patients about their use of and known reactions to natural latex products. Document known food allergies because some foods have allergens that cross-react with latex allergens. In addition, consider your own exposure and risk for reactions to natural latex products.

Avoiding products that contain natural latex proteins can prevent reactions and initial sensitivity. More products, such as surgical gloves, tubing, and vial closures, are now being made from synthetic substances that do not contain latex proteins. One such product is the glove *ElastyLite. It is essential to use latex-free products in the care of a patient with a known latex allergy.* Interventions for the patient who has a type I or a type IV reaction to latex are the same as for reactions caused by other allergens.

TYPE II: CYTOTOXIC REACTIONS

In a type II (cytotoxic) reaction, the body makes special autoantibodies directed against self cells that have some form of foreign protein attached to them. The autoantibody binds to the self cell and forms an immune complex (Fig. 22-5). The self cell is then destroyed along with the attached protein by phagocytosis or lysis (see Chapter 19). Clinical examples of type II reactions include hemolytic anemias, thrombocytopenic purpura, hemolytic transfusion reactions (when a patient receives the wrong blood type during a transfusion), Goodpasture's syndrome, and drug-induced hemolytic anemia.

Treatment of type II cytotoxic reactions begins with discontinuing the offending drug or blood product. Plasmapheresis (filtration of the plasma to remove specific substances) to remove autoantibodies may be beneficial. Otherwise, treatment is symptomatic. Complications such as hemolytic crisis and renal failure can be life threatening.

TYPE III: IMMUNE COMPLEX REACTIONS

In a type III reaction, excess antigens cause immune complexes to form in the blood (Fig. 22-6). These circulating complexes usually lodge in small blood vessel walls. Common sites include the kidneys, skin, joints, and other small blood vessels. The deposited complexes trigger inflammation, and tissue or vessel damage results.

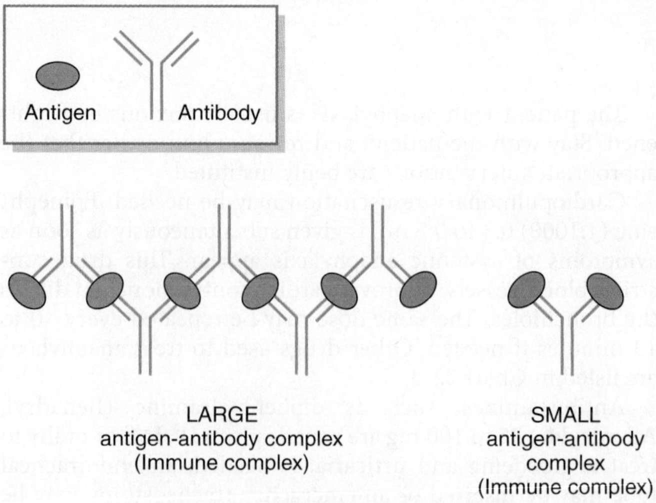
Antigen
Antibody
LARGE
antigen-antibody complex
(Immune complex)
SMALL
antigen-antibody
complex
(Immune complex)

Fig. 22-5 • Antibody-antigen complexes.

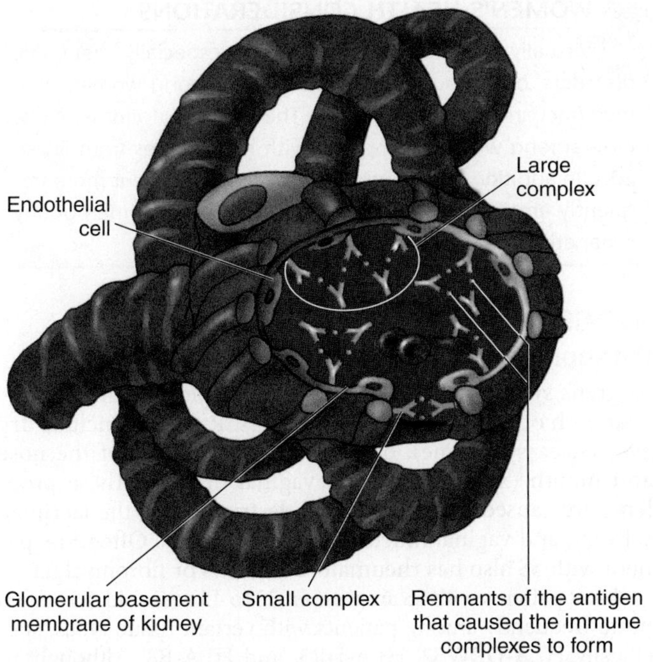
Endothelial cell
Large complex
Glomerular basement membrane of kidney
Small complex
Remnants of the antigen that caused the immune complexes to form

Fig. 22-6 • An immune complex in a type III hypersensitivity reaction.

Many immune complex disorders (mostly connective tissue disorders) are caused by type III reactions. For example, the manifestations of rheumatoid arthritis are caused by immune complexes that lodge in joint spaces followed by destruction of tissue and, later, scarring and fibrous changes. Systemic lupus erythematosus (SLE) has immune complexes lodged in the vessels (vasculitis), the glomeruli (nephritis), the joints (arthralgia, arthritis), and other organs and tissues. (See Chapter 20 for a discussion of SLE.)

Serum sickness is a group of symptoms that occurs after receiving serum or certain drugs. It is caused by a collection of immune complexes deposited in blood vessel walls of the skin, joints, and kidney. The most common causes of serum sickness today are penicillin, other antibiotics, and some animal serum–based drugs. Serum sickness is less common now that vaccines are made with human proteins. Agents known to cause serum sickness include antilymphocyte globulin and antithymocyte globulin, used to treat organ transplant rejection.

The patient with serum sickness has fever, arthralgia (achy joints), rash, lymphadenopathy (enlarged lymph nodes), malaise, and possibly polyarthritis and nephritis, about 7 to 12 days after receiving the causative agent. Teach him or her about the possibility of serum sickness and what symptoms to look for whenever you give a foreign serum. Also keep emergency equipment and drugs close at hand in case he or she has an anaphylactic reaction.

Serum sickness is usually self-limiting, and symptoms subside after several days. Treatment is usually symptomatic; antihistamines are given for itching and aspirin for arthralgias. Prednisone is given if symptoms are severe.

TYPE IV: DELAYED HYPERSENSITIVITY REACTIONS

In a type IV reaction, the reactive cell is the T-lymphocyte (T-cell). Antibodies and complement are not involved. Sensitized T-cells (from a previous exposure) respond to an antigen by releasing chemical mediators and triggering macrophages to destroy the antigen. Unlike a type I reaction, which occurs immediately, a type IV response typically occurs hours to days after exposure. A type IV reaction consists of a local collection of lymphocytes and macrophages, causing edema, induration, ischemia, and tissue damage at the site.

An example of a small type IV reaction is a positive purified protein derivative (PPD) test for tuberculosis. In a patient previously exposed to tuberculosis, an intradermal injection of this agent causes sensitized T-cells to clump at the injection site, release lymphokines, and activate macrophages. Induration and erythema at the site of the injection appear after about 24 to 72 hours.

Other examples of type IV reactions include contact dermatitis, poison ivy skin rashes, local response to insect stings, tissue transplant rejections, and sarcoidosis.

Patch testing for this type of hypersensitivity involves applying test chemicals that contain the allergen(s) to which the patient has been exposed. The patches remain in place for 48 hours. After removal, the skin areas in contact with the chemical are examined closely for the presence of localized redness, swelling, and blisters. If a reaction occurs, the patient is given a list of items containing that chemical to be avoided.

Removal of the offending antigen is the major focus of management. The reaction is self-limiting in 5 to 7 days, and the patient is treated symptomatically. Monitor the reaction site and sites distal to the reaction for circulation adequacy. Diphenhydramine (Benadryl) is of minimal benefit for type IV reactions because histamine is not the main mediator. In addition, IgE does not cause this type of reaction and desensitization does not reduce the response. Corticosteroids or other anti-inflammatory agents can reduce the discomfort and help resolve the reaction more quickly.

TYPE V: STIMULATORY REACTIONS

This type of reaction involves excessive stimulation of a normal cell surface receptor by an autoantibody, resulting in a continuous "turned-on" state for the cell. An example of this type of reaction is Graves' disease, a form of hyperthyroidism. In Graves' disease, an autoantibody binds to the thyroid-stimulating hormone (TSH) receptor sites on the thyroid gland. This binding continually stimulates thyroid cells to produce thyroid hormones, causing the patient to have severe hyperthyroidism (see Chapter 66). The manifestations occur even though the thyroid gland itself is completely normal. In a sense, the tissue responding to the autoantibody is "out of control" from the body's normal feedback system of checks and balances.

For type V reactions involving only one organ, the management focuses on removing enough of the responding (stimulated) tissue to return the function to normal. With Graves' disease, thyroid tissue is either surgically removed or destroyed with radiation. For type V reactions in which antibody stimulation is more widespread, treatment focuses on reducing the production of autoantibodies through immunosuppression.

AUTOIMMUNITY

Autoimmunity is a process whereby a person develops an inappropriate immune response. In this response, antibodies or lymphocytes are directed against healthy normal cells and tissues. For unknown reasons, the immune system fails to recognize certain body cells or tissues as self and thus triggers immune reactions. The responses, both antibody- and cell-mediated, are similar to normal immune responses against invading organisms, but these reactions are now directed against normal body cells. Causes of loss of recognition of self cells are not known.

Examples of diseases that have an autoimmune cause include systemic lupus erythematosus (SLE), polyarteritis nodosa, scleroderma, rheumatoid arthritis, autoimmune hemolytic anemia, rheumatic fever, and Hashimoto's thyroiditis (Table 22-3). Other diseases, such as type 1 diabetes mellitus, may have multiple causes, one of which is autoimmune.

Management of autoimmunities depends on the organ or organs affected. *There is no cure.* Anti-inflammatory drugs and immunosuppressive drugs are commonly used along with symptomatic treatment.

TABLE 22-3 Known or Probable Autoimmune Disorders

Disorder	Autoantigen
SYSTEMIC OR NON-ORGAN SPECIFIC	
Systemic lupus erythematosus	DNA, DNA proteins
Rheumatoid arthritis	IgG, possibly cartilage
Progressive systemic sclerosis	DNA proteins
Mixed connective tissue disorder	DNA proteins
ORGAN SPECIFIC	
Autoimmune hemolytic anemia	Erythrocytes
Autoimmune thrombocytopenic purpura	Platelets
Diabetes mellitus, type I	Islet cells, insulin, insulin receptor
Dermatomyositis	Unknown
Glomerulonephritis	Glomerular basement membranes
Goodpasture's syndrome	Glomerular basement membranes, pulmonary basement membranes
Graves' disease	Thyroid-stimulating hormone receptor
Hashimoto's thyroiditis	Thyroid cell surface
Idiopathic Addison's disease	Adrenal cell
Myasthenia gravis	Acetylcholine receptor, acetylcholine
Pernicious anemia	Intrinsic factor, parietal cell, B_{12} complexes
Psoriasis	Stratum corneum
Reiter's syndrome	Possibly collagen, conjunctival cells
Sjögren's syndrome	Salivary gland cells, vaginal mucous cells, lacrimal gland cells
Uveitis	Uveal tract cells (eye)
Vasculitis	Unknown, possibly collagen or endothelial cells

IgG, immunoglobulin G.

WOMEN'S HEALTH CONSIDERATIONS

Virtually all autoimmune disorders, especially rheumatic disorders, occur much more commonly among women than men (McCance & Huether, 2006). The risk for autoimmune disease among women compared with men ranges from 5:1 to 20:1. In addition, most autoimmune disorders occur more frequently among white women compared with women of any other ethnicity.

SJÖGREN'S SYNDROME

Pathophysiology

Sjögren's syndrome (SS) is a group of problems that often appear with other autoimmune disorders. Problems include dry eyes (sicca syndrome), dry mucous membranes of the nose and mouth (xerostomia), and vaginal dryness. These problems are caused by autoimmune destruction of the lacrimal, salivary, and vaginal mucus-producing glands. Often, the patient with SS also has rheumatoid arthritis or fibromyalgia.

Most patients with SS are women 35 to 45 years old. SS occurs more frequently among patients with certain tissue types, specifically HLA-DRW52, HLA-DR3, and HLA-B8. Although an exact triggering agent has not been identified, viral infection is strongly suspected. The three viruses thought to be triggers for the autoimmune changes leading to SS are the human immune deficiency virus type 1 (HIV-1), human T-cell lymphotrophic virus type 1 (HTLV-1), and Epstein-Barr virus (EBV).

Insufficient tears cause inflammation and ulceration of the cornea. Insufficient saliva decreases digestion of carbohydrates, promotes tooth decay, and increases the incidence of oral and nasal infections. Vaginal dryness increases the incidence of infection and may cause pain during sexual intercourse.

Patient-Centered Collaborative Care

The patient with Sjögren's syndrome (SS) usually has blurred vision, burning and itching of the eyes, and thick mattering in the conjunctiva. Difficulty swallowing food is common, and he or she often has changes in taste sensation. Ask about nosebleeds **(epistaxis)** and frequent upper respiratory infections.

Physical examination reveals enlarged lymph nodes. If rheumatoid arthritis (RA) accompanies SS, the patient has swollen, painful joints and limited joint mobility (see Chapter 20 for a complete discussion of RA). Laboratory assessment may show increased presence of general antinuclear antibodies, anti-SS-A or anti-SS-B antibodies, and elevated levels of IgM rheumatoid factor.

There is no cure for SS. The intensity and the progression of the disorder can be slowed by suppressing immune and inflammatory responses. Drugs used to modulate the immune system in patients with SS include low-dose chemotherapy with methotrexate (Rheumatrex) or cyclophosphamide (Cytoxan). Both drugs have serious long-term side effects, especially on liver and bone marrow function. Other immunosuppressive drugs used to manage SS are corticosteroids, cyclosporine (Neoral, Sandimmune), and hydroxychloroquine (Plaquenil).

A variety of artificial tears and artificial saliva can help reduce the dry eye and dry mouth symptoms. Teach patients to use humidifiers in the home to increase environmental moisture. Use of water-soluble vaginal lubricants and moisturizers can increase patient comfort and reduce the incidence of vaginitis. Some patients relieve dry mouth with systemic pilocarpine (Salagen). This agent mimics the effects of the parasympathetic nervous system, causing increased salivation.

Another intervention for dry eyes is to block the tear outflow channel (nasal punctum). The punctum can be blocked temporarily with small plugs or can be closed surgically. Either method allows the tears produced to remain in contact with the eye longer.

GOODPASTURE'S SYNDROME

Pathophysiology

Goodpasture's syndrome is an autoimmune disorder in which autoantibodies are made against the glomerular basement membrane and neutrophils. The two organs with the most damage are the lungs and the kidney (Bergs, 2005). A person with the disorder may have lung and/or kidney problems. Lung damage is manifested as pulmonary hemorrhage. Kidney damage manifests as glomerulonephritis that may rapidly progress to complete renal failure (see Chapters 70 and 71). Unlike other autoimmune disorders, Goodpasture's syndrome usually occurs in adolescent males or young men (McCance & Huether, 2006). The exact cause or triggering agent is unknown.

Patient-Centered Collaborative Care

Goodpasture's syndrome usually is not diagnosed until serious lung or kidney problems are present. Manifestations include shortness of breath, hemoptysis (bloody sputum), decreased urine output, weight gain, generalized nondependent edema, hypertension, and tachycardia. Chest x-rays show areas of consolidation. The most common cause of death is uremia as a result of renal failure.

Spontaneous resolution of Goodpasture's syndrome has occurred but is rare. Interventions focus on reducing the immune-mediated damage and performing some type of renal supportive therapy.

Drug therapy is the mainstay of treatment for Goodpasture's syndrome. High-dose corticosteroids are most often used. Other drug therapy to suppress the autoimmune response is the same as that for Sjögren's syndrome (SS).

Additional therapy to reduce immune responses involves plasmapheresis (filtration of the plasma to remove some proteins) to remove the autoantibodies. If the lungs and kidneys do not have permanent damage, patients undergoing plasmapheresis have shown clinical improvement. Some patients using plasmapheresis need infusions of intravenous immunoglobulin (IVIG) to maintain antibody protection against infection.

Depending on the level of renal function remaining, the patient may need ongoing dialysis. Therapy usually begins with hemodialysis. For long-term therapy, peritoneal or hemodialysis may be used depending on the patient's health status, ability to self-manage the infusion and drainage systems, and lifestyle (see Chapter 71).

Renal transplantation is an option for some patients with Goodpasture's syndrome. After transplantation, renal function is normal. In rare instances, patients have been disease-free after transplantation. In others, the renal problems are improved but the lung destruction continues. Some of the drugs used to prevent kidney rejection also suppress the autoimmune response.

HUMAN NEEDS NURSING CARE REVIEW

What might you NOTICE if the patient is experiencing an excess protective response in the form of a severe allergic reaction?

- Possible skin rash, blisters, wheals, especially on the skin at the IV site
- Swelling of the face, lips, tongue (angioedema)
- Difficulty breathing, hoarseness, stridor, wheezing
- Cyanosis
- Increasing anxiety

What should you INTERPRET and how should you RESPOND to a patient experiencing inadequate protection as a result of loss of skin integrity?

Perform and interpret physical assessment, including:

- Taking vital signs, especially respiratory rate and depth and blood pressure
- Auscultating all lung fields
- Monitoring oxygen saturation by pulse oximetry
- Checking the accuracy of pulse oximetry readings
- Assessing cognition (mini-mental status exam)
- Assessing for the use of accessory muscles
- Assessing for the presence of thick or excessive secretions
- Assessing the patient's ability to cough and clear the airway

Respond by:

- Removing or discontinuing the offending agent
- Ensuring a patent airway
- Notifying Rapid Response Team
- Applying oxygen, and assessing the patient's responses to this intervention
- Maintaining IV access, changing IV tubing, hanging normal saline
- Keeping the patient's head elevated between 10 and 45 degrees
- Preparing to administer IV diphenhydramine and epinephrine
- Staying with the patient

On what should you REFLECT?

- Observe patient for evidence of drug therapy and oxygen therapy effectiveness (adequate tissue perfusion and oxygenation [see Chapter 29]).
- Think about what may have precipitated this episode and what steps could be taken to either prevent a similar episode or identify it earlier.
- Think about what additional resources could improve the nursing response to this situation.

GET READY FOR THE NCLEX EXAMINATION!

Key Points

Review these Key Points for each NCLEX Examination Client Needs Category.

Safe and Effective Care Environment

- Ensure that only latex-free products are used for a patient who has a known latex allergy.
- Verify that all allergies are documented in a prominent place in the patient's medical record.
- Keep emergency equipment and drugs (epinephrine, Benadryl, cortisone) in or near the room of a patient with known severe allergies or a history of anaphylaxis.

Health Promotion and Maintenance

- Urge all patients with severe allergies or those who have a history of anaphylaxis to wear a medical alert bracelet.
- Teach the patient and family about the manifestations of allergic reactions and when to seek medical advice.

Psychosocial Integrity

- Stay with the patient in anaphylaxis.
- Explain all diagnostic procedures, restrictions, and follow-up care to the patient scheduled for tests related to hypersensitivities.
- Reassure patients who are in anaphylaxis that the appropriate interventions are being instituted.

Physiological Integrity

- Immediately assess the respiratory status and airway of patients who show any symptom of an allergic reaction.
- Immediately discontinue the IV drug of a patient having an anaphylactic reaction to that drug. **Do not** discontinue the IV, but change the IV tubing and hang normal saline.
- Hold the dose of any prescribed drug when a patient develops angioedema.
- Give oxygen to any patient in anaphylaxis.
- Teach the patient who has a known drug allergy which other drugs are likely to stimulate the same reactions.
- Teach the patient who carries an EpiPen how to assemble and use the device. Obtain a return demonstration.

Additional Study Resources

Go to your Companion CD or Evolve at http://evolve.elsevier.com/Iggy/ for *Self-Assessment Questions for the NCLEX Examination.*

Go to Evolve at http://evolve.elsevier.com/Iggy/ for *Prioritization and Delegation Questions for the NCLEX Examination.*

SELECTED BIBLIOGRAPHY

Abbas, A., Lichtman, A., & Pillai, S. (2007). *Cellular and molecular immunology* (6th ed.). Philadelphia: Saunders.

Bergs, L. (2005). Goodpasture syndrome. *Critical Care Nurse, 25*(5), 50-54, 56-58.

Bulechek, G.M., Butcher, H.K., & McCloskey Dochterman, J. (Eds.). (2008). *Nursing interventions classification (NIC)* (5th ed.). St. Louis: Mosby.

Bryant, H. (2007). Anaphylaxis: Recognition, treatment, and education. *Emergency Nurse, 15*(2), 24-28.

Cain, J., Daly, M., & Powers, J. (2007). Act fast against anaphylaxis. *American Nurse Today, 2*(2), 30.

Conboy-Ellis, K., & Braker-Shaver, S. (2007). Intranasal steroids and allergic rhinitis. *The Nurse Practitioner, 32*(4), 44-49.

Fox, R. (2005). Sjögren's syndrome. *Lancet, 366*(9482), 321-331.

Hathaway, L. (2005). Patient-education guide: Anaphylaxis. *Nursing2005, 35*(1), 46-47.

IV rounds: Handling a Type I hypersensitivy reaction. *Nursing2008, 38*(4), 60.

Kemp, S. (2007). Office approach to anaphylaxis: Sooner better than later. *American Journal of Medicine, 160*(8), 664-668.

Laskowski-Jones, L. (2006). First aid for bee, wasp, and hornet stings. *Nursing2006, 36*(7), 58-59.

Lehman, J., & Lieberman, P. (2007). Office-based management of allergic rhinitis in adults. *The American Journal of Medicine, 120*(8), 659-663.

McCance, K., & Huether, S. (2006). *Pathophysiology: The biologic basis for disease in adults and children* (5th ed.). St. Louis: Mosby.

Moorhead, S., Johnson, M., & Maas, M. (Eds.). (2004). *Nursing outcomes classification (NOC)* (3rd ed.). St. Louis: Mosby.

Nussbaum, R., McInnes, R., & Willard, H. (2007). *Thompson & Thompson: Genetics in medicine* (7th ed.). Philadelphia: Saunders.

Pagana, K., & Pagana, T. (2006). *Mosby's manual of diagnostic and laboratory tests* (3rd ed.). St. Louis: Mosby.

Scarlet, C. (2006). Anaphylaxis. *Journal of Infusion Nursing, 29*(1), 39-44.

Cancer Development

23

CHAPTER

M. Linda Workman

LEARNING OUTCOMES

For clinical competence and success on the NCLEX Examination, study this chapter with these Learning Outcomes in mind:

Health Promotion and Maintenance

1. Assist all people to identify behaviors that reduce the risk for cancer development and cancer death.
2. Teach the recommended screening practices and schedules for specific cancer types.

Physiological Integrity

3. Explain why causes of specific cancers can be hard to establish.
4. Use knowledge of basic biology to understand how normal cells can become malignant.
5. Distinguish the features of normal cells from those of benign tumors and cancer cells.
6. Discuss the roles of oncogenes and suppressor genes in cancer development.
7. Compare the cancer development processes of initiation and promotion.
8. Correctly interpret cancer grading, ploidy, and staging reports.
9. Explain the common sites of distant metastasis for cancer and how metastasis contributes to death from cancer.
10. Discuss the role of immunity in protection against cancer.
11. Assess the individual patient's need for genetic testing for cancer predisposition based on family history.

Go to your Companion CD or Evolve at http://evolve.elsevier.com/Iggy/ for *Self-Assessment*
evolve *Questions for the NCLEX Examination* keyed to these Learning Outcomes.

Altered cell growth, such as a mole or a skin tag, is common. Most types of altered cell growth are **benign** (harmless) and do not require intervention. **Malignant cell growth,** or cancer, however, is serious and, without intervention, leads to death. Cancer is a common health problem in the United States and Canada. Nearly 1.5 million people are newly diagnosed with cancer each year (American Cancer Society [ACS], 2008). Some types of cancer can be prevented; others have better cure rates if diagnosed early. As a nurse, you can have a vital impact in educating the public about cancer prevention and early detection methods.

Although cancer is common today, it is not a new disorder. Some types of cancer are more common today, especially among more affluent societies, than in centuries past. Two reasons for this increase are the long life expectancy of people in more affluent countries and increased exposure to substances that cause cancer.

Cancer will occur in about 1 of every 3 persons currently living in North America (ACS, 2008), although cancer risk differs for each person. More than 10 million Americans with a history of cancer are alive today, nearly 5 million of whom are considered cured (ACS, 2008).

PATHOPHYSIOLOGY

Growth of cells and tissues is expected during infancy and childhood, and many human body cells continue to "grow" by **mitosis** (cell division) long after maturation is complete. Such cells are located in tissues in which constant damage or wear is likely and continued cell growth is needed to replace dead tissues. Cells of the skin, hair, mucous membranes, bone marrow, and linings of organs such as the lungs, stomach, intestines, bladder, and uterus, among others, have the ability to divide throughout a person's life span. The growth of these cells is well controlled, ensuring that only the right number of cells is always present in any tissue or organ.

Some tissues and organs stop growing by cell division after development is complete. For example, heart muscle cells no longer divide after fetal life; the number of heart muscle cells is fixed at birth. The size of the heart increases as the person grows because each cell gets larger, but the number of heart muscle cells does not increase. Growth that causes tissue to increase in size by enlarging each cell is **hypertrophy.** Growth that causes tissue to increase in size by increasing the number of cells is **hyperplasia** (Fig. 23-1).

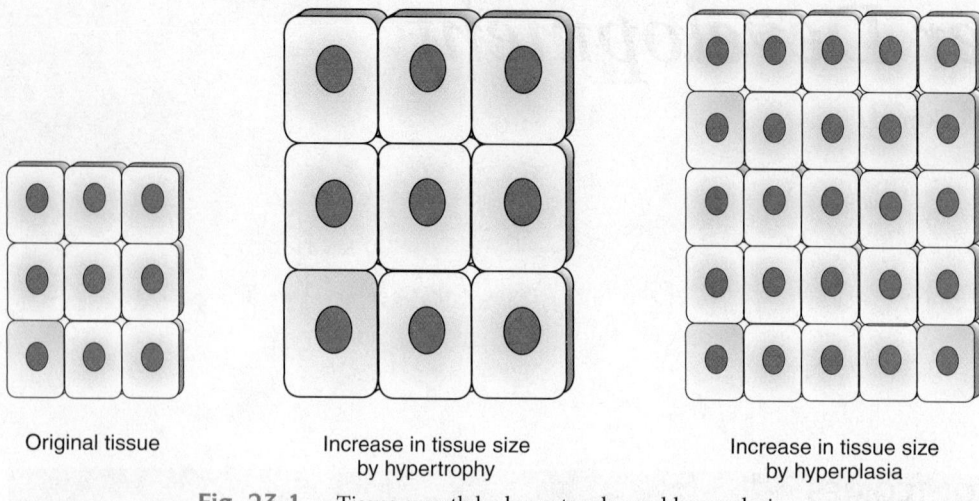
Original tissue
Increase in tissue size by hypertrophy
Increase in tissue size by hyperplasia

Fig. 23-1 • Tissue growth by hypertrophy and hyperplasia.

Any new or continued cell growth not needed for normal development or replacement of dead and damaged tissues is called **neoplasia.** This cell growth is always abnormal even if it causes no harm. Whether the new cells are benign or cancerous, neoplastic cells develop from normal cells (parent cells). Thus cancer cells were once normal cells but changed to no longer look, grow, or function normally. The strict processes controlling normal growth and function have been lost. To understand how cancer cells grow, it is helpful to first understand the regulation and function of normal cells.

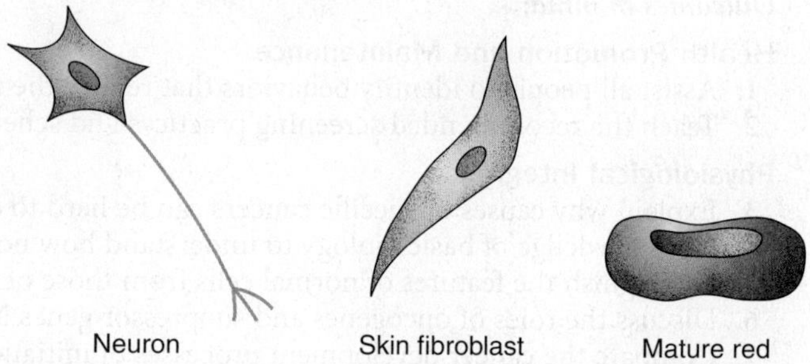
Neuron
Skin fibroblast
Mature red blood cell

Fig. 23-2 • Distinctive morphology of some normal cells.

Biology of Normal Cells

Many different normal cells work together to make the whole person function at an optimal level. For optimal function, each cell must perform in a predictable manner.

Features of Normal Cells

Limited cell division occurs because normal cells divide (undergo mitosis) for only two reasons: (1) to develop normal tissue or (2) to replace lost or damaged normal tissue. Even when they are capable of mitosis, normal cells divide only when body conditions and nutrition are just right.

Apoptosis is programmed cell death. Normal cells have a finite life span. With each round of cell division, the telomeric DNA at the ends of the cell's chromosomes shortens (see Chapter 6). When this DNA is gone, the cell responds to signals for apoptosis. The purpose of apoptosis is to ensure that each organ has an adequate number of cells at their functional peak.

Specific morphology is the feature in which each normal cell type has a distinct and recognizable appearance, size, and shape, as shown in Fig. 23-2.

A small nuclear-to-cytoplasmic ratio means that the nucleus of a normal cell does not take up much space inside the cell. As shown in Fig. 23-2, the size of the normal cell nucleus is small compared with the size of the rest of the cell, including the cytoplasm.

Differentiated function or functions is a feature of normal cells. Every normal cell has at least one special function it performs to contribute to whole-body function. For example, skin cells make keratin, liver cells make bile, cardiac muscle cells contract, nerve cells conduct impulses, and red blood cells make hemoglobin.

Tight adherence occurs because normal cells make proteins that protrude from the membranes, allowing cells to bind closely and tightly together. One such protein is fibronectin, which keeps most normal tissues bound tightly to each other. Exceptions are blood cells. Red blood cells and white blood cells produce no fibronectin and do not usually adhere together.

Nonmigratory is the feature that means normal cells do not wander throughout the body (except for blood cells). This occurs in normal cells because they are tightly bound together, which prevents cell wandering from one tissue into the next.

Orderly and well-regulated growth is a strong feature of normal cells. They do not divide unless body conditions are optimal for cell division. These conditions include the need for more cells, adequate space, and sufficient nutrients and other resources. Cell division **(mitosis),** occurring in a well-recognized pattern, is described by the cell cycle. Fig. 23-3 shows the phases of the cell cycle.

Living cells not actively reproducing are in a reproductive resting state termed G_0. During the G_0 period, cells actively carry out their functions but do not divide. Normal cells spend most of their lives in the G_0 state, just like most humans spend most of their lives in a nonpregnant state.

Mitotic cell division makes one cell divide into two cells. These two cells are identical to each other and to the original cell that started the mitosis. The steps of entering and completing the cell cycle are tightly controlled. Much of this control is regulated by proteins produced by "suppressor genes."

Control of whether a cell enters the cell cycle and completes the cycle to form two new cells depends on the presence and absence of specific proteins. Proteins that promote cells to enter and complete cell division belong to a family of proteins known as *cyclins.* When cyclins are activated, they first allow a cell to

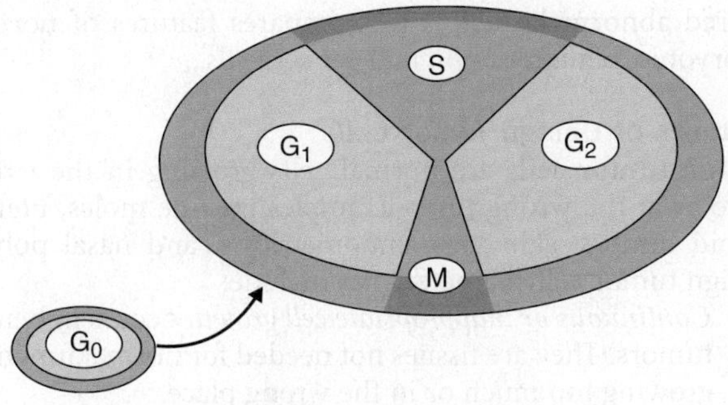
S
G1
G2
M
G0

Fig. 23-3 • The cell cycle.

leave the G_0 state and enter the cycle. These activated cyclins then permit the cell to move through the different phases of the cell cycle and actually divide. The cyclins are the products of oncogenes (see discussion of oncogene activation on p. 407). Proteins produced by suppressor genes regulate the amount of cyclins present in a cell and ensure that cell division occurs only when it is needed. Thus normal cell division represents a balance between the proteins that promote cell division (cyclins) and the proteins that limit cell division (suppressor gene products).

Fig. 23-4 shows the activities of the phases of the cell cycle (described below):

- **G_1.** In this phase, the cell is getting ready for division by taking on extra nutrients, making more energy, and growing extra membrane. The amount of cell fluid (cytoplasm) also increases.
- **S.** Because making one cell into two cells requires twice as much of everything, including DNA, the cell must double its DNA content through DNA synthesis. This process occurs in S phase.
- **G_2.** In this phase, the cell makes important proteins that will be used in actual cell division and in normal physiologic function after cell division is complete.
- **M.** The single cell splits apart into two cells (actual mitosis) during M phase.

Contact inhibition is the stopping of further rounds of cell division when the dividing cell is completely surrounded and touched (contacted) by other cells. Of the normal cells that can divide, each cell divides only when some of its surface is not in direct contact with another cell. Once a normal cell is in direct contact on all surface areas with other cells, it no longer undergoes mitosis. Thus normal cell division is contact inhibited.

Normal chromosomes **(euploidy)** is a feature of most normal human cells. These cells have 23 pairs of chromosomes, the correct number for human beings.

Each normal mature cell has a specific structure and function. The fact that normal mature cells have many different shapes and functions is interesting, considering that all humans started life as a single cell. The function and behavior of that first single cell and its daughter cells are quite different from those of normal adult human cells. Knowledge about these differences has helped in understanding how cancer develops.

Features of Early Embryonic Cells

Rapid and continuous cell division is a normal feature of embryonic cells. These cells spend most of their time within the cell cycle, actively reproducing. The time it takes one embryonic cell to divide into two cells **(generation time)** ranges from 2 to 8 hours. These cells also do not respond to signals for apoptosis. Early embryonic cells have long telomeres that

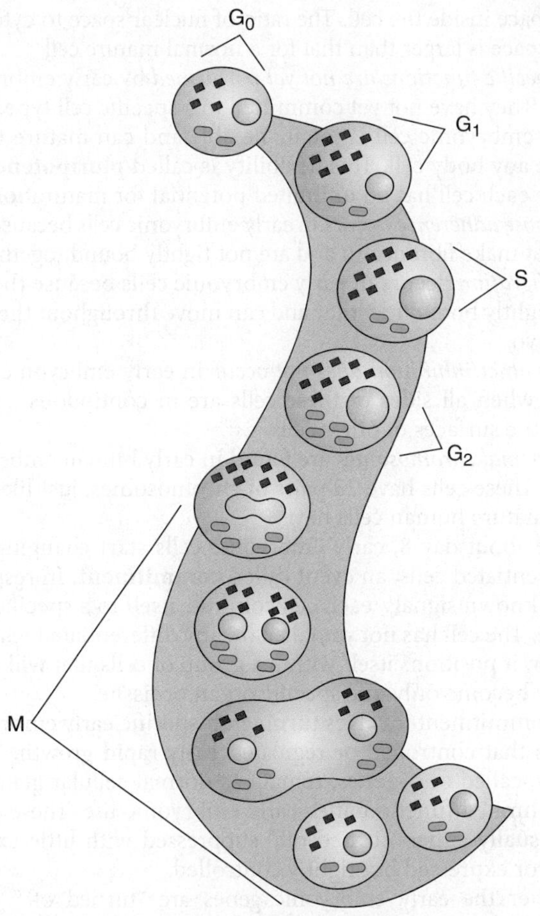
G0
G1
S
G2
M

Fig. 23-4 • Cellular events during mitotic cell division.

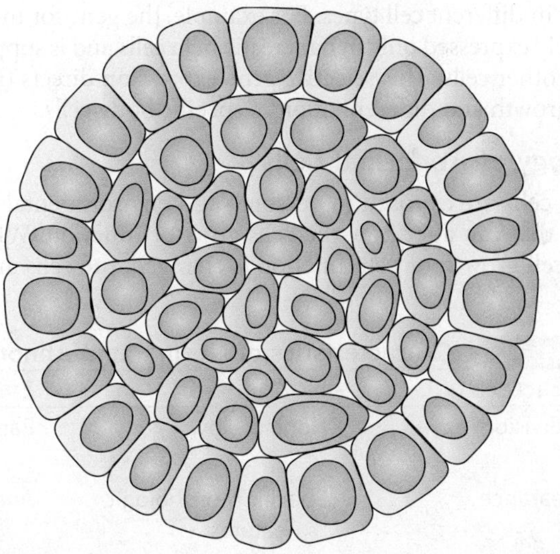

Fig. 23-5 • Embryonic cells at about 5 days after conception.

do not shorten with each cell division. Although some cells during fetal life undergo apoptosis for development of specific structures (e.g., fingers), this is not a feature of embryonic cells.

Anaplasia means "without specific shape or differentiation." Early embryonic cells do not look like the mature cells they will eventually become. They all have the same anaplastic appearance—small and rounded (Fig. 23-5).

A large nuclear-cytoplasmic ratio is a feature of early embryonic cells. The nucleus of these cells is large, taking up most of the space inside the cell. The ratio of nuclear space to cytoplasmic space is larger than that for a normal mature cell.

Specific functions are not yet performed by early embryonic cells. They have not yet committed to a specific cell type. Each early embryonic cell is totally flexible and can mature to become any body cell. This flexibility is called **pluripotency** because each cell has an unlimited potential for maturation.

Loose adherence occurs in early embryonic cells because they do not make fibronectin and are not tightly bound together.

Migration occurs in early embryonic cells because they are not tightly bound together and can move throughout the early embryo.

Contact inhibition does not occur in early embryonic cells, even when all sides of these cells are in continuous contact with the surfaces of other cells.

Normal chromosomes are found in early human embryonic cells. These cells have 23 pairs of chromosomes, just like normal mature human cells have.

At about day 8, early embryonic cells start changing into differentiated cells, an event called **commitment.** In response to unknown signals, each cell commits itself to a specific outcome. The cell has not yet taken on any differentiated features; rather, it positions itself within a group of cells that will eventually become only one specific organ or tissue.

Commitment involves turning off specific early embryonic genes that controlled or regulated early rapid growth. These genes, called **oncogenes,** remain as normal cellular genes but have limited function after early embryonic life. These genes are usually either "turned off," suppressed with little expression, or expressed but tightly controlled.

After the early embryonic genes are "turned off" **(suppressed),** other specific genes that control the expression of differentiated functions must be "turned on" **(expressed)** selectively in different cell types. For example, the gene for insulin is actively expressed only in pancreatic beta cells and is suppressed in all other cells. This selective gene expression directs the normal growth and differentiation of specific body cells.

Biology of Abnormal Cells

Body cells are exposed to personal and environmental conditions that can alter how the cells grow or function. When either cell growth or cell function is changed, the cells are considered abnormal. Table 23-1 compares features of normal, embryonic, benign tumor, and cancer cells.

Features of Benign Tumor Cells

Benign tumor cells are normal cells growing in the wrong place or at the wrong time. Examples include moles, uterine fibroid tumors, skin tags, endometriosis, and nasal polyps. Benign tumor cell characteristics include:

- *Continuous or inappropriate cell growth* occurs in benign tumors. They are tissues not needed for normal function, growing too much or in the wrong place.
- *Specific morphology* occurs with benign tumors. They look like the tissues they come from, retaining the specific morphology of parent cells.
- *A small nuclear-to-cytoplasmic ratio* is a feature of benign tumors just like completely normal cells.
- *Specific differentiated functions* continue to be performed by benign tumors. For example, in endometriosis, one type of benign tumor, the normal lining of the uterus (endometrium) grows in an abnormal place (e.g., on an ovary, on the peritoneum, or in the chest cavity). This displaced endometrium acts just like normal endometrium by changing each month under the influence of estrogen. When the hormone level drops and the normal endometrium sheds from the uterus, the displaced endometrium, wherever it is, also sheds.
- *Tight adherence* of benign tumor cells to each other occurs because they continue to make fibronectin. In addition, many benign tissues are "encapsulated," or surrounded with fibrous connective tissue, helping to hold the benign tissue together.
- *No migration* or wandering of benign tissues occurs because they remain tightly bound and do not invade other body tissues.
- *Orderly growth* with normal growth patterns occurs in benign tumor cells even though their growth is not needed. Growth may continue beyond an appropriate time, but the rate of growth is normal. The benign tumor grows by hyperplastic expansion. *It does not invade.*
- *Normal chromosomes* are usually found in benign tumor cells, although there are exceptions. Most of these cells have 23 pairs of chromosomes, the correct number for humans.

TABLE 23-1 Characteristics of Normal and Abnormal Cells

Characteristic	Normal Cell	Embryonic Cell	Benign Tumor Cell	Malignant Cell
Cell division	None or slow	Rapid, continuous	Continuous or inappropriate	Rapid or continuous
Appearance	Specific morphologic features	Anaplastic	Specific morphologic features	Anaplastic
Nuclear-cytoplasmic ratio	Small	Large	Small	Large
Differentiated functions	Many	None	Many	Some or none
Adherence	Tight	Loose	Tight	Loose
Migratory	No	Yes	No	Yes
Growth	Well regulated	Well regulated	Expansion	Invasion
Chromosomes	Diploid (euploid)	Diploid (euploid)	Diploid (euploid)	Aneuploid*
Mitotic index	Low	High	Low	High*

*Depends on the degree of malignant transformation.

Features of Cancer Cells

Cancer (**malignant**) cells are abnormal, serve no useful function, and are harmful to normal body tissues. Cancers commonly have these features:

- *Rapid or continuous cell division* occurs in many types of cancer cells because they re-enter the cell cycle for mitosis almost continuously. In addition, some cancer cells have a short generation time (2 to 4 hours), but most cancer cells have a generation time similar to that of the parent cells. These cells also do not respond to signals for apoptosis. Most cancer cells have long telomeres and a lot of the enzyme *telomerase,* which maintains telomeric DNA. As a result, cancer cells do not respond to apoptotic signals and have an unlimited life span (are "immortal").
- *Anaplasia* is a feature of cancer cells. They lose the specific appearance of their parent cells. As a cancer cell becomes even more malignant, it becomes smaller and rounded. This appearance change can make diagnosis of cancer type difficult, because many types of cancer cells look alike.
- *A large nuclear-cytoplasmic ratio* is a feature of cancer cells. The nucleus of a cancer cell is larger than that of a normal cell, and the cancer cell is small. The nucleus occupies much of the space within the cancer cell, creating a large nuclear-to-cytoplasmic ratio.
- *Specific functions are lost* partially or completely in cancer cells. *Cancer cells serve no useful purpose.*
- *Loose adherence* is typical for cancer cells because they do not make fibronectin. As a result, cancer cells easily break off from the main tumor.
- *Migration* occurs because cancer cells do not bind tightly together and have many enzymes on their cell surfaces. These features allow the cells to slip through blood vessels and tissues, spreading from the main tumor site to many other body sites. This ability to spread (**metastasize**) is a key feature of cancer cells and a major cause of death. Cancer cells expand and invade other tissues, both close by and more remote from the original tumor. Invasion and persistent growth make untreated cancer deadly.
- *Contact inhibition does not occur* in cancer cells, even when all sides of these cells are in continuous contact with the surfaces of other cells. The persistence of cancer cell division is one factor making the disease so difficult to control.
- *Abnormal chromosomes* (**aneuploidy**) are common in cancer cells as they become more malignant. Chromosomes are lost, gained, or broken; thus cancer cells can have more than 23 pairs or fewer than 23 pairs. In addition, cancer cells may have broken and rearranged chromosomes.

ANIMATION: Metastatic Spread of Breast Cancer ▶

CANCER DEVELOPMENT

Carcinogenesis/Oncogenesis

Carcinogenesis and **oncogenesis** are other names for cancer development. Table 23-2 lists key concepts about cancer development. The process of changing a normal cell into a cancer cell is called **malignant transformation.** This process occurs through the steps of initiation, promotion, progression, and metastasis.

Initiation is the first step in carcinogenesis. Normal cells can become cancer cells if their oncogenes are turned on excessively

TABLE 23-2 Key Concepts Related to Cancer Development

- Neoplastic cells originate from normal body cells.
- Transformation of a normal cell into a cancer cell involves mutation of the genes (DNA) of the normal cell.
- Early embryonic genes that are overexpressed can cause a cell to develop into a tumor.
- Only one cell has to undergo malignant transformation for cancer to begin.
- Benign tumors grow by expansion, whereas malignant tumors grow by invasion.
- Most tumors arise from cells that are capable of cell division.
- A key feature of cancer cells is the loss of apoptosis. These cells have an "infinite" life span.
- Primary prevention of cancer involves avoiding exposure to known causes of cancer.
- Secondary prevention of cancer involves screening for early detection.
- Tobacco use is a causative or permissive factor in 30% of all cancers.
- Tumors that metastasize from the primary site into another organ are still designated as tumors of the originating tissue.

(overexpressed) at any time after early embryonic life. Anything that can penetrate a cell, get into the nucleus, and damage the DNA can change or mutate the genes. Such changes can activate genes that should remain controlled or suppressed and can turn off normal genes. This type of gene change is known as **initiation.** Initiation is an irreversible event that can lead to cancer development. After initiation, a cell can become a cancer cell if the cellular changes that occurred during initiation continue and cell division is not impaired. A cancer cell is not a health threat unless it can divide. If it cannot divide, it cannot form a tumor. *If growth conditions are right, however, widespread metastatic disease can develop from just one cancer cell.*

Substances that change the activity of a cell's genes so that the cell becomes a cancer cell are **carcinogens.** Carcinogens may be chemicals, physical agents, or viruses. Table 23-3 lists known chemical and physical carcinogens. Chapters presenting the care of patients with specific cancers discuss specific carcinogens (when known) within the Etiology sections.

Promotion is the enhancement of growth of an initiated cell. **Promoters** are substances that promote or enhance growth of the initiated cancer cell. Once a normal cell has been initiated by a carcinogen and is a cancer cell, it can become a tumor if its growth is enhanced. Many normal hormones and body proteins, like insulin and estrogen, can act as promoters and make altered cells divide more frequently. The time between a cell's initiation and the development of an overt tumor is called the **latency period,** which can range from months to years. Exposure to promoters can shorten the latency period.

Progression is the continued change of a cancer, making it more malignant over time. Many processes within the tumor must take place for progression to occur. After cancer cells have grown to the point that a detectable tumor is formed (a 1-cm tumor has at least 1 billion cells in it), other events must occur for this tumor to become a health problem. First, the tumor must develop its own blood supply. In the early stages, the tumor receives nutrition only by diffusion. After the tumor reaches 1 cm, however, diffusion is not efficient and cells in the center of the tumor become hypoxic and start to die. To continue to grow and survive, the tumor makes *tumor angiogenesis factor (TAF)*. TAF triggers capillaries and other blood vessels in the area to grow new branches into the tumor. These blood vessels ensure the tumor's continued nourishment and growth.

TABLE 23-3 Known Chemical and Physical Carcinogens

Aflatoxins	Estrogens
Alcoholic beverages	Ether
Aminobiphenyls	Ethylene oxide
Arsenic	Melphalan
Asbestos	Mineral oils
Azathioprine	Myleran
Benzene	Naphthylamine
Benzidine	Nickel
Beryllium	Nitrogen mustard
Cadmium	Nitrosoureas
Chlorambucil	PUVA
Chromium	Radiation (all types)
Coal tar	Silica
Coke oven emissions	Soot
Cyclophosphamide	Sulfuric acid
Cyclosporin A	Tamoxifen
Diethylstilbestrol	Thiotepa
Dioxin	Tobacco smoke (and all other forms)
Drug mixtures containing phenacetin	Vinyl chloride
Dyes containing benzidine	Wood dust
Erionite	

Source: National Toxicology Program. (2005). *Report on carcinogens* (11th ed.). Retrieved September 2007, from http://ntp.niehs.hih.gov/.
PUVA, Psoralen plus ultraviolet A.

As tumor cells continue to divide, some of the new cells change features from the original, initiated cancer cell. Actual colonies or subpopulations within the tumor begin to appear. These cell groups differ from the original cancer cell. Some of the differences provide these cell groups with advantages that allow them to live and divide no matter how the conditions around them change; these differences are thus called *selection advantages.* Changes that a tumor undergoes at this time can allow it to become more malignant. Over time, the tumor cells have fewer and fewer normal cell features.

The original tumor is called the **primary tumor.** It is usually identified by the tissue from which it arose (parent tissue), such as in breast cancer or lung cancer. When primary tumors are located in vital organs, such as the brain or lungs, they can grow excessively and either lethally damage the vital organ or crowd out healthy organ tissue and interfere with that organ's ability to perform its vital function. At other times, the primary tumor is located in soft tissue that can expand without damage as the tumor grows. One such site is the breast. The breast is not a vital organ, and even if it had a large tumor in it, the primary tumor alone would not cause the patient's death. When the tumor spreads from the original site into vital areas, life functions can be disrupted and death may follow.

Metastasis occurs when cancer cells move from the primary location by breaking off from the original group and establishing remote colonies. These additional tumors are called **metastatic** or **secondary tumors.** *Even though the tumor is now in another organ, it is still a cancer from the original altered tissue. For example, when breast cancer spreads to the lung and the bone, it is still breast cancer in the lung and bone—not lung cancer and not bone cancer.* Metastasis occurs through many steps, as shown in Fig. 23-6.

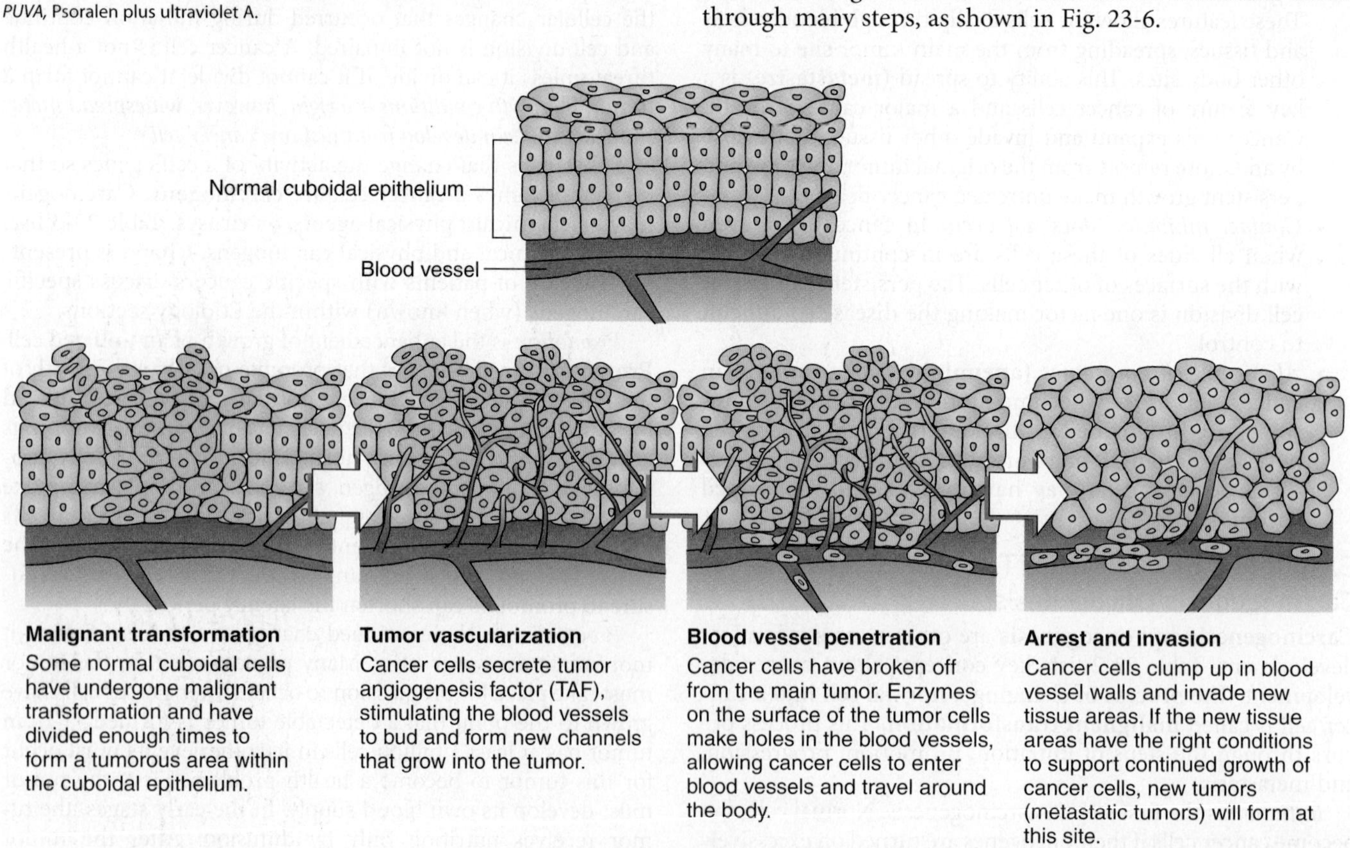
Normal cuboidal epithelium
Blood vessel
Malignant transformation
Some normal cuboidal cells have undergone malignant transformation and have divided enough times to form a tumorous area within the cuboidal epithelium.
Tumor vascularization
Cancer cells secrete tumor angiogenesis factor (TAF), stimulating the blood vessels to bud and form new channels that grow into the tumor.
Blood vessel penetration
Cancer cells have broken off from the main tumor. Enzymes on the surface of the tumor cells make holes in the blood vessels, allowing cancer cells to enter blood vessels and travel around the body.
Arrest and invasion
Cancer cells clump up in blood vessel walls and invade new tissue areas. If the new tissue areas have the right conditions to support continued growth of cancer cells, new tumors (metastatic tumors) will form at this site.

Fig. 23-6 • The steps of metastasis.

Tumors first extend into surrounding tissues. The cancer cells secrete enzymes that open up areas of surrounding tissue. Pressure, created as the tumor increases in size, forces tumor cells to invade new territory.

Spread to distant organs and tissues requires cancer cells to penetrate blood vessels. **Bloodborne metastasis** (tumor cell release into the blood) is the most common cause of cancer spread. Enzymes also make large pores in the patient's blood vessels, allowing tumor cells to enter the blood and circulate throughout the body. Because tumor cells are loosely held together, clumps of cells break off of the primary tumor into blood vessels for transport.

Tumor cells circulate through the blood and enter tissues at remote sites. Clumps of cancer cells can become trapped in capillaries. These clumps damage the capillary wall and allow cancer cells to leave the capillary and enter the surrounding tissue.

When conditions in the remote site can support tumor cell growth, the cells stop circulating (arrest) and invade the surrounding tissues, creating secondary tumors. Table 23-4 lists the common sites of metastasis for specific tumor types.

Another way cancers metastasize is by *lymphatic spread*. Lymphatic spread is related to the number, structure, and location of lymph nodes and vessels. Primary sites that are rich in lymphatics have more early metastatic spread than areas with few lymphatics.

TABLE 23-4 Common Sites of Metastasis for Different Cancer Types

BREAST CANCER	**PROSTATE CANCER**
Bone*	Bone (especially spine and legs)*
Lung*	Pelvic nodes
Liver	**MELANOMA**
Brain	GI tract
LUNG CANCER	Lymph nodes
Brain*	Lung
Bone	Brain
Liver	**PRIMARY BRAIN CANCER**
Lymph nodes	Central nervous system
Pancreas	
COLORECTAL CANCER	
Liver*	
Lymph nodes	
Adjacent structures	

*Most common site of metastasis for the specific malignant neoplasm.

Cancer Classification

Cancers are classified by the type of tissue from which they arise (e.g., glandular, connective). Terms that describe cancer by tissue origin are listed in Table 23-5. Other ways to classify cancer include biologic behavior, anatomic site, and degree of differentiation.

About 100 different types of cancer arise from various tissues or organs. Fig. 23-7 compares cancer distribution by site

TABLE 23-5 Classification of Tumors by Tissue of Origin

Prefix	Tissue of Origin	Benign Tumor	Malignant Tumor*
Adeno	Epithelial glands	Adenoma	Adenocarcinoma
Chondro	Cartilage	Chondroma	Chondrosarcoma
Fibro	Fibrous connective	Fibroma	Fibrosarcoma
Glio	Glial cells (brain)	Glioma	Glioblastoma
Hemangio	Blood vessel	Hemangioma	Hemangiosarcoma
Hepato	Liver	Hepatoma	Hepatocarcinoma Hepatoblastoma
Leiomyo	Smooth muscle	Leiomyoma	Leiomyosarcoma
Lipo	Fat/adipose	Lipoma	Liposarcoma
Lympho	Lymphoid tissues		Malignant lymphomas Hodgkin's lymphoma Non-Hodgkin's lymphoma Burkitt's lymphoma Cutaneous T-cell
Melano	Pigment-producing skin		Melanoma
Meningioma	Meninges	Meningioma	Malignant meningioma Meningioblastoma
Neuro	Nerve tissue	Neuroma Neurofibroma	Neurosarcoma Neuroblastoma
Osteo	Bone	Osteoma	Osteosarcoma
Renal	Kidney		Renal cell carcinoma
Rhabdo	Skeletal muscle	Rhabdomyoma	Rhabdomyosarcoma
Squamous	Epithelial layer of skin, mucous membranes, and organ linings	Papilloma	Squamous cell carcinoma of skin, bladder, lungs, cervix

*Carcinomas are tumors of glandular tissue; sarcomas are tumors of connective tissue; blastomas are tumors of less differentiated, embryonal tissues.

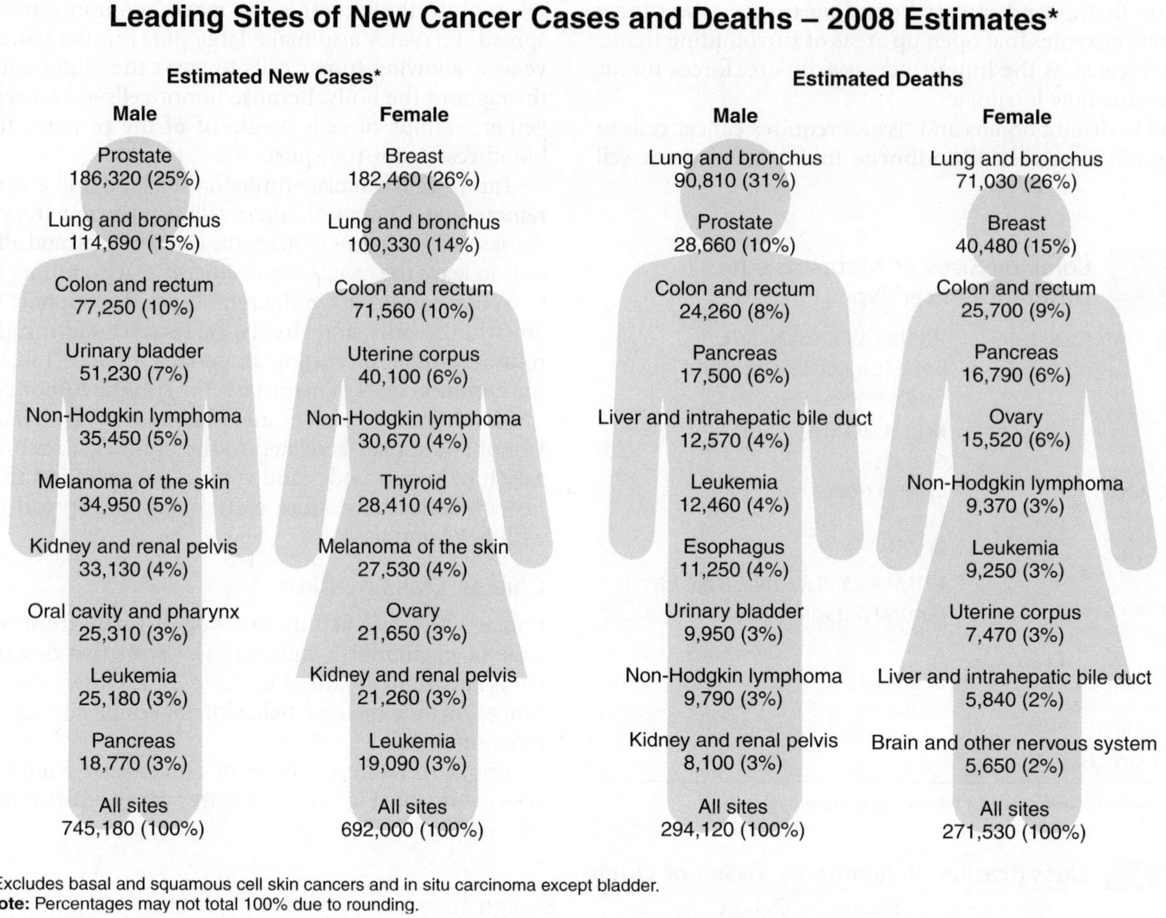
Leading Sites of New Cancer Cases and Deaths – 2008 Estimates*
Estimated New Cases*
Male
Female
Estimated Deaths
Male
Female
Prostate 186,320 (25%)
Lung and bronchus 114,690 (15%)
Colon and rectum 77,250 (10%)
Urinary bladder 51,230 (7%)
Non-Hodgkin lymphoma 35,450 (5%)
Melanoma of the skin 34,950 (5%)
Kidney and renal pelvis 33,130 (4%)
Oral cavity and pharynx 25,310 (3%)
Leukemia 25,180 (3%)
Pancreas 18,770 (3%)
All sites 745,180 (100%)
Breast 182,460 (26%)
Lung and bronchus 100,330 (14%)
Colon and rectum 71,560 (10%)
Uterine corpus 40,100 (6%)
Non-Hodgkin lymphoma 30,670 (4%)
Thyroid 28,410 (4%)
Melanoma of the skin 27,530 (4%)
Ovary 21,650 (3%)
Kidney and renal pelvis 21,260 (3%)
Leukemia 19,090 (3%)
All sites 692,000 (100%)
Lung and bronchus 90,810 (31%)
Prostate 28,660 (10%)
Colon and rectum 24,260 (8%)
Pancreas 17,500 (6%)
Liver and intrahepatic bile duct 12,570 (4%)
Leukemia 12,460 (4%)
Esophagus 11,250 (4%)
Urinary bladder 9,950 (3%)
Non-Hodgkin lymphoma 9,790 (3%)
Kidney and renal pelvis 8,100 (3%)
All sites 294,120 (100%)
Lung and bronchus 71,030 (26%)
Breast 40,480 (15%)
Colon and rectum 25,700 (9%)
Pancreas 16,790 (6%)
Ovary 15,520 (6%)
Non-Hodgkin lymphoma 9,370 (3%)
Leukemia 9,250 (3%)
Uterine corpus 7,470 (3%)
Liver and intrahepatic bile duct 5,840 (2%)
Brain and other nervous system 5,650 (2%)
All sites 271,530 (100%)
*Excludes basal and squamous cell skin cancers and in situ carcinoma except bladder.
Note: Percentages may not total 100% due to rounding.

Fig. 23-7 • Cancer incidence and death by site and gender.

and gender. Cancers are divided into two major categories: solid and hematologic.

Solid tumors develop from specific tissues (e.g., breast cancer, lung cancer). Hematologic cancers arise from blood cell–forming tissues (e.g., leukemias, lymphomas).

Cancer Grading, Ploidy, and Staging

Systems of grading and staging have been developed to help standardize cancer diagnosis, prognosis, and treatment. **Grading** of a tumor classifies cellular aspects of the cancer. **Ploidy** classifies tumor chromosomes as normal or abnormal. **Staging** classifies clinical aspects of the cancer.

Grading is needed because some cancer cells are "more malignant" than others, varying in their aggressiveness and sensitivity to treatment. Some cancer cells barely resemble the tissue from which they arose, are aggressive, and spread rapidly. These cells are a "high-grade" cancer. On the basis of cell appearance and activity, grading compares the cancer cell with the normal parent tissue from which it arose.

Different clinical groups have established different grading systems for different types of cancer cells, but overall, they resemble the standard system listed in Table 23-6. This system rates cancer cells with the lowest rating given to those cells that closely resemble normal cells and the highest rating given to cancer cells that barely resemble normal cells.

Grading the cells is one of the first steps in confirming cancer. Grading is a means of evaluating the patient with cancer for prognosis and appropriate therapy. It also allows health care professionals to evaluate the results of management and compare local, regional, national, and international statistics.

TABLE 23-6 Grading of Malignant Tumors

Grade	Cellular Characteristics
G_x	Grade cannot be determined.
G_1	Tumor cells are well differentiated and closely resemble the normal cells from which they arose. This grade is considered a low grade of malignant change. These tumors are malignant but are relatively slow growing.
G_2	Tumor cells are moderately differentiated; they still retain some of the characteristics of normal cells but also have more malignant characteristics than do G_1 tumor cells.
G_3	Tumor cells are poorly differentiated, but the tissue of origin can usually be established. The cells have few normal cell characteristics.
G_4	Tumor cells are poorly differentiated and retain no normal cell characteristics. Determination of the tissue of origin is difficult and perhaps impossible.

Ploidy is the description of cancer cells by chromosome number and appearance. Normal human cells have 46 chromosomes (23 pairs), the normal diploid number **(euploidy).** When malig-

TABLE 23-7 Staging of Cancer—TNM Classification

	PRIMARY TUMOR (T)
T_x	Primary tumor cannot be assessed
T_0	No evidence of primary tumor
T_{is}	Carcinoma in situ
T_1, T_2, T_3, T_4	Increasing size and/or local extent of the primary tumor
	REGIONAL LYMPH NODES (N)
N_x	Regional lymph nodes cannot be assessed
N_0	No regional lymph node metastasis
N_1, N_2, N_3	Increasing involvement of regional lymph nodes
	DISTANT METASTASIS (M)
M_x	Presence of distant metastasis cannot be assessed
M_0	No distant metastasis
M_1	Distant metastasis

nant transformation occurs, changes in the genes and chromosomes also occur. Some cancer cells gain or lose whole chromosomes and may have structural abnormalities of the remaining chromosomes **(aneuploidy).** The degree of aneuploidy usually increases with the degree of malignancy. Some specific chromosome changes are associated with specific cancers, and their presence is used for diagnosis and prognosis. One example is the "Philadelphia" chromosome abnormality often present in chronic myelogenous leukemia cells (see Chapter 42).

Staging determines the exact location of the cancer and its degree of metastasis at diagnosis. Staging is important because, for most cancers, the smaller the cancer is at diagnosis and the less it has spread, the greater the chances are that treatment will result in a cure. Cancer stage also influences selection of therapy. Staging is done by clinical staging, surgical staging, and pathologic staging. *Clinical staging* assesses the patient's clinical manifestations and evaluates clinical signs for tumor size and possible spread. *Surgical staging* assesses the tumor size, number, sites, and spread by inspection at surgery. *Pathologic staging* is the most definitive type, determining the tumor size, number, sites, and spread by pathologic examination of tissues obtained at surgery.

Specific staging systems include Dukes' staging of colon and rectal cancer and Clark's levels method of staging skin cancer. The American Joint Committee on Cancer developed the **tumor, node, metastasis (TNM)** system to describe the anatomic extent of cancers. The stages guide treatment and are useful for prognosis and comparison of treatment results. The TNM staging systems have specific prognostic value for each solid tumor type. Table 23-7 shows a basic TNM staging system. TNM staging is not useful for leukemia or lymphomas. Staging for these cancers is discussed in Chapter 42.

Tumor growth is assessed in terms of **doubling time** (the amount of time it takes for a tumor to double in size) and **mitotic index** (the percentage of actively dividing cells within a tumor). The smallest detectable tumor is about 1 cm in diameter and contains 1 billion cells. To reach this size, it must undergo at least 30 doublings. A tumor with a mitotic index of less than 10% is a slow-growing tumor; a tumor with an index of 85% is fast growing. Tumors have a wide range of growth rates. Fast-growing tumors, such as lymphomas, may double in 4 weeks; an adenocarcinoma of the lung may double in 20 to 40 weeks.

Cancer Etiology and Genetic Risk

Carcinogenesis takes years and depends on several tumor and patient factors. Three interacting factors influence cancer development: exposure to carcinogens, genetic predisposition, and immune function. These factors account for variation in cancer development from one person to another, even when each person is exposed to the same hazards.

Oncogene activation is the main mechanism of carcinogenesis regardless of the specific cause. These oncogenes were the genes that directed early embryonic development. At about 8 days after conception, these genes should be controlled forever. They are turned on under controlled conditions when cells need to divide for normal growth and replacement of dead or damaged tissues. At other times they are turned off, controlled, or suppressed by "suppressor genes." Suppressor genes can act directly at the DNA level, preventing the oncogene from being overexpressed. Another way that suppressor genes work is by preventing cells from dividing, or maintaining control over the cell cycle.

When a normal cell is exposed to any carcinogen (initiator), the normal cell's DNA can be damaged or mutated. The mutations damage suppressor genes, preventing them from controlling the expression of oncogenes. As a result, the oncogenes are overexpressed and can cause the cells to change from normal cells to cancer cells. When oncogenes are overexpressed in a cell, excessive amounts of cyclins are produced and upset the balance between cell growth enhancement and cell growth limitation. The effect of these excessive cyclins is greater than the effect of the suppressor gene products, thus allowing uncontrolled cell division.

About 70 different oncogenes have been identified. *These oncogenes are not abnormal genes but are part of every cell's normal makeup and were important in early development.* Oncogenes become a problem only if they are activated and overexpressed as a result of exposure to carcinogenic agents or events. Both external and personal factors can activate oncogenes.

External Factors Causing Cancer

External factors, including environmental exposure, are responsible for about 80% of cancer in North America (ACS, 2007b). Environmental carcinogens are chemical, physical, or viral agents that cause cancer. The National Toxicology Program has identified 58 agents known to cause cancer in humans and another 188 agents suspected to be carcinogens (National Toxicology Program, 2005). Table 23-3 lists some known chemical and physical causes of human cancer.

Chemical carcinogenesis can occur from exposures to many known chemicals, drugs, and other products used in everyday life. Hundreds more are suspected of being carcinogenic.

Chemicals vary in how carcinogenic they are. Some substances, such as tobacco and alcohol, appear to be only mildly carcinogenic; it takes long-term exposure to large amounts of these substances before a cancer develops. However, these two substances can act as co-carcinogens; when taken together, they enhance each other's carcinogenic activity.

Not all cells are susceptible to chemical carcinogenesis to the same degree. Normal cells that have the ability to divide are at greater risk for cancer development than are normal cells that are not capable of cell division. For example, cancers commonly arise in bone marrow, skin, lining of the GI tract, ductal cells of the breast, and lining of the lungs. All of these cells normally undergo cell division. Cancers of nerve tissue, cardiac muscle, and skeletal muscle are rare. These cells do not normally undergo cell division.

About 30% of cancers diagnosed in North America are related to tobacco use (ACS, 2007b). Tobacco is the single most important source of preventable carcinogenesis. It contains many different carcinogens and co-carcinogens. Tobacco use both initiates and promotes cancer. The risk for cancer development from tobacco use depends on a person's immune function, amount of tobacco exposure, type of tobacco exposure, and tobacco tar content.

Tissues with the greatest risk for tobacco-induced cancer are those that have direct contact with tobacco or tobacco smoke. Cigarette smoking and tobacco use also promote the development of other cancers. Table 23-8 lists the specific cancers that appear to be associated with tobacco use.

Physical carcinogenesis from physical agents or events causes cancer by the same mechanism as for chemical carcinogens (i.e., DNA damage). Two physical agents that are known to cause cancer are radiation and chronic irritation.

Even small doses of radiation affect cells (National Toxicology Program, 2005). Some effects are temporary and can be repaired. Other effects cannot be repaired and either may be lethal to the damaged cell or induce cancer in the damaged cell. The two types of radiation that cause cancer are ionizing and ultraviolet (UV). Some ionizing radiation is found naturally in such elements as radon, uranium, and radium. Most rocks and soil contain various amounts of uranium and radium. Other sources of ionizing radiation include x-rays for diagnosis and treatment of disease, as well as cosmic radiation. UV radiation is a type of solar radiation, coming from the sun. Other sources of UV radiation include tanning beds and germicidal lights. UV rays do not penetrate deeply, and the most common cancer type caused by UV exposure is skin cancer.

Both ionizing and UV radiation mutate genes. Although radiation exposure induces cancers more often among cells that can divide, it can cause cancer among nondividing cells as well.

Chronic irritation and tissue trauma are suspected to cause cancer. The incidence of skin cancer is higher in the scars of people with burn scars or other types of severe skin injury. Chronically irritated tissues undergo frequent cell division and thus are at an increased risk for spontaneous DNA mutation (Schottenfeld & Beebe-Dimmer, 2006).

Viral carcinogenesis occurs when viruses infect body cells and break the DNA strands. Viruses then insert their own genetic material into the human DNA. Breaking the DNA, along with viral gene insertion, mutates the normal cell's DNA and can either activate an oncogene or damage suppressor genes (National Toxicology Program, 2005). Viruses that cause cancer are **oncoviruses.** Table 23-9 lists cancers of known viral origin.

Dietary factors related to cancer development are poorly understood although dietary practices are suspected to alter cancer risk. Because dietary factors are rarely independent of other possible carcinogenic agents, evidence of dietary contributions to cancer development is clouded. Suspected dietary factors include low fiber intake, high intake of red meat, and high animal fat intake. Preservatives, contaminants, preparation methods, and additives (dyes, flavorings, sweeteners) may have cancer-promoting effects. Chart 23-1 lists foods that have carcinogenic potential and those that are thought to be protective against cancer development.

Personal Factors and Cancer Development

Personal factors, including immune function, age, and genetic risk, also affect whether a person is likely to develop cancer.

Immune function protects the body from foreign invaders and non-self cells (see Chapter 19). Non-self cells include cells that are no longer normal, such as cancer cells. The part of the

TABLE 23-8 Cancer Types Associated with Tobacco Use

• Lung	• Cervical
• Oral cavity	• Kidney
• Pharyngeal	• Bladder
• Laryngeal	• Liver
• Esophagus	• Stomach
• Pancreatic	• Myeloid leukemia

Data from American Cancer Society. (2008). *Cancer facts and figures—2008.* Report No. 00-300M–No. 5008.08. Atlanta: Author.

TABLE 23-9 Cancers Associated with a Known Viral Origin

Virus	Malignancies
Epstein-Barr virus	Burkitt's lymphoma, B-cell lymphoma, nasopharyngeal carcinoma
Hepatitis B virus	Primary liver carcinoma
Hepatitis C virus	Primary liver carcinoma, possibly B-cell lymphomas
Human papillomavirus	Cervical carcinoma, vulvar carcinoma, and other anogenital carcinomas
Human lymphotrophic virus type I	Adult T-cell leukemia
Human lymphotrophic virus type II	Hairy cell leukemia

National Toxicology Program. (2006). *Report on carcinogens* (11th ed.). Available online at http://ntp.niehs.nih.gov.

Chart 23-1 PATIENT AND FAMILY EDUCATION GUIDE

Dietary Habits to Reduce Cancer Risk

- Avoid excessive intake of animal fat.
- Avoid nitrites (prepared lunch meats, sausage, bacon).
- Minimize your intake of red meat.
- Keep your alcohol consumption to no more than one or two drinks per day.
- Eat more bran.
- Eat more cruciferous vegetables, such as broccoli, cauliflower, brussels sprouts, and cabbage.
- Eat foods high in vitamin A (e.g., apricots, carrots, leafy green and yellow vegetables) and vitamin C (e.g., fresh fruits and vegetables, especially citrus fruits).

immune system that protects against cancer is cell-mediated immunity. Natural killer (NK) and helper T-cells provide immune surveillance.

The role of the immune system in protecting against cancer is supported by cancer incidence in immunosuppressed people. Adults older than 60 years have immune systems that function at less-than-optimal levels, and therefore this group has a higher incidence of cancer compared with that of the general population. Organ transplant recipients taking immunosuppressive drugs to prevent organ rejection also have a higher incidence of cancer. In patients with acquired immune deficiency syndrome (AIDS), incidence may be as high as 70%.

Advancing age is the single most important risk factor for cancer (ACS, 2008). As a person ages, immune protection decreases and external exposures to carcinogens accumulate. Manifestations of cancer in older patients may be overlooked as changes of normal aging. Teach older adults to be aware of and report symptoms such as the seven warning signs of cancer (Table 23-10) to health care providers. Health care providers should investigate all manifestations suggestive of disease. Cancer assessment considerations for the older adult are listed in Chart 23-2.

TABLE 23-10 The Seven Warning Signs of Cancer

C	Changes in bowel or bladder habits
A	A sore that does not heal
U	Unusual bleeding or discharge
T	Thickening or lump in the breast or elsewhere
I	Indigestion or difficulty swallowing
O	Obvious change in a wart or mole
N	Nagging cough or hoarseness

Chart 23-2 NURSING FOCUS ON THE OLDER ADULT

Hematologic Assessment

Cancer Type	Assessment Consideration
Colorectal cancer	Ask the patient whether bowel habits have changed over the past year (e.g., in consistency, frequency, color). Is there any obvious blood in the stool? Test at least one stool specimen for occult blood during the patient's hospitalization. Encourage the patient to have a baseline colonoscopy. Encourage the patient to reduce dietary intake of animal fats, red meat, and smoked meats. Encourage the patient to increase dietary intake of bran, vegetables, and fruit.
Bladder cancer	Ask the patient about the presence of: Pain on urination Blood in the urine Cloudy urine Increased frequency or urgency
Prostate cancer	Ask the patient about: Hesitancy Change in the size of the urine stream Pain in the back or legs History of urinary tract infections
Skin cancer	Examine skin areas for moles or warts. Ask the patient about changes in moles (e.g., color, edges, sensation).
Leukemia	Observe the skin for color, petechiae, or ecchymosis. Ask the patient about: Fatigue Bruising Bleeding tendency History of infections and illnesses Night sweats Unexplained fevers
Lung cancer	Observe the skin and mucous membranes for color. How many words can the patient say between breaths? Ask the patient about: Cough Hoarseness Smoking history Exposure to inhalation irritants Shortness of breath Activity tolerance Frothy or bloody sputum Pain in the arms or chest Difficulty swallowing

GENETIC CONSIDERATIONS

Genetic risk for cancer occurs in a small percent of the population; however, people who have a genetic predisposition are at very high risk for cancer development (Strauss-Tranin, 2006). As previously discussed, oncogenes are risk factors related to carcinogenesis. Altered oncogenes are passed on from generation to generation. The development of cancer, however, depends on more than these genes. The oncogene must be overexpressed for cancer to occur. In some people, the sequence of a specific oncogene is different (has been mutated), which may allow it to be activated more easily. In other people, the oncogene is normal but the gene controlling oncogene activity, the suppressor gene, is mutated and allows overexpression of one or more oncogenes, leading to a huge increase in cancer risk.

These variations in gene sequence may be small single nucleotide polymorphisms (SNPs) or may be large areas of mutations. Both types of gene problems can be inherited or can occur as a result of exposure to carcinogens. Patterns of genetic risk for cancer have also been identified, including:

- Inherited predisposition for specific cancers
- Inherited conditions associated with cancer
- Familial clustering
- Chromosomal aberrations

Table 23-11 lists conditions associated with an increased genetic risk for cancer development.

Genetic testing for cancer predisposition is available to confirm or rule out a person's genetic risk for a few specific cancers. These tests are performed on blood, are expensive, and often are not covered by insurance. Genetic testing should not be performed unless a family history clearly indicates the possibility of increased genetic risk and the patient wants to have the test results. *These tests do not diagnose the presence of cancer.*

A variety of issues and potential problems exist with genetic testing for cancer risk. Correct interpretation of the results is critical. Ideally, a genetic counselor is involved in giving the patient information before, as well as after, testing is performed. *A patient's positive test result for a cancer-causing gene mutation shows that he or she is at greatly increased risk for cancer development; however, the cancer still may never develop.*

Other issues regarding genetic testing include who will have access to the information and whether to share the test results with family members. Many patients fear that if they test positive for a cancer-causing gene, they may face discrimination for insurance coverage or in the workplace. Some states have confidentiality safeguards, and others do not. Genetic testing has implications for the entire family, not just the patient being tested. For more information on genetic testing, see Chapter 6.

CULTURAL AWARENESS

The incidence of cancer varies among races. American Cancer Society (ACS) data (2007a) show that African Americans have a higher incidence of cancer than white people do and the death rate is higher for African Americans. Since 1960, the overall incidence among African Americans has increased 27%, whereas for white people it has increased 12%. Cancer sites and cancer-related mortality vary along racial lines as well. One explanation for this difference is that more African Americans have less access to health care. Thus they are more often diagnosed with later stage cancer that is more difficult to cure or control. However, this disparity in health care access does not explain all differences.

Table 23-12 shows common cancers among white, African American, Asian, and Hispanic populations. Understanding these variations can help in planning prevention and early detection strategies that are ethnically specific (Pesquera et al., 2008).

When risks for cancer development are assessed, however, ethnicity and genetic predisposition cannot be considered alone. Behavior and socioeconomic factors must also be assessed. The American Cancer Society (2008, 2007b)

TABLE 23-11 Conditions Associated with a Genetic Predisposition for Cancer

Condition	Specific Cancer Type
Inherited cancers*	Breast cancer Prostate cancer Ovarian cancer
Familial clustering	Breast cancer Melanoma
Bloom syndrome	Leukemia
Familial polyposis	Colorectal cancer
Chromosomal aberrations	
Down syndrome (47 chromosomes)	Leukemia
Klinefelter syndrome (47, XXY)	Breast cancer
Turner syndrome (45, XO)	Leukemia Gonadal carcinoma Meningioma Colorectal cancer

*Not all breast, prostate, or ovarian cancers are inherited.

TABLE 23-12 Racial Differences in Cancer Development

WHITE *COMMON CANCER TYPES*	ASIAN *COMMON CANCER TYPES*
1. Lung	1. Breast
2. Breast	2. Colorectal
3. Colorectal	3. Prostate
4. Prostate	4. Lung
	5. Stomach
AFRICAN AMERICAN *COMMON CANCER TYPES*	**HISPANIC** *COMMON CANCER TYPES*
1. Lung	1. Prostate
2. Prostate	2. Breast
3. Breast	3. Colorectal
4. Colorectal	4. Lung
5. Uterine	

Data from American Cancer Society. (2008). *Cancer facts and figures—2008.* Report No. 00-300M–No. 5008.08. Atlanta: Author.

reports that cancer incidence and survival are often related to socioeconomic factors. These factors include the availability of health care services or the belief that seeking early health care has a positive effect on the outcome of cancer diagnosis.

CANCER PREVENTION

Cancer prevention activities can focus on primary prevention or secondary prevention. **Primary prevention** is the use of strategies to prevent the actual occurrence of cancer. This method of cancer prevention is most effective when there is a known cause for a cancer type. **Secondary prevention** is the use of screening strategies to detect cancer early, at a time when cure or control is more likely.

Primary Prevention

Avoidance of known or potential carcinogens is an effective primary prevention strategy. This method is effective when a cause of cancer is known and avoidance is easily accomplished. For example, teach people to use skin protection during sun exposure to avoid skin cancer. Much lung cancer can be avoided by not using tobacco and by eliminating environmental asbestos exposure. Teach everyone about the dangers of cigarette smoking and other forms of tobacco use. Provide information on smoking cessation strategies and support systems. As more cancer causes are identified, avoidance may become even more effective.

Modifying associated factors appears to have a positive influence in reducing cancer risk. Absolute causes are not known for many cancers, but some conditions appear to increase risk. Examples are the increased incidence of cancer among people who consume alcohol; the association of a diet high in fat and low in fiber with colon cancer, breast cancer, and ovarian cancer; and a greater incidence of cervical cancer among women who have multiple sexual partners (Wells, 2008). Modifying behavior to reduce the associated factor may decrease the risk for cancer development. Therefore teach all people to limit their intake of alcohol to no more than one ounce per day and to include more fruit, vegetables, and whole grains in their diets. Instruct women about the importance of limiting the number of sexual partners and to use safer sex practices to avoid exposure to viruses that can increase the risk for cervical cancer.

Removal of "at risk" tissues reduces cancer risk for a person who has a known high risk for developing a specific type of cancer. Examples include removing moles to prevent conversion to skin cancer, removing colon polyps to prevent colon cancer, and removing breasts to prevent breast cancer. Not all "at risk" tissues can be removed (e.g., those that are part of essential organs).

Chemoprevention is a newer form of potential cancer prevention. This strategy uses drugs, chemicals, natural nutrients, or other substances to disrupt one or more steps important to cancer development. These agents may be able to reverse existing gene damage or halt the progression of the transformation process. Table 23-13 lists agents under investigation for chemoprevention. At this time, only a few agents have been found effective and are commonly prescribed. These include the use of aspirin and celecoxib (Celebrex) to reduce the risk for colon cancer (Bommareddy et al., 2006), the use of vitamin D and tamoxifen to reduce the risk for breast cancer, and the use of lycopene to reduce the risk for prostate cancer (ACS, 2007b; Shukla & Gupta, 2005).

The goal of chemopreventive strategies is prevention of cancer development. Target populations for whom chemoprevention might be effective include:

- Healthy people with no known specific cancer risk
- People at greater-than-normal risk because of increased environmental exposure or decreased immune function
- People with precancerous lesions
- People with a history of cancer

Vaccination is a new method of primary cancer prevention. Currently, the only vaccine approved for cancer prevention is Gardasil, which prevents infection from several forms of the human papilloma virus (HPV). As more viruses are identified as being cancer causing, it is hoped that vaccines will be developed to prevent those viral infections.

TABLE 23-13 Agents Under Investigation for Chemoprevention of Cancer

Category of Prevention	Specific Agents
Prevention of carcinogen formation	Ascorbic acid (vitamin C) Tocopherol (type of vitamin E) Selenium Caffeic acid
Blocking the action of a carcinogen on DNA ("antimutagens")	Carotenoids (vitamin A derivative) Retinoids (vitamin A derivative) Ellagic acid Flavones Oltipraz Butylated hydroxyanisole
Enhancing the elimination of a carcinogen	Isothiocyanate Indole-3-carbinol
Suppression of carcinogenic action	Aspirin Retinoids Lycopene Indomethacin Selenium Steroidal anti-inflammatory agents Protease inhibitors
Antipromotion activity	Carotenoids Lycopene Retinoids Selenium Coumarin Piroxicam Indomethacin Calciferol (vitamin D) Hormone antagonists Tamoxifen Finasteride Evista
Suppression of progression	Danazol Interferon Cysteamine Vorozole

Secondary Prevention

Regular screening for cancer does not reduce cancer incidence but can greatly reduce some types of cancer deaths. Teach all adults the benefits of participating in specific routine screening techniques annually as part of health maintenance. General screening recommendations are listed in chapters discussing cancers by organ system. The age and type of participation in specific screening tests are different for people who have an identified increased risk for a specific cancer type. Examples of recommended screenings include (ACS, 2008, 2007b):

- Yearly mammography for women older than 40 years
- Yearly clinical breast examination for women older than 40 years
- Colonoscopy at age 50 years and then every 10 years
- Yearly fecal occult blood for adults of all ages
- Yearly prostate specific antigen (PSA) test and digital rectal examination (DRE) for men older than 50 years

Because cancer development clearly involves gene changes (either inherited gene mutations or acquired gene damage), researchers have suggested that altering damaged genes could prevent cancer development. Currently, people can be screened for some gene mutations that increase the risk for cancer. Examples of these gene mutations include the *BRCA1* gene, which increases the risk for both breast and ovarian cancer; the *BRCA2* gene, which increases the risk for breast cancer; and the *APC*, *MLH1*, and *MSH2* genes, which increase the risk for colon cancer.

When taking a patient history and the person appears to have a strong family history of either breast cancer or colon cancer, create a three-generation pedigree to more fully explore the possibility of genetic risk. If a pattern of risk emerges, inform the person about the possible benefits of genetic screening and to talk with a genetics professional for more information. Screening can help a person at increased genetic risk for cancer to alter lifestyle factors, participate in early detection methods, or even have at-risk tissue removed. Genetic screening has some personal risks as well as potential benefits (see Chapter 6). Although it is not yet possible to "fix" or remove an abnormal gene in humans, gene therapy in the future is not out of the realm of possibility.

GET READY FOR THE NCLEX EXAMINATION!

Key Points

Review these Key Points for each NCLEX Examination Client Needs Category.

Health Promotion and Maintenance

- Teach patients to use sunscreen and to wear protective clothing during sun exposure.
- Encourage patients to participate in the recommended cancer screening activities for their age-group and cancer risk category.
- Inform all patients who smoke that smoking increases the risk for development of many cancer types.
- Assist anyone interested in smoking cessation to find an appropriate smoking cessation program.
- Assess the patient's knowledge about causes of cancer and his or her screening/prevention practices.
- Assist patients who fear a cancer diagnosis to understand that finding cancer at an early stage increases the chances for cure.
- Teach patients who undergo genetic testing for cancer predisposition about the risks to confidentiality of the test results.
- Ask all patients about their exposures to environmental agents that are known or suspected to increase the risk for cancer.
- Obtain a detailed family history (at least three generations) to assess the patient's risk for familial or inherited cancer.
- Teach anyone, especially older adults, the "seven warning signs of cancer" (see Table 23-10).

Physiological Integrity

- Cancer cells originate from normal body cells.
- Transformation of a normal cell into a cancer cell involves mutation of the genes (DNA) of the normal cell.
- Oncogenes that are overexpressed can cause a cell to develop into a tumor.
- Only one cell has to undergo malignant transformation for cancer to begin.
- Benign tumors grow by expansion, whereas malignant tumors grow by invasion.
- Most tumors arise from cells that are capable of cell division.
- A key feature of cancer cells is the loss of apoptosis. These cells have an "infinite" life span.
- Primary prevention of cancer involves avoiding exposure to known causes of cancer.
- Secondary prevention of cancer involves screening for early detection.
- Tobacco use is a causative factor in 30% of all malignant neoplasms.
- Tumors that metastasize from the primary site into another organ are still designated as tumors of the originating tissue.

Additional Study Resources

Go to your Companion CD or Evolve at http://evolve.elsevier.com/Iggy/ for *Self-Assessment Questions for the NCLEX Examination.*

Go to Evolve at http://evolve.elsevier.com/Iggy/ for *Prioritization and Delegation Questions for the NCLEX Examination.*

SELECTED BIBLIOGRAPHY

Asterisk indicates a classic or definitive work on this subject.

American Cancer Society (ACS). (2008). *Cancer facts and figures—2008.* Report No. 00-300M–No. 5008.08. Atlanta: Author.

American Cancer Society (ACS). (2007a). *Cancer facts and figures for African Americans—2007-2008.* Report No. 8614.07. Atlanta: Author.

American Cancer Society (ACS). (2007b). *Cancer prevention and early detection: Facts & figures—2007.* Report No. 8600.07. Atlanta: Author.

Bommareddy, A., Arasada, B.L., Mathees, D.P., & Dwivedi, C. (2006). Chemopreventive effects of dietary flaxseed on colon tumor development. *Nutrition and Cancer, 54*(2), 216-222.

Bragdon, M., & Scroggs, S. (2006). Cancer prevention. *Clinical Journal of Oncology Nursing, 10*(5), 649-655.

*Frank-Stromborg, M., & Olsen, S. (2001). *Cancer prevention in diverse populations: Cultural implications for health care professionals.* Pittsburgh: Oncology Nursing Society.

Giarelli, E. (2006). Self-surveillance for genetic predisposition to cancer: Behaviors and emotions. *Oncology Nursing Forum, 33*(2), 221-231.

*Hawkins, R. (2001). Mastering the intricate maze of metastasis. *Oncology Nursing Forum, 28*(6), 959-965.

Jegathesan, J., Liebenthal, J.A., Arnett, M.G., Clancy, R.L., & Pierce, J.D. (2005). Apoptosis: Understanding the new molecular pathway. *MEDSURG Nursing, 13*(6), 371-376.

National Toxicology Program. (2005). *Report on carcinogens* (11th ed.). Retrieved September 2007, from http://ntp.niehs.hih.gov/.

Pesquera, M., Yoder, L., & Lynk, M. (2008). Improving cross-cultural awareness and skills to reduce health disparities in cancer. *MEDSURG Nursing, 17*(2), 114-120.

Schottenfeld, D., & Beebe-Dimmer, J. (2006). Chronic inflammation: A common and important factor in the pathogenesis of neoplasia. *CA: A Cancer Journal for Clinicians, 56*(2), 69-83.

Shukla, S., & Gupta, S. (2005). Dietary agents in the chemoprevention of prostate cancer. *Nutrition and Cancer, 53*(1), 18-32.

Strauss-Tranin, A. (2006). The bridge from genomic discoveries to disease prevention. (2006). Oncology Nursing Society Clinical Lectureship. *Oncology Nursing Forum, 33*(5), 891-900.

Wells, S. (2008). Cervical cancer: An overview with suggested practice and policy goals. *MEDSURG Nursing, 17*(1), 43-50.

Workman, L. (2006). The biological basis of cancer. In M. Barton-Burke & G. Wilkes (Eds.), *Cancer therapies* (pp. 1-20). Boston: Jones & Bartlett.

24
CHAPTER

Care of Patients with Cancer

M. Linda Workman

LEARNING OUTCOMES

For clinical competence and success on the NCLEX Examination, study this chapter with these Learning Outcomes in mind:

Safe and Effective Care Environment

1. Apply the principles of asepsis to protect neutropenic patients.
2. Modify the environment to protect patients who have thrombocytopenia.
3. Use personal protective equipment (PPE) when administering chemotherapy or when handling excreta of a patient within 48 hours of receiving chemotherapy.
4. Coordinate with the health care team to adjust the environment for protection of the patient having photodynamic therapy.

Health Promotion and Maintenance

5. Teach patients and family members how to avoid injury and infection when blood counts are low.
6. Teach patients and family members skin protection measures for radiation therapy and photodynamic therapy.
7. Teach patients and family members the proper scheduling of antiemetic therapy to ensure prevention or relief of chemotherapy-induced nausea and vomiting.

Psychosocial Integrity

8. Use effective communication when teaching patients and family members about what to expect during tests and therapeutic procedures.
9. Encourage the patients and family members to express their feelings about the diagnosis of cancer, its prognosis, and treatment.
10. Assess the patient's and family's use of coping strategies related to cancer, cancer treatment, possible role changes, and possible outcomes of the disease and its treatment.
11. Teach patients strategies to improve body image changes that occur as part of cancer treatment.

Physiological Integrity

12. Correctly interpret laboratory data and clinical manifestations to determine the presence of cancer treatment side effects and oncologic emergencies.
13. Prioritize nursing interventions for the patient with neutropenia.
14. Prioritize nursing interventions for the patient with thrombocytopenia.
15. Prioritize nursing care for the patient with radiation-induced skin problems.
16. Ensure personnel safety when working with patients receiving brachytherapy radiation.
17. Prioritize nursing care for the patient with mucositis.
18. Explain the rationale for hormonal manipulation therapy.
19. Discuss the uses of biological response modifiers as supportive cancer therapy.
20. Explain the basis of targeted therapy for cancer.
21. Identify patients at risk for oncologic emergencies.
22. Teach patients and families the manifestations of oncologic emergencies and when to notify the health care provider.

evolve Go to your Companion CD or Evolve at http://evolve.elsevier.com/Iggy/ for *Self-Assessment Questions for the NCLEX Examination* keyed to these Learning Outcomes.

As discussed in Chapter 23, cancer is a common health problem in North America. Most people fear cancer and consider a cancer diagnosis to involve suffering and death. In affluent countries, more than 50% of people diagnosed with cancer are cured and thousands of others live 5 years or longer after the diagnosis (American Cancer Society, 2008). *Regardless of treatment type, cancer always affects a person's physical and psychological functioning.*

Providing care to patients and families experiencing cancer is complex and challenging. This chapter describes the general interventions for cancer and the problems associated with cancer treatment. For specific treatment regimens and patient problems that occur with specific cancer types, consult the chapters in which the cancer is described. Table 24-1 lists common cancer types and the specific locations within this text where the interventions are presented.

GENERAL DISEASE-RELATED CONSEQUENCES OF CANCER

As discussed in Chapter 23, cancer can develop in any organ or tissue but tends to occur more commonly in some tissues than in others. Cancer destroys normal tissue, decreasing function in that tissue or organ. Even when cancers occur in nonvital tissues or organs, they can cause death by **metastasizing** (spreading) into vital organs and disrupting critical physiologic processes (see Chapter 23). Cancers that are left untreated cause:

- Reduced immunity and blood-producing functions
- Altered GI structure and function
- Motor and sensory deficits
- Decreased respiratory function

These impairments cause great physical and emotional distress. Without intervention, cancer invasion of normal tissues leads to death.

TABLE 24-1 Text Location of Specific Cancer Content

Cancer Type	Chapter	Pathophysiology/ Etiology	Treatment & Nursing Interventions
Bladder (urolithial)	69	1575	1576-1577
Brain	47	1060-1061	1062-1065
Breast	73	1663-1665	1671-1681
Cervical	74	1702	1703-1705
Colorectal	59	1293-1294	1296-1302
Esophageal	57	1255-1256	1257-1261
Head and Neck	31	597-598	599-606
Kidney (renal cell carcinoma)	70	1595	1595-1596
Leukemia	42	902-903	905-911
Lung	32	641-642	644-650
Lymphoma	42	913-914	914-915
Ovarian	74	1705	1706-1707
Prostate	75	1719	1721-1725
Skin	27	509	512
Stomach (gastric)	58	1279-1280	1281-1287

REDUCED IMMUNITY AND BLOOD-PRODUCING FUNCTIONS

Impaired immune and hematopoietic function occurs most often in patients with leukemia and lymphoma but also can occur with any cancer that invades the bone marrow. Tumor cells enter the bone marrow and reduce the production of healthy white blood cells, which are needed for normal immune function (see Chapter 19). Thus patients who have cancer, especially leukemia, are at an increased risk for infection.

When cancer invades the bone marrow, it also causes anemia by decreasing the number of red blood cells and causes thrombocytopenia by decreasing the number of platelets. These changes may be caused by the cancer itself, such as in leukemia, or by the cancer treatment, especially chemotherapy. In either case, the patient has weakness and fatigue and is at risk for excessive bleeding.

ALTERED GI STRUCTURE AND FUNCTION

Cancer can alter GI function and impair nutrition. For example, tumors may obstruct or compress structures anywhere along the GI tract, reducing the patient's ability to absorb nutrients and eliminate wastes. Tumors often also increase metabolic rate and increase the need for protein, carbohydrates, and fat at a time when the patient has less energy for meal preparation or eating.

Many tumors spread to the liver, profoundly damaging this organ. The liver has many important functions in metabolism. Reduced liver function leads to malnutrition and death among patients with cancer.

Many patients with cancer have anorexia that often interferes with their ability to meet energy needs. **Cachexia** (extreme body wasting and malnutrition) develops from an imbalance between food intake and energy use (increased catabolism). This problem may occur even when nutritional intake appears adequate. Changes in taste can result from the cancer or the treatment and reduce appetite.

Nutritional support for the patient with cancer, especially one undergoing cancer therapy, is complex and controversial. A diet high in protein and carbohydrates is often prescribed to help him or her maintain weight and to provide the nutrients needed for energy and cellular repair. However, some scientists believe that an excessive intake of protein and vitamins increases the nutrition of the cancer cells and contributes to cancer progression. Patients often believe their cancers can be cured more easily if weight is gained or maintained. Currently no one nutritional plan meets the needs of all patients with cancer.

MOTOR AND SENSORY DEFICITS

Motor and sensory deficits occur when cancers invade bone or the brain or compress nerves. In patients with bone metastases, the primary cancer started in another organ (e.g., the prostate, breast, or lung). The bone sites most often affected are the vertebrae, ribs, pelvis, and femur. The humerus, scapula, sternum, skull, and clavicle are also common sites of cancer spread. Bone metastases cause pain, fractures, spinal cord compression, and hypercalcemia, each of which reduces mobility.

The patient may have sensory changes if the spinal cord is damaged by tumor pressure or if nerves are compressed. Sensory, motor, and cognitive functions are severely impaired when cancer spreads to the brain. Brain metastasis and primary brain tumors also destroy healthy brain tissue, a major cause of cancer death.

CONCEPT MAP Chronic Cancer Pain

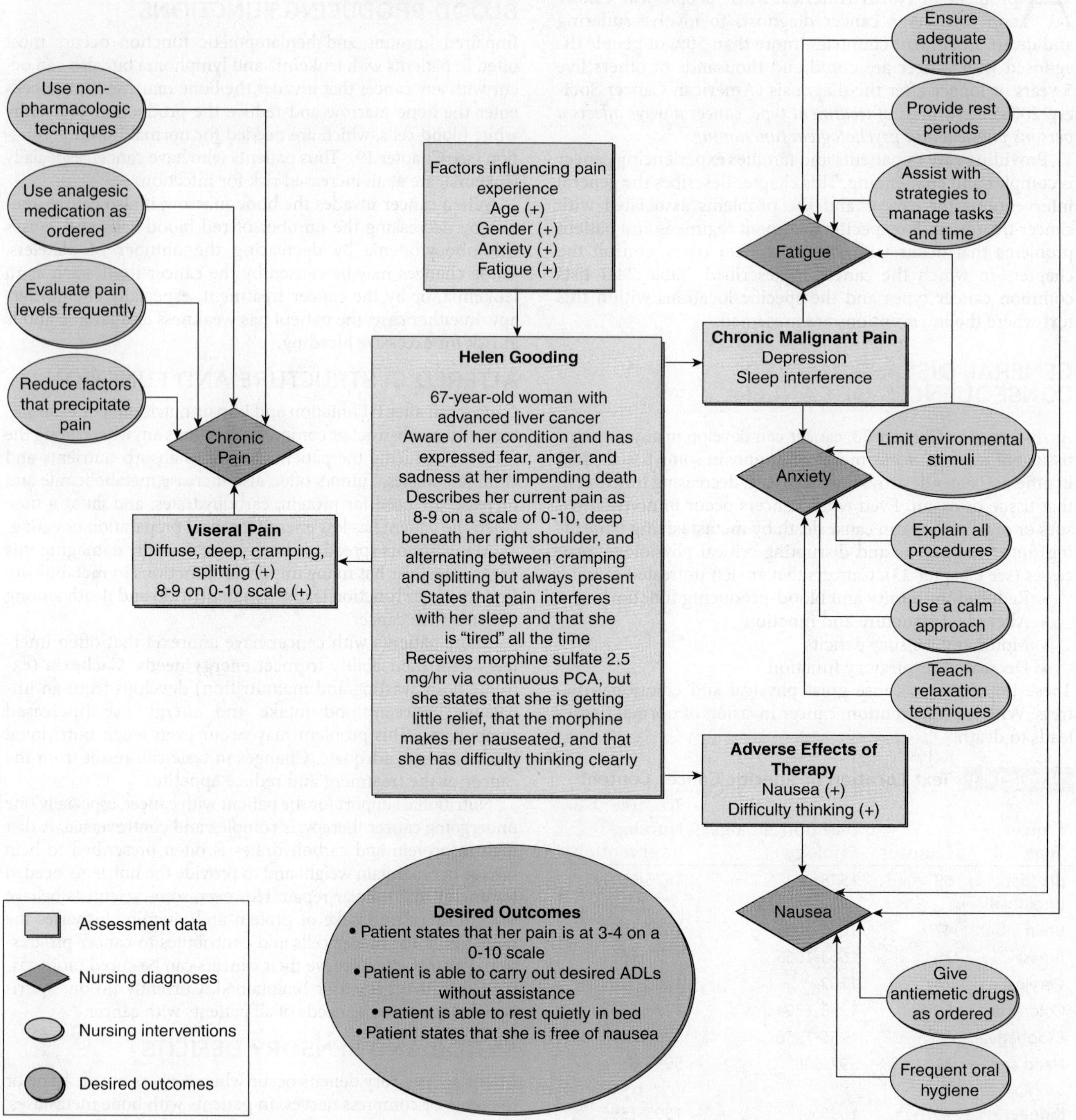
Ensure adequate nutrition
Provide rest periods
Assist with strategies to manage tasks and time
Fatigue
Use non-pharmacologic techniques
Use analgesic medication as ordered
Evaluate pain levels frequently
Reduce factors that precipitate pain
Chronic Pain
Factors influencing pain experience
Age (+)
Gender (+)
Anxiety (+)
Fatigue (+)
Helen Gooding
67-year-old woman with advanced liver cancer
Aware of her condition and has expressed fear, anger, and sadness at her impending death
Describes her current pain as 8-9 on a scale of 0-10, deep beneath her right shoulder, and alternating between cramping and splitting but always present
States that pain interferes with her sleep and that she is "tired" all the time
Receives morphine sulfate 2.5 mg/hr via continuous PCA, but she states that she is getting little relief, that the morphine makes her nauseated, and that she has difficulty thinking clearly
Viseral Pain
Diffuse, deep, cramping, splitting (+)
8-9 on 0-10 scale (+)
Chronic Malignant Pain
Depression
Sleep interference
Limit environmental stimuli
Anxiety
Explain all procedures
Use a calm approach
Teach relaxation techniques
Adverse Effects of Therapy
Nausea (+)
Difficulty thinking (+)
Nausea
Give antiemetic drugs as ordered
Frequent oral hygiene
Desired Outcomes
• Patient states that her pain is at 3-4 on a 0-10 scale
• Patient is able to carry out desired ADLs without assistance
• Patient is able to rest quietly in bed
• Patient states that she is free of nausea
Assessment data
Nursing diagnoses
Nursing interventions
Desired outcomes

Concept Map by Elaine Bishop Kennedy, EdD, RN

The patient with cancer may also have pain. Pain does not always accompany cancer, but it can be a significant problem for those with terminal cancer. The Concept Map on p. 416 presents nursing care issues regarding cancer pain. Chapter 5 provides an in-depth discussion of the causes and management of cancer pain.

DECREASED RESPIRATORY FUNCTION

Cancer can disrupt respiratory function and gas exchange in several ways and often results in death. For example, tumors in the airways cause airway obstruction. If lung tissue is involved, lung capacity is decreased. Tumors can also press on blood and lymph vessels in the chest, blocking blood flow through the chest and lungs and resulting in pulmonary edema and dyspnea. Tumors also can thicken the alveolar membrane and damage pulmonary blood vessels, reducing gas exchange. Thus, with lung cancer or the spread of cancer from other areas into the lungs, patients have hypoxia and poor tissue oxygenation.

CANCER MANAGEMENT

The purpose of cancer management is to prolong survival time or improve quality of life. Although a few spontaneous regressions of cancer have been reported, most patients would die within months of diagnosis without cancer therapy. Therapies for cancer include surgery, radiation, chemotherapy, hormonal manipulation, photodynamic therapy, immunotherapy, gene therapy, and targeted therapy. These therapies may be used separately or, more commonly, in combination to kill cancer cells. The types and amount of therapy used depend on the specific type of cancer, whether the cancer has spread, and the health of the patient. Treatment regimens (protocols) have been established for most types of cancer. These regimens are based on experiments with cancer cells and animals and on experience with other patients with cancer.

SURGERY

Overview

Surgery is the oldest form of cancer treatment and was the first method to cure cancer. Surgery for cancer involves the removal of diseased tissue. If cancer is confined to the removed tissue, surgery alone can result in a "cure" for that cancer. Although many cancers have spread too far at the time of diagnosis for surgery alone to cure, it may still be a useful part of diagnosis, treatment, follow-up, and rehabilitation.

Cancer surgery may be used for prophylaxis, diagnosis, cure, control, palliation, determination of therapy effectiveness, and reconstruction. **Prophylactic surgery** is the removal of "at-risk" tissue to prevent cancer development. It is performed when a patient has either an existing "premalignant" condition or a known family history that strongly predisposes the person to the development of a specific cancer. An example of prophylactic surgery for a premalignant condition is removing a benign mole from a location where continuous irritation or exposure to sunlight occurs. **Diagnostic surgery** (biopsy) is the removal of all or part of a suspected lesion for examination and testing. It provides proof of the presence of cancer. **Curative surgery** is focused on removal of all cancer tissue. Surgery alone can result in a cure rate of 27% to 30% when all visible and microscopic tumor is removed or destroyed. **Cancer control,** or **cytoreductive surgery,** is removing part of the tumor and leaving a known amount of gross tumor. It is also known as "debulking" surgery and alone cannot result in a cure. It decreases the number of cancer cells and increases the chances that other therapies can be successful. **Palliative surgery** is focused on improving the quality of life during the survival time and is not focused on cure. Examples include removal of tumor tissue that is causing pain, obstruction, or difficulty swallowing. The specific procedure used depends on the patient's specific problem. **Second-look surgery** is a "rediagnosis" after treatment. The purpose is to assess the disease status in patients who have been treated and have no symptoms of remaining tumor. The results of this surgery are used to determine whether a specific therapy should be continued or discontinued. This type of surgery is most commonly used with ovarian cancer.

Reconstructive or rehabilitative surgery increases function, enhances appearance, or both. Examples include breast reconstruction after mastectomy, replacement of the esophagus after radiation damage, bowel reconstruction, revision of scars, release of contractures, and placement of penile implants.

Side Effects of Surgical Therapy

Unlike surgery performed for many other reasons, cancer surgery involves the loss of a specific body part or its function. Sometimes whole organs are removed, such as the kidney, lung, breast, testes, arm, or tongue. *Any organ loss reduces function.* The amount of function lost and how much the loss affects patients depend on the location and extent of the surgery. Some cancer surgery results in major scarring or disfigurement. Patients may be anxious about the chances of surviving the cancer and also may be grieving about a loss of body image or a change in lifestyle.

Patient-Centered Collaborative Care

The physical nursing care needs of the patient having surgery for cancer are similar to those related to surgery for other reasons (see Chapters 16, 17, and 18). For cancer surgery, two additional priority care needs are psychosocial support and assisting him or her to achieve or maintain maximum function.

At times, major cancer surgery occurs within days of the diagnosis, before the patient and family have time to adjust. Assess the patient's ability (and the ability of family and significant others) to cope with the uncertainty of cancer and its treatment and with the changes in body image and role. For example, surgery involving the genitals, urinary tract, colon, and rectum may permanently damage these organs, resulting in changes in the patient's means of sexual expression or control of elimination. Procedures to create a urinary or fecal diversion (e.g., a colostomy) may damage nerves, causing erectile dysfunction in men and painful intercourse in women. Removal of a lung permanently reduces the patient's respiratory capacity and forever limits his or her ability to engage in physical activities.

Coordinate with the health care team to provide support for the patient and family. Encourage the patient and family to express their feelings and concerns. Help the patient accept changes in body image by encouraging him or her to look at the surgical site, touch it, and participate in any dressing changes or incisional care required. Provide information about support groups such as those sponsored by the American Cancer Society (www.cancer.org) or specialty cancer organizations. In addition to patient support groups, many of these organizations have separate support groups for spouses and children of the person with cancer. Discuss with the patient

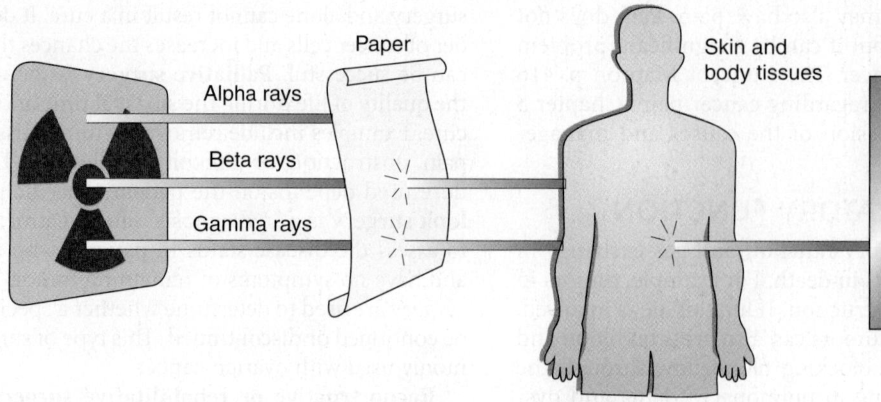
Paper
Alpha rays
Beta rays
Gamma rays
Skin and
body tissues
Lead

Fig. 24-1 • Penetrating capacity of different types of radiation.

the idea of having a person who has coped with the same issues come for a visit. Such visits can be valuable in showing the patient that many aspects of life can be the same after cancer treatment. If the patient is open to this type of support, coordinate the arrangement for such a visit to the hospital or to the patient's home.

Reduced function may be an outcome for some types of cancer surgery. For example, a modified radical mastectomy for breast cancer can lead to muscle weakness and reduced arm function on the side of the surgery. Participation in specific exercises after surgery can minimize functional loss. These exercises can be painful, and the patient needs encouragement to perform them. Teach the patient about the importance of performing and progressing the intensity of the exercises to regain as much function as possible and prevent complications. Coordinate with the physical therapist, occupational therapist, and family members to plan strategies individualized to each patient to regain or maintain optimal function.

RADIATION THERAPY

Overview

The purpose of radiation therapy for cancer is to destroy cancer cells with minimal exposure of the normal cells to the damaging actions of radiation. The effects of radiation are seen only in the tissues in the path of the radiation beam; thus this type of therapy is a *local* treatment. For example, radiation to the chest for breast cancer or lung cancer causes skin changes and hair loss only on the area of the chest actually being irradiated. The person does *not* lose his or her scalp hair. Some effects are apparent within days or weeks, whereas other effects may not be apparent for months to years after radiation therapy is completed.

Most radiation therapy for cancer is ionizing radiation. When cells are exposed to this type of radiation, atoms within the cell are "kicked out" of orbit, resulting in a tremendous release of intracellular energy. Ionizing radiation is given off by many elements, including radium, and any element with an atomic number above 93. In addition, most other elements have **isotopes** (a different form of a specific element that has a slightly different atomic weight and number of neutrons) that also are radioactive. For example, a radioactive isotope of cobalt is used in radiation therapy for cancer. Other radioactive isotopes are used in many diagnostic tests and nuclear medicine procedures.

As a radioactive element breaks down (decays), radiation energy is released in the form of high energy particles (alpha particles and beta particles) and high energy photons (gamma particles). **X-rays** are radiation that is generated by machine. X-ray photons and gamma ray photons are identical in their effects on cells. (However, standard diagnostic x-rays use less intense doses and cause mimimal cell damage.)

Cells damaged by radiation either die outright or become unable to divide. Radiation damage can occur anytime a cell is exposed to radiation and is not confined to cells actively dividing. However, cells in the cell cycle have more damage when exposed to radiation than do nondividing cells.

Three different types of energy, or rays, are produced from radioactive elements: gamma rays, alpha particles, and beta particles. These energies vary in their ability to penetrate tissues and damage cells. Fig. 24-1 shows the penetrating ability of each. *Gamma rays* are used most commonly for radiation therapy because of their ability to deeply penetrate tissues. *Beta particles* have much less ability to penetrate tissues and must be placed within or very close to the cancer cells to be effective as cancer therapy (see discussion of brachytherapy on p. 419). *Alpha particles* are not used as part of radiation therapy for cancer.

The amount of radiation delivered to a tissue is called the **exposure;** the amount of radiation absorbed by the tissue is called the **radiation dose.** The dose is always less than the exposure. Three factors determine the absorbed dose: intensity of exposure, duration of exposure, and closeness of the radiation source to the cells.

The intensity of the radiation decreases with the distance from the radiation source (Fig. 24-2). This factor is known as the *inverse square law*. For example, the radiation dose received at a distance of 2 feet from the radiation source is only one fourth of the dose received at a distance of 1 foot from the radiation source; the dose of radiation received at 3 feet is only one ninth of the dose received at 1 foot.

In theory, if the dose of radiation is high enough, all cells are killed immediately. This does not usually happen with cancer radiation therapy because all cells within a tumor absorb the radiation dose slightly differently. Therefore their overall response to the radiation is slightly different. A few cells die immediately, and more die within the next 24 hours as they attempt to divide. Some cells become sterile as a result of this single treatment. Still other cells repair the radiation-induced damage and recover.

Radiation therapy usually is given as a series of divided doses because of the varying responses of all cancer cells within a given tumor. Small doses of radiation are given on a

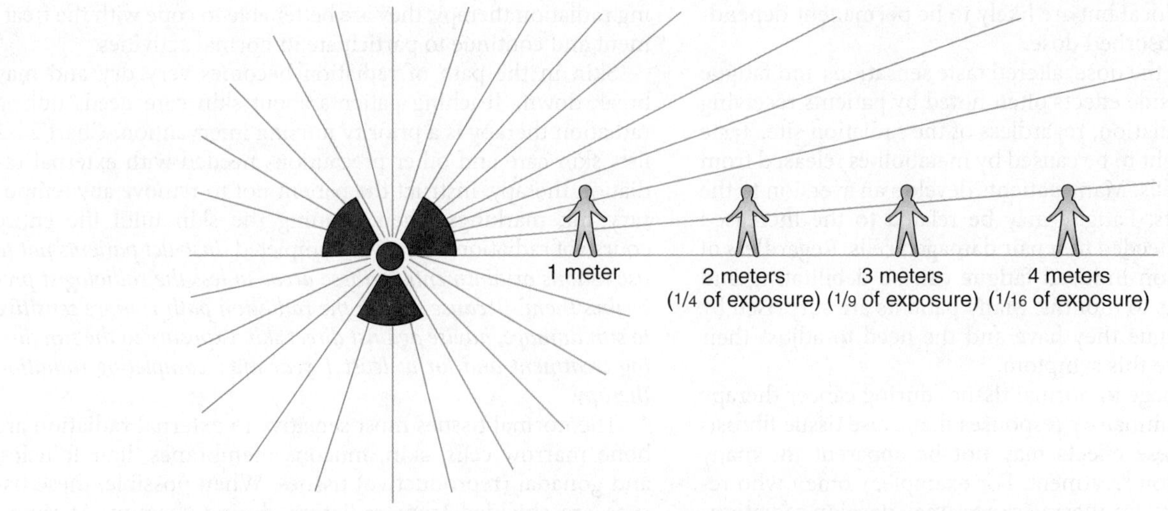
1 meter
2 meters
(1/4 of exposure)
3 meters
(1/9 of exposure)
4 meters
(1/16 of exposure)

Fig. 24-2 • The inverse square law of radiation exposure.

daily basis for a set period of time to allow greater destruction of cancer cells while reducing the damage to normal tissues. The total dose of radiation needed depends on the size and location of the tumor and on the radiation sensitivity of the tumor and surrounding normal tissues. Some normal tissues are more sensitive than others to radiation. For example, healthy breast tissue can tolerate much higher doses of radiation than can the liver. A total dose of 5000 to 6000 **rad** (radiation absorbed dose) might be prescribed for a breast cancer total dose. Only 1200 rad might be prescribed for a primary liver tumor, however, because a higher dose would destroy the liver as well as the tumor.

Radiation Delivery

Two types of delivery are used for cancer therapy: teletherapy and brachytherapy. The type used depends on the patient's general health and on the shape, size, and location of the tumor to be irradiated. The ideal radiation dose is one that can kill the cancer cells with an acceptable level of damage to normal tissues (damage to normal tissues cannot be avoided).

Teletherapy is distant treatment. In teletherapy, the radiation source is external to the patient. *Because the source is external, the patient is not radioactive and is not a hazard to others.*

The exact location of the tumor is determined for greater accuracy of radiation therapy. Once the pattern of radiation delivery is determined, the patient must always be in exactly the same position for all treatments (Camporeale, 2008). Ensure that the patient can get into and maintain this position. Position-fixing devices and markings, either on the patient's body or on the devices, ensure the proper position each day of treatment. These markings may be small permanent "tattoos" or may be ink outlines.

Brachytherapy means "short" or "close" therapy. With brachytherapy, the radiation source comes into direct, continuous contact with the tumor tissues for a specific period of time. This method provides a high dose of radiation in tumor tissues and a limited dose in surrounding normal tissues.

Brachytherapy uses radioactive isotopes either in solid form or within body fluids. Isotopes can be delivered to the tumor tissues in several ways. *With all types of brachytherapy, the radiation source is within the patient. Therefore the patient emits radiation for a period of time and is a hazard to others* (Gosselin & Waring, 2001). When the isotopes used are unsealed and suspended in a fluid, they are given via the oral or IV routes or instilled within body cavities. An example of brachytherapy with soluble isotopes is the ingestion or injection of the radionuclide iodine^{131} (an iodine base with a half-life of 8.05 days) to treat some thyroid cancers. The radioactive iodine concentrates in the thyroid gland and destroys the thyroid cancer cells. *When the isotopes are unsealed, they enter body fluids and eventually are eliminated in waste products, which are radioactive and should not be directly touched by other people. Once the isotope is eliminated, neither the patient nor the body wastes are radioactive. Most of this isotope is eliminated within 48 hours.*

Solid or sealed radiation sources are implanted within or very near the tumor. These radiation sources can be temporary or permanent. Most of the implants emit continuous, low-energy radiation to tumor tissues. Some devices (e.g., seeds or needles) can be placed into the tissues and stay in place by themselves. Other sources must be held in place with special applicators. Some of these devices are so small and the half-life of the isotope so short that the device is permanently left in place (most often for prostate cancer) and does not pose a hazard to other people. Other devices are removed and reused in other patients. *With solid implants, the patient emits radiation while the implant is in place but excreta are not radioactive and do not pose a hazard to anyone.*

Traditional implants deliver "low-dose rates" (LDR) of radiation continuously, and patients are hospitalized for several days. "High-dose rate" (HDR) implant radiation is another delivery type. The patient comes into the radiation therapy department several times a week, and a stronger radiation device is placed for only an hour or so each time. The patient goes home between treatments and is radioactive only when the implant is in place. Chart 24-1 lists the best practices for care of the patient with sealed implant radiation sources and for the safety of the personnel providing the care.

Side Effects of Radiation Therapy

The immediate and long-term side effects of all types of radiation are limited to the tissues exposed to the radiation. Therefore the side effects vary according to the site. Skin changes and hair loss are local but are likely to be permanent depending on the total absorbed dose.

Depending on the dose, altered taste sensations and fatigue are two systemic side effects often noted by patients receiving external beam radiation, regardless of the radiation site. Taste changes are thought to be caused by metabolites released from dead and dying cells. Many patients develop an aversion to the taste of red meats. Fatigue may be related to the increased energy demands needed to repair damaged cells. Regardless of the cause, radiation-induced fatigue can be debilitating and may last for weeks to months. Many patients are surprised by the degree of fatigue they have and the need to adjust their lifestyle to manage this symptom.

Radiation damage to normal tissues during cancer therapy can start the inflammatory responses that cause tissue fibrosis and scarring. These effects may not be apparent for many years after radiation treatment. For example, women who receive HDR therapy for uterine cancer may develop radiation-induced changes in the colon (which also was irradiated) years later, resulting in constipation and obstruction.

Patient-Centered Collaborative Care

Most patients are anxious about radiation and look to the nurse to explain the purpose and side effects of radiation therapy. When patients receive accurate, objective information regarding radiation therapy, they are better able to cope with the treatment and continue to participate in normal activities.

Skin in the path of radiation becomes very dry and may break down. Teaching patients about skin care needs during radiation therapy is a priority nursing intervention. Chart 24-2 lists skin care and other precautions needed with external radiation therapy. Instruct the patient not to remove any temporary ink markings when cleaning the skin until the entire course of radiation therapy is completed. *Instruct patients not to use lotions or ointments in these areas unless the radiologist prescribes them. Because skin in the radiation path is more sensitive to sun damage, advise against direct skin exposure to the sun during treatment and for at least 1 year after completing radiation therapy.*

The normal tissues most sensitive to external radiation are bone marrow cells, skin, mucous membranes, hair follicles, and gonadal (reproductive) tissues. When possible, these tissues are shielded from radiation during therapy. At times, however, they are in the path of radiation and cannot be adequately protected from exposure. Some changes caused by radiation are permanent. The long-term problems vary with the location and dose of radiation received. For example, radiation to the throat and upper chest can cause difficulty in swallowing. Head and neck radiation may damage the salivary glands and cause dry mouth **(xerostomia)** and increase the patient's lifelong risk for tooth decay. Bone exposed to radiation therapy is less dense and breaks more easily. Teach about the types of symptoms that might be expected from the location and dose of radiation received (see Table 24-1 for the location of this information for different cancer types).

Chart 24-1 BEST PRACTICE FOR PATIENT SAFETY & QUALITY CARE

Care of the Patient with Sealed Implants of Radioactive Sources

- Assign the patient to a private room with a private bath.
- Place a "Caution: Radioactive Material" sign on the door of the patient's room.
- If portable lead shields are used, place them between the patient and the door.
- Keep the door to the patient's room closed as much as possible.
- Wear a dosimeter film badge at all times while caring for patients with radioactive implants. The badge offers no protection but measures a person's exposure to radiation and should be used by only one person.
- Wear a lead apron while providing care. Always keep the front of the apron facing the source of radiation (do not turn your back toward the patient).
- Pregnant nurses should not care for these patients; do not allow pregnant women or children younger than 16 years to visit.
- Limit each visitor to one-half hour per day. Be sure visitors are at least 6 feet from the source.
- Never touch the radioactive source with bare hands. In the rare instance that it is dislodged, use a long-handled forceps to retrieve it. Deposit the radioactive source in the lead container kept in the patient's room.
- Save all dressings and bed linens until after the radioactive source is removed. After the source is removed, dispose of dressings and linens in the usual manner. Other equipment can be removed from the room at any time without special precautions and does not pose a hazard to other people.

Chart 24-2 PATIENT AND FAMILY EDUCATION GUIDE

Skin Protection During Radiation Therapy

- Wash the irradiated area gently each day with either water or a mild soap and water as prescribed by your radiologist.
- Use your hand rather than a washcloth to be gentler.
- Rinse soap thoroughly from your skin.
- If there are ink or dye markings that indicate exactly where the beam of radiation is to be focused, take care not to remove them.
- Dry the irradiated area with patting motions rather than rubbing motions; use a clean, soft towel or cloth.
- Use no powders, ointments, lotions, or creams on your skin at the radiation site unless they are prescribed by your *radiologist* or the radiation therapy advanced practice nurse.
- Wear soft clothing over the skin at the radiation site.
- Avoid wearing belts, buckles, straps, or any type of clothing that binds or rubs the skin at the radiation site.
- Avoid exposure of the irradiated area to the sun.
- Protect this area by wearing clothing over it but *not* by applying sunscreen agents during the time you are undergoing the radiation treatments.
- Try to go outdoors in the early morning or evening to avoid the more intense sun rays.
- When outdoors, stay under awnings, umbrellas, and other forms of shade during the times when the sun's rays are most intense (10 AM to 7 PM).
- Avoid heat exposure.

NCLEX EXAMINATION CHALLENGE

The client receiving radiation therapy to the chest for breast cancer asks if she can still play golf during the 6 weeks of her treatment. What is the nurse's best response?

A. "No, your risk for breaking a rib when swinging the golf club hard is greatly increased."
B. "No, you will be too tired to play golf until 2 months after the treatment is completed."
C. "Yes, if you wear a hat or wig to prevent damage to you scalp from sun or wind."
D. "Yes, if you wear a soft, thick shirt to protect your chest skin from sunlight."

evolve For the correct answer, go to http://evolve.elsevier.com/Iggy/.

CHEMOTHERAPY

Overview

Chemotherapy, the treatment of cancer with chemical agents, has a major role in cancer therapy. Chemotherapy is used to cure and to increase survival time. It is used as cancer treatment because it has some selectivity for killing cancer cells over normal cells. This killing effect on cancer cells is related to the ability of chemotherapy to damage DNA and interfere with cell division. Thus the tumors most sensitive to chemotherapy are those that have rapid growth.

As described in Chapter 23, cancer cells can separate from the original tumor, spread to new areas, and establish new cancers at distant sites **(metastasize).** Patients with metastatic cancer will die unless treatment eliminates the metastatic cancer cells along with the original cancer cells. Chemotherapy is useful in treating cancer because its effects are systemic, providing the opportunity to kill metastatic cancer cells that may have escaped local treatment. Chemotherapy used along with surgery or radiation is termed **adjuvant** therapy.

Drugs used for chemotherapy usually are given systemically and exert their cell-damaging **(cytotoxic)** effects against healthy cells as well as cancer cells. The normal cells most affected by chemotherapy are those that divide rapidly, including skin, hair, intestinal tissues, spermatocytes, and blood-forming cells. These drugs are classified by the specific types of action they exert in the cancer cell. Table 24-2 lists categories, drugs, and their potential to induce nausea and vomiting (emetogenic) or to damage surrounding tissue.

TABLE 24-2 Categories of Chemotherapeutic Drugs

Drug	Emetogenic Potential	Tissue Damage Potential
ANTIMETABOLITES		
Capecitabine (Xeloda)	Low	N/A (oral drug)
Cladribine (Leustatin)	Moderate	Bruising
Cytarabine (Cytosar, ara-C)	Moderate	Irritant
Floxuridine (FUDR)	High	Bruising
5-Fluorouracil (Adrucil, Efudex, Fluoroplex)	Moderate	Irritant
Fludarabine (Fludara, FLAMP)	Low	Bruising
Gemcitabine (Gemzar)	Moderate	Bruising
6-Mercaptopurine (Purinethol)	Low	N/A (oral drug)
Methotrexate (Mexate, Folex)	Low - Moderate	Bruising
6-Thioguanine (Lanvis)	Moderate - High	N/A (oral drug)
ANTITUMOR ANTIBIOTICS		
Bleomycin (Blenoxane)	Moderate	Irritant
Dactinomycin (Cosmegen)	High	Vesicant
Daunorubicin (Cerubidine)	High	Vesicant
Doxorubicin (Adriamycin, Rubex)	High	Vesicant
Epirubicin (Ellence)	High	Vesicant
Idarubicin (Idamycin)	Moderate - High	Vesicant
Mitomycin C (Mutamycin)	Moderate	Vesicant
Mitoxantrone (Novantrone)	Low	Irritant
Pentostatin (Nipent)	Moderate - High	Bruising
Plicamycin (Mithracin)	High	Irritant
Valrubicin	N/A	N/A (intravesicular drug)
ANTIMITOTICS		
Docetaxel (Taxotere)	Moderate	Bruising
Etoposide (VP-16, VePesid)	Low	Irritant
Paclitaxel (Taxol)	Moderate	Irritant
Vinblastine (Velban, Velbe, Velsar)	Low - Moderate	Vesicant

Continued

TABLE 24-2 **Categories of Chemotherapeutic Drugs—cont'd**

Drug	Emetogenic Potential	Tissue Damage Potential
ANTIMITOTICS—cont'd		
Vincristine (Oncovin)	Low	Vesicant
Vinorelbine (Navelbine)	Low	Vesicant
ALKYLATING AGENTS		
Altretamine (Hexalen)	Moderate	N/A (oral drug)
Busulfan (Busulfex)	High	Bruising
Carboplatin (Paraplatin)	High	Irritant
Carmustine (BiCNU)	High	Irritant
Chlorambucil (Leukeran)	High	N/A (oral drug)
Cisplatin (Platinol)	High	Irritant
Cyclophosphamide (Cytoxan, Procytox)	High	Bruising
Estramustine (Emcyt, Estracyte)	Moderate	Vesicant
Ifosfamide (IFEX)	High	Bruising
Lomustine (CCNU, CeeNU)	High	N/A (oral drug)
Mechlorethamine (Mustargen)	High	Vesicant
Melphalan (Alkeran)	High	N/A (oral drug)
Oxaliplatin (Eloxatin)	Moderate - High	Vesicant
Streptozocin (Zanosar)	High	Bruising
Temozolomide (Temodar)	Moderate - High	N/A (oral drug)
Thiotepa (Thioplex)	Low	Bruising
TOPOISOMERASE INHIBITORS		
Irinotecan (Camptosar)	Moderate	Irritant
Topotecan (Hycamtin)	Moderate	Irritant
OTHER AGENTS		
Arsenic trioxide (Trisenox)	Moderate	Not known
Asparaginase (Elspar)	Low	Vesicant
Dacarbazine (DTIC)	Moderate - High	Irritant
Hydroxyurea (Hydrea)	Low	N/A (oral drug)
Pegaspargase (Oncaspar)	Low	Bruising
Procarbazine (Matulane, Natulan🍁)	High	N/A (oral drug)

Data from *www.fda.gov/cder/index.html; and www.mdconsult.com/php/82925233-2/homepage.*

Chemotherapy Drug Categories

Antimetabolites are similar to normal metabolites needed for vital cell processes. Most cell reactions require metabolites in order to begin or continue the reaction. Antimetabolites closely resemble normal metabolites and are "counterfeit" metabolites that fool cancer cells into using the antimetabolites in cellular reactions. Because antimetabolites cannot function as proper metabolites, their presence impairs cell division.

Antitumor antibiotics damage the cell's DNA and interrupt DNA or ribonucleic acid (RNA) synthesis. Exactly how the interruptions occur varies with each agent.

Antimitotic agents interfere with the formation of microtubules so cells cannot complete mitosis during cell division. As a result, the cancer cell either does not divide at all or divides only once, resulting in two daughter cells that cannot continue to divide.

Alkylating agents cross-link DNA, making the two DNA strands bind tightly together. This tight binding prevents proper DNA and RNA synthesis, inhibiting cell division.

Topoisomerase inhibitors disrupt an enzyme (topoisomerase) needed for DNA synthesis and cell division. It nicks and straightens the DNA helix, allowing the DNA to be copied, and then reattaches the DNA together. These drugs prevent proper DNA maintenance, causing DNA breakage and cell death.

Other miscellaneous chemotherapy drugs are those with mechanisms of action that are either unknown or do not fit those of other drug categories. Drugs in this category are effective with some tumors.

Combination Chemotherapy

Successful cancer chemotherapy involves giving more than one specific anticancer drug in a timed manner. This technique is called *combination chemotherapy*. Using more than one drug is much more effective in killing cancer cells than using only a single drug. However, the side effects and damage caused to normal tissues also increase with combination chemotherapy.

TABLE 24-3 **Routes of Chemotherapy Administration**

Route	Typical Cancer
Oral	Hodgkin's lymphoma Leukemia (maintenance phase) Small cell lung cancer
Intravenous	Most solid tumors, leukemias Lymphomas
Intra-arterial	Hepatic tumors (primary and metastatic) Head and neck cancers
Isolated limb perfusion	Cancers confined to a limb • Osteogenic sarcoma • Ewing's sarcoma • Rhabdomyosarcoma • Regional melanoma
Intracavitary	Ovarian cancer
• Intraperitoneal	Brain tumors
• Intraventricular	Brain tumors
• Intrathecal	Prophylaxis for acute lymphocytic leukemia
• Intravesical	Bladder tumors

The selection of drugs is based on known tumor sensitivity to the drugs and the degree of side effects expected. For example, most chemotherapy drugs suppress bone marrow activity and immune function to some degree, but some agents cause more bone marrow suppression than others. There is also variation in the timing of drug-induced suppression and neutropenia.

The time when bone marrow activity and white blood cell counts are at their lowest levels after chemotherapy is the **nadir.** It occurs at different times for different drugs. To reduce immunosuppression, combination chemotherapy avoids using drugs with nadirs that occur at or near the same time.

A new approach to chemotherapy selection is checking the patient's genetic profile to determine the likelihood of experiencing dangerous side effects (Miller & McLoed, 2007). This process, known as *pharmacogenomics,* allows a more individualized approach to chemotherapy selection.

Treatment Issues

Dosages for most chemotherapy drugs are calculated according to the type of cancer and the patient's size. Usually, calculations are based on milligrams per square meter of total body surface area (TBSA), which considers both the patient's height and weight.

Chemotherapy drugs are given on a regular basis and are timed to maximize cancer cell kill and minimize damage to normal cells. The schedule may vary somewhat to accommodate a patient's response to therapy, but chemotherapy is usually scheduled every 3 to 4 weeks for a specified number of times (on average, 4 to 12 times). Newer protocols of giving higher doses of chemotherapy more often, called **dose-dense chemotherapy,** are often used for aggressive cancer treatment, especially for breast cancer. This dose-dense chemotherapy also results in more intense side effects than traditional dosing schedules.

Most chemotherapy drugs are given IV, although other routes may be used for specific cancers. Table 24-3 lists routes of chemotherapy administration. The techniques and care needs for different routes are described with the specific cancer type most commonly associated with the specific administration route. Chapter 15 describes the types of venous access devices, many of which are used for chemotherapy.

The IV route is the most preferred route for chemotherapy because the effects of the drugs are rapid and because many of these agents are irritating or damaging to tissues. The standard of care designated by the Oncology Nursing Society (ONS) and supported by the American Society of Clinical Oncologists (ASCO) for safe administration of IV chemotherapy is that administration of these drugs requires special education (Polovich et al., 2005). *Special education for competency does not mean that only an advanced practice nurse can perform this function; however, it does mean that the person should be a registered nurse who has completed an approved chemotherapy course. Responsibility for monitoring the patient during chemotherapy administration, however, rests with all nurses providing care to that patient.*

A major complication of IV infusion is **extravasation,** or the movement of the IV needle so the drug leaks into the surrounding tissues (also called *infiltration*). When the drugs given are **vesicants** (chemicals that damage tissue on direct contact), the results of extravasation can include pain, infection, and tissue loss. Surgical intervention is sometimes needed for severe tissue damage. See Table 24-2 for a listing of known vesicant and irritant chemotherapy drugs.

The most important nursing intervention for extravasation is prevention. Small extravasations resolve without extensive treatment if less than 0.5 mL of the drug has leaked into the tissues. If a larger amount has leaked, extensive tissue damage occurs and surgical intervention may be necessary. *Thus close monitoring of the access site is critical during chemotherapy administration to prevent leakage of larger volumes.* Immediate treatment depends on the specific drug. With some drugs, cold compresses to the area are prescribed; for other agents, warm compresses are used. Antidotes or chemoprotective agents may be injected into the site of extravasation (Schulmeister, 2007). Coordinate with the oncologist and pharmacist to determine the specific antidote needed for the extravasated drug. Chart 24-3 outlines the best practices for documenting an extravasation event.

Most chemotherapy drugs are absorbed through the skin and mucous membranes. As a result, the health care workers who prepare or give these drugs (especially nurses and pharmacists) are at risk for absorbing them. Even at low doses, long-term exposure to chemotherapy drugs can affect health. Anyone preparing, giving, or disposing of chemotherapy drugs or handling excreta from patients within 48 hours of receiving IV chemotherapy should use extreme caution and wear personal protective equipment (PPE). Such equipment includes eye protection, masks, double gloves, or "chemo" gloves, and gown. The Occupational Safety and Health Administration (OSHA) and the Oncology Nursing Society (ONS) have established practice guidelines and protective standards (Polovich, 2003; Polovich et al., 2005).

Side Effects of Chemotherapy

Actual temporary and permanent physical damage can occur to normal tissues from chemotherapy because this treatment is systemic and does not exert its effects only on cancer cells. Known problems include hemorrhagic cystitis, cardiac muscle

Chart 24-3 BEST PRACTICE FOR PATIENT SAFETY & QUALITY CARE

Documentation of Extravasation

- Document the date and time when extravasation was suspected or identified.
- Document the date and time when the infusion was started.
- Record the time when the infusion was stopped.
- Document the exact contents of the infusion fluid and the volume of fluid infused.
- Document the estimated amount of fluid extravasated.
- Diagram the exact insertion site, and indicate whether this is a venous access device, an implanted port, or a tunneled catheter.
- Document the method of administration (pump, controller, etc.; rate of infusion).
- Document the needle type and size.
- Indicate on the diagram the location and number of venipuncture attempts.
- Record the time between the extravasation and the last documented full blood return.
- Identify all agents administered in the previous 24 hours through this site (list agent administered, dosage and volume, and order of administration).
- Take and record the patient's vital signs.
- Ask and record the patient's subjective sensations and symptoms.
- Record all observations of the site, including size, color, and texture.
- Take a photograph of the site.
- Document the administration of neutralizing or antidote agents.
- Document the application of compresses and their temperature.
- Document other nursing interventions.
- Record the patient's responses to nursing interventions.
- Document the prescribing physician notification (including the time).
- Document the written and oral instructions given to the patient about follow-up care.
- Document any consultation request.
- Sign the documentation.

Data modified from Polovich, M., White, J., & Kelleher, L. (Eds.). (2005). *Chemotherapy and biotherapy guidelines and recommendations for practice* (2nd ed.). Pittsburgh: ONS Publishing.

TABLE 24-4 Cytoprotective Drugs Used for Chemoprotection

Agent	Cytotoxic Problem Prevented or Reduced
Amifostine (Ethyol)	Xerostomia
Dexrazoxane (Zinecard)	Cardiomyopathy
Dexrazoxane (Totect)	Tissue damage from anthracycline extravasation
Mesna (MESNEX)	Hemorrhagic cystitis
Pamidronate (Aredia)	Skeletal complications

damage, and loss of bone density. One approach to decrease the impact of chemotherapy on normal tissues is to give the agents with drugs that protect specific healthy cells. These drugs, called **cytoprotectants,** have little effect on cancer cells but do protect some normal tissues (Table 24-4).

Serious short-term side effects occur with aggressive chemotherapy. The side effects on the hematopoietic (blood-producing) system can be life threatening and are the most common reason for changing the dosage or schedule. The suppressive effects on the blood-forming cells of bone marrow cause **anemia** (decreased numbers of red blood cells and hemoglobin), **neutropenia** (decreased numbers of white blood cells leading to immunosuppression), and **thrombocytopenia** (decreased numbers of platelets). Less life-threatening but common distressing side effects include nausea and vomiting, **alopecia** (hair loss), **mucositis** (open sores on mucous membranes), and many skin changes. Other distressing side effects include anxiety, sleep disturbance, altered bowel elimination, and changes in cognitive function. These side effects are referred to as cancer therapy "symptom distress."

Drug therapy often is used to reduce symptom distress for some of these side effects. For other problems, such as alopecia, the side effect cannot be prevented but the patient can be helped to reduce his or her distress from its presence. General nonpharmacologic nursing interventions for many types of symptom distress include distraction, massage, guided imagery, Reiki, aromatherapy, and other forms of complementary therapy.

In addition to physical side effects of therapy, psychosocial issues can occur even during chemotherapy administration. For many chemotherapy regimens, drugs are given over a period ranging from 2 hours to as long as 8 hours. During this time, the patient is confined to a treatment area and is constantly reminded of his or her disease and treatment. Most patients view this time as unpleasant. Distraction methods such as guided imagery, reading, watching television, and talking with visitors have minimal effect on reducing the sense of unpleasantness. A new distraction method, the use of virtual reality during chemotherapy administration, has been shown to help reduce the patient's awareness of the chemotherapy environment and alter the sensations of unpleasantness (see the Evidence-Based Practice box on p. 425). Distraction alone, however, does not reduce the symptom distress experience during and after chemotherapy (Schneider & Hood, 2007).

Patient-Centered Collaborative Care

evolve ONLINE PHARM REVIEW

The priority care issues during chemotherapy are protecting the patient from the life-threatening side effects and managing the distressing symptoms that occur with therapy. For some patients, the symptoms are so unpleasant that they stop treatment.

Bone Marrow Suppression

In addition to killing cancer cells, chemotherapy also destroys some circulating blood cells and reduces replacement of these cells by suppressing bone marrow function. The numbers of

EVIDENCE-BASED PRACTICE

Distraction: It's not just for kids anymore!

Schneider, S., & Hood, L. (2007). Virtual reality: A distraction intervention for chemotherapy. *Oncology Nursing Forum, 34*(1), 39-46.

Receiving IV chemotherapy for cancer, taking anywhere from 1 to 8 hours, is often described by patients as an extremely unpleasant experience. Patients are usually required to stay within a confined area during the treatment because of the tissue-damaging nature of the drugs and the possibility of extravasation or infiltration with movement. Thus patients are in a setting that constantly reminds them of the disease and treatment, with little diversion available to occupy or distract them. Children have been able to derive positive distraction during the chemotherapy experience through the use of virtual reality (VR). This distraction intervention has not been studied for its effectiveness in adult cancer patients undergoing chemotherapy.

The current study sought to determine the usefulness of VR as a distraction in reducing the unpleasant nature of cancer chemotherapy and reducing symptom distress among adults. The study used a randomized cross-over design with 123 adult patients being treated for breast, colon, or lung cancer. Patients either were assigned to use VR during the first round of chemotherapy, followed by chemotherapy treatment rounds without the intervention, or received one or more rounds of chemotherapy with no VR, followed by a round of chemotherapy with VR. One hundred patients completed all aspects of the study. At the end of the chemotherapy sessions with and without VR, subjects completed well-established and reliable instruments measuring symptom distress, state anxiety, and fatigue, as well as an evaluation of VR intervention questionnaire. These instruments were administered again at 48 hours after the chemotherapy sessions.

When using VR, subjects perceived the length of the chemotherapy session to be nearly 25% shorter than it actually was. No person had any adverse effects from the VR, and most stated that it did make the chemotherapy experience more pleasant. Eighty-two percent said they would like to use VR during chemotherapy again. Although symptom distress declined slightly after use of VR compared with the chemotherapy sessions without VR, this difference did not reach statistical significance.

Level of Evidence—4. The study was a well-designed cohort study.

Commentary: Implications for Practice and Research. The use of VR to make the chemotherapy experience more pleasant appears to be a positive distraction without adverse effects. Although some patients can distract themselves by reading, employing guided imagery, and other self-immersion methods, VR may be of greatest benefit to those people who are not as adept at self-immersion. Methods of reducing the unpleasant sensations associated with chemotherapy may help improve treatment outcomes by encouraging patients to continue therapy. Although the initial expense of VR equipment is significant, it may be worth the cost to help make chemotherapy treatments more tolerable. VR is an additional nonpharmacologic intervention nurses can implement when caring for patients receiving cancer chemotherapy. Nurses can advocate with their agency to ensure this intervention is an option for their patients.

all circulating leukocytes, erythrocytes, and platelets are decreased. Reduced leukocyte numbers, especially reduced neutrophils **(neutropenia),** greatly increase the risk for infection. Decreased erythrocytes and platelets cause hypoxia, fatigue, and an increased tendency to bleed.

Infection risk results from neutropenia, placing the patient at extreme risk for sepsis. *This critical problem is the major dose-limiting side effect of cancer chemotherapy and a common cause of death for patients during treatment.* Most chemotherapy drugs suppress bone marrow function to some degree and decrease the patient's protective responses to organism invasion. The severity and duration of the impairment are related directly to the dosage of specific chemotherapeutic drugs. This impairment is temporary, with good recovery of protection within weeks after therapy completion. However, the seriousness of potential infection complications makes this problem a major treatment concern. The infectious processes that occur most commonly are fungal, bacterial, and some residual viral breakthrough. *Most of the infections that develop in a patient with neutropenia result from overgrowth of the patient's own normal flora.*

Infection risk can be managed with the use of biological response modifiers (BRMs) to stimulate bone marrow production of immune system cells. Although not appropriate for all types of cancer, this supportive treatment can reduce the risk for infection during chemotherapy (Moore & Crom, 2006). However, BRMs are expensive and not consistently covered by insurance. This treatment is discussed on pp. 433-434 in the Immunotherapy section. Actual infections are treated with anti-infective drugs, such as antibiotic, antifungal, and antiviral drugs. Just like for any other infection, anti-infective therapy is specific for the organism(s) causing the infection.

Complementary and Alternative Therapies

Many patients with cancer use complementary and alternative therapies to boost immune function and prevent infection. Common therapies include shark cartilage, Echinacea, and megadoses of vitamin C. Although benefit has not yet been determined in clinical trials, the use of these therapies does not appear to have harmful effects.

The priority nursing interventions for the patient with neutropenia are protecting him or her from infection within the health care system and teaching the patient and family how to reduce infection in the home. Total patient assessment, including skin and mucous membrane inspection, lung sounds, mouth assessment, and close inspection of venous access device insertion sites, should be performed every 8 hours by a registered nurse. Explain to the patient the importance of reporting any change in skin and mucous membranes or other health status. Instruct him or her to report any pimple, sore, skin rash, or open area. Other changes to teach him or her to report are the presence of a cough, burning on urination, pain around the venous access site, or new drainage from any location. Good handwashing before contact with the patient is essential for prevention of infection (Siegel & Korniewicz, 2007). Health care workers must use aseptic technique when performing any invasive procedure. Chart 24-4 lists the best practices for infection prevention with neutropenic patients.

When delegating any nursing care activity to unlicensed assistive personnel (UAP) with supervision, teach them the importance of protecting the neutropenic patient from infection. Stress the ways that cross-contamination can occur and how to avoid this source of infection. Also ensure that UAP understand that even when the neutropenic patient is very tired and does not feel well, certain aspects of personal hygiene cannot be deferred. *Teach the importance of mouth care and washing of the axillary and perianal regions at least every 12 hours.*

Monitoring for manifestations of infection is critical for the hospitalized patient with neutropenia. The reduced numbers of neutrophils and other white blood cells can limit the presence of common infection manifestations. Often the patient with neutropenia does not develop a high fever or have purulent drainage even when a severe infection is present. *Any elevation of temperature in a patient with neutropenia is significant and is considered a sign of infection and should be reported to the health care provider immediately.* Hospital units specializing in care for neutropenic patients often have protocols or standard orders that nurses initiate as soon as infection is suspected, *before* a physician examines the patient, because treatment delay can result in sepsis and death. These protocols usually specify what types of cultures to obtain (e.g., blood, urine, sputum, central line, wound), what diagnostic tests to obtain (e.g., chest x-ray), and what antibiotics to immediately start.

Many patients remain at home during periods of neutropenia and are at continuing risk for infection, even though most home environments are likely to have fewer pathogenic organisms. The focus remains on keeping the patient's own normal flora under control and preventing transmission of organisms from other people to him or her. *At no time is the patient an infection hazard to other people; however, other people can be an infection hazard to the patient.* Teach patients and family members precautions to reduce the risk for infection (Chart 24-5).

Anemia (decreased number of circulating red blood cells) and thrombocytopenia (reduced circulating platelets) also result from the bone marrow suppression caused by some chemotherapy drugs. Anemia causes patients to feel fatigued, and some tissues are hypoxic. The cardiac and respiratory systems may not be able to maintain adequate oxygenation. Thrombocytopenia increases the risk for excessive bleeding. When the platelet count is less than 50,000/mm^3, any small trauma can lead to prolonged bleeding. Patients with fewer than 20,000 platelets/mm^3 may have spontaneous and uncontrollable bleeding requiring transfusion therapy (Burruss & Holz, 2005).

The use of biological response modifiers (BRMs) to stimulate bone marrow production of red blood cells and platelets is common for some types of cancer. Erythropoiesis-stimulating agents (ESAs) such as darbepoetin alfa (Aranesp) and epoetin alfa (Epogen, Procrit) can prevent or improve anemia associated with chemotherapy and can reduce the need for transfusion therapy. These drugs, however, do increase the production of many cell types, not just erythrocytes, increasing the patient's risk for hypertension, blood clots, strokes, and heart attacks, especially among older adults (Zarowitz, 2007). In addition, certain types of cancer cells grow faster in the presence of these ESAs, such as head and neck cancer cells, leukemias, and some lymphomas (U.S. Food and Drug Administration, 2007). The basis of dosing for these drugs is now the monitoring of individual patient hemoglobin levels to ensure that just enough red blood cells are produced to avoid the need for transfusion but not to bring hemoglobin or hematocrit levels up to normal.

BRM therapy for thrombocytopenia is the use of oprelvekin (Neumega). This modified version of interleukin 11 (IL-11)

Chart 24-4 BEST PRACTICE FOR PATIENT SAFETY & QUALITY CARE

Care of the Patient with Neutropenia

- Place the patient in a private room whenever possible.
- Use good handwashing technique or use alcohol-based hand rubs before touching the patient or any of the patient's belongings.
- Ensure that the patient's room and bathroom are cleaned at least once each day.
- Do not use supplies from common areas for neutropenic patients. For example, keep a sleeve or box of paper cups in the patient's room and do not share this box with any other patient. Other articles include drinking straws, plastic knives and forks, dressing materials, gloves, and bandages.
- Limit the number of health care personnel entering the patient's room.
- Monitor vital signs every 4 hours, including temperature.
- Inspect the patient's mouth at least every 8 hours.
- Inspect the patient's skin and mucous membranes (especially the anal area) for the presence of fissures and abscesses at least every 8 hours.
- Inspect open areas, such as IV sites, every 4 hours for manifestations of infection.
- Change wound dressings daily.
- Obtain specimens of all suspicious areas for culture (as specified by the agency), and promptly notify the physician.
- Assist the patient in coughing and deep-breathing exercises.
- Encourage activity at a level appropriate for the patient's current health status.
- Change IV tubing daily.
- Keep frequently used equipment in the room for use with this patient only (e.g., blood pressure cuff, stethoscope, thermometer).
- Limit visitors to healthy adults.
- Use strict aseptic technique for all invasive procedures.
- Monitor the white blood cell count, especially the absolute neutrophil count (ANC), daily.
- Avoid the use of indwelling urinary catheters.
- Keep fresh flowers and potted plants out of the patient's room.
- Teach the patient to eat a low-bacteria diet (e.g., avoiding raw fruits or vegetables; undercooked meat, eggs, or fish; pepper and paprika as seasonings sprinkled on food right before eating).

Chart 24-5 PATIENT AND FAMILY EDUCATION GUIDE

Prevention of Infection

During the times your white blood cell counts are low:

- Avoid crowds and other large gatherings of people who might be ill.
- Do not share personal toilet articles, such as toothbrushes, toothpaste, washcloths, or deodorant sticks, with others.
- If possible, bathe daily, using an antimicrobial soap. If total bathing is not possible, wash the armpits, groin, genitals, and anal area twice a day with an antimicrobial soap.
- Clean your toothbrush daily by either running it through the dishwasher or rinsing it in liquid laundry bleach.
- Wash your hands thoroughly with an antimicrobial soap before you eat and drink, after touching a pet, after shaking hands with anyone, as soon as you come home from any outing, and after using the toilet.
- Eat a low-bacteria diet, and avoid salads; raw fruit and vegetables; undercooked meat, fish, or eggs; and pepper and paprika.
- Wash dishes between use with hot, sudsy water, or use a dishwasher.
- Do not drink water, milk, juice, or other cold liquids that have been standing at room temperature for longer than an hour.
- Do not reuse cups and glasses without washing.
- Do not change pet litter boxes.
- Take your temperature at least once a day and whenever you do not feel well.
- Report any of these signs or symptoms of infection to your physician immediately:
  - Temperature greater than 100° F (38° C)
  - Persistent cough (with or without sputum)
  - Pus or foul-smelling drainage from any open skin area or normal body opening
  - Presence of a boil or abscess
  - Urine that is cloudy or foul smelling or that causes burning on urination
- Take all prescribed drugs.
- Do not dig in the garden or work with houseplants.
- Wear a condom (if you are a man) when having sex. If you are a woman having sex with a male partner, ensure that he wears a condom.

increases the production of platelets. The drug causes fluid retention and increases the risk for congestive heart failure and pulmonary edema. Other side effects include conjunctival bleeding, hypotension, and tachycardia. Teach patients taking this drug to weigh themselves daily and keep a record of the weight. Dyspnea should be reported immediately to the health care provider.

The priority for nursing care for the patient with thrombocytopenia is to provide a safe hospital environment. Chart 24-6 lists the best practices for bleeding precautions during hospitalization. Be sure that UAP understand the importance of using bleeding precautions and the need to report any evidence of bleeding immediately.

Teach patients with thrombocytopenia and their families how to avoid injury and excessive bleeding when patients are discharged before the platelet count has returned to normal. Chart 24-7 reviews what specifically to teach patients for how to prevent bleeding and what to do if bleeding occurs.

Chemotherapy-Induced Nausea and Vomiting (CIN)

Nausea and vomiting arise from a variety of local and central nervous system mechanisms. Most chemotherapy drugs are **emetogenic** (vomiting inducing) to some degree, depending on the dose. Most drugs induce nausea and vomiting when the drug is given and for 1 to 2 days afterward. Some drugs, such as cisplatin, induce delayed nausea and vomiting that can continue as long as 5 to 7 days after receiving it. Patients who have chemotherapy-related nausea and vomiting during one round of chemotherapy may begin to have the same symptoms before the next round as a result of sheer anticipation. Once considered the single most distressing side effect of chemotherapy, CIN often can be well controlled with appropriate therapy.

Many antiemetics are available to relieve nausea and vomiting. These drugs vary in the side effects they produce and how well they control chemotherapy-induced nausea and vomiting. One or more antiemetics are usually given before and after chemotherapy. Drugs commonly used short-term to

Chart 24-6 BEST PRACTICE FOR PATIENT SAFETY & QUALITY CARE

Prevention of Injury for the Patient with Thrombocytopenia

- Handle the patient gently.
- Use and teach UAP to use a lift sheet when moving and positioning the patient in bed.
- Avoid IM injections and venipunctures.
- When injections or venipunctures are necessary, use the smallest-gauge needle for the task.
- Apply firm pressure to the needle stick site for 10 minutes or until the site no longer oozes blood.
- Apply ice to areas of trauma.
- Test all urine and stool for the presence of occult blood.
- Observe IV sites every 4 hours for bleeding.
- Instruct alert patients to notify nursing personnel immediately if any trauma occurs and if bleeding or bruising is noticed.
- Avoid trauma to rectal tissues:
  - Instruct UAP not to take temperatures rectally, even on unconscious patients.
  - Do not administer enemas.
  - If suppositories are prescribed, lubricate liberally and administer with caution.
- Measure the patient's abdominal girth daily.
- Instruct the patient and UAP to use an electric shaver rather than a razor.
- When providing mouth care or supervising others in providing mouth care:
  - Use a soft-bristled toothbrush or tooth sponges.
  - Do not use floss.
  - Do not use water pressure gum cleaners.
  - Make certain that dentures fit and do not rub.
- Instruct the patient not to blow the nose or insert objects into the nose.
- Instruct UAP and the patient to wear shoes with firm soles whenever ambulating.
- Keep pathways and walkways clear and uncluttered.

Chart 24-7 PATIENT AND FAMILY EDUCATION GUIDE
Preventing Injury or Bleeding

During the time your platelet count is low:
- Use an electric shaver.
- Use a soft-bristled toothbrush, and do not floss.
- Do not have dental work performed without consulting your cancer health care provider.
- Do not take aspirin or any aspirin-containing products. Read the label to be sure that the product does not contain aspirin or salicylates.
- Do not participate in contact sports or any activity likely to result in your being bumped, scratched, or scraped.
- If you are bumped, apply ice to the site for at least 1 hour.
- Avoid hard foods that would scrape the inside of your mouth.
- Eat warm, cool, or cold foods to avoid burning your mouth.
- Check your skin and mouth daily for bruises, swelling, or areas with small reddish purple marks that may indicate bleeding.
- Notify your cancer health care provider if you:
  - Are injured and persistent bleeding results
  - Have excessive menstrual bleeding
  - See blood in your urine or bowel movement
- Avoid anal intercourse.
- Take a stool softener to prevent straining during a bowel movement.
- Do not use enemas or rectal suppositories.
- Avoid bending over at the waist.
- Do not wear clothing or shoes that are tight or that rub.
- Avoid blowing your nose or placing objects in your nose. If you must blow your nose, do so gently without blocking either nasal passage.
- Avoid playing musical instruments that raise the pressure inside your head, such as brass wind instruments and woodwinds or reed instruments.

control chemotherapy-induced nausea and vomiting are listed in Chart 24-8. *Patient response to antiemetic therapy is highly variable, and the drug combinations should be individualized for best effect.*

Regardless of which drug or drugs are being used to prevent or reduce CIN, they are most effective when used aggressively and on a scheduled basis (Tipton et al., 2007). Just like pain management drug therapy works best when given before pain intensity increases, so does drug therapy for CIN. *Thus the nursing priority is to coordinate with the patient and health care provider to ensure adequate control of CIN. Ensure that premedication with antiemetics is given before each session of IV chemotherapy.* When patients are receiving dose-dense chemotherapy, the intensity of CIN also increases and more or longer antiemetic therapy is needed. Teach patients to continue the therapy as prescribed, even when the nausea and vomiting appear controlled. *When the patient stops taking the drug(s), he or she should start retaking the drug at the first sign of nausea to prevent this side effect from becoming uncontrollable.*

CONSIDERATIONS FOR OLDER ADULTS

At times, older patients have received lower doses of chemotherapy drugs because it was thought that they would not be able to tolerate the side effects of nausea and vomiting. Research indicates that older patients do not have greater nausea and vomiting than do younger patients. Therefore their chemotherapy regimens should not be altered on this basis alone (Cope & Reb, 2006). However, the older adult can become dehydrated more quickly if CIN is not adequately controlled. Teach older adult patients to be proactive with taking their prescribed antiemetics and to contact their health care provider if the CIN either does not resolve within 12 hours or becomes worse.

Complementary and Alternative Therapies

Complementary and alternative therapies may assist the patient with nausea and vomiting to achieve comfort through nonpharmacologic means along with antiemetics. Music, progressive muscle relaxation, guided imagery, acupressure, or distraction may help reduce anxiety and relieve nausea and vomiting. Assess the patient for complications resulting from excessive vomiting, such as dehydration and electrolyte imbalances.

Mucositis

Mucositis (sores in mucous membranes) often develops in the entire GI tract, especially in the mouth (stomatitis). Normally, the lining of the GI tract undergoes rapid cell division and quickly replaces cells. With chemotherapy, mucous membrane cells are killed more rapidly than they are replaced, resulting in sore formation. Mouth sores are painful and interfere with eating and general quality of life (McGuire, 2002). Chart 24-9 lists the best practices for patients with mucositis.

Frequent mouth assessment and oral hygiene are key in managing stomatitis and mucositis. Stress the importance of good and frequent oral hygiene, including teeth cleaning and mouth rinsing. Because most patients with mucositis also have bone marrow suppression and are at risk for bleeding, they must take care to avoid traumatizing the oral mucosa. Instruct them to use a soft-bristled toothbrush or disposable mouth sponges and to avoid using dental floss and water pressure gum cleaners. Encourage them to rinse the mouth with plain water or saline every hour while awake. Teach them to avoid mouthwashes that contain alcohol or other drying agents that may further irritate the mucosa.

Oral hygiene equipment must be kept clean. Remind patients not to share toothbrushes with anyone. Toothbrushes can be cleaned daily by running them through a home dishwasher or by rinsing them with a concentrated solution of liquid bleach or hydrogen peroxide.

Many compounds are available for pain relief from stomatitis or mucositis. Many hospitals offer their own special "swish and spit" mixtures, which contain a local anesthetic combined with anti-inflammatory agents. Tell the patient that these mixtures are not to be swallowed.

Alopecia

Alopecia, hair loss, may occur as whole-body hair loss or may be as mild as only a thinning of the scalp hair. Reassure patients that hair loss is temporary. Hair regrowth usually begins about 1 month after completion of chemotherapy. Inform the patient that the new hair may differ from the original hair in

Chart 24-8 COMMON EXAMPLES OF DRUG THERAPY

Antiemetic Drugs for Chemotherapy-Induced Nausea and Vomiting

Drug/Usual Dosage	Physiologic Purpose	Nursing Interventions	Rationale
SEROTONIN ANTAGONISTS			
Ondansetron (Zofran) 8 mg IV or orally every 8 hr Granisetron (Kytril) 1 mg IV or orally every 12 hr Dolasetron (Anzemet) 100 mg IV or orally 30 minutes before chemo Palonosetron (Aloxi) 0.25 mg IV as a single dose 30 minutes before chemo **Med Error Alert!** Do not confuse Anzemet with Avandamet.	Prevent CIN by blocking the 5-HT3 receptors in the brain (chemotrigger zone) and in the intestines. This action prevents serotonin from binding to the receptors and activating the nausea and vomiting centers.	Teach patient to change positions slowly to avoid falls. Assess the patient for headache.	These drugs may induce bradycardia, hypotension, and vertigo. Headache is a common side effect of drugs from this class.
NEUROKININ RECEPTOR ANTAGONISTS			
Aprepitant (Emend) 3-day oral regimen: *Day 1*, 125 mg 1 hour before chemo *Days 2 and 3*, 80 mg in the morning (no chemo these days)	Reduce CIN by blocking the substance P neurokinin receptor. When used together with a serotonin antagonist and a corticosteroid, both acute and delayed nausea and vomiting are controlled.	Teach patients who are also taking warfarin (Coumadin) to have their INRs checked before and after the 3 days of this therapy. Teach women who are using oral contraceptives to use an additional form of birth control while on this drug.	This drug interferes with the effectiveness of warfarin. The drug reduces the effectiveness of oral contraceptives, increasing the risk for an unplanned pregnancy.
CORTICOSTEROIDS			
Dexamethasone (Decadron) 5-10 mg IV or orally daily	Reduce CIN by decreasing swelling in the brain's chemotrigger zone.	Teach patients to reduce salt intake to about 4 mg daily.	Drug causes fluid retention and hypertension.
PROKINETIC AGENTS			
Metoclopramide (Reglan) 20-40 mg IM or IV twice or three times daily	Reduce CIN by blocking dopamine receptors in the brain's chemotrigger zone.	Teach the patient to avoid driving or operating heavy machinery.	Increased drowsiness is common.
BENZODIAZEPINES			
Lorazepam (Ativan) 1-3 mg orally or IV twice or three times daily	Reduce CIN by enhancing cholinergic effects and by decreasing the person's awareness.	Teach the patient and family that the patient should avoid driving, operating heavy machinery, making legal decisions, and going up and down staircases unassisted.	The drug induces amnesia and profound drowsiness.

CIN, Chemotherapy-induced nausea and vomiting; *INR*, international normalized ratio.

Chart 24-9 BEST PRACTICE FOR PATIENT SAFETY & QUALITY CARE

Mouth Care for Patients with Mucositis

- Examine the patient's mouth (including the roof, under the tongue, and between the teeth and cheek) every 4 hours.
- Document the location, size, and character of fissures, blisters, sores, or drainage.
- Get an order to obtain specimens of sores or drainage for culture.
- Brush the teeth and tongue with a soft-bristled brush or sponges every 8 hours.
- Rinse the mouth with a solution of one-half peroxide and one-half normal saline every 12 hours.
- Avoid the use of alcohol or glycerin-based mouthwashes.
- Encourage the patient to drink 3 or more liters of water per day if another health problem does not require limiting fluid intake.
- Administer antimicrobial drugs as prescribed.
- Administer topical analgesic drugs as prescribed or as needed.
- Help the conscious patient to "swish and spit" room-temperature tap water or normal saline as needed.
- Apply petroleum jelly to the patient's lips after each episode of mouth care and as needed.
- Assist the patient in using "artificial saliva" as needed, if prescribed.
- Urge the patient to avoid using tobacco or drinking alcoholic beverages.
- Assist the patient in menu choices to avoid spicy, salty, acidic, dry, rough, or hard food.
- Cool liquids to prevent burns or irritation.
- If the patient wears dentures, encourage him or her to use them only during meals.
- When not in place, soak dentures in an antimicrobial solution. Rinse thoroughly before placing the dentures in the patient's mouth.
- Offer complete mouth care before and after every meal.

color, texture, and thickness. No known treatment completely prevents alopecia. *The priority nursing interventions for the patient with chemotherapy-induced alopecia are to teach the patient to prevent injury to the scalp and to assist the patient in coping with this body image change.*

The hairless scalp is at risk for injury. Teach the patient to avoid direct sunlight on the scalp by wearing hats or other head coverings. Sunscreen use is essential to prevent sunburn even with minimal sun exposure (many chemotherapy drugs increase sun sensitivity), regardless of skin darkness. This skin can be damaged by helmets, headphones, headsets, and other items that rub the head. Teach the patient to wear some head covering underneath these items. In addition, head coverings during cold weather are needed to reduce body heat loss and prevent hypothermia.

Assist patients in selecting a type of head covering that suits their income and lifestyle. One recommendation is to coordinate wig purchases with the patient's hairdresser or barber. Having very short hair or a shaved head now is common and socially acceptable for men, and many men choose not to wear a wig during chemotherapy. Cutting the hair very short or even shaving the head before chemotherapy begins allows a better wig fit. This practice also removes the uncertainty of when the hair loss will occur.

Suggest that women purchase a wig before therapy begins and have their hairdresser shape the wig to mimic their usual hairstyle so there is less change in appearance. If possible, having two wigs is good so that one can always be clean and ready to wear. High-quality wigs are expensive but can look very much like the patient's own hair. Many local units of the American Cancer Society offer the loan of wigs that other patients have used and then donated to be lent to others with cancer. Patients can disguise hair loss with caps, scarves, and turbans. Some support groups such as the American Cancer Society's "Look Good, Feel Better" program can offer suggestions to help patients improve their appearance at this time.

Changes in Cognitive Function

Some patients being treated with chemotherapy have reported changes in cognitive function, most commonly reduced ability to concentrate, memory loss, and difficulty learning new information during treatment and for months to years after treatment (Bender et al., 2006). Although most types of chemotherapy drugs do not cross the blood-brain barrier and were thought not to affect any part of brain function, the drugs can induce general biochemistry changes that could reduce cognitive function, at least temporarily.

This problem, termed "chemobrain" by patients, has been reported most in women who have had chemotherapy for breast cancer. Changes in cognitive function are not limited either to women or to breast cancer treatment. The fact that it is reported more in this population reflects the issues that breast cancer is very common, it is often treated with high-dose chemotherapy, and most patients with breast cancer survive a long time after therapy.

Recent studies have compared brain structure and cognitive function among groups of women with breast cancer who did not receive chemotherapy, groups of women with breast cancer who did receive chemotherapy, and groups of healthy women. One study found that women receiving chemotherapy, especially with platinum-based drugs, had some shrinkage of both the white matter and the gray matter of the brain (determined by magnetic resonance imaging [MRI]) during chemotherapy and at 1 year after chemotherapy was completed compared with no shrinkage in control subjects (Inagaki et al., 2007). At 3 years after completion of therapy, no differences in brain volumes were found between the chemotherapy and control groups. Two other studies examined cognitive functions and discovered that about 25% of women having chemotherapy experienced decreased cognitive function during and after therapy completion compared with only about 5% of women who did not receive chemotherapy (Schagen et al., 2006).

One puzzling feature of this problem is that only some of the women receiving specific chemotherapy for breast cancer experienced a noticeable reduction in cognitive function. At present, not only is the exact cause of this side effect unclear, so are the personal risk factors. *The priority for nursing care is to support the patient who reports this side effect.* Listen to the patient's concerns, and tell him or her that other patients have also reported such problems. Providing absolute reassurance is difficult because only a few studies using appropriate research methods have examined this issue; however, early results indicate that recovery is likely with time. A common sense approach includes that patients should be warned against also participating in other behaviors that could alter cognitive functioning, such as excessive alcohol intake, recreational drug use, and activities that increase the risk for head injury.

Peripheral Neuropathy

Peripheral neuropathy (PN) is the loss of sensory or motor function of peripheral nerves. Although most commonly seen in patients with long-term diabetes, patients undergoing chemotherapy with nerve-damaging drugs (especially the antimitotics and platinum-based drugs) often have rapid onset of severe PN (Almadrones, 2006; Wickham, 2007). The degree of PN is related to the dosage of the nerve-damaging drugs; higher doses lead to greater neuropathy. This side effect is not new; however, it is more common now as long-term cancer survival has increased. The results of PN on function are widespread, with the most common problems including loss of sensation in the hands and feet, orthostatic hypotension, erectile dysfunction, neuropathic pain, loss of taste discrimination, and severe constipation (Visovsky et al., 2008). PN appears to be a long-term consequence and may be permanent in some people, although this is not yet known. At present, no known interventions prevent PN.

The priority for nursing care of patients experiencing PN is teaching the patient to prevent injury. Loss of sensation increases the patient's risk for injury because he or she may not be aware of excessive heat, cold, or pressure. Just like for patients with diabetes, the risk for injury to the feet is very high. In addition, falls are more likely because the patient cannot feel changes in terrain and because of orthostatic hypotension. Chart 24-10 lists teaching priorities for the patient with chemotherapy-induced peripheral neuropathy.

Some issues, such as erectile dysfunction, may be helped with special devices or drug therapy (see Chapter 75 for a more complete discussion of options for erectile dysfunction). Other issues are not correctable and often affect many aspects of quality of life. For example, the loss of sensation in the hands may make some occupations and leisure activities that require very fine motor skills impossible. For other, such as piano-playing,

Chart 24-10 PATIENT AND FAMILY EDUCATION GUIDE
Chemotherapy-Induced Peripheral Neuropathy

- Protect feet and other body areas where sensation is reduced (e.g., do not walk around in bare feet or stocking feet; always wear shoes with a protective sole).
- Be sure shoes are long enough and wide enough to prevent creating sores or blisters.
- Provide a long break-in period for new shoes; do not wear new shoes for longer than 2 hours at a time.
- Avoid pointed-toe shoes and shoes with heels higher than 2 inches.
- Inspect your feet daily (with a mirror) for open areas or redness.
- Avoid extremes of temperature; wear warm clothing in the winter, especially over hands, feet, and ears.
- Test water temperature with a thermometer when washing dishes or bathing. Use warm water rather than hot water (less than 110° F)
- Use potholders when cooking.
- Use gloves when washing dishes or gardening.
- Do not eat foods that are "steaming hot," allow them to cool before placing them in your mouth.
- Eat foods that are high in fiber (e.g., fruit, whole grain cereals, vegetables).
- Drink two to three liters of fluid (nonalcoholic) daily unless your health care provider has told you to restrict fluid intake.
- Get up from a lying or sitting position slowly. If you feel dizzy, sit back down until the dizziness fades before standing, then stand in place for a few seconds before walking or using the stairs.
- Look at your feet and the floor or ground where you are walking to assess how the ground, floor, or step changes to prevent tripping or falling.
- Avoid using area rugs, especially those that slide easily.
- Use handrails when going up or down steps.

the person may have to watch his or her hands to know just where the keys are and may not be able to control how hard a key is struck. Assess the patient's ability to cope with these changes. Coordinate with an occupational therapist to assist the patient in finding ways to adjust for sensory deficits in performing desired activities or in finding alternative activities.

NCLEX EXAMINATION CHALLENGE

The client is receiving IV chemotherapy over 8 hours on the med-surg unit. The drugs, started by a chemotherapy certified nurse, are being monitored by the unit nurses. After 2 hours, the client reports burning and pain at the IV site. Lowering the IV results in an observable brisk blood return. What is the nurse's best first action?

A. Stop the drug infusion and run normal saline into IV access.
B. Notify the chemotherapy certified nurse who started the infusion.
C. Slow the infusion but continue it since there is a good blood return.
D. Discontinue the infusion, remove the IV, and document the site condition.

evolve For the correct answer, go to http://evolve.elsevier.com/Iggy/.

HORMONAL MANIPULATION

Overview

Hormones are naturally occurring chemicals secreted by endocrine (ductless) glands and picked up by capillaries. Once in the bloodstream, hormones circulate to all body areas but exert their effects only on their specific target tissues. Some hormones make hormone-sensitive tumors grow more rapidly, and some tumors require specific hormones to divide. Thus decreasing the amount of these hormones to hormone-sensitive tumors can slow the cancer growth rate.

Hormonal manipulation can help control some types of cancer for many years. Usually, this therapy does not lead to a cure. The endocrine system usually maintains a delicate hormone balance. When a large amount of one hormone is given, it upsets the balance and disturbs the uptake of other hormones. If a tumor depends on hormone A for growth and a large quantity of hormone B (similar to A) is given to the patient, hormone B will interfere with the tumor's uptake of hormone A or will limit the amount of hormone A produced. As a result, tumor growth is slowed and survival time increases. Table 24-5 lists the drugs commonly used in hormonal manipulation for cancer therapy.

TABLE 24-5 Common Agents Used for Hormonal Manipulation of Cancer

Type of Agent	Example
HORMONE AGONISTS	
Androgen	Fluoxymesterone (Halotestin)
	Testolactone (Teslac)
Estrogen	Chlorotrianisene (Tace)
	Conjugated equine estrogen (Premarin)
	Diethylstilbestrol (DES, Stilphostrol)
	Ethinyl estradiol (Estinyl)
Progestin	Medroxyprogesterone (Amen, Provera)
	Megestrol (Megace)
Luteinizing hormone–releasing hormone (LHRH)	Leuprolide (Eligard, Lupron, Viadur)
	Goserelin (Zoladex)
HORMONE ANTAGONISTS	
Antiandrogens	Bicalutamide (Casodex)
	Flutamide (Eulexin)
Antiestrogens	Fulvestrant (Faslodex)
	Tamoxifen (Nolvadex)
	Toremifene (Fareston)
HORMONE INHIBITORS	
	Aminoglutethimide (Cytadren, Elipten)
	Anastrozole (Arimidex)
	Exemestane (Aromasin)
	Letrozole (Femara)

Some drugs are hormone antagonists that compete with natural hormones at the receptor sites. Often, they are antibodies specific to the receptor. When hormone antagonists are given, they bind to the specific hormone receptor on or in the tumor cell and prevent the needed hormone from binding to the receptor. If a tumor needs a certain hormone to grow and the hormone can enter or activate the cell only through a receptor, hormone antagonists can slow down tumor growth.

A new class of drugs used for hormonal therapy is the hormone inhibitors. These drugs inhibit the production of specific hormones in the normal hormone-producing organs. For example, the aromatase inhibitor *anastrozole* (Arimidex) prevents the production of estrogen in the adrenal gland and reduces blood levels of estrogens.

Side Effects of Hormonal Manipulation

Androgens and the antiestrogen receptor drugs cause masculinizing effects in women. Chest and facial hair may develop, menstrual periods stop, and breast tissue shrinks. Patients may have some fluid retention. For men and women receiving androgens, acne may develop, hypercalcemia is common, and liver dysfunction may occur with prolonged therapy. Women receiving estrogens or progestins have irregular but heavy menses, fluid retention, and breast tenderness. Male and female patients who take estrogen or progestins are at increased risk for deep vein thrombosis.

Feminine manifestations often appear in men who take estrogens, progestins, or antiandrogen receptor drugs. Facial hair thins or disappears, facial skin becomes smoother, body fat is redistributed, and **gynecomastia** (breast development in men) can occur. Testicular and penile atrophy also occurs to some degree. Although sexual function may continue, achieving and maintaining an erection is much more difficult. Teach patients and families about these expected side effects. Encourage them to express their feelings about body image changes. Refer them for counseling, if needed.

PHOTODYNAMIC THERAPY

Overview

Photodynamic therapy (PDT) is the selective destruction of cancer cells through a chemical reaction triggered by different types of laser light. This newer type of therapy can be used to directly destroy some cancers, reduce the size of tumors and then allow more complete tumor removal by surgery, and shrink tumors in airways or the esophagus to relieve obstruction. PDT for cancer therapy is most commonly used for nonmelanoma skin cancers, ocular tumors, GI tumors, and lung cancers located in the airways. It is under investigation for use as therapy combined with other treatment for brain tumors and prostate cancer.

An agent that sensitizes cells to light is injected IV along with a dye. The most common agents used for this purpose are verteporfin and porfimer sodium (Awan & Tarin, 2006). These drugs enter all cells but leave normal cells more rapidly than cancer cells. Usually, within 48 to 72 hours, most of the drug has collected in high concentrations in cancer cells. At this time, a laser light is focused on the tumor. The light activates a chemical reaction within those cells retaining the sensitizing drug that induces irreversible cell damage. Some cells die and slough immediately; others continue to slough for several days. Some lesions require only one exposure to the laser, and others may be re-exposed several days after the first treatment.

Patient-Centered Collaborative Care

The priorities for nursing care of the patient receiving PDT are teaching the patient and family to prevent complications and coordinating changes in the care environment for protection of the patient (Collins & Garner, 2007). *The patient has general sensitivity to light for up to 12 weeks after the photosensitizing drug is injected.* The most intense period of light sensitivity is after injection and before the laser treatment. During this time, the patient is at high risk for sunburn and eye pain.

Teaching must begin before the patient comes for the injection. Specific instructions are listed in Chart 24-11. Instruct the patient to bring clothing, hat, and eye protection to wear on the way home from the injection. Clothing should include gloves, shirts or blouses with long sleeves and high collars, long pants, and socks, to prevent burns from exposure to direct or indirect sunlight (including light through windows) and other intense light sources. Stress that the skin and eyes will remain sensitive for at least 30 days, even among people

Chart 24-11 PATIENT AND FAMILY EDUCATION GUIDE

Photodynamic Therapy

BEFORE PHOTOSENSITIZATION

- Bring protective clothing (e.g., shirts with long sleeves and high collars, long pants or skirt, gloves, socks, wide-brimmed hat) and UV-protective sunglasses with you when you come to be injected with the photosensitizing agent.
- If possible, have someone else drive you home so that you can place a sheet or light blanket over yourself.
- Plan to avoid leaving your home during daylight hours for anywhere from 1 to 3 months.
- Cover all windows with light-blocking shades or heavy drapes/curtains.
- Replace high-wattage light bulbs with lower-wattage ones, and use as few as possible.

AFTER PHOTOSENSITIZATION

- Remember that the photosensitizing effects last from 1 to 3 months.
- Continue to wear all protective clothing, avoid sunlight in any form, and avoid high-wattage indoor lights.
- Drink plenty of water to prevent becoming dehydrated.
- Do not take any newly prescribed or over-the-counter drugs without contacting the physician who performed the photodynamic therapy. Some drugs make the light sensitivity even worse; others interact with the photosensitizing drug.
- When you do start to re-exposure yourself to sunlight and other bright lights, do so slowly. Start out exposing only about 1 inch of your skin to sunlight at a time.
- Start out with only 10 minutes, and increase the time only by about 5 minutes each day.
- Remember that sunscreen will not prevent severe sunburn during this time.
- If you experience pain or blistering, notify the photodynamic therapy health care team.
- Continue to wear dark glasses, even indoors, until you no longer have eye pain when in a normally lighted environment.
- When you no longer are photosensitive, see an ophthalmologist to check whether your retina has any damage.

UV, Ultraviolet.

with very dark skin. Thus the patient will need to use protective measures and be homebound for 1 to 3 months.

When the patient returns for the laser light therapy, the process may occur on an outpatient basis, or for airway lesions, the patient may require several days as an inpatient in an intensive care unit. The nurse coordinates with all other members of the health care team in ensuring that the environment is safe for the patient. Lighting of all types is kept to a minimum. Even the use of a penlight or the sensor on a pulse oximeter can lead to burns for the patient who has been injected with a photosensitizer. Electronic monitoring equipment should have the light intensity of the readout turned down to as low as possible and not facing the patient. When the patient is transported, reducing hallway lighting and avoiding windows are essential. An especially important member of the team to consult is the pharmacist. Any drug the patient is prescribed should be considered for its photosensitizing properties. For example, certain antibiotics (tetracycline and erythromycin) increase photosensitivity as do many antihypertensive drugs. When these drugs are taken by the patient receiving PDT, the intensity of the photosensitivity is increased and the patient's risk for harm also is increased.

IMMUNOTHERAPY: BIOLOGICAL RESPONSE MODIFIERS

Overview

Biological response modifiers (BRMs) modify the patient's biologic responses to tumor cells. The BRMs in current use as cancer therapy are cytokines, which are small protein hormones made by white blood cells. Cytokines made by macrophages, neutrophils, eosinophils, and monocytes are *monokines;* cytokines produced by lymphocytes (especially the T-lymphocytes) are *lymphokines.* Cytokines generally make the immune system work better (see Chapter 19).

Cytokines enhance the immune system. Immune function plays an important role in cancer prevention (see Chapters 19 and 23). Cytokines and other BRMs work as a cancer treatment by stimulating the immune system to recognize cancer cells and take actions to eliminate or destroy them. Some BRMs are also useful in a supporting role, such as colony-stimulating factors that stimulate faster recovery of bone marrow function after treatment-induced suppression.

BRMS as Cancer Therapy

Two common types of BRMs used as cancer therapy are the interleukins (ILs) and interferons (INFs). Some agents can stimulate specific immune system cells to attack and destroy cancer cells; other agents block cancer cell access to an essential function or nutrient.

Interleukins (ILs) are a group of 27 known substances the body makes to help regulate inflammation and immune protection. Some are now synthesized as drugs. ILs help different immune system cells recognize and destroy abnormal body cells. In particular, IL-1, IL-2, and IL-6 appear to "charge up" the immune system and enhance attacks on cancer cells by macrophages, natural killer (NK) cells, and tumor-infiltrating lymphocytes.

Interferons (INFs) are cell-produced proteins that can protect noninfected cells from viral infection and replication. Cancer-related functions of INF include the ability to:

- Slow tumor cell division
- Stimulate the growth and activation of NK cells
- Help cancer cells resume a more normal appearance and function
- Inhibit the expression of oncogenes

INFs have been effective to some degree in the treatment of melanoma, hairy cell leukemia, renal cell carcinoma, ovarian cancer, and cutaneous T-cell lymphoma.

One drug classified as a BRM that has a somewhat different action is thalidomide (Thalomid), which reduces the level of tumor angiogenesis factor (TAF). TAF is needed to maintain blood supply to the tumor. When TAF is reduced, the tumor is poorly nourished and cancer cells die. This drug is approved for treatment of multiple myeloma.

BRMS as Supportive Therapy

BRMs used for supportive therapy during cancer treatment are the colony-stimulating factors (Table 24-6). These factors induce more rapid recovery of the bone marrow after suppression by chemotherapy. This effect has two benefits. First, when bone marrow suppression is shortened or less severe, patients are less at risk for life-threatening infections, anemia, and bleeding. Second, because the colony-stimulating factors allow more rapid bone marrow recovery, patients can receive their chemotherapy on time and may even be able to tolerate higher doses, improving the curative outcome of chemotherapy. These agents, however, can stimulate the growth of leukemia or some lymphoma cells.

Side Effects of Biological Response Modifier Therapy

Patients receiving interleukins have generalized and sometimes severe inflammatory reactions. Fluid shifts and capillary leak are widespread with edema forming in most tissues. Tissue

TABLE 24-6 Common Biological Response Modifiers Used as Supportive Cancer Therapy

Agent	Cell Type Affected	Indications
Sargramostim (Leukine, Prokine)	All granulocytes Neutrophils Eosinophils Monocytes Macrophages	Chemotherapy-induced leukopenia
Filgrastim (Neupogen) Pegfilgrastim (Neulasta)	Neutrophils	Chemotherapy-induced neutropenia
Epoetin alfa (Epogen, Procrit) Darbepoetin alfa (Aranesp)	Erythrocytes	Chemotherapy-induced anemia Chemotherapy-induced fatigue Anemia induced by renal failure
Oprelvekin (Neumega)	Platelets	Chemotherapy-induced thrombocytopenia

swelling affects the function of all organs and can be life threatening. Patients receiving high-dose BRM therapy should receive care in an intensive care or monitoring unit. The effects of BRM therapy are limited to the period of acute drug infusion and resolve when treatment is completed.

Many BRMs induce symptoms of mild inflammation during and immediately after receiving the drug, including fever, chills, rigors, and flu-like general malaise. Problems are worse when higher doses are given, but they seem to become less severe over time. Fever is treated with acetaminophen. Patients with severe rigors (severe shaking chills) are managed with meperidine (Demerol).

Interferon therapy causes peripheral neuropathy similar to that found in patients who have long-standing diabetes mellitus. Some of the problems resulting from the neuropathy include decreased sensory perception, visual disturbances, decreased hearing, unsteady balance and gait, and orthostatic hypotension. It is not known whether the neuropathy is temporary or permanent. (See the discussion of peripheral neuropathy on pp. 430-431.)

Skin rashes, dryness, itching, and peeling occur with many types of BRM therapy. The skin problems are more severe at higher doses and when more than one type of BRM is used at the same time. These reactions are temporary but can cause much discomfort and distress to the patient. Advise patients to apply moisturizers (perfume-free) to the skin and to use mild soap to clean the skin. Involved areas should be protected from the sun with clothing or the use of sunscreen agents. Inform patients to avoid swimming and to refrain from using topical steroid creams on affected areas.

GENE THERAPY

Gene therapy as a cancer treatment is experimental. One method of using gene therapy for cancer is to render the tumor cells more susceptible to damage or death by other treatments. Inserting a viral enzyme gene into brain tumor cells makes them more susceptible to being killed by antiviral agents. Other techniques involve inserting human leukocyte antigen (HLA) genes different from the patient's own HLAs into the tumor cells. This technique makes the patient's immune system cells better able to recognize the cancer cells as foreign and take steps to eliminate or destroy them. Both methods of gene therapy for cancer have shown some success in early-phase clinical trials but are not approved treatments.

Some immune system cells are capable of attacking and killing cancer cells (see Chapter 19). This ability is increased when more of certain cytokines, such as IL-2, are present. Some gene therapy involves inserting additional genes for cytokines into the patient's own immune system cells. These "charged-up" cancer-fighting immune system cells remain active for up to 6 months and can participate in cancer cell–killing episodes.

TARGETED THERAPY

Overview

Targeted therapies combine aspects of gene therapy and immunotherapy. These therapies take advantage of one or more differences in cancer cell growth or metabolism that are either not present or only slightly present in normal cells (Viele, 2005). These differences are a result of specific gene expression in cancer cells. Agents used as targeted therapies often are antibodies that work to disrupt cancer cell division in one of several ways. Some of these drugs "target" and block growth factor receptors, especially the epithelial growth factor receptors (EGFRs) or the vascular endothelial growth factor receptors (VEGFRs). When a cancer cell's growth depends on having the growth factors bind to its specific receptors, blocking the receptor slows or eliminates the cancer cell's growth.

Other agents for targeted therapy may be antibodies directed against cellular substance needed by the cancer cell for growth or a substance in the cell's signal transduction pathway that is important in turning on certain genes for cell growth. Targeted therapy can block these pathways so that the signal for turning on cell division genes does not get through to the cell's nucleus.

Many drugs for targeted therapy have been approved as treatment for certain cancers. *It is important to remember, however, that these drugs will not work unless the cancer cell overexpresses the actual target substance. Thus not all patients with the same cancer type would benefit from the use of targeted therapy.* Each person's cancer cells are evaluated to determine whether the cells have enough of a target to be affected by targeted therapy.

An example of a targeted therapy is trastuzumab (Herceptin). This EGFR antibody binds the excessive amounts of a certain type of EGFR produced by breast cancer cells in response to the activation of the *HER2/neu* gene. Binding this receptor prevents the division of cancer cells and makes them more easily killed by immune system cells. Another monoclonal antibody, rituximab (Rituxan), has a similar effect in some types of lymphoma. Another example of a targeted therapy drug is imatinib mesylate (Gleevec). This drug binds to the energy site of the enzyme *tyrosine kinase* and prevents its activation. The drug is most useful in cancers that overexpress the *ABL1* oncogene, such as Philadelphia chromosome–positive chronic myeloid leukemia. Table 24-7 lists some agents currently used for targeted cancer therapy.

Side Effects of Targeted Therapy

Allergic reactions are an issue in patients receiving monoclonal antibodies. Most of these antibodies were developed in animals and may express some animal proteins. More recently, much of the animal portion of these antibodies was removed. Thus the risk for allergic reactions is reduced but not eliminated. Patients receiving antibodies over time may develop their own antibodies to the drugs, making them less effective and possibly causing severe inflammatory or allergic reactions.

In addition, the EGFR and VEGFR antibodies bind to those specific receptors when the receptors are on normal tissue. Thus side effects occur in those tissues that normally express EGFR, such as the skin, mucous membranes, and lining of the GI tract (Eaby, 2008).

ONCOLOGIC EMERGENCIES

Cancer is a chronic disease. However, a number of acute conditions associated with cancer and its treatment can occur. These conditions, or complications, often require immediate intervention and are thus *oncologic emergencies.* Early diagnosis of such conditions is essential to avoid life-threatening situations. The role of the nurse is to plan and implement interventions to prevent and detect these complications early for immediate treatment.

TABLE 24-7 Examples of Targeted Therapy Agents

Agent	Malignancy
alemtuzumab (Campath)	Chronic lymphocytic leukemia
azacitidine (Vidaza)	Myelodysplastic syndrome
bevacizumab (Avastin)	Colorectal cancer; lung cancer
bortezomib (Velcade)	Lymphoma; multiple myeloma
canertinib	Breast cancer (metastatic)
cetuximab (Erbitux)	Colorectal cancer; head and neck cancer
dasatinib (SPRYCEL)	Chronic myelogenous leukemia resistant to imatinib
epratuzumab (LymphoCide)	Non-Hodgkin's lymphoma
erlotinib (Tarceva)	Pancreatic cancer; lung cancer
galiximab	Non-Hodgkin's lymphoma
gefitinib (Iressa)	Head and neck cancer; lung cancer (no longer approved)
gemtuzumab (Mylotarg)	Acute myelogenous leukemia
imatinib (Gleevec)	Chronic myelogenous leukemia
lapatinib (Tykerb)	Breast cancer (metastatic)
rituximab (Rituxan)	Non-Hodgkin's lymphoma
sorafenib (NEXAVAR)	Renal cell carcinoma
temsirolimus (TORISEL)	Renal cell carcinoma
trastuzumab (Herceptin)	*HER2*-positive breast cancer

SEPSIS AND DISSEMINATED INTRAVASCULAR COAGULATION

Pathophysiology

Sepsis, or *septicemia,* is a condition in which organisms enter the bloodstream. Septic shock is a life-threatening result of sepsis and a common cause of death in patients with cancer. Patients with cancer are at risk for infection and sepsis because their white blood cell counts are often low and their immune function is usually impaired. Chapter 39 describes the pathophysiology of sepsis and septic shock.

Disseminated intravascular coagulation (DIC) is a problem with the blood-clotting process. DIC is triggered by many severe illnesses, including cancer. In patients with cancer, DIC is caused by sepsis (often a gram-negative infection), by the release of thrombin or thromboplastin (clotting factors) from cancer cells, or by blood transfusions. DIC is most often seen in leukemia and in adenocarcinomas of the lung, pancreas, stomach, and prostate.

Extensive, abnormal clotting occurs throughout the small blood vessels of patients with DIC. This widespread clotting uses up the existing clotting factors and platelets. This process is followed by extensive bleeding. Bleeding from many sites is the most common problem and ranges from minimal to fatal hemorrhage. Clots block blood vessels and decrease blood flow to major body organs and result in pain, strokelike manifestations, dyspnea, tachycardia, oliguria (decreased urine output), and bowel necrosis (tissue death). Chapter 39 describes in depth the collaborative management of sepsis-induced DIC.

Patient-Centered Collaborative Care

DIC is a life-threatening problem and has a high mortality rate even when proper therapies are instituted. *Thus the best plan of care for sepsis and DIC is prevention. Identify those patients at greatest risk for sepsis and DIC. Practice strict adherence to aseptic technique during invasive procedures and during contact with nonintact skin and mucous membranes in immunocompromised patients. Teach patients and family members the early manifestations of infection and sepsis and when to seek medical assistance.*

When sepsis is present and DIC is likely, management focuses on reducing the infection and halting the DIC process. IV antibiotic therapy is initiated. During the early phase of DIC, anticoagulants (especially heparin) are given to limit clotting and prevent the rapid consumption of circulating clotting factors. Cryoprecipitated clotting factors are given when DIC has progressed and hemorrhage is the primary problem. See Chapter 39 for a more detailed discussion of the management of DIC.

SYNDROME OF INAPPROPRIATE ANTIDIURETIC HORMONE

Pathophysiology

In healthy people, antidiuretic hormone (ADH) is secreted by the posterior pituitary gland only when more fluid (water) is needed in the body, such as when plasma volume is decreased (see Chapter 13). Certain health problems induce ADH secretion when not needed by the body.

Cancer is the most common cause of the syndrome of inappropriate antidiuretic hormone (SIADH). The cancer most commonly causing SIADH is carcinoma of the lung (especially small cell lung cancer), but SIADH may occur in other types of cancer, especially when tumors are present in the brain. Some tumors actually make and secrete ADH, whereas others stimulate the brain to make and secrete ADH. Drugs often used in patients with cancer also can cause SIADH (e.g., morphine sulfate, cyclophosphamide).

In SIADH, water is reabsorbed to excess by the kidney and put into systemic circulation. The increased water causes hyponatremia (decreased serum sodium levels) and fluid retention. Mild manifestations include weakness, muscle cramps, loss of appetite, and fatigue. Serum sodium levels range from 115 to 120 mEq/L (normal range is 135 to 145 mEq/L). More serious problems occur when even more water is retained, including weight gain, nervous system changes, personality changes, confusion, and extreme muscle weakness. As the sodium level drops toward 110 mEq/L, seizures, coma and death may follow.

Patient-Centered Collaborative Care

SIADH is managed by treating the condition and the cause. Nursing interventions for patients with SIADH aim to ensure patient safety, restore normal fluid balance, and provide supportive care. Management includes fluid restriction (sometimes total fluid intake is reduced to 1 L/day), increased sodium intake, and drug therapy. The drug most often used is demeclocycline, which is taken orally. This drug, an antibiotic, works in opposition to ADH.

A second method for managing SIADH is to reduce or eliminate the underlying cause. Immediate cancer therapy, usually either radiation or chemotherapy, can cause such tumor regression that ADH production returns to normal.

Patient safety includes preventing fluid overload from SIADH from becoming worse, leading to pulmonary edema and heart failure. Any patient with SIADH, regardless of age, is at risk for these complications. The older adult or one who has coexisting cardiac problems, kidney problems, pulmonary problems, or liver problems is at greater risk.

Monitor for indicators of increased fluid overload (increased pulse quality, increasing neck vein distention, presence of crackles in lungs, increasing peripheral edema, reduced urine output) at least every 2 hours. *Pulmonary edema can occur very quickly and can lead to death.* Notify the health care provider of any change that indicates the fluid overload from SIADH either is not responding to therapy or is becoming worse. See Chapter 65 for a more detailed discussion of the patient with SIADH.

SPINAL CORD COMPRESSION

Pathophysiology

Spinal cord compression (SCC) and damage occur either when a tumor directly enters the spinal cord or when the vertebrae collapse from tumor degradation of the bone. Tumors may begin in the spinal cord but more often spread from other areas of the body, such as the lung, prostate, breast, and colon. SCC often causes back pain before neurologic deficits occur. Neurologic problems are specific to the level of spinal compression and can lead to paralysis. If paralysis occurs, it is usually permanent.

Patient-Centered Collaborative Care

Early recognition and treatment of spinal cord compression are key to a positive outcome. Assess the patient for neurologic changes consistent with spinal cord compression. These include back pain, muscle weakness or a sensation of "heaviness" in the arms or legs, numbness or tingling in the hands or feet, loss of ability to distinguish hot and cold, and an unsteady gait. Depending on how low the compression occurs, constipation, incontinence, and difficulty starting or stopping the stream of urine also may be present. A new onset of any of these problems is cause to consider the possibility of SCC. Teach patients and families the manifestations of early SCC, and instruct them to seek help as soon as problems are apparent. If the problem is suspected, magnetic resonant imaging (MRI) is usually ordered immediately.

Treatment is often palliative (Marrs, 2006). Usually, high-dose corticosteroids are given first to reduce swelling around the spinal cord and relieve symptoms. High-dose radiation may be given to reduce the size of the tumor in the area and relieve compression. Radiation also may be used along with chemotherapy to treat the total disease. Surgery may be performed to remove the tumor from the area and rearrange the bony tissue so less pressure is placed on the spinal cord. External back or neck braces may be used to reduce the weight borne by the spinal column and to reduce pressure on the spinal cord or spinal nerves.

HYPERCALCEMIA

Pathophysiology

Hypercalcemia (increased serum calcium level) occurs most often in patients with bone metastasis. Cancer in bone causes the bone to release calcium into the bloodstream. In patients with cancer in other parts of the body (especially the lung, head and neck, kidney, or lymph nodes), the tumor secretes parathyroid hormone, causing bone to release calcium. Decreased mobility and dehydration worsen hypercalcemia.

Early manifestations of hypercalcemia include fatigue, loss of appetite, nausea, vomiting, constipation, and polyuria (increased urine output). More serious problems include severe muscle weakness, loss of deep tendon reflexes, paralytic ileus, dehydration, and electrocardiographic (ECG) changes. The severity of manifestations depends on how high the serum calcium level is and how quickly it developed (see also Chapter 13).

Patient-Centered Collaborative Care

Cancer-induced hypercalcemia develops very slowly for many patients, which allows the body time to adapt to this electrolyte change. As a result, symptoms of hypercalcemia may not be evident until the serum calcium level is greatly elevated. Because adaptation does occur, cancer-induced hypercalcemia is treated only when manifestations are present.

Oral hydration alone may be enough to reduce the serum calcium and relieve symptoms. Normal saline is used when parenteral hydration is needed. Many drugs lower serum calcium levels. Some agents, such oral glucocorticoids, calcitonin, diphosphonate, gallium nitrate, and mithramycin, lower levels quite dramatically. These drugs do not cure hypercalcemia but, instead, reduce serum calcium levels temporarily. When cancer-induced hypercalcemia is life threatening or occurs with renal impairment, dialysis can temporarily reduce serum calcium levels.

SUPERIOR VENA CAVA SYNDROME

Pathophysiology

Superior vena cava (SVC) syndrome occurs when the SVC is compressed or obstructed by tumor growth or by the formation of clots in the vessel (Fig. 24-3). SVC compression can lead to a painful and life-threatening emergency, usually in patients with lymphomas and lung cancer. Patients with cancer of the breast, esophagus, colon, and testes may also be affected.

The manifestations of SVC syndrome result from the blockage of blood flow in the venous system of the head, neck, and upper trunk. A venogram of the upper extremities and the superior vena cava shows a stricture or an occlusion blocking blood flow. Early manifestations occur when the patient arises after a night's sleep and include edema of the face, especially around the eyes, and tightness of the shirt or blouse collar

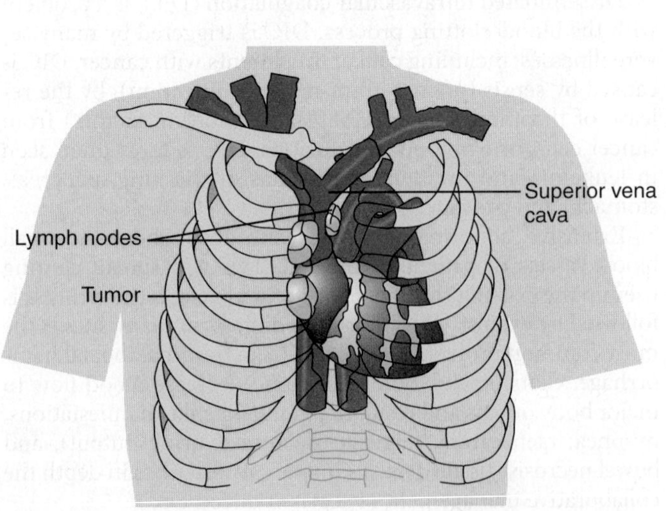
Superior vena cava
Lymph nodes
Tumor

Fig. 24-3 • Compression of the superior vena cava in SVC syndrome.

(Stokes' sign). As the compression worsens, the patient develops edema in the arms and hands, dyspnea, erythema of the upper body, and epistaxis (nosebleeds). Late manifestations include hemorrhage, cyanosis, mental status changes from lack of blood to the brain, decreased cardiac output, and hypotension. Death results if compression is not relieved (Nunnelee, 2007).

Patient-Centered Collaborative Care

SVC syndrome is a late-stage manifestation; the tumor is usually widespread. High-dose radiation therapy to the mediastinal area may be used to provide temporary relief. Surgery is rarely performed for this condition because the tumor may have increased intrathoracic pressure to such a level that it may be impossible to close the chest after the procedure. A metal stent can be placed in the vena cava in an interventional radiation department to relieve swelling. Follow-up angioplasty can keep this stent open for a longer period. (See Chapter 38 for more information on stenting procedures.)

The best treatment results occur when SVC syndrome is in the early stages. Assess each patient for manifestations of SVC syndrome, and notify the physician.

TUMOR LYSIS SYNDROME

Pathophysiology

In tumor lysis syndrome (TLS), large numbers of tumor cells are destroyed rapidly. Their intracellular contents, including potassium and purines (DNA components), are released into the bloodstream faster than the body can eliminate them (Fig. 24-4) (King, 2008; McGraw, 2008). Unlike other oncologic emergencies, TLS is a positive sign that cancer treatment is effective.

Severe or untreated TLS can cause severe tissue damage and death. Serum potassium levels can increase to the point of hyperkalemia, causing severe cardiac dysfunction (see Chapter 13). The large amounts of released purines are converted in the liver to uric acid and released into the blood, causing hyperuricemia. These uric acid crystals precipitate in the kidney, forming sludge in the kidney tubules; this effect blocks the tubules and leads to acute renal failure.

TLS is most often seen in patients receiving radiation or chemotherapy for cancers that are very sensitive to these therapies, including leukemia, lymphoma, small cell lung cancer, and multiple myeloma.

Patient-Centered Collaborative Care

Prevention through hydration is the best management for TLS. Hydration alone can dilute the serum potassium level and increases the kidney filtration rate. As a result, urine flows through the kidney at a greatly increased rate. This action prevents the precipitation of uric acid crystals, increases the excretion of potassium, and mechanically flushes any renal tubular sludge.

With tumors known to be very sensitive to cancer therapy, instruct patients to drink at least 3000 mL (5000 mL is more desirable) of fluid the day before, the day of, and for 3 days after treatment. Some fluids should be alkaline (sodium bicarbonate) to help prevent uric acid precipitation. Stress the importance of keeping fluid intake consistent throughout the 24-hour day, and help patients draw up a schedule of fluid intake.

Because some patients have nausea and vomiting after cancer therapy and may not feel like drinking fluids, stress the importance of following the antiemetic regimen. Instruct patients to contact their health care provider or cancer clinic immediately if nausea and vomiting prevent adequate fluid intake so they can be started on parenteral fluids.

Management becomes more aggressive for patients who become hyperkalemic or hyperuricemic. In addition to increased fluid intake (oral or parenteral), diuretics (especially osmotic types) are given to increase urine flow through the kidney. These agents are given with caution because patients must not become dehydrated. Drugs that increase the excretion of purines, such as allopurinol (Aloprim, Zyloprim) or rasburicase (Elitek), are given. To reduce serum potassium levels for mild to moderate hyperkalemia, sodium polystyrene sulfonate can be given orally or as a retention enema. This treatment does not immediately reduce serum potassium level. For more severe hyperkalemia, IV infusions containing glucose and insulin may be given. Patients who have severe hyperkalemia and hyperuricemia may need dialysis.

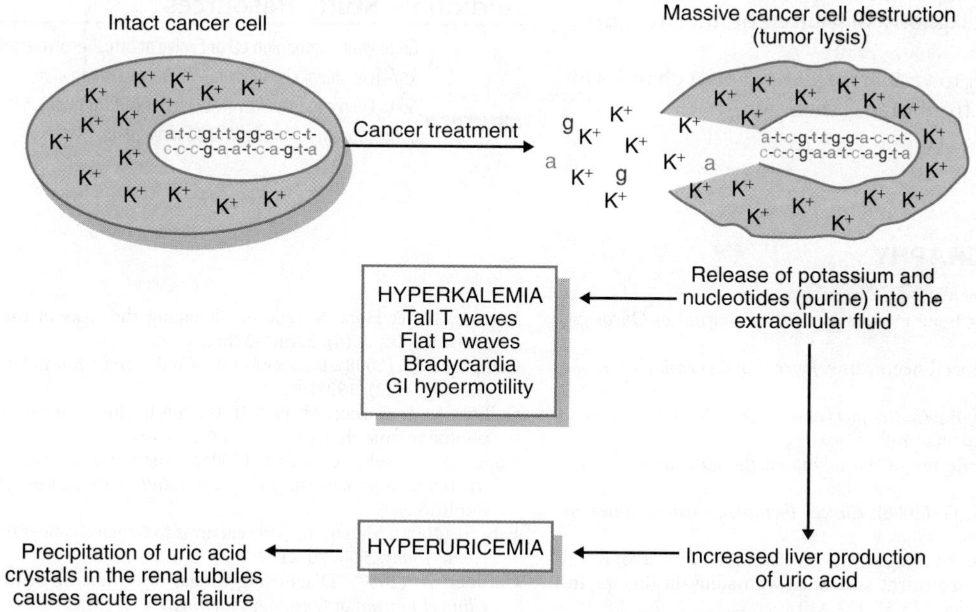

Intact cancer cell
a-t-c-g-t-t-g-g-a-c-c-t-
c-c-c-g-a-a-t-c-a-g-t-a
Cancer treatment
Massive cancer cell destruction (tumor lysis)
Release of potassium and nucleotides (purine) into the extracellular fluid
HYPERKALEMIA
Tall T waves
Flat P waves
Bradycardia
GI hypermotility
Increased liver production of uric acid
HYPERURICEMIA
Precipitation of uric acid crystals in the renal tubules causes acute renal failure

Fig. 24-4 • Pathology of tumor lysis syndrome.

NCLEX EXAMINATION CHALLENGE

The client being treated for lung cancer reports new-onset back pain and asks for pain medication for this problem. What questions should the nurse ask about this issue?

A. "What kinds of pain medications are you taking now and how often are you taking them?"
B. "Do you have any numbness or tingling in your hands or feet or difficulty urinating?"
C. "Can you relate this new back pain to any position or activity that you were performing?"
D. "Have you tried applying heat to your lower back and avoiding bending or lifting?"

evolve For the correct answer, go to http://evolve.elsevier.com/Iggy/.

GET READY FOR THE NCLEX EXAMINATION!

Key Points

Review these Key Points for each NCLEX Examination Client Needs Category.

Safe and Effective Care Environment

- Use aseptic technique during care for open skin areas or any invasive procedure.
- Use good handwashing techniques before providing any care to a patient who is neutropenic.
- Use bleeding precautions for any patient with thrombocytopenia (see Chart 24-6).
- Position shields properly when patients in inpatient settings are receiving brachytherapy.
- Use appropriate personal protection equipment (gowns, gloves, masks, eye protection) when mixing or administering chemotherapeutic agents and when handling excreta of a patient receiving chemotherapy.

Health Promotion and Maintenance

- Teach patients receiving radiation therapy how to care for the skin in the radiation path (see Chart 24-2).
- Identify patients at high risk for infection because of disease or therapy.
- Teach the patient and family about the manifestations of infection and when to seek medical advice.
- Teach patients at risk for bleeding the precautions to take to avoid injury (see Chart 24-7).

Psychosocial Integrity

- Allow the patient the opportunity to express his or her feelings regarding the diagnosis of cancer or the treatment regimen.
- Encourage the patient to verbalize feelings about changes in appearance resulting from cancer therapy.
- Explain all procedures, restrictions, drugs, and follow-up care to the patient and family.
- Offer alternative therapies for relaxation, pain reduction, and distraction, such as massage, music therapy, and guided imagery.
- Help patients use strategies to improve their appearance when alopecia occurs.
- Refer patients and family members to local cancer resources and support groups.

Physiological Integrity

- Assess the venous access device at least every 30 to 60 minutes during chemotherapy administration.
- Assess the patient receiving chemotherapy for manifestations of infection at least every 8 hours.
- Inspect the oral mucosa of patients with neutropenia at least every 8 hours.
- Report any temperature over 100° F (38° C) in a patient with neutropenia.
- Follow agency guidelines for obtaining cultures and diagnostic tests or starting anti-infective therapy in the patient with neutropenic fever.
- Instruct the patient and family in the manifestations of complications and when to seek assistance.
- Pace nonurgent health care activities to reduce the risk for fatigue for patients with anemia.

Additional Study Resources

Go to your Companion CD or Evolve at http://evolve.elsevier.com/Iggy/ for *Self-Assessment Questions for the NCLEX Examination.*

evolve Go to Evolve at http://evolve.elsevier.com/Iggy/ for *Prioritization and Delegation Questions for the NCLEX Examination.*

SELECTED BIBLIOGRAPHY

Asterisk indicates a classic or definitive work on this subject.

Albert, K. (2007). Evaluating bone metastasis. *Clinical Journal of Oncology Nursing, 11*(2), 193-197.

Almadrones, L. (2006). Peripheral neuropathy. *Journal of Gynecologic Oncology Nursing, 16*(1), 5.

American Cancer Society. (2008). *Cancer facts and figures—2008.* Report No. 00-300M–No. 5008.08. Atlanta: Author.

Awan, M., & Tarin, S. (2006). Review of photodynamic therapy. *Surgeon, 4*(4), 231-236.

Barton-Burke, M., & Wilkes, G. (2006). *Cancer therapies.* Boston: Jones & Bartlett.

Bender, C., Sereika, S., Berga, S.L., Vogel, V.G., Brufsky, A.M., Paraska, K.K., et al. (2006). Cognitive impairment associated with adjuvant therapy in breast cancer. *Psycho-oncology, 15*(5), 422-430.

Burruss, N., & Holz, S. (2005). Managing the risks of thrombocytopenia. *Nursing2005, 35*(6), 32hn1-32hn5.

Camporeale, J. (2008). Basics of radiation therapy. *Clinical Journal of Oncology Nursing, 12*(2), 193-195.

Collins, A., & Garner, M. (2007). Caring for lung cancer patients receiving photodynamic therapy. *Critical Care Nurse, 27*(2), 53-60.

Cope, D., & Reb, A. (Eds.). (2006). *An evidence-based approach to the treatment and care of the older adult with cancer.* Pittsburgh: ONS Publishing.

Eaby, B. (2008). Managing skin reactions to targeted cancer therapy. *American Nurse Today, 3*(7), 20-21.

Gardner, A. (2007). Diagnosing fungal infections in neutropenic patients. *Clinical Journal of Oncology Nursing, 11*(1), 29-32.

Gatlin, C., & Schulmeister, L. (2007). When medication is not enough: Nonpharmacologic management of pain. *Clinical Journal of Oncology Nursing, 11*(5), 699-704.

*Gosselin, T., & Waring, J. (2001). Nursing management of patients receiving brachytherapy for gynecologic malignancies. *Clinical Journal of Oncology Nursing, 5*(2), 59-63.

Held-Warmkessel, J. (2005). Managing 3 critical cancer complications. *Nursing2005, 35*(1), 58-63.

Inagaki, M., Yoshikawa, E., Matsuoka, Y., Sugawara, Y., Nakano, T., Akechi, T., et al. (2007). Smaller regional volumes of brain gray and white matter demonstrated in breast cancer survivors exposed to adjuvant chemotherapy. *Cancer, 109*(1), 146-156.

King, J. (2008). What is tumor lysis syndrome? *Nursing2008, 38*(5), 18.

Lavoie-Smith, E., Beck, S., & Cohen, J. (2008). The total neuropathy score: A tool for measuring chemotherapy-induced peripheral neuropathy. *Oncology Nursing Forum, 35*(1), 96-102.

Marrs, J. (2006). Nurse, my back hurts: Understanding malignant spinal cord compression. *Clinical Journal of Oncology Nursing, 10*(1), 114-116.

Matthews, E., Snells, K., & Coats, H. (2006). Intra-arterial chemotherapy for limb preservation in patients with osteosarcoma: Nursing implications. *Clinical Journal of Oncology Nursing, 10*(5), 581-589.

McGraw, B. (2008). At an increased risk: Tumor lysis syndrome. *Clinical Journal of Oncology Nursing, 12*(4), 563-565.

*McGuire, D. (2002). Mucosal tissue injury in cancer therapy. *Cancer Practice, 10*(4), 179-191.

MD Consult. www.mdconsult.com/php/82925233-2/homepage

Mee, C. (2007). Hospice care. *Nursing2007, 37*(11), 43.

Miller, C.R., & McLoed, H. (2007). Pharmacogenomics of cancer chemotherapy–induced toxicity. *Supportive Oncology, 5*(1), 9-14.

Moore, K., & Crom, D. (2006). Hematopoietic support with moderately myelosuppressive chemotherapy regimens: A nursing perspective. *Clinical Journal of Oncology Nursing, 10*(3), 383-388.

Mueller, P., & Glennon, C. (2007). A nurse-developed prechemotherapy education checklist. *Clinical Journal of Oncology Nursing, 11*(5), 715-719.

Nunnelee, J. (2007). Superior vena cava syndrome. *Journal of Vascular Nursing, 25*(1), 2-5.

Oncology Nursing Society. (2006). *Complementary & alternative medicine.* Pittsburgh: ONS Publishing.

*Polovich, M. (Ed.). (2003). *Safe handling of hazardous drugs.* Pittsburgh: ONS Publishing.

Polovich, M., White, J., & Kelleher, L. (Eds.). (2005). *Chemotherapy and biotherapy guidelines and recommendations for practice* (2nd ed.). Pittsburgh: ONS Publishing.

Schagen, S., Muller, M., Boogerd, W., Mellenbergh, G.J., & van Dam, F.S. (2006). Changes in cognitive function after chemotherapy: A prospective longitudinal study in breast cancer patients. *Journal of the National Cancer Institute, 98*(23), 1742-1745.

Schneider, S., & Hood, L. (2007). Virtual reality: A distraction intervention for chemotherapy. *Oncology Nursing Forum, 34*(1), 39-46.

Schulmeister, L. (2007). Totect: A new agent for treating anthracycline extravasation. *Clinical Journal of Oncology Nursing, 11*(3), 387-395.

Siegel, J.H., & Korniewicz, D.M. (2007). Keeping patient safe: An interventional hand hygiene study at an oncology center. *Clinical Journal of Oncology Nursing, 11*(5), 643-646.

Stephenson, N., Swanson, M., Dalton, J., Keefe, F.J., & Engelke, M. (2007). Partner-delivered reflexology: Effects on cancer pain and anxiety. *Oncology Nursing Forum, 34*(1), 127-132.

Tipton, J.M., McDaniel, R.W., Barbour, L., Johnston, M.P., Kayne, M., LeRoy, P., et al. (2007). Putting evidence into practice: Evidence-based interventions to prevent, manage, and treat chemotherapy-induced nausea and vomiting. *Clinical Journal of Oncology Nursing, 11*(1), 69-78.

United States Food and Drug Administration (FDA) (2007). *www.fda.gov/cder/index.html.*

Viele, C. (2005). Keys to unlock cancer: Targeted therapy. *Oncology Nursing Forum, 32*(5), 935-940.

Visovsky, C., Meyer, R., Roller, J., & Poppas, M. (2008). Evaluation and management of peripheral neuropathy in diabetic patients with cancer. *Clinical Journal of Oncology Nursing, 12*(2), 243-247.

Walton, A. (2005). Superior vena cava syndrome: An education sheet for patients. *Clinical Journal of Oncology Nursing, 9*(4), 479-480.

Wickham, R. (2007). Chemotherapy-induced peripheral neuropathy: A review and implications for oncology nursing practice. *Clinical Journal of Oncology Nursing, 11*(3), 361-376.

Wilson, B., & Gardner, A. (2007). Nurses' guide to understanding and implementing the National Comprehensive Cancer Network guidelines for myeloid growth factors. *Oncology Nursing Forum, 34*(2), 347-353.

Zarowitz, B. (2007). Erythropoietic-stimulating agents (ESAs): New safety warning. *Geriatric Nursing, 28*(3), 148-150.

25 CHAPTER

Care of Patients with Infection

Donna D. Ignatavicius

LEARNING OUTCOMES

For clinical competence and success on the NCLEX Examination, study this chapter with these Learning Outcomes in mind:

Safe and Effective Care Environment

1. Explain the Centers for Disease Control and Prevention (CDC) hand hygiene recommendations for health care workers.
2. Control the transmission of infection through hand hygiene and Transmission-Based Precautions.
3. Apply current principles of infection control.

Health Promotion and Maintenance

4. Teach patients, families, and staff about infection control measures.
5. Teach patients and families about antimicrobial therapy.

Psychosocial Integrity

6. Assess patient and family response to Transmission-Based Precautions.

Physiological Integrity

7. Identify patients most at risk for infection, including older adults.
8. Provide information to patient and family about drug therapy for infections.
9. Identify common clinical manifestations of infectious diseases.
10. Interpret laboratory test findings related to infections and infectious diseases.
11. Evaluate nursing interventions for management of the patient with an infection.
12. Explain why multidrug-resistant organisms and other emerging infections are increasing.

Go to your Companion CD or Evolve at http://evolve.elsevier.com/Iggy/ for *Self-Assessment Questions for the NCLEX Examination* keyed to these Learning Outcomes.

The human body has many *protective* systems that promote homeostasis. Physiologic mechanisms are the structural and functional defenses that protect people from stressors such as infection. When these mechanisms fail to work properly or are overcome with microbes, infection can result.

Infections and infectious diseases have been the major cause of millions of deaths worldwide for centuries. Today threats of bioterrorism have been added to the concerns about multidrug-resistant and emerging infections. Global travel and migration have increased exposure to a wider variety of infectious agents than in the past. For example, severe acute respiratory syndrome (SARS), monkeypox, and Avian influenza ("bird flu") have appeared for the first time in the United States during the past decade. However, humans have not gotten any of these diseases yet.

Advancing technology and invasive procedures also introduce microorganisms into the body, often resulting in infection, even though in other environments these microorganisms are harmless. This chapter provides an overview of infection and general principles for prevention and management. Specific infections are described elsewhere in this text.

Overview of the Infectious Process

A **pathogen** is any microorganism (also called an *agent*) capable of producing disease. Infections can be **communicable** (transmitted from person to person, e.g., influenza) or not communicable (e.g., peritonitis). Microorganisms with differing levels of **pathogenicity** (ability to cause disease) surround everyone. **Virulence** is a term for pathogenicity. However, virulence is related more to the frequency with which a pathogen causes disease (degree of communicability) and its ability to invade and damage a host. It can also indicate the severity of the disease.

Many microorganisms live in or on the human host without causing disease. Some microbes are beneficial. Each body location harbors its own characteristic bacteria, or **normal flora.** Normal flora often function to compete with and prevent infection from unfamiliar agents attempting to invade a body site. In some instances, microorganisms that are often pathogenic may be present in the tissues of the host and yet not cause symptomatic disease because of normal flora; this process is called **colonization.**

In the United States, the Centers for Disease Control and Prevention (CDC) collects information about the occurrence and nature of infections and infectious diseases. It then recommends guidelines to health care agencies for infection control and prevention. Certain diseases, such as tuberculosis, must be reported to health departments and the CDC. The infection control practitioner (ICP) for each health care agency is responsible for tracking infections **(surveillance)** and ensuring compliance with federal and local requirements.

Transmission of Infectious Agents

Transmission of infection in health care requires three factors:

- Reservoir (or source) of infectious agents
- Susceptible host with a portal of entry
- Mode of transmission

Reservoirs (sources of infectious agents) are numerous. Animate reservoirs include people, animals, and insects. Inanimate reservoirs include soil, water, other environmental sources, and medical equipment (e.g., IV solutions, urine collection devices). The host's body can be a reservoir; pathogens colonize skin and body substances (e.g., feces, sputum, saliva, wound drainage). A person with an active infection or an asymptomatic **carrier** (one who harbors an infectious agent without active disease) is a reservoir. Examples of *community* reservoirs include sewage, stagnant or contaminated water, and improperly handled foods.

Bacteria like *Neisseria meningitidis* can exist in the respiratory tract while causing no illness. If the bacteria invade the bloodstream or cerebrospinal fluid, they become extremely pathogenic. Another example is *Enterococcus,* which lives as normal flora in the GI system, where it is nonpathogenic and assists in the digestive process. If it enters the bloodstream, *Enterococcus* can cause disease.

Continued multiplication of a pathogen is sometimes accompanied by toxin production. **Toxins** are protein molecules released by bacteria to affect host cells at a distant site. **Exotoxins** are produced and released by certain bacteria into the surrounding environment. Botulism, tetanus, diphtheria, and *Escherichia coli* 0157:H7–related systemic diseases are attributed to exotoxins. **Endotoxins** are produced in the cell walls of certain bacteria and released only with cell lysis. For example, typhoid and meningococcal diseases are caused by endotoxins.

Host factors influence the development of infection (Table 25-1). Host defenses provide the body with an efficient system for *protection* against pathogens. Breakdown of these defense mechanisms may increase the **susceptibility** (risk) of the host to infection.

The patient's *immune status* plays a large role in determining risk for infection. Congenital abnormalities, as well as acquired health problems (e.g., renal failure, steroid dependence, cancer, acquired immune deficiency syndrome [AIDS]), can result in numerous immunologic deficiencies. Depression of the immune system may make the host more susceptible to infection or cripple the ability to combat organisms that have gained entry.

Immunity is resistance to infection; it is usually associated with the presence of antibodies or cells that act on specific microorganisms. **Passive immunity** is of short duration (days or months) and either natural by transplacental transfer from the mother or artificial by injection of antibodies (e.g., immune globulin). **Active immunity** lasts for years and is natural by infection or artificial by stimulation of the body's immune defenses (e.g., vaccination). Chapter 19 discusses the immune system and immunity in detail.

Environmental factors can also influence patients' immune status and thus their susceptibility to or ability to fight infection. Examples include alcohol consumption, nicotine use, inhalation of bone marrow–suppressing toxic chemicals, and certain vitamin deficiencies. Malnutrition, especially protein-calorie malnutrition, places patients at increased risk for infection. Diseases such as diabetes mellitus also predispose a patient to infection. *Older adults have decreased immune systems, as well as other physiologic changes that make them very susceptible to infection* (Chart 25-1).

Medical and surgical interventions may impair normal immune response. Steroid therapy, chemotherapy, and antirejection drugs increase the risk of infection. Medical devices (e.g., intravascular or urinary catheters, endotracheal tubes, synthetic implants) may also interfere with normal host defense mechanisms. Surgery, trauma, radiation therapy, and burns result in nonintact skin. *The body's skin is one of the best barriers or defenses against infection.* When this barrier is broken, infection often results.

Microorganisms may enter the body in a variety of ways, including the respiratory tract, GI tract, genitourinary tract, skin and mucous membranes, and bloodstream.

Pathogens may enter the body through the *respiratory tract.* Microbes in droplets are sprayed into the air when peo-

TABLE 25-1 Host Factors That Influence the Development of Infection

Host Factor	Increased Risk of Infection
Natural immunity	Congenital or acquired immune deficiencies
Normal flora	Alteration of normal flora by antibiotic therapy
Age	Infants and older adults
Hormonal factors	Diabetes mellitus, corticosteroid therapy, and adrenal insufficiency
Phagocytosis	Defective phagocytic function, circulatory disturbances, and neutropenia
Skin/mucous membranes/normal excretory secretions	Break in skin or mucous membrane integrity; interference with flow of urine, tears, or saliva; interference with cough reflex or ciliary action; changes in gastric secretions
Nutrition	Malnutrition or dehydration
Environmental factors	Tobacco and alcohol consumption and inhalation of toxic chemicals
Medical interventions	Invasive therapy, chemotherapy, radiation therapy, and steroid therapy; surgery

Chart 25-1 NURSING FOCUS ON THE OLDER ADULT

Factors That May Increase Risk of Infection in the Older Patient

Factor	Aging-Associated Changes or Conditions
Immune system	Decreased antibody production, lymphocytes, and fever response
Integumentary system	Thinning skin, decreased subcutaneous tissue, decreased vascularity, slower wound healing
Respiratory system	Decreased cough and gag reflexes
Gastrointestinal system	Decreased gastric acid and intestinal motility
Chronic illness	Diabetes mellitus, chronic obstructive pulmonary disease, neurologic impairments
Functional/cognitive impairments	Immobility, incontinence, dementia
Invasive devices	Urinary catheters, feeding tubes, IV devices, tracheostomy tubes
Institutionalization	Increased person-to-person contact and transmission

ple with infected oral or nasal tissues talk, cough, or sneeze. A susceptible host then inhales droplets, and pathogens localize in the lungs or are distributed via the lymphatic system or bloodstream to other areas of the body. Microorganisms that enter the body by the respiratory tract and produce distant infection include influenza virus, *Mycobacterium tuberculosis,* and *Streptococcus pneumoniae.*

Other pathogens enter the body through the GI tract. Some stay there and produce disease (e.g., *Shigella* causing self-limited disease). Others invade the GI tract to produce local and distant infection (e.g., *Salmonella enteritidis*). Some produce limited GI symptoms, causing systemic infection (e.g., *Salmonella typhi*) or profound involvement of other organs (e.g., hepatitis A virus). Millions of foodborne illness cases occur each year in the United States. This type of illness results in many hospitalizations and deaths.

Microorganisms also enter through the genitourinary tract. *Urinary tract infection (UTI) is one of the most common health-care-associated infections (HAIs).* More than half of patients in adult intensive care units (ICUs) have urinary catheters in place. Indwelling urinary catheters are a primary cause of UTIs. *The use of invasive catheters has decreased in long-term care settings because older adults are very susceptible to infections.*

Although intact skin is the best barrier to prevent most infections, some pathogens such as *Treponema pallidum* can enter the body through intact skin or mucous membranes. Most enter through breaks in these normally effective surface barriers. Sometimes a medical procedure creates a break in cutaneous or mucocutaneous barriers, as in catheter-acquired **bacteremia** (bacteria in the bloodstream) and surgical-site infections (SSIs). *Fragile skin of older patients and of those receiving prolonged steroid therapy increases infection risk.*

Microorganisms can gain direct access to the *bloodstream,* especially when invasive devices or tubes are used. The incidence of bloodstream infections (BSIs) continues to increase in hospitals throughout the United States. Central venous catheters (CVCs) are a primary cause of these infections (see Chapter 15 for more discussion of CVC-related BSIs). In the community setting, biting insects can inject organisms into the bloodstream, causing infection (e.g., Lyme disease, West Nile viral encephalitis).

For infection to be *transmitted* from an infected source to a susceptible host, a transport mechanism is required. Microorganisms are transmitted by several routes:

- Contact transmission (indirect and direct)
- Droplet transmission
- Airborne transmission

Contact transmission is the usual mode of transmission of most infections. Many infections are spread by direct or indirect contact. With **direct contact,** the source and host have physical contact. Microorganisms are transferred directly from skin to skin or from mucous membrane to mucous membrane. Often called *person-to-person transmission,* direct contact is best illustrated by the spread of the "common cold."

Indirect contact transmission involves the transfer of microorganisms from a source to a host by passive transfer from a contaminated object. Contaminated articles or hands may be sources of infection. For example, patient-care devices like glucometers and electronic thermometers may transmit pathogens if they are contaminated with blood or body fluids. Uniforms, laboratory coats, and isolation gowns used as part of personal protective equipment may be contaminated as well.

Indirect transmission may involve contact with infected secretions or **droplets.** Droplets are produced when a person talks or sneezes; the droplets travel short distances. Susceptible hosts may acquire infection by contact with droplets deposited on the nasal, oral, or conjunctival membranes. Therefore the CDC recommends that staff stay at least 3 feet (1 m) away from a patient with droplet infection (Siegel et al., 2007). An example of droplet-spread infection is influenza. Unlike airborne droplet nuclei, discussed later, droplets do not stay suspended in the air.

Airborne transmission occurs when small airborne particles containing pathogens leave the infected source and enter a susceptible host. These pathogens can be suspended in the air for a prolonged time. The particles carrying pathogens are usually contained in droplet nuclei or dust; they are usually propelled from the respiratory tract by coughing or sneezing. A susceptible person then inhales the particles directly into the respiratory tract. For example, tuberculosis is spread via airborne transmission.

Preventing the spread of microbes that are transmitted by the airborne route requires the use of special air handling and ventilation systems in an airborne infection isolation room (AIIR). *Mycobacterium tuberculosis* and the varicella-zoster virus (chickenpox) are examples of airborne agents that require one of these systems. In addition to the AIIR, respiratory protection using certified N95 or higher level respirator masks is recommended for health care personnel entering the patient's room (Siegel et al., 2007). The N95 rating means that at least 95% of the inhaled air is filtered.

Other sources of infectious agents include the environment, such as contaminated food, water, or vectors. Vectors are insects that carry pathogens between two or more hosts, such as the deer tick that causes Lyme disease.

The *portal of exit* completes the chain of infection. Exit of the microbe from the host often occurs through the portal of entry. An organism, such as *M. tuberculosis,* enters the respiratory tract and then exits the same tract as the infected host coughs. Some organisms can exit from the infected host by several routes. For example, varicella-zoster virus can spread through direct contact with infective fluid in vesicles and by airborne transmission.

Physiologic Defenses for Infection

Strong and intact host defenses can prevent microbes from entering the body or can destroy a pathogen that has entered. Impaired host defenses may be unable to defend against microbial invasion, allowing entry of organisms that can destroy cells and cause infection. Common defense mechanisms include:

- Body tissues
- Phagocytosis
- Inflammation
- Immune systems

Intact skin forms the first and most important physical barrier to the entry of microorganisms. In addition to providing a mechanical barrier, the skin's slightly acidic pH (resulting from breakdown of lipids into fatty acids), together with normal skin flora, creates an unfriendly environment for many bacteria.

Mucous membranes' mucociliary action provides some mechanical protection against pathogenic invasion. More important, however, mucous membranes are bathed in secretions that inactivate many microorganisms. **Lysozymes,** which dissolve the cell walls of some bacteria, are present in large quantities in many body secretions, particularly in tears and nasal mucus.

Other body systems provide natural barriers to infection. For instance, the healthy respiratory tract clears about 90% of all inhaled material by upper airway filtration, humidification, mucociliary transport, and coughing. Peristaltic action mechanically empties the GI tract of pathogenic organisms. Stomach acid, intestinal secretions, pancreatic enzymes, and bile, together with the competition from normal bowel flora, provide an environment that protects the GI tract from invasion by harmful organisms. In the genitourinary tract, the flushing action of urine eliminates pathogenic organisms. The low pH of urine also maintains a sterile environment, although some microorganisms, such as *Escherichia coli,* thrive in an acid medium.

Phagocytosis occurs when a foreign substance evades the first-line mechanical barriers and enters the body. Various leukocyte types function differently in the immune reaction, but neutrophils bear primary responsibility for phagocytosis. This process of engulfing, ingesting, killing, and disposing of an invading organism is an essential mechanism in host defense. Phagocytic dysfunction dramatically increases a patient's risk for infection.

Inflammation is another important nonspecific defense mechanism for preventing the spread of infection. It occurs when tissue becomes damaged. Damaged cells release enzymes, and polymorphonuclear (PMN) leukocytes (neutrophils) are attracted to the infected site from the bloodstream. One important substance, histamine, increases the permeability of the capillaries in inflamed tissues, thus allowing fluid, proteins, and white blood cells to enter an inflamed area. Other enzymes activate fibrinogen, which causes leaked fluid to clot and prevents its flow away from the damaged site into unaffected tissue, essentially "walling off" the inflamed tissue. The process of phagocytosis disposes of the invading microorganism and often dead tissue. If inflammation is caused by infection, the end products of inflammation form pus, which is then absorbed or exits the body through a break in the skin. Chapter 19 discusses the process of inflammation in more detail.

Specific defense responses to specific microorganisms are provided by the antibody- and cell-mediated immune systems. The **antibody-mediated immune system** produces antibodies directed against certain pathogens. These antibodies inactivate or destroy invading microorganisms as well as protect against future infection from that microorganism. Resistance to other microorganisms is mediated by the action of specifically sensitized T-lymphocytes and is called **cell-mediated immunity.** The components of the immune system work both independently and together to protect against infection. Chapter 19 describes the function of the immune system in detail.

Health Promotion and Maintenance

Infection Control in Inpatient Health Care Agencies

NIC *Infections occur most often in high-risk patients, such as older adults and those who have inadequate immune systems (immunocompromised). Implement interventions to prevent infection and detect signs and symptoms as early as possible.* Chart 25-2 summarizes nursing interventions for infection protection.

Infection acquired in the inpatient health care setting (not present or incubating at admission) is termed a **hospital-acquired infection (HAI).** HAIs can be **endogenous** (from a patient's flora) or **exogenous** (from outside the patient, often from the hands of health care workers). Therefore use of the

Chart 25-2 NIC INTERVENTION ACTIVITIES

The Patient at Risk for Infection

Infection Protection: *Prevention and early detection of infection in a patient at risk*

- Monitor for systemic and localized signs and symptoms of infection.
- Monitor vulnerability to infection.
- Monitor absolute granulocyte count, WBC count, and differential results.
- Screen all visitors for communicable disease.
- Inspect skin and mucous membranes for redness, extreme warmth, or drainage.
- Obtain cultures, as needed.
- Promote sufficient nutritional intake.
- Encourage fluid intake, as appropriate.
- Teach the patient and family about signs and symptoms of infections and when to report them to the health care provider.
- Teach patient and family members how to avoid infections.

NIC intervention activities selected from Bulechek, G.M., Butcher, H.K., & McCloskey Dochterman, J. (Eds.). (2008). *Nursing interventions classification (NIC)* (5th ed.). St. Louis: Mosby. No part of this work is to be altered without prior written permission from the Publisher.

WBC, White blood cell.

less popular term *nosocomial infection* does not imply that an infection was caused by health care (or poor health care delivery) but only that it occurred while receiving health care. HAIs occur in about two million inpatients yearly, causing many deaths. Patients who develop surgical site infection (SSI) have longer and more costly hospital stays and are much more likely to spend time in an ICU (Siegel et al., 2007).

Infection control within a health care facility is designed to reduce the risk of HAIs and thus reduce morbidity and mortality, as recommended in The Joint Commission's National Patient Safety Goals. This goal is consistent with the desire for health care facilities to create a *culture of safety* within their environments (see Chapter 1). Infection control and prevention programs include:

- Facility- and department-specific infection control policies and procedures
- Surveillance and analysis
- Patient and staff education
- Community and interdisciplinary collaboration
- Product evaluation with an emphasis on quality and cost savings

The infection control program of a hospital is coordinated and implemented by a health care professional certified in infection control (CIC) who has clinical and administrative experience. The previous recommendation of one CIC for every 250 occupied acute care beds has been found to be inadequate. Instead, the CDC now recommends one for every 100 occupied acute care beds. Long-term care facilities may not have a practitioner who is dedicated to infection control. However, every facility must designate someone to have the responsibility for coordinating and implementing an infection control program.

Long-term care facilities are unique in that they have a large group of older adults who are together in one setting for weeks to years. Nursing homes, in particular, are required to provide a home-like environment in which residents can move and interact freely. Therefore infection control in these settings can be challenging. As a result, many infectious outbreaks have occurred, such as pneumonia, *Clostridium difficile,* and multidrug-resistant organisms (discussed in the Multidrug-Resistant Organism Infections and Colonization section).

Infection Control in Community-Based Settings

Ambulatory care is the fastest growing segment of the health care system. Less information is available about acquired infections in these settings than in inpatient settings. HAIs in hemodialysis centers and emergency departments are the most common. Infections tend to occur because health care workers do not follow basic infection control principles, especially aseptic technique and injection practices (Siegel et al., 2007).

Methods of Infection Control

All health care workers who come in contact with patients or care areas are involved in some aspect of the infection control program of the agency. Infections can be prevented or controlled in at least five major ways:

- Hand hygiene
- Personal protective equipment (PPE) (also called *barriers*)
- Adequate staffing
- Disinfection/sterilization
- Patient placement and transport

Health care workers' hands are the primary way in which infection is transmitted from patient to patient or staff to patient. **Hand hygiene** refers to both handwashing and alcohol-based hand rubs (ABHRs). In 2002, the CDC released a document entitled "CDC Hand Hygiene Recommendations." These recommendations are summarized in Chart 25-3. *Handwashing is still an important part of hand hygiene, but it is recognized that in some health care settings, sinks may not be readily available.* Despite years of education, health care workers often find it difficult to leave the patient care setting to wash their hands and do not perform hand hygiene on a consistent basis.

Effective **handwashing** includes wetting, soaping, lathering, applying friction under running water for at least 15 seconds, rinsing, and adequate drying. *Friction is essential to remove skin oils and to disperse transient bacteria and soil from hand surfaces.* Performing adequate handwashing takes time that health care workers (HCW) may not feel they have. Handwashing can also cause dry skin, and therefore hand moisturizers are essential to maintain good hand health and hygiene.

Alcohol-based hand rubs have allowed care providers to spend less time seeking out sinks and more time delivering care. However, these hand rubs have their limitations. *If your hands are visibly dirty or soiled or feel sticky or if you have just toileted, wash your hands instead of using alcohol-based rubs.* ABHRs are also ineffective against spore-forming organisms such as *Clostridium difficile,* a common cause of health care–associated diarrhea, especially in older adults taking antibiotics. *Do not use an ABHR before inserting eye drops, ointments, or contact lenses. Alcohol can irritate the patient's eyes causing burning and redness.* The Joint Commission (TJC) requires that health care agencies monitor handwashing practices and the use of ABHRs to make sure that HCWs are performing hand hygiene on a regular basis.

The CDC recommends using antiseptic solutions such as chlorhexidine, povidone-iodine, or PCMX (parachlorometaxylenol) for handwashing in caring for patients who are at high risk (e.g., those who are immunocompromised). The use of these solutions is also recommended after caring for patients who are infected with multidrug-resistant or other virulent organisms.

The CDC guidelines (Centers for Disease Control and Prevention [CDC], 2002a) also address the issue of artificial finger-

Chart 25-3 BEST PRACTICE FOR PATIENT SAFETY & QUALITY CARE

Hand Hygiene

- When hands are visibly soiled or contaminated with proteinaceous material or are visibly soiled with blood or other body fluids, wash hands with soap and water.
- If hands are not visibly soiled, use an alcohol-based hand rub (ABHR) for decontaminating hands or wash hands with soap and water.
- Use either ABHR or wash with soap and water (decontaminate hands) before having direct contact with patients.
- Decontaminate hands before donning sterile gloves to perform a procedure, such as inserting an invasive device (e.g., indwelling urinary catheter).
- Decontaminate hands after contact with a patient's intact skin (e.g., taking a pulse) or with body fluids or excretions/secretions.
- Decontaminate hands after removing gloves.
- Decontaminate hands after contact with inanimate objects (including medical equipment) in the immediate vicinity of the patient.

Data from CDC Hand Hygiene Recommendations (2002).

nails, which have been linked to a number of outbreaks due to poor fingernail health and hygiene. *The guidelines recommend that artificial fingernails and extenders not be worn while caring for patients at high risk for infections, such as those in ICUs or operating suites. Most health care agencies have banned artificial nails for all health care workers providing direct patient care and require that natural nails be short and without nail polish.*

Personal protective equipment (PPE) refers to the use of gloves, isolation gowns, face protection (masks, goggles, face shields), and respirators with N95 or higher filtration (Fig. 25-1). *Gloves are an essential part of infection control and should always be worn as part of Standard Precautions. Either handwashing or use of alcohol-based hand rubs should be done after removing gloves. The combination of hand hygiene and wearing gloves is the most effective strategy for preventing infection transmission!*

Most health care settings in the United States and Canada have switched from latex to non-latex gloves. The U.S. National Institute of Occupational Safety and Health (NIOSH) issued a public warning about potential allergic reactions to those exposed to latex in gloves and other medical products. Reactions include rashes, nasal or eye symptoms, asthma, and (rarely) shock. People with **latex allergy** usually have an allergy to foods such as bananas, kiwis, and avocados. *Hands should be washed after removal of latex gloves to minimize contact time between the skin and proteins in the gloves that may cause allergic reactions.*

Health care workers (HCWs) have not been as strict with wearing gloves as they should because of poor fit or skin dryness, irritation, and dermatitis (Arenas et al., 2005; Kuzu et al., 2005). One possible solution to dry skin is the use of aloe vera–coated gloves. In a study of HCWs in three U.S. and one Canadian hospital, the subjects preferred the aloe vera gloves over gloves without the moisturizer. In addition, they were more compliant with wearing the study gloves because they had less dryness and skin irritation (Korniewicz & Masri, 2007).

Adequate staffing of HCWs is an essential method for preventing infection. In addition to a ratio of one infection control practitioner (ICP) to 100 occupied acute care beds, nurse staffing is critical. The CDC recommends that two methods to ensure adequate infection control (IC) be implemented (Siegel et al., 2007). First, an *infection control nurse liaison* should be designated on every unit of an inpatient facility. This nurse is responsible for implementing new IC policies, increasing staff IC compliance through education, and collaborating with the facility's ICP to monitor for infections. Second, bedside nurse staffing should consists of full-time nurses assigned regularly to the unit rather than float, pool, or agency nurses. Studies have found that infection rates increase when float, pool, or agency nurses are substituted for full-time, regular staff (Siegel et al., 2007).

Sterilization and disinfection have helped invasive procedures become much more common and safe. **Sterilization** means destroying all living organisms and bacterial spores. All items that invade human tissue where bacteria are not commonly found should be sterilized. **Disinfection** does not kill spores and only ensures a reduction in the level of disease-causing organisms. High-level disinfection is adequate when an item is going inside the body where the patient has resident bacteria or normal flora (e.g., GI and respiratory tracts). As with sterilization, no high-level disinfection can occur without first cleaning the item. This can be especially difficult with items that have narrow lumens in which organic debris can become trapped and is not easily visible. For example, endoscopes have been especially challenging to clean and have been linked to a number of infectious outbreaks. Environmental cleaning procedures for patient rooms were also outlined by the CDC in 2007.

Patient placement has been used as a way to reduce the spread of infection. Some studies have suggested that private patient rooms help decrease infections. However, the CDC has not mandated that all patients, even those with infections, have a private room. *The CDC does recommend that private rooms always be used for patients on Airborne Precautions and those in a protective environment (PE).* A PE is architecturally designed and structured to prevent infection from occurring in patients who are at extremely high risk, such as those having stem cell therapy. The CDC also prefers private rooms for patients who are on Contact and Droplet Precautions (Siegel et al., 2007). Many hospitals are increasing their number of private rooms, and some are becoming totally private-room facilities.

Cohorting is another method of patient placement. **Cohorting** is the practice of grouping patients who are colonized or infected with the same pathogen. This method has been used the most with patients who have an outbreak of a multidrug-resistant organism like methicillin-resistant *Staphylococcus aureus* (MRSA). It is particularly effective in long-term care settings.

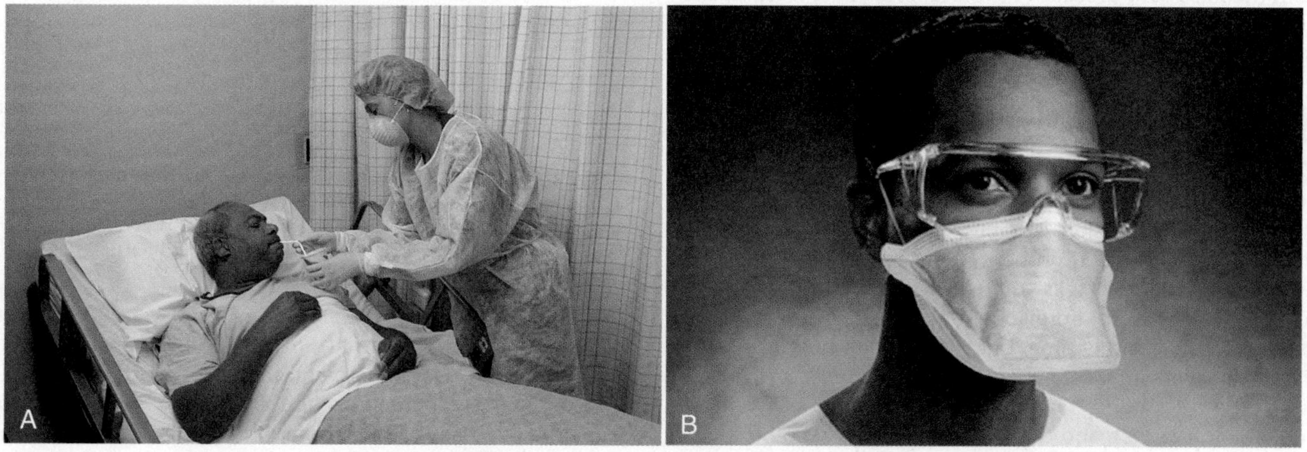
A
B

Fig. 25-1 • **A,** Nurse in personal protective equipment (PPE) caring for a patient in a private room. **B,** N95 respirator mask.

TABLE 25-2 Recommendations for Application of Standard Precautions for the Care of All Patients in All Health Care Settings

Component	Recommendations
Hand hygiene	After touching blood, body fluids, secretions, excretions, contaminated items; immediately after removing gloves; between patient contacts
Personal protective equipment (PPE)	
Gloves	For touching blood, body fluids, secretions, excretions, contaminated items; for touching mucous membranes and nonintact skin
Gown	During procedures and patient-care activities when contact of clothing/exposed skin with blood/body fluids, secretions, and excretions is anticipated
Mask, eye protection (goggles), face shield*	During procedures and patient-care activities likely to generate splashes or sprays of blood, body fluids, secretions, especially suctioning, endotracheal intubation
Soiled patient-care equipment	Handle in a manner that prevents transfer of microorganisms to others and to the environment; wear gloves if visibly contaminated; perform hand hygiene
Environmental control	Develop procedures for routine care, cleaning, and disinfection of environmental surfaces, especially frequently touched surfaces in patient-care areas
Textiles and laundry	Handle in a manner that prevents transfer of microorganisms to others and to the environment
Needles and other sharps	Do not recap, bend, break, or hand-manipulate used needles; if recapping is required, use a one-handed scoop technique only; use safety features when available; place used sharps in puncture-resistant container
Patient resuscitation	Use mouthpiece, resuscitation bag, other ventilation devices to prevent contact with mouth and oral secretions
Patient placement	Prioritize for single-patient room if patient is at increased risk of transmission, is likely to contaminate the environment, does not maintain appropriate hygiene, or is at increased risk of acquiring infection or developing adverse outcome following infection
Respiratory hygiene/cough etiquette (source containment of infectious respiratory secretions in symptomatic patients, beginning at initial point of encounter [e.g., triage and reception areas in emergency departments and physician offices])	Instruct symptomatic persons to cover mouth/nose when sneezing/coughing; use tissues and dispose in no-touch receptacle; observe hand hygiene after soiling of hands with respiratory secretions; wear surgical mask if tolerated or maintain spatial separation, >3 feet if possible

Data from Centers for Disease Control and Prevention, 2007.
*During aerosol-generating procedures on patients with suspected or proven infections transmitted by respiratory aerosols (e.g., SARS), wear a fit-tested N95 or higher respirator in addition to gloves, gown, and face/eye protection.
SARS, Severe acute respiratory syndrome.

Infection control principles for *patient transport* include limiting movement to other areas of the facility, using appropriate barriers like covering infected wounds, and notifying other departments or agencies who are receiving the patient about the necessary precautions (Siegel et al., 2007). Complete and accurate hand-off communication between agencies is also very important to prevent the spread of infection.

DECISION-MAKING CHALLENGE
Coordination of Care

You are working on a medical-surgical unit in a small, rural hospital on the 7 PM-7 AM shift. A patient is admitted from the local nursing home with MRSA in her urine. The nurse in the emergency department (ED) tells you that she is incontinent of both urine and stool due to a previous stroke. No private rooms are available for her at this time, but there is one bed in a semi-private room with an older patient with a fractured leg. No one is likely to be discharged tonight. Your supervisor is busy with a code on another unit, and the ED is too busy to keep her there any longer.

1. Will this patient need to be on Transmission-Based Precautions? Why or why not?
2. Do you need to know anything else about the patient currently in the semi-private room to answer the above question? Why or why not?
3. What PPE should you use to care for this patient?
4. Should your patient have an indwelling urinary catheter to control her urine? Why or why not?
5. What will you teach your unlicensed staff about how to care for this patient?

evolve For suggested answer guidelines, go to http://evolve.elsevier.com/Iggy/.

Centers for Disease Control and Prevention Transmission-Based Guidelines

The 2007 guidelines from the Centers for Disease Control and Prevention (CDC) focus on transmission mechanisms and the precautions needed to prevent the spread of infection. Included in these guidelines are Standard Precautions and Transmission-Based Precautions, including Airborne, Droplet, and Contact Precautions (Tables 25-2 and 25-3).

TABLE 25-3 Transmission-Based Infection Control Precautions

Precautions (In Addition to Standard Precautions)	Examples of Diseases in Category
AIRBORNE PRECAUTIONS	
1. Private room required with monitored negative airflow (with appropriate number of air exchanges and air discharge to outside or through HEPA filter); keep door(s) closed 2. Special respiratory protection: N-95* respirator for known or suspected TB Susceptible persons not to enter room of patient with known or suspected measles or varicella unless immune caregivers are not available Susceptible persons who must enter room must wear N-95 HEPA filter 3. Transport: patient to leave room only for essential clinical reasons, wearing surgical mask	Diseases that are known or suspected to be transmitted by air: Measles (rubeola) *Mycobacterium tuberculosis*, including multidrug-resistant TB (MDRTB) Varicella (chickenpox)†; disseminated zoster (shingles)†
DROPLET PRECAUTIONS	
1. Private room preferred: if not available, may cohort with patient with same active infection with same microorganisms if no other infection present; maintain distance of at least 3 feet from other patients if private room not available 2. Mask: required when working within 3 feet of patient 3. Transport: as above	Diseases that are known or suspected to be transmitted by droplets: Diphtheria (pharyngeal) Streptococcal pharyngitis Pneumonia Influenza Rubella Invasive disease (meningitis, pneumonia, sepsis) caused by *Haemophilus influenzae* type B or *Neisseria meningitidis* Mumps Pertussis
CONTACT PRECAUTIONS	
1. Private room preferred: if not available, may cohort with patient with same active infection with same microorganisms if no other infection present 2. Wear gloves when entering room 3. Wash hands with antimicrobial soap before leaving patient's room 4. Wear gown to prevent contact with patient or contaminated items or if patient has uncontrolled body fluids; remove gown before leaving room 5. Transport: patient to leave room only for essential clinical reasons; during transport, use needed precautions to prevent disease transmission 6. Dedicated equipment for this patient only (or disinfect after use before taking from room)	Diseases that are known or suspected to be transmitted by direct contact: *Clostridium difficile* Colonization or infection caused by multidrug-resistant organisms (e.g., MRSA, VRE) Pediculosis Respiratory syncytial virus Scabies Viral hemorrhagic infections (e.g., Ebola)

Data from Centers for Disease Control and Prevention, 2007.
*Before use: training and fit testing required for personnel.
†Add Contact Precautions for draining lesions.
HEPA, High-efficiency particulate air; *MRSA*, methicillin-resistant *Staphylococcus aureus; VRE*, vancomycin-resistant *Enterococcus*.

Standard Precautions

Standard Precautions reflect that that all body excretions, secretions, and moist membranes and tissues, excluding perspiration, are potentially infectious. The protective measures from the previous Universal Precautions and Body Substance Isolation were combined to better protect health care workers. In 2007, the CDC added two new requirements to these precautions, both of which protect patients (Siegel et al., 2007).

Respiratory hygiene/cough etiquette (RH/CE) is now required because of the widespread SARS outbreaks in 2003. This requirement is directed at patients and visitors with signs of respiratory illness, such as sinus or chest congestion, cough, or rhinorrhea ("runny nose"). The elements for RH/CE include:

- Patient, staff, and visitor education
- Posted signs
- Hand hygiene
- Covering the nose and mouth with a tissue and prompt tissue disposal or using surgical masks (or sneezing/coughing into a shirt sleeve rather than the hand)
- Separation from the person with respiratory infection by more than 3 feet (1 m)

The other requirement is *safe injection practices*. These include using a sterile, single-use disposable needle and syringe for each injection and preventing contamination of injection equipment and medication (Siegel et al., 2007).

Transmission-Based Precautions

Transmission-Based Precautions may also be referred to as *Isolation Precautions*. But, the word *isolation* implies that the patient is physically separated from everyone, which is not always the case.

Airborne Precautions are used for patients known or suspected to have infections transmitted by the airborne transmission route. These infections are caused by organisms that can be suspended in air for prolonged periods. Negative airflow rooms are required to prevent airborne spread of microbes. Enclosed booths with high-efficiency particulate air (HEPA) filtration or ultraviolet light may be used for sputum induction procedures. Tuberculosis, measles (rubeola), and chickenpox (varicella) are examples of airborne diseases.

Droplet Precautions are used for patients known or suspected to have infections transmitted by the droplet transmission route. Such infections are caused by organisms in droplets that may travel 3 feet but are not suspended for long periods. Examples of infectious conditions requiring Droplet Precautions include influenza, mumps, pertussis, and meningitis caused by either *Neisseria meningitidis* or *Haemophilus influenzae* type B.

Contact Precautions are used for patients known or suspected to have infections transmitted by direct contact or contact with items in the environment. Patients with significant multidrug-resistant organism (MDRO) infection or colonization, such as methicillin-resistant *Staphylococcus aureus* (MRSA) or vancomycin-resistant *Enterococcus* (VRE), are placed on Contact Precautions. Other infections requiring Contact Precautions include pediculosis (lice), scabies, respiratory syncytial virus (RSV), and *Clostridium difficile*.

Multidrug-Resistant Organism Infections and Colonizations

Antibiotics have been available for many years. Unfortunately, these drugs were commonly prescribed for conditions that did not need them or were given at higher doses and for longer periods of time than were necessary. As a result, a number of microorganisms have become resistant to certain antibiotics; that is, drugs that were once useful no longer control these infectious agents (multidrug-resistant organisms [MDROs]). For this reason, a culture of safety related to infection control has been mandated by the CDC, the Institute for Healthcare Improvement (IHI), and TJC: Standard Precautions must be strictly followed today in all health care settings to prevent more of these difficult and deadly infections. Descriptions of some examples of MDROs follow.

Methicillin-Resistant *Staphylococcus aureus* (MRSA)

Staphylococcus aureus (S. aureus) is a common bacterium found on the skin and perineum and in the nose of many people. It is usually not infectious when in these areas because the number of bacteria is controlled by good hygiene measures. However, when skin or mucous membranes are not intact, minor infections, like boils or conjunctivitis, may occur. If the organism enters into deep wounds, surgical incisions, the lungs, or bloodstream, more serious infections occur that require strong antibiotics like methicillin.

Within the past 40 years, more and more *S. aureus* infections are not responding to methicillin or other penicillin-based drug. Known as *MRSA,* these infections are one of the fastest growing in health care today. In its 5 Million Lives Campaign, the IHI included reducing MRSA infections as one of its six new goals (Richmond et al., 2007). The CDC estimates that almost 130,000 cases occur in hospitals each year, which lead to 5000 deaths (Siegel et al., 2006). This type of infection is called *hospital-associated MRSA* or *HA-MRSA*. Patients who have HA-MRSA have increased hospital stays at a very high cost. To add to this problem, about 25% of patients may be colonized with the organism, sometimes referred to as a "super bug" (Yamamoto & Marten, 2007). Health care staff members may also be colonized.

MRSA is spread by direct contact and invades hospitalized patients through indwelling urinary catheters, vascular access devices, and endotracheal tubes. It is susceptible to only a few antibiotics, such as vancomycin (Lyphocin, Vancocin) and linezolid (Zyvox). Patients who develop HA-MRSA pneumonia, abscesses, or bacteremia (bloodstream infection [BSI]) can quickly progress to sepsis and death. *Patients most at risk are older adults and those who are immunosuppressed, have a long history of antibiotic therapy, or have invasive tubes or lines. ICU patients are especially at risk.* Assess your patients for risk, and look for possible manifestations. Those who are colonized are not symptomatic. Although controversial, some health care facilities have a MRSA-surveillance program in which each patient's nose is swabbed and cultured for MRSA. Staff may also be cultured. All patients with HA-MRSA infection or colonization should be placed on Contact Precautions.

An emerging infection is community-associated MRSA, or CA-MRSA. This infection develops in community-based health care agencies, such as nursing homes and dialysis centers, and in group facilities or settings, such as prisons, dormitories, and schools. CA-MRSA is a serious illness that causes skin and soft-tissue infections, including abscesses, boils, and blisters. People who get this infection have no risk factors or previous history of MRSA colonization (Yamamoto & Marten, 2007). The best way to decrease the incidence of this growing problem is health teaching. Minocycline (Minocin, Apo-Minocycline♣) and doxycycline (Doryx, Apo-Doxy♣), two older antibiotics, are effective in treating CA-MRSA (Cunha, 2006).

Vancomycin-Resistant Enterococcus (VRE)

Enterococci are bacteria that live in the intestinal tract and are important for digestion. When they move to another area of the body, such as during surgery, they can cause an infection, usually treatable with vancomycin. However, in recent years, over a fourth of these infections have been resistant to the drug and VRE results. Risk factors for this infection include prolonged hospital stays, severe illness, abdominal surgery, enteral nutrition, and immunosuppression. Patients with VRE infections are placed on Contact Precautions.

Unfortunately, VRE can live on almost any surface for days or weeks and still be able to cause an infection. Contamination of toilet seats, door handles, and other objects is very likely for a lengthy period.

Other Multidrug-Resistant Organisms

Although MRSA and VRE have been publicized and extensively studied, other MDROs are emerging. Examples include multidrug-resistant tuberculosis and gonorrhea, both of which are discussed elsewhere in this text. Two other infections, vancomycin-intermediate *S. aureus* (VISA) and vancomycin-resistant *S. aureus* (VRSA), have recently appeared. The first cases of VISA and VRSA have shared some of the same characteristics, including prior MRSA infection, prior and prolonged vancomycin therapy, and renal disease needing dialysis. Two drugs have been effective so far against these two infections—linezolid (Zyvox) and quinupristin-dalfopristin (Synercid). Zyvox resistance has been reported (Todd, 2006a).

DECISION-MAKING CHALLENGE
Legal/Ethical

You are a staff nursing on a vascular surgery unit whose patient population includes many older patients with diabetes. For the past year the rate of infections on this unit, especially staph infections, has been very high. One of the staff nurses is recently separated and has three children. You know that her financial situation is shaky and that she has worked double shifts even when ill. You accidentally find out that she has chronic staphylococcus infections and is probably a carrier. You know that if this information reaches the nurse manager and the infection control department, the staff nurse will probably not be able to work until the infection has cleared—possibly for a month or longer.

1. Are you legally required to do anything with this information? If so, what?
2. Are there any professional or ethical obligations for you? If so, what is the rationale or principle of ethical behavior for this obligation or obligations?
3. If you report this problem to the nurse manager instead of talking with the nurse, what principle of ethical behavior is violated?

evolve For suggested answer guidelines, go to http://evolve.elsevier.com/Iggy/.

Occupational Exposure to Sources of Infection

The **Occupational Safety and Health Administration (OSHA)** is a federal agency that protects workers from injury or illness at their place of employment. Unlike the voluntary guidelines developed by the CDC, OSHA regulations are law. Employers can be fined or disciplined for noncompliance with OSHA regulations. The regulation for prevention of exposure to bloodborne pathogens, such as hepatitis B and hepatitis C or the human immune deficiency virus (HIV), is one example of an OSHA regulation.

Reduction of skin and soft tissue injuries (e.g., needle sticks) is essential to reduce bloodborne pathogen transmission to health care personnel. *OSHA mandates that sharp objects ("sharps") and needles be handled with care.* Many contaminated sharp-object exposures involve nurses. Needleless devices have helped decrease these exposures, especially when caring for patients receiving infusion therapy (see Chapter 15).

Other infection control concerns that nurses and other HCWs have are the possibilities of pandemic influenza, plague, or biologic agent exposure. A large outbreak of one of the MDROs is also worrisome, especially if no drug is sensitive enough for successful management. Nurses fear that they will accidentally bring the infectious agent to their homes and families. *To help prevent this transmission, wear scrubs and change clothes before leaving work. Keep work clothes separate from personal clothes. Take a shower when you get home, if possible, to rid your body of any unwanted pathogens. Be careful not to contaminate equipment that is commonly used, such as your stethoscope or scissors.*

Problems from Inadequate Antimicrobial Therapy

Inadequate antimicrobial therapy may range from an incorrect choice of drug to poor patient adherence. Some infections relapse in a subtle fashion. Drug regimen **noncompliance** (deliberate failure to take the drug) or **nonadherence** (accidental failure to take the drug) prevents contact of harmful microorganisms with sufficient concentrations of the drug and contributes to resistant-organism development.

Some diseases such as tuberculosis (TB) have legal sanctions that require that a patient complete treatment. Patients who are at risk for noncompliance or nonadherence with an anti-TB drug regimen may be placed on *directly observed therapy (DOT).* This means that a health care worker must observe and validate patient compliance with the drug regimen. DOT has been very effective at reducing the spread of multidrug-resistant TB.

Serious complications of infection may also result from incomplete or inadequate antibiotic therapy. Local infections that could be cured without complications, such as cellulitis and pneumonia, may progress to abscess formation if appropriate drug therapy is not continued. Although drug therapy does not always prevent abscess, early therapy may prevent or limit the size of an abscess.

In addition to abscess formation, inadequate therapy may not prevent systemic spread. If the infection is not resolved or if it is treated with drugs that are ineffective for the offending microorganism, the pathogen may enter the bloodstream (septicemia or bloodstream infection [BSI]). Inadequately treated local infections may also lead to BSI with leukocytosis (increased white blood cell count). In severe or advanced cases, leukopenia (decreased white blood cell count) and life-threatening disseminated intravascular coagulation (DIC) may occur. After pathogens invade the bloodstream, no site is protected from invasion.

BSI may progress to **septic shock,** more accurately called *sepsis-induced distributive shock.* In septic shock, insufficient cardiac output is compounded by hypovolemia. Inadequate blood supply to vital organs leads to hypoxia (lack of oxygen) and organ failure. Chapter 39 describes this type of shock and its management in detail.

Patient-Centered Collaborative Care

evolve ONLINE PHARM REVIEW

Assessment

History

The patient's age, history of tobacco or alcohol use, current illness or disease (e.g., diabetes), past and current drug use (e.g., steroids), and poor nutritional status may place him or her at increased risk for infection. Ask the patient about previous vaccinations or immunizations, including the dates of administration.

Determine whether the patient has been exposed to infectious agents. A history of recent exposure to someone with similar clinical symptoms or to contaminated food or water, as well as the time of exposure, assists in identifying a possible source of infection. This information helps determine the incubation period for the disease and thus provides a clue to its cause.

Contact with animals, including pets, may increase exposure to infection. Question the patient about recent animal contact at home or work or in leisure activities (e.g., hiking). Insect bites should be documented.

Obtain a travel history. Travel to areas both within and outside the patient's home country may expose a susceptible person to infectious organisms not encountered in the local community.

A thorough sexual history may reveal behavior associated with an increased risk of sexually transmitted diseases. Obtain a history of IV drug use and a transfusion history to assess the patient's risk for hepatitis B, hepatitis C, and HIV infections.

Identifying the type and location of symptoms may point to affected organ systems. The onset order of symptoms gives clues to the specific problem. Gathering a history of past infection or colonization with multidrug-resistant organisms will help determine which precautions are needed.

Physical Assessment/Clinical Manifestations

Disorders caused by pathogens vary depending on the infection cause and site. Common clinical manifestations are associated with specific sites of infection. Carefully inspect the skin for symptoms of *local* infection at any site *(pain, swelling, heat, redness, pus).* Wounds can easily become infected because the integrity of the skin is broken.

Fever (generally a temperature above 101° F [38° C]), chills, and malaise are primary indicators of a systemic infection. Fever may accompany other noninfectious disorders, and infection can be present without fever. The older adult, whose normal temperature may be 1° to 2° lower than the normal temperature in younger adults, may have a fever at 99° F (37° C). In most patients with an infection, fever **(hyperthermia)** is a normal immune response that can help destroy the pathogen. Assess the patient for these signs and symptoms, and carefully ask about their history and pattern.

Lymphadenopathy (enlarged lymph nodes), pharyngitis, and GI disturbance (usually diarrhea or vomiting) are often associated with infection. To detect enlargement, palpate the cervical, axillary, and other lymph nodes; examine the throat for redness. Ask about changes in stool and if the patient has had any nausea or vomiting.

Psychosocial Assessment

The patient with an infectious disease often has psychosocial concerns. Delay in diagnosis because of the need to await clinical test results produces anxiety. Assess the patient's and family's level of understanding about various diagnostic procedures and the time required to obtain test results. Plan education on infection risk reduction at a time when they are ready to learn.

Feelings of malaise and fatigue often accompany infection. Assess the patient's current level of activity and the impact of these symptoms on family, occupational, and recreational activities.

The potential spread of infection to others is an additional stress associated with the diagnosis of infection. The patient may curtail family and social interactions for fear of spreading the illness. Determine the patient's and family's understanding of the infection, the mode of transmission, and mechanisms that may limit or prevent transmission. Special precautions, although sometimes necessary for preventing transmission of the organism, can be emotionally difficult for the patient and family. Loss of contact with job and social gatherings can lead to depression or anxiety, which may result in a weakening of the immune system. In the inpatient setting, patients have reported dissatisfaction with care and thought that they received less care than other patients (Siegel et al., 2006).

A number of transmissible infectious diseases, especially those identified with social stigmas (e.g., IV drug abuse), are associated with labeling. The patient may feel socially isolated or have guilt related to behavior that increased the risk for infection. Observe carefully for the patient's reaction to labels and how these feelings further affect socialization.

Laboratory Assessment

The definitive diagnosis of an infectious disease requires identification of a microorganism in the tissues of an infected patient. Direct examination of blood, body fluids, and tissues under a microscope may not yield a definitive identification. However, laboratory assessment usually provides helpful information about organisms, such as shape, motility, and reaction to staining agents. Even when direct microscopy does not provide a conclusive specific diagnosis, often enough information is obtained for starting appropriate antimicrobial therapy.

*The best procedure for identifying a microorganism is **culture,*** or isolation of the pathogen by cultivation in tissue cultures or artificial media. Specimens for culture can be obtained from almost any body fluid or tissue. The health care provider usually decides when and where the specimen for culture is taken.

Proper collection and handling of specimens for culture, using Standard Precautions, are essential for obtaining accurate results. Specimens collected must be appropriate for the suspected infection. Be sure that the specimen is of adequate quantity and is freshly obtained and placed in a sterile container to preserve the specimen and microorganism. Label the specimen properly, including the date and time it was collected. Follow your agency's policy if you have any questions about how to perform a culture.

After isolation of a microorganism in culture, antibiotic **sensitivity** testing is performed to determine the effects of various drugs on that particular microorganism. An agent that is killed by acceptable levels of an antibiotic, for example, is considered sensitive to that drug. An organism that is not killed by tolerable levels of an antibiotic is considered resistant to that drug. Preliminary results are usually available in 24 to 48 hours, but the final results generally take 72 hours. *Antibiotic therapy should not begin until after the culture specimen is obtained.*

Newer rapid cultures or assays are beginning to be used in ambulatory care settings to provide quicker assessments of infections. The most popular is the rapid antigen detection test for group A streptococci to rule out "strep throat" in patients who present with pharyngitis (sore, inflamed throat). Other examples of newer tests are those for tuberculosis (TB) and influenza ("flu"), discussed in Chapter 33.

A *complete blood count (CBC) with differential* is often done for the patient with a suspected infection. Five types of leukocytes (white blood cells) are measured as part of the results:

- Neutrophils
- Lymphocytes
- Monocytes
- Eosinophils
- Basophils

In most active infections, especially those caused by bacteria, the total leukocyte count is elevated. Various infections are characterized by changes in the percentages of the different types of leukocytes. The differential count usually shows an increased number of immature neutrophils, or a **shift to the left** ("left shift"). A few infectious diseases, however, such as malaria and infectious mononucleosis, are associated with neutropenia (decreased neutrophils). See Chapter 19 for further discussion.

The *erythrocyte sedimentation rate (ESR)* measures the rate at which red blood cells fall through plasma. This rate is most significantly affected by an increased number of acute-phase reactants, which occurs with inflammation. Thus an elevated ESR (>20 mm/hr) indicates inflammation or infection somewhere in the body. Chronic infection, especially osteomyelitis, and chronic abscesses are commonly associated with an elevated ESR. The ESR is chronically elevated with inflammatory arthritis and other connective tissue diseases as well (see Chapter 20). The effectiveness of therapy is often monitored by a decrease in this value.

Serologic testing is performed to identify pathogens by detecting antibodies to the organism. The antibody titer tends to *increase* during the acute phase of infectious diseases such as hepatitis B. The titer *decreases* as the patient improves.

Many agencies are using DNA microassay analysis for testing genetic differences among bacteria. This test helps to detect antimicrobial genes in nearly all bacteria (Dorrell et al., 2005).

Imaging Assessment

X-ray films may be obtained to determine activity or destruction by an infectious microorganism. Radiologic studies (e.g., chest films, sinus films, joint films, GI studies) are available for diagnosis of infection in a specific body site.

More sophisticated techniques for infection diagnosis include computed tomography (CT) scans and magnetic resonance imaging (MRI). Tomography is helpful in assessing for abscesses. CT scans help identify suspected osteomyelitis and fluid collections that point to possible infection. MRI scans provide a cross-sectional assessment for infection.

Another diagnostic tool for the evaluation of a patient with an infectious disease is ultrasonography. This noninvasive procedure is particularly helpful in detecting infection involving the heart valves.

Scanning techniques using radioactive substances such as gallium can determine the presence of inflammation. Inflammatory tissue is identified by its increased uptake of the injected radioactive material.

Analysis

Common Nursing Diagnoses and Collaborative Problems

The priority nursing diagnoses for patients with an infection or infectious disease are:

1. Hyperthermia related to an increased metabolic state
2. Risk for Social Isolation related to altered state of wellness

The inclusion of other nursing diagnoses depends on the type and extent of the infection. For example, a patient with pneumonia might experience Ineffective Airway Clearance and Fatigue; a patient with a sexually transmitted disease may have Altered Sexuality Patterns.

Additional Nursing Diagnoses and Collaborative Problems

In addition to the priority nursing diagnoses, patients with an infection or infectious disease may have one or more of these diagnoses:

- Acute Pain related to physical injury
- Fatigue related to disease state
- Risk for Deficient Fluid Volume related to hypermetabolic state

The primary additional collaborative problem is Risk for Sepsis, Septic Shock, and Disseminated Intravascular Coagulation (DIC).

Planning and Implementation

Hyperthermia

NOC **Planning: Expected Outcomes.** Patients with an infection or infectious disease are expected to have a return to baseline:

- Temperature
- Apical heart rate
- Respiratory rate

In addition, patients are expected to adhere to their prescribed drug therapy regimen.

Interventions. The primary concern is to provide measures to eliminate the underlying cause of **hyperthermia** (fever) and to destroy the causative microorganism. In collaboration with the health care team, nurses use a variety of methods to manage fever.

Drug Therapy. Drug therapy plays a major role in patient-centered collaborative care of patients with infection. Antimicrobials, also called *anti-infective agents,* are the cornerstone of drug therapy. Antipyretics are used to decrease patient discomfort and reduce fever.

Antibiotics, antiviral agents, and antifungals are common types of *antimicrobials* that are given for infection, depending on its type. In the 1940s, penicillin became the primary antibiotic. Since then, a wide variety of antimicrobial drugs have been developed for the treatment and prevention of infection associated with virtually every class of microorganism. Effective antibiotics are available to treat nearly all bacterial infections, but misuse of antibiotics has contributed to the development of antibiotic-resistant bacteria. A few effective antifungal agents have been developed, but these drugs generally exhibit more toxicity than antibacterial agents. Effective agents are available for the treatment of influenza type A virus infection and HIV, but some viruses, such as HIV, mutate rapidly. These agents have a limited duration of effectiveness.

Effective antimicrobial therapy requires delivery of an appropriate drug, sufficient dosage, proper administration route, and sufficient therapy duration. These four requirements ensure delivery of a concentration of drug sufficient to inhibit or kill infecting microorganisms. Health care providers collaborate on selecting drugs and dosing. Antimicrobials act on susceptible pathogens by:

- Inhibiting cell wall synthesis (e.g., penicillins and cephalosporins)
- Injuring the cytoplasmic membrane (e.g., antifungal agents)
- Inhibiting biosynthesis, or reproduction (e.g., erythromycin, tetracycline, and gentamicin)
- Inhibiting nucleic acid synthesis (e.g., actinomycin)

Teach the drug's actions, side effects, and toxic effects to your patients and their families. Observe and report side effects and adverse events. These reactions vary according to the specific classification of the drug. Most antibiotics can cause nausea, vomiting, and rashes. Stress the importance of completing the entire course of drug therapy, even if symptoms have improved or disappeared. *Before administering an antimicrobial agent, check to see that the patient is not allergic to it (Table 25-4). Be sure to take an accurate allergy history before drug therapy begins.*

Antipyretic drugs, such as acetaminophen (Tylenol, Ace-Tabs🍁), may be given to reduce fever. Because these drugs mask fever, monitoring the course of the disease may be difficult. Therefore, unless the patient is very uncomfortable or if fever presents a significant risk (e.g., in the patient with heart

TABLE 25-4 Allergic Reactions to Antibiotic Therapy

- Flushing
- Wheezing
- Sneezing
- Pruritus
- Urticaria
- Rashes
- Maculopapular to exfoliative dermatitis
- Vascular eruptions
- Erythema multiforme (Stevens-Johnson syndrome)
- Angioneurotic edema
- Serum sickness (headache, fever, chills, hives, malaise, conjunctivitis)
- Anaphylaxis (laryngeal edema, bronchospasm, hypotension, vascular collapse, cardiac arrest)
- Death

Chart 25-4 NIC INTERVENTION ACTIVITIES
The Patient with Infection

Fever Treatment: *Management of a patient with hyperpyrexia caused by nonenvironmental factors*

- Monitor temperature as frequently as is appropriate.
- Monitor blood pressure, pulse, and respiration, as appropriate.
- Monitor skin color and temperature.
- Monitor for decreasing levels of consciousness.
- Monitor for intake and output.
- Monitor for seizure activity.
- Monitor WBC, hemoglobin, and hematocrit values.
- Administer antipyretic medication, as appropriate.
- Cover the patient with a sheet only, as appropriate.
- Administer a tepid sponge bath, as appropriate.
- Encourage increased intake of oral fluids, as appropriate.
- Administer IV fluids, as appropriate.
- Encourage or administer oral hygiene, as appropriate.
- Place patient on hypothermia blanket, as appropriate.
- Monitor temperature closely to prevent treatment-induced hypothermia.

NIC intervention activities selected from Bulechek, G.M., Butcher, H.K., & McCloskey Dochterman, J. (Eds.). (2008). *Nursing interventions classification (NIC)* (5th ed.). St. Louis: Mosby. No part of this work is to be altered without prior written permission from the Publisher.
WBC, White blood cell.

failure, febrile seizures, or head injury), antipyretics are not always prescribed.

Teach patients that they may have waves of sweating after each dose. Sweating may be accompanied by a fall in blood pressure followed by return of fever. These unpleasant side effects of antipyretic therapy can often be alleviated by increasing fluid intake and by regular scheduling of drug administration.

NIC ***Fever Treatment.*** Other interventions to reduce fever may include external cooling and fluid administration. Perform a thorough assessment before and after interventions are implemented (Chart 25-4).

External cooling by hypothermia blankets or ice bags or packs can be effective external mechanisms for reducing a high fever. Alternative cooling methods may be used. Sponging the patient's body with tepid water or applying cool compresses to the skin and pulse points to reduce body temperature is sometimes helpful. *Teach unlicensed assistive personnel (UAP) to observe for and report shivering during any form of external cooling. Shivering may indicate that the patient is being cooled too quickly.*

The use of fans is discouraged because they can disperse airborne- or droplet-transmitted pathogens. Fans can also disturb air balance in negative pressure rooms, making them positive pressure rooms and allowing possible transmission of the agent to those outside the room.

In patients with fever, fluid volume loss is increased from rapid evaporation of body fluids and increased perspiration. As body temperature increases, fluid volume loss increases. Therefore the patient may be at risk for deficient fluid volume, or *dehydration, and require additional fluids either orally or IV. Monitor carefully for signs of dehydration, such as increased thirst, decreased skin turgor, dry mucous membranes, and confusion, especially in older adults. Increase oral fluid intake and provide IV fluids as prescribed.* Chapter 13 discusses interventions for dehydration in detail.

Risk for Social Isolation

Planning: Expected Outcomes. The patient with an infection or infectious disease is expected to cope with feelings of social isolation and to interact with others.

Interventions. Education is the major intervention for meeting this outcome. Teach the patient and family about the mode of transmission of infection and mechanisms that prevent spread to others. Assess coping mechanisms that the patient has used in the past. If he or she is in the hospital, collaborate with the certified hospital chaplain or social worker to help meet the patient's stress, anxiety, or depression.

As part of the health care team, ensure that the patient and family understand the disease process and its cause. If necessary, ensure that the patient and family can state specific ways in which precautions will be used in the home after discharge from the hospital.

Because the patient requiring precautions may feel secluded, encourage staff and family members to maintain contact with the patient. Remind them that the pathogen, not the patient, requires special precautions. Encourage family members and friends to visit and to use appropriate infection control measures. Communication by telephone or e-mail is often effective for continuing contact with loved ones. Television, Internet, and iPods or other MP3 players help bring the outside world into the life of the patient confined to the room.

In the long-term care setting, an outbreak of respiratory or GI infection usually requires limiting visitors, activities, and admissions to the facility. Nurses working in these settings need to be familiar with federal and state regulations regarding managing infections.

Community-Based Care

Patients with infections may be cared for in the home, hospital, nursing home, or ambulatory care setting, depending on the type and severity of the infection. Infections among older adults in nursing homes are common. Residents often have meals together in a communal dining room and participate in group activities. Confused residents may not wash their hands or may enter other resident rooms. Immunizing them against respiratory infections is highly recommended because these illnesses can cause severe complications or death in older adults.

Home Care Management

The patient with an infectious disease such as osteomyelitis who is discharged from the hospital to home may require continued, long-term antibiotic therapy. Emphasize the importance of a clean home environment, especially for the patient who continues to be immunocompromised or who is uniquely susceptible to **superinfection** (i.e., reinfection or a second infection of the same kind) to reduce the chance of infection. Drugs often need to be refrigerated. Ensure that the patient has access to proper storage facilities, and teach him or her to check for signs of improper storage, such as discoloration of the drug.

Ask about the availability of handwashing facilities in the home and check that supplies and instructions are provided as needed. Most people do not know how to wash hands correctly. Demonstrate the procedure with the patient and family, and request a repeat demonstration.

Health Teaching

Explaining the disease and making certain that the patient understands what is causing the illness are the primary purposes of health teaching. Discuss whether the pathogen causing the infection can be spread to others and the modes of transmission.

If the patient has an infectious disease that is potentially transmissible, teach the patient, family, or other home caregivers about precautions. Explain whether any special household cleaning is necessary and, if so, what those special steps include. If syringes with needles are used to administer drug therapy, explain how to dispose safely and legally of needles in the community. Clothing soiled with blood or other body fluids can be washed with bleach or disinfectant (e.g., Lysol). Recommended cleaning measures should be based on actual available equipment and facilities.

For the patient who is discharged to the home setting to complete a course of antimicrobial therapy, the importance of adherence with the planned drug regimen needs to be stressed. Explain the importance of both the timing of doses and the completion of the planned number of days of therapy. The patient (and family as appropriate) should also be taught how the agents need to be taken (e.g., before meals, with meals, without other agents) and the possible side effects. Side effects include those that are expected (e.g., gastric distress after oral administration of erythromycin), as well as more severe adverse reactions (e.g., rash, fever, other systemic signs and symptoms). Teach the patient about allergic manifestations and the need to notify a health care provider if an adverse reaction occurs (see Table 25-4). Also discuss what to do if a drug dose is missed (e.g., doubling the dosage, waiting until the next dose time).

In the past, many patients with severe infection were hospitalized for several weeks or longer to receive IV antimicrobial therapy. Since managed care began, many patients have been discharged with an infusion device to continue drug therapy at home or in other inpatient facilities. The patient, family member, or home care nurse administers the drugs. Chapter 15 describes infusion therapy in the community setting.

The patient is often anxious and fearful that the infection will be transmitted to family members or friends. Teaching the patient and the family ways of preventing the spread of disease allays these fears. Pay careful attention to the patient's and family's concerns. Making concrete suggestions (e.g., "Your wife can wear gloves when changing your dressing") to address specific concerns may reduce these fears.

The patient with an infectious disease associated with lifestyle behaviors, such as sexual activity or IV drug abuse, may have guilt related to the disease. Encourage discussion of feelings associated with the illness, and assist in locating support systems that may help alleviate these feelings, such as clergy or other spiritual or cultural leaders.

Health Care Resources

In unusual instances, a patient who has been hospitalized for an infectious disease may not be able to return to the home setting immediately. In such cases, temporary placement in a skilled nursing facility (SNF) may be needed. Document care requirements, patient history of infection or colonization with multidrug-resistant organisms, medication schedules, and personal needs and preferences on transfer forms. Hand-off communication between the two facilities is required to facilitate a smooth transition from the hospital to the intermediate care setting.

Home care services are often used to teach appropriate administration of drug therapy in the patient's home. Health teaching and wound care may also be needed. These services have proved efficient, effective, psychologically supportive, and less expensive than hospitalization or SNFs.

▪ *Evaluation: Outcomes*

Evaluating the care of the patient with an infection or infectious disease on the basis of the identified nursing diagnoses and collaborative problems is important. The expected outcomes include that the patient:

- Has body temperature and other vital signs within baseline
- Adheres to drug therapy regimen
- Copes with feelings of social isolation
- Interacts with others as appropriate

Specific indicators for these outcomes are listed for each nursing diagnosis under the Planning and Implementation section (see earlier).

NCLEX EXAMINATION CHALLENGE

A postoperative client who had a below-the-knee amputation 2 days ago reports feeling hot and sweaty. His TPR is 100-98-30, and his blood pressure is 156/88. What is the nurse's best action at this time?

A. Call the client's surgeon immediately.
B. Ask the nursing assistant to give him a tepid bath.
C. Give acetaminophen 1000 mg now.
D. Assess his lower extremity surgical site.

evolve For the correct answer, go to http://evolve.elsevier.com/Iggy/.

Critical Issues for the Next Decade: Bioterrorism and Emerging Infections

The main issues related to infection and infection control for the next 5 to 10 years are bioterrorism (Table 25-5), emerging infectious diseases, and multidrug-resistant organisms (MDROs), already discussed. As for any pathogen, strict infection control measures can prevent transmission of these microbes to you and your patients. Some of the most serious infections are briefly described here. Table 25-6 lists more emerging infections that may present as problems in the United States.

TABLE 25-5 Examples of Bioterrorism Agents and General Clinical Management

Pathogen or Agent and Disease Information	Clinical Management*
ANTHRAX (*BACILLUS ANTHRACIS*)	
Cutaneous: 1-7 days after contact, exposed skin itching progressing to papular and vesicular lesions, eschar, edema, ulceration, and sloughing. If untreated, may spread to lymph nodes and bloodstream. Fatality 5%-20%. **Inhalation:** 48 hr after organism or spore inhalation, flu-like illness with possible brief improvement. 2-4 days from initial symptoms, abrupt onset of severe cardiopulmonary illness (dyspnea, tachycardia, fever, diaphoresis, thoracic edema, shock, and respiratory failure). If antibiotics delayed until onset of cardiopulmonary symptoms, mortality high. May be confused with common upper respiratory infection (URI). **Other forms:** Gastrointestinal (GI), meningeal, and sepsis.	**For cutaneous and inhaled anthrax:** No person-to-person spread. Contact Precautions are not needed unless patient presents directly from exposure. Standard Precautions for: Prescribed wound cleansing and management of lesions Ventilator support for respiratory failure Postmortem care
BOTULISM (*CLOSTRIDIUM BOTULINUM* AND NEUROTOXIN)	
Toxin ingestion results in dysphasia, dry mouth, drooping eyelids, and blurred or double vision. Vomiting and constipation or diarrhea may be present initially, extending to symmetric flaccid paralysis in an alert person. Acute bilateral cranial nerve impairment and descending weakness or paralysis follow. Neurologic symptoms after 12-36 hr for foodborne botulism and in 24-72 hr after aerosol exposure. Case fatality up to 10%. Recovery may take months.	Standard Precautions: decontamination of patient is not required. No person-to-person spread. Consider outbreak with suspicion of a single case. Consult with Centers for Disease Control and Prevention (CDC) and health departments. Advise careful cleanup and disposal of suspected contaminated food source *after* consultation with health department about any needed laboratory sampling. Interdisciplinary planning for nutrition and rehabilitation support during lengthy neuromuscular and respiratory recovery.
PLAGUE (*YERSINIA PESTIS*)	
Lymphatic infection: 2-8 days after bites from fleas of an infected rodent (rarely after infected tissue or body fluid contact), onset of fever and chills, painful lymphadenopathy (or bubo—usually inguinal, axillary, or cervical lymph nodes), headache, GI symptoms, and rapidly progressive weakness. 50%-60% fatality if untreated. **Pneumonic:** 1-3 days after aerosolized organism inhalation, fever and chills, productive cough, hemoptysis, rapidly progressive weakness. GI symptoms and bronchopneumonia. Survival unlikely if not treated within 18 hr of symptom onset. **Other forms:** Sepsis with coagulopathy, rarely meningitis.	Droplet Precautions: required for pneumonic plague (until 72 hr of antibiotic therapy). Contact Precautions until decontamination is complete: For any suspected gross contamination. See documentation information listed under Anthrax—above. For prescribed management of bubo(s) if incised to drain. Community and other environmental modifications: Apply insecticide to infested environment and pets (to kill fleas). Reduce food and water supply for rodents. Avoid sick or dead animals.
SMALLPOX (VARIOLA VIRUS) (VARIOLA MAJOR AND MINOR)	
10-17 days after droplet or airborne virus inhalation or contact with bleeding lesions, onset of severe myalgias, headache, and high fever. 2-3 days later, a papular rash appears on face and spreads to extremities (and palms and soles). The rash quickly (simultaneously) becomes vesicular, then painful and pustular (contrasted to varicella rash that crops and concentrates more on trunk with various stages of macules to vesicles seen at one time). Patients are infectious at onset of rash until scabs separate (3 wk). Historically, variola major kills 20%. May be confused with varicella.	Standard, Contact, and Airborne Precautions for patients with vesicular rash pending diagnosis. Same for varicella and variola. Also, avoid contact with organism while handling contaminated clothes and bedding. Wear protective attire (gloves, gown, and N-95 respirator). One case is a public health emergency—highly communicable. Consult CDC and health departments at earliest suspicion. Vaccine does not give reliable lifelong immunity. Previously vaccinated persons are considered susceptible. *Following exposure:* Initiate Airborne Precautions, and observe for unprotected contacts (from days 10-17). Vaccinate within 2-3 days of exposure.
OTHER KEY POINTS	
Assessment: Include account of symptoms, patient's incident (what, where, when, how, others exposed or ill, and officials aware). **Treatment:** Antibiotic-resistance possible. Vaccine and postexposure prophylaxis are subject to change. If any of the above diseases are suspected, consult infection control practitioner for coordination with community health officials and CDC about current recommendations and specimen collection. *If bioterrorism suspected*, Federal Bureau of Investigation (FBI) will coordinate evidence collection and delivery. **Multiple exposures planning:** Emergency and critical care managers must address availability and acquisition of stocks of medications, vaccines, equipment (e.g., ventilators), and communications with officials, as well as public information needs.	

Data from *CDC Emerging Infectious Diseases Journal, 5*(4), July-August 1999. Retrieved January 25, 2008, from www.cdc.gov/ncidod/eid/; and English, J.F., Cundiff, M.Y., Malone, J.D., Pfeiffer, J.A., Bell, M., Steele, L., & Miller, J.M. (1999). *Bioterrorism readiness plan: A template for healthcare facilities* (pp. 11-26). APIC Bioterrorism Task Force and CDC Hospital Infections Program Bioterrorism Working Group (www.apic.org/bioterror/).

*See CDC Transmission-Based Precautions.

TABLE 25-6 Emerging Infectious Diseases in the United States

RECENTLY EMERGING DISEASES
• Severe acute respiratory syndrome (SARS)
• West Nile virus
• Avian influenza
• Hemorrhagic fevers (e.g., Ebola, Marburg)
• Monkeypox
• Bovine spongiform encephalopathy
• Chagas disease
• Vancomycin-intermediate *Staphylococcus aureus* (VISA)
• Vancomycin-resistant *Staphylococcus aureus* (VRSA)
• *Clostridium difficile* (new strain)
OLDER RAPIDLY GROWING DISEASES
• Methicillin-resistant *Staphylococcus aureus* (MRSA)
• Vancomycin-resistant *Enterococcus* (VRE)
• Multidrug-resistant tuberculosis
• *Clostridium difficile*

Preparation for and education about *bioterrorism* has been a major focus of the U.S. government since September 11, 2001. In some cases, vaccines are no longer given for biologic agents like smallpox. Many people in the United States have never been vaccinated, and those who had vaccinations many years ago are not guaranteed to have lifelong immunity. Anthrax, usually seen in animals, may be spread to the skin or inhaled. These infections have a high fatality rate in humans. Plague, once seen centuries ago, is one of the biggest threats because the survival rate is low. Vaccines are being researched and stockpiled by the U.S. government for some of the common biologic agents.

Pandemic infections, such as influenza, are another threat to the population. As recently as the early 1900s, the "Spanish flu" killed millions of people throughout the world. Health care workers are encouraged to have yearly influenza vaccines to prevent common strains of the virus. The federal government and health care agencies around the United States include the risk of pandemic disease in their disaster planning (see Chapter 12). The latest threat of a pandemic is the avian influenza strain (H5N1) or "bird flu" that has caused a pandemic among poultry. Chapter 33 discusses protection from bird flu in more detail. Although this strain is not readily spread to humans, the people who got this disease had contact with infected poultry.

Contaminated food is another source of infection. The incidence of foodborne infections has risen in the United States as reports of contaminated fresh spinach, ground beef, and other foods were found to contain *Escherichia coli (E. coli)* 0157:H7. Many illnesses and thousands of recent deaths in the United States have been caused by this infection. Safer food preparation practices and increased monitoring by federal agencies have resulted from demand for public safety. More information on foodborne illnesses can be found in Chapter 60.

Another pathogen, *Clostridium difficile (C. difficile),* is associated with antibiotic therapy use. An uncommon but virulent strain of this organism has appeared recently in the United States and Canada (Oriola, 2006). *C. difficile* is spread by indirect contact with inanimate objects like medical equipment and commodes, and its toxins cause colon dysfunction and cell death from sepsis. *C. difficile*–associated disease (CDAD) is confirmed by stool culture. Patients who have three or more liquid stools per day for two or more days are suspected of having CDAD. *Older adults are the most at risk for this infection.* Metronidazole (Flagyl) and vancomycin are the drugs of choice.

HUMAN NEEDS NURSING CARE REVIEW

What might you NOTICE if the patient has inadequate protection as a result of infection or infectious disease?

- Flushing and sweating
- Localized skin inflammation (redness, warmth, swelling, pain)
- Open wound (draining or non-draining)
- Report of diarrhea or vomiting
- Report of sore throat
- Fatigue
- Rash
- Acute confusion (in older adults)

What should you INTERPRET and how should you RESPOND to a patient with inadequate protection as a result of infection or infectious disease?

Perform and interpret focused physical assessment findings, including:

- Vital signs
- Skin and/or wound assessment
- Lymph palpation
- Throat inspection

Respond:

- Manage fever if present.
- Take culture of drainage and send to laboratory for analysis.
- Monitor laboratory findings, including complete blood count (CBC) with white blood cell (WBC) differential.
- Place on appropriate Transmission-Based Precautions.
- Teach patients and families about Transmission-Based Precautions and hand hygiene.
- Administer antimicrobial therapy as prescribed.
- Collaborate with the facility's infection control practitioner.
- Teach patients and families about the need to adhere to the drug therapy regimen.
- Follow CDC guidelines and The Joint Commission National Patient Safety Goals (NPSGs).

On what should you REFLECT?

- Monitor the patient's response to drug therapy.
- Monitor the patient's vital signs for return to baseline.
- Evaluate the patient's and family's knowledge of infection, Transmission-Based Precautions, and drug therapy.
- Monitor the staff's compliance with hand hygiene and personal protective equipment (PPE).
- Evaluate the patient's and family's coping ability.
- Think about what else you might do to make the patient more comfortable.
- Decide whether you need to provide alternative or additional interventions or health teaching.

GET READY FOR THE NCLEX EXAMINATION!

Key Points

Review these Key Points for each NCLEX Examination Client Needs Category.

Safe and Effective Care Environment

- Handwashing and alcohol-based hand rubs are two methods of hand hygiene (see Chart 25-3).
- The Centers for Disease Control and Prevention (CDC) recommends a ban on artificial fingernails for health care professionals when they are caring for patients at high risk for infection.
- Infections can be prevented or controlled through hand hygiene, disinfection/sterilization, personal protective equipment (PPE), patient placement, and adequate staffing; proper hand hygiene and gloves are the most important intervention because health care workers' hands are the primary way in which disease is transmitted from patient to patient.
- Standard Precautions are used with all patients in health care settings, assuming that all body excretions and secretions are potentially infectious (see Table 25-2).
- Airborne Precautions are used for patients who have infections transmitted through the air, such as tuberculosis.
- Droplet Precautions are used for patients who have infections transmitted by droplets, such as influenza and certain types of meningitis.
- Contact Precautions are used for patients who have infections transmitted by direct contact or contact with items in the patient's environment.

Health Promotion and Maintenance

- Health teaching about clinical manifestations of infection and drug therapy is important for the patient with an infection being managed at home; some patients may need health care nursing services for IV antimicrobial therapy.
- Teach patients about antimicrobial therapy and protective measures to prevent infection transmission.

Psychosocial Integrity

- Patients who have Transmission-Based Precautions may feel isolated, anxious, or depressed; they may feel neglected and dissatisfied with their care. Help patients cope with these feelings through verbalization and collaboration with the health care team.

Physiological Integrity

- Examples of multiple-resistant organisms include methicillin-resistant *Staphylococcus aureus* (MRSA) and vancomycin-resistant *Enterococcus* (VRE).
- If infections are not treated or are inadequately treated, systemic sepsis (septicemia), septic shock, and disseminated intravascular coagulation (DIC) may result.
- A culture is the most definitive way to confirm and identify microorganisms; sensitivity testing determines which antibiotics will destroy the identified microbes.
- The differential count usually shows a shift to the left (increased number of immature neutrophils) during active infections.
- Antimicrobials and antipyretics are the most common types of drugs used when infection is accompanied by hyperthermia (fever).
- Antipyretics are used only when the fever presents a significant risk or the patient is very uncomfortable, because antipyretics may mask the disease.
- Nursing interventions for fever management are listed in Chart 25-4.
- Critical issues for the next decade include bioterrorism, emerging infectious diseases, and multidrug-resistant organisms (MDROs).

Additional Study Resources

Go to your Companion CD or Evolve at http://evolve.elsevier.com/Iggy/ for *Self-Assessment Questions for the NCLEX Examination.*

Go to Evolve at http://evolve.elsevier.com/Iggy/ for *Prioritization and Delegation Questions for the NCLEX Examination.*

SELECTED BIBLIOGRAPHY

Asterisk indicates a classic or definitive work on this subject.

*Antimicrobial Resistance Interagency Task Force. (2002). *Antimicrobial Resistance Interagency Task Force 2002 annual report on a public health action plan to combat antimicrobial resistance.* Retrieved January 25, 2008, from www.cdc.gov/drugresistance/actionplan/index.htm.

Arenas, M.D., Sanchez-Paya, J., Barril, G., Garcia-Valdecasas, J., Gorriz, J.L., Soriano, A., et al. (2005). A multicentric survey of the practices of hand hygiene in haemodialysis units: Factors affecting compliance. *Nephrology, Dialysis, Transplantation, 20*(6), 1164-1171.

*Celia, F. (2002). Cutaneous anthrax: An overview. *Dermatology Nurse, 14*(2), 89-92.

*Centers for Disease Control and Prevention (CDC). (2001a). Management of occupational exposures to hepatitis B, hepatitis C, and HIV and recommendations for postexposure prophylaxis. *Morbidity and Mortality Weekly Report, 50*(RR-11), 1-42.

*Centers for Disease Control and Prevention (CDC). (2001b). Recognition of illness associated with the intentional release of biologic agent. *Morbidity and Mortality Weekly Report, 50*(41), 893-897.

*Centers for Disease Control and Prevention (CDC). (2002a). Guideline for hand hygiene in health-care settings: Recommendations of the Healthcare Infection Control Practices Advisory Committee and the HICPAC/SHEA/APIC/IDSA Hand Hygiene Task Force. *Morbidity and Mortality Weekly Report, 51*(RR-16), 1-44.

*Centers for Disease Control and Prevention (CDC). (2002b). Guidelines for the prevention of intravascular catheter-related infections, 2002. *Morbidity and Mortality Weekly Report, 51*(RR-10), 1-36.

*Centers for Disease Control and Prevention (CDC). (2002c). *Smallpox response plan and guidelines* (Draft 3.0). Retrieved January 25, 2008, from www.bt.cdc.gov/agent/smallpox/response-plan/index.asp#guidec.

*Centers for Disease Control and Prevention (CDC). (2003). *Food Safety Office.* Retrieved January 25, 2008, from www.cdc.gov/foodsafety/.

Cheek, D.J., McGehee-Smith, H., Cunneen, J., & Cartwright, M. (2005). Sepsis: Taking a deeper look. *Nursing2005, 35*(1), 38-42.

Cunha, B.A. (2006). New uses for older antibiotics: Nitrofurantoin, Amikacin, Colistin, Polymyxin B, Doxycycline, and Minocycline revisited. *Medical Clinics of North America, 90,* 1089-1107.

Davey, V.J. (2007). Questions and answers on pandemic influenza. *AJN, 107*(7), 50-56.

Dorrell, N., Hinchliffe, S.J., & Wren, B.W. (2005). Comparative phylogenomes of pathogenic bacteria by microarray analysis. *Current Opinions in Microbiology, 8*(5), 620-626.

*Gehring, L.L., & Ring, P. (1999). Latex allergy: Creating a safe environment. *MEDSURG Nursing, 8*(6), 358-362.

Kay, M. (2005). Influenza pandemic preparedness. *AJN, 105*(12), 73-74.

Korniewicz, D., & Masri, M.E. (2007). Effect of aloe-vera impregnated gloves on hand hygiene attitudes of health care workers. *MEDSURG Nursing, 16*(4), 247-252.

Kuzu, N., Ozer, F., Aydemir, S., Yalcin, A.N., & Zencir, M. (2005). Compliance with hand hygiene and glove use in a university-affiliated hospital. *Infection Control and Hospital Epidemiology, 26*(3), 312-315.

Lashley, F.R. (2006). Emerging infectious diseases at the beginning of the 21st century. *Online Journal of Issues in Nursing, 11*(1), 1-20.

Metlay, J.P., Powers, J.H., Dudley, M.N., Christiansen, K., & Finch, R.G. (2006). Antimicrobial drug resistance, regulation, and research. *Emerging Infectious Diseases, 12*(2), 183-190.

*Muto, C.A., Jernigan, J.A., Ostrowsky, B.E., Richet, H.M., Jarvis, W.R., Boyce, J.M., et al. (2003). SHEA guideline for preventing nosocomial transmission of multidrug-resistant strains of *Staphylococcus aureus* and *Enterococcus. Infection Control and Hospital Epidemiology 24*(5), 362-386.

*National Institute for Occupational Safety and Health. (1998). *NIOSH alert: Preventing allergic reactions to natural rubber latex in the workplace* (Publication No. 97-135) (updated September 1998, pp. 1, 3, 5-7). Atlanta: U.S. Government Printing Office. Retrieved January 25, 2008, from www.cdc.gov/niosh/latexalt.html.

Oriola, S. (2006). *C. difficile:* A menace in hospitals and homes alike. *Nursing2006, 36*(8), 14-15.

*Osterholm, M.T. (2000). Emerging infections: Another warning. *New England Journal of Medicine, 342*(17), 1280-1281.

Richmond, I., Bernstein, A., Creen, C., Cunningham, C., & Rudy, M. (2007). Reducing harm from MRSA. *Nursing Management, 38*(8), 22-27.

Romero, D.V. (2006). Hand-to-hand combat: Preventing MRSA. *The Nurse Practitioner, 31*(3), 16-23.

Sheff, B. (2005). Avian influenza: Are you ready for a pandemic? *Nursing2005, 35*(9), 26-27.

Siegel, J.D., Rhinehart, E., Jackson, M., Chiarello, L.; the Healthcare Infection Control Practices Advisory Committee. (2006). *Management of multidrug resistant organisms in healthcare settings 2006.* Atlanta: CDC.

Siegel, J.D., Rhinehart, E., Jackson, M., Chiarello, L.; the Healthcare Infection Control Practices Advisory Committee. (2007). *Guidelines for isolation precautions: Preventing transmission of infectious agents in healthcare settings 2007.* Atlanta: CDC.

Todd, B. (2006a). Beyond MRSA: VISA and VRSA. *AJN, 106*(4), 28-30.

Todd, B. (2006b). *Clostridium difficile:* Familiar pathogen, changing epidemiology. *AJN, 106*(5), 33-36.

Todd, B. (2007). Outbreak: *E. coli* 0157:H7. *AJN, 107*(2), 29-32.

Wood, S., Lavieri, M.C., & Durkin, T. (2007). What you need to know about sepsis. *Nursing2007, 37*(3), 46-52.

Yamamoto, L., & Marten, M. (2007). Listen up MRSA, the bug stops here. *Nursing2007, 27*(12), 50-56.

VI

UNIT

Problems of Protection

Management of Patients with Problems of the Skin, Hair, and Nails

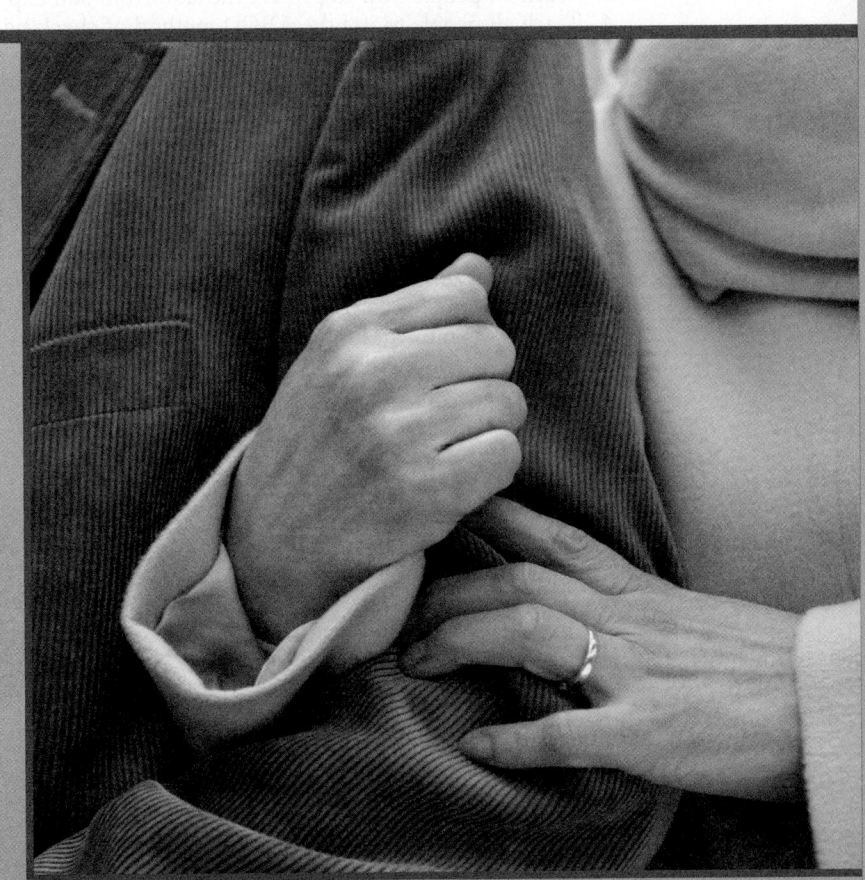

26

CHAPTER

Assessment of the Skin, Hair, and Nails

Janice Cuzzell • M. Linda Workman

LEARNING OUTCOMES

For clinical competence and success on the NCLEX Examination, study this chapter with these Learning Outcomes in mind:

Safe and Effective Care Environment

1. Use knowledge of integumentary changes associated with aging to protect older adult patients from skin injury.
2. Modify techniques to assess skin changes in patients with dark skin.

Health Promotion and Maintenance

3. Teach all people how to protect the skin from sun exposure.
4. Teach all people to use the ABCD method of checking lesions for manifestations of melanoma.
5. Perform health history and risk assessment for skin, hair, and nail problems.

Psychosocial Integrity

6. Use effective communication when teaching patients and family members about what to expect during tests and procedures to assess skin function and skin disease.
7. Reassure patients who have skin changes that are variations of normal.

Physiological Integrity

8. Compare the structures and function of the epidermis, dermis, and subcutaneous tissue.
9. Use proper terminology to communicate skin assessment findings.
10. Distinguish between normal variations and abnormal skin manifestations with regard to skin color, texture, warmth, and moisture.
11. Use the ABCD method of assessing skin lesions for cancer.

evolve Go to your Companion CD or Evolve at http://evolve.elsevier.com/Iggy/ for *Self-Assessment Questions for the NCLEX Examination* keyed to these Learning Outcomes.

The skin, hair, and nails make up the integumentary system. The skin plays a major role in meeting the *human need for protection*. As shown in Fig. 26-1, the skin protects against foreign invasion by providing a first line of defense (the moat), a second line of defense (the castle wall), and even a third line of defense (the knights and soldiers). The normal flora on the surfaces of skin and mucous membranes repels some of the more harmful microorganisms. The intact skin has barrier functions, warning functions, and even fighting functions. Specialized cells called *Langerhans' cells*, present in the skin, engulf any foreign substances (antigens) that invade the body when the skin is injured. These cells then alert the immune system to the presence of the invader.

Although external, the skin is the largest organ of the body and plays a major role in homeostasis. When intact, it helps regulate body temperature and maintains fluid and electrolyte balance. Changes in the skin can communicate information about a person's health and well-being.

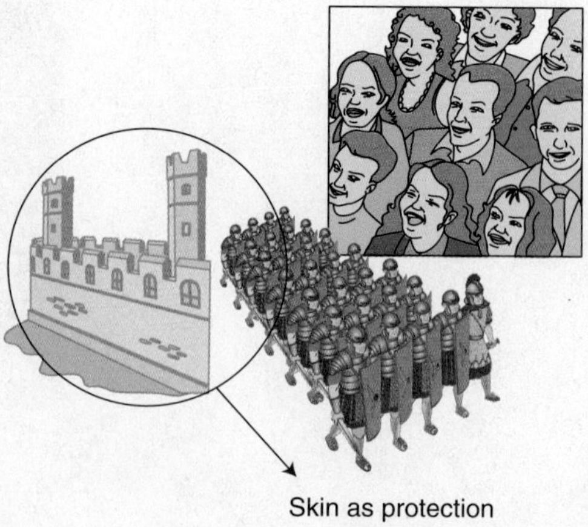
Skin as protection

Fig. 26-1 • Role of the skin in meeting the human need for protection.

Emotional stress, systemic disease, and skin injury or disease can alter the function, appearance, and texture of the skin. Therefore examine the skin for important clues about the patient's health. Because the skin has many sensory receptors, the patient can report subjective skin sensations that might indicate specific health problems. The sensory function of the skin allows the use of touch as a therapeutic intervention to provide comfort, relieve pain, and communicate caring.

ANATOMY AND PHYSIOLOGY REVIEW

Structure of the Skin

As shown in Fig. 26-2, the skin has three layers: fat, dermis, and epidermis. Each layer has unique properties that contribute to the skin's ability to maintain its complex functions.

Subcutaneous fat (adipose tissue) is the innermost layer of the skin, lying over muscle and bone. Fat cells serve as an energy reserve in the event extra calories are needed to power the body. These cells also act as heat insulators for the body. They absorb shock and protect against injury by padding internal structures. Fat distribution varies with body area, age, and gender. Many blood vessels go through the fatty layer and extend into the dermal layer, forming capillary networks that supply nutrients and remove wastes.

The dermis (corium) is the layer above the fat layer. It is composed of connective tissue that contains no cells. The dermis is composed of collagen and elastic fibers that are interwoven to give the skin both flexibility and strength.

Collagen, the main component of dermal tissue, is a protein formed by dermal cells called *fibroblasts.* Collagen production increases in areas of tissue injury and helps form scar tissue. Fibroblasts also produce **ground substance,** a protein lubricant that surrounds the dermal cells and fibers and contributes to the skin's normal suppleness and turgor.

The elasticity of the skin depends on both the amount and quality of the elastic fibers, which are scattered among the collagen fibers. The major component of the elastic fiber is **elastin.**

The dermis has capillaries and lymph vessels for the exchange of oxygen and heat. It is rich in sensory nerves that transmit the sensations of touch, pressure, temperature, pain, and itch.

The epidermis is the outermost skin layer. It is anchored to the dermis by finger-like projections of dermal tissue **(dermal papillae).** The fingers of epidermal tissue that project into the dermis are called **rete pegs.** The epidermis is less than 1 mm thick, but it is the protective barrier between the body and the environment.

The epidermis does not have its own blood supply and receives its nutrients by diffusion from the blood vessels in the dermal layer through the basement membrane. Attached to the basement membrane are the keratinocytes. The basal cells (those keratinocytes capable of cell division and located closest to the basement membrane) continuously divide to form new cells. Older keratinocytes are pushed upward and flattened to form the stratified layers of the epithelium **(malpighian layers).** When these cells reach the outermost skin layer, the **stratum corneum** (horny layer), they are no longer living cells and are shed from the skin. **Keratin,** the protein produced by keratinocytes, makes the horny layer waterproof. A keratinocyte takes about 28 to 45 days to move from the basement membrane to the skin surface.

Vitamin D is activated in the epidermis by ultraviolet (UV) light, such as sunlight. It is then distributed by the blood to the intestinal tract, where it promotes uptake of dietary calcium.

Melanocytes are pigment-producing cells found at the basement membrane. These cells give color to the skin and account for the racial differences in skin tone. Darker skin tones are not caused by increased numbers of melanocytes; rather, the size of the pigment granules (melanin) contained in each cell determines the color. The purpose of melanin is to protect the skin from damage by UV light. For this reasons, people with dark skin are less likely to develop sunburn than lighter-skinned people with the same sun exposure. Freckles,

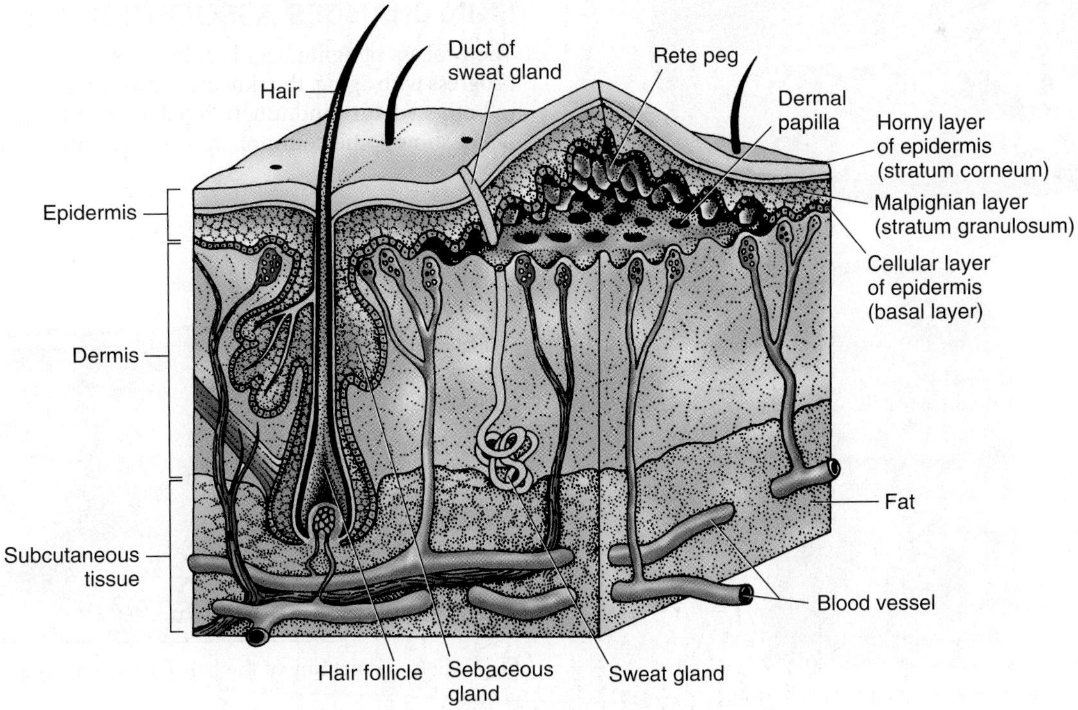
Hair
Duct of sweat gland
Rete peg
Dermal papilla
Horny layer of epidermis (stratum corneum)
Malpighian layer (stratum granulosum)
Cellular layer of epidermis (basal layer)
Epidermis
Dermis
Subcutaneous tissue
Fat
Blood vessel
Hair follicle
Sebaceous gland
Sweat gland

Fig. 26-2 • Anatomy of the skin.

birthmarks, and age spots are caused by patches of melanin within the skin. UV light stimulates the production of melanin, which protects against the harmful effects of sun exposure. Melanin production increases in areas that have endocrine changes or inflammation.

Structure of the Skin Appendages

Hair, a thick protective pelt worn by most mammals, is mainly a cosmetic feature for modern humans. Hair growth varies with race, gender, age, and genetic predisposition. Individual hairs can differ in both structure and rate of growth, depending on body location.

Hair follicles are located in the dermal layer of the skin but are actually extensions of the epidermal layer (see Fig. 26-2). Within each hair follicle, a round column of keratin forms the hair shaft. Hair keratin is tougher than skin keratin. Hair color is genetically determined by a person's rate of melanin production.

Hair growth occurs in cycles, with a growth phase followed by a resting phase. Stressors can alter the growth cycle and result in temporary hair loss. Permanent baldness, such as male pattern baldness, is inherited and is seldom influenced by personal or environmental factors.

Nails on fingers and toes have cosmetic value and serve as useful tools for grasping and scraping. Like hair follicles, the nails are extensions of the keratin-producing epidermal layers of the skin.

The white, crescent-shaped portion of the nail at the lower end of the nail plate is called the **lunula** and is the location of the nail matrix, where nail keratin is formed and nail growth begins (Fig. 26-3). Unlike cyclic hair growth, nail growth is a continuous but slow process. Fingernail replacement requires 3 to 4 months. Toenail replacement may take up to 12 months.

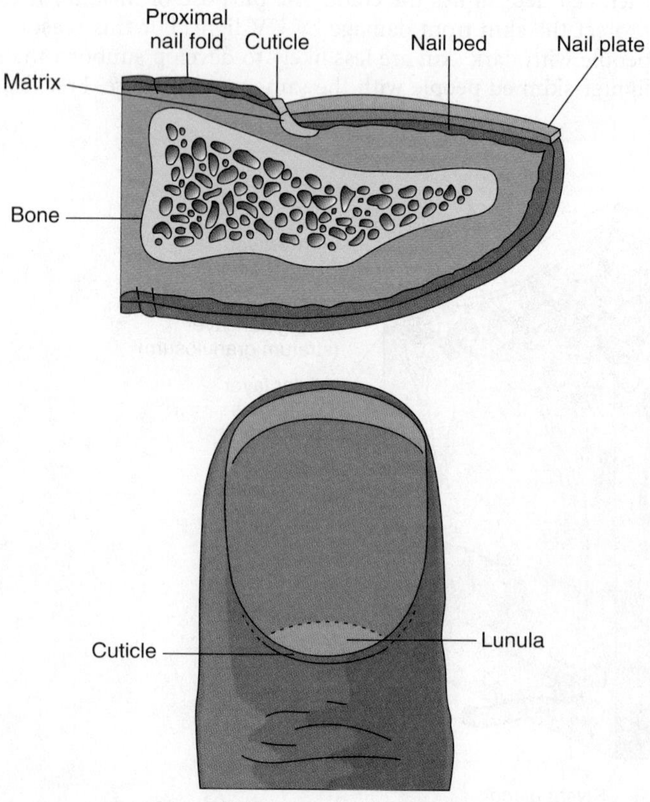
Proximal nail fold
Cuticle
Nail bed
Nail plate
Matrix
Bone
Cuticle
Lunula

Fig. 26-3 • Anatomy of the nail.

The **cuticle,** a layer of keratin at the nail fold, attaches the nail plate to the soft tissue of the nail fold. The nail body is translucent, and the pinkish hue reflects a rich blood supply beneath the nail surface. Nail growth and appearance are often altered during systemic disease or serious illness.

Sebaceous glands are distributed over the entire skin surface except for the palms of the hands and soles of the feet. Most of these glands are connected directly to the hair follicles (Fig. 26-4). The sebaceous glands of the eyelids, nipple areolae, and genitalia are freestanding.

Sebaceous glands produce **sebum,** a mildly bacteriostatic, fat-containing substance. Sebum lubricates the skin and reduces water loss from the skin surface.

Sweat glands of the skin are of two types: eccrine and apocrine. Eccrine sweat glands arise from the epithelial cells. They are found over the entire skin surface and are not associated with the hair follicle. The odorless, colorless, isotonic secretions of these glands are important in the regulation of body temperature. Stimulation of sweat from these glands and the resultant water evaporation can cause the body to lose as much as 10 to 12 liters of fluid in a single day.

Apocrine sweat glands are in direct contact with the hair follicle. They are found mostly in the axillae, nipple areolae, and perineal and periumbilical body areas. The interaction of skin bacteria with the secretions of the apocrine glands causes the distinctive body odor.

Functions of the Skin

The skin is a complex organ responsible for the regulation of many body functions throughout the life span (Table 26-1). In addition to the skin's protective and regulatory functions, its location on the outside of the body makes it an important way to communicate a patient's state of health and body image.

SKIN CHANGES ASSOCIATED WITH AGING

The process of aging begins at birth. As changes in physiology progress with aging, the skin also undergoes age-related changes in both structure and function (Chart 26-1). Figs. 26-5 through 26-12 show some common age-related skin changes.

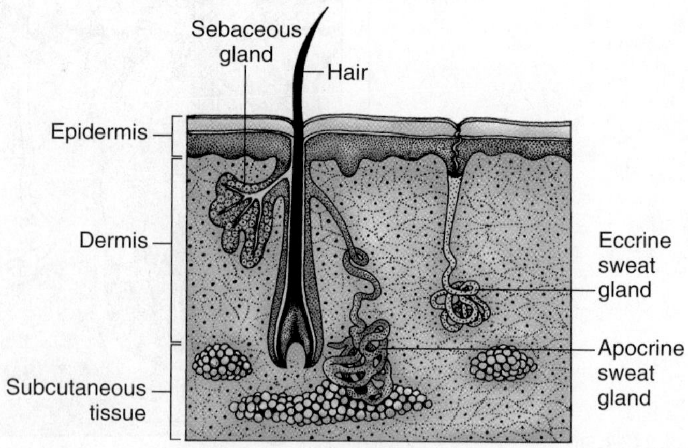
Sebaceous gland
Hair
Epidermis
Dermis
Eccrine sweat gland
Apocrine sweat gland
Subcutaneous tissue

Fig. 26-4 • Anatomy of the hair follicle and sebaceous and sweat glands.

TABLE 26-1 Functions of the Skin

Epidermis	Dermis	Subcutaneous Tissue
PROTECTION		
Keratin provides protection from injury by corrosive materials Inhibits proliferation of microorganisms because of dry external surface Mechanical strength through intercellular bonds	Provides fibroblasts for wound healing Provides mechanical strength Collagen fibers Elastic fibers Ground substance	Mechanical shock absorber Energy reserve
HOMEOSTASIS (WATER BALANCE)		
Low permeability to water and electrolytes prevents systemic dehydration and electrolyte loss	Lymphatic and vascular tissues respond to inflammation, injury, and infection	
TEMPERATURE REGULATION		
Eccrine sweat glands allow dissipation of heat through evaporation of sweat secreted onto the skin surface	Cutaneous vasculature, through dilation or constriction, promotes or inhibits heat conduction from the skin surface	Fat cells act as insulators and assist in retention of body heat
SENSORY ORGAN		
Transmits a variety of sensations through the neuroreceptor system	Encloses an extensive network of nerve endings for relaying sensations to the brain	Contains large pressure receptors
VITAMIN SYNTHESIS		
7-Dehydrocholesterol is present in large concentrations in malpighian cells; photoconversion to vitamin D takes place	No function	No function
PSYCHOSOCIAL		
Body image alterations occur with many epidermal diseases, such as generalized psoriasis	Body image alterations occur with many dermal diseases, such as scleroderma	Body image alterations may result from increases, decreases, and redistribution of body fat stores

Chart 26-1 NURSING FOCUS ON THE OLDER ADULT

Changes in the Integumentary System Related to Aging

Physical Changes	Clinical Findings	Nursing Actions
EPIDERMIS		
Decreased thickness in epidermal layer	Increased skin transparency and fragility	Handle patients carefully. Avoid taping the skin.
Decreased epidermal mitotic activity	Delayed wound healing	Protect open areas to promote wound healing.
Decreased epidermal mitotic homeostasis	Skin hyperplasia, such as hyperkeratoses and skin cancers (especially in sun-exposed areas)	Assess exposed skin areas for sun-induced changes. Assess non–sun-exposed areas to determine base skin features.
Increased epidermal permeability	Increased susceptibility to irritant reactions	Teach patients how to avoid exposure to skin irritants.
Decreased number of Langerhans' cells	Decreased cutaneous inflammatory response	Do not rely on redness and swelling to indicate skin damage.
Decreased number of active melanocytes	Increased sensitivity to sun exposure	Teach patients to wear hats and protective clothing and to use sunscreen when outside.
Hyperplasia of melanocytes at the dermal-epidermal junction (especially in sun-exposed areas)	Mottled hyperpigmentation and hypopigmentation (e.g., liver spots, age spots)	Teach patients to keep track of such spots, but help them to differentiate these "normal" spots from those that need evaluation for malignancy.
Decreased vitamin D production	Increased susceptibility to osteomalacia	Urge patients to take a multiple vitamin or a calcium supplement that contains vitamin D.

Continued

Chart 26-1 NURSING FOCUS ON THE OLDER ADULT

Changes in the Integumentary System Related to Aging—cont'd

Physical Changes	Clinical Findings	Nursing Actions
EPIDERMIS—cont'd		
Flattening of the dermal-epidermal junction	Increased susceptibility to shearing forces, with resultant blisters, purpura, skin tears, and pressure-related skin problems	Avoid pulling or dragging patients. Assist patients confined to bed or chairs to change positions at least every 2 hours.
DERMIS		
Decreased dermal blood flow	Increased susceptibility to dry skin (xerosis)	Teach patients to use moisturizers on the skin and to avoid agents that promote skin dryness.
Decreased vasomotor responsiveness	Increased thermoregulatory alterations (predisposition to heat stroke and hypothermia)	Teach patients to dress for the environmental temperatures and not to rely on skin sensations to tell them they are too hot or too cold.
Decreased dermal thickness	Paper-thin, transparent skin with an increased susceptibility to trauma	Handle patients gently, and avoid the use of tape or tight dressings. Use lift sheets when positioning patients.
Degeneration of elastic fibers	Decreased tone and elasticity (wrinkles)	Use the forehead or chest to test skin turgor.
Benign proliferation of capillaries	Cherry hemangiomas	Teach patients that these are benign.
Reduced number and function of nerve endings	Alterations in sensory perception	Instruct patients to use bath thermometer and to lower the water heater temperature to prevent scalds.
SUBCUTANEOUS LAYER		
Thinning of subcutaneous fat layer	Increased susceptibility to hypothermia	Teach patients to dress warmly in cold weather and to wear hats and gloves when outdoors.
	Decreased resistance to mechanical injury (especially pressure necrosis)	Assist patients confined to bed or chairs to change positions at least every 2 hours.
HAIR		
Decreased number of hair follicles and rate of growth	Increased hair thinning	Suggest wearing hats in cold weather to prevent body heat loss and when in the sun to prevent burning the scalp.
Decreased number of active melanocytes in follicle	Gradual loss of hair color (graying)	Although associated with aging, inform patients that hair color loss can occur at any age.
NAILS		
Decreased rate of growth	Increased susceptibility to fungal infections	Inspect the nails (including toenails) of all older adults. Instruct patients to wear socks and to keep the feet clean, warm, and dry.
Decreased blood flow beneath the nail bed	Longitudinal nail ridges	Use the oral mucosa to assess for cyanosis.
Thickening of the nail	Toenails (especially) thicken and may overhang the toes.	Use fingernails to assess capillary refill. Cut toenails straight across rather than on a curve. Do not use nail appearance alone to determine the presence of a fungal infection. Assess skin in contact with the nail to determine whether the thick nail is irritating it.
GLANDS		
Decreased sebum production despite sebaceous gland hyperplasia	Increased size of pores (especially on nose); large comedones in malar region	Teach patients not to squeeze the pores or comedones to prevent traumatizing the skin.
Decreased eccrine and apocrine gland activity	Increased susceptibility to dry skin	Urge patients to avoid deodorant soaps and to use soaps with a high fat content.
	Decreased perspiration, leading to decreased cooling effect	Do not use sweat production as an indicator of hyperthermia.

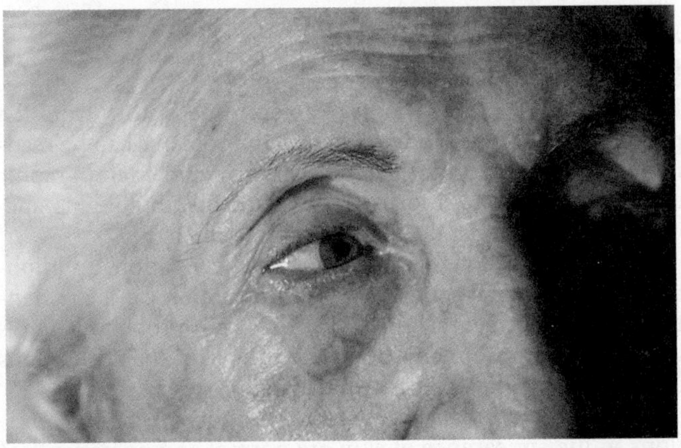

Fig. 26-5 • Eyelid eversion, deepening of the eye orbit, and "bags" under the eye.

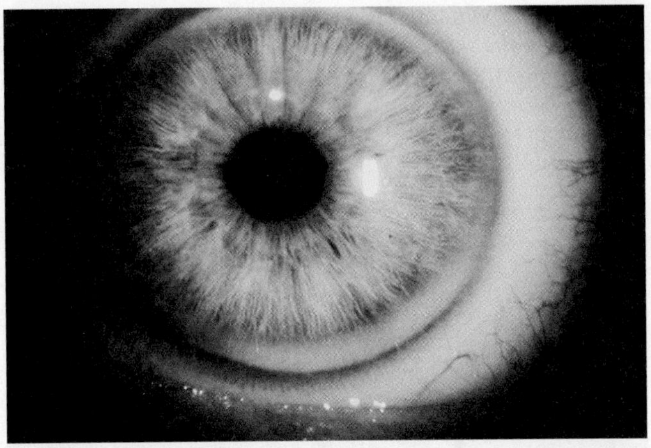

Fig. 26-6 • Arcus senilis of the iris.

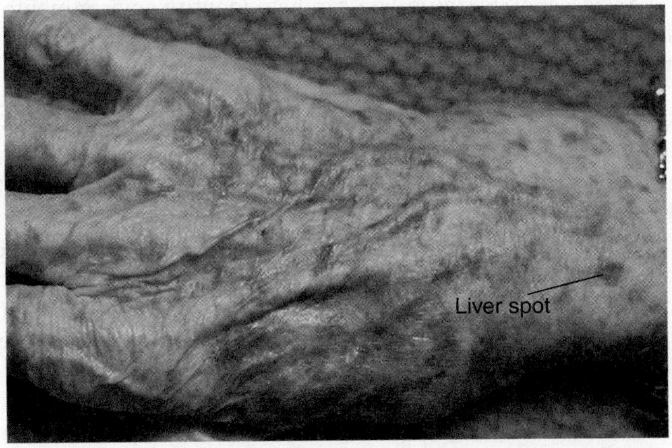
Liver spot

Fig. 26-7 • Paper-thin, transparent skin with actinic lentigo (liver spots).

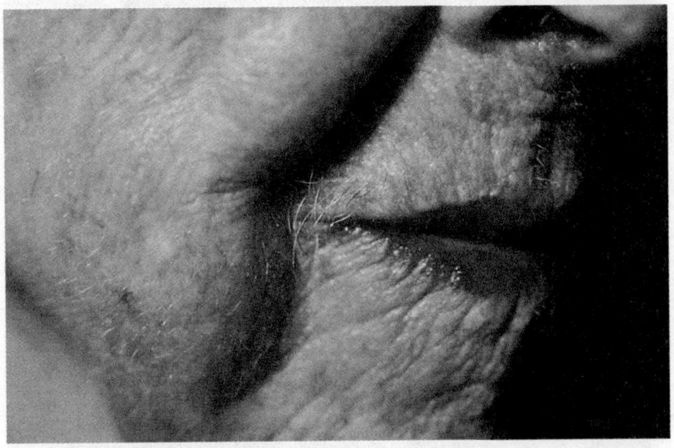

Fig. 26-8 • Wrinkles.

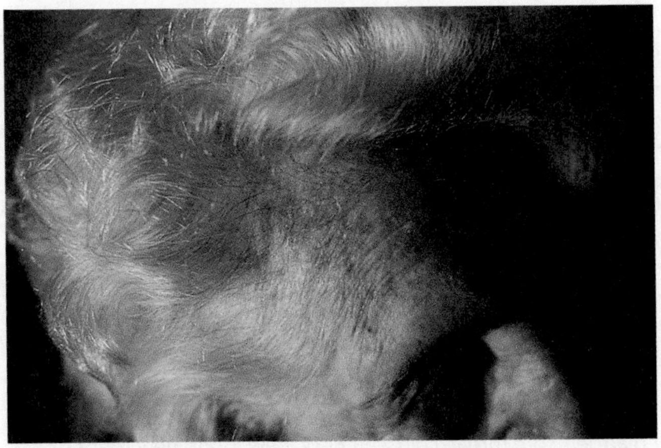

Fig. 26-9 • Graying and thinning of the hair.

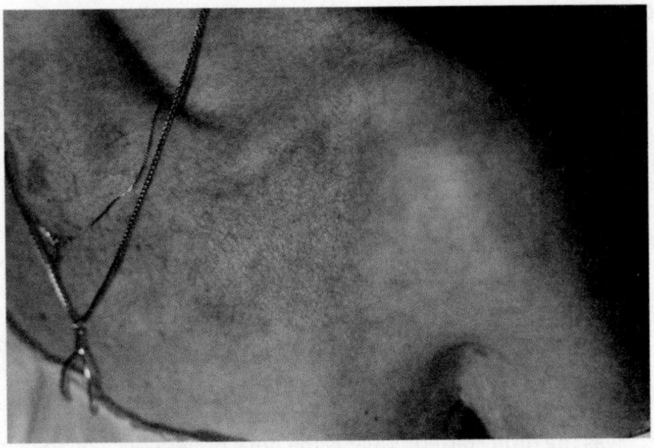

Fig. 26-10 • Xerosis (dry skin).

Individual differences exist in how quickly and to what degree the skin ages. Although genetic background, hormonal changes, and systemic disease may change the appearance of the skin over time, chronic sun exposure is the single most important factor leading to degeneration of the skin components.

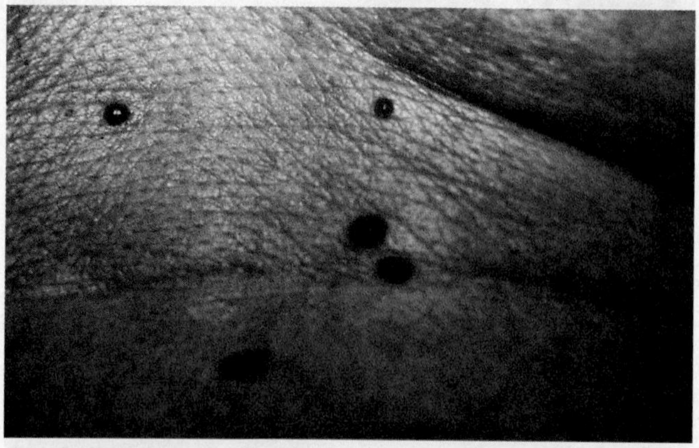

Fig. 26-11 • Senile (cherry) angiomas.

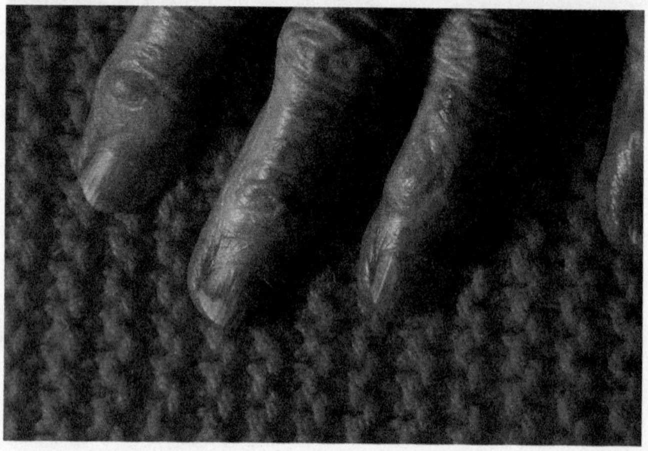

Fig. 26-12 • Nail changes, longitudinal ridges and thickening.

ASSESSMENT METHODS

Patient History

Before examining the skin, take an accurate history from the patient so that actual and potential skin problems can be readily identified. Important data to collect include demographic and socioeconomic information. Chart 26-2 highlights specific questions to ask during a skin assessment.

Demographic data include age, race, occupation, and hobbies or recreational activities. This information can help identify causative or aggravating factors for skin problems. Age is important because many changes in the skin, hair, and nails are normal manifestations of the aging process.

Race and nationality can also be important. Some variations in the appearance of skin are normal among patients of specific races and ethnicities but are abnormal for those of other races or ethnicities.

Information about occupation and hobbies can provide clues to chronic skin exposure to chemicals, irritants, abrasive substances, and other environmental factors that can contribute to skin problems.

Socioeconomic status data can help identify environmental factors that might contribute to skin disease. Recent travel may be a source of skin infections or unusual lesions.

If the patient is well tanned, ask about the amount of time spent in the sun and tanning booths and whether he or she has any skin problems from sun exposure. Use this time to teach the patient about the harmful aspects of sun exposure and how to reduce sun exposure.

Skin problems related to poor hygiene are common. Ask about living conditions, bathing practices, and the availability of running water. Teach people that keeping the skin and hair clean by bathing and shampooing regularly helps maintain the skin's health.

Drug use is important to obtain because prescribed drugs, over-the-counter (OTC) drugs, and herbal preparations or remedies can cause allergies or skin reactions or affect skin function. Ask the patient about any recent use of prescription drugs, OTC drugs (e.g., laxatives, antacids, cold remedies), and herbal preparations or remedies. Determine when each

Chart 26-2 BEST PRACTICE FOR PATIENT SAFETY & QUALITY CARE

Obtaining an Accurate Nursing History of the Patient with a Skin Problem

MEDICAL-SURGICAL HISTORY
- Does the patient have any current or previous medical problems?
- Has the patient undergone any recent or previous surgical procedures?

FAMILY HISTORY
- Is there any family tendency toward chronic skin problems?
- Do any members of the immediate family have recent skin problems?

MEDICATION HISTORY
- Is the patient allergic to any systemic or topical drug? If so, have the patient describe the reaction.
- What prescription drugs has the patient taken recently? When was the drug started? What is the dose or frequency of administration? When was the last dose taken?
- What over-the-counter drugs has the patient taken recently? When was the drug started? What is the dose or frequency of administration? When was the last dose taken?

SOCIAL HISTORY
- What is the patient's occupation?
- What recreational activities does the patient enjoy?
- Has the patient traveled recently?
- What is the patient's nutritional status?

CURRENT HEALTH PROBLEM
- When did the patient first notice the skin problem?
- Where on the body did the problem begin?
- Has the problem gotten better or worse?
- Has a similar skin condition ever occurred before? If so, have the patient describe the typical course and how it was treated.
- Is the problem associated with any of the following: itching, burning, stinging, numbness, pain, fever, nausea and vomiting, diarrhea, sore throat, cold, stiff neck, new foods, new soaps or cosmetics, new clothing or bed linens, or stressful situations?
- Does anything seem to make the problem worse (e.g., sun exposure, drugs, heat or cold, menses)?
- Does anything seem to make the problem better?

drug was started, the dose and frequency of the drug, and the time the last dose was taken. Ask the patient whether skin changes began after starting a new drug. A drug history also helps identify skin changes that result from the treatment of other health problems, such as the changes that occur with long-term steroid or anticoagulant therapy.

Allergies can develop to environmental substances and often have skin manifestations. These allergies may be well documented or have a new onset. Ask about the use of any new personal care product (e.g., shaving products, perfumes, soap, shampoo, lotion, makeup, hair gel, toothpaste), laundry detergents and softeners, and home cleaning products. Determine whether the patient wears gloves to avoid direct contact with cleaning solutions. New clothing may contain chemicals (e.g., stiffeners, anti-wrinkle agents, flame retardants) that come into contact with and irritate the skin. Documenting the body location(s) of the skin problem can help determine its cause.

Nutrition History

Document the patient's weight, height, body build, and food preferences. Poor nutrition, especially protein deficiencies, vitamin deficiencies, and obesity, can increase the patient's risk for skin lesions and delay wound healing. Fat-free diets and chronic alcoholism can lead to vitamin deficiencies and related skin changes. Some skin diseases, such as chronic urticaria and acne, may be worsened by certain foods or food additives.

Hydration status influences overall skin health, and the skin can reflect hydration status. Decreased fluid intake can lead to dry skin. Skin manifestations of severe fluid losses are seen as loose skin that easily forms a tent when pinched together. Fluid overload with edema can stretch the skin, masking wrinkles and allowing the formation of skin "pits" when pressure is applied.

Family History and Genetic Risk

Many skin problems (e.g., psoriasis, skin cancer, keloid formation, eczema) have a familial predisposition or can be inherited. Explore any family tendency of chronic skin problems. Ask about immediate family members' current health status to identify a communicable disease that could be transferred among family members (e.g., ringworm, scabies).

Current Health Problems

Chart 26-2 lists the best practices for obtaining a history from a patient with a skin problem. Begin by gathering information about skin changes and current skin care practices.

If a skin problem is identified, obtain more information about the specific problem, such as:

- When did the patient first notice the rash or skin change?
- Where on the body did the rash begin?
- Has the problem improved or become worse?

If a similar problem has occurred before, ask the patient to describe the course of the skin lesion and how it was treated. Try to link the problem with specific symptoms, such as itching, burning, numbness, pain, fever, sore throat, stiff neck, or nausea and vomiting. Ask him or her to identify anything that seems to make the problem better or worse.

Skin Assessment

Inspection

Skin changes may be related to specific skin diseases and may also reflect a systemic disorder. By using skin assessment skills, you are in a unique position to identify clues about a patient's state of health.

A thorough assessment of the skin is best performed with the patient partially or completely undressed. Incorporate skin examination for actual or potential problems into the routine part of daily care while bathing him or her or assisting with hygiene.

Inspect the patient's skin surfaces in a well-lighted room; natural or bright fluorescent lighting enhances the visibility of subtle skin changes. Although no special equipment is needed, use a penlight to closely inspect lesions and to illuminate the mouth.

Assess each skin surface systematically, including the scalp, hair, nails, and mucous membranes. Give particular attention to the skinfold areas. The moist, warm environment of skinfolds can harbor organisms, such as yeast or bacteria. Observe and document these features:

- Obvious changes in color and vascularity
- Presence or absence of moisture
- Edema
- Skin lesions
- Skin integrity

Check the cleanliness of the various body areas to determine whether the patient's self-care activities need to be evaluated.

Skin color is affected by a number of factors, including blood flow, oxygenation, body temperature, and pigment production. The wide variation in natural skin tones may require different techniques for patients who have darker skin. (See Cultural Awareness, pp. 474-476, for suggestions for assessing patients with darker skin.)

Describe changes in skin color by their appearance (Table 26-2). Document changes in color, and describe whether the changes are general or confined to one body region. Color changes can be seen most easily in the areas of least pigmentation, such as the oral mucosa, sclera, nail beds, and palms and soles. Inspect these areas to help confirm more subtle color changes of general body areas.

Lesions in skin disease are clinically described in terms of primary and secondary lesions (Fig. 26-13). **Primary lesions** are an initial reaction to a problem that alters one of the structural components of the skin. **Secondary lesions** are changes in the appearance of the primary lesion. These changes occur with progression of an underlying disease or in response to a topical or systemic therapeutic intervention. For example, acute dermatitis often occurs as primary vesicles with associated **pruritus** (itching). Secondary lesions in the form of crusts occur as the patient scratches, the vesicles are opened, and the exudate dries. With chronic dermatitis, the skin often becomes **lichenified** (thickened) because of the patient's continual rubbing of the area to relieve itching.

Describe lesions by color, size, location, and shape. Note whether they occur as isolated changes or are grouped and form a distinct pattern. Table 26-3 on p. 471 defines terms used to describe lesions.

Assess each lesion for the following ABCD features that are associated with skin cancer:

Asymmetry of shape
Border irregularity
Color variation within one lesion
Diameter greater than 6 mm

A patient who has a lesion with one or more of the ABCD features should be evaluated by a dermatologist or surgeon. Teach patients these signs, and encourage them to perform total skin self-examination (TSSE) on a monthly basis.

TABLE 26-2 Common Alterations in Skin Color

Alteration	Underlying Cause	Location	Significance
White (pallor)	Decreased hemoglobin level Decreased blood flow to the skin (vasoconstriction)	Conjunctivae Mucous membranes Nail beds Palms and soles Lips	Anemia Shock or blood loss Chronic vascular compromise Sudden emotional upset Edema
	Genetically determined defect of the melanocyte (decreased pigmentation)	Generalized	Albinism
	Acquired patchy loss of pigmentation	Localized	Vitiligo, tinea versicolor
Yellow-orange	Increased total serum bilirubin level (jaundice)	Generalized Mucous membranes Sclera	Increased hemolysis of red blood cells Liver disorders
	Increased serum carotene level (carotenemia)	Perioral Palms and soles Ears and nose Absent in sclera and mucous membranes	Increased ingestion of carotene-containing foods (carrots) Pregnancy Thyroid deficiency Diabetes
	Increased urochrome level	Generalized Absent in sclera and mucous membranes	Chronic kidney disease (uremia)
Red (erythema)	Increased blood flow to the skin (vasodilation)	Generalized	Generalized inflammation (e.g., erythroderma)
		Localized (to area of involvement)	Localized inflammation (e.g., sunburn, cellulitis, trauma, rashes)
		Face, cheeks, nose, upper chest Area of exposure	Fever, increased alcohol intake Exposure to cold
Blue	Increase in deoxygenated blood (cyanosis)	Nail beds Mucous membranes Generalized	Cardiopulmonary disease Methemoglobinemia
	Bleeding from vessels into tissue: Petechiae (1-3 mm) Ecchymosis (>3 mm)	 Localized Localized	 Thrombocytopenia Increased blood vessel fragility
Reddish blue	Increased overall amount of hemoglobin Decreased peripheral circulation	Generalized Distal extremities, nose	Polycythemia vera Inadequate tissue perfusion
Brown	Increased melanin production	Localized (to area of involvement) Pressure points, areolae, palmar creases, and genitalia Face, areolae, vulva, linea nigra	Chronic inflammation Exposure to sunlight Addison's disease Pregnancy; oral contraceptives (melasma)
	Café au lait spots (tan-brown patches) <6 spots >6 spots	 Localized Generalized	 Nonpathogenic Possible neurofibromatosis
	Melanin and hemosiderin deposits (bronze or grayish tan color)	Distal lower extremities Exposed areas or generalized	Chronic venous stasis Hemochromatosis

In describing the location of lesions, determine whether they are generalized or localized. If the lesions are localized, identify the specific body areas involved. This information is important because some diseases have a specific pattern of skin lesions. Involvement of only the sun-exposed areas of the body is important information when a possible cause is being considered. Rashes limited to the skinfold areas (e.g., on the axillae, beneath the breasts, in the groin) may reflect problems related to friction, heat, and excessive moisture.

Edema causes the skin to appear shiny, **taut** (tightly stretched), and paler than uninvolved skin. During skin inspection, document the location, distribution, and color of any areas of edema.

Skin elasticity is also affected by edema. Using moderate pressure, place the tip of the index finger against edematous tissue to determine the degree of indentation, or pitting (see Chapter 13).

Moisture content is assessed by noting the thickness and consistency of secretions. Normally, increased moisture in the

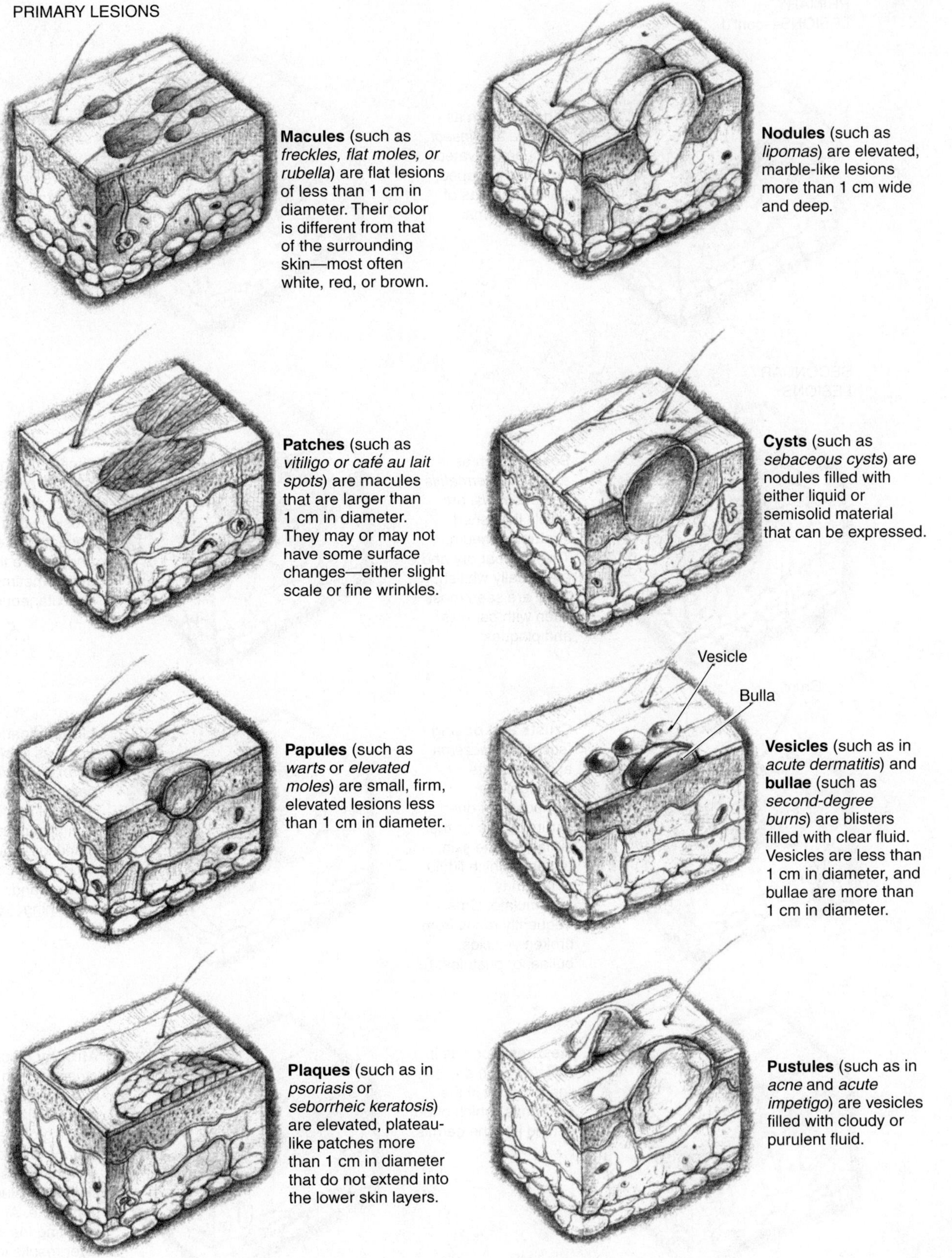
PRIMARY LESIONS
Macules (such as *freckles, flat moles, or rubella*) are flat lesions of less than 1 cm in diameter. Their color is different from that of the surrounding skin—most often white, red, or brown.
Nodules (such as *lipomas*) are elevated, marble-like lesions more than 1 cm wide and deep.
Patches (such as *vitiligo or café au lait spots*) are macules that are larger than 1 cm in diameter. They may or may not have some surface changes—either slight scale or fine wrinkles.
Cysts (such as *sebaceous cysts*) are nodules filled with either liquid or semisolid material that can be expressed.
Vesicle
Bulla
Papules (such as *warts* or *elevated moles*) are small, firm, elevated lesions less than 1 cm in diameter.
Vesicles (such as in *acute dermatitis*) and **bullae** (such as *second-degree burns*) are blisters filled with clear fluid. Vesicles are less than 1 cm in diameter, and bullae are more than 1 cm in diameter.
Plaques (such as in *psoriasis* or *seborrheic keratosis*) are elevated, plateau-like patches more than 1 cm in diameter that do not extend into the lower skin layers.
Pustules (such as in *acne* and *acute impetigo*) are vesicles filled with cloudy or purulent fluid.

Fig. 26-13 • Classification of skin lesions.

Continued

PRIMARY LESIONS—cont'd

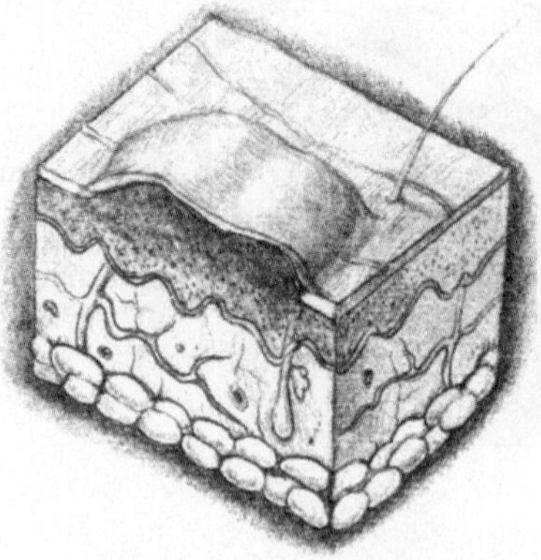

Wheals (such as *urticaria* and *insect bites*) are elevated, irregularly shaped, transient areas of dermal edema.

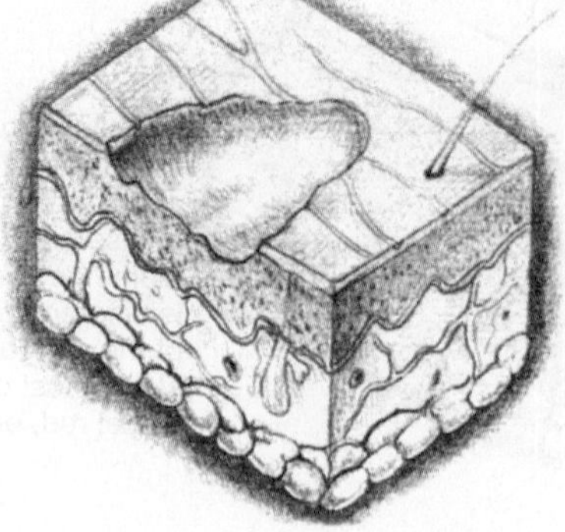

Erosions (such as in *varicella*) are wider than fissures but involve only the epidermis. They are often associated with vesicles, bullae, or pustules.

SECONDARY LESIONS

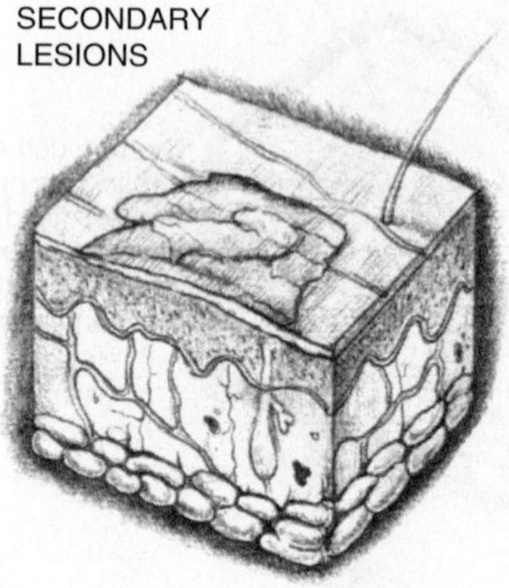

Scales (such as in *exfoliative dermatitis* and *psoriasis*) are visibly thickened stratum corneum. They appear dry and are usually whitish. They are seen most often with papules and plaques.

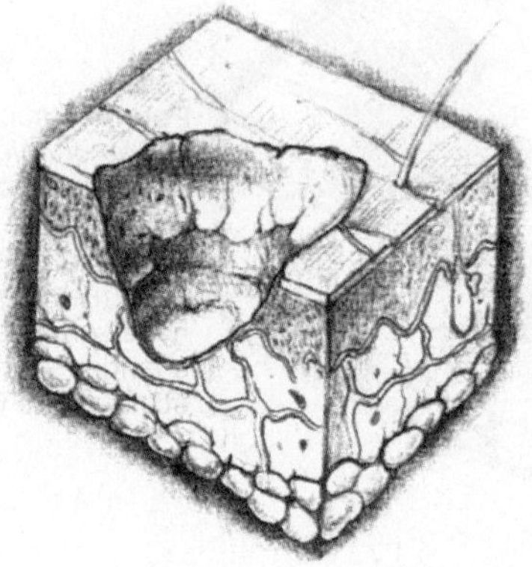

Ulcers (such as *stage 3 pressure sores*) are deep erosions that extend beneath the epidermis and involve the dermis and sometimes the subcutaneous fat.

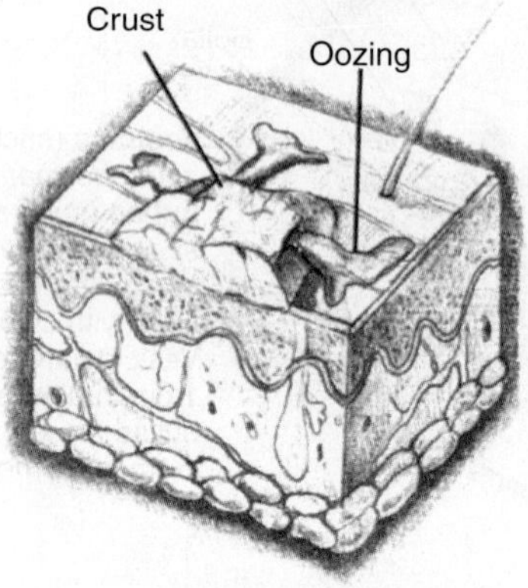
Crust
Oozing

Crusts and oozing (such as in *eczema* and *late-stage impetigo*) are composed of dried serum or pus on the surface of the skin, beneath which liquid debris may accumulate. Crusts frequently result from broken vesicles, bullae, or pustules.

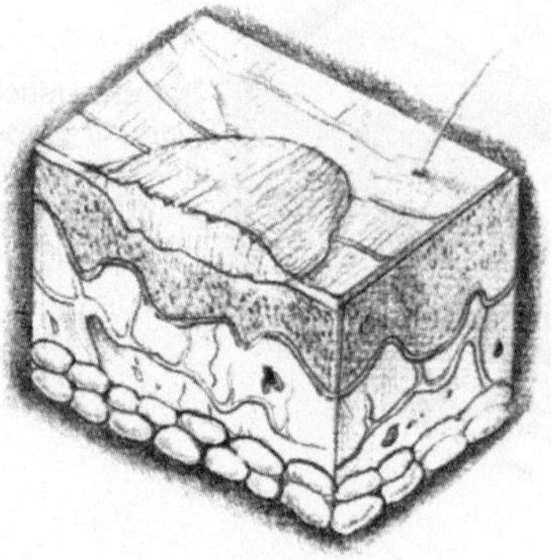

Lichenifications (such as in *chronic dermatitis*) are palpably thickened areas of epidermis with accentuated skin markings. They are caused by chronic rubbing and scratching.

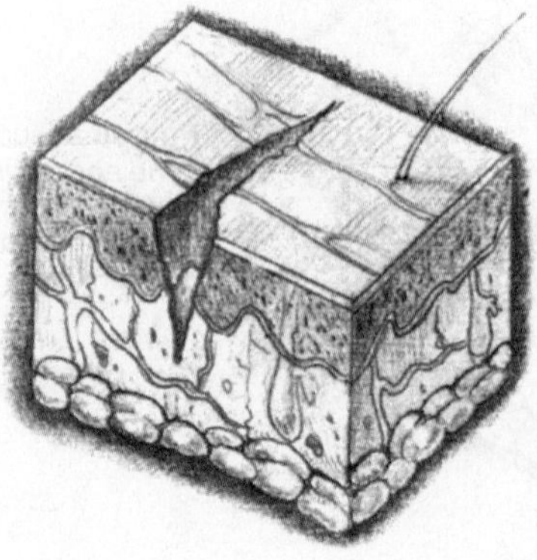

Fissures (such as in *athlete's foot*) are linear cracks in the epidermis, which often extend into the dermis.

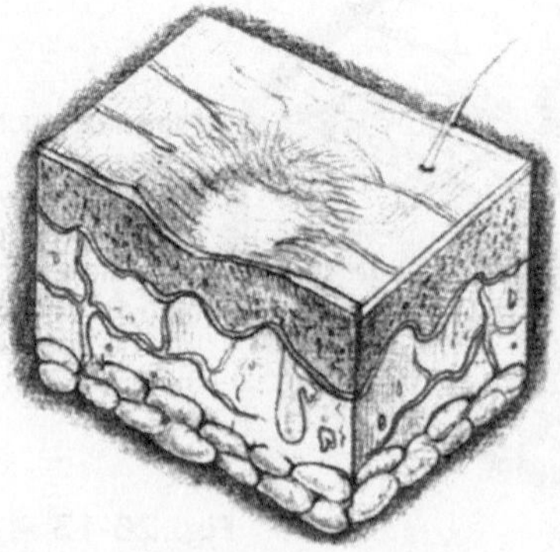

Atrophy (such as *striae* [stretch marks] and *aged skin*) is characterized by thinning of the skin surface with loss of skin markings. The skin is translucent and paper-like. Atrophy involving the dermal layer results in skin depression.

Fig. 26-13, cont'd • Classification of skin lesions.

TABLE 26-3 Terms Commonly Used to Describe Skin Lesion Configurations

annular Ringlike with raised borders around flat, clear centers of normal skin
circinate Circular
circumscribed Well-defined with sharp borders
clustered Several lesions grouped together
coalesced Lesions that merge with one another and appear confluent
diffuse Widespread, involving most of the body with intervening areas of normal skin; generalized
linear Occurring in a straight line
serpiginous With wavy borders, resembling a snake
universal All areas of the body involved, with no areas of normal-appearing skin

form of sweat occurs with increased activity or elevated environmental temperatures. Dampness of skinfold areas occurs as a result of decreased air circulation where the skin surfaces touch. Excess moisture can cause skin breakdown in bedridden and debilitated patients.

Overly dry skin can be caused by factors such as a dry environment, poor skin lubrication, inadequate fluid intake, and the normal processes of aging. Dry skin usually has scaling of the outer surface. Dry skin may be especially marked in areas of limited circulation, such as the feet and lower legs. It is a problem for most adults during the winter months when the air contains less moisture, living in geographic areas with little humidity, and in the hospital environment where humidity is often low.

Vascular changes or markings are classified as normal or abnormal, depending on the cause. Normal vascular markings include birthmarks, cherry angiomas (see Fig. 26-11), spider angiomas, and venous stars. Bleeding into the tissue is abnormal and results in **purpuric lesions** (bleeding under the skin that may progress from red to purple to brownish yellow), petechiae, and ecchymoses.

Petechiae are small, reddish purple lesions (<0.5 mm in diameter) that do not fade or blanch when pressure is applied (Fig. 26-14). They often indicate increased capillary fragility. Petechiae of the lower extremities often occur with stasis dermatitis, a condition frequently seen in patients who have chronic venous insufficiency.

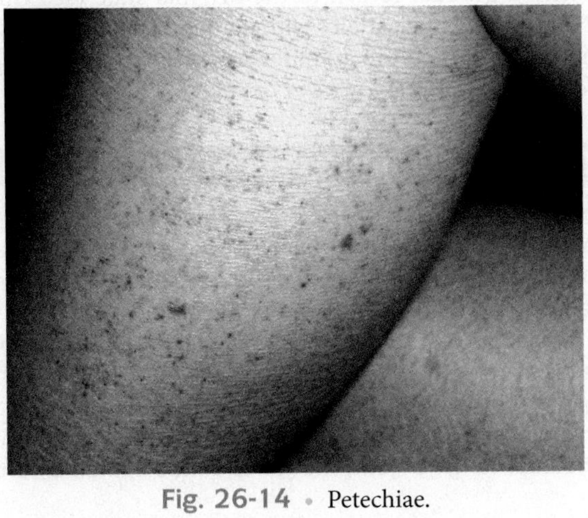

Fig. 26-14 • Petechiae.

Ecchymoses (bruises) are larger areas of hemorrhage that range in size from several millimeters to many centimeters. In older adults, bruising is common after minor trauma to the skin, especially on sun-exposed areas of the body. Certain drugs (e.g., aspirin, warfarin, corticosteroids) and low platelet counts lead to easy or excessive bruising. Anticoagulants and decreased numbers of platelets disrupt clotting action, resulting in ecchymosis.

Integrity of the skin is assessed by first thoroughly examining areas with actual breaks or open areas. For example, skin tears are a common finding in older people as a result of a flattening of the dermal-epidermal junction with aging. The thin, fragile skin is easily damaged by friction or shearing forces, especially if bruising is already present. Look for skin tears in these areas:

- Where constricting clothing rubs against the skin
- On the upper extremities, where the skin is grasped when assisting a patient to ambulate or change position
- Where adhesive tapes or dressings have been applied and removed

Check for the presence of multiple abrasions or early pressure-related skin changes. These findings may indicate previously unrecognized problems in mobility or sensory perception.

Describe breaks in skin integrity by their location, size, color, and distribution, as well as by the presence of drainage or any signs of infection. The evaluation of partial-thickness and full-thickness wounds, including objective criteria that describe progress toward healing, is discussed in Chapter 27.

Cleanliness of the skin is evaluated to gain information about self-care needs. Inspect the hair, nails, and skin closely for excessive soiling and offensive odor. Depending on a patient's degree of self-care deficit, hard-to-reach areas (e.g., perirectal and inguinal skinfolds, axillae, feet) may be less clean than other skin surface areas. Skin can be clean but stained as a result of exposure to chemicals during work or leisure activities.

Patients who have cognitive problems may not pay attention to hygiene measures. Assess the cognitive function of any patient whose hygiene of the skin, hair, or nails appears inadequate.

Tattoos and piercings can cause or mask skin problems and should be carefully examined. Bruises and rashes can occur in tattooed areas but may be difficult to see. Examine newly pierced areas for signs of inflammation or infection. Scars may be present in old tattoos or pierced areas and should be documented. Any areas where tattoos have been removed should be examined for skin changes that may indicate cancer.

Palpation

Skin inspection alone can be misleading, especially in areas of color changes, tattoos, and piercings. Use palpation to gather additional information about skin lesions, moisture, temperature, texture, and turgor (Table 26-4). Wash hands thoroughly before and after palpating a patient's skin. Use gloves to examine nonintact skin, and use Standard Precautions when skin areas are draining.

Palpation confirms the size of the lesions and determines whether they are flat or slightly raised. The consistency of larger lesions can vary from soft and pliable to firm and solid. Subtle changes, such as the difference between a fine **macular** (flat)

TABLE 26-4 Common Clinical Findings in Skin Palpation

Clinical Findings	Cause	Location	Examples of Predisposing Conditions
EDEMA			
Localized	Inflammatory response	Area of injury or involvement	Trauma
Dependent or pitting	Fluid and electrolyte imbalance	Ambulatory: dorsum of foot and medial ankle	Congestive heart failure Renal disease
	Venous and cardiac insufficiency	Bedridden: buttocks, sacrum, and lower back	Hepatic cirrhosis Venous thrombosis or stasis
Nonpitting	Endocrine imbalance	Generalized, but more easily seen over the tibia	Hypothyroidism (myxedema)
MOISTURE			
Increased	Autonomic nervous system stimulation	Face, axillae, skinfolds, palms, and soles	Fever, anxiety, activity Hyperthyroidism
Decreased	Dehydration Endocrine imbalance	Buccal mucous membranes with progressive involvement of other skin surfaces	Fluid loss Postmenopausal status Hypothyroidism Normal aging
TEMPERATURE			
Increased	Increased blood flow to the skin	Generalized Localized	Fever, hypermetabolic states Inflammation
Decreased	Decreased blood flow to the skin	Generalized	Impending shock, sepsis, anxiety Hypothyroidism
		Localized	Interference with vascular flow
TURGOR			
Decreased	Decreased elasticity of the dermis (tenting when pinched)	Abdomen, forehead, or radial aspect of the wrist	Severe dehydration Sudden, severe weight loss Normal aging
TEXTURE			
Roughness or thickness	Irritation, friction	Pressure points (e.g., soles, palms, elbows)	Calluses Chronic eczema Atopic skin diseases
	Sun damage	Areas of sun exposure	Normal aging
	Excessive collagen production	Localized or generalized	Scleroderma Keloids
Softness or smoothness	Endocrine disturbances	Generalized	Hyperthyroidism

rash and a **papular** (raised) rash, may best be determined by palpating with your eyes closed. Ask the patient whether he or she has pain or tenderness during palpation of the skin.

In areas of excess dryness, rub your finger against the skin surface to determine the degree of flaking or scaling. Both generalized and localized changes in skin temperature can be detected by placing the back of a hand on the skin surface. Before assessing for changes in skin temperature, make certain to have warm hands. Cold hands interfere with accurate assessment and are uncomfortable for the patient.

Palpate skin surfaces to assess texture, which differs according to body region and exposure to environmental irritants. For example, areas of long-term sun exposure have a rougher texture than that of protected skin surfaces. The patient whose occupation requires repeated exposure to harsh soaps or chemicals may show skin changes related to this exposure. Increased skin thickness from scarring, lichenification, or edema usually decreases elasticity.

Turgor indicates the amount of skin elasticity. Skin turgor can be altered by a number of factors, including water content and aging. Gently pinch the patient's skin between your thumb and forefinger, and then release. If skin turgor is normal, the skin immediately returns to its original state when released. Poor skin turgor is evidenced by "tenting" of the skin, with a gradual return to the original state (see Chapter 13). Normal loss of elasticity with aging makes the assessment of skin turgor difficult in an older patient. *Assess skin turgor of an older patient on the forehead or chest.*

DECISION-MAKING CHALLENGE
Coordination of Care

You are examining a new resident of an assisted living facility who arrived the evening before. The resident is an 84-year-old woman who is 5 feet tall and weighs 106 pounds. She had a heart valve replaced 2 years ago and has been taking warfarin (Coumadin) ever since. In addition, she takes levothyroxine (Synthroid) for mild hypothyroidism and omeprazole (Prilosec) for gastroesophageal reflux disease (GERD). Her mobility is good although her shoulder range of joint motion is a little limited by arthritis (she cannot raise her arms above her head). You notice that the resident has numerous petechiae on her left arm from 6 inches below the shoulder all the way down to her fingertips. When asked about this, the resident responds that "those spots showed up right after my blood pressure was taken yesterday, but they don't hurt or itch."

1. Where else should you look for petechiae?
2. What other questions should you ask?
3. Is the fact that the petechiae appeared following blood pressure measurement important? Why or why not?
4. Are any of her prescribed drugs relevant to this finding?
5. What is the most likely cause for the petechiae?
6. Should the resident's health care provider be notified, or is documentation of the assessment finding sufficient? (Provide a rationale for your response.)

evolve For suggested answer guidelines, go to http://evolve.elsevier.com/Iggy/.

Hair Assessment

During the skin assessment, inspect and palpate the hair for cleanliness, distribution, quantity, and quality. Hair is normally found in an even distribution over most of the body surfaces, with the hair on the scalp, in the pubic region, and in the axillary folds thicker and coarser than hair on the trunk, arms, and legs. Although color and growth patterns vary, sudden or marked changes in hair characteristics may reflect an underlying disease process. As with skin changes, check any abnormal findings by obtaining an in-depth history of the circumstances surrounding any change.

How well the hair is groomed, including the cleanliness of areas of thicker hair growth, can confirm information already gathered about a patient's social history and health care needs. If the patient has intense itching or scratches continually, examine the scalp and pubis for lice and **nits** (lice eggs). Inspect the scalp for scaling, redness, open areas, crusting, and tenderness.

Dandruff, a collection of patchy or diffuse white or gray scales on the surface of the scalp, is common. The flaking that occurs with dandruff causes many people to mistakenly think the scalp is too dry; however, it is a problem of excessive oil production. Dandruff is mainly a cosmetic problem, but a very oily scalp can induce inflammatory changes with redness and itching. Severe inflammatory dandruff can extend to the eyebrows and the skin of the face and neck. *If severe dandruff is not treated, hair loss can occur.* Teach the patient that dandruff is not caused by dryness and should be treated to prevent hair loss.

Although gradual hair loss occurs with aging, sudden asymmetric or patchy hair loss at any age is of concern. Assess the scalp for distribution and thickness of the hair, and document variations. Body hair loss, especially on the feet or lower legs, may occur as a result of circulatory problems and decreased blood flow to the area.

Hirsutism is excessive growth of body hair or hair growth in abnormal body areas. Increased hair growth across the face and chest in women is a sign of hirsutism. Hirsutism may occur on the face of a woman as part of aging, is one manifestation of hormonal imbalance, and can also occur as a side effect of drug therapy. If hirsutism is present, look for changes in fat distribution and capillary fragility, which can occur in Cushing's disease, and for clitoral enlargement and deepening of the voice, which may indicate ovarian dysfunction.

Nail Assessment

Dystrophic (abnormal) nails may occur with a serious systemic illness or local skin disease involving the epidermal keratinocytes. Assess the fingernails and toenails for color, shape, thickness, texture, and the presence of lesions.

Many variations in color, texture, and grooming of the nails are influenced by factors unrelated to disease, such as occupation. When assessing the older adult, observe for minor variations associated with the aging process (see Fig. 26-12), such as a gradual thickening of the nail plate, the presence of longitudinal ridges, or a yellowish gray discoloration.

Color of the nail plate depends on nail thickness and transparency, amount of red blood cells, arterial blood flow, and pigment deposits (Table 26-5). Fig. 26-15 shows normal variations in nail color. Changes in color can be caused by chemical damage that occurs with some occupations and with the long-term use of nail polish. Regardless of skin color, the healthy nail blanches (lightens) with pressure.

During examination, the patient's fingers and toes should be free of any surface pressure that interferes with local blood flow or alters the appearance of the digits. To differentiate between color changes from the underlying vascular supply and those resulting from pigment deposition, blanch the nail bed to see whether the color changes with pressure. Do this by gently squeezing the end of the finger or toe, exerting downward pressure on the nail bed, and then releasing the pressure. Color caused by vascular alterations changes as pressure is applied and returns to the original state when pressure is released. Color caused by pigment deposition remains unchanged.

Nail shape changes may be related to systemic disease. For example, fingernail clubbing occurs with impaired gas exchange. (See Fig. 32-10 in Chapter 32.)

Assess nail shape by examining the curve of the nail plate and surrounding soft tissue from all angles. Palpate the fingertips to define areas of sponginess, tenderness, or edema. Table 26-6 describes common variations in nail shape.

Thickness of the nail plate can vary with age, trauma, chronic dermatologic disease, or decreased arterial blood flow. In older patients, look for a "heaped-up" appearance of the toenails, which may occur with fungal infection (onychomycosis).

Consistency of the nail is described as hard, soft, or brittle. Nail plates may become hard, with increased thickening. A warm-water soak or lubrication with petroleum jelly is required to soften the nail plates before they can be trimmed.

Soft nail plates, which are thin and bend easily with pressure, are associated with malnutrition, chronic arthritis, myxedema, and peripheral neuritis.

Brittle nails can split, as in the patient with onychomycosis or advanced psoriasis of the fingers and toes. Splitting of the nail plate is also caused by repeated exposure to water and detergents, which damage the plate over time.

Lesions can occur around, on, within, or under the nail. Separation of the nail plate from the nail bed (onycholysis) creates an air pocket beneath the nail plate. The pocket first appears as a grayish white opacity. The color may change as dirt and keratin collect in the pocket, and the area begins to have a bad odor. This problem is common with fungal infections and after trauma. Separation of the nail plate may also occur with psoriasis or with prolonged chemical contact.

TABLE 26-5 Common Alterations in Nail Color

Alteration	Clinical Findings	Significance
White	Horizontal white banding or areas of opacity Generalized pallor of nail beds	Chronic hepatic or renal disease (hypoalbuminemia) Shock Anemia Early arteriosclerotic changes (toenails) Myocardial infarction
Yellow-brown	Diffuse yellow to brown discoloration	Jaundice Peripheral lymphedema Bacterial or fungal infections of the nail Psoriasis Diabetes Cardiac failure Staining from tobacco, nail polish, or dyes Long-term tetracycline therapy Normal aging (yellow-gray color)
	Vertical brown banding extending from the proximal nail fold distally	Normal finding in dark-skinned patients Nevus or melanoma of nail matrix in light-skinned patients
Red	Thin, dark-red vertical lines 1-3 mm long (splinter hemorrhages)	Bacterial endocarditis Trichinosis Trauma to the nail bed Normal finding in some patients
	Red discoloration of the lunula Dark-red nail beds	Cardiac insufficiency Polycythemia vera
Blue	Diffuse blue discoloration that blanches with pressure	Respiratory failure Methemoglobinuria Venous stasis disease (toenails)

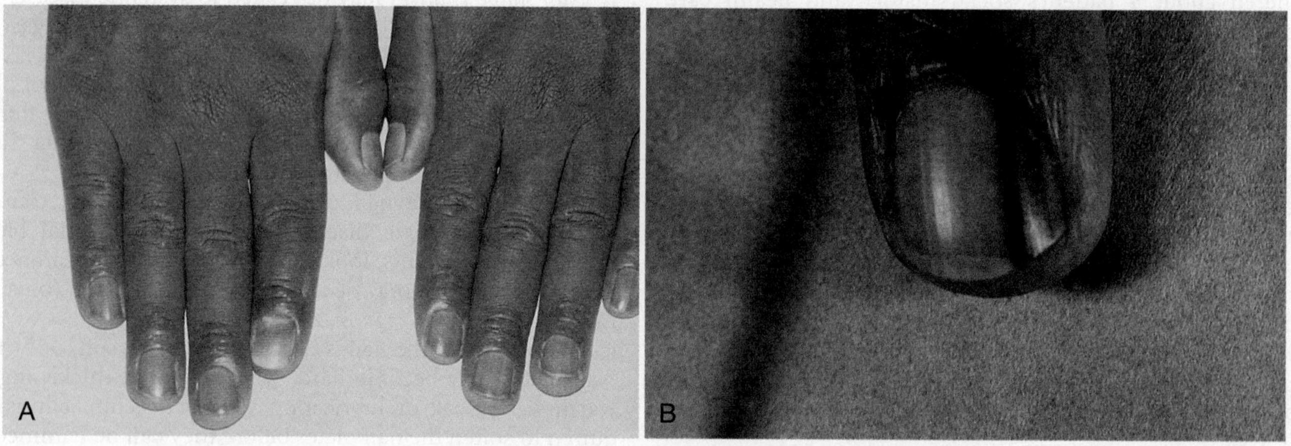
A
B

Fig. 26-15 • **A,** Diffuse nail pigmentation. **B,** Linear nail pigmentation.

Inspect the soft-tissue folds around the nail plate for redness, heat, swelling, and tenderness. **Acute paronychia** (inflammation of the skin around the nail) often occurs with a torn cuticle or an ingrown toenail. If it occurs in an immunocompromised patient, a staphylococcal infection is probable.

Chronic paronychia is more common and is an inflammation that persists for months. People at risk for chronic paronychia are men and women with frequent exposure to water, such as homemakers, bartenders, laundry workers, and nurses.

CULTURAL AWARENESS

Pallor, erythema, cyanosis, and other color changes reflective of the physical state are less visible in patients with naturally dark skin tones. Although physiologic processes are the same for both light-skinned and dark-skinned patients, the amount of skin pigmentation greatly alters how the skin appears in response to physiologic alterations. Consequently, assessment skills to detect the more subtle color changes are needed. Become familiar with the normal appearance of a dark-skinned patient's mucous membranes, nail beds, and skin

TABLE 26-6 Common Variations in Nail Shape

Nail Shape	Clinical Findings		Significance
Normal	Angle of 160 degrees between the nail plate and the proximal nail fold Nail surface slightly convex Nail base firm when palpated	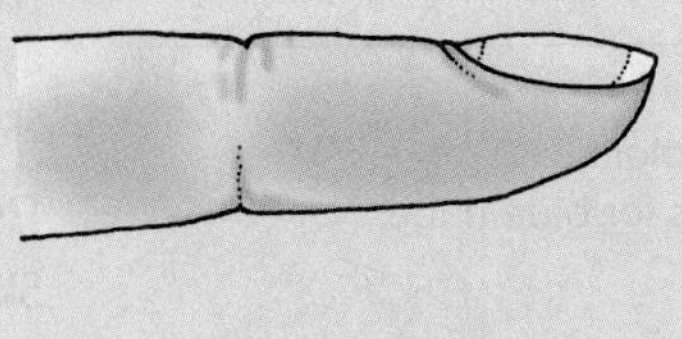	Normal finding
Clubbing			
Early clubbing	Straightening of angle between the nail plate and the proximal nail fold to 180 degrees Nail base spongy when palpated	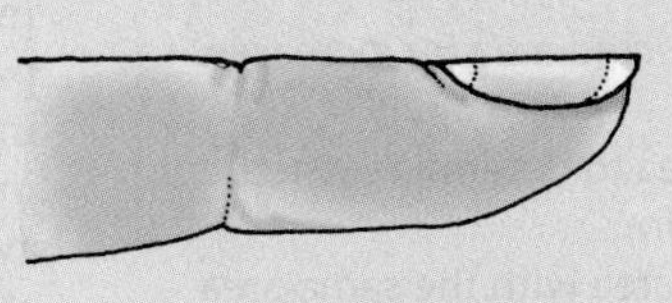	Hypoxia Lung cancer
Late clubbing	Angle between the nail plate and the proximal nail fold exceeds 180 degrees Nail base visibly edematous and spongy when palpated Enlargement of the soft tissue of the fingertips gives a "drumstick" appearance when viewed from above	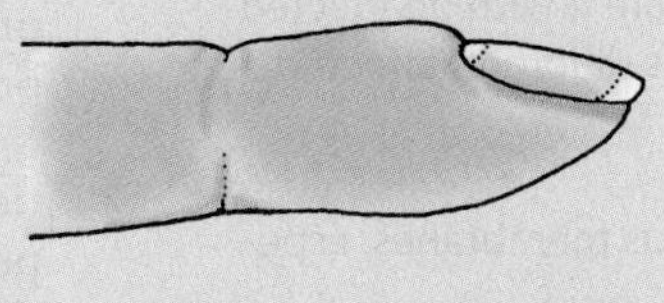	Prolonged hypoxia Emphysema Chronic obstructive pulmonary disease Advanced lung cancer Cystic fibrosis
Spoon nails (koilonychia)			
Early koilonychias	Flattening of the nail plate with an increased smoothness of the nail surface	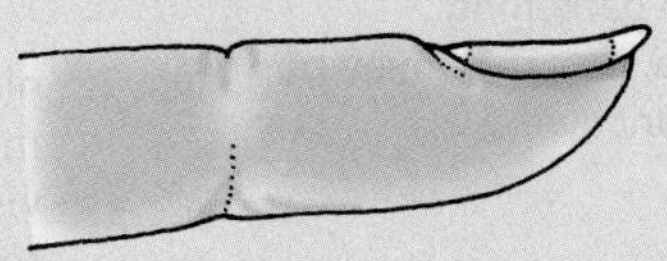	Iron deficiency (with or without anemia) Poorly controlled diabetes >15 yr in duration Local injury Psoriasis Chemical irritants Developmental abnormality
Late koilonychias	Concave curvature of the nail plate		
Beau's grooves	1-mm wide horizontal depressions in the nail plates caused by growth arrest (involves all nails)	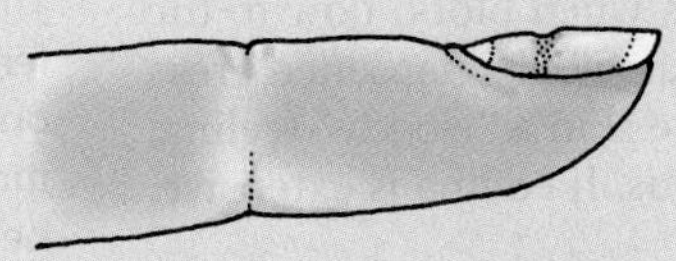	Acute, severe illness Prolonged febrile state Isolated periods of severe malnutrition
Pitting	Small, multiple pits in the nail plate May be associated with plate thickening and onycholysis Most often involves the fingernails (several or all)	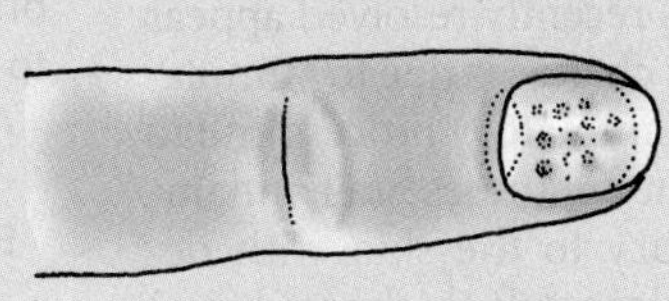	Psoriasis Alopecia areata

tone so that variations from baseline can be identified. Chart 26-3 lists specific assessment techniques for skin manifestations of health problems in people with dark skin.

Skin Assessment Methods for Patients with Dark Skin

Pallor can be detected in people with dark skin by first inspecting the mucous membranes for an ash-gray color. If the lips and the nail beds are not heavily pigmented, they appear paler than normal for that patient. Use good lighting to assess for the absence of the underlying red tones that normally give heavily pigmented skin a healthy glow. With generalized decreased blood flow to the skin, brown skin appears yellow-brown, and very dark brown skin is ash gray.

Cyanosis can be present when gas exchange is impaired. Examine the lips, tongue, nail beds, conjunctivae, and palms and soles for subtle color changes. In a patient with cyanosis, the lips and tongue are gray and the palms, soles, conjunctivae, and nail beds have a bluish tinge. To support these findings, assess for other indicators of hypoxia, including tachycardia, hypotension, changes in respiratory rate, decreased breath sounds, and changes in cognition.

Chart 26-3 **BEST PRACTICE FOR PATIENT SAFETY & QUALITY CARE**

Assessing Changes in Dark Skin

CYANOSIS
- Examine lips and tongue for gray color.
- Examine nail beds, palms, and soles for blue tinge.
- Examine conjunctiva for pallor.

INFLAMMATION
- Compare affected area with nonaffected area for increased warmth.
- Examine the skin of the affected area to determine whether it is shiny or taut or pits with pressure.
- Compare the skin color of affected area with the same area on the opposite side of the body.
- Palpate the affected area and compare it with unaffected area to determine whether texture is different (affected area may feel hard or "woody").

JAUNDICE
- Check for yellow tinge to oral mucous membranes, especially the hard palate.
- Examine the sclera nearest to the iris rather than the corners of the eye.

BLEEDING
- Compare the affected area with the same area on the unaffected body side for swelling or skin darkening.
- If the patient has thrombocytopenia, petechiae may be present on the oral mucosa or conjunctiva.

Inflammation in dark-skinned patients appears as excessive warmth and changes in skin consistency or texture. Use the back of your hand to palpate areas of suspected inflammation for the increased warmth that occurs when blood flow to the skin increases. With the fingertips, palpate for hardened areas deep in the tissue, which may give the skin a "woody" feeling. Inflamed skin is tender and edematous. If edema is extensive, the skin is taut and shiny.

Skin areas where inflammation has recently resolved appear *darker* than the normal skin tone. This change is due to stimulation of the melanocytes during the inflammatory process and to the increased pigment production that continues after inflammation subsides. More extensive injury to the skin with destruction of melanocytes (e.g., deep ulcer, full-thickness burn) may heal with color changes that are *lighter* than the normal skin tone. Unlike acute changes, chronic inflammatory changes are not tender. If scar tissue is present, the skin may feel less supple, especially over the joints. If chronic inflammatory changes are suspected, ask the patient about a history of skin problems in that area of the body.

Jaundice in a patient with dark skin is best assessed by inspecting the oral mucosa, especially the hard palate, for yellow discoloration. Inspection of the conjunctivae and adjacent sclera may be misleading because normal deposits of fat produce a yellowish hue that is visible in contrast to the dark skin around the eyes. Examine the sclera closest to the cornea for a more accurate determination of jaundice. The palms and soles of dark-skinned patients may appear yellow if they are calloused; a callus should not be mistaken for jaundice.

Skin bleeding with purpuric lesions may not be visible in areas of deep pigmentation. Areas of ecchymoses appear darker than normal skin; they may be tender and easily palpable, depending on whether hematoma is present. In most cases, the patient relates a history of trauma to the area that confirms the assessment. Petechiae are rarely visible in dark skin and may be seen only in the oral mucosa and conjunctiva.

Psychosocial Assessment

Skin changes, especially when the face, hair, and hands are involved, often affect a person's body image. Encourage the patient to express his or her feelings about a change in body image or appearance. Assess his or her body language for clues indicating a disturbance in self-concept. For example, the avoidance of eye contact or the use of garments to cover the affected areas communicates concern about physical appearance. Patients with chronic skin diseases often relate a history of social isolation related to a fear of rejection by others or a belief that the skin problem is contagious.

Skin changes linked to poor hygiene are common in patients from low socioeconomic backgrounds, among homeless people, and among those who have reduced cognitive functioning. Assess the patient's overall appearance for excessive soiling, matted hair, body odor, or other self-care deficits. Confirm unsanitary living conditions by obtaining a social history. Patients may relate similar skin problems among family members, friends, and sexual contacts.

If skin problems related to poor hygiene are identified in older patients, also evaluate any physical limitations that might contribute to poor health maintenance. For example, visual or mobility problems can make it difficult for them to see or reach skin surfaces to clean them.

NCLEX EXAMINATION CHALLENGE

The client is a 33-year-old man who is in traction for a fractured femur. The nurse notes that he has significant dandruff and asks one of the UAP to include hair-washing along with the usual morning care. The UAP reports that the client refuses the shampoo because he is afraid that washing his hair will make his scalp even drier and increase the dandruff. What is the nurse's best response to educate UAP and the client?

A. "Even though those flakes look like dry skin, dandruff is a result of excessive oil production."
B. "Use a shampoo for dry hair and do not use the hair dryer to avoid making the problem worse."
C. "I will ask the health care provider to request that a dermatologist be consulted about this problem."
D. "The client has the right to refuse this care, but tell him that his dandruff can be spread to another person."

evolve For the correct answer, go to http://evolve.elsevier.com/Iggy/.

Diagnostic Assessment

Laboratory Assessment

When a fungal, bacterial, or viral pathogen is suspected as the cause of certain skin changes, confirmation by microscopic examination is necessary. *Always wear gloves (use Standard Precautions) when examining skin that is not intact.*

Cultures for fungal infection are obtained when superficial fungal infections are suspected. Using a tongue blade, gently scrape scales from the skin lesions into a clean container and send to the laboratory for culture. Collect fingernail clippings and hair in a similar manner. Unfortunately, waiting for culture results can delay treatment of a superficial fungal infection. For this reason, the specimen is also treated with a potassium hydroxide (KOH) preparation and examined microscopically. Fungal infections show branched hyphae when viewed under a microscope after treatment with KOH. A positive KOH test often eliminates the need for a culture.

For deeper fungal infections, a piece of tissue is obtained for culture. The physician obtains the specimen by punch biopsy (see below in the Skin Biopsy section). When a specimen is needed for cell analysis and special fungal stains, either two specimens are obtained or one specimen is divided before being sent to the laboratory.

Cultures for bacterial infection are obtained from intact primary lesions (bullae, vesicles, or pustules), if possible. Express material from the lesion, collect it with a cotton-tipped applicator, and place the material in a bacterial culture medium specified by the laboratory. For intact lesions, **unroofing** (lifting or puncturing of the outer surface) may be needed using a sterile small-gauge needle before the material can be easily expressed. If crusts are present, remove the crusts with normal saline and swab the underlying exudate.

A biopsy of deep bacterial infections may be required to obtain a specimen for culture. If bacterial cellulitis is suspected, the physician or advanced practice nurse can inject nonbacteriostatic saline deep into the tissue and then aspirate it back; the aspirant is sent for culture.

Cultures for viral infection are indicated if a herpes virus infection is suspected. A cotton-tipped applicator is used to obtain vesicle fluid from intact lesions. Unlike bacterial and fungal specimens, which can remain at room temperature until being transported to the laboratory, viral culture tubes are placed on ice immediately after the specimens are obtained and are transported to the laboratory as soon as possible.

Other Diagnostic Assessment

Other tests for diagnosis of skin problems include biopsy, special noninvasive examination techniques, and skin testing for allergy (discussed in Chapter 27).

Skin Biopsy

A small piece of skin tissue may be obtained for diagnosis or to assess the effectiveness of an intervention. Check with the physician to determine the number, location, and type of skin biopsies to be performed. Depending on the size, depth, and location of the skin changes, the physician may perform a punch biopsy, shave biopsy, or scalpel excision (excisional biopsy).

Punch biopsy is the most common technique. A small, circular, cutting instrument, or "punch," ranging in diameter from 2 to 6 mm, is used. After the site is injected with a local anesthetic, a small plug of tissue is cut and removed. The site may be closed with one or two sutures if it is on the face or leg. Some physicians allow the biopsy site to heal without suturing.

Shave biopsies remove only the portion of the skin elevated above the surrounding tissue when injected with a local anesthetic. A scalpel or razor blade is moved parallel to the skin surface to remove the tissue specimen. Shave biopsies are usually indicated for superficial or raised lesions. Suturing is not needed.

Excisional biopsy is rarely used for skin problems. When needed, larger or deeper specimens are obtained by excision with a scalpel. Deep incisions are made and then sutured after the specimen is removed. Unlike punch and shave biopsies, excisional biopsies involve more discomfort for the patient while the site is healing.

Patient Preparation. Explain to the patient what to expect. Emphasize that a biopsy is a minor procedure with few, if any, complications. If a punch or shave biopsy is planned, reassure him or her that scarring is minimal because of the small size of the tissue removed. If an excisional biopsy is planned, tell him or her that a scar similar to that of a healed surgical incision will result.

Procedure. Establish a sterile field, and assemble all needed supplies and instruments. Local anesthesia is provided by local infiltration using a small-gauge (25-gauge) needle to reduce discomfort during injection. Although preparation of the biopsy site differs according to the physician's preference, the skin is simply wiped with alcohol in most cases.

The most uncomfortable time for the patient is during the injection of a local anesthetic agent, which produces a burning or stinging sensation. Reassure the patient that the discomfort will subside as the anesthetic takes effect. Talking the patient through the procedure with a quiet voice, in combination with a gentle touch, has a calming effect.

After removal, tissue specimens for pathologic study are placed in 10% formalin for fixation. Specimens for culture are placed in sterile saline solution. Bleeding of the biopsy site may be controlled by applying a topical hemostatic agent. If topical treatment does not stop the bleeding, suturing may be used.

Follow-up Care. After bleeding is under control and any sutures have been placed, the site is covered with an adhesive bandage or a dry gauze dressing. Instruct the patient to keep the dressing dry and in place for at least 8 hours. Teach the patient to clean the site daily after the dressing is removed. Tap water or saline can be used to remove any dried blood or crusts. An antibiotic ointment may be prescribed to reduce the risk for infection. The biopsy site may be left open unless a covering is preferred for cosmetic reasons or because the site is an area often soiled. Instruct the patient to report any redness or excessive drainage. Sutures are usually removed 7 to 10 days after biopsy.

Wood's Light Examination

A handheld, long-wavelength ultraviolet (black) light or Wood's light is sometimes used during physical examination. Exposure of some skin infections with this light produces a specific color, such as blue-green or red, that can be used to identify the infection. Hypopigmented skin is more prominent when it is viewed under black light, which makes evaluation of pigment changes in light-skinned patients easier. This examination is always carried out in a darkened room and does not cause discomfort.

Diascopy

Diascopy is a noninvasive and painless technique that eliminates erythema caused by increased blood flow to the skin, thereby easing the inspection of skin lesions. A glass slide or lens is pressed down over the area to be examined, blanching the skin and revealing the shape of the lesions.

HUMAN NEEDS ASSESSMENT REVIEW

What should you expect to NOTICE in a patient with adequate protection related to skin function?

Vital Signs
- Body temperature within normal range

Physical Assessment
- Skin intact (no rashes, abnormal lesions, open areas, or drainage)
- Skin color normal (no cyanosis, pallor, jaundice, inflammation, or areas of uneven pigmentation)
- Skin texture normal (no edema, flaking, scaling, or excessive oiliness)
- Oral mucous membrane and nail beds pink
- Fingertips and nails normal-shaped (no clubbing, nail splitting, or increased nail thickness)
- Body hair distributed evenly over the body, no patchy areas of hair loss
- Scalp free from dandruff

Psychological Assessment
- Patient's eye contact good
- No unusual "hiding" of body areas normally visible in public
- Skin, hair, and nails clean

GET READY FOR THE NCLEX EXAMINATION!

Key Points

Review these Key Points for each NCLEX Examination Client Needs Category.

Safe and Effective Care Environment
- Assist all patients with limited mobility to change positions at least every 2 hours.
- Wash your hands before and after touching any skin lesions.
- Use Standard Precautions when providing care to a patient who has areas of nonintact skin.
- Use lift sheets when moving patients with fragile skin.

Health Promotion and Maintenance
- Encourage all patients to reduce sun exposure and exposure to ultraviolet (UV) light.
- Teach patients to examine all skin areas on a monthly basis for new lesions and changes to existing lesions.
- Encourage all patients to bathe, shampoo the hair, and keep fingernails clean and trimmed.
- Teach all patients the ABCD method of evaluating a lesion for melanoma.

Psychosocial Integrity
- Allow the patient the opportunity to express feelings about a change in body image that results from changes in the skin, hair, or nails.
- Explain all procedures, restrictions, drugs, and follow-up care to the patient and family.
- Check the cognitive function of any patient whose hygiene of the skin, hair, and nails appears inadequate.

Physiological Integrity
- Document any known specific allergies that have skin manifestations.
- Keep skinfold areas on patients clean and dry.
- Position patients who are confined to bed in a way that promotes air circulation to skinfold areas.
- Ask any patient who has started taking a newly prescribed or over-the-counter drug whether he or she has noticed any skin changes that occurred since starting the drug.

Additional Study Resources

Go to your Companion CD or Evolve at http://evolve.elsevier.com/Iggy/ for *Self-Assessment Questions for the NCLEX Examination.*

Go to Evolve at http://evolve.elsevier.com/Iggy/ for *Prioritization and Delegation Questions for the NCLEX Examination.*

SELECTED BIBLIOGRAPHY

Asterisk indicates a classic or definitive work on this subject.

American Cancer Society. (2007). *Cancer facts and figures—2007.* Report No. 00-300M–No. 5008.07. Atlanta: Author.

Anderson, J., Langemo, D., Hanson, D., Thompson, P., & Hunter, S. (2007). What you can learn from a comprehensive skin assessment. *Nursing2007, 37*(4), 65-66.

Fletcher, K. (2005). Skin: Geriatric self-learning module. *MEDSURG Nursing, 14*(2), 138-142.

*Gaskin, F.C. (1986). Detection of cyanosis in the person with dark skin. *Journal of the National Black Nurses Association, 1*(1), 52-60.

Greenhalgh, D.G. (2005). Models of wound healing. *Journal of Burn Care and Rehabilitation, 26*(4), 293-305.

Holloway, S., & Jones, V. (2005). The importance of skin care and assessment. *British Journal of Nursing, 14*(22), 1172-1176.

Jarvis, C. (2008). *Physical examination and health assessment* (5th ed.). Philadelphia: Saunders.

Marks, J., & Miller, J. (2006). *Lookingbill and Marks' principles of dermatology* (4th ed.). Philadelphia: Saunders.

McCance, K., & Huether, S. (2006). *Pathophysiology: The biologic basis for disease in adults and children.* (5th ed.). St. Louis: Mosby.

Meiner, S., & Lueckenotte, A. (Eds.). (2006). *Gerontologic nursing* (3rd ed.). St. Louis: Mosby.

Nazarko, L. (2005). Wound care series. Part Two: Carrying out a thorough assessment. *Nursing & Residential Care, 7*(7), 304-306.

Nussbaum, R., McInnes, R., & Willard, H. (2007). *Thompson & Thompson: Genetics in medicine* (7th ed.). Philadelphia: Saunders.

Pagana, K., & Pagana, T. (2006). *Mosby's manual of diagnostic and laboratory tests* (3rd ed.). St. Louis: Mosby.

Pullen, R. (2007). Assessing skin lesions. *Nursing2007, 37*(8), 44-45.

*Stanley, W. (2003). Nailing a key assessment. *Nursing2003, 33*(8), 50-51.

Wickett, R., & Visscher, M. (2006). Structure and function of the epidermal barrier. *American Journal of Infection Control, 34*(10 Suppl. 2), S98-S110.

Care of Patients with Skin Problems

27 CHAPTER

Janice Cuzzell • M. Linda Workman

LEARNING OUTCOMES

For clinical competence and success on the NCLEX Examination, study this chapter with these Learning Outcomes in mind:

Safe and Effective Care Environment

1. Use principles of infection control to prevent transmission when caring for a patient with a skin infection.
2. Supervise skin care delegated to licensed practical nurses/licensed vocational nurses (LPNs/LVNs) or unlicensed assistive personnel (UAP).
3. Teach the patient with mobility problems and the family how to reduce and relieve skin pressure in the home environment.
4. Ensure that the skin of incontinent patients is kept clean and dry.

Health Promotion and Maintenance

5. Use appropriate risk assessment tools to perform a focused skin assessment and re-assessment to determine risk for pressure ulcer development and adequacy of the skin's protective functions.
6. Teach all people how to perform total self–skin examination (TSSE) to monitor for skin cancer.
7. Teach all people ways to reduce risk for skin cancer.
8. Instruct the patient with a skin infection how to avoid spreading the infection.
9. Assess the ability of the patient with a skin problem to reach the affected area and care for the problem.

Psychosocial Integrity

10. Assess the patient's and family's feelings about a chronic skin condition or visible scar.
11. Support the patient and family in coping with changes in skin integrity and appearance.
12. Encourage the patient with a visible wound or other skin problem to participate in the care of the wound.

Physiological Integrity

13. Compare wound healing by first, second, and third intention.
14. Evaluate wounds for size, depth, presence of infection, and indications of healing.
15. Differentiate the manifestations for stage I through stage IV pressure ulcers.
16. Coordinate with the health care team to plan an individualized strategy for pressure ulcer prevention for a specific patient at increased risk.
17. Identify the key features of psoriasis.
18. Coordinate nursing interventions for care of the patient with psoriasis in the community.
19. Identify key features of melanoma and other skin cancers.

Go to your Companion CD or Evolve at http://evolve.elsevier.com/Iggy/ for *Self-Assessment Questions for the NCLEX Examination* keyed to these Learning Outcomes.

As discussed in Chapter 26, the skin plays an important role in meeting the *human need for protection.* Like the wall surrounding a castle, it provides a strong barrier, in this case to invasion by harmful microorganisms. Skin problems are common, they reduce protection to some degree, and often the cause is not known. In addition to direct functions, the skin reflects other body conditions. Thus problems may truly arise in the skin, or they may be a symptom of a systemic disease or injury. Drugs and other interventions for any health problem can trigger a skin response or reaction. Skin problems can interfere with the medical or surgical treatment of other conditions. Age-related changes and problems caused by immobility, chronic disease, debility, and change in immune function increase the older patient's risk for skin damage.

MINOR SKIN IRRITATIONS

DRYNESS

Pathophysiology

Dry skin **(xerosis)** is a common problem, especially in older patients. It is seen as a fine flaking of the stratum corneum (outermost skin layer). The problem is usually worse on the lower legs where blood flow is poorer. Generalized **pruritus** (itching) often occurs with dry skin. In patients with chronic skin conditions, unrelieved itching causes the patient to scratch and rub the skin in an attempt to relieve the intense itching. These actions may result in secondary skin lesions, excoriations, **lichenification** (thickening), and infection.

Xerosis is worse in areas with dry climates and higher altitudes, such as in the southwestern part of the United States. Central heating and air-conditioning reduce the humidity in the air and increase skin dryness. Wind, cold, and sunlight also worsen the problem. Frequent bathing with harsh soap and hot water further dries the skin, especially if moisturizers are not applied after bathing.

Patient-Centered Collaborative Care

Nursing interventions focus on teaching the patient and family how to maintain healthy skin, to rehydrate the skin, and to relieve itching. Chart 27-1 lists practical ways to avoid overdrying the skin. Remind the patient that bathing with moisturizing soaps, oils, and lotions may reduce dryness. Some soaps and body washes, especially those described as "antimicrobial" and those with perfumes and other scents, may make dry skin worse. Using soap only in soiled or skin-fold areas can also reduce dryness. A 20-minute soak in a warm bath, followed by application of an emollient cream or lotion, can rehydrate the skin and reduce itching. If the patient cannot take a tub bath, teach him or her to wrap the trunk and extremities in warm, moist towels covered by plastic sheeting or a clean garbage bag for 15 to 20 minutes. Skin creams or lotions are more effective when applied to slightly damp skin within 2 to 3 minutes after bathing.

Chart 27-1 PATIENT AND FAMILY EDUCATION GUIDE

Prevention of Dry Skin

- Use a room humidifier during the winter months or whenever the furnace is in use.
- Take a complete bath or shower only every other day (wash face, axillae, perineum, and any soiled areas with soap daily).
- Use tepid water.
- Use a superfatted, nonalkaline soap instead of deodorant soap.
- Rinse the soap thoroughly from your skin.
- If you like bath oil, add the oil to the water at the end of the bath.
- Take care to avoid falls; oil makes the tub slippery.
- Pat rather than rub skin surfaces dry.
- Avoid clothing that continuously rubs the skin, such as tight belts, nylon stockings, or pantyhose.
- Maintain a daily fluid intake of 3000 mL unless contraindicated for another medical condition.
- Do not apply rubbing alcohol, astringents, or other drying agents to the skin.
- Avoid caffeine and alcohol ingestion.

Inform patients that, contrary to popular belief, the cream or lotion is *not* what makes the skin soft and supple. Water is the agent that softens the outer skin layers. Lubricating creams and lotions seal in the moisture provided by water, promoting suppleness and preventing flaking. Some skin lotions are **hydrophilic** (water seeking) and actually draw moisture from the skin, making the dryness worse if they are not applied directly to damp skin.

PRURITUS

Pathophysiology

Pruritus, or itching, is a distressing symptom that may or may not occur with skin disease. It is caused by stimulation of itch-specific nerve fibers at the dermal-epidermal junction. Physical or chemical agents either act directly on these nerve fibers or activate chemical mediators, such as histamine, which then act on the itch receptors.

Itching is a subjective symptom similar to pain. Thus the sensation varies among patients in location and severity. Regardless of the underlying cause, patients usually report that itching is worse at night when there are fewer distractions. Other conditions that make itching worse include poor skin hydration, increased skin temperature, perspiration, and emotional stress.

Patient-Centered Collaborative Care

The priority nursing interventions focus on increasing patient comfort and preventing skin injury. Patients usually try to relieve itching by scratching or rubbing the skin, a response that further stimulates the itch receptors and causes a pattern referred to as the **"itch-scratch-itch" cycle.** When the skin lesions are present with itching, relief can usually be obtained by treatment of the underlying skin disorder with topical or systemic drugs. Systemic diseases, such as liver and venous disorders, can also cause itching without skin lesions. Liver disease often increases the buildup of bilirubin in the skin, which causes itching. Both too little blood flow and too much blood flow to an area (especially the feet and legs) can lead to itching.

Plan care to promote comfort and prevent disruption of skin integrity that can result from vigorous scratching. Because dry skin worsens itching, emphasize proper bathing and skin moisturizing techniques (see Chart 27-1). Encourage patients to keep the fingernails trimmed short, with rough edges filed, to reduce skin damage. Tell patients that wearing mittens or splints at night can help prevent inadvertent scratching during sleep. If the patient cannot perform self-care, teach the family (for home care) and unlicensed assistive personnel (UAP) to trim fingernails and apply mittens or gloves. As always, stress caution not to break the skin or dig into nail corners when trimming the nails of a patient with diabetes.

A cool sleeping environment along with comfort measures such as a cool shower and application of moisturizers may help promote sleep. Additional measures such as using sleep-promoting herbal teas or sedating antihistamines at bedtime (when the side effect of drowsiness is welcome) may provide an uninterrupted night's sleep. Therapeutic baths with colloidal oatmeal preparations or tar extracts may give temporary relief.

If antihistamines are prescribed, closely monitor the patient's response to therapy so that the dosage can be adjusted as needed. The anti-inflammatory properties of topical steroid preparations and other topical agents are increased if the drug is applied to slightly damp skin.

Using topical drugs under an occlusive dressing increases the dose of anti-inflammatory being delivered. Avoid occluding treated areas unless specifically ordered by the physician.

SUNBURN

Sunburn is a first-degree or superficial burn and a very common skin injury. Excessive exposure to ultraviolet (UV) light injures the dermis, stimulating an inflammatory response that dilates the capillaries, leading to redness, tenderness, edema, and occasional blister formation. When large areas of the body are sunburned, systemic inflammatory symptoms, such as headache, nausea, and fever, may be produced.

Erythema (redness) and pain begin within a few hours after sunburn has occurred and increase in intensity for 1 to 2 days before subsiding. Treatment is directed toward comfort and includes cool baths and soothing lotions, such as bland lubricants or refrigerated moisturizing lotions. Antibiotic ointments are used only if blistering of the skin causes infection. If pain is severe, topical corticosteroids may decrease the inflammation temporarily. See Chapter 28 for discussion of prevention and treatment of superficial burns.

URTICARIA

Urticaria (hives) is white or red edematous papules or plaques of various sizes. This problem is usually caused by exposure to allergens (different for different people), which releases histamine in the dermal tissue, causing blood vessel dilation and leakage of plasma protein to form lesions or wheals. The exact cause is rarely identified although drugs, foods, infections, autoimmune diseases, cancer, and physical stimuli often trigger urticaria.

Treatment is aimed at removal of the triggering substance and relief of symptoms. Because the skin reaction is caused by histamine release, antihistamines such as diphenhydramine (Benadryl) are helpful. Teach the patient to avoid overexertion, alcohol consumption, and warm environments (e.g., warm or hot showers), which contribute to blood vessel dilation and make the symptoms worse. In addition, alcohol may increase any sedating effect of antihistamines, increasing the risk for falls and other accidents.

TRAUMA

Pathophysiology

Skin trauma can vary from an aseptic surgical incision to a grossly infected, draining pressure ulcer with deep-tissue destruction. Injury to the skin starts a series of actions to repair the skin and re-establish this protective barrier.

Phases of Wound Healing

Wound healing occurs in three phases: the inflammatory, or "lag," phase; the fibroblastic, or connective tissue repair, phase; and the maturation, or remodeling, phase. Table 27-1 lists the key events of normal wound healing. The length of each phase depends on the type of injury, patient health, and whether the wound is healing by first, second, or third intention (Fig. 27-1).

A wound without tissue loss, such as a clean laceration or a surgical incision, can be closed with sutures or staples. The wound edges are brought together with the skin layers lined up in correct anatomic position **(approximated)** and held in place until healing is complete. Because the wound can be easily closed and dead space eliminated, healing by **first intention** shortens the phases of tissue repair. Inflammation resolves quickly, and connective tissue repair is minimal, resulting in a thin scar.

Deeper tissue injuries or wounds with tissue loss, such as a chronic pressure ulcer or venous stasis ulcer, result in a cavity-like defect that requires gradual filling in of the dead space with connective tissue. This healing occurs by **second intention** and prolongs the repair process.

Wounds with a high risk for infection, such as surgical incisions that enter a nonsterile body cavity or traumatic wounds that occur under unclean conditions, may be intentionally left open for several days. After **debris** (dead cells and tissues) and exudate have been removed (débrided) and inflammation has subsided, the wound is closed by first intention. This type of healing involves delayed primary closure **(third intention)** and results in a scar similar to that found in wounds that heal by first intention. As shown in Table 27-2, healing can be impaired by many factors.

Mechanisms of Wound Healing

When injury occurs, the body restores skin integrity through three processes: re-epithelialization, granulation, and wound contraction. The depth of injury and extent of tissue loss determine how and to what degree each of these processes contributes to wound healing.

Partial-Thickness Wounds

Partial-thickness wounds are more superficial, involving damage to the epidermis and upper layers of the dermis. These wound heal by **re-epithelialization,** the production of new skin cells by undamaged epidermal cells in the basal layer of the dermis and the linings around hair follicles and sweat

TABLE 27-1 Normal Wound Healing

INFLAMMATORY PHASE
- Begins at the time of injury or cell death and lasts 3 to 5 days.
- Immediate responses are vasoconstriction and clot formation.
- After 10 minutes, vasodilation with increased capillary permeability and leakage of plasma (and plasma proteins) into the surrounding tissue.
- Migration of white blood cells (especially macrophages) into the wound.
- Clinical manifestations of local edema, pain, erythema, and warmth.

FIBROBLASTIC PHASE
- Begins about the fourth day after injury and lasts 2 to 4 weeks.
- Fibrin strands form a scaffold or framework.
- Mitotic fibroblast cells migrate into the wound, attach to the framework, divide, and stimulate the secretion of collagen.
- Collagen, together with ground substance, builds tough and inflexible scar tissue.
- Capillaries in areas surrounding the wound form "buds" that grow into new blood vessels.
- Capillary buds and collagen deposits form the "granulation" tissue in the wound, and the wound contracts.
- Epithelial cells grow over the granulation tissue bed.

MATURATION PHASE
- Begins as early as 3 weeks after injury and may continue for a year.
- Collagen is reorganized to provide greater tensile strength.
- Scar tissue gradually becomes thinner and paler in color.
- The mature scar is firm and inelastic when palpated.

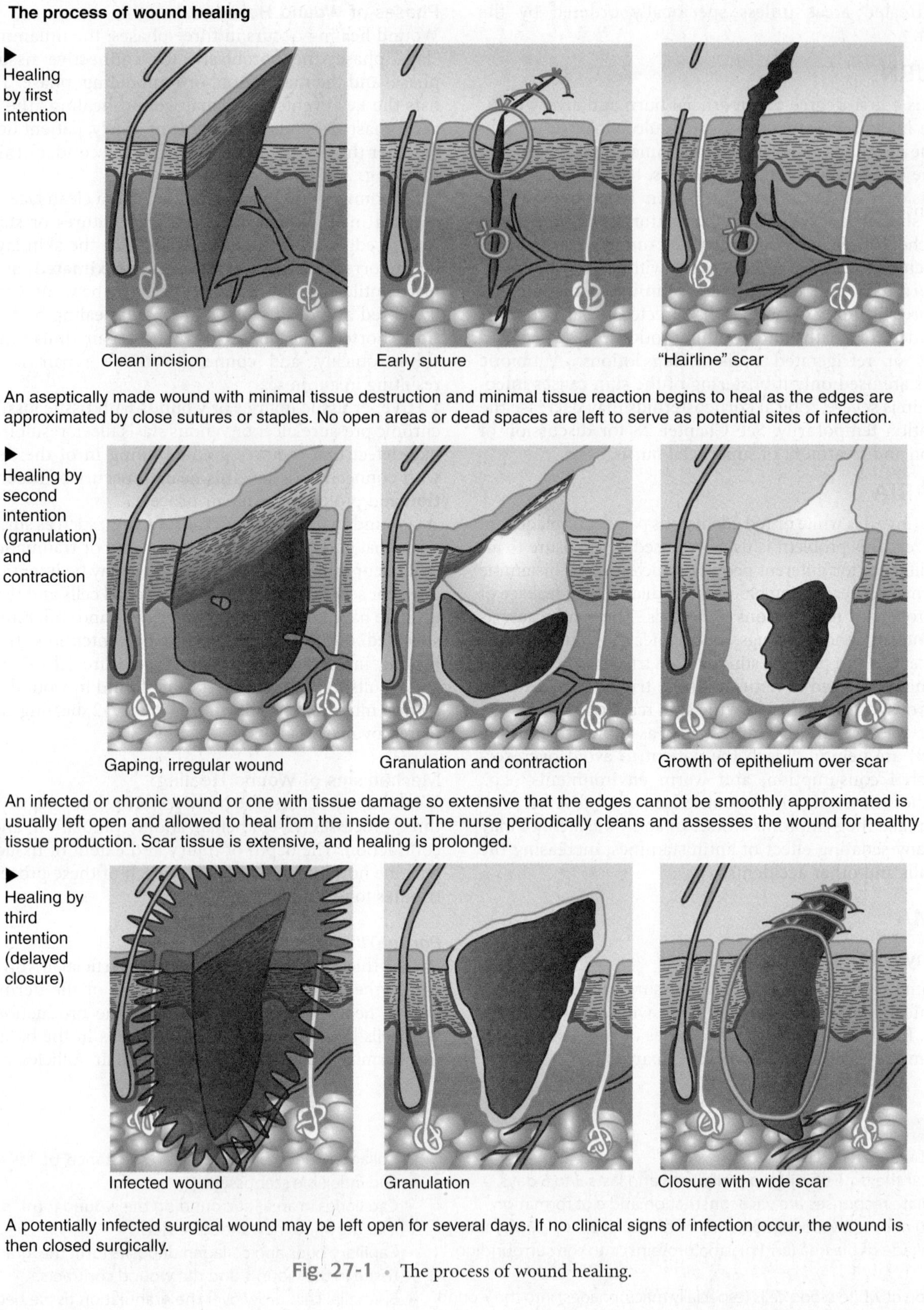
The process of wound healing
Healing by first intention
Clean incision
Early suture
"Hairline" scar
An aseptically made wound with minimal tissue destruction and minimal tissue reaction begins to heal as the edges are approximated by close sutures or staples. No open areas or dead spaces are left to serve as potential sites of infection.
Healing by second intention (granulation) and contraction
Gaping, irregular wound
Granulation and contraction
Growth of epithelium over scar
An infected or chronic wound or one with tissue damage so extensive that the edges cannot be smoothly approximated is usually left open and allowed to heal from the inside out. The nurse periodically cleans and assesses the wound for healthy tissue production. Scar tissue is extensive, and healing is prolonged.
Healing by third intention (delayed closure)
Infected wound
Granulation
Closure with wide scar
A potentially infected surgical wound may be left open for several days. If no clinical signs of infection occur, the wound is then closed surgically.

Fig. 27-1 • The process of wound healing.

TABLE 27-2 **Causes of Impaired Wound Healing**

Cause	Mechanism
ALTERED INFLAMMATORY RESPONSE	
LOCAL	
Arteriosclerosis Diabetes Vasculitis Thrombosis Venous insufficiency Lymphedema Pharmacologic vasoconstriction Irradiated tissue Crush injuries Primary closure under tension	Reduced local tissue circulation, resulting in ischemia, impaired leukocytic response to wounding, and increased probability of wound infection
SYSTEMIC	
Leukemia Prolonged administration of high-dose anti-inflammatory drugs • Corticosteroids • Aspirin	Systemic inhibition of leukocytic response, resulting in impaired host resistance to infection
IMPAIRED CELLULAR PROLIFERATION	
LOCAL	
Wound infection Foreign body Necrotic tissue Repeated injury or irritation Movement of wound (e.g., across a joint) Wound desiccation or maceration	Prolonged inflammatory response, which can result in low tissue oxygen tension and further tissue destruction
SYSTEMIC	
Aging Chronic stress Nutritional deficiencies • Calories • Protein • Vitamins • Minerals • Water Impaired oxygenation • Pulmonary insufficiency • Heart failure • Hypovolemia Cirrhosis Uremia Prolonged hypothermia Coagulation disorders Cytotoxic drugs	Impaired cellular proliferation and collagen synthesis Decreased wound contraction

glands (Fig. 27-2). Skin injury is followed immediately by local inflammation. The inflammatory response causes the formation of a fibrin clot and the release of growth factors that stimulate epidermal cell division (mitosis). New skin cells move into open spaces on the wound surface, where the fibrin clot acts as a frame or scaffold to guide cell movement. Regrowth across the open area **(resurfacing)** is only one cell layer thick at first. As healing continues, the cell layer thickens and stratifies (forms layers) to resemble normal skin. A healed wound re-establishes the protective barrier properties of the skin with keratin production.

In a healthy patient, healing of a partial-thickness wound by re-epithelialization takes about 5 to 7 days. This process occurs most rapidly in tissue that is hydrated and oxygenated and has few organisms present.

Full-Thickness Wounds

In deep partial-thickness and full-thickness wounds, damage extends into the lower layers of the dermis and underlying subcutaneous tissue. As a result, most, if not all, of the epithelial cells at the base of the wound have been destroyed. Thus re-epithelialization is not the major healing process for this type of wound. Removal of the damaged tissue results in a defect that must be filled with scar tissue **(granulation)** for healing to occur. During the proliferative phase of healing, new blood vessels form at the base of the wound and fibro-

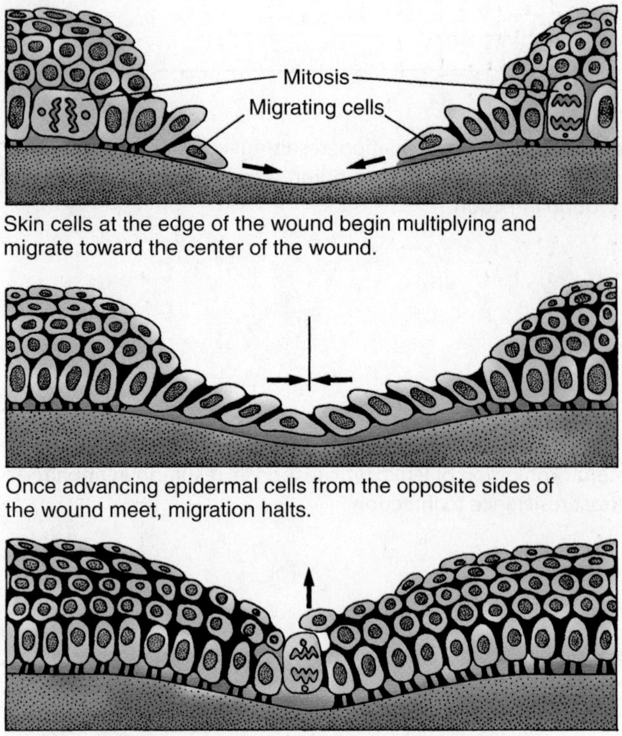
Mitosis
Migrating cells

Skin cells at the edge of the wound begin multiplying and migrate toward the center of the wound.

Once advancing epidermal cells from the opposite sides of the wound meet, migration halts.

Epithelial cells continue to divide until the thickness of the new skin layer approaches normal.

Fig. 27-2 • Re-epithelialization.

blastic cells begin moving into the wound space. Fibroblasts deposit new collagen to replace the damaged tissue.

Some of these fibroblasts take on the features of smooth muscle cells and begin to pull the wound edges inward along the path of least resistance **(contraction)** (see Fig. 27-1). This causes the wound to decrease in size at a uniform rate of about 0.6 to 0.75 mm/day. Complete closure of a wound by contraction depends on the mobility of the surrounding skin as tension is applied to it. If tension in the surrounding skin exceeds the counterforce of wound contraction, healing will be delayed until undamaged epidermal cells at the wound edges can bridge the defect. Unlike re-epithelialization in partial-thickness wounds, which results in the return of a near-normal epithelial barrier, the bridging of epithelial cells across a large area of granulation tissue results in an unstable barrier. A venous leg ulcer is one example of a skin defect that heals poorly by contraction. Re-epithelialization of these chronic wounds often results in a thin epidermal barrier that is easily reinjured.

Re-epithelialization, granulation, and contraction do not continue indefinitely. Natural healing processes can slow down and even stop in the presence of infection, unrelieved pressure, or mechanical obstacles. For example, dead tissue not only supports the overgrowth of organisms but also obstructs collagen deposition and wound contraction. Therefore thorough wound débridement is necessary for healing to occur. In the case of chronic wounds, healing may cease spontaneously and without an obvious cause. In addition, infection in chronic wounds may not show the expected manifestations. Often the only manifestation is failure of the wound to decrease in size or to actually increase in size (Frantz, 2005).

CONSIDERATIONS FOR OLDER ADULTS

As skin ages, the process of wound healing becomes less efficient. Both re-epithelialization and wound contraction slow, and replacement of connective tissue is reduced. Thus the strength of a healed wound in an older adult is reduced and the area is at greater risk for re-injury (Worley, 2006a). When aging skin is further hindered from healing by inadequate nutrition, incontinence, or immobility, any wound in an older adult has a high risk for becoming a chronic wound. Although prevention strategies are best, aggressive treatment of any degree of loss of skin integrity, no matter how small, should be started as soon as it is discovered in an older adult.

Patient-Centered Collaborative Care

Treatment of skin trauma varies with the depth and type of injury. The collaborative management for any type of skin trauma focuses on enhancing wound healing, preventing infection, and restoring function to the area. Management of pressure ulcers presents interventions common to wound healing, as does treatment of burns (see Chapter 28).

PRESSURE ULCERS

Pathophysiology

A **pressure ulcer** is tissue damage caused when the skin and underlying soft tissue are compressed between a bony prominence and an external surface for an extended period. Although they commonly occur over the sacrum, hips, and ankles, *pressure ulcers can occur on any body surface.* For example, nasal cannula tubing that is too tight can cause pressure ulcers behind the ears or in the nares.

Tissue compression from pressure restricts blood flow to the skin, resulting in reduced tissue perfusion and oxygenation, leading to cell death. Ulcers occur most often in people with limited mobility because they cannot change their position to relieve pressure. Sensory impairment is also a contributing factor. Patients who cannot feel or communicate the pain that occurs with unrelieved pressure are more likely to develop pressure ulcers. Once formed, these chronic wounds are slow to heal, resulting in increased morbidity and health care costs. Complications associated with chronic pressure ulcers include sepsis, kidney failure, infectious arthritis, and osteomyelitis (Duhon, 2007).

In addition to pressure, other factors increase the risk for pressure ulcer formation. Friction and shear are mechanical forces that impair skin integrity and set the stage for skin breakdown. Excessive skin moisture, such as urinary incontinence, increases the risk for skin damage when mechanical forces are applied. Nutritional status is also a concern. Protein malnutrition not only makes normal tissue more prone to breakdown but also delays healing (Slachta, 2008).

Mechanical Forces

Pressure occurs as a result of gravity. Dependent tissues in contact with a fixed surface experience varying degrees of pressure. Pressure is determined by the amount of weight exerted at the point of contact, the distribution of weight at the point of contact, and the density of the contacting surface. Excessive or prolonged pressure can compress blood vessels at the point of contact, leading to ischemia, inflammation, and tissue necrosis. Pressure occurs when the patient is positioned on a hard surface that does not diffuse the weight or when he or she remains in the same position too long.

Friction occurs when surfaces rub the skin and irritate or directly pull off epithelial tissue. Such forces are generated when the patient is dragged or pulled across bed linen.

Shear or shearing forces are generated when the skin itself is stationary and the tissues below the skin (e.g., fat, muscle) shift or move (Fig. 27-3). The movement of the deeper tissue layers reduces the blood supply to the skin, leading to skin hypoxia, anoxia, ischemia, inflammation, and necrosis.

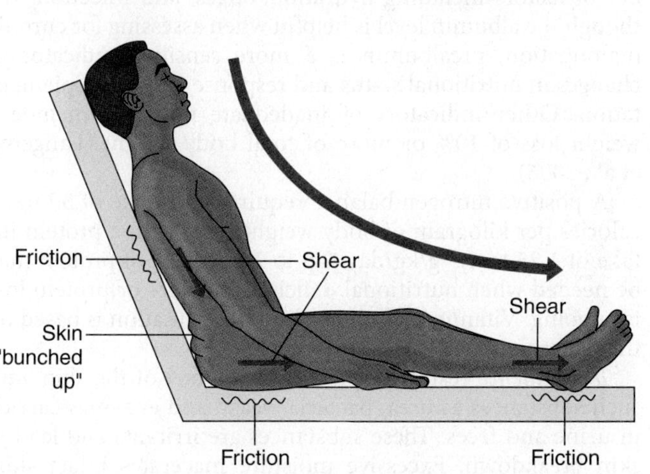
Friction
Shear
Shear
Skin "bunched up"
Friction
Friction

Fig. 27-3 • Shearing forces pulling skin layers away from deeper tissue. The skin is "bunched up" against the back of the mattress while the rest of the bone and muscle in the area presses downward on the lower part of the mattress. Blood vessels become kinked, obstructing circulation and leading to tissue death.

Gravity plays a role in the development of shearing forces. A shear injury usually occurs when a patient is in bed in a semisitting position and gradually slides downward. Often the skin over the sacrum does not slide down at the same pace as the deeper tissues; thus the skin is mechanically "sheared," causing blood vessels to stretch or break and leading to soft-tissue ischemia, although no break in external skin integrity is observed.

CONSIDERATIONS FOR OLDER ADULTS

Older adults are at particular risk for pressure ulcers because of the presence of age-related skin changes. Progressive flattening of cells at the dermal-epidermal junction predisposes older people to skin tears from mechanical shearing forces, such as the removal of tape and friction from tightly applied restraints. In addition, skin moisture and irritation from incontinence and friction over bony prominences can lead to partial-thickness skin destruction and early pressure ulcer formation. **If pressure is unrelieved, tissue destruction progresses to full-thickness injury.**

Incidence/Prevalence

Pressure ulcer development is a problem found among patients in the acute care setting, long-term care facility, and home care setting. Although patient care has improved in many ways and new products are available for prevention and treatment, 3% to 14% of hospitalized patients still experience pressure ulcer formation (Dunleavy, 2008).

Health Promotion and Maintenance

Pressure ulcers can be prevented if the risk is recognized and intervention begins early (Chart 27-2). Key health care team members for pressure ulcer prevention and man-

Chart 27-2 BEST PRACTICE FOR PATIENT SAFETY & QUALITY CARE
Preventing Pressure Ulcers

POSITIONING
- Pad contact surfaces with foam, silicon gel, air pads, or other pressure-relieving pads.
- Do not keep the head of the bed elevated above 30 degrees to prevent shearing.
- Use a lift sheet to move a patient in the bed. Avoid dragging or sliding him or her.
- When positioning a patient on his or her side, do not position directly on the trochanter.
- Reposition an immobile patient at least every 2 hours while in bed and at least every 1 hour while sitting in a chair.
- Do not place a rubber ring or donut under the patient's sacral area.
- When moving an immobile patient from a bed to another surface, use a designated slide board well lubricated with talc or use a mechanical lift.
- Place pillows or foam wedges between two bony surfaces.
- Keep the patient's skin directly off plastic surfaces.
- Keep the patient's heels off the bed surface using bed pillow under ankles.

NUTRITION
- Ensure a fluid intake between 2000 and 3000 mL/day.
- Help the patient maintain an adequate intake of protein and calories.

SKIN CARE
- Perform a daily inspection of the patient's entire skin.
- Document and report any manifestations of skin infection.
- Use moisturizers daily on dry skin, and apply when skin is damp.
- Keep moisture from prolonged contact with skin.
  - Dry areas where two skin surfaces touch, such as the axillae and under the breasts.
  - Place absorbent pads under areas where perspiration collects.
  - Use moisture barriers on skin areas where wound drainage or incontinence occurs.
- ***Do not massage bony prominences.***
- Humidify the room.

SKIN CLEANING
- Clean the skin as soon as possible after soiling occurs and at routine intervals.
- Use a mild, heavily fatted soap or gentle commercial cleanser for incontinence.
- Use tepid rather than hot water.
- In the perineal area, use a disposable cleaning cloth that contains a skin barrier agent.
- While cleaning, use the minimum scrubbing force necessary to remove soil.
- Gently pat rather than rub the skin dry.
- Do not use powders or talcs directly on the perineum.
- After cleansing, apply a commercial skin barrier to those areas in frequent contact with urine or feces.

agement are the certified wound care specialist and the nutritionist.

A pressure ulcer prevention program consists of two steps: (1) identification of high-risk patients and (2) implementation of aggressive intervention for prevention with the use of pressure relief or reduction devices. For patients at risk for pressure ulcers as a result of immobility, including being wheelchair bound, pressure mapping can be used to identify specific risk areas and plan appropriate interventions. The process of pressure mapping involves the use of a computerized tool that measures pressure distribution for a person sitting in a chair or lying on a mattress (Hanson, Thompson, Langemo et al., 2007). The map is displayed as colored areas on the computer screen, based on temperature differences. Shades of red indicate areas of greater heat production associated with greater pressure. Shades of blue indicate cooler skin touch areas under lower pressure. This tool, along with more traditional risk assessment and visual inspection, appears to assist in identifying problem areas even before visual changes occur, allowing better targeted prevention strategies.

Effective risk identification and prevention measures include education of the patient and the caregiver. Documentation of risk assessment, implementation of prevention measures, and education of all people involved in the care of the patient at risk for pressure ulcer formation are key to the plan's success (Dunleavy, 2008). Periodic re-assessment of risk and continuing evaluation of the implemented plan are necessary as patient conditions change.

Identification of High-Risk Patients

All patients admitted to a health care facility or home care agency should be assessed for pressure ulcer risk. The use of a risk assessment tool increases the chances of identifying those patients at greater risk for skin breakdown. The Braden Scale (Fig. 27-4) is the most commonly used skin risk assessment tool. Other factors influencing the risk category for pressure ulcer formation are mental status, activity/mobility, nutritional status, and incontinence.

Mental status changes and decreased sensory perception determine whether the patient is a partner in the prevention of pressure ulcers. When the patient understands that turning and shifting of weight prevent tissue damage, the risk for pressure ulcers decreases. When he or she has a mental status problem because of stroke, head injury, organic brain disease, Alzheimer's disease, or other problem with cognition, the risk for pressure ulcer formation increases.

Independent mobility is a direct factor in the risk for pressure ulcer formation. Patients who have unimpaired mobility and can respond to physical sensation changes are at low risk for pressure ulcer formation. *Any patient, regardless of age, who requires assistance with turning and positioning or who is less aware of physical sensation changes is at high risk for pressure ulcer formation.* Anyone who is confined to bed or a chair is at higher risk than a patient who requires assistance with ambulation.

Nutritional status is a critical risk factor for pressure ulcer development and for successful healing (Slachta, 2008). Intact skin and wound healing depend on a positive nitrogen balance and adequate serum protein levels. The patient in a negative nitrogen balance not only heals more slowly but also is at greater risk for tissue destruction. In addition, draining wounds are a route of protein loss.

Adequate nutrition is critical in the prevention of pressure ulcer formation. A nutritionist should be a part of the pressure reduction team or program.

Nutritional status assessment includes laboratory studies; evaluation of weight and weight change; ability of the patient to consume an adequate diet; and the need for vitamin, mineral, or protein supplementation. *Nutrition is inadequate when the serum albumin level is less than 3.5 mg/dL, the prealbumin level is less than 19.5 mg/dL, or the lymphocyte count is less than 1800/mm^3.* Serum albumin levels are affected by a number of factors including hydration, stress, and infection. Although the albumin level is helpful when assessing for chronic malnutrition, prealbumin is a more sensitive indicator of changes in nutritional status and response to diet supplementation. Other indicators of inadequate nutrition include a weight loss of 10% or more of total body weight (Langemo et al., 2006).

A positive nitrogen balance requires an intake of 30 to 35 calories per kilogram of body weight daily with a protein intake of 1.25 to 1.5 g/kg/day. Up to 2 g/kg/day of protein may be needed when nutritional deficits are severe or protein loss is ongoing. Vitamin and mineral supplementation is based on the patient's nutritional status.

Incontinence results in prolonged contact of the skin with such substances as urea, bacteria, yeast, and enzymes carried in urine and feces. These substances are irritants and lead to skin breakdown. Excessive moisture macerates intact skin, increasing the risk for breakdown. Daily inspection of the skin for any areas of redness or skin breakdown is a major part of pressure ulcer prevention. Maintenance of clean, intact skin also assists in the prevention process. The skin should be washed with a pH-balanced soap to maintain the normal acid level. Creams or lotions are used to lubricate and moisturize the skin. Barrier ointment protection is needed whenever incontinence is present. Absorbent pads or garments must be changed at once with each incontinence episode to avoid prolonged skin contact with urine or feces. *Reddened areas are never massaged directly because this action can damage capillary beds and increase tissue necrosis.*

Pressure-Relieving and Pressure-Reducing Techniques

The cornerstone in the prevention (and treatment) of pressure ulcers is adequate pressure relief. A factor in pressure relief is the **capillary closing pressure,** which is the amount of pressure needed to occlude skin capillary blood flow, in the area at risk. The normal capillary closing pressure ranges from 12 to 32 mm Hg. An effective pressure-relieving device is one that keeps tissue pressure *below* the capillary closing pressure to ensure adequate tissue perfusion and oxygenation. *Most devices have a standardized guaranteed pressure relief reading; however, these readings do not ensure that capillary blood flow for any given patient is adequate. Observe skin color, integrity, and temperature directly to determine capillary flow adequacy.*

Devices are classified according to whether they relieve pressure or merely reduce pressure. In addition, devices are further classified as dynamic or static. Dynamic systems alternate inflation and deflation of the device through the use of electricity. Static devices made of gel, water, foam, or air are in a constant state of inflation that distributes the patient pressure load over a larger area and reduces the pressure any one area experiences.

Patient's name ________		Evaluator's name ________			Date of assessment		
Sensory perception Ability to respond meaningfully to pressure-related discomfort	**1. Completely limited** Unresponsive to painful stimuli (does not moan, flinch, or grasp) because of diminished level of consciousness or sedation OR limited ability to feel pain over most of body surface	**2. Very limited** Responds only to painful stimuli; cannot communicate discomfort except by moaning or restlessness OR has a sensory impairment that limits the ability to feel pain or discomfort over half of the body	**3. Slightly limited** Responds to verbal commands but cannot always communicate discomfort or need to be turned OR has some sensory impairment that limits ability to feel pain or discomfort in one or two extremities	**4. No impairment** Responds to verbal commands; has no sensory deficit that would limit ability to feel or voice pain or discomfort			
Moisture Degree to which skin is exposed to moisture	**1. Constantly moist** Skin is kept moist almost constantly by perspiration, urine; dampness is detected every time the client is moved or turned	**2. Very Moist** Skin is often but not always moist; linen must be changed at least once a shift	**3. Occasionally moist** Skin is occasionally moist, requiring an extra linen change approximately once a day	**4. Rarely moist** Skin is usually dry; linen requires changing only at routine intervals			
Activity Degree of physical activity	**1. Bedfast** Confined to bed	**2. Chairfast** Ability to walk severely limited or nonexistent; cannot bear own weight and must be assisted into chair or wheelchair	**3. Walks occasionally** Walks occasionally during the day but for very short distances, with or without assistance; spends the majority of each shift in bed or chair	**4. Walks frequently** Walks outside the room at least twice a day and inside the room at least once every 2 hours during waking hours			
Mobility Ability to change or control body position	**1. Completely immobile** Does not make even slight changes in body or extremity position without assistance	**2. Very limited** Makes occasional slight changes in body or extremity position but unable to make frequent or significant changes independently	**3. Slightly limited** Makes frequent though slight changes in body or extremity position independently	**4. No limitations** Makes major and frequent changes in position without assistance			
Nutrition Usual food intake pattern	**1. Very poor** Never eats a complete meal; rarely eats more than a third of any food offered; eats two servings or less of protein (meat or dairy products) per day; takes fluids poorly; does not take a liquid dietary supplement OR is NPO or maintained on clear liquids or IV for more than 5 days	**2. Probably inadequate** Rarely eats a complete meal and generally eats only about half of any food offered; protein intake includes only three servings of meat or dairy products per day; occasionally will take a dietary supplement OR receives less than optimal amount of liquid diet or tube feeding	**3. Adequate** Eats over half of most meals; eats a total of four servings of protein (meat, dairy products) each day; occasionally will refuse a meal, but will usually take a supplement if offered OR is receiving tube feeding or total parenteral nutrition, which probably meets most nutritional needs	**4. Excellent** Eats most of every meal; never refuses a meal; usually eats a total of four or more servings of meat and dairy products; occasionally eats between meals; does not require supplementation			
Friction and shear	**1. Problem** Requires moderate to maximum assistance in moving; complete lifting without sliding against sheets is impossible; frequently slides down in bed or chair, requiring frequent repositioning with maximum assistance; spasticity, contractures, or agitation leads to almost constant friction	**2. Potential problem** Moves feebly or requires minimum assistance during a move; skin probably slides to some extent against sheets, chair, restraints, or other devices; maintains relatively good position in chair or bed most of the time but occasionally slides down	**3. No apparent problem** Moves in bed and in chair independently and has sufficient muscle strength to lift up completely during move; maintains good position in bed or chair at all times				
Scoring system: 15-16 = mild risk, 12-14 = moderate risk, <11 = severe risk					Total score		

Fig. 27-4 • The Braden Scale for predicting pressure ulcer risk. *IV,* Intravenous; *NPO,* nothing by mouth.

Pressure relief/reduction products come in many forms, such as specialty beds, mattress replacements, overlays, and assistive devices. Choosing the correct product is important in the success of the prevention plan. Re-evaluate the selected product in use daily for effectiveness in reducing pressure, providing comfort, and eliminating "bottoming out," wherein the patient's bony prominences sink into the mattress or cushion, causing him or her to have pressure even with the product in place.

Pressure-relief devices consistently reduce pressure below capillary closing pressure. These devices are recommended for patients who need:

- Prevention of skin breakdown because they cannot turn (e.g., immobility, loss of sensation)
- Prevention of extension of skin breakdown that has already occurred
- Promotion of healing for breakdown present on several turning surfaces

Pressure-reduction devices lower pressure below that of a standard hospital mattress or chair surface but do not reduce pressure consistently below the capillary closing pressure. These devices are effective for preventing pressure ulcers only when used together with a turning schedule and other skin care measures.

Positioning, as described in Chart 27-2, is critical in reducing pressure. A good plan for positioning is the 30-degree rule. This plan ensures that the patient is positioned and propped so that whatever part of the body is elevated is tilted back at least 30 degrees to the mattress rather than resting directly on a dependent bony prominence. This rule applies to side-lying as well as head-of-bed elevation positions. The patient who requires greater elevation because of respiratory difficulties should be tilted forward even more than 90 degrees, with pillows behind the back to keep pressure off of the sacral/coccyx area. Often positioning is delegated to UAP. Teach UAP the importance of proper positioning and demonstrate how to perform it. Also teach family members to use these techniques in the home.

The patient at risk for pressure ulcers in bed is also at risk while sitting. Carefully assess for proper wheelchair or regular chair cushioning. Collaborate with physical therapists and rehabilitation specialists for selection of these products.

Even with an appropriate mattress or cushion, the patient needs to change or be helped to change positions periodically. Many facilities require turning and positioning every 2 hours. *However, pressure can occur in less time, and the actual turning or repositioning schedule for each patient must be individualized.* When this action is delegated to UAP, teach them the importance of maintaining a repositioning schedule.

Use pillows and other positioning or padding devices to keep heels pressure-free at all times for high-risk patients. Assess heel positioning every 4 hours to ensure that pressure is not redistributed to another high-risk area, such as the sides of the feet. Check heels even more frequently when devices that hide the feet, such as boots, are used, especially if the patient has a peripheral vascular problem.

Patient-Centered Collaborative Care

evolve ONLINE PHARM REVIEW

Assessment

History

When taking a history from the patient with a pressure ulcer, identify the cause of skin loss, as well as factors that may impair healing. Ask about the specific circumstances of the skin loss. Often patients with chronic pressure ulcerations have a history of delayed healing or recurrence of the ulcer after healing has occurred. Because pressure-related skin loss is common among severely debilitated patients, determine whether a patient has any of these contributing factors:

- Prolonged bedrest
- Immobility
- Incontinence
- Diabetes mellitus
- Inadequate nutrition or hydration
- Altered mental status (decreased sensory perception)
- Peripheral vascular disease

Physical Assessment/Clinical Manifestations

Inspect the entire body, including the back of the head, for areas of skin injury or pressure. Give special attention to bony prominences (e.g., the heels, sacrum, elbows, trochanters, posterior and anterior iliac spines) and areas that are vulnerable to excessive moisture. In addition, assess the patient's general appearance for issues related to skin health. Such issues include body weight and the proportion of weight to height because obese persons, as well as thin persons, are at increased risk for malnutrition and pressure ulcer formation. Check overall cleanliness of the skin, hair, and nails. Determine whether any loss of mobility or range of joint motion has occurred. *This assessment should not be delegated to UAP.*

Wound Assessment

The appearance of pressure ulcers changes with the depth of the injury. Chart 27-3 lists the features of the four stages of pressure ulceration, and Fig. 27-5 shows examples.

Assess wounds for location, size, color, extent of tissue involvement, cell types in the wound base and margins, exudate, condition of surrounding tissue, and presence of foreign bodies. Document this initial assessment to serve as a starting point for determining the intervention plan and its effectiveness. How often a wound is assessed is determined by the written policies and procedures at the facility or agency. Weekly documented assessment is the standard in many long-term care facilities; however, daily assessment is needed when the patient is in an acute care setting. *Also assess the wound at each dressing change, comparing the existing wound features with those documented previously to determine the current state of healing or deterioration.*

For intact areas that are red (in lighter-skinned patients), press firmly with fingers at the center of the area and assess whether the area **blanches** (lightens) with pressure. An area that blanches with pressure and then returns to color when pressure is removed indicates color changes related to blood vessel dilation rather than tissue damage or inflammation. When blanching does not occur with pressure, the redness is more likely to be a manifestation of skin injury. Document whether the reddened area blanches with pressure.

Record the location and size of the wound first. Wounds are sized by length, width, and depth using millimeters or centimeters. In standardizing wound size for documentation and communication purposes, assess the wound as a clock face with the 12 o'clock position in the direction of the patient's head and the 6 o'clock position in the direction of the patient's feet. Always measure the length from the 12 o'clock position to the 6 o'clock position and the width between the 9 o'clock posi-

Chart 27-3 KEY FEATURES

Pressure Ulcers

STAGE I

- Skin is intact.
- Area, usually over a bony prominence, is red and does not blanch with external pressure.
- For patients with darker skin that does not blanch:
  - Observable pressure-related alteration of intact skin; changes are compared with an adjacent or opposite area and include one or more of these:
    Skin color (darker or lighted than the comparison area)
    Skin temperature (warmth or coolness)
    Tissue consistency (firm or boggy)
    Sensation (pain, itching)
- The ulcer appears as a defined area of persistent redness in lightly pigmented skin, whereas in darker skin tones, the ulcer may appear with persistent red, blue, or purple hues.

STAGE II

- Skin is not intact.
- There is partial-thickness skin loss of the epidermis or dermis.
- Ulcer is superficial and may be characterized as an abrasion, a blister (open or fluid-filled), or a shallow crater.
- Bruising is *not* present.

STAGE III

- Skin loss is full thickness.
- Subcutaneous tissues may be damaged or necrotic.
- Damage extends down to but not through the underlying fascia; bone, tendon, or muscle are *not* exposed.
- The depth can vary with anatomic location; areas of thin skin (e.g., the bridge of the nose) may show only a shallow crater, whereas thicker tissue areas with larger amounts of subcutaneous fat may show a deep, crater-like appearance.
- Undermining and tunneling may or may not be present.

STAGE IV

- Skin loss is full thickness with exposed or palpable muscle, tendon, or bone.
- Often includes undermining and tunneling.
- Sinus tracts may develop.
- Slough and eschar are often present on at least part of the wound.

UNSTAGEABLE

- Skin loss is full thickness, and the base is completely covered with slough or eschar, obscuring the true depth of the wound.

Data from National Pressure Ulcer Advisory Panel (NPUAP). (February 2007). *Updated staging system.* Website: www.npuap.org

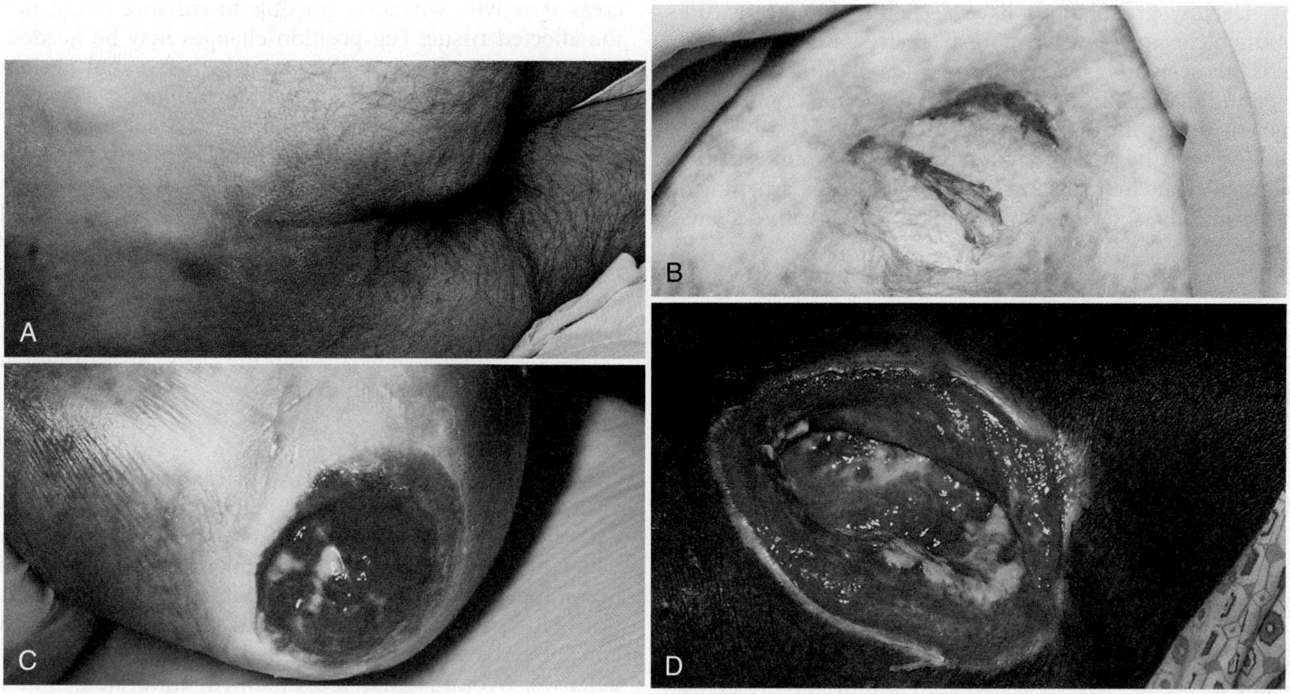

A
B
C
D

Fig. 27-5 • Various stages of pressure ulcers. **A,** Stage I pressure ulcer. **B,** Stage II pressure ulcer. **C,** Stage III pressure ulcer. **D,** Stage IV pressure ulcer.

tion and the 3 o'clock position. Measure depth as the distance from the deepest portion of the wound base to the skin level. Use disposable paper tape measures to obtain the length and width of a wound. Touch the bottom of the wound with a cotton-tipped applicator or swab and mark the place on the swab that is level with the skin surface to obtain wound depth. Then measure the area of the swab between the tip and the mark. When all caregivers use this format, measurement is accurate and wound progress can be determined (Hanson, Langemo, Anderson et al., 2007).

Inspect the wound margins for **cellulitis** (inflammation of the skin cells) extending beyond the area of injury. Progressive tissue destruction, seen as an increase in the size or depth of the ulcer and increased wound drainage, usually indicates impairment in the patient's ability to resist infection if proper measures have been taken to relieve pressure.

Inspect the wound for the presence or absence of necrotic tissue. Because of the depth of tissue destruction, a full-thickness pressure ulcer is often covered by a layer of black, gray, or brown nonviable, denatured collagen called wound **eschar.**

In the early stages of wound healing, the eschar is dry, leathery, and firmly attached to the wound surface. As the inflammatory phase of wound healing begins and removal of wound debris progresses, the eschar starts to lift and separate from the tissue beneath. This nonliving eschar is a good breeding ground for bacteria normally found on the skin surface, as well as those introduced by other means. As bacteria increase, they release enzymes that soften necrotic tissue. This tissue becomes softer and more yellow. In the presence of bacterial colonization, wound exudate increases substantially; the color and odor of wound exudate indicate the major organism present. The features of wound exudate are listed in Table 27-3.

Beneath the separating dead tissue, granulation tissue appears. Early granulation is pale pink, progressing to a beefy red color as it grows and fills the wound. A wound with poor local arterial blood supply appears dry and pale. Venous obstruction causes an excessively moist ulcer surface with a deep reddish purple color (reflective of the deoxygenated blood beneath the ulcer surface).

Palpate the wound to determine the texture of the granulations. Healthy granulations have a slightly spongy texture. Pressure ulcers may involve more extensive tissue destruction than is first seen on inspection. Separation of the skin layers at the wound margins from the underlying granulation tissue is known as **undermining.** Inspect undermined areas for gradual filling with healthy granulations and for wound-healing progress. Palpate the bony prominences for deep hardening of the surrounding soft tissue, which often occurs with deep tissue ischemia.

After ischemia has occurred, continued pressure over the area increases tissue destruction from the deep tissue layers toward the surface, resulting in the formation of tunnels. This "hidden" wound may first have a small opening in the skin with purulent drainage. If such an opening is observed, use a cotton-tipped applicator to probe gently for a much larger tunnel or pocket of necrotic tissue beneath the opening. Additional tunnels may also occur along the main wound. Check all wounds for tunneling and, if present, document the location and length of each tunnel.

TABLE 27-3 Types of Wound Exudate

Characteristics	Significance
SEROSANGUINEOUS EXUDATE	
Blood-tinged amber fluid consisting of serum and red blood cells	Normal for first 48 hr after injury Sudden increase in amount precedes wound dehiscence in wounds closed by first intention
PURULENT EXUDATE	
Creamy yellow pus	Colonization with *Staphylococcus*
Greenish blue pus causing staining of dressings and accompanied by a "fruity" odor	Colonization with *Pseudomonas*
Beige pus with a "fishy" odor	Colonization with *Proteus*
Brownish pus with a "fecal" odor	Colonization with aerobic coliform and *Bacteroides* (usually occurs after intestinal surgery)

Psychosocial Assessment

The patient with pressure ulcers may have an altered body image. Ineffective coping patterns emerge as the patient and family strive to adhere to changes in lifestyle that are needed for healing. In addition, chronic, slow-healing ulcers are often painful and costly to treat.

Assess the patient's and family's knowledge of the treatment goals at each stage of the healing process, as well as adherence to the prescribed treatment regimen. Also assess the patient's skills in cleaning the wound and applying a dressing. Poor adherence to pressure ulcer care procedures may reflect an inability to accept the diagnosis or to cope with the pain, cost, or potential scarring associated with prolonged healing. Depending on the patient's activity level and the location of the ulcer, assistance of a family member or home care nurse may be needed to provide initial care of the pressure ulcer at home.

Explore with the patient specific changes in ADLs that are needed to relieve pressure and promote healing. Promote increased activity whenever possible to enhance circulation to the affected tissue. Leg position changes may be needed for chronic leg ulcers, depending on whether or not peripheral vascular problems contribute to their formation. For patients who have arterial insufficiency, having the legs and feet in a dependent position works with gravity to help ensure adequate blood flow to the lower legs. When arterial blood flow is adequate but venous return is impaired, elevation of the legs may be needed for healing. When the patient is bedridden, frequent repositioning to relieve pressure (every 2 hours in bed, every 1 hour in a chair) can be labor intensive. In the home, repositioning, incontinence management, and dressing changes are often needed around the clock, disrupting family routines and contributing to stress.

Laboratory Assessment

A wound that is exposed is always *contaminated* but is not always *infected. Contamination* is the presence of organisms without any manifestation of infection. The normal immune defenses of the body keep the number of bacteria to a minimum and prevent infection. *Wound infection* is contamination with pathogenic organisms to the degree that growth and spread cannot be controlled by the body's immune defenses. Wounds that are inflamed, indurated, and red; have an odor; and have moderate to heavy exudate should be cultured to identify the causative organism and determine its sensitivity to antibiotics. *The presence of pus as exudate alone does not indicate a local or systemic infection because pus formation occurs when necrotic tissue separates and liquefies.*

If wounds are extensive, if the patient is severely immunocompromised, or if local blood supply to the wound is impaired, bacterial growth may exceed the body's ability to defend against invasion into deeper tissue layers. The result is deep wound infection and eventually bacteremia and sepsis (systemic infection).

Swab cultures are helpful only in identifying the types of bacteria present on the ulcer surface and may be misleading when trying to identify or quantify bacteria in deeper tissues. Wound biopsies allow the numbers of bacteria to be analyzed, but these tests are time consuming, costly, and unavailable in many laboratories. Therefore clinical indicators of infection (cellulitis, progressive increase in ulcer size or depth, changes in the quantity and quality of exudate) and systemic signs of bacteremia (e.g., fever, elevated white blood cell [WBC] count) are used to diagnose an infection.

Other Diagnostic Assessment

Additional laboratory studies are performed on the basis of the suspected cause of the wound. For pressure ulcers to show progress toward healing, the factors contributing to delayed healing must be diagnosed and treated. For example, noninvasive and invasive arterial blood flow studies are indicated if arterial occlusion is suspected in delayed healing of a pressure ulcer on the heel or ankle. Blood tests to establish specific nutritional deficiencies (e.g., prealbumin, albumin, total protein) are helpful in treating the debilitated, malnourished patient with a pressure ulcer.

DECISION-MAKING CHALLENGE
Coordination of Care

The patient is a 90-year-old woman who is an assisted-living resident. She had a stroke 4 years ago and is cognitively intact but requires assistance with ambulating and toileting. She uses a computer about 6 hours per day for e-mail, playing word and card games, and reading the online newspaper. Currently, she has an outbreak of herpes zoster on the left side of the upper back and chest. She has mild to moderate heart failure controlled with furosemide (Lasix, Furoside🍁) and an ACE inhibitor. She weighs 106 pounds and is 5 feet, 2 inches tall.

1. What risk factors does this patient have for pressure ulcer development? How do these factors increase her risk?
2. What additional assessment data should you obtain?
3. Where is she most likely to develop pressure ulcers, and why?
4. Given her diagnoses, level of mobility, and interests, what (if any) position changes should be made, and why?
5. How often should she be assessed for skin changes? (Provide a rationale for your response.)

evolve For suggested answer guidelines, go to http://evolve.elsevier.com/Iggy/.

▪ *Analysis*

Common Nursing Diagnoses and Collaborative Problems

The most common nursing diagnosis for patients with pressure ulcers is Impaired Skin Integrity related to vascular insufficiency and trauma. The most common collaborative problem is Risk for Infection and Wound Extension.

Additional Nursing Diagnoses and Collaborative Problems

In addition to the common nursing diagnoses and collaborative problems, patients with pressure ulcers may have one or more of these:

- Acute Pain or Chronic Pain related to skin trauma, wound infection, and wound treatment
- Disturbed Body Image related to altered appearance
- Ineffective Coping related to the chronicity of the ulcer, alteration in body image, and changes in lifestyle required to promote healing
- Imbalanced Nutrition: Less Than Body Requirements related to inability to ingest food due to biologic, psychological, or economic factors
- Ineffective Tissue Perfusion (Peripheral) related to mechanical reduction of venous or arterial blood flow
- Deficient Knowledge (treatment) related to cognitive limitation or unfamiliarity with information resources

▪ *Planning and Implementation*

The Concept Map on p. 492 addresses care issues related to patients who have or are at risk for pressure ulcers.

Impaired Skin Integrity

NOC **Planning: Expected Outcomes.** The patient with a pressure ulcer is expected to experience complete wound healing and not experience the formation of new pressure ulcers. Indicators include:

- Presence of granulation, re-epithelialization, and scar tissue formation
- Decreased wound size
- Absence of new pressure ulcers

Interventions. Wound care techniques for pressure ulcers vary according to each patient's needs and the physician's preferences. Surgery with aggressive removal of necrotic tissue may be indicated for some patients, whereas a nonsurgical approach to ulcer débridement is preferred for an older patient who has adequate defenses but is too ill or debilitated for surgery.

NIC ***Nonsurgical Management.*** The general NIC interventions for pressure ulcer care are listed in Chart 27-4. Nonsurgical intervention of pressure ulcers is often left to the discretion of the nurse, who coordinates with the health care provider and certified wound care specialist (if available) to select a method of wound dressing on the basis of the identified goal of wound management. Many agencies have guidelines or protocols for wound dressings based, for example, on wound size, depth, and presence of drainage.

Dressings. A properly designed dressing can speed healing by removing unwanted debris from the ulcer surface, protecting exposed healthy tissues, and creating a barrier between the body and the environment until the ulcer is closed. *For a patient with a draining, necrotic ulcer, the dressing must also remove excessive exudate and loose debris without damaging epithelial cells or newly formed granulation tissue. If necrosis is extensive and the eschar is thick, dead tissue must be surgically or chemically removed before further débridement with dressings can be effective.* Depending on the dressing material used, dressings help remove debris either through **mechanical débridement** (mechanical entrapment and detachment of dead tissue) or by **natural chemical débridement** (creating an environment that promotes self-digestion of dead tissues by the bacterial enzymes [autolysis]) (Table 27-4).

After all the dead tissue has been removed, protection of any exposed tendons, bone, and newly formed collagen is critical to pressure ulcer care. The ideal environment for healing is a clean, *slightly* moist ulcer surface with minimal bacterial colonization. Heavy moisture from an excessively draining ulcer or a dressing that is too wet interferes with healing by promoting the growth of organisms and causing maceration (mushiness) of healthy tissue. Likewise, if a clean ulcer surface is exposed to air or if highly absorbent dressing materials are used for prolonged periods, the drying effect can de-

CONCEPT MAP Pressure Ulcer

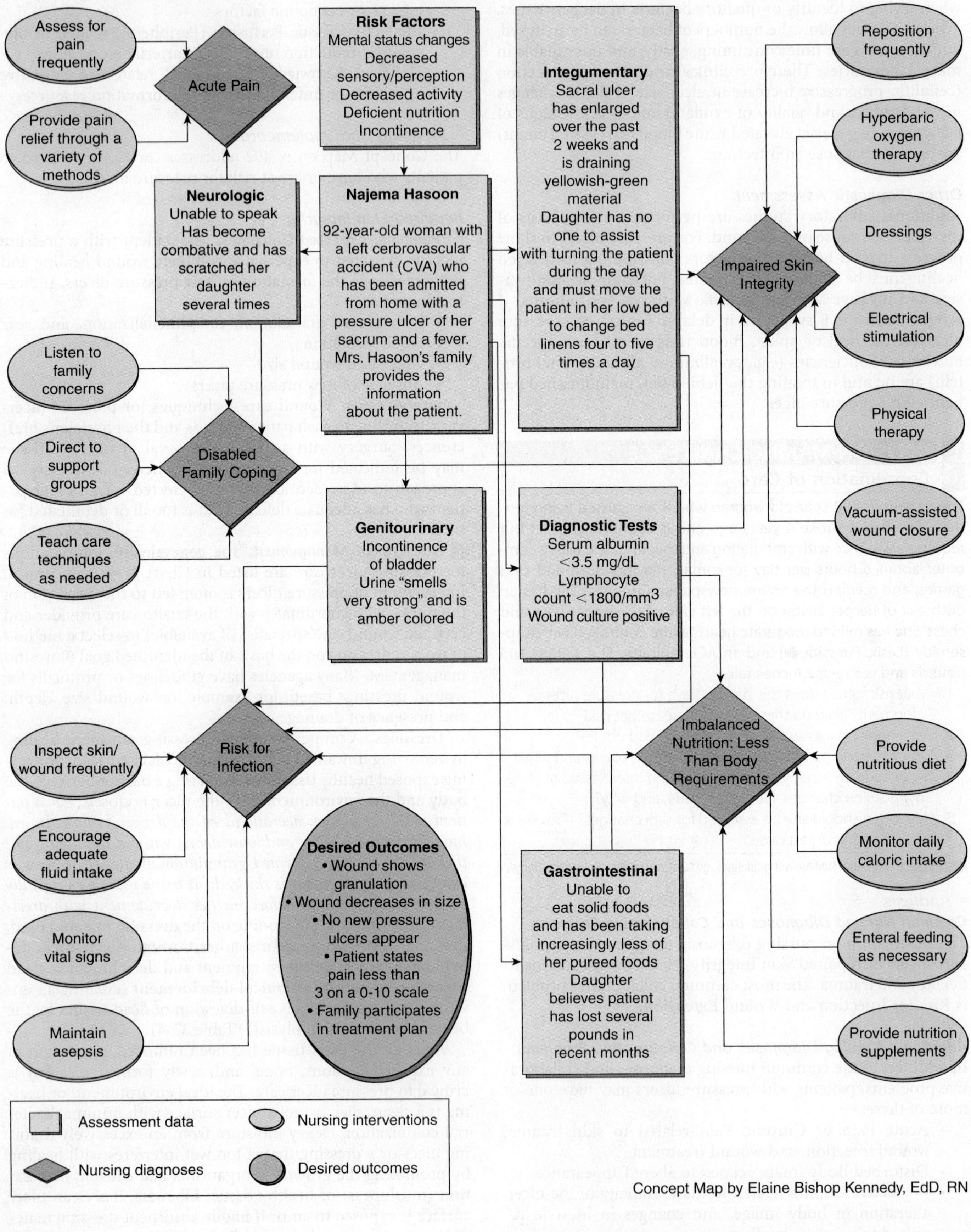
Assess for pain frequently
Acute Pain
Provide pain relief through a variety of methods
Risk Factors
Mental status changes
Decreased sensory/perception
Decreased activity
Deficient nutrition
Incontinence
Neurologic
Unable to speak
Has become combative and has scratched her daughter several times
Najema Hasoon
92-year-old woman with a left cerbrovascular accident (CVA) who has been admitted from home with a pressure ulcer of her sacrum and a fever. Mrs. Hasoon's family provides the information about the patient.
Integumentary
Sacral ulcer has enlarged over the past 2 weeks and is draining yellowish-green material
Daughter has no one to assist with turning the patient during the day and must move the patient in her low bed to change bed linens four to five times a day
Reposition frequently
Hyperbaric oxygen therapy
Dressings
Impaired Skin Integrity
Electrical stimulation
Physical therapy
Vacuum-assisted wound closure
Listen to family concerns
Direct to support groups
Disabled Family Coping
Teach care techniques as needed
Genitourinary
Incontinence of bladder
Urine "smells very strong" and is amber colored
Diagnostic Tests
Serum albumin <3.5 mg/dL
Lymphocyte count <1800/mm3
Wound culture positive
Inspect skin/ wound frequently
Risk for Infection
Imbalanced Nutrition: Less Than Body Requirements
Provide nutritious diet
Monitor daily caloric intake
Encourage adequate fluid intake
Desired Outcomes
• Wound shows granulation
• Wound decreases in size
• No new pressure ulcers appear
• Patient states pain less than 3 on a 0-10 scale
• Family participates in treatment plan
Gastrointestinal
Unable to eat solid foods and has been taking increasingly less of her pureed foods
Daughter believes patient has lost several pounds in recent months
Monitor vital signs
Enteral feeding as necessary
Maintain asepsis
Provide nutrition supplements
Assessment data
Nursing interventions
Nursing diagnoses
Desired outcomes

Concept Map by Elaine Bishop Kennedy, EdD, RN

Chart 27-4 NIC INTERVENTION ACTIVITIES
The Patient with Pressure Ulcers

Pressure Ulcer Care: *Facilitation of healing in pressure ulcers.*
- Describe characteristics of pressure ulcers at regular intervals, including size (L×W×D), stage (I-IV), location, exudate, granulation or necrotic tissue, and epithelialization.
- Monitor color, temperature, edema, moisture, and appearance of surrounding skin.
- Keep the ulcer moist to aid in healing.
- Cleanse the skin around the ulcer with mild soap and water.
- Débride ulcer, as needed.
- Cleanse the ulcer with the appropriate nontoxic solution, working in a circular motion from the center.
- Note characteristics of any drainage.
- Apply dressings, as appropriate.
- Monitor for signs and symptoms of infection in the wound.
- Position every 1 to 2 hours to avoid prolonged pressure.
- Use specialty beds and mattresses, as appropriate.
- Ensure adequate dietary intake.
- Monitor nutritional status.
- Teach individual or family member(s) wound care procedures.
- Initiate consultation services of the enterostomal therapy nurse, as needed.

NIC intervention activities selected from Bulechek, G.M., Butcher, H.K., & McCloskey Dochterman, J. (Eds.). (2008). *Nursing interventions classification (NIC)* (5th ed.). St. Louis: Mosby. No part of this work is to be altered without prior written permission from the Publisher.

TABLE 27-4 Common Dressing Techniques for Wound Débridement

Technique	Mechanism of Action
Wet-to-damp saline-moistened gauze	As with the wet-to-dry technique, necrotic debris is mechanically removed but with less trauma to healing tissue.
Continuous wet gauze	The wound surface is continually bathed with a wetting agent of choice, promoting dilution of viscous exudate and softening of dry eschar.
Topical enzyme preparations	Proteolytic action on thick, adherent eschar causes breakdown of denatured protein and more rapid separation of necrotic tissue.
Moisture-retentive dressing	Spontaneous separation of necrotic tissue is promoted by autolysis.

hydrate surface cells, form scabs, or convert the wound to a deeper injury.

Assess the ulcer for necrotic tissue and the quantity of exudate. Coordinate with the certified wound care specialist to select a dressing material with properties that promote an optimal environment for healing. For example, a material that does not stick to the wound surface and does not remove fragile epithelial cells when it is changed is the dressing of choice for protecting new tissue. Depending on the amount of drainage, select either a hydrophobic or a hydrophilic material:

- A **hydrophobic** (nonabsorbent, waterproof) material is useful when the wound is relatively free of drainage and the purpose is to protect the ulcer from external contamination.
- A **hydrophilic** (absorbent) material draws excessive drainage away from the ulcer surface, preventing maceration.

A variety of synthetic materials with different absorbent properties are available (Table 27-5). Unlike cotton gauze dressings, these may be left intact for extended periods. Biologic and synthetic skin substitutes are available that can also prevent tissue dehydration and promote healing (see Chapter 28). However, the use of these products for chronic wounds is often cost prohibitive.

The frequency of dressing changes depends on the amount of necrotic material or exudate. Dry gauze dressings are changed when "strike through" occurs or when the outer layer of the dressing first becomes saturated with exudate. Gauze dressings used for débridement, such as those placed on a wound wet, allowed to become damp, and then removed, are changed often enough to take off any loose debris or exudate, usually every 4 to 6 hours. *Synthetic dressings are changed when exudate causes the adhesive seal to break and leakage to occur.*

Before reapplying any dressing, gently clean the ulcer surface with saline or a nontoxic wound cleanser as prescribed. If an antibacterial cleanser is prescribed, dilute the agent to reduce tissue toxicity and then rinse and dry the surface thoroughly before applying the dressing.

Physical therapy. The use of daily whirlpool treatments along with dressing changes for débridement can help remove dead tissue. The ulcerated area is immersed in or saturated with warm tap water that contains an antibacterial cleansing agent. Continuous agitation of the water loosens the debris and washes away exudate and particles. During treatment, the ulcer surface is cleansed with a gauze pad. After treatment, the therapist or certified wound care specialist often uses instruments to trim away any obvious bits of dead tissue that are still loosely attached to the ulcer surface.

Drug therapy. Clean, healthy granulation tissue has a blood supply and is capable of providing white blood cells and antibodies to the ulcer surface to combat infection. If extensive necrosis is present or if local tissue defenses are impaired, topical antibacterial agents are often needed to control bacterial growth. (Chapter 28 details the advantages and uses of topical antimicrobial agents.) In the absence of infection, antibiotics are avoided because of the danger of the development of resistant strains of bacteria.

Nutrition therapy. Successful healing of pressure ulcers depends on adequate nutritional stores of calories, protein, vitamins, minerals, and water. Nutritional deficiencies are common among older adults and chronically ill patients. These deficiencies increase the risk for skin breakdown and delayed healing of wounds that are already present. Severe protein deficiency inhibits all stages of the healing process and impairs host defenses against bacterial invasion.

Coordinate with the nutritionist to encourage the patient to eat a well-balanced diet, emphasizing protein, vegetables, fruit, whole grain breads and cereals, and vitamins. Fats are needed in the diet also to ensure formation of cell membranes. (See Chapter 63 for a complete discussion of nursing actions to ensure adequate nutrition.) If the patient cannot eat sufficient amounts of food, other types of feedings may be needed to increase protein and caloric intake (see Chapter 63). Vitamin and mineral supplements are also indicated.

TABLE 27-5 Commonly Used Dressing Materials

	Alginate	Biologic Dressing	Cotton Gauze Dressing	Foam	Hydrocolloidal	Hydrogel Dressing	Adhesive Transparent Film*
Indications	Hemostasis Débridement Absorption Protection	Débridement after eschar removal Protection Test before skin grafts (pigskin and cadaver skin) Burns Dormant, nonhealing wounds that do not respond to other topical therapies	***Continuous Dry*** Absorption Protection (nonadherent contact layer) ***Continuous Wet*** Delivery of topical agent Débridement (autolysis) Protection ***Wet to Damp*** Atraumatic mechanical débridement	Insulation Débridement Absorption Protection	Débridement Absorption Protection	Débridement Absorption Protection	Débridement† Protection (partial-thickness lesions) Secondary (cover) dressing
Advantages	Highly absorbent Biodegradable Easy application Nonadhesive Can be used as packing for deep wounds Can be used for infected wounds	Most "natural" wound covering Reduces pain Conforms to uneven wound surfaces Acts as a catalyst for healing Alternative to autograft	Readily available Good mechanical débridement *if used properly* Effective delivery of topical agents	Absorbent Insulates wound Easy application Nonadhesive (most products) Conforms to uneven wound surfaces	Absorbent Excludes bacteria Waterproof Reduces pain Easy application Easy to store Painless removal	Absorbent Nonadhesive Reduces pain Conducive to use with topical agents Conforms to uneven wound surfaces Amorphous form can be used as a filler Easy to store	Wound visualization Good adhesion Waterproof Reduces pain Cost-effective Easy to store
Disadvantages	Requires secondary dressing to secure Can cause desiccation of tissue if drainage is minimal Foul odor and gelling may be confused with infection	Requires secondary dressing to secure Very expensive Skin substitutes require skill to apply	Delayed healing if used improperly Pain on removal Requires frequent dressing changes	Poor barrier function Requires secondary dressing to secure	Nontransparent Softening and loss of shape with pressure, heat, and friction Odor with dressing removal Expensive Requires use of "fillers" for deep, draining lesions	Poor barrier function Only partial wound visualization Requires secondary dressing to secure Can promote growth of *Pseudomonas* and other microorganisms	Difficult to apply properly Nonabsorbent Adhesive to normal and healing tissue Limited to superficial lesions

*Also available in nonadhesive forms.
†Use with caution in patients with leukopenia or vascular disease.

TABLE 27-5 **Commonly Used Dressing Materials—cont'd**

	Alginate	Biologic Dressing	Cotton Gauze Dressing	Foam	Hydrocolloidal	Hydrogel Dressing	Adhesive Transparent Film*
Dressing changes	When dressing is saturated (every 3-5 days) or more frequently	Topical growth factors: daily Skin substitutes: varies (similar to grafts)	Necrotic base: every 4-6 hr Clean base: every 12-24 hr	When dressing is saturated or more frequently	Necrotic base: every 24 hr Clean base: on leakage of exudates	Necrotic base: every 6-8 hr Clean base: every 24 hr	Necrotic base: every 24 hr Clean base: on leakage of exudate

New technologies. For chronic ulcers that remain open for months, new technologies have had some success. These include electrical stimulation, vacuum-assisted wound closure, hyperbaric oxygen therapy, topical growth factors, and skin substitutes.

Electrical stimulation is the application of a low-voltage current to a wound area to increase blood vessel growth and promote granulation. This treatment is usually performed by a certified wound care specialist. A single electrode can be applied directly to a wound through a sterile dressing, or multiple electrodes can be applied around a wound. The voltage is delivered in "pulses" that may cause the patient to feel a "tingling" sensation. Usually electrical stimulation is performed for 1 hour each day five to seven times per week. This form of treatment is not used with patients who have a pacemaker or who have a wound over the heart.

Vacuum-assisted wound closure (VAC) has been used successfully to reduce or even close chronic ulcers by removing fluids or infectious materials from the wound and enhancing the formation of granulation tissue. This technique requires that a suction tube be covered by a special sponge and sealed in place for 48 hours. During that time, continuous low-level negative pressure is applied through the suction tube. Duration of the treatment is determined by the wound's response. It should not be used in areas where skin cancer is located. Failure of VAC therapy is often due to the inability to maintain an adequate and consistent dressing seal.

Bleeding complications from this procedure can occur if the patient is on anticoagulant therapy or has some degree of reduced tissue health near the wound (e.g., with radiation therapy or poor nutrition). Monitor the patient at least every 2 hours for manifestations of bleeding at or near the wound site while the device is in use (Malli, 2005).

Hyperbaric oxygen (HBO) therapy is the administration of oxygen under high pressure, raising the tissue oxygen concentration. This type of therapy is costly and usually reserved for life- or limb-threatening wounds such as burns, necrotizing soft tissue infections, brown recluse spider bites, osteomyelitis, and diabetic ulcers. The patient is enclosed in a large chamber and exposed to 100% oxygen at pressures greater than normal atmospheric (sea level) pressure. Systemic oxygen enhances the ability of white blood cells to kill bacteria and reduce swelling. Treatment usually lasts from 60 to 90 minutes. Smaller topical oxygen delivery devices are also available. These devices are applied directly over an open wound to promote local tissue oxygenation.

Topical growth factors are biologically active substances that stimulate cell movement and growth. These factors are deficient in chronic wounds, and topical application is being studied as a way to stimulate wound healing. For example, platelet-derived growth factor (PDGF) stimulates the movement of fibroblasts into the wound space. Use of this and other growth factors has been found to be more successful in clean, surgically débrided chronic wounds (Woo et al., 2007).

Skin substitutes are engineered products that aid in the temporary or permanent closure of different types of wounds. These products vary widely in design and application and are used mainly for surgically débrided wounds, such as a full-thickness pressure ulcer before reconstruction with skin grafts or muscle flaps (Woo et al., 2007).

Surgical Management. Surgical management of a pressure ulcer includes removal of necrotic tissue and skin grafting or use of muscle flaps to close wounds that cannot heal by epithelialization and contraction. Not all wounds are candidates for grafting. Those with poor blood flow are unlikely to have successful graft take and heal.

Preoperative care. Before surgery, care is focused on preparing the ulcer to accept a skin graft or muscle flap. Monitor potential donor sites, taking care to maintain the integrity of the donor skin and to avoid minor injuries that may result in infection and graft loss.

Operative procedures. The operative procedures used for surgical management of pressure ulcers include débridement and grafting. One or both of these procedures may be done.

Surgical débridement is the removal of thick, adherent wound crust using a scalpel or scissors. It may be performed to hasten the removal of the dead tissue, a potential source of infection. *The longer open wounds exist, the greater the risk for sepsis or prolonged hospitalization.* Depending on the size and depth of the ulcer and the projected blood loss, débridement can be performed at the bedside or in the treatment room by a wound care specialist or advanced practice nurse. When the wound is large or has a risk for excessive bleeding, débridement is performed in an operating room. In either case, the patient should receive sedation or a local anesthetic before the procedure. Although necrotic tissue does not have sensation, the healthy tissue at the point of attachment may have sensation.

Grafting is used for wound closure when full-thickness ulcers cannot close and when natural healing would result in loss of joint function, an unacceptable cosmetic appearance, or a high potential for wound recurrence. Successful skin grafting requires a clean and granulating or freshly excised ulcer bed. Partial-thickness (split-thickness) or full-thickness strips of skin are removed from the donor area, transferred to the ulcer, and sutured or stapled in place. Full-thickness free grafts and myocutaneous flaps are used to cover deep, massive

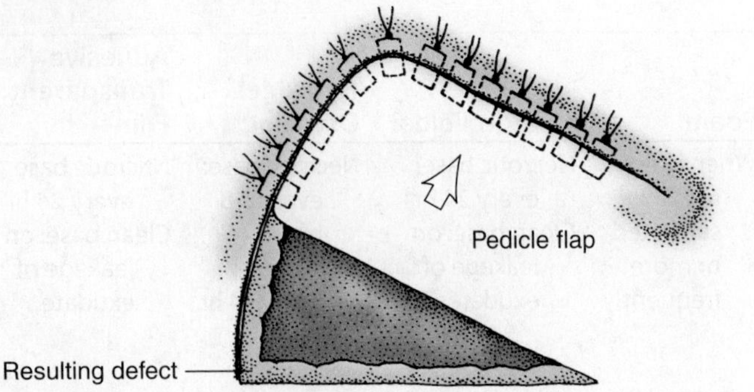
Pedicle flap
Resulting defect

Fig. 27-6 • Full-thickness pedicle flap of skin is separated and rotated to cover the wound. Blood vessels are left intact. The resultant defect is either primarily closed or covered with skin grafts. The flap is held in place with staples or sutures.

ulcers or ulcers in which vital structures, such as bone or tendon, are exposed.

Unlike free grafts, a pedicle flap is a full-thickness flap of skin that is raised and rotated to cover the defect, with one edge of the flap still attached to the site of origin to provide a blood supply (Fig. 27-6). Because all skin layers are removed, full-thickness donor sites are closed surgically or covered with additional split-thickness skin grafts. Partial-thickness donor sites heal spontaneously if infection is avoided.

When extensive surgical débridement has been performed on a large wound that does not have an adequate blood supply for grafting, other closure methods may be needed. If there is sufficient healthy skin around the débrided wound, the edges may be pulled together and surgically closed. Otherwise, the wound is managed with dressings until it closes by contraction and scar formation.

Postoperative care. After surgery, graft sites are immobilized with bulky cotton pressure dressings for 3 to 5 days to allow vascularization, or "take," of the newly grafted skin. Do not disturb the dressing and encourage elevation and complete rest of the grafted area to allow blood vessels to connect the graft with the wound bed. Any activity that might cause movement of the dressing against the body and separation of the graft from the wound is prohibited.

After dressings are removed, monitor the graft for indications of failure to vascularize, nonadherence to the wound, or graft necrosis. If a pedicle flap has been used to cover the wound, inspect the edges of the flap at least every 4 hours for changes in color. *A pale flap with delayed capillary filling when blanched may have inadequate arterial perfusion.* A dusky color or sharp line of color change suggests inadequate venous or lymphatic drainage. Other techniques to monitor trends of blood flow in the graft, depending on the graft's location, include pulse oximetry, Doppler ultrasonography, and transcutaneous oxygen determination.

Nursing care of partial-thickness donor sites aims to protect the area from injury and infection until re-epithelialization can occur and to promote comfort. A pressure dressing is usually placed over the donor area to promote hemostasis. After 24 to 48 hours, this outer dressing is removed, revealing a single wound contact layer of fine-mesh gauze or synthetic mesh material.

Today most donor sites are dressed with moisture-retentive dressings, such as synthetic transparent films. However, if the donor site is treated with dry exposure, promote air circulation to the wound by positioning the patient to avoid pressure on the site and using an overbed cradle to tent the sheets. After the dressing has dried and formed a "scab," keep the wound dry and undisturbed until healing is evident (at 10 to 14 days). As the donor site heals, the gauze and dried blood lift away from the new epithelium beneath. Trimming the separating gauze close to the skin surface reduces the chance of the patient catching the loose end of the dressing on an object and removing the still-adherent gauze before healing is complete.

The donor sites initially may be more painful than graft sites. Administer analgesics as prescribed, and provide other comfort measures as needed. Reposition the patient during the immediate period after surgery to promote comfort only if movement of the graft site can be avoided. Offer or delegate the intervention of back rubs to help relieve muscle spasms that occur with reduced mobility. Pay attention to relieving pressure over unaffected bony prominences that may lead to additional ulcers.

Graft and donor sites on posterior body surfaces present a particular problem. For the graft or flap to become fully vascularized or for the donor sites to dry, the patient must be immobilized in a side-lying or prone position for 7 to 10 days.

An alternative to this positioning is the use of special low-pressure or air-fluidized beds, such as the Clinitron bed, KinAir bed, or FluidAir bed, which not only reduce ischemia of the graft or flap while the patient is supine but also help prevent breakdown of intact skin. A major limitation to the use of these beds is cost, which is usually outweighed by the potential for decreased morbidity and length of hospital or long-term care stay.

Risk for Infection and Wound Extension

NOC **Planning: Expected Outcomes.** The patient with a pressure ulcer is expected to remain free of wound infection or systemic sepsis. Indicators include that the patient will have mild or no:

- White blood cell elevation
- Positive blood culture
- Purulent drainage
- Increase in wound size or depth

Interventions. Priority nursing interventions focus on preventing wound infections and identifying wound infections early to prevent complications.

Monitoring the ulcer's appearance using objective criteria allows evaluation of the response to treatment and early recognition of infection. If an ulcer shows no progress toward healing within 7 to 10 days or worsens, the treatment plan should be re-evaluated. Chart 27-5 outlines objectives of monitoring wounds with and without tissue loss. Patients who are at highest risk for infection are those who are older, have white blood cell disorders, are receiving steroid therapy, or have wounds with a compromised blood supply.

Preventing infection and its complications starts with monitoring the ulcer's progress. Routinely check for manifestations of wound infection: increased redness at the wound margins, edema, purulent and malodorous drainage, and tenderness of the wound margins. Report these signs to the health care provider:

- Sudden deterioration of the ulcer as evidenced by an increase in the size or depth of the lesion
- Changes in the color or texture of the granulation tissue
- Changes in the quantity, color, or odor of exudate

Chart 27-5 BEST PRACTICE FOR PATIENT SAFETY & QUALITY CARE

Monitoring the Wound

Variable	Frequency of Assessment	Rationale
WOUNDS WITHOUT TISSUE LOSS		
EXAMPLES		
Surgical incisions and clean lacerations closed primarily by sutures or staples		
OBSERVATIONS (USING FIRST POSTOPERATIVE DRESSING CHANGE AS BASELINE)		
Check for the presence or absence of increased: Localized tenderness Swelling of the incision line Erythema of the incision line >1 cm on each side of wound Localized heat	At least every 24 hr until sutures or staples are removed	To detect cellulitis (bacterial infections)*
Check for the presence or absence of: Purulent drainage from any portion of the incision site Localized fluctuance (from fluid accumulation) and tenderness beneath a *portion* of the wound when palpated	At least every 24 hr until sutures or staples are removed	To detect abscess formation related to presence of foreign body (suture material) or deeper wound infection*
Check for the presence or absence of approximation (sealing) of wound edges with or without serosanguineous drainage	At least every 24 hr until sutures or staples are removed	To detect potential for wound dehiscence
WOUNDS WITH TISSUE LOSS		
EXAMPLES		
Partial- or full-thickness skin loss caused by pressure necrosis, vascular disease, trauma, etc., and allowed to heal by secondary intention		
OBSERVATIONS		
Wound Size		
Measure wound size at greatest length and width using a metric ruler or, for asymmetric ulcers, by tracing the wound onto a piece of plastic film or sheeting (plastic template) Compare all subsequent measurements against the initial measurement	At least every week, usually every 48-72 hours	To detect increase in wound size and depth secondary to infectious process
Ulcer Base		
Check for the presence or absence of: Necrotic tissue (loose or adherent) Presence or absence of foul odor from wound when dressing is changed Note the frequency of dressing changes or dressing reinforcements owing to drainage.	At least every 24 hr	To detect the need for débridement or the response to treatment (necrotic tissue) and to detect local wound infection (frequent dressing changes and foul odor)
Wound Margins		
Check for the presence or absence of: Erythema and swelling extending outward >1 cm from wound margins Increased tenderness at wound margins	At least every 24 hr or at each dressing change	To detect wound infection*
Systemic Response		
Check for the presence or absence of elevated body temperature or WBCs or positive blood culture	Temperature daily; if elevated, check WBCs and blood culture	To detect bacteremia

*The wounds of patients who are severely immunosuppressed or those wounds with compromised blood supply may not exhibit a typical inflammatory response to local wound infection.

WBCs, White blood cells.

These changes may occur with or without clinical signs of bacteremia, such as fever, an elevated white blood cell count, and positive blood cultures. Use the previously described interventions to prevent the formation of new pressure ulcers and to prevent early-stage ulcers from progressing to deeper wounds (see Chart 27-2).

Maintaining a safe environment can help prevent wound infection. Because of the variety of organisms in the hospital environment, keeping an ulcer totally free of bacteria is impossible. Optimal ulcer management is based on maintaining acceptably low levels of organisms through meticulous wound care and reducing contamination with pathogenic organisms that could lead to sepsis and possible death, especially in older adults. *Teach all personnel to use Standard Precautions and to properly dispose of soiled dressings and linens.*

Community-Based Care

Patients with pressure ulcers may be in acute care, subacute care, long-term care, or home care settings. If pressure ulcer therapy requires hospitalization, most patients with pressure ulcers are discharged before complete wound closure is achieved. Discharge may be to the home setting or to a long-term care facility, depending on the degree of debilitation and other patient factors.

Home Care Management

Care of the ulcer in the patient's home is similar to care in the hospital. Most dressing supplies and pressure-relief devices can be easily obtained at the local pharmacy or medical supply store. If débridement of the ulcer is still needed, a handheld shower device or forceful irrigation of the wound with a 35-mL syringe and 19-gauge angiocatheter can be substituted for whirlpool therapy.

Many patients cannot change their own dressings because of distress over an altered body image or the pain of dressing removal. Others depend on family members or support personnel because of limited physical mobility or inability to reach the wound.

For some patients, drastic changes in daily activities are needed to promote healing. Patients with pressure ulcers on the legs may need frequent rest periods with leg elevation to avoid or reduce edema. Immobile patients with pressure ulcers require around-the-clock repositioning as often as every 2 to 4 hours to prevent further breakdown, which takes its toll on family members or other caregivers. Explain the rationale for activity changes to the patient and family, and explore alternative ways of coping with these changes.

Some patients may need to continue the use of special beds or mattress overlays at home. Although these items can be expensive, their use at home can keep the patient out of other, more-costly health care settings. Coordinate with the case manager to work with the insurance company in providing these important aids for quality patient care.

Health Teaching

Before the patient is discharged, the patient or person who will be performing the wound care should demonstrate facility in removing the dressing, cleaning the wound, and applying the dressing. When choosing a dressing to be used at home, consider the patient's or caregiver's ability to apply the dressing properly. If the patient's finances are limited, also address the cost of the dressing material. Some dressings may be easier to apply and less expensive than other materials. At times, the more expensive dressing materials that require less frequent changing may be preferred. Explain the manifestations of wound infection, and remind the patient and family to report their presence to the health care provider or wound care clinic.

Encourage the patient to eat a balanced diet with frequent high-protein snacks. Discuss diet preferences with the patient, and coordinate with the nutritionist in suggesting foods that promote wound healing. Vitamin and mineral supplements may be prescribed to prevent or treat dietary deficiencies.

If the patient is incontinent, emphasize the need to keep the skin clean and dry. If bowel and bladder training is not possible, discuss the use of absorbent underpads, briefs, and topical moisture barrier creams and ointments as a method to reduce skin exposure to urine and feces.

Health Care Resources

A home care nurse may be needed for a few visits to follow wound progress after the patient is discharged. The hospital nurse provides details of ulcer size and appearance and any special wound care needs in a hand-off report to the nurse in the home, who can then accurately judge changes in ulcer appearance. Chart 27-6 is a guideline for a focused assessment of the patient with pressure ulcers.

To reduce waste and to help decrease the overall cost of treatment, emphasize proper use of dressing materials. Clean tap water and nonsterile supplies are acceptable for treatment of chronic wounds in the home and are less costly than sterile products. Nonsterile dressing materials can often be purchased in bulk from a local medical supply store at reduced cost. Stress the importance of properly cleaning reused items and of handwashing before touching any supplies.

The patient with activity restrictions may need daily assistance from a home care aide. Collaborate with a physical therapist or occupational therapist to help the patient and family continue rehabilitation efforts in the home.

DECISION-MAKING CHALLENGE
Delegation/Supervision

The patient described on p. 491 has developed a stage II pressure ulcer on her left elbow and has stage I changes over her ischial spines. She has asked one of the UAP assisting her today about using a rubber "donut" for sitting when she is using the computer. Also, she would like to use a whirlpool tub daily this week. The UAP brings these requests to you.

1. Is using a rubber donut a good strategy to manage her skin issues over the ischial spines? Why or why not? What will you tell the UAP?
2. What is the probable cause of the ulcer on her left elbow?
3. What care techniques will you teach this patient and the UAP to help heal this ulcer?
4. Is the whirlpool bath a good strategy, and are any special precautions needed?

evolve For suggested answer guidelines, go to http://evolve.elsevier.com/Iggy/.

▪ *Evaluation: Outcomes*

Evaluate the care of the patient with a pressure ulcer on the basis of the identified nursing diagnoses and collaborative problems. The expected outcomes include that the patient will:

- Experience wound healing by secondary intention as evidenced by granulation, epithelialization, and reduction or resolution of wound size

Chart 27-6 HOME CARE ASSESSMENT

The Patient at Risk for Pressure Ulcers

Assess cardiovascular status:
- Presence or absence of peripheral edema
- Hand-vein filling in the dependent position
- Neck-vein filling in the recumbent and sitting positions
- Weight gain or loss

Assess cognition and mental status:
- Level of consciousness
- Orientation to time, place, and person
- Can the patient accurately read a seven-word sentence containing no words more than three syllables?

Assess condition of skin:
- Assess general skin cleanliness
- Observe all skin areas, paying particular attention to bony prominences and those areas in greatest contact with the bed and other firm surfaces
- Measure and record any areas of redness or loss of integrity
- If possible, photograph areas of concern
- Note the presence or absence of skin tenting over the sternum or the forehead
- Note the moistness of skin and mucous membranes
- If wounds are present, remove dressings (noting condition of dressings), cleanse the wound, and compare with previous notations of wound condition:
  - Presence, amount, and nature of exudate
  - Use a ruler to measure wound diameter and depth
  - Amount (%) and type of necrotic tissue
  - Presence of granulation/epithelium
  - Presence or absence of cellulitis
  - Presence or absence of odor

Take the patient's temperature.

Assess the patient's understanding of illness and compliance with treatment:
- Manifestations to report to health care provider
- Mediation plan (correct timing and dose)
- Ambulation or positioning schedule
- Dressing changes/skin care
- Diet modifications (24-hour diet recall)

Assess the patient's nutritional status:
- Change in muscle mass
- Lackluster nails, sparse hair
- Recent weight loss of more than 10% of usual weight
- Impaired oral intake
- Difficulty swallowing
- Generalized edema

- Develop skin thickness in expected range at ulcer area
- Remain infection free

Specific indicators for these outcomes are listed for each nursing diagnosis and collaborative problem under the Planning and Implementation section (see earlier).

COMMON INFECTIONS

Pathophysiology

Skin infections can be bacterial, viral, or fungal. Chart 27-7 lists key features and common locations of each type.

Bacterial Infections

Bacterial skin lesions usually start at the hair follicle, where bacteria easily collect and grow in the warm, moist environment. **Folliculitis** is a superficial infection involving only the upper portion of the follicle and is usually caused by *Staphylococcus.* The rash is raised and red and usually shows small pustules. **Furuncles** (boils) are also caused by *Staphylococcus,* but the infection is much deeper in the follicle (Fig. 27-7). This larger, sore-looking, raised bump may or may not have a pustular "head" at its point. **Cellulitis** is a generalized infection with either *Staphylococcus* or *Streptococcus* and involves the deeper connective tissue.

Minor skin trauma usually occurs before the appearance of folliculitis and furuncles and may or may not contribute to the development of cellulitis. Patients may spread the infection to other parts of their bodies by scratching or rubbing the skin with fingernails that have organisms under them. Furuncles are more likely to occur in areas of heat and moisture, such as in the hair-bearing skin-fold areas. Cellulitis can occur as a result of secondary bacterial infection of an open wound, or it may be unrelated to skin trauma.

An increasingly common skin problem is infection with methicillin-resistant *Staphylococcus aureus* (MRSA) (Leung-Chen, 2008). This infection can range from mild folliculitis to extensive furuncles. It is easily spread to other body areas and to other people by direct contact with infected skin and by contact with articles of clothing, bed linens, athletic equipment, towels, and other objects used by a person with MRSA. The infection does not respond to cleansing with antibacterial soaps or most types of topical and many oral antibiotic therapies (Mendyk, 2008). If MRSA infects a wound or gains access into the blood, deep wound infection, sepsis, organ damage, and death can occur (Holcomb, 2006a). The incidence of the problem is highest among adults living in communal environments, such as dormitories or prisons, and among patients in hospitals or other health care residential settings. (See Chapter 25 for more detailed MRSA discussion.)

Viral Infections

Herpes simplex virus (HSV) infection is the most common viral infection of adult skin. HSV infections are of two types. Type 1 (HSV-1) infections cause the classic recurring cold sore. The severity of the disease increases with age and is worse when the patient is immunosuppressed. Genital herpes, caused by type 2 infection (HSV-2), is also recurrent (see Chapter 76).

After the first infection, the virus remains in the body in a dormant state in the nerve ganglia, and the patient has no symptoms. Reactivation stimulates the virus to travel the pathway of sensory nerves to the skin, where lesions reappear. In healthy people, recurrence of HSV infection is triggered by physical or psychological stressors, such as dry lips, sunburn, trauma, fever, menses, and fatigue. The virus can also be spread by direct contact between an actively infected person and a susceptible host. *Autoinoculation,* or transfer of either viral type from one part of the body to another, is also possible.

The time span between episodes and the severity of each attack vary. Outbreaks of oral herpes simplex usually last 3 to

Chart 27-7 KEY FEATURES

Common Skin Infections

Clinical Manifestations	Distribution
BACTERIAL INFECTIONS	
FOLLICULITIS	
Isolated erythematous pustules occur singly or in groups; hairs grow from centers of many of the lesions. Occasional papules are present. There is little or no associated discomfort. There is no residual scarring.	Areas of hair-bearing skin, especially buttocks, thighs, beard area, and scalp
FURUNCLE	
Small, tender, erythematous nodules become pus filled and more tender over time. Lesions may be single or multiple and also recurrent. Regional lymphadenopathy is sometimes present; fever is rare. Occasional scarring results.	Areas of hair-bearing skin, especially buttocks, thighs, abdomen, posterior neck regions, and axillae
CELLULITIS	
Localized area of inflammation may enlarge rapidly if not treated. Redness, warmth, edema, tenderness, and pain are present. On rare occasions, blisters are present. Cellulitis is often accompanied by lymphadenopathy and fever.	Lower legs, areas of persistent lymphedema, and areas of skin trauma (e.g., leg ulcer, puncture wound)
VIRAL INFECTIONS	
HERPES SIMPLEX	
Grouped vesicles are present on an erythematous base. Vesicles evolve to pustules, which rupture, weep, and crust. Older lesions may appear as punched-out, shallow erosions with well-defined borders. Lesions are associated with itching, stinging, or pain. Secondary bacterial infection with necrosis is possible in immunocompromised patients.	Type 1 classically on the face and type 2 on the genitalia, but either may develop in any area where inoculation has occurred; recurrent infections occur repeatedly in the same skin area
HERPES ZOSTER	
Lesions are similar in appearance to herpes simplex and also progress with weeping and crusting. Grouped lesions present unilaterally along a segment of skin following the pathway of a spinal or cranial nerve (dermatomal distribution). Eruption is preceded by deep pain and itching. Postherpetic neuralgia is common in older adults. Secondary infection with necrosis is possible in immunocompromised patients.	Anterior or posterior trunk following involved dermatome; face, sometimes involving trigeminal nerve and eye
FUNGAL INFECTIONS	
DERMATOPHYTOSIS	
Annular or serpiginous patches are present with elevated borders, scaling, and central clearing. Itching is common. Lesions may be single or multiple.	Anywhere on the body
CANDIDIASIS	
Erythematous macular eruption occurs with isolated pustules or papules at the border (satellite lesions). Candidiasis is associated with burning and itching. Oral lesions (thrush) appear as creamy white plaques on an inflamed mucous membrane. Cracks or fissures at the corners of the mouth may be present.	Skin-fold areas: perineal and perianal region, axillae, beneath breasts, and between the fingers; under wet or occlusive dressings Lesions possibly present on the oral or vaginal mucous membranes

10 days. The patient sheds virus and is contagious for the first 3 to 5 days. The patient may have tingling or burning of the lip before any lesion is evident.

The most common clinical picture of HSV-1 infection is isolated or grouped vesicles on a red base. The infection can occur anywhere on the skin and may be spread by respiratory droplets or by direct contact with an active lesion or virus-containing fluid (e.g., saliva). The lesions are painful and unsightly.

Herpetic whitlow is a form of herpes simplex infection occurring on the fingertips of medical personnel who have come

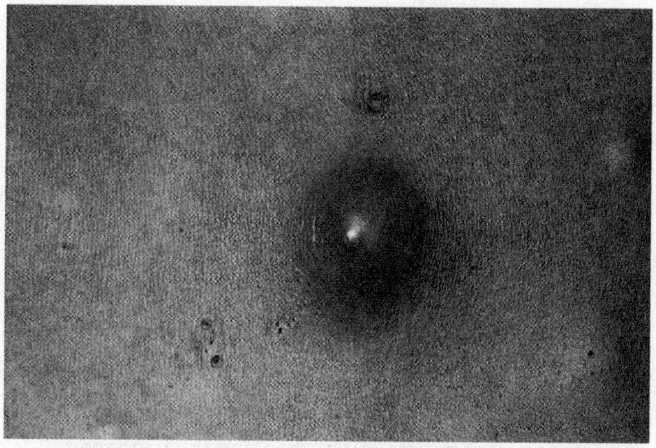

Fig. 27-7 • A furuncle.

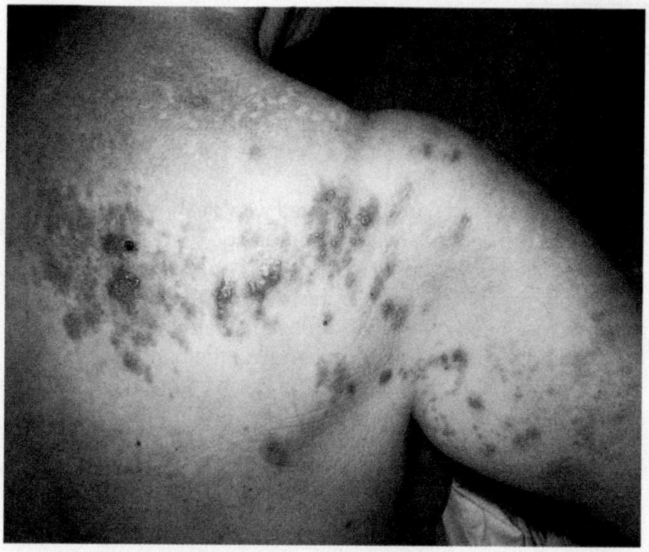

Fig. 27-8 • Herpes zoster.

in contact with viral secretions. This form of herpes can easily be spread to patients. Immunosuppressed patients are at increased risk for severe and persistent eruptions that can lead to life-threatening complications.

Herpes zoster (shingles) is caused by reactivation of the dormant varicella-zoster virus in patients who have previously had chickenpox. The dormant virus resides in the dorsal root ganglia of the sensory cranial and spinal nerves. The lesions of herpes zoster infections are similar to those of herpes simplex, but they have a different distribution pattern (Fig. 27-8). Multiple lesions occur in a segmental distribution on the skin area innervated by the infected nerve. Herpes zoster eruptions usually occur after several days of discomfort, which may vary from minor irritation and itching to severe, deep pain. The eruption usually lasts several weeks. **Postherpetic neuralgia,** severe pain persisting after the lesions have resolved, is a common complication in older patients.

Herpes zoster is a disease of immunosuppression, occurring most often and with greater severity in older people or in anyone who is immunosuppressed for any reason. The disorder can be accompanied by fever and malaise, often progressing to visceral involvement. *It is contagious to people who have not previously had chickenpox and have not been vaccinated against the disease.* Contagion is most likely when the lesions are present as fluid-filled blisters. Keeping patients with these lesions separated from other patients in the environment until the lesions have crusted reduces the risk for transmitting the virus to others. Complications include full-thickness skin necrosis, Bell's palsy, or eye infection, and scarring if the virus is introduced into the eye.

Fungal Infections

Dermatophyte infections, especially superficial infections, can differ in lesion appearance, body location, and species of the infecting organism. The term *tinea* is used to describe dermatophytoses; this term is then followed by the location description. For example *tinea pedis* involves the foot (athlete's foot), *tinea manus* involves the hands, *tinea cruris* involves the groin (jock itch), *tinea capitis* involves the head, and *tinea corporis* involves the rest of the body (ringworm).

Depending on the species, dermatophytes live mainly in the soil, on animals, and on humans. Superficial infection can start only if conditions are right for inoculation and maintenance of the organism in the outer layers of the skin.

Dermatophyte infections occur when the infecting organism comes in contact with impaired skin in a susceptible host. Most infections are spread by direct contact with infected humans or animals. Certain types of infections, such as tinea capitis and tinea corporis, can be transmitted by means of inanimate objects. For example, tinea capitis can be spread by sharing contaminated combs, brushes, hats, pillowcases, and similar objects with people who have poor personal hygiene.

Candida albicans, also known as *yeast infection,* is another common superficial fungal infection of skin and mucous membranes. The organism is present almost everywhere and easily grows in a warm, moist environment. Risk factors for this infection include immunosuppression, long-term antibiotic therapy, diabetes mellitus, and obesity. The incidence is higher in hot, humid climates.

Infected skin has a moist, red, irritated appearance and usually causes itching and burning. Common areas for infection include the perineum, vagina, axillae, under the breasts, and in the mouth (where it is known as *thrush*).

Prevention is aimed at keeping skin-fold areas clean and dry. Turning patients and positioning to enhance airflow also aid in prevention. When the infection is present, meticulous cleanliness and the use of topical antifungal agents are needed. Inspect skin-fold areas as part of the daily skin assessment on any patient with mobility problems. Teach UAP how to position patients for best exposure of infection-prone areas to the air. Stress the importance of changing bed linens and patient gowns whenever they are damp. Report the presence of infection manifestations to the health care provider.

Health Promotion and Maintenance

Prevention of skin infections, especially bacterial and fungal infections, involves avoiding the offending organism and good personal hygiene to remove the organism before infection can occur. *Handwashing and not sharing personal items with others are the best ways to avoid contact with some of the most easily transmitted organisms, including MRSA* (Yamamoto & Marten, 2007). Chart 27-8 highlights strategies to teach patients and family members to prevent spread of the infection to other body areas and to other people.

For older adults who have had chickenpox and are, therefore, at risk for shingles (herpes zoster), a new vaccine has been approved, Zostavax. Its use is recommended for any adult older than 60 years who does not currently have shingles

Chart 27-8 PATIENT AND FAMILY EDUCATION GUIDE
Preventing Spread of MRSA

- Avoid close contact with others, including participation in contact sports, until the infection has cleared.
- Take all prescribed antibiotics exactly as prescribed for the entire time prescribed.
- Keep the infected skin area covered with clean, dry bandages.
- Change the bandage whenever drainage seeps through it.
- Place soiled bandages in a plastic bag, and seal it closed before placing it in the regular trash.
- Wash your hands with soap and warm water before and after touching the infected area or handling the bandages.
- Shower (rather than bathe) daily, using an antibacterial soap.
- Wash all uninfected skin areas before washing the infected area, or use a fresh washcloth to wash the uninfected areas.
- Use each washcloth only once before laundering, and avoid using bath sponges or puffs.
- Sleep in a separate bed from others until the infection is cleared.
- Avoid sitting on or using upholstered furniture.
- Do not share clothing, washcloths, towels, athletic equipment, shavers or razors, or any other personal items.
- Clean surfaces that may have come into contact with your infected skin, drainage, or used bandages (e.g., bathroom counters, shower/bath stalls, toilet seats) with household disinfectant or bleach water mixed daily (1 tablespoon of liquid bleach to 1 quart of water).
- Wash all soiled clothing and linens with hot water and laundry detergent. Dry clothing either in a hot dryer or outside on a clothesline in the sun.
- Urge family members and close friends to shower daily with an antibacterial soap.
- If another person assists you in changing the bandages, make certain he or she uses disposable gloves, pulls them off inside out when finished, places them with the soiled bandages in a sealed bag, and washes his or her hands thoroughly.

MRSA, Methicillin-resistant *Staphylococcus aureus.*

(Laustsen & Neilson, 2007). It is given as a one-time subcutaneous injection of 0.65 mL. The drug should not be given as an IM or IV injection and should not be given to anyone who is immunosuppressed. The most common side effect is an injection site reaction of erythema, pain, tenderness, swelling, warmth, or pruritus.

Patient-Centered Collaborative Care

Assessment

History

To differentiate among the possible causes of the lesions, concentrate on risk factors for each type of infection. If the location and appearance of lesions suggest a bacterial infection, explore any recent history of skin trauma as well as past or current staphylococcal or streptococcal infections. Determine living conditions, home sanitation, personal hygiene habits, and leisure or sport activities. Ask whether fever and malaise are also present.

Lesions appearing on the lips, in the mouth, or in the genital region are more likely to be a possible viral infection. Ask about:

- A history of similar lesions in the same location
- Presence of burning, tingling, or pain
- Recent stress factors that may have precipitated the outbreak
- Recent contact with an infected person

Information that the same type of lesions has occurred before is important in helping differentiate viral from bacterial lesions. If herpes zoster is suspected, ask whether the patient has had chickenpox in the past and about a history of shingles. Also determine whether the patient has received the shingles prevention vaccination, Zostavax.

The type of information you should ask a patient with probable dermatophyte infection depends on the location of the lesions. If tinea corporis or tinea capitis is present, assess the social and environmental factors that may have contributed to infection, such as direct contact with an infected person, poor personal hygiene practices, or frequent contact with animals. If tinea cruris and tinea pedis are suspected, ask the patient about the type and frequency of athletic activities.

Physical Assessment/Clinical Manifestations

Because most skin infections are contagious, take precautions to prevent the spread of infection when performing a physical assessment. Chart 27-7 lists the manifestations of common skin infections.

Laboratory Assessment

When pustules are present in bacterial infections, the infecting organism is confirmed by swab culture of the purulent material. Blood cultures may be helpful, especially if the patient is showing clinical signs of bacteremia.

Viral infections are confirmed by *Tzanck smear* and viral culture. Tzanck smear is a cytologic examination in which cells from the base of a lesion are examined under a microscope. The presence of multinucleated giant cells confirms a viral infection, although the exact virus is not identified.

Fungal infections are confirmed by a potassium hydroxide (KOH) test. Scales from the lesions are scraped, prepared with KOH, and examined under a microscope. The presence of fungal hyphae confirms the diagnosis. In addition to a KOH test, a fungal culture may be needed. Occasionally a skin biopsy is performed to obtain organisms for identification.

Interventions

Most skin infections heal well with nonsurgical management. Surgery may be required when an infectious agent is present in deep tissue layers. The priority nursing interventions focus on patient and family education to prevent infection spread to other body areas or to other people (see Chart 27-8). Meticulous skin care is needed for prevention of infection spread. In some instances, drug therapy is needed.

Skin care with proper cleansing is the most effective intervention. Teach patients with bacterial infections to bathe daily with an antibacterial soap. Instruct them to not squeeze any pustules or crusts but to remove them gently so that topical

Chart 27-9 COMMON EXAMPLES OF DRUG THERAPY
Methicillin-Resistant *Staphylococcus Aureus* (MRSA)

Drug and Dosage	Nursing Implications	Rationale
Vancomycin (Lyphocin, Vancocin) 500 mg IV every 6 hr	Ensure that IV access is patent.	If extravasated, drug is highly tissue damaging.
	Administer drug over at least 60 min and never as a bolus or by IV push.	When given more rapidly, drug causes hypotension, dysrhythmias, and histamine release.
	Observe patient for widespread flushing.	Drug triggers a histamine release causing "red man syndrome."
	Check IV site at least every 2 hr for a change in blood return, redness or pain, or the feeling of hard or "cordlike" veins above the site.	Drug is irritating to veins and can trigger thrombophlebitis.
	Ask the patient about any diarrhea or presence of watery stools.	Drug changes the intestinal flora and can lead to pseudomembranous colitis.
Clindamycin (Cleocin) 150-300 mg orally every 6 hr; 300-600 mg IM or IV 2-4 times daily	When given IV, administer slowly (over 30-60 min).	Rapid administration can induce shock and cardiac arrest.
	Check liver function tests.	Drug can induce liver damage.
	Ask the patient about any diarrhea or presence of watery stools.	Drug changes the intestinal flora and can lead to pseudomembranous colitis.
Linezolid (Zyvox) 400-600 mg orally or IV every 8-12 hr	Take blood pressure at least every 4 hr, especially for anyone who has hypertension.	Drug constricts blood vessels and may trigger hypertensive crisis.
	Check IV site at least every 2 hr for a change in blood return, redness or pain, or the feeling of hard or "cordlike" veins above the site.	Drug is irritating to veins and can trigger thrombophlebitis.
	Ask the patient about any diarrhea or presence of watery stools.	Drug changes the intestinal flora and can lead to pseudomembranous colitis.
	Observe for increased bruising or oozing of blood from gums or at injection sites.	Drug reduces platelet and red blood cell numbers, increasing the risk for bleeding.

drugs can be more easily absorbed. Teach the patient to apply warm compresses twice a day to furuncles or areas of cellulitis to increase comfort.

Applying astringent compresses, such as Burow's solution, to viral lesions for 20 minutes three times a day promotes crust formation and healing. Compresses also relieve the irritation and pain associated with herpetic infection. Teach the patient to avoid constricting garments that might rub the lesions and increase irritation.

Most superficial skin infections resolve more quickly if the involved skin is allowed to dry between treatments. Excessive moisture, especially if occluded by dressings, clothing, or bedding, promotes growth of organisms. If the patient is bedridden, position him or her for optimal air circulation to the area and avoid occlusive dressings or garments.

Isolation Precautions may be needed to reduce the spread of pathogenic organisms to other people. For most superficial bacterial infections, proper handwashing prevents cross-contamination. However, when hospitalized patients are colonized with *Staphylococcus* that is resistant to antibiotic therapy, strict adherence to isolation procedures is necessary.

Of the dermatophyte infections, tinea capitis, tinea corporis, and tinea pedis are most easily transmitted to others. Teach patients to avoid sharing personal items, such as hairbrushes, articles of clothing, or footwear. Repeated infections transmitted by dogs or cats may mean that patients have to get rid of a family pet to control infections.

Drug therapy for superficial infections involves topical agents. Mild bacterial infections of the skin usually resolve with topical antibacterial treatment. Patients with extensive infections, especially if fever or lymphadenopathy is present, require systemic antibiotic therapy. The most common systemic drugs used for bacterial skin infections are penicillins and cephalosporins. For those who are allergic to drugs from these classes, tetracyclines, macrolides, or aminoglycoside antibiotics may be used. For patients infected with MRSA or other drug-resistant organisms, drug therapy may involve IV vancomycin or oral linezolid or clindamycin. Nursing implications related to therapy with these drugs are presented in Chart 27-9.

Acyclovir (Zovirax), valacyclovir (Valtrex), or famciclovir (Famvir) is used for the treatment of viral infections (Wilson, 2007). Topical treatment decreases the numbers of active viruses on the skin surface and reduces pain in primary herpetic infections and localized lesions in immunocompromised patients. Topical treatment is of little benefit in recurrent infection. IV administration is limited to severe primary infections and immunosuppressed patients with symptoms of systemic infection.

Topical antifungal agents are used for patients with dermatophyte and yeast infections. An imidazole cream is applied to the infected skin at least twice a day until the lesions have cleared. To prevent recurrence, therapy is usually continued for 1 to 2 weeks after clearing. In some instances, antifungal powders may also help suppress fungal growth. For widespread or resistant fungal infections, systemic antifungal agents, such as ketoconazole (Nizoral), are given.

CUTANEOUS ANTHRAX

Cutaneous anthrax is an infection caused by the spores of the bacterium *Bacillus anthracis*. In the United States, the most common risk factor is contact with an infected animal. Those most at risk for cutaneous anthrax include farm workers, veterinarians, and tannery and wool workers. This organism has now become a tool for terrorism. *When lesions that are consistent with cutaneous anthrax appear in people who have no exposure to infected animals, consider the possibility of bioterrorism.*

The infection can be confined to the skin, or it may be systemic. At first a raised vesicle appears on an exposed body area such as the head or arms. The lesion may itch and often resembles an insect bite. Within a few days, the center of the vesicle becomes hemorrhagic and sinks inward. An area of necrosis and ulceration begins. Usually this process is painless. The tissue around the wound swells and can become quite edematous. With necrosis, an eschar forms. The two features that distinguish anthrax lesions from insect bites or other skin lesions are that it is painless and that eschar forms regardless of treatment. Patients may have only one lesion, or there may be multiple lesions, usually in the same body area.

Some patients develop glandular symptoms with cutaneous anthrax. The entire area becomes edematous and tender. Fever and chills may be present, as may enlarged lymph nodes.

Diagnosis is made based on the appearance of the lesions, a culture that is positive for the organism, or the presence of anthrax antibodies in the patient's blood. Cultures are most easily obtained in the vesicle stage. Once the eschar is formed, a biopsy may be needed for culture. Blood cultures should be obtained from patients who have a fever.

Oral antibiotics for 60 days are indicated for patients who have no edema or systemic symptoms and whose lesions are not located on the head or neck. The antibiotics of choice are ciprofloxacin (Cipro) or doxycycline (Doryx, Vibramycin). For patients who have a fever, have lesions on the head or neck, are pregnant, or have extensive edema, antibiotics are given IV and then followed by an oral course of 60 days.

PARASITIC DISORDERS

Parasitic skin disorders occur most often in patients with poor hygiene and substandard living conditions or in those who are homeless. Any patient who shows obvious signs of a self-care deficit should be examined for these contagious parasitic infections.

PEDICULOSIS

Pathophysiology

Pediculosis is an infestation by human lice: *pediculosis capitis* (head lice), *pediculosis corporis* (body lice), and *pediculosis pubis* (pubic, or crab, lice). Human lice are oval and 2 to 4 mm long. The female louse lays hundreds of eggs, called *nits,* which are deposited at the hair shaft base in hair-bearing areas.

Patient-Centered Collaborative Care

The most common symptom of pediculosis is itching **(pruritus).** Excoriation from scratching may or may not be present. In addition to causing discomfort, these parasites can also be carriers of disease (e.g., typhus, recurrent fever).

Pediculosis capitis occurs more commonly in women than in men, especially on the sides and back of the scalp. Itching, the result of biting of the scalp by the parasites, is intense. It is most commonly transmitted by children and pets. A secondary infection may also be present from scratching.

Because the louse is difficult to see, examine the scalp for visible white flecks attached to the hair shaft near the scalp—the nits of the female louse. Matting and crusting of the scalp and a foul odor indicate a probable secondary infection.

Pediculosis corporis is caused by lice that live and lay eggs in the seams of clothing. The parasites also cause itching. The only visible sign of infestation may be excoriations on the trunk, abdomen, or extremities (Rushing, 2008).

Pediculosis pubis causes intense itching of the vulvar or perirectal region. Pubic lice, which are more compact and crablike in appearance than body lice, can be contracted from infested bed linens or during sexual intercourse with an infected person. Although these lice are usually found in the genital region, they can also infest the axillae, the eyelashes, and the chest.

The treatment of pediculosis is chemical killing of the parasites with topical sprays, creams, shampoos, such as permethrin (Elimite), lindane (Bio-Well, Kwell, Kwellada), or topical malathion (Ovide, Prioderm). Oral agents may also be used, such as ivermectin (Stromectol). In the case of pediculosis capitis, areas where the patient's head has rested (e.g., on pillows or chair backs) are also treated. Clothing and bed linens should be washed in hot water with detergent or dry-cleaned. The use of a fine-toothed comb helps remove nits from an infested scalp but alone does not cure the infection. In all cases of louse infestation, social contacts are treated when possible.

SCABIES

Scabies is a contagious skin disease caused by mite infestations. Scabies infections are transmitted by close and prolonged contact with an infested companion or infested bedding. Infestation is common among patients with poor hygiene or crowded living conditions. The scabies mite is carried by pets and is found among schoolchildren, homeless people, and institutionalized older patients.

Scabies is manifested by curved or linear ridges in the skin. The itching is more intense than with pediculosis, and patients often report that the itching becomes unbearable at night.

The visible white skin ridges are formed by burrowing of the mite into the outer skin layers. Closely examine the skin between the fingers and on the palms and inner aspects of the wrists, where these ridges are most common. A hypersensitivity reaction to the mite results in excoriated erythematous papules, pustules, and crusted lesions on the elbows, nipples, lower abdomen, buttocks, and thighs and in the axillary folds. Male patients can also have excoriated papules on the penis.

Infestation is confirmed by taking a scraping of a lesion and examining it under the microscope for mites and eggs. Close contacts also should be examined for possible infestation.

Treatment involves the use of scabicides, such as permethrin (Acticin), lindane (Kwell, Kildane, Scabene, Thionex), malathion (Ovide), or benzyl benzoate (Ascabiol) (Idriss & Khachemoune, 2006). Laundering clothes and personal items with hot water and detergent is sufficient to eliminate the mites.

COMMON INFLAMMATIONS

Pathophysiology

The inflammatory skin conditions have a variety of nonspecific manifestations, including severe itching, lesions with indistinct borders, and different distribution patterns. The cause of the eruption may or may not be identifiable. Inflammatory rashes can evolve from acute to chronic conditions.

Most inflammatory rashes are related to allergic immune responses. The responses may be triggered by external skin exposure to allergens or by exposure of the internal environment to allergens and irritants. The result is tissue destruction or skin changes induced by antibodies or cellular mediators of the immune system. (A more detailed description of these immune mechanisms is presented in Chapter 19.)

The specific cause of inflammatory rashes is not always known. When this is the case, the catch-all diagnosis of *nonspecific eczematous dermatitis,* or *eczema,* is often used.

Contact dermatitis is an acute or chronic rash caused either by direct contact with an irritant substance, resulting in toxic injury to the skin, or by contact with an allergen, resulting in a cell-mediated immune reaction.

Atopic dermatitis is a chronic rash that occurs with respiratory allergies and atopic skin disease. The mechanism is unknown, but atopic dermatitis is made worse by factors that include dry or irritated skin, food allergies, chemicals, or stress. (Atopic reactions are described in Chapter 22.)

Patient-Centered Collaborative Care

Because all the inflammatory skin eruptions appear similar, data collected from the patient are needed to identify the cause. Inflammatory skin problems differ from eczematous dermatitis in the chronicity of the disease, the distribution of lesions, and associated symptoms. Chart 27-10 lists the manifestations of many types of inflammatory skin conditions. Diagnosis is based on historical and clinical data.

If the cause of the rash is identified, avoidance therapy is used to reverse the reaction and clear the rash. For example, if a new soap for handwashing causes contact dermatitis of the hands, teach patients to avoid that irritating substance. Even when the cause is unclear, certain irritants may cause the rash to worsen and increase discomfort. Additional interventions promote comfort through suppression of the inflammatory response.

Steroid therapy with topical, intralesional, or systemic steroids is prescribed to suppress inflammation. The vehicle used to deliver a topical steroid depends on the body area involved. Because a side effect of oral corticosteroids (e.g., prednisone) is adrenal suppression, patients receiving long-term therapy must taper their drug dosages rather than stop them abruptly.

Remember that corticosteroids never cure the inflammation. During active disease, these drugs reduce manifestations and relieve associated discomfort. Moisten dressings with warm tap water and place over topical steroids for short periods to increase absorption. Avoid applying topical steroids under occlusive dressings unless specifically prescribed by the health care provider.

Caution all people not to use a topical corticosteroid anywhere, but especially on the face, if an infectious cause of the problem is suspected. Because these drugs suppress the immune response locally, if a skin infection is present, the use of a topical steroid on it will worsen the infection.

Avoid applying oil-based ointments and pastes to the sweaty skin-fold areas because maceration and blocking of

Chart 27-10 KEY FEATURES

Common Inflammatory Skin Conditions

Clinical Manifestations	Distribution
NONSPECIFIC ECZEMATOUS DERMATITIS	
Evolution of lesions from vesicles to weeping papules and plaques. Lichenification occurs in chronic disease. Oozing, crusting, fissuring, excoriation, or scaling may be present. Itching is common.	Anywhere on the body; localized eczema commonly involves the hands or feet.
CONTACT DERMATITIS	
Localized eczematous eruption with well-defined, geometric margins that are consistent with contact by an irritant or allergen. Usually seen in the acute form, but may become chronic if exposure is repeated. Allergy to plants (e.g., poison ivy or oak) classically occurs as linear streaks of vesicles or papules.	Cosmetic/perfume allergy: head and neck. Hair product allergy: scalp. Shoe/rubber allergy: dorsum of feet. Nickel allergy: earlobes. Mouthwash/toothpaste allergy: perioral region. Airborne contact allergy (e.g., paint, ragweed): generalized.
ATOPIC DERMATITIS	
Hallmark in adults is lichenification with scaling and excoriation. Extremely itchy. Face involvement is seen as dry skin with mild to moderate erythema, perioral pallor, and skin folds beneath the eyes (Dennie-Morgan lines). Associated with linear markings on the palms.	Face, neck, upper chest, and antecubital and popliteal fossae.
DRUG ERUPTION	
Bright red erythematous macules and papules are found. Skin blisters in extreme cases. Lesions tend to be confluent in large areas. Moderately itchy. Fever is rare. Dehydration and hypothermia can occur with extensive involvement. Condition clears only after offending drug has been discontinued.	Generalized. Involvement begins on trunk, proceeds distally (legs are the last to be involved).

pores may result in folliculitis. Instead, water-soluble creams are the vehicle of choice for these areas. Lotions and gels prevent matting of the hair and are more appropriate for hairy areas, such as the scalp. Stiff ointments or pastes, such as thick zinc oxide pastes, are used to apply therapy to localized areas because this vehicle clings to the skin where it is applied and resists spreading to uninvolved skin.

Antihistamines provide some relief of itching but may not keep the patient totally symptom free. The sedative effects of antihistamines can be better tolerated if the patient takes most of the daily dose near bedtime. Teach patients to avoid driving or operating heavy machinery if these drugs are taken during the day.

Comfort measures such as cool, moist compresses and lukewarm baths with bath additives have a soothing effect, decrease inflammation, and help débride crusts and scales. Colloidal oatmeal preparations, tar extracts, cornstarch, or oils are often added to baths to relieve itching.

PSORIASIS

Pathophysiology

Psoriasis is a lifelong disorder that has exacerbations and remissions. Even though psoriasis cannot be cured, patients can usually achieve control of symptoms with proper treatment.

Psoriasis is a scaling disorder with underlying dermal inflammation. The problem involves an abnormality in the growth of epidermal cells in the outer skin layers. Normally, cells at the basement membrane of the epidermis take about 28 days to reach the outermost layer, where they are shed. In a person with psoriasis, the rate of cell division is speeded up so that cells are shed every 4 to 5 days.

Although the antigens responsible for psoriasis have yet to be identified, psoriasis appears to be an autoimmune reaction resulting from overstimulation of the immune system. Langerhans' cells in the skin respond to the unknown antigen, leading to T-lymphocyte activation. These cells target the keratinocytes, causing increased cell division and plaque formation.

GENETIC CONSIDERATIONS

A strong genetic predisposition has been recognized in at least 30% of cases (Marks & Miller, 2006), and several genes appear to be involved in expression of the disease. It is likely that the disorder is multifactorial, in that a genetic predisposition exists but environmental factors influence whether or not the disease ever occurs, its severity, and its response to different treatments. Always ask about a family history when assessing the patient with psoriasis.

For many people with psoriasis, there is no family history of the disease. Many environmental factors lead to outbreaks and influence the severity of clinical symptoms, but these vary from person to person. Triggering factors may be local or systemic. A psoriatic lesion may appear after skin trauma (Koebner's phenomenon in which a previously injured area is more susceptible to development of cancer or chronic skin problems), such as surgery, sunburn, or excoriation.

Patients with psoriasis seem to improve in warmer climates, where there is more exposure to sunlight. Systemic factors that can aggravate the disease include infections (severe streptococcal throat infection, *Candida* infection, upper respiratory tract infection), hormonal changes (during puberty and menopause), stress, drugs (lithium, beta-blocking agents, indomethacin, antimalarials), obesity, and the presence of other diseases (Christopher & Meires, 2008).

Some patients with psoriasis also develop a debilitating arthritis. Psoriatic arthritis may be mild or can lead to severe joint changes similar to those seen in rheumatoid arthritis. The association of arthritis with psoriasis strongly suggests that psoriasis is really a systemic connective tissue disorder rather than a simple skin disease. See Chapter 20 for more discussion of connective tissue disorders and arthritis.

Patient-Centered Collaborative Care

Assessment

History

In addition to collecting routine epidemiologic data, ask the patient about any family history of psoriasis, including the age at onset, a description of the disease progression, and the pattern of recurrences. Ask the patient to describe the current flare-up of psoriasis, including whether the onset was gradual or sudden, where the lesions first appeared, whether there have been any changes in severity over time, and whether fever and itching are present. Explore possible precipitating factors, including recent skin trauma, upper respiratory tract infection, recent surgeries, menopause status, past and current use of drugs, and recent stress. Ask about previous interventions and the effectiveness of each in reducing symptoms.

Physical Assessment/Clinical Manifestations

The appearance of psoriasis and its course vary among patients. Typically during flare-ups of the disease, lesions thicken and extend to involve new areas of the body. As psoriasis responds to treatment, lesions become thinner with less scaling.

Psoriasis vulgaris is the most common type of psoriasis and presents as thick, reddened papules or plaques covered by silvery white scales (Fig. 27-9). Borders between the lesions and normal skin are sharply defined. Patches are less red and more moist in skin-fold areas because of sweat-induced maceration. Lesions are usually present in the same areas on both sides of the body. The more common sites are the scalp, elbows, trunk, knees, sacrum, and outside surfaces of the limbs. The facial skin is rarely affected. The patient may have only a few isolated lesions, or the entire skin surface may be affected.

Exfoliative psoriasis (erythrodermic psoriasis) is an explosively eruptive and inflammatory form of the disease with generalized erythema and scaling. It does not form obvious lesions. Examine for signs of dehydration and hypothermia or hyperthermia related to this severe inflammatory reaction. The increased blood vessel dilation and blood flow to the skin can reduce fluid volume through evaporative water loss from the skin surface.

Common Nursing Diagnoses and Collaborative Problems

Nursing diagnoses that may apply to the patient with psoriasis include:

- Impaired Skin Integrity related to immunologic factors
- Disturbed Body Image related to altered appearance
- Ineffective Coping related to the chronicity of the disease and alteration in body image

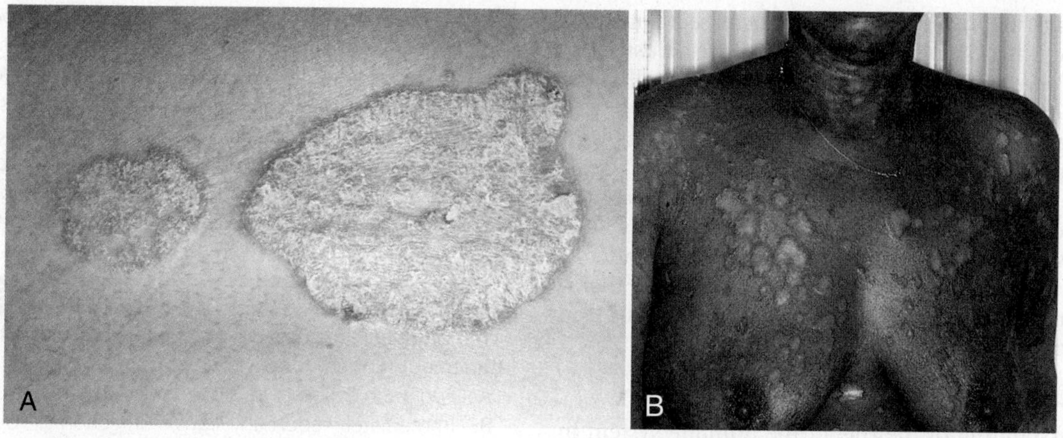
A
B

Fig. 27-9 • **A,** Psoriasis vulgaris in a Caucasian patient. **B,** Psoriasis vulgaris in a dark-skinned patient.

- Deficient Knowledge (Treatment) related to lack of exposure or unfamiliarity of information resources
- Chronic Low Self-Esteem related to alteration in body image
- Social Isolation related to alteration in physical appearance

Interventions

The different approaches to therapy are based on the extent of disease, the patient's distress, the physician's preference, and the response of the psoriasis to treatment. Patients must understand that no cure for psoriasis exists yet. Therapy is aimed at reducing cell proliferation and the inflammation. *Priority nursing strategies include teaching the patient about the disease and its treatment and providing emotional support for the changes in body image often experienced with psoriasis.*

Topical Therapy

The topical agents used to treat psoriasis are topical steroids, topical tar and anthralin preparations, and ultraviolet (UV) light.

Corticosteroids have anti-inflammatory actions. When they are applied to psoriatic lesions, they suppress cell division. The effectiveness of a topical steroid depends on its potency and ability to be absorbed into the skin. The more potent agents are used to treat patients with psoriasis.

Teach patients to enhance the skin penetration of these drugs by applying the steroid directly to the skin and, when possible, use warm, moist dressings and an occlusive outer wrap of plastic (film, gloves, booties, or similar garments) if specifically prescribed.

Tar preparations applied to the skin suppress cell division and reduce inflammation. These drugs are available as solutions, ointments, lotions, gels, and shampoos. The use of coal tar ointments is usually limited to inpatient care and specialized outpatient treatment clinics because these ointments are messy, cause staining, and have an unpleasant odor.

Topical therapy with anthralin (Anthraforte🍁, Drithocreme, Lasan), a hydrocarbon similar in action to tar, also relieves chronic psoriasis. These drugs can be used alone or in combination with coal tar baths and UV light.

Teach the patient to apply the high-potency anthralin, suspended in a stiff paste, to each lesion for short periods (not exceeding 2 hours). The drug is a strong irritant and can cause chemical burns. Remind the patient to check for local tissue reaction and to take care to prevent this drug from coming into contact with uninvolved skin.

Other topical therapies can be effective for many patients with mild to moderate psoriasis. These drugs include calcipotriene (Dovonex), a synthetic form of vitamin D that regulates skin cell division, and tazarotene (Tazorac). Tazorac is **teratogenic** (can cause birth defects) even when used topically. Teach women of childbearing age using this drug to use two forms of contraception.

Ultraviolet Light Therapy

Ultraviolet (UV) radiation is a physical agent commonly used as a topical treatment in many skin conditions, including psoriasis. Ultraviolet B (UVB) light, which produces more energy, is responsible for the obvious biologic effects of the sun, such as burning. Ultraviolet A (UVA) light emits a lower level of energy, requiring longer exposure time before cellular destruction occurs. Although the sun is an inexpensive source of UV radiation, better availability and intensity control occur with the use of artificial light sources. These sources include lamps or cabinets containing UV tubes. *The use of commercial tanning beds is not recommended for the patient with psoriasis.*

Ultraviolet therapy is limited by the potency and distance of the source from the skin, as well as the exposure time. Potency and distance remain constant, and the time of exposure is gradually increased to achieve a mild suntan effect without burning or tenderness. The patient's skin type, ranging from fair to darkly pigmented, affects his or her risk for burning and determines the exposure times. Because of the extremely high intensity of most artificial UVB light sources, treatments are measured in seconds of exposure; patients must wear eye protection during treatment.

Teach patients to inspect the skin carefully each day for signs of overexposure. If patients have tenderness on palpation and have clinical signs of severe erythema or blister formation, notify the physician before therapy is resumed.

Psoralen and UVA (PUVA) treatments involve the ingestion of a photosensitizing agent (psoralen) 2 hours before exposure to UVA light. Because UVA light produces less energy than UVB light, the onset of erythema and skin darkening may be delayed as long as 96 hours after exposure. Treatments are limited to two or three times a week and are not given on consecutive days. Exposure is gradually increased until tanning occurs. As with UVB exposure, dosages are adjusted according to the erythema reaction of normal skin as well as the response of psoriatic lesions.

Teach the patient to observe for generalized redness with edema and tenderness. If these symptoms are present, treatment must be interrupted until they subside. Because of the strong photosensitizing properties of psoralen, patients must wear dark glasses during treatment and for the remainder of the day. Long-term side effects of both UVB and PUVA therapies include premature aging of the skin, actinic keratosis, and an increased risk for skin cancer.

Systemic Therapy

A better understanding of the role of the immune system in the cause of psoriasis has led to biologic therapies to treat moderate to severe plaque disease. Biologic agents alter the acquired immune response, thus preventing overstimulation of keratinocytes (Khachemoune & Guillen, 2006). Although precautions vary with the specific mechanism of action, *these drugs induce immunosuppression and patients are at an increased risk for infection. Instruct them to discontinue the drug and notify the health care provider immediately if manifestations of infection occur.*

Approved biologic agents include alefacept (Amevive), efalizumab (Raptiva), and etanercept (Enbrel). Alefacept is given by IM injection weekly for 12 weeks. Efalizumab is given by subcutaneous injection once weekly. Etanercept is given by subcutaneous injection twice weekly. None of these drugs should be used by patients who are pregnant or breast-feeding. Some patients may be able to give themselves the subcutaneous injections. Demonstrate the proper techniques for drawing up the drug aseptically, selecting an appropriate site, and performing the actual injection. Have the patient perform a return demonstration. Reinforce correct techniques, and help the patient practice until he or she is proficient at the skill.

Other systemic treatment for the patient whose disease is resistant to topical therapy includes a cytotoxic agent, such as low-dose methotrexate (Folex, Mexate). Because of the liver-damaging side effects of methotrexate, liver studies are recommended before therapy is started and at least yearly thereafter. Small doses are usually effective in clearing the lesions. This treatment is avoided for patients who have liver damage, bone marrow suppression, or impaired renal function. In addition, this drug is also teratogenic and should not be used during pregnancy or breast-feeding.

Additional systemic drugs that induce immunosuppression may be used when lesions do not respond to other therapies. Such agents include cyclosporine (Sandimmune) and azathioprine (Imuran). The many health risks associated with these therapies must be considered along with the potential benefits.

Emotional Support

Often patients' self-esteem suffers not only because of the presence of skin lesions but also because of the unpleasantness of some of the treatments. Tar not only looks dirty but also has a very unpleasant odor. Bed linens and pajamas become stained, further discouraging social interaction.

Encourage the patient and family members to express their feelings about having an incurable skin problem that can alter appearance. Urge patients to contact other people with the disorder. Group discussions with family members or significant others can increase the socialization process.

The use of touch takes on an added significance for patients with psoriasis. For example, shake the patient's hand during an introduction or place a hand on the patient's shoulder when explaining a procedure. *Do not wear gloves during these social interactions. Touch, more than any other gesture, communicates acceptance of the person and the skin problem.*

NCLEX EXAMINATION CHALLENGE

What is the teaching priority for the 58-year-old woman started on etanercept (Enbrel) for severe psoriasis?

A. "Avoid sun exposure because this drug increases photosensitivity."
B. "Immediately report any signs of infection to your health care provider."
C. "Be sure to use at least two methods of contraception while taking this drug."
D. "If there is no change in the size of your lesions in a month, stop injecting the drug."

evolve For the correct answer, go to http://evolve.elsevier.com/Iggy/.

BENIGN TUMORS

CYSTS

Cysts are firm, flesh-colored nodules that contain liquid or semisolid material. Unlike cancerous growths, which are hard and firmly attached to underlying structures, a cyst moves and indents on palpation. Often there is a central pore through which the material can be expressed if the lesion is squeezed.

The most common cyst is an epidermal inclusion cyst. These growths are often asymptomatic and can be located anywhere, but they occur most often on the head and trunk. The most common cyst on the scalp is the sebaceous, or pilar, cyst.

If the patient wants to have a cyst removed for appearance or any other reason, surgical excision with primary closure is performed with a local anesthetic agent. The surgeon removes the entire cyst wall during excision to prevent recurrence.

A **pilonidal cyst** is a lesion of the sacral area that often has a sinus track extending into deeper tissue structures. As this cyst fills or becomes infected, it can become tender. An incision and drainage can be performed, but the cyst is likely to refill. The cure for this cyst is surgical removal, and the area heals by second intention.

SEBORRHEIC KERATOSES

Seborrheic keratoses are a common problem of older people. These benign epidermal neoplasms are gradually acquired after middle age and are often mistaken for actinic keratoses or pigmented skin cancers. These growths may occur anywhere but are more commonly found on the face, neck, upper trunk, and arms.

On inspection, seborrheic keratoses appear as multiple "pasted-on" papules or plaques ranging in color from flesh tones to brown or black (Fig. 27-10). The surface of the lesion has a rough, greasy, wartlike texture on palpation.

Seborrheic keratoses are removed only for cosmetic reasons or if a lesion becomes irritated from friction. Cryosurgery or curettage with or without a local anesthetic is performed.

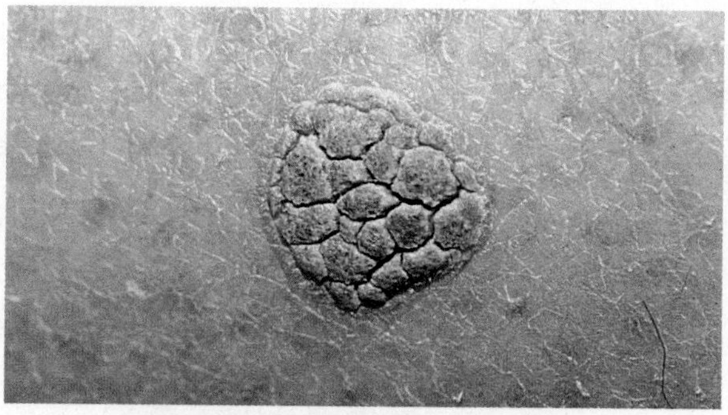

Fig. 27-10 • Seborrheic keratosis.

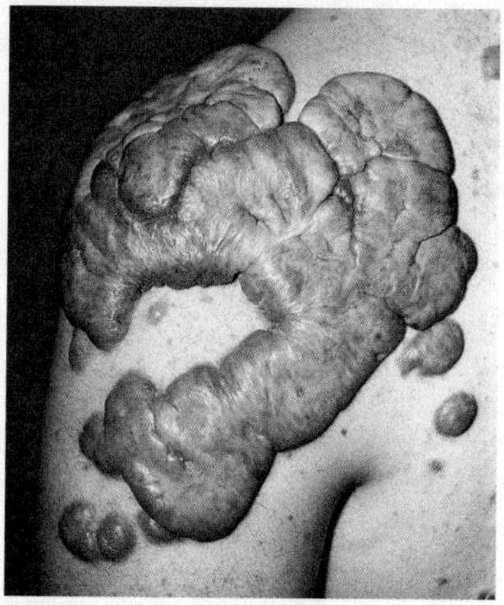

Fig. 27-11 • A keloid.

KELOIDS

A keloid is overgrowth of a scar with an excessive accumulation of collagen and ground substance. Keloids are more common in darker-skinned people and often arise at sites of surgical incisions, burns, and ear piercing (Fig. 27-11).

On physical examination, a keloid is an elevated, protruding lesion that extends beyond the edges of the original injury. These lesions can be cosmetically disfiguring. Treatment is difficult and not always successful. Small lesions may be controlled with intralesional steroid injections. Because surgical excision alone can result in an even larger scar, surgery is usually combined with another form of therapy, such as intralesional steroid injections or low-dose radiotherapy. Pressure dressings or elastic garments worn over the skin for 1 year after excision or steroid injection may also help keep the lesion flat.

NEVI

A **nevus,** or mole, is a benign growth of the pigment-forming cells. These lesions are classified according to their location within the layers of the skin.

Normal nevi have regular, well-defined borders and are uniform in color, ranging from light colors to dark brown. The lesion's surface may be rough or smooth. Because about 50% of malignant melanomas arise from moles, nevi with irregular or spreading borders and those with multiple colors should be considered highly suspicious. Other abnormal findings include sudden changes in the size of the lesion and reports of itching or bleeding.

Unsightly nevi or those subject to repeated irritation or trauma can be removed. Biopsy of any suspicious lesions is performed to rule out malignancy.

SKIN CANCER

Pathophysiology

Overexposure to sunlight is the major cause of skin cancer, although other factors are associated. Because sun damage is an age-related skin finding, screening for suspicious lesions is an important part of physical assessment of the older adult. The most common skin cancers are actinic or solar keratosis, squamous cell carcinoma, basal cell carcinoma, and melanoma. Table 27-6 describes common skin cancers.

Etiology and Genetic Risk

Actinic keratoses are premalignant lesions of the cells of the epidermis. These lesions are common in people with chronically sun-damaged skin. Progression to squamous cell carcinoma may occur if lesions are untreated.

Squamous cell carcinomas are cancers of the epidermis. They can invade locally and are potentially metastatic. Lesions on the ear, lip, and external genitalia are more likely to invade and spread than those found elsewhere on the body (Fig. 27-12). Chronic skin damage from repeated injury or irritation also predisposes to this malignancy.

Basal cell carcinomas arise from the basal cell layer of the epidermis (Fig. 27-13). Early malignant lesions often go unnoticed, and although metastasis is rare, underlying tissue destruction can progress to include vital structures. Genetic predisposition and chronic irritation are risk factors; however, UV exposure is the most common cause.

Melanomas are pigmented cancers arising in the melanin-producing epidermal cells (Fig. 27-14). Risk factors include genetic predisposition, excessive exposure to UV light, and the presence of one or more precursor lesions that resemble unusual moles. *This skin cancer is highly metastatic, and a person's survival depends on early diagnosis and treatment.*

Lighter skin and less pigmentation are genetically inherited traits. Also, a genetic mutation that is inherited in an autosomal-dominant pattern has been found for some cases of familial melanoma. The mutation occurs in a suppressor gene resulting in loss of control of cell growth. Two such mutated genes are *CDKN2A* and *CDK4* (Marks & Miller, 2006).

Incidence/Prevalence

The incidence of skin cancer is highest among light-skinned races and people older than 60 years (American Cancer Society, 2008). The incidence is higher among those who work outdoors, live at higher altitudes or lower latitudes, or spend significant amount of time sunbathing. Occupational exposure to arsenic or other chemical carcinogens also increases risk. The incidence of melanoma has increased during the past 30 years, accounting for 2% of all cancers and 1% of all cancer deaths (American Cancer Society, 2008).

Health Promotion and Maintenance

The single most effective prevention strategy for skin cancer is avoiding or reducing skin exposure to sunlight. However, even when people understand the cause of skin cancer and the seriousness of the disease, preventive behaviors are not always practiced. Common prevention practices include avoiding

TABLE 27-6 Common Skin Cancers

Clinical Manifestations	Distribution	Course
ACTINIC KERATOSIS (PREMALIGNANT)		
Small (1-10 mm) macule or papule with dry, rough, adherent yellow or brown scale Base may be erythematous Associated with yellow, wrinkled, weather-beaten skin Thick, indurated keratoses more likely to be malignant	Cheeks, temples, forehead, ears, neck, backs of hands, and forearms	May disappear spontaneously or reappear after treatment. Slow progression to squamous cell carcinoma is possible.
SQUAMOUS CELL CARCINOMA		
Firm, nodular lesion topped with a crust or with a central area of ulceration Indurated margins Fixation to underlying tissue with deep invasion	Sun-exposed areas, especially head, neck, and lower lip Sites of chronic irritation or injury (e.g., scars, irradiated skin, burns, leg ulcers)	Rapid invasion with metastasis via the lymphatics occurs in 10% of cases. Larger tumors are more prone to metastasis.
BASAL CELL CARCINOMA		
Pearly papule with a central crater and rolled, waxy borders Telangiectasias and pigment flecks visible on close inspection	Sun-exposed areas, especially head, neck, and central portion of face	Metastasis is rare. May cause local tissue destruction. 50% recurrence rate related to inadequate treatment.
MELANOMA		
Irregularly shaped, pigmented papule or plaque Variegated colors, with red, white, and blue tones	Can occur anywhere on the body, especially where nevi (moles) or birthmarks are evident Commonly found on upper back and lower legs Soles of feet and palms in dark-skinned people	Horizontal growth phase followed by vertical growth phase. Rapid invasion and metastasis with high morbidity and mortality.

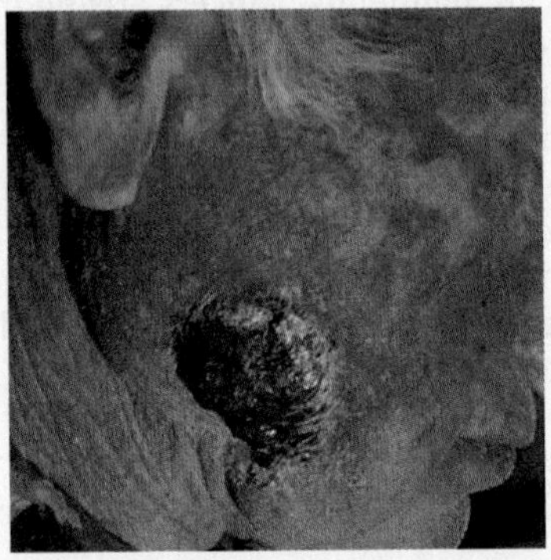

Fig. 27-12 • Squamous cell carcinoma.

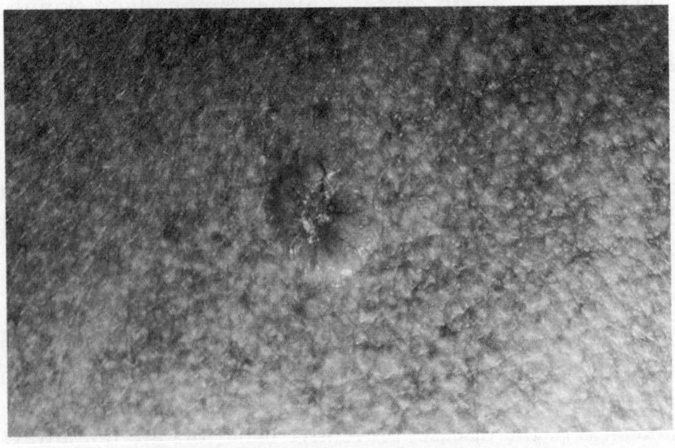

Fig. 27-13 • Basal cell carcinoma.

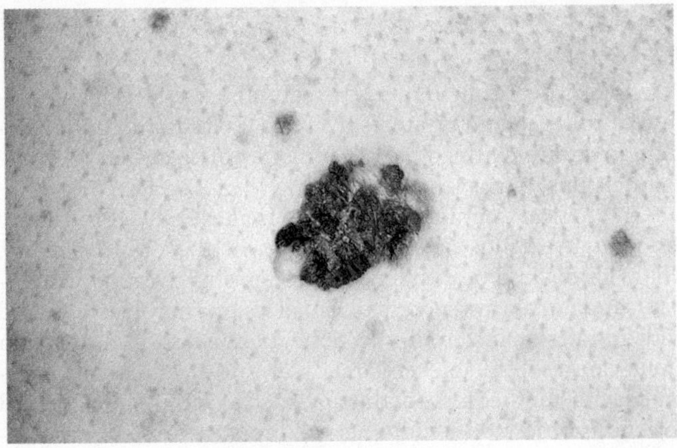

Fig. 27-14 • Melanoma.

direct sunlight, using sunscreen, and wearing protective clothing (including hats) whenever a person is in the sun, to prevent severe sunburn. *Teach all people to avoid tanning beds and salons.* Chart 27-11 lists methods of prevention that patients can use to reduce their risk for skin cancer.

Secondary prevention, early detection, is critical to survival with melanoma. Teach all people to be aware of their skin markings. Keeping a total body spot and lesion map can provide baseline information about suspicious lesions and help identify changes in a lesion or lesions earlier. Once a map is made, the person should systematically inspect his or her body monthly for new lesions and for changes in any existing lesions by performing thorough skin self-examination (TSSE). Often a partner is

EVIDENCE-BASED PRACTICE

Spot check with partners

Loescher, L., Harris, R., Lim, K., & Su, Y. (2006). Thorough skin self-examination in patients with melanoma. *Oncology Nursing Forum, 33*(3), 633-637.

Thorough skin self-examination (TSSE) is instrumental in detecting the presence of melanoma and other skin cancers early when cure is more likely. Patients who have been diagnosed with melanoma remain at increased risk for recurrent skin cancer or development of a new melanoma. Therefore continuing vigilance with TSSE on a monthly basis is needed even after treatment of an existing melanoma is completed. The purpose of this study was to determine to what extent patients previously diagnosed and treated for melanoma participated in this important secondary prevention practice.

Seventy subjects with melanoma being followed at a large National Cancer Institute designated comprehensive cancer center were enrolled in the study and returned all survey materials. Subjects were asked how frequently they examined the skin on all seven body areas included as criteria for TSSE (front of body from waist up, front of thighs and legs, bottom of feet, calves of legs, back of thighs, buttocks and lower back, upper back).

Although 59% responded that they performed TSSE, only 23% met the body area criteria for thorough examination. Those subjects diagnosed with higher stages of disease were more likely to perform TSSE. The main factor in correct performance of TSSE was the inclusion of a partner in the actual examination. The exact role of the partner was not explored. It could be that the partner helped remind the patient to perform the examination as well as served as an examiner and recorder.

Level of Evidence—4. The study was a well-designed cohort study.

Commentary: Implications for Practice and Research. The practice of monthly TSSE has been demonstrated to significantly reduce mortality from melanoma by detecting it at an earlier stage. Patients who have already had melanoma remain at far greater risk for development of new lesions. The two most important implications for nursing are to ensure that patients with melanoma understand their continuing risk and to help them learn to incorporate correct TSSE practice into their lives. The fact that partner participation increases adherence to regular performance of TSSE could be a focus of teaching. Teach the patient and the partner at the same time. Demonstrate how to actually do the examination and exactly what to report.

Chart 27-11 PATIENT AND FAMILY EDUCATION GUIDE

Prevention of Skin Cancer

- Avoid sun exposure between 11 AM and 3 PM.
- Use sunscreens with the appropriate skin protection factor for your skin type.
- Wear a hat, opaque clothing, and sunglasses when you are out in the sun.
- Keep a "body map" of your skin spots, scars, and lesions to detect when changes have occurred.
- Examine your body monthly for possibly cancerous or precancerous lesions.
- Seek medical advice if you note any of these:
  - A change in the color of a lesion, especially if it darkens or shows evidence of spreading
  - A change in the size of a lesion, especially rapid growth
  - A change in the shape of a lesion, such as a sharp border becoming irregular or a flat lesion becoming raised
  - Redness or swelling of the skin around a lesion
  - A change in sensation, especially itching or increased tenderness of a lesion
  - A change in the character of a lesion, such as oozing, crusting, bleeding, or scaling

needed to help evaluate skin spots or lesions on the back. Some people find taking pictures of their skin on a regular basis makes identifying changes easier. Teach everyone to evaluate all skin lesions using the ABCD guide for melanoma (see Chapter 26) and to consult his or her health care provider to examine any lesion having unusual characteristics. When lesions, such as moles, are present, they should be monitored yearly by a dermatologist or other health care professional.

Monthly TSSE is critically important for patients who have already had a melanoma lesion. A recent study found that only about 23% of those who had been treated for melanoma regularly practiced TSSE correctly (Loescher et al., 2006). The major positive influence for TSSE practice was working with a partner in this examination (see the Evidence-Based Practice box above).

Patient-Centered Collaborative Care

Assessment

In addition to age and race, ask the patient about any family history of skin cancer and any past surgery for removal of skin growths. Recent changes in the size, color, or sensation of any mole, birthmark, wart, or scar are also significant. Ask about which geographic regions he or she has lived in and where he or she currently resides. Obtain information about occupational and recreational activities in relation to sun exposure, as well as any occupational history of exposure to chemical carcinogens (e.g., arsenic, coal tar, pitch, radioactive waste, radium). Ask whether any skin lesions are repeatedly irritated by the rubbing of clothing.

Skin that has been injured previously is at greater risk for cancer development, an effect known as *Koebner's phenomenon.* Ask the patient if he or she has ever experienced a severe skin injury that resulted in a scar. Examine all scarred skin areas for the presence of potentially cancerous lesions.

The skin cancers vary in their appearance and distribution. Although most skin cancers appear in sun-exposed areas of the body, inspect the entire skin surface. Systematically examine the skin for any unusual lesions, particularly moles, warts, birthmarks, and scars. Also examine hair-bearing areas of the body, such as the scalp and genitalia. Palpate lesions to determine surface texture. Document the location, size, color, and surface features of all lesions and any subjective reports of tenderness or itching. Use the ABCD method of evaluating all lesions for possible melanoma (see Chapter 26).

Table 27-6 lists facts about common skin cancers. Punch, shave, or excisional biopsy of suspicious lesions is necessary to determine whether a skin lesion is benign or malignant.

Interventions

Surgical and nonsurgical interventions are combined for the effective management of skin cancer. Treatment is determined by the size and severity of the malignancy, the location of the lesion, and the age and general health of the patient.

Surgical Management

Surgical intervention is the most common means of managing any type of skin cancer. It can range from local removal of small lesions, with minimal discomfort and positive cosmetic results, to massive excision of large areas of the skin and underlying tissue for treatment of melanoma.

Cryosurgery involves the local application of liquid nitrogen (−200° C) to isolated lesions, causing cell death and tissue destruction. Local anesthesia is seldom needed because most patients have only minor discomfort during the procedure. Prepare patients for swelling and increased tenderness of the treated area when the skin thaws. Tissue freezing is followed in 1 to 2 days by hemorrhagic blister formation. Instruct patients to clean the sites with hydrogen peroxide to prevent infection. A topical antibiotic may also be prescribed.

Curettage and electrodesiccation may be used for small lesions that are not melanoma. This method can destroy the cancerous cells while minimizing damage to the surrounding uninvolved tissue. After a local anesthetic is given, the surgeon uses a dermal curette to scrape away the cancerous tissue. After curettage is complete, the surgeon places an electric probe on the wound and remnants of the tumor are destroyed by thermal energy.

Wounds created by this treatment heal by second intention, and scarring is usually minimal. Instruct patients in caring for the wound, including cleaning the wound, using prescribed antibacterial drugs, and applying dressings.

Excision is used for biopsy of small lesions. When the diagnosis is melanoma, a sentinel node may be biopsied to determine whether tumor spread has started (see Chapter 23). If the size and location of the lesion permit, surgical excision with primary closure is the preferred method. If the tumor has already been removed several times or if radiation therapy has damaged the surrounding skin, healing by second intention is indicated. This procedure allows the wound to be monitored for cancer recurrence. Skin grafts and flaps are used to repair large defects if tissue destruction is deep.

Mohs' surgery, a specialized form of excision, is used to treat basal and squamous cell carcinomas. The cancerous tissue is sectioned horizontally in layers, and each layer is examined histologically to determine the presence of residual tumor cells. Although the procedure is long and tedious, cure rates are high and there is less removal of healthy tissue compared with other surgical methods.

Wide excision for deeper melanoma or other skin cancers that are large or invasive often involves removing full-thickness skin in the area of the lesion. Depending on tumor depth, subcutaneous tissues and lymph nodes may also be removed. If the remaining skin is easily moved without creating extensive tension, the wound may be just sutured closed. If the remaining skin is tight or the wound is large, skin grafts may be needed to close the surgical wound (see earlier discussion on pp. 495-496).

Nonsurgical Management

Drug therapy may involve topical or systemic chemotherapy, biotherapy, or targeted therapy. Topical chemotherapy with 5-fluorouracil cream is used for treatment of multiple actinic keratoses or for widespread superficial basal cell carcinoma that would require several surgical procedures to eradicate. Therapy is continued for several weeks, and the treated areas become increasingly tender and inflamed as the lesions crust, ooze, and erode. Prepare the patient for an unsightly appearance during therapy, and reassure him or her that the cosmetic result will be positive.

After treatment is discontinued, cool compresses and topical corticosteroid preparations help decrease inflammation and promote comfort.

Systemic chemotherapeutic agents are used in the treatment of skin cancer except when the prognosis is poor, as in advanced melanoma.

Biotherapy with interferon is now an accepted treatment after surgery for melanomas that are at stage III or higher. The patient is first started on high-dose (20,000,000 units/m^2) interferon IV infusions daily for 5 days per week for 4 weeks after the surgical wound is well healed. Maintenance doses of 10,000,000 units/m^2 are continued three times per week for 1 year. The maintenance doses are given subcutaneously, and the patient must learn to self-inject the drug.

Experimental drugs that target lymphocyte control of tumor cell growth are being tried for treatment of metastatic melanoma. One promising type of agent currently in clinical trials is a drug that targets CTLA4 receptor and blocks it, resulting in significant tumor cell regression. Because the receptor is present on certain lymphocytes, the side effects of the drug include inflammation in a wide variety of tissues.

Radiation therapy for skin cancer is limited to older patients with large, deeply invasive basal cell tumors and to those who are poor risks for surgery. Malignant melanoma is resistant to radiation therapy; however, radiation therapy may be helpful for patients with metastatic disease when used in combination with systemic corticosteroids.

NCLEX EXAMINATION CHALLENGE

Which statement made by a client with a skin lesion indicates the need for further teaching?

A. "My wife helps me keep track of all my skin spots and lesions every month."
B. "Usually, I cover this spot with a small bandage so my belt doesn't rub it."
C. "At least I know this spot is not melanoma because it is red, not black."
D. "I should use sunscreen and clothing to protect my skin from sunburn."

evolve For the correct answer, go to http://evolve.elsevier.com/Iggy/.

PLASTIC OR RECONSTRUCTIVE SURGERY

Pathophysiology

The two main types of plastic surgery are aesthetic and reconstructive. **Aesthetic plastic surgery** is cosmetic, with the aim of altering a person's physical appearance. This intervention is sought by those who are unsatisfied with their body image. These procedures are considered elective surgery and are not covered by insurance. They can be very expensive and are most often performed among more affluent people. **Reconstructive plastic surgery** is the correction or improvement of functional defects that have occurred as a result of congenital problems (e.g., cleft lip, syndactyly [webbed fingers or toes]) or trauma and scarring (e.g., skin and joint contractures from burn wounds) or from other types of therapy (e.g., mastectomy for breast cancer therapy). These interventions are sought by patients who cannot perform ADLs as a result of an anatomic problem and are often covered by insurance.

In the United States, the decision to undergo plastic surgery is often a response to social and cultural norms about beauty. Patients become self-conscious about scars, facial lesions, disproportionate anatomic features, or, especially, changes in physical features associated with aging. Loss of skin elasticity and changes in fatty tissue distribution are progressive and especially noticeable around the eyes, near the cheeks, and on the neck. Fine facial wrinkles around the eyes and mouth are one of the first signs of aging. These changes are followed by gradual stretching and downward displacement of the soft tissue of the lower two thirds of the face. Similar changes are seen as skin wrinkling and looseness on the arms, chest, abdomen, buttocks, and thighs. These changes are also seen after dramatic weight loss. Appearance of skin lesions associated with chronic sun exposure also may trouble the aging patient.

Other people may want to change a physical detail associated with specific cultural identity. For example, people have changed eyelid shape, nose size and shape, and lip shape to conform to a more "Caucasian" appearance. Still other people have undergone surgery to increase their sense of belonging to a specific ethnic group. For example, African-American women may have aesthetic surgery to increase the size of their buttocks to conform to cultural norms about beauty and sexuality in the African-American community.

Patient-Centered Collaborative Care

Assessment

History

When taking a history from a patient who elects to have plastic surgery, use a nonjudgmental approach and be careful not to assume the reason for surgery on the basis of physical appearance. Often what might appear to be unsightly to you is of little concern to the patient, who wishes to change something else. Observe for any nonverbal communication that might establish the emotional state of the person or reveal feelings of embarrassment or guilt. Encourage the patient to describe the problem, including why it is bothersome and what he or she expects as a result of the change. Ask about his or her health history and recent medical problems, including obesity and trauma, to predict the amount of surgery needed to correct the defect and potential complications.

Physical Assessment/Clinical Manifestations

The patient seeking plastic surgery may have changes in appearance ranging from minor to significant deformity. Depending on the location of the problem, the patient may need to undress before the examination. Ensure privacy because the patient may be embarrassed by the problem.

Begin the physical assessment by closely examining the area of involvement to determine the extent of the deformity or problem. Have the patient assume different normal sitting and standing postures to provide better visibility of nonfacial defects. Document asymmetry of anatomic features, wrinkling or skin redundancy, scars or disfiguring skin marks, and obvious skin lesions.

Psychosocial Assessment

Regardless of whether a person is having reconstructive surgery or cosmetic surgery, body image and sense of self are always involved. These feelings often are deep-seated and may evoke emotional responses in the person, including shame, anger, resentment, and desperation. A person seeking reconstruction may have felt "different" from other people his or her entire life. A person seeking cosmetic surgery may face ridicule from family or friends about his or her perceived vanity. Use a sensitive, nonjudgmental approach when interacting with the person having or considering plastic surgery. It is important to recognize your own feelings regarding these procedures and to avoid being directive or expressing your own opinions. Often a patient who asks the nurse "Do you think I need this surgery?" is not comfortable with his or her decision.

Assess the patient for his or her sense of self and self-worth. Note whether he or she makes eye contact with you during the interview. Does the patient make any self-deprecating remarks or use the terms *ugly, stupid,* or *not sexy* when referring to himself or herself? If such remarks are made, ask him or her to clarify what is meant. Report concerns to the surgeon.

Address the patient's expectations of plastic surgery. Often people who seek plastic surgery have unrealistic expectations or are uncertain about what they actually want. For example, the patient with minor deformities who is seeking perfection is sure to be disappointed. The patient who wants an operation mainly to please the spouse or partner is also a poor candidate. His or her psychological outlook before surgery should be positive if results are to be therapeutic.

Interventions

Nonsurgical Management

Many techniques to improve skin and general appearance without surgery are available. Some are more invasive than others and have a higher risk for complications. Superficial techniques for skin enhancement include chemical peels, laser resurfacing, and dermabrasion to remove or reduce small scars, fine lines, and other irregular skin surfaces. Dermal filling involves injecting substances to change the contour of a feature or an area. Injection with nerve paralyzing agents (e.g., Botulinum Toxin Type A) can improve appearance temporarily by relaxing muscles beneath the skin surface, which smoothes out some wrinkles and grooves.

Surgical Management

Patients considering cosmetic surgery or reconstructive surgery should "shop" for a reputable surgeon who is certified through the American Board of Plastic Surgery. Not all physicians who are "board certified" are actually certified in this specialty. The patient should meet with the physician who will actually perform the surgery and request referrals to previous patients who have already undergone a similar surgery. It is also a good idea for the patient to contact the state medical board to determine whether the surgeon has had complaints lodged against him or her.

Depending on the planned intervention, surgery is performed either in the outpatient setting with the patient under local anesthesia or in the hospital. Most patients scheduled for plastic surgery have had consultations with their surgeon to discuss the planned intervention, possible complications, and postoperative expectations. The types and complications of common cosmetic procedures are listed in Table 27-7.

Many plastic surgeons use digital imaging both as a visual aid when discussing patients' problems and as a means of documenting before and after surgical intervention. The patient can be shown how the surgery is likely to alter his or her

TABLE 27-7 Common Plastic Surgery Procedures

Description	Indications	Complications
BLEPHAROPLASTY		
Excision of bulging fat and redundant skin of the periorbital area with primary closure	Bags under the eyes	Hematoma Ectropion Corneal injury Visual loss (rare) Wound infection (rare)
BREAST AUGMENTATION (AUGMENTATION MAMMOPLASTY)		
Insertion of synthetic breast-shaped implants through a skin incision	Inadequate breast volume or contour	Hematoma or hemorrhage Wound infection (with gram-positive organisms) Phlebitis
BREAST REDUCTION (REDUCTION MAMMOPLASTY)		
Excision of excessive breast tissue and skin with primary closure	Hypertrophy of breast tissue caused by elevated hormone levels, endocrine abnormalities, or obesity Weight of large breasts can contribute to back pain	Hematoma or hemorrhage Nipple, areola, and skin flap necrosis Wound infection Fat necrosis Wound dehiscence
DERMABRASION		
Abrasive removal of the facial epidermis and portion of the dermis followed by healing by second intention	Moderate to severe acne scar Deep wrinkling Multiple actinic keratoses Hyperpigmentation (postinflammatory or after the use of estrogens)	Hypertrophic scarring Altered skin pigmentation Acne flare Wound infection (rare)
RHINOPLASTY		
Removal of excessive cartilage and tissue from the nose with correction of septal defects if indicated	Disproportionate anatomy Post-traumatic nasal deformity Difficulty breathing through the nose	Hematoma or hemorrhage Ecchymosis and edema (temporary) Wound infection (with gram-positive organisms) Septal perforation Minor skin irritation
RHYTIDECTOMY (FACE-LIFT)		
Removal of excess skin and tissue from the face at the level of the hairline followed by primary closure	Excessive wrinkling or sagging of facial skin	Hematoma or hemorrhage Facial nerve damage (temporary or permanent) Wound infection Ecchymosis and edema (temporary) Skin necrosis Hair loss
LIPOSUCTION (SUCTION LIPECTOMY)		
Removal of subcutaneous fat from localized areas of accumulation such as the hips, abdomen, neck, and arms	Disproportionate distribution of adipose tissue	Hematoma Severe pain Infection Emboli Sagging of skin (if skin is not elastic enough to contract after fat removal)

appearance. Pictures taken of patients are confidential. Showing patients pictures of other patients is done only after proper consent is obtained.

Preoperative Care. The most important nursing action before surgery is teaching the patient what to do before and after surgery to prevent complications and increase the chances for a good outcome. All plastic surgery has a risk for complications and failure. When changing the skin and subcutaneous tissue, the skin is loosened from its connections. This causes significant bleeding, inflammation, and the potential for failure of the tissues to reattach properly. Teach the patient actions to reduce the risk for bleeding and failure of tissue reattachment. These include not smoking or using nicotine in any form because it causes blood vessel constriction and reduces blood flow to the area, delaying attachment and healing. Because of the large amount of blood loss associated with skin (particularly facial) surgery, teach the patient to avoid aspirin and other NSAIDs for several weeks before and after the procedure. Remind them that bruising and swelling can be extensive and that one or more drains in the surgical area may be used to reduce these problems. Hypertension can change blood flow to the skin of the head and neck. Teach the patient with hypertension the importance of maintaining good blood pressure control by adhering to his or her prescribed therapy.

For any plastic surgery, it is important to prevent excessive swelling or skin movement in the operative area. Remind the patient that certain positions and activities may need to be limited after surgery. Stress the importance of following the surgeon's instructions in order to have the best outcome.

Immediate preoperative care is focused on collection of any routine laboratory test data required before general anesthesia and preparation of the operative site. In most cases, the procedure for shaving and washing the skin is dictated by the surgeon's preference.

Patients undergoing facial surgery, specifically **rhytidectomy** (face-lift), are often asked to wash their hair several times with antibacterial soap to decrease bacterial flora near the incision site. Instruct patients to remove any makeup and to avoid using face creams before surgery. If a **rhinoplasty** (reconstruction of the nose) is scheduled, explain the need for nasal packing and review mouth-breathing techniques.

Operative Procedures. Reconstructive procedures vary depending on the location, purpose, and extent of reconstruction. Ironically, in performing plastic surgery, the surgeon must make a wound to correct existing skin deformities.

Postoperative Care. General care after surgery focuses on monitoring for typical postoperative complications (see Chapter 18). Pressure dressings may be applied at the time of surgery and left in place for several days to control hemorrhage and edema formation. Check dressings and any nasal packing for bright red bleeding, and monitor changes in vital signs and level of consciousness indicating active hemorrhage.

Repeated swallowing followed by belching after rhinoplasty is a sign of postnasal bleeding and need to be reported immediately to the surgeon. The patient who has had breast surgery may have drains in place after surgery. Monitor the amount and color of drainage.

Place the patient who has had any facial reconstruction in a semi-Fowler's position to reduce edema and promote comfort. Use lightweight cold compresses to reduce swelling. Check drains to ensure they are unobstructed. Assess for swelling and bruising every 2 hours. Document assessment findings. Remind patients not to increase pressure in the head and neck region, by:

- Staying in an upright position
- Avoiding facial movement such as chewing, talking, smiling
- Avoiding bending over, blowing the nose, sneezing with the mouth closed
- Not bearing down to have a bowel movement

Support garments are used after breast augmentation surgery to reduce edema and tension on the suture line from the weight of the breast tissue. With abdominal reduction surgery, teach the patient to keep the hips flexed to reduce tension on the suture line and to promote tissue attachment.

Monitor for wound infection and progress toward healing. Of particular concern are any areas of skin necrosis or eschar formation near the operative site—a complication from excessive tension on the suture line as a result of edema and blood vessel obstruction. Chart 27-5 lists wound monitoring criteria.

Regardless of the planned procedure, inform the patient to expect edema and discoloration of the operative site. Swelling and bruising alter the facial features and may not resolve for several weeks after surgery. Remind the patient that the true results of surgery will not be visible until healing is complete—usually 6 months to a year or longer after surgery. During this healing time, the patient may become discouraged. Refer him or her to a support group for encouragement (e.g., Cosmetic Surgery and Body Transformation Support Site [www.cosmeticsupport.com]).

OTHER SKIN DISORDERS

ACNE

Acne is a red, pustular eruption that affects the sebaceous glands of the skin. It is a common condition that, despite popular belief, is not confined to adolescents. Lesions result from increased sebum production, which is stimulated by androgenic hormones and obstruction of the sebaceous canal outlet. Debris collection promotes bacterial growth and rupture of the gland into the surrounding dermis with inflammation.

Acne is a progressive disorder that manifests as several types of skin lesions, including non-inflammatory **comedones** (blackheads and whiteheads), inflammatory papules, pustules, and cysts. These lesions are usually present only on the face and upper trunk.

Control of acne is possible, with spontaneous remission occurring over time. However, severe eruptions or chronic inflammation can lead to extensive scarring.

For patients with superficial lesions, topical agents (retinoic acid, benzoyl peroxide, antibiotic solutions) are used. Systemic antibiotics are indicated for those with cystic inflammatory disease. Patients with severe acne may have improvement after receiving isotretinoin (Accutane, Accutane Roche🍁). Side effects include elevated liver function test results; dry, chapped skin; and depression in some patients. The most important concern, however, is the **teratogenic** (can cause birth defects) effect of this drug or any systemic retinoic acid. A pregnancy test is required before therapy, and strict birth control measures must be used during therapy.

LICHEN PLANUS

Lichen planus is a common skin disorder of purple, flat-topped papules that itch. Although viral infections and emotional stress may be possible causes, the actual etiology of lichen planus is not known. The course of the disease can be chronic, or it can resolve spontaneously.

Lesions of lichen planus usually occur over the wrists and the inner surfaces of the forearms, but they may be present also on the lower legs, genitalia, and other body areas. Oral lesions may occur alone or with other skin changes. Unlike the skin lesions, oral lesions have a white, lacelike appearance. These lesions usually occur on the oral mucosa and are often confused with thrush.

Treatment is determined by the symptoms. Topical steroids help reduce inflammation, and antihistamines help relieve itching. Systemic steroids may be prescribed when lesions are widespread, but long-term use is avoided because of the side effects.

PEMPHIGUS VULGARIS

Pemphigus vulgaris is a rare, chronic, blistering disease with high morbidity and mortality. It is caused by an autoimmune disorder that occurs most often during middle and old age.

The acute lesions occur on normal-appearing skin or mucous membrane surfaces as fragile, flaccid bullae. Breaking the bullae leaves partial-thickness wounds that bleed, weep, and eventually form crusts.

Lesions can occur anywhere. The initial lesions usually occur on the oral mucosa, and later lesions form on the trunk. Spread of the disease is seen with the appearance of new lesions on the face and in skin-fold areas while older lesions are in the process of healing. Oral lesions are common and can make chewing and swallowing difficult.

Treatment of pemphigus vulgaris is aimed at suppressing the immune response that causes the blister formation. Systemic steroids and cytotoxic agents are used to bring about remission. Topical antibiotic creams or ointments are used to reduce bacterial infection of the unhealed lesions.

TOXIC EPIDERMAL NECROLYSIS

Toxic epidermal necrolysis (TEN) is a rare acute drug reaction of the skin resulting in diffuse erythema and large blister formation. Mucous membranes are often involved, and systemic toxicity is evident. The most common causative drugs are chemotherapy agents, sulfonamides, pyrazolones, barbiturates, and antibiotics. Removal of the drug is usually followed by gradual healing in 2 to 3 weeks, with widespread peeling of the epidermis.

This problem can occur at any age and as a result of almost any drug therapy. However, older patients with cancer who are receiving chemotherapy, some targeted therapies, and immunotherapy appear to be at greatest risk (Smith, 2007). Other precipitating factors found more commonly among patients with cancer include bone marrow transplantation and neutropenia-induced infections.

The drug thought to be causing a toxic reaction is discontinued, and therapy is aimed at systemic support and prevention of secondary infection. Patients with TEN are often admitted to burn units, where fluid and electrolyte balance, caloric intake, and hypothermia can be closely monitored. Topical antibacterial agents are used to suppress bacterial growth until healing occurs. Systemic steroids are avoided because of the increased risk for infection.

STEVENS-JOHNSON SYNDROME

Stevens-Johnson syndrome is often a drug-induced skin reaction through an immunologic mechanism, similar to toxic epidermal necrolysis (TEN). The disorder may be mild with only skin involvement, or it may be severe and systemic. The skin lesions are widely distributed (including oral and respiratory mucous membranes) and varied in appearance. The patient has a mix of vesicles, erosions, and crusts. With severe involvement, the patient may have respiratory problems, excessive fluid loss, renal failure, and blindness.

Removal of the offending drug is critical. Mild forms of the disorder are usually self-limiting in 10 to 14 days unless the episode was trigger by a bacterial infection. Then, antibiotics are needed (Holcomb, 2007). Severe manifestations require high doses of steroids to suppress the immune and inflammatory reactions. Supportive care may include fluid replacement, mechanical ventilation, and even renal replacement therapy.

LEPROSY

Leprosy (Hansen's disease) is a chronic, contagious, systemic mycobacterial infection of the peripheral nervous system with skin involvement. Although uncommon in the United States, the disease remains a problem in many parts of the world. Most cases in the United States are reported in Florida, Louisiana, Texas, New York, California, and Hawaii. The exact mechanism of infection remains unknown. Studies suggest transmission via the airborne route, by insects, or through direct contact with skin lesions. The clinical course of the disease is either progressive or self-limiting, depending on the immunologic status of the host.

Manifestations of leprosy, including skin changes, are directly related to how resistant the patient is to the mycobacteria:

- Localized (high-immunity) leprosy—one or two isolated, red, anesthetic, hairless plaques that are sometimes scaly
- Generalized (low-immunity) leprosy—widespread, faintly red macules, papules, nodules, and plaques
- Varying degrees of reduced skin sensation of the lesions caused by peripheral nerve damage

Treatment is available on an outpatient basis to control bacterial growth and reduce physical deformities. The most common treatment is a 6- to 12-month course of multiple drug therapy with dapsone (DDS; Avlosulfon), rifampin (Rifadin, Rimactane), clofazimine (Lamprene), ofloxacin (Floxin), and minocycline (Dynacin, Minocin) (World Health Organization, 2007). Other agents that also show some effectiveness include levofloxacin (Levaquin), sparfloxacin (Zagam), and clarithromycin (Biaxin).

HUMAN NEEDS NURSING CARE REVIEW

What might you NOTICE if the patient is experiencing inadequate protection as a result of loss of skin integrity?

- Open skin areas
- Possible presence of drainage
- Sensation changes in or around the area (patient reports pain, itching, or tightness)

What should you INTERPRET and how should you RESPOND to a patient experiencing inadequate protection as a result of loss of skin integrity?

Perform and interpret physical assessment, including:

- Assessing the wound for pain, size, depth, drainage, and presence of infection
- Assessing the skin immediately surrounding the wound for redness and swelling
- Monitoring oxygen saturation by pulse oximetry in the affected extremity (if the open area is on an extremity)
- Assessing the patient for risk factors for wound development (pressure, shear, immobility, reduced cognition, poor nutrition, advanced age, incontinence)
- Assessing the rest of the patient's skin (especially over bony prominences, between skin folds, in the perineal area)

Respond by:

- Documenting wound features
- Cleansing the wound (obtaining cultures, if within agency policy)
- Dressing the wound if drainage is present
- Planning a turning or repositioning schedule
- Teaching UAP or family how to relieve/reduce pressure
- Collaborating with the certified wound care specialist

On what should you REFLECT?

- Observe patient for evidence of restored skin integrity (see Chapter 26).
- Think about what may have precipitated this episode and what steps could be taken to either prevent a similar episode or identify it earlier.
- Think about what additional resources could improve the nursing response to this situation.

GET READY FOR THE NCLEX EXAMINATION!

Key Points

Review these Key Points for each NCLEX Examination Client Needs Category.

Safe and Effective Care Environment

- Assist all patients with limited mobility to change positions at least every 2 hours while awake.
- Evaluate the pressure ulcer risk for all patients on admission and regularly thereafter.
- Be proactive in the use of pressure-relieving devices for any patient who is identified to be at risk for pressure ulcer formation (i.e., requires prolonged bedrest, is an older adult, has some degree of immobility, is incontinent, has some degree of malnutrition, is dehydrated, has decreased sensory perception, or has an altered mental state).
- Wash your hands before and after touching any skin lesions.
- Use Standard Precautions when providing care to a patient who has any areas of nonintact skin.
- Use a lift sheet or mechanical lift to move immobilized older patients rather than pulling or dragging them across bed linens.

Health Promotion and Maintenance

- Encourage all patients to reduce sun exposure and exposure to ultraviolet (UV) light.
- Teach patients how to examine all skin areas on a monthly basis for new lesions and changes to existing lesions. They should keep a record or "body map" of skin lesions.
- Teach patients who have skin scarring from a previous skin injury to examine this area at least monthly for changes related to cancer development or chronic skin conditions.
- Urge all patients to bathe, shampoo the hair, and keep fingernails clean and trimmed on a regular basis.
- Teach all patients the ABCD method of evaluating a lesion for melanoma.
- Keep the skin of patients who are incontinent clean and dry.
- Ensure that women in their childbearing years who are receiving teratogenic drug therapy for a skin problem understand the effects of this therapy and are using two forms of contraception during treatment.

Psychosocial Integrity

- Allow the patient the opportunity to express feelings about a change in body image as a result of changes in the skin, hair, or nails.
- Explain all procedures, restrictions, drugs, and follow-up care to the patient and family.
- Touch the patient who has skin problems to show acceptance.
- Ask the patient who plans to have plastic surgery what he or she expects as a result of the surgery.

Physiological Integrity

- Keep skin-fold areas on patients clean and dry.
- Ask any patient who has started taking a newly prescribed drug whether he or she has noticed any skin changes have occurred since starting the drug.
- Avoid rubbing any area of the skin that has been subjected to pressure.
- Encourage patients with itching to avoid scratching the skin.
- Teach patients to avoid using over-the-counter cortisone preparations on skin lesions until the cause has been identified.
- Teach patients who have a skin infection how to avoid spreading the infection to other parts of their own bodies and to other people.
- Evaluate any open skin area on a patient daily for size, depth, exudate, presence of infection, and indicators of healing.

Additional Study Resources

Go to your Companion CD or Evolve at http://evolve.elsevier.com/Iggy/ for *Self-Assessment Questions for the NCLEX Examination.*

Go to Evolve at http://evolve.elsevier.com/Iggy/ for *Prioritization and Delegation Questions for the NCLEX Examination.*

SELECTED BIBLIOGRAPHY

Asterisk indicates a classic or definitive work on this subject.

American Cancer Society. (2008). *Cancer facts and figures 2008*. Report No. 00-300M–No. 5008.08. Atlanta: Author.

Ayello, E., & Lyder, C. (2007). Protecting patients from harm: Preventing pressure ulcers. *Nursing2007, 37*(10), 36-40.

Baranoski, S. (2006). Pressure ulcers: A renewed awareness. *Nursing2006, 36*(8), 36-41.

Braden, B., & Maklebust, J. (2005). Preventing pressure ulcers with the Braden Scale. *AJN, 105*(6), 70-72.

Bulechek, G.M., Butcher, H.K., & McCloskey Dochterman, J. (Eds.). (2008). *Nursing interventions classification (NIC)* (5th ed.). St. Louis: Mosby.

Calianno, C. (2006a). Wound bed preparation: Laying the foundation for treating chronic wounds, Part I. *Nursing2006, 36*(2), 70-71.

Calianno, C. (2006b). Wound bed preparation: The key to success for chronic wounds, Part II. *Nursing2006, 36*(3), 76-77.

Christopher, G., & Meires, J. (2008). Treating acute onset psoriasis. *The Nurse Practitioner, 33*(7), 8-10.

Cope, D., & Reb, A. (Eds.). (2006). *An evidence-based approach to the treatment and care of the older adult with cancer.* Pittsburgh: Oncology Nursing Society.

*Cuzzell, J. (2002a). Wound assessment and evaluation of wound dressings: Confusion or choice? *Dermatology Nursing, 14*(3), 187-188, 191.

*Cuzzell, J. (2002b). Wound assessment and evaluation: Wound documentation guidelines. *Dermatology Nursing, 14*(4), 265-266.

*Cuzzell, J. (2002c). Wound healing: Translating theory into clinical practice. *Dermatology Nursing, 14*(4), 257-261.

Duhon, J. (2007). Taking the pressure out of pressure ulcer therapy. *RN, 70*(2), 25-31.

Dunleavy, K. (2008). Putting a dent in pressure ulcer rates. *Nursing2008, 38*(1), 20-21.

Fleck, C.A. (2006). Wound assessment parameters and dressing selection. *Advances in skin & wound care, 19*(7), 364-370.

Frantz, R. (2005). Identifying infection in chronic wounds. *Nursing2005, 35*(7), 73.

Hanson, D., Langemo, D., Anderson, J., Hunter, S., & Thompson, P. (2007). Measuring wounds. *Nursing2007, 37*(2), 18-21.

Hanson, D., Thompson, P., Langemo, D., Hunter, S., & Anderson, J. (2007). Pressure mapping: A new path to pressure-ulcer prevention. *American Nurse Today, 2*(11), 10-12.

Holcomb, S. (2006a). Community-associated MRSA: New guidelines for a new age. *The Nurse Practitioner, 31*(9), 8-12.

Holcomb, S. (2006b). Nonmelanoma skin cancer. *Nursing2006, 36*(6), 56-57.

Holcomb, S. (2007). Dodging the bullae: Stevens-Johnson syndrome. *Nursing2007, 37*(6), 64cc1-64cc3.

Idriss, N., & Khachemoune, A. (2006). Scabies. *Dermatology Nursing, 18*(6), 588, 616.

Kent, D. (2007). Getting misty over wound care. *Nursing2007, 37*(9), 36-37.

Khachemoune, A., & Guillen, S. (2006). Psoriasis: Disease management with a brief review of new biologics. *Dermatology Nursing, 18*(1), 40-49.

Langemo, D., Anderson, J., Hanson, D., Hunter, S., Thompson, P., & Posthauer, M.E. (2006). Nutritional considerations in wound care. *Advances in Skin & Wound Care, 19*(6), 297-303.

Laustsen, G., & Neilson, T. (2007). Prevent shingles with Zostavax. *The Nurse Practitioner, 32*(6), 6-7.

Leung-Chen, P. (2008). Everybody's crying MRSA. *AJN, 108*(8), 29-31.

Loescher, L., Harris, R., Lim, K., & Su, Y. (2006). Thorough skin self-examination in patients with melanoma. *Oncology Nursing Forum, 33*(3), 633-637.

Malli, S. (2005). Keep a close eye on vacuum-assisted wound closure. *Nursing2005, 35*(7), 25.

Marks, J.G. Jr., & Miller, J. (2006). *Lookingbill & Mark's principles of dermatology* (4th ed.). Philadelphia: Saunders.

McCance, K., & Huether, S. (2006). *Pathophysiology: The biologic basis for disease in adults and children* (5th ed.). St. Louis: Mosby.

Mendyk, M. (2008). Community-associated MRSA: Coming to a patient near you? *The Nurse Practitioner, 33*(3), 26-32.

National Pressure Ulcer Advisory Panel (NPUAP). (February 2007). *Updated staging system.* Retrieved November 2007, from www.npuap.org.

Novatnack, E., & Schweon, S. (2007). Shingles: What you should know. *RN, 70*(6), 27-31.

Nussbaum, R., McInnes, R., & Willard, H. (2007). *Thompson & Thompson: Genetics in medicine* (7th ed.). Philadelphia: Saunders.

Okan, D., Woo, K., Ayello, E.A., & Sibbald, G. (2007). The role of moisture in wound healing. *Advances in Skin & Wound Care, 20*(1), 39-53.

Pagana, K., & Pagana, T. (2006). *Mosby's manual of diagnostic and laboratory tests* (3rd ed.). St. Louis: Mosby.

Prager, A., & Khachemoune, A. (2006). Basal cell carcinoma. *Dermatology Nursing, 18*(6), 584-585.

Roebuck, H. (2006a). Acne: Intervene early. *The Nurse Practitioner, 31*(10), 24-26, 28, 34, 36, 38, 40, 43.

Roebuck, H. (2006b). For pruritus, combination therapy works best. *The Nurse Practitioner, 31*(3), 12-13.

Roebuck, H. (2006c). Newer treatment options for patients with moderate-to-severe psoriatic disease. *The Nurse Practitioner, 31*(8), 5-7, 11.

Roebuck, H., & Stiegal, M. (2006). The ABCs of melanoma recognition. *The Nurse Practitioner, 31*(6), 11-13.

Rushing, J. (2007). Obtaining a wound culture specimen. *Nursing2007, 37*(11), 18.

Rushing, J. (2008). Assessing a patient for lice infestation. *Nursing2008, 38*(7), 20.

Schweon, S. (2006). MRSA extends its reach. *RN, 69*(2), 33-36.

Shores, J.T., Allen, G., & Gupta, S. (2007). Skin substitutes and alternatives: A review. *Advances in Skin & Wound Care, 20*(9 Pt 1), 493-508.

Slachta, P. (2008). Caring for chronic wounds: A knowledge update. *American Nurse Today, 3*(7) 27-31.

Smith, L. (2007). Toxic epidermal necrolysis. *Clinical Journal of Oncology Nursing, 11*(3), 333-336.

Snow, M. (2006). Shutting down shingles. *Nursing2006, 36*(4), 18-19.

Snow, M. (2007). The truth about scabies. *Nursing2007, 37*(2), 28-30.

Snyder, L. (2008). Wound basics: Type, treatment, and care. *RN, 71*(8), 32-36.

Stotts, N., & Gunningberg, L. (2007). Predicting pressure ulcer risk. *AJN, 107*(11), 40-48.

VanBeuge, S. (2007). Making a stand against malignant melanoma. *American Nurse Today, 2*(8), 18-21.

Wilson, D. (2007). Herpes zoster: Prevention, diagnosis, and treatment. *The Nurse Practitioner, 32*(9), 19-24.

Woo, K., Ayello, E.A., & Sibbald, R.G. (2007). The edge effect: Current therapeutic options to advance the wound edge. *Advances in Skin & Wound Care, 20*(2), 99-117.

World Health Organization. (2007). Leprosy. Retrieved March 15, 2008, from www.who.int/topics/leprosy/en/.

*Worley, C. (2004a). The wound healing process symphony, Part I. *Dermatology Nursing, 16*(1), 67, 72.

*Worley, C. (2004b). The wound healing process symphony, Part II. *Dermatology Nursing, 16*(2), 179-180.

Worley, C. (2006a). Aging skin and wound healing. *Dermatology Nursing, 18*(3), 265-266.

Worley, C. (2006b). So, what do I put on this wound? Making sense of the wound dressing puzzle, Part I. *MEDSURG Nursing, 15*(2), 106-107.

Worley, C. (2006c). So, what do I put on this wound? Making sense of the wound dressing puzzle, Part II. *MEDSURG Nursing, 15*(3), 182-174.

Worley, C. (2006d). So, what do I put on this wound? Making sense of the wound dressing puzzle, Part III. *MEDSURG Nursing, 15*(4), 251-252.

Yamamoto, L., & Marten, M. (2007). Listen up, MRSA, the bug stops here. *Nursing2007, 37*(12), 50-55.

28 CHAPTER

Care of Patients with Burns

Tammy Coffee

LEARNING OUTCOMES

For clinical competence and success on the NCLEX Examination, study this chapter with these Learning Outcomes in mind:

Safe and Effective Care Environment

1. Apply the principles of asepsis to protect burn patients with open wounds.
2. Manage the patient's environment to prevent infection from autocontamination and cross-contamination in patients with burn injuries.

Health Promotion and Maintenance

3. Teach everyone fire prevention strategies.
4. Instruct everyone on the correct use and placement of smoke detectors and carbon monoxide detectors.

Psychosocial Integrity

5. Support the patient and family in coping with permanent changes in appearance and function.
6. Encourage the burn patient with wounds and scars to participate in burn care.
7. Assess the patient's and family's use of coping strategies related to burn injury, treatment, possible role changes, and possible outcomes.
8. Allow patients who have lost family members, homes, or jobs time to grieve for these losses.

Physiological Integrity

9. Identify burn patients at risk for inhalation injury.
10. Compare the manifestations of superficial, partial-thickness, and full-thickness burn injuries.
11. Explain the expected manifestations of neural and hormonal compensation during the resuscitation/emergent phase of burn injury.
12. Prioritize nursing care for the patient during the resuscitation/emergent phase of burn injury.
13. Use laboratory data and clinical manifestations to determine the effectiveness of fluid resuscitation during the resuscitation/emergent phase of burn injury.
14. Prioritize nursing care for the patient during the acute phase of burn injury.
15. Coordinate with the nutritionist to meet the nutritional needs for the patient during the acute phase of burn injury.
16. Evaluate the patient's wound healing during the acute phase of burn injury.
17. Compare pain management for patients in the resuscitation/emergent and acute phases of burn injury.
18. Describe the characteristics of infected burn wounds.
19. Use appropriate positioning and range-of-motion interventions for prevention of mobility problems in the patient with burns.
20. Coordinate nursing care for the patient during the rehabilitation phase of burn injury.

Go to your Companion CD or Evolve at http://evolve.elsevier.com/Iggy/ for *Self-Assessment Questions for the NCLEX Examination* keyed to these Learning Outcomes.

Patients who have burn injuries develop many physiologic, metabolic, and psychological changes. Burn injuries can range from a "sunburn" to major injuries involving all layers of the skin. When the skin is injured, inflammation and fluid loss change the function of most body systems. The burn patient needs comprehensive care for weeks to months to survive the injury, reduce complications, and return to his or her best functional status. A multidisciplinary team of health care providers is needed for best care and patient outcomes. Nurses coordinate the activities of the many professionals involved in providing the best care to burn patients.

INTRODUCTION TO THE BURN PROBLEM

Pathophysiology of Burn Injury

The tissue destruction caused by a burn injury leads to many local and systemic problems. Such problems include fluid and protein losses, sepsis, and changes in metabolic, endocrine, respiratory, cardiac, hematologic, and immune functioning. The extent of local and systemic problems is related to age, general health, extent of injury, depth of injury, and the specific body area injured. Even after healing, the burn injury may cause late complications such as contracture formation and scarring. Therefore the prevention of infection and closure of the burn wound are vitally important. A lack of or delay in wound healing is a key factor for all systemic problems and a major cause of disability and death among patients who are burned.

Skin Changes Resulting from Burn Injury

Anatomic Changes

The skin is the largest organ of the body (see Chapter 26). Each of its two major layers, the epidermis and the dermis, has several sublayers. The epidermis, the outer layer of skin, is a layer of stratified epithelial cells about 0.15 mm thick (somewhat thinner in older adults). This layer can grow back after a burn injury because the epidermal cells surrounding sweat and oil glands and hair follicles extend into dermal tissue and regrow to heal partial-thickness wounds. Together, the sweat and oil glands and the hair follicles are the **dermal appendages.** The depth of the dermal appendages varies from one body area to another. The sweat and oil glands in the palm of the hand and the sole of the foot, for example, extend deep into the dermis. This allows for healing of fairly deep burns in these areas. The epidermis has no blood vessels. Nutrients to this layer diffuse from the second layer of skin, the dermis.

The basement membrane, a thin noncellular protein surface, separates the dermis from the epidermis. The dermis is sometimes called the "true skin" because it is not constantly shed and replaced. The dermis is thicker than the epidermis, ranging in thickness from 0.60 to 1.2 mm. It is made up of collagen, fibrous connective tissue, and elastic fibers. Within the dermis are the blood vessels, sensory nerves, hair follicles, lymph vessels, sebaceous glands, and sweat glands.

When burn injury occurs, skin can regrow as long as parts of the dermis are present. When the entire layer of dermis is burned, all epithelial cells and dermal appendages are destroyed and the skin can no longer restore itself. The subcutaneous tissue lies below the dermis and varies in thickness. With deep burns, the subcutaneous tissues may be damaged, leaving bones, tendons, and muscles exposed.

Functional Changes

The skin has many functions (see Table 26-1 in Chapter 26). It is a protective barrier against injury and microbial invasion from the environment. A burn injury breaks this barrier, greatly increasing the risk for infection.

The skin also helps maintain the delicate fluid and electrolyte balance essential for life. After a burn injury, massive fluid loss occurs through evaporation. Evaporation through burn-injured skin occurs four times as rapidly as from intact skin. The rate of evaporation is in proportion to the total body surface area (TBSA) burned and the depth of injury.

The skin is an excretory organ through sweating. Full-thickness burns destroy the sweat glands, reducing excretory ability.

The skin is a sense organ for pain, pressure, temperature, and touch. These sensations are triggered on the skin in normal daily activities, which allows a person to react to changes in the environment. *All burn injuries are painful.* With partial-thickness burns, nerve endings are exposed, increasing sensitivity and pain. With full-thickness burns, nerve endings are completely destroyed. At first these wounds may not transmit sensation except at wound edges when a sharp stimulus is applied. Despite this destruction, patients often have dull or pressure-type of pain in these areas.

Skin exposed to sunlight activates vitamin D. Partial-thickness burns reduce the activation of vitamin D, and this function is lost completely in full-thickness burns.

The skin helps determine physical identity. The skin's cosmetic quality is part of each person's unique appearance. With a change in appearance through a major burn, psychological problems may develop.

The internal body temperature remains within a narrow range (about 84.2° to 109.4° F [29° to 43° C]) compared with the wide temperature changes in the external environment. Several processes normally adjust to wide differences in external temperature to maintain the narrow range of normal for the internal body temperature. Circulating blood both provides and dissipates heat efficiently. When heat is applied to the skin, the temperature of the layer under the dermis rises rapidly. As soon as the heat source is removed, compensatory processes quickly return the area to a normal temperature. If the heat source is not removed or if it is applied at a rate that exceeds the skin's capacity to dissipate it, cells are destroyed.

The skin can tolerate temperatures up to 104° F (40° C) without injury. At temperatures of 158° F (70° C) and above, cell destruction is so rapid that even brief exposure damages the skin and tissue below the skin. Fig. 28-1 shows the relationship between temperature and exposure time for burn injury.

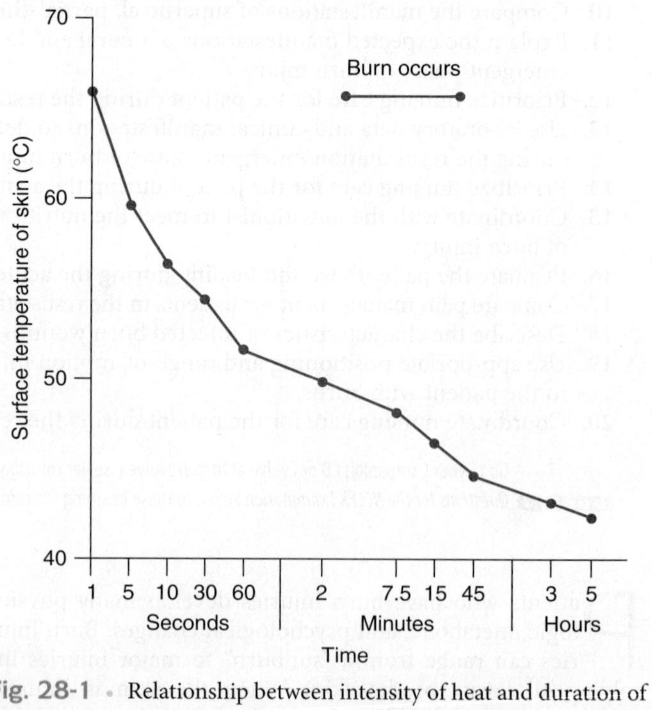

Burn occurs
Surface temperature of skin (°C)
70
60
50
40
1
5
10
30
60
Seconds
2
7.5
15
45
Minutes
3
5
Hours
Time

Fig. 28-1 • Relationship between intensity of heat and duration of exposure. Exposure for prolonged periods causes burns, even with milder temperatures. At more extreme temperatures, tissue damage results after only seconds.

Depth of Burn Injury

The severity of a burn is determined by how much of the body surface area is involved and the depth of the burn. The degree of tissue damage is related to what agent caused the burn and to the temperature of the heat source, as well as how long the skin was exposed to it.

Differences in skin thickness in various parts of the body also affect burn depth. In areas where the skin is thin (e.g., eyelids, ears, nose, genitalia, tops of the hands and feet, fingers, and toes), a short exposure to high temperatures causes a deep burn injury. The skin is thinner in older adults, which increases their risk to greater burn severity, even at lower temperatures of shorter duration.

Burn wounds are classified as superficial-thickness wounds, partial-thickness wounds, full-thickness wounds, and deep full-thickness wounds. The partial-thickness wounds are further divided into superficial and deep subgroups (McCance & Huether, 2006). Table 28-1 lists the clinical differences of these burns.

The American Burn Association (ABA) describes burns as minor, moderate, or major depending on the depth, extent, and location of injury and describes the criteria for referral to a burn center (Table 28-2). Fig. 28-2 shows the tissue layers involved with different depths of injury.

Superficial-Thickness Wounds. Of all burn types, superficial-thickness wounds have the least damage because the epidermis is the only part of the skin that is injured. The epithelial cells

TABLE 28-1 Classification of Burn Depth

Characteristic	Superficial	Superficial Partial-Thickness	Deep Partial-Thickness	Full-Thickness	Deep Full-Thickness
Color	Pink to red	Pink to red	Red to white	Black, brown, yellow, white, red	Black
Edema	Mild	Mild to moderate	Moderate	Severe	Absent
Pain	Yes	Yes	Yes	Yes and no	Absent
Blisters	No	Yes	Rare	No	No
Eschar	No	No	Yes, soft and dry	Yes, hard and inelastic	Yes, hard and inelastic
Healing time	3-5 days	About 2 wk	2-6 wk	Weeks to months	Weeks to months
Grafts required	No	No	Can be used if healing is prolonged	Yes	Yes
Example	Sunburn, flash burns	Scalds, flames, brief contact with hot objects	Scalds; flames; prolonged contact with hot objects, tar, grease, chemicals	Scalds; flames; prolonged contact with hot objects, tar, grease chemicals, electricity	Flames, electricity, grease, tar, chemicals

TABLE 28-2 Classification of Burn Injury and Burn Center Referral Criteria

Characteristics	Comments
MINOR BURNS Deep partial-thickness burns less than 15% TBSA Full-thickness burns less than 2% TBSA No burns of eyes, ears, face, hands, feet, or perineum No electrical burns No inhalation injury No complicated concomitant injury Patient is younger than 60 years and has no chronic cardiac, pulmonary, or endocrine disorder	Patients in this category should receive emergency care at the scene and be taken to a hospital emergency department. A special expertise hospital or designated burn center is not necessary.
MODERATE BURNS Deep partial-thickness burns 15%-25% TBSA Full-thickness burns 2%-10% TBSA No burns of eyes, ears, face, hands, feet, or perineum No electrical burns No inhalation injury No complicated concomitant injury Patient is younger than 60 years and has no chronic cardiac, pulmonary, or endocrine disorder	Patients in this category should receive emergency care at the scene and be transferred either to a special expertise hospital or to a designated burn center.
MAJOR BURNS Partial-thickness burns greater than 25% TBSA Full-thickness burns greater than 10% Any burn involving the eyes, ears, face, hands, feet, perineum Electrical injury Inhalation injury Patient is older than 60 years Burn complicated with other injuries (e.g., fractures) Patient has cardiac, pulmonary, or other chronic metabolic disorders	Patients who meet *any one* of the criteria for a major burn should receive emergency care at the nearest emergency department and then be transferred to a designated burn center as soon as possible.

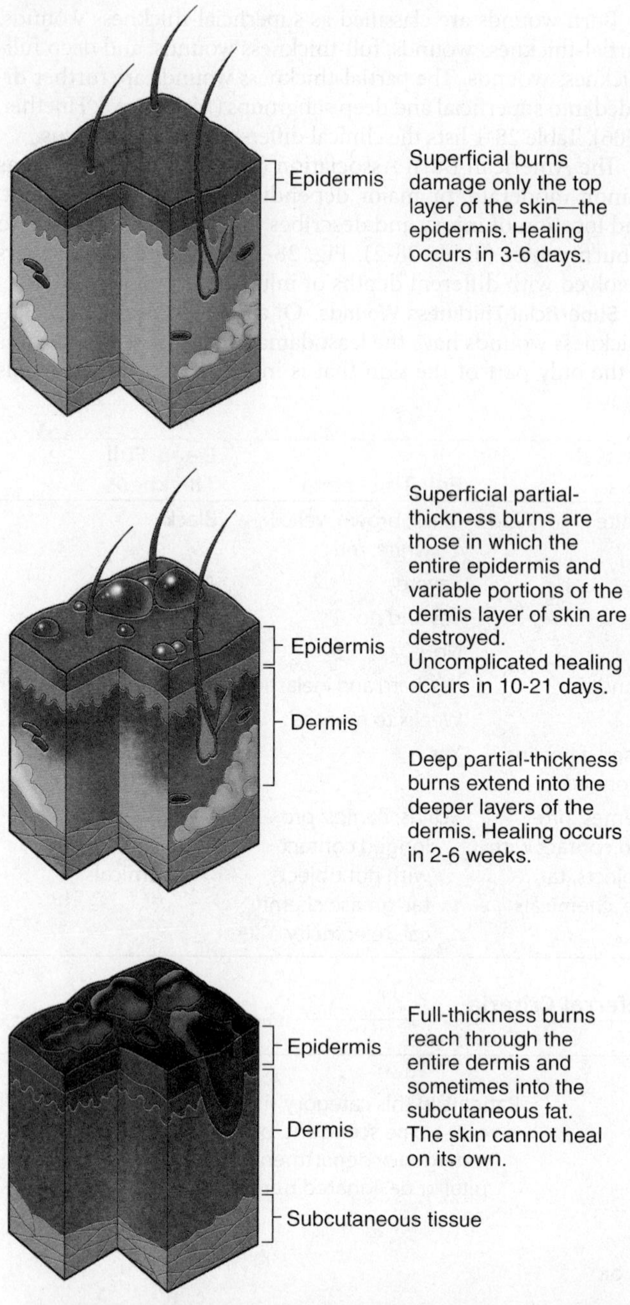
Epidermis
Superficial burns damage only the top layer of the skin—the epidermis. Healing occurs in 3-6 days.
Superficial partial-thickness burns are those in which the entire epidermis and variable portions of the dermis layer of skin are destroyed. Uncomplicated healing occurs in 10-21 days.
Epidermis
Dermis
Deep partial-thickness burns extend into the deeper layers of the dermis. Healing occurs in 2-6 weeks.
Full-thickness burns reach through the entire dermis and sometimes into the subcutaneous fat. The skin cannot heal on its own.
Epidermis
Dermis
Subcutaneous tissue

Fig. 28-2 • The tissues involved in burns of various depths.

and basement membrane, needed for total regrowth, remain present.

Superficial-thickness wounds are caused by prolonged exposure to low-intensity heat (e.g., sunburn) or short (flash) exposure to high-intensity heat. Redness with mild edema, pain, and increased sensitivity to heat occurs as a result. **Desquamation** (peeling of dead skin) occurs for 2 to 3 days after the burn. The area heals rapidly in 3 to 5 days without a scar or other complication.

Partial-Thickness Wounds. A partial-thickness wound involves the entire epidermis and varying depths of the dermis. Depending on the amount of dermal tissue damaged, partial-thickness wounds are further subdivided into superficial partial-thickness and deep partial-thickness injuries.

Superficial partial-thickness wounds are caused by heat injury to the upper third of the dermis, leaving a good blood supply. These wounds are red and moist and **blanch** (lighten) when pressure is applied (Fig. 28-3). The small vessels bringing blood to this area are injured, resulting in the leakage of large amounts of plasma, which in turn lifts off the heat-destroyed epidermis, causing blister formation. The blisters continue to increase in size after the burn as cell and protein breakdown occur. Small blisters are often left intact if they are not present over a joint. Larger blisters are usually opened to promote healing.

Superficial partial-thickness wounds increase pain sensation. Nerve endings are exposed, and any stimulation (touch or temperature change) causes intense pain. With standard care, these burns heal in 10 to 21 days with no scar but some minor pigment changes may occur.

Deep partial-thickness wounds extend deeper into the skin dermis, and fewer healthy cells remain. In these patients, blisters usually do not form because the dead tissue layer is so thick and sticks to the underlying dermis that it does not readily lift off the surface. The wound surface is red and dry with white areas in deeper parts (dry because fewer blood vessels are patent). When pressure is applied to the burn, it may blanch slowly or not at all (Fig. 28-4). Edema is moderate, and pain is less than with superficial burns because more of the nerve endings have been destroyed.

The blood flow to these areas is reduced by blood vessel constriction. Progression to deeper injury can occur from hypoxia and ischemia. Adequate hydration, nutrients, and oxygen are needed for regrowth of skin cells and prevention of conversion to deeper burns. These wounds can convert to full-thickness wounds when tissue damage increases with

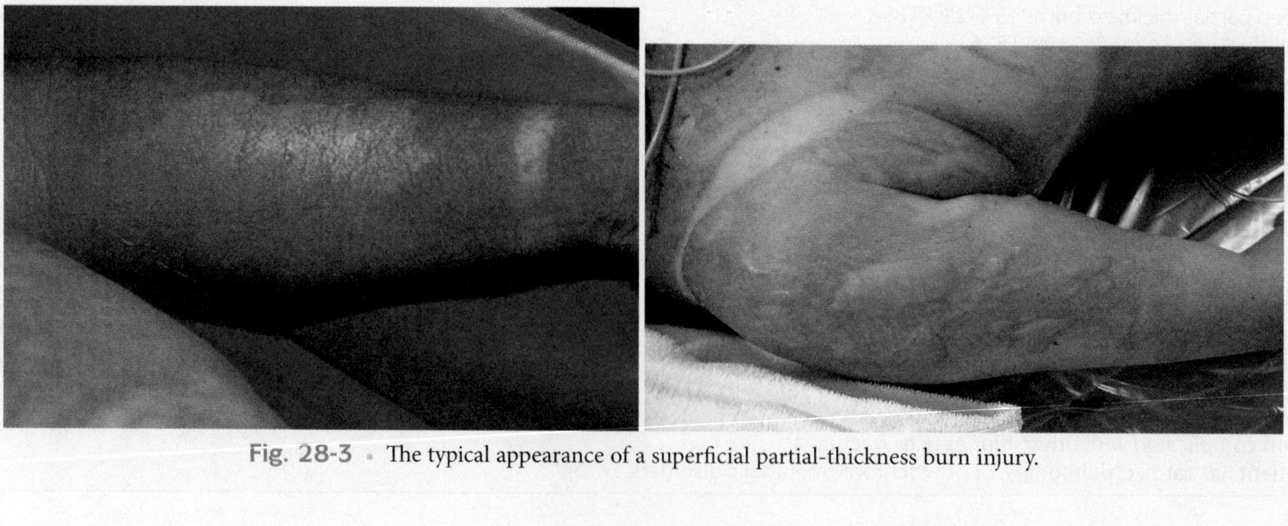

Fig. 28-3 • The typical appearance of a superficial partial-thickness burn injury.

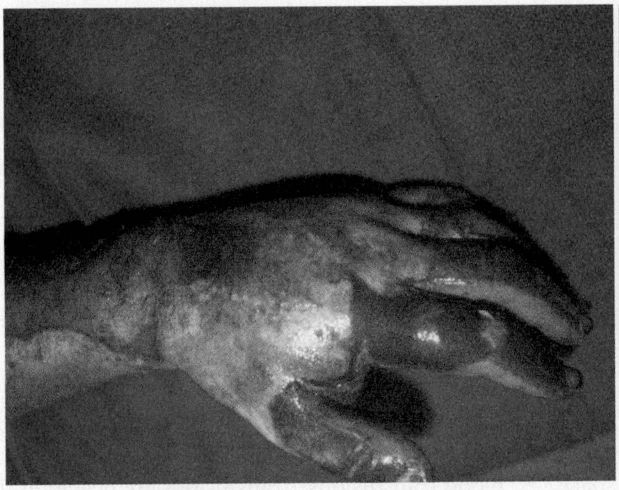

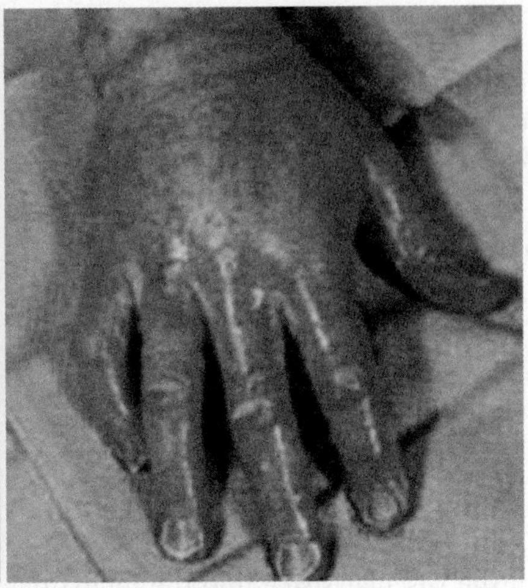

Fig. 28-4 • The typical appearance of a deep partial-thickness burn injury.

infection, hypoxia, or ischemia. Deep partial-thickness wounds generally heal in 3 to 6 weeks, but scar formation results. Surgical intervention with skin grafting can reduce healing time.

Full-Thickness Wounds. A full-thickness wound occurs with destruction of the entire epidermis and dermis, leaving no true skin cells to repopulate (Fig. 28-5). This wound, therefore, does not regrow, and whatever area of the wound is not closed by wound contraction (see Chapter 27) will require grafting.

The full-thickness injury has a hard, dry, leathery *eschar* that forms from coagulated particles of destroyed dermis. *The eschar is dead tissue; it must slough off or be removed from the burn wound before healing can occur.* These thick particles often stick to the lower tissue layer by collagen fibers, which make the eschar removal difficult. Edema is severe under the eschar in a full-thickness wound. When the injury is **circumferential** (completely surrounds an extremity or the chest), blood flow and chest movement for breathing may be reduced by tight eschar. **Escharotomies** (incisions through the eschar) or **fasciotomies** (incisions through eschar and fascia) may be needed to relieve pressure and allow normal blood flow and breathing (see pp. 534-535 of Surgical Management discussion under the Ineffective Tissue Perfusion section).

A full-thickness burn wound may be waxy white, deep red, yellow, brown, or black. Thrombosed vessels may be visible beneath the surface of the burn. These dermal blood vessels are heat coagulated, causing the burned tissue to be **avascular** (without a blood supply). Sensation is reduced or absent in these areas because of nerve ending destruction. Healing time depends on establishing a good blood supply in the injured areas. This process can range from weeks to months.

Deep Full-Thickness Wounds. Deep full-thickness wounds extend beyond the skin into underlying fascia and tissues. These deep injuries damage muscle, bone, and tendons and leave them exposed. These burns occur with flame, electrical, or chemical injuries. The wound is blackened and depressed, and sensation is completely absent (Fig. 28-6). All full-thickness burns need early excision and grafting. Grafting decreases pain and length of stay and hastens recovery. Amputation may be needed when an extremity is involved.

Vascular Changes Resulting from Burn Injury

Circulatory disruption occurs at the burn site immediately after a burn injury. Blood vessels to the burned skin are occluded, and blood flow is reduced or stopped. Damaged macrophages within the tissues release chemicals (mediators) that at first cause blood vessel constriction. Blood vessel thrombosis may occur, causing necrosis, which can lead to deeper injuries in the already damaged areas.

Fluid shift occurs after initial vasoconstriction as a result of blood vessels near the burn, dilating and leaking fluid into the interstitial space (Fig. 28-7). This fluid shift, also known as *third spacing* or *capillary leak syndrome,* is a continuous leak

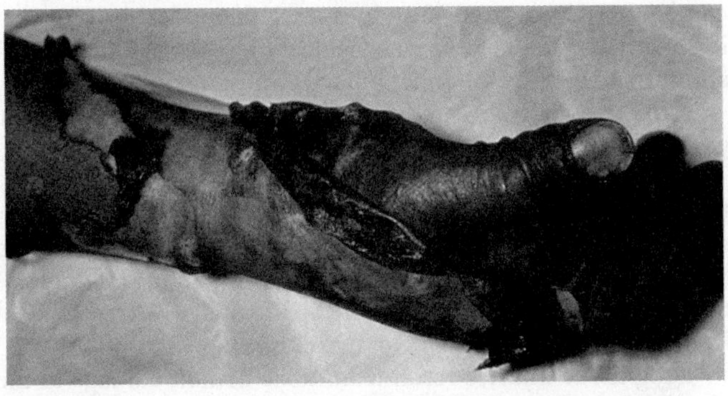

Fig. 28-5 • The typical appearance of a full-thickness burn injury.

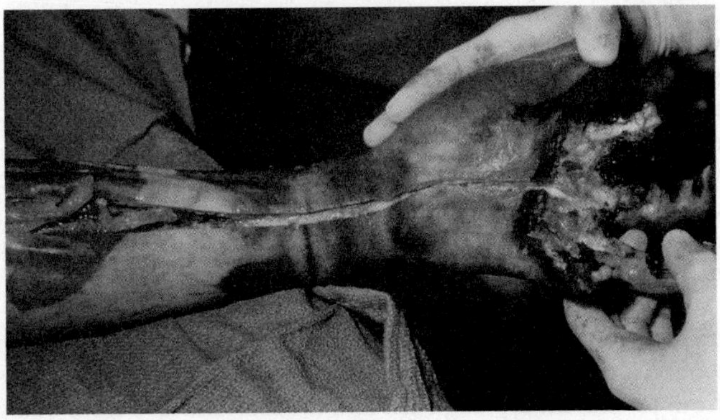

Fig. 28-6 • The typical appearance of a deep full-thickness burn injury.

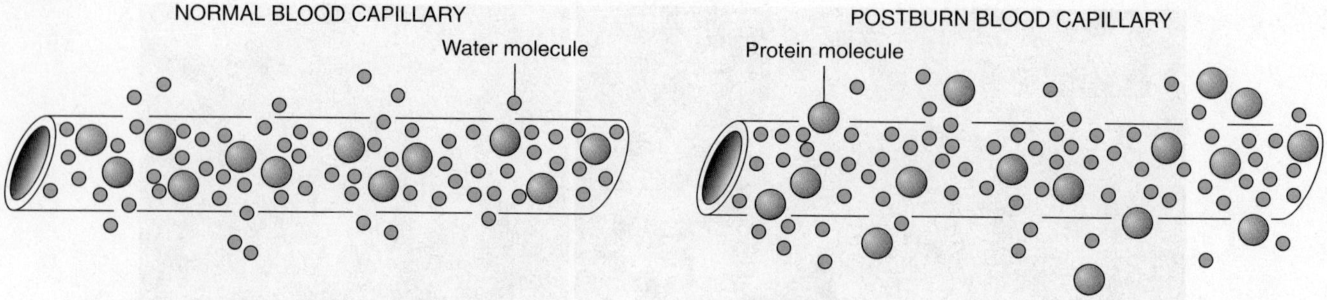
NORMAL BLOOD CAPILLARY
Water molecule
Water is the smallest molecule that can pass through the capillary pores.
POSTBURN BLOOD CAPILLARY
Protein molecule
Permeability is drastically increased, which allows large molecules such as proteins to pass through the capillary pores easily.

Fig. 28-7 • The capillary response to burn injury (early phase). This response is also known as *capillary leak syndrome.*

of plasma from the vascular space into the interstitial space. The loss of plasma fluids and proteins decreases blood volume and blood pressure. Leakage of fluid and electrolytes from the vascular space continues, causing extensive edema, even in areas that were not burned. Fluid shift, with excessive weight gain, usually occurs in the first 12 hours after the burn and can continue for 24 to 36 hours.

The amount of fluid shifted depends on the extent and severity of injury. Capillary leak occurs in both burned and unburned areas when tissue damage is extensive (i.e., more than 20% to 30% total body surface area [TBSA]). Edema develops as plasma and electrolytes escape into the interstitial space. The proteins now in the interstitial space increase the movement of fluids out from the vascular space.

Profound imbalances of fluid, electrolytes, and acid-base occur as a result of the fluid shift and cell damage. These imbalances often include hypovolemia, metabolic acidosis, **hyperkalemia** (high blood potassium levels), and **hyponatremia** (low blood sodium levels). Hyperkalemia occurs as a result of direct cell injury that releases large amounts of cellular potassium. Sodium is retained by the body as a result of the endocrine response to stress. Aldosterone secretion increases, leading to increased sodium reabsorption by the kidney. This sodium, however, quickly passes into the interstitial spaces of the burned area with the fluid shift; therefore, despite the increased amount of sodium in the body, most of the sodium is trapped in the interstitial space and a sodium deficit occurs in the blood. **Hemoconcentration** (elevated blood osmolarity, hematocrit, and hemoglobin) develops from vascular dehydration. This problem increases blood viscosity, reducing flow through small vessels and increasing tissue hypoxia.

Fluid remobilization starts at about 24 hours after injury, when the capillary leak stops and capillary integrity is restored. The diuretic stage begins at about 48 to 72 hours after the burn injury as capillary membrane integrity returns and edema fluid shifts from the interstitial spaces into the intravascular space. Blood volume increases, leading to increased renal blood flow and diuresis unless renal damage has occurred. Body weight returns to normal over the next several days as edema subsides.

During this phase, hyponatremia develops because of increased renal sodium excretion and the loss of sodium from wounds. **Hypokalemia** (low blood potassium level) results from potassium moving back into the cells and also from being excreted in urine output. Anemia often develops as a result of hemodilution, but it is generally not severe enough to require blood transfusions. Transfusions are needed if the patient's hematocrit is less than 20% to 25% and the patient has manifestations of hypoxia. Transfusions are given only when absolutely necessary. Protein continues to be lost from the wounds. Metabolic acidosis is possible because of the loss of sodium bicarbonate in the urine and the increased fat metabolism that occurs because of decreased carbohydrate intake.

Cardiac Changes Resulting from Burn Injury

Heart rate increases and cardiac output decreases because of the initial fluid shifts and hypovolemia that occur after a burn injury. Cardiac output may remain low until 18 to 36 hours after the burn injury. Cardiac output increases with fluid resuscitation and reaches normal levels before plasma volume is restored completely. Proper fluid resuscitation and support with oxygen prevent further complications.

Pulmonary Changes Resulting from Burn Injury

Direct injury to the lung from contact with flames rarely occurs. Rather, respiratory problems are caused by superheated air, steam, toxic fumes, or smoke. Such problems are a major cause of death in patients with burns and are most likely to occur when the burn takes place indoors. Respiratory failure with burn injuries can result from airway edema during fluid resuscitation, pulmonary capillary leak, chest burns that restrict chest movement, and carbon monoxide poisoning.

Respiratory damage from an inhalation injury can occur in the upper and major airways and the lung tissue (Cancio et al., 2007). The upper airway is affected when inhaled smoke or irritants cause edema and obstruct the trachea. Irritants coming in contact with the upper airway often cause a reflex closure of the vocal cords. This protective reflex decreases the amount of smoke and toxic gases entering the lungs. Although air is a poor conductor of heat, some heat does reach the upper airway, causing an inflammatory response that leads to edema of the mouth and throat with the potential of airway obstruction.

More airway injury is caused by the chemicals and toxic gases (rather than heat) that are produced during combustion. The ciliated membranes lining the trachea normally trap bacteria and foreign materials. Smoke and combustion products slow this activity, which allows foreign particles to enter the bronchi. The lining of the trachea and bronchi may slough 48 to 72 hours after injury, enter the airway, narrow the tracheal lumen, and obstruct the lower airways.

Lung tissue injuries result from toxic irritant damage to the alveoli and capillaries. Leaking capillaries cause alveolar edema.

This edema can occur immediately or as late as 1 week after the injury. The fluid that diffuses into the lung tissue spaces contains proteins that form fibrinous membranes and lead to respiratory distress. Progressive pulmonary failure develops, leading to acute pulmonary insufficiency and infection.

Gastrointestinal Changes Resulting from Burn Injury

The fluid shifts and decreased cardiac output that occur after injury divert blood flow to the brain, heart, and liver. As a result, other organs, including the GI tract, have decreased blood flow. Gastric mucosal integrity and motility are impaired. The sympathetic nervous system stress response increases secretion of epinephrine and norepinephrine, which inhibit GI motility and further reduce blood flow to the area. Peristalsis decreases, and a paralytic ileus may develop. Secretions and gases collect in the intestines and stomach, causing abdominal distention.

Curling's ulcer (acute gastroduodenal ulcer that occurs with the stress of severe injury) may develop within 24 hours after a severe burn injury because of reduced GI blood flow and mucosal damage (McCance & Huether, 2006). The mucus lining the stomach normally acts as a barrier to the presence of hydrogen ions secreted into the stomach contents. With decreased gastric mucus production, this barrier is disrupted and hydrogen ion production is increased and ulcers may develop as a result. However, this complication is now less common because of the use of H_2 histamine blockers, drugs that protect GI mucosal tissues, and early enteral feeding.

Metabolic Changes Resulting from Burn Injury

A serious burn injury greatly increases metabolism by increasing secretion of catecholamines, antidiuretic hormone, aldosterone, and cortisol. With this hypermetabolism, the patient's oxygen use and calorie needs are high.

The catecholamines activate the stress response. The increased production (and loss) of heat breaks down protein and fat (a process called **catabolism**), rapidly uses glucose and calories, and increases urine nitrogen loss. The heat and water lost from the burn also increase metabolic and catabolic rates, which increase calorie needs. Depending on the extent of injury, the patient's calorie needs double or triple normal energy needs. These increased rates peak 4 to 12 days after the burn and can remain elevated for months until all wounds are closed.

The hypermetabolic condition also increases core body temperature. The patient loses heat through the burned skin because the protective barrier is lost. Core body temperature increases as a response to the adjustment in temperature regulation by the hypothalamus. A central body temperature control change occurs to adapt to the hypermetabolic state, resulting in the development of a low-grade fever. This change is a "resetting" of the body's normal temperature-control system to a higher baseline body temperature.

Immunologic Changes Resulting from Burn Injury

Burn injury disrupts or destroys the protective barrier of the skin, increasing the risk for infection. The injury activates the inflammatory response and often suppresses immune function (see Chapter 19). All types of immunity are suppressed. Topical and systemic antibiotics, general anesthesia, blood transfusion, and the stress of surgery further reduce immune function.

Compensatory Responses to Burn Injury

Any tissue injury is a stressor and can disrupt homeostasis. Two compensatory (adaptive) responses have immediate benefit: the inflammatory response and the sympathetic nervous system stress response. Together these responses cause changes that result in many of the manifestations seen in the first 2 to 3 days after a burn injury.

Inflammatory compensation can be helpful by triggering healing in the injured tissues. It also is responsible for some of the serious problems that occur with the fluid shift. Inflammatory compensation causes blood vessels to leak fluid into the interstitial space and white blood cells to release chemicals that trigger local tissue reactions. These responses cause the massive fluid shift, edema, and hypovolemia that are seen in the **resuscitation/emergent phase** (first 48 hours) after a burn injury. The extent of the inflammatory response depends on the burn severity. Chapter 19 explains the inflammatory responses in detail.

Inflammatory compensation is immediately helpful to the body when injury occurs. These actions are intended to function on a local and short-term basis. When these actions are widespread or persistent, they can cause severe tissue damage.

Sympathetic nervous system compensation is the stress response that occurs when any physical or psychological stressors are present. Changes caused by sympathetic compensation are most evident in the cardiovascular, respiratory, and GI systems. Fig. 28-8 shows the results of sympathetic nervous system stimulation.

Etiology of Burn Injury

Burn injuries are caused by dry heat (flame), moist heat (scald), contact with hot surfaces, chemicals, electricity, and ionizing radiation. The cause of the injury affects both the prognosis and the treatment.

Dry heat injuries are caused by open flame. The most common flame injuries occur in house fires and explosions. Ignited clothing from an open flame accounts for most of the injuries. Explosions usually result in flash burns because they produce a brief exposure to very high temperatures.

Moist heat (scald) injuries are caused by contact with hot liquids or steam. Scald injuries are more common among older adults than among younger adults. Hot liquid spills usually burn the upper, front areas of the body. Immersion scald injuries usually involve the lower body.

Contact burns occur when hot metal, tar, or grease contact the skin, often leading to a full-thickness injury. Hot metal injuries occur when a body part contacts a hot surface, such as a space heater or iron. They also can occur in industrial settings from molten metals. Tar and asphalt temperatures usually are greater than 400° F, and deep injuries occur within seconds when the skin is immersed in or splashed with them. Hot grease injuries from cooking are usually deep because of the temperature of the grease.

Chemical burns occur as a result of accidents in homes or industry. They can also be the result of a deliberate assault on a person. Tissue injury occurs when chemicals come into direct contact with the skin and epithelial tissues or are ingested. The severity of the injury depends on the duration of contact, the concentration of the chemical, the amount of tissue exposed, and the action of the chemical.

Alkalis found in oven cleaners, fertilizers, drain cleaners, and heavy industrial cleaners damage the tissues by causing

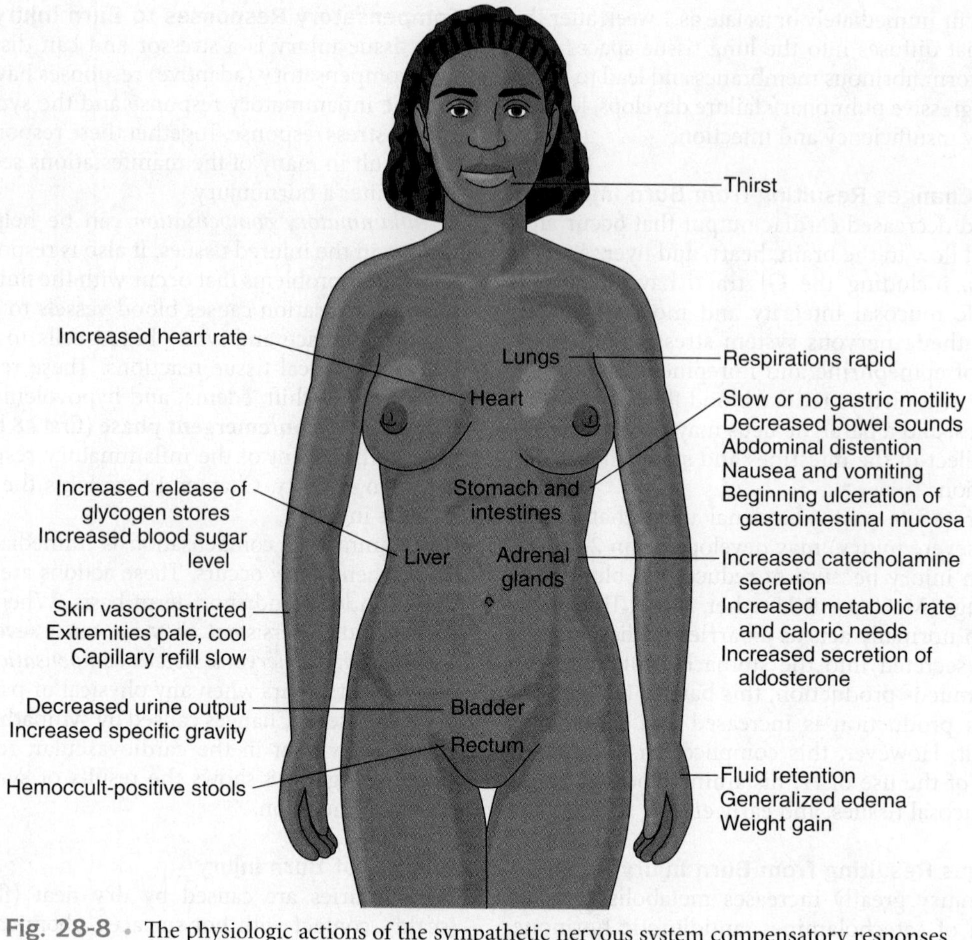
Thirst
Increased heart rate
Lungs
Respirations rapid
Heart
Slow or no gastric motility
Decreased bowel sounds
Abdominal distention
Nausea and vomiting
Beginning ulceration of gastrointestinal mucosa
Increased release of glycogen stores
Increased blood sugar level
Stomach and intestines
Liver
Adrenal glands
Increased catecholamine secretion
Increased metabolic rate and caloric needs
Increased secretion of aldosterone
Skin vasoconstricted
Extremities pale, cool
Capillary refill slow
Decreased urine output
Increased specific gravity
Bladder
Rectum
Hemoccult-positive stools
Fluid retention
Generalized edema
Weight gain

Fig. 28-8 • The physiologic actions of the sympathetic nervous system compensatory responses to burn injury (early phase).

the skin and its proteins to liquefy. This allows for deeper spread of the chemical and more severe burns. Acids found in bathroom cleaners, rust removers, chemicals for swimming pools, and industrial drain cleaners damage tissue by coagulating cells and skin proteins, which can limit the depth of tissue damage. Organic compounds are found in chemical disinfectants and gasoline. They cause damage because they are fat soluble and are easily absorbed through the skin. Once absorbed, they produce toxic effects on the kidneys and liver.

Electrical injuries are burns occurring when an electrical current enters the body (Fig. 28-9). These injuries have been called the "grand masquerader" of burns injuries because the surface injuries may look small but the associated internal injuries can be huge. Electrical injuries are divided into high and low voltage, with high voltage being greater than 1000 volts. Tissue injury from electrical trauma results from electrical energy being converted to heat energy. The extent of injury depends on the type of current, the pathway of flow, the local tissue resistance, and the duration of contact. The skin is the most resistant organ; the greatest resistance is in the epidermis of the skin. At high voltages, the difference in tissue resistance is not important. Although various underlying tissues have different resistance to current flow, once skin resistance is overcome, the body acts as a conductor and current flows throughout the involved body part. Bone has a very high resistance because of its density. Current will flow along the surface of the bone, and the heat generated damages the attached muscle. As a result, deep muscle injury may be present even when superficial muscles appear normal or uninjured.

The longer the electricity is in contact with the body, the greater the damage. The duration of contact is increased by tetanic contractions of the strong flexor muscles in the forearm, which can prevent the person from releasing the electrical source.

It is difficult to know the exact path a current takes in the body. The course of flow is first defined by the locations of the "contact sites," which are the entrance and exit wounds (Fig. 28-10). At first, the wounds may not be obvious. The path of injury may involve many internal tissues between the two contact sites.

Burn injuries from electricity can occur in one of three ways: *thermal burns, flash burns,* or *true electrical injury.* Thermal burns occur when clothes ignite from heat or flames produced by electrical sparks. External burn injuries can occur when the electrical current jumps, or "arcs," between two body surfaces. These injuries usually are severe and deep. True electrical injury occurs when direct contact is made with an electrical source. Internal damage results, and the injuries can be devastating. Damage starts on the inside and goes out; deep-tissue destruction may not be apparent immediately after injury. Organs in the path of the current may become ischemic and necrotic (Arnoldo et al., 2006).

Radiation injuries occur when people are exposed to large doses of radioactive material. The most common type of tissue

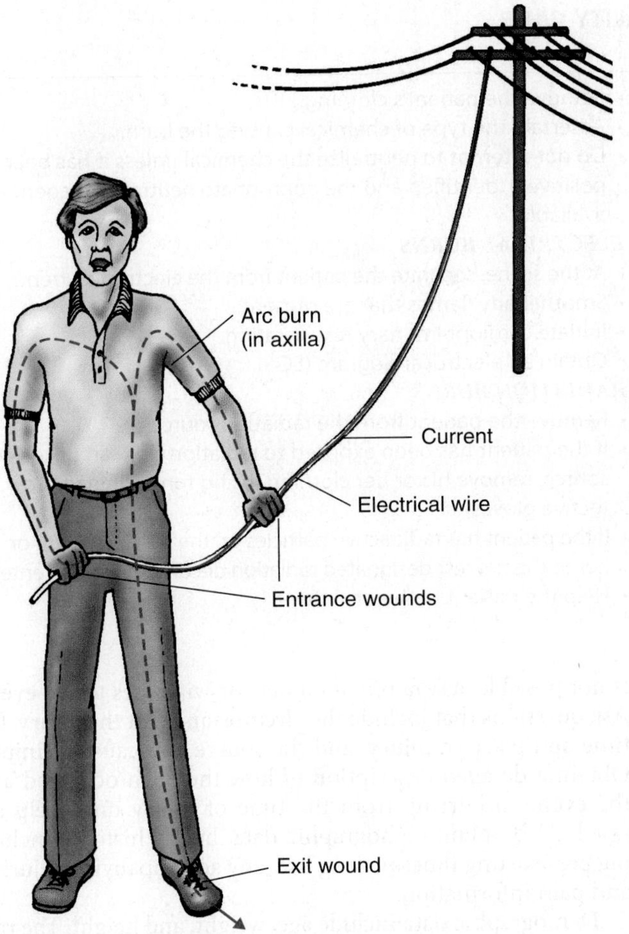
Arc burn
(in axilla)
Current
Electrical wire
Entrance wounds
Exit wound

Fig. 28-9 • The mechanism of electrical injury: Currents passing through the body follow the path of least resistance to the ground.

injury from radiation exposure occurs with therapeutic radiation. This injury is usually minor and rarely causes extensive skin damage.

Radiation exposure is more serious in industrial settings where radioactive energy is produced or radioactive isotopes are used. Injury severity depends on the amount and type of energy deposited over time. Chapter 24 discusses the potential for tissue damage from alpha, beta, and gamma radiation. The severity of injury is determined by the type of radiation, distance from the source, duration of exposure, absorbed dose, and depth of penetration into the body.

Incidence/Prevalence of Burn Injury

Fires and burns are the fifth most common cause of unintentional injury deaths in the United Stares and the third leading cause of fatal home injuries (American Burn Association, 2007). Although the number of fatalities and injuries caused by residential fires has declined gradually over the past several decades, many residential fire-related deaths remain preventable and continue to pose a significant public health problem.

An estimated 4000 fire and burn deaths occur each year (American Burn Association, 2007). This total includes deaths from fires and motor vehicle or aircraft crashes, electricity, chemicals, hot liquids and substances, and any other sources of burn injury. Most deaths occur at the scene of the incident or during transport.

Men experience more burn injuries than women. Death from burn injuries decreases with appropriate intervention. Factors that increase the risk for death include age older than 60 years, a burn greater than 40% TBSA, and the presence of an inhalation injury. When a patient has all three risk factors, the risk for death is very high. Better outcomes from burn injuries occur because of the many therapeutic advances, such as vigorous fluid resuscitation, early burn wound excision, improved critical care monitoring, early enteral nutrition, antibiotics, and the use of specialized burn centers.

HEALTH PROMOTION AND MAINTENANCE

Minor burns are common occurrences, and prevention involves planning and awareness. Teach all people to assess how hot the water is before bathing, showering, or immersing a body part in it. Reinforce the use of potholders when taking food from conventional or microwave ovens. Stress the importance of never adding a flammable substance (e.g., gasoline, kerosine, alcohol, lighter fluid, charcoal starter) to an open flame. Suggest the use of sunscreen agents and protective clothing to avoid sunburn.

House fires also are common and lead to severe burns and death. Teach people to reduce the risk for house fires by never smoking in bed, avoiding smoking when drinking alcohol or taking drugs that induce sleep, and keeping matches or lighters out of the reach of children or anyone who is cognitively impaired. If space heaters must be used, stress the importance of keeping clothing, bedding, and other flammable objects away from them. Remind people to keep the screens and doors closed on the fronts of fireplaces and to have chimneys swept each year to prevent creosote buildup. Also remind patients using home oxygen not to smoke when oxygen is in use (Edelman et al., 2008).

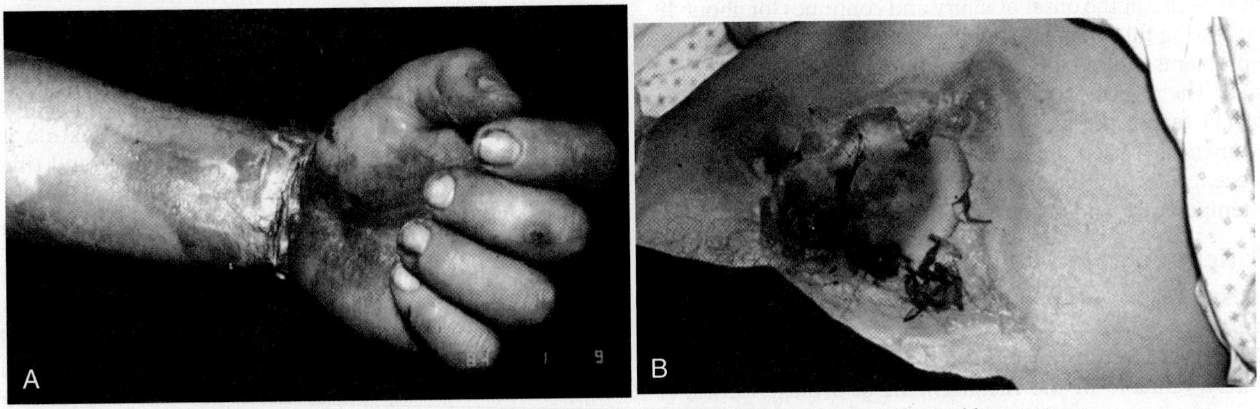
A
B

Fig. 28-10 • Electrical wound contact sites. **A**, Possible entrance site. **B**, Possible exit site.

Chart 28-1 BEST PRACTICE FOR PATIENT SAFETY & QUALITY CARE

Emergency Management of Burns

EMERGENCY CARE

GENERAL MANAGEMENT FOR ALL TYPES OF BURNS
- Assess for airway patency.
- Administer oxygen as needed.
- Cover the patient with a blanket.
- Keep the patient on NPO status.
- Elevate the extremities if no fractures are obvious.
- Obtain vital signs.
- Initiate an IV line, and begin fluid replacement.
- Administer tetanus toxoid for prophylaxis.
- Perform a head-to-toe assessment.

SPECIFIC MANAGEMENT

FLAME BURNS
- Smother the flames.
- Remove smoldering clothing and all metal objects.

CHEMICAL BURNS
- If dry chemicals are present on skin or clothing, DO NOT WET THEM.
- Brush off any dry chemicals present on the skin or clothing.
- Remove the patient's clothing.
- Ascertain the type of chemical causing the burn.
- Do not attempt to neutralize the chemical unless it has been positively identified and the appropriate neutralizing agent is available.

ELECTRICAL BURNS
- At the scene, separate the patient from the electrical current.
- Smother any flames that are present.
- Initiate cardiopulmonary resuscitation.
- Obtain an electrocardiogram (ECG).

RADIATION BURNS
- Remove the patient from the radiation source.
- If the patient has been exposed to radiation from an unsealed source, remove his or her clothing (using tongs or lead protective gloves).
- If the patient has radioactive particles on the skin, send him or her to the nearest designated radiation decontamination center.
- Help the patient bathe or shower.

Leaving a burning building is critical to preventing injury or death. Teach all people to use smoke detectors and carbon monoxide detectors within their home and to ensure that the detectors are in good working order. The number of detectors needed depends on the size of the home. Recommendations are that each bedroom has a separate smoke detector, there should be at least one detector in the hallway of each story, and at least one detector is needed for the kitchen, each stairwell, and each house/home entrance. Teach everyone to develop a planned escape route with alternatives for when a main route is blocked by fire. Reinforce that no one should ever re-enter a burning building to retrieve belongings.

RESUSCITATION/EMERGENT PHASE OF BURN INJURY

Overview

Burns can be a devastating and dehumanizing injury. Events within the first hour after injury can make the difference between life and death for the patient with a burn injury. Immediate care focuses on maintaining an open airway, ensuring adequate breathing and circulation, limiting the extent of injury, and maintaining the function of vital organs. Chart 28-1 outlines the emergency management of a burn injury.

The **resuscitation/emergent phase** is the first phase of a burn injury. It begins at the onset of injury and continues for about 48 hours. During this phase, the injury is evaluated and the immediate problems of fluid loss, edema, and reduced blood flow are assessed. The priority goals of management during this period are to (1) secure the airway, (2) support circulation by fluid replacement, (3) keep the patient comfortable with analgesics, (4) prevent infection through careful wound care, (5) maintain body temperature, and (6) provide emotional support.

Patient-Centered Collaborative Care

evolve ONLINE PHARM REVIEW

Assessment

History

Knowledge of circumstances surrounding the burn injury is extremely valuable in the management of a burn victim. If possible, obtain information directly from the patient. If this is not possible, ask family members or witnesses to the event. Ask questions that include the circumstances of the injury, the time and place of injury, and the source and cause of injury. Obtain a detailed description of how the burn occurred and the events occurring from the time of injury until help arrived. Also obtain demographic data, health history (including pre-existing illness), drug use, any accompanying injuries, and pain information.

Demographic data include age, weight, and height. The rate of serious complications and death from burn injuries is increased among adults older than 50 years. Chart 28-2 lists the age-related differences in older adults' responses to a burn injury. The patient's preburn weight is used to calculate fluid rates, energy requirements, and drug doses. The preburn weight often is referred to as *dry weight,* because it represents the patient's weight before edema begins to form. Calculations based on a weight obtained after fluid replacement is started are not accurate because of water-induced weight gain. Height is important in determining total body surface area (TBSA), which is used to calculate nutritional needs.

A health history, including any pre-existing illnesses, must be known for appropriate treatment to be given. Obtain information from the patient specifically about his or her history of cardiac or renal impairment, chronic alcoholism, substance abuse, and diabetes mellitus; any of these problems influence fluid resuscitation. The physiologic stress seen with a burn can make a mild disease process develop more symptoms or worsen an active process. Obtain a drug history that includes allergies, current drugs, and immunization status from the patient or family. Determine the dose and time the last drug was taken. Ask whether the patient smokes or drinks alcohol daily; these factors can influence treatment and physical responses.

Other injuries are unusual but may occur at the time of the burn. The most common causes of additional injuries are falls and motor vehicle crashes. Such injuries increase the patient's risk for complications or death. Determine whether additional injuries such as fractures, chest injuries, and abdominal trauma are causing pain or discomfort.

Chart 28-2 NURSING FOCUS ON THE OLDER ADULT

Age-Related Changes Increasing Complications from Burn Injury

Age-Related Changes	Complications and Nursing Considerations
Thinner skin, sensory impairment, decreased mobility	Sensory impairment and decreased mobility increase the risk for burn injury. Thinner skin increases the depth of injury even when the exposure to the cause of injury is of shorter duration.
Slower healing time	Longer time with open areas results in a greater risk for infection and metabolic derangements.
More likely to have cardiac impairments	Limits the aggressiveness of fluid resuscitation. Increases the risk for shock and renal failure.
Reduced inflammatory and immune responses	Increases the risk for infection and sepsis. Patient may not have a fever when infection is present.
Reduced thoracic and pulmonary compliance	Increased risk for atelectasis, hypoxia, and other pulmonary complications.
More likely to have pre-existing medical conditions such as diabetes mellitus, renal impairment, or pulmonary impairment	Any of these disorders compromise vital organ function and can interfere with fluid resuscitation efforts or other treatments.

TABLE 28-3 Factors Determining Inhalation Injury or Airway Obstruction

- Patients who were injured in a closed space
- Patients with extensive burns or with burns of the face
- Intra-oral charcoal, especially on teeth and gums
- Patients who were unconscious at the time of injury
- Patients with singed scalp hair, nasal hairs, eyelids, or eyelashes
- Patients who are coughing up carbonaceous sputum
- Changes in voice such as hoarseness or brassy cough
- Use of accessory muscles or stridor
- Poor oxygenation or ventilation
- Edema, erythema, and ulceration of airway mucosa
- Wheezing, bronchospasm

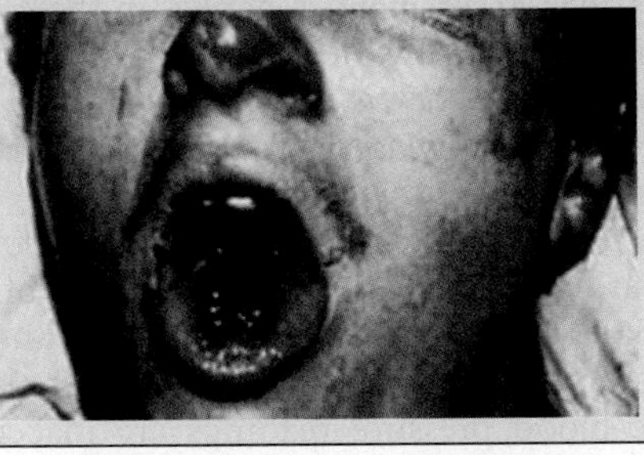

Physical Assessment/Clinical Manifestations

Physical assessment findings in the resuscitation/emergent phase differ greatly from findings later in the course of the injury. Use a systematic approach to ensure that no problem is missed. Although all systems are important, assessment of the respiratory system is critical to prevent life-threatening complications.

Respiratory Assessment. Patients with major burn injuries and those with inhalation injury are at risk for respiratory problems. Therefore continuing airway assessment is a nursing priority. Respiratory manifestations common with a burn injury are listed in Table 28-3.

Direct Airway Injury. Inhalation injuries are present in about 5% to 15% of the patients admitted to burn centers. The degree of inhalation damage depends on the fire source, temperature, environment, and types of toxic gases generated. Ask about the source of the fire, duration of exposure, and whether the fire was in an enclosed space. Assess the respiratory system by inspecting the mouth, nose, and pharynx. Burns of the lips, face, ears, neck, eyelids, eyebrows, and eyelashes are strong indicators that an inhalation injury may be present. Burns inside the mouth and singed nasal hairs also indicate possible inhalation injury. Black particles of carbon in the nose, mouth, and sputum and edema of the nasal septum indicate smoke inhalation, as does a "smoky" smell to the patient's breath.

A change in respiratory pattern may indicate a pulmonary injury. The patient may:

- *Become progressively hoarse*
- *Develop a brassy cough*
- *Drool or have difficulty swallowing*
- *Produce sounds on exhalation that include audible wheezes, crowing, and stridor*

Any of these changes may mean the patient is about to lose his or her airway. Immediately apply oxygen and notify the Rapid Response Team if any of these manifestations are present.

▼ AUDIO CLIP: High- and Low-Pitched Wheezes

Upper airway edema and inhalation injury are most common in the trachea and mainstem bronchi. Auscultation of these areas may reveal wheezes, which are a sign of partial obstruction. *Patients with severe inhalation injuries may have such rapid obstruction that, within a short time, they cannot force air through the narrowed airways. As a result, the wheezing sounds disappear. This finding indicates impending airway obstruction and demands immediate intubation.* Many patients are intubated when an inhalation injury is suspected rather than waiting until obstruction makes endotracheal or nasotracheal intubation difficult or impossible.

Carbon Monoxide Poisoning. Carbon monoxide is one of the leading causes of death from a fire. It is a colorless, odorless, tasteless gas released in the process of combustion. Inhalation injury is a risk for carbon monoxide poisoning.

Carbon monoxide (CO) is rapidly transported across the lung membrane and binds tightly to hemoglobin in place of oxygen to form carboxyhemoglobin (CoHb). In addition, CO causes the oxyhemoglobin dissociation curve to shift to the left, thereby impairing oxygen unloading at the tissue level. This shift results in a substantial reduction in oxygen delivery, given that 98% of the oxygen supplied to the tissues comes bound to hemoglobin. Even though the oxygen-carrying capacity of the hemoglobin is reduced, the blood gas value of partial pressure of arterial oxygen (Pao_2) is normal (Rosenthal, 2006). The vasodilating action of carbon monoxide causes the "cherry red" color in these patients. Manifestations vary with the concentration of CoHb. Table 28-4 lists the effects of carbon monoxide poisoning.

Thermal (Heat) Injury. Except for rare events such as steam inhalation, aspiration of scalding liquid, or explosion of flammable gases under pressure, thermal burns to the respiratory tract are usually limited to the upper airway above the glottis (nasopharynx, oropharynx, and larynx). *Heat damage of the pharynx is often severe enough to produce edema and upper airway obstruction, especially epiglottitis. The problem can occur any time during resuscitation. In the unresuscitated patient, supraglottic edema may be delayed because of the dehydration that occurs with hypovolemia. During fluid resuscitation, however, the tissues rehydrate and then swell from capillary leak. For this reason, when it is known that the upper airways were exposed to heat, intubation may be performed as an early intervention before obstruction occurs. When intubation has not been performed, continuous upper airway assessment for recognition of edema and obstruction is critical to the patient's survival.*

Inhaled steam can injure the lower respiratory tract because water holds heat better than dry air does. The respiratory tract down to the major bronchioles can be damaged by steam. Ulcerations, redness, and edema of the mouth and epiglottis are the first manifestations, with rapid swelling leading to upper airway obstruction. Stridor, hoarseness, and shortness of breath result.

Smoke Poisoning. Smoke poisoning, or chemical injury from the inhalation of combustion by-products, is a common type of inhalation injury. Toxic by-products, especially hydrogen cyanide, are produced when plastics or home furnishings are burned. Cyanide binds to cell energy-making components, thereby inhibiting cell metabolism and cell function.

Pulmonary Fluid Overload. Pulmonary edema can occur even when the lung tissues have not been damaged directly. Other damaged tissues release such large amounts of histamine and other inflammatory mediators causing capillary leak that even lung capillaries leak fluid into the pulmonary tissue spaces.

Circulatory overload from fluid resuscitation may cause left-sided congestive heart failure. This problem creates high pressure within pulmonary blood vessels that pushes fluid into the lung tissue spaces. Excess lung tissue fluid makes gas exchange difficult. *The patient is short of breath and has dyspnea in the supine position. Crackles are heard on auscultation. Elevate the head of the bed to at least 45 degrees, apply humidified oxygen, and notify the burn team or the Rapid Response Team.*

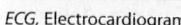

▼ AUDIO CLIP: High- and Low-Pitched Crackles

External Factors. In addition to pulmonary problems, patients with burn injuries may have breathing problems from external factors. The most common external factor affecting breathing is tight eschar from deep circumferential chest burns. The eschar either restricts chest movement or compresses structures in the neck and throat to such an extent that air flow is impaired. Inspect the patient's chest hourly for ease of respiration, amount of chest movement, rate of breathing, and effort required to breathe. Use continuous pulse oximetry to assess breathing effectiveness in maintaining blood oxygen levels.

Cardiovascular Assessment. Changes in the cardiovascular system begin immediately after the burn injury and include shock. *Hypovolemia shock is a common cause of death in the resuscitation/emergent phase in patients with serious injuries.* See Chapter 39 for discussion of shock.

At first, cardiac manifestations are from hypovolemia and decreased cardiac output. Monitor the degree of edema, and assess cardiac status by measuring central and peripheral pulses, blood pressure, capillary refill, and pulse oximetry. Noninvasive blood pressure readings are inaccurate in patients with large burns involving the upper extremities. Thus invasive monitoring may be needed for blood pressure measurement. At first, the patient has tachycardia, decreased blood pressure, and decreased peripheral pulses. Peripheral capillary refill is slow or absent as tissue blood flow decreases. With fluid resuscitation, peripheral edema increases, as does the patient's body weight.

Electrocardiographic (ECG) changes indicate electrical damage to the heart. These changes are most common with electrical burn injuries or with stress that induces a myocardial infarction. Obtain baseline ECG tracings at the time of admission to the hospital or burn center. Continue the ECG monitoring throughout the resuscitation/emergent phase. Compare current ECG tracings with the initial tracings to assess whether the patient is experiencing new-onset conduction abnormalities from the burn injury or the fluid resuscitation.

Renal/Urinary Assessment. Changes in renal function with burn injury are related to decreased renal blood flow and to

TABLE 28-4 Physiologic Effects of Carbon Monoxide Poisoning

Carbon Monoxide Level	Physiologic Effects
1%-10% (normal)	Increased threshold to visual stimuli Increased blood flow to vital organs
11%-20% (mild poisoning)	Headache Decreased cerebral function Decreased visual acuity Slight breathlessness
21%-40% (moderate poisoning)	Headache Tinnitus Nausea Drowsiness Vertigo Altered mental state Confusion Stupor Irritability Decreased blood pressure, increased and irregular heart rate Depressed ST segment on ECG and dysrhythmias Pale to reddish purple skin
41%-60% (severe poisoning)	Coma Convulsions Cardiopulmonary instability
61%-80% (fatal poisoning)	Death

ECG, Electrocardiogram.

the presence of cellular debris. During the fluid shift of the resuscitation/emergent period, blood flow to the kidney may not be adequate for glomerular filtration. As a result, urine output is greatly decreased compared with IV fluid intake. The urine is highly concentrated and has a high specific gravity.

Other substances may be present in the blood that flows through the kidney. Destroyed red blood cells release hemoglobin and potassium. When muscle damage occurs from a major burn or electrical injury, a large oxygen-carrying protein called **myoglobin** is released from damaged muscle and circulates to the kidney. Most damaged cells release proteins that form uric acid. All of these large molecules in the blood may precipitate in the kidney tubular system. This precipitation forms a sludge that blocks kidney blood and urine flow and may cause renal failure.

Assess renal function by accurately measuring urine output hourly and comparing this value with fluid intake. Urine output is decreased during the first 24 hours of the resuscitation/emergent phase. Fluid resuscitation is provided at the rate needed to maintain hourly urine output at 30 to 50 mL or 0.5 mL/kg/hr. Assess response to fluid resuscitation by measuring urine specific gravity, blood urea nitrogen (BUN), serum creatinine, and serum sodium levels in addition to hourly urine output. Examine the urine for color, odor, and the presence of particles or foam.

Skin Assessment. Assess the skin to determine the size and depth of burn injury. The size of the injury is first estimated in comparison with the *total body surface area (TBSA)*. For example, a burn that involves 40% of the TBSA is a 40% burn. The size of the injury is important not only for diagnosis and prognosis but also for calculating drug doses, fluid replacement volumes, and caloric needs.

Inspect the skin to identify injured areas and changes in color and appearance. Except with electrical burns, this initial size assessment usually can be made accurately with specific assessment tools and charts.

The most rapid method for calculating the size of a burn injury in adult patients whose weights are in normal proportion to their heights is the *rule of nines* (Fig. 28-11). With this method, the body is divided into areas that are multiples of 9%. Although the rule of nines is useful at the site of injury and in emergency departments, overestimation of the TBSA involved can easily occur. More complex evaluations using other methods are made in the burn unit.

Because specific treatments are related to the depth of the burn injury, initial assessment of the skin includes estimations of burn depth. Criteria for depth of injury are based on appearance and associated characteristics (see Depth of Burn Injury section, pp. 521-523).

Bedside evaluation of burn depth remains the most common and cost-effective method; however, it is only an estimate. Other methods, such as thermography, the use of vital dyes, indocyanine green (ICG) video angiography, and laser Doppler imaging (LDI) more precisely measure the amount of tissue perfusion of the injured tissue. ICG and LDI are the most accurate of the three methods. Laser Doppler imaging is used more frequently because it is relatively accurate, less invasive, and faster than the other methods (Devgan et al., 2006).

Gastrointestinal Assessment. Although the GI tract usually is not directly injured (except with some chemical burns), changes in function are expected in all burn patients. The decreased blood flow and sympathetic stimulation during the resuscitation/emergent phase reduce GI motility and promote development of a paralytic ileus. Auscultate the abdomen to assess bowel sounds. Bowel sounds are commonly reduced or absent in a patient with severe burns. Other manifestations indicating paralytic ileus include nausea, vomiting, and abdominal distention. Patients with burns of 25% TBSA or who are intubated generally require a nasogastric (NG) tube inserted to prevent aspiration and remove gastric secretions. Assess the tube for placement and patency after insertion. Because of the potential for ulcer formation in the GI tract, each stool and vomitus are examined for the presence of gross blood or other material that indicates partially digested blood ("coffee ground"–appearing crumbs). Test for the presence of occult blood on any vomit or stool.

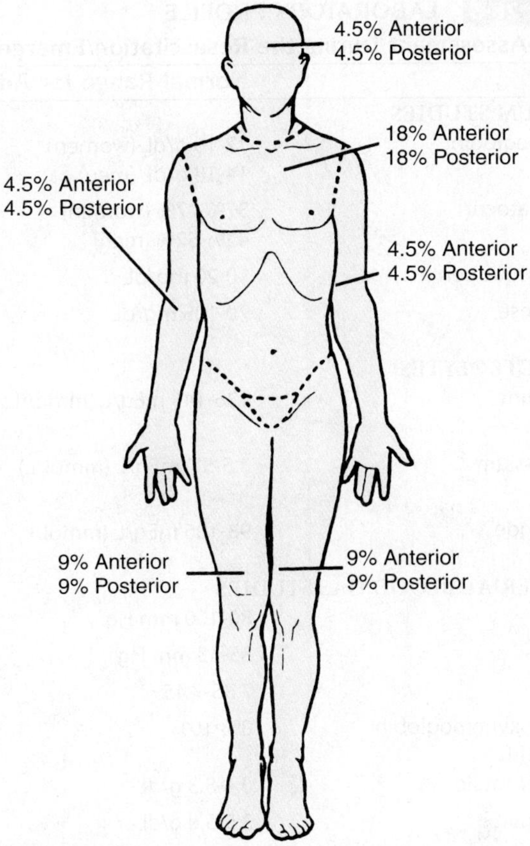
4.5% Anterior
4.5% Posterior
18% Anterior
18% Posterior
4.5% Anterior
4.5% Posterior
4.5% Anterior
4.5% Posterior
9% Anterior
9% Posterior
9% Anterior
9% Posterior

Fig. 28-11 • The rule of nines for estimating burn percentage.

Laboratory Assessment

Changes in laboratory test values are found in different phases of postburn recovery and reflect tissue damage or compensatory responses. However, other changes in specific laboratory findings may suggest complications.

During the resuscitation/emergent phase and before the start of fluid resuscitation, venous blood analysis reflects the fluid shift and direct tissue damage. Baseline laboratory test values and early postburn expected changes are listed in Chart 28-3.

Changes in the total white blood cell (WBC) count and differential count reflect immune function and inflammatory responses to the burn injury. The burn patient's total WBC count, especially the neutrophil percentage, first rises and then drops rapidly, with a "left shift" (see Chapter 19) as the immune

Chart 28-3 LABORATORY PROFILE

Burn Assessment During the Resuscitation/Emergent Phase

Test	Normal Range for Adults	Significance of Abnormal Findings
SERUM STUDIES		
Hemoglobin	12-16 g/dL (women) 14-18 g/dL (men)	Elevated as a result of fluid volume loss
Hematocrit	37%-47% (women) 42%-52% (men)	Elevated as a result of fluid volume loss
Urea nitrogen	10-20 mg/dL	Elevated as a result of fluid volume loss
Glucose	70-105 mg/dL	Elevated as a result of the stress response and altered uptake across injured tissues
ELECTROLYTES		
Sodium	136-145 mEq/L (mmol/L)	Decreased; sodium is trapped in edema fluid and lost through plasma leakage
Potassium	3.5-5.0 mEq/L (mmol/L)	Elevated as a result of disruption of the sodium-potassium pump, tissue destruction, and red blood cell hemolysis
Chloride	98-106 mEq/L (mmol/L)	Elevated as a result of fluid volume loss and reabsorption of chloride in urine
ARTERIAL BLOOD GAS STUDIES		
Pao_2	80-100 mm Hg	Slightly decreased
$Paco_2$	35-45 mm Hg	Slightly increased from respiratory injury
pH	7.35-7.45	Low as a result of metabolic acidosis
Carboxyhemoglobin	0%-10%	Elevated as a result of inhalation of smoke and carbon monoxide
OTHER		
Total protein	6.4-8.3 g/dL	Low; protein exudate is lost through the wound
Albumin	3.5-5.0 g/dL	Low; protein is lost through the wound and through vascular membranes because of increased permeability

system becomes unable to sustain its defenses. If sepsis occurs, the total WBC count may be as low as 2000 cells/mm^3.

Other laboratory tests that provide useful information about the burn patient's status include urine electrolyte assays, urine cultures, liver enzyme studies, and clotting studies. Drug and alcohol screens are obtained if drug or alcohol intoxication is suspected.

CULTURAL AWARENESS

For African-American patients, a sickle cell preparation may be appropriate if sickle status is unknown. The trauma of a burn injury often triggers a sickle cell crisis in patients who have the disease and in those who carry the trait.

Imaging Assessment

Standard x-rays and scans do not provide direct assessment data about the burn wound. These assessments are not performed unless other trauma is suspected.

Other Diagnostic Assessment

In addition to routine laboratory tests, specific studies of involved organs are performed. For example, when burn injuries involve the eye, an ophthalmic evaluation detects corneal damage (see Chapters 48 and 49 for specific eye and vision evaluation procedures).

Specific diagnostic studies are performed when deep organ trauma is suspected. Such studies include IV renograms, computed tomography (CT), ultrasonography, bronchoscopy, and magnetic resonance imaging (MRI).

Analysis

A burned patient has dramatic changes not only in the directly damaged tissues but also in many other body systems. During the course of the illness, most burn patients experience all of the common and many of the additional nursing diagnoses listed in the following sections.

Common Nursing Diagnoses and Collaborative Problems

Priority nursing diagnoses for patients with burn injuries in the resuscitation/emergent phase who have sustained a burn injury greater than 25% of the total body surface area (TBSA) are:

1. Decreased Cardiac Output related to altered stroke volume from an increase in capillary permeability
2. Deficient Fluid Volume related to active fluid volume loss, electrolyte imbalance, and inadequate fluid resuscitation
3. Ineffective Tissue Perfusion (Cerebral, Cardiopulmonary, Renal, Gastrointestinal, and Peripheral) related to hypovolemia from extravascular fluid shifts, decreased cardiac output, constriction of eschar, and edema
4. Ineffective Breathing Pattern related to respiratory distress from upper airway edema, pulmonary edema, airway obstruction, and pneumonia
5. Acute Pain and Chronic Pain related to biologic injury, damaged or exposed nerve endings, débridement, dressing changes, invasive procedures, and donor sites

Primary collaborative problems are:
1. Potential for Pulmonary Edema
2. Potential for Acute Respiratory Distress Syndrome (ARDS)

Additional Nursing Diagnoses and Collaborative Problems
In addition to the common nursing diagnoses and collaborative problems, patients with burn injuries in the resuscitation/emergent phase may have one or more of these:
- Excess Fluid Volume related to massive IV fluid administration
- Ineffective Thermoregulation related to trauma, hypermetabolism, and a loss of the protective barrier
- Disturbed Sensory Perception (Visual, Auditory, and Tactile) related to periorbital edema or ulcerations, hospital environment, noise, infections, and dressings
- Anxiety related to threat of death, initial burn trauma, situational crisis, painful procedures, unfamiliar environment, separation from significant others, and loss of control
- Fear related to pain, knowledge deficit, therapeutic procedures, hospitalization, separation, and social re-entry

Planning and Implementation

Decreased Cardiac Output; Deficient Fluid Volume; Ineffective Tissue Perfusion

NOC **Planning: Expected Outcomes.** With appropriate intervention, the patient is expected to have cardiac output restored to normal. Indicators include these vital signs and assessment parameters:
- Blood pressure at or near the patient's normal range
- Palpable peripheral pulses (or heard with Doppler) in all extremities
- Oxygen saturation, partial pressure of arterial oxygen (Pao_2), partial pressure of arterial carbon dioxide ($Paco_2$), and arterial pH at or near the normal ranges

Interventions. Interventions are aimed at increasing blood fluid volume, supporting compensatory mechanisms, and preventing complications. Nonsurgical management is often sufficient for achieving these aims. Surgical management is required most often for full-thickness burns.

Nonsurgical Management. Fluid volume and tissue blood flow are restored through IV fluid therapy and drug therapy. Priority nursing interventions are carrying out fluid resuscitation and monitoring for indications of effectiveness or complications.

Rapid infusion of IV fluids, known as *fluid resuscitation,* is needed to maintain sufficient blood volume for normal cardiac output, mean arterial pressure, and tissue oxygenation. Chart 28-4 lists NIC intervention activities for fluid resuscitation. Many formulas for calculating fluid requirements exist. Table 28-5 lists those commonly used for the therapy of adult patients. Although the types and amounts of electrolytes, crystalloids, and colloids vary, the purpose of all of these formulas is to prevent shock by maintaining circulating blood fluid volume. The optimal formula and infusion schedules remain controversial.

Resuscitation for a severe burn requires large fluid loads in a short time to maintain blood flow to vital organs. All common formulas recommend that half of the calculated fluid volume for 24 hours be given in the first 8 hours after injury. The other half is given over the next 16 hours for a total of 24 hours. Fluid boluses are avoided because they increase capillary pressure and worsen edema. In the second 24-hour period after a burn injury, the volume and content of the IV fluids are based on the patient's specific fluid volume and electrolyte imbalances and his or her response to treatment. Usually, this resuscitation involves hourly infusion amounts that are greatly in excess of the 125 mL to 150 mL per hour commonly infused for other conditions (Pham et al., 2008).

Fluid replacement formulas are calculated from the time of injury and not from the time of arrival at the hospital. For example, if a burn injury occurred at 8 AM but the patient was not admitted to the hospital until 10 AM, the first 8-hour period would be completed at 4 PM, or 8 hours after the injury. Thus if resuscitation was delayed by 2 hours until admission to the hospital, calculated fluids would need to be given over the next 6-hour period rather than an 8-hour period. All burn resuscitation formulas are used as guides. The patient's response to therapy determines exact fluid requirements. No single formula has been found to provide superior results over another.

The management of extensive burns may require placement of a large-bore central venous catheter so that massive fluid loads can be given. Peripheral lines are less useful be-

Chart 28-4 NIC INTERVENTION ACTIVITIES

The Burn Patient During the Resuscitation/Emergent Phase

Fluid Resuscitation: *Administering prescribed intravenous fluids rapidly*
- Obtain and maintain a large-bore IV.
- Collaborate with physicians to ensure administration of both crystalloids (e.g., lactated Ringer's) and colloids (e.g., Hespan and Plasmanate), as appropriate.
- Administer IV fluids, as prescribed.
- Monitor hemodynamic status.
- Monitor oxygen status.
- Monitor for fluid overload.
- Monitor output of various body fluids (e.g., urine, nasogastric drainage, and chest tube).
- Monitor BUN, creatinine, total protein, and albumin levels.
- Monitor for pulmonary edema and third spacing.

NIC intervention activities selected from Bulechek, G.M., Butcher, H.K., & McCloskey Dochterman, J. (Eds.). (2008). *Nursing interventions classification (NIC)* (5th ed.). St. Louis: Mosby. No part of this work is to be altered without prior written permission from the Publisher.
BUN, Blood urea nitrogen.

TABLE 28-5 Composition of Common Burn Fluid Resuscitation Formulas

Formula	Solution and Amount for the First 24 Hours
Parkland (Baxter)	Crystalloid only (lactated Ringer's) 4 mL/kg/% TBSA burn
Modified Parkland	Crystalloid only (lactated Ringer's) 4 mL/kg/% TBSA burn + 15 mL/m² of TBSA
Modified Brooke	Protenate or 5% albumin in 0.9% saline Lactated Ringer's without dextrose 0.5 mL to 1.5 mL/kg/% TBSA burn

TBSA, Total body surface area.

cause they become dislodged or fluid flow is cut off when massive peripheral edema compresses the IV catheter.

Monitoring patient responses is important to determine the adequacy of fluid resuscitation for hydration and blood perfusion of the brain, heart, and kidneys. Urine output is the most common and most sensitive noninvasive assessment parameter for cardiac output and tissue perfusion (see Chapters 13 and 39). *Regardless of the total amount of fluid calculated as needed to meet the fluid requirements of the patient, the amount of fluid given depends on how much IV fluid per hour is needed to maintain the hourly urine output at 0.5 mL/kg (about 30 mL/hr). Adjustment of the IV fluid rate on the basis of urine output plus serum electrolyte values is known as the* ***titration*** *of fluid. In patients with burns larger than 35% TBSA, the use of urine output and vital signs to guide resuscitation may not be adequate. Invasive monitoring of cardiac and pulmonary function is needed to ensure optimal fluid resuscitation.*

Burn patients often develop severe hypovolemic shock and need invasive cardiac monitoring. Vital parameters such as central venous pressure, pulmonary artery pressures, and cardiac output are obtained on an hourly to continuous basis.

Monitor the ECG activity of patients who have sustained large burns. Nonburn-related dysrhythmias, such as atrial fibrillation, are often present in older patients. Compare current ECG findings with those obtained on admission.

Drug therapy for decreased cardiac output in burn patients is different than that for the heart failure patient. A common mistake in treatment is giving diuretics to increase urine output rather than changing the amount and rate of fluid infused. *Diuretics do not increase cardiac output; they actually decrease circulating volume and cardiac output by pulling fluid from the circulating blood volume to enhance diuresis.* This effect reduces blood flow to other vital organs (especially the heart, lungs, and brain) and greatly increases the risk for severe hypovolemic shock. Therefore diuretics are not generally used to improve urine output for burn patients. An exception is the patient with a burn injury caused by electrical energy. Muscle and deep tissue damage release large protein molecules (myoglobin), which precipitate in and obstruct the renal tubules. Although the diuretic *mannitol* (Osmitrol) is often used in this situation, it should always be given after adequate urine output has been established.

CONSIDERATIONS FOR OLDER ADULTS

In older patients, especially those with cardiac disease, a complicating factor in reduced cardiac output may be heart failure or myocardial infarction. Drugs that increase cardiac output (e.g., dopamine [Intropin]) or that strengthen the force of myocardial contraction (e.g., digoxin [Lanoxin]) may be used along with fluid therapy.

Surgical Management. The surgical procedure for the treatment of inadequate tissue perfusion is *escharotomy.* An incision through the burn eschar relieves pressure caused by the constricting force of fluid buildup under circumferential burns on the extremity or chest and improves circulation. If the pressure is not relieved, arterial compression can occur with a loss of blood flow to the extremity leading to ischemia and possible necrosis. Incisions are made along the length of the extremity and extend into the subcutaneous tissue (Figs. 28-6 and 28-12). This procedure relieves the tourniquet effect of the

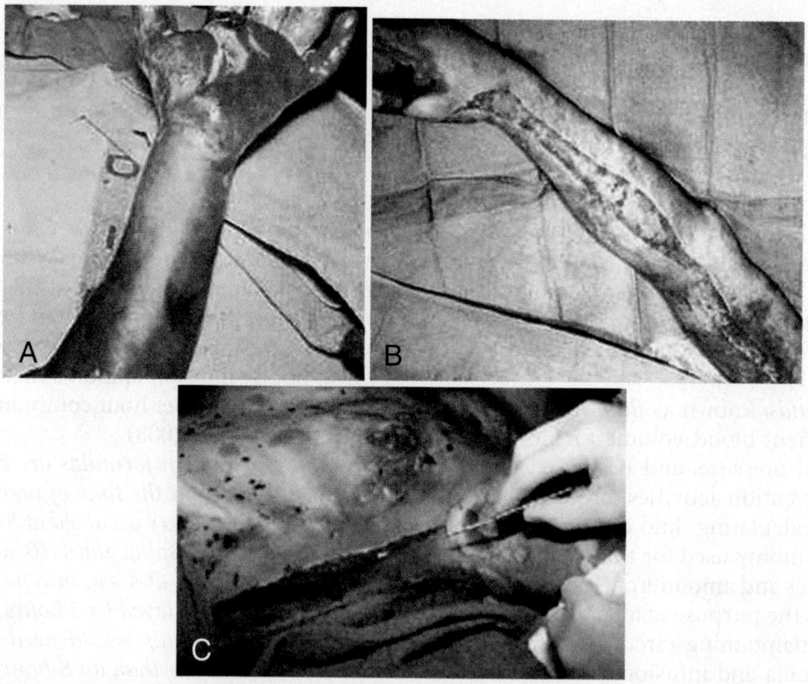

Fig. 28-12 • Escharotomy to release circumferential burn eschar and improve circulation to a distal extremity. **A,** Tight circumferential eschar restricting swelling as edema forms in the tissue beneath the eschar. Edema compresses blood vessels, which inhibits blood flow to the distal extremity. **B,** An escharotomy incision allows outward swelling of edematous tissues. Restricted blood flow through the vessels to the distal extremity is relieved. **C,** An anterior axillary incision is made bilaterally to relieve respiratory distress.

eschar. If tissue pressure remains elevated after escharotomy, a *fasciotomy* (a deeper incision extending through the fascia) may be needed.

Escharotomies are often performed at the bedside. No anesthesia is needed for escharotomy because nerve endings have been destroyed by the burn injury, but sedation and analgesia are given to reduce anxiety. Assure the patient that he or she will be made as comfortable as possible during the procedure. Remove the dressings, and thoroughly cleanse the areas to be incised. After the procedure, apply topical antimicrobial drugs and dressings to the area. Carefully monitor escharotomy sites for bleeding. Fasciotomies should be performed in an operating room with the patient under general anesthesia.

Ineffective Breathing Pattern

NOC **Planning: Expected Outcomes.** With proper intervention, the patient is expected to maintain a patent airway and have an effective breathing pattern. Indicators include that the patient should have either mildly compromised or normal oxygen saturation, PaO_2, $PaCO_2$, and arterial pH.

Interventions. Nursing and medical interventions are aimed at supporting normal pulmonary function and preventing pulmonary problems. Specific plans for pulmonary management depend on the cause of the breathing problem and the status of the respiratory tract. Thus a priority nursing intervention is monitoring the patient's respiratory status.

Nonsurgical Management. Interventions include airway maintenance, promotion of ventilation, monitoring gas exchange, oxygen therapy, drug therapy, positioning, and deep breathing.

Airway maintenance begins at the burn scene in an unconscious patient and may involve only a chin lift or a head-tilt maneuver. *Remember that upper airway edema becomes pronounced 8 to 12 hours after the beginning of fluid resuscitation. These patients often require nasal or oral intubation if crowing, stridor, or dyspnea is present* (Mlcak et al., 2007).

A bronchoscopy is performed to examine the vocal cords and airways of patients at risk for obstruction. Patients with severe smoke inhalation or poisoning may require a bronchoscopy on admission and routinely thereafter for examination of the respiratory tract, deep suctioning of the lungs, and removal of sloughing necrotic tissue. Assess the endotracheal tube hourly to ensure patency and location in intubated patients.

Other causes of airway obstruction are excessive secretions and sloughed tissue from damaged lungs. Suction as indicated based on clinical assessment or clinician order. Vigorous endotracheal or nasotracheal tube suctioning is performed after chest physiotherapy and aerosol treatments. Patients report that deep endotracheal suctioning is extremely painful. Therefore suctioning the endotracheal tube often requires increased analgesia or sedation.

Promoting ventilation includes ensuring that skeletal muscle movement of the chest is adequate for ventilation. Chest movement can be restricted by tight dressings that cover the neck, chest, and abdomen. Observe the patient for ease of respiratory movements, and loosen tight dressings as needed to assist with ventilation.

Monitor for gas exchange by using laboratory tests (e.g., arterial blood gas, carboxyhemoglobin levels) and by assessing for cyanosis, disorientation, and increased pulse rate. Other data to monitor in critically ill patients include chest x-ray findings, pulmonary artery catheter pressures, and central venous pressures.

The possibility of cyanide poisoning is considered in patients involved in house fires. An elevated plasma lactate level is a useful indicator of cyanide toxicity in patients who do not have severe burns.

Oxygen therapy by giving humidified oxygen by facemask, cannula, or hood is used to manage any breathing impairment in the burn patient. Arterial oxygenation less than 60 mm Hg is an indication for intubation and mechanical ventilation. Keep emergency airway equipment at or near the patient's bedside. This equipment includes oxygen, masks, cannulas, manual resuscitation bags, laryngoscope, endotracheal tubes, and equipment for tracheostomy. Chapter 34 addresses specific nursing actions for patients during mechanical ventilation.

Drug therapy with antibiotics is used when pneumonia or other pulmonary infections impair breathing. Drug selection is based on known culture and sensitivity reports or on the specific organisms common to that burn unit. Impaired breathing from cardiac failure and increased pulmonary pressures may be treated with drugs that improve cardiac output and enhance urine output.

When a patient's activity during mechanical ventilation severely compromises respiratory mechanics, it may be necessary to use a paralytic drug, such as atracurium (Tracrium) or vecuronium (Norcuron). This situation is often referred to as "bucking" the ventilator. Paralytic drugs remove all breathing control from the patient, making mechanical ventilation easier. *These drugs do not prevent the patient from seeing and hearing or from experiencing fear, pain, and loss of control. Any patient receiving neuromuscular blockade drugs must also receive drugs for sedation, analgesia, and antianxiety unless clinically contraindicated.* Extreme care must be taken to ensure that all alarms are operative and that patients are checked frequently, because they cannot call for help should they become extubated.

Positioning and deep breathing can improve breathing patterns and oxygenation. Turn the patient frequently, and assist him or her out of bed to a chair as much as possible. Teach the patient to use coughing and deep-breathing exercises. Urge him or her to use incentive spirometry every 2 hours while awake. Chest physiotherapy may be helpful to mobilize lung secretions, depending on the patient's clinical condition and the clinician's prescription.

Surgical Management. A tracheotomy may be needed when long-term intubation is expected. This procedure increases the risk for infection in burn patients even more than in nonburned patients. Emergency tracheotomies are performed when an airway becomes occluded and oral or nasal intubation cannot be achieved.

Other surgical procedures for improving the burn patient's breathing pattern include inserting chest tubes and performing an escharotomy. Chest tubes are used to re-expand the lung when a pneumothorax or hemothorax has occurred (see Chapter 34). Tight eschar on the neck, chest, or abdomen can restrict respiratory movement. Escharotomies (described on pp. 534-535) can relieve this restriction and permit greater respiratory movement.

Acute Pain; Chronic Pain

The pain with burn injuries is both chronic and acute. Many factors contribute to burn pain and may be altered to reduce pain perception. Pain from the actual injury is worse when painful procedures are performed. Many nursing procedures needed by burn patients increase pain. Accurate assessment of the patient's pain before and during procedures is an essential part of pain management.

NOC **Planning: Expected Outcomes.** The pain level of a patient with a burn injury is expected to be alleviated or reduced. Indicators include that the patient should rarely demonstrate these behaviors:

- Reporting pain
- Moaning and crying
- Making facial expressions of pain
- Losing his or her appetite

Interventions. The plan for pain management is tailored to the patient's tolerance for pain, coping mechanisms, and physical status. The priority nursing actions include continually assessing the patient's pain level, using appropriate pain-reducing strategies, and preventing complications.

Nonsurgical Management. Interventions for the patient having pain include drug therapy, complementary therapy measures, and environmental manipulation.

Drug therapy usually requires both opioid analgesics, such as morphine sulfate, hydromorphone (Dilaudid), fentanyl, and non-opioid analgesics. Although these drugs may provide adequate pain relief when no procedures are being performed, they rarely offer more than moderate relief during acutely painful procedures. In addition, they depress respiratory function and reduce intestinal motility. Thus nonpharmacologic interventions also are needed for the burn patient (Faucher & Furukawa, 2006).

During the resuscitation/emergent postburn phase, the IV route is used for giving opioid drugs because of problems with absorption from the muscle and stomach. When these agents are given IM or subcutaneously, they remain in the tissue spaces and do not relieve pain. In addition, when edema is present, all the doses are rapidly absorbed at once when the fluid shift is resolving. This delayed absorption can result in lethal blood levels of analgesics.

Anesthetic agents, such as ketamine (Ketalar), pentobarbital sodium (Nembutal, Novopentobarb♣), and nitrous oxide, also reduce pain. Use strict protocols when giving these agents to prevent serious complications.

Complementary and alternative therapy measures include relaxation techniques, meditative breathing, guided imagery, music therapy, massage, and healing or therapeutic touch. Hypnosis and autohypnosis can be used by lucid, cooperative patients under the direction of trained therapists. Therapeutic touch, acupuncture, and acupressure are used to a limited extent for burn patients; the results are variable. Nontraditional and complementary therapy types of pain intervention are detailed in Chapter 2.

Environmental changes, such as providing a quiet environment, using nonpainful tactile stimulation, and increasing the patient's control can increase comfort. Sleep deprivation increases patients' discomfort. Increasing sleep or rest time in a quiet environment helps reduce the adverse effects of sleep deprivation, replenishes body hormone stores, helps prevent critical care unit psychosis, and restores the diurnal effects of endorphins. Coordinate with all members of the health care team to ensure that most procedures are performed during the patient's waking hours.

Tactile stimulation can reduce pain. Help the patient change positions every 2 hours to reduce pressure on any specific area, improve circulation to painful areas, and ease pain. Massage nonburn areas to reduce pain transmission and stimulate endorphin release. Apply heat and maintain warm room temperatures to prevent shivering.

To reduce anxiety and increase feelings of confidence and independence, encourage the patient to participate in pain control measures. For example, make a contract with him or her that specifies how long a painful procedure will last. This helps patients deal with the pain for that particular period. Patient-controlled analgesia (PCA) also reduces pain. Important issues and techniques for the best use of PCA include giving an initial bolus of 5 to 10 mg of morphine (or equivalent drug), increasing the PCA dose as needed to achieve pain relief, and planning for a change in dosing regimens at night (e.g., giving a bolus dose at bedtime). See Chapter 5 for an in-depth discussion of combination drug therapy for pain management.

Surgical Management. Early surgical excision of the burn wound is used in many burn centers (see the Surgical Excision section on p. 540). Early excision under anesthesia reduces the pain from daily débridement at the bedside or during hydrotherapy.

DECISION-MAKING CHALLENGE
Coordination of Care

The patient is a 42-year-old man admitted directly to the burn center after sustaining an injury while burning trash. He had thrown gasoline on the trash, and the flames shot back, catching his clothes on fire. At the scene he was given oxygen with a 100% non-rebreather mask. He has partial-thickness burns on his entire face, neck, anterior chest, and anterior lower legs. He also has circumferential deep partial-thickness burns to his bilateral forearms and hands. The estimated TBSA burn is 37%. On admission, he is oriented, has no shortness of breath, and states his pain is 10/10. Further assessment reveals singed scalp hair, eyebrows, and nasal hairs. There is no carbonaceous sputum or carbon deposits on the tongue and throughout the mouth and throat. A 20-gauge IV line is present in the right antecubital space, and he has received 200 mL of normal saline. His admission to the burn unit is 1 hour after sustaining the injury.

1. Is this patient at risk for an inhalation injury? Why or why not?
2. Do you need to perform further assessment of the airway? If yes, what would you expect to find on your assessment that would indicate airway obstruction, and why?
3. Once the patient is found to have an adequate airway and level of consciousness, what are the priority interventions to be implemented next?
4. What drugs would you give and by what route would you administer them to control the patient's pain?

evolve For suggested answer guidelines, go to http://evolve.elsevier.com/Iggy/.

Potential for Pulmonary Edema

Planning: Expected Outcomes. With intervention, the patient with a burn injury is expected to be free of pulmonary edema.

Interventions. Pulmonary edema can result from lung injury or from fluid resuscitation and myocardial overload. Even young, healthy people can become fluid overloaded. These patients usually receive digoxin or other agents to improve left ventricular function and prevent or treat pulmonary edema. Diuretics, a mainstay of therapy for pulmonary edema from other causes, may or may not be used in the resuscitation/emergent phase, depending on the patient's blood volume and renal function.

Potential for Acute Respiratory Distress Syndrome

Planning: Expected Outcomes. The patient with a burn injury is expected to:

- Not experience acute respiratory distress
- Have arterial blood gases (ABGs) within normal limits
- Maintain normal lung compliance.

Interventions. Patients who develop acute respiratory distress syndrome (ARDS) as a result of burn injury require thorough assessments and interventions. The interventions are aimed at increasing lung compliance and improving Pa_{O_2} (partial pressure of arterial oxygen) levels. The priority nursing care actions are coordinating respiratory therapy strategies and monitoring the patient's response to these interventions.

In collaboration with the physician and respiratory therapist, give positive end-expiratory pressure (PEEP) to augment the decreased lung volume by providing a continuous positive pressure in the airways and alveoli. This procedure enhances the diffusion of oxygen across the alveolar-capillary membrane. PEEP can be combined with intermittent mandatory volume (IMV) to enhance its effectiveness.

Assess and document the patient's response so that needed ventilator changes can be made. *Document and immediately report any signs of respiratory distress or change in respiratory patterns to the burn team and the respiratory therapist.* Monitor pulse oximetry and ABG levels to assess changes in respiratory status.

Neuromuscular blocking drugs (atracurium) can be used in patients receiving mechanical ventilation to reduce oxygen consumption (see the discussion of specific nursing care under Drug Therapy [Ineffective Breathing Pattern], p. 535).

DECISION-MAKING CHALLENGE
Critical Rescue

The patient who sustained a 37% TBSA burn injury described on p. 536 is started on fluid resuscitation using the Parkland formula as a guide. The laboratory studies sent were complete blood count (CBC), chemistries, ABGs, hepatic panel, urinalysis, prothrombin time (PT), partial thromboplastin time (PTT), and international normalized ratio (INR).

1. What information is needed for this formula? What type of fluid is administered?
2. Using the Parkland formula, calculate the amount of fluid this patient would require for the first 24 hours (he weighs 176 pounds).
3. Laboratory results are: hemoglobin, 20 g/dL; hematocrit, 52%; glucose, 162 mg/dL; blood urea nitrogen, 25 mg/dL. How would you interpret these values, and what should be your next step?
4. What other clinical indicators would you use to assess the adequacy of the fluid resuscitation?
5. What is the most likely cause for the elevated blood glucose level?

evolve For suggested answer guidelines, go to http://evolve.elsevier.com/Iggy/.

ACUTE PHASE OF BURN INJURY

Overview

The acute phase of burn injury begins about 36 to 48 hours after injury and lasts until wound closure is complete. During this phase, a multidisciplinary approach to care is needed. The nurse coordinates care that is directed toward continued assessment and maintenance of the cardiovascular and respiratory systems, as well as toward GI and nutritional status, burn wound care, pain control, and psychosocial interventions.

Patient-Centered Collaborative Care

evolve ONLINE PHARM REVIEW

Assessment

Physical Assessment/Clinical Manifestations

Cardiopulmonary Assessment. In the acute phase of burn injury, the priority nursing interventions are to assess the cardiovascular and respiratory systems to maintain these systems and to identify or prevent complications. At this time, the patient may develop pneumonia that can result in respiratory failure requiring mechanical ventilation. Although cardiovascular problems related to the fluid shift should be resolved, the patient is at risk for infection and sepsis, which affect cardiovascular function. The interventions used in the resuscitation/emergent phase also may be needed for these new problems.

Neuroendocrine Assessment. The increased metabolic demands placed on the body after a severe burn injury can severely deplete nutritional stores. Weigh the patient daily without dressings or splints, and compare it with his or her preburn weight. A 2% loss of body weight indicates a mild deficit. A 10% or more weight loss is important and requires the evaluation and modification of calorie intake. For very accurate calorie requirements, indirect calorimetry may be used. This method determines kilocalories of energy expenditure by measuring oxygen consumption (V_{O_2}) and carbon dioxide production (V_{CO_2}). Measurements are taken while the patient is at rest—usually at least 30 minutes after the most recent dressing changes or other stressful procedures. Indirect calorimetry often is performed shortly after admission and at least once each week until the wounds are closed.

Immune Assessment. The patient with a burn injury is at risk for infection because of open wounds and reduced immune function. *Burn wound sepsis is a serious complication of burn injury, and infection is the leading cause of death during the acute phase of recovery.* Continually assess the patient for signs of local and systemic infections (Table 28-6), including changes in wound appearance, changes in neurologic and GI function, and subtle changes in vital signs. Monitor for manifestations of gram-positive, gram-negative, and fungal infections (Table 28-7). Enforce meticulous handwashing by all health care personnel. Use aseptic technique in caring for wounds and during invasive monitoring to prevent infections.

Musculoskeletal Assessment. Patients with a burn injury are at risk for musculoskeletal problems as a result of other injuries, immobility, healing processes, and treatment. The musculoskeletal status is first evaluated on admission to the hospital or burn center and throughout the acute phase of injury. Assess active and passive range of motion for all joints, including the neck. Give special attention to joints within the burn area. Ranges and limitations are documented for future reference.

Analysis

During the acute phase of the burn injury, the patient with a burn injury has resolution of some earlier problems, may have initial problems that extend into the acute phase, and may develop new problems.

Common Nursing Diagnoses and Collaborative Problems

Priority nursing diagnoses for patients with burn injuries greater than 25% TBSA in the acute phase of recovery are:

1. Impaired Skin Integrity related to burn wound, graft site, or donor site and physical immobilization

2. Risk for Infection related to inadequate primary defenses (wounds), the presence of multiple invasive catheters, reduced immune function, and malnutrition
3. Imbalanced Nutrition: Less Than Body Requirements related to increased metabolic rate; reduced calorie intake; and increased urinary nitrogen losses
4. Impaired Physical Mobility related to open burn wounds, pain, and scars and contractures
5. Disturbed Body Image related to trauma, changes in physical appearance and lifestyle, and alterations in sensory and motor function

The primary collaborative problem is Wound Care Management.

TABLE 28-6 Local and Systemic Signs of Infection

LOCAL SIGNS
- Conversion of a partial-thickness injury to a full-thickness injury
- Ulceration of healthy skin at the burn site
- Erythematous, nodular lesions in uninvolved skin and vesicular lesions in healed skin
- Edema of healthy skin surrounding the burn wound
- Excessive burn wound drainage
- Pale, boggy, dry, or crusted granulation tissue
- Sloughing of grafts
- Wound breakdown after closure
- Odor

SYSTEMIC SIGNS
- Altered level of consciousness
- Changes in vital signs (tachycardia, tachypnea, temperature instability, hypotension)
- Increased fluid requirements for maintenance of a normal urine output
- Hemodynamic instability
- Oliguria
- GI dysfunction (diarrhea, vomiting, abdominal distention, paralytic ileus)
- Hyperglycemia
- Thrombocytopenia
- Change in total white blood cell count (above normal or below normal)
- Metabolic acidosis
- Hypoxemia

Additional Nursing Diagnoses and Collaborative Problems

In addition to the common nursing diagnoses and collaborative problems, patients with burn injuries in the acute phase may have one or more of these:
- Grieving related to loss of significant others, loss of possessions, physical disfigurement, and changes in body image
- Disabled Family Coping related to loss of home, family, or significant others; crises resulting from burn injury; disturbances in normal functions; role changes; and prolonged hospitalization and rehabilitation
- Ineffective Coping related to situational crises, disfigurement, separation, and sensory overload
- Self-Care Deficits (Feeding, Bathing/Hygiene, Dressing/Grooming, Toileting) related to pain; contractures; and loss of function in the hands, extremities, and other body parts
- Sexual Dysfunction related to trauma; perineal, genital, and breast burns; immobility, fatigue, and depression; and disturbance in body image
- Sleep Deprivation related to pain, treatment regimen, and environmental noise
- Social Isolation related to the altered state of wellness, protective isolation treatment regimen, and alterations in physical appearance
- Deficient Knowledge (treatment regimen and healing process) related to unfamiliarity of information resources and cognitive limitation
- Potential for Pneumonia
- Potential for Septicemia

▪ *Planning and Implementation*

Impaired Skin Integrity; Wound Care Management

NOC **Planning: Expected Outcomes.** With appropriate intervention, the patient with a burn injury is expected to have no further loss of skin integrity and have skin integrity restored. Indicators include that the patient:
- Has presence of granulation, re-epithelialization, and scar tissue formation
- Has decreased wound size
- Has no new wounds

Interventions. Interventions aim to preserve the integrity of nonburned skin, enhance wound healing of burned skin, and prevent complications.

Nonsurgical Management. Nonsurgical burn wound management involves removing exudates and necrotic tissue, cleaning the area, stimulating granulation and revasculariza-

TABLE 28-7 Signs and Symptoms of Sepsis Caused by Different Organisms

Sign/Symptom	Gram-Positive	Gram-Negative	Fungal
Onset	Insidious, 2-6 days	Rapid, 12-36 hr	Delayed
Cognition	Severe disorientation and lethargy	Mild disorientation	Mild disorientation
Ileus	Severe	Severe	Mild
Diarrhea	Rare	Severe	Occasional
Temperature	Fever	Hypothermia	Fever
Hypotension	Late	Early	Late
White blood cell count	Neutrophilia	Neutropenia	Neutrophilia
Platelets	Normal	Low	Low

tion, and applying dressings. Restoring skin, whether by natural healing or grafting, starts with the removal of eschar and other cellular debris from the burn wound. This removal is called **débridement.** Nonsurgical treatment allows debris removal through mechanical and enzymatic actions that separate eschar over time. The goal is to have the wound prepare itself for grafting and wound closure by a natural process. Priority nursing interventions are aimed at assessing the wound, providing appropriate wound care, and preventing infection and other complications.

Mechanical débridement. Burn wounds are débrided and cleaned one or two times each day during **hydrotherapy** (the application of water for treatment). Nurses, unlicensed assistive personnel (UAP), and physical therapists perform hydrotherapy daily to débride and examine the wounds. Hydrotherapy can be performed by immersing the patient in a tub, showering him or her on a specially designed shower table, or washing only small areas of the wound at the bedside. Showering enhances wound inspection and allows water temperature to be kept constant.

Nurses and skilled technicians use forceps and scissors to remove loose, nonviable tissue during hydrotherapy. The care of intact blisters is controversial. At most burn units, small blisters are left alone because they are a protective barrier that promotes wound healing. Washcloths or gauze sponges are used to débride soft, "cheesy" eschar. During hydrotherapy, wash burn areas thoroughly and gently with mild soap or detergent and water. Then rinse these areas with room-temperature water.

Enzymatic débridement. Enzymatic débridement can occur naturally by autolysis or artificially by the application of exogenous agents. **Autolysis** is the disintegration of tissue by the action of the patient's own cellular enzymes. This process is seldom used in North America for larger burns because it is slow and results in a prolonged hospital stay, increasing the risk for infection.

Topical enzyme agents, such as collagenase (Santyl), are used for rapid wound débridement. When these agents are applied directly to the burn wound in a once-a-day dressing change, the enzymes digest collagen in necrotic tissues. They require a moist environment within a specific pH range to be active. Polysporin powder is often used with this topical agent to prevent infection.

Dressing the burn wound. After burn wounds are cleaned and débrided, topical antibiotics are reapplied to prevent infection (see pp. 540-541 in the Risk for Infection section). Some type of dressing is then applied to the burn wound. Burn dressings include standard wound dressings, biologic dressings, synthetic dressings, and artificial skin.

Standard wound dressings. Standard wound dressings are multiple layers of gauze applied over the topical agents on the burn wound. The number of gauze layers depends on:

- Depth of the injury
- Amount of drainage expected
- Area injured
- Patient's mobility
- Frequency of dressing changes

The gauze layers are held in place with roller-type gauze bandages applied in a distal to proximal direction or with circular net fabrics. Cover gauze dressings on the patient's extremities with elastic wraps, especially if the patient is ambulatory. Dressings are generally changed and reapplied every 8 to 24 hours after thoroughly cleaning the areas.

Biologic dressings. Biologic dressings are often used for temporary wound coverage and closure. These dressings are skin or membranes obtained from human tissue donors (homograft or allograft) or animals (heterograft or xenograft). When applied over open wounds, a biologic dressing rapidly adheres and promotes healing or prepares the wound for permanent skin graft coverage.

Biologic materials are used in healing partial-thickness and granulating full-thickness wounds that are clean and free of eschar. Table 28-8 lists the advantages and disadvantages of biologic dressings. The type of biologic dressing selected depends on the type of wound to be covered and the availability of the material.

Homografts, also called *allografts,* are human skin obtained from a cadaver and provided through a skin bank. They are fresh or frozen; frozen skin is thawed in a warm bath of sterile normal saline before application. Disadvantages to the use of homografts are the high costs ($750 to $1500 per square foot) and the risk of transmitting a bloodborne infection.

Heterografts, also called *xenografts,* are skin obtained from another species. Pigskin is the most common heterograft and is compatible with human skin. Pigskin is assessed daily for adherence and need for replacement.

Amniotic membrane is another form of biologic dressing used on burn wounds. Its large size, low cost, and availability have helped with its success. In full-thickness injuries, the amniotic membrane adheres to the wound. With partial-thickness areas, the amniotic membrane is effective as a dressing until epithelial cell regrowth occurs. The membrane requires frequent changes because it does not develop a blood supply and it disintegrates in about 48 hours.

TABLE 28-8 Biologic Dressings

USES
- Débridement of untidy wounds after separation of eschar
- Promotion of re-epithelialization of deep partial-thickness wounds
- Temporary coverage after excision of the burn wound
- Protection of granulation tissue between autografts
- Test graft before autografting

ADVANTAGES
- Early adherence to the wound
- Reduction of evaporative heat loss
- Reduction of evaporate water loss
- Prevention of dehydration of granulation tissue
- Reduction of exudate protein losses
- Reduction of pain
- Assistance in wound débridement
- Enhancement of healing with partial-thickness injuries
- Protection of exposed neovascular tissue
- Inhibition of bacterial proliferation

DISADVANTAGES
- Early lysis resulting in bacterial proliferation
- Expensive
- Rejection responses
- Not readily available
- Storage (some may require refrigeration or freezing)
- Possible transmission of diseases, such as hepatitis

Cultured skin can be grown from a small specimen of epidermal cells from an unburned area of the patient's body. The cells are grown in a laboratory to produce cell sheets that can be grafted on the patient to generate a permanent skin surface. The length of time for culturing and growing the skin is prolonged, and the cell sheets are fragile. Take care when applying these sheets to ensure adherence and prevent sloughing. This process is very costly.

Artificial skin is an alternative approach to closure of the burn wound. This substance has two layers, a Silastic epidermis and a porous dermis made from beef collagen and shark cartilage. After the artificial skin is applied to a clean, excised wound surface, fibroblasts move into the collagen part of the artificial skin and create a structure similar to normal dermis. The artificial dermis slowly dissolves and is replaced with normal blood vessels and connective tissue *(neodermis).* The neodermis supports a standard autograft placed over it when the Silastic layer is removed.

Biosynthetic dressings. Biosynthetic wound dressings are a combination of biosynthetic and synthetic materials. Biobrane is commonly used and effective in the treatment of clean superficial partial-thickness burns such as scalds, as a covering for meshed autografts, and as a donor site dressing.

Biobrane is made up of a nylon fabric that is partially embedded into a silicone film. Collagen is incorporated into both the silicone and nylon components. The nylon fabric comes into contact with the wound surface and forms an adherent bond until epithelialization has occurred. The porous silicone film allows exudates to pass through.

Synthetic dressings. Synthetic dressings are made of solid silicone and plastic membranes (e.g., polyvinyl chloride and polyurethane). They may be substituted for antimicrobial, standard, or biologic dressings. Synthetic dressings are applied directly to the surface of a clean or surgically prepared wound and remain in place until they fall off or are removed. Because many of these dressings are transparent or translucent, the wound can be inspected without removing the dressing. Pain is reduced at the site because these agents also prevent contact of the nerve endings with air. These dressings also are used to cover donor sites where skin was obtained for autografting.

Transparent film is the dressing commonly used for the care of donor site wounds. This dressing type promotes faster healing with low infection rates, minimal pain, and reduced cost.

Surgical Management. Surgical management of burn wounds focuses on excision and wound covering. Surgical excision is performed early in the postburn period. Grafting may be performed throughout the acute phase as burn wounds are made ready and donor sites are available. Early grafting reduces the time patients are at risk for infection and sepsis. Wound covering by autografting involves taking healthy skin from an area of the patient's intact skin and transplanting it to an excised burn wound.

Surgical excision. Surgical excision is the most common treatment for full-thickness and deep partial-thickness wounds. The patient is taken to the operating room within the first 5 days after injury and again as needed until all wounds are closed permanently.

The burn wound is excised by either a tangential or a fascial excision technique. In the tangential technique, the surgeon removes very thin layers of the necrotic burn surface until bleeding tissue is encountered. Bleeding indicates that a bed of healthy dermis or subcutaneous fat has been reached.

In the fascial technique, the surgeon cuts away the burn wound to the level of superficial fascia. Fascial excision usually is performed only for very deep and extensive burns. Blood loss is minimal, and grafting is usually successful.

Wound covering. Permanent skin coverage for large full-thickness injuries is achieved by applying an autograft. Skin for an autograft is taken from the patient's own body. The surgeon removes a piece of skin from a remote unburned area of the body and transplants it to cover the burn wound. Skin grafts are generally of split thickness (0.015 inch), and a partial-thickness injury is formed at the site of surgical removal (the donor site). Grafts are placed either on a clean granulated bed or over an area of burn from which dead tissue has just been removed (see also Chapter 27).

The available donor sites for larger burns are small. Patients with larger burns may have only 5% to 20% of the skin surface available to use for covering the 80% to 95% burned area. Coverage is accomplished by:

- Repeated removal of skin from the same donor site, with time allowed between harvests for healing
- Meshing the split-thickness skin grafts (Fig. 28-13) to allow a small graft to cover a larger area. Healing time is slower for a meshed graft because the skin must fill in open meshed areas (interstices), as well as attach to the granulation bed

Risk for Infection

Burn wound infection occurs through **autocontamination,** in which the patient's own normal flora overgrows and invades other body areas, especially the GI tract (Magnotti & Dietch, 2005); and **cross-contamination,** in which organisms from other people or environments are transferred to the patient.

NOC **Planning: Expected Outcomes.** The patient is expected to remain free from infection by cross-contamination and not develop septicemia. Indicators include that the patient will exhibit only mild or none of these manifestations:

- Foul-smelling discharge
- Fever
- Blood culture colonization
- Wound site colonization
- White blood cell count elevation

Interventions. Interventions aim to prevent infection and remove infected tissue.

Nonsurgical Management. Priority nursing interventions include using principles of asepsis to prevent infection transmission, providing a safe environment, and monitoring for early detection of infection. Drug therapy, isolation therapy, and environmental management are strategies for preventing and managing infection.

Drug therapy for infection prevention. Burn wound conditions promote the growth of *Clostridium tetani,* and all burn patients are at risk for this dangerous infection. Tetanus toxoid, 0.5 mL given IM, enhances immunity to *C. tetani.* This agent is routinely given when the patient is admitted to the hospital. Administration of tetanus immune globulin (human) (Hyper-Tet) is recommended when the patient's history of tetanus immunization is not known.

The use of topical antimicrobial drugs is an important intervention for infection prevention in burn wounds. The goal

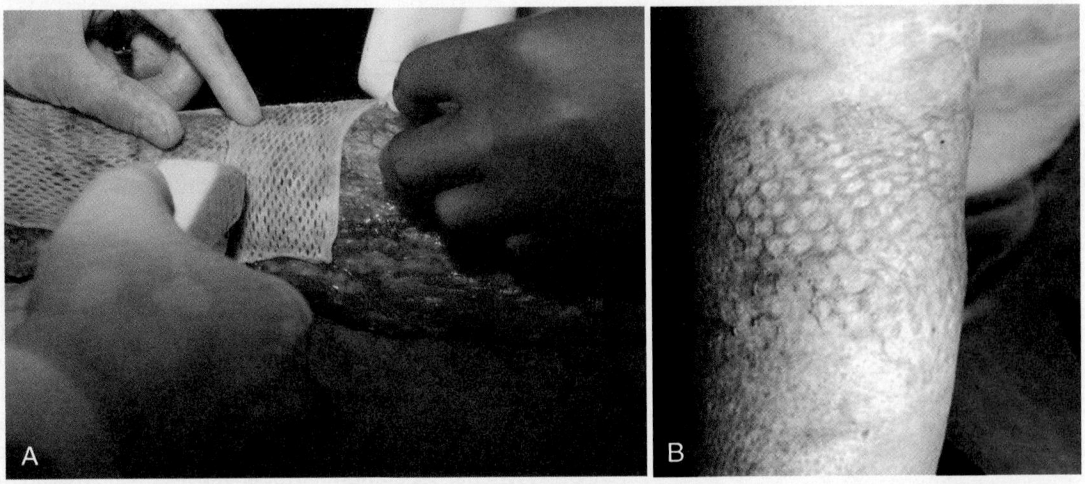
A
B

Fig. 28-13 • The typical appearance of meshed autografts. **A,** Appearance of meshed autograft at application. **B,** Appearance of meshed autograft after healing.

of this therapy is to reduce bacterial growth in the wound and prevent systemic sepsis.

Topical antibiotics are applied by either the *open* or the *closed* technique. With the open technique, use either aseptic or clean methods to apply the agent directly to the burn wound without further dressing the wound. Clean the wound every 8 to 24 hours, and apply fresh antimicrobial agents each time. With the more common closed technique, dress the burn wound after applying the topical agents.

Two of the more commonly used agents are silver sulfadiazine (Silvadene, Flamazine🍁) and mafenide acetate (Sulfamylon). Topical antimicrobial drugs are not applied to freshly grafted areas because they may inhibit cell growth. Chart 28-5 lists the features of many topical antimicrobial agents.

Drug therapy for treatment of infection. Systemic antibiotics are used when burn patients have symptoms of an actual infection, including septicemia. Broad-spectrum antibiotics are given until the results of blood cultures and sensitivity status are available. At that time, antibiotics that are effective against the specific organism(s) causing the infection are used. Because of increased metabolism, burn patients generally require a larger-than-normal dose of these drugs to maintain effective blood levels. For some antimicrobials, serial peak and trough blood levels are monitored to determine the efficacy of treatment and evaluate potential ear and kidney toxicity.

Providing a safe environment. Providing a safe environment can include isolation therapy. More commonly, it involves coordinating all members of the health care team in the use of asepsis and in monitoring for early recognition of actual infection.

Isolation therapy is used in some burn centers with the belief that it reduces cross-contamination. However methods of isolation are varied and controversial. Some burn centers practice no isolation, whereas others use near-total sterile conditions. All isolation methods use proper and consistent handwashing as the most effective technique for preventing infection transmission.

Use of asepsis requires all health care personnel to wear gloves during all contact with open wounds. The use of sterile versus clean gloves for routine wound care varies by agency and is a matter of debate. Regardless of sterility, change gloves when handling wounds on different areas of the body and between handling old and new dressings.

The equipment on burn units is not shared among patients. Disposable items (e.g., pillows, syringes, dishes) are used as much as possible. Assign any equipment used in daily routine care (e.g., thermometers, blood pressure cuffs, stethoscopes) to each patient for the duration of his or her stay. Daily cleaning of the equipment and general housekeeping are essential for infection control. All single-item unit equipment must be cleaned after use on one patient and before use on another. Because *Pseudomonas* has been found in plants, the presence of plants and flowers is prohibited. Some burn units do not permit patients to eat raw foods (e.g., salads, fruit, pepper) to reduce exposure to organisms. Rugs and upholstered articles are difficult to clean and may harbor organisms; their use is also restricted.

Visitors are restricted when the patient is immunosuppressed. Ill people, small children, and other patients should not come into direct contact with the burn patient. Some burn units recommend that all visitors wear protective clothing (gowns, gloves, masks, and shoe and hair covers) in the burn patient's room, but no data support the effectiveness of this approach.

Early detection involves careful monitoring of the burn wounds at each dressing change. Examine the wounds for these signs of infection:

- Pervasive odor
- Color changes—focal, dark red, brown discoloration in the eschar
- Change in texture
- Purulent drainage
- Exudate
- Sloughing grafts
- Redness at the wound edges extending to nonburned skin

Laboratory cultures and biopsies are recommended. Quantitative biopsies of the eschar and granulation tissue are performed routinely and as needed to monitor the growth of organisms. These tests are the gold standard for wound monitoring.

Surgical Management. Infected burn wounds with colony counts of or approaching 10^5 colonies per gram of tissue may

Chart 28-5 COMMON EXAMPLES OF DRUG THERAPY

Burns

Agent	Description	Action	Advantages	Disadvantages	Interventions
Silver sulfadiazine (Silvadene, Thermazene)	Nontoxic salt of silver sulfadiazine in water-based cream	Binds to bacterial cell membranes and interferes with DNA synthesis	Does not cause hypochloremia, hyponatremia, electrolyte imbalance, or kidney disease Painless Wide-spectrum antimicrobial action against gram-positive and gram-negative organisms Long shelf life Delays eschar separation to a lesser degree than do many other topical drugs	Absorbed into eschar less than other drugs May cause rash, pruritus, burning, and leukopenia Not consistently effective for burns covering 60% of the body Not effective against *Pseudomonas*	Watch for signs of infection, such as soupiness of wound area. Watch for allergic reaction causing a drop in white blood cell count. Do not use if reaction to sulfonamide has occurred. Use on deep partial-thickness or full-thickness wounds.
Collagenase (Santyl) with Polysporin powder	Topical enzymatic débriding agent with 250 collagenase units/g of white petroleum	Digests collagen in necrotic tissue	Painless Daily dressing changes No side effects Quick débridement action Easy to apply Not harmful to healthy tissue Specific only to nonviable tissue	Expensive	Apply once a day. Painless. Use on deep partial-thickness wound with eschar. Monitor wounds for infection. May be used with barrier dressing such as Xeroform.
Mafenide acetate (Sulfamylon)	Soft, white, nonstaining, water-based cream Available in solution	Bacteriostatic action against many gram-positive and gram-negative organisms	Effective against *Pseudomonas* Long shelf life Excellent for treating electrical burns Penetrates thick eschar May use as a solution to wet down grafts or wounds	May lead to infection May cause metabolic acidosis, hyperpnea, and rash When applied, may cause pain that lasts 30-40 minutes	Premedicate for pain before application. Monitor blood gas and serum electrolyte levels. Monitor for infection.
Nitrofurazone (Furacin)	Cream, solution, or water-soluble ointment, or foam	Wide-spectrum anti-bacterial	Effective against *Staphylococcus aureus* and some antibiotic-resistant organisms Causes neither pain nor maceration	May cause contact dermatitis (rare) Messy to apply in cream form May cause renal problems if used in extensive burns	Observe carefully for signs of allergic reaction and evidence of superinfection.
Gentamicin sulfate (Garamycin, Gentamar)	Available as a cream or solution for topical use	Antibiotic action against organisms resistant to other drugs	Effective against *Pseudomonas* Does not cause pain	May have ototoxic (ear) and nephrotoxic (kidney) effects May result in resistance by certain organisms	Use with caution in patients with decreased renal function. Monitor serum and urine creatinine clearance before and during treatment.

Chart 28-5 COMMON EXAMPLES OF DRUG THERAPY

Burns—cont'd

Agent	Description	Action	Advantages	Disadvantages	Interventions
Polymyxin B-bacitracin	Topical cream	Wide-spectrum antimicrobial	Painless Effective against many gram-positive and gram-negative organisms Can be used on face Can be placed on healed grafts to lubricate	May cause urticaria, burning, and inflammation Does not penetrate eschar	Apply every 2-8 hr to keep areas moist.

be life threatening, even with antibiotic therapy. Surgical excision of the burn wound may be necessary to control these infections.

Imbalanced Nutrition: Less Than Body Requirements

NOC **Planning: Expected Outcomes.** The patient is expected to maintain adequate nutrient intake for meeting the body's calorie needs. Indicators include that the patient should have mild or no deviations from the normal ranges of:

- Weight/height ratio
- Food intake
- Hematocrit and hemoglobin
- Serum albumin
- Blood glucose

Interventions. Interventions aim to calculate the patient's calorie needs and provide an adequate daily source of calories and nutrients that the patient can ingest and metabolize. Coordinate with a nutritionist to meet the desired outcomes regarding the patient's nutrition status. Therapy begins with calculating the patient's current daily calorie needs. Several formulas and charts are used for this calculation. Nutritional requirements for a patient with a large burn area can exceed 5000 kcal/day (Prelak et al., 2007). In addition to a high-calorie intake, the burn patient requires a diet high in protein for wound healing. Work with the nutritionist and the patient to plan additions to standard nutritional patterns.

Oral nutrition therapy may be delayed for several days after the injury until the GI tract is motile. Nasoduodenal tube feedings are often started soon after admission. Beginning enteral feedings early helps decrease weight loss, gut atrophy, bacterial translocation, and sepsis. These feedings often are started within 4 hours of beginning fluid resuscitation. This type of supplement prevents nutritional deficits in severely burned patients.

Encourage patients who can eat solid foods to ingest as many calories as possible. Consider the patient's preferences for diet planning and food selection. Encourage patients to request food whenever they feel they can eat, not just according to the hospital's standard meal schedule. Offer frequent high-calorie, high-protein supplemental feedings. Keep an accurate calorie count for foods and beverages that are actually ingested by the patient.

Patients who cannot swallow but who have adequate gastric motility may meet calorie and nutrition needs through enteral tube feedings (see Chapter 63). Parenteral nutrition may be given IV when the GI tract is not functional or when the patient's nutritional needs cannot be met by oral and enteral feeding. This method is used as a last resort because it is invasive and can lead to infectious and metabolic complications.

Impaired Physical Mobility

NOC **Planning: Expected Outcomes.** The patient with a burn injury is expected to regain and maintain an optimal ability to move purposefully. Indicators include that the patient should be mildly compromised or not compromised in:

- Muscle movement
- Joint movement
- Walking
- Body positioning performance

Interventions. Interventions aim to maintain the patient's preburn range of joint motion and prevent contracture formation.

Nonsurgical Management. Nonsurgical management includes the nursing interventions of positioning, range-of-motion exercises, ambulation, and pressure dressings.

Positioning is critical for patients with burn injuries because the position of comfort for the patient is often one of joint flexion, which increases the risk for contracture development. Maintain the patient in a neutral body position with minimal flexion. Best practice for the prevention of contractures is listed in Chart 28-6. Splints and other devices may help the patient maintain good positioning. These devices are used most often on the joints of the hands, elbows, knees, neck, and axillae.

Range-of-motion exercises are performed actively at least three times a day. If the patient cannot move a joint actively, perform passive range-of-motion exercises. Give burned hands special attention. Urge the patient to perform active range-of-motion exercises for the hand, thumb, and fingers every hour while he or she is awake.

Ambulation is started as soon as possible after the fluid shifts have resolved. Patients with a variety of attached equipment (IV catheters, nasogastric tubes, ECG leads, extensive dressings) can ambulate with preparation and assistance. This activity is performed two or three times a day and progresses in length each time. Ambulation inhibits bone density loss, strengthens muscles, stimulates immune function, promotes ventilation, and prevents many complications.

Pressure dressings are applied after the graft heals to help prevent contractures and tight hypertrophic scars, which can inhibit mobility. These dressings also inhibit venous stasis and edema formation in areas with decreased lymphatic outflow. Pressure dressings may be elastic wraps or specially designed, custom-fitted, elasticized clothing that provides continuous pressure over burned areas. Fig. 28-14 shows such garments. For best effectiveness, pressure garments must be worn at least 23 hours a day, every day, until the scar tissue is mature (12 to 24 months). These garments can be uncomfortable with itchi-

Chart 28-6 BEST PRACTICE FOR PATIENT SAFETY & QUALITY CARE

Positioning to Prevent Contractures

Affected Body Part	Position of Function	Intervention
Head and neck	Hyperextension	No pillow. Place a towel roll under the patient's neck or shoulder. Neck splint.
Posterior neck	Flexion	Have patient turn the head from side to side.
Upper chest and chest	Shoulder retraction	Place patient in supine position. Place a folded towel under the spine, between the scapulae.
Lateral trunk	Flexion to uninvolved side	Place the patient supine with arm on the affected side up over the head.
Anterior shoulder	Abduction and external rotation	Maintain the upper arm at 90 degrees of abduction from the lateral aspect of the trunk.
Posterior shoulder	Slight flexion and interior rotation	Keep the arm slightly behind the midline.
Axilla	Abduction with 10- to 15-degree forward flexion and external rotation	Support the abducted arm with suspension from IV pole or bedside table. Axilla splint.
Elbow	Extension and supination	Keep the joint in the extended position.
Wrist	30 to 45 degrees of extension	Use a splint.
Fingers		
MP joints	70 to 90 degrees of flexion	Use a splint.
PIP and DIP joints	Extended	Use a splint.
Ankle	90 degrees of dorsiflexion	Use a padded footboard or splint with heels free of pressure.
Legs	15 to 20 degrees of abduction	Place small pillow between legs.
Hip	Extension and neutral rotation	Supine with lower extremity extended. Trochanter roll. Foam wedge along lateral aspect of thigh.

DIP, Distal interphalangeal; *MP*, metatarsophalangeal; *PIP*, proximal interphalangeal.

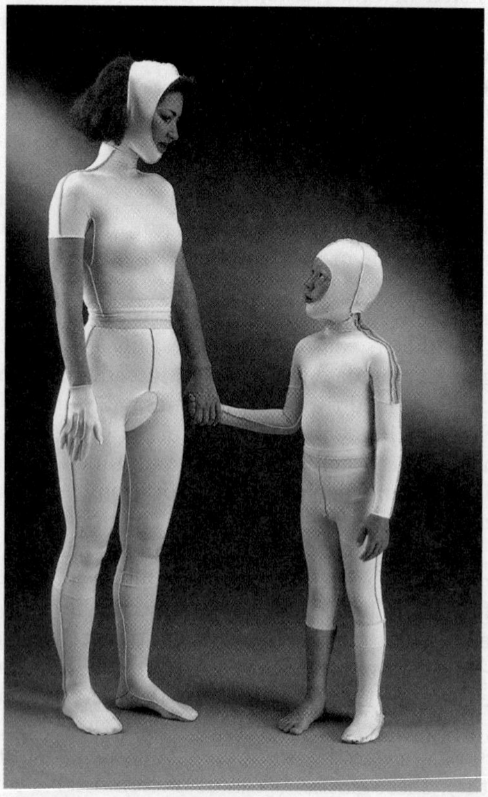

Fig. 28-14 • Models wearing pressure garments.

ness and increased warmth. Reinforce to the patient and family that wearing pressure garments is very beneficial in saving mobility and reducing scarring.

Surgical Management. Surgical management restores mobility rather than prevents immobility. Surgical release of contractures is most commonly performed in the neck, axilla, elbow flexion areas, and hand. Specific surgical procedures to improve movement vary for each patient.

Nursing responsibilities after surgery include interventions to prevent contractures from re-forming, as well as the care of new grafts and suture lines. Constantly reinforce the need for the patient to adhere to exercise and splinting regimens to prevent the recurrence of joint immobility.

Disturbed Body Image

NOC **Planning: Expected Outcomes.** After intervention, the patient with a burn injury is expected to have a positive perception of his or her own appearance and body functions. Indicators include that the patient should consistently demonstrate these behaviors:

- Willingness to touch the affected body part
- Adjustment to changes in body function
- Willingness to use strategies to enhance appearance and function
- Successful progression through the grieving process
- Use of support systems

Interventions. Nonsurgical and surgical interventions can assist patients who have body image disturbances as a result of burn injury.

Nonsurgical Management. Understanding the stages of grief is helpful for the patient, family, and health care professionals. Assess which stage of grief the patient is currently experiencing, and help interpret his or her behaviors. The patient often is unaware of or is confused by his or her feelings. Reassure the patient that feelings of grief, loss, anxiety, anger, fear, and guilt are normal. The patient may be grieving the loss of body parts, appearance, role identity, and social identity. Coordinate with other health care team members (e.g., psychologist, psychiatrist, social worker, clergy or religious leader) in addressing these problems.

Accept the physical and psychological features of the patient. Present patients and families with realistic expected outcomes for the patient's functional capacity and physical appearance. Provide information sessions and counseling for the family to help identify effective patterns of support. Facilitate the patient's use of these systems and the development of new support systems. Make referrals to support groups. To identify the effectiveness of such assistance and possible gaps in support, evaluate support resources throughout the course of illness.

Engaging in decision making and independent activities fosters feelings of self-worth, which are closely linked to body image. To this end, plan and encourage the patient's active participation in self-care activities. Assist family members to understand that it is more beneficial for the patient to perform these activities than to have them performed by someone else. Urge families to include the patient in family decision making to the same degree that he or she participated in this process before the injury.

Surgical Management. Reconstructive and cosmetic surgery can be performed for many years after the burn injury. Restoring function and improving appearance through surgical techniques often increase the patient's feelings of self-worth and promote a positive body image. Many patients have unrealistic expectations of reconstructive surgery and envision an appearance identical or equal in quality to the preburn state. Teach the patient and family about expected cosmetic outcomes.

DECISION-MAKING CHALLENGE
Critical Rescue

A 42-year-old who sustained a 37% TBSA flame burn had topical silver sulfadiazine (Silvadene) applied to his wounds. On the second postburn day, his WBC count dropped from 11,000/mm^3 to 4,000/mm^3 with no left shift. The patient remained afebrile and hemodynamically stable. The fluid resuscitation was successful, and he did not require intubation. On the fifth postburn day, his upper arms were full-thickness injuries rather than partial-thickness, and he underwent grafting with split-thickness meshed grafts to his bilateral upper forearms and hands with skin taken from his thighs. The operative dressings were removed on the third and fifth postoperative days.

1. What is the likely cause of the sudden decrease in the patient's WBC count?
2. What assessment data would indicate the grafts are healing?
3. What is the best position for the upper extremities and hands to prevent contractures?

evolve For suggested answer guidelines, go to http://evolve.elsevier.com/Iggy/.

REHABILITATIVE PHASE OF BURN INJURY
Overview

Although rehabilitation efforts are started from the time of admission, the technical rehabilitative phase begins with wound closure and ends when the patient returns to the highest possible level of functioning. The emphasis during this phase is the psychosocial adjustment of the patient, the prevention of scars and contractures, and the resumption of preburn activity, including resuming work, family, and social roles. This phase may take years or even last a lifetime as patients adjust to permanent limitations that may not be apparent until long after the initial injury.

Patient-Centered Collaborative Care

Although attention is placed first on the physical interventions for the burn injury, psychological care is equally important. Provide psychosocial support to the patient and family throughout hospitalization but more extensively in the rehabilitative phase.

Information from the patient and family aids in the assessment and diagnosis of psychological problems and allows treatment to be instituted. Explore the patient's feelings about the burn injury. It is extremely difficult for patients to concentrate on the many tasks before them when obstacles such as guilt and grief are in the forefront.

Ask the patient or family member whether there is a history of psychological problems. To assist with a future plan of care, assess and document the type of coping mechanisms the patient has used successfully during times of stress. Also assess the patient's family unit and the family members' history of interaction. Identify cultural and ethnic factors, and consider these when planning psychosocial interventions.

Throughout the hospitalization the patient progresses through a variety of stages and exhibits many feelings, including denial, regression, and anger. Accurately assess the patient's feelings during each stage so appropriate plans of care can be developed and carried out.

Community-Based Care

Discharge planning for the patient with a burn injury begins at the time of admission to the hospital or burn center. In most burn centers, the multidisciplinary team meets regularly to plan for discharge. In helping the patient reach mutually established discharge goals, the team evaluates the progress of each discipline. Table 28-9 lists common discharge needs of the patient with burns.

Psychosocial Preparation

During the recovery period and for some time after discharge from the hospital, patients with severe burn injuries are likely to have psychological problems that require intervention. Such problems include post-traumatic stress disorder, sexual dysfunction, and severe depression. Assistance is coordinated with the patient, family, and health care team. Psychosocial assistance is best provided by a professional counselor with experience in helping burn patients.

One specific area to address with the patient is the reaction of others to the sight of healing wounds and disfiguring scars. Patients with facial burns are especially subjected to stares and other reactions from the general public. Visits from friends and short public appearances before discharge may help the patient begin adjusting to this problem. Community reintegration programs can assist the psychosocial and physical recovery of the patient with serious burns.

Home Care Management

The patient with severe burns is discharged from the acute care setting when life-threatening complications are resolved and minimal wound areas remain open. During the first

TABLE 28-9 Needs to Address Before Discharge of the Patient with Burns

- Early patient assessment
- Financial assessment
- Evaluation of family resources
- Weekly discharge planning meeting
- Psychological referral
- Patient and family teaching (home care)
- Designation of principal learners (specific family members or significant others who will help with care)
- Development of teaching plan
- Training for wound care
- Rehabilitation referral
- Home assessment (on-site visit)
- Medical equipment
- Public health nursing referral
- Evaluation of community resources
- Visit to referral agency
- Re-entry programs for school or work environment
- Nursing home placement
- Environmental interventions
- Auditory testing
- Speech therapy
- Prosthetic rehabilitation

weeks at home, the patient usually needs at least daily wound care, physical therapy, nutritional support, symptom management, and drug therapy.

Although the patient usually views going home in a positive light, the problems of physical care and the psychological stresses from changes in appearance, role, function, and lifestyle may overwhelm the patient and family. Successful discharge depends on extensive planning and preparation of the patient, family, and home environment through education and the involvement of appropriate support agencies and services.

Preparation for discharge includes assessment of the family and home care situation from physical and social perspectives. Consider the needs of the patient when evaluating the home for cleanliness; access to bathing facilities, electricity, and running water; stairways; number of occupants; temperature control; and safety. If the burn injuries occurred in a house fire, a new residence may need to be established.

Health Teaching

Education about burn care and living with the consequences of burn injuries begins when the patient is admitted to the hospital or burn center. A weekly plan for patient education is outlined; the goal is progression toward independence for the patient and family. Critical for this goal is teaching patients and family members to perform such care tasks as dressing changes. Allow patients and family members to first observe dressing changes, then to assist in performing the changes, and finally to change the dressings independently under your supervision.

Before discharge, all people who will be involved in the patient's home care participate in discharge planning and teaching sessions. In addition to details about dressing changes, explain:

- Signs and symptoms of infection
- Drug regimens
- Proper use of prosthetic and positioning devices
- Correct application and care of pressure garments
- Comfort measures to reduce pruritus
- Dates for follow-up appointments

Health Care Resources

The health care team evaluates the family in terms of capacity and willingness to assist in providing care to the patient after discharge. A visiting nurse or case manager referral can assist the family with care problems arising at home. In addition, the visiting nurse can help the family determine what special equipment, supplies, or services will be needed. The frequency of home visits depends on the patient's condition and the ability of family members to function as care providers. *It is imperative that the visiting nurse have extensive experience in providing burn care.* The home care nurse may need a brief visit to the patient while in the hospital and observation of burn wound care.

The home care of a patient after a serious burn often involves daily physical therapy and rehabilitation sessions at special centers. Address and resolve transportation problems before the patient is discharged. In some instances, the burn center has arrangements for transportation. Some community volunteer agencies provide transportation by private car.

When rehabilitation is prolonged, the patient may be discharged to a rehabilitation facility. Consult with the rehabilitation team, and provide copies of the care and teaching plans used with the patient.

DECISION-MAKING CHALLENGE
Coordination of Care

A 42-year-old patient who sustained a flame injury and received skin grafting is being prepared for discharge. Although most of his wounds healed without surgery, you notice that he does not look at his wounds during dressing changes. He has not asked any questions regarding scar formation or repigmentation of his skin. The night shift nurse reported to you that the patient was awakened in the middle of the night with a flashback of the accident. Your assessment reveals that he is having an adjustment disorder with the potential of post-traumatic stress disorder.

1. Are these symptoms the patient is experiencing part of the complex systemic response to burn injuries? If so, is this expected at this time? Why or why not?
2. What resources or referrals would be most appropriate for this patient at this time?
3. What other needs should be addressed before discharge?

evolve For suggested answer guidelines, go to http://evolve.elsevier.com/Iggy/.

▪ *Evaluation: Outcomes*

Evaluate the care of the patient with a burn injury on the basis of the identified nursing diagnoses and collaborative problems. The expected outcomes include that the patient should:

- Have cardiac output restored to normal
- Maintain adequate oxygenation and circulation to all vital organs
- Maintain a patent airway
- Have an effective breathing pattern
- Have pain alleviated or reduced
- Experience no further loss of skin integrity
- Have skin integrity restored without complications
- Remain free from infection by cross-contamination

- Not experience septicemia
- Maintain an adequate nutrient intake for meeting the body's calorie needs
- Regain and maintain an optimal ability to move purposefully
- Have a positive perception of his or her own appearance and body functions

Specific indicators for these outcomes are listed for each nursing diagnosis and collaborative problem in the Planning and Implementation section (see earlier).

GET READY FOR THE NCLEX EXAMINATION!

Key Points

Review these Key Points for each NCLEX Examination Client Needs Category.

Safe and Effective Care Environment

- Use strict aseptic technique when caring for patients who have open burn wounds.
- Check ventilator alarms hourly for patients who are receiving paralytic drugs during mechanical ventilation.

Health Promotion and Maintenance

- Encourage all people to have and maintain home smoke and carbon monoxide detectors.
- Warn patients who smoke about not smoking in bed or when taking any substance that induces sedation (drugs or alcohol).
- Instruct patients who have reduced sensation in hands or feet to use a bath thermometer to check water temperature before bathing.
- Teach patients to avoid exposing the burned skin areas to the sun or to temperature extremes.

Psychosocial Integrity

- Allow patients time to grieve over a change in body image.
- Reassure patients that pain will be managed effectively.
- Explain all procedures to the patient.
- Give analgesics, sedatives, and antianxiety drugs to patients receiving paralytic drugs during mechanical ventilation.
- Encourage the patient to actively participate in pain control measures.
- Encourage the patient to look at and touch burned areas.

Physiological Integrity

- Assess the burn patient's airway and adequacy of breathing before assessing any other body system.
- Keep an endotracheal kit or tracheostomy kit at the bedside of any patient with facial burns, burns inside the mouth, singed nasal hairs, or a "smoky" smell to the breath.
- Notify the physician immediately if the patient with an inhalation injury becomes more breathless or audible wheezes disappear.
- Give half of the fluid volume calculated for the first 24 hours after burn injury in the first 8 hours postburn.
- Give prescribed opioid analgesics by the IV route during the resuscitation/emergent phase of burn recovery.
- Position patients to prevent contractures and promote joint function.
- Assist patients to ambulate several times each day as soon as the fluid shifts have resolved.
- Encourage patients to use the prescribed splints and pressure garments to prevent joint immobility.

Additional Study Resources

Go to your Companion CD or Evolve at http://evolve.elsevier.com/Iggy/ for *Self-Assessment Questions for the NCLEX Examination.*

evolve

Go to Evolve at http://evolve.elsevier.com/Iggy/ for *Prioritization and Delegation Questions for the NCLEX Examination.*

SELECTED BIBLIOGRAPHY

Asterisk indicates a classic or definitive work on this subject.

American Burn Association. (2007). National Burn Repository: Summary of the findings 1995-2005. Website: www.ameriburn.org

Arnoldo, B., Klein, M., & Gibran, B.S. (2006). Practice guidelines for electrical burns. *Journal of Burn Care and Research, 27*(4), 439-447.

*Badger, J. (2001). Burns: The psychological aspects. *AJN, 101*(11), 38-44.

Benner, J. (2008). Online support for burn victims. *Nursing2008, 38*(4), 23.

Bulechek, G.M., Butcher, H.K., & McCloskey Dochterman, J. (Eds.). (2008). *Nursing interventions classification (NIC)* (5th ed.). St. Louis: Mosby.

Burd, A., & Chui, T. (2005). Allogenic skin in treatment of burns. *Clinical Dermatology, 23*(4), 276-287.

Cancio, L.C., Batchinsky, A.I., Dubick, M.A., Park, M.S., Black, I.H., Gomez, R., et al. (2007). Inhalation injury: Pathophysiology and clinical care proceedings of a symposium conducted at the Trauma Institute of San Antonio. *Burns, 33*(6), 681-692.

Devgan, L., Bhat, S., Aylward, S., & Spence, R.J. (2006). Modalities for the assessment of burn wound depth. *Journal of Burns and Wounds, 5*, 7-15.

Edelman, D., Maleyko-Jacobs, S., White, M.T., Lucas, C.E., & Ledgerwood, A.M. (2008). Smoking and home oxygen: A preventable public health hazard. *Journal of Burn Care & Research, 29*(1), 119-122.

Faucher, L., & Furukawa, K. (2006). Practice guidelines for the management of pain. *Journal of Burn Care and Research, 27*(5), 659-668.

Herndon, D. (2007). *Total burn care* (3rd ed.). Philadelphia: Saunders.

Laskowski, L. (2006). First aid for burns. *Nursing2006, 36*(1), 41-43.

Magnotti, L., & Deitch, E. (2005). Burns, bacterial translocation, gut barrier function, and failure. *Journal of Burn Care and Rehabilitation, 26*(5), 383-391.

McCance, K., & Huether, S. (2006). *Pathophysiology: The biologic basis for disease in adults and children* (5th ed.). St. Louis: Mosby.

Meiner, S., & Lueckenotte, A. (Eds.). (2006). *Gerontologic nursing,* (3rd ed.). St. Louis: Mosby.

Mlcak, R., Suman, O., & Herndon, D. (2007). Respiratory management of inhalation injury. *Burns, 33*(1), 2-13.

Noble, J., Gomez, M., & Fish, J. (2006). Quality of life and return to work following electrical burns. *Burns, 32*(2), 159-164.

Nowlin, A. (2006). The delicate business of burn care. *RN, 69*(1), 52-57.

Pagana, K., & Pagana, T. (2006). *Mosby's manual of diagnostic and laboratory tests* (3rd ed.). St. Louis: Mosby.

Pham, T., Cancio, L., & Gibran, N. (2008). American Burn Association Practice Guidelines Burn Shock Resuscitation. *Journal of Burn Care & Research, 29*(1), 257-266.

Prelack, K., Dylewski, M., & Sheridan, R. (2007). Practical guidelines for nutritional management of burn injury and recovery. *Burns, 33*(1), 14-24.

Rosenthal, L. (2006). Carbon monoxide poisoning: Immediate diagnosis and treatment are crucial to avoid complications. *AJN, 106*(3), 40-47.

Shakespeare, P. (2005). The role of skin substitutes in treatment of burn injuries. *Clinical Dermatology, 23*(4), 413-418.

HUMAN NEEDS OVERVIEW

Oxygenation and Tissue Perfusion

All cells and tissues need oxygen to live and function. Some cells, such as brain cells and heart muscle cells, are very dependent on oxygen. Without oxygen, brain cells stop functioning and die in about 5 to 10 minutes. Other cells, such as skin cells, can live and function for many hours with low oxygen levels or even without oxygen. Skeletal muscle cells can survive for hours with low levels of oxygen but cannot function for very long without it.

The source of oxygen for all body cells is the air we breathe into our lungs. Delivery of oxygen to the cells and tissues requires the pumping mechanism of the heart and the oxygen-carrying mechanism of the hemoglobin in red blood cells. In health, the need of body tissues for oxygen is balanced by the body's oxygen intake and delivery systems (Fig. 1, *A*). When oxygen needs increase, such as during mild to moderate exercise, oxygen intake through the respiratory system increases to compensate (or adapt) and to keep oxygen delivery to the tissues in balance with their oxygen need (Fig. 1, *B*).

When oxygen need increases as a result of heavy exercise or an illness in which metabolism is increased (and the person has a fever), all oxygen intake and delivery systems must compensate by increasing their activity to match the increased oxygen need. When this compensation is perfect, the increased rate and depth of respiration, along with the increased heart rate and blood pressure, keep oxygen intake and delivery in balance with oxygen need (Fig. 2).

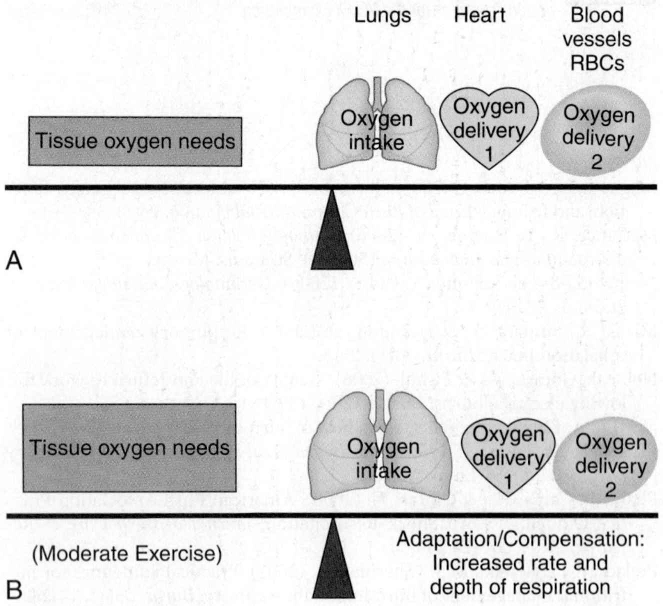

Lungs
Heart
Blood vessels RBCs
Tissue oxygen needs
Oxygen intake
Oxygen delivery 1
Oxygen delivery 2
A
Tissue oxygen needs
Oxygen intake
Oxygen delivery 1
Oxygen delivery 2
(Moderate Exercise)
Adaptation/Compensation: Increased rate and depth of respiration
B

Fig. 1

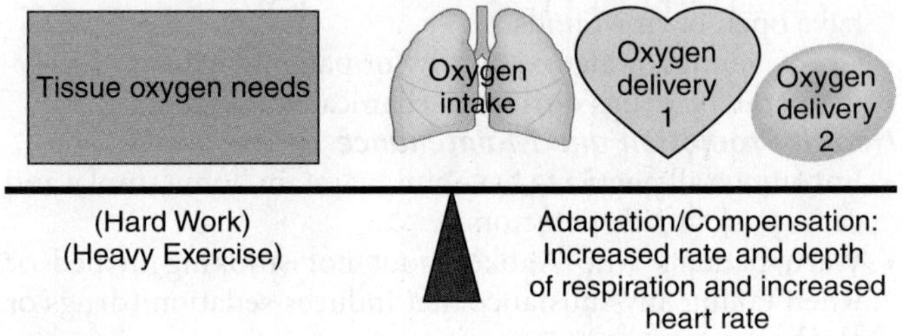

Tissue oxygen needs
Oxygen intake
Oxygen delivery 1
Oxygen delivery 2
(Hard Work)
(Heavy Exercise)
Adaptation/Compensation: Increased rate and depth of respiration and increased heart rate

Fig. 2

Some health problems reduce the body's ability to compensate when oxygen need is greater than basic (basal) levels. For example, in a person with asthma, the lungs may be able to take in enough oxygen to meet basic oxygen needs but cannot adjust or compensate when a greater oxygen intake is needed, such as during mild to moderate exercise (Fig. 3, *A*). In this situation, the heart needs to compensate *more* to increase delivery of the set amount of oxygen taken in by the lungs (Fig. 3, *B*).

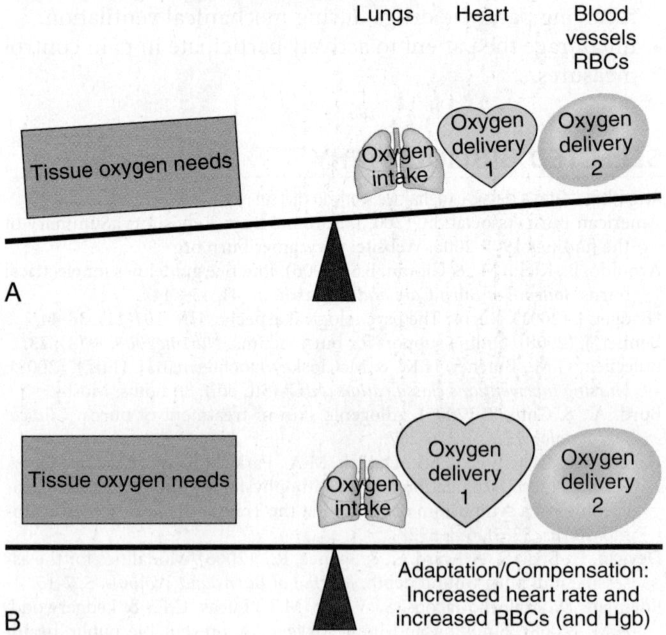

Lungs
Heart
Blood vessels RBCs
Tissue oxygen needs
Oxygen intake
Oxygen delivery 1
Oxygen delivery 2
A
Tissue oxygen needs
Oxygen intake
Oxygen delivery 1
Oxygen delivery 2
Adaptation/Compensation: Increased heart rate and increased RBCs (and Hgb)
B

Fig. 3

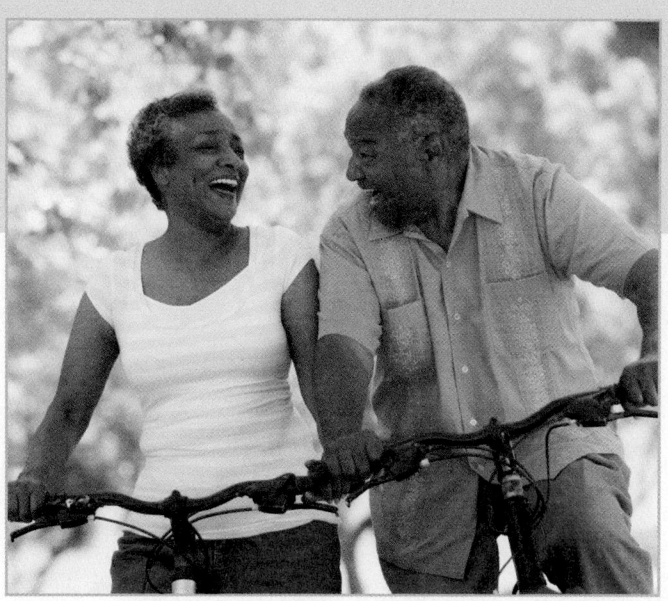

In another situation, when a person has a cardiac problem and the heart rate alone cannot increase oxygen delivery during mild to moderate exercise (Fig. 4, *A*), his or her respiratory rate needs to increase more than usual to keep oxygen delivery in balance with oxygen need.

What happens when any part of the oxygen intake or delivery system has a problem that interferes with ensuring that the cells have enough oxygen? Consider a patient with pneumonia who has great difficulty with oxygen intake to the point that his or her body's basic oxygen need is not met. Even though the oxygen need is at a basic level, the need is unbalanced compared with oxygen intake and delivery. The patient's compensation mechanisms are working (respiratory rate and heart rate are increased) but are not completely effective. How could balance be restored? The best way is to eliminate the pneumonia, which could take days even with proper drug therapy. Other ways involve reducing oxygen need to the lowest possible level by having the patient rest and improving oxygen intake by increasing the percentage of oxygen that he or she breathes (oxygen therapy) (Fig 4, *B*).

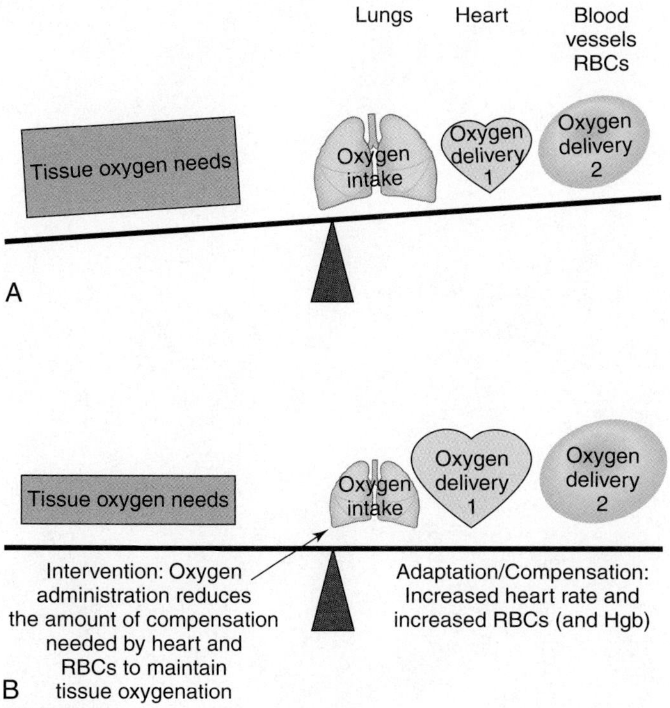

Lungs
Heart
Blood vessels RBCs
Tissue oxygen needs
Oxygen intake
Oxygen delivery 1
Oxygen delivery 2
A
Tissue oxygen needs
Oxygen intake
Oxygen delivery 1
Oxygen delivery 2
Intervention: Oxygen administration reduces the amount of compensation needed by heart and RBCs to maintain tissue oxygenation
Adaptation/Compensation: Increased heart rate and increased RBCs (and Hgb)
B

Fig. 4

VII
UNIT

Problems of Oxygenation

Management of Patients with Problems of the Respiratory Tract

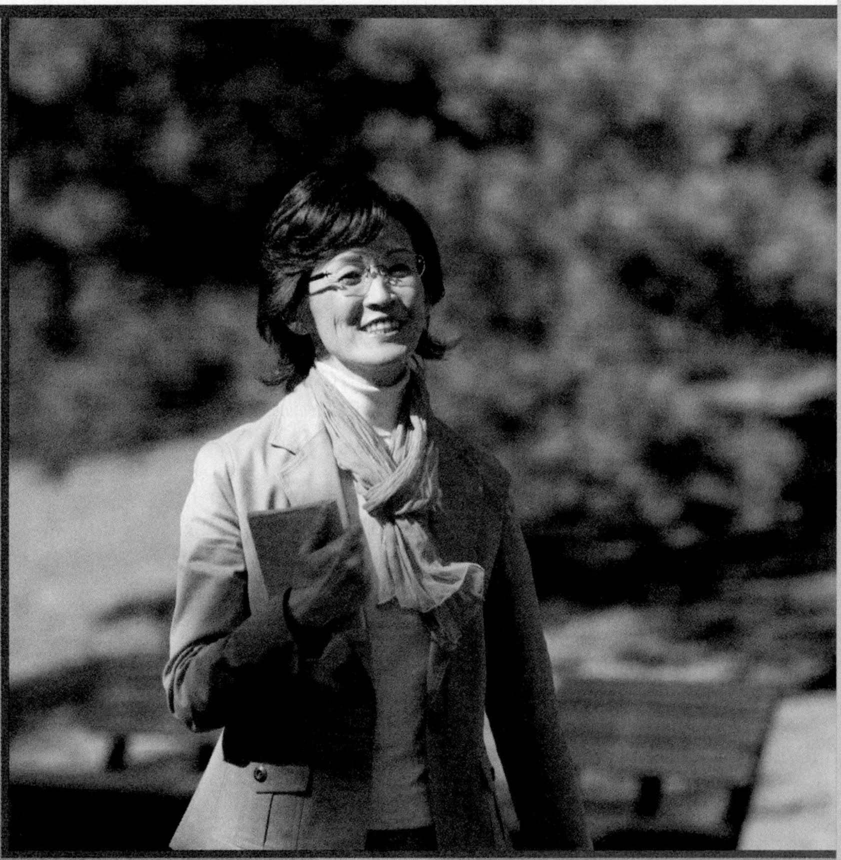

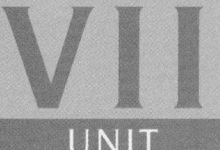

29

CHAPTER

Assessment of the Respiratory System

Harry C. Rees

LEARNING OUTCOMES

For clinical competence and success on the NCLEX Examination, study this chapter with these Learning Outcomes in mind:

Health Promotion and Maintenance

1. Encourage all people to use masks and adequate ventilation when engaging in activities that expose them to inhalation irritants.

Psychosocial Integrity

2. Use effective communication when teaching patients and family members about what to expect during tests and procedures to assess respiratory function and respiratory disease.

Physiological Integrity

3. Assess the patient's endurance in performing ADLs.
4. Perform health history and risk assessment for pulmonary problems.
5. Use concepts of anatomy and appropriate psychomotor skills to apply respiratory assessment techniques correctly.
6. Perform a clinical respiratory assessment, including health history, physical assessment, and psychosocial assessment.
7. Distinguish between normal and abnormal (adventitious) breath sounds.
8. Explain the respiratory changes associated with aging.
9. Calculate the pack-year smoking history for the patient who smokes or who has ever smoked cigarettes.
10. Correctly interpret arterial blood gas values to assess the patient's respiratory status.
11. Explain nursing care needs for the patient after bronchoscopy or open lung biopsy.

Go to your Companion CD or Evolve at http://evolve.elsevier.com/Iggy/ for *Self-Assessment Questions for the NCLEX Examination* keyed to these Learning Outcomes.

The respiratory system includes the upper airways, lungs, lower airways, and alveolar air sacs. This system is important in helping the body *meet its need for oxygenation and tissue perfusion* because the source of the oxygen for all body cells is the air we breathe. All cells need oxygen (O_2) to live, grow, and perform their specific jobs. Air with oxygen enters the nose and mouth and moves through the airways or respiratory tubes (trachea, bronchi, bronchioles) and into the air sacs (alveoli) of the lungs. Once in the air sacs, the oxygen from the air moves into the blood so that it can be carried to all tissues and organs. The waste gas created in the tissues, carbon dioxide (CO_2), moves from the blood into the air sacs so it can be exhaled into the air. So, oxygen intake depends on the respiratory system (Fig. 29-1). All systems depend on adequate oxygen intake for tissue perfusion with oxygen. Thus any problem of the respiratory system affects total body health and well-being. This chapter reviews the normal physiology of the respiratory system and assessment of respiratory status.

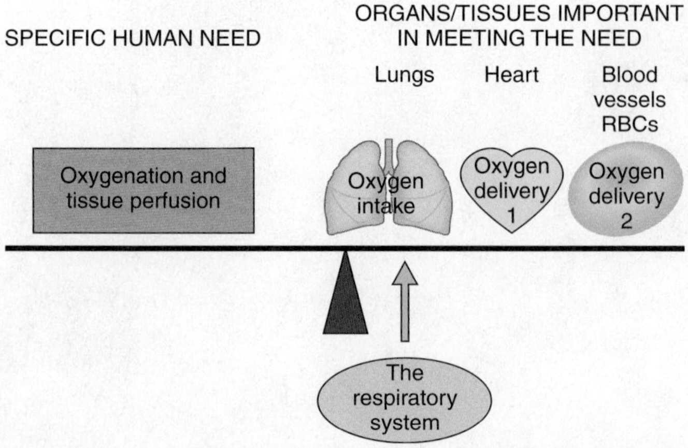
SPECIFIC HUMAN NEED
ORGANS/TISSUES IMPORTANT IN MEETING THE NEED
Lungs
Heart
Blood vessels RBCs
Oxygenation and tissue perfusion
Oxygen intake
Oxygen delivery 1
Oxygen delivery 2
The respiratory system

Fig. 29-1 • Role of the respiratory system in meeting the human need for oxygenation and tissue perfusion.

Lung and breathing problems are common and are the fifth leading cause of death in North America (McCance & Huether, 2006). Some respiratory problems are chronic, and the patient has physical and lifestyle limitations. Many acute health problems, medical therapies, and surgeries adversely affect respiratory function temporarily or permanently.

ANATOMY AND PHYSIOLOGY REVIEW

The purposes of breathing are (1) to provide *oxygen for tissue perfusion* so that cells have enough oxygen to take part in metabolism and (2) to remove carbon dioxide, the major waste product of metabolism. The respiratory system also influences acid-base balance, speech, sense of smell, fluid balance, and temperature control. The lungs are also an excretory organ because they can also break down some toxins and eliminate them from the body during exhalation.

Upper Respiratory Tract

The upper airways consist of the nose, the sinuses, the **pharynx** (throat), and the **larynx** (voice box) (Fig. 29-2).

Nose and Sinuses

The nose is the organ of smell, with receptors from cranial nerve I (olfactory) located in the upper areas. This organ is rigid and contains two passages separated in the middle by the septum. The upper one third of the nose is composed of bone; the lower two thirds is composed of cartilage, allowing some movement. The septum and interior walls of the nasal cavity are lined with mucous membranes that have a rich blood supply. The **anterior nares** (nostrils or external openings into the nasal cavities) are lined with skin and hair, which help keep foreign particles or organisms from entering the lungs. The posterior nares are openings from the nasal cavity into the nasopharynx.

The **turbinates** are three bony projections that protrude into the nasal cavities from the walls of the internal portion of the nose (see Fig. 29-2). Turbinates increase the total surface area for filtering, heating, and humidifying inspired air before it passes into the nasopharynx. Inspired air entering the nose is first filtered in the nares. Particles not filtered out in the nares are trapped in the mucous layer of the turbinates. These particles are moved by **cilia** (hairlike projections) to the oropharynx, where they are either swallowed or expectorated. Inspired air is humidified by contact with the mucous membrane and is warmed by heat from the vascular network.

The **paranasal sinuses** are air-filled cavities within the bones that surround the nasal passages (Fig. 29-3). Lined with

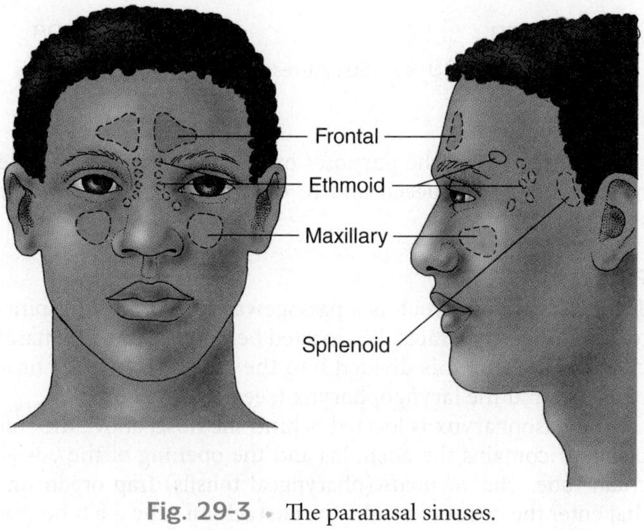

Frontal
Ethmoid
Maxillary
Sphenoid

Fig. 29-3 • The paranasal sinuses.

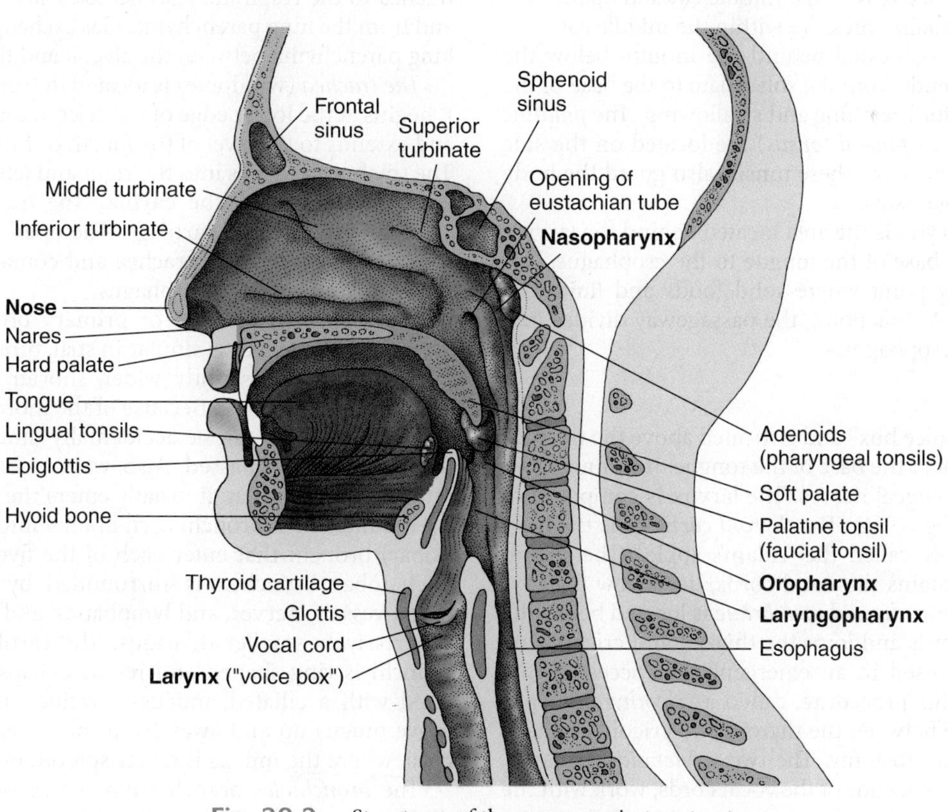

Frontal sinus
Superior turbinate
Sphenoid sinus
Middle turbinate
Opening of eustachian tube
Inferior turbinate
Nasopharynx
Nose
Nares
Hard palate
Tongue
Lingual tonsils
Epiglottis
Hyoid bone
Adenoids (pharyngeal tonsils)
Soft palate
Palatine tonsil (faucial tonsil)
Thyroid cartilage
Oropharynx
Glottis
Laryngopharynx
Vocal cord
Esophagus
Larynx ("voice box")

Fig. 29-2 • Structures of the upper respiratory tract.

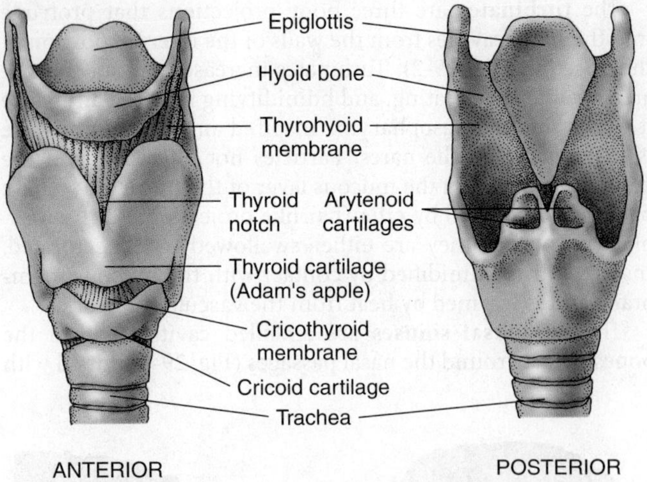
Epiglottis
Hyoid bone
Thyrohyoid membrane
Thyroid notch
Arytenoid cartilages
Thyroid cartilage (Adam's apple)
Cricothyroid membrane
Cricoid cartilage
Trachea
ANTERIOR
POSTERIOR

Fig. 29-4 • Structures of the larynx.

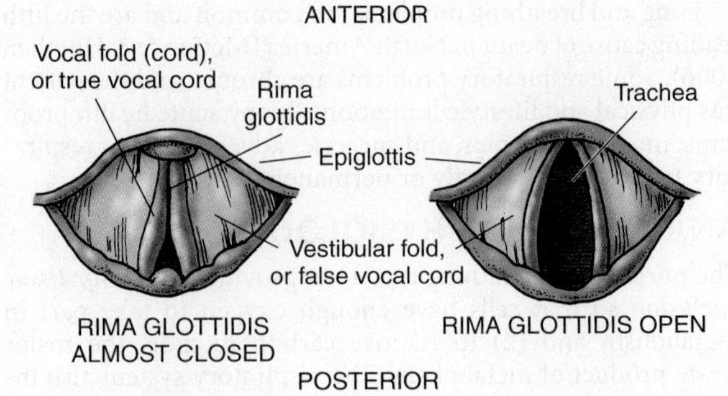
ANTERIOR
Vocal fold (cord), or true vocal cord
Rima glottidis
Trachea
Epiglottis
Vestibular fold, or false vocal cord
RIMA GLOTTIDIS ALMOST CLOSED
RIMA GLOTTIDIS OPEN
POSTERIOR

Fig. 29-5 • Detail of the glottis (two vocal folds and the intervening space, the rima glottidis).

ciliated membrane, the purposes of the sinuses are to provide resonance during speech and to decrease the weight of the skull.

Pharynx

The **pharynx,** or throat, is a passageway for both the respiratory and digestive tracts. It is located behind the oral and nasal cavities. The throat is divided into the nasopharynx, the oropharynx, and the laryngopharynx (see Fig. 29-2).

The nasopharynx is located behind the nose, above the soft palate. It contains the adenoids and the opening of the eustachian tube. The *adenoids* (pharyngeal tonsils) trap organisms that enter the nose or mouth. The **eustachian tube** is a tube that connects the nasopharynx with the middle ear and opens during swallowing to equalize pressure within the middle ear.

The oropharynx is located behind the mouth, below the nasopharynx. It extends from the soft palate to the base of the tongue and is used for breathing and swallowing. The *palatine tonsils* (also known as *faucial tonsils*) are located on the side borders of the oropharynx. These tonsils also guard the body against invading organisms.

The **laryngopharynx** is the area located behind the larynx, extending from the base of the tongue to the esophagus. It is the critical dividing point where solid foods and fluids are separated from air. At this point, the passageway divides into the larynx and the esophagus.

Larynx

The **larynx** is the "voice box" and is located above the trachea, just below the throat at the base of the tongue. It is innervated by the recurrent laryngeal nerves. The larynx is composed of several cartilages (Fig. 29-4). The *thyroid cartilage* is the largest and is commonly called the "Adam's apple." The *cricoid cartilage,* which contains the vocal cords, lies below the thyroid cartilage. The *cricothyroid membrane* is located below the level of the vocal cords and joins the thyroid and cricoid cartilages. This site is used in an emergency for access to the lower airways. In this procedure, called a *cricothyroidotomy,* an opening is made between the thyroid and cricoid cartilage and results in a tracheostomy. The two *arytenoid* cartilages, which attach at the back ends of the vocal cords, work with the thyroid cartilage in vocal cord movement.

Inside the larynx are two pairs of vocal cords: the false vocal cords and the true vocal cords. The **glottis** is the opening between the true vocal cords (Fig. 29-5). The **epiglottis** is a leaf-shaped, elastic structure that is attached along one edge to the top of the larynx. Its hingelike action prevents food from entering the trachea (aspiration) by closing over the glottis during swallowing. The epiglottis opens during breathing and coughing.

Lower Respiratory Tract

Airways

The lower airways consist of the trachea; two mainstem bronchi; lobar, segmental, and subsegmental bronchi; bronchioles; alveolar ducts; and alveoli (Fig. 29-6). The lower respiratory tract (also called the *tracheobronchial tree*) is an inverted treelike structure consisting of muscle, cartilage, and elastic tissues. This system of branching tubes, which decrease in size from the trachea to the respiratory bronchioles, allows gases to move to and from the lung parenchyma. Gas exchange takes place in the lung parenchyma between the alveoli and the lung capillaries.

The trachea (windpipe) is located in front of the esophagus. It begins at the lower edge of the cricoid cartilage of the larynx and extends to the level of the fourth or fifth thoracic vertebra. The trachea branches into the right and left mainstem bronchi at a junction called the **carina.** The trachea contains 6 to 10 C-shaped rings of cartilage. The open portion of the C is the back portion of the trachea and contains smooth muscle that is shared with the esophagus.

The mainstem bronchi, or primary bronchi, begin at the carina. The bronchus is similar in structure to the trachea. The right bronchus is slightly wider, shorter, and more vertical than the left bronchus. Because of the more vertical line of the right bronchus, it can be accidentally intubated when an endotracheal tube is passed. Also, when a foreign object is aspirated from the throat, it usually enters the right bronchus.

The mainstem bronchi each branch into the five secondary (lobar) bronchi that enter each of the five lobes of the lung. Each lobar bronchus is surrounded by connective tissue, blood vessels, nerves, and lymphatics, and each branches into progressively smaller divisions. The cartilage of these lobar bronchi is ring-shaped and resists collapse. The bronchi are lined with a ciliated, mucus-secreting membrane. The cilia move mucus up and away from the lower airway to the trachea, where the mucus is either spit out or swallowed.

The *bronchioles* branch from the secondary bronchi and divide into smaller and smaller tubes, which are the terminal

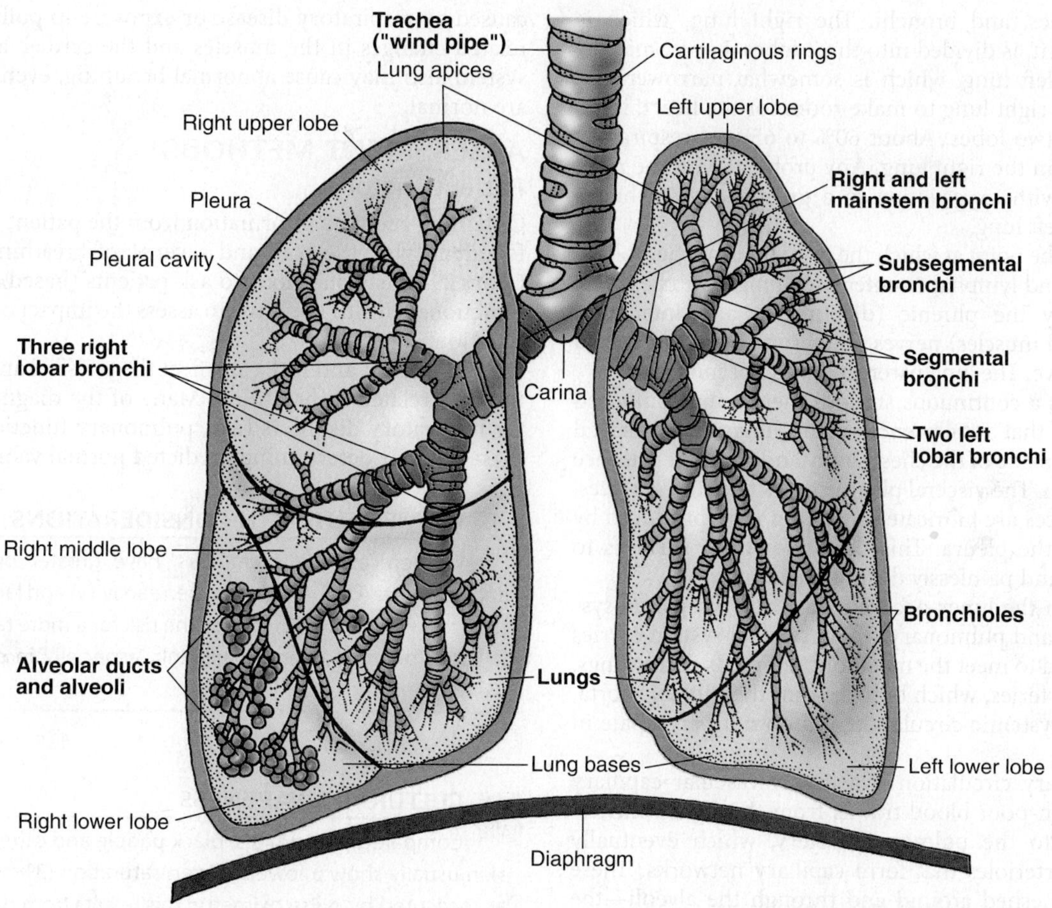
Trachea
("wind pipe")
Lung apices
Cartilaginous rings
Left upper lobe
Right upper lobe
Pleura
Right and left
mainstem bronchi
Pleural cavity
Subsegmental
bronchi
Three right
lobar bronchi
Segmental
bronchi
Carina
Two left
lobar bronchi
Right middle lobe
Bronchioles
Alveolar ducts
and alveoli
Lungs
Lung bases
Left lower lobe
Right lower lobe
Diaphragm

Fig. 29-6 • Structures of the lower respiratory tract (structural size and proportions not drawn to scale).

and respiratory bronchioles (Fig. 29-7). These tubes are less than 1 mm in diameter. They have no cartilage and depend entirely on the elastic recoil of the lung to remain patent. The terminal bronchioles do not participate in gas exchange.

Alveolar ducts branch from the respiratory bronchioles and resemble a bunch of grapes. Alveolar sacs arise from these ducts. The alveolar sacs contain groups of alveoli, which are the basic units of gas exchange (see Fig. 29-7). A pair of healthy adult lungs has about 290 million alveoli, which are surrounded by lung capillaries. These numerous small alveoli share common walls, making a large surface area for gas exchange. In a healthy adult, this surface area is about the size of a tennis court. **Acinus** is a term for the structural unit consisting of a respiratory bronchiole, an alveolar duct, and an alveolar sac.

In the walls of the alveoli, specific cells called *type II pneumocytes* secrete **surfactant,** a fatty protein that reduces surface tension in the alveoli. Without surfactant, **atelectasis** (collapse of the alveoli) occurs. In atelectasis, gas exchange is reduced because alveolar surface area is reduced.

Lungs

The lungs are spongelike, elastic, cone-shaped organs located in the pleural cavity in the chest. The apex (top) of each lung extends above the clavicle; the base (bottom) of each lung lies just above the diaphragm (the major muscle of inspiration). The lungs are composed of millions of alveoli and their related

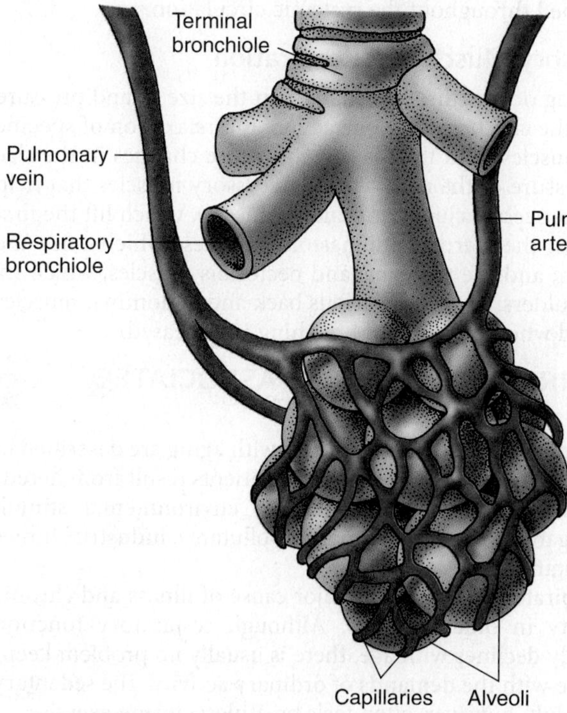
Terminal
bronchiole
Pulmonary
vein
Pulmonary
artery
Respiratory
bronchiole
Capillaries
Alveoli

Fig. 29-7 • The terminal bronchioles and the acinus.

ducts, bronchioles, and bronchi. The right lung, which is larger than the left, is divided into three lobes: upper, middle, and lower. The left lung, which is somewhat narrower and smaller than the right lung to make room for the heart, is divided into only two lobes. About 60% to 65% of respiratory function occurs in the right lung. Any problem with the right lung interferes with *oxygenation* to a greater degree than a problem in the left lung.

The hilum is the point at which the primary bronchus, blood vessels, nerves, and lymphatics enter each lung. The chest wall is innervated by the phrenic (diaphragm) and intercostal (pleura, ribs, and muscles) nerves. The bronchi are innervated by the vagus nerve. The lung parenchyma is not innervated.

The **pleura** is a continuous smooth membrane composed of two surfaces that totally enclose the lungs. The parietal pleura lines the inside of the chest cavity and the upper surface of the diaphragm. The visceral pleura covers the lung surfaces. These two surfaces are lubricated by a thin fluid produced by the cells lining the pleura. This fluid allows the surfaces to glide smoothly and painlessly during breathing.

Blood flow in the lungs occurs through two separate systems: bronchial and pulmonary. The bronchial system carries the blood needed to meet the metabolic demands of the lungs. The bronchial arteries, which branch from the thoracic aorta, are part of the systemic circulation and do not participate in gas exchange.

ANIMATION: Pulmonary Circulation ▶

The pulmonary circulation is a highly vascular capillary network. Oxygen-poor blood travels from the right ventricle of the heart into the pulmonary artery, which eventually branches into arterioles that form capillary networks. These capillaries are meshed around and through the alveoli—the site of gas exchange (see Fig. 29-7). Freshly oxygenated blood travels from the capillaries and through smaller veins to the pulmonary veins and then to the left atrium. From the left atrium, oxygenated blood flows into the left ventricle, where it is pumped throughout the systemic circulation.

Accessory Muscles of Respiration

Breathing occurs through changes in the size of and pressure within the chest cavity. Contraction and relaxation of specific chest muscles (and the diaphragm) cause changes in the size and pressure of the chest cavity. Accessory muscles that help in this process include the scalene muscles, which lift the first two ribs; the sternocleidomastoid muscles, which raise the sternum; and the trapezius and pectoralis muscles, which fix the shoulders. At times, various back and abdominal muscles are used when the work of breathing is increased.

RESPIRATORY CHANGES ASSOCIATED WITH AGING

The respiratory changes that occur with aging are described in Chart 29-1. Many changes in older patients result from heredity and a lifetime of exposure to environmental stimuli (e.g., cigarette smoke, bacteria, air pollutants, industrial fumes and irritants).

Respiratory disease is a major cause of illness and chronic disability in older patients. Although respiratory function normally declines with age, there is usually no problem keeping pace with the demands of ordinary activity. The sedentary older adult, however, often feels breathless during exercise.

It is difficult to determine which respiratory changes in older adults are related to normal aging and which changes are caused by respiratory disease or exposure to pollutants. Age-related changes in the muscles and the cardiac and vascular system also may cause abnormal breathing, even if the lungs are normal.

ASSESSMENT METHODS

Patient History

Obtaining accurate information from the patient is important for identifying the type and severity of breathing problems. Chart 29-2 lists questions to ask patients (based on Gordon's Functional Health Patterns) to assess the impact of pulmonary function.

Age, gender, and race can affect the physical and diagnostic findings related to breathing. Many of the diagnostic studies for respiratory disorders (e.g., pulmonary function tests) use these data for determining predicted normal values.

WOMEN'S HEALTH CONSIDERATIONS

Women, especially smokers, have greater bronchial responsiveness (i.e., bronchial hyperreactivity) and larger airways than men. This factor increases the risk for a more rapid decline in lung function as an older adult, especially in people who were or are smokers.

CULTURAL AWARENESS

Compared with whites, black people and others with dark skin usually show a lower oxygen saturation (3% to 5% lower) as measured by pulse oximetry; this results from deeper coloration of the nail bed and does not reflect true oxygen status.

Explore the home, community, and workplace for environmental factors that could cause or worsen lung disease. Occupational lung diseases include pneumoconiosis, which results from the inhalation of dust (e.g., coal dust, stone dust, silicone dust); toxic lung injury; and hypersensitivity disease (e.g., hypersensitivity to latex). Work history includes the exact dates of employment and a brief job description. Exposure to industrial dusts of any type or to the chemicals found in smoke and fumes may cause breathing disorders. Bakers, coal miners, stone masons, cotton handlers, woodworkers, welders, potters, plastic and rubber manufacturers, printers, popcorn workers, farm workers, and steel foundry workers are at risk for breathing problems. Also at risk are people who have ever worked with asbestos. Use this opportunity to teach patients about the use of masks and adequate ventilation to protect the respiratory system from inhalation irritants.

Ask the patient about the home and living conditions, such as the type of heat used (e.g., gas heater, wood-burning stove, fireplace, kerosene heater). Determine exposure to any irritants (e.g., noxious fumes, chemicals, animals, birds, air pollutants). Ask about hobbies and leisure activities. Hobbies such as painting, working with ceramics, building model airplanes, refinishing furniture, or woodworking may expose the patient to harmful chemicals. Teach patients to wear masks during these exposures and to ensure the area is well ventilated.

Ask patients about their respiratory history (Table 29-1), including smoking history, drug use, travel, and area of residence.

Chart 29-1 NURSING FOCUS ON THE OLDER ADULT

Changes in the Respiratory System Related to Aging

Physiologic Change	Nursing Interventions	Rationales
Alveoli Alveolar surface area decreases. Diffusion capacity decreases. Elastic recoil decreases. Bronchioles and alveolar ducts dilate. Ability to cough decreases. Airways close early.	Encourage vigorous pulmonary hygiene (i.e., encourage patient to turn, cough, and deep breathe), especially if he or she is confined to bed or has had surgery. Encourage upright position.	Potential for mechanical or infectious respiratory complications is increased in these situations. The upright position minimizes ventilation-perfusion mismatching.
LUNGS		
Residual volume increases. Vital capacity decreases. Efficiency of oxygen and carbon dioxide exchange decreases. Elasticity decreases.	Include inspection, palpation, percussion, and auscultation in lung assessments. Help patient actively maintain health and fitness. Assess patient's respirations for abnormal breathing patterns. Encourage frequent oral hygiene.	Inspection, palpation, percussion, and auscultation are needed to detect normal age-related changes. Health and fitness help keep losses in respiratory functioning to a minimum. Periodic breathing patterns (e.g., Cheyne-Stokes) can occur. Oral hygiene aids in the removal of secretions.
PHARYNX AND LARYNX		
Muscles atrophy. Vocal cords become slack. Laryngeal muscles lose elasticity and airways lose cartilage.	Have face-to-face conversations with patient when possible.	Patient's voice may be soft and difficult to understand.
PULMONARY VASCULATURE		
Vascular resistance to blood flow through pulmonary vascular system increases. Pulmonary capillary blood volume decreases. Risk of hypoxia increases.	Assess patient's level of consciousness.	Patient can become confused during acute respiratory conditions.
EXERCISE TOLERANCE		
Body's response to hypoxia and hypercarbia decreases.	Assess for subtle manifestations of hypoxia.	Early assessment helps prevent complications.
MUSCLE STRENGTH		
Respiratory muscle strength, especially the diaphragm and the intercostals, decreases.	Encourage pulmonary hygiene, and help patient actively maintain health and fitness.	Regular pulmonary hygiene and overall fitness help maintain maximal functioning of the respiratory system and prevent illness.
SUSCEPTIBILITY TO INFECTION		
Effectiveness of the cilia decreases. Immunoglobulin A decreases. Alveolar macrophages are altered.	Encourage pulmonary hygiene, and help patient actively maintain health and fitness.	Regular pulmonary hygiene and overall fitness help maintain maximal functioning of the respiratory system and prevent illness.
CHEST WALL		
Anteroposterior diameter increases. Thorax becomes shorter. Progressive kyphoscoliosis occurs. Chest wall compliance (elasticity) decreases. Mobility may decrease. Osteoporosis is possible.	Discuss the normal changes of aging. Discuss the need for increased rest periods during exercise. Encourage adequate calcium intake (especially during a woman's pre-menopause phase).	Patients may be anxious because they must work harder to breathe. Older patients have less tolerance for exercise. Calcium intake helps prevent osteoporosis by building bone in younger patients.

Chart 29-2 RESPIRATORY ASSESSMENT
Using Gordon's Functional Health Patterns

HEALTH PERCEPTION—HEALTH MANAGEMENT PATTERN
- How has your general health been?
- Have you had any colds this past year?
- Have you missed work or school because of illness this past year?
- Do you use cigarettes? For how many years? How many packs per day?

ACTIVITY-EXERCISE PATTERN
- Do you feel you have sufficient energy to perform tasks or routines that are required of you?
- Do you feel you have sufficient energy to do what you would like to do?
- Do you exercise? How often? For how long each time? What type(s) of exercise do you perform?
- What activities do you perform in your spare time?
- What is your ability to perform these tasks?

Feeding______	Grooming______
Bathing______	General mobility______
Toileting______	Cooking______
Bed mobility______	Home maintenance______
Dressing______	Shopping______

FUNCTIONAL LEVELS CODE
Level 0: Full self-care
Level I: Requires use of equipment or device
Level II: Requires assistance or supervision of another person
Level III: Requires assistance or supervision of another person and the use of equipment or devices
Level IV: Is dependent and does not participate

Based on Gordon, M. (2007). *Manual of nursing diagnosis* (11th ed.). Boston: Jones & Bartlett.

TABLE 29-1 Important Aspects to Assess in a Respiratory System History

- Smoking history
- Childhood illnesses
  - Asthma
  - Pneumonia
  - Communicable diseases
  - Hay fever
  - Allergies
  - Eczema
  - Frequent colds
  - Croup
  - Cystic fibrosis
- Adult illnesses
  - Pneumonia
  - Sinusitis
  - Tuberculosis
  - HIV and AIDS
  - Lung disease such as emphysema and sarcoidosis
  - Diabetes
  - Hypertension
  - Heart disease
- Influenza, pneumococcal (Pneumovax) and BCG vaccinations
- Surgeries of the upper or lower respiratory system
- Injuries to the upper or lower respiratory system
- Hospitalizations
- Date of last chest x-ray, pulmonary function test, tuberculin test, or other diagnostic tests and results
- Recent weight loss
- Night sweats
- Sleep disturbances
- Lung disease and condition of family members
- Geographic areas of recent travel
- Occupation and leisure activities

AIDS, Acquired immune deficiency syndrome; *BCG*, bacille Calmette-Guérin; *HIV*, human immune deficiency virus.

Smoking history includes the use of cigarettes, cigars, pipe tobacco, marijuana, and other controlled substances. Ask the patient whether any of these substances are used now or in the past. Assess whether the patient has passive exposure to smoke in the home or workplace. If the patient smokes, ask for how long, how many packs a day, and whether the patient has quit smoking (and how long ago). Document the smoking history in **pack-years** (number of packs smoked per day multiplied by number of years the patient has smoked). Because he or she may have guilt or denial about this habit, assume a nonjudgmental attitude during the interview.

Smoking induces changes in the airways, and these changes lead to varying degrees of airway obstruction. Men who continue to smoke have a more rapid decline in pulmonary function than do nonsmokers. The pulmonary function of patients who have quit smoking for 2 or more years appears to decline less rapidly than in those who continue to smoke.

Drug use, both prescribed drugs and illicit drugs, can affect lung function. Some drugs affect the lungs when taken systemically. Ask about drugs taken for breathing problems and about drugs taken for other conditions. For example, a cough can be a side effect of some antihypertensive drugs (angiotensin-converting enzyme [ACE] inhibitors). Determine which over-the-counter drugs (e.g., cough syrups, antihistamines, decongestants, inhalants, nasal sprays) the patient is using. Also assess the use of complementary and alternative therapies. Ask about past drug use and the reason it was discontinued. For example, the patient may have used many bronchodilator inhalers but may prefer one particular drug for relieving breathlessness. Some drugs for other conditions can cause permanent changes in lung function. For example, patients may have pulmonary fibrosis if they received bleomycin (Blenoxane) as chemotherapy for cancer or amiodarone (Cordarone) for cardiac problems. Illicit drugs, such as marijuana or cocaine, are often inhaled. Any illicit drug can be inhaled or smoked.

Allergies are important to the respiratory history. Ask whether the patient has any known allergies to substances such as foods, dust, molds, pollen, bee stings, trees, grass, animal dander and saliva, or any drugs. Ask him or her to describe specific allergic responses. For example, does he or she wheeze, have trouble breathing, cough, sneeze, or have rhinitis after exposure to the allergen? Has he or she ever been treated for an allergic response? If the patient has received treatment for allergies, ask about what caused the need for treatment, the type of treatment, and the response to treatment. *Document any known allergies and the specific type of allergic response in a prominent place in the patient's medical record.*

Travel and geographic area of residence may be relevant for possible exposure to certain diseases. For example, *histoplas-*

mosis, a fungal disease caused by inhalation of contaminated dust, is found in the central part of the United States and in Central America. *Coccidioidomycosis,* another fungal disease, is found mostly in the western and southwestern parts of the United States, in Mexico, and in portions of Central America, as is Hantavirus.

Nutrition Status

Assess the patient's diet history and nutrition status to determine allergic reactions to certain foods or preservatives. Manifestations range from rhinitis, chest tightness, weakness, **dyspnea** (shortness of breath), urticaria, and severe wheezing to loss of consciousness. Ask about his or her usual food intake and whether any breathing problems occur with eating. Malnutrition may occur if the patient has difficulty breathing while eating or preparing food.

Family History and Genetic Risk

Obtain a family history to assess for respiratory disorders with a genetic component, such as cystic fibrosis, some lung cancers, and alpha$_1$-antitrypsin deficiency (one risk factor for emphysema) (Nussbaum et al., 2007). Patients with asthma often have a family history of allergic symptoms and reactive airways. Ask about a history of infectious disease, such as tuberculosis, because family members may have similar environmental or occupational exposures.

Current Health Problems

Whether the breathing problem is acute or chronic, the current health problem usually includes cough, sputum production, chest pain, and shortness of breath at rest or on exertion. During the interview, explore the present illness in chronologic order. Ask specifically about the onset of the problem, how long it lasts, the location of the problem, how often it occurs, whether the problem has become worse over time, what symptoms occur with it, which actions or interventions provide relief and which ones make it worse, and what treatments have been used.

Cough is a main sign of lung disease. Ask the patient how long the cough has been present and whether it occurs at a specific time of day (e.g., on awakening in the morning, which is common in smokers) or in relation to any physical activity. Determine whether the cough is productive or nonproductive, congested, dry, tickling, or hacking.

Sputum production is an important symptom associated with coughing. Check the duration, color, consistency, odor, and amount of sputum. Sputum may be clear, white, tan, gray, or, if infection is present, yellow or green.

Describe the consistency of sputum as thin, thick, watery, or frothy. Smokers with chronic bronchitis have mucoid sputum. Excessive pink, frothy sputum is common with pulmonary edema. Pneumococcal pneumonia often produces rust-colored sputum, and foul-smelling sputum often occurs with a lung abscess. **Hemoptysis** (blood in the sputum) is most often seen in patients with chronic bronchitis or lung cancer. Patients with tuberculosis, pulmonary infarction, bronchial adenoma, or lung abscess may have grossly bloody sputum.

Quantify sputum by describing its volume in terms such as teaspoon, tablespoon, and cups or fractions of cups. Normally, the bronchial tree can produce up to 3 ounces (90 mL) of sputum per day. Determine whether sputum production is increasing, possibly from external stimuli (e.g., an irritant in the work setting) or an internal cause (e.g., chronic bronchitis or a pulmonary abscess).

Chest pain can occur with other health problems as well as with lung problems. A detailed description of chest pain helps distinguish whether pain is pleural, musculoskeletal, cardiac, or gastrointestinal in origin. Ask the patient whether the pain is continuous or made worse by coughing, deep breathing, or swallowing. Cardiac pain is usually intense and "crushing." It may also radiate to the arm, shoulder, or neck. Pulmonary pain varies depending on the cause. Pain that feels like something is "rubbing" inside is more common with pulmonary pain. The pain may appear only on deep inhalation or be present at the end of inhalation and the end of exhalation. Usually, pulmonary pain is not made worse by touching or pressing over the area.

Dyspnea (difficulty in breathing or breathlessness) is a subjective perception and varies among patients. A patient's feeling of dyspnea may not be consistent with the severity of the presenting problem. Determine the type of onset (slow or abrupt); the duration (number of hours, time of day); relieving factors (changes of position, drug use, activity cessation); and whether wheezing, crackles, or stridor occurs with the breathlessness.

Try to quantify dyspnea by asking whether this symptom interferes with ADLs and, if so, how severely. For example, is the patient breathless while dressing, showering, shaving, or eating? Does dyspnea occur after walking one block or climbing one flight of stairs? Table 29-2 classifies dyspnea with changes in ADL performance. A dyspnea assessment scale may be used to assess dyspnea (see Chapter 32).

Ask about **paroxysmal nocturnal dyspnea (PND),** which is intermittent dyspnea during sleep, and about **orthopnea,** which is a shortness of breath that occurs when lying down but is relieved by sitting up. These two conditions often occur with chronic lung disease and left-sided heart failure. In PND, the patient has a sudden onset of breathing difficulty that is severe enough to awaken him or her from sleep.

Physical Assessment

Assessment of the Nose and Sinuses

▶ VIDEO CLIP: Inspection of the Nose

Inspect the patient's external nose for deformities or tumors, and inspect the nostrils for symmetry of size and shape. Nasal flaring may indicate increased respiratory effort. To observe the interior nose, ask the patient to tilt the head back for a penlight examination. Use a nasal speculum and nasopharyngeal mirror for a more thorough inspection of the nasal cavity.

Inspect for color, swelling, drainage, and bleeding. The mucous membrane of the nose normally appears redder than the oral mucosa, but it is pale, engorged, and bluish gray in patients with allergic rhinitis. Check the nasal septum for bleeding, perforation, or deviation. Some degree of septal deviation is common in most adults and appears as an S shape, tilting toward one side or the other. A perforated septum is present if the light shines through the perforation into the opposite nostril; this condition is often found in cocaine users. Nasal polyps, a common cause of obstruction, are pale, shiny, gelatinous lumps or "bags" attached to the turbinates. Block one naris at a time to check whether air moves through the unblocked side easily.

Assessment of the Pharynx, Trachea, and Larynx

Assessment of the pharynx begins with inspection of the external structures of the mouth. To examine the posterior pharynx, use a tongue depressor to press down one side of the

TABLE 29-2 Correlation of Dyspnea Classification with Performance of ADLs

Classification	ADLs Key
Class I: No significant restrictions in normal activity. Employable. Dyspnea occurs only on more-than-normal or strenuous exertion.	*4:* No breathlessness, normal.
Class II: Independent in essential ADLs but restricted in some other activities. Dyspneic on climbing stairs or on walking on an incline but not on level walking. Employable only for sedentary job or under special circumstances.	*3:* Satisfactory, mild breathlessness. Complete performance is possible without pause or assistance but not entirely normal.
Class III: Dyspnea commonly occurs during usual activities, such as showering or dressing, but the patient can manage without assistance from others. Not dyspneic at rest; can walk for more than a city block at own pace but cannot keep up with others of own age. May stop to catch breath partway up a flight of stairs. Is probably not employable in any occupation.	*2:* Fair, moderate breathlessness. Must stop during activity. Complete performance is possible without assistance, but performance may be too debilitating or time consuming.
Class IV: Dyspnea produces dependence on help in some essential ADLs such as dressing and bathing. Not usually dyspneic at rest. Dyspneic on minimal exertion; must pause on climbing one flight, walking more than 100 yards, or dressing. Often restricted to home if lives alone. Has minimal or no activities outside of home.	*1:* Poor, marked breathlessness. Incomplete performance; assistance is necessary.
Class V: Entirely restricted to home and often limited to bed or chair. Dyspneic at rest. Dependent on help for most needs.	*0:* Performance not indicated or recommended; too difficult.

ADLs, Activities of daily living.

tongue at a time (to avoid stimulating the gag reflex). As the patient says "ah," observe the rise and fall of the soft palate and uvula and inspect for color and symmetry, evidence of discharge (postnasal drainage), edema or ulceration, and enlarged or inflamed tonsils.

Inspect the neck for symmetry, alignment, masses, swelling, bruises, and the use of accessory neck muscles in breathing. Palpate lymph nodes for size, shape, mobility, consistency, and tenderness. Tender nodes are usually movable and suggest inflammation. Malignant nodes are often hard and are fixed to the surrounding tissue.

Gently palpate the trachea for position, mobility, tenderness, and masses. Firm palpation may trigger coughing or gagging. The space on each side of the trachea should be equal. Many lung disorders cause the trachea to deviate from the midline. Tension pneumothorax, large pleural effusion, mediastinal mass, and neck tumors push the trachea *away* from the affected area. Pneumonectomy, fibrosis, and atelectasis pull the trachea *toward* the affected area. Decreased tracheal mobility may occur with cancer or fibrosis of the mediastinum.

The larynx is usually examined by a specialist with a laryngoscope. An abnormal voice, especially hoarseness, may be heard when there are problems of the larynx.

Assessment of the Lungs and Thorax

Inspection

Begin inspection of the chest by assessing the front and back of the thorax. Normal landmarks of the chest front (anterior) and back (posterior) are shown in Fig. 29-8. If possible, have the patient sit up during the assessment. He or she should be undressed to the waist and draped for privacy and warmth. Observe the chest, and compare one side with the other. Work from the top (apex) and move downward toward the base, going from side to side, while inspecting for discoloration, scars, lesions, masses, and spinal deformities such as kyphosis, scoliosis, and lordosis. Assessing from side to side allows you to compare the assessment findings for each lung at the same level.

Observe the rate, rhythm, and depth of inspirations, as well as the symmetry of chest movement. Impaired movement or unequal expansion may indicate disease of the lung or the pleura. Observe the type of breathing (e.g., pursed-lip or diaphragmatic breathing) and the use of accessory muscles.

▶ VIDEO CLIP: Respiratory Excursion

Examine the shape of the patient's chest, and compare the anteroposterior (AP or front-to-back) diameter with the lateral (side-to-side) diameter. This ratio normally is about 1:2, depending on body build. The ratio increases to 1:1 in patients with emphysema, which results in the typical barrel-chest appearance.

Normally the ribs slope downward. Patients with air trapping in the lungs caused by chronic asthma or emphysema have more horizontal ribs. Observe for retraction of muscle between the ribs and at the sternal notch. Retractions are areas that get sucked inward when the patient inhales. This does not occur during normal respiratory effort. Retractions may occur when the patient is working hard to inhale around an obstruction.

Palpation

▶ VIDEO CLIP: Respiratory Excursion, Tactile Fremitus

Palpate the chest after inspection. Palpation is performed to assess respiratory movement symmetry and observable abnormalities, to identify areas of tenderness, and to check vocal or tactile **fremitus** (vibration).

Assess chest expansion by placing your thumbs on the patient's spine at the level of the ninth ribs and extending the fingers sideways around the rib cage. As the patient inhales, both sides of the chest should move upward and outward together in one symmetric movement and move your thumbs apart. On exhalation, the thumbs should come back together as they return to the midline. This same technique can be performed on the anterior chest for patients who cannot sit up or change positions. Decreased movement on one side (unilateral or unequal expansion) may be a result of pain, trauma, or **pneumothorax** (air in the pleural cavity). Respiratory lag or slowed movement on one side occurs with the presence of a pulmonary mass, pleural fibrosis, atelectasis, pneumonia, or a lung abscess.

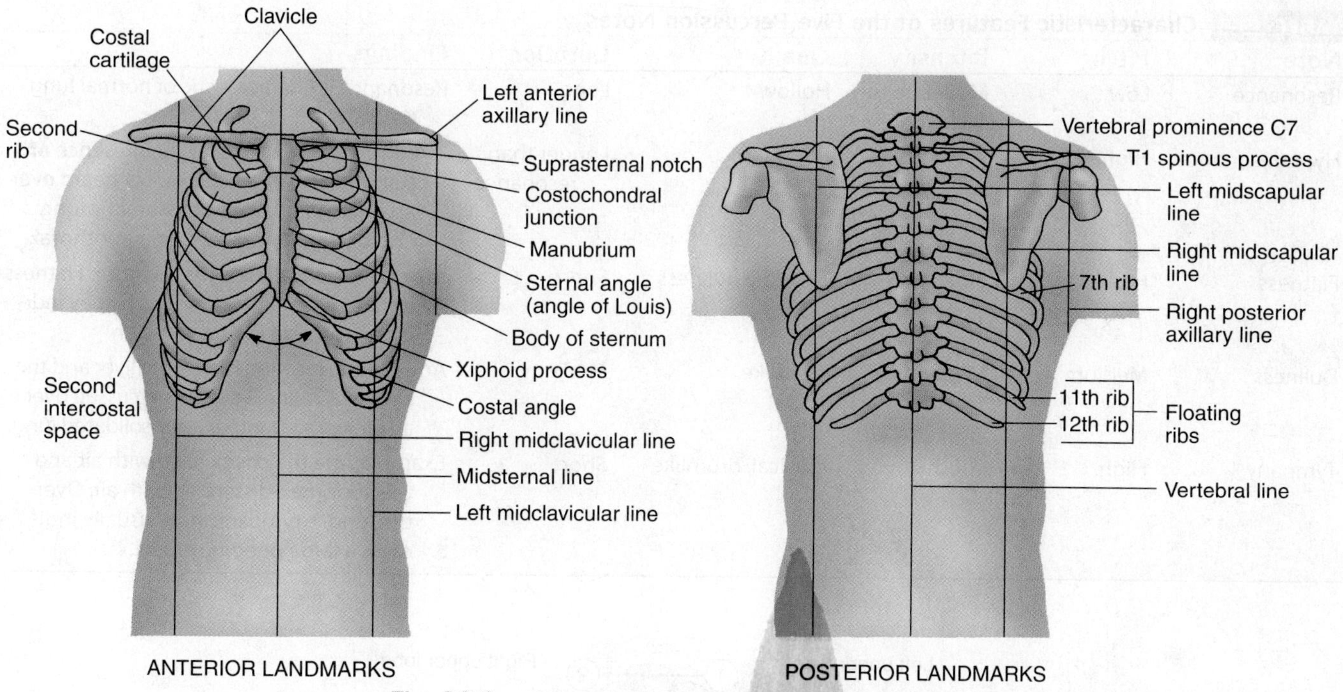
Clavicle
Costal cartilage
Second rib
Left anterior axillary line
Suprasternal notch
Costochondral junction
Manubrium
Sternal angle (angle of Louis)
Body of sternum
Xiphoid process
Second intercostal space
Costal angle
Right midclavicular line
Midsternal line
Left midclavicular line
ANTERIOR LANDMARKS
Vertebral prominence C7
T1 spinous process
Left midscapular line
Right midscapular line
7th rib
Right posterior axillary line
11th rib
12th rib
Floating ribs
Vertebral line
POSTERIOR LANDMARKS

Fig. 29-8 • Anterior and posterior thoracic landmarks.

Palpate any abnormalities found on inspection (e.g., masses, lesions, bruises, swelling). Also palpate for tenderness, particularly if the patient has reported pain. **Crepitus** (air trapped in and under the skin, also known as *subcutaneous emphysema*) is felt as a crackling sensation beneath the fingertips. Document this finding when it occurs around a wound site or a tracheostomy site or if a pneumothorax is suspected.

VIDEO CLIP: Tactile Fremitus ▶

Tactile (vocal) fremitus is a vibration of the chest wall produced when the patient speaks. This vibration can be felt on the chest wall. Fremitus is decreased if the transmission of sound waves from the larynx to the chest wall is slowed. This problem can occur when the pleural space is filled with air (pneumothorax) or fluid **(pleural effusion)** or when the bronchus is obstructed. Fremitus is increased with pneumonia and abscesses because they increase the density of the thorax and enhance transmission of the vibrations.

VIDEO CLIPS: Diaphragmatic Excursion; Percussion, Anterior Thorax ▶

Percussion

Use percussion to assess for pulmonary resonance, the boundaries of organs, and diaphragmatic excursion. Percussion involves tapping the chest wall, which sets the underlying tissues into motion and produces audible sounds (Fig. 29-9).

Percussion produces five different notes (Table 29-3). These sounds assist in determining the density of the underlying structures (i.e., whether the lung tissue contains air or fluid or is solid).

Auscultation

Auscultation includes listening for normal breath sounds, adventitious sounds, and voice sounds. This technique provides information about the flow of air through the tracheobronchial tree and helps identify fluid, mucus, or obstruction in the respiratory system (Bradley, 2007). The diaphragm side of the stethoscope is designed to detect high-pitched sounds.

Begin auscultation with the patient sitting in an upright position. With the stethoscope pressed firmly against the chest wall (clothing can distort or muffle sounds), instruct the patient to breathe slowly and deeply through an open mouth. (Breathing through the nose sets up turbulent sounds that are transmitted to the lungs.) Use a systematic approach, beginning at the lung apices and moving from side to side down through the intercostal spaces to the lung bases (Fig. 29-10). This side-to-side method allows you to compare one lung with the other at the same level. Avoid listening over bony structures while auscultating the thorax on all sides. Listen to a full respiratory cycle, noting the quality and intensity of the breath sounds. Observe the patient for dizziness caused by hyperventilation during auscultation. If dizziness occurs, tell the patient to relax and breathe normally for a few minutes.

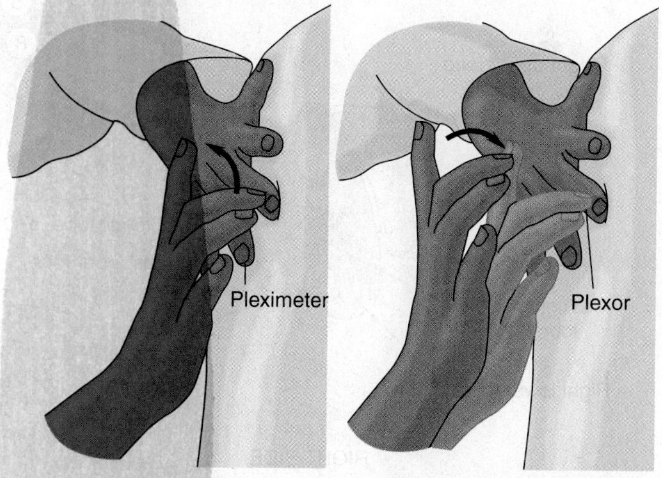
Pleximeter
Plexor

Fig. 29-9 • Percussion technique.

Normal breath sounds are produced as air vibrates while moving through the passages from the larynx to the alveoli. Breath sounds are identified by their location, intensity, pitch, and duration within the respiratory cycle (e.g., early or late

TABLE 29-3 Characteristic Features of the Five Percussion Notes

Note	Pitch	Intensity	Quality	Duration	Findings
Resonance	Low	Moderate to loud	Hollow	Long	Resonance is characteristic of normal lung tissue.
Hyperresonance	Higher than resonance	Very loud	Booming	Longer than resonance	Hyperresonance indicates the presence of trapped air, so it is commonly heard over an emphysematous or asthmatic lung and occasionally over a pneumothorax.
Flatness	High	Soft	Extreme dullness	Short	An example location is the sternum. Flatness percussed over the lung fields may indicate a massive pleural effusion.
Dullness	Medium	Medium	Thudlike	Medium	An example location is over the liver and the kidneys. Dullness can be percussed over an atelectatic lung or a consolidated lung.
Tympany	High	Loud	Musical, drumlike	Short	Examples are the cheek filled with air and the abdomen distended with air. Over the lung, a tympanic note usually indicates a large pneumothorax.

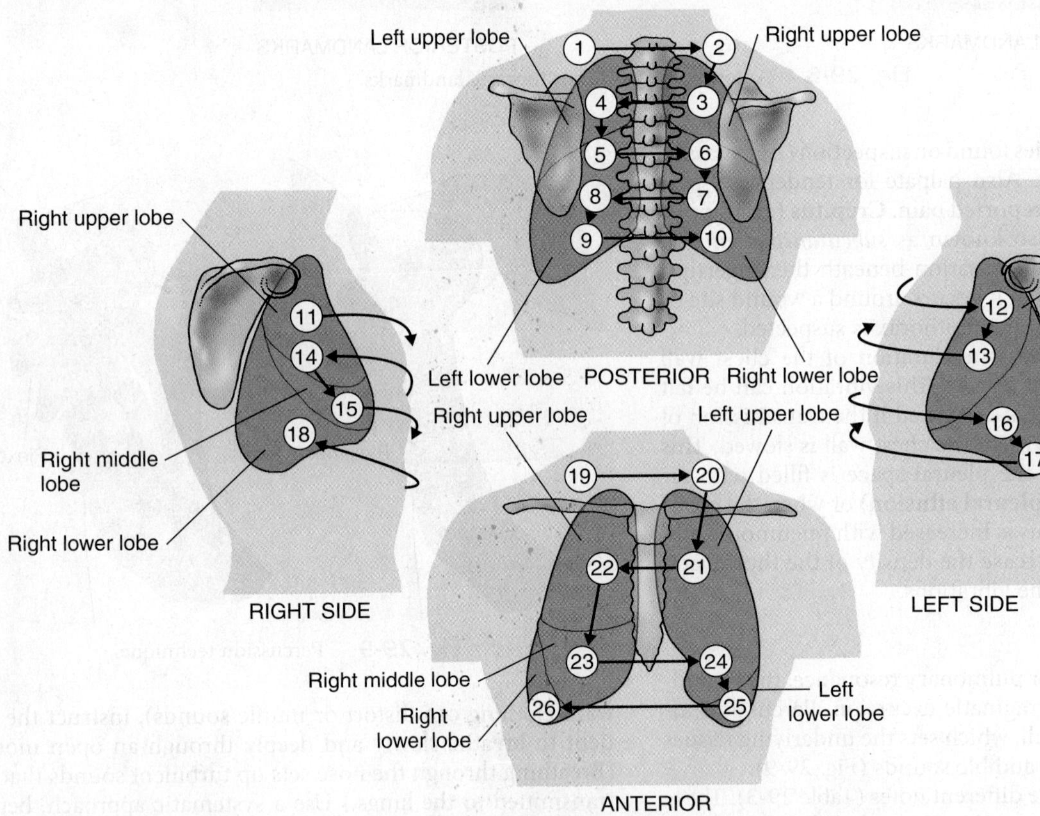

Left upper lobe
Right upper lobe
Left lower lobe
POSTERIOR
Right lower lobe
Right upper lobe
Right middle lobe
Right lower lobe
RIGHT SIDE
Left upper lobe
Left lower lobe
LEFT SIDE
Right upper lobe
Left upper lobe
Right middle lobe
Right lower lobe
Left lower lobe
ANTERIOR

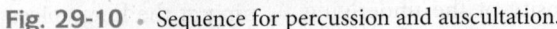

Fig. 29-10 • Sequence for percussion and auscultation.

AUDIO CLIP: Bronchial; Bronchovesicular; and Vesicular Breath Sounds

inspiration and expiration). Normal breath sounds are known as "bronchial" or "tubular" (harsh hollow sounds heard over the trachea and mainstem bronchi), "bronchovesicular" (heard over the branching bronchi), and "vesicular" (soft rustling sound heard in the periphery over small bronchioles) (Table 29-4). Describe these sounds as *normal, increased, diminished,* or *absent.*

When bronchial breath sounds are heard at the lung edges, they are abnormal. This increased sound occurs when the bronchial sounds are transmitted to an area of increased density, such as in patients with atelectasis, tumor, or pneumonia. When heard in an abnormal location, bronchovesicular breath sounds may indicate normal aging or an abnormality such as pulmonary consolidation and chronic airway disease.

Adventitious sounds are additional breath sounds superimposed on normal sounds, and they indicate pathologic changes in the lung. Table 29-5 describes adventitious sounds: crackle, wheeze, rhonchus, and pleural friction rub. Adventitious sounds vary in pitch, intensity, duration, and the phase of the

TABLE 29-4 Characteristics of Normal Breath Sounds

	Pitch	Amplitude	Duration	Quality	Normal Location
Bronchial (tubular, tracheal) 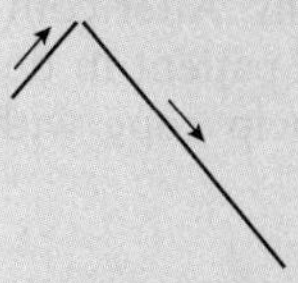	High	Loud	Inspiration < expiration	Harsh, hollow, tubular, blowing	Trachea and larynx
Bronchovesicular 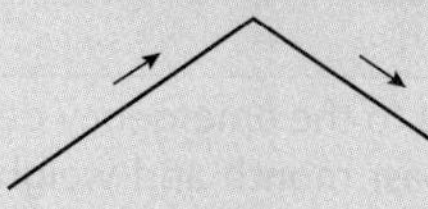	Moderate	Moderate	Inspiration = expiration	Mixed	Over major bronchi where fewer alveoli are located; posterior, between scapulae (especially on right); anterior, around upper sternum in first and second intercostal spaces
Vesicular 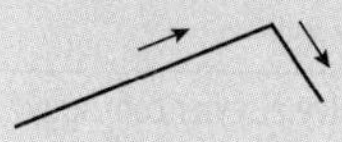	Low	Soft	Inspiration > expiration	Rustling, like the sound of the wind in the trees	Over peripheral lung fields where air flows through smaller bronchioles and alveoli

From Jarvis, C. (2008). *Physical examination and health assessment* (5th ed.). Philadelphia: Saunders.

TABLE 29-5 Characteristic Features of Adventitious Breath Sounds

Adventitious Sound	Occurrence in the Respiratory Cycle	Character	Association
DISCONTINUOUS			
Fine crackles Fine rales High-pitched rales	Either early or late inspiration	Popping, discontinuous sounds caused by air moving into previously deflated airways; sounds like hair being rolled between fingers near the ear "Velcro" sounds late in inspiration usually associated with restrictive disorders	Asbestosis Atelectasis Interstitial fibrosis Bronchitis Pneumonia Chronic pulmonary diseases
Coarse crackles Low-pitched crackles	More common on expiration but may be present early in inspiration	Lower-pitched, coarse, discontinuous rattling sounds caused by fluid or secretions in large airways; likely to change with coughing or suctioning	Bronchitis Pneumonia Tumors Pulmonary edema
CONTINUOUS			
Wheeze	Audible during either inspiration, expiration, or both	Squeaky, musical, continuous sounds associated with air rushing through narrowed airways; may be heard without a stethoscope Arise from the small airways Usually do not clear with coughing	Inflammation Bronchospasm Edema Secretions Pulmonary vessel engorgement (as in cardiac "asthma")
Rhonchus (rhonchi)	Audible during both inspiration and expiration but commonly more prominent on expiration	Lower-pitched, coarse, continuous snoring sounds Arise from the large airways	Thick, tenacious secretions Sputum production Obstruction by foreign body Tumors
PLEURAL FRICTION RUB			
	Heard during both inspiration and expiration, generally at the end of inspiration and the beginning of expiration	Loud, rough, grating, scratching sounds caused by the inflamed surfaces of the pleura rubbing together; often associated with pain on deep inspirations Heard in lateral lung fields	Pleurisy Tuberculosis Pulmonary infarction Pneumonia Lung cancer

AUDIO CLIP: High- and Low-Pitched Crackles; High- and Low-Pitched Wheezes; and Pleural Friction Rub

respiratory cycle in which they occur. Document exactly what you hear on auscultation.

Voice sounds (vocal resonance) through the normally air-filled lung produce a muffled, unclear sound because sound vibrations travel poorly through air. These sounds become louder and more distinct when the sound travels through a solid tissue or liquid. The presence of a consolidated area of the lung, pneumonia, atelectasis, pleural effusion, tumor, or abscess causes increased vocal resonance.

NCLEX EXAMINATION CHALLENGE

The nurse hears bronchial breath sounds over the left lower lobe when auscultating the lungs of a 50-year-old client. Further examination reveals decreased fremitus and dullness to percussion in the same area. What do these findings indicate?

A. Normal physical exam for a 50-year-old
B. An obstruction of the larger airways
C. An area of increased density
D. Subcutaneous emphysema

evolve For the correct answer, go to http://evolve.elsevier.com/Iggy/.

Other Indicators of Respiratory Adequacy

Assess other indicators of respiratory adequacy, because gas exchange affects all body systems. Some indicators (e.g., cyanosis) indicate immediate oxygenation problems. Other changes (e.g., clubbing, weight loss, unevenly developed muscles) reflect long-term oxygenation problems.

Skin and mucous membranes changes, such as pallor or cyanosis, may indicate *inadequate oxygenation.* Areas to assess include the nail beds and the mucous membranes of the oral cavity. Examine the fingers for clubbing (see Fig. 32-10), which indicates hypoxia of long duration.

General appearance includes muscle development and general body build. Long-term respiratory problems limit the ability to maintain body weight and lead to a loss of general muscle mass (McCance & Huether, 2006). Arms and legs may appear thin or poorly muscled. The muscles of the neck and chest may be hypertrophied, especially in the patient with chronic obstructive pulmonary disease (COPD).

Endurance decreases whenever breathing is inadequate for effective gas exchange (McCance & Huether, 2006). Observe how easily the patient moves and whether he or she is short of breath while resting or becomes short of breath when walking 10 to 20 steps. As the patient speaks, note how often he or she pauses for breath between words.

Psychosocial Assessment

Breathing difficulty from any cause often induces anxiety. The patient may be anxious because of reduced oxygen to the brain or because the sensation of not getting enough air is a frightening experience. The thought of having a possible serious respiratory problem, such as lung cancer, can also induce anxiety. Encourage the patient to express his or her feelings and fears about manifestations and their possible meaning.

Assess those aspects of the patient's lifestyle that either can affect respiratory function or are affected by it. Some respiratory problems may become worse with stress. Ask about present life stresses and usual coping mechanisms.

Chronic respiratory disease may cause changes in family roles and relationships, social isolation, financial problems, and unemployment or disability. Discuss coping mechanisms to assess the patient's reaction to these stressors and discover strengths and ineffective behaviors. For example, the patient may react to stress with dependence on family members, withdrawal, or failure to adhere to interventions. After completing the psychosocial assessment, assist the patient in determining the support systems available to help cope with changes resulting from breathing problems.

DECISION-MAKING CHALLENGE
Coordination of Care

The patient is a 48-year-old man who comes to the emergency department with a persistent cough for the past month and weight loss. He has been a one-half pack-a-day smoker for 30 years, although he has tried to quit several times. He appears fatigued and anxious.

1. Calculate the pack-year smoking history for this patient.
2. What questions are important to ask as part of your assessment?
3. What other assessment questions should you ask?

evolve For suggested answer guidelines, go to http://evolve.elsevier.com/Iggy/.

Diagnostic Assessment

Laboratory Assessment

Several laboratory tests (Chart 29-3) are useful in assessing respiratory problems. A red blood cell (RBC) count provides data about the transport of oxygen. The hemoglobin molecule, found in RBCs, transports oxygen to the tissues. A deficiency of hemoglobin could cause hypoxemia.

Arterial blood gas (ABG) analysis assesses *oxygenation* (partial pressure of arterial oxygen [Pao_2]), alveolar ventilation (partial pressure of arterial carbon dioxide [$Paco_2$]), and acid-base balance. Blood gas studies provide information for monitoring treatment results, adjusting oxygen therapy, and evaluating the patient's responses (Swiderski & Byrum, 2007). See Chapter 14 for more details on blood gas analysis.

Sputum specimens obtained by expectoration or tracheal suctioning assist in identifying organisms or abnormal cells, such as in cancer or an allergy. Sputum culture and sensitivity analyses identify bacterial infection and determine which specific antibiotics will be most effective. Sputum cytologic examination helps diagnose malignant lesions by identifying cancer cells. Benign conditions, such as allergy or autoimmunity, may also be identified by cytologic testing. Eosinophils and Curschmann's spirals (a mucus form) are often found by cytologic study in patients with allergic asthma.

Imaging Assessment

Chest x-rays are used for patients with respiratory tract disorders to evaluate the status of the chest and to provide a baseline for comparison with future changes. Standard chest x-rays are performed from **posteroanterior** (PA; back to front) and left lateral (LL) positions. Portable chest x-rays (taken anteroposterior [AP], front to back) cost more, and the films are of lower quality and are more difficult to interpret.

Chest x-rays are used to assess pathologic changes in the lung, such as with pneumonia, atelectasis, pneumothorax, and tumor. They also can be used to detect the presence of pleural fluid and the position and placement of an endotracheal tube or other invasive catheters. These films have limitations, however, and may appear normal, even when severe chronic bronchitis, asthma, or emphysema is present.

Chart 29-3 LABORATORY PROFILE

Respiratory Assessment

Test	Normal Range for Adults	Significance of Abnormal Findings
BLOOD STUDIES		
COMPLETE BLOOD COUNT		
Red blood cells	*Females:* 4.2-5.4 million/mm^3 *Males:* 4.7-6.1 million/mm^3	*Elevated levels* (polycythemia) may be due to the excessive production of erythropoietin, which occurs in response to a hypoxic stimulus, as in COPD, and from living at a high altitude. *Decreased levels* indicate possible anemia, hemorrhage, or hemolysis.
Hemoglobin, total	*Females:* 12-16 g/dL, or 7.4-9.9 mmol/L *Males:* 14-18 g/dL, or 8.7-11.2 mmol/L	Same as for red blood cells.
Hematocrit	*Females:* 37%-47%, or 0.37-0.47 SI units *Males:* 42%-52%, or 0.42-0.52 SI units	Same as for red blood cells.
White blood cell count (leukocyte count, WBC count)	*Total:* 5,000-10,000/mm^3	*Elevations* indicate possible acute infections or inflammations, pneumonia, meningitis, tonsillitis, or emphysema. *Decreased levels* may indicate an overwhelming infection, an autoimmune disorder, or immunosuppressant therapy.
DIFFERENTIAL WHITE BLOOD CELL (LEUKOCYTE) COUNT		
Neutrophils	2500-8000/mm^3 or 55%-70% of total	*Elevations* indicate possible acute bacterial infection (pneumonia), COPD, or inflammatory conditions (smoking). *Decreased levels* indicate possible viral disease (influenza).
Eosinophils	50-500/mm^3 or 1%-4% of total	*Elevations* indicate possible COPD, asthma, or allergies. *Decreased levels* indicate pyogenic infections.
Basophils	25-100/mm^3 or 0.5%-1% of total	*Elevations* indicate possible inflammation; seen in chronic sinusitis, hypersensitivity reactions. *Decreased levels* may be seen in an acute infection.
Lymphocytes	1000-4000/mm^3 or 20%-40% of total	*Elevations* indicate possible viral infection, pertussis, and infectious mononucleosis. *Decreased levels* may be seen during corticosteroid therapy.
Monocytes	100-700/mm^3 or 2%-8% of total	*Elevations:* see Lymphocytes; also may indicate active tuberculosis. *Decreased levels:* see Lymphocytes.
ARTERIAL BLOOD GASES		
Pao_2	80-100 mm Hg *Older adults:* values may be lower	*Elevations* indicate possible excessive oxygen administration. *Decreased levels* indicate possible COPD, asthma, chronic bronchitis, cancer of the bronchi and lungs, cystic fibrosis, respiratory distress syndrome, anemias, atelectasis, or any other cause of hypoxia.
$Paco_2$	35-45 mm Hg	*Elevations* indicate possible COPD, asthma, pneumonia, anesthesia effects, or use of opioids (respiratory acidosis). *Decreased levels* indicate hyperventilation/respiratory alkalosis.
pH	Up to 60 yr: 7.35-7.45 60-90 yr: 7.31-7.42 >90 yr: 7.26-7.43	*Elevations* indicate metabolic or respiratory alkalosis. *Decreased levels* indicate metabolic or respiratory acidosis.
HCO_3^-	21-28 mEq/L	*Elevations* indicate possible respiratory acidosis as compensation for a primary metabolic alkalosis. *Decreased levels* indicate possible respiratory alkalosis as compensation for a primary metabolic acidosis.
Spo_2	95%-100% *Older adults*: values may be slightly lower	*Decreased levels* indicate possible impaired ability of hemoglobin to release oxygen to tissues.

COPD, Chronic obstructive pulmonary disease; *HCO_3^-*, bicarbonate ion; *$Paco_2$*, partial pressure of arterial carbon dioxide; *Pao_2*, partial pressure of arterial oxygen; *Spo_2*, peripheral oxygen saturation.

Sinus and facial x-rays are used to assess fluid levels in the sinus cavities to assist in the diagnosis of acute or chronic sinusitis.

Digital imaging, which uses less radiation, has started to replace most film images. Digital imaging is especially useful to assess lung and chest lesions. A computer enhances the image to give the greatest amount of detail. The image can be adjusted to emphasize a specific area.

Computed tomography (CT) is useful when an x-ray reveals a suspicious lesion, because pulmonary soft tissue densities, tumors, and blood clots can be seen. Chest CT is usually performed with consecutive 5- to 10-mm cross-sectional views of the entire chest. Then, using higher resolution, 1-mm scans are taken of suspicious areas. Chest CTs, especially "spiral CT" scans, can now identify most pulmonary embolisms.

Usually CT scans require a contrast agent injected IV. The contrast enhances the visibility of structures such as tumors, blood vessels, and chambers of the heart. These scans assist in making a diagnosis. Your role in this diagnostic test is to provide information to the patient and to determine whether the patient has any sensitivity to the contrast material. Ask the patient whether he or she has a known allergy to iodine or shellfish.

Ventilation and perfusion scanning ($\dot{V}/\dot{Q}$ scan) can identify the areas of the lung being ventilated and the distribution of blood within the lungs. It is an older test used to support or rule out a diagnosis of pulmonary embolism. This test uses an injected or inhaled radionuclide followed by scanning. The procedure is painless, and the radioactive substance leaves the body in about 8 hours.

Other Noninvasive Diagnostic Assessment

Pulse Oximetry

Pulse oximetry identifies hemoglobin saturation. Usually hemoglobin is almost 100% saturated with oxygen. The pulse oximeter uses a wave of infrared light and a sensor placed on the patient's finger, toe, nose, earlobe, or forehead. Ideal normal pulse oximetry values are 95% to 100%. Normal values are a little lower in older patients and in patients with dark skin. To avoid confusion with the Pao_2 values from arterial blood gases, pulse oximetry readings are recorded as the Spo_2 (arterial oxygen saturation) or Sao_2.

Pulse oximetry can detect desaturation before manifestations (e.g., dusky skin, pale mucosa, pale or blue nail beds) occur (DeMeulenaere, 2007). Causes for low readings include patient movement, hypothermia, decreased peripheral blood flow, ambient light (sunlight, infrared lamps), decreased hemoglobin, edema, and fingernail polish (Rodden et al., 2007). Covering the sensor with a fingertip cut from a glove or changing its position may help accuracy if too much ambient light is present.

Results lower than 91% (and certainly below 86%) are an emergency and require immediate assessment and treatment. When the Spo_2 is below 85%, body tissues have a difficult time becoming oxygenated. An Spo_2 less than 70% is usually life threatening, but in some cases, values below 80% may be life threatening. Pulse oximetry is less accurate at lower values (DeMeulenaere, 2007).

Capnometry and Capnography

Capnometry and capnography are methods that measure the amount of carbon dioxide present in exhaled air, which is an indirect measurement of arterial carbon dioxide levels. These noninvasive tests measure end-tidal carbon dioxide levels ($ETCO_2$) in both intubated patients and those breathing spontaneously. With capnometry, the exhaled air sample is tested with a sensor that changes the CO_2 level into a color or number for analysis. With capnography, the CO_2 level is graphed as a specific waveform along with a number. These methods provide information about CO_2 production, pulmonary perfusion, alveolar ventilation, respiratory patterns, ventilator effectiveness, and possible rebreathing of exhaled air.

The normal pressure of end-tidal carbon dioxide ($PETCO_2$) ranges between 20 and 40 mm Hg, just slightly lower than the normal range of arterial PCO_2. Changes in $PETCO_2$ reflect changes in breathing effectiveness and may occur before hypoxia can be detected using pulse oximetry. Thus the use of both pulse oximetry and $PETCO_2$ for critically ill patients and those with respiratory problems can provide information to direct early intervention.

Factors or conditions that increase $PETCO_2$ above normal levels are those that reflect *inadequate oxygenation,* such as fever, hypoventilation, partial airway obstruction, and rebreathing exhaled air. Factors or conditions that decrease $PETCO_2$ below normal levels are those that reflect poor ventilation, such as hypothermia, poor cardiac output, hypotension, hypovolemia, pulmonary embolism, apnea, total airway obstruction, and tracheal extubation.

Pulmonary Function Tests

Pulmonary function tests (PFTs) evaluate lung function and breathing problems. These tests include lung volumes and capacities, flow rates, diffusion capacity, gas exchange, airway resistance, and distribution of ventilation. The results are interpreted by comparing the patient's data with expected findings for age, gender, race, height, weight, and smoking status.

The PFTs are useful in screening patients for lung disease even before the onset of manifestations (Dinella, 2005). Serial testing (repeated tests over time) provides objective data that may be used as a guide to treatment (e.g., changes in lung function can support a decision to continue, change, or discontinue a specific therapy). PFTs done before surgery may identify the patient at risk for lung complications after surgery. One of the most common reasons for performing such tests is to determine the cause of dyspnea. When performed while the patient exercises, PFTs help determine whether dyspnea is caused by lung or cardiac dysfunction or by muscle weakness. These tests are also useful for determining the effect of occupation on lung function and any related disability.

Patient Preparation. Explain the purpose of the tests for planning care. Advise the patient not to smoke for 6 to 8 hours before testing. According to institutional policy and procedure, bronchodilator drugs may be withheld for 4 to 6 hours before the test. The patient with breathing problems often fears further breathlessness and is anxious before these "breathing" tests. Help reduce anxiety by describing what will happen during and after the testing.

Procedure. PFTs can be performed at the bedside or in the respiratory laboratory by a respiratory therapist or respiratory technician. The patient is asked to breathe through the mouth only. A nose clip may be used to prevent air from escaping. The patient performs different breathing maneuvers while measurements are obtained. Table 29-6 describes the most commonly used PFTs and their purpose.

TABLE 29-6 **Characteristics and Purposes of Pulmonary Function Tests**

Test	Purpose
FVC (forced vital capacity) records the maximum amount of air that can be exhaled as quickly as possible after maximum inspiration.	FVC gives an indication of respiratory muscle strength and ventilatory reserve. FVC is often reduced in obstructive disease (because of air trapping) and in restrictive disease.
FEV_1 (forced expiratory volume in 1 sec) records the maximum amount of air that can be exhaled in the first second of expiration.	FEV_1 is effort dependent and declines normally with age. It is reduced in certain obstructive and restrictive disorders.
FEV_1/FVC is the ratio of expiratory volume in 1 sec to FVC.	This ratio provides a much more sensitive indication of obstruction to airflow. This ratio is the hallmark of obstructive pulmonary disease. It is normal or increased in restrictive disease.
$FEF_{25\%-75\%}$ records the forced expiratory flow over the 25%-75% volume (middle half) of the FVC.	This measure provides a more sensitive index of obstruction in the smaller airways.
FRC (functional residual capacity) is the amount of air remaining in the lungs after normal expiration. FRC test requires use of the helium dilution, nitrogen washout, or body plethysmography technique.	Increased FRC indicates hyperinflation or air trapping, which may result from obstructive pulmonary disease. FRC is normal or decreased in restrictive pulmonary diseases.
TLC (total lung capacity) is the amount of air in the lungs at the end of maximum inhalation.	Increased TLC indicates air trapping associated with obstructive pulmonary disease. Decreased TLC indicates restrictive disease.
RV (residual volume) is the amount of air remaining in the lungs at the end of a full, forced exhalation.	RV is increased in obstructive pulmonary disease such as emphysema.
DLCO (diffusion capacity of carbon monoxide) reflects the surface area of the alveolocapillary membrane. The patient inhales a small amount of CO, holds for 10 sec, and then exhales. The amount inhaled is compared with the amount exhaled.	DLCO is reduced whenever the alveolocapillary membrane is diminished, such as occurs in emphysema, pulmonary hypertension, and pulmonary fibrosis. It is increased with exercise and in conditions such as polycythemia and congestive heart disease.

Follow-up Care. Because many breathing maneuvers are performed during PFTs, observe the patient for increased dyspnea or bronchospasm after these studies. Document whether drugs were given during testing.

Exercise Testing

Exercise increases metabolism and increases gas transport because energy is used. Exercise testing assesses the patient's ability to work and perform ADLs, differentiates reasons for exercise limitation, evaluates disease influence on exercise capacity, and determines whether supplemental oxygen is needed during exercise. These tests are performed on a treadmill or bicycle or by a self-paced 12-minute walking test. The normal patient's exercise is limited by circulatory factors, whereas the pulmonary patient is limited by breathing capacity, gas exchange compromise, or both. Explain exercise testing, and assure the patient that he or she will be closely monitored by trained professionals throughout the test.

Skin Tests

Skin tests are used with other diagnostic data to identify various infectious diseases (e.g., tuberculosis), viral diseases (e.g., mononucleosis, mumps), and fungal diseases (e.g., coccidioidomycosis, histoplasmosis). Allergies and the status of the immune system also can be checked through skin testing. Exposure to the allergen or organism used in testing produces a specific reaction (delayed hypersensitivity reaction) of the patient's immune system. (See Chapters 19 and 22 for further discussion of these tests.)

Other Invasive Diagnostic Assessment

Endoscopic Examinations

Endoscopic studies to assess breathing problems include bronchoscopy, laryngoscopy, and mediastinoscopy. With *laryngoscopy*, a tube for visualization is inserted into the larynx to assess the function of the vocal cords, remove foreign bodies caught in the larynx, or obtain tissue samples for biopsy or culture. A *mediastinoscopy* is the insertion of a flexible tube through the chest wall just above the sternum into the area of the upper chest between the lungs. This procedure is performed in the operating room (OR) with the patient under general anesthesia to examine local structures for the presence of tumors and to obtain tissue samples for biopsy or culture. Most complications are related to the anesthetic agents and bleeding. The most common procedure is the bronchoscopy, described next.

A **bronchoscopy** is the insertion of a tube in the airways, usually as far as the secondary bronchi, for the purpose of viewing airway structures and obtaining tissue samples for biopsy or culture. It is used to diagnose and manage pulmonary diseases. Flexible bronchoscopy can be performed in the ICU with low-dose sedation. Rigid bronchoscopy usually requires general anesthesia and the use of the OR. A flexible bronchoscopy can be used to evaluate the airway, assist with placing or changing an endotracheal tube, collecting specimens, and diagnosing infections. Bronchoscopy is most useful to assist with cancer staging and removal of secretions that are not cleared with normal suctioning procedures.

Patient Preparation. Explain the procedure to the patient, and verify that consent for the procedure was obtained. Goals, risks, and benefits of the procedure must be discussed with the patient or the legal guardian. Patient allergies must be documented. The Joint Commission (TJC) National Patient Safety Goals require that there be a final verification or "time out" (The Joint Commission, 2007). Two patient identifiers are used to confirm the correct patient, and a verification of the procedure must be done before the start of the procedure. Laboratory tests that may be required include a complete blood count (CBC), platelet count, prothrombin time, electrolytes, and chest x-ray. The patient should be on NPO status for 4 to 8 hours before the procedure to reduce the risk for aspiration. Premedication with one of the benzodiazepines may be used to provide both sedation and amnesia. Opioids may also be used alone or in conjunction with the benzodiazepines.

Benzocaine spray as a topical anesthetic to numb the oropharynx is used cautiously, if at all. This agent may induce a condition called **methemoglobinemia,** which is the conversion of normal hemoglobin to methemoglobin (Wesley, 2006). Methemoglobin is an altered iron state that does not carry oxygen, resulting in tissue hypoxia. Other topical anesthetic sprays, such as lidocaine, appear less likely to induce this problem.

The normal blood level of methemoglobin is less than 1%. When this level increases, tissue oxygenation is reduced. Cyanosis occurs with methemoglobin levels between 10% and 20%. Anxiety, tachycardia, and lethargy develop at levels between 20% and 50%. Death can occur when levels reach 50% to 70%. *Methemoglobinemia should be suspected if a patient becomes cyanotic after receiving a topical anesthetic, if he or she does not respond to supplemental oxygen, and if blood is a characteristic chocolate-brown in color. Notify the Rapid Response Team.* It can be reversed with supplemental oxygen and IV administration of 1% methylene blue (1 to 2 mg/kg).

Procedure. The procedure can be done in a bronchoscopy suite (the patient does not need to hospitalized) or can be done at the bedside, especially in an ICU. The bronchoscope is inserted either through the naris or the oropharynx. Maintain IV access, and continuously monitor the patient's pulse, blood pressure, respiratory rate, and oxygen saturation. Apply supplemental oxygen.

Follow-up Care. Monitor the patient until the effects of the sedation have resolved and a gag reflex has returned. Continue to monitor the patient's vital signs, including oxygen saturation, and assess breath sounds every 15 minutes for the first 2 hours. Also assess for potential complications. These may include bleeding, infection, or hypoxemia (possibly related to a pneumothorax or methemoglobinemia).

Thoracentesis

Thoracentesis is the aspiration of pleural fluid or air from the pleural space. It can be used for diagnosis or treatment. Microscopic examination of the pleural fluid helps in making a diagnosis. Pleural fluid may be drained to relieve blood vessel or lung compression and the respiratory distress caused by cancer, empyema, pleurisy, or tuberculosis. Drugs can also be instilled into the pleural space during thoracentesis.

Patient Preparation. Patient preparation is essential before thoracentesis to ensure cooperation during the procedure and to prevent complications. Tell the patient to expect a stinging sensation from the local anesthetic agent and a feeling of pressure when the needle is inserted. Stress the importance of not moving during the procedure (avoiding coughing, deep breathing, or sudden movement) to avoid puncture of the pleura or lung.

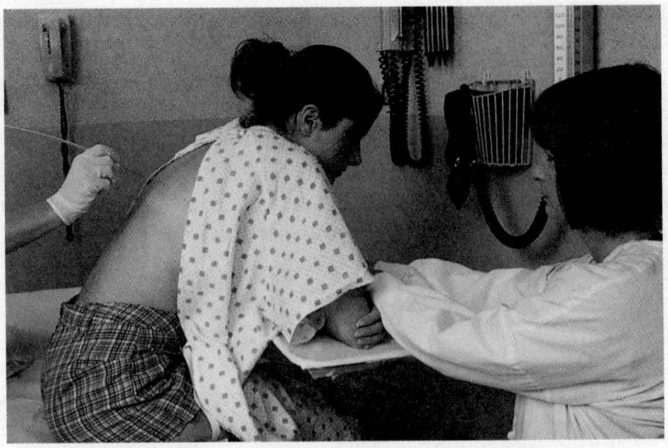

Fig. 29-11 • Position for thoracentesis.

Fig. 29-11 shows the best position for thoracentesis. This position widens the spaces between the ribs and permits easy access to the pleural fluid. Properly position and physically support the patient during the procedure. Use pillows to make the patient comfortable and to provide physical support. When the sitting position is used for the procedure, stand in front of the patient to prevent the table from moving and the patient from falling.

Before the procedure, ask the patient about any allergy to local anesthetic agents. Verify that the patient has signed an informed consent. The entire chest or back is exposed, and the aspiration site is shaved if necessary. The actual site depends on the volume and location of the effusion (determined by x-rays, sonography, and percussion).

Procedure. Thoracentesis is often performed at the bedside by a nurse practitioner or a physician, although computed tomography or ultrasound may be used to guide it. The person performing the procedure and any assistants wear goggles and masks to prevent accidental eye or oral splash exposure to the pleural fluid. After draping the patient and cleaning the skin with an antiseptic agent, a local anesthetic is injected into the selected site. Keep the patient informed of the procedure while observing for shock, pain, nausea, pallor, diaphoresis, cyanosis, tachypnea, and dyspnea.

The short 18- to 25-gauge thoracentesis needle (with an attached syringe) is advanced into the pleural space. Gentle suction is applied as the fluid in the pleural space is slowly aspirated. A vacuum collection bottle is sometimes needed to remove larger volumes of fluid. To prevent re-expansion pulmonary edema, usually no more than 1000 mL of fluid is removed at one time. If a pleural biopsy is to be performed, a second, larger needle with a cutting edge and collection chamber is used. After the needle is withdrawn, pressure is applied to the puncture site and a small sterile dressing is applied.

Follow-up Care. After thoracentesis, a chest x-ray is performed to rule out possible pneumothorax and **mediastinal shift** (shift of central thoracic structures toward one side). Monitor vital signs, and auscultate breath sounds for absent or reduced sounds on the affected side. Check the puncture site and dressing for leakage or bleeding. Also assess for complications, such as reaccumulation of fluid in the pleural space, subcutaneous emphysema, infection, and tension pneumothorax. Urge the patient to breathe deeply to promote expansion of the lung. Document the procedure, including the patient's response; the volume and character of the fluid removed; any specimens sent to the laboratory; the location of the puncture site; and respiratory assessment findings before, during, and after the procedure (Rushing, 2006).

Teach the patient about the manifestations of a **pneumothorax** (partial or complete collapse of the lung), which can occur within the first 24 hours after a thoracentesis. Manifestations include:

- Pain on the affected side that is worse at the end of inhalation and the end of exhalation
- Rapid heart rate
- Rapid, shallow respirations
- A feeling of air hunger
- Prominence of the affected side that does not move in and out with respiratory effort
- Trachea slanted more to the unaffected side instead of being in the center of the neck

Instruct the patient to come to the emergency department immediately if these manifestations occur.

Lung Biopsy

A lung biopsy is performed to obtain tissue for histologic analysis, culture, or cytologic examination. The tissue samples are used to make a definite diagnosis about the type of cancer, infection, inflammation, or lung disease. There are several types of lung biopsies. The site and extent of the lesion determine which one is used. Transbronchial biopsy (TBB) and transbronchial needle aspiration (TBNA) are performed during bronchoscopy. Transthoracic needle aspiration is an approach through the skin (percutaneous) for areas that cannot be reached by bronchoscopy. An open lung biopsy is performed in the operating room.

Patient Preparation. The patient may worry about the outcome of the biopsy and may associate the term *biopsy* with *cancer.* Explain what to expect before and after the procedure, and explore the patient's feelings and fears. To reduce discomfort and anxiety, an analgesic or sedative may be prescribed before the procedure. Inform the patient undergoing percutaneous biopsy that discomfort is reduced with a local anesthetic agent but that pressure may be felt during needle insertion and tissue aspiration. Open lung biopsy is performed in the operating room with the patient under general anesthesia, and the usual preparations before surgery apply (see Chapter 16).

Procedure. Percutaneous lung biopsy may be performed in the patient's room or in the radiology department after an informed consent has been obtained. Fluoroscopy or CT is often used to visualize more clearly the area undergoing biopsy and to guide the procedure. Positioning of the patient is similar to that for thoracentesis. The skin is cleansed with an antiseptic agent, and a local anesthetic is given. Under sterile conditions, a spinal-type 18- to 22-gauge needle is inserted through the skin into the desired area (e.g., tissue, nodule, lymph node) and tissue needed for microscopic examination is obtained. Apply a dressing after the procedure.

An open lung biopsy is performed in the operating room. The patient undergoes a thoracotomy in which lung tissue is exposed. At least two tissue specimens are taken (usually from an upper lobe and a lower lobe site). A chest tube is placed to remove air and fluid so the lung can re-inflate, and then the chest is closed.

Follow-up Care. Monitor the patient's vital signs and breath sounds at least every 4 hours for 24 hours, and assess for signs of respiratory distress (e.g., dyspnea, pallor, diaphoresis, tachypnea). Pneumothorax is a serious complication of needle biopsy and open lung biopsy. Report reduced or absent breath sounds immediately. Monitor for hemoptysis (which may be scant and transient) or, in rare cases, for frank bleeding from vascular or lung trauma.

DECISION-MAKING CHALLENGE
Critical Rescue

The patient is a 45-year-old woman who had a bronchoscopy under local (topical) anesthesia about 15 minutes ago. She tells you that she is thirsty and scared and that her voice seems "squeaky." She also wants to smoke a cigarette because she has not had one for over 12 hours.

Her vital signs taken 10 minutes ago indicate a respiratory rate of 24 and an oxygen saturation of 92%. When you retake her vital signs, her respiratory rate is 28 and her oxygen saturation is 90%.

1. Are these vital signs of concern? Why or why not?
2. What are the possible causes of these changes?
3. Should you give her something to drink now?
4. Should she be allowed to smoke now? Why?
5. What should be your next action?

evolve For suggested answer guidelines, go to http://evolve.elsevier.com/Iggy/.

HUMAN NEEDS ASSESSMENT REVIEW

What should you expect to NOTICE in a patient with adequate oxygenation and tissue perfusion related to respiratory function?

Vital Signs

- Respiratory rate and heart rate within normal range
- Oxygen saturation of 95% or higher

Physical Assessment

- Able to speak a sentence of 12 words without stopping for breath
- Able to walk and talk without stopping for breath
- Skin color normal (no cyanosis, pallor, or jaundice)
- Oral mucous membrane and nail beds pink with rapid capillary refill
- Fingertips and nails normal-shaped, no clubbing
- Anterior to posterior diameter of chest about two-thirds smaller than lateral diameter
- Space between each rib no larger than the breadth of the patient's finger
- Usually breathes in through the nose and out through the mouth or nose
- Breathing quiet

- Air movement heard (with a stethoscope) in all lobes of both lungs
- Sputum production minimal, clear or white
- Muscle development even with no muscle loss on arms and legs
- Weight proportionate to height; does not appear underweight

Psychological Assessment

- Oriented and not confused
- Energy level good, can engage in desired work, recreational, and personal activities

Laboratory Assessment

- Red blood cell, hemoglobin, hematocrit, and white blood cell levels within normal limits for age and gender

GET READY FOR THE NCLEX EXAMINATION!

Key Points

Review these Key Points for each NCLEX Examination Client Needs Category.

Health Promotion and Maintenance

- Encourage all people to use masks and adequate ventilation when exposed to inhalation irritants.

Psychosocial Integrity

- Explain all diagnostic procedures, restrictions, and follow-up care to the patient scheduled for tests.

Physiological Integrity

- Assess the degree to which breathing problems interfere with the patient's ability to perform ADLs.
- Document any known specific allergies that have respiratory manifestations.
- Ask the patient about recent travel.
- Assess the airway and breathing effectiveness for any patient who has shortness of breath or any change in mental status.
- Assess the patient's respiratory status every 15 minutes for at least the first 2 hours after undergoing an endoscopic test for respiratory disorders.

Additional Study Resources

Go to your Companion CD or Evolve at http://evolve.elsevier.com/Iggy/ for *Self-Assessment Questions for the NCLEX Examination.*

Go to Evolve at http://evolve.elsevier.com/Iggy/ for *Prioritization and Delegation Questions for the NCLEX Examination.*

SELECTED BIBLIOGRAPHY

Bradley, R. (2007). Improving respiratory assessment skills. *The Journal for Nurse Practitioners, 3*(4), 276-277.

DeMeulenaere, S. (2007). Pulse oximetry: Uses and limitations. *The Journal for Nurse Practitioners, 3*(5), 312-317.

Dinella, J. (2005). The ins and outs of pulmonary function testing. *Nursing2005, 35*(12), 70-71.

Fernadez, M., Burns, K., Calhoun, B., George, S., Martin, B., & Weaver, C. (2007). Evaluation of a new pulse oximeter sensor. *American Journal of Critical Care, 16*(2), 146-151.

Gordon, M. (2007). *Manual of nursing diagnosis* (11th ed.). Boston: Jones & Bartlett.

Jarvis, C. (2008). *Physical examination and health assessment* (5th ed.). Philadelphia: Saunders.

McCance, K., & Huether, S. (2006). *Pathophysiology: The biologic basis for disease in adults and children* (5th ed.). St. Louis: Mosby.

Meiner, S., & Lueckenotte, A. (Eds.). (2006). *Gerontologic nursing* (3rd ed.). St. Louis: Mosby.

Nussbaum, R., McInnes, R., & Willard, H. (2007). *Thompson & Thompson: Genetics in medicine* (7th ed.). Philadelphia: Saunders.

Pagana, K., & Pagana, T. (2006). *Mosby's manual of diagnostic and laboratory tests* (3rd ed.). St. Louis: Mosby.

Rodden, A., Spicer, L., Diaz, V., & Steyer, T. (2007). Does fingernail polish affect pulse oximeter readings? *Intensive and Critical Care Nursing, 23*(1), 51-55.

Rushing, J. (2006). Assisting with thoracentesis. *Nursing2006, 36*(12), 18.

Swiderski, D., & Byrum, D. (2007). Are you an ABG ace? *American Nurse Today, 2*(4), 18-21.

The Joint Commission. (2007). *National Patient Safety Goals: Hospital/critical access hospital.* Retrieved September 2007, from www.jointcommission.org/patientsafety/.

Wesley, C. (2006). Responding to methemoglobinemia after bronchoscopy. *Nursing2006, 36*(12), 64cc1-64cc2.

Care of Patients Requiring Oxygen Therapy or Tracheostomy

30

CHAPTER

Harry C. Rees

LEARNING OUTCOMES

For clinical competence and success on the NCLEX Examination, study this chapter with these Learning Outcomes in mind:

Safe and Effective Care Environment

1. Act as a patient advocate for patients receiving oxygen or who have tracheostomies.
2. Protect from injury the patient receiving oxygen or who has a tracheostomy.
3. Use medical asepsis when providing tracheostomy care.
4. Verify safe use of appropriate oxygen delivery systems and tracheostomy equipment.

Health Promotion and Maintenance

5. Teach the patient requiring oxygen therapy to not smoke when using oxygen.

Psychosocial Integrity

6. Support the patient and family in coping with changes in breathing status and the need for a tracheostomy.
7. Develop and evaluate an appropriate nonverbal form of communication for a patient with a tracheostomy.

Physiological Integrity

8. Perform a focused respiratory assessment and re-assessment to determine adequacy of oxygenation and tissue perfusion.
9. Administer oxygen therapy by nasal cannula, mask, endotracheal tube, or tracheal tube, and evaluate the patient's response.
10. Apply knowledge of anatomy and physiology to prevent aspiration in a patient with a tracheostomy.
11. Teach the patient and family about home management of oxygen therapy or tracheostomy.
12. Assess for complications of oxygen therapy for those patients whose respiratory efforts are controlled by the hypoxic drive.
13. Use laboratory data and clinical manifestations to determine the presence of hypoxemia or hypercarbia.

Go to your Companion CD or Evolve at http://evolve.elsevier.com/Iggy/ for *Self-Assessment Questions for the NCLEX Examination* keyed to these Learning Outcomes.

All cells and tissues need oxygen to live and function. Three systems—the respiratory system, the cardiovascular system, and the hematologic system—work together to ensure sufficient tissue perfusion with oxygen for cell survival and proper function (see Fig. 29-1). The *human need for oxygenation and tissue perfusion* can go unmet as a result of many problems with the lungs. When a problem occurs in the respiratory system that interferes with adequate oxygenation, both the cardiac system and the hematologic system adjust and work harder to restore balance and maintain oxygenation and tissue perfusion (Fig. 30-1). Oxygen therapy and the use of a tracheostomy are interventions that can help improve *oxygenation and tissue perfusion* and, at the same time, reduce the burden on the cardiovascular and hematologic systems.

OXYGEN THERAPY

Overview

Oxygen (O_2) is a gas that is essential for life, as well as a drug used for relief of **hypoxemia** (low levels of oxygen in the blood) and **hypoxia** (decreased tissue oxygenation). The oxygen content of atmospheric air is about 21%. Oxygen therapy is prescribed when the oxygen needs of the patient cannot be met by atmospheric or "room air" alone. It is used for both acute and chronic breathing problems that cause decreased blood and tissue oxygen levels as indicated by decreased partial pressure of arterial oxygen (Pao_2) levels or by decreased arterial oxygen saturation (Sao_2). Conditions outside the respiratory system that increase oxygen demand, decrease oxygen-carrying capability of the blood, or decrease cardiac output also are indications for oxygen therapy. Such conditions include heart failure, sepsis, fever, some poisons, and decreased hemoglobin levels or poor hemoglobin quality.

The goal of oxygen therapy is to use the lowest *fraction of inspired oxygen* (FiO_2) to have an acceptable blood oxygen level without causing harmful side effects. *Although oxygen improves the* PaO_2 *level, it does not cure the problem or stop the disease process.* The average patient with some degree of hypoxia requires an oxygen flow of 2 to 4 L/min via nasal cannula or up to 40% via Venturi mask. The patient who is hypoxemic and has chronic **hypercarbia** (increased partial pressure of arterial carbon dioxide [$PaCO_2$] levels) needs lower levels of oxygen delivery, usually 1 to 2 L/min via nasal cannula, to prevent decreased respiratory effort. (A low PaO_2 level is this patient's primary drive for breathing.)

Patient-Centered Collaborative Care

Assessment

Arterial blood gas (ABG) analysis is the best measure for determining the need for oxygen therapy and for evaluating its effects. Oxygen need can also be determined by noninvasive monitoring, such as pulse oximetry.

Common Nursing Diagnoses and Collaborative Problems

Nursing diagnoses that may apply to patients requiring oxygen therapy include:

- Anxiety related to hypoxemia
- Acute Confusion related to hypoxemia
- Impaired Spontaneous Ventilation related to oxygen therapy

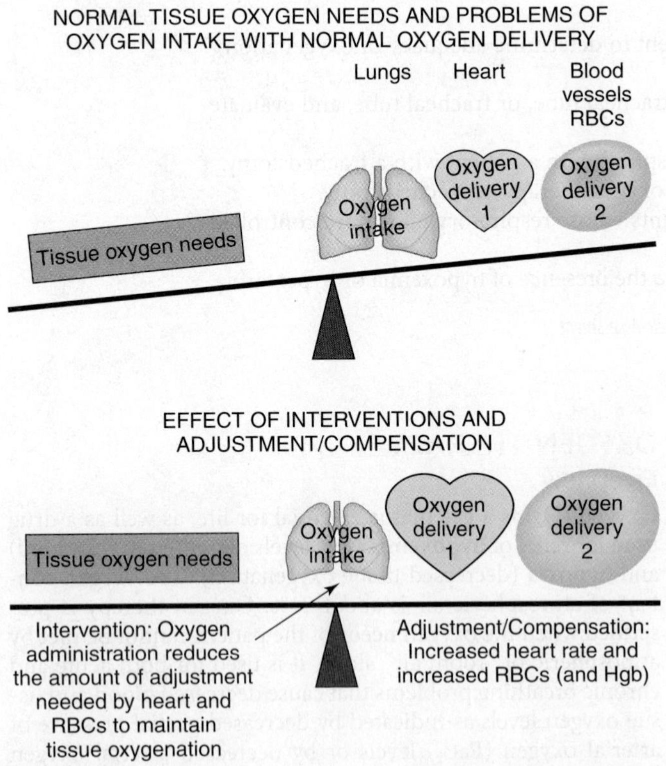
NORMAL TISSUE OXYGEN NEEDS AND PROBLEMS OF OXYGEN INTAKE WITH NORMAL OXYGEN DELIVERY
Lungs
Heart
Blood vessels RBCs
Oxygen intake
Oxygen delivery 1
Oxygen delivery 2
Tissue oxygen needs
EFFECT OF INTERVENTIONS AND ADJUSTMENT/COMPENSATION
Oxygen intake
Oxygen delivery 1
Oxygen delivery 2
Tissue oxygen needs
Intervention: Oxygen administration reduces the amount of adjustment needed by heart and RBCs to maintain tissue oxygenation
Adjustment/Compensation: Increased heart rate and increased RBCs (and Hgb)

Fig. 30-1 • Restoration of adequate oxygenation and tissue perfusion by oxygen delivery adjustments and oxygen therapy when respiratory problems interfere with meeting tissue oxygen needs.

Interventions

Before starting oxygen therapy and while caring for a patient receiving oxygen therapy, you must be knowledgeable about oxygen hazards and complications. Know the rationale and the expected outcome related to oxygen therapy for each patient receiving oxygen. Chart 30-1 lists NIC interventions for patients using oxygen therapy.

Hazards and Complications of Oxygen Therapy

Combustion

Oxygen itself does not burn, but it supports and enhances combustion. Therefore a fire burns more readily in the presence of oxygen. For example, when the oxygen content of the air around a lighted cigarette is nearly 50%, the entire cigarette flames up and can catch items nearby on fire (Edelman et al., 2008). Open fires, even small ones like candles or cigarettes, should not be in the same room during oxygen therapy. Take special precautions during oxygen delivery, including posting a sign on the door of the patient's room. Smoking is prohibited in the patient's room, including at home, when oxygen is in use.

All electrical equipment must be grounded to prevent fires from electrical arcing sparks. Grounded plugs may have three prongs or only two prongs with one prong being wider than the other. Grounded outlets usually have a green or red dot on the plate. Frayed cords must be repaired because they can cause a spark that can ignite a flame. Flammable solutions (containing high concentrations of alcohol or oil) are not used in rooms in which oxygen is in use.

Chart 30-1 NIC INTERVENTION ACTIVITIES

The Patient with Respiratory Problems

Oxygen Therapy: *Administration of oxygen and monitoring of its effectiveness*

- Clear oral, nasal, and tracheal secretions, as appropriate.
- Maintain airway patency.
- Set up oxygen equipment and administer through a heated, humidified system.
- Monitor the oxygen liter flow.
- Monitor position of oxygen delivery device.
- Periodically check oxygen delivery device to ensure that the prescribed concentration is being delivered.
- Monitor the effectiveness of oxygen therapy (e.g., pulse oximetry, ABGs), as appropriate.
- Ensure replacement of oxygen mask/cannula whenever the device is removed.
- Observe for signs of oxygen-induced hypoventilation.
- Monitor for signs of oxygen toxicity and absorption atelectasis.
- Monitor oxygen equipment to ensure that it is not interfering with the patient's attempts to breathe.
- Monitor patient's anxiety related to need for oxygen therapy.
- Monitor for skin breakdown from friction of oxygen device.
- Provide for oxygen when patient is transported.
- Instruct patient and family about use of oxygen at home.
- Arrange for use of oxygen devices that facilitate mobility and teach patient accordingly.

NIC intervention activities selected from Bulechek, G.M., Butcher, H.K., & McCloskey Dochterman, J. (Eds.). (2008). *Nursing interventions classification (NIC)* (5th ed.). St. Louis: Mosby. No part of this work is to be altered without prior written permission from the Publisher.

ABG, Arterial blood gas.

Oxygen-Induced Hypoventilation

Assess for oxygen-induced hypoventilation in the patient whose main respiratory drive is hypoxia (hypoxic drive), such as in the patient with chronic lung disease who also has carbon dioxide retention **(hypercarbia).** The arterial carbon dioxide ($Paco_2$) level for these patients gradually rises over time. The central chemoreceptors in the brain (medulla) are normally sensitive to increased $Paco_2$ levels. When these receptors are active, they stimulate breathing and increase respiratory rate. When the $Paco_2$ increases gradually to above 60 to 65 mm Hg, this normal mechanism no longer functions. The central chemoreceptors lose sensitivity to increased levels of $Paco_2$ and do not respond by increasing the rate and depth of respiration. This loss of sensitivity to high levels of $Paco_2$ is called **CO_2 narcosis.** For these patients, the stimulus to breathe is a *decreased arterial oxygen level.* The low oxygen levels are sensed by peripheral chemoreceptors in the carotid sinus areas and aortic arch. When arterial oxygen (Pao_2) levels drop (hypoxemia), these receptors signal the brain to increase the respiratory rate and depth; this is known as the *hypoxic drive* to breathe.

The hypoxic drive occurs only in the presence of severely elevated $Paco_2$ levels that have occurred slowly, over years (i.e., in the patient who has hypoxemia and hypercarbia). When the patient with low Pao_2 levels and high $Paco_2$ levels receives oxygen therapy, the Pao_2 level increases, removing the stimulation for breathing, and the patient has respiratory depression. (The patient being ventilated mechanically is not at risk for this complication.)

Oxygen therapy is prescribed at the lowest liter flow (usually 1, 2, or 3 L/min) needed to treat the hypoxemia. A system that delivers more precise oxygen levels (e.g., a Venturi mask) is preferred for this patient. However, a patient with chronic obstructive pulmonary disease may not tolerate a facemask.

Closely monitor the respiratory rate and depth while the patient is receiving oxygen. Monitoring is especially important when it is the first time he or she receives oxygen or when the $Paco_2$ levels are not known. Manifestations of hypoventilation are seen during the first 30 minutes of oxygen therapy. The patient's color improves (from ashen or gray to pink) because of an increase in the Pao_2 level before the apnea or respiratory arrest occurs from loss of the hypoxic drive. Therefore carefully monitor the level of consciousness, respiratory pattern and rate, and pulse oximetry for those at risk for oxygen-induced hypoventilation, apnea, and respiratory arrest. *Although oxygen-induced hypoventilation is a serious concern, untreated or inadequately treated hypoxemia is a greater threat to life.*

Oxygen Toxicity

Oxygen toxicity is related to the concentration of oxygen delivered, duration of oxygen therapy, and degree of lung disease present. In general, an oxygen level greater than 50% given continuously for more than 24 to 48 hours may damage the lungs. *Although oxygen toxicity is a serious concern, inadequately treated hypoxemia is a greater threat to life.*

The causes and manifestations of lung injury from oxygen toxicity are the same as those for acute respiratory distress syndrome (ARDS) (see Chapter 34). Initial symptoms include nonproductive cough, substernal chest pain, GI upset, and dyspnea. As exposure to high levels of oxygen continues, the symptoms become more severe with decreased vital capacity, decreased compliance (which results in more dyspnea), crackles, and hypoxemia. Prolonged exposure to high oxygen levels damages lung tissues. Atelectasis, pulmonary edema, hemorrhage, and hyaline membrane formation result. Surviving this critical condition depends on correcting the underlying disease process and decreasing the oxygen amount delivered.

The toxic effects of oxygen are difficult to treat, making prevention a priority. The lowest level of oxygen needed to maintain oxygenation and prevent oxygen toxicity is prescribed. Closely monitor arterial blood gases (ABGs) during oxygen therapy, and notify the physician of Pao_2 levels greater than 90 mm Hg. Also monitor the prescribed oxygen level and length of therapy to identify the patient at higher risk. High oxygen levels are avoided unless absolutely necessary. The use of continuous positive airway pressure (CPAP) with an oxygen mask, bi-level positive airway pressure (BiPAP), or positive end-expiratory pressure (PEEP) on the mechanical ventilator (see Chapter 34) may reduce the amount of oxygen needed. As soon as the patient's condition allows, the prescribed amount of oxygen is decreased.

Absorption Atelectasis

Nitrogen in the air normally helps maintain patent airways and alveoli. Making up 79% of room air, nitrogen prevents alveolar collapse. When high oxygen levels are delivered, nitrogen is diluted, oxygen diffuses from the alveoli into the circulation, and the alveoli collapse. Collapsed alveoli cause atelectasis (called *absorption atelectasis*), which is detected by auscultation. Monitor the patient closely for crackles and decreased breath sounds every 1 to 2 hours when oxygen therapy is started and as often as needed thereafter.

Drying of the Mucous Membranes

When an oxygen flow rate higher than 4 L/min is needed, humidity is added to the delivery system (Fig. 30-2). Ensure that oxygen can be seen bubbling through the water in the humidifier.

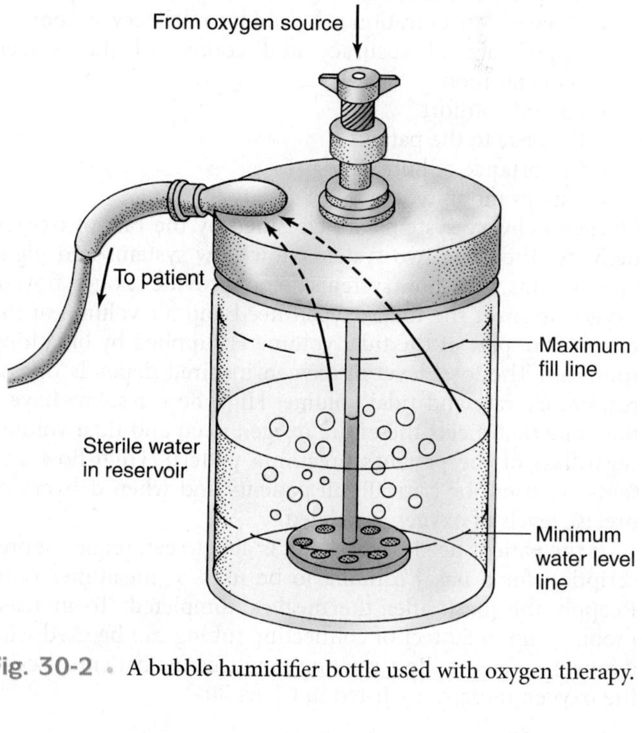
From oxygen source
To patient
Maximum fill line
Sterile water in reservoir
Minimum water level line

Fig. 30-2 • A bubble humidifier bottle used with oxygen therapy.

Oxygen can also be humidified via a large-volume jet nebulizer in mist form (aerosol). A heated nebulizer raises the humidity even more and is used when oxygen is delivered through an artificial airway. Usually the upper airway passages warm the air during breathing, but these passages are bypassed when an artificial airway, such as an endotracheal tube, is in use.

For the patient to receive properly humidified oxygen, the humidifier or nebulizer must have a sufficient amount of sterile water and the flow rate must be adequate. Condensation often forms in the tubing. Remove this condensation as it collects by disconnecting the tubing and emptying the water. Minimize the time the tubing is disconnected because the patient does not receive oxygen during this period. Some humidifiers and nebulizers have a water trap that hangs from the tubing so that the condensation can be drained without disconnecting. *To prevent bacterial contamination, never drain the fluid back into the humidifier or nebulizer.* Check the water level and change the humidifier as needed.

Infection

The humidifier or nebulizer may be a source of bacteria, especially if it is heated. *Pseudomonas aeruginosa* is often the organism involved. Oxygen delivery equipment such as cannulas and masks can also harbor organisms. Change equipment as per policy or protocol, which ranges from every 24 hours for humidification systems to every 7 days or whenever necessary for cannulas and masks.

Oxygen Delivery Systems

Oxygen can be delivered by many systems. Regardless of the type of delivery system used, it is important to understand its indications, advantages, and disadvantages. Use the equipment properly, and ensure appropriate equipment maintenance. Consult a respiratory therapist whenever there is a question or concern about an oxygen delivery system.

The type of delivery system used depends on:

- Oxygen concentration required by the patient
- Oxygen concentration achieved by a delivery system
- Importance of accuracy and control of the oxygen concentration
- Patient comfort
- Expense to the patient
- Importance of humidity
- Patient mobility

Oxygen delivery systems are classified by the rate of oxygen delivery. There are two systems: low-flow systems and high-flow systems. Low-flow systems do not provide enough flow of oxygen to meet the total oxygen need and air volume of the patient. So, part of the tidal volume is supplied by breathing room air. The total level of oxygen inspired depends on the respiratory rate and tidal volume. High-flow systems have a flow rate that meets the entire oxygen need and tidal volume regardless of the patient's breathing pattern. High-flow systems are used for critically ill patients and when delivery of precise levels of oxygen is needed.

If the patient needs a mask but is able to eat, request a prescription for a nasal cannula to be used at mealtimes only. Reapply the mask after the meal is completed. To increase mobility, up to 50 feet of connecting tubing can be used with connecting pieces. Best nursing practices for patients receiving oxygen therapy are listed in Chart 30-2.

Chart 30-2 BEST PRACTICE FOR PATIENT SAFETY & QUALITY CARE

Oxygen Therapy

- Check the physician's prescription with the type of delivery system and liter flow or percentage of oxygen actually in use.
- Obtain a prescription for humidification if oxygen is being delivered at 4 L/min or more.
- Be sure the oxygen and humidification equipment is functioning properly.
- Check the skin around the patient's ears, back of the neck, and face every 4 to 8 hours for pressure points and signs of irritation.
- Ensure that mouth care is provided every 8 hours and as needed; assess nasal and oral mucous membranes for cracks or other signs of dryness.
- Pad the elastic band and change its position frequently to prevent skin breakdown.
- Pad tubing in areas that put pressure on the skin.
- Cleanse the cannula or mask by rinsing with clear, warm water every 4 to 8 hours or as needed.
- Cleanse skin under the tubing, straps, and mask every 4 to 8 hours or as needed.
- Lubricate the patient's nostrils, face, and lips with nonpetroleum cream to relieve the drying effects of oxygen.
- Position the tubing so it does not pull on the patient's face, nose, or artificial airway.
- Ensure that there is no smoking and that no candles or matches are lit in the immediate area.
- Assess and document the patient's response to oxygen therapy.
- Provide the patient with ongoing teaching and reassurance to enhance his or her adherence with oxygen therapy.

Low-Flow Oxygen Delivery Systems

Low-flow delivery systems include the nasal cannula, simple facemask, partial rebreather mask, and non-rebreather mask (Table 30-1). These systems are inexpensive, easy to use, and fairly comfortable. A disadvantage is that the actual amount of oxygen delivered varies and depends on the patient's breathing pattern. The oxygen is diluted with room air (21% oxygen), which lowers the amount of oxygen actually inspired.

Nasal Cannula. The nasal cannula, or nasal prongs (Fig. 30-3), is used at flow rates of 1 to 6 L/min. Oxygen concentrations of 24% (at 1 L/min) to 44% (at 6 L/min) can be achieved. Flow rates greater than 6 L/min do not increase oxygenation because the **anatomic dead space** (places where air flows but the structures are too thick for gas exchange) is full. In addition, high flow rates increase mucosal irritation. With the use of a nasal cannula, an effective oxygen level can be delivered to patients who are nose breathers and those who are mouth breathers.

The nasal cannula is often used for chronic lung disease and for any patient needing long-term oxygen therapy. The patient who retains carbon dioxide rarely is prescribed to receive oxygen at a rate higher than 2 to 3 L/min because of the risk for losing the drive to breathe, thereby increasing the risk for apnea or respiratory arrest. Place the nasal prongs in the nostrils, with the openings facing the patient, following the natural anatomic curve of the nares.

Facemasks. Facemasks for oxygen delivery can deliver a wide range of oxygen flow rates and concentrations.

TABLE 30-1 Comparison of Low-Flow Oxygen Delivery Systems

FiO_2 Delivered	Nursing Interventions	Rationales
NASAL CANNULA		
24%-40% FiO_2 at 1-6 L/min ≈24% at 1 L/min ≈28% at 2 L/min ≈32% at 3 L/min ≈36% at 4 L/min ≈40% at 5 L/min ≈44% at 6 L/min	Ensure that prongs are in the nares properly.	A poorly fitting nasal cannula leads to hypoxemia and skin breakdown.
	Provide water-soluble jelly to nares PRN.	This substance prevents mucosal irritation related to the drying effect of oxygen; promotes comfort.
	Assess the patency of the nostrils.	Congestion or a deviated septum prevents effective delivery of oxygen through the nares.
	Assess the patient for changes in respiratory rate and depth.	The respiratory pattern affects the amount of oxygen delivered. A different delivery system may be needed.
SIMPLE FACEMASK		
40%-60% FiO_2 at 5-8 L/min; flow rate must be set at least at 5 L/min to flush mask of carbon dioxide ≈40% at 5 L/min ≈45%-50% at 6 L/min ≈55%-60% at 8 L/min	Be sure mask fits securely over nose and mouth.	A poorly fitting mask reduces the FiO_2 delivered.
	Assess skin and provide skin care to the area covered by the mask.	Pressure and moisture under the mask may cause skin breakdown.
	Monitor the patient closely for risk of aspiration.	The mask limits the patient's ability to clear the mouth, especially if vomiting occurs.
	Provide emotional support to the patient who feels claustrophobic.	Emotional support decreases anxiety, which contributes to a claustrophobic feeling.
	Suggest to the health care provider to switch the patient from a mask to the nasal cannula during eating.	Use of the cannula prevents hypoxemia during eating.
PARTIAL REBREATHER MASK		
60%-75% at 6-11 L/min, a liter flow rate high enough to maintain reservoir bag two-thirds full during inspiration and expiration	Make sure that the reservoir does not twist or kink, which results in a deflated bag.	Deflation results in decreased oxygen delivered and rebreathing of exhaled air.
	Adjust the flow rate to keep the reservoir bag inflated.	The flow rate is adjusted to meet the pattern of the patient.
NON-REBREATHER MASK		
80%-95% FiO_2 at liter flow to maintain reservoir bag two-thirds full	Interventions as for partial rebreather mask; this patient requires close monitoring.	Rationales as for partial rebreather mask. Monitoring ensures proper functioning and prevents harm.
	Make sure that valves and rubber flaps are patent, functional, and not stuck. Remove mucus or saliva.	Valves should open during expiration and close during inhalation to prevent dramatic decrease in FiO_2. Suffocation can occur if the reservoir bag kinks or if the oxygen source disconnects.
	Closely assess the patient on increased FiO_2 via non-rebreather mask. Intubation is the only way to provide more precise FiO_2.	The patient may require intubation.

FiO_2, Fraction of inspired oxygen.

Simple facemasks are used to deliver oxygen concentrations of 40% to 60% for short-term oxygen therapy or in an emergency (Fig. 30-4). A minimum flow rate of 5 L/min is needed to prevent the rebreathing of exhaled air. Give special attention to skin care under the mask and the elastic strap and to the proper fitting of the mask so that inspired oxygen levels are maintained.

Partial rebreather masks provide oxygen concentrations of 60% to 75% with flow rates of 6 to 11 L/min. It is a mask with a reservoir bag but no flaps (Fig. 30-5). The patient first rebreathes with each breath one third of the exhaled tidal volume, which is high in oxygen and provides a high fraction of inspired oxygen (FiO_2). Be sure that the bag remains slightly inflated at the end of inspiration; otherwise, he or she will not be getting the desired amount of oxygen. If needed, call the respiratory therapist for assistance.

Non-rebreather masks provide the highest oxygen level of the low-flow systems and can deliver an FiO_2 greater than 90%, depending on the patient's breathing pattern. This type of mask is often used with patients whose respiratory status is unstable and who may require intubation.

The non-rebreather mask has a one-way valve between the mask and the reservoir and two flaps over the exhalation ports (Fig. 30-6). The valve allows the patient to draw all needed oxygen from the reservoir bag, and the flaps prevent room air from entering through the exhalation ports (room air would dilute the oxygen concentration). During exhalation, air leaves through these exhalation ports while the one-way valve pre-

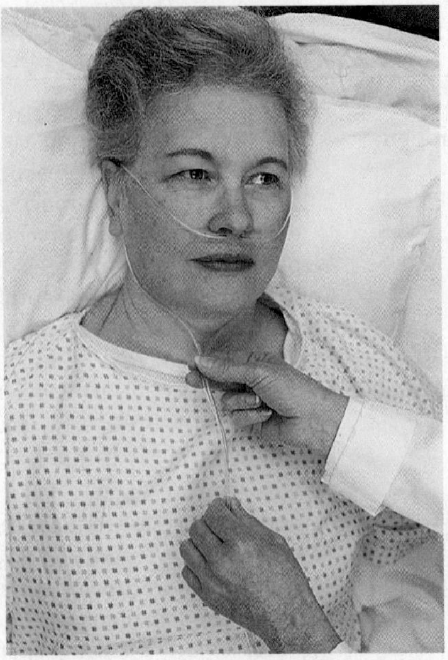

Fig. 30-3 • A nasal cannula (prongs).

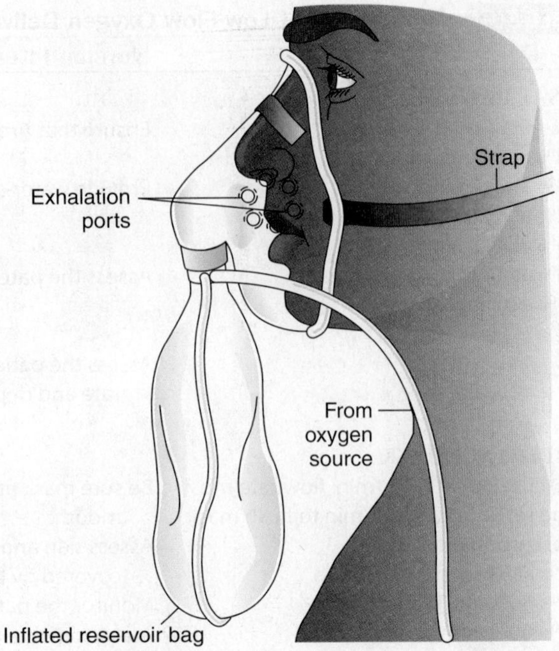
Strap
Exhalation ports
From oxygen source
Inflated reservoir bag

Fig. 30-5 • A partial rebreather mask.

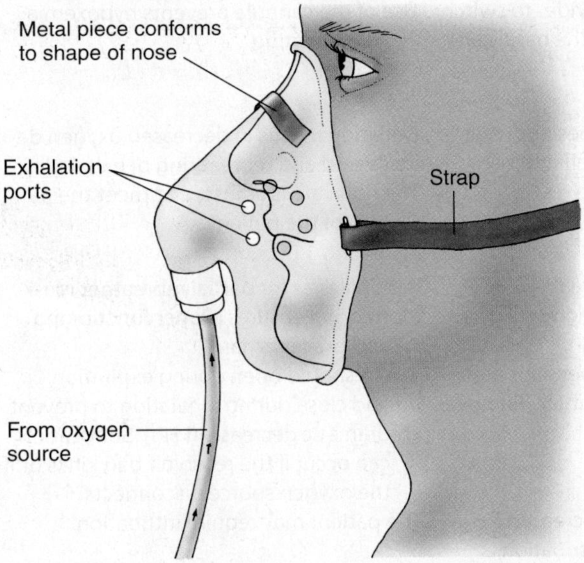
Metal piece conforms to shape of nose
Exhalation ports
Strap
From oxygen source

Fig. 30-4 • A simple facemask used to deliver oxygen.

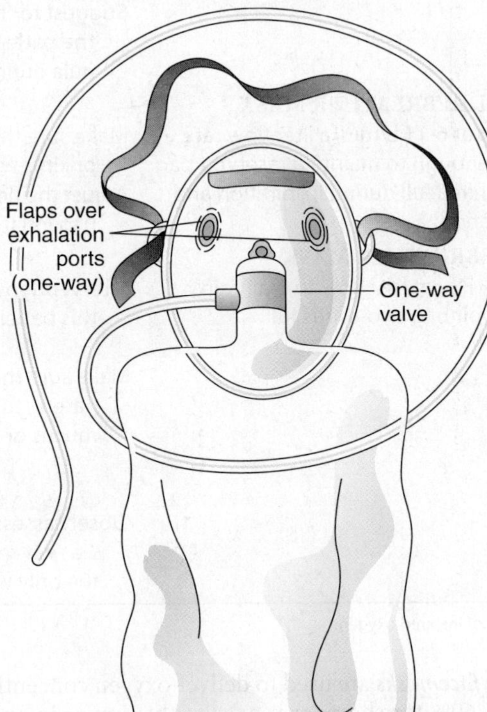
Flaps over exhalation ports (one-way)
One-way valve

Fig. 30-6 • A non-rebreather mask.

vents exhaled air from re-entering the reservoir bag. *It is crucial to ensure that the valve and flaps are intact and functional during each breath.* Some models include only one flap on the mask, or one of the exhalation flaps may be removed for safety purposes. *If the oxygen source should fail or be depleted when both flaps are in place, the patient would not be able to inhale room air.* The flow rate is kept at a level high enough to keep the bag inflated during inhalation—usually 10 to 15 L/minute. Assess for this safety feature at least hourly.

High-Flow Oxygen Delivery Systems

High-flow systems (Table 30-2) include the Venturi mask, aerosol mask, face tent, tracheostomy collar, and T-piece. These devices deliver an accurate oxygen level that meets the patient's oxygen needs when properly fitted. A high-flow system delivers oxygen concentrations from 24% to 100% at 8 to 15 L/min.

Venturi masks (commonly called *Venti masks*) deliver the most accurate oxygen concentration. It works by pulling in a proportional amount of room air for each liter flow of oxygen. An adaptor is located between the bottom of the mask and the oxygen source (Fig. 30-7). Adaptors with holes of different

TABLE 30-2 Comparison of High-Flow Oxygen Delivery Systems

FiO_2 Delivered	Nursing Interventions	Rationales
VENTURI MASK (VENTI MASK)		
24%-50% FiO_2 with flow rates as recommended by the manufacturer, usually 4-10 L/min; provides high humidity	Perform constant surveillance to ensure an accurate flow rate for the specific FiO_2.	An accurate flow rate ensures FiO_2 delivery.
	Keep the orifice for the Venturi adaptor open and uncovered.	If the Venturi orifice is covered, the adaptor does not function and oxygen delivery varies.
	Provide a mask that fits snugly and tubing that is free of kinks.	FiO_2 is altered if kinking occurs or if the mask fits poorly.
	Assess the patient for dry mucous membranes.	Comfort measures may be indicated.
	Change to a nasal cannula during mealtime.	Oxygen is a drug that needs to be given continuously.
AEROSOL MASK, FACE TENT, TRACHEOSTOMY COLLAR		
24%-100% FiO_2 with flow rates of at least 10 L/min; provides high humidity	Assess that aerosol mist escapes from the vents of the delivery system during inspiration and expiration.	Humidification should be delivered to the patient.
	Empty condensation from the tubing.	Emptying prevents the patient from being lavaged with water, promotes an adequate flow rate, and ensures a continued prescribed FiO_2.
	Change the aerosol water container as needed.	Adequate humidification is ensured only when there is sufficient water in the canister.
T-PIECE		
24%-100% FiO_2 with flow rates of at least 10 L/min; provides high humidity	Empty condensation from the tubing.	Condensation interferes with flow rate delivery of FiO_2 and may drain into the tracheostomy if not emptied.
	Keep the exhalation port open and uncovered.	If the port is occluded, the patient can suffocate.
	Position the T-piece so that it does not pull on the tracheostomy or endotracheal tube.	The weight of the T-piece pulls on the tracheostomy and causes pain or erosion of skin at the insertion site.
	Make sure the humidifier creates enough mist. A mist should be seen during inspiration and expiration.	An adequate flow rate is needed to meet the inspiration effort of the patient. If not, the patient will be "air-hungry."

FiO_2, Fraction of inspired oxygen.

sizes allow specific amounts of air to mix with the oxygen. More precise delivery of oxygen results. Each adaptor also determines the needed flow rate. For example, to deliver 24% of oxygen, the flow rate must be 4 L/min. Another type of Venturi mask has one adaptor with a dial that is used to select the amount of oxygen desired. Humidification is not needed with the Venturi mask. This system is best for the patient with chronic lung disease because it delivers a more precise oxygen concentration.

Other high-flow systems include the face tent, aerosol mask, tracheostomy collar, and T-piece. They are often used to provide high humidity with oxygen delivery. A dial on the humidity source regulates the oxygen level being delivered. A face tent fits over the chin, with the top extending halfway across the face. The oxygen level delivered varies, but the face tent, instead of a tight-fitting mask, is useful for facial trauma or burns. An aerosol mask is used when high humidity is needed after extubation or upper airway surgery or for thick secretions. The tracheostomy collar is used to deliver high humidity and the desired oxygen to the patient with a tracheostomy. A special adaptor, called the *T-piece*, is used to deliver any desired FiO_2 to the patient with a tracheostomy, laryngectomy, or endotracheal tube (Fig. 30-8). Adjust the flow rate so that the aerosol appears on the exhalation side of the T-piece.

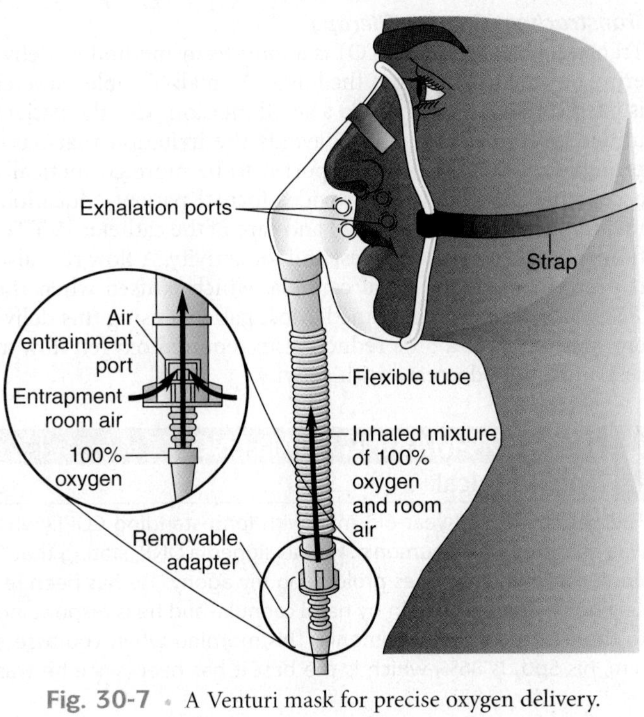
Exhalation ports
Strap
Air entrainment port
Entrapment room air
100% oxygen
Flexible tube
Inhaled mixture of 100% oxygen and room air
Removable adapter

Fig. 30-7 • A Venturi mask for precise oxygen delivery.

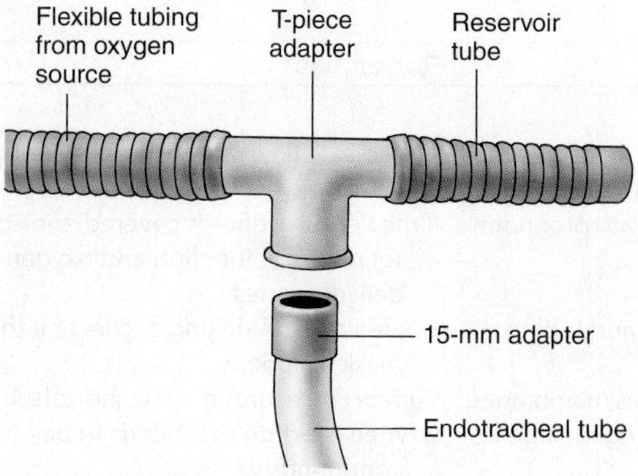

Flexible tubing from oxygen source
T-piece adapter
Reservoir tube
15-mm adapter
Endotracheal tube

Fig. 30-8 • A T-piece apparatus for attachment to an endotracheal or tracheostomy tube.

Noninvasive Positive-Pressure Ventilation

Noninvasive positive-pressure ventilation (NPPV) is a technique using positive pressure to keep alveoli open and improve gas exchange without the need for airway intubation. This type of ventilation can deliver oxygen or may use just room air. A nasal mask or full-face mask delivery system allows mechanical delivery of either bi-level positive airway pressure (BiPAP) or nasal continuous positive airway pressure (CPAP).

For BiPAP, a cycling machine delivers a set inspiratory positive airway pressure each time the patient begins to inspire. As he or she begins to exhale, the machine delivers a lower set end-expiratory pressure. Together, these two pressures improve tidal volume.

Nasal CPAP delivers a set positive airway pressure throughout each cycle of inhalation and exhalation. The effect is to open collapsed alveoli. Patients who may benefit from this form of oxygen or air delivery include those with atelectasis after surgery or cardiac-induced pulmonary edema. This technique is also used for sleep apnea. The effect of this use is to hold open the upper airways (Fig. 30-9).

Transtracheal Oxygen Therapy

Transtracheal oxygen (TTO) is a long-term method of delivering oxygen directly into the lungs. A small, flexible catheter is passed into the trachea via a small incision with the patient under local anesthesia. TTO avoids the irritation that nasal prongs cause. Patients also report it to be more cosmetically acceptable. A TTO team provides formal patient education, including the purpose of TTO and care of the catheter. A TTO flow rate is prescribed for rest and for activity. A flow rate also is prescribed for the nasal cannula, which is used when the TTO catheter is being cleaned. Most patients using this delivery method have a 55% reduction in required oxygen flow at rest and a 30% decrease with activity.

DECISION-MAKING CHALLENGE
Legal/Ethical

The patient is a 68-year-old man with long-standing COPD who was admitted for pneumonia. He has signed a DNR, stating that "I don't want any machines prolonging my agony." He has been receiving oxygen at 3 L/min by nasal cannula, and he is responding to the treatment for pneumonia. This morning when you assess him, his Spo_2 is 86%, which is the best it has been since he was admitted. He tells you that he feels so much better that he hopes he can go home soon. When you come back into the room, his daughter (from out-of-town) has removed the nasal cannula, saying "he shouldn't have this, he is a DNR." The patient is having more respiratory difficulty and his Spo_2 is now 80%.

1. Should you reposition the nasal cannula? Why or why not?
2. Is oxygen therapy a violation of DNR?

evolve For suggested answer guidelines, go to http://evolve.elsevier.com/Iggy/.

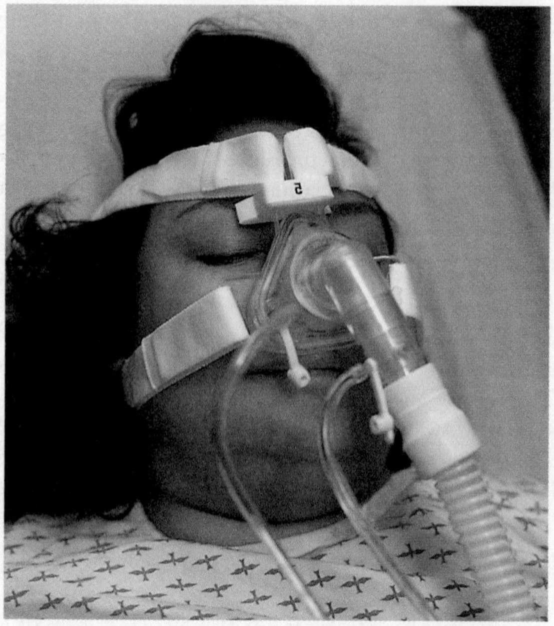

Fig. 30-9 • Nasal continuous positive airway pressure (CPAP).

Community-Based Care
Home Care Management

The patient must be stable and optimally treated before the need for home oxygen is considered. For Medicare to cover the cost of continuous oxygen therapy, the patient must have severe hypoxemia defined as a partial pressure of arterial oxygen (Pao_2) level of less than 55 mm Hg or an arterial oxygen saturation (Spo_2) of less than 88% on room air and at rest. The criteria vary when hypoxemia is caused by cardiac rather than pulmonary problems or when oxygen is needed only at night or with exercise.

After the need for home oxygen therapy is verified, begin a teaching plan about oxygen therapy. Assist the patient to select a durable medical equipment (DME) company to deliver oxygen equipment; also help him or her select a community health nursing agency for follow-up care in the home. The patient is reevaluated for the need for oxygen therapy on a periodic basis.

While providing discharge planning and teaching, be sensitive to the patient's emotional adjustment to oxygen therapy. Encourage the patient to share feelings and concerns. He or she may be concerned about social acceptance. Help him or her realize that adherence to oxygen therapy is important for being able to participate in ADLs and other events that bring enjoyment.

Home Care Preparation

The nurse or respiratory therapist teaches the patient about the equipment needed for home oxygen therapy, including the oxygen source, delivery devices, humidity sources, and safety aspects of using and maintaining the equipment.

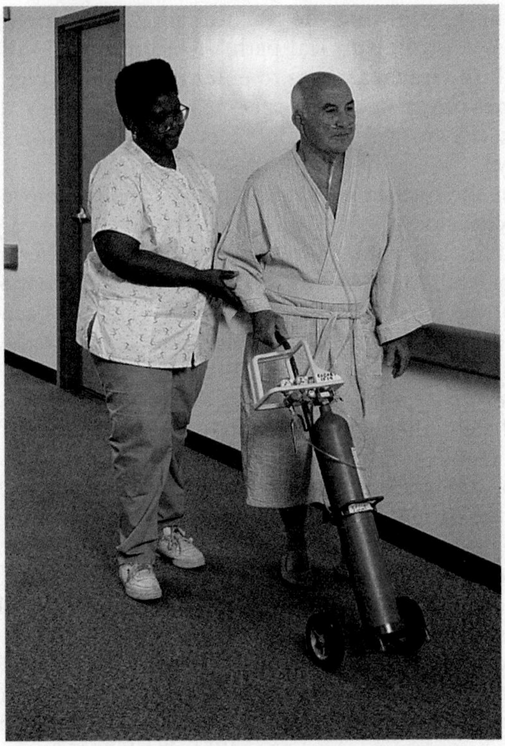

Fig. 30-10 • Small E size oxygen tank (cylinder) for portability.

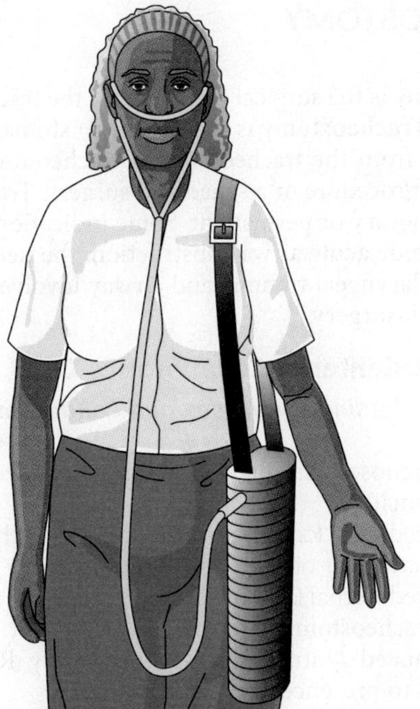

Fig. 30-11 • Liquid oxygen.

Home oxygen therapy is provided in one of three ways: compressed gas in a tank or a cylinder, liquid oxygen in a reservoir, or an oxygen concentrator. Compressed gas in an oxygen tank (green) is the most often used oxygen source. An oxygen tank is economical, and pure oxygen can be delivered at a wide range of flow rates. The large H cylinder may be used as a stationary source, and the small E tank is available for transporting the patient (Fig. 30-10). Teach the patient and family to check the gauge daily to assess the amount of oxygen left in the tank. As a safety precaution, the tanks must always be in a stand or rack. A tank that is accidentally knocked over could suddenly decompress and move around in an uncontrolled manner. Smaller (and lighter) D and C cylinders are available for the patient to carry.

Liquid oxygen for home use is oxygen gas that has been liquefied. A concentrated amount of oxygen is available in a lightweight and easy-to-carry container similar to a Thermos bottle (Fig. 30-11). The patient can fill the portable tank from the large stationary liquid vessel. This type of oxygen lasts longer than gaseous oxygen in a conventional tank of the same size; however, it is expensive and the oxygen evaporates if it is not used continuously.

The **oxygen concentrator** or oxygen extractor is a machine that removes nitrogen, water vapor, and hydrocarbons from room air. Oxygen is concentrated from room air and is delivered at more than 90%. The concentrator, although noisy and large, is the least expensive system and does not need to be filled. It is often used in the home as a stationary system. A smaller version of the machine that can plug into DC electrical outlets can be rented for use during car or boat trips. Liquid oxygen and E tanks are used when the patient leaves home for short trips.

Humidification is rarely needed for any of these oxygen systems. It may be helpful, however, when the flow rate is higher than 4 L/min.

In any of the three home oxygen systems, an oxygen-conserving reservoir-type nasal cannula can be used to reduce oxygen flow needs by about 50%. Two types available are the mustache type and the pendant type. A reservoir for storage of exhaled oxygen is attached to the tubing. The stored oxygen is then delivered back to the patient on the next inhalation. The reservoir sits on top of the upper lip (mustache type) or hangs around the neck (pendant type).

Regardless of the type of oxygen delivery device used, review safety issues with the patient and family. Stress to the patient the importance of not smoking when he or she is using oxygen. Teach that candles, gas burners, and fireplaces (or other open flames) are not to be used in the same room that oxygen is being used.

NCLEX EXAMINATION CHALLENGE

The client is a 64-year-old general surgery client who was weaned off mechanical ventilation this morning. Her Spo_2 after extubation was 97%. Despite her efforts to cough and deep breathe, her Spo_2 is now 88%. Which interventions should the nurse implement? (Select all that apply.)

A. Notify the Rapid Response Team.
B. Assist the client from the supine position to a side-lying position.
C. Confirm her pulse oximeter is correct.
D. Assess the client for breath sounds and for shortness of breath or dyspnea.
E. Administer oxygen therapy at 2 liters per minute via nasal cannula.
F. Administer oxygen at 100% via a non-rebreather mask.

evolve For the correct answer, go to http://evolve.elsevier.com/Iggy/.

TRACHEOSTOMY

Overview

Tracheotomy is the surgical incision into the trachea to create an airway. **Tracheostomy** is the (tracheal) stoma, or opening, that results from the tracheotomy. A tracheotomy can be an emergency procedure or a scheduled surgery. Tracheostomies can be temporary or permanent. Some indications for tracheostomy include acute airway obstruction, the need for airway protection, laryngeal trauma, and airway involvement during head or neck surgery.

Patient-Centered Collaborative Care

Common Nursing Diagnoses and Collaborative Problems

Nursing diagnoses that may apply to patients requiring tracheostomy include:

- Impaired Gas Exchange related to weak chest muscles, obstruction, or other physical problems
- Impaired Verbal Communication related to physical barrier (tracheostomy, intubation)
- Imbalanced Nutrition: Less Than Body Requirements related to presence of endotracheal tube
- Risk for Infection related to invasive procedures
- Impaired Oral Mucous Membrane related to mechanical factors (endotracheal tube)
- Impaired Social Interaction related to communication barriers

Interventions

Preoperative Care

The care for the patient having a tracheostomy is similar to that for a laryngectomy (see Chapter 31). Focus on his or her knowledge deficits through teaching, and discuss tracheostomy care, communication, and speech.

Operative Procedures

Initially, the neck is extended and an endotracheal (ET) tube is placed by the anesthesia provider to maintain the airway. An incision is then made through the anterior skin of the neck, exposing the tracheal rings and moving other tissues out of the surgical path. A second incision is made through the tracheal rings to enter the trachea (Fig. 30-12). The types of incisions and specific techniques vary, depending on the surgeon's preference and the reason for the surgery.

After the trachea is entered, the ET tube is removed while the tracheostomy tube is inserted. The tracheostomy tube is secured in place with sutures and tracheostomy ties (or Velcro tube holders). A chest x-ray is obtained to ensure proper placement of the tube. If intubation is not possible, a tracheotomy can be done with the patient awake under local anesthesia.

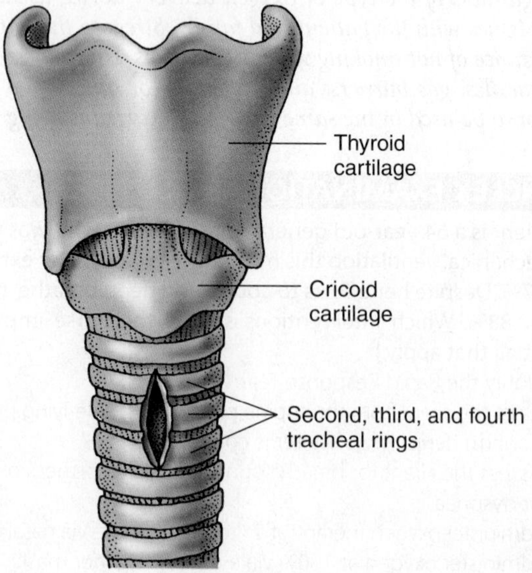
Thyroid cartilage
Cricoid cartilage
Second, third, and fourth tracheal rings

Fig. 30-12 • A vertical tracheal incision for a tracheostomy.

Postoperative Care

Immediately after surgery, focus care on ensuring a patent airway. Confirm the presence of bilateral breath sounds. Conduct a thorough respiratory assessment at least every 2 hours. Assess the patient for complications from the procedure.

Complications

Major complications can arise after surgery. Table 30-3 lists manifestations, management, and prevention of other serious complications of tracheostomy.

Tube obstruction can occur as a result of secretions or by cuff displacement. Indicators of obstruction include difficulty breathing; noisy respirations; difficulty inserting a suction catheter; thick, dry secretions; and unexplained peak pressures (if a mechanical ventilator is in use). Assess the patient at least hourly for tube patency. Prevent obstruction by helping the patient cough and deep breathe, providing inner cannula care, humidifying the oxygen source, and suctioning. If tube obstruction occurs as a result of cuff prolapse over the end of the tracheostomy tube, the physician or advanced practice nurse repositions or replaces the tube.

Tube dislodgement and accidental decannulation can occur when the tube system is not secure. This problem can be prevented by securing the tube in place. This action reduces movement and traction on the tube from oxygen or ventilator tubing or accidental pulling by the patient. *Tube dislodgment in the first 72 hours after surgery is an emergency because the tracheostomy tract has not matured and replacement is difficult. The tube may end up in the subcutaneous tissue instead of in the trachea. If this occurs, first ventilate the patient using a manual resuscitation bag and facemask while another nurse calls for help.*

Ensure that a tracheostomy tube of the same type (including an obturator) and size (or one size smaller) is at the bedside at all times, along with a tracheostomy insertion tray. If decannulation occurs after 72 hours, extend the patient's neck and open the tissues of the stoma to secure the airway. With the obturator inserted into the tracheostomy tube, quickly and gently replace the tube and remove the obturator. Check for airflow through the tube and for bilateral breath sounds. If you cannot secure the airway, notify a more experienced nurse, respiratory therapist, or physician for assistance. Ventilate via a bag-valve mask. *If the patient is in distress, call the Rapid Response Team for help.*

Pneumothorax (air in the chest cavity) can develop during the tracheotomy procedure if the chest cavity is entered. When pneumothorax occurs during tracheotomy, it usually does so at the apex of the lung. Chest x-rays after placement are used to assess for pneumothorax.

TABLE 30-3 **Complications of Tracheostomy**

Complications and Description	Manifestations	Management	Prevention
Tracheomalacia: constant pressure exerted by the cuff causes tracheal dilation and erosion of cartilage.	An increased amount of air is required in the cuff to maintain the seal. A larger tracheostomy tube is required to prevent an air leak at the stoma. Food particles are seen in tracheal secretions. The patient does not receive the set tidal volume on the ventilator.	No special management is needed unless bleeding occurs.	Use an uncuffed tube as soon as possible. Monitor cuff pressure and air volumes closely, and detect changes.
Tracheal stenosis: narrowed tracheal lumen is due to scar formation from irritation of tracheal mucosa by the cuff.	Stenosis is usually seen after the cuff is deflated or the tracheostomy tube is removed. The patient has increased coughing, inability to expectorate secretions, or difficulty in breathing or talking.	Tracheal dilation or surgical intervention is used.	Prevent pulling of and traction on the tracheostomy tube. Properly secure the tube in the midline position. Maintain proper cuff pressure. Minimize oronasal intubation time.
Tracheoesophageal fistula (TEF): excessive cuff pressure causes erosion of the posterior wall of the trachea. A hole is created between the trachea and the anterior esophagus. The patient at highest risk also has a nasogastric tube present.	Similar to tracheomalacia: Food particles are seen in tracheal secretions. Increased air in cuff is needed to achieve a seal. The patient has increased coughing and choking while eating. The patient does not receive the set tidal volume on the ventilator.	Manually administer oxygen by mask to prevent hypoxemia. Use a small, soft feeding tube instead of a nasogastric tube for tube feedings. A gastrostomy or jejunostomy may be performed by the physician. Monitor the patient with a nasogastric tube closely; assess for TEF and aspiration.	Maintain cuff pressure. Monitor the amount of air needed for inflation, and detect changes. Progress to a deflated cuff or cuffless tube as soon as possible.
Trachea-innominate artery fistula: a malpositioned tube causes its distal tip to push against the lateral wall of the tracheostomy. Continued pressure causes necrosis and erosion of the innominate artery. ***This is a medical emergency.***	The tracheostomy tube pulsates in synchrony with the heartbeat. There is heavy bleeding from the stoma. ***This is a life-threatening complication.***	Remove the tracheostomy tube immediately. Apply direct pressure to the innominate artery at the stoma site. Prepare the patient for immediate repair surgery.	Correct the tube size, length, and midline position. Prevent pulling or tugging on the tracheostomy tube. **Immediately notify the physician of the pulsating tube.**

Subcutaneous emphysema occurs when there is an opening or tear in the trachea and air escapes into fresh tissue planes of the neck. Air can also progress throughout the chest and other tissues into the face. Inspect and palpate for air under the skin around the new tracheostomy. *If the skin is puffy and you can feel a crackling sensation, notify the physician immediately.*

Bleeding in small amounts from the tracheotomy incision can be expected for the first few days, but constant oozing is abnormal. Wrap gauze around the tube and pack gauze gently into the wound to apply pressure to the bleeding sites.

Infection can occur at any time. In the hospital, use sterile technique to prevent infection during suctioning and tracheostomy care. Assess the stoma site at least once per shift for purulent drainage, redness, pain, or swelling. Tracheostomy dressings may be used to keep the stoma clean and dry. These dressings resemble a gauze pad (4 × 4) with an area removed to fit around the tube. If tracheostomy dressings are not available, fold standard sterile 4 × 4s to fit around the tube. *Do not cut the dressing because small bits of gauze could then be aspirated through the tube.* Change these dressings often because moist dressings provide a medium for bacterial growth. Careful wound care prevents most local infections.

Tracheostomy Tubes

Many types of tracheostomy tubes are available (Fig. 30-13). The one chosen depends on the specific needs of the patient. Tracheostomy tubes are available in many sizes and are made of various types of materials, such as plastic or metal. The tubes may be reusable; however, most tubes in use today are disposable. A tracheostomy tube may or may not have a cuff. It also may have an inner cannula that can be either disposable or reusable. For patients receiving mechanical ventilation, a cuffed tube is used in acute care settings. A noncuffed tube is

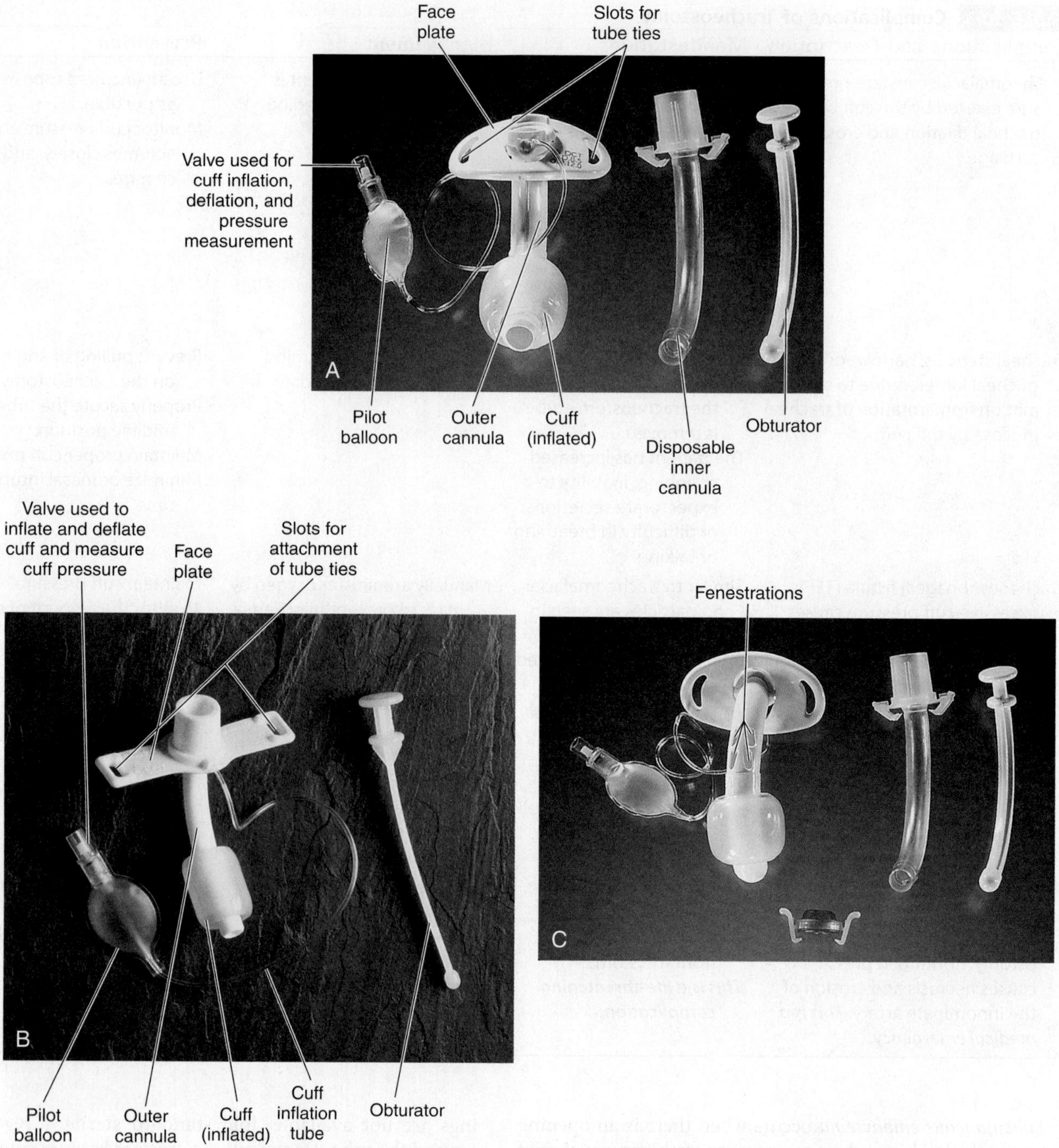
Face plate
Slots for tube ties
Valve used for cuff inflation, deflation, and pressure measurement
A
Pilot balloon
Outer cannula
Cuff (inflated)
Disposable inner cannula
Obturator
Valve used to inflate and deflate cuff and measure cuff pressure
Face plate
Slots for attachment of tube ties
B
Pilot balloon
Outer cannula
Cuff (inflated)
Cuff inflation tube
Obturator
Fenestrations
C

Fig. 30-13 • Tracheostomy tubes. **A,** Dual-lumen cuffed tracheostomy tube with disposable inner cannula. **B,** Single-lumen cannula cuffed tracheostomy tube. **C,** Dual-lumen cuffed fenestrated tracheostomy tube.

used for airway maintenance when mechanical ventilation is not required.

For tubes with a reusable inner cannula, inspect, suction, and clean the inner cannula. During the first 24 hours after surgery, perform cannula care as often as needed, perhaps every 30 to 60 minutes. Thereafter, care is determined by the patient's needs and agency policy. In planning for self-care, teach him or her to remove the inner cannula and check for cleanliness. Also instruct the patient about suctioning and tracheostomy cleaning.

Because breathing and swallowing move the tube, a cuffed tube does not protect against aspiration. Having a cuffed tube inflated may give a false sense of security that aspiration cannot occur during feeding or mouth care. In addition, the pilot balloon does not reflect whether the correct amount of air is present in the cuff.

A fenestrated tube can function in many different ways. When the inner cannula is in place, the fenestration is covered over (closed) and this tube works like a double-lumen tube. With the inner cannula removed and the plug or red stopper

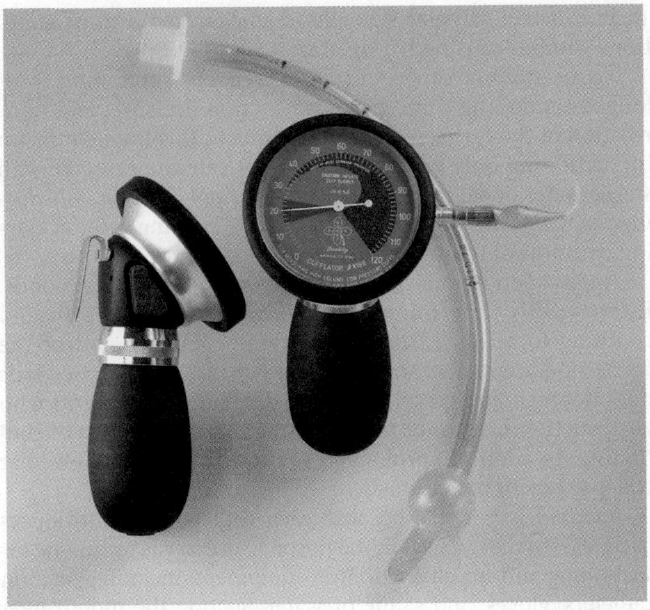

Fig. 30-14 • An aneroid pressure manometer for cuff inflation and measuring cuff pressures.

locked in place, air can pass through the fenestration, around the tube, and up through the natural airway. The patient can then cough and speak. If the patient has trouble with any of these actions, he or she should be evaluated for proper tube placement, patency, size, and fenestration. *Do not cap the tube until the problem is identified and corrected.*

A fenestrated tube may or may not have a cuff. With a cuff, some air flows through the natural airway when the patient is not being mechanically ventilated. *Always deflate the cuff before capping the tube with the decannulation cap; otherwise, the patient has no airway.*

Patients with metal tracheostomy tubes scheduled for magnetic resonance imaging (MRI) need to change to a plastic tube. Metal tubes could be dislodged or heat up with exposure to the magnetic field during the scan.

Care Issues for the Patient with a Tracheostomy

Prevention of Tissue Damage

Tissue damage can occur at the point where the inflated cuff presses against the tracheal mucosa. Mucosal ischemia occurs when the pressure exerted by the cuff on the mucosa exceeds the capillary perfusion pressure. To reduce the risk for tracheal damage, keep the cuff pressure between 14 and 20 mm Hg or 20 and 28 cm H_2O (ideally, 25 cm H_2O or less).

Most cuffs are designed to use a high volume of air while keeping low pressure on the tracheal mucosa. Inflate the cuff to form a seal between the trachea and the cuff while creating the least amount of pressure. If the cuff cannot be inflated to seal well enough, a larger-diameter tube may be needed. A pressure cuff inflator can be used to inflate the cuff to a specified pressure or to check the cuff pressure (Fig. 30-14).

Check the cuff pressure at least once during each shift, especially with the minimal leak technique, and keep the pressure at 14 to 20 mm Hg or 20 to 28 cm H_2O. In rare situations, the cuff pressure is increased to maintain ventilator volumes when peak pressures are greater than 50 mm Hg (65 cm H_2O) and positive end-expiratory pressure (PEEP) is greater than 10 mm Hg (14 cm H_2O). High PEEP values can deflate the cuff over time, and more air may need to be added to maintain a proper seal. Manufacturers have guidelines for the specific volumes for each cuff size. Most cuffs are adequately inflated with less than 10 mL of air.

Although a high cuff pressure causes tracheal damage, other factors may make the damage worse. The patient who is malnourished, dehydrated, hypoxic, older, or receiving corticosteroids has poor tissue healing and is at risk for greater tissue damage. Tube friction and movement are important factors that damage the mucosa. Reduce local airway damage by maintaining proper cuff pressures, stabilizing the tube, suctioning only when needed, and preventing and treating malnutrition, dehydration, and hypoxia.

Air Warming and Humidification

The tracheostomy tube bypasses the nose and mouth, which normally humidify, warm, and filter the air before it reaches the lower respiratory tract. If humidification and warming are not adequate, tracheal damage can occur. Thick, dried secretions can occlude the airways.

To prevent these complications, humidify the air as prescribed. On an ongoing basis, assess for a fine mist emerging from the tracheostomy collar or T-piece during inspiration and expiration. To increase the amount of humidity delivered, a warming device can be attached to the humidification source. At the same time, a temperature probe is placed in the tubing circuit. *The temperature is kept between 98.6° and 100.4° F (37° and 38° C). It should never exceed 104° F (40° C).* Monitor the circuit temperature hourly by feeling the tubing and by checking the probe. Ensure adequate hydration, which also helps liquefy secretions. Increasing the flow rate at the flowmeter also increases the amount of delivered humidity.

Suctioning

Suctioning maintains a patent airway and promotes gas exchange by removing secretions from the patient who cannot cough adequately. Chart 30-3 lists best practices for suctioning. Assess the patient's need for suctioning. Suctioning is needed when audible or noisy secretions, crackles, or wheezes are heard on auscultation or when restlessness, increased pulse or respiratory rates, or mucus in the artificial airway is present. Other indications include patient requests for suctioning or an increase in the peak airway pressure on the ventilator.

◀ ANIMATION: Suctioning

Suctioning is performed most often through an artificial airway but can be accomplished either through the nose or the mouth. Suctioning of both routes is routine for the patient with retained secretions.

Suctioning through the nose has similar complications as suctioning through an artificial airway. Entry through the nose into the throat can be painful. Slow, careful placement of the catheter, with a good understanding of the nasopharyngeal anatomy, can make the procedure less traumatic. Placing a nasopharyngeal airway and suctioning through it helps prevent trauma to the nasal mucosa. Advance the catheter through the nasopharynx and into the laryngopharynx while the patient receives oxygen by mask or nasal cannula. Once the catheter enters the larynx, the patient may cough. On inhalation, insert the catheter through the vocal cords and into the trachea. Occasionally, the catheter can be disconnected from suction and attached to an oxygen source, with the patient receiving oxygen via the catheter.

Chart 30-3 BEST PRACTICE FOR PATIENT SAFETY & QUALITY CARE

Suctioning the Artificial Airway

1. Assess the need for suctioning (routine unnecessary suctioning causes mucosal damage, bleeding, and bronchospasm).
2. Wash hands. Don protective eyewear. Maintain Standard Precautions.
3. Explain to the patient that sensations such as shortness of breath and coughing are to be expected but that any discomfort will be very brief.
4. Check the suction source. Occlude the suction source, and adjust the pressure dial to between 80 and 120 mm Hg to prevent hypoxemia and trauma to the mucosa.
5. Set up a sterile field.
6. Preoxygenate the patient with 100% oxygen for 30 seconds to 3 minutes (at least three hyperinflations) to prevent hypoxemia. Keep hyperinflations synchronized with inhalation.
7. Quickly insert the suction catheter until resistance is met. *Do not apply suction during insertion.*
8. Withdraw the catheter 0.4 to 0.8 inch (1 to 2 cm), and begin to apply suction. Use intermittent suction and a twirling motion of the catheter during withdrawal. *Never suction longer than 10 to 15 seconds.*
9. Hyperoxygenate for 1 to 5 minutes or until the patient's baseline heart rate and oxygen saturation are within normal limits.
10. Repeat as needed for up to three total suction passes.
11. Suction mouth as needed, and provide mouth care.
12. Wash hands.
13. Describe secretions, and document patient's responses.

Suctioning can cause hypoxia, tissue (mucosal) trauma, infection, vagal stimulation, bronchospasm, and cardiac dysrhythmias.

Hypoxia can be caused by these factors in the patient with a tracheostomy:

- Ineffective oxygenation before, during, and after suctioning
- Use of a catheter that is too large for the artificial airway
- Prolonged suctioning time
- Excessive suction pressure
- Too frequent suctioning

Prevent hypoxia by hyperoxygenating the patient with 100% oxygen with a manual resuscitation bag attached to an oxygen source. If the patient can take deep breaths, instruct him or her to do so three or four times with the existing oxygen delivery system before suctioning. If possible, monitor the heart rate or use a pulse oximeter while suctioning to assess tolerance of the procedure. Assess for hypoxia (e.g., increased heart rate and blood pressure, oxygen desaturation, cyanosis, restlessness, anxiety, cardiac dysrhythmias). Oxygen saturation below 90% by pulse oximetry indicates hypoxemia. If hypoxia occurs, stop the suctioning procedure. Using the 100% oxygen delivery system, reoxygenate the patient until baseline parameters return.

ANIMATION: Pulse Oximeter ▶

Use a catheter of the correct size to reduce the risk for hypoxia. The size should not exceed half of the size of the tracheal lumen. In adults, the standard catheter size is 12 Fr or 14 Fr. Correct catheter size allows efficient removal of secretions without causing hypoxemia.

Tissue trauma can result from frequent suctioning, prolonged suctioning time, excessive suction pressure, and nonrotation of the catheter. Prevent trauma to this fragile mucosa by suctioning only when needed. Lubricate the catheter with sterile water or saline before insertion. *Apply suction only during the withdrawal of the catheter.* Use a twirling motion during withdrawal to prevent grabbing of the mucosa.

Apply suction intermittently for only 10 to 15 seconds. Estimate this time frame by holding your own breath and counting to 10 or 15 during suctioning. At the end of the 15 seconds, end the suctioning procedure. Fifteen seconds does not seem long to a healthy person, but most patients who need suctioning cannot tolerate more than 15 seconds of suctioning. In addition, prolonged suctioning can cause alveolar collapse (suction atelectasis).

Infection is possible because each catheter pass introduces bacteria into the trachea. In the hospital, use sterile technique for suctioning and for all suctioning equipment, including suction catheters, gloves, and saline or water. Suction the mouth *after* suctioning the artificial airway. *Never use oral suction equipment for suctioning an artificial airway, because this can introduce oral bacteria into the lungs.* Use clean technique with home suctioning procedures because the number of virulent organisms in the home environment is lower than in the hospital.

Vagal stimulation and bronchospasm are possible during suctioning. Vagal stimulation results in severe bradycardia, hypotension, heart block, ventricular tachycardia, asystole, or other dysrhythmias. *If vagal stimulation occurs, stop suctioning immediately and oxygenate the patient manually with 100% oxygen.* Bronchospasm sometimes occurs when the catheter passes into the airway. The patient may need a bronchodilator to relieve bronchospasm and respiratory distress. In addition, hypoxia caused by suctioning can stimulate a variety of cardiac dysrhythmias. If the patient has cardiac monitoring in place, check the monitor during suctioning.

Tracheostomy Care

Tracheostomy care keeps the tube free of secretions, maintains a patent airway, and provides wound care. This procedure is performed whether or not the patient can clear secretions. Perform tracheostomy care according to agency policy, usually every shift and as needed. Chart 30-4 outlines best practices for tracheostomy care.

Before proceeding with tracheostomy care, assess the patient as shown in Chart 30-5. The need for suctioning and tracheostomy care is determined by the amount and consistency of secretions, medical diagnosis (specifically pulmonary diseases), ability of the patient to cough and deep breathe, need for mechanical ventilation, and wound care. Using a penlight, inspect the inner lumen of a single-lumen tube to assess for the presence of secretions.

Secure tracheostomy tubes in place using either twill tape ties or Velcro tracheostomy tube holders. Both devices require changing when soiled or at least once a day to keep them clean, to prevent infection, and to assess for skin irritation under the ties. A properly secured tie or holder allows space for only one or two fingers to be placed between the tie or holder and the neck. Tube movement causes irritation and coughing, which in turn may cause decannulation. *Keeping the tube secure while changing the ties or holder to prevent ac-*

cidental decannulation is critical. One way to accomplish this safely is to keep the old ties or holder on the tube while applying new ties or a new holder, but a secure hand on the tube is the most reliable method of tube stabilization. Include the patient in this process as a step toward self-care. Fig. 30-15 shows correct placement of a tracheostomy dressing.

Bronchial and Oral Hygiene

Bronchial hygiene promotes a patent airway and prevents infection. Turn and reposition the patient every 1 to 2 hours, support out-of-bed activities, and encourage ambulation. These actions promote lung expansion and gas exchange and help remove secretions. Coughing and deep breathing, combined with the chest percussion, vibration, and postural drainage, promote pulmonary care (see Chapter 32).

Oral hygiene is important to keep the airway patent, to prevent bacterial overgrowth and dental caries, and to promote comfort. Maintain Standard Precautions during the procedure. Avoid using glycerin swabs or mouthwash that contains alcohol to clean the mouth because these products dry the mouth, change its pH, and promote bacterial growth. Instead, use a toothette or soft-bristled toothbrush moistened in water for mouth care. Hydrogen peroxide solutions can help remove crusted matter but may break down healing tissue. Use these agents only with a physician's prescription. Help the patient rinse his or her mouth with normal saline every 4 hours while awake or as often as he or she desires.

Examine the mouth for loss of mucosal integrity or dental problems. Ulcers, bacterial or fungal *(Candida)* growth, and other infections are treated medically. Apply lip balm or water-soluble jelly to prevent cracked lips or skin breakdown and to promote patient comfort. Mouth care helps promote oral health, comfort, and aesthetic appearance. Offering an opportunity for the patient or family member to perform mouth care allows participation in care and increases self-esteem.

Chart 30-4 **BEST PRACTICE FOR PATIENT SAFETY & QUALITY CARE**

Tracheostomy Care

1. Assemble the necessary equipment.
2. Wash hands. Maintain Standard Precautions.
3. Suction the tracheostomy tube if necessary.
4. Remove old dressings and excess secretions.
5. Set up a sterile field.
6. Remove and clean the inner cannula. Use half-strength hydrogen peroxide to clean the cannula and sterile saline to rinse it. If the inner cannula is disposable, remove the cannula and replace it with a new one.
7. Clean the stoma site and then the tracheostomy plate with half-strength hydrogen peroxide followed by sterile saline. Ensure that none of the solutions enters the tracheostomy.
8. Change tracheostomy ties if they are soiled. Secure new ties in place before removing soiled ones to prevent accidental decannulation. If a knot is needed, tie a square knot that is visible on the side of the neck. One or two fingers should be able to be placed between the tie tape and the neck.
9. Wash hands.
10. Document the type and amount of secretions and the general condition of the stoma and surrounding skin. Document the patient's response to the procedure and any teaching or learning that occurred.

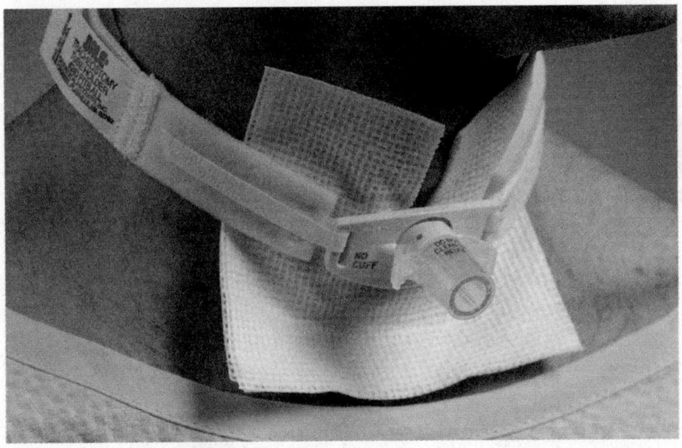

Fig. 30-15 • Placement of tracheostomy gauze dressing and Velcro tracheostomy tube holder.

Chart 30-5 **FOCUSED ASSESSMENT**

The Patient with a Tracheostomy

- Note the quality, pattern, and rate of breathing:
  - Within patient's baseline?
    Tachypnea can indicate hypoxia.
    Dyspnea can indicate secretions in the airway.
- Assess for any cyanosis, especially around the lips, which could indicate hypoxia.
- Check the patient's pulse oximetry reading.
- If oxygen is prescribed, is the patient receiving the correct amount, with the correct equipment and humidification?
- Assess the tracheostomy site:
  - Note the color, consistency, and amount of secretions in the tube or externally.
  - If the tracheostomy is sutured in place, is there any redness, swelling, or drainage from suture sites?
  - If the tracheostomy is secured with ties, what is the condition of the ties? Are they moist with secretions or perspiration? Are the secretions dried on the ties? Is the tie secure?
  - Assess the condition of the skin around the tracheostomy and neck. Be sure to check underneath the neck for secretions that may have drained to the back. Check for any breakdown related to pressure from the ties or from excess secretions.
  - Assess behind the faceplate for the size of the space between the outer cannula and the patient's tissue. Are any secretions collected in this area?
- If the tube is cuffed, check cuff pressure.
- Auscultate the lungs.
- Are a second (emergency) tracheostomy tube and obturator available?

Oral secretions can move down the trachea and collect above the inflated cuff of the endotracheal tube. When the cuff is deflated, the secretions can move into the lungs. The Hi-Lo Evac endotracheal tube has an additional lumen open to the area above the cuff and can help prevent aspiration of oral secretions. The extra lumen allows suctioning of the airway above the cuff before deflating, thus preventing movement of oral secretions deeper into the airway.

Nutrition

Swallowing can be a major problem for the patient with a tracheostomy tube in place. In a normal swallow, the larynx lifts and moves forward to protect itself from the passing stream of food and saliva. Laryngeal lift also opens the upper esophageal sphincter. The tracheostomy tube sometimes tethers the larynx in place, making it unable to move efficiently. The result is difficulty in swallowing. Also, when the tracheostomy tube cuff is inflated, it can balloon backwards and interfere with the passage of food through the esophagus. The wall between the back of the posterior trachea and the front of the esophagus is very thin, allowing this pushing problem.

Instruct the patient to keep the head of the bed elevated for at least 30 minutes after eating. Chart 30-6 outlines best practices to prevent aspiration during swallowing.

Chart 30-6 BEST PRACTICE FOR PATIENT SAFETY & QUALITY CARE

Preventing Aspiration During Swallowing

- Avoid having meals when the patient is fatigued.
- Provide smaller and more frequent meals.
- Provide adequate time; do not "hurry" the patient.
- Provide close supervision if the patient is self-feeding.
- Keep emergency suctioning equipment close at hand and turned on.
- Avoid water and other "thin" liquids.
- Thicken all liquids, including water.
- Avoid foods that generate thin liquids during the chewing process, such as fruit.
- Position the patient in the most upright position possible.
- When possible, completely (or at least partially) deflate the tube cuff during meals.
- Suction after initial cuff deflation to clear the airway and allow maximum comfort during the meal.
- Feed each bite or encourage the patient to take each bite slowly.
- Encourage the patient to "dry swallow" after each bite to clear residue from the throat.
- Avoid consecutive swallows of liquids.
- Provide controlled small volumes of liquids, using a spoon.
- Encourage the patient to "tuck" his or her chin down and forward while swallowing.
- Allow the patient to indicate when he or she is ready for the next bite.
- If the patient coughs, stop the feeding until he or she indicates that the airway has been cleared.
- Continuously monitor tolerance to oral food intake by assessing respiratory rate, ease, pulse oximetry, and heart rate.

Speech and Communication

The patient can speak when there is a cuffless tube, when a fenestrated tracheostomy tube is in place, and when the fenestrated tube is capped or covered. Until natural speech is feasible, teach him or her and the family about other communication means. A writing tablet, a Magic Slate, communication "flash cards" on a ring, a communication board with pictures and letters, hand signals, or a computer, as well as a call light within reach, are used to promote communication and decrease frustration from not being able to speak or be understood. Phrase questions for "yes" or "no" answers to help the patient respond efficiently. Move the patient closer to the nurses' station, and mark the central call light system to indicate that he or she cannot speak.

The inability to talk is a major stressor for the patient. Helping communication is an important nursing function. When the patient can tolerate cuff deflation, he or she places a finger over the tracheostomy tube on exhalation. This forces air up through the larynx, vocal cords, and mouth and allows speech. During the process of decannulation, when the fenestrated tube is "capped," the patient has the benefit of speech without the need to cover the tube.

A device to facilitate speech for the patient with a tracheostomy is a special one-way valve that fits over the tube and replaces the need for finger occlusion. The valve allows him or her to breathe in through the tracheostomy tube. On exhalation, the valve closes so that air is forced through the vocal cords, allowing speech. For this valve to assist in speech, the patient must not be connected to a ventilator, must have the cuff deflated, and must be able to breathe around the tube. Some valves have an extra port for supplemental oxygen without impairing the ability to speak.

Emotional Care

Addressing psychological concerns is an important aspect of nursing care of patients recovering from a tracheostomy. While providing physical care, keep in mind the emotional impact of an artificial airway. Acknowledge the patient's frustration with communication, and allow time for communication. When speaking to him or her, use a normal tone of voice. The tracheostomy tube does not alter hearing or comprehension.

Body Image

The patient may have a change in body image because of deformity, the presence of a stoma or artificial airway, speech changes, a change in the method of eating, or difficulty with speech. Help the patient set realistic goals, starting with involvement in self-care.

Work with the family to ease the patient into a more normal social environment. Provide encouragement and positive reinforcement while demonstrating acceptance and caring behaviors. Assess the family for the need for counseling.

After surgery, the patient may feel shy and socially isolated. He or she can wear loose-fitting shirts, decorative collars, or scarves to cover the tracheostomy tube.

Weaning

Weaning the patient from a tracheostomy tube entails a gradual decrease in the tube size and ultimate removal of the tube. Carefully monitor this process, especially after each change. The physician, nurse practitioner, or respiratory advanced-practice nurse performs the steps in the process.

First, the cuff is deflated as soon as the patient can manage secretions and does not need mechanical ventilation. This change allows him or her to breathe through the tube and through the upper airway. Next, the tube is changed to an uncuffed tube. If this is tolerated, the size of the tube is gradually decreased. When a small fenestrated tube is placed (No. 4 or 6, depending on the size of the airway), the tube is capped so that all air passes through the upper airway and the fenestra, with none passing through the tube. Assess the patient to ensure adequate airflow around the tube when it is capped. The tube may be removed after he or she tolerates more than 24 hours of capping. Place a dry dressing over the stoma (which gradually heals on its own). Usually, a small scar remains.

Another device used for the transition from tracheostomy to natural breathing is a *tracheostomy button*. The button maintains stoma patency and assists spontaneous breathing. The Kistner tracheostomy tube and Olympic tracheostomy button are examples of this type of device. To function, the button must fit properly. A disadvantage is the possibility of decannulation—the tube can dislodge from the trachea but remain in the neck tissues.

DECISION-MAKING CHALLENGE

Critical Rescue

The patient is a 62-year-old man who is 2 days post-op from a radical neck dissection and laryngectomy with a permanent tracheostomy for head and neck cancer. You are performing tracheostomy care now. When you remove the ties to change them, the patient coughs and both the inner and outer cannula pop out from the tracheotomy.

1. What is your first action?
2. Should you attempt to reposition both tubes?
3. Should you call the Rapid Response Team? Provide a rationale for your response.
4. What could have been done differently to prevent this problem?

evolve For suggested answer guidelines, go to http://evolve.elsevier.com/Iggy/.

Community-Based Care

By the time of discharge from the hospital, the patient should be able to provide self-care, which may include tracheostomy care, nutritional care, suctioning, and methods of communication. Although education begins before surgery, most self-care is taught in the hospital. Teach the patient and family how to care for the tracheostomy tube. Review airway care, including cleaning and inspecting for signs of infection. Teach clean suction technique, and review the plan of care.

Instruct the patient to use a shower shield over the tracheostomy tube when bathing to prevent water from entering the airway. Teach him or her to cover the airway with cotton or foam to protect it during the day. Covering the permanent opening filters the air entering the stoma, keeps humidity in the airway, and enhances appearance. Attractive coverings are available in the form of cotton scarves, decorative collars, crocheted bibs, and jewelry. Using colored seam binding for tracheostomy ties after the stoma has matured may enhance overall body image. Shirt or dress color can be matched or coordinated with seam bindings.

Teach the patient to increase humidity in the home. Instruct him or her to instill normal saline into the artificial airway 10 to 15 times a day, as prescribed. Tell him or her to continue using the method of communication that began in the hospital and to wear a medical alert bracelet that identifies the inability to speak.

The health care team assesses specific discharge needs and makes referrals to home care agencies and durable medical equipment companies (for suction equipment and tracheostomy supplies). Clinic or physician follow-up visits occur early after discharge, but the home care nurse also is an important resource for the patient and family. The home care nurse initiates (with a physician's prescription) and coordinates the services of nutritionists, nurses, speech pathologists, and social workers. The home care or hospital nurse informs the patient and family of community resources that can offer support and friendships.

CONSIDERATIONS FOR OLDER ADULTS

Self-managing tracheostomy care and oxygen therapy can be difficult for the older patient who has vision problems or difficulty with upper arm movement. Teach him or her to use magnifying lenses or glasses to ensure the proper setting on the oxygen gauge. Assess his or her ability to reach and manipulate the tracheostomy. If possible, work with a family member who can provide assistance during tracheostomy care.

HUMAN NEEDS NURSING CARE REVIEW

What might you NOTICE if the patient is experiencing inadequate oxygenation and tissue perfusion as a result of respiratory problems?

- Respirations rapid and shallow
- Respirations noisy
- Cannot speak more than 4 or 5 words without pausing for breath
- Change in cognition, acute confusion
- Decreased oxygen saturation by pulse oximetry
- Skin cyanosis or pallor (lighter-skinned patients)
- Cyanosis or pallor of the lips and oral mucous membranes (in patients of any skin color)
- Tachycardia
- Patient appears to strain to catch breath
- Fatigue

What should you INTERPRET and how should you RESPOND to a patient experiencing inadequate oxygenation and tissue perfusion as a result of a respiratory problem?

Perform and interpret physical assessment, including:

- Taking vital signs
- Auscultating all lung fields
- Monitoring oxygen saturation by pulse oximetry
- Checking the accuracy of pulse oximetry readings
- Checking most recent laboratory values for hematocrit, hemoglobin, and ABG levels
- Assessing cognition (mini-mental status exam)
- Assessing for the use of accessory muscles
- Assessing for the presence of thick or excessive secretions
- Assessing the patient's ability to cough and clear the airway

Respond by:

- Applying oxygen and assessing the patient's responses to this intervention
- Keeping the patient's head elevated to about 30 degrees
- Suctioning (oral, pharyngeal, endotracheal, tracheostomy), if needed
- Notifying the physician or Rapid Response Team
- Prioritizing and pacing activities to prevent fatigue

On what should you REFLECT?

- Observe the patient for evidence of restored oxygenation (see Chapter 29)
- Think about what may have precipitated this episode and what steps could be taken to either prevent a similar episode or identify it earlier.
- Think about what additional resources could improve the nursing response to this situation.

GET READY FOR THE NCLEX EXAMINATION!

Key Points

Review these Key Points for each NCLEX Examination Client Needs Category.

Safe and Effective Care Environment

- Never allow water condensation in an oxygen delivery system to drain back into the system.
- Use sterile technique when performing endotracheal or tracheal suctioning.
- Inspect the oral mucous membranes each shift for anyone who has an endotracheal tube.
- Keep a tracheostomy tube (and obturator) and tracheostomy insertion tray at the bedside for the first 72 hours after a tracheotomy has been performed.
- Never use oral suctioning equipment to suction an artificial airway.

Health Promotion and Maintenance

- Monitor the rate and depth of respiration at least every hour for any patient with hypercarbia and CO_2 narcosis who is receiving oxygen by mask or nasal cannula.
- Use aspiration precautions for any patient with an altered level of consciousness or who has an endotracheal tube (see Chart 30-6).
- Teach the patient and family how to perform tracheostomy care (see Chart 30-4).

Psychosocial Integrity

- Allow the patient and family members the opportunity to express fear or anxiety regarding a change in breathing status or the possibility of intubation and mechanical ventilation.
- Teach family members ways to communicate with a patient who is intubated or being mechanically ventilated.
- Reassure patients who are intubated that the loss of speech is temporary.
- Encourage patients with permanent tracheostomies to become involved in self-care.

Physiological Integrity

- Apply oxygen to anyone who is hypoxemic.
- Ensure that oxygen therapy delivered to the patient is humidified appropriately (and warmed, when possible).
- Monitor arterial blood gases (ABGs) and oxygen saturation of all patients receiving oxygen therapy.
- Assess the skin under the mask and under the plastic tubing every shift for patients receiving oxygen by mask.
- Assess the skin of the nares and under the elastic band every shift for patients receiving oxygen by nasal cannula.
- Observe any patient receiving oxygen at greater than a 50% concentration for early symptoms of oxygen toxicity (i.e., nonproductive cough, substernal chest pain, GI upset, dyspnea).
- Use a manual resuscitation bag to ventilate the patient if the tracheostomy tube has dislodged or become decannulated.
- Assess the new tracheostomy stoma site at least once per shift for purulent drainage, redness, pain, and swelling as indicators of infection.
- Keep the tracheal cuff pressure between 14 and 20 mm Hg to prevent tissue injury.
- Secure new tracheostomy ties or tube holders in place before removing the soiled ones to prevent accidental decannulation.

Additional Study Resources

Go to your Companion CD or Evolve at http://evolve.elsevier.com/Iggy/ for *Self-Assessment Questions for the NCLEX Examination.*

evolve Go to Evolve at http://evolve.elsevier.com/Iggy/ for *Prioritization and Delegation Questions for the NCLEX Examination.*

SELECTED BIBLIOGRAPHY

Asterisk indicates a classic or definitive work on this subject.

Beattie, S. (2006). Back to basics with O_2 therapy. *RN, 69*(9), 37-40.

Crimlisk, J., O'Donnell, C., & Grillone, G. (2006). Standardizing adult tracheostomy tube styles. *Dimensions of Critical Care Nursing, 25*(1), 35-43.

Cutler, C., & Davis, N. (2005). Improving oral care in patients receiving mechanical ventilation. *American Journal of Critical Care, 14*(5), 389-394.

Davis, M., & Johnston, J. (2008). Maintaining supplemental oxygen during transport. *AJN, 108*(1), 35-36.

*Dixon, B., & Tasota, F. (2003). Action stat: Inadvertant tracheal decannulation. *Nursing2003, 33*(1), 96.

Edelman, D., Maleyko-Jacobs, S., White, M., Lucas, C., & Ledgerwood, A. (2008). Smoking and home oxygen therapy: A preventable public health hazard. *Journal of Burn Care and Research, 29*(1), 119-122.

Fischer, R. (2007). Prevent fires when using oxygen cylinder regulators. *Nursing2007, 37*(1), 20.

Gavaghan, S., & Jeffries, M. (2006). Your patient's receiving noninvasive positive-pressure ventilation. *Nursing2006, 36*(3), 46-47.

Grams, L., & Spremulli, M. (2008). Assessing a patient for dysphagia. *Nursing2008, 38*(8), 15.

Happ, M.B., Tate, J., & Garrett, K. (2006). Nonspeaking older adults in the ICU. *AJN, 106*(5), 29.

Lynch, M. (2006). Dyspnea. *Clinical Journal of Oncology Nursing, 10*(3), 323-326.

*Mahler, D., Fierro-Carrion, G., & Baird, J. (2003). Evaluation of dyspnea in the elderly. *Clinics in Geriatric Medicine, 19*(1), 19-33.

McCance, K., & Huether, S. (2006). *Pathophysiology: The biologic basis for disease in adults and children* (5th ed.). St. Louis: Mosby.

*McConnell, E. (2002). Providing tracheostomy care. *Nursing2002, 32*(1), 17.

Metheny, N. (2006). Preventing respiratory complications of tube feedings: Evidence-based practice. *American Journal of Critical Care, 15*(4), 360-369.

Pagana, K., & Pagana, T. (2006). *Mosby's manual of diagnostic and laboratory tests* (3rd ed.). St. Louis: Mosby.

Pruitt, B. (2005). Clear the air with closed suctioning. *Nursing2005, 35*(7), 44-45.

Pruitt, B. (2006). Does home respiratory therapy have a place in the hospital? *Nursing2006, 36*(6), 64hn1-64hn3.

Pruitt, B., & Jacobs, M. (2005). Clearing away pulmonary secretions. *Nursing2005, 35*(7), 37-40.

Pullen, R. (2007). Communicating with a patient on mechanical ventilation. *Nursing2007, 37*(4), 22.

Rushing, J. (2006). Using bag-valve-mask ventilation. *Nursing2006, 36*(1), 72.

Serna, E., & McCarthy, M. (2006). Heads up to prevent aspiration during enteral feeding. *Nursing2006, 36*(1), 76-77.

Stoltzfus, S. (2006). The role of noninvasive ventilation. *Dimensions of Critical Care Nursing, 25*(2), 66-70.

31
CHAPTER

Care of Patients with Noninfectious Upper Respiratory Problems

M. Linda Workman

LEARNING OUTCOMES

For clinical competence and success on the NCLEX Examination, study this chapter with these Learning Outcomes in mind:

Safe and Effective Care Environment

1. Supervise care delegated to licensed practical nurses/licensed vocational nurses (LPNs/LVNs) or nursing assistants to patients who have had radical surgeries for head or neck cancer.
2. Act as a patient advocate for patients receiving oxygen or who have tracheostomies.

Health Promotion and Maintenance

3. Assess the patient for risk factors for head and neck cancer.

Psychosocial Integrity

4. Support the patient and family in coping with changes in breathing status and the need for a laryngectomy.
5. Develop and evaluate an appropriate nonverbal form of communication for a patient with a laryngectomy.

Physiological Integrity

6. Perform a focused upper respiratory assessment and re-assessment to determine adequacy of oxygenation and tissue perfusion.
7. Prioritize nursing care needs for the patient after a nasoseptoplasty.
8. Recognize manifestations and care needs of a patient with an anterior nosebleed and of a patient with a posterior nosebleed.
9. Prioritize nursing care needs for a patient with facial trauma.
10. Describe the pathophysiology and the potential complications of sleep apnea.
11. Apply knowledge of anatomy to prevent aspiration in a patient with a tracheostomy.
12. Perform wound care and laryngectomy care.
13. Use correct technique to suction via a tracheostomy or laryngectomy tube.
14. Teach the patient and family about home management of a laryngectomy stoma or tracheostomy.

Go to your Companion CD or Evolve at http://evolve.elsevier.com/Iggy/ for *Self-Assessment Questions for the NCLEX Examination* keyed to these Learning Outcomes.

The upper airway structures include the nose, sinuses, oropharynx, larynx, and trachea. These areas are important to the *human need for oxygenation and tissue perfusion* by providing the entrance site for air, which is the source of oxygen. Problems of the upper airways, especially the larynx and trachea, have the potential to disturb oxygenation and tissue perfusion by interfering with oxygen delivery. The upper airway structures may have specific health problems and also may be affected by other common acute and chronic disorders. Patients with upper respiratory problems are found in the community and many health care settings. *The major nursing priority with disorders of the upper respiratory tract is to promote oxygenation by ensuring a patent airway.*

NONINFECTIOUS DISORDERS OF THE NOSE AND SINUSES

FRACTURE OF THE NOSE

Pathophysiology

Nasal fractures often result from injuries received during falls, sports activities, motor vehicle collisions, or physical assaults. If the bone or cartilage is not displaced, serious complications usually do not result from the fracture and treatment may not be needed. Displacement of either the bone or cartilage, however, can cause airway obstruction or cosmetic deformity and is a potential source of infection.

Patient-Centered Collaborative Care

Assessment

Document any nasal problem, including deviation, malaligned nasal bridge, a change in nasal breathing, crackling of the skin (crepitus) on palpation, midface bruising, and pain. Blood or clear fluid (cerebrospinal [CSF]) rarely drains from one or both nares as a result of a simple nasal fracture. The presence of CSF drainage could indicate a skull fracture. CSF can be differentiated from normal nasal secretions because CSF contains glucose that will test positive with a dipstick. In addition, when CSF dries on a piece of filter paper, a yellow "halo" appears as a ring at the dried edge of the fluid. Although important in evaluating general facial fractures, x-rays are not always useful in the diagnosis of nasal fractures.

Interventions

The health care provider performs a simple **closed reduction** (manipulation of the bones by palpation to position them in proper alignment) of the nasal fracture using local or general anesthesia within the first 24 hours after injury. After 24 hours, the fracture is more difficult to reduce because of edema and scar formation. Simple closed fractures need not be surgically treated. Treatment focuses on pain relief and cold compresses to decrease swelling.

Rhinoplasty

Reduction and surgery may be needed for severe fractures or for those that do not heal properly. **Rhinoplasty** is a surgical reconstruction of the nose for cosmetic purposes and to improve airflow. The patient returns from surgery with packing in both nostrils; this packing prevents bleeding and provides support for the reconstructed nose. The gauze packing is usually treated with an antibiotic ointment, such as bacitracin (Bacitin🍁) to reduce the risk for infection. A "moustache" dressing (or drip pad), often a folded 2 × 2 gauze pad, is usually placed under the nose (Fig. 31-1). A splint or cast may cover the nose for better alignment and protection. The nurse or patient changes the drip pad as necessary.

After surgery, observe for edema and bleeding. Check vital signs every 4 hours until the patient is discharged. *Assessing how often the patient swallows is a priority. Repeated swallowing may indicate posterior nasal bleeding.* Use a penlight to examine the throat for bleeding, and notify the surgeon if bleeding is present. The patient with uncomplicated rhinoplasty is discharged the day of surgery. Instruct him or her and the family about the routine care described below.

Instruct the patient to stay in a semi-Fowler's position and to move slowly. Encourage rest and the use of cool compresses on the nose, eyes, or face to help reduce swelling and bruising. If a general anesthetic was used, the patient may eat soft foods once he or she is alert and the gag reflex has returned. Urge the patient to drink at least 2500 mL/day.

To prevent bleeding, teach the patient to limit Valsalva maneuvers (e.g., forceful coughing or straining during a bowel movement), not to sniff upward or blow the nose, and not to sneeze with the mouth closed for the first few days after the packing is removed. Laxatives or stool softeners may be prescribed to ease bowel movement. Instruct the patient to avoid aspirin and other NSAIDs to prevent bleeding. Prophylactic antibiotics may be prescribed to prevent infection. Recommend the use of a humidifier to prevent drying of the mucosa. Explain that edema and bruising may last for weeks and that the final surgical result will be evident in 6 to 12 months.

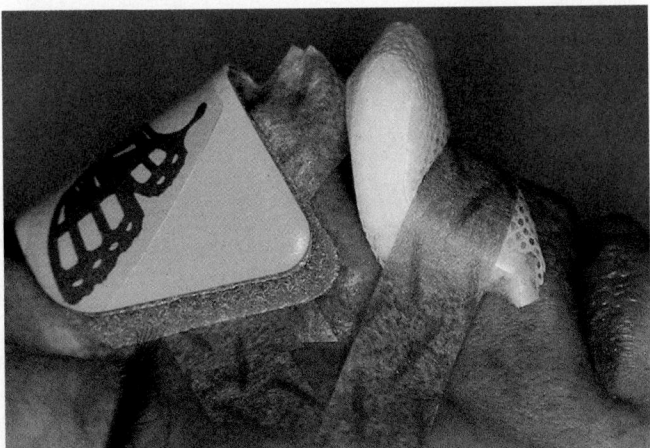

Fig. 31-1 • Immediate postoperative appearance of a patient who has undergone rhinoplasty. Note the splint and gauze drip pad (moustache dressing).

Nasoseptoplasty

Nasoseptoplasty, or **submucous resection (SMR),** may be needed to straighten a deviated septum when chronic symptoms (e.g., "stuffy" nose, snoring, sinusitis) or discomfort occurs. Most adults have a slight nasal septum deviation with no symptoms. Major deviations, however, may obstruct the nasal passages or interfere with airflow and sinus drainage. The deviated section of the cartilage and bone is removed as an ambulatory surgical procedure. The amount resected depends on the type and degree of deformity. Nursing care is similar to that for a rhinoplasty.

EPISTAXIS

Pathophysiology

Epistaxis (nosebleed) is a common problem because of the many capillaries within the nose. Nosebleeds occur as a result of trauma, hypertension, blood dyscrasia (e.g., leukemia), inflammation, tumor, decreased humidity, nose blowing, nose picking, chronic cocaine use, and procedures such as nasogastric suctioning. Men usually are affected more often than women. Older adults tend to bleed most often from the posterior portion of the nose.

Patient-Centered Collaborative Care

The patient often reports that the bleeding started after sneezing or blowing the nose. Document the amount and color of the blood, and take the vital signs. Ask the patient about the number, duration, and causes of previous bleeding episodes. Record this information in the patient's medical record.

Chart 31-1 lists the best practices for emergency care of the patient with a nosebleed. Medical attention is needed if the nosebleed does not respond to these interventions. In such cases, the affected capillaries may be cauterized with silver nitrate or electrocautery and the nose packed. Anterior packing controls bleeding from the anterior nasal cavity.

Posterior nasal bleeding is an emergency because it cannot be easily reached and the patient may lose a lot of blood quickly. Posterior packing, epistaxis catheters (nasal pressure tubes), or a gel tampon is used to stop bleeding that originates in the pos-

Chart 31-1 **BEST PRACTICE FOR PATIENT SAFETY & QUALITY CARE**

Emergency Care of a Patient with an Anterior Nosebleed

EMERGENCY CARE

- Position the patient upright and leaning forward to prevent blood from entering the stomach and possible aspiration.
- Reassure the patient and attempt to keep him or her quiet to reduce anxiety and blood pressure.
- Apply direct lateral pressure to the nose for 5 minutes, and apply ice or cool compresses to the nose and face if possible.
- Maintain Standard Precautions or Body Substance Precautions.
- If nasal packing is necessary, loosely pack both nares with gauze or nasal tampons.
- To prevent rebleeding from dislodging clots, instruct the patient not to blow the nose for several hours after the bleeding stops.
- Seek medical assistance if these measures are ineffective or if the bleeding occurs frequently.

terior nasal region. With packing, the physician positions a large gauze pack in the posterior nasal cavity above the throat, threads the attached string through the nose, and tapes it to the patient's cheek to prevent pack movement. Epistaxis catheters look like very short (about 6 inches) urinary catheters (Fig. 31-2, *A*). These tubes have an exterior balloon along the tube length in addition to an anchoring balloon on the end. The tubes are inserted into both nares. The physician first inflates the anchoring balloon to keep the tubes in place. Then the pressure balloons are inflated carefully for both tubes at the same time to compress bleeding vessels (Fig. 31-2, *B*). Placement of posterior packing or pressure tubes is uncomfortable, and the airway may be obstructed if the pack slips. Most patients who have posterior nasal bleeding are hospitalized.

Observe the patient for respiratory distress and for tolerance of the packing or tubes. Humidity, oxygen, bedrest, and antibiotics may be prescribed. Opioid drugs may be prescribed for pain. Assess patients receiving opioids at least hourly for gag and cough reflexes. Oral care and hydration are important because of mouth breathing. Use pulse oximetry to monitor for hypoxemia. The tubes or packing is usually removed after 1 to 5 days.

After the tubes or packing is removed, teach the patient and family the following interventions to use at home for comfort and safety. Petroleum jelly can be applied to the nares for lubrication and comfort. Nasal saline sprays and humidification add moisture and prevent rebleeding. Instruct the patient to avoid vigorous nose blowing, the use of aspirin or other NSAIDs, and strenuous activities such as heavy lifting for at least 1 month.

NASAL POLYPS

Nasal polyps are benign, grapelike clusters of mucous membrane and connective tissue. They often occur bilaterally and are caused by irritation to the nasal mucosa or sinuses, allergies, or infection (chronic sinusitis). If polyps become too large, airway obstruction may result.

Manifestations of nasal polyps include obstructed nasal breathing, a change in the character of nasal discharge, and a change in speech quality. Patients who have had polyps are at risk for recurrence.

Surgery is the treatment of choice for nasal polyps. The extent of the surgery required depends on the location and type of polyp present.

Benign nasal polyps are treated with nasally inhaled steroids and surgical removal **(polypectomy).** A polypectomy can be performed using either local or general anesthesia. Observe the patient for bleeding after surgery. The nostrils are usually packed with gauze for 24 hours after surgery. Nasal polyps often recur if they are not completely removed.

CANCER OF THE NOSE AND SINUSES

Tumors of the nasal cavities and sinuses are rare and may be either benign or malignant. Malignant tumors can occur at all ages, but the peak incidence is 40 to 45 years of age in men and 60 to 65 years of age in women. Asian Americans have a higher incidence of nasopharyngeal cancer (American Cancer Society [ACS], 2006).

The onset of sinus cancer is slow, and manifestations resemble sinusitis. Thus the patient may have advanced disease at diagnosis. Manifestations of nasal or sinus cancer include persistent nasal obstruction, drainage, bloody discharge, and pain that does not improve after treatment of sinusitis. Local lymph node enlargement often occurs on the side with tumor mass.

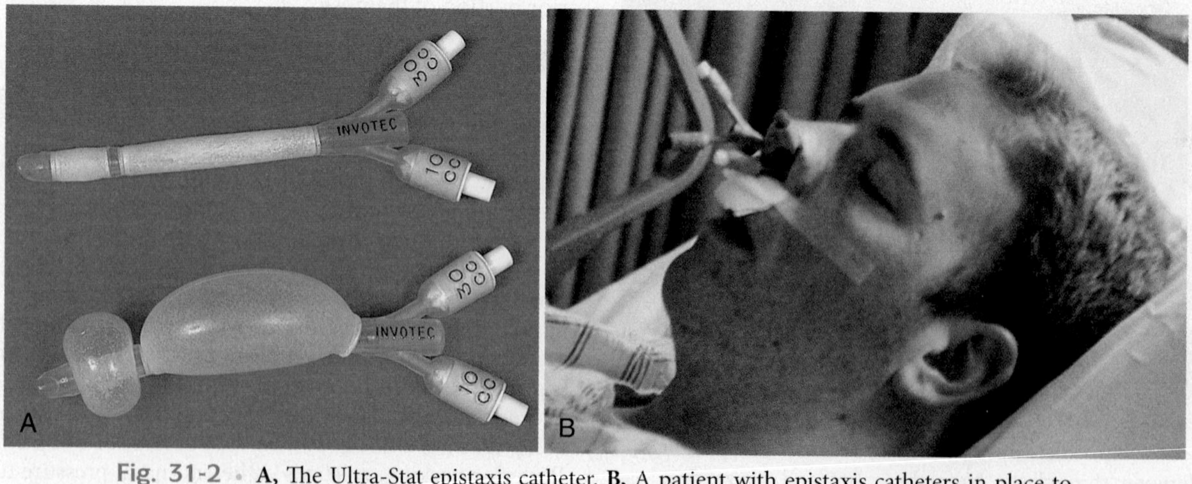
A
B
INVOTEC
INVOTEC
30 cc
10 cc
30 cc
10 cc

Fig. 31-2 • **A,** The Ultra-Stat epistaxis catheter. **B,** A patient with epistaxis catheters in place to control a posterior nasal bleed.

Radiation therapy is the main treatment for nasopharyngeal cancers. Surgical removal is performed if radiation therapy is not successful. The specific surgery depends on tumor size and location and the degree of invasion. Problems after surgery include a change in body image or speech and altered nutrition. These problems are most common when the maxilla and floor of the nose are involved in the surgery. Patients often also have changes in taste and smell.

Provide general postoperative care (see Chapter 18), including maintaining a patent airway, monitoring for hemorrhage, providing wound care, assessing nutritional status, and performing tracheostomy care (if needed). (See Chapter 30 for tracheostomy care.) Perform careful mouth and sinus cavity care with saline irrigations using an electronic irrigation system (e.g., WaterPik, Sonicare) or a syringe. Assess the patient for pain and infection. Collaborate with the nutritionist to help the patient make food selections that promote healing.

FACIAL TRAUMA

Pathophysiology

Facial trauma is described by the specific bones (e.g., mandibular, maxillary, orbital, nasal fractures) and the side of the face involved. Mandibular (lower jaw) fractures can occur at any point on the mandible and are the most common facial fractures. *Le Fort I* is a nasoethmoid complex fracture. *Le Fort II* is a maxillary *and* nasoethmoid complex fracture. *Le Fort III* is a combination of I and II plus an orbital-zygoma fracture, often called "craniofacial disjunction" because it leaves the midface with no connection to the skull. The rich blood supply of the face leads to extensive bleeding and bruising with facial trauma.

Patient-Centered Collaborative Care

Assessment

The first action to take for a patient with facial trauma is airway assessment. Manifestations of airway obstruction include stridor, shortness of breath, dyspnea, anxiety, restlessness, hypoxia, **hypercarbia** (elevated blood levels of carbon dioxide), decreased oxygen saturation, cyanosis, and loss of consciousness. After establishing the airway, assess the site of soft-tissue trauma, bleeding, and possible fractures. Check for soft-tissue edema, facial asymmetry, pain, or leakage of spinal fluid through the ears or nose, indicating a temporal bone or basilar skull fracture. Assess vision and eye movement because orbital and maxillary fractures can entrap the eye. Check behind the ears in the mastoid area for extensive bruising, known as the "battle sign." Because facial trauma can occur with spinal trauma and skull fractures, cranial computed tomography, facial series, and cervical spine films also are obtained.

Interventions

The priority action is to establish and maintain a patent airway. Anticipate the need for emergency intubation, **tracheotomy** (surgical incision into the trachea to create an airway), or **cricothyroidotomy** (creation of a temporary airway by making a small opening in the throat between the thyroid cartilage and the cricoid cartilage). When the patient arrives at a trauma center, care focuses on establishing an airway, controlling hemorrhage, and assessing for the extent of injury. If shock is present, fluid resuscitation and identification of bleeding sites are started immediately.

Time is critical in stabilizing the patient who has head and neck trauma. Early response and treatment by special services (e.g., trauma team, maxillofacial surgeon, general surgeon, otolaryngologist, plastic surgeon, dentist) optimize the patient's recovery.

Stabilizing the fractured segment of a jaw fracture allows the teeth to heal in proper alignment. This process involves **fixed occlusion** (wiring the jaws together in the mouth-closed position). The patient remains in fixed occlusion for 6 to 10 weeks. Antibiotic therapy may be prescribed because of oral wound contamination. Treatment delay, tooth infection, or poor oral care may cause mandibular bone infection. The patient may then require surgical **débridement** (removal of dead tissue within a wound), IV antibiotic therapy, and a longer period with the jaws in a fixed position.

Facial fractures often are repaired with microplating surgical systems such as BoneSource. These shaping plates hold the bone fragments in place until new bone growth occurs. Large areas of skull can be replaced with BoneSource. Bone cells grow into the BoneSource and re-matrix into a stable bone support. The plates may remain in place permanently or may be removed after healing has occurred.

If the mandibular fracture is repaired with titanium plates, teach the patient about oral care, soft-diet restrictions, and follow-up care with a dentist. These plates are permanent and do not interfere with magnetic resonance imaging (MRI) studies.

Fixation methods may use resorbable devices (plates and screws) to hold tissues in place. These devices are made from a plastic-like material that retains its integrity for about 8 weeks and then slowly biodegrades. Resorbable devices are not used when the area has previously been irradiated or for patients who smoke or who have drug or alcohol dependence, uncontrolled diabetes mellitus, immunosuppression, or impaired cardiac function, all of which impair healing.

Inner maxillary fixation (IMF) is another common method of securing a mandibular fracture. The bones are realigned and then wired in place with the bite closed. The physician can repair nondisplaced aligned fractures in a clinic or office using local dental anesthesia. General anesthesia is used to repair displaced or complex fractures or fractures that occur with other facial bone fractures.

After surgery, teach the patient about oral care with an irrigating device, such as a WaterPik or Sonicare. If the patient has inner maxillary fixation, teach self-care with wires in place, including a dental liquid diet. If the patient vomits, watch for aspiration because of the patient's inability to open the jaws to allow ejection of the emesis. Teach him or her how to cut the wires if emesis occurs. *Instruct the patient to keep wire cutters with him or her at all times in case this emergency arises.* If the wires are cut, instruct him or her to return to the surgeon for rewiring as soon as possible to reinstitute fixation.

Nutrition is important for any patient with fractures. Oral needs may be difficult to meet because of oral fixation, pain, and surgery. Collaborate with the nutritionist for patient teaching and support.

NCLEX EXAMINATION CHALLENGE

The client is a 21-year-old man who is in the PACU recovering from an inner maxillary fixation for a mandibular fracture. His jaws are wired together. As the nurse raises the head of his bed, he begins to vomit a large amount of liquid vomitus. What is the nurse's best first action?

A. Administer the prescribed antiemetic by the IV or rectal route.
B. Cut the wires holding his jaws together, and carefully remove them from his mouth.
C. Position him on his side, and suction his mouth with a large-bore catheter.
D. Immediately notify the surgeon, the anesthesiologist, or the Rapid Response Team.

evolve For the correct answer, go to http://evolve.elsevier.com/Iggy/.

NONINFECTIOUS DISORDERS OF THE ORAL PHARYNX AND TONSILS

OBSTRUCTIVE SLEEP APNEA

Pathophysiology

Sleep apnea is a breathing disruption during sleep that lasts at least 10 seconds and occurs a minimum of 5 times in an hour. Although sleep apnea can have a neurologic origin, the most common form occurs as a result of upper airway obstruction by the soft palate or tongue. Factors that contribute to sleep apnea include obesity, a large uvula, a short neck, smoking, enlarged tonsils or adenoids, and oropharyngeal edema. Men are affected more often than women, and the risk increases with age.

During sleep, the muscles relax and the tongue and neck structures are displaced. As a result, the upper airway is obstructed even though chest wall movement is unimpaired. The apnea increases blood carbon dioxide levels and decreases the pH. These blood gas changes stimulate neural centers. The sleeper awakens after 10 seconds or longer of apnea and corrects the obstruction, and respiration resumes. After he or she goes back to sleep, the cycle begins again, sometimes as often as every 5 minutes (Berry, 2008).

This cyclic pattern of disrupted sleep prevents the deep sleep needed for best rest. Thus the person may have excessive daytime sleepiness, an inability to concentrate, and irritability.

Patient-Centered Collaborative Care

Assessment

Patients are often unaware that they have sleep apnea. The disorder should be suspected for any person who has persistent daytime sleepiness or reports "waking up tired," particularly if he or she snores heavily. Other manifestations include irritability and personality changes. In some cases, sleep apnea is diagnosed by family members who observe the problem when the person sleeps in a supine position. A complete health assessment should be performed when excessive daytime sleepiness is a problem.

The most accurate test for sleep apnea is polysomnography (PSG) performed during an overnight sleep study. The patient is directly observed while wearing a variety of monitoring equipment, including an electroencephalograph (EEG), an electrocardiograph (ECG), a pulse oximeter, and an electromyograph (EMG). This test determines the depth of sleep, type of sleep, respiratory effort, oxygen saturation, and muscle movement.

Interventions

Nonsurgical Management

A change in sleeping position or weight loss may be all that is needed to reduce or correct mild sleep apnea. Position-fixing devices that prevent subluxation of the tongue and neck structures also may be effective in preventing obstruction. For more severe sleep apnea, nonsurgical or surgical methods to prevent obstruction may be needed.

A common method to prevent airway collapse is the use of positive-pressure ventilation to hold open the upper airways. A nasal mask or full-face mask delivery system allows mechanical delivery of either bi-level positive airway pressure (BiPAP), autotitrating positive airway pressure (APAP), or nasal continuous positive airway pressure (CPAP). With BiPAP, a machine delivers a set inspiratory positive airway pressure at the beginning of each breath. As the patient begins to exhale, the machine delivers a lower end expiratory pressure. These two pressures hold open the upper airways. With APAP, the machine adjusts continuously, resetting the pressure throughout the breathing cycle to meet the patient's needs. Nasal CPAP delivers a set positive airway pressure continuously during each cycle of inhalation and exhalation. For any positive pressure ventilation through a facemask during sleep, a small electric compressor delivers the positive pressure. Proper fit of the mask over the nose and mouth or just over the nose is key to successful treatment (see Fig. 30-9 in Chapter 30). Although noisy and often annoying, these methods are well accepted by most patients after an initial adjustment period.

One drug has been approved to help manage the daytime sleepiness associated with sleep apnea. Modafinil (Attenace, Provigil) is helpful for patients who have *narcolepsy* (uncontrolled daytime sleep) from sleep apnea by promoting daytime wakefulness. This action does *not* treat the cause of sleep apnea.

Surgical Management

Surgical intervention for sleep apnea may involve a simple adenoidectomy, uvulectomy, or remodeling of the entire posterior oropharynx (uvulopalatopharyngoplasty [UPP]). Both conventional and laser surgeries are used for this purpose. A tracheostomy may be needed for very severe sleep apnea that is not relieved by more moderate interventions.

NONINFECTIOUS DISORDERS OF THE LARYNX

VOCAL CORD PARALYSIS

Vocal fold (cord) paralysis may result from injury, trauma, or disease that affects the larynx, laryngeal nerves, or vagus nerve. Prolonged intubation with an endotracheal (ET) tube may cause temporary or, rarely, permanent paralysis. Laryngeal paralysis may occur in patients with neurologic disorders. Damage to the vagus nerve (by chest injury) or brainstem may lead to nerve dysfunction. The laryngeal nerves may be damaged from trauma or disorders that involve the chest, esophagus, or thyroid. Paralysis of both vocal cords may result from direct injury, stroke involving the brainstem, or total thyroidectomy.

Vocal fold paralysis may affect both cords or only one. When only one vocal cord is involved (most common), the airway remains patent but the voice is affected. Manifestations of open bilateral vocal cord paralysis include hoarseness; a breathy, weak voice; and aspiration of food. *Bilateral closed vocal cord paralysis causes airway obstruction and is a medical emergency if the symptoms are severe and the patient cannot compensate. Stridor is the major manifestation.*

Securing a patent airway is the primary intervention. Place the patient in a high Fowler's position to aid in breathing and proper alignment of airway structures. Assess for upper airway obstruction. *Immediately notify the Rapid Response Team if dyspnea with stridor occurs.* Emergency endotracheal intubation or tracheostomy may be needed.

AUDIO CLIP: Stridor

Various surgical procedures can improve the voice. One simple procedure for open vocal cord paresis involves injecting polytef (Teflon) into the affected cord so it enlarges toward the unaffected cord. This technique improves closure during speaking and eating.

The patient with open vocal cord paralysis is at risk for aspiration because the airway may not close during swallowing. Teach him or her to hold the breath during swallowing. This action allows the larynx to rise, close, and divert food back into the esophagus during swallowing. Also teach him or her to tuck the chin down and tilt the forehead forward during swallowing to prevent aspiration. Indications of aspiration include immediate coughing on swallowing of liquids or solids, a "wet"-sounding voice, and "tearing up" or watery eyes on swallowing. Chest x-rays and laryngeal and chest auscultation are also useful to diagnose aspiration pneumonia.

VOCAL CORD NODULES AND POLYPS

Nodules often appear at the point at which the vocal cords touch during speech. **Nodules** are enlarged, fibrous tissues caused by infectious processes or overuse of the voice. People most affected are those who often speak loudly, such as teachers, coaches, sports fans, and singers.

Vocal cord polyps are chronic, edematous masses. They occur most often in smokers, people with allergies, or those who live in dry climates. Vocal cysts also may occur.

Nodules and polyps are painless. The main manifestation is painless hoarseness because of the loss of coordinated closure of the vocal cords (Fig. 31-3).

Management of cord nodules or polyps is aimed at educating the patient and family. Instruct the patient about tobacco-use hazards, smoking-cessation programs, and the importance of voice rest. Treatment includes not speaking, especially not whispering, and avoiding heavy lifting. Stool softeners are used to avoid bearing down during elimination, which would cause the glottis to close. Humidifying inspired air may soothe the vocal cords and prevent overdrying.

Speech and language therapy is used for behavioral voice changes and helps the patient learn to reduce speech intensity. This therapy may make surgery unnecessary.

If hoarseness is not relieved by voice rest or speech and language therapy, the surgeon may remove the nodules or polyps under direct laryngoscopy. Laser and surgical resection are used to remove the mucous membrane of the affected cord. If both cords are involved, one cord is usually allowed to heal before surgery is performed on the other cord. These procedures are often performed as ambulatory surgery. Thus the patient should be educated before surgery and before he or she goes home.

After surgery the patient must maintain complete voice rest for about 14 days to promote healing. Chart 31-2 lists NIC interventions for communication enhancement. Teach about alternative methods of communication such as a slate board, pen and paper, Magic Slate, or alphabet board. While the patient is an inpatient, place a sign on his or her door, over the bed, and on the intercom system to help implement voice rest.

Chart 31-2 NIC INTERVENTION ACTIVITIES
The Patient with Problems in Vocalization

Communication Enhancement: *Speech Deficit: Assistance in accepting and learning alternate methods for living with impaired speech*

- Provide verbal prompts/reminders.
- Listen attentively.
- Refrain from shouting at the patient with communication disorders.
- Use picture board, if appropriate.
- Use hand gestures, as appropriate.
- Perform prescriptive speech-language therapies during informal interactions with patient.
- Teach esophageal speech, as appropriate.
- Instruct patient and family on use of speech aids (e.g., tracheal-esophageal prosthesis and artificial larynx).
- Encourage patient to repeat words.
- Provide positive reinforcement and praise, as appropriate.
- Carry on one-way conversations, as appropriate.
- Reinforce need for follow-up with speech pathologist after discharge.

NIC intervention activities selected from Bulechek, G.M., Butcher, H.K., & McCloskey Dochterman, J. (Eds.). (2008). *Nursing interventions classification (NIC)* (5th ed.). St. Louis: Mosby. No part of this work is to be altered without prior written permission from the Publisher.

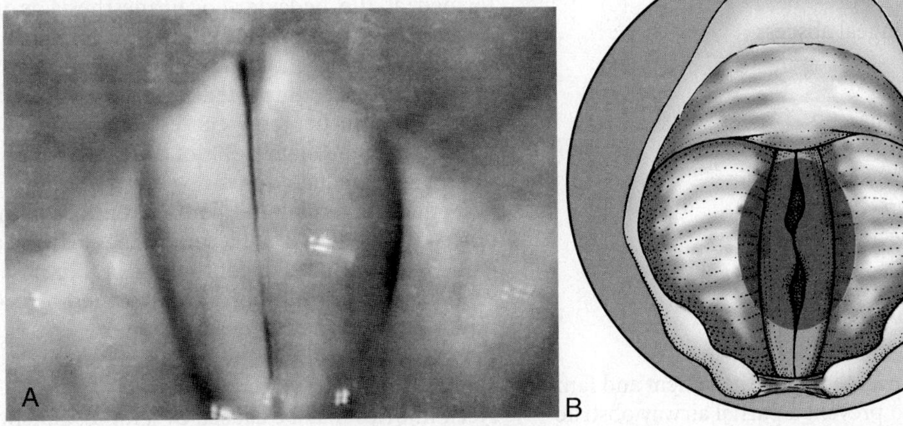
A
B

Fig. 31-3 • **A,** Close-up view of normal vocal cords in phonation. **B,** Vocal cord nodules and polyps prevent approximation of the vocal cords. Hoarseness results.

LARYNGEAL TRAUMA

Laryngeal trauma occurs with a crushing or direct blow injury, fracture, or injury such as that induced by prolonged endotracheal intubation.

Manifestations of laryngeal trauma include difficulty breathing **(dyspnea),** inability to produce sound **(aphonia),** hoarseness, and **subcutaneous emphysema** (air present in the subcutaneous tissue). Bleeding from the airway **(hemoptysis)** may occur, depending on the location of the trauma. The physician performs a direct visual examination by laryngoscopy or fiberoptic laryngoscopy of the larynx to determine the nature and extent of the injury.

Management of patients with laryngeal injuries consists of airway assessment and monitoring vital signs (including respiratory status and pulse oximetry) every 15 to 30 minutes. *Maintaining a patent airway is a priority.* Apply oxygen and humidification as prescribed to maintain adequate oxygen saturation. *If the patient has respiratory difficulty, stay with him or her and instruct other trauma team members or the Rapid Response Team to prepare for an emergency intubation or tracheotomy.* Manifestations of respiratory difficulty include increasing tachypnea, nasal flaring, anxiety, sternal retraction, shortness of breath, dyspnea, restlessness, decreased oxygen saturation, decreased level of consciousness, and stridor.

Surgical intervention is necessary for lacerations of the mucous membranes, cartilage exposure, and paralysis of the cords. Laryngeal repair is performed as soon as possible to prevent laryngeal stenosis and to cover any exposed cartilage. An artificial airway may be needed.

OTHER UPPER AIRWAY DISORDERS

UPPER AIRWAY OBSTRUCTION

Pathophysiology

Upper airway obstruction is a life-threatening emergency in which airflow is interrupted through the nose, mouth, pharynx, or larynx. Early recognition is essential to prevent further complications, including respiratory arrest. Causes of upper airway obstruction include:

- Tongue edema (surgery, trauma, angioedema as an allergic response to a drug)
- Occlusion by the tongue (e.g., with loss of gag reflex, loss of pharyngeal muscle tone, unconsciousness, coma)
- Laryngeal edema
- Peritonsillar and pharyngeal abscess
- Head and neck cancer
- Thick secretions
- Stroke and cerebral edema
- Smoke inhalation edema
- Facial, tracheal, or laryngeal trauma
- Foreign-body aspiration
- Burns of the head or neck area
- Anaphylaxis

Patient-Centered Collaborative Care

Assessment

Upper airway obstruction is frightening to the patient and family. Prompt care is essential to prevent a partial airway obstruction from progressing to a complete obstruction. A patient with a partial obstruction (e.g., caused by limited edema or a small foreign body) may have only subtle or general manifestations such as diaphoresis, tachycardia, and elevated blood pressure. Unexplained or persistent recurrent symptoms warrant evaluation even though the symptoms are vague. To rule out a tumor, foreign body, or infection, diagnostic procedures, such as a chest x-ray, neck films, laryngoscopic examination, and computed tomography, are performed.

Observe for hypoxia and hypercarbia, restlessness, increasing anxiety, sternal retractions, a "seesawing" chest, abdominal movements, or a feeling of impending doom related to actual air hunger. Use pulse oximetry for ongoing monitoring of oxygen saturation. Continually assess for stridor, cyanosis, and changes in level of consciousness.

Interventions

Assess for the cause of the obstruction. When the obstruction is due to the tongue falling back or the accumulation of secretions, slightly extend the patient's head and neck and insert a nasal or an oral airway. Suction to remove obstructing secretions. If the obstruction is caused by a foreign body, perform abdominal thrusts (Fig. 31-4).

Upper airway obstruction may require emergency procedures such as cricothyroidotomy, endotracheal intubation, or tracheotomy. Direct laryngoscopy may be performed before or with these procedures to determine the cause of obstruction. A direct laryngoscopy examination, in a controlled situation, may be used to remove foreign bodies.

Cricothyroidotomy is an emergency procedure often performed outside the hospital by emergency medical personnel or in the emergency department by a physician. A **cricothyroidotomy** is a stab wound at the cricothyroid membrane between the thyroid cartilage and the cricoid cartilage ring (see Fig. 29-4). Any hollow tube—but preferably a tracheostomy tube—can be placed through this opening to keep the new airway open until a tracheotomy can be performed. This procedure is used when it is the *only* way to secure an airway. Another emergency procedure to bypass an obstruction involves the physician inserting a 14-gauge needle directly into the cricoid space to allow air movement into and out of the lungs.

Endotracheal intubation is performed by inserting a tube into the trachea via the nose **(nasotracheal)** or mouth **(orotracheal)** by a physician, nurse anesthetist, or other specially trained personnel.

Tracheotomy is a surgical procedure and takes about 5 to 10 minutes to perform. Ideally it is performed in the OR with the patient under local or general anesthesia. It can be performed at the bedside. Local anesthesia is used if there is concern that the airway will be lost during the induction of anesthesia. A tracheotomy is reserved for the patient who cannot be easily intubated with an endotracheal tube. The emergency tracheotomy can establish an airway in less than 2 minutes. See Chapter 30 for a discussion of care of the patient with a tracheotomy.

Patients receiving mechanical ventilation for upper airway obstruction or respiratory failure may require a tracheostomy after 7 or more days of continuous oral or nasal intubation. In such cases, the procedure is performed to prevent laryngeal injury by the endotracheal tube.

NECK TRAUMA

Neck injuries may be caused by a knife, gunshot, or traumatic accident. The patient with neck trauma may have more than one injury, including cardiovascular, respiratory, intestinal, and neurologic damage. The final outcome of this type of in-

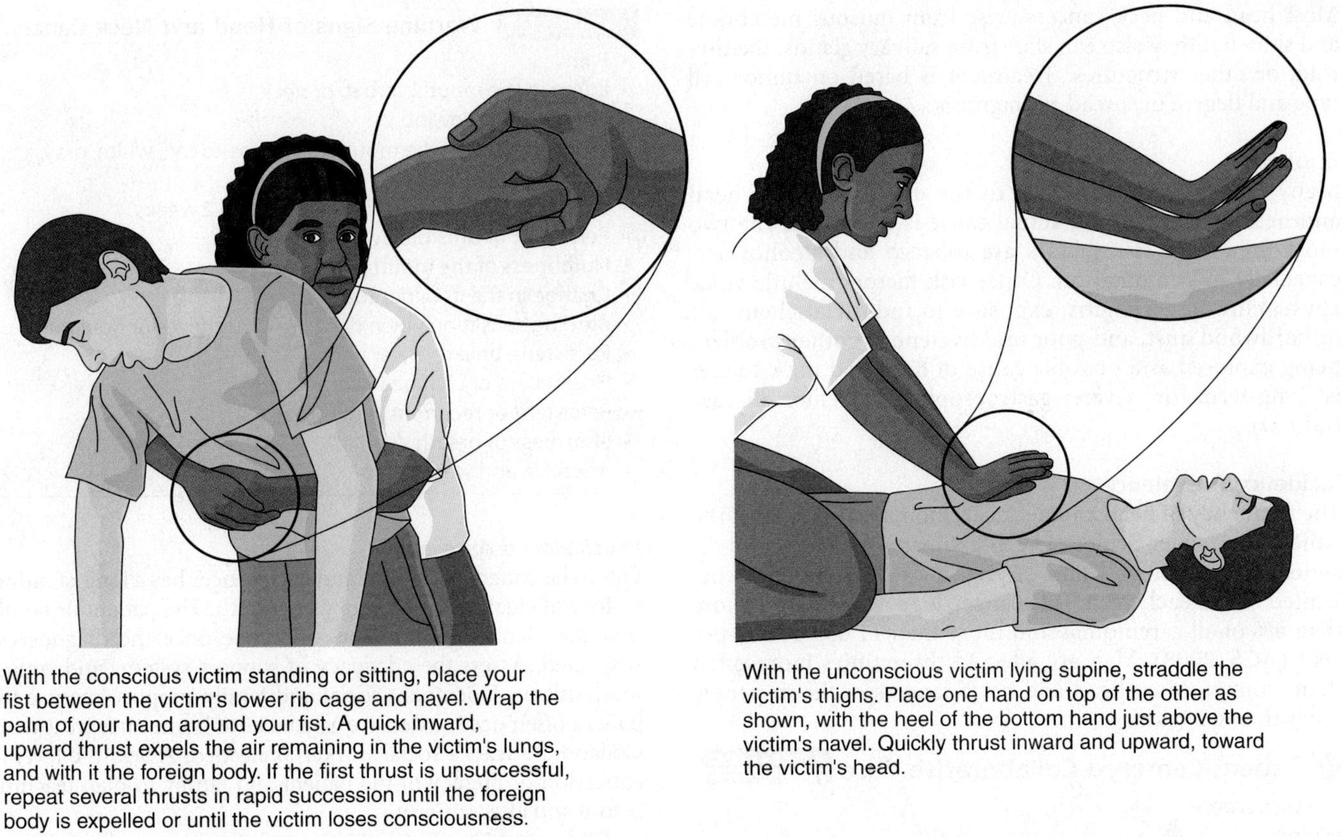
With the conscious victim standing or sitting, place your fist between the victim's lower rib cage and navel. Wrap the palm of your hand around your fist. A quick inward, upward thrust expels the air remaining in the victim's lungs, and with it the foreign body. If the first thrust is unsuccessful, repeat several thrusts in rapid succession until the foreign body is expelled or until the victim loses consciousness.
With the unconscious victim lying supine, straddle the victim's thighs. Place one hand on top of the other as shown, with the heel of the bottom hand just above the victim's navel. Quickly thrust inward and upward, toward the victim's head.

Fig. 31-4 • The abdominal thrust maneuver (formerly known as the *Heimlich maneuver*) for relief of upper airway obstruction caused by a foreign body.

jury depends on the initial assessment and care. Consult a critical care or emergency textbook and see Chapter 47 for more in-depth information.

The priority nursing care for a patient with neck trauma is assessing for and maintaining a patent airway. After airway patency is ensured, then assess for manifestations of bleeding or impending shock.

Perform a neurologic assessment for mental status, sensory level, and motor function. Injury to the carotid artery may result in death, stroke, or paralysis from disruption of blood flow to the brain (see Chapter 43). A carotid angiogram may be needed to rule out vascular injuries.

Esophagus injury may occur with neck trauma. Assess for chest pain and tenderness, oral bleeding, and **crepitus** (crackling sounds when palpating the skin). A barium or meglumine diatrizoate (Gastrografin) swallow may be needed to rule out an esophageal perforation injury.

Cervical spine injuries often occur at the same time as a neck injury (see Chapter 45). Health care personnel must take great care not to make these injuries worse by causing neck movement while establishing the airway using the jaw-thrust maneuver. Prepare to assist in emergency intubation, cricothyrotomy, or tracheotomy to establish a patent airway. Interventions for patients in shock are detailed in Chapter 39.

HEAD AND NECK CANCER

Pathophysiology

Head and neck cancer can disrupt breathing, eating, facial appearance, self-image, speech, and communication. This form of cancer can be devastating, even when treated successfully. The care needs for patients with these problems are complex, requiring a coordinated and comprehensive team approach. The patient can receive appropriate care only after the location and size of the tumor are accurately identified.

Head and neck cancer is curable when treated early. The prognosis for those who have more advanced disease at diagnosis depends on the extent and location of the tumor. Untreated cancer of the head and neck is a fatal disease within 2 years of diagnosis.

Most head and neck cancers (80%) are squamous cell carcinomas of the mucosa that are slow growing, taking several years to develop (ACS, 2008). Often these tumors first appear as deep ulcerations.

The cancer begins when the mucosa is chronically irritated and changes into a tougher mucosa *(squamous metaplasia)*. This tougher mucosa occurs by increasing the mucosal thickness (*acanthosis* or hyperplasia) or by developing a keratin layer *(keratosis)*. At the same time, genes controlling cell growth are damaged, allowing growth enhancement of these abnormal cells, which eventually become malignant. These lesions may then take the form of white, patchy lesions **(leukoplakia)** or red, velvety patches **(erythroplasia)**.

The growth and spread **(metastasis)** of head and neck cancer first occur into nearby structures, such as lymph nodes, muscle, and bone. Systemic spread through the blood and lymphatic systems to distant sites may also occur—usually to the lungs or liver.

The degree of malignancy is determined by cellular analysis. Earlier stage cancers are described as *carcinoma in situ* and *well differentiated.* Without treatment, cancers progress to be *moderately differentiated* and, finally, *poorly differentiated.*

Most head and neck cancers arise from mucous membrane and skin, but they also can start from salivary glands, the thyroid, or other structures. Treatment is based on tumor cell type and degree of spread at diagnosis.

Etiology

Many risk factors contribute to the development of head and neck cancer, but the actual cause is unknown. The two most important risk factors are tobacco and alcohol use, especially in combination. Other risk factors include voice abuse, chronic laryngitis, exposure to industrial chemicals or hardwood dust, and poor oral hygiene. Another problem being explored as a possible cause of head and neck cancer is long-term or severe gastroesophageal reflux disease (GERD).

Incidence/Prevalence

The frequency of head and neck carcinoma is increasing. The American Cancer Society (ACS) estimates 45,000 newly diagnosed cases of oral and laryngeal cancers occur in the United States each year. This cancer type accounts for more than 4% of all carcinomas and more than 11,000 deaths per year (ACS, 2008). Men are affected three times more often than women. Most head and neck cancers occur in people older than 60 years.

Patient-Centered Collaborative Care

evolve ONLINE PHARM REVIEW

Assessment

History

The patient with head and neck cancer may have difficulty speaking because of hoarseness, shortness of breath, tumor bulk, and pain. It is important to be sensitive to these difficulties during the interview.

Ask about tobacco and alcohol use, history of recurrent acute or chronic laryngitis or pharyngitis, oral sores, and lumps in the neck. Calculate the patient's smoking history by the number of packs smoked per day times the number of years the patient has smoked **(pack-years).** Ask about alcohol intake (how many drinks per day and for how many years). These questions may be uncomfortable for both you and the patient but are an important part of the history. Also ask about exposure to environmental or occupational pollutants.

Assess problems related to risk factors. For example, nutrition may be poor because of alcohol intake and impaired liver function. Assess dietary habits and any weight loss. Ask about any chronic lung disease, which may have an impact on the patient's breathing pattern.

Physical Assessment/Clinical Manifestations

Table 31-1 lists the warning signs of head and neck cancer. With laryngeal cancer, painless hoarseness may occur because of tumor size and an inability for the vocal cords to come together for normal speech **(phonation).** Lesions of the vocal cords are the earliest form of laryngeal cancer. Any person who has a history of hoarseness, mouth sores, or a lump in the neck for 3 to 4 weeks should be evaluated for laryngeal cancer.

Inspection and palpation of the head and neck are important parts of the physical examination. An advanced practice nurse or physician may perform a laryngeal examination using a laryngeal mirror or fiberoptic laryngoscope. Lesions may be seen on inspection. The neck is palpated to assess for enlarged lymph nodes.

TABLE 31-1 Warning Signs of Head and Neck Cancer

- Pain
- Lump in the mouth, throat, or neck
- Difficulty swallowing
- Color changes in the mouth or tongue to red, white, gray, dark brown, or black
- Oral lesion or sore that does not heal in 2 weeks
- Persistent or unexplained oral bleeding
- Numbness of the mouth, lips, or face
- Change in the fit of dentures
- Burning sensation when drinking citrus juices or hot liquids
- Persistent, unilateral ear pain
- Hoarseness or change in voice quality
- Persistent or recurrent sore throat
- Shortness of breath
- Anorexia and weight loss

Psychosocial Assessment

Often the patient with head and neck cancer has a long-standing history of cigarette or alcohol use or both. The patient or family may feel denial, guilt, blame, or shame once the diagnosis is suspected. Assess the adequacy of support systems and coping mechanisms. Document social and family support because the patient often needs extensive assistance at home after treatment. Collaborate with a social worker as needed. Assess the level of education or literacy of the patient and family to plan teaching before and after surgery.

Document any family history of cancer, as well as the patient's age, gender, occupation, and ability to perform ADLs. Ask the patient whether his or her occupation requires continual oral communication. Job retraining may be needed if treatment affects speech.

Laboratory Assessment

Diagnostic tests include a complete blood cell count, bleeding times, urinalysis, and blood chemistries. The patient with chronic alcoholism may have low protein and albumin levels from poor nutrition. Renal and liver function tests are performed to rule out cancer spread and to evaluate the patient's ability to metabolize drugs and chemotherapy agents.

Imaging Assessment

Many types of imaging studies, including x-rays of the skull, sinuses, neck, and chest, are useful in diagnosing cancer spread, other tumors, and the extent of tumor invasion. Computed tomography (CT) of the head and neck, with or without contrast media, helps evaluate the tumor's exact location.

Magnetic resonance imaging (MRI) can help differentiate normal from diseased tissue. An MRI is more sensitive than a CT in defining the extent of soft-tissue invasion.

The brain, bone, and liver are evaluated with nuclear imaging, bone scans, single-photon emission computerized tomography (SPECT) scans, and positron emission tomography (PET) scans. These tests help locate additional tumor sites.

Other Diagnostic Assessment

Other helpful tests include direct and indirect laryngoscopy, tumor mapping, and biopsy. *Panendoscopy* (laryngoscopy, nasopharyngoscopy, esophagoscopy, and bronchoscopy) is performed with general anesthesia to define the extent of the tumor. Tumor-mapping biopsies are performed to identify tumor location. Biopsy tissues taken at the time of the panendoscopy confirm the diagnosis and determine the tumor type, cell features, and location. Tumor staging by the TNM (tumor, nodes, metastasis) method (see Chapter 23) is also performed.

▪ *Analysis*

Common Nursing Diagnoses and Collaborative Problems

The primary collaborative problem is Potential for Respiratory Obstruction.

Priority nursing diagnoses for patients with head and neck carcinomas are:

1. Risk for Aspiration related to edema, anatomic changes, or altered protective reflexes
2. Anxiety related to threat of death, change in role status, or change in economic status
3. Disturbed Body Image related to tumor and treatment modalities

Additional Nursing Diagnoses and Collaborative Problems

In addition to the common nursing diagnoses and collaborative problems, patients with head and neck carcinomas may have one or more of these:

- Acute Pain or Chronic Pain related to tumor invasion of tissues and nerves and surgical intervention
- Imbalanced Nutrition: Less Than Body Requirements related to dysphagia, anxiety, tumor process, surgical resection, or chronic alcohol intake
- Impaired Verbal Communication related to tumor invasion, hoarseness, pain, or surgical resection
- Impaired Skin Integrity related to altered circulation, nutritional deficit, tumor invasion, radiation, chemical factors (body secretions or substances), or surgical wound
- Ineffective Coping related to altered body image, communication method, or ineffective social support
- Impaired Social Interaction related to body image disturbance and lifestyle practices
- Deficient Knowledge (treatment regimen and resources) related to lack of exposure to or lack of interest in learning

▪ *Planning and Implementation*

Potential for Respiratory Obstruction

NOC **Planning: Expected Outcomes.** The patient with head and neck cancer is expected to attain and maintain adequate tissue oxygenation. Indicators include:

- Arterial blood gas values within the normal range
- Rate and depth of respiration within the normal range
- Pulse oximetry within the normal range
- Absence of cyanosis or pallor

Interventions. The goal of treatment is to remove or eradicate the cancer while preserving as much normal function as possible. The physician presents the available treatment options. Surgery, radiation, or chemotherapy may each be used alone or in combination. In planning treatment options, the patient's general physical condition, nutritional status, and age; the effects of the tumor on body function; and the patient's personal choice are all considered. Treatment for laryngeal cancer may range from radiation therapy (for a small specific area or tumor) to total laryngopharyngectomy with bilateral neck dissections followed by radiation therapy. The specific treatment depends on the extent and location of the lesion. Voice-conservation procedures are used only if they do not risk incomplete removal of the tumor. Nursing care focuses on the patient's total needs, including preoperative preparation, competent in-hospital care, discharge planning and teaching, and extensive outpatient rehabilitation.

Nonsurgical Management. Monitor the respiratory system by assessing respiratory rate, breath sounds, pulse oximetry, arterial blood gas values, and the results of pulmonary function tests. Respiratory distress may indicate narrowing of the airway related to tumor growth, edema, or both. Position the patient for optimal air exchange. Teach the patient and family about the use of Fowler's and semi-Fowler's positions. Sitting upright in a reclining chair may promote more comfortable breathing. Chapters 5 and 9 provide additional information on palliation and pain control for patients who elect not to have therapy and for those whose therapy has not been effective.

Radiation therapy for treatment of small cancers in specific locations has a cure rate of at least 80%. The cure rate for larger cancers is lower when radiation is used as the only therapy. Standard therapy uses 5000 to 7500 rad (radiation absorbed dose), usually over 6 weeks and in daily or twice-daily doses. Radiation may be used alone or in combination with surgery. Because radiation therapy slows tissue healing, it might not be performed before surgery. Radiation therapy is an outpatient treatment (see Chapter 24). Most patients have hoarseness, dysphagia, skin problems, and dry mouth for a few weeks after radiation therapy.

Hoarseness may become worse. Reassure the patient and family that voice improves within 4 to 6 weeks after completion of radiation therapy. Urge the patient to use voice rest and alternate means of communication until the effects of radiation therapy have passed.

Most patients have a sore throat and difficulty swallowing during radiation therapy to the neck. Gargling with saline or sucking ice may decrease discomfort. Mouthwashes and throat sprays containing a local anesthetic agent such as lidocaine or diphenhydramine can provide temporary relief. Analgesic drugs may be prescribed.

The skin at the site of irradiation becomes red and tender and may peel during therapy. Instruct the patient to avoid exposing this area to sun, heat, cold, and abrasive treatments such as shaving. Teach the patient to wear protective clothing made of soft cotton and to wash this area gently with a mild soap, such as Dove. Stress that only the lotions or powders prescribed by the radiation oncologist should be used on this skin until the area has healed.

If the salivary glands are in the path of irradiation, the patient has a dry mouth **(xerostomia).** This side effect is long-term and may be permanent. Some of the problems from reduced saliva include increased risk for dental caries, increased risk for oral infections, halitosis (bad breath), and taste changes. Although there is no cure for xerostomia, interventions can help reduce the discomfort. Heavy fluid intake, particularly water, and humidification can help ease the discomfort. Some patients benefit from the use of artificial saliva, such as Salivart, or saliva stimulants, such as Salagen and cevimeline (cholinergic drugs). Chewing gum and sucking hard candy may relieve dry mouth temporarily.

Chemotherapy can be used alone or in addition to surgery or radiation for head and neck cancer. Chapter 24 discusses the general care needs of patients receiving chemotherapy.

Surgical Management. Tumor size and location (TNM classification) determines the type of surgery needed for the specific head and neck cancer. Very small, early-stage tumors may be removed by laser therapy or photodynamic therapy;

however, few head and neck tumors are found at this stage and most require extensive traditional surgery. Reconstruction is also determined by the tumor size and amount of tissue to be resected and reconstructed. Surgical procedures for head and neck cancers include laryngectomy (total and partial), tracheostomy, and oropharyngeal cancer resections. The major types of surgery for laryngeal cancer include cord stripping, removal of a vocal cord **(cordectomy)**, partial laryngectomy, and total laryngectomy. If cancer is in the lymph nodes in the neck or if the tumor has a high rate of nodal spread, the surgeon performs a nodal neck dissection along with removal of the primary tumor ("radical neck"). A pathologist evaluates the resected lymph nodes for tumor invasion.

Preoperative care. Teach the patient and family about the tumor. The surgeon explains the surgical procedure and obtains informed consent. Discuss and interpret the implications of such consent with the patient and family.

Explain about self-care of the airway, alternate methods of communication, suctioning, pain control methods, the critical care environment (including ventilators and critical care routines), nutritional support, feeding tubes, and goals for discharge. The patient will need to learn new methods of speech. Help him or her prepare for this change before surgery and to practice the use of an alternate form of communication (e.g., pen and pencil, Magic Slate, picture or alphabet board, or computerized word generator). Determine the communication method most preferred by the patient.

A team approach for planning care and rehabilitation is critical for the best outcome. The team includes nurses, physicians, speech-language pathologists, social workers, nutritionists, respiratory therapists, and occupational and physical therapists. Professionals from all these disciplines help evaluate and prepare the patient who has head and neck cancer. Chapter 16 describes general preoperative assessment and education.

Operative procedures. Table 31-2 lists specific information about the various surgical procedures for laryngeal cancer. Hemilaryngectomy (vertical or horizontal) and supraglottic laryngectomy are types of partial voice conservation laryngectomies.

To protect the airway, a tracheostomy is needed. With a partial laryngectomy, the tracheostomy is usually temporary. With a total laryngectomy, the upper airway is separated from the throat and esophagus, and the trachea is brought out through the skin in the neck and sutured in place, creating a stoma. This airway opening (a laryngectomy stoma) is permanent.

Neck dissection includes the removal of lymph nodes, the sternocleidomastoid muscle, the jugular vein, the 11th cranial nerve, and surrounding soft tissue. Because the 11th cranial nerve (spinal accessory nerve) is cut during this procedure, shoulder drop will be present after surgery. Physical therapy exercises are needed after surgery to help the patient ease the shoulder drop by using other muscle groups.

Postoperative care. Head and neck surgery often lasts 8 hours or longer. Usually the patient spends the immediate period after surgery in the surgical intensive care unit. Monitor airway patency, vital signs, hemodynamic status, and comfort level. Monitor for hemorrhage and other general complications of anesthesia and surgery (see Chapter 18). Take vital signs hourly for the first 24 hours and then every 2 hours or according to agency policy until the patient is stable. After the patient is transferred from the critical care unit, monitor vital signs every 4 hours or according to agency policy. The patient is generally out of bed by the second day.

Complications after surgery include airway obstruction, hemorrhage, wound breakdown, and tumor recurrence. *The first priorities after head and neck surgery are airway maintenance and ventilation.* Other priorities are wound, flap, and reconstructive tissue care; pain management; nutrition; and psychological adjustment, including speech and language therapy.

Airway maintenance and ventilation. Immediately after surgery, the patient may need ventilatory assistance because of a long-term smoking history, chronic lung disease, and a long duration of anesthesia. Most patients wean easily from the ventilator after this type of surgery because the thoracic and abdominal cavities are not entered. During weaning, the patient usually uses a tracheostomy collar (over the artificial airway or open stoma) with oxygen and humidity to help move mucus secretions. Secretions may remain blood-tinged for 1 to 2 days. Use Body Substance Precautions, and report any increase in bleeding to the surgeon. Humidity helps remove crusts and prevent obstruction of the tube with secretions. Some surgeons prescribe instillations of 5 to 10 mL of

TABLE 31-2 Surgical Procedures for Laryngeal Cancer and Their Effect on Voice Quality

Procedure	Description	Resulting Voice Quality
Laser surgery	Tumor reduced or destroyed by laser beam through laryngoscope	Normal/hoarse
Transoral cordectomy	Tumor (early lesion) resected through laryngoscope	Normal/hoarse (high cure rate)
Laryngofissure	No cord removed (early lesion)	Normal (high cure rate)
Supraglottic partial laryngectomy	Hyoid bone, false cords, and epiglottis removed Neck dissection on affected side performed if nodes involved	Normal/hoarse
Hemilaryngectomy or vertical laryngectomy	One true cord, one false cord, and one half of thyroid cartilage removed	Hoarse
Total laryngectomy	Entire larynx, hyoid bone, strap muscles, one or two tracheal rings removed Nodal neck dissection if nodes involved	No natural voice

sterile saline or sodium bicarbonate into the airway every 2 hours; however, this practice is controversial.

A laryngectomy tube is used for patients who have undergone a *total laryngectomy* and need an appliance to prevent scar tissue shrinkage of the skin-tracheal border. This tube is similar to a tracheostomy tube but is shorter and wider with a larger lumen (Fig. 31-5). Laryngectomy tube care is similar to tracheostomy tube care (see Chapter 30) except that the patient can change the laryngectomy tube daily or as needed. A laryngectomy button is similar to a laryngectomy tube but is softer, has a single lumen, and is very short. A button is comfortable for the patient, is easily removed for cleaning, and is available in various sizes and lengths for a custom fit. Provide a Magic Slate or paper and pencil for communication because the patient cannot speak other than mouthing words.

Coughing, deep breathing, and saline instillation are usually effective in clearing secretions. The lack of a surgical incision in the chest or abdomen improves the ability to cough. Instruct the patient how to cough and deep breathe to clear secretions.

Oral secretions can be suctioned by the alert patient using a Yankauer or tonsillar suction or a soft red latex catheter. Teach the patient to suction away from the side of the surgery to prevent wound opening immediately after surgery. Patients can participate in their own care by using a table mirror for visibility. Provide a clean environment for the catheter.

Stoma care after a total laryngectomy is a combination of wound care and airway care. Inspect the stoma with a flashlight. Clean the suture line with half-strength hydrogen peroxide to prevent secretions from forming crusts and obstructing the airway. Perform suture line care every 1 to 2 hours during the first few days after surgery and then every 4 hours thereafter. The mucosa of the stoma and trachea should be bright and shiny and without crusts, similar to the appearance of the oral mucosa.

Wound, flap, and reconstructive tissue care. Tissue "flaps" may be used to close the wound and improve appearance. Commonly used reconstructive flaps are myocutaneous flaps, island flaps, rotation flaps, trapezius flaps, split-thickness skin grafts (STSGs), and free flaps with microvascular anastomosis. Flaps are skin, subcutaneous tissue, and sometimes muscle, taken from other body areas. These flaps may be used for reconstruction after any type of head and neck resection. After neck dissection, the surgeon places an STSG over the exposed carotid artery before covering it with skin flaps or reconstructive flaps.

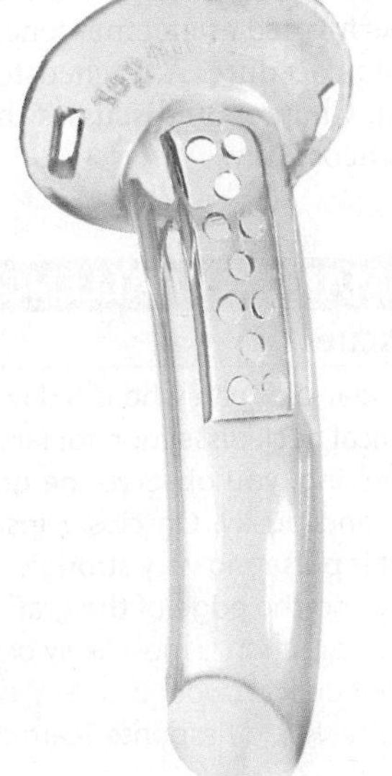

Fig. 31-5 • A laryngectomy tube. Note that the outer cannula is shorter and has a diameter wider than that of a tracheostomy tube.

The first 24 hours after surgery are critical. Evaluate all grafts and flaps hourly for the first 72 hours. Monitor capillary refill, color, drainage, and Doppler activity of the major feeding vessel. Report changes to the surgeon immediately because surgical intervention may be needed. Position the patient so that the side of the head and neck with the flaps is not dependent.

Hemorrhage. Hemorrhage is a possible complication after any surgery, but it is uncommon with laryngectomy. The surgeon often places a closed surgical drain in the neck area to collect blood and drainage for about 72 hours after surgery. The drain also helps maintain the position of the reconstructed skin flaps. Any drain obstruction or equipment malfunction may cause a buildup of blood or serum under the flaps. This collection can impair blood flow to and from the flaps, resulting in flap failure and tissue loss. A sudden stoppage of drainage may indicate a clot obstructing the drain. Monitor drainage, and record its amount and character. Check the patency and functioning of the drainage system. Report any drain malfunction or change in flap appearance to the surgeon. Depending on the surgeon's prescription and the agency's policy, you may need to empty the drainage container or "milk" the drain.

Wound breakdown. Wound breakdown is a common complication caused by poor nutrition, a long smoking history, alcohol use, wound contamination, and previous radiation therapy. Manage wound breakdown with packing and local care as prescribed to keep the wound clean and to stimulate the growth of healthy granulation tissue. Wounds may be extensive, and the carotid artery may be exposed. Split-thickness skin grafts often are placed over the carotid artery for protection in the event of wound dehiscence. As the wound heals, granulation tissue covers the artery and prevents rupture. If granulation is slow and the carotid artery is at risk, another surgical flap may be made to cover the carotid artery and close the wound.

When the carotid artery ruptures, large amounts of bright red blood spurt quickly. It is also possible for the carotid artery to have a small leak, with continuous oozing of bright red blood. Usually, a small leak leads to a complete rupture within a short time. *If a carotid artery leak is suspected, call the Rapid Response Team and do not touch the area because additional pressure could cause an immediate rupture. If the carotid artery ruptures because of drying or infection, immediately place constant pressure over the site and secure the airway. Maintain direct manual, continuous pressure on the carotid artery, and immediately transport the patient to the operating room for carotid resection. Do not leave the patient. Carotid artery rupture has a high risk of stroke and death. Nursing response can save the patient's life.*

Pain management. Pain is caused by the surgical cutting or manipulation of tissue and by nerve compression. Pain should be controlled, and the patient should still be able to participate in his or her care. Morphine (Statex♣) often is given IV by a patient-controlled analgesia (PCA) pump for the first 1 to 2 days after surgery. As the patient progresses, liquid opioid analgesics can be given by feeding tube. Oral drugs for pain and discomfort are started only after the patient can tolerate oral intake. After discharge, the patient still requires pain management, especially if he or she is receiving radiation therapy. An adjunct to the pain regimen may be liquid NSAIDs. These drugs provide excellent pain relief and can be used along with opioid analgesics. Amitriptyline (Elavil) or other tricyclic antidepressants may also be used for the lancinating pain of nerve-root involvement.

Nutrition. A nasogastric, gastrostomy, or jejunostomy tube is placed during surgery for nutritional support while the head and neck heal. Initially the patient receives IV fluids or parenteral nutrition until the intestinal tract has recovered from the effects of anesthesia. After that, nutrients can be given via the feeding tube. The nutritional support team or nutritionist assesses the patient before surgery and is available for consultation after surgery. The common nutrition goal is to provide 35 to 40 kcal/kg of body weight daily. Replacement of protein and water loss is calculated carefully.

The nasogastric tube (the most commonly used type of tube) usually remains in place for 7 to 10 days after surgery. Before removing the tube, assess the patient's ability to swallow if nutrition is to be given by mouth. Aspiration *cannot* occur after a total laryngectomy because the airway and esophagus have been completely separated. Reassure the patient that aspiration will not occur, and stay with him or her during the first few swallowing attempts. Swallowing may be uncomfortable at first, and analgesics may be needed.

Speech and language rehabilitation. The patient's voice quality and speech are altered after surgery. Although this problem has enormous effects on the patient's ability to maintain social interactions, continue employment, and maintain a desired quality of life, it is often poorly addressed while he or she is hospitalized. Working with him or her and the family toward developing an acceptable communication method during the inpatient period is essential for a satisfactory outcome.

Together with the speech and language pathologist (SLP), discuss the principles of speech therapy with the patient and family early in the course of the treatment plan (see Chart 31-2). Voice and speech differences depend on the type of surgical resection (see Table 31-2). Speech production varies with patient practice, amount of tissue removed, and radiation effects, but the speech can be very understandable.

The speech rehabilitation plan for patients who have a total laryngectomy at first consists of writing, using a picture board, or using a computer. The patient then uses an artificial larynx and, ideally, eventually learns esophageal speech. For success, the patient needs encouragement and support from the speech pathologist, hospital team, and family while relearning to speak. This process can be time consuming and requires concentration each time the patient speaks. Having a **laryngectomee** (a person who has had a laryngectomy) from one of the local self-help organizations visit the patient and family is often beneficial. The International Association of Laryngectomees is very active and supportive, as is the American Cancer Society (ACS) Visitor Program.

Common means of speech communication after laryngectomy include esophageal speech, the use of mechanical devices, and the use of a tracheoesophageal fistula (TEF).

Esophageal speech is attempted by most patients who have a total laryngectomy. Sound can be produced this way by "burping" the air swallowed or injected into the esophageal pharynx and shaping the words in the mouth. The voice produced is a monotone; it cannot be raised or lowered and carries no pitch. In the English language, the vocal cords are required for 15 consonants; the remaining 10 consonants can be formed by shaping the mouth. If patients do not have adequate hearing, esophageal speech will be difficult because they need to use their mouth to shape the words as they hear them. Hearing-impaired patients may need hearing aids.

Some patients have intestinal bloating as a result of swallowing air for esophageal speech. Antacids may help reduce bloating sensations. Esophageal speech also helps strengthen the respiratory and abdominal muscles, which aids in clearing secretions and in breathing.

Mechanical devices, called *electrolarynges,* may be used by the patient who cannot attain esophageal speech. Most are battery-powered devices placed against the side of the neck or cheek. The air inside the mouth and throat is vibrated, and the patient moves his or her lips and tongue as usual. Another external device (Cooper-Rand), also battery powered, consists of a plastic tube that is placed in the patient's mouth and vibrates during speech. The quality of speech generated with these devices is robot-like and does not sound natural.

Tracheoesophageal fistulas (TEFs) may be used if esophageal speech is ineffective and if the patient meets strict criteria. A surgical connection (fistula) is created between the trachea and the esophagus using a special catheter. The fistula can be created either at the time of the laryngectomy or later. After the fistula heals, a silicone prosthesis (e.g., the Blom-Singer prosthesis) is inserted in place of the catheter (Fig. 31-6). The patient covers the stoma and the opening of the prosthesis with a finger or opens and closes the opening with a special valve to divert air from the lungs, through the trachea, into the esophagus, and out of the mouth. Lip and tongue movement, not the prosthesis itself, produces speech.

Surgical procedures for other head and neck cancers. The major types of surgeries for other head and neck cancers are called *composite resections.* These resections are a combination of surgical procedures, including partial or total glossectomies, partial mandibulectomies, and, if needed, nodal neck dissections. Tracheostomy may be planned to provide an adequate airway. (See Chapter 56 for more information about oral cancer.)

Tracheotomy. A **tracheotomy** is a surgical incision into the trachea for the purpose of establishing an airway (tracheostomy). It can be performed as an emergency procedure or as a scheduled surgical procedure. A tracheostomy can be temporary or permanent. Chapter 30 discusses the nursing care of a patient with a tracheostomy.

DECISION-MAKING CHALLENGE
Critical Rescue

The patient is a 70-year-old man who is 5 days post-op after a laryngectomy and radical neck dissection for laryngeal cancer. When you change the dressing, you observe the graft over the carotid artery appears dry and dusky. On closer inspection, you notice that the whole graft is pulsating very strongly and some bright red blood is seeping around the edge of the graft.

1. What type of complication is most likely occurring?
2. Should you continue with wound care? Why or why not?
3. Should you call the Rapid Response Team or the surgeon? Why or why not?
4. Should you apply pressure to the graft site? Why or why not?

evolve For suggested answer guidelines, go to http://evolve.elsevier.com/Iggy/.

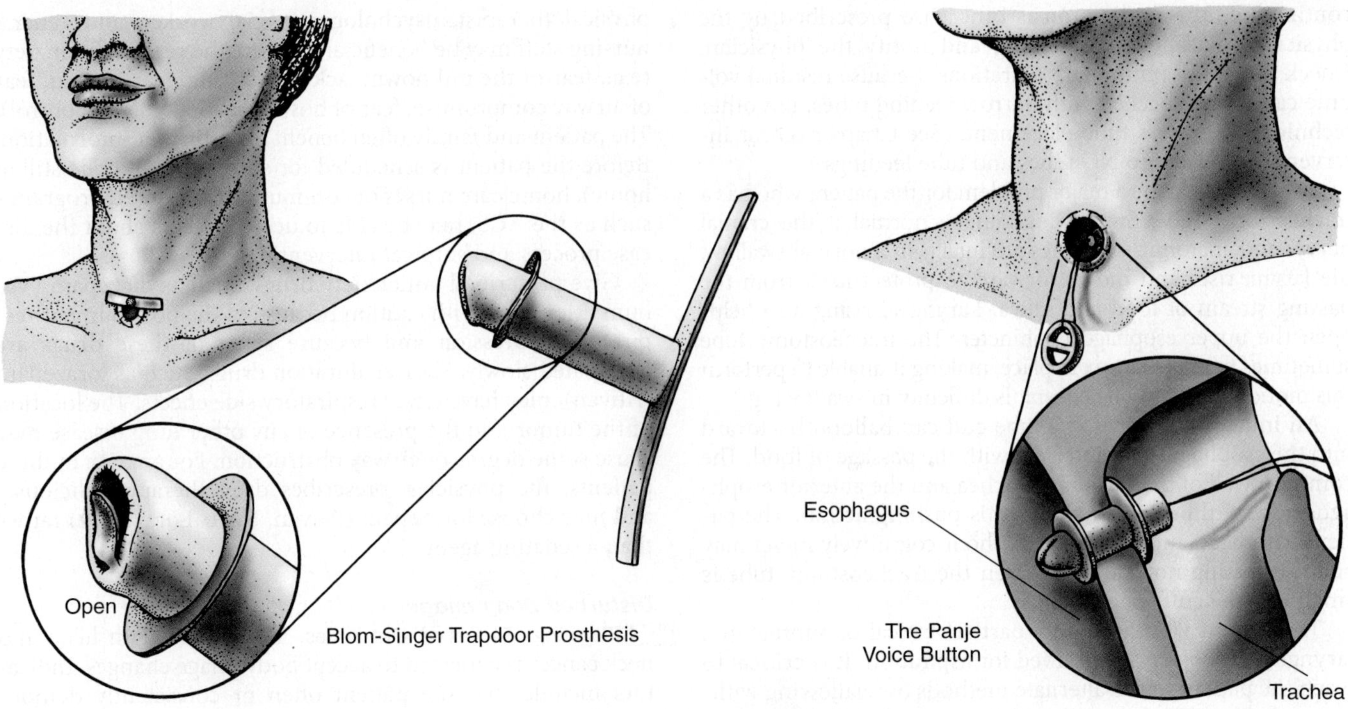
Open
Blom-Singer Trapdoor Prosthesis
Esophagus
The Panje
Voice Button
Trachea

Fig. 31-6 • Examples of tracheoesophageal prostheses.

Risk for Aspiration

NOC Planning: Expected Outcomes. The patient with head and neck cancer is expected not to aspirate food, gastric contents, or oral secretions into the lungs. Indicators include that the patient often or consistently demonstrates these behaviors:

- Positions self upright for eating or drinking
- Selects foods according to swallowing ability
- Chooses liquids and foods of proper consistency

Interventions. The surgical changes in the upper respiratory tract and altered swallowing mechanisms increase the patient's risk for aspiration. Aspiration can result in life-threatening pneumonia, weight loss, prolonged hospitalization, and increased costs. Chart 31-3 lists actions for aspiration prevention.

The presence of a nasogastric (NG) feeding tube may further increase the potential for aspiration because it keeps the lower esophageal sphincter partially open. The one exception is the patient who has undergone a total laryngectomy. In these cases, the airway is separated from the esophagus, making aspiration impossible; such a patient is *not* at risk.

A dynamic swallow study, such as a barium swallow under fluoroscopy, evaluates a patient's ability to protect the airway from aspiration and helps determine the appropriate method of swallow rehabilitation. In many cases, enteral feedings are used either because of the patient's inability to swallow or because of continued aspiration risk.

When an NG tube is in place, help prevent aspiration with the use of routine reflux precautions. These precautions include elevating the head of the bed and strictly adhering to tube feeding regimens, including no bolus feedings at night. Check residual feeding before each bolus feeding (or every 4 to 6 hours with continuous feeding), and evaluate the patient's tolerance of the tube feeding. If the residual volume is high (above 100 mL for bolus feeding or 2 hour's worth of

Chart 31-3 BEST PRACTICE FOR PATIENT SAFETY & QUALITY CARE

Prevention of Aspiration During Swallowing

- Avoid having meals when the patient is fatigued.
- Provide smaller and more frequent meals.
- Provide adequate time; do not "hurry" the patient.
- Provide close supervision if the patient is self-feeding.
- Keep emergency suctioning equipment close at hand.
- Avoid water and other "thin" liquids.
- Thicken liquids.
- Avoid foods that generate thin liquids during the chewing process, such as fruit.
- Position the patient in the most upright position possible.
- When possible, completely (or at least partially) deflate the tube cuff during meals.
- Suction after initial cuff deflation to clear the airway and allow maximum comfort during the meal.
- Feed each bite or encourage the patient to take each bite slowly.
- Encourage the patient to "dry swallow" after each bite to clear residue from the throat.
- Avoid consecutive swallows by cup or straw.
- Provide controlled small volumes of liquids, using a spoon.
- Encourage the patient to "tuck" his or her chin down and move the forehead forward while swallowing.
- Allow the patient to indicate when he or she is ready for the next bite.
- If the patient coughs, stop the feeding until the patient indicates the airway has been cleared.
- Continuously monitor tolerance to oral food intake by assessing respiratory rate, ease, pulse oximetry, and heart rate.

continuous tube feeding, or as otherwise prescribed by the physician), withhold the feeding and notify the physician. Check the pH of pulmonary secretions. Because residual volume cannot be checked with narrow feeding tubes, use other techniques to assess tube placement. (See Chapter 63 for interventions related to NG tubes and tube feedings.)

Swallowing can be a major problem for the patient who has a tracheostomy tube. Swallowing can be normal if the cranial nerves and anatomic structures are intact. In a normal swallow, the larynx rises and moves forward to protect itself from the passing stream of food and saliva. Laryngeal rising also helps open the upper esophageal sphincter. The tracheostomy tube sometimes fixes the larynx in place, making it unable to perform this motion efficiently. The result is difficulty in swallowing.

An inflated tracheostomy tube cuff can balloon backward into the esophagus and interfere with the passage of food. The common wall of the posterior trachea and the anterior esophagus is very thin, which allows this pushing action. The patient with head and neck cancer who is cognitively intact may adapt to eating normal food when the tracheostomy tube is small and the cuff is not inflated.

The patient who has had a partial vertical or supraglottic laryngectomy *must* be observed for aspiration. It is critical to teach the patient to use alternate methods of swallowing without aspirating. The "supraglottic" method of swallowing is especially effective after a partial laryngectomy or base-of-tongue resection (Chart 31-4). To reinforce teaching and learning, place a chart in the patient's room detailing the steps. A dynamic swallow study is performed to guide rehabilitation for swallowing and to evaluate the patient's ability to protect the airway.

Anxiety

NOC **Planning: Expected Outcomes.** The patient with head and neck cancer is expected to have decreased anxiety. Indicators include that the patient often or consistently demonstrates:

- Verbalization of reduced anxiety
- Absence of distress, irritability, and facial tension
- Effective use of coping strategies

Interventions. Conferences with the physician, clinical nurse specialist, nutritionist, speech and language pathologist, physical therapist, psychologist, social worker, and general nursing staff may be beneficial. Explore the reason for anxiety (e.g., fear of the unknown, lack of teaching, fear of pain, fear of airway compromise, fear of hospitalization, loss of control). The patient and family often benefit from further information. Before the patient is scheduled for surgery (and while still at home), home care nurses or community-sponsored programs, such as the ACS, may be able to decrease fears about the disease process and surgical interventions.

Give prescribed antianxiety drugs, such as diazepam (Valium, Meval♣), with caution because of the possibility of respiratory depression and because some of these drugs are eliminated slowly. Shorter-duration drugs, such as lorazepam (Ativan), may have fewer respiratory side effects. The location of the tumor and the presence of any other lung disease may cause some degree of airway obstruction. For anxiety in these patients, the physician prescribes drug therapy judiciously and may choose lorazepam (Ativan, Novo-Lorazem♣) rather than a sedating agent.

Disturbed Body Image

NOC **Planning: Expected Outcomes.** The patient with head and neck cancer is expected to accept body image changes. Indicators include that the patient often or consistently demonstrates:

- Willingness to touch the affected body part
- Willingness to use strategies to enhance appearance
- Participation in self-care
- Interaction with visitors, staff, and family members

Interventions. The patient with head and neck cancer may have a permanent change in body image because of deformity, the presence of a stoma or artificial airway, speech changes, and a change in the method of eating. He or she may not be able to speak at all or have permanent hoarseness or speech deficits. Help him or her set realistic goals, starting with involvement in self-care. Teach the patient alternate communication methods so he or she can functionally communicate in the hospital and after discharge.

Teach the family to ease the patient into a normal social environment. Use positive reinforcement and encouragement while demonstrating acceptance and caring behaviors. The family also may benefit from counseling sessions while the patient is still in the hospital.

After surgery the patient may feel socially isolated because of the change in voice and facial appearance. Loose-fitting, high-collar shirts or sweaters, scarves, and jewelry can be worn to cover the laryngectomy stoma, tracheostomy tube, and other changes related to surgery. Cosmetics may aid in covering disfigurement. Most surgeons try to place the incisions in the natural skin fold lines if doing so does not pose a risk for cancer recurrence.

Community-Based Care

If no complications occur, the patient is usually discharged home or to an extended care facility within 2 weeks. At the time of discharge, he or she or a family member should be able to perform tracheostomy or stoma care and participate in nutrition, wound care, and communication methods.

The patient and family may feel more secure about discharge if they receive a referral to select support groups or a community health agency familiar with the care of patients recovering from head and neck cancer. The nurse coordinates

Chart 31-4 PATIENT AND FAMILY EDUCATION GUIDE

The Supraglottic Method of Swallowing

1. Place yourself in an upright, preferably out-of-bed, position.
2. Clear your throat.
3. Take a deep breath.
4. Place $^1/_2$ to 1 teaspoon of food into your mouth.
5. Hold your breath, or "bear down" (Valsalva maneuver).
6. Swallow twice.
7. Release your breath, and clear your throat.
8. Swallow twice again.
9. Breathe normally.

This method exaggerates the normal protective mechanisms of cessation of respiration during the swallow. The double swallow attempts to clear food that may be pooling in the pharynx, vallecula, and piriform sinuses. This method is used only after a dynamic radiographic swallow study has demonstrated that it is appropriate and safe for the patient.

the efforts of the health care team in assessing the specific discharge needs and making the appropriate referrals to home care agencies. Professionals such as nutritionists, nurses, physical therapists, speech and language pathologists, and social workers may be needed. Coordinate the scheduling for chemotherapy or radiation therapy with the patient and family.

Home Care Management

Extensive home care preparation is needed after a laryngectomy for cancer. The convalescent period is long, and airway management is complicated. The patient or family must be able to take an active role in care.

General cleanliness of the home is assessed by the home care nurse or case manager. For the patient with severe respiratory problems, home changes to allow for one-floor living may be needed. Increased humidity is needed. A humidifier add-on to a forced-air furnace can be obtained. If this cost is not manageable or if the home is heated by radiators, a room humidifier or vaporizer may be used. Be sure to stress that meticulous cleaning of these items is needed to prevent spread of mold or other sources of infection.

A home care nurse often is involved with care after discharge and is an important resource for the patient and family. This nurse assesses the patient and home situation for problems in self-care, complications, adjustment, and adherence to the medical regimen. Chart 31-5 lists assessment areas for the patient in the home after a laryngectomy. This nurse reinforces health care teaching, self-care teaching, and smoking-cessation regimens.

Health Teaching

Education begins before surgery, and most self-care is taught in the hospital. Teach the patient and family how to care for the stoma or tracheostomy or laryngectomy tube, depending on the type of surgery performed. Review incision and airway care, including cleaning and inspecting for signs of infection. Chart 31-6 lists self-care actions for the patient after laryngeal cancer surgery. Many of these actions also apply to any surgery for head and neck cancer.

Stoma care teaching is focused on protection. Instruct the patient to use a shower shield over the tube or stoma when bathing to prevent water from entering the airway. Teach men who use electric shavers to cover the stoma while shaving to keep hair from falling into it. Suggest that the patient wear a protective cover or stoma guard to protect the stoma during the day. For those with permanent stomas after laryngectomy or for those with permanent tracheostomies, covering the opening has a double benefit: (1) filtering the air entering the stoma while keeping humidity in the airway, and (2) enhancing aesthetic appearance. Attractive coverings are available in the form of cotton scarves, crocheted bibs, and jewelry. Using colored seam binding for tracheostomy ties after the stoma has matured may enhance overall body image. Shirt or dress color can be matched or coordinated with seam bindings of various colors.

Instruct the patient how to increase humidity in the home. If prescribed, teach the patient to instill normal saline into the

Chart 31-6 PATIENT AND FAMILY EDUCATION GUIDE

Home Laryngectomy Care

- Avoid swimming, and use care when showering or shaving.
- Lean slightly forward and cover the stoma when coughing or sneezing.
- Wear a stoma guard or loose clothing to cover the stoma.
- Clean the stoma with mild soap and water. Lubricate the stoma with a non–oil-based ointment as needed.
- Increase humidity by using saline in the stoma as instructed, a bedside humidifier, pans of water, and houseplants.
- Obtain and wear a MedicAlert bracelet and emergency care card for life-threatening situations.

Chart 31-5 HOME CARE ASSESSMENT

Patients After Laryngectomy

Assess respiratory status.
- Observe rate and depth of respiration.
- Auscultate lungs.
- Check patency of airway.
- Examine the tracheostomy drainage for amount, color, and character.
- Examine nail beds and mucous membranes for evidence of cyanosis.
- Obtain a pulse oximetry reading.

Assess condition of wound.
- Remove dressings (noting condition of dressings).
- Cleanse the wound.
- Compare with previous notations of wound condition:
  Presence, amount, and nature of exudate
  Presence/absence of cellulitis
  Presence/absence of odor

Assess patient's psychosocial status.
- Ask the patient about passing the time, visitors, and trips outside the house.
- Observe whether the patient communicates responses directly or whether a family member speaks for the patient.
- Observe patient and family member interactions.
- Determine what method of communication the patient has selected, and observe the patient's skill with it.
- Observe whether the patient is wearing pajamas or is dressed in street clothes.

Take the patient's temperature at each home care visit.

Assess the patient's understanding of illness and adherence to treatment.
- Manifestations to report to the health care provider
- Medication plan (correct timing and dose)
- Ambulation or positioning schedule
- Dressing changes/skin care
- Diet modifications (24-hour diet recall)
- Skill in tracheostomy or dressing care

Assess patient's nutritional status.
- Change in muscle mass
- Lackluster nails/sparse hair
- Recent weight loss greater than 10% of usual weight
- Impaired oral intake
- Difficulty swallowing
- Generalized edema

artificial airway 10 to 15 times a day. Stress the importance of keeping well hydrated to prevent secretions from thickening.

Communication involves having the patient continue the selected method of alternate communication that began in the hospital. Instruct him or her to wear a medical alert (Medic-Alert) bracelet and carry a special identification card (Fig. 31-7). For patients with a laryngectomy, this card is available from the local chapters of the International Association of Laryngectomees. The card instructs the reader about providing an emergency airway or resuscitating someone who has a stoma.

Smoking cessation is a difficult but important issue after head and neck cancer surgery because smoking is a major risk factor for this type of cancer. Stress that smoking cessation can reduce the risk for developing other cancers and can increase the rate of healing from surgery.

Smoking cessation is not an easy task, and most patients need continuing support and reinforcement to sustain this action. Chemical and psychological assistance are available for smoking cessation. See Chapter 38 for a detailed discussion of smoking cessation methods.

Psychosocial Preparation

The many changes resulting from a laryngectomy influence physical, social, and emotional functioning. Patients may perceive changes in their quality of life. Begin preparing the patient and family by scheduling a visit from a person who has adjusted to these changes.

The patient who is discharged to home with a permanent stoma, tracheostomy tube, nasogastric (NG) tube, and wounds has an altered body image. Stress the importance of returning to as normal a lifestyle as possible. Most patients can resume many of their usual activities within 4 to 6 weeks after surgery.

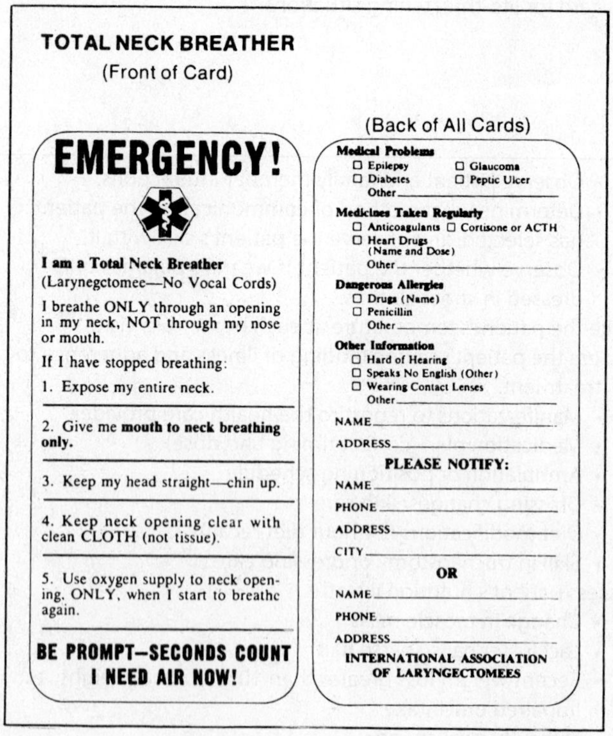
TOTAL NECK BREATHER
(Front of Card)

EMERGENCY!

I am a Total Neck Breather
(Larynegctomee—No Vocal Cords)

I breathe ONLY through an opening in my neck, NOT through my nose or mouth.

If I have stopped breathing:

1. Expose my entire neck.
2. Give me **mouth to neck breathing only.**
3. Keep my head straight—chin up.
4. Keep neck opening clear with clean CLOTH (not tissue).
5. Use oxygen supply to neck opening, ONLY, when I start to breathe again.

BE PROMPT—SECONDS COUNT I NEED AIR NOW!

(Back of All Cards)

Medical Problems
☐ Epilepsy ☐ Glaucoma
☐ Diabetes ☐ Peptic Ulcer
Other ____

Medicines Taken Regularly
☐ Anticoagulants ☐ Cortisone or ACTH
☐ Heart Drugs (Name and Dose)
Other ____

Dangerous Allergies
☐ Drugs (Name)
☐ Penicillin
Other ____

Other Information
☐ Hard of Hearing
☐ Speaks No English (Other)
☐ Wearing Contact Lenses
Other ____

NAME ____
ADDRESS ____

PLEASE NOTIFY:
NAME ____
PHONE ____
ADDRESS ____
CITY ____

OR

NAME ____
PHONE ____
ADDRESS ____

INTERNATIONAL ASSOCIATION OF LARYNGECTOMEES

Fig. 31-7 • Emergency wallet card for identification of laryngectomy.

A longer time is needed after a combination of radiation therapy and surgery and for those patients who also have other chronic diseases such as diabetes mellitus, heart failure, or chronic obstructive pulmonary disease. The patient may be frustrated at times while trying to adjust to changes in appearance, smell, taste, and communication.

The patient with a total laryngectomy cannot produce sounds during laughing and crying. Mucus secretions may appear unexpectedly when these emotions arise or when coughing or sneezing occurs. The mucus can be embarrassing, and the patient needs to be prepared to cover the stoma with a handkerchief or gauze. The patient who has undergone composite resections has difficulty with speech *and* swallowing. He or she may need to deal with tracheostomy and feeding tubes in public places.

Health Care Resources

Inform the patient and family of community organizations (e.g., ACS) and local laryngectomee clubs, which can offer support, information, and friendships. When the patient has problems paying for health care services, equipment, and prescriptions, a visiting nurse agency may be helpful in locating available resources.

In many areas the local unit of the ACS or Canadian Cancer Society can help provide dressing materials and nutritional supplements to patients in need. These organizations may also provide transportation to and from follow-up visits or radiation therapy.

DECISION-MAKING CHALLENGE
Coordination of Care

A patient who had a laryngectomy and radical neck dissection for laryngeal cancer comes back to the clinic 3 weeks after discharge. She lives with her daughter and grandchildren. She tells you that esophageal speech is going well and that her grandsons help her work on "burping" the words out. She also says she has had many visitors and is glad that so many friends are helping her recover. You think she looks thin, and when you weigh her, she weighs 16 lbs less than the day she was discharged from the acute care setting. When you ask her what she is eating, she is a little reluctant but finally tells you she has not been eating much because swallowing is uncomfortable and she is afraid she may choke.

1. Is this weight loss a concern?
2. Are her fears reasonable? Why or why not?
3. What suggestions can you make for improving her nutrition?
4. How could you coordinate her care to meet her needs?

evolve For suggested answer guidelines, go to http://evolve.elsevier.com/Iggy/.

▪ Evaluation: Outcomes

Evaluate the care of the patient with head and neck cancers on the basis of the identified nursing diagnoses and collaborative problems. The expected outcomes are that the patient:

- Maintains a patent airway
- Performs self-care of the artificial airway and wound
- Performs ADLs independently or with minimal assistance
- Attains or maintains adequate nutrition
- Does not aspirate gastric contents or food
- Engages in desired social interactions

Specific indicators for these outcomes are listed for each nursing diagnosis and collaborative problem in the Planning and Implementation section (see earlier).

HUMAN NEEDS NURSING CARE REVIEW

What might you NOTICE if the patient is experiencing inadequate oxygenation and tissue perfusion as a result of upper airway problems?

- Voice changes (nasal quality if the problem is above the palate, "breathy" or "whispery" if the problem is in the larynx or trachea)
- Snoring
- Mouth breathing
- Change in cognition or level of consciousness or acute confusion
- Decreased oxygen saturation by pulse oximetry
- Skin cyanosis or pallor (lighter-skinned patients)
- Cyanosis or pallor of the lips and oral mucous membranes (patients of any skin color)
- Tachycardia and dysrhythmia

What should you INTERPRET and how should you RESPOND to a patient experiencing inadequate oxygenation and tissue perfusion as a result of a respiratory problem?

Perform and interpret physical assessment, including:

- Taking vital signs
- Monitoring oxygen saturation by pulse oximetry
- Checking the accuracy of pulse oximetry readings
- Assessing for the presence of thick or excessive secretions
- Assessing the patient's ability to cough and clear the airway
- Assessing nasal drainage and sputum for color and blood
- Checking most recent laboratory values for white blood cell and ABG levels
- Assessing cognition (mini-mental status exam)
- Assessing hydration status

Respond by:

- Suctioning (oral, pharyngeal, endotracheal, tracheostomy), if needed
- Applying oxygen and assessing the patient's responses to this intervention
- Keeping the patient's head elevated to about 30 degrees
- Notifying physician or Rapid Response Team
- Ensuring venous access

On what should you REFLECT?

- Observe patient for evidence of restored oxygenation (see Chapter 29).
- Think about what may have precipitated this episode and what steps could be taken to either prevent a similar episode or identify it earlier.
- Think about what additional resources could improve the nursing response to this situation.

GET READY FOR THE NCLEX EXAMINATION!

Key Points

Review these Key Points for each NCLEX Examination Client Needs Category.

Safe and Effective Care Environment

- Use sterile technique when performing endotracheal or tracheal suctioning.
- Use Standard Precautions when caring for a patient with epistaxis.

Health Promotion and Maintenance

- Encourage people who smoke to quit smoking or using tobacco in any way.
- Encourage people who use alcohol to reduce their intake of alcoholic beverages.
- Teach patients how to blow the nose without closing off one nostril.
- Use aspiration precautions for any patient with an altered level of consciousness or who has an endotracheal tube (see Chart 31-3).
- Teach the patient and family how to perform tracheostomy care (see Chart 30-4 in Chapter 30).
- Teach patients who have had radiation therapy to the neck or oral cavity to have dental examinations at least every 6 months.

Psychosocial Integrity

- Allow the patient and family members the opportunity to express fear or anxiety regarding a cancer diagnosis or a change in breathing status.
- Teach family members ways to communicate with a patient who cannot speak after surgery for head and neck cancer.
- Encourage patients with permanent tracheostomies or laryngectomies to become involved in self-care.
- Encourage the patient who has had head and neck surgery for cancer to look at the wound and touch the affected area.
- Allow the patient and family to grieve about the loss of function and change in body image.
- Allow time to communicate with the patient who has voice loss as a result of disease or treatment.
- Refer patients and families to the ACS or the Canadian Cancer Society after surgery for head and neck cancer.

Physiological Integrity

- Assess airway patency for any patient who experiences facial or nasal trauma.
- Notify the Rapid Response Team when a patient experiences a posterior nasal bleed.
- Check the airway and packing at least every hour for a patient who has posterior nasal packing placed after nasal surgery or posterior epistaxis.
- Instruct patients who have had mandibular immobilization or fixation after a mandibular fracture to keep wire cutters with them at all times.
- Apply oxygen to any patient who develops stridor.
- Ensure that oxygen therapy delivered to the patient is humidified (and warmed, when possible).
- Use a manual resuscitation bag to ventilate the patient if the tracheostomy tube has dislodged or been decannulated.
- Assess the new tracheostomy stoma site at least once per shift for purulent drainage, redness, pain, and swelling, as indicators of infection.

- Keep the tracheal cuff pressure between 14 and 20 mm Hg to prevent tissue injury.
- Teach patients receiving radiation therapy how to care for the skin in the radiation path (see Chart 24-2 in Chapter 24).

Additional Study Resources

Go to your Companion CD or Evolve at http://evolve.elsevier.com/Iggy/ for *Self-Assessment Questions for the NCLEX Examination.*

evolve Go to Evolve at http://evolve.elsevier.com/Iggy/ for *Prioritization and Delegation Questions for the NCLEX Examination.*

SELECTED BIBLIOGRAPHY

Asterisk indicates a classic or definitive work on this subject.

American Cancer Society (ACS). (2006). *Cancer reference information.* Retrieved October 2007, from www.cancer.org/docroot/CRI/.

American Cancer Society (ACS). (2008). *Cancer facts and figures, 2008.* 01-300M-No. 5008.08. Atlanta: Author.

Armstrong, J., & McCaffery, R. (2006). The effects of mucositis on quality of life in patients with head and neck cancer. *Clinical Journal of Oncology, 10*(1), 53-56.

Beattie, S. (2007). Respiratory distress. *RN, 70*(7), 34-38.

Berry, D. (2008). Case study: Obstructive sleep apnea. *MEDSURG Nursing, 17*(1), 11-16.

Bulechek, G.M., Butcher, H.K., & McCloskey Dochterman, J. (Eds.). (2008). *Nursing interventions classification (NIC)* (5th ed.). St. Louis: Mosby.

*Cady, J. (2002). Laryngectomy: Beyond loss of voice—caring for the patient as a whole. *Clinical Journal of Oncology Nursing, 6*(6), 347-353.

Couch, M., & Senior, B. (2005). Nonsurgical and surgical treatments for sleep apnea. *Anesthesiology Clinics of North America, 23*(3), 525-534.

Dobbin, K. (2006). Wake up to the risks of sleep apnea. *Nursing2006, 36*(11), 64hn1-64hn2.

Gavaghan, S., & Jeffries, M. (2006). Your patient's receiving noninvasive positive-pressure ventilation. *Nursing2006, 36*(5), 46-47.

Gould, L. (2006). Nutrition: Care of head and neck cancer patients with swallowing difficulties. *British Journal of Nursing, 15*(20), 1091-1092, 1094-1096.

Happ, M., Tate, J., & Garrett, K. (2006). Nonspeaking older adults in the ICU. *AJN, 106*(5), 29.

Holman, M. (2005). Obstructive sleep apnea: Implications for primary care. *The Nurse Practitioner, 30*(9), 38-42.

Kucik, C., & Clenney, T. (2005). Management of epistaxis. *American Family Physician, 71*(2), 305-311.

McCance, K., & Huether, S. (2006). *Pathophysiology: The biologic basis for disease in adults and children* (5th ed.). St. Louis: Mosby.

Metheny, N. (2006). Preventing respiratory complications of tube feeding: Evidence-based practice. *American Journal of Critical Care, 15*(4), 360-369.

Moorhead, S., Johnson, M., & Maas, M. (Eds.). (2004). *Nursing outcomes classification (NOC)* (3rd ed.). St. Louis: Mosby.

Pagana, K., & Pagana, T. (2006). *Mosby's manual of diagnostic and laboratory tests* (3rd ed.). St. Louis: Mosby.

Pruitt, B. (2005a). Clear the air with closed suctioning. *Nursing2005, 35*(7), 44-45.

Pruitt, B. (2005b). Clearing away pulmonary secretions. *Nursing2005, 35*(7), 37-41.

Pullen, R. (2007). Communicating with a patient on mechanical ventilation. *Nursing2007, 37*(4), 22.

Randall, D. (2006). Epistaxis packing: Practical pointers for nosebleed control. *Postgraduate Medicine, 119*(1), 77-82.

Schaller, J. (2008). Myths: Facts about obstructive sleep apnea. *Nursing2008, 38*(1), 27.

Schiech, L. (2007). Looking at laryngeal cancer. *Nursing2007, 37*(5), 50-55.

Willard, R., & Dreher, M. (2005). Wake-up call for sleep apnea. *Nursing2005, 35*(3), 46-49.

Care of Patients with Noninfectious Lower Respiratory Problems

32

CHAPTER

M. Linda Workman

LEARNING OUTCOMES

For clinical competence and success on the NCLEX Examination, study this chapter with these Learning Outcomes in mind:

Safe and Effective Care Environment

1. Ensure safe oxygen delivery.
2. Ensure the proper oxygen flow rate for patients with hypercarbia.
3. Use appropriate infection control methods to protect the patient with cystic fibrosis from respiratory infections.
4. Ensure appropriate functioning of the chest tube drainage system after a thoracotomy.

Health Promotion and Maintenance

5. Encourage everyone to not smoke or to quit smoking.
6. Encourage all people who are exposed to inhalation irritants in the workplace or at home to use appropriate protection.
7. Teach patients with chronic airflow limitation how to use a peak flowmeter.
8. Teach patients using aerosol or dry powder inhalers for drug delivery the correct way to use these devices.
9. Teach patients who are using preventive drug therapy for asthma the importance of taking the prescribed drugs daily, even when asthma symptoms are not present.
10. Teach patients with asthma to have their rescue inhalers with them at all times.

Psychosocial Integrity

11. Encourage the patient and family to express their feelings about a change in breathing status.
12. Explain all therapeutic procedures, restrictions, and follow-up care to the patient and his or her family.
13. Teach the patient with activity limitations from respiratory problems how to modify techniques and conserve energy to perform ADLs and desired activities independently.

Physiological Integrity

14. Compare the pathophysiology and clinical manifestations of asthma, bronchitis, and emphysema.
15. Identify risk factors for chronic obstructive pulmonary disease (COPD) and lung cancer.
16. Use laboratory data and clinical manifestations to determine the effectiveness of therapy for impaired gas exchange in a patient with breathing problems.
17. Interpret peak expiratory flow (PEF) readings for the need for intervention.
18. Coordinate care for the patient immediately after lung volume reduction surgery.
19. Compare the side effects of radiation treatment for lung cancer with those of chemotherapy for lung cancer.
20. Coordinate nursing interventions for the patient with chest tubes.

evolve Go to your Companion CD or Evolve at http://evolve.elsevier.com/Iggy/ for *Self-Assessment Questions for the NCLEX Examination* keyed to these Learning Outcomes.

ANIMATION: Asthma

Lower airway problems directly affect gas exchange and have serious consequences for the *human need for oxygenation and tissue perfusion.* Many of these problems are chronic and progressive, requiring major changes in a person's lifestyle. The older patient with a lower airway problem may need special help even before the disorder becomes severe because of age-related changes in breathing effectiveness. Chart 32-1 lists nursing issues for the older patient with a respiratory problem.

CHRONIC AIRFLOW LIMITATION

Chronic airflow limitation (CAL) is a group of chronic lung diseases that include asthma, chronic bronchitis, and pulmonary emphysema. Emphysema and chronic bronchitis, termed **chronic obstructive pulmonary disease (COPD),** are characterized by bronchospasm and dyspnea (see Fig. 32-1). The tissue damage is not reversible and increases in severity, eventually leading to respiratory failure. Asthma, unlike COPD, is an intermittent disease with *reversible* airflow obstruction and wheezing.

More than 40 million Americans suffer from some form of CAL, and 1 million people between the ages of 40 and 65 years have moderate to severe disability from CAL (Centers for Disease Control and Prevention [CDC], 2007). Although some problems are not reversible, good management strategies can help maintain adequate *oxygenation and tissue perfusion,* as well as improve overall health.

ASTHMA

Pathophysiology

Bronchial asthma is an intermittent and reversible airflow obstruction affecting only the airways, not the alveoli (Fig. 32-1). Airway obstruction can occur in two ways: (1) inflammation and (2) airway hyperresponsiveness (sometimes called "twitchy airways"). Inflammation obstructs the **lumen** (i.e., the inside) of airways. Airway hyperresponsiveness obstructs airways by constricting bronchial smooth muscle causing a narrowing of the airway from the outside. Airway inflammation can trigger bronchiolar hyperresponsiveness, and many people with asthma have both problems at the same time. Severe airway obstruction can be fatal. More than 5000 deaths from acute asthma occur in the United States each year (CDC, 2007).

Chart 32-1 NURSING FOCUS ON THE OLDER ADULT

Chronic Respiratory Disorder

- Provide rest periods between such activities as bathing, meals, and ambulation.
- Place the patient in an upright position for meals to prevent aspiration.
- Encourage nutritional fluid intake after the meal to promote increased calorie intake.
- Schedule drugs around routine activities to increase adherence to drug therapy.
- Arrange chairs in strategic locations to allow the patient with dyspnea to walk and rest as needed.
- Encourage prompt access to a health care facility for any manifestation of infection.
- Ensure that the patient has received the pneumococcal vaccine.
- Encourage the patient to have an annual influenza vaccination.

Etiology and Genetic Risk

Asthma may be classified into different types based on the events known to trigger the attacks; however, the pathophysiology is similar for all types of asthma regardless of triggering event. Inflammation of the mucous membranes lining the airways is a key event in triggering an asthma attack. Inflammation occurs in response to the presence of specific allergens; general irritants such as cold air, dry air, or fine airborne particles; microorganisms; and aspirin. Airway hyperresponsiveness can occur with exercise, with an upper respiratory illness, and for unknown reasons (Sims, 2006).

GENETIC CONSIDERATIONS

Asthma from inflammation or hyperresponsive airways may have a genetic component, although a specific gene or mutation has not yet been identified. In addition, genetic variation in the gene that controls the synthesis and activity of beta adrenergic receptors has an impact on drug therapy for asthma. Patients who have a mutation in this gene do not respond as expected to short-acting or long-acting beta agonists and need to have an altered therapy plan (Conboy-Ellis, 2006). Teaching these patients about why their drug therapies are different from standard recommendations is a nursing responsibility that can assist with therapy adherence.

When asthma is well controlled, the airway changes are temporary and reversible. With poor control, chronic inflammation can lead to damage and hyperplasia of the bronchial epithelial cells and of the bronchial smooth muscle. When asthma attacks are frequent, even exposure to low levels of the triggering agent or event may stimulate an attack.

Inflammation triggers asthma for some people when allergens bind to specific antibody molecules (especially immunoglobulin E [IgE]). These molecules are attached to tissue cells called *mast cells* and white blood cells called *basophils.* These cells are filled with granules containing chemicals that can start local inflammatory responses (see Chapters 19 and 22). Some of these chemicals, such as histamine, start an immediate inflammatory response, which can be blocked by drugs like diphenhydramine (Benadryl). Others, such as leukotriene and eotaxin, are slower and cause later, prolonged inflammatory responses, which can be blocked by drugs like montelukast (Singulair), zafirlukast (Accolate), and zileuton (Zyflo). All these chemicals also attract more white blood cells (eosinophils, macrophages, basophils) to the area, which then release even more inflammatory-inducing chemicals (mediators). Inflammation of airway mucous membranes causes blood vessel dilation and capillary leak, leading to tissue swelling with increased secretions and mucus production (McCance & Huether, 2006; Sims, 2006). Inflammation can also occur through general irritation rather than allergic responses. Although some of the same cells and chemicals cause this response, allergy therapy is not useful for general irritation-induced asthma.

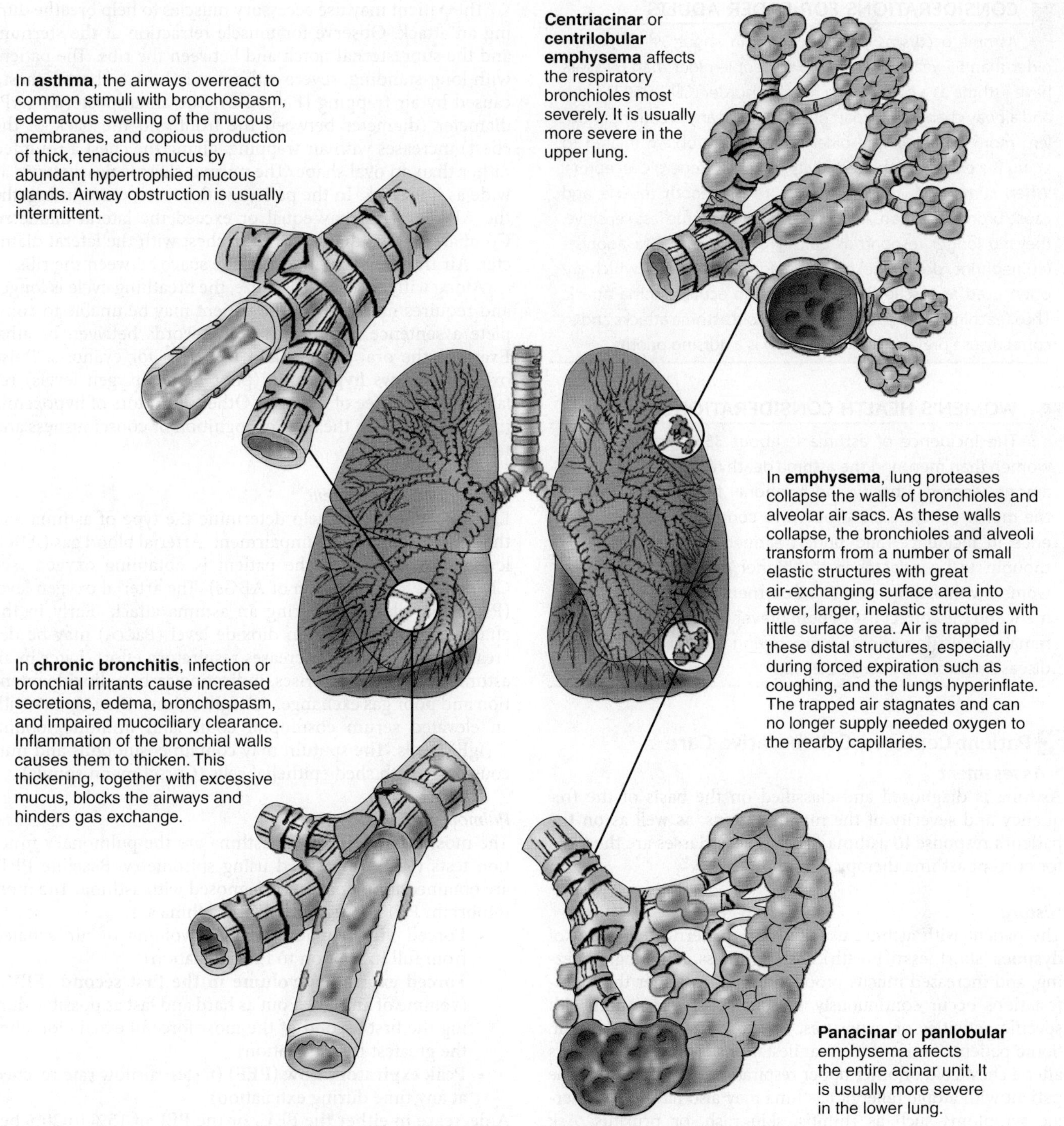
In **asthma**, the airways overreact to common stimuli with bronchospasm, edematous swelling of the mucous membranes, and copious production of thick, tenacious mucus by abundant hypertrophied mucous glands. Airway obstruction is usually intermittent.
Centriacinar or **centrilobular emphysema** affects the respiratory bronchioles most severely. It is usually more severe in the upper lung.
In **emphysema**, lung proteases collapse the walls of bronchioles and alveolar air sacs. As these walls collapse, the bronchioles and alveoli transform from a number of small elastic structures with great air-exchanging surface area into fewer, larger, inelastic structures with little surface area. Air is trapped in these distal structures, especially during forced expiration such as coughing, and the lungs hyperinflate. The trapped air stagnates and can no longer supply needed oxygen to the nearby capillaries.
In **chronic bronchitis**, infection or bronchial irritants cause increased secretions, edema, bronchospasm, and impaired mucociliary clearance. Inflammation of the bronchial walls causes them to thicken. This thickening, together with excessive mucus, blocks the airways and hinders gas exchange.
Panacinar or **panlobular** emphysema affects the entire acinar unit. It is usually more severe in the lower lung.

Fig. 32-1 • The pathophysiology of chronic airflow limitation (CAL).

Bronchospasm is a narrowing of the bronchial tubes through constriction of the smooth muscle around and within the bronchial walls. It occurs in some people as a result of airway hyperresponsiveness when small amounts of pollutants or respiratory viruses stimulate nerve fibers, causing constriction of bronchial smooth muscle. If these substances also stimulate an inflammatory response at the same time, the chemicals released during inflammation also trigger constriction. Severe bronchospasm alone, especially in smaller bronchioles, can profoundly limit airflow to the alveoli.

Aspirin and other NSAIDs can trigger asthma in some people although this response is not a true allergy. It results from increased production of leukotriene when aspirin or NSAIDs suppress other inflammatory pathways.

Incidence/Prevalence

Asthma can occur at any age. About half of adults with asthma also had the disease in childhood. Asthma is more common in urban settings than in rural settings, possibly as a result of more air pollution.

CONSIDERATIONS FOR OLDER ADULTS

Asthma occurs as a new disorder in about 3% of people older than 55 years. Another 3% of people older than 60 years have asthma as a continuing chronic disorder (CDC, 2007). Lung and airway changes as a part of aging make any breathing problem more serious in the older adult. One problem related to aging is a change in the sensitivity of beta-adrenergic receptors. When stimulated, these receptors relax smooth muscle and cause bronchodilation. As these receptors become less sensitive, they no longer respond as quickly or as strongly to agonists (epinephrine, dopamine) and beta-adrenergic drugs, which are often used as rescue therapy during an acute asthma attack. Thus teaching older patients how to avoid asthma attacks and to correctly use preventive drug therapy is a nursing priority.

WOMEN'S HEALTH CONSIDERATIONS

The incidence of asthma is about 35% higher among women than men, and the asthma death rates are also higher among women. Obesity and hormonal fluctuations around the menstrual cycle are thought to contribute to the difference in incidence, and undertreatment of the disease is thought to be a factor in the higher death rate. Teaching women with asthma how to be partners in asthma management and the correct use of both preventive and rescue drugs remains a nursing priority in improving the outcomes of the disease (Ostrom & Goergen, 2006).

Patient-Centered Collaborative Care

Assessment

Asthma is diagnosed and classified on the basis of the frequency and severity of the manifestations, as well as on the patient's response to asthma drugs. These classes are the basis for current asthma therapy (Chart 32-2).

History

The patient with asthma usually has a pattern of episodes of **dyspnea** (shortness of breath), chest tightness, coughing, wheezing, and increased mucus production. Ask whether the manifestations occur continuously, seasonally, in association with specific activities or exposures, or more frequently at night. Some patients notice these manifestations lasting 4 to 8 weeks after a chest cold or other upper respiratory tract infection. The patient with atopic (allergic) asthma may also have other allergic symptoms such as rhinitis, skin rash, or pruritus. Ask whether any other family members have asthma or respiratory problems. Ask about the patient's current or previous smoking habits. If the patient smokes, use this opportunity to teach him or her about smoking cessation (Chart 32-3). Wheezing in nonsmokers is an important symptom in the diagnosis of asthma.

▶ AUDIO CLIP: High- and Low-Pitched Wheezes

Physical Assessment/Clinical Manifestations

The patient with mild to moderate asthma may have no manifestations between asthma attacks. During an acute episode, the most common manifestations are an audible wheeze and increased respiratory rate. The wheeze is louder on exhalation. When inflammation occurs with asthma, coughing may increase.

The patient may use accessory muscles to help breathe during an attack. Observe for muscle retraction at the sternum and the suprasternal notch and between the ribs. The patient with long-standing, severe asthma may have a "barrel chest," caused by air trapping (Fig. 32-2). The anteroposterior (AP) diameter (diameter between the front and the back of the chest) increases with air trapping, giving the chest a rounded rather than an oval shape. The normal chest is nearly twice as wide as it is thick. In the patient with severe, chronic asthma, the AP diameter may equal or exceed the lateral diameter. Compare the AP diameter of the chest with the lateral diameter. Air trapping also increases the space between the ribs.

Along with an audible wheeze, the breathing cycle is longer and requires more effort. The patient may be unable to complete a sentence of more than five words between breaths. Examine the oral mucosa and nail beds for cyanosis. Pulse oximetry shows **hypoxemia** (poor blood oxygen levels) related to the degree of dyspnea. Other indicators of hypoxemia include changes in the level of cognition or consciousness and tachycardia.

Laboratory Assessment

Laboratory tests can help determine the type of asthma and the degree of breathing impairment. Arterial blood gas (ABG) levels show how well the patient is obtaining oxygen (see Chapter 14 for discussion of ABGs). The arterial oxygen level (Pao_2) may decrease during an asthma attack. Early in the attack, the arterial carbon dioxide level ($Paco_2$) may be decreased as the patient increases respiratory effort. Later in an asthma episode, $Paco_2$ rises, indicating carbon dioxide retention and poor gas exchange. Allergic asthma often occurs with an elevated serum eosinophil count and immunoglobulin E (IgE) levels. The sputum may contain eosinophils and mucous plugs with shed epithelial cells (Curschmann spirals).

Pulmonary Function Tests

The most accurate tests for asthma are the pulmonary function tests (PFTs) measured using spirometry. Baseline PFTs are obtained for all patients diagnosed with asthma. The most important PFTs for a patient with asthma are:

- **Forced vital capacity (FVC)** (volume of air exhaled from full inhalation to full exhalation)
- **Forced expiratory volume in the first second (FEV_1)** (volume of air blown out as hard and fast as possible during the first second of the most forceful exhalation after the greatest full inhalation)
- **Peak expiratory flow (PEF)** (fastest airflow rate reached at any time during exhalation).

A decrease in either the FEV_1 or the PEF of 15% to 20% below the expected value for age, gender, and size is common for the patient with asthma. An increase of 12% in these values after treatment with bronchodilators is diagnostic for asthma. Airway responsiveness is tested by measuring the PEF and FEV_1 before and after the patient inhales the drug *methacholine*, which induces bronchospasm in susceptible people.

Other Diagnostic Assessment

Chest x-rays may be used to rule out other causes of dyspnea or to track changes in chest structure over time. For the patient taking theophylline, blood drug levels are used to determine whether a therapeutic level is being maintained.

Chart 32-2 KEY FEATURES

Asthma: The Step System

Clinical Manifestations	Treatment Recommendations
STEP I. MILD INTERMITTENT	
Symptoms or episodes occur less than once a week. Episodes/exacerbations are short, lasting only a few hours. Symptoms are present at night no more frequently than twice per month. PFTs are normal between episodes. During episodes/exacerbations, FEV_1 or PEF is at least 80% of normal. PEF or FEV_1 variability is less than 20%.	No daily drugs needed Use of short-acting inhaled beta agonist during episodes (rescue inhaler) Increased use of rescue inhaler more than 2 days per week (except for aftermath of viral infections or exercise-induced bronchospasms) indicates the need to start the next step in long-term therapy
STEP II. MILD PERSISTENT	
Symptoms or episodes occur more than once per week but not daily. Symptoms are present at night more than twice per month. Episodes/exacerbations affect activity and sleep. During episodes/exacerbations, FEV_1 or PEF is at least 80% of normal. PEF or FEV_1 variability is 20% to 30%.	Use of a daily anti-inflammatory: *Inhaled corticosteroid (ICS) low-dose Inhaled cromolyn Leukotriene antagonist Use of a rescue inhaler for relief during episodes Increased use of rescue inhaler more than 2 days per week (except for aftermath of viral infections or exercise-induced bronchospasms) indicates the need to start the next step in long-term therapy
STEP III. MODERATE PERSISTENT	
Symptoms occur daily. Episodes/exacerbations affect activity and sleep. Symptoms are present at night more than once per week. During episodes/exacerbations, FEV_1 or PEF is only 60% to 80% of normal. PEF or FEV_1 variability is greater than 30%.	*Add a daily long-acting beta agonist to low-dose ICS **or** Continue ICS alone but increase to medium-dose range **or** Add one of the following to low-dose ICS: Leukotriene receptor antagonist Theophylline Zileuton Increased use of rescue inhaler more than 2 days per week (except for aftermath of viral infections or exercise-induced bronchospasms) indicates the need to start the next step in long-term therapy
STEP IV. SEVERE PERSISTENT	
Symptoms occur daily. Episodes/exacerbations are frequent. Symptoms are present at night frequently. Activities are limited. During episodes/exacerbations, FEV_1 or PEF is at 60% or less of normal. PEF or FEV_1 variability is greater than 30%.	*Medium-dose ICS and long-acting beta agonist or Medium-dose ICS and either leukotriene receptor antagonist or theophylline Increased use of rescue inhaler more than 2 days per week (except for aftermath of viral infections or exercise-induced bronchospasms) indicates the need to start the next step in long-term therapy
STEP V. SEVERE PERSISTENT NOT RESPONSIVE TO PREVIOUS STEP	*High-dose ICS and long-acting beta agonist Omalizumab considered for patients with constant exposure to non-seasonal allergens
STEP VI. SEVERE PERSISTENT NOT RESPONSIVE TO PREVIOUS STEP	*High-dose ICS, oral corticosteroids (at lowest possible dose daily or every other day), and long-acting beta agonist Omalizumab considered for patients with constant exposure to non-seasonal allergens

Modified from National Institutes of Health. (2007). *Guidelines for the diagnosis and management of asthma.* Expert panel report 3. Bethesda, MD: U.S. Department of Health and Human Services.

FEV_1, Volume of air blown out as hard and fast as possible during the first second of the most forceful exhalation after the greatest full inhalation; *PEF*, peak expiratory flow; *PFTs*, pulmonary function tests.

*Preferred drug regimen.

Interventions

The goals of asthma therapy are to improve airflow, relieve symptoms, and prevent episodes. Adult asthma is best managed when the patient is an active partner in the management plan. Priority nursing actions focus on patient education about drug therapy and lifestyle management, including exercise, to assist the patient in understanding his or her disease and its treatment.

Patient Education

Asthma is often an intermittent disease. With guided self-care, patients can co-manage this disease, increasing symptom-free periods and decreasing the number and severity of attacks (Ellis, 2008). Good management decreases the number of hospital admissions and increases participation in patient-chosen pleasure, work, and family activities. Self-care requires

Chart 32-3 PATIENT AND FAMILY EDUCATION GUIDE
Smoking Cessation

- Make a list of the reasons you want to stop smoking (e.g., your health and the health of those around you, saving money, social reasons).
- Set a date to stop smoking, and keep it. Decide whether you are going to begin to cut down on the amount you smoke or are going to stop "cold turkey." Whatever way you decide to do it, keep this important date!
- Ask for help from those around you. Find someone who wants to quit smoking and "buddy up" for support. Look for assistance in your community, such as formal smoking cessation programs, counselors, and certified acupuncture specialists or hypnotists.
- Consult your health care provider about nicotine replacement therapy (e.g., patch, gum).
- Remove ashtrays and lighters from your view.
- Talk to yourself! Remind yourself of all the reasons you want to quit.
- Think of a way to reward yourself with the money you save from not smoking for a year.
- Avoid places that might tempt you to smoke. If you are used to having a cigarette after meals, get up from the table as soon as you are finished eating. Think of new things to do at times when you used to smoke (e.g., taking a walk, exercising, calling a friend).
- Find activities that keep your hands busy: needlework, painting, gardening, even holding a pencil.
- Take five deep breaths of clean, fresh air through your nose and out your mouth if you feel the urge to smoke.
- Keep plenty of healthy, low-calorie snacks, such as fruit and vegetables, on hand to nibble on. Try sugarless gum or mints as a substitute for tobacco.
- Drink at least eight glasses of water each day.
- Begin an exercise program with the approval of your health care provider. Be aware of the positive, healthy changes in your body since you stopped smoking.
- List the many reasons why you are glad that you quit. Keep the list handy as a reminder of the positive things you are doing for yourself.
- If you have a cigarette, think about what the conditions were that caused you to light it. Try and think of a strategy to avoid that (or those) conditions.
- Don't beat yourself up for backsliding; just face the next day as a new day.
- Think of each day without tobacco as a major accomplishment. It is!!

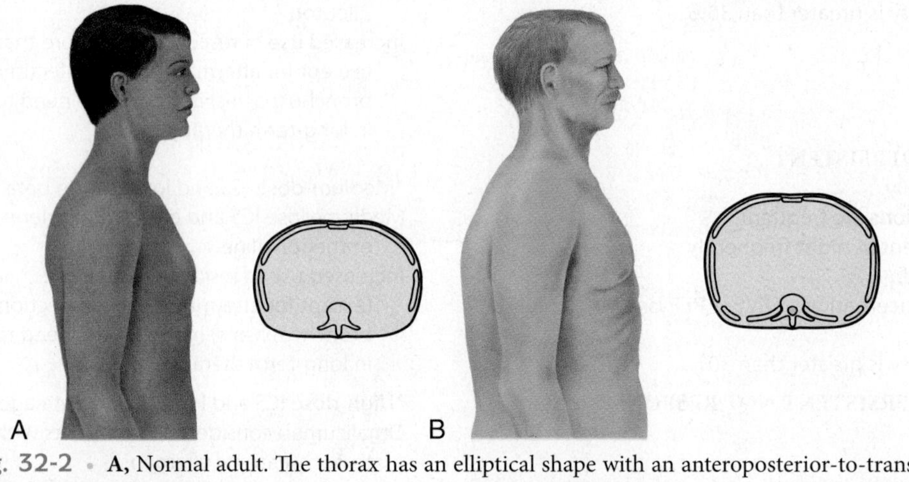
A
B

Fig. 32-2 • **A,** Normal adult. The thorax has an elliptical shape with an anteroposterior-to-transverse diameter of 1:2 or 5:7. **B,** Barrel chest. Note equal anteroposterior-to-transverse diameter and that ribs are horizontal instead of the normal downward slope. This is associated with normal aging and also with chronic emphysema and asthma as a result of hyperinflation of lungs.

extensive education for the patient to be able to self-assess respiratory status, self-treat (including adjusting the frequency and dosage of prescribed drugs), and determine when to consult the health care provider.

Teach the patient to assess symptom severity at least twice daily with a peak flowmeter and adjust drugs to manage inflammation and bronchospasms to prevent or relieve symptoms. Chart 32-4 describes the correct method to use the meter. The patient should first establish a baseline or "personal best" peak expiratory flow (PEF) by measuring his or her PEF twice daily for 2 to 3 weeks when asthma is well controlled and recording the results (Pruitt, 2005). This way, the patient will know when his or her peak flow is reduced to the point that more drugs are needed or that emergency assistance is needed. When the patient has established a "personal best," all other readings are compared with this value in terms of percent of personal best. Some meters are color-coded to help the patient interpret the results. Green zone readings are at least

Chart 32-4 PATIENT AND FAMILY EDUCATION GUIDE

Asthma Management

- Avoid potential environmental asthma triggers, such as smoke, fireplaces, dust, mold, and weather changes (especially warm to cold or sudden barometric changes).
- Avoid medications that could trigger asthma (e.g., aspirin, NSAIDs, beta blockers).
- Avoid food that has been prepared with monosodium glutamate (MSG) or metabisulfite.
- If you experience symptoms of exercise-induced asthma, use your bronchodilator inhaler 30 minutes before exercise to prevent or reduce bronchospasm.
- Be sure you know the proper technique and correct sequence when you use metered dose inhalers.
- Get adequate rest and sleep.
- Reduce stress and anxiety; learn relaxation techniques; adopt coping mechanisms that have worked for you in the past.
- Wash all bedding with hot water to destroy dust mites.
- Monitor your peak expiratory flow rates with a flowmeter at least twice daily using these techniques:
  - Make sure the device reads zero or is at base level.
  - Stand up (unless you have a physical disability).
  - Take as deep a breath as possible.
  - Place the meter in your mouth, and close your lips around the mouthpiece.
  - Blow out as hard and as fast as possible (1-2 sec).
  - Do not cough, spit, or let your tongue block the mouthpiece.
  - Write down the value obtained.
  - Repeat the process two additional times, and record the highest of the three numbers in your chart.
  - Clean your meter as described in the meter's instructions.
- Seek immediate emergency care if you experience any of these:
  - Gray or blue fingertips or lips
  - Difficulty breathing, walking, or talking
  - Retractions of the neck, chest, or ribs
  - Nasal flaring
  - Failure of drugs to control worsening symptoms
  - Peak expiratory rate flow declining steadily after treatment, or a flow rate 50% below your usual flow rate

80% or above the "personal best." This is the ideal range for asthma control and indicates that no increases in drug therapy are needed. Yellow is a range between 50% and 80% of personal best. When a patient has a reading in this range, he or she needs to use the "rescue drug," as prescribed. Within a few minutes after using the rescue drug, another PEF reading should be made to determine whether the rescue is working. Frequent or consistent readings in the yellow zone indicate the need for a change in preventive (control) drugs. Red is a range below 50% of the patient's personal best and indicates serious respiratory obstruction. *Teach the patient who has a reading in the red zone to immediately use the rescue drugs and seek emergency help.*

Education involves a specified drug therapy plan that is tailored to meet the personal pattern of asthma for the patient (Pruitt & Jacobs, 2005). Teach the patient to keep a symptom and intervention diary to learn his or her triggers of asthma symptoms, early cues for impending attacks, and personal response to drugs. Stress the importance of proper use of the asthma action plan for any severity of asthma. Chart 32-4 lists areas to emphasize when teaching the patient with asthma.

Drug Therapy

Pharmacologic management of adult patients with asthma is based on the step category for severity and treatment (see Chart 32-2) (National Institutes of Health, 2007). **Preventive therapy drugs** are those used to change airway responsiveness to prevent asthma attacks from occurring. *They are used every day, regardless of symptoms.* **Rescue drugs** are those used to actually stop an attack once it has started. Some patients may need drug therapy only during an asthma episode. For others, daily drugs are needed to keep asthma episodic rather than a more frequent problem. This therapy involves the use of bronchodilators and various drug types to reduce inflammation. Some drugs reduce the asthma response, and other drugs actually prevent the response. Combination drugs are two agents from different classes combined together for better response. Chart 32-5 lists the most common preferred drugs in each class for preventive and rescue (symptomatic) therapy of asthma. The actions, interventions, and rationales for most drugs within a single class are similar although drug dosages may differ. Be sure to consult a pharmacology text or drug handbook for more information on a specific drug.

Bronchodilators. Bronchodilators increase bronchiolar smooth muscle relaxation. They have no effect on inflammatory processes. Thus when a patient with asthma has airflow obstruction by both bronchospasm and inflammation, at least two types of drug therapy are needed. Bronchodilators work by stimulating the beta$_2$-adrenergic receptors on bronchial smooth muscle in much the same way that the sympathetic nervous system transmitters *epinephrine* and *norepinephrine* do. These drugs include beta$_2$ agonists, cholinergic antagonists, and methylxanthines.

Beta$_2$ agonists bind to the beta$_2$-adrenergic receptors and cause an increase in the intracellular level of a substance called *cyclic adenosine monophosphate (cAMP).* This substance triggers smooth muscle relaxation.

Short-acting beta$_2$ agonists (SABAs) provide rapid but short-term relief. These inhaled drugs are most useful when an attack begins (rescue drug) or as premedication when the patient is about to begin an activity that is likely to induce an asthma attack (Fitzgerald, 2006; National Institutes of Health, 2007). Such agents include albuterol (Proventil, Ventolin), bitolterol (Tornalate), levalbuterol (Xopenex), pirbuterol (Maxair), and terbutaline (Brethaire). When inhaled from either a metered dose inhaler (MDI) or a dry powder inhaler (DPI), the drug is delivered directly to the site of action and systemic effects are minimal (unless the agent is overused or abused). Teach the patient the correct technique to use with an inhaled drug to achieve the greatest benefit from the drug. Chart 32-6 describes the proper way to use an MDI. Fig. 32-3 shows a patient using a "spacer" with an MDI. Chart 32-7

Chart 32-5 COMMON EXAMPLES OF DRUG THERAPY
Asthma Prevention and Treatment

Drug/Usual Dosage	Purpose/Action	Nursing Interventions	Rationale
BRONCHODILATORS			
SHORT-ACTING BETA AGONIST (SABA)			
Albuterol (Proventil, Ventolin) 1-2 inhalations every 4-6 hr (90 mcg/inhaled dose)	Causes bronchodilation by relaxing bronchiolar smooth muscle through binding to and activating pulmonary $beta_2$ receptors. Primary use is a fast-acting "rescue" drug to be used either during an asthma attack or just before engaging in activity that usually triggers an attack.	Teach patient to carry with him or her at all times.	The drug can stop or reduce life-threatening bronchoconstriction, which can occur anytime.
		Teach patient to monitor heart rate.	Excessive use causes systemic symptoms, especially tachycardia.
		When taking this drug with other inhaled drugs, teach patient to use this drug at least 5 minutes before the other inhaled drugs.	The bronchodilation effect of the drug allows better penetration of the other inhaled drugs.
		Teach patient the correct technique for using the MDI or DPI, and obtain a return demonstration.	Correct technique is essential to getting the drug to the site of action. Poor technique allows the drug to escape through the nose and mouth.
LONG-ACTING BETA AGONIST (LABA)			
Salmeterol (Serevent) 2 inhalations every 12 hr (25 mcg/inhalation with MDI) (50 mcg/inhalation with DPI)	Causes bronchodilation by relaxing bronchiolar smooth muscle through binding to and activating pulmonary $beta_2$ receptors. Onset of action is slow with a long duration. Primary use is prevention of an asthma attack.	Teach patient to shake inhaler (MDI) well before using.	Drug separates easily.
		Teach patient to not use this drug with the onset of asthma symptoms or worsening of wheezing.	Drug has slow onset of action and does not relieve or reverse symptoms.
		Teach patient the correct technique for using the MDI or DPI, and obtain a return demonstration.	Correct technique is essential to getting the drug to the site of action. Poor technique allows the drug to escape through the nose and mouth.
CHOLINERGIC ANTAGONIST			
Ipratropium (Atrovent, Apo-Ipravent🍁) 2-4 inhalations 4-6 times daily (18 mcg/inhalation)	Causes bronchodilation by inhibiting the parasympathetic nervous system, allowing the sympathetic system to dominate, releasing norepinephrine that activates $beta_2$ receptors. Purpose is to both rescue and prevent asthma. Drug does not work as well as SABAs but can be used in place of SABAs by patients who cannot tolerate side effects of $beta_2$ agonists.	If patient is to use this as a "rescue" drug, teach him or her to carry it at all times.	The drug can stop or reduce life-threatening bronchoconstriction, which can occur anytime.
		Teach patient to shake MDI well before using.	Drug separates easily.
		Teach patient to drink at least 4 L of fluid daily unless another health problem requires fluid restriction.	Drug causes mouth dryness.
		Teach patient to observe for and report blurred vision, eye pain, headache, nausea, palpitations, tremors, inability to sleep.	These are systemic symptoms of overdose and require intervention.
		Teach patient the correct technique for using the MDI or DPI, and obtain a return demonstration.	Correct technique is essential to getting the drug to the site of action. Poor technique allows the drug to escape through the nose and mouth.

From National Institutes of Health. (2007). *Guidelines for the diagnosis and management of asthma*. Expert panel report 3. Bethesda, MD: U.S. Department of Health and Human Services.
DPI, Dry powder inhaler; *MDI*, metered dose inhaler; *SABA*, short-acting $beta_2$ agonists.

Chart 32-5 COMMON EXAMPLES OF DRUG THERAPY

Asthma Prevention and Treatment—cont'd

Drug/Usual Dosage	Purpose/Action	Nursing Interventions	Rationale
METHYLXANTHINES			
Theophylline (Elixophyllin, Theo-Dur, Uniphyl, Theo-lair, many others) 5 mg/kg IV or 10-12 mg/kg orally as loading dose; 200-800 mg orally daily	Acts like caffeine to cause bronchodilation by relaxing bronchiolar smooth muscles through inhibiting an enzyme that breaks down the intracellular trigger for relaxation. Used to prevent asthma attacks and to stop an attack once it has started.	Understand that a higher dose is required at the beginning of therapy (loading dose) than is used to maintain the effect.	Drug requires a specific blood level to work. A loading dose is required to achieve this level. Then, lower doses are used for maintenance because the drug is eliminated slowly.
		Teach patient to take the daily dose in evenly spaced divided doses.	Maintains an even blood level and has a better effect.
		Teach patient to make and keep appointments to monitor blood levels of the drug.	Drug has a narrow margin of safety and many severe side effects.
		Teach patient not to drink coffee or other caffeinated beverages while on this drug.	Drug is similar to caffeine, and taking it with caffeine increases the risk for toxicity.
ANTI-INFLAMMATORIES			
All of these drugs help improve bronchiolar airflow by decreasing the inflammatory response of the mucous membranes in the airways. *They do not cause bronchodilation.*			
CORTICOSTEROIDS			
Fluticasone (Flovent) 50 mcg by MDI twice daily; 100-250 mcg by DPI daily	Disrupts all known production pathways of inflammatory mediators. The main purpose is to prevent an asthma attack caused by inflammation or allergies.	Teach patient to use the drug daily, even when no symptoms are present.	Maximum effectiveness requires continued use for 48-72 hr and depends on regular use.
		Teach patient to perform good mouth care and to check the mouth daily for lesions or drainage.	Drug reduces local immunity and increases the risk for local infections, especially *Candida albicans* (yeast).
		Teach patient to not use this drug with the onset of asthma symptoms or worsening of wheezing.	Drug has slow onset of action and does not relieve or reverse symptoms.
		Teach patient the correct technique for using the MDI or DPI, and obtain a return demonstration.	Correct technique is essential to getting the drug to the site of action. Poor technique allows the drug to escape through the nose and mouth.
Prednisone (Deltasone, Predone) 1-40 mg orally daily	Not recommended unless asthma symptoms cannot be controlled with any other therapy.	Teach patient about the numerous expected side effects (GI ulceration, fat redistribution, weight gain, hyperglycemia).	Knowing the side effects to expect reduces anxiety.
		Teach patient to avoid anyone who has an upper respiratory infection.	Drug reduces all protective inflammatory responses, increasing the risk for infection.
		Teach patient to avoid activities that lead to injury.	Blood vessels become more fragile, leading to bruising and petechiae.
		Teach patient to take drug with food.	The drug increases the risk for GI ulceration; food helps reduce the risk.
		Teach patient not to suddenly stop taking the drug for any reason. If patient cannot take the oral drug because of vomiting, he or she should receive the drug parenterally.	The drug suppresses adrenal production of corticosteroids, which are essential for life.

Continued

Chart 32-5 COMMON EXAMPLES OF DRUG THERAPY

Asthma Prevention and Treatment—cont'd

Drug/Usual Dosage	Purpose/Action	Nursing Interventions	Rationale
NSAID			
Nedocromil (Tilade) 4 mg by MDI every 6 hr	Stabilizes the membranes of mast cells and prevents the release of inflammatory mediators. Purpose is to prevent asthma attack triggered by inflammation or allergens.	Teach patient to use the drug daily, even when no symptoms are present.	Drug has slow onset of action for asthma prevention and is most effective when taken consistently.
		Teach patient to not use this drug with the onset of asthma symptoms or worsening of wheezing.	Drug does not relieve or reverse symptoms.
		Teach patient the correct technique for using the MDI, and obtain a return demonstration.	Correct technique is essential to getting the drug to the site of action. Poor technique allows the drug to escape through the nose and mouth.
LEUKOTRIENE ANTAGONIST			
Montelukast (Singular) 10 mg orally daily	Blocks the leukotriene receptor, preventing the inflammatory mediator from stimulating inflammation. Purpose is to prevent asthma attack triggered by inflammation or allergens.	Teach patient to use the drug daily, even when no symptoms are present.	Drug has slow onset of action for asthma prevention and is most effective when taken consistently.
		Teach patient not to decrease the dose of or stop taking any other asthma drugs unless otherwise instructed by the health care professional.	This drug is for long-term asthma control and does not replace other drugs, especially corticosteroids and rescue drugs.
IMMUNOMODULATOR			
Omalizumab (Xolair) 150-375 mg subcutaneously every 2-3 wk	Drug is an antibody that binds to the IgE receptors on mast cells and basophils, preventing allergens from triggering the release of inflammatory mediators. Purpose is prevention of allergen-triggered asthma attacks.	Administer drug in a facility equipped to handle anaphylaxis.	Drug is associated with anaphylaxis.
		Do not administer more than 150 mg per injection site.	Larger doses can cause severe injection site reactions with bruising, erythema, warmth, burning, stinging, pruritus, hives, pain, induration, mass, and inflammation lasting up to 7 days.
		Keep patient at the facility for 30-60 min after injection.	Allergic reactions and anaphylaxis are most likely within the first 30-60 min after injection.
		Teach patient not to decrease the dose of or stop taking any other asthma drugs unless otherwise instructed by the health care professional.	This drug may take months before it is effective and, even then, does not stop an attack that has started. It is an additional drug for allergic asthma and does not replace other drugs.

From National Institutes of Health. (2007). *Guidelines for the diagnosis and management of asthma*. Expert panel report 3. Bethesda, MD: U.S. Department of Health and Human Services.

DPI, Dry powder inhaler; *MDI,* metered dose inhaler; *SABA,* short-acting beta$_2$ agonists.

Chart 32-6 PATIENT AND FAMILY EDUCATION GUIDE

How to Use an Inhaler Correctly*

WITH A SPACER

1. Before each use, remove the caps from the inhaler and the spacer.
2. Insert the mouthpiece of the inhaler into the non-mouthpiece end of the spacer.
3. Shake the whole unit vigorously three or four times.
4. Place the mouthpiece into your mouth, over your tongue, and seal your lips tightly around it.
5. Press down firmly on the canister of the inhaler to release one dose of medication into the spacer.
6. Breathe in slowly and deeply. If the spacer makes a whistling sound, you are breathing in too rapidly.
7. Remove the mouthpiece from your mouth, and, keeping your lips closed, hold your breath for at least 10 seconds and then breathe out slowly.
8. Wait at least 1 minute between puffs.
9. Replace the caps on the inhaler and the spacer.
10. At least once a day, clean the plastic case and cap of the inhaler by thoroughly rinsing in warm, running tap water; at least once a week, clean the spacer in the same manner.

WITHOUT A SPACER (PREFERRED TECHNIQUE)

1. Before each use, remove the cap and shake the inhaler according to the instructions in the package insert.
2. Tilt your head back slightly, and breathe out fully.
3. Open your mouth, and place the mouthpiece 1 to 2 inches away.
4. As you begin to breathe in deeply through your mouth, press down firmly on the canister of the inhaler to release one dose of medication.
5. Continue to breathe in slowly and deeply (usually over 3-5 sec).
6. Hold your breath for at least 10 seconds to allow the medication to reach deep into the lungs, and then breathe out slowly.
7. Wait at least 1 minute between puffs.
8. Replace the cap on the inhaler.
9. At least once a day, remove the canister and clean the plastic case and cap of the inhaler by thoroughly rinsing in warm, running tap water.

WITHOUT A SPACER (ALTERNATIVE METHOD)

1. Follow steps 1 and 2 of the preferred technique for using an inhaler without a spacer.
2. Place the mouthpiece into your mouth, over your tongue, and seal your lips tightly around it.
3. Follow steps 4 to 9 of the preferred technique for using an inhaler without a spacer.

*Avoid spraying in the direction of the eyes.

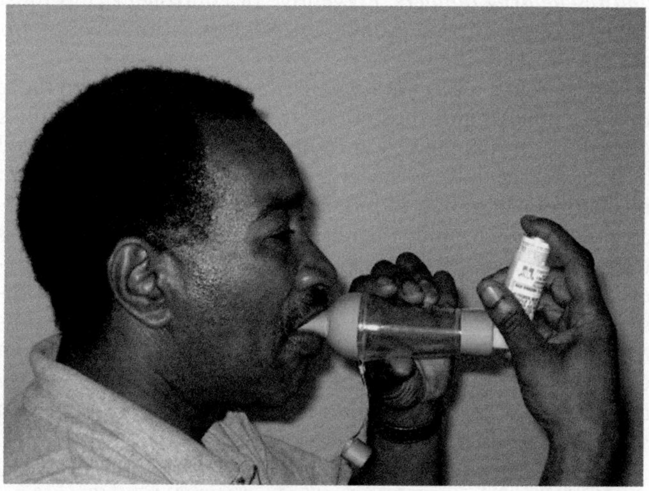

Fig. 32-3 • Patient using an aerosol inhaler with a spacer.

describes the proper care and use of a DPI. Fig. 32-4 shows a patient using a DPI.

Teach the patient to always carry the rescue drug inhaler with him or her and to ensure that enough drug remains in the inhaler to provide a quick dose when needed. Dry powder inhalers indicate the amount of remaining drug; however, aerosol (MDI) inhalers do not. Demonstrate how to check aerosol inhaler drug levels by placing the inhaler in water (Fig. 32-5). Full inhalers sink to the bottom. An empty inhaler floats on its side.

Long-acting beta$_2$ agonists (LABAs) are also delivered by inhaler directly to the site of action—the bronchioles. Proper use of the long-acting agonists can decrease the need to rescue as often with short-acting agonists. Unlike short-acting agonists, long-acting drugs need time to build up an effect but the effects are longer lasting. *Thus these drugs are useful in preventing an asthma attack but have no value during an acute attack. Therefore teach patients not to use LABAs to rescue them during an attack or when wheezing is getting worse but, instead,*

Chart 32-7 PATIENT AND FAMILY EDUCATION GUIDE

How to Use a Dry Powder Inhaler (DPI)

FOR INHALERS REQUIRING LOADING

- First load the drug by:
  - Turning the device to the next dose of drug, or
  - Inserting the capsule into the device, or
  - Inserting the disk or compartment into the device

AFTER LOADING THE DRUG AND FOR INHALERS THAT DO NOT REQUIRE DRUG LOADING

- Read your doctor's instructions for how fast you should breathe for your particular inhaler.
- Place your lips over the mouthpiece, and breathe in forcefully (there is no propellant in the inhaler; only your breath pulls the drug in).
- Remove the inhaler from your mouth as soon as you have breathed in.
- *Never exhale (breathe out) into your inhaler.* Your breath will moisten the powder, causing it to clump and not be delivered accurately.
- *Never wash or place the inhaler in water.*
- *Never shake your inhaler.*
- Keep your inhaler in a dry place at room temperature.
- If the inhaler is preloaded, discard the inhaler after it is empty.
- Because the drug is a dry powder and there is no propellant, you may not feel, smell, or taste it as you inhale.

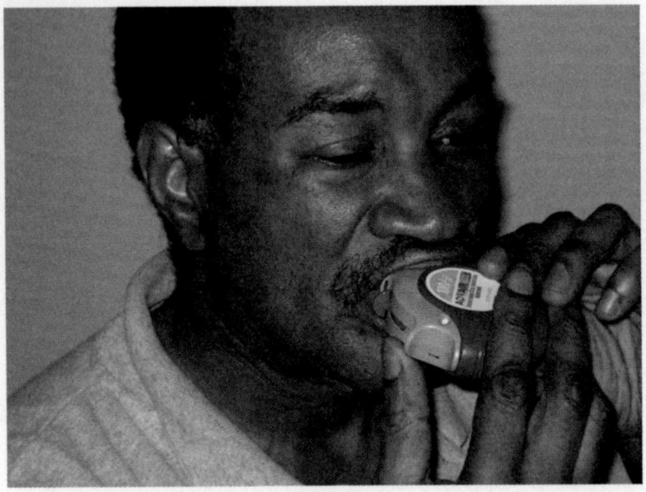
Fig. 32-4 • Patient using a dry powder inhaler (DPI).

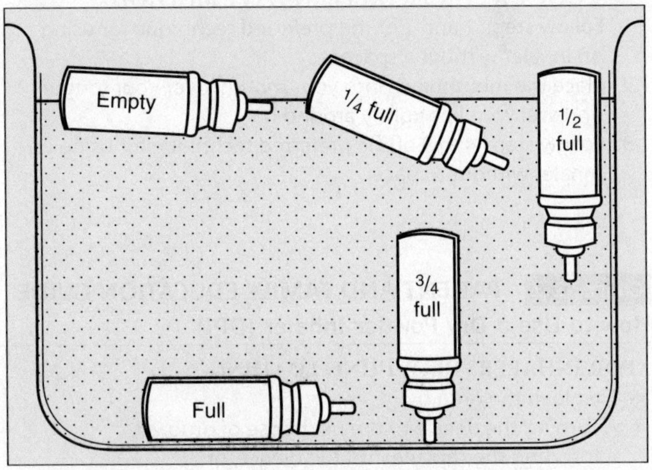
Empty
1/4 full
1/2 full
3/4 full
Full
Fig. 32-5 • Checking the drug level in an aerosol inhaler.

to use a SABA. Relying on LABAs during an attack can lead to worsening of symptoms and death. Examples of LABAs include formoterol (Foradil) and salmeterol (Serevent). *Teach the patient to use these drugs daily as prescribed, even when no symptoms are present.*

Cholinergic antagonists, also called *anticholinergic drugs,* are similar to atropine and block the parasympathetic nervous system. This blockade allows the sympathetic nervous system to dominate, resulting in increased bronchodilation and decreased pulmonary secretions. The most common drug in this class is ipratropium (Atrovent), which is used as an inhalant. Most cholinergic antagonists are short acting and must be used several times a day, although long-acting agents such as tiotropium (Spiriva) are available for use once a day. These drugs are not as effective as $beta_2$ agonists and are recommended as first-line asthma therapy only for those patients who cannot tolerate the side effects of $beta_2$ agonists.

Methylxanthines are used when other types of management are ineffective. The classic drug in this class is theophylline (Theo-Dur). Other drugs include aminophylline (Truphylline), oxtriphylline (Choledyl🍁), and dyphylline (Dilor, Lufyllin). *These drugs are given systemically, have narrow therapeutic ranges, and have many side effects. Blood levels of these drugs need to be monitored closely because the drug level that causes dangerous side effects is not much higher than the level needed to dilate the bronchioles. Teach the patient who takes these drugs daily to keep all appointments for monitoring blood levels of the drug and not to self-increase the dose.* The most dangerous side effects result from excessive cardiac and central nervous system stimulation and include dysrhythmias, hypertension, and seizure activity.

Anti-Inflammatory Agents. Anti-inflammatory agents decrease the inflammatory responses in the airways. Some are given systemically and have more side effects. Others are used as inhalants and have few systemic side effects.

Corticosteroids decrease inflammatory and immune responses in many ways, including by preventing the synthesis of mediators. Inhaled corticosteroids (ICSs) can be helpful in preventing the manifestations of asthma. Newer high-potency steroid inhalers, such as fluticasone (Flovent), budesonide (Pulmicort), and mometasone (Asmanex), may be used once per day for maintenance. Systemic corticosteroids, because of severe side effects, are avoided for mild to moderate intermittent asthma and are used on a short-term basis for moderate asthma. For some patients with severe asthma, daily oral corticosteroids may be needed. *Both inhaled corticosteroids and those taken orally are preventive. They are not effective in reversing symptoms during an asthma attack and should not be used as rescue drugs. Teach patients the difference between ICSs and rescue drug inhalers.* Preventive or controller drugs must be used on a scheduled basis, even when asthma symptoms are not present.

Nonsteroidal anti-inflammatory drugs (NSAIDs), both those that are inhaled and those that are taken orally, are useful as *preventive* asthma therapy and should be taken on a scheduled basis. They include a variety of agents that have different mechanisms of action to reduce airway inflammation. Nedocromil (Tilade) inhibits the release of inflammatory mediators from respiratory cells and white blood cells. Mast cell stabilizers, such as cromolyn sodium (Intal), prevent mast cell membranes from opening when an allergen binds to IgE. Thus these drugs help prevent atopic asthma attacks but are not useful during an acute episode. *The inhaled NSAIDs are not effective in reversing symptoms during an asthma attack and should not be used as rescue drugs.*

Leukotriene antagonists are oral drugs that work in several ways to prevent an asthma episode. Montelukast (Singulair) and zafirlukast (Accolate) block the leukotriene receptor. Zileuton (Zyflo) prevents leukotriene synthesis. *These drugs are not effective in reversing symptoms during an asthma attack and should not be used as rescue drugs.*

Immunomodulators are monoclonal antibodies that prevent allergens from binding to receptor sites on mast cells and basophils. This action prevents allergens from triggering the release of mediators from mast cells and basophils. Thus these drugs help prevent atopic asthma attacks but are not useful during an acute episode. Omalizumab (Xolair) is currently the only drug in this class. It is injected subcutaneously every 2 to 3 weeks. Because there is a relatively high risk of anaphylaxis from this drug, it should be administered only in a setting capable of handling this type of reaction.

Exercise/Activity

Regular exercise, including aerobic exercise, is a recommended part of asthma therapy. Aerobic exercise assists in maintaining cardiac health, enhancing skeletal muscle strength, and promoting ventilation and perfusion. Patients with asthma should examine the conditions that trigger an attack and adjust the exercise routine as needed. Some may need to premedicate with inhaled beta agonists (SABAs) before beginning activity. For others, adjusting the environment may be needed. For example, outdoor ice-skating in cold, dry air can trigger an attack; indoor ice-skating may be less of a problem. Sports that involve more "rest" action, such as baseball, are less likely to trigger symptoms than "nonrest" action sports, such as basketball.

Oxygen Therapy

Supplemental oxygen is often used during an acute asthma attack. Oxygen is delivered by mask, nasal cannula, or endotracheal tube. High flow rates or concentrations may be needed when bronchospasms are severe and limit flow of oxygen through the bronchiole tubes. Heliox, a mixture of helium and oxygen (often 50% helium and 50% oxygen), can help improve oxygen delivery to the alveoli. This gas mixture is lower in density than oxygen alone or oxygen with atmospheric air (which contains nitrogen) and flows even when airway resistance is high (Pruitt, 2007). *Ensure that no open flames (e.g., cigarette smoking, fireplaces, burning candles) or other combustion hazards are in rooms where oxygen is in use.*

Status Asthmaticus

Status asthmaticus is a severe, life-threatening acute episode of airway obstruction that intensifies once it begins and often does not respond to common therapy. The patient arrives in the emergency department with extremely labored breathing and wheezing. Use of accessory muscles for breathing and distention of neck veins are observed. *If the condition is not reversed, the patient may develop pneumothorax and cardiac or respiratory arrest.* The physician immediately prescribes IV fluids, potent systemic bronchodilators, steroids (to decrease inflammation), epinephrine, and oxygen in an attempt to reverse the acute condition. Prepare for emergency intubation. When wheezing decreases, management is similar to that for any patient with asthma.

DECISION-MAKING CHALLENGE
Critical Rescue

The patient is a 42-year-old woman who has had asthma since she was a child. She has always treated her asthma only when symptoms appeared but now is on an asthma management plan for both prevention and treatment. She comes to the emergency department with audible wheezes on inhalation and exhalation. Her PEF and FEV_1 are 40% below her personal best. Her respiratory rate is 34 breaths/min, pulse 122 bpm. She has suprasternal and intercostal retractions. Her asthma management drugs include:

- salmeterol (Serevent) 2 puffs every 12 hr
- terbutaline (Brethaire) 2 puffs PRN
- fluticasone (Flovent) 2 puffs daily
- cromolyn sodium (Intal) 1-2 puffs 4 times per day

Her partner tells you that she has not used any of her inhalers for the past week because the drugs are expensive and she has felt well.

1. Should you start oxygen on this patient? Why or why not?
2. What additional assessment data should you obtain?
3. Which of the patient's current drugs should be administered immediately? Why?
4. What is your interpretation of this patient's immediate condition based on PEF?
5. What teaching priorities are needed for this patient?

evolve For suggested answer guidelines, go to http://evolve.elsevier.com/Iggy/.

CHRONIC OBSTRUCTIVE PULMONARY DISEASE

Pathophysiology

Most patients with emphysema have chronic bronchitis at the same time, but each condition has its own pathophysiologic process (Fig. 32-6).

Emphysema

The two major changes that occur with pulmonary emphysema are loss of lung elasticity and hyperinflation of the lung (see Fig. 32-1). These changes result in dyspnea and the need for an increased respiratory rate.

In the healthy lung, protein degrading enzymes called *proteases* are present to destroy and eliminate protein-based particulate matter and organisms inhaled during breathing. If these proteases are present in higher-than-normal levels, they damage the alveoli and the small airways by breaking down elastin. High protease levels cause the alveolar sacs to lose their elasticity and the small airways to collapse or narrow. Some alveoli are destroyed, and others become large and flabby, with decreased area for effective gas exchange.

An increased amount of air becomes trapped in the lungs. Causes of air trapping are loss of elastic recoil in the alveolar walls, overstretching and enlargement of the alveoli into air-filled spaces called *bullae,* and collapse of small airways (bronchioles). These changes greatly increase the work of breathing. The hyperinflated lung flattens the diaphragm (Fig. 32-7), weakening the effect of this muscle. As a result, the patient

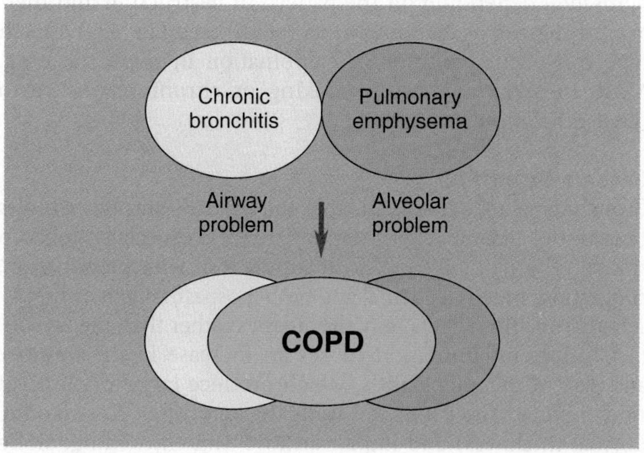
Chronic bronchitis
Pulmonary emphysema
Airway problem
Alveolar problem
COPD

Fig. 32-6 • The interaction of chronic bronchitis and emphysema in chronic obstructive pulmonary disease (COPD).

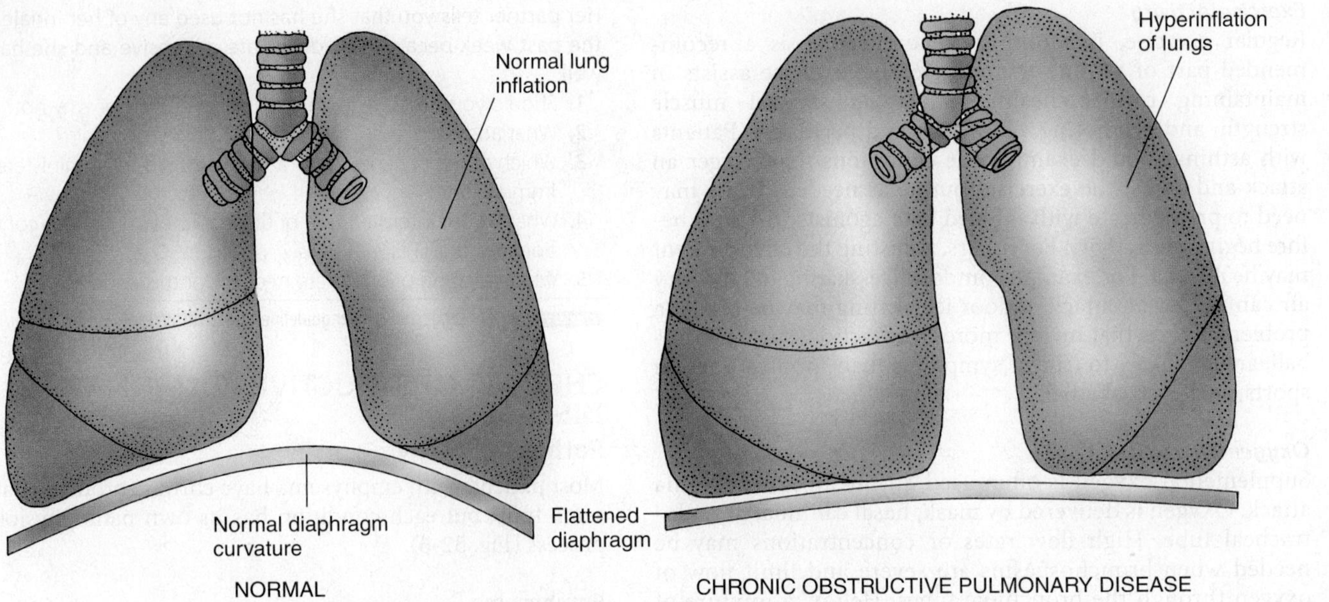
Normal lung
inflation
Normal diaphragm
curvature
NORMAL
Hyperinflation
of lungs
Flattened
diaphragm
CHRONIC OBSTRUCTIVE PULMONARY DISEASE

Fig. 32-7 • Diaphragm shape and lung inflation in the normal patient and in the patient with chronic airflow limitation (CAL).

with emphysema needs to use additional muscles (accessory muscles) in the neck, chest wall, and abdomen to inhale and exhale. This increased effort increases the need for oxygen, making the patient work harder and have an "air hunger" sensation. Often, inhalation starts before exhalation is completed, resulting in an uncoordinated pattern of breathing.

Gas exchange is affected by the increased work of breathing and the loss of alveolar tissue. Although some alveoli enlarge, the curves of alveolar walls decrease and less surface area is available for gas exchange. Often the patient adjusts by increasing the respiratory rate, so arterial blood gas (ABG) values may not show gas exchange problems until the patient has advanced disease. Then carbon dioxide is produced faster than it can be eliminated, resulting in carbon dioxide retention and chronic respiratory acidosis (see Chapter 14). The patient with late-stage emphysema also has a low arterial oxygen (Pao_2) level, because it is difficult for oxygen to move from diseased lung tissue into the bloodstream.

Emphysema is classified as *panlobular, centrilobular,* or *paraseptal* depending on the pattern of destruction and dilation of the gas-exchanging units (acini) (see Fig. 32-1). Each type can occur alone or in combination in the same lung. Most are associated with smoking or chronic exposure to other inhalation irritants.

Chronic Bronchitis

Bronchitis is an inflammation of the bronchi and bronchioles caused by chronic exposure to irritants, especially tobacco smoke. The irritant triggers inflammation, with vasodilation, congestion, mucosal edema, and bronchospasm. Unlike emphysema, bronchitis affects only the airways rather than the alveoli.

Chronic inflammation causes an increase in the number and size of mucous glands, which produce large amounts of thick mucus. The bronchial walls thicken (often to twice the normal thickness) and impair airflow. This thickening, along with excessive mucus, blocks some of the smaller airways and narrows larger ones. Small airways are affected before large airways become involved.

Chronic bronchitis hinders airflow and gas exchange because of mucous plugs and infection narrowing the airways. As a result, the Pao_2 decreases (hypoxemia) and the arterial blood carbon dioxide ($Paco_2$) level increases (respiratory acidosis).

Etiology and Genetic Risk

Cigarette smoking is the most important risk factor for COPD. The patient with an 8–pack-year history usually has obstructive lung changes but no manifestations of disease. The patient with a 20–pack-year history or longer often has early-stage COPD found as changes in pulmonary function tests (PFTs).

The harmful effects of tobacco result in part because inhaled smoke triggers the release of excessive amounts of the proteases from cells in the lungs. These enzymes break down elastin, the major component of alveoli. By impairing the action of cilia, smoking also inhibits the cilia from clearing the bronchi of mucus, cellular debris, and fluid.

In addition to the increased risk for COPD from active smoking, passive smoking (or secondhand smoke) contributes to upper and lower respiratory problems. The risk is greater when exposure occurs in small, confined spaces.

CULTURAL AWARENESS

The prevalence of smoking remains higher among African Americans, blue-collar workers, and less educated people than in the overall population of the United States. Smoking prevalence is highest among Northern Plains American Indians and Alaskan Natives. The overall prevalence of smoking for both men and women has decreased over the past two decades, but the decrease for women has been less than it has for men (American Cancer Society, 2008). Development of culturally appropriate smoking cessation programs as well as research examining barriers to cessation in these populations may help reduce this disparity.

Alpha$_1$-antitrypsin deficiency is a less common but important risk factor for COPD. A special enzyme, alpha$_1$-antitrypsin (AAT), is made by the liver and is normally present in the lungs. One purpose of AAT is to regulate the proteases that are present to break down inhaled pollutants and organisms. AAT, a protease inhibitor, prevents the proteases from working on lung structures.

The production of normal amounts of AAT depends on the inheritance of a pair of normal gene alleles for this protein. The AAT gene is recessive. Thus if one of the pair of alleles is faulty and the other allele is normal, the person makes enough AAT to prevent COPD unless there is significant exposure to cigarette smoke and other precipitating factors. This person, however, is a carrier for AAT deficiency. If both alleles are faulty, COPD develops at a fairly young age even when the person is not exposed to cigarette smoke or other irritants.

About 100,000 Americans have severe AAT deficiency, and many more have mild to moderate deficiencies (Nussbaum et al., 2007). Although an AAT deficiency causes problems in other organs, such as the skin and liver, lung diseases are the most common problem caused by the deficiency.

GENETIC CONSIDERATIONS

The gene for AAT has many known mutations, some of which increase the risk for emphysema. Variation of mutations (polymorphisms) results in different levels of AAT deficiency. This variation is one reason why the disease is more severe for some people than for others. The most serious mutation for an increased risk for emphysema is the Z mutation, although others also increase the risk but to a lesser degree. Table 32-1 shows the most common AAT mutations increasing the risk for emphysema.

Air pollution alone plays a relatively small role in the patient with emphysema and chronic bronchitis. The effect of air pollution is additive to tobacco exposure.

Incidence/Prevalence

The prevalence of chronic bronchitis and emphysema in the United States has been estimated at about 13.5 million (for chronic bronchitis) and 2 million (for emphysema). Chronic obstructive pulmonary disease/chronic airflow limitation (COPD/CAL) is the fourth leading cause of morbidity and mortality in the United States (Global Initiative for Chronic Obstructive Lung Disease [GOLD], 2007).

TABLE 32-1 Characteristics Associated with the Most Common Alpha$_1$-Antitrypsin Gene Mutations

Mutation Genotype	Level of Serum Alpha$_1$-Antitrypsin (% of normal)	Disease Severity
M/S	80%	No detectable disease
S/S	50%-60%	Minimal to no disease expression
M/Z	50%-55%	Minimal to no disease expression
S/Z	30%-35%	Pulmonary disease, early age
Z/Z	10%-15%	Severe COPD, extra-pulmonary involvement

From Workman, M.L., & Winkelman, C. (2008). Genetic influences in common respiratory disorders. *Critical Care Nursing Clinics of North America 20* (2), 171-189.

Complications

COPD affects the *oxygenation and tissue perfusion* to all tissues. Complications of the disorder can result in organ anoxia and tissue death. Major problems occur, such as hypoxemia, acidosis, respiratory infection, cardiac failure, and dysrhythmias.

Hypoxemia and acidosis occur because the patient with COPD is less able to exchange gas, oxygenation decreases and carbon dioxide levels increase. These problems reduce general cellular function.

Respiratory infection risk increases because of the increased mucus and poor oxygenation. The organisms most often causing bacterial infections include *Streptococcus pneumoniae, Haemophilus influenzae,* and *Moraxella catarrhalis.* Acute respiratory infections make COPD manifestations worse by increasing inflammation and mucus production and inducing more bronchospasm. Airflow becomes even more limited, the work of breathing increases, and dyspnea results.

Cardiac failure, especially **cor pulmonale** (right-sided heart failure caused by pulmonary disease), occurs with bronchitis or emphysema. Air trapping, airway collapse, and stiff alveolar walls increase the lung tissue pressure, making blood flow through lung vessels more difficult. The increased pressure makes the workload heavy on the right side of the heart, which pumps blood into the lungs. As the disease progresses, the amount of oxygen in the blood decreases, causing major blood vessels in the lung to constrict. To pump blood through these narrowed vessels, the right side of the heart must generate high pressures. In response to this heavy workload, the right chambers of the heart enlarge and thicken, causing right-sided heart failure with backup of blood into the general venous system. Chart 32-8 lists key features of cor pulmonale.

Cardiac dysrhythmias are common in patients with COPD. They may be a result of hypoxemia (from decreased oxygen to the heart muscle), other cardiac disease, drug effects, or acidosis.

Chart 32-8 KEY FEATURES

Cor Pulmonale

- Hypoxia and hypoxemia
- Increasing dyspnea
- Fatigue
- Enlarged and tender liver
- Warm, cyanotic hands and feet, with bounding pulses
- Cyanotic lips
- Distended neck veins
- Right ventricular enlargement (hypertrophy)
- Visible pulsations below the sternum
- GI disturbances, such as nausea or anorexia
- Dependent edema
- Metabolic and respiratory acidosis
- Pulmonary hypertension

Health Promotion and Maintenance

Health experts agree that the incidence and severity of COPD would be drastically reduced by smoking cessation (Crawford & Harris, 2008). COPD is rare among people who have never smoked cigarettes. Disease progression can be slowed by smoking cessation. Encourage all people who smoke to quit smoking. Chart 32-3 provides tips to teach people about smoking cessation.

Other measures to reduce the incidence of COPD are to avoid inhalation irritants in all environments. Teaching all people to use masks when working in areas with high levels of particulate matter can reduce individual exposure. Proper venting of workplaces and recreation areas that have airborne or particulate matter also reduces exposure.

Patient-Centered Collaborative Care

evolve ONLINE PHARM REVIEW

The Concept Map on p. 625 addresses assessment and nursing care issues related to COPD.

▪ Assessment

History

Ask about risk factors such as age, gender, occupational history, and ethnic-cultural background when taking a history from a patient who may have chronic obstructive pulmonary disease (COPD). COPD is seen more often in older men. Some types of emphysema occur in families, especially those with alpha$_1$-antitrypsin (AAT) deficiency.

Obtain a thorough smoking history, because tobacco use is a major risk factor. Ask about the length of time the patient has smoked and the number of packs smoked daily. Use these data to determine the pack-year smoking history. If the patient smokes, use this opportunity as a teachable moment to discuss smoking cessation strategies (see Chart 32-3).

Ask the patient to describe his or her breathing problems. Assess whether the patient has any difficulty breathing while talking. Can he or she speak in complete sentences, or is it necessary to take a breath between every one or two words? Ask about the presence, duration, or worsening of wheezing, coughing, and shortness of breath. Determine what activities trigger these problems. Assess the patient's cough pattern. If the cough is productive, ask whether sputum is clear or colored and how much is produced each day. Ask the patient to recall the time of day when the sputum production is greatest. Smokers often have a productive cough when they get up in the morning; nonsmokers generally do not. Ask whether sputum production has increased or changed during the past year.

Check the relationship between activity tolerance and dyspnea by asking the patient to compare his or her activity level and shortness of breath now with those of a month ago and a year ago. Likewise, ask about any difficulty with eating and sleeping. Many patients sleep in a semi-sitting position because breathlessness is worse when lying down **(orthopnea).** Ask about usual daily activities and any difficulty with sleeping, bathing, dressing, or sexual activity. Document this initial assessment to serve as a starting point for determining the intervention plan and its effectiveness.

Weigh the patient, and compare this weight with previous weights. Unplanned weight loss occurs with an increase in COPD severity. COPD increases metabolic needs as a result of the increased work of breathing. Dyspnea and mucus production often result in poor food intake and inadequate nutrition. Ask the patient to recall a typical day's meals and fluid intake. When heart failure is present with COPD, general edema with weight gain may occur.

Physical Assessment/Clinical Manifestations

General appearance can provide clues about the patient's respiratory status and energy level. Observe his or her weight in proportion to height, posture, mobility, muscle mass, and overall hygiene. The patient with increasingly severe COPD is thin, with loss of muscle mass in the extremities, although the neck muscles may be enlarged. He or she tends to be slow moving and slightly stooped. Usually the person sits with a forward-bending posture, sometimes with the arms held forward (Fig. 32-8). When dyspnea becomes severe, activity intolerance may be so great that bathing and general grooming are neglected.

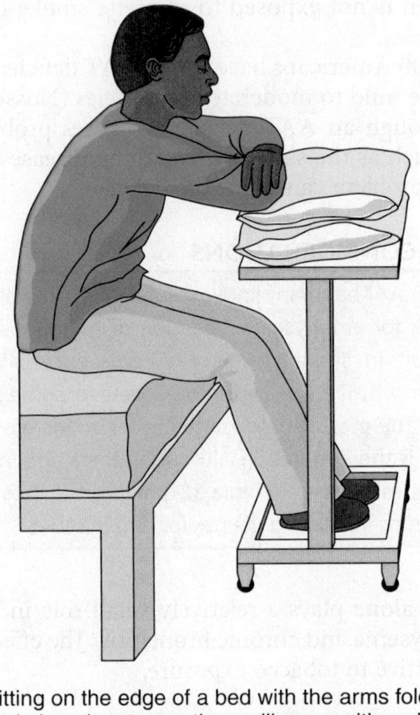

Sitting on the edge of a bed with the arms folded and placed on two or three pillows positioned over a nightstand.

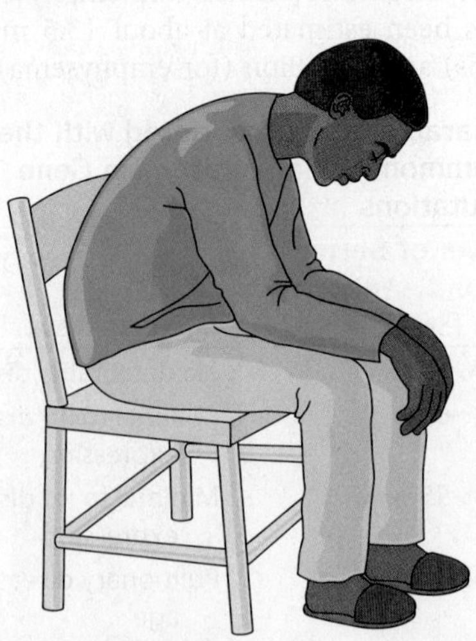

Sitting in a chair with the feet spread shoulder-width apart and leaning forward with the elbows on the knees. Arms and hands are relaxed.

Fig. 32-8 • Orthopnea positions that patients with chronic airflow limitation (CAL) can assume to ease the work of breathing.

CONCEPT MAP Respiratory Acidosis (COPD Related)

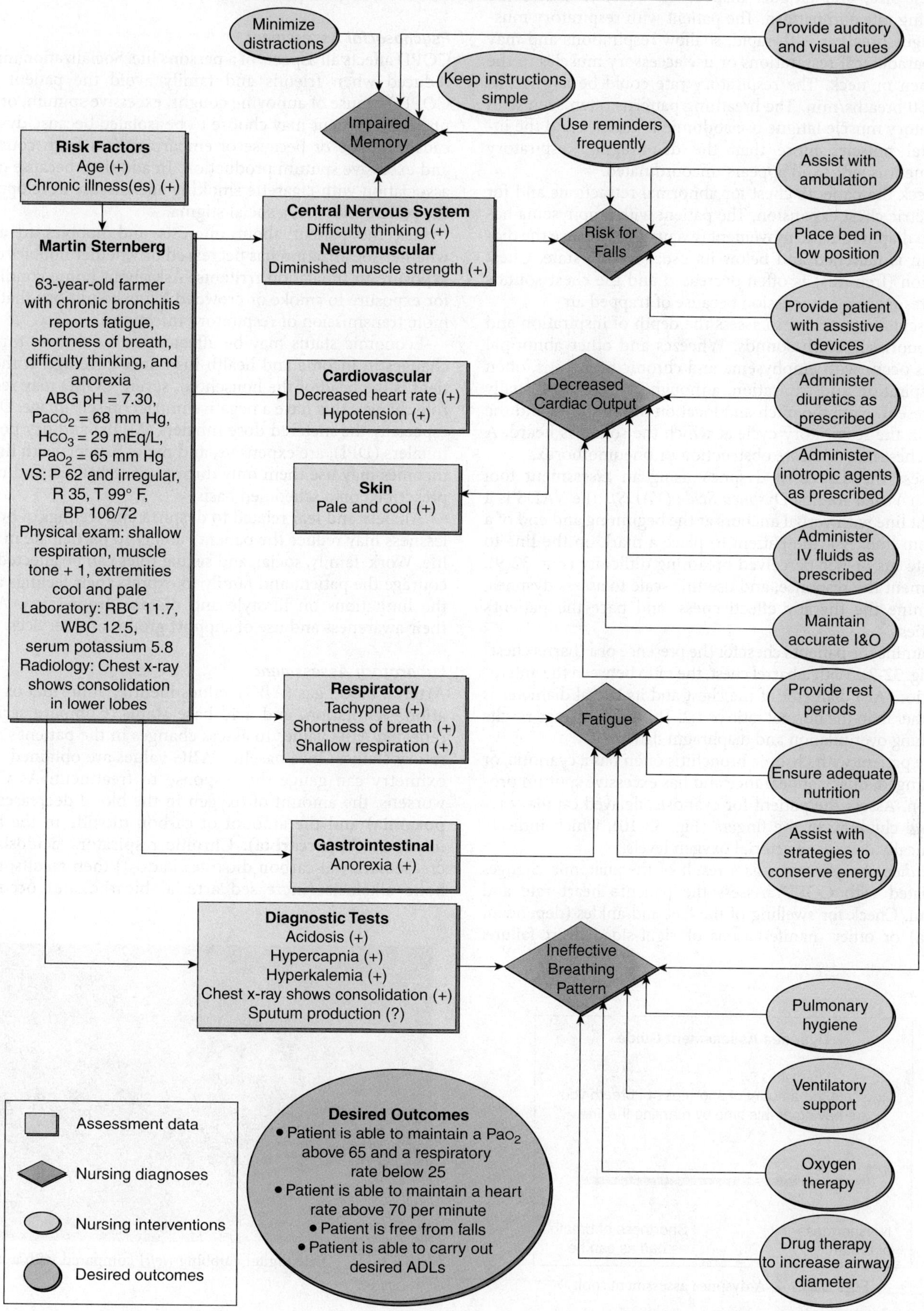
Minimize distractions
Keep instructions simple
Provide auditory and visual cues
Impaired Memory
Use reminders frequently
Risk Factors
Age (+)
Chronic illness(es) (+)
Assist with ambulation
Central Nervous System
Difficulty thinking (+)
Neuromuscular
Diminished muscle strength (+)
Risk for Falls
Place bed in low position
Martin Sternberg
63-year-old farmer with chronic bronchitis reports fatigue, shortness of breath, difficulty thinking, and anorexia
ABG pH = 7.30,
Paco2 = 68 mm Hg,
Hco3 = 29 mEq/L,
Pao2 = 65 mm Hg
VS: P 62 and irregular, R 35, T 99° F, BP 106/72
Physical exam: shallow respiration, muscle tone + 1, extremities cool and pale
Laboratory: RBC 11.7, WBC 12.5, serum potassium 5.8
Radiology: Chest x-ray shows consolidation in lower lobes
Provide patient with assistive devices
Cardiovascular
Decreased heart rate (+)
Hypotension (+)
Decreased Cardiac Output
Administer diuretics as prescribed
Administer inotropic agents as prescribed
Skin
Pale and cool (+)
Administer IV fluids as prescribed
Maintain accurate I&O
Respiratory
Tachypnea (+)
Shortness of breath (+)
Shallow respiration (+)
Fatigue
Provide rest periods
Ensure adequate nutrition
Gastrointestinal
Anorexia (+)
Assist with strategies to conserve energy
Diagnostic Tests
Acidosis (+)
Hypercapnia (+)
Hyperkalemia (+)
Chest x-ray shows consolidation (+)
Sputum production (?)
Ineffective Breathing Pattern
Pulmonary hygiene
Ventilatory support
Assessment data
Nursing diagnoses
Nursing interventions
Desired outcomes
Desired Outcomes
• Patient is able to maintain a Pao2 above 65 and a respiratory rate below 25
• Patient is able to maintain a heart rate above 70 per minute
• Patient is free from falls
• Patient is able to carry out desired ADLs
Oxygen therapy
Drug therapy to increase airway diameter

Concept Map by Elaine Bishop Kennedy, EdD, RN

Respiratory changes occur as a result of obstruction, changes in chest size, and fatigue. Inspect the chest to assess the breathing rate and pattern. The patient with respiratory muscle fatigue breathes with rapid, shallow respirations and may have paradoxical respirations or use accessory muscles in the abdomen or neck. The respiratory rate could be as high as 40 to 50 breaths/min. The breathing patterns often seen with respiratory muscle fatigue use abdominal muscles and the intercostal muscles more than the diaphragm. Respiratory movement is jerky and appears uncoordinated.

Check the patient's chest for abnormal retractions and for symmetric chest expansion. The patient with emphysema has limited diaphragmatic movement (excursion) because the diaphragm is flattened and below its usual resting state. Chest vibration (fremitus) is often decreased and the chest sounds hyperresonant on percussion because of trapped air.

Auscultate the chest to assess the depth of inspiration and any abnormal breath sounds. Wheezes and other abnormal sounds occur with emphysema and chronic bronchitis, often on inspiration and expiration, although crackles are usually not present. Note the pitch and location of the sound and the point in the respiratory cycle at which the sound is heard. A silent chest may indicate obstruction or pneumothorax.

Assess the degree of dyspnea using an assessment tool called a *Visual Analog Dyspnea Scale (VADS)*. The VADS is a straight line with verbal anchors at the beginning and end of a 100-mm line. Ask the patient to place a mark on the line to indicate his or her perceived breathing difficulty (Fig. 32-9). Document the response, and use this scale to assess dyspnea, determine the therapy effectiveness, and pace the patient's activities.

Examine the patient's chest for the presence of a "barrel chest" (see Fig. 32-2). With a barrel chest, the ratio between the anteroposterior (AP) diameter of the chest and its lateral diameter is 2:2 rather than the normal ratio of 1:2. This shape change results from lung overinflation and diaphragm flattening.

The patient with chronic bronchitis often has a cyanotic, or blue-tinged, dusky appearance and has excessive sputum production. Assess the patient for cyanosis, delayed capillary refill, and clubbing of the fingers (Fig. 32-10), which indicate chronically decreased arterial oxygen levels.

Cardiac changes occur as a result of the anatomic changes associated with COPD. Assess the patient's heart rate and rhythm. Check for swelling of the feet and ankles (dependent edema) or other manifestations of right-sided heart failure. Examine nail beds and oral mucous membranes. The patient with later-stage emphysema may have pallor or frank cyanosis.

Psychosocial Assessment

COPD affects all aspects of a person's life. Socialization may be reduced when friends and family avoid the patient with COPD because of annoying coughs, excessive sputum, or dyspnea. The patient may choose to be isolated because dyspnea causes fatigue or because of embarrassment from coughing and excessive sputum production. In addition, because of the association with cigarette smoking and disease development, the patient may feel a social stigma.

Ask the patient about interests and hobbies to assess whether socialization has decreased or whether hobbies cause exposure to inhalation irritants. Ask about home conditions for exposure to smoke or crowded living conditions that promote transmission of respiratory infections.

Economic status may be affected by the disease through changes in income and health insurance coverage. If the patient is the head of the household, severe COPD may require role changes that have a negative impact on self-image. Drugs, especially the metered dose inhalers (MDIs) and dry powder inhalers (DPI), are expensive, and many patients with limited incomes may use them only during exacerbations and not as prescribed on a scheduled basis.

Anxiety and fear related to dyspnea and feelings of breathlessness may reduce the patient's ability to participate in a full life. Work, family, social, and sexual roles can be affected. Encourage the patient and family to express their feelings about the limitations on lifestyle and disease progression. Assess their awareness and use of support groups and services.

Laboratory Assessment

Arterial blood gas (ABG) values identify abnormal oxygenation, ventilation, and acid-base status. Compare serial or repeated ABG values to assess changes in the patient's respiratory status. Once baseline ABG values are obtained, pulse oximetry can gauge the response to treatment. As COPD worsens, the amount of oxygen in the blood decreases **(hypoxemia)** and the amount of carbon dioxide in the blood increases **(hypercarbia).** Chronic respiratory acidosis (increased arterial carbon dioxide [$Paco_2$]) then results; metabolic alkalosis (increased arterial bicarbonate) occurs as

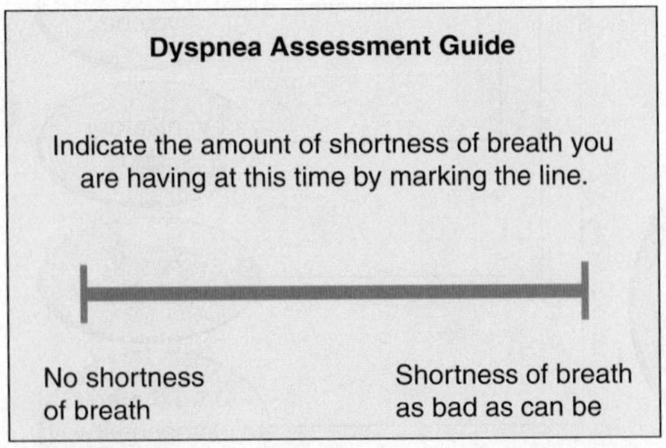
Dyspnea Assessment Guide
Indicate the amount of shortness of breath you are having at this time by marking the line.
No shortness of breath
Shortness of breath as bad as can be

Fig. 32-9 • A dyspnea assessment tool.

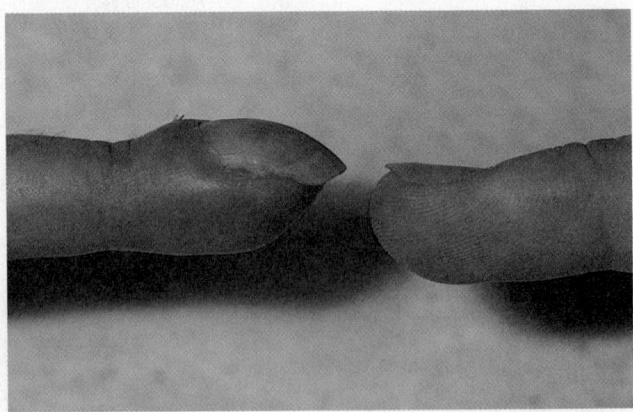

Fig. 32-10 • Late digital clubbing *(left)* compared with a normal digit *(right)*.

compensation by the kidney retention of bicarbonate. This change is seen on ABGs as an elevation of HCO_3^-. Not all patients with COPD are carbon dioxide retainers, even when hypoxemia is present. Carbon dioxide diffuses more easily across lung membranes than does oxygen. Hypercarbia is a problem in advanced emphysema (because the alveoli are affected) rather than in bronchitis (wherein the airways are affected). For more detailed information about acidosis, see Chapter 14.

Sputum samples are obtained for culture from hospitalized patients with an acute respiratory infection. In the community, sputum cultures are rarely obtained. The infection is treated on the basis of manifestations and the common bacterial organisms. A white blood cell count helps confirm the presence of infection.

Other blood tests include hemoglobin and hematocrit to determine polycythemia (a compensatory increase in red blood cells in the chronically hypoxic patient). Serum electrolyte levels are examined because hypophosphatemia, hyperkalemia, hypocalcemia, and hypomagnesemia reduce muscle strength. In patients with a family history of COPD, serum AAT levels may be drawn.

Imaging Assessment

Chest x-rays are obtained to rule out other chest diseases and to check the progress of patients with respiratory infections or chronic disease. With advanced emphysema, chest x-rays show hyperinflation and a flattened diaphragm. They may not be helpful in the diagnosis of early or moderate disease.

Other Diagnostic Assessment

COPD is classified from mild to severe on the basis of manifestations and pulmonary function test (PFT) changes (Table 32-2; see also Table 29-6 in Chapter 29). Airflow rates and lung volume measurements help distinguish airway disease (obstructive disease) from interstitial lung disease (restrictive diseases). PFTs determine lung volumes, flow volume curves, and diffusion capacity. Each test is performed before and after the patient inhales a bronchodilator agent. The person being tested for COPD usually has some manifestations and may be anxious about the potential diagnosis. Encourage the patient to express his or her feelings about testing and the potential impact of the results. Explain the preparations for the procedures (if any), whether pain or discomfort will be involved, and any needed follow-up care.

The lung volumes measured for COPD are vital capacity (VC), residual volume (RV), and total lung capacity (TLC) (see Table 29-6 in Chapter 29). RV is most profoundly affected, although all volumes and capacities change to some degree in COPD. The RV increase reflects the trapped, stale air remaining in the lungs.

Flow volume curves measure the patient's ability to move air into and out from the lungs. The rate of airflow out of the lungs during a rapid, forceful, and complete exhalation from TLC to RV (forced expiratory volume [FEV]) indirectly measures the flow resistance of the lung. A diagnosis of COPD is based mostly on the FEV_1 (the FEV in the first second of exhalation). FEV_1 can also be expressed as a percentage of the forced vital capacity (FVC). As the disease progresses, the ratio of FEV_1 to FVC becomes smaller.

The diffusion test measures how well a test gas (carbon monoxide) diffuses across the alveolar-capillary membrane and combines with the hemoglobin of red blood cells. In emphysema, alveolar wall destruction causes a large decrease in surface area for diffusion of gas into the blood, leading to a decreased diffusion capacity. In bronchitis, even though lung volumes are increased, the diffusion capacity is usually normal.

The patient with COPD has decreased oxygen saturation, often much lower than 90%. Changes in pulse oximetry results below the patient's usual saturation require medical attention.

Peak expiratory flowmeters are used to monitor the effectiveness of the prescribed drugs to relieve obstruction. Peak flow rates increase as obstruction resolves. Teach the patient to self-monitor the peak expiratory flow rates at home and adjust drugs as needed.

TABLE 32-2 Classification of COPD Severity

Stage	Manifestations	Pulmonary Function Test Results
0 (At risk)	±Chronic cough ±Chronic sputum production +Exposure to environmental risk factors	Normal
I (Mild)	+Chronic cough ±Sputum production	FEV_1/FVC <70% FEV_1 <80% of predicted
II (Moderate)	±Dyspnea ±Chronic cough ±Sputum production	FEV_1/FVC <70% FEV_1 <80% but at least <50% of predicted
III (Severe)	+Dyspnea +Chronic cough +Sputum production	FEV_1/FVC <70% FEV_1 <50% but at least <30% of predicted
IV (Very severe)	++Dyspnea ++Chronic cough ++Sputum production	FEV_1/FVC <70% FEV_1 <30% of predicted OR FEV_1 <50% of predicted with respiratory failure

Data from Global Initiative for Chronic Obstructive Lung Disease (GOLD). (2007). *Global strategy of the diagnosis, management, and prevention of chronic obstructive pulmonary disease.* MCR Vision, Inc. Website: www.gold.copd.org.

NCLEX EXAMINATION CHALLENGE

The client has all of the following ABG results. Which one alerts the nurse to the fact that the client has a long-term respiratory problem with CO_2 retention?

A. pH = 7.12
B. HCO_3^- = 31 mEq/L
C. $Paco_2$ = 68 mm Hg
D. Pao_2 = 78 mm Hg

evolve For the correct answer, go to http://evolve.elsevier.com/Iggy/.

Analysis

Common Nursing Diagnoses and Collaborative Problems

These are priority nursing diagnoses for patients with chronic obstructive pulmonary disease (COPD):

1. Impaired Gas Exchange related to alveolar-capillary membrane changes, reduced airway size, ventilatory muscle fatigue, and excessive mucus production
2. Ineffective Breathing Pattern related to airway obstruction, diaphragm flattening, fatigue, and decreased energy
3. Ineffective Airway Clearance related to excessive secretions, fatigue, decreased energy, and ineffective cough
4. Imbalanced Nutrition: Less Than Body Requirements related to dyspnea, excessive secretions, anorexia, and fatigue
5. Anxiety related to dyspnea, a change in health status, and situational crisis
6. Activity Intolerance related to fatigue, dyspnea, and an imbalance between oxygen supply and demand

A primary collaborative problem for patients with COPD is Potential for Pneumonia or Other Respiratory Infections.

Additional Nursing Diagnoses and Collaborative Problems

In addition to the common nursing diagnoses and collaborative problems, patients with COPD may have one or more of these:

- Fatigue related to a change in metabolic energy or hypoxemia
- Deficient Knowledge (disease process, prescribed treatments, activity limitations) related to unfamiliarity with information resources
- Sexual Dysfunction related to extreme fatigue
- Impaired Spontaneous Ventilation related to ventilatory muscle fatigue
- Sleep Deprivation related to dyspnea or an unfamiliar environment (hospitalization)
- Disturbed Thought Processes related to hypoxemia or sleep deprivation
- Ineffective Coping related to high degree of threat, inadequate level of perception of control, changes in lifestyle, situational crisis, or knowledge deficit

Other collaborative problems for patients with COPD include Potential for Respiratory Failure and Potential for Right-Sided Heart Failure.

DECISION-MAKING CHALLENGE
Delegation/Supervision

The patient is a 72-year-old African-American man who is a resident of the nursing home because of severe dyspnea related to long-standing COPD. He is on continuous oxygen by nasal cannula at 2 L/min. The UAP assigned to him reports that he has gained 7 lbs since the last time he was weighed (1 week ago) and that he seemed "grouchy." Results of his last set of vital signs (taken 12 hours ago) are close to his usual results.

1. Who should take his next vital signs—the UAP, the LPN/LVN, or the RN? Provide a rationale for your choice.
2. What should you ask the UAP about this patient?

evolve For suggested answer guidelines, go to http://evolve.elsevier.com/Iggy/.

Planning and Implementation

Impaired Gas Exchange

NOC **Planning: Expected Outcomes.** The patient with COPD is expected to attain and maintain gas exchange at a level within his or her chronic baseline values. Indicators include:

- Maintenance of Spo_2 of at least 88%
- Absence of cyanosis
- Maintenance of cognitive orientation

Interventions. Most patients with COPD use nonsurgical management to improve or maintain gas exchange. Surgical management requires that the patient meet strict criteria.

Nonsurgical Management. The mainstays of nursing management for patients with COPD include airway maintenance, monitoring, drug therapy, cough enhancement, oxygen therapy, and pulmonary rehabilitation. Nursing priorities are teaching the patient to be a partner in COPD management by participating in therapies to improve ventilation and by adhering to prescribed drug therapy.

Airway maintenance is the most important intervention to improve gas exchange. Keep the patient's head, neck, and chest in alignment. Assist him or her to liquefy secretions and clear the airway of secretions.

Monitoring for changes in respiratory status is key to providing prompt interventions to reduce complications. Assess the hospitalized patient with COPD at least every 2 hours, even when the purpose of hospitalization is not COPD management. Provide the prescribed oxygen, assess the patient's response to treatment, and prevent complications.

If the patient's condition continues to worsen despite treatment, more aggressive therapy is needed. Intubation and mechanical ventilation may be needed for patients in respiratory failure, including those who are unable to sustain spontaneous breathing patterns.

Cough enhancement can improve gas exchange by helping increase airflow in the larger airways. Chart 32-9 lists NIC intervention activities to promote cough enhancement.

Oxygen therapy is prescribed for relief of hypoxemia (decreased blood oxygen levels) and hypoxia (decreased tissue oxygenation). The need for oxygen therapy and its effectiveness can be determined by arterial blood gas values and oxygen saturation by pulse oxymetry. The patient with COPD may need an oxygen flow of 2 to 4 L/min via nasal cannula or up to 40% via Venturi mask. *The patient who is hypoxemic and also has chronic hypercarbia requires lower levels of oxygen delivery, usually 1 to 2 L/min via nasal cannula. A low arterial oxygen level is this patient's primary drive for breathing. Do not increase the oxygen flow rate in patients with hypercarbia because this may lower their respiratory rate or even make them stop breathing spontaneously.* Ensure that there are no open flames or other combustion hazards in rooms in which oxygen is in use. More information on oxygen therapy is found in Chapter 30.

Chart 32-9 NIC INTERVENTION ACTIVITIES

The Patient with Chronic Obstructive Pulmonary Disease

Cough Enhancement: *Promotion of deep inhalation by the patient with subsequent generation of high intrathoracic pressures and compression of underlying lung parenchyma for the forceful expulsion of air.*

- Monitor results of pulmonary function tests, particularly vital capacity, maximal inspiratory force, forced expiratory volume in 1 second (FEV_1), and FEV_1/FVC, as appropriate.
- Assist patient to a sitting position with head slightly flexed, shoulders relaxed, and knees flexed.
- Encourage patient to take several deep breaths.
- Encourage patient to take a deep breath, hold it for 2 seconds, and cough two or three times in succession.
- Instruct the patient to inhale deeply several times, to exhale slowly, and to cough at the end of exhalation.
- Instruct patient to follow coughing with several maximal inhalation breaths.

Oxygen Therapy: *Administration of oxygen and monitoring of its effectiveness.*

- Clear oral, nasal, and tracheal secretions, as appropriate.
- Restrict smoking.
- Maintain airway patency.
- Set up oxygen equipment and administer through a heated, humidified system.
- Monitor the oxygen liter flow.
- Monitor position of oxygen delivery device.
- Periodically check oxygen delivery device to ensure that the prescribed concentration is being delivered.
- Monitor the effectiveness of oxygen therapy (e.g., pulse oximetry, ABGs), as appropriate.
- Assure replacement of oxygen mask/cannula whenever the device is removed.
- Monitor patient's ability to tolerate removal of oxygen while eating.
- Observe for signs of oxygen-induced hypoventilation.
- Monitor for signs of oxygen toxicity and absorption atelectasis.
- Monitor oxygen equipment to ensure that it is not interfering with the patient's attempts to breathe.
- Monitor patient's anxiety related to need for oxygen therapy.
- Monitor for skin breakdown from friction of oxygen device.
- Provide for oxygen when patient is transported.
- Instruct patient and family about use of oxygen at home.
- Arrange for use of oxygen devices that facilitate mobility and teach patient accordingly.

NIC intervention activities selected from Bulechek, G.M., Butcher, H.K., & McCloskey Dochterman, J. (Eds.). (2008). *Nursing interventions classification (NIC)* (5th ed.). St. Louis: Mosby. No part of this work is to be altered without prior written permission from the Publisher.
ABG, Arterial blood gas.

Drug therapy for COPD involves the same inhaled and systemic drugs as for asthma. These drugs include beta-adrenergic agents, cholinergic antagonists, methylxanthines, corticosteroids, and NSAIDS (see Chart 32-5). The focus is on long-term control therapy with longer duration drugs, such as arformoterol (Brovana) and tiotropium (Spiriva). The patient with COPD is more likely to be taking systemic agents (in addition to inhaled drugs) than is the patient with asthma. An additional drug class for COPD is the mucolytics, which thin secretions, making them easier to expectorate.

Mucolytic agents are prescribed for the patient with thick, tenacious (sticky) mucous secretions. Nebulizer treatments with normal saline or with a mucolytic agent such as acetylcysteine (Mucosil, Mucomyst♣) or dornase alfa (Pulmozyme) and normal saline help thin secretions and facilitate expectoration. Guaifenesin (Organidin, Naldecon Senior EX) is a systemic mucolytic that is taken orally.

Stepped therapy, which adds drugs as COPD progresses, is recommended for patients with chronic bronchitis or emphysema, although the patient's responses to drug therapy is the best indicator of when drugs or their dosages need changing. The expected outcomes are for the patient to have more awareness of the disease and to participate in symptom management. Newly diagnosed patients and their family members have concerns about being able to use inhalers correctly (Carlson et al., 2006). Teach patients and family members the correct techniques for using inhalers and to care for them properly.

Pulmonary rehabilitation can be used to improve function and endurance in patients with COPD. Patients often respond to the dyspnea of COPD by limiting their activity, even basic ADLs. Over time, the muscles of ventilation and other large muscle groups weaken and are less efficient in the use of oxygen. The result is increased dyspnea with lower activity levels.

Pulmonary rehabilitation involves education and exercise training to prevent general and pulmonary muscle deconditioning. Formal programs are usually at least 6 weeks long; however, many patients can benefit from ongoing exercise. Each patient's exercise program is personalized to reflect his or her current limitations and outcome goals. All exercises should be performed at least 2 or 3 times each week (Bauldoff & Diaz, 2006). The simplest plan involves having the patient walk (indoors or outdoors) daily at a self-paced rate until symptoms limit further walking, followed by a rest period, and then continue walking until 20 minutes of actual walking has been accomplished. As the time during rest periods decreases, the patient can add 5 more minutes of walking time. The benefits of this type of exercise have been shown even for people with severe COPD (GOLD, 2007). Teach patients whose symptoms are severe to modify the exercise by using a walker with wheels or, if needed, to use oxygen therapy during the exercise period.

Exercise conditioning of the large muscle groups or retraining of the ventilatory muscles also may be part of a pulmonary rehabilitation program. Two techniques are isocapneic hyperventilation and resistive breathing. Isocapneic hyperventilation, in which the patient hyperventilates into a machine that controls the levels of oxygen and carbon dioxide, increases endurance. In resistive breathing, the patient breathes against a set resistance. Resistive breathing increases ventilatory muscle strength and endurance.

Surgical Management. Lung transplantation is performed for select patients with end-stage COPD. (See the lung transplantation section under Surgical Management [Cystic Fibrosis], pp. 636-637). The more common surgical procedure for patients with COPD is lung reduction surgery.

Lung transplantation and lung reduction surgery can improve gas exchange in the patient with COPD. Transplantation is a relatively rare procedure because of cost and the scarce availability of donor lungs. For this reasons, the few transplants performed for COPD are usually single lung (GOLD, 2007).

The goal of lung reduction surgery is improvement of gas exchange through removal of hyperinflated lung tissue. These areas of the lungs are filled with stagnant air that is not renewed with some atmospheric air (containing oxygen) during each respiratory cycle. Instead, this stagnant air continues to receive carbon dioxide until the level of carbon dioxide in the hyperinflated alveolus is the same as that in the capillary. Hyperinflated lung areas are useless for gas exchange. After successful lung reduction, most patients have at least a 75% improvement in FEV_1, decreased TLC and RV, and increased activity tolerance. Oxygen therapy may no longer be needed.

Preoperative care. Patients are selected for this procedure on the basis of having end-stage emphysema, minimal chronic bronchitis, and stable cardiac function; being ambulatory and not dependent on a ventilator; not having pulmonary fibrosis, asthma, or late-stage cancer; and having been a nonsmoker for at least 6 months. The patient must complete pulmonary rehabilitation before surgery to maximize lung and muscle function. The patient must reach a state in which he or she is able to walk, without stopping, for 30 minutes at 1 mile/hr and maintain a 90% or better oxygen saturation level.

In addition to standard preoperative testing, the patient having lung reduction surgery has tests to determine the location of greatest lung hyperinflation and poorest lung blood flow. These tests include pulmonary plethysmography, gas dilution, and perfusion scans.

Operative procedures. Usually, lung reduction is performed on both lungs through either a large midline incision or a transverse anterior thoracotomy. Each lung is deflated separately and examined for color and texture differences. Normal lung tissue darkens to purple or gray when deflated and becomes more dense or rubbery in texture. Hyperinflated areas do not deflate, and they remain pink with a spongy texture. After areas to remove have been identified, the surgeon removes as much of this tissue as possible, sealing off and reinforcing the remaining normal lung tissue.

Postoperative care. After lung reduction surgery, the patient needs close monitoring for continuing respiratory problems as well as for usual postoperative complications. In addition to the usual care required after thoracotomy (see Surgical Management [Lung Cancer], pp. 645-649), bronchodilator and mucolytic therapies are maintained. Pulmonary hygiene includes incentive spirometry 10 times per hour while awake, chest physiotherapy starting on the first day after surgery, and hourly pulmonary assessment.

Pain is usually managed by epidural delivery of opioids during the early period after surgery. This type of analgesic delivery reduces pain, limits sedation and cognitive dysfunction, and allows the patient to more fully participate in pulmonary hygiene measures.

DECISION-MAKING CHALLENGE

Critical Rescue

The 72-year-old nursing home resident described earlier is disoriented on an oxygen flow rate of 4 L/min. His vital signs are: P = 112, thready and irregular, R = 12 through pursed lips, BP = 140/110. His fingers are clubbed, he has a "barrel" chest, he has pitting edema of his lower extremities, and his neck veins are flat in the upright position.

1. Which of these assessment findings is important? Why?
2. What additional assessment data should you obtain?
3. Should you increase his oxygen flow rate? Why or why not?

evolve For suggested answer guidelines, go to http://evolve.elsevier.com/Iggy/.

Ineffective Breathing Pattern

NOC **Planning: Expected Outcomes.** The patient with COPD is expected to achieve an effective breathing pattern that decreases the work of breathing. Indicators include:

- Respiratory rhythm within normal limits for the patient's age
- Presence of synchronous thoracoabdominal movement
- Use of accessory muscles appropriate to the patient's activity level
- Increased activity tolerance

Interventions. Before any intervention, assess the patient to determine the breathing pattern, especially the rate, rhythm, depth, and use of accessory muscles. The patient with COPD relies more on accessory muscles than on the diaphragm for breathing. These muscles, however, are less efficient than the diaphragm, and the work of breathing increases. Determine whether there are any contributing factors to the increased work of breathing, such as respiratory infection. Interventions aim to improve the patient's breathing efforts and decrease the work of breathing through the use of specific breathing techniques, positioning, exercise conditioning, and energy conservation.

Breathing techniques, such as diaphragmatic or abdominal and pursed-lip breathing, may be helpful for managing dyspneic episodes (Warren & Livesay, 2006). The patient uses these techniques, shown in Chart 32-10, during all activities. The amount of stale air in the lungs is reduced, and he or she gains confidence and control in managing dyspnea. Teach these techniques when the patient is free of dyspnea.

In diaphragmatic breathing, the patient consciously increases movement of the diaphragm. Lying on the back allows the abdomen to relax. Breathing through pursed lips uses the mild resistance of partially closed lips to prolong exhalation and to increase airway pressure. This technique delays airway compression and reduces air trapping. Pursed-lip breathing can be used during diaphragmatic or abdominal breathing.

Positioning the patient in an upright position with the head of the bed elevated can help alleviate dyspnea by increasing chest expansion, relaxing the chest muscles, and placing the diaphragm in the proper position to contract. This position also conserves energy by supporting the patient's arms and upper body.

Chart 32-10 PATIENT AND FAMILY EDUCATION GUIDE

Breathing Exercises

DIAPHRAGMATIC OR ABDOMINAL BREATHING

- Lie on your back with your knees bent.
- Place your hands or a book on your abdomen to create resistance.
- Begin breathing from your abdomen while keeping your chest still. You can tell if you are breathing correctly if your hands or the book rises and falls accordingly.

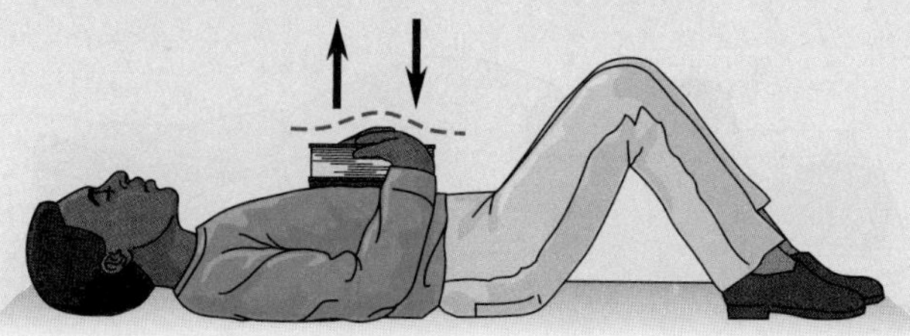

PURSED-LIP BREATHING

- Close your mouth, and breathe in through your nose.
- Purse your lips as you would to whistle. Breathe out slowly through your mouth, without puffing your cheeks. Spend at least twice the amount of time it took you to breathe in.
- Use your abdominal muscles to squeeze out every bit of air you can.
- Remember to use pursed-lip breathing during any physical activity. Always inhale before beginning the activity and exhale while performing the activity. Never hold your breath.

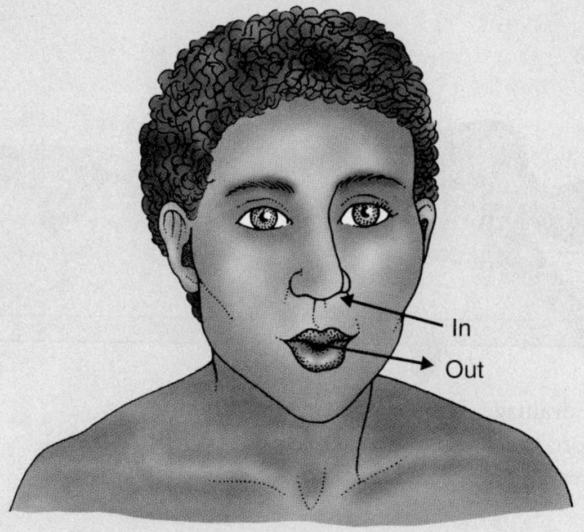
In
Out

Energy conservation is the planning and pacing of activities for maximum tolerance and minimum discomfort. Once the FEV_1 falls below 50% predicted, the patient's ability to perform ADLs is limited. Ask the patient to describe a typical daily schedule. Each activity is divided into its smaller parts to determine whether that task can be performed in a different way or at a different time of the day. Assist him or her to plan and pace daily activities. Rest periods are paced between activities. Help the patient develop a personal chart outlining the day's activities and planned rest periods.

Encourage the patient to avoid working with the arms raised. Activities involving the arms decrease exercise tolerance because the accessory muscles of ventilation are then used to stabilize the arms and shoulders. Many activities involving the arms can be done sitting at a table leaning on the elbows. Teach the patient to adjust work heights to reduce back strain and fatigue. Remind him or her to keep arm motions smooth and flowing to prevent jerky motions that waste energy. Teach about the use of adaptive tools for housework, such as long-handled dustpans, sponges, and dusters, to reduce bending and reaching.

Suggest how the patient can organize work spaces so that items used most often are within easy reach. Measures such as dividing laundry or groceries into small parcels that can be handled easily, using disposable plates to save washing time, and letting dishes dry in the rack also conserve energy. Talking requires energy and use of the lungs; therefore teach the patient not to talk when engaged in other activities that require energy, such as walking. In addition, teach him or her to avoid breath-holding while performing any activity.

Ineffective Airway Clearance

NOC **Planning: Expected Outcomes.** The patient with COPD is expected to maintain a patent airway. Indicators include:

- Coughs effectively
- No occurrence of aspiration
- Maintenance of Spo_2 of at least 88%

Interventions. The patient with COPD often has difficulty with removal of secretions, which results in compromised breathing and poor *oxygenation and tissue perfusion.* Excessive mucus also increases the risk for respiratory infections. Assess breath sounds routinely as part of physical assessment and before and after interventions. Careful use of drugs combined with controlled coughing, hydration, and postural drainage may help in airway clearance. If these measures fail, a tracheostomy may be needed on a temporary or permanent basis.

Controlled coughing at specific times of the day is helpful because the patient with COPD has excessive mucus. Teach him or her to cough on arising in the morning to eliminate mucus that collected during the night. Coughing to clear mucus before mealtimes may facilitate a more pleasant meal. Coughing before bedtime may ensure clear lungs for a less interrupted night's sleep.

To cough effectively, teach the patient to sit in a chair or on the side of a bed with feet placed firmly on the floor. Instruct him or her to turn the shoulders inward and to bend the head slightly downward, hugging a pillow against the stomach. The patient then takes a few deep breaths. After the third to fifth deep breath (in through the nose, out through pursed lips), instruct him or her to bend forward slowly while coughing two or three times from the same breath. Observe the color, consistency, odor, and amount of secretions. On return to a sitting position, the patient takes a comfortable deep breath. The entire coughing procedure is repeated at least twice. After coughing exercises, allow him or her to rest and provide mouth care.

Chest physiotherapy (PT) with postural drainage (Fig. 32-11) helps some patients move secretions into central airways, re-expand lung tissue, and have more efficient use of the ventilatory muscles. It combines chest percussion with vibration to loosen secretions. Postural drainage uses specific positions and gravity to help remove secretions. Because it does not have a proven benefit for all patients with COPD, postural drainage with chest PT is not used routinely in this population.

Suctioning is performed only when abnormal breath sounds are present—not on a routine schedule. For the patient with a

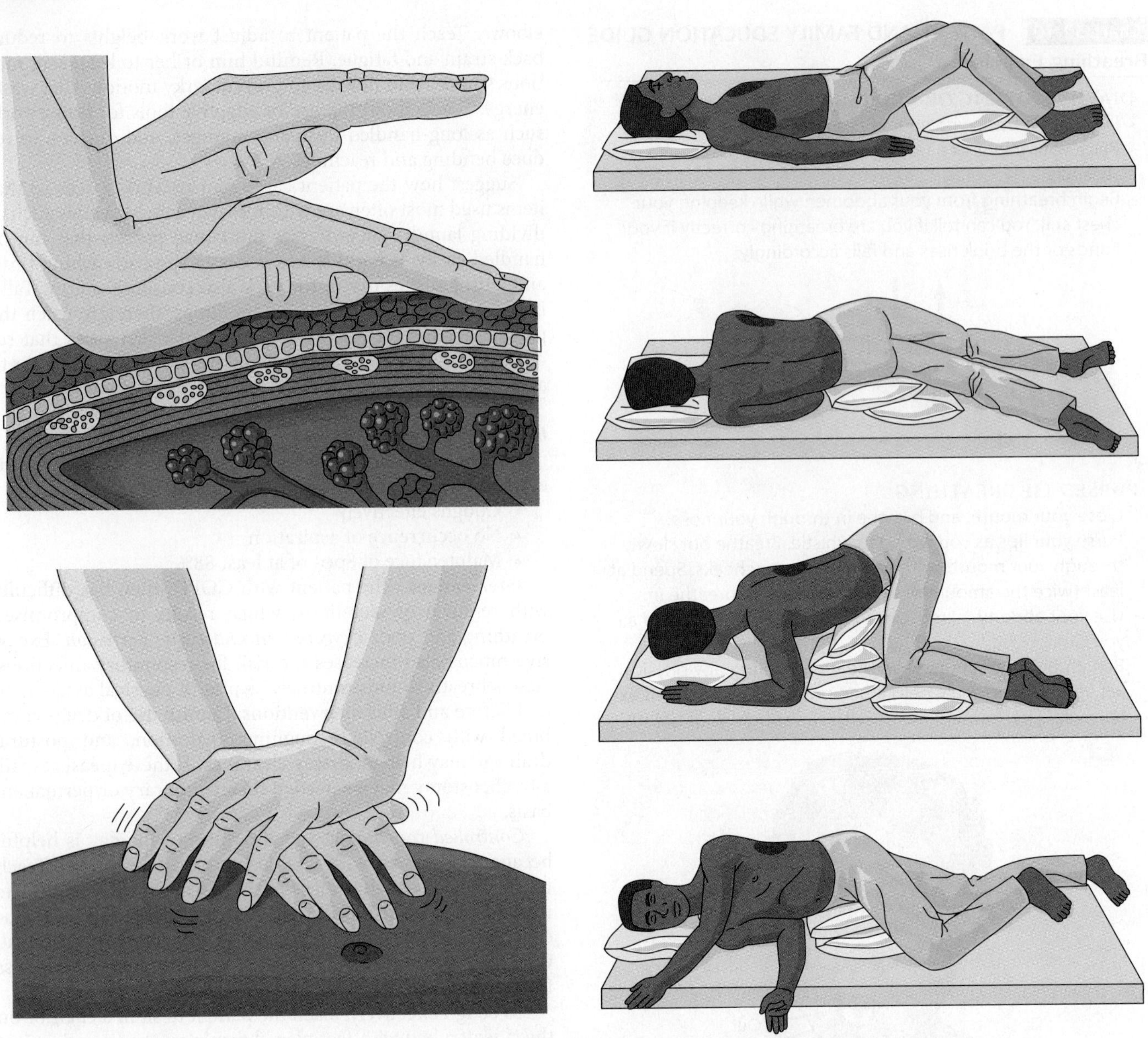

Fig. 32-11 • Chest physiotherapy (chest PT) and postural drainage. *Left,* Percussion and vibration techniques. The nurse may use one or two hands with vibration, which is performed when the patient exhales or coughs. *Right,* Positions for postural drainage of respiratory secretions.

weak cough, weak pulmonary muscles, and inability to expectorate effectively, the nurse or respiratory therapist performs nasotracheal suctioning. Assess the patient for dyspnea, tachycardia, and dysrhythmias during the procedure. Assess for improved breath sounds after suctioning. Suctioning is discussed in detail in Chapter 31.

Positioning may improve airway clearance. Assist the patient who can tolerate sitting in a chair out of bed for 1-hour periods two to three times a day. This position helps move secretions and keeps the diaphragm in a better position for ventilation.

Hydration helps airway clearance by thinning secretions, making them easier to remove by coughing. Unless hydration needs to be avoided for other health problems, teach the patient with COPD to drink at least 2 to 3 L/day. Humidifiers may be useful for those living in a dry climate or those who use dry heat during the winter. Instruct the patient to clean the humidifier daily to prevent the growth of mold spores.

Flutter valve mucus clearance devices can be helpful to assist patients to remove airway secretions (Warren & Livesay, 2006). The device is a small, handheld plastic pipe with a short, fat stem and a perforated lid over the bowl (Fig. 32-12). Inside the bowl is a free-moving steel ball. The patient inhales deeply and exhales forcefully through the device, causing the ball to move and set up vibrations that are transmitted to the patient's chest and airways. The vibrations loosen secretions and allow them to be coughed out more easily.

Imbalanced Nutrition: Less Than Body Requirements

NOC **Planning: Expected Outcomes.** The patient with COPD is expected to achieve and maintain a body weight within 10% of ideal. Indicators include:

- Maintains an appropriate weight/height ratio
- Maintains serum albumin or prealbumin within the normal range

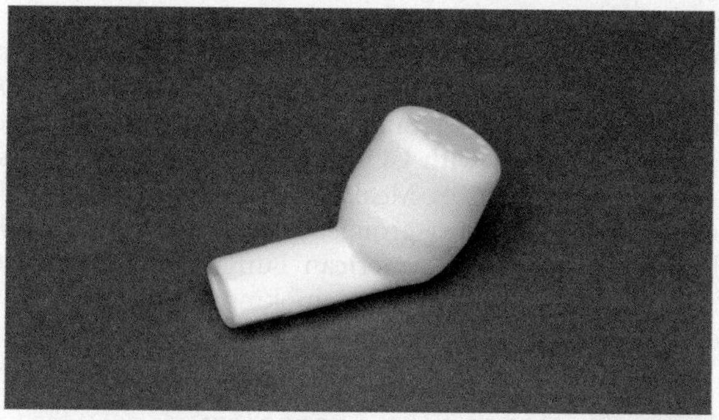

Fig. 32-12 • The FLUTTER flutter-valve mucus clearance device.

Interventions. The patient with COPD often has food intolerance, nausea, early satiety, loss of appetite, and meal-related dyspnea. The increased work of breathing raises calorie and protein needs. These conditions lead to protein-calorie malnutrition for many patients. Malnourished patients lose total body mass, ventilatory muscle mass and strength, lung elasticity, and alveolar-capillary surface area. All of these problems reduce effective breathing.

Identify patients at risk for or who have this complication and request nutritional consultation. Monitor his or her weight and other indicators of nutrition, such as skin condition and serum prealbumin levels.

Dyspnea management is needed because shortness of breath (dyspnea) is the most common problem related to eating. Dyspnea during mealtimes can be reduced by resting before meals. Teach the patient to plan the biggest meal of the day for the time when he or she is most hungry and well rested. Four to six small meals a day may be preferred to three larger ones. Teach the patient to use pursed-lip and abdominal breathing to alleviate dyspnea. Suggest that using a bronchodilator 30 minutes before the meal may be helpful to reduce dyspnea due to bronchospasm.

Food selection can help prevent weight loss and improve appetite. Abdominal bloating and a feeling of fullness often prevent the patient from eating a complete meal. Teach about foods that are easy to chew and not gas-forming. Dry foods stimulate coughing, and foods such as milk and chocolate may increase the thickness of saliva and secretions. Advise the patient to avoid these foods when symptomatic. Inform him or her that caffeinated beverages should be avoided because they increase urine output and may lead to dehydration.

Urge the patient to eat high-calorie, high-protein foods. Dietary supplements, such as Pulmocare, provide nutrition with reduced carbon dioxide production. If early satiety (feeling too "full" to eat) is a problem, advise him or her to avoid drinking fluids before and during the meal.

Anxiety

NOC **Planning: Expected Outcomes.** The patient with COPD is expected to have decreased anxiety. Indicators include that the patient consistently demonstrates these behaviors:

- Identifying factors that contribute to anxiety
- Identifying activities to decrease anxiety
- Verbalizing anxiety is reduced or absent

Interventions. Patients with COPD often have increased anxiety during acute dyspneic episodes, especially if they feel as though they are choking on excessive secretions. Also, anxiety has been shown to cause dyspnea.

Psychological interventions are useful when symptoms are worsened because of anxiety. Help the patient understand this effect and have a plan for dealing with anxiety. Together with the patient, develop a written plan that states exactly what he or she should do if symptoms flare. Having a plan provides confidence and control in knowing what to do, which often helps reduce anxiety. Stress the use of pursed-lip and diaphragmatic breathing techniques during periods of anxiety or panic.

Family, friends, and support groups can be helpful. Recommend professional counseling, if needed, as a positive suggestion, and in no way suggest that this need represents a failure of the patient to cope. Stress that talking with a counselor can help identify techniques to maintain control over the dyspnea and feelings of panic.

Explore other approaches to help the patient control dyspneic episodes and panic attacks. Examples include progressive relaxation, hypnosis therapy, and biofeedback. Biofeedback helps the patient determine the impact of various stimuli on symptoms. Ultimately he or she learns to relax and control these stimuli to avoid the aggravating symptoms. At times, anti-anxiety drug therapy may be needed for severe anxiety.

Activity Intolerance

NOC **Planning: Expected Outcomes.** The patient with COPD is expected to increase activity to a level acceptable to him or her. Indicators include:

- Maintenance of baseline SaO_2 with activity
- Performance of ADLs with no or minimal assistance
- Performance of selected activities with minimal dyspnea or tachycardia
- Participation in family, work, or social activities as desired

Interventions. The patient with COPD often has chronic fatigue. While in the acute phases of the illness, he or she may need extensive help with the ADLs of eating, bathing, and grooming. As the acute problem resolves, encourage the patient to pace activities and provide as much self-care as possible. Teach him or her not to rush through morning activities, because rushing increases dyspnea, fatigue, and hypoxemia. As activity gradually increases, assess the patient's response by noting skin color changes, pulse rate and regularity, blood pressure, and work of breathing. Suggest the use of supplemental oxygen during periods of high energy use, such as bathing or walking.

Potential for Pneumonia or Other Respiratory Infections

NOC **Planning: Expected Outcomes.** The patient with COPD is expected to remain free from serious respiratory infection. Indicators include that the patient consistently demonstrates these behaviors:

- Verbalizes clinical manifestations of respiratory infection
- Describes respiratory infection–monitoring procedures
- Uses prevention activities such as pneumonia and influenza vaccination and crowd avoidance
- Seeks medical assistance when manifestations of respiratory infection first appear

Interventions. Pneumonia is one of the most common complications of COPD. Patients who have excessive secretions or who have artificial airways are at increased risk for respiratory tract infections. The risk is greatly increased for older adults. Teach patients to avoid large crowds, and stress the importance of receiving a pneumonia vaccination and a yearly influenza vaccine ("flu shot") (Bruce & McEvoy, 2007).

Community-Based Care

Home Care Management

Most patients with chronic obstructive pulmonary disease (COPD) are treated in the ambulatory care setting and cared for at home. When pneumonia or a severe exacerbation of the disease develops, the patient usually returns home after treatment. For those with advanced disease, however, 24-hour care may be needed for ADLs and for monitoring for acute episodes or progression of the illness. Patients may not be able to enjoy work or recreational activities because of severe dyspnea and fatigue. If home care is not possible, placement in a long-term care setting may be needed.

Hypoxemic patients can benefit from long-term use of oxygen at home. Home oxygen may be needed only during periods of exercise or sleep if hypoxemia occurs only during these times. Continuous, long-term oxygen therapy can reverse tissue hypoxia and decrease pulmonary vascular resistance. It can also improve cognitive ability and well-being. For more information on home oxygen therapy, see Chapter 30.

Most patients can benefit from a structured pulmonary rehabilitation program. The overall goal of these collaborative programs is to increase a person's ability to compensate for and live with COPD. The patient with COPD is referred to a pulmonary rehabilitation program before illness becomes severe. Those with the least severe functional loss benefit the most.

Collaborate with the case manager to obtain the equipment needed for care at home. Patient needs may include oxygen therapy, a hospital-type bed, a nebulizer, a tub transfer bench, and visits from a home care nurse to continue monitoring the health status, review the drug regimen, and evaluate home care needs.

The patient with COPD faces a lifelong disease with remissions and exacerbations. Explain to the patient and family that he or she may have periods of anxiety, depression, and ineffective coping. The person who was a smoker may also have self-directed anger.

Financial concerns often increase anxiety and interfere with disease management. The condition may worsen to the point that the patient cannot work. Disability benefits through Social Security or private disability insurance plans can help ease the financial burden. Medicare or other health insurers may assist with payment for home oxygen therapy and nebulizer treatments. Coordinate with the social worker or case manager to help the patient make the needed arrangements.

Health Teaching

Patients with COPD need to know as much about the disease as possible so that they can better manage it and themselves. Patients and families should be able to discuss drug therapy, manifestations of infection, avoidance of respiratory irritants, the nutrition therapy regimen, and activity progression. Instruct them to identify and avoid stressors that can worsen the disease.

Teach the patient techniques of pursed-lip breathing, diaphragmatic breathing, positioning, relaxation therapy, energy conservation, and coughing and deep breathing. Two factors that interfere with teaching hospitalized patients are the shortened length of stay and the presence of dyspnea. It may be unrealistic to cover all of the topics in the education checklist during a single hospitalization. The primary nurse or case manager should coordinate teaching with the home care or clinic staff.

Health Care Resources

Provide appropriate referrals as needed. Home care visits may be warranted, particularly if the patient must use home oxygen therapy for the first time. Chart 32-11 lists assessment areas for the patient with COPD at home. Referral to assistance programs, such as Meals on Wheels, can be helpful. Provide a list of support groups, as well as Better Breather clubs sponsored by the American Lung Association. If the patient is having difficulty with smoking cessation and indicates the desire for assistance, make the referrals.

Chart 32-11 HOME CARE ASSESSMENT

The Patient with Chronic Obstructive Pulmonary Disease

ASSESS RESPIRATORY STATUS AND ADEQUACY OF VENTILATION

- Measure rate, depth, and rhythm of respirations.
- Examine mucous membranes and nail beds for evidence of hypoxia.
- Determine use of accessory muscles.
- Examine chest and abdomen for paradoxical breathing.
- Count number of words patient can speak between breaths.
- Determine need and use of supplemental oxygen. (How many liters per minute is the patient using?)
- Determine level of consciousness and presence/absence of confusion.
- Auscultate lungs for abnormal breath sounds.
- Measure oxygen saturation by pulse oximetry.
- Determine sputum production, color, and amount.
- Ask about activity level.
- Observe general hygiene.
- Measure body temperature.

ASSESS CARDIAC STATUS

- Measure rate, quality, and rhythm of pulse.
- Check dependent areas for edema.
- Check neck veins for distention with the patient in a sitting position.
- Measure capillary refill.

ASSESS NUTRITIONAL STATUS

- Weight maintenance, loss, or gain
- Food and fluid intake
- Use of nutritional supplements
- General condition of the skin
- Assess patient's and caregiver's adherence and understanding of illness and treatment, including:
  - Correct use of supplemental oxygen
  - Correct use of inhalers
  - Drug schedule and side effects
  - Manifestations to report to the health care provider indicating the need for acute care
  - Increasing severity of resting dyspnea
  - Increasing severity of usual symptoms
  - Development of new symptoms associated with poor oxygenation
  - Respiratory infection
  - Failure to obtain the usual degree of relief with prescribed therapies
  - Unusual change in condition
  - Use of pursed-lip and diaphragmatic breathing techniques
  - Scheduling of rest periods and priority activities
  - Participation in rehabilitation activities

DECISION-MAKING CHALLENGE
Coordination of Care

The patient is a 67-year-old retired teacher with COPD who lives in a first-floor condo with her husband, who is also a retired teacher. The home care nurse is making a follow-up visit 1 week after the patient returned home after a 4-day hospital stay for exacerbation of symptoms. On arriving at the home, the home care nurse finds the patient upset and crying. When asked what has upset her, she replies that her husband "won't let me do anything around the house because I am so short of breath. I might as well be dead."

1. How should the nurse respond to this statement?
2. What psychosocial assessment of this patient and her situation should be made?
3. Should the visiting nurse include the husband in any part of this discussion? Why or why not?
4. What adjustments in household tasks could this patient make to conserve her energy?

evolve For suggested answer guidelines, go to http://evolve.elsevier.com/Iggy/.

Evaluation: Outcomes

Evaluate the care of the patient with COPD on the basis of the identified nursing diagnoses and collaborative problems. The expected outcomes are that the patient should:

- Attain and maintain gas exchange at a level within his or her chronic baseline values
- Achieve an effective breathing pattern that decreases the work of breathing
- Maintain a patent airway
- Achieve and maintain a body weight within 10% of his or her ideal weight
- Have decreased anxiety
- Increase activity to a level acceptable to him or her
- Avoid serious respiratory infections

Specific indicators for these outcomes are listed for each nursing diagnosis and collaborative problem under the Planning and Implementation section.

CYSTIC FIBROSIS

Pathophysiology

Cystic fibrosis (CF) is a genetic disease that affects many organs and lethally impairs pulmonary function. Although this disorder is present from birth and usually is first seen in early childhood, almost half of all people with cystic fibrosis in the United States are adults (Cystic Fibrosis Foundation, 2007).

The underlying problem of CF is blocked chloride transport in the cell membranes. The error in chloride transport causes the formation of mucus that has little water content and is thick. The thick, sticky mucus causes problems in the lungs, pancreas, liver, salivary glands, and testes. The mucus plugs up glands in these organs, causing atrophy and organ dysfunction. Nonpulmonary problems include pancreatic insufficiency with malnutrition and intestinal obstruction, poor growth, male sterility, and cirrhosis of the liver. These primary problems cause many additional health problems in young adulthood, especially osteoporosis and diabetes mellitus (Cystic Fibrosis Foundation, 2007). The primary cause of death in the patient with CF is respiratory failure.

The pulmonary problems of CF result from the constant presence of thick, sticky mucus and are the most serious complications of the disease. The mucus narrows airways, reducing airflow and interfering with *oxygenation and tissue perfusion*. The constant presence of mucus results in chronic respiratory tract infections, chronic bronchitis, and chronic dilation of the bronchioles (bronchiectasis). Lung abscesses are common. Over time, the bronchioles distend and have increased numbers (hyperplasia) of mucus-producing cells and increased mucus-producing cell size (hypertrophy). Complications include pneumothorax, arterial erosion and hemorrhage, and respiratory failure.

The disorder is most common among white people, and about 4% are carriers. CF is very rare among African Americans and Asians. Males and females are affected equally.

GENETIC CONSIDERATIONS

CF is an autosomal recessive disorder in which both gene alleles must be mutated for the disease to be expressed. The CF gene is located on chromosome 7 and produces a protein that controls chloride movement across cell membranes (Nussbaum et al., 2007). The severity of CF varies greatly; however, life expectancy is always considerably reduced, with an average of 32 years. People with one mutated allele are carriers and have few or no symptoms of CF but can pass the abnormal allele on to their children. Currently, more than 1200 different mutations have been identified. The inheritance of different mutations is thought to be responsible for the wide variation in disease severity.

With improvement in specific testing, people with health problems who were not known to have CF previously may be identified so that therapies can be tailored for better outcomes. In acute care settings, patients with what appear to be acute pulmonary problems who do not respond as expected to proven therapy may, in actuality, have some undiagnosed form of CF that unfavorably influences the clinical course of a superimposed pulmonary problem (Workman & Winkelman, 2008). In this type of case, the nurse should obtain a good history of the patient's previous respiratory problems and his or her response to therapy. The possibility of CF should always be kept in mind when a patient does not respond as expected to standard therapies.

Patient-Centered Collaborative Care

Assessment

Usually, cystic fibrosis (CF) is diagnosed in childhood. The major diagnostic test is sweat chloride analysis (Gardner, 2007). Additional genetic testing can be performed to determine which specific mutation a person may have. This distinction can be important because different mutations result in different degrees of disease severity. The defect in chloride movement prevents absorption of sodium chloride in the sweat glands; thus more chloride than normal is present in the sweat. The sweat chloride test is positive for CF when the chloride level in the sweat ranges between 60 and 200 mEq/L (mmol/L), compared with the normal value of 5 to 35 mEq/L.

Nonpulmonary manifestations include abdominal distention, gastroesophageal reflux, rectal prolapse, foul-smelling stools, and **steatorrhea** (excessive fat in stools). The patient may be malnourished and have many vitamin deficiencies, especially of the fat-soluble vitamins like vitamins A, D, E, and K. As pancreatic function decreases, he or she has symptoms of diabetes mellitus from loss of insulin production. In addition, the adult with CF is usually smaller and thinner than average.

Pulmonary manifestations caused by CF are progressive. The respiratory infections are frequent or chronic with periods of exacerbations. Patients usually have chest congestion, limited exercise tolerance, cough, sputum production, use of accessory muscles, and decreased pulmonary function (especially FVC and FEV_1) (Grossman & Grossman, 2005). Chest x-rays show persistent infiltrate and an increased anteroposterior (AP) diameter.

During an acute exacerbation or when the disease progresses to end stage, the patient has increased chest congestion, reduced activity tolerance, increased crackles, increased cough, increased sputum production (often with hemoptysis), and severe dyspnea. Fatigue increases in proportion with the dyspnea. Arterial blood gas (ABG) studies show acidosis with greatly reduced partial pressure of arterial oxygen (Pao_2), increased partial pressure of arterial carbon dioxide ($Paco_2$), increased bicarbonate levels, and low pH.

When infection is present, the patient has fever, an elevated white blood cell count, and decreased oxygen saturation. Other manifestations of infection include tachypnea, tachycardia, intercostal retractions, weight loss, and increased fatigue.

Interventions

The patient with CF needs daily therapy to slow disease progress and enhance gas exchange. There is no cure for CF.

Nonsurgical Management

The management of the patient with CF is complex and lifelong. Nutritional management focuses on weight maintenance, vitamin supplementation, diabetes management, and pancreatic enzyme replacement. Pulmonary management is focused on preventive maintenance and management of pulmonary exacerbation. Priority nursing interventions focus on teaching about drug therapy, infection prevention, pulmonary hygiene, nutrition, and vitamin supplementation.

Preventive/maintenance therapy involves the use of a regimen of chest physiotherapy, positive expiratory pressure, active cycle breathing technique, and an individualized regular exercise program. Pulmonary function tests (PFTs), especially FEV_1, are monitored regularly. Maintenance drugs include bronchodilators, anti-inflammatory agents, mucolytics, and antibiotics.

Exacerbation therapy is needed when the patient with CF has a change in manifestations from baseline. Such changes include increased chest congestion, decreased activity tolerance, increased or new-onset crackles, and at least a 10% decrease in FEV_1. Other manifestations occurring with exacerbation include increased sputum production with bloody or purulent sputum, increased frequency and duration of coughing, decreased appetite, weight loss, fatigue, decreased Sao_2, and ventilatory muscle retractions. Often infection is present and the patient also has fever, increased lung infiltrate on chest x-ray, and an elevated white blood cell count.

Every attempt is made to avoid having the patient with CF mechanically ventilated. Treatment focuses on airway clearance, increased oxygenation, and antibiotic therapy. Supplemental oxygen is prescribed on the basis of Sao_2 levels. Heliox delivery of 50% oxygen and 50% helium may improve gas exchange and oxygen saturation. The respiratory therapist initiates airway clearance techniques (ACTs) four times a day. Bronchodilator and mucolytic therapies are intensified (higher doses given more frequently than for maintenance). Steroidal anti-inflammatory agents are started or increased.

Depending on the severity of the exacerbation, a 10- to 14-day course of oral antibiotics may be prescribed. If the exacerbation is more severe, aerosolized tobramycin is prescribed. If oral/inhaled antibiotics are not effective or if the exacerbation is very severe, IV antibiotics are used, usually an aminoglycoside, such as tobramycin and colistin or meropenem (Merrem) (Elpern et al., 2007).

A serious bacterial infection for patients with CF is *Burkholderia cepacia*. The organism lives well in the respiratory systems of patients with CF and becomes resistant to antibiotic therapy relatively quickly. It is spread by casual contact from one CF patient to another. For this reason, the Cystic Fibrosis Foundation bans infected patients from participating in any foundation-sponsored events. It is also possible for *B. cepacia* to be transmitted to a CF patient during clinic and hospital visits; thus special infection control measures that limit close contact between persons with CF are needed. These measures include separating CF patients on hospital units and seeing them in the clinic on different days. Strict CF Foundation–approved procedures should be used when cleaning clinic rooms, pulmonary function laboratories, and respiratory therapy equipment to reduce the risk of contamination.

Teach patients about protecting themselves by avoiding direct contact of bodily fluids such as saliva and sputum. Teach them not to routinely shake hands or kiss people in social settings. Handwashing is critical because the organism also can be acquired indirectly from contaminated surfaces, such as sinks and tissues.

As specialized treatment for CF improves and life span increases, other problems may occur. Patients may have bronchiole bleeding from lung arteries. Interventional radiology may be needed to embolize the bleeding arterial branches. Patients with CF may undergo this procedure repeatedly to control hemoptysis. See Chapter 38 for information on interventional radiology vascular procedures.

Surgical Management

The surgical management of the patient with CF involves lung and/or pancreatic transplantation. The patient has reduced manifestations but is at continuing risk for lethal pulmonary infections, especially with anti-rejection drug therapy. Transplantation extends life by 10 to 20 years, depending on other factors.

Fewer lung transplants are performed compared with transplantation of other solid organs. The problem is related to the scarcity of available lungs. In addition, many of the people who could benefit from lung transplantation have serious problems in other organs that make extended surgical procedures dangerous.

Lung transplant procedures include two lobes or a single lung transplantation, as well as double-lung transplantation. The type of procedure is determined by the patient's age and overall condition, the cause of the lung problem, and the life expectancy after transplantation. Usually, the patient with CF has a bilateral lobe transplant from either a cadaver donor or living-related donor.

Preoperative Care. Many factors are considered before lung transplantation surgery. Recipient and donor criteria vary from one program to another, but some criteria are universal.

Recipient criteria for the person who will receive the transplant include that the recipient must have severe, irreversible lung damage. It is important, however, that the patient be well enough to survive the surgery. Usually only those younger than 55 years receive transplants, although transplantation is considered on an individual basis. Exclusion criteria are:

- Severe psychiatric disorders or self-destructive tendency
- Proven history of not adhering or poorly adhering to medical regimens
- Current cancer or cancer within the past 5 years
- Systemic infection
- Irreversible heart, kidney, or liver damage/disease
- Presence of any problem that would be made worse by immunosuppression

Donor criteria, regardless of whether the lung tissue is obtained from a cadaver or from a living-related donor, include:

- Infection free
- Cancer free
- Healthy lung tissue
- Close tissue match with the recipient
- Same blood type as the recipient

When the donor is living-related, additional criteria are:

- Age is younger than 55 years.
- Donor has normal cardiac function.
- Pulmonary function will remain adequate after tissue removal.
- The donor has had no previous chest surgery.
- Donor is psychologically stable.
- Donor has not been coerced into this situation.

The two nursing priorities before surgery are teaching the patient the expected regimen of pulmonary hygiene to be used in the period immediately after surgery and assisting the patient in a pulmonary muscle strengthening/conditioning regimen.

Operative Procedures. The patient may or may not need to be placed on cardiopulmonary bypass, depending on the exact procedure. Those having single-lung or lobe transplantation usually do not need bypass; those having double-lung transplantation usually do.

The most common incision used for lung transplantation is a transverse thoracotomy ("clamshell") for best access. The diseased lung or lungs are removed. The new lobes, lung, or lungs are placed in the chest cavity with **anastomoses** (connections) made to the proper airways (trachea, mainstem bronchus, or secondary bronchus) and blood vessels. Usually, lung transplantation surgery is completed within 4 to 6 hours.

Postoperative Care. The patient is intubated for at least 48 hours. In addition, chest tubes and arterial lines are in place. Much of the care needed is the same as that for any thoracic surgery (see pp. 645-649).

Major problem areas after lung transplantation are bleeding, infection, and transplant rejection. Bleeding is most common in patients who had cardiopulmonary bypass with anticoagulation. Usually the patient remains in the ICU for several days after transplantation.

Anti-rejection drug regimens must be started immediately after surgery, which increases the risk for infection. The drugs generally used for routine long-term rejection suppression after organ transplantation are combinations of very specific immunosuppressants (cyclosporine [Sandimmune]), less specific immunosuppressants (azathioprine [Imuran] or mycophenolate mofetil [CellCept]), and one of the corticosteroids, such as prednisone (Apo-Prednisone♣, Deltasone♣) or prednisolone (Delta-Cortef). Corticosteroids are avoided in the first 10 to 14 days after surgery because of their negative impact on the healing process. (See Chapter 19 for more information on anti-rejection therapy.)

PRIMARY PULMONARY HYPERTENSION

Pathophysiology

Pulmonary hypertension can occur as a complication of other lung disorders. Primary pulmonary hypertension (PPH) occurs in the absence of other lung disorders, and its cause is unknown although exposure to some drugs increases the risk. This disorder is rare and occurs mostly in women between the ages of 20 and 40 years (Widlitz et al., 2007).

GENETIC CONSIDERATIONS

About 50% of patients with the disorder have a genetic mutation in the *BMPR2* gene, which codes for a growth factor receptor (McCance & Huether, 2006). Excessive activation of this receptor allows increased growth of arterial smooth muscle in the lungs, making these arteries thicker. Many more people have mutations in this gene than have PPH. It is thought that these mutations increase the susceptibility to PPH when other, often unknown, environmental factors also are present. Often PPH is not diagnosed until late in the disease process when the lungs and heart have already been significantly damaged. Teach people, especially women, who have a first-degree relative (parent or sibling) with PPH to have regular health checks and to consult a health care provider whenever pulmonary problems are present (Ross, 2007).

The pathologic problem in PPH is blood vessel constriction with increasing vascular resistance in the lung. Pulmonary blood pressure rises and blood flow decreases, leading to poor perfusion and hypoxemia. Eventually, the right side of the heart fails (cor pulmonale) from the continuous workload of pumping against the high pulmonary pressures. Without treatment, death usually occurs within 2 years after diagnosis.

Patient-Centered Collaborative Care

Assessment

The most common early manifestations are dyspnea and fatigue in an otherwise healthy adult. Some patients also have angina-like chest pain. Table 32-3 lists the classification of PPH.

Diagnosis is made from the results of right-sided heart catheterization showing elevated pulmonary pressures. Other test results suggesting pulmonary hypertension include abnormal ventilation-perfusion scans and pulmonary function tests (PFTs) showing reduced functional pulmonary volumes with reduced diffusion capacity, and spiral computed tomography (CT).

Interventions

Nonsurgical interventions that reduce pulmonary pressures and slow the development of cor pulmonale involve drugs that dilate pulmonary vessels and prevent clot formation. Warfarin (Coumadin) therapy is taken daily to achieve an international normalized ratio (INR) of 1.5 to 2.0. Calcium channel blockers, such as nifedipine (Procardia) and diltiazem (Cardizem), have been used to dilate blood vessels. Endothelin-receptor

TABLE 32-3 Severity Classification for Primary Pulmonary Hypertension

Class	Manifestations
I	Pulmonary hypertension diagnosed by pulmonary function tests and right-sided cardiac catheterization No limitation of physical activity Moderate physical activity does not induce dyspnea, fatigue, chest pain, or lightheadedness
II	No manifestations at rest Mild to moderate physical activity induces dyspnea, fatigue, chest pain, or lightheadedness
III	No or slight manifestations at rest Mild (less than ordinary) activity induces dyspnea, fatigue, chest pain, or lightheadedness
IV	Dyspnea and fatigue present at rest Unable to carry out any level of physical activity without manifestations Manifestations of right-sided heart failure apparent (dependent edema, engorged neck veins, enlarged liver)

Data from Eells, P. (2004). Advances in prostacyclin therapy for pulmonary arterial hypertension. *Critical Care Nurse, 24*(2), 42-54.

antagonists, such as bosentan (Tracleer), induce blood vessel relaxation and decrease pulmonary arterial pressure. These agents, however, cause general vessel dilation and some degree of hypotension. Natural and synthetic prostacyclin agents provide the best specific dilation of pulmonary blood vessels. Continuous infusion of epoprostenol (Flolan) or treprostinil (Remodulin) through a small IV pump reduces pulmonary pressures and increases lung blood flow. An alternate therapy that is also effective is the delivery of treprostinil (Remodulin) by subcutaneous infusion through a microinfusion pump.

A critical nursing priority for a patient undergoing this therapy is that, although it is very effective, deaths have been reported if the drug delivery is interrupted even for a matter of minutes. Teach the patient to always have backup drug cassettes and battery packs. If these are not available or if the line is disrupted, the patient should go to the emergency department immediately. The second nursing priority is working with the patient to prevent sepsis. The continuous central line IV setup provides an access for organisms to directly enter the bloodstream. Teach the patient and at least one family member to use strict aseptic technique in all aspects of manipulating the drug delivery system. Also teach him or her to notify the pulmonologist at the first sign of any respiratory or systemic infection.

When the heart has undergone some hypertrophy and cardiac output has fallen, the patient may be started on a regimen of digoxin (Lanoxin) and diuretics. Oxygen therapy is used when dyspnea is continuous or uncomfortable. These therapies do not cure the disorder; they just improve function and reduce symptoms.

Surgical management of primary pulmonary hypertension involves single-lung or whole-lung transplantation. When cor pulmonale also is present, the patient may need a combined heart-lung transplantation. It is not known whether the process of pulmonary vasoconstriction can begin again in the transplanted lungs or if the transplant is a "cure."

NCLEX EXAMINATION CHALLENGE

The client is a 21-year-old nursing student with PPH who is admitted for an emergency appendectomy and is now in the PACU. She has a peripheral venous line in her left arm and a central venous catheter connected to a continuous infusion pump with Flolan. Her postoperative orders indicate that she is to receive 2 g of cephalothin (Keflin) by IVPB immediately. When the drug arrives, her peripheral line is infiltrated. What is the nurse's best action?

A. Infuse the Keflin into the central line along with the Flolan.
B. Disconnect the Flolan for 15 minutes and infuse the Keflin.
C. Restart a peripheral IV and use it to administer the Keflin.
D. Ask whether the Keflin can be given orally since the client is awake.

evolve For the correct answer, go to http://evolve.elsevier.com/Iggy/.

INTERSTITIAL PULMONARY DISEASES

The category of interstitial pulmonary diseases contains a variety of lung disorders, also called *fibrotic lung* diseases, that have some features in common. All affect the alveoli, blood vessels, and surrounding support tissue of the lungs rather than the airways. Thus these disorders are **restrictive** (preventing good expansion and recoil of the gas exchange unit) rather than obstructive. With restrictive disease, the lung tissues thicken, causing reduced gas exchange and "stiff" lungs that do not expand well (Pruitt, 2008). Unlike obstructive problems, air trapping does not occur and the patient does not develop a "barrel chest." Often the onset of these disorders is slow and dyspnea is the most common manifestation.

SARCOIDOSIS

Pathophysiology

Sarcoidosis is a granulomatous disorder of unknown cause that can affect any organ, but the lung is involved most often. It develops over time with growths called **granulomas** forming in the lungs. Granulomas contain lymphocytes, macrophages, epithelioid cells, and giant cells.

Pulmonary sarcoidosis involves autoimmune responses in which the normally protective T-lymphocytes increase and cause damaging actions in lung tissue. Alveolar cells are the targets of the damaging actions. No single cause for T-lymphocyte activation has been identified, although infection and genetic predisposition appear to play a role. Alveolar inflammation **(alveolitis)** occurs from the presence of immune cells in the alveoli. Chronic inflammation causes **fibrosis** (scar tissue formation in the lungs). The fibrosis reduces **lung compliance** (elasticity) and the ability to exchange gases. **Cor pulmonale** (right-sided cardiac failure) is often present, because the heart can no longer pump effectively against the stiff, fibrotic lung.

The disease usually affects young adults. Manifestations include enlarged lymph nodes in the hilar area of the lungs, lung infiltrate on chest x-ray, skin lesions, and eye lesions. The first indication of disease may be an abnormal chest x-ray in an otherwise healthy patient. The most common symptoms include cough, dyspnea, hemoptysis, and chest discomfort. In many patients, the illness resolves permanently. Others may have progressive pulmonary fibrosis and severe systemic disease.

Patient-Centered Collaborative Care

Sarcoidosis is suspected in the patient who has a cough, dyspnea, and abnormal chest x-ray but is otherwise asymptomatic. Other conditions to rule out before diagnosing sarcoidosis are lung infections and cancer. Fiberoptic bronchoscopy may also be used in the diagnosis of this disorder (see Chapter 29).

Sarcoidosis is staged on the basis of x-ray findings. Higher stages have greater damage and more widespread disease. Pulmonary function studies often show a restrictive pattern of decreased lung volumes and impaired diffusing capacity. Irreversible lung changes develop in 10% to 15% of patients. Patients who develop severe restrictive disease may also develop secondary pulmonary hypertension.

The goal of therapy is to lessen symptoms and prevent fibrosis. Management varies. If the patient is asymptomatic and has normal pulmonary function, no treatment is given. Decreased total lung capacity (TLC), diffusing capacity, or forced vital capacity (FVC); involvement of other organs; and hypercalcemia are indicators for treatment.

Corticosteroids are the main type of therapy. Dosages vary from 40 to 60 mg daily with tapering doses over 6 to 8 weeks, to a maintenance dose of 10 to 15 mg daily for 6 months. Further therapy may continue over 12 months. Follow-up and monitoring include assessment of symptom severity, pulmonary function studies, chest x-rays, a complete blood count, serum creatinine, serum calcium, and urinalysis. Teach the patient about side effects of steroid therapy and other aspects of physical care as indicated.

IDIOPATHIC PULMONARY FIBROSIS

Pathophysiology

Idiopathic pulmonary fibrosis is a common restrictive lung disease. The typical patient is an older adult with a history of cigarette smoking or chronic exposure to inhalation irritants such as metal particles, dust, organic chemicals, and wood fires. Unlike sarcoidosis, pulmonary fibrosis is highly lethal. Most patients have progressive disease with few remission periods. Even with proper treatment, patients usually survive less than 5 years after diagnosis.

Pulmonary fibrosis is an example of excessive wound healing. Once lung injury occurs, an inflammatory process begins tissue repair. The inflammation continues beyond normal healing time, causing extensive fibrosis and scarring. These changes thicken alveolar tissues, making gas exchange difficult.

Patient-Centered Collaborative Care

The onset of disease is slow, with early symptoms of mild dyspnea on exertion. Pulmonary function tests show decreased FVC. As the fibrosis progresses, the patient becomes more dyspneic and hypoxemia becomes severe. Eventually, the patient needs high levels of oxygen and often is still hypoxemic. Respirations are rapid and shallow.

The goal of therapy is to slow the fibrotic process and manage dyspnea. Corticosteroids and other immunosuppressants are the mainstays of therapy. Immunosuppressant drugs include cytotoxic drugs such as cyclophosphamide (Cytoxan, Neosar, Procytox🍁), azathioprine (Imuran), chlorambucil (Leukeran), or methotrexate (Folex). These drugs have many side effects, including immunosuppression, nausea, and lung and liver damage and have shown limited benefit. New studies using the combination therapy of corticosteroids, azathioprine, interferon gamma 1b, and *N*-acetylcysteine show promise of slowing disease progression (Burns, 2006). Starting drug therapy early is critical, even though not all patients respond to therapy. Even among those who have a response to therapy, the disease eventually continues to progress and leads to death by respiratory failure.

Lung transplantation is a curative therapy; however, the selection criteria, cost, and availability of organs make this option unlikely for most patients.

The patient and family need support and help with community resources after diagnosis. Nursing care focuses on assisting the patient and family in understanding the disease process and maintaining hope for control of the fibrosis. It is important to prevent respiratory infections. Teach the patient and family about the manifestations of infection, and encourage them to avoid respiratory irritants, crowds, and other people with known infections.

Home oxygen is needed by the time the patient becomes symptomatic because significant fibrosis has already occurred. Teach him or her about oxygen use as a continuous therapy. Fatigue is a major problem. Teach the patient and family about energy conservation measures (see discussion of energy conservation, p. 631 in the Chronic Obstructive Pulmonary Disease section). Activity limitations and rest help reduce the work of breathing and oxygen consumption.

Support the patient's need to be as independent as possible, and encourage him or her to pace activities and accept assistance as needed. The disease is costly because the patient is often unable to work and may need home care.

In the later stages of the disease, the focus is to reduce the sensation of dyspnea. This is often accomplished with the use of oral, parenteral, or nebulized morphine. Provide information about hospice, which supports and coordinates resources to meet the needs of the patient and family when the prognosis for survival is less than 6 months.

OCCUPATIONAL PULMONARY DISEASE

Pathophysiology

Exposure to occupational or environmental fumes, dust, vapors, gases, bacterial or fungal antigens, and allergens can result in a variety of respiratory disorders. Depending on the degree, frequency, and intensity of exposure and on the specific disease, patients may have acute reversible effects or chronic lung disease. All occupational pulmonary diseases are made worse by cigarette smoking; thus smoking cessation efforts are very important.

Many occupational diseases have an onset of symptoms long after the initial exposure to the offending agent. The patient's personal history can provide clues about the presence and cause of occupational pulmonary diseases. Common occupational pulmonary diseases include occupational asthma, pneumoconiosis, diffuse interstitial fibrosis, and extrinsic allergic alveolitis. Chart 32-12 lists the key features of these disorders.

Chart 32-12 KEY FEATURES

Common Occupational Pulmonary Diseases

Disease and Category	Causes and Manifestations
OCCUPATIONAL ASTHMAS	
Latency (allergic) asthma	Airway narrowing related only to workplace exposures Atopic allergic response to industrial irritants Develops after a period of exposure (from several weeks to several years) Characterized by airflow limitation Usually resolves when exposure ceases Obstructive disease
Irritant-induced asthma	Manifestations appear only in the workplace First onset usually occurs within 24 hours of exposure Common irritants are chlorine, ammonia, and phosgene Characterized by sloughing of epithelium, thickening of the basement membranes, and mucosal inflammation Early manifestations include cough, wheeze, and dyspnea High exposures can lead to pulmonary edema, ARDS, and death Most tissue changes are permanent Obstructive and restrictive disease
PNEUMOCONIOSIS	
Silicosis	Chronic fibrosis from long-term inhalation of silica dust Found among people working in mines, stone quarries, and foundries. Also found in people working in these industries: glass-making, pottery, sandblasting, tile and brick making, soap and polishes, and manufacture of filters Characterized by nodule formation between alveoli leading to fibrosis Manifestations include dyspnea on exertion, fatigue, weight loss, reduced lung volume, and upper lobe fibrosis Restrictive disease
Coal Miner's disease (Black Lung disease)	Massive deposits of coal dust in the lungs leading to diffuse fibrosis Develops earlier among miners who smoke Early manifestations are similar to bronchitis Emphysema is a late development Restrictive disease
DIFFUSE INTERSTITIAL FIBROSIS	
Asbestosis	Occurs among people who work in asbestos mines, building construction/remodeling, and shipyards Characterized by diffuse pleural thickening and diaphragmatic calcification Restrictive disease
Talcosis	Occurs among people who work in industries that manufacture paint, ceramics, roofing materials, cosmetics, and rubber goods Restrictive disease
Berylliosis	Occurs among people who work in industries in which metal is heated (steel mills, welding) or metal is machined, creating dust Has a genetic component for increased susceptibility to disease after beryllium exposure Restrictive disease
EXTRINSIC ALLERGIC ALVEOLITIS	
"Farmer's Lung" "Bird Fancier's Lung" "Machine Operator's Lung"	Hypersensitivity pneumonitis as an immunologic response to inhaling dust or chemical that contains bacterial or fungal antigens Characterized by formation of granulomas with central necrosis in the alveoli and surrounding blood vessels Restrictive disease

ARDS, Acute respiratory distress syndrome.

Patient-Centered Collaborative Care

Consider an occupational cause for all patients with new-onset asthma or dyspnea. Obtain a thorough history of occupational exposure and onset of symptoms because there may or may not be a latency period between exposure and onset of symptoms. Determine whether the symptoms are acute or chronic. Ask the patient about the use of inhalation protection and about cigarette smoking. Use this opportunity to teach the patient about ways to quit smoking.

Prevention is important to avoiding disability from occupation-related disease. Teach about the importance of using special respirators and ensuring adequate ventilation when working in potentially harmful environments.

The patient with occupational asthma with a latency period should be removed from the site of exposure, transferred to a job without exposure, and treated with asthma drugs. Nursing care is similar to the care for asthma not caused by the workplace environment. Refer the patient to a social worker, who provides information regarding compensation and pensions.

Nursing interventions for patients with occupational lung restrictive disease are the same as for those with emphysema. Hypoxemic patients require supplemental oxygen. In addition, respiratory therapies to promote sputum clearance are essential.

BRONCHIOLITIS OBLITERANS ORGANIZING PNEUMONIA (BOOP)

Pathophysiology

Bronchiolitis obliterans organizing pneumonia (BOOP) is an inflammatory process that allows connective tissue plugs to form in the lower airways and in the tissue between the alveoli. The lumenal inflammation triggers white blood cell clumping with fibroblast (connective cell) growth that occludes and eventually obliterates these airways and leads to restricted lung volume with decreased vital capacity. Fibrosis is not part of the pathology of BOOP. It is not a true pneumonia, but the manifestations resemble respiratory infection.

No true cause of BOOP has been established although many personal and environmental conditions are associated with it. Suggested triggers include infectious organisms, drugs (chemotherapy agents, certain antibiotics [sulfa-based drugs, cephalosporins, amphotericin B], antiseizure drugs, cocaine, and amiodarone), or the presence of another connective tissue disorder such as rheumatoid arthritis or systemic lupus erythematosis. BOOP is also associated with chest radiation therapy for cancers in the breast or lung.

BOOP is most common in people between 30 and 60 years and affects all races and both genders equally. It is not associated with cigarette smoking or other tobacco use. It is more common among patients who have received solid organ transplants and may be part of an acute rejection episode. Depending on how fast the problem progresses and the degree to which it interferes with gas exchange, BOOP can lead to death.

Patient-Centered Collaborative Care

An event or condition triggers the inflammatory cascade within lower airway lumens, causing manifestations of dyspnea, fever, mild cough, flu-like symptoms, and crackles on auscultation. In some patients, the problem resolves spontaneously. In others, the problem can rapidly progress and be fatal within 3 days of the appearance of manifestations. Usually, manifestations are present for weeks or months and do not improve with standard antibiotic therapy (White & Ruth-Sahd, 2007).

Diagnosis of BOOP is difficult because the manifestations are nonspecific and are similar to many other respiratory problems. Chest x-rays do not differentiate BOOP from any other respiratory problem. Although computed tomography (CT) scans can show more widespread changes in pulmonary tissue, it can only suggest BOOP, not confirm it. Biopsy with histologic findings are needed to confirm a BOOP diagnosis.

The most effective treatment for BOOP is corticosteroid therapy. A short course of the drug for acute disease can reduce manifestations, and the patient may never have a relapse. For patients with more severe disease and those with any type of additional health problem, a year of corticosteroid therapy may be needed (White & Ruth-Sahd, 2007). In this population, BOOP is more of a chronic disease with some degree of permanent restrictive disease. Exacerbations can occur.

LUNG CANCER

Pathophysiology

Lung cancer is a leading cause of cancer-related deaths worldwide. In the United States, more deaths from lung cancer occur each year than from prostate cancer, breast cancer, and colon cancer combined. The American Cancer Society estimates that more than 186,000 new cases of lung cancer are diagnosed each year and that more than 165,000 deaths occur each year from it (American Cancer Society, 2008). The overall 5-year survival for all patients with lung cancer is only 14%. This poor long-term survival is due to the fact that most lung cancers are diagnosed at a late stage, when metastasis is present. Only 15% of patients have small tumors and localized disease at the time of diagnosis (American Cancer Society, 2008).

Despite many advances in cancer treatment, the overall prognosis for lung cancer remains poor unless the tumor can be removed completely by surgery. Treatment of lung cancer is often aimed toward relieving symptoms **(palliation)** rather than cure because of the presence of metastasis.

Most primary lung cancers arise from the bronchial epithelium. These cancers are collectively called *bronchogenic carcinomas.* Lung cancers can be classified according to their histologic cell type as small cell lung cancer (SCLC), epidermoid (squamous cell) cancer, adenocarcinoma, and large cell cancer. The last three types are now referred to as *non–small cell lung cancer (NSCLC)* because of their similar responses to treatment (Walker, 2008). Chapter 23 discusses the general mechanisms and processes of cancer development.

Metastasis (spread) of lung cancer occurs by direct extension, through the blood, and by invading lymph glands and vessels. Tumors in the bronchial tubes can grow and obstruct the bronchus partially or completely. Tumors in other areas of lung tissue can grow so large that they can obstruct the airway by compressing it. Tumors in the edges of the lungs spread and can compress the alveoli, nerves, blood vessels, and lymph vessels. All of these problems interfere with *oxygenation and tissue perfusion.*

The patterns of metastasis depend on the type of tumor cell and the location of the tumor. Lung lymph nodes, as well as more distant lymph nodes, can be invaded.

Hematogenous (bloodborne) metastasis of lung cancer is due to invasion of blood vessels in the lungs. **Emboli** (tumor pieces) spread to distant body areas. These sites include the bone, liver, brain, and adrenal glands.

Additional manifestations, known as *paraneoplastic syndromes,* complicate certain lung cancers. The paraneoplastic syndromes are caused by hormones secreted by tumor cells. Paraneoplastic syndrome commonly occurs with SCLC. Table 32-4 lists the endocrine paraneoplastic syndromes that may occur, most commonly with SCLC.

TABLE 32-4 Endocrine Paraneoplastic Syndromes Associated with Lung Cancer

Ectopic Hormone	Manifestation
Adrenocorticotropic hormone (ACTH)	Cushing's syndrome
Antidiuretic hormone	Syndrome of inappropriate antidiuretic hormone (SIADH) Weight gain General edema Dilution of serum electrolytes
Follicle-stimulating hormone (FSH)	Gynecomastia
Parathyroid hormone	Hypercalcemia
Ectopic insulin	Hypoglycemia

Staging of lung cancer is performed at diagnosis to assess the size and extent of the disease. These factors are correlated to survival rate. The staging of lung cancer is based on the TNM system (T, primary *t*umor; N, regional lymph *n*odes; M, distant *m*etastasis). See Table 23-7 in Chapter 23 for a typical cancer staging system. Higher numbers represent later stages and less chance for cure or long-term survival.

Incidence/Prevalence

Lung cancers occur as a result of repeated exposure to inhaled substances that cause chronic tissue irritation or inflammation. Cigarette smoking is the major risk factor and is responsible for 85% of all lung cancer deaths (American Cancer Society, 2008). The risk for lung cancer is directly related to the total exposure to cigarette smoke as determined by the number of years of smoking and number of packs of cigarettes smoked per day (pack-years). Pipe and cigar smoking also increase risk. The incidence of lung cancer decreases when smoking stops, and after 15 years of smoking cessation, it approaches that of those who have never smoked. About 50,000 ex-smokers, however, develop lung cancer in the United States each year.

Etiology and Genetic Risk

Nonsmokers exposed to "passive," or "secondhand," smoke also have a greater risk for lung cancer than do nonsmokers who are minimally exposed to cigarette smoke. Passive smoke has many of the carcinogens found in inhaled, or "mainstream," tobacco smoke.

Other risk factors for lung cancer include chronic exposure to asbestos, beryllium, chromium, coal distillates, cobalt, iron oxide, mustard gas, petroleum distillates, radiation, tar, nickel, and uranium. Air pollution that contains benzopyrenes and hydrocarbons also increases the risk for lung cancer.

GENETIC CONSIDERATIONS

Lung cancer development varies among people with similar smoking histories, suggesting that genetic factors can influence susceptibility. Differences in a gene product that activates carcinogens (a cancer susceptibility gene) and another gene product that clears carcinogens from the body (a cancer resistance gene) are associated with differences in personal susceptibility to lung cancer. More recent evidence supports the possibility that differences in a gene that regulates cell division, the *Tp53* gene, may be the most important genetic susceptibility link for lung cancer development. Mutations in the alleles of this gene are known to increase the susceptibility to a wide variety of cancers both with and without exposure to environmental risks, including lung cancer development among smokers and nonsmokers (Zhang et al., 2006).

Health Promotion and Maintenance

Primary prevention for lung cancer is directed at reducing tobacco smoking. Educational strategies start with elementary school children to discourage them from beginning to smoke. Nurses are actively involved in encouraging nonsmokers not to begin to smoke, in promoting smoking cessation programs, and in establishing a smoke-free environment. Encourage nonsmokers to avoid passive, or secondhand, smoke by avoiding environmental exposure.

Teach workers in industrial settings about safety precautions, such as wearing specialized masks and protective clothing, to reduce occupational hazards. Encourage people who are at high risk for lung cancer development to seek frequent health examinations. Urge patients being treated for lung cancer to quit smoking. The actual diagnosis of the disease and its treatment time represent "teachable moments."

Secondary prevention by early detection has not been considered feasible in the past with earlier detection not making a difference in long-term survival rates. New data from recent studies indicate that screening people at risk for lung cancer using annual spiral CT scans can detect cancers very early, at stage I, when cure is probable and long-term survival (longer than 5 years) is very likely (Henschke et al, 2006). See the Evidence-Based Practice box on p. 643.)

NCLEX EXAMINATION CHALLENGE

The client is a 56-year-old woman who has smoked 3 packs of cigarettes per day from the time she was 14 years old to when she was 42, and then smoked 2 packs of cigarettes per day from age 42 to the present. How should the nurse calculate this client's pack-year smoking history?

A. 146 pack-years
B. 112 pack-years
C. 86 pack-years
D. 42 pack-years

evolve For the correct answer, go to http://evolve.elsevier.com/Iggy/.

Patient-Centered Collaborative Care

Assessment

History

Ask the patient about risk factors, including smoking, hazards in the workplace, and warning signals (Table 32-5). Have the patient describe how many packs of cigarettes per day he or she has smoked and for how many years to determine the pack-year smoking history.

Ask about the presence of lung cancer manifestations, such as hoarseness, cough, sputum production, hemoptysis, shortness of breath, or change in endurance. Assessing for and documenting these manifestations provide information about the extent of nursing care and teaching the patient needs now

EVIDENCE-BASED PRACTICE

Early diagnosis does make a difference

Henschke, C.I., Yankelevitz, D.F., Libby, D.M., Pasmantier, M.W., Smith, J.P., Miettinen, O.S., et al. (2006). Survival of patients with stage I lung cancer detected on CT screening. *New England Journal of Medicine, 355*(17), 1763-1771.

Overall survival for lung cancer diagnosed at stages III and IV has been poor, triggering clinicians to find a way to screen for lung cancer with the concept of diagnosing it at an earlier stage when cure or control is more likely. Previous noninvasive screening methods, such as sputum cytology and bronchial washings, have not been shown to be effective in early diagnosis. This multicenter, prospective study of more than 27,000 people at risk for lung cancer examined the use of an annual spiral CT scan for identification of early-stage tumors over a 12-year period.

A total of 484 participants were diagnosed with lung cancer, 412 (85%) at stage I. Of these patients, 375 had surgery, 302 within the first month after diagnosis. Of these, 92% were still living 10 years after the initial diagnosis. Eight of the 412 diagnosed at stage I elected not to have any treatment, and all died within 5 years of the diagnosis. For the remaining 102 who either had surgery more than 1 month after diagnosis or elected to receive other therapies (radiation and/or chemotherapy), 88% were still living 10 years after the initial diagnosis. Both groups had better survival than the general expectation of 80% at 10 years for those who are diagnosed at stage I without screening. This group concluded that annual screening of people at risk for lung cancer is an effective method of increasing survival.

Level of Evidence—3. The study was a well-designed controlled study without randomization.

Commentary: Implications for Practice and Research. Although smoking cessation is the best prevention for most types of lung cancer, cigarette smoking is addictive and the habit is very difficult to stop. For those people who are at risk because of a smoking history or occupational exposure, annual spiral CT screening can be a life-saving method of secondary prevention. However, the procedure is expensive and few insurance companies support its use as a screening tool. Even when covered by insurance, participation in screening is low. Nurses should promote this screening method to people who are at risk for lung cancer. In addition, getting involved in processes, such as lobbying and petitioning insurance groups, to promote acceptance and coverage of this screening method also may lead to improved lung cancer survival rates.

TABLE 32-5 Warning Signals Associated with Lung Cancer

- Hoarseness
- Change in respiratory pattern
- Persistent cough or change in cough
- Blood-streaked sputum
- Rust-colored or purulent sputum
- Frank hemoptysis
- Chest pain or chest tightness
- Shoulder, arm, or chest wall pain
- Recurring episodes of pleural effusion, pneumonia, or bronchitis
- Dyspnea
- Fever associated with one or two other signs
- Wheezing
- Weight loss
- Clubbing of the fingers

and can be used later to determine therapy effectiveness. Many manifestations are common and may have been present for years. Ask the patient to describe any recent changes in symptoms or if position affects symptoms.

Assess for chest pain or discomfort, which can occur at any stage of tumor development. Chest pain may be localized or on just one side and can range from mild to severe. Ask about any sensation of fullness, tightness, or pressure in the chest, which may suggest obstruction. A piercing chest pain or pleuritic pain may occur on inspiration. Pain radiating to the arm results from tumor invasion of nerve plexuses in advanced disease.

Physical Assessment/Clinical Manifestations—Pulmonary

Manifestations of lung cancer are often nonspecific and appear late in the disease process. Specific manifestations depend on the type and location of the tumor. Chills, fever, and cough may be related to pneumonitis or bronchitis that occur with obstruction. Assess sputum quantity and quality. Blood-tinged sputum may occur with bleeding from a tumor. Hemoptysis is a later finding in the course of the disease. If infection or necrosis is present, sputum may be purulent and copious.

Breathing patterns may be labored or painful. An obstructive breathing pattern may occur as prolonged exhalation alternating with periods of shallow breathing. Rapid, shallow breathing occurs with pleuritic chest pain and an elevated diaphragm. Inspiratory efforts are reduced in advanced disease. Look for and document the presence of abnormal retractions, the use of accessory muscles, flared nares, stridor, and asymmetric diaphragmatic movement on inspiration. Dyspnea and wheezing may be present with airway obstruction. Ask about the patient's level of dyspnea at rest, with activity, and in the supine position (orthopnea). Determine how much the dyspnea interferes with his or her participation in ADLs, work, recreational activities, and family responsibilities. Ask the patient to compare his or her participation in activities during the past week with that of a month ago and a year ago.

Areas of tenderness or masses may be felt when palpating the chest wall. Increased vibrations felt on the chest wall **(fremitus)** indicate areas of the lung where air spaces are replaced with tumor or fluid. Fremitus is decreased or absent when the bronchus is obstructed. The trachea may be displaced from midline if a mass is present in the area.

Lung areas with masses sound dull or flat rather than hollow or resonant on chest percussion. Breath sounds may change with the presence of a tumor. Wheezes indicate partial obstruction of airflow in passages narrowed by tumors. Decreased or absent breath sounds indicate complete obstruction of an airway by a tumor or fluid. Increased loudness or sound intensity of the voice while listening to breath sounds indicates increased density of lung tissue from tumor compression. A pleural friction rub is heard when inflammation also is present.

AUDIO CLIP: Pleural Friction Rub

Physical Assessment/Clinical Manifestations—Nonpulmonary

Many other systems can be affected by lung cancer and have changes at the time of diagnosis. Heart sounds may be muffled by a tumor or fluid around the heart (cardiac tamponade). Dysrhythmias may occur as a result of hypoxemia or direct pressure of the tumor on the heart. Cyanosis of the lips and fingertips or clubbing of the fingers may be present (see Fig. 32-10).

Bones become thin with tumor invasion and break easily. The patient may have bone pain or pathologic fractures. Handle the patient carefully. Thin bones can fracture with little pressure and without trauma. Even heavy coughing can break a rib.

Late manifestations of lung cancer usually include fatigue, weight loss, anorexia, dysphagia, and nausea and vomiting. *Superior vena cava syndrome may result from tumor pressure in or around the vena cava. This syndrome is an emergency (see Chapter 24) and requires immediate medical attention.* Lethargy and somnolence may develop, and the patient may have confusion or personality changes as a result of brain metastasis. Bowel and bladder tone or function may be affected by tumor spread to the spine and spinal cord.

Psychosocial Assessment

The poor prognosis for lung cancer has made it a much-feared disease. Lung cancer manifestations, especially dyspnea, add to the patient's fear and anxiety. The patient with a history of cigarette smoking may feel guilt and shame. Convey acceptance, and interact with the patient in a nonjudgmental way. Encourage the patient and family to express their feelings about the possible diagnosis of lung cancer.

Few patients with stage III or higher lung cancer are cured or live longer than 5 years after diagnosis. Many are given limited palliative treatment for symptom relief. Fear of pain and death is common.

Other Diagnostic Assessment

The diagnosis of lung cancer is made by direct examination of cancer cells. Cytologic examination of early morning sputum specimens may identify tumor cells; however, cancer cells may not be present in the sputum. When pleural effusion is present, fluid can be obtained by thoracentesis for cytology.

Most commonly, lung lesions are first identified on chest x-rays. Computed tomography (CT) examinations are then used to identify the lesions more clearly. Usually, the entire chest is scanned at 5- to 10-mm slices and the suspicious areas are then scanned at 1- to 2-mm slices for the highest resolution.

Fiberoptic bronchoscopy provides direct visibility of the tracheobronchial tree. Specimens and bronchial brushings can be obtained with this technique, especially when lesions are located within or close to an airway. Needle biopsy during bronchoscopy may be used to obtain cancer cells.

A thoracoscopy may be performed through a video-assisted thoracoscope entering the chest cavity via small incisions through the chest wall. This procedure allows direct visualization of the lung tissue. To identify metastasis in mediastinal lymph nodes, a mediastinoscopy may be performed through a small chest incision.

Other diagnostic studies may be needed to determine how widely the cancer has spread. Such tests include needle biopsy of lymph nodes, direct surgical biopsy, and thoracentesis with pleural biopsy. Magnetic resonance imaging (MRI) and radionuclide scans of the liver, spleen, brain, and bone help determine the location of metastatic tumors. Pulmonary function tests and arterial blood gas (ABG) analysis help determine the overall respiratory status. Positron emission tomography (PET) scanning is becoming the most thorough way to locate metastases. Together, these tests help determine the extent of the cancer and the best methods to treat it.

DECISION-MAKING CHALLENGE
Coordination of Care

The patient is a 51-year-old man who works as a welder and has just been diagnosed with stage II lung cancer. He smoked heavily as a younger man and was able to stop smoking for 5 years when he was diagnosed with Hodgkin's lymphoma 15 years ago. He was successfully treated with chemotherapy and radiation at that time and has not had a recurrence of the lymphoma. Ten years ago he started smoking again and now smokes two packs per day. He and his wife are distraught at the diagnosis, and he is verbally blaming himself for the lung cancer, saying he knows he is going to die.

1. What are this man's risk factors for lung cancer?
2. What should you tell him about his chances of dying?
3. Should you approach him at this distressing time about quitting smoking? Why or why not?

evolve For suggested answer guidelines, go to http://evolve.elsevier.com/Iggy/.

Interventions for Cure

Interventions for the patient with lung cancer can be aimed at curing the disease, increasing survival time, and enhancing quality of life through palliation. Both nonsurgical and surgical interventions are used to achieve these aims. Some patients with lung cancer may undergo interventions for all three aims at different stages in the disease process. Currently, cures are most likely for patients who undergo treatment for stage I or II disease. Cure is rare for patients who undergo treatment for stage III or IV disease, although survival time is increasing, especially for non–small cell lung cancer (Tyson, 2007; Walker, 2008).

Nonsurgical Management

Chemotherapy is often the treatment of choice for lung cancers, especially small cell lung cancer (SCLC). It may be used alone or as adjuvant therapy in combination with surgery for non–small cell lung cancer (NSCLC). The exact combination of drugs used varies depending on the response of the tumor and the overall health of the patient; however, most include platinum-based agents (Tyson, 2007).

Side effects that occur with chemotherapy for lung cancer include chemotherapy-induced nausea and vomiting (CIN), **alopecia** (hair loss), open sores on mucous membranes (**mucositis**), immunosuppression, anemia, **thrombocytopenia** (decreased numbers of platelets), and peripheral neuropathy (PN). Some of these side effects are presented briefly below. Consult Chapter 24 for a thorough discussion of the nursing care needs for patients who have these side effects.

Reassure patients that hair loss is temporary. Hair regrowth begins about 1 month after chemotherapy is completed. Hair loss can be disguised by the use of wigs, scarves, turbans, and caps.

The chemotherapy agents used for lung cancer treatment are **emetogenic** (inducing nausea and vomiting). Many effective antiemetic drugs are available. Usually one or more antiemetics are given before and after chemotherapy. Drugs used to control chemotherapy-induced nausea and vomiting are listed in Chart 24-8 in Chapter 24. Patient response to antiemetic therapy varies, and the drug combinations are individualized for best effect.

Frequent mouth assessment and oral hygiene are key in managing mucositis. Stress the importance of good, frequent oral hygiene, including tooth cleaning and mouth rinsing. Teach patients to use a soft-bristled toothbrush or disposable mouth sponges and to avoid using dental floss and water-pressure gum cleaners.

Immunosuppression, which greatly increases the risk for infection, is the major dose-limiting side effect of chemotherapy for lung cancer. Immunosuppression can be managed by the use of biological response modifiers (BRMs) to stimulate bone marrow production of immune system cells. Teach the patient and family about precautions to take to reduce the patient's chances of developing an infection (see Chart 24-5 in Chapter 24). (See Chapter 24 for more information about chemotherapy and associated nursing care.)

Targeted therapy is now becoming more common in the treatment of later stage lung cancer. As discussed in Chapter 24, these agents take advantage of one or more differences in cancer cell growth or metabolism that is either not present or only slightly present in normal cells. These differences are a result of specific gene expression in cancer cells. Agents used as targeted therapies often are antibodies that work to disrupt cancer cell division in one of several ways. Some of these drugs "target" and block growth factor receptors, especially the epithelial growth factor receptors (EGFR) or the vascular endothelial growth factor receptors (VEGFR). When a lung cancer cell's growth depends on having the growth factors bind to their specific receptors, blocking the receptors at least slows the cancer cell's growth. Two agents most often used for targeted therapy of certain types of non–small cell lung cancer are erlotinib (Tarceva), an oral drug, and bevacizumab (Avastin), which is given IV. Neither drug is used alone as therapy for lung cancer, and bevacizumab tends to intensify common chemotherapy side effects.

Radiation therapy can be an effective treatment for locally advanced lung cancers confined to the chest. Best results are seen when radiation is used in addition to surgery or chemotherapy. Radiation may be performed before surgery to shrink the tumor and make resection easier.

Usually radiation therapy for lung cancer is performed daily for a 5- to 6-week period. Only the areas thought to have cancer are positioned in the radiation path. The immediate side effects of this treatment are skin irritation and peeling, fatigue, nausea, and taste changes. Some patients have esophagitis during therapy, making adequate nutrition more difficult. Teach patients to eat foods that are soft, bland, and high in calories. Consult with a nutritionist to provide a list of foods that are easier to swallow and nutritious. Suggest that the patient drink liquid nutrition supplements, such as Ensure or Boost, between meals to maintain weight and energy levels. Narrowing of the esophagus can occur as a late response to radiation therapy for lung cancer and may require dilation or reconstructive surgery.

Skin care in the radiation-treated area can be difficult. If the area has been marked with a dye to outline the areas for radiation, instruct the patient not to wash off the markings. The use of ink or dye markings is rare, with most cancer centers using small permanent tattoos to mark the area. Instruct patients not to use lotions or ointments on the skin of the chest unless the radiologist prescribes them. Because skin in the radiation path is more sensitive to sun damage, advise patients to avoid direct skin exposure to the sun during treatment and for at least 1 year after radiation is completed. See Chapter 24 for other nursing care issues associated with radiation therapy.

Photodynamic therapy (PDT) may be used to remove small bronchial tumors when they are accessible by bronchoscopy. Once used only for palliation, this therapy is now used also for cure of select lung cancers. The patient is first injected with an agent that sensitizes cells to light. This drug enters all cells but leaves normal cells more rapidly than cancer cells. Usually, within 48 to 72 hours, most of the drug has collected in high concentrations in cancer cells. At this time, the patient goes to the operating room where, under anesthesia and intubation, a laser light is focused on the tumor. The light activates a chemical reaction within those cells retaining the sensitizing drug that induces irreversible cell damage. Some cells die and slough immediately; others continue to slough for several days.

The photosensitizing drug has many effects that require special patient teaching and care both before and after the laser treatment (Collins & Garner, 2007). Chapter 24 describes these issues in detail. In addition to these general care issues, when PDT is used in the airways, the patient usually requires a stay in the ICU for airway management. The sloughing tissue can block the airway as can airway edema from the inflammatory response of the tissues. In addition, the patient is at risk for bronchial hemorrhage, fistula formation, and hemoptysis. A complicating factor in caring for patients who have undergone bronchial PDT is the fact that the patient is now supersensitive to light and will remain so for 30 to 90 days. Thus special precautions are needed along with environmental manipulation to keep the patient safe during his or her hospital stay and during the next 3 months. Chapter 24 discusses environmental safety in detail, and Chart 24-11 in Chapter 24 presents points to teach the patient and family.

Surgical Management

Surgery is the main treatment for stage I and stage II NSCLC. Total removal of a non–small cell primary lung cancer is undertaken in hope of achieving a cure. If complete resection is not possible, the surgeon removes the bulk of the tumor. The specific surgery depends on the stage of the cancer and the patient's overall health and functional status. Lung cancer surgery may involve removal of the tumor only, removal of a lung segment, removal of a lobe **(lobectomy),** or removal of the entire lung **(pneumonectomy).** These procedures can be performed by open thoracotomy or by thoracoscopy with minimally invasive surgery in select patients.

Preoperative Care. The goals of care before surgery are to relieve anxiety and promote the patient's participation (see Chapter 16 for routine preoperative care). Encourage the patient to express fears and concerns, reinforce the surgeon's explanation of the surgical procedure, and provide education related to what is expected after surgery. Teach about the probable location of the surgical incision or thoracoscopy

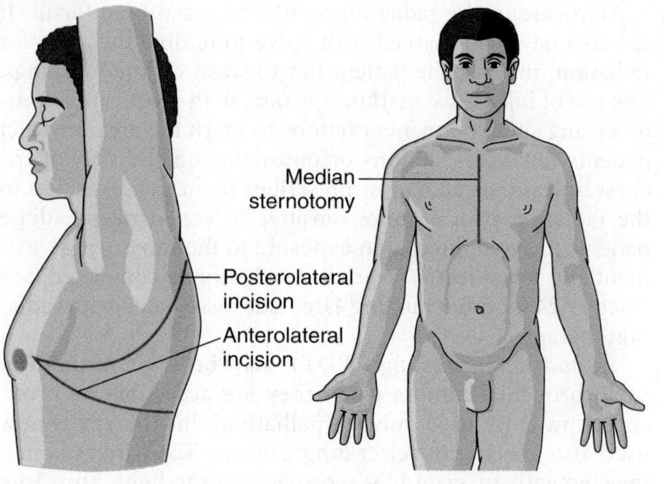
Median
sternotomy
Posterolateral
incision
Anterolateral
incision

Fig. 32-13 • Common incision locations for partial or total pneumonectomy.

openings, shoulder exercises, and the chest tube and drainage system (except after pneumonectomy).

Operative Procedures. Three types of incisions can be made depending on the location of the cancer: posterolateral, anterolateral, and median sternotomy (Fig. 32-13). The incisions are large and are held open with retractors during surgery, contributing to pain after surgery.

A segmental resection **(segmentectomy)** is a lung resection that includes the bronchus, pulmonary artery and vein, and tissue of the involved lung segment or segments, which are divisions of lobes. A **wedge resection** is removal of the peripheral portion of small, localized areas of disease. A **lobectomy** is the removal of an entire lung lobe. A **pneumonectomy** is the removal of an entire lung, including all blood vessels. The bronchus to that lung is severed and sutured.

Removal of a lobe or even an entire lung can be accomplished through video-assisted thoracoscopic surgery (VATS) for select patients. The procedure involves making three small incisions in the chest for placement of the thoracoscope and other instruments. These same openings are used later for placement of drains and chest tubes. The lung section, lobe, or lung is isolated from the airway, which is surgically closed. The lobe or the lung is closed off from the rest of the lung using a double-stapling technique. Then the tissue is encapsulated in an impermeable bag to prevent leakage of tumor tissue and possible seeding of the cancer and is then removed whole through one of the small incisions.

Postoperative Care. Care after surgery for patients who have undergone thoracotomy (except for pneumonectomy) requires closed-chest drainage to drain air and blood that accumulate in the pleural space. A **chest tube,** a drain placed in the pleural space to restore intrapleural pressure, allows reexpansion of the lung (Fig. 32-14). The chest tube also prevents air and fluid from returning to the chest. The drainage system consists of one or more chest tubes or drains, a collection container placed below the chest level, and a water seal to keep air from entering the chest. The drainage system may be a stationary, disposable, self-contained system (Fig. 32-15) or a smaller, portable, disposable, self-contained system (Fig. 32-16). The basic principles of gravity and pressure are the same with both systems. The nursing care priorities for the patient with a chest tube are to ensure the integrity of the system, promote comfort, ensure chest tube patency, and prevent complications.

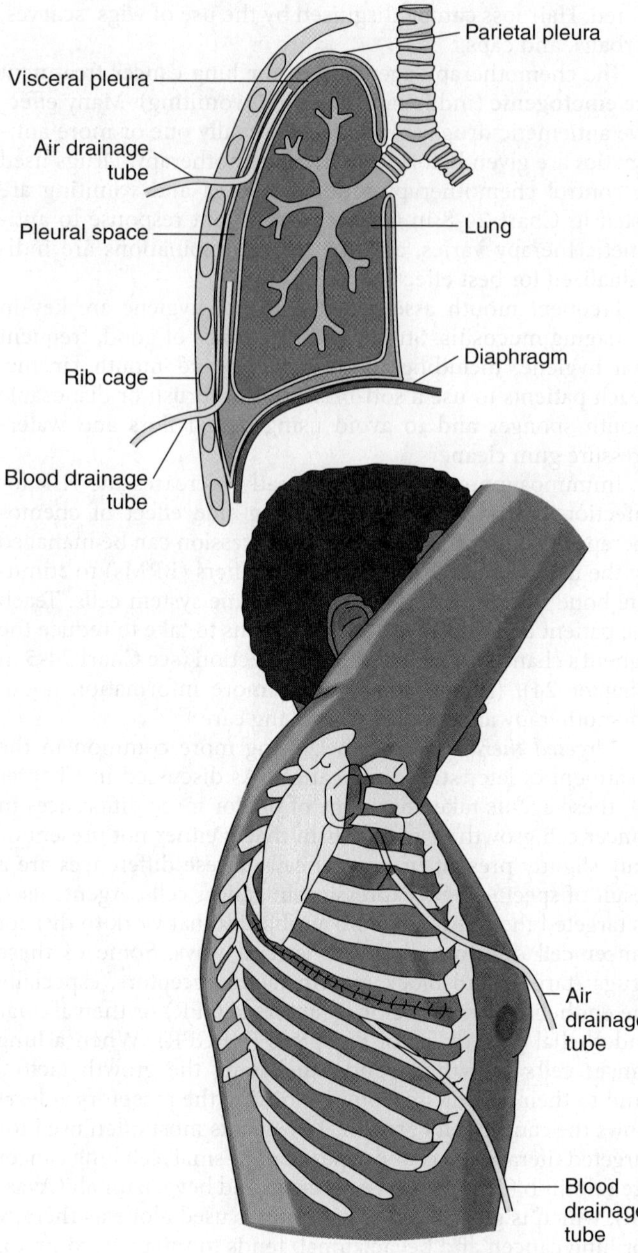
Parietal pleura
Visceral pleura
Air drainage
tube
Pleural space
Lung
Diaphragm
Rib cage
Blood drainage
tube
Air
drainage
tube
Blood
drainage
tube

Fig. 32-14 • Chest tube placement.

Chest Tube Placement and Care. The tip of the tube used to drain air is placed near the front lung apex (see Fig. 32-14). The tube that drains liquid is placed on the side near the base of the lung. After lung surgery, two tubes, anterior and posterior, are used. The puncture wounds are covered with airtight dressings.

The chest tube is connected to about 6 feet of tubing that leads to a collection device placed several feet below the chest. The tubing allows the patient to turn and move without pulling on the chest tube. Keeping the collection device below the chest allows gravity to drain the pleural space. When two chest tubes are inserted, they are joined by a Y-connector near the patient's body; the 6 feet of tubing is attached to the Y-connector.

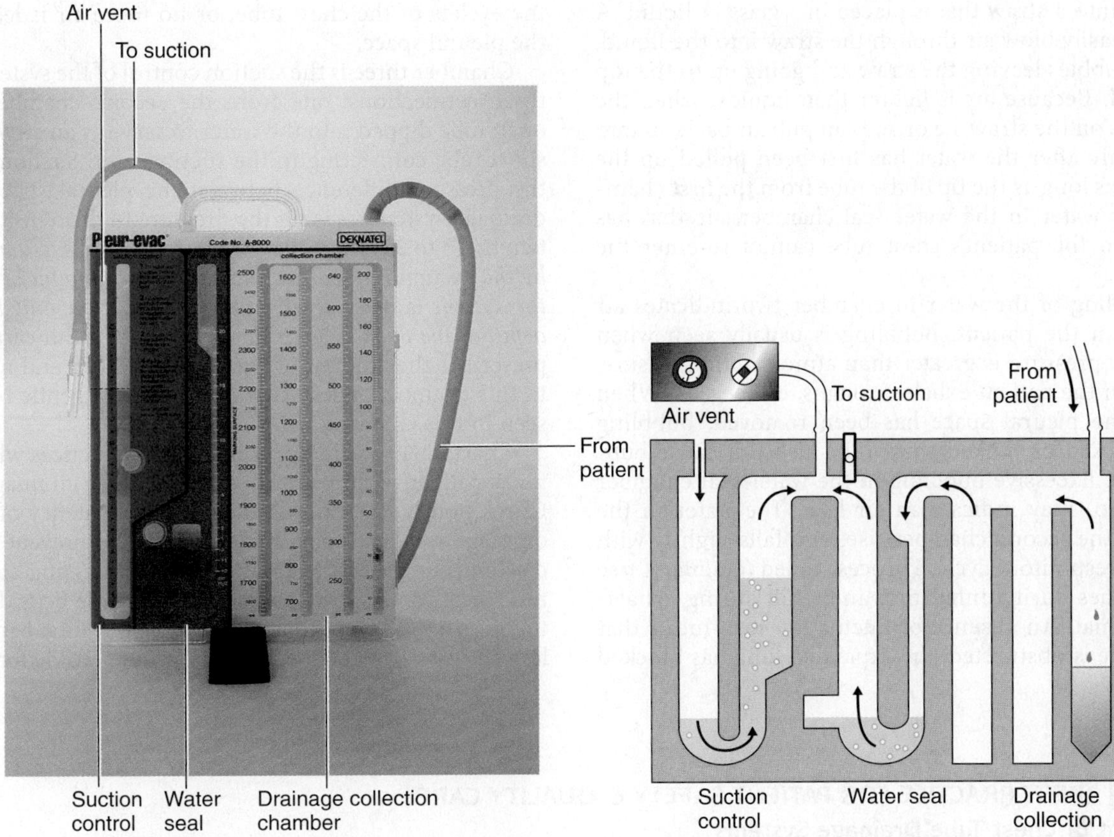
Air vent
To suction
Pleur-evac
Code No. A-6000
DEKNATEL
collection chamber
From patient
Suction control
Water seal
Drainage collection chamber
From patient
To suction
Air vent
From patient
Suction control
Water seal
Drainage collection

Fig. 32-15 • *Left,* The Pleur-Evac drainage system, a commercial three-bottle chest drainage device. *Right,* Schematic of the drainage device.

Stationary chest tube drainage systems usually use a water seal mechanism that acts as a one-way valve to prevent air or liquid from moving back into the chest cavity. The Pleur-Evac system is a common device using a one-piece disposable plastic unit with three chambers. The three chamber are connected to one another. The tube(s) from the patient is(are) connected to the first chamber in the series of three. This chamber is the drainage collection container. The second chamber in the series is the water seal to prevent air from moving back up the tubing system and into the chest. The third chamber, when suction is applied, is the suction regulator.

In setting up the system, chamber one (nearest to the patient) does not at first have fluid in it. The tubing from the patient penetrates shallowly into this chamber, as does the tube connecting chamber one with chamber two.

Chamber one collects the fluid draining from the patient. This fluid is measured hourly during the first 24 hours. *The fluid in chamber one must never fill to the point that it comes into direct contact with either the tube draining from the patient or the tube connecting this chamber to chamber two. If the tubing from the patient enters the fluid, drainage stops and can lead to a tension pneumothorax.*

Chamber two is the water seal that prevents air from entering the patient's pleural space. Air from the pleural space also enters chamber one but moves immediately to chamber two through the connecting tube. This tube must always be under the water level in chamber two to prevent air from returning to the patient. The tube acts as a one-way valve, allowing air to move into the water and preventing air in this chamber from re-entering the tube. This action is similar to

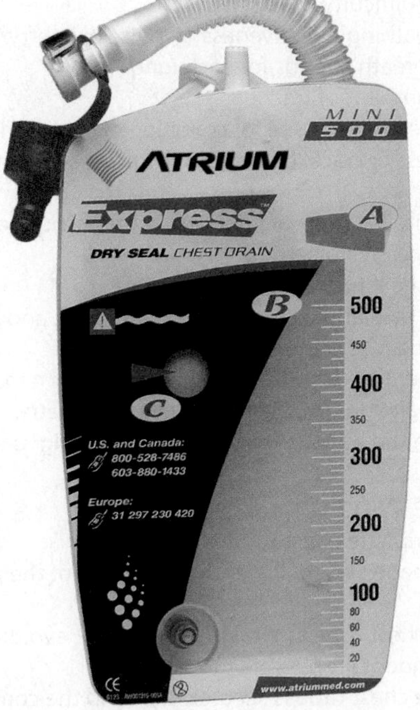
MINI 500
ATRIUM
Express
A
DRY SEAL CHEST DRAIN
B
C
U.S. and Canada:
800-528-7486
603-880-1433
Europe:
31 297 230 420
500
400
300
200
100
www.atriummed.com

Fig. 32-16 • A portable chest drainage system.

blowing air into a straw that is placed in a glass of liquid. A person can easily blow air through the straw into the liquid, as seen by bubbles leaving the straw and going up to the top of the liquid. Because air is lighter than liquids, when the person sucks on the straw, he or she can pull air back up into the straw only after the water has first been pulled up the straw. Thus, as long as the tip of the tube from the first chamber is under water in the water seal chamber, air that has escaped from the patient's chest tube cannot re-enter the patient.

The bubbling of the water in chamber two indicates air drainage from the patient. Bubbling is usually seen when intrathoracic pressure is greater than atmospheric pressure, such as when the patient exhales, coughs, or sneezes. When the air in the pleural space has been removed, bubbling stops. A blocked or kinked chest tube also can cause bubbling to stop. Excessive bubbling in the water seal chamber (chamber two) may indicate an air leak. The water in the long tube of the second chamber rises and falls slightly with the patient's respiratory cycle, a process called *tidaling*. A rise of 2 to 4 inches during inhalation and a fall during exhalation are normal. An absence of fluctuation may mean that the chest tube is obstructed, the expanded lung has blocked the eyelets of the chest tube, or no more air is leaking into the pleural space.

Chamber three is the suction control of the system and has three connections: one from the second chamber; a long, open tube dipped into the water to serve as an air vent; and a short tube connecting to the suction unit. Suction enhances the pressure difference between the pleural space and the drainage system, causing the pressure to drop inside the system by 15 to 20 cm. *Although the amount of suction generated by the suction unit can be increased, the amount of suction in the system is determined not by the suction unit but by the depth of the open tube in the water.* The health care provider prescribes the amount of water to be placed and maintained in this chamber. While suction is applied, gentle bubbling is seen in this chamber.

Chart 32-13 summarizes best safety practices when caring for a patient with a water seal chest tube drainage system. Check hourly to ensure the sterility and patency of any chest drainage system. Tape tubing junctions to prevent accidental disconnections, and keep an occlusive dressing at the chest tube insertion site. Keep sterile gauze at the bedside to cover the insertion site immediately if the chest tube becomes dislodged. Also keep padded clamps at the bedside for use if the

Chart 32-13 BEST PRACTICE FOR PATIENT SAFETY & QUALITY CARE

Management of Chest Tube Drainage Systems

PATIENT

- Ensure that the dressing on the chest around the tube is tight and intact. Depending on agency policy and the surgeon's preference, reinforce or change loose dressings.
- Assess for difficulty breathing.
- Assess breathing effectiveness by pulse oximetry.
- Listen to breath sounds for each lung.
- Check alignment of trachea.
- Check tube insertion site for condition of the skin. Palpate area for puffiness or crackling that may indicate subcutaneous emphysema.
- Observe site for signs of infection (redness, purulent drainage) or excessive bleeding.
- Check to see if tube "eyelets" are visible.
- Assess for pain and its location and intensity, and administer drugs for pain as prescribed.
- Assist patient to deep breathe, cough, perform maximal sustained inhalations, and use incentive spirometry.
- Reposition the patient who reports a "burning" pain in the chest.

DRAINAGE SYSTEM

- Do not "strip" the chest tube.
- Keep drainage system lower than the level of the patient's chest.
- Keep the chest tube as straight as possible, avoiding kinks and dependent loops.
- Ensure the chest tube is securely taped to the connector and that the connector is taped to the tubing going into the collection chamber.
- Assess bubbling in the water seal chamber; should be gentle bubbling on patient's exhalation, forceful cough, position changes.
- Assess for "tidaling."
- Check water level in the water seal chamber, and keep the level at that recommended by the manufacturer.
- Check water level in suction control chamber, and keep at the level prescribed by the surgeon.
- Clamp the chest tube only for brief periods to change the drainage system or when checking for air leaks.
- Check and document amount, color, and characteristics of fluid in the collection chamber, as often as needed according to the patient's condition and agency policy.
- Empty collection chamber or change the system before the drainage makes contact with the bottom of the tube.
- When sample of drainage is needed for culture or other laboratory test, obtain it from the chest tube; after cleansing chest tube, use a 20-gauge (or smaller) needle and draw up specimen into a syringe.

IMMEDIATELY NOTIFY PHYSICIAN OR RAPID RESPONSE TEAM FOR:

- Tracheal deviation.
- Sudden onset or increased intensity of dyspnea.
- Oxygen saturation less than 90%.
- Drainage greater than 70 mL/hr.
- Visible eyelets on chest tube.
- Chest tube falls out of the patient's chest (first, cover the area with dry, sterile gauze).
- Chest tube disconnects from the drainage system (first, put end of tube in a container of sterile water and keep below the level of the patient's chest).
- Drainage in tube stops (in the first 24 hours).

drainage system is interrupted. Position the drainage tubing to prevent kinks and large loops of tubing, which can block drainage and prevent lung re-expansion.

Manipulation of the chest tube should be kept to a minimum. Do not vigorously "strip" the chest tube because this can create up to −400 cm of water negative pressure and damage lung tissue. If any tube manipulation is needed, gentle hand-over-hand "milking" of the tube, with stopping between each hand hold, is used to move blood clots and prevent obstruction (Halm, 2007). Follow agency policies and guidelines on this action.

Assess the patient's respiratory status and document the amount and type of drainage hourly. Usually the drainage in chamber one is not emptied unless the container is so full that the fluid is in danger of coming into contact with the chest drainage tube. The self-contained systems have calibrations on the collection chamber. Record the amount of hourly drainage. Notify the physician of drainage if more than 100 mL/hr occurs. After the first 24 hours, assess drainage at least every 8 hours.

Check the water seal chamber for unexpected bubbling created by an air leak in the system. Bubbling is normal during forceful expiration or coughing because air in the chest is being expelled. Continuous bubbling indicates an air leak that must be identified. Notify the physician if bubbling occurs continuously in the water seal chamber. On the physician's prescription, gently apply a padded clamp briefly on the drainage tubing close to the occlusive dressing. If the bubbling stops, the air leak may be at the chest tube insertion site or within the chest, requiring physician intervention. Air bubbling that does not cease when a padded clamp is applied indicates that the air leak is between the clamp and the drainage system. Release the clamp as soon as this assessment is made.

Mobile or portable chest tube drainage systems are "dry" chest drainage systems that do not use water to form a seal to prevent air from re-entering the patient's lung through the chest tube. Instead, these lightweight devices use a dynamic control "flutter" valve that prevents backflow of air. The flutter valve is a soft rubber tube surrounded by a harder plastic tube. When the patient exhales, air is forced from the chest cavity into the chest tube, under pressure. This pressure forces the soft flutter valve open and air moves into the harder surrounding tube shell (which has a vent for air). When the patient inhales, creating negative pressure in the chest tube, the soft sides of the flutter valve collapse on themselves (like the sides of a deflated balloon when a person sucks on the mouthpiece instead of blowing into the mouthpiece), closing the one-way valve.

Although previously recommended only for use in patients who had a simple, uncomplicated pneumothorax, some mobile chest tube drainage units have larger collection chambers that increase their use. These portable units allow the patient to ambulate more freely and even go home with chest tubes still in place (Carroll, 2005).

NCLEX EXAMINATION CHALLENGE

The client is 1 day post-op after a right lower lobectomy for stage II lung cancer and has two chest tubes in place. He is grimacing and tells the nurse he has intense burning pain in his lower chest. The nurse notes that there is no bubbling on exhalation in the water seal chamber. What is the nurse's best first action?

A. Immediately notify either the Rapid Response Team or the thoracic surgical resident.
B. Administer the prescribed opioid analgesic immediately, and then assess the chest tube system.
C. No action is needed because these responses are normal for the first post-op day after lobectomy.
D. Assist the client to a side-lying position and re-assess the water seal chamber for bubbling.

evolve For the correct answer, go to http://evolve.elsevier.com/Iggy/.

Pain Management. Most patients experience intense pain after an open thoracotomy for at least the first 24 hours. It is considerably less for the patient after lung cancer surgery using minimally invasive techniques. However, pain control is needed in either case for patient comfort and to assist him or her to participate in techniques to reduce the risk of postoperative complications (see Chapter 18). Administer the prescribed drugs for pain, and assess the patient's responses to them. Teach patients using patient-controlled analgesia (PCA) devices to self-administer the drug before pain intensity becomes too severe. Monitor vital signs before and after giving opioid analgesics, especially for the patient who is not being mechanically ventilated. Plan care activities around the timing of analgesia to reduce the stimulation of additional pain.

Respiratory Management. Immediately after surgery the patient is mechanically ventilated. See Chapter 34 for nursing care of the patient receiving mechanical ventilation.

Once the patient is breathing on his or her own, the priorities are to maintain a patent airway, ensure adequate ventilation, and prevent complications. Assess the patient at least every 2 hours for adequacy of ventilation and gas exchange. Check the alignment of the trachea. Assess oxygen saturation and the rate and depth of respiration. Listen to breath sounds in all lobes on the nonoperative side, particularly noting the presence of crackles. Assess the oral mucous membranes for cyanosis and the nail beds for rate of capillary refill. Perform oral suctioning as necessary.

Usually the patient receives oxygen by mask or nasal cannula for the first couple of days after surgery. Warm and humidify the oxygen. Assist the patient to a semi-Fowler's position or up in a chair as soon as possible. Encourage him or her to use the incentive spirometer every hour while awake. If coughing is permitted, help him or her cough by splinting any incision and ensuring that the chest tube does not pull with movement. Ensuring that pain is handled properly increases the patient's ability to cough and deep breathe effectively.

Pneumonectomy Care. After pneumonectomy, the pleural cavity on the affected side is an empty space. The surgeon sometimes inserts a clamped chest tube for only a day because serous fluid may then accumulate in the empty space and create adhesions, which reduce mediastinal shift toward the affected side. Closed-chest drainage is not usually used.

Complications of a pneumonectomy can include empyema and the development of a bronchopleural fistula. Positioning of the patient after pneumonectomy varies according to surgeon preference and the patient's comfort. Some surgeons want the patient placed on the nonoperative side immediately after a pneumonectomy to reduce stress on the bronchial stump incision. Others prefer that the patient be placed on the operative side to allow fluids to fill in the space formerly taken up by the lungs.

Interventions for Palliation

Oxygen therapy is prescribed when the patient is hypoxemic. Even if the hypoxemia is not severe, the physician may prescribe oxygen to relieve dyspnea and anxiety. Humidification is used with oxygen therapy for the patient with lung cancer. (See Chapter 30 for issues related to home oxygen therapy.)

Drug therapy with bronchodilators and corticosteroids is prescribed for the patient with bronchospasm to decrease bronchospasm, inflammation, and edema. Mucolytics may be of use to ease removal of thick mucus and sputum. Bacterial infections are treated with the appropriate antibiotic therapy.

Radiation therapy can help relieve hemoptysis, obstruction of the bronchi and great veins (superior vena cava syndrome), **dysphagia** (difficulty swallowing) from esophageal compression, and pain resulting from bone metastasis. Usually radiation for palliation uses higher doses for shorter periods. Skin care issues and fatigue are the same as those occurring with radiation therapy for cure.

Thoracentesis and pleurodesis are used when pleural effusion is a problem for the patient with lung cancer. The excess fluid increases dyspnea, discomfort, and the risk for infection. The goal of treatment is to remove pleural fluid and prevent its formation. **Thoracentesis** is fluid removal by suction after the placement of a large needle or catheter into the intrapleural space. Fluid removal temporarily relieves hypoxia; however, the fluid can rapidly re-form in the pleural space. When fluid development is continuous and uncomfortable, a continuously draining catheter may be placed into the intrapleural space to collect the fluid.

Another technique to relieve pleural effusion is to insert a chest tube to drain the fluid and to instill a **sclerosing agent,** an agent that is an irritant and causes inflammation. The aim of this technique is to cause a **pleurodesis** (an inflammatory response that causes the pleura to stick to the chest wall). If pleurodesis occurs, it prevents formation of effusion fluid. Liquid sclerosing agents for pleurodesis are instilled after some of the effusion fluid has been removed. The patient is asked to assume a variety of positions to ensure the widest spread of the fluid within the pleural space. Talc pleurodesis involves using a thorascope to deliver talc (in the form of a powder) to the area where the fluid forms. This procedure also causes inflammation and thickening that reduce the formation of effusion fluid.

These procedures can be performed under local anesthesia at the bedside or in an operating room. Usually the patient is also given an analgesic or sedative. Once the sclerosing agent is instilled, the chest tube is clamped to prevent drainage of the agent. Chart 32-14 reviews best practices for care of the patient undergoing pleurodesis.

Dyspnea management is needed because the patient with lung cancer tires easily and is often most comfortable resting in a semi-Fowler's position. Dyspnea is reduced with oxygen, use of a morphine drip, and positioning for comfort. The severely dyspneic patient may be most comfortable sitting in a lounge chair or reclining chair.

Pain management may be needed for chest pain and pain radiating to the arm. With bone metastasis, the patient may also have bone pain. Perform a complete pain assessment with attention to onset, intensity, quality, duration, and the patient's description of the pain. The goal of therapy is to help the patient to be as pain-free and as comfortable as possible.

Pharmacologic management with opioid drugs as oral, parenteral, or transdermal preparations is needed. Nonpharmacologic measures, such as positioning, hot or cold compresses, distractions, and guided imagery, may also be helpful. Prescribed analgesics are most effective when given around the clock. Additional PRN analgesics are used for breakthrough pain. Ongoing assessment and evaluation of the effectiveness of the pain control regimen are primary nursing responsibilities.

Hospice care can be beneficial for the patient in the terminal phase of lung cancer. Hospice programs provide support to the terminally ill patient and the family by meeting physical and psychosocial needs, adjusting the palliative care regimen as needed, making home visits, and providing volunteers for errands and respite care. (See Chapter 9 for a more complete discussion of end-of-life issues.) The American Cancer Society may also be able to provide assistance through support groups for patients and families or through the use of equipment, such as a hospital bed or bedside commode.

Chart 32-14 BEST PRACTICE FOR PATIENT SAFETY & QUALITY CARE

Care of the Patient Undergoing Pleurodesis

- Reinforce explanation of the pleurodesis, and inform the patient that drugs will be used to promote comfort before the procedure. (The physician may administer IV analgesia/sedation immediately before the procedure.)
- Ensure that the chest tube is clamped after instillation of the sclerosing agent.
- Monitor vital signs and respiratory status at the completion of the procedure and then at least every 30 minutes until the effects of the IV drugs have dissipated.
- Thereafter, monitor vital signs every 4 hours for 24 hours. (The patient may have a low-grade fever. Pleurodesis creates pleuritis between the visceral and parietal layers, thus preventing further fluid collection.)
- If a rotation schedule is ordered, assist the patient to the correct position for appropriate time frames and provide reassurance.
- Unclamp the chest tube after completion of the rotation schedule or at the specified time.
- Assess chest tube drainage, and document the amount and character of the drainage.
- Perform a complete respiratory assessment every 2 hours, and observe for manifestations of distress, including those of pneumothorax (rapid respiration, reduced breath sounds on the affected side, dyspnea, decreased oxygen saturation, tracheal deviation, prominence of one side of the chest).
- Analgesics may be administered as needed to promote comfort.
- When drainage has decreased ($<$150 mL in 12-24 hr), the physician may remove the chest tube. Maintain an occlusive dressing at the insertion site for a minimum of 48 hours.

HUMAN NEEDS NURSING CARE REVIEW

What might you NOTICE if the patient is experiencing inadequate oxygenation and tissue perfusion as a result of chronic obstructive respiratory problems?

- Respirations rapid and shallow
- Decreased oxygen saturation by pulse oximetry
- Skin cyanosis or pallor (lighter-skinned patients)
- Cyanosis or pallor of the lips and oral mucous membranes (in patients of any skin color)
- Tachycardia
- Patient appears to work hard to inhale and exhale
- Patient is restless or anxious
- Patient's general appearance is thin compared with height
- Muscles of the neck appear thick
- Arm and leg muscles appear thin
- Fingers are clubbed
- Chest is barrel-shaped (has a round rather than an oval shape with the front to back depth increased)
- Ribs are spaced more than a finger-breadth apart

What should you INTERPRET and how should you RESPOND to a patient experiencing inadequate oxygenation and tissue perfusion as a result of an acute critical respiratory problem?

Perform and interpret physical assessment, including:
- Taking vital signs
- Auscultating all lung fields
- Monitoring oxygen saturation by pulse oximetry
- Checking the accuracy of pulse oximetry readings
- Assessing cognition (Mini-Mental State Examination)
- Assessing for the presence and characteristic of sputum production
- Assessing the patient's ability to cough and clear the airway

Interpret laboratory values, including:
- Elevated red blood cell count, hematocrit, and hemoglobin
- Elevated white blood cell count
- Arterial blood gas values: pH less than 7.35, HCO_3^- more than 24 mm Hg, $Paco_2$ more than 45 mm Hg; Pao_2 less than 80 mm Hg

Respond by:
- Assisting the patient to an upright position, with arms resting on a table or armrests
- Performing or assisting the patient to perform chest physiotherapy/pulmonary hygiene
- Ensuring that oxygen delivery is kept low enough to maintain respirations of no fewer than 16 breaths per minute
- Prioritizing and pacing activities to prevent fatigue
- Administering prescribed inhaled drugs
- Administering respiratory therapy treatments or collaborating with the respiratory therapist to administer these treatments
- Re-assessing respiratory status after respiratory therapy treatment
- Ensuring a fluid intake of at least 3 liters per day

On what should you REFLECT?
- Observe patient for evidence of improved oxygenation (see Chapter 29)
- Think about what may have made the patient's dyspnea worse and what steps could be taken to prevent a similar episode
- Think about what patient teaching focus could help reduce the intensity of dyspnea in the future

GET READY FOR THE NCLEX EXAMINATION!

Key Points

Review these Key Points for each NCLEX Examination Client Needs Category.

Safe and Effective Care Environment
- Avoid high liter flow rates of oxygen for patients with COPD.
- Ensure that no open flames or combustion hazards are in rooms where oxygen is in use.
- Protect the patient with cystic fibrosis from hospital-acquired pulmonary infections.
- Ensure proper function of chest tube drainage equipment.

Health Promotion and Maintenance
- Teach patients who come into contact with inhalation irritants in their workplaces or leisure time activities to use a mask to avoid respiratory contact with these substances.
- Teach anyone who smokes that smoking increases the risk for development of many pulmonary problems.
- Assist patients interested in smoking cessation to find an appropriate smoking cessation program.
- Encourage older adults who are confined to bed for any reason or who are recovering from surgery to turn, cough, and deep breathe at least every 2 hours.
- Encourage all patients older than 50 years and anyone with a respiratory problem to receive a yearly influenza vaccination.
- Teach all patients who smoke the warning signs of lung cancer.

Psychosocial Integrity
- Assess the degree to which breathing problems interfere with the patient's ability to perform ADLs, work, and leisure time activities.
- Encourage the patient and family to express their feelings regarding the diagnosis of cancer or the treatment regimen.
- Allow patients to verbalize feelings about changes in appearance resulting from cancer therapy.
- Explain all diagnostic procedures, restrictions, and follow-up care to the patient scheduled for tests.
- Help patients use strategies to improve their appearance when alopecia occurs.
- Refer patients and family members to local cancer resources and support groups.

Physiological Integrity
- Monitor the rate and depth of respiration at least every hour for any patient with hypercarbia and CO_2 narcosis who is receiving oxygen by mask or nasal cannula.
- Document any known specific allergies that have respiratory manifestations.
- Assess the airway and breathing effectiveness for any patient who experiences shortness of breath or any change in mental status.
- Apply oxygen to anyone who is hypoxemic.
- Ensure that oxygen therapy delivered to the patient is humidified (and warmed, when possible).

- Monitor arterial blood gases and oxygen saturation of all patients receiving oxygen therapy.
- Teach patients receiving radiation therapy how to care for the skin in the radiation path (see Chart 24-2 in Chapter 24).

Additional Study Resources

Go to your Companion CD or Evolve at http://evolve.elsevier.com/Iggy/ for *Self-Assessment Questions for the NCLEX Examination.*

evolve Go to Evolve at http://evolve.elsevier.com/Iggy/ for *Prioritization and Delegation Questions for the NCLEX Examination.*

SELECTED BIBLIOGRAPHY

American Cancer Society. (2008). *Cancer facts and figures—2008.* Report No. 01-300M-No. 5008.08. Atlanta: Author.

Bauldoff, G., & Diaz, P. (2006). Improving outcomes for COPD patients. *The Nurse Practitioner, 31*(8), 26-43.

Bruce, M., & McEvoy, P. (2007). COPD: Your role in early detection. *The Nurse Practitioner, 32*(11), 24-33.

Bulechek, G.M, Butcher, H.K, & McCloskey Dochterman, J. (Eds.). (2008). *Nursing interventions classification (NIC)* (5th ed.). St. Louis: Mosby.

Burns, S. (2006). Ask the experts: Idiopathic pulmonary fibrosis. *Critical Care Nurse, 26*(6), 65-66, 74.

Carlson, M.L., Ivnik, M.A., Dierkhising, R.A., O'Byrne, M.M., & Vickers, K.S. (2006). A learning needs assessment of patients with COPD. *MEDSURG Nursing, 15*(4), 204-212.

Carroll, P. (2005). Keeping up with mobile chest drains. *RN, 68*(10), 26-31.

Centers for Disease Control and Prevention (CDC). (2007). National surveillance for asthma—United States, 1980-2004. *Morbidity and Mortality Weekly Report, 56*(SS08), 1-14, 18-54.

Collins, A., & Garner, M. (2007). Care for lung cancer patients receiving photodynamic therapy. *Critical Care Nurse, 27*(2), 53-60.

Collins, L.G., Haines, C., Perkel, R., & Enck, R.E. (2007). Lung cancer: Diagnosis and management. *American Family Physician, 75*(1), 56-63.

Conboy-Ellis, K. (2006). Asthma: Pathogenesis and management. *The Nurse Practitioner, 31*(11), 24-37.

Cope, D., & Reb, A. (Eds.). (2006). *An evidence-based approach to the treatment and care of the older adult with cancer.* Pittsburgh: Oncology Nursing Society.

Coughlin, A., & Parchinsky, C. (2006). Go with the flow of chest tube therapy. *Nursing2006, 36*(3), 36-41.

Crawford, A., & Harris, H. (2008). COPD: Help your patients breathe easier. *RN, 71*(1), 20-25.

Cystic Fibrosis Foundation. (2007). Retrieved January, 2008, from www.cff.org/.

Ellis, K. (2008). Keeping asthma at bay. *American Nurse Today, 3*(2), 20-25.

Elpern, E., Patel, G., & Balk, R. (2007). Antibiotic therapy for pulmonary exacerbations in adults with cystic fibrosis. *MEDSURG Nursing, 16*(5), 293-298.

Finch, C.K., Tolley, E., James, A., Fisher, K., & Self, T.H. (2007). Gender differences in peak flow meter use. *The Nurse Practitioner, 32*(5), 46-48.

Fitzgerald, M. (2006). Managing bronchospasms with short-acting beta$_2$-agonists. *The Nurse Practitioner, 31*(9), 47-53.

Fox, S., & Lyon, D. (2006). Symptom clusters and quality of life in survivors of lung cancer. *Oncology Nursing Forum, 33*(5), 931-936.

Gardner, J. (2007). What you need to know about cystic fibrosis. *Nursing2007, 37*(7), 52-55.

Global Initiative for Chronic Obstructive Lung Disease (GOLD). (2007). *Global strategy of the diagnosis, management, and prevention of chronic obstructive pulmonary disease.* MCR Vision, Inc. Website: www.gold.copd.org

Grossman, S., & Grossman, L. (2005). Pathophysiology of cystic fibrosis: Implications for critical care nurses. *Critical Care Nurse, 25*(4), 46-51.

Halm, M. (2007). To strip or not to strip: Physiological effects of chest tube manipulation. *American Journal of Critical Care, 16*(6), 609-612.

Henschke, C.I., Yankelevitz, D.F., Libby, D.M., Pasmantier, M.W., Smith, J.P., Miettinen, O.S., et al. (2006). Survival of patients with stage I lung cancer detected on CT screening. *New England Journal of Medicine, 355*(17), 1763-1771.

Hoffman, A.J., Given, B.A., von Eye, A., Gift, A.G., & Given, C.W. (2007). Relationships among pain, fatigue, insomnia, and gender in persons with lung cancer. *Oncology Nursing Forum, 34*(4), 785-792.

McCance, K., & Huether, S. (2006). *Pathophysiology: The biologic basis for disease in adults and children* (5th ed.). St. Louis: Mosby.

Meiner, S., & Lueckenotte, A. (Eds.). (2006). *Gerontologic nursing* (3rd ed.). St. Louis: Mosby.

National Institutes of Health. (2007). *Guidelines for the diagnosis and management of asthma.* Expert panel report 3. Bethesda, MD: U.S. Department of Health and Human Services.

Nussbaum, R., McInnes, R., & Willard, H. (2007). *Thompson & Thompson genetics in medicine* (7th ed.). Philadelphia: Saunders.

Ostrom, N., & Goergen, B. (2006). Asthma management in women. *The Journal for Nurse Practitioners, 2*(7), 450-459.

Pagana, K., & Pagana, T. (2006). *Mosby's manual of diagnostic and laboratory tests* (3rd ed.). St. Louis: Mosby.

Pruitt, B. (2007). Latest advances in respiratory care. *Nursing2007, 37*(7), 56cc1-56cc3.

Pruitt, B. (2008). Loosening the bonds of restrictive lung disease. *Nursing2008, 38*(8), 34-39

Pruitt, B., & Jacobs, M. (2005). Caring for a patient with asthma. *Nursing2005, 35*(2), 48-51.

Pruitt, W. (2005). Teaching your patient to use a peak flow meter. *Nursing2005, 35*(3), 54-55.

Rice, V. (2006). Nursing intervention and smoking cessation: Meta-analysis update. *Heart and Lung, 35*(3), 147-163.

Roman, M. (2007). Asthma. *MEDSURG Nursing, 16*(3), 209-210.

Roman, M., & Mercado, D. (2006). Review of chest tube use. *MEDSURG Nursing, 15*(1), 41-43.

Ross, C. (2007). Pulmonary arterial hypertension: Early recognition and treatment can make a lifetime difference for your patient. *The Journal for Nurse Practitioners, 3*(6), 404-409.

Rushing, J. (2007). Managing a water-seal chest drainage unit. *Nursing2007, 37*(12), 12.

Sarna, L., Cooley, M.E., Brown, J.K., Williams, R.D., Chernecky, C., Padilla, G., et al. (2006). Quality of life and health status of dyads of women with lung cancer and family members. *Oncology Nursing Forum, 33*(6), 1109-1116.

Shuey, K., & Payne, Y. (2005). Malignant pleural effusion. *Clinical Journal of Oncology Nursing, 9*(1), 529-532.

Simon, B. (2007). Lung cancer diagnosis in primary care. *The Nurse Practitioner, 32*(1), 43-48.

Sims, J. (2006). An overview of asthma. *Dimensions of Critical Care Nursing, 25*(6), 264-268.

Song, M., Babbs, A., Studer, S., & Zangle, S. (2008). Course of illness after the onset of chronic rejection in lung transplant recipients. *American Journal of Critical Care, 17*(3), 246-253.

Tyson, L. (2007). Non–small cell lung cancer: New hope for a chronic illness. *Oncology Nursing Forum, 34*(5), 963-970.

Vena, C., Parker, K., Allen, R., Bliwise, D., Jain, S., & Kimble, L. (2006). Sleep-wake disturbances and quality of life in patients with advanced lung cancer. *Oncology Nursing Forum, 33*(4), 761-769.

Walker, S. (2008). Updates in non–small-cell lung cancer. *The Clinical Journal of Oncology Nursing, 12*(4), 587-596.

Wall, M.P. (2007). Predictors of functional performance in community-dwelling people with COPD. *Journal of Nursing Scholarship, 39*(3), 222-228.

Warren, M.L., & Livesay, S. (2006). Taking action against acute COPD. *American Nurse Today, 1*(3), 12-15.

Wells, M., Sarna, L., Cooley, M.E., Brown, J.K., Chernecky, C., Williams, R.D., et al. (2007). Use of complementary and alternative medicine therapies to control symptoms in women living with lung cancer. *Cancer Nursing, 30*(1), 45-55.

White, K., & Ruth-Sahd, L. (2007). Bronchiolitis obliterans organizing pneumonia. *Critical Care Nurse, 27*(3), 53-66.

Widlitz, A., McDevitt, S., Ward, G.R., & Krichman, A. (2007). Practical aspects of continuous intravenous treprostinil therapy. *Critical Care Nurse, 27*(2), 41-50.

Wise, R., & Tashkin, D. (2007). Optimizing treatment of chronic obstructive pulmonary disease: An assessment of current therapies. *American Journal of Medicine, 120*(8 Suppl. A), S4-S13.

Workman, M.L., & Winkelman, C. (2008). Genetic influences in common respiratory disorders. *Critical Care Nursing Clinics of North America* (in press).

Yoder, L. (2006a). An overview of lung cancer symptoms, pathophysiology, and treatment. *MEDSURG Nursing, 15*(4), 231-234.

Yoder, L. (2006b). Lung cancer epidemiology. *MEDSURG Nursing, 15*(3), 171-174.

Zhang X., Miao X., Guo Y., Tan, W., Zhou, Y., Sun, T., et al. (2006). Genetic polymorphisms in cell cycle regulatory genes *MDM2* and *TP53* are associated with susceptibility to lung cancer. *Human Mutation, 27*(1), 110-117.

Care of Patients with Infectious Respiratory Problems

33
CHAPTER

M. Linda Workman

LEARNING OUTCOMES

For clinical competence and success on the NCLEX Examination, study this chapter with these Learning Outcomes in mind:

Safe and Effective Care Environment

1. Explain the physiology of communicable respiratory diseases and the airborne and droplet modes of organism transmission.
2. Apply principles of infection control (e.g., hand hygiene, Isolation Precautions, Airborne Precautions) when providing care to patients with respiratory infections.
3. Use the "ventilator bundle" interventions to prevent ventilator-associated pneumonia.
4. Educate the patient and family about infection control practices for care of a patient who has tuberculosis and lives at home.
5. Prepare to participate in disease-containment activities in the event of an outbreak of H5N1 avian influenza.

Health Promotion and Maintenance

6. Identify adults at highest risk for contracting influenza, pneumonia, tuberculosis, and other respiratory infections.
7. Provide information to everyone about immunization against influenza and pneumonia.
8. Teach everyone the use of specific infection control techniques, especially hand hygiene and Centers for Disease Control and Prevention (CDC) cough/sneeze etiquette, to avoid acquiring and spreading respiratory infections.

Psychosocial Integrity

9. Adjust teaching activities to avoid contributing to patient fatigue.
10. Incorporate behavioral management techniques when reinforcing the need for adherence to drug therapy regimens to treat respiratory infections.

Physiological Integrity

11. Perform focused respiratory assessment and re-assessment.
12. Recognize manifestations of infectious respiratory diseases.
13. Compare the manifestations of pneumonia in the younger adult with those exhibited by the older adult with pneumonia.
14. Provide information to the patient and family about side effects of anti-tuberculosis (TB) therapy and when to notify the health care provider.
15. Administer oxygen therapy to the patient with hypoxemia, and evaluate his or her response.
16. Interpret correctly the TB test results for a person with normal immune function and a person with compromised immune function.

Go to your Companion CD or Evolve at http://evolve.elsevier.com/Iggy/ for *Self-Assessment Questions for the NCLEX Examination* keyed to these Learning Outcomes.

DISORDERS OF THE NOSE AND SINUSES

RHINITIS

Pathophysiology

Rhinitis, an inflammation of the nasal mucosa, is the most common problem of the nose and sinuses. Inflammation can be caused by infection (viral or bacterial) or contact with allergens. Often an allergic rhinitis will make the mucous membranes more susceptible to invasion, and an infection will accompany the allergy. Regardless of the cause, rhinitis is uncomfortable. Usually, however, it does not interfere with the person's ability to meet the *human need for oxygenation and tissue perfusion* because the nose is not the only respiratory passageway.

Allergic rhinitis, often called *hay fever* or *allergies,* is triggered by hypersensitivity reactions to airborne allergens, especially plant pollens or molds. Some episodes are "seasonal" in that they tend to recur at the same time each year and last only a few weeks. *Chronic rhinitis* occurs either intermittently with no seasonal pattern or continuously whenever the person is exposed to allergens such as dust, animal dander, wool, and foods (e.g., seafood). Other causes of rhinitis include a "rebound" nasal congestion from overuse of nose drops or sprays (rhinitis medicamentosa) and chronic nasal inhalation of cocaine.

Acute viral rhinitis (**coryza,** or the common cold) is caused by any one of at least 200 viruses. It spreads from person to person by droplets from sneezing or coughing. Colds are most contagious in the first 2 to 3 days after symptoms appear. Teach everyone to take precautions to avoid spreading infection at this time. Colds are self-limiting unless a bacterial infection occurs at the same time. Complications occur most often in immunosuppressed people and older adults, especially if they live or work in crowded conditions or in group settings (e.g., long-term care facility).

Patient-Centered Collaborative Care

In both acute and chronic allergic rhinitis, the presence of the **allergen** (offending substance) causes a release of natural chemicals, such as histamine, from white blood cells in the nasal mucosa. These chemicals bind to blood vessel receptor sites, causing local blood vessel dilation and capillary leak, leading to edema and swelling of the nasal mucosa. The resulting symptoms include headache, nasal irritation, sneezing, nasal congestion, rhinorrhea (watery drainage from the nose), and itchy, watery eyes.

Viral or bacterial invasion of the nasal passages causes the same local tissue responses as allergic rhinitis. Often the patient also has systemic manifestations, including a sore, dry throat and a low-grade fever.

Management of the patient with any type of rhinitis focuses on symptom relief and patient education. Teach him or her about correct use of the drug therapy prescribed.

Drug therapy, including antihistamines and decongestants, is prescribed but must be used with caution in the older adult because of side effects such as vertigo, hypertension, urinary retention, and insomnia. *Antihistamines* block the chemicals released by white blood cells from binding to receptor sites on blood vessels and nasal tissues, preventing local edema and itching. *Decongestants* work by constricting blood vessels, thus decreasing edema. *Antipyretics* are given if fever is present. *Antibiotics* are prescribed only for bacterial rhinitis. Rhinitis caused by overuse of nose drops or sprays is treated by discontinuing the offending drug. Steroid nasal sprays may be used to decrease the rebound nasal congestion during the first week after discontinuing the drug.

Complementary and alternative therapies may be used to decrease the severity of acute viral rhinitis for some people early in the course of the problem. Common agents used for this purpose are Echinacea, large doses of vitamin C, and zinc preparations such as COLD-EEZE or Zicam. It is not clear how these agents reduce symptom severity or duration of illness, but it is believed they may help increase nonspecific immune function.

Supportive therapy can increase the patient's comfort and help prevent spread of the infection. Instruct the patient about the importance of rest (8 to 10 hours a day) and fluid intake of at least 2000 mL/day (about eight glasses) unless other health problems (e.g., heart failure, chronic kidney disease) limit this amount. Humidifying the air helps relieve congestion. Ways to increase humidity include using a room humidifier, inhaling steam from a pan of boiled water after removing it from the heat, or breathing steamy air in the bathroom after running hot shower water.

The patient is most likely to spread the infection during the first 2 to 3 days after symptoms begin. Teach him or her to reduce the risk of spreading the cold by thoroughly washing hands, especially after nose blowing, sneezing, coughing, rubbing the eyes, or touching the face. Other precautions include staying home from work, school, or places where people gather; covering the mouth and nose with a tissue when sneezing or coughing; disposing properly of used tissues immediately; and avoiding close contact with other people (e.g., kissing, hugging, hand-shaking). Stress the need to avoid close contact with people who are more susceptible to infection, such as older adults, infants, and anyone who has a chronic respiratory problem. An uncomplicated cold typically subsides within 7 to 10 days.

The patient with recurrent allergic rhinitis can have allergy testing to determine the cause. The patient may prevent further episodes by avoiding the allergen or using desensitization therapy. Chapter 22 discusses desensitization in detail.

SINUSITIS

Pathophysiology

Sinusitis is an inflammation of the mucous membranes of one or more of the sinuses. Swelling can obstruct the flow of secretions from the sinuses, which may then become infected. The disorder often follows rhinitis. Other conditions leading to sinusitis include deviated nasal septum, nasal polyps or tumors, inhaled air pollutants or cocaine, facial trauma, nasal intubation, dental infection, or decreased immune function. In chronic sinusitis, the mucous membrane is permanently thickened from repeated inflammation.

The most common organisms causing sinus infection are *Streptococcus pneumoniae, Haemophilus influenzae, Diplococcus,* and *Bacteroides*. Sinusitis most often develops in the maxillary and frontal sinuses. Complications include cellulitis, abscess, and meningitis.

Diagnosis is made on the basis of the patient's history and manifestations. Transillumination (reflection of light through tissues) of the affected sinus is decreased. This can be assessed by having the patient place a lighted penlight tip into the mouth and closing the lips around it in a darkened room. Non-swollen sinuses reflect light through the skin as seen as a red glow on the cheek between the eye and the lip. Sinuses that are swollen or filled with secretions have a reduced or absent glow. Other diagnostic tests for sinusitis include sinus x-rays, endoscopic examination, and computed tomography (CT).

Bacterial sinusitis requiring antibiotic therapy is usually indicated by purulent drainage from one or both nares and lack of response to decongestant therapy (Williamson et al., 2006).

Patient-Centered Collaborative Care

Assess for the manifestations of sinusitis, including nasal swelling and congestion, headache, facial pressure, and pain (usually worse when the head is tilted forward or is in a dependent position). Other manifestations include tenderness to touch over the involved area, low-grade fever, cough, and purulent or bloody nasal drainage.

Nonsurgical Management

Treatment includes the use of broad-spectrum antibiotics (e.g., amoxicillin), analgesics for pain and fever (e.g., acetaminophen [Tylenol, Atasol]), decongestants (e.g., phenylephrine [Neo-Synephrine]), steam humidification, hot and wet packs over the sinus area, and nasal saline irrigations. Teach the patient to increase fluid intake to more than 10 glasses of water or juice per day unless another medical problem requires fluid restriction. If this treatment plan is not successful, he or she may need to be evaluated with sinus films and CT. Surgical intervention may be needed if nonsurgical management fails to provide relief.

Surgical Management

Antral irrigation, also known as *maxillary antral puncture and lavage,* is an outpatient procedure. With the patient under local anesthesia, a large-gauge needle is inserted into the maxillary sinus on the affected side. Fluid or pus is drained from the sinus. The sinus is then irrigated with saline solution, an antibiotic solution, or both.

Other surgical procedures may be used to open the sinus cavities if antral irrigation is not successful. In the Caldwell-Luc procedure, the surgeon makes an incision under the upper lip into the maxillary sinus. The infected mucosa is then removed. With the nasal antral window procedure, the surgeon makes an opening in the front portion of the lower nasal bone to improve drainage through the nares. After either procedure, the patient may have difficulty eating for a few days because of pain and swelling. Chart 33-1 describes the best practices for postoperative care for patients undergoing these procedures. When the ethmoid sinuses need to be opened, the surgeon uses an external incision along the side of the nose from the middle of the eyebrow.

Endoscopic sinus surgery is a common method of diagnosing and treating sinus disorders. Direct inspection of the sinuses through a sinus endoscope is completed with the patient under general anesthesia in a same-day surgical center. The procedure takes only minutes, although the nasal mucosa may take from 4 to 6 weeks to heal. The patient goes home the same day and can return to work in 4 to 5 days. Instruct him or her to use saline nasal sprays frequently (every 2 to 4 hours) to prevent mucosal crusting and promote healing.

DISORDERS OF THE ORAL PHARYNX AND TONSILS

PHARYNGITIS

Pathophysiology

Pharyngitis, or "sore throat," is a common inflammation of the mucous membranes of the pharynx. It accounts for more than 15 million office visits each year in the United States. This condition often occurs with acute rhinitis and sinusitis.

Chart 33-1 BEST PRACTICE FOR PATIENT SAFETY & QUALITY CARE

Postoperative Care for Patients with Sinus Surgery

- Place the patient in the semi-Fowler's position to promote drainage and prevent swelling.
- Perform *gentle* oral hygiene to promote healing and prevent injury to the surgical incision.
- Teach the patient to use ice compresses as prescribed for 24 hours.
- Change the "mustache" dressing under the nose as needed, and record the type and amount of drainage.
- Teach the patient and family to change this dressing.
- Teach the patient to eat soft foods and increase fluid intake.
- Recommend that the patient sleep in a reclining chair or with pillows to keep his or her head at about a 20-degree angle.
- Recommend the use of a room humidifier at night.
- Stress to the patient the need to limit the Valsalva maneuver (no coughing, blowing the nose, or straining at stool) for at least 2 weeks postoperatively to prevent bleeding and tissue damage.
- Teach the patient to take his or her temperature twice daily during the first week after surgery and to report an elevation to 100° F or higher to the surgeon.

Acute pharyngitis can be caused by bacteria, viruses, other organisms, trauma, dehydration, irritants, tobacco use, and alcohol consumption. The most common bacterium causing pharyngitis is group A beta-hemolytic *Streptococcus* (Kamienski, 2007), but most adult cases are caused by a virus. The incidence of infection is highest between late fall and spring, especially in colder climates.

Patient-Centered Collaborative Care

Assessment

The patient with pharyngitis has throat soreness and dryness, throat pain, pain on swallowing (odynophagia), difficulty swallowing (dysphagia), and fever. Viral and bacterial pharyngitis are often difficult to distinguish on physical assessment. When inspecting a throat infected with either virus or bacteria, mild to severe hyperemia (redness) may be seen with or without enlarged tonsils and with or without exudate. Ask about nasal discharge, which can vary from thin and watery to thick and purulent. Lymph node enlargement in the neck occurs with both viral and bacterial pharyngitis. When a tonsillar abscess occurs with pharyngitis, the patient may have a "hot potato" voice—a thickened voice of poor quality.

Bacterial infections are more often associated with enlarged red tonsils, exudate, purulent nasal discharge, and local lymph node enlargement. Chart 33-2 compares the manifestations of viral and bacterial pharyngitis. Viral pharyngitis is contagious for 2 to 3 days. Symptoms usually subside within 3 to 10 days after onset, and the disease is usually self-limiting.

Bacterial pharyngitis, such as group A streptococcal infection, can lead to serious medical complications (Table 33-1), including acute glomerulonephritis and rheumatic fever carditis. Acute glomerulonephritis may occur 7 to 10 days after the acute infection, and rheumatic fever may develop 3 to 5 weeks after the acute infection.

Throat cultures are important in distinguishing viral from a group A beta-hemolytic streptococcal infection; however, the results are not entirely accurate. False-negative cultures

Chart 33-2 **KEY FEATURES**

Acute Viral and Bacterial Pharyngitis

Feature	Viral Pharyngitis	Bacterial Pharyngitis
Temperature	Low-grade or no fever	High temperature (>101° F [38° C], and usually 102°-104° F [39°-40° C])*
Ear manifestations	Retracted or dull tympanic membrane	Retracted or dull tympanic membrane
Throat manifestations	Scant or no tonsillar exudate Slight erythema of pharynx and tonsils	Severe hyperemia of pharyngeal mucosa, tonsils, and uvula Erythema of tonsils with yellow exudate
Neck manifestations	Possible lymphadenopathy	Anterior cervical lymphadenopathy and tenderness
Skin manifestations	No rash	Possible scarlatiniform rash Possible petechiae on chest or abdomen or both
Dysphagia, odynophagia	Present	Present
Other symptoms	No cough Rhinitis Mild hoarseness Headache	No cough Voice characterized by pain on voicing and slurred speech Headache Arthralgia Myalgia
Laboratory data	Complete blood count usually normal White blood cell count usually ≤10,000/mm³ Negative throat culture results	Complete blood count abnormal White blood cell count usually >12,000/mm³* Throat culture results positive for beta-hemolytic streptococcus
Onset	Gradual	Abrupt

*May not be present in adults older than 65 years.

TABLE 33-1 **Complications of Group A Streptococcal Infection**

- Rheumatic fever
- Acute glomerulonephritis
- Peritonsillar abscess
- Retropharyngeal abscess
- Otitis media
- Sinusitis
- Mastoiditis
- Bronchitis
- Pneumonia
- Scarlet fever

can occur, some of which are due to incorrect throat culture technique. The organisms are not uniformly distributed throughout the throat and can be missed during swabbing. To obtain a specimen, rub a sterile cotton swab from a throat culture kit first over the right tonsillar area, moving across the right arch, the uvula, and then across the left arch to the left tonsillar area (Rushing, 2007). Remove the swab without touching the patient's teeth, tongue, or gums. Place the swab back into the tube, cap it, and then crush the glass ampule in the culture tube. Send it to the laboratory as quickly as possible. Results are usually ready in 24 to 48 hours.

Many types of rapid tests and screens for group A beta-hemolytic streptococcal antigen are available. These tests vary in specificity and sensitivity and cost about the same as a culture and sensitivity, but the results are available within minutes. Two common tests are the GenProbe and the Optical Immunoassay (OIA).

A CBC is performed when the patient's condition is severe or does not improve. Patients who need a CBC are those who have high fevers, lethargy, or manifestations of complications. A CBC may indicate other causes of pharyngitis.

When taking a history, ask about the patient's recent contacts (within the past 10 days) with people who have been ill. Specifically ask whether he or she has been ill with symptoms of a cold or upper respiratory tract infection recently. Document any previous history of streptococcal infections, rheumatic fever, valvular heart disease, or penicillin allergy. Because diphtheria *(Corynebacterium diphtheriae)* can cause pharyngitis, ask about and document whether the patient has had a diphtheria immunization.

Interventions

Most sore throats in adults are viral, do not require antibiotic therapy, and respond to supportive interventions. Teach the patient to rest, increase his or her fluid intake, humidify the air, use analgesics for pain, gargle several times each day with warm saline, and use throat lozenges containing mild anesthetics.

The management of bacterial pharyngitis involves the use of antibiotics and the same supportive care provided for viral pharyngitis. For streptococcal infection, an oral penicillin or cephalosporin is prescribed. Drugs from the macrolide class (e.g., azithromycin or erythromycin) are recommended if the patient is allergic to penicillin. *Stress the importance of completing the entire antibiotic prescription, even when symptoms improve or subside.* If the patient cannot tolerate the drug, notify the health care provider so that the antibiotic can be changed. If adherence is a concern or if the patient cannot swallow pills, long-acting penicillin can be given IM in a single dose.

The patient should be re-evaluated if there is no improvement in 3 days or if manifestations are still present after completion of the antibiotic course. Persistent bacterial pharyngitis may occur with immunosuppression. Any patient whose bacterial pharyngitis does not improve with antibiotics should consider human immune deficiency virus (HIV) testing.

A rare complication of pharyngitis in adults is infection of the epiglottis and supraglottic structures (epiglottitis). The epiglottis is a flaplike structure that closes over the trachea during swallowing to prevent aspiration. An inflamed epiglottis can swell and obstruct the airway, causing an emergency that inhibits oxygenation and tissue perfusion. *Any patient with pharyngitis who has stridor or indications of airway obstruction should be immediately evaluated by a health care provider in a setting in which intubation or tracheostomy can be performed quickly and safely* (Rushing, 2007).

AUDIO CLIP: Stridor

Teach the patient how to take his or her oral temperature accurately every morning and evening until the infection resolves. He or she is not contagious after 24 hours of antibiotic therapy. Family members or close contacts who also have a sore throat should be evaluated, and a throat culture may be indicated.

TONSILLITIS

Pathophysiology

Tonsillitis is an inflammation and infection of the tonsils and lymphatic tissues located on each side of the throat. The tonsils are lymphatic tissue shaped like a small almond. Each tonsil is covered by a mucous membrane and has small valleys (crypts) across its surface. Tonsils filter organisms and protect the respiratory tract from infection (McCance & Huether, 2006).

Tonsillitis is a contagious airborne infection. Acute or chronic tonsillitis can occur in any age-group, but it is less common in adults. The infection is usually more severe when it occurs in adolescents or adults.

Acute tonsillitis usually lasts 7 to 10 days and often is caused by bacteria. The most common organism is *Streptococcus.* Other bacterial causes include *Staphylococcus aureus, Haemophilus influenzae,* and *Pneumococcus.* Viruses also cause tonsillitis. Chronic tonsillitis may result from an unresolved acute infection or recurrent infections.

Patient-Centered Collaborative Care

Chart 33-3 lists the manifestations of acute tonsillitis. Diagnostic tests often used to rule out other causes of the sore throat and fever include a CBC, throat culture and sensitivity (C&S) studies, and Monospot test. If respiratory symptoms are present, chest x-rays may be needed. The white blood cell (WBC) count usually is elevated in bacterial infections and normal in viral infections. Throat C&S studies identify the causative organism and direct the choice of drug therapy.

The health care provider prescribes antibiotics (usually penicillin or azithromycin) for 7 to 10 days. Nursing priorities include teaching the patient about supportive care and stressing the importance of completing antibiotic therapy. Teach him or her to rest, increase fluid intake, humidify the air, use analgesics for pain, gargle several times each day with warm saline, and use throat lozenges containing mild anesthetics.

Surgical intervention for tonsillitis may be needed for recurrent acute infections (especially group A beta-hemolytic streptococcal infections), chronic infections that have not responded to antibiotic therapy, a peritonsillar abscess, and enlarged tonsils or adenoids that obstruct the airway. It is usually performed after the patient has recovered from an acute tonsillitis and no infection is present (except with an acute peritonsillar abscess). The procedure may involve complete tonsil removal (for chronic infection) or a partial tonsil removal for obstruction without infection. A common procedure to remove the tonsils is dissection and snare, although laser tonsillectomy, radiothermal ablation tonsillectomy, and tonsil "shaving" are being used increasingly. The adenoids may be removed at the same time. When the patient is an adult, a tonsillectomy and adenoidectomy (T&A) is usually performed with him or her under general anesthesia. After surgery, nursing interventions focus on assessing for airway clearance, providing pain relief, and monitoring for excessive bleeding.

Chart 33-3 KEY FEATURES

Acute Tonsillitis

- Sudden onset of a mild to severe sore throat
- Fever
- Muscle aches
- Chills
- Dysphagia, odynophagia (painful swallowing of food)
- Pain in the ears
- Headache
- Anorexia
- Malaise
- "Hot potato" voice (thickened voice of poor quality)
- Tonsils visually swollen and red with pus
- Tonsils may be covered with a white or yellow exudate
- Purulent drainage may be expressed by pressing a tonsil
- Uvula visually edematous or inflamed
- Cervical lymph nodes usually tender and enlarged

PERITONSILLAR ABSCESS

Peritonsillar abscess (PTA), or *quinsy,* is a complication of acute tonsillitis. The infection spreads from the tonsil to the surrounding tissue, which forms an abscess. The most common cause of PTA is group A beta-hemolytic streptococcus.

Signs of infection are pronounced on examination. Pus forms behind the tonsil and causes one-sided swelling with deviation of the uvula. The swelling may cause the patient to drool, have severe throat pain radiating to the ear, have a voice change, and have difficulty swallowing. He or she may also have a tonic contraction of the muscles of chewing (trismus) and have difficulty breathing.

Outpatient management with antibiotic therapy and percutaneous needle aspiration of the abscess is usually needed. Opioid analgesics may be given IV for the severe pain, and IV steroids may be prescribed to reduce the swelling (Kamienski, 2007). The patient usually improves in 36 hours. *Stress the importance of completing the antibiotic regimen and of coming to the emergency department quickly if symptoms of obstruction appear (drooling and stridor).* Teach him or her about comfort measures (e.g., warm saline gargles or irrigations, an ice collar, analgesics). Hospitalization is required when the airway is in jeopardy or when the infection does not respond to antibiotic therapy. Incision and drainage (I&D) of the abscess, plus additional antibiotic therapy, may be needed. A tonsillectomy may be performed to prevent recurrence.

DISORDERS OF THE LARYNX AND LUNGS

LARYNGITIS

Laryngitis is an inflammation of the mucous membranes lining the larynx and may or may not include edema of the vocal cords. It can occur as a single problem or occur with upper respiratory infections. Laryngitis also can be a manifestation of a related disease process, such as throat or lung cancer. Common causes include exposure to irritating inhalants and pollutants (e.g., chemical agents, tobacco, alcohol, smoke), overuse of the voice, inhalation of volatile gases (e.g., glue, paint thinner, butane), or intubation. An increasingly common cause of recurrent laryngitis is gastroesophageal reflux disease (GERD).

Assess the patient for acute hoarseness, dry cough, and difficulty swallowing. Complete but temporary voice loss (aphonia) also may occur. A laryngeal mirror is used by a physician or advanced practice nurse to examine the larynx visually and to identify inflammation, polyps, edema, or tumor. If suspicious lesions are present, an x-ray, computed tomography (CT), or fiberoptic laryngoscopic examination may be needed. Patients who may have a disorder other than acute laryngitis are referred to an ear, nose, and throat (ENT) specialist (otolaryngologist).

Nursing management is aimed toward symptom relief and prevention. Treatment consists of voice rest, steam inhalations, increased fluid intake, and throat lozenges. The health care provider may prescribe antibiotic therapy and bronchodilators when sinusitis, bronchitis, or other bacterial infection is also present. Teach the patient and family about relief measures, infection prevention, and avoidance of alcohol, tobacco, and pollutants, which can irritate the larynx.

Preventive therapy is aimed toward increasing the patient's and family's awareness of the hazards of tobacco and alcohol use. Emphasize the activities that place an added strain on the larynx, such as singing, cheering, public speaking, heavy lifting, and whispering. Speech-language therapy is used when vocal cord injury occurs with laryngitis and for any voice disorder. For recurrent bouts of laryngitis, further medical and voice evaluations are indicated.

INFLUENZA

Pathophysiology

Influenza, or "flu," is a highly contagious acute viral respiratory infection that can occur in adults of all ages. Epidemics are common and lead to complications of pneumonia or death, especially in older adults or debilitated or immunocompromised patients. Between 5% and 20% of the U.S. population develop influenza each year, and more than 36,000 deaths per year are caused by it (Goldrick & Goetz, 2006). Hospitalization may be required. Influenza may be caused by one of several viruses, usually referred to as *A, B,* and *C.*

The patient with influenza usually has a severe headache, muscle aches, fever, chills, fatigue, weakness, and anorexia. Adults are contagious from 24 hours before symptoms occur and up to 5 days after they begin. Patients who are immunosuppressed may remain contagious for several weeks. Manifestations of sore throat, cough, and rhinorrhea (watery discharge from the nose) generally follow the initial symptoms for a week or longer. Most patients continue to feel fatigued for 1 to 2 weeks after the acute episode has resolved.

Health Promotion and Maintenance

Vaccinations for the prevention of influenza are widely available. The vaccine is changed every year on the basis of which specific viral strains are most likely to pose a problem during the influenza season (i.e., late fall and winter). Usually, the vaccines contain three antigens for the three expected viral strains (trivalent). Influenza vaccinations can be taken as an IM injection (Fluviron, Fluzone) or as a live attenuated influenza vaccine (LAIV) by intranasal spray (FluMist). An **attenuated virus** is a live virus that has been scientifically altered to reduce its ability to cause an infection. The intranasal vaccine is live, and some people develop influenza symptoms after its use. For this reason, its use is recommended only for healthy people up to 49 years of age. People recommended to be vaccinated each year include those older than 50 years, people with chronic illness or immune compromise, those living in institutions, people living with or caring for adults with health problems that put them at risk for severe complications of influenza, and health care personnel providing direct care to patients (Centers for Disease Control and Prevention [CDC], 2007a). The Joint Commission (TJC) recommends that all personnel in hospital settings and other health care institutions be vaccinated annually for influenza as part of meeting National Patient Safety Goal 10 (The Joint Commission [TJC], 2007; Tucker et al., 2008).

Teach the patient who is sick to reduce the risk of spreading the flu by thoroughly washing hands, especially after nose blowing, sneezing, coughing, rubbing the eyes, or touching the face. Other precautions include staying home from work, school, or places where people gather; covering the mouth and nose with a tissue when sneezing or coughing; disposing properly of used tissues immediately; and avoiding close contact with other people (e.g., kissing, hugging, hand-shaking) (Pruitt, 2007). Although handwashing is a good method to prevent transmitting the virus in droplets from sneezing or coughing, many people cannot wash their hands as soon as they have coughed or sneezed. New "etiquette" recommended by the CDC for controlling flu spread is to sneeze or cough into the upper sleeve rather than into the hand (CDC, 2006). (Respiratory droplets on the hands can contaminate surfaces and be transmitted to other people.)

Patient-Centered Collaborative Care

Viral infections do not respond to traditional antibiotic therapy. Antiviral agents may be effective for prevention and treatment of some types of influenza. Amantadine (Symmetrel) and rimantadine (Flumadine) have been effective in the prevention and treatment of influenza A. Ribavirin (Virazole) has been used for severe influenza B. Newer antivirals include zanamivir (Relenza), which is used as an oral inhalant, and oseltamivir (Tamiflu), which is an oral tablet. Both these antivirals prevent viral spread in the respiratory tract by inhibiting a viral enzyme (neuraminidase) that allows the virus to penetrate respiratory cells. These agents may shorten the duration of influenzas A and B if taken within 24 to 48 hours after the onset of manifestations. Both agents also may be used for prevention.

Advise the patient to stay in bed for several days and drink large amounts of fluids unless another medical problem requires fluid restriction (e.g., kidney disease, heart failure).

Saline gargles may ease sore throat pain. Antihistamines may reduce the rhinorrhea. Other supportive and comfort measures are the same as those for acute rhinitis.

DECISION-MAKING CHALLENGE

Coordination of Care

The patient is a 75-year-old woman with severe COPD who lives with her 48-year-old daughter, her daughter's husband, who is 56-years-old, and twin granddaughters age 16. In addition to the COPD, the patient has chronic heart failure after an MI 2 years ago. The daughter is a stay-at-home mom who volunteers on Sundays at the preschool Sunday school program. The son-in-law works nights as a security guard at the local community college.

1. Who in this family should be vaccinated for influenza this year, and with what agent? Provide a rationale for your choices.
2. Which family member(s) is/are most likely to bring influenza home to other family members, and why?
3. What additional precautions should you teach this family to avoid transmitting influenza to the patient?

evolve For suggested answer guidelines, go to http://evolve.elsevier.com/Iggy/.

PNEUMONIA

Pathophysiology

Pneumonia is an excess of fluid in the lungs resulting from an inflammatory process. The inflammation is triggered by many infectious organisms and by inhalation of irritating agents. Infectious pneumonias are categorized as either community-acquired (CAP) or hospital-acquired (nosocomial; known as HAP or HAI), depending on where the patient was exposed to the infectious agent. This distinction is important because hospital-acquired pneumonias are more likely to be resistant to some antibiotics than are CAPs (Flanders et al., 2006).

The inflammation occurs in the interstitial spaces, the alveoli, and often the bronchioles. The process begins when organisms penetrate the airway mucosa and multiply in the alveolar spaces. To do this, they must survive the lung's many defenses against microbial invasion, including the inflammatory response. White blood cells migrate to the area of infection, causing local capillary leak, edema, and exudate. These fluids collect in and around the alveoli, and the alveolar walls thicken. Both events seriously reduce gas exchange and lead to hypoxemia, interfering with *oxygenation and tissue perfusion* and can lead to death. Red blood cells and fibrin also move into the alveoli. The capillary leak spreads the infection to other areas of the lung. If the organisms move into the bloodstream, sepsis results; if the infection extends into the pleural cavity, empyema results.

The fibrin and edema of inflammation stiffen the lung, reducing compliance and decreasing the vital capacity. Alveolar collapse (atelectasis) further reduces the ability of the lungs to oxygenate the blood moving through it. As a result, arterial oxygen tension falls, causing hypoxemia (insufficient oxygen in the blood) and reduced oxygenation and tissue perfusion (McCance & Huether, 2006).

Pneumonia may occur as lobar pneumonia with **consolidation** (solidification, lack of air spaces) in a segment or an entire lobe of the lung or as bronchopneumonia with diffusely scattered patches around the bronchi. The extent of lung involvement after the organism invades depends on the host defenses. Bacteria multiply quickly in a person whose immune system is compromised. Tissue necrosis results when organisms form an abscess that perforates the bronchial wall.

Etiology

In general, people develop pneumonia when their immune systems cannot combat the virulence of the invading organisms. Organisms from the environment, invasive devices, equipment and supplies, staff, or other people can invade the body. Risk factors are listed in Table 33-2. Pneumonia can be caused by bacteria, viruses, mycoplasmas, fungi, rickettsiae, protozoa, and helminths (worms). Noninfectious causes of pneumonia include inhalation of toxic gases, chemicals, and smoke and aspiration of water, food, fluid, and vomitus.

Incidence/Prevalence

In the United States, 2 to 5 million cases of pneumonia occur each year, and it is the seventh leading cause of death (Miskovich-Riddle & Keresztes, 2006). The highest incidence among adults occurs in older adults, nursing home residents, hospitalized patients, and those being mechanically ventilated. Community-acquired pneumonia (CAP) is more common than hospital-acquired pneumonia and occurs in late fall and winter as a complication of influenza. Hospital-acquired pneumonia (HAP) is a common **nosocomial infection** (one that is acquired as a result of transmission during a hospital stay). A specific type of HAP is ventilator-associated pneumonia (VAP). HAP has a 20% to 50% mortality rate; the highest incidence is in those patients infected with *Pseudomonas aeruginosa*, *Acinetobacter*, other "high-risk" organisms, or secondary bacteremia. The mortality rate also is higher in patients who have severe hypoxemia (arterial oxygen <80 mm Hg) and in those who develop widespread atelectasis, pleural effusion, or ventilatory failure.

TABLE 33-2 Risk Factors for Pneumonia

COMMUNITY-ACQUIRED PNEUMONIAS

- Is an older adult
- Has never received the pneumococcal vaccination or received it more than 6 years ago
- Did not receive the influenza vaccine in the previous year
- Has a chronic health problem or other coexisting condition
- Has recently been exposed to respiratory viral or influenza infections
- Uses tobacco or alcohol

HOSPITAL-ACQUIRED PNEUMONIAS

- Is an older adult
- Has a chronic lung disease
- Has presence of gram-negative colonization of the mouth, throat, and stomach
- Has an altered level of consciousness
- Has had a recent aspiration event
- Has presence of endotracheal, tracheostomy, or nasogastric tube
- Has poor nutritional status
- Has immunocompromised status (from disease or drug therapy)
- Uses drugs that increase gastric pH (histamine [H2] blockers, antacids) or alkaline tube feedings
- Is currently receiving mechanical ventilation (ventilator-acquired pneumonia [VAP])

Health Promotion and Maintenance

Of the different types of pneumonia organisms, the most common are 6B, 23F, 14, 9V, 19A, and 19F. All these types plus 17 others are included in the pneumococcal polysaccharide vaccine (PPV23). *Patient education is important in the prevention of pneumonia (Chart 33-4), especially encouraging everyone older than 65 years and those who have a chronic health problem to receive the PPV23.* This vaccine is usually given once; however, some experts believe that older adults and those with chronic health problems could benefit from a second vaccination if more than 5 years have passed since the first vaccination (American Lung Association, 2006).

Other prevention techniques include strict handwashing to avoid the spread of organisms and avoiding large gatherings of people during cold and flu season. Teach the patient who has a cold or the flu to see his or her health care provider if fever lasts more than 24 hours, if the problem lasts longer than 1 week, or if symptoms worsen.

Hospital respiratory therapy equipment should be well maintained and decontaminated or changed as recommended. Use sterile water rather than tap water in GI tubes, and institute Aspiration Precautions as indicated. Specific interventions to prevent aspiration are discussed in Chapter 31.

VAP is on the rise, especially among patients with endotracheal tubes in place for mechanical ventilation (Augustyn, 2007; American Association of Critical-Care Nurses, 2008). Although just having the tube providing a direct connection between the environment and the patient's lower respiratory passageways increases the risk for VAP, the risk can be reduced with conscientious assessment and meticulous nursing care (Hsieh & Tuite, 2006; Tolentino-DelosReyes et al., 2007). Prevention activities can help meet TJC National Patient Safety Goal 7. Three care actions, known as a "ventilator bundle," have been shown to reduce the incidence of VAP—hand hygiene, oral care, and head-of-bed elevation (see the Evidence-Based Practice box on p. 661). Oral care, in particular, can help reduce the risk because many of the most common organisms causing VAP are translocated from the patient's mouth into the respiratory tract (Weitzel et al., 2006). Chart 33-5 lists best practices for preventing VAP.

Chart 33-4 PATIENT AND FAMILY EDUCATION GUIDE

Preventing Pneumonia

- Know whether you are at risk for pneumonia (older than 65 years, have a chronic health problem [especially a respiratory problem], or have limited mobility and are confined to a bed or chair during your waking hours).
- Have the annual influenza vaccine after discussing appropriate timing of the vaccination with your primary health care provider.
- Discuss the pneumococcal vaccine with your primary health care provider, and have the vaccination as recommended.
- Avoid crowded public areas during flu and holiday seasons.
- If you have a mobility problem, cough, turn, move about as much as possible, and perform deep-breathing exercises.
- If you are using respiration equipment at home, clean the equipment as you have been taught.
- Avoid indoor pollutants, such as dust, secondhand (passive) smoke, and aerosols.
- If you do not smoke, do not start.
- If you smoke, seek professional help on how to stop (or at least decrease) your habit.
- Be sure to get enough rest and sleep on a daily basis.
- Eat a healthy, balanced diet.
- Drink at least 3 liters of nonalcoholic fluids each day (unless fluid restrictions are needed because of another health problem).

NCLEX EXAMINATION CHALLENGE

The nurse is providing care to a client who is receiving mechanical ventilation. Which nursing action should be implemented to prevent VAP for this client?

A. Providing oral care every 8 hours.
B. Positioning the client on his or her side.
C. Ensuring the oxygen delivered is humidified.
D. Verifying that the client has received the pneumonia vaccination.

evolve For the correct answer, go to http://evolve.elsevier.com/Iggy/.

Patient-Centered Collaborative Care

evolve ONLINE PHARM REVIEW

The Concept Map on p. 662 addresses assessment and nursing care issues related to patients who have pneumonia. The manifestations of pneumonia differ in older patients compared with younger patients.

Assessment

History

When assessing a patient who may have pneumonia, consider the risk factors for infection (see Table 33-2). Obtain the information from a family member if the patient is confused or too dyspneic. Document age; living, work, or school environment;

Chart 33-5 BEST PRACTICE FOR PATIENT SAFETY & QUALITY CARE

Preventing Ventilator-Associated Pneumonia (VAP)

- If possible, perform oral care with a disinfecting oral rinse right *before* the intubation.
- Do not wear hand jewelry, especially rings, when providing care to ventilator patients.
- Wash hands before and after contact with the patient.
- Provide complete oral care at least every 12 hours.
- Remove subglottic secretions frequently (at least every 2 hours) or continuously (when the endotracheal tube has a separate lumen that opens directly above the tube cuff).
- Keep the head of the bed elevated to at least 30 degrees unless another health problem is a contraindication for this position.
- Verify that an initial x-ray has been obtained to confirm the placement of any nasogastric tube before instilling drugs, fluids, or feedings into the tube.
- Avoid turning the patient or placing him or her in the supine position (even briefly) within an hour after a bolus tube feeding.
- Work with the patient and health care team to assist in the weaning process as soon as possible (see Chapter 34).

Information from Tolentino-DelosReyes, A., Ruppert, S., & Shiao, P. (2007). Evidence-based practice: Use of the ventilator bundle to prevent ventilator-associated pneumonia. *American Journal of Critical Care, 16*(1), 20-27.

diet, exercise, and sleep routines; swallowing problems; presence of a nasogastrointestinal tube; tobacco and alcohol use; past and current use of "street" drugs; and history of drug addiction and injection drug use. Ask the patient about past respiratory illnesses and whether he or she has been exposed to influenza or pneumonia or has had a recent viral infection. Ask about recent skin rashes, insect bites, and exposure to animals.

If the patient has chronic respiratory problems, ask whether respiratory equipment is used in the home. Assess whether the patient's home cleaning level is adequate to prevent infection. Ask him or her when the last influenza or pneumococcal vaccine was received.

Physical Assessment/Clinical Manifestations

First observe the general appearance. Many patients with pneumonia have flushed cheeks, bright eyes, and an anxious expression. The patient may have chest or pleuritic pain or discomfort, myalgia, headache, chills, fever, cough, tachycardia, dyspnea, tachypnea, and sputum production. Severe chest muscle weakness also may be present from sustained coughing.

Observe the patient's breathing pattern, position, and use of accessory muscles. The hypoxic patient may be uncomfortable in a lying position and will sit upright, balancing with the hands. Assess the cough and the amount, color, consistency, and odor of sputum produced.

Crackles are heard with auscultation when fluid is in interstitial and alveolar areas. Wheezing may be heard as a result of inflammation and exudate in the airways. Bronchial breath sounds are heard over areas of density or consolidation. Tactile fremitus is increased over areas of pneumonia, and percussion is dulled in these areas. Chest expansion may be diminished or unequal on inspiration.

In evaluating vital signs, compare the results with baseline values. The patient with pneumonia is likely to be hypotensive with orthostatic changes as a result of vasodilation and dehydration, especially older adults. A rapid, weak pulse may indicate hypoxemia, dehydration, or impending shock. Dysrhythmias may be present as a result of cardiac tissue hypoxia. Common pneumonia manifestations and their causes are listed in Table 33-3.

CONSIDERATIONS FOR OLDER ADULTS

The older adult with pneumonia often has weakness, fatigue, lethargy, confusion, and poor appetite. Fever and cough may be absent, but hypoxemia is usually present. The most common manifestation of pneumonia in the older adult patient is acute confusion from hypoxia rather than fever or cough.

Psychosocial Assessment

The patient with pneumonia often has pain, fatigue, and dyspnea, all of which promote anxiety. Assess anxiety by looking at his or her facial expression and general tenseness of facial and shoulder muscles. Listen to him or her carefully, and use a calm, slow approach to assessment. Because of airway obstruction and muscle fatigue, the patient with dyspnea speaks in broken sentences. Keep the interview short if significant dyspnea or breathing discomfort is present.

▼ AUDIO CLIPS: High- and Low-Pitched Crackles; High- and Low-Pitched Wheezes

EVIDENCE-BASED PRACTICE

Don't neglect basic oral care to prevent VAP

Tolentino-DelosReyes, A., Ruppert, S., & Shiao, P. (2007). Evidence-based practice: Use of the ventilator bundle to prevent ventilator-associated pneumonia. *American Journal of Critical Care, 16*(1), 20-27.

Ventilator-associated pneumonia (VAP) is a serious hospital-acquired infection that results in longer patient stays and significant mortality rates in acute care settings. Prevention of this complication is a focus of TJC National Patient Safety Goal 7, *prevention of healthcare-associated infections.* The Centers for Disease Control and Prevention (CDC) has developed the "ventilator bundle" approach of interventions to prevent VAP. The purpose of the study described in this article was to examine the use of the bundle by nurses before and after an educational intervention; however, its meta-analysis performed on 19 research articles regarding the effectiveness of individual bundle activities on the prevention of VAP is of particular importance in ensuring the use of evidence-based practices. The ventilator bundle for prevention of VAP recommended by the CDC consists of:

- Elevating the head of the bed to between 30 and 45 degrees whenever possible
- Continuously removing subglottic secretions
- Changing the ventilator circuit no more frequently than every 48 hours
- Handwashing before and after contact with each patient

Critical review of research for each action and other factors contributing to VAP development demonstrated that these interventions are effective in preventing VAP when performed in association with the additional modifications or interventions:

- Not wearing hand jewelry (rings) when caring for ventilator patients
- Performing meticulous oral care no less than every 12 hours

Level of Evidence—1. The study provides a meta-analysis of relevant randomized controlled clinical trials.

Commentary: Implications for Practice and Research. Most of the activities recommended by the CDC for prevention of VAP are cost-effective, safe, and feasible. The addition of oral care and not wearing hand jewelry when caring for ventilator patients is also cost-effective, safe, and feasible. The evidence of infections from translocation of mouth organisms to the respiratory tract in particular overwhelmingly supports the need for meticulous oral care, an area often neglected when caring for seriously ill patients. Educating nurses and other care providers in the proper method of providing adequate oral care to patients who are being mechanically ventilated and who may not be alert is essential in preventing VAP.

CONCEPT MAP Bacterial Pneumonia

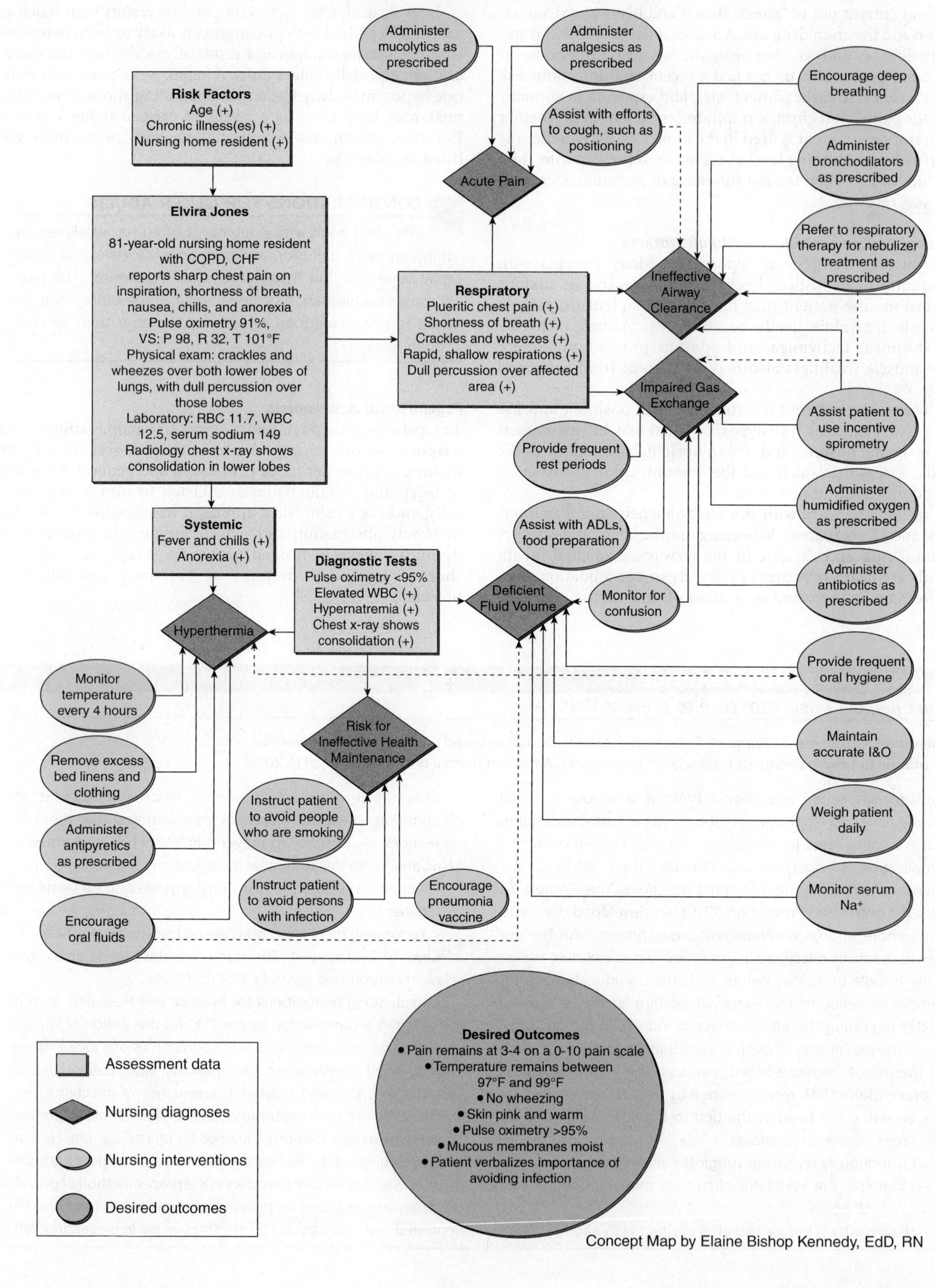
Administer mucolytics as prescribed
Administer analgesics as prescribed
Encourage deep breathing
Risk Factors
Age (+)
Chronic illness(es) (+)
Nursing home resident (+)
Assist with efforts to cough, such as positioning
Administer bronchodilators as prescribed
Acute Pain
Elvira Jones
81-year-old nursing home resident with COPD, CHF reports sharp chest pain on inspiration, shortness of breath, nausea, chills, and anorexia
Pulse oximetry 91%,
VS: P 98, R 32, T 101°F
Physical exam: crackles and wheezes over both lower lobes of lungs, with dull percussion over those lobes
Laboratory: RBC 11.7, WBC 12.5, serum sodium 149
Radiology chest x-ray shows consolidation in lower lobes
Refer to respiratory therapy for nebulizer treatment as prescribed
Respiratory
Plueritic chest pain (+)
Shortness of breath (+)
Crackles and wheezes (+)
Rapid, shallow respirations (+)
Dull percussion over affected area (+)
Ineffective Airway Clearance
Impaired Gas Exchange
Assist patient to use incentive spirometry
Provide frequent rest periods
Administer humidified oxygen as prescribed
Systemic
Fever and chills (+)
Anorexia (+)
Assist with ADLs, food preparation
Diagnostic Tests
Pulse oximetry <95%
Elevated WBC (+)
Hypernatremia (+)
Chest x-ray shows consolidation (+)
Administer antibiotics as prescribed
Deficient Fluid Volume
Monitor for confusion
Hyperthermia
Provide frequent oral hygiene
Monitor temperature every 4 hours
Risk for Ineffective Health Maintenance
Maintain accurate I&O
Remove excess bed linens and clothing
Instruct patient to avoid people who are smoking
Weigh patient daily
Administer antipyretics as prescribed
Instruct patient to avoid persons with infection
Encourage pneumonia vaccine
Monitor serum Na+
Encourage oral fluids
Desired Outcomes
• Pain remains at 3-4 on a 0-10 pain scale
• Temperature remains between 97°F and 99°F
• No wheezing
• Skin pink and warm
• Pulse oximetry >95%
• Mucous membranes moist
• Patient verbalizes importance of avoiding infection
Assessment data
Nursing diagnoses
Nursing interventions
Desired outcomes

Concept Map by Elaine Bishop Kennedy, EdD, RN

Laboratory Assessment

Sputum is obtained and examined by Gram stain, culture, and sensitivity testing; however, the responsible organism often is not identified. A sputum sample is easily obtained from the patient who can cough into a specimen container. Extremely ill patients may need suctioning to obtain a sputum specimen. In these situations, a specimen is obtained by sputum trap (Fig. 33-1) during suctioning. A CBC is obtained to identify **leukocytosis** (an elevated WBC count), which is a common finding except in older adults. Blood cultures may be performed to determine whether the organism has invaded the blood (Coughlin, 2007). An HIV test may be performed. Urine may be examined for blood, pus, or protein, which may occur in the septic patient with pneumonia.

TABLE 33-3 Pathophysiology of Common Clinical Manifestations of Pneumonia

Clinical Manifestation	Pathophysiology
Increased respiratory rate/ dyspnea	Stimulation of chemoreceptors Increased work of breathing as a result of decreased lung compliance Stimulation of J receptors Anxiety Pain
Hypoxemia	Alveolar consolidation Pulmonary capillary shunting
Cough	Fluid accumulation in the receptors of the trachea, bronchi, and bronchioles
Purulent, blood-tinged, or rust-colored sputum	A result of the inflammatory process in which fluid from the pulmonary capillaries and red blood cells moves into the alveoli
Fever	Phagocytes release pyrogens that cause the hypothalamus to increase body temperature
Pleuritic chest discomfort	Inflammation of the parietal pleura causes pain on inspiration

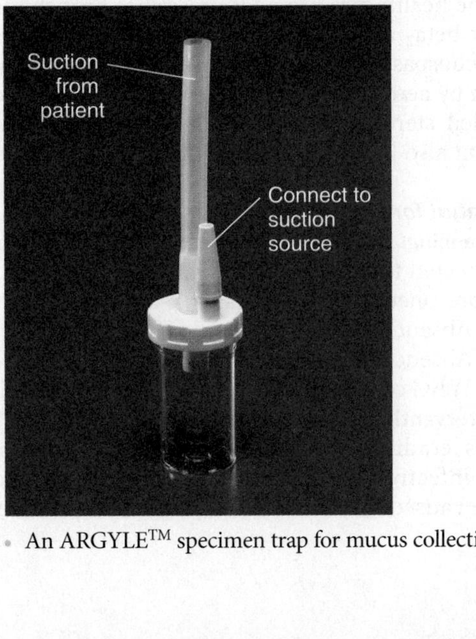
Suction from patient
Connect to suction source

Fig. 33-1 • An ARGYLE™ specimen trap for mucus collection.

In severely ill patients, arterial blood gases (ABGs) may be performed to determine baseline arterial oxygen and carbon dioxide levels and help identify a need for supplemental oxygen. Serum electrolyte, blood urea nitrogen (BUN), and creatinine levels also are assessed. A high BUN level may occur as a result of dehydration. Hypernatremia (high blood sodium levels) occurs with dehydration as a result of fever and decreased fluid intake.

Imaging Assessment

Chest x-ray continues to be the most common diagnostic test for pneumonia but may not show changes until 2 or more days after manifestations are present (Holcomb, 2006). It usually appears on chest x-ray as an area of increased density. It may involve a lung segment, a lobe, one lung, or both lungs. *In the older adult, the chest x-ray is essential for early diagnosis of pneumonia because symptoms are often vague.*

Other Diagnostic Assessment

Pulse oximetry is used to assess for hypoxemia. More invasive tests may be needed, such as transtracheal aspiration, bronchoscopy, or direct needle aspiration of the lung to obtain lower airway specimens. Thoracentesis is most often used in patients who have an accompanying pleural effusion.

DECISION-MAKING CHALLENGE

Delegation/Supervision

The patient is an 82-year-old man with pneumonia who was admitted through the ED. His wife says that he has had a cold for about a week and has been taking over-the-counter cough suppressants. This morning, he said he was too tired to eat breakfast. The wife went to the grocery store and when she returned she found the patient in his pajamas trying to clean the street in front of their home with a vacuum cleaner. When she asked him to come in the house, he did not know which house was his. His admitting vital signs are T, 97.6° F; P, 116, irregular and thready; R, 24 and shallow; BP, 100/56; pulse oximetry, 88%. He is now on your unit.

1. Which person should be assigned to his care today—the UAP, the experienced LPN/LVN, or the RN who is newly licensed? Provide a rationale for your choice.
2. What actions should be taught or stressed to the person assigned to care for this patient?

The admitting orders are: ceftriaxone (Rocephin) 2 g IV piggyback stat, then 1 g every 12 hours; oxygen at 5 L by nasal cannula; vital signs hourly; and 500 mL saline IV bolus stat.

3. What should be performed first, and by whom? Provide a rationale for this choice.

evolve For suggested answer guidelines, go to http://evolve.elsevier.com/Iggy/.

■ ***Analysis***

Common Nursing Diagnoses and Collaborative Problems

Priority nursing diagnoses for patients with pneumonia are:

1. Impaired Gas Exchange related to effects of alveolar-capillary membrane changes
2. Ineffective Airway Clearance related to effects of infection, excessive tracheobronchial secretions, fatigue and decreased energy, chest discomfort, muscle weakness

A primary collaborative problem for the patient with pneumonia is Potential for Sepsis.

Additional Nursing Diagnoses and Collaborative Problems

In addition to the common nursing diagnoses and collaborative problems, patients with pneumonia may have one or more of these:

- Acute Pain related to effects of inflammation of parietal pleura, coughing
- Deficient Fluid Volume related to increased respiratory rate, fever, infection, increased metabolic rate
- Sleep Deprivation related to pain, dyspnea, unfamiliar environment (hospitalization)
- Potential for Pleural Effusion

Planning and Implementation

Impaired Gas Exchange

NOC **Planning: Expected Outcomes.** The patient with pneumonia is expected to have adequate gas exchange. Indicators of adequate gas exchange are:

- Maintenance of Sao_2 of at least 95% or in the patient's normal range
- Absence of cyanosis
- Maintenance of cognitive orientation

Interventions. Interventions to manage impaired gas exchange are similar to those for the patient with chronic airflow limitation (CAL) (see Chapter 32). In pneumonia, oxygen is the gas exchange affected most; therefore hypoxemia is the primary problem. Carbon dioxide retention is not common in pneumonia. Nursing priorities include delivery of oxygen therapy and assisting the patient with bronchial hygiene.

Oxygen therapy is usually delivered by nasal cannula or mask unless the hypoxemia does not improve with these delivery devices. The patient who is confused may not tolerate a facemask. Check the skin under the device and under the elastic band, especially around the ears, for areas of redness or skin breakdown. Other NIC activities for oxygen therapy are listed in Chart 33-6.

Incentive spirometry, also referred to as *sustained maximal inspiration,* is a type of bronchial hygiene used in pneumonia. The objective is to improve inspiratory muscle performance and to prevent or reverse atelectasis (alveolar collapse). Instruct the patient to exhale fully, then place the mouthpiece in his or her mouth, and then take a long, slow, deep breath for 3 to 5 seconds. Evaluate technique, and record the volume of air inspired. Teach the patient to perform 5 to 10 breaths per session every hour while awake.

Ineffective Airway Clearance

NOC **Planning: Expected Outcomes.** The patient with pneumonia is expected to maintain a patent airway. Indicators are:

- Effective cough
- Absence of pallor or cyanosis
- Absence of crackles and wheezes on auscultation
- Pulse oximetry at or above 95%

Interventions. Interventions for ineffective airway clearance for pneumonia are similar to those for COPD or asthma. Because of fatigue, muscle weakness, chest discomfort, and excessive secretions, the patient with pneumonia often has difficulty clearing secretions. Help him or her cough and deep breathe at least every 2 hours. The alert patient may use an incentive spirometer to facilitate deep breathing and stimulate coughing. Chest physiotherapy (CPT or chest PT) is no longer recommended for uncomplicated pneumonia. Dehydration should be avoided, but there is no evidence that hydration helps clear secretions. Encourage the alert patient to drink at least 3 liters of fluid daily unless another health problem requires fluid restriction. Adequate hydration may help thin secretions and make them easier to remove. Monitor intake and output to ensure adequate hydration, especially when fever and tachypnea are present.

Chart 33-6 NIC INTERVENTION ACTIVITIES

The Patient with Pneumonia

Oxygen Therapy: *Administration of oxygen and monitoring of its effectiveness*

- Clear oral, nasal, and tracheal secretions, as appropriate.
- Restrict smoking.
- Maintain airway patency.
- Set up oxygen equipment and administer through a heated, humidified system.
- Monitor the oxygen liter flow.
- Monitor position of oxygen delivery device.
- Instruct patient about importance of leaving oxygen delivery device on.
- Periodically check oxygen delivery device to ensure that the prescribed concentration is being delivered.
- Monitor the effectiveness of oxygen therapy (e.g., pulse oximetry, ABGs), as appropriate.
- Assure replacement of oxygen mask/cannula whenever the device is removed.
- Monitor patient's ability to tolerate removal of oxygen while eating.
- Change oxygen delivery device from mask to nasal prongs during meals, as tolerated.
- Monitor for signs of oxygen toxicity and absorption atelectasis.
- Monitor patient's anxiety related to need for oxygen therapy.
- Monitor for skin breakdown from friction of oxygen device.
- Provide for oxygen when patient is transported.

NIC intervention activities selected from Bulechek, G.M., Butcher, H.K., & McCloskey Dochterman, J. (Eds.). (2008). *Nursing interventions classification (NIC)* (5th ed.). St. Louis: Mosby. No part of this work is to be altered without prior permission from the Publisher.
ABG, Arterial blood gas.

The health care provider prescribes bronchodilators, especially $beta_2$ agonists (see Chart 32-5 in Chapter 32), when bronchospasm is part of the disease process. They are initially given by aerosol nebulizer and then by metered-dose inhaler. Inhaled steroids are used with acute pneumonia when the patient also has bronchial asthma or airway swelling.

Potential for Sepsis

NOC **Planning: Expected Outcomes.** The patient with pneumonia is expected to be free of the invading organism and to return to a pre-pneumonia health status. Indicators are:

- Absence of fever
- Absence of pathogens in blood and sputum cultures
- WBC count and differential within normal limits

Interventions. The key to effective treatment of pneumonia is eradication of the organism causing the infection. Anti-infectives are given for all types of pneumonias except those caused by viruses. The health care provider prescribes

TABLE 33-4 Recommended Drugs for Treatment of Pneumonia in Acute Care Settings

Amikacin (Amikin)	Doxycycline (Adoxa, many others)
Ampicillin/sulbactam (Unasyn)	Gentamicin (Garamycin)
Azithromycin (Zithromax, Zmax)	Imipenem/Cilastatin (Primaxin)
Aztreonam (Azactam)	Levofloxacin (Iquix, Levaquin, Quixin)
Cefuroxime (Ceftin, Kefurox, Zinacef)	Linezolid (Zyvox)
Erythromycin (E-Mycin, E.E.S., many others)	Meropenem (Merrem)
Cefepime (Maxipime)	Metronidazole (Flagyl, many others)
Ceftriaxone (Rocephin)	Moxifloxacin (Avelox, Vigamox)
Cefotaxime (Claforan)	Piperacillin/tazobactam (Zosyn)
Ceftazidime (Ceptaz, Fortaz, Tazicef, Tazidime)	Teicoplanin (Targocid)*
Ciprofloxacin (Ciloxan, Cipro)	Ticarcillin/clavulanate (Timentin)
Clindamycin (Cleocin Phosphate, Cleocin)	Vancomycin (Vancocin)
Clarithromycin (Biaxin)	
Dirithromycin (Dynabac)	

Data from Andriesse, G., & Verhoef, J. (2006). Nosocomial pneumonia: Rationalizing the approach to empirical therapy. *Treatments in Respiratory Medicine, 5*(1), 11-30; Miskovich-Riddle, L., & Keresztes, P. (2006). CAP management guidelines. *The Nurse Practitioner, 31*(1), 43-53.

* Investigational drug.

anti-infective therapy based on whether the pneumonia is community-acquired (CAP) or hospital-acquired (HAP). The exact drug or drugs and their routes of delivery are determined by the severity of the infection, the organism suspected or identified, and whether the patient has other conditions or factors that increase the risk for complications. Table 33-4 lists recommended drugs for treatment of pneumonia. Although standard treatment protocols are recommended, drug therapy choices also reflect the degree of drug resistance in the specific geographic area and in that hospital setting (Andriesse & Verhoef, 2006).

If IV drugs are used, the patient may be able to be switched to oral therapy in 2 or 3 days, depending on the response (e.g., stable clinical condition, afebrile). The course of anti-infective therapy varies with the drug used and the organism(s) involved. Usually anti-infectives are used for 5 to 7 days for a patient with uncomplicated CAP and up to 21 days for an immunocompromised patient or one with HAP.

Drug resistance is becoming increasingly common, especially for infections with *Streptococcus pneumoniae.* This problem is known as *drug-resistant Streptococcus pneumoniae,* or *DRSP.* DRSP is most common among people older than 65 years and among those who became infected as a result of exposure to young children from a day-care environment.

For pneumonia resulting from aspiration of food or stomach contents, interventions focus on prevention of lung damage and treating the infection. Aspiration of acidic substances (e.g., vomitus, stomach contents) can cause widespread inflammation, leading to acute respiratory distress syndrome (ARDS) and permanent lung damage. In these conditions, steroids and NSAIDs are used with antibiotics to reduce the inflammatory response.

NCLEX EXAMINATION CHALLENGE

The 82-year-old client with pneumonia has become increasingly confused, and his Sao_2 has changed from 91% 1 hour ago to 88% now and his respiratory rate has increased from 26 to 32. What is the nurse's first best action?

A. Assist him to a more upright position.
B. Increase the flow rate on his IV piggyback antibiotic.
C. Increase his O_2 flow rate by 2 L and re-assess in 5 minutes.
D. Call the Rapid Response Team or his health care provider.

evolve For the correct answer, go to http://evolve.elsevier.com/Iggy/.

Community-Based Care

The patient needs to continue the anti-infective drugs as prescribed. An important nursing role is to reinforce, clarify, and provide information to the patient and family as indicated.

Home Care Management

No special changes are needed in the home. If the home consists of more than one story, the patient may prefer to stay on one floor for a few weeks, because stair climbing may increase fatigue and dyspnea. Bath and hygiene needs may be met by using a bedside commode if a bathroom is not located on the level the patient is using. Home care needs depend on the patient's level of fatigue, dyspnea, and family and social support.

The long recovery phase of pneumonia, especially in the older patient, can be frustrating and perhaps depressing. Fatigue, weakness, and a residual cough can last for weeks. Some patients fear they will never return to a "normal" level of functioning. It is important to prepare them for the course of the disease and to offer reassurance that complete recovery will occur. Early after discharge, a home health nursing assessment may be helpful (Chart 33-7).

Health Teaching

Review all drugs with the patient and family, and emphasize completing anti-infective therapy. Teach the patient to notify the health care provider if chills, fever, persistent cough, dys-

Chart 33-7 FOCUSED ASSESSMENT

The Patient Recovering from Pneumonia

Ask whether the patient has had any of these:

- New-onset confusion
- Chills
- Fever
- Persistent cough
- Dyspnea
- Wheezing
- Hemoptysis
- Increased sputum production
- Chest discomfort
- Increasing fatigue
- Any other symptoms that have failed to resolve

Assess the patient for:

- Fever
- Diaphoresis
- Cyanosis, especially around the mouth or conjunctiva
- Dyspnea, tachypnea, or tachycardia
- Adventitious or abnormal breath sounds
- Weakness

pnea, wheezing, hemoptysis, increased sputum production, chest discomfort, or increasing fatigue recurs or if symptoms fail to resolve. Stress the importance of getting plenty of rest and gradually increasing exercise.

An important aspect of education for the patient and family is the avoidance of upper respiratory tract infections and viruses. Teach him or her to avoid crowds (especially in the fall and winter when viruses are prevalent), people who have a cold or flu, and exposure to irritants such as smoke. Stress the importance of following his or her health care provider's recommendations for vaccination against influenza and pneumonia. A balanced diet and adequate fluid intake are essential.

Health Care Resources

Inform patients who smoke that smoking is a risk factor for pneumonia. Provide them with information on smoking-cessation classes through the American Lung Association (ALA) and American Cancer Society. The health care provider may prescribe nicotine patches. *Warn the patient of the danger of myocardial infarction if smoking is continued while using the patches.* Urge him or her to enroll in a smoking-cessation program to assist in the nicotine withdrawal process in conjunction with nicotine patches. Provide information booklets on pneumonia provided by the ALA. Urge the patient who has not already been vaccinated against influenza or pneumonia to take this preventive measure when the pneumonia has resolved.

Evaluation: Outcomes

Evaluate the care of the patient with pneumonia on the basis of the identified nursing diagnoses and collaborative problems. The expected outcomes are that he or she:

- Attains or maintains adequate gas exchange
- Maintains patent airways
- Is free of the invading organism
- Returns to his or her pre-pneumonia health status

Specific indicators for these outcomes are listed for each nursing diagnosis and collaborative problem under the Planning and Implementation section (see earlier).

SEVERE ACUTE RESPIRATORY SYNDROME (SARS)

A new respiratory infection was first identified in China early in November 2002. At first appearing as an atypical pneumonia, the infection was termed **severe acute respiratory syndrome,** or **SARS.** In 2003, more than 8600 cases of SARS were reported to the World Health Organization, including 325 cases in North America. Worldwide, more than 700 people died from the disease, with mortality rates highest in less affluent countries (World Health Organization [WHO], 2008).

Pathophysiology

The cause of SARS is a new virus from a family of virus types known as *coronaviruses.* These viruses have ribonucleic acid (RNA) as their genetic material and have many projections that look like a halo or "corona" when examined by electron microscopes. This family of viruses causes many forms of the common cold. The new virus, known as *SARS Co-V,* is a mutated form of the coronavirus and is more virulent than most members of this virus family. The virus infects cells of the respiratory tract, triggering an inflammatory response. It stays in the respiratory passageways rather than spreading into the blood because it grows best at temperatures slightly lower than the normal core body temperature.

The virus is easily spread by airborne droplets from infected people through sneezing, coughing, and talking. It can contaminate surfaces and objects, although it does not survive on nonliving surfaces for long periods. People at greatest risk for SARS are those in close direct contact with an infected person. The portals of entry for infection with the virus are the mucous membranes of the eyes, nose, and mouth.

Patient-Centered Collaborative Care

Assessment

The manifestations of SARS are the same as those of any respiratory infection. Usually, the patient has a fever higher than 100.4° F (38.0° C), a headache, and general body aches. Mild cold symptoms of a runny nose, sore throat, and watery eyes may also be present. Within 2 to 7 days, the patient develops a dry cough and has difficulty breathing. Hypoxia, with cyanosis, low oxygen saturation, and a feeling of breathlessness, indicates more severe illness. Chest x-rays show a pattern similar to pneumonia or other respiratory distress syndromes. Diagnosis is made by the manifestations and the use of a rapid SARS test, the reverse transcriptase-polymerase chain reaction (RT-PCR) that detects SARS-CoV RNA in the blood within 2 days after symptoms begin.

Interventions

No known effective treatment for this infection exists at this time. Standard antibiotic agents and antiviral drugs cannot kill the virus or prevent its replication. Interventions are supportive to allow the patient's own immune system to fight the infection. Oxygen is given when hypoxia or breathlessness is present. Respiratory treatments to dilate the bronchioles and move respiratory secretions are used. If gas exchange is not improved with oxygen therapy alone, intubation and mechanical ventilation may be needed. Antibiotics are used to treat a bacterial pneumonia that may occur with SARS.

Prevention of Infection Spread

Isolating the person with SARS and adhering to strict transmission precautions are effective in containing the infection and preventing an epidemic. These techniques, promoted by the World Health Organization, were successful in preventing a SARS **pandemic,** a general epidemic spread over a wide geographic area and affecting a large proportion of the population. No new cases of SARS have been reported since 2004 (WHO, 2008).

A major nursing responsibility is the prevention infection spread. Handwashing is a key prevention intervention. Gloves may be used but are not a replacement for good handwashing. Use Airborne Precautions and Contact Precautions with patients who are suspected to have SARS. Use gowns and eye protection when coming into direct contact with the patient. Airborne isolation is recommended. When the patient is out of the isolation environment, he or she must wear a mask. If for some reason he or she cannot wear a mask, all other people in the environment should wear a mask.

When performing procedures that normally induce coughing or promote aerosolization of particles (e.g., suctioning, using a positive-pressure facemask, obtaining a sputum culture, giving aerosolized treatments), be sure to protect yourself and other health care workers. Wear a disposable particulate mask respi-

rator (e.g., N-95, N-99, or N-100) and protective eyewear during such procedures. Keep the door to the patient's room closed. Avoid touching your face with contaminated gloves. Wash your hands after you remove the gown, gloves, eyewear, and face shield and whenever you leave the patient's room. Wear clean gloves when disinfecting contaminated surfaces or equipment.

AVIAN INFLUENZA—"BIRD FLU"

Pathophysiology

Many viral infections among animals are not transmitted to humans. Viral infections are common among wild and domestic birds, including chickens and ducks, and usually remain a problem only among birds. A notable exception was the 1918 "Spanish" influenza that resulted in at least 40 million deaths worldwide and perhaps as many as 100 million deaths (Thomas & Noppenberger, 2007). This virus, the H1N1 strain, mutated and became highly infectious to humans. Other Avian viruses have also mutated and caused large epidemics of influenza, including the 1968 and 1997 "Hong-Kong" strains. A new avian virus is the H5N1 strain that has infected millions of birds, especially in Asia, but had not appeared to infect humans. *World health officials are concerned that this strain could mutate to allow first bird-to-human infection and then mutate again to allow person-to-person human infection. This possibility is a major concern because humans have essentially no naturally occurring immunity to this virus and the infection could lead to a worldwide pandemic with very high mortality rates.*

As early as 1997, a few cases of H5N1 infections among humans who had significant contact with infected birds had been discovered. Another small outbreak among humans occurred in 2003.

As of January 2008, 349 cases of H5N1 avian influenza in humans have been reported to the World Health Organization, with a total of 216 deaths (61% mortality rate). These cases have occurred in 14 countries in Asia and the Middle East (WHO, 2008). The majority of human cases have occurred in people who have major contact with infected birds; however, a few of the cases appear to have occurred as a result of person-to-person contact.

The virus spreads in birds by oral-fecal transmission as a result of bird droppings contaminating ponds, lakes, and rivers. The infected bird-to-human transmission is thought to occur by the oral-fecal contamination route. However, because there have been too few cases, it is not known if this is the major transmission route for the person-to-person infections. The rapid onset of symptoms in the patients who contracted the disease from an infected person suggests an airborne droplet route also may promote transmission (Thomas & Noppenberger, 2007). The infection is *not* spread by eating the cooked meat of contaminated birds.

Health Promotion and Maintenance

The prevention of a worldwide pandemic of avian flu is the responsibility of everyone. Health officials have been monitoring the situation with human outbreaks and with testing of both wild and domestic bird species throughout the world. Although vaccine research is ongoing, no effective vaccine is available. Thus the recommended approach to disease prevention is early recognition of new cases and the implementation of community and personal quarantine and social-distancing behaviors to reduce exposure to the virus (WHO, 2008).

Plans for prevention and containment in North America have been developed with the cooperation of most levels of government. When a cluster of cases is discovered in an area, the antiviral drugs oseltamivir (Tamiflu) and zanamivir (Relenza) should be widely distributed. These drugs are not likely to prevent the disease but may reduce the severity of the infection and reduce the mortality rate. The infected patients should be cared for in strict isolation. All nonessential public activities in the area should be stopped. These include public gatherings of any type, attendance at schools, religious services, shopping, and many types of employment. People should stay home and use their emergency preparedness supplies (food, water, and drugs) they have stockpiled for at least 2 weeks (see Chapter 12). Travel to and from this area should be stopped.

Urge all people to pay attention to public health announcements and early warning systems for disease outbreaks. Teach them the importance of starting prevention behaviors immediately upon notification of an outbreak. Teach all people to have a minimum of a 2-week supply of all their prescribed drugs and at least a 2-week supply of nonperishable food and water for each member of the household. They should also have a battery-powered radio (and batteries) to keep informed of updates in an active prevention situation. See Chapter 12 for more information on items to have ready in the home for disaster preparedness. *An avian influenza epidemic is a disaster, and containing it requires the cooperation of all people.*

Patient-Centered Collaborative Care

Care of the patient with avian influenza focuses on supporting the patient and preventing spread of the disease. Both are equally important. The initial manifestations of avian influenza are similar to other respiratory infections—cough, fever, and sore throat. These progress rapidly to shortness of breath and pneumonia. In addition, diarrhea, vomiting, abdominal pain, and bleeding from the nose and gums occur (Sheff, 2006). *Ask whether any patient with these symptoms has recently (within the past 10 days) traveled to areas of the world affected by H5N1. If such travel has occurred, coordinate with the health care team to place the patient in an airborne isolation room with negative air pressure. These precautions remain until the diagnosis of H5N1 is confirmed or ruled out.* Diagnosis is made based on clinical manifestations and positive testing. The most rapid test that is accurate early in the disease course is the H5 polymerase chain reaction test performed at a WHO-approved laboratory. Blood antibody tests also can confirm an H5N1 diagnosis but will not be accurate until the person has been infected for at least 14 days (Pipper et al., 2007).

When providing care to the patient with avian influenza, personal protective equipment is essential. Coordinate the protection activity by ensuring that anyone entering the patient's room for any reason wears a fit-tested respirator (Anderson, 2006). Use other Airborne Precautions and Contact Precautions as described in Chapter 25. Teach other health care workers to self-monitor for disease symptoms, especially of respiratory infection, for at least a week after the last contact with the patient. Use the antiviral drug oseltamivir (Tamiflu) or zanamivir (Relenza) within 48 hours of the first contact with the infected patient. If a vaccine is available, receive it in the recommended two-step process.

No known effective treatment for this infection exists at this time. Standard antibiotic agents and antiviral drugs cannot kill the virus or prevent its replication. Interventions are supportive to allow the patient's own immune system to fight the infection. Oxygen is given when hypoxia or breathlessness is present. Respiratory treatments to dilate the bronchioles and move respiratory secretions are used. If gas exchange is not improved with oxygen therapy alone, intubation and mechanical ventilation may be needed. Antibiotics are used to treat a bacterial pneumonia that may occur with H5N1.

In addition to the need for respiratory support, the patient with H5N1 may have severe diarrhea and need fluid therapy. The transmission precautions may prevent the use of a scale to determine fluid needs by weight changes. Monitor the patient's hydration status, and carefully measure intake and output. The type of fluid prescribed by the health care provider for rehydration therapy varies with the patient's cardiovascular status and the osmolarity of the blood. *The two most important areas to monitor during rehydration are pulse rate and quality and urine output.*

PULMONARY TUBERCULOSIS

Pathophysiology

Tuberculosis (TB) is a highly communicable disease caused by *Mycobacterium tuberculosis.* It is the most common bacterial infection worldwide (WHO, 2008). The organism is transmitted via **aerosolization** (i.e., an airborne route). When a person with active TB coughs, laughs, sneezes, whistles, or sings, droplets become airborne and may be inhaled by others. Far more people are infected with the bacillus than actually develop active TB.

ANIMATION: Tuberculosis ▶

The bacillus multiplies freely when it reaches a susceptible site (bronchi or alveoli). An exudative response occurs, causing a nonspecific pneumonitis. With the development of acquired immunity, further growth of bacilli is controlled in most initial lesions. These lesions usually resolve and leave little or no residual bacilli. Only a small percentage of people initially infected with the bacillus ever develop active TB. The greatest risk for active TB among people who are HIV negative is during the first 2 years after infection.

Cell-mediated immunity develops 2 to 10 weeks after infection and is manifested by a positive reaction to a tuberculin test. The primary infection may be so small that it does not appear on a chest x-ray. The process of infection occurs in this order:

1. The granulomatous inflammation created by the tubercle bacillus in the lung becomes surrounded by collagen, fibroblasts, and lymphocytes.
2. **Caseation necrosis,** necrotic tissue being turned into a granular mass, occurs in the center of the lesion. If this area shows on x-ray, it is called **Ghon tubercle,** or the primary lesion.

Areas of caseation then undergo resorption, degeneration, and fibrosis. These necrotic areas may calcify (calcification) or liquefy (liquefaction). If liquefaction occurs, the liquid material then empties into a bronchus and the evacuated area becomes a cavity (cavitation). Bacilli continue to grow in the necrotic cavity wall and spread via lymph channels into new areas of the lung.

A lesion also may progress by direct extension if bacilli multiply rapidly during inflammation. The lesions may extend through the pleura, resulting in pleural or pericardial effusion. **Miliary** or **hematogenous TB** is the spread of TB throughout the body when a large number of organisms enter the blood. Many tiny, discrete nodules scattered throughout the lung are seen on chest x-ray. The brain, meninges, liver, kidney, or bone marrow can become infected as a result of spread through the blood.

Initial infection is seen more often in the middle or lower lobes of the lung. The local lymph nodes are infected and enlarged. An asymptomatic period usually follows the primary infection and can last for years or decades before clinical symptoms develop. *An infected person is not infectious to others until manifestations of disease occur.*

Secondary TB is a reactivation of the disease in a previously infected person. Reactivation is more likely when defenses are lowered, which may be part of the reason older adults and people with HIV disease are at greater risk for TB. The upper lobes are the most common site of reactivation and are referred to as *Simon's foci.* The American Lung Association's TB classification is shown in Table 33-5.

Etiology

M. tuberculosis is a nonmoving, slow-growing, acid-fast rod transmitted via the airborne route. People who are usually infected are those having repeated close contact with an infectious person who has not yet been diagnosed with TB. The risk of transmission is reduced after the infectious person has received proper drug therapy for 2 to 3 weeks, clinical improvement occurs, and acid-fast bacilli [AFB] in the sputum are reduced.

Incidence/Prevalence

The incidence of TB has been steadily decreasing in the United States, although increases in incidence have been seen in many other countries (CDC, 2007b). In the United States, the people who are at greatest risk for development of TB are:

- Those in constant, frequent contact with an untreated person
- Those who have immune dysfunction or HIV
- People who live in crowded areas such as long-term care facilities, prisons, and mental health facilities
- Older and homeless people
- Abusers of injection drugs or alcohol
- Lower socioeconomic groups
- Foreign immigrants (especially from Mexico, the Philippines, and Vietnam)

TABLE 33-5 American Lung Association Classification of Tuberculosis

Class	Criteria
0	No TB exposure, not infected
1	TB exposure, no evidence of infection
2	TB infection, no disease
3	TB clinically active (patients with completed diagnostic evidence of TB—both a significant reaction to TB skin test and clinical or x-ray evidence of TB)
4	TB: not clinically active (patients with history of TB or abnormal chest x-ray film but no significant TB skin test reaction or clinical evidence)
5	TB: suspect (diagnosis pending); used during diagnostic testing of suspect patients for no longer than 3 months

The incidence of TB among recent immigrants is nearly 10 times that of the native-born American (CDC, 2007b).

Patient-Centered Collaborative Care

Assessment

Early detection of TB depends on subjective findings rather than on observable symptoms. TB has a slow onset, and many patients are not aware of symptoms until the disease is advanced. *A diagnosis of TB should be considered for any patient with a persistent cough or other symptoms compatible with TB, such as weight loss, anorexia, night sweats, hemoptysis, shortness of breath, fever, or chills.*

History

Assess the patient's past exposure to TB. Ask about his or her country of origin and travel to foreign countries where incidence of TB is high. It is important to ask about the results of any previous tests for TB. Also ask whether the patient has had bacillus Calmette-Guérin (BCG) vaccine. The BCG vaccine contains attenuated tubercle bacilli and is used in many countries to produce increased resistance to TB. *Anyone who has received BCG vaccine within the previous 10 years will have a positive skin test that can complicate interpretation.* Usually the size of the skin response decreases each year after BCG vaccination. These patients should be evaluated for TB with a chest x-ray. The effectiveness of BCG vaccine in preventing TB is controversial, and it is not used for this purpose in the United States.

Physical Assessment/Clinical Manifestations

The patient with TB has progressive fatigue, lethargy, nausea, anorexia, weight loss, irregular menses, and a low-grade fever. Manifestations may have been present for weeks or months. Night sweats may occur with the fever. The patient has a cough and mucopurulent sputum, which may be streaked with blood. Chest tightness and a dull, aching chest pain occur with the cough. Ask about, assess for, and document the presence of any of these manifestations to help with diagnosis, to establish a baseline, and to plan nursing interventions.

Physical examination of the chest does not provide conclusive evidence of TB. Dullness with percussion may be heard over involved the lung fields, as may bronchial breath sounds, crackles, and increased transmission of spoken or whispered sounds. Partial obstruction of a bronchus from endobronchial disease or compression by lymph nodes may produce localized wheezing.

Laboratory Assessment

A diagnosis of TB is suggested by the manifestations and a positive smear for acid-fast bacillus. Sputum is obtained, smeared on a slide, and stained with a red dye. After the slide has dried, it is treated with an acid alcohol to remove the stain. TB does not de-stain with this procedure and remains red. *The acid-fast bacillus test is not specific for TB (other organisms are also acid-fast), but it is used as a quick method to determine whether TB precautions should be started until more definitive testing can be completed with either the purified protein derivative two-step procedure or the QuantiFERON-TB Gold.*

Blood analysis by an enzyme-linked immunosorbent assay using the QuantiFERON-TB Gold (QFT-G) is the most sensitive and rapid test for the presence of *M. tuberculosis* (Todd, 2006). Results are ready in 24 hours. Although this test is not recommended for mass or public health screening, it is very useful in the acute care setting to determine whether a symptomatic patient actually has TB.

Sputum culture confirms the diagnosis. Enhanced TB cultures and automated mycobacterial cultures require 1 to 4 weeks to determine a positive or negative result. A newer technique that soon may be in common use and replace sputum culture is the microscopic observation drug susceptibility (MODS) test (Moore et al., 2006). It is an assay that microscopically examines sputum-containing broth for the presence of TB-associated coils and cords. Results are usually available within 7 days. After drugs are started, sputum samples are obtained again to determine therapy effectiveness. Cultures are usually negative after 3 months of treatment.

The tuberculin test (Mantoux test) result is the most commonly used reliable test of TB infection. A small amount (0.1 mL) of purified protein derivative (PPD) is given intradermally in the forearm. An area of induration (not just redness) measuring 10 mm or greater in diameter 48 to 72 hours after injection indicates exposure to and infection with TB. If possible, the site is re-evaluated after 72 hours because the incidence of false-negative readings is greater at 48 hours. *A positive reaction does not mean that active disease is present but indicates exposure to TB or the presence of inactive (dormant) disease.* A reaction of 5 mm or greater is considered positive in people with HIV infection. *A reduced skin reaction or a negative skin test does not rule out TB disease or infection of the very old or anyone who is severely immunocompromised.* Failure to have a skin response because of reduced immune function when infection is present is called **anergy.**

Screening is performed yearly for anyone at high risk for coming into contact with people infected with TB. Screening is particularly important for foreign-born people and migrant workers. Participation in screening programs is enhanced when programs are delivered in a culturally sensitive and nonthreatening manner. Urge anyone who is considered high risk to have an annual TB screening test.

Once a person's skin test is positive for TB, a chest x-ray is needed to detect clinically active TB or old, healed lesions. Caseation and inflammation may be seen on the x-ray if the disease is active. Instruct anyone who has manifestations of TB to seek medical attention. The chest x-rays of HIV-infected patients may be normal or may show infiltrates in any lung zone along with hilar lymph node enlargement.

Common Nursing Diagnoses and Collaborative Problems

Nursing diagnoses and collaborative problems that may apply to patients with TB include:

- Impaired Gas Exchange related to disease progression
- Deficient Knowledge (Infection Control, Therapeutic Regimen, Nutrition) related to lack of exposure or information misinterpretation
- Fatigue related to poor tissue oxygenation and increased metabolism
- Imbalanced Nutrition: Less Than Body Requirements related to increased metabolism, poor appetite, drug regimen, or fatigue
- Social Isolation related to altered state of wellness or changed appearance

Interventions

Combination drug therapy is the most effective method of treating TB and preventing transmission. Active TB is treated with a combination of drugs to which the organism is sensitive. Therapy continues until the disease is under control. The use of multiple-drug regimens destroys organisms as quickly as possible and reduces the emergence of drug-resistant organisms. Current first-line therapy uses isoniazid (INH) and rifampin throughout the therapy; pyrazinamide is added for the first 2 months (Chart 33-8). This protocol shortens the therapy from 6 to 12 months to 6 months. Ethambutol is the recommended fourth drug in first-line therapy. Some of these drugs are now available in two or even three drug combinations. The dosages and precautions are the same as for the individual drugs within the combination. Variations of the first-line drugs along with other drug types are used when the patient does not tolerate the standard first-line therapy (Cohen, 2006; Ruppert, 2007). Nursing interventions focus on patient teaching for drug therapy adherence and infection control.

Strict adherence to the prescribed drug regimen is crucial for suppressing the disease. Thus your major role is teaching the patient about drug therapy and stressing the importance of taking each drug regularly, exactly as prescribed, for as long as it is prescribed. Provide accurate information in multiple formats, such as pamphlets, videos, drug-schedule worksheets. An anxious patient may not absorb information well. You may need to repeat the information and obtain the help of family members. To determine whether the patient understands how to take the drugs, ask him or her to describe the treatment regimen, major side effects, and when to call the health care agency and physician.

The TB drugs may cause the patient to have nausea. Teach him or her to prevent nausea by taking the daily dose at bedtime. Antiemetics may also prevent this problem. Instruct him or her about the need for a well-balanced diet to promote healing. An increased intake of foods that are rich in iron, protein, and vitamins C and B is recommended for the patient with TB. Collaborate with the nutritionist for specialized needs.

The patient with TB may have changes in physical stamina and also faces concerns about the prognosis of the disease. Be realistic in offering a positive outlook for the patient who adheres to the drug regimen. Tell him or her that fatigue will diminish as the treatment progresses. *With current resistant strains of TB, however, emphasize that not taking the drugs as prescribed could lead to an infection that is difficult to treat or has total drug resistance.*

Multidrug-resistant TB (MDR TB) strains are emerging as are strains that are considered extensively drug-resistant (XDR TB), especially among patients who have HIV disease (Trossman, 2008). MDR-TB is an infection that resists INH and rifampin. XDR TB is resistant not only to the first-line anti-tuberculosis drugs but also to the second-line antibiotics, including the fluoroquinolones and at least one of the aminoglycosides. Drug therapy for MDR TB and XDR TB is more limited than standard first-line therapy and requires higher doses for longer periods. *Absolute adherence to therapy for these patients is critical for survival and cure of the disease.*

An area to stress when teaching the patient and family with either MDR TB or XDR TB is that the patient is not resistant to the drugs—the organism is. So, a person who acquires the infection and develops TB from a patient with a resistant strain of bacillus will also have drug-resistant disease. Thus teaching infection control strategies is a priority and should be constantly reinforced.

Other care issues for the patient with TB include teaching about infection prevention and what to expect regarding disease status monitoring and participating in activities. TB is often treated outside the acute care setting, with the patient convalescing in the home setting. Airborne Precautions are not necessary in this setting because family members have already been exposed; however, all members of the household need to undergo TB testing. Teach the patient to cover the mouth and nose with a tissue when coughing or sneezing, to place used tissues in plastic bags, and to wear a mask when in contact with crowds until the drugs suppress infection.

Tell the patient that sputum specimens are needed usually every 2 to 4 weeks once drug therapy is initiated. When the results of three sputum cultures are negative, the patient is no longer infectious and may return to former employment. Remind him or her to avoid exposure to any inhalation irritants because they can cause further lung damage.

The hospitalized patient with active TB is placed on Airborne Precautions (see Chapter 25) in a well-ventilated room. The room should have at least six exchanges of fresh air per minute and should be ventilated to the outside if possible. All health care workers must wear a N95 or high-efficiency particulate air (HEPA) respirator when caring for the patient (Fig. 33-2). When hand and clothing contamination is a risk, implement Standard Precautions by using appropriate barrier protection (i.e., gowns and gloves). Perform thorough handwashing before and after patient care. Precautions are discontinued when the patient is no longer considered infectious.

Community-Based Care

Home Care Management

Most patients with TB are managed outside the hospital; however, patients may be diagnosed with TB while in the hospital if pneumonia is suspected or other complications exist. Discharge may be delayed if the living situation is high risk or if nonadherence is likely. Collaborate with the case manager or social service worker in the hospital or the community health nursing agency to ensure that the patient is discharged to the appropriate environment with continued supervision.

Health Teaching

Teach the patient to follow the drug regimen exactly as prescribed and always to have a supply on hand. Teach about side effects and ways of reducing them to ensure adherence. Remind him or her that the disease is usually no longer contagious after drugs have been taken for 2 to 3 consecutive weeks and clinical improvement is seen; however, *he or she must continue with the prescribed drugs for 6 months or longer as prescribed.* Directly observed therapy (DOT), in which the nurse or other health care provider watches the patient swallow the drugs, may be indicated in some situations. This practice contributes to more treatment successes, fewer relapses, and less drug resistance.

The patient who has weight loss and severe lethargy should gradually resume his or her usual activities. Proper nutrition must be maintained to prevent recurrence of infection.

To help with concerns about the contagious aspect of the infection, provide the patient with information about TB. A key to preventing transmission is identifying those in close

Chart 33-8 COMMON EXAMPLES OF DRUG THERAPY

First-Line Treatment for Tuberculosis

Drug/Usual Dosage	Purpose/Action	Nursing Interventions	Rationales
Isoniazid (INH) 200-300 mg orally daily or 600-900 mg orally twice each week	Kills actively growing mycobacteria outside the cell and inhibits the growth of dormant bacteria inside macrophages and caseating granulomas.	Teach the patient to take the drug on an empty stomach (1 hour before or 2 hours after meals) and to avoid antacids.	Food and antacids slow or prevent absorption of the drug from the GI tract.
		Teach the patient to take a daily multiple vitamin that contains the B-complex vitamins while on this drug.	Drug can deplete the body of this vitamin.
		Remind the patient to avoid drinking alcoholic beverages while on this drug.	The drug can cause liver damage. This effect is potentiated by alcohol.
		Teach the patient to report darkening of the urine, a yellow appearance to the skin or whites of the eyes, and an increased tendency to bruise or bleed.	These manifestations may indicate liver toxicity or failure.
Rifampin (RIF) 500-600 mg orally daily or twice each week	Kills slower-growing organisms, even those that reside in macrophages and caseating granulomas.	Teach the patient to expect the drug to stain the skin and urine and expect all other secretions to have a reddish-orange tinge; also, soft contact lenses will become permanently stained.	This is an expected and harmless side effect of the drug and will clear some time after the patient stops taking the drug.
		Teach women using oral contraceptives to use an additional method of contraception while taking this drug and for 1 month after stopping the drug.	This drug reduces the effectiveness of oral contraceptives, increasing the risk for an unplanned pregnancy.
		Remind the patient to avoid drinking alcoholic beverages while on this drug.	The drug can cause liver damage. This effect is potentiated by alcohol.
		Teach the patient to report darkening of the urine, a yellow appearance to the skin or whites of the eyes, and an increased tendency to bruise or bleed.	These manifestations may indicate liver toxicity or failure.
		Ask the patient about all other drugs in use.	This drug interacts with many drugs.
Pyrazinamide (PZA) 1000-2000 mg orally daily or 3000-6000 mg orally twice each week	Is not inactivated by the acidic environment of macrophages and can effectively kill organisms residing within them.	Ask whether the patient has ever had gout.	This drug increases uric acid formation and will make gout worse.
		Teach the patient to drink at least 8 ounces of water when taking this tablet and to increase fluid intake.	More fluids help prevent uric acid from precipitating and causing gout or kidney problems.
		Teach the patient to wear protective clothing, a hat, and sunscreen when going outdoors in the sunlight.	The drug causes photosensitivity and greatly increases the risk for sunburn.
		Remind the patient to avoid drinking alcoholic beverages while on this drug.	The drug can cause liver damage. This effect is potentiated by alcohol.
		Teach the patient to report darkening of the urine, a yellow appearance to the skin or whites of the eyes, and an increased tendency to bruise or bleed.	These manifestations may indicate liver toxicity or failure.
Ethambutol (EMB) 750-1500 mg orally daily or 2500-5000 mg orally twice each week	Inhibits bacterial RNA synthesis, thus suppressing bacterial growth. It is slow-acting and is bacteriostatic rather than bactericidal. Thus is must be used in combination with other anti-TB drugs.	Remind the patient to avoid drinking alcoholic beverages while on this drug.	The drug induces severe nausea and vomiting when alcohol is ingested.
		Teach the patient to report any changes in vision, such as reduced color vision, blurred vision, or reduced visual fields, immediately to his or her health care provider.	The drug can cause optic neuritis, especially at high doses, and can lead to blindness. When the problem is discovered early, the eye problems are usually reversed when the drug is stopped.
		Ask whether the patient has ever had gout.	This drug increases uric acid formation and will make gout worse.
		Teach the patient to drink at least 8 ounces of water when taking this tablet and to increase fluid intake.	More fluids help prevent uric acid from precipitating and causing gout or kidney problems.

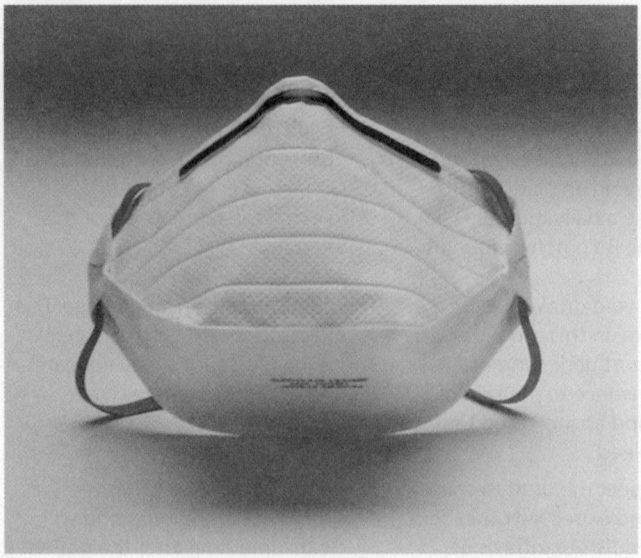

Fig. 33-2 • A high-efficiency particulate air (HEPA) respirator used in the care of patients with active or "rule-out" tuberculosis.

contact with the infected person so that they can be tested and treated if needed. Health care professionals have an important role in this aspect of care. Identified contacts are assessed with a TB test and possibly a chest x-ray to determine TB infection status. Multidrug therapy may be indicated as a preventive strategy for heavily exposed individuals or for those who have other health problems that reduce the immune response.

Health Care Resources

Teach the patient to receive follow-up care by a health care provider for at least 1 year during active treatment. The American Lung Association (ALA) can provide free information to the patient about the disease and its treatment. In addition, Alcoholics Anonymous and other health care resources for patients with alcoholism are available if needed. Assist the patient who uses illicit drugs to locate a drug treatment program. Urge smokers to quit, and assist them in finding an appropriate smoking-cessation program.

DECISION-MAKING CHALLENGE
Coordination of Care

The patient is a 55-year-old migrant worker from Mexico who is working in the orchards of Michigan in September. He is being seen as part of a TB screening program at a mobile clinic sponsored by a local university (staffed by nursing students and medical students under the supervision of their faculty). The patient is thin and has a productive cough that he says he has had for 2 years. He smokes two packs of cigarettes daily and drinks beer on the weekends. On Monday, he, along with all his co-workers at the apple farm, received a PPD test. Today (Wednesday), when you read the test, he has a 2-mm area of induration around the injection site.

1. What risk factors does this patient have for TB?
2. Does the PPD response indicate a negative test, old TB, or currently active TB?
3. What questions should you ask this patient?
4. What follow-up should he receive?
5. What are the teaching priorities for this patient until he is seen again?

evolve For suggested answer guidelines, go to http://evolve.elsevier.com/Iggy/.

LUNG ABSCESS

Pathophysiology

A lung abscess is a localized area of lung destruction caused by liquefaction necrosis, which is usually related to pyogenic bacteria. Patients with this problem often have a history of pneumonia, aspiration of mouth or stomach contents, or obstruction as a result of a tumor or foreign body. Other causes of aspiration leading to lung abscess formation include any condition that alters the ability to swallow, such as alcoholic blackouts, seizure disorders, other neurologic deficits, and swallowing disorders. Bronchial obstruction may cause a necrotizing process in the lung that eventually becomes an abscess.

Multiple abscesses and cavities form in patients with tuberculosis (TB) or fungal infections of the lung. Immunosuppressed patients, such as those receiving chemotherapy or those with a disease such as leukemia or acquired immune deficiency syndrome (AIDS), are at high risk for fungal infections. Most common organisms are anaerobic bacteria, *Staphylococcus* or other gram-positive organisms, or gram-negative or opportunistic infections such as fungi.

Patient-Centered Collaborative Care

Ask the patient about any recent history of influenza, pneumonia, febrile illness, cough, and foul-smelling sputum production. Ask about the sputum color and odor and about any **pleuritic chest pain** (a stabbing pain upon taking a deep breath). Often the patient is febrile, pale, fatigued, and cachectic. Auscultation may reveal decreased breath sounds, and there is dullness on percussion in the involved area. Bronchial breath sounds and crackles are often heard over the site of the lesion. A chest x-ray and sputum samples are needed for the diagnosis.

Nursing diagnoses and interventions for the patient with pneumonia also apply to the patient with a lung abscess. Treatment involves antibiotics and drainage of the abscess. More than one antibiotic may be prescribed. Provide frequent mouth care, and observe for oral overgrowth of *Candida albicans,* especially in older adults.

INHALATION ANTHRAX

Pathophysiology

Inhalation anthrax (also known as *respiratory anthrax*) is a bacterial infection caused by the gram-positive, rod-shaped organism *Bacillus anthracis,* which lives as a spore in contaminated soil. Infection with this organism can occur through the skin, the intestinal tract, or the lungs. *Inhalation anthrax is a rare natural occurrence in the United States, but it has a fatality rate of nearly 100% without treatment. It is not spread by person-to-person contact. Because the inhalation form of the disease is so rare, any occurrence is considered unnatural or an intentional act of bioterrorism.*

This organism first forms a **spore,** an encapsulated organism that is inactive. When many spores are inhaled into the deep parts of the lungs, macrophages engulf them. Once inside the macrophage, the organism leaves its capsule and replicates. The active bacteria produce several toxins that they release into the infected tissues and the blood. These toxins increase the virulence of the organism by creating massive edema in infected tissues, suppressing neutrophil action, causing hemorrhage, and destroying both lung cells and white blood cells. The infected macrophages carry the organisms to the lymph nodes. From these nodes, the organisms can enter the blood and spread rapidly, causing sepsis and meningitis.

Patient-Centered Collaborative Care

Assessment

Inhalation anthrax is a two-stage illness, and manifestations may not begin until as long as 8 weeks after exposure to the organism. Manifestations are listed in Chart 33-9.

The prodromal stage is the first stage and is difficult to distinguish from influenza or pneumonia. Manifestations are nonspecific. In this stage, patients have a fever, some fatigue, mild chest pain, and a dry, harsh cough. *A special feature of inhalation anthrax is that it is not accompanied by upper respiratory manifestations of rhinitis, headache, watery eyes, or sore throat.* Usually, the patient starts to feel better and symptoms improve in 2 to 4 days.

Although diagnosis is difficult at this stage, if the patient begins appropriate antibiotic therapy, the likelihood of survival is high. Diagnostic tests may show a slightly elevated white blood cell count with increasing numbers of band neutrophils. Other indicators of inhalation anthrax that may be detectable at this time are positive Gram stain of the serum and a mediastinal "widening" on chest x-ray as the lymph nodes in the area greatly enlarge. After several days, blood cultures may be positive for the organism and the genetic material of the bacteria may be detected through the amplification process of the polymerase chain reaction (PCR). These more definitive diagnostic tests may not be evident, however, until the disease has progressed to the fulminant stage.

The fulminant stage is the second stage and begins after the patient feels a little better. Usually there is a sudden onset of a feeling of breathlessness. This sensation rapidly progresses to severe respiratory distress, dyspnea, diaphoresis, stridor on inhalation and exhalation, and cyanosis. The patient has a high fever. Mediastinitis and pleural effusions develop. As the disease spreads through the blood, causing septic shock and meningitis, death often occurs within 24 to 36 hours after the onset of breathlessness even if antibiotics are started in this stage.

Chart 33-9 KEY FEATURES

Inhalation Anthrax

Prodromal Stage (early)	Fulminant Stage (late)
Fever	Sudden onset of breathlessness
Fatigue	Dyspnea
Mild chest pain	Diaphoresis
Dry cough	Stridor on inhalation and exhalation
No manifestations of upper respiratory infection	Hypoxia
Mediastinal "widening" on chest x-ray	High fever
	Mediastinitis
	Pleural effusion
	Hypotension
	Septic shock

Interventions

The naturally occurring organism has a cell wall and is sensitive to many antibiotics, including the penicillins and the cephalosporins; however, it is thought that organisms grown for bioterrorism may have been altered to be resistant to these antibiotics. Therefore the antibiotics used for suspected or diagnosed inhalation anthrax include combination therapy with ciprofloxacin, doxycycline, and amoxicillin (Chart 33-10). The same drugs are used individually in oral form for prophylaxis when people have been exposed to inhalation anthrax.

Teach patients with any type of lower respiratory infection to be especially vigilant for changes after they think they are getting well. They need to seek medical attention immediately upon having a setback that starts with breathlessness.

PULMONARY EMPYEMA

Pathophysiology

Empyema is a collection of pus in the pleural space. The most common cause of empyema is pulmonary infection, lung abscess, or infected pleural effusion. Pneumonia or lung abscess can spread across the pleura. Lymph node obstruction can cause a **retrograde** (backward) flood of infected lymph into the pleural space. In addition, a liver abscess or abdominal abscess can spread through the lymphatic system into the lung area. Thoracic surgery and chest trauma can introduce bacteria directly into the pleural space, leading to empyema. Blood from trauma may collect in the pleural space. Poor drainage of this blood promotes infection.

Chart 33-10 COMMON EXAMPLES OF DRUG THERAPY

Prophylaxis and Treatment of Inhalation Anthrax

Prophylaxis	Treatment
Ciprofloxacin (Cipro) 500 mg orally twice daily	Ciprofloxacin (Cipro IV) 400 mg IV every 12 hr
Or	*Or*
Doxycycline (Vibramycin) 100 mg orally twice daily	Doxycycline (Doxy 100) 100 mg IV every 12 hr
Or (if organism is proven susceptible to penicillin)	***Plus** one or two of the following secondary agents (parenteral form; dosage based on patient's weight and age)*
Amoxicillin (Amoxil, Trimox) 500 mg orally every 8 hr	Rifampin (RIF) Clindamycin (Cleocin) Vancomycin (Vancocin, Vancoled)
Prophylaxis must continue for 60 days (or longer if exposure was heavy).	**Treatment with IV drugs continues for at least 7 days. When the response is good and the patient improves, IV drugs are changed to oral agents and are continued for at least 60 days.**

Patient-Centered Collaborative Care

Important history findings include recent febrile illness (including pneumonia), chest pain, dyspnea, cough, and trauma. Observe and document the character of the sputum. Chest wall motion may be reduced on physical examination. If a pleural effusion is present, fremitus may be decreased or absent on palpation, percussion may sound flat, and breath sounds are decreased on auscultation. With compression of lung tissue near the effusion, abnormal breath sounds include bronchial breath sounds, egophony, and whispered pectoriloquy.

Ask about fever, chills, night sweats, and weight loss. If there is cardiac compromise, the patient may be hypotensive because of a mediastinal deviation. Assess the point of maximal impulse (PMI) because it may be displaced on cardiac palpation.

A chest x-ray is ordered, and a sample of the pleural fluid is obtained via thoracentesis for help in making the diagnosis. Empyema fluid is thick, opaque, exudative, and foul smelling. The pleural fluid is sent to the laboratory and is analyzed for color, red blood cell count, white blood cell count and differential, glucose and protein levels, lactate dehydrogenase (LDH), and pH. Gram stains, acid-fast stains, and cytology studies are also performed. A protein level higher than 3 g/100 mL indicates an exudative process.

Therapy for empyema is focused on emptying the empyema cavity, re-expanding the lung, and controlling the infection. Antibiotics appropriate for the identified organism are prescribed. Closed-chest drainage is used to promote lung expansion. The health care provider places one or more chest tubes in the lower parts of the empyema sac. Underwater seal drainage is used without suction initially, but suction may be added if the lung fails to expand with gravity drainage alone. The tube is removed when the lung is fully expanded and the infection is under control. Open thoracotomy and removal of a portion of the pleura may be needed for thick pus or marked pleural thickening. Nursing interventions are similar to those for patients with a pleural effusion, pneumothorax, or infection. Chapter 32 describes these interventions in detail.

HUMAN NEEDS NURSING CARE REVIEW

What might you NOTICE if the patient is experiencing inadequate oxygenation and tissue perfusion as a result of a respiratory infection?

- Respirations rapid and shallow
- Decreased oxygen saturation by pulse oximetry
- Skin cyanosis or pallor (lighter-skinned patients)
- Cyanosis or pallor of the lips and oral mucous membranes (in patients of any skin color)
- Tachycardia
- Patient appears to work hard to inhale and exhale
- Patient is restless, anxious, or confused

What should you INTERPRET and how should you RESPOND to a patient experiencing inadequate oxygenation and tissue perfusion as a result of an acute critical respiratory problem?

Perform and interpret physical assessment, including:
- Taking vital signs
- Auscultating all lung fields
- Monitoring oxygen saturation by pulse oximetry
- Checking the accuracy of pulse oximetry readings
- Assessing cognition (mini-mental status exam)
- Assessing for the presence and characteristic of sputum production
- Assessing the patient's ability to cough and clear the airway

Interpret laboratory values:
- Elevated white blood cell count
- Arterial blood gas values: pH lower than 7.35, HCO_3^- at or below 24 mm Hg, $Paco_2$ at or below 45 mm Hg; Pao_2 below 90 mm Hg

Respond by:
- Administering oxygen
- Assisting the patient to an upright position, with arms resting on a table or armrests
- Performing or assisting the patient to perform chest physiotherapy/pulmonary hygiene
- Prioritizing and pacing activities to prevent fatigue
- Administering prescribed IV, oral, or inhaled drugs
- Administering respiratory therapy treatments or collaborating with the respiratory therapist to administer these treatments
- Re-assessing respiratory status after respiratory therapy treatment
- Ensuring a fluid intake of at least 3 liters per day

On what should you REFLECT?
- Observe patient for evidence of improved oxygenation (see Chapter 29).
- Think about what patient teaching focus could help reduce the occurrence of a respiratory infection in the future.

GET READY FOR THE NCLEX EXAMINATION!

Key Points

Review these Key Points for each NCLEX Examination Client Needs Category.

Safe and Effective Care Environment
- Teach patients with respiratory infections to limit infection spread by washing hands after blowing the nose or using a tissue.
- Remind patients that colds are most easily spread to others during the first 2 to 3 days after symptoms begin.
- Ask any patient with a respiratory infection if he or she is from a foreign country or has recently visited a foreign country.
- Ask patients from other countries whether they have had BCG as a vaccination against TB. Patients who have had

BCG usually have a large, positive reaction to a PPD skin test, making the test less reliable as an indicator of active TB disease.

- Use Airborne Precautions for any patient who has TB or SARS manifestations until proven otherwise.
- Keep the door to the room of any patient with a respiratory infection closed until the cause of the infection is identified.

Health Promotion and Maintenance

- Teach everyone the "etiquette" of sneezing or coughing into the upper sleeve rather than the hand when a tissue is not available.
- Receive a yearly influenza vaccination because you come into contact more frequently with infected people and also because you can have a mild or subclinical case of influenza and spread it to people who are immunocompromised.
- Urge all adults older than 50 years, anyone who has a chronic respiratory problem, anyone who is immunocompromised to any degree, and anyone who lives with a person who is older, immunocompromised, or has a chronic respiratory disease to receive yearly influenza vaccinations.
- Urge all adults older than 50 years, anyone who has a chronic respiratory problem, anyone who is immunocompromised to any degree, and anyone who lives with a person who is older or immunocompromised or has a chronic respiratory disease to receive the pneumonia vaccination.
- Stress to patients that they should complete the drug regimen for any respiratory infection for which anti-infective therapy has been prescribed.
- Urge all people to quit smoking or using tobacco in any form.
- Encourage family members of patients with TB who live at home to ensure good ventilation of the home with open windows whenever possible.
- Teach all people to be prepared for an emergency or disaster by having sufficient food, water, and prescribed drugs for at least 2 weeks (see Chapter 12).
- Teach all people to follow community infection containment procedures if there is a possible outbreak of H5N1 in the area.

Psychosocial Integrity

- Assess any older patient who has acute confusion for pneumonia (remembering that he or she may not have a cough or fever).
- Assure the family of an older adult patient with pneumonia who is confused that the new-onset confusion is temporary.
- Reassure the patient who feels depressed by the degree of fatigue felt and the activity intolerance experienced that the recovery times for influenza and pneumonia are long (weeks to months), especially for the older adult.
- Teach people who may be afraid of contracting inhalational anthrax that this disease is not transmitted by person-to-person contact.
- Inform patients who have a positive TB test that far more people are infected with the bacillus than have active TB disease.
- Assess the likelihood of adherence to the drug regimen for patients with TB.
- Identify patients who may require a directly observed therapy (DOT) program in which they must be directly observed by a health care professional while swallowing the drug.
- Assess the degree of social interaction for patients receiving drug therapy for active TB on an outpatient basis.

Physiological Integrity

- Administer humidified oxygen therapy to patients with hypoxemia.
- Assess the skin under and around a facemask or nasal cannula for evidence of skin breakdown at least every 8 hours.
- Teach all patients with a respiratory infection of bacterial origin to complete all anti-infective therapy as prescribed.
- Urge patients to limit the use of decongestant nasal sprays to no more than 4 days.
- Teach patients with allergic rhinitis to avoid contact with the offending allergen(s).
- Caution older adults using antihistamines that these drugs may make hypertension worse.
- Treat epiglottitis in an adult as an emergency because it can lead to complete respiratory obstruction.
- Assess the patient receiving first-line drug therapy for TB for any manifestation of liver impairment (dark urine, clay-colored stools, anorexia, jaundiced sclera or hard palate).
- Teach women taking rifampin or rifapentine as drug therapy for TB that these drugs reduce the effectiveness of oral contraceptives and that an additional form of birth control should be used while on this therapy.

Additional Study Resources

Go to your Companion CD or Evolve at http://evolve.elsevier.com/Iggy/ for *Self-Assessment Questions for the NCLEX Examination.*

Go to Evolve at http://evolve.elsevier.com/Iggy/ for *Prioritization and Delegation Questions for the NCLEX Examination.*

SELECTED BIBLIOGRAPHY

Asterisk indicates a classic or definitive work on this subject.

American Association of Critical-Care Nurses (AACN). (2008). Ventilator-associated pneumonia. *Critical Care Nurse, 28*(3), 83-85.

American Lung Association. (2006). *Pneumonia fact sheet.* Retrieved January 2008, from www.lungusa.org/site/pp.asp?c=dvLUK9O0E&b=35692#2.

Anderson, E. (2006). Avian flu: Are you prepared to fight a pandemic? *American Association of Occupational Health Nursing Journal, 54*(1), 8-10.

Andriesse, G., & Verhoef, J. (2006). Nosocomial pneumonia: Rationalizing the approach to empirical therapy. *Treatments in Respiratory Medicine, 5*(1), 11-30.

Augustyn, B. (2007). Ventilator-associated pneumonia: Risk factors and prevention. *Critical Care Nurse, 27*(4), 32-39.

Bulechek, G.M., Butcher, H.K., & McCloskey Dochterman, J. (Eds.). (2008). *Nursing interventions classification (NIC)* (5th ed.). St. Louis: Mosby.

*Centers for Disease Control and Prevention (CDC). (2001). Notice to readers: Considerations for distinguishing influenza-like illness from inhalational anthrax. *Morbidity and Mortality Weekly Report, 50*(44), 984-986.

Centers for Disease Control and Prevention (CDC). (2006). *Cover your cough.* Retrieved January 2008, from www.cdc.gov/flu/protect/covercough.htm.

Centers for Disease Control and Prevention (CDC). (2007a). 2007-2008 Prevention & control of influenza: Recommendations of the Advisory Committee on Immunization Practices (ACIP). *Morbidity and Mortality Weekly Report, 56*(RR06), 1-54.

Centers for Disease Control and Prevention (CDC). (2007b). *Trends in tuberculosis, 2006. TB Elimination Division.* Retrieved January 2008, from www.cdc.gov/tb.

Cohen, S. (2006). Diagnosis and treatment of tuberculosis. *The Journal for Nurse Practitioners, 2*(6), 390-396.
Coughlin, A. (2007). Combating community-acquired pneumonia. *Nursing2007, 37*(2), 64hn1-64hn3.
Flanders, S., Collard, H., & Saint, S. (2006). Nosocomial pneumonia: State of the science. *American Journal of Infection Control, 34*(2), 84-93.
Goldrick, B. (2005). Infection in the older adult. *American Journal of Nursing, 105*(6), 31-34.
Goldrick, B., & Goetz, A. (2006). 'Tis the season for influenza. *The Nurse Practitioner, 31*(12), 24-33.
Goldrick, B., & Goetz, A. (2007). Pandemic influenza: What infection control professionals should know. *American Journal of Infection Control, 35*(1), 7-13.
Holcomb, S. (2007). When your patient has pneumonia. *Nursing2007, 37*(6), 48cc1-48cc3.
Hsieh, H-Y., & Tuite, P. (2006). Prevention of ventilator-associated pneumonia: What nurses can do. *Dimension of Critical Care Nursing, 25*(5), 201-208.
Kamienski, M. (2007). When sore throat gets serious. *American Journal of Nursing, 107*(10), 35-38.
*Krouse, J., & Krouse, H. (1999). Introduction to sinus disease: II. Diagnosis and treatment. *ORL—Head and Neck Nursing, 17*(3), 6-17.
Lawson, P. (2005). Zapping VAP with evidence-based practice. *Nursing2005, 35*(5), 66-67.
McCance, K., & Huether, S. (2006). *Pathophysiology: The biologic basis for disease in adults and children* (5th ed.). St. Louis: Mosby.
Miskovich-Riddle, L., & Keresztes, P. (2006). CAP management guidelines. *The Nurse Practitioner, 31*(1), 43-53.
Moore, D.A., Evans, C.A., Gilman, R.H., Caviedas, L., Coronel, J., Vivar, A., et al. (2006). Microscopic-observation drug-susceptibility assay for the diagnosis of TB. *New England Journal of Medicine, 335*(15), 1539-1550.
Pipper, J., Inoue, M., Ng, L.F., Neuzil, P., Zhang, Y., & Novak, L. (2007). Catching bird flu in a droplet. *Nature Medicine, 13*(10), 1259-1263.
Pruitt, B. (2007). Fending off influenza. *Nursing2007, 37*(10), 44-46.
Pruitt, B., & Jacobs, M. (2006). How can you prevent ventilator-associated pneumonia? *Nursing2006, 36*(2), 36-41.
Pullen, R., & Hayes, D. (2007). Administering pneumococcal vaccine. *Nursing2007, 37*(9), 59.
Robinson, S., & Holmes, J. (2006). Preventing nosocomial pneumonia. *American Journal of Nursing, 106*(9), 72A-72-G.
Ruppert, R. (2007). Tuberculosis today: Fighting an ancient adversary. *American Nurse Today, 2*(11), 32-36.
Rushing, J. (2007). Obtaining a throat culture. *Nursing2007, 37*(3), 20.
Sheff, B. (2006). Avian influenza: Poised to launch a pandemic? *Nursing2006, 36*(1), 51-53.
The Joint Commission. (2007). *National Patient Safety Goals.* Website: www.jointcommission.org
Thomas, J., & Noppenberger, J. (2007). Avian influenza: A review. *American Journal of Hospital Systems Pharmacists, 64*(1), 149-165.
Todd, B. (2007). Extensively drug-resistant tuberculosis. *American Journal of Nursing, 107*(6), 29-31.
Todd, B. (2006). The QuantiFERON-TB Gold test. *American Journal of Nursing, 106*(6), 33-37.
Tolentino-DelosReyes, A., Ruppert, S., & Shiao, P. (2007). Evidence-based practice: Use of the ventilator bundle to prevent ventilator-associated pneumonia. *American Journal of Critical Care, 16*(1), 20-27.
Trossman, S. (2008). New interest in an old health threat. *American Nurse Today, 3*(1), 37-38.
Tucker, S., Poland, G., & Jacobson, R. (2008). Requiring influenza vaccination for health care workers. *AJN, 108*(2), 32-34.
Weber, C. (2006). Update on avian influenza pandemic threat. *Urologic Nursing, 26*(1), 67-68.
Weitzel, T., Robinson, S., & Holmes, J. (2006). Preventing nosocomial pneumonia. *AJN, 106*(9), 72A-72G.
Williamson, I., Benge, S., Moore, M., Kumar, S., Cross, M., & Little, P. (2006). Acute sinusitis: Which factors do FPs believe are most diagnostic and best predict antibiotic efficacy? *Journal of Family Practice, 55*(9), 789-796.
World Health Organization (WHO). (2008). *Data and statistics.* Retrieved January 2008, from www.who.int/research/en/.

Care of Critically Ill Patients with Respiratory Problems

34 CHAPTER

John M. Clochesy • Ronald Hickman

LEARNING OUTCOMES

For clinical competence and success on the NCLEX Examination, study this chapter with these Learning Outcomes in mind:

Safe and Effective Care Environment

1. Protect the patient receiving mechanical ventilation.
2. Ensure safe operation of endotracheal tubes, tracheostomy tubes, and mechanical ventilators.
3. Modify the environment to protect patients receiving anticoagulant or fibrinolytic therapy.

Health Promotion and Maintenance

4. Identify hospitalized patients at risk for a pulmonary embolism.
5. Teach people at risk for pulmonary embolism techniques to reduce the risk.
6. Teach patients and family members how to avoid injury during anticoagulation therapy.

Psychosocial Integrity

7. Support the patient and family in coping with changes in breathing status and the need for mechanical ventilation.
8. Develop interventions to communicate effectively with a patient who cannot talk as a result of intubation.
9. Reassure patients experiencing acute respiratory difficulties that appropriate interventions are being implemented.

Physiological Integrity

10. Assess the respiratory status of any patient who develops sudden-onset respiratory difficulty or acute confusion.
11. Use laboratory data and clinical manifestations to evaluate the adequacy of ventilatory interventions.
12. Compare the features of respiratory failure of ventilatory origin with those of respiratory failure of oxygenation origin.
13. Coordinate nursing care for the conscious patient being mechanically ventilated.
14. Maintain a patent airway on anyone who has experienced chest trauma.
15. Schedule essential patient care and diagnostic activities to promote rest and sleep.

Go to your Companion CD or Evolve at http://evolve.elsevier.com/Iggy/ for *Self-Assessment Questions for the NCLEX Examination* keyed to these Learning Outcomes.

Any respiratory problem can progress to a life-threatening emergency and death, even with prompt treatment. These problems severely interfere with the *human need for oxygenation and tissue perfusion* and may overwhelm the normal adaptive responses of the cardiac and blood oxygen delivery systems (Fig. 34-1). *Therefore prompt recognition and interventions are needed to prevent serious complications and death.*

An acute injury or problem that results in severe respiratory impairment can occur at any age. Older adults, however, are more at risk for developing critical respiratory problems. The patient who is short of breath is also anxious and fearful. Be prepared to manage both the physical and emotional needs of the patient during any respiratory emergency.

PULMONARY EMBOLISM

Pathophysiology

A **pulmonary embolism** (PE) is a collection of particulate matter (solids, liquids, or air) that enters venous circulation and lodges in the pulmonary vessels. Large emboli obstruct pulmonary blood flow, leading to reduced oxygenation of the whole body, pulmonary tissue hypoxia, and potential death. Any substance can cause an embolism, but a blood clot is the most common (McCance & Huether, 2006). PE is common,

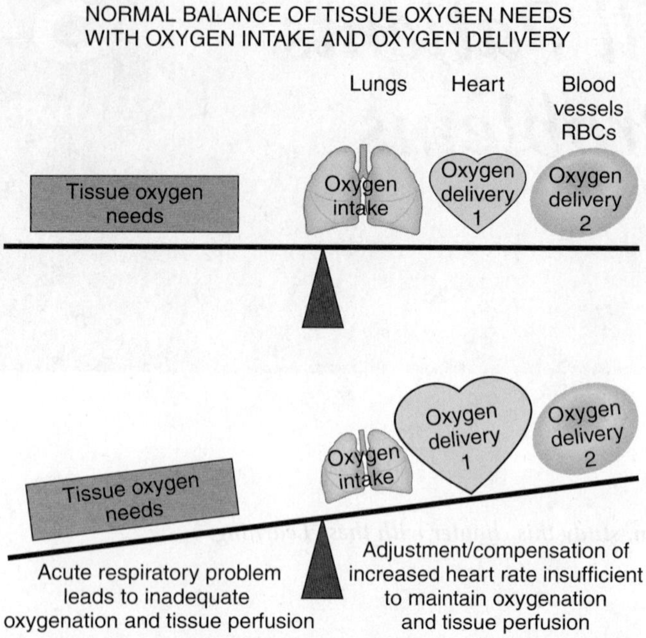
NORMAL BALANCE OF TISSUE OXYGEN NEEDS
WITH OXYGEN INTAKE AND OXYGEN DELIVERY
Lungs
Heart
Blood vessels RBCs
Tissue oxygen needs
Oxygen intake
Oxygen delivery 1
Oxygen delivery 2
Tissue oxygen needs
Oxygen intake
Oxygen delivery 1
Oxygen delivery 2
Acute respiratory problem leads to inadequate oxygenation and tissue perfusion
Adjustment/compensation of increased heart rate insufficient to maintain oxygenation and tissue perfusion

Fig. 34-1 • Rapid-onset acute respiratory problems overwhelm the ability of the cardiac oxygen delivery system to adapt and restore balance. The red blood cell (RBC) oxygen delivery system cannot begin to adapt to the acute respiratory problem.

ANIMATION: Pulmonary Embolism

and many patients die within 1 hour of the onset of symptoms or before the diagnosis has even been suspected.

A PE is the most common acute pulmonary disease among hospitalized patients. In most people with PE, a blood clot from a deep vein thrombosis (DVT) breaks loose from one of the veins in the legs or in the pelvis. The clot breaks off, travels through the vena cava into the right side of the heart, and then lodges in the pulmonary artery or one or more of its branches. Platelets collect on the embolus, triggering the release of substances that cause blood vessel constriction. Widespread pulmonary vessel constriction and pulmonary hypertension impair gas exchange. Deoxygenated blood is moved into the arterial circulation, causing **hypoxemia** (low arterial blood oxygen level), although some patients with PE do *not* have hypoxemia.

Major risk factors for DVT leading to PE are:

- Prolonged immobility
- Central venous catheters
- Surgery
- Obesity
- Advancing age
- Conditions that increase blood clotting
- History of thromboembolism

In addition, smoking, pregnancy, estrogen therapy, heart failure, stroke, cancer (particularly lung or prostate), Trousseau's syndrome, and trauma increase the risk for DVT and PE.

Fat, oil, air, tumor cells, amniotic fluid, foreign objects (e.g., broken IV catheters), injected particles, and infected clots or pus can enter a vein and cause PE. Fat emboli from fracture of a long bone and oil emboli from diagnostic procedures do not impede blood flow in the lungs (Sweeney & Ardisson, 2006); instead, they cause blood vessel injury and acute respiratory distress syndrome (ARDS). Amniotic fluid embolus has a high mortality rate and occurs as a rare complication of childbirth, abortion, or amniocentesis. Septic clots (emboli) often arise from a pelvic abscess, an infected IV catheter, and nonsterile injections of illegal drugs. With septic clots, the toxic effects of the infection are more serious than the venous blockage.

Health Promotion and Maintenance

Although pulmonary embolism (PE) can occur in healthy people and may give no warning, it occurs more often in some situations. Thus prevention of conditions that lead to PE is a major nursing concern. Preventive actions for PE are those that also prevent venous stasis and DVT. Best practices for PE prevention are outlined in Chart 34-1.

Lifestyle changes can help reduce the risk for PE. Urge patients to stop smoking cigarettes, especially women who take oral contraceptives. Reducing weight and becoming more physically active, such as walking one or more miles each day, can reduce risk for PE. Teach patients who are traveling for long periods to drink plenty of water, change positions often, avoid crossing the legs, and get up from the sitting position at least 5 minutes out of every hour. Actions to prevent DVT and PE after surgery are described in Chapters 16 and 18.

For patients known to be at risk for PE, small doses of heparin or a similar drug may be prescribed every 8 to 12 hours. Heparin prevents excessive clotting in patients after trauma or surgery or when restricted to bedrest. Occasionally, a drug to reduce platelet aggregation, such as clopidogrel (Plavix), is used in place of heparin.

Chart 34-1 **BEST PRACTICE FOR PATIENT SAFETY & QUALITY CARE**

Prevention of Pulmonary Embolism

- Start passive and active range-of-motion exercises for the extremities of immobilized and postoperative patients.
- Ambulate patients soon after surgery.
- Use antiembolism and pneumatic compression stockings and devices after surgery.
- Avoid the use of tight garters, girdles, and constricting clothing.
- Prevent pressure under the popliteal space (e.g., with a pillow).
- Perform a comprehensive assessment of peripheral circulation.
- Elevate the affected limb 20 degrees or more above the level of the heart to improve venous return, as appropriate.
- Change patient position every 2 hours, or ambulate as tolerated.
- Prevent injury to the vessel lumen by preventing local pressure, trauma, infection, or sepsis.
- Refrain from massaging or compressing leg muscles.
- Instruct patient not to cross legs.
- Administer prophylactic low-dose anticoagulant and antiplatelet drugs.
- Teach the patient to avoid activities that result in the Valsalva maneuver.
- Administer drugs that will prevent episodes of the Valsalva maneuver, as appropriate.
- Teach the patient and family about precautions.
- Encourage smoking cessation.

Patient-Centered Collaborative Care

evolve ONLINE PHARM REVIEW

Assessment

History

Assess any patient with sudden onset of breathing difficulty about the risk factors for PE, especially a history of DVT, recent surgery, or prolonged immobility.

Physical Assessment/Clinical Manifestations

Respiratory manifestations are outlined in Chart 34-2. Assess the patient for difficulty breathing (dyspnea) occurring with a rapid heart rate and pleuritic chest pain (sharp, stabbing-type pain on inspiration). These symptoms are found in most patients who have PE. Other symptoms vary depending on the size and the type of embolism. Breath sounds may be normal, but crackles usually occur. Often a dry cough is present. **Hemoptysis** (bloody sputum) may result from pulmonary infarction.

Cardiac manifestations include distended neck veins, **syncope** (fainting or loss of consciousness), cyanosis, and hypotension. *Assess for this symptom cluster, and, if present, notify the Rapid Response Team.* Hypotension during massive emboli results from acute pulmonary hypertension and reduced forward blood flow. Often abnormal heart sounds, such as an S_3 or S_4, occur. Electrocardiogram findings are abnormal, nonspecific, and transient. T-wave and ST-segment changes occur in many patients; left-axis or right-axis deviations are also common (Shaughnessy, 2007).

Miscellaneous manifestations can include a low-grade fever and petechiae on the skin over the chest and in the axillae. Some patients have more vague symptoms resembling the flu, such as nausea, vomiting, and general malaise (English, 2006).

Psychosocial Assessment

The onset of symptoms is usually abrupt, making the patient with PE anxious and fearful. Hypoxemia may cause the patient to have a sense of impending doom and increased restlessness. The emergency nature of the disorder and admission to an intensive care unit (ICU) increase the patient's anxiety and fear of death.

Chart 34-2 KEY FEATURES

Pulmonary Embolism

SYMPTOMS

- Dyspnea, sudden onset
- Pleuritic chest pain
- Apprehension, restlessness
- Feeling of impending doom
- Cough
- Hemoptysis

SIGNS

- Tachypnea
- Crackles
- Pleural friction rub
- Tachycardia
- S_3 or S_4 heart sound
- Diaphoresis
- Fever, low-grade
- Petechiae over chest and axillae
- Decreased arterial oxygen saturation (Sao_2)

Laboratory Assessment

The hyperventilation triggered by hypoxia and pain first leads to respiratory alkalosis, indicated by low partial pressure of arterial carbon dioxide ($Paco_2$) values on arterial blood gas (ABG) analysis. The alveolar-arterial (A-a) gradient is increased. The "friendlier" Pao_2-Fio_2 (fraction of inspired oxygen) ratio is commonly used to assess shunt because it does not require use of the complex A-a gradient formula. As blood is shunted without picking up oxygen from the lungs, the $Paco_2$ level starts to rise, resulting in respiratory acidosis. Later, metabolic acidosis results from build up of lactic acid due to tissue hypoxia. (See Chapter 14 for a more detailed discussion of acidosis.)

Even if ABG studies and pulse oximetry show hypoxemia, these results alone are not sufficient for the diagnosis of PE (Clautier, 2007). *A patient with a small embolus may not be hypoxemic, and PE is not the only cause of hypoxemia.*

Imaging Assessment

A chest x-ray may show a PE if it is large. Some lung infiltration may be present around the embolism site. However, the chest x-ray may not show any acute changes. Spiral computed tomography (CT) scans are most often used to diagnose PE (Clautier, 2007).

The physician may perform transesophageal echocardiography (TEE) (see Chapter 35) to help detect PE. Doppler ultrasound studies or impedance plethysmography (IPG) may be used to document the presence of DVT and to support a diagnosis of PE.

DECISION-MAKING CHALLENGE

Critical Rescue

You are assigned to care for a 60-year-old woman who is in the medical intensive care unit (MICU) for community-acquired pneumonia requiring mechanical ventilation. She is a 1 pack per day (ppd) smoker and does not use alcohol or recreational drugs. Before admission, she had several days with shortness of breath (SOB), a productive cough, and generalized fatigue. While in the MICU, she was on strict bedrest because of mechanical ventilatory support. Her drugs include erythromycin for community-acquired pneumonia, hydromorphone (Dilaudid) as needed for pain, and acetaminophen (Tylenol) as needed for fever. Two hours ago, she was extubated, and the mechanical ventilation was discontinued. As you begin your morning physical assessment, you notice that she is agitated, confused, and tachycardic and has tachypneic breathing at 35 times per minute; her oxygen saturation by pulse oximetry is 86%.

1. What should be your first action?
2. What risk factors does she have for a pulmonary embolism?
3. For what other manifestations should you assess?
4. Is oxygen by mask appropriate for this patient? Why or why not?
5. What other actions should you take?

evolve For suggested answer guidelines, go to http://evolve.elsevier.com/Iggy/.

Analysis

Common Nursing Diagnoses and Collaborative Problems

The primary collaborative problem for patients with PE is hypoxemia. Priority nursing diagnoses for patients with PE are:

1. Decreased Cardiac Output related to acute pulmonary hypertension
2. Anxiety related to hypoxemia and life-threatening illness

The secondary collaborative problem is Potential for Bleeding.

Additional Nursing Diagnoses and Collaborative Problems

In addition to the common nursing diagnoses and collaborative problems, patients with PE may have one or more of these:

- Impaired Gas Exchange related to disrupted pulmonary perfusion and increased dead space
- Fatigue related to hypoxemia
- Impaired Oral Mucous Membrane related to oxygen therapy
- Acute Confusion related to hypoxemia
- Sleep Deprivation related to the ICU environment

▪ Planning and Implementation

Hypoxemia

When a patient has a sudden onset of dyspnea and chest pain, immediately notify the Rapid Response Team. Reassure the patient, and assist him or her to a position of comfort with the head of the bed elevated. Prepare for oxygen therapy and blood gas analysis while continuing to monitor and assess for other changes.

NOC **Planning: Expected Outcomes.** The patient with PE is expected to have adequate tissue perfusion in all major organs. Indicators of adequate perfusion are:

- ABGs within normal limits
- Pulse oximetry above 95%
- Cognitive status not compromised
- Absence of pallor and cyanosis

Interventions. Nonsurgical management of PE is most common. In some cases, surgery may be needed in addition to drug therapy. Selected NIC intervention activities for the patient with PE are listed in Chart 34-3.

Nonsurgical Management. Goals of management for PE are to increase gas exchange, improve lung perfusion, reduce risk for further clot formation, and prevent complications. Priority nursing interventions include implementing oxygen therapy, administering anticoagulation or fibrinolytic therapy, monitoring the patient's responses to the interventions, and providing psychosocial support.

Oxygen therapy is important for the patient with PE. The severely hypoxemic patient may need mechanical ventilation and close monitoring with ABG studies. In less severe cases, oxygen may be applied by nasal cannula or mask. Use pulse oximetry to monitor oxygen saturation and determine the degree of hypoxemia.

Monitor the patient continually for any changes in status. Check vital signs, lung sounds, and cardiac and respiratory status at least every 1 to 2 hours. Document increasing dyspnea, dysrhythmias, distended neck veins, and pedal and sacral edema. Assess for crackles and other abnormal lung sounds along with cyanosis of the lips, conjunctiva, oral mucosa, and nail beds.

Drug therapy with anticoagulants may be prescribed to keep the embolus from enlarging and to prevent the formation of new clots. Active bleeding, stroke, and recent trauma are reasons to avoid this therapy. Before proceeding, each patient is evaluated to determine the risk versus the benefit of anticoagulant therapy.

Heparin is usually used unless the PE is massive or occurs with hemodynamic instability. A fibrinolytic drug may then be used to break up the existing clot. Review the patient's partial thromboplastin time (PTT)—also called *activated partial thromboplastin time (aPTT)*—before therapy is started, every 4 hours when therapy begins, and daily thereafter. Therapeutic PTT values usually range between 1.5 and 2.5 times the control value for this problem.

Some fibrinolytic drugs, such as alteplase (Activase, tPA), are used for treatment of PE. Specific criteria for use of these drugs are massive PE (those that obstruct blood flow to a lobe or more than one segment) and emboli that induce hemodynamic instability that includes failure to maintain blood pressure without supportive measures.

Heparin therapy usually continues for 5 to 10 days. Most patients are started on an oral anticoagulant, such as warfarin (Coumadin, Warfilone♣), on the third day of heparin use. Therapy with both heparin and warfarin continues until the patient has an international normalized ratio (INR) of 2.0 to 3.0. To facilitate early discharge, a low-molecular-weight heparin (e.g., dalteparin or enoxaparin) is often used along with the warfarin. Monitor the INR daily. Warfarin use continues for 3 to 6 weeks, but some patients at high risk may take warfarin indefinitely. Charts 34-4 and 34-5 list common drugs used and which laboratory tests to monitor. These drugs and their associated nursing care are discussed also in Chapters 38, 40, and 41.

Anticoagulation and fibrinolytic therapy can lead to excessive bleeding. In addition, even when clotting times are in the desired ranges, the patient may develop another problem that requires invasive therapy and a return to more normal coagulation responses. *Thus it is critical to keep antidotes to anticoagulant drugs on the unit for patients undergoing this therapy. The antidote for heparin is protamine sulfate; the antidote for warfarin is injectable phytonadione, vitamin K_1 (AquaMEPHYTON, Mephyton).* Antidotes for fibrinolytic therapy include clotting factors, fresh frozen plasma, and aminocaproic acid (Amicar).

Chart 34-3 NIC INTERVENTION ACTIVITIES

The Patient with Pulmonary Embolism

Embolus Care: Pulmonary: *Limitation of complications for a patient experiencing or at risk for occlusion of pulmonary circulation*

- Evaluate chest pain (e.g., intensity, location, radiation, duration, and precipitating and alleviating factors).
- Auscultate lung sounds for crackles or other adventitious sounds.
- Monitor respiratory pattern for symptoms of respiratory difficulty (e.g., dyspnea, tachypnea, and shortness of breath).
- Monitor determinants of tissue oxygen delivery (e.g., Pao_2, Sao_2, and hemoglobin levels and cardiac output), if available.
- Monitor for symptoms of inadequate tissue oxygenation (e.g., pallor, cyanosis, and sluggish capillary refill).
- Encourage good ventilation (e.g., incentive spirometry and cough and deep breathe every 2 hours).
- Instruct the patient and/or family regarding diagnostic procedures, as appropriate.
- Monitor side effects of anticoagulant medications, if appropriate.

NIC intervention activities selected from Bulechek, G.M., Butcher, H.K., & McCloskey Dochterman, J. (Eds.). (2008). *Nursing interventions classification (NIC)* (5th ed.). St. Louis: Mosby. No part of this work is to be altered without prior written permission from the Publisher.

$Paco_2$, Partial pressure of arterial carbon dioxide; *Pao_2*, partial pressure of arterial oxygen; *Sao_2*, arterial oxygen saturation.

Chart 34-4 COMMON EXAMPLES OF DRUG THERAPY

Pulmonary Embolism

Drug and Usual Dosage	Purpose	Nursing Interventions	Rationales
Heparin sodium (Hepalean🍁) 5000-10,000 units IV push initially; then dose adjustment is based on PTT, 1300 units/hr on continuous drip or, less preferably, intermittent infusion	To begin anticoagulation to minimize growth of existing clots and to prevent the development of additional clots	Monitor PTT and know expected therapeutic PTT range for each patient.	Ongoing assessment helps detect side effects and prevent complications.
		Report PTT results. Monitor patient for bleeding or bruising.	Reporting and monitoring enable the physician to begin early treatment of a prolonged PTT and excessive bleeding.
		Re-bolus every time infusion is increased.	To maintain anticoagulation within consistent therapeutic levels.
		Do not use with salicylates.	An increased anticoagulation effect can occur with salicylates.
		Monitor platelets daily for thrombocytopenia.	Heparin-induced thrombocytopenia (HIT), a type of arterial thrombosis, can occur.
		Have the antidote *protamine sulfate* available.	Being prepared for an emergency helps prevent further complications.
		Avoid puncture sites, and apply pressure to venipuncture and IM injection sites.	Pressure at puncture sites helps promote clotting.
		Avoid use of firm toothbrushes, straight razors, and rectal thermometers.	Safety measures help prevent bleeding.
Enoxaparin (Lovenox) 1 mg/kg subcutaneously every 2 hr ❗ **Med Error Alert!** Enoxaparin can be given only subcutaneously, NOT intravenously or intramuscularly.	To allow for hospital discharge before complete switch to oral anticoagulants	Same as with unfractionated heparin.	Same as with unfractionated heparin.
Warfarin sodium (Coumadin, Warfilone sodium🍁) 10-15 mg orally for 3 days initially; then dose adjustment is based on INR, usually 5-10 mg orally daily Now available as a parenteral drug for use in hospitalized patients. Dosage is the same as with the oral form of the drug.	To allow for long-term anticoagulation in at-risk patients to prevent the development of future clots	Monitor INR, and know expected therapeutic INR range for each patient.	Ongoing assessment helps detect side effects and prevent complications.
		Report INR results. Monitor the patient for bleeding or bruising.	Reporting enables the physician to begin early treatment of a prolonged INR.
		Monitor for fever and skin rash.	Adverse drug reaction can occur.
		Consult the pharmacist about potential drug interactions.	There are many drug interactions with warfarin.
		Have the antidote *vitamin K (phytonadione)* available.	Being prepared for an emergency helps prevent further complications.
		Apply pressure to venipuncture and IM injection sites.	Pressure at puncture sites helps promote clotting.
		Avoid use of firm toothbrushes, straight razors, and rectal thermometers.	Safety measures help prevent bleeding.
		Teach the patient which foods are high in vitamin K.	Food sources of vitamin K will alter INR.
Alteplase (tissue plasminogen activator, recombinant; tPA; Activase) 100 mg IV infusion over 2 hr	To promote lysis of large pulmonary emboli in those patients who are hemodynamically unstable	Assess for internal and external bleeding.	Bleeding is the most common adverse effect.
		Reconstitute with sterile water without preservative immediately before use.	Recommended preparation ensures drug stability.
		Administer with caution to patients who have been receiving aspirin, dipyridamole, heparin, or other anticoagulants.	Other drugs with anticoagulation effects increase the risk of bleeding.

INR, International normalized ratio; *IVP*, intravenous push, or bolus; *PTT*, partial thromboplastin time.

Chart 34-5 LABORATORY PROFILE

Blood Tests Used to Monitor Anticoagulation Therapy

Test	Normal Range	Significance of Abnormal Findings
Partial thromboplastin time (PTT, aPTT [APTT])	Normal values for each local laboratory may vary. When activator reagents are used by the laboratory, the normal clotting time is shortened. Common normal ranges are 20-30 sec in some laboratories and 30-40 sec in others. Therapeutic range for PE is 1.5-2.5 times the normal value (e.g., if normal is 20-30 sec, then therapeutic range is 40-75 sec).	*Subtherapeutic times* may signify that the patient is not receiving enough heparin to prevent extension of the blood clot. An increase in the dosage or rate of infusion is usually indicated. *Therapeutic times* mean that the clotting time is increased from normal but this increase is indicated in the case of PE. *Prolonged times* in patients with PE (i.e., >75 sec) indicate that the patient is at risk of serious spontaneous bleeding. Heparin is usually held or decreased until the PTT drops back into the therapeutic range.
Prothrombin time (pro time, PT)	11-12.5 sec. Therapeutic range for anticoagulant therapy in PE is 1.5-2 times the normal or control value in seconds. Control values can vary day to day because reagents used may vary. If INR values are reported with the PT, therapeutic range for PE is 2.5-3.0, or 3.0-4.5 for recurrent PE.	*Subtherapeutic values* may signify that the patient is not receiving enough warfarin. An increase in the dosage is usually indicated. *Therapeutic values* mean that the pro time is increased from normal but this increase is indicated in the case of PE. *Prolonged values* in the treatment of PE indicate that the patient is at risk for bleeding. The warfarin dose is usually decreased or held, the patient is instructed to eat foods high in vitamin K, or an injection of vitamin K may be given.

aPTT or *APTT*, Activated partial thromboplastin time; *INR*, international normalized ratio; *PE*, pulmonary embolism.

Surgical Management. Two surgical procedures for the management of PE are embolectomy and inferior vena cava interruption.

Embolectomy is the surgical removal of the embolus from pulmonary blood vessels. It may be performed when fibrinolytic therapy cannot be used for a patient who has massive or multiple large pulmonary emboli with shock. Special thrombectomy catheters that can mechanically break up clots, such as the AngioJet, allow quick and effective reduction of clots with or without the use of thrombolytic drugs.

Inferior vena cava interruption with placement of a vena cava filter is a lifesaving measure by preventing further embolus formation for some patients. Now that some of these filters are removable, the filter can be placed before symptoms develop in patients who are at high risk for clots, such as those who must remain on prolonged bedrest because of illness or injury. These filters can be removed when the risk for clot formation decreases, or they can be left in place permanently. Patients for whom filter placement is considered less risky than drug therapy include those with recurrent or major bleeding while receiving anticoagulants, those with septic PE, and those undergoing pulmonary embolectomy. Placement of a vena cava filter is detailed in Chapter 38.

Decreased Cardiac Output

NOC **Planning: Expected Outcomes.** The patient with PE is expected to have adequate circulation. Indicators of adequate circulation are:

- Maintenance of pulse rate and blood pressure within the normal ranges
- Maintenance of a urine output of at least 30 mL/hr
- Absence of cyanosis

Interventions. In addition to the interventions used for hypoxemia, IV fluid therapy and drug therapy are used to increase cardiac output.

IV fluid therapy involves giving crystalloid solutions to restore plasma volume and prevent shock (see Chapter 39). Continuously monitor the electrocardiogram (ECG) and pulmonary artery and central venous/right atrial pressures of the patient receiving IV fluids because increased fluids can worsen pulmonary hypertension and lead to right-sided heart failure.

Drug therapy with agents that increase myocardial contractility **(positive inotropic agents)** may be prescribed when IV therapy alone does not improve cardiac output. Common drugs include milrinone (Primacor) and dobutamine (Dobutrex). Assess the patient's cardiac status hourly during therapy with inotropic drugs. Vasodilators, such as nitroprusside (Nipride, Nitropress), may be used to decrease pulmonary artery pressure if it is impeding cardiac contractility.

Anxiety

NOC **Planning: Expected Outcomes.** The patient with PE is expected to have a reduction in the level of anxiety. Indicators include that he or she consistently demonstrates these behaviors:

- Statement that anxiety is reduced
- Absence of distress, irritability, and facial tension
- Effective use of coping strategies

Interventions. The patient with PE is anxious and fearful for many reasons. Interventions for reducing anxiety in those with PE include oxygen therapy (see Interventions on p. 680 in the Hypoxemia section), communication, and drug therapy.

Communication is critical in allaying anxiety. Acknowledge the anxiety and the patient's perception of a life-threatening situation. Stay with him or her, and speak calmly and clearly, providing assurance that appropriate measures are being taken. When giving drugs, changing position, taking vital signs, or assessing the patient, explain the rationale and share information.

Drug therapy with an antianxiety drug may be prescribed if the patient's anxiety increases or prevents adequate rest. Unless he or she is intubated and mechanically ventilated, agents that have a sedating effect are avoided.

Potential for Bleeding

NOC **Planning: Expected Outcomes.** The patient with PE is expected to remain free from bleeding. Indicators are:
- Absence of bruising or petechiae
- Maintenance of hematocrit and hemoglobin within the normal range

Interventions. As a result of drug therapy that disrupts clots or prevents their formation, the patient's ability to start and continue the blood-clotting cascade when injured is seriously impaired and the risk for bleeding is high. Priority nursing objectives are ensuring that appropriate antidotes are present on the nursing unit, protecting the patient from situations that could lead to bleeding, and monitoring closely the amount of bleeding that is occurring.

Assess at least every 2 hours for evidence of bleeding in the form of oozing, bruises that cluster, petechiae, or purpura. Examine all stools, urine, drainage, and vomitus visually for gross blood, and test for occult blood. Measure any blood loss as accurately as possible. Measure the patient's abdominal girth every 8 hours. Increases in abdominal girth can indicate internal bleeding. Best practices to prevent bleeding are outlined in Chart 34-6.

Monitor laboratory values daily. Review the complete blood count (CBC) results to determine the patient's risk for bleeding and whether actual blood loss has occurred. If the patient has severe blood loss, packed red blood cells may be prescribed (see the discussion of transfusion therapy in Chapter 42). Monitor the platelet count. A decreasing count may indicate ongoing clotting or development of heparin-induced thrombocytopenia (HIT) caused by the formation of anti-heparin antibodies.

NCLEX EXAMINATION CHALLENGE

The client recovering from a PE is receiving a continuous infusion of heparin IV. When the nurse comes to take vital signs, the client has blood on his pajama jacket and pillow. He is pinching his nose to control a nosebleed. What is the nurse's best first action?

A. Prepare to administer protamine sulfate parenterally.
B. Prepare to administer phytonadione parenterally.
C. Call the physician or Rapid Response Team.
D. Slow the IV, and assess the bleeding.

evolve For the correct answer, go to http://evolve.elsevier.com/Iggy/.

Community-Based Care

The patient with a PE is discharged when hypoxemia and hemodynamic instability have been resolved and adequate anticoagulation has been achieved. Anticoagulation therapy usually continues after discharge.

Home Care Management

Some patients are discharged to home with minimal risk for recurrence and no permanent physiologic changes. Others may have extensive heart or lung damage and need to modify their homes and lifestyles.

Chart 34-6 BEST PRACTICE FOR PATIENT SAFETY & QUALITY CARE

Prevention of Injury for the Patient Receiving Anticoagulant or Fibrinolytic Therapy

- Handle the patient gently.
- Use and teach UAP to use a lift sheet when moving and positioning the patient in bed.
- Avoid IM injections and venipunctures.
- When injections or venipunctures are necessary, use the smallest-gauge needle for the task.
- Apply firm pressure to the needle stick site for 10 minutes or until the site no longer oozes blood.
- Apply ice to areas of trauma.
- Test all urine, vomitus, and stool for the presence of occult blood.
- Observe IV sites every 4 hours for bleeding.
- Instruct alert patients to notify nursing personnel immediately if any trauma occurs and if bleeding or bruising is noticed.
- Avoid trauma to rectal tissues:
  - Instruct UAP not to take temperatures rectally, even on unconscious patients.
  - Do not administer enemas.
  - If suppositories are prescribed, lubricate liberally and administer with caution.
- Instruct the patient and UAP to use an electric shaver rather than a razor.
- When providing mouth care or supervising others in providing mouth care:
  - Use a soft-bristled toothbrush or tooth sponges
  - Do not use floss
  - Check to make certain that dentures fit and do not rub
- Instruct the patient not to blow the nose forcefully or insert objects into the nose.
- Instruct UAP and the patient to wear shoes with firm soles whenever the patient is ambulating.
- Ensure that antidotes to anticoagulation therapy are on the unit.

UAP, Unlicensed assistive personnel.

Patients with extensive lung damage may have activity intolerance and become fatigued easily. The living arrangements may need to be modified so that patients can spend all or most of the time on one floor and avoid climbing stairs. Depending on the degree of impairment, patients may require some or much assistance with ADLs.

Health Teaching

The patient with a PE may continue anticoagulation therapy for weeks, months, or years after discharge, depending on the risks for PE. Teach him or her and the family about Bleeding Precautions, activities to reduce the risk for deep vein thrombosis (DVT) and recurrence of PE, complications, and the need for follow-up care (Chart 34-7).

Health Care Resources

Patients using anticoagulation therapy are usually seen in a clinic or health care provider's office weekly for blood drawing and assessment. Those who are homebound may have a visit from a home care nurse to perform these actions (see Chart 34-8 for a focused assessment guide). Patients with severe dyspnea may need home oxygen therapy. Respiratory therapy

Chart 34-7 PATIENT AND FAMILY EDUCATION GUIDE

Preventing Injury and Bleeding

During the time you are taking anticoagulants:

- Use an electric shaver.
- Use a soft-bristled toothbrush, and do not floss.
- Do not have dental work performed without consulting your health care provider.
- Do not take aspirin or any aspirin-containing products. Read the label to be sure that the product does not contain aspirin or salicylates.
- Do not participate in contact sports or any activity likely to result in your being bumped, scratched, or scraped.
- If you are bumped, apply ice to the site for at least 1 hour.
- Avoid hard foods that would scrape the inside of your mouth.
- Eat warm, cool, or cold foods to avoid burning your mouth.
- Check your skin and mouth daily for bruises, swelling, or areas with small, reddish purple marks that may indicate bleeding.
- Notify your health care provider if you:
  - Are injured and persistent bleeding results
  - Have excessive menstrual bleeding
  - See blood in your urine or bowel movement
- Avoid anal intercourse.
- Take a stool softener to prevent straining during a bowel movement.
- Do not use enemas or rectal suppositories.
- Do not wear clothing or shoes that are tight or that rub.
- Avoid blowing your nose forcefully or placing objects in your nose. If you must blow your nose, do so gently without blocking either nasal passage.
- Avoid playing musical instruments that raise the pressure inside your head, such as brass wind instruments and woodwinds or reed instruments.
- Keep all appointments for laboratory tests.

Chart 34-8 HOME CARE ASSESSMENT

The Patient After Pulmonary Embolism

Assess respiratory status.

- Observe rate and depth of ventilation.
- Auscultate lungs.
- Examine nail beds and mucous membranes for evidence of cyanosis.
- Take a pulse oximetry reading.
- Ask the patient if chest pain or shortness of breath is experienced in any position.
- Ask the patient about the presence of sputum and its color and character.

Assess cardiovascular status.

- Take vital signs, including apical pulse, pulse pressure; assess for presence or absence of orthostatic hypotension and quality and rhythm of peripheral pulses.
- Note presence or absence of peripheral edema.
- Examine hand vein filling in the dependent position.
- Examine neck vein filling in the recumbent and sitting positions.

Assess lower extremities for deep vein thrombosis.

- Examine lower legs and compare with each other for:
  - General edema
  - Calf swelling
  - Surface temperature
  - Presence of red streaks or cordlike, palpable structure
- Measure calf circumference.
- Ask the patient to dorsiflex and plantarflex each foot. Note the ease with which the patient can do this, and ask whether pain is experienced in either position.
- Gently squeeze the calf of each leg laterally and from front to back. Ask the patient whether pain or tenderness is experienced with either maneuver.

Assess for evidence of bleeding.

- Examine the mouth and gums for oozing or frank bleeding.
- Examine all skin areas for bruising or petechiae.
- If the patient voids during the visit, test the urine for occult blood.

Assess cognition and mental status.

- Level of consciousness
- Orientation to time, place, and person
- Can the patient accurately read a seven-word sentence containing no words with more than three syllables?

Assess the patient's understanding of illness and adherence to treatment.

- Manifestations to report to health care provider
- Medication plan (correct timing and dose)
- Bleeding Precautions
- Prevention of deep vein thrombosis

treatments can be performed in the home. The nurse or case manager coordinates arrangements for oxygen and other respiratory therapy to be available if needed at home.

DECISION-MAKING CHALLENGE

Coordination of Care

The patient described on p. 679 with a PE is going home. She will continue warfarin therapy for at least 1 month.

1. What will you tell this patient about warfarin therapy?
2. Is she still at risk for a PE? Why or why not?
3. What should you teach her to help reduce her risk for PE?

evolve For suggested answer guidelines, go to http://evolve.elsevier.com/Iggy/.

■ *Evaluation: Outcomes*

Evaluate the care of the patient with PE on the basis of the identified nursing diagnoses and collaborative problems. The expected outcomes are that he or she:

- Attains and maintains adequate gas exchange and oxygenation
- Does not experience hypovolemia and shock
- Remains free from bleeding episodes
- States that levels of anxiety are reduced
- Uses effective coping strategies

Specific indicators for these outcomes are listed for each nursing diagnosis and collaborative problem under the Planning and Implementation section (see earlier).

ACUTE RESPIRATORY FAILURE

Pathophysiology

Acute respiratory failure is classified by blood gas abnormalities. The critical values are partial pressure of arterial oxygen (Pa_{O_2}) less than 60 mm Hg, arterial oxygen saturation (Sa_{O_2}) less than 90%, or partial pressure of arterial carbon dioxide (Pa_{CO_2}) more than 50 mm Hg occurring with acidemia (pH $<$7.30) (Beattie, 2007). Acute respiratory failure is further defined as *ventilatory failure, oxygenation failure,* or a *combination of both ventilatory and oxygenation failure.* Whatever the underlying problem, the patient in acute respiratory failure is always **hypoxemic** (has low arterial blood oxygen levels).

Ventilatory Failure

Ventilatory failure is the type of problem in oxygen intake (ventilation) and blood delivery (perfusion) that causes a ventilation-perfusion ($\dot{V}/\dot{Q}$) mismatch in which perfusion is normal but ventilation is inadequate. It occurs when the chest pressure does not change enough to permit air movement into and out of the lungs. As a result, too little oxygen reaches the alveoli and carbon dioxide is retained. Both problems lead to hypoxemia.

Ventilatory failure is often the result of these three problems: a physical problem of the lungs or chest wall, a defect in the respiratory control center in the brain, or poor function of the respiratory muscles, especially the diaphragm. The problem is defined by a Pa_{CO_2} level above 45 mm Hg in patients who have otherwise healthy lungs.

Many diseases and problems can result in ventilatory failure. Causes are described as either **extrapulmonary** (involving nonpulmonary tissues but affecting respiratory function) or **intrapulmonary** (disorders of the respiratory tract). Table 34-1 lists common causes of ventilatory failure.

Oxygenation Failure

In oxygenation failure, chest pressure changes are normal and air moves in and out without difficulty but does not oxygenate the pulmonary blood sufficiently. It occurs in the type of ($\dot{V}/\dot{Q}$) mismatch in which air movement and oxygen intake (ventilation) are normal but lung blood flow (perfusion) is decreased.

Many lung diseases and problems can cause oxygenation failure. Problems include impaired diffusion of oxygen at the alveolar level, right-to-left shunting of blood in the pulmonary vessels, $\dot{V}/\dot{Q}$ mismatch, breathing air with a low partial pressure of oxygen (a rare problem), and abnormal hemoglobin that fails to bind oxygen. In one type of $\dot{V}/\dot{Q}$ mismatch, areas of the lungs are still being perfused but gas exchange cannot occur, which leads to hypoxemia. An extreme example of $\dot{V}/\dot{Q}$ mismatch is a right-to-left shunt in which venous blood is shunted into the arterial system without being oxygenated. Normally, less than 5% of cardiac output contains venous blood that has bypassed oxygenation. With a right-to-left shunt, even more venous blood is not oxygenated and applying 100% oxygen does not correct the problem. A classic cause of such a $\dot{V}/\dot{Q}$ mismatch is acute respiratory distress syndrome (ARDS). Table 34-2 lists specific causes of oxygenation failure.

TABLE 34-1 Common Causes of Ventilatory Failure

EXTRAPULMONARY CAUSES

Neuromuscular disorders
- Myasthenia gravis
- Guillain-Barré syndrome
- Poliomyelitis

Spinal cord injuries affecting nerves to intercostal muscles

Central nervous system dysfunction
- Stroke
- Increased intracranial pressure
- Meningitis

Chemical depression
- Opioid analgesics, sedatives, anesthetics

Kyphoscoliosis

Massive obesity

Sleep apnea

External obstruction/constriction

INTRAPULMONARY CAUSES

Airway disease
- Chronic obstructive pulmonary disease (COPD), asthma

Ventilation-perfusion ($\dot{V}/\dot{Q}$) mismatch
- Pulmonary embolism
- Pneumothorax
- Acute respiratory distress syndrome (ARDS)
- Amyloidosis
- Pulmonary edema
- Interstitial fibrosis

TABLE 34-2 Common Causes of Oxygenation Failure

- Low atmospheric oxygen concentration
  - High altitudes, smoke inhalation, carbon monoxide poisoning
- Pneumonia
- Congestive heart failure with pulmonary edema
- Pulmonary embolism (PE)
- Acute respiratory distress syndrome (ARDS)
- Interstitial pneumonitis-fibrosis
- Abnormal hemoglobin
- Hypovolemic shock
- Hypoventilation
- Complications of nitroprusside therapy
  - Thiocyanate toxicity, methemoglobinemia

Combined Ventilatory and Oxygenation Failure

Combined ventilatory and oxygenation failure involves **hypoventilation** (poor respiratory movements). Gas exchange at the alveolar-capillary membrane is poor so that too little oxygen reaches the blood and carbon dioxide is retained. The condition may or may not include poor lung perfusion. When lung perfusion is not adequate, $\dot{V}/\dot{Q}$ mismatch occurs and both ventilation and perfusion are inadequate. This type of respiratory failure leads to a more profound hypoxemia than either ventilatory failure or oxygenation failure alone.

A combination of ventilatory failure and oxygenation failure occurs in patients who have abnormal lungs, such as those who have any form of chronic bronchitis, have emphysema, or are having an asthma attack. The bronchioles and alveoli are diseased (causing oxygenation failure), and the work of breathing increases until the respiratory muscles cannot function effectively (causing ventilatory failure). Acute respiratory failure results. This process can also occur in patients who have cardiac failure along with respiratory failure. This problem is serious because the cardiac system cannot adapt to the hypoxia by increasing the cardiac output.

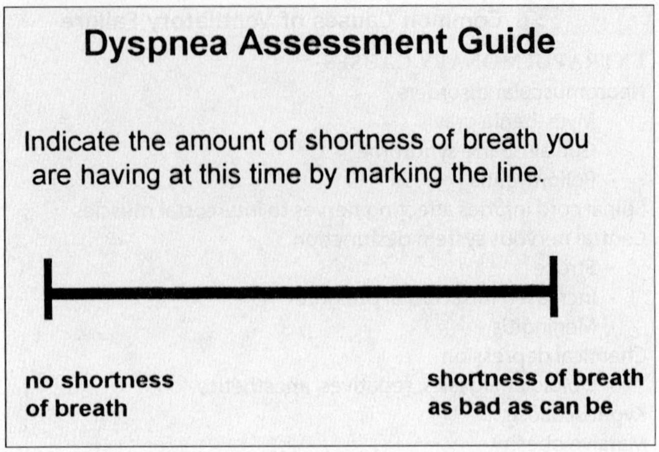
Dyspnea Assessment Guide
Indicate the amount of shortness of breath you are having at this time by marking the line.
no shortness of breath
shortness of breath as bad as can be

Fig. 34-2 • A dyspnea assessment tool.

Patient-Centered Collaborative Care

Assessment

Assess for **dyspnea** (perceived difficulty breathing), the hallmark of respiratory failure. Evaluate dyspnea with the use of a dyspnea assessment guide (Fig. 34-2). Depending on the process, nature, and course of the underlying problem, the patient may or may not be aware of changes in the work of breathing. In addition, he or she needs to be alert enough to perceive the sensation of breathlessness.

Dyspnea is more intense when it develops rapidly. Slowly progressive respiratory failure may first be noticed as dyspnea on exertion (DOE) or when lying down. The patient may have **orthopnea,** finding it is easier to breathe in an upright position. With chronic respiratory problems, a minor increase in dyspnea from baseline may represent severe gas exchange problems.

Assess for a change in the patient's respiratory rate or pattern, a change in lung sounds, and manifestations of hypoxemia (pallor, cyanosis, increased heart rate, restlessness, confusion) and **hypercarbia** (high arterial blood levels of carbon dioxide). Pulse oximetry may show decreased oxygen saturation, but an arterial blood gas (ABG) analysis is needed for the most accurate assessment of oxygenation. The health care provider reviews the ABG studies to identify the degree of hypercarbia and hypoxemia.

Interventions

Oxygen therapy is appropriate for any patient who has acute hypoxemia. It is prescribed in acute respiratory failure to keep the partial pressure of arterial oxygen (Pao_2) level above 60 mm Hg while treating the underlying cause of the respiratory failure (Beattie, 2007). Oxygen therapy is discussed in detail in Chapter 30. If supplemental oxygen does not maintain acceptable Pao_2 levels, mechanical ventilation may be needed.

Help the patient find a position of comfort that allows easier breathing—usually a more upright position. To decrease the anxiety occurring with dyspnea, assist him or her to use relaxation, diversion, and guided imagery. Start energy-conserving measures, such as minimal self-care and no unnecessary procedures. Drugs given systemically or by metered dose inhaler (MDI) may be prescribed to widen the bronchioles and decrease inflammation to promote gas exchange. Teach the patient how to use the inhaler (see Chart 32-6 in Chapter 32) and about the drugs. Encourage deep breathing and other breathing exercises.

ACUTE RESPIRATORY DISTRESS SYNDROME

Pathophysiology

Acute respiratory distress syndrome (ARDS) is acute respiratory failure with these indicators:

- Hypoxemia that persists even when 100% oxygen is given
- Decreased pulmonary compliance
- Dyspnea
- Noncardiac-associated bilateral pulmonary edema
- Dense pulmonary infiltrates on x-ray (ground-glass appearance)

Often ARDS occurs after an acute lung injury (ALI) as a traumatic event in people who have no previous pulmonary disease. The mortality rate is high even when intensive interventions are used. Other terms for ARDS include *noncardiogenic pulmonary edema, adult respiratory distress syndrome,* and *shock lung.*

Despite different causes of ALI in ARDS, the main trigger is a systemic inflammatory response (Winkelman, 2008). For this reason, the manifestations of ARDS are similar regardless of the cause. The major site of injury in the lung is the alveolar-capillary membrane, which is normally permeable to only small molecules. The alveolar-capillary membrane can be injured from conditions such as sepsis, pulmonary embolism, shock, aspiration, or inhalation injury. Lung tissue normally remains relatively dry, but in patients with ARDS, lung fluid increases and contains a high level of proteins (McCance & Huether, 2006).

Other changes occur in the alveoli and respiratory bronchioles. The type II pneumocyte produces surfactant, a substance that maintains the elasticity of lung tissue and prevents alveolar collapse. Surfactant activity is reduced in ARDS either because type II pneumocytes are damaged or because the surfactant is diluted by excess lung fluids. As a result, the alveoli become unstable and tend to collapse unless they are filled with fluid. These fluid-filled or collapsed alveoli cannot exchange gases. As a result, edema forms around terminal airways, which are compressed and closed and can be destroyed. Lung volume is further reduced, and there is even less **compliance** (elasticity). As fluid continues to leak in more lung areas, fluid, protein, and blood cells collect in the alveoli and in the spaces between the alveoli. Lymph channels are compressed, and more fluid collects. Poorly inflated alveoli receive blood but cannot oxygenate it, increasing the shunt. Hypoxemia and ventilation-perfusion ($\dot{V}/\dot{Q}$) mismatch result. Transfusion-related acute lung injury (TRALI) is a noncardiogenic pulmonary edema associated with the activation of the inflammatory response due to a recent transfusion of plasma-containing products (Knippen, 2006). These products include whole blood, packed red blood cells (PRBCs), platelets, and fresh frozen plasma, all of which are associated with TRALI in critically ill adults (Kleinman et al., 2007).

Etiology and Genetic Risk

Acute lung injury (ALI) leading to ARDS has many causes (Table 34-3). Some causes involve direct injury to lung tissue; others do not directly involve the respiratory system. Serious nervous system injury, such as head or spinal trauma, strokes, tumors, and sudden increases in cerebrospinal fluid pressure,

TABLE 34-3 Common Causes of Acute Lung Injury

- Shock
- Trauma
- Serious nervous system injury
- Pancreatitis
- Fat and amniotic fluid emboli
- Pulmonary infections
- Sepsis
- Inhalation of toxic gases (smoke, oxygen)
- Pulmonary aspiration
- Drug ingestion (e.g., heroin, opioids, aspirin)
- Hemolytic disorders
- Multiple blood transfusions
- Cardiopulmonary bypass
- Near-drowning (especially in fresh water)

may cause massive sympathetic discharge. Systemic blood vessel constriction results, with movement of large volumes of blood into lung circulation. Lung pressure increases and injures the lung. Any problems that cause cerebral hypoxia can lead to the same type of lung injury. TRALI is mediated by inflammation. When a patient is being transfused, he or she is being exposed to plasma that contains foreign proteins and antibodies. This exposure activates white blood cells (WBCs) and causes agglutination (clumping) of the foreign proteins and WBCs, which then travel to the lungs. The clumped material injures the pulmonary capillaries, causing capillary leak and additional inflammation (McCance & Huether, 2006).

Other factors produce ARDS by direct injury to the lung. For example, aspiration of gastric contents may obstruct or burn the airway when the gastric contents are highly acidic (pH less than 2.5). With this type of direct injury, type I pneumocytes are destroyed. Injured capillaries allow protein and cells to escape from the blood vessels into lung tissues. Lung radiation, near-drowning, and inhalation of toxic gases all injure the alveolar and capillary tissue layers. Trauma, sepsis, drowning, and burns also cause the release of proteins (thromboplastins), which form fibrin clots in the blood. These clots, together with platelets and leukocytes, are filtered out in the lung. In many cases of ARDS, especially after trauma, clot production is increased and **fibrinolysis** (clot breakdown) is reduced. As a result, small emboli remain in the lung. Disseminated intravascular coagulation (DIC) plays a role in some patients.

GENETIC CONSIDERATIONS

An increased genetic risk is suspected in the development and progression of ARDS. The inflammatory response clearly allows progression of an acute lung injury (ALI) to ARDS; however, not all patients with ALI progress to ARDS. It appears that patients who have hyper-inflammatory responses to injury are more likely to develop ARDS (Workman & Winkelman, 2008) and their inflammatory response is genetically mediated. Ask about the patient's previous responses to infection or injury. If the patient has consistently had greater-than-expected inflammatory responses, he or she may be at increased risk for ARDS after ALI and should be closely monitored for manifestations of the disorder.

Incidence/Prevalence

The actual incidence of ARDS is unknown because it is part of other health problems and is not systematically reported as a separate disorder. A 2006 estimate suggested that 150,000 to 200,000 cases of ARDS occur yearly in the United States (American Lung Association, 2006) although many health care professionals believe this estimate to be low.

Health Promotion and Maintenance

The nursing priority in the prevention of ARDS is early recognition of patients at high risk for the syndrome. Because patients who aspirate gastric contents are at great risk, closely assess and monitor those receiving tube feeding and those with problems that impair swallowing and gag reflexes (Metheny, 2006). Follow meticulous infection control guidelines, including handwashing, invasive catheter and wound care, and Body Substance Precautions. Teach unlicensed assistive personnel (UAP) the importance of always adhering to infection control guidelines. Carefully observe patients who are being treated for any health problem associated with ARDS.

Patient-Centered Collaborative Care

Assessment

Physical Assessment/Clinical Manifestations

Assess the breathing of any patient with a condition that increases the risk for ARDS. Determine whether increased work of breathing is present, as indicated by hyperpnea, grunting respiration, cyanosis, pallor, and retraction **intercostally** (between the ribs) or **substernally** (below the ribs). Document sweating, respiratory effort, and any change in mental status. *No abnormal lung sounds are present on auscultation because the edema of ARDS occurs first in the interstitial spaces and not in the airways.* Monitor vital signs at least hourly to assess for hypotension, tachycardia, and dysrhythmias.

Diagnostic Assessment

The diagnosis of ARDS is established by a lowered partial pressure of arterial oxygen (PaO_2) value, determined by arterial blood gas (ABG) measurements. Because a widening alveolar oxygen gradient (increased fraction of inspired oxygen [FIO_2] does not lead to increased PaO_2 levels) develops with increased shunting of blood, the patient has a progressive need for higher levels of oxygen. He or she does not respond to high concentrations of oxygen (refractory hypoxemia) and often needs intubation and mechanical ventilation. A large difference between the predicted and actual alveolar oxygen tension indicates shunting. Sputum cultures obtained by the health care provider through bronchoscopy and by transtracheal aspiration are used to determine if a lung infection also is present (Taylor, 2005).

The chest x-ray usually shows diffuse haziness or a "whited-out" (ground-glass) appearance of the lung. An ECG rules out cardiac problems and usually reveals no specific changes. Pulmonary artery (Swan-Ganz) catheter placement and hemodynamic monitoring is a diagnostic tool. In the patient with ARDS, the pulmonary capillary wedge pressure (PCWP) is usually low to normal. This pressure differs from that in the patient with cardiac-induced pulmonary edema, in which the PCWP is above 18 mm Hg. Chapter 40 explains hemodynamic monitoring in detail.

Common Nursing Diagnoses and Collaborative Problems

Nursing diagnoses and collaborative problems that may apply to patients with ARDS include:

- Anxiety related to hypoxemia, life-threatening illness, loss of control
- Impaired Gas Exchange related to disrupted pulmonary ventilation and perfusion
- Fatigue related to hypoxemia and systemic inflammation
- Sleep Deprivation related to the intensive care unit (ICU) environment
- Imbalanced Nutrition: Less Than Body Requirements related to presence of endotracheal tube, chemical paralysis, increased metabolic rate
- Risk for Injury related to elevated FiO_2 or barotrauma
- Potential for Ventilator-Associated Pneumonia (VAP)

Interventions

The patient with ARDS often needs intubation and mechanical ventilation with positive end-expiratory pressure (PEEP) or continuous positive airway pressure (CPAP) (Burns, 2005). Sedation and paralysis may be needed for adequate ventilation and to reduce tissue oxygen needs. Because one of the side effects of PEEP is tension pneumothorax, assess lung sounds hourly and suction as often as needed to maintain a patent airway. Positioning may be important in promoting gas exchange, although the exact position is controversial. Some patients do better in the prone position, especially if it is started early in the disease course, although the turning equipment is awkward and care in this position is more difficult (Mancebo et al., 2006; Powers, 2007). Continuously turning the patient to 40 degrees from side to side or using a 90-degree lateral position also appears to improve perfusion (Goldhill et al., 2007; Thomas et al., 2007).

Drug and Fluid Therapy

Corticosteroids may be used in the treatment of ARDS because they decrease white blood cell movement and stabilize the capillary membrane. Their effectiveness, however, has not been determined. It is thought that they may help reduce the fibrosis that occurs in late ARDS. Antibiotics are used to treat infections when organisms are identified.

Many interventions are under investigation, but none has been effective in improving survival. Such interventions include agents that modify the inflammatory responses and oxidative stress (vitamins C and E, *N*-acetylcysteine), nitric oxide, and surfactant replacement.

Recent research shows that patients with ARDS who receive conservative fluid therapy have improved lung function and a shorter duration of mechanical ventilation and ICU length of stay compared with those who receive more liberal fluid therapy (Wiedemann et al., 2006). (See the Evidence-Based Practice box below.) Conservative fluid therapy involves infusing smaller amounts of IV fluid and the use of diuretics

EVIDENCE-BASED PRACTICE

Less fluid is better

Wiedemann, H.P., Wheeler, A.P., Bernard, G.R., Thompson, B.T., Hayden, D., deBoisblanc, B., et al. (2006). Comparison of two fluid-management strategies in acute lung injury. *New England Journal of Medicine, 354*(24), 2564-2576.

Acute lung injury leading to acute respiratory distress syndrome (ARDS) is common and life threatening. The potential adverse outcomes include permanent lung injury and death, although at the onset of the disorder, there is no way of predicting which patients will survive and recover and which will not recover. Pulmonary edema appears to increase the risk for serious consequences; thus conservative fluid resuscitation strategies have been proposed. However, insufficient fluid resuscitation could result in damage and dysfunction to other organs. Thus the optimum fluid management intervention for early intervention for patients with ARDS is unknown.

The purpose of this large, multisite, randomized, controlled study was to determine whether conservative fluid management strategies or liberal fluid management strategies had better outcomes for patients with ARDS in terms of death rates at 60 days, ventilator-free days, and number of days in the ICU. More than 1000 patients with acute lung injury were enrolled in the study and randomly assigned to either the conservative fluid management treatment group or the liberal fluid management treatment group. Overall, the subjects in both groups were similar for age ranges, causes of acute lung injury, gender, and severity of injury. The protocols for fluid management were strictly followed in all settings for both groups.

The death rate at 60 days for the conservative fluid management group was 25.5% and for the liberal fluid management group was 28.28.4%. This difference in favor of conservative fluid management did not reach statistical significance ($p = 0.30$). However, the other outcome measurements did show more favorable results for the conservative fluid management group without increasing the incidence of hypovolemic shock and organ failure. Those subjects in the conservative fluid management group spent 2 fewer days in the ICU and had 2 more ventilator-free days than did those subjects in the liberal fluid management group. These positive outcomes were statistically significant ($p < 0.001$).

Level of Evidence—2. The study was a well-designed, randomized, controlled trial.

Commentary: Implications for Practice and Research. The practice of aggressive fluid resuscitation with liberal IV fluids to prevent hypovolemic shock in patients with acute lung injury may intensify pulmonary edema and contribute to the progression of ARDS. Nurses need to closely monitor patient responses to fluid resuscitation and to coordinate with physicians to adjust fluid replacement volumes to match actual fluid needs to avoid or reduce the degree of pulmonary edema.

to maintain fluid balance, whereas liberal fluid therapy often results in an increasingly positive fluid balance and more systemic edema. For those patients with significant edema, particular care is needed to minimize the development of pressure sores.

Nutrition Therapy

The patient with ARDS is at risk for malnutrition, which further reduces respiratory muscle function and the immune response. Therefore enteral nutrition (tube feeding) or parenteral nutrition is started as soon as possible (Powers, 2007; Pruitt, 2007).

Case Management

Case management of the patient with ARDS focuses on the phases of ARDS rather than on day-to-day care. The course of ARDS and its management are divided into four phases:

Phase 1. This phase includes early changes of dyspnea and tachypnea. Early interventions focus on supporting the patient and providing oxygen.

Phase 2. Patchy infiltrates form from increasing pulmonary edema. Interventions include mechanical ventilation and prevention of complications.

Phase 3. This phase occurs over days 2 through 10, and the patient has progressive hypoxemia that responds poorly to high levels of oxygen. Interventions focus on maintaining adequate oxygen transport, preventing complications, and supporting the failing lung until it has had time to heal.

Phase 4. Pulmonary fibrosis with progression occurs after 10 days. This phase is irreversible and is often called "late" or "chronic" ARDS. Patients who develop this stage and survive it will have some permanent lung damage. Interventions focus on preventing sepsis, pneumonia, and multiple organ dysfunction syndrome (MODS), as well as weaning the patient from the ventilator. The patient in this phase may be ventilator dependent for weeks to months. Care may occur in specialized units or facilities that focus on rehabilitation and long-term weaning. Some patients may not be "weanable" and may go home or to a long-term care facility dependent on mechanical ventilation.

DECISION-MAKING CHALLENGE
Coordination of Care

A 53-year-old woman with known ischemic heart disease is electively hospitalized for a coronary artery bypass graft (CABG) surgery. While in surgery, she received two units of packed red blood cells, fresh frozen plasma, and platelets to correct a clotting problem. On arrival in the ICU, she was attached to mechanical ventilatory support. A chest x-ray and arterial blood gas analysis were obtained. On physical examination, lung sounds are coarse bilaterally. The chest x-ray shows patchy infiltrates bilaterally, and the ABG indicates a respiratory acidosis with a $Paco_2$ of 68 mm Hg.

1. For what type of acute lung injury is this patient at greatest risk?
2. What risk factors for TRALI does the patient have?
3. What actions should you initiate?

evolve For suggested answer guidelines, go to http://evolve.elsevier.com/Iggy/.

THE PATIENT REQUIRING INTUBATION AND VENTILATION

Pathophysiology

With mechanical ventilation, the patient who has severe problems of gas exchange may be supported until the underlying problem improves or resolves. Usually mechanical ventilation is a temporary life-support technique. The need for this support may be lifelong for those with severe restrictive lung disease and those chronic, progressive neuromuscular diseases that reduce effective ventilation.

Mechanical ventilation is most often used for patients with hypoxemia and progressive alveolar hypoventilation with respiratory acidosis. The hypoxemia is usually due to pulmonary shunting of blood when other methods of oxygen delivery do not provide a sufficiently high fraction of inspired oxygen (Fio_2). Mechanical ventilation may be used for patients who need ventilatory support after surgery, those who expend too much energy with the work of breathing and barely maintain adequate gas exchange, or those who have general anesthesia or heavy sedation to allow diagnostic or therapeutic interventions.

Patient-Centered Collaborative Care

▪ *Assessment*

Assess the patient about to be intubated in the same way as for other breathing problems. Once mechanical ventilation has been started, assess the respiratory system on an ongoing basis. Monitor and assess for problems related to the artificial airway or ventilator, as well as for those related to mechanical ventilation.

▪ *Common Nursing Diagnoses and Collaborative Problems*

Nursing diagnoses and collaborative problems that may apply to patients requiring mechanical ventilation include:

- Impaired Verbal Communication related to physical barrier
- Sleep Deprivation related to interruptions for monitoring, noisy environment
- Death Anxiety related to loss of independent breathing ability
- Impaired Oral Mucous Membrane related to presence of endotracheal tube
- Potential for Ventilator-Associated Pneumonia

▪ *Interventions*

Endotracheal Intubation

The patient who needs mechanical ventilation must have an artificial airway. The most common type of airway for a short-term basis is the endotracheal (ET) tube. A tracheostomy is usually considered if the patient needs an artificial airway for longer than 10 to 14 days (see Chapter 30) to reduce tracheal and vocal cord damage. The goals of intubation are to maintain a patent airway, provide a means to remove secretions, and provide ventilation and oxygen.

Endotracheal Tube. An ET tube is a long polyvinyl chloride tube that is passed through the mouth or nose and into the trachea (Fig. 34-3). When properly positioned, the tip of the ET tube rests about 2 cm above the **carina** (the point at which the trachea divides into the right and left mainstem bronchi).

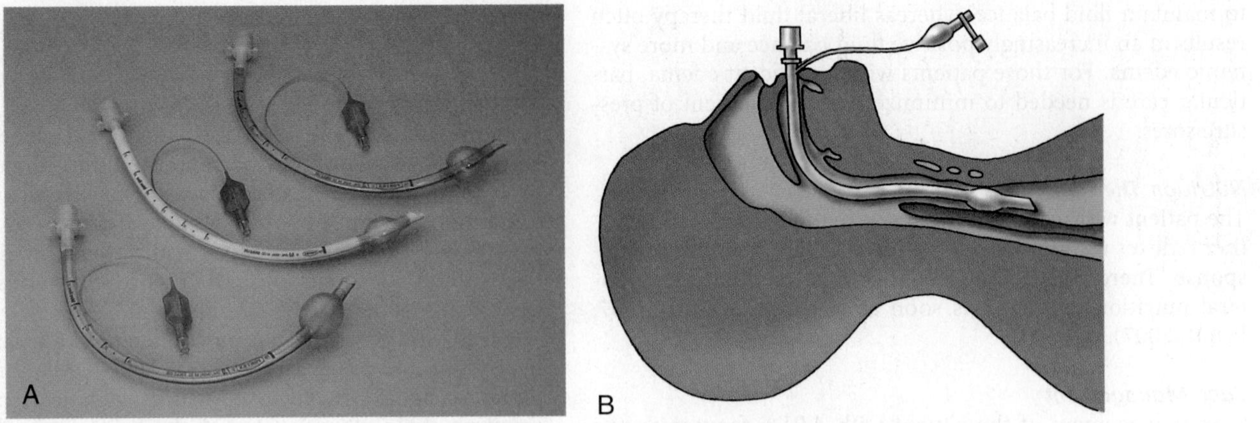
A
B

Fig. 34-3 • **A,** Endotracheal tubes. **B,** Correct placement of an oral endotracheal tube.

Oral intubation is the easiest and quickest method of establishing an airway and is often performed as an emergency procedure. Because of increased problems with sinusitis and otitis media, the nasal route is reserved for facial or oral traumas and surgeries and when oral intubation is not possible. The nasal route is not used if the patient has a blood clotting problem. An anesthesiologist, nurse anesthetist, or pulmonologist usually performs the intubation.

An ET tube has several parts (see Fig. 34-3). The shaft of the tube has a radiopaque line running the length of the tube. This line shows on x-ray and is used to determine correct tube placement. Short horizontal lines (depth markings) are used to place the tube correctly at the naris or mouth (at the incisor tooth) and to identify how far the tube has been inserted.

ANIMATION: Endotracheal Intubation ▶

The cuff at the distal end of the tube is inflated after placement and can create a seal between the trachea and the cuff. The seal ensures delivery of a set tidal volume when mechanical ventilation is used. When the cuff is inflated to an adequate sealing volume, a minimal amount of air can pass around the cuff to the vocal cords, nose, or mouth. Thus the patient cannot talk when the cuff is inflated. The cuff should be inflated using a minimal-leak technique.

The pilot balloon with a one-way valve permits air to be inserted into the cuff and prevents air from escaping. This balloon is a guide for determining whether air is present in the cuff, but it does not show how much or how little air is present.

The adaptor connects the ET tube to ventilator tubing or to other types of oxygen delivery systems. The endotracheal tube size is listed on the shaft of the tube. Adult tube sizes range from 7 to 9 mm. Tube size selected is based on the size of the patient.

Preparing for Intubation. Know the proper procedure for summoning intubation personnel in the facility to the bedside in an emergency situation. Explain the procedure to the patient as clearly as possible. *Basic life support measures, such as obtaining a patent airway and the delivery of 100% oxygen by a manual resuscitation bag with a facemask, are crucial to survival until help arrives.*

In an emergency, bring the code (or "crash") cart, airway equipment box, and suction equipment (often already on the code cart) to the bedside. Maintain a patent airway through positioning and the insertion of an oral or nasopharyngeal airway until the patient is intubated. During intubation, the nurse coordinates the response and continuously monitors for changes in vital signs, signs of hypoxia or hypoxemia, dysrhythmias, and aspiration. Ensure that each intubation attempt lasts no longer than 30 seconds, preferably less than 15 seconds. After 30 seconds, provide oxygen by means of a mask and manual resuscitation bag to prevent hypoxia and cardiac arrest. Suction as necessary.

Verifying Tube Placement. Immediately after an ET tube is inserted, placement should be verified. The most accurate ways to verify placement are by checking end-tidal carbon dioxide levels and by chest x-ray (Metheny, 2006). Assess for breath sounds bilaterally, symmetrical chest movement, and air emerging from the ET tube. If breath sounds and chest wall movement are absent on the left side, the tube may be in the right mainstem bronchus. The person intubating the patient should be able to reposition the tube without repeating the entire intubation procedure.

If the tube is in the stomach, the abdomen may be distended. Continuously monitor chest wall movement and breath sounds until tube placement is verified by chest x-ray.

Stabilizing the Tube. The nurse, respiratory therapist, or anesthesia provider stabilizes the ET tube at the mouth or nose. The tube is marked at the level where it touches the incisor tooth or naris. Two people working together use a head halter technique to secure the tube. Chart 34-9 outlines best practices for securing an oral or nasal ET tube.

An oral airway also may be inserted to keep the patient from biting an oral endotracheal tube. One person stabilizes the tube at the correct position and prevents head movement while a second person applies the tape. After the procedure is completed, verify and document the presence of bilateral and equal breath sounds and the level of the tube.

Nursing Care. Assess tube placement, minimal cuff leak, breath sounds, and chest wall movement regularly. Prevent pulling or tugging on the tube by the patient to prevent dislodgment or "slipping" of the tube, and check the pilot balloon to ensure that the cuff is inflated. Suctioning, coughing, and speaking attempts can cause dislodgment. Neck flexion moves the tube away from the carina; neck extension moves the tube closer to the carina. Rotation of the head also causes the tube to move. Mouth secretions and tongue movement can loosen the tape and change the tube's position. When other measures fail, apply soft wrist restraints, as prescribed, for the patient who is pulling on the tube. *Restraints are used as a last resort to prevent accidental extubation.* Adequate sedation (chemical restraint) may be needed to decrease agitation or prevent extubation. Obtain permission for restraints from the patient or family. More information on airway management is found in Chapter 30.

Chart 34-9 BEST PRACTICE FOR PATIENT SAFETY & QUALITY CARE

Securing an Oral and Nasal Endotracheal Tube

Little evidence is available to provide clinical direction on the best method to secure endotracheal (ET) and nasotracheal tubes; however, adhesive tape is the easiest, least expensive, and most frequently used.

Adhesive tape may be irritating to the skin, and frequent tape changes may disrupt the skin integrity. An additional reported complication is hospital-acquired cutaneous mucomycosis occurring around the surgical tape securing the ET tube. Protecting the skin, especially on the face, is a high priority for patients and nurses. This must be balanced against making sure the ET tube is not dislodged. A simple yet effective method of securing the oral and nasotracheal tube is demonstrated here:

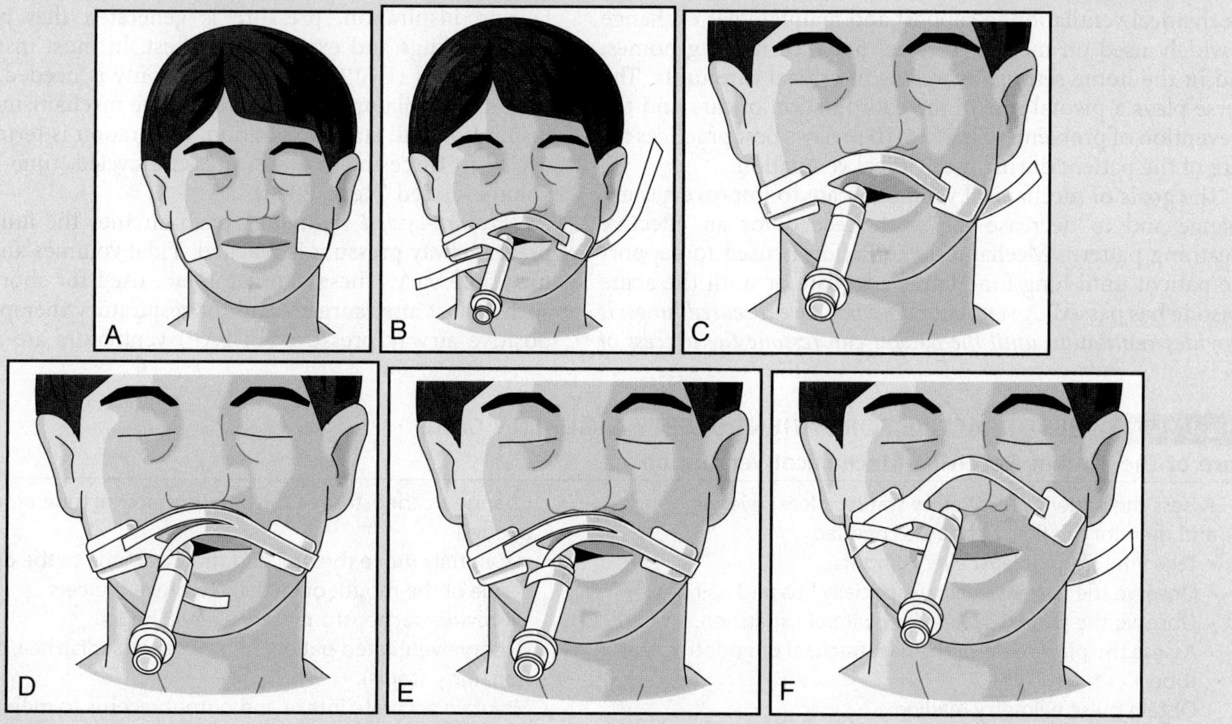
A
B
C
D
E
F

1. Prepare the skin by shaving the cheeks and upper lip, if possible.
2. Protect the skin by applying tincture of benzoin to the skin and ET tube and allow to dry (Mastisol may also be used, but Detachol must be used before removing the tape); then apply a 1 × 3–inch piece of thin DuoDerm or other protective or hydrocolloid membrane to the skin on the cheeks *(A)*.
3. Lay a 30-inch (about $2^1/_2$-foot) piece of adhesive tape on a flat surface, sticky side up. Cover the middle portion of the tape with another piece of tape (about 10 inches long) (sticky side to sticky side) to protect the back of the patient's neck. A tongue blade on each end folded over can keep it from getting tangled or sticking prematurely.
4. Place the tape behind the patient's neck. Remove the tongue blades, and place the tape on the protective membrane up to the end of the mouth on each side. Trim the tape as needed, and split each end of the tape.
5. Place the upper part of one end of the tape on the upper lip. Wrap the lower part of the tape securely around the tube *(B, C)*. Place the upper part of the other end of the tape on the upper lip, and wrap the lower part securely around the tube *(D, E)*. Do not have the tube too far to either side of the mouth, or it can cause skin breakdown in the corner of the mouth or lips.
6. The same method can be used for nasal tubes, but do not tape the tube too tightly to the nose or skin breakdown will occur on the naris *(F)*.
7. Always tape the tube to the upper lip; never the lower. The lower jaw moves too much with attempts to speak or oral care, which will move the tube and cause irritation and discomfort for the patient. The tape should be inspected at least every shift for signs of loosening or skin irritation or breakdown, especially with increased oral secretions. Tightness of the tape should also be checked each shift if swelling in the face and neck occurs or if there is an increase in fluid retention (as in anasarca, sepsis, or acute respiratory distress syndrome).

An additional technique for securing tubing that can decrease ET tube movement and provide a fulcrum for pulling on ventilator tubing is to attach a 6-inch (50-mL) piece of flexible ventilator tubing between the ET tube adaptor and the Y-connector of the ventilator tubing. The procedure for this technique is:

1. Shave the chest or clean with alcohol a portion of the chest at right angles to the angle of Louis. Apply tincture of benzoin, and allow to dry.
2. Prepare Montgomery straps by taking two 6-inch pieces of 2-inch wide adhesive tape. Double-back one end of each piece of tape, and cut a small hole in the ends that are doubled over.
3. Apply the tape to the prepared chest with the ends with the hole over each other. Thread a 12-inch piece of twill (trach) tape through both holes. Position the tubing with the Y-connector over the holes, and tie into place. This procedure allows all pulling on the tubing to place strain on the tape (straps) and not on the face or the tube. Caution should be taken if patients have increased partial pressure of arterial carbon dioxide retention, and end-tidal carbon dioxide monitoring may be useful when weaning.

Complications of an ET or nasotracheal tube can occur during placement, while in place, during extubation, or after extubation (either early or late). Trauma and other problems can occur to the face; eye; nasal and paranasal areas; oral, pharyngeal, bronchial, tracheal, and pulmonary areas; esophageal and gastric areas; and cardiovascular, musculoskeletal, and neurologic systems.

Mechanical Ventilation

Mechanical ventilation to support and maintain gas exchange is widely used on medical-surgical units, in nursing homes, and in the home setting, as well as in critical care units. The nurse plays a pivotal role in the coordination of care and the prevention of problems. Chart 34-10 reviews best practices for care of the patient during mechanical ventilation.

The goals of mechanical ventilation are to improve gas exchange and to decrease the work needed for an effective breathing pattern. Mechanical ventilation is used to support the patient until lung function is adequate or until the acute episode has passed. *A ventilator does not cure diseased lungs; it provides ventilation until the patient can resume the process of breathing.* It is important to remember *why* the patient is using the ventilator so that management efforts also focus on correcting the causes of the respiratory failure. If normal oxygenation, ventilation, and respiratory muscle strength are achieved, mechanical ventilation can be discontinued.

Types of Ventilators. Many types of ventilators are available. The ventilator selected depends on the severity of the disease process and the length of time ventilator support is needed. Most ventilators in use today are positive-pressure ventilators. During inspiration, pressure is generated that pushes air into the lungs and expands the chest. In most instances, an endotracheal (ET) tube or tracheostomy is needed. Positive-pressure ventilators are classified by the mechanism that ends inspiration and starts expiration. Inspiration is terminated or cycled in three major ways: pressure-cycled, time-cycled, or volume-cycled (Rose, 2006).

Pressure-cycled ventilators push air into the lungs until a preset airway pressure is reached. Tidal volumes and inspiratory time vary. These ventilators are used for short periods, such as just after surgery and for respiratory therapy. Bi-level positive airway pressure (Bi-PAP) ventilators are a modern

Chart 34-10 BEST PRACTICE FOR PATIENT SAFETY & QUALITY CARE

Care of the Patient Receiving Mechanical Ventilation

- Assess the patient's respiratory status at least every 4 hours and then for the first 24 hours as needed:
  - Take vital signs at least every 4 hours.
  - Observe the patient's color (especially lips and nail beds).
  - Observe the patient's chest for bilateral expansion.
  - Assess the placement of the nasotracheal or endotracheal tube.
  - Obtain pulse oximetry reading.
  - Evaluate ABGs as indicated.
  - Maintain head of the bed more than 30 degrees when patient is supine in bed to prevent microaspiration and ventilator-associated pneumonia.
- Document pertinent observations in the patient's medical record (chart).
- Check at least every 8 hours to be sure the ventilator setting is as prescribed.
- Check to be sure alarms are set (especially low-pressure and low-exhaled volume).
- If the patient is on PEEP, observe the peak airway pressure dial to determine the proper level of PEEP.
- Observe the exhaled volume digital display to be sure the patient is receiving the prescribed tidal volume.
- Empty ventilator tubings when moisture collects. *Never empty fluid in the tubing back into the cascade.*
- Ensure humidity by keeping delivered air temperature maintained at body temperature.
- Be sure the tracheostomy cuff (or endotracheal cuff) is adequately inflated to ensure tidal volume.
- Auscultate the lungs for crackles, wheezes, equal breath sounds, and decreased or absent breath sounds.
- Observe the patient's need for tracheal, oral, or nasal suctioning every 2 hours. Provide adequate suctioning as needed.
- Observe the patient's mouth around the endotracheal tube for pressure ulcers.
- Perform mouth care every 2 hours.
- Change tracheostomy tape or endotracheal tube tape as needed.
  - Carefully move the oral endotracheal tube to the opposite side of the mouth once daily to prevent ulcers.
  - Provide tracheostomy care every 8 hours.
- Observe ventilated patients for GI distress (diarrhea, constipation, tarry stools).
- Maintain accurate intake and output records to monitor fluid balance.
- Turn the patient at least every 2 hours, and get the patient out of bed as prescribed to promote pulmonary hygiene and prevent complications of immobility.
- Schedule treatments and nursing care at intervals for rest.
- Monitor the patient's progress on current ventilator settings, and make appropriate changes, as indicated.
- Monitor the patient for the effectiveness of mechanical ventilation in terms of his or her physiologic and psychological status.
- Monitor for adverse effects of mechanical ventilation: infection, barotrauma, reduced cardiac output.
- Position the patient to facilitate ventilation/perfusion matching ("good lung down"), as appropriate.
- Monitor the effects of ventilator changes on oxygenation and the patient's subjective response.
- Monitor readiness to wean.
- Explain all procedures and treatments; provide access to a call bell; visit the patient frequently.
- Provide a letter board or pencil and paper for communication. Request consultation with speech therapist for assistance, if necessary.
- Initiate relaxation techniques, as appropriate.
- Administer muscle-paralyzing agents, sedative, and narcotic analgesics, as appropriate.
- Include the patient and his or her family whenever possible (especially during suctioning and tracheostomy care).

ABGs, Arterial blood gases; *PEEP,* positive end-expiratory pressure.

form of pressure-cycled ventilator in which the ventilator provides a preset inspiratory pressure and an expiratory pressure similar to positive end-expiratory pressure (PEEP).

Time-cycled ventilators push air into the lungs until a preset time has elapsed. Tidal volume and pressure vary, depending on the needs of the patient and the type of ventilator.

Volume-cycled ventilators push air into the lungs until a preset volume is delivered. A constant tidal volume is delivered regardless of the pressure needed to deliver the tidal volume. A set pressure limit, however, prevents excessive pressure from being exerted on the lungs. The advantage of this type of ventilator is that a constant tidal volume is delivered regardless of the changing compliance of the lungs and chest wall or the airway resistance.

Microprocessor ventilators are computer-managed positive-pressure ventilators. A computer is built into the ventilator to allow ongoing monitoring of ventilatory functions, alarms, and patient conditions. It often has components of volume-, time-, and pressure-cycled ventilators. This type of ventilator is more responsive to patients who have severe lung disease and those who need prolonged weaning trials. Examples include the Draeger Evita XL (Fig. 34-4) and Puritan-Bennett 840.

Modes of Ventilation. The mode of ventilation is the way in which the patient receives breaths from the ventilator.

Assist-control (AC) ventilation is the mode used most often and is mainly a resting mode. The ventilator takes over the work of breathing for the patient. The tidal volume and ventilatory rate are preset. If the patient does not trigger spontaneous breaths, a minimal ventilatory pattern is established by the ventilator. It is programmed to respond to the patient's inspiratory effort if he or she does begin a breath. In this case, the ventilator delivers the preset tidal volume while allowing the patient to control the rate of breathing.

A disadvantage of the AC mode is that if the patient's spontaneous breathing rate increases, the ventilator continues to deliver a preset tidal volume with each breath. The patient may then hyperventilate, and respiratory alkalosis occurs. Investigate causes of hyperventilation, such as pain, anxiety, or acid-base imbalances, and correct them.

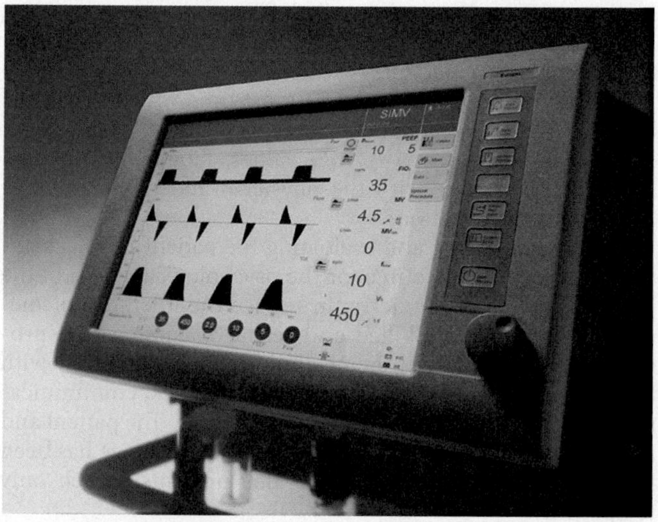
SIMV
10
5
35
4.5
0
10
450

Fig. 34-4 • Display signals, alarms, and control panel of a typical volume-cycled ventilator.

Synchronized intermittent mandatory ventilation (SIMV) is similar to AC ventilation in that tidal volume and ventilatory rate are preset. If the patient does not breathe, a minimal ventilatory pattern is established by the ventilator. Unlike the AC mode, SIMV allows spontaneous breathing at the patient's own rate and tidal volume between the ventilator breaths. It can be used as a main ventilatory mode or as a weaning mode. When used for weaning, the number of mechanical breaths (SIMV breaths) is gradually decreased (e.g., from 12 to 2) and the patient gradually resumes spontaneous breathing. The mandatory ventilator breaths are delivered when the patient is ready to inspire. This action coordinates breathing between the ventilator and the patient.

Bi-level positive airway pressure (BiPAP) provides noninvasive pressure support ventilation by nasal mask or facemask. Although BiPAP is most often used for patients with sleep apnea, it also may be used for patients with respiratory muscle fatigue to avoid more invasive ventilation methods.

Other modes of ventilation, such as pressure support and continuous flow (flow-by), are part of most microprocessor ventilators. Both types decrease the work of breathing and are often used for weaning patients from mechanical ventilation. Other modes are maximum mandatory ventilation (MMV), inverse inspiration-expiration (I/E) ratio, permissive hypercarbia, airway pressure–release ventilation, proportional assist ventilation, high-frequency ventilation, and high-frequency oscillation. Many of these modes use special ventilators, tubing, or airways.

Ventilator Controls and Settings. The volume-cycled ventilator is the most widely used ventilator in the acute care setting. Regardless of the type of volume-cycled ventilator used, the controls and types of settings are universal (see Fig. 34-4). The physician prescribes the ventilator settings, and usually the ventilator is readied or set up by the respiratory department. The nurse assists in connecting the patient to the ventilator and monitors the ventilator settings.

Tidal volume (V_T) is the volume of air the patient receives with each breath. It can be measured on either inspiration or expiration. The average prescribed V_T ranges between 7 and 10 mL/kg of body weight. Adding a zero to the weight of patients in kilograms gives an estimate of tidal volume.

Rate, or breaths/min, is the number of ventilator breaths delivered per minute. The rate is usually set between 10 and 14 breaths/min.

Fraction of inspired oxygen (Fio_2) is the oxygen level delivered to the patient. The prescribed Fio_2 is determined by the arterial blood gas (ABG) value and the patient's condition. Ventilators can provide 21% to 100% oxygen, depending on need.

The oxygen delivered to the patient is warmed to body temperature (98.6° F [37° C]) and humidified to 100%. These processes are needed because upper air passages of the respiratory tree, which normally warm, humidify, and filter air, are bypassed. Humidifying and warming prevent mucosal damage and ease clearance of secretions.

Peak airway (inspiratory) pressure (PIP) indicates the pressure needed by the ventilator to deliver a set tidal volume at a given lung compliance. The PIP value appears on the display on the front or top of the ventilator. It is the highest pressure reached during inspiration. Monitoring trends in PIP reflect changes in resistance of the lungs and resistance in the ventilator. An increased PIP reading means increased airway resistance in the patient or in the ventilator tubing (bronchospasm or pinched tubing), increased amount of secretions, pulmonary edema, or decreased pulmonary compliance (the lungs or chest wall is "stiffer" or harder to inflate). An upper pressure limit is set on the ventilator to prevent barotrauma. When the limit is reached, the high-pressure alarm sounds and the remaining volume is not given.

Continuous positive airway pressure (CPAP) applies positive airway pressure throughout the entire respiratory cycle for spontaneously breathing patients. Sedating drugs are given cautiously or not at all when the patient is receiving CPAP so that respiratory effort is not suppressed. CPAP keeps the alveoli open during inspiration and prevents alveolar collapse during expiration. This process increases functional residual capacity (FRC), improves gas exchange, and improves oxygenation.

The most common use of CPAP is to help in the weaning process. During CPAP, no ventilator breaths are delivered. The ventilator just delivers oxygen and provides monitoring and an alarm system. The respiratory pattern is determined by the patient's efforts. Normal levels of CPAP are 5 to 15 cm H_2O, adjusted to promote adequate oxygenation. If no pressure is set, the patient receives no positive pressure. Thus the patient is then using the ventilator as a T-piece with alarms.

Modifications of CPAP include nasal CPAP and BiPAP. These modifications are used for select problems.

Positive end-expiratory pressure (PEEP) is positive pressure exerted during the expiratory phase of ventilation. PEEP improves oxygenation by enhancing gas exchange and preventing atelectasis. It is used to treat persistent hypoxemia that does not improve with an acceptable oxygen delivery level. PEEP is often added when the partial pressure of arterial oxygen (Pao_2) remains low with an Fio_2 of 50% to 70% or greater.

The need for PEEP indicates a severe gas-exchange problem. *It is important to lower the Fio_2 delivered whenever possible because prolonged use of a high Fio_2 can damage lungs from the toxic effects of oxygen.* PEEP prevents alveoli from collapsing because the lungs are kept partially inflated so that alveolar-capillary gas exchange is promoted throughout the ventilatory cycle. The effect should be an increase in arterial blood oxygenation so that the Fio_2 can be decreased.

PEEP is "dialed in" with the PEEP dial on the control panel. The amount of PEEP is usually 5 to 15 cm H_2O and is read (monitored) on the peak airway pressure dial, the same dial used to read the PIP. When PEEP is added, the dial does not return to zero at the end of exhalation; rather, it returns to a baseline that has been increased from zero by the amount of PEEP applied.

Flow is how fast each breath is delivered and is usually set at 40 L/min. *If a patient is agitated or restless, has a widely fluctuating pressure reading on inspiration, or has other signs of air hunger, the flow may be set too low. Increasing the flow should be tried before using chemical restraints.*

Other settings may be used, depending on the type of ventilator and mode of ventilation. Examples include inspiratory and expiratory cycle, waveform, expiratory resistance, and plateau.

Nursing Management. The use of mechanical ventilation involves a collaborative and complex decision-making process for both the patient and family and the health care team. Address the physical and psychological concerns of the patient and family because the mechanical ventilator often causes them anxiety. Carefully explain the purpose of the ventilator, and acknowledge that the patient might feel some different sensations. Encourage the patient and family to express their concerns. Act as the coach to help and support the patient and family through this experience. In an emergency, explanations may not occur until the emergency has been controlled. Patients undergoing mechanical ventilation in ICUs often experience delirium, or "ICU psychosis." These patients need frequent, repeated explanations and reassurance.

When caring for a ventilated patient, be concerned with the patient first and the ventilator second (Lindgren & Ames, 2005; Manno, 2005). It is vital to understand why mechanical ventilation is needed. Causes such as excessive amounts of secretions, sepsis, and trauma require different interventions to allow ventilator independence. In addition, understand the patient's chronic health problems, especially chronic obstructive pulmonary disease (COPD), left-sided heart failure, anemia, and malnutrition. These problems may slow weaning from mechanical ventilation and require close monitoring and intervention.

Three nursing priorities in caring for the patient during mechanical ventilation are monitoring and evaluating patient responses, managing the ventilator system safely, and preventing complications (Lindgren & Ames, 2005; Manno, 2005).

Monitoring the Patient's Response. A major nursing responsibility is to monitor, evaluate, and document the patient's response to the ventilator. Assess vital signs and listen to breath sounds every 30 to 60 minutes at first. Monitor respiratory parameters (e.g., capnography, pulse oximetry), and check ABG values. Vital signs change during hypercarbia and hypoxemia.

Assess the breathing pattern in relation to the ventilatory cycle to determine whether the patient is tolerating or fighting the ventilator. Assess and record breath sounds, including bilateral equal breath sounds to ensure proper endotracheal (ET) tube placement. To determine the need for suctioning, observe secretions for type, color, and amount.

Assess the area around the ET tube or tracheostomy site at least every 4 hours for color, tenderness, skin irritation, and drainage, and document the findings. Monitoring provides information to guide the patient's activities, such as weaning, physical or occupational therapy, and self-care. Pace activities so that oxygenation and ventilation are adequate. Interpret ABG values to evaluate ventilation, and suggest ventilator settings that help the patient.

Because the nurse spends the most time with the patient, he or she is most likely to be the first person to recognize slight changes in vital signs or ABG values, fatigue, or distress. Promptly coordinate with the physician and implement the appropriate interventions.

While monitoring and evaluating the patient's clinical status, also serve as a resource for the psychological needs of the patient and family. Anxiety can reduce the tolerance of mechanical ventilation. Skilled and sensitive nursing care promotes psychological well-being and promotes synchrony with the ventilator. Because the patient cannot speak, communication can be frustrating and anxiety producing. The patient and family may panic because they believe that the voice has been lost. Reassure them that the ET tube prevents speech only temporarily.

Plan methods of communication to meet the patient's needs. Magic Slates, writing paper, computers, and tracheostomy tubes that permit talking are ways to communicate. Finding a successful means for communication is important because the patient often feels isolated as a result of the inability to speak. Try to anticipate his or her needs and provide easy access to frequently used belongings. Visits from family, friends, and pets and keeping a call light within reach are some ways of giving patients a sense of control over the environment. Urge them to participate in self-care.

Managing the Ventilator System. Ventilator settings are prescribed by the physician, often in conjunction with the respiratory therapist. These settings include tidal volume, respiratory rate, fraction of inspired oxygen (FIO_2), and mode of ventilation (assist-control [AC] ventilation, synchronized intermittent mandatory ventilation [SIMV]), and adjunctive modes, such as positive end-expiratory pressure [PEEP], pressure support, or continuous flow).

Perform and document ventilator checks according to the standards of the unit or facility. Respond promptly to alarms. During a ventilator check, compare the prescribed ventilator settings with the actual settings. Check the level of water in the humidifier and the temperature of the humidifying system to ensure that they are not too high. Temperature extremes damage the airway mucosa. Remove any condensation in the ventilator tubing by draining water into drainage collection receptacles, and empty them every shift. *To prevent bacterial contamination, do not allow tubing moisture and water to enter the humidifier.*

Mechanical ventilators have alarm systems that warn of a problem with either the patient or the ventilator. *Alarm systems must be activated and functional at all times. If the cause of the alarm cannot be determined, ventilate the patient manually with a resuscitation bag until the problem is corrected by another health care professional.* The two major alarms on a ventilator indicate either a high pressure or a low exhaled volume. Table 34-4 lists nursing interventions for various causes of ventilator alarms.

TABLE 34-4 Nursing Interventions for Various Causes of Ventilator Alarms

Cause	Nursing Interventions
HIGH-PRESSURE ALARM (sounds when peak inspiratory pressure reaches the set alarm limit [usually set 10-20 mm Hg above the patient's baseline PIP])	
There is an increased amount of secretions in the airways or a mucous plug.	Suction as needed.
The patient coughs, gags, or bites on the oral ET tube.	Insert oral airway to prevent biting on the ET tube.
The patient is anxious or fights the ventilator.	Provide emotional support to decrease anxiety. Increase the flow rate. Explain all procedures to the patient. Provide sedation or paralyzing agent per the physician's prescription.
Airway size decreases related to wheezing or bronchospasm.	Auscultate breath sounds. Consult with the physician for management of bronchospasm.
Pneumothorax occurs.	Auscultate breath sounds. Consult with the physician about a new onset of decreased breath sounds or unequal chest excursion, which may be due to pneumothorax.
The artificial airway is displaced; the ET tube may have slipped into the right mainstem bronchus.	Assess the chest for unequal breath sounds and chest excursion. Obtain a chest x-ray as ordered to evaluate the position of the ET tube. After the proper position is verified, tape the tube securely in place.
Obstruction in tubing occurs because the patient is lying on the tubing or there is water or a kink in the tubing.	Assess the system, moving from the artificial airway toward the ventilator. Empty water from the ventilator tubing, and remove any kinks.
There is increased PIP associated with deliverance of a sigh.	Coordinate with respiratory therapist or physician to adjust the pressure alarm.
Decreased compliance of the lung is noted; a trend of gradually increasing PIP is noted over several hours or a day.	Evaluate the reasons for the decreased compliance of the lungs. Increased PIP occurs in ARDS, pneumonia, or any worsening of pulmonary disease.
LOW EXHALED VOLUME (OR LOW-PRESSURE) ALARM (sounds when there is a disconnection or leak in the ventilator circuit or a leak in the patient's artificial airway cuff)	
A leak in the ventilator circuit prevents breath from being delivered.	Assess all connections and all ventilator tubings for disconnection.
The patient stops spontaneous breathing in the SIMV or CPAP mode or on pressure support ventilation.	Evaluate the patient's tolerance of the mode.
A cuff leak occurs in the ET or tracheostomy tube.	Evaluate the patient for a cuff leak. A cuff leak is suspected when the patient can talk (air escapes from the mouth) or when the pilot balloon on the artificial airway is flat (see section on tracheostomy tubes in Chapter 30).

ARDS, Acute respiratory distress syndrome; *CPAP*, continuous positive airway pressure; *ET*, endotracheal; *PIP*, peak inspiratory pressure; *SIMV*, synchronized intermittent mandatory ventilation.

Provide proper care of the ET or tracheostomy tube. Maintain a patent airway by suctioning when these are present:

- Secretions
- Increased peak airway (inspiratory) pressure (PIP)
- Rhonchi (wheezes)
- Decreased breath sounds

Careful maintenance of the ET or tracheostomy tube also ensures a patent airway. *Assess the tube's position at least every 2 hours, especially for the patient whose airway is attached to heavy ventilator tubing that may pull on the tracheostomy or ET tube. Position the ventilator tubing in such a way that the patient can move without pulling on the ET or tracheostomy tube. The ET tube can move and slip into the right mainstem bronchus.* To detect changes in the tube's position, mark the level at which the tube touches the patient's teeth or nose. Give mouth care at least every 2 hours for oral hygiene and to prevent loosening of the tape that holds the tube.

Preventing Complications. Most problems are due to the positive pressure from the ventilator. Nearly every body system is affected.

Cardiac problems from mechanical ventilation include hypotension and fluid retention. Hypotension is caused by positive pressure that increases chest pressure and inhibits blood return to the heart. The decreased venous return decreases cardiac output, reflected as hypotension. Hypotension is most often seen in patients who are dehydrated or need high PIP for ventilation. Teach the patient to avoid a **Valsalva maneuver** (bearing down while holding the breath).

Fluid is retained because of decreased cardiac output. The kidneys receive less blood flow, which then stimulates the renin-angiotensin-aldosterone system to retain fluid. Also, humidified air in the ventilator system contributes to fluid retention. If inspired air humidity is not adequate, the airways become dehydrated and the secretions solidify. Monitor the patient's fluid intake and output, weight, hydration, and signs of hypovolemia.

Lung problems during mechanical ventilation include **barotrauma** (damage to the lungs by positive pressure), **volutrauma** (damage to the lung by excess volume delivered to one lung over the other), and acid-base imbalance. Barotrauma includes pneumothorax, subcutaneous emphysema, and pneumomediastinum. Patients at highest risk for barotrauma have chronic airflow limitation (CAL), have blebs, are on PEEP, have dynamic hyperinflation, or require high pressures to ventilate the lungs (because of "stiff" lungs, as seen in acute respiratory distress syndrome [ARDS]). Blood gas abnormalities can be corrected by ventilator changes and adjustment of fluid and electrolyte imbalances.

GI and nutritional problems result from the stress of mechanical ventilation. Stress ulcers occur in many patients receiving mechanical ventilation. These ulcers complicate the patient's nutritional status and, because the mucosa in not intact, increase the risk for systemic infection. Antacids, sucralfate (Carafate, Sulcrate♣), and histamine blockers such as ranitidine (Zantac) or proton-pump inhibitors such as esomeprazole (Nexium) are often prescribed as soon as the patient is intubated. Changes in chest and abdominal cavity pressure can lead to a paralytic ileus. This problem affects absorption of nutrients through the GI system, requiring short-term parenteral nutritional support.

Because many other acute or life-threatening events occur at the same time, nutrition is often neglected. *Malnutrition is an extreme problem for these patients and is a major reason why they cannot be weaned from the ventilator. In malnutrition, the respiratory muscles lose mass and strength. The diaphragm, the major muscle of inspiration, is affected early. When the diaphragm and other respiratory muscles are weakened, ineffective breathing results, fatigue occurs, and the patient cannot be weaned from the ventilator.*

Balanced nutrition, whether by diet, enteral feedings, or parenteral feeding, is essential whenever a ventilator is used (O'Leary-Kelley et al., 2005). Furthermore, nutrition for the patient with chronic obstructive pulmonary disease (COPD) requires that special attention be given to the percentage of carbohydrates in the diet. During metabolism, carbohydrates are broken down to glucose, which then produces energy, carbon dioxide, and water. Excessive carbohydrate loads increase carbon dioxide production, which the patient with COPD may be unable to exhale. Hypercarbic respiratory failure results. Nutritional formulas with a higher fat content (e.g., Pulmocare, Nutri-Vent, intralipids) are calorie sources to combat this problem.

Electrolyte replacement is also important because they have a major impact on muscle function. Closely monitor potassium, calcium, magnesium, and phosphate levels, and replace them as prescribed.

Infections are always a threat for the patient using a ventilator, especially ventilator-associated pneumonia (VAP). The ET or tracheostomy tube bypasses the body's normal process of filtering air and provides a direct access for bacteria to the lower parts of the respiratory system. Often within 48 hours the artificial airway is colonized with bacteria, which promotes pneumonia development. Aspiration of colonized fluid from the mouth or the stomach can be a source of infection. Pneumonia prolongs hospital stay and increases morbidity. *Infection prevention through strict adherence to infection control, especially handwashing, during suctioning and care of the tracheostomy or ET tube, is essential.* To prevent pneumonia, perform oral care every 2 hours and implement pulmonary hygiene, including chest physiotherapy, postural drainage, and turning and positioning (Lawson, 2005; Powers, 2007). More information on VAP can be found in Chapter 33.

Muscle deconditioning and weakness can occur because of immobility. Having the patient get out of bed, ambulate with assistance, and perform exercises not only improves muscle strength but also boosts morale, enhances gas exchange, and promotes oxygen delivery to all muscles.

Ventilator dependence is the inability to wean off the ventilator. This problem can be psychological or physiologic, but more often it has a physiologic basis. The longer a patient uses a ventilator, the more difficult is the weaning process because the respiratory muscles fatigue and cannot assume breathing. The health care team uses every method of weaning before a patient is declared "unweanable."

Collaborate with the physician, social worker or psychologist, and a member of the clergy to discuss with the patient and the family the patient's quality of life, goals, and values. In accordance with this discussion, make arrangements for home ventilation, nursing home placement, or withdrawal of life support (in terminal cases). Special units and facilities are available to maximize the rehabilitation and weaning of ventilator-dependent patients.

Weaning. Weaning is the process of going from ventilatory dependence to spontaneous breathing. The weaning process is

TABLE 34-5 Weaning Methods

SYNCHRONOUS INTERMITTENT MANDATORY VENTILATION
- The patient breathes between the machine's preset breaths/min rate.
- The machine is initially set on an SIMV rate of 12, meaning the patient receives a minimum of 12 breaths/min by the ventilator.
- The patient's respiratory rate will be a combination of ventilator breaths and spontaneous breaths.
- As the weaning process ensues, the physician prescribes gradual decreases in the SIMV rate, usually at a decrease of 1 to 2 breaths/min.

T-PIECE TECHNIQUE
- The patient is taken off the ventilator for short periods (initially 5 to 10 minutes) and allowed to breathe spontaneously.
- The ventilator is replaced with a T-piece (see Chapter 30) or CPAP, which delivers humidified oxygen.
- The prescribed Fio_2 may be higher for the patient on the T-piece than on the ventilator.
- Weaning progresses as the patient can tolerate progressively longer periods off the ventilator.
- Nighttime weaning is not usually attempted until the patient can maintain spontaneous respirations most of the day.

PRESSURE SUPPORT VENTILATION
- PSV allows the patient's respiratory effort to be augmented by a predetermined pressure assist from the ventilator.
- As the weaning process ensues, the amount of pressure applied to inspiration is gradually decreased.
- Another method of weaning with PSV is to maintain the pressure but gradually decrease the ventilator's preset breaths/min rate.

CPAP, Continuous positive airway pressure; *Fio_2*, fraction of inspired oxygen; *PSV*, pressure support ventilation; *SIMV*, synchronized intermittent mandatory ventilation.

prolonged if complications develop. Many problems can be avoided through skillful nursing care. For example, turning and positioning the patient not only promote comfort and prevent skin breakdown but also improve gas exchange and prevent pneumonia and atelectasis. Table 34-5 lists various weaning techniques.

CONSIDERATIONS FOR OLDER ADULTS

The older patient, especially one who has smoked or who has a chronic lung problem such as COPD, is at risk for ventilator dependence and failure to wean. Age-related changes, such as increased chest wall stiffness, reduced ventilatory muscle strength, and decreased lung elasticity, reduce the likelihood of weaning. The usual manifestations of ventilatory failure—hypoxemia and hypercarbia—may be less obvious in the older adult, and other clinical measures of oxygenation, such as a change in mental status, should be used to determine breathing effectiveness.

Extubation. Extubation is the removal of the endotracheal (ET) tube. The tube is removed when the need for intubation has been resolved. Before removal, explain the procedure. Set up the prescribed oxygen delivery system at the bedside, and bring in the equipment for emergency reintubation. Hyperoxygenate the patient, and thoroughly suction both the ET tube and the oral cavity. Then rapidly deflate the cuff of the ET tube and remove the tube at peak inspiration. Immediately instruct the patient to cough. It is normal for large amounts of oral secretions to collect. Give oxygen by facemask or nasal cannula. The fraction of inspired oxygen (Fio_2) is usually prescribed at 10% higher than the level used while the ET tube was in place.

Monitoring after extubation is essential. Monitor the vital signs every 5 minutes at first, and assess the ventilatory pattern for manifestations of respiratory distress (Astle & Smith, 2007). It is common for patients to be hoarse and have a sore throat for a few days after extubation. Teach the patient to sit in a semi-Fowler's position, take deep breaths every half-hour, use an incentive spirometer every 2 hours, and limit speaking right after extubation. These measures help gas exchange, decrease laryngeal edema, and reduce vocal cord irritation. Observe closely for respiratory fatigue and airway obstruction.

Early manifestations of obstruction are mild dyspnea, coughing, and the inability to expectorate secretions. Notify the physician or Rapid Response Team at the onset of these problems, to evaluate the need for reintubation. ***Stridor*** *is a high-pitched, crowing noise during inspiration caused by laryngospasm or edema above or below the glottis. This sound is a late manifestation of a narrowed airway and requires prompt attention. Immediately call the Rapid Response Team.* Racemic epinephrine, a topical aerosol vasoconstrictor, is given, and reintubation may be needed (Pruitt, 2006).

◀ AUDIO CLIP: Stridor

NCLEX EXAMINATION CHALLENGE

The client is a 106-pound woman who is being mechanically ventilated after surgery. The ventilator is volume-cycled and set at 500 mL tidal volume and 16 breaths per minute. Her latest ABGs are pH, 7.48; HCO_3^-, 23 mEq/L; $Paco_2$, 25 mm Hg; Pao_2, 98 mm Hg. How should the nurse interpret this laboratory finding?

A. Normal ABGs indicating adequate ventilation
B. Acute respiratory alkalosis and hyperventilation
C. Acute respiratory acidosis and hypoventilation
D. Chronic respiratory acidosis and hypoventilation

evolve For the correct answer, go to http://evolve.elsevier.com/Iggy/.

CHEST TRAUMA

Chest injuries are responsible for about 16,000 or 25% of traumatic deaths in the United States each year. Many of the injured die before arriving at health care facilities. Relatively few chest injuries require thoracotomy. The remainder can be treated with basic resuscitation, intubation, or chest tube placement. *The first emergency approach to all chest injuries is ABC (airway, breathing, circulation) followed by rapid assessment and treatment of life-threatening conditions.*

Pulmonary Contusion

Pulmonary contusion, a potentially lethal injury, is the most common chest injury seen in the United States. After a contusion, respiratory failure develops over time rather than immediately. This condition most often follows injuries caused by rapid deceleration during vehicular accidents. Hemorrhage occurs in and between the alveoli. The resulting edema decreases lung movement and reduces the area for gas exchange. The patient becomes hypoxemic and dyspneic. The bronchial mucosa is irritated, and secretions increase.

Patients with pulmonary contusion may be asymptomatic at first and can later develop respiratory failure. These patients present with bloody sputum, decreased breath sounds, crackles, and wheezes. At first, the chest x-ray may show no abnormalities. A hazy opacity in the lobes or parenchyma may develop over several days. If there is no disruption of the parenchyma, resorption of the bruise often occurs without treatment.

Treatment includes maintenance of ventilation and oxygenation. Monitor central venous pressure (CVP) closely, and restrict fluid intake as needed. The patient in obvious respiratory distress may need mechanical ventilation with positive end-expiratory pressure (PEEP) to inflate the lungs.

A vicious cycle occurs in which more muscle effort is needed for ventilating a lung with a contusion and the patient becomes progressively hypoxemic. This situation causes him or her to tire easily, have reduced gas exchange, and become more fatigued and hypoxemic. Flail chest may also occur when pulmonary contusion occurs with parenchymal damage. This condition often leads to acute respiratory distress syndrome (ARDS).

Rib Fracture

Rib fractures are a common injury to the chest wall. They most often result from direct blunt trauma to the chest. Direct force applied to the ribs fractures them and drives the bone ends into the chest. Thus there is a risk for deep chest injury, such as pulmonary contusion, pneumothorax, and/or hemothorax.

The patient has pain on movement and splints the chest defensively. Splinting reduces breathing depth and leads to inadequate clearance of pulmonary secretions. If the patient has pre-existing pulmonary disease, the risk for atelectasis and pneumonia increases. Those with injuries to the first or second rib, flail chest, seven or more fractured ribs, or expired volumes of less than 15 mL/kg often have a deep chest injury and a poor prognosis.

Management of uncomplicated rib fractures is simple because the fractured ribs reunite spontaneously. The chest is usually not splinted by tape or other materials. The main focus is to decrease pain so that adequate ventilation is maintained. An intercostal nerve block may be used if pain is severe. Potent analgesics that cause respiratory depression are avoided.

Flail Chest

Flail chest is the inward movement of the thorax during inspiration, with outward movement during expiration. It usually involves one side of the chest and results from multiple rib fractures caused by blunt chest trauma leaving a segment of the chest wall loose. Flail chest often occurs in high-speed vehicular crashes. It is more common in older patients and has a high mortality rate.

The movement of this loose segment becomes opposite of the expansion and contraction movement of the rest of the chest wall. Flail chest can also occur from bilateral separations of the ribs from their cartilage connections to each other anteriorly, without an actual rib fracture. This condition can occur during cardiopulmonary resuscitation on an older adult. Other injuries to the lung tissue under the flail segment may be present. Gas exchange is impaired, as is the ability to cough and clear secretions. Defensive splinting further reduces the patient's ability to exert the extra effort required for breathing and may contribute later to failure to wean.

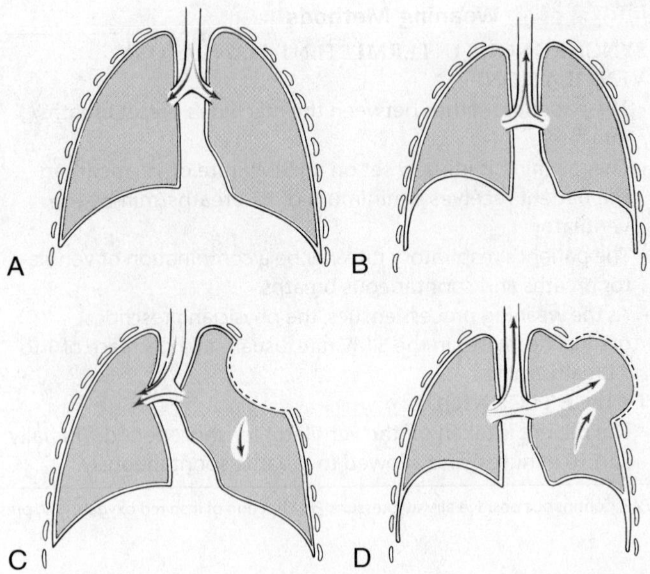
A
B
C
D

Fig. 34-5 • Flail chest. Normal respiration: **A**, Inspiration; **B**, Expiration. Paradoxic motion: **C**, Inspiration. Area of the lung underlying unstable chest wall sucks in on inspiration. **D**, Expiration. Unstable area balloons out. Note movement of mediastinum toward opposite lung during inspiration.

Assess the patient with a flail chest for paradoxic chest movement, dyspnea, cyanosis, tachycardia, and hypotension. **Paradoxic chest movement** is the "sucking inward" of the loose chest area during inspiration and a "puffing out" of the same area during expiration (Fig. 34-5). The patient is often anxious, short of breath, and in pain (McCance & Huether, 2006).

Nursing interventions include humidified oxygen, pain management, promotion of lung expansion through deep breathing and positioning, and secretion clearance by coughing and tracheal aspiration.

The patient with a flail chest may be managed with vigilant respiratory care. Mechanical ventilation may be needed if respiratory failure or shock occurs. Monitor ABG values closely, along with vital capacity. With severe hypoxemia and hypercarbia, the patient is intubated and mechanically ventilated with PEEP. With lung contusion or an underlying pulmonary disease, the risk for respiratory failure increases. Flail chest is stabilized by positive-pressure ventilation rather than surgery. Surgical stabilization is used only in extreme cases of flail chest.

Monitor the patient's vital signs and fluid and electrolyte balance closely so that hypovolemia or shock can be managed immediately. If he or she has a lung contusion, monitor central venous pressure (CVP) and give IV fluids as prescribed. Assess for pain, and intervene to relieve the pain. Analgesic drugs by IV, epidural, or nerve block route may be prescribed. Give psychosocial support to the extremely anxious patient by explaining all procedures, talking slowly, and allowing time for him or her to express feelings and concerns.

Pneumothorax

Any chest injury that allows air to enter the pleural space results in a rise in chest pressure and a reduction in vital capacity. Severity depends on the amount of lung collapse produced. Pneumothorax is often caused by blunt chest trauma and may occur with some degree of hemothorax. The pneumothorax can be open (pleural cavity is exposed to outside air, as through an open wound in the chest wall) or closed. Assessment findings commonly include:

- Reduced breath sounds on auscultation
- Hyperresonance on percussion
- Prominence of the involved side of the chest, which moves poorly with respirations
- Deviation of the trachea away from (closed) or toward (open) the affected side

In addition, the patient may have pleuritic pain, tachypnea, and **subcutaneous emphysema** (air under the skin in the subcutaneous tissues) (Bademan, 2007).

An ultrasound examination or a chest x-ray is used for diagnosis. Chest tubes may be needed to allow the air to escape and the lung to re-inflate.

Tension Pneumothorax

Tension pneumothorax, a rapidly developing and life-threatening complication of blunt chest trauma, results from an air leak in the lung or chest wall (Day, 2006). Air forced into the chest cavity causes complete collapse of the affected lung. Air that enters the pleural space during inspiration does not exit during expiration. As a result, air continues to collect under pressure, compressing blood vessels and limiting venous return. Because this process leads to decreased filling of the heart, cardiac output is reduced. *If not promptly detected and treated, tension pneumothorax is quickly fatal.* Causes of tension pneumothorax are blunt chest trauma, mechanical ventilation with positive end-expiratory pressure (PEEP), closed-chest drainage (chest tubes), and insertion of central venous access catheters.

Assessment findings with tension pneumothorax include:

- Asymmetry of the thorax
- Tracheal movement *away* from midline to the *unaffected* side
- Respiratory distress
- Absence of breath sounds on one side
- Distended neck veins
- Cyanosis
- Hypertympanic sound on percussion over the affected side

Pneumothorax is detectable on a chest x-ray. ABG assays show hypoxia and respiratory alkalosis.

A large-bore needle is inserted by the health care provider into the second intercostal space in the midclavicular line of the affected side as initial treatment for tension pneumothorax. After this measure is completed, a chest tube is placed into the fourth intercostal space and the other end is attached to a water seal drainage system until the lung re-inflates. Chest tubes are discussed in detail in Chapter 32.

Hemothorax

Hemothorax is a common problem occurring after blunt chest trauma or penetrating injuries. A *simple* hemothorax is a blood loss of less than 1500 mL into the chest cavity; a *massive* hemothorax is a blood loss of more than 1500 mL.

Bleeding is caused by injury to the lung tissue, such as lung contusions or lacerations, that can occur with rib and sternal fractures. Massive internal chest bleeding in blunt chest trauma may stem from the heart, great vessels, or the intercostal arteries.

Physical assessment findings vary with the size of the hemothorax. If the hemothorax is small, the patient may not have symptoms. If the hemothorax is larger, the patient may have respiratory distress. In addition, breath sounds are reduced on auscultation. Percussion on the involved side results in a dull sound. Blood in the pleural space is visible on a chest x-ray and confirmed by diagnostic thoracentesis.

Interventions are aimed at removing the blood in the pleural space to normalize pulmonary function and to prevent infection. Front and back chest tubes are inserted to empty the pleural space. Carefully monitor the chest tube drainage. The physician evaluates chest x-rays serially to determine treatment effectiveness.

An open thoracotomy may be needed when there is initial loss of 1500 to 2000 mL of blood from the chest cavity or persistent bleeding at the rate of 200 mL/hr over 3 hours. Monitor the vital signs, blood loss, and overall intake and output. Assess the patient's response to the chest tubes, and infuse IV fluids and blood as prescribed. The blood lost through chest drainage can be autotransfused back into the patient if needed.

Tracheobronchial Trauma

Most tears of the tracheobronchial tree result from severe blunt trauma or rapid deceleration. The tears often involve the mainstem bronchi. Injuries to the trachea usually occur at the junction of the trachea and cricoid cartilage. These injuries are often caused by striking the neck against the dashboard or steering wheel during a car crash. Patients with lacerations of the trachea develop massive air leaks, which cause air to enter the mediastinum and leads to extensive subcutaneous emphysema. Upper airway obstruction may also occur, causing severe respiratory distress and inspiratory stridor. Large tracheal tears are managed by cricothyroidotomy or tracheotomy below the level of injury. A patient with a torn mainstem bronchus may develop a tension pneumothorax rapidly once he or she is intubated and ventilated with positive pressure.

Assess the patient for hypoxemia by ABG assays. Apply oxygen as needed. Depending on the degree of injury, the patient may need mechanical ventilation or surgical repair. Assess vital signs every 15 minutes because the patient is likely to be hypotensive and in shock. Continue to assess for subcutaneous emphysema and listen to the lungs every 1 to 2 hours. Decreased breath sounds or wheezing may indicate further obstruction, atelectasis, or pneumothorax. Care of the patient with a tracheostomy is discussed in Chapter 30.

HUMAN NEEDS NURSING CARE REVIEW

What might you NOTICE if the patient is experiencing inadequate oxygenation and tissue perfusion as a result of respiratory problems?

- Respirations rapid and shallow
- Change in cognition, acute confusion (especially in older adults)
- Decreased oxygen saturation by pulse oximetry
- Skin cyanosis or pallor (lighter-skinned patients)
- Cyanosis or pallor of the lips and oral mucous membranes (in patients of any skin color)
- Tachycardia
- Patient appears to strain to catch breath
- Patient is restless or anxious

What should you INTERPRET and how should you RESPOND to a patient experiencing inadequate oxygenation and tissue perfusion as a result of an acute critical respiratory problem?

Perform and interpret physical assessment, including:

- Taking vital signs
- Auscultating all lung fields
- Monitoring oxygen saturation by pulse oximetry
- Checking the accuracy of pulse oximetry readings
- Checking most recent laboratory values for ABG levels
- Assessing cognition (mini-mental status exam)
- Assessing for the presence of hemoptysis
- Assessing the patient's ability to cough and clear the airway
- Asking the patient if he or she has chest pain
- Checking for the presence of petechiae, especially over the chest

Respond by:

- Applying oxygen with a non-rebreather mask, and assessing the patient's responses to this intervention
- Keeping the patient's head elevated to about 30 degrees
- Suctioning (oral, pharyngeal, endotracheal, tracheostomy), if needed
- Notifying physician or Rapid Response Team
- Staying with the patient
- Calling for the emergency cart to be brought to the patient's bedside
- Reassuring the patient that appropriate interventions are being instituted
- Preparing for intubation
- Using a manual resuscitation bag if the patient's Sao_2 falls below 60% while receiving oxygen by mask
- Starting an IV

On what should you REFLECT?

- Observe patient for evidence of restored oxygenation (see Chapter 29)
- Think about what may have precipitated this episode and what steps could be taken to either prevent a similar episode or identify it earlier.
- Think about what additional resources could improve the nursing response to this situation.

GET READY FOR THE NCLEX EXAMINATION!

Key Points

Review these Key Points for each NCLEX Examination Client Needs Category.

Safe and Effective Care Environment

- Use aseptic technique when caring for a patient requiring pulmonary suctioning.
- Identify patients in your setting who are at risk for developing a pulmonary embolism.
- Use Bleeding Precautions for any patient receiving anticoagulant or fibrinolytic therapy (see Chart 34-6).
- Keep antidotes available when patients are receiving heparin (antidote is protamine) or warfarin (antidote is phytonadione).
- Inspect the mouth and perform oral care every 2 hours for anyone who has an endotracheal tube or is being mechanically ventilated.
- Ensure that alarm systems on mechanical ventilators are activated and functional at all times.

Health Promotion and Maintenance

- Teach patients ways to promote venous return and avoid deep vein thrombosis (DVT), especially when traveling long distances (see Chart 34-1).
- Use Aspiration Precautions for any patient with an altered level of consciousness, poor gag reflex, neurologic impairment, or an endotracheal tube.
- Check the patient with ARDS hourly for oxygen saturation, vital sign changes, or any indication of increased work of breathing such as cyanosis, pallor, and retractions.
- Assess all patients with blunt chest trauma for position of the trachea and bilateral breath sounds.

Psychosocial Integrity

- Allow the patient and family members the opportunity to express feelings and concerns about a change in breathing status or the possibility of intubation and mechanical ventilation.
- Teach family members ways to communicate with a patient who is intubated or being mechanically ventilated.
- Reassure intubated patients that speech loss is temporary.
- Remember that patients who are receiving mechanical ventilation and are being chemically paralyzed usually can hear and can feel pain.

Physiological Integrity

- Notify the physician immediately for any patient who develops sudden-onset respiratory difficulty.
- Check oxygen saturation by pulse oximetry for any patient who has trouble breathing or who develops acute confusion.
- Evaluate arterial blood gas values to determine the severity of hypoxia and the patient's response to therapy.
- Apply oxygen to anyone who is hypoxemic.
- Ensure that oxygen therapy delivered to the patient is humidified (and warmed, when possible).

- Assess lung sounds bilaterally each hour for patients who are receiving PEEP.
- Check all ventilator settings against the prescription at least once per shift.
- Administer drugs for pain to patients who have rib fractures, and encourage deep breaths.
- Maintain a patent airway on all patients who experience trauma.

Additional Study Resources

Go to your Companion CD or Evolve at http://evolve.elsevier.com/Iggy/ for *Self-Assessment Questions for the NCLEX Examination.*

evolve Go to Evolve at http://evolve.elsevier.com/Iggy/ for *Prioritization and Delegation Questions for the NCLEX Examination.*

SELECTED BIBLIOGRAPHY

Asterisk indicates a classic or definitive work on this subject.

American Lung Association. (2006). *Adult (acute) respiratory distress syndrome (ARDS) fact sheet.* Retrieved August 2007, from www.lungusa.org/site/pp.asp?c=dvLUK9O0E&b=35012.

Andrews, P., & Habashi, N. (2007). Understanding high-frequency oscillatory ventilation. *American Nurse Today, 2*(10), 29-32.

Astle, S., & Smith, D. (2007). Taking your patient off a ventilator. *RN, 70*(5), 34-39.

Bademan, E. (2007). Act fast against pneumothorax. *American Nurse Today, 2*(5), 58.

Ballard, N., Robley, L., Barrett, D., Fraser, D., & Mendoza, I. (2006). Patients' recollections of therapeutic paralysis in the intensive care unit. *American Journal of Critical Care, 15*(1), 86-94.

Beattie, S. (2007). Bedside emergency: Respiratory distress. *RN, 70*(7), 34-38.

Bulechek, G.M., Butcher, H.K., & McCloskey Dochterman, J. (Eds.). (2008). *Nursing interventions classification (NIC)* (5th ed.). St. Louis: Mosby.

Burns, S. (2005). Mechanical ventilation of patients with acute respiratory distress syndrome and patients requiring weaning. *Critical Care Nurse, 25*(4), 14-23.

*Burns, S.M. (1999). Weaning from long-term mechanical ventilation. In C.M. Chulay & S.M. Burns (Eds.), *Care of the mechanically ventilated patient series.* Aliso Viejo, CA: American Association of Critical Care Nurses.

Clautier, L. (2007). Diagnosis of pulmonary embolism. *Clinical Journal of Oncology Nursing, 11*(3), 343-348.

*Clochesy, J., Daly, B., & Montenegro, H. (1995). Weaning chronically critically ill adults from mechanical ventilatory support: A descriptive study. *American Journal of Critical Care, 4*(2), 93-99.

Davis, M., & Johnston, J. (2008). Maintaining supplemental oxygen during transport. *AJN, 108*(1), 35-36.

Day, M. (2006). Tension pneumothorax from central line placement. *Nursing2006, 36*(11), 80.

English, J. (2006). Prodromal signs and symptoms of a venous pulmonary embolism. *MEDSURG Nursing, 15*(6), 352-356.

Giuliano, K., & Higgins, T. (2005). New generation pulse oximetry in the care of critically ill patients. *American Journal of Critical Care, 14*(1), 26-37.

Goldhill, D.R., Imhoff, M., McLean, B., & Waldmann, C. (2007). Rotational bed therapy to prevent and treat respiratory complications: A review and meta-analysis. *American Journal of Critical Care, 16*(1), 50-61.

*Happ, M.B. (2001). Communicating with mechanically ventilated patients: State of the science. *AACN Clinical Issues: Advanced Practice in Acute and Critical Care, 12*(2), 247-258.

Happ, M.B., Swigart, V.A., Tate, J.A., Arnold, R.M., Sereika, S.M., & Hoffman, L.A. (2007). Family presence and surveillance during weaning from prolonged mechanical ventilation. *Heart & Lung, 36*(1), 47-57.

Kleinman, S., Gajic, O., & Nunes, E. (2007). Promoting recognition of transfusion-related acute lung injury. *Critical Care Nurse, 27*(4), 49-53.

Knippen, M. (2006). Transfusion-related acute lung injury. *American Journal of Nursing, 106*(6), 61-64.

Lawson, P. (2005). Zapping VAP with evidence-based practice. *Nursing2005, 35*(5), 66-67.

Lindgren, V., & Ames, N. (2005). Caring for patients on mechanical ventilation. *American Journal of Nursing, 105*(5), 50-60.

Mancebo, J., Fernández, R., Blanch, L., Rialp, G., Gordo, F., Ferrer, M., et al. (2006). A multicenter trial of prolonged prone ventilation in severe acute respiratory distress syndrome. *American Journal of Respiratory and Critical Care Medicine, 173*(11), 1233-1239.

Manno, M. (2005). Managing mechanical ventilation. *Nursing2005, 35*(12), 36-41.

McCance, K., & Huether, S. (2006). *Pathophysiology: The biologic basis for disease in adults and children* (5th ed.). St. Louis: Mosby.

Meiner, S., & Lueckenotte, A. (Eds.). (2006). *Gerontologic nursing,* (3rd ed.). St. Louis: Mosby.

Metheny, N. (2006). Preventing respiratory complications of tube feedings: Evidence-based practice. *American Journal of Critical Care, 15*(4), 360-369.

Munro, C.L., Grap, M.J., Elswick, R.K. Jr., McKinney, J., Sessler, C.N., & Hummel, R.S. III. (2006). Oral health status and development of ventilator-associated pneumonia: A descriptive study. *American Journal of Critical Care, 15*(5), 453-460.

O'Leary-Kelley, C.M., Puntillo, K.A., Barr, J., Stotts, N., & Douglas, M.K. (2005). Nutritional adequacy in patients receiving mechanical ventilation who are fed enterally. *American Journal of Critical Care, 14*(3), 222-230.

Pagana, K., & Pagana, T. (2006). *Mosby's manual of diagnostic and laboratory tests* (3rd ed.). St. Louis: Mosby.

Powers, J. (2007). The five P's spell positive outcomes for ARDS patients. *American Nurse Today, 2*(3), 34-38.

Pruitt, B. (2006). Weaning patients from mechanical ventilation. *Nursing2006, 36*(9), 36-41.

Pruitt, B. (2007). Take an evidence-based approach to treating acute lung injury. *Nursing2007, Spring*(Suppl.), 14-18.

Rose, L. (2006). Advanced modes of mechanical ventilation: Implications for practice. *AACN Advanced Critical Care, 17*(2), 145-158.

Shaughnessy, K. (2007). Massive pulmonary embolism. *Critical Care Nurse, 27*(1), 39-50.

Sweeney, J., & Ardisson, M. (2006). What's a fat embolism? *Nursing2006, 36*(11), 22.

Taylor, M. (2005). ARDS diagnosis and management. *Dimensions of Critical Care Nursing, 24*(5), 197-207.

Thomas, P.J., Paratz, J.D., Lipman, J., & Stanton, W.R. (2007). Lateral positioning of ventilated intensive care patients: A study of oxygenation, respiratory mechanics, hemodynamics, and adverse events. *Heart & Lung, 36*(4), 277-286.

Tolentino-DelosReyes, A.F., Ruppert, S.D., & Shiao, S.Y. (2007). Evidence-based practice: Use of the ventilator bundle to prevent ventilator-associated pneumonia. *American Journal of Critical Care, 16*(1), 20-27.

Wiedemann, H.P., Wheeler, A.P., Bernard, G.R., Thompson, B.T., Hayden, D., deBoisblanc, B., et al. (2006). Comparison of two fluid-management strategies in acute lung injury. *New England Journal of Medicine, 354*(24), 2564-2576.

Winkelman, C. (2008). Inflammation and genomics in the critical care unit. *Critical Care Nursing Clinics of North America, 20*(2), 213-221.

Workman, M.L., & Winkelman, C. (2008). Genetic influences in common respiratory disorders. *Critical Care Nursing Clinics of North America, 20*(2), 171-189.

VIII

UNIT

Problems of Cardiac Output and Tissue Perfusion

Management of Patients with Problems of the Cardiovascular System

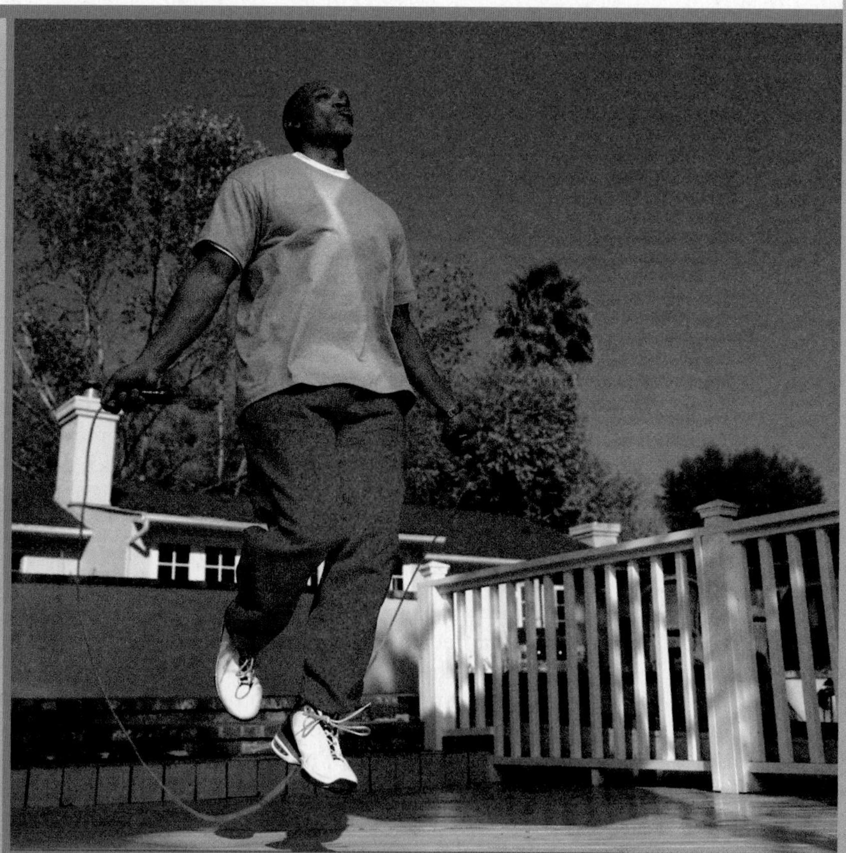

35 CHAPTER

Assessment of the Cardiovascular System

Donna Ignatavicius • Sharon Henry Walicek

LEARNING OUTCOMES

For clinical competence and success on the NCLEX Examination, study this chapter with these Learning Outcomes in mind:

Safe and Effective Care Environment

1. Assess patients for complications of diagnostic tests.

Health Promotion and Maintenance

2. Evaluate patients at risk for cardiovascular (CV) problems.
3. Explain pretest and post-test care associated with diagnostic CV testing.

Psychosocial Integrity

4. Explain psychological responses to CV disease, such as denial.

Physiological Integrity

5. Briefly review the anatomy and physiology of the CV system.
6. Explain nursing implications related to CV changes associated with aging.
7. Describe the unique characteristics of heart disease in women.
8. Perform focused physical assessment for patients with CV problems.
9. Interpret laboratory test findings for patients with suspected or actual CV disease.
10. Evaluate invasive hemodynamic monitoring data.

evolve Go to your Companion CD or Evolve at http://evolve.elsevier.com/Iggy/ for *Self-Assessment Questions for the NCLEX Examination* keyed to these Learning Outcomes.

As the name implies, the cardiovascular (CV) system comprises the heart and blood vessels (both arteries and veins). It is responsible for supplying oxygen to body organs and other tissues *(perfusion).* The heart muscle, called the **myocardium,** must receive sufficient oxygen to pump blood to other parts of the body. The arteries must be patent so that the pumped blood can reach the rest of the body. *Oxygenation* is needed for cells to live and function properly. When diseases or other problems of the CV systems occur, *oxygenation and perfusion* decrease, often resulting in life-threatening events or a risk for these events.

The CV system works with the respiratory and hematologic systems to meet the human need for oxygenation and tissue perfusion (see Fig. 1 of the Human Needs Overview). Any problem in these systems requires the CV system to work harder to meet oxygenation and tissue perfusion needs.

In almost every year since 1900, cardiovascular disease (CVD) has been the number-one cause of death in the United States. Nearly 2500 Americans die of CVD each day, an average of one death every 25 seconds. The disease kills more people than the next four causes of death combined, including cancer, chronic lower respiratory diseases, accidents, and diabetes. *Of particular concern is that CVD is the leading cause of death for women.* In addition, the American Heart Association (AHA) estimates that about one in three adults is living with some form of the disease. About 40% of people who experience a myocardial infarction will die within 1 year from the initial cardiac event (Rosamond et al., 2007).

ANATOMY AND PHYSIOLOGY REVIEW

Heart

Structure

The human heart is a fist-sized, muscular organ located in the mediastinum between the lungs (Fig. 35-1). Each beat of the heart pumps about 60 mL of blood, or 5 L/min. During strenuous physical activity, it can double the amount of blood pumped to meet the increased oxygen needs of the body tissues. The heart is protected by a covering called the *pericardium.* A muscular wall (septum) separates the heart into two halves: right and left. Each half has an upper chamber (atrium) and a lower chamber (ventricle) (Fig. 35-2).

The *right atrium (RA)* receives *deoxygenated* venous blood (venous return) from the body through the superior and inferior venae cavae. It also receives blood from the heart muscle through the coronary sinus. Most of this venous return flows passively from the RA, through the opened tricuspid valve,

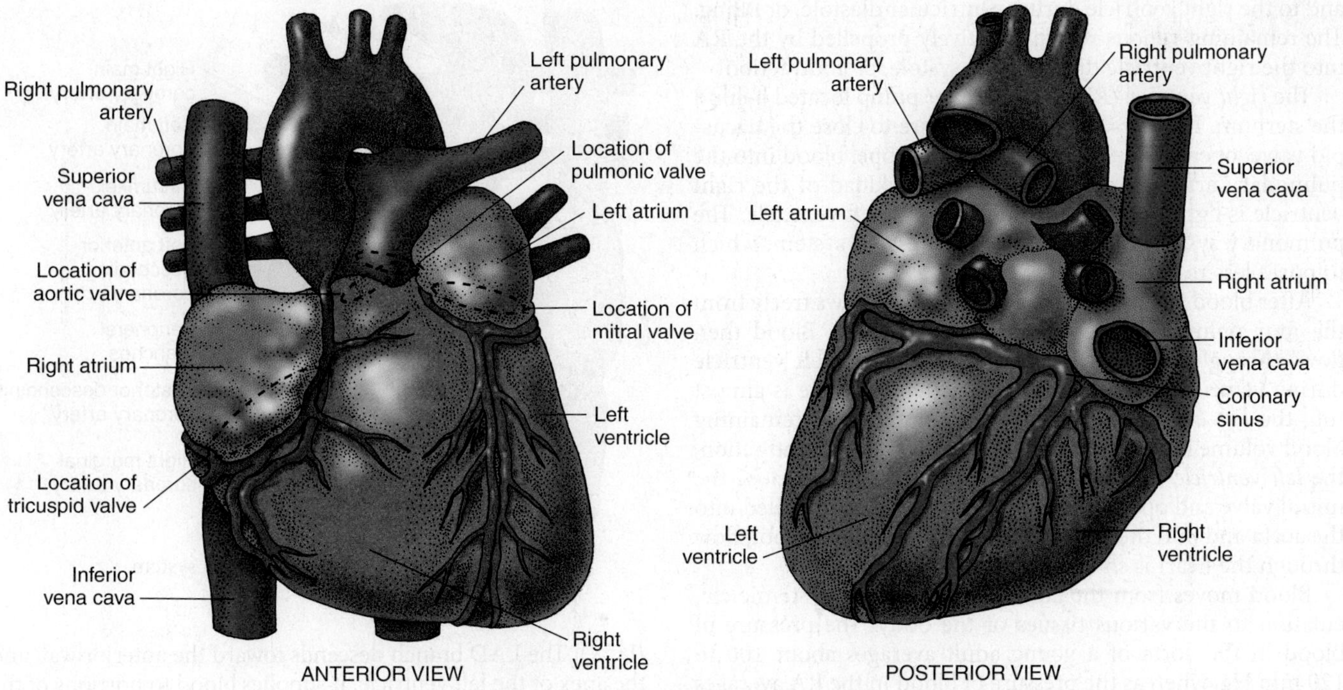
Right pulmonary artery
Superior vena cava
Location of aortic valve
Right atrium
Location of tricuspid valve
Inferior vena cava
Left pulmonary artery
Location of pulmonic valve
Left atrium
Location of mitral valve
Left ventricle
Right ventricle
ANTERIOR VIEW
Left pulmonary artery
Left atrium
Left ventricle
Right pulmonary artery
Superior vena cava
Right atrium
Inferior vena cava
Coronary sinus
Right ventricle
POSTERIOR VIEW

Fig. 35-1 • Surface anatomy of the heart.

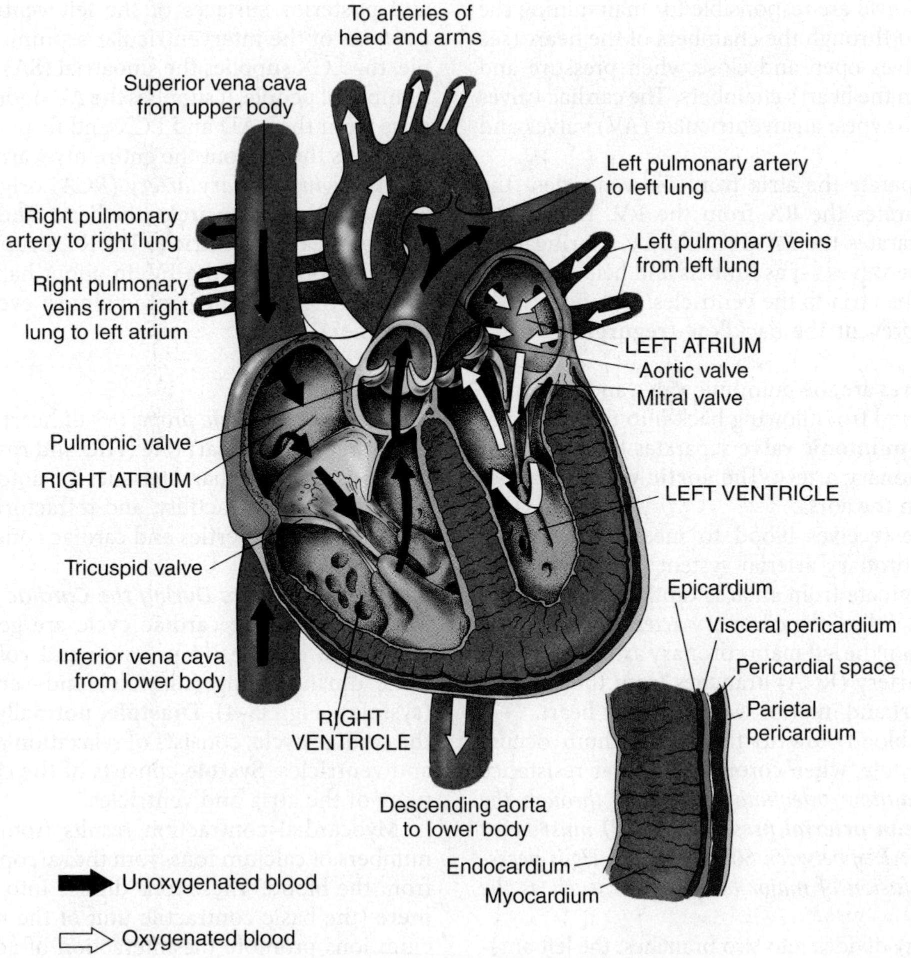
To arteries of head and arms
Superior vena cava from upper body
Left pulmonary artery to left lung
Right pulmonary artery to right lung
Right pulmonary veins from right lung to left atrium
Left pulmonary veins from left lung
LEFT ATRIUM
Aortic valve
Mitral valve
Pulmonic valve
RIGHT ATRIUM
LEFT VENTRICLE
Tricuspid valve
Epicardium
Visceral pericardium
Inferior vena cava from lower body
Pericardial space
Parietal pericardium
RIGHT VENTRICLE
Descending aorta to lower body
Endocardium
Myocardium
Unoxygenated blood
Oxygenated blood

Fig. 35-2 • Blood flow through the heart.

and to the right ventricle during ventricular diastole, or filling. The remaining venous return is actively propelled by the RA into the right ventricle during atrial systole, or contraction.

The *right ventricle (RV)* is a muscular pump located behind the sternum. It generates enough pressure to close the tricuspid valve, open the pulmonic valve, and propel blood into the pulmonary artery and the lungs. The workload of the right ventricle is light compared with that of the left ventricle. The pulmonary system is normally a low-pressure system, which imposes less resistance to flow.

After blood is *reoxygenated* in the lungs, it flows freely from the four pulmonary veins into the left atrium. Blood then flows through an opened mitral valve into the left ventricle during ventricular diastole. When the left ventricle is almost full, the *left atrium (LA)* contracts, pumping the remaining blood volume into the left ventricle. With systolic contraction, the *left ventricle (LV)* generates enough pressure to close the mitral valve and open the aortic valve. Blood is propelled into the aorta and into the systemic arterial circulation. Blood flow through the heart is shown in Fig. 35-2.

Blood moves from the aorta throughout the systemic circulation to the various tissues of the body. The pressure of blood in the aorta of a young adult averages about 100 to 120 mm Hg, whereas the pressure of blood in the RA averages about 0 to 5 mm Hg. These differences in pressure produce a pressure gradient, with blood flowing from an area of higher pressure to an area of lower pressure. The heart and vascular structures are responsible for maintaining these pressures.

The four *cardiac valves* are responsible for maintaining the forward flow of blood through the chambers of the heart (see Fig. 35-2). These valves open and close when pressure and volume change within the heart's chambers. The cardiac valves are classified into two types: atrioventricular (AV) valves and semilunar valves.

The *AV valves* separate the atria from the ventricles. The **tricuspid valve** separates the RA from the RV. The **mitral (bicuspid) valve** separates the LA from the LV. During ventricular diastole, these valves act as funnels and help move the flow of blood from the atria to the ventricles. During systole, the valves close to prevent the backflow **(regurgitation)** of blood into the atria.

The *semilunar valves* are the pulmonic valve and the aortic valve that prevent blood from flowing back into the ventricles during diastole. The **pulmonic valve** separates the right ventricle from the pulmonary artery. The **aortic valve** separates the left ventricle from the aorta.

The heart muscle receives blood to meet its metabolic needs through the coronary arterial system (Fig. 35-3). The coronary arteries originate from an area on the aorta just beyond the aortic valve. All of the coronary arteries feeding the left heart originate from the left main coronary artery (LMCA). The right coronary artery (RCA) branches from the aorta to perfuse the right heart and inferior wall of the left heart.

Coronary artery blood flow to the myocardium occurs primarily during diastole, when coronary vascular resistance is minimized. *To maintain adequate blood flow through the coronary arteries,* ***mean arterial pressure (MAP)*** *must be at least 60 mm Hg. A MAP of between 60 and 70 mm Hg is necessary to maintain perfusion of major body organs, such as the kidneys and brain.*

The *left main artery* divides into two branches: the left anterior descending (LAD) and the left circumflex coronary artery

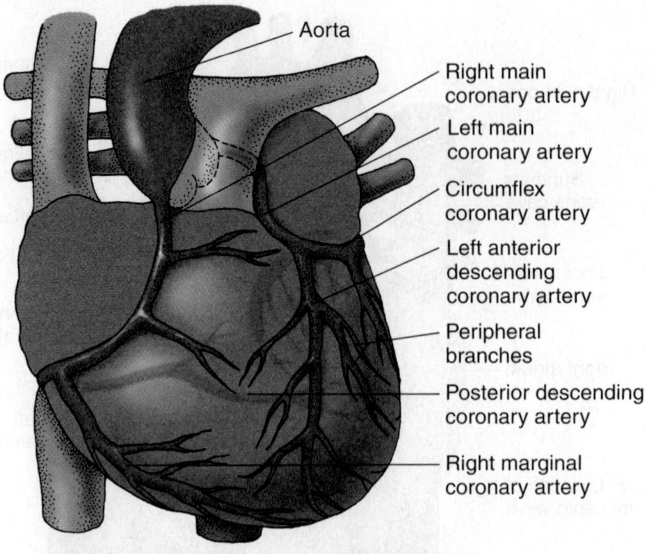
Aorta
Right main coronary artery
Left main coronary artery
Circumflex coronary artery
Left anterior descending coronary artery
Peripheral branches
Posterior descending coronary artery
Right marginal coronary artery

Fig. 35-3 • Coronary arterial system.

(LCX). The LAD branch descends toward the anterior wall and the apex of the left ventricle. It supplies blood to portions of the left ventricle, ventricular septum, chordae tendineae, papillary muscle, and, to a lesser extent, the right ventricle.

The LCX descends toward the lateral wall of the left ventricle and apex. It supplies blood to the left atrium, the lateral and posterior surfaces of the left ventricle, and sometimes portions of the interventricular septum. In about half of people, the LCX supplies the sinoatrial (SA) node. In a very small number of people, it supplies the AV node. Peripheral branches arise from the LAD and LCX and form an abundant network of vessels throughout the entire myocardium.

The *right coronary artery (RCA)* originates from the right sinus of Valsalva, encircles the heart, and descends toward the apex of the right ventricle. The RCA supplies the RA, RV, and inferior portion of the LV. In about half of people, the RCA supplies the SA node, and in almost everyone, the RCA supplies the AV node.

Function

The *electrophysiologic properties* of heart muscle are responsible for regulating heart rate (HR) and rhythm. Cardiac muscle cells possess the characteristics of automaticity, excitability, conductivity, contractility, and refractoriness. Chapter 36 describes these properties and cardiac conduction in detail.

Sequence of Events During the Cardiac Cycle

The phases of the cardiac cycle are generally described in relation to changes in pressure and volume in the left ventricle during filling (diastole) and ventricular contraction (systole) (Fig. 35-4). **Diastole,** normally about two thirds of the cardiac cycle, consists of relaxation and filling of the atria and ventricles. **Systole** consists of the contraction and emptying of the atria and ventricles.

Myocardial contraction results from the release of large numbers of calcium ions from the sarcoplasmic reticulum and from the blood. These ions diffuse into the **myofibril sarcomere** (the basic contractile unit of the myocardial cell). Calcium ions promote the interaction of actin and myosin protein filaments, causing these filaments to link and overlap.

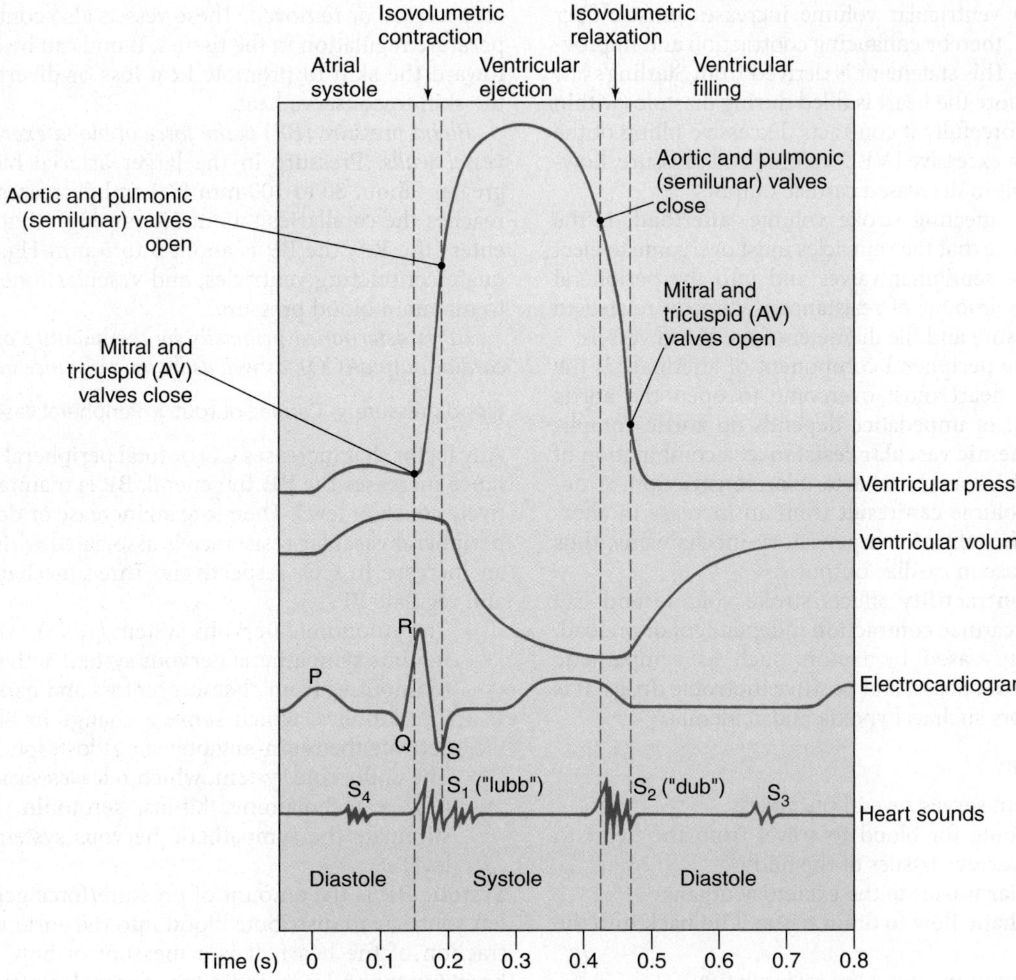
Isovolumetric contraction
Isovolumetric relaxation
Atrial systole
Ventricular ejection
Ventricular filling
Aortic and pulmonic (semilunar) valves close
Aortic and pulmonic (semilunar) valves open
Mitral and tricuspid (AV) valves open
Mitral and tricuspid (AV) valves close
Ventricular pressure
Ventricular volume
R
P
Q
S
Electrocardiogram
S4
S1 ("lubb")
S2 ("dub")
S3
Heart sounds
Diastole
Systole
Diastole
Time (s) 0 0.1 0.2 0.3 0.4 0.5 0.6 0.7 0.8

Fig. 35-4 • Events of the cardiac cycle.

Cross-bridges, or linkages, are formed as the protein filaments slide over or overlap each other. These cross-bridges act as force-generating sites. The sliding of these protein filaments shortens the sarcomeres, producing myocardial contraction.

Cardiac muscle relaxes when calcium ions are pumped back into the sarcoplasmic reticulum, causing a decrease in the number of calcium ions around the myofibrils. This reduced number of ions causes the protein filaments to disengage, the sarcomere to lengthen, and the muscle to relax.

Mechanical Properties of the Heart

The electrical and mechanical properties of cardiac muscle determine the function of the cardiovascular system. The healthy heart can adapt to various pathophysiologic conditions (e.g., stress, infections, hemorrhage) to maintain adequate blood flow to the various body tissues. Blood flow from the heart into the systemic arterial circulation is measured clinically as **cardiac output (CO),** the amount of blood pumped from the left ventricle each minute. *CO depends on the relationship between heart rate (HR) and stroke volume (SV); it is the product of these two variables:*

$$\text{Cardiac output} = \text{Heart rate} \times \text{Stroke volume}$$

In adults, the CO ranges from 4 to 7 L/min. Because CO requirements vary according to body size, the cardiac index is calculated to adjust for differences in body size. The **cardiac index** can be determined by dividing the CO by the body surface area. The normal range is 2.7 to 3.2 L/min/m^2 of body surface area.

Heart rate (HR) refers to the number of times the ventricles contract each minute. The normal resting HR for an adult is between 60 and 100 beats/min. Increases in rate increase myocardial oxygen demand. The HR is extrinsically controlled by the autonomic nervous system (ANS), which adjusts rapidly when necessary to regulate cardiac output. *The parasympathetic (vagus nerve) system slows the HR, whereas sympathetic stimulation increases the heart rate.* An increase in circulating catecholamines (e.g., epinephrine and norepinephrine) usually causes an increase in HR and contractility. Many cardiovascular drugs, particularly beta blockers, block this sympathetic (fight or flight) pattern by decreasing the HR.

Stroke volume (SV) is the amount of blood ejected by the left ventricle during each contraction. Several variables influence SV and, ultimately, CO. These variables include HR, preload, afterload, and contractility.

Preload refers to the degree of myocardial fiber stretch at the end of diastole and just before contraction. The stretch imposed on the muscle fibers results from the volume contained within the ventricle at the end of diastole. *Preload is determined by the amount of blood returning to the heart from both the venous system (right heart) and the pulmonary system (left heart) (left ventricular end-diastolic [LVED] volume).*

An increase in ventricular volume increases muscle-fiber length and tension, thereby enhancing contraction and improving stroke volume. This statement is derived from Starling's law of the heart: The more the heart is filled during diastole (within limits), the more forcefully it contracts. Excessive filling of the ventricles results in excessive LVED volume and pressure, however, and may result in decreased cardiac output.

Another factor affecting stroke volume, **afterload,** is the pressure or resistance that the ventricles must overcome to eject blood through the semilunar valves and into the peripheral blood vessels. The amount of resistance is directly related to arterial blood pressure and the diameter of the blood vessels.

Impedance, the peripheral component of afterload, is the pressure that the heart must overcome to open the aortic valve. The amount of impedance depends on aortic compliance and total **systemic vascular resistance,** a combination of blood viscosity (thickness) and arteriolar constriction. A decrease in stroke volume can result from an increase in afterload without the benefit of compensatory mechanisms, thus leading to a decrease in cardiac output.

Myocardial contractility affects stroke volume and CO and is the force of cardiac contraction independent of preload. Contractility is increased by factors such as sympathetic stimulation, calcium release, and positive inotropic drugs. It is decreased by factors such as hypoxia and acidemia.

Vascular System

The vascular system serves several purposes:

- Provides a route for blood to travel from the heart to nourish the various tissues of the body
- Carries cellular wastes to the excretory organs
- Allows lymphatic flow to drain tissue fluid back into the circulation
- Returns blood to the heart for recirculation

The vascular system is divided into the arterial system and the venous system. In the arterial system, blood moves from the larger arteries to a network of smaller blood vessels, called *arterioles,* which meet the capillary bed. In the venous system, blood travels from the capillaries to the venules and to the larger system of veins, eventually returning in the venae cavae to the heart for recirculation.

Arterial System

The high-pressure blood vessels of the arterial vascular system can be classified according to their size and wall structure. The large arteries, such as the aorta and femoral arteries, follow relatively straight routes and have few branches. Smaller arteries, such as the internal iliac and mesenteric arteries, divide from larger ones and have multiple branches.

Arteries may branch into arterioles or connect with other arteries. The arterioles branch into terminal arterioles, which then join with capillaries and venules to form the capillary network. The exchange of nutrients across the capillary membrane occurs primarily by three processes: osmosis, filtration, and diffusion. (See Chapter 13 for detailed discussions of these processes.)

The arterial system delivers blood to various tissues for oxygen and nourishment. At the tissue level, nutrients, chemicals, and body defense substances are distributed and exchanged for cellular waste products, depending on the needs of the particular tissue. The arteries transport the cellular wastes to the excretory organs (e.g., kidneys and lungs) to be reprocessed or removed. These vessels also contribute to temperature regulation in the tissues. Blood can be either directed toward the skin to promote heat loss or diverted away from the skin to conserve heat.

Blood pressure (BP) is the force of blood exerted against the vessel walls. Pressure in the larger arterial blood vessels is greater (about 80 to 100 mm Hg) and decreases as blood flow reaches the capillaries (about 25 mm Hg). By the time blood enters the RA, the BP is about 0 to 5 mm Hg. Volume, adequate contracting ventricles, and vascular tone are necessary to maintain blood pressure.

BP is determined primarily by the quantity of blood flow or cardiac output (CO), as well as by the resistance in the arterioles:

$$\text{Blood pressure} = \text{Cardiac output} \times \text{Peripheral vascular resistance}$$

Any factor that increases CO or total peripheral vascular resistance increases the BP. In general, BP is maintained at a relatively constant level. Therefore an increase or decrease in total peripheral vascular resistance is associated with a decrease or an increase in CO, respectively. Three mechanisms mediate and regulate BP:

- The autonomic nervous system (ANS), which excites or inhibits sympathetic nervous system activity in response to impulses from chemoreceptors and baroreceptors
- The kidneys, which sense a change in blood flow and activate the renin-angiotensin-aldosterone mechanism
- The endocrine system, which releases various hormones (e.g., catecholamine, kinins, serotonin, histamine) to stimulate the sympathetic nervous system at the tissue level

Systolic BP is the amount of pressure/force generated by the left ventricle to distribute blood into the aorta with each contraction of the heart. It is a measure of how effectively the heart pumps and is an indicator of vascular tone. **Diastolic BP** is the amount of pressure/force against the arterial walls during the relaxation phase of the heart.

BP is regulated by balancing the sympathetic and parasympathetic nervous systems of the *ANS*. Changes in ANS activity are responses to messages sent by the sensory receptors in the various tissues of the body. These receptors, including the baroreceptors, chemoreceptors, and stretch receptors, respond differently to the biochemical and physiologic changes of the body.

Baroreceptors in the arch of the aorta and at the origin of the internal carotid arteries are stimulated when the arterial walls are stretched by an increased BP. Impulses from these baroreceptors inhibit the vasomotor center, which is located in the pons and the medulla. Inhibition of this center results in a drop in BP.

Several 1- to 2-mm collections of tissue have been identified in the carotid arteries and along the aortic arch known as **peripheral chemoreceptors.** These receptors are sensitive primarily to hypoxemia (a decrease in the partial pressure of arterial oxygen [Pao_2]). When stimulated, these chemoreceptors send impulses along the vagus nerves to activate a vasoconstrictor response and raise BP.

The central chemoreceptors in the respiratory center of the brain are also stimulated by **hypercapnia** (an increase in partial pressure of arterial carbon dioxide [$Paco_2$]) and acidosis. The direct effect of carbon dioxide on the central nervous system (CNS), however, is 10 times stronger than the effect of hypoxia on the peripheral chemoreceptors.

Stretch receptors in the vena cava and the right atrium are sensitive to pressure or volume changes. When a patient is hypovolemic, stretch receptors in the blood vessels sense a reduced volume or pressure and send fewer impulses to the CNS. This reaction stimulates the sympathetic nervous system to increase the heart rate (HR) and constrict the peripheral blood vessels.

The *kidneys* also help regulate cardiovascular activity. When renal blood flow or pressure decreases, the kidneys retain sodium and water. BP tends to rise because of fluid retention and activation of the renin-angiotensin-aldosterone mechanism (see Fig. 13-6 in Chapter 13). This mechanism results in vasoconstriction and sodium retention (and thus fluid retention). Vascular volume is also regulated by the release of antidiuretic hormone (vasopressin) from the posterior pituitary gland (see Chapter 13).

Other factors can also influence the activity of the cardiovascular system. Emotional behaviors (e.g., excitement, pain, anger) stimulate the sympathetic nervous system to increase BP and HR. Increased physical activity such as exercise increases BP and pulse rate during the activity. Body temperature can affect the metabolic needs of the tissues, thereby influencing the delivery of blood. In hypothermia, tissues require fewer nutrients and blood pressure falls. In hyperthermia, the metabolic requirement of the tissues is greater and BP and pulse rate rise.

Venous System

The primary function of the venous system is to complete the circulation of blood by returning blood from the capillaries to the right side of the heart. It is composed of a series of veins that are located next to the arterial system. A second superficial venous circulation runs parallel to the subcutaneous tissue of the extremity. These two venous systems are connected by communicating veins that provide a means for blood to travel from the superficial veins to the deep veins. Blood flow is directed toward the deep venous circulation.

Veins have the ability to accommodate large shifts in volume with minimal changes in venous pressure. This flexibility allows the venous system to accommodate the administration of IV fluids and blood transfusions, as well as to maintain pressure during blood loss and dehydration. All veins in the superficial and deep venous systems in the legs (except the smallest and the largest veins) have valves that direct blood flow back to the heart; this prevents retrograde flow (backflow). The force that pushes the blood forward in the veins is skeletal muscle in the extremities. The superior and inferior vena cava are also valveless, which allows unimpeded blood flow return to the heart.

Gravity exerts an increase in **hydrostatic pressure** in the capillaries when the patient is in an upright position, which delays venous return. Hydrostatic pressure is lessened in dependent areas such as the legs when the patient is lying down, and thus there is less hindrance of venous return to the heart.

CARDIOVASCULAR CHANGES ASSOCIATED WITH AGING

A number of physiologic changes in the cardiovascular system occur with advancing age (Chart 35-1). Many of these changes result in a loss of cardiac reserve. Thus these changes are usually not evident when the older adult is resting. They become apparent only when the person is physically or emotionally stressed and the heart cannot meet the increased metabolic demands of the body.

ASSESSMENT METHODS

Patient History

The focus of the patient history is on obtaining information about risk factors and symptoms of cardiovascular disease (Chart 35-2). Assess the patient's age, gender, and ethnic origin. Ask about any chronic disease or illness that the patient may have. The incidence of conditions such as coronary artery disease (CAD) and valvular disease increases with *age*. The incidence of CAD also varies with the patient's *gender*. Men have a higher risk for CAD than women of all ages, except in the oldest age-group of 80 years and older.

WOMEN'S HEALTH CONSIDERATIONS

Postmenopausal women are two to three times more likely than premenopausal women to have CAD. The incidence for the disease in women is about 10 years later than for men and 20 years later for myocardial infarction (MI) and death to occur. After an acute MI, women tend to have a higher mortality rate and suffer more complications when compared with men (Rosamond et al., 2007).

Women with waist and abdominal obesity (greater waist-hip ratio) are more likely to experience cardiovascular disease (CVD) than are women with excess fat in their buttocks, hips, and thighs. Diabetes mellitus is also a major risk factor, especially in women.

Heart disease is the leading cause of diabetes-related death for both men and women. Adults with diabetes have heart disease death rates 2 to 4 times higher than those without diabetes. The risk for stroke is also 2 to 4 times higher among people with diabetes. The number of premature deaths (younger than 65 years) from heart disease is greatest among American Indians and Alaska Natives and lowest among Asians (Rosamond et al., 2007).

Age, gender, ethnic background, and family history of CVD are *nonmodifiable* (uncontrollable) risk factors for CVD. *Modifiable* (controllable) risk factors are personal habits, including cigarette use, physical inactivity, obesity, and psychological variables. Ask the patient about each of these common modifiable risk factors.

Cigarette smoking is a major risk factor for CVD, specifically CAD and peripheral vascular disease (PVD). Three compounds in cigarette smoke have been implicated in the development of CAD: tar, nicotine, and carbon monoxide.

The smoking history should include the number of cigarettes smoked daily, the duration of the smoking habit, and the age of the patient when smoking started. A person who smokes fewer than four cigarettes per day has twice the risk of CVD as a person who does not smoke. Anyone who smokes more than 20 cigarettes per day has four times the risk. Record the smoking history in **pack-years,** which is the number of packs per day multiplied by the number of years the patient has smoked.

Ask about the patient's desire to quit, past attempts to quit, and the methods used. Determine nicotine dependence by asking questions such as:

- How soon after you wake up in the morning do you smoke?
- Do you wake up in the middle of your sleep time to smoke?

Chart 35-1 NURSING FOCUS ON THE OLDER ADULT

Changes in the Cardiovascular System Related to Aging

Change	Nursing Interventions	Rationales
CARDIAC VALVES		
Calcification and mucoid degeneration occur, especially in mitral and aortic valves.	Assess heart rate and rhythm and heart sounds for murmurs. Question patients about dyspnea.	Murmurs may be detected before other symptoms. Valvular abnormalities may result in rhythm changes.
CONDUCTION SYSTEM		
Pacemaker cells decrease in number. Fibrous tissue and fat in the sinoatrial node increase. Few muscle fibers remain in the atrial myocardium and bundle of His. Conduction time increases.	Assess the electrocardiogram (ECG) and heart rhythm for dysrhythmias or a heart rate less than 60 beats/min.	The sinoatrial (SA) node may lose its inherent rhythm. Atrial dysrhythmias occur in many older adults; 80% of older adults experience premature ventricular contractions (PVCs).
LEFT VENTRICLE		
The size of the left ventricle increases. The left ventricle becomes stiff and less distensible. Fibrotic changes in the left ventricle decrease the speed of early diastolic filling by about 50%.	Assess the ECG for a widening QRS complex and a longer QT interval.	Ventricular changes result in decreased stroke volume, ejection fraction, and cardiac output during exercise; the heart is less able to meet increased oxygen demands.
	Assess the heart rate at rest and with activity.	Maximum heart rate with exercise is decreased.
	Assess for activity intolerance.	The heart is less able to meet increased oxygen demands.
AORTA AND OTHER LARGE ARTERIES		
The aorta and other large arteries thicken and become stiffer and less distensible. Systolic blood pressure increases to compensate for the stiff arteries. Systemic vascular resistance increases as a result of less distensible arteries; therefore the left ventricle pumps against greater resistance, contributing to left ventricular hypertrophy.	Assess blood pressure. Note increases in systolic, diastolic, and pulse pressures. Assess for activity intolerance and shortness of breath. Assess the peripheral pulses.	Hypertension may occur and must be treated to avoid target organ damage.
BARORECEPTORS		
Baroreceptors become less sensitive.	Assess the patient's blood pressure with the patient lying and then sitting or standing.	Orthostatic (postural) and postprandial changes occur because of ineffective baroreceptors.
	Assess for dizziness when the patient changes from a lying to a sitting or standing position. Teach the patient to change positions slowly.	Changes may include blood pressure decreases of 10 mm Hg or more, dizziness, and fainting.

- Do you find it difficult not to smoke in places where smoking is prohibited?
- Do you smoke when you are ill?

Three to four years after a patient has stopped smoking, his or her cardiovascular risk appears to be similar to that of a person who has never smoked. Be sure to ask those who do not currently smoke whether they have ever smoked and when they quit. Passive smoke significantly reduces blood flow in healthy young adults' coronary arteries, and the risk of dying increases among those who are exposed to secondhand smoke (Rosamond et al., 2007).

A *sedentary lifestyle* is also a major risk factor for heart disease. Regular physical activity promotes cardiovascular fitness and produces beneficial changes in blood pressure and levels of blood lipids and clotting factors. Unfortunately, few people in the United States engage in the recommended exercise guidelines: 30 minutes daily of light to moderate exercise, which is equivalent to a 30-minute brisk walk. According to the American Heart Association (Rosamond et al., 2007), only about a fourth of people in the United States engage in this much exercise five times a week, and fewer engage in vigorous physical activity (enough to promote cardiopulmonary fitness) three times a week. Encourage increased physical exercise as part of a lifestyle change to reduce the risk for CAD. Ask patients about the type of exercise they perform, how long a period they have participated in the exercise, and the frequency and intensity of the exercise.

About two thirds of American adults are **overweight** when defined as a body mass index (BMI) of 25 to 30. **Obesity,** defined as a BMI greater than 30, is particularly a problem for

Chart 35-2 CARDIOVASCULAR ASSESSMENT

Using Gordon's Functional Health Patterns

HEALTH PERCEPTION–HEALTH MANAGEMENT
- What advice has your health care provider offered you about exercise, diet, or smoking?
- Can you follow that advice?
- What medications (both over-the-counter and prescription) are you supposed to be taking?
- Are you taking them as suggested or prescribed?
- What problems have you had with the medications?

NUTRITION-METABOLIC
- What is your usual daily diet? (Analyze the diet for saturated fat, cholesterol, total calorie, and sodium content.)
- How much fluid do you drink daily? Are you thirsty?
- What do you weigh? When did you last weigh yourself?
- How often do you weigh yourself?
- What is your height?
- Do you know your cholesterol level? What is it?
- How often do you feel nauseated or not interested in eating?
- Do your feet/ankles swell during the day? At night, too?

ELIMINATION
- How often do you urinate in the daytime?
- How often do you wake up at night to urinate?

ACTIVITY/EXERCISE
- What is the most strenuous exercise you did last week?
- How active are you compared with 6 months ago? 1 year ago?
- How often do you feel fatigued or tired?
- Can you climb a flight of stairs and walk a block without feeling short of breath or experiencing chest pain?
- Do you experience leg cramps when you walk or climb stairs?

SLEEP/REST
- Where do you sleep? (In bed? In a lounge chair?)
- How many pillows do you sleep on?
- Do you ever wake up at night short of breath?
- What happens when you wake up short of breath?
- Do you ever wake up at night with pain or cramps in your legs? How do you relieve that sensation?

COGNITIVE/PERCEPTUAL
- How is your memory? What does your family say about your memory?
- How often do you feel dizzy, disoriented, or faint?
- Do you ever have chest discomfort? How often? What precipitates it? What is it like? How do you relieve it? What is its level on a scale of 0 to 10?
- Do you ever have leg or buttock pain? What are its characteristics?
- How do you learn best?

ROLE/RELATIONSHIP
- What is your job?
- What does a day's work entail?
- What are your family responsibilities?
- With whom do you live?
- Who is available to help you?

SEXUALITY/REPRODUCTIVE
- Has your ability to engage in sexual activity changed in the past year? If so, how?
- Do you take any medications that affect your sexual response? If so, what?

COPING/STRESS TOLERANCE
- What do you think has been happening to you?
- How do you respond to being caught in a traffic jam or meeting a deadline?
- What do you do to relax?
- What do you do when you feel stressed?

Based on Gordon, M. (2007). *Manual of nursing diagnosis* (11th ed.). Boston: Jones & Bartlett.

African-American women, Mexican Americans, and native Hawaiians, but the exact cause of this cultural difference is unknown (Rosamond et al., 2007). It is also associated with hypertension, hyperlipidemia, and diabetes; all are known contributors to CVD.

A variety of *psychological factors* make people more vulnerable to the development of heart disease. Those who are highly competitive, overly concerned about meeting deadlines, and often hostile or angry are at higher risk for heart disease. Psychological stress, anger, depression, and hostility are all closely associated with risk of developing heart disease.

You might ask the patient, "How do you respond when you have to wait for an appointment?" Chronic anger and hostility appear to be closely associated with CVD. The constant arousal of the sympathetic nervous system as a result of anger may influence blood pressure, serum fatty acids and lipids, and clotting mechanisms. Observe the patient, and assess his or her response to stressful situations.

Review the patient's medical history, noting any major illnesses such as diabetes mellitus, renal disease, anemia, high BP, stroke, bleeding disorders, connective tissue diseases, chronic pulmonary diseases, heart disease, and thrombophlebitis. These conditions can influence the patient's cardiovascular status.

Ask about previous treatment for CVD, identify previous diagnostic procedures (e.g., electrocardiography [ECG], cardiac catheterization), and request information about any medical or invasive treatment of CVD. It is important to ask specifically about recurrent tonsillitis, streptococcal infections, and rheumatic fever because these conditions may lead to valvular abnormalities of the heart. In addition, inquire about any known congenital heart defects. Many patients with congenital heart problems live into adulthood because of improved treatment and surgeries.

Ask patients about their drug history, beginning with any current or recent use of prescription or over-the-counter (OTC) medications or herbal/natural products (e.g., ginseng). Inquire about known sensitivities to any drug and the nature of the reaction (e.g., nausea, rash). Patients should be asked whether they have recently used cocaine or any IV "street" drugs because these substances may be associated with chest pain or endocarditis.

Ask women whether they are taking oral contraceptives or an estrogen replacement. The incidence of myocardial infarction (MI) and stroke in women older than 35 years who take oral contraceptives is increased but only if they smoke, have diabetes, or have hypertension.

The *social history* includes information about the patient's living situation, including having a domestic partner, other household members, environment, and occupation. Identification of support systems is especially important in exploring the possibility that the patient might have difficulty paying for medications or treatment. People who report an annual household income of less than $10,000 or cannot work have a greater risk for CVD than people who have an income of over $50,000 (Rosamond et al., 2007).

Ask about occupation, including the type of work performed and the requirements of the specific job. For instance, does the job involve physical exertion such as lifting heavy objects? Is the job emotionally stressful? What does a day's work entail? Does the patient's job require him or her to be outside in extreme weather conditions?

Nutrition History

A nutrition history includes the patient's recall of food and fluid intake during a 24-hour period, self-imposed or medically prescribed dietary restrictions or supplementations, and the amount and type of alcohol consumption. The nutritionist reviews the type of foods selected by the patient for the amount of sodium, sugar, cholesterol, fiber, and fat. Collaborate with the nutritionist to explore the patient's attitude toward food, knowledge level of essential and nonessential dietary elements, and willingness to make changes in the diet. Cultural beliefs and economic status can influence the choice of food items and therefore must be considered in this planning. Family members or significant others who are responsible for shopping and cooking should be included in this discussion.

NCLEX EXAMINATION CHALLENGE

A client has received health teaching about lifestyle changes that can help reduce his risk for cardiovascular disease. Which of these statements by the client indicates a need for further teaching by the nurse?

A. "I have to watch what I eat so that I can lose some weight."
B. "I quit smoking last year because I have smoked since I was 12."
C. "I can't do anything about my disease risk because it's in my genes."
D. "I have to take my blood pressure medication as the doctor wants me to."

evolve For the correct answer, go to http://evolve.elsevier.com/Iggy/.

Family History and Genetic Risk

Review the family history, and obtain information about the age, health status, and cause of death of immediate family members. A positive family history for CAD in a first-degree relative (parent, sibling, or child) is a major risk factor. It is *more* important than other factors such as hypertension, obesity, diabetes, or sudden cardiac death. Ninety percent of CAD patients have at least one of these major risk factors: high total cholesterol levels, hypertension, diabetes, and current cigarette use (Rosamond et al., 2007).

GENETIC CONSIDERATIONS

Cardiovascular disease has many contributory factors, including a genetic tendency. Inflammation is an important risk factor for heart disease. Variations in two interleukin genes may identify a patient's predisposition to inflammation and risk for CV disease. This predisposition has been suggested to cause early, aggressive heart disease. Several genes have been reported to be associated with heart disease, stroke, and hypertension, but the impact of each individual gene is not fully understood (Rosamond et al., 2007). Additional discussions about genetic factors are found in other chapters in this unit.

Current Health Problems

Ask the patient to describe his or her health concerns. Expand on the description of these concerns by obtaining information about their onset, duration, sequence, frequency, location, quality, intensity, associated symptoms, and precipitating, aggravating, and relieving factors. Major symptoms usually identified by patients with CVD include chest pain or discomfort, dyspnea, fatigue, palpitations, weight gain, syncope, and extremity pain.

Pain or discomfort, considered a traditional symptom of heart disease, can result from ischemic heart disease, pericarditis, and aortic dissection. Chest pain can also be due to noncardiac conditions such as pleurisy, pulmonary embolus, hiatal hernia, gastroesophageal reflux disease, neuromuscular abnormalities, and anxiety. Thoroughly evaluate the nature and characteristics of the chest pain. Because pain resulting from myocardial ischemia is life threatening and can lead to serious complications, its cause should be considered ischemic (reduced or obstructed blood flow to the myocardium) until proven otherwise. When assessing for symptoms, use alternative terms such as "discomfort," "heaviness," "pressure," and "indigestion."

WOMEN'S HEALTH CONSIDERATIONS

Some patients, especially women, do not experience pain in the chest but instead feel discomfort or indigestion. Women often present with a "triad" of symptoms. In addition to indigestion or feeling of abdominal fullness, feelings of chronic fatigue despite adequate rest and feelings of "inability to catch one's breath" are also common in heart disease. The patient may also describe the sensation as aching, choking, strangling, tingling, squeezing, constricting, or viselike. Others with severe neuropathy may experience few or no traditional symptoms except shortness of breath, despite major ischemia.

Ask the patient to identify when the symptoms were first noticed (onset):

- Did the symptoms begin suddenly or develop gradually (manner of onset)?
- How long did they last (duration)?

If he or she has repeated painful episodes, assess how often the symptoms occur (frequency). If pain is present, ask whether it is different from any other episodes of pain. Ask the patient to describe what activities he or she was doing when it first occurred, such as sleeping, arguing, or running (precipitating factors). If possible, the patient should point to the area where the chest pain occurred (location) and to describe if and how the pain radiated (spread).

In addition, ask how the pain feels and whether it is sharp, dull, or crushing (quality). To understand the severity of the pain, ask the patient to grade it from 0 to 10, with 0 indicating an absence of pain and 10 indicating severe pain (intensity). He or she may also report other signs and symptoms that oc-

TABLE 35-1 **Assessment of Chest Discomfort: How Various Types of Chest Pain Differ**

Onset	Quality and Severity	Location and Radiation	Duration and Relieving Factors
ANGINA			
Sudden, usually in response to exertion, emotion, or extremes, in temperature	Squeezing, viselike pain	Substernal; may spread across the chest and the back and/ or down the arms	Usually the left side of chest without radiation. Usually lasts less than 15 min; relieved with rest, nitrate administration, or oxygen therapy
MYOCARDIAL INFARCTION			
Sudden, without precipitating factors, often in early morning	Intense stabbing, viselike pain or pressure, severe	Substernal; may spread throughout the anterior chest and to the arms, jaw, back, or neck	Continuous or no chest discomfort; relieved with morphine, cardiac drugs, and oxygen therapy
PERICARDITIS			
Sudden	Sharp, stabbing, moderate to severe	Substernal; usually spreads to the left side or the back	Intermittent; relieved with sitting upright, analgesia, or administration of anti-inflammatory agents
PLEUROPULMONARY			
Variable	Moderate ache, worse on inspiration	Lung fields	Continuous until the underlying condition is treated or the patient has rested
ESOPHAGEAL-GASTRIC			
Variable	Squeezing, heartburn, variable severity	Substernal; may spread to the shoulders or the abdomen	Variable; may be relieved with antacid administration, food intake, or taking a sitting position
ANXIETY			
Variable, may be in response to stress or fatigue	Dull ache to sharp stabbing; may be associated with numbness in fingers	Usually last 30 min or longer or is relieved with opioids	Usually lasts a few minutes

cur at the same time (associated symptoms), such as dyspnea, diaphoresis, nausea, and vomiting. Other factors that need to be addressed are those that may have made the chest pain worse (aggravating factors) or less intense (relieving factors). Chest pain can arise from a variety of sources (Table 35-1). By obtaining the appropriate information, you can help identify the source of the chest discomfort.

Dyspnea (difficult or labored breathing) can occur as a result of both cardiac and pulmonary disease. It is experienced by the patient as uncomfortable breathing or shortness of breath. When obtaining the history, ask what factors precipitate and relieve dyspnea, what level of activity produces dyspnea, and what the patient's body position was when dyspnea occurred.

Dyspnea that is associated with activity, such as climbing stairs, is referred to as ***dyspnea on exertion (DOE)****. This is usually an early symptom of heart failure and may be the only symptom experienced by women.*

The patient with advanced heart disease may experience **orthopnea** (dyspnea that appears when he or she lies flat). Several pillows may be needed to elevate the head and chest, or a recliner to prevent breathlessness may be used. *The severity of orthopnea is measured by the number of pillows or the amount of head elevation needed to provide restful sleep.* This symptom is usually relieved within a matter of minutes by sitting up or standing.

Paroxysmal nocturnal dyspnea (PND) develops after the patient has been lying down for several hours. In this position, blood from the lower extremities is redistributed to the venous system, which increases venous return to the heart. A diseased heart cannot compensate for the increased volume and is ineffective in pumping the additional fluid into the circulatory system. Pulmonary congestion results. The patient awakens abruptly, often with a feeling of suffocation and panic. He or she sits upright and dangles the legs over the side of the bed to relieve the dyspnea. This sensation may last for 20 minutes.

Fatigue may be described as a feeling of tiredness or weariness resulting from activity. The patient may report that an activity takes longer to complete or that he or she tires easily after activity. Although fatigue in itself is not diagnostic of heart disease, many people with heart failure are limited by leg fatigue during exercise. Fatigue that occurs after mild activity and exertion usually indicates inadequate cardiac output (due to low stroke volume) and anaerobic metabolism in skeletal muscle. *It can also accompany other symptoms or may be an early indication of heart disease in women.*

Ask about the time of day the patient experiences fatigue and the activities that he or she can perform. Fatigue resulting from decreased cardiac output is often worse in the evening. Ask whether the patient can perform the same activities as he or she could perform a year ago or the same activities as others of the same age. Often he or she limits activities in response to fatigue and, unless questioned, is unaware how much less active he or she has become.

A feeling of fluttering or unpleasant feeling in the chest caused by an irregular heartbeat is referred to as **palpitations.** They may result from a change in heart rate or rhythm or from an increase in the force of heart contractions. Rhythm disturbances that may cause palpitations include paroxysmal supraventricular tachycardia, premature contractions, and sinus tachycardia. Those that occur during or after strenuous physical activity, such as running and swimming, may indicate overexertion or possibly heart disease. Noncardiac factors that may precipitate palpitations include anxiety, stress, fatigue, insomnia, hyperthyroidism, and the ingestion of caffeine, nicotine, or alcohol. Ask the patient about specific factors that cause the patient's palpitations.

A sudden weight increase of 2.2 pounds (1 kg) can result from excess fluid (1 L) in the interstitial spaces. Weight gain is the best indicator of fluid retention. This condition is commonly known as **edema.** It is possible for weight gains of up to 10 to 15 pounds (4.5 to 6.8 kg, or 4 to 7 L of fluid) to occur before edema is apparent. Ask whether the patient has noticed a tightness of shoes, indentations from socks, or tightness of rings.

Syncope refers to a brief loss of consciousness. The most common cause is decreased perfusion to the brain. Any condition that suddenly reduces cardiac output, resulting in decreased cerebral blood flow, can lead to a syncopal episode. Conditions such as cardiac rhythm disturbances, especially ventricular dysrhythmias, and valvular disorders, such as aortic stenosis, may trigger this symptom. **Near-syncope** refers to dizziness with an inability to remain in an upright position. Explore the circumstances that lead to dizziness or syncope.

CONSIDERATIONS FOR OLDER ADULTS

Syncope in the aging person may result from hypersensitivity of the carotid sinus bodies in the carotid arteries. Pressure applied to these arteries while turning the head, shrugging the shoulders, or performing a Valsalva maneuver (bearing down during defecation) may stimulate a vagal response. A decrease in blood pressure and heart rate can result, which can produce syncope. This type of syncopal episode may also result from postural (orthostatic) or postprandial (after eating) hypotension.

Extremity pain may be caused by two conditions: ischemia from atherosclerosis and venous insufficiency of the peripheral blood vessels. Patients who report a moderate to severe cramping sensation in their legs or buttocks associated with an activity such as walking have **intermittent claudication** related to decreased arterial tissue perfusion. *Claudication pain is usually relieved by resting or lowering the affected extremity to decrease tissue demands or to enhance arterial blood flow.* Leg pain that results from prolonged standing or sitting is related to venous insufficiency from either incompetent valves or venous obstruction. This pain may be relieved by elevating the extremity.

Functional History

After the history of the patient's cardiovascular status is obtained, he or she may be classified according to the New York Heart Association's Functional Classification (Table 35-2) or other system. The four classifications (I, II, III, and IV) depend on the degree to which ordinary physical activities (routine ADLs) are affected by heart disease. The Killip Classification provides a more objective description of the hemodynamics of heart failure and is described in Chapter 40. Recently, a new classification of heart failure has been established based on the patient's symptoms. This new system is further described in Chapter 40 as well.

Physical Assessment

A thorough physical assessment is the foundation for the nursing database and the formation of nursing diagnoses and collaborative problems. Any changes noted during the course of illness can be compared with this initial database. Evaluate the patient's vital signs on admission to the hospital or during the initial visit to the clinic or health care provider's office.

General Appearance

Physical assessment begins with the patient's general appearance. Assess general build and appearance, skin color, distress level, level of consciousness, shortness of breath, position, and verbal responses.

Patients can have left- or right-sided heart failure, or both. They can also be diagnosed with systolic and/or diastolic heart failure. *As a result, poor cardiac output and decreased cerebral perfusion may cause confusion, memory loss, and slowed verbal responses, especially in older adults.* Patients with chronic heart failure may also appear malnourished, thin, and cachectic. Late signs of severe right-sided heart failure are ascites, jaundice, and **anasarca** (generalized edema) as a result of prolonged congestion of the liver. Heart failure may also cause fluid retention and may be manifested by obvious generalized dependent edema. Chapter 37 differentiates right and left failure and systolic from diastolic heart failure in detail.

TABLE 35-2 New York Heart Association Functional Classification of Cardiovascular Disability

CLASS I
- Patients with cardiac disease but without resulting limitations of physical activity
- Ordinary physical activity does not cause undue fatigue, palpitation, dyspnea, or anginal pain

CLASS II
- Patients with cardiac disease resulting in slight limitation of physical activity
- They are comfortable at rest
- Ordinary physical activity results in fatigue, palpitation, dyspnea, or anginal pain

CLASS III
- Patients with cardiac disease resulting in marked limitation of physical activity
- They are comfortable at rest
- Less than ordinary physical activity causes fatigue, palpitation, dyspnea, or anginal pain

CLASS IV
- Patients with cardiac disease resulting in inability to carry on any physical activity without discomfort
- Symptoms of cardiac insufficiency or of the anginal syndrome may be present, even at rest
- If any physical activity is undertaken, discomfort is increased

Excerpted from The New York Heart Association. (1964). *Diseases of the heart and blood vessels: Nomenclature and criteria for diagnosis* (6th ed.). Boston: Little, Brown.

Skin

Skin assessment includes color and temperature. The best areas in which to assess circulation include the nail beds, mucous membranes, and conjunctival mucosa, because small blood vessels are located near the surface of the skin.

If there is normal blood flow or adequate perfusion to a given area in *light-colored skin,* it appears pink, perhaps rosy, in *color* and it is warm to the touch. *Decreased perfusion is manifested as cool, pale, and moist skin. Pallor is characteristic of anemia and can be seen in areas such as the nail beds, palms, and conjunctival mucous membranes in any patient.*

A bluish or darkened discoloration of the skin and mucous membranes in *light-skinned* people is referred to as **cyanosis.** This condition results from an increased amount of deoxygenated hemoglobin. It is not an early sign of decreased perfusion but occurs later with other symptoms. *Dark-skinned patients may experience cyanosis as a graying of the same tissues.*

Central cyanosis involves decreased oxygenation of the arterial blood in the lungs and appears as a bluish tinge of the conjunctivae and the mucous membranes of the mouth and tongue. Central cyanosis may indicate impaired lung function or a right-to-left shunt found in congenital heart conditions. Because of impaired circulation, there is marked desaturation of hemoglobin in the peripheral tissues, which produces a bluish or darkened discoloration of the nail beds, earlobes, lips, and toes.

Peripheral cyanosis occurs when blood flow to the peripheral vessels is decreased by peripheral vasoconstriction. Constriction results from a low cardiac output or an increased extraction of oxygen from the peripheral tissues. Peripheral cyanosis localized in an extremity is usually a result of arterial or venous insufficiency. **Rubor** (dusky redness) that replaces pallor in a dependent foot suggests arterial insufficiency.

Skin *temperature* can be assessed for symmetry by touching different areas of the body with the dorsal (back) surface of the hand or fingers. Decreased blood flow results in decreased skin temperature. It is lowered in several clinical conditions, including heart failure, peripheral vascular disease, and shock.

Extremities

Assess the patient's hands, arms, feet, and legs for skin changes, vascular changes, clubbing, and edema. Skin mobility and turgor are affected by fluid status. Dehydration and aging reduce skin turgor, and edema decreases skin elasticity. Vascular changes in an affected extremity may include paresthesia, muscle fatigue and discomfort, numbness, pain, coolness, and loss of hair distribution from a reduced blood supply. Fig. 32-1 in Chapter 32 shows late clubbing.

Clubbing of the fingers and toes is caused by chronic oxygen deprivation in body tissues. It is common in patients with advanced chronic pulmonary disease, congenital heart defects, and cor pulmonale (right-sided heart failure). The angle of the normal nail bed is 160 degrees. With **clubbing,** the nail straightens out to an angle of 180 degrees, and the base of the nail becomes spongy. Fig. 35-5 describes assessment of clubbing.

Peripheral edema is a common finding in patients with cardiovascular problems. The location of edema helps determine its potential cause. Bilateral edema of the legs may be seen in those with heart failure or chronic venous insufficiency. Abdominal and leg edema can be seen in patients with heart disease and cirrhosis of the liver. Localized edema in one extremity may be the result of venous obstruction (thrombosis) or lymphatic blockage of the extremity (lymphedema). Edema may also be noted in dependent areas, such as the sacrum, when a patient is confined to bed. In other patients, edema results from third spacing when plasma proteins decrease. Dependent foot and ankle edema is also a common side effect of certain antihypertensive drugs, such as amlodipine (Norvasc).

Document the location of edema as precisely as possible (e.g., midtibial or sacral) and the number of centimeters from an anatomic landmark. The extent of edema can be assessed as mild, moderate, or severe (or 1+, 2+, 3+, or 4+). However, these values are not precise and are very unreliable. Determine whether the edema is **pitting** (the skin can be indented) or nonpitting.

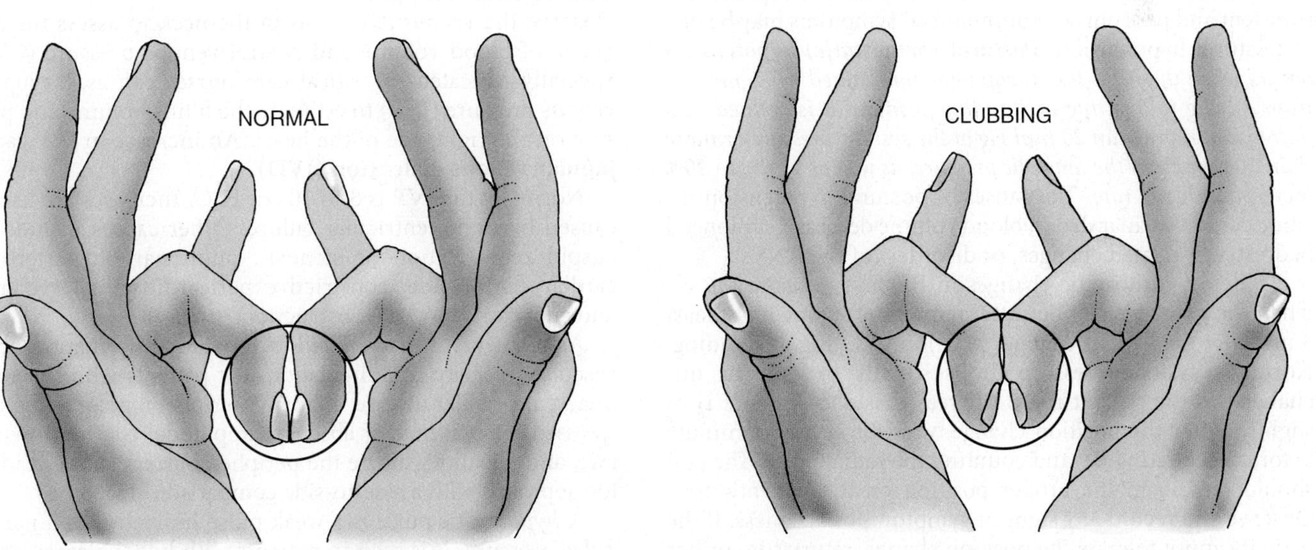
NORMAL
CLUBBING

Fig. 35-5 • Assessment of clubbing. The patient places the fingernails of the ring fingers together and holds them up to a light. If the examiner can see a diamond shape between the nails, there is no clubbing. Clubbing is identified by the absence of the diamond shape.

Blood Pressure

Arterial blood pressure is measured *indirectly* by sphygmomanometry. This technique of measurement is described in detail in nursing skills textbooks.

The National High Blood Pressure Education Program Joint National Committee (JNC) on Prevention, Detection, Evaluation, and Treatment of High Blood Pressure (2003) defines **hypertension** as a systolic pressure of 140 mm Hg or higher or a diastolic pressure of 90 mm Hg or higher, or taking drugs to control blood pressure. A blood pressure that exceeds 135/85 mm Hg increases the workload of the left ventricle and oxygen consumption of the myocardium. About one of every five Americans has hypertension.

More than one fourth of adults in the United States have prehypertension. ***Prehypertension** includes blood pressure (BP) readings of 120 to 139 mm Hg systolic or 80 to 89 mm Hg diastolic without antihypertensive drug therapy. Prehypertensive patients are at a high risk for developing hypertension. Normal BP is a systolic blood pressure less than 120 mm Hg and diastolic blood pressure less than 80 mm Hg.* Although the cause of hypertension is not known for most people, it can be effectively controlled with lifestyle modification and/or drug therapy. This disease is a major contributor to the development of CAD and heart failure. *According to the American Heart Association, the prevalence of hypertension in African Americans and other blacks in the United States is among the highest in the world. These patients are at increased risk of stroke, heart disease, and end-stage kidney disease* (Rosamond et al., 2007).

A BP less than 90/60 mm Hg may be inadequate for providing proper and sufficient nutrition to body cells. In certain circumstances, such as shock and hypotension, the Korotkoff sounds are less audible or are absent. In these cases, palpate the BP, use an ultrasonic device (Doppler device), or obtain a direct measurement by arterial catheter. When BP is palpated, only the systolic pressure can be determined. More information on *direct* measurement of arterial pressure is available in the Hemodynamic Monitoring section on p. 726.

Patients may report dizziness or light-headedness when they move from a flat, supine position to a sitting or a standing position at the edge of the bed. Normally these symptoms are transient and pass quickly; pronounced symptoms may be due to postural hypotension. ***Postural (orthostatic) hypotension** occurs when the BP is not adequately maintained while moving from a lying to a sitting or standing position. It is defined as a decrease of more than 20 mm Hg of the systolic pressure or more than 10 mm Hg of the diastolic pressure, as well as a 10% to 20% increase in heart rate.* The causes of postural hypotension include cardiovascular drugs, blood volume decrease, prolonged bedrest, age-related changes, or disorders of the ANS.

To detect orthostatic changes in BP, first measure the BP when the patient is supine. After remaining supine for at least 3 minutes, the patient changes position to sitting or standing. Normally systolic pressure drops slightly or remains unchanged as the patient rises, whereas diastolic pressure rises slightly. After the position change, wait for at least 1 minute before auscultating BP and counting the radial pulse. The cuff should remain in the proper position on the patient's arm. Observe and record any signs or symptoms of dizziness. If the patient cannot tolerate the position change, return him or her to the previous position of comfort.

Paradoxical blood pressure is an exaggerated decrease in systolic pressure by more than 10 mm Hg during the inspiratory phase of the respiratory cycle (normal is 3 to 10 mm Hg). Certain clinical conditions that potentially alter the filling pressures in the right and left ventricles may produce a paradoxical BP. Such conditions include pericardial tamponade, constrictive pericarditis, and pulmonary hypertension. During inspiration, the filling pressures normally decrease slightly. However, decreased fluid volume in the ventricles resulting from these pathologic conditions produces a marked reduction in cardiac output. The procedure for assessing a paradoxical BP is found in Chapter 37, Chart 37-10.

The difference between the systolic and diastolic values is referred to as **pulse pressure.** This value can be used as an indirect measure of cardiac output. Narrowed pulse pressure is rarely normal and results from increased peripheral vascular resistance or decreased stroke volume in patients with heart failure, hypovolemia, or shock. It can also be seen in those with mitral stenosis or regurgitation. An increased pulse pressure may occur in patients with slow heart rates, aortic regurgitation, atherosclerosis, hypertension, and aging.

The **ankle-brachial index (ABI)** can be used to assess the vascular status of the lower extremities. A BP cuff is applied to the lower extremity just above the malleolus. The systolic pressure is measured by Doppler ultrasound at both the dorsalis pedis and posterior tibial pulses. The higher of these two pressures is then divided by the higher of the two brachial pulses to obtain the ABI.

Normal values for the ABI are 1.00 or higher because BP in the legs is usually higher than BP in the arms. ABI values less than 0.80 usually indicate moderate vascular disease, whereas values less than 0.50 indicate severe vascular compromise. Although used primarily to help identify peripheral vascular disease, the ABI may be effective as a risk factor in predicting other CV disease in women, especially coronary artery disease (Pearson, 2007) (see the Evidence-Based Practice box on p. 717).

A **toe brachial pressure index (TBPI)** may be performed instead of or in addition to the ABI to determine arterial perfusion in the feet and toes. TBPI is the toe systolic pressure divided by the brachial (arm) systolic pressure.

Venous and Arterial Pulses

Observe the *venous pulsations* in the neck to assess the adequacy of blood volume and central venous pressure (CVP). Specially educated or critical care nurses can assess jugular venous pressure (JVP) to estimate the filling volume and pressure on the right side of the heart. An increase in JVP causes **jugular venous distention (JVD).**

Normally the JVP is 3 to 10 cm H_2O. Increases are usually caused by right ventricular failure. Other causes include tricuspid regurgitation or stenosis, pulmonary hypertension, cardiac tamponade, constrictive pericarditis, hypervolemia, and superior vena cava obstruction.

VIDEO CLIP: Pulses, Lower Extremities

Assessment of *arterial pulses* provides information about vascular integrity and circulation. For patients with suspected or actual vascular disease, all major peripheral pulses should be assessed for presence or absence, amplitude, contour, rhythm, rate, and equality. Palpate the peripheral arteries in a head-to-toe approach with a side-to-side comparison (Fig. 35-6).

A *hypokinetic* pulse is a weak pulse indicative of a narrow pulse pressure. It is seen in patients with hypovolemia, aortic stenosis, and decreased cardiac output. A *hyperkinetic* pulse is a large, "bounding" pulse caused by an increased ejection of blood. It occurs in patients with a high cardiac output (with

EVIDENCE-BASED PRACTICE

Are ankle-brachial index values correlated with cardiovascular risks in women?

Pearson, T.L. (2007). Correlation of ankle-brachial index values with carotid disease, coronary disease, and cardiovascular risk factors in women. *Journal of Cardiovascular Nursing, 22*(6), 436-439.

Ankle-brachial index (ABI) values have been used to help identify patients with peripheral arterial disease (PAD) for a number of years. Previous research has found a relationship between PAD and cardiac mortality and morbidity. The purpose of this study was to explore the correlation of a low ABI with coronary artery disease (CAD); carotid artery stenosis (CAS); and selected risk factors, such as smoking, hypercholesterolemia, and diabetes. Participants in this descriptive study were 810 healthy women. Data on risk factors were collected using a questionnaire; carotid artery stenosis was determined by ultrasound. The study found a significant correlation between ABI and CAS, suggesting that atherosclerosis occurs in multiple vessels at one time. The researchers believed that a self-report for risk factors influenced the lack of significant correlation between them and ABI values.

Level of Evidence—6. This study was descriptive using a convenience sample.

Commentary: Implications for Practice and Research. Although this study was descriptive and exploratory, it suggests that ABI may be correlated with cardiovascular (CV) diseases other than PAD. ABI is a simple procedure to perform and not invasive like other CV diagnostic tests. Additional research is needed to validate these findings and determine if ABI is associated with CV disease risk or occurrence.

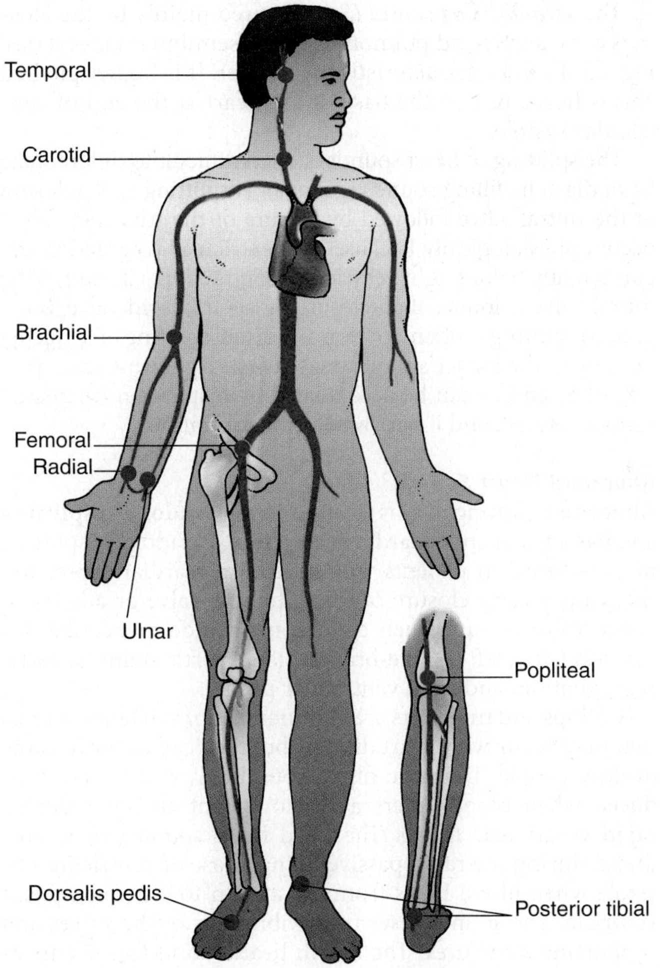
Temporal
Carotid
Brachial
Femoral
Radial
Ulnar
Popliteal
Dorsalis pedis
Posterior tibial

Fig. 35-6 • Pulse points for assessment of arterial pulses.

exercise, sepsis, or thyrotoxicosis) and in those with increased sympathetic system activity (with pain, fever, or anxiety).

In **pulsus alternans,** a weak pulse alternates with a strong pulse despite a regular heart rhythm. It is seen in patients with severely depressed cardiac function. They may be asked to hold their breath to exclude any false readings. You can palpate the brachial or radial arteries to assess this condition, but it is more accurately assessed by auscultation of blood pressure.

Auscultation of the major arteries (e.g., carotid and aorta) is necessary to assess for bruits. **Bruits** are swishing sounds that may occur from turbulent blood flow in narrowed or atherosclerotic arteries. Assess for the absence or presence of bruits by placing the bell of the stethoscope over the skin of the carotid artery while the patient holds his or her breath. Normally there are no sounds if the artery has uninterrupted blood flow. A bruit may develop when the internal diameter of the vessel is narrowed by 50% or more, but this does not indicate the severity of disease in the arteries. Once the vessel is blocked 90% or greater, the bruit often cannot be heard.

▶ VIDEO CLIP: Carotid Artery

Precordium

Assessment of the precordium (the area over the heart) involves inspection, palpation, percussion, and auscultation. *In most settings, the medical-surgical nurse seldom performs precordial palpation and percussion. Critical care nurses and advanced practice nurses are qualified to perform the complete assessment.* Therefore only inspection and auscultation are described here. Begin by placing the patient in a supine position, with the head of the bed slightly elevated for comfort. Some patients may require elevation of the head of the bed to 45 degrees for ease and comfort in breathing.

▶ VIDEO CLIP: Auscultatory Landmarks

Inspection

A cardiac examination is usually performed in a systematic order, beginning with inspection. Inspect the chest from the side, at a right angle, and downward over areas of the precordium where vibrations are visible. Cardiac motion is of low amplitude, and sometimes the inward movements are more easily detected by the naked eye.

Examine the entire precordium (Fig. 35-7), and note any prominent pulses. Movement over the aortic, pulmonic, and tricuspid areas is abnormal. Pulses in the mitral area (the apex of the heart) are considered normal and are referred to as the **apical impulse,** or the **point of maximal impulse (PMI).** The PMI should be located at the left fifth intercostal space (ICS) in the midclavicular line. If it appears in more than one ICS

▶ VIDEO CLIP: Anterior Chest

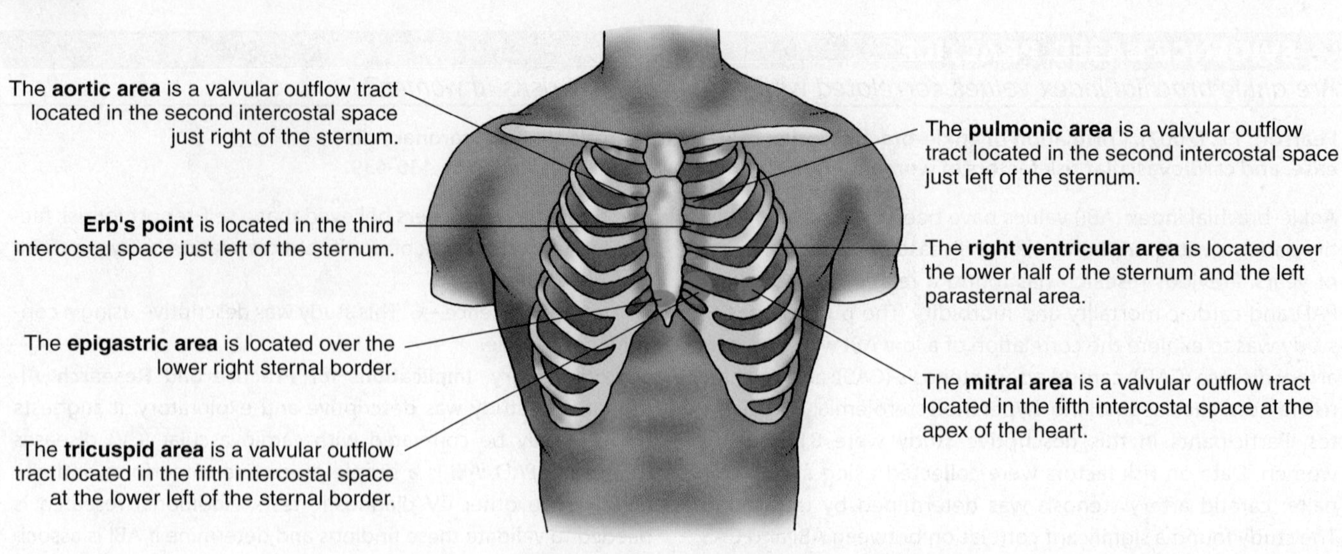
The **aortic area** is a valvular outflow tract located in the second intercostal space just right of the sternum.
Erb's point is located in the third intercostal space just left of the sternum.
The **epigastric area** is located over the lower right sternal border.
The **tricuspid area** is a valvular outflow tract located in the fifth intercostal space at the lower left of the sternal border.
The **pulmonic area** is a valvular outflow tract located in the second intercostal space just left of the sternum.
The **right ventricular area** is located over the lower half of the sternum and the left parasternal area.
The **mitral area** is a valvular outflow tract located in the fifth intercostal space at the apex of the heart.

Fig. 35-7 • Areas for myocardial inspection and auscultation.

and has shifted lateral to the midclavicular line, the patient may have left ventricular hypertrophy.

Auscultation

Auscultation evaluates heart rate and rhythm, cardiac cycle (systole and diastole), and valvular function. The technique of auscultation requires a good-quality stethoscope and extensive clinical practice. Identifying specific abnormal heart sounds is most important in critical care and telemetry. Some hospitals are equipped with monitored beds in every unit, but telemetry is used only when needed.

VIDEO CLIP: Auscultation with Diaphragm and Bell ▶

Listen to heart sounds in a systematic order. Examination usually begins at the aortic outflow tract area and progresses slowly to the apex of the heart. The diaphragm of the stethoscope is pressed tightly against the chest to listen for high-frequency sounds and is useful in listening to the first and second heart sounds and high-frequency murmurs. Repeat the progression from the base to the apex of the heart using the bell of the stethoscope, which is held lightly against the chest. The bell can screen out high-frequency sounds and is useful in listening for low-frequency gallops (diastolic filling sounds) and murmurs.

Attention is given to the areas in Fig. 35-7 (except the epigastric area). Auscultation allows for assessment of heart rate and rhythm, murmurs, extrasystolic sounds, and rubs in the presence of a current or suspected cardiac problem.

Normal Heart Sounds

AUDIO CLIP: S_1 ▶

ANIMATION: Heart Valves and Sounds ▶

The *first heart sound* (S_1) is created by the closure of the mitral and tricuspid valves (atrioventricular valves) (see Fig. 35-4). When auscultated, S_1 is softer and longer; it is of a low pitch and is best heard at the lower left sternal border or the apex of the heart. It may be identified by palpating the carotid pulse while listening. S_1 marks the beginning of ventricular systole and occurs right after the QRS complex on the electrocardiogram (ECG).

S_1 can be accentuated or intensified in conditions such as exercise, hyperthyroidism, and mitral stenosis. A decrease in sound intensity occurs in patients with mitral regurgitation and heart failure. If you have difficulty hearing heart sounds, have the patient lean forward or roll to his or her left side.

◀ AUDIO CLIP: S_2

The *second heart sound* (S_2) is caused mainly by the closing of the aortic and pulmonic valves (semilunar valves) (see Fig. 35-4). S_2 is characteristically shorter. It is higher pitched and is heard best at the base of the heart at the end of ventricular systole.

The splitting of heart sounds is often difficult to differentiate from diastolic filling sounds (gallops). A splitting of S_1 (closure of the mitral valve followed by closure of the tricuspid valve) occurs physiologically because left ventricular contraction occurs slightly before right ventricular contraction. Closure of the mitral valve is louder than closure of the tricuspid valve, however, so splitting is often not heard. Normal splitting of S_2 occurs because of the longer systolic phase of the right ventricle. Splitting of S_1 and S_2 can be accentuated by inspiration (increased venous return), and it narrows during expiration.

Abnormal Heart Sounds

Abnormal splitting of S_2 is referred to as **paradoxical splitting** and has a wider split heard on expiration. Paradoxical splitting of S_2 is heard in patients with severe myocardial depression that causes early closure of the pulmonic valve or a delay in aortic valve closure. Such conditions include myocardial infarction (MI), left bundle-branch block, aortic stenosis, aortic regurgitation, and right ventricular pacing.

◀ AUDIO CLIPS: Third and Fourth Heart Sounds

Gallops and murmurs are common abnormal heart sounds that may occur with heart disease, but they can occur in some healthy people. Diastolic filling sounds (S_3 and S_4) are produced when blood enters a noncompliant chamber during rapid ventricular filling. The third heart sound (S_3) is produced during the rapid passive filling phase of ventricular diastole when blood flows from the atrium to a noncompliant ventricle. The sound arises from vibrations of the valves and supporting structures. The fourth heart sound (S_4) occurs as blood enters the ventricles during the active filling phase at the end of ventricular diastole.

S_3 is called a **ventricular gallop,** and S_4 is referred to as **atrial gallop.** These sounds can be caused by decreased compliance of either or both ventricles. Left ventricular diastolic filling sounds are best heard with the patient on his or her left side. The bell of the stethoscope is placed at the apex and at the left lower sternal border during expiration.

An S_3 heart sound is most likely to be a normal finding in children or those younger than 30 years of age. An S_3 gallop in patients older than 35 years is considered abnormal and represents a decrease in left ventricular compliance. It can be detected as an early sign of heart failure or as a ventricular septal defect.

An atrial gallop (S_4) may be heard in patients with hypertension, anemia, ventricular hypertrophy, MI, aortic or pulmonic stenosis, and pulmonary emboli. *It may be heard also with advancing age because of a stiffened ventricle.*

The presence of both S_3 and S_4, called a *summation* or a *quadruple gallop,* is an indication of severe heart failure. If the quadruple rhythm is present and the patient has tachycardia, the two sounds may fuse to produce a rhythm that sounds like a horse galloping.

AUDIO CLIPS: Systolic and Diastolic Murmurs

Murmurs reflect turbulent blood flow through normal or abnormal valves. They are classified according to their timing in the cardiac cycle: *systolic* murmurs (e.g., aortic stenosis and mitral regurgitation) occur between S_1 and S_2, whereas *diastolic* murmurs (e.g., mitral stenosis and aortic regurgitation) occur between S_2 and S_1. Murmurs can occur during presystole, midsystole, or late systole or diastole or can last throughout both phases of the cardiac cycle. They are also graded according to their intensity, depending on their level of loudness (Table 35-3).

AUDIO CLIPS: Types of Murmurs

Although you are not expected to grade murmurs as a medical-surgical nurse, describe their location based on where they are best heard. Some murmurs transmit or radiate from their loudest point to other areas, including the neck, the back, and the axilla. The configuration is described as crescendo (increases in intensity) or decrescendo (decreases in intensity). The quality of murmurs can be further characterized as harsh, blowing, whistling, rumbling, or squeaking. They are also described by pitch—usually high or low.

AUDIO CLIP: Pericardial Friction Rub

A **pericardial friction rub** originates from the pericardial sac and occurs with the movements of the heart during the cardiac cycle. Rubs are usually transient and are a sign of inflammation, infection, or infiltration. They may be heard in patients with pericarditis resulting from MI, cardiac tamponade, or post-thoracotomy.

NCLEX EXAMINATION CHALLENGE

A middle-aged client who has a diagnosis of cardiovascular disease is admitted to the telemetry unit for an abnormal heart rhythm and chest discomfort. What physical assessment findings should the nurse expect for this client? (Select all that apply.)

A. Headache
B. Palpitations
C. Irregular heart rate
D. Diarrhea
E. Fatigue
F. Hypercapnia

evolve For the correct answer, go to http://evolve.elsevier.com/Iggy/.

TABLE 35-3 Grading of Heart Murmurs

Grade I	Very faint	Grade V	Very loud, accompanied by a palpable thrill, and audible with the stethoscope partially off the patient's chest
Grade II	Faint but recognizable		
Grade III	Loud but moderate in intensity	Grade VI	Extremely loud, may be heard with the stethoscope slightly above the patient's chest, accompanied by a palpable thrill
Grade IV	Loud and accompanied by a palpable thrill		

Psychosocial Assessment

To most people, the heart is a symbol of their ability to exist, survive, and love. A patient with a heart-related illness, whether acute or chronic, usually perceives it as a major life crisis. The patient and family confront not only the possibility of death but also fears about pain, disability, lack of self-esteem, physical dependence, and changes in family dynamics. Assess the meaning of the illness to the patient and family by asking, "What do you understand about what happened to you (or the patient)?" and "What does that mean to you?" When they perceive the stressor as overwhelming, formerly adequate support systems may no longer be effective. In these circumstances, the patient and family members attempt to cope to regain a sense or feeling of control.

Coping behaviors vary among patients and their families. Those who feel helpless to meet the demands of the situation may exhibit behaviors such as disorganization, fear, and anxiety. Ask them, "Have you ever encountered such a situation before?" "How did you manage that situation?" and "To whom can you turn for help?" The answers to these questions often reassure the patient and family that they have encountered difficult situations in the past and have the ability and resources to cope with them.

A common and normal response is denial, which is a defense mechanism that enables the patient to cope with threatening circumstances. He or she may deny the current cardiovascular condition, may state that it was present but is now absent, or may be excessively cheerful. Denial becomes maladaptive when the patient is noncompliant or does not adhere to the interdisciplinary plan of care.

Family members and significant others may be more anxious than the patient. Often they recall all events of the illness, are unprotected by denial, and are afraid of recurrence. Disagreements may occur between the patient and family members over adherence to appropriate follow-up care.

Diagnostic Assessment

Laboratory Assessment

Assessment of the patient with cardiovascular dysfunction includes examination of the blood for abnormalities. The examination is performed to help establish a diagnosis, detect concurrent disease, assess risk factors, and monitor response to treatment. Normal values for serum cardiac enzymes and serum lipids are listed in Chart 35-3.

Serum Markers of Myocardial Damage

Events leading to cellular injury cause a release of enzymes from intracellular storage, and circulating levels of these enzymes are dramatically elevated. Acute myocardial infarction (MI), also known as *acute coronary syndrome,* can be confirmed by abnormally high levels of certain proteins or isoenzymes. These serum studies are commonly referred to as *car-*

Chart 35-3 LABORATORY PROFILE

Cardiovascular Assessment

Normal Range	Significance of Abnormal Findings
SERUM CARDIAC ENZYMES	
Creatine kinase (CK) *Females:* 30-135 units/L *Males:* 55-170 units/L Values higher after exercise	Elevations indicate possible brain, myocardial, and skeletal muscle necrosis or injury.
CK-MM (CK_3) 100% of total CK	Elevations occur with muscle injury.
CK-MB (CK_2) 0% of total CK	Elevations occur with myocardial injury or after percutaneous transluminal angioplasty and intracoronary streptokinase infusion.
CK-BB (CK_1) 0%	Elevations occur with brain tissue injury.
SERUM LIPIDS	
Total lipids 400-1000 mg/dL	Elevation indicates increased risk of coronary artery disease (CAD).
Cholesterol 122-200 mg/dL, or 3.16-6.5 mmol/L *Older adult (>70 yr):* 144-280 mg/dL	Elevation indicates increased risk of CAD.
Triglycerides *Females:* 35-135 mg/dL *Males:* 40-160 mg/dL *Older adult (>65 yr):* 55-260 mg/dL	Elevation indicates increased risk of CAD.
Plasma high-density lipoproteins (HDLs) *Females:* mean, 40 mg/dL *Males:* mean, 40 mg/dL Older adult range increases with age	Elevations protect against CAD.
Plasma low-density lipoproteins (LDLs) 60-180 mg/dL *Older adult (>65 yr):* 92-221 mg/dL	Elevation indicates increased risk of CAD.
HDL:LDL ratio 3:1	Elevated ratios may protect against CAD.
VLDL 25%-50%	Elevated level indicates risk of CAD.
C-reactive protein (CRP) <1.0 mg/dL	Elevation may indicate tissue infarction or damage.
SERUM MARKERS	
Troponins Cardiac troponin T <0.20 ng/mL Cardiac troponin I <0.03 ng/mL	Elevations indicate myocardial injury or infarction.
Myoglobin <90 mcg/L	Elevation indicates myocardial infarction.

VLDL, Very-low-density lipoproteins.

diac markers and include troponin, creatine kinase–MB, and myoglobin.

Troponin is a myocardial muscle protein released into the bloodstream with injury to myocardial muscle. Troponins T and I are not found in healthy patients, so any rise in values indicates cardiac necrosis or acute MI. Specific markers of myocardial injury, troponins T and I, have a wide diagnostic time frame, making them useful for patients who present several hours after the onset of chest pain. Even low levels of troponin T are treated aggressively because of increased risk of death from cardiovascular disease (CVD). Obtaining cardiac markers at the bedside in the emergency department can be done as "point of care" (POC) testing for patients experiencing or at risk for acute MI, with results available within 15 to 20 minutes. These markers are evaluated in addition to clinical signs and symptoms and ECG changes when identifying at-risk patients.

Creatine kinase (CK) is an enzyme specific to cells of the brain, myocardium, and skeletal muscle. The appearance of CK in the blood indicates tissue necrosis or injury, with levels following a predictable rise and fall during a specified period. Cardiac specificity must be determined by measuring isoenzyme activity. There are three isoenzymes of CK: CK-MM is the predominant isoenzyme of skeletal muscle; CK-MB is found in myocardial muscle; and CK-BB occurs in the brain. CK-MB activity is most specific for MI and shows a predictable rise and fall during 3 days; a peak level occurs about 24 hours after the onset of chest pain.

Treatment modalities for early intervention after acute MI and acute ischemia require more rapid diagnosis of MI. An assay using monoclonal anti–CK-MB antibodies (stat CK) can detect myocardial necrosis accurately 3 hours after emergency department admission when examined with an ECG. Two subforms of CK-MB (CK-MB_1 and CK-MB_2) have also been identified. Abnormal elevations of these CK subforms may occur as early as 2 hours after MI. They remain elevated for up to 12 hours after MI and appear to be very sensitive and specific early diagnostic markers of MI.

Another early marker of an MI is myoglobin. **Myoglobin,** a low-molecular-weight heme protein found in cardiac and skeletal muscle, is the earliest marker detected—as early as 2 hours after an MI with rapid decline after 7 hours. Because myoglobin is not cardiac specific and is found in skeletal and cardiac muscle, its clinical usefulness is more limited than troponin.

Serum Lipids

Elevated lipid levels are considered a risk factor for coronary artery disease (CAD). *Cholesterol, triglycerides,* and the protein components of *high-density lipoproteins (HDL)* and *low-density lipoproteins (LDL)* are evaluated to assess the risk for CAD. The desired ranges for lipids are (Pagana & Pagana, 2006):

- Total cholesterol less than 200 mg/dL
- Triglyceride less than 150 mg/dL
- HDL more than 40 mg/dL ("good" cholesterol)
- LDL less than 70 mg/dL in high-risk cardiovascular patients, less than 100 mg/dL in patients with moderate risk factors

Each of the lipoproteins contains varying proportions of cholesterol, triglyceride, protein, and phospholipid. HDL contains mainly protein and 20% cholesterol, whereas LDL is mainly cholesterol. Elevated LDL levels are positively correlated with CAD, whereas elevated HDL levels are negatively correlated and appear to be a protective factor. LDL pattern size is of significant importance in determining risk for CVD. LDL pattern A is associated with non–insulin resistance; normal glucose, insulin, and HDL levels; and a normal blood pressure. LDL pattern B is associated with insulin resistance; increased glucose, insulin, and triglyceride levels; and hypertension.

A fasting blood sample for the measurement of serum cholesterol levels is preferable to a nonfasting sample. If triglycerides are to be evaluated with cholesterol, the health care provider requests the specimen after a 12-hour fast

Lipoprotein-a, or Lp(a), is a modified form of LDL, the most common familial lipoprotein disorder in patients with premature coronary artery disease. Lp(a) is atherogenic (increases atherosclerotic plaques) and prothrombotic (increases clots). Therefore the desired outcome is a value less than 30 mg/dL. The patient should be fasting and avoid smoking before the test (Pagana & Pagana, 2006).

Other Serum Tests

Homocysteine is an amino acid that is produced when proteins break down. A certain amount of homocysteine is present in the blood, but elevated values may be an independent risk factor for the development of CVD. Although the relationship between homocysteine and CVD remains controversial, elevated levels of homocysteine may increase the risk of disease as much as smoking and hyperlipemia, especially in women. High-risk patients who have a personal or family history of premature heart disease should be screened. A level less than 14 mmol/dL is considered optimal (Pagana & Pagana, 2006).

Inflammation is a common and critical component to the development of atherothrombosis. **Highly sensitive C-reactive protein (hsCRP)** has been the most studied marker of inflammation. Any inflammatory process can produce CRP in the blood. Elevations are seen also with hypertension, infection, and smoking. A level less than 1 mg/dL is considered low risk; a level over 3 mg/dL places the patient at high risk for heart disease. The most useful time to measure CRP appears to be for risk assessment in middle-aged or older persons.

Microalbuminuria, or small amounts of protein in the urine, has been shown to be a clear marker of widespread endothelial dysfunction in cardiovascular disease (along with elevated CRP). It should be screened annually in all patients with hypertension, metabolic syndrome, or diabetes mellitus. Microalbuminuria has also been used as a marker for renal disease, particularly in patients with hypertension and diabetes.

Blood coagulation studies evaluate the ability of the blood to clot. They are important in patients with a greater tendency to form thrombi (e.g., those with atrial fibrillation, prosthetic valves, or infective endocarditis). These tests are also essential for monitoring patients receiving anticoagulant therapy (e.g., during cardiac surgery, during treatment of an established thrombus). 🛡

Prothrombin time (PT) and *international normalized ratio (INR)* are used when initiating and maintaining therapy with oral anticoagulants, such as sodium warfarin (Coumadin, Warfilone🍁). They measure the activity of prothrombin, fibrinogen, and factors V, VII, and X. INR is the most reliable way to monitor anticoagulant status in warfarin therapy. The therapeutic ranges vary significantly based on the reason for the anticoagulation and the patient's history.

Partial thromboplastin time (PTT) is assessed in patients who are receiving heparin (Hepalean🍁). It measures deficiencies in all coagulation factors except VII and XIII.

Arterial blood gas (ABG) determinations are often obtained in patients with CVD. Determination of tissue oxygenation, carbon dioxide removal, and acid-base status is essential to appropriate intervention and treatment. (See Chapter 14 for a complete discussion of ABGs.)

Fluid and electrolyte balance is essential for normal cardiovascular performance. Cardiac manifestations often occur when there is an imbalance in either fluids or *electrolytes* in the body. For example, the cardiac effects of hypokalemia (low serum potassium level) include increased electrical instability, ventricular dysrhythmias, and an increased risk of digitalis toxicity. The effects of hyperkalemia on the myocardium include slowed ventricular conduction, peaked T waves on the ECG, and contraction followed by asystole (cardiac standstill).

Cardiac manifestations of hypocalcemia are ventricular dysrhythmias, a prolonged QT interval, and cardiac arrest. Hyper-

TABLE 35-4 Indications for Cardiac Catheterization

- To confirm suspected heart disease, including coronary artery disease, myocardial disease, valvular disease, and valvular dysfunction
- To determine the location and extent of the disease process
- To assess:
  - Stable, severe angina unresponsive to medical management
  - Unstable angina pectoris
  - Uncontrolled heart failure, ventricular dysrhythmias, or cardiogenic shock associated with acute myocardial infarction, papillary muscle dysfunction, ventricular aneurysm, or septal perforation
- To determine best therapeutic option (percutaneous transluminal coronary angioplasty, stents, coronary artery bypass graft, valvulotomy versus valve replacement)
- To evaluate effects of medical or invasive treatment on cardiovascular function, percutaneous transluminal coronary angioplasty, or coronary artery bypass graft patency

calcemia shortens the QT interval and causes AV block, digitalis hypersensitivity, and cardiac arrest. Serum sodium values reflect fluid balance and may be decreased, indicating a fluid excess in patients with heart failure (dilutional hyponatremia).

Because magnesium regulates some aspects of myocardial electrical activity, hypomagnesemia has been implicated in some forms of ventricular dysrhythmias known as *torsades de pointes.* Hypomagnesemia prolongs the QT interval, causing this specific type of ventricular tachycardia. Chapter 13 describes these electrolytes in more detail.

The *erythrocyte (red blood cell [RBC]) count* is usually decreased in rheumatic fever and infective endocarditis. It is increased in heart diseases characterized by inadequate tissue oxygenation.

Decreased *hematocrit and hemoglobin* levels (e.g., caused by hemorrhage or hemolysis from prosthetic valves) indicate anemia and can lead to angina or aggravate heart failure. Vascular volume depletion with hemoconcentration (e.g., hypovolemic shock and excessive diuresis) results in an elevated hematocrit.

The *leukocyte (white blood cell [WBC]) count* is typically elevated after an MI and in various infectious and inflammatory diseases of the heart (e.g., infective endocarditis and pericarditis). An increased WBC has been implicated as a strong independent risk factor for stroke and heart disease, particularly in postmenopausal women, even in the absence of obesity, hypertension, smoking, diabetes, or older age.

Other Diagnostic Assessment

Posteroanterior (PA) and left lateral *x-ray* views of the chest are routinely obtained to determine the size, silhouette, and position of the heart. In acutely ill patients, a simple anteroposterior (AP) view may be obtained at the bedside. Cardiac enlargement, pulmonary congestion, cardiac calcifications, and placement of central venous catheters, endotracheal tubes, and hemodynamic monitoring devices are assessed by x-ray.

Angiography of the arterial vessels, or **arteriography,** is an invasive diagnostic procedure that involves fluoroscopy and the use of contrast media. This procedure is performed when an arterial obstruction, narrowing, or aneurysm is suspected. The interventional radiologist performs selective arteriography to evaluate specific areas of the arterial system. For example, a coronary arteriography, which is performed during left-sided cardiac catheterization, assesses arterial circulation within the heart. It can also be performed on arteries in the extremities, mesentery, and cerebrum. Angiography is discussed under the appropriate associated diseases elsewhere in this text.

TABLE 35-5 Complications of Cardiac Catheterization

RIGHT-SIDED HEART CATHETERIZATION
- Thrombophlebitis
- Pulmonary embolism
- Vagal response

LEFT-SIDED HEART CATHETERIZATION AND CORONARY ARTERIOGRAPHY
- Myocardial infarction
- Stroke
- Arterial bleeding or thromboembolism
- Dysrhythmias

RIGHT-SIDED OR LEFT-SIDED HEART CATHETERIZATION*
- Cardiac tamponade
- Hypovolemia
- Pulmonary edema
- Hematoma or blood loss at insertion site
- Reaction to contrast medium

*In addition to those cited for each procedure.

Cardiac Catheterization

The most definitive but most invasive test in the diagnosis of heart disease is cardiac catheterization. **Cardiac catheterization** may include studies of the right or left side of the heart and the coronary arteries. Some of the most common indications for cardiac catheterization are listed in Table 35-4.

Patient Preparation. Assessment of the patient's physical and psychosocial readiness and knowledge level is an important aspect of preparation because many patients have anxiety and fear about cardiac catheterization.

Review the purpose of the procedure, inform the patient about the length of the procedure, state who will be present, and describe the appearance of the catheterization laboratory. Tell the patient about the sensations he or she may experience during the procedure, such as palpitations (as the catheter is passed up to the left ventricle), a feeling of heat or a hot flash (as the medium is injected into either side of the heart), and a desire to cough (as the medium is injected into the right side of the heart). Written, electronic, or illustrated materials or DVDs may be used to assist in understanding.

The risks of cardiac catheterization are usually explained by the cardiologist. The risks vary with the procedures to be performed and the patient's physical status (Table 35-5). Several complications may follow coronary arteriography, such as:
- Myocardial infarction (MI)
- Stroke
- Arterial bleeding

- Thromboembolism
- Lethal dysrhythmias
- Arterial dissection
- Emergent coronary artery bypass surgery
- Death

The cardiologist or radiologist obtains a written informed consent from the patient or responsible party before the procedure.

The patient is admitted to the hospital on the day of the catheterization procedure. He or she may be admitted earlier if there is renal dysfunction. Fluids and acetylcysteine (Mucomyst) may be given 12 to 24 hours before the procedure for renal protection. Contrast-induced renal dysfunction can result from vasoconstriction and the direct toxic effect of the contrast agent on the renal tubules. Hydration and the administration of acetylcysteine pre- and post-study help eliminate or minimize contrast-induced renal toxicity.

Standard preoperative tests are performed, which usually include a chest x-ray, complete blood count, coagulation studies, and 12-lead ECG. The patient receives nothing by mouth after midnight or has only a liquid breakfast if the catheterization is to take place in the afternoon. The catheterization site is shaved and antiseptically prepared according to agency policy.

Before the procedure, take the patient's vital signs, auscultate the heart and the lungs, and assess the peripheral pulses. Question him or her about any history of allergy to iodine-based contrast agents. Be sure that the signed informed consent is completed. An antihistamine or steroid may be given to a patient with a positive history or to prevent a reaction. A mild sedative is usually administered before the procedure. If the patient normally takes a digitalis preparation or diuretic, it is usually withheld before the catheterization. Analysis of electrolytes, blood urea nitrogen (BUN), creatinine, coagulation profile, and CBC is essential before and after the procedure, and abnormalities are discussed with the physician.

Procedure. The patient is taken to the cardiac catheterization laboratory (sometimes referred to as the "cath lab"), placed in the supine position on the x-ray table, and securely strapped to the table. Inform him or her that this precaution is necessary because the table turns like a cradle during the procedure. The physician injects a local anesthetic at the insertion site. During the procedure, the patient is instructed to report any chest pain, pressure, or other symptoms to the staff.

The *right side of the heart* is catheterized first and may be the only side examined. The cardiologist inserts a catheter through the femoral vein to the inferior vena cava or through the basilic vein to the superior vena cava. The catheter is advanced through either the inferior or the superior vena cava and, guided by fluoroscopy, is advanced through the right atrium, through the right ventricle, and, at times, into the pulmonary artery (Fig. 35-8). Intracardiac pressures (right atrial, right ventricular, pulmonary artery, and pulmonary artery wedge pressures) and blood samples are obtained. A contrast medium is usually injected to detect any cardiac shunts or regurgitation from the pulmonic or tricuspid valves.

In a *left-sided heart catheterization,* the cardiologist advances the catheter against the blood flow from the femoral or brachial artery up the aorta, across the aortic valve, and into the left ventricle. Alternatively, he or she may pass the catheter from the right side of the heart through the atrial septum, using a special needle to puncture the septum. Intracardiac pressures and blood samples are obtained. The pressures of the left atrium, left ventricle, and aorta, as well as mitral and aortic valve status, are evaluated. The cardiologist injects contrast dye into the ventricle; cineangiograms (rapidly changing films) evaluate left ventricular motion. Calculations are made regarding end-systolic volume, end-diastolic volume, stroke volume, and ejection fraction.

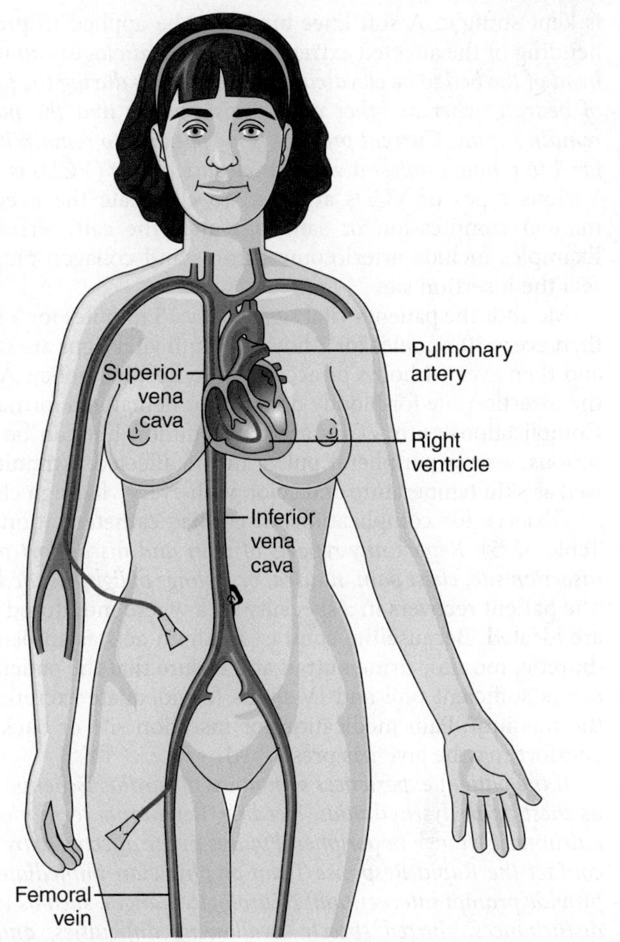
Pulmonary artery
Superior vena cava
Right ventricle
Inferior vena cava
Femoral vein

Fig. 35-8 • Right-sided heart catheterization. The catheter is inserted into the femoral vein and advanced through the inferior vena cava (or, if into an antecubital or basilic vein, through the superior vena cava), right atrium, and right ventricle, and into the pulmonary artery.

The technique for *coronary arteriography* is the same as for left-sided heart catheterization. The catheter is advanced into the aortic arch and positioned selectively in the right or left coronary artery. Injection of a contrast medium permits viewing the coronary arteries. By assessing the flow of the medium through the coronary arteries, information about the site and severity of coronary lesions is obtained.

An alternative to injecting a medium into the coronary arteries is **intravascular ultrasonography (IVUS),** which introduces a flexible catheter with a miniature transducer at the distal tip to view the coronary arteries. The transducer emits sound waves, which reflect off the plaque and the arterial wall to create an image of the blood vessel. IVUS is more reliable than angiography in indicating plaque distribution and composition, arterial dissection, and degree of stenosis of the occluded artery.

Follow-up Care. After cardiac catheterization, the patient is typically restricted to bedrest and the insertion site extremity is kept straight. A soft knee brace can be applied to prevent bending of the affected extremity. *Some cardiologists allow the head of the bed to be elevated up to 30 degrees during the period of bedrest, whereas other cardiologists prefer that the patient remain supine. Current practice is for patients to remain in bed for 4 to 6 hours unless a vascular closure device (VCD) is used.* Various types of VCDs are used to eliminate the need for manual compression or sandbags after the catheterization. Examples include arteriotomy sutures and collagen plugs to seal the insertion site.

Monitor the patient's vital signs every 15 minutes for 1 hour, then every 30 minutes for 2 hours or until vital signs are stable, and then every 4 hours or according to hospital policy. Assess the insertion site for bloody drainage or hematoma formation. Complications with VCDs are not common but can be very serious. Assess peripheral pulses in the affected extremity, as well as skin temperature and color, with every vital sign check.

Observe for complications of cardiac catheterization (see Table 35-5). *Report any reports of pain and discomfort at the insertion site, chest pain, nausea, or feelings of light-headedness.* The patient recovers in a specialty area where monitored beds are located. Because the contrast medium acts as an osmotic diuretic, monitor urine output and ensure that the patient receives sufficient oral and IV fluids for adequate excretion of the medium. Pain medication for insertion site or back discomfort may be given as prescribed.

If the patient experiences symptoms of cardiac ischemia such as chest pain, dysrhythmias, bleeding, hematoma formation, or a dramatic change in peripheral pulses in the affected extremity, contact the Rapid Response Team or physician immediately to provide prompt intervention! Neurologic changes, such as visual disturbances, slurred speech, swallowing difficulties, and extremity weakness, should also be reported immediately.

Review home instructions and risk factor modification with the patient before discharge. Remind the patient to:

- Limit activity for several days, including avoiding lifting and exercise.
- Leave the dressing in place for at least the first day at home.
- Observe the insertion site over the next few weeks for increased swelling, redness, warmth, and pain. Bruising or a small hematoma is expected.

DECISION-MAKING CHALLENGE

Delegation/Supervision

An older adult has returned from the cardiac cath lab with an IV and vascular closure device at the insertion site. She is confused and restless and says she is thirsty. Her BP has been low with an average of 96/50, and her pulse has been between 80 and 92. She was not confused before the procedure. You are a new RN graduate assigned to her care. There is one nursing technician working in the recovery area.

1. What assessments will you perform at this time and why?
2. Why is this patient confused? Think of all the possibilities.
3. The patient's vital signs have to be monitored frequently. Should you delegate this task to the nursing technician (NT)? Why or why not?
4. What other nursing tasks and activities could be delegated to the NT?
5. What health teaching does this patient and her family need?

evolve For suggested answer guidelines, go to http://evolve.elsevier.com/Iggy/.

Electrocardiography

The electrocardiogram (ECG) is a routine part of every cardiovascular evaluation and is one of the most valuable diagnostic tests. Various forms are available: resting ECG, continuous ambulatory ECG (Holter monitoring), exercise ECG (stress test), signal-averaged ECG, and 30-day event monitoring. The resting ECG provides information about cardiac dysrhythmias, myocardial ischemia, the site and extent of MI, cardiac hypertrophy, electrolyte imbalances, and the effectiveness of cardiac drugs. Other forms are described in Chapter 36. The normal ECG pattern and a detailed discussion of the interpretation of abnormal patterns are also found in Chapter 36.

Electrophysiologic Studies

An **electrophysiologic study (EPS)** is an invasive procedure during which programmed electrical stimulation of the heart is used to cause and evaluate lethal dysrhythmias and conduction abnormalities. Patients who have survived cardiac arrest, have recurrent tachydysrhythmias, or experience unexplained syncopal episodes may be referred for EPS. Induction of the dysrhythmia during EPS helps find an accurate diagnosis and aids in effective treatment. These procedures have risks similar to those for cardiac catheterization and are performed in a special catheterization laboratory, where conditions are strictly controlled and immediate treatment is available for any adverse effects. Chapter 36 describes this diagnostic study in detail.

Exercise Electrocardiography (Stress Test)

The **exercise electrocardiography** test (also known as *exercise tolerance*, or **stress test**) assesses cardiovascular response to an increased workload. The stress test helps determine the functional capacity of the heart and screens for asymptomatic coronary artery disease. Dysrhythmias that develop during exercise may be identified, and the effectiveness of antidysrhythmic drugs can be evaluated.

Patient Preparation. Because risks are associated with exercising, the patient must be adequately informed about the purpose of the test, the procedure, and the risks involved. Written consent must be obtained. Anxiety and fear are common before stress testing. Therefore assure the patient that the procedure is performed in a controlled environment in which prompt nursing and medical attention is available.

The patient is instructed to get plenty of rest the night before the procedure. He or she may have a light meal 2 hours before the test but should avoid smoking or drinking alcohol or caffeine-containing beverages on the day of the test. The cardiologist decides whether the patient should stop taking any cardiac medications. Usually, cardiovascular drugs such as beta blockers or calcium channel blockers are withheld on the day of the test to allow the heart rate to increase during the stress portion of the test. Patients are advised to wear comfortable, loose clothing and rubber-soled, supportive shoes. Instruct them to tell the physician if symptoms such as chest pain, dizziness, shortness of breath, and an irregular heartbeat are experienced during the test.

Before the stress test, a resting 12-lead ECG, cardiovascular history, and physical examination are performed to check for any ECG abnormalities or medical factors that might interfere with the test. Check to see that all emergency supplies such as cardiac drugs, a defibrillator, and other necessary resuscitation equipment are available in the room in which the stress test is performed. It is important to be proficient in the use of resuscitation equipment when assisting the physician because chest pain, dysrhythmias, and other ECG changes may occur.

Procedure. The technician places electrodes on the patient's chest and attaches them to a multilead monitoring system. Note baseline blood pressure (BP), heart rate (HR), and respiratory rate. The two major modes of exercise available for stress testing are pedaling a bicycle ergometer and walking on a treadmill. A bicycle ergometer has a wheel operated by pedals that can be adjusted to increase the resistance to pedaling. The treadmill is a motorized device with an adjustable conveyor belt. It can reach speeds of 1 to 10 miles/hr and can also be adjusted from a flat position to a 22-degree incline.

After the patient is shown how to use the bicycle or to walk on the treadmill, he or she begins to exercise. During the test, the BP and ECG are closely monitored as the resistance to cycling or the speed and incline of the treadmill are increased. The patient exercises until one of these findings occurs:

- A predetermined HR is reached and maintained.
- Signs and symptoms such as chest pain, fatigue, extreme dyspnea, vertigo, hypotension, and ventricular dysrhythmias appear.
- Significant ST segment depression or T wave inversion occurs.
- The 20-minute protocol is completed.

Follow-up Care. After the test, the nurse or other qualified health care team member monitors the ECG and BP until the patient has completely recovered. After recovery, he or she can return home if the test was performed on an ambulatory basis. Advise him or her to avoid a hot shower for 1 to 2 hours after the test because this may cause hypotension. If he or she does not recover but continues to have pain or ventricular dysrhythmias or appears medically unstable, admission to a telemetry unit for observation is needed.

For patients who cannot exercise because of conditions such as peripheral vascular disease or arthritis, pharmacologic stress testing with agents such as dobutamine may be indicated. The nursing considerations are similar to those for the patient who has undergone an exercise ECG.

Echocardiography

As a noninvasive, risk-free test, echocardiography is easily performed at the bedside or on an ambulatory care basis. **Echocardiography** uses ultrasound waves to assess cardiac structure and mobility, particularly of the valves. It helps assess and diagnose cardiomyopathy, valvular disorders, pericardial effusion, left ventricular function, ventricular aneurysms, and cardiac tumors.

There is no special *preparation* for echocardiography. Inform the patient that the test is painless and takes 30 to 60 minutes to complete. The patient is instructed to lie quietly during the test and on his or her left side with the head elevated 15 to 20 degrees.

During an echocardiogram, a small transducer lubricated with gel to facilitate movement and conduction is placed on the patient's chest at the level of the third or fourth intercostal space near the left sternal border. The transducer transmits high-frequency sound waves and receives them as they are reflected from different structures. These echoes are usually videotaped simultaneously with the echocardiogram and can be recorded on graph paper for a permanent record.

After the images are taped, cardiac measurements that require several images can be obtained. Routine measurements include chamber size, ejection fraction, and flow gradient across the valves. There is no specific *follow-up care* for a patient who has undergone an echocardiogram.

A slightly more aggressive form of echocardiogram is a **pharmacologic stress echocardiogram** using either dobutamine or dipyridamole. This test is usually used when patients cannot tolerate exercise. Dobutamine (Dobutrex) increases the heart's contractility; dipyridamole (Persantine, Apo-Dipyridamole♣) is a coronary artery dilator. Patients are required to be NPO status for 3 to 6 hours before the test except for sips of water with medications. The technician ensures that IV access is present before the procedure and monitors BP and pulse continuously throughout the procedure. After the procedure, vital signs are monitored until BP returns to baseline and the pulse rate slows to less than 100 beats/min.

Transesophageal Echocardiography

Echocardiograms may also be performed transesophageally (through the esophagus). **Transesophageal echocardiography (TEE)** examines cardiac structure and function with an ultrasound transducer placed immediately behind the heart in the esophagus or stomach. The transducer provides especially detailed views of posterior cardiac structures such as the left atrium, mitral valve, and aortic arch. Preparation and follow-up are similar to that for an upper GI endoscopic examination (see Chapter 55).

Myocardial Nuclear Perfusion Imaging

The use of radionuclide techniques in cardiovascular assessment is called **myocardial nuclear perfusion imaging (MNPI).** Cardiovascular abnormalities can be viewed, recorded, and evaluated using radioactive tracer substances. These studies are useful for detecting myocardial infarction (MI) and decreased myocardial blood flow and for evaluating left ventricular ejection. Conducting myocardial nuclear imaging tests, in conjunction with exercise or the administration of vasodilating agents such as dipyridamole (Persantine, Apo-Dipyridamole♣), allows clearer identification of how the heart responds to stress.

Inform the patient that these tests are noninvasive. Because the amount of radioisotope is small, radiation exposure risks are minimal. If a dilating agent is to be used, advise the patient to avoid cigarettes and caffeinated food or drinks for 4 hours before administration of the vasodilator.

Common tests in nuclear cardiology include technetium (^{99m}Tc) pyrophosphate scanning, thallium imaging, and multigated cardiac blood pool imaging.

For the *technetium scan,* a small dose of ^{99m}Tc pyrophosphate is injected into the antecubital vein. The patient waits at least 2 hours while the kidneys clear the unbound technetium. A gamma-scintillation camera scans the heart to identify the areas of increased uptake of the radioisotope. The radioisotope accumulates in damaged myocardial tissue and is referred to as a "hot spot." This test helps detect an acute MI and define its location and size, but it does not show an old infarction.

For *thallium imaging,* a small dose of thallium-201 (^{201}Tl) is injected into the antecubital vein. A nuclear camera takes images of the heart 10 minutes later to detect areas of normal blood flow and intact cells, which rapidly take up the thallium. Necrotic or ischemic tissue does not take up the radioisotope and appears as "cold spots" on the scan. Scanning is repeated in 2 to 4 hours to evaluate thallium clearance.

Thallium imaging may be performed with the patient at rest or during an exercise test. Dipyridamole (Persantine, Apo-Dipyridamole♣) is administered before the Persantine thallium test. Dobutamine hydrochloride (Dobutrex) may be given instead. By causing vasodilation, these drugs simulate the effects of exercise and are used for patients who cannot exercise on a bike or treadmill. They may cause flushing, headache, dyspnea, and chest tightness for a few moments after injection.

Thallium imaging performed during an exercise test may demonstrate perfusion deficits not apparent at rest. First, the stress test procedure is performed. After the patient reaches maximum activity level, a small dose of ^{201}Tl is injected IV. The patient continues to exercise for about 1 to 2 minutes, after which the scanning is performed. Nuclear cardiologists often compare the resting and stress images to differentiate between fixed and reversible defects in the myocardium.

Thallium imaging is used to assess myocardial scarring and perfusion, to detect the location and extent of an acute or chronic MI, to evaluate graft patency after coronary bypass surgery, and to evaluate antianginal therapy, thrombolytic therapy, or balloon angioplasty.

Cardiac blood pool imaging is a noninvasive test for evaluating cardiac motion and calculating ejection fraction. It uses a computer to synchronize the patient's electrocardiogram (ECG) with pictures taken by a gamma-scintillation camera. The technician attaches the patient to an ECG and injects a small amount of ^{99m}Tc IV. The radioisotope is not taken up by tissue but remains "tagged" to red blood cells in the circulation. The camera may take pictures of the radioactive material as it makes its first pass through the heart.

During **multigated blood pool scanning,** the computer breaks the time between R waves on the ECG into fractions of a second, called "gates." The camera records blood flow through the heart during each of these gates. By analyzing the information from multiple gates, the computer can evaluate the ventricular wall motion and calculate ejection fraction (percentage of the left ventricular volume that is ejected with each contraction) and ejection velocity. Areas of decreased, absent, or paradoxical movement of the left ventricle may also be identified.

Positron emission tomography (PET) scans are used to compare cardiac perfusion and metabolic function and differentiate normal from diseased myocardium. The technician administers the first radioisotope (nitrogen-13-ammonia) and then begins a 20-minute scan to detect myocardial perfusion. Next, the technician administers a second radioisotope (fluoro-18-deoxyglucose). After a pause, a second scan is performed to detect the metabolically active myocardium, which is using glucose.

The two scans are compared. In a normal heart, performance and metabolic function will match. In an ischemic heart, there will be a mismatch—a reduction in perfusion and increased glucose uptake by the ischemic myocardium. The scanning procedure takes 2 to 3 hours, and the patient may be asked to use a treadmill or exercise bicycle in conjunction with the scan.

Depending on which test is performed, the patient may report fatigue or discomfort at the antecubital injection site. If a stress test was paired with the study, he or she will need follow-up care for the stress test.

Magnetic Resonance Imaging

Magnetic resonance imaging (MRI) is a noninvasive diagnostic option. An image of the heart or great vessels is produced through the interaction of magnetic fields, radio waves, and atomic nuclei showing hydrogen density. Simply put, the radio waves "bounce off" the body tissue being examined. Because each tissue has its own density, the computer image clearly differentiates between different types of tissues. MRI permits determination of cardiac wall thickness, chamber dilation, valve and ventricular function, and blood movement in the great vessels. Improved MRI techniques allow coronary artery blood flow to be mapped with nearly the accuracy of a cardiac catheterization.

Before an MRI, ensure that the patient has removed all metallic objects, including watches, jewelry, clothing with metal fasteners, and hair clips. Depending on the type of MRI, patients with pacemakers or implanted defibrillators should not undergo an MRI because the magnetic fields can deactivate them. However, some of the newer machines do not cause this problem. A few patients experience claustrophobia during the 15 to 60 minutes required to complete the scan.

Electronic-Beam Computed Tomography Scan

Electronic-beam computed tomography (EBCT) is a valuable tool in cardiovascular diagnostics. This test helps determine whether calcifications are present in the arteries; calcifications are a common component of arterial plaque. The 64-slice CT is used to determine the **coronary artery calcium (CAC) score,** which is a measure of the amount of coronary artery calcification. The test cannot predict the site of future events or determine the severity of the risk. According to the American Heart Association (AHA) clinical expert consensus document on calcium scoring, a CAC score of greater than 400 requires intensive preventive therapies (Greenland et al., 2007).

Hemodynamic Monitoring

Hemodynamic monitoring is an invasive system used in critical care areas to provide quantitative information about vascular capacity, blood volume, pump effectiveness, and tissue perfusion. It directly measures pressures in the heart and great vessels. These procedures are usually performed for more seriously ill patients and can provide more accurate measurements of blood pressure, heart function, and volume status.

Hemodynamic monitoring does involve significant risks, although complications are uncommon. Therefore informed consent is required. After obtaining consent, the nurse prepares a pressure-monitoring system. The components of this system are a catheter with an infusion system, a transducer, and a monitor. The catheter receives the pressure waves (mechanical energy) from the heart or the great vessels. The transducer converts the mechanical energy into electrical energy, which is displayed as waveforms or numbers on the monitor. Patency of the catheter is maintained with a slow continuous flush of normal saline, usually infused at 3 to 4 mL/hr under pressure to prevent the backup of blood and occlusion of the catheter.

To prepare the transducer, balance and calibrate it according to hospital policy and the manufacturer's specifications. Finally, identify the phlebostatic axis (Chart 35-4) and level the transducer to it. When the monitoring system is prepared, the physician inserts the catheter.

A pulmonary artery catheter is a multi-lumen catheter with the capacity to measure right atrial and indirect left atrial pressures or pulmonary artery wedge pressure (PAWP), also known as the **pulmonary artery occlusive pressure (PAOP).** A cardiac output measurement may also be obtained, as well as cardiac index and systemic and pulmonary vascular resistance.

The physician explains the procedure and advises the patient and family about the risks. He or she then obtains written patient consent for the procedure. Although this system is used to guide therapy, it is not itself a treatment. Ask the patient to remain still and in the supine or Trendelenburg position for insertion of the catheter.

The physician inserts a balloon-tipped catheter percutaneously through a large vein, usually the internal jugular or subclavian, and directs it to the right atrium (RA). When the catheter tip reaches the RA, the physician inflates the balloon. The catheter advances with the flow of blood through the tricuspid valve, into the right ventricle, past the pulmonic valve, and into a branch of the pulmonary artery. The balloon is deflated after the catheter tip reaches the pulmonary artery. Waveforms are viewed on the monitor as the pulmonary artery catheter is advanced (Fig. 35-9). A chest x-ray is used to check the location of the catheter.

Right atrial pressure is measured by a pressure sensor on the catheter inside the RA. Normal RA pressure ranges from 1 to 8 mm Hg. Increased RA pressures may occur with right ventricular failure, whereas low RA pressures usually indicate hypovolemia.

Normal pulmonary artery pressure (PAP) ranges from 15 to 26 mm Hg systolic/5 to 15 mm Hg diastolic (mean, 15) and is constantly visible on the monitor. When the balloon at the catheter tip is inflated, the catheter advances and wedges in a branch of the pulmonary artery. The tip of the catheter can sense pressures transmitted from the left atrium, which reflect left ventricular end-diastolic pressure (LVEDP). The pressure measured during balloon inflation is called the **pulmonary artery wedge pressure (PAWP).** PAWP closely reflects left atrial pressure and LVEDP in patients with normal left ventricular function, normal heart rates, and no mitral valve disease. The PAWP is a mean pressure and normally ranges between 4 and 12 mm Hg.

Elevated PAWP measurements may indicate left ventricular failure, hypervolemia, mitral regurgitation, or intracardiac shunt. A decreased PAWP is seen with hypovolemia or afterload reduction. Individual values may be less important than the trend in values.

The critical care nurse obtains and records RA pressure, PAP, and PAWP at appropriate intervals (usually every 1 to

Chart 35-4 **BEST PRACTICE FOR PATIENT SAFETY & QUALITY CARE**

Identification of the Phlebostatic Axis

1. Position the patient supine.
2. Palpate the fourth intercostal space at the sternum.

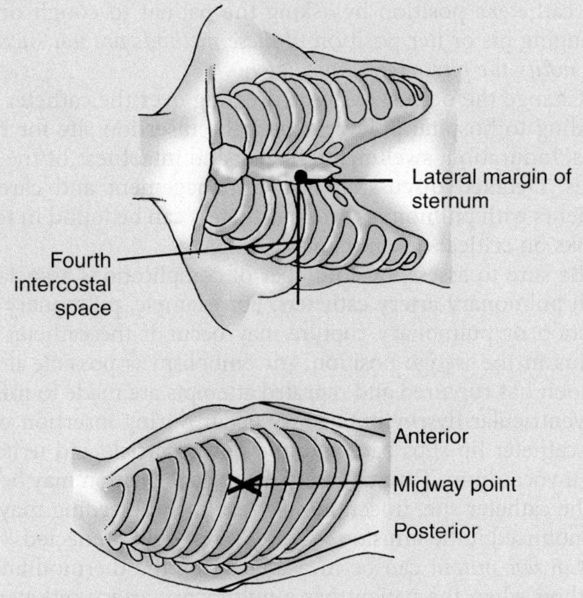

Lateral margin of sternum
Fourth intercostal space
Anterior
Midway point
Posterior

3. Follow the fourth intercostal space to the side of the patient's chest.
4. Determine the midway point between anterior and posterior.
5. Find the intersection between the midway point and the line from the fourth intercostal space, and mark it with an X in indelible ink. This is the phlebostatic axis.

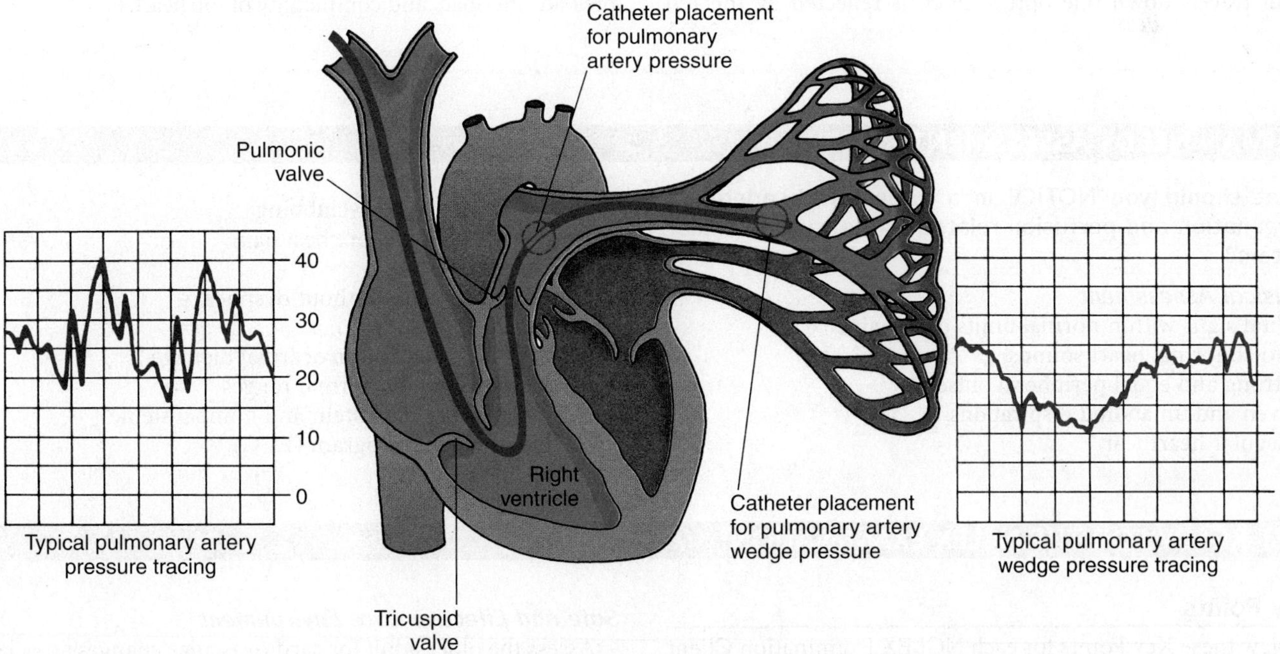

Catheter placement for pulmonary artery pressure
Pulmonic valve
40
30
20
10
0
Typical pulmonary artery pressure tracing
Right ventricle
Tricuspid valve
Catheter placement for pulmonary artery wedge pressure
Typical pulmonary artery wedge pressure tracing

Fig. 35-9 • Cardiac pressure waveforms can be seen on the monitor.

4 hours). The trend of these pressures helps guide medical therapy. During pressure recording, it is important that the transducer be at the level of the phlebostatic axis. The patient is usually supine with the head elevated up to 45 degrees during hemodynamic readings, although the position may not affect results (Giuliano et al., 2003). If the balloon remains in the wedge position after PAWP measurement, try to change the catheter's position by asking the patient to cough or by changing his or her position. *If these methods are not successful, notify the physician immediately.*

Change the occlusive sterile dressing over the catheter according to hospital policy. Inspect the insertion site for redness, induration, swelling, drainage, and intactness of the sutures. Detailed discussion of the management and care of patients with pulmonary artery catheters can be found in textbooks on critical care nursing.

Be sure to assess for a number of complications associated with pulmonary artery catheters. For example, pulmonary infarction or pulmonary rupture may occur if the catheter remains in the wedge position. Air embolism is possible if the balloon has ruptured and repeated attempts are made to inflate it. Ventricular dysrhythmias may occur during insertion or if the catheter tip slips back into the right ventricle and irritates the myocardium. Thrombus and embolus formation may occur at the catheter site. Infection may result, and bleeding may be pronounced if the infusion system becomes disconnected.

Cardiac output can be measured using the thermodilution method when the patient has a pulmonary artery catheter. A specified amount (5 or 10 mL) of iced or room-temperature IV solution (normal saline or dextrose in water) is injected into the proximal port of the catheter. The solution mixes with the blood in the RA and travels with the flow of blood through the heart. A temperature-sensitive device located on the tip of the catheter in the pulmonary artery registers and senses the change in blood temperature. This information is transmitted to a cardiac output computer, which displays a digital value.

Mixed venous oxygen saturation (Svo_2) reflects the balance between the patient's oxygen supply and demand. Svo_2 may be measured with a pulmonary artery catheter with fiberoptics. Light travels down one optical fiber, is reflected by the red blood cells according to the oxygen saturation of the hemoglobin, and returns to an optical module for interpretation and continuous display. The normal range for Svo_2 is 60% to 80%. Using Svo_2 monitoring individualizes the plan of care so that the Svo_2 remains in the normal range and the patient's oxygen supply and demand are in balance.

Direct measurement of *arterial BP* is done by invasive arterial catheter in critically ill patients. The physician or specially trained nurse inserts an intra-arterial catheter into the radial or femoral artery. After the physician has inserted the catheter, it is attached to pressure tubing. A normal saline flush solution is infused constantly under pressure to maintain the integrity of the system. A transducer attached to the tubing allows continuous direct monitoring of the arterial BP. Direct measurements of BP are usually 10 to 15 mm Hg greater than indirect (cuff) measurements. The arterial catheter may also be used to obtain blood samples for arterial blood gas values and other blood tests.

Because the arterial vasculature is a high-pressure system, frequent assessment of the arterial site and infusion system is essential. *Note any bleeding around the intra-arterial catheter or any loose connections, and correct the situation immediately.* Collateral circulation must be assessed by Doppler before and while the arterial catheter is in place. Carefully monitor color, pulse, and temperature distal to the insertion site for any early signs of circulatory compromise. Complications of systemic intra-arterial monitoring include pain, infection, arteriospasm, or obstruction at the site with the potential for distal infarction, air embolism, and hemorrhage.

Unlike conventional hemodynamic monitoring, **impedance cardiography (ICG)** is a flexible and fast-acting noninvasive monitoring system that consists of four ICG electrodes, four electrocardiogram (ECG) electrodes, and a portable ICG monitor. Simply stated, it measures the total impedance (resistance) to the flow of electricity in the heart. ICG can be used in any setting: in the intensive care unit (ICU), in the emergency department (ED), and in the home. It is used to assess, plan, and individualize the treatment plan for patients with heart failure, severe trauma, or fluid management. The system provides measures of thoracic fluid, left ventricular function (cardiac output and cardiac index), preload, afterload, and contractility of the heart.

HUMAN NEEDS ASSESSMENT REVIEW

What should you NOTICE in a patient with adequate oxygenation and perfusion related to the cardiovascular system?

Physical Assessment

- Vital signs within normal limits or baseline
- No abnormal heart sounds
- Strong and equal peripheral pulses
- Even and unlabored respirations
- Regular heartbeat
- No pallor, cyanosis, or clubbing
- No syncope, fatigue, or chest pain
- No edema
- Can perform ADLs without dyspnea

Diagnostic Assessment

- No serum markers of myocardial damage
- Serum lipids within normal ranges
- Normal C-reactive protein and homocysteine
- Normal electrocardiogram (ECG)

GET READY FOR THE NCLEX EXAMINATION!

Key Points

Review these Key Points for each NCLEX Examination Client Needs Category.

Safe and Effective Care Environment

- Assess the older adult for cardiovascular changes associated with aging as described in Chart 35-1.

- Assess patients for allergy to iodine-based contrast media before having diagnostic tests requiring a contrast agent.
- After invasive cardiovascular diagnostic testing, such as angiography and cardiac catheterization, monitor the insertion site for bleeding and hematoma formation.
- Assess vital signs carefully in patients having invasive cardiovascular testing; report new dysrhythmias after testing.

Health Promotion and Maintenance

- Identify patients at risk for cardiovascular disease, especially those with hyperlipidemia, hypertension, excess weight, physical inactivity, smoking, psychological stress, a positive family history, and diabetes.
- Teach patients how to reduce the risk of heart disease through exercise, diet modification, smoking cessation, and medications, as needed.
- Inform patients that genetics and other nonmodifiable risk factors, such as family history and gender, contribute to the development of CAD.

Psychosocial Integrity

- Discuss with the patient any feelings or concerns he or she might have about the stress of cardiac illness, diagnostic testing, or other issues, and use therapeutic measures to decrease anxiety.
- Recognize that denial is a common and normal response to help patients cope with threatening circumstances.
- Be aware that coping behaviors of those who have cardiovascular problems vary from patient to patient.
- Allow the patient to express feelings about an actual or perceived loss of health or social status related to cardiovascular disease.

Physiological Integrity

- Assess the patient's report of pain to differentiate the pain of angina and myocardial infarction (MI) from other noncardiac causes; *discomfort, indigestion, squeezing, heaviness,* and *viselike* are common terms used to describe chest pain of cardiac origin.
- Recall that syncope is a transient loss of consciousness and is common in older adults.
- Use jugular venous pressure to assess the filling volume and pressure on the right side of the heart.
- Assess for bruits, which are swishing sounds that develop in narrowed arteries.
- Auscultate the heart for normal first and second sounds, as well as for abnormalities such as an S_3, S_4, murmur, or gallop.
- Monitor serum markers of myocardial damage and other cardiac-related laboratory tests as listed in Chart 35-3.
- Assess patients having cardiac catheterizations for potential complications as listed in Table 35-5.
- Directly assess cardiac pressures and cardiac output when patients have invasive hemodynamic monitoring systems.

Additional Study Resources

Go to your Companion CD or Evolve at http://evolve.elsevier.com/Iggy/ for *Self-Assessment Questions for the NCLEX Examination.*

evolve Go to Evolve at http://evolve.elsevier.com/Iggy/ for *Prioritization and Delegation Questions for the NCLEX Examination.*

SELECTED BIBLIOGRAPHY

Asterisk indicates a classic or definitive work on this subject.

Arsianian-Engoren, C. (2007). Black, Hispanic, and white women's perception of heart disease. *Progress in Cardiovascular Nursing, 22*(1), 13-19.

Bern, L., Brandt, M., Mbelu, N., Asonye, U., Fisher, T., Shaver, Y., et al. (2007). Differences in blood pressure values obtained with automated and manual methods in medical inpatients. *MEDSURG Nursing, 16*(6), 356-362.

*Beyerle, K. (2002). Point of care testing of cardiac markers aids patient experiencing or at risk for acute myocardial infarction. *Nursing Management, 33*(9), 37-39.

*Bonham, P.A. (2003). Determining the toe brachial pressure index. *Nursing2003, 33*(9), 54-55.

Cheek, D., & Tester, J. (2008). Women and heart disease: What's new? *Nursing2008, 38*(1), 37-42.

Crean, C.A. (2007). How can electrophysiology help your patient? *Nursing2007, 37*(7), 60-61.

*DeVon, H.A., & Zerwic, J.J. (2003). The symptoms of unstable angina: Do women and men differ? *Nursing Research, 52*(2), 108-118.

Gibson, D. (2007). Vascular closure devices: What you know can prevent serious complications. *American Nurse Today, 2*(7), 11-14.

*Giuliano, K.K, Scott, S.S., Brown, V., & Olson, M. (2003). Backrest angle and cardiac output measurement in critically ill patients. *Nursing Research, 52*(4), 242-248.

Greenland, P., Bonow, R.O., Brundage, B.H., Budoff, M.J., Eisenberg, M.J., Grundy, S.M., et al. (2007). ACCF/AHA clinical expert consensus document on coronary artery calcium scoring by computed tomography in global cardiovascular risk assessment and in evaluation of patients with chest pain. *Circulation, 115*(3), 402-426.

Jarvis, C. (2008). *Physical examination and health assessment* (5th ed.). St. Louis: Mosby.

Lloyd-Jones, D.M., Liu, K., Tian, L., & Greenland, P. (2006). Narrative review: Assessment of C-reactive protein in risk prediction for cardiovascular disease. *Annals of Internal Medicine, 145*(1), 35-42.

Marchiondo, K. (2007). Transesophageal imaging and interventions: Nursing implications. *Critical Care Nurse, 27*(2), 25-35.

*Mehta, M. (2003). Assessing cardiovascular status. *Nursing2003, 33*(1), 56-57.

*Natarajan, S., Liao, Y., Cao, G., Lipsitz, S.R., & McGee, D.L. (2003). Sex differences in risk for coronary heart disease mortality associated with diabetes and established coronary heart disease. *Archives of Internal Medicine, 163*(14), 1735-1740.

*National Cholesterol Education Program. (2002). *Third report of the Expert Panel on Detection, Evaluation, and Treatment of High Blood Cholesterol in Adults (Adult Treatment Panel III).* NIH Publication No. 02-5215. Bethesda: National Heart, Lung, and Blood Institute.

*National High Blood Pressure Education Program. (2003). *The seventh report of the Joint National Committee on Prevention, Detection, Evaluation, and Treatment of High Blood Pressure.* NIH Publication No. 03-5233. Bethesda: National Heart, Lung, and Blood Institute.

*New York Heart Association Criteria Committee. (1964). *Diseases of the heart and blood vessels: Nomenclature and criteria for diagnosis* (6th ed.). Boston: Little, Brown.

Ott, L.K. (2008). Assessing blood flow with CT angiography. *Nursing2008, 38*(1), 26.

Pagana, K.D., & Pagana, T.J. (2006). *Manual of diagnostic and laboratory tests* (3rd ed.). St. Louis: Mosby.

Pearson, T.L. (2007). Correlation of ankle-brachial index values with carotid disease, coronary disease, and cardiovascular risk factors in women. *Journal of Cardiovascular Nursing, 22*(6), 436-439.

Rosamond, W., Flegal, K., Furie, K., Go, A., Greenlund, K., Haase, N., et al. (2007). Heart disease and stroke statistics 2008 update: A report from the American Heart Association Statistics Committee and Stroke Statistics Committee. *Circulation, 117,* e-1-39. Retrieved January 13, 2008, from www.circulationaha.org.

*Siomko, A.J. (2000). Demystifying cardiac markers. *AJN, 100*(1), 36-41.

*Turner, M.A. (2000). Monitoring hemodynamics noninvasively. *Nursing2000, 30*(5), 32cc1-32cc8.

*Valli, G., & Giardina, E.G. (2002). Benefits, adverse effects and drug interactions of herbal therapies with cardiovascular effects. *Journal of American College of Cardiology, 39*(7), 1083-1095.

36

CHAPTER

Care of Patients with Dysrhythmias

Pamela C. Zickafoose

LEARNING OUTCOMES

For clinical competence and success on the NCLEX Examination, study this chapter with these Learning Outcomes in mind:

Safe and Effective Care Environment

1. Provide a safe environment for patients and staff when using a cardiac defibrillator.

Health Promotion and Maintenance

2. Teach patients and their families about drug therapy used for common dysrhythmias.
3. Educate patients and families about procedures and other interventions for common dysrhythmias.

Physiological Integrity

4. Identify typical physical assessment findings associated with common dysrhythmias.
5. Explain how to perform an electrocardiogram (ECG) test.
6. Analyze an ECG rhythm strip to identify normal sinus rhythm and common or life-threatening dysrhythmias.
7. Plan collaborative care for patients experiencing common dysrhythmias.
8. Explain the purpose and types of pacing used as interventions for patients with dysrhythmias.
9. Connect and maintain pacing devices.
10. Explain how to perform emergency care procedures, such as cardiopulmonary resuscitation (CPR) and automated external defibrillation.
11. Plan community-based care for a patient after pacemaker or implantable cardioverter/defibrillator insertion.

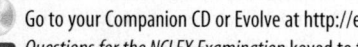

Go to your Companion CD or Evolve at http://evolve.elsevier.com/Iggy/ for *Self-Assessment Questions for the NCLEX Examination* keyed to these Learning Outcomes.

Cardiac dysrhythmias are abnormal rhythms of the heart's electrical system that can affect its ability to effectively pump *oxygenated* blood throughout the body. Some dysrhythmias are life threatening, and others are not. They are the result of disturbances of cardiac electrical impulse formation, conduction, or both. When the heart does not work effectively as a pump, *perfusion* to vital organs and peripheral tissues can be impaired, resulting in organ dysfunction or failure.

Many diseases, especially coronary artery disease (CAD), electrolyte imbalances, changes in oxygenation, and drug toxicity can cause abnormal heart rhythms. Dysrhythmias can occur in people of any age but occur most often in older adults. To provide collaborative patient-centered care using best practices, a *basic* understanding of cardiac electrophysiology, the conduction system of the heart, and the principles of electrocardiography is needed as a medical-surgical nurse. Specialty nurses and advanced practice nurses have a more in-depth knowledge as they manage patients with these cardiac problems in critical care areas.

REVIEW OF CARDIAC ELECTROPHYSIOLOGY

Electrophysiologic Properties

The electrophysiologic properties of cardiac cells regulate heart rate and rhythm. Specialized cardiac muscle cells possess unique properties: automaticity, excitability, conductivity, and contractility.

Automaticity (pacing function) is the ability of cardiac cells to generate an electrical impulse spontaneously and repetitively. Normally, only primary pacemaker cells (sinoatrial [SA] node, atrioventricular [AV] junction) possess the ability to generate an electrical impulse. Under certain conditions, such as myocardial ischemia (decreased blood flow), electrolyte imbalance, hypoxia, drug toxicity, and infarction (cell death), any cardiac cell may generate electrical impulses independently and create dysrhythmias. Disturbances in automaticity may involve either an increase or a decrease in pacing function.

Excitability is the ability of non-pacemaker heart cells to respond to an electrical impulse generated from pacemaker cells and to depolarize. **Depolarization** occurs when the normally negatively charged cells within the heart muscle develop a positive charge.

Conductivity is the ability to transmit an electrical stimulus from cell membrane to cell membrane. As a result, excitable cells depolarize in rapid succession from cell to cell until all cells have depolarized. *The wave of depolarization causes the deflections of the electrocardiogram (ECG) waveforms that are recognized as the P wave and the QRS complex.* Disturbances in conduction result when conduction is too rapid or too slow, when the pathway is totally blocked, or when the electrical impulse travels an abnormal pathway.

Contractility is the ability of atrial and ventricular muscle cells to shorten their fiber length in response to electrical stimulation, generating sufficient pressure to propel blood forward. *Contractility is the mechanical activity of the heart.*

ANIMATION: Conduction of Heart Impulses

Cardiac Conduction System

The cardiac conduction system consists of specialized cells (Fig. 36-1). It is responsible for the generation and conduction of electrical impulses that cause atrial and ventricular depolarization. The conduction system consists of the sinoatrial node, atrioventricular junctional area, and bundle branch system.

The conduction system begins with the **sinoatrial (SA) node** (also called the *sinus node*), located close to the surface of the right atrium near its junction with the superior vena cava. *The SA node is the heart's primary pacemaker.* It can spontaneously and rhythmically generate electrical impulses at a rate of 60 to 100 beats per minute and therefore has the greatest degree of automaticity.

The SA node is richly supplied by the sympathetic and parasympathetic nervous systems, which increase and decrease the rate of discharge of the sinus node, respectively. This process results in changes in the heart rate.

Impulses from the sinus node move directly through atrial muscle and lead to atrial depolarization, which is *reflected in a P wave on the ECG*. Atrial muscle contraction should follow. Within the atrial muscle are slow and fast conduction pathways leading to the atrioventricular (AV) node.

The **atrioventricular (AV) junctional** area consists of a transitional cell zone, the AV node itself, and the bundle of His. The AV node lies just beneath the right atrial endocardium, between the tricuspid valve and the ostium of the coronary sinus. Here T-cells (transitional cells) cause impulses to slow down or to be delayed in the AV node before proceeding to the ventricles. This delay is *reflected in the PR segment on the ECG*. This slow conduction provides a short delay, allowing the atria to contract and the ventricles to fill. The contraction is known as "atrial kick" and contributes additional blood volume for a greater cardiac output. The AV node is also controlled by both the sympathetic and the parasympathetic nervous systems. The bundle of His connects with the distal portion of the AV node and continues through the interventricular septum.

The *bundle of His* extends as a right bundle branch down the right side of the interventricular septum to the apex of the right ventricle. On the left side, it extends as a left bundle branch, which further divides.

At the ends of both the right and the left bundle branch systems are the Purkinje fibers. These fibers are an interweaving network located on the endocardial surface of both ventricles, from apex to base. The fibers then partially penetrate into the myocardium. **Purkinje cells** make up the bundle of His, bundle branches, and terminal Purkinje fibers. These cells are responsible for the rapid conduction of electrical impulses throughout the ventricles, leading to ventricular depolarization and the subsequent ventricular muscle contraction. A few nodal cells in the ventricles also occasionally demonstrate automaticity, giving rise to ventricular beats or rhythms.

ELECTROCARDIOGRAPHY

ANIMATION: Events Represented by the ECG

The **electrocardiogram (ECG)** provides a graphic representation, or picture, of cardiac electrical activity. The cardiac electrical currents are transmitted to the body surface. Electrodes, consisting of a conductive gel on an adhesive pad, are placed on specific sites on the body and attached to cables connected to an ECG machine or to a monitor. The cardiac electrical current is transmitted via the electrodes and through the lead

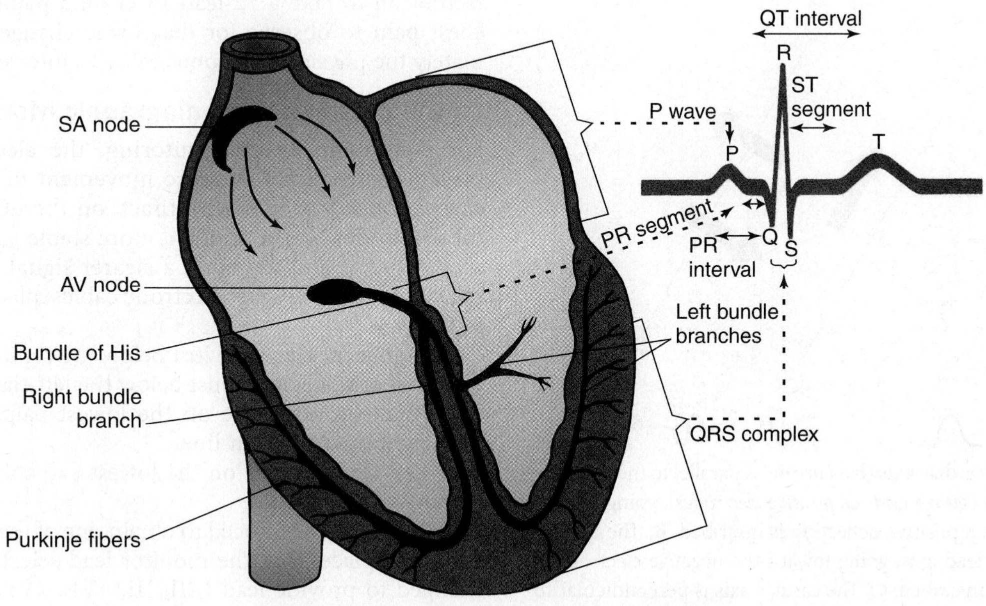

QT interval
R
ST
segment
P wave
P
T
SA node
PR segment
PR
Q
S
interval
AV node
Left bundle
branches
Bundle of His
Right bundle
branch
QRS complex
Purkinje fibers

Fig. 36-1 • The cardiac conduction system.

wires to the machine or monitor, which displays the cardiac electrical activity.

A lead provides one view of the heart's electrical activity. Multiple leads, or views, can be obtained. Electrode placement is the same for male and female patients.

Lead systems are made up of a positive pole and a negative pole. An imaginary line joining these two poles is called the **lead axis.** The direction of electrical current flow in the heart is the **cardiac axis.** The relationship between the cardiac axis and the lead axis is responsible for the deflections seen on the ECG pattern:

- The baseline is the **isoelectric** line. It occurs when there is no current flow in the heart after complete depolarization and also after complete repolarization. Positive deflections occur above this line, and negative deflections occur below it. Deflections represent depolarization and repolarization of cells.
- If the direction of electrical current flow in the heart (cardiac axis) is toward the positive pole, a **positive deflection** (above the baseline) is viewed (Fig. 36-2, *A*).
- If the direction of electrical current flow in the heart (cardiac axis) is moving away from the positive pole toward the negative pole, a **negative deflection** (below the baseline) is viewed (Fig. 36-2, *B*).
- If the cardiac axis is moving neither toward nor away from the positive pole, a biphasic complex (both above and below baseline) will result (Fig. 36-2, *C*).

Lead Systems

The standard 12-lead ECG consists of 12 leads (or views) of the heart's electrical activity. Six of the leads are called *limb leads* because the electrodes are placed on the four limbs in the frontal plane. The remaining six leads are called *chest (precordial) leads* because the electrodes are placed on the chest in the horizontal plane.

Standard bipolar *limb leads* consist of three leads (I, II, and III) that each measures the electrical activity between two points and a fourth lead (right leg) that acts as a ground electrode. Of the three measuring leads, the right arm is always negative, the left leg is always positive, and the left arm can be either positive or negative.

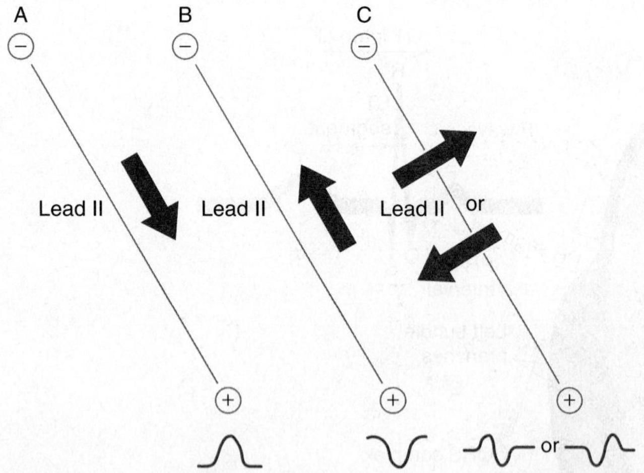
A
B
C
Lead II
Lead II
Lead II
or
or

Fig. 36-2 • **A,** The cardiac axis *(bold arrow)* is parallel to the lead axis *(the line between the negative and the positive electrodes),* going toward the positive electrode; a positive deflection is inscribed. **B,** The cardiac axis is parallel to the lead axis, going toward the negative electrode; a negative deflection is inscribed. **C,** The cardiac axis is perpendicular to the lead axis, going neither toward the positive electrode nor toward the negative electrode; a biphasic deflection is inscribed.

Other lead systems include the 18-lead ECG, which adds six leads placed on the horizontal plane on the right side of the chest to view the right side of the heart. This is sometimes referred to as a "right-sided ECG." The extra leads are sometimes placed on the back.

Unipolar limb leads consist of a positive electrode only. The unipolar limb leads are aVR, aVL, and aVF, with *a* meaning augmented. *V* is a designation for a unipolar lead. The third letter denotes the positive electrode placement: *R* for right arm, *L* for left arm, and *F* for foot (left leg). The positive electrode is at one end of the lead axis. The other end is the center of the electrical field, at about the center of the heart (Table 36-1).

There are six unipolar (or V) *chest leads,* determined by the placement of the chest electrode. The four limb electrodes are placed on the extremities, as designated on each electrode (right arm, left arm, right leg, and left leg). The fifth (chest) electrode on a monitor system is the positive, or exploring, electrode and is placed in one of six designated positions to obtain the desired chest lead. With a 12-lead ECG, four leads are placed on the limbs and six are placed on the chest, eliminating the need to move any electrodes about the chest.

Positioning of the electrodes is crucial in obtaining an accurate ECG. Comparisons of ECGs taken at different times will be valid only when electrode placement is accurate and identical at each test. Positioning is particularly important when working with patients with chest deformities or large breasts. Patients may be asked to move the breasts to ensure proper electrode placement.

While obtaining a 12-lead ECG, remind the patient to be as still as possible in a semi-reclined position, breathing normally. Any repetitive movement will cause artifact and could lead to inaccurate interpretation of the ECG.

Nurses are sometimes responsible for obtaining 12-lead ECGs, but more commonly, technicians are trained to perform this skill. Remind the technician to notify the nurse or physician of any suspected abnormality. A nurse may direct a technician to take a 12-lead ECG on a patient experiencing chest pain to observe for diagnostic changes, but it is ultimately the physician's responsibility to interpret the ECG.

Continuous Electrocardiographic Monitoring

For continuous ECG monitoring, the electrodes are not placed on the limbs because movement of the extremities causes "noise," or motion artifact, on the ECG signal. Place the electrodes on the trunk, a more stable area, to minimize such artifacts and to obtain a clearer signal. If the monitoring system provides five electrode cables, place the electrodes as follows:

- Right arm electrode just below the right clavicle
- Left arm electrode just below the left clavicle
- Right leg electrode on the lowest palpable rib, on the right midclavicular line
- Left leg electrode on the lowest palpable rib, on the left midclavicular line
- Fifth electrode placed to obtain one of the six chest leads

With this placement, the monitor lead select control may be changed to provide lead I, II, III, aVR, aVL, or aVF or one chest lead. The monitor automatically alters the polarity of the electrodes to provide the lead selected.

TABLE 36-1 **Electrode Placement for 12 Leads**

Lead	Negative Electrode	Positive Electrode	Ground Electrode
I	Right arm or under the right clavicle	Left arm or under the left clavicle	Right leg or lowest rib, left midclavicular line
II	Right arm or under the right clavicle	Left leg or lowest rib, left midclavicular line	Right leg or under the left clavicle
III	Left arm or under the left clavicle	Left leg or lowest rib, left midclavicular line	Right leg or under the right clavicle
aVR	Average potential of left arm (or under the left clavicle) and left leg (or lowest rib, left midclavicular line)	Right arm or under the right clavicle	Right leg or lowest rib, right midclavicular line
aVL	Average potential of right arm (or under the right clavicle) and left leg (or lowest rib, left midclavicular line)	Left arm or under the left clavicle	Same as for aVR
aVF	Average potential of right arm (or under the right clavicle) and left arm (or under the left clavicle)	Left leg or lowest rib, left midclavicular line	Same as for aVR
V_1	Average potential of right arm, left arm, and left leg	Fourth intercostal space (ICS), right sternal border	Same as for aVR
V_2	Same as for V_1	Fourth ICS, left sternal border	Same as for aVR
V_3	Same as for V_1	Midway between V_2 and V_4	Same as for aVR
V_4	Same as for V_1	Fifth ICS, left midclavicular line	Same as for aVR
V_5	Same as for V_1	Horizontal to V_4, left anterior axillary line	Same as for aVR
V_6	Same as for V_1	Horizontal to V_4, left midaxillary line	Same as for aVR

The clarity of continuous ECG monitor recordings is affected by skin preparation and electrode quality. To ensure the best signal transmission and to decrease skin impedance, clean the skin and shave the area if needed. Make sure the area for electrode placement is dry. The gel on each electrode must be moist and fresh. Attach the electrode to the lead cable and then to the contact site. The contact site should be free of any lotion, tincture, or other substance that increases skin impedance. Electrodes cannot be placed on irritated skin or over scar tissue. The application of electrodes may be done by unlicensed assistive personnel (UAP), but the nurse must determine which lead to select and check for correct electrode placement. Assess the quality of the ECG rhythm transmission to the monitoring system.

The ECG cables can be attached directly to a wall-mounted monitor (a hard-wired system) if the patient's activity is restricted to bedrest and sitting in a chair, as in a critical care unit. For an ambulatory patient, the ECG cable is attached to a battery-operated transmitter (a **telemetry** system) held in a pouch. The ECG is transmitted via antennae located in strategic places, usually in the ceiling, to a remote monitor. Telemetry allows freedom of movement within a certain area without losing transmission of the ECG.

Some acute care facilities have monitor technicians (monitor "techs") who are educated in ECG rhythm interpretation and are responsible for:

- Watching a bank of monitors on a unit
- Printing ECG rhythm strips routinely and as needed
- Interpreting rhythms
- Reporting the patient's rhythm and significant changes to the nurse

The technical support is particularly helpful on a telemetry unit that does not have monitors at the bedside. *The nurse remains ultimately responsible for accurate ECG rhythm interpretation, as well as for patient assessment and management.*

Some units have full-disclosure monitors, which continuously store ECG rhythms in memory up to a certain amount of time, allowing nurses and health care providers to access and print them for more thorough patient assessment and management. Routine strips, as well as any changes in rhythm, are printed and documented in the patient's record.

The health care provider is responsible for determining when monitoring can be suspended, such as during showering. He or she also determines whether monitoring is needed during off-unit testing procedures and for transportation to other facilities.

Prehospital personnel, such as paramedics and emergency medical technicians (EMTs) with advanced training, frequently monitor ECG rhythms at the scene and on the way to a health care facility. They function under medical direction and protocols but may also be communicating with a nurse in the emergency department.

The ECG strip is printed on graph paper (Fig. 36-3), with each small block measuring 1 mm in height and width. ECG recorders and monitors are standardized at a speed of 25 mm/sec. Time is measured on the horizontal axis. At this speed, each small block represents 0.04 second. Five small blocks make up one large block, defined by darker bold lines and representing 0.20 second. Five large blocks represent 1 second, and 30 large blocks represent 6 seconds. Vertical lines in the top margin of the graph paper are usually 15 large blocks apart, representing 3-second segments (Fig. 36-4).

Electrocardiographic Complexes, Segments, and Intervals

Complexes that make up a normal ECG consist of a P wave, a QRS complex, a T wave, and possibly a U wave. Segments include the PR segment, the ST segment, and the TP segment.

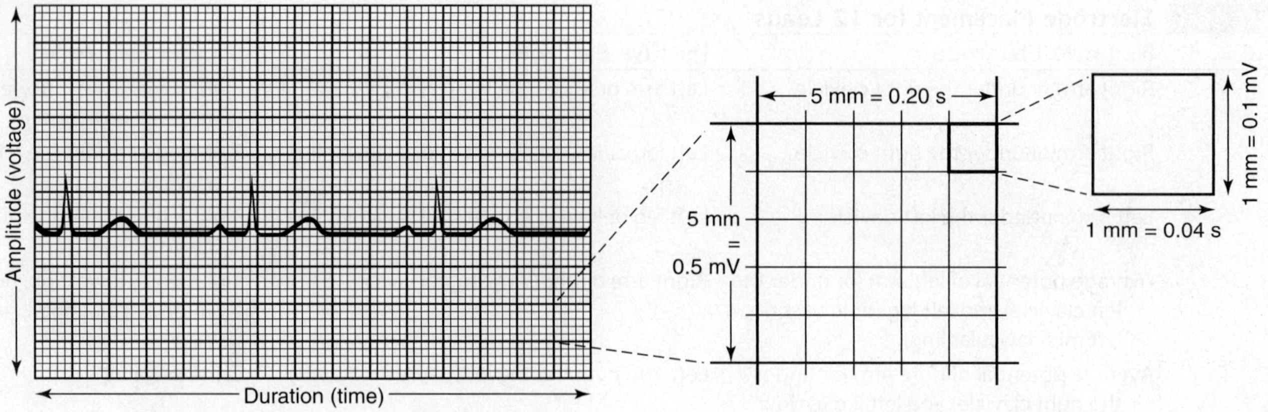
Amplitude (voltage)
Duration (time)
5 mm = 0.20 s
5 mm
=
0.5 mV
1 mm = 0.04 s
1 mm = 0.1 mV

Fig. 36-3 • Electrocardiographic waveforms are measured in amplitude (voltage) and duration (time).

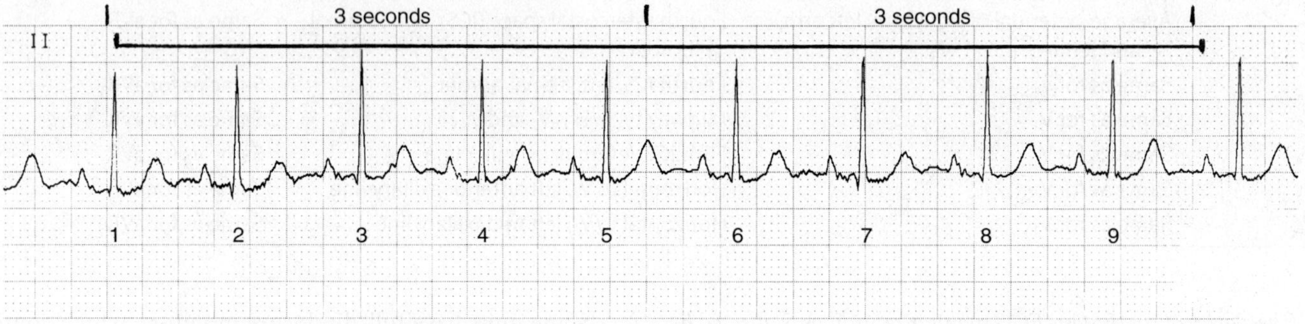
3 seconds
3 seconds
II
1
2
3
4
5
6
7
8
9

Fig. 36-4 • Each segment between the dark lines *(above the monitor strip)* represents 3 seconds when the monitor is set at a speed of 25 mm/sec. To estimate the ventricular rate, count the QRS complexes in a 6-second strip and then multiply that number by 10 to estimate the rate for 1 minute. In this example, there are 9 QRS complexes in 6 seconds. Therefore the heart rate can be estimated to be 90 beats/min.

Intervals include the PR interval, the QRS duration, and the QT interval (Fig. 36-5).

The **P wave** is a deflection representing atrial depolarization. The shape of the P wave may be a positive, negative, or biphasic (both positive and negative) deflection, depending on the lead selected. When the electrical impulse is consistently generated from the sinoatrial (SA) node, the P waves have a consistent shape in a given lead. If an impulse is then generated from a different (ectopic) focus, such as atrial tissue, the shape of the P wave changes in that lead, indicating that an ectopic focus has fired.

The **PR segment** is the isoelectric line from the end of the P wave to the beginning of the QRS complex, when the electrical impulse is traveling through the atrioventricular (AV) node, where it is delayed. It then travels through the ventricular conduction system to the Purkinje fibers.

The **PR interval** is measured from the beginning of the P wave to the end of the PR segment. It represents the time required for atrial depolarization as well as the impulse delay in the AV node and the travel time to the Purkinje fibers. It normally measures from 0.12 to 0.20 second (five small blocks).

The **QRS complex** represents ventricular depolarization. The shape of the QRS complex depends on the lead selected. The Q wave is the first negative deflection and is not present in all leads. When present, it is small and represents initial ventricular septal depolarization. When the Q wave is abnormally present in a lead, it represents myocardial necrosis (cell death). The R wave is the first positive deflection. It may be small, large, or absent, depending on the lead. The S wave is a negative deflection following the R wave and is not present in all leads.

The **QRS duration** represents the time required for depolarization of both ventricles. It is measured from the beginning of the QRS complex to the J point (the junction where the QRS complex ends and the ST segment begins). It normally measures from 0.04 to 0.10 second (up to three small blocks).

The **ST segment** is normally an isoelectric line and represents early ventricular repolarization. It occurs from the J point to the beginning of the T wave. Its length varies with changes in the heart rate, the administration of medications, and electrolyte disturbances. It is normally not elevated more than 1 mm or depressed more than 0.5 mm from the isoelectric line. Its amplitude is measured at a point 1.5 to 2 mm after the J point. ST elevation or depression can be caused by myocardial injury, ischemia or infarction, conduction abnormalities, or the administration of medications.

The **T wave** follows the ST segment and represents ventricular repolarization. It is usually positive, rounded, and slightly asymmetric. If an ectopic stimulus excites the ventricles during this time, it may cause ventricular irritability, lethal dysrhythmias, and possible cardiac arrest in the vulnera-

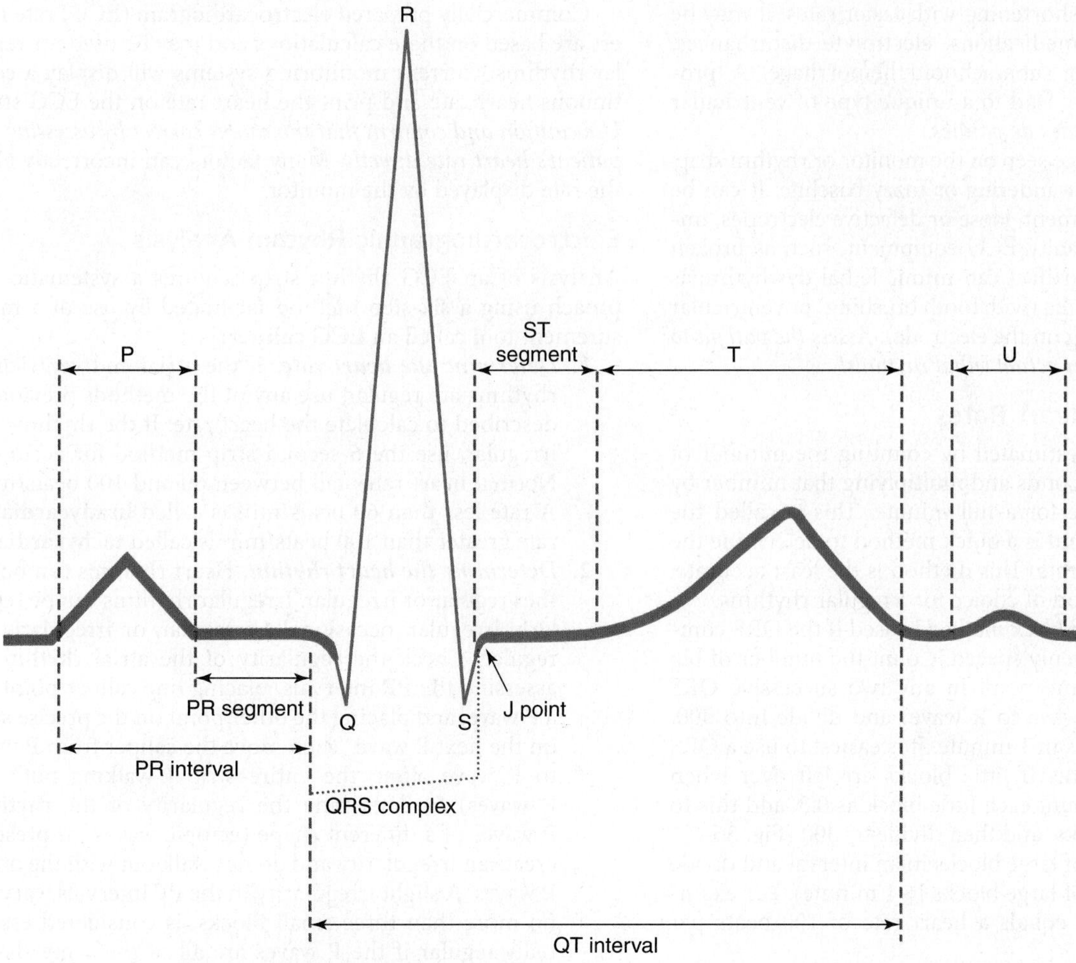
R
P
ST
segment
T
U
PR segment
Q
S
J point
PR interval
QRS complex
QT interval

P wave:	Represents atrial depolarization.
PR segment:	Represents the time required for the impulse to travel through the AV node, where it is delayed, and through the bundle of His, bundle branches, and Purkinje fiber network, just before ventricular depolarization.
PR interval:	Represents the time required for atrial depolarization as well as impulse travel through the conduction system and Purkinje fiber network, inclusive of the P wave and PR segment. It is measured from the beginning of the P wave to the end of the PR segment.
QRS complex:	Represents ventricular depolarization and is measured from the beginning of the Q (or R) wave to the end of the S wave.
J point:	Represents the junction where the QRS complex ends and the ST segment begins.
ST segment:	Represents early ventricular repolarization.
T wave:	Represents ventricular repolarization.
U wave:	Represents late ventricular repolarization.
QT interval:	Represents the total time required for ventricular depolarization and repolarization and is measured from the beginning of the QRS complex to the end of the T wave.

Fig. 36-5 • The components of a normal electrocardiogram.

ble heart. This is known as the *R-on-T phenomenon.* T waves may become tall and peaked, inverted (negative), or flat as a result of myocardial ischemia, potassium or calcium imbalances, medications, or autonomic nervous system effects.

The **U wave,** when present, follows the T wave and may result from slow repolarization of ventricular Purkinje fibers. It is of the same polarity as the T wave, although generally it is smaller. It is not normally seen in all leads and is more common in lead V_3. An abnormal U wave may suggest an electrolyte abnormality (particularly hypokalemia) or other disturbance. Correct identification is important so that it is not mistaken for a P wave. If in doubt, notify the health care provider and request that a potassium level be obtained.

The **QT interval** represents the total time required for ventricular depolarization and repolarization. The QT interval is measured from the beginning of the QRS complex to the end of the T wave. This interval varies with the patient's age and gender and changes with the heart rate, lengthening with slower heart rates and shortening with faster rates. It may be prolonged by certain medications, electrolyte disturbances, Prinzmetal's angina, or subarachnoid hemorrhage. A prolonged QT interval may lead to a unique type of ventricular tachycardia called *torsades de pointes.*

Artifact is interference seen on the monitor or rhythm strip, which may look like a wandering or fuzzy baseline. It can be caused by patient movement, loose or defective electrodes, improper grounding, or faulty ECG equipment, such as broken wires or cables. Some artifact can mimic lethal dysrhythmias like ventricular tachycardia (with tooth brushing) or ventricular fibrillation (with tapping on the electrode). *Assess the patient to differentiate artifact from actual lethal rhythms!*

Determination of Heart Rate

The heart rate can be estimated by counting the number of QRS complexes in 6 seconds and multiplying that number by 10 to calculate the rate for a full minute. This is called the *6-second strip method* and is a quick method to determine the mean or average heart rate. This method is the least accurate; however, it is the method of choice for irregular rhythms.

For accuracy, the *big block method* is used if the QRS complexes are regular or evenly spaced. Count the number of big blocks between the same point in any two successive QRS complexes (usually R wave to R wave) and divide into 300. There are 300 big blocks in 1 minute. It is easiest to use a QRS that falls on a dark line. If little blocks are left over when counting big blocks, count each little block as 0.2, add this to the number of big blocks, and then divide by 300 (Fig. 36-6).

Count the number of large blocks in an interval and divide into 300 (the number of large blocks in 1 minute). For example, three large blocks equals a heart rate of 100 beats per minute (300/3 = 100).

Another method (called the *memory method*) relies on memorizing this sequence: 300, 150, 100, 75, 60, 50, 43, 37, 33, 30. This is the big block method with the math already done. Find a QRS complex that falls on the dark line representing 0.2 second or a big block, and count backwards to the next QRS complex. Each dark line is a memorized number. This is the method most widely used in hospitals for calculating heart rates for regular rhythms.

Commercially prepared electrocardiogram (ECG) rate rulers are based on these calculations and may be used for regular rhythms. Current monitoring systems will display a continuous heart rate and print the heart rate on the ECG strip. *Use caution and confirm that the rate is correct by assessing the patient's heart rate directly.* Many factors can incorrectly alter the rate displayed by the monitor.

Electrocardiographic Rhythm Analysis

Analysis of an ECG rhythm strip requires a systematic approach using a six-step method facilitated by use of a measurement tool called an **ECG caliper:**

1. ***Determine the heart rate.*** If the atrial and ventricular rhythms are regular, use any of the methods previously described to calculate the heart rate. If the rhythms are irregular, use the 6-second strip method for accuracy. Normal heart rates fall between 60 and 100 beats/min. A rate less than 60 beats/min is called **bradycardia.** A rate greater than 100 beats/min is called **tachycardia.**
2. ***Determine the heart rhythm.*** Heart rhythms can be either regular or irregular. Irregular rhythms can be regularly irregular, occasionally irregular, or irregularly irregular. Check the regularity of the atrial rhythm by assessing the PP intervals, placing one caliper point on a P wave, and placing the other point on the precise spot on the next P wave. Then move the caliper from P wave to P wave along the entire strip ("walking out" the P waves) to determine the regularity of the rhythm. P waves of a different shape (ectopic waves), if present, create an irregularity and do not walk out with the other P waves. A slight irregularity in the PP intervals, varying no more than three small blocks, is considered essentially regular if the P waves are all of the same shape. This alteration is caused by changes in intrathoracic pressure during the respiratory cycle.

   Check the regularity of the ventricular rhythm by assessing the RR intervals, placing one caliper point on a portion of the QRS complex (usually the most prominent portion of the deflection) and the other point on the precise spot of the next QRS complex. Move the caliper from QRS complex to QRS complex along the entire strip

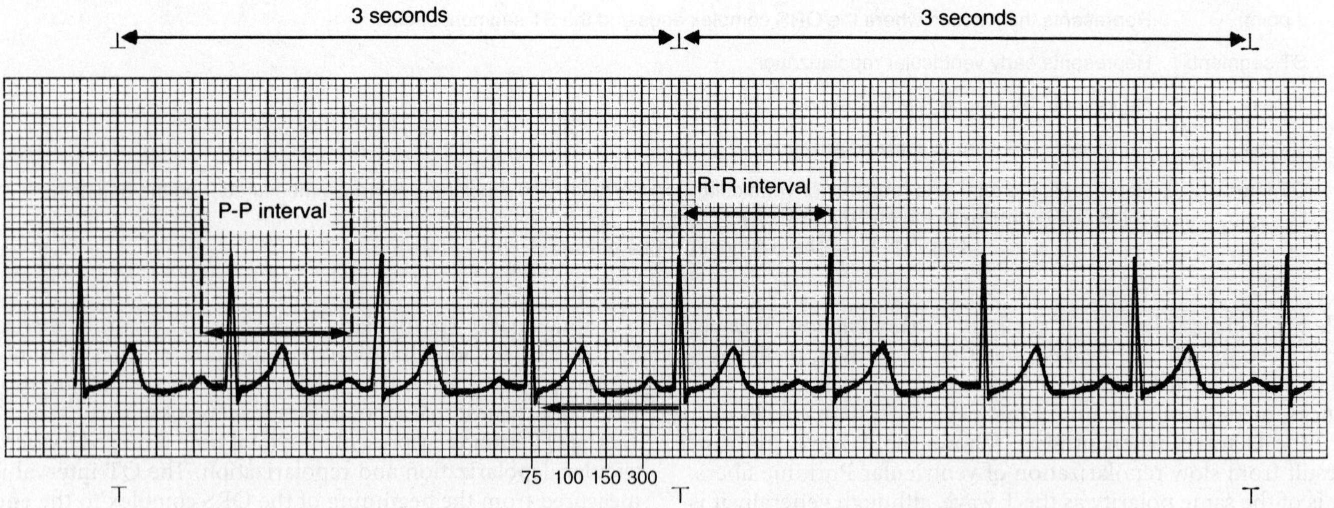
3 seconds
3 seconds
R-R interval
P-P interval
75 100 150 300

Fig. 36-6 • In this example, the heart rate using the big block method is 300 ÷ 4 big blocks (between QRS complexes), or 75 beats/min. The memory method is also demonstrated with a heart rate of 75 beats/min.

(walking out the QRS complexes) to determine the regularity of the rhythm. QRS complexes of a different shape (ectopic QRS complexes), if present, create an irregularity and do not walk out with the other QRS complexes. A slight irregularity of no more than three small blocks between intervals is considered essentially regular if the QRS complexes are all of the same shape.

3. ***Analyze the P waves.*** Check that the P wave shape is consistent throughout the strip, indicating that atrial depolarization is occurring from impulses originating from one focus, normally the SA node. Determine whether there is one P wave occurring before each QRS complex, establishing that a relationship exists between the P wave and the QRS complex. This relationship indicates that an impulse from one focus is responsible for both atrial and ventricular depolarization. The nurse may observe more than one P wave shape, more P waves than QRS complexes, absent P waves, or P waves coming after the QRS, each indicating that a dysrhythmia exists. Ask these five questions when analyzing P waves:
   - Are P waves present?
   - Are the P waves occurring regularly?
   - Is there one P wave for each QRS complex?
   - Are the P waves smooth, rounded, and upright in appearance, or are they inverted?
   - Do all the P waves look similar?
4. ***Measure the PR interval.*** Place one caliper point at the beginning of the P wave and the other point at the end of the PR segment. The PR interval normally measures between 0.12 and 0.20 second. The measurement should be constant throughout the strip. The PR interval cannot be determined if there are no P waves or if P waves occur after the QRS complex. Ask these three questions about the PR interval:
   - Are PR intervals greater than 0.20 second?
   - Are PR intervals less than 0.12 second?
   - Are PR intervals constant across the ECG strip?
5. ***Measure the QRS duration.*** Place one caliper point at the beginning of the QRS complex and the other at the J point, where the QRS complex ends and the ST segment begins. The QRS duration normally measures between 0.04 and 0.10 second. The measurement should be constant throughout the entire strip. Check that the QRS complexes are consistent throughout the strip. When the QRS is narrow (0.10 second or less), this indicates that the impulse was not formed in the ventricles and is referred to as *supraventricular* or *above the ventricles.* When the QRS complex is wide (greater than 0.10 second), this indicates that the impulse is either of ventricular origin or of supraventricular origin with aberrant conduction, meaning deviating from the normal course or pattern. More than one QRS complex pattern or occasionally missing QRS complexes may be observed, indicating a dysrhythmia.

   Ask these questions to evaluate QRS intervals:
   - Are QRS intervals less than or greater than 0.12 second?
   - Are the QRS complexes similar in appearance across the ECG paper?
6. ***Interpret the rhythm.*** Using steps 1 to 5, you can interpret the cardiac rhythm and differentiate normal and abnormal cardiac rhythms.

NORMAL RHYTHMS

Normal sinus rhythm (NSR) is the rhythm originating from the sinoatrial (SA) node (dominant pacemaker) that meets these ECG criteria (Fig. 36-7):

- *Rate:* Atrial and ventricular rates of 60 to 100 beats/min
- *Rhythm:* Atrial and ventricular rhythms regular
- *P waves:* Present, consistent configuration, one P wave before each QRS complex
- *PR interval:* 0.12 to 0.20 second and constant
- *QRS duration:* 0.04 to 0.10 second and constant

Sinus arrhythmia is a variant of NSR. It results from changes in intrathoracic pressure during breathing. In this context, the term *arrhythmia* does not mean an absence of rhythm, as the term suggests. Instead, the heart rate increases slightly during inspiration and decreases slightly during exhalation. This irregular rhythm is frequently observed in healthy children as well as adults.

Sinus arrhythmia has all the characteristics of NSR except for its irregularity. The PP and RR intervals vary, with the difference between the shortest and the longest intervals being greater than 0.12 second (three small blocks):

- *Rate:* Atrial and ventricular rates are between 60 and 100 beats/min.
- *Rhythm:* Atrial and ventricular rhythms are irregular, with the shortest PP or RR interval varying at least 0.12 second from the longest PP or RR interval.

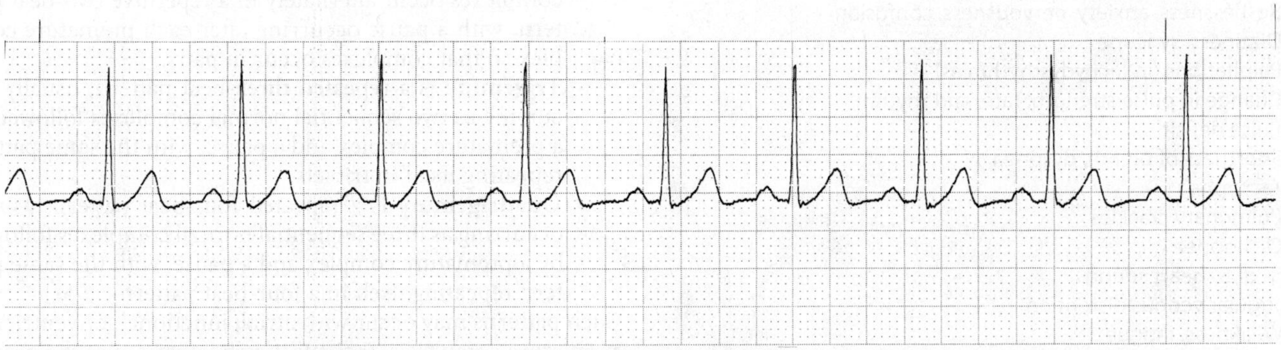

Fig. 36-7 • Normal sinus rhythm. Both atrial and ventricular rhythms are essentially regular (a slight variation in rhythm is normal). Atrial and ventricular rates are both 83 beats/min. There is one P wave before each QRS complex, and all the P waves are of a consistent morphology, or shape. The PR interval measures 0.18 second and is constant; the QRS complex measures 0.06 second and is constant.

- *P waves:* One P wave before each QRS complex; consistent configuration.
- *PR interval:* Normal, constant.
- *QRS duration:* Normal, constant.

Sinus arrhythmias occasionally are due to nonrespiratory causes, such as digitalis or morphine. These drugs enhance vagal tone and cause decreased heart rate and irregularity unrelated to the respiratory cycle.

DYSRHYTHMIAS

Overview

Any disorder of the heartbeat is called a **dysrhythmia.** Historically, the term *arrhythmia* has been used in the literature. Although the terms are often used interchangeably, *dysrhythmia* is more accurate.

Dysrhythmias result from:

- A disturbance in the relationship between electrical conductivity and the mechanical response of the myocardium
- A disturbance in impulse formation (either from an abnormal rate or from an ectopic focus)
- A disturbance in impulse conduction (delays and blocks)
- The combination of several mechanisms

Although many dysrhythmias have no clinical manifestations, many others have serious consequences if not treated. A summary of key features is found in Chart 36-1.

Dysrhythmia Terminology

Tachydysrhythmias are heart rates greater than 100 beats per minute. They are a major concern in the adult patient with coronary artery disease (CAD). Coronary artery blood flow occurs mostly during diastole when the aortic valve is closed and is determined by diastolic time and blood pressure in the root of the aorta. Tachydysrhythmias are serious because they:

- Shorten the diastolic time and therefore the coronary perfusion time (the amount of time available for blood to flow through the coronary arteries to the myocardium).
- Initially increase cardiac output and blood pressure. However, a continued rise in heart rate decreases the ventricular filling time because of a shortened diastole, decreasing the stroke volume. Consequently, cardiac output and blood pressure will begin to decrease, reducing aortic pressure and therefore coronary perfusion pressure.
- Increase the work of the heart, increasing myocardial oxygen demand.

The patient with a tachydysrhythmia may have:

- Palpitations
- Chest discomfort (pressure or pain from myocardial ischemia or infarction)
- Restlessness and anxiety
- Pale, cool skin
- Syncope ("blackout") from hypotension

Tachydysrhythmias may also lead to heart failure. Presenting symptoms of heart failure may include dyspnea, lung crackles, distended neck veins, fatigue, and weakness (see Chapter 37).

Bradydysrhythmias occur when the heart rate is less than 60 beats per minute. These rhythms can also be significant because:

- Myocardial oxygen demand is reduced from the slow heart rate, which can be beneficial.
- Coronary perfusion time may be adequate because of a prolonged diastole, which is desirable.
- Coronary perfusion pressure may decrease if the heart rate is too slow to provide adequate cardiac output and blood pressure; this is a serious consequence.

Therefore the patient may tolerate the bradydysrhythmia well if the blood pressure is adequate. If the blood pressure is not adequate, symptomatic bradydysrhythmias may lead to myocardial ischemia or infarction, dysrhythmias, hypotension, and heart failure.

Premature complexes are early rhythm complexes. They occur when a cardiac cell or cell group, other than the sinoatrial (SA) node, becomes irritable and fires an impulse before the next sinus impulse is produced. The abnormal focus is called an *ectopic focus* and may be generated by atrial, junctional, or ventricular tissue. After the premature complex, there is a pause before the next normal complex, creating an irregularity in the rhythm. The patient with premature complexes may be unaware of them or may feel **palpitations** or a "skipping" of the heartbeat. If premature complexes, especially those that are ventricular, become more frequent, the patient may experience symptoms of decreased cardiac output.

Premature complexes may occur *repetitively in a rhythmic fashion:*

- **Bigeminy** exists when normal complexes and premature complexes occur alternately in a repetitive two-beat pattern, with a pause occurring after each premature complex so that complexes occur in pairs.
- **Trigeminy** is a repeated three-beat pattern, usually occurring as two sequential normal complexes followed by a premature complex and a pause, with the same pattern repeating itself in triplets.
- **Quadrigeminy** is a repeated four-beat pattern, usually occurring as three sequential normal complexes followed by a premature complex and a pause, with the same pattern repeating itself in a four-beat pattern.

Such patterns may occur with atrial, junctional, or ventricular premature complexes. Patients may be unaware of the premature beats, or they may feel palpitations.

Escape complexes or *escape rhythms* may occur when the SA node fails to discharge or is blocked or when a sinus impulse fails to depolarize the ventricles because of an atrioventricular (AV) nodal block. Escape complexes or rhythms serve as a secondary

Chart 36-1 KEY FEATURES

Sustained Tachydysrhythmias and Bradydysrhythmias

- Chest discomfort, pressure, or pain, which may radiate to the jaw, the back, or the arm
- Restlessness, anxiety, nervousness, confusion
- Dizziness, syncope
- Palpitations (in tachydysrhythmias)
- Change in pulse strength, rate, and rhythm
- Pulse deficit
- Shortness of breath, dyspnea
- Tachypnea
- Pulmonary crackles
- Orthopnea
- S_3 or S_4 heart sounds
- Jugular venous distention
- Weakness, fatigue
- Pale, cool, skin; diaphoresis
- Nausea, vomiting
- Decreased urine output
- Delayed capillary refill
- Hypotension

or escape pacemaker and are seen after a pause. Such impulses may originate from AV junctional or ventricular tissue. They stop when the SA node or the AV node can function normally. If there are pauses followed by escape beats or rhythms, patients may feel light-headed, dizzy, or faint during the pause.

Classification of Dysrhythmias

Dysrhythmias are classified according to their site of origin. The sites include the SA node, atrial tissue, AV node, junctional tissue, and ventricular tissue. Dysrhythmias may be caused by a disturbance in impulse formation or by conduction delays or blocks. The incidence and the prevalence of dysrhythmias are not known because they usually result from an underlying condition, such as heart disease. *The incidence increases with age.*

Sinus Dysrhythmias

The sinus node is the **pacemaker** in all sinus dysrhythmias. Innervation from sympathetic and parasympathetic nerves is normally in balance to ensure a normal sinus rhythm (NSR). An imbalance increases or decreases the rate of SA node discharge either as a normal response to activity or physiologic changes or as a pathologic response to disease.

Sinus Tachycardia. Sympathetic nervous system stimulation or vagal inhibition results in an increased rate of SA node discharge, which increases the heart rate. When the rate of SA node discharge is more than 100 beats per minute, the rhythm is called *sinus tachycardia* (Fig. 36-8, *A*). Sinus tachycardia, with temporary heart rates of 200 to 220 beats per minute, may be normal in infants and children. The rate gradually decreases until age 10 years. From age 10 years to adulthood, the heart rate normally does not exceed 100 beats per minute except in response to activity and then usually does not exceed 160 beats per minute. Rarely does the heart rate reach 180 beats per minute.

Sinus tachycardia initially increases cardiac output and blood pressure. However, continued increases in heart rate decrease coronary perfusion time, diastolic filling time, and coronary perfusion pressure while increasing myocardial oxygen demand.

Increased sympathetic stimulation is a normal response to physical activity but may also be caused by anxiety, pain, stress, fear, fever, anemia, hypoxemia, hyperthyroidism, and pulmonary embolism. Drugs such as catecholamines, atropine, caffeine, alcohol, nicotine, aminophylline, and thyroid medications may also increase the heart rate. In some cases, sinus tachycardia is a compensatory response to decreased cardiac output or blood pressure, as occurs in hypovolemic shock, myocardial infarction (MI), infection, and heart failure.

The patient may be asymptomatic except for an increased pulse rate. However, if the rhythm is not well tolerated, he or she may have symptoms. Assess for fatigue, weakness, shortness of breath, orthopnea, neck vein distention, decreased oxygen saturation, and decreased blood pressure. Also assess for restlessness and anxiety from decreased cerebral perfusion and for decreased urine output from impaired renal perfusion. The patient may also have anginal pain and palpitations. The ECG pattern may show T-wave inversion or ST-segment elevation or depression in response to myocardial ischemia.

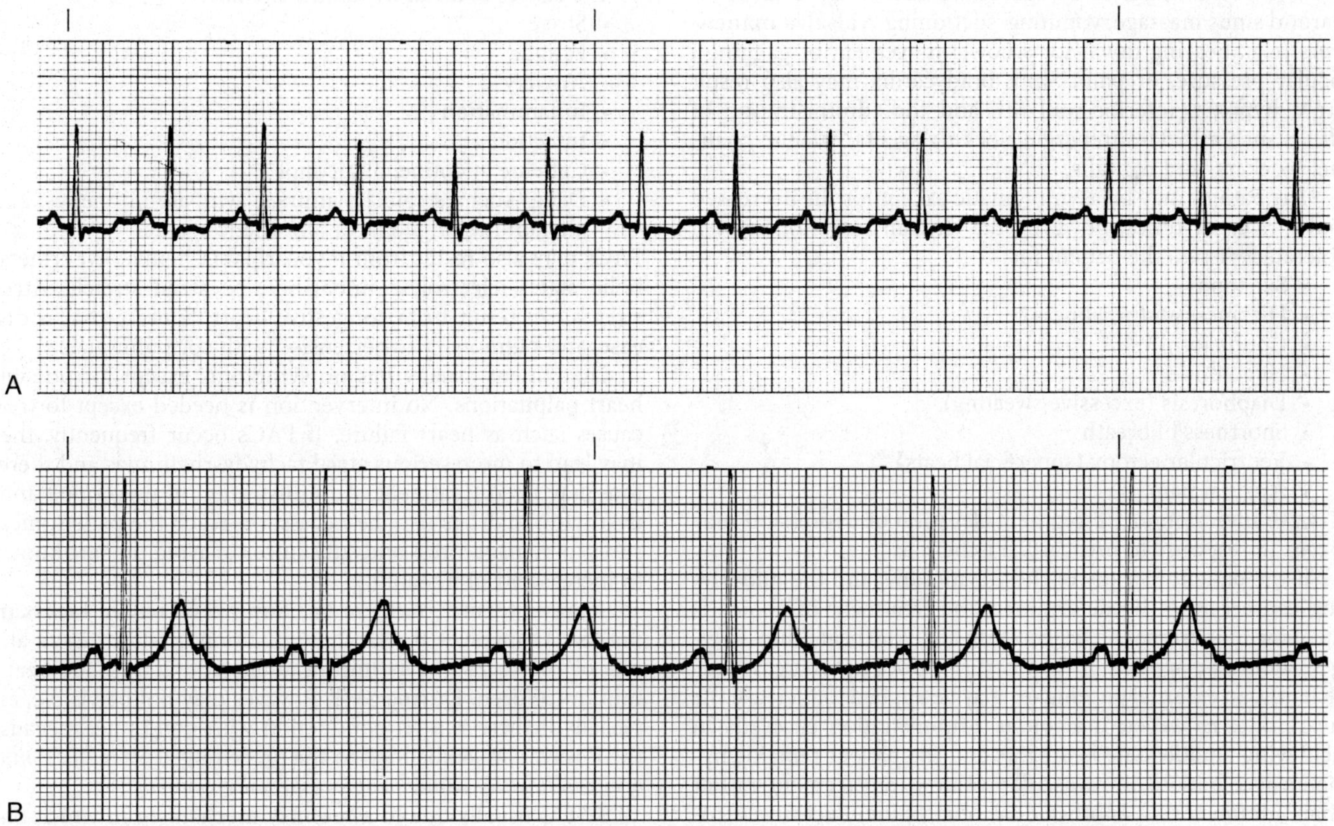
A
B

Fig. 36-8 • Sinus rhythms. **A,** Sinus tachycardia (heart rate, 110 beats/min; PR interval, 0.12 second; QRS complex, 0.08 second). **B,** Sinus bradycardia (heart rate, 52 beats/min; PR interval, 0.18 second; QRS complex, 0.08 second).

Collaborate with the health care provider to identify the cause of sinus tachycardia and select the appropriate treatment. The desired outcome is to decrease the heart rate to normal levels by treating the underlying cause. For example, if the patient has angina, administer oxygen, help him or her rest, and administer nitroglycerin or morphine as prescribed. IV diuretics may be given for decompensated heart failure. Begin intravascular volume replacement for hypovolemia, or administer antipyretics and antibiotics to the patient with fever and infection. Teach the patient to remain on bedrest if the tachycardia is causing hypotension or weakness.

Collaborate with the respiratory therapist, when indicated, to oxygenate and suction the patient who has hypoxemia (decreased arterial oxygen) from excessive airway secretions. Beta-adrenergic blocking agents may also be prescribed for the patient with too much sympathetic nervous system stimulation. Provide emotional support and health teaching about these interventions for the patient and family.

Sinus Bradycardia. Excessive vagal stimulation (parasympathetic system) to the heart causes a decreased rate of sinus node discharge. This stimulus slows the heart rate and decreases the speed of conduction through the heart. When the sinus node discharge rate is less than 60 beats/min in adults, the rhythm is called **sinus bradycardia** (Fig. 36-8, *B*). Sinus bradycardia increases coronary perfusion time, but it may decrease coronary perfusion pressure. However, myocardial oxygen demand is *decreased.*

Well-conditioned athletes have a hypereffective heart, in which the strong heart muscle provides an adequate stroke volume while not requiring a higher heart rate for a normal cardiac output. Excessive vagal stimulation may result from carotid sinus massage, vomiting, suctioning, **Valsalva maneuvers** (e.g., bearing down for a bowel movement or gagging), ocular pressure, or pain. Sinus bradycardia may also result from hypoxia, inferior wall MI, and the administration of drugs such as beta-adrenergic blocking agents, calcium channel blockers, and digitalis.

The patient may be asymptomatic except for the decreased pulse rate. At times, however, the rhythm may not be well tolerated. Assess the patient for:

- Syncope
- Dizziness and weakness
- Confusion
- Hypotension
- Diaphoresis (excessive sweating)
- Shortness of breath
- Ventricular ectopy (superficial beats)
- Anginal pain

T-wave inversion or ST-segment elevation or depression may occur in response to myocardial ischemia.

If the patient has any of these symptoms and the underlying cause cannot be determined, the treatment of choice is atropine to increase the heart rate to about 60 beats/min. Oxygen should be applied. If the heart rate does not increase sufficiently, an external pacemaker may be applied to increase the heart rate. However, if atropine administration succeeds in achieving an adequate heart rate and the patient remains hypotensive, initiate intravascular volume replacement rather than administering another dose of atropine. Excessive atropine may induce tachycardia and myocardial ischemia. If a medication is suspected to be the cause, withhold the drug and notify the physician.

DECISION-MAKING CHALLENGE
Critical Rescue

A 60-year-old male patient is admitted with chest pain to the telemetry unit where you work. While having a bowel movement on the bedside commode, the patient becomes short of breath and diaphoretic. The ECG waveform shows bradycardia.

1. What other assessment findings should you anticipate?
2. Why does this patient probably have bradycardia?
3. Does this dysrhythmia need treatment? Why or why not? What intervention would you implement first?
4. What is the drug treatment of choice for symptomatic bradycardia? How does this drug increase heart rate?

evolve For suggested answer guidelines, go to http://evolve.elsevier.com/Iggy/.

Atrial Dysrhythmias

With atrial dysrhythmias, the focus of impulse generation shifts away from the sinus node to the atrial tissue, which acts as an ectopic pacemaker for one or more beats. The shift changes the axis (direction) of atrial depolarization, resulting in a P-wave shape that differs from normal P waves. The most common atrial dysrhythmias are premature atrial complexes, supraventricular tachycardia, atrial flutter, and atrial fibrillation.

Premature Atrial Complexes. A **premature atrial complex (PAC)** occurs when atrial tissue becomes irritable. This ectopic focus fires an impulse before the next sinus impulse is due. The premature P wave may not always be clearly visible because it can be hidden in the preceding T wave. Examine the T wave closely for any change in shape, and compare with other T waves. A PAC is usually followed by a pause.

The causes of atrial irritability include:

- Stress
- Fatigue
- Anxiety
- Inflammation
- Infection
- Caffeine, nicotine, or alcohol
- Drugs such as catecholamines, sympathomimetics, amphetamines, digitalis, or anesthetic agents

PACs may also result from myocardial ischemia, hypermetabolic states, electrolyte imbalance, or atrial stretch. Atrial stretch can result from congestive heart failure, valvular disease, and pulmonary hypertension with cor pulmonale.

The patient usually has no symptoms except for possible heart palpitations. No intervention is needed except to treat causes such as heart failure. If PACs occur frequently, they may lead to more serious atrial tachydysrhythmias and therefore may need treatment. Administration of prescribed antidysrhythmic drugs may be necessary. Teach the patient measures to manage stress and substances to avoid that are known to increase atrial irritability.

Supraventricular Tachycardia. Supraventricular tachycardia (SVT) involves the rapid stimulation of atrial tissue at a rate of 100 to 280 beats/min in adults and 200 to 300 beats/min in children. During SVT, P waves may not be visible, especially if there is a 1:1 conduction with rapid rates, because the P waves are embedded in the preceding T wave. *SVT may occur in healthy young people, especially women.*

SVT is usually due to a re-entry mechanism in which one impulse circulates repeatedly throughout the atrial pathway, restimulating the atrial tissue at a rapid rate. The term **paroxysmal supraventricular tachycardia (PSVT)** is used when the rhythm is intermittent. It is initiated suddenly by a premature complex such as a PAC and terminated suddenly with or without intervention.

The clinical manifestations depend on the duration of the SVT and the rate of the ventricular response. In patients with a sustained rapid ventricular response, assess for palpitations, chest pain, weakness, fatigue, shortness of breath, nervousness, anxiety, hypotension, and syncope. Cardiovascular deterioration may occur if the rate does not sustain adequate blood pressure. In that case, SVT can result in angina, heart failure, and cardiogenic shock. With a nonsustained or slower ventricular response, the patient may be asymptomatic except for occasional palpitations.

If SVT occurs in a healthy person and stops on its own, no intervention may be needed other than eliminating identified causes. If it continues, the patient should be studied in the electrophysiology laboratory. The preferred treatment for recurrent SVT is radiofrequency catheter ablation. In sustained SVT with a rapid ventricular response, the desired outcomes of treatment are to decrease the ventricular response, convert the dysrhythmia to a sinus rhythm, and treat the cause. Vagal stimulation (e.g., carotid massage) may be successful, but often temporarily, and must be performed only by a physician.

Administer oxygen and prescribed antidysrhythmic drugs, such as diltiazem (Cardizem) or adenosine (Adenocard), which slow the ventricular rate by increasing the AV block (Chart 36-2). In the severely compromised patient, the nurse may assist the physician in attempting atrial overdrive pacing or in delivering a synchronized electrical shock (cardioversion) to re-establish an organized rhythm and regain cardiac stability.

Chart 36-2 COMMON EXAMPLES OF DRUG THERAPY
Common Dysrhythmias

Drug	Usual Dosage	Nursing Interventions	Rationales
CLASS I DRUGS			
TYPE IA			
Procainamide hydrochloride (Pronestyl)	50 mg/kg/day orally in 4 divided doses	Monitor BP.	Hypotension warrants drug discontinuation.
Used for AF, WPW, PVCs, VT	20-30 mg IV, not to exceed 17 mg/kg, followed by infusion of 1-4 mg/min	Monitor for widening QRS complex, prolonged QT or PR interval, or heart block.	Toxic side effects necessitate stopping procainamide administration.
Disopyramide phosphate (Norpace)	100-200 mg orally every 6 hr	Monitor BP.	Hypotension is a common side effect.
Used for AF, WPW, PSVT, PVCs, VT		Watch for shortness of breath and weight gain.	Disopyramide can cause heart failure in a patient with CAD.
		Monitor for widening QRS complex, prolonged QT or PR interval, or heart block.	Toxic side effects necessitate stopping disopyramide administration.
TYPE IB			
Lidocaine (Xylocaine) Used for PVCs, VT, VF	1-1.5 mg/kg IV bolus, then 0.5-0.75 mg/kg IV boluses every 5-10 min to a loading dose of 3 mg/kg, followed by 2-4 mg/min infusion For VF or pulseless VT: 1-1.5 mg/kg IV bolus every 3-5 min to a loading dose of 3 mg/kg, followed by 2-4 mg/min infusion	Watch for confusion, paresthesias, slurring of speech, drowsiness, or seizure activity.	CNS adverse effects predominate; they may require a decrease in dosage or discontinuation of the infusion.
Mexiletine hydrochloride (Mexitil)	200-300 mg orally every 8 hr with food	Monitor BP and heart rate.	Hypotension and bradycardia may occur.
Used for PVCs, VT, VF	125-250 mg IV bolus for 5-10 min 0.5-1.5 mg/min infusion	Assess for tremors, blurred vision, dizziness, ataxia, or confusion.	CNS adverse reactions predominate.
Tocainide hydrochloride (Tonocard) Used for PVCs, VT, VF	400 mg orally every 8 hr initially 400-800 mg orally every 8 hr Maximum of 2.4 g daily	Watch for tremors.	Tremors indicate that the maximum dose is being approached.
	Take with food	Monitor heart rate and BP.	Bradycardia and hypotension may occur.
		Teach patient to report shortness of breath, wheezing, chest pain, or cough, as well as dyspnea and distended neck veins or swelling of the extremities.	Pulmonary fibrosis is a serious side effect, which necessitates discontinuation of the drug; the drug may also cause CHF.

Continued

Chart 36-2 COMMON EXAMPLES OF DRUG THERAPY

Common Dysrhythmias—cont'd

Drug	Usual Dosage	Nursing Interventions	Rationales
TYPE IC			
Flecainide acetate (Tambocor) Used for AF, PSVT, life-threatening ventricular dysrhythmias	100 mg orally twice daily Maximum dose of 400 mg	Monitor for an increase in frequency and severity of dysrhythmias.	Flecainide can induce dysrhythmias.
		Monitor heart rate and BP.	Bradycardia and hypotension may occur.
		Monitor for CHF, dizziness, visual disturbances, paresthesias, and tremors.	Side effects may require a decrease in dosage or discontinuation of the drug.
Propafenone hydrochloride (Rythmol) Used for PAF, WPW, life-threatening ventricular dysrhythmias	150-300 mg orally every 8 hr	Monitor for an increase in dysrhythmias.	Propafenone can induce dysrhythmias.
		Monitor heart rate and BP.	Bradycardia and hypotension may occur.
		Monitor for CNS effects, dizziness, anxiety, ataxia, insomnia, confusion, and seizures, as well as CHF and GI distress.	Side effects may require a decrease in dosage or discontinuation of the drug.
CLASS II DRUGS			
Propranolol hydrochloride (Inderal, Apo-Propranolol🍁) Used for AF, atrial flutter, PSVT, PVCs	10-80 mg orally four times daily before meals 0.1 mg/kg slow IV bolus divided into 3 equal doses given at intervals of 2-3 min at rate of 1 mg/min	Monitor heart rate and BP.	Bradycardia and decreased BP are expected effects.
		Assess for shortness of breath or wheezing.	$Beta_2$-blocking effects on the lungs can cause bronchospasm.
		Assess for insomnia, fatigue, and dizziness.	Side effects may require decrease in dosage or discontinuation of the drug.
Acebutolol hydrochloride (Sectral) Used for AF, atrial flutter, PSVT, PVCs	600-1200 mg orally daily	Monitor heart rate and BP.	Bradycardia and decreased BP are expected effects.
		Assess for shortness of breath or wheezing.	$Beta_2$-blocking effects on the lungs can cause bronchospasm.
		Assess for insomnia, fatigue, and dizziness.	Side effects may require a decrease in dosage or discontinuation of the drug.
Esmolol hydrochloride (Brevibloc) Used for AF, atrial flutter, PSVT, PVCs	Initially, 500 mcg/kg/min for 1 min, then 50 mcg/kg/min for 4 min IV Titrate up if necessary	Monitor heart rate and BP.	Bradycardia and decreased BP are expected effects.
		Assess for shortness of breath or wheezing.	$Beta_2$-blocking effects on the lungs can cause bronchospasm.
		Assess for insomnia, fatigue, and seizures.	Side effects may require a decrease in dosage or discontinuation of the drug.
Sotalol hydrochloride (Betapace) Used for AF, PAF, PSVT, life-threatening ventricular dysrhythmias	Initial dose of 80 mg orally twice daily Dosage may be increased every 2-3 days, if necessary, to 240-320 mg daily in 2-3 divided doses	Assess ECG rhythm for torsades de pointes and other serious new ventricular dysrhythmias.	Sotalol may have proarrhythmic effects.
		Assess for fatigue, bradycardia, dyspnea, CHF, chest pain, hypotension, dizziness, hypoglycemia, nausea, and vomiting.	Adverse reactions may warrant drug discontinuation.
		Sotalol should not be administered to patients with hypokalemia or hypomagnesemia before correction of these imbalances.	Hypokalemia or hypomagnesemia may prolong the QT interval and cause torsades de pointes.
		Sotalol is contraindicated in patients with bronchial asthma, sinus bradycardia, or second- and third- degree AV block (unless a functioning pacemaker is present), prolonged QT syndrome, cardiogenic shock, or CHF.	Sotalol has beta-blocking (class II) effects and class III effects.

Chart 36-2 COMMON EXAMPLES OF DRUG THERAPY

Common Dysrhythmias—cont'd

Drug	Usual Dosage	Nursing Interventions	Rationales
CLASS III DRUGS			
Amiodarone hydrochloride (Cordarone) Used for AF, PAF, PSVT, life-threatening ventricular dysrhythmias	800-1600 mg orally daily in divided doses for 1-3 wk, then 600-800 mg daily for 1 mo, then 200-600 mg daily (average of 400 mg daily) Rapid loading dose: 150 mg IV over first 10 min (15 mg/min); slow loading dose: 360 mg IV over next 6 hr (1 mg/min); maintenance infusion: 540 mg IV over next 18 hr (0.5 mg/min), then 720 mg/24 hr (0.5 mg/min)	Use volumetric infusion pump and polyvinyl chloride (PVC) tubing with in-line filter, and infuse via central line.	Drug is irritating to peripheral vasculature; drug is more stable in glass bottle.
		Rapid-loading IV dose must not be administered faster than 10 min. Must stay with patient and monitor heart rate and BP.	Hypotension may occur. It should be treated by slowing the infusion and other standard therapy. Cordarone should not be discontinued unless necessary.
		Continually monitor ECG rhythm during IV infusion; measure QT and QT_c.	Bradycardia and AV block may occur and are treated by slowing the infusion rate and providing pacemaker therapy, if necessary. May cause a worsening of ventricular dysrhythmias.
		Assess the patient's knowledge of the treatment regimen and side effects.	Drug has major side effects, which make noncompliance a problem; patients may take the drug for $1^1/_2$-3 mo before full clinical effects are apparent.
		Monitor heart rate, BP, and cardiac rhythm when initiating therapy.	Bradycardia, hypotension, and worsening dysrhythmia can occur.
		Teach patients to report any muscle weakness, tremors, or difficulty with ambulation.	Muscle-related side effects usually develop during the first week of treatment.
		Teach patients to report shortness of breath, cough, pleuritic pain, or fever.	Pulmonary side effects may indicate drug-induced pulmonary toxicity.
		Teach patients to report any visual disturbances and to wear sunglasses outdoors in the daytime if they have photophobia.	Corneal pigmentation occurs in most patients but generally does not interfere with vision; if it does, the dosage is decreased.
		Teach patients to use barrier sunscreens.	Photosensitivity reactions may occur.
		Teach patients to report any signs of thyroid problems or hepatotoxicity.	Thyroid problems or hepatotoxicity may occur, necessitating a decrease in dosage or discontinuation of the drug.
Ibutilide fumarate (Corvert) Used for AF, atrial flutter	1 mg IV over 10 min for patients >60 kg; 0.01 mg/kg over 10 min for patients <60 kg May repeat dose 10 min after completion of first infusion if necessary	Stop infusion as soon as dysrhythmia is terminated, or in event of sustained or nonsustained VT, or marked prolongation of QT or QT_c.	Drug may cause potentially fatal dysrhythmias.
		Observe patients with continuous ECG monitoring and measure QT or QT_c for at least 4 hr after infusion or until QT_c has returned to baseline.	Acute ventricular dysrhythmias must be promptly identified and treated. Patient may develop heart blocks.
		Patients with atrial fibrillation of >2-3 days' duration must be adequately anticoagulated for at least 2 wk.	Atrial fibrillation is associated with formation of thrombi in atrial chambers.
		Hypokalemia and hypomagnesemia must be corrected before Corvert infusion.	This is important to reduce potential for proarrhythmic effects.

Continued

Chart 36-2 COMMON EXAMPLES OF DRUG THERAPY

Common Dysrhythmias—cont'd

Drug	Usual Dosage	Nursing Interventions	Rationales
CLASS III DRUGS—cont'd			
Dofetilide (Tikosyn) Used for AF, atrial flutter	125-500 mcg orally twice daily	Teach patients to change positions slowly.	Orthostatic hypotension is a common side effect of the drug.
		Inform patients that dosages will be adjusted, depending on their creatinine clearance level.	The patient must have adequate creatinine clearance to prevent drug toxicity.
		Monitor patients on telemetry for several days; observe for and report bradycardia and hypotension.	Bradycardia and hypotension are common side effects.
CLASS IV DRUGS			
Verapamil hydrochloride (Calan, Isoptin♣) Used for AF, atrial flutter, PSVT	2.5-5 mg IV for 1-2 min for narrow-complex SVT or PSVT; after 15-30 min may give 5-10 mg IV for 1-2 min, if necessary, and repeat to a maximum of 20 mg 80-120 mg orally every 6-8 hr	Monitor heart rate and BP.	Bradycardia and hypotension are common side effects.
		Teach patients to remain recumbent for at least 1 hr after IV administration.	Hypotension may occur; may be reversed with calcium chloride ($CaCl_2$), 0.5-1 g slow IV.
		Teach patients to change positions slowly when receiving oral therapy.	Dizziness and orthostatic hypotension often occur until tolerance develops.
		Teach patients to report dyspnea, orthopnea, distended neck veins, or swelling of the extremities.	Heart failure may occur, necessitating a decrease in dosage or discontinuation of the drug.
Diltiazem hydrochloride (Cardizem) Used for AF, atrial flutter, PSVT	0.25 mg/kg IV for 2 min After 15 min, give 0.35 mg/kg IV for 2 min 5-15 mg/hr IV infusion	Monitor heart rate and BP.	Bradycardia and hypotension are common side effects.
		Teach patients to remain recumbent for at least 1 hr after IV administration.	Hypotension may occur.
		Teach patients to report dyspnea, orthopnea, distended neck veins, or swelling of the extremities.	Heart failure may occur, necessitating a decrease in dosage or discontinuation of the drug.
OTHER DRUGS			
Digoxin (Lanoxin, Novodigoxin♣) Used for CHF, AF, atrial flutter, PSVT	Rapid digitalization: 0.5-1 mg orally or IV initially; 0.125-0.5 mg orally every 6 hr or IV until a total of 1-1.5 mg is reached Maintenance: 0.125-0.25 mg orally or IV daily or every other day (may be less for older adults)	Assess apical heart rate for 1 min before each dose.	Decreased heart rate is an expected response, but bradycardia may indicate toxicity.
		Assess for sudden increase in heart rate and change of rhythm from regular to irregular, or irregular to regular.	Changes in heart rate or rhythm may indicate toxicity.
		Teach patients to report anorexia, nausea, vomiting, diarrhea, paresthesias, confusion, or visual disturbances.	Side effect can indicate toxicity.
		Monitor serum potassium levels.	Hypokalemia increases the risk of toxicity and ventricular dysrhythmias.
		Monitor serum creatinine levels.	Impaired renal function can cause toxicity; the dosage is altered if this occurs.

Chart 36-2 COMMON EXAMPLES OF DRUG THERAPY

Common Dysrhythmias—cont'd

Drug	Usual Dosage	Nursing Interventions	Rationales
OTHER DRUGS—cont'd			
Atropine sulfate Used for bradycardia	0.5-1 mg IV bolus may be repeated every 3-5 min, if necessary, to a maximum of 0.04 mg/kg For asystole, PEA, or EMD: 1 mg IV bolus every 3-5 min, if necessary, to a total of 0.04 mg/kg	Monitor heart rate and rhythm after administration. Assess for chest pain after administration. Assess for urinary retention and dry mouth after administration. Avoid using in patients with acute angle-closure glaucoma.	Increased heart rate is expected. Increased heart rate may cause ischemia in patients with CAD. Atropine is an anticholinergic agent. Atropine increases intraocular pressure.
Adenosine (Adenocard) Used for PSVT, WPW	6 mg IV for 1-3 sec followed by 20-mL saline flush; may repeat in 1-2 min, if necessary, at 12 mg IV for 1-3 sec with 20-mL flush; may repeat 12 mg IV after 1-2 min if necessary	Monitor heart rate and rhythm after administration. Assess patients for facial flushing, shortness of breath, dyspnea, and chest pain. Assess patients for recurrence of PSVT or ventricular ectopy.	A short period of asystole is common after administration; bradycardia and hypotension may occur. These side effects commonly occur. Recurrence of PSVT is common; PVCs may occur.
Magnesium sulfate Used for torsades de pointes	1-2 g diluted in 100 mL of D_5W administered IV for 1-2 min for VF or VT 1-2 g in 50-100 mL of D_5W for 5-60 min for loading dose; 0.5-1 g/hr for 24 hr for supplementation	Assess ECG rhythm for conversion to sinus rhythm. Assess patients for facial flushing, hypotension, and respiratory and CNS depression.	Hypomagnesemia may precipitate refractory VF. Magnesium sulfate causes vasodilation and respiratory and CNS depression.

AF, Atrial fibrillation; *AV*, atrioventricular; *BP*, blood pressure; *CAD*, coronary artery disease; *CHF*, congestive heart failure; *CNS*, central nervous system; D_5W, 5% dextrose in water; *EMD*, electromechanical dissociation; *PAF*, paroxysmal atrial fibrillation/flutter; *PEA*, pulseless electrical activity; *PSVT*, paroxysmal supraventricular tachycardia; *PVC*, premature ventricular complex; *SVT*, supraventricular tachycardia; *VF*, ventricular fibrillation; *VT*, ventricular tachycardia; *WPW*, Wolff-Parkinson-White.

Atrial Fibrillation

Pathophysiology. **Atrial fibrillation (AF)** is the most common dysrhythmia seen in clinical practice. More than 2 million Americans have AF. It is responsible for a third of hospitalizations for cardiac rhythm disturbances (Bentz, 2006). Incidence of AF increases with age. More than 80% of AF patients are older than 65 years, and prevalence of the dysrhythmia is expected to double over the next 50 years. AF causes serious problems in older people, leading to heart failure and/or stroke. Risk factors include hypertension (HTN) (the biggest risk factor), diabetes mellitus, male gender, congestive heart failure, and valvular disease (Chen-Scarabelli, 2005). Alcohol intake may trigger temporary episodes, as well as cardiac surgery, electrocution, MI, pericarditis, myocarditis, and pulmonary embolism. Treatment of the underlying disorder will often eliminate these temporary AF episodes (Bentz, 2006).

In patients with AF, multiple rapid impulses from many atrial foci depolarize the atria in a totally disorganized manner at a rate of 350 to 600 times per minute. The result is a chaotic rhythm with no clear P waves, no atrial contractions, loss of atrial kick, and an irregular ventricular response (Fig. 36-9, *A*). The atria merely quiver in fibrillation (commonly called "A fib"). Often the ventricles beat with a rapid rate in response to the numerous atrial impulses. Heart dilation and blood pooling in the atria can lead to thrombus formation, and this increases the risk of stroke or other embolic events. The rapid and irregular ventricular rate decreases ventricular filling and reduces cardiac output, further impairing the heart's perfusion ability.

Patient-Centered Collaborative Care. AF may be intermittent or chronic. Symptoms depend on the ventricular rate. If the ventricular rate is rapid, the presenting symptoms may be similar to those described earlier for supraventricular tachycardia. Because of loss of atrial kick, however, the patient in uncontrolled AF is at greater risk for an inadequate cardiac output. Assess the patient for fatigue, weakness, shortness of breath, distended neck veins, dizziness, decreased exercise tolerance, anxiety, syncope, palpitations, chest discomfort or pain, and hypotension.

The patient is also at risk for pulmonary embolism. Thrombi may form within the right atrium and then move through the right ventricle to the lungs. Assess for shortness of breath, chest pain, hemoptysis (blood-tinged sputum), and a feeling of impending doom.

In addition, the patient is at risk for systemic emboli, particularly an embolic stroke, which may cause severe neurologic impairment or death. Be sure to assess for manifestations of stroke, such as changes in mentation or level of consciousness, speech, sensory function, and motor function.

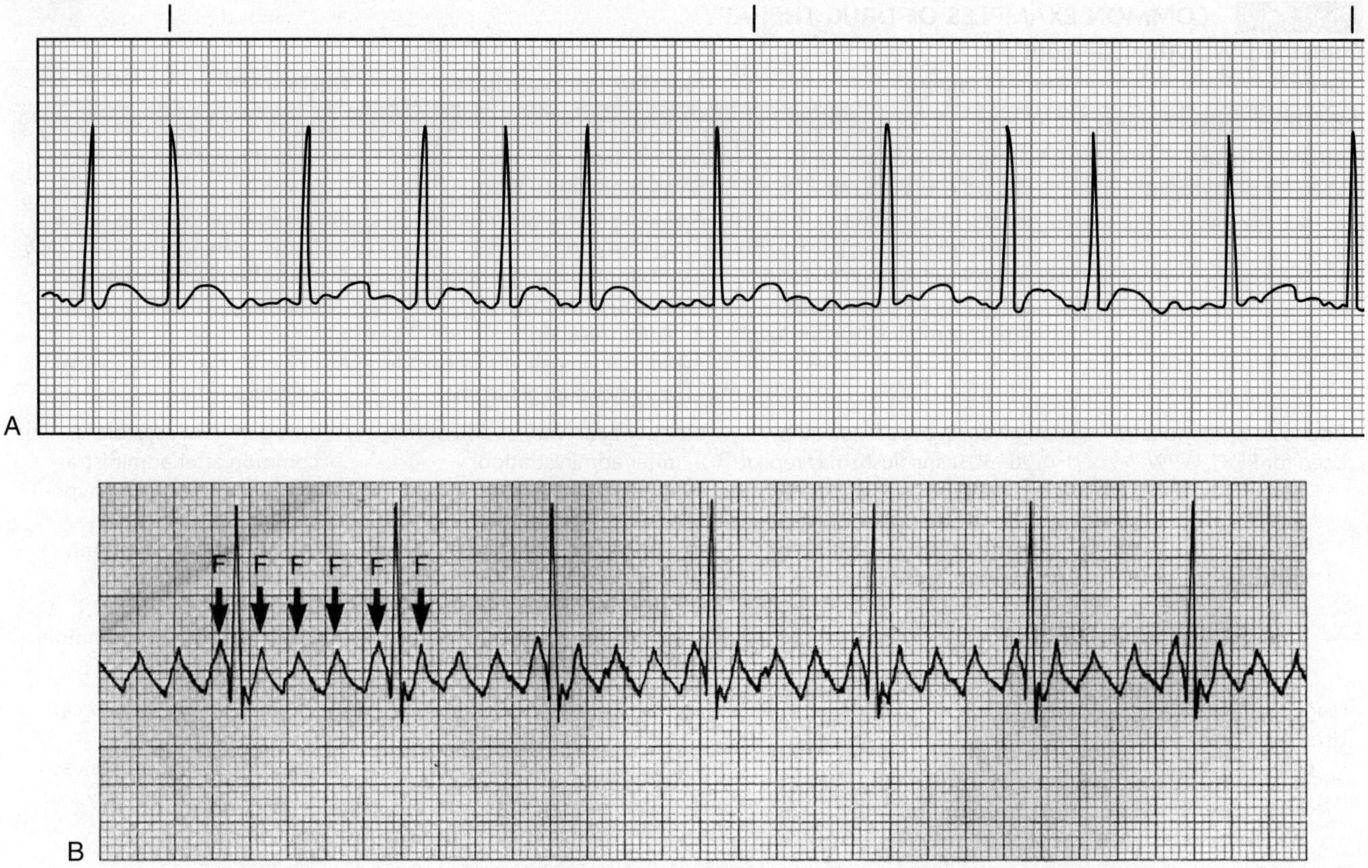
A
F
F
F
F
F
F
B

Fig. 36-9 • Atrial dysrhythmias. **A,** Atrial fibrillation. Note wavy baseline with atrial electrical activity and irregular ventricular rhythm. **B,** Atrial flutter with 4:1 block. The atrial rate is 280 beats/min; the ventricular rate is 70 beats/min.

Assess pulses, urine output, and back pain. Report any of these symptoms to the health care provider immediately. Patients with AF who have valvular disease are particularly at risk for thromboemboli.

Traditional interventions include antidysrhythmic drugs to slow the ventricular conduction or to convert the AF to normal sinus rhythm (NSR). Examples of these drugs are calcium channel blockers like diltiazem (Cardizem), or amiodarone (Cordarone) for more difficult-to-control AF. In addition, the nurse may give anticoagulants, such as heparin, enoxaparin (Lovenox), and sodium warfarin (Coumadin), for patients at high risk for emboli.

Cardioversion is the electrical treatment of choice. Before elective cardioversion, the health care provider prescribes anticoagulation therapy for about 6 weeks to prevent a thromboembolic event if the rhythm is successfully converted. To assess for the presence of atrial clots, a contraindication for cardioversion, the physician may order a transesophageal echocardiogram (TEE) before attempting emergency cardioversion (see Chapter 35). When AF has persisted more than 12 months, it is not likely to convert to a sinus rhythm by drug therapies and may fail to respond to electrical cardioversion, which is discussed on p. 756.

AF resistant to medical therapies may be treated with *radiofrequency catheter ablation.* Pulmonary vein ablation creates scar tissue that blocks impulses and disconnects the pathway of the abnormal rhythm. This treatment has proven effective for paroxysmal AF with a single focus and is becoming increasingly more common. Patients with AF with a rapid ventricular rate not responsive to drug therapy may have AV nodal ablation performed to totally disconnect the conduction from the atria to the ventricles. However, this treatment requires implantation of a permanent ventricular pacemaker. *Bi-ventricular pacing* may be another alternative for patients with heart failure and conduction disorders. Bi-atrial pacing, anti-tachycardia pacing, and implantable atrial defibrillators are other methods used to suppress or resolve AF. All of these methods are discussed on pp. 757-758.

Patients in AF with decompensated heart failure (discussed in Chapter 37) may benefit from the **maze procedure,** an open-chest surgical technique often performed with coronary artery bypass grafting (CABG). Before this procedure, electrophysiologic mapping studies are done to confirm the diagnosis of AF. The surgeon places a maze of sutures in strategic places in the atrial myocardium, pulmonary artery, and possibly the superior vena cava to prevent electrical circuits from developing and continuing AF. Sinus impulses can then depolarize the atria before reaching the AV node and preserve the atrial kick. Postoperative care is similar to that after other open-heart surgical procedures (see Chapter 40).

DECISION-MAKING CHALLENGE
Delegation/Supervision

A 78-year-old woman with palpitations and shortness of breath is admitted to the telemetry unit. She had a cardiac catheterization 2 years ago for chest pain, but no heart problems were found. The monitor "tech" reports that she now has atrial fibrillation (AF) with a rapid ventricular response.

1. What is your best response to the "tech?"
2. What other physical assessment findings would you expect for this patient?
3. What drug therapy should you anticipate administering to this patient? Why is it given?
4. What part of this patient's care can be safely delegated to the patient care assistant?
5. For what complications should you observe, and why might they occur in this patient?

evolve For suggested answer guidelines, go to http://evolve.elsevier.com/Iggy/.

Atrial Flutter. **Atrial flutter** is rapid atrial depolarization occurring at a rate of 250 to 350 times per minute (see Fig. 36-9, B). The atrioventricular (AV) node blocks the number of impulses that reach the ventricles as a protective mechanism. Atrial flutter may be caused by rheumatic or ischemic heart disease, heart failure (HF), AV valve disease, pre-excitation syndromes, septal defects, pulmonary emboli, thyrotoxicosis, alcoholism, or pericarditis.

The clinical manifestations depend on the rate of ventricular response. Assess the patient for palpitations, weakness, fatigue, shortness of breath, nervousness, anxiety, syncope (loss of consciousness), angina, and evidence of heart failure and shock. Carotid sinus massage may temporarily decrease the ventricular rate to facilitate rhythm interpretation, but it can be performed only by the physician. The patient with a normal ventricular rate is usually asymptomatic.

The collaborative management outcomes are the same as those for SVT and AF. Administer oxygen and prescribed drugs, such as ibutilide (Corvert), amiodarone (Cordarone), and diltiazem (Cardizem), to slow the rapid ventricular response.

If the patient is severely compromised, cardioversion is the treatment of choice. Rapid atrial overdrive pacing may be attempted or radiofrequency catheter ablation may be necessary if the patient does not respond to these therapies. These therapies are discussed on pp. 756-757.

Junctional Dysrhythmias

Nodal cells in the AV junctional area can generate electrical impulses and are therefore secondary or latent pacemaker cells. They have a slower rate of discharge, usually 40 to 60 beats/min, and are usually suppressed. Occasionally these cells do generate impulses as an escape pacemaker when the sinus node is excessively slow, or the cells may do so as irritable rhythms. These rhythms are most commonly temporary, and patients usually remain stable.

Ventricular Dysrhythmias

The ventricles have the fewest nodal cells and are the slowest pacemaker. However, irritable ventricular cells may generate electrical impulses and fire prematurely. Because the impulse originates in and depolarizes one ventricle first and then spreads to depolarize the other, the resulting QRS complex is wide, measuring greater than 0.12 second. The QRS complex is bizarre or oddly shaped, looking different from the normal QRS complexes. The atrial rhythm typically remains regular unless the underlying rhythm is sinus arrhythmia, discussed on p. 737 in the Normal Rhythms section.

Idioventricular Rhythm (Ventricular Escape Rhythm). During an **idioventricular rhythm** (ventricular escape rhythm), the ventricular nodal cells pace the ventricles. Because their rate of firing is slow, the rate is usually less than 40 beats/min. If P waves are seen, they are independent of the QRS complexes.

Idioventricular rhythm is seen as a rhythm in the dying heart, where downward displacement of the pacemaker has occurred. **Pulseless electrical activity (PEA)** is characterized by no palpable pulse and therefore no *perfusion,* although electrical activity is displayed on the monitor. Common causes of PEA are:

- Hypovolemia
- Hypoxia
- Acidosis
- Hyperkalemia or hypokalemia
- Hypothermia
- Drug overdose
- Tension pneumothorax
- Coronary or pulmonary thrombosis
- Cardiac tamponade

Because idioventricular pacemakers are unstable, unreliable, and slow, the patient is hypotensive and in shock. Assess the patient's airway, breathing, circulation, level of consciousness, and oxygenation. He or she may become pulseless and therefore in cardiac arrest requiring CPR.

Emergency Care: Idioventricular Rhythms. Begin cardiopulmonary resuscitation (CPR) and get assistance unless there is a do-not-resuscitate (DNR) order. The team may start advanced cardiac life support (ACLS) measures, including epinephrine administration, intravascular volume replacement, and other measures. The physician may then use a pacemaker or discontinue resuscitation efforts.

Premature Ventricular Complexes. **Premature ventricular complexes (PVCs)** result from increased irritability of ventricular cells and are seen as early ventricular complexes followed by a pause. When multiple PVCs are present, the QRS complexes may be unifocal or uniform, meaning that they are of the same shape (Fig. 36-10, *A*) or multifocal or multiform, meaning that they are of different shapes (Fig. 36-10, *B*). PVCs frequently occur in repetitive rhythms, such as bigeminy (two), trigeminy (three), and quadrigeminy (four). Two sequential PVCs are a pair, or couplet. Three or more successive PVCs are usually called **nonsustained ventricular tachycardia (NSVT).**

Premature ventricular contractions are common, and their frequency increases with age. PVCs may be insignificant or may occur with myocardial ischemia or MI, CHF, chronic hypoxemia, chronic airway limitation (CAL), anemia, hypokalemia, or hypomagnesemia. The administration of catecholamines, sympathomimetic drugs, and digitalis, as well as acidosis, anesthesia, stress, nicotine intake, ingestion of caffeine and alcohol, infection, trauma, or surgery, can also cause PVCs. *Postmenopausal women often find that caffeine causes palpitations and PVCs.*

The patient may be asymptomatic or may experience palpitations or chest discomfort caused by increased stroke volume

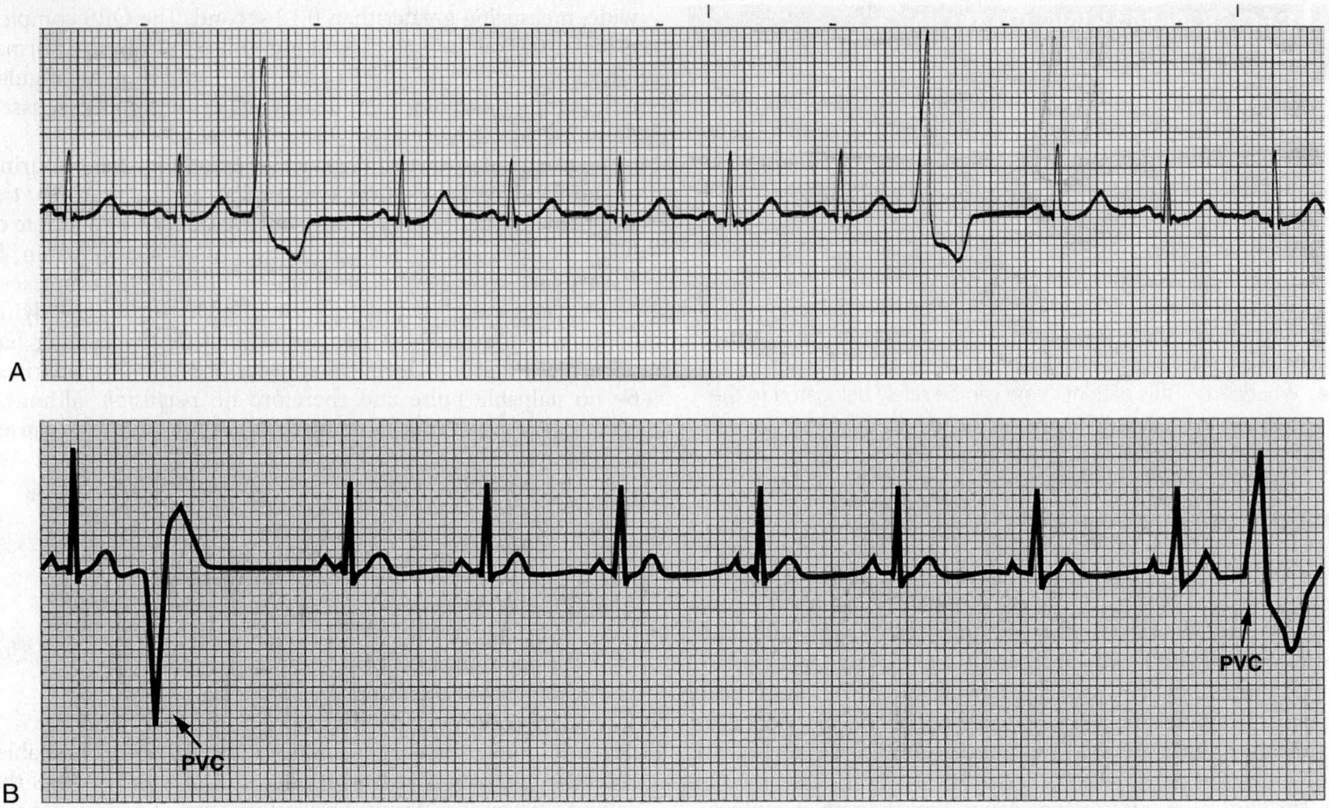
A
B
PVC
PVC

Fig. 36-10 • Ventricular dysrhythmias. **A,** Normal sinus rhythm with unifocal premature ventricular complexes (PVCs). **B,** Normal sinus rhythm with multifocal PVCs (one negative and the other positive).

of the normal beat after the pause. Peripheral pulses may be diminished or absent with the PVCs themselves because the decreased stroke volume of the premature beats may *decrease peripheral perfusion. Because other rhythms also cause widened QRS complexes, assess whether the premature complexes perfuse to the extremities. Palpate the carotid, brachial, or femoral arteries while observing the monitor for widened complexes or auscultating for the apical heart sounds.* With acute MI, PVCs may be considered warning dysrhythmias, possibly triggering ventricular tachycardia (VT) or ventricular fibrillation (VF).

If there is no underlying heart disease, PVCs are not usually treated other than by eliminating any contributing cause (e.g., caffeine, stress). With acute myocardial ischemia or MI, PVCs are managed by administering oxygen and amiodarone (Cordarone) as prescribed. Potassium is given for replacement therapy if hypokalemia is the cause. People with more than 5000 PVCs in a 24-hour period are usually placed on beta blockers.

Ventricular Tachycardia. Ventricular tachycardia (VT), sometimes referred to as "V tach," occurs with repetitive firing of an irritable ventricular ectopic focus, usually at a rate of 140 to 180 beats/min or more (Fig. 36-11). VT may result from increased automaticity or a re-entry mechanism. It may be intermittent (nonsustained VT) or sustained, lasting longer than 15 to 30 seconds. The sinus node may continue to discharge independently, depolarizing the atria but not the ventricles, although P waves are seldom seen in sustained VT.

Ventricular tachycardia may occur in patients with ischemic heart disease, MI, cardiomyopathy, hypokalemia, hypomagnesemia, valvular heart disease, heart failure, drug toxicity, hypotension, or ventricular aneurysm. In patients who go into cardiac arrest, VT is commonly the initial rhythm before deterioration into ventricular fibrillation (VF) as the terminal rhythm.

Clinical manifestations of sustained VT partially depend on the ventricular rate. Slower rates are better tolerated. *In some patients, VT causes cardiac arrest. Assess the patient's airway, breathing, circulation, level of consciousness, and oxygenation level.*

For the *stable* patient with sustained VT, administer oxygen and confirm the rhythm via a 12-lead ECG. Amiodarone, lidocaine, or magnesium sulfate may be given. Current ACLS guidelines state that elective cardioversion is highly recommended for stable VT. The physician may prescribe an oral antidysrhythmic agent, such as mexiletine (Mexitil) or sotalol (Betapace, Sotacor♣) to prevent further occurrences. *Unstable* VT without a pulse is treated the same way as ventricular fibrillation, described next.

Ventricular Fibrillation

Pathophysiology. **Ventricular fibrillation (VF),** sometimes called "V fib," is the result of electrical chaos in the ventricles and is *life threatening!* Impulses from many irritable foci fire in a totally disorganized manner so that ventricular contraction cannot occur. There are no recognizable ECG deflections (Fig. 36-12, A). The ventricles merely quiver, consuming a tremendous amount of oxygen. *There is no cardiac output or pulse and therefore no cerebral, myocardial, or systemic perfusion. This rhythm is rapidly fatal if not successfully ended within 3 to 5 minutes.*

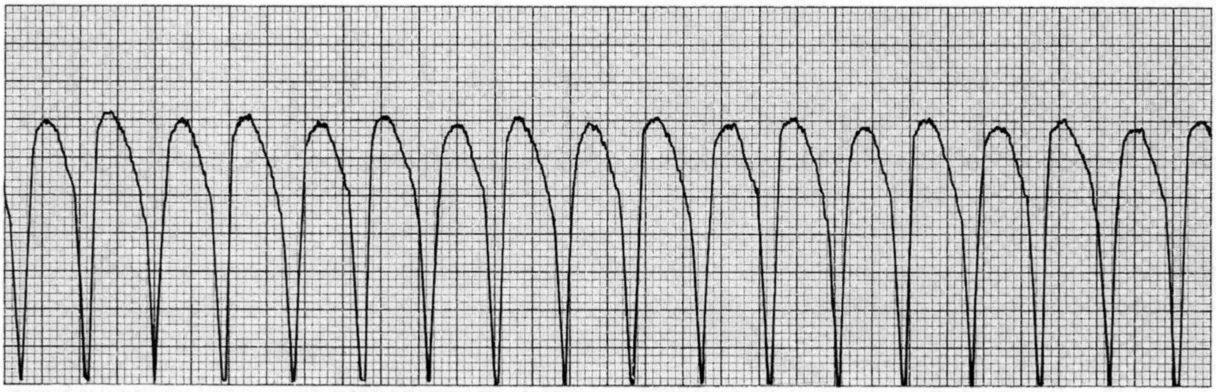

Fig. 36-11 • Ventricular dysrhythmias. Sustained ventricular tachycardia at a rate of 166 beats/min.

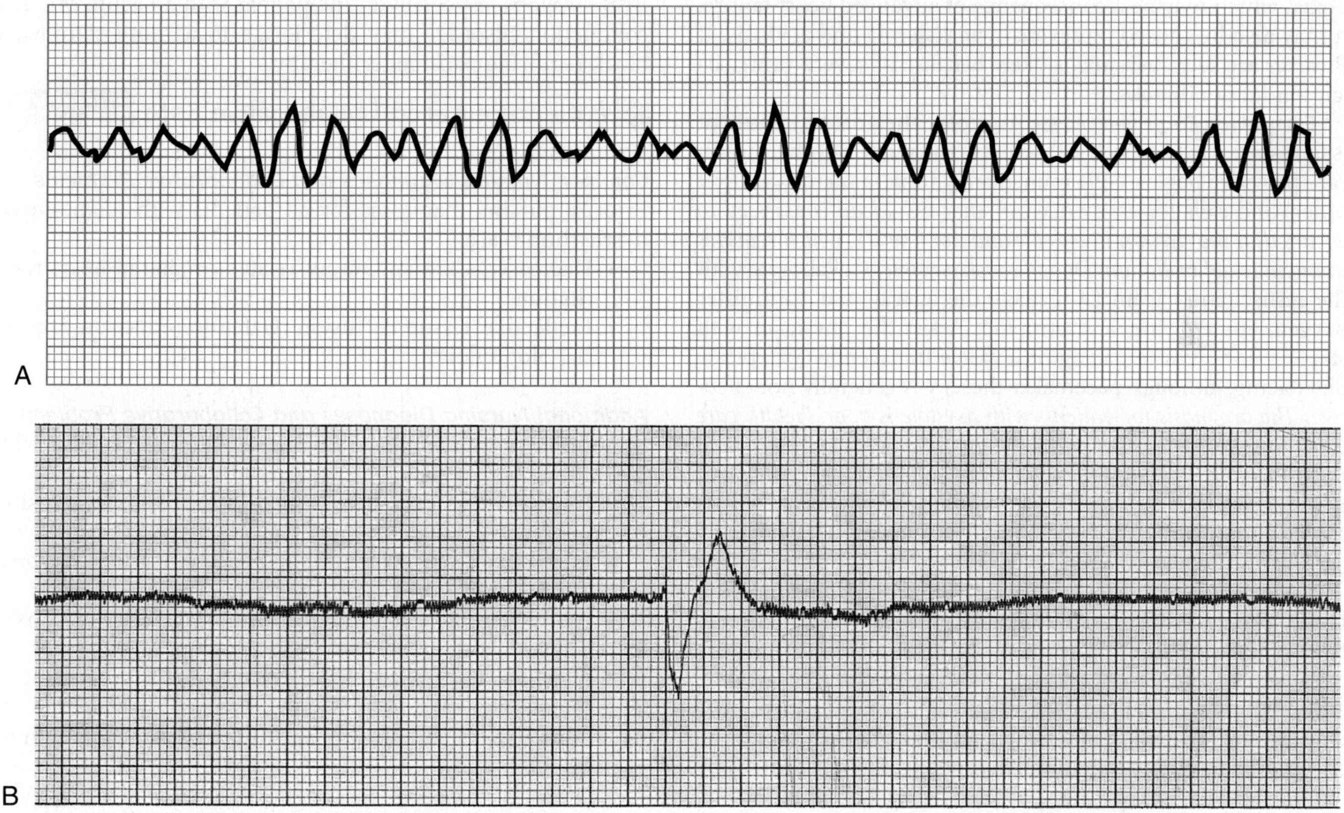

Fig. 36-12 • Ventricular dysrhythmias. **A,** Coarse ventricular fibrillation. **B,** Ventricular asystole with one idioventricular complex.

VF may be the first manifestation of coronary artery disease (CAD). Patients with myocardial infarction (MI) are at great risk for VF. It may also occur in those with hypokalemia, hypomagnesemia, hemorrhage, antidysrhythmic therapy, rapid supraventricular tachycardia (SVTs), or shock. Surgery or trauma may cause VF as well.

Patient-Centered Collaborative Care. When VF begins, the patient becomes faint, immediately loses consciousness, and becomes pulseless and apneic (no breathing). There is no blood pressure, and heart sounds are absent. Respiratory and metabolic acidosis develop. Seizures may occur. Within minutes, the pupils become fixed and dilated and the skin becomes cold and mottled. *Death results without prompt intervention.*

Emergency care: ventricular fibrillation. The goals of treatment are to resolve VF promptly and convert it to an organized rhythm. *Therefore the priority is to defibrillate the patient immediately according to ACLS protocol.* If a defibrillator is not readily available, CPR must be continued until the defibrillator arrives. An automatic external defibrillator (AED) is frequently used because it is simple for both medical and lay personnel. Defibrillation is discussed on p. 756.

If the VF does not end after one defibrillator shock, the nurse and resuscitation team resume CPR and provide airway management for about 2 minutes. *High-quality CPR and defibrillation is now the recommended treatment for VF.* The team also gives oxygen and drug therapy, including vasopressin, epinephrine, amiodarone, procainamide (Pronestyl), lidocaine, and magnesium sulfate, alternating with defibrillation. If VF is successfully converted to an organized rhythm, supportive therapy is continued.

Ventricular Asystole. **Ventricular asystole,** sometimes called *ventricular standstill,* is the complete absence of any ventricular rhythm (Fig. 36-12, *B*). There are no electrical impulses in the ventricles and therefore *no* ventricular depolarization, no QRS complex, no contraction, no cardiac output, and no pulse, respirations, or blood pressure. *The patient is in full cardiac arrest.* The sinoatrial (SA) node, in some cases, may continue to fire and depolarize the atria, with only P waves seen on the ECG. The sinus impulses, however, do not conduct to the ventricles, and QRS complexes remain absent. In most cases, the entire conduction system is electrically silent, with no P waves seen on the ECG.

Ventricular asystole usually results from myocardial hypoxia, which may be a consequence of advanced heart failure. It may also be caused by severe hyperkalemia and acidosis. If P waves are seen, asystole is likely because of severe ventricular conduction blocks.

Emergency Care: Ventricular Asystole. The goal of treatment is to restore cardiac electrical activity. The nurse or other health care provider begins CPR immediately (unless there is a DNR order) and calls for assistance. *Another ECG lead is assessed to ensure that the rhythm is asystole and not fine VF, which requires immediate defibrillation. Do not shock asystole.* Collaborate with the resuscitation team to manage the airway and administer oxygen, epinephrine, and atropine. Assist the physician with starting noninvasive pacing or invasive transvenous or epicardial pacing, although pacemaker therapy is generally not effective. *The prognosis for patients with asystole is poor. Health care providers should consider ending resuscitation efforts if there is no response after standard interventions have been implemented and when cessation is approved by an authorized physician. Nurses should know the criteria for terminating CPR and ACLS based on current facility and state legal policies.*

An emerging clinical practice is allowing or encouraging family presence at resuscitation attempts. This can be a positive experience for family members and significant others because it promotes closure after the death of a loved one. Although there may be staff resistance and some limits to family presence, overall it is a beneficial practice that should be considered in all resuscitation attempts.

Atrioventricular Blocks

Atrioventricular (AV) blocks exist when supraventricular impulses are excessively delayed or totally blocked in the AV node or intraventricular conduction system. Conduction may be temporarily or permanently abnormal for a number of reasons. The SA node continues to function normally, and atrial depolarizations and P waves occur regularly. Because of the conduction dysfunction, ventricular depolarizations and QRS complexes are either delayed or blocked.

The degrees of heart blocks include:

- In *first-degree* AV block, all sinus impulses eventually reach the ventricles.
- In *second-degree* heart block, some sinus impulses reach the ventricles but others do not because they are blocked.
- In *third-degree* heart block (complete heart block), none of the sinus impulses reach the ventricles. The ventricles are therefore depolarized by a second, independent pacemaker.

AV blocks are differentiated by their PR intervals. Interventions depend on the severity of the block. Oxygen, drug therapy, pacing, and/or permanent pacemakers may be used, depending on the degree of the AV block.

Bundle Branch Blocks

Bundle branch block (BBB) is a conduction delay or block within one of the two main bundle of His branches. The underlying rhythm is usually sinus in origin (e.g., sinus rhythm with bundle branch block). BBB may be a temporary or a permanent conduction disorder. Right or left BBBs are occasionally seen in patients with normal hearts. More commonly they are seen in patients with cardiovascular disease, such as congenital heart disease, rheumatic heart disease, and ventricular hypertrophy.

Although shown on an ECG, no clinical manifestations are specifically related to BBB. Notify the physician when a new BBB develops, especially in the patient with an acute MI. The conduction disorder may deteriorate to a more significant block requiring pacemaker therapy.

Patient-Centered Collaborative Care

evolve ONLINE PHARM REVIEW

Analysis

Common Nursing Diagnoses and Collaborative Problems

Priority nursing diagnoses for all patients with *symptomatic* dysrhythmias are:

- Decreased Cardiac Output related to altered heart rate/rhythm
- Ineffective Tissue Perfusion related to reduction of arterial blood flow

Additional Nursing Diagnoses and Collaborative Problems

In addition to the common nursing diagnoses, patients with dysrhythmias may have one or more of these:

- Impaired Gas Exchange related to ventilation-perfusion imbalance
- Ineffective Coping related to uncertainty and situational crisis
- Activity Intolerance related to imbalance between oxygen supply/demand
- Deficient Knowledge related to cause and treatment of dysrhythmia

An additional collaborative problem is Potential for Pulmonary Edema.

Planning and Implementation

Decreased Cardiac Output and Ineffective Tissue Perfusion

NOC **Planning: Expected Outcomes.** The patient with dysrhythmias is expected to have adequate blood flow ejected from the left ventricle to support systemic perfusion pressure. Indicators include that the patient will have a normal or baseline:

- Apical heart rate
- Systolic and diastolic blood pressure
- Activity tolerance
- Cognitive status
- Skin color
- Peripheral pulses
- Ejection fraction

Additional indicators include that the patient will *not* have:

- Dysrhythmias
- Abnormal heart sounds
- Angina
- Dyspnea

Chart 36-3 NIC INTERVENTION ACTIVITIES

The Patient with Dysrhythmias

Cardiac Care: *Limitation of complications resulting from an imbalance between myocardial oxygen supply and demand for a patient with symptoms of impaired cardiac function*

- Evaluate chest pain (e.g., intensity, location, radiation, duration, and precipitating and alleviating factors).
- Perform a comprehensive appraisal of peripheral circulation (e.g., check peripheral pulses, edema, capillary refill, color, and temperature of extremity).
- Monitor cardiovascular status.
- Document cardiac dysrhythmias.
- Monitor vital signs frequently.
- Evaluate the patient's response to ectopy or dysrhythmias.
- Monitor appropriate laboratory values (e.g., cardiac enzymes, electrolyte levels).
- Provide antiarrhythmic therapy according to unit policy (e.g., antiarrhythmic medication, cardioversion, or defibrillation), as appropriate.
- Monitor patient's response to antiarrhythmic medications.
- Arrange exercise and rest periods to avoid fatigue.
- Monitor the patient's activity tolerance.
- Monitor for dyspnea, fatigue, tachypnea, and orthopnea.
- Promote stress reduction.
- Instruct the patient on the importance of immediately reporting any chest discomfort.
- Offer spiritual support to the patient and/or family (e.g., contact clergy), as appropriate.

- Fatigue
- Pulmonary edema

Interventions. The nurse's major priority for care is to assess for complications and monitor the patient for response to treatment (Chart 36-3). Interventions are specific to the type of dysrhythmia, the cause, the effect it has on cardiac output, and the risk it presents to the patient.

NIC ***Cardiac Care.*** Monitor or direct UAP to monitor the patient's electrocardiographic (ECG) rhythm. Assess for manifestations associated with dysrhythmias, such as abnormal pulse rate and rhythm, palpitations, chest pain, syncope, decreased blood pressure, and dyspnea.

Assess the patient's apical and radial pulses for a full minute for any irregularity, which may occur with premature beats, escape beats, atrial fibrillation (AF), or second-degree heart blocks. If the apical pulse rate differs from the radial pulse rate, a pulse deficit exists and suggests that *not all beats are perfusing.* Clinical manifestations of sustained tachydysrhythmias and bradydysrhythmias are summarized in Chart 36-1.

Assess the psychosocial impact of dysrhythmias on patients and families and the effectiveness of their coping skills. Assessment of the patient's past and current history is essential because dysrhythmias are associated with both acute and chronic disorders, as well as with medical and surgical therapies. Review the interpretation of the patient's 12-lead ECG and other diagnostic tests.

Nonsurgical Management. Nonsurgical management of dysrhythmias includes drug therapy, vagal maneuvers, temporary pacing, cardioversion, cardiopulmonary resuscitation (CPR), defibrillation, and catheter ablation. The Joint Commission's 2007 National Patient Safety Goals (NPSGs) include standardizing and limiting the number of drug concentrations used by organizations, identifying and listing look-alike/sound-alike medications to prevent errors, and labeling all medications and medication containers. Many types of drugs are given to manage dysrhythmias.

Drug therapy. Drug therapy for dysrhythmias often includes those from one or more classes of antidysrhythmic agents (see Chart 36-2). The **Vaughn-Williams classification** is commonly used to categorize drugs according to their effects on the action potential of cardiac cells (classes I though IV). Other drugs also have antidysrhythmic effects but do not fit the Vaughn-Williams classification.

Class I antidysrhythmics are membrane-stabilizing agents used to decrease automaticity. The three subclassifications in this group include type IA drugs, which moderately slow conduction and prolong repolarization, prolonging the QT interval. These drugs are used to treat or to prevent supraventricular and ventricular premature beats and tachydysrhythmias, but they are not as commonly used as other drugs. An example is procainamide hydrochloride (Pronestyl). Type IB drugs shorten repolarization. These drugs are used to treat or prevent ventricular premature beats, ventricular tachycardia (VT), and ventricular fibrillation (VF). Examples include lidocaine and mexiletine hydrochloride (Mexitil). Type IC drugs markedly slow conduction and widen the QRS complex. These agents are used primarily to treat or to prevent recurrent, life-threatening ventricular premature beats, VT, and VF. Examples include flecainide acetate (Tambocor) and propafenone hydrochloride (Rythmol).

Class II antidysrhythmics control dysrhythmias associated with excessive beta-adrenergic stimulation by competing for receptor sites and thereby decreasing heart rate and conduction velocity. Beta-adrenergic blocking agents, such as propranolol (Inderal) and esmolol hydrochloride (Brevibloc), are class II drugs. They are used to treat or to prevent supraventricular and ventricular premature beats and tachydysrhythmias. Sotalol hydrochloride (Betapace, Sotacor🍁) is an antidysrhythmic agent with both non-cardioselective beta-adrenergic blocking effects (class II) and action potential duration prolongation properties (class III). It is an oral agent recommended for the treatment of documented ventricular dysrhythmias, such as VT, that are life threatening.

Class III antidysrhythmics lengthen the absolute refractory period and prolong repolarization and the action potential duration of ischemic cells. Class III drugs include amiodarone (Cordarone) and ibutilide (Corvert) and are used to treat or prevent ventricular premature beats, VT, and VF.

Class IV antidysrhythmics slow the flow of calcium into the cell during depolarization, thereby depressing the automaticity of the sinoatrial (SA) and atrioventricular (AV) nodes, decreasing the heart rate, and prolonging the AV nodal refractory period and conduction. Calcium channel blockers, such as verapamil hydrochloride (Calan, Isoptin🍁) and diltiazem hydrochloride (Cardizem), are class IV drugs. They are used to treat supraventricular tachycardia (SVT), atrial flutter, and atrial fibrillation (AF) to slow the ventricular response.

Other drugs, such as digoxin, atropine, adenosine, and magnesium sulfate, may be used to treat dysrhythmias. Digoxin (Lanoxin, Novodigoxin🍁) increases vagal tone, slowing AV nodal conduction. It is useful in treating chronic AF

Chart 36-4 COMMON EXAMPLES OF DRUG THERAPY

Cardiac Arrest

Drug	Usual Dosage	Nursing Interventions	Rationales
Epinephrine (Adrenalin) Used for asystole, VF, VT, PEA, hypotension, anaphylaxis	1-mg IV bolus followed by 20-mL saline flush every 3-5 min If this fails, consider 2-5 mg IV bolus every 3-5 min; 1-mg, 3-mg, and 5-mg IV boluses (3 min apart); or 0.1 mg/kg IV bolus every 3-5 min If necessary give endotracheally with dose at least 2-2$^{1}/_{2}$ times the IV dose	Monitor for return of rhythm and pulse when used for asystole or VF.	Return of rhythm and pulse is the expected response.
		Assess for tachycardia, dysrhythmias, or hypertension.	Adverse reactions can occur with a dramatic response.
		Assess for the development of coarse VF when given during the VF.	This may improve the response to defibrillation.
Amiodarone hydrochloride (Cordarone) Used for AF, PAF, PSVT, life-threatening ventricular dysrhythmias	300 mg IV push for cardiac arrest in VF/pulseless VT 150 mg IVP over 10 min (15 mg/min), followed by 360 mg IV over next 6 hr (1 mg/min), followed by 540 mg IV over next 18 hr (0.5 mg/min) After first 24 hr, continue maintenance infusion of 720 mg/24 hr (0.5 mg/min)	Monitor for return of rhythm and pulse when used for recurrent unstable VT or VF.	Return of rhythm and pulse is the expected response.
		Use with extreme caution in patients receiving other antidysrhythmics.	Amiodarone reduces the hepatic and renal clearance of certain antiarrhythmics, specifically procainamide, quinidine, and flecainide.
		Use caution in patients with pulmonary, hepatic, or thyroid disease.	Amiodarone can cause fatal toxicity, especially in patients receiving more than 600 mg daily.
		Perform continuous cardiac monitoring while the patient is receiving the loading dose.	There is a slow onset of antiarrhythmic effect and a high risk of life-threatening arrhythmias.
Dopamine hydrochloride (Intropin) Used for hypotension, shock, CHF, renal failure	2.5-5 mcg/kg/min IV infusion; titrate to desired clinical response 1-2 mcg/kg/min for renal and mesenteric vasodilation 2-10 mcg/kg/min for beta-adrenergic effects 10-20 mcg/kg/min for alpha-adrenergic effects	Assess patients for increased BP.	Increased BP is the expected response.
		Monitor for tachycardia, dysrhythmias, or hypertension.	Adverse reactions may occur.
		Monitor IV site for infiltration.	Extravasation of drug can occur, causing necrosis.
		Assess for urine output <30 mL/hr, pallor, cyanosis, pain, or numbness in the extremities.	Dosages >10 mcg/kg/min cause vasoconstriction of renal and peripheral blood vessels; dosages of 2-5 mcg/kg/min may improve urine output by causing renal vasodilation and improving renal blood flow.

and atrial flutter by controlling the rate of ventricular response. However, digoxin does not convert AF to sinus rhythm. Atropine is a parasympatholytic or vagolytic agent. It is used to treat vagally induced symptomatic bradydysrhythmias. Adenosine is an endogenous nucleoside that slows AV nodal conduction to interrupt re-entry pathways. Magnesium sulfate is an electrolyte administered to treat refractory VT or VF because these patients may be hypomagnesemic, with increased ventricular irritability. The drug is also used for a life-threatening VT called **torsades de pointes** that often results from certain antidysrhythmics, such as amiodarone.

In addition to antidysrhythmics, several other *drugs are used during cardiac arrest* (Chart 36-4). *Epinephrine (Adrenalin) is a first-line agent in all cardiac arrests.* It is given mainly for its alpha-adrenergic effects to increase vasomotor tone for myocardial and cerebral perfusion. Its beta-adrenergic effects may stimulate the heart and increase myocardial contractility to improve cardiac output. Vasopressin has potent vasoconstricting effects and is equivalent to epinephrine in VF and pulseless VT. It has a long half-life and is given one time as an IV bolus of 40 units. Dopamine hydrochloride (Intropin) is generally used for its beta-adrenergic effects after cardiac arrest but may be used for its alpha-adrenergic effects during resuscitation. Dobutamine hydrochloride (Dobutrex) is a beta-adrenergic agent used to improve myocardial contractility and increase cardiac output.

Norepinephrine (Levophed) or phenylephrine hydrochloride (Neo-Synephrine) may be used for its alpha-adrenergic effects to increase vasomotor tone and increase perfusion pres-

Chart 36-4 COMMON EXAMPLES OF DRUG THERAPY
Cardiac Arrest—cont'd

Drug	Usual Dosage	Nursing Interventions	Rationales
Dobutamine hydrochloride (Dobutrex) Used for short-term management of cardiac decompensation	2-20 mcg/kg/min IV infusion	Assess for increased BP.	Increased BP is the expected response.
		Assess for hypertension and dysrhythmias.	Adverse reactions may occur.
Norepinephrine (Levophed) Used for cardiogenic shock and hypotension	0.5-1 mcg/min IV infusion, titrate to desired effect, up to 8-30 mcg/min	Assess for increased BP.	Increased BP is the expected response.
		Monitor for bradycardia.	Reflex bradycardia may occur with a rise in BP.
		Monitor for hypertension and dysrhythmias.	Adverse reactions may occur with a dramatic response.
		Administer drug through central IV line.	Extravasation can occur.
		Assess for urine output <30 mL/hr, pallor, cyanosis, pain, or numbness in the extremities.	Norepinephrine is a powerful vasoconstrictor.
		Assess for chest pain after resuscitation.	Norepinephrine increases myocardial oxygen demand.
Sodium bicarbonate Used for acid-base imbalance, metabolic acidosis	1 mEq/kg IV bolus given after the first 10 min of cardiac arrest if necessary 0.5 mEq/kg IV bolus every 10 min thereafter if necessary	Assess arterial blood gas values for metabolic acidosis.	Administration without evidence of metabolic acidosis can result in alkalosis, which can hinder resuscitation efforts.
Isoproterenol (Isuprel) Used for bradycardia, torsades de pointes, beta blocker OD	2-10 mcg/min IV infusion; titrate to desired clinical response	Assess for increased heart rate.	Increased heart rate is the expected response.
		Assess for tachycardia, hypotension, or hypertension.	Adverse reactions may occur with a dramatic response.
		Assess for chest pain after resuscitation.	Isoproterenol increases myocardial oxygen demand.
		Monitor for ventricular dysrhythmias.	Isoproterenol increases ventricular irritability, especially in patients who are hypokalemic or who are receiving digitalis.
Calcium chloride ($CaCl_2$) Used for hyperkalemia, hypocalcemia, calcium channel or beta blocker OD	2-4 mg/kg IV slowly; may repeat every 10 min if necessary	Calcium chloride is indicated only for cardiac arrest associated with hyperkalemia, hypocalcemia, or calcium channel blocker toxicity.	Calcium chloride may cause cellular damage and cerebrovascular spasm.
Vasopressin Used for VF, asystole, PEA, shock	40 units IV bolus, one time	Monitor for return of rhythm and pulse when used for VF or pulseless VT.	Return of rhythm and pulse is the expected response.

AF, Atrial fibrillation; *BP*, blood pressure; *CHF*, congestive heart failure; IVP, IV push; *PAF*, paroxysmal AF; *PSVT*, paroxysmal supraventricular tachycardia; *OD*, overdose; *PEA*, pulseless electrical activity; *VF*, ventricular fibrillation; *VT*, ventricular tachycardia.

sure. Sodium bicarbonate, along with regular insulin and calcium chloride, may be administered during cardiac arrest for patients who are hyperkalemic. It may also be used, if necessary, to treat a documented base deficit metabolic acidosis, as occurs in diabetic ketoacidosis or tricyclic antidepressant overdose. In addition to hyperkalemia, calcium chloride is given for hypocalcemia or calcium channel blocker toxicity because the conditions may cause cell damage and cerebrovascular vasospasm. Isoproterenol (Isuprel) is indicated to increase the heart rate in heart transplant patients, but pacing is preferred.

Vagal maneuvers. Vagal maneuvers induce vagal stimulation of the cardiac conduction system, specifically the SA and

AV nodes. Although not as common today, vagal maneuvers may be attempted to treat supraventricular tachydysrhythmias and include carotid sinus massage and Valsalva maneuvers. The results of these interventions, however, are often temporary and may cause "rebound" tachycardia or severe bradycardia. Further therapy must be initiated.

In **carotid sinus massage,** the physician massages over one carotid artery for a few seconds, observing for a change in cardiac rhythm. This intervention causes vagal stimulation, slowing SA and AV nodal conduction. Prepare the patient for the procedure, instruct him or her to turn the head slightly away from the side to be massaged, and observe the cardiac monitor for a change in rhythm. An ECG rhythm strip is recorded before, during, and after the procedure. After the procedure, assess vital signs and the level of consciousness. *Complications include bradydysrhythmias, asystole, VF, and cerebral damage. Because of these risks, carotid massage is not commonly performed. A defibrillator and resuscitative equipment must be immediately available during the procedure.*

To stimulate a *vagal reflex,* the health care provider instructs the patient to bear down as if straining to have a bowel movement. Assess the patient's heart rate, heart rhythm, and blood pressure; observe the cardiac monitor; and record an ECG rhythm strip before, during, and after the procedure to determine the effect of therapy.

Unintended vagal stimulation sometimes occurs. Therefore be very cautious when performing procedures that may accidentally cause it. For example, tracheal suctioning, enema administration, and rectal temperature checks can stimulate the vagus nerve and decrease the heart rate. Instruct the patient not to strain during bowel movements and to avoid constipation through proper diet and exercise. Stool softeners may be prescribed. Instruct the patient to prevent gagging during oral hygiene, which can also trigger a vagal response. Monitor the heart rate and rhythm of a patient who is vomiting, because a vagal reflex can result. Some patients experience a vagal response when raising their arms above their head and must be reminded to avoid this movement. Tight collars and neckties can also trigger vagal responses.

Temporary pacing. **Temporary pacing** is a nonsurgical intervention that provides a timed electrical stimulus to the heart when either the impulse initiation or the conduction system of the heart is defective. The electrical stimulus then spreads throughout the heart to depolarize the cells, which should be followed by contraction and cardiac output. Electrical stimuli may be delivered to the right atrium or right ventricle (single-chamber pacemakers) or to both (dual-chamber pacemakers).

When a pacing stimulus is delivered to the heart, a spike (or pacemaker artifact) is seen on the monitor or ECG strip. The spike should be followed by evidence of depolarization (i.e., a P wave, indicating atrial depolarization, or a QRS complex, indicating ventricular depolarization). This pattern is referred to as *capture,* indicating that the pacemaker has successfully depolarized, or captured, the chamber.

Temporary pacing is used for patients with symptomatic, atropine-refractory bradydysrhythmias (particularly second-degree heart block type II and third-degree heart block) or for patients with asystole. Temporary pacing may also be initiated prophylactically in stable patients with left bundle branch block in certain situations, such as insertion of a pulmonary artery catheter.

A different type of pacing may be used to treat symptomatic tachydysrhythmias. Occasionally **atrial overdrive pacing** is attempted to terminate atrial tachydysrhythmias, such as atrial flutter or atrial fibrillation (AF). Overdrive pacing is accomplished by rapidly pacing the atrium to capture the heart and control depolarization, followed by no pacing, in the hope that the sinus node will regain control of the heart. Ventricular overdrive pacing may be done to end ventricular tachydysrhythmias in much the same way. This procedure is usually performed by the physician or advanced practice nurse who is specially trained. *Have emergency equipment available in case the patient becomes more unstable or goes into cardiac arrest.*

The two basic modes of pacing are synchronous (demand) pacing and asynchronous (fixed-rate) pacing. Temporary pacing is *usually* done in the synchronous (demand) pacing mode. The pacemaker's sensitivity is set to sense the patient's own beats. When the patient's heart rate is above the rate set on the pulse generator, the pacemaker does not fire. When the patient's heart rate is less than the generator setting, the pacemaker provides electrical impulses.

The **asynchronous (fixed-rate) pacing mode** is used when the patient is asystolic or profoundly bradycardic, which may occur after open-heart surgery. When the pulse generator is set in an asynchronous mode, it does not sense any heart beats. The pacemaker continues to fire at a fixed rate as set on the generator. This continued firing is not a problem as long as the patient remains asystolic or has a rate slower than the pacemaker rate, because all beats come from the pacemaker and there is no competition from the patient's beats. If the patient's rate increases and equals or exceeds the pacemaker rate, however, competition (undersensing) is noted. The danger is that a pacemaker stimulus may reach the heart during the vulnerable period of repolarization (R-on-T phenomenon, with the pacer spike falling on the T wave) and possibly cause ventricular fibrillation (VF). If this occurs, set the pacemaker to a synchronous mode to avert potential problems.

The two basic types of *temporary* pacing are noninvasive (external) temporary pacing and invasive temporary pacing. **Noninvasive temporary pacing (NTP)** is accomplished through the application of two large external electrodes. The electrodes are attached to an external pulse generator, which can operate on alternating current (AC) or battery power. The generator emits electrical pulses, which are transmitted through the electrodes and then transcutaneously to stimulate ventricular depolarization when the patient's heart rate is slower than the rate set on the pacemaker.

Noninvasive temporary pacing is used as an emergency measure to provide demand ventricular pacing in a profoundly bradycardic or asystolic patient until invasive pacing can be used or the patient's heart rate returns to normal. It may be used prophylactically when performing procedures or transporting patients at risk for bradydysrhythmias. However, it is used only as a temporary measure to maintain heart rate and perfusion until a more permanent method of pacing is used.

Depending on the facility, nurses on telemetry units may perform noninvasive temporary pacing. In a nonemergent situation, explain NTP to the patient and family and prepare the equipment. Wash the skin with soap and water. Do not rub the skin or apply alcohol or tinctures on the skin because electrical current flows from the patches through the skin and causes discomfort. Apply the electrodes on the chest according to package instructions, with one placed on the upper chest to the right of the sternum and one placed over the heart apex. The electrode cannot be placed over female breast tissue. Displace the breast tissue to position the electrode underneath the breast.

Turn the pacer on, set the pacing rate as ordered, and establish the stimulation threshold (the lowest current that achieves capture with each pacing spike followed by a QRS complex). Set the current milliamperes (mA) output 2 mA above the dose at which consistent capture is observed. The rate should be adjusted according to patient response. The QRS complex is wide because one ventricle depolarizes first, followed by the other.

Palpate the right radial or carotid pulse, and assess the blood pressure using the patient's right arm, ensuring that each paced beat is perfused. Vital signs are not taken on the left side of the body because they may not be accurate, particularly if a high milliamperage is used.

The most common complication of NTP is discomfort from muscle stimulation, skin irritation, and diaphoresis (excessive sweating) from the patch electrodes. Be sure that the electrodes are in good contact with the skin and in the best location to achieve the lowest threshold. Give analgesics or sedatives as prescribed to provide comfort.

An **invasive temporary pacemaker** system consists of an external battery-operated pulse generator and pacing electrodes, or lead wires. These wires attach to the generator on one end and are in contact with the heart on the other end. Electrical pulses, or stimuli, are emitted from the negative terminal of the generator, flow through a lead wire, and stimulate the cardiac cells to depolarize. The current seeks ground by returning through the other lead wire to the positive terminal of the generator, thus completing a circuit. The intensity of electrical current is set by selecting the appropriate current output, measured in milliamperes.

Patients do not usually feel invasive pacemaker stimuli. However, they occasionally feel an uncomfortable sensation from the stimuli if strong electrical currents (high milliamperage) are delivered by the pacemaker. The discomfort may be alleviated by decreasing the current if possible.

Complications of invasive temporary pacing may be serious and include:

- Infection or hematoma at the pacemaker wire insertion site
- Ectopic complexes (usually premature ventricular complexes [PVCs]) caused by irritability from the pacing wire in the ventricle, use of high current, or undersensing with pacemaker competition
- Loss of capture, noted by the presence of a pacing stimulus or spike but no QRS complex
- Undersensing or pacemaker competition, noted when pacing stimuli occur at a fixed rate in the presence of an adequate intrinsic rhythm
- Oversensing, noted when the pacemaker fails to fire in the presence of an inadequate intrinsic rhythm
- Electromagnetic interference, noted by altered generator variables
- Stimulation of the chest wall or diaphragm, noted by rhythmic contraction of the chest wall muscles or hiccups with the use of high current or from lead wire perforation, which could cause cardiac tamponade

For patient safety, when the metal external ends of lead wires are not attached to a pulse generator, insulate the wire ends to prevent microshock. The fingertips of rubber gloves work well for this purpose, and the wire ends may then be looped and covered with nonconductive tape. All electrical equipment in the room must be properly grounded using a three-pronged plug. Report faulty electrical equipment, such as frayed or broken electrical wire, to the biomedical engineering department. Neither the patient nor the bed should be in contact with such equipment. The risk is that ungrounded electrical current may conduct through the lead wire, stimulate the heart, and cause ventricular fibrillation (VF). Remember to wear rubber gloves when touching any of the wires. Static electricity may be conducted from your hands to the patient, causing dysrhythmias if gloves are not worn.

Cardiopulmonary resuscitation. Management of the patient in cardiac arrest depends on prompt recognition and therapeutic interventions for successful reversal of a potentially fatal event.

When cardiac arrest occurs, cardiac output stops. The underlying rhythm is usually ventricular tachycardia (VT), ventricular fibrillation (VF), or asystole. Without cardiac output, the patient is pulseless and becomes unconscious because of inadequate cerebral *perfusion and oxygenation.* Shortly after cardiac arrest, respiratory arrest occurs.

Cardiopulmonary resuscitation (CPR), also known as *basic cardiac life support (BCLS),* must be initiated immediately to help prevent brain damage and death. When finding an unresponsive patient, confirm unresponsiveness and call 911 or the emergency response team *before initiating CPR.* The initial priorities are ABC:

- Maintain a patent **a**irway.
- Ventilate (**b**reathing) with a mouth-to-mask device.
- Start chest **c**ompressions.

Reduce the risk of health care–associated infections by using Standard Precautions. As soon as help arrives, a board is placed under the patient who is not on a firm surface. To make room for the resuscitation team and the crash cart, ask that the area be cleared of movable items and unnecessary personnel.

An area that has been researched recently is the effectiveness of ventilation and complications associated with CPR. Several new recommendations for improved CPR have been suggested. In the health care setting, devices such as the ResQPOD are being used to regulate pressures in the thorax to prevent complications such as pneumothorax. It is used only when the pulse is absent. The American Heart Association's guidelines support the use of this device to increase circulation during CPR by refilling the heart after each chest compression.

Another area of research is the support of hands-only CPR, especially when the cardiac arrest occurs outside the hospital setting. Evidence suggests that chest compressions by themselves may be as effective as compressions *with* ventilation. Although not yet incorporated into the CPR guidelines, the recommendations are (Sayre et al., 2008):

- Bystanders (laypeople) not trained in CPR should use only hands-only CPR.
- Bystanders trained in CPR who are confident in their ability to provide rescue breathing should use either the standard CPR procedure OR the hands-only technique.
- Bystanders trained in CPR who are *not* confident in their ability to provide rescue breathing should use only the hands-only technique.

Additional clinical research is needed before the CPR guidelines may change.

Complications of standard CPR include:

- Rib fractures
- Fracture of the sternum

- Costochondral separation
- Lacerations of the liver and spleen
- Pneumothorax
- Hemothorax
- Cardiac tamponade
- Lung contusions
- Fat emboli

The desired outcome of resuscitation is the rapid return of a pulse, blood pressure, and consciousness. This is rarely achieved by CPR and basic measures alone. More definitive therapy must be initiated as soon as possible with advanced cardiac life support (ACLS) measures, including defibrillation, if needed.

Advanced cardiac life support. *Whereas all nurses and other health care personnel should learn CPR, special training is required to perform ACLS.* When the AED or crash cart arrives, apply ECG electrodes to the patient's chest and turn on the monitor. Direct the team to continue CPR, and continue to coordinate the personnel who respond to the emergency. *If the patient is in VF or pulseless VT, the immediate priority is to defibrillate! After defibrillation, CPR is resumed. CPR must continue at all times except during defibrillation. The term "push hard and push fast" is used to improve circulation during resuscitation.*

An oropharyngeal airway is inserted to facilitate proper ventilation. A manual resuscitation bag (MRB) with mask is attached to an oxygen flowmeter set at 10 to 15 L/min. Direct the person managing the airway to ventilate the lungs with the MRB, maintaining the proper head-tilt or chin-lift position of the patient. Start two large-bore IV lines if the patient does not have any infusing normal saline. These lines provide access for emergency drug administration. Suction equipment is also set up, with a tonsillar suction tube for suctioning vomitus and a suction catheter for endotracheal suctioning. Check carotid or femoral pulses with or without chest compressions, blood pressure, and pupils every few minutes. Document all assessments and findings, therapeutic measures, and the patient's responses throughout the resuscitation.

Additional measures include endotracheal intubation with ventilation and oxygenation, IV administration of emergency cardiac drugs, and occasionally external pacing. Chest compressions are continued as long as the patient remains pulseless or until a physician decides to terminate resuscitation attempts.

If ACLS is successful and the patient has a return of spontaneous circulation (ROSC), clinical evidence indicates that *therapeutic hypothermia* helps protect the nervous system, especially the brain. This therapy is indicated for patients who had VF, VT pulseless activity, or asystole and should be started as soon as possible after ROSC. The patient is cooled quickly with a cooling blanket, hypothermia pads, or other method to reach the target of 89.6° to 93.2° F (32° to 34° C). Maintain this temperature for 24 hours before slowly rewarming the patient at a rate of 0.5° to 1° C per hour (Pyle et al., 2007). Cardiovascular support with drug therapy and other treatments are used as needed during this process.

NCLEX EXAMINATION CHALLENGE

A client's ECG monitor shows asystole. He becomes unresponsive and is not breathing. What is the nurse's first priority?

A. Begin chest compressions.
B. Establish an airway.
C. Ventilate with a breathing mask.
D. Elevate the head of the bed.

evolve For the correct answer, go to http://evolve.elsevier.com/Iggy/.

Cardioversion. Cardioversion is a *synchronized* countershock that may be performed in emergencies for unstable ventricular or supraventricular tachydysrhythmias or electively for stable tachydysrhythmias that are resistant to medical therapies. If the patient has been taking digoxin, the drug is withheld for up to 48 hours before an elective cardioversion. Digoxin increases ventricular irritability and puts the patient at risk for VF after the countershock. For elective cardioversion for atrial flutter or fibrillation, the patient must take anticoagulants for 4 to 6 weeks before the procedure to prevent clots from moving from the heart to the brain or lungs.

The shock depolarizes a large amount of myocardium during the cardiac depolarization. It is intended to stop the re-entry circuit and allow the sinus node to regain control of the heart. Emergency equipment must be available during the procedure. The physician, advanced practice nurse, or other qualified nurse explains the procedure to the patient and family. Assist the patient in signing a consent form unless the procedure is an emergency for a life-threatening dysrhythmia. Because he or she is usually conscious, a short-acting anesthetic agent should be administered for sedation.

One electrode is placed to the left of the precordium, and the other is placed on the right next to the sternum and below the clavicle. The defibrillator should be set in the synchronized mode. This avoids discharging the shock during the T wave, which may increase ventricular irritability, causing ventricular fibrillation (VF). Charge the defibrillator to the energy level requested, usually starting at a low rate. *For safety, be sure that the oxygen delivery device has been removed and turned away from the patient. Oxygen supports combustion, and a fire may result if there is arcing from the electrodes.*

The health care provider loudly and clearly asks all personnel to clear contact with the patient and the bed, as required for electrical safety. Ensure that all personnel have cleared contact before the shock is delivered.

After cardioversion, assess the patient's response and heart rhythm. Therapy is repeated as requested, if necessary, until the desired result is obtained or alternative therapies are considered. If the patient's condition deteriorates into VF after cardioversion, check to see that the synchronizer is turned off so that immediate defibrillation can be administered.

Nursing care after cardioversion includes:

- Maintaining a patent airway
- Administering oxygen
- Assessing vital signs and the level of consciousness
- Administering antidysrhythmic drug therapy, as prescribed
- Monitoring for dysrhythmias
- Assessing for chest burns from electrodes
- Providing emotional support
- Documenting the results of cardioversion

Defibrillation. Defibrillation, an *asynchronous* countershock, depolarizes a critical mass of myocardium simultaneously to stop the re-entry circuit, allowing the sinus node to regain control of the heart. *Early defibrillation is critical in resolving pulseless VT or VF. It must not be delayed for any reason after the equipment and skilled personnel are present. The earlier defibrillation is performed, the greater the chance of survival.*

Effective CPR should continue until a defibrillator is available. Newer biphasic defibrillators allow a lower direct current shock and cause less damage to the myocardium. Therefore they are replacing older monophasic defibrillators in most facilities. The defibrillator is charged to 120 to 200 joules (biphasic) or 360 joules (monophasic) for one countershock from the defibrillator. Before defibrillation, loudly and clearly command all personnel to clear contact with the patient and the bed and check to see they are clear before the shock is delivered. Resume CPR immediately after the shock, and continue CPR for 5 cycles or about 2 minutes. Then reassess the rhythm, and if VF or pulseless VT continues, charge the defibrillator to give a second shock at the same energy level previously used. Resume CPR after the shock, and continue with the ACLS protocol. Nursing care for defibrillation is the same as for cardioversion.

Automatic external defibrillation. The American Heart Association promotes the use of automatic external defibrillators (AEDs) for use by laypersons and health care professionals responding to cardiac arrest emergencies (Fig. 36-13). These devices are found in many public places such as malls and commercial jets. The patient in cardiac arrest must be on a firm, dry surface. The rescuer places two large adhesive-patch electrodes on the patient's chest in the same positions as for defibrillator electrodes. The rescuer stops CPR and commands anyone present to move away, ensuring that no one is touching the patient. This measure eliminates motion artifact when the machine analyzes the rhythm. The rescuer presses the "analyze" button on the machine. After rhythm analysis, which may take up to 30 seconds, the machine either advises that a shock is necessary or advises that a shock is not indicated. *Shocks are recommended for VF or pulseless VT only.*

If a shock is indicated, issue a command to clear all contact with the patient and press the charge button. Once the AED is charged, press the shock button and the shock will be delivered according to ACLS protocol. The shock is delivered through the patches, so it is hands-off defibrillation, which is safer for the rescuer. The rescuer then resumes CPR until the AED instructs to "stop CPR" to analyze the rhythm. If the rhythm is VF or VT and another shock is indicated, the AED will instruct the rescuer to charge and deliver another shock. Newer AEDs perform rhythm analysis and defibrillation without the need for a rescuer to press a button to analyze or to shock the victim. It is essential that ACLS be provided as soon as possible. Use of AEDs allows for earlier defibrillation. Therefore there is a greater chance of successful rhythm conversion and patient survival.

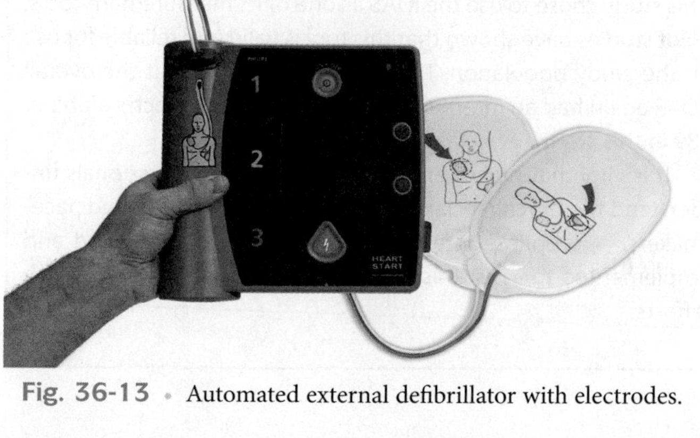
1
2
3
HEART START
Fig. 36-13 • Automated external defibrillator with electrodes.

Radiofrequency catheter ablation. Radiofrequency catheter ablation is an invasive procedure that may be used to destroy an irritable focus causing a supraventricular or ventricular tachydysrhythmia. The patient must first undergo electrophysiologic studies and mapping procedures to locate the focus. Then radiofrequency waves are delivered to abolish the irritable focus. When ablation is performed in the AV nodal or His bundle area, damage may also occur to the normal conduction system, causing heart blocks and requiring implantation of a permanent pacemaker.

Surgical Management. Patients who have life-threatening dysrhythmias may require surgical treatment for long-term management. The type of treatment depends on the nature of the dysrhythmia. Procedures include permanent pacing, coronary artery bypass grafting (CABG), aneurysmectomy, insertion of an implantable cardioverter/defibrillator, and open-chest cardiac massage.

Permanent pacemaker insertion is performed to treat conduction disorders that are not temporary, including complete heart block. These pacemakers are usually powered by a lithium battery and have an average life span of 10 years. After the battery power is depleted, the generator must be replaced by a procedure done with the patient under local anesthesia. Some pacemakers are nuclear-powered and have a life span of 20 years or longer. Other pacemakers can be recharged externally. Combination pacemaker/defibrillator devices are also available.

A newer type of pacemaker may be utilized to coordinate contractions between the right and left ventricles. In addition to pacing used in the right side of the heart, an additional lead is placed in the left lateral wall of the left ventricle through the coronary sinus. This procedure allows synchronized depolarization of the ventricles and is used in patients with moderate to severe heart failure to improve functional ability.

The surgeon usually implants the pulse generator in a surgically made subcutaneous pocket at the shoulder in the right or left subclavicular area, which creates a visible bulge. The leads are introduced transvenously via the cephalic or the subclavian vein to the endocardium on the right side of the heart. After the procedure, monitor the ECG rhythm to check that the pacemaker is working correctly. Assess the implantation site for bleeding, swelling, redness, tenderness, and infection. The dressing over the site should remain clean and dry. The patient should be afebrile and have stable vital signs. The physician prescribes initial activity restrictions, which are then gradually changed. Complications of permanent pacemakers are similar to those of temporary invasive pacing.

Pacemaker checks are done on an ambulatory care basis at regular intervals. Reprogramming may be needed if pacemaker problems develop. The pulse generator is interrogated using an electronic device to determine the pacemaker settings and battery life.

For patients who live far from the pacemaker clinic or physician's office, pacemaker information can be sent by telephone. The patient attaches ECG electrodes to the wrists or chest and places the telephone receiver in a transmitting unit. The sound signals are relayed via telephone lines to the clinic or office, where they are converted and recorded as the ECG rhythm strip and information about the pacemaker variables. Stress the need to keep clinic appointments for more detailed pacemaker checks and reprogramming, if necessary, as well as for assessment.

Coronary artery bypass grafting (CABG) is performed if the cause of the dysrhythmia is coronary artery insufficiency that is unresponsive to medical therapy. This procedure is described in Chapter 40.

Ventricular aneurysms are a complication of myocardial infarction (MI) and may be the source of intractable ventricular tachydysrhythmias. The surgeon *resects the* ***aneurysm***, a ballooning portion of the ventricular wall. Resection of the area eliminates the dangerous irritable focus and thus the cause of the dysrhythmias. Care of the patient is similar to that for CABG, described in Chapter 40.

The *implantable cardioverter/defibrillator (ICD)* is indicated for patients who have experienced one or more episodes of spontaneous sustained ventricular tachycardia (VT) or ventricular fibrillation (VF) not caused by an MI. Collaborate with the physician and the electrophysiology nurse to prepare the patient for this procedure. A psychological profile is done to determine whether the patient can cope with the discomfort and fear associated with internal defibrillation from the ICD. Many patients report anxiety or other psychological distress, especially when ICD shocks occur (Sears & Conti, 2006). Several nursing assessment tools have been developed and tested to determine the patient's adjustment after an ICD (see the Evidence-Based Practice box below).

The leads of the device are introduced through the skin, and the generator is implanted in the left pectoral area, similar to a permanent pacemaker insertion procedure. This procedure is performed in the electrophysiology laboratory. If ICD therapies are not successful and the patient remains in VF or pulseless VT, the qualified nurse or health care provider must promptly externally defibrillate.

The generator may be activated or deactivated by the physician placing a magnet over the implantation site for a few moments. The patient requires close monitoring in the postoperative period for dysrhythmias and complications such as bleeding and cardiac tamponade. The nurse must know whether the ICD is activated or deactivated. Care of the patient is similar to that after implantation of a permanent pacemaker.

When external chest compressions and ACLS measures are unsuccessful in resuscitating the patient in cardiac arrest, the physician may perform *open-chest cardiac massage* using a thoracotomy or sternotomy approach in post–cardiac surgery patients. Internal defibrillation may also be performed. This procedure is a drastic measure that frequently results in devastating consequences for the patient *and is therefore used as a last resort.*

Community-Based Care

For many patients, dysrhythmias are a disorder resulting from chronic cardiac and pulmonary diseases. Patients may be cared for in a variety of settings, including the acute care hospital, subacute unit, traditional nursing home, or their own home. They are admitted to the hospital when they experience life-threatening or potentially life-threatening dysrhythmias, often associated with an acute disorder. Others can be managed with office or clinic visits or in other settings.

Home Care Management

Patients discharged from the hospital may have considerable needs, often more related to their underlying chronic diseases than to their dysrhythmias. A case manager or care coordinator can assess the need for health care resources and coordinate access to services.

The focus of the home care nurse's interventions is assessment and health teaching. Patients and families often fear recurrence of a life-threatening dysrhythmia. Patients with an ICD may dread or fear the activation of the device. The community-based nurse provides the patient and family members with an opportunity to verbalize their concerns and fears. Provide emotional support as well as information about support groups and referrals in the community. Assess the patient for possible side effects of antidysrhythmic agents or complications from a pacemaker or ICD.

Health Teaching

The patient who has had a dysrhythmia caused by an acute problem, such as electrolyte imbalance or MI, is taught about prevention, early recognition, and management of that disor-

EVIDENCE-BASED PRACTICE

How do patients with implanted cardiac devices adjust?

Beery, T.A., Baas, L.S., & Henthorn, C. (2007). Self-reported adjustment to implanted cardiac devices. *Journal of Cardiovascular Nursing, 22*(6), 516-524.

This cross-sectional design study provides information about how patients who have implanted devices (implantable cardioverter/defibrillators [ICDs] and pacemakers) can adjust to this change in their daily lives. A convenience sample of 174 men and women was recruited from two large midwestern U.S. cities. Subjects completed the Implanted Device Adjustment Scale (IDAS), the SF-36 quality-of-life measure, and several tools about mood. Perceived adjustment was good regardless of age, gender, type of device, and whether a shock was delivered. The results of the IDAS were weakly correlated with the mental component of the SF-36 but not the physical component. Patients with ICDs were more fearful and anxious than those with pacemakers.

Level of Evidence—6. The evidence was obtained from a single descriptive study.

Commentary: Implications for Practice and Research. Previous studies have shown that patients with ICDs have anxiety and fear related to having implanted cardiac devices. The authors of this study chose to use the IDAS as one of its measurement tools. Pilot studies have shown that this tool is valid and reliable for use in the study population. The researchers found that the overall IDAS again had an internal consistency with Cronbach's alpha of .89 in this study.

It is vital that nurses and other health care professionals understand the psychosocial implications of having ICDs and pacemakers. Appropriate interventions need to be developed and implemented to assist this group of patients in further research efforts.

der. Teach the patient and family about lifestyle modifications designed to prevent, decrease, or control the occurrence of dysrhythmias, as outlined in Chart 36-5. This teaching may be provided in the acute care setting, physician's office, health care clinic, or home setting.

Patients and their families must have a thorough understanding of the prescribed *drug therapy*, including antidysrhythmic agents. Pharmacies provide written instructions with filled prescriptions. Teach patients and families the generic and trade names of their drugs, as well as the drugs' purposes, using basic terms that are easily understood. Clear instructions regarding dosage schedules and common side effects are important (see Chart 36-2). Emphasize the importance of reporting these side effects and any dizziness, nausea, vomiting, chest discomfort, or shortness of breath to the health care provider. Chart 36-6 highlights special considerations for older adults receiving antidysrhythmic therapy.

Teach all patients and their family members how to take a pulse. Remind them to report any signs of a change in heart rhythm, such as a significant decrease in pulse rate, a rate more than 100 beats/min, or increased rhythm irregularity.

Patients who have a *permanent pacemaker* are given written and verbal information about the type and settings of their pacemaker. Teach the patient to report any pulse rate lower than that set on the pacemaker. Review the proper care of the pacemaker insertion site and the importance of reporting any fever or any redness, swelling, or drainage at the pacemaker insertion site. If the surgical incision is near either shoulder, teach and demonstrate range-of-motion exercises to perform to prevent shoulder stiffness.

Instruct patients with pacemakers to keep handheld cellular phones at least 6 inches away from the generator, with the handset on the ear opposite the side of the generator. Teach them to avoid sources of strong electromagnetic fields, such as magnets and telecommunications transmitters. These may cause interference and could change the pacemaker settings, causing a malfunction. Magnetic resonance imaging (MRI) is usually contraindicated, depending on the machine's technology. Remind patients to carry a pacemaker identification card and to wear a medical alert bracelet. Chart 36-7 outlines the major points for patient and family teaching after the insertion of a permanent pacemaker.

Patients with an *implantable cardioverter/defibrillator (ICD)* usually continue to receive antidysrhythmic drugs after discharge from the hospital. Provide clear instructions about the purposes of drug therapy, the dosage schedules, special instructions, and side effects that need to be reported. If patients experience an internal defibrillator shock, they must sit or lie down immediately and notify the physician. Some describe the experience of a shock as a quick thud or kick in the chest, whereas others relate severe discomfort similar to that of external defibrillation. Usually the shock is not as severe because the heart is sandwiched by the defibrillation pads, thus requiring less electrical current to convert the dysrhythmia. Inform family members that they may feel an electrical shock if they are touching the patient during delivery of the shock but that it is not harmful. Provide information about how to access the emergency medical services (EMS) system in the community. Recommend resources for the family to learn how to perform cardiopulmonary resuscitation (CPR).

Remind patients with an ICD to avoid sources of strong electromagnetic fields, such as large electrical generators and radio or television transmitters. These may inhibit tachydysrhythmia detection and therapy or may cause pacing or shocks. MRI is contraindicated for patients with ICDs. Handheld cellular phones must be at least 6 inches away from the generator, with the handset held to the ear opposite the side of the ICD. If the pulse generator emits a beeping sound or provides some other indicator, the patient must move away from the area as quickly as possible to prevent deactivation of the device. Teach the patient with an ICD to carry an ICD identification card and wear a medical alert bracelet. Chart 36-8 highlights the important points for teaching patients and family members and significant others.

Chart 36-5 PATIENT AND FAMILY EDUCATION GUIDE

How to Prevent or Decrease Dysrhythmias

FOR PATIENTS AT RISK FOR VASOVAGAL ATTACKS CAUSING BRADYDYSRHYTHMIAS

- Avoid doing things that stimulate the vagus nerve, such as raising your arms above your head, applying pressure over your carotid artery, applying pressure on your eyes, bearing down or straining during a bowel movement, and stimulating a gag reflex when brushing your teeth or putting objects in your mouth.

FOR PATIENTS WITH PREMATURE BEATS AND ECTOPIC RHYTHMS

- Take the medications that have been prescribed for you, and report any adverse effects to your physician.
- Stop smoking, avoid caffeinated beverages as much as possible, and drink alcohol only in moderation.
- Learn ways to manage stress and avoid getting too tired.

FOR PATIENTS WITH ISCHEMIC HEART DISEASE

- If you have an angina attack, treat it promptly with rest and nitroglycerin administration as prescribed by your physician. This decreases your chances of experiencing a dysrhythmia.
- If chest pain is not relieved after taking the amount of nitroglycerin that has been prescribed for you, seek medical attention promptly. Also, seek prompt medical attention if the pain becomes more severe or you experience other symptoms, such as sweating, nausea, weakness, and palpitations.

FOR PATIENTS AT RISK FOR POTASSIUM IMBALANCE

- Know the symptoms of decreased potassium levels, such as muscle weakness and cardiac irregularity.
- Eat foods high in potassium, such as tomatoes, beans, prunes, avocados, bananas, strawberries, and lettuce.
- Take the potassium supplements that have been prescribed for you.

NCLEX EXAMINATION CHALLENGE

A client with third-degree heart block is discharged to home with a permanent pacemaker. Which of these statements by the client indicates a need for further discharge teaching?

A. "I shouldn't get too close to any telephones, especially cellular ones."
B. "If my pulse is too low, I should set the pacemaker to the same rate."
C. "I will get an ID bracelet and card so everyone will know I have a pacemaker."
D. "I have to stay away from magnetic areas and MRI machines."

evolve For the correct answer, go to http://evolve.elsevier.com/Iggy/.

Chart 36-6 NURSING FOCUS ON THE OLDER ADULT

Dysrhythmias

Older adults are at increased risk for dysrhythmias because of changes in their cardiac conduction system. The sinoatrial node has fewer pacemaker cells. There is a loss of fibers in the bundle branch system. Therefore older adults are at risk for sinus node dysfunction and may require pacemaker therapy. The most common dysrhythmias are premature atrial contractions, premature ventricular contractions, and atrial fibrillation. Dysrhythmias tend to be more serious in older patients because of underlying heart disease, causing cardiac decompensation. Consequently, blood flow to organs, which may already be decreased because of the aging process, is further compromised, leading to multisystem organ dysfunction. Special nursing considerations for the older patient with dysrhythmias are:

- Evaluate the patient with dysrhythmias immediately for the presence of a life-threatening dysrhythmia or hemodynamic deterioration.
- Assess the patient with a dysrhythmia for angina, hypotension, heart failure, and decreased cerebral and renal perfusion.
- Consider these causes of dysrhythmias when taking the patient's history: hypoxia, drug toxicity, electrolyte imbalances, heart failure, and myocardial ischemia or infarction.
- Assess the patient's level of education, hearing, learning style, and ability to understand and recall instructions to determine the best approaches for teaching.
- Assess the patient's ability to read written instructions.
- Teach the patient the generic and trade names of prescribed antidysrhythmic drugs, as well as their purposes, dosage, side effects, and special instructions for their use.
- Provide clear written instructions in basic language and easy-to-read print.
- Provide a written drug dosage schedule for the patient, considering all the drugs the patient is taking and possible drug interactions.
- Assess the patient for possible side effects or adverse reactions to drugs considering age and health status.
- Teach the patient to take his or her pulse and to report significant changes in heart rate or rhythm to the health care provider.
- Inform the patient of available resources for blood pressure and pulse checks, such as blood pressure clinics, home health agencies, and cardiac rehabilitation programs.
- Instruct the patient on the importance of keeping follow-up appointments with the health care provider and reporting symptoms promptly.
- Include the patient's family members or significant other in all teaching whenever possible.
- Teach the patient to avoid drinking caffeinated beverages, to stop smoking, to drink alcohol only in moderation, and to follow his or her prescribed diet.

Chart 36-7 PATIENT AND FAMILY EDUCATION GUIDE

Permanent Pacemakers

- Follow the instructions for pacemaker site skin care that have been specifically prepared for you. Report any fever or redness, swelling, or drainage from the incision site to your physician.
- Keep your pacemaker identification card in your wallet, and wear a medical alert bracelet.
- Take your pulse for 1 full minute at the same time each day, and record the rate in your pacemaker diary. Take your pulse any time you feel symptoms of a possible pacemaker failure, and report your heart rate and symptoms to your physician.
- Know the rate at which your pacemaker is set and the basic functioning of your pacemaker. Know what rate changes to report to your physician.
- Do not apply pressure over your generator. Avoid tight clothing or belts.
- You may take baths or showers without concern for your pacemaker.
- Inform other physicians and dentists that you have a pacemaker. Certain tests they may wish to perform (e.g., magnetic resonance imaging) could affect or damage your pacemaker.
- Know the indications of battery failure for your pacemaker as you were instructed, and report these findings to your physician if they occur.
- Do not operate electrical appliances directly over your pacemaker site because this may cause your pacemaker to malfunction.
- Do not lean over electrical or gasoline engines or motors. Be sure that electrical appliances or motors are properly grounded.
- Avoid all transmitter towers for radio, television, and radar. Radio, television, other home appliances, and antennas do not pose a hazard.
- Be aware that antitheft devices in stores may cause temporary pacemaker malfunction. If symptoms develop, move away from the device.
- Inform airport personnel of your pacemaker before passing through a metal detector, and show them your pacemaker identification card. The metal in your pacemaker will trigger the alarm in the metal detector device.
- Stay away from any arc welding equipment.
- Be aware that it is safe to operate a microwave oven unless it does not have proper shielding (old microwave ovens) or is defective.
- Report any of these symptoms to your physician if you experience them: difficulty breathing, dizziness, fainting, chest pain, weight gain, and prolonged hiccupping. If you have any of these symptoms, check your pulse rate and call your physician.
- If you feel symptoms when near any device, move 5 to 10 feet away from it and then check your pulse. Your pulse rate should return to normal.
- Keep all of your physician and pacemaker clinic appointments.
- Take all medications prescribed for you as instructed.
- Follow your prescribed diet.
- Follow instructions on restrictions on physical activity, such as no sudden, jerky movement for 8 weeks to allow the pacemaker to settle in place.

Chart 36-8 PATIENT AND FAMILY EDUCATION GUIDE

Implantable Cardioverter/Defibrillator

- Follow the instructions for implantable cardioverter/defibrillator (ICD) site skin care that have been specifically prepared for you.
- Report to your physician any fever or redness, swelling, soreness, or drainage from your incision site.
- Do not wear tight clothing or belts that could cause irritation over the ICD generator.
- Avoid activities that involve rough contact with the ICD implantation site.
- Keep your ICD identification card in your wallet, and consider wearing a medical alert bracelet.
- Know the basic functioning of your ICD device and its rate cutoff, as well as the number of consecutive shocks it can deliver.
- Avoid magnets directly over your ICD because they can inactivate the device. If beeping tones are coming from the ICD, move away from the electromagnetic field immediately (within 30 seconds) before the inactivation sequence is completed, and notify your physician.
- Inform all physicians and dentists caring for you that you have an ICD implanted because certain diagnostic tests and procedures must be avoided to prevent ICD malfunction. These include diathermy, electrocautery, and nuclear magnetic resonance tests.
- Avoid other sources of electromagnetic interference, such as devices emitting microwaves (not microwave ovens); transformers; radio, television, and radar transmitters; large electrical generators; metal detectors, including handheld security devices at airports; antitheft devices; arc welding equipment; and sources of 60-cycle (Hz) interference. Also avoid leaning directly over the alternator of a running motor of a car or boat.
- Report to your physician symptoms such as fainting, nausea, weakness, blackout, and rapid pulse rates.
- Take all medications prescribed for you as instructed.
- Follow instructions on restrictions on physical activity, such as not swimming, driving motor vehicles, or operating dangerous equipment.
- Follow your prescribed diet.
- Keep all physician and ICD clinic appointments.
- Sit or lie down immediately if you feel dizzy or faint to avoid falling if the ICD discharges.
- Post emergency telephone numbers.
- Know how to contact the local emergency medical services (EMS) systems in your community. Inform them in advance that you have an ICD so that they can be prepared if they need to respond to an emergency call for you.
- Know how to perform cough cardiopulmonary resuscitation (CPR) as instructed.
- Encourage family members to learn how to perform CPR. Family members should know that if they are touching you when the device discharges, they may feel a slight shock but that this is not harmful to them.
- Follow instructions on what to do if the ICD successfully discharges, after which you feel well. This may include maintaining a diary of the date, the time, activity preceding the shock, symptoms, the number of shocks delivered, and how you feel after the shock. The physician may wish to be notified each time the device discharges.
- Avoid strenuous activities that may cause your heart rate to meet or exceed the rate cutoff of your ICD because this causes the device to discharge inappropriately.
- Notify your physician for information regarding access to health care if you are leaving town or are relocating.

Health Care Resources

The cardiac rehabilitation nurse typically provides written and oral information about dysrhythmias, antidysrhythmic drugs, pacemakers, and ICDs, as well as information about cardiac exercise programs, educational programs, and support groups. The office or ambulatory care nurse may also provide information about resources. Teach the patient how to contact the local chapter of the American Heart Association (www.americanheart.org) or the provincial chapter of the Heart and Stroke Foundation in Canada (www.heartandstroke.ca) for information about dysrhythmias, pacemakers, and CPR training.

Manufacturers of pacemakers and ICDs provide helpful booklets and videotapes to give patients and their families a better understanding of these therapies. Teach patients how to use telephonic systems for transmission of their rhythms to the ambulatory care setting or health care provider's office. Stress the importance of keeping scheduled appointments for visits with the cardiologist and pacemaker or ICD clinic. Instruct patients to contact the local ambulance or paramedic services and emergency facilities to let them know that they have these devices implanted. Encourage the patient and family to attend pacemaker or ICD support groups.

Evaluation: Outcomes

Evaluate the care of the patient with dysrhythmias on the basis of the identified nursing diagnoses and collaborative problems. The primary expected outcome is that the patient will have adequate blood flow from the left ventricle to support systemic blood pressure. Specific indicators for these outcomes are listed for each nursing diagnosis in the Planning and Implementation section (see earlier).

HUMAN NEEDS NURSING CARE REVIEW

What might you NOTICE if the patient is experiencing inadequate oxygenation and tissue perfusion as a result of dysrhythmias?

- Report of chest discomfort or pain
- Report of dizziness or syncope
- Shortness of breath
- Weakness and fatigue
- Decreased urine output
- Pale, cool skin
- Diaphoresis
- Anxiety or restlessness

What should you INTERPRET and how should you RESPOND to a patient experiencing inadequate oxygenation and perfusion as a result of dysrhythmias?

Perform and interpret physical assessment, including:

- Taking vital signs (may have hypotension and weak pulse)
- Checking for pulse deficit
- Asking if patient has palpitations
- Checking capillary refill (decreased)
- Listening to lung and heart sounds
- Assessing cognition
- Taking an ECG
- Checking oxygen saturation

Respond by:

- Applying oxygen
- Keeping the head of the bed elevated unless patient is very hypotensive
- Maintaining or starting an IV line
- Notifying the health care provider or Rapid Response Team
- Giving drug therapy as prescribed
- Assisting with other procedures as needed, for example, defibrillation

On what should you REFLECT?

- Evaluate patient's response to drug therapy.
- Observe for evidence of increased oxygenation and perfusion.
- Think about what else you could have done to assist the patient with this problem.

GET READY FOR THE NCLEX EXAMINATION!

Key Points

Review these Key Points for each NCLEX Examination Client Needs Category.

Safe and Effective Care Environment

- Be very careful to protect patients and staff to prevent electrical injury when assisting with invasive pacemakers, cardioversion, and defibrillation.
- Use infection control precautions during resuscitation efforts for a patient with a dysrhythmia.

Health Promotion and Maintenance

- Teach patients with dysrhythmias the correct drug, dose, route, time, and side effects of prescribed medications, and teach them to notify their physicians if adverse effects occur (see Chart 36-2).
- Teach family members where to learn cardiopulmonary resuscitation (CPR) to decrease their anxiety while living with a patient with dysrhythmias.
- Teach patients the importance of adhering to their prescribed cardiac regimen, such as checking their pulse to ascertain pacemaker function.

Physiological Integrity

- Assess patients with dysrhythmias for a decrease in cardiac output resulting in inadequate oxygenation and perfusion to vital organs (see Chart 36-1).
- Monitor patients with dysrhythmias, including conducting a physical assessment and health history, as well as interpreting ECG rhythm strips. Report significant changes to the health care provider.
- Perform and interpret common dysrhythmias, especially bradycardia, tachycardia, atrial fibrillation and ventricular fibrillation (VF), premature ventricular contractions (PVCs), and asystole, using ECG analysis (see Figs. 36-1 through 36-12).
- Use the special considerations when caring for older adults with dysrhythmias, as described in Chart 36-6.
- Noninvasive pacing is an emergency measure to provide demand ventricular pacing in patients with profound bradycardia or asystole. Teach patients to expect possible discomfort.
- Identify and intervene in life-threatening situations by providing cardiopulmonary resuscitation, electrical therapy, or drug administration.
- Automated external defibrillators are used by medical and lay personnel as an essential intervention for VF.
- Do not perform CPR while the patient is being defibrillated.
- Use Charts 36-7 and 36-8 to educate patients with permanent pacemakers or ICDs.

Additional Study Resources

Go to your Companion CD or Evolve at http://evolve.elsevier.com/Iggy/ for *Self-Assessment Questions for the NCLEX Examination.*

evolve Go to Evolve at http://evolve.elsevier.com/Iggy/ for *Prioritization and Delegation Questions for the NCLEX Examination.*

SELECTED BIBLIOGRAPHY

Aehlert, B. (2006). *ECGs made easy.* St. Louis: Mosby.

Aehlert, B. (2007). *Rapid ACLS* (2nd ed.). St. Louis: Mosby.

Alspach, G. (2006). 2005 Guidelines for CPR and ECG: New, but improved? *Critical Care Nurse, 26*(1), 8-13.

American Heart Association. (2005). 2005 Guidelines for cardiopulmonary resuscitation and emergency cardiovascular care: International consensus on science. *Circulation, 112*(Suppl.), IV-1-IV-205.

American Heart Association. (2006). *Handbook of emergency cardiovascular care for healthcare providers.* Dallas, TX: American Heart Association.

Anderson, C. (2005). The body electric: A review of literature on implantable cardioverter defibrillators. *Collegian, 12*(4), 29-35.

Atwood, D. (2005). Home Study Program. Using an algorithm to easily interpret basic cardiac rhythms. *AORN Journal, 82*(5), 758-772.

Beasley, B., & West, M. (2006). *Understanding 12-lead EKGs: A practical approach* (2nd ed.). Upper Saddle River, NJ: Pearson Education.

Beery, T.A., Bass, L.S., & Henthorn, C. (2007). Self-reported adjustment to implanted cardiac devices. *Journal of Cardiovascular Nursing, 22*(6), 516-524.

Bentz, B. (2006). Gaining control over A-fib. *RN, 69*(12), 35-38.

Berenbom, L., Weiford, B., Vacek, J., Emert, M., Hall, W., Andrews, M., et al. (2005). Differences in outcomes between patients treated with single- versus dual-chamber implantable cardioverter defibrillators: A substudy of the Multicenter Automatic Defibrillator Implantation Trial II. *Annals of Noninvasive Electrocardiology, 10*(4), 429-435.

Brantman, L., & Howie, J. (2006). Use of amiodarone to prevent atrial fibrillation after cardiac surgery. *Critical Care Nurse, 26*(1), 48-59.

Bulechek, G.M., Butcher, H.K., & McCloskey Dochterman, J. (Eds.). (2008). *Nursing interventions classifications (NIC)* (5th ed.). St. Louis: Mosby.

Chapman, E., Parameshwar, J., Jenkins, D., Large, S., & Tsui, S. (2007). Psychosocial issues for patients with ventricular assist devices: A qualitative pilot study. *American Journal of Critical Care, 16*(1), 72-81.

Chen-Scarabelli, C. (2005). Supraventricular arrhythmias: An electrophysiology primer. *Progress in Cardiovascular Nursing, 20*(1), 24-31.
Cotter, J., Bixby, M., & Morse, B. (2006). Helping patients who need a permanent pacemaker. *Nursing2006, 36*(8), 50-54.
Coughlin, R.M. (2007). Recognizing ventricular arrhythmias and preventing sudden cardiac death. *American Nurse Today, 2*(5), 38-44.
Craig, K., & Hopkins-Pepe, L. (2006). Understanding the new AHA guidelines, Part II. *Nursing2006, 36*(5), 52-53.
Deneke, T., Khargi, K., Grewe, P., Calcum, B., Laczkovics, A., Keyhan-Falsafi, A., et al. (2006). Catheter ablation of regular atrial arrhythmia following surgical treatment of permanent atrial fibrillation. *Journal of Cardiovascular Electrophysiology, 17*(1), 18-24.
Dougherty, C.M., Johnston, S.K., & Thompson, E.A. (2007). Reliability and validity of the self-efficacy expectations and outcome expectation after implantable cardioverter defibrillator implantation scales. *Applied Nursing Research, 20*(4), 116-124.
Drew, B.J., & Funk, M. (2006). Practice standards for ECG monitoring in hospital settings: Executive summary and guide for implementation. *Critical Care Nursing Clinics of North America, 18*(2), 157-168.
Dunbar, S. (2005). Psychosocial issues of patients with implantable cardioverter defibrillators. *American Journal of Critical Care, 14*(4), 294-303.
Fugate, J. (2006). Pharmacologic management of cardiac emergencies. *Journal of Infusion Nursing, 29*(3), 147-150.
Geiter, H. (2007). *E-Z ECG rhythm interpretation.* Philadelphia: F.A. Davis.
Gever, M. (2005). Procainamide: Test your drug IQ. *Nursing, 35*(5), 32cc4.
Goldenberg, I., & Moss, A. (2007). Treatment of arrhythmias and use of implantable cardioverter-defibrillators to improve survival in elderly patients with cardiac disease. *Clinics in Geriatric Medicine, 23*(1), 205-219.
Goldich, G. (2006a). Understanding the 12-lead ECG, Part I. *Nursing2006, 36*(11), 36-42.
Goldich, G. (2006b). Understanding the 12-lead ECG, Part II. *Nursing2006, 36*(12), 36-42.
Gura, M. (2006). Implantable cardioverter defibrillator therapy. *Journal of Cardiovascular Nursing, 20*(4), 276-287.
Humphreys, M. (2006). Pericardial conditions: Signs, symptoms and electrocardiogram changes. *Emergency Nurse, 14*(1), 30-36.
Huszar, R.J. (2007a). *Basic dysrhythmias: Interpretation and management* (3rd ed.). St. Louis: Mosby.
Huszar, R.J. (2007b). *Pocket guide to basic dysrhythmias: Interpretation and management* (3rd ed.). St. Louis: Mosby.
Lange, S., & Nguyen, Q.N. (2006). Cables and electrodes can burn patients during MRI. *Nursing2006, 36*(11), 18.
Maiocco, G. (2005). Review: Magnesium prophylaxis after cardiac surgery reduces the risk of arrhythmia and atrial fibrillation. *Evidence-Based Nursing, 8*(2), 55.
Mutchner, L. (2007). The ABCs of CPR again. *AJN, 107*(1), 60-68.
O'Brien, M., Langberg, J., Valderrama, A., Kerkendoll, K., Roneiko, N., & Dunbar, S. (2005). Implantable cardioverter defibrillator storm: Nursing care issues for patients and families. *Critical Care Nursing Clinics of North America, 17*(1), 9-16.
Pyle, K., Pierson, G., Lepman, D., & Hewett, M. (2007). Keeping cardiac arrest patients alive with therapeutic hypothermia. *American Nurse Today, 2*(7), 32-37.
Rocca, J.D. (2007). Atrial fibrillation. *Nursing2007,* 37(4), 37-44.
Sayre, M.R., Berg, R.A. Cave, D.M., Page, R.L., Potts, J., White, R.D., et al. (2008). Hands-only (compression-only) cardiopulmonary resuscitation: A call to action for bystander response to adults who experience out-of-hospital sudden cardiac arrest. *Circulation, 117*(21), 2162-2167.
Sears, S.F., & Conti, J.B. (2006). Psychological aspects of cardiac devices and recalls in patients with implantable cardioverter defibrillators. *American Journal of Cardiology, 98,* 565-567.
Sherrod, M., Albarez, Y., Brookshire, A., & Cheek, D. (2007). A woman's worst enemy. *American Nurse Today, 2*(2), 25-29.
Smallwood, A. (2005). Nurse-led elective cardioversion: An evidence-based practice review. *Nursing in Critical Care, 10*(5), 231-241.
Strzyzewski, N. (2006). Common errors made in resuscitation of respiratory and cardiac arrest. *Plastic Surgical Nursing, 26*(1), 10-16.
Thygerson, A., Gulli, B., & Krohmer, J. (2007). *First Aid, CPR, and AED* (5th ed.). Sudbury, MA: Jones & Bartlett.

37

CHAPTER

Care of Patients with Cardiac Problems

Donna D. Ignatavicius • Sharon Henry Walicek

LEARNING OUTCOMES

For clinical competence and success on the NCLEX Examination, study this chapter with these Learning Outcomes in mind:

Safe and Effective Care Environment

1. Evaluate the status of patients with end-stage heart disease regarding advance directives.
2. Provide the patient with heart failure (HF) and the family information on discharge to home, hospice, or other community-based setting.
3. Collaborate with the interdisciplinary team when providing care to patients with cardiac problems.
4. Identify community resources for patients with cardiac problems and their families.

Health Promotion and Maintenance

5. Perform a comprehensive assessment of patients experiencing cardiac problems.
6. Provide special care needs of older adults with heart failure.
7. Teach patients about actions to maintain health and prevent worsening HF.

Psychosocial Integrity

8. Assess the patient and family response to living with chronic HF and possible transplantation.

Physiological Integrity

9. Explain the pathophysiology of HF.
10. Compare and contrast left-sided and right-sided HF.
11. Identify common nursing diagnoses and collaborative problems for patients with HF.
12. Explain how common drug therapies improve cardiac output and prevent worsening of HF.
13. Assess patients for adverse effects of drug therapy for cardiac problems.
14. Monitor the laboratory values for patients with cardiac problems.
15. Intervene to improve the patient's cardiovascular status when needed.
16. Provide emergency care for patients experiencing life-threatening complications, such as cardiac tamponade and pulmonary edema.
17. Identify essential focused assessments used by the home care nurse for patients with heart failure.
18. Compare and contrast common valvular disorders.
19. Describe surgical management for patients with valvular disease.
20. Develop a teaching/learning plan for patients with valvular disease.
21. Differentiate between common cardiac inflammations and infections—endocarditis, pericarditis, and rheumatic carditis.
22. Provide postoperative care for patients having a heart transplant.
23. Identify clinical assessment findings for patients with cardiomyopathy.

evolve Go to your Companion CD or Evolve at http://evolve.elsevier.com/Iggy/ for *Self-Assessment Questions for the NCLEX Examination* keyed to these Learning Outcomes.

Although most people do not consider heart disease an incurable illness, more die from heart disease than from the next seven leading causes of death combined. This health problem is the most common reason for hospital stays in patients older than 65 years in the United States. When the heart is diseased, it cannot effectively pump an adequate amount of arterial blood to the rest of the body. Arterial blood carries *oxygen* and nutrients to vital organs, such as the kidneys and brain, and peripheral tissues. When these organs and other body tissues are not adequately *perfused,* they may not function properly.

Long-term survival depends on adherence to therapy and a collaborative patient-centered approach to ensure the best management of the illness and the highest possible quality of life. As discussed in Chapter 1, the Institute for Healthcare Improvement (IHI) included as one of its outcomes to deliver reliable, evidence-based care for congestive heart failure to prevent readmissions to the hospital. This outcome is one of 12 interventions to save patient lives and prevent medical harm.

HEART FAILURE

Heart failure, sometimes referred to as **pump failure,** is a general term for the inability of the heart to work effectively as a pump. It results from a number of acute and chronic cardiovascular problems that are discussed later in this chapter and elsewhere in the cardiovascular unit.

Pathophysiology

Types of Heart Failure

The major types of heart failure are:

- Left-sided heart failure
- Right-sided heart failure
- High-output failure

Because the two ventricles of the heart represent two separate pumping systems, it is possible for one to fail by itself for a short period. *Most heart failure begins with failure of the left ventricle and progresses to failure of both ventricles.* Typical causes of **left-sided heart (ventricular) failure** include hypertensive, coronary artery, and valvular disease involving the mitral or aortic valve. Decreased tissue perfusion from poor cardiac output and pulmonary congestion from increased pressure in the pulmonary vessels indicate left ventricular failure (LVF).

ANIMATION: Congestive Heart Failure ▶

Left-sided heart failure was formerly referred to as **congestive heart failure (CHF);** however, not all cases of LVF involve fluid accumulation. In the clinical setting, though, the term *CHF* is still commonly used. Left-sided failure may be acute or chronic and mild to severe. It can be further divided into two subtypes: systolic heart failure and diastolic heart failure.

Systolic heart failure (systolic ventricular dysfunction) results when the heart cannot contract forcefully enough during systole to eject adequate amounts of blood into the circulation. Preload increases with decreased contractility, and afterload increases as a result of increased peripheral resistance (e.g., hypertension) (McCance & Huether, 2006). The **ejection fraction** (the percentage of blood ejected from the heart during systole) drops from a normal of 50% to 70% to below 40% with ventricular dilation. As it decreases, tissue perfusion diminishes and blood accumulates in the pulmonary vessels. Manifestations of systolic dysfunction may include symptoms of inadequate tissue perfusion or pulmonary and systemic congestion. Systolic heart failure is often called "forward failure" because cardiac output is decreased and fluid backs up into the pulmonary system. Because these patients are at high risk for sudden cardiac death, patients with an ejection fraction of less than 30% are considered candidates for an implantable cardioverter/defibrillator (ICD; also known as an internal cardioverter/defibrillator) (see Chapter 36).

In contrast, **diastolic heart failure (heart failure with preserved left ventricular function)** occurs when the left ventricle cannot relax adequately during diastole. Inadequate relaxation or "stiffening" prevents the ventricle from filling with sufficient blood to ensure an adequate cardiac output. Although ejection fraction is more than 40%, the ventricle becomes less compliant over time because more pressure is needed to move the same amount of volume as compared with a healthy heart. Diastolic failure represents about 20% to 40% of all heart failure, primarily in older adults and in women who have chronic hypertension and undetected coronary artery disease. Clinical manifestations and management of diastolic failure are similar to those of systolic dysfunction (McCance & Huether, 2006).

Right-sided heart (ventricular) failure may be caused by left ventricular failure, right ventricular MI, or pulmonary hypertension. In this type of heart failure (HF), the right ventricle cannot empty completely. Increased volume and pressure develop in the venous system, and peripheral edema results.

High-output heart failure can occur when cardiac output remains normal or above normal, unlike left- and right-sided heart failure, which are typically low-output states. High-output failure is caused by increased metabolic needs or hyperkinetic conditions, such as septicemia (fever), anemia, and hyperthyroidism. This type of heart failure is not as common as other types.

Classification and Staging of Heart Failure

The American College of Cardiology (ACC) and American Heart Association (AHA) have developed evidence-based guidelines for staging and managing heart failure as a chronic, progressive disease. These guidelines do not replace the New York Heart Association (NYHA) functional classification system, which is used to describe symptoms a patient may exhibit (see Table 35-2 in Chapter 35).

The ACC/AHA staging system when compared with the NYHA system categorizes patients as:

A. Patients at high risk for developing heart failure (Class I NYHA)
B. Patients with cardiac structural abnormalities or remodeling who have not developed HF symptoms (Class I NYHA)
C. Patients with current or prior symptoms of heart failure (Class II or III NYHA)
D. Patients with refractory end-stage heart failure (Class IV NYHA)

Another popular method for staging HF is the Killip Classification System, which is based on the heart's hemodynamic ability. Table 40-3 in Chapter 40 outlines this system.

Compensatory Mechanisms

When cardiac output is insufficient to meet the demands of the body, compensatory mechanisms operate to improve cardiac output (Fig. 37-1). Although these mechanisms may initially increase cardiac output, they eventually have a damaging effect on pump function. Major compensatory mechanisms include:

- Sympathetic nervous system stimulation
- Renin-angiotensin system (RAS) activation
- Other chemical responses
- Myocardial hypertrophy

Stimulation of the Sympathetic Nervous System

In heart failure (HF), *stimulation of the sympathetic nervous system* (i.e., increasing catecholamines) as a result of tissue hypoxia represents the most immediate compensatory mechanism. Stimulation of the adrenergic receptors causes an increase in heart rate (beta adrenergic) and blood pressure from vasoconstriction (alpha adrenergic).

Because cardiac output (CO) is the product of heart rate (HR) and stroke volume (SV), an increase in HR results in an

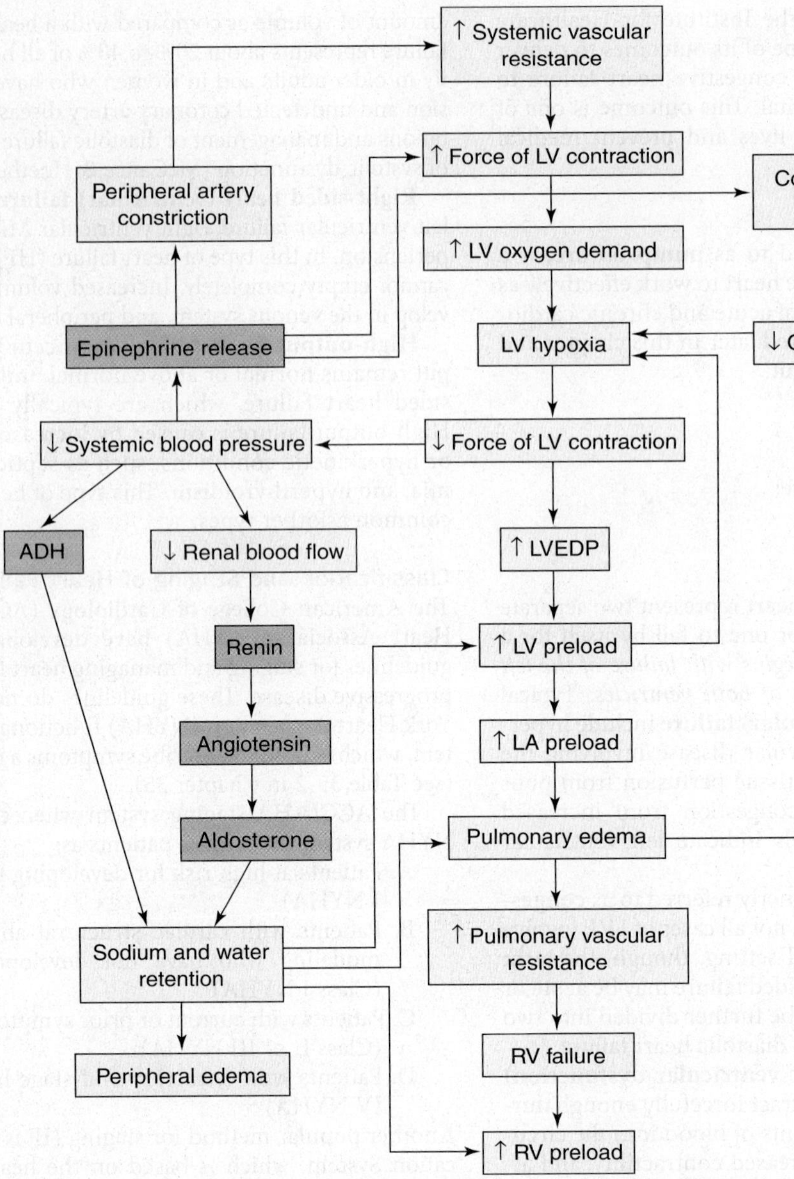
↑ Systemic vascular resistance
↑ Force of LV contraction
Peripheral artery constriction
Coronary artery constriction
↑ LV oxygen demand
Epinephrine release
LV hypoxia
↓ Oxygen supply
↓ Systemic blood pressure
↓ Force of LV contraction
ADH
↓ Renal blood flow
↑ LVEDP
Renin
↑ LV preload
Angiotensin
↑ LA preload
Aldosterone
Pulmonary edema
↑ Pulmonary vascular resistance
Sodium and water retention
RV failure
Peripheral edema
↑ RV preload

Fig. 37-1 • Left-sided heart failure from elevated systemic vascular resistance. Left heart failure leads to right heart failure. Systemic vascular resistance and preload are exacerbated by renal and adrenal mechanisms. *ADH,* Antidiuretic hormone; *LA,* left atrial; *LV,* left ventricular; *LVEDP,* left ventricular end-diastolic pressure; *RV,* right ventricular.

immediate *increase in cardiac output.* The HR is limited, though, in its ability to compensate for decreased CO. If it becomes too rapid, diastolic filling time is limited and CO may start to decline. An increase in HR also significantly increases oxygen demand by the myocardium. If the heart is poorly perfused because of arteriosclerosis, HF may worsen.

Stroke volume (SV) is also *improved* by sympathetic stimulation. Sympathetic stimulation increases venous return to the heart, which further stretches the myocardial fibers causing dilation. According to Starling's law, increased myocardial stretch results in more forceful contraction. More forceful contractions increase SV and CO. After a critical point is reached within the cardiac muscle, further volume and stretch reduce the force of contraction and cardiac output.

Sympathetic stimulation also results in *arterial vasoconstriction.* Vasoconstriction has the benefit of maintaining blood pressure and improving tissue perfusion in low-output states. However, constriction of the arteries increases **afterload,** the resistance against which the heart must pump. Afterload is the major determinant of myocardial oxygen requirements. As it increases, the left ventricle requires more energy to eject its contents and SV may decline.

Renin-Angiotensin System Activation

Reduced blood flow to the kidneys, a common occurrence in low-output states, results in activation of the renin-angiotensin system (RAS). Vasoconstriction becomes more pronounced in response to angiotensin II, and aldosterone secretion causes sodium and water retention. Preload and afterload increase. Angiotensin II contributes to **ventricular remodeling** resulting in progressive myocyte (myocardial cell) contractile dysfunction over time (McCance & Huether, 2006).

Other Chemical Responses

In addition to the sympathetic nervous system and RAS responses, other mechanisms are activated when a patient experiences heart failure (HF). Most of these actions contribute to worsening of the condition.

In those who have had an MI, heart muscle cell injury causes an *immune response.* Pro-inflammatory cytokines, such as tumor necrosis factor (TNF) and interleukins (IL-1 and IL-6), are released, especially with left-sided HF. These substances contribute to ventricular remodeling.

Natriuretic peptides are neurohormones that work to promote vasodilation and diuresis through sodium loss in the renal tubules. The **B-type natriuretic peptide (BNP)** is produced and released by the ventricles when the patient has fluid overload as a result of HF. It increases with age and has a greater concentration in women (Kincade & Frazier, 2006). People who are obese have lower BNP levels compared with those who are not (Kreiger, 2007).

Low cardiac output (CO) causes decreased cerebral perfusion. As a result, the posterior pituitary gland secretes *vasopressin* (antidiuretic hormone [ADH]). The hormone causes vasoconstriction and fluid retention, which worsen HF.

Endothelin is secreted by endothelial cells when they are stretched. As the myocardial fibers are stretched in patients with HF, this potent vasoconstrictor is released, which increases peripheral resistance and hypertension. HF worsens as a result of these actions.

Myocardial Hypertrophy

Myocardial hypertrophy (enlargement of the myocardium), with or without chamber dilation, is another compensatory mechanism. The walls of the heart thicken to provide more muscle mass, which results in more forceful contractions, further increasing cardiac output. Cardiac muscle, however, may hypertrophy more rapidly than collateral circulation can provide adequate blood supply to the muscle. Often a hypertrophied heart is slightly oxygen deprived.

All the compensatory mechanisms contribute to an increase in the consumption of myocardial oxygen. When the demand for oxygen increases and the myocardial reserve has been exhausted, clinical manifestations of HF develop.

Etiology

Heart failure (HF) is caused by systemic hypertension in 75% of cases. About a third of patients experiencing MI also develop HF. The next most common cause is structural heart changes, such as valvular dysfunction, particularly pulmonic or aortic stenosis, which leads to pressure or volume overload on the heart. Common direct causes and risk factors for HF are listed in Table 37-1.

CONSIDERATIONS FOR OLDER ADULTS

The use of certain drugs can also lead to heart failure (HF), especially in older adults. Long-term use of NSAIDs, such as ibuprofen (Motrin), cause fluid and sodium retention. Many older adults take these drugs for arthritic pain and inflammation. Thiazolidinediones (TZDs) (e.g., pioglitazone [Actos]) used for diabetics also cause fluid and sodium retention. These drugs should be used with caution in the older adult population.

TABLE 37-1 Common Causes and Risk Factors for Heart Failure

- Hypertension
- Coronary artery disease
- Cardiomyopathy
- Substance abuse (alcohol and illicit/prescribed drugs)
- Valvular disease
- Congenital defects
- Cardiac infections and inflammations
- Dysrhythmias
- Diabetes mellitus
- Smoking/Tobacco use
- Family history
- Hyperkinetic conditions (e.g., hyperthyroidism)

Right-sided HF in the absence of left-sided HF is usually the result of pulmonary problems, such as chronic obstructive pulmonary disease (COPD) or pulmonary hypertension. Acute respiratory distress syndrome (ARDS) may also cause right-sided HF.

Incidence/Prevalence

Over five million people in the United States have HF, and about 550,000 new cases occur each year. African Americans are affected twice as often as Euro-Americans, probably because they have many risk factors that can lead to HF (www.americanheart.org). The disease is a major cause of disability and death after myocardial infarction, often due to nonadherence with the treatment plan and recommended lifestyle changes.

CONSIDERATIONS FOR OLDER ADULTS

Heart failure has been referred to as a U.S. epidemic, although it is a major problem worldwide (Rasmusson et al., 2006). One of the U.S. *Healthy People 2010* objectives is to reduce by 50% the number of hospitalizations of older adults with HF as the principal diagnosis. Interventions aimed at patient and family education can help meet this objective (Table 37-2). As the "baby boomer" population reaches 65 years of age, the numbers of hospital stays and deaths are likely to dramatically increase.

Patient-Centered Collaborative Care

evolve ONLINE PHARM REVIEW

▪ *Assessment*

History

When obtaining a history, keep in mind the many conditions that can lead to HF. Carefully question the patient about his or her medical history, including hypertension, angina, MI, rheumatic heart disease, valvular disorders, endocarditis, and pericarditis. Ask about the patient's perception of his or her activity tolerance, breathing pattern, sleeping pattern, urinary pattern, and fluid volume status, as well as his or her knowledge about HF.

Left-Sided Heart Failure. With left ventricular systolic dysfunction, cardiac output (CO) is diminished, leading to impaired tissue perfusion, anaerobic metabolism, and unusual fatigue. Assess activity tolerance by asking whether the patient

TABLE 37-2 Meeting *Healthy People 2010* Objectives

CARDIAC DISEASE

Objective 12.6: To reduce hospitalizations of older adults with heart failure as the principal diagnosis.

- For patients hospitalized for heart failure, collaborate with the case manager for discharge planning, including adequate support in the community.
- Provide a continuing plan of care for patients and their families or other caregivers when the patient is discharged from the hospital.
- If the patient is discharged to home, call to check that he or she has no impending signs and symptoms of heart failure (the case manager may make calls).
- Teach the patient and family or other caregiver about when to call the health care provider for health changes so the patient can be treated at home.
- Ensure that the interdisciplinary team provides the patient with follow-up care in the home or nursing home.

can perform normal ADLs or climb flights of stairs without fatigue or dyspnea. Many patients with heart failure (HF) experience weakness or fatigue with activity or have a feeling of heaviness in their arms or legs. Ask about their ability to perform simultaneous arm and leg work (e.g., walking while carrying a bag of groceries). Such activity may place an unacceptable demand on the failing heart. Ask the patient to identify his or her most strenuous activity in the past week. Many people unconsciously limit their activities in response to fatigue or dyspnea and may not realize how limited they have become.

Perfusion to the myocardium is often impaired with left ventricular failure, especially with cardiac hypertrophy. The patient may report chest discomfort or may describe palpitations, skipped beats, or a fast heartbeat.

As the amount of blood ejected from the left ventricle diminishes, hydrostatic pressure builds in the pulmonary venous system and results in fluid-filled alveoli and pulmonary congestion. Thus cough is often an early manifestation of HF. The patient in early HF describes the cough as irritating, nocturnal (at night), and usually nonproductive. *As HF becomes very severe, he or she may begin expectorating frothy, pink-tinged sputum—a sign of life-threatening pulmonary edema.*

Dyspnea also results from rising pulmonary venous pressure and pulmonary congestion. Carefully question about the presence of dyspnea and when and how it developed. The patient may refer to dyspnea as "trouble in catching my breath," "breathlessness," or "difficulty in breathing."

As **exertional dyspnea** develops (also called *dyspnea upon* or *on exertion [DUE/DOE]*), the patient often stops previously tolerated levels of activity because of shortness of breath. Dyspnea at rest in the recumbent (lying flat) position is known as **orthopnea.** Ask how many pillows are used to sleep or whether the patient sleeps in an upright position in a bed, recliner, or other type of chair.

Patients who describe sudden awakening with a feeling of breathlessness 2 to 5 hours after falling asleep have **paroxysmal nocturnal dyspnea (PND).** Sitting upright, dangling the feet, or walking usually relieves this condition.

Right-Sided Heart Failure. Signs of systemic congestion occur as the right ventricle fails, fluid is retained, and pressure builds in the venous system. Edema develops in the lower legs and ascends to the thighs and abdominal wall. Patients may notice that their shoes fit more tightly, or their shoes or socks may leave indentations on their swollen feet. They may have removed their rings because of swelling in their fingers and hands. Ask about weight gain. An adult may retain 4 to 7 liters of fluid (10 to 15 lb [4.5 to 6.8 kg]) before pitting edema occurs.

GI reports of nausea and anorexia may be a direct consequence of liver engorgement resulting from fluid retention. *In advanced HF, ascites and an increased abdominal girth may develop from the pronounced liver congestion.* Another finding related to fluid retention is diuresis at rest. At rest, fluid in the peripheral tissue is mobilized and excreted and the patient describes frequent awakening at night to urinate.

Obtain a careful nutritional history, questioning about the use of salt and the types of food consumed. Ask about daily fluid intake. Patients with HF may experience increased thirst and drink excessive fluid (4000 to 5000 mL) because of sodium retention.

Physical Assessment/Clinical Manifestations

Manifestations of HF depend on the type of failure, the ventricle involved, and the underlying cause. Impaired tissue perfusion, pulmonary congestion, and edema dominate the picture of left ventricular failure (Chart 37-1). Conversely, systemic venous congestion and peripheral edema are associated with right ventricular failure (Chart 37-2).

Left-Sided Heart Failure. Left ventricular failure is associated with decreased cardiac output and elevated pulmonary venous pressure. It may appear clinically as weakness, fatigue,

Chart 37-1 KEY FEATURES

Left-Sided Heart Failure

DECREASED CARDIAC OUTPUT
- Fatigue
- Weakness
- Oliguria during the day (nocturia at night)
- Angina
- Confusion, restlessness
- Dizziness
- Tachycardia, palpitations
- Pallor
- Weak peripheral pulses
- Cool extremities

PULMONARY CONGESTION
- Hacking cough, worse at night
- Dyspnea/breathlessness
- Crackles or wheezes in lungs
- Frothy, pink-tinged sputum
- Tachypnea
- S_3/S_4 summation gallop

Chart 37-2 KEY FEATURES

Right-Sided Heart Failure

SYSTEMIC CONGESTION
- Jugular (neck vein) distention
- Enlarged liver and spleen
- Anorexia and nausea
- Dependent edema (legs and sacrum)
- Distended abdomen
- Swollen hands and fingers
- Polyuria at night
- Weight gain
- Increased blood pressure (from excess volume) or decreased blood pressure (from failure)

dizziness, confusion, pulmonary congestion, breathlessness, oliguria (scant urine output), or death. Decreased blood flow to the major body organs can cause dysfunction, especially renal failure. Nocturia may occur when the patient is at rest.

Obtain the patient's vital signs. When obtaining blood pressure (BP), note the presence or absence of an auscultatory gap or orthostatic (postural) hypotension. The **proportional pulse pressure** is calculated as follows:

$$\frac{\text{Systolic BP} - \text{Diastolic BP}}{\text{Systolic BP}}$$

A proportional pulse pressure less than 25% indicates severely compromised cardiac output (CO). The pulse may be tachycardic, or it may alternate in strength **(pulsus alternans).** Take the apical pulse for a full minute, noting any irregularity in heart rhythm. *An irregular heart rhythm resulting from premature atrial contractions (PACs), premature ventricular contractions (PVCs), or atrial fibrillation (AF) is common in HF (see Chapter 36).* The sudden development of an irregular rhythm may further compromise CO. Carefully monitor the patient's respiratory rate, rhythm, and character, as well as oxygen saturation. The respiratory rate typically exceeds 20 breaths/min.

Assess whether the patient is oriented to person, place, and time. A short mental status examination may be used if there are concerns about orientation. Objective data are important because in daily conversation many people are skillful at covering up memory losses. Older adults are frequently disoriented or confused when the heart fails because of brain hypoxia (decreased oxygen).

Increased heart size is common with a displacement of the apical impulse to the left. A third heart sound, **(S_3) gallop**, an early diastolic filling sound indicating an increase in left ventricular pressure, may be heard on auscultation. This sound is often the first sign of HF. A fourth heart sound (S_4) also can occur; it is not a sign of failure but is a reflection of decreased ventricular compliance.

Auscultate for crackles and wheezes of the lungs. Late inspiratory crackles and fine profuse crackles that repeat themselves from breath to breath and do not diminish with coughing indicate HF. Crackles are produced by intra-alveolar fluid and are often noted first in the dependent areas of the lungs. *They usually develop in the bases and spread upward as the condition worsens.* Identify the precise location of the crackles. Wheezes indicate a narrowing of the bronchial lumen caused by engorged pulmonary vessels.

Right-Sided Heart Failure. Right ventricular failure is associated with increased systemic venous pressures and congestion. On inspection, assess the neck veins for distention and measure abdominal girth. Hepatomegaly (liver engorgement), hepatojugular reflux, and ascites may also be assessed. Abdominal fluid can reach volumes of more than 10 liters.

Assess for dependent edema. In ambulatory patients, edema is in the ankles and legs. When patients are restricted to bedrest, the sacrum is dependent and edema accumulates there. *Edema is an extremely unreliable sign of HF, and therefore accurate daily weights are needed to document fluid retention. Weight is the most reliable indicator of fluid gain or loss.*

Psychosocial Assessment

Heart failure (HF) is usually a chronic, debilitating disease. Anxiety and frustration are common. Symptoms such as dyspnea increase the patient's anxiety level.

Patients with HF, especially those with advanced disease, are at high risk for depression. It is not certain whether the functional impairments contribute to the depression or depression affects functional ability. Hospitalized patients may be depressed, particularly those who have been rehospitalized for an acute episode of HF. Some, however, do not have depression until they are in the community. Lifestyle changes and quality of life issues can cause depression many months after the initial diagnosis of HF (Thomas et al., 2008).

Assess patients and their families for anxiety and depression. Ask them about their usual methods of coping, as well as any history of depression. If anxiety or depression is present, notify the health care provider for further assessment. In many hospitals, social workers, certified clinical chaplains, or psychologists administer specific assessment tools to determine the extent of the problem. Some patients need drug therapy and nonpharmacologic modalities, such as cognitive behavior therapy, biofeedback, or relaxation training.

Hope is a major indicator of well-being for patients with HF. Those who are hopeful tend to feel better and are more socially involved. Asking patients about their activities and the significant people in their life and how often they can interact with them provides clues about patient and family coping.

Laboratory Assessment

Electrolyte imbalance may occur from complications of HF or as side effects of drug therapy, especially diuretic therapy. Regular evaluations of a patient's *serum electrolytes,* including sodium, potassium, magnesium, calcium, and chloride, are essential. Any impairment of renal function resulting from inadequate perfusion causes elevated blood urea nitrogen and serum creatinine and decreased creatinine clearance levels. *Urinalysis* may reveal proteinuria and high specific gravity. *Hemoglobin* and *hematocrit* tests should be performed to identify HF resulting from anemia. If the patient has fluid volume excess, the hematocrit levels may appear low as a result of hemodilution.

B-type natriuretic peptide (BNP) is used for diagnosing HF (in particular, diastolic HF) in patients with acute dyspnea. As discussed earlier, it is part of the body's response to decreased cardiac output from either left or right ventricular dysfunction. An increase in BNP best differentiates between the dyspnea of HF and that associated with lung dysfunction (Kincade & Frazier, 2006). However, patients with atrial dysrhythmias and renal disease may also have elevated BNP levels (Kreiger, 2007).

Microalbuminuria is an early indicator of decreased compliance of the heart and occurs before the BNP rises. It serves as an "early warning detector" that lets the health care provider know that the heart is experiencing early signs of decreased compliance, long before symptoms occur.

CONSIDERATIONS FOR OLDER ADULTS

Thyroxine (T_4) and thyroid-stimulating hormone (TSH) levels should be determined in patients who are older than 65 years, have atrial fibrillation, or have evidence of thyroid disease. Heart failure (HF) may be caused or aggravated by hypothyroidism or hyperthyroidism.

Arterial blood gas (ABG) values often reveal hypoxia (low oxygen level) because oxygen does not diffuse easily through fluid-filled alveoli. Respiratory alkalosis may occur because of hyperventilation; respiratory acidosis may occur because of carbon dioxide retention. Metabolic acidosis may indicate an accumulation of lactic acid.

Imaging Assessment

Chest x-rays can be helpful in diagnosing left ventricular failure. Typically the heart is enlarged (cardiomegaly), representing hypertrophy or dilation. Pleural effusions develop less often and generally reflect biventricular failure. *Echocardiography is considered the best tool in diagnosing heart failure.* Cardiac valvular changes, pericardial effusion, chamber enlargement, and ventricular hypertrophy can be diagnosed using this noninvasive technique. The test can also be used to determine ejection fraction.

Radionuclide studies (thallium imaging or technetium pyrophosphate scanning) can also indicate the presence and cause of HF. Multigated angiographic (MUGA) scans provide information about left ventricular ejection fraction and velocity, which are typically low in patients with HF.

Other Diagnostic Assessment

An *electrocardiogram* (ECG) is also performed. It may show ventricular hypertrophy, dysrhythmias, and any degree of myocardial ischemia, injury, or infarction. It is *not* helpful in determining the presence or extent of HF.

Pulmonary artery catheters allow the assessment of cardiac function and volume status in acutely ill patients. These measurements can confirm the diagnosis and guide the management of HF. Right atrial pressure may be normal or elevated in left ventricular failure and is elevated in right ventricular failure. Pulmonary artery pressure (PAP) and pulmonary artery wedge pressure (PAWP) are elevated in left-sided HF because volumes and pressures are increased in the left ventricle. (See Chapter 35 for a more detailed description of these diagnostic assessments.)

Analysis

Common Nursing Diagnoses and Collaborative Problems

The priority nursing diagnoses for patients with HF include:

1. Impaired Gas Exchange related to ventilation/perfusion imbalance
2. Decreased Cardiac Output related to altered contractility, preload, and afterload
3. Activity Intolerance related to an imbalance between oxygen supply and demand

The primary collaborative problem is Potential for Pulmonary Edema.

Additional Nursing Diagnoses and Collaborative Problems

In addition to the common nursing diagnoses and collaborative problems, patients with HF may have:

- Excess Fluid Volume related to compromised regulatory mechanism
- Acute Confusion related to delirium
- Ineffective Therapeutic Regimen Management related to social support deficits, complexity of therapeutic regimen, or knowledge deficit
- Anxiety related to stress, change in health status and role function, or threat of death
- Ineffective Tissue Perfusion (Cerebral) related to mechanical reduction of arterial blood flow
- Impaired Physical Mobility related to limited cardiovascular endurance
- Risk for Ineffective Tissue Perfusion (Renal) related to hypovolemia

Some patients are also at risk for these collaborative problems:

- Potential for Pneumonia
- Potential for Depression
- Potential for Dysrhythmias

Planning and Implementation

The patient-centered collaborative care that patients with HF need depends in large part on their disease stage.

Impaired Gas Exchange

NOC **Planning: Expected Outcomes.** The patient with HF is expected to have adequate pulmonary tissue perfusion. Indicators include normal or baseline:

- Pulmonary artery pressure (PAP)
- Respiratory function
- Respiratory rate
- ABGs and pH
- Oxygen saturation

Interventions. The purpose of collaborative care is to promote an optimal spontaneous breathing pattern that increases oxygenation and maintains a normal carbon dioxide level in the blood.

NIC *Ventilation assistance* is essential for the patient with heart failure (Chart 37-3). Monitor or have assistive personnel monitor the patient's respiratory rate, rhythm, and quality every 1 to 4 hours. Auscultate breath sounds every 4 to 8 hours. The oxygen content of the blood is often decreased in patients who have pulmonary congestion. *Provide the necessary amount of supplemental oxygen within a range prescribed by the health care provider to maintain oxygen saturation at 90% or greater.*

If the patient has dyspnea, place him or her in a high Fowler's position with pillows under each arm to maximize chest expansion and improve oxygenation. Repositioning and performing coughing and deep-breathing exercises every 2 hours help improve oxygenation and prevent atelectasis. Collaborate with the respiratory therapist, if available, to plan the most effective methods for assisting with ventilation.

Decreased Cardiac Output

NOC **Planning: Expected Outcomes.** The patient with HF is expected to have improved and increased cardiac pump effectiveness. Indicators include normal or baseline:

- Systolic and diastolic blood pressure
- Apical pulse rate
- Ejection fraction
- Peripheral pulses
- Skin color
- Urine output
- Cognitive status

Interventions. Interventions are directed at optimizing the two major components of cardiac output (CO): stroke volume (SV) (determined by preload, afterload, and contractility) and heart rate (HR).

Nonsurgical Management. Nonsurgical management relies primarily on a variety of drugs (Table 37-3). If drug therapy is ineffective, other nonsurgical options are available.

Chart 37-3 NIC INTERVENTION ACTIVITIES

The Patient with Heart Failure

Ventilation Assistance: *Promotion of an optimal spontaneous breathing pattern that maximizes oxygen and carbon dioxide exchange in the lungs.*

- Monitor respiratory and oxygenation status.
- Initiate and maintain supplemental oxygen, as prescribed.
- Position to alleviate dyspnea.
- Auscultate breath sounds, noting areas of decreased or absent ventilation and presence of adventitious sounds.
- Position to minimize respiratory efforts (e.g., elevate the head of the bed, and provide overbed table for patient to lean on).
- Monitor the effects of position change on oxygenation: ABG, Sao_2, Svo_2, end-tidal CO_2, Q_{sp}/Q_t, A-aDO_2 levels.

Hemodynamic Regulation: *Optimization of heart rate, preload, afterload, and contractility.*

- Monitor and document heart rate, rhythm, and pulses.
- Monitor peripheral pulses, capillary refill, and temperature and color of extremities.
- Monitor pulmonary capillary/pulmonary artery wedge pressure and central venous/right atrial pressure, if appropriate.
- Administer vasodilator and/or vasoconstrictor medication, as appropriate.
- Administer positive inotropic/contractility medications.
- Maintain fluid balance by administering IV fluids or diuretics, as appropriate.
- Monitor intake/output, urine output, and patient weight, as appropriate.
- Monitor electrolyte levels.
- Auscultate heart sounds.

Energy Management: *Regulation of energy use to treat or prevent fatigue and optimize function.*

- Monitor cardiorespiratory response to activity (e.g., tachycardia, other dysrhythmias, dyspnea, diaphoresis, pallor, hemodynamic pressures, and respiratory rate).
- Determine patient's physical limitations.
- Encourage alternate rest and activity periods.
- Arrange physical activities to reduce competition for oxygen supply to vital body functions (e.g., avoid activity immediately after meals).
- Encourage physical activity (e.g., ambulation or performance of activities of daily living, consistent with patient's energy resources).
- Monitor patient's oxygen response (e.g., pulse rate, cardiac rhythm, and respiratory rate) to self-care or nursing activities.
- Teach patient and significant other techniques of self-care that will minimize oxygen consumption (e.g., self-monitoring and pacing techniques for performance of activities of daily living).

NIC intervention activities selected from Bulechek, G.M., Butcher, H.K., & McCloskey Dochterman, J. (Eds.). (2008). *Nursing interventions classification (NIC)* (5th ed.). St. Louis: Mosby.

A-aDO₂, Alveolar-arterial oxygen pressure difference; *ABG*, arterial blood gas; *CO_2*, carbon dioxide; Q_{sp}/Q_t, physiologic blood flow per minute/cardiac output per minute; *Sao_2*, saturation of arterial oxygen; *Svo_2*, saturation of venous oxygen.

TABLE 37-3 **Commonly Used Drug Classifications for Patients with Systolic Heart Failure**

Angiotensin-converting enzyme (ACE) inhibitors or angiotensin-receptor blockers (ARBs)
Diuretics
- High-ceiling
- Potassium-sparing

Human B-type natriuretic peptides
Nitrates
Inotropics
- Beta-adrenergic agonists
- Phosphodiesterase inhibitors
- Calcium sensitizers
- Digitalis

Beta-adrenergic blockers

NIC **Hemodynamic regulation.** Interventions to improve stroke volume include reducing afterload, reducing preload, and improving cardiac muscle contractility. A major role of the nurse is to give medications as prescribed, monitor for their therapeutic and adverse effects, and teach the patient and family about drug therapy. A variety of classes of drugs that reduce afterload and preload are used to manage heart failure (see Table 37-3).

Drugs that reduce afterload. By relaxing the arterioles, arterial vasodilators can reduce the resistance to left ventricular ejection (afterload) and improve CO. These drugs do not cause excessive vasodilation but reverse some of the inappropriate or excessive vasoconstriction common in HF.

Angiotensin-converting enzyme (ACE) inhibitors and angiotensin-receptor blockers (ARBs). Patients with even mild heart failure (HF) resulting from left ventricular dysfunction should be given a trial of ACE inhibitors or ARBs. Both ACE inhibitors such as enalapril (Vasotec), fosinopril (Monopril), and ramipril (Altace), and ARBs such as valsartan (Diovan), irbesartan (Avapro), and losartan (Cozaar) improve function and quality of life for patients with HF. ACE inhibitors are the first-line drug of choice, but some health care providers may prefer to start the patient on an ARB because ACE inhibitors can cause a nagging, dry cough. For patients with *acute* HF, the health care provider may prescribe an IV push ACE inhibitor such as Vasotec IV.

The ACE inhibitors and ARBs suppress the renin-angiotensin system (RAS), which is activated in response to decreased renal blood flow. ACE inhibitors prevent conversion of angiotensin I to angiotensin II, resulting in arterial resistance, arterial dilation, and increased SV. ARBs block the effect of angiotensin II receptors and thus decrease arterial resistance and arterial dilation. In addition, these drugs block aldosterone, which prevents sodium and water retention, thus decreasing fluid overload. *Both ACEs and ARBs work more effectively for Euro-Americans than for African-American populations.* Volume-depleted patients should receive a low starting dose, or the fluid volume should be restored before beginning the prescribed drug. Monitor for hyperkalemia, a potential adverse drug effect in patients who have renal dysfunction.

ACE inhibitors and ARBs are started slowly and cautiously. The first dose may be associated with a rapid drop in blood pressure (BP). Patients at risk for hypotension usually have an initial systolic BP less than 100 mm Hg, are older than 75 years, have a serum sodium level less than 137 mEq/L, or are volume depleted. Monitor BP for several hours after the initial dose and each time the dose is increased.

Clarify with the health care provider the guidelines for administering these drugs. For example, many clinicians maintain patients with HF at a systolic BP ranging from 90 to 110 mm Hg. In this case, assess for orthostatic hypotension, acute confusion, poor peripheral perfusion, and reduced urine output. Monitor serum potassium levels for hyperkalemia and serum creatinine, which can indicate renal dysfunction. Additional nursing implications for selected ACE inhibitor/ARB drugs are described in Chapter 38 on p. 801 in the Drug Therapy section.

Human B-type natriuretic peptides. Human B-type natriuretic peptides (hBNPs) such as nesiritide (Natrecor) are often used to treat *acute* HF. Endogenous BNP is released in response to decreased CO and causes *natriuresis,* or loss of sodium in the renal tubules, as well as vasodilation. Natrecor lowers pulmonary capillary wedge pressure (PCWP) and improves renal glomerular filtration. It is given as an IV bolus over 60 seconds followed with a continuous infusion for up to 48 hours. *When giving this drug, monitor BP and pulse carefully because significant decreases in BP may occur.* Although the patient's systolic BP may be between 90 and 100, he or she is usually asymptomatic. *Give Natrecor through a separate infusion line because it is incompatible with heparin and most other parenteral medications. Expect an increase in the serum BNP after drug administration.*

Interventions that reduce preload. Ventricular fibers contract less forcefully when they are overstretched, such as in a failing heart. Interventions aimed at reducing preload attempt to decrease volume and pressure in the left ventricle, increasing ventricular muscle stretch and contraction. Preload reduction is appropriate for HF accompanied by congestion with total body sodium and water overload.

Nutrition therapy. In HF, nutrition therapy is aimed at reducing sodium and water retention. In collaboration with the nutritionist, the health care provider may restrict sodium intake in an attempt to decrease fluid retention. Many patients need to omit table salt (no added salt) from their diet, thus reducing sodium intake to about 3 g daily.

If salt intake must be reduced further, the patient may need to eliminate all salt in cooking, as well as high-sodium foods (e.g., ham, bacon, pickles), thus reducing sodium intake to 2 g daily. Collaborate with the nutritionist to help the patient select foods that meet such a restricted therapeutic diet. An appropriate sodium restriction is important to prevent recurrence of acute heart failure.

Few patients are placed on severe fluid restrictions. However, patients with excessive aldosterone secretion may experience thirst and drink 3 to 5 liters of fluid each day. As a result, their fluid intake may be limited to a more normal 2 liters daily. Adherence to these simple strategies varies. *Supervise unlicensed assistive personnel (UAP) to ensure that they limit the prescribed intake and accurately record intake and output.*

Weigh the patient daily, or delegate this activity to UAP and supervise that it is done. *Keep in mind that 1 kg of weight gain or loss equals 1 liter of retained or lost fluid. The same scale should be used every morning before breakfast for the most accurate assessment of weight.* Monitor for a decrease in weight, an expected outcome because excess fluid is excreted from the body.

Drug therapy. Common drugs prescribed to reduce preload are diuretics and venous vasodilators. Morphine sulfate is given to reduce anxiety, decrease preload and afterload, slow respirations, and reduce the pain associated with a myocardial infarction (MI). Additional drugs are used for patients who have special needs.

The health care provider adds *diuretics* to the regimen when diet and fluid restrictions have not been effective in managing the symptoms of systemic or pulmonary congestion. *Diuretics are the first-line drug of choice in older adults with HF and fluid overload* (Aronow, 2006). These drugs enhance the renal excretion of sodium and water by reducing circulating blood volume, decreasing preload, and reducing systemic and pulmonary congestion.

The type and dosage of diuretic prescribed depend on the degree of HF and renal function. High-ceiling (loop) diuretics, such as furosemide (Lasix, Furoside♣, Novosemide♣), torsemide (Demadex), and bumetanide (Bumex), are most effective for treating fluid volume overload.

CONSIDERATIONS FOR OLDER ADULTS

Loop diuretics continue to work even after excess fluid is removed. As a result, some patients, especially older adults, can become dehydrated. Observe the patient for manifestations of dehydration in the older adult, especially acute confusion and decreased urinary output.

Although these drugs continue to work after excess fluid is removed, they are needed to ensure effective diuresis for many patients in HF. For those with *acute* HF, Lasix or Bumex can be given by IV push (IVP). Lasix can be given in doses of 20 to 40 mg IV and increased by 20 mg every 2 hours until the desired diuresis is obtained. The usual IV initial dose for Bumex is 1 to 2 mg once or twice daily, but it is more often given in a continuous infusion of 10 mg over 24 hours.

The practitioner may initially use a thiazide diuretic such as hydrochlorothiazide (HCTZ) (HydroDIURIL, Urozide♣) and metolazone (Zaroxolyn) for *older adults* with *mild* volume overload. Zaroxolyn is a long-acting agent and is therefore often given every second, third, or fourth day, depending on patient need and tolerance.

Unlike loop diuretics, the action of thiazides is self-limiting (i.e., diuresis decreases after edema fluid is lost). Therefore the dehydration that may occur with loop diuretics is not common with these drugs. Patients also prefer thiazides because of the gradual onset of diuresis.

As HF progresses, many patients develop diuretic resistance with refractory edema. The health care provider may choose to manage this problem by prescribing both types of diuretics.

Monitor for and prevent potassium deficiency (hypokalemia) from diuretic therapy. The signs of hypokalemia are nonspecific neurologic and muscular symptoms, such as generalized weakness, depressed reflexes, and irregular heart rate.

Some practitioners also prescribe a potassium-sparing diuretic such as spironolactone (Aldactone) for patients at risk for dysrhythmias. Although not as effective as other diuretics, Aldactone helps retain potassium and thus decrease the risk of ventricular dysrhythmias.

If the patient's serum potassium level is less than 4.0 mEq/L, the health care provider has several alternatives:

- Add a potassium-sparing diuretic to the regimen (e.g., spironolactone [Aldactone])
- Request that patients further increase their intake of potassium-rich foods
- Prescribe a potassium supplement

Patients being managed with ACE inhibitors or ARBs and diuretics at the same time may not experience hypokalemia. However, if their kidneys are not functioning well, they may develop hyperkalemia (elevated serum potassium level). Review the patient's serum creatinine level. If the creatinine is greater than 1.8, notify the health care provider before administering supplemental potassium.

The health care provider may prescribe *venous vasodilators* (e.g., nitrates) for the patient with HF who has persistent dyspnea. Significant constriction of venous and arterial blood vessels occurs to compensate for reduced CO. Constriction reduces the volume of fluid that the vascular bed can hold and increases preload. Venous vasodilators may benefit by:

- Returning venous vasculature to a more normal capacity
- Decreasing the volume of blood returning to the heart
- Improving left ventricular function

Nitrates may be administered IV, orally, or topically. IV nitrates are used most often for *acute* HF. These drugs cause primarily venous vasodilation but also a significant amount of arteriolar vasodilation. Monitor the patient's blood pressure when starting nitrate therapy or increasing the dosage. Patients may initially report headache, but assure them that they will develop a tolerance to this effect and that the headache will cease or diminish. Acetaminophen (Tylenol, Exdol♣) can be given to help relieve discomfort.

Unfortunately, tolerance to the vasodilating effects develops when nitrates are given around-the-clock. To prevent this tolerance, the health care provider may prescribe at least one 12-hour nitrate-free period out of every 24 hours (usually overnight). Nitrates such as isosorbide (Imdur, ISMO) are prescribed to provide nitrate-free periods and reduce the problem of tolerance. Chapter 40 discusses nitrates in more detail.

Drugs that enhance contractility. Contractility of the heart can also be enhanced with drug therapy. Positive inotropic drugs are most commonly used, but vasodilators and beta-adrenergic blockers may also be administered. For chronic HF, low-dose beta blockers are most commonly used. Digoxin (Lanoxin) may be prescribed to improve symptoms, thereby decreasing dyspnea and improving functional activity. This older and long-used drug is very inexpensive. In some settings, nesiritide (Natrecor) may be administered for end-stage HF, although this drug is very expensive (see discussion of Natrecor for acute HF on p. 772).

Digoxin. Although not commonly used today, digoxin (Lanoxin, Novodigoxin♣), a cardiac glycoside, has been demonstrated to *provide symptomatic benefits* for patients in *chronic* heart failure (HF) with sinus rhythm and atrial fibrillation. Digoxin (sometimes called "dig") therapy reduces exacerbations of HF and hospitalizations when added to a regimen of ACE inhibitors or ARBs, beta blockers, and diuretics. It may increase mortality due to drug toxicity, however, especially in older adults.

The potential benefits of digoxin include:

- Increased contractility
- Reduced heart rate (HR)
- Slowing of conduction through the atrioventricular node
- Inhibition of sympathetic activity while enhancing parasympathetic activity

Digoxin is erratically absorbed from the GI tract. Many drugs, especially antacids, interfere with its absorption. It is eliminated primarily by renal excretion. Older patients should be maintained on lower doses of the drug than younger patients.

Increased cardiac automaticity occurs with toxic digitalis levels or in the presence of hypokalemia, resulting in ectopic beats (e.g., premature ventricular contractions [PVCs]). *Changes in potassium level, especially a decrease, causes patients to be more sensitive to the drug and cause toxicity.*

The clinical manifestations of ***digitalis toxicity*** *are often vague and nonspecific and include anorexia, fatigue, and changes in mental status, especially in older adults. Toxicity may cause nearly any dysrhythmia, but PVCs are most commonly noted. Assess for early signs of toxicity such as bradycardia and loss of the P wave on the ECG. Carefully monitor the apical pulse rate and heart rhythm of patients receiving digoxin.* The health care provider determines the desirable HR to achieve. Some physicians prefer a rate less than 60 beats per minute. Report the development of either an irregular rhythm in a patient with a previously regular rhythm or a regular rhythm in a patient with a previously irregular one. Monitor serum digoxin and potassium levels (hypokalemia potentiates digitalis toxicity) to identify toxicity. Older adults are more likely than other patients to become toxic because of decreased renal excretion.

Any drug that increases the workload of the failing heart also increases its oxygen requirement. Be alert for the possibility that the patient may experience angina (chest pain) in response to digoxin.

CONSIDERATIONS FOR OLDER ADULTS

For older adults who have HF, the selection and dosing for cardiac drugs should be individualized. For example, after correction of any hyponatremia or volume depletion, ACE inhibitors should be started in low doses and slowly increased to therapeutic levels. Digoxin increases the mortality rate in women with HF, especially older women (Aronow, 2006).

Other inotropic drugs. Patients experiencing *acute* heart failure (HF) are candidates for IV drugs that increase contractility. For example, *beta-adrenergic agonists,* such as dobutamine (Dobutrex), are used for short-term treatment of *acute* episodes of HF. Dobutamine improves cardiac contractility and thus cardiac output and myocardial-systemic perfusion.

A more potent drug used for *acute* HF, milrinone (Primacor), functions as a vasodilator/inotropic medication with phosphodiesterase activity. Also known as a *phosphodiesterase inhibitor,* this drug increases cyclic adenosine monophosphate (cAMP), which enhances the entry of calcium into myocardial cells to increase contractile function. Like the beta-adrenergic drugs, Primacor is given IV.

Levosimendan (Simdax) is a calcium-sensitizing medication and a positive inotropic drug. It appears to bind to troponin C in the heart muscle and therefore increases the contraction of the heart. Simdax is used most often in patients who have had or are at high risk for myocardial infarction. Chapter 40 discusses inotropic drugs in more detail.

NCLEX EXAMINATION CHALLENGE

An older adult taking digoxin and furosemide for chronic heart failure is admitted to the emergency department (ED) with an apical pulse of 52. She is disoriented to time and place and states that she "can't see very well." What is the nurse's first action?

A. Call the ED physician immediately.
B. Draw a serum digoxin level.
C. Assess for signs of hypokalemia.
D. Establish the client's airway.

evolve For the correct answer, go to http://evolve.elsevier.com/Iggy/.

Beta-adrenergic blockers. Beta blockers improve the condition of some patients in HF. It appears that prolonged exposure to increased levels of sympathetic stimulation and catecholamines worsens cardiac function. Beta-adrenergic blockade reverses this effect, improving morbidity, mortality, and quality of life for patients in HF.

Beta blockers must be started slowly for HF. Patients in *acute* HF should not be started on these drugs. Carvedilol (Coreg), metoprolol (Lopressor, Betaloc♣), and bisoprolol (Zebeta) are approved for treatment of *chronic* HF. The first dose is extremely low, and the patient is monitored either in the hospital or in the health care provider's office to assess for bradycardia or hypotension.

Instruct the patient to weigh daily and to report any signs of worsening HF immediately. The health care provider gradually titrates the drug dose upward. The patient is evaluated at least weekly for changes in BP, pulse, activity tolerance, and orthopnea. A modest drop in BP is acceptable if he or she remains asymptomatic and can stand without experiencing dizziness or a further drop in BP. The resting HR should remain between 55 and 60 and increase slightly with exercise. Activity tolerance improves, and less orthopnea is experienced. Most patients with mild and moderate HF demonstrate improved ejection fraction, decreased hospital admissions, and improvement in symptoms when beta blockers are added to their treatment regimens. The benefits of beta-blocker therapy are seen over a long period and not immediately.

For patients with *diastolic* HF, drug therapy has not been as effective. Calcium channel blockers, ACE inhibitors, and beta blockers have been used with various degrees of success.

Other nonsurgical options. In addition to drug therapy, nonsurgical options, both noninvasive and invasive, may be used and include:

- Continuous positive airway pressure (CPAP)
- Cardiac resynchronization therapy (CRT)
- Investigative gene therapy

Continuous positive airway pressure (CPAP) is a respiratory treatment that improves obstructive sleep apnea in patients with HF. It also improves cardiac output (CO) and ejection fraction (EF) by decreasing afterload and preload, blood pressure (BP), and dysrhythmias. Sleep apnea is directly correlated with coronary artery disease as a result of diminished oxygen supply to the heart during apneic episodes. This respiratory problem is discussed in detail in Chapter 31.

Cardiac resynchronization therapy (CRT), also called *biventricular pacing,* uses a permanent pacemaker alone or is combined with an implantable cardioverter/defibrillator. Electrical stimulation causes more synchronous ventricular contractions to improve EF, CO, and mean arterial pressure. This modality is indicated for patients with class III or IV HF and an EF of less than 35%. CRT improves the patient's ability to perform ADLs. Chapter 36 discusses pacing in more detail.

Gene therapy may be indicated for patients in end-stage HF who are not candidates for heart transplantation. This therapy replaces damaged genes with normal or modified genes by a series of injections of growth factor into the left ventricle. Although still investigative, this therapy has resulted in improved exercise tolerance and regrowth of cardiac cells.

Surgical Management. Heart transplantation is still the ultimate choice for end-stage HF (see discussion on p. 789). Several surgical procedures are available to improve CO in patients who are *not* candidates for a transplant or are awaiting transplant.

Ventricular assist devices. Patients with debilitating end-stage heart failure are often sent home on drug therapy and referred to hospice. However, ventricular assist devices (VADs) can dramatically improve the lives of many patients (Stahovich et al., 2007). In this procedure, a mechanical pump is implanted to work with the patient's own heart (Fig. 37-2). Both left and right VADs are available, depending on the type of heart failure the patient has. Those with end-stage kidney disease, severe chronic lung disease, clotting disorders, and infections that do not respond to antibiotics are not candidates for this surgery. Postoperative complications include bleeding, infective endocarditis, ventricular dysrhythmias, and stroke. Nursing care is similar to that described for cardiac surgery in Chapter 40.

These devices can be used short-term while awaiting heart transplantation (a "bridge-to-transplant" procedure) or long-term (destination therapy). Most patients survive with a VAD until a transplant is available. Patients who have long-term devices have an increased length of life and an improved quality of life (Richards & Stahl, 2007).

Other surgical therapies. Heart failure causes ventricular remodeling, or dilation, which worsens as the disease progresses. Several new therapies are used to reshape the left ventricle in patients with HF. Perioperative care is similar to

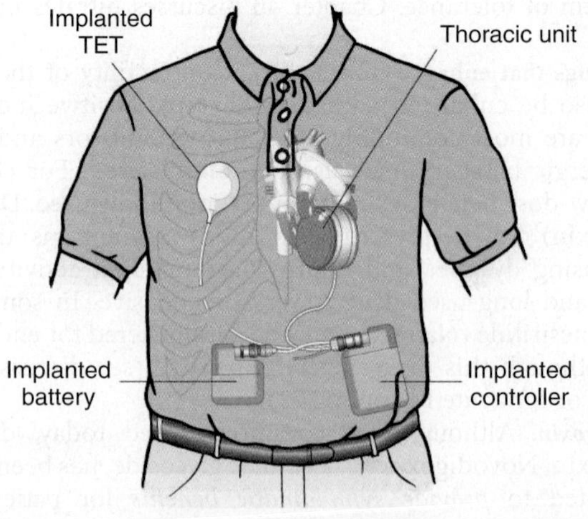
Implanted
TET
Thoracic unit
Implanted
battery
Implanted
controller

Fig. 37-2 • The AbioCor System has four main parts that are implanted inside the body. *TET,* Transtelephonic electrocardiographic transmission device.

that for the patient experiencing a coronary artery bypass graft (CABG) (see Chapter 40). The most common ventricular reconstructive procedures include:

- Partial left ventriculectomy (PLV)
- Endoventricular circular patch
- Acorn cardiac support device
- Myosplint

Also known as **heart reduction surgery,** PLV (sometimes referred to as the *Batista procedure*) involves removing a triangle-shaped section of the weakened heart in the left lateral ventricle to reduce the ventricle's diameter and decrease wall tension. In **endoventricular circular patch cardioplasty,** the surgeon removes portions of the cardiac septum and left ventricular wall and grafts a circular patch (synthetic or autologous) into the opening. This procedure provides a more normal shape to the left ventricle to improve EF and CO.

The **acorn cardiac support device** is a polyester mesh jacket that is placed over the ventricles to provide support and to avoid overstretching the myocardial muscle. The material for the jacket has been used for other procedures, such as vascular grafts. The jacket appears to reduce hypertrophy of the heart muscle and assists with improvement of the EF.

The **myosplint** has recently been approved for use in the United States. Electrical stimulation of several tension pads (splints) on the outside of the ventricle changes it to a more normal shape to improve function.

Activity Intolerance

NOC **Planning: Expected Outcomes.** The patient with HF is expected to take actions to manage energy for initiating and sustaining activity. Indicators include that the patient:

- Balances activity and rest
- Uses naps to restore energy
- Recognizes energy limitations
- Organizes activities to conserve energy
- Adapts lifestyle to energy level
- Reports adequate endurance for activity

Interventions. The purpose of interdisciplinary interventions is to regulate energy to prevent fatigue and optimize function (see Chart 37-3).

NIC The patient in severe HF initially requires physical and emotional rest for *energy management*. On the first day of hospitalization, he or she may sit up in a chair for meals and perform basic leg exercises while out of bed. Nursing care should be organized to allow periods of rest. Collaborate with the interdisciplinary team to observe and document the patient's physiologic response to activity.

As the patient's condition improves, the physical therapist (PT) starts ambulation, usually on hospital day 2. The PT or nurse checks the BP, pulse, and oxygen saturation before and after the activity. A BP change of more than 20 mm Hg or a pulse increase of more than 20 beats per minute may indicate that the activity is too stressful. Other indications of activity intolerance include dyspnea, fatigue, and chest pain. Ask a patient displaying any of these symptoms to rate how hard he or she has been working on a scale of 1 to 20, with 20 being the maximum perceived exertion. If the patient rates the exertion more than 12, counsel him or her to slow down. If activity is tolerated, the PT steadily increases the activity level until the patient is ambulating 200 to 400 feet several times per day.

If the patient is able, the PT (or assistive nursing or PT personnel) might time him or her for 6 minutes while walking at a comfortable pace. The distance the patient can walk can be used to determine his or her functional level and activity plan.

Potential for Pulmonary Edema

Planning: Expected Outcomes. The patient with HF is expected to not develop cardiogenic pulmonary edema. Indicators include that he or she will have:

- No adventitious breath sounds
- Vital signs within normal limits
- ABG values within normal limits

Interventions. Monitor for manifestations of acute pulmonary edema, a life-threatening event that can result from severe HF (with fluid overload), acute MI, mitral valve disease, and possibly dysrhythmias. In pulmonary edema, the left ventricle fails to eject sufficient blood and pressure increases in the lungs because of the accumulated blood. The increased pressure causes fluid to leak across the pulmonary capillaries and into the lung airways and tissues.

Assess for early manifestations, such as crackles in the lung bases, dyspnea at rest, disorientation, and confusion, especially in older patients. Documentation of the precise location of the crackles is essential because the level of the fluid ascends as the pulmonary edema worsens. The patient in acute pulmonary edema is also typically extremely anxious, tachycardic, and struggling for air. As pulmonary edema becomes more severe, he or she may have a moist cough productive of frothy, blood-tinged sputum and his or her skin may be cold, clammy, or cyanotic. Chart 37-4 lists the major clinical manifestations of this complication.

The patient diagnosed with pulmonary edema is admitted to the acute care hospital, often in a critical care unit. Reassure the patient that his or her distress will decrease with proper management. *If the patient is not hypotensive, place him or her in a sitting (high Fowler's) position with his or her legs down to decrease venous return to the heart. The priority nursing action is to administer high-flow oxygen therapy at 5 to 6 L/min by facemask or at 10 to 15 L/min by non-rebreather mask with reservoir (Bixby, 2005). Apply a pulse oximeter and cardiac monitor to keep the patient's oxygen saturation above 90%.* If supplemental oxygen does not resolve the patient's respiratory distress, collaborate with the respiratory therapist, if available, for more aggressive therapy, such as continuous positive airway pressure (CPAP) ventilation. Intubation and mechanical ventilation are used if needed.

If the patient's systolic blood pressure is above 100, give sublingual nitroglycerin (NTG) to decrease afterload and preload every 5 minutes for three doses while establishing IV

Chart 37-4 KEY FEATURES

Pulmonary Edema

- Crackles
- Dyspnea at rest
- Disorientation or acute confusion (especially in older adults as early symptom)
- Tachycardia
- Hypertension or hypotension
- Reduced urinary output
- Cough with frothy, pink-tinged sputum
- Premature ventricular contractions and other dysrhythmias
- Anxiety
- Restlessness
- Lethargy

Chart 37-5 HOME CARE ASSESSMENT

The Patient with Heart Failure

Assess for signs of heart failure, including:
- Changes in vital signs (heart rate >100 beats/min at rest, new atrial fibrillation, blood pressure <90 or >150 systolic)
- Indications of poor tissue perfusion
  - Fatigue
  - Angina
  - Activity intolerance
  - Changes in mental status
  - Pallor or cyanosis
  - Cool extremities
- Indications of congestion
  - Presence of cough or dyspnea
  - Weight gain
  - Jugular venous distention and peripheral edema

Assess functional ability, including:
- Performance of ADLs
- Mobility and ambulation (review frequency and duration of walking, development of symptoms, and pulse rate)
- Cognitive ability

Assess nutritional status, including:
- Food and fluid intake
- Intake of sodium-rich foods
- Alcohol consumption
- Skin turgor

Assess home environment, including:
- Safety hazards, especially related to oxygen therapy
- Structural barriers affecting functional ability
- Social support (family, home health services)

Assess the patient's adherence and understanding of illness and its treatment, including:
- Signs and symptoms to report to health care provider
- Dosages, effects, and side or toxic effects of medications
- When to report for laboratory and health care provider visits
- Ability to accurately weigh self on scale
- Presence of advance directive
- Use of home oxygen, if appropriate

Assess patient and caregiver coping skills

access for additional drug therapy (Bixby, 2005). The physician prescribes rapid-acting diuretics, such as Lasix or Bumex. Lasix is given IV over 1 to 2 minutes, usually at a starting dose of 40 mg, with another 40 mg repeated if needed in 30 minutes. Each increment of 40 mg of Lasix should be administered over 1 to 2 minutes to avoid ototoxicity. Bumex may be administered 1 to 2 mg IVP or as a continuous infusion to provide consistent fluid removal over 24 hours. Monitor vital signs frequently, every 30 to 60 minutes.

If the patient's blood pressure is adequate, IV morphine sulfate may be prescribed, 1 to 2 mg at a time, to reduce venous return (preload), decrease anxiety, and reduce the work of breathing. Monitor respiratory rate and BP closely. Other drugs, such as IV NTG and drugs to treat HF, may be administered. Monitor the patient's vital signs closely (especially BP) while these drugs are being given.

Community-Based Care

Patients who are not adequately prepared for discharge or do not have good community support and follow-up for self-management are at high risk for recurrent hospital admissions for heart failure (HF). Collaborate with the case manager or care coordinator to assess the patient's needs for health care resources. An inability to obtain help in activities such as food shopping and obtaining medications is a major contributor to hospital readmission. If home support is available, the patient may be discharged home in the care of a family member or other caregiver. Home care nurses may direct the care and aides may provide assistance with ADLs for a short time. If the patient has multiple health problems or has been severely compromised by heart disease, he or she may require admission to a skilled unit for either transitional or long-term care.

Home Care Management

The focus of the home care nurse's interventions is assessment and health teaching, which are reimbursable by Medicare and other third-party payers. Chart 37-5 lists the major areas of home health assessment.

Patients with chronic HF need to make many adjustments in their lifestyles. They must adhere to a medical regimen that includes dietary restrictions, activity prescriptions, and drug therapy. They need careful, concise explanations of the self-management plan. The community-based nurse in any setting encourages the patient to verbalize fears and concerns about his or her illness and assists in exploring coping skills. Patient participation in self-management can help alleviate and control symptoms.

Health Teaching

Health teaching is essential for promoting self-management (also called *self-care*). Riegel et al. (2007) reported the results of a study of patients with HF to determine the factors that influence adherence to self-care (see the Evidence-Based Practice box on p. 777). Many patients are readmitted to hospitals because they do not maintain their prescribed treatment plan, including lifestyle changes.

Most hospitals are using extensive discharge health teaching packets with videos, CDs, and easy-to-read information about heart failure and the importance of adhering to specific self-management strategies at home. One standardized and commonly used self-management plan called *MAWDS* is outlined in Table 37-4.

Several types of programs are available for continuing follow-up of patients with HF at home to evaluate the effectiveness of hospital discharge health teaching. For example, a nurse-led intervention in New York resulted in improved self-management for ambulatory care patients after hospital discharge. Nurses provided health teaching and gave every patient a scale for daily weights. Patients were instructed to report any symptom of worsening heart failure to their health care provider. Nurses made frequent phone calls to check on self-management adherence for the next 12 months. At the end of this period, patients in the study group had fewer hospitalizations than a comparison group who did not have the follow-up nursing intervention (Mennick, 2006).

EVIDENCE-BASED PRACTICE

What factors help determine which patients with heart failure will manage their care at home?

Riegel, B., Dickson, V.V., Goldberg, L.R., & Deatrick, J.A. (2007). Factors associated with the development of expertise in heart failure self-care. *Nursing Research, 56*(4), 235-243.

The purpose of this qualitative and quantitative study was to describe how expertise in self-care for heart failure (HF) develops. The convenience sample was 29 patients with chronic disease who were interviewed about HF self-care, surveyed to measure factors that influence self-care, and tested for cognitive functioning. After data analysis, the subjects were rated as poor, good, or expert in HF self-care.

The results showed that only 10% of the sample were expert in self-care. Patients who rated as poor in self-care reported more depression, sleepiness, cognitive problems, and poorer family support and functioning than the experts. Experts had fewer health-related problems and strong family support. The researchers concluded that family support is a strong factor associated with successful self-care.

Level of Evidence—6. The research was a small descriptive study that used a convenience sample of 29 patients.

Commentary: Implications for Practice and Research. One large limitation was that the study did not describe the demographics of the subjects (e.g., how many were men and how many were women, their ages, and racial/ethnic origins). The assumption is that all the subjects were white and most were men. However, this study did validate other literature regarding the need for strong family support to adhere to lifestyle changes and a complex treatment plan. Nurses need to be sure to include whomever patients designate as family or support systems when providing health teaching for self-management. Additional studies should be conducted to examine other factors, such as depression and sleepiness that occurred in the poor self-care managers.

TABLE 37-4 Heart Failure Self-Management Health Teaching (MAWDS)

Medications:
- Take medications as prescribed, and do not run out.
- Know the purpose and side effects of each drug.
- Avoid NSAIDs.

Activity:
- Stay as active as possible, but don't overdo it.
- Know your limits.
- Be able to carry on a conversation while exercising.

Weight:
- Weigh each day at the same time on the same scale to monitor for fluid retention.

Diet:
- Limit daily sodium intake to 2 to 3 grams as prescribed.
- Limit daily fluid intake to 2 liters.

Symptoms:
- Note any new or worsening symptoms, and notify the health care provider immediately.

Ambulatory care clinics for heart failure patients are also becoming increasingly common. Their purpose is to offer assessments, drug therapy, and health teaching. Crowder (2006) reported the results of a qualitative study of 15 patients enrolled in an outpatient congestive heart failure (CHF) clinic. She found that the subjects wished they had enrolled in the clinic earlier before their disease had further progressed. Patient outcomes, including function and quality of life, improved as a result of being followed up in an ambulatory care setting.

Activity Schedule. Encourage patients with HF to stay as active as possible and to develop a regular exercise regimen. Those who are more active appear to have better outcomes. The primary outcome is development of a regular exercise routine (e.g., home walking program). However, teach the patient not to overdo it. Medicare and third-party payers typically do not reimburse for cardiac rehabilitation for HF, and paying for a cardiac rehabilitation program out of pocket is expensive.

Although most patients appear to benefit from exercise programs, those with persistent crackles and uncontrolled edema despite medical therapy are not encouraged to exercise until their HF is stabilized. When exercise is indicated, teach the patient to begin walking 200 to 400 feet per day. At home the patient should try to walk at least three times a week and should slowly increase the amount of time walked (perhaps 10 minutes a week) over several months. If chest pain or severe dyspnea occurs while exercising or the patient has fatigue the next day, he or she is probably advancing the activity too quickly and should slow down. Encourage him or her to keep an exercise diary that documents the time and duration of each exercise session, as well as HR and any symptoms that occur with exercise.

Indications of Worsening or Recurrent Heart Failure. Many patients who are readmitted to hospitals for treatment of HF fail to seek medical attention promptly when symptoms recur. Instruct the patient and caregiver to immediately report to the health care provider the occurrence of any of these symptoms:
- Rapid weight gain (3 lb in a week or 1 to 2 lb overnight)
- Decrease in exercise tolerance lasting 2 to 3 days
- Cold symptoms (cough) lasting more than 3 to 5 days
- Excessive awakening at night to urinate
- Development of dyspnea or angina at rest or worsening angina
- Increased swelling in the feet, ankles, or hands

Drug Therapy. Provide oral, written, and video instructions about the drug regimen. Teach the caregiver and patient how to count a pulse rate, especially if the patient is on digoxin or beta blockers. Chart 37-6 lists instructions for the patient taking either of these drugs at home.

Advise the patient taking diuretics to take them in the morning to avoid waking during the night for voiding. After determining whether he or she has a weight scale and can use it, emphasize the importance of weighing each morning. Although this simple intervention can greatly assist in managing HF, most patients do not weigh themselves regularly. Emphasize the relationship between weight gain, fluid retention, and HF. Daily weights indicate whether the patient

Chart 37-6 PATIENT AND FAMILY EDUCATION GUIDE

Beta Blocker/Digoxin Therapy

- Establish same time of day to take this medication everyday.
- Continue taking this medication unless your health care provider tells you to stop.
- Do not take digoxin at the same time as antacids or cathartics (laxatives).
- Take your pulse rate before taking each dose of digoxin. Notify your health care provider of a change in pulse rate (60 to 100 beats/min is normal) or rhythm, as well as increasing fatigue, muscle weakness, confusion, or loss of appetite (signs of digoxin toxicity).
- If you forget to take a dose, it may be delayed a few hours. However, if you do not remember it until the next day, you should take only your usual daily dose.
- Report for scheduled laboratory tests (e.g., potassium and digoxin levels).
- If potassium supplements are prescribed, continue the dose until told to stop by your health care provider.

is losing or retaining fluid. Some motivated patients are taught to use a sliding scale to adjust their daily diuretic dose depending on their daily weight, similar to the way a diabetic patient adjusts an insulin dose based on the capillary glucose level.

Teach patients taking ACE inhibitors or ARBs to move slowly when changing positions, especially from a lying to a sitting position. Remind them to report dizziness, lightheadedness, and cough to the health care provider.

Serum potassium level and renal function must be monitored at least every few months for patients taking diuretics and ACE inhibitors or ARBs. Diuretics, especially loop diuretics such as Lasix and Bumex, deplete potassium and often cause hypokalemia. Conversely, ACE inhibitors, ARBs, or potassium-sparing diuretics may result in potassium retention. If potassium levels drop below 4.0 mEq/L, the health care provider may prescribe potassium supplements or add potassium-sparing diuretics such as spironolactone (Aldactone). Provide information about potassium-rich foods to include in the diet for patients at risk for hypokalemia.

Nutrition Therapy. Remind patients with chronic HF to restrict their dietary sodium. In collaboration with the home care nurse or nutritionist, provide written instructions on low- or restricted-sodium diets. A 3-g sodium diet is recommended for *mild to moderate* disease. Remind the patient to avoid salty foods and table salt. Patients usually find this diet palatable and fairly easy to follow.

A 2-g sodium diet is needed for patients with *severe* HF. They should not add salt during or after meal preparation, avoid milk and milk products, use few canned or prepared foods, and read food labels to determine sodium content. This diet is not easily tolerated for many patients, and the cost of low-sodium foods is a financial burden. Therefore the home care nurse or nurse and nutritionist in the patient's post-hospital setting should assess for adherence.

Some patients prefer to use commercial salt substitutes. Most salt substitutes contain potassium. The patient's renal status and serum potassium level need to be considered before these products can be recommended. Lemon, garlic, and herbs can be used to enhance the flavor of low-salt foods.

Advance Directives. About 50% of deaths from HF are sudden—many without any warning or worsening of symptoms. Assess whether the patient has written advance directives. If not, provide information about them during his or her hospital stay. Because most of these deaths occur at home, it is important for the health care provider or home care nurse to discuss advance directives with the patient and family. The family should be prepared to act in agreement with the patient's wishes in the event of cardiac arrest. If resuscitation is desired, the family should know how to activate the emergency medical system (EMS) and how to provide cardiopulmonary resuscitation (CPR) until an ambulance arrives. If CPR is not desired, the patient, family, and nurse plan how the family will respond. For some patients with end-stage disease, hospice care is an option. Chapter 9 discusses hospice and end-of-life care in detail.

Health Care Resources

A home care nurse, ambulatory care clinic, or nurse-led follow-up program may be needed to assess the patient's adherence to medication and nutrition therapy and to monitor for worsening or recurrent HF. Patients with activity limitations often benefit from the services of a home care aide. Although participation in structured cardiac rehabilitation programs has been shown to be beneficial, referrals to such programs are not widespread because coverage is usually not provided by third-party payers. Many larger hospitals use teleconferencing devices to monitor chronic CHF patients at home. They not only monitor the heart but also auscultate lung and heart sounds and can observe the patient through a video monitor.

In addition to home care support, other resources are available for patient education and family support. The American Heart Association is an excellent community resource for pamphlets, books, cookbooks, and videotapes or DVDs related to HF and heart disease. The organization also provides referrals to various local support groups for patients and their caregivers.

For equipment needs (e.g., home oxygen therapy, hospital bed), medical supply companies provide setup and maintenance services. Chapter 30 provides a detailed description of home oxygen therapy.

DECISION-MAKING CHALLENGE

Critical Rescue

A 76-year-old woman with hypertension, diabetes mellitus, osteoarthritis in her knees and feet, and chronic heart failure was discharged to home last week to live with her daughter and son-in-law. She is alert and oriented but needs help with most of her ADLs. The patient has been very careful with her diet and has avoided high-sodium foods and excess fluids. Today her weight is 3 pounds more than 2 days ago. She has noticed that she is more tired over the past few days and has "trouble catching my breath" when she uses her walker. Her daughter decides to take her to the physician where you are the office nurse.

1. What additional assessment should you perform when you interview this patient in the office?
2. What is the significance of the change in her condition at home?
3. What is your priority action at this time and why?
4. What drug(s) might she receive to help manage her health problem?

evolve For suggested answer guidelines, go to http://evolve.elsevier.com/Iggy/.

■ *Evaluation: Outcomes*

Evaluate the care of the patient with HF on the basis of the identified nursing diagnoses and collaborative problems. The expected outcomes include that the patient will:

- Have adequate pulmonary tissue perfusion
- Have increased cardiac pump effectiveness
- Take actions to manage energy
- Be free of pulmonary edema

Specific indicators for these outcomes are listed for each nursing diagnosis and collaborative problem in the Planning and Implementation section (see earlier discussion).

VALVULAR HEART DISEASE

Pathophysiology

Acquired valvular dysfunctions include mitral stenosis, mitral regurgitation, mitral valve prolapse, aortic stenosis, and aortic regurgitation (Chart 37-7). The tricuspid valve is affected infrequently, primarily following endocarditis in IV drug abusers.

Mitral Stenosis

Mitral stenosis usually results from rheumatic carditis, which can cause valve thickening by fibrosis and calcification. Rheumatic fever is the most common cause of the problem. As cases of rheumatic fever have decreased, so has the incidence of mitral stenosis. Nonrheumatic causes include atrial myxoma (tumor), calcium accumulation, and thrombus formation (McCance & Huether, 2006).

In mitral stenosis, the valve leaflets fuse and become stiff and the chordae tendineae contract and shorten. The valve opening narrows, preventing normal blood flow from the left atrium to the left ventricle. As a result of these changes, left atrial pressure rises, the left atrium dilates, pulmonary artery pressures increase, and the right ventricle hypertrophies.

Pulmonary congestion and right-sided HF occur initially. Later, when the left ventricle receives insufficient blood volume, preload is decreased and cardiac output (CO) falls.

People with mild mitral stenosis are usually asymptomatic. As the valvular orifice narrows and pressure in the lungs increases, the patient experiences dyspnea on exertion, orthopnea, paroxysmal nocturnal dyspnea (sudden dyspnea at night), palpitations, and dry cough. Hemoptysis and pulmonary edema appear as pulmonary hypertension and congestion progress. Right-sided HF can cause hepatomegaly, neck vein distention, and pitting edema late in the disorder.

On palpation, the pulse may be normal, rapid, or irregularly irregular (as in atrial fibrillation). Because the development of atrial fibrillation indicates that the patient may decompensate, the physician should be notified immediately of the development of an irregularly irregular rhythm. A rumbling, apical diastolic murmur is noted on auscultation.

Mitral Regurgitation (Insufficiency)

The fibrotic and calcific changes occurring in **mitral regurgitation** (insufficiency) prevent the mitral valve from closing completely during *systole.* Incomplete closure of the valve allows the backflow of blood into the left atrium when the left ventricle contracts (Todd & Higgins, 2005). During *diastole,* regurgitant output again flows from the left atrium to the left ventricle along with the normal blood flow. The increased volume must be ejected during the next systole. To compensate for the increased volume and pressure, the left atrium and ventricle dilate and hypertrophy.

Rheumatic heart disease is the major cause of mitral regurgitation. When it results from rheumatic heart disease, it usually coexists with some degree of mitral stenosis; it affects women more often than men. Nonrheumatic causes, more

Chart 37-7 KEY FEATURES

Valvular Heart Disease

Mitral Stenosis	Mitral Regurgitation	Mitral Valve Prolapse	Aortic Stenosis	Aortic Regurgitation
Fatigue Dyspnea on exertion Orthopnea Paroxysmal nocturnal dyspnea Hemoptysis Hepatomegaly Neck vein distention Pitting edema Atrial fibrillation Rumbling, apical diastolic murmur	Fatigue Dyspnea on exertion Orthopnea Palpitations Atrial fibrillation Neck vein distention Pitting edema High-pitched holosystolic murmur	Atypical chest pain Dizziness, syncope Palpitations Atrial tachycardia Ventricular tachycardia Systolic click	Dyspnea on exertion Angina Syncope on exertion Fatigue Orthopnea Paroxysmal nocturnal dyspnea Harsh, systolic crescendo-decrescendo murmur	Palpitations Dyspnea Orthopnea Paroxysmal nocturnal dyspnea Fatigue Angina Sinus tachycardia Blowing, decrescendo diastolic murmur

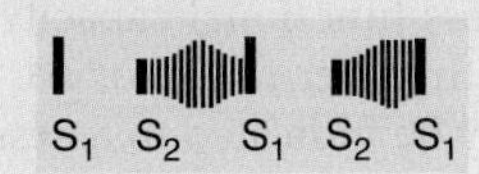
S_1 S_2 S_1 S_2 S_1

S_1 S_2S_3 S_1 S_2S_3
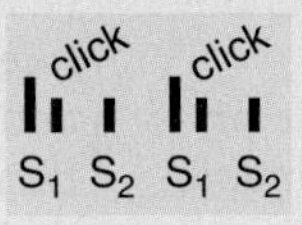
click
click
S_1 S_2 S_1 S_2
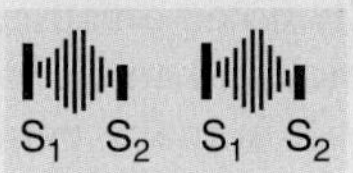
S_1 S_2 S_1 S_2
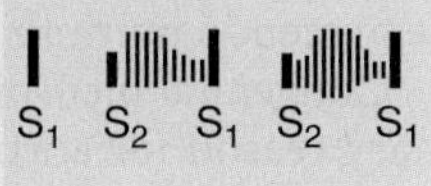
S_1 S_2 S_1 S_2 S_1

common in men, include papillary muscle dysfunction or rupture resulting from ischemic heart disease, infective endocarditis, and a congenital anomaly.

Mitral regurgitation usually progresses slowly; patients may remain symptom-free for decades. Symptoms begin to occur when the left ventricle fails in response to chronic blood volume overload. They include fatigue and chronic weakness as a result of reduced CO. Dyspnea on exertion and orthopnea develop later. A significant number of patients report anxiety, atypical chest pains, and palpitations. Assessment may reveal normal BP, atrial fibrillation, or changes in respirations characteristic of left ventricular failure.

When right-sided HF develops, the neck veins become distended, the liver enlarges (hepatomegaly), and pitting edema is noted. A high-pitched systolic murmur at the apex, with radiation to the left axilla, is heard on auscultation. Severe regurgitation often exhibits a third heart sound (S_3).

Mitral Valve Prolapse

Mitral valve prolapse (MVP) occurs because the valvular leaflets enlarge and prolapse into the left atrium during systole. This abnormality is usually benign but may progress to pronounced mitral regurgitation.

Most patients with MVP are asymptomatic. However, some may report chest pain, palpitations, or exercise intolerance. Chest pain is usually atypical with patients describing a sharp pain localized to the left side of the chest. Dizziness, **syncope** ("blackouts"), and palpitations may be associated with atrial or ventricular dysrhythmias.

A normal HR and BP are usually found on physical examination. A midsystolic click and a late systolic murmur may be audible at the apex. The intensity of the murmur is not related to the severity of the prolapse.

The etiology of MVP is variable and has been associated with conditions such as Marfan syndrome and other congenital cardiac defects (see Chapter 20 for a discussion of Marfan syndrome). Usually, however, no other cardiac abnormality is found. A familial occurrence is well established.

Aortic Stenosis

Aortic stenosis is the most common cardiac valve dysfunction in the United States and is often considered a disease of "wear and tear." In **aortic stenosis,** the aortic valve orifice narrows and obstructs left ventricular outflow during systole. This increased resistance to ejection or afterload results in ventricular hypertrophy. As stenosis worsens, cardiac output becomes fixed and cannot increase to meet the demands of the body during exertion. Symptoms then develop. Eventually the left ventricle fails, blood backs up in the left atrium, and the pulmonary system becomes congested. Right-sided HF can occur late in the disease. *When the surface area of the valve becomes 1 cm or less, surgery is indicated on an urgent basis!*

The classic symptoms of aortic stenosis result from the fixed cardiac output: dyspnea, angina, and syncope occurring on exertion. When cardiac output falls in the late stages of the disease, the patient experiences marked fatigue, debilitation, and peripheral cyanosis. A narrow pulse pressure is noted when the BP is measured. A diamond-shaped, systolic crescendo-decrescendo murmur is usually noted on auscultation.

Congenital bicuspid or unicuspid aortic valves are the primary reason for aortic stenosis in many patients. Rheumatic aortic stenosis occurs with rheumatic disease of the mitral valve and develops in young and middle-aged adults. Atherosclerosis and degenerative calcification of the aortic valve are the major causative factors in older adults. *Aortic stenosis has become the most common valvular disorder in all countries with aging populations.*

Aortic Regurgitation (Insufficiency)

In patients with **aortic regurgitation,** the aortic valve leaflets do not close properly during diastole and the *annulus* (the valve ring that attaches to the leaflets) may be dilated, loose, or deformed. This allows flow of blood from the aorta back into the left ventricle during diastole. The left ventricle, in compensation, dilates to accommodate the greater blood volume and eventually hypertrophies.

Patients with aortic regurgitation remain asymptomatic for many years because of the compensatory mechanisms of the left ventricle. As the disease progresses and left ventricular failure occurs, the major symptoms are exertional dyspnea, orthopnea, and paroxysmal nocturnal dyspnea. Palpitations may be noted with severe disease, especially when the patient lies on the left side. Nocturnal angina with diaphoresis often occurs.

On palpation, the nurse notes a "bounding" arterial pulse. The pulse pressure is usually widened, with an elevated systolic pressure and diminished diastolic pressure. The classic auscultatory finding is a high-pitched, blowing, decrescendo diastolic murmur.

Aortic insufficiency usually results from nonrheumatic conditions such as infective endocarditis, congenital anatomic aortic valvular abnormalities, hypertension, and Marfan syndrome (a rare, generalized, systemic disease of connective tissue).

Patient-Centered Collaborative Care

Assessment

A patient with valvular disease may suddenly become ill or may slowly develop symptoms over many years. Collect information about the patient's family health history, including valvular or other forms of heart disease to which he or she may be genetically predisposed. Question about attacks of rheumatic fever and infective endocarditis, the specific dates when these occurred, and the use of antibiotic prophylaxis against the recurrence of rheumatic fever. Also question the patient about a history of IV drug abuse. Discuss the patient's fatigue level and tolerated activity level, the presence of angina or dyspnea, and the occurrence of palpitations, if present.

As part of the physical assessment, obtain vital signs, inspect for signs of edema, palpate and auscultate the heart and lungs, and palpate the peripheral pulses. Assessment findings are summarized in Chart 37-7.

For valvular heart disease, *echocardiography* is the diagnostic procedure of choice because it is an excellent noninvasive tool for defining cardiac structure, movement of the valve leaflets, and size and function of the cardiac chambers. Transesophageal echocardiography (TEE) or transthoracic echocardiography (TTE) is the gold standard for assessing most valve problems (Todd & Higgins, 2005). Exercise tolerance testing (ETT) and stress echocardiography are sometimes performed to evaluate symptomatic response, assess functional capacity, and enhance auscultatory findings. With either mitral or aortic stenosis, cardiac catheterization may be indicated to assess the severity of the stenosis and its other effects on the heart.

In patients with mitral stenosis, the chest x-ray shows left atrial enlargement, prominent pulmonary arteries, and an enlarged right ventricle. In those with mitral regurgitation (insufficiency), the chest x-ray reveals an increased cardiac shadow, indicating left ventricular and left atrial enlargement.

In the later stages of aortic stenosis, the chest x-ray may show left ventricular enlargement and pulmonary congestion. Left atrial and left ventricular dilation appear on the chest x-ray of patients with aortic regurgitation (insufficiency). If HF is present, pulmonary venous congestion is also evident.

The health care provider also requests an ECG to assess abnormalities such as left ventricular hypertrophy, as seen with mitral regurgitation and aortic regurgitation, or right ventricular hypertrophy, as seen in severe mitral stenosis. *Atrial fibrillation is a common finding in both mitral stenosis and mitral regurgitation and may develop in aortic stenosis because of left atrial dilation.*

Common Nursing Diagnoses and Collaborative Problems

Nursing diagnoses that may apply to patients with valvular heart disease include:

- Decreased Cardiac Output related to altered stroke volume
- Impaired Gas Exchange related to ventilation/perfusion imbalance
- Activity Intolerance related to inability of the heart to meet metabolic demands during activity
- Acute Pain related to physiologic injury agent (hypoxia)

Interventions

Management of valvular heart disease depends on which valve is affected and the degree of valve impairment. Some patients can be managed with yearly monitoring and drug therapy, whereas others require invasive procedures or heart surgery.

Nonsurgical Management

Nonsurgical management focuses on drug therapy and rest. During the course of valvular disease, left ventricular failure with pulmonary or systemic congestion may develop. Diuretics, beta blockers, digoxin, and oxygen are often administered to improve the symptoms of heart failure (HF). Nitrates are administered cautiously to patients with aortic stenosis because of the potential for syncope associated with a reduction in left ventricular volume (preload). Vasodilators such as calcium channel blockers may be used to reduce the regurgitant flow for patients with aortic or mitral stenosis.

Prophylactic antibiotic therapy is required for all patients with valve disease before any invasive procedure. Procedures that require antibiotic coverage include bronchoscopy, endoscopy, sigmoidoscopy, colonoscopy, genitourinary instrumentation, surgery, and dental procedures of any type.

A major concern in valvular heart disease is maintaining cardiac output if atrial fibrillation develops. With mitral valvular disease, left ventricular filling is especially dependent on atrial contraction. When atrial fibrillation develops, there is no longer a single coordinated atrial contraction. Cardiac output can decrease, and HF may occur. Ineffective atrial contraction may also lead to the stasis of blood and thrombi in the left atrium. Monitor the patient for the development of an irregular rhythm, and notify the primary care provider if it develops. (See Chapter 36 for a detailed explanation of atrial fibrillation.)

The primary care provider usually starts therapy to first control the heart rate to maintain cardiac output (<100 is considered a controlled ventricular response) and then attempt to restore normal sinus rhythm. If that goal is unsuccessful, the drugs slow ventricular rate. The physician might elect to convert a patient from atrial fibrillation to sinus rhythm using IV diltiazem (Cardizem, Apo-Diltiaz🍁) or amiodarone (Cordarone, Pacerone). Monitor the patient on a unit where both cardiac rhythm and BP can be closely watched. Synchronized countershock (cardioversion) may be attempted if atrial fibrillation is rapid, the patient decompensates, and the rhythm is unresponsive to medical treatment (see Chapter 36).

If the patient remains in atrial fibrillation, low-dose amiodarone (Cordarone) is often prescribed to slow ventricular rate. Procainamide hydrochloride (Pronestyl hydrochloride, Procanbid) may be added to the regimen. A beta-blocking agent (e.g., metoprolol) may also be considered to slow the ventricular response.

For valvular heart disease and chronic atrial fibrillation, anticoagulation with sodium warfarin (Coumadin, Warfilone🍁) is usually a part of the medical treatment plan to prevent thrombus formation. Thrombi may form in the atria or on defective valve segments, resulting in systemic emboli. If a portion breaks off and travels to the brain, one or more strokes may occur. Assess the patient's baseline neurologic status, and monitor for changes. A TEE is often done before synchronized cardioversion to ensure that thrombi are not present that could embolize when this therapy is administered.

Rest is often an important part of treatment. Activity may be limited because cardiac output (CO) cannot meet increased metabolic demands and angina or HF can result. A balance of rest and exercise is needed to prevent muscle atrophy.

Surgical Management

Surgical repair or replacement of heart valves has a major effect on the prognosis of valvular heart disease. Correct timing is crucial. Repair or replacement of the valve is usually performed after symptoms of left ventricular failure have developed but before irreversible dysfunction occurs. *Surgical therapy is the only definitive treatment of aortic stenosis and is recommended when angina, syncope, or dyspnea on exertion develops.*

Reparative Procedures. Reparative procedures are becoming more popular because of continuing problems with thrombi, endocarditis, and left ventricular dysfunction after valve replacement. Reparative procedures do not result in a normal valve, but they usually "turn back the clock," resulting in a more functional valve and an improvement in cardiac output. Turbulent blood flow through the valve may persist, and degeneration of the repaired valve is possible.

Balloon valvuloplasty, an invasive nonsurgical procedure, is possible for stenotic mitral and aortic valves; however, careful selection of patients is needed. It may be the initial treatment of choice for people with noncalcified, mobile mitral valves. Patients selected for *aortic* valvuloplasty are usually older and are at high risk for surgical complications or have refused operative treatment. The benefits of this procedure for aortic stenosis tend to be short lived, rarely lasting longer than 6 months.

When performing *mitral* valvuloplasty, the physician passes a balloon catheter from the femoral vein, through the atrial septum, and to the mitral valve. The balloon is inflated to enlarge the mitral orifice. For aortic valvuloplasty, the physician inserts the catheter through the femoral artery and advances it to the aortic valve, where it is inflated to enlarge the orifice. The procedure usually offers immediate relief of symptoms because the balloon has dilated the orifice and improved leaflet mobility. The results are comparable with those of surgical commissurotomy for appropriately selected patients.

After valvuloplasty, observe the patient closely for bleeding from the catheter insertion site and institute post-angiogram precautions. Bleeding is likely because of the large size of the catheter. Also observe for signs of a regurgitant valve by closely monitoring heart sounds, CO, and heart rhythm. Because vegetations (thrombi) may have been dislodged from the valve, observe for any indication of systemic emboli (see Infective Endocarditis, p. 783).

Direct (open) commissurotomy is accomplished with cardiopulmonary bypass during open heart surgery. The surgeon visualizes the valve, removes thrombi from the atria, incises the fused commissures (leaflets), and débrides calcium from the leaflets, widening the orifice.

Mitral valve annuloplasty (reconstruction) is the reparative procedure of choice for most patients with acquired mitral insufficiency. To make the annulus (the valve ring that attaches to and supports the leaflets) smaller, the physician may suture the leaflets to an annuloplasty ring or take tucks in the patient's annulus. Leaflet repair is often performed at the same time. Elongated leaflets may be shortened, and shortened leaflets may be repaired by lengthening the chordae that bind them in place. Perforated leaflets may be patched with synthetic grafts.

Annuloplasty and leaflet repair result in an annulus of the appropriate size and in leaflets that can close completely. Thus regurgitation is eliminated or markedly reduced.

Replacement Procedures. The development of a wide variety of *prosthetic* (synthetic) and *biologic* (tissue) valves has improved the surgical therapy and prognosis of valvular heart disease. Although prosthetic valves are durable, all patients must receive oral anticoagulation because of the possibility of clot formation.

Biologic valves may be **xenograft** (from other species), such as a porcine valve (from a pig) (Fig. 37-3) or a bovine valve (from a cow). Because tissue valves are associated with little risk of clot formation, long-term anticoagulation is *not* indicated. Xenografts are not as durable as prosthetic valves and usually must be replaced every 7 to 10 years. The durability of the graft is related to the age of the recipient. Calcium in the blood, which is present in larger quantities in younger patients, breaks down the valves. The older the patient, the longer the xenograft will last. Valves donated from human cadavers and **pulmonary autographs** (relocation of the patient's own pulmonary valve to the aortic position [Ross procedure]) are also being used for valve replacement.

An aortic valve is replaced with a mechanical valve for most symptomatic adults with aortic stenosis and aortic insufficiency. A tissue valve cannot be used because of the high pressure within the aorta.

Preoperative Care. Patients undergoing valve surgery have open heart surgery similar to the procedure for a coronary artery bypass graft (CABG) (see Chapter 40). Ideally, surgery is an elective and planned procedure. Inform the patient and family about the management of postoperative pain, incision care, and strategies to prevent respiratory complications (see Chapters 16 and 18). Teach patients receiving oral anticoagulants to stop taking them before surgery, usually at least 72 hours before the procedure. Patients also need to have a preoperative dental examination. If dental caries or periodontal disease is present, these problems must be resolved before valve replacement.

Postoperative Care. Nursing interventions for open heart surgery for valve disorders are similar to those for a CABG (see Chapter 40). However, a few significant differences depend in part on the type of valvular surgery. Patients with mitral stenosis often have pulmonary hypertension and stiff lungs. Monitor respiratory status closely during weaning from the ventilator. Be especially alert for bleeding in those with aortic valve replacements because of a higher risk for postoperative hemorrhage.

Patients with valve replacements are also more likely to have significant reductions in CO after surgery, especially those with aortic stenosis or left ventricular failure from mitral valve disease. Carefully monitor cardiac output (CO), and identify indications of heart failure. High filling pressures—pulmonary artery wedge pressure (PAWP) greater than 18 mm Hg—may be required to maintain an acceptable CO in the immediate postoperative period. Patients who have had valve replacements with prosthetic valves require lifetime prophylactic anticoagulation therapy to prevent thrombus formation.

Community-Based Care

The patient with valvular heart disease may be discharged home on medical therapy or postoperatively after valve repair or replacement. Because fatigue is a common problem, ensure

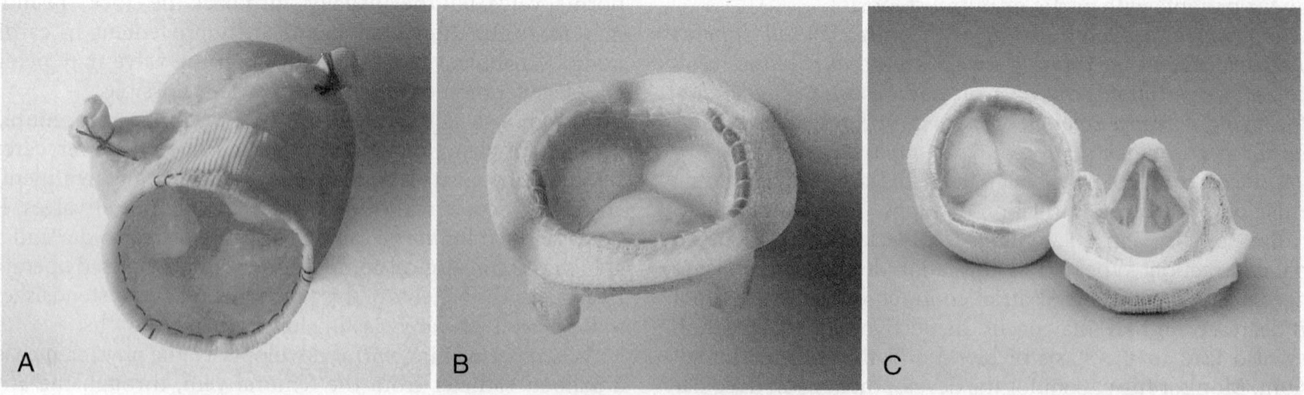

Fig. 37-3 • Examples of biologic (tissue) heart valves. **A,** Freestyle, a stentless pig valve with no frame. **B,** Hancock II, a stented pig valve. **C,** Carpentier-Edwards pericardial bioprosthesis.

that the home environment can provide rest while moving the patient toward increased activity levels. Some older adults with aortic stenosis live in long-term care settings.

Home Care Management

A home care nurse may be needed to help the patient adhere to drug therapy and activity schedules and to detect any problems, particularly with anticoagulant therapy. Patients who have undergone surgery may require a nurse for assistance with incision care. A home care aide may assist with ADLs if the patient lives alone or is older.

Health Teaching

The teaching plan for the patient with valvular heart disease includes:

- The disease process and the possibility of heart failure
- Drug therapy, including diuretics, vasodilators, beta blockers, calcium channel blockers, antibiotics, and anticoagulants
- The prophylactic use of antibiotics
- A plan of activity and rest to conserve energy

Because patients with defective or repaired valves are at risk for infective endocarditis, teach them to adhere to the precautions described for endocarditis. *Remind them to inform all health care providers of the valvular heart disease history. Tell providers that they require antibiotic administration before all invasive procedures and tests.* Health teaching for the patient is described in Chart 37-8.

Teach patients taking anticoagulants how to manage their drug therapy successfully, including nutritional considerations (if taking warfarin) and the prevention of bleeding. For example, the patient should be taught to avoid foods high in vitamin K and to use an electric razor to avoid skin cuts. In addition, teach him or her to report any bleeding or excessive bruising to the health care provider. Patients who have had prosthetic valve replacement need to take anticoagulants for the rest of their lives.

For patients who have surgery, reinforce how to care for the sternal incision and instruct them to watch for and report any fever, drainage, or redness at the site. Most patients can usually return to normal activity after 6 weeks but should avoid heavy physical labor with their upper extremities for 3 to 6 months to allow the incision to heal. Those who have had valvular surgery should also avoid invasive dental procedures for 6 months because of the potential for endocarditis. Some procedures may be done with caution but only if the patient takes a course of antibiotic therapy. Those with prosthetic valves need to avoid any procedure using magnetic resonance unless the newest technology is available. Remind patients to obtain a medical alert bracelet, card, or necklace to indicate they have a valve replacement and are taking anticoagulants.

Patients with valvular heart disease may have complicated medication schedules, as well as long-term antibiotic or anticoagulant therapy. These circumstances potentially can lead to nonadherence to self-management. Provide clear, concise instructions about drug therapy, and discuss the risks associated with nonadherence. Patients with a failed valve or those who do not follow the treatment plan are at high risk for heart failure. Teach them to report any changes in cardiovascular status, such as dyspnea, syncope, dizziness, edema, and palpitations.

The psychological response to valve surgery is similar to that after coronary artery bypass surgery. Patients may experience an altered self-image as a result of the required lifestyle changes or the visible medial sternotomy incision. In addition, those with prosthetic valves may need to adjust to a soft but audible clicking sound of the prosthetic valve. Encourage patients to verbalize their feelings about the prosthetic heart valve. Patients may display a variety of emotions postoperatively, especially when they get home.

Chart 37-8 PATIENT AND FAMILY EDUCATION GUIDE

Valvular Heart Disease

- Notify all your health care providers that you have a defective heart valve.
- Remind the health care provider of your valvular problem when you have any dental work (cleaning, filling, extraction), any examination by instrument (cystoscopy, endoscopy, sigmoidoscopy), or any other invasive procedure (arteriogram, surgery).
- Request antibiotic prophylaxis before and after these procedures if the health care provider does not offer it.
- Clean all wounds and apply antibiotic ointment to prevent infection.
- Notify your health care provider immediately if you experience fever, petechiae (pinpoint red dots on your skin), or shortness of breath.

Health Care Resources

The American Heart Association's Mended Hearts, Inc. (www.mendedhearts.org) is a community resource that provides information about valvular heart disease. A wallet-sized card can be obtained to identify the patient as needing prophylactic antibiotics. An identification bracelet or necklace that states the name of the drugs the patient is taking should also be worn.

NCLEX EXAMINATION CHALLENGE

A client is preparing for discharge after a mitral valve replacement. Which of these statements by the client indicates a need for further health teaching?

A. "I have to be careful and stay away from people who have colds."
B. "I won't have any dental work for 6 months after I go home."
C. "I need to take my Coumadin for the next 2 weeks."
D. "I need to tell doctors that I have a replaced valve."

evolve For the correct answer, go to http://evolve.elsevier.com/Iggy/.

INFLAMMATIONS AND INFECTIONS

INFECTIVE ENDOCARDITIS

Pathophysiology

Infective endocarditis (previously called *bacterial endocarditis*) refers to a microbial infection (e.g., viruses, bacteria, fungi) involving the endocardium. A healthy, defective, or prosthetic valve can be affected, but infection may occur also in apparently healthy endocardium or in septal defects. The most common infective organism is *Streptococcus viridans* or *Staphylococcus aureus.*

Infective endocarditis occurs primarily in patients who abuse IV drugs, have had valve replacements, have experienced systemic infection, or have structural cardiac defects. With a cardiac defect, blood may flow rapidly from a high-pressure area to a low-pressure zone, eroding a section of endocardium. Platelets and fibrin adhere to the denuded endocardium, forming a vegetative lesion. During bacteremia, bacteria become trapped in the low-pressure "sinkhole" and are deposited in the vegetation. Additional platelets and fibrin are deposited, which causes the vegetative lesion to grow. The endocardium and valve are destroyed. Valvular insufficiency may result when the lesion interferes with normal alignment of the valve. If vegetations become so large that blood flow through the valve is obstructed, the valve appears stenotic and then is very likely to *embolize* (i.e., cause emboli to be released).

Possible ports of entry for infecting organisms include:

- The oral cavity (especially if dental procedures have been performed)
- Skin rashes, lesions, or abscesses
- Infections (cutaneous, genitourinary, GI, systemic)
- Surgery or invasive procedures, including IV line placement

Patient-Centered Collaborative Care

Assessment

Because the mortality rate remains high, early detection of infective endocarditis is essential. Unfortunately, many patients (especially older adults) are misdiagnosed. Clinical manifestations usually occur within 2 weeks of a bacteremia (Chart 37-9).

Assessment usually reveals a recurrent fever. Most patients have temperatures from 99° to 103° F (37.2° to 39.4° C). As a result of physiologic changes associated with aging, however, many older adults remain afebrile. The severity of symptoms may depend on the virulence of the infecting organism.

Physical Assessment/Clinical Manifestations

Assess the patient's *cardiovascular status.* Almost all patients with infective endocarditis develop murmurs. Carefully auscultate the precordium, noting and documenting any new murmurs (usually regurgitant in nature) or any changes in the intensity or quality of an old murmur. An S_3 or S_4 heart sound also may be heard.

Heart failure (HF) is the most common complication of infective endocarditis. Assess for right-sided HF (as evidenced by peripheral edema, weight gain, and anorexia) and left-sided HF (as evidenced by fatigue, shortness of breath, and crackles on auscultation of breath sounds). See discussion of HF earlier in this chapter.

Chart 37-9 KEY FEATURES

Infective Endocarditis

- Fever associated with chills, night sweats, malaise, and fatigue
- Anorexia and weight loss
- Cardiac murmur (newly developed or change in existing)
- Development of heart failure
- Evidence of systemic embolization
- Petechiae
- Splinter hemorrhages
- Osler's nodes (on palms of hands and soles of feet)
- Janeway's lesions (flat, reddened maculas on hands and feet)
- Positive blood cultures

Arterial embolization is a major complication in up to half of patients with infective endocarditis. Fragments of vegetation break loose and travel randomly through the circulation. When the left side of the heart is involved, vegetation fragments are carried to the spleen, kidneys, GI tract, brain, and extremities. When the right side of the heart is involved, emboli enter the pulmonary circulation.

Splenic infarction with sudden abdominal pain and radiation to the left shoulder can also occur. When performing an *abdominal assessment,* note rebound tenderness on palpation. The classic pain described with renal infarction is flank pain that radiates to the groin and is accompanied by hematuria or pyuria. Mesenteric emboli may result in the patient reporting diffuse abdominal pain, often after eating, and abdominal distention.

Whereas about a third of patients have *neurologic changes,* others have signs and symptoms of pulmonary problems. Emboli to the central nervous system cause either transient ischemic attacks (TIAs) or a stroke. Confusion, reduced concentration, and aphasia or dysphagia may occur. Pleuritic chest pain, dyspnea, and cough are symptoms of pulmonary infarction related to embolization.

Petechiae (pinpoint red spots) occur in many patients with endocarditis. Examine the mucous membranes, the palate, the conjunctivae, and the skin above the clavicles for small, red, flat lesions. Assess the distal third of the nail bed for **splinter hemorrhages,** which appear as black longitudinal lines or small red streaks.

Other Diagnostic Assessment

A positive *blood culture* is a prime diagnostic test. Both aerobic and anaerobic specimens are obtained for culture. Some slow-growing organisms may take 3 weeks and require a specialized medium to isolate. Therefore cultures are monitored by the laboratory for 3 to 4 weeks. Low hemoglobin and hematocrit levels may also be present.

Echocardiography has improved the ability to diagnose infective endocarditis accurately. Transesophageal echocardiography (TEE) allows visualization of cardiac structures that are difficult to see with transthoracic echocardiography (TTE). TEE provides good resolution and is very sensitive for discovering valvular abnormalities, thereby enabling the clinician to diagnose infective endocarditis more accurately (see Chapter 35).

The most reliable criteria then for diagnosing endocarditis include positive blood cultures, a new regurgitant murmur, and evidence of endocardial involvement by echocardiography.

Interventions

Care of the patient with endocarditis usually includes antimicrobials, rest balanced with activity, and supportive therapy for HF. If these interventions are successful, surgery is usually not required.

Nonsurgical Management

The major component of treatment for endocarditis is drug therapy. Other interventions help prevent the life-threatening complications.

Antimicrobials are the main treatment, with the choice of drug depending on the specific organism involved. Because vegetations surround and protect the offending microorganism, an appropriate drug must be given in a sufficiently high dose to ensure its destruction. Antimicrobials are usually given IV, with the course of treatment lasting 4 to 6 weeks. For most bacterial cases, the ideal antibiotic is one of the penicillins or cephalosporins.

Patients may be hospitalized for several days to institute IV therapy and then are discharged for continued IV therapy at home. After hospitalization, most patients who respond to therapy may continue it at home when they become afebrile, have negative blood cultures, and have no signs of HF or embolization.

Anticoagulants are of no value in preventing embolization from vegetations. Because they may result in bleeding, they are avoided unless they are required to prevent thrombus formation on a prosthetic valve.

The patient's activities are balanced with *adequate rest.* Explain proper oral and general body hygiene. Consistently use appropriate aseptic technique to protect the patient from contact with potentially infective organisms. Nursing assessment for signs of HF (e.g., rapid pulse, fatigue, cough, dyspnea) continues throughout the antimicrobial regimen.

Surgical Management

The cardiac surgeon may be consulted if antibiotic therapy is ineffective in sterilizing a valve, if refractory HF develops secondary to a defective valve, if large valvular vegetations are present, or if multiple embolic events occur. Current surgical interventions for infective endocarditis include:

- Removing the infected valve (either biologic or prosthetic)
- Repairing or removing congenital shunts
- Repairing injured valves and chordae tendineae
- Draining abscesses in the heart or elsewhere

Preoperative and postoperative care of patients having surgery involving the valves is similar to that described earlier for valve replacement (pp. 781-782).

Community-Based Care

Community-based care for patients with infective endocarditis is essential to resolve the problem, prevent relapse, and avoid complications. Patients and families need to be motivated and have the knowledge, physical ability, and resources to administer IV antibiotics at home. Collaborate with the home care nurse to complete health teaching started in the hospital and to monitor patient adherence and health status.

In collaboration with the case manager, the home care nurse and pharmacist arrange for appropriate supplies to be available to the patient at home. Supplies include the prepared antibiotic, IV pump with tubing, alcohol wipes, IV access device, normal saline solution, and a saline flush solution drawn up in syringes. A saline lock, peripherally inserted central catheter (PICC) line, or central catheter is positioned at a venous site that is easily accessible to the patient or a family member.

Teach the patient and family how to administer the antibiotic and care for the infusion site while maintaining aseptic technique. The patient or family member should demonstrate this technique before the patient is discharged from the hospital. Emphasize the importance of maintaining a blood level of the antibiotic by administering the antibiotics as scheduled. After stabilization at home, the case manager or other nurse contacts the patient every week to determine whether he or she is adhering to the antibiotic therapy and whether any problems have been encountered.

Encourage proper hygiene, particularly oral hygiene. Advise patients to use a soft toothbrush, to brush their teeth at least twice per day, and to rinse the mouth with water after brushing. They should not use irrigation devices or floss the teeth because bacteremia may result. Teach them to clean any open skin areas well and apply an antibiotic ointment.

Patients must remind health care providers (including their dentists) of their endocarditis. Teach patients to request prophylactic antibiotics for every invasive procedure, especially dental care.

Instruct patients to note any indications of endocarditis such as fever. Remind them to monitor and record their temperature daily for up to 6 weeks. Teach them to report fever, chills, malaise, weight loss, increased fatigue, sudden weight gain, or dyspnea to their primary care provider.

PERICARDITIS

Pathophysiology

Acute pericarditis is an inflammation or alteration of the pericardium (the membranous sac that encloses the heart). The problem may be fibrous, serous, hemorrhagic, purulent, or neoplastic. Acute pericarditis is most commonly associated with:

- Malignant neoplasms
- Idiopathic causes
- Infective organisms (bacteria, viruses, or fungi)
- Post–myocardial infarction (MI) syndrome (Dressler's syndrome)
- Post-pericardiotomy syndrome
- Systemic connective tissue disease
- Renal failure

The cause of the pericarditis determines its presentation. Acute viral pericarditis commonly follows a respiratory infection. In a small percentage of patients who experience an MI, **Dressler's syndrome** occurs from 1 to 12 weeks after the infarction. This syndrome is characterized by pericarditis, fever, and pericardial and pleural effusions. **Post-pericardiotomy syndrome** occurs in some patients after cardiac surgery.

Chronic constrictive pericarditis occurs when chronic pericardial inflammation causes a fibrous thickening of the pericardium. It is caused by tuberculosis, radiation therapy, trauma, renal failure, or metastatic cancer. In chronic constrictive pericarditis, the pericardium becomes rigid, preventing adequate filling of the ventricles and eventually resulting in cardiac failure.

Patient-Centered Collaborative Care

Assessment

Assessment findings include substernal precordial pain that radiates to the left side of the neck, the shoulder, or the back. Pain is classically grating and oppressive and is aggravated by breathing (mainly on inspiration), coughing, and swallowing. The pain is worse when the patient is in the supine position and may be relieved by sitting up and leaning forward. Ask specific questions to evaluate chest discomfort because it is important that the pain of pericarditis be differentiated from that of an acute MI (see Chapter 40).

A pericardial friction rub may be heard with the diaphragm of the stethoscope positioned at the left lower sternal border. This scratchy, high-pitched sound is produced when the inflamed, roughened pericardial layers create friction as their surfaces rub together.

Patients with chronic constrictive pericarditis have signs of right-sided HF, elevated systemic venous pressure with jugular distention, hepatic engorgement, and dependent edema. Exertional fatigue and dyspnea are common complications. Thickening of the pericardium is seen on echocardiography or a computed tomography (CT) scan.

Patients with acute pericarditis may have an elevated white blood cell count and usually have a fever. Therefore blood culture and sensitivity may be analyzed in the laboratory. The ECG usually shows ST-T spiking with the onset of inflammation, which returns to baseline with treatment. Atrial fibrillation is also common. Echocardiograms may be used to determine a pericardial effusion.

Interventions

Pain Management

The patient may be hospitalized for symptom relief. The health care provider usually prescribes NSAIDs for pain. Patients who do not obtain relief within 48 to 96 hours and who do not have bacterial pericarditis may receive corticosteroid therapy. Assess for outcomes of pain management, and assist the patient to assume positions of comfort—usually sitting upright and leaning slightly forward. If the pain is not relieved within 24 to 48 hours, notify the primary care provider.

The various causes of pericarditis require specific therapies. For example, bacterial pericarditis (acute) usually requires antibiotics and pericardial drainage. The usual clinical course of acute pericarditis is short term (2 to 6 weeks), but episodes may recur. Chronic pericarditis caused by malignant disease may be treated with radiation or chemotherapy, whereas uremic pericarditis is treated by hemodialysis. The definitive treatment for chronic constrictive pericarditis is surgical excision of the pericardium **(pericardiectomy).**

A significant complication of pericarditis is **pericardial effusion,** which occurs when the space between the parietal and visceral layers of the pericardium fills with fluid. This complication puts the patient at risk for **cardiac tamponade,** or excessive fluid within the pericardial cavity. Tamponade restricts diastolic ventricular filling, and cardiac output drops. Findings of cardiac tamponade include:

- Jugular venous distention
- **Paradoxical pulse,** also known as pulsus paradoxus (systolic blood pressure 10 mm Hg higher or more on expiration than on inspiration) (Chart 37-10)
- Decreased cardiac output
- Muffled heart sounds
- Circulatory collapse

ANIMATION: Pericardial Tamponade

Emergency Care: Acute Cardiac Tamponade

Acute cardiac tamponade may occur when small volumes (20 to 50 mL) of fluid accumulate rapidly in the pericardium. If the fluid accumulates slowly, the pericardium may stretch to accommodate several hundred milliliters of fluid. Report any suspicion of this complication to the physician immediately. *Cardiac tamponade is an emergency!* The physician may initially manage the decreased cardiac output (CO) with increased fluid volume administration while awaiting an echocardiogram or x-ray to confirm the diagnosis. Unfortunately, these tests are not always helpful because the fluid volume around the heart may be too small to visualize. Hemodynamic monitoring in a specialized critical care unit usually demonstrates compression of the heart, with all pressures (right atrial, pulmonary artery, and wedge) being similar and elevated (plateau pressures).

Chart 37-10 BEST PRACTICE FOR PATIENT SAFETY & QUALITY CARE

Care of the Patient with Pericarditis

- Assess the nature of the patient's chest discomfort. (Pericardial pain is typically substernal. It is worse on inspiration and decreases when the patient leans forward.)
- Auscultate for a pericardial friction rub.
- Assist the patient to a position of comfort.
- Provide anti-inflammatory agents as prescribed.
- Explain that anti-inflammatory agents usually decrease the pain within 48 hours.
- Avoid the administration of aspirin and anticoagulants because these may increase the possibility of tamponade.
- Auscultate the blood pressure carefully to detect paradoxical blood pressure (pulsus paradoxus), a sign of tamponade.
    - Palpate the blood pressure, and inflate the cuff above the systolic pressure.
    - Deflate the cuff gradually, and note when sounds are first audible on expiration.
    - Identify when sounds are also audible on inspiration.
    - Subtract the inspiratory pressure from the expiratory pressure to determine the amount of pulsus paradoxus (>10 mm Hg is an indication of tamponade).
- Inspect for other indications of tamponade, including jugular venous distention with clear lungs, muffled heart sounds, and decreased cardiac output.
- Notify the physician if tamponade is suspected.

The physician may elect to perform a **pericardiocentesis** to remove fluid and relieve the pressure on the heart. Under echocardiographic or fluoroscopic and hemodynamic monitoring, the cardiologist inserts an 8-inch (20.3-cm), 16- or 18-gauge pericardial needle into the pericardial space. The physician and the nurse monitor the needle's position, recognizing that ST-wave and T-wave changes indicate myocardial injury and that the needle must be withdrawn slightly. When the needle is properly positioned, a catheter is inserted and all available pericardial fluid is withdrawn. A pericardial drain may be temporarily placed. Monitor the pulmonary artery, wedge, and right atrial pressures during the procedure. The pressures should return to normal as the fluid compressing the heart is removed, and the clinical manifestations of tamponade should resolve. In situations in which the cause of the effusion is unknown, pericardial fluid specimens may be sent to the laboratory for cell count, culture and sensitivity tests, and cytology.

After the pericardiocentesis, closely monitor the patient for the recurrence of tamponade. Pericardiocentesis alone often does not resolve acute tamponade. *Be prepared to provide adequate fluid volumes to increase CO and to prepare the patient for emergency sternotomy if tamponade recurs.*

If the patient has a recurrence of tamponade or recurrent effusions or adhesions from chronic pericarditis, a portion or all of the pericardium may need to be removed to allow adequate ventricular filling and contraction. The surgeon may create a pericardial window, which involves removing a portion of the pericardium to permit excessive pericardial fluid to drain into the pleural space. In more severe cases, removal of the toughened encasing pericardium (pericardiectomy) may be necessary.

RHEUMATIC CARDITIS

Pathophysiology

Rheumatic carditis, also called *rheumatic endocarditis,* is a sensitivity response that develops after an upper respiratory tract infection with group A beta-hemolytic streptococci, which occurs in almost half of patients with rheumatic fever. The precise mechanism by which the infection causes inflammatory lesions in the heart is not established; however, inflammation is evident in all layers of the heart. The inflammation results in impaired contractile function of the myocardium, thickening of the pericardium, and valvular damage.

Rheumatic carditis is characterized by the formation of Aschoff bodies (small nodules in the myocardium that are replaced by scar tissue). A diffuse cellular infiltrate also develops and appears to be responsible for the HF. The pericardium becomes thickened and covered with exudate, and a serosanguineous pleural effusion may develop. The most serious damage occurs to the endocardium, with inflammation of the valve leaflets developing. Hemorrhagic and fibrous lesions form along the inflamed surfaces of the valves, resulting in stenosis or regurgitation primarily of the mitral and aortic valves (McCance & Huether, 2006).

Patient-Centered Collaborative Care

Rheumatic carditis is one of the major indicators of rheumatic fever. The common clinical manifestations are:

- Tachycardia
- **Cardiomegaly** (enlarged heart)
- Development of a new murmur or a change in an existing murmur
- Pericardial friction rub
- Precordial pain
- Electrocardiogram (ECG) changes (prolonged PR interval)
- Indications of heart failure (HF)
- Evidence of an existing streptococcal infection

Primary prevention is extremely important. Teach all patients to remind their health care providers to provide appropriate antibiotic therapy if they develop the indications of streptococcal pharyngitis:

- Moderate to high fever
- Abrupt onset of a sore throat
- Reddened throat with exudate
- Enlarged and tender lymph nodes

Penicillin is the antibiotic of choice for treatment. Erythromycin (Eryc, Erythromid🍁) is the alternative for penicillin-sensitive patients.

The signs of rheumatic carditis must be recognized promptly, and antibiotic therapy is started immediately for secondary prevention. Teach the patient to continue the antibiotic administration for the full 10 days to prevent reinfection. Suggest ways to manage the fever, such as maintaining hydration and taking antipyretics. Encourage the patient to get adequate rest.

Emphasize tertiary prevention in patient education, explaining that a recurrence of rheumatic carditis is probable with reinfection by streptococcus. Thus antibiotic therapy is essential for streptococcal infection. Antibiotic prophylaxis is necessary for the rest of his or her life to prevent infective endocarditis (see Infective Endocarditis, p. 783).

CARDIOMYOPATHY

Pathophysiology

Cardiomyopathy is a subacute or chronic disease of cardiac muscle, and the cause may be unknown. Cardiomyopathies are classified into four categories on the basis of abnormalities in structure and function: dilated cardiomyopathy, hypertrophic cardiomyopathy, restrictive cardiomyopathy, and arrhythmogenic right ventricular cardiomyopathy (Table 37-5).

Dilated cardiomyopathy (DCM) is the structural abnormality most commonly seen. DCM involves extensive damage to the myofibrils and interference with myocardial metabolism. Ventricular wall thickness is normal, but both ventricles are dilated (left ventricle is usually worse) and systolic function is impaired. Decreased CO from inadequate pumping of the heart causes the patient to experience dyspnea on exertion (DOE), decreased exercise capacity, fatigue, and palpitations. Causes may include alcohol abuse, chemotherapy, infection, inflammation, and poor nutrition.

The cardinal features of **hypertrophic cardiomyopathy (HCM)** are asymmetric ventricular hypertrophy and disarray of the myocardial fibers. Left ventricular hypertrophy leads to a stiff left ventricle, which results in diastolic filling abnormalities. Obstruction in the left ventricular outflow tract is seen in most patients with HCM. In about half of patients, HCM is transmitted as a single-gene autosomal dominant trait (McCance & Huether, 2006). Some patients die without any symptoms, whereas others have DOE, syncope, dizziness, and palpitations. Many athletes who die suddenly probably had hypertrophic cardiomyopathy (Bruce, 2005).

Restrictive cardiomyopathy, the rarest of the cardiomyopathies, is characterized by stiff ventricles that restrict filling during diastole. Symptoms are similar to left or right heart failure (HF) or both. The disease can be primary or caused by endocardial or myocardial disease such as sarcoidosis or amyloidosis. The prognosis for this type of cardiomyopathy is poor, with half of patients dying within 2 years of diagnosis (Bruce, 2005).

Arrhythmogenic right ventricular cardiomyopathy (dysplasia) results from replacement of myocardial tissue with fibrous and fatty tissue. Although the name implies right ventricle disease, about a third of patients also have left ventricle (LV) involvement. This disease has a familial association and most often affects young adults. Some patients have symptoms, and others do not.

Patient-Centered Collaborative Care

Assessment

Findings in cardiomyopathy depend on the structural and functional abnormalities. For example, left ventricular or biventricular failure is characteristic of *dilated* cardiomyopathy (DCM). Some patients with DCM are asymptomatic for months to years and have left and/or right ventricular dilation confirmed on x-ray examination or echocardiography. Others experience sudden, pronounced symptoms of left ventricular failure, such as progressive dyspnea on exertion, orthopnea, palpitations, and activity intolerance. Right-sided HF develops late in the disease and is associated with a poor prognosis. Atrial fibrillation occurs in some patients and is associated with embolism.

The clinical picture of *hypertrophic* cardiomyopathy (HCM) results from the hypertrophied septum causing a reduced stroke

TABLE 37-5 **Pathophysiology, Signs and Symptoms, and Treatment of Common Cardiomyopathies**

	HYPERTROPHIC CARDIOMYOPATHY	
Dilated Cardiomyopathy	**Nonobstructed**	**Obstructed**
PATHOPHYSIOLOGY		
Fibrosis of myocardium and endocardium Dilated chambers Mural wall thrombi prevalent	Hypertrophy of all walls Hypertrophied septum Relatively small chamber size	Same as for nonobstructed except for obstruction of left ventricular outflow tract associated with the hypertrophied septum and mitral valve incompetence
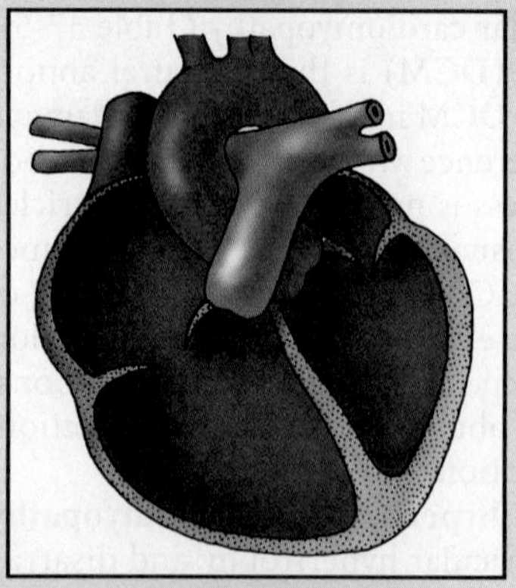		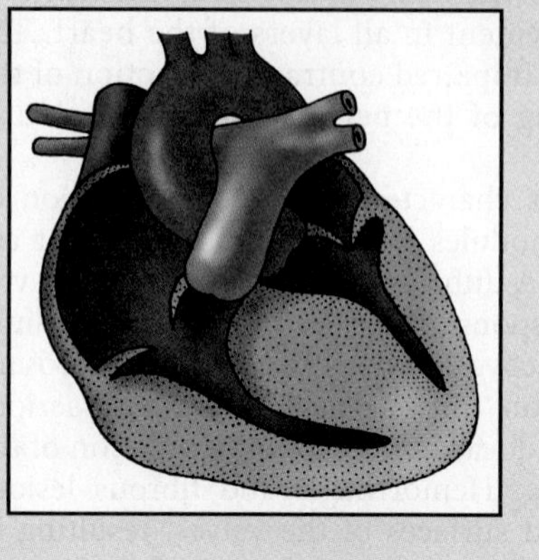
SIGNS AND SYMPTOMS		
Fatigue and weakness Heart failure (left side) Dysrhythmias or heart block Systemic or pulmonary emboli S_3 and S_4 gallops Moderate to severe cardiomegaly	Dyspnea Angina Fatigue, syncope, palpitations Mild cardiomegaly S_4 gallop Ventricular dysrhythmias Sudden death common Heart failure	Same as for nonobstructed except with mitral regurgitation murmur Atrial fibrillation
TREATMENT		
Symptomatic treatment of heart failure Vasodilators Control of dysrhythmias Surgery: heart transplant	For both: Symptomatic treatment Beta blockers Conversion of atrial fibrillation Surgery: ventriculomyotomy or muscle resection with mitral valve replacement Nitrates and other vasodilators ***contraindicated*** with the obstructed form	

volume (SV) and cardiac output (CO). Most patients are asymptomatic until late adolescence or early adulthood. The primary symptoms of HCM are exertional dyspnea, angina, and syncope. The chest pain is atypical in that it usually occurs at rest, is prolonged, has no relation to exertion, and is not relieved by the administration of nitrates. A high incidence of ventricular dysrhythmias is associated with HCM. Sudden death occurs and may be the first manifestation of the disease.

Echocardiography, radionuclide imaging, and angiocardiography during cardiac catheterization are performed to diagnose and differentiate cardiomyopathies.

▪ *Interventions*

The treatment of choice for the patient with cardiomyopathy varies with the type of cardiomyopathy and may include both medical and surgical interventions.

Nonsurgical Management

The care of patients with dilated or restrictive cardiomyopathy is initially the same as for HF. Drug therapy includes the use of diuretics, vasodilating agents, and cardiac glycosides to increase CO. Because patients are at risk for sudden death, teach them to report any palpitations, dizziness, or fainting, which might indicate a dysrhythmia. Antidysrhythmic drugs or implantable cardiac defibrillators may be used to control life-threatening dysrhythmias. To block inappropriate sympathetic stimulation and tachycardia, beta blockers (e.g., metoprolol) are used. If cardiomyopathy has developed in response to a toxin, further exposure to that toxin must be avoided. Alcohol ingestion causes cardiac depressant effects and must be avoided also.

Management of obstructive HCM includes administering negative inotropic agents such as beta-adrenergic blocking agents (carvedilol) and calcium antagonists (diltiazem). They decrease the outflow obstruction that accompanies exercise and also decrease HR, resulting in less angina, dyspnea, and syncope. Vasodilators, diuretics, nitrates, and cardiac glycosides are contraindicated in patients with obstructive HCM because vasodilating and positive inotropic effects may worsen the obstruction (Bruce, 2005). Strenuous exercise is also prohibited because it can increase the risk of sudden death.

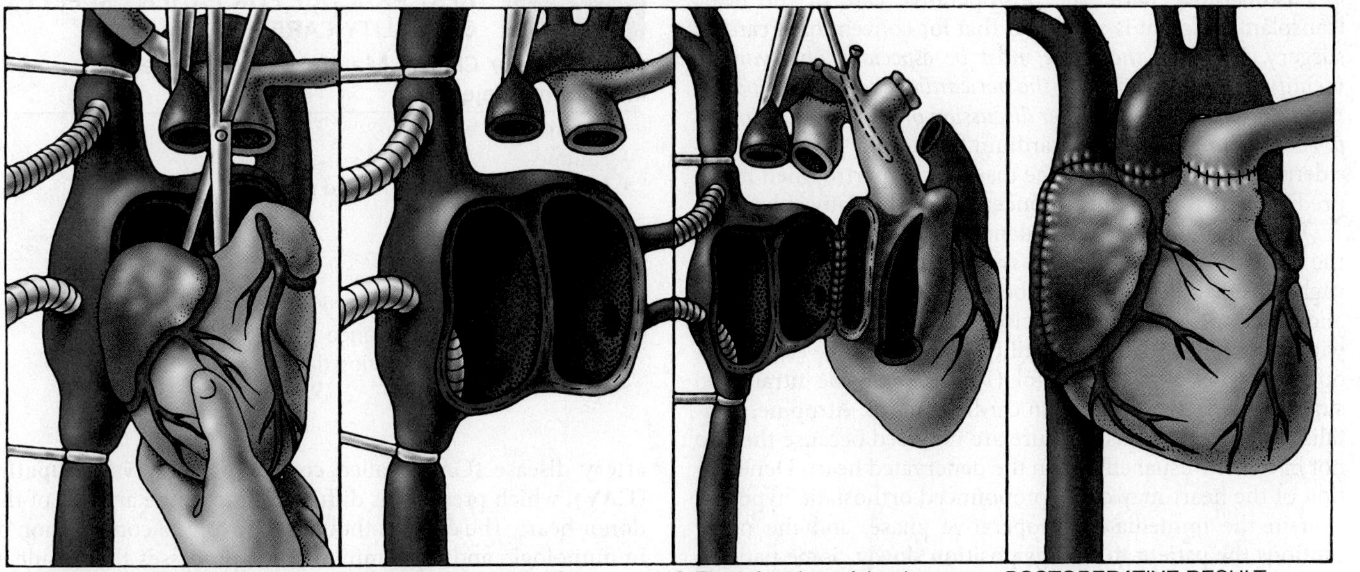

1. After the recipient is placed on cardiopulmonary bypass, the heart is removed.
2. The posterior walls of the recipient's left and right atria are left intact.
3. The left atrium of the donor heart is anastomosed to the recipient's residual posterior atrial walls, and the other atrial walls, the atrial septum, and the great vessels are joined.

POSTOPERATIVE RESULT

Fig. 37-4 • One technique for heart transplantation.

Surgical Management

The type of surgery performed depends on the type of cardiomyopathy. The most commonly used surgical treatment for obstructive HCM involves excising a portion of the hypertrophied ventricular septum to create a wider outflow tract (**ventriculomyomectomy;** also called *ventricular septal myectomy*). This procedure results in long-term improvement in activity tolerance for most patients.

Percutaneous alcohol septal ablation is an option for patients with HCM. Absolute alcohol is injected into a target septal branch of the left anterior descending coronary artery to produce a small septal infarction. This procedure also widens the LV outflow tract (Bruce, 2005).

The patient with arrhythmogenic right ventricular cardiomyopathy who does not respond to drug therapy may have a radiofrequency catheter ablation or placement of an implantable defibrillator (see Chapter 36 for discussion of these procedures).

Heart transplantation (surgical replacement with a donor heart) is the treatment of choice for patients with severe DCM and may be considered for patients with restrictive cardiomyopathy. The procedure may be done also for end-stage heart disease due to coronary artery disease, valvular disease, or congenital health disease.

Preoperative Care. Criteria for candidate selection for heart transplantation include:

- Life expectancy less than 1 year
- Age generally less than 65 years
- New York Heart Association (NYHA) class III or IV
- Normal or only slightly increased pulmonary vascular resistance
- Absence of active infection
- Stable psychosocial status
- No evidence of current drug or alcohol abuse

Once the candidate is eligible and a heart is available, provide preoperative care as described in Chapter 16.

DECISION-MAKING CHALLENGE

Legal/Ethical

A well-known former professional football player is admitted for his second heart transplant for end-stage heart failure. The media have reported for the past 6 months that he has a long history of smoking and drug and alcohol use. His surgeon states that the patient has recently completed treatment for substance abuse and is eligible for another transplant.

1. What ethical issues are involved in this situation? Should this patient have priority over other eligible patients?
2. One of your peers tells you that she thinks the patient doesn't deserve a second chance. How should you respond to her statement?
3. Why do you think the surgeon is planning to perform a second transplant for this patient?

evolve For suggested answer guidelines, go to http://evolve.elsevier.com/Iggy/.

Operative Procedures. The surgeon transplants a heart from a donor with a comparable body weight and ABO compatibility into a recipient less than 6 hours after procurement. In the most common procedure **(bicaval technique),** the intact right atrium of the donor heart is preserved by anastomoses at the patient's (recipient's) superior and inferior vena cavae. In the more traditional **orthotopic** technique, cuffs of the patient's right and left atria are attached to the donor's atria. Anastomoses are made between the recipient and donor atria, aorta, and pulmonary arteries (Fig. 37-4). Because the remaining remnant of the recipient's atria contains the sinoatrial (SA) node, two unrelated P waves are visible on the ECG.

Postoperative Care. The postoperative care of the heart transplant recipient is similar to that for conventional cardiac surgery. *However, the nurse must be especially observant to identify occult bleeding into the pericardial sac with the potential for tamponade (see earlier discussion of this complication on p. 786).* The recipient's pericardium has usually stretched considerably to accommodate the diseased, hypertrophied heart, predisposing the patient to concealed postoperative bleeding.

The transplanted heart is denervated (disconnected from the body's autonomic nervous system) and is unresponsive to vagal stimulation. The HR is between 90 and 110 beats/min and responds slowly to exercise, stress, or position change with increases in HR, contractility, and CO. In the early postoperative phase, isoproterenol (Isuprel) may be titrated to support the HR and maintain cardiac output. Atropine, digitalis, and carotid sinus pressure are not used because they do not have their usual effects on the denervated heart. Denervation of the heart may cause pronounced orthostatic hypotension in the immediate postoperative phase, and the nurse cautions the patient to change position slowly. Some patients also require a permanent pacemaker that is rate responsive to his or her activity level. The purpose is to increase CO and improve activity tolerance.

To suppress natural defense mechanisms (especially T- and B-cell function) and prevent transplant rejection, patients require immunosuppressants for the rest of their lives. The foundation of immunosuppressant therapy is a combination of drugs that work on various parts of the immune system. Chapter 19 describes transplant rejection and prevention in detail.

After surgery, perform comprehensive cardiovascular and respiratory assessments frequently according to agency or heart transplant physician protocol. Chart 37-11 lists the signs and symptoms of rejection that are specific to heart transplant. Report any of these manifestations immediately. To detect rejection, the heart transplant physician performs right endomyocardial biopsies at regularly scheduled intervals and whenever symptoms occur.

Nurses must be very careful about handwashing and aseptic technique because patients are immunosuppressed from drug therapy. *Infection is the major cause of death.* It usually develops in the immediate post-transplant period or during treatment for acute rejection.

About 72% of patients survive 5 years after transplantation; most return to NYHA class I or II status (Hoffman et al., 2006). Many of the surviving patients have a form of coronary artery disease (CAD) called **coronary artery vasculopathy (CAV),** which presents as diffuse plaque in the arteries of the donor heart. The cause is thought to involve a combination of immunologic and non-immunologic processes that result in vascular endothelial injury and an inflammatory response (Hoffman et al., 2006). Because the heart is denervated, patients do not usually experience angina. Regularly scheduled exercise tolerance tests and angiography are required to identify CAV. Only a small percentage of patients with CAV benefit from revascularization procedures like balloon angioplasty or coronary artery bypass surgery, although stents are beginning to show some promise in managing these patients. Retransplantation may be done in select patients.

To delay the development of CAV, encourage patients to follow lifestyle changes similar to those with primary CAD (see Chapter 40). The physician may prescribe a calcium channel blocker such as diltiazem (Cardizem) to prevent coronary spasm and closure. Stress the importance of strict adherence with nutritional modifications and drug regimens. Teach the patient the importance of participating in a regular exercise program. Collaborate with the physical therapist to plan the most appropriate exercise plan for the patient.

Discharge planning involves a collaborative interdisciplinary approach. Patients require extensive health teaching for self-management and community resources for support. Counseling and support groups can help patients cope with their fear of organ rejection. Drug therapy adherence is crucial to prevent this problem. Continuing, community-based care for patients with a heart transplant is similar to that for heart failure as discussed on p. 776.

Chart 37-11 BEST PRACTICE FOR PATIENT SAFETY & QUALITY CARE

Assessing for Clinical Manifestations of Heart Transplant Rejection

- Shortness of breath
- Fatigue
- Fluid gain (edema, increased weight)
- Abdominal bloating
- New bradycardia
- Hypotension
- Atrial fibrillation or flutter
- Decreased activity tolerance
- Decreased ejection fraction (late sign)

HUMAN NEEDS NURSING CARE REVIEW

What might you NOTICE if a patient is experiencing inadequate oxygenation and tissue perfusion as a result of heart failure?

- Report of shortness of breath, especially on exertion
- Report of dizziness
- Report of weight gain within days
- Syncope
- Dyspnea on exertion
- Report of palpitations
- Report of fatigue and weakness
- Disorientation or acute confusion (especially in older adults)
- Peripheral or abdominal ascites

What should you INTERPRET and how should you RESPOND to a patient experiencing inadequate oxygenation and tissue perfusion as a result of heart failure?

Perform and interpret physical assessment, including:

- Taking vital signs
- Monitoring oxygen saturation by pulse oximetry
- Performing a complete cardiovascular assessment

- Performing a complete respiratory assessment (listen for crackles or wheezes)
- Weighing patient
- Assessing cognition
- Assessing for pain or other symptoms

Respond by:

- Seeing health care provider immediately or calling 911 if patient is not in hospital setting.... OR
- Notifying physician or Rapid Response Team in hospital setting
- Raising the head of the bed to a sitting position
- Giving oxygen
- Maintaining or starting IV line
- Administering furosemide IV push (IVP) as prescribed
- Monitoring intake and output
- Giving ACE inhibitors or ARBs as prescribed IV or orally

On what should you REFLECT?

- Observe patient for increased urinary output.
- Monitor for decreased respiratory distress.
- Continue to monitor for improvement.
- Think about the possible cause(s) of the patient's heart failure.
- Think about your response to the patient.
- Develop a teaching plan for the patient to help prevent worsening or recurrent acute episodes of heart failure.

GET READY FOR THE NCLEX EXAMINATION!

Key Points

Review these Key Points for each NCLEX Examination Client Needs Category.

Safe and Effective Care Environment

- Provide information about continuing care for patients with heart failure (HF) after discharge to the community.
- Assess whether patients with end-stage HF have advance directives. If not, provide information about them.
- Collaborate with members of the health care team when developing and implementing a plan of care for patients with heart failure.
- Teach patients about community support groups and resources such as the American Heart Association.

Health Promotion and Maintenance

- Provide teaching about self-management at home for patients with HF (see Table 37-4).
- Monitor older adults who are taking digoxin for manifestations of toxicity. Monitor potassium levels to check for hypokalemia (see Chart 37-6).
- Teach patients taking ACE inhibitors or ARBs to change positions slowly to avoid orthostatic hypotension, especially older adults.
- Teach the patient with valvular dysfunction, cardiac infection, or cardiomyopathy the necessity of taking preventive antibiotic therapy before any invasive procedure.

Psychosocial Integrity

- Assess the patient for depression resulting from altered self-concept and anxiety.
- Assess the patient's coping skills.

Physiological Integrity

- Assess the patient for manifestations of right- and left-sided HF (see Charts 37-1 and 37-2).
- Weigh daily and record intake and output of patients with HF.
- Assess for early signs and symptoms of pulmonary edema (e.g., crackles in the lung bases, dyspnea at rest, disorientation, confusion), especially in older adults.
- Assess for symptoms of worsening HF: rapid weight gain (3 lb in a week), a decrease in exercise tolerance lasting 2 to 3 days, cold symptoms (cough) lasting more than 3 to 5 days, nocturia, development of dyspnea or angina at rest, or unstable angina.
- Monitor the HF patient on beta blockers carefully for hypotension and bradycardia.
- Monitor the pulse of patients taking digitalis preparations before administration, and report to the health care provider a pulse that is not within the desired parameters.
- Monitor for manifestations of pulmonary edema as listed in Chart 37-4.
- Place the patient in a sitting position and provide oxygen therapy at a high flow rate (unless otherwise contraindicated) if pulmonary edema is suspected.
- Recognize that home care nurses perform focused physical assessments for cardiac patients as delineated in Chart 37-5.
- Monitor the patient with valvular dysfunction for atrial fibrillation, which may lead to hemostasis and mural thrombi. Monitor for an irregularly irregular cardiac rhythm, and administer warfarin as indicated.
- Assess neurovascular status frequently because emboli from valvular disease may cause strokes.
- Differentiate major types of cardiomyopathy as described in Table 37-5.
- Observe for symptoms of heart transplant rejection as listed in Chart 37-11.
- Provide care for patients with pericarditis as outlined in Chart 37-10.

Additional Study Resources

Go to your Companion CD or Evolve at http://evolve.elsevier.com/Iggy/ for *Self-Assessment Questions for the NCLEX Examination.*

evolve

Go to Evolve at http://evolve.elsevier.com/Iggy/ for *Prioritization and Delegation Questions for the NCLEX Examination.*

SELECTED BIBLIOGRAPHY

Asterisk indicates a classic or definitive work on this subject.

Aronow, W.S. (2006). Heart failure update: Treatment of heart failure with a normal left ventricular ejection fraction in the elderly. *Geriatrics, 61*(8), 16-20.

*Artinian, N.T. (2003). The psychosocial aspects of heart failure. *AJN, 103*(12), 32-42.

*Ayers, D.M.M. (2004). Heart failure. *Nursing2004, 34*(11), 46-47.

Bixby, M. (2005). Turn back the tide of cardiogenic pulmonary edema. *Nursing2005, 35*(5), 56-60.

*Bond, A.E., Nelson, K., Germany, C.L., & Smart, A.N. (2003). The left ventricular assist device. *AJN, 103*(1), 32-41.

Bruce, J. (2005). Getting to the heart of cardiomyopathy. *Nursing2005, 35*(8), 44-47.

*Carelock, J., & Clark, A.P. (2003). Heart failure: Pathophysiologic mechanisms. *AJN, 101*(12), 26-35.

Chojnowski, D. (2007). Taking aim at heart failure. *Nursing2007, 37*(11), 50-53.

*Colbert, K., & Greene, M.H. (2003). Nesiritide (Natrecor): A new treatment for acutely decompensated congestive heart failure. *Critical Care Nursing Quarterly, 26*(1), 40-44.

Crowder, B.F. (2006). Improved symptom management through enrollment in an outpatient congestive heart clinic. *MEDSURG Nursing, 15*(1), 27-35.

Dakin, C.L. (2008). New approaches to heart failure in the ED. *AJN, 108*(3), 68-71.

Ellis, W.M. (2005). Getting to the heart of HF core measures. *Nursing2005, 35*(12), 68-69.

*Guido, G.W. (2000). Heart transplant from an ethical perspective. *Critical Care Clinics of North America, 12*(1), 111-119.

Hayes, D.D. (2007). Mitral valve prolapse. *Nursing2007, 37*(1), 51.

Heffelfinger, P.M. (2007). Cardiac resynchronization therapy. *Nursing2007, 37*(3), 53.

*Hoercher, K.J., Vacha, C.J., & McCarthy, P.M. (2002). Left ventricular splints and wraps for end-stage heart failure: A new approach in the new millennium. *Journal of Cardiovascular Nursing, 16*(3), 82-86.

Hoffman, F.M., Nelson, B.J., Drangstveit, M.B., Flynn, B.M., Watercott, E.A., & Zirbes, J.M. (2006). Caring for transplant recipients in a nontransplant setting. *Critical Care Nurse, 26*(2), 53-74.

*Kearney, K. (2000). Emergency: Digitalis toxicity. *AJN, 100*(6), 51-52.

Kincade, E., & Frazier, S.K. (2006). BNP assays: Predicting the future of CHF patients. *The Nurse Practitioner, 31*(12), 36-41.

*Konick-McMahan, J., Bixby, J., & McKenna, C. (2003). Heart failure in older adults: Providing nursing care to improve outcomes. *Journal of Gerontological Nursing, 29*(12), 35-41.

Kreiger, G. (2007). A basic guide to understanding plasma B-type natriuretic peptide in the diagnosis of congestive heart failure. *MEDSURG Nursing, 16*(2), 75-78.

Lindgren, T.G., Fukuoka, Y., Rankin, S.H., Cooper, B.A., Carroll, D., Munn, Y.L. (2008). Cluster analysis of elderly cardiac patients' prehospital symptomatology. *Nursing Research, 57(1)*, 14-23.

McCance, K.L., & Huether, S.E. (2006). *Pathophysiology: The biologic basis for disease in adults and children* (5th ed.). St. Louis: Mosby.

Mennick, F. (2006). A nurse-led program for patients with heart failure. *AJN, 106*(11), 20.

Rasmusson, K.D., Hall, J.A., & Renlund, D.G. (2006). Heart failure epidemic boiling to the surface. *The Nurse Practitioner, 31*(11), 12-21.

Richards, N.M., & Stahl, M.A. (2007). Ventricular assist devices in the adult. *Critical Care Nurse Quarterly, 30*(2), 104-118.

Riegel, B., Dickson, V.V., Goldberg, L.R., & Deatrick, J.A. (2007). Factors associated with the development of expertise in heart failure self-care. *Nursing Research, 56*(4), 235-243.

*Smith, A.L., & Brown, C.S. (2003). New advances and novel treatments in heart failure. *Critical Care Nursing Quarterly, 26*(2), 3-15.

Stahovich, M., Chillcott, S., & Dembitsky, W.P. (2007). The next treatment option: Using ventricular assist devices for heart failure. *Critical Care Nurse Quarterly, 30*(4), 337-346.

Thomas, S. A., Chapa, D. V., Friedman, E., Durden, C., Ross, A., Lee, M. C. Y., et al. (2008). Depression in patients with heart failure: Prevalence, pathophysiological mechanisms, and treatment. *Critical Care Nurse, 28*(2), 40-55.

Todd, B.A., & Higgins, K. (2005). Recognizing aortic and mitral valve disease. *Nursing2005, 35*(6), 58-64.

*Tokarczyk, T.R. (2003). Cardiac transplantation as a treatment option for the heart failure patient. *Critical Care Nursing Quarterly,* 26(1), 61-68.

Wingate, S., & Wiegland, D. L.-M. (2008). End-of-life care in the critical care unit for patients with heart failure. *Critical Care Nurse, 28*(2), 84-94.

*Wisniewski, A. (2004). Muscle up your knowledge of myocarditis. *Nursing2004, 34*(10), 17.

Care of Patients with Vascular Problems

38

CHAPTER

Donna D. Ignatavicius • Sharon Henry Walicek

LEARNING OUTCOMES

For clinical competence and success on the NCLEX Examination, study this chapter with these Learning Outcomes in mind:

Safe and Effective Care Environment

1. Collaborate with interdisciplinary health care team members when providing care for patients with vascular problems.

Health Promotion and Maintenance

2. Identify risk factors for vascular problems.
3. Encourage patient participation in lifestyle modifications to prevent vascular problems.

Physiological Integrity

4. Explain the pathophysiology of arteriosclerosis and atherosclerosis, including the factors that cause arterial injury.
5. Interpret essential laboratory data related to risk for atherosclerosis.
6. Discuss the role of nutrition therapy in the management of patients with arteriosclerosis.
7. Describe the differences between essential and secondary hypertension.
8. Develop a collaborative plan of care for a patient with essential hypertension.
9. Provide information to patients on adverse effects of drugs for hypertension and when to notify the health care provider.
10. Compare assessment findings typically present in patients with peripheral arterial and peripheral venous disease.
11. Identify when venous thromboembolism (VTE) and complications of VTE occur.
12. Implement nursing interventions to help prevent VTE.
13. Describe the nurse's role in monitoring patients who are receiving anticoagulants.
14. Monitor for complications of vascular surgery.
15. Perform a focused vascular assessment.
16. Compare Raynaud's and Buerger's disease.

Go to your Companion CD or Evolve at http://evolve.elsevier.com/Iggy/ for *Self-Assessment Questions for the NCLEX Examination* keyed to these Learning Outcomes.

Disorders of the cardiovascular system cause many problems and may lead to complete shutdown of all body organs and eventually death. Although these health problems can affect any part of the human body, including the heart, brain, and kidneys, the *peripheral* vascular system and its associated diseases are described here. When peripheral blood vessels are diseased or damaged, especially in the legs, arterial blood flow is impaired, preventing distal areas like the feet from being adequately *perfused* and *oxygenated.* The result can be ischemia and necrosis or cell death. Venous disease causes blood to back up into the distal areas and can lead to edema and thromboses (clots) that can be become emboli, a life-threatening complication.

ARTERIOSCLEROSIS AND ATHEROSCLEROSIS

Pathophysiology

Arteriosclerosis is a thickening, or hardening, of the arterial wall that is often associated with aging. **Atherosclerosis,** a type of arteriosclerosis, involves the formation of plaque within the arterial wall and is the leading risk factor for cardiovascular disease. Usually the disease affects the larger arteries, such as the coronary artery beds; the aorta; carotid and vertebral arteries; renal, iliac, and femoral arteries; or any combination of these.

The exact pathophysiology of atherosclerosis is not known, but the condition is thought to occur from blood vessel damage

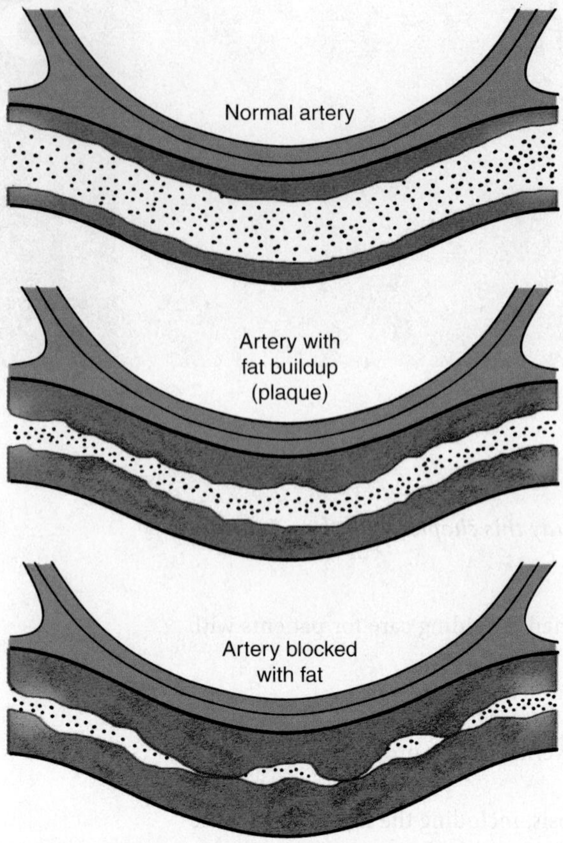
Normal artery
Artery with
fat buildup
(plaque)
Artery blocked
with fat

Fig. 38-1 • Pathophysiology of atherosclerosis.

that causes an inflammatory response (see the discussion of inflammation in Chapter 19) (Fig. 38-1). After the vessel becomes inflamed, a fatty streak appears on the intimal surface (inner lining) of the artery.

Next, a stable or unstable plaque develops. *Stable* plaque is a white, glistening, fibrous elevation that covers a lipid (primarily cholesterol) core. By contrast, *unstable* plaque has a liquid lipid core. At this stage, it is elevated enough to partially or completely reduce or block the blood flow of an artery.

In the final stage, the fibrous lesions become calcified, hemorrhagic, ulcerated, or thrombosed and affect all layers of the vessel. The rate of progression of the process may be influenced by genetic factors, certain chronic diseases (e.g., diabetes mellitus), and lifestyle habits, including smoking, eating habits, and level of exercise. When *stable* plaque ruptures, thrombosis and vessel constriction obstruct the lumen, causing inadequate perfusion to distal tissues. *Unstable* plaque rupture causes more severe damage. After the rupture occurs, the exposed underlying tissue causes platelet adhesion and rapid thrombus (clot) formation. The thrombus may suddenly block a blood vessel, resulting in ischemia and infarction (e.g., myocardial infarction) (McCance & Huether, 2006).

Endothelial (intimal) injury of the major arteries of the body can be caused by many factors. Elevated levels of **lipids** (fats) like low-density lipoprotein cholesterol (LDL-C) and decreased levels of high-density lipoprotein cholesterol (HDL-C) can cause chemical injuries to the vessel wall. (See Chapter 35, which describe lipids in more detail.) Chemical injury can also be caused by elevated levels of toxins in the bloodstream, which may occur with renal failure or by carbon monoxide circulating in the bloodstream from cigarette smoking. The vessel wall can be weakened by the natural process of aging or by diseases such as hypertension.

Genetic predisposition and diabetes have a major effect on the development of atherosclerosis. Some patients have familial **hyperlipidemia,** an elevation of serum lipid levels. In these people, the liver makes excessive cholesterol and other fats. In some people with hereditary atherosclerosis, however, the blood cholesterol level is normal. The reason for the development and progression of plaque in these patients is not understood.

Patients with severe diabetes mellitus frequently have premature and severe atherosclerosis from microvascular damage. The premature atherosclerosis occurs because diabetes promotes an increase in LDL-C and triglycerides (lipids) in plasma. In addition, arterial damage may result from the effect of hyperglycemia.

Other factors are indirectly related to atherosclerosis development. A list of direct and indirect risk factors is found in Table 38-1.

It is not known exactly how many people have atherosclerosis, but small plaques are almost always present in the arteries of young adults. The incidence can be better quantified by assessing the number of cardiovascular diseases (CVDs) that result from atherosclerosis. An estimated 81 million U.S. adults have one or more types of CVD. Coronary artery disease affects 16 million people, and stroke affects another 6 million. About half of those with CVD are older than 60 years, and many more are middle-aged (American Heart Association [AHA], 2008). The number of people affected by atherosclerosis is likely to increase as the population ages, especially as 79 million "baby boomers" soon turn 60.

Patient-Centered Collaborative Care

Assessment

Physical Assessment/Clinical Manifestations

Because of the high incidence of hypertension in patients with atherosclerosis, assess the blood pressure in both arms. Perform a complete cardiovascular assessment because associated heart disease is often present.

Palpate pulses at all of the major sites on the body, and note any differences. Carotid arteries are palpated separately because of the risk of blocking blood flow to the brain. Also palpate for temperature differences in the lower extremities, and check capillary filling. Prolonged capillary filling (>3 seconds in young to middle-aged adults; >5 seconds in older adults) generally indicates poor circulation, *although this indicator is not the most reliable.* An extremity in a person with severe athero-

TABLE 38-1 Risk Factors for Atherosclerosis

- Low HDL-C
- High LDL-C
- Increased triglycerides
- Genetic predisposition
- Diabetes mellitus
- Obesity
- Sedentary lifestyle
- Smoking
- Stress
- African American or Hispanic

HDL-C, High-density lipoprotein cholesterol; *LDL-C,* low-density lipoprotein cholesterol.

sclerotic disease may be cool or cold with a diminished or absent pulse.

Many patients with vascular disease have a bruit in the larger arteries, which can be heard with a stethoscope or Doppler probe. A **bruit** is a turbulent, swishing sound, which can be soft or loud in pitch. It is heard as a result of blood trying to pass through a narrowed artery. A bruit is considered abnormal, but it does not indicate the severity of disease. Bruits often occur in the carotid, aortic, femoral, and popliteal arteries. A decrease in intensity or a complete loss of a pulse may indicate an arterial occlusion (blockage).

Laboratory Assessment

Patients with atherosclerosis often have elevated lipids, including cholesterol and triglycerides. Total serum *cholesterol* levels should be below 200 mg/dL. Elevated cholesterol levels are confirmed by HDL and LDL measurements. Increased low-density lipoprotein cholesterol (LDL-C) ("bad" cholesterol) levels indicate that a person is at an increased risk for atherosclerosis. Low high-density lipoprotein cholesterol ("good" cholesterol) (HDL-C) levels also indicate an increased risk. A desirable LDL-C level is one below 100 mg/dL for healthy people and below 70 mg/dL for those diagnosed with CVD or who are diabetic. A desirable HDL-C level is 40 mg/dL or above.

Triglyceride levels may also be elevated with atherosclerosis and is an emerging lipid risk factor by the Adult Treatment Panel Report No. 3 (ATP III) released by the National Heart, Lung, and Blood Institute (National Cholesterol Education Program, 2002). A level of 150 mg/dL or above indicates **hypertriglyceridemia.** Women should have a level below 135 mg/dL (Pagana & Pagana, 2006). Elevated triglycerides are considered a marker for other lipoproteins. They also suggest **metabolic syndrome,** which increases the risk for coronary heart disease (see Table 40-1 and discussion in Chapter 40).

Homocysteine is a sulfur-containing amino acid derived from dietary protein. Although controversial, there may be a positive correlation between increased homocysteine levels and the development of peripheral vascular disease (PVD), coronary artery disease (CAD), stroke, and venous thrombosis. High serum levels of homocysteine may block production of nitric oxide on the vascular endothelium, making the cell walls less elastic and permitting plaque to build up. Elevated homocysteine levels may be lowered by a diet enriched with B-complex vitamins, particularly folic acid. Some health care providers may recommend homocysteine screening for high-risk patients who have a family history of premature cardiovascular disease, angina, or elevated cholesterol. Other laboratory tests that may be performed to rule out CVD are discussed in Chapter 40.

Interventions

Atherosclerosis progresses for years before clinical manifestations occur. Adults who are at risk for the disease can often be identified through cholesterol screening and history. Because of the high incidence in the United States, low-risk people 20 years of age and older are advised to have their total serum cholesterol level evaluated at least once every 5 years. More frequent measurements are suggested for people with multiple risk factors and those older than 40 years.

Recent testing and management recommendations from the National Cholesterol Education Program (NCEP) and ATP guidelines have a major preventive focus for people with multiple risk factors. In need of major lifestyle changes, these groups of high-risk patients, termed "coronary heart disease equivalents," include:

- Those with diabetes but without signs of vascular disease
- People with a Framingham Heart Study 10-year absolute risk score of over 20% for coronary heart disease events
- Those identified with multiple metabolic risk factors

The new category groups these people at the same risk level as those who already have vascular disease.

Interventions for patients with atherosclerosis or those at high risk for the disease focus on lifestyle changes. Teach patients about the need to make daily changes by avoiding or minimizing modifiable risk factors. *Modifiable risk factors* are those that can be changed or controlled by the patient, such as smoking, weight management, and exercise. Nutrition is one of the most important parts of the risk-reduction plan. Chapter 40 describes how to manage modifiable risk factors in detail in the Health Promotion and Maintenance section, p. 850. If lipoprotein levels do not improve after lifestyle changes, the health care provider may prescribe drug therapy to lower cholesterol and/or triglycerides.

Nutrition Therapy

Emphasize the importance of nutrition for patients at risk for atherosclerosis. For those with elevated homocysteine levels, encourage a diet including enriched or fortified cereals that contain 100% of the daily requirement of folic acid, pyridoxine (vitamin B_6), and cyanocobalamin (vitamin B_{12}). If nutritional changes do not decrease homocysteine levels, multivitamins containing 0.4 mg of folic acid, 2 mg of pyridoxine, and 6 mcg of cyanocobalamin may be added.

The Nutrition Committee of the American Heart Association (AHA) has established *Dietary Guidelines for Healthy Adults* to outline the best strategies for a *heart-healthy diet.* Formerly known as *Step One Diet* and *Step Two Diet,* the revised guidelines focus on the need to achieve and maintain a healthy weight and make appropriate food choices. The major guidelines of the AHA for healthy Americans older than 2 years replace the *Step One Diet.* To decrease serum cholesterol level, a total fat intake of less than 30% of total calories should be consumed. Less than 10% of total caloric intake should be from saturated fat, up to 10% of total calories should be from polyunsaturated fat, and 10% to 15% should come from monounsaturated fat. The Step One diet limits cholesterol intake to less than 300 mg daily.

In collaboration with the nutritionist, teach the patient about the types of fat content in food. Meats and eggs contain mostly saturated fats. Because canola (rapeseed) oil is rich in monounsaturated fat and safflower and sunflower oil are rich in polyunsaturated oils, they are recommended over highly saturated oils such as palm or coconut oil. Cholesterol is found also in animal sources such as meat and eggs.

The focus of cholesterol management is an aggressive approach to lowering LDL-C values and raising HDL-C levels. Having an LDL-C value of less than 100 mg/dL is optimal; values of 100 to 129 mg/dL are near or less than optimal. Patients with LDL-C values of 130 to 159 mg/dL (borderline high) are advised to follow a fat-modified diet and regular exercise regimen and increase omega-3 fatty acids in their diet or as a supplement. Increased fiber of 25 to 35 g in the daily diet is also recommended. In collaboration with the nutritionist, teach patients with LDL-C values of 160 mg/dL or greater (high or very high) to follow a more structured nutritional plan aimed at decreasing saturated fat and cholesterol and, if appropriate, promoting weight loss.

For high-risk people, such as those with high cholesterol, diabetes, or CVD, the AHA recommends the NCEP Therapeutic Lifestyle Changes (TLC) diet, which outlines appropriate medical nutrition therapy. Formerly called the *Step Two Diet,* recommendations include testing the patient's serum cholesterol levels and then retesting 6 and 12 weeks after the initial nutritional intervention. If the cholesterol level has not significantly decreased, the patient may be referred to a nutritionist (registered dietitian) for instruction on the NCEP—TLC diet, which limits saturated fat to less than 7% of total calories and cholesterol to less than 200 mg/day.

Drug Therapy

For patients with elevated total and LDL-C levels that do not respond adequately to dietary intervention, the health care provider prescribes one or more lipid-lowering agents (Table 38-2). Drug choice depends on the serum lipid levels. Because most of these drugs can produce major side effects, they are generally given only when nonpharmacologic management has been unsuccessful.

A class of drugs known as *3-hydroxy-3-mathylglutaryl coenzyme A (HMG-CoA) reductase inhibitors (statins)* successfully reduces total cholesterol in most patients when used for an extended period. These drugs are also referred to as *antihyperlipoproteinemics.* Examples include lovastatin (Mevacor), simvastatin (Zocor), and atorvastatin (Lipitor), which lower both LDL-C and triglyceride levels. Statins reduce cholesterol synthesis in the liver and increase clearance of LDL-C from the blood. *Therefore they are contraindicated in patients with active liver disease or during pregnancy because they can cause muscle myopathies and marked decreases in liver function. Statin drugs are discontinued if the patient has muscle cramping or elevated liver enzyme levels.*

A different type of lipid-lowering agent, ezetimibe (Zetia), may be used in place of or in combination with statin-type drugs. This drug inhibits the absorption of cholesterol through the small intestine. Vytorin is a combination drug containing ezetimibe and simvastatin. This drug works two ways—by reducing the absorption of cholesterol and by decreasing the amount of cholesterol synthesis in the liver. Other statin combinations have been developed to improve lipid levels, such as Advicor, a combination of niacin and lovastatin. Aspirin and pravastatin are now combined as Pravigard. Amlodipine (Norvasc) and atorvastatin are combined as Caduet to decrease blood pressure while decreasing triglycerides (TGs), increasing HDL, and lowering LDL. Combining drugs may improve adherence for the patient who is often taking multiple drugs.

Complementary and Alternative Therapy

Nicotinic acid or niacin (Niaspan), a B vitamin, may lower LDL-C and very-low-density lipoprotein (VLDL) cholesterol levels and increase HDL-C levels in some patients. It is used as a single agent or in combination with an acid-binding resin drug or a statin. Low doses are recommended because many patients experience flushing and a very warm feeling all over. Higher doses can result in an elevation of hepatic enzymes.

Omacor (omega-3 fatty acids) has been approved by the Food and Drug Administration (FDA) as an adjunct to nutrition to reduce TGs that are greater than 500 mg/dL. This drug also decreases plaque growth and inflammation and reduces clot formation (Harris et al., 2008).

HYPERTENSION

Pathophysiology

Hypertension is a systolic blood pressure at or above 140 mm Hg and/or a diastolic blood pressure at or above 90 mm Hg in people who do not have diabetes mellitus. Patients with diabetes and heart disease should have a blood pressure below 130/90 (Rosendorf et al., 2007).

In 2003, the Seventh Report of the Joint National Committee on Prevention, Detection, Evaluation, and Treatment of High Blood Pressure made significant changes in classifying blood pressure in adults. The new classification for **"normal" adult blood pressure** is less than 120 mm Hg systolic *and* less than 80 mm Hg diastolic. Adults with a blood pressure (BP) of 120 to 139 mm Hg systolic *or* 80 to 89 mm Hg diastolic, considered "normal" under previous guidelines, are now classified as pre-hypertensive. These patients need lifestyle changes to prevent cardiovascular complications (Table 38-3). The relationship between hypertension and cardiovascular events is direct and independent of other risk factors. The higher the patient's blood pressure is, the greater the chance for coronary, cerebral, renal, and peripheral vascular disease. Control of hypertension, however, has resulted in major decreases in cardiovascular morbidity and mortality (Table 38-4).

▶ ANIMATION: Physiology of Blood Pressure

TABLE 38-2 Commonly Used Drugs for Atherosclerosis

HMG-CoA reductase inhibitors (statins):
- Lovastatin (Mevacor)
- Atorvastatin (Lipitor)
- Simvastatin (Zocor)
- Fluvastatin (Lescol)
- Rosuvastatin (Crestor)
- Pravastatin (Pravachol)

Fibric acids:
- Gemfibrozil (Lopid)
- Fenofibrate (Tricor)
- Advicor (combination of niacin [fibric acid] and lovastatin)
- Zetia
- Lovaza

TABLE 38-3 Blood Pressure Classification

Classification	Blood Pressure Measurement	Blood Pressure Readings
Normal	Systolic	<120 mm Hg
	and diastolic	<80 mm Hg
Prehypertension	Systolic	120-139 mm Hg
	or diastolic	80-89 mm Hg
Stage 1: Hypertension	Systolic	140-159 mm Hg
	or diastolic	90-99 mm Hg
Stage 2: Hypertension	Systolic	≥160 mm Hg
	or diastolic	≥100 mm Hg

From Joint National Committee. (2003). *The Seventh Report of the Joint National Committee on Prevention, Detection, Evaluation, and Treatment of High Blood Pressure.* NIH Publication No. 03-5233. Bethesda, MD: National Heart, Lung, and Blood Institute.

TABLE 38-4 Meeting *Healthy People 2010* Objectives

BLOOD PRESSURE

Objective 12.11: Increase the proportion of adults with high blood pressure who are taking action to help control their blood pressure.

- Teach adults with high blood pressure the importance of controlling sodium intake, including reading food labels for sodium content and avoiding high-sodium foods, such as bacon, ham, and processed snacks.
- Refer overweight adults to a support group or weight-reduction program.
- Teach about the importance of exercise and increased physical activity to reduce blood pressure.
- For the adult who smokes, teach about the relationship between cardiovascular disease and smoking. Refer the person to a smoking cessation program.
- Participate in community or health care agency health fairs to screen for hypertension and provide community education.
- Teach all adults to have their blood pressure taken at least once every 2 years. For those with hypertension, monitor blood pressure as recommended by the health care provider.

Isolated systolic hypertension (ISH) is a major health threat, especially for older adults. For years, emphasis was placed on the diastolic BP (DBP) reading, and attempts were made to lower this number to under 80. However, as people age, the systolic BP (SBP) becomes more significant because it is a better indicator than DBP of risk for heart disease and stroke. Research has shown that DBP rises until age 55 years and then declines, whereas SBP continues to rise. ISH is defined as a SBP reading at or above 140 with a DBP below 90. For older adults, it is the most common form of hypertension and has no symptoms (Nash, 2006).

The systemic arterial pressure is a product of cardiac output (CO) and total peripheral vascular resistance (PVR). Cardiac output is determined by the stroke volume and heart rate ($CO = SV \times HR$). Control of peripheral vascular resistance (i.e., vessel constriction or dilation) is maintained by the autonomic nervous system and circulating hormones, such as norepinephrine and epinephrine. Consequently, any factor that increases peripheral vascular resistance, heart rate, or stroke volume increases the systemic arterial pressure. Conversely, any factor that decreases peripheral vascular resistance, heart rate, or stroke volume decreases the systemic arterial pressure.

Stabilizing mechanisms exist in the body to exert an overall regulation of systemic arterial pressure and to prevent circulatory collapse. Four control systems play a major role in maintaining blood pressure: the arterial baroreceptor system, regulation of body fluid volume, the renin-angiotensin/aldosterone system, and vascular autoregulation.

The *arterial baroreceptors* are found primarily in the carotid sinus, aorta, and wall of the left ventricle. They monitor the level of arterial pressure and counteract a rise in arterial pressure through vagally mediated cardiac slowing and vasodilation with decreased sympathetic tone. Therefore reflex control of circulation elevates the systemic arterial pressure when it falls and lowers it when it rises. Why baroceptor control fails in hypertension is unknown. There is evidence for upward resetting of baroreceptor sensitivity so that pressure measures are inadequately sensed even though pressure decreases are not.

Changes in *fluid volume* also affect the systemic arterial pressure. If there is an excess of sodium and/or water in a person's body, the blood pressure rises through complex physiologic mechanisms that change the venous return to the heart, producing a rise in cardiac output. If the kidneys are functioning adequately, a rise in systemic arterial pressure produces diuresis and a fall in pressure. Pathologic conditions change the pressure threshold at which the kidneys excrete sodium and water, thereby altering the systemic arterial pressure.

Renin, angiotensin, and aldosterone also regulate blood pressure (see discussion in Chapter 13). The kidney produces renin, an enzyme that acts on angiotensinogen (a plasma protein substrate) to split off angiotensin I, which is converted by an enzyme in the lung to form angiotensin II. Angiotensin II has strong vasoconstrictor action on blood vessels and is the controlling mechanism for aldosterone release. Aldosterone then works on the collecting tubules in the kidneys to reabsorb sodium. Sodium retention inhibits fluid loss, thus increasing blood volume and subsequent blood pressure.

Inappropriate secretion of renin may cause increased peripheral vascular resistance in essential (primary) hypertension. In high blood pressure, renin levels should fall because the increased renal arteriolar pressure should inhibit renin secretion. For most people with essential hypertension, however, renin levels are normal.

The process of *vascular autoregulation,* which keeps perfusion of tissues in the body relatively constant, appears to be important in causing hypertension. This mechanism is poorly understood.

Sustained BP elevation in patients with essential (primary) hypertension results in damage to vital organs. Essential hypertension produces medial hyperplasia (thickening) of the arterioles. As the blood vessels thicken and perfusion decreases, body organs are damaged. These changes can result in myocardial infarctions, strokes, peripheral vascular disease (PVD), or renal failure.

Malignant hypertension is a severe type of elevated blood pressure that rapidly progresses. A person with this health problem usually has symptoms such as morning headaches, blurred vision, and dyspnea and/or symptoms of uremia (accumulation in the blood of substances ordinarily eliminated in the urine). Patients are often in their 30s, 40s, or 50s with their systolic blood pressure greater than 200 mm Hg. The diastolic blood pressure is greater than 150 mm Hg or greater than 130 mm Hg when there are pre-existing complications. Unless intervention occurs promptly, a patient with malignant hypertension may experience renal failure, left ventricular failure, or stroke.

Etiology and Genetic Risk

Hypertension can be essential (primary) or secondary (Table 38-5). Essential hypertension accounts for 85% to 90% of all cases.

Essential Hypertension

Although there is no known cause for **essential hypertension,** many risk factors are associated with this disease:

- Age greater than 60 years
- A family history of hypertension
- Excessive calorie consumption

TABLE 38-5 Etiology of Hypertension

ESSENTIAL (PRIMARY)
- No known cause
- Associated risk factors:
  - Family history of hypertension
  - High sodium intake
  - Excessive calorie consumption
  - Physical inactivity
  - Excessive alcohol intake
  - Low potassium intake

SECONDARY
- Renal vascular and renal parenchymal disease
- Primary aldosteronism
- Pheochromocytoma
- Cushing's disease
- Coarctation of the aorta
- Brain tumors
- Encephalitis
- Psychiatric disturbances
- Pregnancy
- Drugs:
  - Estrogen (e.g., oral contraceptives)
  - Glucocorticoids
  - Mineralocorticoids
  - Sympathomimetics

- Physical inactivity
- Excessive alcohol intake
- Hyperlipidemia
- African-American ethnicity
- High intake of salt or caffeine
- Reduced intake of potassium, calcium, or magnesium
- Obesity
- Smoking
- Stress

A family history of hypertension is a major risk factor. In families with hypertension, there may be a defect in renal secretion of sodium or a heightened sympathetic nervous system response to stress.

Secondary Hypertension

Specific disease states and drugs can increase a person's susceptibility to hypertension. A person with this type of elevation in blood pressure has **secondary hypertension.**

Renal disease is one of the most common causes of secondary hypertension. Hypertension can develop when there is any sudden damage to the kidneys. Renovascular hypertension is associated with narrowing of one or more of the main arteries carrying blood directly to the kidneys, known as *renal artery stenosis (RAS).* Many patients have been able to reduce the categories as well as the doses of their antihypertensive drugs when the narrowed arteries are dilated through angioplasty with stent placement. All patients requiring three or four categories of antihypertensive drugs at high doses should be screened for RAS.

Dysfunction of the adrenal medulla or the adrenal cortex can also cause secondary hypertension. Adrenal-mediated hypertension is due to primary excesses of aldosterone, cortisol, and catecholamines. In *primary aldosteronism,* excessive aldosterone causes hypertension and hypokalemia (low potassium levels). It usually arises from benign adenomas of the adrenal cortex. *Pheochromocytomas* originate most commonly in the adrenal medulla and result in excessive secretion of catecholamines. In *Cushing's syndrome,* excessive glucocorticoids are excreted from the adrenal cortex. The most common cause of Cushing's syndrome is either adrenocortical hyperplasia or adrenocortical adenoma.

Drugs that can cause secondary hypertension include estrogen, glucocorticoids, mineralocorticoids, sympathomimetics, cyclosporine, and erythropoietin. *The use of estrogen-containing oral contraceptives is probably the most common cause of secondary hypertension in women.* Discontinuation of drugs capable of causing hypertension often reverses this problem.

Incidence/Prevalence

One in every three American adults has high blood pressure or is being treated for hypertension (AHA, 2008). The disease shortens life expectancy. A higher percentage of men than women have hypertension until age 45 years. From 45 to 54 years, women have a slightly higher percentage of hypertension than men. After age 54 years, women have a much higher percentage of the disease (AHA, 2008).

CULTURAL AWARENESS

The prevalence of hypertension in African Americans in the United States is among the highest in the world and is constantly increasing. When compared with Euro-Americans, they develop high BP (HBP) earlier in life, making them much more likely to die from strokes, heart disease, and kidney disease (AHA, 2008). The reason for these differences is not known, but genetics and environmental factors may play a role. Those who live in very rural or urban areas may have difficulty accessing health care or may have transportation problems. In some urban areas, people are afraid to leave their homes because of neighborhood crime (Artinian et al., 2007).

Health Promotion and Maintenance

Teach patients ways to decrease risk factors for hypertension. Risk factor prevention and lifestyle changes are discussed under the nursing diagnosis of Deficient Knowledge on p. 800.

Patient-Centered Collaborative Care

evolve ONLINE PHARM REVIEW

Assessment

History

During history taking, review the patient's risk factors for hypertension. Collect data on the patient's age; ethnic origin or race; family history of hypertension; average dietary intake of calories, sodium- and potassium-containing foods, and alcohol; and exercise habits. Also assess any past or present history of renal or cardiovascular disease and current use of drug therapy or illicit drugs.

Physical Assessment/Clinical Manifestations

When a diagnosis of hypertension is made, most people have no symptoms. However, they may experience headaches, dizziness, or fainting as a result of the elevated blood pressure. Some patients also have facial flushing (redness). Obtain blood pressure readings in both arms. Two or more readings are taken at each visit, with the average of the read-

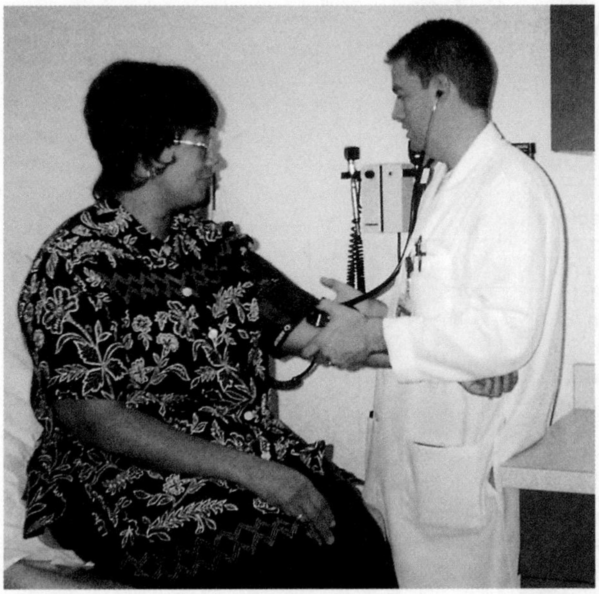

Fig. 38-2 • Blood pressure screening during history and physical examination.

ings used as the value for the visit (Fig. 38-2). To detect postural (orthostatic) changes, also take readings with the patient in the supine (lying) or sitting position and at least 2 minutes later when standing. **Orthostatic hypotension** is a decrease in blood pressure (20 mm Hg systolic and/or 10 mm Hg diastolic) when the patient changes position from lying to sitting.

Funduscopic examination of the eyes to observe vascular changes in the retina is done by a skilled practitioner. The appearance of the retina can be a reliable index of the severity and prognosis of hypertension.

Physical assessment is helpful in diagnosing several conditions that produce secondary hypertension. The presence of abdominal bruits is typical of patients with renal vascular disease. Tachycardia, sweating, and pallor may suggest a pheochromocytoma (adrenal medulla tumor). Coarctation of the aorta is evidenced by elevation of blood pressure in the arms, with normal or low blood pressure in the lower extremities. Femoral pulses are also delayed or absent.

Psychosocial Assessment

Assess for psychosocial stressors that can worsen hypertension and affect the patient's ability to adhere to treatment. Evaluate job-related, economic, and other life stressors, as well as the patient's response to these stressors. Some patients may have difficulty coping with the lifestyle changes needed to control hypertension. Be sure to assess past coping strategies.

Diagnostic Assessment

Although no laboratory tests are diagnostic of essential hypertension, several laboratory tests can assess possible causes of secondary hypertension. Renal disease can be diagnosed by the presence of protein, red blood cells, pus cells, and casts in the urine; elevated levels of blood urea nitrogen (BUN); and elevated serum creatinine levels. The creatinine clearance test directly indicates the glomerular filtration ability of the kidneys. The normal value is 107 to 139 mL/min for men and 87 to 107 mL/min for women (Pagana & Pagana, 2006). Decreased levels indicate renal disease.

Urinary test results are positive for the presence of catecholamines in patients with a pheochromocytoma (tumor of the adrenal medulla). An elevation in levels of serum corticoids and 17-ketosteroids in the urine is diagnostic of Cushing's disease.

No specific x-ray studies can diagnose hypertension. Routine chest radiography may help recognize cardiomegaly (heart enlargement).

An electrocardiogram (ECG) determines the degree of cardiac involvement. Left atrial and ventricular hypertrophy is the first ECG sign of heart disease resulting from hypertension. Left ventricular remodeling can be detected on the 12-lead ECG (see Chapter 40 for discussion of remodeling).

▪ *Analysis*

Common Nursing Diagnoses and Collaborative Problems

The priority nursing diagnoses for patients with hypertension include:

1. Deficient Knowledge related to information misinterpretation or unfamiliarity with information resources
2. Risk for Ineffective Therapeutic Regimen Management related to nonadherence to treatment

Additional Nursing Diagnoses and Collaborative Problems

In addition to the common nursing diagnoses, patients may have:

- Ineffective Tissue Perfusion (Renal, Cerebral, Cardiopulmonary, Peripheral) related to decreased blood flow
- Risk for Imbalanced Nutrition: More Than Body Requirements related to learned eating behaviors, ethnic and cultural values, lack of social support for weight loss, and/or imbalance between activity level and caloric intake
- Fatigue related to altered body chemistry (drugs) and disease state
- Sexual Dysfunction related to altered body function from drug therapy
- Ineffective Coping related to inadequate level of perception of control
- Excess Fluid Volume related to compromised regulatory mechanism
- Risk for Noncompliance related to knowledge and skill relevant to the regimen behavior

These collaborative problems may also apply for some patients with hypertension:

- Potential for Cerebrovascular Hemorrhage
- Potential for Myocardial Infarction
- Potential for Retinal Hemorrhage

▪ *Planning and Implementation*

Deficient Knowledge

NOC **Planning: Expected Outcomes.** The patient with hypertension is expected to have an understanding about a specific treatment regimen. Indicators include that the patient will be able to describe:

- Specific disease process
- Rationale for treatment regimen
- Self-care responsibilities for ongoing treatment
- Self-monitoring techniques
- Expected effects of treatment
- Benefits of disease management

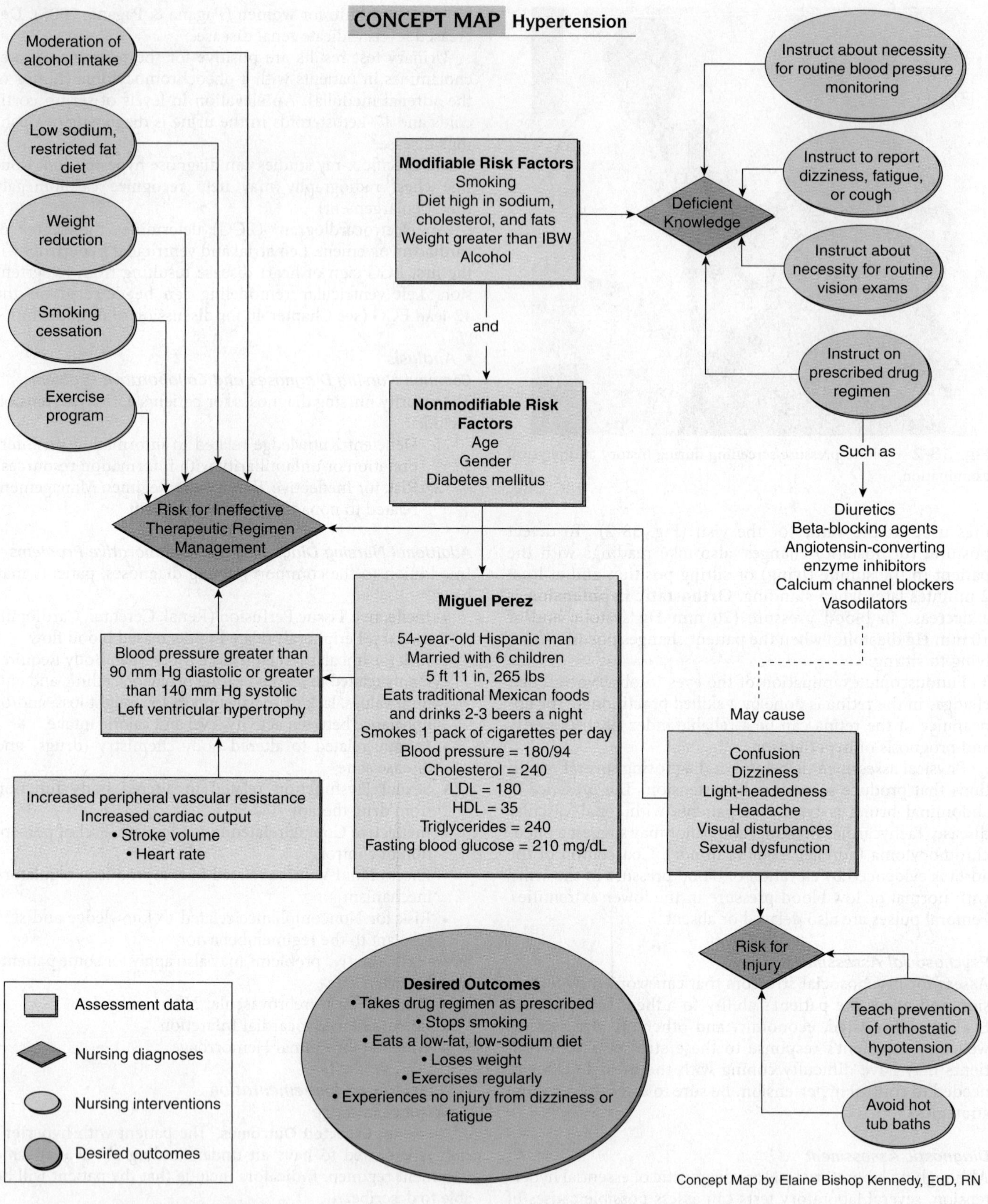
CONCEPT MAP Hypertension
Moderation of alcohol intake
Low sodium, restricted fat diet
Weight reduction
Smoking cessation
Exercise program
Risk for Ineffective Therapeutic Regimen Management
Modifiable Risk Factors
Smoking
Diet high in sodium, cholesterol, and fats
Weight greater than IBW
Alcohol
and
Nonmodifiable Risk Factors
Age
Gender
Diabetes mellitus
Deficient Knowledge
Instruct about necessity for routine blood pressure monitoring
Instruct to report dizziness, fatigue, or cough
Instruct about necessity for routine vision exams
Instruct on prescribed drug regimen
Such as
Diuretics
Beta-blocking agents
Angiotensin-converting enzyme inhibitors
Calcium channel blockers
Vasodilators
Miguel Perez
54-year-old Hispanic man
Married with 6 children
5 ft 11 in, 265 lbs
Eats traditional Mexican foods and drinks 2-3 beers a night
Smokes 1 pack of cigarettes per day
Blood pressure = 180/94
Cholesterol = 240
LDL = 180
HDL = 35
Triglycerides = 240
Fasting blood glucose = 210 mg/dL
Blood pressure greater than 90 mm Hg diastolic or greater than 140 mm Hg systolic
Left ventricular hypertrophy
Increased peripheral vascular resistance
Increased cardiac output
• Stroke volume
• Heart rate
May cause
Confusion
Dizziness
Light-headedness
Headache
Visual disturbances
Sexual dysfunction
Risk for Injury
Teach prevention of orthostatic hypotension
Avoid hot tub baths
Desired Outcomes
• Takes drug regimen as prescribed
• Stops smoking
• Eats a low-fat, low-sodium diet
• Loses weight
• Exercises regularly
• Experiences no injury from dizziness or fatigue
Assessment data
Nursing diagnoses
Nursing interventions
Desired outcomes
Concept Map by Elaine Bishop Kennedy, EdD, RN

Interventions. Lifestyle changes are considered the foundation of hypertension control. If the modifications are unsuccessful, the health care provider considers the use of antihypertensive drugs (see the Concept Map above). There is no surgical treatment for essential hypertension. However, surgery may be indicated for certain causes of secondary hypertension, such as renal vascular disease, coarctation of the aorta, and pheochromocytoma.

Lifestyle Modifications. In collaboration with the health care team, recommend:
- Sodium restriction
- Weight reduction

TABLE 38-6 Drug Classes Used for Hypertension Management
• Thiazide (low-ceiling) diuretics
• Loop (high-ceiling) diuretics
• Potassium-sparing diuretics
• Calcium channel blockers
• Beta-adrenergic blockers (cardioselective and noncardioselective)
• Angiotensin-converting enzyme (ACE) inhibitors
• Angiotensin II receptor blockers (ARBs)
• Aldosterone receptor antagonists

- Moderation of alcohol intake
- Exercise
- Relaxation techniques
- Tobacco and caffeine avoidance

Strategies to help patients make these changes are discussed in Chapter 40.

Drug Therapy. Drug therapy is individualized for each patient, with consideration given to culture, age, concomitant illness, severity of blood pressure elevation, and cost of drugs and follow-up.

According to the Seventh Report of the Joint National Committee on Prevention, Detection, Evaluation, and Treatment of High Blood Pressure 2003 guidelines, most patients with hypertension need two or more drugs to adequately control blood pressure. Because of the lower cost and effectiveness of thiazide-type diuretics, they are usually the drugs of choice for patients with uncomplicated hypertension, as a single agent or in combination with other classes of drugs. However, teach men that they may experience decreased libido (desire for sex) and decreased sexual performance.

In the largest hypertensive trial done to date, Antihypertensive and Lipid-Lowering Treatment to Prevent Heart Attack Trial (ALLHAT), the use of diuretics has been practically unmatched in preventing the cardiovascular complications of hypertension. Calcium channel blockers, angiotensin-converting enzyme (ACE) inhibitors, angiotensin II receptor antagonists, and aldosterone receptor antagonists also can be tried. Alpha blockers should not be used for initial therapy. *Once-a-day drug therapy is best, especially for the older adult, because the more doses required each day, the higher the risk that a patient will not follow the treatment regimen.* Examples of commonly used drug classes for hypertension are listed in Table 38-6.

Diuretics. Three basic types of diuretics are used to decrease blood volume and lower blood pressure:

- Thiazide (low-ceiling) diuretics such as hydrochlorothiazide (HydroDIURIL, Urozide🍁) prevent sodium and water reabsorption in the distal tubules while promoting potassium excretion.
- Loop (high-ceiling) diuretics such as furosemide (Lasix, Furoside🍁) depress sodium reabsorption in the ascending loop of Henle and promote sodium and potassium excretion.
- Potassium-sparing diuretics such as spironolactone (Aldactone, Novospiroton🍁) act on the distal tubule to inhibit reabsorption of sodium ions in exchange for potassium, thereby retaining potassium. When used, they are typically in combination with another diuretic to conserve potassium. These drugs are fairly weak but can provide a synergistic effect, as well as spare potassium.

Diuretics are the drugs of choice for patients who have asthma, chronic airway limitation, chronic renal disease, and select cases of heart failure. Caution is indicated in using thiazide diuretics in hypertensive patients with gout or with a history of significant hyponatremia, because these problems can worsen.

Diuretics enhance the antihypertensive effectiveness when using multiple drug therapy combinations and are inexpensive. Adherence to the drug regimen is enhanced because the drug can usually be prescribed on a once-a-day or, at most, twice-a-day schedule. However, the frequent voiding that occurs after a person takes a diuretic may interfere with daily activities. *The most frequent side effect associated with diuretics is hypokalemia (low potassium levels). Monitor the serum potassium level and assess for irregular pulse and muscle weakness, which may indicate hypokalemia. Teach patients taking potassium-depleting diuretics to eat foods high in potassium, such as bananas and orange juice.* However, many people need a potassium supplement to maintain adequate serum potassium levels. Assess for hypokalemia and hyperkalemia for patients taking potassium-sparing diuretics. Hyperkalemia can occur also if they are taking angiotensin-converting enzyme (ACE) inhibitors and/or angiotensin II receptor blockers (ARBs). Both of these electrolyte disturbances are characterized by weakness and an irregular pulse and are described in detail in Chapter 13.

Other antihypertensive drugs. *Calcium channel blockers* such as verapamil hydrochloride (Calan) and amlodipine (Norvasc) lower blood pressure by interfering with the transmembrane flux of calcium ions. This results in vasodilation, which *decreases* blood pressure.

ACE inhibitors are also used as single or combination agents in the treatment of hypertension. These drugs block the action of the angiotensin-converting enzyme as it attempts to convert angiotensin I to angiotensin II, one of the most powerful vasoconstrictors in the body. As a result, the vessels constrict less, which helps control blood pressure. ACE inhibitors include captopril (Capoten) and enalapril (Vasotec).

Instruct the patient receiving an ACE inhibitor for the first time to get out of bed slowly to avoid the severe hypotensive effect that can occur with initial use. Orthostatic hypotension may occur with subsequent doses, but it is less severe. If dizziness continues or there is a significant decrease in the systolic blood pressure (more than a change of 20 mm Hg), notify the health care provider or teach patients to notify their provider. The older patient is at the greatest risk for postural hypotension because of the cardiovascular changes associated with aging. If a cough develops, the drug is discontinued.

Angiotensin II receptor antagonists, also called *angiotensin II receptor blockers (ARBs),* make up a group of drugs that selectively block the binding of angiotensin II to its receptor in the vascular and adrenal tissues by competing directly with angiotensin II but not inhibiting ACE. Examples of drugs in this group are candesartan (Atacand) and losartan (Cozaar). ARBs can be used alone or in combination with other antihypertensive drugs. They are excellent options for patients who report a nagging cough associated with ACE inhibitors and for those with hyperkalemia. In addition, these drugs do not require initial adjustment of the dose for older adults or for any patient with renal impairment. Like the ACEs, the ARBs are not as effective in African Americans unless these drugs are taken with diuretics or another category such as a beta blocker or calcium channel blocker (AHA, 2008).

Aldosterone receptor antagonists block the hypertensive effect of the mineralocorticoid hormone *aldosterone.* Aldosterone increases sodium reabsorption by the kidney and is a significant contributor to hypertension, cardiac and vascular remodeling, and heart failure. Eplerenone (Inspra) lowers blood pressure by blocking aldosterone binding at the mineralocorticoid receptor sites in the kidney, heart, blood vessels, and brain. The recommended dosage is 50 mg daily, which can be increased to 100 mg daily. Generally well tolerated, eplerenone has dose-related adverse effects of hypertriglyceridemia, hyponatremia, and hyperkalemia. Using ACE inhibitors or ARBs at the same time increases the risk of hyperkalemia. Monitor potassium levels carefully, initially every 2 weeks for the first few months and then monthly thereafter.

When taking eplerenone, itraconazole (Sporanox) and ketoconazole (Nizoral) should not be taken. Drug interactions are common. Patients taking erythromycin, fluconazole (Diflucan), saquinavir (Fortovase), and verapamil (Isoptin) can take eplerenone but with a reduction in dosage by half to 25 mg daily. Teach patients that grapefruit juice and the popular herb *St. John's wort* can also increase the chance of adverse effects. Like for all antihypertensives, remind patients not to get up quickly, drive, or climb stairs until they are familiar with the effects of the drug.

Beta-adrenergic blockers are categorized as cardioselective (working only on the cardiovascular system) and non-cardioselective. Cardioselective beta blockers may be prescribed to lower blood pressure by blocking beta receptors in the heart and peripheral vessels, reducing the cardiac rate and output. By blocking these receptors, the drugs decrease heart rate and myocardial contractility. Common side effects of beta blockers include fatigue, weakness, depression, and sexual dysfunction, although the potential for side effects depends on the "selective" blocking effects of the drug. Non-cardioselective beta blockers are usually not prescribed for patients with respiratory disorders because they prevent normal dilation of the bronchi. This can cause pulmonary vasoconstriction and respiratory compromise.

Patients with diabetes who take beta blockers may not have the usual manifestations of hypoglycemia because the sympathetic nervous system is blocked. The body's responses to hypoglycemia such as gluconeogenesis may also be inhibited by certain beta blockers.

Beta blockers are the drug of choice for hypertensive patients with ischemic heart disease (IHD) because the heart is the most common target of end-organ damage with hypertension. If this drug is not tolerated, a long-acting calcium channel blocker can be used. In patients with unstable angina or myocardial infarction (MI), beta blockers or calcium channel blockers should be used initially in combination with ACE inhibitors or ARBs, with addition of other drugs if needed to control the blood pressure. Best practice for controlling hypertension in post–myocardial infarction (MI) patients includes a combination therapy of beta blockers, ACE inhibitors or ARBs (not as common), and aldosterone antagonists plus intense management of lipids and the use of aspirin. Low-dose aspirin should be considered only once the blood pressure is controlled because of the increased risk for hemorrhagic stroke in patients with uncontrolled hypertension.

A new class of drugs, *renin inhibitors,* is effective for mild to moderate hypertension. Aliskiren (Tekturna) is an example and can be used alone or with a thiazide diuretic. Renin is an enzyme produced in the kidneys that causes vasoconstriction, increases peripheral resistance, and increases cardiac output. The result is an increase in blood pressure. Renin inhibitors prevent renin from producing this action. Side effects are minimal and not common, although respiratory distress may occur.

Central alpha agonists act on the central nervous system, preventing reuptake of norepinephrine and resulting in lower peripheral vascular resistance and blood pressure. Clonidine (Catapres) is most commonly used in this drug classification and is usually given as a transdermal patch, providing control of blood pressure for as long as 7 days. Side effects include sedation, postural hypotension, and impotence. This group of drugs is not indicated for first-line management of hypertension.

Alpha-adrenergic antagonists, such as prazosin (Minipress), doxazosin (Cardura), and terazosin (Hytrin), dilate the arterioles and veins. These drugs can lower blood pressure quickly, but their use is limited because of frequent and bothersome side effects. Cardura and Hytrin may be prescribed when patients have benign prostatic hypertrophy (enlargement) (BPH) because of the dilating effect of the vessels, thus decreasing hypertrophy and improving blood flow.

Risk for Ineffective Therapeutic Regimen Management

NOC **Planning: Expected Outcomes.** The patient with hypertension is expected to take personal actions to promote wellness, recovery, and rehabilitation based on professional advice. Indicators include that the patient will consistently:

- Discuss prescribed treatment regimen with health care professional
- Perform treatment regimen as prescribed
- Monitor treatment and drug responses
- Keep appointments with health care professional

Interventions. Patients who require pharmacologic treatment to control essential hypertension usually need to take drug therapy for the rest of their lives. Frequently, however, some stop taking their prescribed drugs because they have no symptoms and have troublesome side effects.

In the hospital setting, collaboration with the pharmacist is helpful to discuss the goals of therapy with the patient, including potential side effects, to help identify potential problems. Assist the patient in tailoring the therapeutic regimen to his or her lifestyle and daily schedule.

Patients who do not adhere to antihypertensive treatment are at great risk for target organ damage and *hypertensive crisis* (malignant hypertension) (Chart 38-1). Patients in hypertensive crisis are admitted to critical care units, where they receive IV antihypertensive therapy such as nitroprusside (Nipride), nicardipine (Cardene IV), fenoldopam (Corlopam), or labetalol (Normodyne). These drugs act quickly as vasodilators to decrease blood pressure (BP). Hospitalization for complications of hypertension can be costly in medical expenses, lost income, and deterioration in the quality of life.

Community-Based Care

Home Care Management

Many people do not successfully take drug therapy as prescribed without some intervention designed to enhance adherence. There is no one cause of poor adherence. Patients often stop taking their drugs with the assumption that the hypertension is under control because they have no symptoms. Some just forget to take their doses. Others may think they are not sick enough. Many patients assume that once their blood pressure returns to normal levels, they no longer need medication. They may also stop because of adverse side effects or cost. Evidence-based approaches can be used to improve adherence to taking drugs. Reviewing instructions and sending home written instructions appear to have the most impact on improving short-term adherence but less impact on long-term therapy. Self-administration of drugs is a behavior that must be learned, and most health care professionals have little training in how to assist others in behavior modification. Develop a plan with the patient, and identify what you will do to encourage adherence and how other health care providers can also support this expected outcome.

Chart 38-1 **BEST PRACTICE FOR PATIENT SAFETY & QUALITY CARE**

Emergency Care of Patients with Hypertensive Crisis

EMERGENCY CARE

ASSESS
- Severe headache
- Extremely high blood pressure
- Dizziness
- Blurred vision
- Disorientation

INTERVENE
- Place patient in a semi-Fowler's position.
- Administer oxygen.
- Administer IV nitroprusside (Nitropress), nicardipine (Cardene IV), or other infusion drug as prescribed (for nitroprusside, cover infusion bag to prevent drug breakdown by light).
- Monitor blood pressure every 5 to 15 minutes until the diastolic pressure is below 90 and not less than 75; then monitor blood pressure every 30 minutes.
- Observe for neurologic or cardiovascular complications, such as seizures; numbness, weakness, or tingling of extremities; dysrhythmias; or chest pain.

The patient should obtain an ambulatory blood pressure monitoring (ABPM) device for use at home so that the pressure can be checked. Evaluate the patient's and family's ability to use this device. If weight reduction is a desired outcome, suggest having a scale in the home for weight monitoring. For patients who do not want to self-monitor, are not able to self-monitor, or have "white-coat" syndrome when they go to their health care provider (causing elevated BP), continuous ABPM may be used. The monitor is worn for 24 hours or longer while patients perform their normal daily activities. Blood pressure is automatically taken every 15 to 30 minutes and recorded for review later. The advantage of this technique is that the health care provider can view the changes in BP readings throughout the 24-hour period to get a picture of a true BP value (Pickering et al., 2006).

Artinian and her colleagues studied the effect of nurse-managed telemonitoring of blood pressure among urban African Americans. Each patient's blood pressure was monitored at home and then transmitted via telephone using a toll-free number (see the Evidence-Based Practice box below).

Health Teaching

Instruct the patient about sodium restriction, weight maintenance or reduction, alcohol restriction, stress management, and exercise. If necessary, also explain about the need to stop using tobacco, especially smoking. Provide oral and written information about the indications, dosage, times for administration, side effects, and drug interactions for antihypertensives. Stress that medication must be taken as prescribed and that when all of it has been consumed, the prescription must be renewed on a continual basis. Suddenly stopping drugs such as beta blockers can result in angina (chest pain), myocardial infarction (MI), or rebound hypertension.

Also urge patients to report unpleasant side effects, such as excessive fatigue, cough, or sexual dysfunction. In many instances, an alternative drug can be prescribed to minimize certain side effects.

EVIDENCE-BASED PRACTICE

Does a community nurse–managed blood pressure telemonitoring program help lower blood pressure?

Artinian, N., Flack, J.M., Nordstrom, C.K., Hockman, E.M., Washington, O.G., Jen, K-L.C., et al. (2007). Effects of nurse-managed telemonitoring on blood pressure at 12-month follow-up among urban African Americans. *Nursing Research, 56*(5), 312-322.

Hypertension is one of the most important risk factors for cardiovascular disease and is increasing, especially among African Americans. This study used a convenience sample recruited from free blood pressure screening programs in an urban area. The subjects were randomized into two groups: the control (usual care) group (n = 193); and an intervention group (n = 194). The intervention group had usual care plus blood pressure (BP) telemonitoring at home. The subjects monitored their BP at home and then transmitted it over the phone using a toll-free number. Data were collected at 3-, 6-, and 12-month follow-ups. After the intervention nurses received the BP readings, they contacted subjects to review goals and provide telecounseling about lifestyle modification and drug adherence. As a result of this program, the nurse-managed intervention group had clinically and statistically significant reductions in both systolic and diastolic BP when compared with the control group who received usual care.

Level of Evidence—5. The subjects were randomized into two groups, and other intervening variables were controlled.

Commentary: Implications for Practice and Research. Lack of adherence to lifestyle modifications and drug therapy for hypertension is a growing problem. This study tested an intervention in a high-risk group to demonstrate that nursing interventions can help control the disease. Although subjects lived in one urban area, the number of subjects in each group was large. This study should be repeated in rural areas and with other racial/ethnic groups.

Nurses should continue to find ways to promote health in the community. For those who work in inpatient settings, help patients locate community resources that can help with follow-up care.

Hypertension is a chronic illness. Allow patients to verbalize feelings about the disease and its treatment. Advise them that their involvement in the collaborative plan of care can lead to control of the disease and can prevent complications.

Health Care Resources

A home care nurse may be needed for follow-up to monitor the blood pressure. Evaluate the patient's or family's ability to obtain accurate BP measurements, and assess adherence with treatment. The American Heart Association (www.aha.org), the Red Cross, or a local pharmacy may be used for free blood pressure checks if patients cannot buy equipment to monitor their blood pressure. Health fairs are also available in most locations.

▪ ***Evaluation: Outcomes***

Evaluate the care of the patient with hypertension on the basis of the identified nursing diagnoses and collaborative problems. The expected outcomes are that the patient will:

- Understand a specific treatment regimen
- Take personal action to promote wellness, recovery, and rehabilitation based on professional advice

Specific indicators for these outcomes are listed for each nursing diagnosis under the Planning and Implementation section (see earlier).

NCLEX EXAMINATION CHALLENGE

An older adult is starting hydrochlorothiazide (HydroDIURIL) 25 mg and enalapril (Vasotec) 5 mg daily. What is the nurse's first priority for health teaching?

A. Teach the client to change positions slowly when getting out of bed.
B. Review foods high in potassium, including bananas and orange juice.
C. Remind the client to expect increased urine output at night.
D. Tell the client that blood pressure monitoring will be needed.

evolve For the correct answer, go to http://evolve.elsevier.com/Iggy/.

PERIPHERAL ARTERIAL DISEASE

Peripheral vascular disease (PVD) includes disorders that change the natural flow of blood through the arteries and veins of the peripheral circulation. It affects the legs much more frequently than the arms. Generally, a diagnosis of PVD implies arterial disease (peripheral arterial disease [PAD]) rather than venous involvement. Some patients have both arterial and venous disease. The cost of the disease is very high and is expected to rise as "baby boomers" age and obesity in the United States increases.

Pathophysiology

PAD is a result of systemic atherosclerosis. It is a chronic condition in which partial or total arterial occlusion (blockage) deprives the lower extremities of *oxygen* and nutrients. PAD in the legs is sometimes referred to as *lower extremity arterial disease (LEAD)*. Atherosclerosis leads to blockage of the arteries that supply the lower legs and feet. The tissues below the blockage (obstruction) cannot live without an adequate *oxygen* and nutrient supply.

Obstructions are classified as inflow or outflow, according to the arteries involved and their relationship to the inguinal ligament (Fig. 38-3). *Inflow* obstructions involve the distal end of the aorta and the common, internal, and external iliac arteries. They are located above the inguinal ligament. *Outflow* obstructions involve the femoral, popliteal, and tibial arteries and are below the superficial femoral artery (SFA). Gradual inflow occlusions may not cause significant tissue damage. Gradual outflow occlusions typically do.

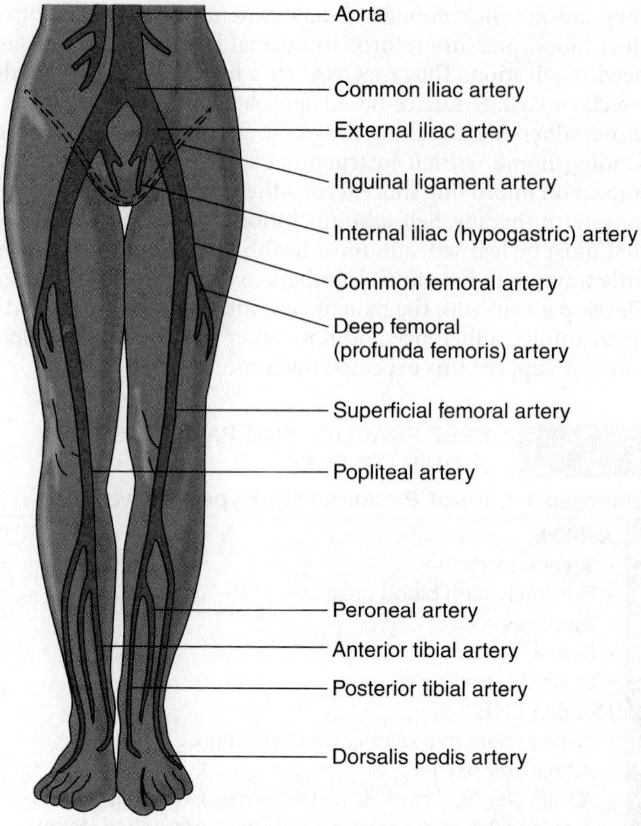
Aorta
Common iliac artery
External iliac artery
Inguinal ligament artery
Internal iliac (hypogastric) artery
Common femoral artery
Deep femoral
(profunda femoris) artery
Superficial femoral artery
Popliteal artery
Peroneal artery
Anterior tibial artery
Posterior tibial artery
Dorsalis pedis artery

Fig. 38-3 • Common locations of inflow and outflow lesions.

Because atherosclerosis is the most common cause of chronic arterial obstruction, the risk factors for atherosclerosis apply to PAD as well. Common risk factors include hypertension, hyperlipidemia, diabetes mellitus, cigarette smoking, obesity, and familial predisposition. Advancing age also increases the risk of disease related to atherosclerosis. Patients with PAD have an increased risk for developing chronic angina, MI, or stroke and are much more likely to die within 10 years compared with those who do not have the disease.

About 10 to 12 million people in the United States have PAD, most of them older than 65 years (AHA, 2008). Diagnosis of the disease is improving because measurement of the ankle-brachial index (ABI) is becoming more common. However, many patients are not diagnosed unless they develop leg pain. African Americans are affected more often than any other group, most likely because they have many of the risk factors such as diabetes and hypertension (AHA, 2008). It generally occurs in men older than 45 years and in postmenopausal women.

Patient-Centered Collaborative Care

▪ ***Assessment***

The clinical course of chronic PAD can be divided into four stages (Chart 38-2). Patients do not experience symptoms in the early stages of disease.

Chart 38-2 KEY FEATURES

Chronic Peripheral Arterial Disease

STAGE I: ASYMPTOMATIC
- No claudication is present.
- Bruit or aneurysm may be present.
- Pedal pulses are decreased or absent.

STAGE II: CLAUDICATION
- Muscle pain, cramping, or burning occurs with exercise and is relieved with rest.
- Symptoms are reproducible with exercise.

STAGE III: REST PAIN
- Pain while resting commonly awakens the patient at night.
- Pain is described as numbness, burning, toothache-type pain.
- Pain usually occurs in the distal portion of the extremity (toes, arch, forefoot, or heel), rarely in the calf or the ankle.
- Pain is relieved by placing the extremity in a dependent position.

STAGE IV: NECROSIS/GANGRENE
- Ulcers and blackened tissue occur on the toes, the forefoot, and the heel.
- Distinctive gangrenous odor is present.

Physical Assessment/Clinical Manifestations

Most patients initially seek medical attention for a classic leg pain known as **intermittent claudication** (a term derived from a word meaning "to limp"). Usually they can walk only a certain distance before a cramping, burning muscle discomfort or pain forces them to stop. The pain stops after rest. When patients resume walking, they can walk the same distance before the pain returns. Thus the pain is considered reproducible. As the disease progresses, they can walk only shorter and shorter distances before pain recurs. Ultimately, pain may occur even while at rest. Ask the patient about the nature of leg pain to determine whether the manifestation is present.

Rest pain, which may begin while the disease is still in the stage of intermittent claudication, is a numbness or burning sensation, often described as feeling like a toothache that is severe enough to awaken patients at night. It is usually located in the toes, the foot arches, the forefeet, the heels and, rarely, in the calves or ankles. Patients can sometimes get pain relief by keeping the limb in a dependent position (below the heart). Those with rest pain often have advanced disease that may result in limb loss.

Patients with **inflow disease** have discomfort in the lower back, buttocks, or thighs. Patients with *mild* inflow disease have discomfort after walking about two blocks. This discomfort is not severe but causes them to stop walking. It is relieved with rest. Patients with *moderate* inflow disease experience pain in these areas after walking about one or two blocks. The discomfort is described as being more like pain, but it eases with rest most of the time. *Severe* inflow disease causes severe pain after walking less than one block. These patients usually have rest pain.

Patients with **outflow disease** describe burning or cramping in the calves, ankles, feet, and toes. Instep or foot discomfort indicates an obstruction below the popliteal artery. Those with *mild* outflow disease experience discomfort after walking about five blocks. This discomfort is relieved by rest. Patients with *moderate* outflow disease have pain after walking about two blocks. Intermittent rest pain may be present. Those with *severe* outflow disease usually cannot walk more than one-half block and usually experience rest pain. They may hang their feet off the bed at night for comfort and report more frequent rest pain than do those with inflow disease.

Specific findings for PAD depend on the severity of the disease. Observe for loss of hair on the lower calf, ankle, and foot; dry, scaly, dusky, pale, or mottled skin; and thickened toenails. With severe arterial disease, the extremity is cold and gray-blue (cyanotic) or darkened. Pallor may occur when the extremity is elevated. Dependent **rubor** (redness) may occur when the extremity is lowered. Muscle atrophy can accompany prolonged chronic arterial disease.

CULTURAL AWARENESS

Because only severe cyanosis is evident in the skin of dark-skinned patients, to detect cyanosis assess their skin and nail beds for a dull, lifeless color. The soles of the feet and the toenails are less pigmented and allow detection of cyanosis or duskiness in the lower extremities.

Palpate all pulses in both legs. The most sensitive and specific indicator of arterial function is the quality of the posterior tibial pulse, because the pedal pulse is not palpable in a small percentage of people. The strength of the pulse should be compared bilaterally. Several scales are available for grading pulse strength.

Note early signs of ulcer formation or complete ulcer formation, a complication of PAD. Arterial and venous stasis ulcers differ from diabetic ulcers (Chart 38-3). Initially, **arterial ulcers** are painful and develop on the toes (often the great toe), between the toes, or on the upper aspect of the foot. With prolonged occlusion, the toes can become gangrenous. Typically, the ulcer is small and round with a "punched out" appearance and well-defined borders. Skin lesions are discussed in further detail in Chapter 27.

Imaging Assessment

Arteriography of the lower extremities may be done if stenting of the narrowed vessel is planned or to determine the exact amount of narrowing or occlusion before peripheral bypass surgery. This procedure involves injecting contrast medium into the arterial system, and the risks, which include hemorrhage, thrombosis, embolus, and death, are serious. The procedure for this test is described in Chapter 35.

Other Diagnostic Assessment

Noninvasive testing for arterial disease has become a more common method of diagnosis. It provides information about the arterial system with minimal risk.

Using a Doppler probe, *segmental systolic blood pressure measurements* of the lower extremities at the thigh, calf, and ankle are an inexpensive, noninvasive method of assessing PAD. Normally, blood pressure readings in the thigh and calf are higher than those in the upper extremities. With the presence of arterial disease, these pressures are lower than the brachial pressure.

With *inflow* disease, pressures taken at the thigh level indicate the severity of disease. Mild inflow disease may cause a difference of only 10 to 30 mm Hg in pressure on the affected

Chart 38-3 KEY FEATURES

Lower Extremity Ulcers

Feature	Arterial Ulcers	Venous Ulcers	Diabetic Ulcers
History	Patient reports claudication after walking about 1-2 blocks Rest pain usually present Pain at ulcer site Two or three risk factors present	Chronic nonhealing ulcer No claudication or rest pain Moderate ulcer discomfort Patient reports of ankle or leg swelling	Diabetes Peripheral neuropathy No reports of claudication
Ulcer location and appearance	End of the toes Between the toes Deep Ulcer bed pale, with even edges Little granulation tissue	Ankle area Brown pigmentation Ulcer bed pink Usually superficial, with uneven edges Granulation tissue present	Plantar area of foot Metatarsal heads Pressure points on feet Deep Pale, with even edges Little granulation tissue
	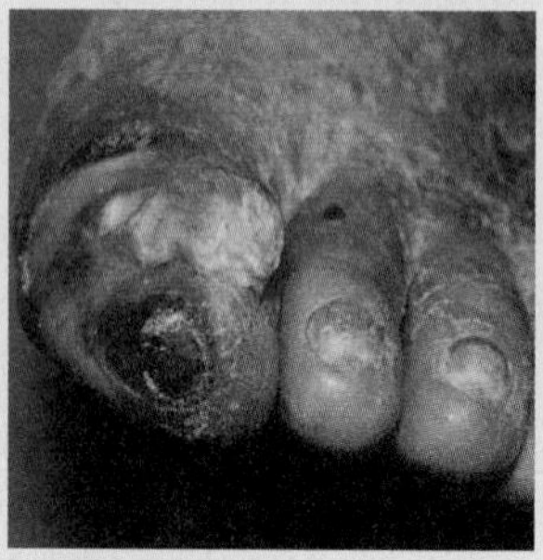	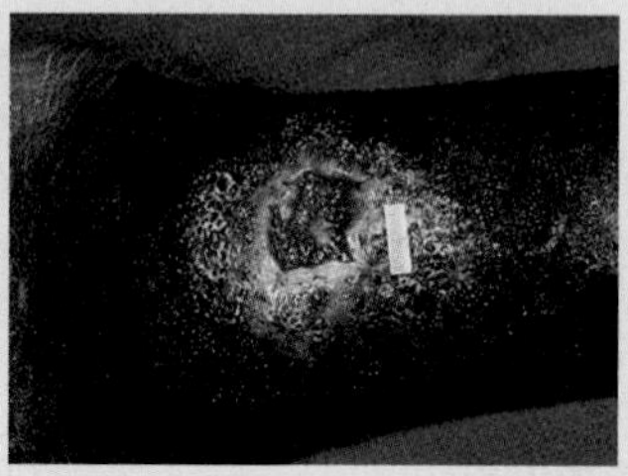	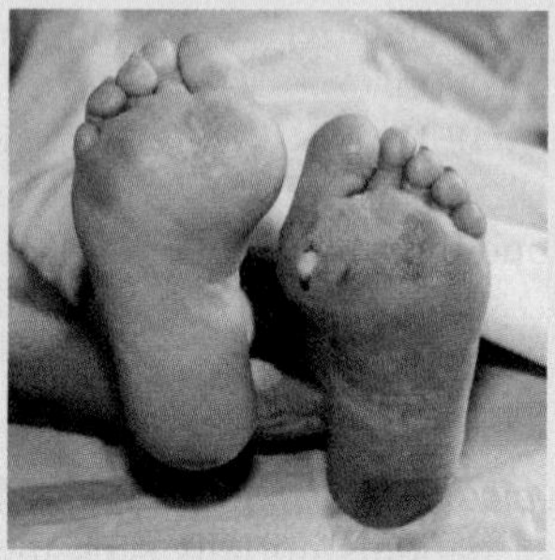
Other assessment findings	Cool or cold foot Decreased or absent pulses Atrophy of skin Hair loss Pallor with elevation Dependent rubor Possible gangrene When acute, neurologic deficits noted	Ankle discoloration and edema Full veins when leg slightly dependent No neurologic deficit Pulses present May have scarring from previous ulcers	Pulses usually present Cool or warm foot Painless
Treatment	Treat underlying cause (surgical, revascularization) Prevent trauma and infection Patient education, stressing foot care	Long-term wound care (Unna boot, damp-to-dry dressings) Elevate extremity Patient education Prevent infection	Rule out major arterial disease Control diabetes Patient education regarding foot care Prevent infection

Photographs of venous ulcer and diabetic ulcer from Bryant, R., & Nix, D. (2007). *Acute and chronic wounds: Current management concepts* (3rd ed.). Philadelphia: Saunders. Photograph of arterial ulcer from Libby, P., Bonow, R.O., Mann, D.L., & Zipes, D.P. (2008). *Braunwald's heart disease: A textbook of cardiovascular medicine* (8th ed.). Philadelphia: Saunders.

side compared with the brachial pressure. Severe inflow disease can cause a pressure difference of more than 40 to 50 mm Hg. The ankle pressure is normally equal to or more than the brachial pressure.

To evaluate *outflow* disease, compare ankle pressure with the brachial pressure, which provides a ratio known as the **ankle-brachial index (ABI).** The value can be derived by dividing the ankle blood pressure by the brachial blood pressure. *An ABI of less than 0.9 in either leg is diagnostic of PAD.* As an alternative, particularly for diabetics, a toe-brachial index (TBI) may be performed in a certified vascular laboratory (Sieggreen, 2006).

Exercise tolerance testing (by chemical stress test or treadmill) may give valuable information about claudication (muscle pain) without rest pain. The technician obtains resting pulse volume recordings and has the patient walk on a treadmill until the symptoms are reproduced. At the time of symptom onset or after about 5 minutes, the technician obtains another pulse volume recording. Normally, there may be an increased waveform with minimal, if any, drop in the ankle pressure. In patients with arterial disease, the waveforms are decreased (dampened) and there is a decrease in the ankle pressure of 40 to 60 mm Hg for 20 to 30 seconds in the affected limb. If the return to normal pressure is delayed (longer than 10 minutes), the results suggest abnormal arterial flow in the affected limb.

Plethysmography can also be performed to evaluate arterial flow in the lower extremities. The measurement provides graphs or tracings of arterial flow in the limb. If an occlusion is present, the waveforms are decreased to flattened, depending on the degree of occlusion.

▪ *Interventions*

First determine whether the altered tissue perfusion is of arterial or venous origin. An accurate assessment often provides this information, but in some people both conditions may exist. In this case, each disease must be considered separately when interventions are planned.

Nonsurgical Management

Exercise, position changes, promotion of vasodilation, drug therapy, and invasive nonsurgical procedures are used to increase arterial flow to the affected limb.

Using Exercise and Positioning. *Exercise* may improve arterial blood flow to the affected limb through buildup of the collateral circulation. **Collateral circulation** provides blood to the affected area through smaller vessels that develop and compensate for the occluded vessels. Exercise is individualized for each patient, but people with severe rest pain, venous ulcers, or gangrene should not participate. Others with PAD can benefit from exercise that is started gradually and slowly increased. Instruct the patient to walk until the point of claudication, stop and rest, and then walk a little farther. Eventually, he or she can walk longer distances as collateral circulation develops. Collaborate with the health care provider and physical therapist in determining an appropriate exercise program. Exercise rehabilitation has been used to relieve symptoms but requires a motivated patient. Supervised sessions are generally not reimbursed by health care insurance.

Positioning to promote circulation has been somewhat controversial. Some patients have swelling in their extremities. *Because swelling prevents arterial flow, feet should be elevated. Teach them to avoid raising their legs above the heart level because extreme elevation slows arterial blood flow to the feet.*

In severe cases, patients with PAD and swelling may sleep with the affected leg hanging from the bed or sit upright in a chair for comfort. *Instruct all patients with the disease to avoid crossing their legs and avoid wearing restrictive clothing (e.g., garters to hold up nylon stockings, particularly common among older women), which interfere with blood flow. Teach them the importance of inspecting their feet daily for color or other changes.*

Promoting Vasodilation. Vasodilation can be achieved by providing warmth to the affected extremity and preventing long periods of exposure to cold. Encourage the patient to maintain a warm environment at home and to wear socks or insulated shoes at all times. *Caution him or her to never apply direct heat to the limb such as with the use of heating pads or extremely hot water. Sensitivity is decreased in the affected limb. Burns may result.*

Encourage patients to prevent exposure of the affected limb to the cold because cold temperatures cause vasoconstriction (decreasing of the diameter of the blood vessels) and therefore decrease arterial blood flow. They should also drink adequate fluids to prevent increased blood viscosity.

Emotional stress, caffeine, and nicotine also can cause vasoconstriction. *Emphasize that complete abstinence from smoking or chewing tobacco is the most effective method of preventing vasoconstriction.* The vasoconstrictive effects of each cigarette may last up to 1 hour after the cigarette is smoked.

Drug Therapy. For patients with chronic PAD, prescribed drugs include hemorheologic and antiplatelet agents. Pentoxifylline (Trental) is a hemorheologic agent that increases the flexibility of red blood cells. It decreases blood viscosity by inhibiting platelet aggregation and decreasing fibrinogen and thus increases blood flow in the extremities. Many patients report limited improvement in their daily lives after taking pentoxifylline. Moreover, those with extremely limited endurance for walking have reported improvement to the point that they can perform some activities (e.g., walk to the mailbox or dining room) that were previously impossible.

Antiplatelet agents, such as aspirin (acetylsalicylic acid, Ancasal🍁) and clopidogrel (Plavix), are commonly used. Aspirin 325 or 81 mg daily may be recommended for patients with chronic PAD. However, the evidence shows that clopidogrel is better than aspirin for reducing the risk for myocardial infarction (MI), ischemic stroke, and vascular death. Patients with PAD and no contraindications to platelet therapy should receive either aspirin or clopidogrel.

Controlling hypertension can improve tissue perfusion by maintaining pressures that are adequate to perfuse the periphery but not constrict the vessels. Teach about the effect of blood pressure on the circulation, and instruct in methods of control. For example, patients taking beta blockers may have drug-related claudication or a worsening of symptoms. The health care provider closely monitors those who are receiving beta blockers.

Percutaneous Transluminal Angioplasty. A nonsurgical but invasive method of improving arterial flow is **percutaneous transluminal angioplasty (PTA).** One or more arteries are dilated with a balloon catheter advanced through a cannula, which is inserted into or above an occluded or stenosed artery. When the procedure is successful, it opens the vessel and improves arterial blood flow. In addition, **stents** (wirelike devices) may be used along with the PTA to help keep the vessel open. Patients who are candidates for PTA must have occlusions or stenoses that are accessible to the catheter. The physician often uses this procedure for those who are poor surgical candidates, who cannot withstand general anesthesia, or for whom amputation may be inevitable. Reocclusion may occur after this procedure, and the procedure may be repeated. Some patients are occlusion-free for up to 3 to 5 years, whereas others may experience reocclusion within a year.

During PTA, intravascular stents may be placed to ensure adequate blood flow in a stenosed vessel. Candidates for stents are patients with stenosis of the common or external iliac arteries. These devices are cost-effective and result in shorter hospital stays and earlier recoveries.

Laser-Assisted Angioplasty. Another invasive procedure is **laser-assisted angioplasty.** A laser probe is advanced through a cannula similar to that used for PTA. Laser-assisted angioplasty is usually reserved for smaller occlusions in the distal superficial femoral, proximal popliteal, and common iliac arteries. Heat from the laser vaporizes the arteriosclerotic plaque to open the occluded or stenosed artery. If significant stenosis remains after the artery is opened, a balloon catheter may be inserted to further dilate the artery. Preparation of the patient for PTA or laser-assisted angioplasty is similar to that for diagnostic angiography.

The priority for postprocedure nursing care is observing for bleeding at the puncture site. Closely observe vital signs, and perform frequent checks of the distal pulses in both limbs. Patients are typically restricted to bedrest, with the limb straight for about 6 to 8 hours before ambulation unless special collagen plugs are used to seal the vessel. Many receive anticoagulant therapy such as heparin during the procedure and for a short time after the procedure. Some type of antiplatelet drug is prescribed for 1 to 3 months after the procedure. However, patients usually take aspirin on a permanent basis.

Atherectomy. The technique of mechanical rotational abrasive **atherectomy** is used to improve blood flow to ischemic limbs in people with PAD. The rotational atherectomy device (rotablator) is a high-speed rotary metal burr ranging in size from 1.25 to 4.5 mm in diameter. The distal half of the burr is embedded with fine abrasive bits, which at speeds of 100,000 to 120,000 rotations per minute result in fine-particle destruction of tissue. The rotablator is designed to preferentially scrape "hard" surfaces (e.g., plaque) while minimizing damage to the vessel surface.

Surgical Management

Patients with severe rest pain or claudication that interferes with the ability to work or threatens loss of a limb become surgical candidates. **Arterial revascularization** is the surgical procedure most commonly used to increase arterial blood flow in an affected limb.

Surgical procedures are classified as inflow or outflow. Inflow procedures involve bypassing arterial occlusions above the superficial femoral arteries (SFAs). Outflow procedures involve surgical bypassing of arterial occlusions at or below the SFAs. For those who have both inflow and outflow problems, the inflow procedure (for larger arteries) is done before the outflow repair.

Inflow procedures include aortoiliac, aortofemoral, and axillofemoral bypasses. Outflow procedures include femoropopliteal and femorotibial bypasses. Inflow procedures are more successful, with less chance of reocclusion or postoperative ischemia. Outflow procedures are less successful in relieving ischemic pain and are associated with a higher incidence of reocclusion.

Graft materials for the bypasses are selected on an individual basis. For outflow procedures, the preferred graft material is the patient's own saphenous vein. However, some patients experience coronary artery disease and may need this vein for coronary artery bypass. When the saphenous vein is not usable, the cephalic or basilic arm veins may be used.

Grafts made of synthetic materials, such as polytetrafluoroethylene (PTFE), GORE-TEX, and Dacron, have also been used when autogenous veins were not available. Although synthetic grafts have achieved adequate patency in arteries above the knee, they have failed to achieve satisfactory results in infrapopliteal outflow vessels. In addition, autogenous veins are often not long enough for use in these vessels. Composite grafts constructed from multiple vein segments offer even better patency to arteries below the knee.

Preoperative Care. Preparing the patient for surgery is similar to procedures described for general or epidural anesthesia (see Chapter 16). Documentation of vital signs and peripheral pulses provides a baseline of information for comparison during the postoperative phase. Depending on the surgical procedure, the patient may have an IV line, urinary catheter, central venous catheter, and/or arterial line. To prevent postoperative infection, antibiotic therapy is typically given before the procedure.

Operative Procedures. The anesthesia provider places the patient under general, epidural, or spinal anesthesia. Epidural or spinal induction is preferred for older adults to decrease the risk of cardiopulmonary complications in this age-group. If arterial bypass is to be accomplished by autogenous grafts, the surgeon removes the veins through an incision. The blocked artery is then exposed through an incision, and the replacement vein or synthetic graft material is sutured above and below the occlusion to increase blood flow around the occlusion.

For *aortoiliac* and *aortofemoral* bypass surgery, the surgeon makes a midline incision into the abdominal cavity to expose the abdominal aorta, with additional incisions in each groin (Fig. 38-4). Graft material is tunneled from the aorta to the groin incisions, where it is sutured in place.

In an *axillofemoral* bypass (Fig. 38-5), the surgeon makes an incision beneath the clavicle and tunnels graft material subcutaneously with a catheter from the chest to the iliac crest, into a groin incision, where it is sutured in place. Neither the thoracic nor the abdominal cavity is entered. For that reason, the axillofemoral bypass is used for high-risk patients who cannot tolerate a procedure requiring abdominal surgery.

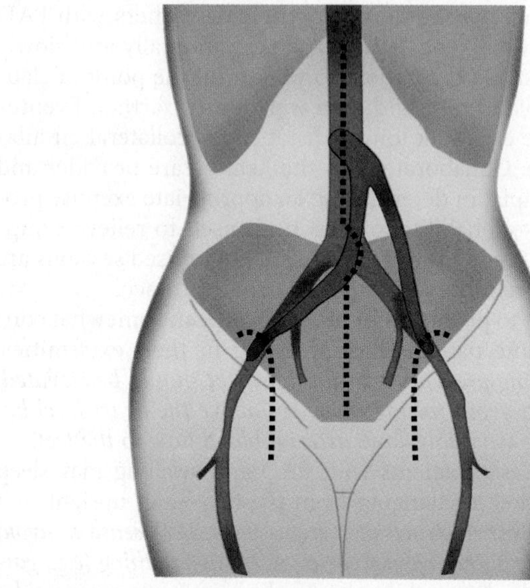

Fig. 38-4 • In aortoiliac and aortofemoral bypass surgery, a midline incision into the abdominal cavity is required, with an additional incision in each groin.

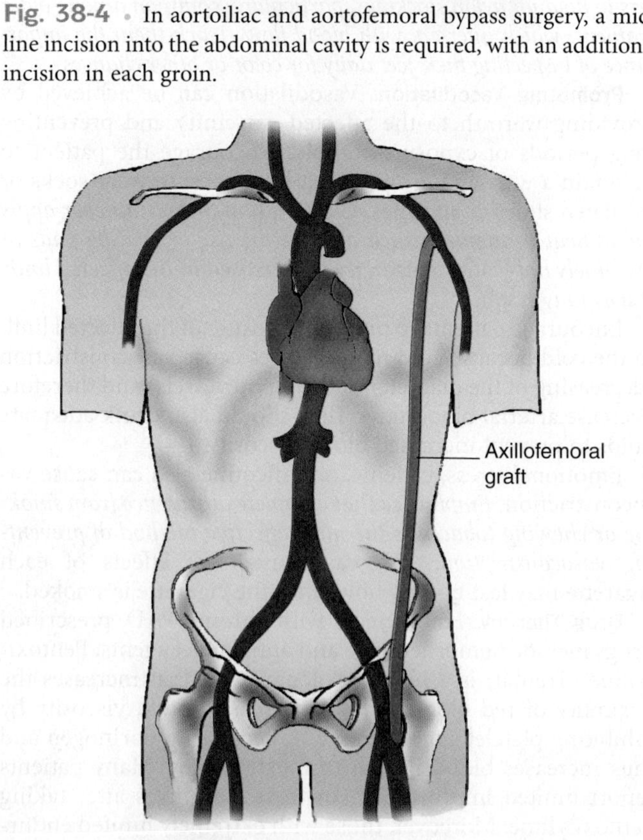
Axillofemoral graft

Fig. 38-5 • An axillofemoral bypass graft.

Postoperative Care. *Graft occlusion is an important complication to detect after surgery, which often occurs within the first 24 hours.* Therefore nursing assessment is crucial.

Monitor the patency of the graft by checking the extremity every 15 minutes for the first hour and then hourly for changes in color, temperature, and pulse intensity. Warmth, redness, and edema of the affected extremity are often expected outcomes of surgery as a result of increased blood flow. Immediately postoperatively, the operating suite or postanesthesia care unit (PACU) nurse marks the site where the distal (dorsalis pedis or posterior tibial) pulse is best palpated or heard by Doppler ultrasonography. This information is communicated to the nursing staff on the critical care unit where the patient will be sent. "Hand-off" reporting is essential to promote safety and quality care.

Observe for report of pain, which may be one of the first indicators of postoperative graft occlusion. Many people experience a throbbing pain caused by the increased blood flow to the extremity. Because this sensation is different from ischemic pain, be sure to assess the type of pain that is experienced. Pain from occlusion may be masked by patient-controlled analgesia.

To promote graft patency, monitor the patient's blood pressure and notify the surgeon if the pressure increases or decreases beyond normal limits. Hypotension may indicate hypovolemia, which can increase the risk of clotting. Range of motion of the affected limb is usually limited, with bending of the hip and knee contraindicated. Consult with the surgeon on a case-by-case basis regarding limitations of movement, including turning. Patients are usually restricted to bedrest for at least 18 to 24 hours after surgery.

Coughing and deep breathing every 1 to 2 hours and using an incentive spirometer are essential. Patients who have undergone aortoiliac or aortofemoral bypass are allowed nothing by mouth (NPO) for at least 1 day after surgery. Those who have undergone bypass surgery of the lower extremities not involving the aorta or abdominal wall (femoropopliteal or femorotibial bypass) may remain NPO status until the first postoperative day, when they are allowed clear liquids.

If manifestations of graft occlusion occur, notify the surgeon immediately! Perfusion through the graft must be resolved promptly to avoid ischemic injury to the limb. Emergency **thrombectomy** (removal of the clot), which the surgeon may perform at the bedside, is the most common treatment for acute graft occlusion. Thrombectomy is associated with excellent results in prosthetic grafts. Results of thrombectomy in autogenous vein grafts are not as successful and often necessitate graft revision and even replacement.

Local intra-arterial thrombolytic (clot-dissolving) therapy with an agent such as tissue plasminogen activator (t-PA) or an infusion of a platelet inhibitor such as abciximab (ReoPro) may be used for acute graft occlusions. This therapy is provided in select settings in which health care providers are experts in its use. Other antiplatelet drugs such as the glycoprotein IIb/IIIa inhibitors *tirofiban (Aggrastat)* and *eptifibatide (Integrilin)* may be used as alternatives. The physician considers these therapies when the surgical alternative (e.g., thrombectomy with or without graft revision or replacement) carries high morbidity or mortality rates or when surgery for this type of occlusion has traditionally yielded poor results. Closely assess the patient for manifestations of bleeding if thrombolytics are used.

Compartment syndrome occurs when tissue pressure within a confined body space becomes elevated and restricts blood flow. The resulting ischemia can lead to tissue damage and eventually tissue death. Assess the motor and sensory function of the affected extremity. Assess for increasing pain, swelling, and tenseness. Report any of these symptoms to the health care provider immediately.

Graft or wound infections can be life threatening and can endanger the patient's limb. Use sterile technique when in contact with the incision, and observe for symptoms of infection at or around the graft and incision sites. Assess the area for induration, erythema, tenderness, warmth, edema, or drainage. Also monitor for fever and leukocytosis (increased serum white blood cell count). Notify the surgeon if any of these symptoms occur.

Community-Based Care

Peripheral arterial disease (PAD) is a chronic, long-term problem with frequent complications. Patients may benefit from a case manager who can follow them across the continuum of care. The desired outcome is that the patient can be maintained in the home.

Management at home often requires an interdisciplinary team approach, including several home care visits. Chart 38-4 outlines the assessment highlights for home care patients with peripheral vascular disease (PVD).

Instruct patients on methods to promote vasodilation. Teach them to avoid raising their legs above the level of the heart unless venous stasis is also present. Provide written and oral instructions on foot care and methods to prevent injury and ulcer development (Chart 38-5).

Patients who have had surgery require additional instruction on incision care (see Chapter 18). Encourage all patients to avoid smoking and to limit dietary fat intake to less than 30% of the total daily calories. Remind them to drink adequate fluids to prevent dehydration.

Patients with chronic arterial obstruction may fear recurrent occlusion or further narrowing of the artery. They often fear that they might lose a limb or become debilitated in other

Chart 38-4 HOME CARE ASSESSMENT

The Patient with Peripheral Vascular Disease

Assess tissue perfusion to affected extremity(ies), including:
- Distal circulation, sensation, and motion
- Presence of pain, pallor, paresthesias, pulselessness, paralysis, poikilothermia (coolness)
- Ankle-brachial index

Assess adherence to therapeutic regimen, including:
- Following foot care instructions
- Quitting smoking
- Maintaining dietary restrictions
- Participating in exercise regimen
- Avoiding exposure to cold and constrictive clothing

Assess ability to manage wound care and prevent further injury, including:
- Use of compression stockings or compression pumps as directed
- Use of various dressing materials
- Signs and symptoms to report to nurse

Assess coping ability of patient and family members.

Assess home environment, including:
- Safety hazards, especially related to falls

Chart 38-5 PATIENT AND FAMILY EDUCATION GUIDE

Foot Care for the Patient with Peripheral Vascular Disease

- Keep your feet clean by washing them with a mild soap in room-temperature water.
- Keep your feet dry, especially the ankles and between the toes.
- Avoid injury to your feet and ankles. Wear comfortable, well-fitting shoes. Never go without shoes.
- Keep your toenails clean and filed. Have someone cut them if you cannot see them clearly. Cut your toenails straight across.
- To prevent dry, cracked skin, apply a lubricating lotion to your feet.
- Prevent exposure to extreme heat or cold. Never use a heating pad on your feet.
- Avoid constricting garments.
- If a problem develops, see a podiatrist or physician.
- Avoid extended pressure on your feet or ankles, such as occurs when you lean against something.

ways. Indeed, chronic PAD may worsen, especially in those with diabetes mellitus. Reassure them that participation in prescribed exercise, nutrition therapy, and drug therapy, along with cessation of smoking, can limit further formation of atherosclerotic plaques.

Patients with arterial compromise may need assistance with ADLs if activity is limited by pain. They may need to limit or avoid stair climbing, depending on the severity of disease. Patients who have undergone surgery or need to limit activity usually need temporary help with daily activities by the family or other caregiver.

Patients who must limit activity because of PAD may benefit from the assistance of a home care aide. Those who have undergone surgery may require a home care nurse to assist with incision care. In collaboration with the case manager, arrange for home care resources before discharge.

ACUTE PERIPHERAL ARTERIAL OCCLUSION

Pathophysiology

Although chronic peripheral arterial disease (PAD) progresses slowly, the onset of **acute arterial occlusions** may be sudden and dramatic. An **embolus** (piece of clot that travels and lodges in a new area) is the most common cause of peripheral occlusions, although a local thrombus may be the cause. Occlusion may affect the upper extremities but it is more common in the lower extremities. Emboli originating from the heart are the most common cause of acute arterial occlusions. Most patients with an embolic occlusion have had an acute myocardial infarction (MI) and/or atrial fibrillation within the previous weeks.

Patient-Centered Collaborative Care

Patients with an acute arterial occlusion describe severe pain below the level of the occlusion that occurs even at rest. The affected extremity is cool or cold, pulseless, and mottled. Small areas on the toes may be blackened or gangrenous. *Those with acute arterial insufficiency often present with the "six P's" of ischemia:*

- *Pain*
- *Pallor*
- *Pulselessness*
- *Paresthesia*
- *Paralysis*
- *Poikilothermia (coolness)*

The health care provider must initiate treatment promptly to avoid permanent damage or loss of an extremity. Anticoagulant therapy with unfractionated heparin (UFH, Hepalean♣) is usually the first intervention to prevent further clot formation. A bolus of up to 10,000 units may be prescribed. The patient may undergo angiography.

A surgical *thrombectomy* or *embolectomy* with local anesthesia may be performed to remove the occlusion. The physician makes an incision, which is followed by an **arteriotomy** (a surgical opening into an artery). The physician then inserts a catheter into the artery and retrieves the embolus. It may be necessary to close the artery with a patch graft.

Postoperatively, monitor the affected extremity for improvement in color, temperature, and pulse and monitor other extremities for manifestations of new thrombi or emboli. Pain should significantly diminish after the surgical procedure, although mild incisional pain remains. Watch closely for complications caused by reperfusing the artery after thrombectomy or embolectomy, which include spasms and swelling of the skeletal muscles. Swelling of the skeletal muscles can result in compartment syndrome, which causes edema, pain on passive movement, poor capillary refill, numbness, and muscle tenseness. **Fasciotomy** (surgical opening into the tissues) may be necessary to prevent further injury and save the limb.

The use of systemic thrombolytic therapy for acute arterial occlusions has been disappointing because bleeding complications may outweigh the benefits obtained. Local intra-arterial thrombolytic therapy with alteplase (Activase) or t-PA and the use of platelet inhibitors, such as abciximab (ReoPro), have emerged as alternatives to surgical treatment in selected settings. *When thrombolytics are given, monitor for manifestations of bleeding, bruising, or hematoma.* When a patient receives any platelet inhibitor, platelet counts need to be monitored for the first 3, 6, and 12 hours after the start of the infusion. *If the platelet count decreases to below 100,000/mm³, the abciximab infusion needs to be readjusted or discontinued. If any of these complications occur, notify the physician immediately.*

ANEURYSMS OF CENTRAL ARTERIES

Pathophysiology

An **aneurysm** is a permanent localized dilation of an artery, which enlarges the artery to at least two times its normal diameter. It may be described as *fusiform* (a diffuse dilation affecting the entire circumference of the artery) or *saccular* (an outpouching affecting only a distinct portion of the artery). Aneurysms may also be described as *true* or *false.* In true aneurysms, the arterial wall is weakened by congenital or acquired problems. False aneurysms occur as a result of vessel injury or trauma to all three layers of the arterial wall.

Dissecting hematomas, traditionally called *dissecting aneurysms,* are more accurately described as *aortic dissections* (see the later discussion on p. 814). They differ from aneurysms in that they are formed when blood accumulates in the wall of an artery.

Aneurysms tend to occur at specific anatomic sites (Fig. 38-6), most commonly in the abdominal aorta. They often occur at a point where the artery is not supported by skeletal muscles or on the lines of curves or flexion in the arterial tree.

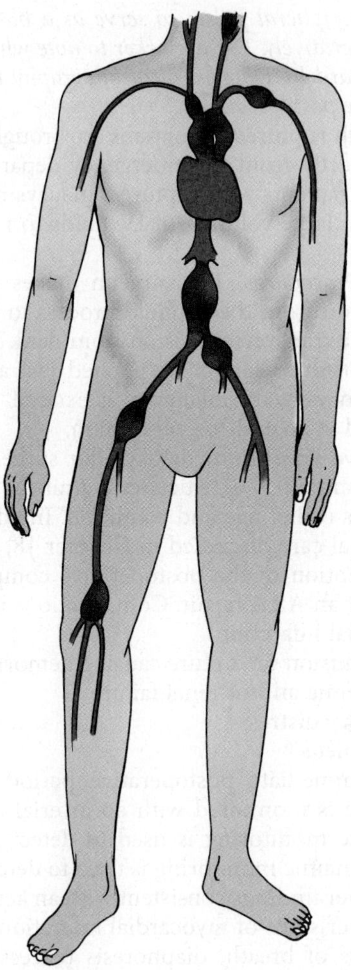

Fig. 38-6 • Common anatomic sites of arterial aneurysms.

An aneurysm forms when the middle layer (media) of the artery is weakened, producing a stretching effect in the inner layer (intima) and outer layers of the artery. As the artery widens, tension in the wall increases and further widening occurs, thus enlarging the aneurysm. Hypertension (high blood pressure) produces more tension and enlargement within the artery. As the aneurysm grows, the risk of arterial rupture increases. When *dissecting* aneurysms occur, the aneurysm enlarges, blood is lost, and blood flow to organs is diminished.

ANIMATION: Abdominal Aortic Aneurysm ▶

Abdominal aortic aneurysms (AAAs) account for most aneurysms and are commonly asymptomatic. Most of these are located between the renal arteries and the aortic bifurcation. Of all AAAs greater than 6 cm in diameter, about half rupture within 1 year.

Thoracic aortic aneurysms (TAAs) are not quite as common and are frequently misdiagnosed. They are typically discovered when advanced imaging is used to assess other conditions. TAAs commonly develop between the origin of the left subclavian artery and the diaphragm. They are located in the descending, ascending, and transverse sections of the aorta. They can also occur in the aortic arch and are very difficult to manage surgically.

Aneurysms can cause symptoms by exerting pressure on surrounding structures or by rupturing. *Rupture is the most frequent complication and is life threatening because abrupt and massive hemorrhagic shock results.* Thrombi within the wall of an aneurysm can also be the source of emboli in distal arteries below the aneurysm.

Atherosclerosis is the most common cause of aneurysms, with hypertension, hyperlipidemia, and cigarette smoking being contributing factors. Family history may also play a role. Syphilis (a sexually transmitted disease), Marfan syndrome (a connective tissue disease), and Ehlers-Danlos syndrome (a rare genetic disorder) are other causes of AAAs. Chronic inflammation (aortitis) and blunt trauma, usually from motor vehicle crashes, can cause aneurysms in the descending thoracic aorta (Irwin, 2007).

About 15,000 people in the United States die each year of abdominal aneurysms (Irwin, 2007). Thoracic aortic aneurysms occur most often in older adults and have a high mortality rate even with surgical intervention. AAAs are more common in men than in women, but the reason is unknown.

Patient-Centered Collaborative Care

Assessment

Most patients with abdominal or thoracic aneurysms are asymptomatic when their aneurysms are first discovered by routine examination or during imaging study performed for another reason. However, a few patients do have symptoms that bring them to their health care provider or the emergency department.

Physical Assessment/Clinical Manifestations

Because there may be symptoms, assess patients with a known or suspected *abdominal aortic aneurysm (AAA)* for abdominal, flank, or back pain. Pain is usually described as steady with a gnawing quality, unaffected by movement, and lasting for hours or days.

A pulsation in the upper abdomen slightly to the left of the midline between the xyphoid process and the umbilicus may be present. A detectable aneurysm is at least 5 cm in diameter. *Auscultate for a bruit over the mass, but avoid palpating the mass because it may be tender and there is a risk of rupture!* If expansion and impending rupture of an AAA are suspected, assess for severe pain of sudden onset in the back or lower abdomen, which may radiate to the groin, buttocks, or legs.

Patients with a rupturing AAA are critically ill and in hemorrhagic (hypovolemic) shock. Signs include hypotension, diaphoresis, decreased level of consciousness, oliguria (scant urine output), loss of pulses distal to the rupture, and dysrhythmias. Retroperitoneal hemorrhage is manifested by hematomas in the flanks (lower back). Rupture into the abdominal cavity causes abdominal distention.

When a *thoracic aortic aneurysm* is suspected, assess for back pain and manifestations of compression of the aneurysm on adjacent structures. Signs include shortness of breath, hoarseness, and difficulty swallowing. TAAs are not often detected by physical assessment, but occasionally a mass may be visible above the suprasternal notch. Assess the patient with suspected rupture of a thoracic aneurysm for sudden and excruciating back or chest pain. Hypovolemic shock also occurs with TAA (see Chapter 39).

Imaging Assessment

An abdominal x-ray or a lateral x-ray of the spine often shows an AAA. The "eggshell" appearance of the aneurysm supports the diagnosis.

Computed tomography (CT) scanning is the standard tool for assessing the size and location of an abdominal or thoracic aneurysm. A thoracic aneurysm can be diagnosed by chest x-ray. Aortic arteriography is usually performed for patients who are to undergo surgical repair of a thoracic aneurysm. Ultrasonography is a noninvasive technique that provides an accurate diagnosis, as well as information about the size and location of an AAA.

Interventions

The size of the aneurysm and the presence of symptoms determine patient management.

Nonsurgical Management

The goal of nonsurgical management is to monitor the growth of the aneurysm and maintain the blood pressure at a normal level to decrease the risk of rupture.

Because elevated blood pressure can increase the rate of aneurysmal enlargement, hypertension is an important risk factor for rupture. Patients with hypertension are treated with antihypertensive drugs to decrease the rate of enlargement and the risk for early rupture.

For those with small or asymptomatic aneurysms, frequent ultrasound or CT scans are necessary to monitor the growth of the aneurysm. Emphasize the importance of following through with scheduled tests to monitor the growth. Also explain the clinical manifestations of aneurysms that need to be promptly reported.

Surgical Management

Surgical management of an aneurysm may be an elective or an emergency procedure. *For patients with a rupturing abdominal aortic or a thoracic aneurysm, emergency surgery is performed.*

Patients with TAAs measuring 2.8 inches (7 cm) or more in diameter and those with smaller aneurysms that are producing symptoms are advised to have elective surgery. Those with smaller aneurysms that are not causing symptoms are treated nonsurgically until symptoms occur or the aneurysm enlarges.

The most common surgical procedure for AAA has traditionally been a resection or repair **(aneurysmectomy)**. However, the mortality rate for elective resection is high and markedly increases for emergency surgery.

Endothelial stent grafts have improved mortality rates and shortened the hospital stay for select patients who need AAA repair. The stents (wirelike devices) are inserted percutaneously (through the skin), avoiding abdominal incisions and therefore decreasing the risk of a prolonged postoperative recovery. Postoperative care is similar to care required after an arteriogram (angiogram).

Abdominal Aortic Aneurysm Resection. In an AAA resection, the physician excises (cuts out) the aneurysm from the abdominal aorta to prevent or repair the rupture. The goal is to secure stable aortic integrity and tissue perfusion throughout the body.

Preoperative Care. Preoperative care is similar to that for patients undergoing any surgery with general anesthesia (see Chapter 16). A bowel preparation and emphasis on coughing and deep breathing are very important. Because significant blood loss may occur during AAA resection, patients planning elective surgery may be advised to bank their blood for autologous (self) transfusions during and after surgery.

Assess all peripheral pulses to serve as a baseline for comparison postoperatively. Use a marker to note where the pulse is palpated or heard by Doppler ultrasonography to facilitate locating the pulse postoperatively.

Patients with ruptured aneurysms are brought to the operating suite directly from the emergency department. Preoperative care of patients with ruptured aneurysms involves administration of large volumes of IV fluids to maintain tissue perfusion.

Operative Procedures. The surgeon makes a midline abdominal incision from the xyphoid process to the symphysis pubis or a wide transverse incision from flank to flank to expose the aneurysm. Clamps are applied just above and just below the aneurysm, the aneurysm is excised, and a Dacron graft is sutured in an end-to-end fashion.

Postoperative Care. Immediately after surgery, the patient is typically admitted to a critical care unit for 24 hours, depending on his or her age and condition. In addition to providing the usual care discussed in Chapter 18, assess for and assist in prevention of the postoperative complications that can occur after an AAA repair. Complications include:

- Myocardial infarction
- Graft occlusion or rupture causing hemorrhage
- Hypovolemia and/or renal failure
- Respiratory distress
- Paralytic ileus

During the immediate postoperative period, the patient's blood pressure is monitored with an arterial catheter. Continuous cardiac monitoring is used to detect any dysrhythmias. Hemodynamic monitoring is used to detect low cardiac output and other findings consistent with an acute *myocardial infarction*. Other signs of myocardial infarction include chest pain, shortness of breath, diaphoresis (excessive sweating), anxiety, and restlessness.

A major priority for nursing care is to assess for signs of graft occlusion or rupture. Assess vital signs and circulation every 15 minutes for the first hour and then hourly, with assessment of pulses distal to the graft site (including the posterior tibial and dorsalis pedis pulses). Report signs of *graft occlusion or rupture*, including:

- Changes in pulses
- Cool to cold extremities below the graft
- White or blue extremities or flanks
- Severe pain
- Abdominal distention
- Decreased urine output

Limit elevation of the head of the bed to 45 degrees or less to avoid flexion of the graft.

Hypovolemia and renal failure may occur because of blood loss during surgery or before if rupture occurred. Assess urine output via a Foley catheter hourly. If urine output is less than 50 mL/hr, notify the surgeon. Although advances in surgical technique have decreased the risk of renal failure after clamping during surgery, renal failure may occur. Renal failure caused by acute tubular necrosis (ATN) is more common after emergency surgery. In addition to monitoring urine output, in collaboration with the physician, monitor serum creatinine and blood urea nitrogen (BUN) levels daily.

Assess respiratory rate and depth every hour and auscultate breath sounds every 4 hours to monitor for *respiratory complications*. The patient may be mechanically ventilated. However, early extubation is preferred if he or she is stable. Administer opioids for pain as prescribed. If the patient remains intubated, turn and suction him or her as needed. Teach him or her to use firm abdominal support of the incision with a pillow or bath blanket during coughing exercises. After extubation, assist the patient to a bedside chair within 24 hours. Early mobility decreases the risk of atelectasis and deep vein thrombosis.

Paralytic ileus after AAA repair is expected for 2 to 3 days. Patients usually have a nasogastric tube set to low suction until they begin to pass flatus. Listen for bowel sounds every 8 hours, and report their return and reports of flatus to the physician. Some surgeons begin to introduce fluids or soft food to stimulate peristalsis. Prolonged absence of flatus and presence of abdominal distention may indicate a paralytic ileus or a bowel infarction.

Thoracic Aortic Aneurysm Repair. Repair of thoracic aneurysms is tailored to each patient. The procedure depends on the type and location of the aneurysm. Total cardiopulmonary bypass (CPB) is necessary for excision of aneurysms in the ascending aorta, and partial bypass is often used during excision of aneurysms in the descending aorta.

The care of the patient undergoing thoracic aneurysm resection is similar to that for the patient having thoracic surgery. Chapter 34 describes thoracic surgery in detail.

The surgeon uses either a thoracotomy or a median sternotomy approach to enter the thoracic cavity. A Dacron graft or prosthesis is sewn onto the aorta in place of the excised TAA. Saccular aneurysms, which have an outpouching from a distinct portion of the arterial wall, can sometimes be removed without aortic resection. Newer procedures do not remove the aneurysm. Instead, the surgeon cuts into the aneurysm and inserts a graft. The walls of the aneurysm are wrapped around the graft for stability.

The care of a patient who has undergone TAA repair is similar to that for other chest surgeries. Patients who have undergone CPB receive care similar to that described in Chapter 40. Assess for and assist in the prevention of postoperative complications that can occur after a thoracic aneurysm repair. Complications include:

- Hemorrhage
- Ischemic colitis
- Cerebral and spinal cord ischemia (causing paraplegia)
- Respiratory distress
- Infection
- Cardiac dysrhythmias

Assess vital signs at least hourly, reporting any signs of hemorrhage (e.g., a decrease in blood pressure, an increase in pulse rate, rapid respirations, diaphoresis) to the physician immediately. Assess for bleeding or separation at the graft site by noting significant increases in chest drainage from the chest tubes.

Accidental interruption of the blood supply to the spinal cord during thoracic aneurysm repair can result in paraplegia. Assess the patient hourly for sensation and motion in all extremities, and report changes immediately!

After TAA repair, patients are especially likely to develop *respiratory distress* from atelectasis or pneumonia. This problem occurs as a result of both CPB and incisional discomfort. Both atelectasis and pneumonia may cause shallow breathing and poor cough effort. These patients are often mechanically ventilated at least overnight after surgery.

Hospital-acquired infection is a major concern for any vascular surgery. The patient usually receives IV antibiotics and may be discharged to home to continue oral antibiotic therapy. The Joint Commission (TJC) and other groups have placed a major emphasis on preventing infection while patients are in the hospital.

Assess all patients recovering from TAA repair for cardiac *dysrhythmias.* The stress of the thoracic surgery, added to the increased incidence of arteriosclerosis in this group, may predispose patients to a myocardial infarction, cardiac dysrhythmias, or heart failure.

Endovascular Repair of Abdominal Aortic Aneurysms. The repair of AAAs with **endovascular stent grafts** is an alternative for some patients. Those selected for endovascular repair of AAAs are generally at high risk for major abdominal surgery. Some patients may be referred for endovascular repair before the aneurysm reaches the recommended diameter for elective surgery.

Different designs of endovascular stent grafts are used, depending on the anatomic involvement of the aneurysm. The stent graft is flexible with either Dacron or polytetrafluoroethylene (PTFE) material. It is inserted through a skin incision into the femoral artery by way of a catheter-based system. The catheter is advanced to a level above the aneurysm away from the renal arteries. The graft is released from the catheter, and the stent graft is placed with a series of hooks. This procedure is done in collaboration with the vascular surgeon, interventional radiologist, operating room team, and, at some centers, vascular medicine physician.

The endovascular repair of AAAs has decreased the length of hospital stay for patients requiring repair of abdominal aneurysms. However, the patient needs to be closely monitored, in the hospital and at home, for the development of complications after the procedure. Expert nursing care is required to allow for early identification of problems, and complications require timely surgical intervention. In addition, coordination and collaboration with the health care team are required for discharge planning and follow-up care for patients at home.

Complications for stent repair include:

- Conversion to open surgical repair
- Bleeding
- Aneurysm rupture
- Peripheral embolization
- Misplacement of the stent graft

NCLEX EXAMINATION CHALLENGE

When assessing a client who just returned from an abdominal aortic aneurysm repair, which assessment finding requires immediate intervention?

A. Absent bowel sounds in all quadrants
B. Blood pressure of 104/72 and pulse of 96
C. Urine output of 60 mL/hr
D. Severe abdominal pain and distention

evolve For the correct answer, go to http://evolve.elsevier.com/Iggy/.

Community-Based Care

Most patients are discharged to home after aneurysm repair. However, in the absence of family or other support systems, the postoperative patient may be discharged to a transitional care or long-term care facility for rehabilitation.

If discharged to home, the patient must follow instructions regarding activity level and incisional care. Because stair climbing may be restricted initially, he or she may need a bedside commode if the bathroom is inaccessible.

For patients who have not undergone surgical aneurysm repair, the teaching plan emphasizes the importance of compliance with the schedule of CT scanning to monitor the size of the aneurysm. *Teach patients receiving treatment for hypertension about the importance of continuing to take prescribed drugs. Instruct them about the signs and symptoms that must promptly be reported to the health care provider, which include:*

- *Abdominal fullness or pain or back pain*
- *Chest or back pain, shortness of breath, difficulty swallowing, or hoarseness*

Teach the patient who has undergone surgical repair about activity restrictions, wound care, and pain management. Patients may not engage in activities that involve lifting heavy objects (usually more than 15 to 20 pounds [6.8 to 9.1 kg]) for 6 to 12 weeks postoperatively. Advise them to use caution for activities that involve pulling, pushing, or straining. Those who usually engage in vigorous activities should discuss them with their health care provider. Most patients are restricted from driving a car for several weeks after discharge.

In collaboration with the case manager or social worker, assess the availability of transportation to and from appointments for patients needing CT monitoring. Those who have undergone surgery may require the services of a home care nurse for initial assistance with dressing changes. A home care aide may be needed to assist with ADLs, depending on the patient's support system.

ANEURYSMS OF THE PERIPHERAL ARTERIES

Although femoral and popliteal aneurysms are not common, they are often associated with an aneurysm in another location of the arterial tree (see Fig. 38-6). To detect a popliteal aneurysm, a pulsating mass is seen in the popliteal space. To detect a femoral aneurysm, observe a pulsatile mass over the femoral artery. Both extremities are evaluated because more than one femoral or popliteal aneurysm may be present.

The patient may have symptoms of limb ischemia (decreased blood flow), including diminished or absent pulses, cool to cold skin, and pain. Pain also may be present if an adjacent nerve is compressed. The recommended treatment for either type of aneurysm, regardless of the size, is surgery because of the risk of thromboembolic complications.

To treat a femoral aneurysm, the surgeon removes the aneurysm and restores circulation using a Dacron graft or an autogenous saphenous vein graft. Most surgeons prefer to bypass rather than resect a popliteal aneurysm.

After surgery, monitor for lower limb ischemia. Palpate pulses below the graft to assess graft patency. Often, Doppler ultrasonography is necessary to assess blood flow when pulses are not palpable. *Report sudden development of pain or discoloration of the extremity immediately to the physician because it may indicate graft occlusion.*

AORTIC DISSECTION

Pathophysiology

Aortic dissection has traditionally been referred to as a *dissecting aneurysm.* However, because this condition is more accurately described as a *dissecting hematoma,* the term *aortic dissection* is more commonly used.

Aortic dissection is thought to be caused by a sudden tear in the aortic intima, opening the way for blood to enter the aortic wall. Degeneration of the aortic media may be the primary cause for this condition, with hypertension being an important contributing factor.

Aortic dissection is not common but is a life-threatening problem. It is often associated with connective tissue disorders such as Marfan syndrome. It occurs also in older people, peaking in adults in their 50s and 60s. Men are more commonly affected than women (Scheetz, 2006).

Because the circulation of any major artery arising from the aorta can be impaired in patients with aortic dissection, this condition is highly lethal and represents an emergency situation. Although the ascending aorta and descending thoracic aorta are the most common sites, dissections can also occur in the abdominal aorta and other arteries.

Patient-Centered Collaborative Care

Assessment

The most common symptom is pain. It is described as "tearing," "ripping," and "stabbing" and tends to move from its point of origin. Depending on the site of dissection, the patient may feel pain in the anterior chest, back, neck, throat, jaw, or teeth.

Diaphoresis (excessive sweating), nausea, vomiting, faintness, and apprehension are also common. Blood pressure is usually elevated unless complications such as cardiac tamponade or rupture have occurred. In these cases, the patient becomes rapidly hypotensive. A decrease or absence of peripheral pulses is common, as is aortic regurgitation, which is characterized by a musical murmur better heard along the right sternal border. Neurologic deficits such as an altered level of consciousness, paraparesis, and strokes also can occur.

Chest x-ray, computed tomography (CT), magnetic resonance imaging (MRI), and aortic angiography may be used to confirm the diagnosis. However, MRI scanning is very time-consuming and may not be the test of choice. Transthoracic echocardiography (TTE) or transesophageal echocardiography (TEE) may be performed at the bedside for patients who cannot be moved (Scheetz, 2006).

Interventions: Emergency Care

The expected outcomes for emergency care are:

- Elimination of pain
- Reduction of systolic blood pressure to 100 to 120 mm Hg
- Decrease in the velocity of left ventricular ejection

The physician prescribes IV sodium nitroprusside (Nitropress, Nipride) or fenoldopam (Corlopam) by continuous drip initially to lower the blood pressure. If this regimen is not effective, nicardipine hydrochloride (Cardene) may be used.

Subsequent treatment depends on the location of the dissection. Patients receive continued medical treatment for uncomplicated distal dissections and surgical treatment for proximal dissections. For those receiving long-term medical treatment, the systolic blood pressure must be maintained at or below 130 to 140 mm Hg. Beta blockers (e.g., propranolol) and calcium channel antagonists (amlodipine) are indicated.

Patients receiving surgical intervention for a proximal dissection always require cardiopulmonary bypass (CPB) (see Chapter 40). The surgeon removes the intimal tear and sutures edges of the dissected aorta. Usually, a prosthetic graft is used.

BUERGER'S DISEASE

Pathophysiology

Buerger's disease (thromboangiitis obliterans) is an uncommon occlusive disease limited to the medium and small arteries and veins. The distal upper and lower limbs are the most frequently affected. Typically, Buerger's disease is identified in young adult men who smoke. Larger arteries such as the femoral and brachial become involved in the late stages of the disease. The veins are less commonly involved.

The disease often extends into the tissues around the vessels, resulting in fibrosis and scarring that bind the artery, vein, and nerve firmly together. Cessation of cigarette smoking usually arrests the disease process. Continued smoking causes occlusion in the more proximal vessels.

The cause of Buerger's disease is unknown although there is a strong association with tobacco smoking. A familial or genetic predisposition and autoimmune etiologic factors are also possible.

Patient-Centered Collaborative Care

Assessment

The first clinical manifestation of Buerger's disease is usually **claudication** (muscle pain caused by an inadequate blood supply) of the arch of the foot. Intermittent claudication may occur in the lower extremities. The pain may be ischemic, occurring in the digits while the patient is at rest. Often there is an aching pain that is more severe at night. Intermittent shocklike pain can be the result of ischemic neuropathy. Patients often have increased sensitivity to cold and report coldness and numbness. On physical examination, pulses are often diminished in the distal extremities and the extremities are cool and red or cyanotic in the dependent position.

A diagnosis of Buerger's disease is based on a physical finding of peripheral ischemia. Ulcerations and gangrene may be seen in the digits. The ulcerations are usually sharply demarcated. The gangrenous lesion can be small or can affect the entire digit.

Arteriograms can be useful in delineating the degree of disease in the arteries. Commonly, arteriography reveals multiple segmental occlusions in the smaller arteries of the forearm, hand, leg, and foot. Plethysmographic studies of the fingers or toes may be diagnostic of the disease in the early stages. These studies can also be useful in following the progression of the disease in more proximal arteries (see Chapter 35 for discussion of these tests).

Interventions

Nursing interventions are directed at:

- Preventing the progression of the disease
- Avoiding vasoconstriction
- Promoting vasodilation
- Relieving pain
- Managing ulceration and gangrene

To prevent the progression of Buerger's disease, complete abstinence from tobacco in all forms is essential. Teach the patient to avoid extreme cold or prolonged exposure to cold to prevent vasoconstriction. Instruct him or her about drugs that may be used for vasodilation (e.g., nifedipine [Procardia]). The treatment for Buerger's disease is similar to that for peripheral arterial disease (PAD) (see the discussion of Interventions on p. 807 in the Peripheral Arterial Disease section).

SUBCLAVIAN STEAL

Subclavian steal occurs in the upper extremities as a result of a subclavian artery occlusion or stenosis. The result is altered blood flow and ischemia in the arm. Subclavian steal can occur in people at any age but is more common in those with risk factors for atherosclerosis. Symptoms include tiredness in the arm with exertion, paresthesias, dizziness, and exercise-induced pain in the forearms when the arms are elevated.

Physical assessment usually reveals a significant difference in the blood pressures between the arms. A difference greater than 20 mm Hg is considered significant. Another important finding is a subclavian bruit, which can occur on the affected side. The subclavian pulse may be decreased on the occluded side compared with the opposite side. The affected arm may also be discolored or cyanotic. However, this finding generally occurs only in severe cases.

Surgery is the recommended intervention for cyanosis or pain. One of three procedures may be used: endarterectomy of the subclavian artery, carotid-subclavian bypass, or dilation of the subclavian artery with placement of a vascular stent.

Postoperative nursing care of the patient includes monitoring of the arterial flow in the affected arm. Check brachial and radial pulses frequently, and observe for ischemic changes. Observe the arm for edema, redness, or any other signs.

THORACIC OUTLET SYNDROME

Thoracic outlet syndrome is a compression of the subclavian artery at the thoracic outlet by anatomic structures such as a rib or muscle. The arterial wall may be damaged, producing thrombosis or embolization to distal arteries of the arms. The three common sites of compression in the thoracic outlet are:

- The interscalene triangle
- Between the coracoid process of the scapula and the pectoralis minor tendon
- Most common, the costoclavicular space

Thoracic outlet syndrome is more common in women and in those whose occupations require holding their arms up or leaning over, such as baseball players, golfers, and swimmers. It is also seen in people who have had trauma (e.g., whiplash) or clavicular fracture. Patients generally report neck, shoulder, and arm pain that may be intermittent. They may also have numbness and moderate edema of the extremity. The pain and numbness are worse when the arm is placed in certain positions such as over the head or out to the side. Some patients may have overdeveloped neck and shoulder muscles, and the affected arm may appear cyanotic.

Collaborative care includes physical therapy, exercises, and avoiding aggravating positions such as elevating the arms. Surgical management involves resection of the anatomic structure that is compressing the artery. It is performed only if a patient has severe pain, has lost hand function, or is responding poorly to conservative treatment.

RAYNAUD'S PHENOMENON

Pathophysiology

Raynaud's phenomenon is caused by vasospasm of the arterioles and arteries of the upper and lower extremities, usually unilaterally. *Raynaud's disease* occurs bilaterally. The two terms are sometimes used interchangeably. Although they are related, there are some differences. Raynaud's phenomenon usually occurs in people older than 30 years. Raynaud's disease can occur between the ages of 17 and 50 years. Raynaud's phenomenon can occur in either gender, but Raynaud's disease is more common in women.

The pathophysiology is the same for both entities. The etiology is unknown. Patients often have an associated systemic connective tissue disease such as systemic lupus erythematosus or progressive systemic sclerosis (see Chapter 20).

As a result of vasospasm, the superficial skin vessels are constricted and blanching of the extremity occurs, followed by cyanosis. When the vasospasm is relieved, the tissue becomes reddened or hyperemic (Fig. 38-7). The patient's extremities are numb and cold, and he or she may report pain and swelling. Ulcers may also be present. These attacks are intermittent and can be aggravated by cold or stress. In severe cases, the attack lasts longer and gangrene of the digits can occur.

Patient-Centered Collaborative Care

Management involves relieving or preventing the vasoconstriction by drug therapy. Commonly prescribed drugs are nifedipine (Procardia), cyclandelate (Cyclospasmol), and phenoxybenzamine (Dibenzyline). These vasodilating agents may help relieve the symptoms, but they can cause uncomfortable side effects such as facial flushing, headaches, hypotension, and dizziness.

For severe symptoms that are not reduced by drugs, a lumbar sympathectomy may be performed. The surgeon cuts the sympathetic nerve fibers that cause vasoconstriction of blood vessels in the legs. This method is effective for foot symptoms. For the upper extremities, a similar procedure—sympathetic ganglionectomy—may provide symptom relief. The long-term effectiveness of these treatments is questionable.

Patient education is important in prevention of complications. Explain methods to prevent vasoconstriction, such as minimizing exposure to cold, reducing caffeine intake, smoking cessation (if the patient smokes), and decreasing stress. *Teach the patient to wear warm clothes, socks, and gloves when exposed to cool or cold temperatures. He or she should keep the home at a comfortably warm temperature and wear gloves to the grocery store.* Help the patient identify stressors, and provide suggestions for reducing them. (See Chapter 20 for further discussion of Raynaud's disease as it relates to connective tissue disease.)

POPLITEAL ENTRAPMENT

Popliteal entrapment causes ischemic symptoms in the affected leg or foot because of anatomic compression of the popliteal artery. It occurs in young people, most often in men. Patients report intermittent claudication (muscle pain caused by decreased blood flow) of one or both legs.

Physical examination may reveal ischemic changes of the affected leg with normal function of the unaffected limb. When the patient is at rest, the nurse may note diminished distal pulses, although this is a rare finding. Diagnosis of popliteal entrapment is possible only after an accurate history, physical examination, and arteriography.

The recommended management is surgical repair of the anatomic compression. Reconstruction of the popliteal artery may be necessary to restore arterial blood flow to the limb. Nursing care involves preventing complications and evaluating the patency of the graft or artery after surgery. Observe for ischemic changes and evaluate distal pulses at least every hour initially and then every 4 hours. Follow agency or physician protocol for specific requests based on the patient's needs.

PERIPHERAL VENOUS DISEASE

To function properly, veins must be patent (open) with competent valves. Vein function also requires the assistance of the surrounding muscle beds to help pump blood toward the heart. If one or more veins are not operating properly, they become distended and clinical manifestations occur.

Three distinct problems alter the blood flow in veins:

- Thrombus formation *(venous thrombosis)* can lead to pulmonary embolism (PE), a life-threatening complication. **Venous thromboembolism (VTE)** is the current term that includes both deep vein thrombosis and PE.
- Defective valves lead to *venous insufficiency* and *varicose veins,* which are not life threatening but are problematic.
- Skeletal muscle lacks contractility.

VENOUS THROMBOEMBOLISM

Pathophysiology

Venous thromboembolism (VTE) is one of health care's greatest challenges and includes both thrombus and embolus complications. A **thrombus** (also called a *thrombosis*) is a blood

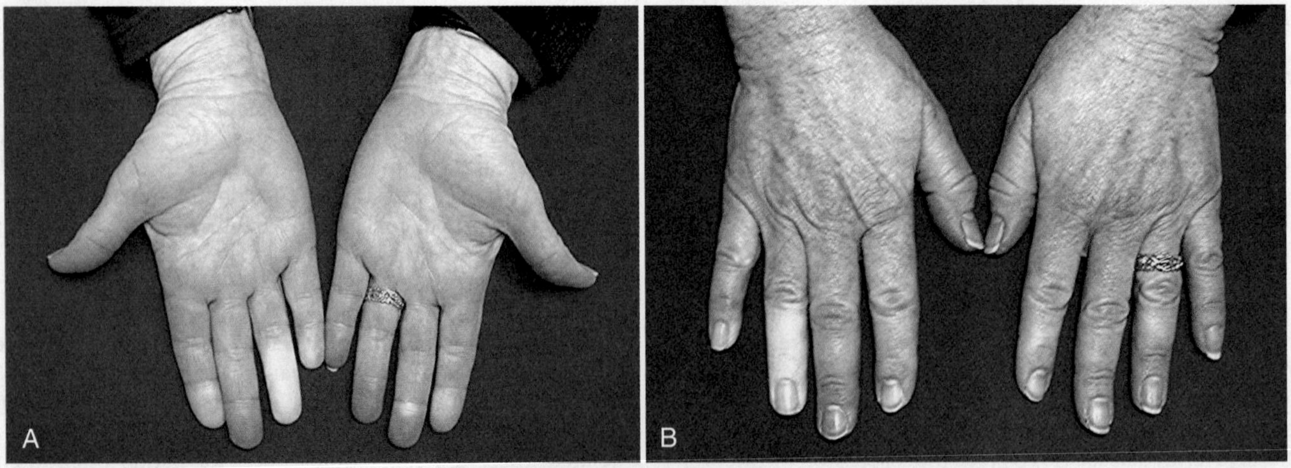
A
B

Fig. 38-7 • Color changes of Raynaud's syndrome.

clot believed to result from an endothelial injury, venous stasis, or hypercoagulability. The thrombosis may not be specifically attributable to one element, or it may involve all three elements. It is often associated with an inflammatory process. When a thrombus develops, inflammation occurs around the clot, thickening the vein wall and consequently possibly leading to embolization (the formation of an **embolus**).

Thrombophlebitis refers to a thrombus that is associated with inflammation. **Phlebothrombosis** is a thrombus without inflammation. Thrombophlebitis can occur in superficial veins. However, it most frequently occurs in the deep veins of the lower extremities.

Deep vein thrombophlebitis, commonly referred to as **deep vein thrombosis (DVT),** not only is most common but also is more serious than superficial thrombophlebitis because it presents a greater risk for pulmonary embolism (PE). In PE, a dislodged blood clot travels to the pulmonary artery. DVT develops most often in the legs but can occur also in the upper arms as a result of increased use of central venous devices.

Thrombus formation has been associated with stasis of blood flow, endothelial injury, and/or hypercoagulability, known as **Virchow's triad.** The precise cause of these events remains unknown. However, a few predisposing factors have been identified. Thrombosis has commonly occurred in people undergoing certain surgical procedures.

The highest incidence of clot formation occurs in patients who have undergone hip surgery, total knee replacement, or open prostate surgery. Other conditions that seem to promote thrombus formation are ulcerative colitis, heart failure, and immobility. Complications of immobility occur during prolonged bedrest such as when a patient is confined to bed for an extensive illness. People who sit for long periods (e.g., on an airplane) are also at risk for VTE.

Phlebitis (vein inflammation) associated with invasive procedures such as IV therapy can predispose patients to thrombosis. Severe infections, systemic lupus erythematosus, polycythemia vera, oral contraceptives, and trauma have also been linked to thrombosis. Cancer, especially adenocarcinoma of the visceral organs, is the most common malignancy associated with DVT. Cancer has been discovered in nearly all people with fatal PEs who did not have other predisposing factors.

Millions of people in the United States are affected by DVT each year, and many die from pulmonary embolism. The largest number of deaths occurs in older adults. African Americans have a high rate of death resulting from PE because of predisposing risk factors and coexisting diseases, such as certain cancers and chronic renal and cardiac failure.

Health Promotion and Maintenance

In the *community,* if a person has a history of VTE, these precautions should be taken:

- Avoid oral contraceptives.
- Drink adequate fluids to avoid dehydration.
- Exercise legs during long periods of bedrest or sitting.

In the *inpatient setting,* interventions to prevent VTE include:

- Patient education
- Leg exercises
- Early ambulation
- Adequate hydration
- Graduated compression stockings (not as commonly used today)
- Intermittent pneumatic compression, such as sequential compression devices (SCDs)
- Venous plexus foot pump

Patient-Centered Collaborative Care

Assessment

People with DVT may have symptoms or may be asymptomatic. *The classic signs and symptoms of DVT are calf or groin tenderness and pain and sudden onset of unilateral swelling of the leg.* Pain in the calf on dorsiflexion of the foot (positive Homans' sign) appears in only a small percentage of patients with DVT, and false-positive findings are common. *Therefore checking a Homans' sign is not advised!* Examine the area described as painful, comparing this site with the other limb. *Gently* palpate the site, observing for **induration** (hardening) along the blood vessel and for warmth and edema. Redness may also be present (Fig. 38-8).

Localized edema in one extremity may suggest thrombophlebitis. Some experts suggest to measure and compare right and left calf and thigh circumferences for changes over time as an indicator of DVT or venous insufficiency. However, serial leg measurements are not the most reliable indicator of DVT.

DVT can occur also in the arm from an indwelling IV catheter or from compression injuries to the arm or subclavian vein by a rib. Although diagnostic tests are available, physical examination findings are often adequate for diagnosis. If a definitive diagnosis is lacking from physical assessment findings alone, diagnostic tests (e.g., duplex ultrasonography, Doppler flow studies, impedance plethysmography) may be performed.

The preferred diagnostic test for DVT is *venous duplex ultrasonography,* a noninvasive test. *Doppler flow studies* may also be useful in the diagnosis, but they are more sensitive in detecting proximal rather than distal DVT. Normal venous circulation creates audible signals, whereas thrombosed veins produce little or no sound. The accuracy of the scanning depends on the technical skill of the health care professional performing the test. If the test is negative but a DVT is still suspected, a venogram may be needed to make an accurate diagnosis. However, venograms are not performed frequently today because of complications from the contrast medium, including sensitivity and acute renal failure.

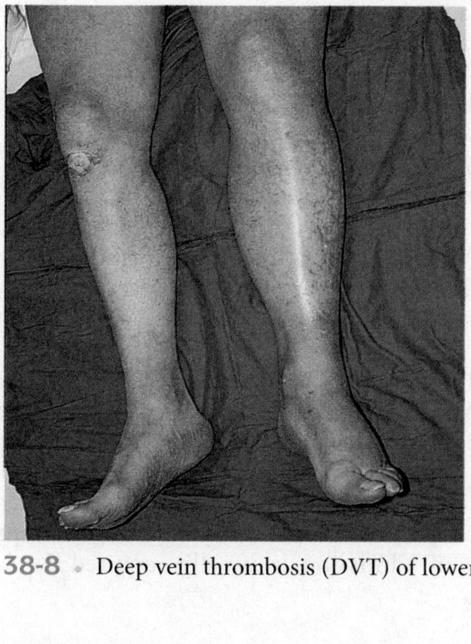

Fig. 38-8 • Deep vein thrombosis (DVT) of lower leg.

Impedance plethysmography assesses venous outflow and can detect most DVTs that are located above the popliteal vein. However, it is not helpful in locating clots in the calf and is less sensitive than Doppler studies.

Magnetic resonance direct thrombus imaging (MRI), another noninvasive test, is useful in finding a DVT in the proximal deep veins and is better than traditional venography in finding DVT in the inferior vena cava or pelvic veins.

A D-dimer test is a global marker of coagulation activation and measures fibrin degradation products produced from fibrinolysis (clot breakdown). The test is used for the diagnosis of DVT when the patient has few clinical signs and stratifies patients into a high-risk category for reoccurrence. Useful as an adjunct to noninvasive testing, a negative D-dimer test can exclude a DVT without an ultrasound.

Common Nursing Diagnoses and Collaborative Problems

Nursing diagnoses that may apply to patients with DVT include:

1. Risk for Ineffective Tissue Perfusion (Peripheral) related to interruption of venous blood flow
2. Acute Pain related to physical injury agent (thrombus)

The most common collaborative problem is Potential for Embolism.

Interventions

The focus of managing thrombophlebitis is to prevent complications such as pulmonary emboli, prevent further thrombus formation, and prevent an increase in size of the thrombus. Deep vein thrombophlebitis (thrombosis) is the most common type of thrombophlebitis. Patients with DVT are often hospitalized for treatment, although this practice is changing as a result of the use of newer drugs.

Nonsurgical Management

DVT is usually treated medically using a combination of rest, drug therapy, and preventive measures. Prevention of DVT is crucial for patients at risk. Preventive measures are listed on p. 817 in the Health Promotion and Maintenance section.

Rest. Supportive therapy for DVT includes bedrest and elevation of the extremity. Teach the patient to elevate his or her legs when in bed and in a chair. To help prevent chronic venous insufficiency, instruct patients with active and resolving DVT to wear knee- or thigh-high compression or elastic stockings for an extended period.

Some health care providers prescribe intermittent or continuous warm, moist soaks to the affected area. *Do not massage the affected extremity to prevent the thrombus from dislodging and becoming an embolus.* All patients are evaluated for signs and symptoms of pulmonary embolism (PE), which include shortness of breath and chest pain. Emboli may also travel to the brain or heart, but these complications are not as common as PE. Chapter 34 describes PE manifestations in detail.

Drug Therapy. *Anticoagulants are the drugs of choice for actual DVT and for patients at risk for DVT.* The conventional treatment has been IV unfractionated heparin followed by oral anticoagulation with warfarin (Coumadin). However, unfractionated heparin can be problematic because each patient's response to the drug is unpredictable and hospital admission is usually required for laboratory monitoring and dose adjustments. The use of low–molecular weight heparin (LMWH) is changing the management of both DVT and PE.

Unfractionated Heparin Therapy. Many patients with a confirmed diagnosis of an existing blood clot are started on a regimen of IV unfractionated heparin (UFH, Hepalean🍁) therapy. UFH is an anticoagulant agent that at low doses interacts with antithrombin III to produce selective inhibition of clotting factors IIa (thrombin) and Xa. At higher doses, it inhibits practically all clotting factors. The ultimate result is inhibition of fibrin formation. The physician prescribes UFH to prevent the formation of other clots, which often develop in the presence of an existing clot, and to prevent enlargement of the existing clot. Over a long period, the existing clot is slowly absorbed by the body.

Before UFH administration, a baseline prothrombin time (PT), activated partial thromboplastin time (APTT or aPTT), International Normalized Ratio (INR), complete blood count (CBC) with platelet count, urinalysis, stool for occult blood, and creatinine level are required. Notify the physician if the platelet count is below 120,000/mm^3.

UFH is initially given in a bolus IV dose of about 80 to 100 units/kg of body weight or 5000 units followed by continuous infusion. The infusion is regulated by a reliable electronic pump that protects against accidental free flow of solution. The physician or clinical pharmacist prescribes concentrations of UFH (in 5% dextrose in water) and the number of units or milliliters per hour needed to maintain a therapeutic aPTT (usually 18-20 units/kg/hr or at least 30,000 units over 24 hours). aPTT is measured at least daily, and results are reported to the health care provider as soon as results are available to allow adjustment of heparin dosage. Therapeutic levels of aPTTs are usually 1½ to 2 times normal control levels. *Notify the physician if the value is greater than 70 seconds, or follow hospital protocol for reporting critical laboratory values. Assess patients for signs and symptoms of bleeding, which include hematuria, frank or occult blood in the stool, ecchymosis (bruising), petechiae, an altered level of consciousness, or pain.*

UFH can also decrease platelet counts. Mild reductions are common and are resolved with continued heparin therapy. Severe platelet reductions, although rare, result from the development of antiplatelet bodies within 6 to 14 days after the beginning of treatment. Platelets aggregate into "white clots" that can cause thrombosis, usually in the form of an acute arterial occlusion. The provider discontinues heparin administration if severe **heparin-induced thrombocytopenia (HIT)** (platelet count <150,000), or "white clot syndrome," occurs. LMWH is used more commonly today because of the complications involved with UFH.

Bivalirudin (Angiomax) and lepirudin (Refludan) are highly selective direct thrombin inhibitors that may be used as alternatives to heparin or for patients who have had HIT. Like heparin, these drugs increase the risk for bleeding. An oral anticoagulant like warfarin (Coumadin) may also be substituted for heparin if necessary.

Ensure that protamine sulfate, the antidote for heparin, is available if needed for excessive bleeding. Chart 38-6 highlights information important to nursing care and patient education associated with anticoagulant therapy.

To *prevent* DVT, heparin may be given in low doses subcutaneously for high-risk patients, especially after orthope-

Chart 38-6 **BEST PRACTICE FOR PATIENT SAFETY & QUALITY CARE**

The Patient Receiving Anticoagulant Therapy

- Carefully check the dosage of anticoagulant to be administered, even if the pharmacy prepared the drug.
- Monitor the patient for signs and symptoms of bleeding, including hematuria, frank or occult blood in the stool, ecchymosis, petechiae, altered mental status (indicating possible cranial bleeding), or pain (especially abdominal pain, which could indicate abdominal bleeding).
- Monitor vital signs frequently for decreased blood pressure and increased pulse (indicating possible internal bleeding).
- Have antidotes available as needed (e.g., protamine sulfate for heparin; vitamin K for warfarin [Coumadin, Warfilone]).
- Monitor activated partial thromboplastin time (aPTT) for patients receiving unfractionated heparin. Monitor prothrombin time (PT) or International Normalized Ratio (INR) for patients receiving warfarin or low-molecular weight heparin (LMWH).
- Apply prolonged pressure over venipuncture sites and injection sites.
- When administering *subcutaneous* heparin, apply pressure over the site and do not massage.
- Teach the patient going home while taking an anticoagulant to:
  - Use only an electric razor
  - Take precautions to avoid injury; for example, do not use tools such as hammers or saws, where accidents commonly occur
  - Report signs and symptoms of bleeding, such as blood in the urine or stool, nosebleeds, ecchymosis, or altered mental status
  - Take the prescribed dosage of drug at the precise time that it was prescribed to be given
  - Not stop taking the drug abruptly; the physician usually tapers the anticoagulant gradually

dic surgery. However, other drugs are used more often, including:

- Low–molecular weight heparin (e.g., enoxaparin [Lovenox]) (drug class of choice after orthopedic surgery)
- Selective factor Xa inhibitors (e.g., fondaparinux [Arixtra])
- Warfarin (Coumadin, Warfilone♣)

Low–Molecular Weight Heparin. Subcutaneous low-molecular weight heparins (LMWHs) such as enoxaparin (Lovenox), dalteparin (Fragmin), and ardeparin (Normiflo) have a consistent action and are preferred for prevention and treatment of DVT. Danaparoid (Orgaran) is also classified as an LMWH but is actually a heparinoid. LMWHs bind less to plasma proteins, blood cells, and vessel walls, resulting in a longer half-life and more predictable response. These drugs inhibit thrombin formation because of reduced factor IIa activity and enhanced inhibition of factor Xa and thrombin.

Some patients taking LMWH may be safely managed at home with daily visits from a home care nurse. Candidates for home therapy must have stable DVT or PE, low risk for bleeding, adequate renal function, and normal vital signs. They must be willing to learn self-injection or have a family member, friend, or home care nurse administer the subcutaneous injections.

Some health care providers place the patient on a regimen of IV unfractionated heparin (UFH) for several days and then follow up with an LMWH. In this case, the UFH is discontinued at least 30 minutes before the first LMWH injection. The usual dose of enoxaparin is 1 mg/kg of body weight, not to exceed 90 mg, and is repeated every 12 hours. If the patient's creatinine level is greater than 2 mg/dL (indicating renal insufficiency), the health care provider lowers the dose. Dalteparin can be given once daily at 200 units/kg of body weight and does not require dose adjustment for renal insufficiency. The usual dose of ardeparin is 50 units/kg of body weight and is given every 12 hours.

Monitor the INR daily. Assess all stools for occult blood. The aPTTs are not checked on an ongoing basis because the doses of LMWH are not adjusted.

Warfarin Therapy. If the patient is receiving continuous UFH, warfarin (Coumadin), an oral anticoagulant, may be added at least 5 days later. Patients receiving LMWH are placed on the oral drug after the first dose. Warfarin works in the liver to inhibit synthesis of the four vitamin K–dependent clotting factors and takes 3 to 4 days before it can exert therapeutic anticoagulation. The heparin continues to provide therapeutic anticoagulation until this effect is achieved. IV heparin is then discontinued.

Therapeutic levels of warfarin are monitored by measuring PT and/or the INR. Because PTs are often inconsistent and misleading, the INR was developed. Most laboratories report both results. Most patients receiving warfarin should have an INR between 1.5 and 2.0 to prevent future DVT and to minimize the risk of stroke or hemorrhage. For patients with additional cardiovascular problems, the desired INR may higher. Warfarin therapy should be started with low doses, at least 5 mg, and gradually titrated up according to the INR. Patients usually receive this drug for 3 to 6 months or longer after an episode of DVT if no precipitating factors were discovered, with recurrence, or if there are continuing risk factors.

Nursing assessment for bleeding is similar to that described for patients receiving heparin. *Ensure that vitamin K, the antidote for warfarin, is available in case of excessive bleeding* (see Chart 38-6). However, anticoagulation is not possible for 3 weeks after vitamin K administration.

Thrombolytic Therapy. The use of systemic thrombolytic therapy for DVT is effective in dissolving thrombi quickly and completely. The greatest advantage is thought to be the prevention of valvular damage and venous insufficiency, or "post-phlebitis syndrome." However, because of increased bleeding risk, thrombolytic therapy is contraindicated after surgery and after trauma, strokes, or spinal injuries. To be most effective, thrombolytic therapy must be started within 5 days after the onset of symptoms.

Thrombolytic drugs such as recombinant tissue plasminogen activator (t-PA) and platelet inhibitors such as abciximab (ReoPro), tirofiban (Aggrastat), and eptifibatide (Integrilin) may be effective in dissolving a clot or preventing new clots during the first 24 hours. Infusion given via a catheter can be injected directly into the thrombus. Compared with giving systemic thrombolytic dosing, this approach decreases the concentration needed and reduces the chance of bleeding. Thrombolytic drugs, such as alteplase and reteplase, are used to treat peripheral vascular occlusion. Reteplase is a plasminogen activator that penetrates the clot and causes lysis. *It is not compatible with heparin and should not be given in the same IV line.* Reteplase has been used successfully in treating coronary thrombosis. Use in peripheral vascular occlusion is experimental. *The most serious complication from thrombolytic therapy is intracerebral bleeding. Be aware of the importance of thrombolytic therapy, its indications, and its implications for nursing care. Closely monitor patients for signs and symptoms of bleeding, including a decreased level of consciousness.*

DECISION-MAKING CHALLENGE
Critical Rescue

A middle-aged woman is a consultant who has traveled every week by plane for 15 years. Recently she noticed redness and swelling in her left mid-calf with swollen ankles. The area is very painful, especially when she climbs stairs. The patient has a history of smoking and hypertension. She sees her health care provider, who admits her immediately to the hospital.

1. Why do you think this patient was admitted on an urgent basis to the hospital?
2. What risk factors does she have that predispose her to this health problem?
3. What type of drug do you think will be prescribed for her, and what are your nursing responsibilities when giving this drug?
4. What other nursing care, including health teaching, will this patient require?
5. During her second hospital day, the patient reports chest pain and shortness of breath. What is your priority action, and why do you think she has these symptoms?

evolve For suggested answer guidelines, go to http://evolve.elsevier.com/Iggy/.

Surgical Management

A deep vein thrombus is rarely removed surgically unless there is a massive occlusion that does not respond to medical treatment and the thrombus is of recent (1 to 2 days) onset. **Thrombectomy** is the most common surgical procedure for removing the clot. Preoperative and postoperative care of patients undergoing thrombectomy are similar to the care for those undergoing arterial surgery (see p. 808 in the Peripheral Arterial Disease section).

Inferior Vena Caval Interruption. Recurrent deep vein thrombosis (DVT) or pulmonary emboli that do not respond to medical treatment and for patients who cannot tolerate anticoagulation, **inferior vena caval interruption** may be indicated to prevent pulmonary emboli.

Preoperative care is similar to that provided for patients receiving local anesthesia (see Chapter 16). If they have recently been taking anticoagulants, collaborate with the physician about interrupting this therapy in the preoperative period to avoid hemorrhage.

The surgeon usually inserts a filter device, or "umbrella," into the femoral vein. The device is meant to trap emboli in the inferior vena cava before they progress to the lungs. Holes in the device allow blood to pass through, thus not significantly interfering with the return of blood to the heart. Popular inferior vena caval filters include the bird's nest filter and the Greenfield filter.

Postoperatively, inspect the groin insertion site for bleeding and signs or symptoms of infection. Other postoperative nursing care is similar to that for any patient undergoing local surgery (see Chapter 18).

Ligation or External Clips. If an inferior vena caval filter is not successful in preventing pulmonary emboli or if the filter becomes blocked with thrombi, the surgeon may perform ligation or insert external clips on the inferior vena cava to prevent pulmonary emboli.

Preoperative care for patients undergoing ligation of the vena cava or placement of an external clip is similar to that for an abdominal laparotomy. If the patient is receiving anticoagulation therapy, collaborate with the surgeon about temporary interruption of therapy.

Ligation and insertion of external clips in the inferior vena cava are often performed through an abdominal laparotomy. In a ligation, the surgeon ties off the inferior vena cava to block emboli. Application of an external clip narrows the inferior vena cava to four serrated transverse slits, 3 to 5 mm in diameter. If laparotomy is performed, the external clip procedure is preferred because there are fewer hemodynamic or venous complications and a low frequency of recurrent pulmonary emboli associated with its use.

Postoperative care for the patient with inferior vena caval ligation or external clip placement is similar to that for an abdominal laparotomy.

Community-Based Care

Patients recovering from thrombophlebitis or DVT are usually ambulatory when they are discharged from the hospital. The primary focus of planning for discharge is to educate the patient and family about the hazards of anticoagulation therapy.

Teach patients recovering from DVT to stop or avoid smoking and to avoid the use of oral contraceptives to decrease the risk of recurrence. Alternative forms of birth control may be used. Most patients are discharged on a regimen of warfarin (Coumadin, Warfilone♣) or low-molecular weight heparin (LMWH). Instruct patients and their families to avoid potentially traumatic situations, such as participation in contact sports. Provide written and oral information about the signs and symptoms of bleeding (see Chart 38-6). Reinforce the need to report any of these manifestations to the health care provider immediately.

The anticoagulant effect of warfarin may be reversed by omitting one or two doses of the drug or by the administration of vitamin K. In case of injury, teach patients to apply pressure to bleeding wounds and to seek medical assistance immediately. Encourage them to carry an identification card or wear a medical alert bracelet that states that they are taking warfarin or any other anticoagulant.

Also instruct patients to tell their dentist and other health care providers that they are taking warfarin before receiving treatment or prescriptions. Prothrombin times are affected by many prescription and over-the-counter drugs such as NSAIDs. The action of warfarin is also affected by high-fat and vitamin K–rich foods, such as cabbage, cauliflower, broccoli, asparagus, turnips, spinach, kale, fish, and liver. Therefore instruct patients to eat a well-balanced diet with moderate amounts of vitamin K and to avoid taking additional drugs without consulting a health care provider (Chart 38-7). Teach patients also to prevent dehydration and to avoid alcohol and sitting for prolonged periods.

In collaboration with the case manager (CM) or other discharge planner, arrange for patients to obtain a device to self-monitor INR at home. This device is similar to a glucometer for glucose testing and requires a fingerstick blood sample applied to a test strip or plastic cuvette, which is then inserted into the machine. Self-monitoring can be used as either the testing alone or for self-management, in which the patient

Chart 38-7 PATIENT AND FAMILY EDUCATION GUIDE

Food and Drugs That Interfere with Warfarin (Coumadin)

Eat small amounts of foods rich in vitamin K each day, including any of these:

- Broccoli
- Cauliflower
- Spinach
- Kale
- Green leafy vegetables
- Brussels sprouts
- Cabbage
- Liver

If possible, avoid:

- Allopurinol
- NSAIDs
- Acetaminophen
- Vitamin E
- Histamine blockers
- Cholesterol-reducing drugs
- Antibiotics
- Birth control pills
- Antidepressants
- Thyroid drugs
- Antifungal infections
- Other anticoagulants
- Corticosteroids
- Herbs, such as St. John's wort, garlic, ginseng, *Ginkgo biloba*

uses the test results to adjust drug dosages based on a dosing protocol (Pence & McErlane, 2005). If the patient cannot use a monitoring device, teach a family member or other caregiver how to perform the procedure. If the patient lives alone, collaborate with the CM to arrange for follow-up laboratory appointments to have blood drawn at frequent intervals—usually every week until the patient's values are stabilized.

Patients receiving subcutaneous LMWH injections at home need instruction on self-injection. Teach the appropriate caregiver and family members or friends, if necessary, to administer the injections.

Patients who have experienced DVT may fear recurrence of a thrombus. They may also be concerned about treatment with warfarin and the risk for bleeding. Assure them that the prescribed treatment will help resolve this problem and that ongoing assessment of PTs and INRs decreases the risks of bleeding.

Patients discharged on a regimen of warfarin need access to a pharmacy to renew prescriptions and obtain a medical alert bracelet. They also need access to a laboratory for frequent monitoring of PTs and INRs unless they are self-monitoring.

VENOUS INSUFFICIENCY

Pathophysiology

Venous insufficiency occurs as a result of prolonged venous hypertension that stretches the veins and damages the valves. Valvular damage can lead to a backup of blood and further venous hypertension, resulting in edema. Because the patient cannot eliminate waste products, they build up within the tissues. With time, this stasis (stoppage) results in venous stasis ulcers, swelling, and cellulitis.

The veins cannot function properly when thrombosis occurs or when valves are not working correctly. Venous hypertension can occur in people who stand or sit in one position for long periods (e.g., teachers, office personnel). Obesity can also cause chronically distended veins, which lead to damaged valves. Thrombus formation can contribute to valve destruction. Chronic venous insufficiency also often occurs in patients who have had thrombophlebitis. In severe cases, venous ulcers develop.

Venous leg ulcer disease is a major cause of death, pain, and health care costs. Most venous ulcer care is delivered in the community setting by home care nurses or through self-management.

Patient-Centered Collaborative Care

Assessment

Venous insufficiency may result in edema of both legs. There may be **stasis dermatitis** or reddish-brown discoloration along the ankles, extending up to the calf. In people with long-term venous insufficiency, **stasis ulcers** often form. They can result from the edema or from minor injury to the limb. Ulcers typically occur over the malleolus, more often medially (inner ankle) than laterally (outer ankle). The ulcer usually has irregular borders. In general, these ulcers are chronic and difficult to heal (see Chart 38-3). Many people live with ulcers for years, and recurrence is common. Some may lose one or both legs if ulcers are not controlled.

Interventions

The focus of treating venous insufficiency is to decrease edema and promote venous return from the affected leg. Patients are not usually hospitalized for venous insufficiency alone unless it is complicated by an ulcer or another disorder is occurring at the same time.

Nonsurgical Management

Treatment of chronic venous insufficiency is nonsurgical unless it is complicated by a venous stasis ulcer that requires surgical débridement. The goals of managing venous stasis ulcers are to heal the ulcer, prevent infection, and prevent stasis with recurrence of ulcer formation. Collaborate with the wound care nurse or wound, ostomy, and continence nurse to make recommendations for ulcer care. A nutritionist can suggest dietary supplements, such as zinc and vitamins A and C, as well as high-protein foods, to promote wound healing.

Patients with chronic venous insufficiency wear elastic or compression stockings, which fit from the middle of the foot to just below the knee or to the thigh. Stockings should be worn during the day and evening. Legs should be elevated for at least 20 minutes four or five times per day. When the patient is in bed, remind him or her to elevate the legs above the level of the heart (Chart 38-8).

Coordinate with the physician about the use of intermittent sequential pneumatic compression or foot plexus pumps for patients with past or present venous stasis ulcers. If an open venous ulcer is present, the device may be applied over a dressing such as an Unna boot. Instruct the patient to apply the pump as directed during the period of healing. Because of the high incidence of venous ulcer recurrence, encourage patients with chronic venous insufficiency whose ulcers have healed to continue compression therapy for life.

Venous stasis ulcers are slightly more manageable than ulcers resulting from arterial disease. They are chronic in

Chart 38-8 PATIENT AND FAMILY EDUCATION GUIDE

Venous Insufficiency

ELASTIC STOCKINGS

- Wear elastic stockings as prescribed, usually during the day and evening.
- Put the stockings on upon awakening and before getting out of bed.
- When applying the stockings, do not "bunch up" and apply like socks. Instead, place your hand inside the stocking and pull out the heel. Then place the foot of the stocking over your foot and slide the rest of the stocking up. Be sure that rough seams on the stocking are on the outside, not next to your skin.
- Do not push stockings down for comfort, because they may function like a tourniquet and further impair venous return.
- Put on a clean pair of stockings each day. Wash them by hand (not in a washing machine) in a gentle detergent and warm water.
- If the stockings seem to be "stretched out," replace them with a new pair.

DOS AND DON'TS

- Elevate your legs for at least 20 minutes four or five times a day. When in bed, elevate your legs above the level of your heart.
- Avoid prolonged sitting or standing.
- Do not cross your legs. Crossing at the ankles is acceptable for short periods.
- Do not wear tight, restrictive pants. Avoid girdles and garters.

nature, with some patients having the same ulcer for years. Ulcers often heal, only to recur in the same area several years later.

Two types of occlusive dressings are used for venous stasis ulcers: oxygen-permeable dressings and oxygen-impermeable dressings. Because the role of atmospheric oxygen in wound healing is controversial, opinions vary with regard to which type of dressing is preferred. An oxygen-permeable polyethylene film and an oxygen-impermeable hydrocolloid dressing (e.g., DuoDerm) are common. Hydrocolloid dressings are left in place for a minimum of 3 to 5 days for best effect. Use medical aseptic technique when changing dressings. If the wound is infected, use Contact Precautions in addition to Standard Precautions.

Artificial skin products can be used for difficult-to-heal venous leg ulcers. These first-generation products are very expensive but are laying the foundation in the field, with costs anticipated to come down in the future. Except for cultured epithelial autografts, artificial skins are only temporary. Artificial skin serves as a biologic cover to secrete growth factors to promote more growth factor secretion from the patient's own skin to speed the wound healing process.

If the patient is ambulatory, an **Unna boot** may be used. An Unna boot dressing is constructed of gauze that has been moistened with zinc oxide. Apply the boot to the affected limb, from the toes to the knee, after the ulcer has been cleaned with normal saline solution. It is then covered with an elastic wrap and hardens like a cast. This promotes venous return and prevents stasis. The Unna boot also forms a sterile environment for the ulcer. The physician or advanced practice nurse changes the boot about once a week. Instruct the patient to report increased pain, which indicates that the boot may be too tight.

The health care provider may prescribe topical agents, such as Accuzyme, to chemically débride the ulcer, eliminating necrotic tissue and promoting healing. If an infection or cellulitis develops, systemic antibiotics are necessary.

Surgical Management

Surgery for chronic venous insufficiency is not usually performed because it is not successful. Attempts at transplanting vein valves have had limited success. Surgical débridement of venous ulcers is similar to that performed for arterial ulcers.

Community-Based Care

The goal for the patient with chronic venous insufficiency is to be managed in the home. For patients with frequent acute complications and repeated hospital admissions, case management can help meet appropriate clinical and cost outcomes.

Help patients plan for opportunities and facilities that allow for elevation of the lower extremities in and outside the home. In addition, collaborate with the wound specialist to plan care of the ulcers at home.

Instruct patients with chronic venous stasis to:

- Avoid standing still if possible
- Elevate their legs when sitting
- Avoid crossing their legs
- Avoid wearing tight girdles, tight pants, and narrow-banded knee-high socks

The physician prescribes antiembolism stockings. Teach patients to apply these stockings before they get out of bed in the morning and to remove them just before going to bed at night (see Chart 38-8). Also advise them that they will probably need to wear these stockings for the rest of their lives.

To improve circulation and aid in weight reduction, collaborate with the physical therapist to prescribe an exercise program on an individual basis. Encourage all patients to maintain an optimal weight and consult with the nutritionist to plan a weight-reduction diet.

Patients with venous stasis disease, especially those with venous stasis ulcers, may require long-term emotional support to assist them in meeting long-term needs. They may also need assistance in coping with necessary lifestyle adjustments, such as changes in occupation.

Patients with venous stasis ulcers may need the assistance of a home care nurse to perform dressing changes. Those with Unna boots need weekly transportation to their health care provider for dressing changes. Collaborate with the case manager to arrange for a sequential compression device in the home if the health care provider prescribes one.

VARICOSE VEINS

Pathophysiology

Varicose veins are distended, protruding veins that appear darkened and tortuous. They can occur in anyone, but they are common in adults older than 30 years whose occupations require prolonged standing. Varicose veins are frequently seen also in patients with systemic problems (e.g., heart disease), obesity, and a family history of varicose veins.

As the vein wall weakens and dilates, venous pressure increases and the valves become incompetent (defective). The incompetent valves enhance the vessel dilation, and the veins become tortuous and distended. The patient may report pain, especially after standing, and may experience a feeling of fullness in the legs. Nursing assessment reveals distended, protruding veins.

The Trendelenburg test assists with the diagnosis. Place the patient in a supine position with elevated legs. As he or she sits up, the veins would normally fill from the distal end. However, if there are varicosities, the veins fill from the proximal end.

Patient-Centered Collaborative Care

Conservative measures are the treatment of choice, including wearing elastic stockings and elevating the extremities as much as possible. Patients who continue to have pain or unsightly veins, despite this treatment, may opt for either sclerotherapy or surgical removal of the vein.

Sclerotherapy is performed on small or a limited number of varicosities. The physician injects a sclerosing solution directly into the vein, or he or she may use a laser device. A pressure dressing may be applied over the sclerosed vein to keep vessels free of blood for 24 to 72 hours. The surgeon performs an incision and drainage of trapped blood in the sclerosed vein 14 to 21 days after injection, followed by application of a second pressure dressing for 12 to 18 hours.

Varicose veins are surgically removed when they are larger than 4 mm in diameter or are in clusters. The stab avulsion technique may be used if the saphenous veins are competent. The surgeon exposes varices through 2- to 3-mm stab incisions, grasping the veins with hooks and dividing and removing each vein.

The surgeon may need to strip (remove) affected veins if the saphenous vein is affected. The surgeon threads a long wire through an incision above an affected vein, pulling it down through the vein and out through an incision below the vein. After this procedure, the legs are bandaged with firm elastic bandages.

After surgery, assess the groin and entire leg for bleeding through the elastic bandage. Instruct the patient to keep the legs elevated and to perform range-of-motion exercises of the legs at least hourly. Patients are ambulatory and are often discharged from the hospital by the first postoperative day. At this time, instruct them to continue to wear elastic stockings, walk, limit sitting, avoid standing in one place, and elevate their legs when sitting.

Application of radiofrequency (RF) energy is a new technique done as an alternative to surgery. The vein is heated from the inside by the RF energy and shrinks. Collateral veins nearby take over.

Laser treatment is another alternative to surgery. Performed by interventional radiologists, the endovenous laser treatment uses a laser fiber to heat and close the main vessel that is contributing to the varicosity.

PHLEBITIS

Phlebitis is an inflammation of the superficial veins caused by an irritant such as peripheral IV therapy (see Chapter 15). The patient has a reddened, warm area radiating up the arm. Pain, soreness, and swelling may also occur.

Management involves application of warm, moist soaks, which dilate the vein and promote circulation. Sometimes a heating unit is used to keep the soaks warm. Apply the soaks, making sure that the temperature is not hot enough to burn the patient, and assess for complications, such as tissue necrosis, infection, or pulmonary embolus. After a few days of conservative therapy, the inflammation usually subsides. Elastic stockings may be prescribed if the phlebitis occurs in a leg.

VASCULAR TRAUMA

Many types of trauma can result in vascular injury. Vascular injuries include punctures, lacerations, and transections. Acute blunt or penetrating trauma may result in a false aneurysm or hematoma. Arteriovenous fistulas may be seen after penetrating injuries. The more common causes of penetrating injuries to the blood vessels are gunshot and knife wounds.

Blunt trauma, which is less common, can result from high-speed automobile crashes as a result of the shearing force of rapid deceleration. Vascular trauma can also occur during arterial puncture for arteriographic or hemodynamic studies in which a dissection, hematoma, or occlusive lesion occurs.

The history and physical examination aid in establishing the diagnosis of vascular injury. Ask the patient or family about the mechanism of injury, the site of injury, the amount of blood loss, and symptoms present after the injury.

Assess for circulatory, sensory, and motor impairment, but be aware that, despite significant trauma, impairment may not be apparent, especially if deep vessels have been injured. Arteriography provides essential information about the vascular injury. Emergency or urgent surgical intervention is needed for ischemia to maximize successful revascularization.

Management of vascular injuries is often initiated in a hospital emergency department. Careful patient triage is crucial. The most important principles in the management of vascular trauma are establishing a patent airway, controlling bleeding, and restoring blood flow.

The method of repair varies with the type of vascular injury. Techniques include vein bypass grafting, lateral suture repair, thrombectomy (excision of blood clot), resection with end-to-end anastomosis, and vein patch grafting.

HUMAN NEEDS NURSING CARE REVIEW

What might you NOTICE if the patient is experiencing inadequate oxygenation and tissue perfusion as a result of vascular problems?

- Redness and swelling in lower leg (venous)
- Pallor, cyanosis (darkened), mottling, or rubor in lower leg (arterial)
- Report of pain/cramping in lower legs or hands (at rest or during activity)

- Ulcers on ankles, feet, or digits
- Pulsating mass in abdomen (abdominal aortic aneurysm)
- Decreased level of consciousness (LOC), diaphoresis, decreased urine output (rupturing aortic aneurysm)

What should you INTERPRET and how should you RESPOND to a patient experiencing inadequate oxygenation and tissue perfusion as a result of coronary artery disease?

Perform and interpret physical assessment, including:
- Taking vital signs
- Assessing peripheral pulses
- Assessing capillary refill
- Checking for sensation and temperature
- Completing a pain assessment
- Assessing ulcer

Respond by:
- Notifying physician immediately or calling Rapid Response Team if aortic rupture suspected
- Monitoring vital signs
- Giving oxygen if aneurysm rupture suspected
- Starting an IV line if aneurysm rupture suspected
- Documenting abnormal peripheral vascular assessment findings
- Elevating legs if swollen unless arterial blood flow is poor

On what should you REFLECT?
- Think about how you responded.
- Continue to monitor patient for changes in peripheral blood flow, including pulse assessments.
- Observe patient for decreased report of pain

GET READY FOR THE NCLEX EXAMINATION!

Key Points

Review these Key Points for each NCLEX Examination Client Needs Category.

Safe and Effective Care Environment
- In collaboration with the health care team, plan care for the patient with atherosclerosis and hypertension including the nutritionist and pharmacist.
- To reduce the risk of injury, caution patients about orthostatic hypotension when taking antihypertensive drugs.

Health Promotion and Maintenance
- In collaboration with the nutritionist, assist the patient to incorporate healthy eating behaviors to lower cholesterol and saturated fats and increase fresh fruits, vegetables, and fiber in the diet. For overweight patients, assist in a weight-reduction plan. Teach patients taking statin-type drugs to report adverse effects to their health care provider.
- Teach patients ways to prevent deep vein thrombosis and subsequent embolism. In the hospital setting, provide measures, such as wearing compression stockings, to prevent or manage DVT.
- Assess the patient for modifiable and nonmodifiable risk factors for vascular disease, and teach health promotion behaviors to the patient and family. Pay particular attention to the patient with a family history of cardiovascular disease (see Table 38-1).

Physiological Integrity
- Remember that risk factors such as smoking increase the pathophysiologic process of atherosclerosis.
- Closely observe the patient receiving anticoagulants or thrombolytics for signs of bleeding, and monitor appropriate laboratory values for desired outcome values.
- Monitor for decreased serum potassium levels when patients are taking thiazide or loop diuretics.
- Teach patients to move slowly when changing position if taking any of the antihypertensive drugs listed in Table 38-6.
- Teach patients taking any of the statins in Table 38-2 to report muscle cramping to their health care provider. The patient's liver enzymes are monitored carefully.
- Provide emergency care for the patient having a hypertensive crisis as described in Chart 38-1.
- Recognize that clinical manifestations of peripheral vascular disease (PVD) depend on whether it affects the arteries or veins. In addition to pallor, rubor, or cyanosis, key features of chronic peripheral arterial disease are listed in Chart 38-2.
- Vasodilating drugs or surgery is used for arterial vascular diseases.
- Deep vein thrombosis is the most common type of peripheral vascular problem. When symptoms are present, they include swelling, redness, localized pain, and warmth.
- Teach patients about self-care when they have venous insufficiency.
- Assess for venous and arterial ulcers as described in Chart 38-3.
- Teach foot care for patients with PVD as outlined in Chart 38-5.
- Teach patients about precautions for anticoagulant therapy as described in Chart 38-6. Teach about food and drugs that interfere with warfarin (Coumadin) as listed in Chart 38-7.
- Monitor for indications of aneurysm rupture: diaphoresis, nausea, vomiting, pallor, hypotension, tachycardia, severe pain, and decreased level of consciousness.
- Essential hypertension is called *primary hypertension* and is not caused by another health problem or drug. Secondary, or nonessential, hypertension is caused by other health problems or drug therapy (see Table 38-5).

Additional Study Resources

Go to your Companion CD or Evolve at http://evolve.elsevier.com/Iggy/ for *Self-Assessment Questions for the NCLEX Examination.*

Go to Evolve at http://evolve.elsevier.com/Iggy/ for *Prioritization and Delegation Questions for the NCLEX Examination.*

SELECTED BIBLIOGRAPHY

Asterisk indicates a classic or definitive work on this subject.

*ALLHAT Officers and Coordinators for the ALLHAT Collaborative Research Group. (2002a). Major outcomes in high-risk hypertensive patients randomized to angiotensin-converting enzyme inhibitor or calcium channel blocker vs diuretic. The Antihypertensive and Lipid-Lowering Treatment to Prevent Heart Attack Trial (ALLHAT). *Journal of the American Medical Association, 288*(23), 2981-2997.

*ALLHAT Officers and Coordinators for the ALLHAT Collaborative Research Group. (2002b). Major outcomes in moderately hypercholesterolemic, hypertensive patients randomized to pravastatin vs usual care. The Antihypertensive and Lipid-Lowering Treatment to Prevent Heart Attack Trial (ALLHAT-LLT). *Journal of the American Medical Association, 288*(23), 2998-3007.

American Heart Association (AHA). (2008). *Heart Disease and Stroke Statistics-2008 Update.* Dallas: American Heart Association.

Aronow, W.S. (2007). Peripheral arterial disease: Management of peripheral arterial disease in the elderly. *Geriatrics, 62*(1), 19-25.

Artinian, N., Flack, J.M., Nordstrom, C.K., Hockman, E.M., Washington, O.G., Jen, K-L.C., et al. (2007). Effects of nurse-managed telemonitoring on blood pressure at 12-month follow-up among urban African Americans. *Nursing Research, 56*(5), 312-322.

Bartley, M.K. (2006). Keep venous thromboembolism at bay. *Nursing2006, 36*(10), 36-43.

Beck, D.M. (2006). Venous thromboembolism (VTE) prophylaxis: Implications for medical-surgical nurses. *MEDSURG Nursing, 15*(5), 282-286.

Bergen, J.J., Schmid-Schonbein, G.W., Smith, P.D.C., Nicolaides, A.N., Boisseau, M.R., & Eklof, B. (2006). Chronic venous disease. *New England Journal of Medicine, 355*(5), 488-498.

*Bussard, M.E. (2002). Reteplase: Nursing implications for catheter-directed thrombolytic therapy for peripheral vascular occlusions. *Critical Care Nurse, 22*(3), 57-63.

Croce, H.D. (2007). Aortic dissection. *RN, 70*(3), 26-32.

*Day, M.W. (2003). Recognizing and managing deep vein thrombosis. *Nursing2003, 33*(5), 36-42.

*Douglas, J.G., Bakris, G.L., Epstein, M., Ferdinand, K.C., Ferrario, C., Flack, J.M., et al. (2003). Consensus Statement of the Hypertension in African Americans Working Group of the International Society on Hypertension in Blacks. Management of high blood pressure in African Americans. *Archives of Internal Medicine, 163*(5), 525-541.

*Eichinger, S., Minar, E., Bialonczyk, C., Hirschl, M., Quehenberger, P., Schneider, B., et al. (2003). D-dimer levels and risk of recurrent venous thromboembolism. *Journal of the American Medical Association, 290*(8), 1071-1074.

Fink, J.A., & Kaboli, P.J. (2006). *Prophylaxis of venous thromboembolism in surgical patients.* 48-56. Accessed October 2006, from www.patientcare-online.com

Francis, J.L., & Drexler, A.J. (2005). Striking back at heparin-induced thrombocytopenia. *Nursing2005, 35*(9), 48-51.

Harris, W.S., Miller, M., Tighe, A.P., Davidson, M.H., & Schaefer, E.J. (2008). Omega-3 fatty acids and coronary heart disease: Clinical and mechanistic perspectives. *Atherosclerosis, 197*(1), 12-24.

*Hess, C.T. (2003). Managing your patient's arterial ulcer. *Nursing2003, 33*(5), 17.

Irwin, G.H. (2007). How to protect a patient with aortic aneurysm. *Nursing2007, 37*(2), 36-42.

Jarvis, C. (2008). *Physical examination and health assessment* (5th ed.). St. Louis: Mosby.

*Joint National Committee. (2003). *The Seventh Report of the Joint National Committee on Prevention, Detection, Evaluation, and Treatment of High Blood Pressure.* NIH Publication No. 03-5233. Bethesda, MD: National Heart, Lung, and Blood Institute.

Karppanen, H., & Mervaala, E. (2006). Sodium intake and hypertension. *Progress in Cardiovascular Diseases, 49*(2), 59-75.

*Malacaria, B., & Feloney, C.D.H. (2003). Going with the flow of anticoagulant therapy. *Nursing2003, 33*(3), 36-42.

McCance, K.L., & Huether, S.E. (2006). *Pathophysiology: The biologic basis for disease in adults and children* (5th ed.). St. Louis: Mosby.

Nash, D.T. (2006). Systolic hypertension: Combination therapy as one approach to treating a persistent condition. *Geriatrics, 61*(12), 22-28.

*National Cholesterol Education Program. (2002). *Third Report of the Expert Panel on Detection, Evaluation, and Treatment of High Blood Cholesterol in Adults (Adult Treatment Panel III).* NIH Publication No. 02-5215. Bethesda, MD: National Heart, Lung, and Blood Institute.

Pagana, K.D., & Pagana, T.J. (2006). *Mosby's manual of diagnostic and laboratory tests* (3rd ed.). St. Louis: Mosby.

Pence, C., & McErlane, K. (2005). Anticoagulation self-monitoring. *AJN, 105*(10), 62-65.

Pickering, T.G., Phil, D., Shimbo, M.D., & Haas, D. (2006). Ambulatory blood-pressure monitoring. *New England Journal of Medicine, 354*(22), 2368-2374.

Reilly, A. (2005). Raynaud's phenomenon. *AJN, 105*(8), 57-64.

Rice, K.L. (2005). How to measure ankle/brachial index. *Nursing2005, 25*(1), 56-57.

Rosendorff, C., Black, H.R., Cannon, C.P., Gersh, B.J., Gore, J., Izzo, J.L. Jr., et al. (2007). Treatment of hypertension in the prevention and management of ischemic heart disease: A scientific statement from the AHA Council for High Blood Pressure Research and the Councils on Clinical Cardiology and Epidemiology and Prevention. *Circulation, 115*(21), 2761-2788.

Scheetz, L. (2006). Aortic dissection. *AJN, 106*(4), 55-57.

Sieggreen, M. (2006). A contemporary approach to peripheral arterial disease. *The Nurse Practitioner, 31*(7), 14-26.

Turner, L. (2006). Keeping warfarin in balance. *Nursing2006, 36*(11), 43-46.

*Woods, A. (2004). Loosening the grip of hypertension. *Nursing2004, 34*(12), 36-43.

39 CHAPTER

Care of Patients with Shock

M. Linda Workman

LEARNING OUTCOMES

For clinical competence and success on the NCLEX Examination, study this chapter with these Learning Outcomes in mind:

Safe and Effective Care Environment

1. Evaluate patient risk for hypovolemic shock or sepsis and septic shock.
2. Ensure vital sign measurements are accurate, and monitor them for changes indicating the presence of shock.
3. Apply principles of infection control to prevent infection and sepsis in susceptible patients.

Health Promotion and Maintenance

4. Teach all people to avoid dehydration.
5. Teach all people to use safety devices to avoid trauma.
6. Instruct all patients going home after surgery or invasive procedures to seek immediate attention for persistent manifestations of early shock.
7. Teach all patients who have a local infection to seek medical attention when manifestations of systemic infection appear.

Psychosocial Integrity

8. Assess the vital signs, especially pulse and oxygen saturation, for any patient who has a sudden change in mental status, including increased anxiety, apprehension, or agitation.
9. Reassure the patient in shock that the appropriate interventions are being implemented.

Physiological Integrity

10. Compare the risk factors, causes, and manifestations of different types of shock.
11. Identify the manifestations associated with shock progression.
12. Use laboratory data and clinical manifestations to determine the effectiveness of therapy for shock.
13. Describe the actions, side effects, and nursing implications of drug therapy for shock.
14. Coordinate the nursing care for the patient experiencing any stage of hypovolemic shock.
15. Explain the role of systemic inflammatory response syndrome (SIRS) in the manifestations and progression of sepsis and septic shock.
16. Coordinate the nursing care for the patient with sepsis or septic shock.

Go to your Companion CD or Evolve at http://evolve.elsevier.com/Iggy/ for *Self-Assessment Questions for the NCLEX Examination* keyed to these Learning Outcomes.

OVERVIEW

Organs, tissues, and cells need a continuous supply of oxygen to function properly. The lungs first bring oxygen into the body, and the cardiovascular system (heart, blood, and blood vessels) delivers oxygen to all tissues and removes cellular wastes (Fig. 39-1). **Shock** is widespread abnormal cellular metabolism that occurs when the human need for *oxygenation and tissue perfusion* is not met to the level needed to maintain cell function (McCance & Huether, 2006). It is a condition rather than a disease and represents the "whole-body" response that occurs when too little oxygen is delivered to the tissues. All body organs are affected by shock and either work harder to adapt and compensate for reduced oxygenation (see Fig. 39-1) or fail to function because of hypoxia. Shock is a "syndrome" because the cellular, tissue, and organ events that occur in response to its presence happen in a predictable sequence.

Any problem that impairs oxygen delivery to tissues and organs can start the syndrome of shock and lead to a life-threatening emergency. Most often, shock is a result of cardiovascular problems and changes. Patients in acute care settings are at higher risk, but shock can occur in any setting. For example, older patients in long-term care settings are at risk for sepsis and shock related to urinary tract infections. When adaptive adjustments (compensation) or health care interventions are not effective and shock

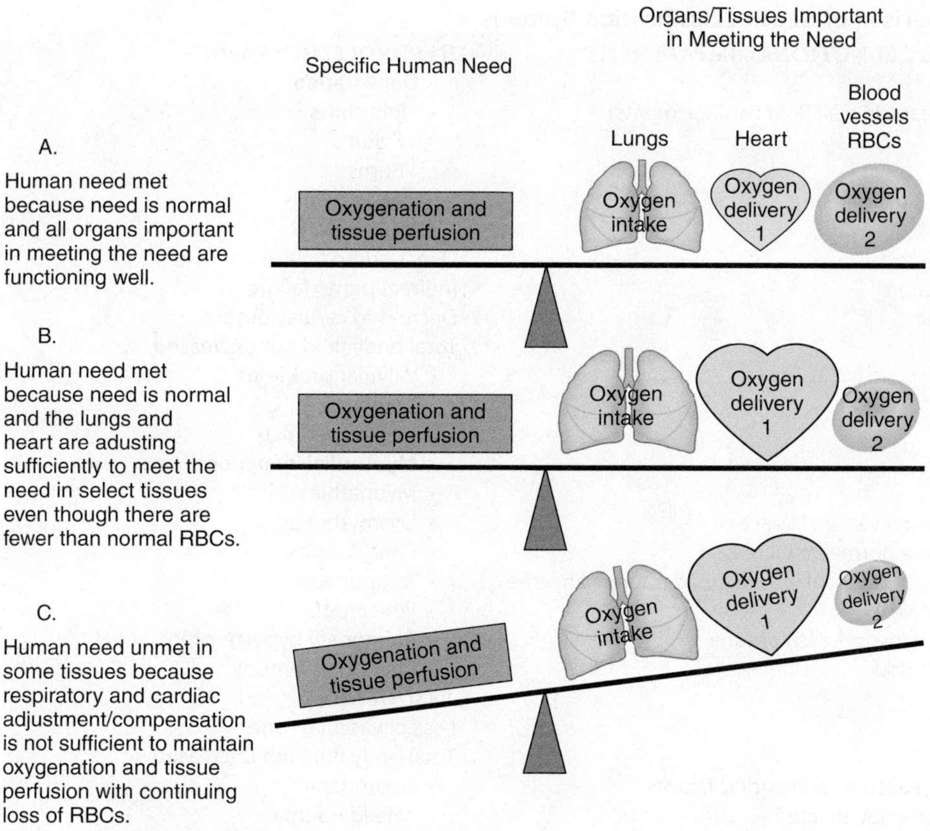
Specific Human Need
Organs/Tissues Important in Meeting the Need
Lungs
Heart
Blood vessels RBCs
A.
Human need met because need is normal and all organs important in meeting the need are functioning well.
Oxygenation and tissue perfusion
Oxygen intake
Oxygen delivery 1
Oxygen delivery 2
B.
Human need met because need is normal and the lungs and heart are adusting sufficiently to meet the need in select tissues even though there are fewer than normal RBCs.
Oxygenation and tissue perfusion
Oxygen intake
Oxygen delivery 1
Oxygen delivery 2
C.
Human need unmet in some tissues because respiratory and cardiac adjustment/compensation is not sufficient to maintain oxygenation and tissue perfusion with continuing loss of RBCs.
Oxygenation and tissue perfusion
Oxygen intake
Oxygen delivery 1
Oxygen delivery 2

Fig. 39-1 • Human need for oxygenation and tissue perfusion affected by hypovolemic shock and adjustment/compensation.

progresses, severe hypoxia can lead to cell loss, multiple organ dysfunction syndrome (MODS), and death.

Shock is usually classified by the functional impairment it causes (hypovolemic shock, cardiogenic shock, distributive shock, and obstructive shock) (Kelley, 2005) or by the origin of the problem (hypovolemic, cardiogenic, vasogenic, and septic shock). Table 39-1 compares both classification systems and common problems leading to each shock category.

Many manifestations of shock are similar regardless of what starts the process or which tissues are affected first. These common manifestations result from physiologic adjustments (adaptive or compensatory mechanisms) made by the sympathetic nervous system, the endocrine system, and the cardiovascular system that attempt to ensure continued oxygenation of vital organs. Manifestations unique to any one type of shock result from specific tissue dysfunction. The common features of shock are listed in Chart 39-1.

Review of Oxygenation and Tissue Perfusion

Oxygenation and tissue perfusion depend on how much oxygen from arterial blood perfuses the tissue. Tissue and organ perfusion is related to mean arterial pressure (MAP). Because the cardiovascular system is a closed but continuous circuit, the factors that influence MAP include:

- Total blood volume
- Cardiac output
- Size of the vascular bed

Total blood volume and cardiac output are directly related to MAP, so increases in either total blood volume or cardiac output *raise* MAP. Decreases in either total blood volume or cardiac output *lower* MAP.

The size of the vascular bed is inversely (negatively) related to MAP. This means that increases in the size of the vascular bed *lower* MAP and decreases *raise* MAP (Fig. 39-2). Blood vessels, especially small arteries and veins connected to capillaries, can increase in diameter by relaxing the smooth muscle in vessel walls **(dilation)** or decrease in diameter by contracting the muscle **(vasoconstriction).** When blood vessels dilate and total blood volume remains the same, blood pressure decreases and blood flow is slower. When blood vessels constrict and total blood volume remains the same, blood pressure increases and blood flow is faster.

Blood vessels contain nerves from the sympathetic division of the autonomic nervous system. Some nerves continuously stimulate vascular smooth muscle so that the blood vessels are normally partially constricted. This state of partial blood vessel constriction is called **sympathetic tone.** Increases in sympathetic stimulation constrict blood vessel smooth muscle even more, raising MAP. Decreases in sympathetic tone relax blood vessel smooth muscle, dilating blood vessels and lowering MAP.

Blood flow to organs varies and adjusts to changes in tissue oxygen needs. The body can selectively increase blood flow to some areas while reducing blood flow to others. Some organs, such as the skin and skeletal muscles, can tolerate low levels of oxygen for hours without dying or being damaged. Other organs (e.g., heart, brain, liver, pancreas) tolerate **hypoxic** (low levels of tissue oxygenation) conditions poorly, and even just

TABLE 39-1 Comparison of Shock Classification Systems

CLASSIFICATION BY FUNCTIONAL IMPAIRMENT	***HYPOVOLEMIC—cont'd***
HYPOVOLEMIC	• Dehydration
Total body fluid decreased (in all fluid compartments)	• Fluid shifts
• Hemorrhage	Trauma
• Dehydration	Burns
CARDIOGENIC	Anaphylaxis
Direct pump failure	***CARDIOGENIC***
Fluid volume not affected	Direct pump failure
• Myocardial infarction	Indirect pump failure
• Valvular problems	Decreased cardiac output
Stenosis	Total body fluid not decreased
Incompetence	• Valvular problems
• Myopathies	Stenosis
• Dysrhythmias	Incompetence
• Cardiac arrest	• Myocardial infarction
DISTRIBUTIVE	• Myopathies
Fluid shifted from central vascular space	• Dysrhythmias
Total body fluid volume normal or increased	• Cardiac arrest
• Neural-induced loss of vascular tone (head trauma, anesthesia, opioids, sedatives)	• Tamponade
• Chemical-induced loss of vascular tone	• Pericarditis
Sepsis (Septic Shock)	• Pulmonary hypertension
Anaphylaxis	• Pulmonary emboli
Capillary leak	***VASOGENIC***
OBSTRUCTIVE	Loss of vascular tone
Cardiac function decreased by noncardiac factors	Total body fluid not decreased
Total body fluid volume not affected	• Neurogenic
Central volume decreased	Head trauma
• Pulmonary hypertension	Vasovagal response
• Tension pneumothorax	Drugs affecting the central nervous system (anesthesia, opioids, sedatives)
• Pericarditis	• Vessel dilation
• Thoracic tumor	Anaphylaxis
• Tamponade	Inflammation
CLASSIFICATION BY SITE OF ORIGIN	***SEPTIC***
HYPOVOLEMIC	Loss of vascular tone
Central vascular volume decreased	Eventual reduced cardiac output
Total body fluid may or may not be decreased	Seen as a more intense type of vasogenic shock
• Hemorrhage	• Infection

a few minutes without adequate oxygen results in serious damage and cell death.

Types of Shock

Types of shock and their causes vary because shock is a manifestation of a pathologic condition rather than a disease state. Specific problems leading to different types of shock are listed in Table 39-2. *More than one type of shock can be present at the same time.* For example, trauma caused by a car crash may trigger hemorrhage (leading to hypovolemic shock) and a myocardial infarction (leading to cardiogenic shock).

Hypovolemic shock occurs when too little circulating blood volume causes a MAP decrease, resulting in the body's total need for oxygen not being met. Common problems leading to hypovolemic shock are hemorrhage (external or internal) and dehydration. A complete discussion of the pathophysiology and management of hypovolemic shock begins on p. 830.

Cardiogenic shock occurs when the actual heart muscle is unhealthy and pumping is directly impaired. Myocardial infarction is the most common cause of direct pump failure. Other causes are listed in Table 39-2. Any type of pump failure decreases cardiac output and MAP. Chapter 40 discusses the pathophysiology and collaborative care for the person with cardiogenic shock due to myocardial infarction.

Distributive shock is the type of shock that occurs when blood volume is not lost from the body but is distributed to the interstitial tissues where it cannot circulate and deliver oxygen. It can be caused by a loss of sympathetic tone, blood vessel dilation, pooling of blood in venous and capillary beds, and increased blood vessel permeability (capillary leak). All these factors can decrease mean arterial pressure (MAP) and may be started by nerve changes (neural-induced) or the presence of chemicals (chemical-induced).

Neural-induced distributive shock is a loss of MAP that occurs when sympathetic nerve impulses controlling blood vessel smooth muscle are decreased and the smooth muscles of blood vessels relax, causing vasodilation. This blood vessel dilation can be a normal local response to injury, but shock results when the vasodilation is widespread or systemic (King & Olson, 2007). Common problems that can cause a systemic loss of sympathetic tone are listed in Table 39-2.

Chart 39-1 KEY FEATURES

Shock

CARDIOVASCULAR MANIFESTATIONS
- Decreased cardiac output
- Increased pulse rate
- Thready pulse
- Decreased blood pressure
- Narrowed pulse pressure
- Postural hypotension
- Low central venous pressure
- Flat neck and hand veins in dependent positions
- Slow capillary refill in nail beds
- Diminished peripheral pulses

RESPIRATORY MANIFESTATIONS
- Increased respiratory rate
- Shallow depth of respirations
- Decreased $Paco_2$
- Decreased Pao_2
- Cyanosis, especially around lips and nail beds

NEUROMUSCULAR MANIFESTATIONS

EARLY
- Anxiety
- Restlessness
- Increased thirst

LATE
- Decreased central nervous system activity (lethargy to coma)
- Generalized muscle weakness
- Diminished or absent deep tendon reflexes
- Sluggish pupillary response to light

RENAL MANIFESTATIONS
- Decreased urine output
- Increased specific gravity
- Sugar and acetone present in urine

INTEGUMENTARY MANIFESTATIONS
- Cool to cold
- Pale to mottled to cyanotic
- Moist, clammy
- Mouth dry; pastelike coating present

GASTROINTESTINAL MANIFESTATIONS
- Decreased motility
- Diminished or absent bowel sounds
- Nausea and vomiting
- Constipation

$Paco_2$, Partial pressure of arterial carbon dioxide; *Pao_2*, partial pressure of arterial oxygen.

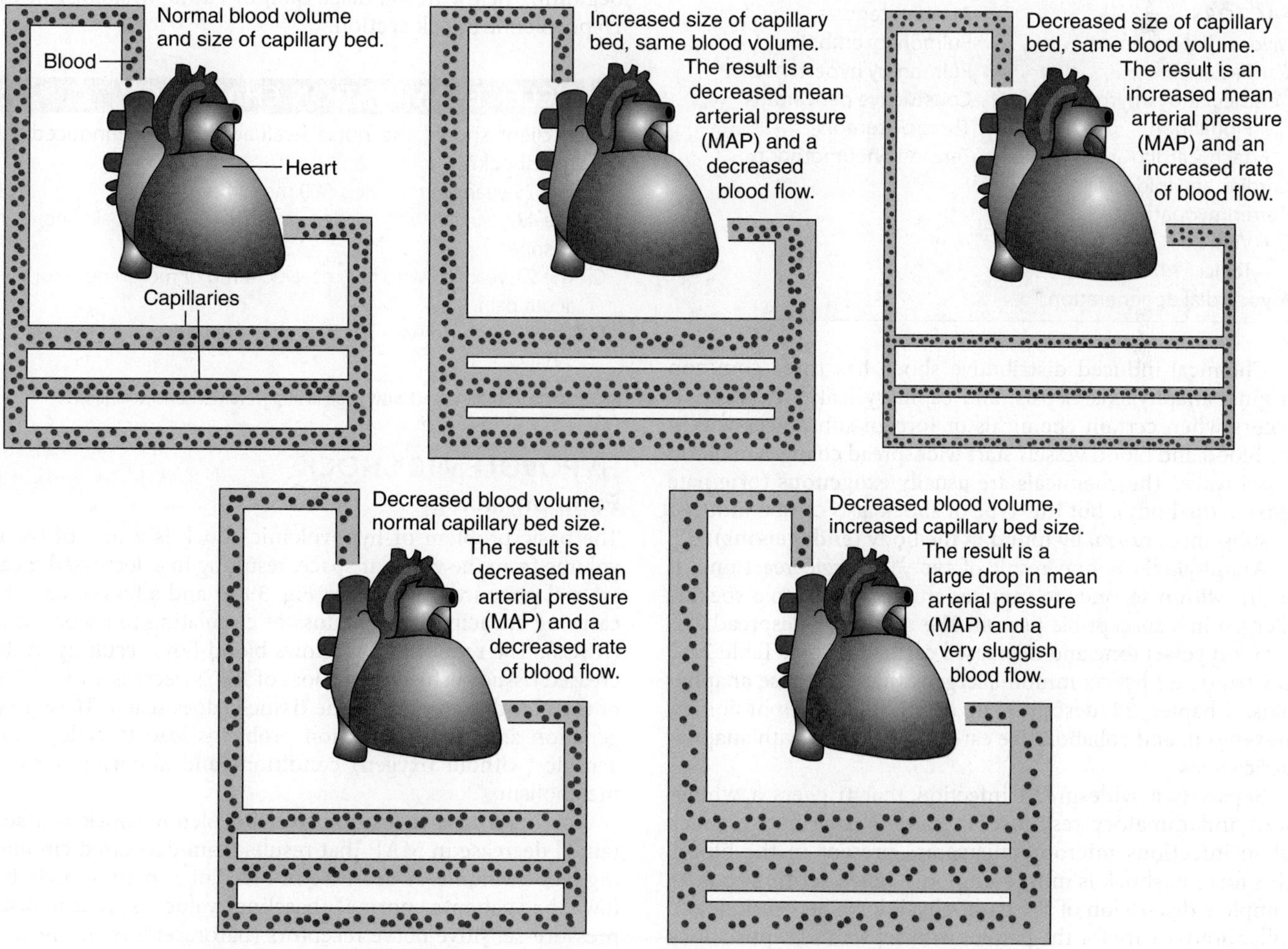
Normal blood volume and size of capillary bed.
Blood
Heart
Capillaries
Increased size of capillary bed, same blood volume. The result is a decreased mean arterial pressure (MAP) and a decreased blood flow.
Decreased size of capillary bed, same blood volume. The result is an increased mean arterial pressure (MAP) and an increased rate of blood flow.
Decreased blood volume, normal capillary bed size. The result is a decreased mean arterial pressure (MAP) and a decreased rate of blood flow.
Decreased blood volume, increased capillary bed size. The result is a large drop in mean arterial pressure (MAP) and a very sluggish blood flow.

Fig. 39-2 • Interaction of blood volume and the size of the capillary bed affecting mean arterial pressure.

TABLE 39-2 Causes of Shock

HYPOVOLEMIC SHOCK ***OVERALL CAUSE*** Body fluid depletion Hemorrhage • Trauma • GI ulcer • Surgery • Inadequate clotting Hemophilia Liver disease Malnutrition Bone marrow suppression Cancer Anticoagulation therapy Dehydration • Vomiting • Diarrhea • Heavy diaphoresis • Diuretic therapy • Nasogastric suction • Diabetes insipidus • Hyperglycemia	**DISTRIBUTIVE SHOCK** ***OVERALL CAUSE*** Decreased vascular volume or tone ***SPECIFIC CAUSE OR RISK FACTORS*** Neural-induced • Pain • Anesthesia • Stress • Spinal cord injury • Head trauma Chemical-induced • Anaphylaxis • Sepsis • Capillary leak Burns Extensive trauma Hepatic dysfunction Hypoproteinemia
CARDIOGENIC SHOCK ***OVERALL CAUSE*** Direct pump failure ***SPECIFIC CAUSE OR RISK FACTORS*** Myocardial infarction Cardiac arrest Ventricular dysrhythmias • Fibrillation • Tachycardia Cardiac amyloidosis Cardiomyopathies • Viral • Toxic Myocardial degeneration	**OBSTRUCTIVE SHOCK** ***OVERALL CAUSE*** Indirect pump failure ***SPECIFIC CAUSE OR RISK FACTORS*** Cardiac tamponade Arterial stenosis Pulmonary embolus Pulmonary hypertension Constrictive pericarditis Thoracic tumors Tension pneumothorax

Chemical-induced distributive shock has three common origins: anaphylaxis, sepsis, and capillary leak syndrome. It occurs when certain chemicals or foreign substances within the blood and blood vessels start widespread changes in blood vessel walls. The chemicals are usually **exogenous** (originate outside the body), but this type of shock also can be induced by substances normally found in the body **(endogenous).**

Anaphylaxis is one result of type I allergic reactions. It begins within seconds to minutes after exposure to a specific allergen in a susceptible person. The result is widespread loss of blood vessel tone and decreased cardiac output. Table 22-2 in Chapter 22 lists common allergens that can cause anaphylaxis. Chapter 22 describes in detail the pathophysiology, prevention, and collaborative care of the patient with anaphylactic shock.

Sepsis is a widespread infection that triggers a whole-body inflammatory response. It leads to distributive shock when infectious microorganisms are present in the blood. This form of shock is most commonly called **septic shock.** A complete discussion of the pathophysiology, prevention, and collaborative care for the patient with sepsis and septic shock begins on p. 838.

Capillary leak syndrome is the response of capillaries to the presence of biologic chemicals (mediators) that change blood vessel integrity and allow fluid to shift from the blood in the vascular space into the interstitial tissues. Once in the interstitial tissue, these fluids are stagnant and cannot deliver oxygen or remove tissue waste products. These fluid shifts result from increased size of capillary pores, loss of plasma osmolarity, and increased hydrostatic pressure in the blood. Problems causing fluid shifts include severe burns, liver disorders, ascites, peritonitis, paralytic ileus, severe malnutrition, large wounds, hyperglycemia, kidney disease, hypoproteinemia, and trauma.

Obstructive shock is caused by problems that impair the ability of the normal heart muscle to pump effectively. The heart itself remains normal, but conditions outside the heart prevent either adequate filling of the heart or adequate contraction of the healthy heart muscle. The most common causes of obstructive shock are pericarditis and cardiac tamponade (see Table 39-2). The assessment and care of the person with cardiac tamponade are presented in detail in Chapter 37 (pericarditis) and Chapter 40 (as a complication after cardiac bypass graft surgery).

Although the causes and initial manifestations associated with the different types of shock vary, eventually the effects of hypotension and ***anaerobic cellular metabolism*** *(metabolism without oxygen) result in the common key features of shock listed in Chart 39-1.* The origin of these features is explained beginning below in the discussion of Pathophysiology in the Hypovolemic Shock section.

NCLEX EXAMINATION CHALLENGE

Which client should the nurse evaluate for neural-induced distributive shock?

A. The 25-year-old receiving 500 mg of penicillin IV.
B. The 47-year-old with sudden-onset severe chest pain and dyspnea.
C. The 21-year-old who has received 4 mg of morphine IV for acute pain.
D. The 82-year-old who has had severe vomiting and diarrhea for 2 days.

evolve For the correct answer, go to http://evolve.elsevier.com/Iggy/.

HYPOVOLEMIC SHOCK

Pathophysiology

The basic problem of hypovolemic shock is a loss of blood volume from the vascular space, resulting in a decreased mean arterial pressure (MAP) (see Fig. 39-2) and a loss of oxygen-carrying capacity from the loss of circulating red blood cells (RBCs). The reduced MAP slows blood flow, resulting in decreased tissue perfusion. The loss of RBCs decreases the ability of the blood to oxygenate the tissue it does reach. These oxygenation and tissue perfusion problems lead to cellular anaerobic (without oxygen) conditions and abnormal cellular metabolism.

The main trigger leading to hypovolemic shock is a sustained decrease in MAP that results from decreased circulating blood volume. A decrease in MAP of 5 to 10 mm Hg below the patient's normal baseline value is detected by pressure-sensitive nerve receptors (baroreceptors) in the aortic arch and carotid sinus. This information is transmitted to

TABLE 39-3 Adaptive Responses and Events During Hypovolemic Shock

INITIAL STAGE
Decrease in baseline mean arterial pressure (MAP) of 5-10 mm Hg
Increased sympathetic stimulation
• Mild vasoconstriction
• Increase in heart rate
NONPROGRESSIVE STAGE
Decrease in MAP of 10-15 mm Hg from the patient's baseline value
Continued sympathetic stimulation
• Moderate vasoconstriction
• Increased heart rate
• Decreased pulse pressure
Chemical compensation
• Renin, aldosterone, and antidiuretic hormone secretion
Increased vasoconstriction
Decreased urine output
Stimulation of the thirst reflex
Some anaerobic metabolism in nonvital organs
• Mild acidosis
• Mild hyperkalemia
PROGRESSIVE STAGE
Decrease in MAP of >20 mm Hg from the patient's baseline value
Anoxia of nonvital organs
Hypoxia of vital organs
Overall metabolism is anaerobic
• Moderate acidosis
• Moderate hyperkalemia
• Tissue ischemia
REFRACTORY STAGE
Severe tissue hypoxia with ischemia and necrosis
Release of myocardial depressant factor from the pancreas
Buildup of toxic metabolites
Multiple organ dysfunction syndrome (MODS)
Death

brain centers, which stimulate adjustments (adaptive or compensatory mechanisms). These mechanisms ensure continued blood flow and oxygen delivery to vital organs while limiting blood flow to less vital areas. Moving oxygenated blood into selected areas while bypassing others ("shunting") causes the manifestations of shock.

If the events that caused the initial decrease in MAP are halted at this point, the adaptive (compensatory) mechanisms can return the body tissues to a normal perfused and oxygenated state, even without outside intervention. If the initiating events continue and MAP decreases further, some tissues function under anaerobic conditions. This condition increases lactic acid levels and other harmful metabolites (e.g., protein-destroying enzymes, oxygen free radicals). These substances cause electrolyte and acid-base imbalances with tissue-damaging effects and depressed heart muscle activity. These effects are temporary and reversible if the cause of shock is corrected within 1 to 2 hours after onset. When shock conditions continue for longer periods without help, the resulting acid-base imbalance, electrolyte imbalances, and increased metabolites cause so much cell damage in vital organs that multiple organ dysfunction syndrome (MODS) occurs and full recovery from shock is no longer possible. Table 39-3 summarizes the adaptive responses and events during the progression of shock.

Stages of Shock

The syndrome of shock progresses in four stages when the conditions that cause shock remain uncorrected and poor cellular oxygenation continues. These stages are:

1. Initial stage
2. Nonprogressive stage
3. Progressive stage
4. Refractory stage

The stages are defined on the basis of how well compensatory mechanisms are working, the severity of the clinical manifestations, and whether tissue damage is reversible.

Initial Stage of Shock (Early Stage)

The **initial** (early) stage of shock is present when the patient's baseline MAP is decreased by less than 10 mm Hg. During this stage, adaptive (compensatory) mechanisms are so effective at returning MAP to normal levels that oxygenated blood flow to all vital organs is maintained. The cellular change in this stage is increased anaerobic metabolism with production of lactic acid, although overall cellular metabolism is still aerobic. The adaptive responses of vascular constriction and increased heart rate are effective, and both cardiac output and MAP are maintained within the normal range. Because vital organ function is not disrupted, the manifestations of shock are difficult to detect. *A heart and respiratory rate increased from the patient's baseline level or a slight* ***increase*** *in diastolic blood pressure may be the only objective manifestation of this early stage of shock.*

Nonprogressive Stage of Shock (Compensatory Stage)

The **nonprogressive** (compensatory) **stage of shock** occurs when MAP decreases by 10 to 15 mm Hg from baseline. Kidney and hormonal adaptive (compensatory) mechanisms are activated because cardiovascular adjustments alone are not enough to maintain MAP and supply needed oxygen to the vital organs.

The kidneys and baroreceptors sense an ongoing decrease in MAP and trigger the release of renin, antidiuretic hormone (ADH), aldosterone, epinephrine, and norepinephrine. Kidney compensation occurs through the actions of renin, aldosterone, and ADH. Renin, secreted by the kidney, starts the reactions to decrease urine output, increase sodium reabsorption, and cause widespread blood vessel constriction (see Fig. 13-6 in Chapter 13). ADH is secreted by the posterior pituitary gland. ADH increases water reabsorption in the kidney, further reducing urine output, and also causes blood vessel constriction in the skin and other less vital tissue areas. Together these actions adapt or adjust (compensate) for shock by maintaining the fluid volume within the central blood vessels.

Tissue hypoxia occurs in nonvital organs (e.g., skin, GI tract) and in the kidney, but it is not great enough to cause permanent damage. Because some metabolism is anaerobic, acid-base and electrolyte changes occur in response to the buildup of metabolites. Changes include **acidosis** (low blood pH) and **hyperkalemia** (increased blood potassium level).

Manifestations of the nonprogressive stage of shock include both subjective and objective changes resulting from decreased tissue perfusion. Subjective changes include thirst sensation and anxiety. Objective changes may include restlessness, tachycardia, increased respiratory rate, decreased urine output, falling systolic blood pressure, rising diastolic blood pressure, narrowing pulse pressure, cool extremities, and a 2% to 5% decrease in oxygen saturation measured by pulse oximetry. *Comparing these changes with the values and manifestations obtained earlier is critical to identifying this stage of shock.*

If the patient is stable and adaptive mechanisms are supported by medical and nursing interventions, he or she can remain in this stage for hours without having permanent damage. *Stopping the conditions that started the shock at this stage and providing supportive interventions can prevent the shock from progressing.* The cellular effects of this stage are reversible when nurses recognize the problem and coordinate with the health care team to start appropriate interventions.

Progressive Stage of Shock (Intermediate Stage)

The **progressive stage of shock** occurs when there is a sustained decrease in MAP of more than 20 mm Hg from baseline. In this stage, adaptive or compensatory mechanisms are functioning but can no longer deliver sufficient oxygen, even to vital organs. In fact, these helpful mechanisms use large amounts of oxygen in some tissues (e.g., the heart), which worsens the problem of general poor oxygenation. Vital organs develop hypoxia, and less vital organs become **anoxic** (no oxygen) and **ischemic** (cell dysfunction or death from lack of oxygen). As a result of poor oxygenation and a buildup of toxic metabolites, some tissues have severe cell damage and die.

Manifestations of the progressive stage of shock include a *worsening* of both subjective and objective changes resulting from decreased tissue perfusion. *Therefore continuous monitoring and comparison with earlier findings is critical at this stage to assess therapy effectiveness.* Subjective changes include severe thirst sensation and deeper anxiety. The patient may express a sense of "something bad" about to happen. He or she may have some immediate confusion. Objective changes are a rapid, weak pulse; low blood pressure; pallor to cyanosis of oral mucous membranes and nail beds; cool and moist skin; anuria; and a 5% to 20% decrease in oxygen saturation measured by pulse oximetry. Laboratory data at this stage may show a low pH, rising lactic acid level, and rising potassium level.

The progressive stage of shock is a life-threatening emergency. Vital organs can tolerate this situation for only a short time before being damaged permanently. Immediate interventions are needed to reverse the effects of this stage of shock. Tolerance varies from person to person and depends on age and pre-existing health. The patient's life usually can be saved if the conditions causing shock are corrected within 1 hour or less of the onset of the progressive stage.

Refractory Stage of Shock (Irreversible Stage)

The **refractory stage** or **irreversible stage** of shock occurs when too much cell death and tissue damage result from too little oxygen reaching the tissues. Vital organs have overwhelming damage. This stage is termed *refractory* because the body can no longer respond effectively to interventions and shock continues. The remaining cells metabolize anaerobically. *Therapy is not effective in saving the patient's life, even if the cause of shock is corrected and MAP temporarily returns to normal.* So much tissue damage has occurred with widespread release of toxic metabolites and destructive enzymes that cell damage in vital organs continues despite aggressive interventions. Manifestations are a rapid loss of consciousness; nonpalpable pulse; cold, mottled, or dusky extremities; slow, shallow respirations; and unmeasurable oxygen saturation.

Multiple Organ Dysfunction Syndrome

The sequence of cell damage caused by the massive release of toxic metabolites and enzymes is termed **multiple organ dysfunction syndrome (MODS).** Once the damage has started, the sequence becomes a vicious cycle as more dead cells break open and release harmful metabolites. The metabolites trigger small clots *(microthrombi)* to form. The clots block tissue oxygenation and damage more cells, thus continuing the devastating cycle. MODS occurs first in the liver, heart, brain, and kidney. The most profound change is damage to the heart muscle. One cause of this damage is the release of myocardial depressant factor (MDF) from the ischemic pancreas.

Etiology

Hypovolemic shock occurs when too little circulating blood volume causes a MAP decrease that results in the body's total need for oxygen not being met. Common problems leading to hypovolemic shock are hemorrhage (external or internal) and dehydration.

Hypovolemic shock caused by external hemorrhage is common after trauma and surgery. Hypovolemic shock caused by internal hemorrhage occurs with blunt trauma, GI ulcers, and poor control of surgical bleeding. External and internal hemorrhage can be caused by any problem that reduces the levels of clotting factors (see Table 39-2). Hypovolemia as a result of dehydration can be caused by any problem that decreases fluid intake or increases fluid loss (see Table 39-2).

Incidence/Prevalence

The exact incidence of hypovolemic shock is not known because it is a response rather than a disease. It is a common complication among hospitalized patients in emergency departments and after surgery or invasive procedures.

Health Promotion and Maintenance

Although hypovolemic shock often occurs as a complication of surgical intervention or trauma, primary prevention is possible. Teach all people to prevent dehydration by having an adequate fluid intake during exercise and when in hot, dry environments. Urge people to prevent trauma and hemorrhage by using proper safety equipment and seat belts and being aware of hazards in the home or workplace.

Secondary prevention of hypovolemic shock is a major nursing responsibility. Keep in mind that just being a patient in the acute care setting is a risk factor. Identify patients at risk for dehydration, and assess for early manifestations. This is especially important for those who have reduced cognition or reduced mobility or who are on NPO status (Mattiace, 2008).

Assess all patients who have invasive procedures or trauma for obvious or occult bleeding. Compare pulse quality and rate with baseline. Compare urine output with fluid intake. Check vital signs for patients who have persistent thirst. Assess for shock in any patient who develops a change in mental status, an increase in pain, or an increase in anxiety. Chart 39-2 lists NIC interventions for the early detection of shock among hospitalized patients.

When patients have invasive procedures or ambulatory surgery and then go home, teach them and their families the manifestations of shock. Stress the importance of seeking immediate help for obvious heavy bleeding, persistent thirst, decreased urine output, light-headedness, or a sense of im-

Chart 39-2 NIC INTERVENTION ACTIVITIES

Prevention of Shock Progression

Shock Prevention: *Detecting and treating a patient for impending shock*

- Monitor for early compensatory shock responses (e.g., normal blood pressure, narrowed pulse pressure, mild orthostatic hypotension [15 to 25 mm Hg], slight delayed capillary refill, pale/cool skin or flushed skin, slight tachypnea, nausea and vomiting, increased thirst, or weakness).
- Monitor possible sources of fluid loss (e.g., chest tube, wound, and nasogastric drainage; diarrhea; vomiting; and increasing abdominal girth and extremity girth, hematemesis, or hematochezia).
- Monitor circulatory status (e.g., blood pressure, skin color, skin temperature, heart sounds, heart rate and rhythm, presence and quality of peripheral pulses, and capillary refill).
- Monitor for signs of inadequate tissue oxygenation (e.g., apprehension, increased anxiety, changes in mental status, agitation, oliguria, and cool, mottled periphery).
- Monitor pulse oximetry.
- Monitor laboratory values, especially Hgb and Hct levels, clotting profile, ABG, lactate level, electrolyte levels, cultures, and chemistry profile.
- Note bruising, petechiae, and condition of mucous membranes.
- Note color, amount, and frequency of stools, vomitus, and nasogastric drainage.
- Test urine for blood, and protein, as appropriate.
- Place patient in supine, legs elevated position.
- Administer IV and/or oral fluids, as appropriate.
- Insert and maintain a large-bore IV access, as appropriate.
- Administer oxygen and/or mechanical ventilation, as appropriate.

NIC intervention activities selected from Bulechek, G.M., Butcher, H.K., & McCloskey Dochterman, J. (Eds.). (2008). *Nursing interventions classification (NIC)* (5th ed.). St. Louis: Mosby.

pending doom (a feeling that something bad is happening or going to happen).

Patient-Centered Collaborative Care

The Concept Map on p. 834 addresses assessment and nursing care issues related to hypovolemic shock.

Assessment

History

Collect data on risk factors and causative factors related to hypovolemic shock. If the patient is alert and stable, question him or her directly. If the patient is not alert or if his or her condition is not stable, collect information from family members. *Age* is important because hypovolemic shock from trauma is more common in young adults and other types of shock are more common in older adults. Ask patients specific questions about recent illness, trauma, procedures, or chronic health problems that may lead to shock. These problems include GI ulcers, general surgery, hemophilia, liver disorders, prolonged vomiting, and prolonged diarrhea. Ask about the use of drugs such as aspirin, diuretics, and antacids that may cause changes leading to hypovolemic shock or may indicate the presence of a problem that can contribute to shock.

Ask about fluid intake and output during the previous 24 hours. *Information about urine output is especially important because urine output is reduced during the first stages of shock, even when fluid intake is normal.*

Assess the patient for obvious signs or factors that can lead to shock. Areas to examine for signs of hemorrhage include the gums, wounds, and sites of dressings, drains, and vascular accesses. Also check *under* the patient for blood. Observe for any swelling or skin discoloration that may indicate an internal hemorrhage.

Physical Assessment/Clinical Manifestations

Most manifestations of hypovolemic shock are caused by the changes resulting from compensatory efforts. **Adaptive** or **compensatory mechanisms** are physiologic adjustments or responses that try to keep an adequate blood flow to vital organs. Signs of shock are first evident as changes in cardiovascular function. As shock progresses, changes in the renal, respiratory, integumentary, musculoskeletal, and central nervous systems become evident. *When a patient is at risk for or is suspected of having hypovolemic shock, a registered nurse should perform the assessment and obtain vital signs rather than a licensed practical nurse/licensed vocational nurse (LPN/LVN) or unlicensed assistive personnel (UAP).* Ensure that vital sign measurements are accurate, and monitor them for trends indicating shock.

Cardiovascular changes that occur with shock start with decreased mean arterial pressure (MAP) leading to adaptive (compensation) responses. Thus the earliest clinical signs of hypovolemic shock are cardiovascular.

Assess the central and peripheral pulses for rate and quality. In the initial stage of hypovolemic shock, the pulse rate increases to keep cardiac output and MAP at normal levels, even though the actual **stroke volume** (amount of blood pumped out from the heart) per beat is decreased. *Increased heart rate is the earliest manifestation of shock.* Because stroke volume is decreased, the peripheral pulses are difficult to palpate and are easily blocked with light pressure. As hypovolemic shock progresses, peripheral pulses may be absent.

Changes in systolic blood pressure are not always present in the initial stage of shock and should not be used as the main indicator of shock presence or progression. When assessing the blood pressure of a patient at risk for shock, consider his or her normal baseline blood pressure. Although a blood pressure of 90/50 mm Hg may indicate severe shock in one person, it may be the normal blood pressure for another healthy adult.

When vasoconstriction is present, diastolic pressure increases but systolic pressure remains the same. As a result, the **pulse pressure,** which is the difference between the systolic and diastolic pressures, is smaller (sometimes called "narrower"). Monitor blood pressure for changes from baseline levels and for changes from the previous measurement. For

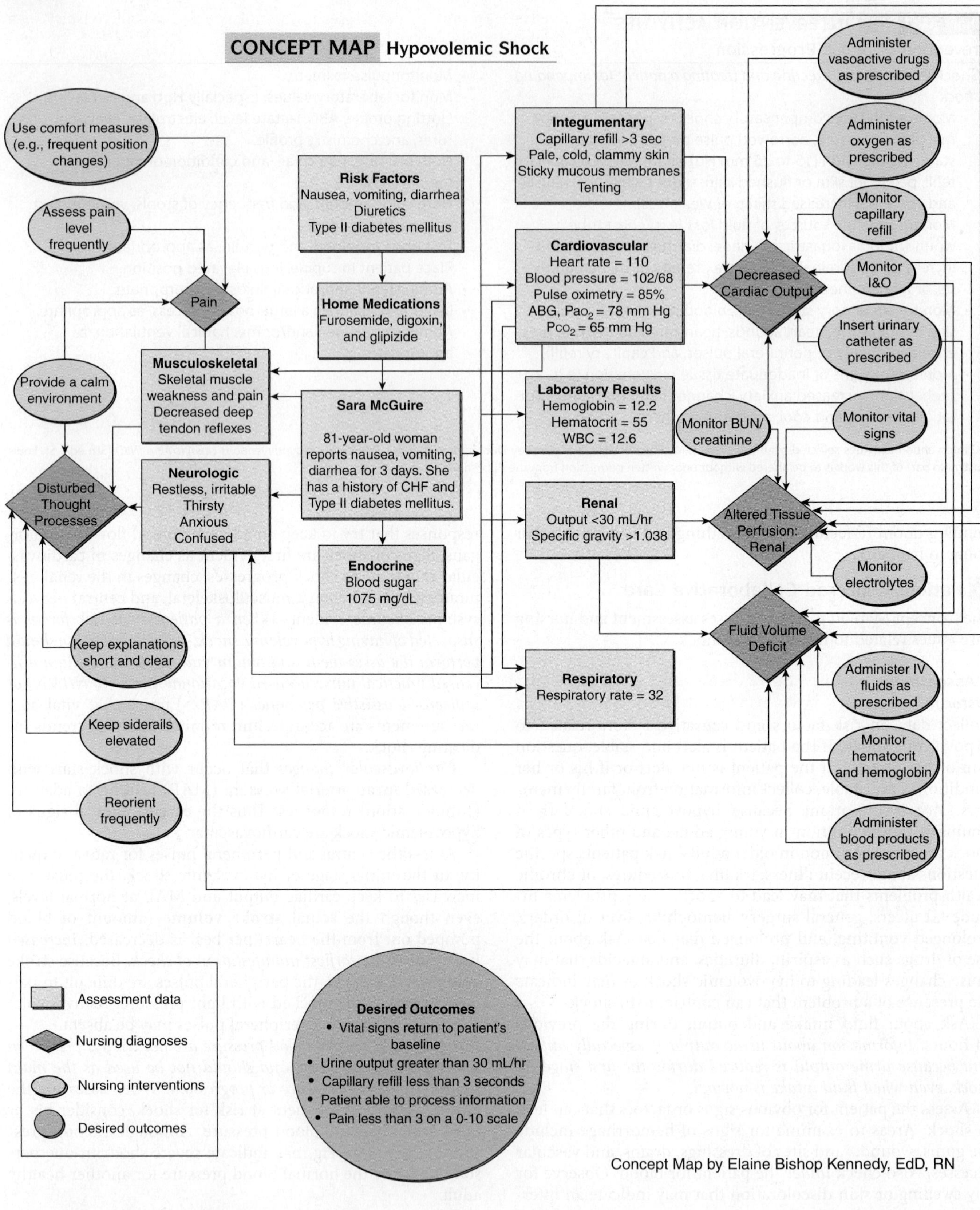
CONCEPT MAP Hypovolemic Shock
Use comfort measures (e.g., frequent position changes)
Assess pain level frequently
Pain
Provide a calm environment
Disturbed Thought Processes
Keep explanations short and clear
Keep siderails elevated
Reorient frequently
Risk Factors
Nausea, vomiting, diarrhea
Diuretics
Type II diabetes mellitus
Home Medications
Furosemide, digoxin, and glipizide
Musculoskeletal
Skeletal muscle weakness and pain
Decreased deep tendon reflexes
Sara McGuire
81-year-old woman reports nausea, vomiting, diarrhea for 3 days. She has a history of CHF and Type II diabetes mellitus.
Neurologic
Restless, irritable
Thirsty
Anxious
Confused
Endocrine
Blood sugar 1075 mg/dL
Integumentary
Capillary refill >3 sec
Pale, cold, clammy skin
Sticky mucous membranes
Tenting
Cardiovascular
Heart rate = 110
Blood pressure = 102/68
Pulse oximetry = 85%
ABG, Pao_2 = 78 mm Hg
Pco_2 = 65 mm Hg
Laboratory Results
Hemoglobin = 12.2
Hematocrit = 55
WBC = 12.6
Renal
Output <30 mL/hr
Specific gravity >1.038
Respiratory
Respiratory rate = 32
Administer vasoactive drugs as prescribed
Administer oxygen as prescribed
Monitor capillary refill
Monitor I&O
Decreased Cardiac Output
Insert urinary catheter as prescribed
Monitor BUN/creatinine
Monitor vital signs
Altered Tissue Perfusion: Renal
Monitor electrolytes
Fluid Volume Deficit
Administer IV fluids as prescribed
Monitor hematocrit and hemoglobin
Administer blood products as prescribed
Assessment data
Nursing diagnoses
Nursing interventions
Desired outcomes
Desired Outcomes
• Vital signs return to patient's baseline
• Urine output greater than 30 mL/hr
• Capillary refill less than 3 seconds
• Patient able to process information
• Pain less than 3 on a 0-10 scale

Concept Map by Elaine Bishop Kennedy, EdD, RN

accuracy, use the same equipment on the same extremity. Validate an electronic reading with a manual reading.

Systolic pressure decreases as shock progresses and cardiac output decreases. A reduced systolic pressure narrows the pulse pressure even further. When shock continues and interventions are not adequate, compensation fails and both systolic and diastolic pressures decrease. At this stage, blood pressure is difficult to hear. Palpation or a Doppler device may be needed to detect the systolic blood pressure.

Oxygen saturation is assessed through pulse oximetry. Pulse oximetry values between 90% and 95% occur with the nonprogressive stage of shock, and values between 75% and

80% occur with the progressive stage of shock. *Any value below 70% is considered a life-threatening emergency and may signal the refractory stage of shock.*

Respiratory changes with shock are an adaptive or compensatory response to help maintain oxygenation when tissue perfusion is decreased. Assess the rate, depth, and ease of respiration, and auscultate the lungs for abnormal breath sounds. Respiratory rate increases during hypovolemic shock to ensure that oxygen intake is increased so that it can be delivered to critical tissues. When shock progresses to the stage at which lactic acidosis is present, the respiratory depth also increases.

Renal and urinary changes occur with shock to adapt or compensate for decreased MAP by saving body water through decreased filtration and increased water reabsorption. Assess urine for volume, color, specific gravity, and the presence of blood or protein. *A decrease in urine output is a sensitive indicator of early shock. Measure urine output at least every hour. In severe shock, urine output is decreased (compared with fluid intake) or even absent.* Of the four vital organs (heart, brain, liver, and kidney), only the kidney can tolerate hypoxia and anoxia for up to 1 hour without permanent damage. When hypoxia or anoxia persists beyond this time, patients are at risk for acute tubular necrosis (ATN) and kidney failure.

Skin changes occur in shock because of reduced blood flow in the skin. An early adaptive or compensatory mechanism for hypovolemic shock is blood vessel constriction in the skin, which reduces skin perfusion. This allows more blood to circulate to the vital organs, which cannot tolerate low oxygen levels.

Assess the skin for temperature, color, and degree of moisture. With shock, it feels cool or cold to the touch and is moist. As shock progresses, color changes are first evident in the mucous membranes and in the skin around the mouth. Pallor or cyanosis is best assessed in the oral mucous membranes in dark-skinned patients. Color changes in patients with lighter skin are noted first in the extremities and then in the central trunk area. The skin feels clammy or moist to the touch, not because sweating increases but because the normal fluid lost through the skin does not evaporate quickly on cold skin (Ecklund & Ecklund, 2007). As shock progresses, skin becomes mottled. Lighter-skinned patients have an overall grayish blue color, and darker-skinned patients appear darker, without an underlying reddish glow.

Evaluate capillary refill time by pressing on the patient's fingernail until it blanches and then observing how fast the nail bed resumes color when pressure is released. Normally the nail bed capillaries resume color as soon as pressure is released. With shock, capillary refill is slow or is sometimes absent. Capillary refill may not be a reliable indicator for peripheral blood flow in older patients or those with anemia, diabetes mellitus, or peripheral vascular disease.

Central nervous system changes with shock often first manifest as thirst. This sensation is caused by stimulation of the thirst centers in the brain in response to decreased blood volume.

Assess the patient's level of consciousness (LOC) and orientation to person, place, and time. Most causes of hypovolemic shock do not interfere with nerve impulse transmission. The central nervous system changes of hypovolemic shock are caused by cerebral hypoxia. In the initial and nonprogressive stages, patients may be restless or agitated and may be anxious or have a feeling of impending doom that has no obvious cause. As hypoxia progresses, confusion and lethargy occur. Lethargy progresses to somnolence and loss of consciousness as cerebral hypoxia worsens.

Skeletal muscle changes during shock are muscle weakness and pain in response to tissue hypoxia and anaerobic metabolism. These are later manifestations of shock. Weakness is generalized and has no specific pattern. The electrolyte changes of shock worsen muscle weakness by decreasing action potentials. Then deep tendon reflexes are decreased or absent.

Assess muscle strength by having the patient squeeze your hand and by trying to keep his or her arms flexed while you attempt to straighten them. Assess deep tendon reflexes by lightly tapping the patellar tendons and Achilles tendons with a reflex hammer and observing the degree of reflexive movement.

Psychosocial Assessment

Changes in mental status and behavior may be early signs of shock. Observe the patient closely, and document behavior. Assess current mental status by evaluating LOC and noting whether the patient is asleep or awake. If the patient is asleep, attempt to awaken him or her and document how easily he or she is aroused. If the patient is awake, determine whether he or she is oriented to person, time, and place. Avoid asking questions that can be answered with a "yes" or a "no" response. Consider these points during assessment:

- Is it necessary to repeat questions to obtain a response?
- Does the response answer the question asked?
- Does the patient have difficulty making word choices?
- Is the patient irritated or upset by the questions?
- Can the patient concentrate on a question long enough to answer appropriately, or is the attention span limited?

If possible, talk with family members to determine whether the patient's behavior and mental status are typical or represent a change.

Laboratory Assessment

Although no single laboratory finding confirms or rules out shock, changes in laboratory data may support the diagnosis of hypovolemic shock. (Chart 39-3 lists common laboratory findings occurring with hypovolemic shock.) As shock progresses, arterial blood gas values become abnormal. The pH decreases, the partial pressure of arterial oxygen (Pao_2) decreases, and the partial pressure of arterial carbon dioxide ($Paco_2$) increases. Changes in other laboratory values may occur with specific causes of hypovolemic shock.

Hematocrit and hemoglobin levels decrease if shock is caused by hemorrhage. When shock is caused by dehydration or a fluid shift, hematocrit and hemoglobin levels are elevated.

▪ Common Nursing Diagnoses and Collaborative Problems

Nursing diagnoses that may apply to patients with hypovolemic shock include:

- Ineffective Tissue Perfusion (General) related to hypovolemia
- Deficient Fluid Volume related to active fluid volume loss
- Decreased Cardiac Output related to hypovolemia
- Anxiety related to potential for death
- Disturbed Thought Processes related to decreased cerebral perfusion

Chart 39-3 LABORATORY PROFILE

Hypovolemic Shock

Test	Normal Range for Adults	Significance of Abnormal Findings
pH (arterial)	7.35-7.45	Decreased: insufficient tissue oxygenation causing anaerobic metabolism and acidosis
Pa_{O_2}	80-100 mm Hg	Decreased: anaerobic metabolism
Pa_{CO_2}	35-45 mm Hg	Increased: anaerobic metabolism
Lactic acid (arterial)	0.3-0.8 mmol/L	Increased: anaerobic metabolism with buildup of metabolites
Hematocrit	*Females:* 37%-47% *Males:* 42%-52%	Increased: fluid shift, dehydration Decreased: hemorrhage
Hemoglobin	*Females:* 12-16 g/dL *Males:* 14-18 g/dL	Increased: fluid shift, dehydration Decreased: hemorrhage
Potassium	3.5-5.0 mEq/L or mmol/L	Increased: dehydration, acidosis

Data from Pagana, K., & Pagana, T. (2002). *Mosby's manual of diagnostic and laboratory tests* (2nd ed.). St. Louis: Mosby.
Pa_{CO_2}, Partial pressure of arterial carbon dioxide; *Pa_{O_2}*, partial pressure of arterial oxygen.

DECISION-MAKING CHALLENGE

Critical Rescue

The patient is a 53-year-old man who had an open reduction of his right forearm after falling from a tree while trimming it. His only health problems are mild hypertension and being 15 pounds underweight for his height. His history includes that he smokes two packs of cigarettes and drinks a six-pack of beer daily. When he comes to the day surgery recovery unit, his vital signs are: BP, 142/90; pulse, 86; respirations, 18; pulse oximetry, 97%. The dressing around his forearm is dry and intact. The fingers of his right hand are warm and pink with good capillary refill. When you call his name, he responds although he does not open his eyes.

1. Are any indications of shock currently present? Provide a rationale for your answer.

It is now 15 minutes later and the patient's BP is 140/92; pulse, 92; respirations, 18. Pulse oximetry is 95%. The dressing is dry and intact, his fingers are slightly cool, and capillary refill is slightly slower than during the previous assessment. He is awake and tells you that his right arm hurts and that he is thirsty. You administer the prescribed analgesic by injection.

2. Are any indications of shock currently present? Provide a rationale for your answer.
3. What should you check regarding the coolness of the fingers?
4. Should you give him sips of water? Why or why not?

In another 15 minutes his vital signs have changed: BP, 132/96; pulse, 100; respirations, 22. He tells you that the pain is much better but that he is very thirsty and feels light-headed and a little nauseated. He then belches twice. His postoperative orders read that the IV can be removed when 1000 mL has infused if he is stable.

5. Are any of the changes in vital signs a cause for concern? If so, which ones?
6. Could the changes in vital signs be related to either his pain or the analgesic? Why or why not?
7. Given his surgery, where should you look for bleeding?
8. Should you remove his IV at this time? Why or why not?
9. Should you wait 15 minutes before retaking his vital signs?

You retake his vital signs in 10 minutes: BP, 106/80; pulse, 112; respirations, 26. Pulse oximetry is 90%. Just as you start to check his capillary refill, he says "Josey (his wife's name), bring me a bucket, I am going to be sick." With that he vomits a large amount of bright red blood.

10. Which vital sign changes are consistent with shock?
11. Which stage of shock is present?
12. What is the most likely cause of the bleeding?
13. Is there anything a nurse could have done differently to identify shock earlier?

evolve For suggested answer guidelines, go to http://evolve.elsevier.com/Iggy/.

Chart 39-4 BEST PRACTICE FOR PATIENT SAFETY & QUALITY CARE

The Patient in Hypovolemic Shock

- Ensure a patent airway.
- Start an IV catheter, or maintain an established catheter.
- Administer oxygen.
- Elevate the patient's feet, keeping his or her head flat or elevated to a 30-degree angle.
- Examine the patient for overt bleeding.
- If overt bleeding is present, apply direct pressure to the site.
- Administer drugs as prescribed.
- Increase the rate of IV fluid delivery.
- Do not leave the patient.

Interventions

Medical and nursing interventions for patients in hypovolemic shock focus on reversing the shock, restoring fluid volume to the normal range, and preventing complications through supportive and drug therapies. The nursing role of monitoring is critical to determine whether the patient is responding to therapy or whether shock is progressing and a change in intervention is needed. Surgery may be needed to correct the problem leading to hypovolemic shock. Chart 39-4 lists best practices for patients in hypovolemic shock.

Nonsurgical Management

The goals of shock management are to maintain tissue oxygenation, increase vascular volume to normal range, and support compensatory mechanisms. Oxygen therapy, fluid replacement therapy, and drug therapy are useful for this problem.

Chart 39-5 COMMON EXAMPLES OF DRUG THERAPY
Hypovolemic Shock

Drug/Usual Dosage	Purpose/Action	Nursing Interventions	Rationales
VASOCONSTRICTORS			
Dopamine (Intropin, Revimine♣) 5-20 mcg/kg/min IV Norepinephrine (Levophed), initial dose 0.5-1 mcg/min IV, to maintain systolic BP between 90 and 100 mm Hg Phenylephrine HCl 0.1-0.5 mg IV every 15 min	Improve blood flow by increasing peripheral resistance, increasing venous return to the heart, and improving myocardial contractility.	Assess the patient for chest pain.	Drug increases myocardial oxygen consumption.
		Monitor urine output hourly.	Higher doses decrease renal perfusion and urine output.
		Assess blood pressure every 15 min.	Hypertension is a sign of overdose.
		Assess the patient for headache.	Headache is an early symptom of drug excess.
		Assess every 30 min for extravasation, and check extremities for color and perfusion.	If the drug gets into the tissues, it can cause severe vasoconstriction, tissue ischemia, and tissue necrosis.
		Assess for chest pain.	Drug can cause rapid onset of vasoconstriction in the myocardium and impair cardiac oxygenation
INOTROPIC AGENTS			
Dobutamine (Dobutrex) 1.0-20 mcg/kg/min IV as a continuous infusion Milrinone (Primacor) 50 mcg/kg bolus over 10 min; 0.3-0.75 mcg/kg/min continuous IV infusion	Drugs directly stimulate adrenergic receptor sites on the heart muscle ($beta_1$ receptors) and improve heart muscle cell contraction.	Assess for chest pain.	Drug increases myocardial oxygen consumption and can cause angina or infarction.
		Assess blood pressure every 15 min.	Hypertension is a sign of overdose.
AGENTS ENHANCING MYOCARDIAL PERFUSION			
Sodium nitroprusside (Nitropress, Nipride♣) 0.25-10 mcg/kg/min IV	Improves blood flow to the myocardium by dilating the coronary arteries. This effect is primary and rapid but short.	Protect drug container from light.	Light degrades drug quickly.
		Assess blood pressure at least every 15 min.	The vasodilating effect can cause systemic vasodilation and hypotension, especially in older adults.

Oxygen therapy is useful whenever shock is present. Oxygen can be delivered by mask, hood, nasal cannula, nasopharyngeal tube, endotracheal tube, or tracheostomy tube. Oxygen is given in liters per minute (L/min) (when using a cannula) or concentration by percentage (when using a mask).

IV therapy or fluid resuscitation is a mainstay of management for hypovolemic shock. Crystalloids and colloids are the two types of fluids used for volume replacement during hypovolemia. Crystalloid solutions contain nonprotein substances (e.g., minerals, salts, sugars). Colloid solutions contain large molecules (usually proteins or starches) (see Chapter 13).

Crystalloid fluids are given to help maintain an adequate fluid and electrolyte balance. Two common solutions are normal saline and Ringer's lactate. Normal saline (0.9% sodium chloride in water) is the fluid replacement solution of choice used to increase plasma volume (Beattie, 2007) and can also be infused with any blood product. Ringer's lactate contains sodium, chloride, calcium, potassium, and lactate dissolved in water. This isotonic solution expands volume, and the lactate buffers any acidosis. *Do not infuse this solution with blood or blood products because the calcium induces clotting of the infusing blood.*

Protein-containing colloid fluids help restore osmotic pressure and fluid volume. Blood and blood products are often used for this purpose when shock is caused by blood loss. These fluids include whole blood, packed red blood cells, plasma, plasma fractions, and synthetic plasma expanders.

Whole blood and packed red blood cells increase hematocrit and hemoglobin levels along with fluid volume. Whole blood is used to replace large volumes of blood loss because it increases volume and improves the oxygen-carrying capacity of the blood. Packed red cells are given for moderate blood loss because they restore the red blood cell deficit and improve oxygen-carrying capacity without adding excessive fluid volume. Chapter 42 discusses nursing care issues when giving blood or blood products.

Human plasma, an acellular blood product containing some clotting factors, is given to restore osmotic pressure when hematocrit and hemoglobin levels are within normal ranges. Plasma protein fractions (e.g., Plasmanate) and synthetic plasma expanders (e.g., hetastarch [hydroxyethyl starch, Hespan]) increase plasma volume and are used as early treatment for hypovolemic shock before a cause has been established.

Drug therapy may be needed if the volume deficit is severe and the patient does not respond sufficiently to the replacement of fluid volume and blood products. The actions of drugs for shock increase venous return, improve cardiac contractility, or improve cardiac perfusion by dilating the coronary vessels (Miller, 2007). Chart 39-5 lists the drugs used to treat hypovolemic shock.

Vasoconstricting drugs stimulate venous return by constricting blood vessels and decreasing venous pooling of blood. These actions increase cardiac output and mean arterial pressure (MAP), which help improve tissue perfusion and oxygenation. Such agents include dopamine (Intropin, Revimine♣) and norepinephrine (Levophed). These drugs can produce serious side effects, and their dosages must be carefully calculated on the basis of the patient's size and response to treatment (Cooper, 2008) (see Chart 39-5).

Inotropic drugs directly stimulate adrenergic receptor sites on the heart muscle ($beta_1$ receptors) and improve heart muscle cell contraction. Thus greater recoil occurs and more blood leaves the left ventricle during contraction. Some of these drugs also stimulate the ventricles. Drugs with these actions include dobutamine (Dobutrex) and milrinone (Primacor).

Drugs enhancing myocardial perfusion help ensure that the heart is well perfused, especially when giving drugs to improve cardiac contraction, so that aerobic metabolism is maintained in the heart cells and maximum contractility can occur. Drugs that dilate coronary blood vessels while minimally dilating systemic vessels are used for this purpose. A common drug with this action is sodium nitroprusside (Nitropress, Nipride♣). *Care is taken because these drugs can cause systemic vasodilation and increase shock if the patient is volume depleted.*

Monitoring vital signs and level of consciousness is a major nursing action to determine the patient's condition and the effectiveness of therapy. Monitor:

- Pulse
- Blood pressure
- Pulse pressure
- Central venous pressure (CVP)
- Respiratory rate
- Skin and mucosal color
- Oxygen saturation
- Mental status
- Urine output

Assess these parameters at least every 15 minutes until the shock is controlled and the patient's condition improves. Hemodynamic monitoring in critical care settings includes intra-arterial monitoring, mixed venous oxygen saturation (Svo_2), pulmonary artery monitoring, and pulmonary capillary wedge pressures.

Insertion of a CVP catheter allows pressure to be monitored in the patient's right atrium or superior vena cava while providing venous access. Changes in CVP reflect hypovolemic shock. As circulating volume decreases, the amount of blood returning to the right atrium also decreases, causing the CVP to decrease from baseline levels.

Intra-arterial catheters allow continuous monitoring of blood pressure and are an access for arterial blood sampling. Intra-arterial catheters are inserted into an artery (radial, brachial, femoral, or dorsalis pedis). The catheter is attached to pressure tubing and a transducer. The transducer converts pressure in the artery into an electrical signal that is seen as a visible waveform on an oscilloscope and as digital numeric value.

Surgical Management

The nonsurgical interventions described on pp. 836-838 are used to stabilize the patient's hemodynamic status. After a cause has been established, surgical intervention may be needed to correct the cause of shock. Such procedures include vascular repair or revision, surgical hemostasis of major wounds, closure of bleeding ulcers, and chemical scarring (chemosclerosis) of varicosities.

Community-Based Care

Hypovolemic shock is a complication of another condition and is resolved before patients are discharged from the acute care setting. Because more patients are receiving treatment on an outpatient basis and are being discharged earlier from acute care settings, especially after surgery and other invasive procedures, more patients at home are at increased risk for hypovolemic shock. Teach patients and family members the early manifestations of shock (increased thirst, decreased urine output, light-headedness, unexplained sense of apprehension) and to seek immediate medical attention if they appear.

SEPSIS AND SEPTIC SHOCK

Pathophysiology

Sepsis and septic shock is a complex type of distributive shock that usually begins as a bacterial or fungal infection and progresses to a dangerous condition over a period of days. The typical progression of septic shock is outlined in Fig. 39-3. *Note that as progression occurs, the pathologic problems occur faster and to a greater degree. Thus control of sepsis and prevention of septic shock through appropriate intervention are easier to achieve early in the course of the syndrome. Failure to recognize and intervene in early sepsis is the major contributing factor for progression to septic shock and death* (Aherns, 2007; Cheek et al., 2005; Kleinpell et al., 2006).

Infection

When infection is confined to a local area, it does not lead to sepsis and shock. As described in Chapter 19, in the person whose immune system and inflammatory responses are effective, the presence of organism invasion first starts a helpful, nonspecific series of local responses to confine and eliminate the organism and to prevent the infection from becoming worse or widespread.

The white blood cells (WBCs) in the area of invasion secrete cytokines to trigger a local inflammatory response and bring more phagocytic WBCs to the area to fight and kill the invading organisms. The results of this local response constrict the small veins and dilate the arterioles in the area of

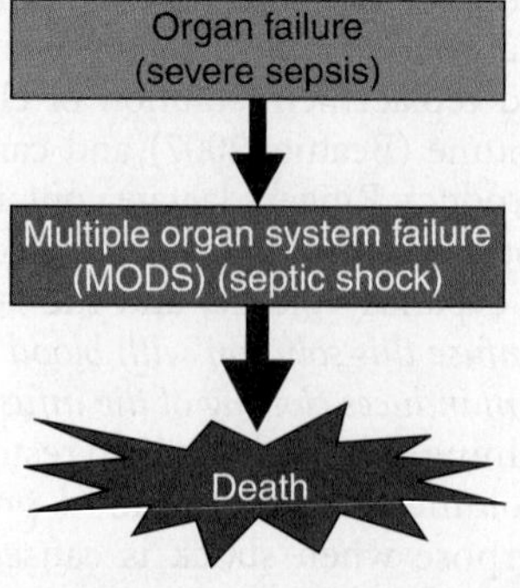
Local infection
Systemic infection
(early sepsis)
SIRS (systemic inflammatory
response syndrome)
Organ failure
(severe sepsis)
Multiple organ system failure
(MODS) (septic shock)
Death

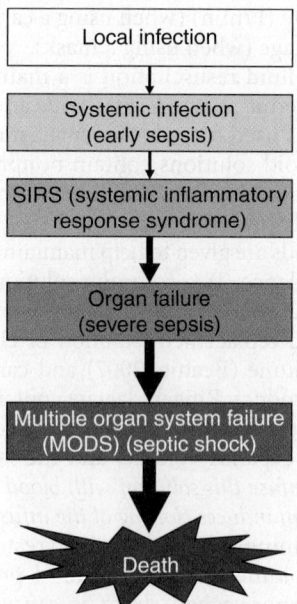

Fig. 39-3 • Common progression of events leading to septic shock.

injury. These blood vessel changes cause redness and warmth of the locally infected tissues and increase blood flow to the area to deliver more nutrients.

Blood flow to the area increases **(hyperemia),** and **edema** (swelling) forms at the site of injury or invasion. Capillary leak also occurs, allowing blood plasma to leak into the tissues. This response causes swelling and pain. Edema at the site of injury or invasion protects the area from further injury by creating a cushion of fluid. The extra fluid also can dilute any toxins or organisms that have entered the area. The duration of these responses depends on the size and severity of the infection, but usually they subside within a few days, when the infection has been managed by these responses. *An important feature of the benefit of these responses is that they are limited only to the area of infection and stop as soon as they are no longer needed.* The patient does not have fever, tachycardia, decreased oxygen saturation, or reduced urine output.

Sepsis

Sepsis is a widespread infection coupled with a more general inflammatory response, known as *systemic inflammatory response syndrome (SIRS),* that is triggered when an infection escapes local control. With the organisms and their toxins or endotoxins in the bloodstream at this point and entering other body areas, the inflammatory responses become an enemy, leading to extensive tissue and vascular changes that further impair oxygenation and tissue perfusion. At the tissue level, the WBCs are producing many pro-inflammatory cytokines, especially interleukin-1 (IL-1), interleukin-6 (IL-6), and tumor necrosis factor-alpha (TNF-A) (Abbas et al., 2007). (See Chapter 19 for a discussion of cytokines.) As a result, there is widespread vasodilation and pooling of blood in some tissues. The patient has mild hypotension, a urine output that is lower than expected for fluid intake, and an increased respiratory rate. These actions result in a hypodynamic state with decreased cardiac output. The patient's temperature can vary depending on the duration of sepsis and on his or her WBC function. Some patients have a low-grade fever and others have a high fever. Still others may have a lower than normal body temperature. The fever and hypotension result directly from SIRS. The reduced urine output and increased respiratory rate are the adaptive (compensatory) responses to impaired oxygenation and tissue perfusion. Usually in this stage, the patient has the elevated WBC count expected with a systemic infection.

Microthrombi begin to form within the capillaries of some organs, causing some cell hypoxia and reducing organ function. This problem is hard to detect, but if sepsis is stopped at this point, the organ damage is completely reversible. The microthrombi increase the number of cells that are operating under anaerobic conditions, which results in the generation of more toxic metabolites. These cause more cell damage and increase the production of pro-inflammatory cytokines, leading to an intensifying or amplification of the SIRS and a vicious repeating cycle of poor oxygenation and tissue perfusion (Fig. 39-4). Although these manifestations are subtle, they do indicate early sepsis and will usually progress unless intervention occurs at this time.

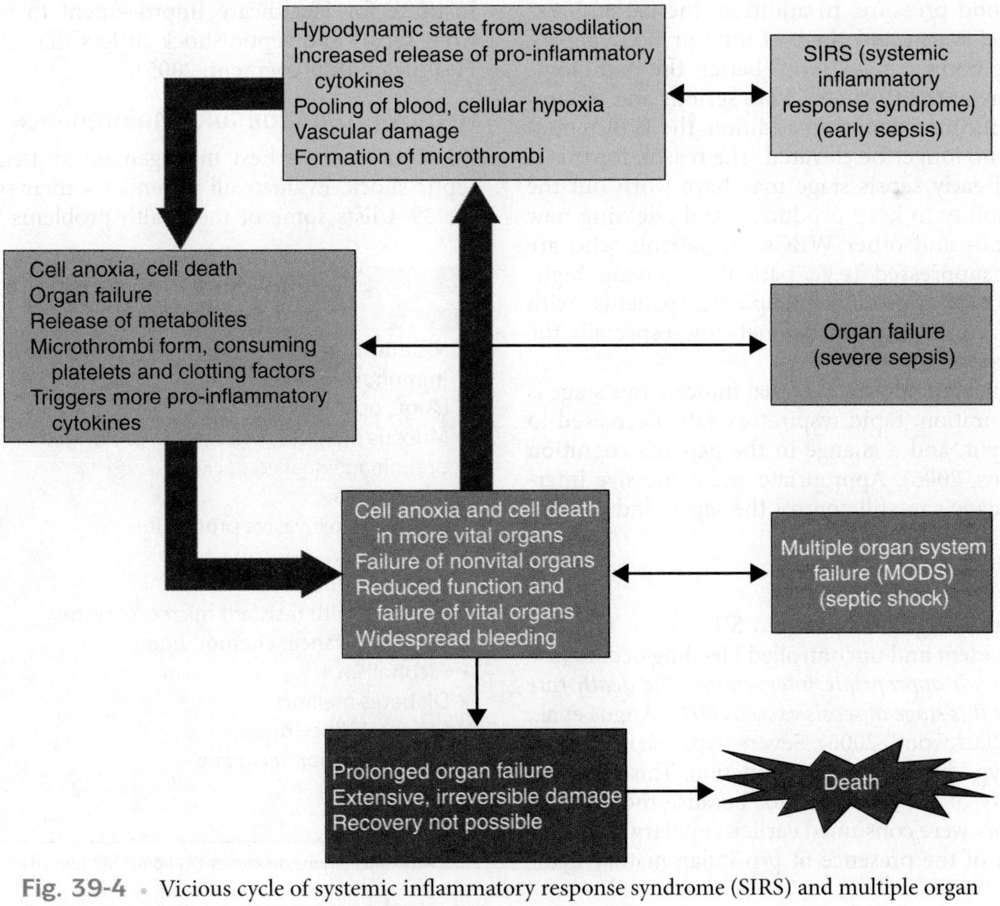
Hypodynamic state from vasodilation
Increased release of pro-inflammatory cytokines
Pooling of blood, cellular hypoxia
Vascular damage
Formation of microthrombi
SIRS (systemic inflammatory response syndrome) (early sepsis)
Cell anoxia, cell death
Organ failure
Release of metabolites
Microthrombi form, consuming platelets and clotting factors
Triggers more pro-inflammatory cytokines
Organ failure (severe sepsis)
Cell anoxia and cell death in more vital organs
Failure of nonvital organs
Reduced function and failure of vital organs
Widespread bleeding
Multiple organ system failure (MODS) (septic shock)
Prolonged organ failure
Extensive, irreversible damage
Recovery not possible
Death

Fig. 39-4 • Vicious cycle of systemic inflammatory response syndrome (SIRS) and multiple organ dysfunction syndrome (MODS) in septic shock.

Unfortunately, this early hypodynamic state has a relatively short duration and can be missed by the patient as well as health care providers. When early sepsis is identified and treated aggressively at this stage, the cycle of progression is stopped and the outcome is good. When early sepsis is not identified and treated at this stage, it almost always progresses to severe sepsis, which is much harder to control.

Severe Sepsis

Severe sepsis is the progression of sepsis with an amplified inflammatory response (see Fig. 39-4). All tissues are involved and all have some degree of hypoxia, although some organs are experiencing cell death and dysfunction at this time. Microthrombi formation is widespread, using much of the available platelets and clotting factors. This condition is known as *disseminated intravascular coagulation (DIC).* In addition, the amplified SIRS and cytokine release increase capillary leakiness, injure cells (especially endothelial cells of blood vessels), and increase cell metabolism. Damage to endothelial cells reduces anticlotting actions and triggers the formation of even more small clots. Anaerobic metabolism continues, and cell uptake of oxygen is poor. In addition, the continued stress response triggers the continued release of glucose from the liver and the patient also has hyperglycemia. The more severe the response, the higher the blood glucose level.

Despite the severity of this stage and the fact that it may be present for 24 hours or more, it is often missed. One of the reasons it may be missed is that the cardiac function is hyperdynamic in this phase. The pooling of blood and the widespread capillary leak stimulate the heart, and cardiac output is *increased* with a more rapid heart rate and an elevated systolic blood pressure. In addition, the patient's extremities may feel warm and there is little or no cyanosis. Even though the patient may "look" better, the pathologic changes occurring at the tissue level are serious and by now have caused significant damage. In addition, the WBC count at this time may no longer be elevated. The reason for this is that a prolonged early sepsis stage may have worn out the bone marrow's ability to keep producing and releasing new mature neutrophils and other WBCs. In patients who are already immunosuppressed (e.g., patients receiving high-dose chemotherapy, transplant recipients, patients with AIDS), the WBC count may be extremely low, especially the segmented neutrophils.

The major clinical manifestations that indicate this stage is lower oxygen saturation, rapid respiratory rate, decreased to absent urine output, and a change in the patient's cognition and affect (Aherns, 2006). Appropriate and aggressive interventions at this stage can still control the sepsis and prevent septic shock.

Septic Shock

Septic shock is the stage of sepsis and SIRS when multiple organ failure is evident and uncontrolled bleeding occurs (see Fig. 39-4). *Even with appropriate intervention, the death rate among patients in this stage of sepsis exceeds 60%* (Angus et al., 2001; Riddell & Blackwood, 2006). Severe hypovolemic shock is present with hypodynamic cardiac function. This is the result of an inability of the blood to clot because the platelets and clotting factors were consumed earlier, capillary leak continues as a result of the presence of pro-inflammatory cytokines, and cardiac contractility is poor from cellular ischemia and the presence of myocardial depressant factor. The clinical manifestations resemble the late stage of hypovolemic shock.

Etiology and Genetic Risk

The major cause of sepsis is a bacterial infection that escapes local control, although in immunocompromised patients, fungal infections also can lead to sepsis. Common organisms causing sepsis include gram-negative bacteria (*Pseudomonas aeruginosa, Escherichia coli,* and *Klebsiella pneumoniae*) and gram-positive bacteria (*Staphylococcus* and *Streptococcus*). Table 39-4 lists some of the health problems that increase the risk for sepsis and septic shock.

Although infection is part of sepsis, some people are at greater risk based on genetic variations. These variations lead to differences in the ability of the immune system to kill or clear microorganisms, as well as differences in how rapidly and to what extent SIRS is triggered (Papathanassoglou et al., 2006). At present it is not feasible to test for these genetic differences, but at some point they will be used to assess risk and modify interventions.

Incidence/Prevalence

Sepsis and septic shock are common events in the United States. More than 750,000 cases occur annually and result in over 200,000 deaths (Angus, 2001). The incidence is increasing as a result of more drug-resistant organisms and the fact that patients are discharged from the hospital "quicker and sicker." Sepsis takes time to develop, and the patient may be discharged before manifestations are obvious. This high incidence has resulted in a nationwide response initiated by the Institute for Healthcare Improvement to reduce death rate from sepsis and septic shock to less than 25% (Institute for Healthcare Improvement, 2005).

Health Promotion and Maintenance

Prevention is the best management strategy for sepsis and septic shock. Evaluate all patients for their risk for sepsis. Table 39-4 lists some of the health problems that increase the

TABLE 39-4 Conditions Predisposing to Sepsis and Septic Shock

- Malnutrition
- Immunosuppression
- Large, open wounds
- Mucous membrane fissures in prolonged contact with bloody or drainage-soaked packing
- GI ischemia
- Exposure to invasive procedures
- Malignancy
- Older than 80 years
- Infection with resistant microorganisms
- Receiving cancer chemotherapy
- Alcoholism
- Diabetes mellitus
- Chronic kidney disease
- Transplantation recipient
- Hepatitis
- HIV/AIDS

AIDS, Acquired immune deficiency syndrome; *HIV,* human immune deficiency.

risk for septic shock. Use aseptic technique during invasive procedures and when working with nonintact skin and mucous membranes in immunocompromised patients. Remove indwelling urinary catheters and IV access lines as soon as they are no longer needed.

Early detection of sepsis before progression to septic shock is a major nursing responsibility. Because sepsis can be a complication of many conditions found in acute care settings, always consider its possibility. Assess vital signs often (at least twice per shift) for changes from baseline levels. Review laboratory data for changes in serum lactate levels, in total WBC count, and in the differential. The hallmark of sepsis is an increasing serum lactate level, a normal or low total WBC count, and a decreasing segmented neutrophil level with a rising band neutrophil level. This change is called a **left shift** (see Chapter 19).

Early detection can be made by patients and families, as well as health care personnel. This is especially important for patients discharged to home after invasive procedures or surgery. Teach patients the manifestations of local infection (local redness, pain, swelling, purulent drainage, loss of function) and of early sepsis (fever, urine output less than intake, lightheadedness). Teach them how to use a thermometer and to take the temperature twice a day and whenever they are not feeling well. Urge those with symptoms of early sepsis to immediately contact their health care provider. Teach them that if antibiotics are prescribed to take these drugs as prescribed and to complete the entire course.

Patient-Centered Collaborative Care

evolve ONLINE PHARM REVIEW

Assessment

Sepsis and septic shock differ from other types of shock in many ways. First, the entire syndrome may occur over many hours to days and the manifestations usually are less obvious. The chance for recovery is good when the patient is recognized as being in early sepsis and appropriate interventions are started. Septic shock, on the other hand, has a rapid downhill course, and chances for recovery are relatively poor. Identifying patients in the earlier stages of sepsis can make the greatest difference in survival. Second, the cause of sepsis is often less obvious than for other types of shock.

History

Collect data about risk factors and causative factors related to septic shock. Age is important because sepsis develops more easily among older, debilitated patients who are immunosuppressed. Chart 39-6 lists factors that increase the older adult's risk for shock. Ask about recent illness, trauma, invasive procedures, or chronic conditions that may lead to sepsis. Check which drugs the patient has used in the past week. Some drugs may directly cause changes leading to shock. Also, a drug regimen may indicate a disease or problem that can contribute to sepsis. These drugs include aspirin and aspirin-containing drugs, antibiotics, and cancer therapy drugs.

Chart 39-6 NURSING FOCUS ON THE OLDER ADULT

Risk Factors for Shock

HYPOVOLEMIC SHOCK
- Diuretic therapy
- Diminished thirst reflex
- Immobility
- Use of aspirin-containing products
- Use of integrative therapies such as *Ginkgo biloba*
- Anticoagulant therapy

CARDIOGENIC SHOCK
- Diabetes mellitus
- Presence of cardiomyopathies

DISTRIBUTIVE SHOCK
- Diminished immune response
- Reduced skin integrity
- Presence of cancer
- Peripheral neuropathy
- Strokes
- Institutionalization (hospital or extended-care facility)
- Malnutrition
- Anemia

OBSTRUCTIVE SHOCK
- Pulmonary hypertension
- Presence of cancer

Physical Assessment/Clinical Manifestations

Manifestations of sepsis and septic shock occur over many hours, and some change during the progression. Table 39-5 summarizes specific manifestations and laboratory changes from normal during the different stages of sepsis and septic shock.

Cardiovascular changes differ in the different stages of sepsis and septic shock. Cardiac output and blood pressure are lower (hypodynamic) in early sepsis and in septic shock. In severe sepsis, cardiac output is higher as are heart rate and blood pressure (hyperdynamic), although this is indication of a worsening condition rather than an improvement. Increased cardiac output is reflected by tachycardia, increased stroke volume, a normal-to-elevated systolic blood pressure, and a normal CVP. Increased cardiac output and vasodilation make the skin color appear normal with pink mucous membranes and the skin may feel warm to the touch. This situation is temporary, and eventually the cardiac output is greatly reduced.

TABLE 39-5 Changes in Selected Parameters During Sepsis and Septic Shock

Parameter	Normal	Early Sepsis	Late Sepsis	Septic Shock
Cardiac output	Normal 3-5 L/min	Decreased	Increased	Greatly decreased
Stroke volume	Normal 60-80 mL	Decreased	Increased	Greatly decreased
Serum lactate (arterial)	<2 mmol/L	Normal to slightly increased	2-4 mmol/L	>4 mmol/L
Blood glucose	<110 mg/dL	110-120 mg/dL	120-150 mg/dL	>150 mg/dL
Oxygen saturation	95%-100%	<95%	<85%	<80%

As sepsis progresses, DIC may occur with formation of thousands of small clots in the tiny capillaries of the liver, kidney, brain, spleen, and heart. These small clots reduce oxygenation in those organs, causing hypoxia and ischemia that may be seen as decreasing oxygen saturation with pulse oximetry.

The huge number of small clots uses clotting factors and fibrinogen faster than they can be produced by the liver. This problem makes patients much more susceptible to hemorrhage, which occurs in the septic shock stage. Coupled with the continued capillary leak, the bleeding causes hypovolemia and cardiac output, blood pressure, and pulse pressure decrease dramatically. The manifestations of this phase are the same as those of the later stages of hypovolemic shock.

Respiratory changes are first caused by the adaptive or compensatory mechanisms to try and maintain oxygenation with a rate increase. As tissue hypoxia becomes more profound and metabolic acidosis is present, the depth of respiration also increases. The lungs are susceptible to damage, and the life-threatening lung complication of acute respiratory distress syndrome (ARDS) may occur in septic shock. ARDS in septic shock is caused by the continued systemic inflammatory response syndrome (SIRS) increasing the formation of oxygen free radicals, which damage the lung cells. Oxygen free radicals also can form as a result of oxygen therapy and in response to release of oxidizing enzymes from damaged cells. *The presence of ARDS in a patient with septic shock has a high mortality rate.*

Skin changes differ at different stages of sepsis. In the hypodynamic stages, blood is shunted away from the skin by vasoconstriction and pallor, cyanosis, or mottling may be present. In the hyperdynamic stage, the skin is warm and no cyanosis is evident. When sepsis progresses to septic shock and circulation is severely compromised, the skin is cool and clammy and pallor, mottling, or cyanosis is present. In patients with DIC, petechiae and ecchymoses can occur anywhere. Blood may ooze from the gums, other mucous membranes, and venipuncture sites, as well as around IV catheters.

A renal urinary change that indicates any type of sepsis or shock problem is urine output that is less than expected considering fluid intake. When a patient who has no known kidney or bladder problem suddenly starts having a low urine output, be suspicious of sepsis or septic shock. The reduced output is caused at first by the capillary leak and low circulating volume. As sepsis progresses and hypoxemia worsens, hormonal changes reduce urine output as does kidney cell dysfunction.

Psychosocial Assessment

The indicator that patients may be in the beginning of severe sepsis is often a change in affect or behavior. Compare the patient's current behavior, verbal responses, and general affect with those assessed earlier in the day or the day before. They may seem just slightly different in their reactions to greetings, comments, or jokes. They may be less patient than usual or act restless or fidgety. Patients may make statements such as, "I feel as if something is wrong, but I don't know what." If this behavior is a change from prior assessments, consider the possibility of sepsis and shock.

Laboratory Assessment

No single laboratory test confirms the presence of sepsis and septic shock. The presence of bacteria in the blood supports the diagnosis of sepsis although this finding may not be present in up to 30% of patients with sepsis (Kleinpell, 2005). Obtain specimens of urine, blood, sputum, and any drainage for culture to identify the causative organisms. Other abnormal laboratory findings that occur with septic shock include changes in the WBC count; the differential leukocyte count may show a left shift. Hematocrit and hemoglobin levels usually do not change until late in septic shock. At that point, the hematocrit and hemoglobin levels, fibrinogen levels, and platelet count are low from the DIC. The serum lactate level is above normal when hypoxemia is severe enough to cause acidosis, and the serum bicarbonate levels are lower than normal. Unfortunately, these parameters may take time to change and cannot be relied on as sensitive indicators of the patient's worsening condition (Aherns, 2007).

Another indicator of sepsis and septic shock is a low blood level of **activated protein C.** This protein is an enzyme that helps prevent inappropriate clot formation. It is activated when it binds to healthy endothelial cells of blood vessels. In sepsis, the endothelial cells injured by endotoxins cannot activate protein C and thousands of small clots form in the capillaries of vascular organs. Decreasing levels of activated protein C indicate the beginning of severe sepsis even before other manifestations are evident.

Other biologic indicators of sepsis and septic shock are changes in plasma D-dimer levels and specific cytokine (interleukin-6 [IL-6] and interleukin-10 [IL-10]) levels. Plasma D-dimer levels rise during sepsis as the fibrin in clots is broken down. IL-6 is a pro-inflammatory cytokine, and IL-10 is an anti-inflammatory cytokine. In sepsis, IL-6 levels rise and IL-10 levels either remain normal or decrease.

The actual diagnosis of sepsis is difficult to make, yet the best outcome depends on an early diagnosis and the imple-

TABLE 39-6 Systemic Inflammatory Response Syndrome (SIRS) Criteria

- Temperature of more than 100.4° F (38° C) or less than 96.8° F (36° C)
- Heart rate of more than 90 beats per minute
- Respiratory rate of more than 20 breaths per minute or a $Pa{CO_2}$ level of less than 32 mm Hg
- Abnormal white blood cell count (>12,000/mm³ or <4000/mm³ or >10% bands)
- Sepsis is considered to be present if two or more SIRS criteria are present along with any known infection and one or more of these clinical manifestations:
  - Hypotension
  - Urine output less than expected for fluid intake
  - Positive fluid balance
  - Decreased capillary refill
  - Hyperglycemia (>120 mg/dL in the absence of known diabetes)
  - Unexplained change in mental status

Modified from American College of Chest Physicians (ACCP) and the Society of Critical Care Medicine (SCCM).

$Pa{CO_2}$, Partial pressure of arterial carbon dioxide.

mentation of appropriate aggressive interventions. In general, sepsis is considered to exist when an infection is present along with any two of the established SIRS criteria, with any one of the additional clinical manifestations (Table 39-6).

Planning and Implementation

A common collaborative problem for patients with septic shock is Potential for Multiple Organ Dysfunction Syndrome (MODS).

NOC Planning: Expected Outcomes

The patient with sepsis or septic shock is expected to have normal aerobic cellular metabolism. Indicators include:

- Arterial blood gases (pH, Pa_{O_2}, and Pa_{CO_2}) within the normal range
- Maintenance of a urine output of at least 20 mL/hr
- Maintenance of mean arterial blood pressure within 10 mm Hg of baseline
- Absence of multiple organ dysfunction syndrome (MODS)
- States measures to reduce the risk for sepsis

Interventions

Interventions for sepsis and septic shock focus on identifying the problem as early as possible, correcting the conditions causing shock, and preventing complications. The Institute for Healthcare Improvement has recommended the use of a sepsis resuscitation bundle for treatment of sepsis. A "bundle" is a group of two or more specific interventions that have been shown to be effective when applied together or in sequence. The sepsis resuscitation bundle and management bundle are presented in Table 39-7.

Oxygen therapy is useful whenever poor tissue perfusion and poor oxygenation are present. Oxygen is delivered in the same ways as for hypovolemic shock. However, the patient with septic shock is most likely to be mechanically ventilated. Care of the patient being mechanically ventilated is discussed in detail in Chapter 34.

Drug therapy to enhance cardiac output and restore vascular volume is essentially the same as that used in hypovolemic shock (see Chart 39-5). In addition, drug therapy is needed to combat sepsis, adrenal insufficiency, hyperglycemia, and clotting problems.

Although septic shock can be caused by any organism, the most common agents are gram-negative bacteria. When blood cultures have identified specific bacteria, IV antibiotics with known activity against the bacteria are given, although antibiotic therapy must begin before organisms are identified, preferably within 1 hour of a sepsis diagnosis (Powers & Jacobi, 2006). Multiple drugs with wide activity are prescribed, based on the site of infection and the most common geographic infections when the actual causative organism is not known. Drugs and drug categories commonly used for septic shock include vancomycin, aminoglycosides, systemic penicillin or cephalosporins, macrolides, and quinolones.

The stress of severe sepsis causes adrenal insufficiency in many patients. Adrenal support involves providing the patient with low-dose corticosteroids during the treatment period for at least 7 days. The most common drugs used for this purpose are IV hydrocortisone and oral fludrocortisone (Florinef).

Patients with sepsis or septic shock usually have elevated blood glucose levels (>150 mg/dL), which is associated with a poor outcome. Insulin therapy is used to maintain blood glucose levels ideally within the upper limits of normal (80 to 110 mg/dL) or at least lower than 150 mg/dL.

During severe sepsis, patients have microvascular abnormalities and form many small clots. In the past, heparin therapy was used to limit unneeded clotting and to prevent the consumption of clotting factors. Current therapy involves the use of activated protein C to manage microvascular abnormalities and prevent bleeding.

Synthetic activated protein C has been shown to stop the inflammatory responses during sepsis, preventing small clot formation and halting the progression of the disorder before

TABLE 39-7 Bundles for Resuscitation and Management of Severe Sepsis

SEPSIS RESUSCITATION BUNDLE

1. Measure serum lactate levels.
2. Obtain blood cultures *before* administering antibiotics.
3. Administer broad-spectrum antibiotic therapy within 1 to 3 hours of establishing diagnosis.
4. If either hypotension or a serum lactate level greater than 4 mmol/L (36 mg/dL) is present, institute:
   a. IV delivery of 20 mL/kg of crystalloid fluids (or the colloid equivalent)
   b. If hypotension does not respond to initial fluid resuscitation by increasing the mean arterial pressure (MAP) to at least 65 mm Hg, start IV vasopressor therapy
5. If hypotension persists despite fluid resuscitation and vasopressor therapy and either septic shock is present or the serum lactate level remains greater than 4 mmol/L (36 mg/dL), use these parameters to monitor therapy effectiveness:
   a. Central venous pressure (CVP) of at least 8 mm Hg
   b. Central venous oxygen saturation (Scv_{O_2}) of at least 70% or a mixed venous oxygen saturation (Sv_{O_2}) of at least 65%

SEPSIS MANAGEMENT BUNDLE

1. When septic shock is present, administer low-dose steroids (200 to 300 mg hydrocortisone IV daily in divided doses) in accordance with intensive care unit (ICU) protocol.
2. Administer drotrecogin alfa (activated) for patients meeting ICU and drotrecogin criteria.
3. Administer insulin to maintain blood glucose levels at least lower than 150 mg/dL.
4. Use mechanical ventilation to maintain inspiratory plateau pressures less than 30 cm H_2O.

Adapted from Institute for Healthcare Improvement and Surviving Sepsis Campaign, 2005.

septic shock occurs. Drotrecogin alfa (Xigris) is the only currently approved drug with this activity. It is given as a continuous infusion over 4 days in patients who are considered at high risk for death (Riddell & Blackwood, 2006). *The drug has many serious complications and, because it disrupts clotting activity, is not given to patients with other bleeding problems.* In addition, the drug is very expensive, with a single dose costing over $7000.

Blood replacement therapy is used when septic shock progresses to hemorrhage. This therapy may involve the use of clotting factors (cryoprecipitate), fresh frozen plasma (FFP), whole blood, or packed red blood cells. Chapter 42 discusses in detail the care of the patient during blood replacement.

Chart 39-7 HOME CARE ASSESSMENT
The Patient at Risk for Sepsis

Assess the patient for any clinical manifestations of infection, including:
- Temperature, pulse, respiration, and blood pressure
- Color of skin and mucous membranes
- The mouth and perianal area for fissures or lesions
- Any nonintact skin area for the presence of exudates, redness, increased warmth, swelling
- Any pain, tenderness, or other discomfort anywhere
- Cough or any other symptoms of a cold or the flu
- Urine; or ask patient whether urine is dark or cloudy, has an odor, or causes pain or burning during urination

Assess patient's and caregiver's adherence to and understanding of infection prevention techniques.

Assess home environment, including:
- General cleanliness
- Kitchen and bathroom facilities, including refrigeration
- Availability and type of soap for handwashing
- Presence of pets, especially cats, rodents, or reptiles

Community-Based Care

Sepsis should be resolved before patients are discharged from the acute care setting. Because more patients are receiving treatment on an outpatient basis and are being discharged earlier from acute care settings, more patients at home are at increased risk for infection and septic shock.

Home Care Management

Evaluate the home environment for safety regarding infection hazards. Note the general cleanliness, especially in the kitchen and bathrooms. Chart 39-7 lists focused patient and environmental assessment data to obtain during a home visit.

Health Teaching

Protecting frail patients from infection and sepsis at home is an important nursing function. Teach about the importance of self-care strategies, such as good hygiene, handwashing, balanced diet, rest and exercise, skin care, and mouth care. If patients or family members do not know how to take a temperature or read a thermometer, teach them and obtain a return demonstration. Teach patients and families to notify the health care provider immediately if fever or other signs of infection appear. General recommendations for Infection Precautions for patients at risk for sepsis are listed in Chart 39-8.

▪ *Evaluation: Outcomes*

Evaluate the care of the patient with sepsis or septic shock. The expected outcome is that the patient will maintain normal aerobic cellular metabolism. Specific indicators for these outcomes are listed for the collaborative problem under the Planning and Implementation section (see earlier).

Chart 39-8 PATIENT AND FAMILY EDUCATION GUIDE
Infection Precautions

- Avoid crowds and other large gatherings of people, who might be ill.
- Do not share eating utensils or personal toilet articles (e.g., toothbrushes, toothpaste, washcloths, deodorant sticks) with others.
- If possible, bathe daily.
- Wash the armpits, groin, genitals, and rectal area at least twice a day with an antimicrobial soap.
- Clean your toothbrush daily by either running it through the dishwasher or rinsing it in liquid laundry bleach.
- Wash your hands thoroughly with an antimicrobial soap before you eat or drink, after touching a pet, after shaking hands with anyone, as soon as you come home from any outing, and after using the toilet.
- Wash dishes between use with hot, sudsy water, or use a dishwasher.
- Do not drink water that has been standing for longer than 15 minutes.
- Do not reuse cups and glasses without washing them.
- Do not change pet litter boxes.
- Take your temperature at least once a day.
- Refrigerate and prepare food appropriately. Do not eat raw or undercooked meat, fish, poultry, or eggs.
- Report any of the following signs or symptoms of infection to your physician immediately:
  - Temperature greater than 100° F (38° C)
  - Persistent cough (with or without sputum)
  - Pus or foul-smelling drainage from any open skin area or normal body opening
  - Presence of a boil or abscess
  - Urine that is cloudy or foul-smelling or causes burning on urination
- Do not dig in the garden or work with houseplants.
- Use antibacterial cleansers to clean kitchen and bathroom surfaces at least twice each week. If you clean these areas yourself, wear rubber or vinyl work gloves while cleaning.
- Use a condom when having sex.
- Take all drugs as prescribed.

HUMAN NEEDS NURSING CARE REVIEW

What might you NOTICE if the patient is experiencing inadequate oxygenation and tissue perfusion as a result of hypovolemic shock?

- Pulse rapid and thready
- Pulse pressure narrowed
- Respirations rapid and shallow
- Oxygen saturation by pulse oximetry decreased
- Skin cyanosis or pallor (lighter-skinned patients)
- Skin cool and clammy
- Cyanosis or pallor of the lips and oral mucous membranes (in patients of any skin color)
- Patient is restless or anxious
- Patient has a urine output that is less than expected compared with fluid intake
- Patient states he or she is thirsty

What should you INTERPRET and how should you RESPOND to a patient experiencing inadequate oxygenation and tissue perfusion as a result hypovolemic shock?

Perform and interpret physical assessment, including:

- Taking vital signs
- Auscultating all lung fields
- Monitoring oxygen saturation by pulse oximetry
- Checking the accuracy of pulse oximetry readings
- Assessing cognition (mini-mental status exam)
- Checking incisions, body orifices, and under the patient for signs of active bleeding
- Assessing the skin for bruises and petechiae
- Examining all body areas for swelling or discoloration that could indicate internal bleeding

Interpret laboratory values:

- Arterial blood gas values: pH lower than 7.35
- Elevated serum lactate levels
- Hemorrhage:
  - Decreased hematocrit and hemoglobin
  - Decreased total red blood cell and platelet counts
- Dehydration:
  - Elevated red blood cell count, hematocrit, and hemoglobin
  - Elevated white blood cell count

Respond by:

- Applying oxygen
- Assisting the patient to shock position (head and chest flat or elevated to no more than 30 degrees; legs elevated)
- Notifying the Rapid Response Team
- Ensuring placement of venous access
- Increasing IV fluid infusion rate

On what should you REFLECT?

- Observe patient for evidence of improved circulation and oxygenation (see Chapter 35).
- Think about what may have caused the hypovolemia.
- Think about how the nurse may have identified the problem sooner.

GET READY FOR THE NCLEX EXAMINATION!

Key Points

Review these Key Points for each NCLEX Examination Client Needs Category.

Safe and Effective Care Environment

- Use strict aseptic techniques when performing invasive procedures, changing dressings, and handling nonintact skin.
- Use good handwashing techniques before providing any care to a patient who is either immunocompromised or immune deficient.

Health Promotion and Maintenance

- Identify patients at high risk for infection due to age, disease, work environment, or leisure activities.
- Teach the patient and family about the clinical manifestations of infection and when to seek medical advice.

Psychosocial Integrity

- Assess all patients at risk for shock for a change in affect, reduced cognition, altered level of consciousness, and increased anxiety.
- Stay with the patient in shock.
- Explain all diagnostic and treatment procedures to the patient and family.
- Reassure patients who are in shock that the appropriate interventions are being instituted.

Physiological Integrity

- Assess the immunocompromised patient every shift for infection.
- Assess the skin integrity of the patient with reduced immune function at least every shift.
- Immediately assess vital signs of patients who have a change in level of consciousness, increased thirst, or anxiety.
- Assess for changes in pulse rate and quality rather than blood pressure as an indicator of shock.
- Give oxygen to any patient in shock.
- Assess hourly urine output to evaluate adequacy of treatment for hypovolemic shock.

Additional Study Resources

Go to your Companion CD or Evolve at http://evolve.elsevier.com/Iggy/ for *Self-Assessment Questions for the NCLEX Examination.*

Go to Evolve at http://evolve.elsevier.com/Iggy/ for *Prioritization and Delegation Questions for the NCLEX Examination.*

SELECTED BIBLIOGRAPHY

Asterisk indicates a classic or definitive work on this subject.

Abbas, A., Lichtman, A., & Pillai, S. (2007). *Cellular and molecular immunology* (6th ed.). Philadelphia: Saunders.

Aherns, T. (2006). Hemodynamics in sepsis. *AACN Advanced Critical Care, 17*(4), 435-445.

Aherns, T. (2007). Sepsis: Stopping an insidious killer. *American Nurse Today, 2*(1), 36-39.

*Angus, D., Linde-Zwirble, W., Lidicker, J., Clermanit, G., Carcillo, J., & Pinsky, M. (2001). Epidemiology of severe sepsis in the United States: Analysis of incidence, outcome, and associated costs of care. *Critical Care Medicine, 29*(7), 1303-1310.

Atkinson, M., & Ryzner, D. (2007). Sepsis signposts: Can you spot them? *American Nurse Today, 2*(10), 20-22.

Beattie, S. (2007). Bedside emergency: Hemorrhage. *RN, 70*(8), 30-34.

Bridges, E., & Dukes, S. (2005). Cardiovascular aspects of septic shock: Pathophysiology, monitoring, and treatment. *Critical Care Nurse, 25*(2), 14-40.

Cheek, D.J., McGehee-Smith, H., Cunneen, J., & Cartwright, M. (2005). Sepsis: Taking a deeper look. *Nursing2005, 35*(1), 38-42.

Cooper, B. (2008). Review and update on inotropes and vasopressors. *AACN Advanced Critical Care, 19*(1), 5-15.

Duhon, J. (2006). When organs fail one by one. *RN, 69*(5), 44-49.

Ecklund, M., & Ecklund, C. (2007). How to recognize and respond to hypovolemic shock. *American Nurse Today, 2*(4), 28-31.

Giuliano, K. (2007). Physiological monitoring for critically ill patients: Testing a predictive model for the early detection of sepsis. *American Journal of Critical Care, 16*(2), 122-131.

Institute for Healthcare Improvement. (2005). *Critical care: Sepsis bundle.* Retrieved February 2008, from www.ihi.org.

Kelley, D. (2005). Hypovolemic shock: An overview. *Critical Care Nursing Quarterly, 28*(1), 2-19.

King, K., & Olson, D. (2007). What you should know about neurogenic shock. *American Nurse Today, 2*(2), 36-39.

Kleinpell, R. (2005). Working out the complexities of severe sepsis. *The Nurse Practitioner, 30*(4), 43-48.

Kleinpell, R., Graves, B., & Ackerman, M. (2006). Incidence, pathogenesis, and management of sepsis. *AACN Advanced Critical Care, 17*(4), 385-393.

Laskowski-Jones, L. (2006). First aid for bleeding wounds. *Nursing2006, 36*(9), 50-51.

Lee, C. (2006). Role of exogenous arginine vasopressin in the management of catecholamine refractory septic shock. *Critical Care Nurse, 26*(6), 17-23.

Mattiace, R. (2008). Preventing hypovolemic shock. *American Nurse Today, 3*(3), 28.

McCance, K., & Huether, S. (2006). *Pathophysiology: The biologic basis for disease in adults and children* (5th ed.). St. Louis: Mosby.

Miller, J. (2007). Keeping your patient hemodynamically stable. *Nursing2007, 37*(5), 36-41.

Pagana, K., & Pagana, T. (2006). *Mosby's manual of diagnostic and laboratory tests* (3rd ed.). St. Louis: Mosby.

Papathanassoglou, E., Giannakopoulou, M., & Bozas, E. (2006). Genomic variations and susceptibility to sepsis. *AACN Advanced Critical Care, 17*(4), 395-422.

Powers, J., & Jacobi, J. (2006). Pharmacologic treatment related to severe sepsis. *AACN Advanced Critical Care, 17*(4), 423-432.

Riddell, A., & Blackwood, B. (2006). Severe sepsis: Patient management focusing on administration of drotrecogin alfa (activated) infusion. *Nursing in Critical Care, 11*(1), 7-15.

*Stengle, J., & Dries, D. (1994). Sepsis in the elderly. *Critical Care Nursing Clinics of North America, 6*(2), 421-427.

Todd, B. (2006). Preventing bloodstream infection. *AJN, 106*(1), 29-30.

Wood, S., Lavieri, M., & Durkin, T. (2007). What you need to know about sepsis. *Nursing2007, 37*(3), 46-51.

Care of Patients with Acute Coronary Syndromes

40
CHAPTER

Vicki Brownrigg • Sharon Henry Walicek • Donna D. Ignatavicius

LEARNING OUTCOMES

For clinical competence and success on the NCLEX Examination, study this chapter with these Learning Outcomes in mind:

Safe and Effective Care Environment

1. Maintain continuity of care between health care agencies or hospital and home when discharging patients who have had cardiac interventions or surgeries.

Health Promotion and Maintenance

2. Encourage patient participation in cardiovascular risk modification programs and lifestyle changes.
3. Provide care that meets the special needs of older adults having coronary artery bypass graft (CABG) surgery.

Psychosocial Integrity

4. Assess patient and family responses to acute coronary events, especially myocardial infarction (MI).

Physiological Integrity

5. Compare and contrast the clinical manifestations of stable angina, unstable angina, and MI.
6. Differentiate between modifiable and nonmodifiable risk factors for coronary artery disease (CAD).
7. Interpret physical and diagnostic assessment findings in patients who have CAD.
8. Prioritize nursing care for patients who have chest pain.
9. Teach patients and families about drug therapy for CAD.
10. Explain the nursing care for patients who have thrombolysis for an MI.
11. Develop a plan of care for the patient who has a percutaneous transluminal coronary angioplasty.
12. Provide postoperative care for the patient who has CABG surgery.
13. Differentiate between traditional CABG surgery, minimally invasive direct coronary artery bypass, off-pump CABG, and transmyocardial laser revascularization.

Go to your Companion CD or Evolve at http://evolve.elsevier.com/Iggy/ for *Self-Assessment Questions for the NCLEX Examination* keyed to these Learning Outcomes.

Coronary artery disease (CAD), also called *coronary heart disease (CHD)* or simply *heart disease,* is the single largest killer of American men and women in all ethnic groups. When the arteries that supply the myocardium (heart muscle) are diseased, the heart cannot pump blood effectively to adequately perfuse vital organs and peripheral tissues. The organs and tissues need oxygen in arterial blood for survival. When *oxygenation* and *perfusion* are impaired, the patient can have life-threatening clinical manifestations and possibly death.

The incidence of CAD has declined over the past decade. This decline is due to many factors, including increasingly effective treatment and an increased awareness and emphasis on reducing major cardiovascular risk factors (e.g., hypertension, smoking, high cholesterol). Some coronary events occur in patients without traditional risk factors.

Pathophysiology

Coronary artery disease (CAD) is a broad term that includes chronic stable angina and acute coronary syndromes. It affects the arteries that provide blood, oxygen, and nutrients to the myocardium. When blood flow through the coronary arteries is partially or completely blocked, ischemia and infarction of the myocardium may result. Ischemia occurs when *insufficient oxygen* is supplied to meet the requirements of the myocardium. **Infarction** (necrosis, or cell death) occurs when severe ischemia is prolonged and *decreased perfusion* causes irreversible damage to tissue.

Chronic Stable Angina Pectoris

Angina pectoris means "strangling of the chest." It is caused by a temporary imbalance between the coronary arteries' ability to supply oxygen and the cardiac muscle's demand for *oxy-*

gen. ***Ischemia*** *(lack of oxygen) that occurs with angina is limited in duration and does not cause permanent damage of myocardial tissue.*

Angina may be of two main types: stable angina and unstable angina. **Chronic stable angina (CSA)** is chest discomfort that occurs with moderate to prolonged exertion in a pattern that is familiar to the patient. The frequency, duration, and intensity of symptoms remain the same over several months. CSA results in only slight limitation of activity and is usually associated with a *fixed* atherosclerotic plaque. It is usually relieved by nitroglycerin or rest and often is managed with drug therapy. Rarely does CSA require aggressive treatment. Unstable angina is discussed in the following Acute Coronary Syndromes section.

Acute Coronary Syndromes

The term **acute coronary syndrome (ACS)** is used to describe patients who have either *unstable* angina or an acute myocardial infarction. In ACS, it is believed that the atherosclerotic plaque in the coronary artery *ruptures,* resulting in platelet aggregation ("clumping"), thrombus (clot) formation, and vasoconstriction (Fig. 40-1). The amount of disruption of the atherosclerotic plaque determines the degree of coronary artery obstruction (blockage) and the specific disease process. The artery has to have at least 40% plaque accumulation before it starts to block blood flow.

Historically, an acute myocardial infarction (MI) was diagnosed by the presence of ST-segment elevation on the 12-lead electrocardiogram (ECG) (see discussion of the normal ECG

◀ ANIMATION: Acute Coronary Syndrome

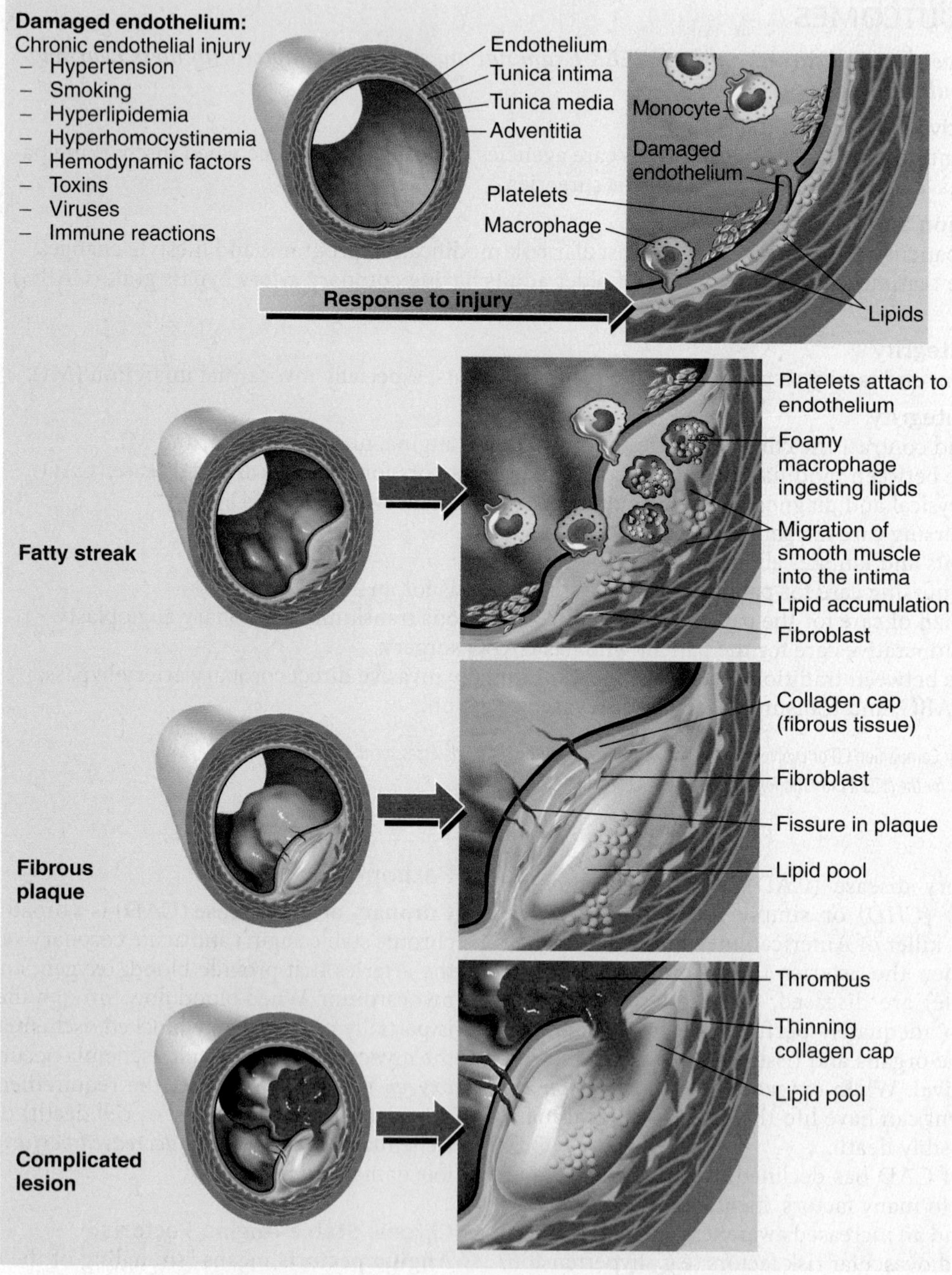

Damaged endothelium:
Chronic endothelial injury
– Hypertension
– Smoking
– Hyperlipidemia
– Hyperhomocystinemia
– Hemodynamic factors
– Toxins
– Viruses
– Immune reactions
Endothelium
Tunica intima
Tunica media
Adventitia
Monocyte
Damaged endothelium
Platelets
Macrophage
Lipids
Response to injury
Platelets attach to endothelium
Foamy macrophage ingesting lipids
Migration of smooth muscle into the intima
Lipid accumulation
Fibroblast
Fatty streak
Collagen cap (fibrous tissue)
Fibroblast
Fissure in plaque
Lipid pool
Fibrous plaque
Thrombus
Thinning collagen cap
Lipid pool
Complicated lesion

Fig. 40-1 • A cross section of an atherosclerotic coronary artery.

in Chapter 36). However, all patients do not present with this finding. Instead, they are classified into one of three categories according to the presence or absence of ST-segment elevation on the ECG and positive troponin markers (see Chapter 35 for discussion of troponins):

- ST-elevation MI (STEMI) (traditional manifestation)
- Non–ST-elevation MI (NSTEMI) (common in women)
- Unstable angina

Between 10% and 30% of patients with *unstable* angina progress to having an MI in 1 year, and 29% die of MI in 5 years (American Heart Association [AHA], 2008).

Unstable Angina Pectoris

Unstable angina (the most commonly used term) is chest pain or discomfort that occurs at rest or with exertion and causes severe activity limitation. An increase in the number of attacks and in the intensity of the pain indicates unstable angina. The pain may last longer than 15 minutes or may be poorly relieved by rest or nitroglycerin. Unstable angina describes a variety of disorders, including *new-onset angina, variant (Prinzmetal's) angina,* and *pre-infarction angina.*

New-onset angina describes the patient who has his or her first angina symptoms, usually after exertion or other increased demands on the heart. **Variant (Prinzmetal's) angina** is chest pain or discomfort resulting from coronary artery spasm and typically occurs after rest. **Pre-infarction angina** refers to chest pain that occurs in the days or weeks before an MI.

Myocardial Infarction

The most serious acute coronary syndrome is myocardial infarction (MI), often referred to as *acute MI* or *AMI.* Undiagnosed or untreated angina can lead to this very serious health problem.

Myocardial infarction (MI) occurs when myocardial tissue is abruptly and severely deprived of oxygen. When blood flow is quickly reduced by 80% to 90%, ischemia develops. Ischemia can lead to injury and necrosis of myocardial tissue if blood flow is not restored. Most MIs are the result of atherosclerosis of a coronary artery, rupture of the plaque, subsequent thrombosis, and **occlusion** (blockage) of blood flow. Other factors may be involved, however, such as coronary artery spasm, platelet aggregation, and emboli from mural thrombi (thrombi lining the walls of the cardiac chambers).

Often MIs begin with infarction (necrosis) of the subendocardial layer of cardiac muscle. This layer has the longest myofibrils in the heart, the greatest *oxygen* demand, and the poorest *oxygen* supply. Around the initial area of infarction (zone of necrosis) in the subendocardium are two other zones: (1) the zone of injury, tissue that is injured but not necrotic; and (2) the zone of ischemia, tissue that is oxygen deprived. This pattern is illustrated in Fig. 40-2.

Infarction is a dynamic process that does not occur instantly. Rather, it evolves over a period of several hours. **Hypoxia** (decreased oxygen) from ischemia may lead to local vasodilation of blood vessels and acidosis. Potassium, calcium, and magnesium imbalances, as well as acidosis at the cellular level, may lead to changes in normal conduction and contractile functions. Catecholamines (epinephrine and norepinephrine) released in response to hypoxia and pain may increase the heart's rate, contractility, and afterload. These factors increase *oxygen* requirements in tissue that is already oxygen deprived.

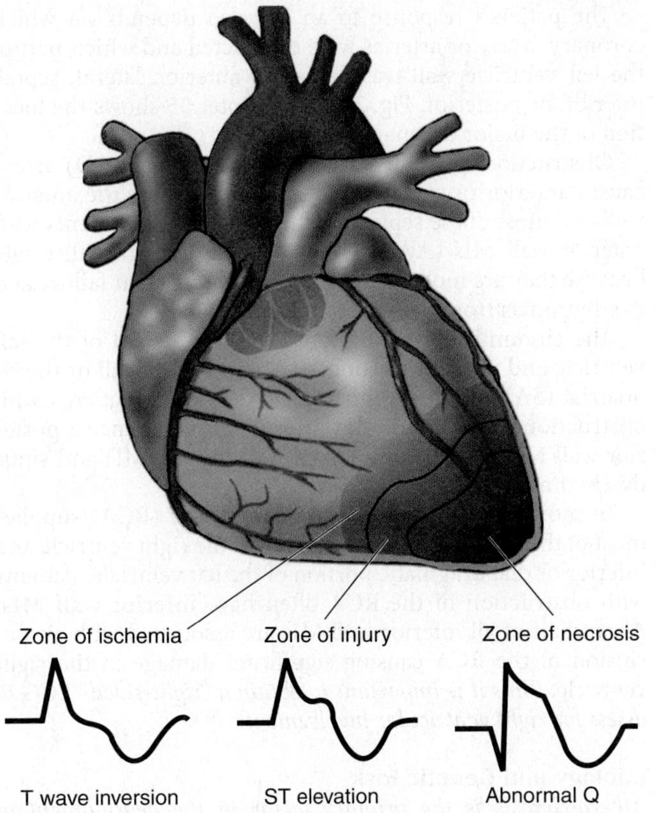

Zone of ischemia
Zone of injury
Zone of necrosis
T wave inversion
ST elevation
Abnormal Q

Fig. 40-2 • Electrocardiographic changes and patterns associated with myocardial infarction.

This may lead to life-threatening ventricular dysrhythmias. The area of infarction may extend into the zones of injury and ischemia. The actual extent of the zone of infarction depends on three factors: collateral circulation, anaerobic metabolism, and workload demands on the myocardium.

The infarction may involve only the subendocardium (called a **subendocardial MI**) or may spread to the epicardium or to all three layers of cardiac muscle. When all three layers are involved, the MI is termed **transmural.** Subendocardial MIs have less effect on wall motion and cardiac output than do transmural infarctions. When fewer grams of myocardium are affected, the characteristic "Q" wave on the ECG, which may also indicate an old infarction, may not appear.

Obvious physical changes do not occur in the heart until 6 hours after the infarction, when the infarcted region appears blue and swollen. *These changes explain the need for intervention within the first 4 to 6 hours of symptom onset.* After 48 hours, the infarcted area turns gray with yellow streaks as neutrophils invade the tissue and begin to remove the necrotic cells. By 8 to 10 days after infarction, granulation tissue forms at the edges of the necrotic tissue. Over a 2- to 3-month period, the necrotic area eventually develops into a shrunken, thin, firm scar. Scar tissue permanently changes the size and shape of the entire left ventricle **(ventricular remodeling).** Remodeling may decrease left ventricular function, cause heart failure, and increase morbidity and mortality. The scarred tissue does not contract nor does it conduct electrically. Thus this area is often the cause of chronic ventricular dysrhythmias surrounding the infarcted zone.

The patient's response to an MI also depends on which coronary artery or arteries were obstructed and which part of the left ventricle wall was damaged: anterior, lateral, septal, inferior, or posterior. Fig. 35-3 in Chapter 35 shows the location of the major coronary arteries.

Obstruction of the left anterior descending (LAD) artery causes anterior or septal MIs because it perfuses the anterior wall and most of the septum of the left ventricle. Patients with anterior wall MIs (AWMIs) have the highest mortality rate because they are most likely to have left ventricular failure and dysrhythmias from damage to the left ventricle.

The circumflex artery supplies the lateral wall of the left ventricle and possibly portions of the posterior wall or the sinoatrial (SA) and atrioventricular (AV) nodes. Patients with obstruction of the circumflex artery may experience a posterior wall MI (PWMI) or a lateral wall MI (LWMI) and sinus dysrhythmias.

In most people, the right coronary artery (RCA) supplies most of the SA and AV nodes, as well as the right ventricle and inferior or diaphragmatic portion of the left ventricle. Patients with obstruction of the RCA often have **inferior wall MIs.** About half of all inferior wall MIs are associated with an occlusion of the RCA causing significant damage to the right ventricle. *Thus it is important to obtain a "right-sided" ECG to assess for right ventricular involvement.*

Etiology and Genetic Risk

Atherosclerosis is the primary factor in the development of CAD. Numerous risk factors contribute to atherosclerosis and subsequently to CAD (also see Chapter 38).

Nonmodifiable risk factors are personal characteristics that cannot be altered or controlled. These risk factors, which interact with each other, include age, gender, family history, and ethnic background. People with a family history of CAD are at high risk for developing the disease. These factors are discussed in more detail in Chapter 35.

WOMEN'S HEALTH CONSIDERATIONS

Age is the most important risk factor for developing CAD in women. The older a women is, the more likely she will have the disease. When compared with men, women are, on average, 10 years older when they have CAD. In addition, women who have MIs have a greater risk of dying during hospitalization. When they are older than 50 years, women are more likely than men to die within 1 year after their MI (Redberg, 2006).

Modifiable risk factors are lifestyle choices that can be controlled by the patient, such as smoking and obesity. These factors are described later on this page in the Health Promotion and Maintenance section and in more detail in Chapter 35.

Incidence/Prevalence

According to the American Heart Association (AHA) (2008), 64% of women and 50% of men who had a myocardial infarction (MI) ("heart attack") were not aware that they had CAD. The average age of a person having a first MI is 64.5 years for men and 70.4 years for women (AHA, 2008).

Every 26 seconds, a person in the United States has a major coronary event. Every minute, someone will die of one. Many people die from coronary heart disease without being hospitalized. Most of these are sudden deaths caused by cardiac arrest.

WOMEN'S HEALTH CONSIDERATIONS

Premenopausal women have a lower incidence of MI than men. However, for postmenopausal women in their 70s or older, the incidence of MI equals that of men. Family history is also a risk factor for women; those whose parents had CAD are more susceptible to the disease.

Many patients who survive MIs are not able to return to work. CAD is the leading cause of premature, permanent disability in the United States, accounting for about 20% of disability allowances by the Social Security Administration.

Health Promotion and Maintenance

Ninety-five percent of sudden cardiac arrest victims die before reaching the hospital, largely because of ventricular fibrillation ("v fib"). To help combat this problem, *automatic external defibrillators (AEDs)* are found in many public places, such as in shopping centers and on airplanes. Employees are taught how to use these devices if a sudden cardiac arrest occurs. Some patients with diagnosed CAD have AEDs in their homes or at work.

Health promotion efforts are directed toward controlling or altering modifiable risk factors for CAD. Some of these factors have a genetic basis, which is described elsewhere in this text. Common risk factors include:

- Elevated serum lipid levels
- Tobacco use
- Limited physical activity
- Hypertension
- Diabetes mellitus
- Obesity
- Excessive alcohol
- Stress

People who have one or more of these risk factors should modify or eliminate them to decrease their chances of CAD. *For patients at risk for coronary artery disease (CAD), especially MI, assess specific risk factors and implement an individualized patient teaching plan.*

CULTURAL AWARENESS

Several groups have a higher genetic risk for CAD than others. African-American and Hispanic women have higher CAD risk factors than white women of the same socioeconomic status. Of American Indians and Alaskan Natives 18 years of age and older, about 64% of men and 81% of women have one or more CAD risk factors (hypertension [HTN], smoking, high cholesterol, excess weight, or diabetes mellitus). The leading cause of death for both men and women in the Euro-American population is cardiac disease, even though they may not have genetic predispositions to developing cardiovascular risk factors.

Elevated Serum Lipid Levels

The risk of CAD rises as serum cholesterol and triglyceride levels increase. In addition to measuring the total serum cholesterol, low-density lipoprotein (LDL), high-density lipoprotein

(HDL), and triglyceride (TG) levels are important in assessing risk for CAD. LDL cholesterol is the "bad" type, and HDL cholesterol is referred to as "good" because it has protective properties. *Elevated levels of LDL combined with low levels of HDL increase the risk of MI.* Also, total serum cholesterol levels put the patient at a higher risk of developing an MI. According to the AHA (2008), a 10% reduction in serum cholesterol may result in a 30% reduction in the incidence of CAD and MI. The *fasting* total cholesterol should be below 200 mg/dL. The goal for LDL levels in patients who are at high risk or have existing CAD is less than 70 mg/dL. For patients at low or moderate risk, LDL should also be substantially less than 100 mg/dL (AHA, 2008). HDL cholesterol levels should be above 40 mg/dL, although this recommendation may soon be changed to a higher level. The recommended triglyceride level is less than 135 mg/dL in women and 150 mg/dL in men (Pagana & Pagana, 2006).

Approaches to decrease lipids are focused on diet, exercise, and drug therapy that lowers cholesterol and triglyceride levels. Teach patients with elevated lipid levels to reduce intake of saturated fats to less than 7% of total calories, avoid *trans* fatty acids, and take in less than 200 mg per day of cholesterol. Daily physical activity and weight management are also important to reduce lipid levels. Drug therapy to decrease cholesterol is discussed in detail in Chapter 38 in the Arteriosclerosis and Atherosclerosis section.

Complementary and Alternative Therapies

Teach patients that adding omega-3 fatty acids from fish and plant sources has been effective in reducing lipid levels, stabilizing atherosclerotic plaques, and reducing sudden death from an MI (Harris et al., 2007). The preferred source of omega-3 acids is from fish three times a week or a daily fish oil nutritional supplement (at least 1 g) containing eicosapentaenoic acid (EPA) and docosahexaenoic acid (DHA) (AHA, 2008). Although not as useful in reducing CAD as fish oil, sources of plant-derived omega-3 acids include flaxseed, flaxseed oil, walnuts, and canola oil (Psota et al., 2006). Flaxseed oil, containing alpha linolenic acid, also may be taken as a daily nutritional supplement.

Garlic supplements may also have a small effect on reducing lipid levels, but they have not been shown to prevent MI. Patients often take a number of other supplements, such as vitamin E, coenzyme Q10, Pantesin, and vitamin B complex to decreased the risk of heart disease. None of these substances has been found to be helpful in reducing coronary artery disease (see the Evidence-Based Practice box below).

Tobacco Use

In the United States, an estimated 23.4% of men and 18.5% of women smoke cigarettes, putting them at increased risk of MI (AHA, 2008). About five million U.S. men and women chew

EVIDENCE-BASED PRACTICE

What is the role of dietary supplements in the prevention and treatment of coronary artery disease?

Knox, J., & Gaster, B. (2007). Dietary supplements for the prevention and treatment of coronary artery disease. *Journal of Alternative and Complementary Medicine, 13*(1), 83-95.

The combination of the occurrence and mortality associated with coronary artery disease (CAD) and the widespread use of dietary supplements by patients diagnosed with CAD led the researchers to conduct this study of the efficacy of dietary supplements for the prevention and treatment of coronary artery disease.

This was a systematic review of studies of 15 dietary supplements marketed for the prevention and/or treatment of CAD, hypertension, and/or hypercholesterolemia. Studies were identified by searching the databases ProQuest, MEDLINE, and Cochrane Library from May 2004 through April 2006. Additional studies were identified though the reference lists of the papers obtained through the initial search. Inclusion criteria included double-blinded, placebo-controlled, randomized clinical trials (RCTs) with duration longer than 1 week. Included studies investigated the outcomes of the identified supplement on hypercholesterolemia, hypertension, or cardiac events. Combination therapies were excluded because of the inability to isolate the effect of single supplements in the combined products. Only papers published in English were included. The quality of the selected papers was evaluated based on the Jadad et al. scoring tool, a validated tool awarding points for randomization, blinding, and handling of subjects that dropped out of the studies. Of the 15 supplements identified in the review, there were little data to support the efficacy of these supplements for the prevention and treatment of CAD. Moreover, most of the studies were found to be of poor quality. The strongest evidence identified was for the use of policosanol and garlic for hyperlipidemia.

Level of Evidence—1. This was a well-conducted systematic review of randomized clinical trials. However, it was noted by the researchers that many of the RCTs reviewed were of poor quality.

Commentary: Implications for Practice and Research. Although there is a growing body of evidence (and greater body of marketing information without evidence) regarding the use of dietary supplements for the treatment and prevention of coronary artery disease, the available data are inconclusive and often based on poorly designed studies. Nurses need to be aware of the limitations of the current evidence both for and against the efficacy of dietary supplements taken to either treat or prevent CAD. Even the evidence supporting the use of garlic for hyperlipidemia is of question because of the odor associated with this supplement, which made blinding of the subjects difficult. Another concern identified by the researchers was the variable makeup of the products being studied, making any generalizations to all products with the supplements invalid. It is clear that additional research of high quality is needed to determine the efficacy of dietary supplements in the care of patients with CAD and that greater standardization of these products is needed before being able to generalize any results of these studies.

tobacco, with the highest rates in the South and rural areas. Tobacco use and **passive smoking** from "second-hand smoke" (also called *environmental smoke*) substantially reduce blood flow in the coronary arteries.

Tobacco use, especially cigarette smoking, accounts for over one third of deaths from CAD. It enhances the process of atherosclerosis through mechanisms that are still poorly understood. Nicotine begins the release of catecholamines, resulting in an increased heart rate and peripheral vasoconstriction. This action causes increases in blood pressure (BP), cardiac afterload, and oxygen consumption. Cigarette smoking has also been found to cause endothelial dysfunction and increased vessel wall thickness. This process increases the risk for clot formation and vessel occlusion. The resulting hypertension may exacerbate the atherosclerotic process by increasing vessel wall permeability. Another problem with cigarette smoking is the production of carbon monoxide, which has been found to decrease the oxygen content in arterial blood. The good news is that when cigarette smoking is stopped, the risk for CAD decreases. A person who stops smoking may decrease the risk of CAD by as much as 80% in 1 year. Reducing the tar and nicotine content of the cigarettes smoked does not reduce the risk of CAD (AHA, 2008).

Ask about tobacco use, and advise the tobacco user and family members who smoke to quit using this harmful substance. Teach all patients to avoid environmental tobacco smoke at work and at home if at all possible. Additional information about tobacco use and smoking cessation is found in Chapters 32 and 35.

Physical Activity

Physical inactivity may be the most important risk factor for the general population. Less-active, less-fit persons have a 30% to 50% greater risk of developing high BP, which predisposes to CAD. Physical inactivity is more common among women than men, among African Americans and Hispanics than Euro-Americans, among older adults than younger adults, and among the less affluent than the more affluent (AHA, 2008). The causes for these differences are not known. Teach patients that regular physical activity helps maintain body weight and muscle mass while optimizing BP and lipid values.

Moderate-intensity activities like walking are associated with a major reduction in CAD risk. However, intense exercising may contribute to plaque rupture and increase the number of cardiac episodes. Teach patients that participating in exercise for 30 minutes a day can reduce hypertension and increase secretions of endorphins. It also leads to decreased smoking and eating, improved metabolism, and a stronger feeling of well-being. Other benefits include decreased blood clotting and higher plasma HDL levels, increased heart volume, increased cardiac capillary blood flow, and decreased heart rate. Physical activity does not increase collateral circulation or reduce the size of existing plaques.

Other Factors

One in three Americans has *hypertension* (HTN). This disease increases the workload of the heart, which increases the risk of MI. The cause of primary HTN is not known. However, it is easily detected and usually controllable. About half of patients having a first MI have a BP greater than 160/95 mm Hg. Ways to manage hypertension and therefore reduce the risk of CAD are described in Chapter 38.

CULTURAL AWARENESS

The prevalence of hypertension (HTN) among African Americans and whites in the southeastern United States is greater than among those in other regions of the country. Blacks have the highest prevalence in the United States and are among the highest in the world. They develop HTN earlier in life, and the average blood pressures are much higher than in other groups (AHA, 2008). The causes for differences are not known but may be related to genetics or diet.

Diabetes mellitus (DM) is a major risk factor for heart disease. A woman with diabetes mellitus is twice as likely to develop CAD than a woman without DM. Heart disease is the leading cause of diabetic-related death in both men and women. Most adults with diabetes also have hypertension.

Obesity is strongly associated with the development of hypertension, diabetes, and increased serum lipid levels. Women with fat deposited around their waists are at the highest risk for CAD. Teach the importance of weight management to help prevent these chronic and potentially life-threatening diseases.

Alcohol may help prevent or contribute to the development of CAD, depending on the amount consumed. Excessive consumption, described as having more than 3 ounces (90 mL) per day, can lead to increased heart disease, hypertension, and metabolic syndrome. A lower amount may help prevent CAD (Lucas et al., 2005).

CULTURAL AWARENESS

Modifiable risk factors vary for people of different racial and ethnic backgrounds. Some of the differences may be explained by lack of access to health care for some groups or by genetic factors. American Indians, for example, have the highest percentage of smokers among women and men. However, many of these people have poor access to care or have language barriers in a predominantly English-speaking, Euro-American health care system. Nutritional preferences may also explain some of the differences. For instance, according to the AHA (2008), high cholesterol is more common in African-American and Hispanic populations. Diets higher in fat and cholesterol are often less expensive and may be a factor in explaining differences, and obesity is more common in these groups. Genetic factors may also contribute to the differences among ethnic groups.

A person's response to *emotional stress* may also be associated with heart disease. Work stress, in particular, may be associated with left ventricular hypertrophy. During times of stress, increased heart rate increases the work of the heart, thus causing changes in the left ventricle.

Metabolic syndrome, also called *syndrome X,* has been recognized as a risk factor for cardiovascular (CV) disease and is being aggressively researched (Johnson & Weinstock, 2006). Patients who have three of the factors in Table 40-1 are diagnosed with **metabolic syndrome.** This health problem increases the risk for developing diabetes and CAD. About 47 million

TABLE 40-1 Indicators of Risk Factors for Metabolic Syndrome

Risk Factor	Indicator
Hypertension	**Either** blood pressure of 130/85 mm Hg or higher **or** taking antihypertensive drug(s)
Decreased HDL-C (usually with high LDL-C) level	**Either** HDL-C <40 mg/dL for men or <50 mg/dL for women **or** taking an anticholesterol drug
Increased level of triglycerides	**Either** 150 mg/dL or higher **or** taking an anticholesterol drug
Increased fasting blood glucose (due to diabetes, glucose intolerance, or insulin resistance)	**Either** 110 mg/dL or higher **or** taking antidiabetic drug(s)
Large waist size (excessive abdominal fat causing central obesity)	40″ (102 cm) or greater for men or 35″ (89 cm) or greater for women
Increased pro-thrombotic state	Increased fibrinogen or plasma activator inhibitor (blood-clotting factors)
Increased pro-inflammatory state	Increased C-reactive protein, a marker for inflammation

people in the United States have metabolic syndrome (AHA, 2008). This increase is likely due to physical inactivity and the current obesity epidemic (Johnson & Weinstock, 2006). Management is aimed at reducing risks, managing hypertension, and preventing complications.

Elevated levels of serum *homocysteine,* an amino acid, have been associated with an increased incidence of CAD. However, research findings are not consistent regarding its risk. Vitamin B supplements have been thought to decrease homocysteine. The evidence about the value of vitamin B is inconclusive and controversial, requiring future research (Lonn, 2007).

Patients with multiple modifiable risk factors have several times the risk of CAD as those without these characteristics. Although many factors place a person at risk for heart disease, there are well-documented, effective ways of promoting cardiovascular health. *The most important interdisciplinary intervention is health teaching* (Chart 40-1).

WOMEN'S HEALTH CONSIDERATIONS

Women continue to lack knowledge about CAD and how to prevent it. Those who have knowledge of health promotion behaviors (HPB) often do not practice them on a regular basis. Thanavaro et al. (2006) found that women need help with identifying barriers to HPB. The authors recommend that health teaching for women should begin in their early 20s to modify their risk for CAD, especially for those who smoke and have a family history of CAD.

Patient-Centered Collaborative Care

evolve ONLINE PHARM REVIEW

Assessment

History

If symptoms of CAD are present at the time of the interview, delay collecting data until interventions for symptom relief, vital sign instability, and dysrhythmias are started and discomfort resolves. If the patient had pain, ask about how he or she has managed the discomfort and other symptoms and which drugs he or she may be taking. When the patient is *pain free,* obtain information about family history and modifiable risk factors, including eating habits, lifestyle, and physical activity levels. Ask about a history of smoking and how much alcohol is consumed each day. Collaborate with the nutritionist to assess current body mass index (BMI) and weight.

Physical Assessment/Clinical Manifestations

Rapid assessment of the patient with chest pain or other presenting symptoms is crucial. It is important to differentiate among the types of chest pain and to identify the source. Question the patient to determine the characteristics of the discomfort. Appropriate questions to ask concerning the discomfort include onset, location, radiation, intensity, duration, and precipitating and relieving factors.

Ask the patient if the pain is in the chest, epigastric area, jaw, back, shoulder, or arm. Ask him or her to rate the pain on a scale of 0 to 10, with 10 being the highest level of discomfort. Some patients describe the discomfort as tightness, a burning sensation, pressure, or indigestion.

WOMEN'S HEALTH CONSIDERATIONS

Many women of any age experience atypical angina. **Atypical angina** manifests as indigestion, pain between the shoulders, an aching jaw, or a choking sensation that occurs with exertion. It has often been diagnosed as panic disorder, stress, menopause-related problems, GI disease, or hypochondriasis (Shaw et al., 2006).

Chart 40-2 compares and contrasts angina and infarction pain. Because angina pain is ischemic pain, it usually improves when the imbalance between oxygen supply and demand is resolved. For example, rest reduces tissue demands

Chart 40-1 PATIENT AND FAMILY EDUCATION GUIDE

Prevention of Coronary Artery Disease

SMOKING
- If you smoke, quit.
- If you don't smoke, don't start.

DIET
- Consume sufficient calories for your body to include:
  - Less than 7% from saturated fats
  - Avoiding *trans* fatty acids
- Limit your cholesterol intake to less than 200 mg/day.
- Limit your sodium intake as specified by your health care provider.

CHOLESTEROL
- Have your lipid levels checked regularly.
- If your cholesterol and LDL levels are elevated, follow your health care provider's advice.

PHYSICAL ACTIVITY
- If you are middle-aged or older or have a history of medical problems, check with your health care provider before starting an exercise program.
- Appropriate exercise should be enjoyable, burn 400 calories per session, and sustain a heart rate of 120 to 150 beats/min, depending on your age.
- Exercise periods should be at least 20 to 30 minutes long with 10-minute warm-up and 5-minute cool-down periods.
- If you cannot exercise moderately three to five times each week, walk daily for 30 minutes at a comfortable pace.
- If you cannot walk 30 minutes daily, walk any distance you can (e.g., park farther away from a site than necessary; use the stairs, not the elevator, to go one floor up or two floors down).

DIABETES
- Manage your diabetes with your health care provider.

BLOOD PRESSURE
- Have your blood pressure checked regularly.
- If your blood pressure is elevated, follow your health care provider's advice.
- Continue to monitor your blood pressure at regular intervals.

OBESITY
- Avoid severely restrictive or fad diets.
- Restrict intake of saturated fats, simple sugars, and cholesterol-rich foods.
- Increase your physical activity.

LDL, Low-density lipoprotein.

Chart 40-2 KEY FEATURES

Angina and Myocardial Infarction

Angina	Myocardial Infarction
Substernal chest discomfort: • Radiating to the left arm • Precipitated by exertion or stress (or rest in variant angina) • Relieved by nitroglycerin or rest • Lasting <15 min	Pain or discomfort: • Substernal chest pain radiating to the left arm • Pain or discomfort in jaw, back, shoulder, or abdomen • Occurring without cause, usually in the morning • Relieved only by opioids • Lasting 30 min or more
Few, if any, associated symptoms	Frequent associated symptoms: • Nausea/vomiting • Diaphoresis • Dyspnea • Feelings of fear and anxiety • Dysrhythmias • Fatigue • Palpitations • Epigastric distress • Anxiety • Dizziness • Disorientation/acute confusion • Feeling "short of breath"

and nitroglycerin improves oxygen supply. Discomfort from an MI does not usually resolve with these measures. *Also note any associated symptoms, including nausea, vomiting, diaphoresis, dizziness, weakness, palpitations, and shortness of breath.*

CONSIDERATIONS FOR OLDER ADULTS

The presence of associated symptoms without chest discomfort is significant. In up to 40% of all patients with MI, primarily older women and patients with diabetes, chest pain or discomfort may be mild or absent. Instead, they have associated symptoms. *Some older patients may think they are having indigestion and therefore not recognize that they are having an MI. Others report shortness of breath as the only symptom.* The major manifestation of MI in people older than 80 years may be disorientation or acute confusion due to poor cardiac output.

Assess *blood pressure* and *heart rate.* Interpret the patient's cardiac rhythm and presence of *dysrhythmias.* Sinus tachycardia with premature ventricular contractions (PVCs) frequently occurs in the first few hours after an MI.

Next assess *distal peripheral pulses* and *skin temperature.* The skin should be warm with all pulses palpable. In the patient with unstable angina or MI, poor cardiac output may be manifested by cool, diaphoretic ("sweaty") skin and diminished or absent pulses. *Auscultate for an S_3 gallop, which often indicates heart failure—a serious and common complication of MI.* Also assess the *respiratory rate* and breath sounds for signs of heart failure. An increased respiratory rate is common because of anxiety and pain, but *crackles or wheezes* may indicate *left-sided* heart failure. An S_4 heart sound is a common finding in the patient who has had a previous MI or hypertension. Assess for the presence of *jugular venous distention* and *peripheral edema.*

The patient with MI may experience a *temperature elevation* for several days after infarction. Temperatures as high as 102° F (39° C) may occur in response to myocardial necrosis, indicating the inflammatory response.

Psychosocial Assessment

Denial is a common early reaction to chest discomfort associated with angina or MI. On average, the patient with an acute MI waits more than 2 hours before seeking medical attention. Often he or she rationalizes that symptoms are due to indigestion or overexertion. In some situations, denial is a normal part of adapting to a stressful event. However, denial that interferes with identifying a symptom such as chest discomfort can be harmful. Explain the importance of reporting any discomfort to the health care provider.

Fear, depression, anxiety, and anger are other common reactions of many patients and their families. Assist in identifying these feelings. Encourage them to explain their understanding of the event, and clarify any misconceptions.

CULTURAL AWARENESS

African Americans and women tend to delay seeking treatment for MI and therefore have higher mortality rates than Euro-Americans. One contributing factor to this delay is a greater incidence of dyspnea as an acute symptom among these groups rather than the classic pain more typical of other groups.

Laboratory Assessment

Although there is no single ideal test to diagnose MI, the most common laboratory tests include troponins T and I, creatine kinase-MB (CK-MB), and myoglobin. These cardiac markers are specific for MI and cardiac necrosis. Troponins T and I and myoglobin rise quickly. CK-MB is the most specific marker for MI but does not peak until about 24 hours after the onset of pain. These tests are described in more detail in Chapter 35.

Imaging Assessment

Unless there is associated cardiac dysfunction (e.g., valve disease) or heart failure, a chest x-ray is not diagnostic for angina or MI.

Thallium scans use radioisotope imaging to assess for ischemia or necrotic muscle tissue related to angina or myocardial infarction (MI). Areas of decreased or absent perfusion, referred to as *cold spots,* identify ischemia or infarction. Thallium may be used with the exercise tolerance test. Dipyridamole (Persantine) thallium scanning (DTS) may also be used.

Contrast-enhanced cardiovascular magnetic resonance (CMR) may also be done as a noninvasive approach to detect MI. *Echocardiography* may be used to visualize the structures of the heart.

Use of the 64-slice **computed tomography coronary angiography (CTCA)** has been found to be helpful in diagnosing coronary artery disease in symptomatic patients identified as having a "low- or intermediate-pretest probability" risk for CAD. This new generation of high-speed CT scanners is becoming a highly reliable, noninvasive way to evaluate CAD (Meijboom, 2007).

Other Diagnostic Assessment

Twelve-lead electrocardiograms (ECGs) allow the health care provider to examine the heart from varying perspectives. By identifying the lead(s) in which ECG changes are occurring, the health care provider can identify both the occurrence and the location of ischemia (angina) or necrosis (infarction). In addition to the traditional 12-lead ECG, the health care provider may request a "right-sided" or 18-lead ECG to determine whether ischemia or infarction has occurred in the right ventricle.

An ischemic myocardium does not repolarize normally. Thus 12-lead ECGs obtained during an angina episode reveal ST depression, T-wave inversion, or both. **Variant angina,** caused by coronary vasospasm (vessel spasm), usually causes elevation of the ST segment during angina attacks. These ST and T-wave changes usually subside when the ischemia is resolved and pain is relieved. However, the T wave may remain flat or inverted for a period of time. If the patient is not experiencing angina at the moment of the test, the ECG is usually normal unless he or she has evidence of an old MI.

When infarction occurs, one of three ECG changes is usually observed: ST-elevation MI (STEMI), T-wave inversion, or non–ST-elevation MI (NSTEMI). An abnormal Q wave (wider than 0.04 seconds or more than one-third the height of the QRS complex) may develop, depending on the amount of myocardium that has necrosed. Women having an MI often present with an NSTEMI or T-wave inversion.

The Q wave may develop because necrotic cells do not conduct electrical stimuli. Hours to days after the MI, the ST-segment and T-wave changes return to normal. However, when the Q wave exists, it may become permanent. The Q waves may disappear after a number of years, but their absence does not necessarily mean that the patient has not had an MI.

After the acute stages of an angina episode or MI, the health care provider often requests an *exercise tolerance test (stress test)* on a treadmill to assess for ECG changes consistent with ischemia, evaluate medical therapy, and identify those who might benefit from invasive therapy. Pharmacologic stress-testing agents such as dobutamine (Dobutrex) may be used instead of the treadmill. Treadmill exercise testing is only moderately accurate for women when compared with men (Redberg, 2006).

Cardiac catheterization may be performed to determine the extent and exact location of coronary artery obstructions. It allows the cardiologist and cardiac surgeon to identify patients who might benefit from percutaneous transluminal angioplasty (PCTA) and stent placement or from coronary artery bypass grafting (CABG). Each of the diagnostic tests in this section is described in detail in Chapter 35.

▪ *Analysis*

The patient with coronary artery disease (CAD) may have either angina or MI. If MI is suspected or cannot be completely ruled out, the patient is admitted to a telemetry unit for continuous monitoring or to a critical care unit if hemodynamically unstable.

Common Nursing Diagnoses and Collaborative Problems

The priority nursing diagnoses for patients with CAD are:

1. Acute Pain related to imbalance between myocardial oxygen supply and demand
2. Ineffective Tissue Perfusion (Cardiopulmonary) related to interruption of arterial blood flow
3. Activity Intolerance related to fatigue caused by imbalance between oxygen supply and demand
4. Ineffective Coping related to effects of acute illness and major changes in lifestyle

For the patient experiencing an MI, the most important collaborative problems include:

1. Potential for Dysrhythmias
2. Potential for Heart Failure
3. Potential for Recurrent Symptoms and Extension of Injury

Additional Nursing Diagnoses and Collaborative Problems

In addition to the common nursing diagnoses and collaborative problems, patients with CAD may have one or more of these nursing diagnoses and collaborative problems:

- Ineffective Sexuality Pattern related to pain and effects of illness
- Impaired Physical Mobility related to pain or fear of movement
- Potential for Acute Renal Failure

Planning and Implementation

Astute assessment skills, timely analysis of troponin, and analysis of the 12-lead ECG (or 18-lead ECG for a suspected right ventricular infarction) are essential to ensure appropriate patient care management. This is particularly important since the average time a patient waits before seeking treatment is 2 hours and 20 minutes. This delay lessens the 4- to 6-hour window of opportunity for the most advantageous treatment with percutaneous intervention.

Acute Pain

Planning: Expected Outcomes. The patient with CAD is expected to state that pain, *if present*, is relieved. Older women and patients with diabetes often do not have the characteristic chest pain and may have silent (no pain or discomfort) myocardial ischemia or silent MI.

CONSIDERATIONS FOR OLDER ADULTS

Absence of chest pain in older adults with MI may be due to cognitive impairment or inability to verbalize pain sensation. However, in most cases, it is probably due to increased collateral circulation. Silent myocardial ischemia increases the incidence of new coronary events and should be treated aggressively.

Interventions. The purpose of collaborative management is to eliminate discomfort by providing pain relief measures, decreasing myocardial oxygen demand, and increasing myocardial oxygen supply.

Emergency Measures. Evaluate any report of pain, obtain vital signs, ensure an IV access, and notify the health care provider of the patient's condition. Chart 40-3 summarizes the emergency interventions for the patient with symptoms of CAD.

Pain relief helps increase the oxygen supply and decrease myocardial oxygen demand. The American Heart Association (AHA) recommends several pain management strategies, including morphine sulfate and oxygen. *Give morphine as the priority in managing pain in patients having an MI!*

Drug Therapy. At home or in the hospital, the patient may take nitroglycerin to relieve episodic anginal pain. Aspirin 325 mg, an antiplatelet drug, may also be taken daily to prevent clots that further block coronary arteries. This drug is discussed on p. 859 in the Ineffective Tissue Perfusion section.

Chart 40-3 BEST PRACTICE FOR PATIENT SAFETY & QUALITY CARE

Emergency Care of the Patient with Chest Discomfort

EMERGENCY CARE

- Assess airway, breathing, and circulation (ABCs). Defibrillate as needed.
- ***Provide continuous ECG monitoring.***
- Obtain the patient's description of pain or discomfort.
- Obtain the patient's vital signs (blood pressure, pulse, respiration).
- Assess/provide vascular access.
- Consult chest pain protocol or notify the physician or Rapid Response Team for specific intervention.
- Obtain a 12-lead ECG if indicated.
- Provide pain relief medication and aspirin as prescribed.
- Administer oxygen therapy to maintain oxygen saturation ≥95%.
- Remain calm. Stay with the patient if possible.
- Assess the patient's vital signs and intensity of pain 5 minutes after administration of medication.
- Remedicate with prescribed drugs (if vital signs remain stable), and check the patient every 5 minutes.
- Notify the physician if vital signs deteriorate.

Nitroglycerin (NTG), a nitrate often referred to as "nitro," increases collateral blood flow, redistributes blood flow toward the subendocardium, and dilates the coronary arteries. In addition, it decreases myocardial oxygen demand by peripheral vasodilation, which decreases both preload and afterload. Teach the patient to hold the tablet under the tongue and drink 5 mL of water, if necessary, to allow the tablet to dissolve. NTG spray is also available and is more quickly absorbed. Pain relief should begin within 1 to 2 minutes and should be clearly evident in 3 to 5 minutes. After 5 minutes, recheck the patient's pain intensity and vital signs. If the BP is less than 100 mm Hg systolic or 25 mm Hg lower than the previous reading, lower the head of the bed and notify the health care provider. If the patient is experiencing some but not complete relief and vital signs remain stable, another NTG tablet or spray may be used. In 5-minute increments, a total of three doses may be administered in an attempt to relieve angina pain. If the patient uses NTG spray instead of the tablet, teach him or her to sit upright and spray the dose under the tongue. NTG topical patches should be placed below the nipple line to decrease discomfort.

Angina usually responds to NTG. The patient typically states that the pain is relieved or markedly diminished. When simple measures, such as taking three sublingual nitroglycerin tablets one after the other, do not relieve chest discomfort, the patient may be experiencing an MI. *Immediately inform the health care provider and prepare the patient for transfer to a specialized unit where close monitoring and appropriate management can be provided. If the patient is at home or in the community, call 911 for transfer to the closest emergency department.*

In a specialized unit, the health care provider may prescribe IV NTG for management of the chest pain. Begin the drug infusion slowly, checking the BP and pain level every 3 to 5 minutes. The nitroglycerin dose is increased until the pain is relieved, the BP falls excessively, or the maximum prescribed dose is reached (Chart 40-4).

Chart 40-4 COMMON EXAMPLES OF DRUG THERAPY

Coronary Artery Disease (Nitrates, Beta Blockers, and Antiplatelet Agents)

Drug	Usual Dosage	Nursing Interventions	Rationales
NITRATES			
Nitroglycerin (Nitrostat, NitroQuick)	0.3-0.4 mg sublingually every 5 min; up to 3 tablets over 15 min	Instruct patients to lie down with the head of the bed at a level of comfort when taking the sublingual form.	Hypotension can be dramatic, immediate, and intensified by the upright position.
Nitrolingual translingual spray	0.4 mg/metered spray	Monitor BP. Pay attention to orthostatic changes.	A decrease in BP occurs with vasodilation.
		Instruct patients to allow the sublingual tablet to dissolve and to avoid swallowing the tablet.	The sublingual dose is absorbed through the sublingual mucous membranes.
		Check the expiration date on sublingual tablets and sprays. Tablets should be replaced every 3-5 mo.	The efficacy of the tablets decreases with time.
		Determine whether pain is relieved.	Additional medication may be required to relieve pain.
		Monitor for headache.	Vasodilation is generalized.
		Do not administer to patients taking drugs used to treat sexual dysfunction (e.g., sildenafil, tadalafil, vardenafil).	Very serious (possibly fatal) interactions may occur.
Isosorbide dinitrate (Isordil, Iso-Bid)	2.5 mg sublingually every 4-6 hr; 5-40 mg orally four times daily	Instruct patients taking sublingual forms to lie down before administration.	The hypotensive effect can be dramatic and immediate with sublingual administration.
	40-80 mg sustained-release tablet every 8-12 hr	Monitor BP, and assess for dizziness.	A decrease in BP occurs with vasodilation.
Isosorbide mononitrate (Imdur)	60-mg extended-release tablet daily	Schedule sustained-release form with an 8- to 12-hr dose-free interval.	Tolerance may develop.
Nitroglycerin patch (Minitran, Nitro-Dur, Nitrek)	Transdermally started at 5 mg/24 hr (10-cm^2 system)	Remove the patch from the patient before defibrillation.	The patient may develop a burn.
		Rotate application sites.	Rotation prevents skin irritation.
		Apply the patch to a clean, dry, hairless area.	The drug is better absorbed when the skin is clean, dry, and hairless.
		Remove patch after 12-14 hr each day.	Removal prevents drug tolerance.
BETA BLOCKERS			
Carvedilol (Coreg, Coreg CR)	12.5-25 mg twice daily for Coreg; 40-80 mg once daily for Coreg CR	Assess heart rate before administration.	Beta-blocking effects cause a decrease in heart rate.
		Monitor BP.	The hypotensive effect is due to a decrease in cardiac output, suppressed renin activity, and beta-blocking effects.
		Observe for signs of heart failure.	Heart failure may occur as a result of a decrease in cardiac output.
		Assess for shortness of breath and wheezing.	$Beta_2$-blocking effects in the lungs can cause bronchoconstriction.
Metoprolol (Lopressor, Toprol XL, Betaloc🍁), a cardioselective beta-adrenergic blocker	*Angina:* 25-100 mg daily *MI:* 100 mg twice daily; 5 mg IV over 2 min may be repeated twice for a total of 15 mg	Assess heart rate before administration; do not administer if heart rate <50-60 beats/min.	Beta blockers may cause further decreases in heart rate.
		Monitor BP, and hold for systolic <90-100 mm Hg.	Decreased BP pressure is an anticipated effect.
		Assess patients for cough, shortness of breath, edema, and weight gain.	These are indications of heart failure.

BP, Blood pressure; *MI*, myocardial infarction; *AV*, Atrioventricular; *SA*, sinoatrial.

Continued

Chart 40-4 COMMON EXAMPLES OF DRUG THERAPY

Coronary Artery Disease (Nitrates, Beta Blockers, and Antiplatelet Agents)—cont'd

Drug	Usual Dosage	Nursing Interventions	Rationales
ANTIPLATELET AGENTS			
Aspirin (Empirin, Apo-ASA♣, Ecotrin)	81-325 mg orally daily	Suggest that patients take the daily dose with food.	Gastric irritation may occur.
		Question patients about ringing in the ears.	Tinnitus may occur with aspirin toxicity.
		Emphasize to patients that aspirin is an important cardiac medication and should be continued unless they are told to stop.	Studies document significantly better survival rates for patients with coronary artery disease receiving aspirin.
Clopidogrel (Plavix) **Med Error Alert!** Do not confuse Plavix with Paxil	*Recent MI:* 75 mg daily *Acute coronary syndrome:* 300 mg, then 75-150 mg daily	Teach patients to take drug with food.	Drug can cause diarrhea and other GI disturbances.
		Inform patients to report any usual bleeding or bruising.	Drug prevents platelet aggregation, thus slowing down clot formation.

BP, Blood pressure; *MI,* myocardial infarction; *AV,* Atrioventricular; *SA,* sinoatrial.

When pain or other symptoms have subsided and the patient is stabilized, the health care provider may change the drug to an oral or topical nitrate. During administration of long-term oral and topical nitrates, an 8- to 12-hour nitrate-free period should be maintained to prevent tolerance. The patient may initially report a headache. Give acetaminophen (Tylenol, Exdol♣) before the nitrate to ease some of this discomfort.

The health care provider usually prescribes *morphine sulfate (MS)* to relieve discomfort that is unresponsive to nitroglycerin. Morphine relieves MI pain, decreases myocardial oxygen demand, relaxes smooth muscle, and reduces circulating catecholamines. It is usually administered in 2- to 10-mg doses IV every 5 to 15 minutes until the maximum prescribed dose is reached or the patient experiences relief or signs of toxicity. Adverse effects of morphine include respiratory depression, hypotension, bradycardia, and severe vomiting. Treatment for morphine toxicity consists of administering naloxone (Narcan) 0.2 to 0.8 mg IV, vasopressor drugs, IV fluids, and oxygen therapy. Monitor the patient's vital signs and cardiac rhythm every few minutes.

These strategies are often enough to relieve the pain. If they are not adequate, additional interventions identified in the Ineffective Tissue Perfusion (Cardiopulmonary) section may be attempted.

Other Interventions. Several other interventions may be used with drug therapy to relieve chest pain. Supplemental oxygen may increase the amount of oxygen available to myocardial tissue. Therefore oxygen is often prescribed and administered at a flow of 2 to 4 L/min by nasal cannula titrated to maintain an arterial oxygen saturation (Sao_2) of 95% or higher. If the BP is stable, assist the patient in assuming any position of comfort. Placing the patient in semi-Fowler's position often enhances comfort and tissue oxygenation. A quiet, calm environment and explanations of interventions often reduce anxiety and help relieve chest pain. If needed, teach the patient to take several deep breaths to increase oxygenation.

DECISION-MAKING CHALLENGE
Critical Rescue

A 55-year-old female patient visits an urgent care center with a report of burning epigastric pain. She states that she believes it is a bad case of heartburn that "just won't go away." Assessment findings reveal slight shortness of breath, diaphoresis, and nausea and vomiting. Vital signs are BP, 122/78; P, 82; R, 20; T, 98.2° F. She is 5 feet, 2 inches tall and weighs 188 pounds. Her tentative diagnosis is to "r/o MI."

1. What additional data and assessments should you collect at this time?
2. What intervention would you implement first? What intervention would you implement second?
3. How might this patient's initial symptoms differ from those of a male patient who has an MI?
4. When she has recovered from this event, what health teaching might she need?

evolve For suggested answer guidelines, go to http://evolve.elsevier.com/Iggy/.

Ineffective Tissue Perfusion (Cardiopulmonary)

NOC **Planning: Expected Outcomes.** The patient with coronary artery disease (CAD) is expected to have adequate blood flow through the coronary vasculature to maintain heart function. Indicators include that the patient will have functional or baseline:

- Ejection fraction
- Pulmonary wedge pressure
- Cardiac biomarkers
- Apical heart rate
- Systolic and diastolic blood pressure

Interventions. Because myocardial infarction (MI) is a dynamic process, restoring perfusion to the injured area (usually within 4 to 6 hours) often limits the amount of extension and improves left ventricular function. Complete, sustained reperfusion of coronary arteries in the first few hours after an MI has decreased mortality rates.

Drug Therapy. *Aspirin (ASA)* therapy is recommended by the American College of Cardiology and the AHA. It inhibits both platelet aggregation and vasoconstriction, thereby decreasing the likelihood of thrombosis. The antiplatelet effect of ASA begins within 1 hour of use and continues for several days. Administer 162 to 325 mg non–enteric-coated aspirin every day to all patients with suspected CAD unless absolutely contraindicated. Instruct the patient to chew and swallow the drug and continue taking the drug unless adverse effects occur. *Observe for bleeding tendencies, such as nosebleeds or blood in the stool. The drug should be discontinued if bleeding occurs. If the patient has new-onset angina at home, teach him or her to chew aspirin 325 mg (4 "baby aspirins" that are 81 mg each) immediately and call 911!*

Thrombolytic therapy using **fibrinolytics** dissolves thrombi in the coronary arteries and restores myocardial blood flow. Examples of these agents, which target the fibrin component of the coronary thrombosis, include:

- Tissue plasminogen activator (t-PA, alteplase [Activase]) (IV or intracoronary)
- Reteplase (Retavase) (IV or intracoronary)
- Tenecteplase (TNK) (IV push [IVP])

Intracoronary fibrinolytics may be delivered during cardiac catheterization. Thrombolytic agents are most effective when administered within the first 6 hours of a coronary event. They are used in men and women, young and old.

Thrombolytic therapy is given in a unit where the patient can be continuously monitored. It is indicated for chest pain of longer than 30 minutes' duration that is unrelieved by nitroglycerin, with indications of transmural ischemia and injury as shown by the ECG. Contraindications include recent abdominal surgery or stroke because bleeding may occur when fresh clots are lysed (broken down or dissolved). Table 40-2 lists the current contraindications to thrombolytic therapy.

Patients who weigh less than 143 pounds (65 kg) may need to have their dose of thrombolytic adjusted to lessen the likelihood of bleeding. *During administration, immediately report any indications of bleeding to the health care provider. After administration, observe for signs of bleeding by:*

- *Documenting the patient's neurologic status (in case of intracranial bleeding)*
- *Observing all IV sites for bleeding and patency*
- *Monitoring clotting studies*
- *Observing for signs of internal bleeding (watching hemoglobin and hematocrit)*
- *Testing stools, urine, and emesis for occult blood*

Glycoprotein (GP) IIb/IIIa inhibitors target the platelet component of the thrombus. Abciximab (ReoPro), eptifibatide (Integrilin), and tirofiban (Aggrastat) are administered IV to prevent fibrinogen from attaching to activated platelets at the site of a thrombus. These medications are used in acute coronary syndromes (especially unstable angina, NSTEMI, and non–Q-wave MI). They are also given before and during percutaneous transluminal coronary angioplasty (PTCA) to maintain patency of the newly opened artery and with fibrinolytic agents after MI. If the GP IIb/IIIa inhibitors are used with a fibrinolytic agent, the dose of the thrombolytic is reduced by 25% to 50% to decrease the risk of bleeding. *When giving GP IIb/IIIa inhibitors, assess the patient closely for bleeding or hypersensitivity reactions. If either occurs, notify the health care provider immediately.*

Once-a-day *beta-adrenergic blocking agents* (e.g., metoprolol XL [Toprol XL], carvedilol CR [Coreg CR]), sometimes just called *beta blockers (BBs),* decrease the size of the infarct, the occurrence of ventricular dysrhythmias, and mortality rates in patients with MI. The physician usually prescribes a cardioselective beta-blocking agent within the first 1 to 2 hours after an MI if the patient is hemodynamically stable. Beta blockers slow the heart rate and decrease the force of cardiac contraction (see Chart 40-4). Thus these agents prolong the period of diastole and increase myocardial perfusion while reducing the force of myocardial contraction. With beta blockade, the heart can perform more work without ischemia. During beta-blocking therapy, monitor for:

- Bradycardia
- Hypotension
- Decreased level of consciousness (LOC)
- Chest discomfort

Assess the lungs for crackles (indicative of heart failure) and wheezes (indicative of bronchospasm). Hypoglycemia, depression, nightmares, and forgetfulness are also problems with beta blockade, especially in older patients. Many of these side effects decrease with time. *Do not give BBs if the pulse is below 60 or the systolic BP is below 100 without first checking with the health care provider.*

Health care providers frequently prescribe *angiotensin-converting enzyme (ACE) inhibitors* or *angiotensin receptor blockers (ARBs)* within 48 hours of an MI to prevent ventricular remodeling and the development of heart failure. Both ACE inhibitors and ARBs increase survival after an MI. Monitor the patient for decreased urine output, hypotension,

TABLE 40-2 Contraindications to Thrombolytic Therapy

ABSOLUTE

- Any prior intracranial hemorrhage
- Known structural cerebral vascular lesion (e.g., arteriovenous malformations)
- Known malignant intracranial neoplasm (primary or metastatic)
- Ischemic stroke within 3 months EXCEPT acute ischemic stroke within 3 hours
- Suspected aortic dissection
- Active bleeding or bleeding diathesis (excluding menses)
- Significant closed-head or facial trauma within 3 months

RELATIVE

- History of chronic, severe, poorly controlled hypertension
- Severe uncontrolled hypertension on presentation (SBP >180 mm Hg or DBP >110 mm Hg)*
- History of prior ischemic stroke within 3 months, dementia, or known intracranial pathology not covered in contraindications
- Traumatic or prolonged (≥10 minutes) CPR or major surgery (within 3 weeks)
- Recent (within 2-4 weeks) internal bleeding
- Noncompressible vascular punctures
- For streptokinase/anistreplase: prior exposure (>5 days ago) or prior allergic reaction to these agents
- Pregnancy
- Active peptic ulcer
- Current use of anticoagulants; the higher the INR, the higher risk of bleeding

*Could be an absolute contraindication in low-risk patients with MI.
CPR, Cardiopulmonary resuscitation; *DBP,* diastolic blood pressure; *INR,* international normalized ratio; *MI,* myocardial infarction; *SBP,* systolic blood pressure.

and cough. Check for changes in serum potassium, creatinine, and blood urea nitrogen. (Chapter 38 provides a more detailed discussion of ACE inhibitors and ARBs.)

For patients with angina, the health care provider may prescribe calcium channel blockers to enhance vasodilation and myocardial perfusion. These drugs are indicated for patients with variant angina or for those who are hypertensive and continue to have angina despite therapy with beta blockers (unstable angina). They are not indicated after an MI. Monitor the patient for hypotension and peripheral edema, and review the frequency of angina episodes.

Calcium channel blockers are also used for chronic stable angina (CSA). When they are not successful in managing CSA, *ranolazine (Ranexa)* may be added to the drug regimen. This drug has anti-angina and anti-ischemic properties and is often effective in relieving the pain associated with CSA (Zerumsky & McBride, 2006).

Percutaneous Transluminal Coronary Angioplasty (PTCA). For some patients having an MI, primary PTCA with stent (metallic mesh) placement may be used to reopen the thrombosed coronary artery. Percutaneous intervention has been associated with excellent return of blood flow through the coronary artery when it can be performed within 2 to 3 hours of the onset of symptoms by an interventional cardiologist. Many community hospitals can now perform emergent PTCA. When primary PTCA is not available, patients should receive immediate thrombolytic agents if they are appropriate candidates and then be transferred to a facility that can perform PTCA. This procedure is described in detail on p. 865 of this chapter.

Patients who receive fibrinolytics require PTCA for more definitive treatment such as stent placement. Therefore, if criteria for PTCA are met, it is more advantageous to go directly to the catheterization lab where definitive treatment, not just clot resolution, can be performed.

Monitor the patient for indications that the clot has been lysed (dissolved) and the artery reperfused. These indications include:

- Abrupt cessation of pain or discomfort
- Sudden onset of ventricular dysrhythmias
- Resolution of ST-segment depression or T-wave inversion
- A peak at 12 hours of markers of myocardial damage

After clot lysis with thrombolytics, large amounts of thrombin are released into the system, increasing the risk of vessel reocclusion. To maintain the patency of the coronary artery after thrombolytic therapy, the health care provider usually prescribes aspirin and IV heparin. Maintain the heparin infusion for 3 to 5 days as prescribed, and monitor the activated partial thromboplastin time (aPTT). The target aPTT range is usually $1\frac{1}{2}$ to $2\frac{1}{2}$ times the control sample. The heparin antifactor Xa assay (heparin assay) test may be used instead of the aPTT in some clinical facilities. Low–molecular-weight heparin (LMWH) (enoxaparin [Lovenox]) may be substituted for IV heparin.

Activity Intolerance

Planning: Expected Outcomes. The patient with coronary artery disease (CAD) is expected to walk at least 200 feet four times a day without chest discomfort or shortness of breath.

Interventions. Activity intolerance is reduced by a planned program of cardiac rehabilitation implemented primarily by the nurse and physical therapist and continued after discharge.

NIC **Cardiac rehabilitation** is the process of actively assisting the patient with cardiac disease in achieving and maintaining a vital and productive life while remaining within the limits of the heart's ability to respond to increases in activity and stress (Chart 40-5). It can be divided into three phases. *Phase 1* begins with the acute illness and ends with discharge from the hospital. *Phase 2* begins after discharge and continues through convalescence at home. *Phase 3* refers to long-term conditioning.

In the acute phase (phase 1), promote rest and ensure limited mobility. Assistance may be needed for some ADLs, such as ambulation to the bathroom. Patients progress at their own rate to increasing levels of activity depending on their clinical status, age, and physical capabilities.

The next step in phase 1 is independent ambulation of the patient in the room and to the bathroom. Encourage progressive ambulation in the hallway, usually 50, 100, and then 200 feet three times a day. In addition, the patient may begin showering for 5 or 10 minutes with warm water. A chair should be available to facilitate rest and maintain balance.

Assess the patient's heart rate, blood pressure (BP), respiratory rate, and level of fatigue with each higher level of activity. Decreases greater than 20 mm Hg in the systolic BP, changes of 20 beats per minute in the pulse rate, and reports of dyspnea or chest pain indicate intolerance of activity. If these manifestations develop, notify the health care provider and do not advance the patient to the next level. Older adults with CAD often have needs and concerns different from those of younger adults, as described in Chart 40-6.

Ineffective Coping

NOC **Planning: Expected Outcomes.** The patient with CAD is expected to take personal actions to manage stressors related to CAD. Indicators include that the patient will consistently:

- Identify effective coping patterns
- Verbalize a sense of control
- Report a decrease in stress
- Verbalize acceptance of the situation
- Seek information concerning illness and treatment
- Modify lifestyle as needed
- Adapt to life changes

Interventions. Assess the patient's level of anxiety while allowing expressions of any apprehension, and attempt to define its origin. Simple, repeated explanations of therapies, expectations, and surroundings, as well as patient progress, may help relieve anxiety.

NIC Identify the patient's current *coping* mechanisms. The most common are denial, anger, and depression. Denial allows the patient to decrease a threat and use problem-focused coping mechanisms. The patient may avoid discussing what has happened and yet comply with treatment regimens. This type of denial decreases anxiety and should not be discouraged. *However, denial that results in a patient who refuses to follow treatment regimens can be harmful.* Because this behavior is usually due to extreme anxiety or fear, threats only worsen the behavior. Remain calm, and avoid confronting the patient. Clearly indicate when a behavior is not acceptable and is potentially harmful as a result of noncompliance.

Anger may represent an attempt to regain control of life. Encourage the patient to verbalize the source of frustration, and provide opportunities for decision making and control.

Chart 40-5 NIC INTERVENTION ACTIVITIES

The Patient with Coronary Artery Disease and Acute Coronary Syndrome

Pain Management: *Alleviation of pain or a reduction in pain to a level of comfort that is acceptable to the patient.*

- Perform a comprehensive assessment of pain to include location, characteristics, onset/duration, frequency, quality, intensity or severity of pain, and precipitating factors.
- Verify level of discomfort with patient, note changes in the medical record, inform other health professionals working with the patient.
- Ensure that patient receives attentive analgesic care.
- Determine the needed frequency of making an assessment of patient comfort, and implement monitoring plan.
- Evaluate the effectiveness of the pain control measures used while performing thorough ongoing assessment of the pain experience.

Cardiac Care: Acute: *Limitation of complications for a patient recently experiencing an episode of an imbalance between myocardial oxygen supply and demand resulting in impaired cardiac function.*

- Evaluate chest pain (e.g., intensity, location, radiation, duration, and precipitating and alleviating factors).
- Monitor cardiac rhythm and rate.
- Auscultate heart sounds.
- Auscultate lungs for crackles or other adventitious sounds.
- Monitor neurological status.
- Monitor intake/output, urine output, and daily weight, if appropriate.
- Administer medications to relieve/prevent pain and ischemia, if needed.

Cardiac Care: Rehabilitative: *Promotion of maximum functional activity level for a patient who has experienced an episode of impaired cardiac function that resulted from an imbalance between myocardial oxygen supply and demand.*

- Monitor the patient's activity tolerance.
- Maintain ambulation schedule, as tolerated.
- Instruct the patient and family on the exercise regimen, including warm-up, endurance, and cool-down, as appropriate.
- Instruct the patient and family on any lifting/pushing weight limitations, if appropriate.
- Encourage realistic expectations for the patient and family.

Coping Enhancement: *Assisting a patient to adapt to perceived stressors, changes, or threats that interfere with meeting life demands and roles.*

- Appraise the patient's understanding of the disease process.
- Use a calm, reassuring approach.
- Provide an atmosphere of acceptance.
- Assist the patient in developing an objective appraisal of the event.
- Help patient to identify the information he or she is most interested in obtaining.
- Provide factual information concerning diagnosis, treatment, and prognosis.
- Foster constructive outlets for anger and hostility.
- Explore with the patient previous methods of dealing with life problems.
- Support the use of appropriate defense mechanisms.

NIC intervention activities selected from Bulechek, G.M., Butcher, H.K., & McCloskey Dochterman, J. (Eds.). (2008). *Nursing interventions classification (NIC)* (5th ed.). St. Louis: Mosby. No part of this work is to be altered without prior written permission from the Publisher.

Collaborate with the certified spiritual chaplain in the hospital to help the patient cope with the situation.

Depression may be a response to grief and loss of function. Listen as the patient verbalizes feelings of loss, being careful not to offer false or general reassurances. Acknowledge depression, but encourage the patient to perform ADLs and other activities within restrictions. Chart 40-5 summarizes four major NIC intervention activities for patients with CAD.

Potential for Dysrhythmias

Planning: Expected Outcomes. The patient with CAD is expected to resume a normal sinus rhythm or normal rhythm and to be hemodynamically stable.

Interventions. *Dysrhythmias are the leading cause of prehospital death in most patients with myocardial infarction (MI).* Even in the early period of hospitalization, most patients with MI experience some abnormal cardiac rhythm. When a dysrhythmia develops:

- Identify the dysrhythmia.
- Assess hemodynamic status.
- Evaluate for discomfort.

Dysrhythmias are treated when they are causing hemodynamic compromise, are increasing myocardial oxygen requirements, or predispose to lethal ventricular dysrhythmias.

Typical dysrhythmias for the patient with an *inferior* MI are bradycardias and second-degree AV blocks resulting from

Chart 40-6 NURSING FOCUS ON THE OLDER ADULT

Coronary Artery Disease

- Recognize that chest pain may not be evident in the older patient. Examples of associated symptoms are unexplained dyspnea, confusion, or GI symptoms.
- Although older adults have a greater reduction in mortality rate from myocardial infarction (MI) with the use of thrombolytics, they also have the most severe side effects. Monitor older patients receiving thrombolytics extremely carefully.
- Dysrhythmia may be a normal age-related change rather than a complication of MI. Determine whether the dysrhythmia is causing significant symptoms. Then notify the physician.
- If beta blockers are used, assess the patient carefully for the development of side effects. Exacerbation of the depression some older adults have is a significant problem with beta blockade.
- Plan slow, steady increases in activity. Older adults with minimal previous exercise show particular benefit from a gradual increase in activity.
- Older adults should plan longer warm-up and cool-down periods when participating in an exercise program. Their pulse rates may not return to baseline until 30 minutes or longer after exercise.

ischemia of the AV node. These rhythms tend to be intermittent. Monitor the cardiac rhythm and rate and the hemodynamic status. If the patient becomes hemodynamically unstable, a temporary pacemaker may be necessary.

The patient with an *anterior* MI is likely to exhibit ventricular irritability (premature ventricular contractions [PVCs]). Third-degree or bundle branch block is a serious complication in this patient because it indicates that a large portion of the left ventricle is involved. The health care provider may insert a pacemaker. Observe the patient closely to detect the development of heart failure. Appropriate interventions for dysrhythmias are described in Chapter 36.

Potential for Heart Failure

Planning: Expected Outcomes. The patient with coronary artery disease (CAD) is expected to regain hemodynamic stability as evidenced by:

- BP and pulse rate within acceptable range and adequate for metabolic demands
- Adequate urine output
- Mental alertness
- Clear lungs on auscultation
- Palpable peripheral pulses

Interventions. Decreased cardiac output related to heart failure is a relatively common complication after an MI resulting from left ventricular dysfunction, rupture of the intraventricular septum, papillary muscle rupture with valvular dysfunction, or right ventricular infarction. The most severe form of heart failure, *cardiogenic shock,* discussed later on this page, accounts for most in-hospital deaths after an MI. The type of management used to increase cardiac output depends on the location of the MI and the type of heart failure that resulted from the infarction.

Managing Left Ventricular Failure. When a patient with MI experiences damage to the left ventricle, rupture of the intraventricular septum, or tear of a papillary muscle, the amount of blood that the heart can eject is reduced. When volume and pressure are markedly increased in the pulmonary vasculature, pulmonary complications develop.

Nursing assessment and monitoring. Assess for manifestations of left ventricular failure and pulmonary edema by listening for crackles and identifying their location in the lung fields. Wheezing, tachypnea, and frothy sputum may also occur with pulmonary edema. Auscultate the heart, paying particular attention to the presence of an S_3 heart sound.

Monitor for these signs of inadequate organ *perfusion* that may result from decreased cardiac output:

- A change in orientation or mental status
- Urine output less than 30 mL/hr
- Cool, clammy extremities with decreased or absent pulses
- Unusual fatigue
- Recurrent chest pain

In specialized units, hemodynamic monitoring requiring the insertion of a pulmonary artery catheter may be started to assess the patient's preload, afterload, and cardiac output. Obtain and record hemodynamic measurements, which include:

- Right atrial pressure
- Pulmonary artery systolic and diastolic pressures
- Pulmonary artery wedge pressure (PAWP) (a measure of preload)
- Pulmonary vascular resistance
- Systemic vascular resistance (a measure of afterload)
- Cardiac output
- Central venous pressure (CVP)
- Cardiac index

Single values of these measurements are less significant than the trend of values combined with the patient's clinical manifestations. They help health care providers identify heart failure and guide the administration of fluids and vasoactive drugs.

Classification of postmyocardial infarction heart failure. Killip categorized heart failure after an MI into four classes based on prognosis (Table 40-3). This system complements the ACC/AHA heart failure classification of function assessment discussed in Chapter 37.

Patients with *class I* heart failure often respond well to reduction in preload with IV nitrates and diuretics. Monitor the urine output hourly, check vital signs hourly, continue to assess for signs of heart failure, and review the serum potassium level.

Patients with *class II* and *class III* heart failure may require diuresis and more aggressive medical intervention, such as afterload reduction and/or enhancement of contractility. IV nitroprusside or nitroglycerin may be used to decrease both preload and afterload. These drugs are given as continuous infusions in specialized units where the PAWP and BP can be closely monitored. The BP can drop in response to excessive vasodilation.

Patients in *classes II* and *III* are usually started on once-a-day beta blockers (usually Toprol XR or Coreg CR). Dosing is titrated depending on goal achievement and drug tolerance. Other drugs, including ACE inhibitors and ARBs, are commonly prescribed to promote ventricular remodeling. These drugs are described in Chart 40-4 and in Chapters 37 and 38.

Positive inotropes, such as dobutamine (Dobutrex) and milrinone (Primacor), increase the force of cardiac contraction. They are administered by continuous IV infusion. The effects of these drugs on the blood vessels and heart rate vary and may be dose dependent. The infusions are titrated to promote cardiac output. *Use caution when giving these drugs because of the potential risk for increasing myocardial oxygen consumption and further decreasing cardiac output. Monitor the patient frequently, paying particular attention to the development of chest pain.*

Class IV heart failure is cardiogenic shock. In **cardiogenic shock,** necrosis of more than 40% of the left ventricle occurs. Most patients have a stuttering pattern of chest pain, resulting in piecemeal extension of the MI. Monitor for manifestations of cardiogenic shock, which include:

- Tachycardia
- Hypotension
- BP less than 90 mm Hg or 30 mm Hg less than the patient's baseline

TABLE 40-3 Killip Classification of Heart Failure

Class	Description
I	Absent crackles and S_3
II	Crackles in the lower half of the lung fields and possible S_3
III	Crackles more than halfway up the lung fields and frequent pulmonary edema
IV	Cardiogenic shock

- Urine output less than 30 mL/hr
- Cold, clammy skin with poor peripheral pulses
- Agitation, restlessness, or confusion
- Pulmonary congestion
- Tachypnea
- Continuing chest discomfort

Early detection is essential because established cardiogenic shock has a high mortality rate.

Drug therapy. Medical interventions aim to relieve pain and decrease myocardial oxygen requirements through preload and afterload reduction (see Chart 40-4 and Chart 40-7). The health care provider prescribes IV morphine, which is used to decrease pulmonary congestion and relieve pain. Oxygen is administered. Intubation and mechanical ventilation may be necessary.

Use the information gained from hemodynamic monitoring to titrate drug therapy. Preload reduction may be cautiously attempted with diuretics or nitroglycerin, as described for patients with Killip class III heart failure. (See Chapter 35 for a complete discussion of preload and afterload.) Monitor systolic pressure continuously because vasodilation may result in a further decline in BP. Vasopressors and positive inotropes may be used to maintain organ perfusion, but these drugs increase myocardial oxygen consumption and can worsen ischemia. Use extreme caution in giving drug therapy.

Intra-aortic balloon pump. When patients do not respond to drug therapy with improved tissue perfusion, decreased workload of the heart, and increased cardiac contractility, an **intra-aortic balloon pump (IABP)** may be inserted. The IABP is an invasive intervention that is used to improve myocardial perfusion during an acute MI, reduce preload and afterload, and facilitate left ventricular ejection.

The health care provider can insert the device percutaneously or through a surgical cutdown. Inflation of the IABP during diastole augments the diastolic pressure and improves coronary perfusion by increasing blood flow to the arteries. Deflation of the balloon just before systole reduces afterload at the time of systolic contraction. This action facilitates empty-

Chart 40-7 COMMON EXAMPLES OF DRUG THERAPY

Commonly Used Intravenous Vasodilators and Inotropes

Drug	Usual Dosage	Nursing Interventions	Rationales
NITRATES			
Nitroprusside sodium (Nipride, Nitropress)	IV only by infusion device Begin with 0.4-0.5 mcg/kg/min May increase gradually to 10 mcg/kg/min	Monitor BP every 2-5 min when initiating therapy. If BP drops excessively, elevate the legs, decrease the dose, and increase fluids per unit policy. Monitor PAWP, SVR, BP, heart rate, urine output frequently. Titrate medication to obtain the desired effect.	This agent is a potent, rapidly reversible vasodilator acting on both peripheral venous and arterial musculature. BP may drop in 2 min.
		Protect from light.	This agent is light sensitive.
		Maintain dose at less than 3 mcg/kg/min if possible.	Doses higher than 3 mcg/kg/min are associated with thiocyanate or cyanide toxicity.
		In patients requiring doses higher than 3 mcg/kg/min for longer than 24-36 hr, monitor for metabolic acidosis, confusion, or hyperreflexia. Examine blood thiocyanate level.	These are indications of the toxic effects of cyanide.
Nitroglycerin (Tridil)	IV only by infusion device started at 5 mcg/kg/min and gradually increased in increments of 5 every 3-5 min; if no response after 20 mcg/kg/min, increase by 10-20 mcg until desired response	Monitor BP every 1-3 min when initiating therapy. If BP drops excessively, elevate the legs and decrease the dose according to unit policies. Monitor RAP, PAWP, SVR, BP, heart rate, and urine output frequently. Titrate medication to obtain the desired effect.	This agent dilates coronary arteries. It is a more potent systemic vasodilator than an arterial vasodilator. BP may drop in 1 min.
		Intermittent administration of IV nitroglycerin should be considered.	Tolerance may develop rapidly to nitroglycerin administered by continuous IV.
		Monitor patients for headache.	Headache is a frequent side effect of initial nitroglycerin therapy.

BP, Blood pressure; *ECG*, electrocardiogram; *I&O*, input and output; *PAWP*, pulmonary artery wedge pressure; *RAP*, right atrial pressure; *SVR*, systemic vascular resistance.

Continued

Chart 40-7 COMMON EXAMPLES OF DRUG THERAPY

Commonly Used Intravenous Vasodilators and Inotropes—cont'd

Drug	Usual Dosage	Nursing Interventions	Rationales
NITRATES—cont'd			
Milrinone (Primacor)	IV bolus 50 mcg/kg given over 10 min; start infusion of 0.375-0.75 mcg/kg/min; reduce dose in renal impairment	Assess BP and pulse every 5 min. If BP drops 30 mm Hg, stop infusion and call health care provider.	Hypotension is a common adverse effect.
		Monitor I&O and weight.	The drug causes diuresis.
Fenoldopam (Corlopam)	0.01-1.6 mcg/kg/min IV	Assess BP and pulse every 5 min, then every 1 hr × 2, then every 4 hr, or according to agency policy.	Same as for milrinone.
		Monitor I&O, and assess for signs of dehydration.	
		Observe IV site for extravasation.	
SYMPATHOMIMETICS			
Dopamine (Intropin)	IV only by infusion device Starting dose 2-5 mcg/kg/min	Determine the reason for use and the expected result.	This agent is a dose-dependent activator of alpha, beta, and dopaminergic receptors.
	Titrate up to 50 mcg/kg/min	Observe the patient's heart rate, ECG, BP, PAWP, SVR, cardiac output, and urine output every 5 min to every 1 hr.	2-5 mcg/kg/min stimulates dopaminergic receptors, which promotes renal and mesenteric blood flow.
		Titrate the dose carefully to maintain the dose range and obtain the desired effect.	5 mcg/kg/min stimulates beta receptors. This increases heart rate and contractility more than 10-15 mcg/kg/min, alpha effects predominate. This causes peripheral constriction.
		Infuse through a central catheter.	Extravasation can cause tissue necrosis and sloughing.
		Monitor patients for ectopy and angina.	These are adverse effects.
Dobutamine (Dobutrex)	IV only by infusion device, 2-10 mcg/kg/min. May increase to 40 mcg/kg/min.	Observe patients continuously during administration.	This agent is a very strong $beta_1$-receptor activator and a moderately strong $beta_2$-activator.
		Titrate the drug on the basis of heart rate, ECG findings, BP, PAWP, cardiac output, SVR, and urine output.	
		Monitor for atrial and ventricular ectopy.	Dysrhythmias are an adverse effect.

BP, Blood pressure; *ECG,* electrocardiogram; *I&O,* input and output; *PAWP,* pulmonary artery wedge pressure; *RAP,* right atrial pressure; *SVR,* systemic vascular resistance.

ing of the left ventricle and improves cardiac output. The balloon catheter is attached to a pump console, which is triggered by an ECG tracing and arterial waveform.

Immediate reperfusion. Immediate reperfusion is an invasive intervention that shows some promise for managing cardiogenic shock. The patient is taken to the cardiac catheterization laboratory, and an emergency left-sided heart catheterization is performed. If he or she has a treatable occlusion or occlusions, the surgeon performs a percutaneous transluminal coronary angioplasty (with stent placement) in the catheterization laboratory or the patient is transferred to the operating suite for a coronary artery bypass graft (CABG).

Managing Right Ventricular Failure. Conditions other than left ventricular failure may result in decreased cardiac output after an MI. In about a third of patients with inferior MIs, right ventricular infarction and failure develop. In this instance, the right ventricle fails independently of the left. Decreased cardiac output with a paradoxical pulse, clear lungs, and jugular venous distention occurs when the patient is in semi-Fowler's position.

A right ventricular MI may be documented by echocardiography and by an ECG using right-sided precordial leads. The desired outcome of management is to improve right ventricular stroke volume by increasing right ventricular fiber stretch or preload. To enhance right ventricular preload, give sufficient fluids (as much as 200 mL/hr) to increase right atrial pressure to 20 mm Hg. *Monitor the pulmonary artery wedge pressure (PAWP)—attempting to maintain it below 15 to 20 mm Hg—and auscultate the lungs to assess for left-sided heart failure. If symptoms of this complication occur, notify the health care provider immediately.*

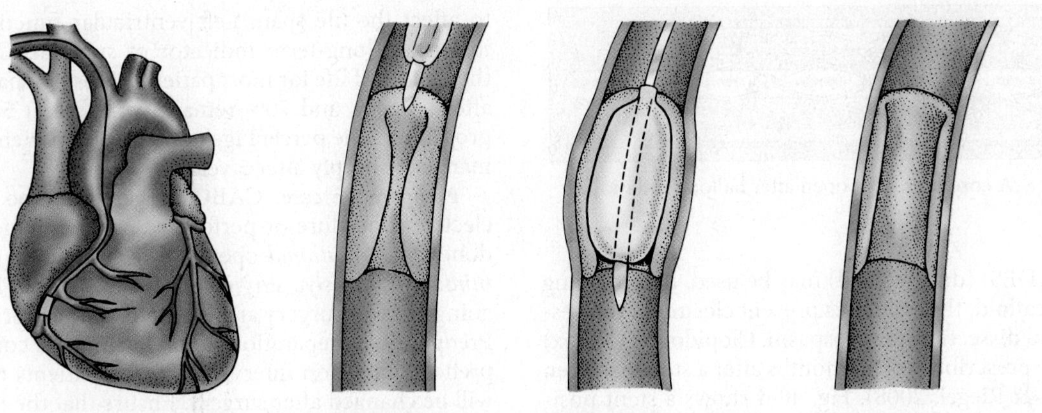
1. The balloon-tipped catheter is positioned in the artery.
2. The uninflated balloon is centered in the obstruction.
3. The balloon is inflated, which flattens plaque against the artery wall.
4. The balloon is removed, and the artery is left unoccluded.

Fig. 40-3 • Percutaneous transluminal coronary angioplasty.

Potential for Recurrent Symptoms and Extension of Injury

Planning: Expected Outcomes. The initial desired outcome for treating the patient with acute coronary syndrome (ACS) is to stop the continuing ischemic process and prevent or minimize serious adverse events such as MI (if unstable angina), MI extension, or death. The patient is expected to experience minimal angina while engaging in ADLs and an exercise program.

Interventions. *Recurrent discomfort despite medical therapy is one of the major indications for surgical management of CAD.* Patients who continue to have chest discomfort despite medical therapy or who have ischemia during a stress test may require invasive correction by PTCA or CABG to resolve angina or prevent MI. Before invasive treatment, a left-sided cardiac catheterization with coronary angiogram is performed to document that the lesions are correctable and that left ventricular pump function is adequate.

Percutaneous Transluminal Coronary Angioplasty. **Percutaneous transluminal coronary angioplasty (PTCA),** most commonly done before stent placement, is an invasive but nonsurgical technique. It is performed to reduce the frequency and severity of discomfort for patients with angina and to bridge patients to coronary bypass graft surgery. Because of the artery's normal elasticity and "memory" to retain its original shape, the artery often re-occludes if a stent is not used as part of the procedure.

Patients who are most likely to benefit from PTCA have single- or double-vessel disease with discrete, proximal, noncalcified lesions (clots). This procedure often does not work for complex clots. When identifying which lesions are treatable with PTCA, the cardiologist considers the clot's complexity and location, as well as the amount of myocardium at risk. Although treating lesions located in the left main artery places a large amount of myocardial tissue at risk if the vessel closes quickly, these lesions are now being treated more with PTCA and stent placement. In the past, coronary artery bypass grafting (CABG) was the intervention used for these patients. PTCA may also be used for the patient with an evolving acute MI, either alone or with thrombolytic therapy or glycoprotein (GP) IIb/IIIa inhibitor, to reperfuse the damaged myocardium.

Before the procedure, the patient receives an initial dose of clopidogrel (Plavix), an antiplatelet drug. The dosage amount depends on whether the patient received thrombolytics. The physician performs the angioplasty under fluoroscopic guidance in the cardiac catheterization laboratory. A balloon-tipped catheter is introduced through a guidewire to the coronary artery occlusion. The physician activates a compressor that inflates the balloon to force the plaque against the vessel wall, thus dilating the wall, and reduces or eliminates the occluding clot. Balloon inflation may be repeated until angiography indicates a decrease in the stenosis (narrowing) to less than 50% of the vessel's diameter (Fig. 40-3).

After the procedure, IV heparin is administered in a continuous infusion to prevent thrombus formation. IV or intracoronary nitroglycerin or diltiazem (Cardizem) is given to prevent coronary vasospasm. PTCA initially reopens the vessel in most appropriately selected patients. Within the first 24 hours, however, a small percentage of patients have re-stenosis. At 6 months, a larger number have one or more blockages.

After the procedure, monitor for potential problems including acute closure of the vessel (causes chest pain), bleeding from the insertion site, and reaction to the contrast medium used in angiography. Also monitor for hypotension, hypokalemia, and dysrhythmias. Report any of these findings to the physician immediately.

The health care provider usually prescribes a long-term nitrate and dual antiplatelet therapy with aspirin and clopidogrel (Plavix) for patients after PTCA. A beta blocker and an ACE inhibitor or ARB are added for patients who have had primary angioplasty after an MI. Many patients continue to have infusions of GP IIb/IIIa inhibitors during the initial hours after PTCA. Some may experience hypokalemia after the procedure and require careful monitoring and potassium supplements. The nursing interventions for patients receiving these drugs are described in Chart 40-4. Provide careful explanations of drug therapy and any recommended lifestyle changes.

Other Procedures. Other techniques being used to ensure continued patency of the vessel are laser angioplasty (the laser breaks up the clot), atherectomy, and stents. **Atherectomy** devices can either excise and retrieve plaque or emulsify it. One of the advantages of this procedure is that it creates a less bulky vessel with better elastic recoil. **Stents** are expandable metal mesh devices that are used to maintain the patent lumen created by angioplasty or atherectomy. Bare metal or drug-

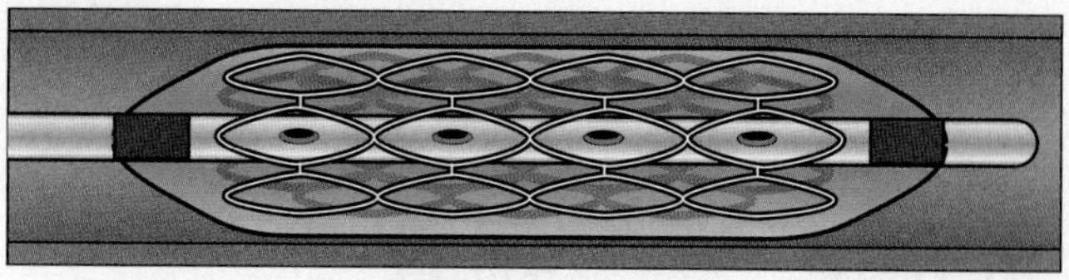

Fig. 40-4 • A coronary stent open after balloon inflation.

eluting stents (DES) (drug-coated) may be used. By providing a supportive scaffold, these devices prevent closure of the vessel from arterial dissection or vasospasm. Clopidogrel (Plavix) and aspirin are prescribed for 12 months after a stent has been placed (Moser & Riegel, 2008). Fig. 40-4 shows a stent positioned in a coronary artery.

Another procedure that may be performed is rheolytic thrombectomy (e.g., AngioJet, Vortex), which uses low-pressure, high-speed saline jets to break up the clot. The EndiCOR X-SIZER lances and aspirates a clot simultaneously.

Injecting vascular endothelial growth factor (VEGF) during angioplasty has increased perfusion to the wall of the heart. Also, VEGF helps initiate new blood vessel growth and development, which results in increased blood supply to cardiac muscle.

ANIMATION: Coronary Artery Bypass Graft ▶

Coronary Artery Bypass Graft Surgery. Over 500,000 **coronary artery bypass graft (CABG)** surgeries are performed in the United States each year. It is the most common type of cardiac surgery and the most common procedure for older adults. Almost half of all CABGs are done for patients older than 65 years. The occluded coronary arteries are bypassed with the patient's own venous or arterial blood vessels or synthetic grafts. *The internal mammary artery (IMA) is the current graft of choice because it has a 90% patency rate at 12 years after the procedure.*

CABG is indicated when patients do not respond to medical management of CAD or when disease progression is evident. Because of the development of drug-eluting stents (DESs), patients who previously had no option other than CABG have been able to have their vessels revascularized without surgery. The decision for surgery is based on the patient's symptoms and the results of cardiac catheterization. Candidates for surgery are patients who have:

- Angina with greater than 50% occlusion of the left main coronary artery that cannot be stented
- Unstable angina with severe two-vessel disease, moderate three-vessel disease, or small-vessel disease in which stents could not be introduced
- Ischemia with heart failure
- Acute MI with cardiogenic shock
- Signs of ischemia or impending MI after angiography or PTCA
- Valvular disease
- Coronary vessels unsuitable for PTCA

The vessels to be bypassed should have proximal clots blocking more than 70% of the vessel's diameter but with good distal runoff. Bypass of less occluded vessels may result in poor perfusion through the graft and early obstruction. CABG is most effective when adequate ventricular function remains and the ejection fraction is close to or greater than 50%. Patients with lower ejection fractions are subject to develop more complications.

For most patients, the risk is low and the benefits of bypass surgery are clear. Surgical treatment of CAD does not appear to affect the life span. Left ventricular function is the most important long-term indicator of survival. CABG improves the quality of life for most patients. Most are pain free at 1 year after surgery, and 70% remain pain free at 5 years after the procedure. The percentage of patients experiencing some pain increases sharply after 5 years.

Preoperative care. CABG surgery may be planned as an elective procedure or performed as an emergency. It may be done as a *traditional* operative technique or performed as a *minimally invasive surgical (MIS)* technique. Patients undergoing elective surgery are admitted on the morning of surgery. Preoperative preparations and teaching are completed during prehospitalization interviews. Teach patients that their drugs will be changed after surgery. Ensure that the necessary drugs have been administered before surgery.

Familiarize the patient and family with the cardiac surgical–critical care unit (sometimes referred to as the "open heart" unit), and prepare them for postoperative care. If the procedure is elective, demonstrate and have the patient return a demonstration of how to splint the chest incision, cough, deep breathe, and perform arm and leg exercises. Stress that:

- The patient should report any pain to the nursing staff.
- Most of the pain will be in the site where the vessel was harvested. (With the use of endovascular vessel harvesting (EVH) and small one or two 1-inch incisions, the pain and edema are less than for previously performed procedures.)
- Analgesics will be given for pain.
- Coughing and deep breathing are essential to prevent pulmonary complications.
- Early ambulation is important to decrease the risk of venous thrombosis and possible embolism.

For the traditional surgical procedure, explain that the patient will have a sternal incision, possibly a large leg incision, one, two or three chest tubes, an indwelling urinary catheter, pacemaker wires, and hemodynamic monitoring. An endotracheal tube will be connected to a ventilator for several hours postoperatively. Tell the patient and family that the patient will not be able to talk while the endotracheal tube is in place. When describing the postoperative course, emphasize that close monitoring and the use of sophisticated equipment are standard treatment.

Preoperative anxiety is common. An appropriate nursing assessment should identify the level of anxiety and the coping methods patients have used successfully in the past. Some patients may find it helpful to define their fears. Common sources of fear include fear of the unknown, fear of bodily harm, and fear of death.

In elective procedures, patients may benefit from detailed information about the surgery. Others may feel overwhelmed by so much material. Some patients need to discuss their feelings in detail or describe the experiences of people they know who have undergone CABG. Assess patients' anxiety level and help them cope.

Operative procedures. Coronary artery bypass surgery is performed with the patient under general anesthesia for both cardiopulmonary bypass and off-pump surgery. For the *traditional operative procedure,* the cardiac surgical team begins the procedure with a median sternotomy incision and visualization of the heart and great vessels. Another surgical team may begin harvesting the vein if it is to be used for the graft. Synthetic grafts may be used instead.

Cardiopulmonary bypass (CPB) is used to provide oxygenation, circulation, and hypothermia during induced cardiac arrest. Blood is diverted from the heart to the bypass machine, where it is heparinized, oxygenated, and returned to the circulation through a cannula placed in the ascending aortic arch or femoral artery (Fig. 40-5). During bypass, the patient's core temperature remains between 95° F (35° C) (cold cardioplegia) and normal temperature (warm cardioplegia). Although cooling decreases the rate of metabolism and demand for oxygen, keeping the heart "warm" decreases postoperative complications that were more common when cold cardioplegia was used. The heart is perfused with a potassium solution, which decreases myocardial oxygen consumption and causes the heart to stop during diastole. This process ensures a motionless operative field and prevents myocardial ischemia.

Once the heart is arrested, the grafting procedure can begin. The surgeon uses the IMA, a saphenous vein, or both, or a radial artery to bypass blockages in the coronary arteries (Fig. 40-6). The distal end of the vessel graft is dissected and attached below the clot in the coronary artery. If the surgeon uses a venous graft or the radial artery, it is anastomosed (sutured) proximally to the aorta and distally to the coronary artery just beyond the occlusion, thus improving myocardial perfusion. After flow rates through the grafts are measured, the heart is rewarmed slowly. The cardioplegic solution is flushed from the heart. The heart regains its rate and rhythm, or it may be defibrillated to return it to a normal rhythm. When the procedure is completed, the patient may be rewarmed (if cold cardioplegia was used) and weaned from the bypass machine while the grafts are observed for patency and leakage. The surgeon may place atrial and ventricular pace-

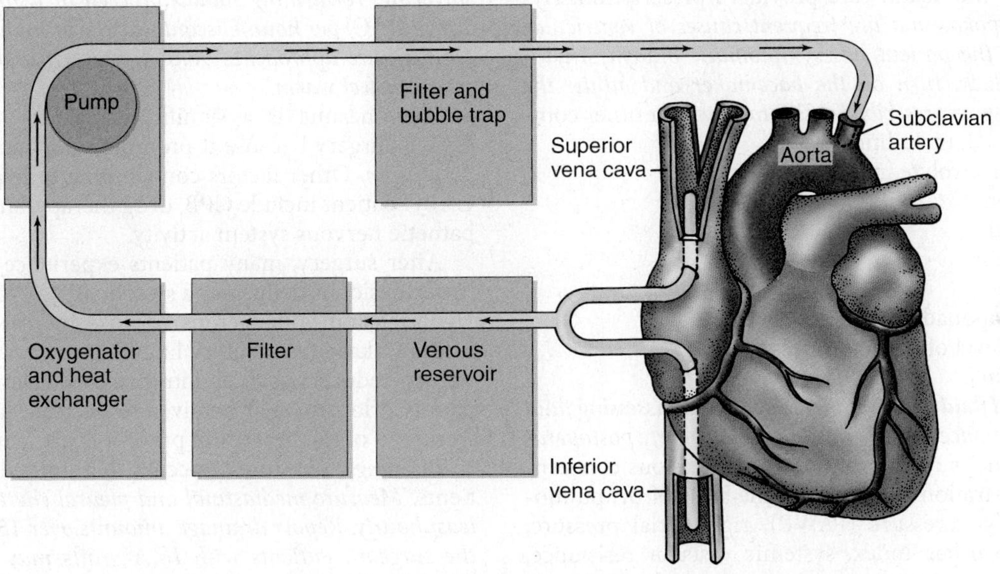
Pump
Filter and bubble trap
Subclavian artery
Superior vena cava
Aorta
Oxygenator and heat exchanger
Filter
Venous reservoir
Inferior vena cava

Fig. 40-5 • Heart-lung bypass circuitry used during cardiopulmonary bypass.

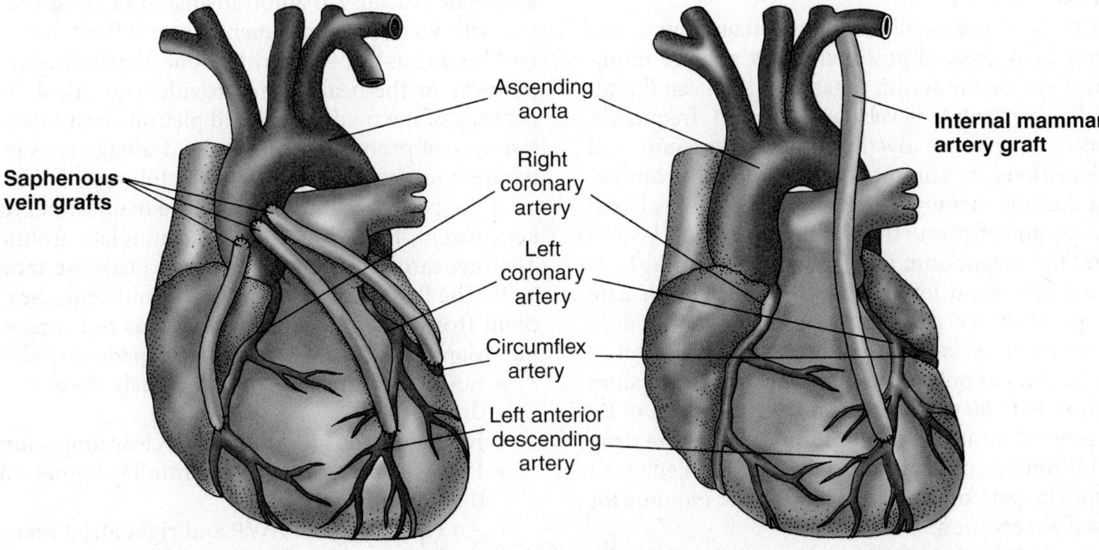
Saphenous vein grafts
Ascending aorta
Right coronary artery
Left coronary artery
Circumflex artery
Left anterior descending artery
Internal mammary artery graft

Fig. 40-6 • Two methods of coronary artery bypass grafting. The procedure used depends on the nature of the coronary artery disease, the condition of the vessels available for grafting, and the patient's health status.

maker wires and mediastinal and pleural chest tubes. Finally, the surgeon closes the sternum with wire sutures.

Postoperative care. After traditional surgery, the patient is transported to a post–open heart surgery unit and undergoes mechanical ventilation for 3 to 6 hours. *He or she requires highly skilled nursing care from a nurse qualified to provide post–cardiac surgery care, including routine postoperative care described in Chapter 18. Be sure to use sterile technique when changing sternal or donor site dressings.*

Connect the mediastinal tubes to water-seal drainage systems, and ground the epicardial pacer wires by connecting them to the pacemaker generator. Monitor pulmonary artery and arterial pressures, as well as the heart rate and rhythm, which are displayed on a monitor.

Closely assess the patient for dysrhythmias, such as ventricular ectopic rhythms, bradydysrhythmias, atrial fibrillation, or heart block. Manage symptomatic dysrhythmias according to unit protocol or the health care provider's prescription. *Hypoxemia and hypokalemia are frequent causes of ventricular dysrhythmias. If the patient has symptomatic bradydysrhythmias or heart block, turn on the pacemaker and adjust the pacemaker settings as prescribed.* Also, monitor for other complications of CABG, including:

- Fluid and electrolyte imbalance
- Hypotension
- Hypothermia
- Hypertension
- Bleeding
- Cardiac tamponade
- Decreased level of consciousness
- Anginal pain

Management of fluid and electrolyte imbalance. *Assessing fluid and electrolyte balance is a high priority in the early postoperative period.* Edema is common. However, decisions concerning fluid administration are made on the basis of BP, pulmonary artery wedge pressure (PAWP), right atrial pressure, cardiac output, cardiac index, systemic vascular resistance, blood loss, and urine output. An experienced specialized nurse interprets the assessment findings and adjusts fluid administration on the basis of standing unit policies or specific prescription from the physician.

Serum electrolytes (especially calcium, magnesium, and potassium) may be decreased postoperatively and are monitored carefully. Because the serum potassium level can fluctuate dramatically, electrolyte levels are checked frequently, since imbalances can cause dysrhythmias. Potassium and magnesium depletions are common and may result from hemodilution or diuretic therapy. Calcium replacement is based on the *ionized* serum calcium. The desired potassium level is 4.0 mEq/L, and the magnesium level should be 2.2 mEq/L.

If the serum potassium level is depleted, the health care provider may prescribe IV potassium replacement. The dose of potassium given exceeds the usual recommended level of no more than 20 mEq of potassium per hour. For a potassium bolus, as much as 40 to 80 mEq may be mixed in 100 mL of IV solution and given at a rate up to 40 mEq per hour. The drug must be given through a central catheter and controlled by an infusion pump. The patient is placed on a cardiac monitor for intense, focused observation.

Management of other complications. *Hypotension* (systolic BP <90 mm Hg) is a major problem because it may result in the collapse of the graft. Decreased preload (decreased PAWP) can result from hypovolemia or vasodilation. If the patient is hypovolemic, it might be appropriate to increase fluid administration or administer blood. The health care provider may manage the patient with volume replacement followed by vasopressor therapy to increase the BP. However, if hypotension is the result of left ventricular failure (increased PAWP), IV inotropes might be needed.

Hypothermia is a common problem after surgery. Although warm cardioplegia is now the usual operative procedure used, it is not uncommon for the body temperature to drift downward after the patient leaves the surgical suite. Monitor the body temperature, and institute rewarming procedures if the temperature drops below 96.8° F (36° C). Rewarming may be accomplished with warm blankets, lights, or thermal blankets. The danger of rewarming patients too quickly is that they may begin shivering, resulting in metabolic acidosis, increased myocardial oxygen consumption, and hypoxia. *To prevent shivering, rewarming should proceed at a rate no faster than 1.8° F (1° C) per hour. Discontinue the procedure when the body temperature approaches 98.6° F (37° C) and the patient's extremities feel warm.*

Hypothermia is a significant risk for the patient after CABG surgery because it promotes vasoconstriction and *hypertension.* Other factors contributing to hypertension in the CABG patient include CPB, drug therapy, and increased sympathetic nervous system activity.

After surgery, many patients experience hypertension (if hypertension is defined as a systolic BP >140 to 150 mm Hg). Hypertension is dangerous because increased pressure promotes leakage from suture lines and may cause bleeding. Afterload reducers such as nitroprusside (Nipride) or fenoldopam (Corlopam) may be given to decrease afterload, ease the workload of the heart, and prevent heart failure.

Bleeding after surgery occurs to a limited extent in all patients. *Measure mediastinal and pleural chest tube drainage at least hourly. Report drainage amounts over 150 mL per hour to the surgeon. Patients with IMA grafts may have more chest drainage than those with saphenous vein grafts.* To access the IMA, the pleural space has to be entered and requires a pleural chest tube with the mediastinal tubes, making pulmonary assessment crucial. An autotransfusion of chest drainage to assist with volume management when 500 mL has accumulated or 4 hours has elapsed may be done, depending on the clinical pathway or the health care provider's protocol. Maintain the patency of the mediastinal and pleural chest tubes. One effective way of promoting chest tube drainage is to prevent a dependent loop from forming in the tubing.

If the patient is bleeding and the mediastinal tubes are not kept patent, fluid (blood) may accumulate around the heart. The myocardium is compressed, and **cardiac tamponade** results. The fluid compresses the atria and ventricles, preventing them from filling adequately and thus reducing cardiac output. Manifestations of cardiac tamponade include:

- Sudden cessation of previously heavy mediastinal drainage
- Jugular venous distention but clear lung sounds
- Pulsus paradoxus (BP >10 mm Hg higher on expiration than on inspiration)
- An equalizing of PAWP and right atrial pressure
- Cardiovascular collapse

Tamponade can be confirmed by echocardiogram or chest x-ray. Pericardiocentesis may not be appropriate for tamponade after CABG because the blood in the pericardium may have clotted. Volume expansion and emergency sternotomy with drainage are the treatments of choice.

The patient may also demonstrate *changes in level of consciousness,* which may be permanent or transient (short-term). Transient changes related to anesthesia, CPB, air emboli, or hypothermia occur in many patients. Neurologic deficits may include slowness to arouse, memory loss, and confusion.

Patients with transient neurologic deficits usually return to baseline neurologic status within 4 to 8 hours. Permanent deficits associated with an intraoperative stroke may be manifested by:
- Abnormal pupillary response
- Failure to awaken from anesthesia
- Seizures
- Absence of sensory or motor function

Check the patient's neurologic status every 30 to 60 minutes until he or she has awakened from anesthesia. Then check every 2 to 4 hours or per agency policy.

Pain management. Differentiate between sternotomy pain, which is expected after CABG, and *anginal pain,* which might indicate graft failure. Typical sternotomy pain is localized, does not radiate, and often becomes worse when the patient coughs or breathes deeply. He or she may describe the pain as sharp, aching, or burning. Pain may stimulate the sympathetic nervous system, which increases the heart rate and vascular resistance while decreasing cardiac output. Administer enough of the prescribed analgesic in adequate doses to control pain. During the process of weaning the patient from mechanical ventilation, however, it may be necessary to use short-acting analgesics and to limit pain medication because of the respiratory depressant effects of analgesia.

Transfer from the special care unit. Mechanical ventilation is usually provided for 3 to 6 hours after surgery until the patient is breathing adequately and is hemodynamically stable. During the first day, the patient usually has pacemaker wires, hemodynamic monitoring lines, and mediastinal tubes removed. He or she is then transferred to an intermediate care unit. *All CABG patients, especially those with IMA grafts, are at high risk for atelectasis, the number-one complication. Encourage them to splint, cough, turn, and deep breathe to expectorate secretions. Early ambulation after surgery is essential.* Two hours after extubation (removal of the endotracheal tube), patients should be dangled as tolerated and turned side to side. Within 4 to 8 hours after extubation, help patients out of bed into a chair. By the first day after surgery, they should be out of bed in a chair and ambulating 25 to 100 feet three times a day as tolerated. Continue to monitor for decreased cardiac output, pain, dysrhythmias, oxygen saturation, and infection during these activities.

Monitor the neurovascular status of the donor arm of patients whose radial artery was used as a graft in CABG. Assess the hand color, temperature, pulse (both ulnar and radial), and capillary refill every hour initially. In addition, check the fingertips, hand, and arm for sensation and mobility at least every 4 hours. IV nitroglycerin is often given for the first 24 hours postoperatively to promote vasodilation in the donor arm and therefore maintain circulation.

Many patients have supraventricular dysrhythmias (especially atrial fibrillation) during the postoperative period, usually on the second or third postoperative day. Examine the monitor pattern for atrial fibrillation. When auscultating the heart, listen for an irregular rhythm.

Sternal wound infections develop between 5 days and several weeks after surgery in a small number of patients and are responsible for increased costs and longer length of stays. Be alert for **mediastinitis** (infection of the mediastinum) by observing for:
- Fever continuing beyond the first 4 days after CABG
- Instability (bogginess) of the sternum
- Redness, induration, swelling, or drainage from suture sites
- An increased white blood cell count

The health care provider may perform a needle biopsy to confirm a sternal infection. Surgical débridement, antibiotic wound irrigation, and IV antibiotics are usually indicated. If sternal osteomyelitis has developed, 4 to 6 weeks of IV antibiotics are required. Prophylactic use of mupirocin (Bactroban) intranasally may be prescribed to decrease the incidence of sternal wound infection.

Postpericardiotomy syndrome is a source of chest discomfort for some post–cardiac surgery patients. The syndrome is characterized by pericardial and pleural pain, pericarditis, a friction rub, an elevated temperature and white blood cell count, and dysrhythmias. Postpericardiotomy syndrome may occur days to weeks after surgery and seems to be associated with blood remaining in the pericardial sac. Observe for the development of pericardial or pleural pain. For most patients, the syndrome is mild and self-limiting. However, they may require treatment similar to that for pericarditis. Be prepared to detect acute cardiac (pericardial) tamponade (see Chapter 37).

NCLEX EXAMINATION CHALLENGE

After receiving the change-of-shift report, which client should the nurse assess first? The client with:

A. Stable angina who had chest pain relieved with two nitroglycerin tablets 1 hour ago
B. Unstable angina having substernal chest pain, nausea, sweating, and anxiety
C. Stable vital signs who returned from the percutaneous coronary intervention lab 30 minutes ago
D. An acute MI transferred from the coronary care unit earlier today reporting a headache

evolve For the correct answer, go to http://evolve.elsevier.com/Iggy/.

Minimally Invasive Direct Coronary Artery Bypass. The **minimally invasive direct coronary artery bypass (MIDCAB)** (also known as *"keyhole" surgery*) may be indicated for patients with a lesion of the left anterior descending (LAD) artery. In one of the most common MIDCAB procedures, a 2-inch left thoracotomy incision is made and the fourth rib is removed. Then, the left internal mammary artery (IMA) is dissected and attached to the still-beating heart below the level of the lesion. Cardiopulmonary bypass (CPB) is not required.

After surgery, assess for chest pain and ECG changes (Q waves and ST-segment and T-wave changes in leads V_2 to V_6) because occlusion of the IMA graft occurs acutely in about 10% of patients. *If there is any question of acute graph closure, immediately notify the health care provider.* Patients tend to have more incisional pain after MIDCAB than after traditional CABG surgery, but the pain can usually be managed with oxycodone or codeine. *Because they have a thoracotomy incision and a chest tube or smaller-lumen vacuum chest device, they are encouraged to cough, deep breathe, and use an incentive spirometer for a week postoperatively.* Most patients spend less than 6 hours in a critical care unit and are discharged in 2 or 3 days.

Endovascular (Endoscopic) Vessel Harvesting (EVH). Regardless of whether the traditional CABG or the MIDCAB is performed, the donor vessel may be obtained using an endoscope rather than a large surgical incision. The radial artery or a vein in the leg may be taken using this method. Instead of a large, painful incision, the patient has one or two very small incisions in the leg or arm. This procedure has decreased hospital length of stay, postoperative complications, and pain.

Transmyocardial Laser Revascularization. **Transmyocardial laser revascularization** is a procedure for patients with unstable angina and inoperable CAD with areas of reversible myocardial ischemia. After a single-lung intubation, a left anterior thoracotomy is performed and the heart is visualized. A laser is used to create 20 to 24 long, narrow channels through the left ventricular muscle to the left ventricle. These channels will eventually allow oxygenated blood to flow during diastole from the left ventricle to nourish the muscle. After surgery, the patient is transported to a critical care unit, where hemodynamic monitoring is used to assess for anginal episodes and bleeding disturbances.

Off-Pump Coronary Artery Bypass. Off-pump coronary artery bypass (OPCAB) is a procedure in which open heart surgery is performed without the use of a heart-lung bypass machine. Advantages include shorter hospital stays and decreased mortality rate, risk of infection, and cost. OPCAB does have some risk, such as increased skill and steeper learning curve for surgeons to master the technique and inaccessible surgery sites.

Robotic Heart Surgery. Robotic heart surgery is a new step toward less invasive open heart surgery. Surgeons operate endoscopically through very small incisions in the chest wall. Use of robotics provides surgeons with capabilities that simplify the surgical process, eliminates tremors that can exist with human hands, increases the ability to reach otherwise inaccessible sites, and improves depth perception and visual acuity.

Other advantages of robotic procedures include shorter hospital stays (average stay is 2 to 3 days), less pain because of smaller incisions, no need for heart-lung bypass machine, less anxiety for the patient, and greater patient acceptance. The use of robotics also allows surgeons to perform telesurgery, performing heart procedures over long distances.

Disadvantages include computer failure, limited numbers of surgeons skilled in these techniques, and the length of surgery time (the time is about 50 minutes longer than the conventional surgery).

Community-Based Care

Home Care Management

Case management is most appropriate for patients who meet high-cost, high-volume, and high-risk criteria. Patients with coronary artery disease (CAD) clearly meet all these criteria. Clinical pathways and case management programs for those with CAD are used in most U.S. hospitals. By focusing on cardiovascular risk reduction and improving the continuity of care, health care professionals have reduced the length and cost of hospital stays. Posthospital case management should reduce hospital readmission rates and improve patient health.

Patients who have experienced a myocardial infarction (MI), angina, or coronary artery bypass graft (CABG) surgery are usually discharged to home or to a transitional care setting with drug therapy and specific activity prescriptions. Depending on the procedure, hospital stays may be 3 to 5 days for patients with MI or those undergoing CABG and only 1 to 3 days for those undergoing percutaneous transluminal coronary angioplasty (PTCA) or newer surgeries. Therefore patients are still recovering when they are discharged from the hospital and need continuing care.

Patients should not be discharged to home alone. Assess whether he or she has family or friends to provide assistance. In some cases, a home care nurse may be needed (Chart 40-8). Older adults are often living alone when coronary events occur and may have a greater need for home assistance after CABG surgery (Chart 40-9). Patients who were residents in long-term care may be returned there after hospitalization for unstable angina, MI, or CABG surgery.

Cardiac rehabilitation is available in most communities for patients after an MI or CABG surgery, but only a small percentage participate in structured rehabilitation programs. The most frequently cited reasons for nonparticipation are lack of insurance coverage, a physician's decision that it is unnecessary, and the patient's decision that it is not necessary. Those who participate in these programs report greater improvement in exercise tolerance and improved ability to control stress. However, no difference in their return to work has been seen.

Health Teaching

The need for health teaching depends in part on the treatment plan or type of procedure that the patient received. Because hospital stays are short and patients are quite ill during hospi-

Chart 40-8 HOME CARE ASSESSMENT

The Patient Who Has Had a Myocardial Infarction

Assess cardiovascular function, including:
- Current vital signs (compare with previous to identify changes)
- Recurrence of discomfort (characteristics, frequency, onset)
- Indications of heart failure (weight gain, crackles, cough, dyspnea)
- Adequacy of tissue perfusion (mentation, skin temperature, peripheral pulses, urine output)
- Indications of serious dysrhythmia (very irregular pulse, palpitations with fainting or near fainting)

Assess coping skills, including:
- Is patient displaying denial, anger, or fear?
- Is the caregiver providing adequate support?
- Are the patient and caregiver disagreeing about treatment?

Assess functional ability, including:
- Activity tolerance (examine the patient's activity diary: review distance, duration, frequency, and symptoms occurring during exercise)
- Activities of daily living (is any assistance needed?)
- Household chores (who performs them?)
- Does patient plan to return to work? When?

Assess nutritional status, including:
- Food intake (review patient's intake of fats and cholesterol)

Assess patient's understanding of illness and treatment, including:
- How to treat chest discomfort
- Signs and symptoms to report to health care provider
- Dosage, effects, and side effects of medications
- How to advance and when to limit activity
- Modification of risk factors for coronary artery disease

talization, most in-hospital education programs concentrate on the skills essential for self-care after discharge.

As part of home visits or a cardiac rehabilitation program, identify the additional educational needs of the patient and family and their readiness to learn. Develop a teaching plan, which usually includes education about the normal anatomy and physiology of the heart, the pathophysiology of angina and MI, risk factor modification, activity and exercise protocols, cardiac drugs, and when to seek medical assistance. Teach patients that myocardial healing after an MI begins early and is usually complete in 6 to 8 weeks. Remind those who have undergone traditional CABG that the sternotomy should heal in about 6 to 8 weeks but upper body exercise needs to be limited for several months.

Patients who have undergone CABG require instruction on incision care for the sternum and the graft site. Teach them to inspect the incisions daily for any redness, swelling, or drainage. The leg of a saphenous vein donor site is often edematous. Instruct patients to avoid crossing legs, to wear elastic stockings until the edema subsides, and to elevate the surgical limb when sitting in a chair. Teach patients who have had a radial artery graft to open and close the hand vigorously 10 times every 2 hours.

Risk Factor Modification. Modification of risk factors is a necessary part of a patient's management and involves changing his or her health maintenance patterns. Such modifications may include tobacco cessation, altered nutritional habits, regular exercise, BP control, and blood glucose control. Each of these factors has been discussed earlier in this chapter in the Health Promotion and Maintenance section.

For patients who use tobacco, explain its negative effects, especially cigarette smoking. Many patients choose to quit smoking soon after an MI. Chapter 38 also provides information on this lifestyle change.

The mainstays of cholesterol control are nutritional therapy and anti-hyperlipidemic agents, as described in Chapter 38. Teach patients to avoid adding salt when beginning a meal. A reduction of 80 mg/day of sodium can reduce the systolic blood pressure (SBP) by 5 mm Hg and 3 mm Hg for the diastolic blood pressure (DBP). Maintain adequate dietary potassium, calcium, and magnesium intake. Increasing potassium may reduce the SBP by 8 mm Hg. Booklets and cookbooks that can assist the patient in learning to cook with reduced fats, oils, and salt are available from the American Heart Association (AHA).

Collaborate with the physical therapist to establish an activity and exercise schedule as part of rehabilitation, depending on the cardiac procedure that was performed. Instruct the patient to remain near home during the first week after discharge and to continue a walking program. Patients may engage in light housework or any activity done while sitting and that does not precipitate angina. During the second week, they are encouraged to increase social activities and possibly to return to work part-time. By the third week, they may begin to lift objects as heavy as 15 pounds (e.g., 2 gallons of milk) but should avoid lifting or pulling heavier objects for the first 6 to 8 weeks. Chart 40-10 lists suggested instructions for activity level.

Patients may begin a simple walking program by walking 400 feet twice a day at the rate of 1 mile/hr the first week after discharge and increasing the distance and rate as tolerated, usually weekly, until they can walk 2 miles at 3 to 4 miles per hour. Teach them to take their pulse reading before, halfway through, and after exercise. Teach the patient to stop exercising if the target pulse rate is exceeded or if dyspnea or angina develops.

After a limited exercise tolerance test, the physical therapist or nurse encourages the patient to join a formal exercise program, ideally one that assists him or her in monitoring cardiovascular progress. The program should include 5- to 7-minute warm-up and cool-down periods, as well as 30 minutes of aerobic exercise. The patient should engage in aerobic exercise a minimum of three (and preferably five) times a week.

Complementary and Alternative Therapies. Additional therapies can aid in reducing the patient's anxiety about progressive activity both in the immediate postoperative period and during the rehabilitation phase. Many patients who have had cardiac surgery or other invasive procedures use complementary and alternative therapies. However, they often do not share with their health care providers that they use these therapies. Techniques such as progressive muscle relaxation, guided imagery,

Chart 40-9 NURSING FOCUS ON THE OLDER ADULT
Coronary Artery Bypass Graft Surgery

- Be aware that perioperative mortality rates are higher for the older patient than for the patient younger than 60 years.
- Monitor neurologic and mental status carefully because older adults are more likely to have transient neurologic deficits after coronary artery bypass graft (CABG) surgery than younger adults are.
- Observe for side effects of cardiac drugs because older patients are more likely to develop toxic effects from positive inotropes (dobutamine) and potent antihypertensives (nitroglycerin or nitroprusside).
- Monitor the patient closely for dysrhythmias because older adults are more likely to have dysrhythmias, such as atrial fibrillation or supraventricular tachycardia, after CABG surgery.
- Be aware that recuperation after CABG surgery is slower for older patients and that their average length of hospital stay is longer.
- Teach the patient and family that during the first 2 to 5 weeks after discharge, fatigue, chest discomfort, and lack of appetite may be particularly bothersome for older adults.
- Teach patient to let someone know where he or she is walking outside.

Chart 40-10 PATIENT AND FAMILY EDUCATION GUIDE
Activity for the Patient with Coronary Artery Disease

- Begin by walking the same distance at home as in the hospital (usually 400 feet) three times each day.
- Carry nitroglycerin with you.
- Check your pulse before, during, and after the exercise.
- Stop the activity for a pulse increase of more than 20 beats/min, shortness of breath, angina, or dizziness.
- Exercise outdoors when the weather is good.
- Gradually increase the walking until the distance is 1/4 mile twice daily (usually the end of the second week).
- After an exercise tolerance test and with your physician's approval, walk at least three times each week, increasing the distance by 1/2 mile every other week, until the total distance is 2 miles.
- Avoid straining (lifting, pushups, pull-ups, and straining at bowel movements).

music therapy, pet therapy, and therapeutic touch may decrease anxiety, reduce depression, and increase compliance with activity and exercise regimens after heart surgery.

Sexual Activity. Sexual activity is often a subject of great concern to patients and their partners. Inform the patient and his or her partner that engaging in their usual sexual activity is unlikely to damage the heart. Patients can resume sexual intercourse on the advice of the health care provider, usually after an exercise tolerance assessment. In general, those who can walk one block or climb two flights of stairs without symptoms can usually safely resume sexual activity.

Suggest that initially these patients have intercourse after a period of rest. They might try having intercourse in the morning when they are well rested or wait 1½ hours after exercise or a heavy meal. The position selected should be comfortable for both the patient and his or her partner so that no undue stress is placed on the heart or suture line.

Drug Therapy. Assess patients with diabetes mellitus for their ability to control hyperglycemia. Review the prescribed dosage of insulin or oral antidiabetic drugs with the patient and family. The patient and/or family should demonstrate accurate testing of blood for glucose levels and the technique for insulin administration, if used.

Teach the patient about the type of prescribed cardiac drugs, the benefit of each drug, potential side effects, and the correct dosage and time of day to take each drug. Drug regimens vary considerably. However, many patients with angina are discharged while taking aspirin, a beta blocker, a calcium channel blocker, an anti-hyperlipidemic agent, and a nitrate. Those who have experienced an MI may require aspirin, a beta blocker, an anti-hyperlipidemic agent, and an ACE inhibitor and/or an ARB. The regimen can be complex. Determine whether the patient can comply with the instructions.

Use of sublingual or spray nitroglycerin (NTG) deserves special attention. Teach the patient to carry NTG at all times. Keep the tablets in a glass, light-resistant container. The drug should be replaced every 3 to 5 months before it loses its potency or stops producing a tingling sensation when placed under the tongue. Chart 40-11 gives instructions for management of chest discomfort at home.

NCLEX EXAMINATION CHALLENGE

A client with chronic stable angina receives discharge teaching from the nurse. Which statement by the client indicates a need for further teaching?

A. "I need to take my nitroglycerin tablets to prevent any serious problems."
B. "At the first sign of chest discomfort, I will stop any activity and sit down."
C. "I will call 911 if my chest discomfort continues after taking 3 nitroglycerin tablets."
D. "I understand I must follow up with my health care provider regularly."

evolve For the correct answer, go to http://evolve.elsevier.com/Iggy/.

Seeking Medical Assistance. Teach patients to notify their health care provider if they have:

- Heart rate remaining less than 50 after arising
- Wheezing or difficulty breathing
- Weight gain of 3 pounds in 1 week or 1 to 2 pounds overnight

Chart 40-11 PATIENT AND FAMILY EDUCATION GUIDE

Management of Chest Pain at Home

- Keep fresh nitroglycerin available for immediate use.
- At the first indication of chest discomfort, cease activity and sit or lie down.
- Place one nitroglycerin tablet or spray under your tongue, allowing the tablet to dissolve.
- Wait 5 minutes for relief.
- If no relief results, repeat the nitroglycerin and wait 5 more minutes.
- If there is no relief, repeat and wait 5 more minutes.
- If there is still no relief, call 911 for transportation to a health care facility.
- Carry a medical identification card or wear a bracelet or necklace that identifies a history of heart problems.

- Persistent increase in NTG use
- Dizziness, faintness, or shortness of breath with activity

Remind them to always call 911 for transportation to the hospital if they have:

- Chest discomfort that does not improve after 20 minutes or 3 NTG tablets
- Extremely severe chest or epigastric discomfort with weakness, nausea, or fainting
- Other associated symptoms that are particular to them, such as fatigue and nausea

Health Care Resources

The AHA is an excellent source for booklets, films, CDs, DVDs, cookbooks, and professional service referrals for the patient with CAD. Many local chapters have their own cardiac rehabilitation programs.

Within the community, cardiac rehabilitation programs may be affiliated with local hospitals, community centers, or other facilities, such as clinics. Many shopping malls open before shopping hours to allow a measured walking program indoors. This opportunity is particularly popular with older patients because it provides a good support group and allows for an appropriate place to exercise in inclement weather.

Mended Hearts is a nationwide program with local chapters that provides education and support to CABG patients and their families. Smoking-cessation programs and clinics and weight-reduction programs are located within the community. Many hospitals also sponsor health fairs, BP screening, and risk factor modification programs.

Evaluation: Outcomes

Evaluate the patient with CAD on the basis of the identified nursing diagnoses and collaborative problems. The expected outcomes are that the patient will:

- State that discomfort or other symptoms are alleviated
- Have adequate blood flow through the coronary vasculature to ensure heart function
- Walk 200 feet four times a day without discomfort, shortness of breath, or other symptoms of CAD
- Take personal actions to manage stressors related to CAD

Specific indicators for these outcomes are listed for each nursing diagnosis and collaborative problem in the Planning and Implementation section (see earlier).

HUMAN NEEDS NURSING CARE REVIEW

What might you NOTICE if the patient is experiencing inadequate oxygenation and tissue perfusion as a result of coronary artery disease?

- Report of pain (chest, shoulder, arm, jaw, back, or abdomen)
- Report of persistent indigestion
- Dyspnea
- Diaphoresis
- Report of nausea
- Vomiting
- Anxious behavior
- Report of palpitations
- Report of fatigue
- Disorientation or acute confusion (especially in older adults)

What should you INTERPRET and how should you RESPOND to a patient experiencing inadequate oxygenation and tissue perfusion as a result of coronary artery disease?

Perform and interpret physical assessment, including:

- Taking vital signs
- Monitoring oxygen saturation by pulse oximetry
- Taking 12-lead ECG
- Assessing level of consciousness and cognition
- Conducting complete pain assessment
- Drawing blood for laboratory assessment (e.g., troponins)
- Auscultating breath sounds for crackles or wheezes (left-sided heart failure)
- Auscultating heart for abnormal heart sounds
- Assessing for peripheral edema (right-sided heart failure)

Respond by:

- Calling 911 if patient is not in hospital setting OR notifying physician or Rapid Response Team in hospital setting
- Ensuring that patient rests
- Giving oxygen
- Giving nitroglycerin tablet
- Maintaining or starting IV line
- Administering morphine sulfate if MI suspected or diagnosed

On what should you REFLECT?

- Observe patient for decreased report of pain and associated symptoms.
- Continue to monitor oxygen.
- Continue to monitor for dysrhythmias and vital signs.
- Think about what could have precipitated this coronary event.
- Think about how you responded.
- Develop teaching plan for the patient to help prevent further episodes.

GET READY FOR THE NCLEX EXAMINATION!

Key Points

Review these Key Points for each NCLEX Examination Client Needs Category.

Safe and Effective Care Environment

- Collaborate with members of the interdisciplinary health care team members (e.g., physical therapist, case manager, home care providers) when caring for the cardiac patient. Ensure effective communication among all health care providers, especially when transferring the patient from the hospital to community-based settings.

Health Promotion and Maintenance

- Assist patients in securing personal medical identification alert devices that provide information regarding their heart conditions.
- In collaboration with the interdisciplinary health care team, assess the patient for activity tolerance and help design an appropriate exercise regimen.
- Teach the patient about the signs and symptoms of cardiovascular disease and when to seek medical assistance.
- Assess the patient for risk factors of coronary artery disease (CAD), such as obesity, smoking, positive family history, cholesterol management, and the diagnosis and treatment of hypertension.
- Teach patients about the importance of decreasing their risk for CAD.
- Be sure that older adults have adequate support at home after discharge from the hospital. Refer patients and families to appropriate community programs and support groups.

Psychosocial Integrity

- Allow patients to verbalize and express feelings of fear, anxiety, anger, denial, and grief regarding their CAD.
- Address the needs of the family and significant others, and provide teaching and information regarding the disease process. Clarify any misconceptions.

Physiological Integrity

- Explain to patients the need to make lifestyle changes for modifiable risk factors. Nonmodifiable risk factors like age and family history cannot be changed (see Chart 40-1).
- Teach patients that angina is the pain associated with decreased blood flow to the heart muscle. An MI indicates necrosis of heart muscle tissue (see Chart 40-2).
- Identify and interpret diagnostic values for cardiac markers, such as troponins and myoglobin, and other indicators of CAD.
- Monitor patients receiving thrombolytics and anticoagulants, such as heparin, for bleeding.
- For patients undergoing invasive cardiac procedures, assess for signs and symptoms of active bleeding.
- Interpret and assess the patient with CAD for dysrhythmias.
- Evaluate the patient for pain characteristics (e.g., type, location, duration, cause, intensity, and measures taken to relieve symptoms).
- Teach patients and their families about drug therapy, including how to use nitroglycerin if they have chest or other cardiac-related pain (see Chart 40-4).

- Identify and assess for complications for post-cardiac surgery patients, especially fluid and electrolyte imbalance, bleeding, hypothermia, hypertension, and angina pain.
- Provide emergency care for the patient with chest pain as described in Chart 40-3.

SELECTED BIBLIOGRAPHY

Asterisk indicates a classic or definitive work on this subject.

American Heart Association (AHA). (2008). *Heart disease and stroke statistics—2008 update*. Dallas, TX: American Heart Association. Retrieved February 1, 2008, from www.americanheart.org/downloadable/heart/1200078608862HS_Stats%202008.final.pdf.

Anderson, J.L. (2007). ACC/AHA 2007 guidelines for the management of patients with unstable angina/non ST-elevation myocardial infarction. Executive summary: A report of the American College of Cardiology/American Heart Association Task Force on Practical Guidelines (Writing Committee to revise the 2002 guidelines for the management of patients with unstable angina/non-ST elevation myocardial infarction). *Journal of the American College of Cardiology, 50*(7), 652-726.

*Antman, E.M., Anbe, D.T., Armstrong, P.W., Bates, E.R., Green, L.A., Hand, M., et al. (2004). ACC/AHA guidelines for the management of patients with ST-elevation myocardial infarction. Executive summary: A report of the American College of Cardiology/American Heart Association Task Force on Practice Guidelines (Writing Committee to revise the 1999 guidelines for the management of patients with acute myocardial infarction). *Circulation, 110*(5), 588-636.

Boden, W.E., O'Rourke, R.A., Teo, K.K., Hartigan, P.M., Maron, D.J., Kostuk, W.J., et al. (2007). Optimal medical therapy with or without PCI for stable coronary disease. *New England Journal of Medicine, 356*(15), 1503-1516.

Bønaa, K.H., Njølstad, I., Ueland, P.M., Schirmer, H., Tverdal, A., Steigen, T., et al. (2006). Homocysteine lowering and cardiovascular events after acute myocardial infarction. *New England Journal of Medicine, 354*(15), 1578-1588.

Bosen, D.M., & Mackavich, S.D. (2006). Managing mediastinitis after cardiac surgery. *Nursing2006, 36*(8), 64cc1-6.

Bulechek, G.M., Butcher, H.K., & McCloskey Dochterman, J. (Eds.). (2008). *Nursing interventions classification (NIC)* (5th ed.). St. Louis: Mosby.

Eschiti, V.S. (2005). Cardiovascular disease research in Native Americans. *Journal of Cardiovascular Nursing, 30*(3), 155-161.

Grundy, S.M., Cleeman, J.I., Daniels, S.R., Donato, K.A., Eckel, R.H., Franklin, B.A., et al. (2005). Diagnosis and management of the metabolic syndrome: An American Heart Association/National Heart, Lung, and Blood Institute Scientific Statement. *Circulation, 112*(17), 2735-2752.

Harris, W.S., Miller, M., Tighe, A.P., Davidson, M.H., & Schaefer, E.J. (2007). Omega-3 fatty acids and coronary heart disease risk: Clinical and mechanistic perspectives. *Atherosclerosis*. Retrieved February 20, 2008, from www.ncbi.nlm.nih.gov.

Hayman, L.L., & Hughes, S. (2008). Progress in prevention: Preventing heart disease—a global challange and a call to action. *Journal of Cardiovascular Nursing, 23*(1), 65-66.

Johnson, L.W., & Weinstock, R.S. (2006). The metabolic syndrome: Concepts and controversy. *Mayo Clinic Proceedings, 81*(12), 1615-1620.

Katz, A. (2007). Sexuality and myocardial infarction. *AJN, 107*(3), 49-52.

*Kip, K.E., Marroquin, O.C., Kelley, D.E., Johnson, B.D., Kelsey, S.F., Shaw, L.J., et al. (2004). Clinical importance of obesity versus metabolic syndrome I cardiovascular risk in women: A report from the Women's Ischemia Syndrome Evaluation (WISE) study. *Circulation, 109*(6), 706-713.

Knox, J., & Gaster, B. (2007). Dietary supplements for the prevention and treatment of coronary artery disease. *Journal of Alternative and Complementary Medicine, 13*(1), 83-95.

Lins, S., Guffey, D., VanRiper, S., & Kline-Rogers, E. (2006). Decreasing vascular complications after percutaneous coronary interventions: Partnering to improve outcomes. *Critical Care Nurse, 26*(6), 38-46.

Lonn, E. (2007). Homocysteine in the prevention of ischemic health disease, stroke and venous thromboembolism: Therapeutic target or just another distraction? *Current Opinions in Hematology, 14*(5), 481-487.

Lucas, D.L., Brown, R.A., Wassef, M., & Giles, T.D. (2005). Alcohol and the cardiovascular system: Research challenges and opportunities. *Journal of the American College of Cardiology, 45*(12), 1916-1923.

McCance, K., & Huether, S. (2008). *Pathophysiology: The biologic basis for disease in adults* (5th ed.). St. Louis: Mosby.

Meijboom, W.B., van Mieghem, C.A., Mollet, N.R., Pugliese, F., Weustink, A.C., van Pelt, N., et al. (2007). 64-slice computed tomography coronary angiography in patients with high, intermediate, or low pretest probability of significant coronary artery disease. *Journal of the American College of Cardiology, 50*(15), 1469-1475.

Moser, D.K., & Riegel, B. (2008). *Cardiac nursing: A companion to Braunwald's heart disease*. St. Louis: Mosby.

Mullen-Fortino, M., & O'Brien, N. (2008). Caring for a patient after coronary artery bypass graft surgery. *Nursing 2008, 38*(3), 46-52.

National Heart, Lung, and Blood Institute (NHLBI). (2006). *Getting the message: Heart disease is the #1 killer of women*. Retrieved February 1, 2008, from www.nhlbi.nih.gov/health/hearttruth/whatis/message.htm.

Nissen, S.E., Tuzcu, E.M., Schoenhagen, P., Crowe, T., Sasiela, W.J., Tsai, J., et al. (2005). Statin therapy, LDL cholesterol, C-reactive protein, and coronary artery disease. *New England Journal of Medicine, 352*(1), 29-38.

Opie, L.H., & Gersh, B.J. (2005). *Drugs for the heart*. Philadelphia: Saunders.

Pagana, K.D., & Pagana, T.J. (2006). *Mosby's manual of diagnostic and laboratory tests* (3rd ed.). St. Louis: Mosby.

Psota, T.L., Gebauer, S.R., & Kris-Ehterton, P. (2006). Dietary omega-3 fatty acid intake and cardiovascular risk. *American Journal of Cardiology, 98*(4A), 3i-18i.

Redberg, R.F. (2006). What's different about the evaluation of chest pain in women? *Patient Care*. Retrieved December 14, 2007, from www.patientcareonline.com.

*Robinson, A.W. (2002). Older women's experiences if living alone after heart surgery. *Applied Nursing Research, 15*(3), 118-125.

Ryan, C.J., DeVon, H.A., Horne, R., King, K.B., Milner, K., Moser, D.K., et al. (2007). Symptom clusters in acute myocardial infarction. *Nursing Research, 56*(2), 72-81.

Scordo, K.A. (2005). Noninvasive diagnosis of coronary artery disease in women. *Journal of Cardiovascular Nursing, 20*(6), 420-426.

Serruys, P.W., Kutryk, J., & Onig, A. (2006). Coronary artery stents. *New England Journal of Medicine, 354*(5), 483-495.

Shaw, L.J., Bairey Merz, C.N., Pepine, C.J., Reis, S.E., Bittner, V., Kelsey, S.F., et al. (2006). Insights from the NHLBI-sponsored Women's Ischemia Syndrome Evaluation (WISE) study. Part I: Gender differences in traditional and novel risk factors, symptom evaluation, and gender-optimized diagnostic strategies. *Journal of the American College of Cardiology, 47*(Suppl. 3), S4-S20.

Thanavaro, J.L., Moore, S.M., Anthony, M., Narsavage, G., & Delicath, T. (2006). Predictors of health promotion behavior in women without prior history of coronary artery disease. *Applied Nursing Research, 19*(3), 149-155.

Weil, K.M. (2007). On guard for intra-aortic balloon pump problems. *Nursing2007, 37*(7), 28.

Wung, S.F. (2007). Discriminating between right coronary artery and circumflex artery occlusion by using a noninvasive 18-lead electrocardiogram. *American Journal of Critical Care, 16*(1), 63-71.

Zerumsky, K., & McBride, B.F. (2006). Ranolazine in the management of chronic stable angina. *American Journal of Health-System Pharmacists, 63*(23), 2331-2338.

Additional Study Resources

Go to your Companion CD or Evolve at http://evolve.elsevier.com/Iggy/ for *Self-Assessment Questions for the NCLEX Examination.*

evolve Go to Evolve at http://evolve.elsevier.com/Iggy/ for *Prioritization and Delegation Questions for the NCLEX Examination.*

IX
UNIT

Problems of Tissue Perfusion

Management of Patients with Problems of the Hematologic System

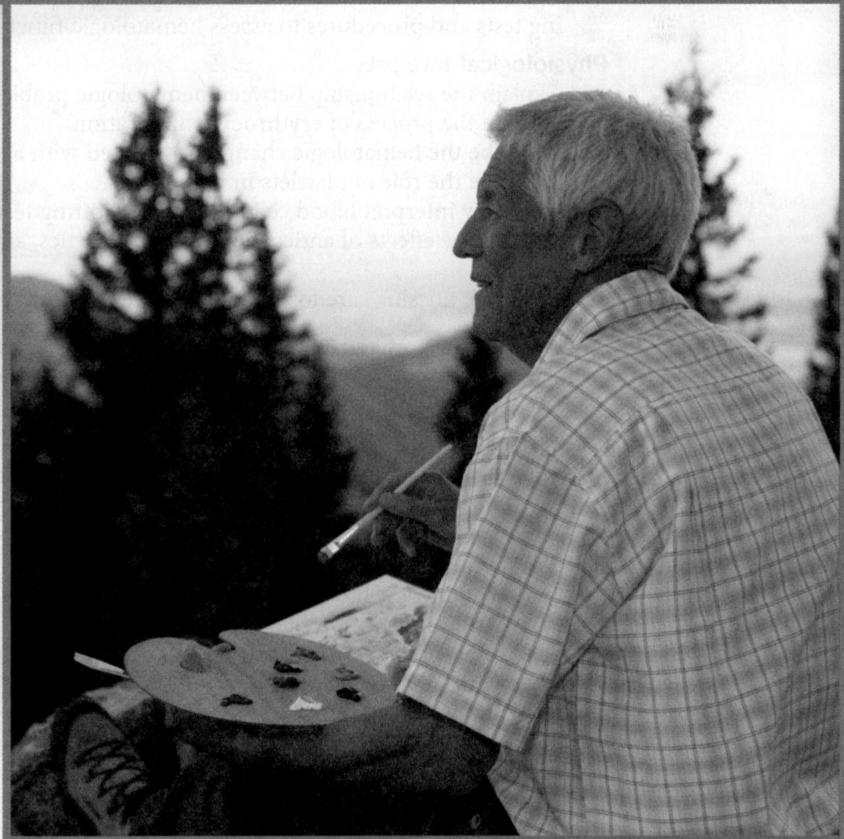

41 CHAPTER

Assessment of the Hematologic System

M. Linda Workman

LEARNING OUTCOMES

For clinical competence and success on the NCLEX Examination, study this chapter with these Learning Outcomes in mind:

Safe and Effective Care Environment

1. Verify that the patient has given informed consent for a bone marrow aspiration or biopsy.

Health Promotion and Maintenance

2. Assess the patient's endurance in performing ADLs.
3. Perform a clinical health history and risk assessment for hematologic function.

Psychosocial Integrity

4. Use effective communication when teaching patients and family members about what to expect during tests and procedures to assess hematologic function.

Physiological Integrity

5. Explain the relationship between hematologic problems and the need for oxygen.
6. Explain the process of erythrocyte maturation.
7. Describe the hematologic changes associated with aging.
8. Describe the role of platelets in hemostasis.
9. Correctly interpret blood cell counts and clotting tests to assess hematologic status.
10. Explain the effects of anticoagulants, fibrinolytics, and inhibitors of platelet activity on hematologic function.
11. Prioritize nursing care for the patient after bone marrow aspiration.

Go to your Companion CD or Evolve at http://evolve.elsevier.com/Iggy/ for *Self-Assessment Questions for the NCLEX Examination* keyed to these Learning Outcomes.

The hematologic system is the blood, blood cells, lymph, and organs involved with blood formation or blood storage. This system is important in helping the body meet the *human need for oxygenation and tissue perfusion,* because the blood itself is one of the oxygen delivery systems (Fig. 41-1). All systems depend on blood circulation for tissue perfusion with oxygen. Thus any problem of the hematologic system affects total body health and well-being. This chapter, together with Chapter 19, reviews the normal physiology of the hematologic system and assessment of hematologic status.

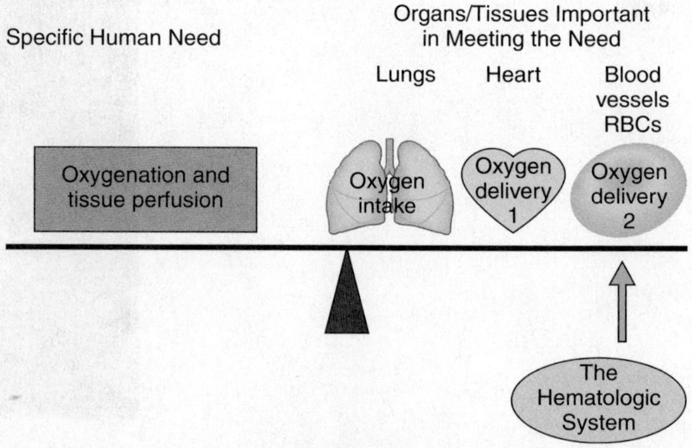
Specific Human Need
Organs/Tissues Important in Meeting the Need
Lungs
Heart
Blood vessels RBCs
Oxygenation and tissue perfusion
Oxygen intake
Oxygen delivery 1
Oxygen delivery 2
The Hematologic System

Fig. 41-1 • Role of the hematologic system in meeting the human need for oxygenation and tissue perfusion.

ANATOMY AND PHYSIOLOGY REVIEW

Bone Marrow

Bone marrow is the blood-forming (hematopoietic) organ. It produces most of the cells of the blood, including red blood cells (RBCs, erythrocytes), white blood cells (WBCs), and platelets. Bone marrow is involved also in the immune responses (see Chapter 19).

Each day the bone marrow in a healthy adult releases about 2.5 billion RBCs, 2.5 billion platelets, and 1 billion WBCs (leukocytes) per kilogram of body weight. Although blood is produced in many bones during childhood, this function is limited to the marrow of flat bones (sternum, skull, pelvic and shoulder girdles) and the ends of long bones in adults. As a person ages, fatty tissue slowly replaces active bone marrow. In older adults, the amount of fatty marrow increases and only a small portion of the remaining marrow continues to produce blood.

The bone marrow first produces stem cells. These blood stem cells are immature, unspecialized (undifferentiated) cells that are capable of becoming any one of several types of blood cells: RBCs, WBCs, or platelets, depending on the body's needs (Fig. 41-2).

The next stage in blood cell production is the committed stem cell (also called the *precursor cell*). A committed stem cell enters one growth pathway and can at that point specialize (differentiate) into only one cell type. Committed stem cells actively divide but require the presence of a specific growth factor for specialization. For example, erythropoietin is a growth factor made in the kidneys that is specific for the RBC. Many different growth factors influence WBC and platelet growth (see Chapters 19, 24, and 42 for a more in-depth discussion of cytokines and growth factors).

Blood Components

Blood is composed of plasma and cells. Plasma is part of the body's extracellular fluid. It is similar to the interstitial fluid found between tissue cells, but plasma contains much more protein. The three major types of plasma proteins are albumin, globulins, and fibrinogen.

Albumin increases the osmotic pressure of the blood, preventing the plasma from leaking into the tissues. Globulins have many functions, such as transporting other substances and protecting the body against infection. Globulins are also the main proteins of antibodies. Fibrinogen is an inactive protein that is activated to form fibrin. Fibrin molecules assemble together to form structures important in the blood clotting process.

The blood cells include RBCs, WBCs, and platelets. These cells differ in structure, site of maturation, and function.

Red blood cells **(erythrocytes)** are the largest proportion of blood cells. Mature RBCs have no nucleus and have a biconcave disk shape. Together with a flexible membrane, this feature allows RBCs to change their shape without breaking as they pass through narrow, winding capillaries. The number of RBCs a person has varies with gender, age, and general health, but the normal range is from 4,200,000 to 6,100,000/mm^3.

As shown in Figs. 41-2 and 41-3, RBCs start out as stem cells, enter the myeloid pathway, and progress in stages to mature RBCs (i.e., erythrocytes). Healthy, mature RBCs have a life span of about 120 days after being released into the blood. As RBCs age, their membranes become more fragile. These old cells are trapped and destroyed in the tissues, spleen, and liver. Some parts of destroyed RBCs (e.g., iron) are recycled and used to make new RBCs.

The RBCs produce hemoglobin (Hgb). Each normal mature RBC contains thousands of hemoglobin molecules. The heme part of each hemoglobin molecule needs a molecule of iron. Only when the heme molecule is complete with iron can it transport up to four molecules of oxygen. *Therefore iron is an essential part of hemoglobin.* The globin portion of hemoglobin carries carbon dioxide. RBCs also are buffers and help maintain acid-base balance.

The most important feature of hemoglobin is its ability to combine loosely with oxygen. With only a small drop in oxygen level in the tissues, a greater increase in the transfer of oxygen from hemoglobin to tissues occurs. This transfer is also known as **oxygen dissociation** and is important in helping meet body tissue needs for oxygen. Some problems change the speed and amount of oxygen released to the tissues.

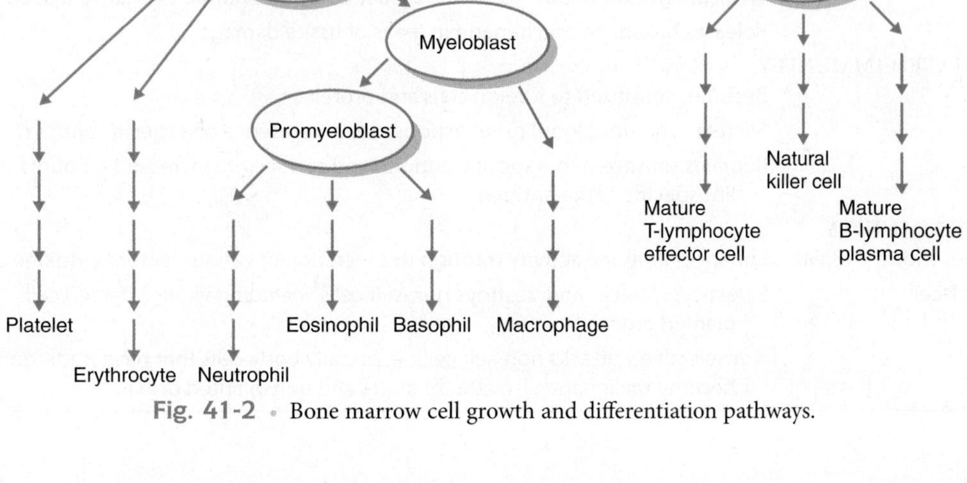
Pluripotent stem cell
Committed myeloid stem cell
Committed lymphoid stem cell
Myeloblast
Promyeloblast
Natural killer cell
Mature T-lymphocyte effector cell
Mature B-lymphocyte plasma cell
Platelet
Eosinophil
Basophil
Macrophage
Erythrocyte
Neutrophil

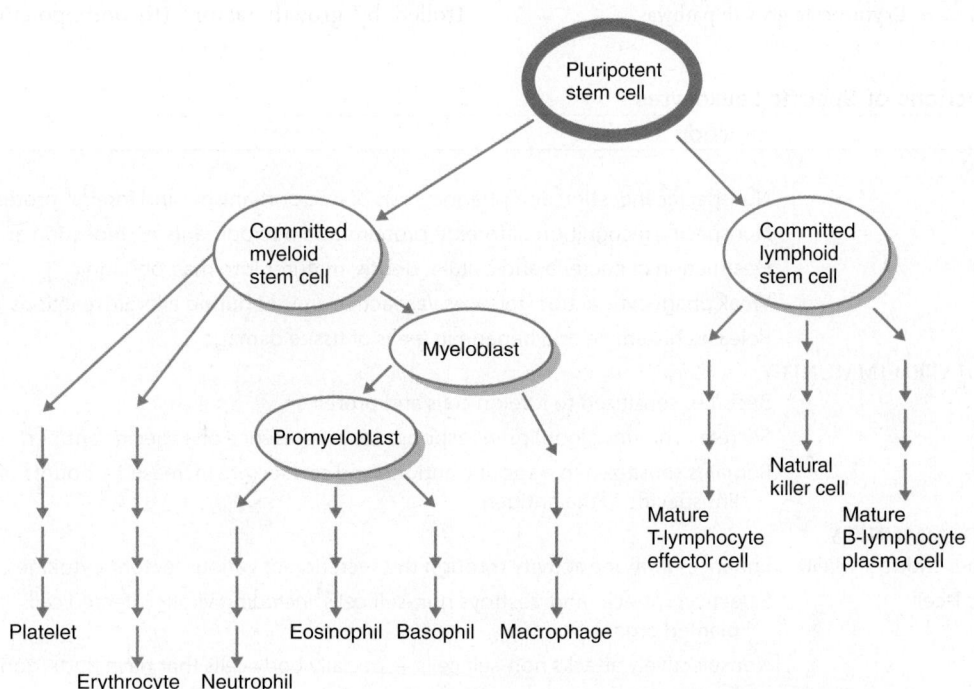

Fig. 41-2 • Bone marrow cell growth and differentiation pathways.

The total number of RBCs a person has is carefully controlled to ensure that enough RBCs are present for good oxygenation without having too many cells that could "thicken" the blood and slow its flow. Thus RBC production or **erythropoiesis** (selective growth of stem cells into mature erythrocytes) must be properly balanced with RBC destruction or loss. When balanced, this process helps meet the *body's need for tissue perfusion by ensuring adequate delivery of oxygen.* The trigger for RBC production is an increase in the need for tissue oxygenation. The kidney produces the RBC growth factor *erythropoietin* at the same rate as RBC destruction or loss occurs to maintain a constant normal level of circulating RBCs. When tissue oxygenation is less than normal **(hypoxia),** the kidney releases more erythropoietin. This growth factor then stimulates the bone marrow to increase RBC production. When tissue oxygenation is normal or high, the kidney reduces erythropoietin levels, slowing the production of RBCs. Synthetic erythropoietin (Procrit, Epogen, EPO) has the same effect on bone marrow as the naturally occurring erythropoietin.

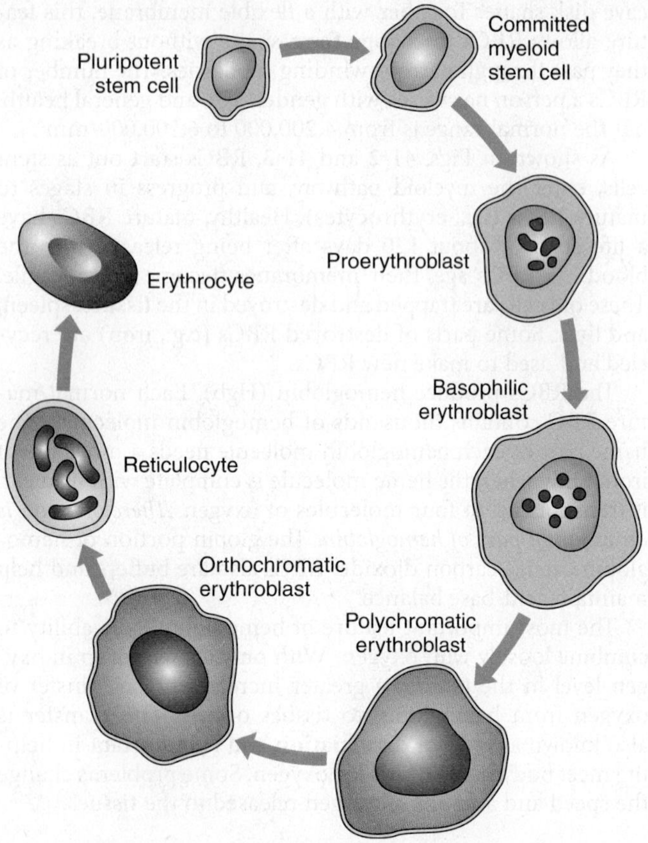
Pluripotent stem cell
Committed myeloid stem cell
Proerythroblast
Basophilic erythroblast
Polychromatic erythroblast
Orthochromatic erythroblast
Reticulocyte
Erythrocyte

Fig. 41-3 • Erythrocyte growth pathway.

Many substances are needed to form hemoglobin and RBCs, including iron, vitamin B_{12}, folic acid, copper, pyridoxine, cobalt, and nickel. A lack of any of these substances can lead to anemia. Anemia is the result of any problem that reduces the function or the number of RBCs to the point that tissue oxygen needs are not completely met.

White blood cells (WBCs), or leukocytes, perform actions important for protection through inflammation and immunity (Table 41-1). The many types of WBCs all have specialized functions. Many WBCs are formed in the bone marrow and are part of the hematologic system. WBC function is presented in Chapter 19 because these cells provide immunity and protect against invasion and infection.

Platelets are the third type of blood cells. They are the smallest of the blood cells, formed as fragments of a giant precursor cell in the bone marrow, the megakaryocyte. Fig. 41-2 shows the overall blood cell growth pathways, and Fig. 41-4 shows platelet development.

Platelets stick to injured blood vessel walls and form platelet plugs that can stop the flow of blood from the injured site. They also produce substances important to blood clotting (coagulation). Platelets help keep blood vessels intact by beginning the repair of damage to small blood vessels. They perform most of their functions by **aggregation** (clumping).

Bone marrow production of platelets also is precisely controlled by growth factors (thrombopoietin). After platelets

TABLE 41-1 Functions of Specific Leukocytes

Leukocyte	Function
INFLAMMATION	
Neutrophil	Nonspecific ingestion and phagocytosis of microorganisms and foreign protein
Macrophage	Nonspecific recognition of foreign proteins and microorganisms; ingestion and phagocytosis
Monocyte	Destruction of bacteria and cellular debris; matures into macrophage
Eosinophil	Weak phagocytic action; releases vasoactive amines during allergic reactions
Basophil	Releases histamine and heparin in areas of tissue damage
ANTIBODY-MEDIATED IMMUNITY	
B-lymphocyte	Becomes sensitized to foreign cells and proteins
Plasma cell	Secretes immunoglobulins in response to the presence of a specific antigen
Memory cell	Remains sensitized to a specific antigen and can secrete increased amounts of immunoglobulins specific to the antigen
CELL-MEDIATED IMMUNITY	
T-lymphocyte helper/inducer T-cell	Enhances immune activity through the secretion of various factors, cytokines, and lymphokines
Cytotoxic-cytolytic T-cell	Selectively attacks and destroys non-self cells, including virally infected cells, grafts, and transplanted organs
Natural killer cell	Nonselectively attacks non-self cells, especially body cells that have undergone mutation and become malignant; also attacks grafts and transplanted organs

leave the bone marrow, they are stored in the spleen and then released slowly to meet the body's needs. Normally, 80% of platelets circulate and 20% are stored in the spleen. Each platelet has a life span of 1 to 2 weeks.

Accessory Organs of Blood Formation

The spleen and liver are important accessory organs for blood production. They help regulate the growth of blood cells and form factors that ensure proper blood clotting.

The *spleen* is located under the diaphragm to the left of the stomach. It contains three types of tissue: white pulp, red pulp, and marginal pulp. These tissues all help balance blood cell production with blood cell destruction and assist with immunity. White pulp is filled with WBCs, especially lymphocytes and macrophages. It is a major site of antibody production. As whole blood filters through the white pulp, unwanted cells (e.g., bacteria, old RBCs) are removed. Red pulp contains enlarged blood vessels (sinuses) that store RBCs and platelets. Marginal pulp contains the ends of many arteries and other blood vessels.

The spleen destroys old or imperfect RBCs, breaks down the hemoglobin released from these destroyed cells, stores platelets, and filters antigens. A patient who has had a splenectomy has reduced immune functions. Thus, after a splenectomy, patients are less able to rid themselves of disease-causing organisms and are at greater risk for infection and sepsis.

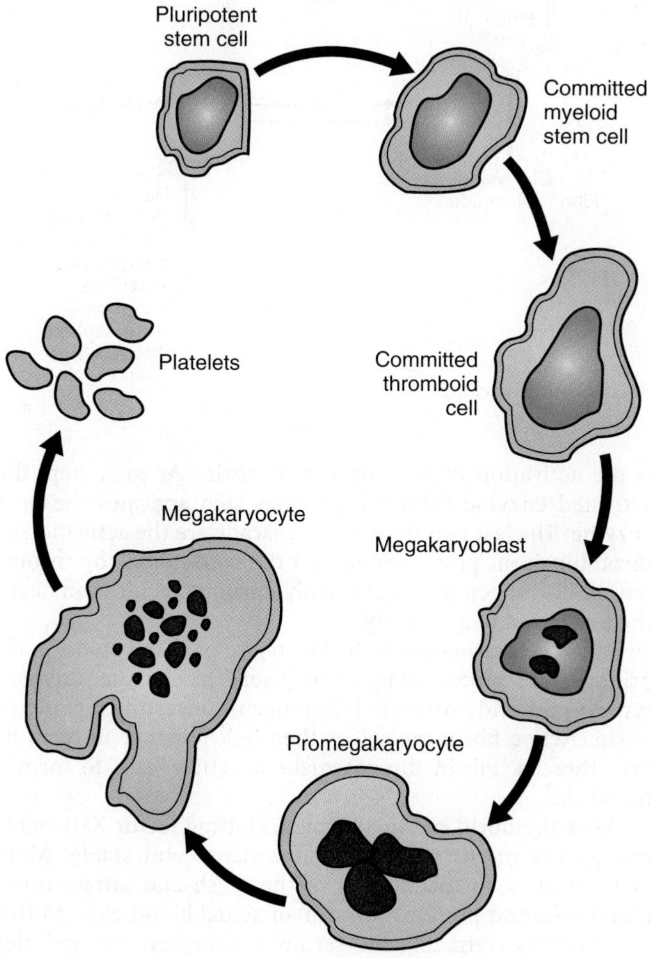
Pluripotent stem cell
Committed myeloid stem cell
Committed thromboid cell
Megakaryoblast
Promegakaryocyte
Megakaryocyte
Platelets

Fig. 41-4 • Platelet growth pathway.

The *liver* is the site for production of prothrombin and most of the blood clotting factors. In addition, proper liver function and bile production are important in forming vitamin K in the intestinal tract. (Vitamin K is needed to produce blood clotting factors VII, IX, and X and prothrombin.) Large quantities of whole blood and blood cells can be stored in the liver. The liver also converts bilirubin (one end product of hemoglobin breakdown) to bile and stores extra iron within the protein *ferritin.*

Hemostasis/Blood Clotting

Hemostasis is the process of controlled blood clotting. With proper hemostasis, localized blood clotting occurs in damaged blood vessels to prevent excessive blood loss while blood continues to circulate to all other areas for tissue perfusion. This important function is a complex process that balances blood clotting actions with anti-clotting actions. When injury occurs, hemostasis begins with the formation of a platelet plug and continues with a series of events that eventually cause the formation of a fibrin clot. Intrinsic and extrinsic factors are involved in blood clotting. Three processes result in blood clotting: platelet aggregation with formation of a platelet plug, the blood clotting cascade, and the formation of a complete fibrin clot.

Platelet aggregation begins forming a platelet plug by having platelets clump together. This process is essential for blood clotting. Platelets normally circulate as individual cell-like structures. They are not attracted to each other and do not clump together until activated. Activation causes platelet membranes to become sticky, allowing them to clump together. When platelets clump, they form large, semisolid plugs in blood vessel lumens and walls, disrupting local blood flow. *These platelet plugs are not clots and cannot provide complete hemostasis.*

Substances that cause platelets to clump include adenosine diphosphate (ADP), calcium, thromboxane A_2, and collagen. Platelets themselves secrete some of these substances, whereas other substances that activate platelets are external to the platelet. Platelet plugs start the cascade reaction that ends with local blood clotting. When too few platelets are present, blood clotting is impaired, increasing the person's risk for bleeding and hemorrhage.

Blood clotting is a cascade triggered by the formation of a platelet plug. Platelet plugs can occur from both intrinsic and extrinsic factors. The beginning of the blood clotting cascade is rapidly amplified or enhanced. That is, the final result is much larger than the triggering event. In this sense, the cascade works like a landslide. A few small pebbles rolling down a steep hillside can dislodge large rocks and pieces of soil, causing a final enormous movement of earth. Just like landslides, cascade reactions are hard to stop once set into motion.

Intrinsic factors are problems or substances directly in the blood itself that first make platelets clump and then trigger the blood clotting cascade (Fig. 41-5). These conditions include circulating debris and prolonged venous stasis. Continuing the cascade to the point of blood clotting requires having sufficient amounts of all the different clotting factors and cofactors (Table 41-2).

Extrinsic factors are those outside of the cell that can also induce platelet plugs to form. These are usually the result of changes in the blood vessels rather than in the blood. The most common extrinsic event is trauma that damages blood

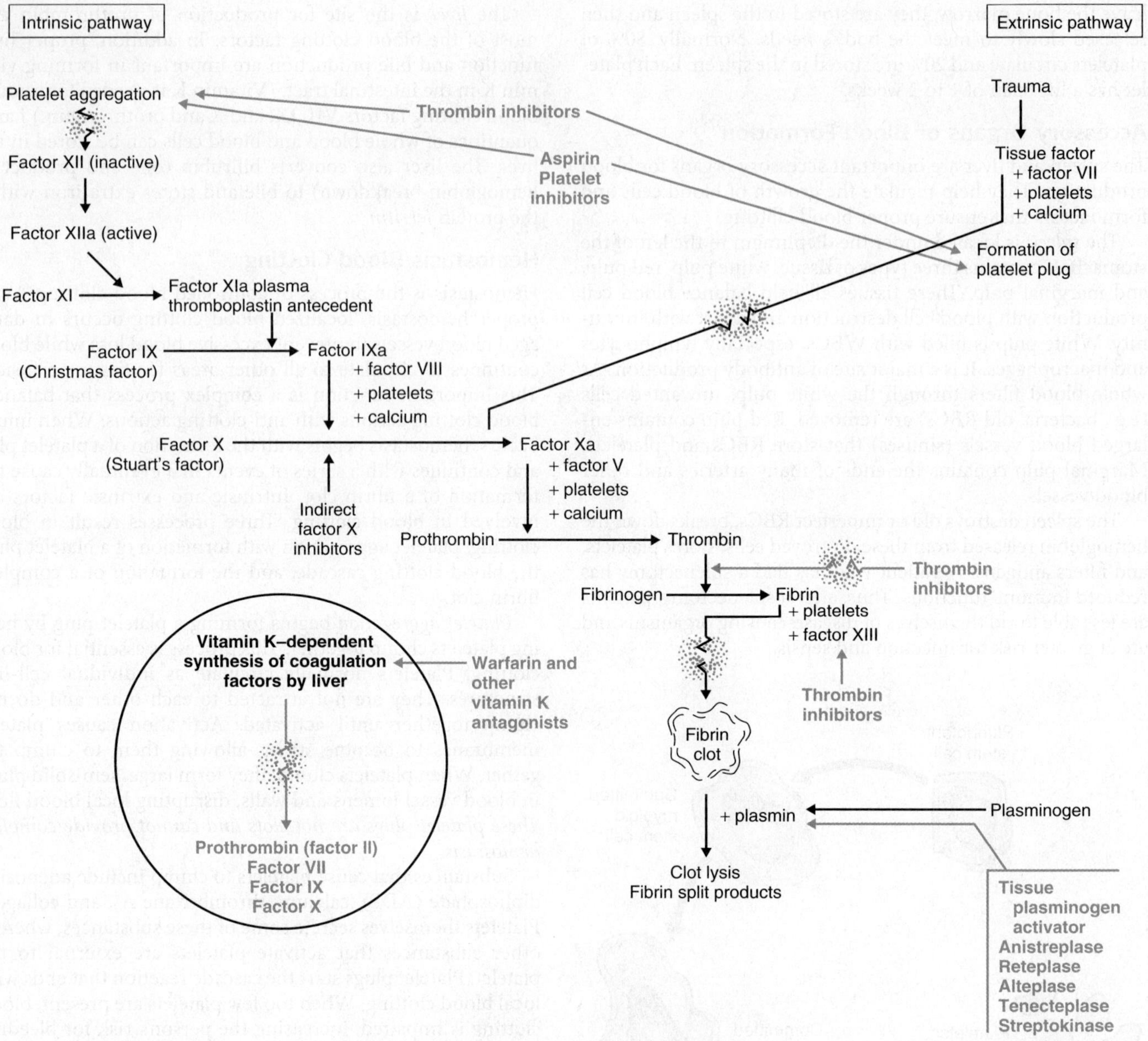

Intrinsic pathway
Extrinsic pathway
Platelet aggregation
Thrombin inhibitors
Trauma
Factor XII (inactive)
Aspirin
Platelet
inhibitors
Tissue factor
+ factor VII
+ platelets
+ calcium
Factor XIIa (active)
Formation of
platelet plug
Factor XI
Factor XIa plasma
thromboplastin antecedent
Factor IX
(Christmas factor)
Factor IXa
+ factor VIII
+ platelets
+ calcium
Factor X
(Stuart's factor)
Factor Xa
+ factor V
+ platelets
+ calcium
Indirect
factor X
inhibitors
Prothrombin
Thrombin
Thrombin
inhibitors
Fibrinogen
Fibrin
+ platelets
+ factor XIII
Vitamin K–dependent
synthesis of coagulation
factors by liver
Warfarin and
other
vitamin K
antagonists
Thrombin
inhibitors
Fibrin
clot
+ plasmin
Plasminogen
Prothrombin (factor II)
Factor VII
Factor IX
Factor X
Clot lysis
Fibrin split products
Tissue
plasminogen
activator
Anistreplase
Reteplase
Alteplase
Tenecteplase
Streptokinase

Fig. 41-5 • Summary of blood-clotting cascade.

vessels and exposes the platelets to collagen. Collagen then activates platelets and causes clumping. The platelet plug is formed within seconds of the trauma. The blood clotting cascade is started sooner by this pathway because some of the steps of the intrinsic pathway are bypassed. Other blood vessel changes that can trigger platelets to clump include inflammation, bacterial toxins, or foreign proteins.

Whether the platelet plugs are formed because of abnormal blood (intrinsic factors) or by exposure to inflamed or damaged blood vessels (extrinsic factors), the end result of the cascade is the same: *formation of a fibrin clot and local blood coagulation.*

The steps of the cascade between the formation of a platelet plug and the formation of a fibrin clot depend on the presence of specific clotting factors. In addition, calcium and more platelets are needed at every step.

Clotting factors (see Table 41-2) are inactive enzymes that become activated in a sequence. The last part of the sequence is the activation of fibrinogen into fibrin. At each step, the activated enzyme from the previous step activates the next enzyme. The last two steps in the cascade are the activation of thrombin from prothrombin and the conversion (by thrombin) of fibrinogen into fibrin. Only fibrin molecules can begin the formation of a true clot.

Fibrin clot formation is the last phase of blood clotting. Fibrinogen is a protein made in the liver. The enzyme *thrombin* removes the end portions of fibrinogen, converting it to active fibrin. Active fibrin molecules then link together to form fibrin threads. Fibrin threads make a netlike base to form a blood clot.

After the fibrin mesh is formed, clotting factor XIII tightens up the mesh, making it more dense and stable. More platelets stick to the threads of the mesh and attract other blood cells and proteins to form an actual blood clot. As this clot tightens (retracts), the serum is squeezed out and clot formation is complete.

TABLE 41-2 **The Clotting Factors**

Factor	Action
I: Fibrinogen	Factor I is converted to fibrin by the enzyme *thrombin.* Individual fibrin molecules form fibrin threads, which are the scaffold for clot formation and wound healing.
II: Prothrombin	Factor II is the inactive precursor of thrombin. Prothrombin is activated to thrombin by coagulation factor X (Stuart-Prower factor). After it is activated, thrombin converts fibrinogen (coagulation factor I) into fibrin and activates factors V and VIII. Synthesis is vitamin K–dependent.
III: Tissue thromboplastin	Factor III interacts with factor VII to initiate the extrinsic clotting cascade.
IV: Calcium	Calcium (Ca^{2+}), a divalent cation, is a cofactor for most of the enzyme-activated processes required in blood coagulation. Calcium also enhances platelet aggregation and makes red blood cells clump together.
V: Proaccelerin	Factor V is a cofactor for activated factor X, which is essential for converting prothrombin to thrombin.
VI: Discovered to be an artifact	No factor VI is involved in blood coagulation.
VII: Proconvertin	Factor VIII activates factors IX and X, which are essential in converting prothrombin to thrombin. Synthesis is vitamin K–dependent.
VIII: Antihemophilic factor	Factor VII together with activated factor IX enzymatically activates factor X. In addition, factor VIII combines with another protein (von Willebrand's factor) to help platelets adhere to capillary walls in areas of tissue injury. A lack of factor VIII is the basis for classic hemophilia (hemophilia A).
IX: Plasma thromboplastin component (Christmas factor)	Factor IX, when activated, activates factor X to convert prothrombin to thrombin. This factor is essential in the common pathway between the intrinsic and extrinsic clotting cascades. A lack of factor IX is the basis for hemophilia B. Synthesis is vitamin K–dependent.
X: Stuart-Prower factor	Factor X, when activated, converts prothrombin into thrombin. Synthesis is vitamin K–dependent.
XI: Plasma thromboplastin antecedent	Factor XI, when activated, assists in the activation of factor IX. However, a similar factor must exist in tissues. People who are deficient in factor XI have mild bleeding problems after surgery but do not bleed excessively as a result of trauma.
XII: Hageman factor	Factor XII is critically important in the intrinsic pathway for the activation of factor XI.
XIII: Fibrin-stabilizing factor	Factor XIII assists in forming cross-links among the fibrin threads to form a strong fibrin clot.

Anti-Clotting Forces

Because blood clotting occurs through a rapid cascade process, in theory it keeps forming fibrin clots whenever the cascade is set into motion until all blood throughout the entire body has coagulated. Such widespread clotting would lead to death. Therefore, whenever the blood clotting cascade is started, anti-clotting forces are also started to limit clot formation only to damaged areas so that normal blood flow is maintained everywhere else. When blood clotting and anti-clotting actions are normal and balanced, clotting occurs only where it is needed and normal blood flow elsewhere is maintained. The anti-clotting forces involve two types of actions. One action ensures that activated clotting factors are present only in limited amounts. The other action prevents over-enlargement of the fibrin clot, a process called **fibrinolysis.**

When the blood clotting cascade is activated, certain anti-clotting substances are also activated. Known anti-clotting proteins include protein C, protein S, and antithrombin III. Protein C and protein S increase the breakdown of clotting factors V and VIII. Antithrombin III inactivates thrombin and clotting factors IX and X. These actions prevent clots from becoming too large or forming in an area where blood clotting is not needed. A person who has a deficiency of any of these anti-clotting factors has an increased risk for pulmonary embolism, myocardial infarction, and strokes.

Fibrinolysis limits the size of blood clots by dissolving fibrin clot edges with special enzymes (Fig. 41-6). The process starts by activating plasminogen to plasmin. Plasmin, an enzyme, then digests fibrin, fibrinogen, and prothrombin, controlling the size of the fibrin clot.

HEMATOLOGIC CHANGES ASSOCIATED WITH AGING

Aging changes the cellular and plasma components of blood (Meiner & Lueckenotte, 2006). Chart 41-1 lists assessment tips for older adults. The older adult has a decreased blood volume with lower levels of plasma proteins. The lower plasma protein level may be related to a low dietary intake of proteins and reduced protein production by the older liver.

As bone marrow ages, it produces fewer blood cells. Total red blood cell (RBC) and white blood cell (WBC) counts (especially lymphocyte counts) are lower among older adults (Edwards & Baird, 2005). Platelet counts do not appear to change with age. Lymphocytes become less reactive to antigens and lose immune function. Antibody levels and responses are lower and slower in older adults. The WBC count does not rise as high in response to infection in older people as it does in younger people.

Hemoglobin levels also change with age. Hemoglobin levels in men and women fall after middle age. Iron-deficient diets may play a role in this reduction.

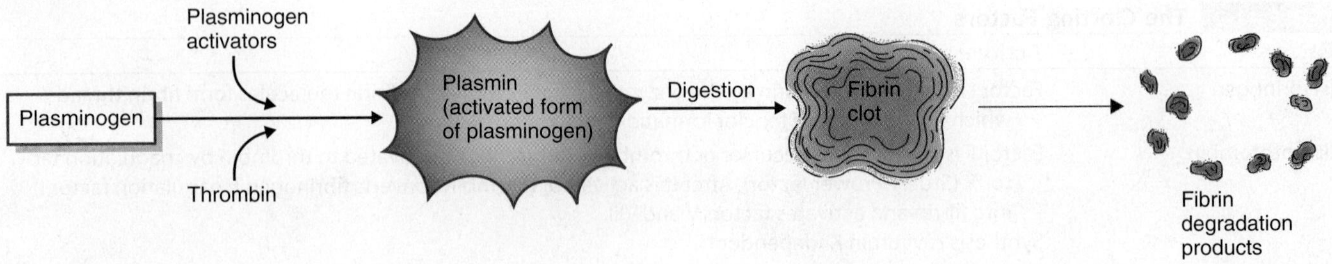
Plasminogen activators
Plasminogen
Thrombin
Plasmin (activated form of plasminogen)
Digestion
Fibrin clot
Fibrin degradation products

Fig. 41-6 • The process of fibrinolysis.

Chart 41-1 NURSING FOCUS ON THE OLDER ADULT

Hematologic Assessment

Findings in Hematologic Disorders	Normal Changes in the Older Adult	Significance/Alternatives
NAIL BEDS (FOR CAPILLARY REFILL)		
Pallor or cyanosis may indicate a hematologic disorder.	Thickened or discolored nails make viewing skin color beneath the nails impossible.	Use another body area, such as the lip, to assess central capillary refill.
HAIR DISTRIBUTION		
Thin or absent hair on the trunk or extremities may indicate poor circulation to a particular area.	Progressive loss of body hair is a normal facet of aging.	A relatively even pattern of hair loss that has occurred over an extended period is not significant.
SKIN MOISTURE		
Skin dryness may indicate any of a number of hematologic disorders.	Skin dryness is a normal result of aging.	Skin moisture is not usually a reliable indicator of an underlying pathologic condition in the older adult.
SKIN COLOR		
Skin color changes, especially pallor and jaundice, are associated with some hematologic disorders.	Pigment loss and skin yellowing are common changes associated with aging.	Pallor in an older adult may not be a reliable indicator of anemia. Laboratory testing is required. Yellow-tinged skin in an older adult may not be a reliable indicator of increased serum bilirubin levels. Laboratory testing is required.

Chart 41-2 HEMATOLOGIC ASSESSMENT

Using Gordon's Functional Health Patterns

ACTIVITY-EXERCISE PATTERN

- How does your energy level seem to you compared with last year at this time?
- Do you feel rested after a typical night's sleep?
- Have you experienced any dizziness or light-headedness?
- Does your heart ever seem to pound?
- How much exercise do you get? How often? What type?
- Do you feel you have enough energy to do what you want or need to do?

NUTRITION-METABOLIC PATTERN

- Have you noticed any change in your skin lately?
- How easily do you bruise?
- Do your gums ever bleed? Under what conditions?
- How much meat do you eat in a week?
- How often do you eat salads or other green leafy vegetables?
- Are you taking any vitamin or mineral supplements?
- Do your feet and hands usually feel warm or cold?
- Has your weight changed by 5 pounds or more this year?
- How often do you take aspirin or any other NSAID?
- What drugs do you take daily?

Modified from Gordon, M. (2007). *Manual of nursing diagnosis* (11th ed.). Boston: Jones & Bartlett.

NCLEX EXAMINATION CHALLENGE

Which nursing diagnosis or collaborative problem is most appropriate for the majority of adult clients over the age of 75 years as a result of normal changes related to aging and not to drug therapy?

A. Decreased Cardiac Output related to hypervolemia
B. Risk for Injury related to increased bleeding tendency
C. Fatigue related to decreased oxygen-carrying capacity
D. Risk for allergic reactions related to increased leukocyte activity

evolve For the correct answer, go to http://evolve.elsevier.com/Iggy/.

ASSESSMENT METHODS

Patient History

Chart 41-2 lists questions based on Gordon's Functional Health Patterns to ask during assessment of hematologic function. Age and gender are important to consider when assessing the patient's hematologic status. Bone marrow function and immune activity decrease with age.

WOMEN'S HEALTH CONSIDERATIONS

At all ages, women have lower blood cell counts than do men. This difference is greater during menstrual years because blood loss from menstruation may occur slightly faster than blood cell production. This gender difference also may be related to a blood dilution caused by fluid retention from female hormones.

TABLE 41-3 Drugs Impairing the Hematologic System

Generic Name	Common Trade Names
DRUGS CAUSING BONE MARROW SUPPRESSION	
Altretamine	Hexalen, Hexastat♣
Amphotericin B	Fungizone
Azathioprine	Imuran
Chemotherapeutic agents	
Chloramphenicol	Chloromycetin, Novochlorocap♣
Chromic phosphate	Phosphocol
Colchicine	(Generic only)
Didanosine	Videx
Eflornithine	Ornidyl
Foscarnet sodium	Foscavir
Ganciclovir	Cytovene
Interferon alfa	Actimmune, Alferon, Intron-A, Roferon-A, Wellferon
Pentamidine	Pentam 300, NebuPent, Pentacarinat♣
Sodium iodide	Iodopen
Zalcitabine	HIVID
Zidovudine	AZT, Retrovir, Novo-AZT♣
DRUGS CAUSING HEMOLYSIS	
Acetohydroxamic acid	Lithostat
Amoxicillin	Amoxil, Augmentin, Apo-Amoxi♣
Chlorpropamide	Diabinese, Glucamide, Novo-Propamide♣
Doxapram	Dopram
Glyburide	DiaBeta, Micronase, Euglucon♣
Mefenamic acid	Ponstel, Ponstan♣
Menadiol diphosphate	Synkayvite
Methyldopa	Aldomet, Dopamet♣
Nitrofurantoin	Macrodantin, Novo-Furantoin♣
Penicillin G benzathine	Bicillin, Crystapen
Penicillin V	Pen-Vee K, Pen Vee, Nu-Pen-VK♣
Primaquine	(Generic only)
Procainamide hydrochloride	Procan-SR, Promine, Pronestyl
Quinidine polygalacturonate	Cardioquin, Quinalan, Novoquinidin♣
Quinine	Legatrin, Quindan
Sulfonamides	Sulfamethoxazole (Gantanol), sulfisoxazole (Gantrisin, Novo-Soxazole♣)
Tolbutamide	Oramide, Orinase, Apo-Tolbutamide♣, Mobenol♣
Vitamin K	AquaMEPHYTON, Konakion
DRUGS DISRUPTING PLATELET ACTION	
Aspirin	Anacin, Ascriptin, Bufferin, Ecotrin, Entrophen♣, Riphen♣, Triaphen♣
Carbenicillin	Geopen, Pyopen♣

Continued

Personal factors to include in hematologic assessment are liver function, the presence of known immunologic or hematologic disorders, current drug use, dietary patterns, and socioeconomic status. Because the liver makes clotting factors, ask about manifestations that may indicate liver problems, such as jaundice, anemia, and gallstones. Previous radiation therapy for cancer may result in some permanent impairment of hematologic function if marrow-forming bones were in the radiation path.

It is also important to collect information about occupation, hobbies, and the location of housing. This information may indicate an exposure to agents or chemicals that affect bone marrow growth and hematologic function.

Check all drugs that the patient is using or has used in the past 3 weeks. Ask about the use of antibiotics, because prolonged antibiotic therapy can lead to clotting problems or bone marrow depression. Table 41-3 lists drugs known to change hematologic function.

TABLE 41-3 Drugs Impairing the Hematologic System—cont'd

Generic Name	Common Trade Names
DRUGS DISRUPTING PLATELET ACTION—cont'd	
Carindacillin	Geocillin
Dipyridamole	Persantine, Apo-Dipyridamole♣, Novo-Dipiradol♣
Ibuprofen	Advil, Motrin
Moxalactam	Moxam
Naproxen	Aleve, Anaprox, Naprosyn
Oxaprozin	Daypro
Pentoxifylline	Trental
Sulfinpyrazone	Anturane, Antazone♣, Novopyrazone♣
Ticarcillin	Ticar
Ticlopidine	Ticlid
Valproic acid	Dalpro, Depakene, Epival♣

Ask the patient about use of "blood thinners" and NSAIDs. If these types of drugs have been prescribed, it is a strong indication that the person either has a blood clotting problem or has a health problem that requires changing blood clotting activity. Such drugs include anticoagulants, fibrinolytics, and platelet inhibitors. Many patients refer to these drugs as *blood thinners* although they do not cause any change in the thickness or viscosity of the blood. Fig. 41-5 shows where in the blood clotting cascade these agents work.

Anticoagulant drugs work by interfering with one or more steps involved in the blood clotting cascade. Thus these agents *prevent* new clots from forming and limit or prevent extension of formed clots. *Anticoagulants cannot break down existing clots.* These drugs are classified as thrombin inhibitors, vitamin K antagonists, and indirect factor X inhibitors.

Fibrinolytic drugs (also known as *thrombolytic drugs*) selectively break down fibrin threads already present in the formed blood clot. The mechanism to start fibrin degradation is activation of the inactive tissue protein *plasminogen* to its active form, *plasmin.* Plasmin directly attacks and degrades the fibrin molecule, having fewer effects on the fibrinogen molecule. Thus the action of fibrinolytic drugs is the selective breakdown of formed fibrin clots with less effect on clot formation.

The use of fibrinolytic drugs results in the best clot breakdown with less disruption of blood clotting. These drugs are the first-line therapy for problems caused by small, localized, formed clots such as myocardial infarction (MI), limited arterial thrombosis, and thrombotic strokes. For some problems, such as MI, these drugs are given only within the first 6 hours after the onset of symptoms. This time limitation is not related to drug activity because fibrinolytic agents can break down clots older than 6 hours. Rather, the tissue that has been anoxic for more than 6 hours as a result of an acute event is not likely to benefit from this therapy, making the risks to the patient greater than the advantages.

Platelet inhibitors are drugs that either prevent platelets from becoming active or prevent activated platelets from clumping together. The most widely used drug for this effect is aspirin, which inhibits the production of substances that can trigger platelet activation, such as thromboxane. Other drugs change the platelet membrane, reducing its "stickiness," or prevent activators from binding to platelet receptor sites.

Nutrition Status

Diet can alter cell quality and affect blood clotting. Ask patients to record everything eaten during the previous week. Use this information to determine the causes of anemias and of protein, mineral, or vitamin deficiencies. Diets high in fat and carbohydrates and low in protein, iron, and vitamins can cause many types of anemia and decrease the functions of all blood cells.

Ask the patients about alcohol consumption. Chronic alcoholism can cause nutritional deficiencies and liver impairment, both of which reduce blood clotting.

Certain dietary habits can enhance blood clotting. Diets high in vitamin K, found in leafy green vegetables, may increase the rate of blood clotting. Assess the amount of salads and other raw vegetables that the patient eats and whether he or she routinely takes supplemental vitamins. Also assess the amount of calcium in the diet or in supplements.

Assess the patient's ability to understand and follow instructions related to diet, procedures and tests, and prescribed drugs or diets. Ask about personal resources, such as finances and social support. A person with a poor income may have a diet low in iron and protein because food sources of these substances are often more expensive.

Family History and Genetic Risk

An accurate family history is important because many disorders affecting blood and blood clotting are inherited (Nussbaum et al., 2007). Ask whether anyone in the family has had hemophilia, frequent nosebleeds, postpartum hemorrhages, excessive bleeding after tooth extractions, or heavy bruising after relatively mild trauma. Ask whether any family member has sickle cell disease or sickle cell trait. Although sickle cell disease is seen most often among African Americans, anyone can have the trait.

Current Health Problems

Determine whether the patient has had swelling of lymph nodes or excessive bruising or bleeding and whether the bleeding was spontaneous or induced by trauma. Ask about the amount and duration of bleeding after routine dental work. Determine whether a woman has menorrhagia (excessive menstrual flow). Ask her to estimate the number of pads or tampons used during the most recent menstrual cycle and whether this amount represents a change from her usual pattern of menstrual flow. Ask whether clots are present in menstrual blood. If the patient has had menstrual clots, ask her to estimate clot size using coins or fruit for comparison ("clots are dime-sized" or "clots are the size of lemons").

Assess whether the patient has shortness of breath on exertion, palpitations, frequent infections, fevers, recent weight loss, headaches, or paresthesias. Any or all of these symptoms may occur with hematologic disease.

The single most common symptom of anemia is fatigue. This problem occurs because oxygen delivery to cells is less than normal oxygen needs. The cells use oxygen to produce the high-energy chemical *adenosine triphosphate (ATP)* needed to perform most cellular work. When oxygen delivery to cells is reduced, all cellular work decreases and fatigue increases. Ask patients about feeling tired, needing more rest, or losing endurance during normal activities. Ask them to compare their activities during the past month with those of the same month a year ago. Determine whether they have other symptoms of anemia, such as vertigo, tinnitus, and a sore tongue.

Physical Assessment

Assess the whole body because blood problems may cause oxygen delivery to be less than what is needed for normal *oxygenation and tissue perfusion* in all systems. Some assessment findings associated with hematologic problems are less reliable when seen in the older adult (see Chart 41-1). Equipment needed for physical assessment of hematologic function includes a stethoscope, a blood pressure cuff, and a pen light.

Skin Assessment

Inspect the color of the skin for pallor or jaundice and of the mucous membranes and nail beds for pallor or cyanosis. Pallor of the gums, conjunctivae, and palmar creases indicates decreased hemoglobin levels and poor tissue oxygenation. Assess the gums for active bleeding in response to light pressure or brushing the teeth with a soft-bristled brush and for any lesions or draining areas. Inspect for petechiae and large bruises (ecchymoses). **Petechiae** are pinpoint hemorrhagic lesions in the skin. Bruises may cluster together. For hospitalized patients, determine whether there is bleeding from sites such as nasogastric tubes, endotracheal tubes, central lines, peripheral IV sites, or Foley catheters. Check the skin turgor, and ask about itching because dry skin or itching can indicate hematologic disease.

CULTURAL AWARENESS

Pallor and cyanosis are more easily detected in people with darker skin by examining the oral mucous membranes and the conjunctiva of the eye. Jaundice can be seen more easily on the roof of the mouth. Petechiae may be visible only on the palms of the hands or the soles of the feet. Bruises can be seen as darker areas of skin and palpated as slight swellings or irregular skin surfaces. Ask the patient about pain when skin surfaces are touched lightly or palpated. (Chapter 26 provides tips for assessing darker skin.)

Head and Neck Assessment

Check for pallor or ulceration of the mouth mucosa. The tongue may be completely smooth in pernicious anemia and iron deficiency anemia or smooth and beefy red in nutritional deficiencies. These manifestations may occur with fissures at the corners of the mouth. Assess for jaundice of the sclera.

Inspect and palpate all lymph node areas. Document any lymph node enlargement, including whether palpation of the enlarged node causes pain. It is important to determine whether the enlarged node moves or remains fixed in position with palpation.

Respiratory Assessment

When blood problems reduce oxygen delivery, the lungs work harder to make adjustments that can maintain tissue perfusion. Assess the rate and depth of respiration while the patient is at rest, as well as during and after mild physical activity (e.g., walking 20 steps in 10 seconds). Note whether the patient can complete a 10-word sentence without stopping for a breath. Assess whether the patient is fatigued easily, has shortness of breath at rest or on exertion, or needs extra pillows to sleep comfortably at night. Many anemias cause these symptoms as a result of respiratory changes made as adjustments to reduced oxygen delivery to tissues.

Cardiovascular Assessment

When blood problems reduce oxygen delivery, the heart works harder to make adjustments that maintain tissue perfusion. Observe for chest heaves, distended neck veins, edema, or signs of phlebitis. Use a stethoscope to listen for murmurs, gallops, irregular rhythms, and abnormal blood pressure (BP). Systolic BP tends to be lower than normal in patients with anemia. If the patient has excessive red blood cells, BP is higher than normal. Severe anemias can cause enlargement of the right ventricle and heart disease as the heart tries to adjust to compensate for a continuous reduction in oxygen delivery.

Renal and Urinary Assessment

The kidneys have many blood vessels, and bleeding problems may present as gross or occult hematuria (blood in the urine). Inspect a voided sample of urine for color. Hematuria may appear as grossly bloody red or dark brownish gold urine. Test the urine for proteins with a urine test dipstick because protein and blood in the urine increase its protein content.

Musculoskeletal Assessment

Rib or sternal tenderness is an important sign of leukemia (cancer of the blood). This manifestation occurs when the bone marrow greatly overproduces cells, increasing the pressure in the bones. Examine the skin over superficial bones, including the ribs and sternum, by applying firm pressure with the fingertips. Assess the range of joint motion, and document any swelling, joint pain, or motion limitation.

Abdominal Assessment

The normal adult spleen usually is *not* palpable. An enlarged spleen, however, occurs with many hematologic problems. An enlarged spleen may be detected by percussion, although palpation is more reliable. The spleen lies just beneath the abdominal wall, under the ribs on the left side. When it is enlarged, the spleen can be identified by its movement during respiration. During palpation, have the patient lie in a relaxed, supine position while you stand on the patient's right and palpate the left upper quadrant. *Palpate gently and cautiously because an enlarged spleen may be tender and easily ruptured.*

Palpating the edge of the liver in the right upper quadrant of the abdomen can detect hepatic enlargement, which often occurs with hematologic problems. The normal liver may be palpable as much as 4 to 5 centimeters below the right costal margin but usually is not palpable in the epigastrium.

A common cause of anemia among older adults is a chronically bleeding GI ulcer or polyp. If the ulcer is located in the stomach or the small intestine, obvious blood may not be visible in the stool or such a small amount is passed each day that the patient is not aware of it. Therefore obtain a stool specimen for occult blood testing.

Central Nervous System Assessment

Examining cranial nerves and testing neurologic function are important in hematologic assessment because some problems cause specific changes. Vitamin B_{12} deficiency impairs cerebral, olfactory, spinal cord, and peripheral nerve function, and severe chronic deficiency may cause permanent neurologic degeneration. Many neurologic problems can develop in patients who have leukemia as a result of bleeding, infection, or tumor spread. When the patient with a suspected bleeding disorder has any head trauma, expand the assessment to include frequent neurologic checks and mental status examinations (see Chapter 43).

Other manifestations that occur with impaired hematologic function include fever, chills, and night sweats.

Psychosocial Assessment

The patient with hematologic problems may have a chronic illness (e.g., hemophilia or cancer) or an acute episode of a chronic disease (e.g., pernicious anemia). In either case, each person brings his or her own coping style to the illness. Develop a rapport with the patient, and learn what coping mechanisms he or she has used successfully during past illnesses or crises.

Ask the patient and family members about social support networks, community resources, and financial health. A problem in any of these areas can interfere with the patient's adherence to therapy and, ultimately, recovery.

Diagnostic Assessment

Laboratory Assessment

In hematologic disease, the most definitive signs are often the laboratory test results. Chart 41-3 lists laboratory data used to assess hematologic function.

Tests of Cell Number and Function

A peripheral blood smear is made by taking a drop of blood and spreading it over a slide. It can be read by an automated calculator or a by a technologist with a microscope. This rapid test can provide important information on the sizes, shapes, and approximate proportions of different blood cell types within the peripheral blood.

A complete blood count (CBC) includes a number of studies: red blood cell (RBC) count, white blood cell (WBC) count, and hematocrit (Hct) and hemoglobin (Hgb) levels. The RBC count measures circulating RBCs in 1 mm^3 of blood. The WBC count measures all leukocytes present in 1 mm^3 of blood. To determine the percentages of different types of leukocytes circulating in the blood, a WBC count with differential leukocyte count is performed. The hematocrit is calculated as the percentage of RBCs in the total blood volume. The hemoglobin level is the total amount of hemoglobin in blood.

The CBC can measure other features of the RBCs, including mean corpuscular volume (MCV), mean corpuscular hemoglobin (MCH), and mean corpuscular hemoglobin concentration (MCHC). MCV measures the average volume or size of a single RBC and is useful for classifying anemias. When the MCV is elevated, the cell is larger than normal (macrocytic), as seen in megaloblastic anemias. When the MCV is decreased, the cell is smaller than normal (microcytic), as seen in iron deficiency anemia. The MCH is the average amount of hemoglobin by weight in a single RBC. The MCHC measures the average amount of hemoglobin by percentage in a single RBC. When the MCHC is decreased, the cell has a hemoglobin deficiency and is hypochromic (a lighter color), as in iron deficiency anemia.

Reticulocyte count is another hematologic test helpful in determining bone marrow function. A reticulocyte is an immature RBC that still has its nucleus. An elevated reticulocyte count indicates that RBCs are being produced by the bone marrow at a faster rate than they can mature. Normally only about 2% of circulating RBCs are reticulocytes. An elevated reticulocyte count is desirable in an anemic patient or after hemorrhage because this indicates that the bone marrow is responding appropriately to a decrease in the total RBC mass. An elevated reticulocyte count without a precipitating cause usually indicates health problems, such as polycythemia vera (a malignant condition in which the bone marrow overproduces RBCs).

Hemoglobin electrophoresis detects abnormal forms of hemoglobin, such as hemoglobin S in sickle cell disease. Hemoglobin A is the major type of hemoglobin in the normal RBC from an adult. Decreased hemoglobin A levels with increasing levels of other types of hemoglobin indicate some hematologic problems, such as sickle cell disease.

Leukocyte alkaline phosphatase (LAP) is an enzyme produced by normal mature neutrophils. Elevated LAP levels occur during episodes of infection or stress. An elevated neutrophil count without an elevation in LAP level occurs with some types of leukemia.

Coombs' tests, both direct and indirect, are used for blood typing. The direct test detects the presence of antibodies (also called *antiglobulins*) against RBCs that may be attached to a person's RBCs. Although healthy people can make these antibodies, in certain diseases (e.g., systemic lupus erythematosus, mononucleosis, lymphomas) these antibodies are directed against the patient's own RBCs. The presence of these antibodies usually causes a hemolytic anemia.

The indirect Coombs' test detects the presence of circulating antiglobulins. The test is used to determine whether the patient has serum antibodies to the type of RBCs that he or she is about to receive by blood transfusion.

Serum ferritin, transferrin, and the total iron-binding capacity (TIBC) tests measure iron levels. Abnormal levels of iron and TIBC occur with hematologic problems, including iron deficiency anemia.

The serum ferritin test measures the amount of iron present as free iron in the plasma. The amount of serum ferritin is related to the amount of intracellular iron and represents 1% of the total body iron stores. Therefore the serum ferritin level provides a means to assess total iron stores. People with serum ferritin levels within 10 grams of the normal range for their gender have adequate iron stores; people with levels 10 grams or more lower than the normal range have inadequate iron stores and have difficulty recovering from any blood loss.

Chart 41-3 LABORATORY PROFILE

Hematologic Assessment

Test	Range	International Reference Units	Significant of Abnormal Findings
Red blood cell (RBC) count	*Females:* 4.2-5.4 million/mm³ *Males:* 4.7-6.1 million/µL	4.2-5.4 × 10¹² cells/L 4.7-6.1 × 10¹² cells/L	*Decreased levels* indicate possible anemia or hemorrhage. *Increased levels* indicate possible chronic hypoxia or polycythemia vera.
Hemoglobin (Hgb)	*Females:* 12-16 g/dL *Males:* 14-18 g/dL	112-160 g/dL 140-180 g/dL	Same as for RBC
Hematocrit (Hct)	*Females:* 37%-47% *Males:* 42%-52%	0.37-0.47 fraction 0.42-0.52 fraction	Same as for RBC.
Mean corpuscular volume (MCV)	80-95 mm³	Same as reference range	*Increased levels* indicate macrocytic cells, possible anemia. *Decreased levels* indicate microcytic cells, possible iron deficiency anemia.
Mean corpuscular hemoglobin (MCH)	27-31 pg/cell	Same as reference range	Same as for MCV.
Mean corpuscular hemoglobin concentration (MCHC)	32-36 g/dL cells	320-370 g/L	*Increased levels* may indicate spherocytosis or anemia. *Decreased levels* may indicate iron deficiency anemia or a hemoglobinopathy.
White blood cell (WBC) count	5000-10,000/mm³	5.0-10.0 × 10⁹ cells/L	*Increased levels* are associated with infection, inflammation, autoimmune disorders, and leukemia. *Decreased levels* may indicate prolonged infection or bone marrow suppression.
Reticulocyte count	0.5%-0.2% of RBCs	0.005-0.20 fraction	*Increased levels* may indicate chronic blood loss. *Decreased levels* indicate possible inadequate RBC production.
Total iron-binding capacity (TIBC)	250-460 mcg/dL	45-82 µmol/L	*Increased levels* indicate iron deficiency. *Decreased levels* may indicate anemia, hemorrhage, hemolysis.
Iron (Fe)	*Females:* 60-160 mcg/dL *Males:* 80-180 mcg/dL	11-29 µmol/L 14-32 µmol/L	*Increased levels* indicate iron excess, hemochromocytosis, liver disorders, megaloblastic anemia. *Decreased levels* indicate possible iron deficiency anemia, hemorrhage.
Serum ferritin	*Females:* 10-150 ng/mL *Males:* 12-300 ng/mL	Same as reference range	Same as for iron.
Platelet count	150,000-400,000/mm³	150-400 × 10⁹/L	*Increased levels* may indicate polycythemia vera or malignancy. *Decreased levels* may indicate bone marrow suppression, autoimmune disease, hypersplenism.
Hemoglobin electrophoresis	Hgb A₁: 95%-98% Hgb A₂: 2%-3% Hgb F: 0.8%-2% Hgb S: 0% Hgb C: 0%	>0.95 fraction 0.020-0.030 fraction <0.02 fraction 0.0 fraction 0.0 fraction	*Variations* indicate hemoglobinopathies.
Direct Coombs' and indirect Coombs' test	Negative	Negative	*Positive findings* indicate antibodies to RBCs.
Prothrombin time (PT)	11-12.5 sec	Patient PT/normal PT (INR)	*Increased time* indicates possible deficiency of clotting factors V and VII. *Decreased time* may indicate vitamin K excess.
Bleeding time	1-9 min	Same as reference range	*Increased time* may indicate inadequate platelet function or number, clotting factor deficiencies.
Fibrin degradation products	<10 mcg/mL	<10 mg/L	*Increased levels* may indicate disseminated intravascular coagulation of fibrinolysis.

INR, International normalized ratio; *pg*, pictogram.

Transferrin is a protein that transports dietary iron from the intestines to cell storage sites. Transferrin is not easily measured, but by measuring the amount of iron that can be bound to serum transferrin indirectly, one can determine whether an adequate amount of transferrin is present. This test is the total iron-binding capacity (TIBC) test. In healthy people, only about 30% of the transferrin is bound to iron in the blood. TIBC is measured by taking a sample of blood and adding measured amounts of iron to it. TIBC is calculated when the blood no longer binds the iron but allows it to precipitate. TIBC increases when a person is deficient in serum iron and stored iron levels. Such a value indicates that an adequate amount of transferrin is present but less than 30% of it is bound to serum iron.

Tests Measuring Bleeding and Coagulation

Capillary fragility test measures how easily capillaries are damaged. The intracapillary pressure in the arm is increased by occluding venous outflow or by applying controlled negative pressure to a skin area. A blood pressure cuff is usually inflated to a pressure halfway between the systolic and diastolic pressures. This pressure is maintained for 5 minutes, and the petechiae that appear below the cuff are counted. Normally, 5 to 10 petechiae appear. When the number of petechiae that form increases, the cause of excessive bleeding or bruising is capillary fragility rather than poor platelet action.

Bleeding time test evaluates vascular and platelet activity during hemostasis. A special spring-loaded lancet that makes a uniform wound depth is applied to the forearm while a blood pressure cuff remains inflated at 40 mm Hg. Blood is blotted from the site at 30-second intervals, and the time required for the bleeding to stop is recorded. Normal bleeding time ranges from 1 to 9 minutes.

Prothrombin time (PT) measures how long blood takes to clot. This test reflects how much of the clotting factors II, V, VII, and X is present and how well they are functioning. When enough of these clotting factors are present and functioning, the PT shows blood clotting between 11 and 13 seconds or within 85% to 100% of the time needed for a control sample of blood to clot. PT is prolonged when one or more clotting factors is deficient, such as when liver disease is present. Sodium warfarin (Coumadin, Warfilone🍁) therapy is also monitored using PT levels. Usually warfarin therapy is considered appropriate when the PT is prolonged by 1.5 to

EVIDENCE-BASED PRACTICE

Save your patient an extra needle stick

Prue-Owens, K. (2006). Use of peripheral venous access devices for obtaining blood samples for measurement of activated partial thromboplastin times. *Critical Care Nurse, 26*(1), 30-38.

The purposes of the present nursing study were (1) to determine the accuracy of activated partial thromboplastin times (aPTTs) from a peripheral venous access device (VAD) flushed with saline in patients receiving continuous IV heparin therapy and (2) to determine the minimum discard volume needed to ensure that blood samples obtained from peripheral VADs would provide an accurate test result when compared with samples obtained by venipuncture.

The literature review for the present study included a meta-analysis of previous clinical evidence supporting the practice of obtaining blood samples through an existing access flushed with 0.9% saline at established intervals for patency. Conclusions from these previous studies included that tests other than aPTT were accurate when obtained from these lines, that samples obtained from tunneled catheters were not accurate, and that a common discard of 5 mL should be standard.

This prospective, quasi-experimental study included a convenience sample of 23 patients between the ages of 18 and 75 years who had a functional VAD and were receiving continuous IV heparin therapy. A total of 55 pairs of blood samples (one from the patient's VAD and one from a separate venipuncture on the same patient) were obtained and compared. One third of the VAD samples were obtained after a discard of 1 mL plus the 0.5 mL estimated "dead space," one third after a discard of 2 mL plus the dead space, and one third after a discard of 3 mL plus the dead space. Each sample was sent to the laboratory where the technologists were blinded to the source of the sample. All samples were analyzed in duplicate. The results showed no significant differences in aPTTs determined by samples obtained from separate venipunctures and those obtained from the VADs after any of the discard volumes used in the study. Thus the study supports obtaining blood samples for aPTT from an existing VAD after a 1 mL discard plus dead space volume, saving patients the pain and anxiety of additional venipunctures.

Level of Evidence—3. The study was well designed and prospective, without randomization. In addition, a meta-analysis of previous research on the topic was provided.

Commentary: Implications for Practice and Research. The design of the study was appropriate to answer the research questions posed. Study strengths include its prospective design, that the sample of subjects included both men and women, that the blood analysis was performed in duplicate on each sample, and that the technologists performing the analyses were blinded as to the source of the blood samples. The limitations include that the sample size was small, that potential subjects older than 75 years were excluded from the study, that the "dead space" of the VAD was only estimated and not measured, and that only one type of VAD with an extension set was used. Thus generalizability is somewhat limited. Future studies that measure the actual dead space in specific VADs and studies that include subjects older than 75 years to validate these results among older adults are needed.

Venipuncture for regularly scheduled blood tests, some as frequent as every 4 to 6 hours, can be painful and stressful. Establishing that results of tests performed on blood samples obtained through VADs are not different from those obtained from the same patients at the same time by separate venipuncture allows nurses to obtain blood samples from VADs, thus saving patients the pain and anxiety associated with standard venipuncture for the purposes of blood drawing only.

2.0 times the patient's normal PT value, depending on the specific reason for the warfarin therapy.

The PT test is now used less often to assess how fast blood clots because control blood is taken from different people and may not be the same even in one laboratory from one day to the next. To reduce PT errors as a result of control blood variation or in some of the chemicals used in the test, the international normalized ratio is used to assess clotting time.

International normalized ratio (INR) measures the same process as the PT in a slightly different way: by establishing a normal mean or standard for PT. The INR is calculated by dividing the patient's PT by the established standard PT. A normal INR ranges between 0.7 and 1.8. When using the INR to monitor warfarin therapy, the goal is usually to maintain the patient's INR between 2.0 and 3.0 regardless of the actual PT in seconds. The desired INR range for any patient, however, is individualized for specific patient factors.

Partial thromboplastin time (PTT) assesses the intrinsic clotting cascade and the action of factors II, V, VIII, IX, XI, and XII. PTT is prolonged whenever any of these factors is deficient, such as in hemophilia or disseminated intravascular coagulation (DIC). Because factors II, IX, and X are vitamin K–dependent and are produced in the liver, liver disease can decrease their levels and prolong the PTT. Heparin (Calciparin, Hepalean♣) therapy is monitored by PTT. Desired therapeutic ranges for anticoagulation are 1.5 to 2.0 times normal values.

Controversy exists as to whether this test is accurate when the blood sample is taken through a vascular access device (e.g., a normal saline lock) instead of through a separate new venipuncture, especially when the patient also is receiving heparin therapy. With an appropriate discard, samples obtained through vascular access devices accurately reflect the patient's activated partial thromboplastin time (aPTT) (see the Evidence-Based Practice box at left).

Platelet aggregation, or the ability to clump, is tested by mixing the patient's plasma with a substance called *ristocetin.* The degree of clumping is noted. Aggregation can be impaired in von Willebrand's disease and during the use of drugs such as aspirin, anti-inflammatory agents, psychotropic agents, and platelet inhibitors.

DECISION-MAKING CHALLENGE
Critical Rescue

The patient is a 55-year-old woman who is on warfarin therapy because of atrial fibrillation. Her INRs have been very inconsistent, ranging from 0.6 to 3.5. Last week, her INR was 0.7 and she was told to double her warfarin dose. When she comes to the clinic today, you take her vital signs including blood pressure. When you come back to draw blood for the INR, the arm you used to measure her blood pressure looks dark to you. On close inspection you see that her arm is covered with petechiae from where the blood pressure cuff was located down to her wrist.

1. Should you draw a blood sample for the INR? If so, what technique would you use?
2. What other assessment data should you obtain?
3. Is this manifestation likely to be related to her atrial fibrillation, or is it likely to be related to the warfarin therapy?
4. What is your priority action, and why?

evolve For suggested answer guidelines, go to http://evolve.elsevier.com/Iggy/.

Imaging Assessment

Assessment of the patient with a suspected hematologic problem can include radioisotopic imaging. Isotopes are used to evaluate the bone marrow for sites of active blood cell formation and sites of iron storage. Radioactive colloids are used to determine organ size and liver and spleen function.

The patient is given a radioactive isotope IV about 3 hours before the procedure. The patient is then taken to the nuclear medicine department for the scan, where he or she must lie still for about an hour. No special patient preparation or follow-up care is needed for these tests.

Standard x-rays may be used to diagnose some hematologic problems. For example, multiple myeloma causes classic bone destruction, with a "Swiss cheese" appearance on x-ray.

Bone Marrow Aspiration and Biopsy

Bone marrow aspiration or biopsy is often performed to evaluate the patient's hematologic status when other tests show persistent abnormal findings. Results can provide important information about bone marrow function, including the production of all blood cells and platelets. Bone marrow aspiration and bone marrow biopsy are similar invasive procedures. In a bone marrow aspiration, cells and fluids are suctioned from the bone marrow. In a bone marrow biopsy, solid tissue and cells are obtained by coring out an area of bone marrow with a large-bore needle.

A physician's request and a signed informed consent from the patient are obtained before a bone marrow aspiration or biopsy is performed. Bone marrow aspiration may be performed by a physician, an advanced practice nurse, or a physician assistant, depending on the agency's policy and regional law. The procedure may be performed at the patient's bedside, in an examination room, or in a laboratory.

After learning what specific tests will be performed on the marrow, check the facility's procedure manual and the hematology laboratory to determine how to handle the specimen. Some tests require that heparin or other solutions be added to the specimen.

Patient Preparation

Most patients are anxious or fearful before a bone marrow aspiration. Patients who have had a bone marrow aspiration in the past may have less anxiety or more anxiety, depending on their previous experience. You can help reduce anxiety and allay fears by providing accurate information and emotional support (Rushing, 2006). Some patients like to have their hand held during the procedure.

Explain the procedure to the patient, and tell him or her that you will stay during the entire procedure. Occasionally a friend or family member is permitted to be present to hold the patient's hand and provide additional emotional support. If a local anesthetic is used, tell the patient that the injection will feel like a stinging or burning sensation. Tell him or her to expect a heavy sensation of pressure and pushing while the needle is being inserted. Some patients also can hear a crunching sound or feel a scraping sensation as the needle punctures the bone. Explain that a brief sensation of painful pulling will be experienced as the marrow is being aspirated by mild suction in the syringe. If a biopsy is performed, the patient may feel more pressure and discomfort as the needle is rotated into the bone.

Assist the patient onto an examining table, and expose the site (usually the iliac crest). If this site is not available or if more marrow is needed, the sternum can be used. If the iliac crest is the site, place the patient in the prone position or, occasionally, in the side-lying position. Depending on the tests to be performed on the specimen, a laboratory technician may also be present to ensure proper handling of the specimen.

Procedure

The procedure usually lasts from 5 to 15 minutes. Patients may have pain. The type and the amount of anesthesia or sedation depend on the physician's preference, the patient's preference and previous experience with bone marrow aspiration and biopsy, and the setting.

A local anesthetic agent is injected into the skin around the site. The patient may also receive a mild tranquilizer or a rapid-acting sedative, such as midazolam (Versed), lorazepam (Ativan, Apo-Lorazepam♣, Novo-Lorazem♣), or etomidate (Amidate). Some patients do well with guided imagery or autohypnosis.

Aspiration or biopsy procedures are invasive, and sterile precautions are observed. The skin over the site is cleaned with a disinfectant. For an aspiration, the needle is inserted with a twisting motion and the marrow is aspirated by pulling back on the plunger of the syringe. When sufficient marrow has been aspirated to ensure accurate analysis, the needle is rapidly withdrawn while the tissues are supported at the site. For a biopsy, a small skin incision is made and the biopsy needle is inserted through the skin opening. Pressure and several twisting motions are needed to ensure coring and loosening of an adequate amount of marrow tissue. Apply external pressure to the site until hemostasis is ensured. A pressure dressing or sandbags may be applied to reduce bleeding at the site.

Follow-up Care

Cover the site with a dressing after bleeding is controlled, and closely observe it for 24 hours for signs of bleeding and infection. A mild analgesic (aspirin-free) may be given for discomfort, and ice packs can be placed over the site to limit bruising. Instruct the patient to inspect the site every 2 hours for the first 24 hours and to note the presence of active bleeding or bruising. Advise him or her to avoid contact sports or any activity that might result in trauma to the site for 48 hours.

Information obtained from bone marrow aspiration or biopsy reflects the degree and quality of bone marrow activity present. The counts made on a marrow specimen can indicate whether different cell types are present in the expected quantities and proportions. In addition, bone marrow aspiration or biopsy can confirm the spread of cancer cells from other tumor sites.

DECISION-MAKING CHALLENGE

Coordination of Care

The patient is a 25-year-old man who had a bone marrow aspiration 8 hours ago to determine a possible cause of profound anemia. He was sent home after the test with instructions to keep an ice pack on the site for a few hours and not to engage in heavy physical activity or take aspirin. He calls to say that after 4 hours of icing and taking 400 mg of ibuprofen, he felt "pretty good" and walked to a local bar to meet his friends. He had two beers and played pool for a couple hours and then walked home. Now the site (his right iliac crest) is throbbing and he has a 12-inch bruise all around it.

1. Should he come back to the hematology unit to be seen? Why or why not?
2. What factors may have contributed to bleeding at the site?
3. In considering the instructions he was given, could anything have been clarified to reduce the risk for bleeding?

evolve For suggested answer guidelines, go to http://evolve.elsevier.com/Iggy/.

HUMAN NEEDS ASSESSMENT REVIEW

What should you expect to NOTICE in a patient with adequate oxygenation and tissue perfusion related to hematologic function?

Vital Signs

- Heart rate and respiratory rate within normal range
- Blood pressure within normal range

Physical Assessment

- Able to speak a sentence of 12 words without stopping for breath
- Able to walk and talk without stopping for breath
- Skin color normal (no cyanosis, pallor, or jaundice)
- Oral mucous membrane and nail beds pink with rapid capillary refill
- Gums pink, no petechiae or bleeding
- Appropriate distribution of body hair, especially on legs and feet
- Warm hands and feet, no dependent edema
- Creases on palms of the hand (when stretched) red (or brown in people with dark skin)
- Skin clear with no large bruises or petechiae
- Lower eyelid conjunctive red
- Urine output just about equal to fluid intake
- Urine clear and yellow

Psychological Assessment

- Oriented and not confused
- Energy level good, able to engage in desired work, recreational, and personal activities

Laboratory Assessment

- Red blood cell, hemoglobin, hematocrit, white blood cell, and platelet levels within normal limits for age and gender
- Reticulocyte count less than 2%

GET READY FOR THE NCLEX EXAMINATION!

Key Points

Review these Key Points for each NCLEX Examination Client Needs Category.

Safe and Effective Care Environment

- Use good handwashing techniques before providing any care to any patient, especially one who is either immunocompromised or immune deficient.
- Verify that a patient having a bone marrow aspiration or biopsy has signed an informed consent statement.

Health Promotion and Maintenance

- Teach people to avoid unnecessary contact with environmental chemicals or toxins. If contact cannot be avoided, teach people to use safety precautions.
- Instruct patients about the importance of eating a diet with adequate amounts of foods that are good sources of iron, folic acid, and vitamin B_{12}.

Psychosocial Integrity

- Explain all procedures, restrictions, drugs, and follow-up care to the patient and family.
- Ask patients about their activity level and whether they are satisfied with the energy they have for activities.
- Support the patient during a bone marrow aspiration or biopsy.

Physiological Integrity

- Tissue oxygenation and perfusion rely on normal hematologic function for oxygen delivery.
- The most common manifestation of a hematologic problem is fatigue.
- Remember that a platelet plug and a fibrin clot are not the same.
- Understand the effects of age and gender on red blood cell, hematocrit, and hemoglobin levels.
- Apply an ice pack to the needle site after a bone marrow aspiration or biopsy.
- Check the needle site at least every 2 hours after a bone marrow aspiration or biopsy. If the patient is going home, teach the patient and family how to assess the site for bleeding and when to seek help.
- Instruct patients to avoid activities that may traumatize the site after a bone marrow aspiration or biopsy.

Additional Study Resources

Go to your Companion CD or Evolve at http://evolve.elsevier.com/Iggy/ for *Self-Assessment Questions for the NCLEX Examination.*

evolve

Go to Evolve at http://evolve.elsevier.com/Iggy/ for *Prioritization and Delegation Questions for the NCLEX Examination.*

SELECTED BIBLIOGRAPHY

Asterisk indicates a classic or definitive work on this subject.

Beattie, S. (2007). Bone marrow aspiration and biopsy. *RN, 70*(2), 41-43.

Cranwell-Bruce, L. (2007). Anticoagulation therapy: Reinforcing patient education. *MEDSURG Nursing, 16*(1), 55-58.

Edwards, N., & Baird, C. (2005). Interpreting laboratory values in older adults. *MEDSURG Nursing, 14*(4), 220-229.

Gordon, M. (2007). *Manual of nursing diagnosis* (11th ed.). Boston: Jones & Bartlett.

Jarvis, C. (2008). *Physical examination and health assessment* (5th ed.). Philadelphia: Saunders.

McCance, K., & Huether, S. (2006). *Pathophysiology: The biologic basis for disease in adults and children* (5th ed.). St. Louis: Mosby.

Meiner, S., & Lueckenotte, A. (Eds.). (2006). *Gerontologic nursing,* (3rd ed.). St. Louis: Mosby.

Nussbaum, R., McInnes, R., & Willard, H. (2007). *Thompson & Thompson: Genetics in medicine* (7th ed.). Philadelphia: Saunders.

Pagana, K., & Pagana, T. (2006). *Mosby's manual of diagnostic and laboratory tests* (3rd ed.). St. Louis: Mosby.

Prue-Owens, K. (2006). Use of peripheral venous access devices for obtaining blood samples for measurement of activated partial thromboplastin times. *Critical Care Nurse, 26*(1), 30-38.

Rushing, J. (2006). Assisting with bone marrow aspiration and biopsy. *Nursing2006, 36*(3), 68.

Turka, J. (2005). Understanding international normalized ratio (INR). *Nursing2005, 35*(8), 18-19.

*Woodrow, P. (2003). Assessing blood results in older people: Haematology and liver function tests. *Nursing Older People*, 15(3), 29-31.

42

CHAPTER

Care of Patients with Hematologic Problems

Katherine L. Byar

LEARNING OUTCOMES

For clinical competence and success on the NCLEX Examination, study this chapter with these Learning Outcomes in mind:

Safe and Effective Care Environment

1. Apply the principles of asepsis to protect immunocompromised patients.
2. Modify the environment to protect patients who have thrombocytopenia.
3. Identify appropriate community resources for the patient with a serious hematologic problem or recovering from a stem cell transplant.
4. Plan continuity of care between the hospital and community-based agencies for the patient having a stem cell transplant.
5. Verify patient identification before any form of transfusion therapy.

Health Promotion and Maintenance

6. Teach patients ways to prevent leukemia or lymphoma by avoiding known environmental causative agents.
7. Identify patients at increased risk for infection and hemorrhage.
8. Assess the patient's endurance in performing ADLs.
9. Coordinate with a nutritionist to teach patients with dietary deficiency–related anemia about the appropriate food sources for anemia prevention.
10. Teach patients and family members how to avoid injury and infection when blood counts are low.

Psychosocial Integrity

11. Encourage the patients and family members to express their feelings about the diagnosis of a serious hematologic problem, its prognosis, and treatment.
12. Use effective communication when teaching patients and family members about what to expect during tests and therapeutic procedures.
13. Use complementary and alternative therapies along with drug therapy to improve patient comfort.

Physiological Integrity

14. Identify three clinical manifestations common to patients who have any type of anemia.
15. Explain the pattern of inheritance for sickle cell disease.
16. Prioritize nursing care for the patient who has sickle cell disease.
17. Identify the risk factors for the development of leukemia, lymphoma, and myelodysplastic syndromes.
18. Correctly interpret laboratory data and clinical manifestations to determine the presence of infection in a patient who has neutropenia.
19. Prioritize nursing interventions for the patient with neutropenia.
20. Prioritize nursing interventions for the patient with thrombocytopenia.
21. Prioritize nursing responsibilities during transfusion therapy.
22. Identify patients at risk for complications of transfusion therapy.

Go to your Companion CD or Evolve at http://evolve.elsevier.com/Iggy/ for *Self-Assessment Questions for the NCLEX Examination* keyed to these Learning Outcomes.

Hematologic problems result from the impaired production, the impaired function, or the abnormal destruction of any type of blood cell. Problems of the hematologic system can affect many tissues and organs by interfering with the *human need for oxygenation and tissue perfusion.* The type and severity of the disorder determine the impact it has on the health of patients. This chapter discusses mild hematologic disorders and those that are potentially life threatening, such as sickle cell disease and leukemia.

RED BLOOD CELL DISORDERS

Red blood cells (RBCs), also known as **erythrocytes,** are the major cell in the blood. Tissue *oxygenation* depends on keeping the circulating number of RBCs within the normal range for the person's age and gender. It also depends on the ability of RBCs to perform their normal functions. RBC disorders include problems in production, function, and destruction. Problems may result in poor function of RBCs, decreased numbers of RBCs **(anemia),** or an excess of RBCs **(polycythemia).**

ANEMIA

Anemia is a reduction in either the number of RBCs, the amount of hemoglobin, or the **hematocrit** (percentage of packed RBCs per deciliter [dL]) of blood). It is a clinical sign, not a specific disease, because it occurs with many health problems. Anemia can result from dietary problems, genetic disorders, bone marrow disease, or excessive bleeding. GI bleeding is the most common reason for anemia in adults.

There are many types and causes of anemia. Some are caused by a deficiency in one or more of the components needed to make fully functional RBCs. Such anemias can be caused by deficiencies of iron, vitamin B_{12}, folic acid, or intrinsic factor. Other causes include a decreased rate of RBC production and increased RBC destruction. Table 42-1 lists common causes of many anemias. Despite the many causes of anemia, the effects of anemia on the patient (Chart 42-1) and the nursing care needed are similar for all types of anemia (Coyer & Lash, 2008).

TABLE 42-1 Common Causes of Anemia

Type of Anemia	Common Causes
Sickle cell disease	Autosomal recessive inheritance of two defective gene alleles for hemoglobin synthesis
Glucose-6-phosphate dehydrogenase (G6PD) deficiency anemia	X-linked recessive deficiency of the enzyme *G6PD*
Autoimmune hemolytic anemia	Abnormal immune function in which a person's immune reactive cells fail to recognize his or her own red blood cells as self cells
Iron deficiency anemia	Inadequate iron intake caused by • Iron-deficient diet • Chronic alcoholism • Malabsorption syndromes • Partial gastrectomy Rapid metabolic (anabolic) activity caused by • Pregnancy • Adolescence • Infection
Vitamin B_{12} deficiency anemia	Dietary deficiency Failure to absorb vitamin B_{12} from intestinal tract as a result of • Partial gastrectomy • Pernicious anemia
Folic acid deficiency anemia	Dietary deficiency Malabsorption syndromes Drugs • Oral contraceptives • Anticonvulsants • Methotrexate
Aplastic anemia	Exposure to myelotoxic agents • Radiation • Benzene • Chloramphenicol • Alkylating agents • Antimetabolites • Sulfonamides • Insecticides Viral infection (unproven) • Epstein-Barr virus • Hepatitis B • Cytomegalovirus

Chart 42-1 KEY FEATURES

Anemia

INTEGUMENTARY MANIFESTATIONS
- Pallor, especially of the ears, the nail beds, the palmar creases, the conjunctivae, and around the mouth
- Cool to the touch
- Intolerance of cold temperatures
- Nails become brittle and may lose the normal convex shape; over time, nails become concave and fingers assume club-like appearance

CARDIOVASCULAR MANIFESTATIONS
- Tachycardia at basal activity levels, increasing with activity and during and immediately after meals
- Murmurs and gallops heard on auscultation when anemia is severe
- Orthostatic hypotension

RESPIRATORY MANIFESTATIONS
- Dyspnea on exertion
- Decreased oxygen saturation levels

NEUROLOGIC MANIFESTATIONS
- Increased somnolence and fatigue
- Headache

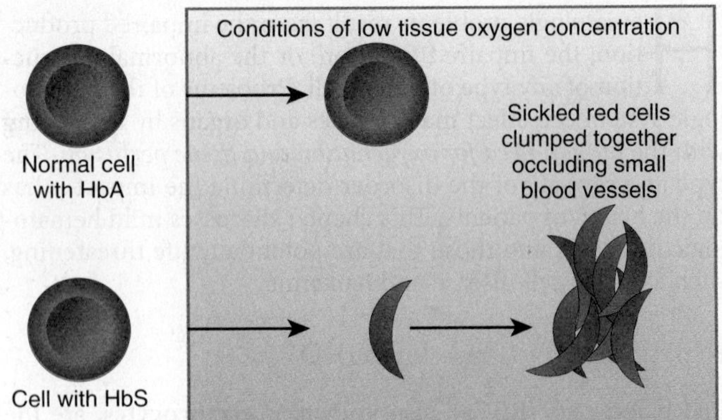
Conditions of low tissue oxygen concentration
Normal cell with HbA
Sickled red cells clumped together occluding small blood vessels
Cell with HbS

Fig. 42-1 • Red blood cell actions under conditions of low tissue oxygenation. (*HbA*, Hemoglobin A; *HbS*, hemoglobin S).

ANEMIAS RESULTING FROM INCREASED DESTRUCTION OF RED BLOOD CELLS

Sickle Cell Disease

Pathophysiology

Sickle cell disease is a genetic disorder that results in chronic anemia, pain, disability, organ damage, increased risk for infection, and early death. There is a difference between sickle cell disease state and sickle cell trait. In addition, there is great variation among patients in how severe the disease is and when complications start.

The main problem in this disorder is the formation of abnormal hemoglobin chains. In healthy adults, the normal hemoglobin molecule has two alpha chains and two beta chains of amino acids. This normal adult hemoglobin is called **hemoglobin A (HbA).** Normal adult hemoglobin usually is 98% to 99% HbA, with a small percentage of a fetal form of hemoglobin (HbF).

In sickle cell disease, at least 40% (and often much more) of the total hemoglobin contains an abnormality of the beta chains, known as *hemoglobin S (HbS).* HbS is sensitive to changes in the oxygen content of the RBC. When RBCs having large amounts of HbS are exposed to decreased oxygen states, the abnormal beta chains contract and pile together within the cell, distorting the shape of the RBC. These cells assume a sickle shape, become rigid, and clump together, causing the RBCs to become "sticky" and fragile. These clumps form masses of sickled RBCs that block blood flow (Fig. 42-1). This blood vessel obstruction leads to further tissue **hypoxia** (reduced oxygen supply) and more sickle-shaped cells, which then leads to more blood vessel obstruction and ischemia in the affected tissues. Repeated episodes of ischemia lead to progressive organ damage from anoxia and infarction. Conditions that cause sickling include hypoxia, dehydration, infections, venous stasis, pregnancy, alcohol consumption, high altitudes, low environmental or body temperatures, acidosis, strenuous exercise, and anesthesia.

Usually, sickled cells go back to normal shape when the low oxygen condition is removed and proper *tissue perfusion* resumes. Although the cells then appear normal, at least some of the hemoglobin remains twisted, decreasing cell flexibility. The cell membranes become damaged over time, and cells are permanently sickled. The membranes of cells with HbS are more fragile and more easily broken. The average life span of an RBC containing 40% or more of HbS is about 12 to15 days, much less than the 120-day life span of normal RBCs. This reduced RBC life span causes **hemolytic** (blood cell–destroying) anemia in patients with sickle cell disease.

The patient with sickle cell disease has periodic episodes of extensive cellular sickling, called **crises.** The crises have a sudden onset and can occur as often as weekly or as seldom as once a year. Many patients are in good health much of the time, with crises occurring only in response to conditions that cause local or systemic **hypoxemia** (deficient oxygen in the blood).

Repeated blockages of larger blood vessels have long-term damaging effects on tissues and organs. Most effects occur as a result of tissue hypoxia, anoxia, ischemia, and cell death. Tissues and organs begin to have small infarcted areas. Eventually, so many healthy cells are destroyed that organ failure results. Organs most often affected in this way are the spleen, liver, heart, kidney, brain, bones, and retina.

Etiology and Genetic Risk

Sickle cell disease is a genetic disorder with an autosomal recessive pattern of inheritance (see Chapter 6). The formation of the beta chains of hemoglobin depends on a pair of gene alleles (alternate forms of a gene). A mutation in these alleles leads to the formation of HbS instead of HbA. In sickle cell disease, the patient has two HbS gene alleles, one inherited from each parent, usually resulting in 80% to 100% of the total hemoglobin containing HbS. Patients with sickle cell disease have severe manifestations of the disease even when triggering conditions are mild. If a patient with sickle cell disease has children, each child will inherit one of the two abnormal gene alleles and at least have sickle cell trait.

In *sickle cell trait,* one normal gene allele and one abnormal gene allele are inherited, so only half of the hemoglobin chains produced will be abnormal. The patient is a carrier of the HbS gene allele (Fig. 42-2). The patient can pass the trait on to his or her children, but the patient has only mild manifestations of the disease under severe precipitating conditions because less than 40% of the hemoglobin is abnormal.

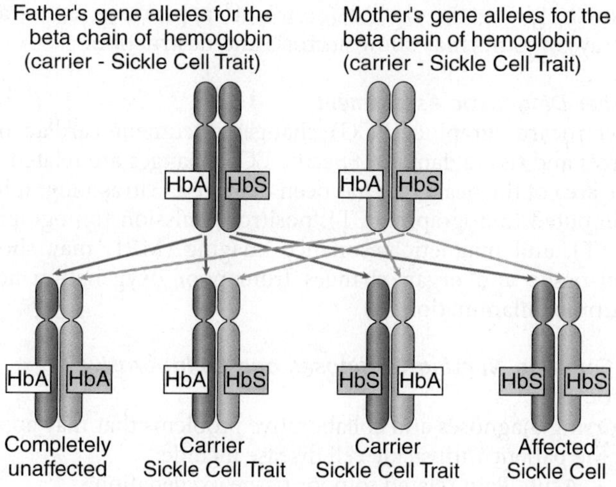
Father's gene alleles for the beta chain of hemoglobin (carrier - Sickle Cell Trait)
Mother's gene alleles for the beta chain of hemoglobin (carrier - Sickle Cell Trait)
HbA HbS
HbA HbS
HbA HbA
HbA HbS
HbS HbA
HbS HbS
Completely unaffected
Carrier Sickle Cell Trait
Carrier Sickle Cell Trait
Affected Sickle Cell
Fig. 42-2 • Inheritance pattern for sickle cell disease.

Incidence/Prevalence

Sickle cell trait and different forms of sickle cell disease occur in people of all races and ethnicities but less often among white people. In the United States, about 70,000 people have sickle cell disease, most commonly African Americans (Sickle Cell Information Center, 2007). Sickle cell disease occurs in 1 in 400 African Americans, and 1 in 12 to 1 in 15 (8%) African Americans are carriers of one sickle cell gene allele and have sickle cell trait (Nussbaum et al., 2007).

Patient-Centered Collaborative Care

Assessment

History

An adult with sickle cell disease usually has a long-standing diagnosis of the disorder. An adult with sickle cell trait usually has no symptoms or abnormal laboratory findings other than the presence of hemoglobin S. This person may be unaware that he or she has a problem until an acute illness is present or when anesthesia is administered.

Ask him or her about previous crises, what led to the crises, severity, and usual treatments. Explore recent contact with ill people and activities to determine what caused the current crisis. Ask the patient about symptoms of infection as the cause of a crisis, such as sore throat, cough, GI changes, or pain and burning upon urination.

Review all activities and events during the past 24 hours, including food and fluid intake, exposure to temperature extremes, drugs taken, exercise, trauma, stress, recent airplane travel, and ingestion of alcohol or other recreational drugs. Ask about changes in sleep and rest patterns, ability to climb stairs, and any activity that induces shortness of breath. Determine his or her perceived energy level using a scale ranging from 0 to 10 (0 = not tired with plenty of energy; 10 = total exhaustion) to assess the degree of fatigue. This activity review provides important information about fatigue, activity tolerance, and participation in ADLs.

Physical Assessment/Clinical Manifestations

Pain is the most common symptom of sickle cell crisis. Jaundice may also be present with RBC destruction and release of bilirubin. Other manifestations vary with the site of tissue damage.

Cardiovascular changes, including the risk for high-output heart failure, occur because of the anemia. Assess the patient for shortness of breath and general fatigue or weakness. Other problems may include murmurs and the presence of an S_3 heart sound. Assess his or her cardiac and vascular status by comparing peripheral pulses, temperature, and capillary refill in all extremities. Extremities distal to blood vessel occlusion are cool to the touch with slow capillary refill and may have reduced or absent pulses. The heart rate may be rapid and the blood pressure low to average, with a decreased pulse pressure, because breakage of RBCs leads to anemia. Anemia results in a less viscous (thinner) blood that moves more rapidly through the heart and blood vessels under lower pressures than does normally viscous blood.

Priapism is a prolonged penile erection. This complication can occur in men who have sickle cell disease as a result of vascular engorgement in erectile tissue. The condition is very painful and can last for hours. During the priapism episode, the patient usually cannot urinate.

Skin changes include pallor or cyanosis because of poor *oxygenation* from decreased *perfusion* and anemia. Examine the lips, tongue, nail beds, conjunctivae, palms, and soles of the feet at least every 8 hours for subtle color changes. With cyanosis, the lips and tongue are gray and the palms, soles, conjunctivae, and nail beds have a bluish tinge.

Another skin manifestation of sickle cell disease is jaundice. Bilirubin, present inside RBCs, is released when fragile cells are damaged, leading to jaundice. Assess for jaundice in patients with darker skin by inspecting the roof of the mouth for a yellow appearance. Yellow-tinged sclera may be misleading because of normal deposits of fat that appears yellowish in contrast to the dark skin around the eye. Examine the sclera closest to the cornea to assess jaundice more accurately. The palms and soles of dark-skinned patients may appear yellow if callous and could be mistaken for jaundice. Jaundice often causes intense itching.

Despite the anemia, patients with sickle cell disease usually are not iron deficient. In fact, with increased RBC production and destruction, iron released from the cells may increase the pigmentation of the skin.

As many as 75% of adults with sickle cell disease have open sores or ulcers on the lower legs that are caused by poor *tissue perfusion.* The outer sides and inner aspect of the ankle or the shin are common ulcer sites. Inspect the legs and feet for open lesions or darkened areas that may indicate necrotic tissue. These lesions often become necrotic or infected, requiring débridement and antibiotic therapy. Skin grafting may be needed when ulcers fail to heal.

Abdominal changes include major organ damage to the spleen and liver. These organs are usually the first to be damaged from many episodes of hypoxia and ischemia. In crisis, abdominal pain is diffuse and steady, involving the back and legs (Sickle Cell Information Center, 2007). Bowel sounds should be present with normal activity. Palpate the liver and spleen for enlargement. The liver or spleen may feel firm and enlarged with a nodular or "lumpy" texture in later stages of the disease. Check for guarding or rebound tenderness to palpation. A rapidly enlarging liver or spleen that occurs with increasing jaundice may indicate blood trapping in those organs.

Renal and urinary changes are common as a result of poor perfusion and decreased tissue oxygenation. Chronic kidney disease occurs as a result of anoxic damage to the kidney nephrons. With early damage, the kidneys are less effective at filtration and reabsorption. The urine contains protein, and the patient may unable to concentrate urine. Eventually, the kidneys fail, resulting in little or no urine output. The buildup of toxic waste product in the blood leads to death.

Musculoskeletal changes occur because arms and legs are common sites of blood vessel occlusion in sickle cell disease. Joints also may be damaged from hypoxic episodes and have necrotic degeneration. Inspect the arms and legs for symmetry, and record any areas of swelling or color difference. Ask patients to move all joints. Record the range of motion and any pain with movement.

Central nervous system (CNS) changes may occur in sickle cell disease. During crises, patients may have a low-grade fever. If the CNS has infarcts or repeated episodes of hypoxia, patients may have seizures or manifestations of a stroke. Assess hand grasps on both sides. Also assess the patient's gait and coordination.

Psychosocial Assessment

Psychosocial assessment is important because behavioral changes are early manifestations of cerebral hypoxia from poor *tissue perfusion*. Observe the patient, and document behavior. Ask family members whether the current behavior and mental status are usual for the patient.

Sickle cell disease is a painful, life-limiting disorder that can be passed on to one's children. Assess the patient's psychosocial needs in terms of new factors, established support systems, use of coping patterns, and disease progression. Ask the patient about how he or she views the disease and what changes in lifestyle have been made as limitations increased.

Laboratory Assessment

The diagnosis of sickle cell disease is based on the large percentage of hemoglobin S (HbS) seen on electrophoresis. A person who has sickle cell trait usually has less than 40% HbS, and the patient with sickle cell disease may have 80% to 100% HbS. This percentage does not change during crises. Another indicator of sickle cell disease is the number of RBCs with permanent sickling. This value is less than 1% among people who do not have sickle cell disease, is 5% to 50% among people with sickle cell trait, and may exceed 90% among patients with sickle cell disease.

Other laboratory tests can indicate complications of the disease, especially during crises. The hematocrit of patients with sickle cell disease is low (between 20% and 30%) because the life span of the RBC is so much shorter than normal and because many cells are destroyed. This value decreases even more during crises or when the bone marrow fails to produce cells during stress (aplastic crisis). The reticulocyte count is high, indicating anemia of long duration. It is high because the bone marrow is releasing immature red blood cells (reticulocytes) to make up for the low hematocrit and resulting tissue hypoxia. Often the total bilirubin levels are high in patients with sickle cell disease because bilirubin is released from damaged and dead red blood cells.

The total white blood cell (WBC) count is usually high in patients with sickle cell disease. This elevation is related to chronic inflammation caused by tissue hypoxia and ischemia.

Imaging Assessment

Bone changes occur as a result of chronically stimulated marrow and low bone oxygen levels. The skull may show changes on x-ray as a result of bone surface cell destruction and new growth, giving the skull a "crew cut" appearance on x-ray. X-rays of joints may show necrosis and destruction.

Other Diagnostic Assessment

Electrocardiographic (ECG) changes document cardiac infarcts and tissue damage. Specific ECG changes are related to the area of the heart that has been damaged. Ultrasonography, computed tomography (CT), positron emission tomography (PET), and magnetic resonance imaging (MRI) may show soft-tissue and organ changes from poor oxygenation and chronic inflammation.

▪ Common Nursing Diagnoses and Collaborative Problems

Nursing diagnoses and collaborative problems that may apply to the patient with sickle cell disease include:

- Acute Pain related to poor tissue oxygenation
- Chronic Pain related to joint destruction
- Potential for Sepsis
- Potential for Multiple Organ Dysfunction and Death

▪ Interventions

Acute Pain; Chronic Pain

The most common problem of sickle cell disease is pain. The pain with sickle cell crisis is the result of tissue injury caused by poor oxygenation from obstructed blood flow. At times, patients have mild pain episodes that can be managed at home. However, pain is often severe enough to require hospitalization and large doses of opioid analgesics. Acute pain episodes have a sudden onset, usually involving the chest, back, abdomen, and extremities (Dorman, 2005). Complications of sickle cell disease, such as bone necrosis, can cause severe, chronic pain, requiring large doses of opioid analgesics.

Ask the patient whether the pain is typical of past pain episodes. If not, other pain causes or disease complications must be explored. Use of a pain rating scale can help proper pain management. Ask the patient to rate pain on a scale ranging from 0 to 10, and evaluate the effectiveness of interventions based on the ratings.

Concerns about substance abuse can lead to inadequate pain treatment in these patients. Opioid addiction is rare, occurring in only 2% to 5% of patients with sickle cell disease. Treatment of pain is based on past pain history, previous drug use, disease complications, and current pain assessment. Health care providers need to be aware of their own attitudes when caring for this population. If substance abuse is suspected, the treatment of addiction is incorporated into the patient's overall treatment plan. Management of substance abuse and sickle cell disease poses many challenges, because the patient usually cannot be expected to be totally opioid-free. Addicted patients with acute pain crisis may need opioids for short periods.

Drug therapy for patients in acute sickle cell crisis often starts with at least 48 hours of IV analgesics. (Chart 42-2 lists best practices for nursing care of the patient in sickle cell crisis.) Morphine and hydromorphone (Dilaudid) are given IV on a routine schedule or by infusion pump using patient-controlled analgesia (PCA) (see Chapter 5). Once relief is obtained, the IV dose can be tapered and the drug given orally. Avoid "as needed" (PRN) schedules because they do not provide adequate relief. Avoid IM injections because absorption is impaired by poor perfusion and sclerosed skin. Moderate pain may be

Chart 42-2 BEST PRACTICE FOR PATIENT SAFETY & QUALITY CARE

Care of the Patient in Sickle Cell Crisis

- Administer oxygen.
- Administer pain medication as prescribed.
- Hydrate the patient with normal saline IV and with beverages of choice (without caffeine) orally.
- Remove any constrictive clothing.
- Encourage the patient to keep extremities extended to promote venous return.
- Do not raise the knee gatch of the bed.
- Elevate the head of the bed no more than 30 degrees.
- Keep room temperature at or above 72° F (22.2° C).
- Avoid taking blood pressure with external cuff.
- Check circulation in extremities every hour:
  - Pulse oximetry of fingers and toes
  - Capillary refill
  - Peripheral pulses
  - Toe temperature

treated with oral doses of opioids or NSAIDs. (See Chapter 5 for more information on pain management.)

Hydroxyurea (Droxia) has been successfully used to reduce the number of sickling and pain episodes. Hydroxyurea works by stimulating fetal hemoglobin (HbF) production. HbF is present during fetal development, but its production is turned off before birth. Increasing the level of HbF reduces sickling of red blood cells in patients with sickle cell disease. However, this drug is associated with an increased incidence of leukemia. Long-term complications should be discussed with the patient before this therapy is started. Hydroxyurea also suppresses bone marrow function, and regular follow-up to monitor complete blood counts (CBCs) for drug toxicity is important. *Hydroxyurea also causes birth defects. Thus sexually active women of childbearing age should use at least two methods of birth control while taking this drug.*

Hydration by the oral or IV route helps reduce the duration of pain episodes. Urge the patient to drink water or juices. Hypotonic fluids, such as dextrose 5% in water (D_5W) or dextrose 5% in 0.45% sodium chloride, are infused at 250 mL/hr for 4 hours. Hypotonic fluids are used because the patient's blood volume is usually hypertonic as a result of dehydration. Using hypotonic fluids can help bring the patient's blood osmolarity back down to the normal range of 270 to 300 mOsm. The IV rate is then reduced to 125 mL/hr if more hydration is needed.

Complementary therapies and other measures, such as keeping the room warm, using distraction and relaxation techniques, positioning with support for painful areas, aroma therapy, therapeutic touch, and warm soaks or compresses, all help reduce pain perception. *Do not assume that these methods alone will provide adequate pain relief. Analgesics are needed to manage sickle cell pain.*

Potential for Sepsis

The patient with sickle cell disease is at greater risk for bacterial infection because of decreased spleen function resulting from anoxic damage to the spleen. Over time, the spleen may become completely nonfunctional. Interventions aim at preventing infection, controlling infection, and starting treatment early for specific infections. The patient who develops a fever should have diagnostic testing for sepsis including CBC with differential, blood cultures, reticulocyte count, urine culture, and a chest x-ray. Usually these patients are started on prophylactic antibiotics.

Prevention and early detection strategies are used to protect the patient in sickle cell crisis from infection. Frequent, thorough handwashing is of the utmost importance. Any person with an upper respiratory tract infection who must enter the patient's room wears a mask. Use strict aseptic technique for all invasive procedures. Coordinate with all members of the health care team to ensure adherence to these strategies.

Continually assess the patient for infection, and monitor the daily CBC with differential WBC count. Inspect the mouth every 8 hours for lesions indicating fungal or viral infection. Listen to the lungs every 8 hours for crackles, wheezes, or reduced breath sounds. Each time the patient voids, inspect the urine for odor and cloudiness, and ask about urgency, burning, or pain during urination. Take vital signs at least every 4 hours to assess for fever or supervise this action when performed by others.

Drug therapy is a major defense against the infections that develop in the patient with sickle cell disease. Prophylactic therapy with twice-daily oral penicillin reduces the number of pneumonia and other streptococcal infections. Urge the patient to receive yearly influenza vaccinations and to receive the pneumonia vaccine. Drug therapy for an actual infection can control infection and prevent sepsis. Drugs used depend on the sensitivity of the specific organism causing the infection, as well as on the extent of the infection.

Potential for Multiple Organ Dysfunction

Continued blood vessel occlusion by clumping of sickled cells increases the risk for multiple organ dysfunction. Management of sickle cell disease focuses on prevention of blood vessel occlusion and promotion of oxygenation.

The patient in sickle cell crisis is admitted to the acute care hospital. Assess for adequate *perfusion* to all body areas. Remove restrictive clothing, and instruct the patient to avoid flexing the knees and hips.

Hydration is needed because dehydration increases cell sickling and must be avoided. Assist him or her in maintaining adequate hydration. The patient in acute crisis needs an oral or IV intake of at least 200 mL/hr.

Oxygen is given during crises because lack of oxygen is the main cause of sickling. Ensure that oxygen therapy is nebulized to prevent dehydration. Monitor oxygen saturation using pulse oximetry. Patients with low oxygen saturation should have an arterial blood gas (ABG) drawn and a chest x-ray.

Transfusion with RBCs can be helpful to increase HbA levels and dilute HbS levels. During transfusion, monitor the patient for complications of the procedure (discussed on pp. 920-921 in the Transfusion Reactions section).

Transfusions are prescribed cautiously to prevent iron overload from repeated transfusions. Iron overload damages the heart, liver, and endocrine organs. Monitor the patient's serum ferritin, serum iron (Fe), and total iron-binding capacity (TIBC). Deferoxamine mesylate (Desferal, Desferrioxamine) or deferasirox (Exjade) may be prescribed to treat transfusion-induced iron overload.

In some treatment centers, hematopoietic stem cell transplantation (HSCT) is performed to correct abnormal hemoglobin permanently. Because HSCT is expensive and may result in chronic and life-threatening complications, its risks and benefits need to be considered for each patient.

DECISION-MAKING CHALLENGE
Coordination of Care

A 21-year-old African-American man who has a history of sickle cell disease is brought to the emergency department at midnight. He and his family are from out of town and flew in earlier in the day. The patient tells you he has joint and back pain. He is very fearful because the pain is getting progressively worse. He rates his pain as a 9 on a 0 to 10 scale. He is pale, and his vital signs are normal except for slight tachycardia. He is still nauseated from the motion sickness induced by the plane trip. He says that he has been able to drink only about 2 cups of liquids today.

1. What questions related to pain would you ask this patient?
2. What drugs would you expect this patient to receive and by which route?
3. What diagnostic tests would you expect to be requested for this patient?
4. What nursing assessments would be most important for you to make at this time?
5. What factor or factors could have triggered this crisis episode?

evolve For suggested answer guidelines, go to http://evolve.elsevier.com/Iggy/.

Community-Based Care

Sickle cell disease becomes worse over time. Rarely is there a true remission, although the number of crisis episodes may be reduced. Care focuses on teaching the patient and family how to prevent crises and complications (Chart 42-3). The patient with sickle cell disease may receive care in different settings, including acute care, subacute care, extended or assistive care, and home care.

Chart 42-3 PATIENT AND FAMILY EDUCATION GUIDE
Prevention of Sickle Cell Crisis

- Drink at least 3 to 4 liters of liquids every day.
- Avoid alcoholic beverages.
- Avoid smoking cigarettes or using tobacco in any form.
- Contact your health care provider at the first sign of illness or infection.
- Be sure to get a "flu shot" every year.
- Ask your health care provider about taking the pneumonia vaccine.
- Avoid temperature extremes of hot or cold.
- Be sure to wear socks and gloves when going outside on cold days.
- Avoid planes with unpressurized passenger cabins.
- Avoid travel to high altitudes (e.g., cities like Denver and Santa Fe).
- Ensure that any health care professional who takes care of you knows you have sickle cell disease, especially the anesthesia provider and radiologist.
- Consider genetic counseling and screening.
- Avoid strenuous physical activities.
- Engage in mild, low-impact exercise at least three times a week when you are not in crisis.

Teach the patient to avoid specific activities that lead to hypoxia and hypoxemia. Stress the recognition of the early symptoms of crisis so that interventions can be started early to prevent pain, complications, and permanent tissue damage. He or she is often given opioid analgesics for self-management of sickle cell crises at home. Teach the patient and family about the correct use of these drugs. In addition, counsel patients about the hereditary aspects of sickle cell disease and provide information about prenatal diagnosis, birth control methods, and pregnancy options.

WOMEN'S HEALTH CONSIDERATIONS

Pregnancy in women with sickle cell disease may be life threatening. Patients who have damage to vital organs are advised against becoming pregnant. Usually, barrier methods of contraception (cervical cap, diaphragm, or condoms with or without spermicides) are recommended for women with sickle cell disease. The use of oral contraceptives (OCs) is controversial, because OCs may increase clot formation, especially among smokers, predisposing them to crises. The risks versus benefits of OCs must be examined for each patient.

Glucose-6-Phosphate Dehydrogenase Deficiency Anemia

Pathophysiology

Many forms of **hemolytic** (blood cell–destroying) anemia are present from birth as a result of defects or deficiencies of one or more enzymes in red blood cells (RBCs). More than 200 such disorders are known. Most of these enzymes are needed to complete some critical step in RBC energy production. The most common type of inherited hemolytic anemia is the deficiency of the enzyme *glucose-6-phosphate dehydrogenase (G6PD).* This disease is inherited as an X-linked recessive disorder and affects about 10% of all African Americans (McCance & Huether, 2006).

G6PD stimulates reactions in glucose metabolism. Because RBCs contain no **mitochondria** (sites of production of adenosine triphosphate [ATP]), metabolism of glucose is needed to generate energy in these cells. Newly produced RBCs from patients with G6PD deficiency have sufficient levels of G6PD. However, as the cells age, the level decreases rapidly. Cells with reduced amounts of G6PD break more easily during exposure to some drugs (e.g., sulfonamides, aspirin, quinine derivatives, chloramphenicol, dapsone, high doses of vitamin C, and thiazide diuretics) and exposure to benzene and other toxins.

The patient usually does not have symptoms until exposed to these agents or until a severe infection develops. After exposure to any of these agents, patients have acute breakage of RBCs lasting from 7 to 12 days. During this acute phase, anemia and jaundice develop. The hemolytic reaction is limited because only older RBCs, containing less G6PD, are destroyed.

Patient-Centered Collaborative Care

It is critical that the drug or toxin responsible for the hemolytic reaction be identified and totally removed. Donated blood is screened for this deficiency before transfusion because cells deficient in G6PD can be hazardous for the recipient.

Hydration is important during an episode of hemolysis to prevent debris and hemoglobin from collecting in the kidney tubules, which can lead to acute renal failure. Osmotic diuretics, such as mannitol (Osmitrol), may help prevent this complication. Transfusions are needed when anemia is present and kidney function is normal (see the Transfusion Therapy section beginning on p. 917).

Immunohemolytic Anemia

The most common types of hemolytic anemias in North America are the immunohemolytic anemias, also referred to as *autoimmune hemolytic anemias* (McCance & Huether, 2006). Acquired hemolytic syndromes result from increased RBC destruction occurring in response to trauma, malarial infection, exposure to certain chemicals or drugs, and autoimmune reactions. All increase the rate of RBC destruction by causing membrane **lysis** (breakage).

In immunohemolytic anemia, immune system products (e.g., antibodies) attack a person's own RBCs for unknown reasons. Some hemolytic anemias occur with other autoimmune disorders (e.g., systemic lupus erythematosus). Regardless of the cause, RBCs are viewed as non-self by the immune system and then are attacked and destroyed.

The two types of immunohemolytic anemia are warm antibody anemia and cold antibody anemia. **Warm antibody anemia** occurs with immunoglobulin G (IgG) antibody excess. These antibodies are most active at 98.6° F (37° C) and may be triggered by drugs, chemicals, or other autoimmune problems. **Cold antibody anemia** has complement protein fixation on immunoglobulin M (IgM) and occurs most at 86° F (30° C). This problem often occurs with a Raynaud's-like response in which the arteries in the hands and feet constrict profoundly in response to cold temperatures or stress.

Management depends on symptom severity. Steroid therapy to suppress immune function is the first line of treatment and is temporarily effective in most patients. Splenectomy and more intense immunosuppressive therapy with cyclophosphamide (Cytoxan, Procytox♣) and azathioprine (Imuran) may be used if steroid therapy fails. Plasma exchange therapy to remove attacking antibodies is effective for patients who do not respond to immunosuppressive therapy.

ANEMIAS RESULTING FROM DECREASED PRODUCTION OF RED BLOOD CELLS

Anemias caused by decreased RBC production occur in response to many problems. Some are caused by failure of the bone marrow to produce healthy RBCs. Anemias also are caused by failure of the body to make or absorb a substance needed for RBC production.

CONSIDERATIONS FOR OLDER ADULTS

Older patients often have restricted diets and may be unable to eat meat because of tooth loss or economic reasons and thus are at risk for iron deficiency anemia. Ask about a family history of anemia. B_{12} deficiency anemia often occurs in patients 50 to 80 years of age and may result from an inherited genetic mutation.

Iron Deficiency Anemia

Adults usually have between 2 and 6 g of iron, depending on the size of the person and the amount of hemoglobin in the cells. About two thirds of this iron is contained in hemoglobin. The other one third is stored in the bone marrow, spleen, liver, and muscle. With iron deficiency, the iron stores are depleted first, followed by the hemoglobin stores. As a result, RBCs are small **(microcytic)** and the patient has mild symptoms of anemia, including weakness and pallor. In iron deficiency anemia, serum ferritin values are less than 10 ng/mL (normal range is 12 to 300 ng/mL).

Iron deficiency anemia is common and can result from blood loss, poor GI absorption of iron, and an inadequate diet. The problem is a decreased iron supply for the developing RBC. Iron deficiency anemia is most common in women, older adults, and people with poor diets.

Any adult with iron deficiency should be evaluated for abnormal bleeding, especially from the GI tract. The management of iron deficiency anemia involves increasing the oral intake of iron from food sources (e.g., red meat, organ meat, egg yolks, kidney beans, leafy green vegetables, and raisins). An adequate diet supplies about 10 to 15 mg of iron per day. However, only 5% to 10% of dietary iron is absorbed. This amount is enough to meet the needs of men and of women after childbearing age but is not sufficient to supply the greater needs of menstruating women. If iron losses are mild, oral iron supplements, such as ferrous sulfate, are started. This treatment should cause the hemoglobin level to rise about 2 g/dL in 4 weeks. Treatment continues until the hemoglobin level returns to normal. Instruct patients to take the iron supplement between meals for better absorption and to reduce GI distress. When iron deficiency anemia is severe, iron solutions can be given IM. These solutions must be given using the Z-track best practice method outlined in Chart 42-4.

Chart 42-4 BEST PRACTICE FOR PATIENT SAFETY & QUALITY CARE

Administering Intramuscular Medications by the Z-Track Method

- Draw the drug up into the syringe using aseptic technique.
- Add 0.25 mL of air to the syringe.
- Discard the needle used to draw up the drugs.
- Place a new needle (22-gauge, 2 to 3 inches long) on the syringe.
- Make certain that the injection site is in bright light.
- *Select the dorsal gluteal site ONLY if injecting iron dextran. The ventrogluteal site is recommended for all other IM injections.*
- Identify appropriate landmarks for administration into the upper, outer quadrant.
- Once the site is selected, pull the skin and subcutaneous tissues sideways away from the muscle.
- Clean the site while holding the skin and subcutaneous tissues off to the side.
- Insert the needle deeply into the muscle tissue.
- Aspirate to determine needle placement.
- Iron dextran is black; look very closely to determine whether blood is being aspirated into the syringe.
- If blood is aspirated, withdraw the needle and begin the procedure again from the first step.
- If no blood is aspirated, inject the drug slowly, followed by injection of the air bubble.
- Quickly withdraw the needle.
- Release the skin and subcutaneous tissue.
- *Do not massage the injection site.*

Vitamin B_{12} Deficiency Anemia

Production of RBCs depends on adequate **DNA** synthesis in the precursor cells so that cell division and growth into functional RBCs can occur. All cell division requires adequate amounts of folic acid to make DNA. One function of vitamin B_{12} is to activate the enzymes that move folic acid into the cell where DNA synthesis occurs. Vitamin B_{12} deficiency causes anemia by inhibiting folic acid transport and reducing DNA synthesis in precursor cells. These precursor cells then undergo improper DNA synthesis and increase in size. Only a few are released from the bone marrow. This type of anemia is called *megaloblastic* or **macrocytic anemia** because of the large size of these abnormal cells.

Vitamin B_{12} deficiency results from poor intake of foods containing vitamin B_{12}. This can occur with vegetarian diets or diets lacking dairy products. Problems such as small bowel resection, diverticula, tapeworm, or overgrowth of intestinal bacteria can lead to poor absorption of vitamin B_{12}. Anemia resulting from failure to absorb vitamin B_{12} **(pernicious anemia)** is caused by a deficiency of **intrinsic factor** (a substance normally secreted by the gastric mucosa), which is needed for intestinal absorption of vitamin B_{12}.

Vitamin B_{12} deficiency anemia may be mild or severe, usually develops slowly, and produces few symptoms. Patients usually have pallor and jaundice, as well as **glossitis** (a smooth, beefy-red tongue), fatigue, and weight loss. Because vitamin B_{12} is needed for normal nerve function, patients with pernicious anemia may also have **paresthesias** (abnormal sensations) in the feet and hands and poor balance.

When anemia is caused by a dietary deficiency, the aim of management is to increase the intake of foods rich in vitamin B_{12} (animal proteins, eggs, nuts, dairy products, dried beans, citrus fruit, leafy green vegetables). Vitamin supplements may be prescribed when anemia is severe. Vitamin B_{12} and folic acid levels are monitored. Patients who may have pernicious anemia are tested using the Shilling test, which measures the presence of vitamin B_{12} in the urine after the patient is given an oral dose of radioactive vitamin B_{12}. If the patient does not absorb the radioactive vitamin B_{12} because of pernicious anemia, it cannot get into the urine. Patients who have pernicious anemia are given vitamin B_{12} injections weekly at first and then monthly for the rest of their lives. A new drug, cyanocobalamin (CaloMist), that delivers vitamin B_{12} by nasal spray has just been approved to maintain vitamin levels after the patient's deficiency has first been treated by the traditional injection method.

Folic Acid Deficiency Anemia

Folic acid deficiency can also cause anemia. Manifestations are similar to those of vitamin B_{12} deficiency, but nervous system functions remain normal because folic acid deficiency does not affect nerve function. The absence of neurologic problems helps distinguish folic acid deficiency from vitamin B_{12} deficiency. The disease develops slowly, and symptoms may be attributed to other problems or diseases.

Three common causes of folic acid deficiency are poor nutrition, malabsorption, and drugs. Poor nutrition, especially a diet lacking green leafy vegetables, liver, yeast, citrus fruits, dried beans, and nuts, is the most common cause. Malabsorption syndromes, such as Crohn's disease, are the second most common cause. Chronic alcohol abuse with malnutrition is another cause. Anticonvulsants and oral contraceptives can slow or prevent the absorption and conversion of folic acid to its active form, leading to folic acid deficiency and anemia.

Prevention is aimed at identifying high-risk patients, such as older, debilitated patients with alcoholism; patients at risk for malnutrition; and those with increased folic acid requirements. A diet rich in foods containing folic acid and vitamin B_{12} prevents a deficiency. By assessing dietary habits for all patients, you can determine which patients are at risk for diet-induced anemias. This type of anemia is treated with scheduled folic acid replacement therapy.

Aplastic Anemia

Pathophysiology

Aplastic anemia is a deficiency of circulating red blood cells (RBCs) because of failure of the bone marrow to produce these cells. It is caused by an injury to the immature precursor cell for red blood cells, known as the **pluripotent stem cell.** Although aplastic anemia sometimes occurs alone, it usually occurs with **leukopenia** (a reduction in white blood cells [WBCs]) and **thrombocytopenia** (a reduction in platelets). These three problems occur together because the damaged bone marrow loses the ability to produce any of these cells. **Pancytopenia** (a deficiency of all three cell types) is common in aplastic anemia. Disease onset may be slow or rapid.

The most common type of the disease is acquired aplastic anemia. It can be caused by long-term exposure to toxic agents and drugs (see Table 41-3 in Chapter 41), ionizing radiation, or infection. In about 50% of cases, the cause of aplastic anemia is unknown. The disease may follow viral infection, but it is not known exactly how the bone marrow is damaged. People with Fanconi's anemia may also have hereditary aplastic anemia.

Patient-Centered Collaborative Care

Assess for symptoms of bone marrow failure and poor *oxygenation* such as weakness, pallor, and petechiae or ecchymosis. A complete blood count (CBC) shows severe macrocytic anemia, leukopenia and thrombocytopenia. A bone marrow biopsy may show replacement of marrow-forming cells with fat.

Blood transfusions are the mainstay of management for patients with aplastic anemia. Transfusion is used only when the anemia causes disability or when bleeding is life threatening because of low platelet counts. Unnecessary transfusion increases the chances for developing immune reactions to platelets and shortens the life span of the transfused cell. This therapy is discontinued as soon as the bone marrow begins to produce RBCs.

Immunosuppressive therapy helps patients who have the types of aplastic anemia with a disease course similar to that of autoimmune problems. Drugs such as prednisone, antithymocyte globulin (ATG), and cyclosporine (Sandimmune) have brought about partial or complete remissions. In more severe cases, chemotherapy drugs such as cyclophosphamide (Cytoxan, Procytox♣) have been shown to be effective.

Splenectomy (removal of the spleen) may be needed for patients with an enlarged spleen that is either destroying normal RBCs or suppressing their development. Hematopoietic stem cell transplantation replaces defective stem cells and can cure the disorder (Afable & Lyon, 2008). Cost, availability, and complications limit this treatment of aplastic anemia.

POLYCYTHEMIA

In polycythemia, the number of red blood cells (RBCs) in the blood is *greater* than normal. The blood of a patient with polycythemia is **hyperviscous** (thicker than normal blood). The problem may be temporary (occurring as a result of other conditions) or chronic. One type of polycythemia, polycythemia vera (PV), is fatal if left untreated.

POLYCYTHEMIA VERA

Pathophysiology

Polycythemia vera (PV) is a disease with a sustained increase in blood hemoglobin levels to 18 g/dL, an RBC count of 6 million/mm^3, or a hematocrit of 55% or greater. PV is a cancer of the RBCs with three major hallmarks: massive production of RBCs, excessive leukocyte production, and excessive production of platelets. Extreme **hypercellularity** (cell excess) of the peripheral blood occurs in people with PV.

The patient's facial skin and mucous membranes have a dark, flushed **(plethoric)** appearance. These areas appear purplish or cyanotic because the blood in these tissues is poorly oxygenated. Most patients have intense itching caused by dilated blood vessels and poor *tissue oxygenation*. Blood viscosity is increased, resulting in hypertension. Superficial veins are visibly distended. The thick blood moves more slowly through all tissues and places increased demands on the heart, resulting in hypertension. In some highly vascular areas, blood flow may become so slow that stasis occurs. Vascular stasis causes **thrombosis** (clot formation) within the smaller vessels, occluding blood vessels. The blood vessel occlusion leads to tissue hypoxia, anoxia and, later, to infarction and necrosis. Tissues most at risk for this problem are the heart, spleen, and kidneys, although infarction and damage can occur in any organ or tissue.

Because the actual number of cells in the blood is greatly increased and the cells are not completely normal, cell life spans are shorter. The shorter life spans and increased cell production cause a rapid turnover of circulating blood cells. This rapid turnover increases the amount of cell debris (released when cells die) in the blood, adding to the general "sludging" of the blood. This debris includes uric acid and potassium, which cause the symptoms of gout and **hyperkalemia** (elevated serum potassium level).

Other manifestations of PV are related to abnormal RBCs. Even though the number of RBCs is greatly increased, their oxygen-carrying capacity is impaired, and patients have poor *oxygenation* with severe hypoxia. Patients with PV also have bleeding problems because of platelet impairment.

Patient-Centered Collaborative Care

Polycythemia vera is a malignant disease that progresses in severity over time. If left untreated, few people with PV live longer than 2 years after diagnosis. With treatment by repeated phlebotomies (two to five times per week), the patient may live 10 to 15 years or longer. (**Phlebotomy** is the blood drawing with removal of the patient's RBCs to decrease the number of RBCs and reduce blood viscosity.) Increasing hydration and promoting venous return help prevent clot formation. Therapy aims to prevent clot formation and includes the use of anticoagulants. Chart 42-5 lists health tips for patients with PV.

As the disease progresses, drug therapy is used to control it, although aggressive IV chemotherapy is no longer recommended because of its increased risk for inducing leukemia. Aspirin therapy may be used to decrease clot formation. However, the benefits must be weighed against the increased risk for GI bleeding associated with this therapy. Hydroxyurea, an oral chemotherapy drug, may be prescribed for severe manifestations of the disease.

Chart 42-5 PATIENT AND FAMILY EDUCATION GUIDE

Polycythemia Vera

- Drink at least 3 liters of liquids each day.
- Avoid tight or constrictive clothing, especially garters or girdles.
- Wear gloves when outdoors in temperatures lower than 50° F (10° C).
- Keep all health care–related appointments.
- Contact your physician at the first sign of infection.
- Take anticoagulants as prescribed.
- Wear support hose or stockings while you are awake and up.
- Elevate your feet whenever you are seated.
- Exercise slowly and only on the advice of your physician.
- Stop activity at the first sign of chest pain.
- Use an electric shaver.
- Use a soft-bristled toothbrush to brush your teeth.
- Do not floss between your teeth.

MYELODYSPLASTIC SYNDROMES

Pathophysiology

Myelodysplastic syndromes (MDSs) are a group of disorders caused by the formation of abnormal cells in the bone marrow. These abnormal cells are usually destroyed shortly after they are released into the blood. As a result, patients with MDS have a decrease in all blood cell lines. Anemia is the most common problem, occurring in 90% of patients with MDS, although **neutropenia** (low white blood cell [WBC] count) and **thrombocytopenia** (low platelet count) are also often present.

MDS can occur at any age. However, the disease is most common in people age 60 years or older. Although not officially a type of cancer, MDS has cancer-like features and is considered to be a *precancerous* state. Like cancer, MDS arises from a single population of abnormal cells. About 30% of all patients with MDS do eventually develop acute leukemia. There are many sub-types of MDS, and problems can range from unresponsive anemia to **cytopenia** (low blood cell counts) with increased numbers of blast cells (immature WBC cells).

The exact cause of MDS is not clear. Risk factors include normal physiologic changes associated with aging, chemical exposures (pesticides, benzene), tobacco smoke, and exposure to radiation or chemotherapy drugs. Diagnosis is made by examination of the chromosomes and the genes within the chromosomes (cytogenetic testing) of the bone marrow cells. Peripheral blood smears are used to assess the level of cell maturation and the proportion of abnormal cells.

Patient-Centered Collaborative Care

Treatment for MDS focuses on symptom management and supportive care. Supportive care of the patient with MDS includes blood transfusions for anemia and platelet transfusions for severe thrombocytopenia. Erythropoietin may be given in addition to transfusions. The use of frequent transfusions may result in iron overload and organ damage (Kurtin, 2006). Chelation therapy may be needed to reduce the iron overload before damage to the liver and heart occurs. **Chelation** is the chemical binding of iron and its removal from the body. This therapy is indicated for patients who receive more than 20 units of red blood cell transfusions or for those whose serum ferritin levels are greater than 2500 mcg/L. Drugs used for management of iron overload include deferasirox (Exjade) and deferoxamine mesylate (Desferal, Desferrioxamine).

WHITE BLOOD CELL DISORDERS

As discussed in Chapter 19, white blood cells (WBCs), or **leukocytes,** provide protection from infection and cancer development. This protection depends on maintaining normal numbers and ratios of the different mature, circulating WBCs. When any one type of WBC is present in either abnormally high or abnormally low amounts, immune function is altered to some degree, as are oxygen transport and blood clotting, placing patients at risk for many complications. This section covers the changes and nursing care for patients with disorders involving overgrowth of specific types of WBCs. (See Chapter 21 for the problems and care needs for patients with immune deficiency.)

LEUKEMIA

Pathophysiology

Leukemia is a type of cancer with uncontrolled production of immature WBCs (usually blast cells) in the bone marrow. As a result, the bone marrow becomes overcrowded with immature, nonfunctional cells and production of normal blood cells is greatly decreased. Leukemia may be **acute,** with a sudden onset and short duration, or **chronic,** with a slow onset and symptoms that persist for years.

Leukemias are classified by cell type. Leukemic cells coming from the lymphoid pathways (see Fig. 19-3 in Chapter 19) are typed as **lymphocytic** or **lymphoblastic.** Leukemias in which the abnormal cells come from the myeloid pathways are typed as **myelocytic** or **myelogenous.** Several subtypes exist for each of these diseases, which are classified according to the degree of maturity of the abnormal cell and the specific cell type involved. Biphenotypic leukemia is acute leukemia that shows both lymphocytic and myelocytic features.

With leukemia, cancer occurs in the stem cells or early precursor leukocyte cells, causing excessive growth of a specific type of immature leukocyte. These cells are abnormal, and their excessive production in the bone marrow stops normal bone marrow production of RBCs, platelets, and mature leukocytes. Anemia, thrombocytopenia, and leukopenia result. Often the number of immature, abnormal WBCs in the blood is greatly elevated, and these cells cannot provide infection protection. Leukemic cells can also be found in the spleen, liver, lymph nodes, and central nervous system. Without treatment, the patient will die of infection or hemorrhage. For patients with acute leukemia, these changes occur rapidly and, without intervention, progress to death. Chronic leukemia may be present for years before changes appear.

Etiology and Genetic Risk

The exact cause of leukemia is unknown, although many genetic and environmental factors are involved in its development. The basic problem involves damage to genes controlling cell growth. This damage then changes cells from a normal to a **malignant** (cancer) state. Analysis of the bone marrow of a patient with acute leukemia shows abnormal chromosomes about 50% of the time (McCance & Huether, 2006). Possible risk factors for the development of leukemia include ionizing radiation, exposure to chemicals and drugs, bone marrow **hypoplasia** (reduced production of blood cells), genetic factors, immunologic factors, environmental factors, and the interaction of these factors.

Ionizing radiation exposures such as radiation therapy for cancer treatment or heavy radiation exposure (e.g., the atomic bomb at Hiroshima or the nuclear accident at Chernobyl) increase the risk for leukemia development, particularly acute myelogenous leukemia (AML).

Chemicals and drugs have been linked to leukemia development because of their ability to damage DNA. Previous treatment for cancer that included melphalan, doxorubicin, etoposide, and cyclophosphamide poses risks for leukemia development about 5 to 8 years after treatment. Table 41-3 in Chapter 41 lists chemicals and drugs that damage the hematologic system.

Bone marrow hypoplasia can increase leukemia risk by reducing or changing the rate of bone marrow cell production. Disorders that have marrow hypoplasia and may lead to leukemia development include Fanconi's anemia and myelodysplastic syndromes.

Genetic factors influence leukemia development. There is an increased incidence of the disease among patients with hereditary conditions such as Down syndrome, Bloom syndrome, Klinefelter syndrome, and Fanconi's anemia. Identical siblings of patients with leukemia have a higher incidence of leukemia than does the general population.

Immunologic factors, especially immune deficiencies, may promote the development of leukemia. Leukemia related to immune deficiency may be a result of immune surveillance failure, or the same mechanisms that cause the immune deficiency may also trigger cancer in the WBCs.

Interaction of many host and environmental factors may result in leukemia. Because each person tolerates the interaction of these factors differently, it is difficult to determine the origin of any specific leukemia.

Incidence/Prevalence

Leukemia accounts for 2% of all new cases of cancer and 4% of all deaths from cancer (American Cancer Society, 2008). The incidence depends on many factors, including the type of WBC affected, age, gender, race, and geographic locale.

In the United States, about 44,000 new cases of leukemia occur each year (American Cancer Society, 2008). Leukemia is classified into any one of four types based on the cell type affected and how fast the disease progresses:

- *Acute myelogenous leukemia (AML)* is the most common form of adult-onset leukemia. *Acute promyelocytic leukemia (APL)* is a subtype of AML that makes up about 10% of adult-onset AML.
- *Acute lymphocytic leukemia (ALL)* makes up about 10% of adult-onset leukemias but is most common in children. In adults with ALL, the Philadelphia chromosome, usually the hallmark of chronic myelogenous leukemia, is a common chromosome abnormality.
- *Chronic myelogenous leukemia (CML)* makes up about 20% of adult-onset leukemias, occurring more often in people older than 50 years. A major feature of CML is the

presence of the Philadelphia chromosome abnormality in the leukemic cells. CML has three phases (Rogers, 2005):
- The chronic phase is often a slowly progressing (indolent) course during which the patient may have mild symptoms and respond to standard treatments. The bone marrow usually shows less than 10% blast cells at this time.
- The accelerated phase features spleen enlargement and progressive manifestation, such as intermittent fevers, night sweats, and unexplained weight loss. The patient usually does not respond to standard treatment, and the bone marrow may contain 10% to 30% blast cells and promyelocytes. This phase typically lasts 6 to 12 months.
- The blast phase indicates a transformation to a very aggressive acute leukemia. The bone marrow contains more than 30% blast cells. The promyelocytes and blast cells commonly spread to other tissues and organs.

- *Chronic lymphocytic leukemia (CLL)* is a rare type of leukemia that occurs most often in people older than 50 years and appears to have a hereditary component. Average survival time ranges from less than 19 months for patients diagnosed with advanced disease to more than 10 years for patients diagnosed with early-stage disease.

Patient-Centered Collaborative Care

evolve ONLINE PHARM REVIEW

Assessment

History

Ask the patient about exposure to risk factors and related genetic factors. Age is important because the risk for adult-onset leukemia increases with age. Occupation and hobbies may also reveal exposure to agents that increase the risk for leukemia. Previous illnesses and the medical history may reveal exposure to ionizing radiation or drugs that increase risk.

Changes in immune function increase the risk for infection in the patient with leukemia. Even when his or her blood may show a normal level of WBCs or even a high level, these cells are immature and cannot protect him or her from infection. Ask about the frequency and severity of infections, such as colds, influenza, pneumonia, bronchitis, or unexplained fevers, during the past 6 months.

Platelet function is reduced with leukemia. Ask about any excessive bleeding episodes, such as:
- A tendency to bruise easily
- Nosebleeds
- Increased menstrual flow
- Bleeding from the gums
- Rectal bleeding
- Hematuria (blood in the urine)
- Prolonged bleeding after minor abrasions or cuts

If the patient has experienced such an episode, ask whether this type and extent of bleeding is his or her usual response to injury or represents a change.

The patient with leukemia often has weakness and fatigue from anemia and from the increased metabolism of the leukemic cells. Ask whether any of these have occurred:
- Headaches
- Behavior changes
- Increased somnolence
- Decreased alertness
- Decreased attention span
- Lethargy, muscle weakness
- Loss of appetite
- Weight loss
- Increased fatigue

Listing activities in the previous 24 hours may reveal information about activity intolerance, changes in behavior, and unexplained fatigue. Determine how long the patient has had any of these debilitating symptoms.

Physical Assessment/Clinical Manifestations

Leukemia affects all blood cells, and blood influences the health and function of all organs and systems. Thus many body areas and systems cells may be affected (Chart 42-6). The following manifestations occur with acute leukemia. Some of these findings may be present also in the patient with chronic leukemia in the blast phase.

Cardiovascular changes are usually related to the adjustments the heart needs to make when *tissue perfusion* with oxygen is reduced because of anemia. The heart rate is increased, and blood pressure is decreased. **Murmurs** (abnormal blood flow sounds through the heart) and **bruits** (abnormal blood flow sounds heard over arteries) may be heard. Capillary refill is slow.

Respiratory changes are related to reduced *tissue oxygenation* from anemia and to infection. Respiratory rate increases as anemia becomes more severe. If respiratory infections are present, the patient may have coughing and shortness of breath. Abnormal breath sounds are heard on auscultation.

Skin changes include pallor and coolness to the touch as a result of reduced *tissue perfusion* related to anemia. Pallor is most evident on the face, around the mouth, and in the nail beds. The conjunctiva of the eye also is pale, as are the creases on the palm of the hand (most evident when the skin over the palm of the hand is stretched). **Petechiae** (raised red spots)

Chart 42-6 KEY FEATURES

Acute Leukemia

INTEGUMENTARY MANIFESTATIONS
- Ecchymoses
- Petechiae
- Open infected lesions
- Pallor of the conjunctiva, nail beds, palmar creases, and around the mouth

GASTROINTESTINAL MANIFESTATIONS
- Bleeding gums
- Anorexia
- Weight loss
- Enlarged liver and spleen

RENAL MANIFESTATIONS
- Hematuria

CARDIOVASCULAR MANIFESTATIONS
- Tachycardia at basal activity levels
- Orthostatic hypotension
- Palpitations

RESPIRATORY MANIFESTATIONS
- Dyspnea on exertion

NEUROLOGIC MANIFESTATIONS
- Fatigue
- Headache
- Fever

MUSCULOSKELETAL MANIFESTATIONS
- Bone pain
- Joint swelling and pain

may be present on any area of skin surface, especially the legs and feet. The petechiae may be unrelated to any obvious trauma. Inspect for skin infections or injured areas that have failed to heal. Inspect the mouth for gum bleeding and any sore or lesion that may indicate infection.

Intestinal changes may be related to an increased bleeding tendency and to fatigue. Weight loss, nausea, and anorexia are common. Examine the rectal area for fissures, and test the stool for occult blood. Many patients with leukemia have reduced bowel sounds and are constipated. Enlargement of the liver and spleen and abdominal tenderness also may be present from leukemic cells invading abdominal organs.

Central nervous system (CNS) changes include cranial nerve disturbances, headache, and papilledema from leukemic invasion of the CNS. With advanced disease, seizures and coma may occur.

Miscellaneous changes can include bone and joint tenderness as the marrow is damaged and the bone resorbs. Leukemic cells invade lymph nodes, causing enlargement.

Psychosocial Assessment

The patient with newly diagnosed leukemia is very anxious and fearful of the disease outcome. Current therapies have greatly improved the prognoses of leukemia. Spend time with the patient and family to assess what the diagnosis means to them and what they expect in the future. Without knowing the patient's expectations and feelings, you cannot teach him or her and provide individualized support.

A diagnosis of leukemia has serious consequences for a person's lifestyle. Hospitalization for initial treatment often lasts weeks and may result in boredom, loneliness, isolation, and financial stress. Assess coping patterns, including activities that the patient finds enjoyable and methods that help the patient relax. After initial therapy, the patient may be able to resume work, depending on his or her occupation. Often the patient must make adjustments for changes in functional status. Often he or she is hospitalized repeatedly for complications.

Laboratory Assessment

The patient with acute leukemia usually has decreased hemoglobin and hematocrit levels, a low platelet count, and an abnormal white blood cell (WBC) count. The WBC count may be low, normal, or elevated. The patient with a high WBC count at diagnosis has a poorer prognosis.

The definitive test for leukemia is an examination of cells obtained from bone marrow aspiration and biopsy. The bone marrow is full of leukemic **blast phase cells** (immature cells that are dividing). The proteins **(antigens)** on the surfaces of the leukemic cells help diagnose the type of leukemia. These proteins are "markers" of certain types of leukemia or may indicate prognosis. Such markers include the T11 protein, terminal deoxynucleotidyl transferase (TDT), the common acute lymphoblastic leukemia antigen (CALLA), and the CD33 antigen.

Blood clotting times and factors are usually abnormal with acute leukemia. Reduced levels of fibrinogen and other clotting factors are common. Whole-blood clotting time (Lee-White clotting test) is increased, as is the activated partial thromboplastin time (aPTT).

Chromosome analysis (cytogenetic studies) of the leukemic cells may identify marker chromosomes to help diagnose the type of leukemia, predict the prognosis, and determine therapy effectiveness. An example is the Philadelphia chromosome, which is important in the diagnosis and treatment of chronic myelogenous leukemia (CML).

Imaging Assessment

Specific manifestations determine the need for specific tests. For example, in a patient with dyspnea, a chest x-ray is needed to determine whether leukemic infiltrates are present in the lung. Skeletal x-rays may help determine whether bone **resorption** (loss of bone minerals and density) is present.

DECISION-MAKING CHALLENGE
Delegation/Supervision

The patient is a 56-year-old woman who has been recently diagnosed with AML. Her past medical history includes breast cancer at 42 years of age, for which she was treated with lumpectomy, chemotherapy, and radiation. She also has hypertension. She is admitted to your unit to begin induction chemotherapy.

1. What risk factors would predispose this patient to development of AML?
2. What are some of the physical findings you would expect to see when examining her?
3. What abnormalities would you expect when reviewing her laboratory tests and bone marrow biopsy?
4. What routine vital signs and assessments could be delegated to an LPN/LVN and to UAP? Provide rationales for your choices.

evolve For suggested answer guidelines, go to http://evolve.elsevier.com/Iggy/.

Analysis

Common Nursing Diagnosis and Collaborative Problems

Priority nursing diagnoses for adult patients with acute myelogenous leukemia (AML), the most common type of adult leukemia, are:

1. Risk for Infection related to decreased immune response
2. Risk for Injury related to thrombocytopenia
3. Fatigue related to decreased tissue oxygenation and increased energy demands

The primary collaborative problem is Potential for Antineoplastic Therapy Adverse Effects.

Additional Nursing Diagnosis and Collaborative Problems

In addition to the common nursing diagnoses and collaborative problems, patients with AML may have one or more of these:

- Impaired Skin Integrity related to prolonged immobility
- Impaired Oral Mucous Membrane related to effects of chemotherapy and pancytopenia
- Self-Care Deficit (Total) related to progressive debilitation and weakness
- Imbalanced Nutrition: Less Than Body Requirements related to anorexia, nausea, and vomiting
- Death Anxiety related to uncertainty of prognosis
- Powerlessness related to an inability to control disease progression
- Interrupted Family Processes related to acute, life-threatening illness of a family member
- Ineffective Role Performance related to perceived inability to fulfill parental and other family roles and prolonged hospitalization
- Deficient Diversional Activity related to prolonged hospitalization

Planning and Implementation

Risk for Infection

NOC **Planning: Expected Outcomes.** The patient with leukemia is expected to remain free from infection. Indicators include:

- Absence of fever and foul-smelling or purulent drainage
- Absence of cough, chest pain, and dyspnea
- Absence of urinary frequency, urgency, or pain and burning

Interventions. *Infection is a major cause of death in the patient with leukemia* because the white blood cells are immature and cannot function, and sepsis is a common complication. Infection occurs through both **autocontamination** (normal flora overgrows and penetrates the internal environment) and **cross-contamination** (organisms from another person or the environment are transmitted to the patient). The three most common sites of infection are the skin, respiratory tract, and intestinal tract.

Gram-negative bacteria are the most common cause of infection, although other infections do occur. Interventions aim to halt infection and control infections early. Chart 42-7 lists areas to assess for the patient at risk for infection.

Drug Therapy for Acute Leukemia. Drug therapy for patients with AML is divided into three distinctive phases: induction, consolidation, and maintenance.

Induction therapy is intense and consists of combination chemotherapy started at the time of diagnosis. The goal of this therapy is to achieve a rapid, complete remission of all manifestations of disease. Agencies and physicians differ in drugs used and the treatment schedule. A commonly prescribed course of aggressive chemotherapy includes continuous IV cytosine arabinoside for 7 days together with a brief infusion of daunorubicin for the first 3 days, sometimes referred to as a "7 plus 3" regimen. A side effect of this therapy is severe bone marrow suppression, making the patient even more at risk for infection than before the treatment started.

Prolonged hospitalizations are common while the patient is immunosuppressed. Recovery of bone marrow function requires at least 2 to 3 weeks, during which time the patient must be protected from life-threatening infections. Other side effects include nausea, vomiting, diarrhea, **alopecia** (hair loss), **stomatitis** (mouth sores), kidney toxicity, liver toxicity, and cardiac toxicity. (See Chapter 24 for information on effects of anticancer agents.) Older patients have a greater infection-related death rate during this phase than do younger patients.

Consolidation therapy often consists of another course of either the same drugs used for induction at a different dosage or a different combination of chemotherapy drugs. This treatment occurs early in remission, and its intent is to cure. Consolidation therapy may be either a single course of chemotherapy or repeated courses.

Maintenance therapy may be prescribed for months to years after successful induction and consolidation therapies. It is used for patients with acute lymphocytic leukemia (ALL) and acute promyelocytic leukemia (APL). The purpose is to maintain the remission achieved through induction and consolidation. Maintenance drugs for ALL are milder and are often given orally for 2 to 5 years. Not all types of leukemia respond to maintenance therapy.

Drug Therapy for Chronic Leukemia. Imatinib mesylate (Gleevec) is the main treatment for CML that is Philadelphia

Chart 42-7 FOCUSED ASSESSMENT

Hospitalized or Home Care Patients with Potential or Actual Risk for Infection

GENERAL CONDITION

- Age
- History of allergies
- History of chemotherapy, radiation therapy, or other immunosuppressive therapies, such as steroid use
- Chronic diseases
- History of febrile neutropenia and associated symptoms
- Nutritional status
- Functional status—problems with immobility
- Tobacco use—cigarettes, pipe, cigars, oral
- Recreational drug use
- Alcohol use
- Prescribed and over-the-counter drug use
- Baseline and ongoing vital signs—blood pressure, heart rate, respiratory rate, and temperature

SKIN AND MUCOUS MEMBRANES

- Thorough inspection of all skin surfaces with special attention to axilla, perineum (particularly the anorectal area), and under breasts; inspection of skin for color, vascularity, bleeding, lesions, edema, moist areas, excoriation, irritation, erythema; general condition of hair and nails, pressure areas, swelling, pain, tenderness, biopsy or surgical sites, wounds, enlarged lymph nodes, catheters, or other devices
- Inspection of oral cavity, including lips, tongue, mucous membranes, gingiva, teeth, and throat—color, moisture, bleeding, ulcerations, lesions, exudate, mucositis, stomatitis, plaque, swelling, pain, tenderness, taste changes, amount and character of saliva, ability to swallow, changes in voice, dental caries, patient's oral hygiene routine
- History of current skin disorders or problems with mucous membranes

HEAD, EYES, EARS, NOSE

- Pain, tenderness, exudate, crusting, enlarged lymph nodes

CARDIOPULMONARY

- Respiratory rate and pattern, breath sounds (presence/absence, adventitious sounds), quantity and characteristics of sputum, shortness of breath, use of accessory muscles, dysphagia, diminished gag reflex, tachycardia, blood pressure

GASTROINTESTINAL

- Pain, diarrhea, bowel sounds, character and frequency of bowel movements, constipation, rectal bleeding, hemorrhoids, change in bowel habits, sexual practices, erythema, ulceration

GENITOURINARY

- Dysuria, frequency, urgency, hematuria, pruritus, pain, vaginal or penile discharge, vaginal bleeding, burning, lesions, ulcerations, characteristics of urine

CENTRAL NERVOUS SYSTEM

- Cognition, level of consciousness, personality, behavior

MUSCULOSKELETAL

- Tenderness, pain, loss of function

Modified from Dean, G.E., Haeuber, D., & Rivera, L.M. (1996). Infection. In M. Grant, M. Frank-Stromborg, S.B., Baird, & R. McCorkle, et al. (Eds.), *Cancer nursing: A comprehensive textbook* (2nd ed., p. 975). Philadelphia: Saunders.

chromosome positive. It is targeted therapy that prevents the activation of an enzyme (tyrosine kinase) needed for growth of CML cells. This drug is well tolerated and has been shown to be most effective at inducing remission for early stages of CML. Other drugs used to treat CML include interferon alpha, which reduces the growth and division of leukemic cells, but its use is limited because of intolerable side effects, such as flu-like symptoms and fevers. Leukemic cells with mutations other than the Philadelphia chromosome are usually resistant to imatinib mesylate. Clinical trials with dasatinib (Sprycel) are being conducted for patients whose leukemia becomes nonresponsive to imatinib mesylate.

Treatment of chronic lymphocytic leukemia (CLL) with standard chemotherapy can cause remissions but does not cure the disease. Because CLL appears incurable and therapy has sometimes severe adverse reactions, treatment is often delayed until the patient has disease symptoms. Many available options include treatment with an alkylating agent such as chlorambucil with or without prednisone; fludarabine; and combined chemotherapy such as CVP (cyclophosphamide, vincristine, prednisone). Rituximab, a monoclonal antibody, is often combined with these treatments or used as a single agent (Rogers, 2005).

Drug Therapy for Infection. Drug therapy is the main defense against infections that develop in patients undergoing therapy for AML. Drugs used depend on the sensitivity of the organism causing the infection, as well as infection severity. Drugs for infection are classified as antibacterial, antiviral, or antifungal.

Antibiotic and antibacterial drugs used for prevention or treatment of infection in patients with AML usually include an aminoglycoside antibiotic (amikacin, gentamicin, and tobramycin) and a penicillin, or a third-generation cephalosporin (ceftazidime). Additional powerful antibiotics used may include vancomycin in cases of methicillin-resistant *Staphylococcus aureus* or if indwelling venous catheter infection is suspected.

Systemic antifungal drugs are used when a fungal infection has been diagnosed or is strongly suggested or when a neutropenic patient remains febrile 4 to 7 days after starting antibiotic therapy. Common antifungal drugs include amphotericin B, ketoconazole (Nizoral), voriconazole (Vfend), fluconazole (Diflucan), and nystatin (Mycostatin, Nadostine♣, Nilstat).

Antiviral drugs are used in patients with leukemia to prevent and treat viral infections. Acyclovir is given at the start of chemotherapy, especially for patients who are cytomegalovirus (CMV) positive. If a viral infection is suspected or diagnosed, drug treatments may include ganciclovir, foscarnet, or steroids. The antivirals, although helpful in combating severe infections, have serious adverse effects, especially **ototoxicity** (impaired hearing and/or balance) and **nephrotoxicity** (impaired kidney function). Carefully monitor the patient treated with such drugs for signs of hearing impairment and renal insufficiency.

NIC ***Infection Protection.*** A major objective in caring for the patient with leukemia is protection from infection. All personnel must use extreme care during all nursing procedures. Frequent, thorough handwashing is of the utmost importance. Anyone with an upper respiratory tract infection who must enter the patient's room must wear a mask. Observe strict asepsis when changing dressings or accessing a central venous catheter. Maintain strict aseptic technique in the care of these catheters at all times.

If possible, ensure that the patient is in a private room to reduce cross-contamination. Other precautions are used, such as not allowing standing water in vases, denture cups, or humidifiers in the patient's room, because they are breeding grounds for organisms.

Some facilities prescribe a "minimal bacteria diet" during the neutropenic period. Any uncooked foods, such as raw fruits and vegetables, and pepper are removed from the diet because they contain large numbers of organisms. Whether patients benefit from this diet is not known.

Some facilities place the immunosuppressed patient in a room with a high-efficiency particulate air (HEPA) filtration or laminar airflow system. These systems decrease the number of airborne pathogens. It is not known whether these systems benefit patients.

Continually assess the patient for the presence of infection. This task is difficult because manifestations may not be obvious in the patient with leukopenia. The development of fever and the formation of pus (both indicators of infection) depend on the presence of WBCs. The patient with leukopenia may have a severe infection without pus and with only a low fever.

Monitor the patient's daily CBC with differential WBC count and absolute neutrophil count (ANC). Inspect the mouth during every shift for lesions and mucosa breakdown. Assess the lungs every 8 hours for crackles, wheezes, and reduced breath sounds. Assess all urine for odor and cloudiness. Ask him or her about any urgency, burning, or pain on urination.

Take vital signs at least every 4 hours to assess for fever. A temperature elevation of even 0.5° F (or 0.5° C) above baseline is significant for a patient with leukopenia and indicates infection until it has been proved otherwise.

Many hospital units that specialize in the care of patients with neutropenia have specific protocols for antibiotic therapy if infection is suspected. Usually, the health care provider is notified immediately and specific specimens are obtained for culture. Obtain blood for bacterial and fungal cultures from peripheral sites and from the central venous catheter. Obtain urine specimens, sputum specimens, and specimens from open lesions for culture. Chest x-rays are taken. After the specimens are obtained, the patient begins IV antibiotics.

Skin care is important for preventing infection in the patient with leukemia because the skin may be the only intact defense. Teach him or her about hygiene, and urge daily bathing. If the patient is immobile, turn him or her every hour and apply skin lubricants.

Perform pulmonary hygiene every 2 to 4 hours. Listen to the lungs for crackles, wheezes, and reduced breath sounds. Urge the patient to cough and deep breathe or to perform sustained maximal inhalations every hour while awake.

DECISION-MAKING CHALLENGE
Critical Rescue

The patient described on p. 904 has completed induction therapy for 7 days. A few days later, she develops a fever of 102° F. She does have an indwelling catheter.

1. What assessments should you make at this time?
2. Should you call the hospital's Rapid Response Team? Why or why not?

3. What infection protection measures should be instituted for this patient?
4. What is the most likely source of the patient's infection? Should you assume this IS the ONLY source of infection? Why or why not?

evolve For suggested answer guidelines, go to http://evolve.elsevier.com/Iggy/.

Hematopoietic Stem Cell Transplantation. Hematopoietic stem cell transplantation (HSCT), sometimes called *bone marrow transplantation (BMT),* is standard treatment for the patient with leukemia who has a closely matched donor and who is in temporary remission after induction therapy. HSCT is used also for lymphoma, multiple myeloma, aplastic anemia, sickle cell disease, and many solid tumors.

The bone marrow is the actual site of production of leukemic cells. It can be difficult to ensure that all leukemic cells have been eradicated during induction therapy. Therefore before HSCT, additional chemotherapy with or without total body irradiation are given to purge (condition or clean) the marrow of leukemic cells. *These treatments are lethal to the bone marrow, and without replacement of stem cells by transplantation, the patient would die of infection or hemorrhage.*

After conditioning, new healthy stem cells are given to the patient. The new cells go to the marrow and then begin the process of hematopoiesis, which results in normal, properly functioning cells and, ideally, a permanent cure.

BMT units are commonplace, even in community hospital settings. With long-term survival after transplantation increasing, nurses can expect to be caring for these people—if not during the actual transplantation or recovery period, then during and after the recovery period, in a variety of health care settings.

HSCT started with the use of **allogeneic bone marrow transplantation** (transplantation of bone marrow from a sibling or matched unrelated donor) and has advanced to the use of human leukocyte antigen (HLA)–matched stem cells from the umbilical cords of unrelated donors. Transplants are classified by the source of stem cells. In **autologous transplants,** patients receive their own stem cells (which were collected before high-dose therapy). **Syngeneic transplants** are those with the stem cells taken from the patient's own identical sibling. In **allogeneic transplants,** a closely HLA-matched sibling or an unrelated but matched donor provides the stem cells. Stem cells for transplantation may be obtained by bone marrow harvest, peripheral stem cell pheresis, or umbilical cord blood stem cell banking. Table 42-2 lists the types of transplants.

Transplantation has five phases: stem cell obtainment, conditioning regimen, transplantation, engraftment, and posttransplantation recovery.

Obtaining the stem cells. Stem cells are taken either from the patient directly (autologous stem cells) or from an HLA-matched person (allogeneic stem cells). For allogeneic transplant, a donor is selected from family members tested for HLA type. The best results occur when the donor is an HLA-identical sibling. However, transplant can be successful also between those with closely matched HLA types. The chance of matching with any given sibling is 25%.

Donor registries keep records of potential donors who can provide stem cells for patients who do not have a family member HLA match. The chance of matching with an unrelated donor is 1 in 5000.

TABLE 42-2 Classification of Transplants

Type of Transplant	Sources of Stem Cells
AUTOLOGOUS	
Self-donation	Bone marrow harvest Peripheral stem cell pheresis Umbilical cord blood
SYNGENEIC	
Patient's HLA identical twin	Bone marrow harvest Peripheral stem cell pheresis
ALLOGENEIC	
HLA-matched relative, usually a sibling	Bone marrow harvest Peripheral stem cell pheresis Umbilical cord blood
Unrelated HLA-matched donor	
Mismatched or partially HLA-matched family member or unrelated donor (donor registries)	

HLA, Human leukocyte antigen.

CULTURAL AWARENESS

About 70% of people on the bone marrow donor lists are white. The chance of finding an HLA-matched unrelated donor is estimated at 30% to 40% for white people, but for African Americans the chance is less than 20% because there are fewer African Americans among registered donors. Although blood types are common in all racial groups, tissue types can be very different among racial and ethnic groups. Nationally, efforts are made to publicize the need for donors from all cultural backgrounds. Research in this area has identified several potential barriers to stem cell donation among African Americans. These include fear or not trusting the system, concern about costs to the donor, and concern that the recipient may be a drug abuser or person who would not appreciate the sacrifice of a donation. Targeted education efforts may reduce these barriers (see the Evidence-Based Practice box on p. 908).

Bone marrow harvesting occurs after a suitable donor is identified by tissue typing. The procedure occurs in the operating room, where marrow is removed through multiple aspirations from the iliac crests. About 500 to 1000 mL of marrow is aspirated. This amount is about 5% to 10% of the donor's marrow supply and regrows within a few weeks. The marrow is then filtered and, if autologous, is treated to rid the marrow of any remaining cancer cells. Allogeneic marrow is transfused into the recipient immediately. Autologous marrow is frozen for later use.

Monitor the donor for manifestations of fluid loss, assess for complications of anesthesia, and manage pain. During surgery, donors may lose a large amount of fluid in addition to the volume of marrow taken. Donors are hydrated with saline infusions before and immediately after surgery. Occasionally the donor may need an RBC transfusion. Assess the harvest sites to ensure that the dressings are dry and intact and that the donor is not bleeding excessively.

Marrow donation is usually a same-day surgical procedure. Teach the donor to inspect the harvest sites for bleeding and

EVIDENCE-BASED PRACTICE

Talk up stem cell donation as a "helpful" thing to do

Glasgow, M., & Bello, G. (2007). Bone marrow donation: Factors influencing intentions in African Americans. *Oncology Nursing Forum, 34*(2), 369-377.

Successful allogenic stem cell transplantation depends on a close tissue type match between donor cells and the recipient. Although all tissue types are found in people of every race and ethnicity, some are much more common in one race than in others. African Americans often have a tissue type that is less common among whites and other races. The fact that only a small proportion of donors in the national donor registry are African Americans makes finding a match for non-related donors less likely. This study sought to determine what factors positively influence African-American participation in bone marrow registry and what factors are barriers to such participation.

This study used a two-phase approach to answering the research questions. In the first phase, focus groups of African-American adults were interviewed to establish questions to use regarding the intention to register as a stem cell donor. The focus groups were conducted in the presence of African-American nurses who served as cultural advisors and interpreters of cultural meaning. From these qualitative data, a 65-item tool was developed to obtain quantitative data regarding intent to donate and associated influencing factors. After validity and reliability were established for the tool, it was completed by 220 subjects. Most subjects were female (69%), had a high school education or less, had an income level of less than $20,000 per year, and were Baptist.

The results of this exploratory study indicated that seven factors influenced the intention of these subjects to register as potential bone marrow (stem cell) donors. The positive factors included "helping others," "approval of people," and "value of knowledge." The negative factors included "fear or not trusting," "external influences," and "concern about resources."

Level of Evidence—4. The study was a well-designed cohort study.

Commentary: Implications for Practice and Research. The design of the study was appropriate to begin to answer the questions posed. Study strengths included its cultural sensitivity, the prospective nature, and the sample size. Limitations included that there was little diversity among the subjects with regard to education, religion, and socioeconomic status.

The negative factors are areas that nurses can help change. Much of the fear and distrust were related to getting a disease during the procedure (HIV) and being responsible for the costs related to donation. Nurses can provide reassurance that neither issue is a fact. Another negative factor was that the subjects were concerned that they would not know the donor. The concern was that their donation could go to a person who abused drugs or did not live a healthy lifestyle and that the donation would then be "wasted." Again, education programs provided by nurses could focus on the "helping people" aspect rather than on the possibility of a perceived "undeserving" recipient.

to take analgesics for pain. Pain at the harvest sites (hip) is common and is managed with oral non–aspirin-containing analgesics. Some donors may require opioid analgesics for pain control.

Peripheral blood stem cell (PBSC) harvesting requires three phases: mobilization, collection by pheresis, and reinfusion. **PBSCs** are stem cells that have been released from the bone marrow and circulate within the blood. Although there are fewer stem cells in peripheral blood than in bone marrow, their numbers can be artificially increased. During the mobilization phase, chemotherapy or hematopoietic growth factors are given to the patient for an autologous collection and hematopoietic growth factors alone are given to the donor for an allogeneic collection. These agents increase the numbers of stem cells and WBCs in the peripheral blood. The stem cells are then collected by **pheresis** (withdrawing whole blood, filtering out the cells, and returning the plasma to the patient). One to five pheresis procedures, each lasting 2 to 4 hours, are needed to obtain enough stem cells for transplantation. The cells are frozen and stored for reinfusion after the patient's conditioning regimen is completed.

Monitor the patient or donor closely during pheresis. Complications include catheter clotting and hypocalcemia (caused by anticoagulants). Low calcium levels may cause numbness or tingling in the fingers and toes, abdominal or muscle cramping, or chest pain. Oral calcium supplements may be used to manage these symptoms. Monitor vital signs at least every hour during pheresis. The patient may become hypotensive from fluid loss during the procedure.

Cord blood harvesting involves obtaining stem cells from umbilical cord blood of newborns. This blood has a high concentration of stem cells. Umbilical stem cells are obtained via a simple blood draw from the placenta. After birth, before the placenta detaches, a syringe is used to withdraw 40 to 150 mL of blood from the umbilical vein of the placenta. The syringes are placed in a kit and returned to the Cord Blood Registry for processing and storage. The stem cells may be used later for an unrelated recipient or stored in case the infant develops a serious illness later in life and needs them. The cost of banking and processing umbilical cord stem cells is about $1500, with an additional charge of $200 per year for storage. Umbilical stem cells can last for years when stored properly in liquid nitrogen.

Conditioning regimen. Fig. 42-3 outlines the timing and steps involved in transplantation. The day the patient receives the stem cells is day T-0. Before transplantation, the conditioning days are counted in reverse order from T-0, just like a rocket countdown. After transplantation, days are counted in order from the day of transplantation.

The patient first undergoes a conditioning regimen, which varies with the diagnosis and type of transplant to be received. The conditioning regimen serves two purposes: (1) to "wipe

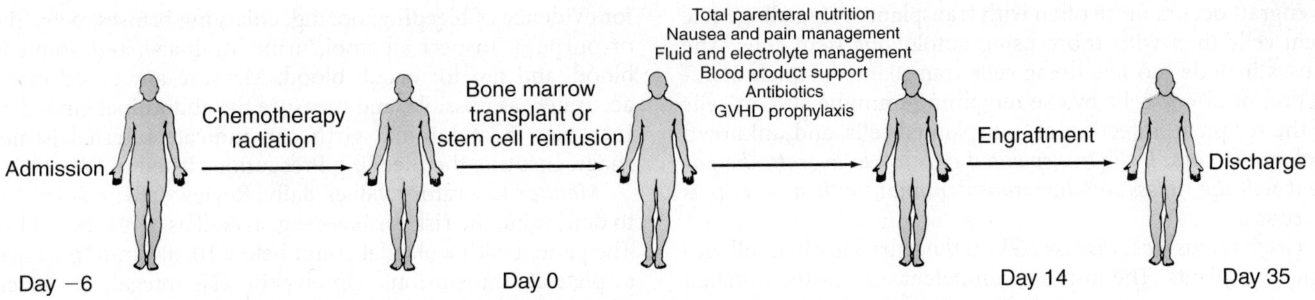
Total parenteral nutrition
Nausea and pain management
Fluid and electrolyte management
Blood product support
Antibiotics
GVHD prophylaxis
Chemotherapy
radiation
Bone marrow
transplant or
stem cell reinfusion
Engraftment
Admission
Discharge
Day −6
Day 0
Day 14
Day 35

Fig. 42-3 • Timing and steps of allogeneic stem cell transplantation. (*GVHD,* Graft-versus-host disease.)

out" the patient's own bone marrow, thus preparing him or her for optimal graft take; and (2) to give higher-than-normal doses of chemotherapy and/or radiotherapy to rid the person of cancer cells (myeloablation). Usually a period of 5 to 10 days is required. The regimen usually includes high-dose chemotherapy and sometimes includes total-body irradiation (TBI). Each conditioning regimen is individually tailored, with the patient's specific disease, overall health, and previous treatment considered. A typical conditioning regimen for an adult with acute myelogenous leukemia (AML) receiving an allogenic HSCT for treatment is:

- *Days T-5 through T-4:* High-dose chemotherapy to obliterate the patient's own bone marrow cells and to kill off any remaining leukemic cells. Specific agents include busulfan, carmustine, cyclophosphamide, cytosine arabinoside, etoposide, and melphalan. The dosages are much higher than those used for normal chemotherapy.
- *Days T-3 through T-1:* Delivery of TBI. The total radiation dose for TBI is 1200 rads given as 200 rads twice daily over 3 days.

Because of the problems and risk for death associated with this conditioning regimen, a non-myeloablative approach may be used instead. Non-myeloablative regimens use lower doses of chemotherapy and/or lower doses of TBI that allow for recovery of a recipient's own immune system. The use of non-myeloablative conditioning regimens decreases the chemotherapy side effects but relies on the development of graft-versus-host disease (GVHD) for the control of the cancer. In contrast, myeloablative conditioning regimens use high doses of chemotherapy with or without radiation therapy to completely destroy a recipient's bone marrow, allowing for replacement by a new immune system (Laffan & Biedrzycki, 2006). There are many variations in non-myeloablative conditioning regimens.

During conditioning, bone marrow and normal tissues respond immediately to the chemotherapy and radiation. *The patient has all of the expected side effects associated with both therapies. When chemotherapy is given in high doses, these side effects are more intense than those seen with standard doses. Side effects include nausea and vomiting, mucositis, capillary leak syndrome, diarrhea, and bone marrow suppression.*

Late effects from the conditioning regimen are also common, occurring as late as 3 to 10 years after transplantation. These problems include veno-occlusive disease (VOD), skin toxicities, cataracts, lung fibrosis, second cancers, cardiomyopathy, endocrine complications, and neurologic complications.

Transplantation. Day T-0 is the day of transplantation. The transplantation itself is very simple. Frozen marrow, PBSCs, or umbilical cord blood cells are thawed and then infused through the patient's central catheter like an ordinary blood transfusion. *However, blood administration tubing is not used because the cells could get caught in the filter and not enter the patient's body.*

Side effects of all types of stem cell transfusions are similar. The patient may have fever and hypertension as a reaction to the preservative used in stem cell storage. To prevent these reactions, acetaminophen (Tylenol), hydrocortisone, and diphenhydramine (Benadryl) are given before the infusion. Antihypertensives or diuretics may be needed to treat fluid volume changes. The patient may have red urine for a short time as a result of red blood cell breakage in the infused stem cells.

Engraftment. The transfused PBSCs and marrow cells circulate briefly in the peripheral blood. The stems cells find their way to the marrow-forming sites of the patient's bones and establish residency there. How the donated stem cells "home in" on the bone marrow sites is not yet understood.

Engraftment, the successful "take" of the transplanted cells in the patient's bone marrow, is key to the whole transplantation process. For the donated marrow or stem cells to "rescue" the patient after large doses of chemotherapy or radiotherapy have wiped out his or her own bone marrow, the transfused stem cells must survive and grow in the patient's bone marrow sites. Engraftment takes 8 to 12 days for peripheral blood stem cell transplantation and 12 to 28 days for bone marrow stem cell transplantation. To aid engraftment, growth factors, such as granulocyte colony-stimulating factor or granulocyte-macrophage colony-stimulating factor, may be given. When engraftment occurs, the patient's WBC, RBC, and platelet counts begin to rise.

Prevention of complications. The period after transplantation is difficult. Infection and bleeding are severe problems because the patient remains without any natural immunity until the transfused stem cells grow and engraft. The nursing care for this patient is the same as for the patient during induction therapy for AML. Helping the patient maintain hope through this long recovery period is difficult. Complications are often severe and life threatening. Help the patient have a positive attitude and be involved in his or her own recovery.

In addition to the problems related to the period of **pancytopenia** (too few circulating blood cells), other complications of HSCT include failure to engraft, development of graft-versus-host disease (GVHD), and development of veno-occlusive disease (VOD).

Failure to engraft occurs when the donated stem cells fail to grow in the bone marrow and function properly. This issue is discussed in advance with the patient and the donor. Failure to engraft occurs more often with transplants using allogeneic stem cells than with those using autologous stem cells. The causes include too few living cells transplanted, attack or rejection of donor cells by the remaining immune system cells of the recipient, infection of transplanted cells, and unknown biologic factors. *If the transplanted cells fail to engraft, the patient will die unless another transplantation with stem cells is successful.*

Graft-versus-host disease (GVHD) occurs mostly in allogeneic transplants. The immunocompetent cells of the donated marrow recognize the patient's (recipient) cells, tissues, and organs as foreign and start an immunologic attack against them. The graft is actually trying to attack the host tissues and cells.

Although all host tissues can be attacked and harmed, the tissues usually damaged are the skin, intestinal tract, and liver. About 25% to 50% of all allogeneic BMT recipients have some degree of GVHD, and more than 15% of the patients who develop GVHD die of its complications. The presence of some GVHD indicates successful engraftment.

Management of GVHD involves limiting the activity of donor T-cells by using drugs to suppress immune function such as cyclosporine, tacrolimus, methotrexate, corticosteroids, mycophenolate mofetil, and antithymocyte globulin. Care is taken to avoid suppressing the new immune system to the extent that either infection risk increases or the new cells stop engrafting.

Veno-occlusive disease (VOD) is the blockage of liver blood vessels by clotting and inflammation (phlebitis). This problem occurs in up to 20% of patients who undergo BMT. Problems usually begin within the first 30 days after transplantation. Patients who received high-dose chemotherapy, especially alkylating agents, are at risk for life-threatening liver complications. Manifestations include jaundice, pain in the right upper quadrant, ascites, weight gain, and liver enlargement.

There is no known way of opening the liver vessels. Thus treatment is supportive. Early detection improves the chance for survival. Fluid management is also crucial. Assess the patient daily for weight gain, fluid retention, increases in abdominal girth, and hepatomegaly.

Risk for Injury

Normal bone marrow production of platelets is severely limited with acute myelogenic leukemia (AML), leading to thrombocytopenia. The patient is at great risk for excessive bleeding in response to minimal trauma. Thrombocytopenia can also be caused by induction therapy for AML or high-dose chemotherapy for transplantation.

NOC **Planning: Expected Outcomes.** The patient with leukemia is expected to remain free from bleeding. Indicators include:

- Maintenance of hematocrit and hemoglobin within normal limits
- Absence of frank bleeding, petechiae, or ecchymosis

Interventions. The patient's platelet count is decreased as a side effect of chemotherapy. During the period of greatest bone marrow suppression (the **nadir**), the platelet count may be very low (less than 10,000/mm^3). He or she is at extreme risk for bleeding once the platelet count falls below 50,000/mm^3, and spontaneous bleeding often occurs when the platelet count is lower than 20,000/mm^3.

Bleeding Precautions are used to protect the patient from injury with bleeding. Assess him or her at least every 4 hours for evidence of bleeding: oozing, enlarging bruises, petechiae, or purpura. Inspect all stool, urine, drainage, and vomit for blood, and test for occult blood. Measure any blood loss as accurately as possible, and measure the abdominal girth daily. Increases in abdominal girth can indicate internal hemorrhage. Institute the Bleeding Precautions listed in Chart 42-8.

Monitor laboratory values daily. Review CBC results daily to determine the risk for bleeding, as well as actual blood loss. The patient with a platelet count below 10,000/mm^3 may need a platelet transfusion. Oprelvekin (Neumega), a platelet (thrombopoietic) growth factor, may be prescribed to induce platelet growth after the completion of chemotherapy. For the patient with severe blood loss, packed RBCs may be prescribed (see discussion on p. 919 in the Red Blood Cell Transfusions section).

Fatigue

Normal production of red blood cells is limited in leukemia, causing anemia, which results in fatigue. Also, leukemic cells have high rates of metabolism, increasing fatigue in the anemic patient with leukemia. Anemia may also occur as a side effect of chemotherapy treatment.

NOC **Planning: Expected Outcomes.** The patient with leukemia is expected to have no increase in fatigue. Indicators include that the patient consistently demonstrates these behaviors:

- Participation in self-care
- Recognition of symptoms of fatigue and alteration of activity before fatigue becomes excessive

Chart 42-8 BEST PRACTICE FOR PATIENT SAFETY & QUALITY CARE

The Patient with Thrombocytopenia

- Handle the patient gently.
- Use a lift sheet when moving and positioning in bed.
- Avoid IM injections and venipunctures.
- When injections or venipunctures are necessary, use the smallest-gauge needle for the task.
- Apply firm pressure to the needle stick site for 10 minutes or until the site no longer oozes blood.
- Apply ice to areas of trauma.
- Test all urine and stool for the presence of occult blood.
- Observe IV sites every 2 hours for bleeding.
- Avoid trauma to rectal tissues:
  - Do not take temperatures rectally.
  - Do not give enemas.
  - Administer well-lubricated suppositories with caution.
  - Advise patient not to have anal intercourse.
- Measure abdominal girth daily.
- Advise the patient to use an electric shaver.
- Teach the patient to avoid mouth trauma:
  - Use soft-bristled toothbrush or tooth sponges.
  - Do not floss between teeth.
  - Avoid dental work, especially extractions.
  - Avoid hard foods.
  - Make sure that dentures fit and do not rub.
- Encourage the patient not to blow the nose or insert objects into the nose.
- Advise the patient to avoid contact sports.
- Teach the patient to wear shoes with firm soles when ambulating.

NIC Interventions. Interventions aim to reduce fatigue through energy management and improving RBC counts.

Nutrition therapy is needed to assist the patient to eat enough calories to meet at least basal energy requirements. However, increasing food intake can be difficult when he or she is fatigued. Collaborate with a nutritionist to provide small, frequent meals high in protein and carbohydrates. Food items that are liquid or semisolid require less effort to eat.

Blood transfusions are sometimes indicated for the patient with fatigue. Transfusions increase the blood's oxygen-carrying capacity and replace missing RBCs. For the patient with fatigue related to anemia, packed RBCs are the blood component choice. (See Chart 42-13 on p. 918 for nursing care during transfusions.)

Drug therapy with colony-stimulating factors is used to reduce the severity and duration of anemia and neutropenia after intensive chemotherapy. For anemia, subcutaneous injections of epoetin alfa (Epogen or Procrit) weekly or every 2 weeks or darbepoetin alfa (Aranesp) subcutaneously weekly to every 3 weeks may be given. These growth factors boost the production of RBCs. The agents cause a stinging sensation when injected. Assess for side effects such as hypertension, headaches, fever, **myalgia** (muscle aches), and rashes. (See Chapter 24 for information on hematopoietic growth factors.)

Energy management is needed to help conserve the patient's energy (Chart 42-9). Examine the patient's schedule of prescribed and routine activities. Assess those activities that do not have a direct positive effect on the patient's condition in terms of their usefulness. If the benefit of an activity is less than its worsening of fatigue, coordinate with other members of the health care team about eliminating or postponing it. Activities that may be postponed include physical therapy and invasive diagnostic tests not needed for assessment or treatment of current problems.

Chart 42-9 NIC INTERVENTION ACTIVITIES

The Patient with Leukemia or the Patient Undergoing Bone Marrow/Stem Cell Transplantation

Energy Management: *Regulating energy use to treat or prevent fatigue and optimize function*

- Determine patient's/significant other's perception of causes of fatigue.
- Encourage verbalization of feelings about limitations.
- Monitor nutritional intake to ensure adequate energy resources.
- Monitor/record patient's sleep pattern and number of sleep hours.
- Limit number of visitors and interruptions by visitors, as appropriate.
- Provide calming diversionary activities to promote relaxation.
- Encourage an afternoon nap, if appropriate.
- Avoid care activities during scheduled rest periods.
- Plan activities for periods when the patient has the most energy.
- Monitor patient's oxygen response (e.g., pulse rate, cardiac rhythm, and respiratory rate) to self-care or nursing activities.
- Instruct patient/significant other to recognize signs and symptoms of fatigue that require reduction in activity.

NIC intervention activities selected from Bulechek, G.M., Butcher, H.K., & McCloskey Dochterman, J. (2008). *Nursing interventions classification (NIC)* (5th ed.). St. Louis: Mosby.

Community-Based Care

The patient with leukemia is discharged after induction chemotherapy and recovery of blood cell production. Follow-up care continues on an outpatient basis. Although many transplant centers discharge patients after engraftment, some centers give high-dose chemotherapy and stem cell infusion on an outpatient basis. This plan involves daily clinic visits and frequent follow-up by nurses in the home care setting.

Home Care Management

Planning for home care for the patient with leukemia begins as soon as remission is achieved. Assess the available support mechanisms. Many patients need a visiting nurse to assist with dressing changes for central venous catheters, nutritional infusions, and platelet infusions and to answer questions. Home transfusion therapy for blood components may be needed.

Coordination of the home care team is critical for the patient receiving stem cell transplantation in the home setting. Potential candidates are evaluated in advance. Criteria include a knowledgeable caregiver, a clean home environment, location near the hospital, telephone access, and emotional stability on the part of the patient and caregiver.

Home care nurses give chemotherapy and monitor the patient for complications. Nurses visit the patient once or twice per day and spend between 4 and 8 hours per day in the home. The patient receives the stem cell transplant infusion in the outpatient clinic. Nursing care is similar to that provided in the hospital. If complications such as sepsis or VOD occur, the patient is admitted to the inpatient facility.

Health Teaching

Instruct the patient and family about the importance of continuing therapy and medical follow-up. Many patients go home with a central venous catheter in place and need instructions about its care. Chart 42-10 lists guidelines for central venous catheter care at home. These guidelines may be altered depending on the home setting, assistance available, and agency policy.

Chart 42-10 PATIENT AND FAMILY EDUCATION GUIDE

Home Care of the Central Venous Catheter

- To maintain patency, flush the catheter briskly with saline once a day and after completing infusions.
- Change the Luer-Lok cap on each catheter lumen weekly.
- Change the dressing every other day:
  - Use clean technique with thorough handwashing.
  - Clean the exit site with alcohol and povidone-iodine (Betadine) or with chlorhexidine.
  - Apply antibacterial ointment to the site, if prescribed.
  - Cover the site with dry sterile gauze dressing, taped securely, or with transparent adherent dressing.
- To prevent tension, always tape the catheter to yourself.
- Look for and report any signs of infection (redness, swelling, or drainage at the exit site)
- In case of a break or puncture in the catheter lumen, immediately clamp the catheter between yourself and the opening. *Notify your physician immediately.*

Protecting the patient from infection at home is just as important as it was during hospitalization. (See Chart 42-7 for focused assessment for the patient at risk for infection.) Urge the patient to use proper hygiene and to avoid crowds or others with infections. Neither the patient nor any household member should receive live virus immunization (poliomyelitis, measles, or rubella) for 2 years after transplantation or while taking immunosuppressive drugs. Instruct the patient to continue mouth care regimens at home. Stress that the patient should immediately notify the physician if he or she has a fever or any other sign of infection. Chart 42-11 lists guidelines for patients for infection prevention.

Many patients return home still at risk for bleeding because platelet recovery is slower than recovery of white blood cells (WBCs). Reinforce safety and bleeding precautions, and emphasize that these precautions must be followed until the platelet count is above 50,000/mm³. Teach the patient and family to assess for petechiae, avoid trauma and sharp objects, apply pressure to wounds for 10 minutes, and report blood in the stool or urine or headache that does not respond to acetaminophen. Chart 42-12 lists guidelines for patients at risk for bleeding.

Psychosocial Preparation

A diagnosis of leukemia threatens self-esteem and the family role. The patient faces the possibility of death, and treatment causes major changes in self-image. Changes occur in his or her body image, level of independence, and lifestyle. Some feel threatened by the environment, seeing everything as potentially infectious. Patients who are cared for in protective isolation may feel lonely and isolated. Help the patient and family define priorities, understand the illness and its treatment, and find hope. Make referrals to support groups sponsored by organizations such as the American Cancer Society ("I Can Cope" and "Make Today Count").

Health Care Resources

The patient with limited social support may need help at home until strength and energy return. A home care aide may suffice for some patients, whereas for others a visiting nurse may be needed to reinforce teaching. The patient may also need equipment for ADLs and ambulation. Assess financial resources. Cancer treatment is expensive, and you will need to coordinate with the social services department to ensure that insurance is adequate. If the patient is uninsured, explore other sources, such as drug company–sponsored compassionate aid programs. The Leukemia and Lymphoma Society of America offers limited financial help, sponsors support groups, and provides information for patients and families.

Prolonged outpatient contact and follow-up are necessary, and patients need transportation to the outpatient facility. Many local units of the American Cancer Society offer free transportation to patients with cancer, including leukemia.

Chart 42-11 PATIENT AND FAMILY EDUCATION GUIDE

Prevention of Infection

- Avoid crowds and other large gatherings of people who might be ill.
- Do not share personal toilet articles, such as toothbrushes, toothpaste, washcloths, or deodorant sticks, with others.
- If possible, bathe daily.
- Wash the armpits, groin, genitals, and anal area at least twice a day with an antimicrobial soap.
- Clean your toothbrush daily by either running it through the dishwasher or rinsing it in liquid laundry bleach and water.
- Wash your hands thoroughly with an antimicrobial soap before you eat or drink, after touching a pet, after shaking hands with anyone, as soon as you come home from any outing, and after using the toilet.
- Eat a low-bacteria diet, and avoid salads, raw fruits and vegetables, undercooked meat, pepper, and paprika.
- Wash dishes between uses with hot, sudsy water, or use a dishwasher.
- Do not drink water that has been standing for longer than 15 minutes.
- Do not reuse cups and glasses without washing.
- Avoid changing pet litter boxes. If unavoidable, use gloves or wash hands immediately.
- Avoid keeping turtles and reptiles as pets.
- Do not feed pets raw or undercooked meat.
- Take your temperature at least twice a day.
- Report any of these manifestations of infection to your physician immediately:
  - Temperature greater than 100° F (38° C)
  - Persistent cough (with or without sputum)
  - Pus or foul-smelling drainage from any open skin area or normal body opening
  - Presence of a boil or abscess
  - Urine that is cloudy or foul smelling, or burning on urination
- Take all drugs as prescribed.
- Do not dig in the garden or work with houseplants.
- Avoid travel to areas of the world with poor sanitation or inadequate health care facilities.

Chart 42-12 PATIENT AND FAMILY EDUCATION GUIDE

The Patient at Risk for Bleeding

- Use an electric shaver
- Use a soft-bristled toothbrush, and do not floss.
- Do not have dental work done without consulting your doctor.
- Do not take aspirin or any aspirin-containing products. Read the label to be sure that the product does not contain aspirin or salicylates.
- Do not participate in contact sports or any activity likely to result in your being bumped, scratched, or scraped.
- If you are bumped, apply ice to the site for at least 1 hour.
- Notify your doctor if you:
  - Experience an injury and persistent bleeding results
  - Have excessive menstrual bleeding
  - See blood in your urine or bowel movement
  - Have a headache that does not respond to acetaminophen
- Avoid anal intercourse.
- Take a stool softener to prevent straining during a bowel movement.
- Do not use enemas or rectal suppositories.
- Avoid bending over at the waist.
- Do not wear clothing or shoes that are tight or that rub.
- Avoid blowing your nose or placing objects in your nose. If you must blow your nose, do so gently without blocking either nasal passage.

NCLEX EXAMINATION CHALLENGE

The client is 22 days post-transplant from an allogeneic stem cell transplantation. The client has been having 6 to 10 watery stools per day for the past 3 days. Which additional assessment by the nurse supports the possibility of graft-versus-host disease (GVHD)?

A. The skin turgor on the client's arms and hands is poor.
B. Today's platelet count is 5000/mm^3, and the WBCs are low.
C. There is some peeling of skin on the client's palms.
D. The client's urine output is less than 800 mL in 24 hours.

evolve For the correct answer, go to http://evolve.elsevier.com/Iggy/.

Evaluation: Outcomes

Evaluate the care of the patient with leukemia on the basis of the identified nursing diagnoses and collaborative problems. The expected outcomes include that the patient will:

- Remain free of infection and sepsis
- Not experience episodes of bleeding
- Be able to balance activity and rest
- Use energy conservation techniques
- Adapt lifestyle to energy level

Specific indicators for these outcomes are listed for each nursing diagnosis and collaborative problem in the Planning and Implementation section.

MALIGNANT LYMPHOMAS

Lymphomas are cancers of the lymphoid tissues. They are the abnormal overgrowth of one type of leukocyte, the lymphocyte. They differ from leukemia in the degree of maturation of the affected cells and the location of cancer cell production. Lymphomas are cancers of committed lymphocytes rather than stem cell precursors (as in leukemia). This growth occurs in lymphoid tissues scattered throughout the body, especially the lymph nodes and spleen, rather than in the bone marrow. Lymphomas are solid tumors rather than cellular suspensions within the blood and bone marrow. There are two major categories of lymphoma among adults: Hodgkin's lymphoma (HL) and non-Hodgkin's lymphoma (NHL).

HODGKIN'S LYMPHOMA

Pathophysiology

Hodgkin's lymphoma (HL) is a cancer that can affect any age-group. However, it appears to peak in two different age-groups: (1) in teens and young adults, and (2) in adults in their 50s and 60s (McCance & Huether, 2006). HL affects younger men and women equally, but the disease is more prevalent in men in the older group.

The exact cause of HL is uncertain. Possible causes include viral infections (i.e., Epstein-Barr virus [EBV], human T-cell leukemia/lymphoma virus [HTLV], and human immune deficiency virus [HIV]) and exposure to chemical agents. There appears to be an increase incidence of HL in siblings of patients with the disease. Most cases of the disease, however, occur in people without identifiable risk factors, and most people with presumptive risk factors do not get the disease.

This cancer usually starts in a single lymph node or a single chain of nodes. The tissue in the node becomes cancerous. These nodes contain a specific cancer cell type, the **Reed-Sternberg cell,** a marker for HL. HL generally spreads from one group of lymph nodes to the next in an orderly fashion, unlike non-Hodgkin's lymphoma.

Patient-Centered Collaborative Care

Assessment

The most common assessment finding is a large but painless lymph node or nodes, often in the neck. A distinctive rare finding in HL is pain in the lymph nodes that is brought on or made worse with ingestion of alcohol. The patient may also have constitutional symptoms called "B symptoms" that may include fevers (>101.5° F [>38° C]), drenching night sweats, and unexplained weight loss (>10% of normal body weight). The presence of these symptoms often means a poorer prognosis. Most patients have no symptoms at time of diagnosis, and specific manifestations often depend on the site and extent of disease.

Diagnosis and subtype are established when biopsy of a node or mass reveals Reed-Sternberg cells (McCance & Huether, 2006). HL is then classified into one of several different subtypes on the basis of the World Health Organization (WHO) classification system.

After diagnosis, the next evaluation of the patient with HL is staging to determine the extent of disease. Staging must be detailed and accurate because the treatment regimen is determined by the extent of disease. Staging usually includes a history and physical examination, CBC, electrolyte panel, renal and liver function tests, erythrocyte sedimentation rate (ESR), and a bone marrow aspiration and biopsy. Computed tomography (CT) of the neck, chest, abdomen, and pelvis is performed as part of the staging process. Positron emission tomography (PET) may be included to assess for areas of disease not detected by CT. PET scans are helpful after treatment to assess disease response to therapy. After staging procedures are complete, the stage of the disease is determined by the Ann Arbor Staging Criteria (Table 42-3).

TABLE 42-3 Staging Criteria for Hodgkin's Lymphoma

Stage	Manifestation Criteria
Ia	Disease is present only in a single lymph node region or in only one non–lymph node site.
Ib	Disease location is the same as Ia. In addition, the patient has some or all of these manifestations: persistent fever, night sweats, weight loss of more than 10% of normal body weight.
IIa	Disease is present in two or more separate lymph node regions on the same side of the diaphragm or two in two non–lymph node sites on the same side of the diaphragm.
IIb	Disease location is the same as IIa. In addition, the patient has some or all of these manifestations: persistent fever, night sweats, weight loss of more than 10% of normal body weight.
IIIa	Disease extends to lymph node regions on both sides of the diaphragm.
IIIb	Disease location is the same as IIIa. In addition, the patient has some or all of these manifestations: persistent fever, night sweats, weight loss of more than 10% of normal body weight.
IIIc	Same as IIIb along with disease present in the spleen.
IV	Disease is present in many body areas, including in one or more non–lymph node tissues and organs.

Interventions

Hodgkin's lymphoma (HL) is one of the most treatable types of cancer. Generally, for stage I and stage II disease, the treatment is external radiation of involved lymph node regions. With more extensive disease, radiation and combination chemotherapy are used to achieve remission. (See Chapter 24 on general care of patients receiving radiation and chemotherapy.)

Nursing management of the patient undergoing treatment for HL focuses on the side effects of therapy, especially:

- Drug-induced pancytopenia, which increases the risk for infection, anemia, and bleeding
- Severe nausea and vomiting, which impair nutritional status
- Skin problems at the site of radiation
- Constipation or diarrhea
- Impaired liver function either by metastasis to the liver or by chemotherapy drugs
- Permanent sterility for male patients receiving radiation to the abdominopelvic region in the pattern of an inverted Y in combination with specific chemotherapy drugs (The patient is informed of this side effect and given the option to store sperm in a sperm bank before treatment.)
- Secondary cancer development as a result of HL treatment (Long-term follow-up includes screening for recurrence, as well as the possible development of a secondary cancer.)

NON-HODGKIN'S LYMPHOMA

Pathophysiology

Non-Hodgkin's lymphoma (NHL) includes all lymphoid cancers that do not have the Reed-Sternberg cell. There are more than 12 subtypes of NHL, including low-grade, intermediate, and high-grade lymphomas. NHL generally spreads through the lymphatic system in a less orderly way than HL. It represents 3% of all cancer-related deaths in the United States, and about 63,000 new cases are diagnosed each year (American Cancer Society, 2008). The incidence of NHL has nearly doubled over the past three decades. The disease is more common in men, white people, and older adults (Rogers, 2006).

The exact cause of NHL is unknown. However, several theories suggest NHL may be associated with autoimmune conditions such as Sjögren syndrome, celiac disease, rheumatoid arthritis, and systemic lupus erythematosus (Ramos-Casals et al., 2005; Zhong, 2006). Immune suppression has also been associated with an increase risk. The disease is more common among solid organ transplantation recipients on immunosuppressive therapy and patients infected with HIV. Chronic infection from *Helicobacter pylori* is associated with a type of lymphoma called *mucosa-associated lymphoid tissue (MALT) lymphoma,* and Epstein-Barr viral infection has been associated with Burkitt's lymphoma (Rogers, 2006). NHL may be related to inherited problems that result in gene damage. Gene damage may result in loss of tumor suppressor gene function, allowing cancer development to occur. There is an increased risk of NHL among people exposed to pesticides, insecticides, and dust.

Patients usually have lymphadenopathy or extranodal involvement at the time of diagnosis. The most common extranodal sites are the GI tract, skin, bone marrow, sinuses, thyroid, or central nervous system (CNS) (Rogers, 2006). Enlarged lymph nodes may be the only symptom of lymphoma because these nodes can arise from lymphoid cells in any tissue and can spread to any organ. Painless swelling of the cervical, axillary, inguinal, and femoral nodes is most often seen. The diagnosis of NHL can be made only after the biopsy of an involved lymph node is reviewed by a hematopathologist.

Lymphoma is not a single disease but, rather, a group of diseases. The specific subtype of lymphoma must be classified because treatment decision varies depending on the subtype of lymphoma. Lymphomas are classified using the World Health Organization (WHO) classification system. The classification system is based on cytology, immunophenotyping by flow cytometry, and genetic (chromosomal translocations and molecular rearrangements) and clinical features. NHLs are broadly classified as B-cell or T-cell lymphomas, depending on the lymphocyte lineage that gave rise to the cancer. B-cell lymphomas are most common (about 90% of NHLs) and T-cell lymphomas make up only about 10% of NHLs (Kasamon & Swinnen, 2004).

Staging is similar to that for Hodgkin's lymphoma (HL). In addition, lactate dehydrogenase (LDH) levels are also evaluated to measure tumor growth rates. This test is also a prognostic indicator. Beta-2 microglobulin levels have been shown to predict response to treatment and time to treatment failure. Cerebrospinal fluid is evaluated when paranasal sinuses, testicular, parameningeal, orbit, CNS, paravertebral, or HIV lymphoma has been diagnosed (National Comprehensive Cancer Network [NCCN], 2005). The stage of NHL is determined by the Ann Arbor Staging Classification (see Table 42-3).

Patients with **indolent** (slow-growing) lymphomas, such as follicular lymphomas, usually have painless lymphadenopathy at diagnosis. Patients with more aggressive B-cell lymphomas may have large abdominal or mediastinal masses at diagnosis that become symptomatic within a short period after they develop. Constitutional symptoms ("B symptoms") such as fevers greater than 101.5° F (>38° C), drenching night sweats, and unintentional weight loss greater than 10% of body weight in the past 6 months occur in about one third of patients with aggressive lymphomas and rarely in indolent lymphomas. Bone marrow involvement in indolent lymphomas is common.

Patient-Centered Collaborative Care

Treatment options for patients with NHL vary based on several factors. These include the subtype of the tumor, international prognostic index (IPI) score, stage of the disease, performance status, and overall tumor burden. Special consideration for patients with multiple additional health problems is important, especially among older adult patients. Many new therapies have evolved over the past decade for various subtypes of NHL. These treatment options include combinations of chemotherapy drugs alone or in combination with monoclonal antibodies (e.g., rituximab and alemtuzumab), localized radiation therapy, radiolabeled antibodies (^{131}I tositumomab and ^{90}Y ibritumomab tiuxetan), hematopoietic stem cell transplantation, and other newer investigational agents, such as vaccine therapy or proteasome inhibitors (i.e., bortezomib) (Long & Versa, 2006).

Nursing care needs are similar to those for patients with HL, with additional organ-specific problems considered if the disease is widespread. With the use of biotherapy common for NHL, close monitoring for infusion-related reactions is needed during and after the delivery of monoclonal antibodies (see Chapter 24 for general care of patients undergoing treatment with biotherapy). Patient and family education are important in the management and prevention of acute and long-term complications.

MULTIPLE MYELOMA

Pathophysiology

Multiple myeloma is a white blood cell (WBC) cancer that involves a more mature lymphocyte called a *plasma cell.* There is overgrowth of B-lymphocyte plasma cells in the bone marrow. These cells normally make antibodies. When they become cancerous, these plasma cells overproduce antibodies (gamma globulins). Thus the disorder is called a "gammopathy." Similar to the leukemias, when the myeloma cells are overproduced, fewer functional red blood cells (RBCs), WBCs, and platelets are produced.

In addition to the excess antibodies, multiple myeloma cells also produce excess cytokines that increase the cancer cell growth rates and destroy bone. The excess antibodies are released into the blood, increasing the serum protein levels and clogging blood vessels in the kidney and other organs. Without treatment, the disease causes progressive bone destruction, bleeding problems, kidney failure, immunosuppression, and death.

Multiple myeloma accounts for about 12,000 deaths per year in the United States (American Cancer Society, 2008). The disease is rare in people younger than 40 years. The median age at time of diagnosis is 65 years (Mangan, 2005). The incidence is higher in American blacks than in whites, with a significantly higher incidence in men.

The cause of multiple myeloma is unknown. Possible risk factors include radiation exposure, chemical exposure, and infection with human herpes virus 8 (HHV-8). This cancer can be distinguished by changes in immunoglobulin structure that begin even before transformation to cancer occurs. When a single clone of cells becomes large enough to make enough of the specifically altered immunoglobulin, the type can be seen and recognized as a unique "spike" pattern on a serum electrophoresis test of plasma proteins. Although many different clones of cells may form at first, one becomes dominant and all cancer cells are derived from that dominant population. This is known as the *monoclonal origin of the abnormal cells* and makes the abnormal immunoglobulin produced by these cells a monoclonal immunoglobulin. Most monoclonal immunoglobulins in myeloma are the immunoglobulin G (IgG) type of paraprotein (60%) or the immunoglobulin A (IgA) type of paraprotein (20%) (Mangan, 2005).

Patient-Centered Collaborative Care

Assessment

About 20% of patients have no symptoms at time of the diagnosis. An elevation of serum total protein or a detection of a monoclonal protein (also known as *paraprotein*) in the blood or urine may be the only finding. Other possible manifestations include fatigue, anemia, bone pain, pathologic fractures, recurrent bacterial infections, and renal dysfunction. More rare problems include hypercalcemia and hyperviscosity syndrome (Mangan, 2005).

A positive finding of a serum monoclonal protein is not sufficient to make a diagnosis of multiple myeloma. About 1% of the population produce a monoclonal protein in the blood but do not have multiple myeloma. This condition is labeled *monoclonal gammopathy of undetermined significance* or *MGUS.* MGUS is a premalignant condition. Patients with MGUS usually have a monoclonal protein concentration below 3 g/dL, less than 5% plasma cells in the bone marrow, absent or only a small amount monoclonal protein in the urine, and no bone lytic lesions, anemia, hypercalcemia, or renal insufficiency. Follow-up of patients with MGUS is important because a small percentage eventually will develop multiple myeloma.

Multiple myeloma is distinguished from MGUS by having more than 10% of the bone marrow infiltrated with plasma cells, the presence of a monoclonal protein in the serum or urine, and the presence of osteolytic bone lesions.

The staging system for multiple myeloma divides patients into stages and prognostic groups on the basis of the serum B2-microglobulin and albumin levels. Other factors that help predict the outcome include age, performance status, serum creatinine, lactate dehydrogenase level (LDH), C-reactive protein, hemoglobin level, platelet count, and cytogenetics abnormalities found in the bone marrow biopsy.

The patient usually first notices fatigue, easy bruising, and bone pain. Symptoms, such as bone fractures, hypertension, infection, hypercalcemia, and fluid imbalance, may occur as the disease progresses. Diagnosis is made by x-ray findings of bone thinning with areas of bone loss that resemble Swiss cheese, immunoglobulin levels, electrophoresis of plasma proteins, and the presence of Bence-Jones protein (protein composed of incomplete antibodies) in the urine. A bone marrow biopsy is performed to evaluate and diagnose the disease and also to determine chromosome abnormalities. An abnormality of chromosome 11 predicts a longer survival, and absence of chromosome 13 is a poor prognostic factor.

Interventions

Treatment options vary. For minimal disease, watchful waiting may be an option instead of chemotherapy. Standard treatment for multiple myeloma is chemotherapy. Agents are chosen based on whether the patient is eligible for an autologous stem cell transplant. If he or she is eligible, drug therapy is used to reduce tumor burden before transplantation. These drugs regimens include dexamethasone alone, dexamethasone with thalidomide, or bortezomib alone or in combination with either thalidomide or dexamethasone. For patients who are not eligible for an autologous stem cell transplantation because of age or additional health problems, standard chemotherapy drugs such as melphalan, prednisone, vincristine, cyclophosphamide, doxorubicin, and carmustine are usually effective. Drugs such as thalidomide and lenalidomide (Revlimid) show promise in controlling the disease.

Despite therapy, multiple myeloma remains incurable. Because most patients with multiple myeloma have local or generalized bone pain, analgesics and alternative approaches for pain management, such as relaxation techniques, aromatherapy, or hypnosis, are used for pain relief. The bone disease of multiple myeloma is treated with bisphosphonates (pamidronate, zoledronic acid), which inhibit bone resorption and can help reduce the skeletal complications.

COAGULATION DISORDERS

Coagulation disorders are bleeding disorders with increased bleeding resulting from defects in one or more components regulating the blood clotting system. Bleeding disorders may be spontaneous or traumatic, localized or generalized, lifelong or acquired. They can arise from a defect in the clotting processes at the vascular, platelet, or clotting factor level.

PLATELET DISORDERS

Platelets have a vital role in blood clotting. Blood clotting always starts with platelets sticking together and forming a platelet plug. Any condition that either reduces the number of platelets or interferes with their ability to adhere (stick to one another, blood vessel walls, collagen, or fibrin threads) can result in increased bleeding. Platelet disorders can be inherited, acquired, or temporarily induced by drugs that limit platelet production or inhibit aggregation.

Reduction of platelets below the level needed for normal blood clotting is called **thrombocytopenia.** It may occur as a result of other conditions or treatments that suppress general bone marrow activity. The problem also can occur from limited platelet formation or an increased rate of platelet destruction in the spleen. The two thrombocytopenic conditions affecting adults are autoimmune thrombocytopenic purpura and thrombotic thrombocytopenic purpura.

AUTOIMMUNE THROMBOCYTOPENIC PURPURA

Pathophysiology

Autoimmune thrombocytopenic purpura is also called *idiopathic thrombocytopenic purpura (ITP).* The total number of circulating platelets is greatly reduced in ITP, even though platelet production in the bone marrow is normal.

Patients with this disorder make an antibody directed against the surface of their own platelets (an antiplatelet antibody). This antibody coats the surface of the platelets, making them more likely to be destroyed by macrophages. The spleen contains a large number of macrophages, and the blood vessels of the spleen are long and twisted. Both of these conditions allow antibody-coated platelets to be destroyed in the spleen. When the rate of platelet destruction exceeds the rate of platelet production, the number of circulating platelets decreases and blood clotting slows.

Although the cause of this disorder is autoimmune, the trigger for the production of autoantibodies is unknown. ITP is most common among women between the ages of 20 and 40 years and among people who have other autoimmune disorders (McCance & Huether, 2006).

Patient-Centered Collaborative Care

Assessment

Manifestations of ITP are at first seen in the skin and mucous membranes: large **ecchymoses** (bruises) or a petechial rash on the arms, legs, upper chest, and neck. Mucosal bleeding occurs easily. If the patient has had significant blood loss, anemia may also be present.

A rare complication is an intracranial bleed–induced stroke. Assess for neurologic function and mental status. Ask family members whether the patient's behavior and responses to questions are typical or represent a change.

ITP is diagnosed by a decreased platelet count and large numbers of megakaryocytes in the bone marrow. Antiplatelet antibodies may be detected in the blood, although this is not a specific test. If the patient has had any episodes of bleeding, hematocrit and hemoglobin levels may be low.

Interventions

As a result of the decreased platelet count, the patient is at great risk for bleeding. Interventions include therapy for the underlying condition and protection from trauma-induced bleeding episodes. Treatment is often limited to those patients with platelet counts lower than 50,000/mm^3, those who are bleeding, and those who are at high risk for bleeding.

Drug therapy to control ITP includes drugs that suppress immune function to some degree. Drugs such as corticosteroids or azathioprine (Imuran) are used to inhibit immune system production of antiplatelet autoantibodies. IV immunoglobulin and IV anti-Rho can be used to prevent the destruction of antibody-coated platelets. More aggressive therapy involves low doses of chemotherapy drugs.

Platelet transfusions are used when platelet counts are less than 20,000/mm^3 and the patient has an acute life-threatening bleeding episode. Transfusions are not performed routinely because the donated platelets are just as rapidly destroyed by the spleen as the patient's own platelets. (See discussion on p. 920 in the Platelet Transfusions section.)

Maintaining a safe environment helps protect the patient from conditions that can lead to bleeding. Closely monitor the amount of bleeding that is occurring. (For nursing care actions, see the discussion of Risk for Injury on p. 910 in the Leukemia section.)

Surgical management with a splenectomy may be needed for the patient who does not respond to drug therapy. (The spleen is the site of excessive platelet destruction.) After splenectomy, the patient is at increased risk for infection because the spleen performs many protective immune functions.

THROMBOTIC THROMBOCYTOPENIC PURPURA

Thrombotic thrombocytopenic purpura (TTP) is a rare disorder in which platelets clump together abnormally in the capillaries and too few platelets remain in circulation. The patient has inappropriate clotting, yet the blood fails to clot properly when trauma occurs. The cause of TTP appears to be an autoimmune reaction in blood vessel cells (endothelial cells) that makes platelets clump together in very small blood vessels. As a result, tissues become ischemic, leading to kidney failure, myocardial infarction, and stroke. Untreated, this disorder is often fatal within 3 months.

Treatment for the patient with TTP focuses on preventing platelet clumping and stopping the underlying autoimmune process. Treatment consists of plasma pheresis and the infusion of fresh frozen plasma. This treatment provides platelet aggregation inhibitors. Drugs that inhibit platelet clumping, such as aspirin, alprostadil (Prostin), and plicamycin, also may be helpful. Immunosuppressive therapy reduces the intensity of this disorder.

CLOTTING FACTOR DISORDERS

Coagulation or bleeding disorders can result from a clotting factor defect. Defects include the inability to produce a specific clotting factor, production of low quantities of clotting factors, or production of a less active form of clotting factors.

Most clotting factor disorders are genetic problems of one clotting factor. Acquired clotting factor disorders usually are related to a damaged liver that cannot produce proper amounts of clotting factors. Common disorders that result from defects at the clotting factor level include hemophilias

A and B and von Willebrand's disease. Disseminated intravascular coagulation (DIC) often occurs with septic shock (see Chapter 39).

HEMOPHILIA

Pathophysiology and Genetics of the Disorder

Hemophilia is actually two different hereditary bleeding disorders resulting from clotting factor deficiencies. Hemophilia A (classic hemophilia) is a deficiency of factor VIII and accounts for 80% of cases of hemophilia. Hemophilia B (Christmas disease) is a deficiency of factor IX and accounts for 20% of cases. The incidence of both disorders is 1 in 10,000 (McCance & Huether, 2006).

GENETIC CONSIDERATIONS

Hemophilia is an X-linked recessive trait. Women who are **carriers** (can pass on the gene without actually having the disorder) have a 50% chance of passing the hemophilia gene to their daughters (who then are carriers) and to their sons (who then have hemophilia). Hemophilia A affects mostly males, none of whose sons will have the gene for hemophilia and all of whose daughters will be carriers. About 30% of patients with hemophilia have no family history. It is thought that their disease is the result of a new gene mutation.

The bleeding disorder of hemophilia A is so severe that before blood transfusions were available, children with hemophilia rarely lived past age 3 years. With transfusion and factor VIII therapy, survival time has increased so that now the disease is seen among adult patients.

The clinical pictures of hemophilias A and B are identical. The patient has abnormal bleeding in response to any trauma because of a deficiency of the specific clotting factor. Patients with hemophilia do not bleed more often or even more rapidly than those without the disease, but they do bleed for a longer period. Hemophiliacs form platelet plugs at the bleeding site, but the clotting factor deficiency impairs the formation of stable fibrin clots. This allows excessive bleeding, which may be mild, moderate, or severe, depending on the degree of factor deficiency.

Patient-Centered Collaborative Care

Assessment of the patient with hemophilia shows:

- Excessive bleeding from minor cuts, bruises, or abrasions (from abnormal platelet function)
- Joint and muscle hemorrhages that lead to disabling long-term problems
- A tendency to bruise easily
- Prolonged and potentially fatal hemorrhage after surgery

The laboratory test results for a patient with hemophilia show a prolonged partial thromboplastin time (PTT), a normal bleeding time, and a normal prothrombin time (PT). The most common problem that occurs with hemophilia is degenerating joint function as a result of chronic bleeding into the joints, especially the hip and knee.

The bleeding problems of hemophilia A are managed by either regularly scheduled infusions of factor VIII cryoprecipitate (Bioclate, Helixate, ReFacto) or intermittent infusions as needed (see Cryoprecipitate Transfusions section, p. 920). The cost of cryoprecipitate is prohibitive for many people with hemophilia. In addition, because the precipitated clotting factors mostly are made from pooled human serum, a low risk for viral contamination remains, even with the use many techniques to purify the drug. Infectious complications of hemophilia therapy include hepatitis B, hepatitis C, cytomegalovirus, and HIV.

TRANSFUSION THERAPY

Any blood component may be removed from a donor and transfused to a recipient (Leighton, 2008). More than 98% of the blood supply in the United States comes from volunteer donors. Most donors give a single unit of blood at a site convenient to their work or home. Blood components may be transfused individually or collectively, with varying degrees of benefit to the recipient. Table 42-4 lists indications for transfusion therapy.

PRETRANSFUSION RESPONSIBILITIES

Nursing actions during transfusions aim at prevention or early recognition of adverse transfusion reactions. Preparation of the patient for transfusion therapy is critical, and institutional

TABLE 42-4 Indications for Treatment with Blood Components

Component	Volume	Infusion Time	Indications
Packed red blood cells (PRBCs)	200-250 mL	2-4 hr	Anemia; hemoglobin <6 g/dL, 6-10 g/dL, depending on symptoms
Washed red blood cells (WBC-poor PRBCs)	200 mL	2-4 hr	History of allergic transfusion reactions Hematopoietic stem cell transplant patients
Platelets			
Pooled	About 300 mL	15-30 min	Thrombocytopenia, platelet count <20,000 Patients who are actively bleeding with a platelet count <80,000
Single donor	200 mL	30 min	History of febrile or allergic reactions
Fresh frozen plasma	200 mL	15-30 min	Deficiency in plasma coagulation factors Prothrombin or partial thromboplastin time 1.5 times normal
Cryoprecipitate	10-20 mL/ unit	15-30 min	Hemophilia VIII or von Willebrand's disease Fibrinogen levels <100 mg/dL
White blood cells (WBCs)	400 mL	1 hr	Sepsis, neutropenic infection not responding to antibiotic therapy

blood product administration procedures must be carefully followed. Before administering any blood product, review the agency's policies and procedures. Chart 42-13 lists best practices for transfusion therapy.

Legally, a prescription from the health care provider is needed to administer blood or its components. The prescription specifies the type of component, the volume, and any special conditions the physician judges to be important. Verify the prescription for accuracy and completeness. In many hospitals, a separate consent form must be obtained before a transfusion is performed.

A blood specimen is obtained for crossmatching (testing of the donor's blood and the recipient's blood for compatibility). The procedure and responsibility for obtaining this specimen are specified by hospital policy. The laboratory requires at least 45 minutes to complete the crossmatch testing. Usually, a new crossmatching specimen is required at least every 72 hours.

Blood components are viscous (thick), requiring that a larger needle (at least 20-gauge) be used, whenever possible, for venous access. Both Y tubing and straight tubing sets are used for blood component infusion. A blood filter (about 170 μm) to remove sediment from the stored blood products is included with blood administration sets and must be used to transfuse most blood products. In massive transfusion, a microaggregate filter (20 to 42 μm) may be used.

Use normal saline as the solution to administer with blood products. Ringer's lactate and dextrose in water are not used for infusion with blood products because they cause clotting or hemolysis of blood cells. *Never add to or infuse other drugs with blood products because they may clot the blood during transfusion.*

Before the transfusion, the priority action is to determine that the blood component delivered is correct and that identification of the patient is correct. Check the physician's prescription together with another registered nurse to determine the patient's identity and whether the hospital identification band name and number are identical to those on the blood component tag. *The patient's room number is not an acceptable form of identification* (The Joint Commission, 2007). Some facilities use a bar code–point of care (BC-POC) system, similar to drug dispensing systems, in an attempt to improve patient safety and reduce identification errors (Dohnalek, 2007).

Chart 42-13 BEST PRACTICE FOR PATIENT SAFETY & QUALITY CARE

Transfusion Therapy

Nursing Actions	Rationales
BEFORE INFUSION	
1. Assess laboratory values.	Many institutions have specific guidelines for blood product transfusions (e.g., platelet count <20,000 or hemoglobin <6 g/dL).
2. Verify the medical prescription.	Legally, a physician's prescription is required for transfusions. The prescription should state the type of product, dose, and transfusion time.
3. Assess the patient's vital signs, urine output, skin color, and history of transfusion reactions.	Determine whether the patient can tolerate infusion. Baseline information may be needed to help identify transfusion reactions.
4. Obtain venous access. Use a central catheter or at least a 20-gauge needle if possible.	The larger-bore needle allows cells to flow more easily without occluding the lumen of the catheter.
5. Obtain blood products from a blood bank. Transfuse immediately.	Once a blood product has been released from the blood bank, the product should be transfused as soon as possible (e.g., red blood cell transfusions should be completed within 4 hours of removal from refrigeration).
6. With another registered nurse, verify the patient by name and number, check blood compatibility, and note expiration time.	Human error is the most common cause of ABO incompatibility reactions.
DURING INFUSION	
7. Administer the blood product using the appropriate filtered tubing.	Filters are needed to remove aggregates and possible contaminants.
8. If the blood product needs to be diluted, use only normal saline solution.	Hemolysis occurs if any other IV solution is used.
9. Remain with the patient during the first 15 to 30 minutes of the infusion.	Hemolytic reactions occur most often within the first 50 mL of the infusion.
10. Infuse the blood product at the prescribed rate.	Fluid overload is a potential complication of rapid infusion.
11. Monitor vital signs.	Vital sign changes often indicate transfusion reactions.
AFTER INFUSION	
12. When the transfusion is completed, discontinue infusion and dispose of the bag and tubing properly.	Bloodborne pathogens may be spread inadvertently through improper disposal.
13. Document.	The patient record should indicate the type of product infused, product number, volume infused, time of infusion, and any adverse reactions.

Examine the blood bag label, the attached tag, and the requisition slip to ensure that the ABO and Rh types are compatible. Check the expiration date, and inspect the product for discoloration, gas bubbles, or cloudiness, all indicators of bacterial growth or hemolysis.

TRANSFUSION RESPONSIBILITIES

Before starting the transfusion, explain the procedure to the patient. Take vital signs, including temperature, immediately before starting the transfusion. Begin the infusion slowly. *Remain with the patient for the first 15 to 30 minutes.* Any severe reaction usually occurs with infusion of the first 50 mL of blood. Ask the patient to report unusual sensations such as chills, shortness of breath, hives, or itching. Assess vital signs 15 minutes after starting the transfusion to detect signs of a reaction. If there are none, the infusion rate can be increased to transfuse 1 unit in about 2 hours (depending on the patient's cardiac status). Take vital signs at least every hour throughout the transfusion or as specified by agency policy.

Blood components without large amounts of RBCs can be infused more quickly. The identification checks are the same as for RBC transfusions. It may be necessary to infuse blood products at a slower rate for older patients. Best practices related to the nursing care needs of older patients during transfusion therapy are listed in Chart 42-14.

Chart 42-14 BEST PRACTICE FOR PATIENT SAFETY & QUALITY CARE

The Older Adult Receiving a Transfusion

- Assess the patient's circulatory, renal, and fluid status before initiating the transfusion.
- Use no larger than a 19-gauge needle.
- Try to use blood that is less than 1 week old. (Older blood cell membranes are more fragile, break easily, and release potassium into the circulation.)
- Take vital signs (especially pulse, blood pressure, and respiratory rate) every 15 minutes throughout the transfusion. Changes in these parameters can indicate fluid overload and may also be the only indicators of adverse transfusion reactions.

OVERLOAD

- Rapid bounding pulse
- Hypertension
- Swollen superficial veins

TRANSFUSION REACTION

- Rapid thready pulse
- Hypotension
- Increased pallor, cyanosis
- Administer blood slowly, taking 2 to 4 hours for each unit of whole blood, packed red blood cells, or plasma.
- Avoid concurrent fluid administration into any other IV site.
- If possible, allow 2 full hours after the administration of 1 unit of blood before administering the next unit.

Electrolyte imbalances are possible as a result of transfusions, especially with packed red blood cells or with whole blood. Potassium is the main electrolyte inside cells. During transfusions, some cells are damaged, releasing potassium and raising the patient's serum potassium level above normal (**hyperkalemia**). This problem is more likely when the blood being transfused has been frozen or is several weeks old.

TYPES OF TRANSFUSIONS

Red Blood Cell Transfusions

RBCs are given to replace cells lost as a result of trauma or surgery. Patients with problems that destroy RBCs or impair RBC maturation also may benefit from RBC transfusions. Packed RBCs, supplied in 250-mL bags, are a concentrated source of RBCs and are the most common component given to RBC-deficient patients. This type of blood product is used for patients who have a hemoglobin level less than 8 g/dL or who are hypoxemic.

Blood transfusions are actually transplantations of tissue from one person to another. The donor and recipient blood must thus be carefully checked for compatibility to prevent lethal reactions (Table 42-5). Compatibility is determined by two different antigen systems (cell surface proteins): the ABO system antigens and the Rh antigen, present on the membranes of RBCs.

RBC antigens are inherited. For the ABO system, a person inherits one of these:

- A antigen (type A blood)
- B antigen (type B blood)
- Both A and B antigens (type AB blood)
- Neither A nor B antigens (type O blood)

Within the first few years of life, circulating antibodies develop against the blood type antigens that person did not inherit. For example, a person with type A blood forms antibodies against type B blood. A person with type O blood has not inherited either A or B antigens and will form antibodies against RBCs with either A or B antigens. If RBCs that have an antigen are infused into a recipient who does not share that antigen, the infused blood is recognized by the recipient's antibodies as non-self and the recipient then has a reaction to the transfused products.

The Rh antigen system is slightly different. An Rh-negative person is born without the Rh-antigen on his or her RBCs and does not form antibodies unless he or she is specifically sensitized to it. Sensitization can occur with RBC transfusions from an Rh-positive person or from exposure during pregnancy and birth. Once an Rh-negative person has been sensi-

TABLE 42-5 Compatibility Chart for Red Blood Cell Transfusions

	RECIPIENT			
Donor	**A**	**B**	**AB**	**O**
A	X		X	
B		X	X	
AB			X	
O	X	X	X	X

tized and antibody development has occurred, any exposure to Rh-positive blood can cause a transfusion reaction. Antibody development can be prevented by giving Rh-immune globulin as soon as exposure to the Rh antigen is suspected. *People who have Rh-positive blood can receive an RBC transfusion from an Rh-negative donor, but Rh-negative people should not receive Rh-positive blood.*

Platelet Transfusions

Platelets are given to patients with platelet counts below 10,000 mm^3 and to patients with thrombocytopenia who are actively bleeding or are scheduled for an invasive procedure. Platelet transfusions are usually pooled from as many as 10 donors and do not have to be of the same blood type as the patient has. For patients who are going to receive a hematopoietic stem cell transplant (HSCT) or who need multiple platelet transfusions, single-donor platelets may be prescribed. Single-donor platelets are taken from just one donor and decrease the amount of antigen exposure to the recipient, helping prevent the formation of platelet antibodies. The chances of allergic reactions to future platelet transfusions are thus reduced.

Platelet infusion bags usually contain 300 mL for pooled platelets and 200 mL for single-donor platelets. Platelets are fragile and must be infused immediately after being brought to the patient's room, usually over a 15- to 30-minute period. A special transfusion set with a smaller filter and shorter tubing is used. *Standard transfusion sets are not used with platelets, because the filter traps the platelets and the longer tubing increases platelet adherence to the lumen.* Additional platelet filters help remove white blood cells (WBCs) from the platelet concentrate. These filters are connected directly to the platelet transfusion set and are used for patients who have a history of febrile reactions or who need multiple platelet transfusions.

Take the vital signs before the infusion, 15 minutes after the infusion starts, and at its completion. The patient may be given diphenhydramine (Benadryl) and acetaminophen (Tylenol) before the transfusion to reduce the chances of a reaction. He or she can become febrile and have **rigors** (severe chills) during transfusion, but these symptoms are not a true transfusion reaction.

Plasma Transfusions

Plasma infusions may be given fresh to replace blood volume. More commonly, plasma is frozen immediately after donation, forming **fresh frozen plasma (FFP).** Freezing preserves the clotting factors, and the plasma can then be used for patients with clotting disorders. Infuse FFP immediately after thawing while the clotting factors are still active. Patients who are actively bleeding with a prothrombin time (PT) or partial thromboplastin time (PTT) greater than 1.5 times normal are candidates for an FFP infusion.

ABO compatibility is required for transfusion of plasma products. The infusion bag contains about 200 mL. Infuse FFP as rapidly as the patient can tolerate, generally over a 30- to 60-minute period, through a regular Y set or straight-filtered tubing.

Cryoprecipitate Transfusions

Cryoprecipitate is a product derived from plasma. Clotting factors VIII and XIII, von Willebrand's factor, and fibrinogen are precipitated from pooled plasma to produce cryoprecipitate. Patients with a fibrinogen level of less than 100 mg/dL are candidates for a cryoprecipitate infusion. Give this highly concentrated blood product to patients with clotting factor disorders at a volume of 10 to 15 mL/unit. Although cryoprecipitate can be infused, it is usually given by IV push within 3 minutes. Dosages are individualized, and it is best if the cryoprecipitate is ABO compatible.

Granulocyte (White Blood Cell) Transfusions

At some centers, neutropenic patients with infections receive white blood cell (WBC) replacement transfusions. This practice is controversial because the potential benefit to the patient must be weighed against the potential severe reactions that often occur with WBC transfusions. The surfaces of WBCs contain many antigens that can cause severe reactions when infused into a patient whose immune system recognizes these antigens as non-self. In addition, transfused WBCs have a short life span and provide minimal protection when infused into another person.

WBCs are suspended in 400 mL of plasma and should be infused over a 45- to 60-minute period. Agency policies often require more strict monitoring of patients receiving WBCs. A physician may need to be present in the hospital unit, and vital signs may need to be taken every 15 minutes throughout the transfusion. Amphotericin B infusion and WBC transfusions should be separated by 4 to 6 hours. The reasons for this are (1) the drug can bind to the membranes of the WBCs and destroy them, and (2) the drug induces fevers and chills, which would be difficult to differentiate from a transfusion reaction.

TRANSFUSION REACTIONS

Patients can develop any of these transfusion reactions: febrile, hemolytic, allergic, or bacterial reactions; circulatory overload; or transfusion-associated graft-versus-host disease (GVHD). To prevent complications, remain alert during transfusions to detect reactions early and initiate appropriate treatment.

Febrile transfusion reactions occur most often in the patient with anti-WBC antibodies, a situation that can develop after multiple transfusions. The recipient develops chills, tachycardia, fever, hypotension, and tachypnea. Giving leukocyte-reduced blood or single-donor HLA-matched platelets reduces the risk for this type of reaction. WBC filters may be used to trap WBCs and prevent their infusion into the patient.

Hemolytic transfusion reactions are caused by blood type or Rh incompatibility. When blood containing antigens different from the patient's own antigens is infused, antigen-antibody complexes are formed in his or her blood. These complexes destroy the transfused cells and start inflammatory responses in the blood vessel walls and organs. The reaction may be mild, with fever and chills, or life threatening, with disseminated intravascular coagulation (DIC) and circulatory collapse. Other manifestations include:

- Apprehension
- Headache
- Chest pain
- Low back pain
- Tachycardia
- Tachypnea
- Hypotension
- Hemoglobinuria
- A sense of impending doom

The onset of a hemolytic reaction may be immediate or may not occur until subsequent units have been transfused.

Allergic transfusion reactions are most often seen in patients with a history of allergy. They may have urticaria, itching, bronchospasm, or anaphylaxis. Onset of this type of reaction usually occurs during or up to 24 hours after the transfusion. Patients with a history of allergy can be given leukocyte-reduced or washed RBCs in which the WBCs and plasma have been removed. This procedure reduces the possibility of an allergic reaction.

Bacterial transfusion reactions occur as a result of infusion of contaminated blood products. Usually a gram-negative organism is the source because these bacteria grow rapidly in blood stored under refrigeration. Symptoms include tachycardia, hypotension, fever, chills, and shock. The onset of a bacterial transfusion reaction is rapid. (See Chapter 39 for care of the patient with septic shock.)

Circulatory overload can occur when a blood product is infused too quickly. This complication is most common with whole-blood transfusions or when the patient receives multiple transfusions. Older adults are most at risk for this problem (see Chart 42-14). Symptoms include:

- Hypertension
- Bounding pulse
- Distended jugular veins
- Dyspnea
- Restlessness
- Confusion

You can both manage and prevent this complication by monitoring intake and output, infusing blood products more slowly, and giving diuretics. (See Chapter 13 for management of patients with fluid overload.)

Transfusion-associated graft-versus-host disease (TA-GVHD) is a rare but life-threatening problem that can occur in both immunosuppressed and immunocompetent patients. Its cause in immunosuppressed patients is similar to that of GVHD that occurs with allogeneic stem cell transplantation, discussed on p. 910, in which donor T-cell lymphocytes attack host tissues.

Manifestations usually occur within 1 to 2 weeks and include thrombocytopenia, anorexia, nausea, vomiting, chronic hepatitis, weight loss, and recurrent infection.

TA-GVHD has an 80% to 90% mortality rate but can be prevented by using irradiated blood products. Irradiation destroys T-cells and their cytokine products.

NCLEX EXAMINATION CHALLENGE

The client is receiving a unit of packed red blood cells. Vital signs are stable 15 minutes into the infusion, and he states he is feeling fine, just a little cold. The nurse tells him that the blood and fluid being infused are cooler than body temperature and that is probably what is making him feel cold. After 45 minutes, the client is shaking with chills. His pulse is rapid and thready, and his blood pressure is 88/40, a change from the 122/76 obtained at the last check. What is the nurse's best first action?

A. Increase the infusion rate
B. Stop the blood transfusion
C. Call the Rapid Response Team
D. Continue the infusion but at a slower rate

evolve For the correct answer, go to http://evolve.elsevier.com/Iggy/.

AUTOLOGOUS BLOOD TRANSFUSIONS

Autologous blood transfusions involve collection and infusion of the patient's own blood. This type of transfusion eliminates compatibility problems and reduces the risk for transmitting bloodborne diseases. The four types of autologous blood transfusions are preoperative autologous blood donation, acute normovolemic hemodilution, intraoperative autologous transfusion, and postoperative blood salvage.

Autologous blood donation before surgery is the most common type of autologous blood transfusion and involves collecting whole blood from the patient, dividing it into components, and storing it for later use (e.g., after a scheduled surgical procedure). As long as hematocrit and hemoglobin levels are within a safe range, the patient can donate blood on a weekly basis until the prescribed amount of blood is obtained. Fresh packed RBCs may be stored for 40 days. For patients with rare blood types, blood may be frozen for up to 10 years. Autologous blood donation may not be used with some cardiac problems and bacteremia.

Acute normovolemic hemodilution involves withdrawal of a patient's RBCs and volume replacement just before a surgical procedure. The goal is to decrease RBC loss during surgery. The blood is stored at room temperature for up to 6 hours and reinfused after surgery. This type of autologous transfusion is not used with anemic patients or those with poor kidney function.

Intraoperative autologous transfusion and blood salvage after surgery are the recovery and reinfusion of a patient's own blood from an operative field or from a bleeding wound. Special devices collect, filter, and drain the blood into a transfusion bag. This blood is used for trauma or surgical patients with severe blood loss. The salvaged blood must be reinfused within 6 hours.

Transfuse autologous blood products using the guidelines previously described. Although the patient receiving autologous blood is not at risk for most types of transfusion reactions, circulatory overload or bacterial transfusion reactions can still occur.

HUMAN NEEDS NURSING CARE REVIEW

What might you NOTICE if the patient is experiencing inadequate oxygenation and tissue perfusion as a result of hematologic problems?

- Skin cyanosis or pallor (lighter-skinned patients)
- Cyanosis or pallor of the lips and oral mucous membranes (in patients of any skin color)
- Tachycardia
- Tachypnea and dyspnea
- Slow capillary refill
- Cool to cold extremities
- Change in cognition, acute confusion
- Decreased oxygen saturation by pulse oximetry

- Decreased urine output
- Presence of bruises or petechiae
- Bleeding of the gums, around IV sites, at sites of venipuncture

What should you INTERPRET and how should you RESPOND to this patient experiencing inadequate oxygenation and tissue perfusion as a result of a hematologic problem?

Perform and interpret physical assessment, including:
- Taking vital signs
- Monitoring oxygen saturation by pulse oximetry
- Checking for blood in stool, urine, vomitus
- Checking for bleeding in the mouth, around IV sites, drains, urinary catheters
- Checking most recent laboratory values for hematocrit and hemoglobin levels and platelet and RBC counts
- Assessing cognition (mini-mental status exam)

Respond by:
- Applying oxygen
- Keeping the patient's head elevated to about 30 degrees
- Handling the patient gently
- Keeping the patient warm (blankets)
- Applying firm pressure to areas actively bleeding
- Notifying physician or Rapid Response Team
- Instituting Bleeding Precautions
- Maintaining or initiating IV therapy
- Preparing to administer blood or blood products
- Keeping venipunctures to a minimum
- Prioritizing and pacing activities to prevent fatigue

On what should you REFLECT?
- Observe patient for evidence of restored tissue perfusion (see Chapter 41).
- Think about what may have precipitated this episode and what steps could be taken to either prevent a similar episode or identify it earlier.
- Think about what additional resources could improve the nursing response to this situation.

GET READY FOR THE NCLEX EXAMINATION!

Key Points

Review these Key Points for each NCLEX Examination Client Needs Category.

Safe and Effective Care Environment
- Use aseptic technique during all central line dressing changes or any invasive procedure.
- Use Standard Precautions for all patients regardless of age, gender, race or ethnicity, sexual orientation, education level, and profession.
- Use good handwashing techniques before providing any care to a patient who is either immunocompromised or immune deficient.
- Use Bleeding Precautions for any patient with thrombocytopenia or pancytopenia (see Chart 42-8).
- Verify with another registered nurse prescriptions for transfusion of blood products.
- Use at least two forms of identification for the patient who is to receive a blood product transfusion (name and identification number). *Do not use a room number to identify the patient.*

Health Promotion and Maintenance
- Teach people to avoid unnecessary contact with environmental chemicals or toxins. If contact cannot be avoided, teach people to use safety precautions.
- Identify patients at high risk for infection because of disease or therapy.
- Teach the patient and family about the manifestations of infection and when to seek medical advice.
- Instruct patients who have anemia as a result of dietary deficiency which foods are good sources of iron, folic acid, and vitamin B_{12}.
- Teach precautions to take to avoid injury (see Chart 42-12) to patients at risk for bleeding.

Psychosocial Integrity
- Allow the patient the opportunity to express his or her feelings regarding the diagnosis of leukemia or lymphoma or the treatment regimen.
- Explain all procedures, restrictions, drugs, and follow-up care to the patient and family.
- Offer alternative therapies for relaxation, pain reduction, and distraction, such as massage, music therapy, and guided imagery.
- Refer patients and family members to local cancer resources and support groups.
- Reassure patients having pain that using opioid analgesics for needed pain relief is not drug abuse.

Physiological Integrity
- Teach the patient about any drugs to be continued after discharge from the hospital.
- Instruct the patient and family in the manifestations of complications and when to seek assistance.
- Pace nonurgent health care activities to reduce the risk for fatigue among patients with anemia or pancytopenia.
- Assess patients in the induction phase of chemotherapy and those after BMT every 8 hours for manifestations of infection.
- Assess the skin integrity of the perianal region of a patient with leukemia after every bowel movement.
- Administer analgesics on a schedule rather than PRN.
- Use normal saline as the solution infusing with blood products.
- Transfuse blood products more slowly to older patients or those who have a cardiac problem.
- Remain with the patient during the first 15 minutes of infusion of any blood product.
- Do not administer any drugs with infusing blood products.

Additional Study Resources

Go to your Companion CD or Evolve at http://evolve.elsevier.com/Iggy/ for *Self-Assessment Questions for the NCLEX Examination.*

Go to Evolve at http://evolve.elsevier.com/Iggy/ for *Prioritization and Delegation Questions for the NCLEX Examination.*

SELECTED BIBLIOGRAPHY

Asterisk indicates a classic or definitive work on this subject.

Afable, M., & Lyon, D. (2008). Severe fatigue: Could it be aplastic anemia? *Clinical Journal of Oncology Nursing, 12*(4), 569-573.

American Cancer Society. (2008). *Cancer facts and figures 2008.* Report No. 01-300M–No. 5008.08. Atlanta: Author.

Anderson, K.C., Alsina, M., Bensinger, W., Biermann, J.S., Chanan-Kahn, A., Comenzo, R.L., et al. (2007). Multiple myeloma: Clinical practice guidelines in oncology. *Journal of the National Comprehensive Cancer Network, 5*(2), 118-147.

Anderson-Reitz, L. (2006). Dose-dense chemotherapy for aggressive non-Hodgkin lymphoma. *Cancer Nursing, 29*(3), 198-206.

Ault, P. (2007). Overview of second-generation tyrosine kinase inhibitors for patients with imatinib-resistant chronic myelogenous leukemia. *Clinical Journal of Oncology Nursing, 11*(1), 125-129.

Barber, F.D. (2006). Multiple myeloma: Early recognition by primary care nurse practitioners. *The Journal for Nurse Practitioners, 2*(10), 665-672.

Bulechek, G.M., Butcher, H.K., & McCloskey Dochterman, J. (Eds.). (2008). *Nursing interventions classification (NIC)* (5th ed.). St. Louis: Mosby.

Burruss, N., & Holz, S. (2005). Managing the risks of thrombocytopenia. *Nursing2005, 35*(6), 32hn1-32hn5.

*Byar, K. (2004). Educating patients about radioimmunotherapy with yttrium-90 ibritumomab tiuxetan (Zevalin). *Seminars in Oncology Nursing, 20* (Suppl. 1), 20-25.

Campbell, P., & Green, A. (2006). The myeloproliferative disorders. *New England Journal of Medicine, 355*(23), 2452-2466.

Coyer, S., & Lash, A. (2008). Pathophysiology of anemia and nursing care implications. *MEDSURG Nursing, 17*(2), 77-83, 91.

D'Antonio, J. (2005). Chronic myelogenous leukemia. *Clinical Journal of Oncology Nursing, 9*(5), 535-538,

Demakos, E.P., & Linebaugh, J.A. (2005). Advances in myelodysplastic syndrome: Nursing implications of azacitidine. *Clinical Journal of Oncology Nursing, 9*(4), 417-423.

Dohnalek, L. (2007). Blood transfusions: How technology can improve patient safety. *American Nurse Today, 2*(5), 46-47.

Dorman, K. (2005). Sickle cell crisis! Managing the pain. *RN, 68*(12), 33-36.

Doss, D. (2006). Advances in oral therapy in the treatment of multiple myeloma. *Clinical Journal of Oncology Nursing, 10*(4), 514-520.

*Durie, B., & Salmon, S. (1975). A clinical staging system for multiple myeloma. Correlation of measured myeloma cell mass with presenting clinical features, response to treatment, and survival. *Cancer,* 36, 842-854.

Galbizo, E., & Williams, L. (2006). Chronic graft-versus-host disease. *Oncology Nursing Forum, 33*(5), 881-883.

Garrett, D., & Yoder, L. (2007). An overview of stem cell transplant as a treatment for cancer. *MEDSURG Nursing, 16*(3), 183-189.

Glasgow, M., & Bello, G. (2007). Bone marrow donation: Factors influencing intentions in African Americans. *Oncology Nursing Forum, 34*(2), 369-377.

Gould, S., Cimino, M.J., & Gerber, D.R. (2007). Packed red blood cell transfusion in the intensive care unit: Limitations and consequences. *American Journal of Critical Care, 16*(1), 39-49.

Holcomb, S. (2005a). Anemia. *Nursing2005, 35*(3), 53.

Holcomb, S. (2005b). Recognizing and managing anemia. *The Nurse Practitioner, 20*(12), 16-31.

The Joint Commission. (2007). *National Patient Safety Goals Patient Identification.* Retrieved May 20, 2008, from www.jointcommission.org.

*Kasamon, Y., & Swinnen, L. (2004). Treatment advances in adult Burkitt lymphoma and leukemia. *Current Opinion in Oncology*, 16, 429-435.

Khattab, A.D., Rawlings, B., & Ali, I.S. (2006). Care of patients with haemoglobin abnormalities: Nursing management. *British Journal of Nursing, 15* (19), 1057-1062.

Kurtin, S. (2006). Advances in the management of low- to intermediate-risk myelodysplastic syndrome: Integrating the National Comprehensive Cancer Network guidelines. *Clinical Journal of Oncology Nursing, 10*(2), 197-208.

Kyles, D. (2007). Is your patient having a transfusion reaction? *Nursing2007, 37*(4), 64hn1-64hn4.

Laffan, A., & Biedrzycki, B. (2006). Immune reconstitution: The foundation for safe living after an allogeneic hematopoietic stem cell transplantation. *Clinical Journal of Oncology Nursing, 10*(6), 787-794.

Leighton, S. (2008). The spin on apheresis. *Nursing2008, 38*(4), 29-31.

Long, J., & Versa, L. (2006). Treatment approaches and nursing considerations for non-Hodgkin's lymphoma. *Seminars in Oncology Nursing, 22*(2), 97-106.

*Lynn, A., Williams, M., Sickler, J., & Burgess, S. (2003). Treatment of chronic lymphocytic leukemia with alemtuzumab: A review for nurses. *Oncology Nursing Forum, 30*(4), 689-696.

Mangan, P. (2005). Recognizing multiple myeloma. *The Nurse Practitioner, 30*(3), 14-27.

Mangan, P. (2006). Teach your patient about multiple myeloma. *Nursing2006, 36*(4), 64hn1-64hn4.

Mason, S. (2006). Mucosa-associated lymphoid tissue (MALT) lymphoma. *Seminars in Oncology Nursing, 22*(2), 73-79.

McCance, K., & Huether, S. (2006). *Pathophysiology: The biologic basis for disease in adults and children* (5th ed.). St. Louis: Mosby.

Moorhead, S., Johnson, M., & Maas, M. (Eds.). (2004). *Nursing outcomes classification (NOC)* (3rd ed.). St. Louis: Mosby.

Mullen, E., & Wang, M. (2007). Recognizing hyperviscosity syndrome in patients with Waldenström macroglobulinemia. *Clinical Journal of Oncology Nursing, 11*(1), 87-95.

Munson, B.L. (2005). Myths & facts…about polycythemia vera. *Nursing2005, 35*(5), 28.

National Comprehensive Cancer Network (NCCN). (2005). *Clinical practice guidelines in oncology: Non-Hodgkin's lymphoma.* Jenkintown, PA: National Comprehensive Cancer Network, pp. 1-62. Retrieved March 3, 2007, from www.nccn.org.

Nussbaum, R., McInnes, R., & Willard, H. (2007). *Thompson & Thompson: Genetics in medicine* (7th ed.). Philadelphia: Saunders.

Pacholok, S. (2007). Simple steps to stamp out vitamin B_{12} deficiency. *Nursing2007, 37*(1), 67-69.

Pfadt, E., & Carlson, D. (2005). Transfusion-associated graft-versus-host disease. *Nursing2005, 35*(2), 88.

Pullen, R. (2005). Administering medication by the Z-track method. *Nursing2005, 35*(7), 24.

Ramos-Casals, M., De Vita, S., & Tzioufas, A.G. (2005). Hepatitis C virus, Sjögren's syndrome, and B-cell lymphoma: Linking infection, autoimmunity, and cancer. *Autoimmunity Reviews, 4*(1), 8-15.

*Riley, M.B., & Byar, K. (2004). The rationale for and background of radioimmunotherapy: An emerging therapy for B-cell non-Hodgkin's lymphoma. *Seminars in Oncology Nursing, 20* (Suppl. 1), 1-7.

Robinson, P. (2005). Is surgery safe for a patient with hemophilia? *Nursing2005, 35*(5), 32hn1-32hn3.

Rogers, B. (2005). Lymphoma & leukemia. *Nursing2005, 35*(7), 56-63.

Rogers, B. (2006). Overview of non-Hodgkin's lymphoma. *Seminars in Oncology Nursing, 22*(2), 67-72.

Saria, M., & Gosselin-Acomb, T. (2007). Hematopoietic stem cell transplantation: Implications for critical care nurses. *Clinical Journal of Oncology Nursing, 11*(1), 53-63.

Sickle Cell Information Center. (2007). Emory University. Atlanta, GA. Website: www.scinfo.org

*Simmons, P. (2003). A primer for nurses who administer blood products. *MEDSURG Nursing, 12*(3), 184-192.

Steingass, S. (2006). Hematopoietic cell transplantation in non-Hodgkin's lymphoma. *Seminars in Oncology Nursing, 22*(2), 107-116.

Todd, K.H. (2006). Sickle cell disease related pain: Crisis and conflict… second in a series. *Journal of Pain, 7*(7), 453-458.

Weaver, B., & McDonald, M. (2006). What you need to know about transfusing platelets. *Nursing2006, 36*(6), 26-27.

Williams, L. (2007). Whatever it takes: Informal caregiving dynamics in blood and marrow transplantation. *Oncology Nursing Forum, 34*(2), 379-387.

Zarowitz, B. (2007). Erythropoietic-stimulating agents (ESAs): New safety warning. *Geriatric Nursing, 28*(3), 148-150.

Zhong, Y. (2006). Non-Hodgkin lymphoma: What primary care professionals need to know. *The Journal for Nurse Practitioners, 2*(5), 309-315, 338.

HUMAN NEEDS OVERVIEW

Mobility, Sensation, and Cognition

The term *mobility* means movement. When referring to physical mobility, it means the ability of the body to move. Mobility is needed for ADL performance and many body functions, including digestion, elimination, circulation, and muscle integrity. In some cases, it helps keep a person *safe* by being able to move to prevent injury.

Mobility is primarily accomplished through the integration of the neurologic and musculoskeletal body systems. Adequate energy from food is needed to nourish the cells of these systems to promote proper function and energy.

Sensation refers to receiving sensory input from the cells of the skin (feeling), eyes (seeing), and ears (hearing) and accurately interpreting this input in the neurons of the central nervous system (CNS). Therefore sensation is also needed to keep the body *safe*. For example, if a person cannot feel water temperature, a burn may result. If vision is impaired, a fall may occur.

Cognition refers to mental processes and intellectual function and is controlled by certain neurons in the gray matter of the brain. These cells are very sensitive to serum glucose and oxygen levels. If either of these substances falls below the amounts needed, the cells cannot function properly, resulting in diminished cognitive ability and a decreased level of consciousness.

Appropriate judgment and decision making are needed to keep a person *safe*. These cognitive processes also allow a person to perform day-to-day activities such as knowing when to eat or how to drive a car.

One or all of these three human needs may be unmet as a result of disease, injury, surgery, or drugs. Problems of the neurologic, sensory, and musculoskeletal systems most commonly affect the need for mobility, sensation, and cognition. The interrelationship of these needs can be compared to a computer and its parts.

As seen in Fig. 1, the computer's central processing unit (CPU), or processor, is the brain of the machine (the *cognitive* center). Much like the spinal cord, it works with the motherboard to send and receive messages (input and output). The connected pins and wires

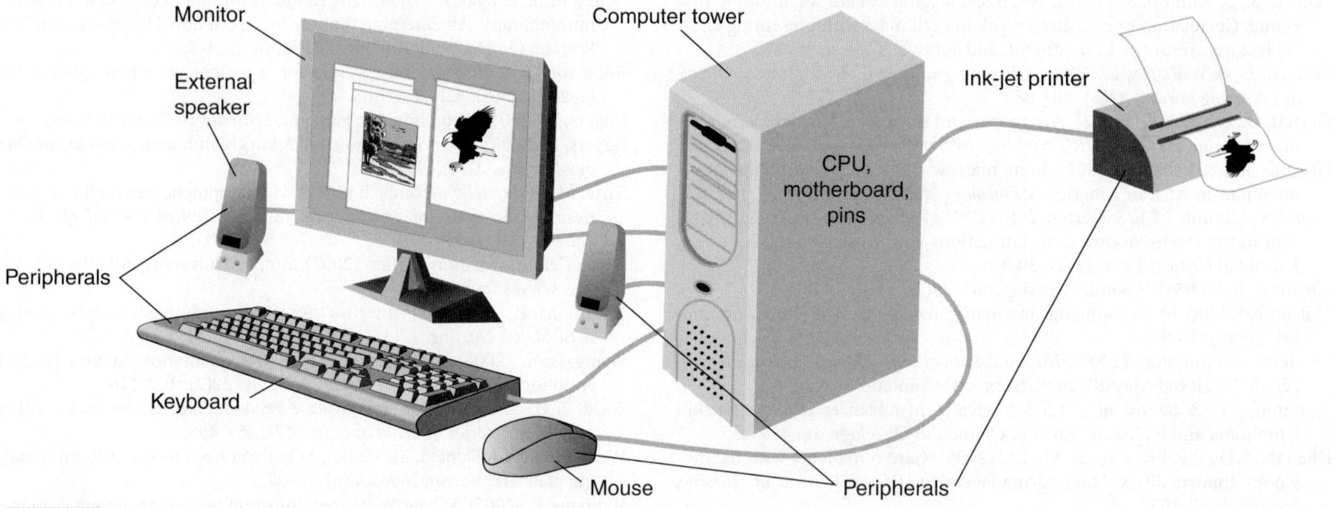

Monitor
Computer tower
External speaker
Ink-jet printer
CPU, motherboard, pins
Peripherals
Keyboard
Mouse
Peripherals

Fig. 1

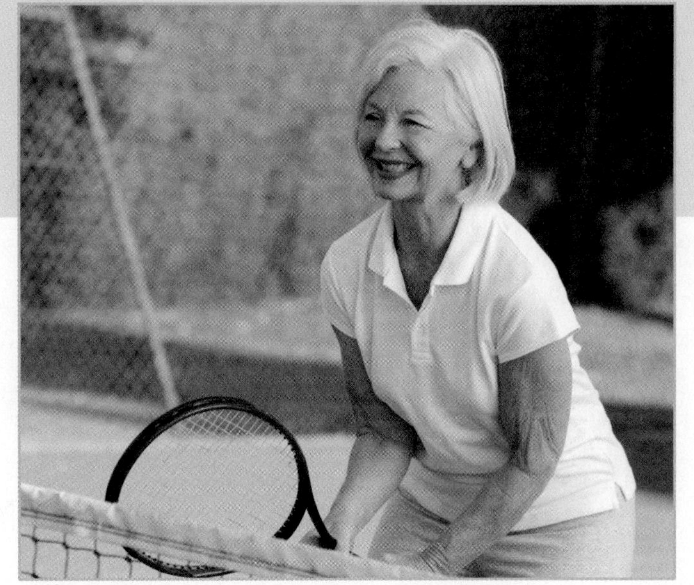

function like the spinal nerves. Peripherals such as the mouse and keyboard are similar in function to the peripheral nervous system (PNS) *(sensation)* and musculoskeletal system *(mobility)*. When all of these parts are working properly, the computer functions without any problems.

However, when the CPU (brain) does not work properly (decreased cognition), the motherboard (spinal cord) and/or peripherals (PNS and muscles) may not function as they should (decreased mobility and sensation). If the motherboard (spinal cord) is broken, no information is sent to or from any of the other parts of the computer. In both cases, there is no display on the monitor (Fig. 2).

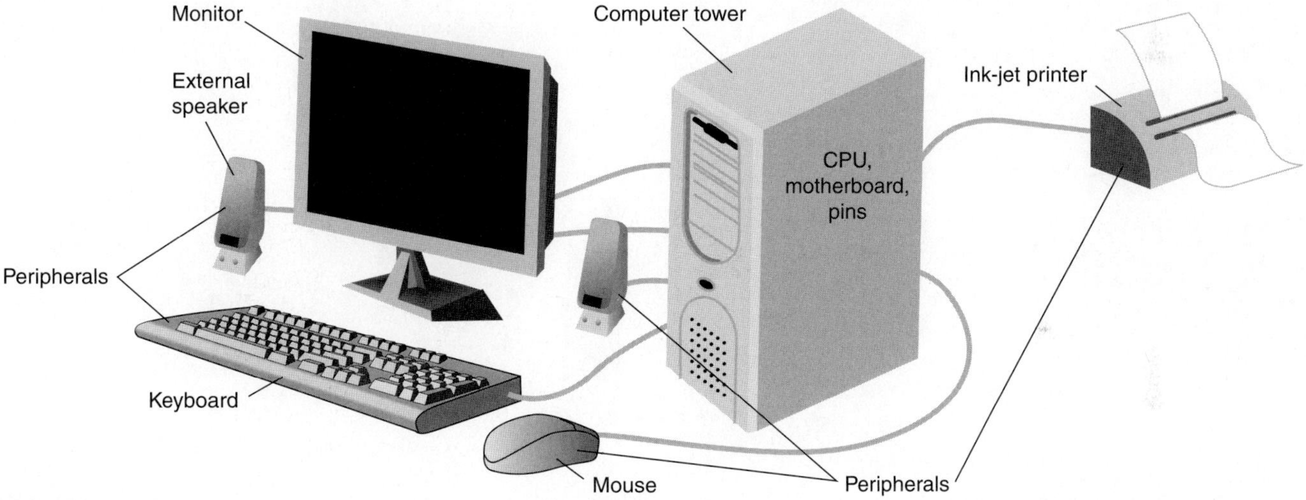

Monitor
Computer tower
External speaker
Ink-jet printer
CPU, motherboard, pins
Peripherals
Keyboard
Mouse
Peripherals

Fig. 2

X

UNIT

Problems of Mobility, Sensation, and Cognition

Management of Patients with Problems of the Nervous System

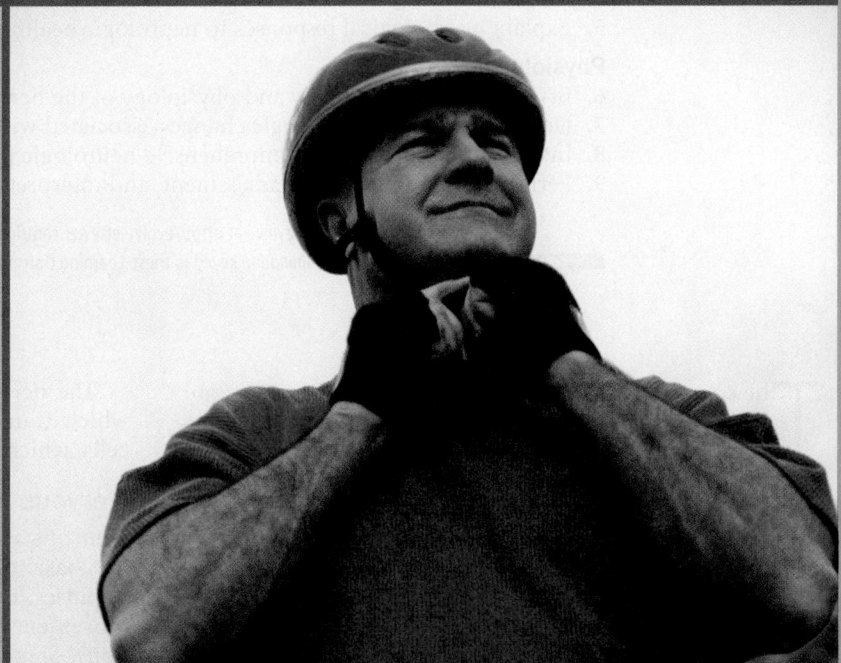

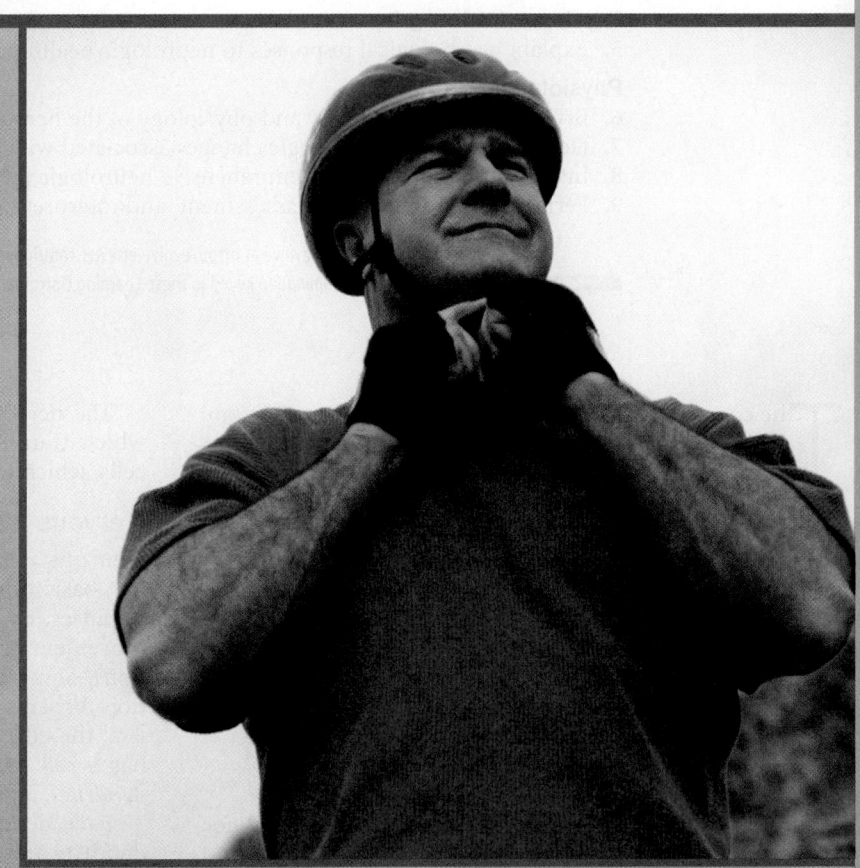

43 CHAPTER

Assessment of the Nervous System

Kathy A. Hausman

LEARNING OUTCOMES

For clinical competence and success on the NCLEX Examination, study this chapter with these Learning Outcomes in mind:

Safe and Effective Care Environment

1. Determine a patient's allergy to contrast media before diagnostic testing.
2. Assess patients for complications of neurologic diagnostic tests.

Health Promotion and Maintenance

3. Identify factors that place patients at risk for neurologic health problems.
4. Explain pre- and post-test care associated with neurologic diagnostic testing.

Psychosocial Integrity

5. Explain psychological responses to neurologic health problems.

Physiological Integrity

6. Briefly review the anatomy and physiology of the nervous system.
7. Describe common physiologic changes associated with aging that affect the nervous system.
8. Interpret findings from a comprehensive neurologic physical assessment.
9. Perform a rapid neurologic assessment, and interpret findings.

evolve Go to your Companion CD or Evolve at http://evolve.elsevier.com/Iggy/ for *Self-Assessment Questions for the NCLEX Examination* keyed to these Learning Outcomes.

The complex nervous system controls *mobility, sensation,* and *cognition.* In addition, through the autonomic nervous system (ANS) it innervates many other body systems to make them function. For example, the sacral spinal nerves (part of the ANS) stimulate the detrusor muscle to contract when the urinary bladder is full.

Health problems involving trauma and diseases of the brain can impair the human needs for mobility, sensation, and/or cognition. When the spine or peripheral nervous system is affected, mobility and/or sensation is often impaired. The primary role of the nurse is to help restore these human needs or to assist the patient to adapt to their deficits.

ANATOMY AND PHYSIOLOGY REVIEW

The major divisions of the nervous system are the central nervous system (CNS) and the peripheral nervous system (PNS). The brain and spinal cord are the major components of the CNS. The PNS is composed of 12 pairs of cranial nerves, 31 pairs of spinal nerves, and the autonomic nervous system. The autonomic nervous system is further subdivided into sympathetic and parasympathetic fibers.

The nervous system contains two types of cells: neurons, which transmit or conduct nerve impulses; and neuroglial cells, which have an interdependent role with the neuron.

Nervous System Cells: Structure and Function

Neurons

The basic unit of the nervous system, the neuron, transmits impulses, or "messages." Some neurons are **motor** (causing movement or mobility), and some are **sensory** (causing sensation). Some process information, and some retain information. When a neuron receives an impulse from another neuron, the effect may be excitation or inhibition. Each neuron has a *cell body,* or *soma;* short, branching processes called *dendrites;* and a single *axon* (Fig. 43-1).

Each dendrite synapses with another cell body, axon, or dendrite and brings information *to* the cell body from other neurons by an *afferent pathway.* An *efferent pathway* sends messages *from* the neuron's cell body to other neurons through an axon. Only one axon is attached to each neuron, which may extend long distances, often down the entire spinal cord.

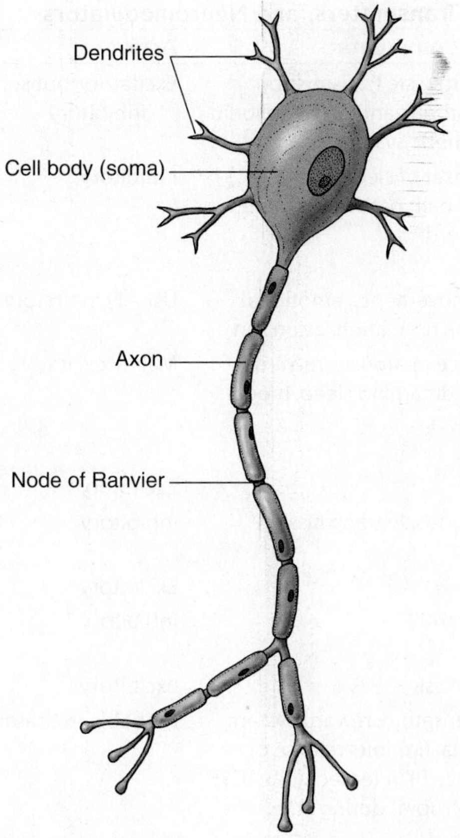
Dendrites
Cell body (soma)
Axon
Node of Ranvier

Fig. 43-1 • The structure of a typical neuron.

Many axons are covered by a **myelin sheath**—a white, lipid covering. Myelinated axons appear whitish and therefore are also called **white matter.** Nonmyelinated axons have a grayish cast and are called **gray matter.** Myelinated axons have gaps in the myelin called *nodes of Ranvier.* The nodes of Ranvier play a major role in impulse conduction (see Fig. 43-1). When the myelin is impaired, the impulses cannot travel from the brain to the rest of the body, such as in patients with multiple sclerosis.

The enlarged, distal end of each axon is called the *synaptic* or *terminal knob.* Within the synaptic knobs are the mechanisms for manufacturing, storing, and releasing a transmitter substance. Each neuron produces a specific **neurotransmitter** substance, or chemical (e.g., acetylcholine or serotonin), that can either enhance or inhibit the impulse but cannot do both. Other substances, although not specifically identified as neurotransmitters, are considered probable transmitters or neuromodulators. Table 43-1 summarizes what is currently known about the major chemicals of the nervous system.

Impulses are transmitted to their eventual destination through synapses, or spaces between neurons. There are two distinct types of synapses: *neuron to neuron* and *neuron to muscle* (or gland). Between the terminal knob and the next cell is a small space called the *synaptic cleft.* The knob, the cleft, and the portion of the cell to which the impulse is being transmitted make up the **synapse.**

Several factors affect the transmission of an impulse, such as distance and strength. Synapses on or near the body of the cell have greater influence than those farther along the dendrite. The strength of the stimulus can also be influenced by other mechanisms, such as inhibition by another neuron, inadequate supply of transmitter substance, and extracellular fluid (ECF) changes. Lack of oxygen or the effects of hypnotics and anesthetics can quickly depress nerve cell activity. For example, in older adults, lack of oxygen to the brain often causes changes in mental state.

Changes in the pH of ECF also affect neuron transmission. For example, acidosis depresses nerve cell activity. Alkalosis, on the other hand, excites nerve cells (see Chapter 13). Increased nerve cell activity occurs with the use of some drugs, such as caffeine (in coffee), theophylline (in tea and some asthma drugs), and theobromine (in cocoa).

Neuroglial Cells

Neuroglial cells, which vary in size and shape, provide protection, structure, and nutrition for the neurons. They are classified into four types: astroglial cells, ependymal cells, oligodendrocytes, and microglial cells. These cells are also part of the blood-brain barrier and help regulate cerebrospinal fluid (CSF).

Central Nervous System: Structure and Function

The central nervous system (CNS) is composed of the *brain,* which directs the regulation and function of the nervous system and all other systems of the body, and the *spinal cord,* which starts reflex activity and transmits impulses to and from the brain.

Brain

The **meninges** form the protective covering of the brain and the spinal cord. The outside layer is the *dura mater.* The **subdural space** is located between the dura mater and the middle layer, the *arachnoid.* The *pia mater* is the most inner layer. Situated between the arachnoid and pia mater is the **subarachnoid space,** where CSF circulates. A potential space, referred to as the *epidural space,* is located between the skull and the outer layer of the dura. This area also extends down the spinal cord and is important in the delivery of epidural analgesia and anesthesia.

The dura also lies between the cerebral hemispheres and the cerebellum and is called the *tentorium.* It helps decrease or prevent the transmission of force from one hemisphere to another and protect the lower brainstem when head trauma occurs. Clinical references may be made to a lesion (e.g., a tumor) as being **supratentorial** (above the tentorium) or **infratentorial** (below the tentorium).

The brain is composed of several parts: cerebrum, diencephalon, hypophysis (pituitary gland), cerebellum, and brainstem. Each part is briefly described here.

Major Parts of the Brain

◀ ANIMATION: Physiology of the Brain

The right and left hemispheres of the *cerebrum* are joined by the corpus callosum. The *left* hemisphere is the dominant hemisphere in most people (even in many left-handed people). Within the deeper structures of the cerebrum are the right and left lateral ventricles. At the base of the cerebrum near the ventricles is a group of neurons called the *basal ganglia,* which regulate the human needs for *mobility.*.

Located in the frontal lobe, the **motor cortex** controls voluntary movement. Corticospinal tracts, also called *pyramidal tracts,* begin in the motor cortex and travel through the brain before crossing in the medulla. This crossing explains how right motor cortex damage affects the movement in the left side of the body and vice versa, such as in many patients who

TABLE 43-1 Sites, Functions, and Actions of Transmitters, Probable Transmitters, and Neuromodulators

Transmitter Substance	Site	Function/Comments	Action
Acetylcholine	Brain, brainstem, basal ganglia, autonomic nervous system	Nerve and muscle transmission Parasympathetic and preganglionic sympathetic system	Excitatory, but some inhibitory
Serotonin	Medial brainstem, hypothalamus, dorsal horn of spinal cord	Possible onset of sleep, mood control; pain pathway inhibitor in spinal cord	Inhibitory
CATECHOLAMINES			
Dopamine	Substantia nigra to basal ganglia	Complex movements, emotional response regulation, attention	Usually inhibitory
Norepinephrine (epinephrine parallels)	Hypothalamus, brainstem, reticular formation, cerebellum, sympathetic nervous system	Maintenance of arousal, reward system, dreaming sleep, mood regulation	Mainly excitatory
AMINO ACIDS			
Aspartate	Brain, spinal cord interneurons	Sensation	Excitatory
Gamma-aminobutyric acid (GABA)	Brain, brainstem, basal ganglia, autonomic nervous system	Nerve and muscle transmission	Inhibitory
Glutamate	Sensory pathways	Sensation	Excitatory
Glycine	Spinal cord interneurons	Muscle control	Inhibitory
PEPTIDES*			
Substance P	Brain, neurons in spinal cord	Pain transmission	Excitatory
Endorphins, enkephalins	Thalamus, hypothalamus, spinal cord, pituitary	Pleasure sensation, reward system, analgesia, (inhibits release of substance P), released with ACTH (corticotropin) during stress	Probably excitatory
GASES			
Nitric acid	Neurons	Not stored in specific site; made by enzymes as needed; released by diffusion	Excitatory
Carbon monoxide	Neurons	Function not well understood	Questionable

*Other peptides under investigation as probable transmitters are vasopressin (ADH), gastrin, cholecystokinin, glucagon, insulin, somatostatin, angiotensin, melanocyte-stimulating hormone (MSH), luteinizing hormone–releasing hormone (LH-RH), and thyrotropin-releasing hormone (TRH). Prostaglandins, also under investigation, are thought to be modulators.

have cerebral strokes. The cerebrum is divided into lobes by sulci (fissures). These lobes work together and are connected by nerve fibers. The name and main function of each lobe is listed in Table 43-2.

Two important speech areas of the cerebrum are Broca's area and Wernicke's area. **Broca's area** (speech area), also located in the frontal lobe, is responsible for the formation of words, or speech. **Wernicke's area** (language area) is located in the temporal lobe and allows processing of words into coherent thought and understanding of written or spoken words.

The *diencephalon,* which lies below the cerebrum, includes the thalamus, hypothalamus, and epithalamus (Fig. 43-2). The **thalamus** is the major "relay station," or "central switchboard," for the CNS. The **hypothalamus** plays a major role in autonomic nervous system control (controlling temperature and other functions) and intellectual function (cognition). The epithalamus contains the roof of the third ventricle and the pineal gland.

The *hypophysis (pituitary gland)* has two lobes, each releasing specific hormones into the circulation under the regulation of the hypothalamus. The pituitary is often referred to as the "master gland" because of its control of numerous hormonal functions. However, the hypothalamus actually controls its functions.

The *cerebellum* receives immediate and continuous information about the condition of the muscles, joints, and tendons. Cerebellar function enables a person to:

- Keep an extremity from overshooting an intended target
- Move from one skilled movement to another in an orderly sequence
- Predict distance or gauge the speed with which one is approaching an object
- Control voluntary movement
- Maintain equilibrium

Unlike the motor cortex, cerebellar control of the body is **ipsilateral** (situated on the same side). The right side of the cerebellum controls the right side of the body, and the left cerebellum controls the left side of the body.

The brainstem includes the midbrain, pons, and medulla. The functions of these structures are presented in Table 43-3. Throughout the brainstem are special cells that constitute the **reticular activating system (RAS),** which controls awareness and alertness. For example, this tissue awakens a person from sleep when presented with a stimulus like loud noise, when there is pain, or when it is time to awaken. The reticular formation area has many connections with the cerebrum, the rest of the brainstem, and the cerebellum.

TABLE 43-2 Brain Lobe Main Functions

FRONTAL LOBE
- The primary motor area (also known as the *motor "strip"* or *cortex*)
- Broca's speech center on the dominant side
- Voluntary eye movement
- Access to current sensory data
- Access to past information or experience
- Affective response to a situation
- Regulates behavior based on judgment and foresight
- Judgment
- Ability to develop long-term goals
- Reasoning, concentration, abstraction

PARIETAL LOBE
- Understand sensation, texture, size, shape, and spatial relationships
- Three-dimensional (spatial) perception
- Important for singing, playing musical instruments, and processing nonverbal visual experiences
- Perception of body parts and body position awareness
- Taste impulses for interpretation

TEMPORAL LOBE
- Auditory center for sound interpretation
- Complicated memory patterns
- Wernicke's area for speech

OCCIPITAL LOBE
- Primary visual center

LIMBIC LOBE
- Emotional and visceral patterns connected with survival
- Learning and memory

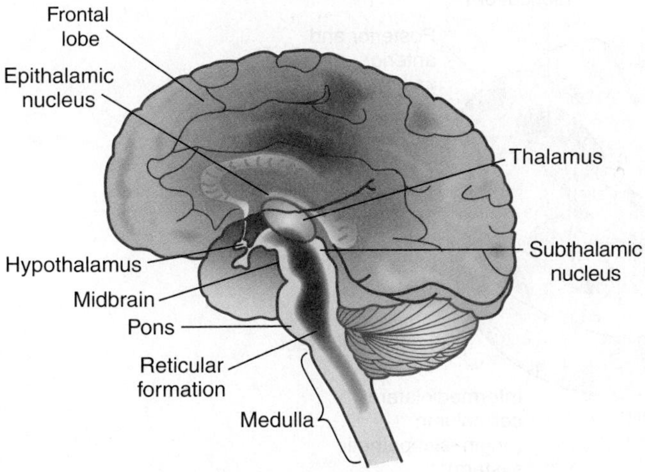

Frontal lobe
Epithalamic nucleus
Thalamus
Hypothalamus
Subthalamic nucleus
Midbrain
Pons
Reticular formation
Medulla

Fig. 43-2 • The structures of the brainstem and diencephalon.

Circulation in the Brain

Circulation in the brain originates from the carotid and vertebral arteries (Fig. 43-3). The internal carotid arteries branch into the anterior cerebral artery (ACA) and middle cerebral arteries (MCA), the largest ones. The two posterior vertebral arteries become the basilar artery, which then divides into two posterior cerebral arteries. The anterior, middle, and posterior cerebral arteries are joined together by small communicating arteries to form a ring at the base of the brain known as the **circle of Willis.**

The *middle* cerebral artery supplies the lateral surface of the cerebrum from about the mid-temporal lobe upward (i.e., the area for hearing and upper body motor and sensory neurons). The *anterior* cerebral artery supplies the midline, or medial, aspect of the same area (i.e., the lower body motor and sensory neurons). The *posterior* cerebral arteries supply the area from the mid-temporal region down and back (occipital lobe), as well as much of the brainstem. When blood flow is interrupted in any of these arteries (e.g., by a clot), the area of the brain being supplied is affected and may not function as it should.

The *blood-brain barrier (BBB)* seems to exist because the endothelial cells of the cerebral capillaries are joined tightly together. This barrier keeps some substances in the bloodstream out of the cerebrospinal circulation and out of brain tissue. Substances that can pass through the BBB include oxygen, glucose, carbon dioxide, alcohol, anesthetics, and water. Large molecules such as albumin, any substance bound to albumin, and many antibiotics are prevented from crossing the barrier.

Cerebrospinal fluid (CSF) also circulates, surrounds, and cushions the brain and spinal cord. While moving through the subarachnoid space, the fluid is continuously produced by the choroid plexus, reabsorbed by the arachnoid villi, and then channeled into the superior sagittal sinus. Expanded areas of subarachnoid space, where there are large amounts of CSF, are called *cisterns.* The largest one is the lumbar cistern, the site of lumbar puncture, from the level of the second lumbar vertebra to the second sacral vertebra (L2-S2).

TABLE 43-3 Brainstem Functions

MEDULLA
- Cardiac-slowing center
- Respiratory center
- Cranial nerves IX (glossopharyngeal), X (vagus), XI (accessory), and XII (hypoglossal) emerge from the medulla, as do portions of cranial nerves VII (facial) and VIII (acoustic)

PONS
- Cardiac acceleration and vasoconstriction centers
- Pneumotaxic center helps control respiratory pattern and rate
- Four cranial nerves originate from the pons: V (trigeminal), VI (abducens), VII (facial), and VIII (acoustic)

MIDBRAIN
- Contains the cerebral aqueduct or aqueduct of Sylvius
- Location of periaqueductal gray, which may abolish pain when stimulated
- Cranial nerve nuclei III (oculomotor) and IV (trochlear) located here

Spinal Cord

The spinal cord controls body movement *(mobility);* regulates organ function; processes sensory information from the extremities, trunk, and many internal organs *(sensation);* and transmits information to and from the brain. It contains H-shaped **gray matter** (neuron cell bodies) that is surrounded by **white matter** (myelinated axons). The white matter is divided into posterior, lateral, and anterior columns. Groups of cells in the white matter (ascending and descending tracts) have been fairly well identified (Fig. 43-4).

Ascending Tracts

Ascending tracts originate in the spinal cord and end in the brain. Three groups of ascending tracts are important for understanding the patient with neurologic problems: spinotha-

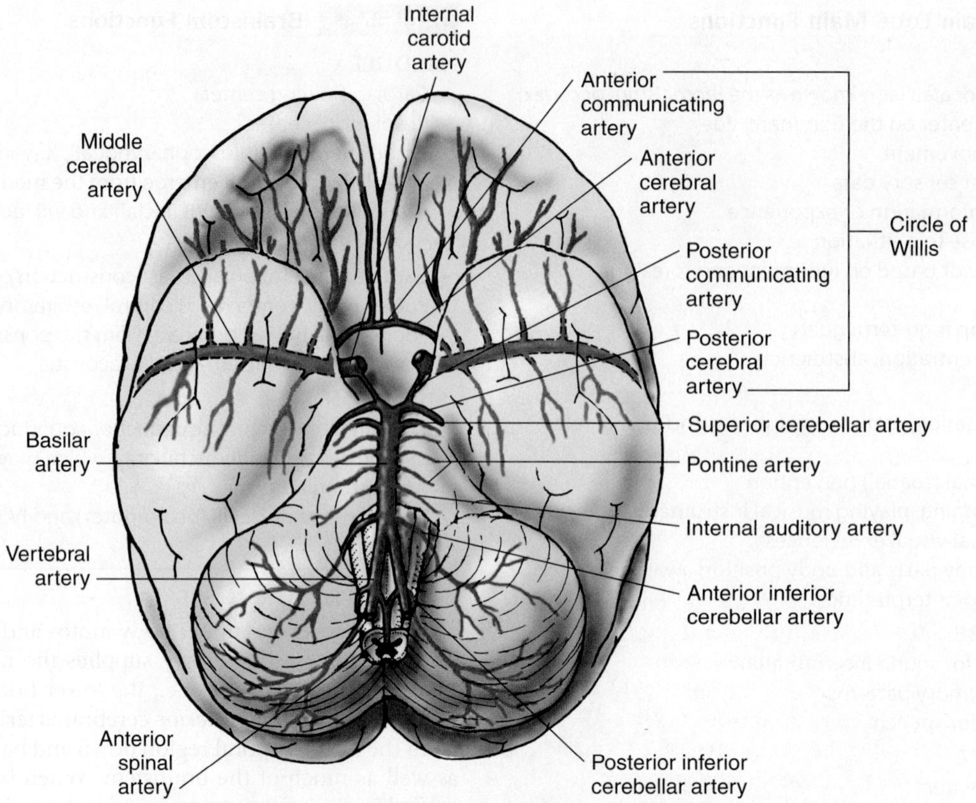
Internal carotid artery
Anterior communicating artery
Middle cerebral artery
Anterior cerebral artery
Circle of Willis
Posterior communicating artery
Posterior cerebral artery
Superior cerebellar artery
Basilar artery
Pontine artery
Internal auditory artery
Vertebral artery
Anterior inferior cerebellar artery
Anterior spinal artery
Posterior inferior cerebellar artery

Fig. 43-3 • Cerebral circulation and the circle of Willis at the base of the brain.

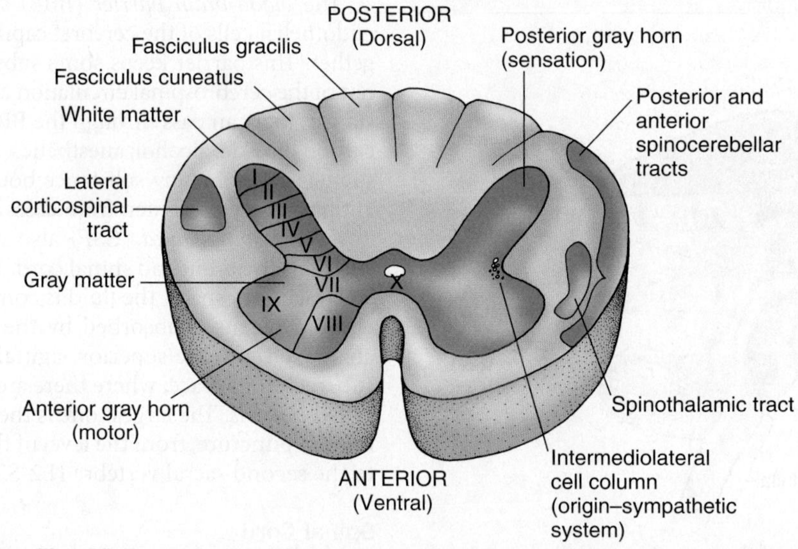
POSTERIOR (Dorsal)
Fasciculus gracilis
Fasciculus cuneatus
White matter
Posterior gray horn (sensation)
Posterior and anterior spinocerebellar tracts
Lateral corticospinal tract
I
II
III
IV
V
VI
VII
VIII
IX
X
Gray matter
Anterior gray horn (motor)
Spinothalamic tract
ANTERIOR (Ventral)
Intermediolateral cell column (origin–sympathetic system)

Fig. 43-4 • A cross section of the spinal cord showing the common tracts.

lamic tracts, spinocerebellar tracts, and fasciculi gracilis and cuneatus (posterior white columns).

As the name indicates, *spinothalamic* tracts begin in the spinal cord with most ending in the thalamus. These tracts carry sensations of pain, temperature, light touch, and pressure. The axon fibers from the cells cross to the opposite side and then continue up to the thalamus. Some branches end in the medulla and pons.

Spinocerebellar tracts begin in the spinal cord and end in the cerebellum. The *posterior* spinocerebellar tract transmits impulses of **proprioception** (awareness of position and movements of body parts) or movement, mostly from the lower extremities. The impulses enter the posterior gray horn and synapse with tract cells in lamina VII. Spinocerebellar axons then form the tract on the *same,* or ipsilateral, side. This tract begins at the second lumbar level and ascends to the medulla and then to the cerebellum.

The *anterior* spinocerebellar tract begins lower in the lumbar spine than does the posterior tract. These fibers cross immediately and ascend as an opposite-side tract, transmitting proprioceptive impulses from the lower extremities. The fibers cross again in the midbrain on their way to the cerebellum.

Because these fibers have crossed the midline twice, the sensations end on the side on which they started.

The *posterior white columns* transmit this information to the thalamus:

- The sensation of proprioception from muscles, joints, and tendons
- Vibratory sense
- Light touch from the skin
- Localization

Most of the fibers ascend on the *same* side as their origin to the medulla, where they cross and then synapse in the thalamus, with termination in the parietal lobe. This tract allows a person to feel an exact point of pressure on the skin. Recognition of pressure includes the shape of an object (with eyes closed), movement across the skin (a number being written), and awareness of two points of touch close together (two-point discrimination).

Descending Tracts

Descending tracts *begin* in the brain and *end* in the spinal cord. The major descending tract of importance for understanding neurologic problems is the lateral *corticospinal,* or *pyramidal,* tract. The corticospinal tract originates in the motor cortex of the frontal lobe and portions of the parietal lobe. The lateral tract fibers cross to the opposite side at the level of the medulla. After crossing, the fibers descend and synapse with interneurons of the gray matter in the spinal cord. These few fibers connect directly with lower motor neurons (LMNs). The cervical spine has a high concentration of fibers synapsing with interneurons, which possibly reflects the complexity of hand and finger movements.

The motor neurons of the other descending tracts and the basal ganglia used to be referred to as an *extrapyramidal system.* It was thought that pyramidal neurons caused voluntary muscle activity and that extrapyramidal neurons caused automatic or nonvoluntary muscle action. However, all of the descending tracts and the basal ganglia are necessary for *mobility.* The term *extrapyramidal* is still often used clinically, meaning *abnormal spontaneous movement.*

Peripheral Nervous System: Structure and Function

The peripheral nervous system (PNS) is composed of the spinal nerves, cranial nerves, and autonomic nervous system.

There are 31 pairs of spinal nerves (8 cervical, 12 thoracic, 5 lumbar, 5 sacral, and 1 coccygeal) exiting from the spinal cord. Each of the nerves has a posterior and an anterior branch. The posterior branch carries sensory information (sensation) to the cord *(afferent pathway).* The anterior branch transmits motor impulses (mobility) to the muscles of the body *(efferent pathway).*

Each spinal nerve is responsible for the muscle innervation and sensory reception of a given area of the body. The cervical and thoracic spinal nerves are relatively close to their areas of responsibility, whereas the lumbar and sacral spinal nerves are some distance from theirs. Because the spinal cord ends between L1 and L2, the axons of the lumbar and sacral cord extend downward before exiting at the appropriate intervertebral foramen. The area controlled by each spinal nerve is roughly reflected in the dermatomes. **Dermatomes** represent sensory input from spinal nerves to specific areas of the skin (Fig. 43-5). For example, the patient with an injury to cervical spinal nerves C6 and C7 has sensory changes in the thumb, index finger, middle finger, middle of the palm, and back of the hand.

Sensory receptors throughout the body monitor and transmit impulses of pain, temperature, touch, vibration, pressure, visceral sensation, and proprioception. Sensory receptors also monitor and transmit the sensations of the special senses—vision, taste, smell, and hearing.

The cell bodies of the anterior spinal nerves are located in the anterior gray matter (anterior horn) of each level in the spinal cord. The anterior motor neurons are also referred to as *lower motor neurons.* As each nerve axon leaves the spinal cord, it joins other spinal nerves to form **plexuses** (clusters of nerves). Plexuses continue as trunks, divisions, and cords and finally branch into individual peripheral nerves.

The **reflex arc** is a closed circuit of spinal and peripheral nerves and therefore requires no control by the brain (Fig. 43-6).

Reflexes consist of sensory input from:

- Skeletal muscles, tendons, skin, organs, and special senses
- Small cells in the spinal cord lying between the posterior and anterior gray matter (interneurons)
- Anterior motor neurons, along with the muscles they innervate

There are 12 *cranial nerves.* Their name, number, origin, type, and function are summarized in Table 43-4. Cranial nerve function is an important part of the nursing assessment of the patient with a neurologic problem. For example, cranial nerves II, III, IV and VI are important for assessment of the patient with a stroke.

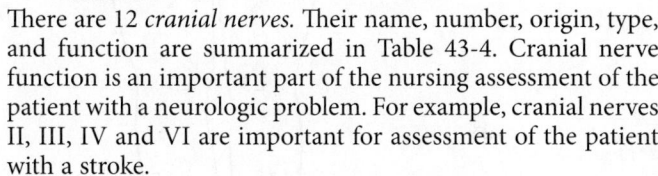

◀ ANIMATION: Cranial Nerves

Autonomic Nervous System: Structure and Function

The **autonomic nervous system (ANS)** is composed of two parts: the sympathetic nervous system (SNS), or the "fight or flight system"; and the parasympathetic nervous system (PNS). ANS functions are not usually under conscious control but may be altered in some people by using biofeedback and other methods.

The SNS cells originate in the gray matter of the spinal cord from T1 through L2 or L3. This part of the ANS is considered *thoracolumbar* because of its anatomic location. The SNS stimulates the functions of the body needed for "fight or flight" (e.g., heart and respiratory rate). It also inhibits those functions not needed in this situation.

The PNS cells originate in the gray matter of the sacral area of the spinal cord (from S2 through S4) plus portions of cranial nerves III, VII, IX, and X *(craniosacral).* The PNS can slow body functions when needed.

Parasympathetic fibers to the organs have some sensory ability in addition to motor function. Sensations of irritation, stretching of an organ, or a decrease in tissue oxygen are transmitted to the thalamus through pathways not yet fully understood. Because pain from internal organs is often felt below the body wall innervated by the spinal nerve, it is presumed that there are connections between the viscera and body structure that relay pain sensations.

NEUROLOGIC CHANGES ASSOCIATED WITH AGING

Neurologic changes associated with aging often affect mobility and sensation. *Motor changes* in late adulthood can cause slower movement and response time and decreased sensation

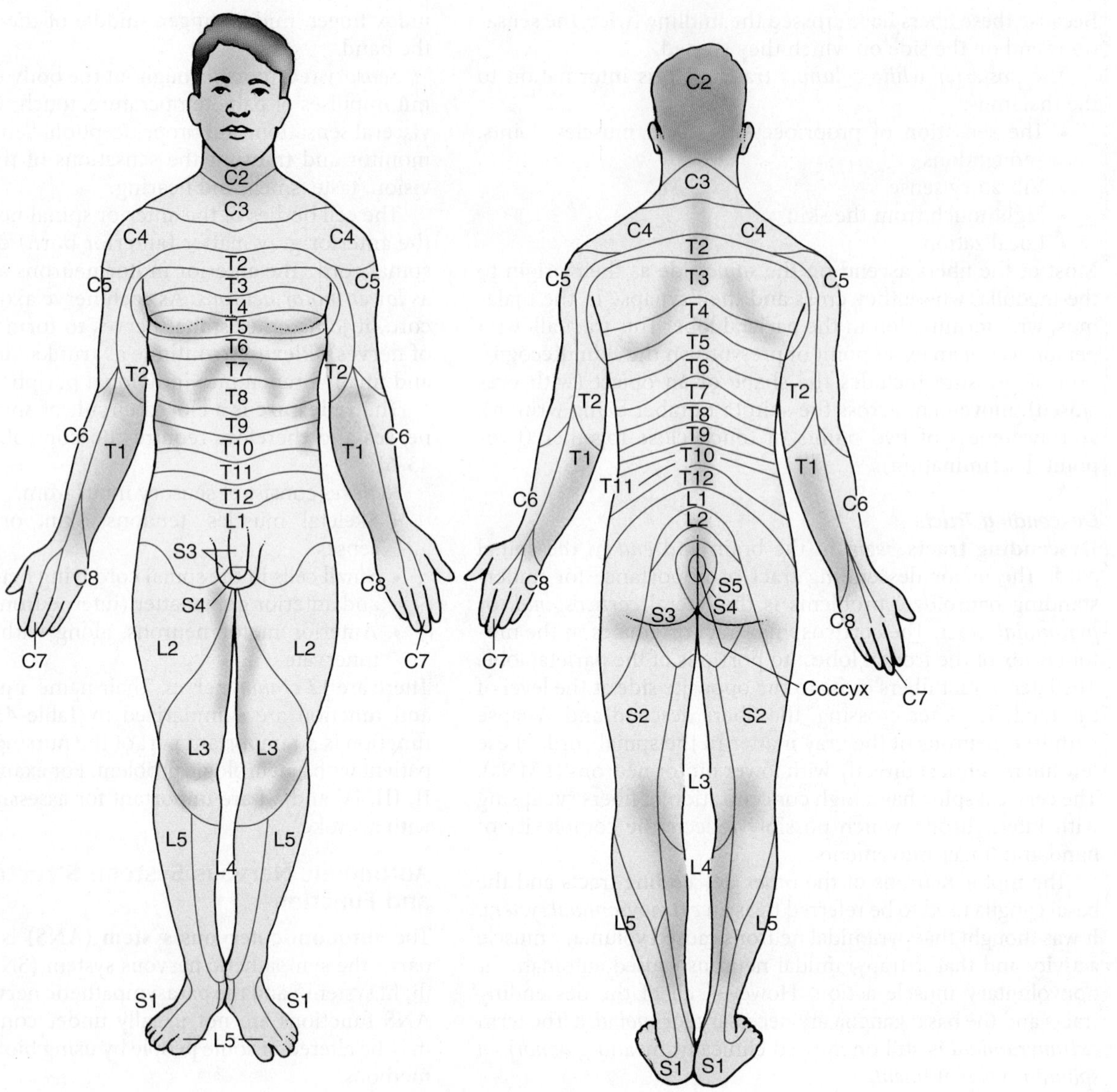
C2
C3
C4
C4
C5
C5
T2
T3
T4
T5
T6
T7
T8
T9
T10
T11
T12
T2
T2
C6
C6
T1
T1
L1
S3
S4
C8
C8
C7
C7
L2
L2
L3
L3
L5
L5
L4
S1
S1
L5
C2
C3
C4
C4
C5
C5
T2
T3
T4
T5
T6
T7
T8
T9
T10
T11
T12
L1
L2
T2
T2
T1
T1
C6
C6
S5
S4
S3
C8
C8
Coccyx
C7
C7
S2
S2
L3
L4
L5
L5
S1
S1

Fig. 43-5 • Dermatomes (cutaneous innervation of spinal nerves).

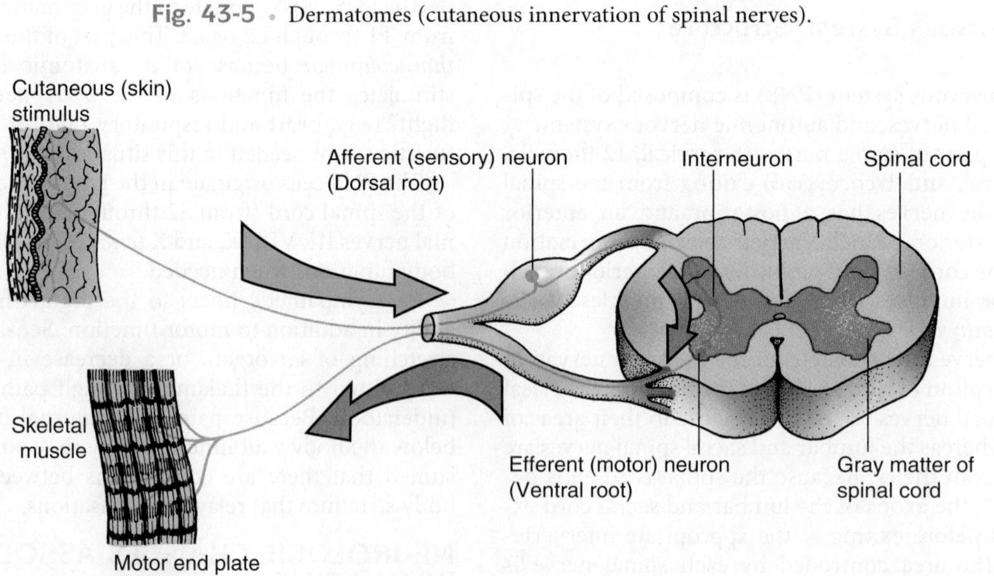
Cutaneous (skin) stimulus
Afferent (sensory) neuron (Dorsal root)
Interneuron
Spinal cord
Skeletal muscle
Efferent (motor) neuron (Ventral root)
Gray matter of spinal cord
Motor end plate response (contraction)

Fig. 43-6 • An example of reflex activity. Stimulation of skin results in involuntary muscle contraction (reflex arc).

TABLE 43-4 Origins, Types, and Functions of the Cranial Nerves

Cranial Nerve	Origin	Type	Function
I: Olfactory	Olfactory bulb	Sensory	Smell
II: Optic	Midbrain	Sensory	Central and peripheral vision
III: Oculomotor	Midbrain	Motor to eye muscles	Eye movement via medial and lateral rectus and inferior oblique and superior rectus muscles; lid elevation via the levator muscle
		Parasympathetic-motor	Pupil constriction; ciliary muscles
IV: Trochlear	Lower midbrain	Motor	Eye movement via superior oblique muscles
V: Trigeminal	Pons	Sensory	Sensation from skin of face and scalp and mucous membranes of mouth and nose
		Motor	Muscles of mastication (chewing)
VI: Abducens	Inferior pons	Motor	Eye movement via lateral rectus muscles
VII: Facial	Inferior pons	Sensory	Pain and temperature from ear area; deep sensations from the face; taste from anterior two thirds of the tongue
		Motor	Muscles of the face and scalp
		Parasympathetic-motor	Lacrimal, submandibular, and sublingual salivary glands
VIII: Vestibulocochlear	Pons-medulla junction	Sensory	Hearing Equilibrium
IX: Glossopharyngeal	Medulla	Sensory	Pain and temperature from ear; taste and sensations from posterior one third of tongue and pharynx
		Motor	Skeletal muscles of the throat
		Parasympathetic-motor	Parotid glands
X: Vagus	Medulla	Sensory	Pain and temperature from ear; sensations from pharynx, larynx, thoracic and abdominal viscera
		Motor	Muscles of the soft palate, larynx, and pharynx
		Parasympathetic-motor	Thoracic and abdominal viscera; cells of secretory glands; cardiac and smooth muscle innervation to the level of the splenic flexure
XI: Accessory	Medulla (anterior gray horn of the cervical spine)	Motor	Skeletal muscles of the pharynx and larynx and sternocleidomastoid and trapezius muscles
XII: Hypoglossal	Medulla	Motor	Skeletal muscles of the tongue

(Chart 43-1). Any problems that affect the nerves, bones, muscles, or joints also affect motor and therefore ADL ability. The older adult may have tremors without rigidity, and deep tendon reflexes may be hypoactive. Balance and coordination may be impaired as a result.

Sensory changes in older adults can also affect their daily activities. Pupils decrease in size, which restricts the amount of light entering the eye, and adapt more slowly. Older adults need increased lighting to see. Touch sensation decreases, which may lead to falls because the older person may not feel small objects or a step underfoot. Vibration sense may be lost in the ankles and feet. (See the discussion on fall prevention in Chapter 3.) Hearing also decreases, especially for high-pitched sounds.

Cognitive functions of perceiving, registering, storing, and using information often change as a normal part of aging (Milisen et al., 2006). Therefore it is important to differentiate between these expected findings and those of dementia, depression, and delirium (3Ds). Failure to correctly diagnosis pathologic cognitive problems may lead to a poor patient outcome.

Intellect does not decline as a result of aging. However, a person with certain health problems may have a decrease in cognitive level. *Cognitive decline is frequently caused by drug interactions or toxicity or by an inadequate oxygen supply to the brain.* Some older adults may need more time than a younger person to process questions, learn new information, solve problems, or complete analogies.

Subtle memory changes are typical for many older people. Long-term memory seems better than recall (recent) or immediate (registration) memory. Older adults may need more time to retrieve information. These changes may be partly due to the loss of cerebral neurons, which is associated with the aging process.

Insomnia, anxiety, and depression in late adulthood may cause changes in mental status. Circadian rhythm disorders may lead to wakefulness until later at night, with extended sleeping in the morning (a pattern opposite that of most health care facility routines). Many older adults require less sleep than do their younger counterparts.

Mental status may also decline as a result of infection. *Often this change in mental status is a key early sign of an infectious process in the older patient, especially urinary tract infection.*

ASSESSMENT METHODS

Patient History

During your introduction, note the patient's appearance and assess his or her speech, affect, and motor function. If he or she seems to have cognitive deficits or has trouble speaking or hearing, ask a family member or significant other to stay during the interview to help obtain an accurate history. Be sure

Chart 43-1 NURSING FOCUS ON THE OLDER ADULT

Changes in the Nervous System Related to Aging

Physiologic Changes	Nursing Implications	Rationales
Slower processing time	Provide sufficient time for the affected older adult to respond to questions and/or direction.	Differentiate normal findings from neurologic deterioration.
Recent memory loss	Reinforce teaching by repetition and written teaching aids.	Greatest loss of brain weight is in the white matter of the frontal lobe. Intellect is not impaired, but the learning process is slowed. Repetition helps the patient learn new information and recall it when needed.
Decreased touch sensation	Remind the patient to look where his or her feet are placed when walking. Instruct the patient to wear shoes that provide good support when walking. If the patient is unable, change his or her position frequently (every hour) while he or she is in bed or the chair.	Decreased sensation may cause the patient to fall.
Change in perception of pain	Ask the patient to describe the nature and specific characteristics of pain. Monitor additional assessment variables to detect possible health problems.	Accurate and complete nursing assessment ensures that the interventions will be appropriate for the older adult (see Chapter 3).
Change in sleep patterns	Ascertain sleep patterns and preferences. Ask if sleep pattern interferes with ADLs. Adjust the patient's daily schedule to his or her sleep pattern and preference as much as possible (e.g., evening versus morning bath).	Most older adults require less sleep than do younger adults. However, frequent rest periods are needed.
Altered balance and/or decreased coordination	Instruct the patient to move slowly when changing positions. If needed, advise the patient to hold on to handrails when ambulating. Assess the need for an ambulatory aid, such as a cane.	The patient may fall if moving too quickly. Assistive and adaptive aids provide support and prevent falls.
Increased risk for infection	Monitor carefully for infection.	Structural deterioration of microglia, the cells responsible for cell-mediated immune response in the central nervous system (CNS).

that glasses, contact lenses, and hearing aids are available if the patient wears any of these aids. Charts 43-2 and 43-3 summarize the information that should be included in the history.

Ask the patient about his or her medical history to determine its association with the current health problem. Inquire about the ability to perform ADLs. Knowing the level of daily activity helps establish a baseline for later comparison as the patient improves or worsens. Ask whether the patient is right-handed or left-handed. This information is important for several reasons:

- The patient may be somewhat stronger on the dominant side, which is expected.
- The effects of cerebral injury or disease are more pronounced if the dominant hemisphere is involved.

Family History and Genetic Risk

Ask about family medical history such as stroke or myocardial infarction (MI) (heart attack). Some diseases occur more often in certain cultural groups and may be caused by a genetic influence or other reason. For example, it has been long established that Huntington disease is inherited. A number of other neurologic diseases have a genetic basis, such as neuromuscular disorders, migraine headaches, and epilepsy. These genetic risks are described with specific neurologic diseases found later in this unit.

Current Health Problems

Obtain information from the patient about current health problems as outlined in Charts 43-2 and 43-3.

Physical Assessment

Perform a focused assessment based on the patient's current health problems. Compare each assessment with the patient's baseline, as well as between right and left sides and between upper and lower extremities. Most of the assessment can be performed with the patient sitting or lying down. *Two types of neurologic assessments may be performed—a complete assessment and a "rapid" assessment.* The method chosen depends

Chart 43-2 BEST PRACTICE FOR PATIENT SAFETY & QUALITY CARE

Establishing a Nursing Database: History

DEMOGRAPHIC DATA
- Age
- Gender

PAST MEDICAL HISTORY
- Patient's medical history
- Family's medical history
- Previous injuries or congenital problems
- Chronic diseases
  - Hypertension
  - Diabetes mellitus
  - Lung disease
- Previous neurologic problems
  - Headaches
  - Seizures
  - Head or spine trauma
  - Eye problems
  - Stroke

CURRENT HISTORY
- Current symptoms
  - Blurred vision
  - Headache
  - Speech or swallowing difficulty
  - Numbness, tingling
  - Weakness, clumsiness
  - Bowel or bladder difficulties
  - Nausea or vomiting
  - Personality changes
  - Seizures
  - Disorientation or other change in mental status
- Allergies
  - Food
  - Medications
  - Environment
- Pain tolerance
  - Medications taken for pain
  - Behaviors to reduce pain
- Medications
  - Prescribed
  - Illicit
  - Over-the-counter
- ADLs

SOCIAL HISTORY
- Usual recreational activities
- Level of physical activity each day
- Hobbies
- Alcohol consumption and use of recreational drugs
- Smoking, use of any tobacco products
- Sleep habits
  - Changes in pattern, duration, or intensity
- Work history
  - Exposure to toxic agents
- Ethnic and cultural background
- Handedness (right or left)
- Educational background

Chart 43-3 NEUROLOGIC ASSESSMENT

Using Gordon's Functional Health Patterns

HEALTH PERCEPTION–HEALTH MANAGEMENT PATTERN
- How would you describe your general health?
- Has your health changed significantly over the past few weeks or months?
- Have you had to miss any work because of changes in your health?

COGNITIVE-PERCEPTUAL PATTERN
- Have you noticed any changes in your vision? Hearing? Memory?
- Do you feel you are having any difficulty in making decisions? In learning?
- Are you experiencing any discomfort? Pain? Weakness?

ACTIVITY-EXERCISE PATTERN
- Do you have enough energy for your activities?
- What is your perceived ability for (code for level according to key below):

Feeding?	Level 0: Full self-care
Bathing?	Level I: Requires use of equipment or device
Toileting?	Level II: Requires assistance or supervision of another person
Bed mobility?	
Dressing?	Level III: Requires assistance or supervision of another person and equipment or device
Grooming?	
General mobility?	
Cooking?	Level IV: Is dependent and does not participate
Home maintenance?	
Shopping?	

Based on Gordon, M. (2007). *Manual of nursing diagnosis* (11th ed.). Boston: Jones & Bartlett.

Chart 43-4 BEST PRACTICE FOR PATIENT SAFETY & QUALITY CARE

Assessment of Mental Status
- Are the patient's answers appropriate?
- Is the patient's behavior and facial expression appropriate?
- Is the speech pattern of normal tone, rate, rhythm, and volume?
- Are the answers complete?
- Is the patient's appearance neat or untidy? Appropriate for age and weather conditions?
- Is the patient cooperative, euphoric, hostile, anxious, withdrawn, or guarded?
- Is the patient experiencing hallucinations or delusions?
- Is the patient's posture and hygiene appropriate for the situation?
- Is the patient drowsy?

on the information needed, the time available with the patient, and your clinical skill level. Advanced practice nurses (APNs) and other health care providers usually perform the complete assessment, although parts of it can be done by any qualified health care professional. It is important that you understand each component of the assessment and what the results might indicate. The complete assessment is described first.

Assessment of Mental Status

While collecting the history data, make observations about the patient's mental status, speech, and behavior as noted in Chart 43-4. An organized head-to-toe physical assessment begins with the mental status.

Level of Consciousness and Orientation

Determine level of consciousness (LOC) by observing the patient's responsiveness and mental status. *A change in LOC is the **first** indication that central neurologic function has declined! The patient who is described as **alert** is awake and responsive. A patient may be alert but not oriented to person, place, or time. Patients who are less than alert are labeled lethargic, stuporous, or comatose. A **lethargic** patient is drowsy or sleepy but is easily awakened. One who is arousable only with vigorous or painful stimulation is **stuporous**. The **comatose** patient is unconscious and cannot be aroused.*

To best identify the patient's level of cognitive function or state of consciousness, describe behavior as response to stimulation. If alert, ask him or her questions to determine orientation. Varying the sequence of questioning on repeated assessments prevents the patient from memorizing the answers. Responses that indicate orientation include:

- The patient's ability to relate the onset of symptoms
- The name of his or her physician/nurse practitioner/ nurse
- The year and month
- His or her address
- The name of the referring physician or health care agency

Advanced age, time of day, drug therapy, and the need for sleep, glucose, or oxygen may affect these responses.

Memory and Attention

Memory is one of the most important parts of the neurologic assessment. If the patient cannot remember, most of the verbal assessment tests are not useful. *Loss of memory, especially recent memory, tends to be an early sign of neurologic problems.* Three types of memory can be tested: long-term (remote) memory, recall (recent) memory, and immediate memory.

Remote, or long-term, **memory** can be tested by asking patients about their birth date, schools attended, the city of birth, or anything from the past that can be verified. Nurses often ask the maiden name of the patient's mother, which is sometimes listed on the admission form and can be checked.

Recall (recent) **memory** can be tested during the history and checked on the medical record:

- The accuracy of the medical history
- Dates of clinic or physician appointments
- The time of admission
- Health care providers seen within the past few days
- Mode of transportation to the hospital or clinic

Immediate (new) **memory** is tested by giving the patient two or three unrelated words, such as "apple," "street," and "chair," and asking him or her to repeat the words to make sure they were heard. After about 5 minutes, while continuing with the examination, ask the patient to repeat the words. An alternative to this method is to give a three-step command and observe whether it is carried out correctly. For example, "Pick up the paper, fold it in half, and draw a square on it."

To assess *attention*, ask the patient to repeat a series of three numbers, such as 4, 7, and 3. The series is increased by one number with each successful repetition until seven or eight digits are achieved. If the patient has difficulty at any level (cannot repeat the series), repeat the numbers. If the patient cannot repeat, stop the procedure. Next, ask the patient to repeat the numbers backward, starting again with three digits and increasing by one each time. Normally, a person should be able to repeat five to eight digits forward and four to six backward. Education, occupation, interest, culture, anxiety, and depression affect mental status, and what is considered "normal" may not be so for a particular patient.

The serial-seven test to determine attention may also be used. The patient is asked to count backward from 100 by 7 (the examiner stops when the patient reaches 65 successfully). Depending on education and other factors, it may be better to ask the person to subtract by three or to add forward by five. Clinical judgment and assessment skills are used when deciding which of these tests to use.

Language and Higher Levels of Cognition

If desired, most *language* and *copying* skills can be assessed during the initial interview. The patient demonstrates understanding by following directions on admission (e.g., getting undressed). If he or she hesitates, indicating word searching, point to objects and ask the patient to name them, such as the door or bed.

The advanced practice nurse (APN) or speech-language pathologist (SLP) tests reading comprehension by writing a simple command and giving it to the patient (e.g., "close your eyes"). Writing can be tested by asking the patient to write a sentence. The clinician must remember that some patients cannot read or write and must modify the examination accordingly. Copying ability is usually tested by having the patient copy something that has been drawn, such as a cross, circle, diamond, or square.

Higher intellectual functions are assessed by asking about favorite hobbies, current events, the names of the last few presidents. Abstract reasoning can be evaluated by asking the meaning of proverbs (e.g., "A stitch in time saves nine" or "A rolling stone gathers no moss"). *People from countries other than the United States or young adults may be unfamiliar with some of these abstract statements.* Consult a professional language interpreter to assist with language and speech assessment.

Begin to assess the patient's judgment during the interview. Did he or she make rational decisions in dealing with his or her symptoms? Ask questions such as "What would you do if stopped for speeding?" and "What would you do if there was a fire in the wastepaper basket?" *Remember that testing of cognition (general knowledge, abstraction, and judgment) is influenced by culture.* For example, in some cultures (e.g., Nigerian, Chinese), men make all decisions or answer these questions for their wives or other female family members.

Assessment of Cranial Nerves

▼ VIDEO CLIPS: Smell and Central Vision

Cranial nerves are typically tested to establish a baseline from which to compare progress or deterioration. However, they are not routinely tested unless the patient has a suspected problem affecting one or more of the cranial nerves (see Table 43-4). The testing of cranial nerve III is usually a part of the rapid neurologic assessment described on p. 942. Adding the specific cranial nerves to be tested on the flow sheet of a patient with a problem affecting the cranial nerves helps ensure continued comparison and assessment.

Assessment of Sensory Function

▼ VIDEO CLIP: Sensory Evaluation

The assessment of sensory function is done for patients with problems affecting the spinal cord or spinal nerves, such as trauma, intervertebral disk disease, Guillain Barré syndrome (GBS), tumor, infection, stenosis, or transverse myelitis. The sensory assessment includes pain, superficial and deep sensation, light touch, and proprioception. *Pain and light touch are the most commonly assessed.*

The acuity level of the patient determines how often the sensory assessment is done. For example, patients with acute spinal cord trauma or ascending GBS are assessed every hour until stable and then every 4 hours. As the condition improves, sensory assessment may be needed only once each shift. Findings are documented according to agency protocol. A special spinal cord assessment flow sheet may be used to document sensory and/or motor findings for the patient with a spinal cord injury.

Pain and temperature sensations are transmitted by the same nerve endings. Therefore if one sensation is tested and found to be intact, it can safely be assumed that the other is intact. Testing temperature sensation can usually be accomplished using a cold reflex hammer and the warm touch of the hand for patients with known or suspected spinal problems.

Assess for *pain sensation* with any sharp or dull object, such as a cotton-tipped applicator or paper clip. Demonstrate what will be done while the patient's eyes are open. Then, ask him or her to keep eyes closed and to indicate whether the touch is sharp or dull. The sharp and dull ends should be changed at random so he or she does not anticipate the next type of sensation. Not all areas need to be tested unless a spinal cord injury has occurred. If testing begins on the hands and feet, there is no need to test the other parts of the extremities because the tracts transmitting pain and temperature sensations are intact. Compare reactions on each side. A sensation reported as dull when the stimulus was actually sharp requires further testing. A patient with sensory loss as a result of diabetes mellitus or peripheral vascular disease may or may not be aware of the loss until tested. Some patients with chronic illness may report that they have had sensory losses for a long time.

VIDEO CLIP: Light Touch ▶

Light *touch discrimination* is likely to be normal if pain and temperature sensations are intact. Touch discrimination and two-point discrimination may be performed as part of a complete neurologic examination by the physician or APN.

For testing **touch discrimination,** the patient closes his or her eyes. The practitioner touches him or her with a finger and asks that he or she point to the area touched. This procedure is repeated on each extremity at random rather than at sequential points. Next, the practitioner touches the patient on each side of the body on corresponding sites at the same time. The patient should be able to point to both sites.

The clinician then touches the patient in two places on the same extremity with two objects, such as cotton-tipped applicators. A person can normally identify two points fairly close together depending on the location of the stimuli. When an area is heavily innervated, the *two-point discrimination will feel closer.*

Abnormal sensory findings may have a peripheral nervous system (PNS) or a central nervous system (CNS) cause. The neuropathies of diabetes, malnutrition, and vascular problems have a PNS cause and generally involve the entire extremity or both extremities. Damage to a specific spinal nerve may not result in significant sensory loss because the spinal nerves overlap. Injury to several nearby spinal nerves is manifested as decreased or absent sensation in the dermatomes of those nerves.

CNS problems can occur within the spinal cord, the brainstem, the cerebellum, and the cerebral cortex. Sensory deficits from spinal cord damage vary with the location of the damage. Involvement of only the posterior column leads to lost **proprioception** (position sense) below the level of the damage on the same side or on both sides (if both the right and left posterior columns are involved). A lesion involving only the right spinothalamic tract results in a loss of pain and temperature sensation below the lesion on the *left* side. Problems in the brainstem, thalamus, and cortex generally result in loss of sensation on the **contralateral** (opposite) side of the body. Cerebellar lesions affect sensation on the *same* side of the body.

Assessment of Motor Function

Throughout the physical assessment, observe the patient for involuntary tremors or movements. Describe these movements as accurately as possible, such as "pill-rolling with the thumbs and fingers at rest" or "intention tremors of both hands" (tremors that occur when the patient tries to do something). These abnormalities can indicate certain diseases, such as multiple sclerosis, or the effects of selected psychotropic drugs.

Measure the patient's hand *strength* by asking him or her to grasp and squeeze two fingers of each of your hands. Then compare the grasps for equality of strength. As another means of evaluating strength, try to withdraw the fingers from the patient's grasp and compare the ease or difficulty. He or she should release the grasps on command—another assessment of consciousness and the ability to follow commands.

To test the patient's strength against resistance, ask him or her to resist your bending or straightening of the arm, hand, leg, or foot being tested (Fig. 43-7). A five-point rating scale is commonly used (see Chapter 52, Table 52-2). Test results are sometimes recorded as 5/5, 3/5, and so forth, indicating the criteria that were used and the status of the patient at that testing. Always evaluate and compare strength on each side. Later testing results are compared with previous results to indicate any change.

Cerebral motor or *brainstem* integrity may also be assessed. Ask the patient to close his or her eyes and hold the arms perpendicular to the body with the palms up for 15 to 30 seconds. If there is a cerebral or brainstem reason for muscle weakness, the arm on the weak side will start to fall, or "drift," with the palm pronating (turning inward). This is called a **pronator drift.** The same can be done for the lower extremities, with the

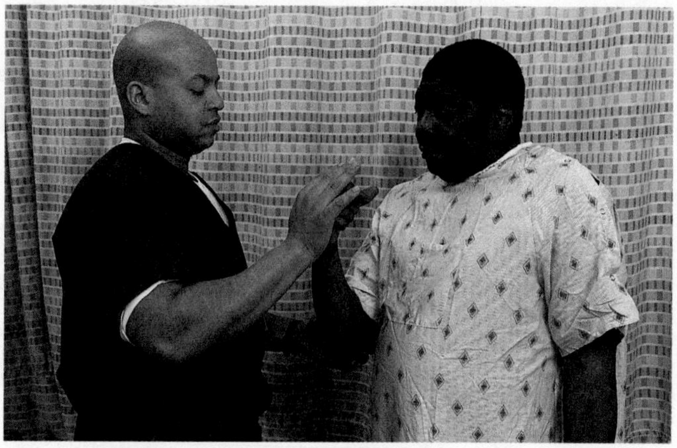

Fig. 43-7 • Testing for strength against resistance.

patient lying on his or her stomach with the legs bent upward at the knees. However, it is easier for most patients to sit on the side of the bed and extend the legs outward.

Assessment of Cerebellar Function

VIDEO CLIP: Fine Motor Coordination

Most of the assessment of cerebellar function can be performed with the patient sitting on the side of the bed or examining table. Fine *coordination* of muscle activity is tested. If cerebellar problems are suspected or diagnosed, ask the patient to perform these tasks with his or her eyes closed:

- Run the heel of one foot down the shin of the other leg, and repeat with the other leg (the patient should be able to do this smoothly and keep the heel on the shin).
- Place the hands palm-up and then palm-down on each thigh, repeating as fast as possible (this can normally be done rapidly).
- With arms out at the side, touch the finger to the nose two or three times, with eyes open and then with eyes closed (this can be done with alternating arms or with each arm individually).

For the last part of the cerebellar assessment, the *ambulatory* patient stands for testing of *gait and equilibrium*. Gait and equilibrium are usually tested at the end or beginning of the entire neurologic assessment. Ask the patient to walk across the room, turn, and return. Observe for uneven steps, difficulty walking, and so forth. To evaluate balance, ask him or her to stand on one foot and then on the other. Tiptoe walking and heel-to-toe walking can also demonstrate gait problems. For patients with sciatic nerve involvement, pain may worsen when they walk on their toes or heels.

To test equilibrium, ask the patient to stand with arms at the sides, feet and knees close together, and eyes open. Check for swaying, and then ask him or her to close his or her eyes and maintain position. The examiner should be close enough to prevent falling if the patient cannot stay erect. If he or she sways with the eyes closed but not when the eyes are open (the **Romberg sign**), the problem is probably **proprioceptive** (awareness of body position). If the patient sways with the eyes both open and closed, the neurologic disturbance is probably *cerebellar* in origin.

If the patient cannot perform any of these activities smoothly, the problem is manifested on the same side as the cerebellar lesion. If both lobes of the cerebellum are involved, the incoordination affects both sides of the body (bilateral).

Assessment of Reflex Activity

VIDEO CLIP: Deep Tendon Reflex

The health care provider, including the APN, may assess deep tendon reflexes (DTRs) and superficial (cutaneous) reflexes. The **deep tendon reflexes** of the biceps, triceps, brachioradialis, and quadriceps muscles and of the Achilles tendon can be tested as part of the routine neurologic assessment. Striking the tendon with the reflex hammer should cause contraction of the muscle (Fig. 43-8). The appropriate muscle contraction indicates an intact reflex arc. The tendon is tapped quickly but not with too much force. If the patient is tensing the muscle, the reflexes will not respond. Having the patient interlock his or her hands and pull outward will help decrease muscle tensing so the reflex can be tested.

The **cutaneous (superficial) reflexes** usually tested are the plantar reflexes and sometimes the abdominal reflexes. The plantar reflex is tested with a pointed (but not sharp) object, such as the handle end of the reflex hammer or the rounded end of bandage scissors. The normal response is plantar flexion of all toes. Dorsiflexion of the great toe and fanning of the other toes **(Babinski's sign)** is abnormal in anyone older than 2 years and represents the presence of central nervous system (CNS) disease. The term "positive Babinski's sign" (abnormal response) and "negative Babinski's sign" (normal response) are clinically used terms but are not correct. **Babinski's sign** is a pathologic, or abnormal, reflex. Health care providers may also use the terms "upgoing" or "downgoing" to refer to the toes of the stimulated foot. "Upgoing" toes is an abnormal response that

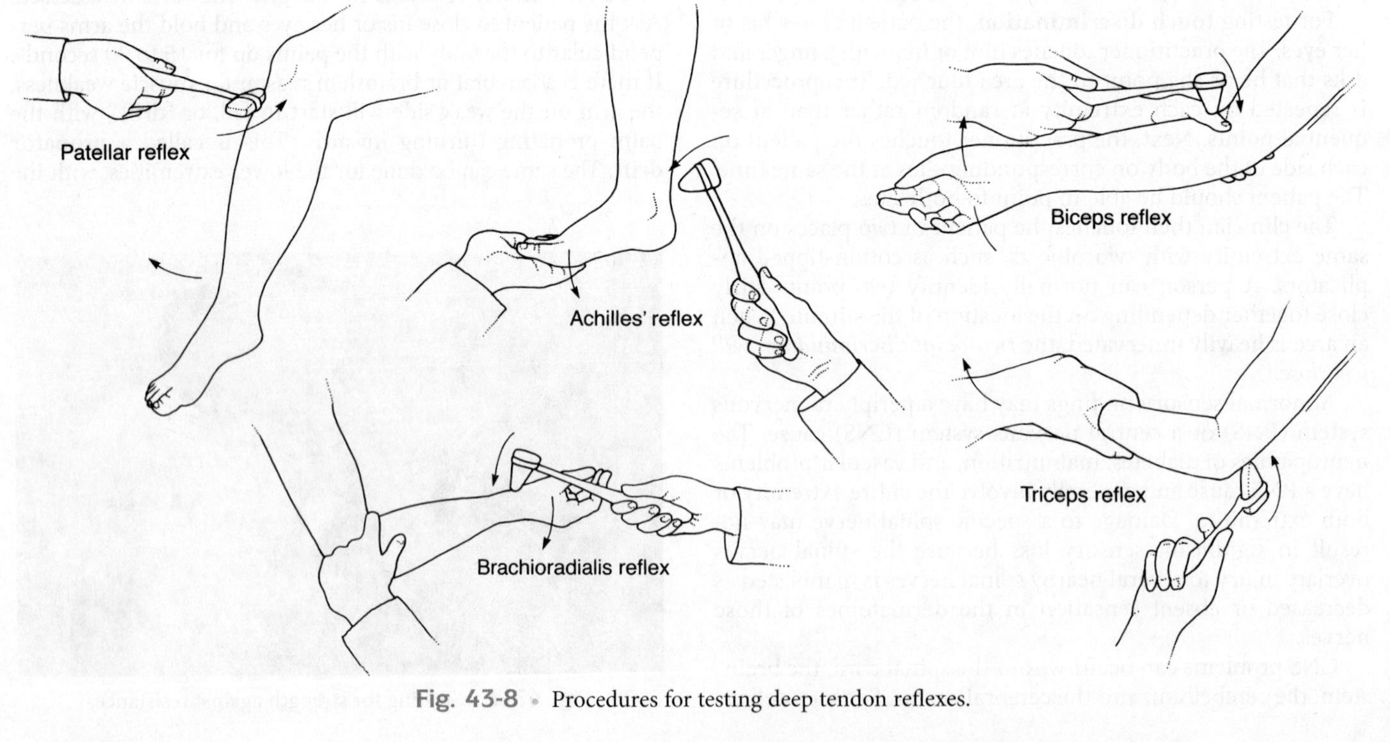
Patellar reflex
Achilles' reflex
Biceps reflex
Triceps reflex
Brachioradialis reflex

Fig. 43-8 • Procedures for testing deep tendon reflexes.

indicates the presence of pathology in the CNS. Babinski's sign can occur with drug and alcohol intoxication, after a seizure, or in patients with multiple sclerosis or liver disease.

To test the abdominal reflex, stroke the patient's abdomen in all four quadrants diagonally toward the umbilicus. The umbilicus should deviate toward the stimulus, but obesity may mask the reflex. The abdominal reflex can be absent in both upper and lower motor neuron disease.

Hyperactive reflexes indicate possible upper motor neuron disease, tetanus, or hypocalcemia. *Hypoactive* reflexes may result from lower motor neuron disease (damage to the spinal cord), disease of the neuromuscular junction, muscle disease, or health problems such as diabetes mellitus, hypothyroidism, or hypokalemia.

Asymmetry of reflexes is an important finding because it probably indicates a disease process. The results of reflex testing are recorded by the use of a stick figure and a scale of 0 to 4 (Fig. 43-9). A score of 2 is considered normal, although scores of 1 (hypoactive) or 3 (stronger than normal) may be normal for a particular patient. **Clonus** is the sudden, brief, jerking contraction of a muscle or muscle group often seen in seizures.

Rapid Neurologic Assessment

A rapid neurologic assessment, or "neuro check," is completed when the patient is admitted to a health care facility on an emergent basis. It is also part of ongoing patient assessment and performed in the event of a sudden change in neurologic status. The typical flow sheet contains data related to level of consciousness, orientation, movement of arms and legs, and pupil size and reaction to light. *Be sure to document all aspects of the rapid neurologic assessment.*

As part of the flow sheet or on a separate form, the **Glasgow Coma Scale (GCS)** (Fig. 43-10) is used in most health care agencies to help describe the patient's level of consciousness (LOC). This tool has been shown to be very reliable for most patients. Some agencies use the GCS along with other assessment findings for a more comprehensive picture of the patient's condition.

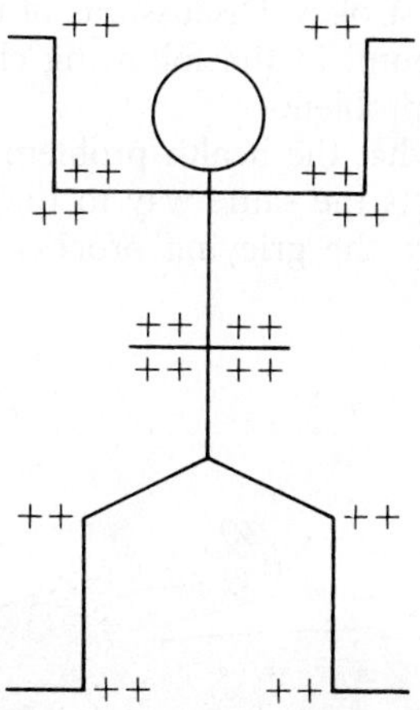

0 Absent, no response
1 (+) Weaker than normal, hypoactive
2 (+ +) Normal
3 (+ + +) Stronger or more brisk than normal
4 (+ + + +) Hyperactive
(Note: 1 and 3 may be normal for some individuals)

Fig. 43-9 • A stick figure and scale for recording reflex activity.

The GCS establishes baseline data in each of these areas: eye opening, motor response, and verbal response. The patient is assessed and assigned a numerical score for each of these areas. A score of 15 represents normal neurologic functioning. A score of 7 represents a comatose state. Thus the lower the score, the lower the patient's LOC. For patients who are intubated and cannot talk, record their score with a "t" after the number. The best possible score for this patient would be 11t.

Use the most appropriate stimulus for getting a response. If the patient is not awake and responding to commands, it may be necessary to use painful stimuli to obtain the best response. The patient's response to central pain (brain response) is assessed first. On the basis of this response, peripheral pain may then be assessed. Failure to apply painful stimuli appropriately may lead to an incorrect conclusion about the patient's neurologic status.

To apply vigorous stimuli, start with the least noxious irritation or pressure and proceed to more painful stimulation if the patient does not respond. Begin each phase of the assessment by speaking in a normal voice. If no response is obtained, use a loud voice. If the patient does not respond, gently shake him or her. The shaking should be similar to that used in attempting to wake up a child. If that is unsuccessful, apply painful stimuli using one of these methods:

- Supraorbital (over eyes) pressure
- Trapezius muscle squeeze
- Mandibular (jaw) pressure
- Sternal (breastbone) rub

GLASGOW COMA SCALE*

Eye Opening	
Spontaneous	4
To sound	3
To pain	2
Never	1
Motor Response	
Obeys commands	6
Localizes pain	5
Normal flexion (withdrawal)	4
Abnormal flexion	3
Extension	2
None	1
Verbal Response	
Oriented	5
Confused conversation	4
Inappropriate words	3
Incomprehensible sounds	2
None	1

* The highest possible score is 15

Fig. 43-10 • The Glasgow Coma Scale.

First, apply supraorbital pressure by placing a thumb under the orbital rim in the middle of the eyebrow and pushing upward. *This technique is not used if the patient has orbital or facial fractures.*

A second technique to elicit pain is to pinch or squeeze the trapezius muscle located at the angle of the shoulder and neck muscle. If the patient remains unresponsive, apply pressure to the jaw using your index and middle fingers. If the patient does not respond, make a fist and rub the knuckles of your hand against the sternum in a twisting motion. The tissue in this area is tender, and bruising is not unusual. Therefore do not use this technique for older adults or for patients who bruise easily (e.g., those on anticoagulant therapy).

The patient may respond to painful stimuli in several ways. Although the initial response to pain may be abnormal flexion or extension, continued application of pain for no more than 20 to 30 seconds may demonstrate that he or she can localize or withdraw. If the patient does not respond after 20 to 30 seconds, stop applying the painful stimulus.

In addition to using the GCS, observe the patient for other signs of altered mental status. These changes include reports of headache; restlessness, irritability, or being unusually quiet; slurred speech; and a change in the level of orientation.

Decerebrate or decorticate posturing, as well as pinpoint or dilated and nonreactive pupils, is a late mental deterioration sign. Notify the health care provider immediately of any change in mental status to possibly prevent further decline! **Decortication** is abnormal posturing seen in the patient with lesions that interrupt the corticospinal pathways (Fig. 43-11, *A*). The patient's arms, wrists, and fingers are flexed with internal rotation and plantar flexion of the legs. **Decerebration** is abnormal posturing and rigidity characterized by extension of the arms and legs, pronation of the arms, plantar flexion, and opisthotonos (body spasm in which body is bowed forward) (Fig. 43-11, *B*). Decerebration is usually associated with dysfunction in the brainstem area.

VIDEO CLIP: Pupil Responses ▶

Assess the patient's pupils as part of ongoing "neuro checks." Pupil constriction is a function of cranial nerve III. ***P****upils should be* ***e****qual in size,* ***r****ound and* ***r****egular in shape, and react to* ***l****ight and* ***a****ccommodation* **(PERRLA).** Estimate the size of both pupils using a millimeter ruler. Patients who have had eye surgery for cataracts or glaucoma often have irregularly shaped pupils. Those using eyedrops for either cataracts or glaucoma may have unequal pupils if only one eye is being treated, and the pupillary response may be altered.

To test for pupil constriction, ask the patient to close his or her eyes. Bring a penlight in from the side of the patient's head, and shine the light in the eye being tested as soon as the patient opens his or her eyes. The pupil being tested should constrict **(direct response).** The other pupil should also constrict slightly **(consensual response).** To test accommodation, ask the patient to focus on a distant object and then immediately look at an object 4 to 5 inches from the nose. The eyes should converge, and the pupils should constrict.

NCLEX EXAMINATION CHALLENGE

During a client's neurologic assessment, the nurse finds that he is very drowsy but is easily aroused. He can state his name but is unsure where he is and what today's date is. Which description of the client should the nurse document? Client is:

A. "Stuporous and disoriented."
B. "Lethargic and oriented."
C. "Alert and oriented."
D. "Lethargic and disoriented."

evolve For the correct answer, go to http://evolve.elsevier.com/Iggy/.

Psychosocial Assessment

Patients vary in their responses to a suspected or actual health problem, often depending on whether it is acute or chronic. Response is also influenced by the *mobility, sensory,* and/or *cognitive* impairments that temporarily or permanently result from neurologic disease or injury. For example, patients who have a mild stroke and no lasting neurologic deficits are more likely to be less depressed than patients who cannot walk as a result of spinal cord injury.

Age may also be a factor in how a patient accepts the illness. For instance, a young adult who has a motorcycle accident causing a traumatic brain injury (TBI) may react differently than an older adult who has a spinal injury. In some cases, the patient's emotional responses result from the health problem itself, especially for TBI patients.

Men may feel differently about their illness than women. Male patients who have had strokes are more often depressed than women with strokes. Discussions of these response differences can be found in the following chapters on specific neurologic health problems.

Regardless of what the health problem is, do not assume that everyone reacts the same way to their illness or injury. Patients experience the grieving process and may fluctuate

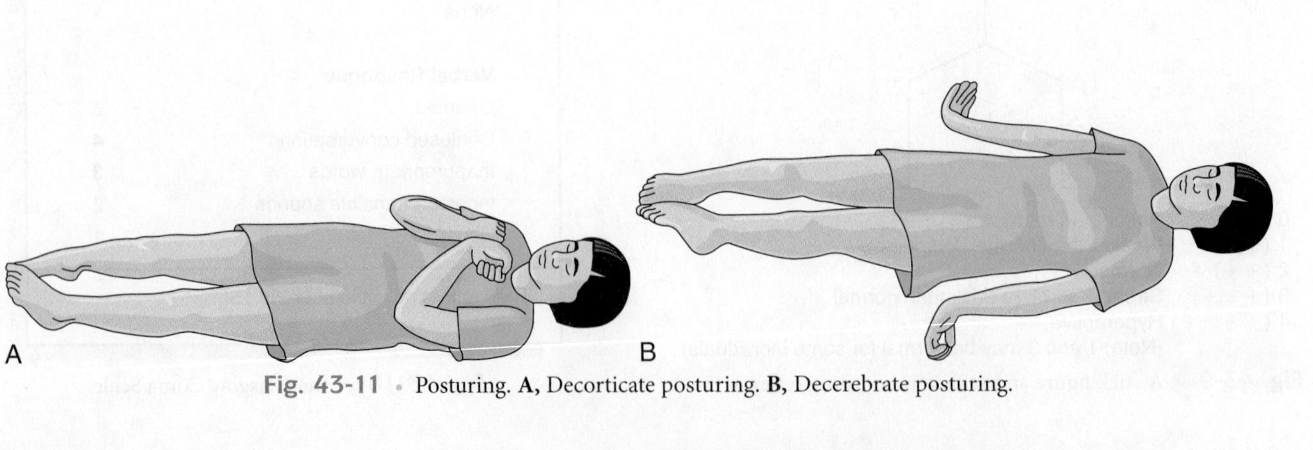
A
B
Fig. 43-11 • Posturing. **A,** Decorticate posturing. **B,** Decerebrate posturing.

between denial, anger, and depression. Encourage patients to express their feelings. Refer them to the appropriate support services if needed. Assess support systems, including family members and friends, if available. Document your assessment and interventions.

Diagnostic Assessment

Laboratory Assessment

For patients with a neurologic problem resulting from a systemic infection, blood cultures are necessary to identify the pathogen. Although the cause of infection must be determined for any patient, this is especially true for those with existing CNS disease. The blood-brain barrier is often not intact in neurologic disease, and the patient is more likely to get an infection of the nervous system, such as meningitis or encephalitis.

Imaging Assessment

Plain X-Rays

Plain *x-rays* of the skull and spine are used to determine bony fractures, curvatures, bone erosion, bone dislocation, and possible calcification of soft tissue, which can damage the nervous system. Several views are taken—anteroposterior, lateral, oblique, and, when necessary, special views of the facial bones. *In head trauma and multiple injuries, one of the first priorities is to rule out cervical spine fracture.*

Explain that the x-ray procedure for the skull and spine is similar to that for a chest x-ray procedure. The patient must remain still during the procedure. Remind him or her that the exposure to radiation is minimal. If the patient is in traction and a portable x-ray unit is not available, the nurse may need to accompany him or her to assist with positioning. Any patient who cannot walk from a wheelchair to the x-ray table should be transferred to the radiology department on a stretcher. The patient is positioned for each of the desired views and is asked not to move just before each x-ray. Follow-up care is not required.

Cerebral Angiography

Cerebral angiography (arteriography) is done to visualize the cerebral circulation to detect blockages in the arteries or veins in the brain, head, or neck. It is not done as often today due to more recent advances in technology. A contrast medium is injected into an artery (usually the femoral) to identify aneurysms, traumatic injuries, strictures/occlusions, tumors, blood vessel displacement from edema, and arteriovenous (AV) malformations. Chart 43-5 lists the precautions that must be taken for patients having any test using contrast media. Table 43-5 describes patient preparation and follow-up nursing care for cerebral angiography and other imaging tests.

The patient is placed on an examining table and made as comfortable as possible. At this time, dentures and hearing aids must be removed. He or she is then connected to cardiac monitoring throughout the procedure. Sedation is usually not used, although the patient may be given medication for relaxation.

The interventional radiologist or other specially trained physician numbs an area at the groin and inserts a catheter into the femoral artery. Under fluoroscopic guidance, the catheter is advanced into a carotid or vertebral artery. Then the physician injects iodinated contrast material into each vessel while recording images from different angles over the head and neck.

Chart 43-5 BEST PRACTICE FOR PATIENT SAFETY & QUALITY CARE

Precautions for the Injection of Contrast Agent for Diagnostic Testing

Special precautions are taken for patients who will receive a contrast agent as part of their diagnostic test. These measures include:

- Following agency guidelines regarding informed consent
- Determining whether the patient has any food or fluid restrictions before the test
- Asking the patient about allergies to contrast agents, shellfish, or iodine
- Determining risk factors for contrast-induced nephropathy (renal damage)
  - Pre-existing renal disease
  - Diabetic nephropathy
  - Heart failure
  - Dehydration

Assess for drugs that interfere with renal perfusion, such as metformin. Interventions include:

- Notifying the health care provider if the patient has reported a risk factor
- Checking the patient's creatinine level (Patients with a level greater than 1.5 mg/dL are more at risk for contrast-induced nephropathy.) Notify the patient's health care provider of results.
- Documenting the date, time, and name of the physician or nurse practitioner notified of the potential allergy and what actions he or she prescribed, if any

After all the vessels have been imaged, the radiologist reviews all the images and consults with the referring physician to decide whether the patient could benefit from any therapeutic radiologic procedure to treat the problem. An arterial closure device is typically used to seal the artery and prevent bleeding.

The x-ray images are stored on a computer. With older equipment, a two-dimension or picture of the vessels is produced. Most radiographic systems now come with software to create three-dimensional images of the blood vessels in the head and/or neck. These systems can also display a "subtracted image" made from two images—one just before the contrast was injected and one with the contrast in the artery. The risks for the procedure are contrast reaction (including hives and flushing), thrombosis (clotting), and bleeding from the entry site. Patients with known contrast sensitivity are pre-treated with steroids.

Computed Tomography

Computed tomography (CT) scanning is an accurate, quick, easy, noninvasive, painless, and least expensive method of diagnosing neurologic problems (see Chart 43-5 and Table 43-5). With the aid of a computer, pictures are taken at many horizontal levels, or slices, of the brain or spinal cord. The cross-sectional slices build up three-dimensional pictures of the brain or spinal cord. A contrast medium may be used to enhance the image. CT scans distinguish bone, soft tissue (e.g., the brain, vascular system, and ventricular system), and fluids such as cerebrospinal fluid (CSF) or blood. Tumors, infarctions, hemorrhage, hydrocephalus, and bone malformations can also be

TABLE 43-5 Preparation and Follow-up for Selected Diagnostic Procedures

Test	Patient Care Preparation	Patient Care Follow-up
Cerebral angiography	Determine whether the patient is allergic to iodinated contrast agents, and follow the guideline in Chart 43-5. Ensure that the patient is NPO 4 to 6 hours before the test. Reinforce these important points: • Your head is immobilized during the procedure • Do not move during the procedure • You will feel a warm or hot sensation when the dye is injected—this is normal • You will be able to talk to the physician—let him or her know if you are in pain or have any concerns Assess and document neurologic signs, vital signs, and neurovascular checks.	Follow agency policy regarding care of the injection site, which may include: • Check dressing for bleeding and swelling around site • Apply ice pack to site • Keep the extremity straight and immobilized • Maintain pressure dressing for 2 hours Check the extremity for adequate circulation to include skin color and temperature, pulses distal to the injection site, and capillary refill. If bleeding is present, maintain manual pressure on the site and notify the physician immediately. Assess vital signs and "neuro" signs per orders. Increase oral or IV fluid intake unless contraindicated. Document assessments and interventions.
Computed tomography (CT) 3-Dimensional CT scan CT angiography Xenon CT Intrathecal contrast-enhanced CT	Follow the guidelines listed in Chart 43-5 if a contrast agent is to be given. Determine if the patient is claustrophobic if a closed CT scan is used. Inform the radiology staff or physician to determine if sedation is necessary. Instruct the patient to remove hairpins, hairpieces, or wigs. Identify the need for preprocedural sedation if the patient cannot tolerate a closed CT scan. Inform the patient that the scanner may make noise or knocking sounds. Reassure the patient that he or she will be able to communicate with the technician throughout the procedure. If contrast is used, the patient may feel a warm or cool sensation after the dye is injected. Occasionally the patient may report a slight metallic taste. A lumbar puncture is performed before an intrathecal contrast-enhanced CT.	Monitor the patient for a delayed allergic response if contrast medium was used.
Positron emission tomography (PET)	Follow preparation as listed for CT. Instruct the patient to withhold caffeine, alcohol, and tobacco for 24 hours before the test. Ensure that the patient has been NPO status for 4 to 12 hours before the procedure (if the patient is diabetic, no insulin is given before the test). Do not give any glucose solutions and any other drugs that alter glucose metabolism. Insert two IV lines.	The radioisotope is eliminated in the urine; no special precautions required. Encourage the patient to increase fluid intake unless contraindicated.
Single-photon emission computed tomography (SPECT)	Patient preparation is similar to that for PET/CT. Determine whether the patient has recently had other nuclear medicine screenings, which may leave traces of the radiopharmaceutical agent. Follow the guidelines listed in Chart 43-5 regarding use of a contrast agent.	The patient can return to his or her previous activity level.

TABLE 43-5 Preparation and Follow-up for Selected Diagnostic Procedures—cont'd

Test	Patient Care Preparation	Patient Care Follow-up
Magnetic resonance imaging (MRI) Magnetic resonance angiography (MRA) Magnetic resonance spectroscopy (MRS)	Follow the information for CT scan. No metal objects may enter the MRI room. Ask the patient about any metal implants including any type of pacemaker device, implantable pumps, or stimulating devices. Instruct the patient to remove all metal objects (jewelry, earrings, body piercings, hairpins, watches, rings, pens). Check with the radiologist regarding tattoos. Do not enter the MRI room unless you have checked with the radiology technician and are sure that neither you nor the patient has any metal device. Ensure all equipment and supplies are free of metal.	No special postprocedure or follow-up care is required.
Lumbar puncture	Explain the procedure, noting that some discomfort may be felt when the local anesthetic is injected or that pain may occur in the leg(s) when the spinal needle is inserted. Place the patient in the fetal position, and remind him or her to remain still. If needed, keep the patient from moving.	Obtain vital signs and complete neurologic checks. Follow agency policy regarding bedrest and remaining flat. Encourage the patient to increase fluid intake unless contraindicated. Monitor for complications, especially increased intracranial pressure (severe headache, nausea, vomiting, photophobia, change in level of consciousness). Observe the needle insertion site for leakage. Notify the physician if it occurs. Provide drug for headache. Notify the physician if drug does not relieve pain.

identified. A CT scan may be performed after a myelogram. (See Chapter 52 for a brief discussion of this test.)

The patient is placed on a movable table in a head-holding device. He or she must remain completely still during the test, which may be difficult. The table is positioned in the machine—a large, donut-shaped structure. Depending on the scan, the patient may be completely enclosed or in a more open situation. A noncontrast series of pictures are taken first. Then, if needed, the patient is withdrawn from the scanner and given an injection of the iodinated contrast medium. The scan is then repeated. Each set of head scans takes less than 5 minutes in newer scanners. Spinal studies take about 10 minutes per body section (cervical, thoracic, lumbar) and are less likely to require contrast injection.

Most patients with new neurologic symptoms have both a pre-contrast and post-contrast study of the head. Contrast-enhanced CT is especially useful in locating and identifying tumor types and abscesses. For situations in which bleeding is the only concern (e.g., in trauma patients), contrast scans are not usually required.

After a standard CT scan, imaging software digitally removes images of soft tissue so that only images of bone remain. Through the use of this technology, bone deformities, trauma, and birth defects are more easily identified.

CT angiography involves administering contrast dye IV before the CT scan. It is used to identify blockages or narrowing of blood vessels, aneurysms, and other blood vessel abnormalities.

Xenon computed tomography is performed to evaluate blood flow to brain tissue. The patient breathes xenon, a colorless, odorless gas, while undergoing a standard CT scan.

An intrathecal contrast-enhanced CT scan is performed to diagnose disorders of the spine and spinal nerve roots. A lumbar puncture is performed so that a small amount of spinal fluid can be removed and mixed with contrast dye and injected. The patient is positioned to allow for the contrast medium to move around the spinal cord and nerve roots as needed. The patient may have a headache after the procedure. Follow facility policy regarding patient positioning after the procedure.

Magnetic Resonance Imaging

Magnetic resonance imaging (MRI) produces images that are better than the CT scan. It does not use ionizing radiation but, instead, relies on magnetic fields. Multiple sets of images are taken that are used to determine normal and abnormal anatomy. Images may be enhanced with the use of gadolinium, a non–iodine-based contrast medium. MRIs of the spine have largely replaced CT scans and myelography for evaluation. Some facilities have a *functional MRI (fMRI)* machine that can assess blood flow to the brain rather than merely show its anatomical structure.

In addition to the traditional MRI, a *magnetic resonance angiography (MRA), magnetic resonance spectroscopy (MRS)* or *diffusion imagining (DI)* may be requested. MRA is used to evaluate blood flow and blood vessel abnormalities such as an arterial blockage, intracranial aneurysms, and AV malformations. MRS is used to detect abnormalities in the brain's biochemical processes, such as that which occurs in epilepsy, Alzheimer's disease, and brain attack (stroke). DI uses MRI techniques to evaluate ischemia in the brain to determine the location and severity of a stroke.

Newer, open-sided units ("open MRI") now produce adequate images for those patients who do not want standard MRI scanners. MRI has been contraindicated for patients with cardiac pacemakers, other implanted pumps or devices, and ion-containing metal aneurysm clips. However, extensive trials are testing ways to safely scan some patients with pacemakers. Other implanted devices, such as vascular stents, intravascular catheter (IVC) filters, and metal vascular embolic devices, may be scanned immediately or after a certain period of time, depending on manufacturers' recommendations. MRI may also be contraindicated in patients who are confused or agitated, have unstable vital signs, are on continuous life support, or have older tattoos (which contain lead). New physiologic monitoring systems made specifically for the scanner allow some patients who are unstable to be scanned. A comprehensive online list of medical devices tested for MRI safety and compatibility can be found at www.mrisafety.com. Medical personnel must remove any medical devices they are carrying or wearing and ensure that only approved devices are allowed in the MRI room (see Chart 43-5 and Table 43-5).

Positron Emission Tomography

Positron emission tomography (PET) is a diagnostic tool that is not available in all medical centers (see Table 43-5). Its benefit over a CT scan or MRI is that it provides information about the *function* of the brain, specifically glucose and oxygen metabolism and cerebral blood flow. Current CT scanners provide information about the *structure* of the central nervous system (CNS). The newest PET machines are combination CT-PET scanners that fuse images together to produce better information about the type and location of brain dysfunction.

The physician or nuclear medicine technologist injects the patient with IV deoxyglucose, which is tagged to an isotope. The isotope emits activity in the form of positrons, which are scanned and converted into a color image by computer. The more active a given part of the brain, the greater the glucose uptake. This test is used to evaluate drug metabolism and detect areas of metabolic alteration that occur in dementia, epilepsy, psychiatric and degenerative disorders, neoplasms, and Alzheimer's disease. The level of radiation is equivalent to that of five or six x-rays but much less than exposure during CT.

Teach the patient that he or she will be NPO the night before morning testing and 4 hours before afternoon testing. Patients with diabetes have their test in the morning before taking their antidiabetic drugs. During this 2- to 3-hour procedure, the patient may be blindfolded and have earplugs inserted for all or part of the test. He or she is asked to perform certain mental functions to activate different areas of the brain. Older adults and patients with mental health/behavioral health problems may be too anxious to have a PET scan.

Single-Photon Emission Computed Tomography

The limitation of PET may be overcome through the use of **single-photon emission computed tomography (SPECT).** This test uses a radiopharmaceutical agent that enables radioisotopes to cross the blood-brain barrier. The agent is administered by IV injection. Gamma-emitting radionuclides have longer half-lives, therefore eliminating the need for a cyclotron near the scanner. Although SPECT is less expensive than PET, the resolution of the images is limited. SPECT is particularly useful in studying cerebral blood flow, amnesia, neoplasms, head trauma, persistent vegetative state, or brain death. The test is contraindicated in women who are breast-feeding (see Table 43-5).

The patient is injected with the material about 1 hour before the actual scan by the radiologist, certified nuclear medicine technologist, or specially trained RN. The patient is positioned on an x-ray table in a quiet dark room for the actual scans. Several gamma cameras scan his or her head. When completed, the images are downloaded to a computer.

Magnetoencephalography

Magnetoencephalography (MEG) is a noninvasive imaging technique used to measure the magnetic fields produced by electrical activity in the brain via extremely sensitive devices such as superconducting quantum interference devices (SQUIDs). MEG is somewhat similar to electroencephalography (EEG). The advantage is greater accuracy because of the minimal distortion of the signal. This allows for more usable and reliable localization of brain function. The brain can be observed "in action" rather than just viewing a still MRI image. These machines are not widely available because of their extremely high cost.

NCLEX EXAMINATION CHALLENGE

A diabetic client is scheduled to have an MRI with contrast medium for her cervical spine neck pain. What is the most important action for the nurse to implement prior to this client's test?

A. Remind the client that she will be NPO.
B. Instruct her to force fluids after the test.
C. Ask her about allergies to iodine, shellfish, and other contrast medium.
D. Teach her about how the test will be performed.

evolve For the correct answer, go to http://evolve.elsevier.com/Iggy/.

Other Diagnostic Assessment

Electromyography

Electromyography (EMG) is used to identify nerve and muscle disorders as well as spinal cord disease. (See Chapter 46 for a description of patient preparation, procedure, and follow-up care.) Electromyography and electroneurography or nerve conduction velocity studies (NCVSs) are usually used together and are referred to as *electromyoneurography.*

Electroencephalography

Electroencephalography (EEG) records the electrical activity of the cerebral hemispheres (Chart 43-6). Each graphic recording represents the voltage changes in various areas of the brain (determined by recording the difference between two electrodes). The EEG may be normal even when a pathologic condition is present. The test is performed to:

- Determine the general activity of the cerebral hemispheres
- Determine the origin of seizure activity (epilepsy)
- Determine cerebral function in pathologic conditions other than epilepsy, such as tumors, abscesses, cerebrovascular disease, hematomas, injury, metabolic diseases, degenerative brain disease, and drug intoxication
- Differentiate between organic and hysterical or feigned blindness or deafness

Chart 43-6 **BEST PRACTICE FOR PATIENT SAFETY & QUALITY CARE**

The Patient Having an Electroencephalogram

- Thoroughly explain the procedure to the patient.
- If the order is for the patient to be "sleep deprived," remind the patient to wake up about 2 to 3 AM and to stay awake for the rest of the night.
- Instruct the patient to avoid central nervous system depressants or stimulants. Withhold anticonvulsants only if instructed by the physician. Monitor the patient carefully for seizures if medication is withheld.
- Instruct the patient not to drink caffeine-containing fluids, such as coffee or tea, on the day of the test.
- Reassure the patient that the test is not dangerous or uncomfortable.
- Ask the patient to wash his or her hair on the morning of the test. Instruct the patient not to apply sprays or oils after the hair has been washed. The patient should remove all hairpins, ribbons, and other hair accessories.
- Inform the patient that he or she will need to wash the hair after the test to remove the electrode glue.

- Monitor cerebral activity during surgical anesthesia
- Diagnose sleep disorders (all-night EEG)
- Determine brain death

The patient is placed on a reclining chair or bed. According to an internationally accepted procedure, 16 to 24 electrodes are usually attached to the scalp with a jelly-like substance and connected to the machine. The physician or EEG technician places glue over the electrodes to prevent slippage. The patient must lie still with his or her eyes closed during the initial recording. The rest of the test engages the patient in certain activities: hyperventilation, photic stimulation, and sleep. A portable EEG may be performed at the bedside if necessary, but the preference is for the EEG to be done in a very quiet room.

Hyperventilation produces cerebral vasoconstriction and alkalosis, which increases the likelihood of seizure activity. The patient is asked to breathe deeply 20 to 30 times for 3 minutes. In *photic stimulation,* a strobe light (bright light) is placed in front of the patient. Frequencies of 1 to 20 flashes per second are used with the patient's eyes open and then closed. If the patient's seizures are photosensitive in origin, the EEG will show waves corresponding to each flash of light or waves indicating seizure activity. *Sleep* is either natural or induced by an oral or IV sedative. EEG waves indicative of temporal lobe epilepsy can be demonstrated best during sleep.

Throughout the test, which takes 40 to 60 minutes, the technician watches the patient closely and records any movement. These movements alter the record and must be labeled as artifacts. Examples of artifacts are tongue movement, eye blinking, muscle tenseness, and nervousness.

Evoked Potentials

Evoked potentials (also called *evoked response*) measure the electrical signals to the brain generated by hearing, touch, or sight. These tests are used to assess sensory nerve problems and confirm neurologic conditions including multiple sclerosis, brain tumor, acoustic neuroma (small tumors of the inner ear), and spinal cord injury. Evoked potentials are also used to test sight and hearing (especially in infants and young children), monitor brain activity among coma patients, and confirm brain death.

One set of electrodes is attached to the patient's scalp using conducting paste, and the second set is attached to the part of the body to be tested. A stimulus is applied, and the amount of time it takes for the impulse generated by stimuli to reach the brain is recorded. Under normal circumstances, the process of signal transmission is instantaneous.

Auditory evoked potentials (also called *brainstem auditory evoked response*) are used to assess high-frequency hearing loss, diagnose any damage to the acoustic nerve and auditory pathways in the brainstem, and detect acoustic neuromas. The patient sits in a soundproof room and wears headphones. Clicking sounds are delivered one at a time to one ear while a masking sound is sent to the other ear.

Visual evoked potentials detect loss of vision from optic nerve damage (in particular, damage caused by multiple sclerosis). The patient sits close to a screen and is asked to focus on the center of a shifting checkerboard pattern. Only one eye is tested at a time. The other eye is either kept closed or covered with a patch.

Somatosensory evoked potentials measure response from stimuli to the peripheral nerves and can detect nerve or spinal cord damage or nerve degeneration from multiple sclerosis and other degenerating diseases. Tiny electrical shocks are delivered by electrode to a nerve in an arm or leg.

Cerebral Blood Flow Evaluation

Cerebral blood flow (CBF) can be measured in many areas of the brain with the use of radioactive substances. It is particularly useful in evaluating cerebral vasospasm. Explain the test, and ask the physician if central nervous system (CNS) depressants and stimulants should be withheld for 24 hours before the test.

Because *xenon* readily diffuses into brain tissue, it is the most common choice as an inhaled or injected tracer. The xenon travels through the vessels of the brain, where it is detected by external scintillation counters placed on the skull. Normal CBF is 50 to 55 mm/min/100 g of cerebral tissue. The patient receives various stimuli during the test. Increases in local blood flow can be seen with any neuronal activity, such as reading, hand movement, seizures, and temperature elevation (up to 107.6° F [42° C]). Local blood flow decreases with neurodegenerative disease, comas of metabolic origin, increased intracranial pressure (ICP), or subarachnoid hemorrhage. Follow-up care for this test is not required.

Lumbar Puncture

Lumbar puncture (spinal tap) is the insertion of a spinal needle into the subarachnoid space between the third and fourth (sometimes the fourth and fifth) lumbar vertebrae (see Table 43-5). A lumbar puncture is used to:

- Obtain cerebrospinal fluid (CSF) pressure readings with a manometer
- Obtain CSF for analysis
- Check for spinal blockage caused by a spinal cord lesion
- Inject contrast medium or air for diagnostic study
- Inject spinal anesthetics
- Inject certain drugs
- Reduce mild to moderate increased ICP in certain conditions

Because of the danger of sudden release of CSF pressure, a lumbar puncture is not done for patients with symptoms indicating increased ICP. The procedure is also not performed in patients with skin infections at or near the puncture site because of the danger of introducing infective organisms into the CSF.

The health care provider cleans the skin site thoroughly. The injection site is determined, and the local anesthetic is injected. In a few minutes, a spinal needle is inserted between the third and fourth lumbar vertebrae. Instruct the patient to inform the provider if there is shooting pain or a tingling sensation. After determining proper placement in the subarachnoid space by removing the stylet and seeing CSF, the patient is asked to relax as much as possible so the pressure reading will be accurate. Opening and closing pressure readings are taken and recorded. Three to five test tubes of CSF are usually collected and numbered sequentially. After specimen collection, the needle is withdrawn, slight pressure is applied, and an adhesive bandage strip is placed over the insertion site. Be sure that the patient does not move. If the patient is restless or cannot cooperate, two people may need to assist instead of one. Consider this possibility before beginning the procedure.

Examination of CSF has been a useful diagnostic tool for some time. Recent technical advances are increasing the number of analyses that can be done on CSF. The normal characteristics of CSF and some of the more common abnormalities are given in Table 43-6. Gram-stain smears can test for particular types of meningitis, such as tubercular meningitis. CSF can be cultured, and sensitivity studies determine the best choice of antibiotic if an infection is diagnosed. A specific test for neurosyphilis is the fluorescent treponemal antibody absorption (FTA-ABS) test. Cytologic studies of CSF can identify tumor cells.

TABLE 43-6 Significance of Cerebrospinal Fluid Findings

Findings	Significance
PRESSURE	
Less than 20 cm H_2O	Normal range
COLOR/APPEARANCE	
Clear, colorless	Normal
Pink-red to orange	Red blood cells present
Yellow	Bilirubin present owing to hemolysis of red blood cells; possible causes include subarachnoid hemorrhage, jaundice, increased cerebrospinal fluid (CSF) protein, hypercarotenemia, or hemoglobinemia
Brown	Methemoglobin present, indicating previous meningeal hemorrhage
Unclear or hazy	Cell count is elevated
CELLS	
0-5 small lymphocytes/mm^3	Normal
More than 5 lymphocytes/mm^3	Reaction to infection, tumor, chemical substance, or blood
PROTEINS	
TOTAL	
15-45 mg/dL *(up to 70 mg/dL in older adults)*	Normal
45-100 mg/dL	Paraventricular tumor
50-200 mg/dL	Viral infection
More than 500 mg/dL	Bacterial infection, Guillain-Barré syndrome
Less than 15 mg/dL	Meningismus, pseudotumor cerebri, hyperthyroidism, normal finding after lumbar puncture
IMMUNE GAMMA GLOBULIN (IGG, THE MOST IMPORTANT PROTEIN)	
3%-12% of total protein	Normal
More than 12% of total protein	Multiple sclerosis, neurosyphilis, or viral infection
ALBUMIN/GLOBULIN RATIO	
8:1	Normal
GLUCOSE	
50-75 mg/dL or 60%-70% of blood glucose level	Normal
Less than 50 mg/dL (usually accompanied by the presence of pathologic organisms)	Bacterial, fungal, or viral meningitis; central nervous system (CNS) leukemia; or cancer
OTHER CHARACTERISTICS	
LACTIC ACID	
10-25 mg/dL	Normal
More than 25 mg/dL	Systemic acidosis or increased CSF glucose metabolism
GLUTAMINE	
6-15 mg/dL	Normal
More than 15 mg/dL	Hepatic coma or cirrhosis of liver
LACTATE DEHYDROGENASE	
10% of serum level or 2.0-7.2 units/mL	Normal
More than 10% of serum level	Bacterial meningitis, inflammatory diseases of CNS

Complications of lumbar puncture, although not common, include brainstem herniation (discussed in Chapter 47), infection, CSF leakage, and hematoma formation.

Transcranial Doppler Ultrasonography

Intracranial hemodynamics can be evaluated through the use of the transcranial Doppler (TCD). It uses sound waves to measure blood flow through the arteries. The test is particularly valuable in evaluating cerebral vasospasm or narrowing of arteries. TCD is safe and repeatable and is an inexpensive alternative to angiography.

Muscle and Nerve Biopsies

Muscle or *nerve biopsies* are used to diagnose neuromuscular disorders. They may also reveal if a person is a carrier of a defective gene that could be passed on to children. Under local anesthesia, an incision is made into the skin or a hollow needle is inserted through the skin to remove a small sample of muscle or nerve. A CT scan or MRI is performed before a *brain biopsy.* This procedure involves injection of a local anesthetic into the scalp, drilling a small hole through the skull, and inserting a hollow needle into the site of the lesion. Muscle, nerve, and brain biopsy samples are analyzed under a microscope to identify abnormalities.

GET READY FOR THE NCLEX EXAMINATION!

Key Points

Review these Key Points for each NCLEX Examination Client Needs Category.

Safe and Effective Care Environment

- When caring for older adults, remind them to move slowly and use caution when ambulating. Older adults have an altered balance and decreased coordination (see Chart 43-1).
- For tests that use contrast media, use precautions as listed in Chart 43-5.
- Check for bleeding after patients have an angiography. If bleeding is observed, call the radiologist immediately.
- Before MRI, check for devices such as pacemakers, vascular stents, and implanted pumps.

Health Promotion and Maintenance

- Reinforce teaching and use teaching aids for older adults who typically have recent memory loss.
- Explain what patients should expect before diagnostic testing for neurologic structure and function.
- Encourage patients who receive contrast media or isotopes to push fluids to increase elimination of the material.
- Teach patients having an EEG to follow the precautions listed in Chart 43-6.

Psychosocial Integrity

- Assess the mental status of patients as part of the neurologic assessment, including orientation.
- Remember that a change in level of consciousness (LOC) is the first indicator of neurologic decline.
- Assess the patient's reaction to the neurologic disease or injury.
- Assess the patient's memory because loss of memory, especially recent memory, tends to be an early sign of neurologic problems.

Physiological Integrity

- Take a patient history, including information listed in Charts 43-2 and 43-3.
- Evaluate the patient's sensory and motor abilities, as well as gait, balance, and coordination.
- Use the Glasgow Coma Scale as one measure of neurologic functioning—the lower the score, the poorer the function. Assess for mental status changes (see Chart 43-4).
- Check pupils for size, shape, and reaction. Pupils should be equal in size, round and regular in shape, and reactive to light and accommodation.
- Be aware that decerebrate or decorticate posturing and pinpoint or dilated nonreactive pupils are late signs of neurologic deterioration.
- Provide pre-test and post-test nursing care for patients having neurologic diagnostic testing, as outlined in Table 43-5.
- Follow best practice guidelines in Chart 43-6 when caring for a patient having an EEG.
- Assist with patient positioning during a lumbar puncture (fetal position preferred).
- Recall that normal cerebrospinal fluid (CSF) is clear and colorless with few cells.

Additional Study Resources

Go to your Companion CD or Evolve at http://evolve.elsevier.com/Iggy/ for *Self-Assessment Questions for the NCLEX Examination.*

evolve

Go to Evolve at http://evolve.elsevier.com/Iggy/ for *Prioritization and Delegation Questions for the NCLEX Examination.*

SELECTED BIBLIOGRAPHY

Asterisk indicates a classic or definitive work on this subject.

Bolek, B. (2006). Facing cranial nerve assessment. *American Nurse Today, 1*(2), 21-22.

Gambrell, M. (2004). Seizures 101. *Nursing2004, 34*(8), 36-41.

Gordon, M. (2007). *Manual of nursing diagnosis* (11th ed.). Boston: Jones & Bartlett.

*Hinkle, J. (2002). SPECT: A powerful imaging tool. *AJN, 102*(3), 24A-24G.

Jarvis, C. (2007). *Physical examination and health assessment* (4th ed.). Philadelphia: Saunders.

*Lower, J. (2002). Facing neuron assessment fearlessly. *Nursing2002, 32*(2), 58-65.

*Lower, J. (2003). Using pain to assess neurologic response. *Nursing2003, 33*(60), 56-57.

Milisen, K., Braes, T., Fick, D.M., & Foreman, M.D. (2006). Cognitive assessment and differentiating the 3 D's (dementia, depression, delirium). *Nursing Clinics of North America, 41*(1), 1-21.

Pagana, K.D., & Pagana, T.J. (2006). *Mosby's manual of diagnostic and laboratory tests* (3rd ed.). St. Louis: Mosby.

Photo Guide. (2006). Assessing the cranial nerves. *Nursing2006, 36*(11), 47-49.

Rushing, J. (2007). Assisting with lumbar puncture. *Nursing2007, 37*(1), 23.

Solomon, E.P. (2009). *Introduction to human anatomy and physiology* (3rd ed.). Philadelphia: Saunders.

Thompson, H.J. (2006). *Neurological assessment of the older adult: A guide for nurses.* Chicago: American Association of Neuroscience Nurses.

44 CHAPTER

Care of Patients with Problems of the Central Nervous System: The Brain

Kathy A. Hausman • Donna D. Ignatavicius

LEARNING OUTCOMES

For clinical competence and success on the NCLEX Examination, study this chapter with these Learning Outcomes in mind:

Safe and Effective Care Environment

1. Provide health teaching for hospital discharge to home or other setting for patients with chronic problems of the brain.
2. Collaborate with interdisciplinary health care team members when caring for patients with Parkinson disease (PD) and Alzheimer's disease (AD).
3. Protect patients with AD, PD, and seizures from injury.
4. Implement seizure precautions for patients at risk for acute seizures or status epilepticus.
5. Identify community resources for patients with PD and AD.

Health Promotion and Maintenance

6. Teach patients with chronic headaches about complementary and alternative therapies.
7. Teach patients in highly populated areas ways to prevent meningitis.
8. Identify triggers for patients with chronic headaches.

Psychosocial Integrity

9. Encourage family involvement in developing the plan of care for patients with chronic brain disorders.
10. Identify ways to help prevent caregiver stress when caring for patients with AD and other chronic neurodegenerative diseases.
11. Adapt communication techniques for patients with dementia.

Physiological Integrity

12. Compare the assessment findings of migraine, cluster, and tension headaches.
13. Prioritize care for patients with migraine headaches.
14. Differentiate the common types of seizures, including presenting clinical manifestations.
15. Prioritize care for patients experiencing acute seizures and status epilepticus.
16. Provide care for a patient having a seizure.
17. Provide care for patients with bacterial meningitis and encephalitis.
18. Assess for abnormal neurologic findings in patients with chronic brain problems.
19. Develop a community-based plan of care for a patient with PD and AD.
20. Provide health teaching for patients and family about drug therapy for patients with chronic brain problems.
21. Provide care for patients with AD.
22. Develop a teaching plan for caregivers of patients with AD.
23. Identify the need for genetic counseling for patients who have Huntington disease.

evolve Go to your Companion CD or Evolve at http://evolve.elsevier.com/Iggy/ for *Self-Assessment Questions for the NCLEX Examination* keyed to these Learning Outcomes.

The brain is part of the central nervous system (CNS) that functions as the body's center for controlling mobility (movement), sensation, and cognition. Health problems involving damage of the brain can be acute or chronic. These problems often affect the patient's level of independence and quality of life. This chapter discusses acute CNS infections and common *chronic* neurodegenerative diseases of the brain that may impair the human needs for *mobility* and *cognition*. Care of patients with chronic disorders requires coordination by nurses and other members of the interdisciplinary health care team. The patient and family are also vital members of the team in making decisions about the plan of care.

HEADACHES

Almost everyone has had a headache at some time in his or her life. Some headaches are related to "colds," allergies, or stress and are temporary. Others can be very serious and potentially life threatening. For example, an abnormal neurologic assessment together with symptoms of a cluster headache may indicate a serious neurologic problem. Patients with these symptoms are referred immediately to their health care provider or the emergency department.

Although there are many types and causes of headaches, the focus of this section is on the three most common types that cause people to seek medical attention: migraine headaches, cluster headaches, and tension headaches. Patients are usually managed in the ambulatory care setting by the primary health care provider. However, it is not unusual for the person in severe pain to seek treatment in the emergency department.

As part of the nursing assessment, ask patients about the pattern of their headaches. For example:

- When do the headaches occur?
- How often?
- How long do they last?
- Do certain foods, alcohol, or other things trigger the headaches?
- Have there been any recent changes in your headaches?
- How do you treat the headaches? Does this treatment work?
- How often and what drug or herbal remedy do you take?

Other questions include:

- Is there a family history of headaches?
- Where do the headaches begin? Do they spread to other areas?
- Do you experience other symptoms with the headaches, such as weakness or changes in speech?
- How does this impact your activities of daily living?

Patients are encouraged to keep a headache diary, which may help identify the type of headache they are experiencing. Teach them to notify their health care provider if the severity, intensity, or nature of the headache increases or changes. Encourage them to report whether the headache is associated with unusual visual changes and whether the prescribed drug is no longer effective.

MIGRAINE HEADACHE

Pathophysiology

A **migraine headache** is a chronic, episodic disorder with multiple subtypes. It is classified as a *long-duration headache* because it usually lasts longer than 4 hours. Migraines tend to be familial and may have a genetic basis, although only a few genes have been identified for less common types. For instance, mutations in the *ATP1A2* gene are linked to a rare type of migraine called *familial hemiplegic migraine* (Sanchez-del-Rio et al., 2006).

Women are affected more often than men, making migraines the ninth leading cause of disability in women (Jung, 2007). Women with anxiety and depressive personalities seem to be predisposed to migraines and other chronic health problems (Tan et al., 2007).

Several theories have emerged regarding the causes of migraines, which may involve vascular, genetic, neurologic (central neuronal hyperexcitability), chemical, and environmental factors. It is generally agreed that migraine headaches are mediated via the trigeminal vascular system and its central projections. Blood vessels in the brain overreact to a triggering event, causing spasm in the arteries at the base of the brain. This response is followed by arterial constriction and a decrease in cerebral blood flow. Cerebral hypoxia may occur. Platelets clump together, and serotonin, a vasoconstrictor, is released. Other arteries dilate, which triggers the release of **prostaglandins** (chemicals that cause inflammation and swelling) and other substances that increase sensitivity to pain. Recent research findings suggest a role of excessive synaptic glutamate release or decreased removal of glutamate and potassium from the synaptic cleft (Sanchez-del-Rio et al., 2006).

Many patients find that certain factors, or *triggers* (e.g., caffeine, red wine), tend to cause migraine headache attacks. Each patient is different regarding which environmental factors trigger headaches. For some patients, getting emotionally upset or angry can lead to an attack.

Patient-Centered Collaborative Care

Assessment

Migraines fall into three categories: migraines with aura, migraines without aura, and atypical migraines. An **aura** is a sensation such as visual changes that signals the onset of a headache or seizure. In a migraine, the aura occurs immediately before the migraine episode. *Most headaches are migraines without aura.* The key features of migraines are listed in Chart 44-1. **Atypical migraines** are less common and include menstrual and cluster migraines. The stages of migraine may include:

- Prodrome (or prodromal) phase, in which the patient has specific symptoms such as food cravings or mood changes
- Aura phase (if present), which generally involves visual changes, flashing lights, or **diplopia** (double vision)
- Headache phase, which may last a few hours to a few days
- Termination phase, in which the intensity of the headache decreases
- Postprodrome phase, in which the patient is often fatigued, may be irritable, and has muscle pain

The diagnosis of migraine headache is based on the patient's history and on physical, neurologic, and psychological assessment. The typical migraine is described as a unilateral, frontotemporal, *throbbing* pain in the head that is often worse behind one eye or ear. It is often accompanied by a sensitive scalp, anorexia, **photophobia** (sensitivity to light), **phonophobia** (sensitivity to noise), and nausea with or without vomiting. The pain and associated symptoms can last from 4 to 72 hours. Patients tend to have the same clinical manifestations each time they have a migraine headache. Some may have to refrain from regular activities for several days if they cannot control or relieve the pain in its early stage.

Some physicians recommend screening migraine patients with the Minnesota Multiphasic Personality Inventory-2 (www.pearsonassessments.com/tests/mmpi_2.htm) to identify personality traits and possible mental health/behavioral health problems (Tan et al., 2007). Neuroimaging such as magnetic resonance imaging (MRI) may be indicated if the patient has other neurologic findings, a history of seizures, findings not consistent with a migraine, or a change in the severity of the symptoms or frequency of the attacks.

Neuroimaging is also recommended in patients older than 50 years with a new onset of headaches, especially women. New evidence suggests that women with a history of mi-

Chart 44-1 KEY FEATURES

Migraine Headaches

PHASES OF MIGRAINE WITH AURA (CLASSIC MIGRAINE)

FIRST, OR PRODROME, PHASE

Aura develops over a period of several minutes and lasts no longer than 1 hour.

Well-defined transient focal neurologic dysfunction exists.

Pain may be preceded by:
- Visual disturbances
- Flashing lights
- Lines or spots
- Shimmering or zigzag lights

Pain may be preceded by a variety of neurologic changes, including:
- Numbness, tingling of the lips or tongue
- Acute confusional state
- Aphasia
- Vertigo
- Unilateral weakness
- Drowsiness

SECOND PHASE

Headache is accompanied by nausea and vomiting.

Pain usually begins in the temple. It increases in intensity and becomes throbbing within 1 hour.

THIRD PHASE

Pain changes from throbbing to dull.

Headache, nausea, and vomiting usually last from 4 to 72 hours. (Older patients may have aura without pain, known as a visual migraine.)

MIGRAINE WITHOUT AURA (COMMON MIGRAINE)

Migraine begins without an aura before the onset of the headache.

Pain is aggravated by performing routine physical activities.

Pain is unilateral and pulsating.

One of these symptoms is present:
- Nausea and/or vomiting
- **Photophobia** (light sensitivity)
- **Phonophobia** (sound sensitivity)

Headache lasts for 4 to 72 hours.

Migraine often occurs in the early morning, during periods of stress, or in those with premenstrual tension or fluid retention.

ATYPICAL MIGRAINE

Status migrainous
- Headache lasts longer than 72 hours.

Migrainous infarction
- Neurologic symptoms are not completely reversible within 7 days.
- Ischemic infarct is noted on neuroimaging.

Unclassified
- Headache does not fulfill all of the criteria to be classified a migraine.

graines with visual symptoms may have an increased risk for stroke. This risk increases if a migraine with visual symptoms occurred in the past year. Teach women older than 50 years who have migraines about the risk factors for cardiovascular disease. Encourage them to notify their health care provider if they experience symptoms such as facial drooping, arm weakness, or difficulties with speech.

Common Nursing Diagnoses and Collaborative Problems

Nursing diagnoses that often apply to patients with migraine headaches include:
- Acute Pain related to biologic and chemical factors
- Anxiety and Fear related to the potential of developing a headache, inability to perform ADLs during the headache period, loss of employment, change in social patterns
- Activity Intolerance related to pain and nausea

Interventions

Migraine headaches are often not diagnosed or managed following current best practices. Therefore the National Headache Foundation has recommended the "Three R" approach for patients and health care providers (www.headaches.org):
- *Recognize* migraine symptoms
- *Respond* and see the health care provider
- *Relieve* pain and associated symptoms

The priority for care of the patient having migraines is pain management. This outcome may be achieved by abortive and preventive therapy. Drug therapy, trigger management, and complementary and alternative therapies are the major approaches to care. Provide detailed patient and family education regarding the collaborative plan of care.

Abortive Therapy

Abortive therapy is aimed at alleviating pain during the aura phase (if present) or soon after the headache has started. *Drug therapy* is prescribed to manage migraine headaches. Some of the drugs being used have major side effects, contraindications, and nursing implications. The health care provider must consider any other medical conditions that the patient has when prescribing drug therapy. In general, the patient is started on a low dose that is increased until the desired clinical effect is obtained. Table 44-1 lists commonly used drugs for migraine headaches. Many new drugs are being investigated for this painful and often debilitating health problem.

Mild migraines may be relieved by acetaminophen (APAP) (Tylenol, Abenol🍁). NSAIDs such as ibuprofen (Motrin) and naproxen (Naprosyn) may also be prescribed. In the United States, the Food and Drug Administration (FDA) has approved several over-the-counter (OTC) anti-inflammatory drugs for migraines, including Advil Migraine Capsules, Motrin Migraine Pain Caplets, and Excedrin Migraine Tablets or Caplets (contain APAP, aspirin, and caffeine). Caffeine narrows blood vessels by blocking adenosine, which dilates vessels and increases inflammation. Antiemetics may be prescribed to relieve nausea and vomiting. Metoclopramide (Reglan, Clopra) may be administered with NSAIDs to promote gastric emptying and decrease vomiting.

For more *severe* migraines, drugs such as triptan preparations, ergotamine derivatives, and isometheptene combinations are needed. A potential side effect of these drugs is **rebound headache,** also known as **medication overuse headache,** in which another headache occurs after the drug relieves the initial migraine.

TABLE 44-1 **Commonly Used Drugs for Migraine Headache**

NONSPECIFIC ANALGESICS
• Acetaminophen
• Isometheptene
• Butalbital
NONSTEROIDAL ANTI-INFLAMMATORY DRUGS (NSAIDs)
• Ibuprofen
• Naproxen
BETA BLOCKERS
• Propranolol
• Timolol
ERGOTAMINE PREPARATIONS
• Ergotamine with caffeine (oral or suppository) (Cafergot [Migergot])
• Ergotamine sublingual (SL) (Ergomar SL)
• Dihydroergotamine (DHE) nasal spray (Migranal)
TRIPTAN PREPARATIONS
• Almotriptan (Axert)
• Eletriptan (Relpax)
• Rizatriptan (Maxalt)
• Zolmitriptan (Zomig)
• Sumatriptan (Imitrex)
• Frovatriptan (Frova)
ISOMETHEPTENE COMBINATION
• Midrin
ANTIEPILEPTIC DRUGS (AEDS)
• Divalproex (Depakote)
• Topiramate (Topamax)

Triptan preparations relieve the headache and associated symptoms by activating the 5-HT (serotonin) receptors on the cranial arteries, the basilar artery, and the blood vessels of the dura mater to produce a vasoconstrictive effect. Examples include zolmitriptan (Zomig) and eletriptan (Relpax). Sumatriptan (Imitrex) is also available in tablets, as an injection, and in a nasal spray. For many patients, these drugs are highly effective for pain, nausea, vomiting, and light and sound sensitivity with few side effects. Most are contraindicated in patients with actual or suspected ischemic heart disease, cerebrovascular ischemia, hypertension, and peripheral vascular disease and in those with Prinzmetal's angina because of the potential of coronary vasospasm. Patients respond differently to drugs, and several types or combinations may be tried before the headache is relieved.

Teach patients taking triptan drugs to take them as soon as migraine symptoms develop. Instruct patients to report chest pain or tightness to their health care providers immediately because they may develop angina. Remind them to use contraception (birth control) while taking the drugs because they may not be safe for women who are pregnant. Teach them to expect common side effects that include flushing, tingling, and a hot sensation. These annoying sensations tend to subside after the patient's body gets used to the drug. Triptan drugs should not be taken with selective serotonin reuptake inhibitor (SSRI) antidepressants or St. John's wort, an herb used commonly for depression.

Ergotamine preparations such as Cafergot are taken at the start of the headache. The patient may take up to six tablets in 24 hours or use a rectal suppository. Dihydroergotamine (DHE) may be given IV, IM, or as a nasal spray (Migranal) with an antiemetic if pain control and relief of nausea are not achieved with other drugs. DHE should not be given within 24 hours of a triptan drug.

Midrin is a combination drug containing APAP, isometheptene, and dichloralphenazone. It is the most common *isometheptene combination* given for treating migraines and is an excellent option when ergotamine preparations are not tolerated or do not work.

Other drugs that have been prescribed to relieve migraine pain include opioids and barbiturates. *These drugs should be avoided if at all possible because they are addictive. Some opioids actually cause a migraine.*

Preventive Therapy

Prevention strategies are used when a migraine occurs more than twice per week, substantially interferes with ADLs, or is not relieved with acute treatment. Unless otherwise contraindicated, the health care provider may initially prescribe an NSAID, beta-adrenergic blocker, or antiepileptic drug (AED). Propranolol (Inderal, Apo-Propranolol♣, Novopranol♣) and timolol (Blocadren, Apo-Timol♣) are the only beta blockers approved for migraine prevention. These drugs can lower blood pressure and decrease pulse rate. *Teach patients, especially older adults, how to take their pulse, and encourage them to report bradycardia or clinical manifestations of heart failure such as fatigue and shortness of breath to their health care provider.*

Topiramate (Topamax) is the most common AED used for migraines, but it should be used in low doses. Reports of suicides have been associated with this drug when it is used in larger doses, most often with patients who have bipolar disorder.

In addition to drug therapy, *trigger avoidance and management* are important strategies for preventing migraine episodes. For example, some patients find that avoiding tyramine-containing products, such as pickled products, caffeine, beer, wine, preservatives, and artificial sweeteners, reduces their headaches. Others have identified specific factors that trigger an attack for them. Help patients identify triggers that could cause migraine episodes, and teach them to avoid them once identified (Chart 44-2).

Complementary and Alternative Therapies

Many patients use complementary and alternative therapies as adjuncts to drug therapy. Yoga, meditation, massage, exercise, biofeedback, and relaxation techniques are helpful in preventing or treating migraines for some patients. For example, at the beginning of a migraine attack, the patient may be able to reduce pain by lying down and darkening the room. He or she may want both eyes covered and a cool cloth on the forehead. If the patient falls asleep, he or she should remain undisturbed until awakening.

Acupuncture and acupressure may be effective in relieving pain for some patients. A number of herbs are also used for headaches, both for prevention and pain management. Teach patients that all herbs and nutritional remedies should be approved by their health care provider before use because they could interact with prescribed medication. Table 44-2 lists some commonly used natural remedies and herbs for migraines.

Health Teaching

Teach patients about the importance of taking preventive drugs regularly. Remind them to avoid triggers and use complementary and alternative therapies to help them relax and avoid a

Chart 44-2 PATIENT AND FAMILY EDUCATION GUIDE

Factors That May Trigger a Migraine Attack

Teach patients to avoid the foods, medications, and other factors that may trigger a migraine attack.

Food and beverages (tyramine-containing):
- Alcoholic drinks: beer, wine, and hard liquor
- Aged cheese
- Caffeine found in beverages such as coffee, tea, cola
- Chocolate
- Foods with yeast such as pastry and fresh breads
- Monosodium glutamate (MSG)
- Nitrates (food preservatives), pickled or fermented foods
- Nuts
- Artificial sweeteners
- Smoked fish

Drugs:
- Cimetidine (Tagamet)
- Estrogens
- Nitroglycerin
- Nifedipine (Procardia, Nifed♣)

Other factors:
- Anger, conflict
- Fatigue
- Hormonal fluctuations, such as menstruation, pregnancy, and menopause
- Light glare
- Missed meals
- Psychological stress
- Sleep problems
- Smells, such as tobacco smoke
- Travel to different altitudes

TABLE 44-2 Commonly Used Herbs to Prevent Migraine Headaches

- Feverfew (*Tanacetum parthenium*) (most commonly used)
- Bay (*Laurus nobilis*)
- Willow (*Salix*)
- Ginger (*Zingiber officinale*)
- Red pepper (*Capsicum*)
- Valerian (*Valeriana officinalis*)
- Dong Quai (*Angelica sinensis*)
- *Ginkgo biloba*
- Lavender
- Lemon balm (*Melissa officinalis*)
- Peppermint
- Magnesium
- Purslane (*Portulaca oleracea*)

headache. Teach patients who have migraine headaches to practice a healthy lifestyle. Emphasize the importance of healthy habits such as avoiding smoking, exercising regularly, eating a balanced diet, and getting adequate rest and sleep.

CLUSTER HEADACHE

Pathophysiology

Cluster headaches are manifested by brief intense unilateral pain that generally occurs in the spring and fall. It is classified as the *most common chronic short-duration headache* with pain lasting less than 4 hours. Also referred to as *histamine cephalalgia*, it is far less common than migraines. Men are affected three to four times more often than women (McGeeney, 2005). The cause and mechanism of cluster headaches are not known but have been attributed to vasoreactivity and oxyhemoglobin desaturation. Neuroimaging studies suggest that cluster headaches are related to an overactive hypothalamus. Positron emission tomography (PET) scans and magnetic resonance imaging (MRI) demonstrate an increase in neuronal hypothalamic density and hypothalamic size in patients with cluster headaches (McGeeney, 2005). There may be a small genetic link, diet has no effect, and the disorder is unrelated to personality type.

Patient-Centered Collaborative Care

Assessment

Question the patient about prescribed drugs for both the prevention and relief of the headache, as well as OTC drugs and herbs he or she may be taking. Interventions used by the patient may include relaxation techniques, meditation, acupuncture, or massage therapies. Ask the patient to recall a typical week's activities and any recent changes in lifestyle. Ask him or her to identify bedtimes and waking times to help assess changes in activity or lack of continuity in the sleep-wake cycle.

The pain of these unilateral (one-sided) oculotemporal or oculofrontal headaches is often described as excruciating, boring, and *nonthrobbing*. The intense pain is felt deep in and around the eye. The headaches last from 8 to 24 hours each day at the same time for about 4 to 12 weeks (hence the term *cluster*), followed by a period of remission for 9 months to a year. This episodic form is the most common, although there is a chronic, intractable form in which there may not be a remission for more than a year. The average duration of each headache is 30 to 90 minutes.

The pain may radiate to the forehead, temple, or cheek. It may also radiate, but to a lesser extent, to the ear and neck. The temporal artery may be prominent and tender. The patient often paces, walks, or sits and rocks during an attack. A cluster is the only headache type in which this behavior occurs. During periods of remission, alcohol does not cause a headache (as it does during the headache period). The onset of the pain is associated with relaxation, napping, or rapid eye movement (REM) sleep.

The headache usually occurs with:
- **Ipsilateral** (same side) tearing of the eye
- **Rhinorrhea** ("runny nose") or congestion
- **Ptosis** (drooping eyelid)
- Eyelid edema
- Facial sweating
- **Miosis** (constriction of pupils)

The ptosis may become permanent. Assess for possible bradycardia, flushing or pallor of the face, increased intraocular pressure, and increased skin temperature. Nausea and vomiting may also occur. The patient may become restless and agitated from the intense pain of the headache.

Interventions

The health care provider typically prescribes some of the same types of drugs used for migraines, such as triptans, ergotamine preparations, and antiepileptic drugs (see discussion of drug therapy in the Migraine Headache section). Additional drugs include calcium channel blockers, especially verapamil

(Calan), lithium, and corticosteroids. OTC capsaicin, available as a nasal spray (civamide), melatonin, and glucosamine are also used by some patients. Provide health teaching about drug therapy.

During the periods of attack, teach the patient to wear sunglasses and to sit facing away from the window to help decrease exposure to light and glare. If the health care provider prescribes oxygen, 100% oxygen via mask at 7 to 10 L/min is typically administered with the patient in a sitting position. Administer the oxygen for 15 to 30 minutes and discontinue it when the headache is relieved. Oxygen reduces cerebral blood flow and inhibits activity of the carotid bodies, which are sensitive to oxygen levels in the body. *Patients may use oxygen at home. Teach them about the precautions that must be taken when oxygen is used (see Chapter 30).*

To prevent future attacks brought on by precipitating factors (bursts of anger, prolonged anticipation, excessive physical activity, and excitement), discuss their relationship to the onset of cluster headaches. Explain the need for and importance of a consistent sleep-wake cycle.

Surgical intervention may be recommended for patients with *chronic* drug-resistant cluster headaches. Invasive ambulatory care procedures, such as *percutaneous stereotactic rhizotomy (PSR),* are performed with varying success rates. Information about this procedure is found in Chapter 46 in the Trigeminal Neuralgia section. Long-term high-frequency electrical stimulation of the posterior hypothalamus, also known as *deep brain stimulation,* may reduce or eliminate pain (see discussion on p. 969 in the Parkinson Disease section). It has not been approved by the FDA but is being investigated. Both of these procedures have major complications that can cause permanent brain or nerve damage. Therefore they are done as a last resort.

TENSION HEADACHE

Tension headaches are the most *common type of chronic long-duration headache,* lasting more than 4 hours. As the name implies, they are caused by stress and tension. Tension headaches are characterized by neck and shoulder muscle tenderness and bilateral pain at the base of the skull and in the forehead. They appear similar to migraine headaches, and distinguishing between the two can be very difficult. The classic signs of nausea, vomiting, photophobia (light sensitivity), phonophobia (noise sensitivity), and aggravation of the headache with activity that are typical of migraines may also occur with tension headaches.

Management of tension headaches includes non-opioid analgesics such as acetaminophen and NSAIDs. A combination of ibuprofen plus caffeine may be more effective in relieving pain than NSAIDs alone. Muscle relaxants, such as tizanidine (Zanaflex), and divalproex (Depakote), an antiepileptic drug, may help prevent these headaches. Some patients also need antianxiety or antidepressant drugs. Opioids and barbiturates may be used on a short-term basis, but they are very addictive and should be used sparingly. Teach patients about expected side effects of drug therapy.

Complementary and Alternative Therapies

Peppermint oil applied topically or taken orally works for some patients to control pain. Although not scientifically proven, it may relax the smooth muscle of the blood vessels (Barclay, 2007). Teach patients that therapies such as massage, yoga, and meditation may decrease anxiety and prevent headaches. Acupuncture and acupressure may help relieve them.

Health teaching also includes the importance of lifestyle changes. Talk to the patient about developing a routine sleeping pattern. Ask him or her about food intake, and provide information if needed about a healthy diet. Collaborate with the patient to develop a plan to incorporate exercise into his or her daily routine. Provide the patient with a list of community resources and activities to help recognize stress and participate in techniques to break the stress cycle (Graner, 2007).

NCLEX EXAMINATION CHALLENGE

A client with a known history of migraines is admitted to the emergency department with a severe throbbing frontal headache and photophobia. What is the nurse's first action when caring for this client?

A. Provide a darkened room and quiet environment.
B. Interview the client about what triggered the headache.
C. Give sumatriptan (Imitrex) injection immediately.
D. Provide an emesis basin and tissues.

evolve For the correct answer, go to http://evolve.elsevier.com/Iggy/.

SEIZURES AND EPILEPSY

Pathophysiology

A **seizure** is an abnormal, sudden, excessive, uncontrolled electrical discharge of neurons within the brain that may result in a change in level of consciousness (LOC), motor or sensory ability, and/or behavior. A single seizure may occur for no known reason. Some seizures are caused by a pathologic condition of the brain, such as a tumor. In this case, once the underlying problem is treated, the patient is often asymptomatic.

Epilepsy is defined by the National Institute of Neurological Disorders and Stroke as two or more seizures experienced by a person. It is a chronic disorder in which repeated unprovoked seizure activity occurs. It may be caused by an abnormality in electrical neuronal activity, an imbalance of neurotransmitters, especially gamma aminobutyric acid (GABA), or a combination of both.

Types of Seizures

The International Classification of Epileptic Seizures recognizes three broad categories of seizure disorders: generalized seizures, partial seizures, and unclassified seizures.

Generalized Seizures

Six types of **generalized seizures** may occur and involve *both* cerebral hemispheres. The **tonic-clonic seizure** lasting 2 to 5 minutes begins with a **tonic** phase that causes stiffening or rigidity of the muscles, particularly of the arms and legs, and immediate loss of consciousness. **Clonic** or rhythmic jerking of all extremities follows. The patient may bite his or her tongue and may become incontinent of urine or feces. Fatigue, acute confusion, and lethargy may last up to an hour after the seizure.

Occasionally, only tonic or clonic movement may occur. A **tonic seizure** is an abrupt increase in muscle tone, loss of consciousness, and autonomic changes lasting from 30 seconds to several minutes. The **clonic seizure** lasts several minutes and causes muscle contraction and relaxation.

The **absence seizure** is more common in children and tends to run in families. It consists of brief (often just seconds) periods of loss of consciousness and blank staring as though the person is daydreaming. The patient's eyes may flutter and **automatisms** (involuntary behaviors) such as lip smacking and picking at clothes may also occur. He or she is not aware of these behaviors. The patient returns to baseline immediately after the seizure. Left undiagnosed or untreated, the seizures may occur frequently throughout the day, interfering with school or other daily activity.

The **myoclonic seizure** causes a brief jerking or stiffening of the extremities that may occur singly or in groups. Lasting for just a few seconds, the contractions may be symmetric (both sides) or asymmetric (one side).

In an **atonic (akinetic) seizure,** the patient has a sudden loss of muscle tone, lasting for seconds, followed by **postictal** (after the seizure) confusion. In most cases, these seizures cause the patient to fall, which may result in injury. This type of seizure tends to be most resistant to drug therapy.

Partial Seizures

Partial seizures, also called *focal* or *local* seizures, begin in a part of *one* cerebral hemisphere. They are further subdivided into two main classes: complex partial seizures and simple partial seizures. In addition, some partial seizures can become generalized tonic-clonic, tonic, or clonic seizures. Partial seizures are most often seen in adults and generally are less responsive to medical treatment when compared with other types.

Complex partial seizures may cause loss of consciousness **(syncope),** or "black out," for 1 to 3 minutes. Characteristic automatisms may occur as in absence seizures. The patient is unaware of the environment and may wander at the start of the seizure. In the period after the seizure, he or she may have **amnesia** (loss of memory). Because the area of the brain most often involved in this type of epilepsy is the temporal lobe, complex partial seizures are often called *psychomotor* seizures or *temporal lobe* seizures.

CONSIDERATIONS FOR OLDER ADULTS

Complex partial seizures are most common among older adults and account for nearly 40% of all diagnosed seizures in this group (Vacca & Olson, 2007). These seizures are difficult to diagnose because symptoms appear similar to dementia, psychosis, or Alzheimer's disease (AD), especially in the **postictal stage** (after the seizure). New-onset seizures in older adults are typically associated with conditions such as hypertension, cardiac disease, diabetes mellitus, stroke, and Alzheimer's disease.

The patient with a **simple partial seizure** remains conscious throughout the episode. He or she often reports an **aura** (unusual sensation) before the seizure takes place. This may consist of a "déjà vu" (already seen) phenomenon, perception of an offensive smell, or sudden onset of pain. During the seizure, the patient may have one-sided movement of an extremity, experience unusual sensations, or have autonomic symptoms. Autonomic changes include a change in heart rate, skin flushing, and epigastric discomfort.

Unclassified Seizures

Unclassified, or **idiopathic,** seizures account for about half of all seizure activity. They occur for no known reason and do not fit into the generalized or partial classifications.

Etiology and Genetic Risk

Primary or **idiopathic epilepsy** is not associated with any identifiable brain lesion or other specific cause. **Secondary seizures** result from an underlying brain lesion, most commonly a tumor or trauma. They may also be caused by:

- Metabolic disorders
- Acute alcohol withdrawal
- Electrolyte disturbances (e.g., hyperkalemia, water intoxication, hypoglycemia)
- High fever
- Stroke
- Head injury
- Substance abuse
- Heart disease

Seizures resulting from these problems are not considered epilepsy. Various risk factors can trigger a seizure, such as increased physical activity, emotional stress, excessive fatigue, alcohol or caffeine consumption, or certain foods or chemicals.

GENETIC CONSIDERATIONS

Several genetic links that may contribute to seizures have been identified:

- Defective genes for channels that regulate neuronal signals affect the flow of ions into and out of the cells.
- Patients with progressive myoclonus are missing the cystatin B protein.
- An abnormally active version of a gene that increases resistance to antiepileptic drugs has been identified in patients who cannot obtain seizure control with varied and multiple drugs.
- An abnormal gene that controls neuronal migration can lead to areas of misplaced or abnormally formed neurons or dysplasia.

Patient-Centered Collaborative Care

Assessment

Question the patient or family about how many seizures the patient has had, how long they last, and any pattern of occurrence. Ask the patient or family to describe the seizures that the patient has had. Clinical manifestations vary depending on the type of seizure experienced, as described earlier. Ask about the presence of an aura before seizures begin **(preictal phase).** Question whether the patient is taking any prescribed drugs or herbs or has had head trauma or high fever. Assess any alcohol and/or illicit drug history. Ask about any other medical condition such as a previous stroke or hypertension.

Diagnosis is based on the history and physical examination. A variety of diagnostic tests are performed to rule out other causes of seizure activity and to confirm the diagnosis of epilepsy. Typical diagnostic tests include an electroencephalogram (EEG), computed tomography (CT) scan, MRI, or positron emission tomography (PET) scan. These tests are described in Chapter 43. Laboratory studies are performed to identify metabolic or other disorders that may cause or contribute to seizure activity.

Common Nursing Diagnoses and Collaborative Problems

Nursing diagnoses and collaborative problems that often apply to patients with epilepsy include:

- Risk for Injury related to seizure activity
- Ineffective Coping related to uncertainty and inadequate level of perception of control
- Risk for Ineffective Breathing Pattern related to neuromuscular dysfunction
- Potential for Status Epilepticus

Interventions

Removing or treating the underlying condition or cause of the seizure manages *secondary* epilepsy and seizures that are not considered epileptic. *In most cases, primary epilepsy is successfully managed through drug therapy.*

Nonsurgical Management

Most seizures can be completely or almost completely controlled through the administration of **antiepileptic drugs (AEDs),** sometimes referred to as *anticonvulsants,* for specific types of seizures.

Drug Therapy. Drug therapy is the major component of management (Chart 44-3). The health care provider intro-

Chart 44-3 COMMON EXAMPLES OF DRUG THERAPY

Antiepileptic Drugs

Drug	Indication for Use	Nursing Interventions
Carbamazepine (Tegretol, Tegretol-XR, Carbatrol)	Partial, generalized tonic-clonic seizures	Monitor for headache, dizziness, diplopia or blurred vision, N/V, and leukopenia. Monitor CBC. Do not crush or chew sustained-release capsules.
Clonazepam (Klonopin)	Absence, myoclonic, and akinetic seizures	Monitor results of liver function tests.
Clorazepate dipotassium	Adjunctive management of partial seizures	Give with food. Monitor blood pressure.
Diazepam (Valium, Apo-Diazepam🍁), lorazepam (Ativan), Diastat (Valium rectal gel delivery system)	Status epilepticus	Monitor airway, breathing, circulation (ABCs).
Divalproex (Depakote), valproic acid (Depakene)	All types of seizures	Monitor for hair loss, tremor, increased liver enzymes, bruising, and N/V. Monitor CBC, PT, PTT, and AST.
Ethosuximide (Zarontin)	Absence seizures	Watch for N/V, skin rash, lethargy, and anorexia. Monitor CBC and liver function tests. (Drug used infrequently.)
Felbamate (Felbatol)	Adjunctive therapy for intractable complex partial seizures	Note that aplastic anemia and liver failure are major sequelae of treatment. Patient must sign consent for use, acknowledging risk for aplastic anemia and liver failure. Monitor CBC. Monitor liver function tests. Watch for anorexia and weight loss.
Gabapentin (Neurontin)	Partial seizures	Watch for increased appetite and weight gain. Monitor for ataxia, irritability, dizziness, and fatigue.
Lamotrigine (Lamictal)	Partial seizures	Watch for diplopia, headaches, dizziness, drowsiness, ataxia, N/V, and life-threatening rash when given with valproic acid.
Levetiracetam (Keppra) **Med Error Alert!** Do not confuse Keppra with Kaletra, an antiretroviral drug used to treat HIV.	Adjunct management of partial seizures	Monitor renal function carefully. Notify health care provider for gait or coordination problems.
Oxcarbazepine (Trileptal)	Partial seizures	Monitor for hyponatremia.
Phenobarbital (Barbita, Luminal)	Generalized tonic-clonic seizures, partial seizures	Note that this is less desirable than other antiepileptic drugs (AEDs) because of sedation. Be aware that overdose can be fatal. Monitor for drowsiness, sleep disturbances, cognitive impairment, and depression.

AST, Aspartate aminotransferase; *CBC,* complete blood count; *N/V,* nausea and vomiting; *PT,* prothrombin time; *PTT,* partial thromboplastin time.

Continued

Chart 44-3 COMMON EXAMPLES OF DRUG THERAPY

Antiepileptic Drugs—cont'd

Drug	Indication for Use	Nursing Interventions
Phenytoin (Dilantin), fosphenytoin (Cerebyx)	All types, except absence, myoclonic, and atonic seizures; for status epilepticus	Monitor for gastric distress, gingival hyperplasia, anemia, ataxia, and nystagmus. Check CBC and calcium levels; monitor for therapeutic drug levels (10-20 mcg/mL) and toxic levels (>30 mcg/mL). For IV phenytoin, flush catheter with saline before and after administration. For fosphenytoin, use phenytoin equivalent for dosing.
Primidone (Mysoline, Sertan♣)	Partial seizures, generalized tonic-clonic seizures	Monitor for vertigo and lethargy. Watch for drug interactions with phenobarbital and isoniazid.
Tiagabine (Gabitril)	Partial seizures	Monitor for dizziness, weakness, nervousness, psychomotor slowing, nystagmus, and paresthesias. Administer with food.
Topiramate (Topamax)	Adjunctive therapy for intractable partial seizures	Monitor for ataxia, confusion, dizziness, and fatigue. Be aware of increased risk for renal calculi.
Valproate (Depakote), valproate sodium injection (Depacon)	Simple and complex absence seizures Adjunct therapy for partial complex and generalized tonic-clonic seizures	Monitor for hair loss, tremor, increased liver enzymes, bruising, and N/V. Monitor CBC, PT, PTT, AST.
Zonisamide (Zonegran)	Adjunctive therapy for partial seizures	Monitor CBC, platelets, and renal function. Assess mental status, especially memory.

AST, Aspartate aminotransferase; *CBC*, complete blood count; *N/V*, nausea and vomiting; *PT*, prothrombin time; *PTT*, partial thromboplastin time.

CONSIDERATIONS FOR OLDER ADULTS

The health care provider considers these desirable effects when prescribing antiepileptic drugs for the older adult (Vacca & Olson, 2007):

- Minimal possibility of toxicity
- Low side effects
- Oral route for dosing
- Easily metabolized and absorbed
- Long half-life with infrequent dosing to prevent missed dose
- Readily excreted
- Minimal protein binding because they lose protein and a therapeutic dose may be toxic to them
- Minimal to no weight gain to prevent complications that may be associated with heart disease

duces one antiepileptic drug (AED) at a time to achieve seizure control. If the chosen drug is not effective, the dosage may be increased or another drug introduced. At times, seizure control is achieved only through a combination of drugs. The dosages are adjusted to achieve therapeutic blood levels without causing major side effects.

Teach patients to take their drugs on time to maintain therapeutic blood levels and maximum effectiveness. Be aware of drug-drug and drug-food interactions. Instruct the patient to avoid drugs and foods that might interfere with the absorption or metabolism of the AED. For instance, warfarin (Coumadin, Warfilone♣) should not be given with phenytoin (Dilantin). Document side and adverse effects of the prescribed drugs, and report to the health care provider.

Health Teaching. Provide an educational program for the patient and family (Chart 44-4). Ask them what they understand about the disorder, and correct any misinformation. As new information is presented, be sure that the patient and family can understand it. Refer patients and families to the Epilepsy Foundation of America (www.epilepsyfoundation.org) for more information and community support groups.

Emphasize that AEDs must not be stopped even if the seizures have stopped. Discontinuing these drugs can lead to the recurrence of seizures or the life-threatening complication of status epilepticus (discussed on p. 959). Some patients may stop therapy because they do not have the money to purchase the drugs. Refer limited-income patients to the social services department for assistance or to a case manager to locate other resources.

Teach patients the importance of having their serum drug levels monitored to ensure a therapeutic level, and assess for high levels that could indicate toxicity. Collaborate with the case manager about transportation needs, if necessary.

A balanced diet, proper rest, and stress reduction techniques usually minimize the risk of breakthrough seizures. Encourage the patient to keep a seizure diary to determine whether there are factors that tend to be associated with seizure activity. Patients should follow state law concerning allowances for driving a motor vehicle.

All states prohibit discrimination against people who have epilepsy. Patients who work in occupations in which a seizure might cause serious harm to themselves or others (e.g., construction workers, operators of dangerous equipment, pilots, railroad engineers) may need other employment. They may need to decrease or modify strenuous or potentially dangerous physical activity to avoid harm, although this varies with each

Chart 44-4 PATIENT AND FAMILY EDUCATION GUIDE

Instructions for the Patient with Epilepsy

- Drug therapy information:
  - Name, dosage, time of administration
  - Actions to take if side effects occur
  - Importance of taking drug as prescribed and not missing a dose
  - What to do if a dose is missed or cannot be taken
  - Importance of having blood drawn for therapeutic or toxic levels as requested by the health care provider
- **Do not take any medication, including over-the-counter drugs, without asking your health care provider.**
- Wear a medical alert bracelet or necklace or carry an ID card indicating epilepsy.
- Follow up with your neurologist, physician, or other health care provider as directed.
- Be sure a family member or significant other knows how to help you in the event of a seizure and knows when your health care provider or emergency medical services should be called.
- Investigate and follow state laws concerning driving and operating machinery.
- Avoid alcohol and excessive fatigue.
- Contact the Epilepsy Foundation (www.epilepsyfoundation.org) or other organized epilepsy group for additional information. Epilepsy Canada (www.epilepsy.ca) also provides resources and support.

person. Various local, state, and federal agencies can help with finances, living arrangements, and vocational rehabilitation.

Seizure Precautions. *Precautions are taken to prevent the patient from injury if a seizure occurs. Specific seizure precautions vary depending on health care agency policy. Be sure that oxygen and suctioning equipment with an airway are readily available. If the patient does not have an IV access, insert a saline lock, especially for those patients who are at significant risk for generalized tonic-clonic seizures.* The saline lock provides ready access if IV drug therapy must be given to stop the seizure.

Siderails should be in the "up" position at all times. Siderails are rarely the source of significant injury, and the effectiveness of the use of padded siderails to maintain safety is debatable. Padded siderails may embarrass the patient and the family. Follow agency policy about the use of siderails because they are now classified as a restraint device. Other methods to protect the patient, such as placing a mattress on the floor, may be used instead of siderails.

Padded tongue blades do not belong at the bedside and should NEVER be inserted into the patient's mouth because the jaw may clench down as soon as the seizure begins! Forcing a tongue blade or airway into the mouth is more likely to chip the teeth and increase the risk of aspirating tooth fragments than prevent the patient from biting the tongue. Furthermore, improper placement of a padded tongue blade can obstruct the airway.

Seizure Management. The actions taken during a seizure should be appropriate for the type of seizure (Chart 44-5). For example, for a simple partial seizure, observe the patient and document the time that the seizure lasted. Redirect the patient's attention away from an activity that could cause injury. Turn the patient on the side during a generalized tonic-clonic or complex partial seizure because he or she may lose consciousness. If possible, turn the patient's head to the side to prevent aspiration and allow secretions to drain. Remove any objects that might injure the patient.

Chart 44-5 BEST PRACTICE FOR PATIENT SAFETY & QUALITY CARE

Care of the Patient During a Tonic-Clonic or Complete Partial Seizure

- Protect the patient from injury.
- Do not force anything into the patient's mouth.
- Turn the patient to the side to keep the airway clear.
- Loosen any restrictive clothing the patient is wearing.
- Maintain the patient's airway and suction as needed.
- Do not restrain or try to stop the patient's movement; guide movements if necessary.
- Record the time the seizure began and ended.
- At the completion of the seizure:
  - Take the patient's vital signs.
  - Perform neurologic checks.
  - Keep the patient on his or her side.
  - Allow the patient to rest.
  - Document the seizure (see Chart 44-6).

It is not unusual for the patient to become cyanotic during a generalized tonic-clonic seizure. The cyanosis is generally self-limiting, and no treatment is needed. Some health care providers prefer to give the high-risk patient (e.g., older adult, critically ill or debilitated patient) oxygen by nasal cannula or facemask during the postictal phase. *He or she is not restrained because this may cause injury and may worsen the situation, causing more seizure activity. For any type of seizure, carefully observe the seizure and document assessment findings* (Chart 44-6).

Emergency Care: Acute Seizure and Status Epilepticus Management. Seizures occurring in greater intensity, number, or length than the patient's usual seizures are considered *acute.* They may also appear in clusters that are different from the patient's typical seizure pattern. Treatment with lorazepam (Ativan, Apo-Lorazepam🍁) or diazepam (Valium, Meval🍁, Vivol🍁, Diastat [rectal diazepam gel]) may be given to stop the clusters to prevent the development of status epilepticus. IV phenytoin (Dilantin) or fosphenytoin (Cerebyx) may be added.

***Status epilepticus** is a medical emergency and is a prolonged seizure lasting longer than 5 minutes or repeated seizures over the course of 30 minutes. It is a potential complication of all types of seizures. Seizures lasting longer than 10 minutes can cause death!* Common causes of status epilepticus include:

- Sudden withdrawal from antiepileptic drugs
- Infections
- Acute alcohol or drug withdrawal
- Head trauma
- Cerebral edema
- Metabolic disturbances

Convulsive status epilepticus must be treated promptly and aggressively! Establish an airway and notify the health care provider immediately if this problem occurs! Establishing an airway is the priority for this patient's care. Intubation by an anesthesia provider or respiratory therapist (RT) may be necessary. Administer oxygen as indicated by the patient's condition. If not already in place, establish IV access with a large-bore catheter, and start 0.9% sodium chloride. The patient is usually placed

Chart 44-6 FOCUSED ASSESSMENT

Seizures: Nursing Observations and Documentation

How often the seizures occur
- Date, time, and duration of the seizure

Description of each seizure
- Tonic, clonic
- Staring spells, blinking
- Automatism

Whether more than one type of seizure occurs

Sequence of seizure progression
- Where the seizure began
- Body part first involved

Observations during the seizure
- Changes in pupil size and any eye deviation
- Level of consciousness
- Presence of apnea, cyanosis, and salivation
- Incontinence of bowel or bladder during the seizure
- Eye fluttering
- Movement and progression of motor activity
- Lip smacking or other automatism
- Tongue or lip biting

How long the seizures last

When the last seizure took place

Whether the seizures are preceded by an aura
- Dizziness, numbness, or visual disturbances
- Gustatory (taste) or auditory disturbances

What the patient does after the seizure
- Feels drowsy or weak
- May resume normal behavior
- May be unaware that the seizure took place

How long it takes for the patient to return to pre-seizure status

in the intensive care unit for continuous monitoring and management.

Blood is drawn to determine arterial blood gas levels and to identify metabolic, toxic, and other causes of the uncontrolled seizure. Brain damage and death may occur in the patient with tonic-clonic status epilepticus. Left untreated, metabolic changes result, leading to hypoxia, hypotension, hypoglycemia, cardiac dysrhythmias, or lactic (metabolic) acidosis. Further harm to the patient occurs when muscle breaks down and myoglobin accumulates in the kidneys, which can lead to renal failure and electrolyte imbalance. *This is especially likely in the older adult.*

The drugs of choice for treating status epilepticus are IV push lorazepam (Ativan, Apo-Lorazepam♣) or diazepam (Valium). Diazepam rectal gel (Diastat) may be used instead. Lorazepam is usually given as 4 mg over a 2-minute period. This procedure may be repeated, if necessary, until a total of 8 mg is reached. *Monitor the patient for respiratory distress, and have endotracheal intubation equipment readily available. Collaborate with the RT to manage this patient.*

To prevent additional tonic-clonic seizures or cardiac arrest, a loading dose of IV phenytoin (Dilantin) is given and oral doses administered as a follow-up after the emergency is resolved. Initially, give phenytoin at no more than 50 mg/min using an infusion pump. An alternative to phenytoin is fosphenytoin (Cerebyx), a water-soluble phenytoin prodrug. It is compatible with most IV solutions. It also causes fewer cardiovascular complications than phenytoin and can be given in an IV dextrose solution. After administration, fosphenytoin converts to phenytoin in the body. Therefore the FDA requires the dosage to be written as a phenytoin equivalent (PE); 150 mg of fosphenytoin equals 100 mg of phenytoin. Give fosphenytoin at a rate of 100 to 150 mg/min IV piggyback.

Serum drug levels should be checked every 6 to 12 hours after the loading dose and then 2 weeks after oral phenytoin has started. Teach the patient about the side and adverse effects of any AED that is prescribed (see Chart 44-3).

NCLEX EXAMINATION CHALLENGE

The physician prescribes a loading dose of 18 mg/kg IV phenytoin (Dilantin) to be given at 50 mg/min. The client weighs 176 pounds. The nurse sets the pump for the drug to be infused over _____ minutes (round to the nearest whole number).

evolve For the correct answer, go to http://evolve.elsevier.com/Iggy/.

Surgical Management

Patients who cannot be managed effectively with drug therapy may be candidates for surgery, including vagal nerve stimulation (VNS) and conventional surgical procedures. VNS is a fairly new procedure that has been very successful for many patients with epilepsy.

Vagal Nerve Stimulation. Vagal nerve stimulation (VNS) may be performed for control of continuous simple or complex partial seizures. Patients with generalized seizures are not candidates for surgery because VNS may result in severe neurologic deficits. The stimulating device (much like a cardiac pacemaker) is surgically implanted in the left chest wall. An electrode lead is attached to the left vagus nerve, tunneled under the skin, and connected to a generator. The procedure usually takes 2 hours with the patient under general anesthesia. The stimulator is activated by the physician either in the operating room or, more commonly, 2 weeks after surgery. Programming is adjusted gradually over a period of time. The pattern of stimulation is individualized to the patient's tolerance. The generator runs continuously, stimulating the vagus nerve according to the programmed schedule.

The patient can activate the VNS with a handheld magnet when experiencing an aura, thus aborting the seizure. Patients experience a change in voice quality, which signifies that the vagus nerve has been stimulated. They usually report a relief in intensity and duration of seizures and an improved quality of life.

Observe for complications after the procedure such as hoarseness (most common), cough, dyspnea, neck pain, or dysphagia (difficulty swallowing). Teach the patient to avoid MRIs and microwaves, shortwave radios, and ultrasound diathermy, a physical therapy treatment.

Conventional Surgical Procedures. A small percentage of patients with epilepsy cannot be fully controlled with drug therapy or VNS. When all other options are exhausted, conventional surgery may be needed to improve the patient's quality of life. The largest group of conventional surgical candidates includes those with complex partial seizures in the frontal or temporal lobe.

Before surgery, the patient is admitted to a special inpatient observation unit. While there, he or she has continuous electroencephalogram (EEG) recording, close observation, and in many hospitals, video monitoring at all times except during personal care activities. The patient is taken off all AEDs. After the seizure area is identified, electrodes may be surgically implanted into the brain tissue to identify the extent of the focal area. This step is followed by additional continuous EEG and video monitoring, as well as close observation by the nursing staff. The area is surgically removed if vital areas of brain function will not be affected.

Preoperative care is similar to that described for patients undergoing a craniotomy (see Chapter 47). Preoperative diagnostic tests include MRI and single-photon emission computed tomography (SPECT)/positron emission tomography (PET) scans as described in Chapter 43. An intracarotid amobarbital test (Wada test) and neuropsychological testing are also done. The Wada test assesses hemispheric lateralization of language and memory after injection of amobarbital, a short-acting anesthetic. This procedure establishes the safety of surgery to preserve language memory. Neuropsychological testing evaluates memory, visuospatial function, language function, and intelligence quotient (IQ) to identify deficiencies in the brain that might correspond to areas believed to be the epileptic region. It is also used to compare preoperative and postoperative cognitive functioning.

Another surgical approach, the *partial corpus callosotomy,* may be used to treat tonic-clonic or atonic seizures in patients who are not candidates for other surgical procedures. The surgeon sections the anterior two thirds of the corpus callosum, preventing neuronal discharges from passing between the two hemispheres of the brain. This surgery usually reduces the number and severity of the seizures, making them more likely to respond to more conventional drug therapy. This procedure is not as commonly done as other surgeries but is very successful for some patients.

INFECTIONS

MENINGITIS

Pathophysiology

ANIMATION: Meningitis ▶

Meningitis is an inflammation of the meninges that surround the brain and spinal cord. Bacterial and viral organisms are most often responsible for meningitis, although fungal meningitis and protozoal meningitis also occur. *Viral meningitis is usually self-limiting, and the patient has a complete recovery. Bacterial meningitis is potentially life threatening.* Regardless of the causative organism, symptoms are the same.

The organisms responsible for meningitis enter the central nervous system (CNS) via the bloodstream at the blood-brain barrier. Direct routes of entry occur as a result of penetrating trauma, surgical procedures, or a ruptured cerebral abscess. **Otorrhea** (ear discharge) or **rhinorrhea** (nasal discharge, or "runny nose"), which may be caused by a basilar skull fracture, may lead to meningitis as a result of the direct communication of cerebrospinal fluid (CSF) with the environment. The invading organisms travel throughout the CNS via the subarachnoid space. The organism produces an inflammatory response in the pia mater, the arachnoid, the CSF, and the ventricles. The **exudate** (pus) formed may spread to both cranial and spinal nerves, causing further neurologic deterioration. Increased intracranial pressure (ICP) may occur as a result of blockage of the flow of CSF, change in cerebral blood flow, or thrombus (blood clot) formation.

Viral Meningitis

Viral meningitis, the most common type, is sometimes referred to as **aseptic meningitis.** It often results from a variety of viral illnesses, including measles, mumps, herpes simplex, and herpes zoster. The formation of exudate that is common in bacterial meningitis does not occur, and no organisms are obtained from the CSF. Inflammation occurs over the cerebral cortex, the white matter, and the meninges. The susceptibility of the brain tissue to the virus varies depending on which type of cell is involved. The herpes simplex virus alters cellular metabolism, which quickly results in necrosis of the cells. Other viruses cause an alteration in the production of enzymes or neurotransmitters, which results in cell dysfunction and possible neurologic defects.

Clinical manifestations of viral meningitis include fever, **photophobia** (light sensitivity), headache, myalgias (muscle aches), and nausea. Herpes simplex type 2 may cause genital lesions. A maculopapular rash is seen when the causative organism is an enterovirus. Treatment is symptomatic. If genital lesions are present, acyclovir may be prescribed.

Fungal Meningitis

Cryptococcus neoformans meningitis is the most common fungal infection that affects the CNS of patients with acquired immune deficiency syndrome (AIDS). Fulminant invasive fungal sinusitis is also a recognized cause of fungal meningitis. The clinical manifestations vary because the compromised immune system affects the inflammatory response. For example, some patients have fever and others do not. Almost all of them have headache, nausea, and vomiting and show a decline in mental status. Treatment is symptomatic and includes IV antifungal agents.

Bacterial Meningitis

Bacterial meningitis is a medical emergency with a mortality rate of about 25%. It occurs most often in fall and winter when upper respiratory tract infections commonly occur. The most frequently involved organisms responsible for bacterial meningitis include *Streptococcus pneumoniae* (pneumococcal disease) and *Neisseria meningitidis* (Table 44-3).

Meningococcal meningitis is the only type of bacterial meningitis that occurs in outbreaks. It is most likely to occur in areas of high population density, such as college dormitories, military barracks, and crowded living areas. The number of outbreaks on college campuses has been decreasing over the past few years because many states require students to be vaccinated against meningitis. *Teach people who live in highly populated areas the importance of getting the meningitis polysaccharide vaccine (Menomune) to prevent infection by certain groups of meningococcal bacteria.*

The number of cases of Haemophilus influenzae and pneumococcal meningitis has also decreased. Teach patients who are at risk for influenza ("flu") and pneumonia to have vaccines as recommended by their health care provider. Encourage all older

TABLE 44-3 Common Bacteria That Cause Meningitis

- *Neisseria meningitidis* (meningococcal)
- *Streptococcus pneumoniae* (pneumococcal)
- Streptococci, group A
- *Staphylococcus aureus*
- *Escherichia coli*
- *Klebsiella*
- *Proteus*
- *Pseudomonas*
- *Listeria monocytogenes*
- *Haemophilus influenzae* (not as common because of immunization)

adults and those with chronic illnesses of any age to have these protective immunizations to prevent meningitis. Teach people to contact the Meningitis Foundation of America (www.meningitisfoundationofamerica.com) for more information.

Usually, the patient has a predisposing condition such as otitis media, pneumonia, acute or chronic sinusitis, or sickle cell anemia that increases the likelihood of meningitis. A brain or spinal surgery may also contribute to the development of meningitis. Populations likely to have the disease include patients who are immune suppressed or have infections elsewhere in the body and older adults, especially those with chronic debilitating diseases. In rare cases, tongue piercing has been associated with infections, including meningitis.

Patient-Centered Collaborative Care

Assessment

Perform a complete neurologic and neurovascular assessment to detect clinical manifestations associated with a diagnosis of meningitis or suspected meningitis as outlined in Chart 44-7.

Physical Assessment/Clinical Manifestations

Presenting signs and symptoms of meningitis result from meningeal irritation. Assess for fever, headache, and altered mental status. The patient may also report photophobia and have signs of increased intracranial pressure (ICP), such as decreasing level of consciousness. Although the classic **nuchal rigidity** (stiff neck) and positive Kernig's and Brudzinski's signs have been traditionally used to diagnose meningitis, these findings occur in only a small percentage of patients with a definitive diagnosis. Seizures may also occur, particularly in bacterial meningitis. Older adults, patients who are immune compromised, and those who have been inadequately treated with antibiotics may not have fever.

Assess the patient for complications, including increased ICP resulting from the presence of exudate (pus), which can lead to hydrocephalus and cerebral edema. *Left untreated, increased ICP can lead to herniation of the brain and death (see Chapter 47).*

Seizure activity may be caused by irritation of the cerebral cortex. Because of abnormal stimulation of the hypothalamic area, excessive amounts of antidiuretic hormone (ADH) (vasopressin) are produced. This results in water retention and dilution of serum sodium caused by increased sodium loss by the kidneys. This syndrome of inappropriate antidiuretic hormone (SIADH) production may lead to further increases in ICP.

Assess the patient's vascular status by:

- Observing the color and temperature of the extremities
- Determining the presence of peripheral pulses
- Identifying any indicators of abnormal bleeding

Septic emboli in the blood may block circulation in the small vessels of the hands and feet, leading to gangrene. Excessive fibrinolysis (breakdown of fibrin clots) that occurs in bacteremia and infections from viruses, fungi, or protozoa may lead to disseminated intravascular coagulation (DIC). Involvement of the cerebral arteries, veins, and venous sinuses may lead to seizures and hemiparesis.

Laboratory Assessment

The most significant laboratory test used in the diagnosis of meningitis is the analysis of the cerebrospinal fluid (CSF). Patients older than 60 years, those who are immune compromised, or those who have signs of increased ICP usually have a CT scan before the lumbar puncture. If there will be a delay in obtaining the CSF, blood is drawn for culture and sensitivity. A broad-spectrum antibiotic should be given before the lumbar puncture. The CSF is analyzed for cell count, differential count, and protein. Glucose concentrations are determined, and culture, sensitivity, and Gram stain studies are performed.

Counterimmunoelectrophoresis (CIE) may be performed to determine the presence of viruses or protozoa in the CSF. CIE is also indicated if the patient has received antibiotics before the CSF was obtained. To identify a possible bacterial source of infection, specimens for culture are obtained and Gram stains of the urine, throat, and nose are also performed. Table 44-4 compares CSF findings in bacterial meningitis and in viral meningitis.

A complete blood count (CBC) is performed. The white blood cell (WBC) count is usually elevated well above the normal value. Serum electrolyte values are also assessed. Dilutional hyponatremia may occur as a result of SIADH, a complication of bacterial meningitis.

Chart 44-7 KEY FEATURES

Meningitis

- Decreased (or change in) level of consciousness
- Disoriented to person, place, and year
- Pupil reaction and eye movements
  - Photophobia
  - Nystagmus
  - Abnormal eye movements
- Motor response
  - Normal early in disease process
  - Hemiparesis, hemiplegia, and decreased muscle tone possible later
  - Cranial nerve dysfunction, especially CN III, IV, VI, VII, VIII
- Memory changes
  - Attention span (usually short)
  - Personality and behavior changes
  - Bewilderment
- Severe, unrelenting headaches
- Generalized muscle aches and pain
- Nausea and vomiting
- Fever and chills
- Tachycardia
- Red macular rash (meningococcal meningitis)

TABLE 44-4 Cerebrospinal Fluid Findings in Bacterial and Viral Meningitis

Finding	Bacterial Meningitis	Viral Meningitis
Appearance	Cloudy, turbid	Clear
White blood cells	Increased	Increased
Protein	Increased	Increased, slightly elevated
Glucose	Decreased	Most often normal, but may be decreased
CSF pressure	Elevated	Varies

Other Diagnostic Assessment

X-rays of the chest, air sinuses, and mastoids are obtained to determine the presence of infection. A CT or MRI scan may be performed to identify increased ICP, the presence of a brain abscess, or developing hydrocephalus.

Interventions

The most important nursing intervention for patients with meningitis is the accurate monitoring and recording of their neurologic status, vital signs, and vascular assessment. Best practices for nursing care are listed in Chart 44-8. Standard Precautions are appropriate for all patients with meningitis unless the patient has a bacterial type that is transmitted by droplets, such as *Neisseria meningitides* and *Haemophilus influenzae.* Patients with these infections should be placed on Droplet Precautions *in addition to* Standard Precautions. When possible, place the patient on Droplet Precautions in a private room. Stay at least 3 feet from the patient unless wearing a mask. Patients who are transported outside of the room should wear a mask and follow Respiratory Hygiene/Cough Etiquette (see Chapter 25). Teach visitors about the need for these precautions.

Monitoring Neurologic Status

Assess the patient's neurologic status and vital signs at least every 4 hours or more often if clinically indicated. *The priority for care is to monitor for early neurologic changes that may indicate increased ICP, such as decreased level of consciousness (LOC).* The patient is also at risk for seizure activity, and care should be provided as discussed in Interventions on p. 959 in the Seizures and Epilepsy section.

Cranial nerve testing is included as part of the routine neurologic assessment because of possible cranial nerve involvement. Particular attention is given to cranial nerves III, IV, VI, VII, and VIII (see Chapter 43). *A sixth cranial nerve defect (inability to move the eyes laterally) may indicate the development of* ***hydrocephalus*** *(excessive accumulation of CSF within the brain's ventricles). Other indicators of hydrocephalus include signs of increased ICP and urinary incontinence. Urinary incontinence results from decreasing LOC.*

Chart 44-8 BEST PRACTICE FOR PATIENT SAFETY & QUALITY CARE

Care of the Patient with Meningitis

- Follow ABCs (airway, breathing, circulation).
- Take vital signs and perform neurologic checks every 2 to 4 hours, as required.
- Perform cranial nerve assessment, with particular attention to cranial nerves III, IV, VI, VII, and VIII, and monitor for changes.
- Manage pain with drug and nondrug methods.
- Perform vascular assessment, and monitor for changes.
- Give drugs and IV fluids as prescribed, and document the patient's response.
- Record intake and output carefully to maintain fluid balance and prevent fluid overload.
- Monitor body weight to identify fluid retention early.
- Monitor laboratory values closely; report abnormal findings to the physician or nurse practitioner promptly.
- Position carefully to prevent pressure ulcers.
- Perform range-of-motion exercises every 4 hours as needed.
- Decrease environmental stimuli:
  - Provide a quiet environment.
  - Minimize exposure to bright lights from windows and overhead lights.
  - Maintain bedrest with head of bed elevated 30 degrees.
- Maintain Transmission Precautions per hospital policy (for bacterial meningitis).
- Monitor for and prevent complications:
  - Increased intracranial pressure
  - Vascular dysfunction
  - Fluid and electrolyte imbalance
  - Seizures
  - Shock

Drug Therapy

To avoid life-threatening complications, the health care provider prescribes a broad-spectrum antibiotic until the results of the culture and Gram stain are available. After this information is available, the appropriate anti-infective drug to treat the specific type of meningitis is given. Treatment of bacterial meningitis generally requires a 2-week course of IV antibiotics. Drug therapy should begin within 1 to 2 hours after it is prescribed. Monitor and document the patient's response.

The patient with bacterial meningitis may experience increased ICP, and seizure activity may occur. Drugs used by the physician to treat these complications include hyperosmolar agents and antiepileptic drugs (AEDs). Controversy exists as to whether steroids are helpful in the treatment of all adults with meningitis. They are, however, recommended for patients with *Streptococcus pneumoniae* meningitis. People who have been in close contact with a patient with *Neisseria meningitides* should have prophylaxis (preventive) treatment with rifampin (Rifadin, Rofact🍁), ciprofloxacin (Cipro), or ceftriaxone (Rocephin). Preventive treatment with rifampin may be prescribed for those in close contact with a patient with *Haemophilus influenzae* meningitis.

Monitoring for Complications

Perform a complete vascular assessment every 4 hours or more often, if indicated, to detect early vascular compromise from septic emboli. This severe complication is most often seen in circulation to the hand. Assess the patient's temperature, color, pulses, and capillary refill in the fingernails. If vascular compromise is not noticed and left untreated, gangrene can develop quickly, possibly leading to loss of the involved arm. The health care team monitors the patient for other complications, including septic shock, coagulation disorders, acute respiratory distress syndrome, and septic arthritis. These health problems are discussed elsewhere in this textbook.

ENCEPHALITIS

Pathophysiology

Encephalitis is an inflammation of the brain tissue and often the surrounding meninges. It affects the cerebrum, the brainstem, and the cerebellum. A viral agent most often causes the disease, although bacteria, fungi, or parasites may also be involved (e.g., malaria). *Viral encephalitis can be life threatening or lead to persistent neurologic problems such as learning disabilities, epilepsy, memory, or fine motor deficits.* It is always caused by a viral infection elsewhere in the body. The virus travels to the central nervous system (CNS) via the bloodstream, along peripheral or cranial nerves, or in the meninges (e.g., varicella zoster).

After the virus invades the brain tissue, it begins to reproduce, causing an inflammatory response. Unlike in meningitis, this response does not cause exudate (pus) formation. Inflammation extends over the cerebral cortex, the white matter, and the meninges, causing degeneration of the neurons of the cortex. Demyelination of axons occurs in the involved area because the white matter is destroyed. This leads to hemorrhage, edema, necrosis (cell death), and the development of small lacunae (hollow cavities) within the cerebral hemispheres. Widespread edema can cause compression of blood vessels leading to a further increase in intracranial pressure (ICP). Death may occur from herniation and increased ICP.

Arboviruses can be transmitted to humans through the bite of an infected mosquito or tick. The most common types of encephalitis caused by arboviruses are eastern or western equine encephalitis, St. Louis encephalitis, California encephalitis, and West Nile virus.

West Nile virus has gained attention in the United States because it has spread rapidly throughout the country and is a potentially serious illness. This infection is generally mild, and usually the patient is asymptomatic. However, a small percentage of patients develop severe disease. The incubation period is 2 to 15 days after being bitten by an infected mosquito. Other possible sources of transmission include blood products, breast milk, or an organ transplant. Diagnostic tests to determine the presence of West Nile virus include enzyme-linked immunosorbent assay and West Nile virus–specific IgM antibody in the blood or CSF.

In mild cases, the patient has no symptoms or has mild flu-like symptoms (e.g., fever, body aches, nausea, vomiting). About 1 in 150 people develops serious symptoms that may include high fever, severe headache, decreased level of consciousness, tremors, vision loss, seizures, and muscle weakness or paralysis. These manifestations may last for several weeks, and neurologic deficits may be permanent. A few patients die from the disease.

Echovirus, coxsackievirus, poliovirus, herpes zoster, and viruses that cause mumps and chickenpox are the common *enteroviruses* associated with encephalitis. *Herpes simplex virus type 1* (HSV1) encephalitis is the most common nonepidemic type of encephalitis in North America. Patients with this disease often have a history of cold sores. The mortality rates for HSV1 encephalitis are very high compared with those for other types of encephalitis.

Amebic meningoencephalitis is caused by the amebae *Naegleria* and *Acanthamoeba.* Both are found in warm freshwater areas and can enter the nasal mucosa of people swimming in ponds or lakes. The *amebae* may also be found in soil and decaying vegetation. Although this infection has not often been seen in the past, the incidence in North America is increasing, perhaps because ponds and lakes are becoming more polluted.

Patient-Centered Collaborative Care

Assessment

The typical patient with encephalitis has a fever and reports nausea, vomiting, and a stiff neck. Assess for other clinical manifestations, including:

- High fever
- Changes in mental status (e.g., agitation)
- Motor dysfunction (e.g., dysphagia [difficulty swallowing])
- Focal (specific) neurologic deficits
- Photophobia (light sensitivity) and phonophobia (noise sensitivity)
- Fatigue
- Symptoms of increased ICP (e.g., decreased LOC)

Assess LOC using the Glasgow Coma Scale (see Chapter 43) or other agency-approved assessment tool. The patient may be lethargic, stuporous, or comatose. Mental status changes are more extensive in the patient with encephalitis than with meningitis. Changes include acute confusion, irritability, and personality and behavior changes (especially noted in the presence of herpes simplex). Signs of meningeal irritation include the presence of nuchal (neck) rigidity and motor changes that vary from a mild weakness to hemiplegia. The patient may have muscle tremors, spasticity, an ataxic gait (postencephalitic parkinsonism), myoclonic jerks, and increased deep tendon reflexes. Seizure activity is common. Nausea, vomiting, headache, and vertigo also may occur.

Observe for cranial nerve involvement, such as ocular palsies (paralysis), facial weakness, and nystagmus (involuntary lateral eye movements). The herpes zoster lesion affects cranial and spinal nerve root ganglia, which is clinically manifested by a rash, severe pain, itching, burning, or tingling in the areas innervated by these nerves.

In severe cases of encephalitis, the patient may have increased ICP resulting from cerebral edema, hemorrhage, and necrosis of brain tissue. Monitor vital signs for indications of a widened pulse pressure, bradycardia, and irregular respirations. The pupils become increasingly dilated and less responsive to light. Left untreated, increased ICP leads to herniation of the brain tissue and possibly death (see Chapter 47).

A CSF specimen may be obtained, depending on the patient's condition, to determine the specific offending organism. A polymerase chain reaction (PCR) test may be used to detect viral DNA or ribonucleic acid (RNA) in the CSF. Specificity and sensitivity in diagnosing encephalitis are excellent, especially with herpes simplex virus (HSV). The test is rapid and noninvasive, replacing the brain biopsy for diagnosis.

Interventions

Teach people who live in mosquito-infested areas to protect themselves and their families from West Nile virus infections. Chart 44-9 lists measures for preventing this infection. There is no curative treatment for West Nile viral encephalitis.

Nursing interventions for encephalitis are similar to those for meningitis with the exception of drug therapy. Supportive nursing care and prompt recognition and treatment of increased ICP are essential components of management. *Main-*

Chart 44-9 PATIENT AND FAMILY EDUCATION GUIDE

Protecting the Patient and Family from West Nile Virus

- Limit your time outside between dusk and dawn when mosquitoes are out.
- Wear protective clothing, including long sleeves and pants.
- Use an insect repellent containing DEET when outdoors.
- Remove areas of standing water from flower pots, trash cans, and rain gutters.
- Check window and door screens for holes that need repair.
- Keep hot tubs and pools clean and properly chlorinated.

tain a patent airway to prevent the development of atelectasis or pneumonia, which can lead to further brain hypoxia (lack of oxygen).

Provide supportive nursing care for the patient who is immobile, stuporous, or comatose. Delegate and supervise unlicensed assistive personnel (UAP) to turn, cough, and deep breathe the patient at least every 2 hours. Perform deep tracheal suctioning even in the presence of increased ICP if respiratory status is compromised. Assess vital signs and neurologic signs every 2 hours or more frequently if clinically indicated. Elevate the head of the bed 30 to 45 degrees unless contraindicated (e.g., after lumbar puncture or in the patient with severe hypotension). Keep the patient's room darkened and quiet to promote comfort and decrease agitation. Remind UAP to provide safety measures such as keeping the bed in the lowest position.

Acyclovir (Zovirax) is the antiviral drug of choice for the treatment of herpes encephalitis and is associated with a significantly lower mortality rate than vidarabine (Vira-A). Drug therapy is most effective if begun early before the patient becomes stuporous or comatose. This change usually occurs within 4 to 6 days after the initial neurologic symptoms. No specific drug therapy is available for infection by arboviruses or enteroviruses.

Provide patient and family support. Families need health teaching to understand how to care for their loved ones. They are often fearful that the patient may not return to his or her baseline. Collaborate with a certified chaplain, social worker, or case manager to provide additional emotional support and counseling.

Patients with encephalitis and permanent neurologic deficits are usually discharged to a rehabilitation setting or a long-term care facility. Those with minimal neurologic problems are discharged to the home setting.

PARKINSON DISEASE

Pathophysiology

ANIMATION: Parkinson Disease ▶

Parkinson disease (PD), also referred to as *Parkinson's disease* and *paralysis agitans,* is a progressive neurodegenerative disease that is the third most common neurologic disorder of older adults. It is a debilitating disease affecting motor ability and is characterized by four cardinal symptoms: tremor, rigidity, **bradykinesia** or **akinesia** (slow movement/no movement), and postural instability. Most people have *primary,* or idiopathic, disease. A few patients have *secondary* parkinsonian symptoms from conditions such as brain tumors and certain anti-psychotic drugs.

Motor activity occurs as a result of integrating the actions of the cerebral cortex, basal ganglia, and cerebellum. The basal ganglia are a group of neurons located deep within the cerebrum at the base of the brain near the lateral ventricles. When the basal ganglia are stimulated, muscle tone in the body is inhibited and voluntary movements are refined. The secretion of two major neurotransmitters accomplishes this process: dopamine and acetylcholine (ACh).

Dopamine is produced in the substantia nigra, as well as in the adrenal glands, and is transmitted to the basal ganglia along a connecting neural pathway for secretion when needed. *ACh* is produced and secreted by the basal ganglia, as well as in the nerve endings in the periphery of the body. ACh-producing neurons transmit *excitatory* messages throughout the basal ganglia. Dopamine *inhibits* the function of these neurons, allowing control over voluntary movement. This system of checks and balances allows for refined, coordinated movement, such as picking up a pencil and writing.

Widespread degeneration of the *substantia nigra* then leads to a decrease in the amount of dopamine in the brain. When dopamine levels are decreased, a person loses the ability to refine voluntary movement. The large number of excitatory ACh-secreting neurons remain active, creating an imbalance between excitatory and inhibitory neuronal activity. The resulting excessive excitation of neurons prevents a person from controlling or initiating voluntary movement.

Not only does PD interfere with movement as a result of dopamine loss in the brain, it also reduces the sympathetic nervous system influence on the heart and blood vessels. This loss results in the orthostatic hypotension frequently seen in the patient with PD.

PD is separated into stages according to the symptoms and degree of disability (Table 44-5). Stage 1 is mild disease with unilateral limb involvement, whereas the patient with stage 5 disease is completely dependent in all ADLs. Other classifications refer simply to mild, moderate, and severe disease.

Etiology and Genetic Risk

Although the exact cause of PD is not known, it is probably due to environmental and genetic factors. Exposure to pesticides, herbicides, industrial chemicals and metals, as well as drinking well water, being over the age of 40, and have reduced estrogen levels, are known risk factors for the development of PD.

GENETIC CONSIDERATIONS

A number of inherited forms of the disease are associated with gene mutation. Genetic mutation has been identified in some families with PD. Of the nine genes identified, the *parkin 1* gene on chromosome 4 has been the most studied. In the presence of a genetic mutation, alpha-synuclein, a major component of Lewy bodies, is produced and thought to contribute to neuronal death (McCarron, 2006).

TABLE 44-5 Stages of Parkinson Disease

STAGE 1: INITIAL STAGE
• Unilateral limb involvement
• Minimal weakness
• Hand and arm trembling
STAGE 2: MILD STAGE
• Bilateral limb involvement
• Masklike facies
• Slow, shuffling gait
STAGE 3: MODERATE DISEASE
• Postural instability
• Increased gait disturbances
STAGE 4: SEVERE DISABILITY
• Akinesia
• Rigidity
STAGE 5: COMPLETE ADL DEPENDENCE

Incidence/Prevalence

PD affects more than 1.5 million people in the United States. As the population ages, the number of those affected is expected to dramatically increase. Men are affected more often than women. Symptoms of idiopathic PD typically begin in people between 40 and 70 years of age with a peak onset in the 60s. Young-onset PD typically occurs in people 21 to 40 years of age. The disease progresses faster in patients who are older at diagnosis (McCarron, 2006).

Patient-Centered Collaborative Care

Assessment

Collect data related to the time and progression of symptoms noticed by the patient or the family. The older adult, who may assume that these behaviors are normal changes associated with aging, may ignore early signs and symptoms such as *resting* tremors, bradykinesia (slowed movement), and problems with muscular rigidity. Tremors are usually noticed in the upper extremities first and may increase with stress. Slow voluntary movements and reduced automatic movements may be manifested by a change in the patient's handwriting. Chart 44-10 summarizes the clinical manifestations of Parkinson disease. Assess the patient for **rigidity,** or resistance to passive movement of the extremities, which is classified as:

- Cogwheel, manifested by a rhythmic interruption of the muscle movement
- Plastic, defined as mildly restrictive movement
- Lead pipe, or total resistance to movement

Rigidity is present early in the disease process and progresses over time. Observe the patient's ability to relax a muscle or move a selected muscle group.

Changes in facial expression or a **masklike facies** with wide-open, fixed, staring eyes are caused by rigidity of the facial muscles (Fig. 44-1). This rigidity can lead to difficulties in chewing and swallowing, particularly if the pharyngeal muscles are involved. As a result, the patient may have inadequate

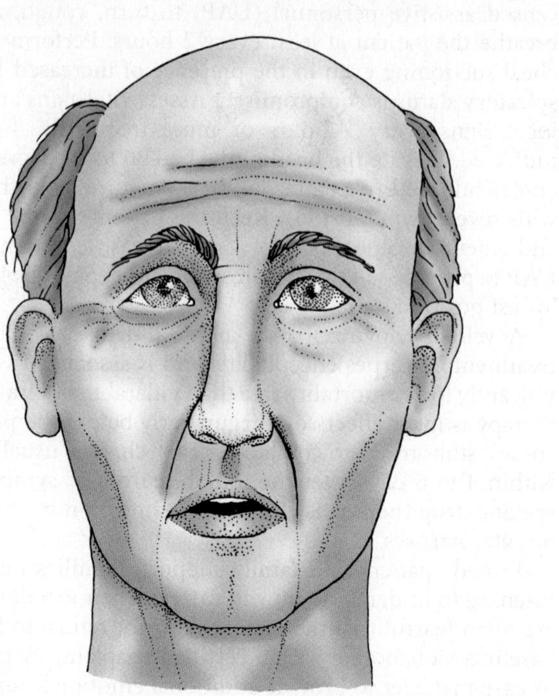

Fig. 44-1 • The masklike facial expression typical of patients with Parkinson disease.

Chart 44-10 KEY FEATURES

Parkinson Disease

- Posture
  - Stooped posture
  - Flexed trunk
  - Fingers abducted and flexed at the metacarpophalangeal joint
  - Wrist slightly dorsiflexed
- Gait
  - Slow and shuffling
  - Short, hesitant steps
  - Propulsive gait
  - Difficulty stopping quickly
- Motor
  - **Bradykinesia** (slow movement)
  - Muscular rigidity
  - Akinesia
  - Tremors
  - "Pill-rolling" movement
  - Masklike facies
  - Difficulty chewing and swallowing
  - Uncontrolled drooling, especially at night
  - Fatigue
  - Difficulty getting into and out of bed
  - Reduced arm swinging on one side of the body when walking
  - Micrographia (change in handwriting or handwriting gets smaller)
- Speech
  - Soft, low-pitched voice
  - **Dysarthria** (slurred speech)
  - **Echolalia** (automatic repetition of what another person says) and repetition of sentences
  - **Hypophonia** (soft voice), change in voice volume or articulation
- Autonomic dysfunction
  - Orthostatic hypotension
  - Excessive perspiration
  - Oily skin
  - Seborrhea
  - Flushing
  - Changes in skin texture
  - Blepharospasm (eyelid spasm)
- Psychosocial assessment
  - Emotionally labile
  - Depressed
  - Paranoid
  - Easily upset
  - Rapid mood swings
  - Cognitive impairments (i.e., dementia)
  - Delayed reaction time
  - Sleep disturbances

nutrition. Uncontrolled drooling may occur. Some patients develop dementia later as the disease progresses. In addition to changes in voluntary movement, many patients experience autonomic nervous system symptoms, such as excessive perspiration and orthostatic hypotension. Orthostatic hypotension was originally thought to be a side effect of levodopa therapy. However, it is probably related to loss of sympathetic innervation in the heart and blood vessel response.

The diagnosis of PD is made on the basis of clinical findings after other neurologic diseases are eliminated as possibilities. There are no specific diagnostic tests. Analysis of cerebrospinal fluid (CSF) may show a decrease in dopamine levels although the results of other studies are usually normal. Other diagnostic tests may be done such as an MRI, single-photon emission computed tomography (SPECT), or a positron emission test (PET).

Common Nursing Diagnoses and Collaborative Problems

Nursing diagnoses that often apply to patients with Parkinson disease include:

- Impaired Physical Mobility related to neuromuscular impairment
- Risk for Falls related to decreased muscle strength, muscle rigidity, and orthostatic hypotension
- Risk for Self-Care Deficit related to neuromuscular impairment
- Risk for Impaired Verbal Communication related to facial muscle rigidity
- Chronic Confusion related to dementia
- Risk for Imbalanced Nutrition: Less Than Body Requirements related to dysphagia

Interventions

In addition to the health care provider, physical and/or occupational therapist, speech-language pathologist, nutritionist, and case manager, collaborate with the patient and family to develop an interdisciplinary treatment plan. In some cases, palliative surgery may be performed to assist the patient to remain mobile for as long as possible. Chart 44-11 summarizes best practices for nursing management of the patient with PD.

Chart 44-11 BEST PRACTICE FOR PATIENT SAFETY & QUALITY CARE

Care of the Patient with Parkinson Disease

- Allow the patient extra time to respond to questions.
- Administer medications promptly on schedule to maintain continuous therapeutic drug levels.
- Provide medication for pain, tingling in limbs as needed.
- Monitor for side effects of medications, especially orthostatic hypotension, hallucinations, and acute confusional state (delirium).
- Collaborate with physical and occupational therapists to keep the patient as mobile and as independent as possible in ADLs.
- Allow the patient time to perform ADLs and mobility skills.
- Implement interventions to prevent complications of immobility, such as constipation, pressure ulcers, and contractures.
- Schedule appointments and activities late in the morning to prevent rushing the patient, or schedule them at the time of the patient's optimal level of functioning.
- Teach the patient to speak slowly and clearly. Use alternative communication methods, such as a communication board. Refer to speech-language pathologist.
- Monitor the patient's ability to eat and swallow. Monitor actual food and fluid intake. Collaborate with the nutritionist.
- Provide high-protein, high-calorie foods or supplements to maintain weight.
- Recognize that Parkinson disease affects the patient's body image. Focus on the patient's strengths.
- Assess for depression and anxiety.
- Assess for insomnia or sleeplessness.

Nonsurgical Management

Drug therapy is an essential part of management, which decreases signs and symptoms and allows the patient to provide self-care and have a reasonable quality of life. One of the most important desired outcomes is that the patient will improve *mobility (movement),* a basic human need.

Drug Therapy. Drugs are prescribed to treat the symptoms of PD with the purpose of increasing the patient's functional abilities. An equally important goal is to prescribe drugs with minimal long-term side effects. Many questions and controversies remain about which drugs to use, when to start therapy, and how to prevent complications. Drug administration is closely monitored, and the health care provider adjusts the dosage or changes therapy as the patient's condition requires. Teach the patient and family how to monitor for and report adverse effects of drug therapy.

Dopamine agonists mimic dopamine by stimulating dopamine receptors in the brain. They are typically the most effective during the first 3 to 5 years of use. The benefit of these agents is fewer incidents of **dyskinesias** (problems with movement) and **"wearing off" phenomenon** (loss of response to the drug) when compared with other drugs. This problem is characterized by periods of good mobility ("on") alternating with periods of poor mobility ("off"). Patients report that their most distressing symptom is "off time" (Backer, 2006).

Examples of dopamine agonists are apomorphine (Apokyn [a morphine derivative]), pramipexole (Mirapex), and ropinirole (Requip). Another drug in this class, rotigotine, is available as a continuous transdermal patch (Neupro) to maintain a consistent level of dopamine. *Dopamine agonists are associated with adverse effects such as orthostatic (postural) hypotension, hallucinations, sleepiness, and drowsiness. Remind patients to avoid operating heavy machinery or driving if they have any of these symptoms. Teach them to change from a lying or sitting position to standing by moving slowly. The health care provider should not prescribe drugs in this class to older adults because of their severe adverse drug effects.*

Almost all patients are on Sinemet, a combination *levodopa-carbidopa* drug, at some point in their disease. It may be the initial drug of choice if the patient's presenting symptoms are severe or interfere with work or school. Both an immediate-release (IR) and controlled-release (CR) form of Sinemet in varying doses are available. The levodopa agents are less expensive than the dopamine agonists and are better at improving motor function. Long-term use leads to dyskinesia (inability to perform voluntary movement). Teach the patient and family to give the drug before meals to increase absorption and transport across the blood-brain barrier.

Catechol *O*-methyltransferases (COMTs) are enzymes that inactivate dopamine. Therefore COMT *inhibitors* block this activity, thus prolonging the action of levodopa. One example is entacapone (Comtan), which is often used in combination with levodopa. Stalevo is a combination of levodopa, carbidopa, and entacapone. The benefit of these combinations is that the disease is treated in several ways with one drug. However, they are not beneficial for those patients who need more specific dosages of individual drugs.

Monamine oxidase type B (MAO-B) inhibitors (MAOIs) are more popular for use in patients with early or mild symptoms of PD. Entacapone (Comtan) and selegiline (Deprenyl, Eldepryl) are often given with levodopa for early or mild disease. A newer MAOI for PD is rasagiline mesylate (Azilect), which can be given as a single drug or with levodopa. These drugs slow the main type (B) of monamine oxidase in the brain, increasing dopamine concentrations and helping reduce the clinical manifestations of PD.

Teach patients taking MAOIs about the need to avoid foods, beverages, and drugs that contain tyramine, including aged, smoked, or cured foods and sausage. Remind them to also avoid red wine and beer to prevent severe headache and life-threatening hypertension (Thomure, 2006). Patients should continue these restrictions for 14 days after the drug is discontinued.

When other drugs are no longer effective, bromocriptine mesylate (Parlodel), a *dopamine receptor antagonist,* may be prescribed to promote the release of dopamine. It may be used alone or in combination with carbidopa/levodopa (Sinemet). Some providers may prescribe Parlodel early in the course of treatment. It is especially useful in the patient who has experienced side effects such as dyskinesias or orthostatic hypotension while receiving Sinemet.

Amantadine (Symmetrel) is an *antiviral drug* that has anti-Parkinson benefits. It may be given early in disease to reduce symptoms. It is also prescribed with Sinemet to reduce dyskinesias. Rivastigmine (Exelon) is a *cholinesterase inhibitor* that is used only when patients with PD have dementia. This drug works to improve the transmission of acetylcholine in the brain by delaying its destruction by the enzyme acetylcholinesterase.

For severe motor symptoms such as tremors and rigidity, one of the older *anticholinergic* drugs may be prescribed. Examples are benztropine (Cogentin) and procyclidine (Kemadrin). *These drugs should be avoided in older adults because they can cause acute confusion, urinary retention, constipation, dry mouth, and blurred vision. For these reasons, they are not prescribed today as often as in the past. Newer and safer drugs are now available.*

For the patient on any long-term drug therapy regimen, drug tolerance or *drug toxicity* often develops. Drug toxicity may be evidenced by delirium (acute confusion), cognitive impairment, decreased effectiveness of the drug, or hallucinations. Delirium may be difficult to assess in the patient who is already suffering from chronic dementia as a result of PD or another disease. If possible, compare the patient's current cognitive and behavioral status with his or her baseline before drug therapy began.

When drug tolerance is reached, the drug's effects do not last as long as previously. The treatment of PD drug toxicity or tolerance includes:

- A reduction in drug dosage
- A change of drug or in the frequency of administration
- A drug holiday (particularly with levodopa therapy)

During a **drug holiday,** which typically lasts up to 10 days, the patient receives no drug therapy for PD. Carefully monitor the patient for symptoms of PD during this time and document assessment findings.

Exercise and Ambulation. *A "freezing" gait and postural instability are major problems for patients with PD.* Nontraditional exercise programs, such as yoga and tai chi, may help elevate mood, as well as improve mobility, in the early stage of the disease. Early in the disease process, collaborate with physical and occupational therapists to plan and implement a program to keep the patient mobile and flexible by incorporating active and passive range-of-motion (ROM) exercises, muscle stretching, and activity. Remind the patient to avoid concentrating on his or her feet when walking to prevent falls.

Self-Management. In collaboration with the rehabilitation team, encourage the patient to participate as much as possible in self-management, including ADLs. The team makes the environment conducive to independence in activity and as stress-free and safe as possible. Occupational and physical therapists provide training in ADLs and the use of adaptive devices, as needed, to facilitate independence. The occupational therapist (OT) evaluates the patient for the need for adaptive devices (e.g., special utensils for eating).

Injury Prevention. Patients with PD tend to not sleep well at night because of drug therapy and the disease itself. Some patients nap for short periods during the day and may not be aware that they have done so. This sleep misperception may put the patient at risk for injury. For example, he or she may fall asleep while driving an automobile. Therefore teach the patient and family to monitor the patient's sleeping pattern and discuss whether he or she can operate machinery or perform other potentially high-risk tasks safely.

Nutrition. Collaborate with the nutritionist (registered dietitian [RD]) to evaluate the patient's food intake and ability to eat. The patient's intake of calcium, vitamin K, and other nutrients is evaluated, especially in the patient who is susceptible to falling or has difficulty swallowing. The RD considers the patient's bowel habits and adjusts the diet if constipation occurs. If the patient has trouble swallowing, collaborate with the speech-language pathologist (SLP) for an extensive swallowing evaluation. Based on these findings and the patient interview, an individualized nutritional plan is developed. Usually a soft diet or thick, cold fluids, such as milk shakes, are more easily tolerated.

Small, frequent meals or a commercial powder, such as Thick-It, added to liquids may assist the patient who has difficulty swallowing. Elevate the patient's head to allow easier swallowing and prevent aspiration. Remind UAP and teach the family to be careful when serving or feeding the patient. The SLP can be very helpful in recommending specific feeding strategies. Be sure that UAP record food intake daily or as needed. The patient loses weight because of altered food intake and the increased number of calories burned secondary to muscle rigidity. Teach the family to weigh the patient once a week so that adjustments to the diet can be made as indicated. As the disease progresses and swallowing becomes more of a problem, supplemental feedings become the main source of nutrition to maintain weight, with meals and other foods taken as the patient can tolerate.

Communication. Collaborate with the SLP if the patient has speech difficulties. Together with the health care team, patient, and family, develop a communication plan. The SLP teaches exercises to strengthen muscles used for breathing, speech, and swallowing. Teach the patient to speak slowly and clearly and to pause and take deep breaths at times during each sentence. Teach the family the importance of avoiding unnecessary environmental noise to increase the listener's ability to hear and understand the patient. Ask the patient to repeat words that the listener does not understand. Have the listener watch the patient's lips and nonverbal expressions for cues as to the meaning of conversation. Remind the patient to organize his or her thoughts before speaking and use facial expression and gestures, if possible, to assist with communication. In addition, he or she should exaggerate words to increase the listener's ability to understand. If the patient cannot communicate verbally, he or she can use alternative methods of communication, such as a communication board, mechanical voice synthesizer, computer, or personal digital assistant (PDA). The SLP assesses the ability to use these devices before a decision is made about which method to use. Some older patients may not want to use electronic methods to communicate.

Psychosocial Support. Although not all patients with PD have dementia, impaired cognitive function and memory deficits are common. Some patients also experience changes in gait and tremors that are uncontrollable. In the late stages of the disease, they cannot move without assistance, have difficulty talking, have minimal facial expression, and may drool. Patients often state that they are embarrassed, and they tend to avoid social events or groups of people. They should not be forced into situations in which they feel ashamed of their appearance. Encourage them to undertake activities that do not require small-muscle dexterity, such as light, modified aerobic exercises.

Collaborate with the social worker or case manager to help the family with financial and health insurance issues, as well as respite care or permanent placement if needed. Refer the patient and family to social and state agencies, as well as support groups as needed (e.g., the National Parkinson Foundation [www.parkinson.org]).

Teach the family to emphasize the patient's abilities or strengths and provide positive reinforcement when he or she meets expected outcomes. The patient, the family or significant other, and the rehabilitation team mutually set realistic outcomes that can be achieved.

The long-term management of PD presents a special challenge in the home care setting. A case manager may be required to coordinate interdisciplinary care and provide support for the patient and family. Impaired mobility affects the patient's daily lifestyle, including sexuality. The case manager or home care nurse uses a holistic approach to ensure that psychosocial, as well as physical, needs are addressed.

As the disease progresses and drug effectiveness decreases, refer the family to a palliative care organization or hospice. Referral sources can be obtained from the Center to Advance Palliative Care (www.capc.org), which advocates applying the principles of palliative care to chronic disease (Bunting-Perry, 2006). Chapter 9 discusses palliative and hospice care in detail.

Surgical Management

Several options are available if surgery for the patient with PD is needed. Surgery is a last resort when drugs are not effective in symptom management. The most common surgeries are stereotactic pallidotomy and thalamotomy, although newer surgical procedures are being tried. Deep brain stimulation may also be done.

Stereotactic Pallidotomy/Thalamotomy. **Stereotactic pallidotomy** (opening into the pallidum within the corpus striatum) can be a very effective treatment for controlling the symptoms associated with PD. First, the target area within the pallidum is identified by a CT or MRI scan. Next, the stereotactic head frame is placed on the patient. IV sedation is given, and a burr hole is made into the cranium. An electrode or cylindric rod is inserted into the target area. The target area receives a mild electrical stimulation, and the patient's reaction is assessed for reduction of tremor and rigidity. If this result does not occur or if unexpected visual, motor, or sensory symptoms appear, the probe is repositioned. When the probe is in the ideal location, a permanent lesion (scarring) is made to destroy the tissue. The patient is monitored in the postanesthesia care unit (PACU) for about 1 hour and is then returned to the inpatient unit for continuing postoperative care.

As an alternative to stereotactic pallidotomy, the surgeon may perform a **thalamotomy** (opening into the thalamus of the brain for the stimulation) for treatment of tremor through thermocoagulation (high-frequency currents to destroy tissue) of brain cells. This procedure is effective for a limited number of patients. Because bilateral procedures have increased surgical complication rates, only unilateral (one-sided) surgery is done to benefit the side of the body that is most affected by the disease.

Deep Brain Stimulation. Deep brain stimulation (DBS) may be used when drug therapy is no longer effective in controlling the patient's symptoms. A thin electrode is implanted in the thalamus or subthalamus and then connected to a "pacemaker" that delivers electrical current to interfere with "tremor" cells. The electrodes are connected to an implantable pulse generator (IPG) that is placed underneath the skin in the patient's chest, similar to a cardiac pacemaker. The patient uses a magnet placed over the IPG to adjust the settings and to check the battery status. He or she continues on drug therapy after the procedure, but a smaller dosage may be needed to control symptoms.

Fetal Tissue Transplantation. Fetal tissue transplantation is an experimental and highly controversial procedure. Fetal substantia nigra tissue, either human or pig, is transplanted into the caudate nucleus of the brain. Preliminary reports suggest that patients show clinical improvement in motor symptoms without dyskinesias after receiving the transplanted tissue. Long-term results are yet to be seen or studied.

ALZHEIMER'S DISEASE

Pathophysiology

Alzheimer's disease (AD), also known as *dementia, Alzheimer type (DAT),* is a chronic, progressive, degenerative disease that accounts for 60% of the dementias occurring in people older than 65 years. It is less commonly seen in people in their 40s and 50s, which is referred to as *early dementia, Alzheimer type,* or *presenile dementia, Alzheimer type.* AD is manifested by loss of memory, judgment, and visuospatial perception and by a change in personality. Over time, the patient becomes increasingly cognitively impaired. Severe physical deterioration takes place and death occurs as a result of complications of immobility.

Structural Changes in the Brain

The brain of the older adult usually weighs less and occupies less space in the cranial vault than does the brain of a younger person. Other changes in the brain that occur with aging include widening of the cerebral sulci, narrowing of the gyri, and enlargement of the ventricles. In the presence of AD, these normal changes are greatly accelerated. Brain weight is reduced further. *Marked atrophy of the cerebral cortex and loss of cortical neurons occur.* The cerebral sulci and fissures, as well as the ventricles, are enlarged more than those of persons of the same age without AD. These areas of the brain are particularly affected:

- Precentral gyrus of the frontal lobe
- Superior temporal gyrus
- Hippocampus
- Substantia nigra

Microscopic changes of the brain found in people with AD include neurofibrillary tangles, amyloid-rich senile or neuritic plaques, and granulovascular degeneration. **Neurofibrillary tangles** are a classic finding at autopsy in the brains of patients with AD. They consist of tangled masses of fibrous tissue throughout the neurons. The same tangles and chemical changes are found in people with Down syndrome.

Neuritic plaques are composed of degenerating nerve terminals and are found particularly in the hippocampus, an important part of the limbic system. Deposited within the plaques are increased amounts of an abnormal protein called *beta amyloid.* Significant progress is occurring in defining the role of beta amyloid in the development of AD.

Although *vascular degeneration* occurs in the normally aging brain, its presence is significantly increased in patients with AD. Vascular degeneration accounts for at least partial loss of the ability of nerve cells to function properly. Cell deterioration and death may lead to hemorrhage. This pathologic change contributes to the mortality associated with this disorder.

Chemical Changes in the Brain

In addition to the structural changes in the brain associated with AD, abnormalities in the neurotransmitters (acetylcholine [ACh], norepinephrine, dopamine, serotonin) may occur. High levels of beta amyloid are associated with reduced ACh by as much as 75%, which leads to a decrease in the amount of acetyltransferase in the hippocampus. This loss is major because the decrease in acetyltransferase interferes with cholinergic innervation to the cerebral cortex. This results in impaired cognition, recent memory, and the ability to acquire new memories. The exact role of reduced neurotransmitters in the development of AD is not well understood.

Etiology and Genetic Risk

The exact cause of AD is unknown. It is well established that *age, gender (women more than men), and family history are the most important risk factors* (Nussbaum et al., 2007). Several other theories and risk factors have been proposed: genetics, chemical imbalances, environmental agents, and immunologic changes. Other risk factors include ethnicity and lower educational level. Compared with Euro-Americans, African Americans have a fourfold risk of developing the disease and Hispanics tend to develop the disease earlier than other groups (Reyes et al., 2006). The cause of these differences is not yet known.

GENETIC CONSIDERATIONS

There is little doubt that many patients with AD have a genetic predisposition to the development of the disease. The patients who seem to have this predisposition have familial AD (FAD). Studies of families are ongoing to determine the exact genetic pathway that is responsible. Most cases of early onset of AD are associated with mutations in genes.

Early-onset FAD (autosomal dominant AD) seems to be related to a rapid decrease in beta amyloid plaque formation, which is caused by defective genes, such as the beta-amyloid precursor gene *(APP)*, the presenilin 1 gene *(PSEN1)*, and the presenilin 2 gene *(PSEN2)*. Late-stage AD research focuses on the role of apolipoprotein E *(APOE)* on chromosome 19 (Nussbaum et al., 2007). People with Down syndrome often develop dementia with clinical manifestations of AD. Down syndrome is a congenital condition resulting from abnormalities of chromosome 21.

Environmental agents, especially certain viruses such as herpes zoster and herpes simplex, and metals such as zinc and copper have also been suggested as causes. Patients who have experienced a head injury or repeated head trauma (e.g., boxers) may be more at risk for AD, and at an earlier age, than others.

Incidence/Prevalence

There is a significant increase in both the incidence and prevalence of AD after 65 years of age although it may affect anyone older than 40 years. The number of people in the United States with AD is estimated at 4.5 million. By the year 2050, that number is projected to increase to 14 million (Yaari & Correy-Bloom, 2007). Its impact on health care costs, including direct and indirect medical and social service costs, is estimated to be greater than $110 billion per year (Reyes et al., 2006).

Health Promotion and Maintenance

There are no proven ways to prevent AD. Current research activities are focusing on eating a balanced diet, eating dark-colored fruits and vegetables, using soy products, and consuming sufficient amounts of folate and vitamins B_{12}, C, and E. These substances have been associated with less risk of developing AD. Walking, swimming, and other exercise not only increase tone and muscle strength but also have been shown to decrease mental decline in AD, as well as other dementias.

Patient-Centered Collaborative Care

evolve ONLINE PHARM REVIEW

Assessment

History

The patient with Alzheimer's disease (AD) often presents with cognitive impairment, although many other disorders, drugs, and environmental factors can cause changes in cognition as well. A thorough history and physical examination are necessary to differentiate AD from other, possibly reversible causes (Table 44-6). Obtain information from family members or significant others because the patient may be unaware of the problems, denying their existence or covering them up. However, it is interesting to note that family members often do not recognize or may deny early changes in their loved one.

The most important information to be obtained is the onset, duration, progression, and course of the symptoms. Question the patient and the family about changes in memory or increasing forgetfulness and about the ability to perform ADLs. Ask about current employment status, work history, and ability to

TABLE 44-6 Causes of Cognitive Impairment in the Older Adult

NEUROLOGIC CAUSES
• Vascular insufficiency
• Infections
• Trauma
• Tumors
• Normal-pressure hydrocephalus
CARDIOVASCULAR CAUSES
• Myocardial infarction
• Dysrhythmias
• Heart failure
• Cardiogenic shock
• Endocarditis
PULMONARY CAUSES
• Infection
• Pneumonia
• Hypoventilation
METABOLIC CAUSES
• Electrolyte imbalance
• Acidosis/alkalosis
• Hypoglycemia/hyperglycemia
• Acute renal failure and chronic kidney disease
• Fluid volume deficit; urinary tract infections
• Hepatic failure
DRUG INTOXICATION
• Misuse of prescribed medications
• Side effects of medications
• Incorrect use of over-the-counter medications
• Ingestion of heavy metals
NUTRITIONAL DEFICIENCIES
• B vitamins
• Vitamin C
• Hypoproteinemia
ENVIRONMENTAL CAUSES
• Hypothermia/hyperthermia
• Unfamiliar environment
• Sensory deprivation/overload
PSYCHOLOGICAL CAUSES
• Depression
• Anxiety
• Pain
• Fatigue
• Grief
• Paranoia

fulfill household responsibilities, including cleaning, grocery shopping, and preparing meals. Inquire about changes in driving ability, ability to handle routine financial transactions, and language and communication skills. In addition, document any changes in personality and behavior.

There is increasing evidence that altered smell is associated with the development of AD. Therefore ask about changes in the ability to smell or changes in the sense of smell. The history taking concludes with a review of the patient's medical history. Of particular importance is a history of head trauma, viral illness, or exposure to metal or toxic waste, as well as any family history of AD or Down syndrome.

Physical Assessment/Clinical Manifestations

Stages of Alzheimer's Disease. The clinical manifestations associated with AD can be grouped into three broad stages on the basis of the progress of the disease (Chart 44-12). The patient does not necessarily progress from one stage to the next in an orderly fashion. A stage may be bypassed, or he or she may exhibit symptoms of one or several stages. Each patient exhibits different disease stages and clinical manifestations. Consequently, most authorities now use broader terms such as *early (mild), middle (moderate),* and *late (severe)* stages.

The primary focus of the neurologic assessment of patients with AD is to identify abnormalities in cognition, including language, personality, and behavior. Physical manifestations of neurologic impairment (seizures, tremors, or ataxia) tend to occur late in the disease process.

Changes in Cognition. Cognition refers to the ability of the brain to process, store, retrieve, and use information. Therefore assess the patient for deficits in these abilities:

- Attention and concentration
- Judgment and perception
- Learning and memory
- Communication and language
- Speed of information processing

One of the first symptoms of AD is short-term memory impairment. New memory and defects in information retrieval result from dysfunction in the hippocampal, frontal, or parietal region. Alterations in communication abilities, such as **apraxia** (inability to use objects correctly), **aphasia** (inability to speak or understand), **anomia** (inability to find words), and **agnosia** (loss of sensory comprehension), are due to dysfunction of the temporal and parietal lobes. Frontal lobe impairment causes problems with judgment, an inability to make decisions, decreased attention span, and a decreased ability to concentrate. As the disease progresses to a later stage, the patient loses all cognitive abilities, is totally unable to communicate, and becomes less aware of the environment.

To assess cognitive status, the nurse or other health care provider can use one of several assessment tools. One of the most popular tools is Folstein's Mini-Mental State Examination (MMSE), also known as the "mini-mental." The MMSE assesses five major areas—orientation, registration, attention and calculation, recall, and speech-language (including reading). Fig. 44-2 lists examples of the questions asked on this test. The patient performs certain cognitive tasks that are scored and added together for a total score of 0 to 30. The lower the score is, the greater the severity of the dementia. It is not unusual for a patient with advanced AD to score below 5.

Although the MMSE is used frequently, the patient must be able to read. For the patient who cannot read or for a quicker screening test, the set test can be used, which is especially useful for the older adult. The patient is asked to name 10 items in each of four sets or categories: fruits, animals, colors, and towns (FACT). Other categories can be used, if needed. The patient receives 1 point for each item for a possible maximum score of 40. Patients who score above 25 do not have dementia. Although this assessment is more comprehensive and easy to administer, it should not be used for patients with hearing impairments or speech and language problems.

Changes in Behavior and Personality. One of the most difficult aspects of AD that families, significant others, and

Chart 44-12 KEY FEATURES

Alzheimer's Disease

EARLY (MILD), OR STAGE I (FIRST SYMPTOMS UP TO 4 YEARS)
- Independent in ADLs
- No social or employment problems initially
- Denies presence of symptoms
- Forgets names; misplaces household items
- Short-term memory loss; difficulty recalling new information
- Subtle changes in personality and behavior
- Loss of initiative; less engaged in social relationships
- Mild cognitive impairment, problems with judgment
- Decreased performance, especially when stressed
- Unable to travel alone to new destinations
- Decreased sense of smell

MIDDLE (MODERATE), OR STAGE II (2 TO 3 YEARS)
- Impairment of all cognitive functions
- Problems with handling or unable to handle money and finances
- Disorientation to time, place, and event
- Possible depression, agitated
- Increasingly dependent in ADLs
- Visuospatial deficits: difficulty driving, gets lost
- Speech and language deficits: less talkative, decrease in use of vocabulary, increasingly non-fluent, and eventually aphasic
- Incontinent
- Wandering; trouble sleeping

LATE (SEVERE), OR STAGE III
- Completely incapacitated; bedridden
- Totally dependent in ADLs
- Motor and verbal skills lost
- General and focal neurologic deficits
- Agnosia (loss of facial recognition)

Orientation to Time
"What is the date?"

Registration
"Listen carefully, I am going to say three words. You say them back after I stop. Ready? Here they are... HOUSE (pause), CAR (pause), LAKE (pause). Now repeat those words back to me." [Repeat up to 5 times, but score only the first trial.]

Naming
"What is this?" [Point to a pencil or pen.]

Reading
"Please read this and do what it says." [Show examinee the words on the stimulus form.]
CLOSE YOUR EYES

A

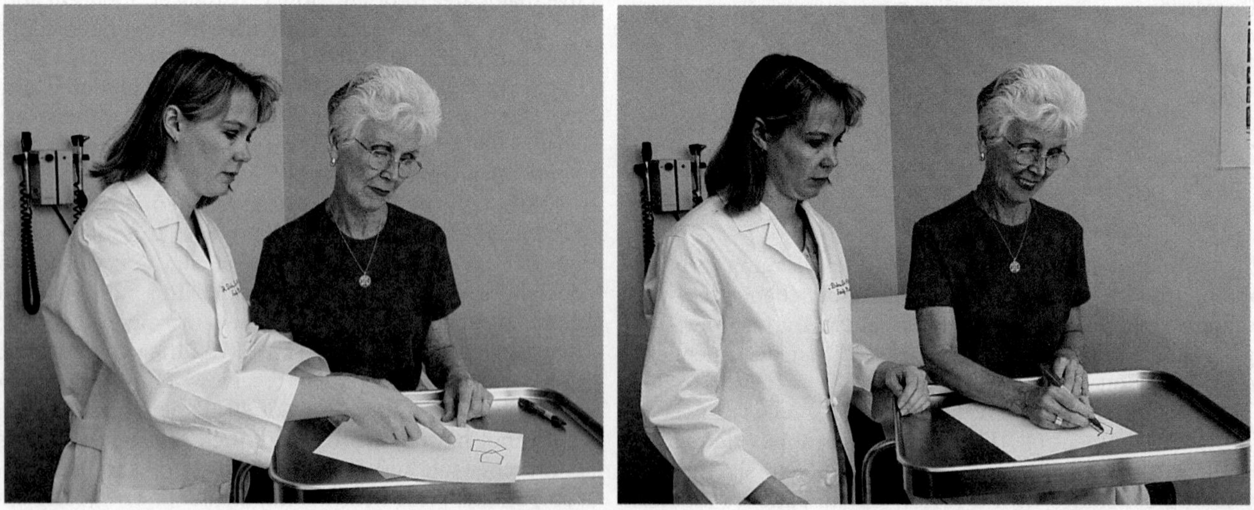

B

Fig. 44-2 • **A,** Examples of questions that are asked on the Mini-Mental State Examination. **B,** Copying is one of the tasks on the MMSE.

health care professionals cope with is the behavioral changes that can occur in advanced disease. Assess the patient for:

- Aggressiveness, especially verbal and physical abusive tendencies
- Rapid mood swings
- Increased confusion at night or when light is not adequate **(sundowning)** or in excessively fatigued patients

The patient may wander and become lost or may go into other rooms to rummage through another's belongings. Hoarding or hiding objects is also common. For example, patients may hoard washcloths in the long-term care setting.

For some patients with dementia, emotional and behavioral problems occur with the primary disease. They may experience paranoia (suspicious behaviors), delusions, hallucinations, and depression. Document these behaviors, and ensure the patient's safety. (Refer to a mental health/behavior health nursing textbook for a complete discussion of these disorders.)

Although drug therapy is not effective in treating dementia, certain drugs may help control the emotional and psychiatric manifestations (e.g., depression, anxiety, paranoia, aggression) associated with the primary disease.

Changes in Self-Management Skills. Observe for changes in the patient's self-management skills, such as:

- Decreased interest in personal appearance
- Selection of clothing that is inappropriate for the weather or event
- Loss of bowel and bladder control
- Decreased appetite or ability to eat

Over time, the patient becomes less mobile and muscle contractures develop. He or she eventually becomes totally immobile and requires total physical care. The patient is then unable to meet the human needs of mobility and cognition.

Psychosocial Assessment

In people with AD, the cognitive changes and biochemical and structural dysfunctions affect personality and behavior. In the early stage, patients often recognize that they are experiencing memory or cognitive changes and may attempt to hide the problems. They begin the grieving process because of anticipated loss, experiencing denial, anger, bargaining, and depression at varying times. Older patients typically think the changes are part of "old age."

As the disease progresses, patients begin to display major changes in emotional and behavioral affect. Of particular importance is the need for an assessment of the patients' reactions to changes in routine or environment. For example, a hospital admission is very traumatic for most patients with dementia. It is not unusual for them to exhibit a catastrophic response or overreact to any change by becoming excessively aggressive or abusive. This is referred to as traumatic relocation syndrome.

As patients become unaware of their behavior, the focus of the psychosocial assessment shifts to the family or significant others. The health care team assesses their ability to cope with the chronicity and progression of the disease and identifies possible support systems.

Laboratory Assessment

No laboratory test can confirm the diagnosis of AD. Definitive diagnosis is made on the basis of brain tissue examination at autopsy, which confirms the presence of neurofibrillary tangles and neuritic plaques.

Genetic testing, specifically for *apolipoprotein E4 (Apo E4)*, may be helpful as an ancillary test (not a predictive test) for the differential diagnosis of AD. *Amyloid beta protein precursor (soluble)* (sBPP) may be measured for patients to diagnose AD and other types of dementia. A decrease in the patient's sBPP in the cerebrospinal fluid (CSF) supports the diagnosis because the amyloid tends to deposit in the brain and is not circulating in the CSF (Pagana & Pagana, 2006).

A variety of other laboratory tests may be performed to rule out other treatable causes of dementia or delirium, including:

- Complete blood count (CBC)
- Serum electrolyte levels, blood urea nitrogen, and glucose
- Vitamin B_{12} levels
- Folate levels
- Thyroid and liver function tests
- Serologic test for syphilis
- Toxicity screening tests; heavy metal screen
- Alcohol screening tests

Imaging Assessment

A CT, PET, or SPECT scan may be performed to rule out other causes of disease. The CT scan typically shows cerebral atrophy and ventricular enlargement, wide sulci, and shrunken gyri in the later stages of the disease. An MRI scan can also rule out other causes of neurologic disease The PET and SPECT scans show a significant decrease in metabolic activity in the brains of people with AD.

Other Diagnostic Assessment

The electroencephalogram (EEG) shows slow-wave delta activity seen in the second and third stages of AD.

To more clearly identify the nature and extent of the patient's cognitive impairment, the neurologist or neuropsychologist administers several neuropsychological tests. The tests selected depend on clinician preference and the ability of the patient to participate in testing. All of the tests focus on cognitive ability and may be repeated over time to measure changes.

▪ *Analysis*

Common Nursing Diagnoses and Collaborative Problems

The priority nursing diagnoses for patients with Alzheimer's disease (AD) are:

1. Chronic Confusion related to Alzheimer's disease
2. Risk for Injury related to wandering, elder abuse or mistreatment
3. Disturbed Sleep Pattern related to changes in sleep phases, anxiety, and/or depression
4. Compromised Family Coping and Caregiver Role Strain related to the patient's prolonged progression of disability and the patient's increasing care needs

Additional Nursing Diagnoses and Collaborative Problems

In addition to the common nursing diagnoses, patients with AD may have one or more of these problems:

- Impaired Verbal Communication related to aphasia
- Imbalanced Nutrition: Less Than Body Requirements related to self-care deficit and/or anorexia
- Total Urinary Incontinence and Bowel Incontinence related to cognitive and self-care deficits
- Social Isolation related to personality and behavior changes

- Risk for Impaired Physical Mobility related to progression of disability
- Risk for Impaired Skin Integrity related to immobility and/or impaired nutritional status
- Self-Care Deficit (Total) related to cognitive deficit
- Sexual Dysfunction related to immobility and chronic confusion
- Risk for Other-Directed Violence and Risk for Self-Directed Violence related to behavior changes
- Hopelessness related to inability to control the progression of disease

Planning and Implementation

The priority for interdisciplinary care is safety! Chronic confusion and physical deficits place the patient with AD at a high risk for injury.

Chronic Confusion

NOC **Planning: Expected Outcomes.** In the very early stages of the disease, the patient with AD is expected to maintain the ability to perform complex mental processes. Indicators include that the patient will be able to:

- Communicate clearly and appropriately
- Comprehend the meaning of events and situations
- Be attentive and concentrate
- Be oriented to person, place, and time
- Process information
- Make appropriate decisions

As the disease progresses, patients cannot meet these criteria. Instead, the desired outcome is to maintain cognitive function for as long as possible to keep them safe and increase quality of life.

Interventions. The health care provider should answer the patient's questions truthfully concerning the diagnosis of AD. In this way, the patient can more fully participate in the interdisciplinary plan of care. Interventions are the same whether he or she is cared for at home, in an adult day care center, in an assisted living center, in a long-term care facility, or in a hospital admitted with another medical condition. *The patient with memory problems always benefits best from a structured and consistent environment.*

Many variables, including physical illness and environmental factors, can worsen or exacerbate (worsen) the clinical manifestations of AD (Table 44-7). The patient with AD frequently has other medical problems such as cardiovascular disease, arthritis, renal insufficiency, and pulmonary disease. Changes in vision and hearing also may be present. Managing these conditions helps the patient's functional abilities.

NIC ***Cognitive Stimulation and Memory Training.*** The purpose of cognitive stimulation and memory training is to reinforce or promote desirable cognitive function and facilitate memory (Chart 44-13). An individualized cognitive therapy program may provide some benefit to the patient.

Structuring the Environment. Collaborate with the health care team to identify conditions in the environment that can be changed to increase the patient's ability to function. The two most important actions are *preventing overstimulation* and *providing a structured and orderly environment.*

Teach the family to keep environmental distractions and noise to a minimum. The patient's home, hospital room, or nursing home room should not have pictures on the wall or other decorations that could be misinterpreted as people or animals that could harm the patient. An abstract painting or wallpaper might look like a fire or an explosion and scare the patient. The room should have adequate, nonglare lighting and no potentially frightening shadows.

In addition to disturbed sleep, other negative effects of high noise levels include decreased nutritional intake, changes in blood pressure and pulse rates, and feelings of increased stress and anxiety. The patient with AD is especially susceptible to

TABLE 44-7 Factors That Can Worsen Alzheimer's Disease

- Stroke
- Subdural hematoma
- Space-occupying lesion
- Decrease in blood supply to the brain
- Myocardial infarction
- Dysrhythmias
- Hypoglycemia
- Impaired renal function
- Impaired hepatic function
- Infection
- Impaired vision and hearing
- Sudden changes in surroundings
- Pain and discomfort
- Drugs
- Physical or chemical restraint

Chart 44-13 NIC INTERVENTION ACTIVITIES

The Patient with Alzheimer's Disease

Cognitive Stimulation: *Promotion of awareness and comprehension of surroundings by utilization of planned stimuli.*

- Offer environmental stimulation through contact with varied personnel.
- Present change gradually.
- Provide a calendar.
- Allow for rest periods.
- Use repetition to present new material.
- Present information in small, concrete portions.
- Use touch therapeutically.

Memory Training: *Facilitation of memory.*

- Discuss with patient/family any practical memory problems experienced.
- Stimulate memory by repeating patient's last expressed thought, as appropriate.
- Reminisce about past experiences with patient, as appropriate.
- Implement appropriate memory techniques such as visual imagery, mnemonic devices, memory games, and memory cues, association techniques, making lists, using computers, using nametags, or rehearsing information.
- Provide for orientation training, such as patient rehearsing personal information and dates, as appropriate.
- Provide for picture recognition memory, as appropriate.
- Encourage patient to participate in group memory training programs, as appropriate.
- Monitor patient's behavior during therapy.

NIC intervention activities selected from Bulechek, G.M., Butcher, H.K., & McCloskey Dochterman, J. (Eds.). (2008). *Nursing interventions classification (NIC)* (5th ed.). St. Louis: Mosby.

these changes and needs to have as much undisturbed sleep at night as possible. Fatigue increases confusion and behavioral manifestations such as agitation and aggressiveness.

When a patient is in a new setting or environment, collaborate with the staff and admitting department to select a room that is in the quietest area of the unit and away from obvious exits, if possible. A private room may be needed if the patient has a history of agitation or wandering. The television should remain off unless the patient turns it on or requests that it be turned on.

Objects such as furniture, a hairbrush, and eyeglasses should be kept in the same place. Establish a daily routine, and follow it as much as possible. Arrange for a communication board for scheduled activities and other information to promote orientation such as the day of the week, the month, and the year. Pictures of people familiar to the patient can also be placed on this board.

Orientation and Validation Therapy. Explain changes in routine to the patient before they occur, repeating the explanation immediately before the changes take place. Clocks and single-date calendars also help the patient maintain day-to-day orientation to the environment in the early stages of the disease process. *For the patient with early disease, reality orientation is usually appropriate. Teach family members and health care staff to frequently reorient the patient to the environment. Remind the patient what day and time it is, where he or she is, and who you are.*

For the patient in the later stages of AD, reality orientation does not work and often increases agitation. The health care team uses validation therapy for the patient with moderate or severe AD. In ***validation therapy,*** *the staff member recognizes and acknowledges the patient's feelings and concerns.* For example, if the patient is looking for a deceased mother, ask him or her to talk about what Mother looks like and what she might be wearing. This response does not argue with the patient but also does not reinforce the patient's belief that Mother is still living.

Promoting Self-Management. As the disease progresses, altered thought processes affect the ability to perform ADLs. Encourage the patient to perform as much self-care as possible and to maintain independence in daily living skills as long as possible. For example, in the home setting, complete clothing outfits that can be easily removed and put on (e.g., shirt, slacks, underwear, socks) and placed on a single hanger are preferred for patient selection. When possible, the patient should participate in meal preparation, grocery shopping, and other household routines. Many patients develop **apraxia,** the inability to make purposeful movements, as the disease progresses.

The occupational and physical therapists provide a complete evaluation and assistance in helping the patient become more independent. Adaptive devices, such as grab bars in the bathtub or shower area, an elevated commode, and adapted eating utensils, may enable him or her to maintain independence in grooming, toileting, and feeding. The physical therapist prescribes an exercise program to improve physical health and functionality.

Promoting Bowel and Bladder Continence. The patient may remain continent of bowel and bladder for long periods if taken to the bathroom or given a bedpan or urinal every 2 hours. Toileting may be needed more often during the day and less frequently at night. UAP or home caregiver encourages the patient to drink adequate fluids to promote optimal voiding. A patient may refuse to drink enough fluids because of a fear of incontinence. Assure the patient that he or she will be toileted on a regular schedule to prevent incontinent episodes.

When patients with AD are in the hospital or other unfamiliar place, they may get out of bed unassisted during the night and fall while trying to locate the bathroom. Do not use siderails unless absolutely necessary. If the patient climbs over the siderail and falls, the injury is likely to be worse than if the bed had been left in the lowest position and the siderails left down (Cotter & Evans, 2008). In both acute and long-term care settings, bed rails are considered a physical restraint and are not used unless they increase patient mobility. Chapter 3 discusses fall prevention in detail.

Maintain a clear path between the bed and bathroom at all times. For patients who are too weak to walk to the bathroom, a bedside commode may be used. Some patients may void in unusual places, such as the sink or a wastebasket. As a reminder of where they should toilet, place a picture of the commode on the bathroom door. Depending on written signs for identification is useless because most patients lose their ability to read as the disease progresses.

Assisting with Facial Recognition. As the disease progresses, the patient may experience **prosopagnosia,** an inability to recognize oneself and other familiar faces. Encourage the family to provide pictures of family members and close friends that are labeled with the person's name on the picture. In addition, advise the family to reminisce with the patient about pleasant experiences from the past. Use *reminiscence therapy* while assisting the patient with ADLs or performing a treatment or assessment. Refer to a personal item in the room to help the patient begin to talk about its meaning in the present and in the past.

It is not unusual for the patient to talk to his or her image in the mirror. This behavior should be allowed as long as it is not harmful. If the patient becomes frightened by the mirror image, remove or cover the mirror. In some long-term care or assisted living settings, a picture of the patient is placed on the room door to help with facial recognition and to help the patient locate his or her room. This picture also helps the staff locate the patient in case of elopement (running away).

Promoting Communication. Use **redirection** by attracting the patient's attention to promote communication. Keep the environment as free from distractions as possible. Speak directly to the patient in a distinct manner. Sentences should be clear and short. Remind the patient to perform one task at a time, and allow sufficient time for completion. It may be necessary to break each task down into many small steps (Chart 44-14).

As the disease progresses, the patient is unable to perform tasks when asked. Show the patient what needs to be done, or provide cues to remind him or her how to perform the task. When possible, explain and demonstrate the task that the patient is asked to perform.

Patients with AD typically have specific speech and language problems, such as:

- **Aphasia** (difficulty speaking and understanding language)
- **Anomia** (difficulty findings words to name an object)
- **Apraxia** (difficulty recognizing words)

Recognize that emotional and physical behaviors may be a form of communication. Interpret the meaning of these behaviors to address them. For example, restlessness may indi-

Chart 44-14 BEST PRACTICE FOR PATIENT SAFETY & QUALITY CARE

Promoting Communication with the Patient with Advanced Alzheimer's Disease

- Ask simple, direct questions that require only a "yes" or "no" answer if the patient can communicate.
- Provide instructions with pictures in a place that the patient will see if he or she can read them.
- Use simple, short sentences and one-step instructions.
- Use gestures to help the patient understand what is being said.
- Validate the patient's feelings.
- Limit choices; too many choices causes frustration and increased confusion.
- Never assume that the patient is totally confused and cannot understand what is being communicated.
- Try to anticipate the patient's needs and interpret nonverbal communication.

cate urinary retention, pain, infection, or hypoxia (lack of oxygen to the brain).

Drug Therapy. **Cholinesterase inhibitors** are drugs approved for treating AD symptoms. They work to improve cholinergic neurotransmission in the brain by delaying the destruction of acetylcholine (ACh) by the enzyme acetylcholinesterase. This action slows the onset of cognitive decline in some patients. None of these drugs alters the course of the disease. Examples include donepezil (Aricept), galantamine (Reminyl), and rivastigmine (Exelon).

Memantine (Namenda) is the first of a new class of drugs that is a low to moderate affinity ***N*-methyl-D-aspartate (NMDA) receptor antagonist.** Overexcitation of NMDA receptors by the neurotransmitter *glutamate* may play a role in AD. This drug therefore blocks excess amounts of glutamate that can damage nerve cells. It is indicated for advanced AD and has been shown to slow the pace of deterioration. Namenda may help maintain patient function for a few months longer. Some patients also have improved memory and thinking skills. This drug can be given with donepezil (Aricept), a cholinesterase inhibitor.

Some patients with AD develop depression and may be treated with **antidepressants.** Selective serotonin reuptake inhibitors (SSRIs), such as paroxetine (Paxil) and sertraline (Zoloft), are usually prescribed. *Tricyclic antidepressants, such as amitriptyline (Elavil, Levate♣), should not be used because of their anticholinergic effect, especially for older adults. Anticholinergic drugs frequently cause serious side effects, including increased confusion, urinary retention, and constipation.*

Psychotropic drugs, also called *antipsychotic* or *neuroleptic drugs,* should be reserved for patients with emotional and behavioral health problems that sometimes accompany dementia, such as hallucinations and delusions. In clinical practice, however, these drugs are sometimes incorrectly used for agitation, combativeness, or restlessness. *Psychotropic drugs are considered chemical restraints because they decrease mobility and patients' self-management ability. Therefore most geriatricians recommend that these drugs be used as a last resort and with caution in low doses for a specific emotional or behavioral health problem.* The specific drug prescribed depends on side effects, the condition of the patient, and expected outcomes. Follow agency policy and The Joint Commission standards concerning the use of chemical restraints.

Complementary and Alternative Therapies. A number of complementary and alternative therapies, such as the use of *Ginkgo biloba,* are being researched that may prevent AD, slow its occurrence, or slow its progression in older adults. Art, massage, dance, and music therapy are often used in long-term care settings to minimize agitation. Chapters 2 and 3 discuss these therapies, especially for older adults.

Risk for Injury

NOC **Planning: Expected Outcomes.** The patient with Alzheimer's disease (AD) is expected to remain free from physical harm and not injure anyone else. A safe home environment is also expected for those patients at home or in a homelike environment, such as assisted-living. Indicators include that there will be adequate:

- Provision of lighting
- Placement of handrails
- Safe storage of drugs
- Provision of assistive devices in accessible locations
- Arrangement of furniture to reduce risks

Interventions. Many patients with AD tend to wander and may easily become lost. In later stages of the disease, some patients may become severely agitated and physically or verbally abusive to others.

Coping with Restlessness and Wandering. Many patients with AD tend to wander and become temporarily lost in the community. *The patient should always wear an identification badge or bracelet when at home.* The badge should include how to contact the primary caregiver. In an inpatient setting, check the patient frequently and place him or her in a room that can be monitored easily. The room should be away from exits and stairs. Some health care agencies place large stop signs or red tape on the floor in front of exits. Others have installed alarm systems to indicate when a patient is opening the door or getting out of a bed or chair.

Teach the family to enroll the patient in the Safe Return Program—a national, government-funded program of the Alzheimer's Association (www.alz.org) that assists in the identification and safe, timely return of people with dementia. The program includes registration of the patient and a 24-hour hotline to be called to assist in finding a lost patient. If a patient wanders and becomes lost, the family (or health care institution) should immediately notify the police department. An up-to-date picture of the patient makes it easier for local authorities, the public, and neighbors to identify the missing patient. Devices using radio wave beacons and a global positioning system (GPS) have been developed to help families and law enforcement officials find a lost patient more easily. These devices include shoes with a GPS unit implanted, jewelry that is hard to remove, and bracelets. Caution families that these devices are not foolproof. Just like cell phones, there are some areas where the signal from the patient may not be picked up easily if at all.

Restlessness may be decreased if the patient is taken for frequent walks. If the patient begins to wander, he or she is redirected. For example, if the patient insists on going shopping for clothes, the patient is redirected to his or her closet to select clothing that will not be recognized as his or her own. This type of activity can be repeated a number of times because the patient has lost short-term memory.

In any setting, keep the patient busy with structured activities. In a health care agency, an activity therapist or volunteer may work with patients as a group or individually to determine the type of activity that is appropriate for the stage of the disease. Puzzles, board games, and art activities are often appropriate. Music and art therapy are becoming very popular in acute and long-term care for patients with dementia.

Physical restraints, such as waist belts and geri-chairs with lapboards, should be applied only as a last resort because they often increase the restlessness and cause agitation. Federal regulations in long-term care facilities in the United States mandate that all residents have the right to be free of both physical and chemical restraints. In addition, all health care agencies accredited by The Joint Commission are required to use alternatives to restraints before resorting to any physical or chemical restraint.

Ensuring Safety. Patients with AD may become injured because they cannot recognize objects or situations as harmful. Remove or secure all potentially dangerous objects (e.g., knives, drugs, cleaning solutions). Patients are often unaware that their driving ability is impaired and usually want to continue this activity even if their driver's license has been suspended or they are unsafe. Automobile keys must be secured, but the patient should be told why they were taken. (See Chapter 3 for more discussion on older adult driving.)

Late in the disease process, the patient may experience seizure activity. If he or she is cared for at home, teach caregivers what action to take when a seizure occurs. (See discussion of Interventions on p. 959 in the Seizures and Epilepsy section.)

Minimizing Agitation. Talking calmly and softly and attempting to redirect the patient to a more positive behavior or activity is an effective strategy when he or she is agitated. Use calm, positive statements, and reassure the patient that he or she is safe. Statements such as "I'm sorry that you are upset," "I know it's hard," and "I will have someone stay with you until you feel better" may help.

Actions to *avoid* when the patient is agitated include raising the voice, confrontation, arguing, reasoning, taking offense, or explaining. Teach the caregiver to not show alarm or make sudden movements out of the person's view. If the patient remains agitated, ensure his or her safety and leave the room after explaining that you will return later. Frequent visual checks must be done during this time. If the patient is connected to any type of tubing or other device, he or she may try to disconnect it or pull it out. These devices should be used cautiously in the patient with dementia. If IV access, for example, is needed, the catheter or cannula is placed in an area that the patient cannot easily see or it should be covered.

Another way to manage this problem is to provide a diversion. For example, if the patient is doing an activity or holding an item such as a stuffed animal or other special item, he or she might be less likely to pay attention to medical devices. Additional strategies to minimize behavioral problems, especially at home, are listed in Table 44-8.

Drugs may be used only if other modalities fail to control the patient's agitation and the behavior may lead to the patient or other being harmed. For example, risperidone (Risperdal) and lorazepam (Ativan) should be used with caution because of their significant potential side effects (e.g., sedation, increased confusion).

Recognizing Abuse or Mistreatment. Patients who are cared for at home are at high risk for neglect or abuse. The Joint Commission requires all patients to be assessed for neglect and abuse on admission to a health care facility. Patients with mild AD may not report these concerns for fear of retaliation. Those with severe AD may not have the ability to report the abuse. Asking questions such as "Who cooks for you?," "Do you get help when you need it?," or "Do you wait long for help to the bathroom?" may be less stressful for the patient to answer. Chapter 3 discusses this problem in detail.

Disturbed Sleep Pattern

Planning: Expected Outcomes. The patient with AD is expected to sleep through the night and be awake most of the day.

Interventions. The patient with AD often has difficulty sleeping at night but tends to nap frequently during the day. Suggest ways to enhance sleep to the family or other caregiver. One way to establish the usual day-night pattern is to keep the patient very active during the day. A daily routine that consists

TABLE 44-8 Minimizing Behavioral Problems at Home

Carefully evaluate the patient's environment.
- Ensure environment is safe:
  - Remove throw rugs.
  - Consider replacing tile floors with non-slippery floors.
  - Arrange furniture and room decorations to maximize the patient's safety when walking.
  - Minimize clutter in all rooms in and outside of the house.
  - Install night lights in patient's room, bathroom, and hallway.
  - Install and maintain smoke alarms, fire alarms, and natural gas detectors.
- Install safety devices for the bathroom.
- Install alarm system or bells on outside doors; place safety locks on doors and gates.
- Ensure that door locks cannot be easily opened by the patient.

Assist the patient to remain oriented as long as possible.
- Place single-date calendars in patient's room and in kitchen.
- Use large-face clocks with a neutral background.

Communicate with the patient based on his or her ability to understand.
- As the disease progresses, use simple language and explain activity before the patient needs to carry it out.
- Break complex tasks down to simple steps.

Encourage the patient to be as independent as possible in ADLs.
- Place complete outfits for the day on hangers; have the patient select one to wear.
- Develop and maintain a predictable routine (e.g., meals, bedtime, morning routine)

When a problem behavior occurs, use distraction to divert patient to another activity.

Minimize excessive stimulation.
- Take the patient on outings when crowds are small.
- If crowds cannot be avoided, minimize the amount of time the patient is present in a crowd. For example, at family gatherings, provide a quiet room for the patient to rest throughout the visit.

Arrange for a day care program if possible.

Register the patient with the Alzheimer's Association Safe Return Program (www.alz.org).

of a balance between passive activities and those requiring more strenuous exercise, such as walking or stretching activities, usually helps promote sleep at night. The patient may want to take a nap in the late afternoon, but this should be discouraged if possible. In the last stage of the disease, the patient may sleep during much of the day and night.

To promote sleep, teach the family to establish a before-bedtime ritual. The routine usually consists of personal hygiene activities (e.g., bathing, toileting, brushing teeth) and measures to reduce noise and eliminate distractions. A back rub or small snack may help the patient prepare for sleep.

The patient's treatment and drug regimen schedules are adjusted to provide for uninterrupted sleep. If more conventional measures fail to cause sleep, the health care provider may prescribe a *mild* antianxiety agent.

Compromised Family Coping; Caregiver Role Strain

NOC **Planning: Expected Outcomes.** The family or other caregivers of the patient with Alzheimer's disease (AD) are expected to have a positive perception of their own health status and life circumstances. Indicators include that they will be satisfied with their:

- Physical health
- Psychological health
- Lifestyle
- Performance of usual roles
- Social support
- Availability of respite

Interventions. The patient with moderate and severe AD requires continual 24-hour supervision and caregiving. Severe cognitive changes leave the patient unable to manage finances, property, or personal care. The family needs to seek legal counsel regarding the patient's competency and the need to obtain guardianship or a durable medical power of attorney when necessary. Refer the family to the local AD support group for literature and information concerning the disease and related problems.

Family members and other caregivers must be aware of their own health and stress levels. Signs of stress include anger, social withdrawal, anxiety, depression, lack of concentration, sleepiness, irritability, and health problems. When signs of stress occur, the caregiver should be referred to his or her health care provider or should seek one on his or her own. It is not unusual for the caregiver to refuse to accept help from others even for a few brief hours. Initially, the caregiver may be more comfortable accepting help for just a few minutes a day so he or she could shower, enjoy a cup of tea, or take a brief walk.

Refer all families to their local chapter of the Alzheimer's Association (www.alz.org) in the United States or to the Alzheimer Society of Canada (www.alzheimer.ca). These organizations provide information and support services to patients and their families, including seminars, audiovisual aids, and publications.

Community-Based Care

Home Care Management

AD is a chronic, progressive condition that eventually leaves the patient completely disoriented and totally dependent on others for all aspects of care. In the early stages, patients may be cared for at home with little need for outside intervention. Whenever possible, the patient and family should be assigned a case manager who can assess their needs for health care resources and find the best placement throughout the continuum of care.

The patient usually begins to withdraw from friends and social events as memory impairment and personality and behavior changes occur. The family may begin to decrease their own social activities as the demands of the patient's care take more of their time. Emphasize to the family the importance of maintaining their own social contacts and leisure activities. Many family members experience caregiver stress, which affects their physical, mental, and emotional health. Chart 44-15 lists strategies for reducing caregiver stress. Chapter 3 discusses caregiver role strain and interventions in more detail.

It is now possible in most areas of the United States and Canada for families to arrange respite care. The patient may be placed in a respite facility or nursing home for the weekend or for several weeks to give the family a rest from the constant care demands. The family may also be able to obtain respite care in the home through a home care agency or assisted-living facility. Remind the family that respite care is for a short period—it is not permanent placement. Some health care agencies have opened adult day care centers or specialty units for patients with AD. In the day care center, patients spend all or part of the day at the facility and participate in activities as their condition permits. Although these centers are usually open only on weekdays, this arrangement allows the caregiver to work or participate in other activities. If patients require 24-hour care, they may be placed in a specialty unit of a long-term care or assisted-living facility.

Teach the family how to be prepared in case the patient becomes restless, agitated, abusive, or combative. In addition, the family can learn how to use reality orientation or validation therapy, depending on the stage of the disease.

Health Teaching

Usually the patient with AD is cared for in the home until late in the disease process unless they can afford private pay care. Because health insurance coverage in the United States and

Chart 44-15 BEST PRACTICE FOR PATIENT SAFETY & QUALITY CARE

Reducing Caregiver Stress

- Maintain realistic expectations for the person with Alzheimer's disease (AD).
- Take each day one at a time.
- Try to find the positive aspects of each incident or situation.
- Use humor with the person who has AD.
- Use the resources of the Alzheimer's Association, including attending local support group meetings.
- Explore alternative care settings early in the disease process for possible use later.
- Establish advance directives with the AD patient early in the disease process.
- Set aside time each day for rest or recreation away from the patient, if possible.
- Seek respite care periodically for longer periods of time.
- Take care of yourself by watching your diet, exercising, and getting plenty of rest.
- Be realistic about what you or they can do, and accept help from family, friends, and community resources.
- Use relaxation techniques.

family finances are not sufficient to cover the services of a private duty nurse or home care aide, family members typically provide the care. The patient plan of care developed by the nurse or case manager, in conjunction with the family, must be reasonable and realistic for the family to implement.

Review how to assist with bathing, dressing, toileting, and other self-management activities. The occupational therapist teaches the family and the patient how to use adaptive equipment, such as a brace, a sling, a cane, or modified eating utensils. The patient may have difficulty chewing, swallowing, or tasting foods and may not be able to eat without assistance.

The family and the nutritionist should develop a diet plan to increase the patient's nutritional intake. In the late stage of AD, the patient's intake often decreases and he or she loses weight.

Provide information to the family on what to do in the event of a seizure and how to protect the patient from injury. Instruct them to notify the health care provider if the seizure is prolonged or if the patient's seizure pattern changes.

Review with the family or other caregiver the name, time, and route of administration; the dosage; and the side effects of all drugs. Remind the family to check with the health care provider before using any over-the-counter drugs or herbs because they may interact with prescribed drug therapy.

Emphasis is placed on the need for the patient to have an established exercise program to maintain mobility for as long as possible, as well as to prevent complications of immobility. In collaboration with the family, the physical therapist (PT) develops an individualized exercise program. The PT may continue to work with the patient at home until goals are achieved, depending on the payer source.

Remind the family or other caregiver to take special precautions to maintain the patient safely at home. The environment must be uncluttered, consistent, and structured. All hazardous items (e.g., cooking range and oven, power tools) are removed, secured, or "locked out." All electrical sockets not in use should be covered with safety plugs. Teach families to install handrails and grab bars in the bathroom. Handrails should be along all stairways, and a guardrail should be placed around porches or open stairwells. Because the patient may have a tendency to wander, especially at night, the family may want to install alarms to all outside doors, the basement, and the patient's bedroom. All outside and basement doors should have deadbolt locks to prevent the patient from going outside unsupervised. Remind the family to adjust the temperature of the water to prevent accidental burns. Night lights should be used in the patient's bedroom, hallway, and bathroom to prevent fear and to help with orientation.

Health Care Resources

When the patient can no longer be cared for at home, referral to an assisted-living or long-term care facility may be needed. Early in the course of the disease, advise the family that placement might be needed in the late stages of the disease or sooner. This allows the family to begin to search for an appropriate facility before a crisis develops and immediate placement is needed. A number of facilities specialize in the care of patients with AD and other dementias. These units generally have a high staff-to-patient ratio and are architecturally designed to meet the special needs of this type of patient. The national office of the Alzheimer's Association publishes an outline of criteria for a dementia unit. In the advanced stage of the disease, the patient may need referral to hospice services for total care. (See the discussion of end-of-life and hospice care in Chapter 9.)

Evaluation: Outcomes

Evaluate the care of the patient with Alzheimer's disease (AD) on the basis of the identified nursing diagnoses. The expected outcomes include that the patient and/or family will:

- Have the ability to maintain complex mental processes *(early AD)* or maintain current cognitive status
- Remain free from injury and have a safe home environment
- Sleep through the night and be awake at appropriate times
- Meet basic human needs (e.g., nutrition, mobility)

The caregiver will have a positive perception of his or her health status and life circumstances. Specific indicators for these outcomes are listed for each nursing diagnosis in the Planning and Implementation section (see earlier).

DECISION-MAKING CHALLENGE
Coordination of Care

An 82-year-old woman has had Alzheimer's disease for 3 years and has been independent, lives alone, and drives a car. Recently her only daughter came to visit and found that her house was not neat and clean as usual. Her mother's hair was dirty and not brushed, and she looked very thin. She was wearing two shoes of different styles. Her daughter became very distressed at her mother's condition and realized that the AD was progressing. There are no other siblings or family members available to help with her mother's care. She decides to call the home care agency where you work for help.

1. How will you respond to this patient's daughter?
2. What services or resources are available for this patient?
3. How could you help coordinate care for this patient?
4. How will you support the distressed daughter?

evolve For suggested answer guidelines, go to http://evolve.elsevier.com/Iggy/.

HUNTINGTON DISEASE
Pathophysiology

Huntington disease (HD) is a hereditary disorder transmitted as an autosomal dominant trait at the time of conception. This movement disorder causes both neurologic and behavioral symptoms.

GENETIC CONSIDERATIONS

Huntington disease is a single gene disorder caused by a mutation in the HD gene *(IT 15)* located on chromosome 4. The mutation is a multiple repeat of the specific base triplet CAG, increasing the length of the gene. An autosomal dominant trait with high penetrance means that a person who inherits just one mutated allele has nearly a 100% chance of developing the disease (McCance & Huether, 2006). This gene mutation has different expressions, depending on whether it is inherited from the mother or father. People who inherit the mutation from their fathers have an earlier onset and a shorter life expectancy than do those who inherit from their mothers. In addition, there is some variation in the disease, depending on the size (length) of the mutation. The longer the mutation, the more severe the disease is at an earlier age (McCance & Huether, 2006).

It is estimated that 25,000 people in the United States have HD, and another 20,000 to 50,000 are thought to carry the gene (www.hdsa.org). Men and women are equally affected, and symptoms begin between 35 and 50 years of age, striking at a highly productive time in life. The clinical onset of HD is gradual. The two main symptoms of the disease are progressive mental status changes, leading to dementia, and **choreiform movements** (rapid, jerky movements) in the limbs, trunk, and facial muscles. Dementia is related to the destruction of neurons within the cerebral cortex. It may also be associated with excessive amounts of dopamine found within the cerebral cortex and limbic systems of those affected. Two structures within the basal ganglia are involved in the development of HD: the caudate nucleus and the putamen. Both structures have close connections to the cerebral cortex and are closely associated with neurotransmitters. Neurotransmitters are secreted at the synapse, or junction, of one neuron with another, and it is through their specific excitation or inhibition of neurons that fine, controlled, integrated motor activity occurs.

In HD, there is a decrease in the amount of *gamma-aminobutyric acid (GABA),* an inhibitory neurotransmitter in the basal ganglia. GABA depletion causes increased activity of the thalamus and other parts of the brain. There may also be an increase in *glutamate,* a major excitatory neurotransmitter. The result of these chemical changes in the brain is brisk, jerky, purposeless movements, particularly of the hands, face, tongue, and legs, which the patient cannot stop (McCance & Huether, 2006).

There are three stages of HD, each lasting roughly 5 years, corresponding to the average 15-year course of the disease. Stage 1 is the onset of neurologic or psychological symptoms. Stage 2 is characterized by an increasing dependence on others for care. Stage 3 results in loss of independent function.

The diagnosis of HD is made on the basis of a family history of the disease and clinical assessment. The triad of dominant inheritance, choreoathetosis (neuromuscular symptoms), and dementia is the hallmark of the disease. The symptoms exhibited by the patient vary in range and severity, age of onset, and rate of progression. Observe for clinical manifestations, which include chorea (jerky movements), poor balance, hesitant or explosive speech, dysphagia (difficulty swallowing), impaired respiration, and bowel and bladder incontinence. Mental status changes include decreased attention span, poor judgment, memory loss, personality changes, and dementia (later in the disease process). Perform a complete neurologic assessment.

Patient-Centered Collaborative Care

There is no known cure or treatment for HD. The only way to prevent transmission of the gene is for those affected to avoid having biologic children. Genetic counseling is important for children of patients with the disease. People at risk for the disease can be tested to determine whether the gene mutation is present. Before the testing procedure is undertaken, counseling is necessary to ensure that the patient has voluntarily decided in favor of testing and is not being pressured by family or friends. In addition, counseling helps determine whether the benefits of knowing the results outweigh the risks of a positive result (e.g., depression or suicide).

Psychotropic agents may be used to manage movement abnormalities that interfere with ADLs or are functionally disabling. They are also used to help control agitation, hallucinations, or psychotic delusions. Drug therapy may be used to treat other symptoms such as depression, anxiety, or obsessive-compulsive behaviors. Many of the drugs used to treat HD may cause side effects that may be difficult to differentiate from signs of HD.

A number of clinical trials are being conducted to find other drugs or supplements that may decrease HD symptoms. Examples include the CoQ10 enzyme, growth factors, glutamate blockers, and antidepressants, such as sertraline (Zoloft).

The care of the patient with HD is managed by the collaborative efforts of the family and health care team and includes:

- Speech-language pathologist (SLP) who helps with communication, swallowing, and drooling
- Nutritionist who plans meals based on the SLP's recommendations and the patient's likes and dislikes
- Physical and occupational therapists who determine exercise conditioning and assistive devices
- Nurses or home health care aides who provide supportive care
- Case manager and social worker who coordinate care and help with referrals to community resources (e.g., Huntington Disease Society of America [www.hdsa.org]) and health care agencies for placement as needed

HUMAN NEEDS NURSING CARE REVIEW

What might you NOTICE if the patient is experiencing impaired mobility and cognition as a result of an acute CNS infection or chronic brain disorder?

- Headache
- Acute or chronic confusion
- Sleepiness or lethargy
- Inability to perform ADLs
- Inability to ambulate or alteration in gait
- Continuing weight loss
- Inability to communicate effectively
- Report of photophobia or phonophobia
- One or more seizures
- Extremity tremors, rigidity, or jerky movements

What should you INTERPRET and how should you RESPOND to a patient experiencing impaired mobility and cognition as a result of an acute CNS infection or chronic brain disorder?

Perform and interpret physical assessment, including:

- Assessing neurologic status, especially level of consciousness (LOC) and mental status
- Taking vital signs (high fever may indicate infection)
- Performing a comprehensive pain assessment
- Assessing ability to communicate
- Assessing nutritional status

Respond by:
- Notifying health care provider or Rapid Response Team if seizure or sudden change in LOC or mental status
- Ensuring an adequate airway
- Protecting patient from injury
- Managing pain
- Giving oxygen (for status epilepticus)
- Reorienting patient
- Assisting with ADLs if needed
- Collaborating with health care team members (e.g., PT, OT, SLP, nutritionist)

On what should you REFLECT?
- Think about how you responded.
- Continue to monitor for improving mental status and changes in LOC.
- Assess triggers or other causes for acute event.
- Develop teaching plan for patient and family for self-management.
- Think about what resources the patient and family may need.

GET READY FOR THE NCLEX EXAMINATION!

Key Points

Review these Key Points for each NCLEX Examination Client Needs Category.

Safe and Effective Care Environment
- For a patient having a tonic-clonic or complete partial seizure, protect the patient from injury.
- For patients who have had one or more seizures, place on "seizure precautions," which includes having oxygen and suctioning emergency equipment available, starting an IV access, and keeping the siderails up at all times. Indicate the reasons for the siderails to meet The Joint Commission requirements.
- Implement interventions for seizures as listed in Chart 44-5. Patients with status epilepticus have a life-threatening complication. Lorazepam and diazepam are the major drugs used for this emergency.
- Monitor for drug toxicity when patients are taking medications for Parkinson disease, especially levodopa combinations such as Sinemet. Delirium and decreased drug effectiveness are the most common indicators of toxicity.
- Collaborate with the health care team in discharge planning and health teaching for patients who have chronic neurodegenerative diseases such as Alzheimer's disease.
- Help patients and families identify community resources for chronic brain disorders, including the Alzheimer's Association and the National Parkinson Foundation.
- Observe patients with Alzheimer's disease closely because they tend to wander and make inappropriate decisions. Safety is a priority for these patients.

Health Promotion and Maintenance
- Teach patients with migraine headaches about triggers that could cause an attack, such as caffeine, wine, and pickled products.
- Teach patients with cluster headaches about precipitating factors, such as anger episodes, excitement, and excessive physical activity.
- In addition to prescribed drug therapy, encourage patients with headaches to use complementary and alternative therapies to help relieve pain, such as ice, darkened room, and relaxation techniques.
- Teach the patient with epilepsy the importance of continuing prescribed antiepileptic drugs (AEDs), even if he or she is seizure-free. Additional instructions for the patient and family are listed in Chart 44-4.
- Encourage people who are in areas of high population density, such as college dormitories and crowded living areas, to become immunized against meningococcal meningitis. Teach older adults and those with chronic illness to have influenza and pneumonia vaccines.
- Teach people who enjoy outdoor activities to avoid areas where mosquitoes and ticks are likely to populate, especially near lakes and wooded areas. If they are in contact with these areas, remind them (especially older adults) to use insect repellent and keep skin exposure at a minimum.

Psychosocial Integrity
- Remind caregivers of patients with chronic neurologic diseases, such as Alzheimer's disease, to find ways to cope with their stress to remain physically and psychologically healthy, as suggested in Chart 44-15.
- Teach caregivers of patients with dementia to use validation therapy, rather than reality orientation. Acknowledge the patient's feelings and concerns.
- Involve patients and families in developing a continuing plan of care to meet expected outcomes and maintain quality of life.
- Adapt communication techniques for the patient with dementia as outlined in Chart 44-14.

Physiological Integrity
- Assess for characteristic clinical manifestations in patients with classic migraine headaches as listed in Chart 44-1.
- Recall that the pain of cluster headaches is usually accompanied by ipsilateral (same side) eye tearing, rhinorrhea, congestion, ptosis, facial sweating, eyelid edema, and/or miosis.
- Recognize that generalized seizures, such as the tonic-clonic seizure, involve both cerebral hemispheres. Partial seizures, also called *focal* or *local seizures,* usually involve only one hemisphere.
- During a seizure, document patient's body movements and other assessments as described in Chart 44-6.
- Monitor for side and adverse effects of antiepileptic drugs (AEDs) as listed in Chart 44-3.
- Assess for clinical manifestations of meningitis as listed in Chart 44-7.
- For patients with meningitis, carefully monitor neurologic status, including vital signs and neurovascular checks. Observe for signs and symptoms of increased intracranial pressure (ICP).
- Assess level of consciousness (LOC) as a priority in patients with encephalitis.
- Assess for key features of Parkinson disease as described in Chart 44-10.

- Keep in mind that newer surgical procedures, such as deep brain stimulation, and experimental stem cell therapies are becoming available as options to control symptoms of Parkinson disease.
- Assess cognitive and functional abilities of the patient with Alzheimer's disease, recognizing that it is a progressive dementia with several stages as listed in Chart 44-12.
- Recall that both familial Alzheimer's disease has a genetic predisposition.
- For patients with Alzheimer's disease, recall that the newer drugs seem to improve function and cognition (cholinesterase inhibitors, such as donepezil [Aricept]) or slow the disease process (Memantine) but they do not cure the disease.
- Administer psychotropic drugs to patients with Alzheimer's disease who also have mental/behavioral health problems, such as depression and severe agitation.
- Remember that Huntington disease is a chronic, hereditary illness that is transmitted as an autosomal dominant trait at the time of conception. Refer patients with the disease for genetic counseling.

Additional Study Resources

Go to your Companion CD or Evolve at http://evolve.elsevier.com/Iggy/ for *Self-Assessment Questions for the NCLEX Examination.*

evolve Go to Evolve at http://evolve.elsevier.com/Iggy/ for *Prioritization and Delegation Questions for the NCLEX Examination.*

SELECTED BIBLIOGRAPHY

Abou Khaled, K.J., & Hirsh, L.J. (2007). Advances in the management of seizures and status epilepticus in critically ill patients. *Critical Care Clinics, 22*, 637-659.

Backer, J.H. (2006). The symptom experience of patients with Parkinson's disease. *Journal of Neuroscience Nursing, 38*(1), 51-57.

Barclay, L. (2007). Peppermint oil may relieve digestive symptoms, headaches. Retrieved June 11, 2008, from *www.medscape.com/viewarticle/555147.*

Boggs, W. (2007). Noncognitive measures predict progression to Alzheimer disease. *Neurology, 68*, 1588-1595.

Bunting-Perry, L.K. (2006). Palliative care in Parkinson's disease: Implications for neuroscience nursing. *Journal of Neuroscience Nursing, 38*(2), 106-113.

Cotter, V.T. (2006). Alzheimer's disease: Issues and challenges in primary care. *Nursing Clinics of North America, 41*(1), 83-93.

Cotter, V.T., & Evans, L.K. (2008). Try this: Avoiding restraints in older adults with dementia. *AJN, 108*(3), 45-46.

Graner, B. (2007). Break the cycle of stress with PBR³. *American Nurse Today, 2*(5), 56-57.

Howland, R.H. (2007). What is vagal nerve stimulation? *Journal of Psychosocial Nursing and Mental Health Services, 44*(8), 11-14.

Jung, S. (2007). The impact of migraines: A case study. *Journal of Neuroscience Nursing, 39*(4), 213-216.

Lawes, R. (2007). Uncovering the layers of meningitis and encephalitis. *Nursing Made Incredibly Easy, 5*(4), 26-34.

Matthews, C., Miller, L., & Mott, M. (2007). Getting ahead of meningitis and encephalitis. *Nursing2007, 107*(11), 37-42.

McCance, K.L., & Huether, S.E. (2006). *Pathophysiology: The biologic basis for disease in adults and children* (5th ed.). St. Louis: Mosby.

McGeeney, B.E. (2005). Cluster headache pharmacotherapy. *American Journal of Therapeutics, 12*(4), 351-358.

McCarron, K. (2006). The shakedown on Parkinson's disease. *Nursing Made Incredibly Easy, 4*(6), 40-50.

Miller, C.A. (2008). Communication difficulties in hospitalized older adults with dementia. *AJN, 108*(3), 58-66.

Moloney, M.F., Strickland, O.L., DeRossett, S.E., Melby, M.K., & Dietrich, A.S. (2007). The experiences of midlife women with migraines. *Journal of Nursing Scholarship, 38*(3), 278-285.

Nussbaum, R.L., McInnes, R.R., & Willard, H.F. (2007). *Thompson & Thompson genetics in medicine* (7th ed.). Philadelphia: Saunders.

Overstreet, M. (2005). West Nile virus. *Nursing2005, 35*(8), 64.

Pagana, K.D., & Pagana, T.J. (2006). *Manual of diagnostic and laboratory tests* (3rd ed.). St. Louis: Mosby.

Reyes, P.F., Nowak, L.A., & Rice, S.G. (2006). Alzheimer's disease: Clinical diagnosis and treatment. *Arrow Quarterly, 22*(1), 9-14.

Sanchez-del-Rio, M., Reuter, U., & Moskowitz, M. (2006). New insights into migraine pathophysiology. *Current Opinion in Neurology, 19*(3), 294-298.

Schutte, D.L. (2006). Alzheimer disease and genetics: Anticipating the questions. *AJN, 106*(12), 40-46.

Sharer, J. (2008). Tackling sundowning in a patient with Alzheimer's disease. *MEDSURG Nursing, 17*(1), 27-30.

Smith, M., & Buckwalter, K. (2005). Behaviors associated with dementia. *AJN, 105*(7), 40-52.

Tan, H.J., Suganthi, C., Dhachayani, S., Rizal, A.M., & Raymond, A.A. (2007). The coexistence of anxiety and depressive personality traits in migraine. *Singapore Medical Journal, 48*(4), 307-310.

Thomure, A. (2006). Helping your patient manage Parkinson's disease. *Nursing2006, 36*(8), 20-21.

Tocco-Blackmer, S. (2007). Overcoming the fear of tonic-clonic seizures. *American Nurse Today, 2*(5) 10-12.

Vacca, V.M., & Olson, A. (2007). Epilepsy in the elderly. *Advance for Nurses MD/DC/VA, 2*, 39-40.

Vandeweerd, C., Paveza, G.J., & Fulmer, T. (2006). Abuse and neglect in older adults with Alzheimer's disease. *Nursing Clinics of North America, 41*(1), 83-93.

Welsh, M. (2008). Treatment challenges in Parkinson's disease. *The Nurse Practitioner, 33*(7), 32-38.

Yaari, R., & Correy-Bloom, J. (2007). Alzheimer's disease. *Seminars in Neurology, 27*(1), 32-41.

Zia, W.C., & Lewin, J.J. (2007). Advances in the management of central nervous system infections in the ICU. *Critical Care Clinics, 22*(4), 661-694.

Care of Patients with Problems of the Central Nervous System: The Spinal Cord

45

CHAPTER

Kathy A. Hausman • Donna D. Ignatavicius

LEARNING OUTCOMES

For clinical competence and success on the NCLEX Examination, study this chapter with these Learning Outcomes in mind:

Safe and Effective Care Environment

1. Educate the patient on ways to prevent back and neck pain, including the need for ergonomics in the workplace.
2. Prioritize the nursing care of the patient with a spinal cord injury (SCI).
3. Collaborate with the health care team when providing care for patients with SCI.
4. Initiate consultations as needed for patients with SCI.
5. Integrate advance directives in the plan of care for patients with amyotrophic lateral sclerosis.
6. Identify community resources for patients with spinal cord health problems and their families.

Health Promotion and Maintenance

7. Counsel patients with SCI and their partners on sexuality issues as needed.
8. Provide discharge information to the patient and family after a lumbar or cervical laminectomy.
9. Perform a comprehensive health assessment of the patient with a spinal cord injury.

Psychosocial Integrity

10. Assess the coping strategies and response of patients with spinal cord problems and their families.
11. Describe the impact of spinal cord health problems on patients and their families.

Physiological Integrity

12. Assess the patient with spinal cord health problems for mobility, gait, strength, and sensation.
13. Implement interventions to prevent complications of immobility when caring for the patient with spinal cord health problems.
14. Use precautions to prevent injury when moving a patient with a spinal cord problem.
15. Apply knowledge of pathophysiology when caring for a patient having autonomic dysreflexia.
16. Explain the clinical manifestations and management options associated with spinal cord tumors.
17. Explain the pathophysiology of multiple sclerosis (MS) and amyotrophic lateral sclerosis (ALS).
18. Explain the role of drug therapy in managing patients with spinal cord problems.
19. Provide postoperative care for patients having spinal cord surgery, including monitoring for complications.

Go to your Companion CD or Evolve at http://evolve.elsevier.com/Iggy/ for *Self-Assessment Questions for the NCLEX Examination* keyed to these Learning Outcomes.

The spinal cord and its nerves play a major role in maintaining the human needs of *mobility* and *sensation.* This chapter focuses on back pain, spinal cord injuries and tumors, and diseases that affect the spinal cord, such as multiple sclerosis (MS) and amyotrophic lateral sclerosis (ALS). These health problems share a common characteristic of impaired *mobility* associated with decreased motor function. As a result, the patient's ability to perform ADLs is often affected. *Sensory* function also may be impaired, either temporarily or permanently. The spinal cord itself may be damaged, or the spinal nerves leading from the cord to the extremities may be affected. In some cases, both the spinal cord and nerves are involved.

BACK PAIN

Back pain is one of the most common reasons for visiting a health care provider. Disabling low back pain is the single greatest cause of injury in the working population. The lumbosacral (lower back) and cervical (neck) vertebrae are most commonly affected because these are the areas where the vertebral column is the most flexible. *Acute* back pain is usually self-limiting. If the pain continues for 3 months or if repeated episodes of pain occur, the patient has *chronic* back pain.

LUMBOSACRAL BACK PAIN (LOW BACK PAIN)

Pathophysiology

Lumbosacral back pain, referred to as **low back pain (LBP),** is more common than cervical pain. Acute pain is caused by muscle strain or spasm, ligament sprain, disk (also spelled "disc") degeneration, or herniation of the nucleus pulposus from the center of the disk. Herniated disks occur most often between the fourth and fifth lumbar vertebrae (L4-5) but may occur at other levels. A bulging or **herniated nucleus pulposus (HNP)** in the lumbosacral area can press on the adjacent spinal nerve (usually the sciatic nerve), causing severe burning or stabbing pain down into the leg or foot. The specific area of pain depends on the level of herniation. Muscle spasms of the affected leg also may occur.

In addition to pain, numbness and tingling may be felt in the affected leg because spinal nerves have both motor and sensory fibers. The HNP may press on the spinal cord itself, causing leg weakness and bowel and bladder dysfunction. Sacral spinal nerves are part of the reflex system for the bowel and bladder. They also contain parasympathetic nerve fibers, which help control bowel and bladder function.

Back pain may also be caused by **spondylolysis,** a defect in one of the vertebrae usually in the lumbar spine. **Spondylolisthesis** occurs when one vertebra slips forward on the one below it, often as a result of spondylolysis. This problem causes pressure on the nerve roots, leading to pain in the lower back and into the buttocks. Pain or numbness may also occur in the leg and foot. **Spinal stenosis,** a narrowing of the spinal canal, is typically seen in people older than 60 years. This narrowing may be caused by infection, trauma, herniated disk, and arthritis and disk degeneration. Most adults older than 50 years have some degree of degenerative disk disease although they may not be symptomatic.

Acute back pain usually results from injury or trauma. The patient typically hyperflexes or twists the back during a vehicular crash, or the injury occurs when the patient lifts a heavy object. Obesity places increased stress on the back muscles and can cause back pain. Smoking has been linked to disk degeneration, possibly caused by constriction of blood vessels that supply the spine. Congenital spinal conditions and scoliosis can also lead to back discomfort. Older adults are at high risk for both acute and chronic LBP. Small, petite, Euro-American women are at high risk for vertebral compression fractures, which cause severe pain and decreased mobility. Chart 45-1 provides a list of specific factors that can cause this problem in the older adult.

Chart 45-1 NURSING FOCUS ON THE OLDER ADULT

Factors Contributing to Low Back Pain

- Changes in support structures
  - Spinal stenosis
  - Hypertrophy of the intraspinal ligaments
  - Osteoarthritis
- Changes in vertebral support and malalignment
  - Scoliosis
  - Lordosis
- Vascular changes
  - Diminished blood supply to the spinal cord or cauda equina caused by arteriosclerosis
  - Blood dyscrasias
- Intervertebral disk degeneration

Health Promotion and Maintenance

Many of the problems related to acute back pain can be prevented by recognizing the cause of back pain and taking appropriate preventive measures. For example, good posture, proper lifting techniques, and exercise can significantly decrease the incidence of low back pain. Nurses and other direct care staff members who move and lift patients are at a very high risk for LBP.

The U.S. Occupational Safety and Health Administration (OSHA) mandated that all industries develop and implement a plan to decrease musculoskeletal injuries among their workers. One way to meet this requirement is to develop an ergonomic plan for the workplace. **Ergonomics** is an applied science in which the workplace is designed to increase worker comfort (thus reducing injury) while increasing efficiency and productivity. An example is equipment design for office furniture that can help reduce back injuries. Chart 45-2 summarizes various ways to prevent LBP.

Chart 45-2 PATIENT AND FAMILY EDUCATION GUIDE

Prevention of Low Back Pain and Injury

- Use proper body mechanics, with specific attention to bending, lifting, and sitting.
- Assess the need for assistance with your household chores or other activities.
- Participate in a regular exercise program, especially one that promotes back strengthening, such as swimming and walking.
- Do not wear high-heeled shoes.
- Use good posture when sitting, standing, and walking.
- Avoid prolonged sitting or standing. Use a footstool and ergonomic chairs and tables to lessen back strain. Be sure that equipment in the workplace is ergonomically designed to prevent injury.
- Keep weight within 10% of ideal body weight. Ensure adequate calcium intake.
- Stop smoking. If you are not able to stop, cut down on the number of cigarettes or decrease the use of other forms of tobacco.

Patient-Centered Collaborative Care

Assessment

Physical Assessment/Clinical Manifestations

The patient's primary concern is continuous pain. Some patients have so much pain that they walk in a stiff, flexed posture, or they may be unable to bend at all. They may walk with a limp, indicating possible sciatic nerve impairment. Walking on the heels or toes often causes severe pain in the affected leg, the back, or both.

Conduct a complete pain assessment as discussed in Chapter 5. Record the patient's current pain score, as well as the worst and best score since the pain began. Ask if pain occurs or gets worse at night or during rest. Determine if a recent injury to the back has occurred. It is not unusual for the patient to say "I just turned around and felt my back go out."

Inspect the patient's back for vertebral alignment and for tenderness and swelling caused by muscle spasm. Painful muscle spasm in the back and affected leg is common because the compressed nerve becomes inflamed and irritates nearby muscle tissue. Patients report stabbing, continuous pain in the muscle closest to the affected disk. They often describe a sharp, burning posterior thigh or calf pain that may radiate to the ankle or toes along the path of one or more spinal nerves. Pain usually does not extend the entire length of the limb. Patients may also report the same type of pain in the middle of one buttock. The pain is often aggravated by sneezing, coughing, or straining. Driving a vehicle is particularly painful.

Ask whether **paresthesia** (tingling sensation) or numbness is present in the involved leg. Both extremities may be checked for sensation by using a pin or paper clip and a cotton ball for comparison of light and deep touch. The patient may feel sensation in both legs but may experience a stronger sensation on the unaffected side. Those with severe problems may lose both bowel and bladder control from sacral spinal nerve involvement.

If the sciatic nerve is compressed, severe pain occurs when the patient's leg is held straight and lifted upwards. Foot, ankle, and leg weakness may accompany lower back pain. To complete the neurologic assessment, evaluate the patient's muscle tone and strength. Muscles in the extremity or in the back atrophy in severe, chronic conditions. The patient has difficulty with movement, and certain movements cause more pain than others.

Other information that may indicate more serious neurologic problems includes a history of fever and chills, recurrent skin or urinary tract infections, progressive motor and sensory loss, and difficulty with urination or having a bowel movement. In addition, patients older than 50 years and those with osteoporosis, immunosuppression, long-term use of steroids, or IV drug abuse require more thorough diagnostic studies.

Diagnostic Assessment

Imaging studies for patients who report mild nonspecific back pain may not be done depending on the nature of the pain. Patients with severe or progressive neurologic deficits or who are thought to have other underlying conditions (e.g., cancer, infection) require complete diagnostic assessment. X-rays of the spine, magnetic resonance imaging (MRI), or a computed tomography (CT) scan may be performed, with or without contrast media, to determine the cause of the pain. Some physicians may request a myelogram, but this test is done less often today. For patients having surgery, some physicians request a diskogram of the affected disk, especially when the level of the injury is not certain.

Electro-diagnostic testing, such as electromyography (EMG) and nerve-conduction studies, may help distinguish motor neuron diseases from peripheral neuropathies and **radiculopathies** (spinal nerve root involvement). These tests are especially useful in chronic diseases of the spinal cord or associated nerves. Chapter 43 describes these tests in more detail.

Interventions

Management of patients with back pain varies with the severity and chronicity of the problem. Most patients with acute LBP need only a short-term treatment regimen. The health care provider starts with conservative measures. If these are unsuccessful, surgery may be needed. Some patients have continuous or intermittent chronic pain that must be managed for an extended period, perhaps for their entire lives.

Nonsurgical Management

Nonsurgical conservative management of LBP includes positioning, drug therapy, heat therapy, physical therapy, and weight control.

The **Williams position** is typically more comfortable and therapeutic for the patient with LBP from a bulging or herniated disk. In this *position,* the patient lies in the semi-Fowler's position with a pillow under the knees to keep them flexed or sits in a recliner chair. This position relaxes the muscles of the lower back and relieves pressure on the spinal nerve root. Most patients also find that they have to change position frequently. Prolonged standing, sitting, or lying down increases back pain. If the patient must stand for a long time for work or other reason, shoe insoles or special floor pads may help decrease pain.

A firm mattress or a backboard placed under a soft mattress may provide back support for some patients. A flat position is sometimes helpful for the patient with a muscle injury. However, a flat position may aggravate the pain caused by disk trauma or disease.

The health care provider prescribes acetaminophen, muscle relaxants, and NSAIDs for acute LBP. Opioid analgesics are no more effective than nonsteroidal analgesics and should be avoided if at all possible. If they must be used, the course of therapy should be short to prevent adverse drug events. Short-term oral steroids in tapering doses may be prescribed for some patients to rapidly reduce inflammation.

Some patients may need an epidural injection for pain relief. A corticosteroid and an anesthetic are injected to reduce inflammation in the affected area. During a facet joint injection, fluoroscopy is used to insert a needle into the epidural space surrounding the facet and a corticosteroid is injected to coat the nerve roots and outside lining of the joints.

Patients having chronic back pain may require an antiepileptic drug (AED) such as gabapentin (Neurontin) and oxcarbazepine (Trileptal) to treat neuropathic (chronic nerve) pain. Most of the drugs in this class can cause hyponatremia (low serum sodium), and some cause weight gain. Older patients should be monitored very carefully for symptoms of hyponatremia, including generalized skeletal muscle weakness, headache, and diarrhea.

Some patients with back pain may have temporary relief from *heat* application. Heat increases blood flow to the affected area and promotes the healing of injured nerves. Moist heat from heat packs or hot towels applied for 20 to 30 minutes at least four times per day is often recommended. Hot showers or baths also are often beneficial. The physical therapist (PT) may provide deep heat therapy, such as ultrasound treatments and diathermy. Collaborate with the PT to monitor the effects of heat treatment by assessing the patient's skin condition and relief of pain. Some patients may receive **phonophoresis,** which is the application of a topical drug (e.g., lidocaine, hydrocortisone) followed by continuous ultrasound for 10 minutes. This procedure pushes the medication into the subcutaneous tissue and provides longer-lasting pain relief.

The *physical therapist* also works with the patient to develop an individualized exercise program. The type of exercises prescribed depends on the location and nature of the injury and the type of pain. The patient does not begin exer-

Chart 45-3 PATIENT AND FAMILY EDUCATION GUIDE

Typical Exercises for Chronic or Postoperative Low Back Pain

EXTENSION EXERCISES

- **Stomach lying:** Lie face down with a pillow under your chest; lift legs straight up (alternate legs) (may not be tolerated).
- **Upper trunk extension:** Lie face down with your arms at your sides, and lift your head and neck.
- **Prone pushups:** Lie face down on a mat and, keeping your body stiff, push up to extend your arms.

FLEXION EXERCISES

- **Pelvic tilt:** Lying on your back with your knees bent, tighten your abdominal muscles to push your lower back against the mat.
- **Semi–sit-ups:** Lying on your back with your knees bent, raise your upper body at a 45-degree angle and hold this position for 5 to 10 seconds.
- **Knee to chest:** Lying on your back with your knees bent, tighten your abdominal muscles to push your lower back against the mat. Now bring one or both knees to your chest and hold this position for 5 to 10 seconds.

cises until acute pain is reduced by other means. Several specific exercises for LBP are listed in Chart 45-3. Water therapy combined with exercise may be helpful for patients with chronic pain. The water provides muscle resistance during exercise to prevent atrophy.

Weight control often helps reduce chronic lower back pain by decreasing the work on the vertebrae caused by excess weight. If the patient's weight exceeds the ideal by more than 10%, caloric restriction is necessary. Health care providers must be sensitive when reinforcing the need for patients to lose weight to prevent or to lessen chronic back pain. When appropriate, the patient is referred to a nutritionist to plan and implement an appropriate calorie-restricted diet plan. Positive reinforcement and self-esteem building are integral to the nutrition plan.

Complementary and Alternative Therapies

The patient may find that other nontraditional and complementary therapies provide short-term pain relief. Patients with low back muscle injuries or *mild* nerve involvement may find relief of pain from chiropractic therapies. These therapies involve manipulative maneuvers of the spine to promote alignment and prevent or treat pressure on nerve roots. Distraction, imagery, acupuncture, and music therapy are examples of pain-relief therapies for acute and chronic pain. Chapters 2 and 5 describe these techniques in detail.

Surgical Management

Surgery is usually performed if conservative measures fail to relieve back pain or if neurologic deficits continue to progress. An orthopedic surgeon or neurosurgeon can perform these surgeries. Two major types of surgery are performed, depending on the severity and exact location of pain: minimally invasive surgery (MIS) and conventional open surgical procedures. MIS is not done if the disk is pressing into the spinal cord (central cord involvement).

Preoperative Care. Preoperative care for the patient preparing for lumbar surgery is similar to that for any patient undergoing surgery (see Chapter 16). Teach the patient about:

- Techniques to get into and out of bed
- Turning and moving in bed
- Sensations, such as numbness and tingling, that may occur in the affected leg or in both legs
- Home care activities and restrictions

Many patients are discharged to home within 24 hours or the next day after surgery. Therefore, before surgery, teach family members or other caregiver how to assist the patient and what restrictions the patient must follow at home.

A bone graft is done if the patient has a spinal fusion. The surgeon explains from where the bone for grafting will be obtained. The patient's own bone is used whenever possible, but additional bone from a bone bank may be needed. The surgeon provides verbal and written information about the type and the source of bone for surgery. Be sure that the patient signs an informed consent form before surgery. While the bone graft heals, the patient may wear a back brace for 4 to 6 weeks after surgery. In this case, the brace is fitted before surgery. Provide information about the importance of wearing the brace as instructed during the healing process, how to take it off and put it on while maintaining spinal alignment, and how to clean it.

Operative Procedures. *Minimally invasive surgeries (MISs)* have the advantage of being associated with less muscle injury, decreased blood loss, and decreased postoperative pain. The primary advantage of these surgical procedures is a shortened hospital stay and the possibility of an ambulatory procedure. Spinal cord and nerve complications are also less likely. Several specific procedures are commonly performed.

A local anesthetic is given for the *percutaneous lumbar diskectomy*, also called *microendoscopic diskectomy (MED)* or *percutaneous endoscopic diskectomy (PED)*. The surgeon uses fluoroscopy to insert an endoscope (arthroscope) next to the affected disk. A special cutting tool or laser probe is threaded through the cannula for removal or destruction of *disk pieces* that are compressing the nerve root. A newer procedure combines the MED with *laser thermodiskectomy* to also shrink the herniated disk. Inpatient hospitalization is not necessary for this procedure.

A *microdiskectomy* involves microscopic surgery directly through a 1-inch incision. This procedure allows easier identification of anatomic structures, improved precision in removing small fragments, and decreased tissue trauma and pain.

Laser-assisted laparoscopic lumbar diskectomy combines a laser with modified standard disk instruments inserted through the laparoscope using an umbilical ("belly button") incision. The procedure may be used to treat herniated disks that are bulging but do not involve the vertebral canal. The primary risks of this surgery are infection and nerve root injury. The patient is typically discharged in 24 hours but may go home the same day.

The most common *conventional open procedures* are diskectomy, laminectomy, and spinal fusion. These procedures involve an incision to expose anatomic landmarks for extensive muscle and soft-tissue dissection. Major complications include nerve injuries, **diskitis** (disk inflammation), and dural tears (tears in the dura covering the spinal cord).

As the name implies, a *diskectomy* is removal of a herniated disk. A *laminectomy* involves removal of part of the laminae and facet joints to obtain access to the disk space. When repeated laminectomies are performed or the spine is unstable, the surgeon may perform a **spinal fusion (arthrodesis)** to stabilize the affected area. Chips of bone are removed, typically from the iliac crest, or obtained from donor bone and are grafted between the vertebrae for support and to strengthen the back. Metal implants (usually titanium pins, screws, plates, or rods) may be required to ensure the fusion of the spine. Before closing, the surgeon may give an **intrathecal** (spinal) dose of morphine to decrease postoperative pain.

Interbody cage fusion is a newer spinal implant. A cage-like device is implanted into the space where the disk was removed. Bone graft tissue is packed around the device. Like instrumentation and fusion, the bone graft grows into and around the cage and creates a stable spine at that level.

An adjunct for patients for whom fusion may be difficult is the placement of an implantable **direct current stimulation (DCS)** device to promote bone fusion. External bone stimulators may also be effective for healing bone fusions.

Postoperative Care. Postoperative care depends on the type of surgery that was performed. In the postanesthesia care unit (PACU), vital signs and level of consciousness are monitored frequently, the same as for any surgery. Best practices for PACU care are discussed in Chapter 18.

Minimally Invasive Surgery. Patients go home the same day or the day after surgery with a Band-Aid or Steri-Strips over their small incision. Those having a microdiskectomy may also have a clear or gauze dressing over the bandage. Most patients notice less pain immediately after surgery, but mild oral analgesics are needed for pain control while nerve tissue heals over the next few weeks. In collaboration with the health care provider and physical therapist, teach the patient to follow the prescribed exercise program, which begins immediately after discharge. Patients should start walking routinely every day. Complications of MIS are rare.

Conventional Open Surgery. Early postoperative nursing care focuses on preventing and assessing complications that might occur in the first 24 to 48 hours (Chart 45-4). As for any patient undergoing surgery, take vital signs at least every 4 hours during the first 24 hours to assess for fever and for hypotension, which could indicate bleeding or severe pain. Perform a neurologic assessment every 4 hours. Of particular importance are movement, strength, and sensation in the extremities.

Carefully check the patient's ability to void. Pain and a flat position in bed make voiding difficult, especially for men. An inability to void may indicate damage to the sacral spinal nerves, which control the detrusor muscle in the bladder. Opioid analgesics have also been associated with difficulty voiding. The patient with a diskectomy or laminectomy typically gets out of bed with assistance on the evening of surgery, which may help with voiding.

Pain control may be achieved with patient-controlled analgesia (PCA) with morphine. The route is changed to oral administration after the patient is able to take fluids or the next morning.

Inspect and teach the family how to check the surgical dressing for blood or any other type of drainage. Clear drainage may mean cerebrospinal fluid (CSF) leakage. The loss of a large amount of fluid may cause the patient to report having a sudden headache. Report signs of any drainage to the surgeon immediately. Bulging at the incision site may be due to a CSF leak or a hematoma, both of which should also be reported to the surgeon.

Chart 45-4 BEST PRACTICE FOR PATIENT SAFETY & QUALITY CARE

Assessing and Managing the Patient with Major Complications of Lumbar Spinal Surgery

Complication	Assessment/Interventions
Cerebrospinal fluid (CSF) leakage	Observe for clear fluid on or around the dressing. Report CSF leakage immediately to the surgeon. (The patient is usually kept on flat bedrest for several days while the dural tear heals.)
Fluid volume deficit	Monitor intake and output; monitor drain output, which should not be more than 250 mL in 8 hr during the first 24 hr. Monitor vital signs carefully for hypotension and tachycardia.
Acute urinary retention	Assist the patient to the bathroom or a bedside commode as soon as possible postoperatively. Assist male patients to stand at the bedside as soon as possible postoperatively.
Paralytic ileus	Monitor for flatus or stool. Assess for abdominal distention, nausea, and vomiting.
Fat embolism syndrome (FES) (more common in people with spinal fusion)	Observe for and report chest pain, dyspnea, anxiety, and mental status changes (particularly common in older adults). Note petechiae around the neck, upper chest, buccal membrane, and conjunctiva. Monitor arterial blood gas values for decreased Pao_2.
Persistent or progressive lumbar radiculopathy (nerve root pain)	Report pain not responsive to opioids. Document the location and nature of pain. Administer analgesics as prescribed.
Infection (e.g., wound, diskitis, hematoma)	Monitor the patient's temperature carefully (a slight elevation is normal). Increased temperature elevation or a spike after the second postoperative day is possibly indicative of infection. Report increased pain or swelling at the wound site or in the legs. Give antibiotics as prescribed if infection is confirmed. Use clean technique for dressing changes.

Empty the surgical drain, usually a Jackson-Pratt or Hemovac, and record the amount of drainage every 8 hours. The surgeon usually removes the drain in 24 to 36 hours.

Correct turning of the patient in bed is especially important. Teach the patient to log roll every 2 hours from side to back and vice versa. In **log rolling,** the patient turns as a unit while his or her back is kept as straight as possible. A turning sheet may be used for obese patients. Either turning method may require additional assistance, depending on how much the patient can assist and on his or her weight. Instruct the patient to keep his or her back straight when getting out of bed. He or she should sit in a straight-back chair with the feet resting comfortably on the floor.

Teach the patient to deep breathe every 2 hours to prevent atelectasis (alveolar collapse) and pneumonia. Until the patient can ambulate independently, he or she wears graduated compression stockings, sequential compression devices (SCDs), or pneumatic compression boots (PCBs) to prevent deep vein thrombosis (DVT) and possible pulmonary emboli. *Older adults are especially likely to develop these complications of immobility.*

When a spinal fusion is performed in addition to a laminectomy, more care is taken with mobility and positioning. The patient may or may not require bedrest for 24 hours, with the nurse or unlicensed assistive personnel (UAP) log rolling him or her every 2 hours. For the conventional fusion, inspect both the iliac and spinal incision dressings for drainage and make sure they are intact. A brace or other type of thoracolumbar support may be worn when the patient is out of bed, although this is not as common today. Remind the patient to avoid prolonged sitting or standing.

Community-Based Care

The patient with back pain who does not undergo surgery is typically managed at home. If back surgery is performed, the patient is usually discharged to home with support from family or significant others. For older adults without a community support system, a short-term stay in a nursing home or transitional care unit may be needed. Collaborate with the case manager or discharge planner, patient, and family to determine the most appropriate placement.

Home Care Management

Inform the patient and family members or significant other that the patient should have a firm mattress to provide support for the entire vertebral column. A bed board or large piece of plywood placed under a soft mattress may suffice. After *conventional open back surgery,* the patient may be limited in the number of times he or she is allowed to climb stairs each day. However, daily walking is encouraged. The patient can usually return to work in 4 to 6 weeks, depending on the nature of the job and the extent and type of surgery. Some patients may not return for 3 to 6 months if their jobs are physically strenuous. Weight that may be lifted is initially limited to 5 pounds. The amount is gradually increased as healing occurs. Driving is not permitted for several weeks until the surgeon re-evaluates the patient.

Patients having any of the MIS procedures may resume normal activities within a few days up to 3 weeks after surgery, depending on the specific procedure that was done and the condition of the patient. He or she may take a shower on the third or fourth day after surgery. Teach the patient to remove the outer clear or gauze dressing, if any is in place, but leave the Steri-Strips in place for a week or so or until they fall off.

Health Teaching

The patient with an acute episode of back pain typically returns to his or her usual activities but may fear a recurrence. Remind the patient that he or she may never have another episode if caution is used. However, continuous or repeated pain can be frustrating and tiring. Encourage the patient and family members to set short-term goals and to take steps toward recovering slowly.

After surgery, in collaboration with the nutritionist and physical therapist, instruct the patient to:

- Continue with a weight-reduction diet, if needed.
- Stop smoking, if applicable.
- Use moist heat as needed.
- Perform strengthening exercises as started preoperatively and in the hospital setting.

The physical therapist reviews and demonstrates the principles of body mechanics and muscle-strengthening exercises. The patient is then asked to demonstrate these principles (Chart 45-5). Formal physical therapy usually begins about 2 weeks after surgery. Teach the patient the importance of keeping all appointments and following the prescribed exercise plan.

The health care provider may want the patient to continue taking anti-inflammatory drugs and muscle relaxants. Remind the patient and family about the possible side effects of drugs and what to do if they occur.

In a few patients, back surgery is not successful. This situation, referred to as **failed back surgery syndrome (FBSS),** is a complex combination of organic, psychological, and socioeconomic factors. Repeated surgical procedures often discourage these patients, who must continue pain management after multiple operations. Nerve blocks and other chronic pain–management modalities may be needed on a long-term basis (see Chapter 5).

Ziconotide (Prialt) is used for severe chronic back pain and FBBS and is given by intrathecal (spinal) infusion with a surgically implanted pump. It is the first available drug in a new class called *N-type calcium channel blockers (NCCBs).* NCCBs seem to selectively block calcium channels on those nerves that usually transmit pain signals to the brain. Ziconotide is also used for patients with cancer, AIDS, and unremitting pain from other nervous system disorders. It can be given with

Chart 45-5 PATIENT AND FAMILY EDUCATION GUIDE

Use of Proper Body Mechanics to Prevent Back Injury After Surgery

- Size up the load to determine the number of persons needed to perform the task.
- When lifting an object, keep your back straight and do not bend at the waist; lift with your large thigh muscles.
- Push objects rather than pull them.
- Do not twist your back.
- Avoid prolonged sitting or standing. Use a footstool to lessen back strain.
- Sit in chairs with good support. Sleep on a firm mattress.
- Avoid shoulder stooping; maintain proper posture.
- Do not walk or stand in high-heeled shoes for prolonged periods (for women).

opioid analgesics but should not be given to patients with severe mental health/behavioral health problems because it can cause psychosis. If symptoms such as hallucinations and delusions occur, the drug should be stopped immediately.

Health Care Resources

Assist the patient in identifying support systems (e.g., family, church groups, clubs) after back surgery or FBSS. For example, a spouse may help the patient with exercises or perform the exercises with the patient. Members of a church group may help run errands and do household chores.

The patient with back pain may continue physical therapy on an ambulatory basis after discharge. For unresolved pain, the patient may be referred to pain specialists or clinics, which are usually found in large metropolitan hospitals. A case manager may be assigned to the patient to help with resource management and utilization.

CERVICAL NECK PAIN

Pathophysiology

Cervical neck pain most often results from a bulging or herniation of the nucleus pulposus (HNP) in an intervertebral disk. As seen in Fig. 45-1, the disk tends to herniate laterally where the annulus fibrosus is weakest and the posterior longitudinal ligament is thinned. The result is spinal nerve root compression, with resulting motor and sensory manifestations, typically in the neck, upper back (over the shoulder), and down the affected arm. The disk between the fifth and sixth cervical vertebrae (C5-6) is affected most often.

If the disk does not herniate, nerve compression may be caused by osteophyte (bony spur) formation from osteoarthritis. The osteophyte presses on the intervertebral foramen, which results in a narrowing of the disk and pressure on the nerve root. As with sciatic nerve compression, the patient with cervical nerve compression may have either continuous or intermittent chronic pain. When the disk herniates centrally, pressure on the spinal cord occurs.

Cervical pain—acute or chronic—may also occur from muscle strain, ligament sprain resulting from aging or poor posture, lifting incorrectly, tumor, or infection. The typical history of the patient includes a report of pain when moving the neck, which radiates to the shoulder and down the arm. The pain may interrupt sleep and may be accompanied by a headache or numbness and tingling in the affected arm. To determine the exact cause of the pain, the health care provider requests diagnostic tests, such as MRI, plain x-rays of the neck, electromyography, or a combination of these. A diskogram may be done to determine the exact level of injury if it is not evident.

Patient-Centered Collaborative Care

Conservative treatment for neck pain is the same as described for low back pain except the exercises focus on the shoulders and neck. The physical therapist teaches the patient the correct techniques for performing "shoulder shrug," "shoulder squeeze," and "seated rowing." If these treatments do not work, some health care providers prescribe a soft collar to stabilize the neck, especially at night. Using the collar longer than 10 days leads to increased pain and decreased muscle strength and range of motion. For that reason, some health care providers do not recommend collars for cervical disk problems.

If conservative treatment is ineffective, surgery may be required, most often using a *conventional open surgical approach.* A neurosurgeon usually performs this surgery because of the complexity of the nerves and other structures in that area of the spine. Depending on the cause and the location of the herniation, either an anterior or posterior approach is used. An anterior cervical diskectomy and fusion (ACDF) is commonly performed. The patient is fitted with a large brace before surgery. Routine preoperative and postoperative care is the same as that described in Chapters 16 and 18.

The priority for care in the immediate postoperative period is maintaining an airway and ensuring that the patient has no problem with breathing. Swelling from the surgery can narrow the trachea, causing a partial obstruction. Chart 45-6 summarizes best practices for postoperative care and discharge planning.

Complications of ACDF can occur from the brace or the surgery itself. The initial brace is worn for 4 to 6 weeks, depending on the patient. When it is removed, a soft collar is worn for several more weeks, or longer if needed. Potential complications of the anterior surgical approach can be found in Chart 45-7.

Some patients may be candidates for minimally invasive surgery (MIS), such as percutaneous cervical diskectomy through an endoscope, with or without laser thermodiskectomy to shrink the herniated portion of the disk. The care for these patients is very similar to that for the patient with low back pain who has MIS (see discussion of surgical management of patients with low back pain on p. 986).

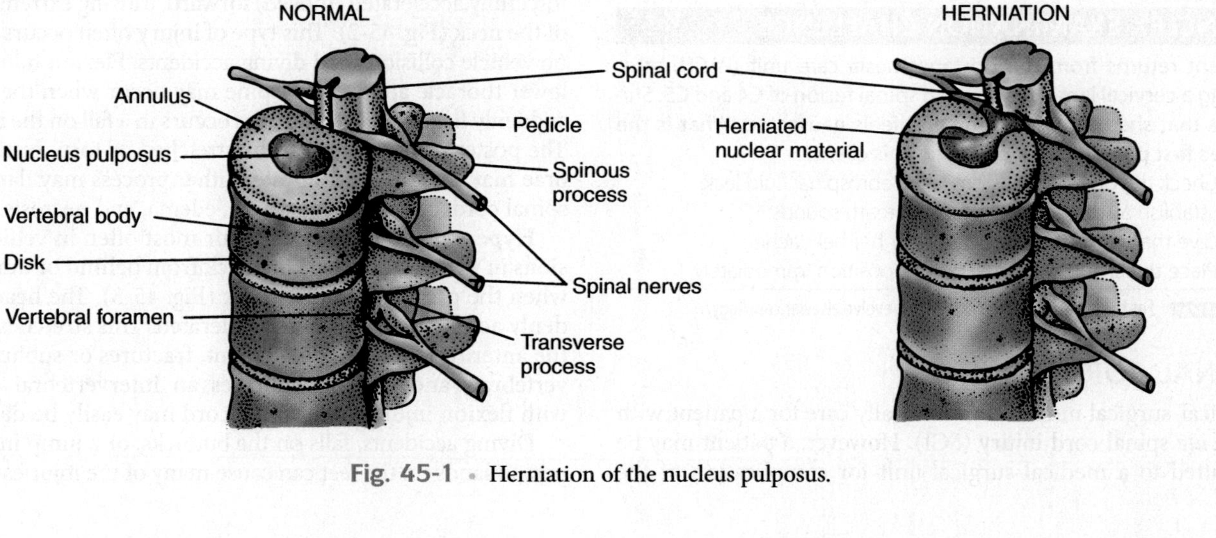
NORMAL
HERNIATION
Spinal cord
Annulus
Pedicle
Herniated nuclear material
Nucleus pulposus
Spinous process
Vertebral body
Disk
Spinal nerves
Vertebral foramen
Transverse process

Fig. 45-1 • Herniation of the nucleus pulposus.

Chart 45-6 BEST PRACTICE FOR PATIENT SAFETY & QUALITY CARE

Care of the Patient After an Anterior Cervical Diskectomy and Fusion

POSTOPERATIVE INTERVENTIONS

- Assess airway, breathing, and circulation (ABCs) (first priority!).
- Check for bleeding and drainage at the incision site.
- Monitor vital signs and neurologic status frequently.
- Check for swallowing ability.
- Monitor intake and output.
- Assess the patient's ability to void (may be a problem secondary to opiates).
- Manage pain adequately.
- Assist the patient with ambulation within a few hours of surgery, if he or she is able.

DISCHARGE TEACHING

- Be sure that someone stays with the patient for the first few days after surgery.
- Review drug therapy.
- Teach care of the incision.
- Review activity restrictions:
  - No lifting
  - No driving until physician permission
  - No strenuous activities
- Walk every day.
- Call the surgeon if symptoms of pain, numbness, and tingling worsen or if swallowing becomes difficult.
- Wear brace or collar per surgeon's prescription.

Chart 45-7 KEY FEATURES

Postoperative Complications of Cervical Diskectomy and Fusion

- Hoarseness due to laryngeal injury; may be temporary or permanent
- Temporary dysphagia; may last few days to several months; usually not severe
- Esophageal, tracheal, or vertebral artery injury
- Wound infection
- Injury to the spinal cord or nerve roots
- Dura mater tears with associated cerebrospinal fluid leaks
- Pseudoarthrosis caused by nonunion of fusion
- Graft and screw loosening if a fusion was performed

NCLEX EXAMINATION CHALLENGE

A client returns from the postanesthesia care unit (PACU) after having a cervical laminectomy and spinal fusion of C4 and C5. She states that she has a headache and feels nauseated. What is the nurse's first priority when caring for this client?

A. Check the dressing for signs of cerebrospinal fluid leak.
B. Establish an airway, and listen to breath sounds.
C. Give the client pain medication for her headache.
D. Place the client in a semi-Fowler's position immediately.

evolve **For the correct answer, go to http://evolve.elsevier.com/Iggy/.**

SPINAL CORD INJURY

Medical-surgical nurses do not usually care for a patient with an *acute* spinal cord injury (SCI). However, a patient may be admitted to a medical-surgical unit for complication of the injury or other medical conditions. Caring for a patient with a SCI requires a patient-centered collaborative approach and involves nearly every health care team member to help meet the patient's expected outcomes.

Despite increased awareness and newer treatments for SCI, the effects of spinal trauma cannot be reversed. However, research continues to find ways to decrease the devastating effects of paralysis. Recent work with stem cells from a variety of sources shows promise in improving motor functions (Divani et al., 2007). Other findings indicate that a combination approach of cell transplant, growth of new neurons, drug therapy, and surgery may be the key to restoring some if not all of the patient's lost motor and sensory function.

Pathophysiology

ANIMATION: Spinal Cord Structure

Loss of motor function *(mobility), sensation,* reflex activity, and bowel and bladder control often result from an SCI. In addition, the patient may experience significant behavior and emotional problems as a result of changes in body image, role performance, and self-concept.

The SCIs are classified as complete or incomplete. A **complete spinal cord injury** is one in which the spinal cord has been severed or damaged in a way that eliminates all innervation below the level of the injury. Injuries that allow some function or movement below the level of the injury are described as an **incomplete spinal cord injury.**

Mechanisms of Injury

When enough force is applied to the spinal cord, the resulting damage causes many neurologic deficits. Sources of force include direct injury to the vertebral column (fracture, dislocation, and subluxation [partial dislocation]) or penetrating trauma (gunshot or knife wounds). Although in some cases the cord itself may remain intact, at other times the cord undergoes a destructive process caused by a contusion (bruise) or compression.

The causes of SCI can be divided into primary and secondary mechanisms of injury. Four *primary* mechanisms may result in an SCI:

- Hyperflexion
- Hyperextension
- Axial loading, or vertical compression
- Excessive rotation

Penetrating injuries to the cord may also occur.

A **hyperflexion** injury occurs when the head is suddenly and forcefully accelerated (moved) forward, causing extreme flexion of the neck (Fig. 45-2). This type of injury often occurs in head-on vehicle collisions and diving accidents. Flexion injury to the lower thoracic and lumbar spine may occur when the trunk is suddenly flexed on itself, such as occurs in a fall on the buttocks. The posterior ligaments can be stretched or torn, or the vertebrae may fracture or dislocate. Either process may damage the spinal cord, causing hemorrhage, edema, and necrosis.

Hyperextension injuries occur most often in vehicle collisions in which the vehicle is struck from behind or during falls when the patient's chin is struck (Fig. 45-3). The head is suddenly accelerated and then decelerated. This stretches or tears the anterior longitudinal ligament, fractures or subluxates the vertebrae, and perhaps ruptures an intervertebral disk. As with flexion injuries, the spinal cord may easily be damaged.

Diving accidents, falls on the buttocks, or a jump in which a person lands on the feet can cause many of the injuries attribut-

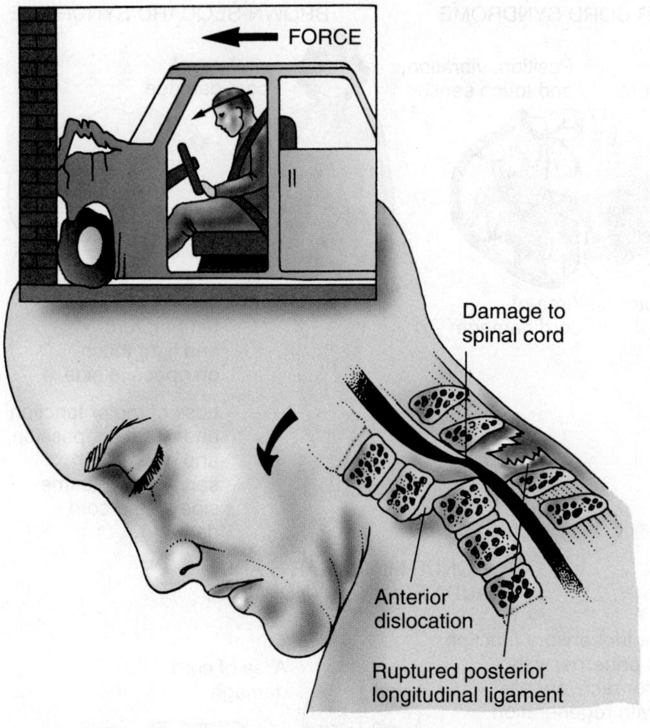
FORCE
Damage to spinal cord
Anterior dislocation
Ruptured posterior longitudinal ligament

Fig. 45-2 • Hyperflexion injury of the cervical spine.

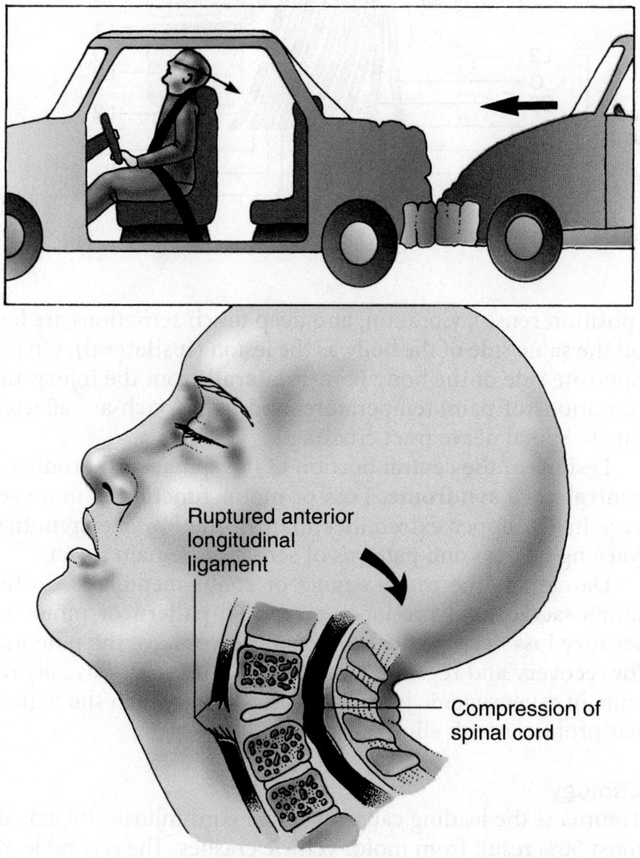
Ruptured anterior longitudinal ligament
Compression of spinal cord

Fig. 45-3 • Hyperextension injury of the cervical spine.

able to **axial loading** (vertical compression) (Fig. 45-4). A blow to the top of the head can cause the vertebrae to shatter. Pieces of bone enter the spinal canal and damage the cord. **Rotation** injuries are caused by turning the head beyond the normal range.

Penetrating injuries to the spinal cord are classified by the speed of the object (e.g., knife, bullet) causing the injury. Low-speed or low-impact injuries cause damage directly at the site or local damage to the spinal cord or spinal nerves. In contrast, high-speed injuries that occur from gunshot wounds cause both direct and indirect damage.

Secondary injury worsens the primary injury. Secondary injuries include:

- Hemorrhage
- Ischemia (lack of blood flow)
- Hypovolemia (decreased circulating blood volume)
- Neurogenic shock (a *medical emergency*)

The spinal cord may be contused, lacerated, or compressed by the injury. Petechial hemorrhage into the central gray matter and later into the white matter may result. Edema occurs when the cord is compressed by hemorrhage or bony fragments. Hemorrhage and loss of blood vessel tone (dilation) after *severe* cord injury may result in hypovolemia. In some patients, especially those with cervical spine injury, a type of hypovolemic shock called *neurogenic shock* may occur (McCance & Huether, 2006).

Extent of Injury

Incomplete SCIs are more common than complete lesions. A patient experiencing an incomplete lesion typically has a mixed pattern of partial motor, sensory, and reflex function. Specific syndromes result from incomplete lesions (Fig. 45-5). A "pure" syndrome may not be seen. *Cervical injuries* may produce:

- Anterior cord syndrome
- Posterior cord syndrome

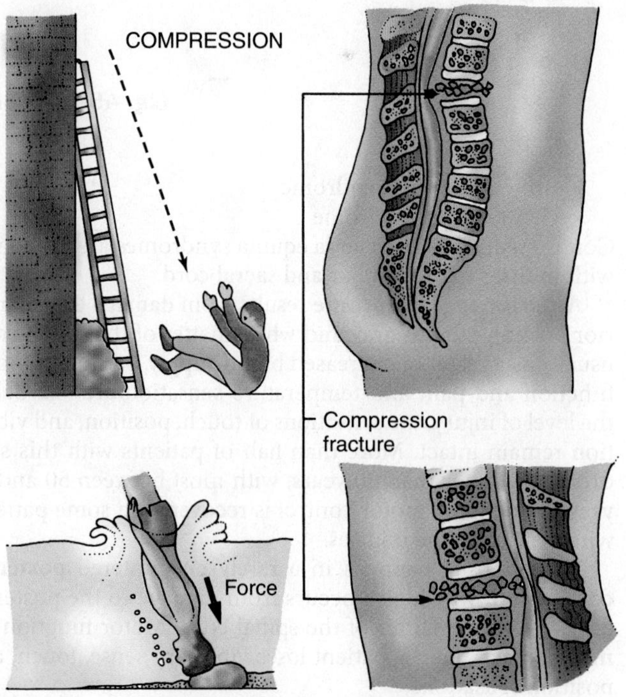
COMPRESSION
Compression fracture
Force

Fig. 45-4 • Axial loading (vertical compression) injury of the cervical spine and the lumbar spine.

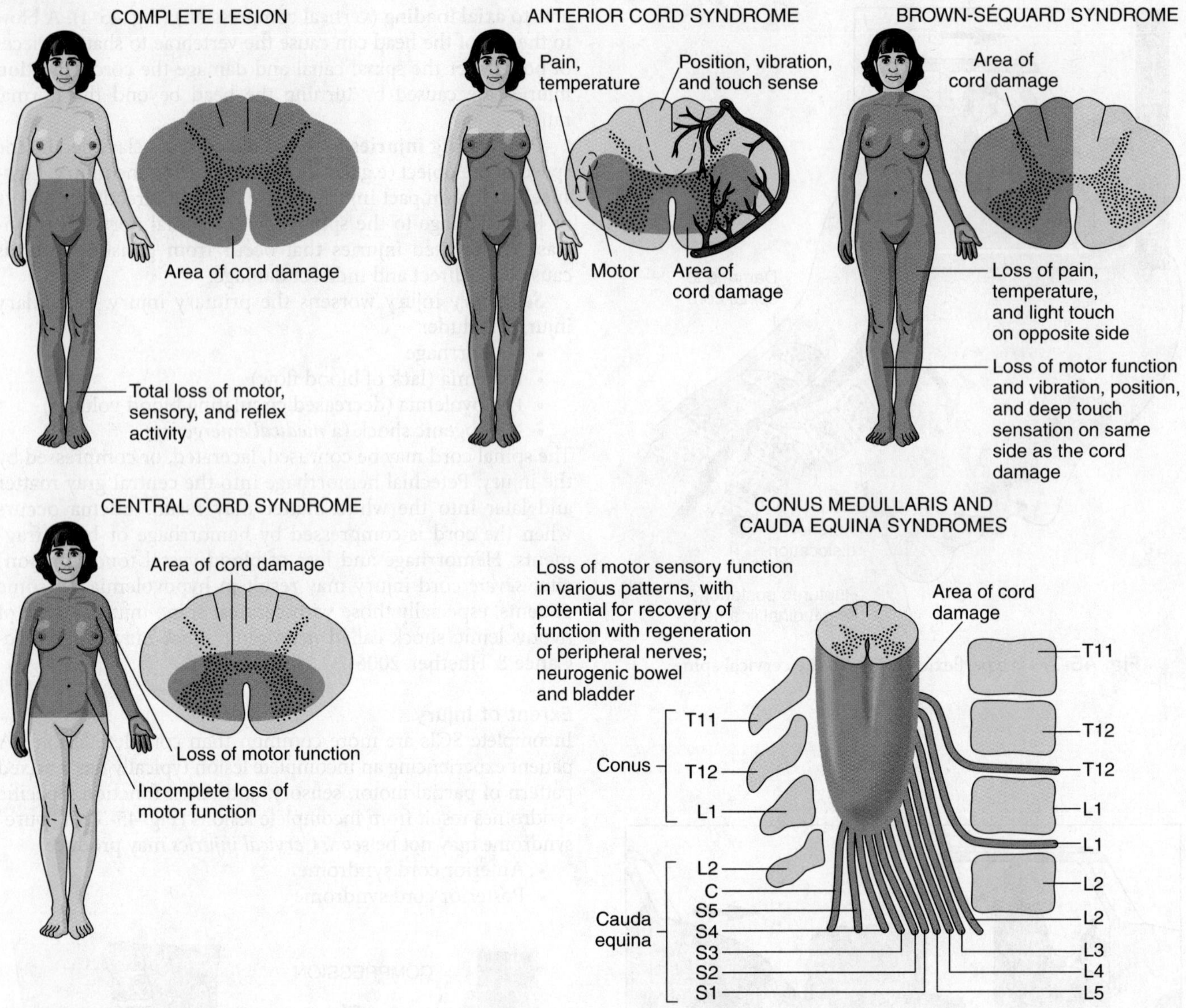
COMPLETE LESION
Area of cord damage
Total loss of motor, sensory, and reflex activity
ANTERIOR CORD SYNDROME
Pain, temperature
Position, vibration, and touch sense
Motor
Area of cord damage
BROWN-SÉQUARD SYNDROME
Area of cord damage
Loss of pain, temperature, and light touch on opposite side
Loss of motor function and vibration, position, and deep touch sensation on same side as the cord damage
CENTRAL CORD SYNDROME
Area of cord damage
Loss of motor function
Incomplete loss of motor function
CONUS MEDULLARIS AND CAUDA EQUINA SYNDROMES
Loss of motor sensory function in various patterns, with potential for recovery of function with regeneration of peripheral nerves; neurogenic bowel and bladder
Area of cord damage
Conus
T11
T12
L1
Cauda equina
L2
C
S5
S4
S3
S2
S1
T11
T12
T12
L1
L1
L2
L2
L3
L4
L5

Fig. 45-5 • Common spinal cord syndromes.

- Brown-Séquard syndrome
- Central cord syndrome

Conus medullaris and cauda equina syndromes are associated with injuries to the lumbar and sacral cord.

Anterior cord syndrome results from damage to the anterior portion of both gray and white matter of the spinal cord, usually as a result of decreased blood supply. Although motor function and pain and temperature sensation are lost below the level of injury, the sensations of touch, position, and vibration remain intact. More than half of patients with this syndrome are older than 40 years, with most between 50 and 70 years. Functional motor control is recovered in some patients with cervical spine injuries.

The opposite happens in a rarely encountered **posterior cord lesion,** which also occurs from damage to the posterior gray and white matter of the spinal cord. Motor function remains intact, but the patient loses vibratory sense, touch, and position sensation.

Brown-Séquard syndrome results from penetrating injuries that cause hemisection of the spinal cord or injuries that affect half of the spinal cord. Motor function, **proprioception** (position sense), vibration, and deep touch sensations are lost on the same side of the body as the lesion **(ipsilateral).** On the opposite side of the body **(contralateral)** from the injury, the sensations of pain, temperature, and light touch are affected due to spinal nerve tract crossing.

Lesions of the central portion of the spinal cord produce a **central cord syndrome.** Loss of motor function is more severe in the upper extremities than in the lower extremities. Varying degrees and patterns of sensation remain intact.

Damage to the *cauda equina* or conus medullaris (in the lumbosacral area) produces a variable pattern of motor or sensory loss because the peripheral nerves have the potential for recovery and regrowth. In addition, this injury usually results in a neurogenic bowel and bladder in which the patient has problems with elimination.

Etiology

Trauma is the leading cause of spinal cord injuries (SCIs); almost 50% result from motor vehicle crashes. The second leading cause is falls, followed by acts of violence and sports/recreation accidents (Fisher, 2007). Falls are particularly likely among older adults. Spinal cord damage in adults can also result from diseases such as tumors.

Incidence/Prevalence

Between 250,000 and 400,000 people in the United States have SCIs, and about 14,000 new injuries occur each year. The patient may be hospitalized for 3 months or longer, including acute care and rehabilitation. Life expectancy has increased, but it is still below that of people without an SCI. Patients usually die from complications of immobility or infection.

The mean age at time of injury is the late 30s. Peak incidence of injury occurs in the summer or warmer months. Men make up most of the SCI patients, and most are white. Cervical cord injuries are more common than thoracic or lumbosacral ones.

Patient-Centered Collaborative Care

evolve ONLINE PHARM REVIEW

Assessment

History

When obtaining a history from a patient with an SCI, gather as much data as possible about how the accident occurred and the probable mechanism of injury. Questions include the location and position of the patient immediately after the injury, the symptoms that occurred after the injury, and the changes that have occurred since the initial signs and symptoms. If possible, ask prehospital rescue personnel about the type of immobilization devices used and whether any problems occurred during stabilization and transport to the hospital. Review the chart regarding the medical treatment given at the scene of injury or in the emergency department (ED) (e.g., drugs, IV fluids). Communicate with the ED nurse as he or she "hands off" the patient. Use the situation, background, assessment, recommendation (SBAR) communication technique to collect valuable information for continuing patient care. (See Chapter 1 for how to use SBAR.)

Obtain the patient's medical history, including a history of arthritis of the spine, congenital deformities, osteoporosis or osteomyelitis, cancer, and previous injury or surgery of the neck or back. These health problems may cause or contribute to an SCI. A detailed history of any respiratory problems is particularly important if the patient has experienced a cervical SCI.

Physical Assessment/Clinical Manifestations

Initial Assessment. Assessing the ABCs (airway, breathing, circulation) is the priority for any trauma patient. *Therefore the first priority for the patient with an SCI is to assess the patient's airway, breathing pattern, and circulation status.* The airway may be compromised because of foreign body obstruction from the tongue or teeth due to facial trauma, injury to the larynx, or mandibular (jaw) fracture (Harris & Sethi, 2006). After an airway is established, assess the patient's breathing pattern. The patient with a cervical SCI is at high risk for respiratory compromise because the cervical spinal nerves (C3-5) innervate the phrenic nerve, which controls the diaphragm. A significant head injury, pneumothorax (air in the chest cavity), hemothorax (blood in the chest cavity), and/or fractured ribs may also cause respiratory distress. Injuries to the occiput (back of the head) and C2 are more likely to occur in the older adult who fell from a low height. Endotracheal intubation with mechanical ventilation may be necessary to prevent respiratory arrest.

Assess for indications of intra-abdominal *hemorrhage* or hemorrhage or bleeding around fracture sites. Indicators of hemorrhage include hypotension and tachycardia with a weak and thready pulse.

Use the Glasgow Coma Scale (see Chapter 43) or other agency-approved assessment tool to assess the patient's *level of consciousness (LOC)*. Cognitive impairment as a result of an associated traumatic brain injury (TBI) or substance abuse is common in patients with traumatic SCIs. Perform a detailed assessment of the patient's motor and sensory status to assist in determining the level of injury and serve as baseline data for future comparison. The level of injury is the lowest neurologic segment with intact or normal motor and sensory function. **Tetraplegia** (also called *quadriplegia*) (paralysis) and **quadriparesis** (weakness) involve all four extremities, as seen with cervical cord and upper thoracic injury. **Paraplegia** (paralysis) and **paraparesis** (weakness) involve only the lower extremities, as seen in lower thoracic and lumbosacral injuries or lesions.

Spinal shock, also called **spinal shock syndrome,** occurs immediately as a concussion response to the injury. The patient has flaccid paralysis and loss of reflex activity below the level of the lesion. It often lasts less than 48 hours but may continue for several weeks (McCance & Huether, 2006). Muscle spasticity begins in patients with cervical or high thoracic injuries when spinal shock is resolved.

Assessment of Sensory and Motor Ability. *Sensation* is carried from the peripheral nerves to the spinal cord and up to the cerebral cortex through several specific tracts. Injury to the spinal cord may prevent those impulses from reaching the brain. To test sensory abilities, ask the patient to close his or her eyes. Touch the skin with a clean safety pin or cotton-tipped applicator, and ask whether he or she can feel the pinprick or light touch. Compare bilateral responses. Follow the sensory distribution of the skin dermatomes (see Fig. 43-5 in Chapter 43), with the examination beginning in the area of reported loss of sensation and ending where sensation becomes normal. For example, sensation of the top of the foot and calf of the leg is spinal skin segment (dermatome) levels L3, L4, and L5. The area at the level of the umbilicus is T10, the clavicle (collarbone) is C3 or C4, and finger sensation is C7 and C8. The patient may report a complete sensory loss, **hypoesthesia** (decreased sensation), or **hyperesthesia** (increased sensation).

The patient's proprioceptive (position sense) function may be assessed. Request that the patient again close his or her eyes. Next move one of his or her fingers or toes up or down. Ask the patient to identify the position of the digits.

In addition to performing a routine motor evaluation of the patient, selected muscles are tested in a more systematic fashion (Chart 45-8). Many scales are available to measure motor function. The American Spinal Injury Association (ASIA) recommends a five-point grading scale, with 0 being no movement and 5 being normal strength (see Table 52-2 in Chapter 52). Ask the patient to flex and extend the elbows, elevate both arms off the bed, flex and extend the wrists and fingers, and touch each finger to the thumb. Patients with spinal injuries at the fifth or sixth cervical vertebra often can flex but not extend their arms. Observe the patient's ability to move the lower extremities. Ask him or her to wiggle the toes, flex and extend the feet and knees, and move one or both hips.

The advanced practice nurse or health care provider may also test deep tendon reflexes (DTRs), including the biceps (C5), triceps (C7), patella (L3), and ankle (S1). It is not unusual for these reflexes, as well as all movement or sensation, to be absent immediately after the injury because of spinal

Chart 45-8 **BEST PRACTICE FOR PATIENT SAFETY & QUALITY CARE**

Assessing Motor Function in the Patient with a Spinal Cord Injury

- To assess C4-5, apply downward pressure while the patient shrugs his or her shoulders upward.
- To assess C5-6, apply resistance while the patient pulls up his or her arms.
- To assess C7, apply resistance while the patient straightens his or her flexed arms.
- To assess C8, make sure the patient is able to grasp an object and form a fist.
- To assess L2-4, apply resistance while the patient lifts his or her legs from the bed.
- To assess L5, apply resistance while the patient dorsiflexes his or her feet.
- To assess S1, apply resistance while the patient plantar flexes his or her feet.

shock. After shock has resolved, the reflexes may return if the lesion is incomplete or involves upper motor neurons.

Cardiovascular and Respiratory Assessment. *Cardiovascular* dysfunction results from disruption of sympathetic fibers of the autonomic nervous system (ANS), especially if the injury is above the sixth thoracic vertebra. Bradycardia, hypotension, and hypothermia occur because of loss of sympathetic input. These changes may lead to cardiac dysrhythmias. *A systolic blood pressure below 90 mm Hg requires treatment because lack of perfusion to the spinal cord could worsen the patient's condition.* In addition, the lack of sympathetic or hypothalamic control causes the patient to lose thermoregulatory functions. As a result, the body tends to assume the temperature of the environment and attempts to compensate by increasing extracellular fluid.

A patient with a cervical SCI is at risk for *respiratory* problems resulting from immobility or from an interruption of spinal innervation to the respiratory muscles. In collaboration with the respiratory therapist (RT), if available, perform a complete respiratory assessment, including pulse oximetry for arterial oxygen saturation. The RT should also evaluate vital capacity and minute volume as part of the assessment. These tests are repeated as the patient's clinical status requires.

Gastrointestinal and Genitourinary Assessment. Assess the patient's *abdomen* for manifestations of internal bleeding, distention, or paralytic ileus. Hemorrhage may result from the trauma, or it may occur later from a stress ulcer or the administration of steroids. Monitor for abdominal pain and changes in bowel sounds. Paralytic ileus may develop within 72 hours of hospital admission. During the period of spinal shock, peristalsis decreases, leading to a loss of bowel sounds and gastric distention. This lack of or interference with autonomic innervation may lead to a reflex or hypotonic bowel.

Autonomic dysfunction initially causes an areflexic (neurogenic) bladder (no reflex ability for bladder contraction), which later leads to urinary retention. The patient is at risk for urinary tract infection from an indwelling urinary catheter; intermittent catheterizations; or bladder distention, stasis, and/or overflow.

Other Assessment. Assess the patient's muscle tone and size. Muscle wasting results from the long-term flaccid paralysis seen in patients with **lower motor neuron (LMN)** lesions (usually lower thoracic or lumbosacral injuries). Incomplete lesions or **upper motor neuron** (UMN) lesions (usually cervical and upper thoracic injuries) cause muscle spasticity, which can lead to contractures after spinal shock has resolved.

Observe the condition of the patient's skin, especially over pressure points, at least twice daily. Assess any reddened area carefully and monitor it daily for change. A pressure-reducing mattress or special bed is used to prevent skin breakdown.

Another complication of prolonged immobility is **heterotopic ossification** (bony overgrowth, often into muscle). Assess for swelling, redness, warmth, and decreased range of motion (ROM) of the involved extremity. Changes in the bony structure are not visible until several weeks after initial symptoms appear.

Psychosocial Assessment

If possible, obtain information about the patient's pre-injury psychosocial status and usual methods of coping with illness, difficult situations, and disappointments. Determine the patient's level of independence or dependence and his or her comfort level in discussing feelings and emotions with family members or close friends. Patients who are emotionally secure and have a positive self-image, supportive family, and financial and job security often adapt best to their injury. Information about the patient's spiritual and religious beliefs or cultural background also assists the nurse in developing the plan of care. The patient with an SCI must cope with changes in body image, self-esteem, independence, role relationships, and sexuality.

In addition, assess family members or significant others to determine how well they are coping with the patient's injury and their role changes. The patient and family must be prepared for extensive rehabilitation and changes in lifestyle. Financial constraints and the possibility of long-term care of the patient may cause additional stress.

Laboratory Assessment

The health care provider requests routine laboratory studies for the patient with an SCI to establish baseline data or to prepare for surgery. A urinalysis is used to check for the presence of blood in the urine after trauma. End tidal carbon dioxide levels or arterial blood gas analysis is done to monitor the respiratory status of a patient at risk for respiratory insufficiency. The findings should be within normal limits unless the patient has a history of heavy smoking or pre-injury pulmonary disease or has respiratory failure. Failure is indicated by decreased oxygen levels, increased carbon dioxide levels, and respiratory acidosis.

Check laboratory values for low hemoglobin count, leukocytosis (increased white blood cells [WBCs]), lymphocytopenia (decreased lymphocytes), and thrombocytopenia (decreased platelets), which can occur in patients with cervical spine injuries. These abnormalities may be related to lack of autonomic innervation to the hematopoietic system (Furlan et al., 2006). Observe patients for clinical signs and symptoms of these changes, such as increased bleeding tendency.

Imaging Assessment

If available, spiral computed tomography (CT) or multi-slice CT should be obtained as soon as possible, especially for the patient who has sustained multiple trauma. Otherwise, CT or magnetic resonance imaging (MRI) is performed to determine the degree and extent of damage to the spinal cord and to detect the presence of blood and bone within the spinal column. The health care provider requests a complete x-ray series of the spine to identify vertebral fractures, subluxation, or dislocation.

Analysis

Common Nursing Diagnoses and Collaborative Problems

The most common nursing diagnoses for patients with a spinal cord injury (SCI) are:

- Ineffective Tissue Perfusion (Spinal Cord) related to interruption of arterial flow
- Ineffective Airway Clearance, Ineffective Breathing Pattern, and Impaired Gas Exchange related to spinal cord injury
- Impaired Physical Mobility and/or Self-Care Deficit (the level depends on the extent and level of the injury) related to decreased or absent muscle control
- Impaired Urinary Elimination and/or Constipation related to sensory/motor impairment
- Impaired Adjustment related to disability or health status change requiring change in lifestyle

Additional Nursing Diagnoses and Collaborative Problems

In addition to the common nursing diagnoses, patients with an SCI may have one or more of these problems:

- Risk for Impaired Skin Integrity related to physical immobilization
- Acute Pain related to physical injury
- Risk for Injury related to altered mobility
- Imbalanced Nutrition: Less Than Body Requirements related to hypermetabolism or inability to absorb nutrients
- Sexual Dysfunction related to altered body function

Collaborative problems include:

- Potential for Deep Vein Thrombosis (DVT)
- Potential for Sepsis
- Potential for Neurogenic Shock
- Potential for Atelectasis, Pneumonia

Planning and Implementation

The desired outcome of treatment is to stabilize the vertebral column as needed, manage damage to the spinal cord, and prevent secondary effects of injury.

Ineffective Tissue Perfusion (Spinal Cord)

Planning: Expected Outcomes. The patient with an SCI is expected to demonstrate adequate spinal cord tissue perfusion as evidenced by no further deterioration in neurologic status.

Interventions. If the patient has a fractured vertebra, the primary concern of the health care team is to reduce and immobilize the fracture to prevent further damage to the spinal cord from bone fragments. Nonsurgical techniques include traction, external fixation, or braces, but surgery may be necessary to stabilize the spine and prevent further spinal cord damage.

Nonsurgical Management. Assess the patient's neurologic status, vital signs, pulse oximetry, and pain score at least every 4 hours. *Document your assessments carefully and in detail, particularly changes in motor or sensory function in the extremities. Failure to do so may prevent other staff members from quickly recognizing deterioration in neurologic status.*

Observe for manifestations of *neurogenic shock,* which may occur within 24 hours after injury, most commonly in patients with injuries above T6. This potentially life-threatening problem results from disruption in the communication pathways between upper motor neurons and lower motor neurons. **Neurogenic shock** is a type of hypovolemic shock causing:

- Severe bradycardia
- Warm, dry skin
- Severe hypotension

Notify the physician immediately if these symptoms occur, because this problem is an emergency! Neurogenic shock is treated symptomatically by restoring fluids to the circulating blood volume.

NIC **Positioning: neurologic.** Regardless of the level of SCI, keep the patient in proper body alignment to prevent further cord injury or irritability (Chart 45-9). Devices such as traction, orthoses, or collars may be used to keep the spine immobilized during healing and rehabilitation.

Immobilization for cervical injuries. The patient may be placed in fixed skeletal traction to realign the vertebrae, facilitate bone healing, and prevent further injury, often after surgi-

Chart 45-9 NIC INTERVENTION ACTIVITIES

The Patient with a Spinal Cord Injury

Airway Management: *Facilitation of patency of air passages.*

- Position patient to maximize ventilation potential.
- Identify patient requiring actual/potential airway insertion.
- Insert oral or nasopharyngeal airway, as appropriate.
- Perform chest physical therapy, as appropriate.
- Remove secretions by encouraging coughing or by suctioning.
- Encourage slow, deep breathing; turning; and coughing.
- Instruct how to cough effectively.
- Assist with incentive spirometer, as appropriate.
- Auscultate breath sounds, noting areas of decreased or absent ventilation and presence of adventitious sounds.
- Perform endotracheal or nasotracheal suctioning, as appropriate.
- Administer humidified air or oxygen, as appropriate.
- Regulate fluid intake to optimize fluid balance.
- Position to alleviate dyspnea.
- Monitor respiratory and oxygenation status, as appropriate.

Positioning: Neurologic: *Achievement of optimal, appropriate body alignment for the patient experiencing or at risk for spinal cord injury or vertebral irritability.*

- Immobilize or support the affected body part, as appropriate.
- Place in the designated therapeutic position.
- Maintain proper body alignment.
- Position with head and neck in alignment.
- Turn using the log roll technique.
- Apply an orthosis collar.
- Instruct on orthosis collar care, as needed.
- Apply and maintain a splinting or bracing device.
- Monitor skin integrity under bracing device/orthosis collar.
- Instruct on pin site care, as needed.
- Monitor traction pin insertion site.
- Perform traction/orthosis device pin insertion site care.
- Monitor traction device setup.

NIC intervention activities selected from Bulechek, G.M., Butcher, H.K., & McCloskey Dochterman, J. (Eds.). (2008). *Nursing interventions classification (NIC)* (5th ed.). St. Louis: Mosby. No part of this work is to be altered without prior written permission from the Publisher.

cal stabilization. The most commonly used device for immobilization of the cervical spine is the halo fixation device. Cervical tongs (e.g., Gardner-Wells, Crutchfield) are used less often today. Either device is inserted by the physician into the outer aspect of the skull. For patients not having surgery, the addition of traction helps reduce the fracture.

The halo fixator is a static traction device (Fig. 45-6). Four pins (or screws) are inserted into the skull. The metal halo ring may be attached to a plastic vest or cast when the spine is stable, allowing increased patient mobility. *Never move or turn the patient by holding or pulling on the halo device. Do not adjust the screws holding it in place. Check the patient's skin frequently to ensure that the jacket is not causing pressure. Pressure is avoided if one finger can be inserted easily between the jacket and the patient's skin.*

Monitor the patient's neurologic status for changes in movement or decreased strength. If skeletal traction is used, maintain the patient in alignment. Ensure that the ropes for the traction remain within the pulley and hang freely.

Common complications of the halo device are pin loosening, local infection, and scarring. More serious complications include osteomyelitis (cranial bone infection), subdural abscess, and instability. Monitor the insertion sites of the halo device or tongs for signs of infection. Hospital policy is followed for pin site care, which may specify the use of solutions such as hydrogen peroxide and saline. Xeroform dressings may also be used. *Monitor vital signs for indications of possible infections, such as osteomyelitis, and report any changes to the physician immediately.*

Immobilization for thoracic and lumbar/sacral injuries. Nonsurgical treatment of an upper thoracic injury is often challenging. Most surgeons choose to stabilize the spine by surgery (open reduction, internal fixation [ORIF]) and then place the patient in a halo fixation device. Prolonged bedrest is seldom recommended. For lower thoracic, lumbar, and sacral injuries, immobilization of the spine is typically accomplished with a brace worn when the patient is out of bed. Lightweight, custom-fit thoracic lumbar sacral orthoses (TLSOs) are preferred to prevent prolonged periods of immobility.

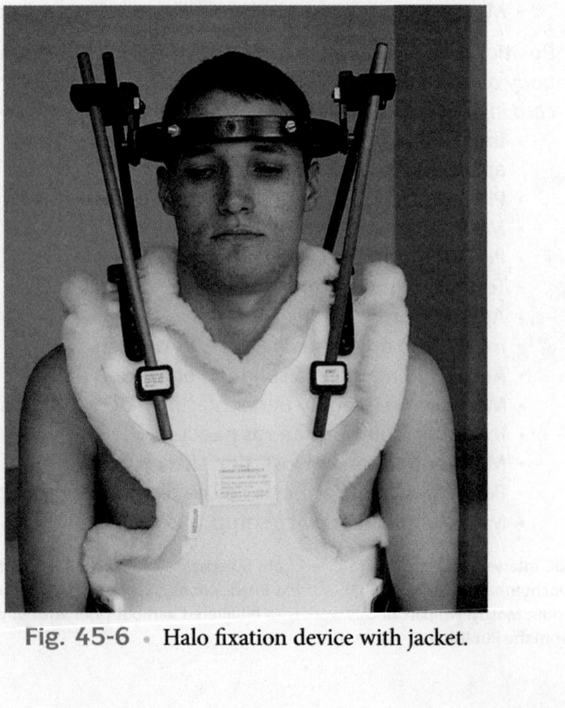

Fig. 45-6 • Halo fixation device with jacket.

DECISION-MAKING CHALLENGE
Coordination of Care

A 21-year-old patient is admitted to the ED with a possible thoracic spinal injury as a result of a motor vehicle crash. He and his friends were drag racing on the interstate when he hit a car on the side of the road and flipped his car. He is very angry, crying, and in severe pain. When you enter the treatment room, you find his girlfriend screaming at him for being "so stupid" and crying hysterically. His mother and father are on the way from another state to be with him and are expected to arrive in about 3 hours.

1. What should you do when you enter the room to assess this patient?
2. What members of the health care team could you call to help in this situation and why?
3. During your assessment, what is your priority and why?
4. When the parents arrive several hours later, they demand to see the physician, who is busy with another patient. How would you respond to them when you are also very busy with several patients? Who might you contact to help you in this situation?

evolve For suggested answer guidelines, go to http://evolve.elsevier.com/Iggy/.

Drug therapy. *Methylprednisolone (Solu-Medrol)* may be prescribed depending on physician preference and the condition of the patient. This drug decreases inflammation, such as that caused by injury to spinal cord and nerve tissue. Monitor the patient receiving IV methylprednisolone closely for adverse drug events, including infection, elevated serum glucose, and stress ulcers. *Dextran,* a plasma expander, may be used to increase capillary blood flow within the spinal cord and to prevent or treat hypotension. *Atropine sulfate* is used to treat bradycardia if the pulse rate falls below 50 to 60 beats per minute. Hypotension, if severe, is treated with inotropic and sympathomimetic agents such as dopamine hydrochloride (Intropin) and isoproterenol.

Centrally acting skeletal muscular relaxants, such as tizanidine (Zanaflex, Sirdalud), may help control severe muscle spasticity (usually upper motor neuron [UMN] injuries). However, these drugs cause severe drowsiness and sedation in most patients and may not be effective in reducing spasticity. As an alternative to these drugs, *intrathecal baclofen (Lioresal) (ITB)* therapy may be prescribed. This drug is administered through a programmable, implantable infusion pump and intrathecal catheter directly into the cerebrospinal fluid. The pump is surgically placed in a subcutaneous pouch in the lower abdomen. Common adverse effects include sedation, fatigue, dizziness, and changes in mental status. *Seizures and hallucinations may occur if ITB is suddenly withdrawn.*

Other drugs to prevent or treat complications of immobility may be needed *later* during the rehabilitative phase. For example, celecoxib (Celebrex) may be prescribed to prevent or treat **heterotopic ossification** (bony overgrowth). Early and continued exercise may decrease the incidence of this complication. Chapter 8 discusses complications of immobility and drug therapy in more detail.

Surgical Management. Emergency surgery may be indicated if there is evidence of spinal cord compression. The procedure is usually necessary to remove bone fragments, hematomas, or penetrating objects such as a bullet. A **decom-**

pressive laminectomy (removal of one or more laminae) allows for cord expansion from edema if more conventional measures fail to prevent neurologic deterioration.

Additional surgical procedures to stabilize and support the spine may be performed at the discretion of the surgeon, depending on the patient's condition and the extent of the injury. Typical procedures include a spinal fusion and the insertion of metal or steel rods, such as Harrington rods, to stabilize thoracic spinal injuries. After surgery, the patient usually wears a brace, a corset, or a TLSO to keep the operative area immobilized during recovery.

After surgery, assess the patient's neurologic status and vital signs at least every hour for the first 4 to 6 hours after surgery and then, if the patient is stable, every 4 hours. Assess for complications of surgery, such as hematoma and edema. Look for swelling under the skin.

The patient is also at risk for cardiovascular instability because of a loss of sympathetic innervation. In some cases, the patient may require a pacemaker. Log roll the patient when he or she is being moved to maintain skeletal alignment, or place on a special bed such as a kinetic treatment table. Monitor the patient's cardiovascular status carefully, especially with position changes. A complete discussion of general postoperative nursing care is found in Chapter 18.

Ineffective Airway Clearance; Ineffective Breathing Pattern; Impaired Gas Exchange

NOC **Planning: Expected Outcomes.** The patient with an SCI is expected to have airway patency, alveolar exchange to maintain blood gas concentrations, and adequate ventilation. Indicators include:

- Ease of breathing
- Normal respiratory rate and rhythm
- End tidal carbon dioxide levels within normal limits
- Oxygen saturation of 95% or greater
- No adventitious breath sounds

Interventions. *Airway management is the priority for a patient with cervical spinal cord injury!* Patients with injuries at or above T6 are especially at risk for respiratory complications and pulmonary embolus during the first 5 days after injury (Berlly & Shem, 2007). These complications are due to impaired functioning of the intercostal muscles and decreased mobility. Depending on the level of injury, intubation or tracheotomy with mechanical ventilation may be needed. *Closely monitor the patient for clinical manifestations of life-threatening respiratory complications, such as pneumonia, pulmonary emboli, and atelectasis. These problems decrease the life expectancy of SCI patients and have replaced renal failure as the leading cause of death.* Assess breath sounds every 4 hours during the first few days after injury, and document and report any adventitious or diminished sounds. Monitor vital signs carefully, and watch for changes in respiratory pattern.

Teach the patient who is tetraplegic to cough by placing his or her hands on either side of the rib cage or upper abdomen below the diaphragm. This technique is sometimes called "assisted coughing," "quad cough," or **"cough assist."** As the patient inhales, push upward to help expand the lungs and cough.

Encourage the patient to use an incentive spirometer. The nurse or respiratory therapist performs a respiratory assessment every 8 hours to determine the effectiveness of these strategies. In some cases it may be necessary to perform oral or nasal suctioning if the patient cannot clear the airway of secretions effectively.

Impaired Physical Mobility; Self-Care Deficit

NOC **Planning: Expected Outcomes.** The patient with an SCI is expected to be free from complications of immobility and perform the most basic physical tasks and personal care activities as independently as possible with or without assistive/adaptive devices. Indicators include that the patient will have no complications of immobility, such as:

- Pressure ulcers
- Deep vein thrombosis
- Contracted joints
- Osteoporotic bone fracture
- Orthostatic (postural) hypotension

Additional indicators include that the patient will be able to perform these activities:

- Transfer from bed to chair (using a lift or sliding board method)
- Have bed and wheelchair mobility
- Eat and drink
- Dress completely
- Bathe and groom
- Provide oral hygiene

Interventions. The patient with an SCI is especially at risk for pressure ulcers, contractures, and deep vein thrombosis (DVT) or pulmonary emboli. Proper positioning not only helps prevent complications but also provides alignment to prevent further spinal cord injury or irritability.

When sitting in a chair, the patient is repositioned or taught to reposition himself or herself more often than every hour. In that position, most of the weight is placed on one area—the ischial tuberosities. *Special pressure-relief devices, such as gel pads, may be used in the wheelchair or the bed, but these do not eliminate the need for regular turning and repositioning.* Chapter 8 discusses in detail the prevention of complications associated with immobility.

Patients with cervical cord injuries are especially at high risk for orthostatic (postural) hypotension, but anyone who is immobilized may have this problem. If the patient changes from a lying position to a sitting or standing position too quickly, he or she may experience hypotension, which could result in dizziness and falls. Because of interrupted sympathetic innervation, the blood vessels do not constrict quickly enough to push blood up into the brain. This causes dizziness or light-headedness and possible falls with syncope ("blackout").

The most important part of promoting self-management is setting realistic expected outcomes on the basis of the patient's potential mobility and functional level. Even patients with a cervical SCI often learn how to perform most ADLs independently in specialized rehabilitation programs. See Chapter 8 for a detailed discussion of interventions to promote mobility and ADLs.

Impaired Urinary Elimination and/or Constipation

NOC **Planning: Expected Outcomes.** The patient with an SCI is expected to achieve control of elimination of urine and stool. Indicators include that the patient will:

- Have a predictable pattern of voiding
- Void more than 150 mL each time
- Empty the bladder completely
- Manage clothing

- Have no urinary incontinence or use leg bag
- Have no urinary infection
- Have control of bowel movements
- Experience ease of stool passage

Interventions. Patients with SCIs have reflex or neurogenic loss of bowel and bladder control. Many can become continent if they rigorously adhere to an established program. The type of program depends on the usual elimination pattern and whether the injury involved upper motor neurons (UMNs) or lower motor neurons (LMNs). A urologic evaluation may be needed to identify bladder type.

Patients with injuries to the lumbosacral area usually have an LMN (flaccid) bladder and bowel. Patients with **flaccid bladders** may achieve emptying of the bladder by performing a Valsalva maneuver or tightening the abdominal muscles. These techniques are not successful for all LMN injuries. To determine the effectiveness of these maneuvers, use a bedside **bladder ultrasound** device to measure bladder residual. This device is discussed in Chapter 69.

Some patients rely solely on intermittent catheterization two or three times daily to empty the bladder. Obese patients and those with very-high-level SCIs may need an indwelling urinary catheter for a period of time. External urinary catheters connected to a leg bag may be used for men.

The patient with any SCI is at risk for long-term renal complications, such as hydronephrosis, renal failure, and kidney stones. Urinary tract infections (UTIs) are common because organisms are introduced into the urinary tract by urinary catheters. Patients with an SCI may not be aware of the infection because they cannot feel dysuria, urgency, or back pain. They must rely on other signs and symptoms, such as foul-smelling urine or fever.

The essential elements of a bowel program include stool softeners, increased fluid intake (unless medically contraindicated), high-fiber diet, and a consistent time for elimination. Rectal digital stimulation is done only if requested by the health care provider because it could cause a vagal response, manifested by severe bradycardia and syncope.

Emergency Care. Observe the patient with an upper SCI (above the level of T6) for signs of autonomic dysreflexia (hyperreflexia). Although it does not occur frequently, **autonomic dysreflexia** is an excessive, uncontrolled sympathetic output. It is characterized by severe hypertension, bradycardia, severe headache, nasal stuffiness, and flushing (Chart 45-10). The cause of this syndrome is a noxious stimulus—usually a distended bladder or constipation. *This is a neurologic emergency and must be promptly treated to prevent a hypertensive stroke!* Chart 45-11 lists emergency care for autonomic dysreflexia.

Chart 45-10 KEY FEATURES

Autonomic Dysreflexia

- Sudden onset of severe, throbbing headache
- Severe, rapidly occurring hypertension
- Bradycardia
- Flushing above level of lesion (face and chest)
- Pale extremities below level of lesion
- Nasal stuffiness
- Sweating
- Nausea
- Blurred vision
- Piloerection
- Feeling of apprehension

Impaired Adjustment

NOC **Planning: Expected Outcomes.** The patient with an SCI is expected to develop an adaptive psychosocial response to a significant life change. Indicators include that the patient will demonstrate:

- Setting realistic goals
- Maintaining self-esteem
- Reporting feeling useful
- Verbalizing optimism about the present and future
- Identifying effective coping strategies

Interventions. Information obtained from the psychosocial assessment is used by the interdisciplinary team to identify strategies to help the patient adjust to the disability. Invite the patient to ask questions, and answer them openly and honestly. Questions about prognosis and potential for complete recovery are referred to the health care provider because the timing and extent of recovery are different for each patient.

Collaborate with the case manager or discharge planner for a review of the patient's insurance and financial status. Many insurance policies do not cover extended rehabilitation services. Therefore other sources, including private foundations and donations, may be needed.

Community-Based Care

Case managers are ideal care coordinators to act as SCI patient advocates. In some settings, case managers begin working with patients in the emergency department to establish a positive image of SCI rehabilitation. Rehabilitation begins in the critical care unit when patients are hemodynamically stable and spinal shock has subsided. They are usually transferred from the acute care setting to a rehabilitation setting, where they learn more about self-care, mobility skills, and bladder and bowel retraining. The length of stay in the rehabilitation hospital or unit is typically 1 to 2 months, depending on the medical complications that may occur, such as infections.

Psychosocial adaptation is one of the critical factors in determining the success of rehabilitation. The case manager or

Chart 45-11 BEST PRACTICE FOR PATIENT SAFETY & QUALITY CARE

Emergency Care of the Patient Experiencing Autonomic Dysreflexia: Immediate Interventions

EMERGENCY CARE

- Place patient in sitting position (first priority!).
- Page/notify health care provider.
- Loosen tight clothing on the patient.
- Assess for and treat the cause.
- Check the urinary catheter tubing (if present) for kinks or obstruction.
- If a urinary catheter is not present, check for bladder distention and catheterize immediately if indicated.
- Place anesthetic ointment on tip of catheter before insertion.
- Check the patient for fecal impaction; if present, disimpact immediately using anesthetic ointment.
- Check the room temperature to ensure that it is not too cool or drafty.
- Monitor blood pressures every 10 to 15 minutes.
- Give nitrates or hydralazine (Apresoline, Novo-Hylazin🍁) as prescribed.

acute care nurse can help the patient prepare for discharge or transfer to a rehabilitation hospital. Assist in verbalizing feelings and fears about body image, self-concept, role performance, self-esteem, and sexuality. The patient should be told about the expected reactions of those outside the security of the hospital environment. Role-playing or anticipating responses to potential problems is helpful. For example, the patient can practice answering questions from children about why he or she is in a wheelchair or cannot move certain parts of the body.

Many patients are concerned about their ability to have sexual intercourse and have children. Most hospitals do not have psychological social workers or counselors to discuss sexuality issues. Rehabilitation programs often include a sexuality/intimacy counselor as part of the interdisciplinary team approach to patient care.

NCLEX EXAMINATION CHALLENGE

A client had a cervical spinal fusion and halo fixation device with jacket placed 2 days ago. He reports to you that he has a severe headache, and he has perspiration on his forehead. His face is flushed, and he reports nausea. What is the nurse's first action in caring for this client?

A. Provide an emesis basin in case he vomits.
B. Report his symptoms to the physician.
C. Check his bladder for distention
D. Raise the head of his bed now.

evolve For the correct answer, go to http://evolve.elsevier.com/Iggy/.

Home Care Management

If the patient is discharged home or returns home for a weekend visit from the rehabilitation setting, the environment must be assessed to ensure that it is free from hazards and can accommodate the patient's special needs (e.g., a wheelchair). The occupational or physical therapist, in collaboration with rehabilitation and the home care nurse, usually assesses the patient's temporary or permanent home environment. Ease of accessibility is particularly important at the entrance of the home as well as the bathroom, kitchen, and bedroom. The height of the patient's bed may need to be adjusted to allow a smooth transfer into or out of the bed.

All adaptive devices that the patient will use at home should be requested and delivered to the rehabilitation facility. This enables the nurse and other therapists to ensure that the items fit correctly and that the patient and family know how to use them correctly.

Health Teaching

The teaching plan for the patient with an SCI includes:

- Mobility skills (including skin care)
- ADLs skills
- Bowel and bladder retraining program
- Drug therapy
- Sexuality education

This information should be reinforced with written handouts, CDs, DVDs, or other patient education material that the patient and family members can use after discharge to the home. Chart 45-12 provides information about aging for middle-aged and older adults with a spinal cord injury.

Mobility and Activities of Daily Living. It is essential that the patient learn mobility skills so that he or she can move on sidewalks, carpeting, and other flooring surfaces. The patient must also be able to use sidewalk curbs while walking independently with crutches or a cane or while in a wheelchair.

Some patients are discharged home or to a rehabilitation setting with a halo vest. A halo vest has a significant physical and psychological impact on patients. Physically, patients find it difficult to perform mobility skills and ADLs independently, especially dressing, bathing, and feeding. From a psychological perspective, patients perceive an altered body image. Teach the patient or other caregiver going home or to a rehabilitation setting how to care for and adjust to the halo device (Chart 45-13).

The ADLs training for the patient with an SCI includes a structured exercise program to promote strength and endurance. The occupational therapist instructs the patient in the correct use of all adaptive equipment. In collaboration with the therapists, instruct family members or the caregiver in transfer skills, feeding, bathing, dressing, positioning, and skin care as discussed briefly in this chapter and in more detail in Chapter 8.

Drug Therapy. Teach the patient and his or her family or other caregiver about the name, purpose, dosage, timing of ad-

Chart 45-12 NURSING FOCUS ON THE OLDER ADULT

What Patients Need to Know About Aging with Spinal Cord Injury

Nursing Intervention	Rationales
Get flu shots annually, tetanus shots every 10 years, and the pneumonia vaccine as required.	Respiratory complications are the most common cause of death after spinal cord injury (SCI).
For women, have annual Papanicolaou (Pap) smears and mammograms.	Limitations in movement may make breast self-examination difficult. All older women should have an annual Pap smear.
Take measures to prevent osteoporosis, such as increasing calcium intake, exercising, and avoiding caffeine and smoking.	Women older than 50 years often lose bone density, which can result in fractures.
Practice meticulous skin care, including moisturizing and drinking plenty of water.	As a person ages, skin becomes dry and less elastic, predisposing the patient to pressure ulcers.
Take measures to prevent constipation, such as drinking adequate fluids, eating a healthy diet with fiber, and exercising.	Constipation is a problem for most patients with SCI, and they are more likely to develop the problem later in life.
Modify activities if joint pain occurs; use a powered rather than a manual wheelchair. Ask the health care provider about treatment options.	Arthritis occurs in more than half of people older than 65 years. Patients with SCI are more likely to develop arthritis as a result of added stress on the upper extremities when using a wheelchair.

Chart 45-13 PATIENT AND FAMILY EDUCATION GUIDE
Use of a Halo Device*

- Be aware that the weight of the halo device alters balance. Be careful when leaning forward or backward.
- Wear loose clothing, preferably with hook and loop (Velcro) fasteners or large openings for head and arms.
- Bathe in the bathtub, or take a sponge bath. (Some physicians allow showers.)
- Wash under the lambswool liner of the vest to prevent rashes or sores; use powders or lotions sparingly under the vest.
- Have someone change the liner if it becomes odorous.
- Support the head with a small pillow when sleeping to prevent unnecessary pressure and discomfort.
- Try to resume usual activities to the extent possible; keep as active as possible. (The weight of the device may cause fatigue or weakness.) However, avoid contact sports or swimming.
- Do not drive because vision is impaired with the device.
- Keep straws available for drinking fluids.
- Cut meats and other food into small pieces to facilitate chewing and swallowing.
- Before going outside in cold temperatures, wrap the pins with cloth to prevent the metal from getting cold.
- Have someone clean the pin sites as recommended by physician or hospital protocol.
- Observe the pin sites daily for redness, drainage, or loosening; report changes to the physician.
- Increase fluids and fiber in the diet to prevent constipation.
- Use a position of comfort during sexual activity.

*Home care instructions may vary depending on hospital or physician preference.

ministration, and side effects of all drugs. They should also understand the possible interaction of prescribed drugs with over-the-counter drugs or alcohol and illegal drugs. Some patients report continuous neuropathic pain and are placed on an antiepileptic drug (AED) such as gabapentin (Neurontin).

Sexuality and Intimacy. Sexual function after spinal cord injury depends on the level and extent of injury. Incomplete lesions allow some control over sensation and motor ability. Complete lesions disconnect the messages from the brain to the rest of the body, and vice versa. However, men with injuries above T6 are often able to have erections by stimulating reflex activity. For example, stroking the penis will cause an erection. Ejaculation is less predictable, and may be mixed with urine. However, urine is sterile, so the patient's partner will not get an infection.

Women with SCI have a different challenge because they have indwelling urinary catheters more commonly than men with SCI. However, some women do become pregnant and have full-term children. For others, ovulation stops in response to the injury. In this case, alternate methods for pregnancy, such as in vitro fertilization, may be an option. Some women also report vaginal dryness. Recommend a water-soluble lubricant for both partners to promote comfort.

For patients who choose not to have intercourse, intimate pleasure can be achieved in other ways, including kissing, hugging, fondling, masturbation, and oral sex. Variations in positioning may be needed to accommodate weak or paralyzed parts of the body. An understanding partner can help the patient adjust to his or her physical changes.

Health Care Resources

Refer the patient and family to local, state or province, and national organizations for more information and support for patients with SCI. These organizations include the National Spinal Cord Injury Association (www.spinalcord.org). Many excellent consumer-oriented books, journals, and DVDs are also available. Support groups may help the patient and family adjust to a changed lifestyle and provide solutions to commonly encountered problems.

A full-time caretaker or personal assistant is sometimes required if the patient with tetraplegia returns home. The caretaker may be a family member or a nursing assistant employed to help provide care and companionship. A patient who is paraplegic is often able to function without assistance after an appropriate rehabilitation program.

▪ *Evaluation: Outcomes*

Evaluate the care of the patient with an SCI on the basis of the identified nursing diagnoses and collaborative problems. The expected outcomes are that the patient:

- Exhibits no deterioration in neurologic status
- Maintains a patent airway, an alveolar exchange to maintain blood gases, and adequate ventilation
- Is free from complications of immobility
- Performs basic ADLs as independently as possible with or without the use of assistive/adaptive devices
- Achieves control of elimination of stool and urine
- Develops an adaptive psychosocial response to a significant life change

Specific indicators for these outcomes are listed for each nursing diagnosis under the Planning and Implementation section (see earlier).

SPINAL CORD TUMORS

Pathophysiology

Spinal cord tumors occur most often in the thoracic area, followed by an almost equal number in the lumbar and cervical regions. Signs and symptoms depend on the location of the tumor and its speed of growth. Tumors that involve the bones of the vertebral column usually occur as a result of metastasis (cancer spread) from other areas of the body.

The pathologic effects of a spinal cord tumor are more often related to compression of the cord than to invasion of the spinal cord itself. As the tumor expands within the vertebral column, it compresses the cord or the spinal nerve roots. Further growth leads to movement of the cord. In addition, a large tumor may affect the blood supply to the cord by compression or obstruct the normal flow of cerebrospinal fluid (CSF). Venous occlusion by the tumor may lead to spinal cord congestion and infarction (tissue death).

The appearance of neurologic signs and symptoms is related to the rate of tumor growth. The spinal cord can often accommodate a slowly growing lesion. With time, the cord may become significantly misshapen and displaced, but the patient has surprisingly few symptoms. On the other hand, a rapidly growing tumor quickly leads to spinal cord compression and edema and the development of neurologic symptoms, such as numbness and paralysis.

Primary spinal cord tumors involve the epidural vessels, spinal meninges, or glial cells of the cord. Their cause is unknown. Anatomically, spinal cord tumors may be extramedullary or intramedullary. **Intramedullary tumors** account for a small number of spinal cord tumors and are usually cancerous. They start within the spinal cord itself, in the central gray matter and the anterior commissure. **Extramedullary tumors,** representing most spinal cord tumors, are found within the spinal dura but outside the cord. They are further defined anatomically as extradural and intradural tumors. *Extradural or epidural* tumors occur between the vertebrae and the spinal dura. They develop in the surrounding bone and cause destruction of the vertebral bodies. *Intradural* tumors are located within the dura and originate from the pia-arachnoid, spinal roots, or ligaments.

Tumors involving the bones of the vertebrae typically develop as a consequence of *metastatic* tumors from the lungs, breasts, prostate, colon, and uterus.

Patient-Centered Collaborative Care

Assessment

Physical Assessment/Clinical Manifestations

The clinical manifestations of a spinal cord tumor depend on its location (Chart 45-14) and rate of growth. The most common problem is pain. Pain results from spinal cord compression, infiltration of the spinal tracts, or irritation of the spinal roots. Assess the quality, severity, and intensity of the pain. In addition, ask the patient to describe factors that worsen and relieve the pain. **Radicular** (nerve root) pain is stabbing or dull, with intermittent episodes of sharp, piercing pain. The pain may increase during coughing, straining, or sneezing. Lying flat may increase the pain as a consequence of stretching the involved spinal nerve roots.

Involvement of the corticospinal tract may lead to mobility problems. Assess for weakness, clumsiness, spasticity, and hyperactive reflexes, and compare responses on both sides of the body. Other presenting signs include ataxia (staggered gait), hypotonia (decreased muscle tone), and a positive Babinski's reflex. Spastic paralysis occurs most often, although a flaccid paralysis may be present in a tumor that affects the spinal roots, an intramedullary tumor in the lumbosacral area, or an extramedullary tumor.

Determine sensory loss on each side of the body, and compare the responses. Early symptoms include a slowly progressive numbness or tingling, pain, and temperature loss. The sensory deficit is further marked by a decreased touch perception, an inability to sense vibration, and a loss of position sense. The patient often reports a tight, bandlike feeling around the trunk. Brown-Séquard syndrome or central cord syndrome may be manifested.

Loss of bladder control often occurs before a loss of bowel control. Assess for urinary hesitancy, dribbling, incontinence, urgency, or acute retention. Bowel dysfunction is manifested by constipation. Keep in mind that the patient is often embarrassed to admit to bladder or bowel dysfunction.

A lesion in the sacral area may cause a decrease in genital sensation and thus affect the patient's sexual function and enjoyment. Men may be unable to have an erection or to ejaculate.

Chart 45-14 KEY FEATURES

Spinal Cord Tumors

GENERAL MANIFESTATIONS
- Pain
- Sensory loss or impairment
- Motor loss or impairment
- Sphincter disturbance (bladder before bowel)

CERVICAL MANIFESTATIONS

HIGH CERVICAL
- Respiratory distress
- Diaphragm paralysis
- Occipital headache
- Quadriparesis
- Stiff neck
- Nystagmus
- Cranial nerve dysfunction

LOW CERVICAL
- Pain in the arms and the shoulders
- Weakness
- Paresthesia
- Motor loss
- Horner's syndrome
- Increased reflexes

THORACIC MANIFESTATIONS
- Sensory loss
- Spastic paralysis
- Positive Babinski's sign
- Bladder and bowel dysfunction
- Pain in the chest and the back
- Muscle atrophy
- Muscle weakness in the legs
- Foot drop

LUMBOSACRAL MANIFESTATIONS
- Low back pain
- Paresis
- Spastic paralysis
- Sensory loss
- Bladder and bowel dysfunction
- Sexual dysfunction
- Decreased-to-absent ankle and knee reflexes

Diagnostic Assessment

Routine x-ray examinations or tomographic scans of the spine are obtained to detect a narrowing of the spinal canal, destruction of the vertebrae, or the presence of calcification. A myelogram may be useful when a block is incomplete; it indicates the level, extent, and boundaries of a tumor. This test is being performed less today because of newer imaging techniques.

An MRI scan with and without enhancement provides more detail of the pathologic condition of the spinal cord than either a CT scan or myelography. EMG may help make a differential diagnosis to rule out multiple sclerosis (MS) or amyotrophic lateral sclerosis (ALS).

Interventions

Nursing care of the patient with a spinal cord tumor includes obtaining the vital signs and checking neurologic status at least every 4 hours and more often as clinically indicated. As for any patient with a spinal cord problem, report any change in motor and sensory status immediately to the physician.

Surgical Management

The primary management of a spinal cord tumor is surgery. The desired outcome of surgical intervention is to remove as much of the tumor as possible. Often, this is not possible and other treatment is needed (e.g., radiation therapy). *Emergency surgery is done if the patient has a rapid loss of motor and sensory function or a loss of bladder and bowel control. Surgical decompression may be performed to maintain bladder, bowel, or motor function and to preserve quality of life—even with a poor prognosis.*

The neurosurgeon performs a laminectomy and surgical decompression and total or partial resection of the tumor. Depending on the extent of the tumor, a spinal fusion may be necessary. Rarely, a cordotomy or a palliative sectioning of sensory roots is done to control intractable pain.

After surgery, assess the patient's vital signs and neurologic status every 1 to 2 hours until they are stable and then every 4 hours. The patient is log rolled (turned as a unit) and repositioned every 2 hours. Inspect the incision site for drainage, especially of cerebrospinal fluid (CSF), and signs of infection. The patient with a cervical cord tumor must also be carefully monitored for respiratory compromise. Postoperative nursing care for a patient undergoing a laminectomy is discussed on p. 987 under Postoperative Care in the Low Back Pain section.

Nonsurgical Management

Radiation therapy may be necessary, depending on the tumor type. It is usually used with low-grade malignant tumors that are not completely removed, with metastatic tumors, or with recurrent tumors when there is no other treatment option. The spinal cord cannot tolerate high doses of radiation. Overexposure to radiation may lead to spinal damage, which develops over 6 to 12 months. It is manifested by progressive spinal cord degeneration and neurologic deficits such as Brown-Séquard syndrome. With time, the patient experiences spastic paralysis, loss of sensation, and bowel and bladder dysfunction. Death may occur. Care of the patient undergoing radiation therapy is described in detail in Chapter 24.

The use of chemotherapy in the treatment of spinal cord tumors is very limited. The drugs that are given tend to be alkylating agents, effective for some central nervous system (CNS) tumors because they cross the blood-brain barrier. Some patients may receive carmustine (NCNU) or lomustine (CCNU). In some cases, combination chemotherapy with procarbazine, vincristine, and carmustine is used (PVC therapy). Chemotherapy may also be used as an adjunctive therapy for tumors metastasized to the spinal cord from other primary sites, such as the breast. Meningeal involvement may benefit from intrathecal (spinal) chemotherapy. Chapter 24 describes the general nursing care associated with giving chemotherapy.

Community-Based Care

Home Care Management

Collaborate with the patient and his or her family members or significant others to identify and suggest ways to eliminate potential hazards in the home. If needed, make a referral to a home care nurse, social worker, or case manager to assess the need for structural alterations to the home. Alterations may be needed to accommodate ambulatory aids (e.g., a walker) and to help the patient to perform ADLs.

Some patients may be discharged from the acute care hospital to a rehabilitation setting, where they can learn to function as independently as possible. Chapter 8 describes rehabilitation in detail.

Health Teaching

The teaching plan for the patient with a spinal cord tumor depends on his or her level of dysfunction. With decompression of the tumor, the severity of the patient's symptoms often lessens. Deficits that may remain include mobility and sensory loss. Learning mobility skills can enable the patient to negotiate movement on sidewalks, carpeting, and other flooring surfaces. The patient must also be able to negotiate sidewalk curbs independently. The physical or occupational therapist instructs the patient in the correct use of all adaptive equipment. Review the individualized bowel and bladder program with the patient, family member, or other caregiver. Chapter 8 describes these programs and the rehabilitation process in detail.

The goal of sexuality education in the acute care setting is to answer questions and correct any misinformation. Unless the nurse has had specific training or experience in sexuality counseling of people with spinal cord tumors or injuries, more detailed questions should be directed to a sexuality counselor.

Health Care Resources

The prognosis for the patient with malignant tumors or metastatic tumors is poor. Determine what the physician and family members have told the patient about diagnosis and prognosis. Encourage the patient to verbalize feelings and fears about prognosis, body image, self-concept, role performance, and self-esteem.

Refer patients and family members to local, state or province, and national organizations for people with spinal cord injuries. These groups often have information and support groups for patients with spinal cord tumors. Refer patients with a malignancy to the American Cancer Society (www.cancer.org). Referral to support groups may also assist families with helping the patient adapt to lifestyle changes. The Canadian Cancer Society (www.cancer.ca) offers similar services.

MULTIPLE SCLEROSIS

Multiple sclerosis (MS) is a chronic autoimmune disease that affects the myelin sheath and conduction pathway of the central nervous system (CNS). It is one of the leading causes of neurologic disability in young adults. This chronic disease is characterized by periods of remission and **exacerbation** (flare). Patients progress at different rates and over different lengths of time. However, as the severity and duration of the disease progress, the periods of exacerbation become more frequent. Patients with MS have a normal life expectancy as long as the effects of the disease are treated.

A major concern reported by most patients is how long it takes to establish a diagnosis of MS. Many have been to several health care providers, given different diagnoses and treatment, and/or been told their symptoms were related to stress and anxiety. All too often the patient and family are relieved to finally have a diagnosis but express anger and frustration that it prevented the start of appropriate treatment. Therefore establish open and honest communication with the patient and allow him or her to share frustrations, anger, and anxiety.

Pathophysiology

Multiple sclerosis is characterized by an inflammatory response that results in diffuse random or patchy areas of plaque in the white matter of the CNS. When this occurs, the myelin sheath is damaged and its thickness is reduced, or **demyelinated.** Myelin is responsible for the electrochemical transmission of impulses between the brain and spinal cord and the rest of the body. Impulses are still transmitted but are not as effective as before. Over time, they may be completely blocked. The white fiber tracts (axons) that connect the neurons in the brain and spinal cord are generally involved in MS. The areas particularly affected include optic nerves, pyramidal tracts, posterior columns, brainstem nuclei, and the periventricular region of the brain. Eventually, with repeated exacerbations of the disease, damage to the axons becomes permanent.

Major types of MS include (McCance & Huether, 2006):

- Relapsing-remitting
- Primary progressive
- Secondary progressive
- Progressive-relapsing

The classic picture of the **relapsing-remitting** type of **MS (RRMS)** occurs in most of the cases. The course of the disease may be mild or moderate, depending on the degree of disability. Symptoms develop and resolve in a few weeks to months, after which the patient returns to baseline.

Primary progressive MS (PPMS) involves a steady and gradual neurologic deterioration without remission of symptoms. The patient has progressive disability with no acute attacks. Patients with this type of MS tend to be between 40 and 60 years of age at onset of the disease.

Secondary progressive MS (SPMS) begins with a relapsing-remitting course that later becomes steadily progressive. Functioning continues to decline with no clear times of remission.

Progressive-relapsing MS (PRMS) is characterized by frequent relapses with some partial recovery but not a return to baseline. Progressive, cumulative symptoms and deterioration occur over several years.

Etiology and Genetic Risk

The exact cause of MS remains unknown and is very complex. Research continues on viral, immunologic, and genetic and environmental etiologic factors. Viruses are well recognized as causes of demyelination and inflammation. Therefore it may be possible that a virus or other infectious agent is the triggering factor in MS. Although a number of viruses have been studied, no single virus has been identified as causing MS in genetically predisposed people.

Genetic predisposition is determined by a pattern of antigens, in particular HLA DR2 and DQ6 (Nussbaum et al., 2007). The disease tends to occur among family members, especially siblings.

According to the National Multiple Sclerosis Society (www.nationalmssociety.org):

- Having a first-degree relative such as a parent or sibling with MS increases a person's risk of developing the disease.
- There is a higher prevalence of certain genes in populations with higher rates of MS.
- Common genetic factors have been found in some families in which there is more than one person with MS.
- Many genetic alterations contribute to the development of MS; not all patients with MS have the same alterations.
- The environment may also contribute to the development of MS. The disease is seen more often in the colder climates of the northeastern, Great Lakes, and Pacific northwestern states, as well as in Canada.

Incidence/Prevalence

MS usually occurs in people between the ages of 20 and 40 years, but cases may occur in those younger than 15 years and older than 50 years. Over 500,000 people in the United States are currently affected. Women are affected about twice as often as men (McCance & Huether, 2006).

Patient-Centered Collaborative Care

Assessment

History

Multiple sclerosis (MS) often looks like other neurologic diseases, which can make the diagnosis difficult and prolonged. As a result, patients often see many health care providers and undergo a variety of diagnostic tests and treatments. Obtaining a thorough history is essential for accurate diagnosis. Ask about a history of vision, mobility, and sensory changes, all of which are early indicators of MS. Symptoms are often vague and nonspecific in the early stages of the disease. Of significance is the patient's report that symptoms were first noticed several years earlier but that medical attention was not sought because the symptoms disappeared. Ask about the progression of symptoms. Pay particular attention to whether the symptoms are intermittent or are becoming progressively worse. Document the date (month and year) when the patient first noticed the clinical manifestations.

Next, ask about factors that aggravate the symptoms, such as fatigue, stress, overexertion, temperature extremes, or a hot shower or bath. Ask the patient and the family about any personality or behavioral changes that have occurred (e.g., euphoria [very elated mood], poor judgment, attention loss). In addition, determine whether there is a family history of MS.

Physical Assessment/Clinical Manifestations

Multiple sclerosis produces a wide variety of manifestations (Chart 45-15). Any myelinated fibers of the brain and spinal cord may be affected. To determine a patient's specific manifestations, perform a complete neurologic assessment, as described in Chapter 43.

First assess the patient's ability to move. The patient often reports increased fatigue and stiffness of the extremities, particularly the legs. Fatigue is one of the most disabling manifestations, affecting almost all patients with MS. Unlike fatigue in others, MS fatigue is associated with continuous sensitivity to temperature.

Chart 45-15 KEY FEATURES

Multiple Sclerosis

- Muscle weakness and spasticity
- Fatigue
- Intention tremors
- Dysmetria (inability to direct or limit movement)
- Numbness or tingling sensations (paresthesia)
- Hypalgesia (decreased sensitivity to pain)
- Ataxia (decreased motor coordination)
- Dysarthria (slurred speech)
- Dysphagia (difficulty swallowing)
- Diplopia (double vision)
- Nystagmus (involuntary eye movements)
- Scotomas (changes in peripheral vision)
- Decreased visual and hearing acuity
- Tinnitus, vertigo (ringing in the ears, dizziness)
- Bowel and bladder dysfunction
- Alterations in sexual function, such as impotence
- Cognitive changes, such as memory loss, impaired judgment, and decreased ability to solve problems or perform calculations

Flexor spasms at night may awaken the patient from sleep. Further examination reveals increased or hyperactive deep tendon reflexes, clonus, positive Babinski's reflex, and absent abdominal reflexes. Gait may be unsteady because of leg weakness and spasticity.

Significant cerebellar findings include **intention tremor** (tremor when performing an activity), **dysmetria** (inability to direct or limit movement), and dysdiadochokinesia (inability to stop one motor impulse and substitute another). Motor movements are often clumsy. The patient may lose balance easily and may exhibit signs of poor coordination.

During examination of the cranial nerves and brainstem function, ask the patient if he or she has or has had episodes of tinnitus (ringing in the ears), vertigo (dizziness), and hearing loss. Assess for facial weakness and dysphagia. Speech problems include dysarthria (slurred speech) and slow, scanning speech.

Typical clinical findings from assessment of the patient's visual acuity, visual fields, and pupils include:

- Blurred vision
- **Diplopia** (double vision)
- Decreased visual acuity
- **Scotomas** (changes in peripheral vision)
- **Nystagmus** (involuntary, rapid eye movements)

Sensory findings include hypalgesia (diminished sensitivity to pain), paresthesia, facial pain, and decreased temperature perception. The patient may report numbness, tingling, burning, or crawling sensations.

If demyelination of the spinal cord has occurred, the patient may experience bowel and bladder dysfunctions as well as alterations in sexuality. The patient may have an areflexic bladder or may experience frequency, urgency, or nocturia. Ask the patient if he or she has constipation or incontinence. Inquire about problems with sexuality, including impotence, difficulty sustaining an erection, and decreased vaginal secretion.

Psychosocial Assessment

Assess the patient for mental status changes. Cognitive changes are usually seen late in the course of the disease and include decreased short-term memory, concentration, and ability to perform calculations; inattentiveness; and impaired judgment.

After the initial diagnosis of MS, the patient is often anxious. Apathy, emotional lability, and depression are common problems that occur later. The patient may be euphoric or giddy, either as a result of the disease itself or because of the drugs used to treat the disease. Assess the patient's previously used coping and stress management skills in preparing him or her for a chronic, usually debilitating disease. Depression is the most frequent psychiatric disorder diagnosed in people with MS.

Laboratory Assessment

No single specific procedure is definitively diagnostic for MS. However, the collective results of a variety of tests are usually conclusive. Changes may be evident during an acute attack. Abnormal cerebrospinal fluid (CSF) findings include an elevated protein level and a slight increase in the white blood cell count. CSF electrophoresis reveals an increase in the myelin basic protein and the presence of oligoclonal (IgG) bands. IgG bands are seen in most patients with MS.

Other Diagnostic Assessment

The McDonald criteria may be used to diagnose MS. Criteria include (Vijay, 2007):

- Two events or "attacks" separated in time and space
- MRI evidence consistent with MS
- CSF findings
- Analysis of evoked potentials as a means of identifying a second attack

The health care provider usually requests a CT scan, which may show an increased density in the white matter and MS plaques. MRI demonstrates the presence of plaques and is considered diagnostic for MS. A complete diagnostic evaluation is necessary to exclude other disease.

Results of visual, auditory, and brainstem evoked potential studies are often abnormal. EMG findings may be grossly abnormal in people with advanced disease.

The diagnosis of MS is made by the exclusion of other neurologic diseases by laboratory and neuroimaging assessment. Specific criteria, including the presence of neurologic dysfunction that occurs over time in more than one area of the central nervous system (CNS), is also diagnostic.

Common Nursing Diagnoses and Collaborative Problems

Nursing diagnoses that may apply to patients with MS include:

- Fatigue related to disease state
- Activity Intolerance related to generalized weakness
- Disturbed Sensory Perception (Visual) related to altered sensory reception
- Impaired Physical Mobility related to neuromuscular impairment
- Impaired Urinary Elimination related to sensory-motor impairment
- Chronic Pain related to chronic physical disability
- Self-Care Deficit related to neuromuscular impairment
- Disturbed Thought Processes related to disease state
- Imbalanced Nutrition: Less Than Body Requirements related to difficulty swallowing
- Sexual Dysfunction related to altered body function

Interventions

The purpose of management is to modify the disease's effects on the immune system, prevent exacerbations, manage symptoms, and improve function. Like for other spinal cord diseases, care of the patient with MS requires the collaborative efforts of the interdisciplinary team.

The patient with MS is often weak and easily fatigued. The Concept Map on p. 1005 illustrates the common problems and interventions for the patient with MS. Teach the patient the importance of planning activities and allowing sufficient time to complete activities. For example, the patient should check that all items needed for work are gathered before leaving the house. Items used on a daily basis should be easily accessible.

Drug Therapy

Current therapies for MS are designed to treat a dysfunctional immune system. A variety of medications are used to treat and control the disease, decrease specific symptoms, and attempt to slow its progression.

The National Multiple Sclerosis Society recommends early and continuous treatment of relapsing-remitting MS with *one* or more of these drugs:

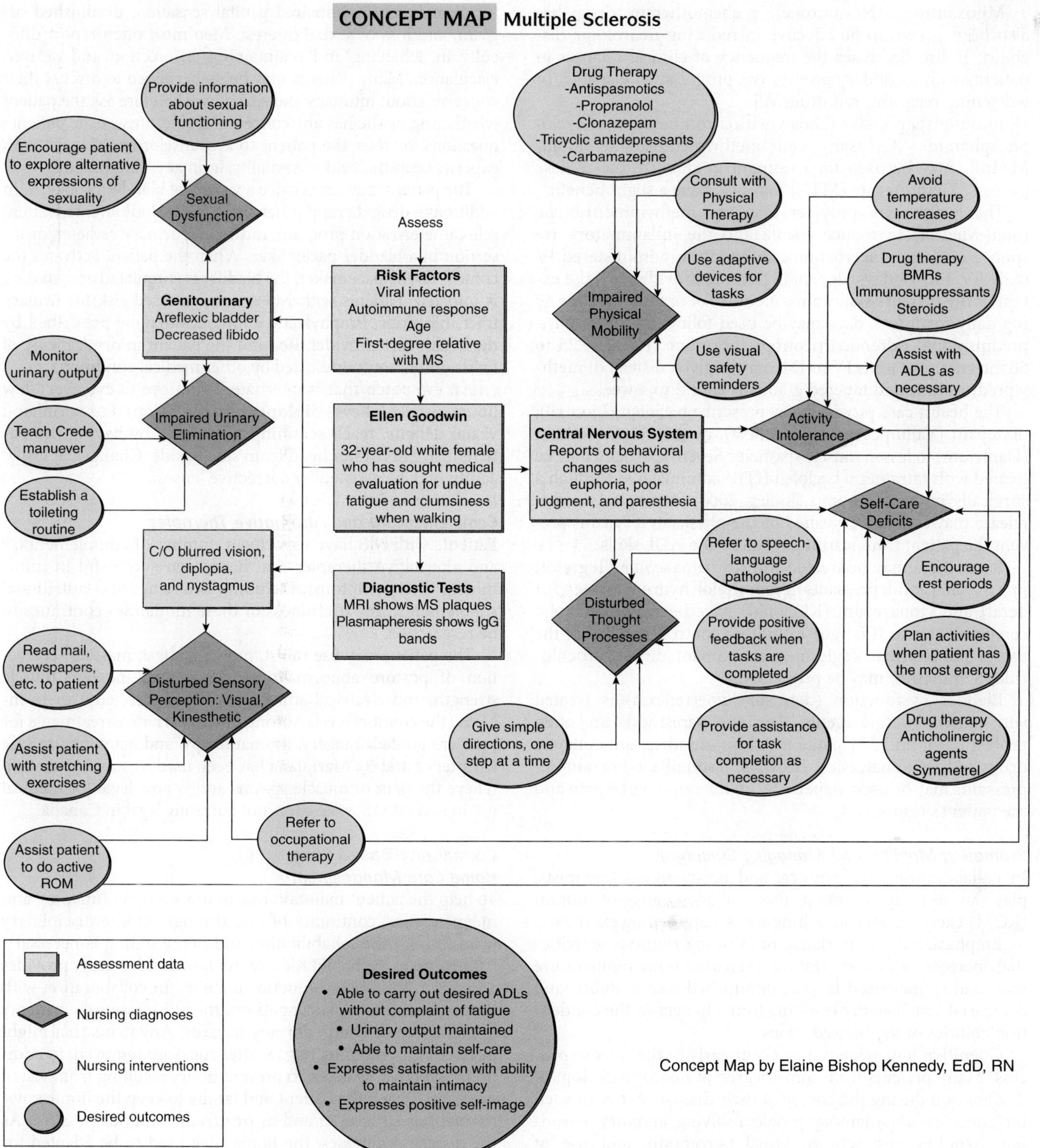
CONCEPT MAP Multiple Sclerosis
Provide information about sexual functioning
Encourage patient to explore alternative expressions of sexuality
Sexual Dysfunction
Assess
Risk Factors
Viral infection
Autoimmune response
Age
First-degree relative with MS
Genitourinary
Areflexic bladder
Decreased libido
Monitor urinary output
Impaired Urinary Elimination
Teach Crede manuever
Establish a toileting routine
Ellen Goodwin
32-year-old white female who has sought medical evaluation for undue fatigue and clumsiness when walking
C/O blurred vision, diplopia, and nystagmus
Diagnostic Tests
MRI shows MS plaques
Plasmapheresis shows IgG bands
Read mail, newspapers, etc. to patient
Disturbed Sensory Perception: Visual, Kinesthetic
Assist patient with stretching exercises
Refer to occupational therapy
Assist patient to do active ROM
Drug Therapy
-Antispasmotics
-Propranolol
-Clonazepam
-Tricyclic antidepressants
-Carbamazepine
Consult with Physical Therapy
Avoid temperature increases
Use adaptive devices for tasks
Impaired Physical Mobility
Drug therapy
BMRs
Immunosuppressants
Steroids
Use visual safety reminders
Assist with ADLs as necessary
Activity Intolerance
Central Nervous System
Reports of behavioral changes such as euphoria, poor judgment, and paresthesia
Self-Care Deficits
Refer to speech-language pathologist
Encourage rest periods
Disturbed Thought Processes
Provide positive feedback when tasks are completed
Plan activities when patient has the most energy
Give simple directions, one step at a time
Provide assistance for task completion as necessary
Drug therapy
Anticholinergic agents
Symmetrel
Assessment data
Nursing diagnoses
Nursing interventions
Desired outcomes
Desired Outcomes
• Able to carry out desired ADLs without complaint of fatigue
• Urinary output maintained
• Able to maintain self-care
• Expresses satisfaction with ability to maintain intimacy
• Expresses positive self-image
Concept Map by Elaine Bishop Kennedy, EdD, RN

- Interferon beta (Avonex, Betaseron, or Rebif), an immunomodulator that modifies the course of the disease and has antiviral effects
- Natalizumab (Tysabri), the first monoclonal antibody approved for MS that binds to WBCs to prevent further damage to the myelin
- Glatiramer acetate (Copaxone), a synthetic protein that is similar to myelin-based protein

Natalizumab has recently been associated with significant liver damage in some patients. Carefully monitor liver enzymes and teach patients and their families to have frequent laboratory tests to assess for changes.

Mitoxantrone (Novantrone), a chemotherapy drug, has also been shown to be effective in reducing neurologic disability. It also decreases the frequency of clinical relapses in patients with secondary progressive, progressive-relapsing, or worsening relapsing-remitting MS.

Immunosuppressive therapy with a combination of cyclophosphamide (Cytoxan) and methylprednisolone (Solu-Medrol) may be used for treatment to stabilize the disease process. Methotrexate (MTX) may also have a slight benefit.

The health care provider may use methylprednisolone (Solu-Medrol) to reduce edema and the inflammatory response in acute exacerbations. One gram is administered IV daily for 3 to 14 days, depending on the provider and the extent of the patient's symptoms. A course of oral prednisone 60 mg daily for 5 to 7 days may be used following the methylprednisolone. Adrenocorticotropic hormone (ACTH), 25 to 60 international units IV or IM, may be given instead of methylprednisolone and tapered gradually over 2 to 4 weeks.

The health care provider may prescribe baclofen (Lioresal), diazepam (Valium, Apo-Diazepam♣), or dantrolene sodium (Dantrium) to lessen muscle spasticity. Severe spasticity may be treated with intrathecal baclofen (ITB) administered through a surgically implanted pump (Ridley, 2006). A surgical tendon release may also be performed by the physician if spasms prevent the patient from learning mobility and ADL skills.

Paresthesia may be treated with carbamazepine (Tegretol) or tricyclic antidepressants. Propranolol hydrochloride (Inderal) and clonazepam (Klonopin) have been used to treat cerebellar ataxia. If fatigue cannot be controlled through the use of nonpharmacologic measures, amantadine hydrochloride (Symmetrel) may be prescribed.

Bladder dysfunction (detrusor hyperreflexia) is treated with anticholinergic agents. Pain and paresthesia are often problems for the MS patient. Antispasmodics, antiepileptic drugs (AEDs), analgesics, NSAIDs, tranquilizers, or antidepressants may be used, depending on the cause of the pain and the patient's response.

Promoting Mobility and Managing Symptoms

In collaboration with physical and occupational therapists, plan an exercise program that includes range-of-motion (ROM) exercises and stretching and strengthening exercises.

Emphasize the importance of avoiding rigorous activities that increase body temperature. Increased body temperature may lead to increased fatigue, diminished motor ability, and decreased visual acuity resulting from changes in the conduction abilities of the injured axons.

Cognitive impairment may occur early in the disease process. Many patients have some degree of neuropsychological dysfunction during the course of their disease. Areas affected include attention, memory, problem solving, auditory reasoning, handling distractions, visual perception, and use of speech. To assist the patient with orientation, place a single-date calendar in the patient's room. Give or encourage the patient to use written lists or recorded messages. To maintain an organized environment, encourage the patient to keep frequently used items in familiar places.

If the patient experiences dysarthria (slurred speech), refer to the speech-language pathologist (SLP) for evaluation and treatment. It is not unusual for the patient with dysarthria also to have dysphagia (difficulty swallowing). The SLP will do a swallowing evaluation. Further diagnostic testing may be indicated.

Women report impaired genital sensation, diminished orgasm, and loss of sexual interest. Men most often report difficulty in achieving and maintaining an erection and delayed ejaculation. Many patients may be embarrassed to discuss their concerns about intimacy and sexuality. Therefore ask the patient whether he or she has any concerns. If able, answer the patient's questions, or refer the patient to a counselor or urologist with experience in the field of sexuality, intimacy, and disability.

The patient may experience a variety of bladder problems. In addition to drug therapy, other measures include an intermittent self-catheterization program, indwelling urinary catheter, or insertion of a bladder pacemaker. When the patient activates the control on the pacemaker, the bladder is stimulated and voiding is initiated. Patients with MS are at increased risk for urinary tract infections. Prophylactic antibiotics may be prescribed by the health care provider. Remind the patient to drink plenty of fluids unless contraindicated by other medical conditions.

An eye patch that is alternated from eye to eye every few hours usually relieves **diplopia** (double vision). For peripheral visual deficits, teach scanning techniques by having the patient move his or her head from side to side. Changes in visual acuity may be assisted by corrective lenses.

Complementary and Alternative Therapies

Patients with MS have reported a number of complementary and alternative therapies that have been successful in minimizing their symptoms, including bee stings and nutritional supplements. The usefulness of these modalities continues to be researched.

The patient may use moist, moderate heat; massage; correction of posture abnormalities; exercises to increase muscle strength; and electrical stimulation of the affected area to increase the comfort level. Among other alternative treatments for pain are guided imagery, aromatherapy, and acupuncture (see Chapters 2 and 5). Marijuana has been used by some patients to relieve the pain of muscle spasms and is now legal for medical use in several U.S. states. It is not currently legal in Canada.

Community-Based Care

Home Care Management

To help the patient maintain maximum strength, function, and independence, continuity of care through an interdisciplinary team in both the rehabilitation and home setting is necessary. Admission to a rehabilitation center is brief but usually provides a program to improve functional ability. In collaboration with the case manager and occupational therapist, assess the patient's home before discharge for any hazards. Any items that might interfere with mobility (e.g., scatter rugs) are removed. In addition, care must be taken to prevent injury resulting from vision problems. Teach the patient and family to keep the home environment as structured and as free from clutter as possible. As the disease progresses, the home may need to be adapted for wheelchair accessibility. Any necessary assistive/adaptive device should be readily available before discharge from the hospital.

Health Teaching

The health care provider explains to the patient and family the development of MS and the factors that may exacerbate the symptoms. Emphasize the importance of avoiding overexertion, stress, extremes of temperatures (fever, hot baths, overheating, and excessive chilling), humidity, and people with upper respiratory tract infections. Explain all medications to be taken on discharge, including the time and route of administration, dosage, purpose, and side effects. Teach the patient how to differentiate expected side effects from adverse or allergic reactions, and provide the name of a resource person to call if questions or problems occur. Provide written instructions as a resource for the patient and caregivers at home.

The physical therapist develops an exercise program appropriate for the patient's tolerance level. The patient is instructed in techniques for self-care, daily living skills, and the use of required adaptive equipment, such as walkers and electric carts. Include information related to bowel and bladder management, skin care, nutrition, and positioning techniques. Chapter 8 describes in detail these aspects of chronic illness and rehabilitation.

Teach patients about the importance of obtaining adequate rest and avoiding undue stress. It is equally important for them to engage in regular social activities. Often patients are anxious and worry about how long the remission will last or when the disease will progress.

Because personality changes are not unusual, teach the family or significant others strategies to enable them to cope with these changes. For example, the family may develop a nonverbal signal to alert the patient to potentially inappropriate behavior (e.g., a talkative person may be reminded to be quiet if a family member displays a prearranged signal). This action avoids embarrassment for the patient.

Health Care Resources

Resources required by the patient depend on the course of the disease and the complications that occur. Patients often are able to live completely independently or may need some assistance. In severe disease, placement in an assisted-living or long-term care facility may be the best alternative. The population of young and middle-aged residents in these settings is increasing as people with chronic, disabling diseases live longer.

Refer the patient and family members or significant others to the local chapter of the National Multiple Sclerosis Society (www.nationalmssociety.org). Other community resources include meal delivery services (e.g., Meals on Wheels), transportation services for the disabled, and homemaker services.

AMYOTROPHIC LATERAL SCLEROSIS

Pathophysiology

Amyotrophic lateral sclerosis (ALS), also known as **Lou Gehrig's disease,** is an adult-onset upper and lower motor neuron disease. It is characterized by progressive weakness, muscle wasting, and spasticity eventually leading to paralysis. Beginning in one area of the body, motor weakness and deterioration spread until the entire body is involved, including the ability to talk, swallow, and breathe. As a result of loss of lower motor neurons (LMNs) found in the spinal cord and brainstem, the muscles they connect to weaken, atrophy, and die.

Loss or death of upper neurons (found in the brain) breaks their connections with LMN, and spasticity occurs in the muscles. Death typically occurs within 3 years of diagnosis due to respiratory failure (Murphy et al., 2007). There is no known cause, no cure, no specific treatment, no standard pattern of progression, and no method of prevention. Unlike with many other neural degenerative diseases, the sensory and autonomic nervous systems are not involved. Cognitive and behavioral dysfunction may occur although the exact cause and extent of this has not been established (Murphy et al., 2007).

Amyotrophic lateral sclerosis may occur at any age, but it is not common. The usual age of onset is between 40 and 70 years. The incidence increases with each decade of life. ALS is more common in men than in women. More recently diagnosed patients appear to have slower disease progression than patients seen before 2001, which has been suggested to be due to lifestyle and environmental changes (Czaplinski et al., 2006).

The cause of the disease is unknown. Researchers are exploring interactions of genetic, viral, and environmental factors as potential causes.

Patient-Centered Collaborative Care

Assessment

The clinical manifestations of ALS include fatigue, muscle atrophy, and weakness. Early symptoms are listed in Chart 45-16.

Along with the motor changes, cognitive changes may be noted in thinking and planning processes. As the disease progresses, muscle atrophy, particularly of the trapezius and sternocleidomastoid muscles, develops. Eventually the respiratory muscles become involved, leading to respiratory compromise, pneumonia, and death.

Diagnosis is based on clinical and diagnostic test findings and by ruling out other causes of the motor changes. There is no specific test to diagnose ALS, but creatine kinase (CK) is increased. The electromyogram (EMG) demonstrates fibrillations and fasciculations of the muscles. A muscle biopsy specimen typically demonstrates small, angulated, atrophic fibers. Other diagnostic studies reveal motor strength deficits in serial muscle testing; abnormal pulmonary function test results, such as a decreased vital capacity (<2 L); and dysphagia (difficulty swallowing).

Interventions

There is no known cure for ALS, but an interdisciplinary approach is needed for maintaining optimum functioning and end-of-life care.

Riluzole (Rilutek) is the only drug approved by the Food and Drug Administration for use with ALS patients. It is not a cure, but it does extend survival time. The usual dose is 50 mg twice daily on an empty stomach. The patient is monitored for liver toxicity from the drug by frequent measures of liver enzymes, such as alanine aminotransferase (ALT) and aspartate aminotransferase (AST). Teach him or her the importance of keeping all follow-up appointments.

The health care provider also prescribes medication for pain, fatigue, spasticity, excessive secretions, sleep disturbances, and other complications as they occur. The interdisciplinary team collaborates with the patient and family to develop an individualized plan of care. The physical therapist and occupational therapist evaluate the patient's home and recommend modifications as the disease progresses. An exer-

Chart 45-16 KEY FEATURES

Early Clinical Manifestations of Amyotrophic Lateral Sclerosis

- Tongue atrophy
- Weakness of the hands and arms
- Beginning muscle atrophy of the arms
- **Fasciculations** (twitching) of the face
- Nasal quality of speech
- **Dysarthria** (slurred speech)
- **Dysphagia** (difficulty swallowing)
- Fatigue while talking

cise and mobility program is developed and special equipment is obtained as needed to help with ADLs and mobility. Other interventions are directed toward preventing complications of immobility and promoting comfort.

The speech-language pathologist (SLP) evaluates the patient for speech and swallowing problems and makes recommendations as needed. The SLP teaches patients various adaptive strategies, such as techniques to help them speak louder and more clearly. He or she works with the patient and family to develop a communication system to be used when the patient can no longer verbally communicate.

A nutrition consult is made to help with planning meals that the patient can swallow. The family is taught how to ensure that the patient obtains sufficient nutrients, fiber, and fluids. When the patient can no longer swallow, a feeding tube may be placed, depending on the patient's decision or advance directives. The nutritionist can recommend the appropriate enteral feedings.

For symptomatic treatment of dyspnea and/or intractable pain, opioids alone or in combination with benzodiazepines if anxiety is present may be prescribed. Titrating the dosages against the clinical symptoms is less likely to cause life-threatening respiratory depression. For treating terminal restlessness and confusion because of hypercapnia, neuroleptics may be used, (e.g., chlorpromazine [Thorazine, Chlorpromanyl♣] 12.5 mg every 4 to 12 hours orally, IV, or rectally).

At some point the patient will require respiratory support. Intermittent positive-pressure ventilation [IPPV] or bi-level positive airway pressure [BIPAP]) may be used to aid breathing during sleep or full time. Mechanical ventilation enables the patient to breathe and prolongs survival; it will not alter progression of the disease. For this reason, many patients elect not to be placed on a mechanical ventilator, according to their wishes or advance directives.

Refer the patient to a hospice program. The hospice team works closely with the family to ensure the patient's comfort. They collaborate with the health care provider to ensure that the patient has the needed medication and pain control, as well as quality of life for the patient and family.

The hospice nurse also provides ongoing support and counseling to the patient and the family as they begin to cope with the impact of this terminal disease. Teach the patient about the need for advance directives, such as a living will. Chapter 9 discusses end-of-life issues and hospice services in detail. Community resources include clinics and other support services run by the ALS Association (www.alsa.org) or the Muscular Dystrophy Association (www.mda.org).

HUMAN NEEDS NURSING CARE REVIEW

What might you NOTICE if the patient is experiencing inadequate mobility and sensation as a result of spinal cord health problems?

- Weakness or paralysis of one or more extremities
- Report of decreased sensation in one or more extremities
- Muscle spasticity or flaccidity
- Forward bent position when ambulating
- Limp or altered gait
- Bladder incontinence or retention
- Bowel incontinence or retention
- Report of pain in back and/or in one or more extremities
- Difficulty breathing

What should you INTERPRET and how should you RESPOND to a patient experiencing inadequate mobility and sensation as a result of spinal cord health problems?

Perform and interpret physical assessment, including:

- Assessing airway patency and breathing pattern
- Assessing level of consciousness
- Taking vital signs
- Performing a complete physical assessment
- Performing a complete neurologic assessment
- Assessing level of pain

Respond by:

- Establishing an airway as needed
- Stabilizing the spine by positioning until surgery or other treatment is provided
- Preparing for imaging assessment tests
- Providing pain medication as prescribed
- Inserting an indwelling urinary catheter
- Collaborating with health care team, especially the physical therapist and the occupational therapist, if needed

On what should you REFLECT?

- Monitor patient for changes in condition, including deterioration of neurologic status.
- Consider how to best collaborate with the health care team when caring for patients with spinal cord injury or illness.
- Think about family reaction to the injury or illness and what additional resources could have been used or should be used in the future.

GET READY FOR THE NCLEX EXAMINATION!

Key Points

Review these Key Points for each NCLEX Examination Client Needs Category.

Safe and Effective Care Environment

- To help prevent back injury, use proper body mechanics as described in Chart 45-5.
- For patients who have back surgery, observe the incision site for bleeding and cerebrospinal fluid leakage (clear fluid).
- Log roll patients having spinal surgery, especially those who have fusions.
- For patients with an SCI, assess airway *first!*
- Observe patients with spinal injuries and diseases for complications of immobility.
- Monitor respiratory status carefully in patients with amyotrophic lateral sclerosis. Patients experience respiratory failure in terminal stages of the disease. Consider their advance directives to assist in planning care.

Health Promotion and Maintenance

- Teach patients who have had spinal surgery to avoid lifting and driving and to use proper body mechanics.
- Teach overweight and obese patients the importance of losing weight to reduce back pain and strain.
- Refer patients to appropriate resources, such as a sexuality counselor or urologist for sexual dysfunction resulting from illness or disease. Counsel them as needed about sexuality issues.
- Assess patients with spinal cord injury and disease for the need for adaptive/assistive devices to become independent in ADLs.
- Implement bowel and bladder retraining programs for patients with SCI and spinal diseases.

Psychosocial Integrity

- Recognize that spinal cord injury and progressive neurologic diseases, such as MS, require the patient to adjust to major life changes.
- Determine patient and family coping strategies to help patients adjust to spinal trauma or disease.
- Encourage patients to share their feelings about life-altering SCI or neurodegenerative disease.
- Refer patients with spinal cord cancer to appropriate resources, such as the American Cancer Society and its support groups.

Physiological Integrity

- Assess pain level in patients with back injury, including the nature of the pain and location.
- Provide complete neurologic assessment of patients with spinal cord health problems, including muscle assessment as described in Chart 45-8.
- Implement drug and non-drug interventions for back pain, including analgesics, NSAIDs, and muscle relaxants. Suggest heat as an adjunct to medication.
- Provide postoperative care and discharge teaching for patients having cervical neck surgery as listed in Chart 45-6.
- Implement interventions to prevent complications associated with immobility, including turning, early ambulation or transfers out of bed, and incentive spirometry.
- Monitor patients with cervical spinal injuries for manifestations of autonomic dysreflexia (see Chart 45-10).
- Provide emergency care for patients who experience autonomic dysreflexia as listed in Chart 45-11.
- Assess patients with multiple sclerosis for clinical manifestations as listed in Chart 45-15. Fatigue is the most common symptom.
- Provide supportive care for the patient with amyotrophic lateral sclerosis. Refer to hospice in the terminal stage of the disease.

Additional Study Resources

Go to your Companion CD or Evolve at http://evolve.elsevier.com/Iggy/ for *Self-Assessment Questions for the NCLEX Examination.*

Go to Evolve at http://evolve.elsevier.com/Iggy/ for *Prioritization and Delegation Questions for the NCLEX Examination.*

SELECTED BIBLIOGRAPHY

Amato, M.P., Portaccio, E., & Zipoli, V. (2006). Are there protective treatments for cognitive decline in MS? *Journal of Neurological Science, 245*(1-2), 183-186.

American Association of Neuroscience Nurses. (2007). *Cervical spine surgery: A guide to preoperative and postoperative patient care.* Chicago: Author.

Arnold, F.M., Filardi, T.Z., Strang, R.D., & McMahon, J.K. (2006). Early neurologic assessment of the patient with spinal cord injury. *Topics in Spinal Cord Injury Rehabilitation, 12*(1), 38-48.

Arzbaecher, J. (2007). Spinal metastasis in glioblastoma multiforme: A case study. *Journal of Neuroscience Nursing, 39*(1), 21-25.

Berlly, M., & Shem, K. (2007). Respiratory management during the first five days after spinal cord injury. *Journal of Spinal Cord Medicine, 30*(4), 309-318.

Bonner, S. (2008). My aching back. *Nursing Made Incredibly Easy, 6*(1), 19-31.

Carpico, B. (2007). Suspected cervical spine injury. *Nursing2007, 37*(3), 88.

Copeland, B. (2007). Surgical versus nonsurgical treatment for back pain. *New England Journal of Medicine, 357*(12), 1255.

Cortez, R., & Levi, A.D. (2007). Acute spinal cord injury. *Current Treatment Options in Neurology, 9*(2), 115-125.

Czaplinski, A., Yen, A.A., Simpson, E., & Appel, S.H. (2006). Slower disease progression and prolonged survival in contemporary patients with amyotrophic lateral sclerosis: Is the natural history of amyotrophic lateral sclerosis changing? *Archives of Neurology, 63*(8), 1139-1143.

Divani, A.A., Hussain, M.S., Magal, E., Heary, R.F., & Qureshi, A.I. (2007). The use of stem cells' hematopoietic stimulating factors therapy following spinal cord injury. *Annals of Biomedical Engineering, 35*(10), 1647-1656.

Dolinak, D., & Balraj, E. (2007). Autonomic dysreflexia and sudden death in people with traumatic spinal cord injury. *American Journal of Forensic Medicine and Pathology, 28*(2), 95-98.

Fisher, D. (2007). Is it upper or lower motor neuron disease? *Nursing Made Incredibly Easy, 5*(2), 64.

Fisher, C.G., Noonan, V.K., & Dvorak, M.F. (2006). Changing face of spine trauma care in North America. *Spine, 31*(Suppl. 11), S2-S8.

Foley, F.W., Coyle, P.K., Hutchinson, B., Kobelt, G.K., & Conner, C.S. (2007). *Multiple sclerosis treatment: The impact on quality of life.* Colorado: Consensus Medical Communications.

Fraser, C., & McGurl, J. (2007). Psychometric testing of the Americanized version of the Guy's Neurological Disability Scale. *Journal of Neuroscience Nursing, 39*(1), 13-19.

Furlan, J.C., & Fehlings, M.G. (2007). Role of screening tests for deep venous thrombosis in asymptomatic adults with acute spinal cord injury: An evidence-based analysis. *Spine, 32*(17), 1908-1916.

Furlan, J.C., Krassioukov, A.V., & Fehlings, M.G. (2006). Hematologic abnormalities within the first week after acute isolated traumatic cervical spinal cord injury: A case controlled cohort study. *Spine, 31*(23), 2674-2683.

Harris, M.B., & Sethi, R.K. (2006). The initial assessment and management of the multiple-trauma patient with an associated spine injury. *Spine, 31*(Suppl. 11), S9-S15.

International Multiple Sclerosis Genetics Consortium, Hafler, D.A., Compston, A., Sawcer, S., Lander E.S., Daly, M.J., et al. (2007). Risk alleles for multiple sclerosis identified by a genomewide study. *New England Journal of Medicine,* 357(9), 851-862.

Jansen, D.E., Krol, B., Groothoff, J.W., & Post, D. (2006). Evaluation of a transmural care model for multiple sclerosis patients. *Journal of Neuroscience Nursing, 38*(5), 384-389.

King, K.J. (2007). What you should know about neurogenic shock. *American Nurse Today, 2,* 36-39.

Koopman, W.J., Benbow, C.L., & Vandervoort, M. (2006). Top 10 needs of people with multiple sclerosis and their significant others. *Journal of Neuroscience Nursing, 38*(5), 369-373.

Logroscino, G., & Armon, C. (2007). Amyotrophic lateral sclerosis: A global threat with a possible difference in risk across ethnicities. *Neurology, 68*(13), E17.

McCance, K.L., & Huether, S.E. (2006). *Pathophysiology: The biologic basis for diseases in adults and children.* St. Louis: Mosby.

Mowery, K. (2007). The challenge of assessing and diagnosing acute abdomen in tetraplegics: A case study. *Journal of Neuroscience Nursing, 39*(1), 5-8.

Murphy, J., Henry, R., & Lomen-Hoerth, C. (2007). Establishing subtypes of the continuum of frontal lobe impairment in amyotrophic lateral sclerosis. *Archives of Neurology, 64*(3), 330-334.

Nakamura, M., Chiba, K., Ishii, K., Ogawa, Y., Takaishi, H., Matsumoto, M., et al. (2006). Surgical outcomes of spinal cord astrocytomas. *Spinal Cord, 44*(12), 740-745.

Nussbaum, R.L., McInnes, R.R., & Willard, H.F. (2007). *Thompson & Thompson genetics in medicine.* Philadelphia: Saunders.

Oken, B.S., Flegal, K., Zajdel, D., Kishiyama, S.S., Lovera, J., Bagert, B., et al. (2006). Cognition and fatigue in multiple sclerosis: Potential effects of medications with central nervous system activity. *Journal of Rehabilitation Research & Development, 43*(1), 83-90.

Orrell, R.W. (2007). Understanding the causes of amyotrophic lateral sclerosis. *New England Journal of Medicine, 357*(8), 822-823.

Poelstra, K.A., Vaccaro, A.R., Rao, S., Patel, D., Brown, A.K., Whang, P.G., et al. (2006). Emergency transport and radiographic evaluation following spinal cord injury. *Topics in Spinal Cord Injury Rehabilitation, 12*(1), 22-37.

Porterfield, S.S., & Hawkins, T. (2007). 2006 Conference Abstracts: Building better bowel programs: The OT and nurse connection. *Spinal Cord Injury Nursing, 24*(1). Retrieved February 20, 2008, from www.unitedspinal.org/

Rao, R.D., Currier, B.L., Albert T.J., Bono, C.M., Marawar, S.V., Poelstra, K.A., et al. (2007). Degenerative cervical spondylosis: Clinical syndromes, pathogenesis, and management. *Journal of Bone and Joint Surgery, 89*(6), 1360-1378.

Ridley, B. (2006). Intrathecal baclofen therapy: Challenges in patients with multiple sclerosis. *Rehabilitation Nursing, 31*(4), 158-164.

Sabin, K.L., & Penckofer, S.M. (2007). Patient expectations of quality of life following lumbar spinal surgery. *Journal of Neuroscience Nursing, 39*(3), 180-189.

Saulino, M., & Jacobs, B.W. (2006). The pharmacological management of spasticity. *Journal of Neuroscience Nursing, 38*(6), 456-459.

Sherwood, P.R., Crago, E.A., Spiro, R.M., & Okonkwo, D. (2007). Cervical spine injuries: Preserving function, improving outcomes. *American Nurse Today, 2*(9), 26-29.

Stankoff, B., Mrejen, S., Tourbah, A., Fontaine, B., Lyon-Caen, O., Lubetzki, C., et al. (2007). Age at onset determines the occurrence of the progressive phase of multiple sclerosis. *Neurology, 68*(10), 779-781.

Vacca, V.M. (2007). Acute paraplegia. *Nursing2007, 37*(6), 64.

Vijay, S. (2007). *The current and emerging landscape of MS treatment.* Retrieved March 30, 2007, from www.medscape.com

White, C.P., White, M., & Russell, C.S. (2007). Multiple sclerosis patients talking with healthcare providers about emotions. *Journal of Neuroscience Nursing, 39*(2), 89-101.

Whiteside, J.W. (2006). Management of head and neck injuries by the sideline physician. *American Family Physician, 74*(8), 1357-1362.

Care of Patients with Problems of the Peripheral Nervous System

46
CHAPTER

Kathy A. Hausman • Donna D. Ignatavicius

LEARNING OUTCOMES

For clinical competence and success on the NCLEX Examination, study this chapter with these Learning Outcomes in mind:

Safe and Effective Care Environment

1. Collaborate with interdisciplinary health care team members when providing care for patients with Guillain-Barré syndrome (GBS) and myasthenia gravis (MG).
2. Identify community resources for peripheral nervous system (PNS) disorders for patients and families.

Health Promotion and Maintenance

3. Provide information to patients and families on common side effects and administration of drugs for PNS disorders.

Psychosocial Integrity

4. Plan interventions for patients with GBS and MG for promoting communication.

Physiological Integrity

5. Perform focused neurologic assessments for patients with PNS disorders.
6. Compare and contrast the pathophysiology and etiology of GBS and MG.
7. Prioritize nursing care for the patient with GBS or MG.
8. Differentiate between a myasthenic crisis and a cholinergic crisis.
9. Identify specific nursing actions regarding drug administration for the patient with MG.
10. Perform a risk assessment for patients with GBS and MG.
11. Assess patients having a thymectomy for postoperative complications.
12. Plan and implement postoperative care for the patient undergoing peripheral nerve repair.
13. Identify risk factors for restless legs syndrome.
14. Compare trigeminal neuralgia and facial paralysis assessment findings.
15. Explain the role of drug therapy in managing the patient with trigeminal neuralgia and facial paralysis.
16. Prioritize care for patients with trigeminal neuralgia.

Go to your Companion CD or Evolve at http://evolve.elsevier.com/Iggy/ for *Self-Assessment Questions for the NCLEX Examination* keyed to these Learning Outcomes.

The peripheral nervous system (PNS) is composed of the spinal nerves, cranial nerves, and part of the autonomic nervous system. Its function is to provide communication from the brain and spinal cord to other parts of the body. Neuropathy or peripheral neuropathy (PN) is a global word that refers to any disease, disorder, or damage to the PNS. These health problems may be acute, such as Guillain-Barré syndrome, or chronic, such as diabetic neuropathy. Typical clinical manifestations of neuropathy include pain, muscle cramps, and muscle weakness.

Acquired neuropathies are grouped into three broad categories: inflammatory, traumatic, or systemic. *Inflammatory* neuropathies such as Guillain-Barré syndrome can affect the entire peripheral nervous system. Trigeminal neuralgia is a type of neuropathy caused by *trauma* or damage to a single nerve—the trigeminal nerve. Examples of *systemic* neuropathy are diabetic PN and chemotherapy-induced PN. Neuropathies that are part of or caused by systemic diseases or treatments are discussed elsewhere in this text. All of these PNS health problems cause impairments in the human needs of *mobility, sensation*, or both.

GUILLAIN-BARRÉ SYNDROME

Pathophysiology

ANIMATION: Guillain-Barré Syndrome

Guillain-Barré syndrome (GBS) is an uncommon disorder affecting middle-aged men slightly more that women. Euro-Americans have the disease more often than other racial or ethnic groups (Atkinson et al., 2006). GBS may be referred to by a variety of other names, such as *acute idiopathic polyneuritis* and *polyradiculoneuropathy.* As a result of **demyelination**

(destruction of the myelin sheath) of the peripheral nerves, *progressive motor weakness* and *sensory abnormalities* occur. Symptoms typically begin in the legs and spread to the arms and upper body. This is referred to as an **ascending paralysis.** Paralysis can increase in intensity until the muscles cannot be used at all and the patient is almost totally immobile. As a result, some patients require mechanical ventilation because of weak or paralyzed respiratory muscles.

Most patients report an acute illness before the development of GBS symptoms, such as gastroenteritis caused by *Campylobacter jejuni* bacteria. Three theories support a viral link to the development of GBS. First, a viral illness creates an autoimmune response that interferes with T–suppressor cell circuits. Second, the causative viral antigen has similar cell surface markers as myelin and the body mistakenly attacks itself. Finally, a direct invasion of the spinal and cranial nerves occurs (Atkinson et al., 2006).

GBS, then, is the result of a variety of related immune-mediated pathological processes. The immune system starts to destroy the myelin sheath that surrounds the axons of the peripheral nerves or attacks the axons themselves. Segmental demyelination (the destruction of myelin between the nodes of Ranvier) is the major pathologic finding in GBS. This destruction affects the transmission of impulses from node to node by slowing it down. Also, the brain receives fewer sensory signals, affecting the patient's ability to feel textures, heat, and pain. On the other hand, the brain may receive altered signals that cause the tingling or "crawling-skin" sensation many patients report.

On microscopic examination, groups of lymphocytes are seen at the points of myelin breakdown, yet the axons usually remain intact. In some instances, secondary damage to the cell body, the neurilemma, or the axon occurs. This can delay recovery or result in permanent neurologic deficits.

Three stages make up the *acute* course of GBS:

- The *acute or initial period* (1 to 4 weeks), which begins with the onset of the first symptoms and ends when no further deterioration occurs
- The *plateau period* (several days to 2 weeks)
- The *recovery phase* (usually 4 to 6 months, maybe up to 2 years), which is thought to coincide with remyelination and axonal regeneration (Some patients do not completely recover and have permanent neurologic deficits, referred to as *chronic GBS.*)

The exact cause of GBS remains unclear. The patient often relates a history of acute illness, trauma, surgery, or immunization 1 to 3 weeks before the onset of neurologic manifestations. Other risk factors include an upper respiratory tract infection or GI illness and positive antibodies to cytomegalovirus or Epstein-Barr virus (EBV). It is believed that the precipitating event or illness causes a limited malfunction of the immune system, which sensitizes the T-cells to the patient's myelin. In response to several antigens, some patients apparently form a demyelinating antibody that has a direct toxic effect on nerves or attracts a cellular immune response. This ultimately destroys the myelin. Other factors associated with the development of GBS are listed in Table 46-1.

Patient-Centered Collaborative Care

evolve ONLINE PHARM REVIEW

Assessment

Obtain a complete health history. Ask the patient to describe GBS symptoms in chronologic order, if possible. Question about the presence of pain, which is common if the patient has **paresthesias** (unpleasant sensations such as burning, stinging, and prickly feeling).

Manifestations of GBS depend on the degree of weakness and the progression of symptoms. Although features vary (Chart 46-1), most people report a sudden onset of muscle weakness and pain. Typically, the disease does not affect level of consciousness, cerebral function, or pupillary constriction or dilation. The clinical variations of GBS (Table 46-2) reflect the areas of earliest or most severe involvement.

With any of the variants, *cranial nerve* involvement most often affects the facial nerve (cranial nerve VII). Assess the

TABLE 46-1 Factors Associated with Development of Guillain-Barré Syndrome

- Acute illness
- Gastrointestinal illness
- *Campylobacter jejuni* bacteria
- Human immune deficiency virus infection
- *Mycoplasma pneumoniae*
- Surgery
- Upper respiratory infection
- Virus
  - Cytomegalovirus
  - Epstein-Barr virus
  - Varicella-zoster virus
- Vaccination
  - Flu
  - Group A *Streptococcus*
  - Rabies
- Drugs
  - Captopril
  - Danazol
  - Penicillamine
- Systemic lupus erythematosus
- Hodgkin's disease

Chart 46-1 KEY FEATURES

Guillain-Barré Syndrome

MOTOR MANIFESTATIONS

- Ascending symmetric muscle weakness → flaccid paralysis without muscle atrophy
- Decreased or absent deep tendon reflexes (DTRs)
- Respiratory compromise (dyspnea, diminished breath sounds, decreased tidal volume and vital capacity) and respiratory failure
- Loss of bowel and bladder control (less common)
- Ataxia

SENSORY MANIFESTATIONS

- Paresthesias
- Pain (cramping)

CRANIAL NERVE MANIFESTATIONS

- Facial weakness
- Dysphagia
- Diplopia
- Difficulty speaking

AUTONOMIC MANIFESTATIONS

- Labile blood pressure
- Cardiac dysrhythmias
- Tachycardia

TABLE 46-2 Clinical Variants of Guillain-Barré Syndrome

ASCENDING GBS
- Most common clinical pattern.
- Weakness, paresthesias, and leg pain begin in the lower extremities and progress upward to include the trunk and arms or affect the cranial nerves.
- Symptoms of an ascending flaccidity or weakness that evolves over hours to several days (1 to 10 days).
- Mild paresis to total quadriplegia.
- Some degree of respiratory compromise.
- Deep tendon reflexes are absent in limbs that become paralyzed.

PURE MOTOR GBS
- Identical to the ascending variant except sensory manifestations are absent and the patient is generally in much less pain.

DESCENDING GBS
- Initially experiences weakness of the face or **bulbar** muscles of the jaw, the sternocleidomastoid muscles (head rotators), and the muscles of the tongue, pharynx, and larynx.
- Weakness progresses downward to involve the limbs.
- May quickly affect the respiratory function
  - Breathlessness during speech
  - Shallow respirations
  - Dyspnea
  - Decreased tidal volume
- Often includes **ophthalmoplegia** (paralysis or weakness of the eye muscles), causing diplopia.
- If the papillary response to light is affected, functional blindness may result.
- Numbness is more common in the hands than in the feet.
- Deep tendon reflexes are decreased or absent.

MILLER FISHER VARIANT
- A rare polyneuropathy.
- Triad of ophthalmoplegia, areflexia (absence of reflexes), and severe ataxia (defective muscle coordination).
- Motor strength and sensory function are normal.
- Pupillary response to light is occasionally affected by the ophthalmoplegia, which results in functional blindness.

patient's ability to smile, frown, whistle, or drink from a straw. In addition to monitoring the functions of cranial nerve VII, assess the patient for dysphagia (difficulty swallowing). Less frequently affected cranial nerves include the glossopharyngeal (IX), vagus (X), accessory (XI), and hypoglossal (XII) nerves. The patient's inability to cough, gag, or swallow results from the involvement of cranial nerves IX and X. Monitor the patient closely for varying blood pressure (hypertensive and hypotensive episodes or orthostatic hypotension), bradycardia, heart block and, possibly, asystole. These symptoms are part of *autonomic dysfunction,* which is linked to vagus nerve (X) deficit. Assess cranial nerve XI (accessory) by asking the patient to shrug the shoulders. Hypoglossal nerve (XII) deficit is evidenced by an inability to stick the tongue out straight.

In addition to determining the usual roles and responsibilities, occupation, motivation, and available support systems, assess the patient's ability to cope with this devastating illness and the accompanying fear and anxiety. In general, GBS is self-limiting and the paralysis is temporary. It is not unusual for the patient to have depression throughout the recovery period, though, due to a feeling of powerlessness.

Although no single clinical or laboratory finding confirms the diagnosis of GBS, the health care provider may perform a lumbar puncture (LP) to evaluate *cerebrospinal fluid (CSF).* An increase in CSF protein level without an increase (or only a slight to moderate increase) in cell count is common. However, high protein levels may not occur until after 1 to 2 weeks of illness, reaching a peak in 4 to 6 weeks. The CSF lymphocyte count is normal.

Peripheral blood tests may show a moderate *leukocytosis* early in the illness. The number of leukocytes rapidly returns to normal if there are no complications or concurrent illness.

Electrophysiologic studies (EPSs) demonstrate demyelinating neuropathy. The degree of abnormality found on testing does not always correlate with clinical severity. Within 3 weeks of symptoms, nerve conduction velocities are depressed. In some cases, denervated potentials (fibrillations) develop later in the illness. Electromyographic (EMG) findings, which reflect peripheral nerve function, are normal early in the illness. Electrophysiologic changes appear only after denervation of muscle has been present for 4 weeks or longer. Nerve conduction velocity (NCV) testing is performed with the EMG. Nerve damage or disease may still exist despite normal NCV results. These tests are described in Chapter 43.

A magnetic resonance imaging (MRI) or computed tomography (CT) scan may be requested to rule out other causes of motor weakness. Respiratory function is often compromised in patients with GBS. Therefore vital capacity may be decreased, and arterial blood gas (ABG) values may be abnormal (decreased partial pressure of arterial oxygen [Pao_2], increased partial pressure of arterial carbon dioxide [$Paco_2$], or increased pH).

Common Nursing Diagnoses and Collaborative Problems

The nursing diagnoses that typically apply for patients with GBS include:

1. Ineffective Breathing Pattern, Ineffective Airway Clearance, and Impaired Gas Exchange related to respiratory muscle weakness or paralysis, inability to cough and deep breathe effectively, and immobility
2. Impaired Physical Mobility and Self-Care Deficit related to weakness, paralysis, and ataxia
3. Acute Pain related to paresthesias
4. Impaired Verbal Communication related to intubation or paralysis of the muscles required for speech
5. Powerlessness, Anxiety, and Fear related to the inability to perform ADLs and usual role responsibilities

Interventions

Drug Therapy and Plasmapheresis

The health care provider follows best practice guidelines from the American Academy of Neurology for the treatment of GBS (Cosi & Versino, 2006). These include:

- Treat with either plasma exchange (PE, also known as *plasmapheresis*) *or* immunoglobulin. There is no benefit to combine these treatments.
- Implement PE for nonambulatory adult patients who seek treatment within 4 weeks of the development of symptoms. It is also recommended for ambulatory patients seen within 2 weeks of onset of symptoms.

- Use IV immunoglobulin (IVIG) for ambulatory patients who seek treatment within 2 weeks of onset of symptoms.
- Do not use corticosteroids unless medically necessary to treat other diseases.

Plasmapheresis removes the circulating antibodies thought to be responsible for the disease. In this procedure, plasma is selectively separated from whole blood. The blood cells are returned to the patient without the plasma. Plasma usually replaces itself, or the patient is transfused with colloidal substitute such as albumin. Fresh frozen plasma is generally not used because of the associated risk of infection and allergic pulmonary edema. This procedure should be done within several days after the onset of the illness, although some patients benefit up to 30 days after the onset of symptoms. The patient usually receives three to four treatments, 1 to 2 days apart. Some patients may require a second round of treatment if they deteriorate after the first plasmapheresis.

Nursing interventions for the patient undergoing plasmapheresis include providing information and reassurance, weighing the patient before and after the procedure, and administering proper care to the shunt, if used. Proper shunt care includes:

- Checking for shunt patency
- Assessing for bruits every 2 to 4 hours
- Keeping double bulldog clamps at the bedside
- Observing the puncture site for bleeding or ecchymosis (bruising)

Observe for signs of complications throughout the procedure (Chart 46-2). Atropine is prescribed in case bradycardia (very slow heart rate, usually below 60 beats/min) occurs.

IVIG has been shown to be as effective as plasmapheresis. It is safer and immediately available. Side effects of immunoglobulin therapy range from minor annoyances (e.g., chills, mild fever, myalgia, headache) to major complications (e.g., anaphylaxis, aseptic meningitis, retinal necrosis, acute renal failure). A serum IgA is drawn before administration of the medication. Infuse IVIG slowly when it is started. Observe for side and adverse effects, and report their occurrence to the health care provider. The rate of administration can be increased based on the patient's tolerance and on agency protocol.

Chart 46-2 BEST PRACTICE FOR PATIENT SAFETY & QUALITY CARE

Preventing and Managing Complications of Plasmapheresis

Complication	Nursing Interventions
Trauma or infection at vascular access site	Keep the site clean and dry. Monitor the site for redness, swelling, drainage, or other signs of infection.
Hypovolemia with resultant hypotension, tachycardia, dizziness, and diaphoresis	Monitor fluid and electrolyte status and vital signs. Administer fluids as prescribed. Provide an explanation of side effects, and reassure the patient.
Hypokalemia and hypocalcemia	Monitor fluid and electrolyte balance. Administer replacement electrolytes as prescribed. Observe for cardiac dysrhythmias.
Temporary circumoral and distal extremity paresthesias, muscle twitching, nausea, and vomiting related to administration of citrated plasma	Add calcium gluconate or calcium chloride to exchange fluids as prescribed. Provide explanations, comfort measures, and reassurance.

NIC Monitoring Respiratory Status and Managing the Airway

The priority nursing intervention for the patient with GBS is to maintain adequate respiratory function (Chart 46-3). In the initial phase of the disease, monitor the patient closely (usually in a critical care unit) for signs of respiratory distress, such as dyspnea, air hunger, adventitious breath sounds, decreased oxygen saturation, and cyanosis. In addition, assess respiratory rate, rhythm, and depth every 1 to 2 hours. In collaboration with the respiratory therapist (RT), check vital capacity every 2 to 4 hours and auscultate the lungs at 4-hour intervals. Monitor the patient's ability to cough and swallow for any change. Assess cognitive status, especially in older adults; a decline often indicates hypoxia.

The purpose of *airway management* is to promote airway patency and gas exchange. Elevate the head of the bed to at least 45 degrees or higher as determined by the patient's response and level of dyspnea. The need for suctioning the patient is based on assessment data. During suctioning, the patient is at risk for vagal nerve stimulation that could lead to bradycardia and cardiac arrest. Monitor the color, consistency, and amount of secretions obtained. Chest physiotherapy, often performed by the RT, and frequent position changes are combined with breathing exercises (coughing and deep breathing) to prevent pneumonia and atelectasis. Encourage the patient to use the incentive spirometer to expand the lungs every few hours. Oxygen may be administered by nasal cannula at a flow rate prescribed by the health care provider.

ABG values or end-tidal carbon dioxide are frequently monitored for acid-base abnormalities; pulse oximetry reveals decreasing oxygen saturation. A decrease in vital capacity to less than 15 to 20 mL/kg (or less than two thirds of the patient's normal) and the inability to clear secretions may be indications for elective intubation. *Keep equipment for performing an endotracheal intubation at the bedside, and have a mechanical ventilator readily available in case of respiratory emergency.*

Managing Cardiac Dysfunction

Both the sympathetic and parasympathetic systems may be affected. Place the patient on a cardiac monitor because of the risk for dysrhythmias. Monitor vital signs closely. Hypertension is treated with a beta blocker or nitroprusside (Nitropress). Hypotension is treated with IV fluids and placing the patient in a supine position unless he or she is in extreme respiratory distress. Atropine may be prescribed to treat bradycardia.

Improving Mobility and Preventing Complications of Immobility

Collaborate with the patient, family, physical and occupational therapists (PT/OT), speech-language pathologist (SLP), and nutritionist to develop interventions that prevent complications of immobility and to address deficits in self-care. Assess the patient's motor (muscle) function every 2 to 4 hours as part of the neurologic assessment. The interventions prescribed for mobility and self-management and to prevent complications

Chart 46-3 NIC INTERVENTION ACTIVITIES

The Patient with Guillain-Barré Syndrome

Respiratory Monitoring: Collection and analysis of patient data to ensure airway patency and adequate gas exchange.

- Monitor rate, rhythm, depth, and effort of respirations.
- Monitor breathing patterns: bradypnea, tachypnea, hyperventilation, Kussmaul respirations, Cheyne-Stokes respirations, apneustic breathing, Biot's respiration, and ataxic patterns.
- Auscultate breath sounds, noting areas of decreased/absent ventilation and presence of adventitious sounds.
- Monitor PFT values, particularly vital capacity, maximal inspiratory force, forced expiratory volume in 1 second (FEV_1), and FEV_1/FVC, as available.
- Monitor mechanical ventilator readings, noting increases in inspiratory pressures and decreases in tidal volume, as appropriate.
- Monitor for increased restlessness, anxiety, and air hunger.
- Note changes in Sao_2, Svo_2, end tidal CO_2, and changes in ABG values, as appropriate.
- Monitor patient's ability to cough effectively.
- Monitor for dyspnea and events that decrease and worsen it.
- Monitor chest x-ray reports.
- Place the patient on side, as indicated, to prevent aspiration; log roll if cervical aspiration suspected.
- Institute respiratory therapy treatments (e.g., nebulizer), as needed.

Airway Management: Facilitation of patency of air passages.

- Position patient to maximize ventilation potential.
- Identify patient requiring actual/potential airway insertion.
- Perform chest physical therapy, as appropriate.
- Remove secretions by encouraging coughing or by suctioning.
- Instruct how to cough effectively.
- Auscultate breath sounds, noting areas of decreased or absent ventilation and presence of adventitious sounds.
- Perform endotracheal or nasotracheal suctioning, as appropriate.
- Administer humidified air or oxygen, as appropriate.
- Administer aerosol treatments, as appropriate.
- Administer ultrasonic nebulizer treatments, as appropriate.
- Position to alleviate dyspnea.
- Monitor respiratory and oxygenation status, as appropriate.

NIC intervention activities selected from Bulechek, G.M., Butcher, H.K., McCloskey Dochterman, J. (Eds.). (2008). *Nursing interventions classification (NIC)* (5th ed.). St. Louis: Mosby.

ABG, Arterial blood gas; *CO_2*, carbon dioxide; *FEV_1*, forced expiratory volume in 1 second; *FVC*, forced vital capacity; *PFT*, pulmonary function test; *Sao_2*, arterial oxygen saturation; *Svo2*, venous oxygen saturation.

depend on the degree of motor deficit. The PT and OT provide assistive devices and instructions for their use.

To ensure safety, assist the patient with ambulation, transfers from bed to chair, position changes, and maintenance of proper body alignment until he or she is able to perform these activities independently. Encourage maximum independence. Perform active or passive range-of-motion (ROM) exercises every 2 to 4 hours, or delegate this activity to unlicensed assistive personnel (UAP) with supervision. Teach family members these techniques. (See Chapter 8 for detailed discussion of ways to improve physical mobility and self-care, as well as ways to prevent immobility consequences.) Monitor the patient's responses, including fatigue level. Provide adequate rest periods between activities and therapy sessions.

Decreased gastric motility, dysphagia, and depression can cause malnutrition. Collaborate with the nutritionist to develop an individualized plan. The patient may require little assistance with feeding or may be totally dependent. If he or she cannot safely swallow food or liquids, enteral nutrition via feeding tube is prescribed. Weigh the patient three times a week, and monitor serum prealbumin each week.

Malnutrition places patients at risk for pressure ulcers, especially when they are immobile. Therefore pay special attention to skin care, including interventions to prevent skin breakdown. Instruct UAP to turn the patient a minimum of every 2 hours. Assess the skin for any areas of redness that may lead to pressure ulcers. If the bed does not have a pressure-reducing mattress, use a mattress overlay to help prevent skin breakdown. Document changes in his or her skin condition every 8 to 12 hours while in the acute care setting and at least daily in a transitional care or rehabilitation setting. If an ulcer develops, implement aggressive interventions to manage the wound. Chapters 8 and 27 discuss pressure ulcer care in detail.

Because pulmonary emboli and deep vein thromboses are common complications of immobility, the health care provider may prescribe prophylactic anticoagulant therapy, such as subcutaneous heparin or Lovenox. Antiembolism stockings and sequential compression stockings may be used to promote venous return. Be sure that stockings are removed at least once every 24 hours for 15 to 30 minutes. Other prevention measures are determined by agency policy or health care provider preference. Chapter 8 describes additional interventions to prevent complications of immobility and promote self-care.

Managing Pain

Assess the severity and nature of the patient's pain, which is often worse at night. The patient may have paresthesia or hyperesthesia (extreme sensitivity to touch), deep muscle aches, and muscle stiffness. The typical pain experienced is often not relieved by medications other than opiates, which can be administered via a patient-controlled analgesia (PCA) pump or continuous IV drip. Other drugs that are given include gabapentin (Neurontin) or tricyclic antidepressants. *Older adults should not receive tricyclic drugs because they cause serious side effects such as urinary retention and blurred vision.* Document the patient's response to pain medication, and notify the health care provider if pain relief is not sufficient. Other pain control measures include frequent repositioning, massage, ice, heat, relaxation techniques, guided imagery, hypnosis, and distractions (e.g., music, visitors). Chapter 5 discusses these modalities and other pain-relief measures in detail.

Promoting Communication

The patient may have difficulty communicating because the muscles required for the production of speech are weak, or he or she may be mechanically ventilated because the respiratory muscles are paralyzed. In either case, collaborate with the speech-language pathologist to develop a communication system. A simple technique involves eye blinking or moving a finger to indicate "yes" and "no." A communication board or flash cards can be used with the letters of the alphabet or a list of common requests, such as the need to be repositioned or the need for pain medication. Computer or personal digital assistant (PDA) technology may also be used. Both the staff and the visitors must know how the patient's communication system operates.

Providing Emotional Support

Teach the patient and family about the illness, and explain all diagnostic tests and treatments. Assess the patient and family for verbal and nonverbal behaviors that indicate powerlessness, anxiety, fear, and grieving. Encourage the patient to verbalize feelings about the illness and its effects, if possible, while fostering hope. Assess previous decision-making patterns, roles, and responsibilities. Ask the patient and family to describe their usual lifestyles and the situations in which they coped effectively to help identify personal factors that influence coping ability.

Refer patients who need further psychosocial support to the social worker, certified hospital chaplain or appropriate spiritual resource, and local support groups. If necessary, obtain a psychological consultation for further evaluation and intervention.

Community-Based Care

The severity and course of Guillain-Barré syndrome (GBS) are extremely variable, which makes the prognosis difficult to predict. The most likely residual deficits at discharge are related to motor status and mobility, self-management, and possibly sensory alteration and disturbed self-concept. For patients who have total quadriparesis (weakness in all four extremities) or respiratory paralysis, the course of the rehabilitation phase is even more variable and may require weeks to years. The expected outcome of the recovery phase is to move from dependence to independence, if possible.

Planning for discharge begins on admission. The patient may be discharged to home or to a rehabilitation unit. In collaboration with the discharge planner or case manager (CM), the nurse makes appropriate referrals to a rehabilitation setting, home care agency, and/or community agencies for assistance in the home setting after discharge.

Include a family member in the education process throughout the patient's hospitalization and in the discharge process. Provide them with both oral and written instructions to improve mobility, use adaptive-assistive devices, and prevent skin breakdown.

If the patient is discharged to home while still needing assistive devices, the CM in collaboration with the interdisciplinary health care team makes certain that the necessary equipment has been delivered after evaluating the home setting. Home care management for patients with GBS is similar to that for those who have had a stroke or spinal cord injury, depending on the nature of the neurologic deficit.

Self-help and support groups for patients with chronic illness are common. Refer the patient and family to these groups, if indicated. For example, the Guillain-Barré Foundation International (www.gbsi.com) provides resources and information for patients and their families. The psychosocial adjustment needed may be minimal or dramatic, depending on the patient's residual deficit, age, gender, usual roles and responsibilities, usual coping strategies, available support systems, and occupation. Help the patient identify other support systems, such as church members, friends, or spiritual resources.

MYASTHENIA GRAVIS

Pathophysiology

Myasthenia gravis (MG) is a chronic disease characterized by fatigue and weakness primarily in muscles innervated by the cranial nerves, as well as in skeletal and respiratory muscles. This autoimmune disease of the neuromuscular junction may take many forms—from mild disturbances of the ocular muscles to a rapidly developing, generalized weakness that may lead to death from respiratory failure. It has remissions and exacerbations (worsening or "flare-ups"). The peak age at onset is between 20 and 30 years. Women are affected three times more often than are men (www.myasthenia.org).

MG is caused by an autoantibody attack on the acetylcholine receptors (AChR) in the muscle end plate membranes. As a result, nerve impulses are not transmitted to the skeletal muscle at the neuromuscular junction, and the muscles cannot contract.

Although the disease is not hereditary, there is a small familial incidence. Evidence also suggests a relationship between MG and hyperplasia (overgrowth) of the thymus gland. The thymus gland is often abnormal. **Thymoma** (encapsulated thymus gland tumor) occurs in a few cases, but most of the remaining cases show hyperplasia of the thymus. There is also a very strong association between MG and hyperthyroidism. D-penicillamine, interferon-alpha, and bone marrow transplantation have been associated with drug-induced (iatrogenic) autoimmune MG.

Patient-Centered Collaborative Care

▪ *Assessment*

Physical Assessment/Clinical Manifestations

Although the onset of MG is usually insidious (slow), some instances of fairly rapid development have been caused by infection, emotional upset, pregnancy, or anesthesia. Ask about any history of these events. A temporary increase in weakness may be noted after vaccination, menstruation, and exposure to extremes in environmental temperature.

In addition to the biographic data and history, ask the patient if he or she noticed the rapid onset of fatigue. Note reports of muscle weakness that increases on exertion or as the day wears on and improves with rest. Ask the patient to describe his or her symptoms, specifically noting the affected muscle groups and any limitation or inability in performing ADLs.

Additional areas of inquiry include any history of **ptosis** (drooping eyelids), **diplopia** (double vision), or **dysphagia** (difficulty chewing or swallowing) and the type of diet best tolerated. Assess the patient about a history of respiratory difficulty, choking, or voice weakness. Other areas of assessment include asking about any difficulty holding up the head, brushing teeth, combing hair, or shaving. Inquiry is made about the presence of paresthesias or aching in weakened muscles. Finally, ask about a history of thymus gland tumor.

The most common symptoms are related to involvement of the levator palpebrae or extraocular muscles (Chart 46-4). Assess for ptosis, diplopia, and weak or incomplete eye clo-

Chart 46-4 KEY FEATURES

Myasthenia Gravis

MOTOR MANIFESTATIONS

- Progressive muscle weakness (proximal) that usually improves with rest
- Poor posture
- Ocular palsies
- Ptosis
- Weak or incomplete eye closure
- Diplopia
- Respiratory compromise
- Loss of bowel and bladder control
- Fatigue

SENSORY MANIFESTATIONS

- Muscle achiness
- Paresthesias
- Decreased smell and taste

sure. These symptoms may last only a few days at the onset and then resolve, only to return weeks or months later. Pupillary responses to light and accommodation are usually normal.

For most patients, the muscles of facial expression, chewing, and speech are affected (**bulbar** involvement). Note the patient's smile, which may be transformed into a snarl. The jaw may hang so that the patient must prop it up with the hand. Chewing and swallowing difficulties, choking, and regurgitation of fluids through the nose may lead to considerable weight loss. Ask about the patient's nutritional intake and any recent weight loss. He or she may have more difficulty eating after talking. After extended conversations, the voice may become weaker or exhibit a nasal twang. In some patients, the tongue has fissures (ulcers).

Less often involved are the muscles of the shoulders, the flexors of the neck, and the hip flexors. Because limb weakness is more often *proximal* (closer to the body), the patient may have difficulty climbing stairs, lifting heavy objects, or raising the arms overhead. Neck weakness may be mild or severe enough to cause difficulty in holding the head erect. Among the trunk muscles, the erector spinae are most commonly affected. This results in difficulty maintaining a sitting or walking posture.

In the most advanced cases of MG, all muscles are weakened, including those associated with respiratory function and the control of bladder and bowel function. In these severe cases, ask about bowel and bladder function. Assess respiratory function frequently.

Muscle atrophy, although rarely severe, occurs in a small percentage of patients with myasthenia gravis (MG). The tendon reflexes should be assessed, but they are not often affected. Assess for pain, although this is seldom a major concern. Some patients report that their weakened muscles ache. If present, paresthesias (painful tingling sensations) affecting the muscles of the face, hands, and thighs are not associated with any loss of sensation. Lost or decreased sensations of smell and taste have been reported. Consciousness is not altered.

In **Eaton-Lambert syndrome,** a form of myasthenia often seen with small cell carcinoma of the lung, the muscles of the trunk and the pelvic and shoulder girdles are most commonly affected. Although weakness increases after exertion, muscle strength may temporarily increase during the first few contractions, followed by rapid decline. Diagnosis is confirmed by electromyography (EMG). Management differs somewhat from that of other types of MG. Treatment includes removing the tumor, managing the cancer, and administering drug therapy to release acetylcholine (ACh). Additional therapies may include plasmapheresis and immunosuppressive therapy (discussed later).

Other Diagnostic Assessment

Because the incidence of MG is rare, diagnosis may be delayed or missed. An experienced clinician can diagnose the disease from the history and physical examination findings. MG may be immediately confirmed by the patient's response to cholinergic drugs. A standard series of laboratory studies is usually performed for patients with known or suspected MG. *Thyroid function* should be tested because **thyrotoxicosis** (excessive thyroid hormone) is present in a small number of myasthenic patients. *Serum protein electrophoresis* evaluates the patient for immunologic disorders. Immunologic-based diseases, such as rheumatoid arthritis, systemic lupus erythematosus, and polymyositis, are associated with the disease.

Testing for *acetylcholine receptor (AChR) antibodies* has become an important diagnostic criterion, because they are elevated in most patients with MG. A positive antibody test result confirms the diagnosis, but a negative finding does not rule out the disease.

Some patients with MG have a thymoma, and therefore patients are assessed for this condition. The thymus, an H-shaped gland located in the upper mediastinum beneath the sternum, is one organ in which AChR antibodies are formed. Although a thymoma can often be seen on routine frontal and lateral chest *x-rays,* a *CT scan* is also done.

Tensilon Testing. Pharmacologic tests with the cholinesterase inhibitors *edrophonium chloride (Tensilon)* and *neostigmine bromide (Prostigmin)* may be performed. Tensilon is used most often for testing because of its rapid onset and brief duration of action. This drug inhibits the breakdown of ACh at the postsynaptic membrane, which increases the availability of ACh for excitation of postsynaptic receptors. To perform the test, the physician first estimates the strength of cranial muscles. Initially, 2 mg (0.2 mL) is injected IV; if this is tolerated, an additional 8 mg (0.8 mL) is injected after 30 seconds. Within 30 to 60 seconds of the first dose, most myasthenic patients show a marked improvement in muscle tone that lasts 4 to 5 minutes. False-positive test results may be caused by increased muscle effort by the patient. False-negative findings may be seen if the tested muscle is extremely weak or refractory to the drug.

Tensilon testing may also be used to help determine whether increasing weakness in the previously diagnosed myasthenic patient is due to a **cholinergic crisis** (too much cholinesterase inhibitor drugs) or a **myasthenic crisis** (too little cholinesterase inhibitor drugs). In a cholinergic crisis, muscle tone does not improve after giving Tensilon. Instead, weakness may actually increase and **fasciculations** (muscle twitching) may be seen around the eyes and face. *The Tensilon test poses a danger of ventricular fibrillation and cardiac arrest, but these reactions rarely occur. Be sure that atropine sulfate, the antidote for Tensilon, is available in case these complications occur.*

Electromyography. A common diagnostic test performed by the physician or technician is electromyography (EMG). Although electrical testing of the normal neuromuscular junction produces no change in the amplitude (force) of muscle contraction, the amplitude of the muscle's response diminishes with progressive stimulation. A decrease in amplitude of more than 10% between the first and fifth responses generally indicates the defective neuromuscular transmission characteristic of, but not unique to, MG. Several muscles may be tested to increase the likelihood of detecting an abnormality. Testing may be performed after exercise or exposure of the muscle to curare or to ischemia.

Single-fiber EMG is even more sensitive in detecting defects of neuromuscular transmission. This test compares the stability of the firing of one muscle fiber with that of another fiber innervated by the same motor neuron. The time interval between the two firings normally shows a minor degree of variability, called *jitter.* Defective transmission increases jitter or actually blocks successive discharges.

NCLEX EXAMINATION CHALLENGE

The nurse is assessing a client admitted with myasthenia gravis. Which of these focused assessment findings are likely to be present in clients with this disease? (Select all that apply.)

A. Ascending paralysis
B. Ptosis
C. Dysphagia
D. Distal muscle weakness
E. Hypertension
F. Dysarthria

evolve For the correct answer, go to http://evolve.elsevier.com/Iggy/.

Common Nursing Diagnoses and Collaborative Problems

Nursing diagnoses that typically apply to patients with myasthenia gravis include:

- Risk for Ineffective Breathing Pattern and Ineffective Airway Clearance related to intercostal muscle weakness
- Self-Care Deficit related to fatigue and muscle weakness
- Activity Intolerance related to fatigue
- Impaired Verbal Communication related to muscle weakness

Interventions

The classic presentation of MG is muscle weakness that increases when the patient is fatigued and limits his or her *mobility* and ability to participate in activities. Management for this disease fall into two categories:

- Treatment that affects the symptoms of MG without influencing the actual course of the disease (anticholinesterases or cholinergic drugs)
- Therapeutic efforts for inducing remission, such as the administration of immunosuppressive drugs or corticosteroids, plasmapheresis, and thymectomy (removal of the thymus gland)

Nonsurgical Management

Although not all patients with MG have respiratory compromise, ongoing assessment and maintenance of respiratory function are nursing care priorities.

Respiratory Support. Both myasthenic crisis and cholinergic crisis increase muscle weakness and the patient's risk for respiratory compromise. The diaphragm and intercostal muscles may be affected, which inhibits the patient's ability to maintain adequate ventilation, breathe deeply, and cough effectively. In addition, dysphagia may result in the aspiration of foods, fluids, or saliva, which worsens the respiratory problems. Because of their respiratory muscle involvement, many of these patients have an increased risk of lung infections.

The patient who cannot cough effectively may require oropharyngeal or nasopharyngeal suctioning. If needed, teach the assisted-cough technique, similar to that used by patients who are quadriplegic. Collaborate with the respiratory therapist (RT) to provide chest physiotherapy consisting of postural drainage, percussion, and vibration to mobilize secretions. *Keep a manual resuscitation (breathing) bag (e.g., Ambu), equipment for oxygen administration, and endotracheal intubation equipment at the bedside in case of respiratory distress!*

Because breathing difficulty or the inability to breathe easily is frightening, be aware of the patient's mental and emotional status during periods of respiratory compromise. Monitor his or her response to drug therapy for muscle weakness. Monitor for pulmonary congestion that can lead to respiratory complications like pneumonia and atelectasis.

As an alternative to mechanical ventilation, BIPAP (bi-level positive airway pressure) should be tried first in patients with acute respiratory failure from MG crisis while awaiting improvement from IV immunoglobulin (IVIG) therapy or plasma exchange. Repeat blood gas measurements and clinical assessment after using the device for a few hours are used to determine its effects.

Promoting Mobility. Assess the patient's muscle strength before and after periods of activity. Provide assistance as necessary to prevent the patient from becoming fatigued. Schedule him or her for tests, treatments, and other activities early in the day or during the energy peaks after giving the prescribed drugs. Assist the patient in planning the periods of rest necessary for avoiding excess fatigue.

During periods of maximum weakness, provide assistance for ambulation, transfers from bed to chair or toilet/commode, position changes, and maintenance of body alignment. Active or passive ROM exercises are performed every 2 to 4 hours with assistance of the nurse, UAP, or family. Assess bony prominences for skin breakdown at least every 2 hours. Teach family members how to perform this skill. Pressure-reducing devices or mattresses are used to help prevent pressure ulcers. Collaborate with the physical and occupational therapists to develop a program for the patient to assist with mobility, self-care, and energy conservation techniques. Chapter 8 discusses other interventions for preventing complications of immobility.

Drug Therapy. Two groups of drugs are typically prescribed for the treatment of myasthenia gravis (MG): anticholinesterases and immunosuppressants. *Give these medications on time to maintain blood levels and thus improve muscle strength.* Monitor and document the patient's response to drug therapy. Provide information for the patient and the family about the indications for, effectiveness of, and side effects of the drugs used in the treatment of MG.

Cholinesterase Inhibitor Drugs. *Cholinesterase (ChE) inhibitor drugs are the first-line management of MG.* These drugs are also referred to as *anticholinesterase drugs* or *antimyasthenics.* They enhance neuromuscular impulse transmission by preventing the decrease of ACh by the enzyme *ChE.* This increases the response of the muscles to nerve impulses and improves muscle strength. The ChE inhibitor drug of choice is pyridostigmine (Mestinon, Regonol). Expect day-to-day variations in dosage depending on the patient's changing symptoms.

Administer ChE inhibitors with a small amount of food to help alleviate GI side effects. *Instruct the patient to eat meals 45 minutes to 1 hour after taking these drugs to avoid aspiration. This is very important if the patient has bulbar involvement.* Drugs containing magnesium, morphine or its derivatives, curare, quinine, quinidine, procainamide, or hypnotics or sedatives should be avoided because they may increase the patient's weakness. Antibiotics such as neomycin, kanamycin, polymyxin B, and certain tetracyclines impair transmitter release and also increase myasthenic symptoms.

A potential adverse effect of ChE inhibitors is cholinergic crisis. Sudden increases in weakness and the inability to clear secretions, swallow, or breathe adequately indicate that the patient is experiencing crisis. Teach the patient and family to monitor for these two types of crises:

1. Myasthenic crisis—an exacerbation (flare-up or worsening) of the myasthenic symptoms caused by not enough anticholinesterase drugs
2. Cholinergic crisis—an acute exacerbation of muscle weakness caused by too many anticholinesterase drugs

Because myasthenic and cholinergic crises have many common characteristics, the type of crisis the patient is experiencing must be identified for effective treatment to be provided (Table 46-3). Monitor carefully for early detection of these emergencies if the patient is in a health care setting.

Emergency care: myasthenic crisis. Myasthenic crisis is often caused by some type of infection. For other patients, increasing muscle weakness leads to an overdose of anticholinesterase drugs. As a result, the patient may experience a *mixed* crisis. The Tensilon test (described on p. 1017), although not always conclusive, is an important procedure for differentiation. *Tensilon produces a temporary improvement in myasthenic crisis but no improvement or worsening of symptoms in cholinergic crisis.*

The priority for nursing management of the patient in myasthenic crisis is maintaining adequate respiratory function. The acutely ill patient may need intensive nursing care for monitoring and maintenance of body functions. He or she may require mechanical ventilation. Cholinesterase-inhibiting drugs are withheld because they increase respiratory secretions and are usually ineffective for the first few days after the crisis begins. Drug therapy is restarted gradually and at lower dosages.

Emergency care: cholinergic crisis. In *cholinergic* crisis, do not give anticholinergic drugs while the patient is maintained with mechanical ventilation. Atropine 1 mg IV may be given and repeated, if necessary. When atropine is prescribed, observe the patient carefully. Secretions can be thickened by the drug, which causes more difficulty with airway clearance and possibly the development of mucous plugs. Unless complications such as pneumonia or aspiration develop, the patient in crisis improves rapidly after the appropriate drugs have been given. Continue to provide assistance as necessary because he or she tires easily after minimal exertion.

Immunosuppression. Immunosuppression may be accomplished with the use of corticosteroids or chemotherapeutic agents. Prednisone is given initially to produce remission and to control and improve symptoms. The drug is tapered over a period of weeks to months. Some patients may need continuous low-dose therapy because of exacerbations of symptoms. For ocular MG, corticosteroid treatment that does not cause significant systemic complications may significantly reduce the prevalence of generalized myasthenia gravis after 2 years on the drug. IV immunoglobulins (IVIG) may also be used for acute disease management or as a long-term option for disease refractory to other treatment.

Plasmapheresis. **Plasmapheresis** is a method by which antibodies are removed from the plasma to decrease symptoms. Six exchanges occur over a 2-week period with follow-up exchanges weekly or monthly as needed. This procedure is usually done on an ambulatory care basis. Nursing management of the patient undergoing plasmapheresis is presented in the earlier discussion of Guillain-Barré syndrome, p. 1014.

Promoting Self-Care. Generalized weakness and fatigue affect the patient's ability to participate in ADLs. Impaired fine motor control and shoulder weakness, which results in difficulty raising the arms, can compound the problem. Self-care deficits may be complete or partial depending on the severity of the illness, the patient's response to drugs, and his or her ability to tolerate activity without excessive fatigue.

To establish limitations, assess the patient's ability to perform ADLs. Although he or she is encouraged to perform activities as independently as possible, assistance is provided as needed to avoid frustration and fatigue. *For maximizing independence and making attempts at self-management suc-*

TABLE 46-3 Characteristics of Myasthenic and Cholinergic Crises

Myasthenic Crisis	Cholinergic Crisis	Mixed Crisis
Increased pulse and respiration	Nausea	Apprehension
Rise in blood pressure	Vomiting	Restlessness
Anoxia	Diarrhea	Dyspnea
Cyanosis	Abdominal cramps	Dysphagia (difficult swallowing)
Bowel and bladder incontinence	Blurred vision	Dysarthria (painful joints)
Decreased urine output	Pallor	Increased lacrimation (tearing)
Absence of cough and swallow reflex	Facial muscle twitching	Increased salivation
	Pupillary miosis	Diaphoresis
	Hypotension	Generalized weakness

cessful, plan activities to follow the administration of medication. Monitor and document the patient's response to or tolerance of activity, providing alternating periods of activity and rest. *Rest is critical because increased fatigue can precipitate a crisis.* In addition, occupational and physical therapists evaluate him or her for assistive-adaptive devices. In collaboration with the nurse, they teach the patient and family energy conservation techniques and ideas for making work and self-management easier after discharge from the hospital.

Assisting with Communication. Weakness of the speech and facial muscles often results in dysarthric (slurred) and nasal speech. Thus it may be difficult for myasthenic patients to make their speech understood by others.

In collaboration with the speech-language pathologist (SLP), determine the patient's ability to communicate. Instruct the patient to speak slowly while attempting to lip-read. Repeat what the patient says to check that it is correct. Questions that can be answered with "yes" or "no" or by gestures may be used along with other communication systems such as eye blinking, notebook and pencil, computer, PDA, and picture, letter, or word boards.

Providing Nutritional Support. The patient with myasthenia gravis (MG) may have difficulty maintaining an adequate intake of food and fluid because the muscles needed for chewing and swallowing become weakened and tire easily. In collaboration with the nutritionist, occupational therapist, and speech-language pathologist, evaluate the patient's nutritional status and his or her ability to receive adequate oral nutrition. Small, frequent meals and high-calorie snacks are often well tolerated. Monitor the effectiveness of the nutrition program by recording the patient's calorie counts, intake and output, serum prealbumin levels, and daily weights (Chart 46-5). If he or she cannot swallow, a feeding tube may be used.

Maintaining Eye Protection. The patient's inability to completely close the eyes may lead to corneal abrasions and further decrease vision and comfort. During the day, apply artificial tears to keep the corneas moist and free from abrasion. A lubricant gel and shield may be applied to the eyes at bedtime to provide more extensive coverage. To help relieve diplopia, cover the eyes with a patch for 2 to 3 hours at a time, one eye at a time. At times, patients tape their eyes shut at night.

Chart 46-5 BEST PRACTICE FOR PATIENT SAFETY & QUALITY CARE

Improving Nutrition in Patients with Myasthenia Gravis

- Assess the patient's gag reflex and ability to chew and swallow.
- Provide frequent oral hygiene as needed.
- Collaborate with the nutritionist, speech-language pathologist, and occupational therapist to plan and implement meals that the patient can eat and enjoy.
- Offer small, frequent meals.
- Cut food into small bites, and encourage the patient to eat slowly.
- Observe patient for choking, nasal regurgitation, and aspiration.
- Provide high-calorie snacks or supplements (e.g., puddings).
- Keep the head of the bed elevated during meals and for 30 to 60 minutes after the patient eats.
- Avoid liquids because they can easily cause choking and aspiration; provide a soft diet.
- Monitor food intake carefully.
- Weigh the patient daily.
- Monitor serum prealbumin levels.
- Administer anticholinesterase drugs, as prescribed: 45 to 60 minutes before meals.

Surgical Management

For patients with MG, **thymectomy** (removal of the thymus gland) is usually performed early in the disease. The procedure is not always immediately effective, and it may take several years for remission to occur—if it occurs at all. Those who have surgery within 2 years of the onset of myasthenic symptoms show the most improvement.

Provide routine preoperative care as discussed in Chapter 16. Because there is no way to predict whether remission or improvement will occur, it is important to avoid making promises, but be optimistic. Immediately before surgery, pyridostigmine (Mestinon) may be given with a small amount of water to keep the patient stable during and after surgery. If steroids have been used, they are also given before surgery and are tapered during the postoperative period. Antibiotics are administered immediately before or during the surgery. Plasmapheresis may be used before and after surgery to decrease circulating antibodies more quickly.

One of two surgical approaches may be used: the transcervical incision (minimal access technique) or the sternal split. The *transcervical approach* is becoming more popular because it allows more rapid recovery with less discomfort after surgery, especially if done using the video-assisted thoracoscopic (VATS) technique (Maat, 2008). However, this procedure is used only for patients who do not have a thymoma. Only a small dressing and an IV line are needed after surgery.

The older *sternal split* procedure is preferred when patients have a thymoma. It allows the surgeon to directly see the mediastinum and areas around the thymus. When thymoma is present, all surrounding involved structures (i.e., the pericardium, the innominate vein, a portion of the superior vena cava, and a portion of the lung) are removed. A single chest tube is placed in the anterior mediastinum. The patient is usually admitted to the critical care unit after surgery. Thymoma should be considered as a potentially malignant tumor requiring prolonged follow-up. The presence of myasthenic weakness can still complicate its management.

Although patients with adequate respiratory function may be extubated immediately after surgery, most require a gradual weaning from the ventilator. Prolonged ventilatory assistance is rare. *After the patient is extubated, pay special attention to pulmonary hygiene.* Suctioning is performed as necessary. Encourage the patient to turn, cough, and breathe deeply and to use incentive spirometry every 2 hours. *In addition to monitoring respiratory function and providing bronchial hygiene, observe for signs of pneumothorax or hemothorax, such as:*

- *Chest pain*
- *Sudden shortness of breath*
- *Diminished or delayed chest wall expansion*
- *Diminished or absent breath sounds*
- *Restlessness or a change in vital signs (decreasing blood pressure or a weak, rapid pulse)*

Report any of these signs and symptoms to the surgeon immediately! Provide oxygen to the patient, and raise the head of the bed to at least 45 degrees.

For the sternal surgical technique, provide chest tube care (see Chapter 34). Both surgical approaches require sterile technique for wound care. Observe the patient for signs of infection, such as increasing or purulent drainage; redness, warmth, or swelling around the wound; and elevated temperature. Patient and family teaching is needed about follow-up care before discharge from the hospital.

NCLEX EXAMINATION CHALLENGE

When caring for a client with myasthenia gravis, which of these nursing activities may be safely delegated to a nursing assistant? (Select all that apply.)

A. Feeding dinner to the client
B. Teaching the family about drug therapy
C. Assisting with client communication
D. Consulting with the physical therapist
E. Assisting with ambulation
F. Recording food and fluid intake

evolve For the correct answer, go to http://evolve.elsevier.com/Iggy/.

Community-Based Care

The patient with myasthenia gravis (MG) may be cared for in a variety of settings, including the home, transitional care, rehabilitation setting, or long-term care facility. The patient discharged from the hospital may be weak and may require the assistance of a family member, home care nurse, physical therapist, occupational therapist (OT), and/or home care aide.

Home Care Management

Patients with MG are often managed at home. They are hospitalized for diagnostic evaluation, myasthenic or cholinergic crisis resulting in respiratory failure, or periods of exacerbation when respiratory function is threatened.

Unless the patient requires assistive devices, little preparation of the home setting is required. In collaboration with physical and occupational therapists, the case manager (CM) and nurse make certain that the necessary equipment has been delivered and properly installed. In addition, they teach the patient and family members how to use the equipment safely. If the patient becomes wheelchair dependent, the discharge planner, CM, or OT checks on any necessary modifications to the home (e.g., the installation of ramps or widening of doorways) that have been completed. The health care team must make sure that all of the patient's continuing care needs can be met wherever he or she is transferred after discharge from the hospital.

Health Teaching

The more the patient and family know about the disease and the drugs used for treatment, the less likely it is that complications will develop. Encourage the patient and the family to ask questions. Discuss the episodic nature of the disease, including factors that increase the risk for exacerbation, such as infection, stress, surgery, hard physical exercise, sedatives, and enemas or strong cathartics (Table 46-4). Teach the patient the importance of collaborating with the health care team to monitor muscle strength, ability to perform ADLs, and the need to adjust drug therapy.

Stress the importance of lifestyle adaptations such as avoiding heat (e.g., sauna, hot tubs, sunbathing), crowds, overeating, erratic changes in sleep habits, or emotional extremes. Teach the signs of exacerbation, such as increased weakness, increased diplopia, ptosis, and problems with chewing or swallowing. Remind the patient to plan activities to allow for rest periods and to conserve energy.

TABLE 46-4 Factors Precipitating or Worsening Myasthenia Gravis

- Various drugs, including:
  - Strong cathartics
  - Antidysrhythmics
  - Beta-blocking agents
  - Antibiotics
  - Antirheumatic drugs
  - Antispasmodics
  - Antihistamines
  - Opioids
  - Phenytoin (Dilantin)
  - Antidepressants (tricyclics)
- Rheumatoid arthritis
- Alcohol
- Hormonal changes
- Stress
- Infection
- Seasonal temperature changes
- Heat
- Surgery
- Enemas

Provide the drug regimen in a written format that includes the names, purposes, dosages, scheduled dosage times, and side effects of the drugs. Explain that the drugs are normally taken before activities such as eating, participating in sports, or working. Stress the importance of maintaining therapeutic blood levels by taking the medications on time and as prescribed and not missing or postponing doses (Chart 46-6). In addition, inform the patient of the side effects of anticholinesterase drugs. Advise him or her to avoid drugs such as morphine, curare, quinine, quinidine, procainamide, mycin-type antibiotics, and drugs containing magnesium. In preparing the patient for discharge, explain the signs and symptoms of myasthenic and cholinergic crises and the need to contact the physician or other health care professional whenever either type of crisis is suspected. *Because respiratory compromise often occurs in myasthenic patients, encourage family members to learn resuscitation procedures. A manual resuscitation bag, suctioning equipment, and oxygen should be available in the home for patients susceptible to crises. Teach family members in the proper use of equipment.*

The episodic nature of MG, the potential or actual loss of independence, and body image changes (e.g., the inability to smile) affect the patient's adjustment. During discharge planning, the CM considers factors such as age, gender, usual roles and responsibilities, available support systems, occupation, and financial status. Because the patient's and family's need for psychosocial adjustment may range from minimal to dramatic, the CM remains sensitive to their needs and provides information and support. Encourage family members or significant others to discuss their feelings with one another.

Health Care Resources

In collaboration with the health care provider, patient, and family, the staff nurse or CM may initiate referrals to home care agencies and to local self-help groups for people who have chronic illnesses and for their families. The Myasthenia Gravis Foundation (www.myasthenia.org) has education and research programs and provides assistance with financial aid and community resources. Support groups are also available. Teach the patient the importance of obtaining and wearing a medical alert (MedicAlert) bracelet or necklace and to carry identification at all times.

Chart 46-6 PATIENT AND FAMILY EDUCATION GUIDE

Helpful Hints for Teaching Patients with Myasthenia Gravis About Drug Therapy

- Keep prescribed drugs and a glass of water at your bedside if you are weak in the morning.
- Wear a watch with an alarm function (or beeper) to remind you to take your drugs.
- Post your drug schedule so others know it.
- Plan strenuous activities, when possible, when the drug peaks.
- Keep an extra supply of drugs in your car or at work. Be sure they are secured.
- Do not take any over-the-counter drugs without checking with your health care provider.

PERIPHERAL NERVE TRAUMA

Pathophysiology

The peripheral nerves are subject to injuries associated with mechanical or vehicular accidents, sports, the injection of particular drugs, military conflicts or wars, and acts of violence (e.g., knife or gunshot wounds). Specific mechanisms of injury include:

- Partial or complete severance of a nerve or nerves
- Contusion, stretching, constriction, or compression of a nerve or nerves
- Ischemia to nerves
- Electrical, thermal, or radiation injury to one or more nerves

Most commonly affected are the median, ulnar, and radial nerves of the arms and the peroneal, femoral, and sciatic nerves of the legs (Fig. 46-1).

After a nerve is cut or damaged, the nerve distal to the injury degenerates and retracts within 24 hours. Motor and sensory dysfunction below the injury coincide with the loss of electrical excitability as the nerve fibers degenerate. Recovery occurs as Schwann cells of the neurilemma regenerate from both the proximal and distal stumps. Dividing mitotically,

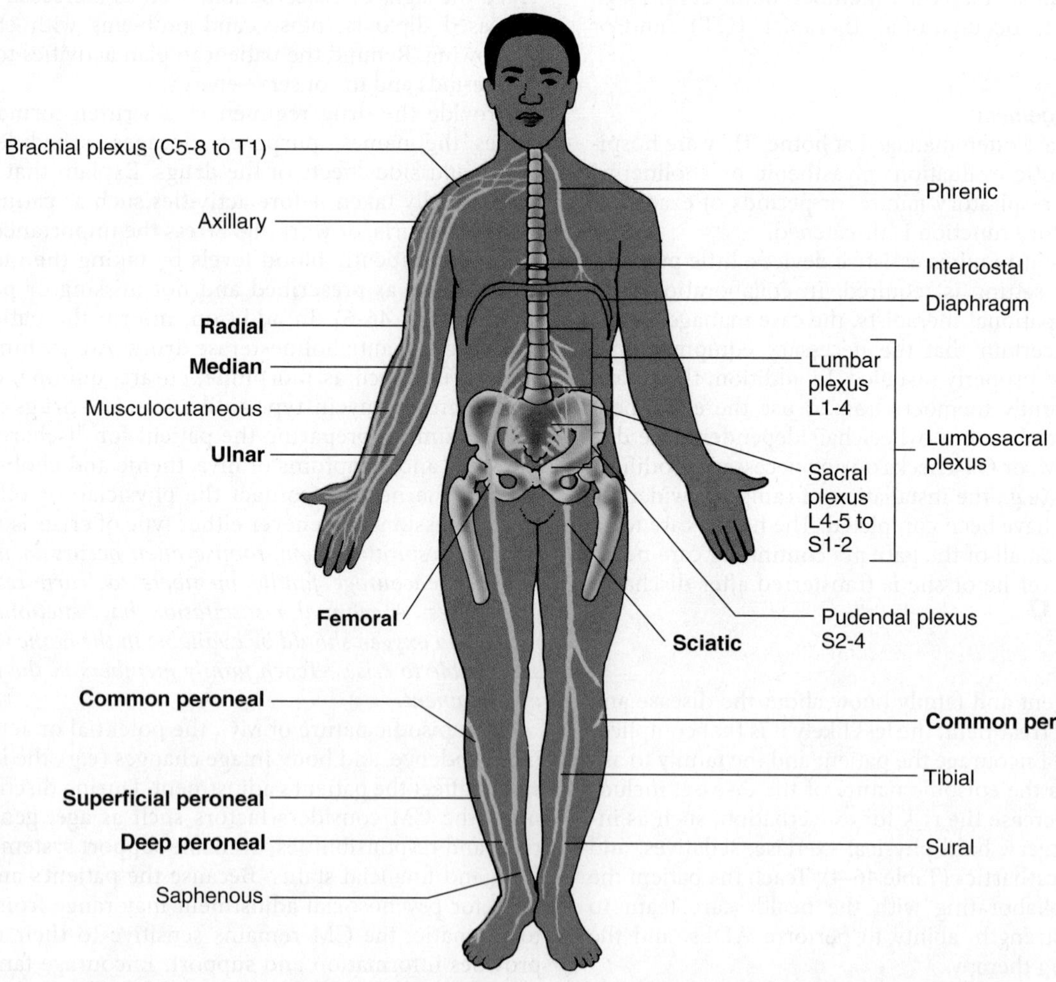
Brachial plexus (C5-8 to T1)
Axillary
Radial
Median
Musculocutaneous
Ulnar
Femoral
Common peroneal
Superficial peroneal
Deep peroneal
Saphenous
Phrenic
Intercostal
Diaphragm
Lumbar plexus L1-4
Lumbosacral plexus
Sacral plexus L4-5 to S1-2
Pudendal plexus S2-4
Sciatic
Common peroneal
Tibial
Sural

Fig. 46-1 • Distribution of selected peripheral nerves in the body. The nerves most commonly affected by trauma are highlighted in bold type.

these cells form neurilemmal cords, which act as guidelines for the regenerating axon. Tiny unmyelinated sprouts are generated at the proximal axon and grow 1 to 4 mm each day. Some can cross the transected gap through guidance by the neurilemma to find their way to the distal stump. The better aligned the union, the more normal the functional return (Fig. 46-2). Reinnervation is always a slow process.

Successfully realigned nerves remyelinate, grow to their former size, and eventually have conduction velocities at most of their former capacity. Successful reinnervation is slowed by infection and increasing age. Disorganization of the nerve or mismatched realignments may result in functional weakness, unintentional muscle movements, and poor sensation.

Some sensory function may return before the regeneration process can occur. This is because nerves above the injured neurons are stimulated to produce collateral innervation to the affected areas. These collaterals occur before the axon has regenerated sufficiently.

Patient-Centered Collaborative Care

Assessment

The patient may relate a history of extremity or pelvic trauma, penetrating injury, recent surgery, or the use of crutches. Peripheral nerve trauma is especially common in wartime combat. In addition to weakness or flaccid *paralysis,* the patient may report *burning sensations* below the trauma or pain that increases with touch or environmental stimulation. Observe for skin and nail changes of the affected extremities.

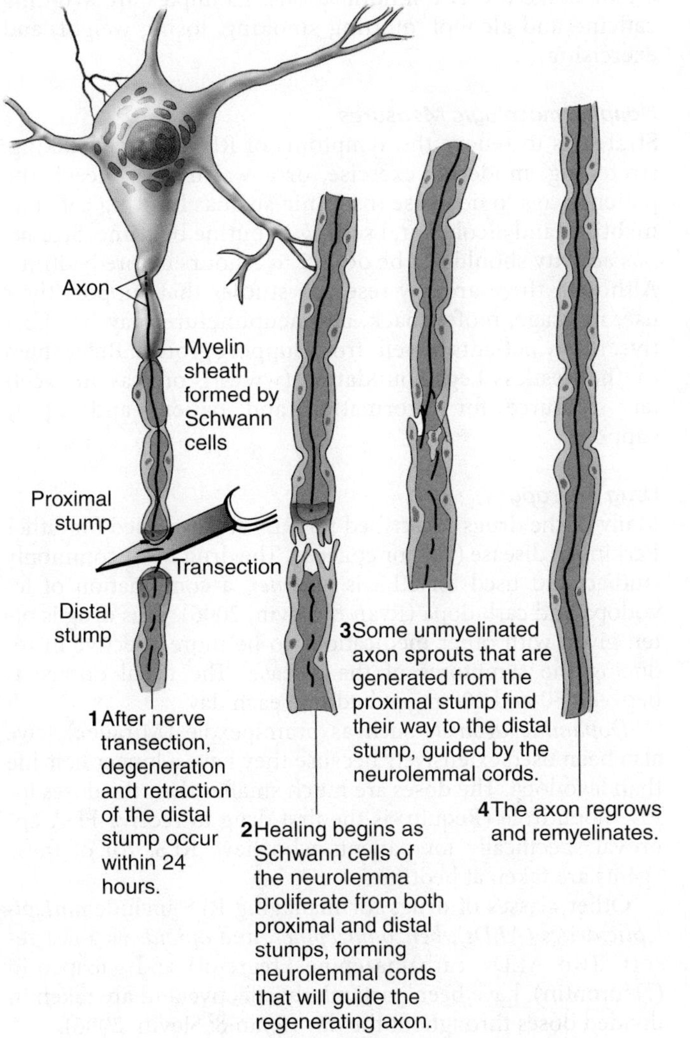
Axon
Myelin sheath formed by Schwann cells
Proximal stump
Transection
Distal stump
1 After nerve transection, degeneration and retraction of the distal stump occur within 24 hours.
2 Healing begins as Schwann cells of the neurolemma proliferate from both proximal and distal stumps, forming neurolemmal cords that will guide the regenerating axon.
3 Some unmyelinated axon sprouts that are generated from the proximal stump find their way to the distal stump, guided by the neurolemmal cords.
4 The axon regrows and remyelinates.

Fig. 46-2 • Regeneration of peripheral nerve after injury.

Perform a physical assessment to determine which neurologic functions are intact. In acute trauma, the injury should first be evaluated by the physician to determine whether movement is contraindicated. If movement is not contraindicated, the patient's motor function is assessed by putting the limb through the normal range of motion. Any abnormal movements, tremor, atrophy, contractions, paresis or paralysis, and weak or absent deep tendon reflexes are documented. Ask the patient about abnormal sensations.

After complete denervation, the extent of vasomotor function is reflected in skin temperature, skin color, and edema. A warm phase and a cold phase have been identified. During the **warm phase,** the extremity is warm and the skin appears flushed or rosy. Over 2 to 3 weeks, this phase is gradually superseded by a **cold phase,** during which the skin appears cyanotic, mottled, or reddish blue and feels cool compared with the unaffected extremity. Use the dorsal surface of the hand to compare skin temperatures because the abundance of temperature receptors in this area provides more accurate assessments. Edema may be noted immediately after injury or later as a result of surgical procedures. Record any evidence of trophic changes (e.g., scaling of skin, brittleness of nails, loss of body hair). This initial assessment serves as the baseline for comparison during subsequent examinations, which are performed every 2 to 4 hours or less frequently as the patient's condition indicates.

Interventions

Interventions for the patient with peripheral nerve trauma depend on the location as well as the type and degree of injury. If the nerve trauma results from a primary lesion, such as a tumor, the underlying problem is addressed first.

The health care provider may prescribe immobilization of the involved area by splint, cast, or traction to provide the rest needed to limit and resolve any inflammation. The purpose of surgical management is to restore the function of the damaged nerve. There are usually no special preoperative interventions for the patient undergoing peripheral nerve repair. Chapter 16 describes the general care of the patient before surgery.

If the nerve is lacerated or transected, surgery may be indicated. Restorative procedures include resecting and suturing to realign the severed nerve ends, nerve grafts, and nerve and tendon transplants.

The timing of procedures to repair nerves has been controversial. In the past, a repair delay of 3 to 8 weeks after injury allowed associated injuries to heal, after which the surgeon could better assess the extent of nerve damage. Although microsurgery and the use of lasers now allow primary nerve repair at the time of injury, the surgeon's judgment in selecting the optimal time and surgical procedure remains crucial.

After an injury, the two severed nerve segments contract and may form scar tissue. Before surgical anastomosis, the surgeon dissects these stumps to remove any damaged nerve tissue. This further decreases the lengths of the ends to be joined. To compensate for this shortening and to avoid excessive tension on the sutured nerve, the involved extremity is positioned in exaggerated flexion. The surgeon aligns the segments under magnification, bringing the nerve fiber ends together, and then sutures the nerve tissue.

After suturing, the extremity is placed in a cast to maintain the flexed position and to avoid tension on the suture line. Ten to 14 days after nerve repair, the entire dressing is removed, the joint flexion is eased, and a new splint may be applied for an additional 2 weeks. At that time, a removable splint may be applied and physical therapy begun. Protection of the nerve sutures is continued for a minimum of 6 weeks.

If a large segment of nerve has been damaged and direct anastomosis would be impossible without stretching the nerve, the surgeon may insert a *nerve graft.* Motor and sensory axons may regenerate through the graft, joining the nerve segments through the two sites of anastomosis. The results of grafting are not usually as favorable as with direct reanastomosis. Immobilization by splints or casts to facilitate healing of the surgical sites is essential.

Splints are usually held in place with elastic wrapping or hook-and-loop (Velcro) closures, which can become too tight if edema develops. *Perform frequent neurovascular assessments, including checking the skin around the splints and casts (hourly, initially) for tightness, warmth, and color. If the patient reports discomfort, tingling, or coolness or if the color is blanched, the cast or splint may be too tight (constricted). Inform the physician immediately about constriction and any indication of drainage under a splint or cast.*

Skin care is essential. Atrophy of the epidermis and underlying tissue causes the skin to become more fragile and more susceptible to injury and breakdown. Decreased skin nutrition and vascularity associated with denervation cause delayed healing, which further worsens the problem. Thoroughly examine the skin for evidence of irritation or injury, and assist or instruct the patient to wash and dry the involved areas carefully. If the skin is dry, lanolin or cocoa butter may be used as a lubricant. *Because sensation may be absent or inhibited, teach the patient to protect the involved areas from temperature extremes and other sources of potential trauma.*

Physical or occupational therapy is the major approach for rehabilitation after surgical repair. Reinforce and help the patient perform the exercises learned in these therapy sessions. Because the regeneration of nerves and subsequent return of sensory and motor function may be extremely slow and produce pain, the patient may become discouraged and depressed. If the disability is permanent, he or she needs encouragement and assistance to cope with the changes in body image, self-esteem, and lifestyle.

RESTLESS LEGS SYNDROME

Pathophysiology

Restless legs syndrome (RLS) is characterized by leg paresthesias (burning, prickly sensation) associated with an irresistible urge to move. The most common type is associated with peripheral and central nerve damage in the legs and spinal cord. Many of those affected with *primary RLS* have a positive family history, indicating a possible genetic basis. The incidence is higher in patients who have diabetes mellitus type 2 and chronic kidney disease. Other potential risk factors include:

- Vitamin and mineral deficiencies
- Polyneuropathies
- Peripheral nerve disease
- Advanced age
- Smoking
- Lack of exercise
- Pinched nerve
- Obesity
- Drugs such as lithium, dopamine antagonists, and selective serotonin reuptake inhibitors
- Caffeine and alcohol

Patient-Centered Collaborative Care

Assessment

The patient reports intense burning or "crawling-type" sensations in the legs and therefore feels the need to move them repeatedly. These symptoms are worse in the evening and at night and when the patient is still for a period of time. Patients feel they need to move to relieve the symptoms. Many move their legs periodically while sleeping. For that reason, they often refer to themselves as "night walkers."

Interventions

The management of RLS is symptomatic and involves treating the underlying cause or contributing factor, if known. Both nonpharmacologic measures and drug therapy are used. Teach patients to avoid as many risk factors as possible or make lifestyle modifications. Examples are avoiding caffeine and alcohol, quitting smoking, losing weight, and exercising.

Nonpharmacologic Measures

Strategies to relieve the symptoms of RLS include walking, stretching, moderate exercise, or a warm bath. Teach the patient ways to decrease insomnia such as limiting caffeine, nicotine, and alcohol and setting a routine bedtime. Strenuous activity should not be done 2 to 3 hours before bedtime. Although there are few research studies that support their use, massage, biofeedback, and acupuncture may be effective. Many patients benefit from support groups. Refer them to The Restless Legs Foundation (www.rls.org) as an excellent resource for information and patient and family support.

Drug Therapy

Many of the drugs prescribed for RLS are also used for either Parkinson disease (PD) or epilepsy. The drug most commonly studied and used for RLS is *Sinemet,* a combination of levodopa and carbidopa (Ryan & Slevin, 2006). This drug is often given with other medications to be more effective in reducing the symptoms of the disease. The usual dosage is between 50 and 200 mg at bedtime each day.

Dopamine agonists such as pramipexole (Mirapex) have also been used extensively because they have a longer half-life than levodopa. The doses are much smaller than the doses for PD. Ropinirole (Requip) is the first drug to receive FDA approval specifically for patients who have RLS. All of these agents are taken at bedtime.

Other classes of drugs for managing RLS include *antiepileptic drugs (AEDs), benzodiazepines, and opioids* as a last resort. Two AEDs, carbamazepine (Tegretol) and gabapentin (Neurontin), have been particularly effective and are taken in divided doses throughout the day (Ryan & Slevin, 2006).

DISEASES OF THE CRANIAL NERVES

Patients with cranial nerve disease may be seen in any practice settings. The cranial nerves may be affected in association with other disorders of the nervous system or as a result of trauma. The most common disorders, those affecting cranial nerves V (trigeminal) and VII (facial), are discussed here.

TRIGEMINAL NEURALGIA

Pathophysiology

Trigeminal neuralgia (TN) is also known as *tic douloureux.* It:

- Is a disease that affects the trigeminal, or fifth cranial, nerve
- Occurs more often in people older than 50 years and in women more often than men (Alexander, 2007)
- Causes a specific type of facial pain, which occurs in sudden, intense facial spasms
- Is usually provoked by minimal stimulation of a trigger zone
- Is unilateral (one-sided) and confined to the area innervated by the trigeminal nerve, most often the second and third branches (Fig. 46-3)

Patients younger than 30 years with pain in more than one branch of the trigeminal nerve may be further evaluated to rule out the possibility of a tumor or multiple sclerosis.

The cause of trigeminal neuralgia is thought to be related to impaired inhibitory mechanisms in the brainstem caused by excessive firing of irritated fibers in the trigeminal nerve. In addition, trauma and infection of the teeth, jaw, or ear may be contributing factors.

Patient-Centered Collaborative Care

Assessment

TN is a chronic pain syndrome. It can be categorized into two types of pain: classic and atypical. When describing classic pain, patients use terms such as "excruciating," "sharp," "shooting," "piercing," "burning," and "jabbing." Between bursts of pain, which last from seconds to minutes, there is usually no pain. Often no sensory or motor deficits are found on examination, but the condition can be agonizing for the patient. The fear of precipitating attacks often causes patients to avoid talking, smiling, eating, or attending to hygienic needs such as shaving, washing the face, and brushing the teeth. The pain can cause uncontrollable facial twitching.

The course of trigeminal neuralgia involves bouts of classic pain for several weeks or months followed by spontaneous remissions. The length of these remissions may vary from days to years, but attack-free periods tend to become shorter as the patient grows older. Symptoms rarely disappear permanently.

By contrast, patients describe atypical pain as a continuous burning sensation that involves the entire face. He or she may not have any remission periods. Some patients experience both types of pain (Alexander, 2007).

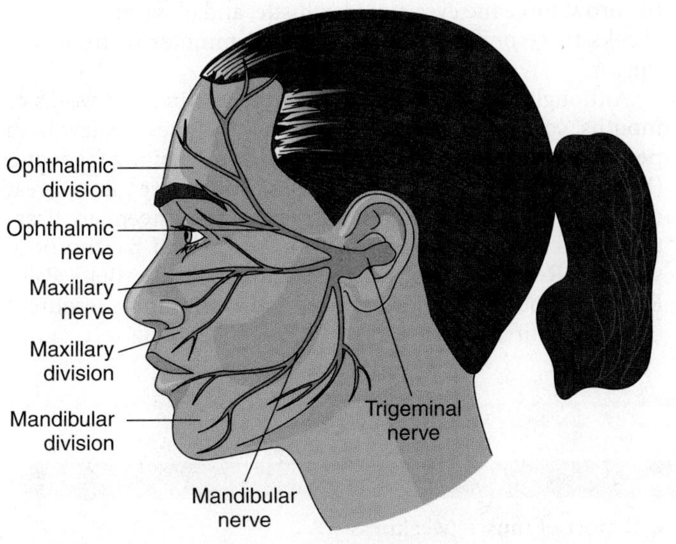
Ophthalmic division
Ophthalmic nerve
Maxillary nerve
Maxillary division
Mandibular division
Trigeminal nerve
Mandibular nerve

Fig. 46-3 • Distribution of the trigeminal nerve and its three divisions: ophthalmic, maxillary, and mandibular.

Interventions

The priority for care of the patient with TN is pain management. Specific interventions are determined by the amount of pain he or she is experiencing. Drug therapy is the first choice, but surgery may be needed for some patients.

Nonsurgical Management

The first choice for drug therapy is antiepileptic drugs, such as carbamazepine (Tegretol) and gabapentin (Neurontin). These drugs are discussed in the Seizures and Epilepsy section in Chapter 44. Muscle relaxants such as baclofen (Lioresal, Kemstro) may also be prescribed. Lidocaine or calcitonin intranasal spray may produce temporary pain relief. Opioids and NSAIDs are not very effective for most patients.

Surgical Management

Surgery is performed if the patient cannot tolerate the side effects of drug therapy or if it is not effective in controlling pain. Surgical procedures include percutaneous stereotactic rhizotomy and microvascular decompression and are performed by a neurosurgeon. Both procedures have a risk for complications such as facial numbness or weakness and recurrence of pain.

In addition to the general preoperative care provided to all patients, the surgeon thoroughly explains the surgical benefits and any expected neurologic deficits. Ensure that the patient understands the procedure to be performed and any risks or complications.

Percutaneous stereotactic rhizotomy (PSR) is performed as an ambulatory care procedure under general anesthesia. The surgeon passes a hollow needle through the inside of the patient's cheek into the trigeminal nerve fibers. A heating current (radiofrequency thermocoagulation) goes through the needle to destroy some of the fibers. The entire nerve is not destroyed. The advantages of this procedure include long-term pain relief, tolerance by older adults, absence of facial paralysis, and preservation of the sensation of touch. Puncturing the internal carotid artery is a possible complication. The affected side is permanently insensitive to pain.

As an option to heat, a balloon microcompression may be performed. The balloon compresses the trigeminal nerve root. A glycerol injection may also be used as an option, but it is not done as commonly as thermocoagulation.

In some patients, a small artery compresses the trigeminal nerve as it enters the pons. Surgical relocation of this artery (**microvascular decompression**) may relieve the pain of TN without compromising facial sensation. This procedure is more invasive, requiring a craniotomy. Though not common, complications include aseptic meningitis, cerebrospinal fluid leak, ataxia, **ipsilateral** (same side) hearing loss, and facial nerve damage. Older adults and patients with other medical problems may not be candidates for this procedure.

In addition to general postoperative care described in Chapter 18, apply an ice pack to the PSR operative site on the cheek and jaw for 3 to 4 hours. Perform a focused cranial nerve assessment to assess whether other nerves have been damaged (e.g., facial nerve). Discourage the patient from chewing on the affected side until paresthesias resolve. A soft diet is usually prescribed. Teach the patient to avoid rubbing the eye on the affected side because the protective mechanism of pain will no longer warn of injury. Instruct him or her to inspect the eye daily for redness or irritation and report any change or blurred vision to the physician. Stress the importance of regular dental examinations because the absence of pain may not warn the patient of potential problems.

In addition to general post-craniotomy care for patients who have microvascular decompression, monitor the patient for signs of complications including headache, cranial nerve dysfunction, and bleeding. Assess his or her corneal reflex, extraocular muscles, and facial nerve, and report abnormal findings to the surgeon. Document all changes promptly.

Psychosocial considerations for the patient with trigeminal neuralgia include disappointment with ineffective drug protocols or surgical procedures, as well as the fear that the pain may recur with any activity. The patient may fail to move the face in an attempt to prevent pain. This behavior may be misinterpreted by others as withdrawal or depression. Refer patients and their families to the Trigeminal Neuralgia Association (TNA) (www.fpa-support.org) for more information and support.

FACIAL PARALYSIS

Pathophysiology

Facial paralysis, or **Bell's palsy,** is an acute paralysis of cranial nerve VII but may also affect cranial nerves V (trigeminal) and VIII (vestibulocochlear [auditory]). The condition is also known as *cranial polyneuritis.* Although the incidence may be slightly higher among people with diabetes, Bell's palsy occurs in all ages and at all times of the year.

Acute maximum paralysis is attained within 48 hours in about half the patients and within 5 days in almost all of them. Pain behind the ear or on the face may occur before paralysis by a few hours or days. The disorder involves a drawing sensation and paralysis of all facial muscles on the affected side. The patient cannot close his or her eye, wrinkle the forehead, smile, whistle, or grimace. He or she may also lose the ability for the eye to tear or may have excessive tearing. The face appears masklike and sags. Taste is usually impaired to some degree, but this symptom seldom persists beyond the second week of paralysis. Tinnitus (ringing in the ears) may also occur.

The cause of Bell's palsy is believed to be the result of an inflammatory process triggered by a formerly dormant herpes simplex virus type 1 (HSV-1). Infections or exposure to cold may trigger the HSV-1 to cause symptoms of the disease. Patients are rarely hospitalized, but the nurse may encounter them in community-based settings such as clinics, physicians' offices, or emergency departments.

Patient-Centered Collaborative Care

Medical management often includes corticosteroids, 30 to 60 mg daily, during the first week after the onset of symptoms, but their use is controversial (Carlson & Pfadt, 2005). Antiviral drugs such as acyclovir (Zovirax) may be prescribed for 7 to 10 days after symptoms begin. Mild analgesics may help relieve the pain. Nursing care is directed toward managing the major neurologic deficits and providing psychosocial support. Because the eye does not close, the cornea must be protected from drying and subsequent ulceration or abrasion. Teach the patient to manually close the eyelid at intervals and to instill artificial tears four times daily. The eye may be patched or taped closed at bedtime.

The patient may be unable to chew, sip fluids through a straw, or control drooling on the affected side. Thus mealtime may become a problem. Encourage him or her to eat and drink using the unaffected side of the mouth. Frequent, small meals may be better tolerated, and patients may require a soft diet. Explain how to use simple techniques of massage; the application of warm, moist heat; and facial exercises.

A facial sling may prevent drooping of the affected side. As muscle tone improves, teach the patient to grimace, wrinkle the brow, force the eyes closed, whistle, and blow air out of the cheeks three or four times daily for 5 minutes in front of a mirror.

Although most patients recover fully within a few weeks or months, some may experience residual weakness. A few have permanent neurologic deficits. For chronic pain, gabapentin (Neurontin) may be prescribed. These patients require a great deal of support because body image and self-esteem are drastically affected. Provide both information and psychosocial support. Refer patients and their families to the Bell's Palsy Research Foundation for support and community resources (www.angelfire.com).

HUMAN NEEDS NURSING CARE REVIEW

What might you NOTICE if a patient is experiencing impaired mobility and/or sensation as a result of acute or chronic peripheral nervous system disorders?

- Report of loss of sensation in extremities or face
- Report of muscle weakness
- Inability to ambulate
- Inability to move legs and/or arms
- Difficulty breathing

- Report of burning, tingling sensations in extremities
- Report of pain in extremities or face
- Ptosis

What should you INTERPRET and how should you RESPOND to a patient experiencing impaired mobility and/or sensation as a result of peripheral nervous system disorders?

Perform and interpret physical assessment, including:

- Performing a complete neurologic assessment
- Assessing a patient's airway and breathing ability (if difficulty breathing is noticed)
- Performing a comprehensive pain assessment

Respond by:

- Notifying health care provider or contacting Rapid Response Team if patient has problems with breathing or experiences a sudden change in neurologic status
- Establishing an airway and promoting ease in breathing (e.g., putting patient in sitting position, providing oxygen)
- Having emergency equipment like ventilator and tracheostomy set available for patient who has respiratory compromise
- Assisting with ambulation and ADLs as needed
- Providing analgesics and other pain-relief measures

On what should you REFLECT?

- Continue to observe patient for changes in muscle weakness, paralysis, and respiratory function.
- Monitor patient for decreased report of pain and associated symptoms.
- Think about ways to promote independence in mobility and self-care.
- Think about health care team members with whom you will need to collaborate to improve mobility.
- Develop a teaching plan for the patient and family for continuing care.

GET READY FOR THE NCLEX EXAMINATION

Key Points

Review these Key Points for each NCLEX Examination Client Needs Category.

Safe and Effective Care Environment

- Collaborate with members of the interdisciplinary team, including the health care provider, physical and occupational therapists, speech-language pathologist, and nutritionist for care of patients with Guillain-Barré syndrome (GBS) and myasthenia (MG).
- Refer patients with peripheral nervous system (PNS) disorders to community support groups and health care organizations, such as the Restless Legs Syndrome Foundation and the Myasthenia Gravis Foundation.

Health Promotion and Maintenance

- Teach patients on cholinesterase inhibitor drugs and their families about clinical manifestations of cholinergic and myasthenic crises as listed in Table 46-3.
- Reinforce the need for patients with MG to take their drugs on time.

Psychosocial Integrity

- Provide alternatives to promote communication for patients with GBS and MG, including speaking slowly, lip-reading, and communication boards or electronic technology.

Physiological Integrity

- Assess for changes in respiratory status and muscle function for patients with GBS and MG.
- Recall that patients with GBS have ascending paralysis, sensory changes, cranial nerve involvement, and autonomic manifestations as a result of demyelination of neurons (see Chart 46-1).
- Note that patients with MG have an autoimmune disease in which muscle weakness, including ocular symptoms, is the result of attacks on the acetylcholine receptors at neuromuscular junctions (see Chart 46-4).
- Prevent and manage common complications of plasmapheresis as described in Chart 46-2.
- Teach patients which factors can worsen or exacerbate MG as listed in Table 46-4.
- Remember that the priority for care for patients with GBS and MG is respiratory monitoring and airway management (see Chart 46-3).
- Assess patients with GBS and MG for the risk for complications of immobility, such as pressure ulcers; take measures to prevent these problems.
- For patients having a thymectomy, maintain adequate respiratory function and observe for complications such as pneumothorax or hemothorax (e.g., chest pain, shortness of breath).
- Perform frequent neurovascular assessments for patients having a peripheral nerve repair.
- Teach patients with restless legs syndrome to minimize risk factors for the disorder, including quitting smoking, exercising, and losing weight.
- Recall that trigeminal neuralgia (TN) affects primarily the fifth cranial nerve (although others may be involved). Facial paralysis (Bell's palsy) affects cranial nerve VII.
- The priority for care of the patient with TN is pain management.
- After surgery for TN, perform a focused cranial nerve assessment to determine damage to the nerves, such as CN VII.

Additional Study Resources

Go to your Companion CD or Evolve at http://evolve.elsevier.com/Iggy/ for *Self-Assessment Questions for the NCLEX Examination.*

Go to Evolve at http://evolve.elsevier.com/Iggy/ for *Prioritization and Delegation Questions for the NCLEX Examination.*

SELECTED BIBLIOGRAPHY

Alexander, D.M. (2007). Facing the pain of trigeminal neuralgia. *Nursing2007, 37*(7), 18-20.

Ali, M.I. (2006). Mechanical ventilation in patients with Guillain-Barré syndrome. *Respiratory Care, 51*(12), 1403-1407.

Atkinson, S.B., Carr, R., Maybee, P., & Haynes, D. (2006). The challenges of managing and treating Guillain-Barré syndrome during the acute phase. *Dimensions of Critical Care Nursing, 25*(6), 256-263.

Bershad, E.M., Feen, E.S., & Suarez, J.I. (2008). Myasthenia gravis crisis. *Southern Medical Journal, 101*(1), 63-69.

Carlson, D.S., & Pfadt, E. (2005). When your patient has acute facial paralysis. *Nursing2005, 35*(4), 54-55.

Chavis, P.S. (2007). Immunosuppressive or surgical treatment for ocular myasthenia gravis. *Archives of Neurology, 64*(12), 1792-1794.

Cosi, V., & Versino, M. (2006). Guillain-Barré syndrome. *Neurological Sciences, 27*(Suppl. 1), S47-S51.

Cup, E.H. (2007). Exercise therapy and other types of physical therapy for patients with neuromuscular diseases: A systematic review. *Archives of Physical Medicine and Rehabilitation, 88*(11), 1452-1464.

Dhar, R. (2008). The morbidity and outcome of patients with Guillain-Barré syndrome admitted to the intensive care unit. *Journal of the Neurological Sciences, 264*(1-2), 121-128.

Feasby, T. (2007). Guidelines on the use of intravenous immune globulin for neurologic conditions. *Transfusion Medicine Reviews, 21*(Suppl. 1), S57-S107.

Garssen, M.P.J.,van Koningsveld, R., & van Doorn, P.A. (2007). Treatment of Guillain-Barré syndrome with mycophenolate mofetil: A pilot study. *Journal of Neurology, Neurosurgery, and Psychiatry, 78*(9), 1010-1012.

Haldeman, D., & Zulkosky, K. (2008). The ascension of Guillain-Barré syndrome. *Critical Care Insider,* Spring, 2-6.

Hampton, T. (2007). Novel therapies target myasthenia gravis. *Journal of the American Medical Association, 298*(2), 163-164.

Jaretzki, A. (2007). Evaluation of results of thymectomy for MG requires accepted standards. *Annals of Thoracic Surgery, 84*(1), 360-361.

Kernich, C.A. (2008). Myasthenia gravis: Maximizing function. *The Neurologist, 14*(1), 75-76.

Leung, N. (2008). Guillain-Barré syndrome in elderly people. *Journal of the American Geriatrics Society, 56*(2), 1381-1382.

Maat, A.P. (2008). Inclusion of the transcervical approach in the video-assisted thoracoscopic-extended thymectomy (VATET) for myasthenia gravis: A prospective trial. *Surgical Endoscopy, 22*(1), 265.

Petty, R. (2007). Lambert-Eaton myasthenic syndrome. *Journal of Neurology, Neurosurgery, and Psychiatry, 78*(8), 265-268.

Ryan, M., & Slevin, J.T. (2006). Restless legs syndrome. *American Journal of Health-System Pharmacy, 63*(17), 1599-1612.

Slack, C.B., & Landis, C.A. (2006). Improving outcomes for restless legs syndrome. *The Nurse Practitioner, 31*(5), 27-37.

Care of Critically Ill Patients with Neurologic Problems

47

CHAPTER

Donna D. Ignatavicius • Kathy A. Hausman

LEARNING OUTCOMES

For clinical competence and success on the NCLEX Examination, study this chapter with these Learning Outcomes in mind:

Safe and Effective Care Environment

1. Collaborate with health care team members when planning and providing care for critically ill patients with neurologic problems.
2. Prioritize care for patients with a stroke or traumatic brain injury (TBI).
3. Identify community resources for patients with severe neurologic problems and their families.
4. Maintain continuity of care between the hospital and community-based agencies for patients discharged with a stroke, head injury, or brain tumor.

Health Promotion and Maintenance

5. Teach the patient about risk factors for having a stroke.
6. Perform a comprehensive health assessment of patients who have a stroke.

Psychosocial Integrity

7. Assess the family's response to a brain cancer diagnosis and treatment options.
8. Provide support to the patient and family coping with life changes that often result from a TBI or stroke.
9. Assess the needs of patients with stroke who have altered sensory perception.

Physiological Integrity

10. Differentiate clinical manifestations and management of patients with a transient ischemic attack (TIA) and stroke.
11. Perform a focused neurologic assessment of patients who are critically ill.
12. Assess the patient on thrombolytic therapy or anticoagulants for potential adverse effects.
13. Evaluate care of the patient with a stroke.
14. Assess patients for adverse responses to TBI, such as increased intracranial pressure (ICP).
15. Implement interventions to prevent increasing ICP.
16. Provide care for the patient experiencing increased ICP.
17. Provide postoperative care for the patient having a craniotomy.
18. Prevent and monitor for postoperative complications of a craniotomy.
19. Explain the role of chemotherapy, radiation, and surgery in the management of patients with brain tumors.
20. Explain the primary focus for management of patients with a brain abscess.

Go to your Companion CD or Evolve at http://evolve.elsevier.com/Iggy/ for *Self-Assessment Questions for the NCLEX Examination* keyed to these Learning Outcomes.

Some neurologic problems can cause patients to become critically ill or die. Stroke, head injury, brain tumor, and brain abscess are examples that can lead to life-threatening increased intracranial pressure (ICP). Permanent neurologic dysfunction or death may be prevented by early recognition and aggressive management of this complication by the health care team. Serious and severe neurologic problems cause varying degrees of impaired *mobility, sensation, and cognition.* These impairments may be temporary or permanent and mild or severe depending on the nature of the health problem.

TRANSIENT ISCHEMIC ATTACK AND REVERSIBLE ISCHEMIC NEUROLOGIC DEFICIT

Ischemic strokes often follow warning signs such as a **transient ischemic attack (TIA)** (also called a *silent stroke*) or a **reversible ischemic neurologic deficit (RIND)** (Chart 47-1). Both warning signs cause temporary neurologic dysfunction resulting from a *brief* interruption in cerebral blood flow, possibly due to cerebral vasospasm or systemic arterial hypertension. The difference between a TIA and an RIND is the length of time the patient is symptomatic. A TIA lasts a few minutes to fewer than 24 hours, whereas RIND symptoms last longer than 24 hours but less than a week. Typically, symptoms of a TIA resolve within 30 to 60 minutes. It is not unusual for symptoms to resolve by the time the patient reaches the emergency department (ED). Both TIAs and RINDs may damage the brain tissue with repeated insults, as seen on magnetic resonance imaging (MRI) or computed tomography (CT). Multiple TIAs indicate a high stroke risk.

Upon admission to the ED, the patient is stabilized as necessary. A complete neurologic assessment is performed, and routine laboratory work, electrocardiogram, and CT scan are done. Patients older than 65 years and those with diabetes, symptoms lasting longer than 10 minutes, or motor or speech difficulties often are admitted. At discharge, the patient is usually placed on anticoagulant therapy (e.g., clopidogrel [Plavix]) unless medically contraindicated. As part of the discharge processes, ensure that the patient is aware of bleeding precautions and the actions to take should bleeding occur. Anticoagulant therapy is discussed in detail in Chapter 38 in the Venous Thromboembolism section. Reinforce the need to follow up with the health care provider and to complete any diagnostic tests requested on an ambulatory care basis.

STROKE (BRAIN ATTACK)

Pathophysiology

A **stroke** is caused by a change in the normal blood supply to the brain. The National Stroke Association now uses the term **brain attack** to better describe a stroke. Both terms are used in clinical practice. *Any stroke is a medical emergency that strikes suddenly, and it should be treated immediately to prevent neurologic deficit and permanent disability.*

Chart 47-1 KEY FEATURES

Transient Ischemic Attack

VISUAL DEFICITS
- Blurred vision
- Diplopia (double vision)
- Blindness in one eye
- Tunnel vision

MOTOR DEFICITS
- Weakness (arm, hand, or leg)
- Gait disturbance (ataxic)

SENSORY DEFICITS
- Numbness (face, arm, or hand)
- Vertigo

SPEECH DEFICITS
- Aphasia
- Dysarthria (slurred speech)

Stroke is the second most common cause of death and major disability worldwide. Although the number of stroke deaths has decreased during the past several years in the United States, stroke remains the third most common cause of death and the primary cause of adult disability. The direct and indirect costs of stroke are more than $41 billion each year (Kulchycki & Edlow, 2006).

Pathophysiologic Changes in the Brain

The brain cannot store oxygen or glucose and therefore must receive a constant flow of blood to provide these substances for normal function. In addition, blood flow is important for the removal of metabolic waste (e.g., carbon dioxide, lactic acid). If blood supply to any part of the brain is interrupted for more than a few minutes, cerebral tissue dies **(infarction).** The result is varying degrees of disability, depending on the location and amount of brain tissue affected. Brain metabolism and blood flow after a stroke are affected around the infarction as well as in the **contralateral** (opposite side) hemisphere. Effects of a stroke on the contralateral (nonaffected) side may be due to brain swelling and further changes in blood flow throughout the brain.

Types of Strokes

Strokes are generally classified as ischemic (occlusive) or hemorrhagic (Fig. 47-1). Most ischemic strokes are either thrombotic or embolic in origin (Table 47-1).

Ischemic Stroke

An **ischemic stroke** is caused by the occlusion of a cerebral artery by either a thrombus or an embolus. A stroke that is caused by a **thrombus** (clot) is referred to as a *thrombotic stroke,* whereas a stroke caused by an **embolus** (dislodged clot) is referred to as an *embolic stroke.* Most strokes are ischemic.

Thrombotic Stroke. Thrombotic strokes account for more than half of all strokes and are commonly associated with the development of atherosclerosis of the blood vessel wall. Atherosclerosis is the process by which plaques develop on the inner wall of the affected arterial vessel. Chapter 38 describes this health problem, including its pathophysiology, in more detail.

Rupture of one or more plaques exposes foam cells to clot-promoting elements in the blood. The end result is clot formation. If the clot is of sufficient size, it may interrupt blood flow

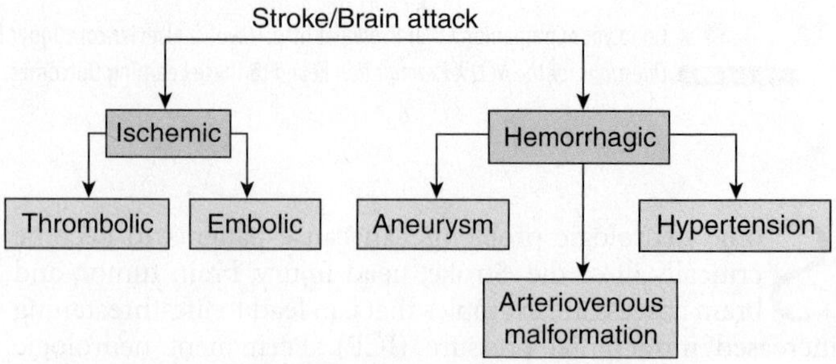
Stroke/Brain attack
Ischemic
Hemorrhagic
Thrombolic
Embolic
Aneurysm
Hypertension
Arteriovenous malformation

Fig. 47-1 • Types of stroke/brain attack.

to the brain tissue supplied by the vessel, causing an occlusive stroke. This process may occur over many years because collateral circulation to the involved area develops to compensate for the occlusion. The **bifurcation** (point of division) of the common carotid artery and the vertebral arteries at their junction with the basilar artery are the most common sites involved. Because of the gradual occlusion (blockage) of the arteries, thrombotic strokes tend to have a *slow* onset.

Embolic Stroke. An embolic stroke is caused by an embolus or a group of emboli that break off from one area of the body and travel to the cerebral arteries via the carotid artery or vertebrobasilar system. The usual source of emboli is the heart. Emboli can occur in patients with nonvalvular atria fibrillation, ischemic heart disease, rheumatic heart disease, and mural thrombi after a myocardial infarction (MI) or insertion of a prosthetic heart valve. Another source of emboli may be plaque that breaks off from the carotid sinus or internal carotid artery. Emboli tend to become lodged in the smaller cerebral blood vessels at their point of bifurcation or where the lumen narrows.

The middle cerebral artery (MCA) is most commonly involved in an embolic stroke. As the emboli occlude the vessel, ischemia develops and the patient experiences the clinical manifestations of the stroke. However, the occlusion may be temporary if the embolus breaks into smaller fragments, enters smaller blood vessels, and is absorbed. For these reasons, embolic strokes are characterized by the *sudden* development and rapid occurrence of neurologic deficits. The symptoms may resolve over several hours or a few days. Conversion of an occlusive stroke to a hemorrhagic stroke may occur because the arterial vessel wall is also vulnerable to ischemic damage from blood supply interruption. Sudden hemodynamic stress may result in vessel rupture, causing bleeding directly within the brain tissue.

Hemorrhagic Stroke

The second major classification of stroke is hemorrhagic stroke. In this type of stroke, vessel integrity is interrupted and bleeding occurs into the brain tissue or into the spaces surrounding the brain (ventricular, subdural, and subarachnoid). Hemorrhage into the brain tissue generally results from a ruptured aneurysm (localized weakening and distortion of vessel wall); rupture of an arteriovenous malformation; or, more commonly, severe hypertension. Amphetamine abuse also causes hemorrhagic stroke; cocaine abuse is associated with both hemorrhagic and ischemic stroke (Jeffrey, 2007b).

◀ ANIMATION: Subarachnoid Hemorrhage

An **aneurysm** is an abnormal ballooning or blister along a normal artery. A congenital aneurysm is a developmental defect in the media and elastica (adventitia or outer layer) of the vessel wall. The child is born with the defect, which may or may not rupture. A secular aneurysm, the most common type, develops in a weak spot on the artery wall, usually along the posterior circulation such as the basilar artery, vertebral artery, or the superior cerebral artery. After a traumatic injury or from plaque formation, a dissecting aneurysm may occur. Also occurring after a traumatic aneurysm is the pseudoaneurysm, a dilation of an artery. A mycotic aneurysm is caused by an infectious agent, for example secondary to bacterial endo-

TABLE 47-1 Differential Features of the Types of Stroke

	ISCHEMIC		
Feature	**Thrombotic**	**Embolic**	**Hemorrhagic**
Evolution	Intermittent or stepwise improvement between episodes of worsening Completed stroke	Abrupt development of completed stroke Steady progression	Usually abrupt onset
Onset	Daytime Gradual (minutes to hours)	Daytime Sudden	Daytime Sudden, may be gradual if caused by hypertension
Level of consciousness	Preserved (patient is awake)	Preserved (patient is awake)	Deepening stupor or coma
Contributing associated factors	Hypertension Atherosclerosis	Cardiac disease	Hypertension Vessel disorders
Prodromal symptoms	Transient ischemic attack		
Neurologic deficits	Deficits during the first few weeks Slight headache Speech deficits Visual problems Confusion	Maximum deficit at onset Paralysis Expressive aphasia	Focal deficits Severe, frequent
Cerebrospinal fluid	Normal; possible presence of protein	Normal	Bloody
Seizures	No	No	Usually
Duration	Improvements over weeks to months Permanent deficits possible	Rapid improvements	Variable Permanent neurologic deficits possible

carditis. Larger aneurysms are more likely to rupture than smaller ones.

Aneurysm rupture causes bleeding into the subarachnoid space, the ventricles, and/or intracerebral tissue. **Vasospasm,** a sudden and periodic constriction of a cerebral artery, often results from a cerebral hemorrhage due to an aneurysm rupture. Blood flow to distal areas of the brain supplied by the artery is markedly diminished, which leads to cerebral ischemia and infarction and further neurologic dysfunction.

An **arteriovenous malformation (AVM)** is an uncommon abnormality that occurs during embryonic development. It is a tangled or spaghetti-like mass of malformed, thin-walled, dilated vessels (Fig. 47-2). The congenital absence of a capillary network forms an abnormal communication between the arterial and venous systems. The vessels may eventually rupture, causing bleeding into the subarachnoid space or into the intracerebral tissue, because normally the capillary network lowers the pressure between the arterial and venous systems. In the absence of the capillary network, the thin-walled veins are subjected to arterial pressure.

Elevated blood pressure leads to changes within the arterial wall that leave it likely to rupture. Damage to the brain occurs from bleeding, causing distortion or displacement. Brain tissue edema is a direct irritant to brain tissue. Hemorrhagic strokes occur more often with sudden, dramatic blood pressure elevations, such as those seen with cocaine abuse.

Etiology and Genetic Risk

Major risk factors that increase the likelihood of strokes are listed in Chart 47-2. Cigarette smoking doubles the risk for strokes (Sauerbeck, 2006). Most of these factors have a familial or genetic predisposition and are discussed elsewhere in this text. For example, relative stroke risk increases with a strong family history of hypertension or atherosclerotic disease. Close blood relatives of a patient with an aneurysm may be at higher risk for intracranial aneurysms and should consider diagnostic testing and follow-up.

Incidence/Prevalence

It is estimated that there are more than 4.7 million stroke survivors in the United States. About 730,000 strokes occur each year, and more than 150,000 deaths result. About 25% of strokes occur in people younger than 65 years (www.americanheart.org). The number of strokes occurring in the younger population is increasing as a result of chronic IV drug abuse. Those using crack cocaine experience an increased incidence of stroke resulting from changes in the clotting mechanism caused by the drugs, spasm of cerebral vessels, or hemodynamic stress from the sudden increase in systolic blood pressure.

Some patients who have had strokes have another one within 1 year. Strokes tend to occur more often in the southern United States ("stroke belt"), which is probably related to the larger older population, tobacco use, obesity, and a high-fat diet.

Health Promotion and Maintenance

People with predisposing health conditions should be aware that they could have a stroke unless they change their lifestyle. Teach them the importance of seeking professional health care and adhering to the recommended treatment plan. Also remind them that other risk factors contribute to health problems such as arteriosclerosis and atherosclerosis, including a sedentary lifestyle and high-fat diet (see Chart 47-2). Recommend a diet high in fruits and vegetables and low in saturated and *trans* fats. Light to moderate alcohol consumption may reduce the risk of stroke, but a higher consumption may increase it. Additional information about lifestyle modifications, such as weight control and smoking cessation, can be found elsewhere in this text.

Patient-Centered Collaborative Care evolve ONLINE PHARM REVIEW

Assessment

History

An accurate history is important in the diagnosis of a stroke. The information obtained assists in identifying the area of the brain involved, as well as the cause. Obtain a history of the patient's activity when the stroke began. Ischemic strokes often occur during sleep, whereas hemorrhagic strokes tend to occur during activity. Next ask the patient or a family member how the symptoms progressed. Be sure to document the history of the stroke's onset. Symptoms of an embolic or hemorrhagic stroke tend to occur abruptly, whereas thrombotic strokes generally have a more gradual progression. Determine the severity of the symptoms, such as whether they worsened after the initial onset (hemorrhagic stroke) or began to improve (embolic stroke). It is important to determine whether the symptoms come and go, possibly indicating a transient ischemic attack (TIA) or a reversible ischemic neurologic deficit (RIND).

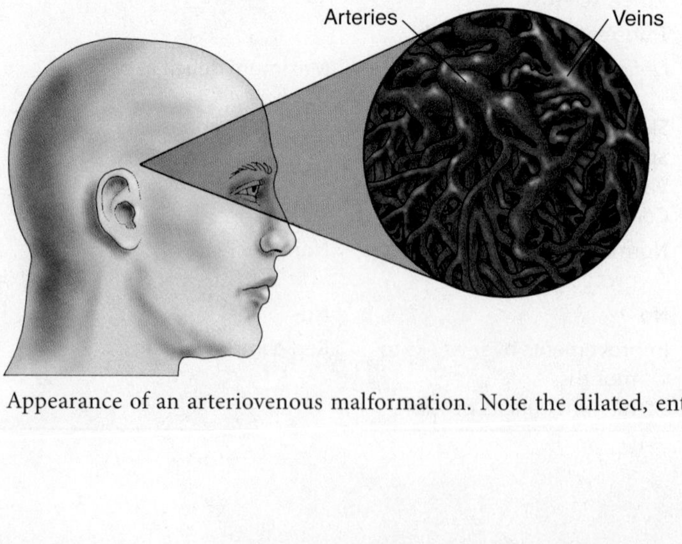
Arteries
Veins

Fig. 47-2 • Appearance of an arteriovenous malformation. Note the dilated, entangled blood vessels.

During the interview, observe the patient's level of consciousness (LOC) and assess for indications of intellectual or memory impairments or difficulties with speech or hearing. Question the patient or family member about the presence of any sensory or motor changes, visual problems, problems with balance or gait, and changes in reading or writing abilities.

In addition, ask about the patient's medical history with specific attention directed toward a history of head trauma, diabetes, hypertension, heart disease, anemia, and obesity. Obtain a list of current medications, including prescribed, over-the-counter (OTC), and recreational (illicit) drugs. To complete the history, obtain data about the patient's social history, including education, employment, travel, leisure activities, and personal habits (e.g., smoking, diet, exercise pattern, drug and alcohol use).

The patient with a cerebral aneurysm often reports the onset of a sudden, severe headache described as "the worst headache of my life." Additional symptoms include nausea and vomiting, photophobia, cranial neuropathy, stiff neck, and change in mental status. There may also be a family history of aneurysms.

Physical Assessment/Clinical Manifestations

*The patient must be evaluated within 10 minutes of arrival in the ED. The same standard applies to patients already hospitalized for other medical conditions who have a stroke. The priority is assessment of ABCs—**a**irway, **b**reathing, and **c**irculation.*

Perform a neurologic assessment. Specific manifestations depend on the extent and location of the ischemia and the arteries involved (Chart 47-3). Physicians and nurses at primary

Chart 47-2 PATIENT AND FAMILY EDUCATION GUIDE

Common Risk Factors for Developing a Stroke

- Atrial fibrillation or heart murmur
- Arteriosclerosis/atherosclerosis
- Previous stroke or transient ischemic attack (TIA)
- Heart surgery
- Valvular heart disease
- Diabetes mellitus
- Smoking
- Substance abuse (particularly cocaine)
- Obesity
- Sedentary lifestyle
- Oral contraceptive use
- Elevated serum cholesterol, lipoprotein, triglyceride, low-density lipoprotein (LDL)
- Previous stroke or TIA
- Heavy alcohol use
- Sudden discontinuation of antihypertensive drugs (causes hemorrhagic stroke)
- Genetic/familial tendency
- Migraines
- Older age
- Male
- African American, Hispanic, or American Indian
- Sickle cell anemia
- Use of phenylpropanolamine (PPA), which is found in antihistamine drugs (causes catastrophic strokes, primarily in young and middle-aged women)
- Brain trauma

Chart 47-3 KEY FEATURES

Stroke Syndromes

MIDDLE CEREBRAL ARTERY STROKES
- Contralateral hemiparesis: arm > leg
- Contralateral sensory deficit
- Homonymous hemianopsia
- Unilateral neglect or inattention
- Aphasia, anomia, alexia, agraphia, and acalculia
- Impaired vertical sensation
- Spatial deficit
- Perceptual deficit
- Visual field deficit
- Altered level of consciousness: drowsy to comatose

POSTERIOR CEREBRAL ARTERY STROKES
- Perseveration (word or action repetition)
- Aphasia, amnesia, alexia, agraphia, visual agnosia, and ataxia
- Loss of deep sensation
- Decreased touch sensation
- Stupor; coma

INTERNAL CAROTID ARTERY STROKES
- Contralateral hemiparesis
- Sensory deficit
- Hemianopsia, blurred vision, blindness
- Aphasia (dominant side)

INTERNAL CAROTID ARTERY STROKES
- Headache
- Bruit

ANTERIOR CEREBRAL ARTERY STROKES
- Contralateral hemiparesis: leg > arm
- Bladder incontinence
- Personality and behavior changes
- Aphasia and amnesia
- Positive grasp and sucking reflex
- Perseveration
- Sensory deficit (lower extremity)
- Memory impairment
- Apraxic gait

VERTEBROBASILAR ARTERY STROKES
- Headache and vertigo
- Coma
- Memory loss and confusion
- Flaccid paralysis
- Areflexia, ataxia, and vertigo
- Cranial nerve dysfunction
- Disconjugate gaze
- Visual deficits (uniorbital) and homonymous hemianopsia
- Sensory loss: numbness

stroke centers or units use a specialized stroke scale such as the National Institutes of Health Stroke Scale (NIHSS) to assess their patients (www.strokecenter.org/trials/scales/nihss). This tool is lengthy but very comprehensive.

Cognitive Changes. The patient may have a variety of cognitive problems in addition to changes in LOC. LOC varies depending on the extent of increased intracranial pressure (ICP) caused by the stroke and on the location of the stroke. Assess for:

- Denial of the illness
- Spatial and **proprioceptive** (awareness of body position in space) dysfunction
- Impairment of memory, judgment, or problem-solving and decision-making abilities
- Decreased ability to concentrate and attend to tasks

Dysfunction in one or more of these areas may be severe depending on the hemisphere involved (Chart 47-4).

The *right* cerebral hemisphere is more involved with visual and spatial awareness and proprioception. A person who has a stroke involving the right cerebral hemisphere is often unaware of any deficits and may be disoriented to time and place. Personality changes include impulsivity (poor impulse control) and poor judgment. The *left* cerebral hemisphere, the dominant hemisphere in all but about 15% to 20% of the population, is the center for language, mathematic skills, and analytic thinking. Therefore a left hemisphere stroke results in **aphasia** (inability to use or comprehend language), **alexia** or **dyslexia** (reading problems), **agraphia** (difficulty with writing), and **acalculia** (difficulty with mathematic calculation). A complete assessment of these problems is performed by a speech and language pathologist (SLP).

Motor Changes. The motor examination provides information about which part of the brain is involved. A *right* **hemiplegia** (paralysis on one side of the body) or **hemiparesis** (weakness on one side of the body) indicates a stroke involving the *left* cerebral hemisphere because the motor nerve fibers cross in the medulla before entering the spinal cord and periphery. On the other hand, a *left* hemiplegia or hemiparesis indicates a stroke in the *right* cerebral hemisphere. If the brainstem or cerebellum is affected, the patient may experience hemiparesis or quadriparesis and **ataxia** (gait disturbance).

In collaboration with the physical and occupational therapists, assess the patient's muscle tone. The patient with **hypotonia,** or **flaccid paralysis,** cannot overcome the forces of gravity, and the extremities tend to fall to the side. The extremities feel heavy, and muscle tone is inadequate for balance, equilibrium, or protective mechanisms. **Hypertonia (spastic paralysis)** tends to cause fixed positions or contractures of the involved extremities. Range of motion (ROM) of the joints is restricted, and shoulder subluxation may easily occur from either spasticity or flaccidity. Also assess proprioception (position sense), head and trunk control, balance, coordination, and gait. The patient who has had a stroke may also be unable to use an object correctly **(agnosia)** or carry out a purposeful motor activity **(apraxia).**

Loss of neurologic control by the cerebral cortex causes a spastic (upper motor neuron) uninhibited bladder. Bowel function may also be affected. Assess the patient for incontinence or retention of urine and stool.

Sensory Changes. The sensory examination evaluates the patient's response to touch and painful stimuli. In addition to diminished motor function, decreased sensation typically occurs on the affected side of the body.

Evaluate for indications of **neglect syndrome,** which is particularly common with strokes in the *right* cerebral hemi-

Chart 47-4 KEY FEATURES

Left and Right Hemisphere Strokes

Feature	Left Hemisphere*	Right Hemisphere
Language	Aphasia Agraphia Alexia	Impaired sense of humor
Memory	Possible deficit	Disorientation to time, place, and person Inability to recognize faces
Vision	Inability to discriminate words and letters Reading problems Deficits in the right visual field	Visual spatial deficits Neglect of the left visual field Loss of depth perception
Behavior	Slowness Cautiousness Anxiety when attempting a new task Depression or a catastrophic response to illness Sense of guilt Feeling of worthlessness Worries over future Quick anger and frustration Intellectual impairment	Impulsiveness Lack of awareness of neurologic deficits Confabulation Euphoria Constant smiling Denial of illness Poor judgment Overestimation of abilities (risk for injury)
Hearing	No deficit	Loss of ability to hear tonal variations

*Location for speech in all but 15% to 20% of people.

sphere. In this syndrome, the patient is unaware of the existence of his or her left or paralyzed side. The typical picture is that of the patient sitting in a wheelchair and leaning to the left with the arm caught in the wheelchair wheel. When questioned, the patient often states that everything is fine and believes that he or she is sitting up straight in the chair. Another typical example of neglect syndrome is the patient who washes or dresses only one side of the body.

Another important part of the nursing assessment focuses on visual ability. Infarction or ischemia involving the carotid artery may cause pupil constriction or dilation, **ptosis** (eyelid drooping), visual field deficits, or pallor and petechiae of the conjunctiva. **Amaurosis fugax,** a brief episode of blindness in one eye, results from retinal ischemia caused by ophthalmic or carotid artery insufficiency. **Hemianopsia,** or blindness in half of the visual field, results from damage to the optic tract or occipital lobe. Most often this deficit occurs as **homonymous hemianopsia,** in which there is blindness in the same side of both eyes (Fig. 47-3). The patient with this condition must turn his or her head to scan the complete range of vision. Otherwise, he or she does not see half of the visual field. For example, the patient eats only half of a meal because that is the only portion seen. Patients with brainstem or cerebellar damage may have abnormal eye movements, such as nystagmus (involuntary movements of the eyes).

Cranial Nerve Function. Assess the patient's ability to chew, which reflects the function of cranial nerve (CN) V. Assessment of the patient's ability to swallow reflects the function of CNs IX and X. In addition, note any facial paralysis or paresis (CN VII), absent gag reflex (CN IX), or impaired tongue movement (CN XII). The patient who has difficulty chewing or swallowing foods and liquids **(dysphagia)** is at risk for aspiration pneumonia and may become constipated or dehydrated from inadequate fluid intake.

Cardiovascular Assessment. Patients with embolic strokes may have a heart murmur, dysrhythmias, or hypertension. It is not unusual for the patient to be admitted to the hospital with a blood pressure greater than 180 to 200/110 to 120 mm Hg. Although a somewhat higher blood pressure (150/100 mm Hg) is needed to maintain cerebral perfusion after a stroke, pressures above this limit may lead to another stroke.

Psychosocial Assessment

The typical patient with a stroke is older than 60 years, is hypertensive, and has varying degrees of motor weakness and level of consciousness. Language and cognitive deficits, as well as behavior and memory problems, may also occur.

Assess the patient's reaction to the illness, especially in relation to changes in body image, self-concept, and ability to perform ADLs. In collaboration with the patient's family and

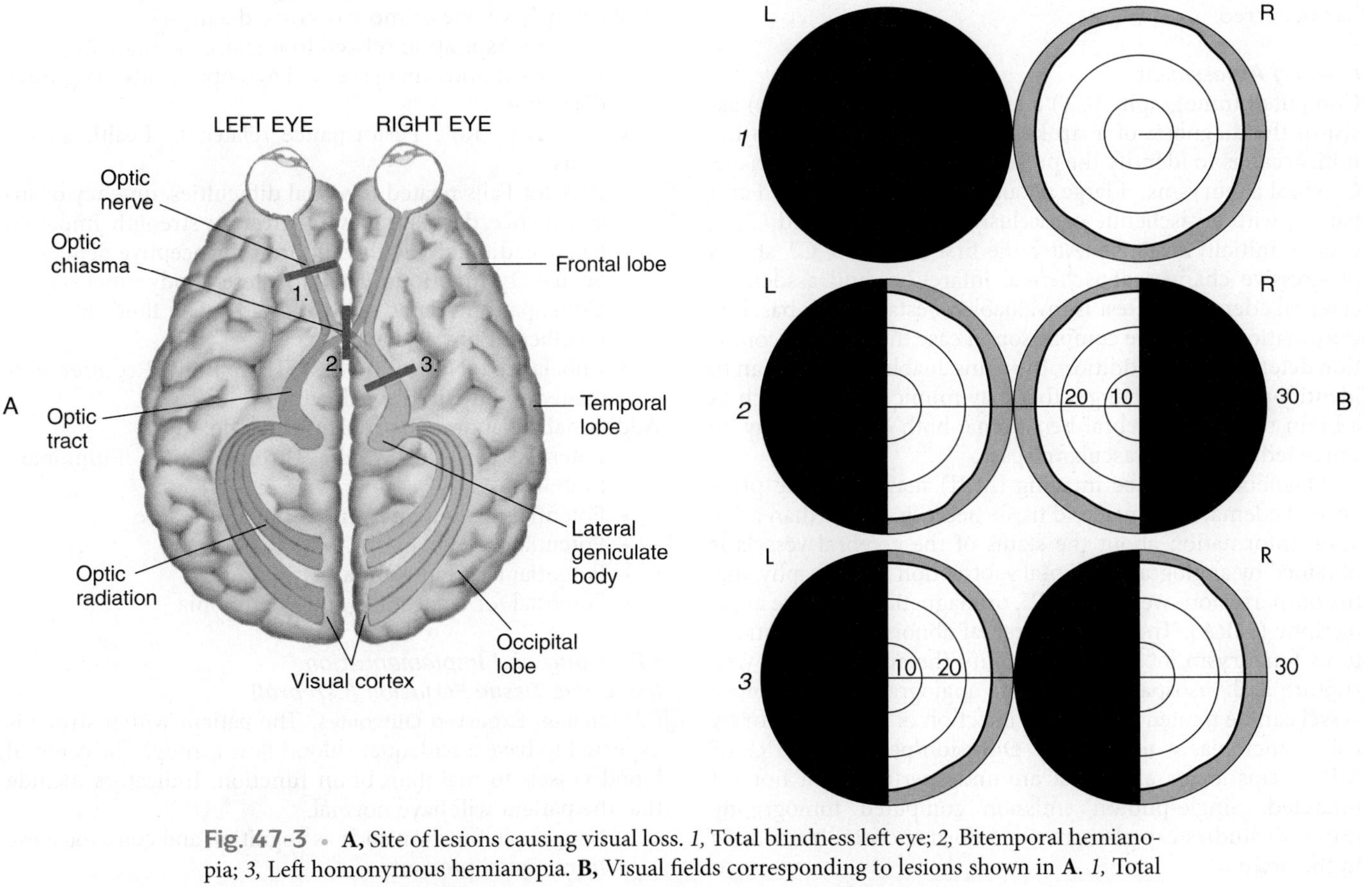
LEFT EYE
RIGHT EYE
Optic nerve
Optic chiasma
1.
2.
3.
Frontal lobe
A
Optic tract
Temporal lobe
Lateral geniculate body
Optic radiation
Occipital lobe
Visual cortex
L
R
1
2
20
10
30
B
3
10
20
30

Fig. 47-3 • **A,** Site of lesions causing visual loss. *1,* Total blindness left eye; *2,* Bitemporal hemianopia; *3,* Left homonymous hemianopia. **B,** Visual fields corresponding to lesions shown in **A**. *1,* Total blindness left eye; *2,* Bitemporal hemianopia; *3,* Left homonymous hemianopia.

friends, identify any problems with coping or personality changes.

Ask about the patient's financial status and occupation, because these aspects may be altered by the residual neurologic deficits of the stroke. Patients who do not have disability or health insurance may worry about how their family will cope financially with the disruption in their lives. Early involvement of social services, certified hospital chaplain, or psychological counseling may enhance coping skills.

Assess for **emotional lability,** especially if the frontal lobe of the brain has been affected. In such cases, the patient laughs and then cries unexpectedly for no apparent reason. Explain these uncontrollable emotions to the family or significant others so they do not feel responsible for these reactions.

Laboratory Assessment

Clinical history and presentation are usually enough to identify a stroke once it has occurred. No definitive laboratory tests confirm its diagnosis. Elevated hematocrit and hemoglobin levels are often associated with a severe or major stroke as the body attempts to compensate for lack of oxygen to the brain. An elevated white blood cell (WBC) count may indicate the presence of an infection, possibly subacute bacterial endocarditis, or a response to physiologic stress, as well as inflammation. The health care provider typically requests a prothrombin time (PT) or international normalized ratio (INR), as well as a partial thromboplastin time (PTT), to establish baseline information in case anticoagulation therapy is started. These diagnostic tests may also provide supportive evidence that a hemorrhagic stroke has occurred.

Imaging Assessment

Computed tomography (CT) and CT angiography (CTA) assist in the diagnosis of a stroke. The primary purpose of the initial scan is to identify the presence of cerebral hemorrhage. Cerebral aneurysms, if large enough, may be identified. For a patient with an ischemic or occlusive stroke, the head CT is usually initially negative. After the first 24 hours, CT shows progressive changes of ischemia, infarction, and associated cerebral edema. This test is invaluable in establishing baseline information for future comparison in case the patient's condition deteriorates. In addition, the scans enable the physician to identify pathologic changes that may mimic a stroke, such as a brain tumor or cerebral hematoma, both of which may be unrelated to cerebrovascular disease.

Magnetic resonance imaging (MRI) may show the presence of edema, ischemia, and tissue necrosis earlier than a CT scan. Information about the status of the cerebral vessels is obtained by angiography, digital subtraction angiography, diffusion/perfusion–weighted MRI, or magnetic resonance angiography (MRA). These studies reveal abnormal vessel structures (aneurysm location) or identify the area of vessel wall rupture and vasospasm. Following angiography, a narrowed vessel can be treated by catheter injection of papaverine or by using angioplasty techniques. Diffusion/perfusion MRI or MRA helps locate areas that are underperfused but not yet infarcted. Single-photon emission computed tomography (SPECT) studies can also provide information on blood flow in the brain.

Other Diagnostic Assessment

To assist in the determination of a cardiac cause of a stroke, the health care provider may request an electrocardiogram (ECG), a Holter monitor test, cardiac enzymes evaluation, and an echocardiogram. As with other cardiovascular diseases, it is not unusual to find these changes on the ECG: inverted T wave, ST depression, and prolongation of the QT interval in the cardiac cycle.

▪ *Analysis*

Common Nursing Diagnoses and Collaborative Problems

The most common nursing diagnoses for patients with a stroke are:

1. Ineffective Tissue Perfusion (Cerebral) related to interruption of arterial blood flow and a possible increase in ICP
2. Impaired Swallowing related to neuromuscular impairment
3. Impaired Physical Mobility and Self-Care Deficit related to neuromuscular impairment or cognitive impairment
4. Impaired Verbal Communication related to decreased circulation in the brain
5. Total Urinary Incontinence and Bowel Incontinence related to neurologic dysfunction
6. Disturbed Sensory Perception related to altered sensory reception, transmission, and integration
7. Unilateral Neglect related to effects of disturbed perceptual abilities or hemianopsia

Additional Nursing Diagnoses and Collaborative Problems

In addition to the common nursing diagnoses, patients with stroke may have one or more of these diagnoses:

- Risk for Aspiration related to impaired swallowing
- Disturbed Body Image related to biophysical or cognitive disability
- Ineffective Role Performance related to health alterations
- Risk for Falls related to visual difficulties, urgency or incontinence, decreased lower extremity strength, impaired balance, difficulty with gait, or proprioceptive deficits
- Sexual Dysfunction related to altered body function
- Constipation related to lack of adequate fluid intake or insufficient physical activity
- Imbalanced Nutrition: Less Than Body Requirements related to impaired swallowing

Additional collaborative problems include:

- Potential for Deep Vein Thrombosis or Pulmonary Embolism
- Potential for Increased Intracranial Pressure
- Potential for Seizures
- Potential for Hypoxemia
- Potential for Atelectasis and Pneumonia

▪ *Planning and Implementation*

Ineffective Tissue Perfusion (Cerebral)

NOC **Planning: Expected Outcomes.** The patient with a stroke is expected to have an adequate blood flow through the cerebral blood vessels to maintain brain function. Indicators include that the patient will have normal:

- Neurologic function such as cognition and consciousness
- Intracranial pressure

- Systolic blood pressure
- Diastolic blood pressure

Interventions. Interventions are determined primarily by the type and extent of the stroke. For select patients with ischemic strokes, early intervention with systemic thrombolytic therapy to dissolve the clot is indicated to address neurologic deficits if implemented within 3 hours of the onset of stroke.

Thrombolytic Therapy. **Intravenous (systemic) thrombolytic therapy** (also called *fibrinolytic therapy*) for an acute ischemic stroke (AIS) dissolves the cerebral artery occlusion to re-establish blood flow and prevent cerebral infarction. Recombinant tissue plasminogen activator (rtPA [Retavase]) is the only drug approved at this point for the treatment of acute ischemic stroke. Thrombolytics activate plasminogen, which degrades the thrombus by breaking down fibrin.

Patients must meet strict eligibility criteria for rtPA administration, including giving the drug within 3 hours after the first stroke symptoms. Thrombolytic therapy is explained to the patient and/or family member, and informed consent is obtained. The dosage of the drug is based on the patient's actual weight. Each hospital has strict protocols for mixing and administering rtPA and for monitoring the patient before and after rtPA administration. In addition to frequent monitoring of vital signs, carefully observe for signs of intracerebral hemorrhage and other signs of bleeding during drug administration. Other best practice interventions are listed in Chart 47-5.

Intra-arterial thrombolysis has the advantage of delivering the thrombolytic agent directly into the thrombus within 6 hours of the stroke's onset. It is particularly beneficial for some patients who have an occlusion of the middle cerebral artery (Adams et al., 2007).

Nonsurgical Management. Nursing interventions are initially aimed at monitoring for neurologic changes or complications associated with stroke. The Plan of Care on pp. 1038-1043 highlights the most important aspects of care for patients who are critically ill as a result of severe neurologic problems. Some patients may have worsening of their neurologic status within 24 to 48 hours after their stroke. A major complication is increased intracranial pressure (ICP) (Chart 47-6). Perform a neurologic assessment when the patient is admitted to the hospital. Reassess him or her every 1 to 4 hours (depending on severity of the condition) using the approved stroke scale.

NIC **Intracranial pressure monitoring.** *The patient is most at risk for increased ICP resulting from edema during the first 72 hours after onset of the stroke (Chart 47-7). Be alert for symptoms of increased ICP, and report any deterioration in the patient's*

Text continues on p. 1043.

Chart 47-5 BEST PRACTICE FOR PATIENT SAFETY & QUALITY CARE

Nursing Interventions After IV Administration of rtPA

- Infuse 0.9 mg/kg (maximum dose 90 mg) over 60 minutes with 10% of the dose given as a bolus over 1 minute.
- Admit the patient to a critical care or specialized stroke unit.
- Perform neurologic assessments, including vital signs, every 15 minutes during infusion and every 30 minutes after that for at least 6 hours; monitor hourly for 24 hours after treatment.
- If systolic blood pressure is 180 mm Hg or greater or diastolic is 105 mm Hg or greater, give antihypertensive drugs as prescribed.
- Do not place invasive tubes, such as NG tubes or indwelling urinary catheters, until patient is stable to prevent bleeding.
- Discontinue the infusion if the patient reports severe headache or has severe hypertension, nausea, and/or vomiting; notify the health care provider immediately.
- Obtain a follow-up CT scan after 24 hours of treatment before starting antiplatelet or anticoagulant drugs.

Chart 47-6 KEY FEATURES

Increased Intracranial Pressure (ICP)

- Decreased level of consciousness (LOC) (lethargy to coma)
- Behavior changes: restlessness, irritability, and confusion
- Headache
- Nausea and vomiting
- Change in speech pattern
- Aphasia
- Slurred speech
- Change in sensorimotor status
- Pupillary changes: dilated and nonreactive pupils ("blown pupils") or constricted and nonreactive pupils
- Cranial nerve dysfunction
- Ataxia
- Seizures (usually within first 24 hrs after stroke)
- Cushing's triad
- Severe hypertension
- Widened pulse pressure
- Bradycardia
- Abnormal posturing
  - Decerebrate (extensor)
  - Decorticate (flexion)

Chart 47-7 NIC INTERVENTION ACTIVITIES

The Patient with a Stroke

Intracranial Pressure Monitoring: Measurement and interpretation of patient data to regulate intracranial pressure.

- Assist with ICP monitoring device insertion.
- Provide information to family/significant others.
- Calibrate and level the transducer.
- Set alarms.
- Record ICP pressure readings.
- Note patient's change in response to stimuli.
- Monitor cerebral perfusion pressure.
- Monitor patient's ICP and neurologic response to care activities.
- Monitor intake and output.
- Monitor insertion site for infection.
- Monitor temperature and WBC count.
- Administer pharmacologic agents to maintain ICP within specified range.
- Space nursing care to minimize ICP elevation.
- Notify health care provider of elevated ICP that does not respond to treatment protocols.

NIC intervention activities selected from Bulechek, G.M., Butcher, H.K., McCloskey Dochterman, J. (Eds.). (2008). *Nursing interventions classification (NIC)* (5th ed.). St. Louis: Mosby. No part of this work is to be altered without prior written permission from the Publisher.

ICP, Intracranial pressure; *WBC*, white blood cell.

PLAN OF CARE Medical Diagnosis: Critically Ill Neurologic Problem Affecting the Brain/Postoperative Craniotomy

NURSING DIAGNOSIS NO. 1: **Decreased Intracranial Adaptive Capacity**

Related Factors

Decreased cerebral perfusion = <60-70 mm Hg
Sustained increase in intracranial pressure (ICP) = >15-20 mm Hg
Systemic hypotension with intracranial hypertension
Brain injuries

Defining Characteristics

Baseline ICP ≥10-15 mm Hg
Disproportionate increase in ICP after a single environmental or nursing maneuver stimulus

Expected Outcomes

Baseline ICP remains ≤15-20 mm Hg
ICP remains stable after nursing activities or environmental stimuli
Remains oriented to time, place, person, and situation
Level of consciousness (LOC) remains stable
No evidence of neurologic compromise

Nursing Interventions	Rationales
NIC Cerebral Perfusion Promotion	
Monitor neurologic status and vital signs.	A decrease or change in LOC is typically the first sign of deterioration in neurologic status. Fever increases metabolic demands, cerebral blood flow (CBF), and ICP.
Calculate and monitor cerebral perfusion pressure (CPP).	A CPP ≥60-70 mm Hg is needed to provide adequate oxygenation and nutrition to brain tissue.
Monitor the patient's ICP and neurologic response to care activities.	ICP may elevate in response to stimulation from care activities. An elevation in ICP decreases CPP.
Monitor central venous pressure (CVP) if central venous access is present. Also perform regular physical examinations to assess fluid balance (edema, rales/crackles on lung auscultation), as well as jugular venous distention.	CVP measures fluid status. ICP elevates with fluid overload.
Monitor pulmonary artery wedge pressure (PAWP) and pulmonary artery pressure (PAP).	Elevated PAWP and PAP indicate ineffective pumping force of the heart and increased fluid pressure in the lungs, upper extremities, head, and neck.
Monitor respiratory status (e.g., rate, rhythm, and depth of respirations; Po_2, Pco_2, pH, and bicarbonate levels).	Adequate gas exchange is required for tissue oxygenation.
Maintain Pco_2 level at 35 mm Hg to avoid hypercarbia.	CO_2 is a powerful vasodilator, which causes cerebral vasodilation and increases ICP.
Monitor $Paco_2$, Sao_2, and hemoglobin levels and cardiac output, if available.	$Paco_2$, Sao_2, and hemoglobin levels and cardiac output are determinants of tissue oxygen delivery.
Administer colloid, blood products, and crystalloid, as appropriate.	Volume expanders maintain hemodynamic parameters.
Administer and titrate vasoactive drugs, as prescribed.	Vasoactive drugs maintain hemodynamic parameters.
Maintain serum glucose level within normal range.	The brain does not store glucose and needs a constant supply for cellular energy. Hypoglycemia can cause brain damage. Hyperglycemia is associated with increased morbidity and mortality.
Consult with the physician to determine optimal head-of-bed (HOB) placement (e.g., 0, 15, or 30 degrees), and monitor the patient's responses to head positioning.	The patient's head should be positioned to best facilitate drainage of blood and cerebrospinal fluid.
Avoid neck flexion or extreme hip/knee flexion.	Absence of neck or hip flexion enhances venous drainage, which prevents increased ICP.
Administer and monitor the effects of osmotic and loop-active diuretics and corticosteroids.	Osmotic diuretics are used to treat cerebral edema by pulling fluid out of edematous brain tissue. A loop-active diuretic may be used to counteract rebound from the osmotic diuretic.
Administer pain medication, as appropriate.	Pain may increase ICP and other stress-related complications.
Test stool and nasogastric (NG) drainage for blood.	Patients receiving anticoagulant drugs should be observed for signs of bleeding.
NIC Intracranial Pressure Monitoring	
Maintain ICP monitoring system; observe waveforms.	If the system is not maintained properly, changes in ICP will be missed.

D Indicates nursing activities that can be delegated to unlicensed assistive nursing personnel at the discretion of the nurse.

PLAN OF CARE Medical Diagnosis: Critically Ill Neurologic Problem Affecting the Brain/Postoperative Craniotomy—cont'd

NURSING DIAGNOSIS NO. 1: Decreased Intracranial Adaptive Capacity—cont'd

Nursing Interventions	Rationales
NIC Intracranial Pressure Monitoring—cont'd	
Check the patient for nuchal rigidity or other meningeal signs.	Nuchal rigidity indicates irritation of the meninges and may indicate inflammation or infection, such as meningitis.
Administer antibiotics.	Antibiotics will treat an infectious process and lower the risk of systemic or intracranial infection.
Record ICP pressure readings, and analyze waveforms.	ICP pressure readings and the characteristics of the waveforms provide indicators of changes in CPP, ICP, and intracranial compliance.
Other Interventions	
Give simple, clear explanations.	Increased ICP may affect cognition and make information processing difficult.
Keep surroundings as quiet and calm as possible.	Stimulation may cause ICP to increase.
Continuing Care Considerations	
Provide the patient and family with written explanations and instructions.	Brain injury and/or anxiety may affect cognition.

NURSING DIAGNOSIS NO. 2: Disturbed Thought Processes

Related Factors

Neurologic impairment
Hypoxia, acute
Cognitive deficit
Memory problems

Defining Characteristics

Cannot recall factual information
Cannot recall recent events
Cannot learn or retain new skills or information
Observed or reported experience of forgetting

Expected Outcomes

Can recall factual information
Can recall recent or past events
Can learn or retain new skills or information
No verbal report or observation of forgetting
Can perform previously learned skill (specify)
Has cognitive functions that remain stable
No verbal report or observation of impaired memory
No verbal report or observation of diminished ability to learn

Nursing Interventions	Rationales
NIC Memory Training	
Discuss with the patient and family any memory problems experienced.	Determines the extent of memory problems and the patient's and family's response to those difficulties.
Reminisce about past experiences with the patient, as appropriate.	Reminiscing about past experiences may assist the patient to remember problem-solving skills and techniques previously used.
Orient to environment, date, time, event, location, etc.	Orientation helps the patient communicate more effectively with others.
Keep items in the same place.	Reduces confusion and frustration.
Protect from sensory overload, and allow frequent rest periods.	Reduces confusion and agitation.
Implement visual imagery, mnemonic devices, memory games, memory cues, association techniques, list making, computers, name tags, or rehearsing of information.	Appropriate memory techniques can assist the patient with storage and retrieval of information.
D Assist in associated learning tasks, as appropriate.	Practice learning and recalling verbal and pictorial information as presented help the patient exercise memory and information retrieval.
Provide for orientation training, as appropriate.	The patient can rehearse personal information and dates to improve retention of key information.
D Have the patient engage in games such as matching pairs of cards, as appropriate.	Matching games provide an opportunity for concentration.
Question the patient about a recent outing or other recent notable event.	Questioning the patient about a recent event provides an opportunity to use memory for recent events.

Continued

PLAN OF CARE Medical Diagnosis: Critically Ill Neurologic Problem Affecting the Brain/Postoperative Craniotomy—cont'd

NURSING DIAGNOSIS NO. 2: **Disturbed Thought Processes—cont'd**

Provide for picture recognition memory, as appropriate.	Pictures trigger memories from storage areas of the brain that are different from those used for speech.
Structure the teaching methods according to the patient's organization of information.	The patient's organization of information will determine the logical sequence of learning for him or her.
Encourage the patient to participate in group memory training programs, as appropriate.	Group support and understanding of memory difficulties make memory problems less threatening.
Monitor the patient's behavior during therapy.	The patient may get agitated and frustrated during therapy, which signals the need to stop the session.
Other Interventions	
D Encourage the patient to use previously learned skills.	Distant memory may remain intact and provide a sense of control to the patient.
Assist the family to understand that assaultive behavior may be the result of poor memory.	Aggressive or combative behavior by the patient may signal a threat to self-esteem from memory loss.
Request a neuropsychology consult.	Evaluation will identify specific cognitive deficits on which the treatment plan is based.
Continuing Care Considerations	
Collaborate with the patient and family to manage tasks that may be difficult for the patient (e.g., paying bills).	The patient may need to have financial or other protection.

NURSING DIAGNOSIS NO. 3: **Impaired Physical Mobility**

Related Factors

Discomfort
Sensoriperceptual impairment
Musculoskeletal impairment
Neuromuscular impairment
Intolerance to activity

Defining Characteristics

Limited ability to perform gross motor skills
Limited ability to perform fine motor skills
Uncoordinated or jerky movement
Limited range of motion
Difficulty turning

Expected Outcomes

Has full or improved range of motion in all joints
Has smooth, coordinated movements
Can turn without assistance
Has stable posture during performance of activities of daily living (ADLs)
Has no movement-induced tremor
Has skin that remains intact with no bruising or rashes
Can perform fine motor skills
Can perform gross motor skills

Nursing Interventions	Rationales
NIC Exercise Therapy: Joint Mobility	
Collaborate with physical therapy in developing and executing an exercise program.	The physical therapist is the primary health care professional responsible for developing and executing an exercise program.
Initiate pain control measures before beginning joint exercise.	Initiating pain control measures before joint exercise increases the likelihood of patient comfort and willingness to engage in the exercise.
D Dress the patient in nonrestrictive clothing.	Nonrestrictive clothing permits full range of joint motion.
D Encourage active range-of-motion exercises according to regular, planned schedule.	Regular periods of active range-of-motion exercise maximize the exercise benefit to joints.
Assist the patient to develop a schedule for active range-of-motion exercises.	Regular exercise maximizes the benefit of the exercise.
D Encourage ambulation, if appropriate.	Ambulation is a form of active joint exercise and also improves cardiovascular tone.

D Indicates nursing activities that can be delegated to unlicensed assistive nursing personnel at the discretion of the nurse.

PLAN OF CARE Medical Diagnosis: Critically Ill Neurologic Problem Affecting the Brain/Postoperative Craniotomy—cont'd

NURSING DIAGNOSIS NO. 3: **Impaired Physical Mobility—cont'd**

NIC Positioning	
Premedicate the patient before turning, as appropriate.	Premedicating the patient before turning will increase patient comfort and decrease resistance to repositioning from fear of pain.
DPlace the patient in the designated therapeutic position.	The designated therapeutic position should cause no undue stress on muscles or joints.
DPosition the patient in proper body alignment.	Proper body alignment preserves the functionality of muscles and bony skeleton.
DMinimize friction and shearing forces when positioning and turning the patient.	Friction and shearing forces will damage the skin and underlying tissues.
DTurn using the log-roll technique.	The log-roll technique keeps the spinal column in alignment during the turn, which prevents injury to the spinal nerves.
Apply a foot board to the bed.	A foot board will prevent foot drop.
DElevate the head of the bed, as appropriate.	The head of the bed may be elevated to provide countertraction or for comfort if permitted.
DTurn the patient as indicated by skin condition.	Patients should be turned at least every 2 hours and have small position shifts more frequently to prevent pressure injury.
DPlace frequently used objects within reach.	Placing frequently used objects within reach permits the patient safe and convenient access.
Other Interventions	
Instruct the patient in the use of assistive devices.	The patient will need instruction to properly use canes, crutches, walkers, splints, or other assistive devices.
Continuing Care Considerations	
Refer the patient to rehabilitative services, as appropriate.	Ongoing support from physical therapists, occupational therapists, and others may be needed to help the patient resume ADLs.
Refer the patient to a vocational counselor, as appropriate.	Long-term physical impairment may require the patient to change employment.
Collaborate with community organizations to inform the public about injury prevention.	Injury prevention saves the person and society as a whole an enormous economic burden.

NURSING DIAGNOSIS NO. 4: **Impaired Swallowing**

Related Factors

- Aspiration pneumonia
- Decreased weight
- Impaired oral hygiene
- Decreased food and fluid intake

Expected Outcomes

- Does not aspirate
- Maintains adequate nutrition intake
- Achieves and maintains weight
- Maintains oral hygiene
- Patient and caregiver demonstrate correct feeding techniques

Nursing Interventions	Rationales
NIC Swallowing Therapy	
Consult with a speech-language pathologist (SLP) and nutritionist (registered dietitian [RD]).	Based on diagnostic studies (e.g., barium swallow, video fluoroscopy) the SLP collaborates with the RD to develop the best diet for the patient.
Obtain daily weights.	This information allows changes in diet to be instituted quickly.
Count calories.	
Monitor laboratory work and consult with the health care team about the need for diet adjustment.	
Provide the patient with supplements such as milkshakes and Ensure, as needed.	Supplements may be needed to meet caloric and protein requirements.
Offer foods such as beef broth and sweet, sour, or salty foods if tolerated.	These foods stimulate saliva production and facilitate the swallowing process.
Provide soft or semisoft foods and fluids. Add powdered thickener (Thick-It) to thicken foods.	Thickened foods and fluids make liquids more manageable and help prevent aspiration.

Continued

PLAN OF CARE Medical Diagnosis: Critically Ill Neurologic Problem Affecting the Brain/Postoperative Craniotomy—cont'd

NURSING DIAGNOSIS NO. 4: Impaired Swallowing—cont'd

Position the patient for meals sitting in a chair or up straight in bed. Position the head and neck slightly forward and flexed. Tell the patient to place food in the back of the mouth on the unaffected side. Keep the patient in the upright position for 30 minutes after eating.	Proper positioning helps prevent aspiration by facilitating swallowing.
Monitor for aspiration including coughing, dyspnea, and cyanosis. Keep suction equipment at the bedside.	Early recognition and treatment of aspiration may prevent aspiration pneumonia.

NURSING DIAGNOSIS NO. 5: Risk for Infection

Related Factors

Invasive procedures and monitoring
Insufficient knowledge to avoid exposure to pathogens
Trauma or injury
Tissue destruction and increased environmental exposure
Increased environmental exposure to pathogens
Immunosuppression (steroids)

Expected Outcomes

Vital signs within normal range for age and condition
Blood work within normal range
Surgical incision, wounds, invasive monitoring insertion sites (e.g., IVs, CVP) free of infection
Breath sounds normal for age and other medical conditions
Adequate fluid and caloric intake either orally or via gastric tube or total enteral nutrition (TEN)

Nursing Interventions	Rationales
NIC Infection Protection	
Monitor for systemic and localized signs and symptoms of infection. Monitor vital signs every 4 hours.	Elevated temperature, pulse, and respirations indicate systemic infection. Redness, heat, swelling, and pain indicate local infection.
Wash hands before, between, and after patient care. Assist the patient to wash hands as needed.	Handwashing is the single most effective method to prevent infection.
Monitor absolute granulocyte count, white blood cell (WBC) count, and differential results.	Elevations in these laboratory tests demonstrate the body's response to infection.
Obtain cultures, as needed (e.g., sputum, blood, urine, wound).	Purulent wound drainage indicates infection. A culture will identify the causative agent and indicate the appropriate antibiotic therapy.
Inspect the condition of any surgical incision, wound, or invasive monitoring insertion site.	A surgical incision may be slightly reddened and swollen from tissue damage but remain free of the purulent drainage, excess swelling, or excess local pain that indicates infection.
Follow agency policy regarding rotating IV sites and removal of invasive monitoring devices.	Asepsis will minimize patient exposure to pathogenic agents and thus minimize the incidence of infection.
Obtain a dietary consult. Monitor intake and output. Count calories, as needed. Provide high-protein supplements, as needed.	Protein and other nutrients are needed to decrease the risk of infection and promote healing.

NURSING DIAGNOSIS NO. 6: Impaired Verbal Communication

Related Factors

Aphasia
Agnosia

Expected Outcomes

Improves communication skills
Can communicate without being frustrated and angry

D Indicates nursing activities that can be delegated to unlicensed assistive nursing personnel at the discretion of the nurse.

PLAN OF CARE Medical Diagnosis: Critically Ill Neurologic Problem Affecting the Brain/Postoperative Craniotomy—cont'd

NURSING DIAGNOSIS NO. 6: **Impaired Verbal Communication—cont'd**

Nursing Interventions	Rationales
NIC Active Listening	
Talk to the patient, not to the visitors.	
Face the patient, make eye contact, speak slowly and clearly.	Facing the patient makes it easier for him or her to hear and understand spoken words.
Do not interrupt when the patient attempts to speak; do not finish the patient's words; allow time for the patient to answer.	
Provide music or other visual stimuli that are meaningful to the patient.	
Assist the patient to adjust to limitations caused by communication problems.	

neurologic status to the health care provider immediately! The first sign of increased ICP is a declining level of consciousness (LOC). Management of increased ICP, including drug therapy, is discussed on p. 1055 under Interventions in the Traumatic Brain Injury section.

The head of the bed (HOB) should be flat or elevated no more than 30 degrees. The rationale is to increase blood flow to the ischemic brain. The physician, clinical pathway, or other plan of care may designate the desired HOB position. Maintain the head in a midline, neutral position to help promote venous drainage from the brain.

In collaboration with other team members, plan care to avoid activities and procedures that may increase ICP, particularly if the patient has indications of cerebral edema. Extreme hip and neck flexion should be avoided. Extreme hip flexion may increase intrathoracic pressure, which may make ICP more difficult to control. Extreme neck flexion interferes with venous drainage from the brain, also making ICP more difficult to control.

Additional nursing considerations include avoiding the clustering of nursing procedures (e.g., giving a bath followed immediately by changing the bed linen) within a short time. This is because the effect on ICP elevation is more dramatic when multiple activities are clustered within a narrow time interval. Hyperoxygenating the patient before suctioning may also be appropriate to avoid even transient hypoxemia and resultant ICP elevation from dilation of cerebral arteries. Fully assess the need for suctioning, because it increases ICP. A quiet environment is particularly important for the patient experiencing a headache, which is common with an aneurysm or increased ICP. The patient may have **photophobia** (sensitivity to light). Therefore the room lights should be kept low.

Monitor vital signs closely, at least every 2 to 4 hours. Notify the health care provider if the blood pressure exceeds acceptable levels. Generally, the health care provider allows the patient to be slightly hypertensive (150/100 mm Hg) to promote cerebral tissue perfusion. A higher blood pressure could lead to a hemorrhagic stroke or rebleeding of an aneurysm (if present). Carefully monitor the patient's temperature, because fever may cause increased ICP. Hypothermia may cause decreased cerebral perfusion.

Patients admitted to a critical care unit are connected to a cardiac monitor and observed for dysrhythmias. The critical care nurse performs a cardiac assessment, with particular attention directed toward auscultation of heart sounds to identify the presence of cardiac murmurs or atrial fibrillation (AF). Murmurs or AF may place the patient at increased risk for emboli. Close physical assessment for indications of hemodynamic stability is indicated. Invasive hemodynamic monitoring may be needed to monitor and evaluate physiologic stability and response to therapy.

Drug therapy. The drugs prescribed depend on the type of stroke and the resulting neurologic dysfunction. In general, the purposes of drug therapy are to prevent further thrombotic episodes (anticoagulation) and to protect the neurons from hypoxia.

Anticoagulants/antiplatelets. Although previously widely used, anticoagulants are controversial and are not considered current best practice by the American Stroke Association for acute ischemic strokes or for preventing future strokes (Adams et al., 2007). Sodium heparin and other anticoagulants, such as warfarin (Coumadin, Warfilone♣), are **high-alert drugs** that can cause bleeding, including intracerebral hemorrhage.

However, an *initial* dose of 325 mg of enteric-coated or other form of aspirin (Ecotrin, Ancasal♣) is recommended within 24 to 48 hours after stroke onset. Aspirin should not be given within 24 hours of rtPA administration. These drugs are antiplatelet drugs and prevent blood clotting by reducing platelet adhesiveness (clumping). These drugs can cause bruising, hemorrhage, and liver disease over a long-term period. Teach the patient to report any unusual bruising or bleeding to the health care provider. The 2007 best practice guidelines for the treatment of acute ischemic stroke recommend *against* the use of clopidogrel (Plavix) or ticlopidine hydrochloride (Ticlid) alone or in combination with aspirin (Adams et al., 2007). Unlike aspirin, these antiplatelet drugs have not been studied for their use after a stroke.

Other drugs. To treat seizures, lorazepam (Ativan), a benzodiazepine, may be administered with close neurologic and cardiopulmonary monitoring. For long-term antiseizure therapy, the health care provider may also prescribe antiepileptic drugs (AEDs), such as phenytoin (Dilantin), gabapentin (Neurontin), or topiramate (Topamax). Neuroprotective drugs such as calcium channel blockers (e.g., nimodipine [Nimotop]) may be given to treat or prevent cerebral vasospasm after a subarachnoid hemorrhage. Vasospasm, which usually occurs between 4 and 14 days after the stroke, slows blood flow to the area and worsens ischemia. Calcium channel blockers work by relaxing the smooth muscles of the vessel wall and reducing the incidence and severity of the spasm. Neurologic functioning may improve, and further deterioration from ischemia is then prevented. In addition, these drugs dilate collateral vessels to ischemic areas of the brain. Although these neuroprotective and vasodilating drugs are sometimes used, the American Stroke Association does not recommend them (Adams et al., 2007). Stool softeners, analgesics for pain, and anti-anxiety drugs may also be prescribed as needed for symptom management. Stool softeners also prevent the Valsalva maneuver during defecation to prevent increased ICP.

Monitoring for other complications. Monitor the patient with an aneurysm or arteriovenous malformation (AVM) for signs and symptoms of hydrocephalus and vasospasm. **Hydrocephalus** (increased cerebrospinal fluid [CSF] within the ventricular and subarachnoid spaces) may occur as a result of blood in the CSF. This prevents CSF from being reabsorbed properly by the arachnoid villi. Cerebral edema, which interferes with the flow of CSF out from the ventricular system, may also develop. Eventually the ventricles become enlarged. If hydrocephalus is left untreated, increased intracranial pressure (ICP) results. Observe for clinical manifestations of hydrocephalus, which are similar to those of ICP elevation, including a change in the LOC. Clinical findings may also include headache, pupil changes, seizures, poor coordination, gait disturbances (if ambulatory), and behavior changes.

Clinical manifestations of vasospasm may include decreased LOC, motor and reflex changes, and increased neurologic deficits (e.g., cranial nerve dysfunction, motor weakness, and aphasia). The symptoms may fluctuate with the occurrence and degree of vasospasm present.

Rebleeding or rupture is a common complication for the patient with an aneurysm or AVM. It may occur within 24 hours of the initial bleed or rupture and up to 7 to 10 days later. Assess for severe headache, nausea and vomiting, a decreased LOC, and additional neurologic deficits. Potential consequences of aneurysm re-bleeding may be catastrophic.

Carotid artery angioplasty with stenting. With the development and refinement of vascular stents, carotid artery angioplasty with stenting (CAS) has become very common. This interventional radiology procedure is done under local anesthesia or moderate sedation. It may be performed by a cardiovascular surgeon or interventional radiologist.

A device called a **distal/embolic protection device (DSP/ESP)** has made this procedure very safe. The DSP is placed beyond the stenosis through a catheter inserted into the femoral artery (groin). It catches any clot debris that breaks off during the CAS. Placement of a carotid stent is performed to open a blockage in the carotid artery typically at the division of the common carotid artery into the internal and external carotid arteries. Throughout the procedure, the patient's neurologic and cardiovascular status are assessed. CAS is less invasive, causes less blood loss, requires shorter hospital stays (overnight) and recovery time, and has fewer complications than a carotid endarterectomy (Strimike, 2007). Postprocedure care is the same as that provided for a carotid endarterectomy (see Surgical Management on p. 1045).

Other nonsurgical techniques. New early techniques are being tried for patients who are not candidates for thrombolytic therapy. For example, hypothermia treatment started during the first few hours after onset of a stroke may help preserve neurologic function in select patients. Techniques for cooling need further evaluation with well-structured research to identify optimal patient selection criteria, target temperature, and duration of therapy. Neuroprotective drugs such as sodium channel blockers, opioid antagonists, free radical scavengers, magnesium, estrogens, gamma-aminobutyric acid (GABA) antagonists, glutamate receptor antagonists, and membrane stabilizers are being tested as a therapy for stroke. A clot-dissolving substance in vampire bat saliva (Ancrod) is also being tested and may be used to develop a new drug to treat occlusive strokes. No conclusive results have been demonstrated, and research is ongoing (Adams et al., 2007). Stem cell and tissue transplants are also being investigated for their potential benefit in replacing dead or damaged neurons and restoring otherwise lost brain function (Hinkle, 2007).

The usual treatment of an *arteriovenous malformation (AVM)* uses interventional therapy to block abnormal arteries or veins and prevent bleeding from the vascular lesion. The same procedure may be performed to occlude the vessels surrounding an aneurysm. Under fluoroscopic guidance, the physician inserts a microcatheter into the carotid artery, typically using a femoral artery approach, and threads it to the vessel to be embolized. The physician then injects an embolic agent, such as platinum coils, detachable silicone balloons, liquid acrylic, or polyvinyl alcohol, to embolize the involved arteries (Fig. 47-4). If the AVM is large, the physician may elect to occlude the artery gradually to allow for a

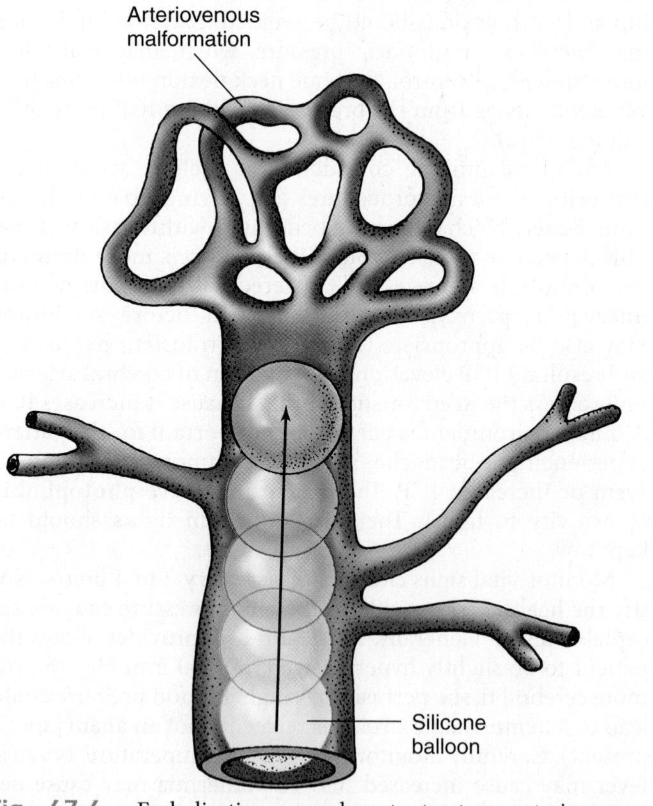
Arteriovenous malformation
Silicone balloon

Fig. 47-4 • Embolization procedure to treat an arteriovenous malformation. The embolic agent travels to the area to cause vessel thrombosis.

slow change in the blood supply to the surrounding brain. In this case, the embolization procedure is carried out over 1 to 2 weeks.

For clipping small aneurysms, a minimally invasive procedure using an endoscope (lighted tube) may be used. Other procedures that do not require a cranial incision are classified as *interventional radiology.* For example, an interventional neuroradiologist can direct a small catheter into the femoral artery and advance the catheter into the aneurysm. Specially designed, detachable platinum wire coils are placed into the aneurysm, which helps seal the area with a clot. It is predicted that this method will soon treat most intracranial aneurysms, thus avoiding craniotomies and their complications.

Surgical Management. Some patients are candidates for surgery to prevent or treat strokes. The surgical procedure depends on the cause of the stroke.

Carotid endarterectomy is a widely used surgical procedure to prevent progressing stroke in symptomatic patients with recurrent TIAs or carotid stenosis. The purpose of a **carotid endarterectomy** is to remove atherosclerotic plaque from the inner lining of the carotid artery. The procedure opens the artery enough to re-establish blood flow and decrease stroke risk.

The patient usually stays in the hospital for two nights unless complications occur or the patient is older. Postprocedure care involves monitoring vital signs, neurologic status, and peripheral pulses. Check the incision site for bleeding. Complications are not common, although stroke is possible. Monitor the patient for cerebral hyperperfusion, which may occur because of increased vascular pressure (from the open artery) and lead to intracranial hemorrhage (stroke). Before discharge, teach the patient to report these symptoms to the health care provider as soon as possible:

- Severe headache
- Change in brain function (e.g., drowsiness, decreased cognition)
- Muscle weakness
- Severe neck pain
- Neck swelling
- Hoarseness or difficulty swallowing (due to nerve damage)

In an **extracranial-intracranial bypass,** the surgeon performs a craniotomy (surgical opening into the brain through the skull) and bypasses the blocked artery by making a graft or a bypass from the first artery to the second artery. This procedure establishes blood flow around the blocked artery and re-establishes blood flow to the involved areas. The two most common techniques are the superficial middle temporal artery-to-middle cerebral artery (STA-MCA) graft and the occipital-to-posterior inferior cerebellar artery (PICA) bypass. Studies show that immediate surgery is associated with a high risk of intracranial hemorrhage and no improvement in outcome except in the patient with an embolus to the middle cerebral artery (Adams et al., 2007).

Whenever possible, an AVM is also totally removed via a craniotomy. The surgeon ligates the group of vessels and removes the defect. Gamma radiation delivered through the gamma knife (see discussion on p. 1062 under Stereotactic Radiosurgery) produces fibrous thickening of the endothelial lining of the vessels to prevent further vessel enlargement and ultimately eliminate the lesion from the cerebral circulation. Improved microsurgical techniques have significantly reduced morbidity and mortality rates, and these procedures are becoming the treatment of choice in many medical centers.

Cerebral aneurysms may be repaired via a craniotomy as soon as the patient's condition is stabilized. Surgery may be postponed for patients with ruptured aneurysms that caused stupor or coma, because their condition makes them high-risk surgical candidates. During surgery, the aneurysm is clipped or a clamp is placed at the base, or neck, of the aneurysm to prevent blood from entering the area. If the aneurysm does not have a neck, it may be wrapped with muscle, muslin, or a plastic coating to reinforce the wall and prevent rebleeding. Timing of the surgery and specific interventions are usually determined by individual physician preferences. Visitors may be limited, and measures to decrease the patient's stress and increase comfort are usually initiated.

For some patients who have hemorrhagic strokes, blood clots may be removed via a craniotomy to relieve intracranial pressure (ICP). Particular indications for clot removal would be a progressively worsening neurologic examination and extension of the intracranial lesion with significant ICP elevation. The care of the patient having a craniotomy is discussed on p. 1063.

Impaired Swallowing

NOC **Planning: Expected Outcomes.** The patient with a stroke is expected to have safe passage of fluids and solids from the mouth to the stomach. Indicators include that the patient will have the best possible ability to:

- Maintain food in the mouth
- Handle oral secretions
- Chew
- Deliver bolus to hypopharynx in time with swallow reflex
- Clear oral cavity

Interventions. Before the patient is given any liquids, food, and medication, he or she must be screened for the ability to swallow. Follow agency guidelines for the screening procedure. Observe for facial drooping, drooling, impaired voluntary cough, hoarseness, incomplete mouth closure, or cranial nerve palsies. Next check the gag and cough reflex. If the patient does not pass this swallowing screen, collaborate with the speech-language pathologist (SLP) to conduct a bedside swallowing screening and evaluation. He or she may recommend a modified barium swallow (video fluoroscopy) to identify specific structures that are impaired during swallowing. *Ensure that the patient remains completely NPO until the SLP determines that the patient can tolerate liquids or foods without aspirating.* Based on the complete swallowing evaluation, the SLP makes recommendations for feeding for the staff to follow. Remind all unlicensed personnel and the family about the need to follow these precautions exactly as they are written.

Some patients can swallow without difficulty but are at risk for aspiration because they are easily distracted and impulsive. These patients require a distraction-free environment with minimal disruption from television, visitors, or environmental noise. Observe for indications of fatigue, because this can significantly interfere with the desire and ability to eat.

NCLEX EXAMINATION CHALLENGE

An older client is admitted to the critical care unit after a left carotid endarterectomy this morning. Which nursing assessment finding is the most important to report to the surgeon?

A. Nausea when moving in bed
B. Blood pressure of 148/86 mm Hg
C. Pain rated at 5 on a 1-10 scale
D. Increasing drowsiness

evolve For the correct answer, go to http://evolve.elsevier.com/Iggy/.

Impaired Physical Mobility; Self-Care Deficit

NOC **Planning: Expected Outcomes.** The patient with a stroke is expected to be able to move purposefully in his or her own environment independently, with or without an assistive device. Indicators include that the best possible outcome for the patient will be achieved in these areas:

- Balance and coordination
- Gait
- Transfer performance

The patient is also expected to perform basic personal care activities and household tasks. Indicators include that the patient will be able to function as independently as possible in:

- Bathing self
- Dressing self
- Feeding self
- Maintaining personal cleanliness
- Toileting
- Performing household tasks

Interventions. Patients who have had a stroke often have flaccid or spastic paralysis. It is not unusual for the patient to have a spastic arm and flaccid leg on the affected side. The affected leg often regains function more quickly than the arm. Patients begin rehabilitation as soon as possible to regain function and prevent complications of immobility, such as pneumonia, atelectasis, and pressure ulcers.

Another major complication of impaired physical mobility is the development of deep vein thrombosis (DVT). This risk is highest in older patients and those with a severe stroke. Provide care to prevent this complication by applying sequential compression stockings or pneumatic compression boots, changing the patient's position frequently, and ambulating the patient if possible. Always report any indications of DVT to the health care provider, and document assessments in the patient's chart. Chapter 38 discusses DVT in detail.

The rehabilitation therapists evaluate the patient's ability to perform basic ADLs and household tasks that will be performed at home. After a thorough evaluation, collaborate with them to develop a plan of care to promote patient independence, with or without assistive or adaptive devices. Therapy begins in the hospital setting and continues after discharge in most cases. Chapter 8 describes interventions for improving mobility and promoting self-management.

Impaired Verbal Communication

NOC **Planning: Expected Outcomes.** Ideally, the patient with a stroke is expected to receive, interpret, and express spoken, written, and nonverbal messages. However, some patients may need to develop strategies for alternative methods of communication, such as pictures or nonverbal language.

Interventions. Language or speech problems are usually the result of a stroke involving the dominant hemisphere. The left cerebral hemisphere is the speech center in most patients. Speech and language problems may be the result of aphasia or dysarthria. Although aphasia is caused by cerebral hemisphere damage, **dysarthria** is due to a loss of motor function to the tongue or to the muscles of speech, causing slurred speech. Involvement of the speech-language pathologist (SLP) as early as possible in the hospitalization greatly increases the patient's chances for optimal recovery. Remind patients to practice their exercises for dysarthria to strengthen their facial and oral muscles.

Aphasia can be classified in a number of ways. Most commonly, it is classified as expressive, receptive, or mixed (Table 47-2). **Expressive (Broca's, or motor) aphasia** is the result of damage in Broca's area of the frontal lobe. It is a motor speech problem in which the patient generally understands what is said but cannot communicate verbally. He or she also has difficulty writing but may be able to write. Rote speech and automatic speech such as responses to a greeting are often intact. The patient is aware of the deficit and may become frustrated and angry. Reassure patients and remind them to talk slowly.

Receptive (Wernicke's, or sensory) aphasia is due to injury involving Wernicke's area in the temporoparietal area. The patient cannot understand the spoken and often the written word. Although he or she may be able to talk, the language is often meaningless. Neologisms (made-up words) are common parts of speech.

Usually the patient has some degree of dysfunction in the areas of both expression and reception. This is known as *mixed aphasia.* Reading and writing ability are equally affected. Few patients have just expressive *or* receptive aphasia. In most cases, though, one type is dominant.

To help communicate with the patient with aphasia, use these guiding principles:

- Present one idea or thought in a sentence (e.g., "I am going to help you get into the chair").
- Use simple one-step commands rather than ask patients to do multiple tasks.
- Speak slowly but not loudly; use cues or gestures as needed.
- Avoid "yes" and "no" questions for patients with expressive aphasia, because they often give automatic responses that may be incorrect.
- Use alternative forms of communication if needed, such as a computer, communication board, or flash cards (often with pictures).

TABLE 47-2 Types of Aphasia

EXPRESSIVE
• Referred to as *Broca's,* or *motor, aphasia*
• Difficulty speaking
• Difficulty writing
RECEPTIVE
• Referred to as *Wernicke's,* or *sensory, aphasia*
• Difficulty understanding spoken words
• Difficulty understanding written words
• Speech often meaningless
• Made-up words
MIXED
• Combination of difficulty understanding words and speech
• Difficulty with reading and writing
GLOBAL
• Profound speech and language problems
• Often no speech or sounds that cannot be understood

For more specific communication strategies for your patient, collaborate with the SLP.

Total Urinary Incontinence; Bowel Incontinence

NOC **Planning: Expected Outcomes.** The patient with a stroke is expected to control elimination of urine and stool. Indicators include that the patient will consistently demonstrate the ability to:

- Recognize the urge to void and defecate
- Maintain predictable pattern of urinary and bowel elimination
- Respond to urge in timely manner
- Get to toilet between urge and passage of urine or stool
- Empty bladder and bowel completely

Interventions. The patient may be incontinent of urine and stool because of an altered level of consciousness, impaired innervation, or an inability to communicate the need to urinate or defecate. Before beginning an education program to correct these problems, the cause must first be established. Typically, the patient who has had a stroke can regain both bowel and bladder control in time. To begin a bladder training program, place the patient on the bedpan or the commode or offer the urinal every 2 hours. Encourage a total fluid intake of at least 2000 mL daily unless contraindicated because of renal or cardiac health problems. A bedside bladder ultrasound is used to check for residual urine after voiding in the early phase of the bladder training program to ensure that the patient is emptying the bladder. Retained urine can lead to a urinary tract infection.

Before establishing a bowel training program, determine the patient's normal time for bowel elimination and any routine that helps promote a stool. This routine is followed, if possible, and the patient is placed on the commode or toilet at the same time as the previous schedule at home. Collaborate with the nutritionist to provide a diet high in bulk and fiber. Encourage the patient to drink apple or prune juice to help promote bowel elimination. A stool softener (Colace) may be prescribed. Suppositories may also assist in re-establishing a bowel routine. Chapter 8 provides a complete discussion of bowel and bladder training programs.

If the patient has an indwelling urinary catheter, it should be removed as soon as possible to prevent the development of bacteremia and sepsis. The patient with a fever or an older adult who becomes increasingly confused should be evaluated for a urinary tract infection.

Disturbed Sensory Perception

Planning: Expected Outcomes. The major concern of patients with sensory or perceptual changes is adapting to the deficits. Therefore the patient with a stroke is expected to adapt to sensory or perceptual changes in vision, proprioception (position sense), and sensation and to be free from injury.

Interventions. Patients with right hemisphere brain damage typically have difficulty with visual-perceptual or spatial-perceptual tasks. They have problems with depth and distance perception and with discrimination of right from left or up from down. Because of these problems, they have difficulty performing routine ADLs. Caregivers help the patient adapt to these disabilities by using frequent verbal and tactile cues and by breaking down tasks into discrete steps. Always approach the patient from the unaffected side, which should face the door of the room.

Place objects within the patient's field of vision. A mirror may help visualize more of the environment. If the patient has **diplopia** (double vision), a patch may be placed over the affected eye. Remind the nursing staff to ensure a safe environment by removing clutter from the room.

The patient with a left hemisphere lesion generally has memory deficits and may show significant changes in the ability to carry out simple tasks. To assist with memory problems, reorient the patient to the month, year, day of the week, and circumstances surrounding hospital admission. Establish a routine or schedule that is as structured, repetitious, and consistent as possible. Provide information in a simple, concise manner. A step-by-step approach is often most effective because the patient can master one step before moving to the next. When possible, ask the family to bring in pictures and other familiar objects.

The patient may be unable to plan and execute tasks in an organized manner. Apraxia, or the inability to perform previously learned motor skills or commands, may be present. Typically, the patient with apraxia exhibits a slow, cautious, and hesitant behavior style. The physical therapist assists the patient in compensating for loss of position sense.

Unilateral Neglect

Planning: Expected Outcomes. The patient with stroke is expected to adjust and use techniques to compensate for one-sided neglect.

Interventions. Unilateral neglect, or neglect syndrome, occurs most commonly in patients who have had a right cerebral stroke. However, it can occur in any patient who experiences hemianopsia, in which the vision of one or both eyes is affected. This problem places the patient at additional risk for injury, especially falls, because of an inability to recognize his or her physical impairment or because of a lack of proprioception (position sense).

Teach the patient to touch and use both sides of the body. For example, encourage the patient to wash both the affected and unaffected sides of the body. When dressing, remind the patient to dress the affected side first. If hemianopsia is present, teach the patient to turn his or her head from side to side to expand the visual field. This scanning technique is also useful when the patient is eating or ambulating.

Community-Based Care

The patient with a stroke may be discharged within 2 to 3 days to home, a rehabilitation center, or a skilled nursing facility (SNF), depending on the extent of the disability and the availability of family or caregiver support. Some patients have no significant neurologic dysfunction and are able to return home and live independently or with minimal support. Other patients are able to return home but require ongoing assistance with ADLs, as well as supervision to prevent accidents or injury. Speech, physical, and/or occupational therapy may continue in the home or on an ambulatory care basis. Patients admitted to a rehabilitation unit/facility or SNF require continued or more complex nursing care as well as extensive physical, occupational, recreational, speech-language, or cognitive therapy, which is coordinated by a case manager. The expected outcome for rehabilitation is to maximize the patient's abilities in all aspects of life. Jeong and Kim (2007) tested a community-based intervention to keep stroke patients active and improve their mood (see the Evidence-Based Practice box on p. 1048).

Some patients who have strokes have severe brain damage. They have profound neurologic impairments and require palliative care.

EVIDENCE-BASED PRACTICE

Community-based rehabilitation for stroke patients

Jeong, S., & Kim, M.T. (2007). Effects of a theory-driven music and movement program for stroke survivors in a community setting. *Applied Nursing Research, 20*(3), 125-131.

Stroke remains the number-one cause of death and disability in South Korea. The quality of life for stroke survivors depends largely on the patient's functional health status. The researchers recruited a small group of subjects for a neighborhood community health center in a large metropolitan city. The 36 participants were randomized into two groups: the experimental group (18) and the control group (18). The experimental group received an 8-week rhythmic auditory stimulation (RAS) music-movement program conducted 2 hours each week. The control group received only referral information about the usual care available in the community. The results showed that the RAS program increased range of motion and joint flexibility, improved mood state, and increased frequency and quality of interpersonal relationships. The participants enjoyed taking the program with other stroke survivors, which increased their sociability.

Level of Evidence—6. This study is an example of a descriptive study, although the small convenience sample was randomized into two groups.

Commentary: Implications for Practice and Research. Although this study was done in South Korea, it has implications for working with stroke survivors in the United States and other countries. The Joint Commission requires continuity of care to ensure that patients leaving the hospital can have their needs met in the community. A program such as the RAS has multiple physical and psychosocial benefits. Community health nurses can develop programs such as this one to help stroke patients have an improved quality of life. More studies are needed with larger groups in other locations.

Home Care Management

Collaborate with the case manager to plan the patient's discharge. Coordinate with rehabilitation therapists to identify needs for assistive or adaptive and safety equipment. The extent of this assessment depends on the patient's disabilities. The home of the patient with hemiparesis should be free from scatter rugs or other obstacles in the walking pathways. The bathtub and toilet should be equipped with grab bars. Antiskid patches or strips should be placed in the bathtub to prevent slipping. The PT or OT works with the patient and the family or significant others to obtain all needed assistive devices and home modifications *before* the patient is discharged from the hospital, rehabilitation setting, or SNF. Appointments for outpatient speech, physical, and occupational therapy are arranged before discharge for continuing care.

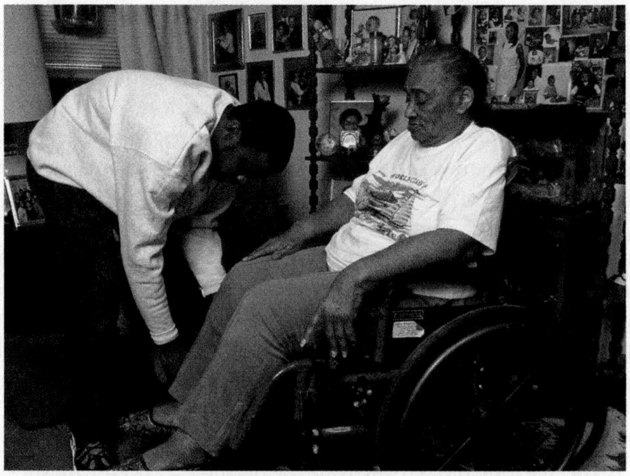

Fig. 47-5 • Son adjusting his mother's wheelchair.

Health Teaching

As part of the discharge process, educate the family about depression that may occur within the 3 months after a stroke. The strongest predictors of post-stroke depression (PSD) are a history of depression, severe stroke, and post-stroke physical or cognitive impairment. Patients may not exhibit typical signs of depression because of their cognitive, physical, and emotional impairments. PSD is associated with increased morbidity and mortality, especially in older men.

The teaching plan for the patient with a stroke also includes drug therapy, ambulation/transfer skills, communication skills, safety precautions, nutritional management, activity levels, and self-management skills. Health teaching should focus on tasks that must be performed by the patient and the family after hospital discharge. Provide both written and verbal instruction in all these areas. Return demonstrations assist in evaluating the family members' competency in tasks required for the patient's care (Fig. 47-5).

The patient must take the prescribed drugs to prevent another stroke and control hypertension. Teach the patient and the family the name of each drug, the dosage, the timing of administration and how to take it, and possible side effects. In collaboration with the PT and OT, teach the patient how to climb stairs safely, if he or she is able; transfer from the bed to a chair; get into and out of a car; and use any aids for mobility. The patient and family members are also taught how to use any equipment needed to increase independence in self-management skills. Provide important information regarding what to do in an emergency and whom to call for nonemergency questions.

Families may feel overwhelmed by the continuing demands placed on them. Depending on the location of the lesion, the patient may be anxious, slow, cautious, hesitant, and lack initiative (left hemisphere lesions) or he or she may be impulsive and seemingly unaware of any deficit. Family members and other caregivers need to spend time away from the patient on a routine basis to continue to provide full-time care without sacrificing their own physical and emotional health. Refer the family to social services or other community resources for further support, counseling, and possible respite care.

Health Care Resources

Available resources include a variety of publications from the American Heart Association (www.americanheart.org), including *Stroke: A Guide for Families* and *Stroke: Why Do They*

Behave That Way? The National Stroke Association (www.stroke.org) also provides publications and videotapes for caregivers and patients. *Recovering After a Stroke: A Patient and Family Guide* is available from the Agency for Healthcare Research and Quality (www.ahrq.gov), formerly the Agency for Health Care Policy and Research. Refer the patient and family members or significant others to local stroke support groups.

For patients who require palliative end-of-life care, refer the family to hospice care. Chapter 9 gives a detailed description of end-of-life care and advance directives.

Evaluation: Outcomes

Evaluate the care of the patient with stroke on the basis of the identified nursing diagnoses and collaborative problems. The expected outcomes are that the patient:

- Has an adequate blood flow through the cerebral vasculature to maintain brain function
- Moves purposefully in his or her own environment with or without assistive devices
- Learns to adapt to sensory and perceptual changes
- Adjusts and uses techniques to compensate for one-sided neglect
- Receives, interprets, and expresses messages or develops strategies for alternative communication methods
- Has safe passage of fluids and solids from the mouth to the stomach
- Controls elimination of urine and stool

Specific indicators for these outcomes are listed for each nursing diagnosis under the Planning and Implementation section (see earlier).

TRAUMATIC BRAIN INJURY

Pathophysiology

A head injury occurs as the result of a blow or jolt to the head or as a result of penetration of the head by a bullet or other foreign object. As a result, the normal functioning of the brain is disrupted. Regardless of the severity of injury, the patient may have short-term or long-term physical, cognitive, financial, and emotional consequences.

Various terms are used to describe the brain injuries that occur when a mechanical force is applied either directly or indirectly to the brain. A force produced by a blow to the head is a *direct* injury, whereas a force applied to another body part with a rebound effect to the brain is an *indirect* injury. The brain responds to these forces by movement within the rigid cranial vault. It may also rebound or rotate on the brainstem, causing diffuse axonal injury (shearing injuries). The brain may be contused (bruised) or lacerated/torn as it moves over the inner surfaces of the cranium, which are irregularly shaped and sharp. Damage most commonly occurs to the frontal and temporal lobes.

Movement or distortion within the cranial cavity is possible because of multiple factors. The first factor is how the brain is supported by cerebrospinal fluid (CSF) within the cranial cavity. When external force is applied to the head, the brain can be injured by the internal surfaces of the skull and meninges. The second factor is the consistency of brain tissue, which is very fragile and prone to injury. Brain injury can also be categorized as primary or secondary.

Primary Brain Injury

Primary brain damage occurs at the time of injury and results from the physical stress (force) within the tissue caused by open or closed trauma. An **open head injury** occurs when the skull is fractured or when it is pierced by a penetrating object. The integrity of the brain and the dura is violated, and there is exposure to outside, or environmental, contaminants. Damage may occur to the underlying vessels, dural sinus, brain, and cranial nerves. A **closed head injury** is the result of blunt trauma; the integrity of the skull is not violated. It is the more serious of the two types of injury, and the damage to brain tissue depends on the degree and mechanisms of injury.

Brain injury may also be described as mild, moderate, or severe. A Glasgow Coma Scale (GCS) score of 13 to 15 and a loss of consciousness for up to 15 minutes reflect a *mild TBI (MTBI)*. A *moderate TBI* often includes a period of loss of consciousness (LOC) up to 6 hours and may occur with other systemic injury and a GCS score of 9 to 12. A short critical care stay may be needed for close monitoring. After injury, these patients may have difficulty with work, learning, and role function. *Severe head injury* (GCS score of 3 to 8 and loss of consciousness for longer than 6 hours) is more serious and requires management in critical care with ongoing monitoring of hemodynamic stability and intracranial pressure (ICP).

The incidence of *minor* head injuries is difficult to estimate because most are not reported. However, they account for most of all diagnosed head injuries. Often patients do not seek medical care because they deny that anything is wrong, do not have any health insurance, or may feel guilty over the circumstances of the injury.

Symptoms include a wide array of physical and cognitive problems that range from persistent headache, dizziness, and drowsiness to other symptoms listed on Chart 47-8. These symptoms usually resolve within 72 hours. In some cases the symptoms persist and may last days, weeks, or months. For other patients, severe physical and cognitive problems remain despite relatively mild initial symptoms and normal diagnostic test findings. This cluster of symptoms is also referred to as *post-concussion syndrome.*

Open Head Injury

The types of fractures associated with an open head injury are linear, depressed, open, and comminuted. A **linear fracture** is a simple, clean break in which the impacted area of bone

Chart 47-8 KEY FEATURES

Traumatic Brain Injury

- Amnesia (loss of memory)
- Seizure
- Loss of consciousness or sleepiness/drowsiness
- Restlessness or irritability
- Disorientation or confusion
- Scalp bruising and tenderness
- Personality changes
- Diplopia
- Gait changes
- Severe head injury:
  - Pupil changes
  - Bradycardia
  - Papilledema
  - High blood pressure/widened pulse pressure
  - Hypotension and tachycardia (hypovolemic shock)
  - Nuchal rigidity (cerebrospinal fluid [CSF] leak)

bends inward and the area around it bends outward. Linear fractures are the most common type of skull fracture. In a **depressed fracture,** the bone is pressed inward into the brain tissue to at least the thickness of the skull. In an **open fracture,** the scalp is lacerated, creating a direct opening to the brain tissue. A **comminuted fracture** involves fragmented bone with depression into the brain tissue.

A unique fracture is a *basilar skull fracture.* It occurs at the base of the skull, usually extending into the anterior, middle, or posterior fossa and results in cerebrospinal fluid (CSF) leakage from the nose or ears. This fracture has the potential for hemorrhage caused by damage to the internal carotid artery; damage to cranial nerves (CN) I, II, VII, and VIII; and infection.

Most penetrating injuries to the skull are caused by gunshot wounds (GSWs) and knife injuries. The degree of injury to brain tissue depends on the velocity (speed), mass, shape, and direction of impact. High-velocity injuries produce the greatest damage to brain tissue. As with any open head injury, the patient with a penetrating injury is at high risk for infection from the object that pierced the skull and from other environmental contaminants.

Closed Head Injury

Closed head injuries are caused by blunt trauma and lead to concussions, contusions, and lacerations of the brain. A **contusion** is a bruising of the brain tissue and is most commonly found at the site of impact (coup injury) or in a line opposite the site of impact **(contrecoup injury)** (Fig. 47-6). The base of the frontal and temporal lobes is most often involved. A **concussion** is a shaky movement of the brain and may be mild or more severe. Some patients lose consciousness for a short time.

The damage to the brain may be mild, as occurs in a concussive injury, or it may be more severe, causing diffuse axonal injury or widespread injury to the white matter of the brain. **Diffuse axonal injury (DAI)** is usually related to high-speed acceleration/deceleration as with automobile crashes. In this injury, significant damage occurs to axons in the white matter. Damage may also be found in the corpus callosum, midbrain, cerebellum, and upper brainstem. Depending on severity, small areas of hemorrhage and enlargement of the lateral ventricles may be seen on computed tomography (CT). Severe DAI may present with immediate coma, and most survivors require long-term care.

A **laceration** causes actual tearing of the cortical surface vessels, which may lead to secondary hemorrhage and significant cerebral edema and inflammation. This condition is more serious than a contusion.

Types of Force

Other factors that must be considered in the dynamics of head injury are the type of force and the mechanisms of injury involved. An *acceleration* injury is caused by an external force contacting the head, suddenly placing the head in motion. A *deceleration* injury occurs when the moving head is suddenly stopped or hits a stationary object (Fig. 47-7). These forces

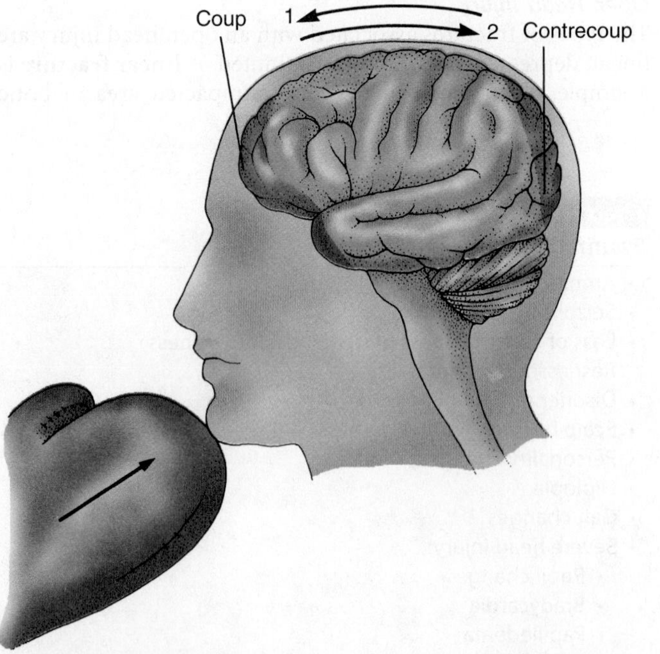
Coup
1
2 Contrecoup

Fig. 47-6 • Coup (site of impact) injury to frontal area of brain, and contrecoup injury to frontal and temporal areas of the brain.

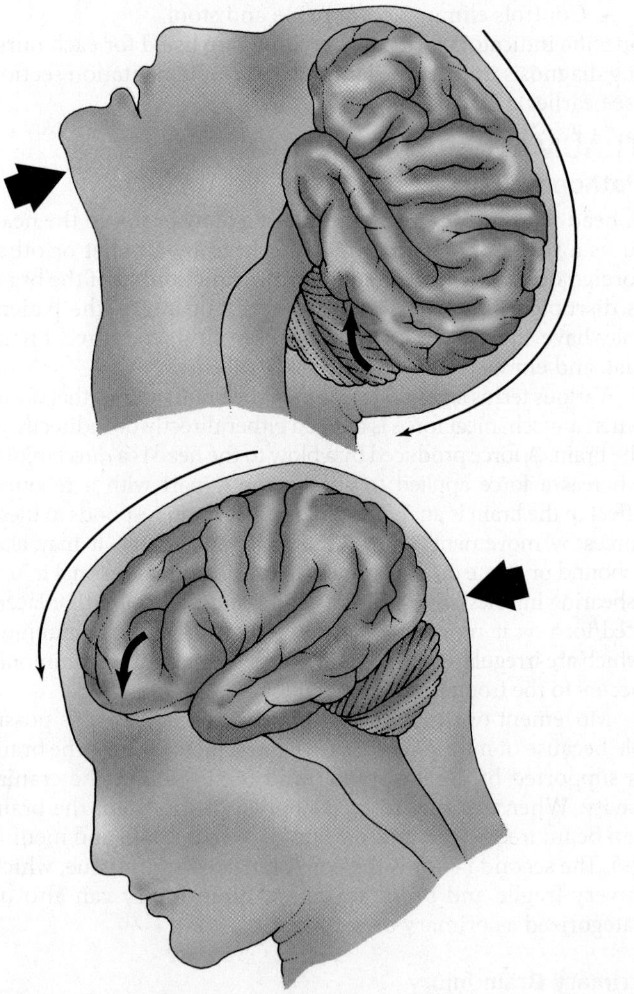

Fig. 47-7 • Head movement during acceleration-deceleration injury, which is typically seen in motor vehicle crashes.

may be sufficient to cause the cerebrum to rotate about the brainstem, resulting in shearing, straining, and distortion of the brain tissue, particularly of the axons in the brainstem and cerebellum. Small areas of hemorrhage may develop around the blood vessels that sustain the impact of these forces (stress), with destruction of adjacent brain tissue. Particularly affected are the basal nuclei and the hypothalamus.

Secondary Injury

Secondary injury to brain injury includes any processes that occurs *after* the initial injury and worsen or negatively influence outcome. They result from physiologic, vascular, and biochemical events that are an extension of the primary injury and involve cellular changes that contribute to tissue injury. The most common response is hypotension, hypoxia, ischemia, and cerebral edema. Damage to the brain tissue occurs primarily because the delivery of oxygen and glucose to the brain is interrupted.

Increased Intracranial Pressure

The cranial contents include brain tissue, blood, and cerebrospinal fluid (CSF). These components are encased in the relatively rigid skull. Within this space, there is little room for any of the components to expand or increase in volume. Through the processes of accommodation and compliance, ICP is maintained at its normal level of 10 to 15 mm Hg despite periodic increases in pressure that occur with straining during defecation, coughing, or sneezing. Any increase in the volume of one component must be compensated for by a decrease in the volume of one of the other components.

As a first response to an increase in the volume of any of these components, the CSF is shunted or displaced from the cranial compartment to the spinal subarachnoid space or the rate of CSF absorption is increased. An additional response, if needed, is a decrease in cerebral blood volume by movement of cerebral venous blood into the sinuses. As long as the brain can compensate for the increase in volume and remain compliant, increases in ICP are minimal.

Increased ICP is the leading cause of death from head trauma in patients who reach the hospital alive. It occurs when compliance no longer takes place and the brain cannot accommodate further volume changes. As ICP increases, cerebral perfusion decreases, leading to tissue hypoxia, a decrease in serum pH level, and an increase in the level of carbon dioxide. This process causes cerebral vasodilation, edema, and a further increase in ICP, and the cycle continues. If the condition remains untreated, the brain may herniate downward toward the brainstem or laterally from a unilateral lesion within one cerebral hemisphere, causing irreversible brain damage and possibly death **(brain herniation syndromes).**

Two types of edema may cause increased ICP: vasogenic edema and cytotoxic edema. A third type (interstitial edema) occurs in the presence of acute brain swelling. *Vasogenic* edema is seen most often as a cause of increased ICP in the adult. It involves an increase in the volume of brain tissue. This increase is caused by an abnormal permeability of the walls of the cerebral vessels, which allows protein-rich plasma infiltrate to leak into the extracellular space of the brain. The fluid collects primarily in the white matter.

Cytotoxic, or cellular, edema may occur as a result of a hypoxic insult, which causes a disturbance in cellular metabolism, the sodium pump, and active ion transport. The brain is quickly depleted of available oxygen, glucose, and glycogen and converts to anaerobic metabolism. The sodium pump fails, and sodium enters the cells and pulls water from the extracellular space. The serum sodium level decreases to less than 120 mEq/L (hyponatremia). As a result, an abnormal accumulation of fluid in the brain cells and a decrease in the extracellular fluid space occur. Cytotoxic edema may lead to vasogenic edema and a further increase in ICP.

Interstitial edema occurs with acute brain swelling and is associated with elevated blood pressure or increased CSF pressure. Edema develops rapidly in the perivascular and periventricular white space and can be controlled through measures to reduce blood pressure, decrease CSF pressures, or increase the **cerebral perfusion pressure (CPP).** The CPP is the pressure gradient over which the brain is perfused. It is influenced by oxygenation, cerebral blood volume, blood pressure, cerebral edema, and ICP and is determined by subtracting the mean ICP from the mean arterial pressure. *Maintenance of a CPP above 70 mm Hg is generally accepted as an expected outcome of therapy.*

Hemorrhage

Hemorrhage, which causes a brain hematoma (collection of blood) or clot, may occur as part of the primary injury and begin at the moment of impact. It may also arise later from vessel damage. Classically, bleeding is caused by vascular damage from the shearing force of the trauma or direct physical damage from skull fractures or penetrating injury. *All hematomas are potentially life threatening because they act as space-occupying lesions and are surrounded by edema.* Three major types of hemorrhage after TBI are **epidural, subdural,** and **intracerebral hemorrhage.** Subarachnoid hemorrhage may also occur. The pathophysiology of hemorrhage is discussed on p. 1031 in the Stroke section.

An **epidural hematoma** results from arterial bleeding into the space between the dura and the inner skull (Fig. 47-8). It is often caused by a fracture of the temporal bone, which houses the middle meningeal artery. Patients with epidural hematomas have "lucid intervals" that last for minutes during which time the patient is awake and talking. This follows a momentary unconsciousness that occurs within minutes of the injury. After the initial interval, symptoms progress very quickly with potentially catastrophic ICP elevation and structural changes. The patient becomes increasingly symptomatic, loses consciousness, and may become increasingly unstable. An epidural hematoma is a neurosurgical emergency!

A **subdural hematoma (SDH)** results from venous bleeding into the space beneath the dura and above the arachnoid (see Fig. 47-8). It occurs most often from a tearing of the bridging veins within the cerebral hemispheres or from a laceration of brain tissue. Bleeding from this injury occurs more slowly than from an epidural hematoma. SDHs are subdivided into acute, subacute, and chronic. An acute SDH presents within 48 hours after impact; the subacute SDH, between 48 hours and 2 weeks; and the chronic SDH, from 2 weeks to several months after injury. SDHs have the highest mortality rate.

An intracerebral hemorrhage (ICH) is the accumulation of blood within the brain tissue caused by the tearing of small arteries and veins in the subcortical white matter (see Fig. 47-8). A subarachnoid hemorrhage (SAH) is the most common type of ICH. It may act as a space-occupying lesion and may

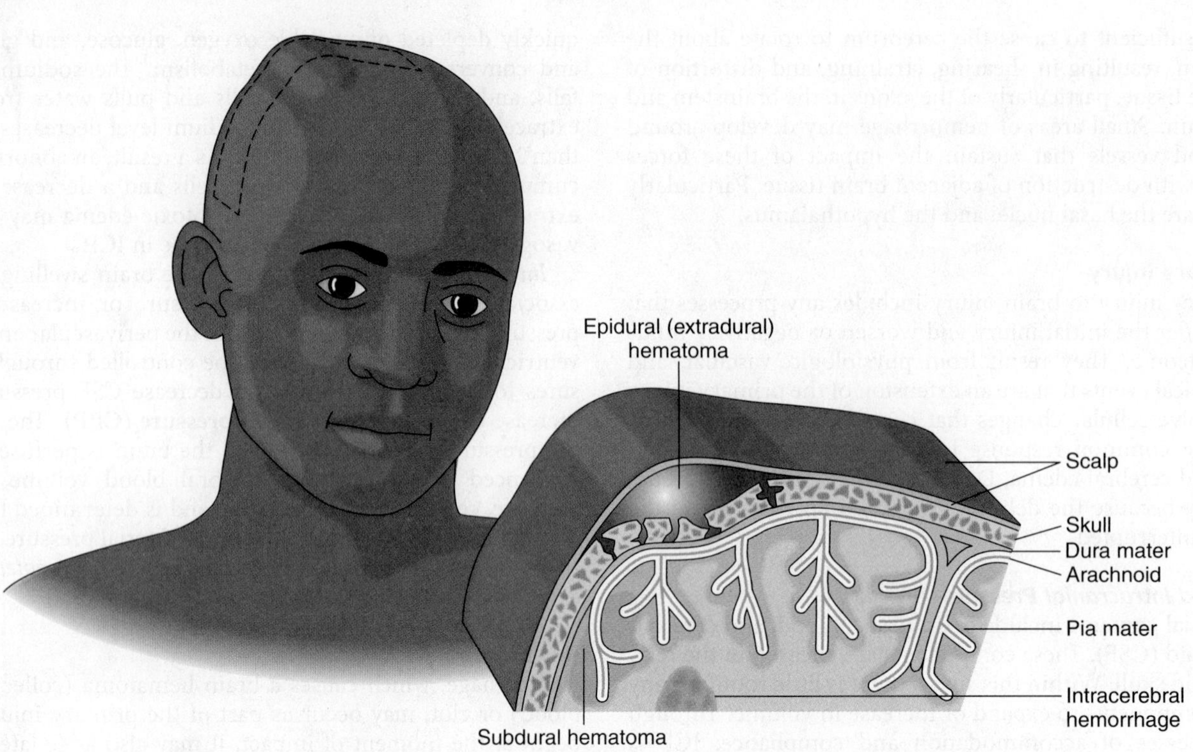

Epidural (extradural) hematoma
Scalp
Skull
Dura mater
Arachnoid
Pia mater
Intracerebral hemorrhage
Subdural hematoma

Fig. 47-8 • Epidural hematoma (outside the dura mater of the brain), subdural hematoma (under the dura mater), and intracerebral hemorrhage (within the brain tissue).

be potentially devastating, depending on its location. ICH may also produce significant brain edema and ICP elevations. A brainstem hemorrhage occurs as a result of direct trauma, fractures, or torsion injuries to the brainstem.

Hydrocephalus

Hydrocephalus is an abnormal increase in CSF volume. It may be caused by impaired reabsorption of CSF at the arachnoid villi (from subarachnoid hemorrhage or meningitis). This is called a *communicating hydrocephalus.* It may also be caused by interference or blockage with CSF outflow from the ventricular system (from cerebral edema, tumor, or debris). The ventricles may dilate from the relative increase in CSF volume. Ultimately, if not treated, this increase may lead to increased ICP.

Brain Herniation

In the presence of increased ICP, the brain tissue may shift and herniate downward. Of the several types of herniation syndromes (Fig. 47-9), uncal herniation is one of the most clinically significant because it is life threatening. It is caused by a shift of one or both areas of the temporal lobe, known as the **uncus.** This shift creates pressure on the third cranial nerve. *Late findings include dilated and nonreactive pupils, ptosis (drooping eyelids), and a rapidly deteriorating level of consciousness. Central herniation* is caused by a downward shift of the brainstem and the diencephalon from a supratentorial lesion. It is clinically manifested by Cheyne-Stokes respirations, pinpoint and nonreactive pupils, and potential hemodynamic instability. All herniation syndromes are potentially life threatening, and the physician must be notified immediately when they are suspected.

Etiology

The most common causes of traumatic brain injury (TBI) in the United States are falls and motor vehicle crashes. In many cases, alcohol and drugs are contributing factors to the event. Acts of violence and sports-related injuries are the next most common causes. The United States is seeing increasing numbers of survivors of head injury secondary to blast injuries as a result of active duty in wartime

Incidence/Prevalence

Each year over a million people in the United States have some type of TBI. Of these, many require hospitalization and some die. According to the Brain Injury Association of America, over 5 million people are currently living with TBI (www.biausa.org). Summer and spring months, evenings, nights, and weekends are associated with the greatest number of injuries. Young males are more likely than young females to have a TBI. Men tend to play more sports, take more risks when driving, and consume large amounts of alcohol. Falls occur most often in older adults.

DECISION-MAKING CHALLENGE
Critical Rescue

A 74-year-old man is admitted to the emergency department (ED) after a fall from a ladder. A nursing history reveals that he was helping a friend fix his roof while drinking several beers on a very hot day. On assessment you find that he is alert and oriented but reports that his head is sore. No swelling, bruising, or bleeding is evident. His vital signs are within normal limits except for his blood pressure, which is 184/106. He has a history of hypertension

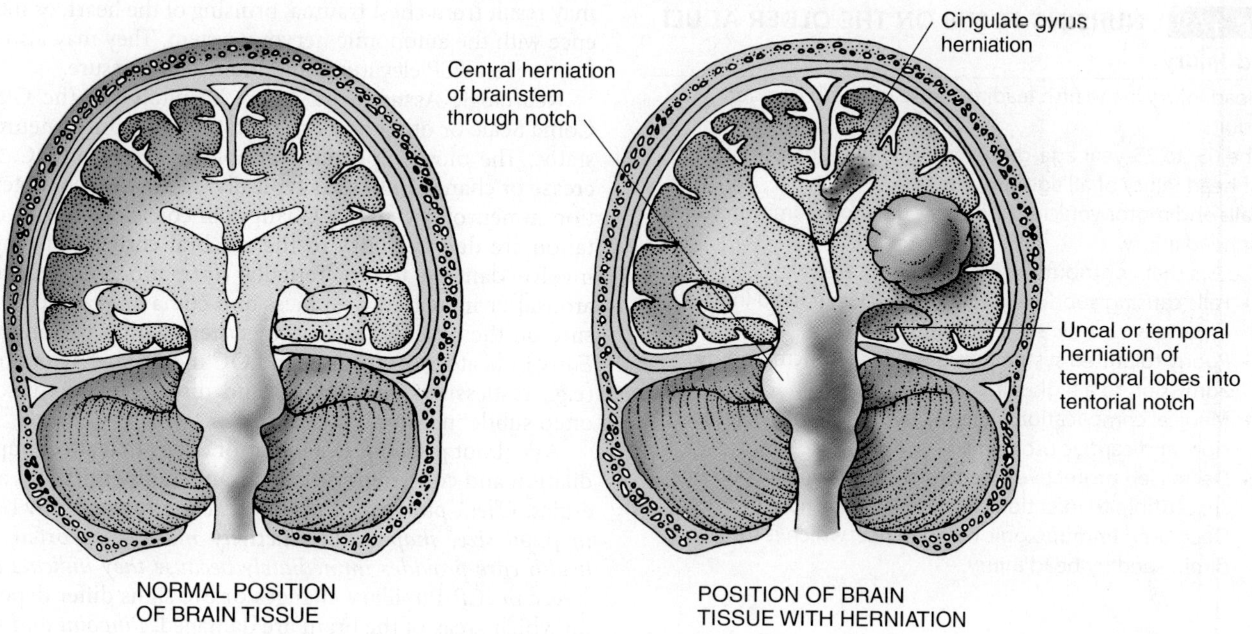
Central herniation
of brainstem
through notch
Cingulate gyrus
herniation
Uncal or temporal
herniation of
temporal lobes into
tentorial notch
NORMAL POSITION
OF BRAIN TISSUE
POSITION OF BRAIN
TISSUE WITH HERNIATION

Fig. 47-9 • Herniation syndromes.

and diabetes mellitus, which are controlled by drug therapy and diet. His wife tells you that he doesn't always take his medication and that he drinks "a lot."

1. What other assessment data do you need at this time?
2. For what health problems should you carefully monitor and why?
3. What risk factors does he have for these problems?
4. While waiting for the CT scan, the patient begins to vomit profusely. What action should you take at this time and why?

evolve For suggested answer guidelines, go to http://evolve.elsevier.com/Iggy/.

Health Promotion and Maintenance

Prevention of falls is particularly important, especially for older adults. People need to be aware of environmental factors that may increase the likelihood of falls such as throw rugs and inadequate lighting. When possible, they should have safety equipment installed in bathtubs and showers. Remind them that balance and coordination may decrease as a result of aging.

Nurses should educate the public on ways to decrease the incidence of TBI by using safe practices such as wearing seat belts. Helmets should be used for skateboarding and bicycle and motorcycle riding. Teach the importance of following driving laws to avoid speeding and other violations.

Patient-Centered Collaborative Care

Assessment

History

Obtaining an accurate history from a patient who has sustained a TBI may be difficult because of either the seriousness of the injury or the presence of amnesia. It is not unusual for the patient to experience **amnesia** (loss of memory) for the events before or after the injury. The patient with a serious head injury is often admitted to the hospital unconscious or in a confused and combative state. If the patient cannot provide information, the history can be obtained from rescue workers or witnesses to the injury. Always ask when, where, and how the injury occurred. Did the patient lose consciousness; if so, for how long? Has there been a change in the level of consciousness (LOC)? If trauma is related to drug or alcohol consumption, it may be difficult to differentiate neurologic changes from head trauma from those produced by intoxication.

Obtain as much information about the events as possible immediately after the injury. Patients with a severe injury may have several different presentations. The patient may be completely unresponsive after the injury. Alternatively, the patient may first be responsive and deteriorate rapidly within a few minutes to several hours. In another typical presentation, the patient is unconscious for a few minutes as a result of the primary brain injury, returns to a normal level of consciousness, and then rapidly deteriorates from secondary insult to the brain.

Determine whether the patient had any seizure activity before or after the injury and whether there is a history of a seizure disorder. It is important to obtain precise information about the circumstances of falls, particularly in the older patient (Chart 47-9). Other pertinent information includes hand dominance, any diseases of or injuries to the eyes, and any allergies to drugs or food, particularly seafood. People allergic to seafood are often allergic to the IV contrast media used in diagnostic tests. Inquire about a history of alcohol or drug use and abuse because these substances may mask the symptoms of increased ICP. The Joint Commission requires all patients to be screened for abuse and neglect when they are admitted to any type of health care facility.

Physical Assessment/Clinical Manifestations

No two injuries are alike. The patient with a TBI may have a variety of manifestations depending on the severity of injury and the resulting increase in intracranial pressure (ICP) (see Chart 47-6). Underlying neurologic problems may be masked by drugs or alcohol. Assess for signs of increased ICP, hypotension, hypoxia, or hypercapnia (increased blood levels of carbon dioxide). The early detection of subtle changes in the

Chart 47-9 NURSING FOCUS ON THE OLDER ADULT

Head Injury

- Head injury is the fifth leading cause of death in older adults.
- The 65- to 75-year age-group has second highest incidence of head injury of all age-groups.
- Falls and motor vehicle crashes are the most common cause of head injury.
- Factors that contribute to high mortality are:
  - Falls causing subdural hematomas (closed head injuries), especially chronic subdural hematomas
  - Poorly tolerated systemic stress, which is increased by admission to a high-stimuli environment
  - Medical complications, such as hypotension, hypertension, and cardiac problems
  - Decreased protective mechanisms, which make patients susceptible to infections (especially pneumonia)
  - Decreased immunologic competence, which is further diminished by head injury

patient's neurologic status enables the health care team to prevent or treat potentially life-threatening complications.

Airway and Breathing Pattern Assessment. *The first priority is the assessment of the patient's ABCs—airway, breathing, and circulation.* Because TBI is associated with cervical spinal cord injuries, all patients with head trauma are treated as though they have cord injury until x-ray studies prove otherwise. *Older adults are especially prone to cervical injuries at the first or second vertebral level, a life-threatening problem.* Assess for indicators of spinal cord injury, such as loss of motor and sensory function, tenderness along the spine, and abnormal head tilt. Monitor for respiratory problems and diaphragmatic breathing, as well as diminished or absent reflexes. The upper cervical spinal nerves innervate the diaphragm to control breathing.

Although hypoxia (decreased oxygen) and hypercapnia (increased carbon dioxide) are best detected through Sao_2 and end-tidal volume carbon dioxide measurement, observe chest wall movement and listen to breath sounds. Any sign of respiratory problems should be reported immediately to the physician. In some cases, an endotracheal tube is inserted for mechanical ventilation. Injuries to the brainstem may cause a change in the patient's breathing pattern, such as Cheyne-Stokes respirations, central neurogenic hyperventilation, and/or apnea.

Vital Signs Assessment. The mechanisms of autoregulation are often impaired as the result of a TBI. The more serious the injury, the more severe is the impact on autoregulation. Monitor the patient's blood pressure and pulse to detect possible changes in cerebral blood flow. The patient may have hypotension or hypertension. **Cushing's triad,** a classic but late sign of increased ICP, is manifested by severe hypertension with a widened pulse pressure and bradycardia. As ICP increases, the pulse becomes thready, irregular, and rapid. Cerebral blood flow increases in response to hypertension. Vasogenic edema may occur, further increasing ICP.

Hypotension and tachycardia suggest hypovolemic shock. This decrease in blood volume may lead to decreased cerebral perfusion pressure and eventually to ischemia and infarct of the brain tissue. Hypovolemic shock is usually due to intra-abdominal bleeding or bleeding into the soft tissue around major fractures—not to intracranial bleeding. Cardiac dysrhythmias may result from chest trauma, bruising of the heart, or interference with the autonomic nervous system. They may also result from severe ICP elevations and brainstem pressure.

Neurologic Assessment. Many hospitals use the Glasgow Coma Scale or other assessment tool to document neurologic status. The most important variable to assess is LOC. A decrease or change in LOC is typically the first sign of deterioration in neurologic status. Changes in consciousness or orientation are due to injury to the cerebral cortex and may also involve damage to the reticular formation. A decrease in arousal or increased sleepiness and coma are caused by pressure on the reticular activating system within the brainstem. *Early* indicators of a change in LOC include behavior changes (e.g., restlessness, irritability) and disorientation, which are often subtle in nature.

Ask about previous eye injury or drugs that affect pupillary dilation and constriction, such as anticholinergics and adrenergics. *Check pupils for size and reaction to light. Any changes in pupil size, shape, and reactivity must be reported to the health care provider immediately because they indicate an increase in ICP.* Pupillary changes or eye signs differ depending on which areas of the brain are damaged. *Pinpoint and nonresponsive pupils are indicative of brainstem dysfunction at the level of the pons.* Of particular importance is the **ovoid pupil,** which is regarded as the midstage between a normal-size pupil and a dilated pupil. In some agencies, a portable automated pupillometer is used to measure pupil size and reaction rather than manual examination.

Asymmetric (uneven) pupils, loss of light reaction, or unilateral or bilateral dilated pupils are treated as herniation of the brain from increased ICP until proven differently. *Pupils that are fixed (nonreactive) and dilated are a poor prognostic sign, resulting from a marked increase in ICP. Patients with this problem are sometimes referred to as having "blown" pupils.*

Check gross vision if the patient's condition permits. Have the patient read any printed material (e.g., the nurse's name tag) or count the number of fingers that you hold within the patient's visual field. Loss of vision is usually caused by injury to the occipital lobe, which produces temporary cortical blindness.

If the patient can cooperate, the health care provider or neurosurgical nurse tests *cranial nerves* (CN) III, IV, and VI. Extraocular movements may be diminished because of increased ICP and hydrocephalus. Damage to the optic chiasm or optic tract may cause visual-field deficits or **diplopia** (double-vision). In the unconscious patient, additional oculocephalic and oculovestibular tests are performed to test the integrity of the brainstem and of CN III, VI, and VII.

Monitor for additional late signs of increased ICP (see Chart 47-6). These include severe headache, nausea, vomiting, seizures, and papilledema (seen by ophthalmoscopic examination). ***Papilledema,*** *also known as a* ***choked disc,*** *is edema and hyperemia (increased blood flow) of the optic disc. It is always a sign of increased ICP.* Headache and seizures are a response to the injury and may or may not be associated with increased ICP. *Always remember that the patient with a head injury is at risk for potentially devastating ICP elevations hours or days after the event!*

Assess for bilateral *motor* responses. The patient's motor loss or dysfunction usually appears contralateral (opposite side) to the site of the lesion, similar to a stroke. For example, a left-sided hemiparesis reflects an injury to the right cerebral hemisphere. A deterioration in motor function or the development of abnormal posturing (**decerebrate** or **decorticate posturing**) or flaccidity is another indicator of increased ICP (see Fig. 43-11 in Chapter 43). These changes are due to dysfunction within the pyramidal (motor) tracts of the spinal cord. Assess for brainstem or cerebellar injury, which may cause **ataxia** (loss of balance), decreased or increased muscle tone, and weakness. Remember that changes in motor function may also be an indicator of a spinal cord injury.

Carefully observe the patient's ears and nose for any signs of cerebrospinal fluid (CSF) leaks that result from a basilar skull fracture. CSF placed on a white absorbent background can be distinguished from other fluids by the "halo" sign, a yellowish stain surrounded by bloody drainage. If it is present, it tests positively for glucose when a strip testing method (Dipstix) is used. *However, this method of determining a CSF leak is not always reliable.* If there is a CSF leak, assess for **nuchal rigidity** (stiff neck), which may indicate infection or blood in the CSF. Nuchal rigidity is not checked until a spinal cord injury has been ruled out.

Palpate the patient's head carefully to detect the presence of fractures or hematomas. Look for areas of ecchymosis (bruising), tender areas of the scalp, and lacerations.

Psychosocial Assessment

Patients with a mild head injury may still have symptoms of disability 1 year or longer after injury. *Long-term effects are not common. The person who has had a moderate or severe head injury, however, is never the same as before the injury.* These patients have varying degrees of personality changes manifested by temper outbursts, depression, risk-taking behavior, and denial of disability. They may become talkative and develop a very outgoing personality. Memory, especially recent or short-term memory, is affected and should not be confused with problems of aphasia. The ability to learn new information and concentration may be affected. The patient may have problems with insight and planning. All these problems may lead to difficulties within the family structure and with social and work-related interactions. Assess coping strategies that have been used in the past to determine the patient's ability to adapt to the changes in physical and cognitive abilities.

Assess family dynamics, particularly if the patient is discharged to the family's care directly from the acute care hospital. The family or significant others must also cope with changes in the patient's physical appearance and cognitive abilities. Many families become angry with the patient for being injured, especially when his or her behavior or their own behavior resulted in an injury that could have been prevented. They may feel guilty that they did not or were not able to prevent the injury. The family or significant others may feel overwhelmed by the complexity of care required and the long recovery period. Both the family and the patient need to develop coping strategies to deal with the potential role reversals and role changes caused by the injury.

Laboratory Assessment

There are no laboratory tests to diagnose a primary brain injury. However, several laboratory tests are used to diagnose or indicate measures to prevent secondary brain insult. The health care provider requests arterial blood gases, complete blood count (CBC), and serum glucose and electrolyte levels. These tests are performed to monitor hemodynamic status, identify electrolyte imbalance, and detect infection. Severe electrolyte imbalances can also contribute to secondary injury, as well as increase the risk of seizures. A toxicology screen and an electrocardiogram (ECG) are often requested.

Imaging Assessment

The health care provider immediately requests computed tomography (CT) scanning to identify the extent and scope of injury to the brain. This diagnostic test can identify the presence of a lesion that requires surgical intervention, such as epidural or subdural hematoma. Radiography and CT scanning of the cervical spine and the skull are done to rule out fractures and dislocations. A chest x-ray is done to identify fractured ribs or other chest injuries. A flat plate of the abdomen, abdominal ultrasound, or abdominal CT may be obtained to assist in the diagnosis of abdominal bleeding or bowel laceration.

Magnetic resonance imaging (MRI) is particularly useful in the diagnosis of diffuse axonal injury, but it is not recommended for patients with ICP monitoring devices or other invasive monitoring devices.

Other Diagnostic Assessment

As the patient's condition stabilizes, the physician may request other diagnostic tests to identify the extent of injury to the brain. For example, the integrity of the cerebral vessels is measured through the use of Doppler flow studies or an arteriogram. Cerebral perfusion is measured by cerebral blood flow studies. Evoked potentials provide information on the functioning sensory pathways and may be useful in predicting outcome.

Interventions

The patient with a *severe* head injury is admitted to the critical care unit or a trauma center. Patients with *moderate* head injuries are admitted to either the general nursing unit or the critical care unit, where they are closely observed for at least 24 hours. Those with *mild* TBI may possibly be sent home from the emergency department with instructions (Chart 47-10).

Nonsurgical Management

As with any critically injured patient, priority is given to maintaining a patent airway, breathing, and circulation. Specific nursing interventions for the patient with a head injury are directed toward preventing or detecting increased ICP, promoting fluid and electrolyte balance, and monitoring the effects of treatments and drug therapy. Providing health teaching and emotional support for the patient and family is a vital part of the plan of care.

Increased ICP Prevention and Detection. Take and record the patient's *vital signs* every 1 to 2 hours or more often based on patient acuity. The health care provider may prescribe drug therapy to prevent severe hypertension or hypotension. The patient in the critical care unit is connected to a cardiac monitor to detect any cardiac dysrhythmias. Nonspecific ST-segment or T-wave changes may occur, possibly in response to stimulation of the autonomic nervous system or an increase in the level of circulating catecholamines such as epinephrine. Document and report cardiac irregularities to the health care provider.

The patient with a head injury is often admitted with a fever—a defense mechanism in the presence of trauma or an indication of inflammatory response. Fever as a consequence of infection may develop later in the course of the disease. A

Chart 47-10 PATIENT AND FAMILY EDUCATION GUIDE

Minor Head Injury

- If the person is sleeping, wake him or her every 3 to 4 hours for the first 2 days, asking his or her name, where he or she is, and the name of the caregiver.
- Expect the person to report headache, nausea, or dizziness for at least 24 hours. If these symptoms are severe or do not improve, contact the physician immediately or take the person back to the emergency department.
- For a headache, give acetaminophen (Tylenol) every 4 hours as needed.
- Avoid giving the person sedatives, sleeping pills, or alcoholic beverages for at least 24 hours unless the physician instructs otherwise.
- Do not allow the person to engage in strenuous activity for at least 48 hours.
- Do not allow nose blowing or ear cleaning for 48 hours.
- If any of these symptoms occur, take the person back to the emergency department immediately:
  - Blurred vision
  - Drainage from the ear or nose
  - Weakness
  - Slurred speech
  - Progressive sleepiness
  - Vomiting
  - Worsening headache
  - Unequal pupil size
- Keep follow-up appointments with the health care provider.

third cause of fever is a central fever caused by hypothalamic damage. It is manifested by an absence of sweating and no diurnal (night and day) variation. This type of fever is high and lasts several days to weeks. In addition, it responds better to cooling (e.g., hypothermia blanket, sponge bath) than to the administration of antipyretic drugs such as acetaminophen (Tylenol, Ace-Tabs♣). *Fever from any cause is associated with higher morbidity and mortality rates.*

Prophylactic *hyperventilation* during the first 20 hours after injury is usually avoided because it may produce ischemia by causing cerebral vasoconstriction. The result is a decrease in cerebral blood volume and ICP. In acute neurologic deterioration, however, it may be used for brief periods of ICP elevations.

The patient who requires mechanical breathing assistance is ventilated to maintain a partial pressure of arterial carbon dioxide ($Paco_2$) of about 35 to 38 mm Hg. One major outcome is to prevent hypercarbia (increased carbon dioxide). *Carbon dioxide is a very potent vasodilator that can contribute to increases in ICP. Arterial oxygen levels (Pao_2) are maintained between 80 and 100 mm Hg to prevent cerebral vasodilation resulting from hypoxemia. Monitor arterial blood gas values at least twice daily and after each change in the ventilator setting.*

Pulmonary secretions tend to pool as the result of a decreased LOC, ineffective cough, or altered breathing pattern. The secretions may be thick because of the diuretics or fluid intake restriction that may be used to prevent cerebral edema. Collaborate with the respiratory therapist to provide chest physiotherapy as needed based on patient assessment. Pay close attention to the ICP response.

Carefully observe the patient with increased ICP when suctioned. If the patient is intubated, manually hyperventilate him or her with 100% oxygen before each pass of the catheter. Overly aggressive hyperventilation with endotracheal suctioning may be dangerous, though, because of the cerebral vasoconstriction caused by even transient hypocapnia (low arterial carbon dioxide levels). This may increase the risk of cerebral ischemia as a secondary event. Allow the patient to rest a few minutes after suctioning to prevent increased ICP. Lidocaine given IV or endotracheally may be used to suppress the cough reflex; coughing increases ICP.

Position the patient to avoid extreme flexion or extension of the neck and to maintain the head in the midline, neutral position. Log roll the patient during turning to avoid extreme hip flexion, and keep the head of the bed elevated at least 30 degrees or as recommended by the health care provider. Head positioning should be based on both intracranial pressure (ICP) and systemic blood pressure. If increasing head elevation lowers ICP but also significantly lowers systemic blood pressure, the patient does not benefit and may actually be harmed. Base head elevation on cerebral perfusion pressure when possible. Carefully position the head of the bed in the older patient. The dura is tightly adhered to the skull and may pull away from the brain, leading to a subdural hematoma.

Patients with *severe* TBI often die. As the deterioration begins, keep in mind that the patient may be a potential organ donor. *Before* brain death is declared, contact the local organ procurement organization. Determine if the patient consented to be an organ donor. This information is typically on a driver's license or other state-issued card or advance directive. The patient's wishes should be followed unless he or she has a medical condition that prevents organ donation. The physician discusses the severity of the patient's condition and the possibility of organ donation with the family. Some families may not agree with the patient's decision, which can cause an ethical dilemma. Health care agencies have ethics committees that can help with these situations.

Criteria for brain death include (Peiffer, 2007):

- Glasgow Coma Scale <3
- Apnea
- No pupillary response
- No gag and cough reflexes
- No oculovestibular reflex (no eye movement after ice water is placed in ears)
- No corneal reflex
- No oculocephalic reflex ("doll's eyes")

DECISION-MAKING CHALLENGE

Legal/Ethical

A 24-year-old male was riding a motorcycle at a high rate of speed when he failed to yield to another vehicle. He sustained a major closed head injury and was admitted to the trauma unit with a Glasgow Coma Scale of 3. His grandmother is his only living relative and was his guardian when he was growing up. She tells you that they have been extremely close ever since his mother died from breast cancer when he was 5 years old. The address of his father is not known because he left the family when the patient was an infant. The neurologist determines that the patient is brain dead and is an excellent candidate for organ donation. His driver's license indicates that he wants to be an organ donor, but his grandmother begins to scream at you when she is told of his wishes. She refuses to let his organs be donated.

1. What legal/ethical dilemma is present in this situation?
2. What ethical principle helps guide how to resolve this dilemma?
3. What is your role in this situation?
4. How can you help the patient's grandmother at this time?

evolve For suggested answer guidelines, go to http://evolve.elsevier.com/Iggy/.

Drug Therapy. *Glucocorticoids* (dexamethasone [Decadron, Dexasone]) and methylprednisolone sodium succinate [Solu-Medrol, Medrol]) have no benefit in the management of increased ICP as a result of head injury or cerebral infarction. Instead, mannitol (Osmitrol), an osmotic diuretic, is used to treat cerebral edema by pulling water out of the extracellular space of the edematous brain tissue. It is most effective when given in boluses rather than as a continuous infusion. Furosemide (Lasix), a loop diuretic, is often used as adjunctive therapy to reduce the incidence of rebound from mannitol. It also enhances the therapeutic action of mannitol. Furosemide also reduces edema and blood volume, decreases sodium uptake by the brain, and decreases the production of CSF at the choroid plexus.

Administer *mannitol* through a filter in the IV tubing or, if given by IV push, draw it up through a filtered needle to eliminate microscopic crystals. For the patient receiving either osmotic or loop diuretics, monitor for intake and output, severe dehydration, and indications of acute renal failure, weakness, edema, and changes in urine output. Serum electrolyte and osmolarity levels are measured every 6 hours. Mannitol is used to obtain a serum osmolarity of 310 to 320 mOsm/L, depending on physician preference and the desired outcome of therapy. Insert an indwelling urinary catheter to maintain strict measurement of output. Check the patient's serum and urine osmolarity daily.

Opioids such as morphine sulfate or fentanyl may be used with ventilated patients to decrease agitation and control restlessness if the agitation is caused by pain. Fentanyl has fewer effects on blood pressure and heart rate than morphine and may therefore be a safer agent to manage pain. These agents may be reversed with naloxone (Narcan), but opioid reversal should be avoided if at all possible to reduce risk of withdrawal and rebound pain and agitation. Sedatives such as lorazepam (Ativan) and midazolam (Versed) may be used for anxiety to promote comfort and treat agitation. Sedatives and opioids may mask the neurologic assessment and potentially lower blood pressure. Therefore they should be administered in small incremental doses to a predetermined endpoint with close assessment of hemodynamic stability and neurologic status.

Neuromuscular blocking agents (NMBAs), such as vecuronium bromide or cisatracurium (Nimbex), may be used for the patient after head trauma if the patient is experiencing dangerous agitation or if the increased activity is causing ICP elevations. These agents have no analgesic and sedative effects and *must never be used without aggressive sedation/analgesia.* NMBAs are associated with an increased risk of pneumonia and other complications. Therefore they are not used as routinely today.

Antiepileptic drugs, such as phenytoin (Dilantin), to prevent seizures that occur initially more than 7 days **(late-onset seizures)** after injury are not recommended. However, they may be recommended as an option to prevent seizure activity that may occur within 7 days after injury **(early-onset seizures).** Acetaminophen (Tylenol, Ace-Tabs♣) and aspirin (acetylsalicylic acid [ASA], Ancasal♣) are given to patients who are febrile (temperature greater than 101° F [38° C]) to reduce fever.

Induction of Barbiturate Coma. Barbiturate coma (coma induced by barbiturates) has been used for intracranial hypertension (increased ICP) that cannot be controlled by other means. Either pentobarbital sodium (Nembutal, Novopentobarb♣) or thiopentone is the drug of choice. These drugs decrease the metabolic demands of the brain and cerebral blood flow, stabilize cell membranes, decrease the formation of vasogenic edema, and produce a more uniform blood supply. The provider adjusts the dosage to maintain complete unresponsiveness. Barbiturate coma is optimally managed using hemodynamic assessment, ICP monitoring, and electroencephalographic (EEG) monitoring to document endpoints. As a consequence, it is difficult to recognize subtle or obvious neurologic changes. The patient requires mechanical ventilation, sophisticated hemodynamic monitoring, and ICP monitoring. Complications of barbiturate coma include decreased GI motility, cardiac dysrhythmias from hypokalemia, hypotension, and fluctuations in body temperature.

Fluid and Electrolyte Management. The patient with TBI is at risk for diabetes insipidus (DI) and the syndrome of inappropriate antidiuretic hormone (SIADH) because the pituitary gland may be injured or compressed from cerebral edema (see Chapter 65). In the patient with multiple trauma, fluid overload can occur and cerebral edema can worsen from the rapid administration of IV fluids or plasma expanders. Fluid management may be titrated to optimize volume resuscitation but minimize brain swelling and ICP elevation. ICP is also influenced by the response to diuretic therapy and laboratory values. Check urine specific gravity every 1 to 4 hours. Monitor serum and urine osmolarity and electrolytes at least daily.

Nutrition Management. The patient with a *major* head injury after the acute phase of management may have changes in these areas:

- Sense of smell
- Ability to taste, swallow, or feel the presence of food within the oral cavity
- Vision, pain, and temperature sensation

As a result, he or she is at risk for nutritional deficits that may interfere with the healing process.

The patient who is moderately to severely injured usually has a decreased LOC, at least temporarily. As a result, the patient is unable to chew or swallow and must receive nutrition and fluids by other methods. If LOC does not improve, long-term nutritional support by enteral feeding is used. A small-lumen nasogastric or nasoduodenal tube or a percutaneous endoscopic gastrostomy (PEG) tube is inserted for continuous or intermittent feeding. Small-bore tubes decrease the risk for aspiration in a patient who is at high risk. For care of the patient receiving enteral feeding, see Chapter 63.

With the use of either type of tube, be sure that unlicensed assistive personnel (UAP) weigh the patient daily. Collaborate with the nutritionist to determine whether caloric needs are being met, and monitor serum prealbumin levels to assess adequacy of protein intake. Assess the patient daily for signs of dehydration, such as dry mucous membranes and weight loss.

For the patient who can take food and fluids by mouth, ensure that mealtime is a pleasant experience. Position the patient to maximize swallowing ability. The speech-language pathologist (SLP) identifies strategies to prevent food from accumulating in the cheek of the affected side. In general, patients who have swallowing problems can tolerate or swallow soft or semisoft foods and liquids (mechanical soft or dental diet, junior baby foods, custards, scrambled eggs) better than thin liquids (water, juice, milk). Powdered thickener (e.g., Thick-It) may be added to thicken foods for better consistency. Supplements such as milkshakes and commercial products may be needed to meet the patient's caloric and protein requirements. Collaborate with the nutritionist and SLP to create a nutritional plan appropriate for the patient with dysphagia.

Sensory, Cognitive, and Behavioral Management. If a large lesion of the parietal lobe is present, the patient may experience a loss of sensation for pain, temperature, touch, and proprioception (position sense), which prevents an appropriate response to environmental stimuli. A hazard-free environment is necessary to prevent injury (e.g., from burns if the patient's coffee is too hot). In collaboration with the therapist, integrate a sensory stimulation program into the comatose or stuporous patient's routine care activities. Sensory stimulation is done to facilitate a meaningful response to the environment. Present visual, auditory, or tactile stimuli one at a time, and explain the purpose and the type of stimulus presented. For example, show a picture of the patient's mother and say, "This is a picture of your mother." The picture is shown several times, and the same words are used to describe the picture. If auditory tapes or DVDs are used, they should not be longer than 10 to 15 minutes. If the stimulus is presented for a longer period, it simply becomes "white" noise, or meaningless background noise.

Patients with a milder injury may be disoriented and have a short-term memory loss. Always introduce yourself before any interaction. Keep explanations of procedures and activities short and simple, and give them immediately before and throughout patient care. To the extent possible, maintain a sleep-wake cycle with scheduled rest periods. Orient the patient to time (day, month, and year) and place, and explain the reason for the hospitalization. Reassure the patient that he or she is safe. Ask the family to bring in familiar objects, such as pictures. Provide orientation cues within the environment, such as a large clock with numbers or a single-date calendar.

An overwhelming majority of brain injury survivors have cognitive impairments, or thinking problems. Cognitive impairments interfere with the brain-injured patient's ability to function effectively in school, at work, and in his or her personal life. *Cognitive rehabilitation* is a way of helping brain-injured patients regain function in areas that are essential for a return to independence and a reasonable quality of life. However, these services are not widely available or accessible.

The patient is at risk for seizure activity. Keep the bed in low position with the side rails up. Hand mittens may be applied if the patient attempts to pull out the IV line or nasogastric tube. Restraining any extremity increases agitation and fear. Use alternatives to restraints first according to hospital policy. For example, covering the patient's IV site may prevent dislodgment. Keeping the patient's hands busy with activity pillows or puzzles accomplishes the same purpose.

Orient the patient to the surroundings as needed, and provide a quiet environment. Closely monitor the patient's response to television programs or the radio. Often he or she cannot distinguish the programs from what is happening within his or her own environment.

Surgical Management

The physician may elect to insert an intracranial pressure (ICP) monitoring device to evaluate the patient's ICP more closely using minimally invasive surgery (MIS). All devices are inserted through a *burr hole* (also known as a *keyhole craniotomy*) that is placed in the skull using a twist drill. Each device is connected to an electronic transducer that converts ICP to electronic impulses and provides information that can be viewed using a monitor at the patient's bedside. The monitor can record the pressure waves and provide a digital readout of the pressure.

Various types of devices for monitoring ICP are used. An **intraventricular catheter (IVC)** is a small tube that is inserted into the anterior horn of the lateral ventricle of the nondominant cerebral hemisphere. The advantages of this system are that cerebrospinal fluid (CSF) can be drained to decrease ICP and specimens can be obtained for laboratory analysis. The **subarachnoid screw or bolt** is a hollow device placed into the subarachnoid space for direct pressure measurement. A disadvantage of the system is that CSF cannot be drained to treat increased ICP. However, it is less invasive, which lowers the risk for infection (Table 47-3) (Schollenberger et al., 2006).

An **epidural catheter** or sensor is a transducer that is placed between the skull and the dura, leaving the dura intact. A similar device is the *subdural catheter,* which is placed under the dura mater. Its major advantage is the decreased risk for infection from an open dural space. The *fiberoptic transducer-tipped pressure sensor* is also a commonly used device for ICP monitoring. It is easily transported and can be placed in the subdural or subarachnoid space, in the ventricle, or directly into brain tissue.

Even though ICP is monitored both through nursing assessment and with a variety of devices, ischemia after TBI remains a problem. Therefore two other techniques are being used to better determine the level of oxygen in the patient's brain: The LICOX Brain Tissue Oxygen Monitoring System and the jugular venous bulb catheter. These devices are especially useful in patients with subarachnoid hemorrhage. The *LICOX catheter* is inserted into the white matter of the brain in the frontal lobe to continuously measure the partial pressure of brain tissue oxygenation ($pBto_2$). Lung function and a high arterial partial pressure of oxygen increase the $pBto_2$, and vice versa. Although normal values are controversial among clinicians, most practitioners want the pressure to be greater than 20 mm Hg. The *jugular catheter* measures oxygen in the internal jugular vein as an indicator of the cerebral oxygen level. The critical care nurse follows the agency's protocols for the management of these devices (Bader, 2006).

In extreme cases in which the patient's ICP cannot be controlled, the physician may elect to perform a **craniotomy** (incision into the cranium) to remove ischemic tissue or the tips of the temporal lobes. The removal of nonvital brain tissue allows expansion of brain tissue without further increasing ICP. A craniotomy may also be performed to remove epidural or subdural hematomas. Care of the patient with a craniotomy is discussed on p. 1063 under Postoperative Care in the Brain Tumors section.

TABLE 47-3 Advantages and Disadvantages of Intracranial Pressure Monitoring Devices

Monitoring Device	Advantages	Disadvantages
Intraventricular catheter (IVC)	Allows accurate measurement of intracranial pressure (ICP) Allows drainage or sampling of cerebrospinal fluid (CSF) Allows instillation of contrast media Provides reliable evaluation of cerebral compliance	Provides additional site for potential infection Most invasive method for monitoring ICP Must be balanced and recalibrated frequently Catheter can become occluded by blood or tissue Insertion can be difficult with small or collapsed ventricles CSF leakage can occur around insertion site
Subarachnoid bolt or screw	Lower infection rates than with IVC Quickly and easily placed Can be used with small or collapsed ventricles Does not penetrate brain parenchyma	Tendency for dampened waveform Less accurate at high ICP May become occluded by blood or tissue Must be balanced and recalibrated frequently (i.e., every 4 hr and whenever patient is repositioned) Baseline drift and tendency for dampened waveform Does not provide for CSF sampling
Subdural/epidural catheter or sensor	Least invasive Decreased risk for infection Easily and quickly placed	Increasing baseline drift over time; therefore accuracy and reliability are questionable Does not provide for CSF sampling or drainage
Fiberoptic transducer-tipped catheter	Can be placed in subdural or subarachnoid space, in ventricle, or into brain tissue Easily transported Requires zeroing only once (during insertion) Baseline drift to 1 mm Hg/day Decreased risk of infection Less waveform artifact No need to adjust transducer to patient's position Easy to insert	Does not provide for CSF sampling or drainage Cannot be recalibrated after placement Probe needs periodic replacement Fragile fiberoptic cable easily damaged and broken

Community-Based Care

The patient with a *minor* or *moderate* head injury recovers at home after discharge from the emergency department (ED) or hospital. The patient with a *major* head injury requires long-term case management and ongoing rehabilitation after hospitalization. A number of specialized head injury rehabilitation facilities are available in the United States and Canada. Communicate the patient's plan of care, including drug therapy (reconciliation), to the nurse in the rehabilitation facility to ensure continuity of care.

Home Care Management

The major desired outcome for rehabilitation after head injury is to maximize the patient's ability to return to his or her highest level of functioning. Activities such as occupational therapy (OT), physical therapy (PT), and speech-language therapy may continue in the home after discharge from the rehabilitation facility. Adaptation of the home environment to accommodate the patient safely may be needed. For example, smoke and fire alarms must function properly because the patient with a head injury often loses the sense of smell. This information can be obtained from the admission data or by a home visit. Home adaptations and referrals to outside agencies are completed before discharge.

Health Teaching

Collaborate with the case manager (CM) to provide the patient and family with both written and verbal instructions for discharge. The teaching plan includes a review of seizure precautions and strategies to adapt to sensory dysfunction. Discuss issues related to personality or behavior problems that may arise and how to cope with them. Explain the purpose, dosage, schedule, and route of administration of drug therapy. Teach the family to encourage the patient to participate in activities as tolerated. Demonstrations and return demonstrations of care activities help family members become more skillful. Stress the importance of regular follow-up visits with therapists and other health care providers.

Patients with personality and behavior problems respond best to a structured and consistent environment. Instruct the family to develop a home routine that provides structure, repetition, and consistency. Remind the family about the importance of reinforcing positive behaviors rather than negative behaviors.

Teach the patient who has sustained a *minor* head injury (e.g., a concussion) that **post-concussion syndrome** may occur. This syndrome is a group of clinical manifestations including, but not limited to:

- Personality changes
- Irritability
- Headaches
- Dizziness
- Restlessness
- Nervousness
- Insomnia
- Memory loss
- Depression

A few patients have these problems for weeks, months, or even years to the extent that they interfere with daily activities such as employment. The prolonged pattern is classified as post-trauma syndrome. The exact cause is not known.

Most patients with *moderate to severe* TBI are discharged with physical and cognitive disabilities. Changes in personality and behavior are very common. The family must learn to cope with the patient's increased fatigue, irritability, temper outbursts, depression, and memory problems. These patients often require constant supervision at home, and eventually families feel socially isolated. Teach the family about the importance of regular respite care, either in a structured day-care respite program or through relief provided by a friend or neighbor. Family members, particularly the primary caretaker, may become depressed and have feelings of loneliness. In addition, they may feel angry with the patient because of the additional responsibilities (financial and emotional) that his or her care has placed on them. To help the family cope with these problems, suggest that they join and actively participate in a local head injury support group.

Health Care Resources

Collaborate with the CM to refer families and patients to local chapters of the Brain Injury Association of America (BIAA) (www.biausa.org) and the National Brain Injury Foundation (NBIF) (www.nbif.org) for information and support. The BIAA has a number of helpful publications on preventing and living with TBI. Other resources include religious, spiritual, and cultural leaders.

BRAIN TUMORS

Brain tumors can arise anywhere within the brain structures and are named according to the cell or tissue where they are located; however, cerebral tumors are the most common. *Primary* tumors originate within the central nervous system (CNS) and rarely **metastasize** (spread) outside this area. *Secondary* brain tumors result from metastasis from other areas of the body, such as the lungs, breast, kidney, and GI tract.

Pathophysiology

Complications of Cerebral Tumors

Regardless of location, the tumor expands and invades, infiltrates, compresses, and displaces normal brain tissue. This leads to one or more of these problems:

- Cerebral edema/brain tissue inflammation
- Increased intracranial pressure (ICP)
- Neurologic deficits
- Hydrocephalus
- Pituitary dysfunction

Cerebral edema (vasogenic edema) results from changes in capillary endothelial tissue permeability that allow plasma to seep into the extracellular spaces. This leads to *increased ICP* and, depending on the location of the tumor, brain herniation syndromes. A variety of *neurologic deficits* result from edema, infiltration, distortion, and compression of surrounding brain tissue. The cerebral blood vessels may become compressed because of edema and increased ICP. This compression leads to ischemia (decreased blood flow) of the area supplied by the vessel. In addition, the tumor may enter the walls of the vessel, causing it to rupture and hemorrhage into the tumor bed or other brain tissue. Some patients who have brain tumors have seizure activity from interference with the brain's normal electrical activity.

Increased ICP may also result from *hydrocephalus* (increased cerebrospinal fluid [CSF]) related to obstruction of the flow of CSF or displacement of the lateral ventricles by the expanding lesion. Typically, a tumor obstructs the aqueduct of Sylvius or one of the ventricles or pushes into the subarachnoid space. Posterior fossa tumors may block the flow of CSF from the fourth ventricle to the foramen of Luschka or Magendie.

Pituitary dysfunction may occur as the tumor compresses the pituitary gland and causes the syndrome of inappropriate antidiuretic hormone (SIADH) or diabetes insipidus (DI). These disorders result in severe fluid and electrolyte imbalances and can be life threatening. (See Chapter 65 for a complete description.)

Classification of Tumors

Brain tumors are usually classified as benign, malignant (cancerous), or metastatic (Table 47-4). They may or may not be treated, depending on their location. Benign (noncancerous) tumors are generally associated with a favorable outcome. Malignant or metastatic tumors require more aggressive intervention including surgery, radiation, and/or chemotherapy.

A second classification system is based on location. **Supratentorial** tumors are located within the cerebral hemispheres. Located beneath the tentorium (fold of dura mater) is the **infratentorial** area—the area of the brainstem structures and cerebellum.

A third classification system depends on the cellular or anatomic origins of the tumor. The nervous system is composed of two types of cells: (1) neurons, which are responsible for nerve impulse conduction; and (2) neuroglial cells, which provide support, nourishment, and protection for neurons. Four specific types of neuroglial cells are astrocytes, oligodendroglia, ependymal cells, and microglia. When classifying gliomas according to this system, tumors are named by their cell type. For example, an astrocytoma is a tumor of astrocytes. Gliomas are *malignant* tumors.

Meningiomas arise from the coverings of the brain (the meninges). They are the most common *benign* tumor. This tumor is in a capsule, globular, and well outlined and causes

TABLE 47-4 Classification of Brain Tumors

BENIGN
• Acoustic neuroma
• Meningioma
• Pituitary adenoma
• Astrocytoma
Grade 1 (may undergo changes and become malignant)
• Chondroma
• Craniopharyngioma
• Hemangioblastoma
MALIGNANT
• Astrocytoma
Grade 2
Grade 3
Grade 4 (also known as *glioblastoma multiforme*)
• Oligodendroglioma
• Ependymoma
• Medulloblastoma
• Chondrosarcoma
• Glioma
• Lymphoma

compression and displacement of nearby brain tissue. Although complete removal of the tumor is possible, it tends to recur.

Pituitary tumors that occur in the anterior lobe account for up to one fourth of brain tumors and may cause endocrine dysfunction. The most common type of pituitary tumor is the adenoma. These tumors are *benign* and often occur in young and middle-aged adults. The presenting symptoms include visual disturbances and hypopituitary signs, such as loss of body hair, diabetes insipidus (DI), infertility, visual field defects, and headaches.

Acoustic neuromas arise from the sheath of Schwann cells in the peripheral portion of cranial nerve VIII. They are also referred to as *cerebellar pontine angle (CPA) tumors* to describe their anatomic location. Acoustic neuromas compress brain tissue and tend to surround nearby cranial nerves (VII, V, IX, X), making surgical removal difficult without causing permanent cranial nerve dysfunction. Women are twice as likely as men to have acoustic neuromas. Common symptoms include hearing loss, **tinnitus** (ringing in the ears), and dizziness or vertigo.

Metastatic, or secondary, tumors account for many brain tumors. Cancer cells from the lung, breast, colon, pancreas, and kidney can travel to the brain via the blood and the lymphatic system. Multiple metastatic lesions are fairly common.

Etiology

The exact cause of brain tumors is unknown. Several areas under investigation include genetic changes, heredity, errors in fetal development, ionizing radiation, electromagnetic fields, environmental hazards, nutrition, viruses, and injury. The use of cellular phones has been investigated as a cause of brain tumors, but findings are not confirmed.

Incidence/Prevalence

Brain tumors account for fewer than 2% of all cancer deaths. About 21,000 people each year are diagnosed with a primary malignant brain tumor in the United States, and two thirds of them die from the disorder (www.acs.org). Many more have metastatic lesions. Brain tumors in the adult population are seen primarily in patients 40 to 70 years of age, and the survival rate is low compared with that of other cancers.

Patient-Centered Collaborative Care

Assessment

When possible, obtain a history from both the patient and the family, including current signs and symptoms. A complete neurologic assessment is needed to establish baseline data and to determine the nature and extent of neurologic deficits.

The clinical manifestations of brain tumors vary with the site of the tumor (Chart 47-11). In general, assess for these symptoms of a brain tumor, which include:

- Headaches that are usually more severe on awakening in the morning
- Nausea and vomiting
- Visual symptoms
- Seizures
- Changes in mentation or personality
- **Papilledema** (swelling of the optic disc)

Neurologic deficits result from the destruction, distortion, or compression of brain tissue. *Supratentorial (cerebral)* tumors usually result in paralysis, seizures, memory loss, cognitive impairment, language impairment, or vision problems. *Infratentorial* tumors produce ataxia, autonomic nervous system dysfunction, vomiting, drooling, hearing loss, and vision impairment. As the tumor grows, ICP increases and the symptoms become progressively more severe.

Chart 47-11 KEY FEATURES

Common Brain Tumors

CEREBRAL TUMORS

- Headache (most common feature)
- Vomiting unrelated to food intake
- Changes in visual acuity and visual fields; diplopia (visual changes caused by papilledema)
- Hemiparesis or hemiplegia
- Hypokinesia (decreased motor ability)
- Hyperesthesia, paresthesia, decreased tactile discrimination
- Seizures
- Aphasia
- Changes in personality or behavior

BRAINSTEM TUMORS

- Hearing loss (acoustic neuroma)
- Facial pain and weakness
- Dysphagia, decreased gag reflex
- Nystagmus
- Hoarseness
- Ataxia and dysarthria (cerebellar tumors)

Diagnosis is based on the history, neurologic assessment, clinical examination, and results of neurodiagnostic testing. Noninvasive diagnostic studies such as CT, MRI, and skull films are conducted first. These tests identify the size, location, and extent of the tumor. The MRI may be used for initial diagnostic evaluation and is a more sensitive diagnostic study, whereas the CT is often used for follow-up during the course of illness.

Cerebral angiography is usually not indicated to diagnose a brain tumor but may be used to provide additional information about blood supply to the tumor. Electroencephalography (EEG), lumbar puncture (LP), brain scan, and positron emission tomography (PET) may be indicated to provide further information about the size, location, and characteristics of the tumor. *To prevent brain herniation, LP should not be performed if the patient is exhibiting signs of ICP elevation.* Laboratory tests may also be requested to evaluate endocrine function, renal status, and electrolyte balance.

Interventions

Interventions depend on the type, size, and location of the tumor. For example, a small benign tumor may be periodically monitored through CT and MRI scanning to assess its growth. Malignant tumors may be managed by chemotherapy, radiation, and/or surgery.

Nonsurgical Management

The outcome of treatment of brain tumors is to decrease tumor size, improve quality of life, and improve survival time. The type of treatment selected depends on the tumor size and location, patient symptoms and general condition, and whether the tumor has occurred again. In addition to traditional interventions, a number of experimental treatment modalities are being investigated. These include blood-brain barrier disruption, recombinant DNA, monoclonal antibodies, new chemotherapeutic drugs, and immunotherapy. For example, an antitenascin radioactive monoclonal antibody treatment (81C6) that is directly injected into the cavity where the tumor was removed is being investigated. The antibodies deliver radiation directly into the brain but are less potent than traditional radiation.

Traditional *radiation therapy* may be used alone, after surgery, or in combination with chemotherapy and surgery. Chapter 24 discusses radiation treatment for patients with cancer.

Drug Therapy. The health care provider may prescribe a variety of drugs to treat the tumor, manage the patient's symptoms, and prevent complications. *Chemotherapy* may be given alone, in combination with radiation and surgery, and with tumor progression. Although these drugs may control tumor growth or decrease tumor burden, the benefit does not last. Chemotherapy usually involves more than one agent that may be given orally, IV, intra-arterially, and/or intrathecally through an Ommaya reservoir placed in a cranial ventricle. In electrochemotherapy, electric voltage carries agents into the tumor. When given systemically, the drug must be lipid soluble to cross the blood-brain barrier.

Commonly used oral drugs are CCNU (lomustine), temozolomide (Temodar), procarbazine (Matulane), and methotrexate (MTX). Vincristine (Oncovin) may be given IV in combination with other drugs. Side effects of these drugs are similar to those of any chemotherapeutic drug. Chapter 24 describes general nursing implications for care of a patient receiving chemotherapy.

Direct drug delivery to the tumor is an emerging practice. Disk-shaped drug (Gliadel) wafers may be placed directly into the cavity created during surgical tumor removal (interstitial chemotherapy). The major drug in the wafer is BCNU (carmustine). This therapy is usually used for newly diagnosed high-grade malignant gliomas, but recurrent tumors may also be treated with this method. Other drugs used are molecularly targeted. Examples include erlotinib (Tarceva), gefitinib (Iressa), and bevacizumab (Avastin).

Analgesics, such as codeine and acetaminophen (Tylenol, Ace-Tabs🍁), are given for headache. Dexamethasone (Decadron) is usually given to control cerebral edema. Glucocorticoids may be used for the treatment of edema resulting from brain tumors. Phenytoin (Dilantin) or other antiepileptic drugs may be given to prevent or treat seizure activity. Histamine blockers such as ranitidine hydrochloride (Zantac, Apo-Ranitidine🍁) or proton pump inhibitors such as pantoprazole (Protonix) are given to decrease gastric acid secretion and prevent the development of stress ulcers.

Stereotactic Radiosurgery. Stereotactic radiosurgery (SRS) is an alternative to traditional surgery. Several techniques are used, including the modified linear accelerator using accelerated x-rays (LINAC), a particle accelerator using beams of protons (cyclotron), and isotope seeds implanted in the tumor (brachytherapy). The gamma knife and CyberKnife are the newest treatments.

The gamma knife is a SRS procedure that uses a single high dose of ionized radiation to focus multiple beams of gamma radiation produced by the radioisotope *cobalt-60* to destroy intracranial lesions selectively without damaging surrounding healthy tissue (Fig. 47-10). Combining neurodiagnostic imaging tools—including MRI, CT, magnetic resonance angiography (MRA), and angiography—with the gamma knife allows for precise localization of deep-seated or anatomically difficult lesions. Treatment usually takes less than an hour, and patients require only overnight hospitalization. Advantages of this technique include its noninvasive nature; a lower risk than the traditional craniotomy; surgical precision; and decreased cost, morbidity, length of hospital stay, and recovery time. A disadvantage is that the device requires an uncomfortable rigid head frame. In another system called the *CyberKnife,* no frame is needed.

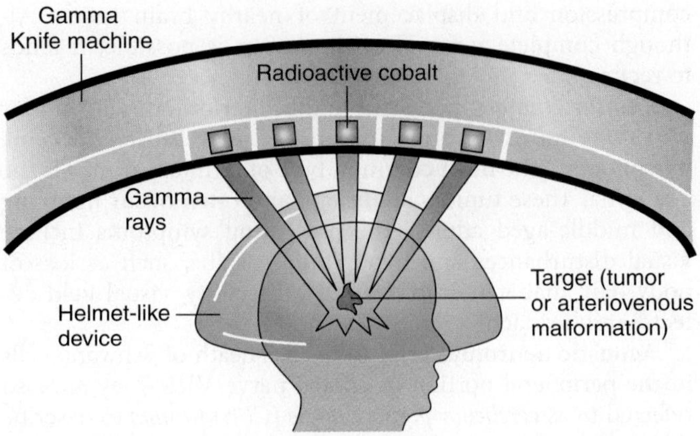
Gamma
Knife machine
Radioactive cobalt
Gamma
rays
Helmet-like
device
Target (tumor
or arteriovenous
malformation)

Fig. 47-10 • A gamma knife treatment. The treatment beams are widely dispersed over the surface of the head to prevent damage to healthy brain tissue. The beams are intense only at the point of target.

Both procedures are used primarily for brain tumors or arteriovenous malformations (AVMs) that are in a difficult location and therefore not removable by craniotomy. Tumors typically treated in this manner are acoustic neuromas, meningiomas, and metastatic tumors. These procedures may also be used with patients who refuse conventional surgery, for patients whose age and physical condition do not allow general anesthesia, as an adjunct to radiation therapy, and for recurrent or residual AVM or tumors after embolization or craniotomy.

Surgical Management

Brain biopsy may be done to determine the specific pathology of the tumor. *Then, a* ***craniotomy*** *(incision into the cranium) may be performed to improve symptoms related to the lesion or to decrease pressure from the tumor.* The challenge for the neurosurgeon is to remove the tumor as completely as possible without damaging normal tissue. Complete removal is possible with some *benign* tumors, which results in a "surgical cure." Postoperatively, the patient is admitted to the critical care unit.

Preoperative Care. The patient having a craniotomy is typically very anxious about having his or her head opened and the brain exposed. Concerns are centered on (1) the possibility of increased neurologic deficits after the surgery and (2) self-image when part or all of the head is shaved. Provide reassurance that the surgeon will spare vital parts of the brain while removing or decreasing the size of the tumor. Teach the patient and family about what to expect immediately after surgery and throughout the recovery period. Some patients require short- or long-term rehabilitation.

Check that the patient has not had alcohol, tobacco, anticoagulants, or NSAIDs for at least 5 days before surgery. Some neurosurgeons require a week or longer. Be sure that the patient has been NPO for at least 8 hours. Other preoperative care is similar to that for any patient having surgery as described in Chapter 16.

Operative Procedures. Surgery is performed under local or general anesthesia or sedation. Small tumors that are easily located may be removed by *minimally invasive surgery (MIS).* For example, the trans-nasal approach using endoscopy can be performed for pituitary tumors. The patient has a short hospital stay and few complications after surgery. Stereotactic surgery using a rigid head frame can be done for tumors that are easily reached. This procedure requires only burr holes and local anesthesia because the brain has no sensory neurons for pain. Laser surgery can also be done.

For a *craniotomy*, the surgeon makes an incision along or behind the hairline after placing the patient's head in a skull fixation device. Several burr holes are drilled into the skull, and a saw is used to remove a piece of bone (bone flap) to expose the tumor area. The flap is stored carefully until the end of the procedure. The tumor is located using imaging technology and removed or debulked (decreased in size). After the tumor removal, the bone flap is replaced and held by small screws or bolts. A drain or monitoring device may be inserted. The surgeon creates a soft dressing "cap" over the top of the head to keep the surgical area clean.

Postoperative Care. *The focus of postoperative care is to monitor the patient to detect changes in status and to prevent or minimize complications, especially increased intracranial pressure (ICP). (See the Plan of Care on pp. 1038-1043.) Assess neurologic and vital signs every 15 to 30 minutes for the first 4 to 6 hours after surgery and then every hour.* If the patient is stable for 24 hours, the frequency of these checks may be decreased to every 2 to 4 hours, depending on the agency's policy or the patient's condition. *Potential neurologic deficits include a decreased level of consciousness (LOC), motor weakness or paralysis, aphasia (speech and/or language problems), visual changes, and personality changes.* Periorbital (around the eye) edema and ecchymosis of one or both eyes are not unusual and are treated with cold compresses to decrease swelling. Irrigate the affected eye with warm saline solution or artificial tears to improve patient comfort. If the patient is still recovering from anesthesia, has a decreased LOC, or may not be able to protect the airway, he or she may remain intubated and have controlled mechanical ventilation.

The patient in the critical care unit is routinely connected to the cardiac monitor. Dysrhythmias may occur after surgery, or they may result from fluid and electrolyte imbalance. Other nursing interventions include strict recording of the patient's intake and output and possibly fluid restriction to 1500 mL daily as clinically indicated. Teach unlicensed assistive personnel (UAP) to perform gentle range-of-motion exercises to all extremities at least every 2 to 3 hours. Delegate and supervise turning, coughing, and deep breathing every 2 hours. To prevent the development of deep vein thrombosis, maintain sequential compression stockings or pneumatic compression boots until the patient ambulates.

Positioning. For patients who have undergone supratentorial surgery, elevate the head of the bed 30 degrees or as tolerated to promote venous drainage from the head. *Position the patient to avoid extreme hip or neck flexion and maintain the head in a midline, neutral position to prevent increased ICP.* The patient may be turned side to side or remain supine. If a large tumor has been removed, place the patient on the nonoperative side to prevent displacement of the cranial contents by gravity. The patient with an *infratentorial* (brainstem) craniotomy should be kept flat and positioned on either side for 24 to 48 hours. This position prevents pressure on the neck-area incision site. It also prevents pressure on the internal tumor excision site from higher cerebral structures. Make sure that the patient remains NPO status for 24 hours, because edema around the medulla and lower cranial nerves may cause vomiting and aspiration.

Monitoring the Dressing. Check the head dressing every 1 to 2 hours for signs of drainage. Mark the area of drainage once during each shift for baseline comparison, although this practice is controversial. A small or moderate amount of drainage is expected. Some patients may have a Hemovac, Jackson-Pratt, or other surgical drain in place for 24 hours after surgery. Measure the drainage every 8 hours, and record the amount and color. A typical amount of drainage is 30 to 50 mL every 8 hours. Follow the manufacturer's and neurosurgeon's instructions to maintain suction within the drain. *Monitor for excessive amounts of drainage. A saturated head dressing or drainage greater than 50 mL/8 hr should be reported immediately to the surgeon. Observe for manifestations of hypovolemic shock and lay the patient flat.*

Monitoring Laboratory Values. The usual laboratory studies monitored postoperatively include complete blood count (CBC), serum electrolyte levels and osmolarity, coagulation studies, and arterial blood gas (ABG) measurements. The patient's hematocrit and hemoglobin concentration may be abnormally low from blood loss during surgery or elevated if the blood was replaced. Hyponatremia (low serum sodium) may occur as a result of fluid volume overload, syndrome of inappropriate antidiuretic hormone (SIADH), or steroid administration. Hypokalemia (low serum potassium) may cause cardiac irritability. Weakness, a change in LOC, and confusion are symptoms of hyponatremia and hypokalemia. Hypernatremia may be caused by meningitis, dehydration, or diabetes insipidus (DI). It is manifested by muscle weakness, restlessness, extreme thirst, and dry mouth. Additional signs of dehydration such as decreased urinary output, thickened lung secretions, and hypotension may be present. *Untreated hypernatremia can lead to seizure activity. DI should be considered if the patient voids large amounts of very dilute urine with an increasing serum osmolarity and electrolyte concentration.*

Ventilating the Patient. Often the patient is mechanically ventilated and hyperventilated for the first 24 to 48 hours after surgery to help prevent increased ICP and improve cerebral oxygen levels. The desired outcome of controlled ventilation is to keep the partial pressure of arterial carbon dioxide ($Paco_2$) at about 35 mm Hg, with normal arterial oxygen levels. This is designed to avoid cerebral vasodilation from hypercarbia (increased carbon dioxide) with the resulting rise in ICP. If the patient is awake or attempting to breathe at a rate other than that set on the ventilator, drugs such as fentanyl citrate or midazolam (Versed) are given to treat pain and anxiety, as well as to promote rest and comfort. Suction the patient as needed. Remember to hyperoxygenate the patient carefully before suctioning.

Drug Therapy. Drugs routinely given postoperatively include antiepileptic drugs, histamine blockers, proton pump inhibitors, and corticosteroids, such as dexamethasone (Decadron). Analgesics such as codeine are given for pain, and acetaminophen is given for fever or mild pain. Some physicians may elect to administer prophylactic antibiotics to prevent infection.

NCLEX EXAMINATION CHALLENGE

A client had a frontal craniotomy to remove a brain tumor 2 days ago. Which of these client care activities can the nurse safely delegate to the unlicensed nursing technician?

A. Emptying the Jackson-Pratt drain
B. Positioning and turning the client
C. Suctioning the client as needed
D. Assessing the client for dysphagia

evolve For the correct answer, go to http://evolve.elsevier.com/Iggy/.

TABLE 47-5 Postoperative Complications of Craniotomy

- Increased intracranial pressure (ICP)
- Hematomas
  - Subdural hematoma
  - Epidural hematoma
- Subarachnoid hemorrhage
- Hypovolemic shock
- Hydrocephalus
- Respiratory complications
  - Atelectasis
  - Hypoxia
  - Pneumonia
  - Neurogenic pulmonary edema
- Wound infection
- Meningitis
- Fluid and electrolyte imbalances
  - Dehydration
  - Hyponatremia
  - Hypernatremia
- Seizures
- Cerebrospinal fluid (CSF) leak
- Cerebral edema

Preventing Postoperative Complications. Postoperative complications are listed in Table 47-5. The major complication of supratentorial surgery is increased ICP from cerebral edema, hemorrhage, or obstruction of the normal flow of cerebrospinal fluid (CSF).

Symptoms of *increased ICP* include severe headache, deteriorating LOC, restlessness, irritability, and dilated or pinpoint pupils that are slow to react or nonreactive to light. Treatment of increased ICP is the same as that described on p. 1055 under Interventions in the Traumatic Brain Injury section.

Subdural and epidural *hematomas and intracranial hemorrhage* are manifested by severe headache, a rapid change in LOC, progressive neurologic deficits, and herniation syndromes (brain tissue shifting, often downward). Bleeding into the posterior fossa may lead to sudden cardiovascular and respiratory arrest. Treatment of a hematoma requires surgical removal. An intracranial hemorrhage is treated with aggressive medical management (e.g., osmotic diuretics, ICP monitoring).

Hydrocephalus (increased CSF in the brain) is caused by obstruction of the normal CSF pathway from edema, an expanding lesion such as a hematoma, or blood in the subarachnoid space. Rapidly progressive hydrocephalus produces the classic symptoms of increased ICP. Slowly progressive hydrocephalus is manifested by headache, decreased LOC, irritability, blurred vision, and urinary incontinence. An intraventricular catheter (**ventriculostomy**) may be placed as an emergency procedure to drain CSF for rapidly deteriorating neurologic function. If long-term treatment is required for chronic hydrocephalus, a surgical shunt is inserted to drain CSF to another area of the body. A ventriculoperitoneal or, less often, a ventriculoatrial or lumbar peritoneal shunt procedure is usually performed. A major complication of the shunting procedure is a subdural hematoma from the tearing of bridging veins. An external lumbar drain may also be used temporarily. Additional information about shunts may be found in neuroscience nursing textbooks.

Respiratory complications include atelectasis, pneumonia, and neurogenic pulmonary edema. Prevent atelectasis and pneumonia by turning the patient frequently and encouraging him or her to take frequent deep breaths to expand the lungs each hour. Humidified air and incentive spirometry are also useful techniques. Other treatment modalities include endotracheal or oral tracheal suctioning and chest physiotherapy. However, these measures may cause an increase in ICP.

Although not common, *neurogenic pulmonary edema* is a life-threatening complication of traumatic brain injury (TBI), brain tumors, and brain surgery. Its symptoms are the same as those of acute pulmonary edema, but there are no associated cardiac problems. In spite of aggressive treatment, most patients with neurogenic pulmonary edema do not survive.

Wound infections occur more often in older and debilitated patients and in patients with a history of diabetes, long-term steroid use, obesity, and previous infections. The patient may contribute to the problem by rubbing or scratching the wound. If infection is present, the wound appears reddened and puffy. It may begin to separate, is sensitive to touch, and feels warm. The patient may or may not be febrile. Treatment is based on the degree and extent of the infection. A localized infection may be treated by cleaning it with an antiseptic and applying local antibiotics. For more severe infections, systemic antibiotic administration is needed. If the underlying bone is involved, it may need to be removed.

Meningitis is an inflammation of the meninges and may occur as a result of surgery or wound infection, a cerebrospinal fluid (CSF) leak, or contamination during surgery. (See the discussion of meningitis in Chapter 44 for a more complete explanation of this complication.)

Complications related to *fluid and electrolyte imbalance* include DI, SIADH, and cerebral salt wasting (CSW). DI is seen most often after supratentorial surgery, especially procedures involving the pituitary gland or hypothalamus. Failure of the posterior pituitary gland to release antidiuretic hormone (ADH) leads to failure of the renal tubules to reabsorb water. The patient's urine output increases dramatically (it may be up to 10 L/day), and the urine specific gravity drops to below 1.005. Urine osmolarity decreases, whereas serum osmolarity increases. The patient may become dehydrated, and hypovolemic shock may develop rapidly if this condition is left untreated. Fluid therapy to replace urinary losses and prevent dehydration may be accomplished by having the patient increase oral intake or use IV fluids. Hormonal replacement may also be necessary, especially if fluid loss is greater than 6 L/24 hr. Aqueous vasopressin is short-acting, lasting only 6 to 8 hours. Desmopressin acetate (DDAVP) may be administered for long-term replacement therapy.

Syndrome of inappropriate antidiuretic hormone (SIADH) occurs when the posterior pituitary gland releases too much ADH, causing water retention. The urine output decreases dramatically, with a urine output of less than 20 mL/hr. Sodium concentration in the urine is normal or elevated, whereas the serum sodium level falls. Other indications of SIADH are loss of thirst, weight gain, irritability, muscle weakness, and decreased LOC. SIADH is treated by fluid restriction, which is usually sufficient to correct the hyponatremia. Slow, controlled IV infusion of 3% hypertonic sodium may be needed for severe hyponatremia (<118 mEq/L).

Cerebral salt wasting (CSW) is thought to result from the influence of atrial natriuretic factor (ANF). ANF cells are located in the hypothalamus and the right atrium and regulate fluid volume. CSW is believed to be the primary cause of hyponatremia in the neurosurgical population. It is characterized by hyponatremia, decreased serum osmolarity, and decreased blood volume. Serum vasopressin and ANF levels can differentiate CSW and SIADH. CSW is treated with the replacement of sodium and isotonic fluid volume.

Patients with complications related to fluid and electrolyte imbalance undergo strict measurement of their intake and output. An accurate daily weight measurement is an essential aspect of nursing care. Carefully assess for indications of fluid overload or dehydration during treatment. Serum electrolyte levels and osmolarity are measured daily (or more often if clinically indicated).

Community-Based Care

The patient with a brain tumor is managed at home if possible. Maintaining a reasonable quality of life is an important outcome for recovery and rehabilitation. Unless the patient has a significant degree of disability, no special preparation for home care is needed. Patients with hemiparesis need assistance to ensure that their home is accessible according to their method of mobility (e.g., cane, walker, wheelchair). The environment should be made safe to prevent falls. For example, teach caregivers to remove scatter rugs and to place grab bars in the bathroom.

Information about the selection of rehabilitation or chronic care facility, if needed, can be obtained from the case manager (CM) or discharge planner. The selected facility should have experience in providing care for neurologically impaired patients. A psychologist should be available to provide input in the evaluation of the cognitive disabilities that the patient may have.

It is very important that the patient and family fully understand the importance of any recommended follow-up health care appointments. The discharge summary should state the name of the person who has been given the follow-up information.

Health teaching includes drug therapy and who to call if adverse drug events occur. Remind the patient to avoid taking any over-the-counter drugs unless approved by the health care provider.

Teach the patient to maintain a program of regular physical exercise within the limits of any disabilities. Referral to the nutritionist may be needed to ensure adequate caloric intake for the patient receiving radiation or chemotherapy.

Seizures are a potential complication that can occur at any time for as long as 1 year or more after surgery. Provide the patient and the family with information about seizure precautions and what to do if a seizure occurs.

Refer the patient and the family or significant others to the American Brain Tumor Association (www.abta.org) or the National Brain Tumor Foundation (www.braintumor.org). The American Cancer Society (www.cancer.org) is also an appropriate community resource for patients with malignant tumors. Home care agencies are available to provide both the physical and rehabilitative care that the patient may need at home. Hospice services and palliative care may be needed if he or she is terminally ill. (See Chapter 9 for additional information.) Brain tumor support groups may also be a valuable asset to the patient and family.

BRAIN ABSCESS

A **brain abscess** is a purulent infection of the brain in which pus forms in the extradural, subdural, or intracerebral area of the brain. The causative organisms are usually bacteria that invade the brain directly or indirectly. Cerebral abscesses may be a complication of meningitis.

Pathophysiology

In general, organisms from the ear, sinus, or mastoid area enter the brain by traveling along the wall of the cerebral veins, and therefore they may spread to any area of the brain. At times, the organisms (especially those from the ear) destroy the bone, form a tract, and enter the brain directly. Septic emboli (dislodged clots) from the heart, the lungs, or a dental or peritonsillar abscess may break off and enter the systemic circulation. These organisms may become lodged in a cerebral vessel and produce a localized infection. Penetrating trauma, open head injuries, and neurosurgical procedures provide a potential means for the direct entry of an organism into the brain. In the past 20 years, the number of patients with a brain abscess as a consequence of immunosuppression, organ transplantation, and acquired immune deficiency syndrome (AIDS) has increased.

The organisms cause a local infection, and acute inflammation surrounds the involved area. Within a few days, necrosis of the tissue takes place, pus forms, and the tissue liquefies. This is followed by the development of cerebral edema from localized vascular congestion and tissue swelling in response to inflammation. During the subsequent few weeks, the area becomes encapsulated, first by fibrous granulation tissue and later by collagenous connective tissue. The abscess usually occurs deep within the cerebral hemisphere and involves the white matter of the brain. Occasionally the abscess does not become encapsulated but, instead, spreads through the brain tissue to the subarachnoid space and ventricular system.

The organism varies with the source of the abscess. *Streptococci* are the most common organisms and are often found with other anaerobes such as *Bacteroides*. *Enterobacteriaceae* such as *Escherichia coli* and *Proteus* organisms may also be combined with *Streptococcus*. Yeast and fungi also cause cerebral abscess formation, particularly in patients who are immunosuppressed. *Toxoplasma gondii* is one of the most commonly seen central nervous system (CNS) opportunistic infection in the AIDS population.

Most brain abscesses occur in the frontal and temporal lobes. A few affected patients have more than one abscess. Mortality rates vary up to more than one half of patients with abscesses. Those that occur in immune suppressed patients are associated with a higher mortality rate.

Patient-Centered Collaborative Care

Assessment

Physical Assessment/Clinical Manifestations

The clinical manifestations of a brain abscess begin slowly and are similar to some of the manifestations of meningitis. The patient may have headache, fever, and neurologic deficits or nonspecific signs and symptoms. Perform a neurologic assessment. The patient may be mildly lethargic or somewhat confused. The pupillary response to light is normal in the early stages. As increased intracranial pressure (ICP) progresses, the pupils may become sluggish, unequal, dilated, and nonresponsive to light. The patient's level of consciousness (LOC) declines to a state in which he or she loses the ability to interact with the environment. Airway and respiratory function may also be altered.

Examination of the patient's visual fields often reveals a **temporal field blindness** (decrease in peripheral vision laterally). If the abscess affects the cerebral hemispheres, nystagmus and a disconjugate gaze may be evident. Motor examination reveals a generalized weakness. More significant motor problems, such as hemiplegia, may be apparent in the presence of a frontal lobe abscess. An ataxic gait is seen with a cerebellar abscess. Sensory impairment varies, although the patient often exhibits no sensory deficits. The patient may have varying degrees of aphasia (impaired communication ability) in the presence of a frontal or temporal lobe abscess. Seizure activity may occur because of irritation of the cortical tissue. Late in the disease process, more severe symptoms of increased ICP occur and include severe headache, decreased LOC (possibly coma), a widened pulse pressure, bradycardia, and irregular respirations. The patient with AIDS often presents with systemic infection, CNS involvement, and lymphoma.

Some patients may have atypical presentations, including older adults (age-related compromise in immune function), those receiving steroid therapy or immune-modulating drugs, and patients with later stages of human immune deficiency virus (HIV) infection (immune system compromise). In the earlier stages, the inflammatory response is responsible for much of the clinical presentation, particularly if cerebral abscess formation results from meningitis. The risk is that the patient may progress to severe abscess formation before the onset of "classic" manifestations.

Diagnostic Assessment

The white blood cell (WBC) count and erythrocyte sedimentation rate (ESR) are usually elevated, indicating the presence of infection. If the abscess is encapsulated, the WBC count may be normal. Obtain specimens for aerobic and, when possible, anaerobic cultures of the blood, ear, nose, and throat to determine the primary source of infection.

The health care provider requests a CT scan to determine the presence of cerebritis, hydrocephalus, or a midline shift. MRI is also useful in detecting the presence of an abscess early in the course of the disease. An EEG can localize the lesion in most cases and shows high-voltage, slow-wave activity; electro-cerebral silence may be noted in the area of the abscess. Radiography of the sinuses and the mastoid is often indicated. A lumbar puncture may be performed if meningitis is also suspected and the patient does not have ICP elevation.

▪ *Interventions*

Drug therapy is prescribed by the physician to treat the abscess. Typically used antibiotics include penicillin G benzathine (Bicillin) and nafcillin sodium (Nafcil, Unipen). Metronidazole (Flagyl, Novonidazol♣) or vancomycin may be used if an anaerobic organism is the causative agent. Antibiotic dosing may be increased to ensure adequate CNS penetration. These agents are particularly useful in the early stages (cerebritis) of abscess formation. A combination of antibiotics is used, particularly if the abscess resulted from septic emboli. Antiepileptic drugs such as phenytoin (Dilantin) may be used to prevent seizures. The drug regimen is strictly followed to maintain therapeutic blood levels. Give analgesics to treat headache.

The physician may surgically drain an encapsulated abscess via a burr hole to reduce the mass effect of the lesion. In certain cases a craniotomy may be performed to remove the abscess. The decision to perform surgery is based on the patient's general condition, the stage of abscess development, and the site of the abscess. Provide routine preoperative and postoperative care for the patient undergoing a craniotomy, as discussed on p. 1063 under Postoperative Care in the Brain Tumors section.

The patient with a brain abscess is discharged to home if few or no neurologic deficits are present. Patients with severe dysfunction are usually transferred to long-term care or a rehabilitation facility. Some patients have permanent neurologic deficits.

HUMAN NEEDS NURSING CARE REVIEW

What might you NOTICE if the patient is experiencing impaired mobility, sensation, and cognition as a result of severe acute neurologic health problems affecting the brain?

- Decreased level of consciousness (LOC)
- Inability to communicate (aphasia)
- Impaired swallowing (dysphagia)
- Weakness or paralysis of one side of the body (hemiparesis or hemiplegia)
- Alteration in gait
- Inability to perform ADLs
- Report of nausea and vomiting
- Report of impaired visual acuity or fields
- Ptosis (eyelid drooping)
- Unilateral body neglect
- Report of decreased peripheral sensation
- Inability to make appropriate judgments; confusion
- Impaired memory
- Report of severe headache

What should you INTERPRET and how should you RESPOND to a patient experiencing impaired mobility, sensation, and cognition as a result of severe neurologic health problems affecting the brain?

Perform and interpret physical assessment, including:

- *Assess airway, breathing, and circulation (ABC) status.*
- Assess neurologic status, especially LOC and mental state.
- Take vital signs (high blood pressure or widened pulse pressure may indicate increased intracranial pressure [ICP]).
- Assess functional status.
- Assess for swallowing and nutrition status.

Respond by:

- Notifying health care provider or Rapid Response Team if patient is having increased ICP.

- Ensuring an adequate airway.
- Giving oxygen to perfuse the brain.
- Establishing IV access.
- Protecting the patient from injury.
- Collaborating with health care team members as needed to meet patient's needs.
- Assisting with ADLs and mobility as needed.

On what should you REFLECT?

- Think about how you responded.
- Continue to monitor neurologic status.
- Monitor for indications of secondary brain insult as patient is treated.
- Think about what health teaching is needed for the patient and family.
- Provide emotional support for the patient and family.
- Think about what other interventions you could implement in caring for the patient.

GET READY FOR THE NCLEX EXAMINATION!

Key Points

Review these Key Points for each NCLEX Examination Client Needs Category.

Safe and Effective Care Environment

- When caring for a patient with a stroke or traumatic brain injury (TBI), assess airway, breathing, and circulation status first and implement interventions to maintain them.
- Monitor patients with critical neurologic health problems for manifestations of increasing intracranial pressure (ICP) as described in Chart 47-6.
- Be aware that the first sign of increased ICP is a *decrease* in level of consciousness (LOC).
- Collaborate with members of the health care team when managing patients with critical neurologic health problems, including the physical and occupational therapists, nutritionist, and social worker.
- Coordinate continuity of care with the hospital case manager or discharge planner when discharging or transferring patients to community-based agencies or home.
- Teach patients and families about community organizations, such as the National Stroke Association and the Brain Injury Association of America.

Health Promotion and Maintenance

- Conduct a complete health assessment for patients with a stroke, with an emphasis on neurologic status.
- Teach patients and families about risk factors for stroke as listed in Chart 47-2.

Psychosocial Integrity

- Assess the emotional reactions of families to a brain cancer diagnosis, and help them cope by providing information and referrals to support systems.
- Teach patients and their families about community resources to help them cope with life changes, especially community support groups that are provided by state and national organizations.
- Assess patients with strokes for sensory perceptual changes such as unilateral neglect and impaired vision; help patients adapt to these changes, such as turning their head from side to side to see the entire meal tray.

Physiological Integrity

- Recall the differences between a transient ischemic attack and a brain attack (stroke) (see Charts 47-1, 47-3, and 47-4).
- Assess the patient's ability to perform ADLs, including the ability to eat because of swallowing problems.
- Assess for types of aphasia as delineated in Table 47-2.
- Monitor the patient on thrombolytic therapy or anticoagulants for bleeding and abnormal coagulation studies.
- Provide best practices for thrombolytic therapy administration as listed in Chart 47-5.
- Provide best practices for ICP monitoring as listed in Chart 47-7.
- Evaluate the collaborative care of the stroke patient by helping him or her achieve the highest level of functioning in the community or long-term health care agency.
- Assess for manifestations of TBI as outlined in Chart 47-8.
- Teach patients with minor head injury and their families to monitor for neurologic changes as listed in Chart 47-10.
- Assess for manifestations of brain tumors as listed in Chart 47-11.
- Recognize that the desired outcome for the patient with a brain tumor is to remove it if possible. Other methods may be used to decrease its size, including chemotherapy, radiation, and surgery.
- The mainstay of management for patients with brain abscess is systemic antibiotic therapy.

Additional Study Resources

Go to your Companion CD or Evolve at http://evolve.elsevier.com/Iggy/ for *Self-Assessment Questions for the NCLEX Examination.*

evolve Go to Evolve at http://evolve.elsevier.com/Iggy/ for *Prioritization and Delegation Questions for the NCLEX Examination.*

SELECTED BIBLIOGRAPHY

Adams, H.P. Jr., del Zoppo, G., Alberts, M.J., Bhatt, D.L., Brass, L., Furlan, A., et al. (2007). Guidelines for the early management of adults with ischemic stroke: A guideline from the American Heart Association/American Stroke Association Stroke Council, Clinical Cardiology Council, Cardiovascular Radiology and Intervention Council, and the Atherosclerotic Peripheral Vascular Disease and Quality of Care Outcomes in Research Interdisciplinary Work Groups. *Stroke, 38*(5), 1655-1711.

Aschkenasy, M.T., & Rothenhaus, T.C. (2006). Trauma and falls in the elderly. *Emergency Medicine Clinics of North America, 24*(2), 413-432.

Bader, M.K. (2006) Recognizing and treating ischemic insults to the brain: The role of brain tissue oxygen monitoring. *Critical Care Nursing Clinics of North America, 18*(2), 243-256.

Batchelor, T.T., & Byrne, T.N. (2006). Supportive care of brain tumor patients. *Hematology Clinics of North America, 20*(6), 1137-1361.

Boner, T. (2006). Hypotension and TIA. *Journal of Neuroscience Nursing, 38*(1), 5.

Change, S.D. (2005). The CyberKnife®: Potential in patients with cranial and spinal tumors. *American Journal of Cancer, 4*(6), 383-393.

Collins, C. (2007). Pathophysiology and classification of acute stroke. *Nursing Standard, 21*(28), 35-39.

Cook, A.M. (2006). Self-care needs of caregivers dealing with stroke. *Journal of Neuroscience Nursing, 38*(1), 31-36.

Correa, D.D. (2006). Cognitive functions in brain tumor patients. *Hematology Clinics of North America, 20*(6), 1363-1367.

Fox, S.W., Mitchell, S.A., & Booth-Jones, M. (2006). Cognitive impairments in patients with brain tumors: Assessment and intervention in the clinic setting. *Clinical Journal of Oncology Nursing, 10*(2), 169-176.

Frizzell, J.P. (2005). Acute stroke: Pathophysiology, diagnosis and treatment. *AACN Clinical Issues: Advanced Practice in Acute Critical Care, 16*(4), 421-440.

Gordon, B.M. (2007). Pharmacological management of secreting pituitary tumors. *Journal of Neuroscience Nursing, 39*(1), 52-57.

Gramitto, M., & Galitz, D. (2008). Update on stroke: The latest guidelines. *The Nurse Practitioner, 33*(1), 39-47.

Hinkle, J.L. (2007). Acute ischemic stroke review. *Journal of Neuroscience Nursing, 39*(5), 285-293, 310.

Jeffrey, S. (2007a). Less preventive treatment after hemorrhagic stroke. *Medscape Medical News.* Retrieved March 24, 2008, from www.medscape.com/viewarticle.

Jeffrey, S. (2007b). Stimulant abuse may increase stroke among young adults. *Medscape Medical News.* Retrieved March 24, 2008, from www.medscape.com/viewarticle.

Jeong, S., & Kim, M.T. (2007). Effects of a theory-driven music and movement program for stroke survivors in a community setting. *Applied Nursing Research, 20*(3), 125-131.

Kulchycki, L.K., & Edlow, J.A. (2006). Geriatric neurologic emergencies. *Emergency Medicine Clinics of North America, 24*(2), 273-298.

Lemke, D.M. (2007). Sympathetic storming after severe traumatic brain injury. *Critical Care Nurse, 27*(1), 30-37.

Liechty, J.A., & Heinzekehr, J.B. (2007). Caring for those without words: A perspective on aphasia. *Journal of Neuroscience Nursing, 39*(5), 316-318.

Marks, J.P. (2006). A critical pathway for meeting the needs of families of patients with severe traumatic brain injury. *Journal of Neuroscience Nursing, 38*(2), 84-89.

Mathiesen, C., Tavianini, H.D., & Palladino, K. (2006). Best practices in stroke rapid response: A case study. *MEDSURG Nursing, 15*(6), 364-369.

McCaffery, C. (2006). Quick! My patient is having an ischemic stroke. *Nursing2006, 36*(7), 56cc1-4.

Morrison, K. (2007). Improving the care of stroke patients. *American Nurse Today, 2*(4), 38-44.

Palmieri, R.L. (2006). Carotid artery stenosis paves the way for a stroke. *Nursing2006, 36*(6), 36-42.

Palmieri, R.L. (2007). Responding to primary brain tumor. *Nursing 2007, 37*(1), 36-43.

Peiffer, K.M.Z. (2007). Brain death and organ procurement. *AJN, 107*(3), 58-66.

Petchprapai, N., & Winkelman, C. (2007). Mild traumatic brain injury: Determinants and subsequent quality of life. A review of the literature. *Journal of Neuroscience Nursing, 39*(5), 260-272.

Presciutti, M. (2006). Nursing priorities in caring for patients with intracerebral hemorrhage. *Journal of Neuroscience Nursing, 38*(Suppl. 4), 296-299.

Richardson, J. (2006). Successful implementation of the National Institutes of Health Stroke Scale on a stroke/neurovascular unit. *The Journal of Neuroscience Nursing, 38*(Suppl. 4), 309-315.

Sauerbeck, L.R. (2006). Primary stroke prevention. *AJN*, 106(11), 40-48.

Schiess, N., & Nath, A. (2007). Management of brain abscess. *Journal of Pharmacy Practice, 20*(2), 158-159.

Schollenberger, J., Rehwoldt, M., & Barnhill, B. (2006). Brain monitors. *RN, 69*(1), 44-50.

Strimike, C.L. (2007). Carotid artery stents: Opening the way to safer stroke prevention. *American Nurse Today, 2*(1), 12-14.

Zink, E.K., & McQuillan, K. (2005). Managing traumatic brain injury. *Nursing2005, 35*(9), 36-44.

XI

UNIT

Problems of Sensation

Management of Patients with Problems of the Sensory System

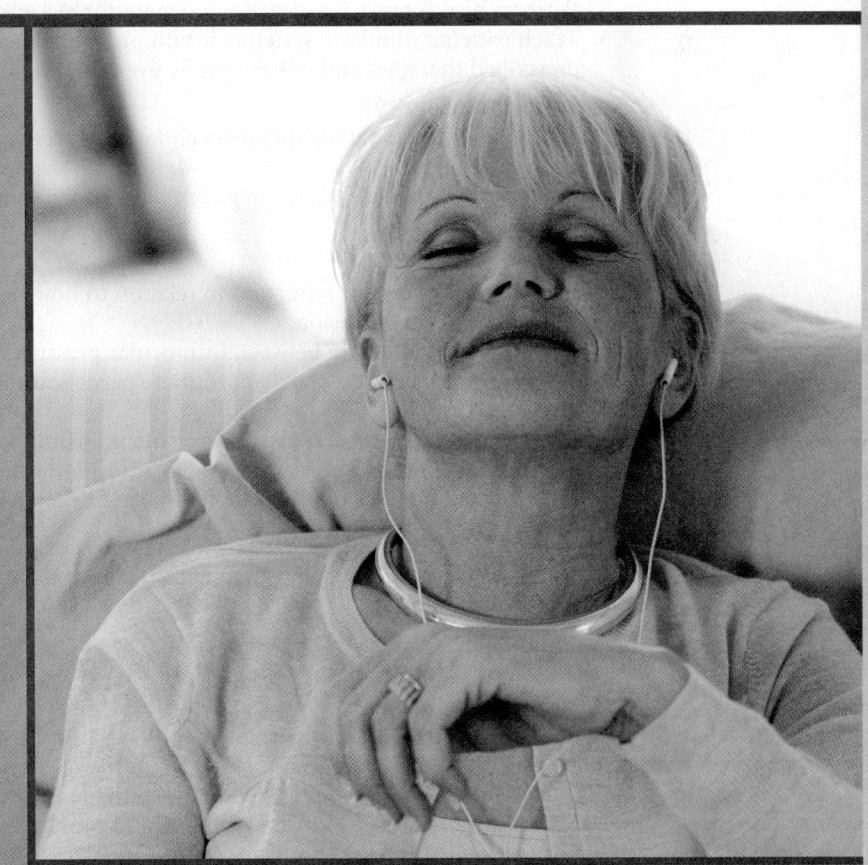

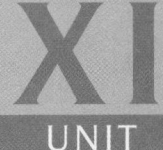

48
CHAPTER

Assessment of the Eye and Vision

M. Linda Workman

LEARNING OUTCOMES

For clinical competence and success on the NCLEX Examination, study this chapter with these Learning Outcomes in mind:

Safe and Effective Care Environment

1. Use aseptic technique when touching the eyelids or external eye structures.
2. Use appropriate technique when instilling eyedrops or eye ointments.
3. Verify that informed consent has been obtained before invasive tests of the eye or vision are performed.

Health Promotion and Maintenance

4. Teach all people the use of eye protection equipment and strategies.
5. Perform health history and risk assessment for eye and vision problems.
6. Teach patients who have systemic health problems that may affect eye health and vision to adhere to prescribed therapies and to have yearly eye examinations by an ophthalmologist.

Psychosocial Integrity

7. Teach patients and family members about what to expect during tests and procedures to assess vision and eye problems.
8. Provide the opportunity for the patient and family to express their feelings about a possible change in vision.

Physiological Integrity

9. Explain the concept of refraction in relation to how the cornea, lens, aqueous humor, and vitreous humor contribute to vision.
10. Explain the relationship between intraocular pressure and eye health.
11. Use concepts of anatomy and appropriate psychomotor skills to apply eye and vision assessment methods correctly.
12. Perform a clinical eye and vision assessment, including health history and psychosocial assessment.
13. Explain the eye changes associated with aging and their impact on vision.
14. Interpret the findings of visual acuity by the Snellen chart.

Go to your Companion CD or Evolve at http://evolve.elsevier.com/Iggy/ for *Self-Assessment Questions for the NCLEX Examination* keyed to these Learning Outcomes.

The eye, along with the brain, is the organ that allows vision. Vision is one of the five senses and is important for communicating with the world. Many people consider vision to be the most important sense in meeting the *human need for sensation and cognition*. It is used to assess surroundings, allow independence, warn of danger, appreciate beauty, work, play, and interact with other people.

Vision begins with the eye, where light is changed into nerve impulses. These impulses are sent to the brain, where images are fully perceived. Many systemic conditions, as well as eye problems, can affect the eye and change vision temporarily or permanently. Changes in the eye and vision can provide information about the patient's general health status and problems that might occur in self-care.

ANATOMY AND PHYSIOLOGY REVIEW

Structure

The eyeball, a round, ball-shaped organ, is located in the front part of the eye orbit. The **orbit** is the bony socket of the skull that surrounds and protects the eye along with the attached muscles, nerves, vessels, and tear-producing glands.

Layers of the Eyeball

The eye has three layers, or coats (Fig. 48-1). The external layer is the **sclera** (the opaque tissue making up the "whites" of the eye) and the transparent cornea on the front of the eye.

The middle layer, or **uvea,** is heavily pigmented. This layer consists of the choroid, the ciliary body, and the iris. The choroid, a dark brown membrane between the sclera and the retina, lines most of the sclera. The choroid has many blood vessels that supply nutrients to the retina.

The ciliary body connects the choroid with the iris and secretes aqueous humor. The **iris** is the colored portion of the external eye; its center opening is the **pupil.** The muscles of the iris contract and relax to control pupil size and the amount of light entering the eye.

The innermost layer is the **retina,** a thin, delicate structure made up of sensory receptors that transmit impulses to the optic nerve. The retina contains blood vessels and two types of photoreceptors called *rods* and *cones.* The rods work at low light levels and provide peripheral vision. The cones are active at bright light levels and provide color and central vision.

The **optic fundus** is the area at the inside back of the eye that can be seen with an ophthalmoscope. This area contains the **optic disc,** a creamy pink to white depressed area in the retina where the optic nerve enters and exits the eyeball. The optic disc is sometimes called the "blind spot" because it contains only nerve fibers and no photoreceptor cells. To one side of the optic disc is a small, yellowish pink area called the *macula lutea.* The center of the macula is the *fovea centralis,* where vision is the most acute.

Refractive Structures and Media

Light waves pass through these structures on the way to the retina: cornea, aqueous humor, lens, and vitreous humor. Each of these structures has a different density, which causes the light waves to bend **(refract)** to some degree and focus images on the retina. These structures are the eye's refracting media.

The **cornea** is the clear layer that forms the external coat on the front of the eye (see Fig. 48-1). The **aqueous humor** is a clear, watery fluid that fills the anterior and posterior chambers of the eye. Aqueous humor is continually produced by the ciliary processes and passes from the posterior chamber, through the pupil, and into the anterior chamber. This fluid drains through the canal of Schlemm into the blood to maintain a balanced intraocular pressure (IOP), the pressure within the eye (Fig. 48-2).

The **lens** is a circular, convex structure that lies behind the iris and in front of the vitreous body. It is normally transparent. The lens bends the rays of light entering through the pupil so that they focus properly on the retina. The curve of the lens changes to focus on near or distant objects. A cataract is a lens that has lost its transparency.

The **vitreous body** is a clear, thick gel that fills the vitreous chamber (the space between the lens and the retina). This gel transmits light and maintains eye shape.

The eye is a hollow organ and must be kept in the shape of a ball for vision to occur. To maintain this shape, the gel in the posterior segment (vitreous humor) and the fluid in the anterior segment (aqueous humor) must be present in set amounts that apply pressure inside the eye to keep it inflated (McCance & Huether, 2006). This pressure is known as **intraocular pressure** or **IOP.** IOP has to be just right. If the pressure is too low, the eyeball is soft and collapses, preventing light from getting to the light-sensitive receptors in the back of the eye on the retina. If the pressure becomes too high, the extra pressure presses on blood vessels in the eye and prevents blood from flowing through them, a condition called glaucoma. Without good perfusion through retinal blood vessels inside the eye, the photoreceptors are inadequately oxygenated and eventu-

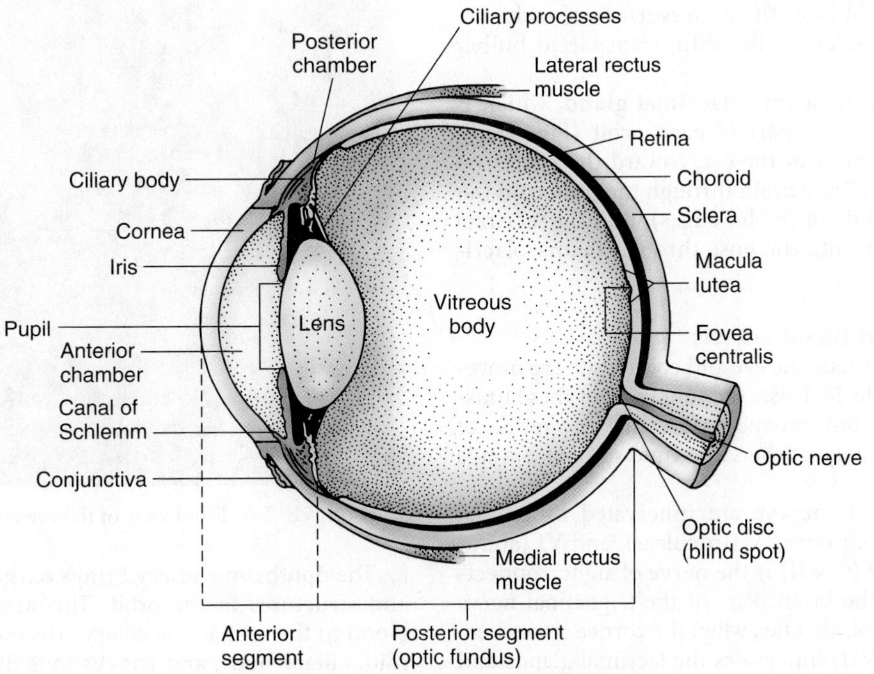
Ciliary processes
Posterior chamber
Lateral rectus muscle
Retina
Ciliary body
Choroid
Cornea
Sclera
Iris
Macula lutea
Vitreous body
Lens
Pupil
Fovea centralis
Anterior chamber
Canal of Schlemm
Optic nerve
Conjunctiva
Optic disc (blind spot)
Medial rectus muscle
Anterior segment
Posterior segment (optic fundus)

Fig. 48-1 • Anatomic features of the eye.

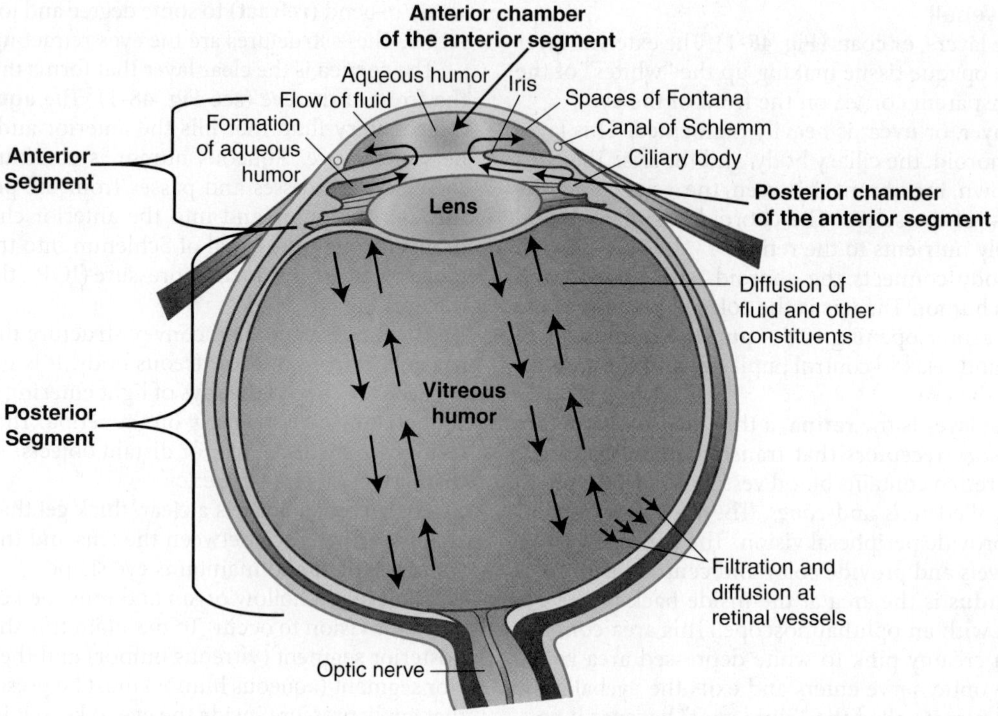
Anterior chamber
of the anterior segment
Aqueous humor
Iris
Flow of fluid
Spaces of Fontana
Formation
of aqueous
humor
Canal of Schlemm
Ciliary body
Anterior
Segment
Lens
Posterior chamber
of the anterior segment
Diffusion of
fluid and other
constituents
Vitreous
humor
Posterior
Segment
Filtration and
diffusion at
retinal vessels
Optic nerve

Fig. 48-2 • Flow of aqueous humor.

ally die. When too many have died, vision is lost and the person is permanently blind.

External Structures

The eyelids are thin, movable folds of skin that protect the eyes, shut out light during sleep, and keep the cornea moist. The upper eyelid is larger than the lower one. The **canthus** is the place where the two eyelids meet at the corner of the eye.

The **conjunctivae** are the mucous membranes of the eye. The palpebral conjunctiva is a thick membrane with many blood vessels that lines the undersurface of each eyelid. Located over the sclera is the thin, transparent bulbar conjunctiva.

Tears are produced by a small **lacrimal gland,** which is located in the upper outer part of each orbit (Fig. 48-3). Tears flow across the front of the eye, toward the nose, and into the inner canthus. They drain through the **punctum** (an opening at the nasal side of the lid edges), into the lacrimal duct and sac, and then into the nose through the nasolacrimal duct.

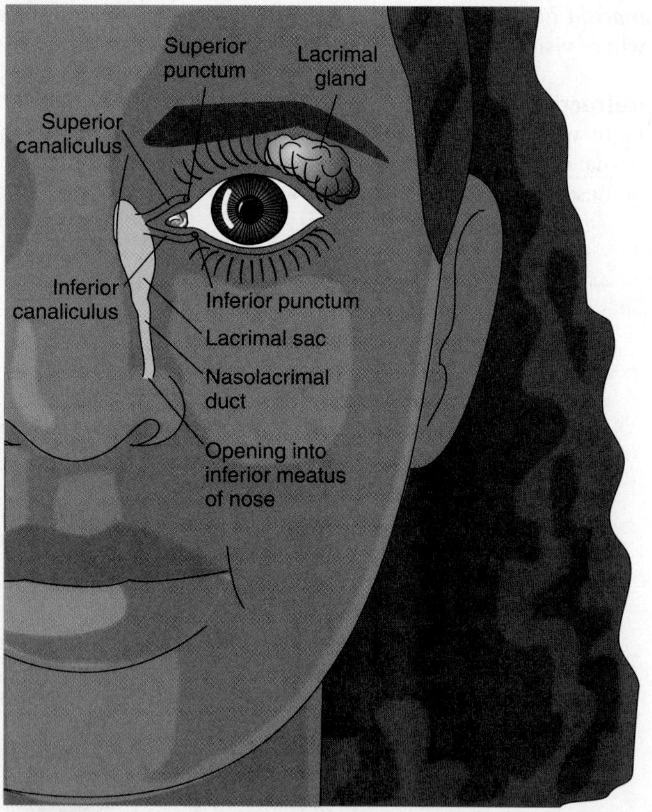
Superior
punctum
Lacrimal
gland
Superior
canaliculus
Inferior
canaliculus
Inferior punctum
Lacrimal sac
Nasolacrimal
duct
Opening into
inferior meatus
of nose

Fig. 48-3 • Front view of the eye and adjacent structures.

Muscles, Nerves, and Blood Vessels

Six voluntary muscles rotate the eye and coordinate eye movements (Fig. 48-4). Table 48-1 lists the functions of these muscles. Coordinated eye movements ensure that the retina of each eye receives an image at the same time so only a single image is seen.

The muscles around the eye are innervated by cranial nerves (CN) III (oculomotor), IV (trochlear), and VI (abducens). The **optic nerve** (CN II) is the nerve of sight, connecting the optic disc to the brain. Part of the trigeminal nerve (CN V) stimulates the blink reflex when the cornea is touched. The facial nerve (CN VII) innervates the lacrimal glands and muscles controlling lid closure.

The ophthalmic artery brings oxygenated blood to the eye and structures in the orbit. This artery branches to supply blood to the retina. The ciliary arteries supply the sclera, choroid, ciliary body, and iris. Venous drainage occurs through the two ophthalmic veins.

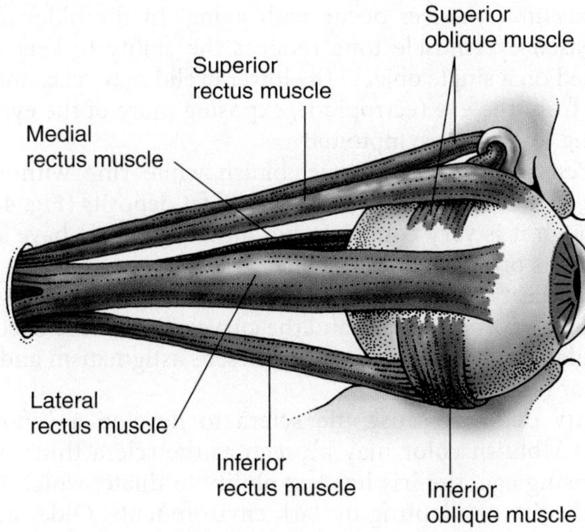
Superior
oblique muscle
Superior
rectus muscle
Medial
rectus muscle
Lateral
rectus muscle
Inferior
rectus muscle
Inferior
oblique muscle

Fig. 48-4 • The extraocular muscles.

TABLE 48-1 Functions of Ocular Muscles
SUPERIOR RECTUS MUSCLE
• Together with the lateral rectus, this muscle moves the eye diagonally upward toward the side of the head.
• Together with the medial rectus, this muscle moves the eye diagonally upward toward the middle of the head.
LATERAL RECTUS MUSCLE
• Together with the medial rectus, contraction of this muscle holds the eye in a straight position.
• Contracting alone, this muscle turns the eye toward the side of the head.
MEDIAL RECTUS MUSCLE
• Contracting alone, this muscle turns the eye toward the nose.
INFERIOR RECTUS MUSCLE
• Together with the lateral rectus, this muscle moves the eye diagonally downward toward the side of the head.
• Together with the medial rectus, this muscle moves the eye diagonally downward toward the middle of the head.
SUPERIOR OBLIQUE MUSCLE
• Contracting alone, this muscle pulls the eye downward.
INFERIOR OBLIQUE MUSCLE
• Contracting alone, this muscle pulls the eye upward.

NCLEX EXAMINATION CHALLENGE

The client asks why keeping IOP in the normal range is so important. What is the nurse's best response to this question?

A. "An increased IOP clouds the lens of the eye, leading to cataracts and blindness."
B. "An increased IOP reduces eye blood flow, leading to glaucoma and blindness."
C. "A reduced IOP changes the shape of the eyeball, leading to nearsightedness."
D. "A reduced IOP changes the shape of the eyeball, leading to farsightedness."

evolve For the correct answer, go to http://evolve.elsevier.com/Iggy/.

Function

The four eye functions that provide clear images of near and far objects are refraction, pupillary constriction, accommodation, and convergence.

Refraction involves bending light rays from the outside world into the eye. The different curved surfaces and refractive media of the eye allow light to pass through to the retina. Each surface and media bends (refracts) light differently to focus an image on the retina. **Emmetropia** is the perfect refraction of the eye: with the lens at rest, light rays from a distant source (6 m or more) are focused into a sharp image on the retina. Fig. 48-5 shows the normal refraction of light within the eye. Images fall on the retina inverted and reversed left to right. For example, an object in the lower nasal visual field strikes the upper outer area of the retina.

Errors of refraction are common. **Hyperopia** (also called *hypermetropia* or *farsightedness*) occurs when the eye does not refract light enough. As a result, images actually fall (converge) behind the retina (see Fig. 48-5). Vision beyond 20 feet is normal, but near vision is poor. Hyperopia is corrected with a convex lens in eyeglasses or contact lenses.

Myopia (nearsightedness) occurs when the eye overrefracts or overbends the light. As a result, images are focused in front of the retina (see Fig. 48-5). Near vision is normal, but distance vision is poor. Myopia is corrected with a biconcave lens in eyeglasses or contact lenses.

Astigmatism is a refractive error caused by unevenly curved surfaces on or in the eye, especially of the cornea. These uneven surfaces distort vision.

Pupillary constriction and dilation control the amount of light that enters the eye. If the level of light to one or both eyes is increased, both pupils constrict (become smaller). The amount of constriction depends on how much light is available and how well the retina can adapt to light changes. Pupillary

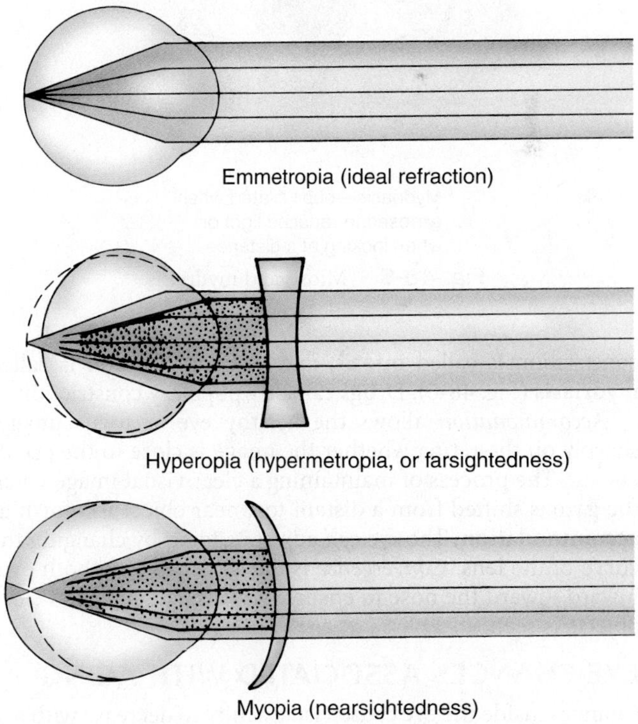
Emmetropia (ideal refraction)
Hyperopia (hypermetropia, or farsightedness)
Myopia (nearsightedness)

Fig. 48-5 • Refraction and correction in emmetropia, hyperopia, and myopia.

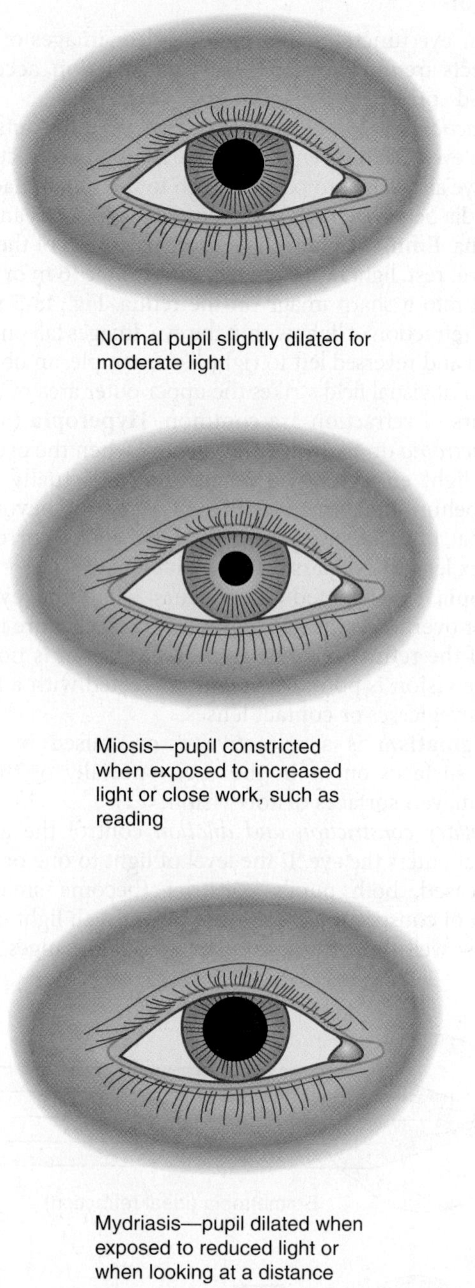
Normal pupil slightly dilated for moderate light
Miosis—pupil constricted when exposed to increased light or close work, such as reading
Mydriasis—pupil dilated when exposed to reduced light or when looking at a distance

Fig. 48-6 • Miosis and mydriasis.

constriction is called **miosis,** and pupillary dilation is called **mydriasis** (Fig. 48-6). Drugs can alter pupillary constriction.

Accommodation allows the healthy eye to focus images sharply on the retina whether the image is close to the eye or distant. The process of maintaining a clear visual image when the gaze is shifted from a distant to a near object is known as **accommodation.** The eye can adjust its focus by changing the curve of the lens. *Convergence* is the ability to turn both eyes inward toward the nose to ensure only a single image of close objects is seen.

EYE CHANGES ASSOCIATED WITH AGING

Changes inside the eye cause visual acuity to decrease with age (Meiner & Lueckenotte, 2006). Age-related changes of the nervous system and in the eye support structures also reduce visual function (Chart 48-1).

Structural changes occur with aging. In the older adult, decreased eye muscle tone reduces the ability to keep gaze focused on a single object. The lower eyelid may relax and fall away from the eye (ectropion), exposing more of the eye and leading to dry-eye symptoms.

Arcus senilis, an opaque, bluish white ring within the outer edge of the cornea, is caused by fat deposits (Fig. 48-7). Although it is very common, not all older people have arcus senilis. Its presence does not affect vision.

The clarity and shape of the cornea change with age. After age 65, the cornea flattens and the curve of its surface becomes irregular. This change causes or worsens astigmatism and distorts or blurs vision.

Fatty deposits cause the sclera to develop a yellowish tinge. A bluish color may be seen as the sclera thins. With increasing age, the iris has less ability to dilate, which leads to difficulty in adapting to dark environments. Older adults may need additional light for reading and to avoid tripping over objects.

Functional changes also occur with aging. The lens yellows with aging, reducing the ability of the eye to transmit and focus light. The aging lens hardens, shrinks, and loses elasticity. As the lens loses elasticity, the ability of the eye to accommodate is gradually lost. The **near point of vision** (the closest distance at which the eye can see an object clearly) increases. Near objects (especially reading material) must be placed farther from the eye to be seen clearly. This age-related change is called **presbyopia.** In addition, the **far point of vision** (farthest point at which an object can be distinguished) decreases. Thus the older person has a narrower visual field.

As a person ages, general color perception decreases, especially among the colors of green, blue, and violet. More light is needed to stimulate the visual receptors. Intraocular pressure (IOP) is slightly higher in older adults.

Health Promotion and Maintenance

Vision is important to everyday function and quality of life. Many vision and eye problems can be avoided, and others can be corrected or managed if discovered early. Nurses can make a difference in preserving vision and eye function by teaching all people about eye protection methods, adequate nutrition, and the importance of regular eye examinations.

The risk for cataract formation and cancer of the eye (ocular melanoma) is increased with exposure to ultraviolet (UV) light. Teach people to protect the eyes by using sunglasses that filter UV light whenever they are outdoors. Also explain that UV protection should be used in tanning parlors and in work environments that have UV exposure (Sitzman, 2006).

Vision can be affected by injury, and eye injury also increases the risk for both cataract formation and glaucoma. Urge all people to wear eye and head protection during work in occupations that involve particulate matter, fluid or blood spatter, high temperatures, or sparks (Sackett & Schenning, 2003). Eye and head protection should be worn during participation in sports, such as baseball, or any activity that increases the risk for the eye being hit by objects in motion. In addition, because excessive eye rubbing can traumatize the delicate outer eye surfaces, teach people to avoid this activity.

Eye infections can lead to vision loss. Although the eye surface is not a sterile environment, the sclera and cornea have no separate blood supply and thus are at risk for infection because the immunities in the blood do not reach these structures. Teach everyone to wash their hands before touching the

Chart 48-1 NURSING FOCUS ON THE OLDER ADULT

Changes in the Eye and Vision Related to Aging

Structure/Function	Change	Implication
Appearance	Eyes appear "sunken."	Do not use eye appearance as an indicator for hydration status.
	Arcus senilis forms.	Reassure patient this change does not affect vision.
	Sclera yellows or appears blue.	Do not use sclera to assess for jaundice.
Cornea	Cornea flattens, which blurs vision.	Encourage older adults to have regular eye examinations and wear prescribed corrective lenses for best vision.
Ocular muscles	Muscle strength is reduced, making it more difficult to maintain an upward gaze or maintain a single image.	Reassure patient this is a normal happening and to refocus gaze frequently to maintain a single image.
Lens	Elasticity is lost, increasing the near point of vision (making the near point of best vision farther away).	Encourage patient to wear corrective lenses for reading.
	Lens hardens, compacts, and forms a cataract.	Stress the importance of yearly vision checks and monitoring for when intervention is needed.
Iris	Decrease in ability to dilate results in small pupil size and poor adaptation to darkness.	Teach older adults the need for good lighting for best vision to avoid tripping and bumping into objects.
Pupil	Pupil size is smaller, reducing the ability to see in dim light.	Teach older adults the need for good lighting for best vision to avoid tripping and bumping into objects.
Color vision	Discrimination among greens, blues, and violets decreases.	The patient may not be able to use "dipstick" or other color-indicator monitors of health status.
Tears	Tear production is reduced, resulting in dry eyes, discomfort, and increased risk for corneal damage or eye infections.	Teach patient to use saline eyedrops on a schedule to reduce dryness. Teach patient to increase humidity in the home.

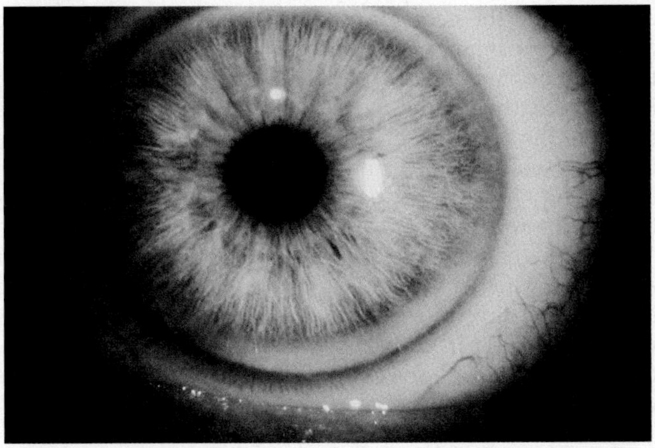

Fig. 48-7 • Arcus senilis of the iris.

eye or eyelid. Teach people who use eyedrops about the proper technique to use these drugs (Chart 48-2) and to not share eyedrops with others. If an eye has a discharge, teach the patient to use a separate eyedrop bottle for this eye and to wash the unaffected eye before washing the affected eye.

Other health problems, especially diabetes mellitus and hypertension, can have serious adverse effects on vision. Teach patients who have these health problems about the importance of controlling blood glucose levels and managing blood pressure to reduce the risk for vision loss. Explain that yearly consultation with an ophthalmologist is needed to ensure coordination with their regular health care provider to slow or prevent eye complications.

Teach all people who have a refractive error to have an eye examination yearly. Young adults who do not have vision problems may need an eye examination only every 3 to 5 years unless a problem develops. Adults older than 40 years should have an eye examination yearly that includes assessment of intraocular pressure and visual fields, because the risk for both glaucoma and cataract formation increases with age. *Anyone who has an eye injury or a suspected infection of the eye should see a health care provider immediately.*

NCLEX EXAMINATION CHALLENGE

Which intervention for safety should the nurse teach an older adult who is taking an oral drug that keeps her pupils constricted?

A. "Open drapes or curtains and turn lights on to increase room lighting."
B. "Do not drink caffeinated beverages because they will make the problem worse."
C. "Keep your eyes closed when showering or bathing to prevent water from entering the eyes."
D. "Avoid bending from the waist or coughing to prevent a sudden increase in blood pressure."

evolve For the correct answer, go to http://evolve.elsevier.com/Iggy/.

ASSESSMENT METHODS

Patient History

Collect information from the patient to determine whether problems with the eye or vision have an impact on daily functioning. Chart 48-3 lists some questions to ask when assessing eye and vision history.

Chart 48-2 PATIENT AND FAMILY EDUCATION GUIDE
Using Eyedrops

- Check the name, strength, expiration date, color, and clarity of the eyedrops to be instilled.
- If both eyes are to receive the same drug and one eye is infected, use two separate bottles and carefully label each bottle with "right" or "left" for the correct eye.
- Wash your hands.
- Remove the cap from the bottle.
- Tilt your head backward, open your eyes, and look up at the ceiling.
- Using your nondominant hand, gently pull the lower lid down against your cheek, forming a small pocket.
- Hold the eyedrop bottle (with the cap off) like a pencil, with the tip pointing down, with your dominant hand.
- Rest the wrist holding the bottle against your mouth or upper lip.
- Without touching any part of the eye or lid with the tip of the bottle, gently squeeze the bottle and release the prescribed number of drops into the pocket you have made with your lower lid.
- Gently release the lower lid.
- Close your eye gently (without squeezing the lids tightly).
- Gently press and hold the corner of the eye nearest the nose to close off the punctum and prevent the drug from being absorbed systemically.
- Without pressing on the lid, gently blot away any excess drug or tears with a tissue.
- Keep the eye closed for about 1 minute.
- Place the cap back on the bottle.
- Check to see whether the drug needs to be kept in the refrigerator.
- Wash your hands again.

Chart 48-3 EYE AND VISION ASSESSMENT
Using Gordon's Functional Health Patterns

COGNITION PERCEPTUAL PATTERN
- Do you have any difficulty seeing objects at a distance?
- Do you have any difficulty reading fine print or doing close work?
- Do you wear eyeglasses or contact lenses?
- What type of light do you use for reading?
- Do you wear sunglasses or a hat when outdoors?
- Do you have frequent headaches?
- Have you noticed any change in your ability to see things at night?
- When did you last have your eyes examined?
- Do you go to an ophthalmologist or an optometrist?
- When were you last tested for glaucoma?

Based on Gordon, M. (2007). *Manual of nursing diagnosis* (11th ed.). Boston: Jones & Bartlett.

Age is an important factor to consider when assessing the visual processes and eye structure. The incidence of glaucoma and cataract formation increases with aging. Presbyopia commonly begins in the 40s.

Gender also may be important. For example, retinal detachments are more common in men and dry-eye syndromes are more common in women.

TABLE 48-2 Systemic Conditions and Common Drugs Affecting the Eye and Vision

SYSTEMIC CONDITIONS AND DISORDERS
- Diabetes mellitus
- Hypertension
- Lupus erythematosus
- Sarcoidosis
- Thyroid dysfunction
- Acquired immune deficiency syndrome
- Cardiac disease
- Multiple sclerosis
- Pregnancy

DRUGS
- Antihistamines
- Decongestants
- Antibiotics
- Opioids
- Anticholinergics
- Cholinergic agonists
- Sympathomimetics
- Oral contraceptives
- Chemotherapy agents
- Corticosteroids
- Carbonic anhydrase inhibitors
- Beta blockers

Occupation and leisure activities can affect vision over time. Ask the patient about his or her work and specifically how the eyes are used. In some occupations, such as computer programming, constant exposure to monitor screens may lead to eyestrain and the need for eyeglasses. Machine operators are at risk for eye injury because of the high speeds at which particles can be thrown at the eye. Ask the patient who works in industrial settings about the use of protective eyewear, such as goggles. Chronic exposure to infrared or ultraviolet light may cause photophobia and cataract formation. Use this time as an opportunity to teach the patient about the use of eye protection during work.

Ask whether the patient plays sports and what types of sports and whether eye protection is used. Even when the eye is not struck directly, a blow to the head near the eye, such as with a baseball, can damage external eye structures, the eye, the connections with the brain, or the area of the brain where vision is perceived.

Systemic medical problems can affect vision or cause complications. Check whether the patient has any condition listed in Table 48-2. Ask about past accidents, injuries, surgeries, or blows to the head that may have led to the present problem. Specifically ask about previous laser surgeries because patients often do not classify laser treatment as surgery.

Drugs, even systemic drugs, can affect vision and the eye (see Table 48-2). Ask about the use of any prescription or over-the-counter drugs, especially decongestants and antihistamines, which tend to dry the eye and may increase intraocular pressure (IOP). Many patients do not consider over-the-counter eyedrops to be drugs. Record the name, strength, dose, and scheduling for all drugs the patient uses. Manifestations of ocular drug effects include **pruritus** (itching), foreign body sensation, redness, tearing, **photophobia** (sensitivity to light), and the development of cataracts or glaucoma.

Nutrition History

Because some ocular problems are caused by or made worse with vitamin deficiencies, ask the patient about his or her food choices. For example, vitamin A deficiency can cause eye dryness, keratomalacia, and blindness. On the other hand, nutrients and antioxidants such as lutein and beta carotene may help maintain retinal function. A diet rich in red, orange, and dark green vegetables and fruit is important to eye health. Teach all people to eat five to ten servings of these foods every day.

Family History and Genetic Risk

Ask the patient about a family history of eye problems. Some conditions, such as a refractive error, show a familial tendency. In addition, some genetic problems lead to visual impairment in adulthood (Nussbaum et al., 2007). When a patient tells you that other relatives, especially first-degree relatives (parents, siblings, and children), have eye problems, be sure to record the gender of the affected person, his or her relationship to the patient, the exact nature of the problem, and the age that the problem was first noted.

Current Health Problems

Ask the patient about the onset of visual changes. Did the change occur rapidly or slowly? *A patient with a sudden or persistent loss of vision within the past 48 hours should be seen immediately by an ophthalmologist, as should the patient experiencing trauma, a foreign body in the eye, sudden ocular pain, or sudden redness.* Determine whether the same symptoms are present to the same degree in both eyes.

Ask these questions if ocular injury or eye trauma is involved:

- How long ago did the injury occur?
- What was the patient doing when it happened?
- If a foreign body was involved, what was its source?
- Was any first aid administered at the scene? If so, what actions were taken?

Physical Assessment

Inspection

Look for head tilting, squinting, or other noticeable actions that offer clues to compensatory stances for attaining clear vision. For example, patients with double vision may cock the head to the side in an attempt to focus the two images into one or they may close one eye to see more clearly.

VIDEO CLIP: External Eye ▶

Assess for symmetry in the appearance of the eyes. Check the eyes to determine whether they are equal distance from the nose, are the same size, and have the same degree of prominence. Assess the eyes for their placement in the orbits and for symmetry of movement. **Exophthalmos** (proptosis) is protrusion of the eye. **Enophthalmos** is the sunken appearance of the eye.

Examine the eyebrows and eyelashes for hair distribution, and determine the direction of the eyelashes. Eyelashes normally point outward and away from the eyelid. Assess the eyelids for **ptosis** (drooping), redness, lesions, or swelling. The lids normally close completely, with the upper and lower lid edges touching. When the eyes are open, the upper lid covers a small portion of the iris. The edge of the lower lid lies below the line between the cornea and sclera. No sclera should be visible between the eyelid and the iris.

Scleral and corneal assessment requires a penlight. Examine the sclera for color; it is usually white. A yellow color may indicate jaundice or systemic problems. In dark-skinned people, the normal sclera may appear yellow and small, pigmented dots may be visible (Jarvis, 2008).

The cornea is best observed by directing a light at it from the side using several angles. The cornea should be transparent, smooth, shiny, and bright. Any cloudy areas or specks may be the result of accidents or injuries.

Assess the blink reflex by bringing a fist quickly toward the patient's face; patients with vision will blink. This reflex can also be assessed by expelling a syringe full of air toward the eyes. The patient blinks if the reflex is intact.

Pupillary assessment involves examining each pupil separately and comparing the results. This examination is also part of the rapid neurologic assessment. The pupils are usually round and of equal size. About 5% of people normally have a noticeable difference in the size of their pupils, which is known as **anisocoria** (Jarvis, 2008). Pupil size varies in people exposed to the same amount of light. Pupils are smaller in older adults. People with myopia have larger pupils. People with hyperopia have smaller pupils. The normal pupil diameter is between 3 and 5 mm. Smaller pupils reduce vision in low light conditions.

◀ VIDEO CLIP: Pupil Responses

Observe the pupils for their response to light. Increasing light causes constriction, whereas decreasing light causes dilation. Constriction of both pupils is the normal response to direct light and to accommodation. Assess pupillary reaction to light by asking the patient to look straight ahead while quickly bringing the beam of a penlight in from the side and directing it at the right pupil. Constriction of the right pupil is a direct response to shining the penlight into that eye. Constriction of the left pupil when light is shined at the right pupil is known as a **consensual response.** Assess the responses for each eye.

Evaluate each pupil for speed of reaction. The pupil should immediately constrict when a light is directed at it. This rapid response is termed *brisk.* If the pupil takes more than 1 second to constrict, the response is termed *sluggish.* Pupils that fail to react are termed *nonreactive* or *fixed.* Compare the reactivity speed of right and left pupils, and document any difference.

In assessing for accommodation, hold the index finger about 18 cm from the patient's nose and move it toward the nose. The patient's eyes normally converge during this movement, and the pupils constrict equally. When accommodation stops, the pupils begin to enlarge and return to their normal size.

Vision Testing

Vision is measured by various tests. First test each eye separately, and then test both eyes together. Patients who wear corrective lenses are tested both without and with their lenses.

◀ VIDEO CLIP: Central Vision

Visual acuity tests measure both distance and near vision. The Snellen chart, or "eye chart," is a simple tool to measure distance vision. This chart has letters, numbers, pictures, or a single letter presented in various positions (Fig. 48-8). The chart with one letter in different positions is used for patients who cannot read, who do not speak the language used at the facility, or who cannot speak but do have adequate cognition. Have the patient stand 20 feet from the chart, cover one eye, and use the other eye to read the line that appears most clear. If the patient can do this accurately, ask him or her to read the next lower line. Repeat this sequence to the last line on which the patient can correctly identify most characters. Repeat the procedure with the other eye. Record findings as a comparison between what the patient can read at 20 feet and the distance at which a

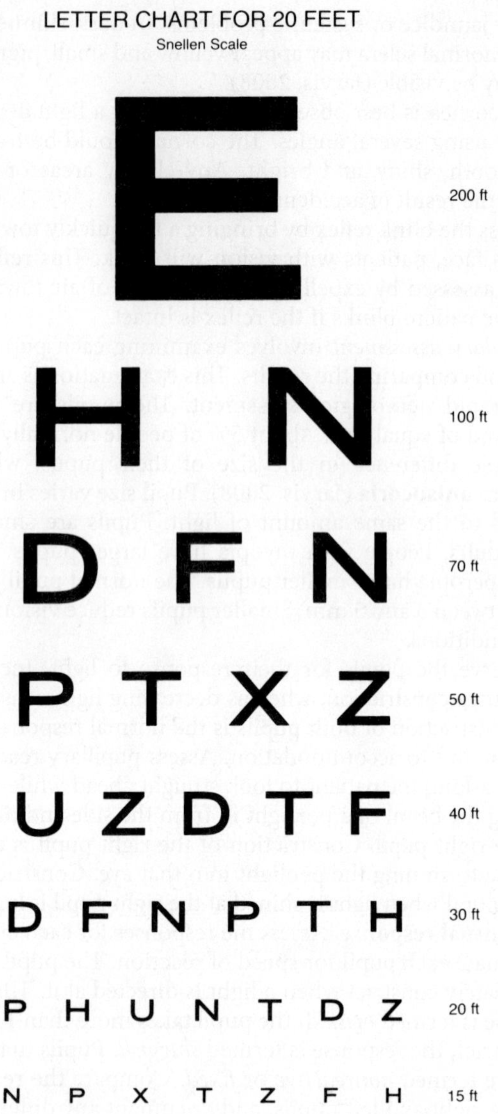
LETTER CHART FOR 20 FEET
Snellen Scale
E
200 ft
H N
100 ft
D F N
70 ft
P T X Z
50 ft
U Z D T F
40 ft
D F N P T H
30 ft
P H U N T D Z
20 ft
N P X T Z F H
15 ft

Fig. 48-8 • A typical Snellen chart.

person with normal vision can read the same line. For example, 20/50 means that the patient can see at 20 feet from the chart what a "healthy eye" can see at 50 feet.

For patients who are in a confined space that does not permit a 20-foot distance to the eye chart or who cannot see the 20/400 character, assess visual acuity by holding fingers in front of their eyes and asking them to count the number of fingers. Acuity is recorded as "count fingers vision at 5 feet," or the farthest distance at which fingers are counted correctly.

Patients who cannot count fingers are tested for hand motion (HM) acuity. Stand about 2 to 3 feet in front of the patient. Ask him or her to cover the eye not being tested. Direct a light onto your hand from behind the patient. Demonstrate the three possible directions in which the hand can move during the test (stationary, left-right, or up-down). Move your hand slowly (1 second per motion), and ask the patient, "What is my hand doing now?" Repeat this procedure five times. Visual acuity is recorded as HM at the farthest distance at which the patient correctly identifies most of the hand motions.

If the patient cannot detect hand movement, test acuity by measuring light perception (LP). Ask the patient first to cover

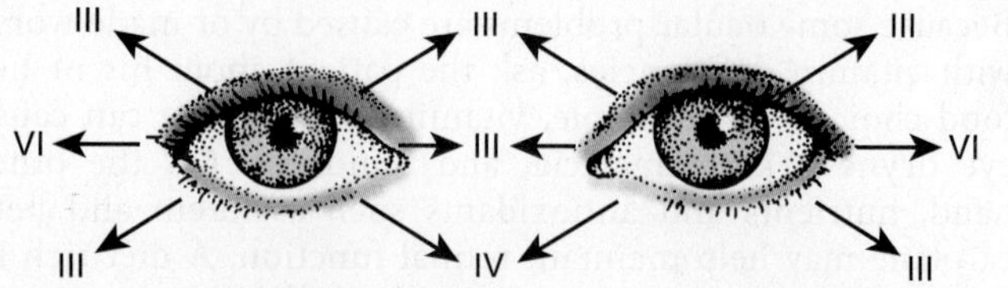
III
III
III
VI
III
VI
III
IV
III

Fig. 48-9 • Checking extraocular movements in the six cardinal positions indicates the functioning of cranial nerves III, IV, and VI.

the left eye. In a darkened room, direct the beam of a penlight at the patient's right eye from a distance of 2 to 3 feet for 1 to 2 seconds. Instruct the patient to say "on" when the beam of light is perceived and "off" when it is no longer detected. If the patient identifies the presence or absence of light three times correctly, acuity is recorded as LP.

Near vision is tested for patients who have difficulty reading without using glasses or other means of vision correction. Use a small, handheld miniature chart called a *Rosenbaum Pocket Vision Screener,* or a *Jaeger card.* Ask the patient to hold the card 14 inches away from his or her eyes and read the characters. Test each eye separately and then together. Record the value of the lowest line on which the patient can identify more than half the characters.

Visual field testing is used to determine the degree of peripheral vision. It can be performed formally with a computerized machine or informally with a "confrontation test" for a crude but rapid check of peripheral vision. During the confrontation test, sit facing the patient and ask him or her to look directly into your eyes while you look into the patient's eyes. Cover your right eye, and have the patient cover his or her left eye so that you both have the same visual field. Then move a finger or an object from a nonvisible area into the patient's line of vision. The patient with normal peripheral vision should notice the object at about the same time you do. Repeat this examination by covering your left eye and the patient covering his or her right eye. Note any areas in which you can see but the patient cannot.

Extraocular muscle function is assessed using the corneal light reflex and the six cardinal positions of gaze. These tests not only assess smoothness of eye movements but also test the function of cranial nerves III, IV, and VI.

The corneal light reflex determines alignment of the eyes. After asking the patient to stare straight ahead, shine a penlight at both corneas from a distance of 12 to 15 inches. The bright dot of light reflected from the shiny surface of the cornea should be in a symmetric position (e.g., at the 1 o'clock position in the right eye and at the 11 o'clock position in the left eye). An asymmetric reflex indicates a deviating eye and possible muscle imbalance.

Use the six cardinal positions of gaze to assess muscle function (Fig. 48-9). The eye will not turn to a particular position if the muscle is weak or if the controlling nerve is affected. Ask the patient to hold his or her head still and to move the eyes to follow a small object such as a pen. Move the object to the patient's right (lateral), upward and right (temporal), down and right, left (lateral), upward and left (temporal), and down and left (see Fig. 48-9). While the patient moves the eyes to these positions, note whether both eyes move in a parallel manner and any deviation of movement. **Nystagmus,** an involuntary and rapid twitching of the eyeball, is a normal find-

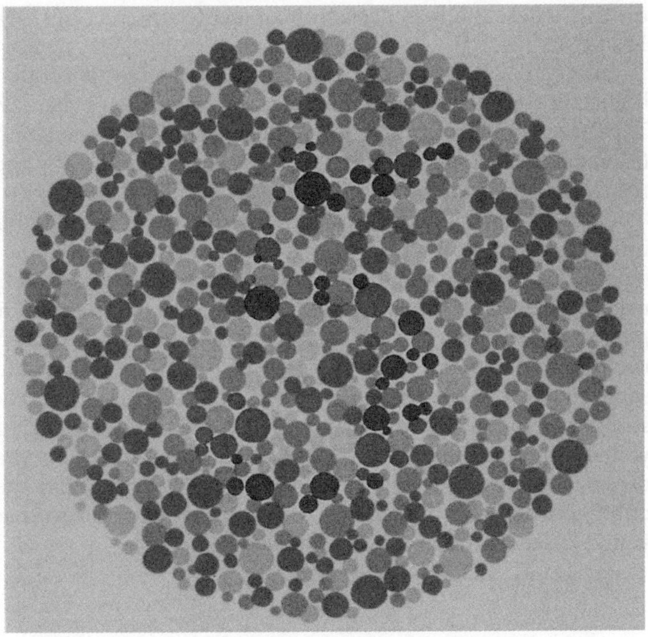

Fig. 48-10 • An Ishihara chart for testing color vision.

ing for the far lateral gaze. It may also be caused by abnormal nerve function or prolonged reduced vision.

Color vision is most commonly tested using the **Ishihara chart,** which shows numbers composed of dots of one color within a circle of dots of a different color (Fig. 48-10). Test each eye separately by asking the patient what numbers he or she sees on the chart. Reading the numbers correctly indicates normal color vision.

Psychosocial Assessment

A patient with changes in visual perception may be anxious or fearful about a possible loss of vision. Patients with severe visual defects may be unable to perform ADLs and may need to change their leisure activities. The sense of dependency resulting from reduced vision can affect self-esteem. Ask the patient how he or she feels about the vision changes, and assess the effectiveness of coping techniques. Discuss his or her concerns with family members to determine whether support is available. Also assess the patient's knowledge and use of services for the visually impaired. Provide information about local resources and services for reduced vision.

Diagnostic Assessment

Laboratory Assessment

Cultures and smears of corneal or conjunctival swabs and scrapings help diagnose infections. Obtain a sample of the exudate for culture before antibiotics or topical anesthetics are instilled. Take swabs from the conjunctivae and any ulcerated or inflamed areas.

Imaging Assessment

Computed tomography (CT) is a useful diagnostic tool for looking at the eyes, bony structures around the eye, and the extraocular muscles. CT is also used for detecting tumors in the orbital space. The use of contrast dye is common unless trauma is suspected. Usually two sets of CT scans are performed—one set taken in the supine position (called *axial images*) and one set taken with the head tipped back as far as possible (called *coronal images*). The coronal images provide the "front view" needed to determine the extent of many eye problems. Tell the patient that this test is not painful but does require that he or she be positioned in a confined space and must keep the head still during the procedure.

Magnetic resonance imaging (MRI) has replaced CT in many settings for looking at the orbits and the optic nerves. MRI is also useful for evaluating ocular tumors. MRI cannot be used to evaluate injuries involving metal in the eyes. *Metal in the eye is an absolute contraindication for MRI.*

Radioisotope scanning is used to locate tumors and lesions in various body organs. Isotope studies differentiate an intraocular tumor from a hemorrhage, especially in the choroid layer.

After the informed consent process, the patient receives a tracer dose of the radioactive isotope, either orally or by injection. He or she is asked to lie still and breathe normally. The scanner measures the radioactivity emitted by the radioactive atoms concentrated in the area being studied. Patients who are anxious or agitated may require sedation.

Assure the patient that the amount of radioisotope used is small and that he or she is not radioactive. No other special follow-up care is required.

Ultrasonography is used to examine the orbit and eye with high-frequency sound waves. This noninvasive test aids in the diagnosis of trauma, intraorbital tumors, proptosis, and choroidal or retinal detachments. It is also used to determine gross outline changes in the eye and the orbit in patients with cloudy corneas or lenses that limit direct examination of the fundus. Ultrasonography helps calculate the length of the eye, one of the measurements used to determine the strength of the intraocular lens implant needed after cataract removal.

Inform the patient that this test is painless because anesthetic drops are instilled into the lower lid. He or she sits upright with the chin in the chin rest. The probe is touched against the patient's anesthetized cornea, and sound waves are bounced through the eye. The sound waves create a reflective pattern on a computer screen that can be examined for abnormalities. No special follow-up care is needed. Remind the patient not to rub or touch the eye until the effects of the anesthetic drops have worn off.

Other Diagnostic Assessment

Many tests are used to examine specific eye structures but are not needed for routine vision assessment. Such tests may be indicated for those with special risks, symptoms, or exposures. These tests are performed only by physicians, optometrists, or advanced practice nurses.

Slit-lamp examination magnifies the anterior eye structures (Fig. 48-11). The patient leans on a chin rest to stabilize the head. A narrow beam (slit) of light is aimed so that only a narrow segment of the eye is brightly lighted. The examiner can then locate the position of any abnormality in the cornea, lens, or anterior vitreous humor. The slit beam also may help identify the presence of cells in the aqueous humor.

Corneal staining consists of placing fluorescein or other topical dye into the conjunctival sac. The dye outlines irregularities of the corneal surface that are not easily visible. This test is used for corneal trauma, problems caused by a contact lens, or the presence of foreign bodies, abrasions, ulcers, or other corneal disorders.

This procedure is noninvasive and is performed under aseptic conditions. The dye is applied topically to the eye, and the eye is then viewed through a blue filter. Nonintact areas of the cornea stain a bright green color.

Tonometry measures intraocular pressure (IOP) using a tonometer. Normal IOP readings are 10 to 21 mm Hg. About 5% of patients with healthy eyes have a slightly higher pressure. Tonometer readings are indicated for all patients older than 40 years. Adults with a family history of glaucoma should have their IOP measured once or twice a year. Several methods and instruments are available to measure IOP. One instrument, the Tono-Pen, is designed for use by patients in the home to measure IOP daily. Some involve direct contact with the eye, whereas others use a noncontact technique (Figs. 48-12 and 48-13).

Intraocular pressure varies throughout the day. It is often higher in the morning but may peak at any time of the day. Therefore always document the time of IOP measurement and teach patients who are measuring IOP at home to perform the measurement at the same time or times each day.

Ophthalmoscopy allows viewing of the eye's external and interior structures with an instrument called an *ophthalmoscope.* This examination can be performed by any nurse but is usually performed by a physician, advanced practice nurse, or physician assistant. It is easiest to examine the fundus when the room is dark, because the pupil will dilate. Stand on the same side as the eye being examined. Tell the patient to look straight ahead at an object on the wall behind you. Placing your thumb on the patient's eyebrow can help you know the distance from the ophthalmoscope to the patient. Hold the ophthalmoscope firmly against your face and align it so that your eye sees through the sight hole (Fig. 48-14).

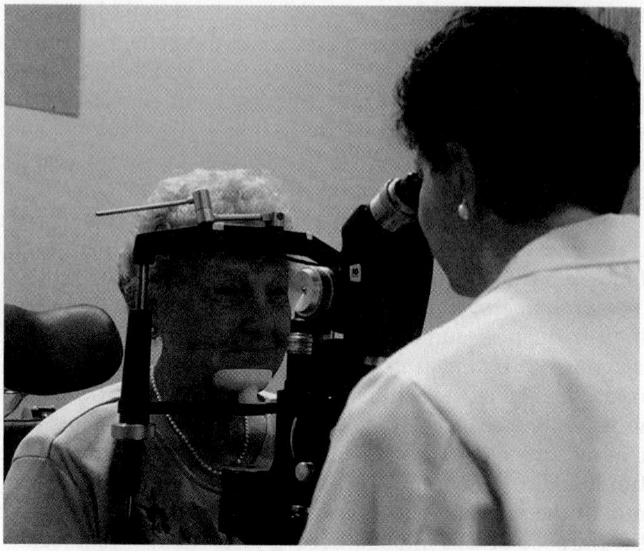

Fig. 48-11 • Slit-lamp ocular examination.

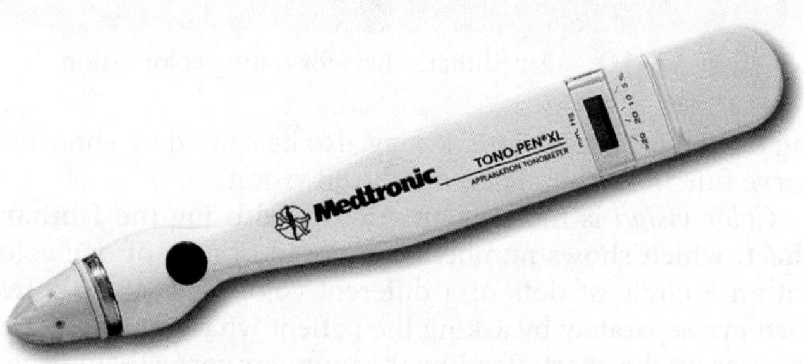
Medtronic
TONO-PEN®XL
APPLANATION TONOMETER

Fig. 48-12 • The Tono-Pen.

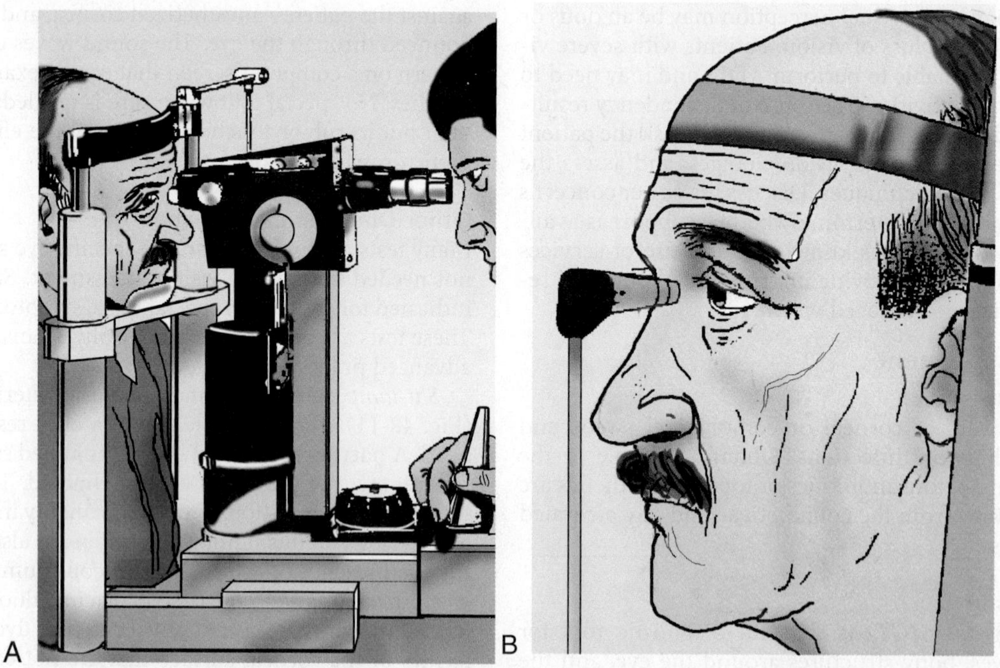
A
B

Fig. 48-13 • Common methods of intraocular pressure evaluation. **A,** The air-puff tonometer can be used for screening large numbers of patients and is the method used by most ophthalmologists. **B,** Goldman's applanation tonometer, used with a slit lamp, is the standard instrument for glaucoma diagnosis and management.

When using the ophthalmoscope, move toward the patient's eye from about 12 to 15 inches away and to the side of his or her line of vision. As you direct the ophthalmoscope at the pupil, a red glare **(red reflex)** should be seen in the pupil as a reflection of the light on the retina. An absent red reflex may indicate a lens opacity or cloudiness of the vitreous. Move toward the patient's pupil while following the red reflex. The retina should then be visible through the ophthalmoscope. Examine the optic disc, optic vessels, fundus, and macula. Table 48-3 lists the features that can be observed in each structure.

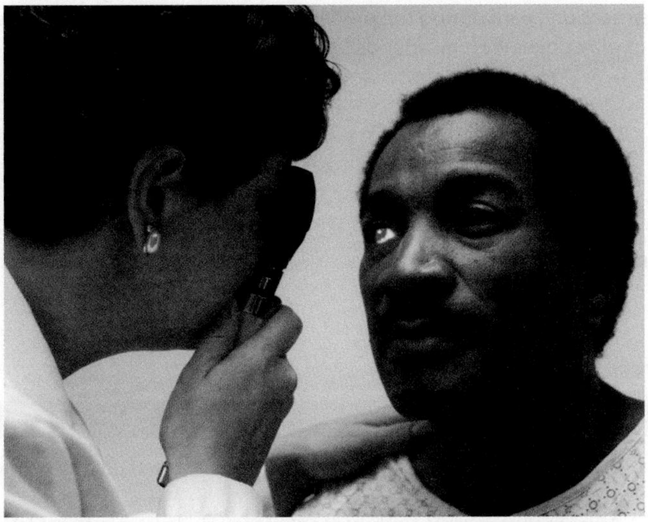

Fig. 48-14 • Proper technique for direct ophthalmoscopic visualization of the retina.

TABLE 48-3 Structures Assessed by Direct Ophthalmoscopy

RED REFLEX
- Presence or absence

OPTIC DISC
- Color
- Margins (sharp or blurred)
- Cup size
- Presence of rings or crescents

OPTIC BLOOD VESSELS
- Size
- Color
- Kinks or tangles
- Light reflection
- Narrowing
- Nicking at arteriovenous crossings

FUNDUS
- Color
- Tears or holes
- Lesions
- Bleeding

MACULA
- Presence of blood vessels
- Color
- Lesions
- Bleeding

The use of an ophthalmoscope may make a confused patient or one who does not understand the language more anxious. Avoid using an ophthalmoscope with a confused patient. When working with a patient who does not speak the language used at the facility, use an interpreter, when possible, to ensure the patient's understanding and cooperation with the examination.

Fluorescein angiography, which is performed by a physician or an advanced practice nurse, provides a detailed image of eye circulation. Photographs are taken in rapid succession after the dye is given IV. This test is useful for assessing problems of retinal circulation (e.g., diabetic retinopathy, retinal hemorrhage, macular degeneration) or for diagnosing intraocular tumors.

Explain the procedure to the patient, and instill mydriatic eyedrops (cause pupil dilation) 1 hour before the test. Chart 48-4 lists the best practice for correct eyedrop instillation. Check that the informed consent has been signed by the patient or responsible person. Warn that the dye may cause the skin to appear yellow for several hours after the test. The stain is eliminated through the urine, which also changes color.

Chart 48-4 BEST PRACTICE FOR PATIENT SAFETY & QUALITY CARE

Instillation of Eyedrops

- Check the name, strength, expiration date, color, and clarity of the eyedrops to be instilled.
- Check to see whether only one eye is to have the drug or if both eyes are to receive the drug.
- If both eyes are to receive the same drug and one eye is infected, use two separate bottles and carefully label each bottle with "right" or "left" for the correct eye.
- Wash your hands.
- Put on gloves if secretions are present in or around the eye.
- Explain the procedure to the patient.
- Have the patient sit in a chair, and you stand behind the patient.
- Ask the patient to tilt the head backward, with the back of the head resting against your body and looking up at the ceiling.
- Gently pull the lower lid down against the patient's cheek, forming a small pocket.
- Hold the eyedrop bottle (with the cap off) like a pencil, with the tip pointing down.
- Rest the wrist holding the bottle against the patient's check.
- Without touching any part of the eye or lid with the tip of the bottle, gently squeeze the bottle and release the prescribed number of drops into the pocket you have made with the patient's lower lid.
- Gently release the lower lid.
- Tell the patient to close the eye gently (without squeezing the lids tightly).
- Gently press and hold the corner of the eye nearest the nose to close off the punctum and prevent the drug from being absorbed systemically.
- Without pressing on the lid, gently blot away any excess drug or tears with a tissue.
- Remove your gloves, and place the cap back on the bottle.
- Ask the patient to keep the eye closed for about 1 minute.
- Wash your hands again.

Intravenous access must be obtained. After the needle is in the vein, 5 mL of a 10% solution of fluorescein is injected. A digital camera is set up with equipment to photograph retinal and choroidal blood vessels as the dye passes through them. The results can be viewed immediately on a computer screen. The procedure takes only a few minutes because the vessels fill quickly.

Encourage patients to drink fluids to help eliminate the dye. Remind them that any yellow or green staining of the skin will disappear in a few hours. After the test, the urine will be bright green until the dye is excreted. Teach the patient to wear dark glasses and avoid direct sunlight until pupil dilation returns to normal, because the bright light will cause eye pain.

Electroretinography is the process of graphing the retina's response to light stimulation. This test is helpful in detecting and evaluating blood vessel changes from disease or drugs. The graph is obtained by placing a contact lens electrode on an anesthetized cornea. Lights at varying speeds and intensities are flashed, and the neural response is graphed. The measurement from the cornea is identical to the response that would be obtained if electrodes were placed directly on the retina.

DECISION-MAKING CHALLENGE

Coordination of Care

The patient is an 86-year-old man who lives alone at home and is scheduled to have fluorescein angiography tomorrow. He still drives and performs all of his own housekeeping responsibilities. In addition, he drives his neighbor, who is blind, to a sheltered workshop every day. The patient calls today with some concerns about whether he will be able to drive himself to and from the procedure, pain during the procedure, and whether he will be able to play poker with his friends later tomorrow night after the test.

1. Should he drive himself to and from the procedure? Why or why not?
2. What should you tell him regarding the preparation and actual fluorescein angiography procedures?
3. What should you teach him about altering his usual activities during the first 24 hours after the procedure?

evolve For suggested answer guidelines, go to http://evolve.elsevier.com/Iggy/.

HUMAN NEEDS ASSESSMENT REVIEW

What should you expect to NOTICE in a patient with adequate sensation related to the eye and vision?

Physical Assessment

- Eyes are symmetrical on the face on a line about even with the tops of the ears.
- Eyes are clear with no drainage or open areas.
- Patient does not squint or tilt the head.
- Patient uses both eyes to read or see at a distance (does not close one eye to improve vision).
- Patient startles when a sudden move is made at the face.
- Patient blinks 5 to 10 times per minute.
- Pupils are the same size in each eye.
- Both pupils constrict when a light is shined at only one eye.
- Appearance is neat with buttons properly buttoned and hair parts straight.
- Patient comments on the presence of art or unusual visual objects in the immediate environment.
- Patient walks without hesitation into a room without bumping into objects in his or her path.

Psychological Assessment

- Patient is oriented and is not confused.
- Patient makes eye contact when speaking.

GET READY FOR THE NCLEX EXAMINATION!

Key Points

Review these Key Points for each NCLEX Examination Client Needs Category.

Safe and Effective Care Environment

- Wash your hands before moving a patient's eyelids.
- If a patient has discharge from one eye, examine the eye without the discharge first.
- Wear gloves when examining any eye with drainage.
- Avoid performing an examination using an ophthalmoscope on a confused patient.

Health Promotion and Maintenance

- Teach patients not to rub their eyes.
- Identify patients at risk for eye injury as a result of work environment or leisure activities.
- Encourage all patients to wear eye protection when they are performing yard work, working in a woodshop or metal shop, or using chemicals or are in any environment in which drops or particulate matter is airborne.

Psychosocial Integrity

- Encourage the patient the opportunity to express his or her feelings regarding a possible change in vision status.
- Refer patients newly diagnosed with permanent vision impairment to local resources and support groups.
- Explain all diagnostic procedures, restrictions, and follow-up care to the patient scheduled for tests.

Physiological Integrity

- Ask the patient about vision problems in any other members of the family, because some vision problems have a genetic component.
- Test the visual acuity of both eyes immediately of any person who experiences an eye injury or any sudden change in vision.

Additional Study Resources

Go to your Companion CD or Evolve at http://evolve.elsevier.com/Iggy/ for *Self-Assessment Questions for the NCLEX Examination.*

Go to Evolve at http://evolve.elsevier.com/Iggy/ for *Prioritization and Delegation Questions for the NCLEX Examination.*

SELECTED BIBLIOGRAPHY

Asterisk indicates a classic or definitive work on this subject.

Davis, G. (2006). Anatomy of the eye in relation to common drug therapies. *Nurse Prescribing, 4*(7), 274-278.

Gordon, M. (2007). *Manual of nursing diagnosis* (11th ed.). Boston: Jones & Bartlett.

Jarvis, C. (2008). *Physical examination and health assessment* (5th ed.). Philadelphia: Saunders.

McCance, K., & Huether, S. (2006). *Pathophysiology: The biologic basis for disease in adults and children* (5th ed.). St. Louis: Mosby.

Meiner, S., & Lueckenotte, A. (Eds.). (2006). *Gerontologic nursing* (3rd ed.). St. Louis: Mosby.

Nussbaum, R., McInnes, R., & Willard, H. (2007). *Thompson & Thompson: Genetics in medicine* (7th ed.). Philadelphia: Saunders.

Pagana, K., & Pagana, T. (2006). *Mosby's manual of diagnostic and laboratory tests* (3rd ed.). St. Louis: Mosby.

Rushing, J. (2007). Administering eyedrops. *Nursing2007, 37*(5), 18.

*Sackett, C., & Schenning, S. (2003). Eye safety in the workplace. *Insight (American Society of Ophthalmic Registered Nurses), 27*(4), 101-102.

Sitzman, K. (2006). Promoting eye health: Prevention and detection of cataracts. *American Association of Occupational Health Nurses, 54*(4), 188.

*Vaughan, D., Asbury, T., & Riordan-Eva, P. (Eds.). (2004). *General ophthalmology* (16th ed.). New York: McGraw-Hill.

49 CHAPTER

Care of Patients with Eye and Vision Problems

M. Linda Workman

LEARNING OUTCOMES

For clinical competence and success on the NCLEX Examination, study this chapter with these Learning Outcomes in mind:

Safe and Effective Care Environment

1. Use aseptic technique when performing an eye examination or instilling drugs into the eye.
2. Apply the principles of infection control when caring for a patient with an eye infection.
3. Orient the patient with reduced vision to his or her immediate environment.
4. Ensure that all members of the health care team are aware of a patient's visual limitations and need for assistance.

Health Promotion and Maintenance

5. Encourage all people, especially those older than 40 years, to have an annual eye examination including measurement of intraocular pressure.
6. Teach patients and family members how to correctly instill ophthalmic drops and ointment into the eye.
7. Teach the patient and family how to alter the home environment for patient safety.

Psychosocial Integrity

8. Teach patients and family members about what to expect during procedures to correct vision and eye problems.
9. Provide the opportunity for the patient and family to express their feelings about a change in vision.
10. Refer the patient with reduced vision and the family to local services for the blind.
11. Teach the patient techniques for performing ADLs and self-care independently.

Physiological Integrity

12. Explain the consequences of increased intraocular pressure (IOP).
13. Identify common actions, conditions, and positions that increase IOP.
14. Prioritize educational needs for the patient after cataract surgery with lens replacement.
15. Prioritize educational needs for patients with primary open-angle glaucoma.
16. Describe the mechanisms of action and nursing implications of drug therapy for glaucoma.
17. Identify the nursing care priorities for the donor when corneal donation is planned.

Go to your Companion CD or Evolve at http://evolve.elsevier.com/Iggy/ for *Self-Assessment Questions for the NCLEX Examination* keyed to these Learning Outcomes.

Many conditions affect vision. Some conditions occur gradually, such as cataracts, and others can result from an acute insult or illness. Even when reduced vision is temporary, the human need for sensation is not met completely and the patient must make some changes in function or lifestyle.

EYELID DISORDERS

The eyelid is composed of thin skin attached to small muscles. It protects the eye surface and spreads tears. Eyelid problems can be related to changes in the structure, function, or position of the eyelid. Lid structure may also be altered by age.

BLEPHARITIS

Blepharitis, an inflammation of the eyelid edges, occurs most often in the older adult and those with dry-eye syndrome (see Keratoconjunctivitis Sicca, p. 1087). Reduced tear production often leads to bacterial infection of the eye structures, because tears inhibit bacterial growth.

Patients usually have itchy, red, and burning eyes. **Seborrhea** (greasy, itchy scaling) of the eyebrows and eyelids is often present. On close inspection, greasy scales and mattering may be seen where the eyelashes exit the eyelid.

Blepharitis is controlled with eyelid care using warm, moist compresses followed by gentle scrubbing with dilute baby shampoo. Instruct the patient to avoid rubbing the eyes because, if infection is present, this action can spread the infection to other eye structures.

ENTROPION

An **entropion** is the turning inward of the eyelid causing the lashes to rub against the eye. Entropion can be caused by eyelid muscle spasms or by scarring and deformity of the eyelid as a result of trauma. Entropion occurs often among older adults because of age-related loss of tissue support.

The patient usually reports "feeling something in my eye." Pain and tears may also be present. The eyelid is turned inward, and the conjunctiva is red. Corneal abrasion may result from constant irritation.

Surgery corrects eyelid position by either tightening the orbicular muscles and moving the eyelid to a normal position or by preventing inward rotation of the eyelid. After surgery, the eye is covered with a patch and the patient is discharged a few hours later.

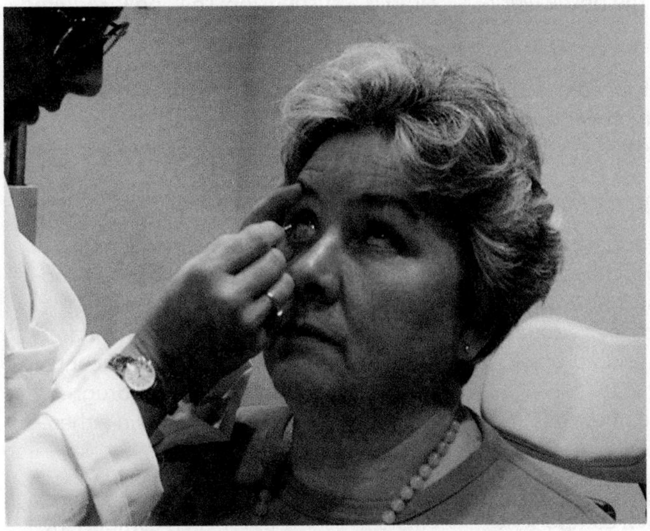

Fig. 49-1 • Application of ophthalmic ointment.

Demonstrate instillation of eyedrops, and evaluate the patient's ability to instill the drops. Instruct the patient to leave the patch in place until he or she is seen by the ophthalmologist and to report any pain or drainage under the patch. Teach the patient or family member how to clean the suture line with a cotton swab and the prescribed solution. A small amount of antibiotic ointment may be applied (Fig. 49-1). Chart 49-1 describes how to apply ophthalmic ointment. Chart 49-2 lists information on common ophthalmic drugs for eye inflammation and infection.

ECTROPION

An **ectropion** is the turning outward and sagging of the eyelid, which often occurs with aging. It is caused by relaxation of the orbicular muscle. This lid position reduces the washing action of tears, leading to corneal drying and ulceration.

Patients often have constant tears and a sagging lower eyelid. Surgery can restore proper lid alignment. After surgery, the eye is covered with a patch and the patient is discharged. Nursing care is the same as for an entropion.

HORDEOLUM

A hordeolum, or *stye*, can be external or internal. An external **hordeolum** is an infection of the sweat glands in the eyelid at the place where the eyelashes exit from the eyelid. A red, swollen, tender area is found on the skin surface side of the eyelid. An internal hordeolum is caused by an infection of the eyelid sebaceous glands. The most common causative organisms are *Staphylococcus aureus, Staphylococcus epidermidis,* and *Streptococcus.* The hordeolum usually affects only one eyelid at a time. Vision is not affected.

Small, beady, swollen areas may be on the skin side of the eyelid or on the conjunctival side of the eyelid. As the hordeolum fills with purulent material, it becomes painful.

Chart 49-1 BEST PRACTICE FOR PATIENT SAFETY & QUALITY CARE

Instillation of Ophthalmic Ointment

- Check the name, strength, and expiration date of the ointment to be instilled. Be sure it is an ophthalmic (eye) preparation and not a general topical ointment.
- Check to see whether only one eye is to have the drug or if both eyes are to receive the drug.
- If both eyes are to receive the same drug and one eye is infected, use two separate tubes and carefully label each tube with "right" or "left" for the correct eye.
- Wash your hands.
- Put on gloves if secretions are present in or around the eye.
- Explain the procedure to the patient.
- Have the patient sit in a chair, and you stand behind the patient.
- Ask the patient to tilt the head backward, with the back of the head resting against your body and looking up at the ceiling.
- Gently pull the lower lid down against the patient's cheek, forming a small pocket.
- Hold the tube (with the cap off) like a pencil, with the tip pointing down.
- Rest the wrist holding the tube against the patient's cheek.
- Without touching any part of the eye or lid with the tip of the tube, gently squeeze the tube and release about a $^1/_4$- to $^1/_2$-inch thin strip of ointment into the pocket you have made with the patient's lower lid. Start at the nose side of the pocket, and move toward the outer edge of the pocket.
- Gently release the lower lid.
- Tell the patient to close the eye gently (without squeezing the lids tightly).
- With the patient's eye closed, gently wipe away any excess ointment with a tissue.
- Tell the patient that sight in that eye will be blurred while the ointment is present in the eye and that he or she should not drive or operate heavy machinery until the ointment is removed.
- Remove your gloves, and place the cap back on the tube.
- Ask the patient to keep the eye closed for about 1 minute.
- Wash your hands again.
- To remove ointment from the eye, wear gloves if drainage is present.
- Then ask the patient to close the eye; wipe the closed lids with a clean tissue from the corner of the eye nearest the nose outward. If you are wiping the same eye twice, use a different area of the tissue or use a new one.

Chart 49-2 COMMON EXAMPLES OF DRUG THERAPY

Eye Inflammation and Infection

Drug	Nursing Interventions*†	Rationales
Med Error Alert! All of these drugs are administered by the eye instillation route, not the oral route. Oral administration of these agents can cause systemic side effects in addition to not having the correct effect on the eyes.		
TOPICAL ANESTHETICS		
Proparacaine HCl, or proxymetacaine (AK-Taine, Alcaine, Ocu-Caine, Ophthetic)	Remind the patient not to rub or touch the eye while it is anesthetized.	Touching may injure the eye.
Tetracaine HCl, cocaine HCl (Pontocaine)	Patch the eye if the patient leaves the facility before the anesthetic wears off.	The use of a patch prevents injury, such as corneal abrasion.
	Instruct the patient not to use discolored solution.	Discoloration is a sign of altered drug composition.
	Teach the patient to store the bottle tightly closed.	Air may cause drug contamination and oxidation.
TOPICAL STEROIDS		
Prednisolone acetate (Ocu-Pred, Ophtho-Tate🍁) Prednisolone phosphate (Inflamase)	Tell the patient to shake the bottle vigorously before use.	Drug is a suspension; shaking is required to distribute the drug evenly in the solution.
Dexamethasone (Dexair, Dexotic, Maxidex) Betamethasone (Betnesol)	Teach the patient to check for corneal ulceration (pain, reduced vision, secretions).	Steroid use predisposes the patient to local infection.
Fluorometholone (Fluor-Op, Liquifilm)	Warn the patient not to share eyedrops with others.	Disease transmission is possible when sharing eyedrops.
ANTI-INFECTIVE AGENTS		
Gentamicin (Genoptic, Gentak Alcomicin🍁) Tobramycin (Tobrex) Ciprofloxacin (Ciloxan)	Teach the patient the importance of using the drug exactly as prescribed, even if he or she needs to use it hourly.	Bacterial and fungal eye infections worsen rapidly and can lead to blindness if not treated adequately.
Erythromycin (Ilotycin) Chlortetracycline (Aureomycin) Sulfisoxazole (Gantrisin)	Teach the patient how to clean exudate from the eyes before using drops.	Cleansing decreases the risk of contaminating the drug and increases contact of the conjunctiva with the drug.
Ofloxacin (Ocuflox) Levofloxacin (Quixin)	Reinforce the importance of completing the prescribed drug regimen.	Adherence is critical to maintain a therapeutic level of drug.
ANTIBIOTIC-STEROID COMBINATIONS		
Tobramycin with dexamethasone (TobraDex) Neomycin sulfate with polymyxin B sulfate and dexamethasone (Maxitrol)	This is the same as for each component alone.	This is the same as for each component alone.
TOPICAL ANTIVIRAL AGENTS		
Trifluridine (Viroptic) Vidarabine (Vira-A)	Teach the patient to refrigerate the drug and protect it from light.	Drug stability is affected by warm temperatures and light.
	Teach the patient to assess for itching lids and burning eyes.	Sensitivity to these drugs is common.
ANTIFUNGAL AGENTS		
Amphotericin B Natamycin (Natacyn)	Teach the patient to assess for itching lids and burning eyes.	Sensitivity to these drugs is common.
NONSTEROIDAL ANTI-INFLAMMATORY AGENTS		
Flurbiprofen (Ocufen) Diclofenac (Voltaren)	Teach the patient to check for bleeding in the eye.	These drugs disrupt platelet aggregation.
Bromfenac (Xibrom) Ketorolac (Acular)	Teach the patient not to wear soft contact lenses during therapy with these drugs.	These drugs interact with contact lens materials and increase the risk for infection.

*When instilling eyedrops, teach patients to use nasal punctal occlusion to reduce the risk for systemic absorption and side effects.

†When more than one topical ophthalmic drug is prescribed, teach patients to separate the instillation of each drug by at least 5 minutes.

Chart 49-3 PATIENT AND FAMILY EDUCATION GUIDE

Application of an Ocular Compress

- Wash your hands.
- Fold a clean washcloth into fourths.
- Soak the washcloth with running tap water that is warm to your inner wrist. (If cool compresses are needed, follow the same steps using cold running tap water.)
- Place the cloth over your closed eye.
- Keep the cloth in place with minimal pressure until the cloth cools (or warms, if cool compresses are prescribed).
- Refold the washcloth so that a different "fourth" will be held against the eye.
- Resoak the cloth with running tap water.
- Repeat applications three times for as many times each day as prescribed by your health care provider.

Treatment includes the use of warm compresses four times a day and an antibacterial ointment. When the lesion opens, the purulent material drains and the pain subsides.

Nursing interventions include applying compresses and instructing the patient in this application. Chart 49-3 describes the proper technique for application of an eye compress.

After compresses have been applied, instill antibiotic ointment. Advise the patient that ointments may cause blurred vision, and teach him or her to remove the ointment from the eyes before driving or operating machinery. To remove the ointment, teach the patient to close the eye and then gently wipe the closed eyelid from the nasal side of the eye outward.

CHALAZION

A **chalazion** is an inflammation of a sebaceous gland in the eyelid. It begins with redness and tenderness (similar to the hordeolum), followed by a gradual *painless* swelling at the gland. In its fully developed state, no inflammatory signs are present. Most chalazia protrude on the inside of the eyelid. The patient has eye fatigue, light sensitivity, and excessive tears.

Treatment includes the use of warm compresses for 15 minutes four times a day, followed by instillation of ophthalmic ointment. If the chalazion is large enough to affect vision, is cosmetically displeasing to the patient, or recurs frequently, it may be removed surgically.

After surgery, antibiotic ointment is instilled and the eye is covered with a patch. Best practices for application of a nonpressure eye patch are described in Chart 49-4.

Instruct the patient to leave the eye patch in place for about 6 hours and then remove the patch and apply warm, wet compresses. Instill antibiotic eyedrops after use of the compresses. Teach him or her to immediately report increasing redness, purulent drainage, or reduced vision to the ophthalmologist.

KERATOCONJUNCTIVITIS SICCA

Pathophysiology

The lacrimal system moistens the eye surface with tears and removes tears from the eye. Problems arise from reduced tear production, infection, or inflammation in the lacrimal system.

Keratoconjunctivitis sicca, or dry-eye syndrome, results from changes in tear composition, lacrimal gland malfunction, or altered tear distribution. Decreased tear production can also occur with the use of some drugs, such as antihistamines, beta-adrenergic blocking agents, or anticholinergic drugs. Diseases associated with decreased tear production include rheumatoid arthritis, leukemia, sarcoidosis, and multiple sclerosis. Radiation or chemical burns to the eye also decrease tear production. Injury to the facial nerve (cranial nerve VII) inhibits tears. Eye dryness may follow vision-enhancing surgery.

Patient-Centered Collaborative Care

The patient may feel as if a foreign body is in the eye, burning and itching eyes, and photophobia (sensitivity to light). The corneal light reflex is dulled or distorted. Tears may contain strands of mucus.

Treatment depends on the severity of the manifestations. Restasis, a cyclosporine ophthalmic emulsion, may be prescribed to increase tear production. Artificial tears (HypoTears, Refresh) are prescribed for daytime use to reduce dryness and can be used as often as necessary. A lubricating ointment (Lacri-Lube SOP, Refresh P.M.) is used at night. If the dry-eye syndrome is caused by an abnormal eyelid position or function, surgery may be needed.

CONJUNCTIVAL DISORDERS

The conjunctiva is a thin mucous membrane that covers and protects the eye. Because of its location, the conjunctiva is subject to trauma and infection.

HEMORRHAGE

Conjunctival blood vessels are fragile and can break with increased pressure during sneezing, coughing, or vomiting. Hemorrhages may also occur with hypertension, trauma, or blood clotting problems.

The small, well-defined area of hemorrhage is bright red under the conjunctiva. The patient is usually concerned about its appearance although no pain or visual impairment occurs with the hemorrhage. It resolves within 14 days without treatment.

CONJUNCTIVITIS

Conjunctivitis is an inflammation or infection of the conjunctiva. Inflammation occurs from exposure to allergens or irritants and is not contagious. Infectious conjunctivitis occurs with bacterial or viral infection and is readily transmitted from person to person (Saligan & Yeh, 2008).

Manifestations of allergic conjunctivitis include edema, a sensation of burning, engorgement of blood vessels ("bloodshot" appearance), excessive tears, and itching.

Treatment includes the instillation of vasoconstrictors and corticosteroid eyedrops (see Chart 49-2). Teach women patients to avoid using makeup around the eye until all symptoms have subsided.

Bacterial conjunctivitis, or "pink eye," is usually caused by *Staphylococcus aureus, Haemophilus influenzae,* or *Pseudomonas aeruginosa.* Manifestations include blood vessel dilation, mild conjunctival edema, tears, and discharge. The discharge is watery at first and then becomes thicker, with shreds of mucus.

Cultures of the drainage are obtained to identify the organism. Medical treatment is aimed at eliminating the infection with topical antibiotics.

Chart 49-4 BEST PRACTICE FOR PATIENT SAFETY & QUALITY CARE

Application of an Eye Patch

NONPRESSURE EYE PATCH

1. Assemble the equipment:
   - Eye patch
   - Skin preparation pad
   - Nonallergenic paper tape
2. Explain the procedure to the patient.
3. Wash your hands.
4. Apply a skin preparation to the patient's forehead and cheek.
5. Instruct the patient to close both eyes gently.
6. Place a patch over the closed eyelid.

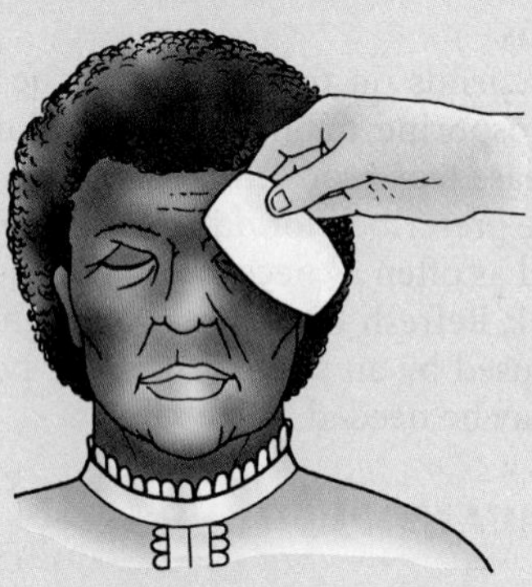

7. Apply tape from the cheek to the middle of the forehead in a diagonal line.

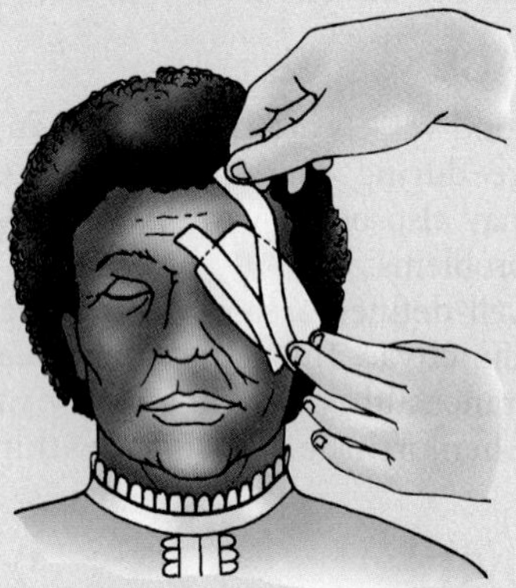

8. Cover the patch with overlapping pieces of tape.

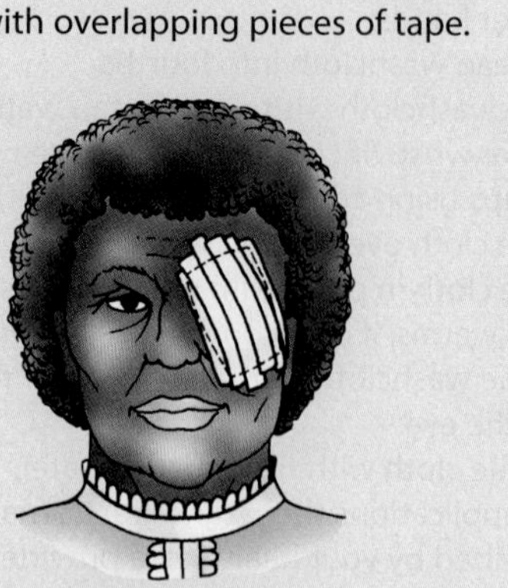

PRESSURE EYE PATCH

1. Assemble the equipment:
   - Two eye patches for each eye requiring treatment
   - Skin preparation pad
   - Nonallergenic paper tape

2-5. Follow corresponding steps under Nonpressure Eye Patch.

6. Fold one eye patch in half, place it over the closed eyelid, and apply a second eye patch (unfolded) over the folded one.

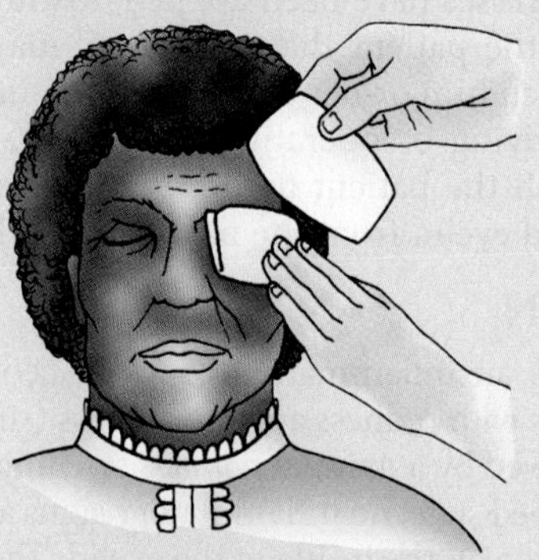

7, 8. Follow corresponding steps under Nonpressure Eye Patch.

Nursing interventions focus on preventing the spread of the disease to the other eye or to other people. Document the amount, color, and type of drainage. Review hygiene with the patient, including handwashing after touching the eye and before instilling eyedrops. Warn the patient not to touch the unaffected eye without first washing the hands and to avoid sharing washcloths and towels with others.

TRACHOMA

Trachoma is a chronic, bilateral scarring form of conjunctivitis caused by *Chlamydia trachomatis.* It is the chief cause of preventable blindness in the world. The incidence is highest in warm, moist climates where sanitation is poor.

The incubation period is 5 to 14 days. At first, trachoma resembles bacterial conjunctivitis. Manifestations include tears, photophobia, and edema of the eyelids and conjunctiva. Follicles form on the upper eyelid conjunctiva. As the disease progresses, the eyelid scars and turns inward, causing the eyelashes to damage the cornea.

Specimens are obtained for culture to identify the causative organism. A 4-week course of oral or topical tetracycline (Achromycin, Apo-Tetra♣) or erythromycin (Apo-Erythro-EC♣, E-Mycin, E.E.S.) is given. Azithromycin (Zithromax) can be used once per week for 1 to 3 weeks.

Nursing interventions focus on infection control. Teach the patient to wash the hands before and after touching the eyes. Teach him or her to keep washcloths separate from those of unaffected people and to launder them separately. In addition, stress the importance of completing the entire course of antibiotics.

CORNEAL DISORDERS

For a sharp image to be focused on the retina, the cornea must be transparent and intact. Corneal problems lead to visual impairment. These problems may be caused by irritation or infection (keratitis) with ulceration of the corneal surface, degeneration of the cornea (keratoconus), or deposits in the cornea (dystrophies). All corneal problems reduce the refracting power of the cornea, and some can lead to blindness.

CORNEAL ABRASION, ULCERATION, AND INFECTION

Pathophysiology

A **corneal abrasion** is a scrape or scratch of the cornea that disrupts the integrity of this structure. This painful condition can be caused by the presence of a small foreign body, trauma, or, most commonly, contact lens use. Other causes or conditions that promote loss of corneal integrity include malnutrition, dry-eye syndromes, and some cancer therapies (Camp-Sorrell, 2007). The abrasion provides a portal of entry for organisms, leading to corneal infection. Bacterial, protozoal, and fungal infections can lead to **corneal ulceration,** which is a deeper disruption of the corneal epithelium, extending into the stromal layer. *This problem is an emergency because the cornea has no separate blood supply and cannot defend itself from infections that have the potential to permanently impair vision.* The increased use of homemade contact lens solutions and the use of large-volume containers of solutions that can easily become contaminated have led to a dramatic rise in the incidence of corneal ulcers infected with *Pseudomonas aeruginosa* and fungi.

Patient-Centered Collaborative Care

The patient with a corneal disorder usually has pain, reduced vision, photophobia, and eye secretions. Cloudy or purulent (pus-filled) fluid may be present on the eyelids or eyelashes. Wear gloves when examining the eye.

The entire cornea may look hazy or cloudy with a patchy area of ulceration. When fluorescein stain is used, the patchy areas appear green. Microbial culture and corneal scrapings can help determine which organism is causing a corneal ulcer. Usually, anti-infective therapy is started before the organism is identified because of the serious potential for vision loss. For culture, obtain swabs from the ulcer and its edges. For corneal scrapings, the cornea is anesthetized with a topical agent and a physician or advanced practice nurse removes samples from the center and edge of the ulcer with a sterile spatula.

Antibiotics, antifungals, and antivirals are prescribed to reduce or eliminate the organisms. Usually, a broad-spectrum antibiotic is prescribed first and may be changed when culture results are known. Steroids may be used with antibiotics to reduce the inflammatory response in the eye. Drugs can be given topically as eyedrops, injected subconjunctivally, or injected IV. Chart 48-4 in Chapter 48 lists best practices for instilling eyedrops.

The patient is usually discharged to home, and the priority nursing interventions are to begin the drug therapy, to ensure patient understanding of the drug therapy regimen, and to prevent infection spread.

Often, the anti-infective therapy involves instilling eyedrops *every hour* for the first 24 hours. Teach the patient how to apply the eyedrops correctly. (See Chart 48-2 in Chapter 48.) Use a small bottle of sterile saline to demonstrate the technique, and obtain a return demonstration. If the patient is unable to safely self-apply the drugs, teach another family member how to do it.

If the eye infection occurs with a corneal abrasion or ulcer, usually only one eye is affected. Teach the patient not to use the drug in the unaffected eye. In addition, teach him or her to wash hands after touching the affected eye and before touching or doing anything to the healthy eye. If both eyes are infected, separate bottles of drugs are needed for each eye. Teach the patient to clearly label the bottles "right eye" and "left eye" and not to switch the drugs from eye to eye. Also teach him or her to completely care for one eye, then wash the hands, and using the drugs for the remaining eye, care for that eye. Teach the patient not to wear contact lenses during the entire time that these drugs are being used because the eye then has fewer protections against infection or injury. In addition, the drugs can cloud or damage the contact lenses.

Stress the importance of applying the drug as often as prescribed, even at night. Stopping the infection at this stage can save the patient's vision in the infected eye. Also instruct the patient to make and keep all follow-up appointments; usually the patient should be seen again in 24 hours or less.

The type of anti-infective used and the frequency of application often change when the organism is identified and the infection is responding to the therapy. Drugs may need to be used for 3 or more weeks to ensure eradication of the infection. Warn women to avoid using makeup around the eye until the infection has cleared to prevent spread of infection. Instruct patients to discard all open containers of contact lens solutions and bottles of eyedrops, because these may be contaminated. Patients may need to avoid the use of contact lenses for weeks or months until the infection is gone and the ulcer is completely healed.

KERATOCONUS AND CORNEAL OPACITIES

Pathophysiology

The cornea can permanently lose it shape, become scarred or cloudy, or become thinner. When these conditions occur, refraction may be reduced or lost and images are not focused sufficiently for the person to have useful vision. Keratoconus, degeneration of the corneal tissue resulting in abnormal corneal shape, can occur with trauma or may occur as part of an inherited disorder (Fig. 49-2). Inadequately treated corneal infections and severe trauma can damage and scar the cornea and lead to severe visual impairment that cannot be improved by nonsurgical interventions.

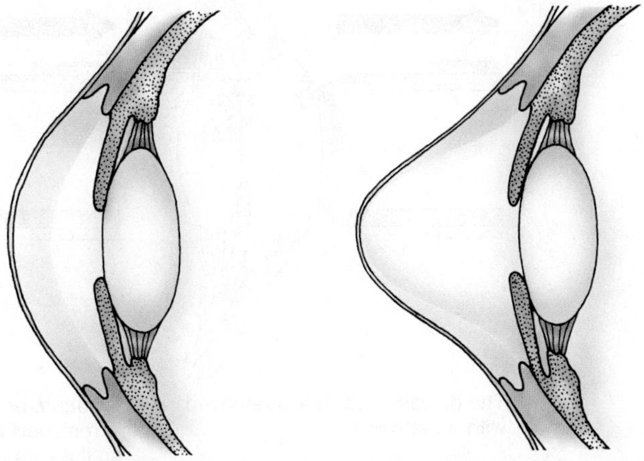
Normal
Keratoconus

Fig. 49-2 • Profiles of a normal eyeball and one with keratoconus.

Patient-Centered Collaborative Care

Treatment for a permanent corneal disorder that obscures vision is aimed at restoring corneal clarity and enhancing the patient's ability to use the remaining vision. The intervention is a **keratoplasty** (corneal transplant)—the surgical removal of diseased corneal tissue and replacement with tissue from a human donor cornea. This process restores vision by removing corneal deformities and replacing them with healthy corneal tissue.

Preoperative care may be short, with little time for teaching because corneal transplantation is performed when the donor tissue becomes available. Usually the patient is quite anxious. Use a calm approach to assess the patient's knowledge of the surgery and of expected care before and after surgery.

Examine the eyes for signs of infection, and report any redness, drainage, or edema to the ophthalmologist. Instill antibiotic drops into the eye to reduce the risk for infection. IV access is obtained before surgery.

Operative procedures are known as *keratoplasties* and are usually performed with local anesthesia in an ambulatory surgical setting. The transplant may involve the entire depth of corneal tissue (penetrating keratoplasty), which is most common, or only certain layers of the corneal tissue (lamellar keratoplasty). The nerves around and behind the eye are numbed so that the patient cannot move or see out of the eye. The surgeon removes the center 7 to 8 mm of the diseased cornea (Fig. 49-3) with a trephine, an instrument that works like a cookie cutter. The same trephine is used to cut the tissue graft from the donor cornea so that the graft will be a perfect fit. The donor corneal graft is sutured into place on the eye. Fig. 49-4 shows the eye after transplantation. The procedure usually takes about an hour, and the patient remains in the recovery area for 1 to 2 hours after the procedure before being discharged to home.

Postoperative care involves extensive patient teaching. After the procedure is completed, a subconjunctival antibiotic injection is given and an antibiotic ointment instilled. The eye is covered with a pressure patch and a protective shield. This dressing is left in place until the next day, when the patient returns to the surgeon.

Notify the ophthalmologist of changes in vital signs or of drainage on the dressing. Instruct the patient to lie on the nonoperative side to reduce intraocular pressure (IOP). During the early period after surgery, he or she cannot see out of the affected eye because of the eye patch and shield.

Show the patient or family member how to apply a patch, and obtain a return demonstration. The patch may need to be worn during the day for the first 3 to 5 days. Teach the patient to wear the shield at night for the first month after surgery and whenever he or she is around small children or pets. Complications after surgery include bleeding, wound leakage, infection, and graft rejection. Teach the patient the correct way to instill eyedrops, and obtain a return demonstration. Show pictures of what the eye and sutures should look like. Teach him or her to examine the eye (or have a family member do the examination) daily for the presence of infection or graft rejection. The presence of purulent discharge, a continuous

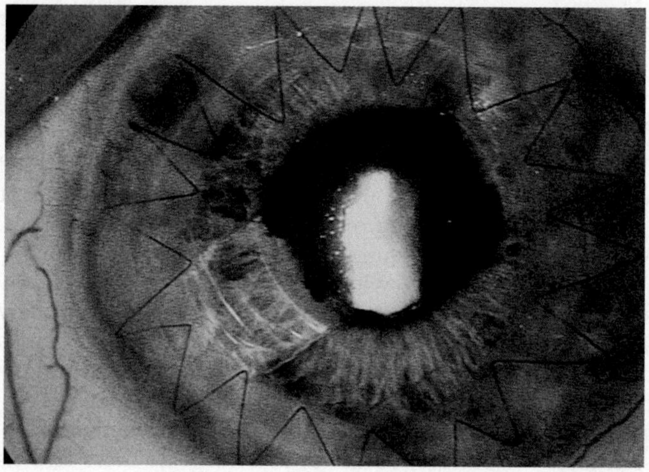

Fig. 49-4 • The appearance of the eye with sutures in place after corneal transplantation.

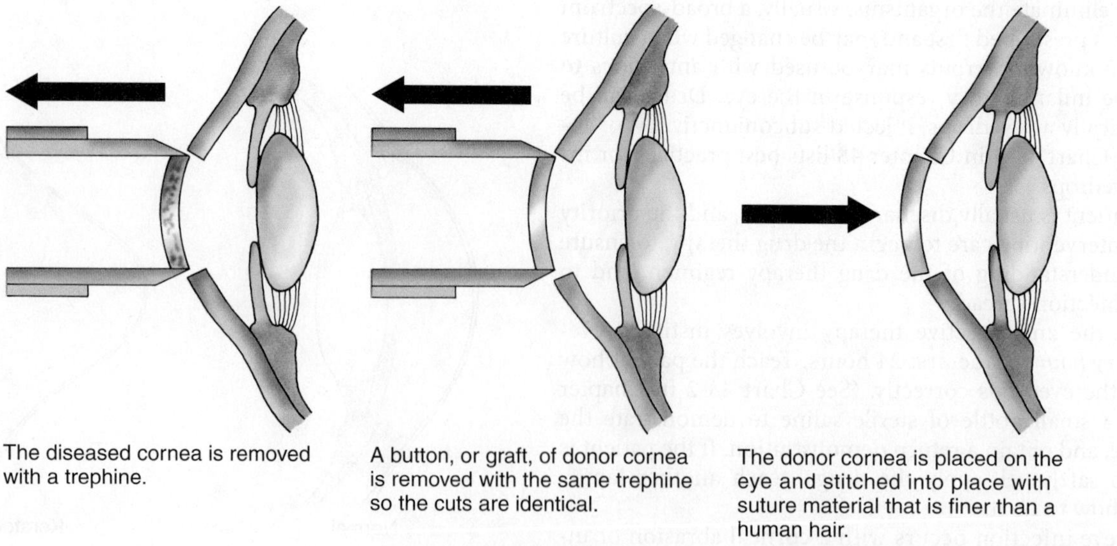
The diseased cornea is removed with a trephine.
A button, or graft, of donor cornea is removed with the same trephine so the cuts are identical.
The donor cornea is placed on the eye and stitched into place with suture material that is finer than a human hair.

Fig. 49-3 • The steps involved in corneal transplantation (penetrating keratoplasty).

leak of clear fluid from around the graft site (not tears), or excessive bleeding should be reported immediately to the surgeon. Other changes that may represent complications include decreased vision, increased reddening of the eye, pain, increased sensitivity to light, and the presence of light flashes or "floaters" in the field of vision. Teach the patient to report any of these manifestations to the surgeon if they develop after the first 48 hours and persist for more than 6 hours.

The eye should be protected from any activity that can increase the pressure on, around, or inside the eye. Teach the patient to avoid jogging, running, dancing, and any other activity that promotes rapid or jerky head motions for several weeks after surgery. Other activities that may raise intraocular pressure (IOP) and should be avoided are listed in Table 49-1. Returning to work depends on the type of work. Patients who have sedentary jobs, such as secretaries, may return to work in as little as 1 week, whereas those who perform heavy lifting and other types of manual labor may need to be off work for 6 to 8 weeks.

Although the cornea has no blood supply, graft rejection is possible. Inflammation starts in the donor cornea near the graft edge and moves toward the center. Vision is reduced, and the cornea becomes cloudy. Frequent applications of topical corticosteroids and other immunosuppressants are used to stop the rejection process. If rejection continues, the graft becomes opaque and blood vessels branch into the opaque tissue.

Eye donation is a common procedure and needed for continuing the service of corneal transplantation. Corneal tissue is obtained from a local eye or tissue bank. An eye bank obtains its supply of corneal tissue from volunteer donors. These donors must be free of infectious disease or cancer at the time of death. If a deceased patient is a potential eye donor, follow these steps:

- Raise the head of the bed 30 degrees.
- Instill antibiotic eyedrops, such as Neosporin or tobramycin.
- Close the eyes, and apply a *small* ice pack to the closed eyes.
- Contact the family and physician to discuss eye donation.

DECISION-MAKING CHALLENGE
Critical Rescue

The patient is a 25-year-old woman who has worn soft contact lenses for the past 12 years. She and her twin sister live together and have started making their own contact lens solutions to save money. Last week, the patient had an eyelash in her eye under the lid and rubbed at it for days trying to remove it. Now it is late Friday night and she calls the ED, saying that she has tremendous eye pain in the right eye and an area that is draining greenish yellow material. She asks whether she should come to the ED tonight or should she try to see her own ophthalmologist tomorrow or Monday.

1. Should she be seen tonight, or should she wait a day or two? Provide a rationale for your response.
2. What risk factors does she have for a corneal ulcer?
3. What should you tell her about infection control even before she arrives at the ED?
4. What will be the teaching priorities for this patient?

evolve For suggested answer guidelines, go to http://evolve.elsevier.com/Iggy/.

TABLE 49-1 Activities That Increase Intraocular Pressure

- Bending from the waist
- Lifting objects weighing more than 10 lbs
- Sneezing, coughing
- Blowing the nose
- Straining to have a bowel movement
- Vomiting
- Having sexual intercourse
- Keeping the head in a dependent position
- Wearing tight shirt collars

CATARACT

Pathophysiology

The lens is a biconvex, transparent, refractive elastic structure suspended behind the iris. A cataract is an opacity of the lens that distorts the image projected onto the retina (Fig. 49-5). With aging, the lens gradually loses water and increases in density (Meiner & Lueckenotte, 2006, Whiteside et al., 2006). This increased density occurs as older lens fibers are compressed and new fibers are produced in the outer layers. Lens proteins dry out and form crystals. As the density of the lens increases, it becomes opaque with a painless loss of transparency. Both eyes may have cataracts; however, the rate of progression in each eye is usually different.

Etiology and Genetic Risk

Cataracts are classified by nature or by onset. They may be present at birth or develop at any time. Cataracts may be age related or caused by trauma or exposure to toxic agents. They also occur with other diseases and ocular disorders (Table 49-2).

Incidence/Prevalence

Cataracts develop in 5 to 10 million people worldwide every year. The age-related cataract is the most common type. Some degree of cataract formation is expected in all people older than 70 years (Vaughan et al., 2004).

Health Promotion and Maintenance

Although most cases of cataracts in North America are age related, the onset of cataract formation occurs earlier with heavy sun exposure or exposure to other sources of ultraviolet

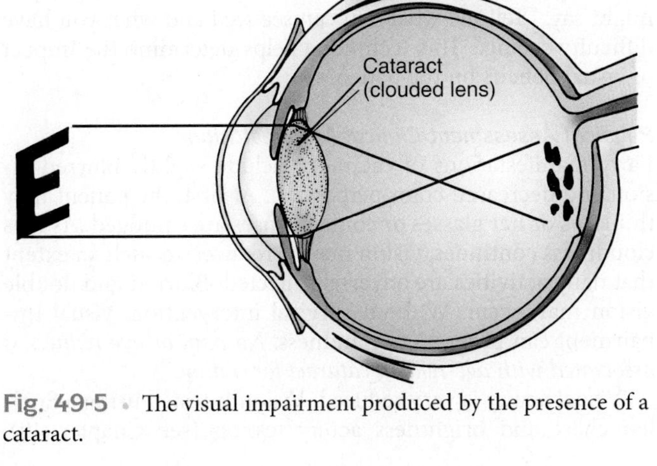
Cataract
(clouded lens)
E

Fig. 49-5 • The visual impairment produced by the presence of a cataract.

TABLE 49-2 Common Causes of Cataracts

AGE-RELATED CATARACTS
• Lens water loss and fiber compaction
TRAUMATIC CATARACTS
• Blunt injury to eye or head
• Penetrating eye injury
• Intraocular foreign bodies
• Radiation exposure, therapy
TOXIC CATARACTS
• Corticosteroids
• Phenothiazine derivatives
• Miotic agents
ASSOCIATED CATARACTS
• Diabetes mellitus
• Hypoparathyroidism
• Down syndrome
• Chronic sunlight exposure
COMPLICATED CATARACTS
• Retinitis pigmentosa
• Glaucoma
• Retinal detachment

light. Teach people to reduce the risk for cataract by wearing sunglasses that limit penetration of ultraviolet light whenever they are out in bright sunlight. Also, cataracts are caused by direct eye injury. Urge all people to wear eye and head protection during sports, such as baseball, or any activity that increases the risk for the eye being hit by objects in motion (Boyd-Monk, 2005; Sitzman, 2006).

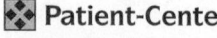

Patient-Centered Collaborative Care

evolve ONLINE PHARM REVIEW

Assessment

History

Age is important because cataracts are most prevalent in the older adult. Ask about these predisposing factors:

- Recent or past trauma to the eye
- Exposure to radioactive materials, x-rays, or ultraviolet light
- Systemic disease (e.g., diabetes mellitus, hypoparathyroidism, Down syndrome, atopic dermatitis)
- Prolonged use of corticosteroids, chlorpromazine, or miotic drugs
- Intraocular disease (e.g., recurrent uveitis)

Ask the patient to describe his or her vision. For example, you might say, "Tell me what you can see well and what you have difficulty seeing." This technique helps determine the impact of visual deficits on the patient.

Physical Assessment/Clinical Manifestations

Early manifestations of cataracts include slightly blurred vision and decreased color perception. At first, the patient may think his or her glasses or contact lenses are smudged. As lens cloudiness continues, vision may be reduced to such an extent that daily activities are adversely affected. Blurred and double vision may occur. Without surgical intervention, visual impairment can progress to blindness. *No pain or eye redness is associated with age-related cataract formation.*

Visual acuity is very reduced. Vision is tested using a Snellen chart and brightness acuity testing (see Chapter 48).

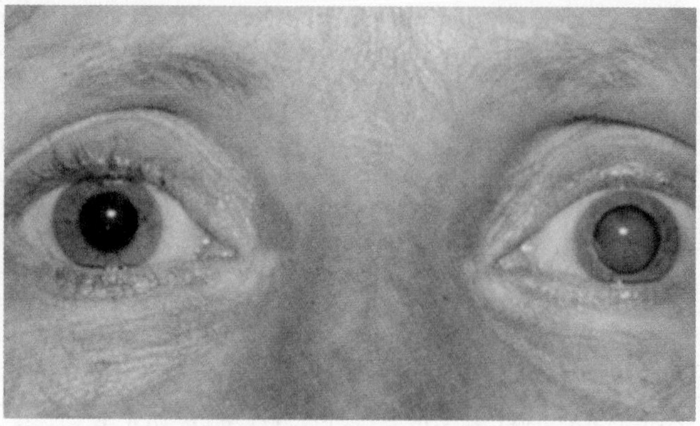

Fig. 49-6 • The appearance of an eye with a mature cataract.

Evaluate the patient's acuity under various lighting conditions, which can help determine the degree of visual disability.

Examine the lens with the direct ophthalmoscope, and describe any observed densities by size, shape, and location. As the cataract matures, the opacity makes it difficult to see the retina and the red reflex may be absent. When this occurs, the pupil is white (Fig. 49-6).

Psychosocial Assessment

Loss of vision is gradual, and the patient may not be aware of the change until reading or driving is affected. Fear of losing one's eyesight can be overwhelming, and the patient may have great anxiety during an eye evaluation. He or she may have old or inaccurate information about cataract surgery and the degree of sight that can be restored. Encourage the patient and family to express feelings and concerns about the reduced vision.

Analysis

Common Nursing Diagnoses and Collaborative Problems

The most common nursing diagnosis for patients with cataracts is Disturbed Sensory Perception (Visual) related to altered sensory reception.

Additional Nursing Diagnoses and Collaborative Problems

In addition to the most common nursing diagnosis, patients with cataracts may have one or more of these:

- Fear related to sensory impairment, loss of eyesight, scheduled surgery, or inability to regain eyesight
- Risk for Injury related to decreased vision
- Social Isolation related to reduced visual acuity, fear of injury, or fear of embarrassment
- Self-Care Deficit (Dressing/Grooming) related to perceptual impairment
- Deficient Knowledge (Cataract Pathophysiology and Treatment) related to lack of information or misconceptions
- Impaired Home Maintenance related to age, limited vision, or activity restrictions imposed by surgery

DECISION-MAKING CHALLENGE

Coordination of Care

The patient is an 82-year-old widower who lives in a retirement village. He has had cataracts for about 10 years, with the right one advancing faster than the left, and wants the surgery because his vision is too poor to pass the driving test. (The retirement community's minibus brought him to the clinic.) He takes his meals in the dining facility and has weekly housekeeping/laundry service. He plays golf daily, using a golf cart, and plays cards every evening. He is scheduled for surgery next week and is in the clinic today for preoperative teaching. In addition to cataracts, he has osteoarthritis of both knees and is on hormonal therapy for prostate cancer. His drugs include aspirin 650 mg twice daily, losartan (Cozaar) 50 mg daily for moderate hypertension, and a multiple vitamin.

1. Should any of these drugs be changed before surgery? Which one(s) and why?
2. What are the priority areas of assessment for this patient? Provide a rationale for your choices.
3. What community resources should you check for this patient?

evolve For suggested answer guidelines, go to http://evolve.elsevier.com/Iggy/.

▪ Planning and Implementation

Disturbed Sensory Perception (Visual)

NOC **Planning: Expected Outcomes.** The patient with cataracts is expected to have Vision Compensation Behavior as indicated by consistent demonstration of these behaviors:

- Monitors symptoms of vision deterioration
- Positions self to advantage vision
- Uses adequate lighting for activity being performed
- Wears eyeglasses or contact lenses correctly
- Cares for eyewear correctly
- Uses vision assistive devices

The patient is also expected to have Sensory Function: Vision as indicated by an increase to mild deviation from the normal range in:

- Central visual acuity and visual fields (left and right)
- Peripheral visual acuity and visual fields (left and right)
- Response to visual stimuli

Interventions. Surgery is the only "cure" for cataracts. However, patients often live with reduced vision for years before the cataract is removed. After vision is reduced to the extent that ADLs are affected, the surgery should be performed as soon as possible. Delaying this intervention increases the risk for falls and other negative events (Hodge et al., 2007). (See the Evidence-Based Practice box below.) Interventions for enhanced communication, safety, and independence before surgery are described on pp. 1106-1107 of Patient-Centered Collaborative Care in the Reduced Vision section.

Preoperative Care. The health care provider has the responsibility (1) of giving the patient accurate information so that he or she can make informed decisions about treatment and (2) of obtaining informed consent. Reinforce this information, and teach about the nature of cataracts, their progression, and their treatment.

Because cataract surgery is usually an ambulatory care procedure and most patients are older, adequate preoperative teaching is problematic. Assess how the patient's vision affects ADLs, especially dressing, eating, and ambulating.

Stress that care after surgery requires the instillation of different types of eyedrops several times a day for 2 to 4 weeks. Careful assessment of eye appearance is also needed. If the patient is unable to perform these tasks, help him or her make arrangements for this care.

An IV infusion may or may not be started in the operating room. A sedative is given before surgery, and a series of ophthalmic drugs are instilled just before surgery to dilate the pupils and cause vasoconstriction. Other eyedrops are instilled to induce paralysis to prevent lens movement. When the patient is in the surgical area, a local anesthetic is injected into the muscle cone behind the eye for anesthesia and eye paralysis.

EVIDENCE-BASED PRACTICE

Delays in cataract surgery increase the risk for negative events

Hodge, W., Horsley, T., Albiani, D., Baryla, J., Belliveau, M., Buhrmann, R., et al. (2007). The consequences of waiting for cataract surgery: A systematic review. *Canadian Medical Association Journal, 176*(9), 1285-1290.

In North America, cataract surgery is the most common procedure performed on adults. Surgical results are thought to enhance quality of life and allow older adults to live independently for a longer period. Some people wait for long periods after a cataract diagnosis to have the surgery for many reasons, including social policy limitations, financial limitations, and personal misconceptions. This study sought to determine whether a 6-month or longer delay in cataract surgery with lens replacement was associated with any negative effects.

This systematic review examined 27 studies of patient outcomes after cataract surgery. Comparisons were made between the outcomes of those patients who had the surgery within 6 weeks of cataract diagnosis and those whose surgeries were delayed by 6 months or longer. The studies examined included 2 randomized controlled trials with 511 subjects, 3 prospective cohort studies, and 22 descriptive studies.

The results indicated that visual impairment worsened with longer wait periods and patient safety suffered, particularly with the increased incidence of falls. Patients also reported a decrease in overall quality of life during the longer wait period. Longer wait periods were not associated with poorer visual restoration.

Level of Evidence—1. The study provides a meta-analysis of 27 relevant clinical studies including 2 randomized controlled clinical trials (RCTs) and 5 prospective cohort studies.

Commentary: Implications for Practice and Research. Although limited by the small number of RCTs in the data evaluated, the strengths of this review include the large numbers of patients and the diverse countries in which the original studies were conducted. In some situations, government policy and insurance practices determine the wait period for cataract surgery. Nurses can help lobby for changes in these practices based on serious negative events that can occur during the wait period that can have an impact on health care costs and independent living for older adults. In those situations in which the patient instigates the delay, nurses can be instrumental in shortening the delay by allaying misconceptions and helping older adults plan the surgical event with family members or outside assistance for transportation and drug administration.

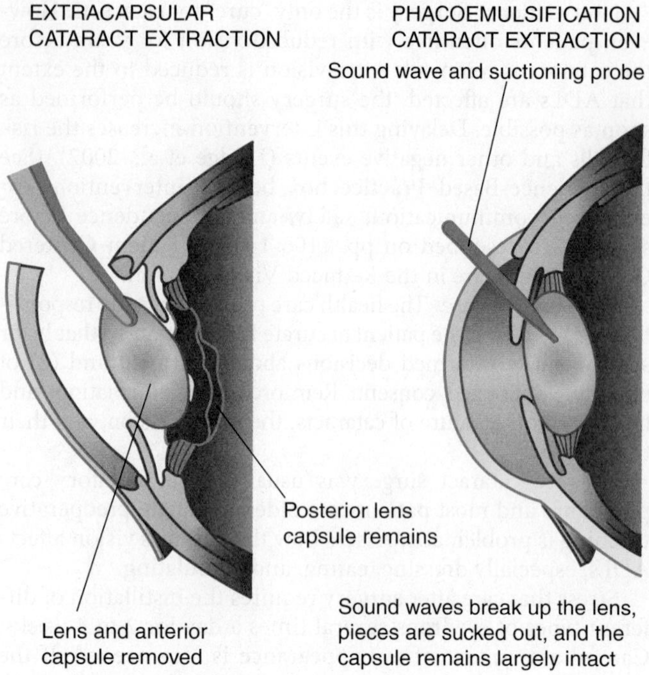
EXTRACAPSULAR CATARACT EXTRACTION
PHACOEMULSIFICATION CATARACT EXTRACTION
Sound wave and suctioning probe
Posterior lens capsule remains
Sound waves break up the lens, pieces are sucked out, and the capsule remains largely intact
Lens and anterior capsule removed

Fig. 49-7 • Surgical approaches to lens removal for cataracts.

Operative Procedures. Extraction of the lens can be extracapsular or, more commonly, performed by phacoemulsification (Fig. 49-7). With *extracapsular removal,* the front portion of the capsule is opened with a small incision and the lens is removed whole. With *phacoemulsification,* a probe is inserted through the capsule and high-frequency sound waves break the cataractous lens into small pieces, which are then removed by suction. In this procedure, the capsule remains intact and the replacement intraocular lens (IOL) is placed inside it. Without a lens replacement, the eye has no accommodative power and has lost most of its refractive ability.

A replacement lens is needed to focus light rays in the retina. Usually, a small, clear, plastic lens is implanted at the time of cataract removal. Replacement lenses can be selected to allow correction of a specific refractive error. Some patients have distant vision restored to 20/20 and may need glasses only for reading or close work. Some replacement lenses have multiple focal planes and may correct all vision for a patient to the extent that glasses or contact lenses are not needed at all or are only minimally needed. Lens replacement surgery is now performed for people who do not have cataracts but who want corrected vision.

Postoperative Care. Immediately after surgery, antibiotics are given subconjunctivally. Usually an antibiotic plus steroid ointment also is instilled. The eye is usually left unpatched, and often the patient is discharged within an hour after surgery. Teach him or her to wear dark glasses outdoors or in brightly lit environments until the pupil responds to light. Teach the patient and family members how to instill the prescribed eyedrops. (See Chart 48-2 in Chapter 48.) Work with them in creating a written schedule for the timing and the order of eyedrops administration. Stress the importance of keeping all follow-up appointments.

Teach the patient that mild eye itching is normal, as is a "bloodshot appearance." The eyelid may be slightly swollen. However, significant swelling or bruising is abnormal. Cool compresses may be beneficial. Discomfort at the site is controlled by a mild analgesic such as acetaminophen (Abenol♣, Tylenol) or acetaminophen with oxycodone (Endocet♣, Percocet, Tylox). Remind him or her to avoid aspirin because of its effects on blood clotting.

Pain early after surgery may indicate a complication, such as increased IOP or hemorrhage. Teach the patient to contact the ophthalmologist if pain occurs with nausea or vomiting.

To reduce increases in IOP (the major complication after surgery), teach the patient and family about activity restrictions. Activities that can cause a sudden rise in IOP are listed in Table 49-1.

Another major complication is infection. Teach the patient and family to observe for increasing redness of the eye, a change in visual acuity, tears, and photophobia. Creamy white, dry, crusty drainage on the eyelids and lashes is normal. However, yellow or green drainage indicates infection and must be reported.

Most patients experience a dramatic improvement in vision as early as the day of surgery. Caution them that final best vision will not be present until 4 to 6 weeks after surgery. However, vision is not expected to become worse after the procedure. *Teach the patient to report any reduction in vision immediately to the ophthalmologist.*

NCLEX EXAMINATION CHALLENGE

The client who has just had cataract removal and lens replacement in his right eye asks whether he can play cards this evening and go golfing tomorrow. What is the nurse's best response?

A. "Golfing is fine, but you need to refrain from playing cards for 1 week."
B. "Playing cards is fine, but you need to refrain from golfing for about 2 weeks."
C. "You should neither play cards nor play golf for at least 2 weeks."
D. "Neither activity is restricted."

evolve For the correct answer, go to http://evolve.elsevier.com/Iggy/.

Community-Based Care

The patient is usually discharged within 2 hours after cataract surgery. Nursing interventions focus on helping the patient and family with plans for return to the home, assisted-living, or extended-care setting.

Home Care Management

If the patient has difficulty instilling eyedrops, a supportive neighbor, friend, or family member can be taught the procedure. Adaptive equipment that positions the bottle of eyedrops directly over the eye can also be purchased. Eyedrops are often prescribed for 4 to 6 weeks after cataract surgery.

Health Teaching

Review these indications of complications after cataract surgery with the patient and family before discharge:

- Sharp, sudden pain in the eye
- Bleeding or increased discharge
- Lid swelling
- Decreased vision
- Flashes of light or floating shapes

Remind the patient to avoid activities that might increase IOP (see Table 49-1). The patient may wash his or her hair a day or two after surgery but only with the head tilted back, such as in a beauty salon or barber shop, to avoid getting water in the eye. Teach him or her to stand in the shower with the face away from the showerhead for the first week after surgery.

Teach the patient about activity restrictions. Cooking and light housekeeping are permitted, but vacuuming should be avoided for several weeks because of the forward flexion involved and the rapid, jerky movements required. Advise him or her to refrain from driving, operating machinery, and participating in certain sports, such as golf, until given specific permission from the ophthalmologist. Chart 49-5 lists items to cover in the focused assessment of a patient in the home environment after cataract surgery.

Health Care Resources

If the patient lives alone and has no family or significant others, arrange for a home care nurse to assess him or her and the home situation. If the patient is unable to instill eyedrops independently, a friend, neighbor, or family member can be taught this technique.

Evaluation: Outcomes

Evaluate the care of the patient with cataracts on the basis of the identified nursing diagnoses. The expected outcomes include that the patient will:

- Demonstrate Vision Compensation Behavior
- Remain free from injury

The patient who had cataract surgery will:

- Have improved Sensory Perception (Visual)
- Recognize manifestations of complications

Specific indicators for these outcomes are listed for each nursing diagnosis under the Planning and Implementation section (see earlier).

Chart 49-5 HOME CARE ASSESSMENT

The Patient After Cataract Surgery

Assess the eye and vision:
- Visual acuity in both eyes using a Jaeger card
- Visual fields of both eyes
- Compare operative eye with nonoperative eye for presence or absence of:
  - Redness
  - Tearing
  - Drainage

Ask the patient about:
- Pain in or around the operative eye
- Any change in visual acuity (decreased or improved) in the operative eye
- Whether any of these has been noticed in the operative eye:
  - Dark spots
  - Increase in the number of floaters
  - Bright flashes of light

Assess the home environment for:
- Safety hazards (especially tripping and falling hazards)
- Kitchen hazards
- Level of room lighting

Assess patient adherence with and understanding of treatment and limitations, such as:
- Signs and symptoms to report
- Drug regimen
- Activity restrictions

Assess functional ability:
- Activities of daily living
- Adherence to drug regimen

GLAUCOMA

Pathophysiology

Glaucoma is a group of ocular diseases resulting in increased IOP. Intraocular pressure (IOP) is the fluid pressure within the eye. As described in Chapter 48, the eye is a hollow organ. For the eye to function properly, the gel in the posterior segment (vitreous humor) and the fluid in the anterior segment (aqueous humor) must be present in set amounts that apply pressure inside the eye to keep it ball-shaped.

The gel-like vitreous humor is made as the eyes form and grow. Once eye growth is complete, this gel does not change in volume. The aqueous humor, however, is continuously made from blood plasma. The ciliary bodies located behind the iris and just in front of the lens make and secrete this fluid (see Fig. 48-2 in Chapter 48). The fluid flows through the pupil into the bulging area in front of the iris. At the outer edges of the iris beneath the cornea, blood vessels collect this fluid and return it to the blood. Usually about 1 mL of aqueous humor is present at all times in the front part of each eye, but it is continuously made and reabsorbed at a rate of about 5 mL daily. *A normal IOP of 10 to 21 mm Hg is maintained when there is a balance between production and outflow of aqueous humor. If the IOP becomes too high, the extra pressure presses on blood vessels in the eye and prevents blood flow, resulting in poorly oxygenated photoreceptors. These sensitive nerve tissues become ischemic and die. When too many have died, sight is lost and the person is permanently blind.* Tissue damage usually starts in the periphery and moves inward toward the fovea centralis. Left untreated, glaucoma can result in blindness. Glaucoma is commonly painless, and the patient may be unaware of a gradual reduction in vision (Halvorson, 2005).

There are several causes and types of glaucoma (Table 49-3). It is classified as primary, secondary, or associated. In primary glaucoma, the most common form, the structures involved in circulation and reabsorption of the aqueous humor undergo direct pathologic change.

Primary open-angle glaucoma (POAG), the most common form of primary glaucoma, usually affects both eyes and is asymptomatic in the early stages. Outflow of aqueous hu-

TABLE 49-3 Common Causes of Glaucoma

PRIMARY GLAUCOMA
- Aging
- Heredity
- Central retinal vein occlusion

SECONDARY GLAUCOMA
- Uveitis
- Iritis
- Neovascular disorders
- Trauma
- Ocular tumors
- Degenerative disease
- Eye surgery

ASSOCIATED GLAUCOMA
- Diabetes mellitus
- Hypertension
- Severe myopia
- Retinal detachment

mor through the chamber angle is reduced. Because the fluid cannot leave the eye at the same rate it is produced, IOP gradually increases. **Angle-closure glaucoma** (also called *closed-angle glaucoma, narrow-angle glaucoma,* or *acute glaucoma*) is less common, has a sudden onset, and is an emergency. The basic problems are a narrowed angle and forward displacement of the iris. Movement of the iris against the cornea narrows or closes the chamber angle, obstructing the outflow of aqueous humor. This can happen suddenly and without warning.

Glaucoma is a common cause of blindness in affluent countries. It is age-related, occurring in about 10% of people older than 80 years (McCance & Huether, 2006).

Patient-Centered Collaborative Care

Primary open-angle glaucoma (POAG) develops slowly, usually without symptoms. The gradual loss of visual fields may go unnoticed because central vision is unaffected. At times, the patient may have foggy vision, reduced accommodation, mild aching in the eyes, or headaches and may require fre-

CONCEPT MAP Glaucoma

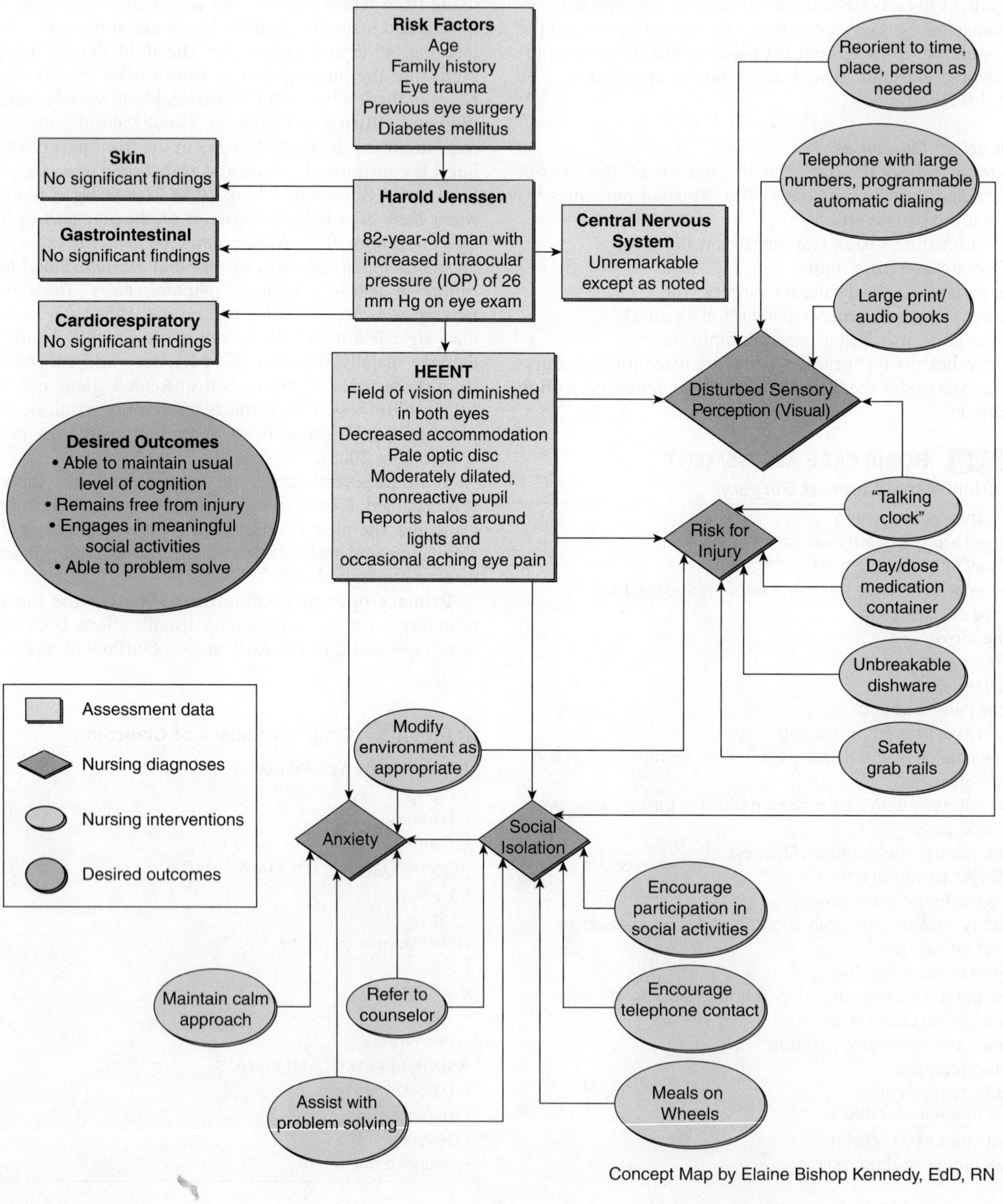
Risk Factors
Age
Family history
Eye trauma
Previous eye surgery
Diabetes mellitus
Skin
No significant findings
Harold Jenssen
82-year-old man with increased intraocular pressure (IOP) of 26 mm Hg on eye exam
Central Nervous System
Unremarkable except as noted
Gastrointestinal
No significant findings
Cardiorespiratory
No significant findings
Reorient to time, place, person as needed
Telephone with large numbers, programmable automatic dialing
Large print/ audio books
HEENT
Field of vision diminished in both eyes
Decreased accommodation
Pale optic disc
Moderately dilated, nonreactive pupil
Reports halos around lights and occasional aching eye pain
Disturbed Sensory Perception (Visual)
Desired Outcomes
• Able to maintain usual level of cognition
• Remains free from injury
• Engages in meaningful social activities
• Able to problem solve
Risk for Injury
"Talking clock"
Day/dose medication container
Unbreakable dishware
Safety grab rails
Assessment data
Nursing diagnoses
Nursing interventions
Desired outcomes
Modify environment as appropriate
Anxiety
Social Isolation
Encourage participation in social activities
Maintain calm approach
Refer to counselor
Encourage telephone contact
Assist with problem solving
Meals on Wheels

Concept Map by Elaine Bishop Kennedy, EdD, RN

quent changes in eyeglass prescriptions (Kowing & Kester, 2007). Late manifestations occur after irreversible damage to optic nerve function and include seeing halos around lights, losing peripheral vision, and experiencing decreased visual acuity not correctable with eyeglasses. The Concept Map on p. 1096 addresses assessment and collaborative care issues for patients who have glaucoma.

Assessment

Physical Assessment/Clinical Manifestations

Ophthalmoscopic examination of the patient with glaucoma shows cupping and atrophy of the optic disc. It becomes wider and deeper and turns white or gray.

To determine the extent of peripheral field losses, visual fields are measured. In POAG, the visual fields first show a small crescent-shaped defect that gradually progresses to a larger field defect.

The manifestations of acute angle-closure glaucoma differ from those of open-angle glaucoma. The onset of symptoms is acute, and the patient has sudden, severe pain around the eyes that radiates over the face. Headache or brow pain, nausea, and vomiting also may occur. Other manifestations include seeing colored halos around lights and sudden blurred vision with decreased light perception. The sclera may appear reddened and the cornea foggy. Ophthalmoscopic examination reveals a shallow anterior chamber, cloudy aqueous humor, and a moderately dilated, nonreactive pupil.

Other Diagnostic Assessments

Tonometry shows an elevated intraocular pressure (IOP). If an elevated reading is found during routine screening examination, take several readings over a period of time at various times of the day to determine a pattern, because IOP varies during the day. In open-angle glaucoma, the tonometry reading is between 22 and 32 mm Hg (normal is 10 to 21 mm Hg). In angle-closure glaucoma, the tonometry reading may be 30 mm Hg or higher.

Perimetry is a commonly used test to screen the visual fields. During this computerized test, the patient is asked to look straight ahead and then indicate, by pressing a control button, when a moving light enters the peripheral vision. This process draws a "map" of the person's peripheral vision and any deficits.

Gonioscopy is a test performed when a high IOP is found and determines whether open-angle or closed-angle glaucoma is present. It uses a special lens that eliminates the corneal curve, is painless, and allows visualization of the angle where the iris meets the cornea.

Optic nerve imaging is commonly used for those people with ocular hypertension or who are at risk for glaucoma from other problems. Three different common computerized methods can assess the thickness and contours of the optic nerve for changes that indicate damage as a result of high IOP. These tests are scanning laser polarimetry, confocal laser ophthalmoscopy, and optical coherence tomography (OCT). Usually one type of test is selected and used on a regular basis for a person at risk for glaucoma to detect, over time, changes that indicate loss of optic nerve fibers. These noninvasive imaging techniques are fast and painless.

Interventions

Nonsurgical Management

Blindness from glaucoma can be prevented by early detection, lifelong treatment, and a regimen of close monitoring and follow-up care. Some degree of vision loss occurs, although use of topical agents that reduce ocular hypertension has been found to delay or prevent damage from glaucoma. Chart 49-6 lists ways to assist the older patient with impaired vision to remain as independent as possible.

Drug therapy for glaucoma focuses on reducing IOP through these mechanisms:

- Constricting the pupil so that the ciliary muscle is contracted, allowing better circulation of the aqueous humor to the site of absorption
- Reducing the production or increasing the absorption of aqueous humor

Eyedrop drugs are the mainstay of control for glaucoma. They do not improve lost vision but prevent more damage by decreasing IOP. The five most common classes of drugs to manage glaucoma are the prostaglandins agonists, adrenergic agonists, beta-adrenergic blockers, cholinergic agonists, and carbonic anhydrase inhibitors (Davis, 2006). Most eye drops cause tearing, mild burning, and blurred vision for a few minutes after instilling the drug. The sclera may also become red and itchy. Specific drug actions and nursing interventions are listed in Chart 49-7.

The priority nursing intervention for the patient on drug therapy for glaucoma is teaching. Provide written instructions similar to those in Chart 48-2 in Chapter 48. The benefit of drug therapy is achieved only when the drugs are used on the prescribed schedule, usually every 12 hours. Teach patients the importance of instilling the drops on time and not skipping doses. When more than one drug is prescribed, teach him or her to wait 10 to 15 minutes between drug instillations to prevent one drug from "washing out" or diluting another drug. Also teach the technique of punctal occlusion (placing pressure on the corner of the eye near the nose) immediately after eyedrop instillation to prevent systemic absorption of the drug. Stress the need for good handwashing, keeping the eyedrop container tip clean, and avoiding touching the tip to any part of the eye.

Systemic osmotic drugs may be given for angle-closure glaucoma as part of emergency treatment to rapidly reduce IOP. These agents include oral glycerin (Osmoglyn) and IV mannitol (Osmitrol).

Surgical Management

Surgery is used when drugs for the patient with open-angle glaucoma are not effective at controlling IOP. The two most common procedures are laser trabeculoplasty and filtering microsurgery. A *laser trabeculoplasty* burns the trabecular meshwork, scarring it and causing the meshwork fibers to tighten. Fiber tightening increases the size of the spaces between the fibers, improving outflow of aqueous humor and reducing IOP. *Filtering microsurgery* creates a drainage hole in the iris between the posterior and anterior chambers. Both of these surgeries are performed as ambulatory procedures.

If glaucoma fails to respond to the common surgical therapies or if the drainage hole does not remain open, a "shunt" or glaucoma drainage device may be implanted. These are most often used for glaucoma caused by trauma. The implanted device usually has a small tube or filament connected to a flat plate positioned on the outside of the eye in the eye orbit. (The plate is not visible on the front part of the eye.) The open part of the fine tube is placed into the front chamber of the eye, just in front of the iris. The fluid then drains through the tube (or along the outside of the tube) into the area around the flat plate where it collects and is reabsorbed into the bloodstream.

Chart 49-6 NURSING FOCUS ON THE OLDER ADULT

Promote Independent Living in Patients with Impaired Vision

DRUGS

- Having a neighbor, relative, friend, or visiting nurse visit once a week to measure the proper drugs for each day may be helpful.
  - If the patient is to take drugs more than once each day, it is helpful to use a container of a different shape (with a lid) each time. For example, if the patient is to take drugs at 9 AM, 1 PM, and 9 PM, the 9 AM drugs would be placed in a round container, the 1 PM drugs in a square container, and the 9 PM drugs in a triangular container.
  - It is helpful to place each day's drug containers in a separate box with raised letters on the side of the box spelling out the day.
- "Talking clocks" are available for the patient with low vision.
- Some drug boxes have alarms that can be set for different times.

COMMUNICATION

- Telephones with large, raised block numbers may be helpful. The best models are those with black numbers on a white phone or white numbers on a black phone.
- Telephones that have a programmable, automatic dialing feature are very helpful. Programmed numbers should include those for the fire department, police, relatives, friends, neighbors, and 911.

SAFETY

- It is best to leave furniture the way the patient wants it and not move it.
- Throw rugs are best eliminated.
- Appliance cords should be short and kept out of walkways.
- Lounge-style chairs with built-in footrests are preferable to footstools.
- Nonbreakable dishes, cups, and glasses are preferable to breakable ones.
- Cleansers and other toxic agents should be labeled with large, raised letters.
- Hook-and-loop (Velcro) strips at hand level may help mark the locations of switches and electrical outlets.

FOOD PREPARATION

- Meals on Wheels is a service that many older adults find helpful. This service brings meals at mealtime, cooked and ready to eat. The cost of this service varies, depending on the patient's ability to pay.
- Many grocery stores offer a "shop by telephone" service. The patient can either complete a computer booklet indicating types, amounts, and brands of items desired, or the store will complete this booklet over the telephone by asking the patient specific information. The store then delivers groceries to the patient's door (many stores also offer a "put away" service) and charges the patient's bank card.
- A microwave oven is a safer means of cooking than a standard stove, although many older patients are afraid of microwave ovens. If the patient has and will use a microwave oven, others can prepare meals ahead of time, label them, and freeze them for later use. Also, many microwavable complete frozen dinners that comply with a variety of dietary restrictions are available.
- Friends or relatives may be able to help with food preparation. Often relatives do not know what to give an older person for birthdays or other gift-giving occasions. One suggestion is a homemade prepackaged frozen dinner that the patient enjoys.

PERSONAL CARE

- Handgrips should be installed in bathrooms.
- The tub floor should have a nonskid surface.
- Male patients should use an electric shaver rather than a razor.
- Choosing a hairstyle that is becoming but easy to care for (avoiding parts) helps in independent living.
- Home hair care services may be available.

DIVERSIONAL ACTIVITY

- Some patients can read large-print books, newspapers, and magazines (available through local libraries and vision services).
- Books, magazines, and some newspapers are available on audiotape.
- Patients experienced in knitting or crocheting may be able to create items fashioned from straight pieces, such as afghans.
- Card games, dominoes, and some board games that are available in large, high-contrast print may be helpful for patients with low vision.

The most serious complication after glaucoma surgery is choroidal hemorrhage. If IOP is too low, fluid may enter the suprachoroid space and cause a choroidal detachment. Extra fluid in this space may break blood vessels located there. Manifestations of choroidal hemorrhage include:

- Acute pain deep in the eye
- Decreased vision
- Vital sign changes

DECISION-MAKING CHALLENGE

Legal/Ethical

The patient is a 72-year-old man with colorectal cancer having surgery today for placement of an implanted venous access device for chemotherapy. You remember him from his last ambulatory surgery. He lists all the prescribed drugs he is currently taking but does not mention the eyedrops he was using 6 months ago for his glaucoma. When you ask him about this omission he tells you that he stopped taking the eyedrops a few months ago and is now "curing his glaucoma" by drinking 6 cups of green tea and taking 5000 mg of vitamin C each day. He asks you not to tell his oncologist because "he isn't into alternative medicine."

1. What assessment should you perform or ask related to the glaucoma?
2. How should you respond to the patient's request not to tell his oncologist about the change in glaucoma treatment? Provide a rationale for your response.
3. What should you tell him about his choice of glaucoma therapy?

evolve For suggested answer guidelines, go to http://evolve.elsevier.com/Iggy/.

VITREOUS HEMORRHAGE

The vitreous is the gel that fills the posterior two thirds of the eye and maintains the eye's shape. Vitreous hemorrhage (bleeding into the vitreous cavity) may result from aging, sys-

Chart 49-7 COMMON EXAMPLES OF DRUG THERAPY (EYEDROPS)

Categories for Management of Glaucoma

Category and Drug	Purpose/Actions	Nursing Implications	Rationales
PROSTAGLANDIN AGONISTS			
Bimatoprost (Lumigan) Latanoprost (Xalatan) Travoprost (Travatan) Unoprostone isopropyl (Rescula)	Drugs lower IOP by dilating the blood vessels in the trabecular mesh of the eye, where the aqueous humor is reabsorbed, collecting more aqueous humor and allowing more fluid to leave the eye.	Teach the patient to check the cornea for abrasions or other signs of trauma.	Drugs should not be used when the cornea is not intact.
		Remind the patient that, over time, the eye color darkens and eyelashes elongate in the eye receiving the drug.	Knowing the side effects in advance reassures the patient that their presence is expected and normal.
		If only one eye is to be treated, teach the patient *not* to place drops in the other eye to try to make the eye colors similar.	Using the drug in an eye with normal IOP can cause a *lower-than-normal* IOP, which reduces vision.
		Warn the patient that using higher doses than are prescribed can reduce the effectiveness of the drug in controlling the glaucoma.	Drug action is based on blocking receptors, which can increase in number when the drug is overused.
ADRENERGIC AGONISTS			
Apraclonidine (Iopidine) Brimonidine tartrate (Alphagan) Dipivefrin hydrochloride (Propine) Epinephryl borate (Epifrin, Epinal, Eppy/N)	These drugs bind to receptors in the eye, reducing the amount of aqueous humor produced by the ciliary bodies. In addition, the pupil of the eye is dilated and flow of the fluid through the pupil is improved. Both these actions reduce the amount of fluid present in the eye at any one time, lowering the intraocular pressure.	Ask whether the patient is taking any antidepressants from the MAO inhibitor class, such as phenelzine (Nardil) or tranylcypromine (Parnate).	These enzyme inhibitors increase blood pressure as do the adrenergic agonists. When taken together, the patient may experience hypertensive crisis.
		Teach the patient to wear dark glasses outdoors and also indoors when lighting is bright.	The pupil dilates (mydriasis) and remains dilated, even when there is plenty of light, causing discomfort.
		Teach the patient not to use the eyedrops with contact lenses in place and to wait 15 minutes after using the drug to put in the lenses.	These drugs are absorbed by the contact lens, which can become discolored or cloudy.
BETA-ADRENERGIC BLOCKERS			
Betaxolol hydrochloride (Betopic) Carteolol (Cartrol, Ocupress) Levobetaxolol (Betaxon) Levobunolol (Betagan) Metipranolol (OptiPranolol) Timolol (Betamol, Timoptic)	By selectively blocking beta-adrenergic receptors in the eye, less aqueous humor is produced by the ciliary bodies. The fluid also appears to be absorbed slightly faster as a result of this drug therapy. Both actions reduce IOP.	Ask whether the patient has moderate to severe asthma or COPD.	If these drugs are absorbed systemically, they constrict pulmonary smooth muscle and narrow airways.
		Warn diabetic patients to check their blood glucose levels more often when taking these drugs.	These drugs induce hypoglycemia and also mask the hypoglycemic symptoms.
		Teach patients who also take oral beta blockers to check their pulse at least twice per day and to notify the health care provider if the pulse is consistently below 58 beats per minute.	These drugs potentiate the effects of systemic beta blockers and can cause an unsafe drop in heart rate and blood pressure.
CHOLINERGIC DRUGS			
Carbachol (Carboptic, Isopto Carbachol, Miostat) Echothiophate (Phospholine Iodide) Pilocarpine (Adsorbocarpine, Akarpine, Isopto Carpine, Ocu-Carpine, Ocusert, Piloptic, Pilopine, Pilostat)	These drugs lower IOP by decreasing the amount of aqueous humor produced and by improving flow of the fluid. They make the pupil smaller (miosis) but, at the same time, make more room between the iris and the lens, allowing the fluid to flow through the pupil better even though it is smaller.	Teach the patient not to use more eyedrops than are prescribed and to report increased salivation or drooling to the health care provider.	These drugs are readily absorbed by conjunctival mucous membranes and can cause systemic side effects of headache, flushing, increased saliva, and sweating.
		Teach the patient to use good light when reading and to take care in darker rooms.	The pupil of the eye will not open more to let in more light, and it may be harder to see objects in dim light. This problem can increase the risk for falls.

Continued

Chart 49-7 COMMON EXAMPLES OF DRUG THERAPY (EYEDROPS)

Categories for Management of Glaucoma—cont'd

Category and Drug	Purpose/Actions	Nursing Implications	Rationales
CARBONIC ANHYDRASE INHIBITORS			
Brinzolamide (Azopt) Dorzolamide (Trusopt)	Drugs reduce IOP by directly inhibiting production of aqueous humor from the zonules of the ciliary bodies. They do not affect the flow or absorption of the fluid.	Ask whether the patient has an allergy to sulfonamide antibacterial drugs.	Drugs are similar to the sulfonamides, and if a patient is allergic to the sulfonamides, an allergy is likely with these drugs, even as eyedrops.
		Teach the patient to shake the drug before applying.	Drug separates on standing.
		Teach the patient not to use the eyedrops with contact lenses in place and to wait 15 minutes after using the drug to put in the lenses.	These drugs are absorbed by the contact lens, which can become discolored or cloudy.
COMBINATION DRUGS			
Brimonidine tartrate and timolol maleate (Combigan)	Same as for each drug alone.	Same as for each drug alone.	Same as for each drug alone.

COPD, Chronic obstructive pulmonary disease; *IOP,* intraocular pressure; *MAO,* monamine oxidase.

temic diseases, or trauma, or it may occur spontaneously. With aging, the vitreous may spontaneously detach from the retina. Torn blood vessels allow bleeding into the vitreous. Diseases that disrupt the retinal blood vessels, such as hypertension and diabetes mellitus, also cause blood leakage into the vitreous.

The main manifestation of vitreous hemorrhage is reduced visual acuity. The degree of reduced vision varies with the severity of the hemorrhage. A mild hemorrhage may cause the patient to see a red haze or "floaters." A moderate hemorrhage may cause the patient to see "black streaks" or "tiny black dots." Severe hemorrhage may reduce visual acuity to hand motion. Eye examination shows a reduced red reflex because light rays are blocked from reaching the retina. Ultrasonography is used to determine the location and extent of the hemorrhage.

A vitreous hemorrhage may absorb slowly with no treatment. Leaking blood vessels can be sealed with laser therapy. If the hemorrhage is still present several weeks to months later, a **vitrectomy** (surgical removal of the vitreous) may be indicated.

UVEITIS

Pathophysiology

The uveal tract has three related parts: the iris, the ciliary body, and the choroid. A common problem within these structures is inflammation, or **uveitis.** Uveitis may occur in the anterior or posterior portion of the eye.

Anterior uveitis is inflammation of the iris, inflammation of the ciliary body, or both. The cause of anterior uveitis is unknown but often follows exposure to allergens, infectious agents, trauma, or systemic disease (rheumatoid arthritis, herpes simplex, herpes zoster). It can follow any local or systemic bacterial infection. Manifestations include aching around the eye; tearing; blurred vision; photophobia; a small, irregular, nonreactive pupil; and a "bloodshot" appearance of the sclera.

Posterior uveitis is the common term for **retinitis** (inflammation of the retina) and **chorioretinitis** (inflammation of both the choroid and the retina). Posterior uveitis occurs with tuberculosis, syphilis, and toxoplasmosis.

The onset of symptoms is slow and painless. Visual impairment in the affected eye results from fluid, fibrin, and cells leaking into the vitreous cavity. The pupil is small, nonreactive, and irregularly shaped. Black dots are visible against the red background of the fundus. Lesions appear as grayish yellow patches on the retinal surface.

Patient-Centered Collaborative Care

Treatment of uveitis includes resting the ciliary body with a cycloplegic drug to paralyze ciliary muscles and dilate the pupil. The pupil is dilated to prevent adhesions between the iris and the lens. Steroid drops are given hourly to reduce the inflammation and to prevent adhesion of the iris to the cornea and lens. Ocular injections of steroids are used in posterior uveitis or when topical steroids have been ineffective. Analgesics that contain neither aspirin nor opioids are prescribed for pain. Systemic antibiotic therapy may be started for posterior uveitis or when infection is present with anterior uveitis.

Cool or warm compresses are applied for ocular pain. Darkening the room and wearing sunglasses reduce the discomfort of photophobia. Because of blurred vision from the cycloplegic drops, instruct the patient not to drive or operate machinery. Review the manifestations of bacterial and fungal ulcers and those of increased intraocular pressure (IOP).

RETINAL DISORDERS

MACULAR DEGENERATION

Pathophysiology

Macular degeneration is the deterioration of the macula (the area of central vision) and can be atrophic (age-related) or exudative. Age-related macular degeneration (AMD) has two types. The most common type is *dry* AMD, caused by gradual blockage of retinal capillaries, allowing retinal cells in the macula to become ischemic and necrotic. Rod and cone photoreceptors die. Central vision declines, and patients describe mild blurring and distortion at first. Eventually, the person loses all central vision (Bourla & Young, 2006). This type of degeneration is more common and progresses at a faster rate among smokers than among nonsmokers. Current research findings suggest that the risk for atrophic macular degeneration can be reduced by increasing long-term dietary intake of antioxidants and the carotenoids *lutein* and *zeaxanthin*. The same dietary treatments appear to slow the progression of macular degeneration. Another cause of AMD is the growth of new blood vessels in the macula, which have thin walls and leak blood and fluid (*wet* AMD).

Exudative macular degeneration is also *wet* but can occur at any age. The condition can occur only in one eye or in both eyes. In addition, the person with AMD can also develop exudative macular degeneration. Patients with exudative (wet) degeneration have a sudden decrease in vision after a serous detachment of pigment epithelium in the macula. Newly formed blood vessels invade this injured area and cause fluid and blood to collect under the macula (like a blister), resulting in scar formation and visual distortion.

Patient-Centered Collaborative Care

Treatment of dry AMD aims to help the patient maximize remaining vision. The loss of central vision reduces the ability to read, write, recognize safety hazards, and drive. Suggest alternative strategies (e.g., large-print books, public transportation) and referrals to community organizations that provide a wide range of adaptive equipment. See pp. 1106-1107 of Patient-Centered Collaborative Care in the Reduced Vision section for a complete discussion of patient care needs.

Management of patients with exudative or wet macular degeneration is geared toward slowing the process and identifying further changes in visual perception. Fluid and blood may resorb in some patients with exudative degeneration. Laser therapy to seal the leaking blood vessels in or near the macula can limit the extent of the damage. Another method used with some success at sealing or destroying the leaking retinal blood vessels is photodynamic therapy (PDT). In this treatment, the patient is given an IV agent to increase photosensitivity (Verteporfin). After the agent is absorbed, a special laser light is applied in the specific area to activate the agent. Activation causes local formation of oxygen radicals that occlude the leaking vessels and prevent excessive formation of new vessels (Schmidt-Luggen, 2006). This treatment outcome is enhanced when agents that prevent new blood vessel growth, such as ranibizumab (Lucentis), are also used in combination with PDT (Kaiser, 2007).

The photosensitizer used in PDT increases the sensitivity of the eye and the skin to sunlight and other bright lights. The length of the increased sensitivity depends on how much of the photosensitizer was used, but it may remain for weeks. During this time, the patient is at high risk for skin and retinal burns. Teaching the patient proper precautions is critical for prevention of injury. Chart 24-11 in Chapter 24 lists precautions to teach patients before, during, and after PDT.

RETINAL HOLES, TEARS, AND DETACHMENTS

Pathophysiology

A **retinal hole** is a break in the retina. These holes can be caused by trauma or can occur with aging. A **retinal tear** is a more jagged and irregularly shaped break in the retina. It can result from traction on the retina. A **retinal detachment** is the separation of the retina from the epithelium. Detachments are classified by the nature of their development.

Rhegmatogenous detachments occur following a hole or tear in the retina caused by mechanical force, creating an opening for the vitreous to move under the retina. When sufficient fluid collects in this space, the retina detaches. *Traction* detachments occur when the retina is pulled away from the support tissue by bands of fibrous tissue in the vitreous. *Exudative* detachments are caused by fluid collecting under the retina. These often occur with a systemic disease or with ocular tumors. No retinal break occurs.

Patient-Centered Collaborative Care

The onset of a retinal detachment is usually sudden and painless because no pain fibers are located in the retina. Patients may suddenly see bright flashes of light **(photopsia)** or floating dark spots in the affected eye. During the initial phase of the detachment or if the detachment is partial, the patient may describe the sensation of a curtain being pulled over part of the visual field. The visual field loss corresponds to the area of detachment.

On ophthalmoscopic examination, detachments are seen as gray bulges or folds in the retina that quiver. Depending on the cause of the detachment, a hole or tear also may be seen at the edge of the detachment.

If a retinal hole or tear is discovered before it causes a detachment, the defect may be closed or sealed. Closure prevents fluid from collecting under the retina and reduces the risk for a detachment. Treatment involves creating an inflammatory response that will bind the retina and choroid together around the break. The inflammatory response can be created with the application of **cryotherapy** (a freezing probe), **photocoagulation** (laser), or **diathermy** (high-frequency current).

Spontaneous reattachment of the retina is rare. Surgical repair is usually needed to place the retina in contact with the underlying structures. A common repair procedure is scleral buckling.

Preoperative Care

The patient is usually anxious and fearful about a possible permanent loss of vision. *Nursing priorities include providing information and reassurance to allay fears.*

Teach the patient to restrict activity and head movement before surgery to prevent further tearing or detachment and to promote drainage of any fluid under the retina. An eye patch is placed over the affected eye to reduce eye movement. Topical drugs are given before surgery to inhibit pupil constriction and accommodation.

Operative Procedures

The surgery is performed with the patient under general anesthesia. In scleral buckling, the ophthalmologist repairs wrinkles or folds in the retina so that the retina can assume its normal smooth position. To promote reattachment, a small piece of silicone is placed against the sclera and held in place by an encircling band (Fig. 49-8). This device keeps the retina in contact with the choroid and sclera to promote attachment. Any fluid under the retina is drained.

Either a gas or silicone oil is placed inside the eye to promote retinal reattachment. These agents press against the retina to hold it in place until healing occurs.

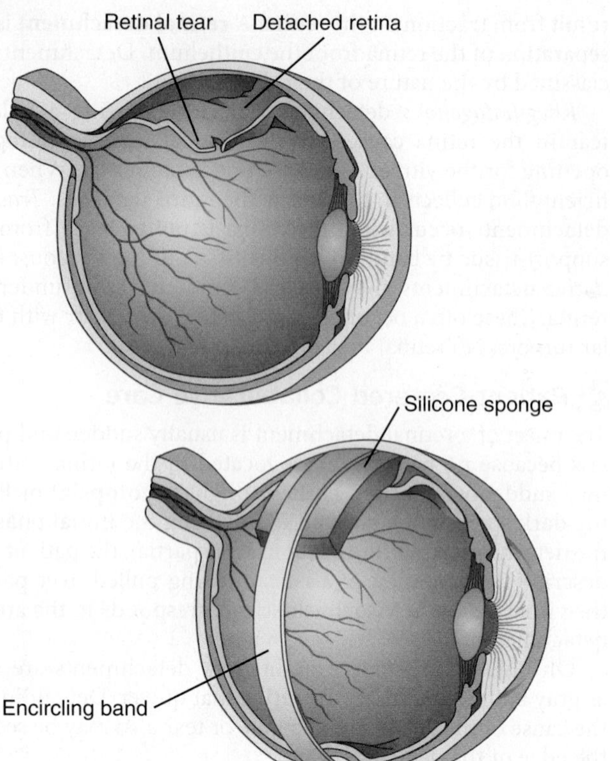
Retinal tear
Detached retina
Silicone sponge
Encircling band

Fig. 49-8 • The scleral buckling procedure for repair of retinal detachment.

Postoperative Care

After surgery, an eye patch and shield are applied. Monitor the patient's vital signs, and check the eye patch and shield for any drainage.

Activity after surgery varies. If gas or oil has been placed in the eye, position the patient on his or her abdomen. Teach the patient to lie with the head turned so that the affected eye is facing up, for several days or until the gas has been absorbed. As an alternative, he or she can sit on the side of the bed and place the head on an over-the-bed table.

Nausea and pain may occur after surgery. Give analgesics and antiemetics as prescribed. Teach the patient to report any sudden increase in pain or pain occurring with nausea. Report these symptoms to the surgeon immediately because they may indicate the development of complications. Remind the patient to avoid activities that increase intraocular pressure (IOP) (see Table 49-1).

Teach the patient to avoid reading, writing, and close work, such as sewing, in the first week after surgery because these activities cause rapid eye movements and promote detachment. Teach him or her the manifestations of infection and detachment (sudden reduced visual acuity, eye pain, pupil that does not respond to light by constricting). Instruct the patient to notify the surgeon immediately if these manifestations occur.

RETINITIS PIGMENTOSA

Several types of retinal disorders can cause progressive degeneration of the retina and lead to blindness. Retinitis pigmentosa (RP) is a condition in which retinal nerve cells degenerate and the pigmented cells of the retina grow and move into the sensory areas of the retina, causing further degeneration.

GENETIC CONSIDERATIONS

Different forms of retinitis pigmentosa can be inherited as an autosomal dominant (AD) trait, an autosomal recessive (AR) trait, or an X-linked recessive trait (Nussbaum et al., 2007). Mutations in more than 20 genes have been identified as being responsible for retinitis pigmentosa, and gene testing for nearly 800 mutations of the AR and AD forms of the problem is commercially available.

The most common early manifestation of retinitis pigmentosa is night blindness, often occurring in childhood. Over time, decreased visual acuity progresses to total blindness. Examination of the retina shows heavy pigmentation in a lacy pattern. Cataracts may accompany this disorder.

No current therapy has proved effective in preventing the degenerative process. The ingestion of 15,000 international units of vitamin A daily has been moderately effective in slowing the progression of the disorder in some patients (Foundation Fighting Blindness, 2008). Other treatments under investigation include retinal microchip implantation and the use of stem cell therapy.

REFRACTIVE ERRORS

Pathophysiology

The ability of the eye to focus images on the retina depends on the length of the eye from front to back and the refractive power of the lens system. **Refraction** is the bending of light rays. Problems in either eye length or refraction can result in refractive errors.

Myopia is nearsightedness. The refractive ability of the eye is too strong for the eye length. Images are bent and fall in front of, not on, the retina. **Hyperopia,** also called *hypermetropia,* is farsightedness. The refractive ability of the eye is too weak, causing images to be focused behind the retina. A short eye length may contribute to the development of hyperopia.

Presbyopia is the age-related problem in which the lens loses its elasticity and is less able to alter its shape to focus the eye for close work. As a result, images fall behind the retina. This problem usually begins in people in their 30s and 40s. **Astigmatism** occurs when the curve of the cornea is uneven. Because light rays are not refracted equally in all directions, the image does not focus on the retina.

Patient-Centered Collaborative Care

Refractive errors are diagnosed through a process known as **refraction.** The patient is asked to view an eye chart while lenses of different strengths are systematically placed in front of the eye. With each lens strength, he or she is asked whether the lenses sharpen or worsen vision. The strength of the lens needed to focus the image on the retina is expressed in measurements called *diopters.*

Nonsurgical Management

Errors of refraction can be corrected with a lens that focuses light rays on the retina (see Fig. 48-5 in Chapter 48). Hyperopic vision is corrected to bring the image forward onto the retina with a concave lens. Myopic vision is corrected with a convex lens to move the focused image back to the retina.

Eyeglasses are used to correct refractive errors. Advantages of eyeglasses are ease of use, durability, availability, and relatively low cost. Disadvantages include a change in appearance, the weight of the frame on the nose, and reduced peripheral vision (vision is corrected only when the patient looks through the center of the lens).

Contact lenses also correct refractive errors. Round plastic disks rest against the cornea and fit under the eyelid. Hard contact lenses correct errors in two ways—by changing the shape of the cornea and by providing direct refraction. Changing corneal shape increases its refracting ability. Direct refraction from the contact lens places the specific refractive power and shape needed in front of the eye so that light rays are correctly focused onto the retina.

Complications of hard contact lens wear include corneal edema, which occurs when the lenses are worn for an extended period. Corneal abrasions can result from overwear, which dries the cornea and causes minute breaks, or from the irritation of the contact lens against the cornea.

Soft contact lenses are larger but better tolerated than hard contact lenses. They resemble the thickness of plastic wrap and can be worn for longer periods because this type of lens allows greater corneal access to moisture and oxygen. Most problems with wearing soft lenses are related to lens deterioration, deposits in the lens, and failure to follow correct lens care practices.

There are two types of soft contact lenses: daily-wear lenses (worn during waking hours) and extended-wear lenses. Extended-wear contact lenses can be worn continuously for several days to several weeks, depending on the patient's environment, activities, and tolerance of the lenses.

Surgical Management

Surgery is a popular alternative for the treatment of refractive errors. The most common vision-enhancing surgeries are laser in-situ keratomileusis (LASIK), placement of Intacs corneal ring segments, and lens replacement. (See surgical intervention for cataracts on p. 1094). All surgical procedures are much more expensive than eyeglasses or any type of contact lens. These procedures, performed as ambulatory surgery, are rarely covered by insurance.

Laser in-situ keratomileusis (LASIK) is a very popular procedure for correcting nearsightedness, farsightedness, and astigmatism using the excimer laser. The superficial layers of the cornea are lifted temporarily as a flap, and brief but powerful laser pulses reshape the deeper corneal layers. After reshaping the deeper layers, the corneal flap is placed back into its original position.

Usually both eyes are treated at the same time, although some people with presbyopia elect to have only one eye corrected for near vision (monovision). Most patients have improved vision within an hour after surgery. Complete healing to best vision may take up to 4 weeks. The outer corneal layer is not damaged. Pain is minimal, and the process can correct a wide variety of refractive errors.

After LASIK correction of refractive errors, many patients no longer require eyeglasses or contact lenses. Overcorrection or undercorrection is possible, however, and some patients may need a mild prescription for a continued refractive error.

Complications include corneal clouding, chronic dry eyes, and refractive errors. Some patients have developed blurred vision and other refractive errors months to years after this surgery as a result of keratectasia. This problem is related to the formation of the corneal flap during surgery and laser-thinning of the cornea. The cornea then becomes unstable and does not refract appropriately.

Intacs corneal ring placement enhances vision for nearsightedness. This surgery does not involve the use of a laser and has the advantage of being reversible. With this procedure, the shape of the cornea is changed by placing a flexible ring in the outer edges of the cornea (outside of the optical zone).

The procedure is performed on both eyes during one surgery under local anesthesia. Improvement to best vision is immediate. Overcorrection or undercorrection of refraction is possible. However, removal, replacement, or adjustment of ring tightness can enhance satisfaction. In addition, replacements can be made if the patient's vision changes further as a result of aging. Because the ring is applied to the cornea outside of the optical zone, the risk for corneal clouding or scarring is lower than with other surgical procedures.

TRAUMA

Trauma to the eye or orbital area can result from almost any activity. Care varies depending on the area of the eye affected and whether the globe of the eye has been penetrated.

HYPHEMA

A **hyphema** is a hemorrhage in the anterior chamber. It occurs when a force is applied to the eye and breaks the blood vessels. If the hyphema is large, it may block the pupil and reduce vision, possibly causing pain and photophobia. Hemolysis of the blood occurs, and the blood is filtered out of the eye through the trabecular meshwork. If the blood particles obstruct the meshwork, increased intraocular pressure (IOP) results.

The patient with a hyphema is treated by bedrest in semi-Fowler's position to use gravity as an aid in keeping the hyphema away from the optical center of the cornea. Minimal or no sudden eye movements are permitted for 3 to 5 days to decrease the risk for rebleeding. Cycloplegic eyedrops may be prescribed to place the eye at rest, and the eye is protected by a patch and shield. Television and reading are restricted. A hyphema usually resolves in 5 to 7 days.

CONTUSION

A contusion of the eyeball and surrounding tissue is caused by traumatic contact with a blunt object. The force of the blow pushes the eye back in the socket. The globe is compressed, and stretching of the ocular soft tissues occurs, which can damage and possibly rupture the globe. Results of the injury may not be seen immediately. These results include edema of the eyelids, subconjunctival hemorrhage, corneal edema, and hyphema.

Periorbital ecchymosis, or "black eye," a common contusion injury, is usually caused by blunt trauma. Bleeding into the soft tissue occurs, creating the bruise. The color fades gradually and disappears in 10 to 14 days. Visual acuity is usually not affected, although orbital pain, photophobia, eyelid edema, and diplopia may be present.

Treatment begins at the time of injury. Ice is applied immediately. The patient should have a thorough eye examination to rule out any other eye injuries.

FOREIGN BODIES

Eyelashes, dust, fingernails, dirt, and airborne particles can come in contact with the conjunctiva or cornea and irritate or abrade the surface. If nothing is seen on the cornea or conjunctiva, the eyelid is everted to examine the conjunctiva. The patient usually has a feeling of something being in the eye and may have blurred vision. Pain occurs if the corneal surface is injured. Tearing and photophobia may be present.

Evaluation of vision is done before treatment (Boyd-Monk, 2005). The eye of any patient with a suspected corneal abrasion is examined with fluorescein, followed by irrigation with normal saline (0.9%) to gently remove the particles. Best practices for ocular irrigation are listed in Chart 49-8.

After the foreign body is removed and if an eye patch is applied, tell the patient how long the patch must be left in place (patching over corneal abrasions is controversial). Follow-up with the ophthalmologist is needed.

LACERATIONS

Lacerations are wounds caused by sharp objects and projectiles. The injury can occur to any part of the eye, but the most commonly injured areas are the eyelids and the cornea.

Initially, close the eye and apply a small ice pack to decrease bleeding. The patient should receive medical attention as soon as possible. If the patient can open the eye, check visual acuity and clean the eyelids. Minor lacerations of the eyelid can be sutured in an emergency department, an urgent care center, or an ophthalmologist's office. A microscope is needed in the operating room if the patient has a laceration that involves the eyelid margin, affects the lacrimal system, involves a large area, or has jagged edges.

Corneal lacerations are an emergency because eye contents may prolapse through the laceration. Manifestations include severe eye pain, photophobia, tearing, decreased visual acuity, and inability to open the eyelid. If the laceration is the result of a penetrating injury, an object may be seen protruding from the eye. *The object is removed only by the ophthalmologist, because it may be holding eye structures in place.*

Antibiotics are given to reduce the risk for infection. Depending on the depth of the laceration, scarring may develop. If the scar alters vision, a corneal transplant may be needed later. If the eye contents have prolapsed through the laceration or if the injury is severe, **enucleation** (surgical eye removal) may be indicated.

PENETRATING INJURIES

Patients with penetrating eye injuries have the poorest chance of retaining vision in the injured eye. Glass, high-speed metal or wood particles, BB pellets, and bullets are common causes of penetrating injuries. The particles can enter the eye and lodge in or behind the eyeball.

The patient usually has some eye pain and says he or she "suddenly felt something hit my eye." An entrance wound may be visible. Depending on the location of the entrance and the resting place of the projectile, vision may be affected.

X-rays and computed tomography (CT) scans of the orbit are usually performed. Computer-generated reconstructions of the CT images are created to study this complex area to ensure the orbit is intact and to look for fractures that might entrap orbital muscles. *Magnetic resonance imaging (MRI) is contraindicated because the procedure may move any metal-containing projectile and cause more injury.*

Surgery is usually needed to remove the foreign object. In some cases, foreign bodies need to be removed by a vitrectomy. IV antibiotics are started before surgery to reduce the risk for infection. A tetanus booster is given if necessary.

Assess and document visual acuity. If the patient cannot see print, determine whether he or she can count fingers or see hand motions. If the patient cannot see movement, assess his or her ability to see light.

OCULAR MELANOMA

Pathophysiology

Melanoma is the most common malignant eye tumor in adults (American Cancer Society, 2008). This tumor occurs most often in the uveal tract among people in their 30s and 40s and is associated with exposure to UV light. Because of its rich blood supply, a melanoma can spread easily. Spread occurs by

Chart 49-8 BEST PRACTICE FOR PATIENT SAFETY & QUALITY CARE

Ocular Irrigation

1. Assemble equipment:
   - Normal saline IV (1000-mL bag)
   - Macrodrip IV tubing
   - IV pole
   - Eyelid speculum
   - Topical anesthetic (proparacaine hydrochloride)
   - Gloves
   - Collection receptacle (emesis basin works well)
   - Towels
   - pH paper
2. Quickly obtain a history from the patient while flushing the tubing with normal saline:
   - Nature and time of the injury
   - Type of irritant or chemical (if known)
   - Type of first aid administered at the scene
   - Any allergies to the "caine" family of medications
3. Evaluate the patient's visual acuity *before* treatment:
   - Ask the patient to read your name tag with the affected eye while covering the good eye.
   - Ask the patient to "count fingers" with the affected eye while covering the good eye.
4. Put on gloves.
5. Place a strip of pH paper in the cul-de-sac of the patient's affected eye to test the pH of the agent splashed into the eye and to know when it has been washed out.
6. Instill proparacaine hydrochloride eyedrops as prescribed.
7. Place the patient in a supine position with the head turned slightly toward the affected eye.
8. Have the patient hold the affected eye open, or position an eyelid speculum.
9. Direct the flow of normal saline across the affected eye from the nasal corner of the eye toward the outer corner of the eye.
10. Assess the patient's comfort during the procedure.
11. If both eyes are affected, irrigate them simultaneously using separate personnel and equipment.

extension through the sclera or invasion of other eye structures into nearby tissue and the brain.

Patient-Centered Collaborative Care

Manifestations of melanoma may not be readily apparent; the tumor may be discovered during a routine examination. Blurring of vision may occur if the macular area is invaded. Visual acuity is reduced if the tumor grows inward toward the center of the eye from the choroid and alters the visual pathway. Increased intraocular pressure (IOP) can result if the tumor invades the canal of Schlemm and obstructs flow of aqueous humor. A change in iris color may occur if the tumor infiltrates the iris. Sudden loss of a portion of the visual field may result from tumor invasion of the space under the retina, producing retinal detachment.

Diagnostic tests for a melanoma depend on the size and tumor growth rate. Ultrasonography or MRI is performed to determine the tumor's location and size. Treatment also depends on the tumor's size and growth rate, as well as the condition of the other eye. Small lesions of the iris not affecting the iris root are monitored until growth is observed. Tumors of the choroid are treated by surgical enucleation or by radiation therapy with a radioactive plaque.

Enucleation (surgical removal of the entire eyeball) is the most common surgery for ocular melanoma and is performed under general anesthesia. After the eye is removed, a ball implant is inserted to provide a base for the socket prosthesis and to ensure the best cosmetic result.

The implant is covered with surrounding tissue, muscles, and conjunctiva. A plastic conformer is placed over the conjunctiva to maintain the shape of the eyelids until a prosthesis can be fitted. After the dressing is removed, a pressure patch is placed over the eye for 24 hours.

Until the prosthesis is fitted (about 1 month after surgery), an antibiotic-steroid ointment is inserted into the cul-de-sac once daily. Best practices for the insertion and removal of the prosthesis are listed in Chart 49-9.

Chart 49-9 BEST PRACTICE FOR PATIENT SAFETY & QUALITY CARE

Insertion and Removal of an Ocular Prosthesis

INSERTION

1. Assemble equipment:
   - Prosthesis
   - Gloves
   - Towel
2. Explain the procedure to the patient.
3. Wash your hands.
4. Cover the work area with a cloth or towel.
5. Don gloves.
6. Remove the prosthesis from its container, and rinse it with tepid water.
7. Lift the patient's upper lid using your nondominant hand.

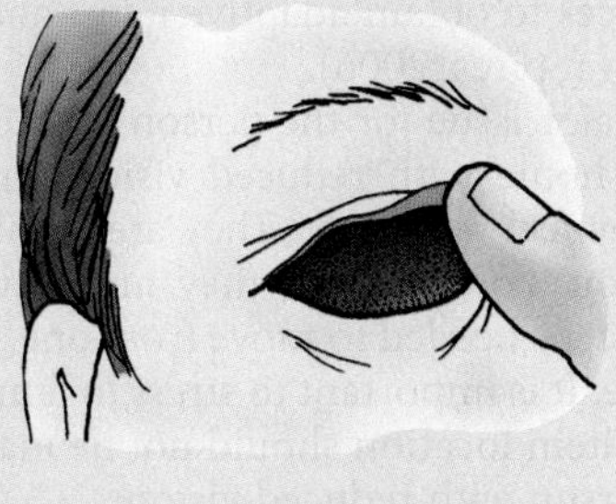

8. Place the prosthesis between the thumb and forefinger of your dominant hand. The notched end of the prosthesis should be closest to the patient's nose.

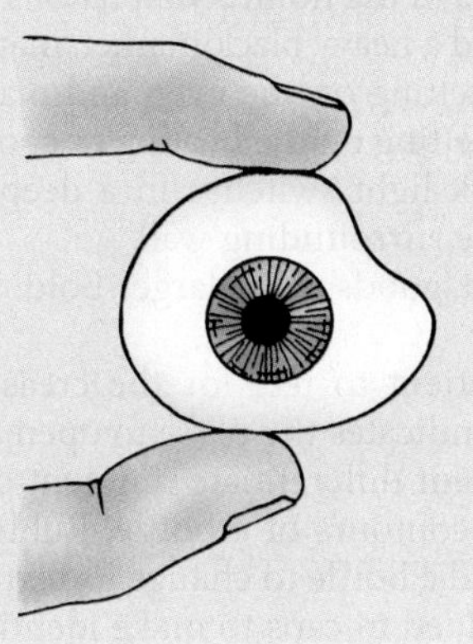

9. Insert the prosthesis with the top edge slipping under the upper lid. Continue until most of the iris is covered by the upper lid.

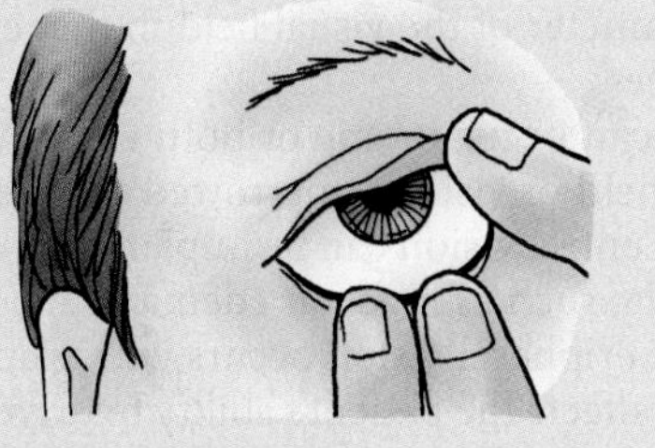

10. Gently release the upper eyelid.
11. Retract the lower lid slightly until the bottom edge of the prosthesis slips behind it.

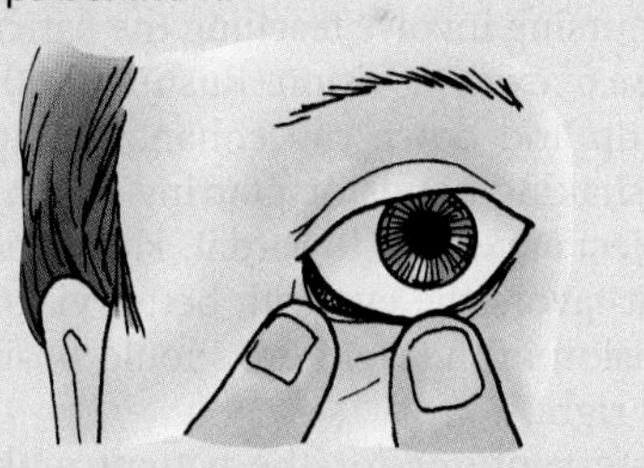

12. Release your hands slowly.

REMOVAL

1. Assemble equipment:
   - Normal saline–filled, labeled container
   - Gloves
2. Explain the procedure to the patient.
3. Wash your hands.
4. Don gloves.
5. Instruct the patient to sit up and tilt the head slightly downward.
6. Place your hand against the patient's cheek, palm side up.
7. Pull the lower lid slightly down and laterally.
8. Allow the prosthesis to slide out onto your hand, or pull gently if necessary.
9. Place the prosthesis in a container filled with normal saline labeled with the patient's name. Cover the container.

Radiation therapy is an "eye-sparing" procedure that can reduce the size and thickness of melanomas but rarely eliminates the tumors completely. The radioactive plaque—a round, flat disk about the size of a dime and containing a radioactive material—is sutured to the sclera overlying the tumor site. The length of time the plaque remains sutured to the sclera depends on the size of the tumor and the dose of radiation to be delivered.

Complications of radiation therapy include vascular changes, retinopathy, glaucoma, necrosis of the sclera, and cataract formation. Vitreous hemorrhage may develop as the tumor becomes smaller and pulls or breaks blood vessels.

While the plaque is in place, the eye may or may not be covered with a patch. Cycloplegic eyedrops and an antibiotic-steroid combination are given. Teach the patient how to instill eyedrops.

REDUCED VISION

Pathophysiology

Different forms of reduced vision may affect any or all aspects of vision, including color, light, image, movement, and acuity. Some periods of reduced vision may be temporary, such as when cataracts obscure vision but surgery has not yet been performed. Patients are legally blind if their best visual acuity with corrective lenses is 20/200 or less in the better eye or if the widest diameter of the visual field in that eye is no greater than 20 degrees.

Blindness can occur in one or both eyes. When one eye is affected, the field of vision is narrowed and depth perception is impaired. Central vision can be impaired by diseases involving the macula, such as macular edema or macular degeneration. Loss of peripheral vision occurs with glaucoma. The loss of side vision affects the patient's ability to drive and awareness of hazards in the periphery.

Patient-Centered Collaborative Care

Priorities for nursing involve teaching the patient techniques to make better use of existing vision (Rushing, 2007b). Moving the head slightly up and down can enhance a three-dimensional effect. When shaking hands or pouring water, the patient can line up the object and move toward it. He or she should choose a position that favors the eye with better vision. For example, people with vision in the right eye should position people and items on their right.

Nursing interventions for the patient with reduced sight focus on communication, safety, ambulation, self-care, and support (Watkinson, 2005). Chart 49-10 lists ways to help patients with reduced vision to function as independently as possible.

Communication is important in helping the patient remain independent and connected to the world. Reduced vision is a common occurrence, and many adaptive devices have been developed to help the person living with reduced vision maintain independence. Many towns and cities now have auditory traffic signals so that persons with reduced vision can know when it is safe to cross a street. Curbs in these areas may have high-contrast color paint to let the person know when to step up or down. Libraries have large-print books and books on tape. "Talking" clocks, watches, and timers are available. Playing cards, games, restaurant menus, calendars, and instruction booklets are available in large print sizes. Computer keyboards with high contrast and larger letters in the keys are available, as are large screens. Direct the patient with reduced vision to the local resources to obtain adaptive items and to learn how best to use them (Spires, 2006).

Safety is a major issue for the person with reduced vision. For patients at home with reduced vision, the home is the place where they feel most safe. They are familiar with room and item location. For example, they may have counted the number of footsteps needed to move from one area to another within the home. It is important to stress to family and friends that changes in item location should not be made without input from the person with reduced vision.

Even people who have experienced gradually reduced vision over time and who use Vision Compensation Behaviors in the home may benefit from having a person with vision assist in making adaptations in the home. Adaptations may include:

- Using tape and a heavy black marker, mark the 350-degree temperature setting on the oven and mark the 70-degree temperature setting on the heating or cooling thermostat.
- Paint or mark light switches in a deep color that contrasts with the surrounding wall.
- Label canned goods with large, bold, black letters on white tape.
- Teach the patient to feel for the crease in paper milk cartons that indicates the place to open the spout.
- Help the patient differentiate different drugs by altering the shape or contours of a bottle. Rubber bands can be wound around a bottle to change its texture. Raised symbols can be glued to caps to make identification easier.

Chart 49-10 NIC INTERVENTION ACTIVITIES

The Patient with Reduced Vision

Communication Enhancement: Visual Deficit: *Assistance in accepting and learning alternate methods for living with diminished vision*

- Identify yourself when you enter the patient's space.
- Note patient's reaction to diminished vision (e.g., depression, withdrawal, denial).
- Accept patient's reaction to diminished vision.
- Assist patient in setting new goals to learn how to "see" with other senses.
- Build on patient's remaining vision, as appropriate.
- Walk one or two steps ahead of the patient, with patient's hand on your elbow.
- Describe environment to patient.
- Do not move items in patient's room without informing patient.
- Read mail, newspaper, and other pertinent information to patient.
- Identify items on food tray in relation to numbers on a clock.
- Fold paper money in different ways for easy identification.
- Inform patient where to locate radio or talking books.
- Provide a magnifying glass or prism eyeglasses, as appropriate, for reading.
- Provide braille reading material, as appropriate.
- Initiate occupational therapy referral, as appropriate.
- Refer patient with visual problems to appropriate agency.

The patient is most at risk for safety problems in an unfamiliar or changing environment. When a person with reduced vision must be hospitalized, promote safety and independence by orienting him or her to the new environment.

Most people with reduced vision had full sight at some time and thus have a background knowledge regarding size and shape that can be used when providing information. Many blind people have some degree of sight. When talking with a person who has limited sight or is blind, always use a normal tone of voice unless he or she is has a hearing problem.

First orient the patient to the immediate environment, including the size of the room. Use one object in the room, such as a chair or hospital bed, as the focal point during your description. Guide the person to the focal point, and orient him or her to the environment from that point. For example, you might say, "To the left of the bed is a chair." Then describe all other objects in relation to the focal point. Go with the patient to other important areas, such as the bathroom, so that he or she can learn their locations. Highlight the location of the toilet, sink, and toilet paper holder. *Never leave the patient with reduced vision in the center of an unfamiliar room.*

Patients with reduced vision prefer to establish the location of important objects, such as the call light, water pitcher, and clock. Once their location has been fixed, do not move these items without the patient's consent. Do not move the location of chairs, stools, and wastebaskets without consulting the patient.

At mealtime, set up food on the tray using clock placement. For example, "There is sliced ham at the 6 o'clock position; peas are located at the 3 o'clock position; to the right of the plate is coffee; salt and pepper are next to the coffee."

Ambulation with a patient who has reduced vision involves allowing him or her to grasp your arm at the elbow. Keep the arm close to your body so that he or she can detect your direction of movement. Alert the patient when obstacles are in the path ahead.

Patients may use a cane to detect obstacles, such as furniture, walls, or curbs. The cane is held in the dominant hand several inches off the floor and sweeps the ground where his or her foot will be placed next. The laser cane sends out signals to help detect obstacles.

Self-care and the ability to control the environment are important. Knock on the door before entering the hospital room or any other environment of a patient with reduced vision. State your name and the reason for visiting when entering the room. Coordinate with other members of the health care team to ensure this etiquette is used consistently. Mark the door to the room to indicate it is occupied by a patient with reduced vision.

Support is needed, especially when the reduced vision is of sudden onset and may be permanent. Patients' reactions to the loss of sight are similar to the reaction to loss of a body part. Allow the newly blind person a period of grieving for the "dead" (nonseeing) eye. He or she may feel hopeless and angry. With time, anger usually gives way to acceptance. The ability to cope may begin within days, but some patients mourn for months or years.

Patients benefit from the honest support that you can provide. They need to hear that it is normal to mourn, to cry, and to feel the loss. Help them move toward acceptance by encouraging the mastery of one task at a time and by providing positive reinforcement for each success.

HUMAN NEEDS NURSING CARE REVIEW

What might you NOTICE if the patient is experiencing reduced sensation as a result of vision problems?

Assessment

- Patient squints or tilts the head when viewing objects or print at a distance.
- Patient closes one eye to read or see at a distance.
- Patient moves reading materials either very close to his or her face or as far away from the face as he or she can reach.
- Patient may not startle when a sudden move is made at the face.
- Pupils are unequal and may not react to light.
- Eyes do not focus on a distant object and track it as it is moved closer to the face.
- Red reflex may be absent or present only in one eye.
- Appearance is disheveled with buttons not properly buttoned, clothing colors or patterns not complementary, and hair parts uneven.
- Patient does not make eye contact and turns head toward sounds rather than sights.
- Patient does not comment on the presence of art or unusual visual objects in the immediate environment.
- Patient walks with hesitation into a room or bumps into objects in his or her path.
- Patient may seem confused about time and place.

What should you INTERPRET and how should you RESPOND to a patient experiencing reduced sensation as a result of vision problems?

Interpret by:

- Assessing visual acuity with a Snellen chart, counting fingers, hand motion, or light perception.
- Asking the patient to describe the objects in the room and their colors.
- Asking the patient what he or she can see well and what is more difficult to see.

Respond by:

- Orienting the patient to the immediate surroundings.
- Offering your arm for the patient to hold when he or she is moving to a different location.
- Not leaving the patient alone in the center of a strange room.
- Asking him or her what assistance is needed for independent activity.
- Assessing the immediate environment for safety hazards and removing the hazard.

GET READY FOR THE NCLEX EXAMINATION!

Key Points

Review these Key Points for each NCLEX Examination Client Needs Category.

Safe and Effective Care Environment

- Use Contact Precautions with any patient who has drainage from the eye or tear duct.
- Avoid performing an ophthalmoscopic examination on a confused or uncooperative patient.
- Orient the patient with reduced vision to his or her immediate surroundings, including how to call for help and where the bathroom is located.
- Identify the room of a patient with reduced vision (without identifying the patient).

Health Promotion and Maintenance

- Identify people at risk for visual impairment as a result of work environment or leisure activities, and teach them specific ways to protect the eyes.
- Encourage all patients to wear eye protection when they are performing yard work, are working in a woodshop or metal shop, are using chemicals, or are in any environment in which drops or particulate matter is airborne.
- Encourage all adult patients older than 40 years to have an eye examination with measurement of intraocular pressure every year.
- Encourage everyone to use polarizing sunglasses whenever outdoors in bright sunlight.
- Teach all patients to wash their hands before and after touching the eyes.

Psychosocial Integrity

- Use a normal tone of voice to talk with a patient who has a vision problem and normal hearing.
- Knock on the door before entering the room of a patient with reduced vision, and introduce yourself.
- Allow the patient and family the opportunity to express their feelings and concerns regarding a change in vision.
- Refer patients newly diagnosed with visual impairment to appropriate local resources and support groups.
- Explain all diagnostic procedures, restrictions, and follow-up care to the patient scheduled for tests.

Physiological Integrity

- Ask the patient about vision problems in any other members of the family, because many vision problems have a genetic component.
- Teach patients the proper technique to use for self-instillation of eyedrops and eye ointment.
- Stress the importance of completing an antibiotic regimen when an infection is present in the eye.
- Teach patients who are at risk for increased intraocular pressure what activities to avoid (see Table 49-1).
- Teach patients with an infection of the eye or eyelid not to rub the eye (to avoid infecting the other eye).
- *Never attempt to remove any object protruding from the eye.*

Additional Study Resources

Go to your Companion CD or Evolve at http://evolve.elsevier.com/Iggy/ for *Self-Assessment Questions for the NCLEX Examination.*

Go to Evolve at http://evolve.elsevier.com/Iggy/ for *Prioritization and Delegation Questions for the NCLEX Examination.*

SELECTED BIBLIOGRAPHY

Asterisk indicates a classic or definitive work on this subject.

American Cancer Society. (2008). *Cancer facts and figures 2008.* Report No. 00-300M–No. 5008.08. Atlanta: Author.

Bourla, D., & Young, T. (2006). Age-related macular degeneration: A practical approach to a challenging disease. *Journal of the American Gerontological Society, 54*(7), 1130-1135.

Boyd-Monk, H. (2005). Bringing common eye emergencies into focus. *Nursing2005, 35*(12), 46-51.

Camp-Sorrell, D. (2007). Eye infection: What's the culprit? *Clinical Journal of Oncology Nursing, 11*(2), 189-190.

Covell, C.A., Graziano, J.A., Rich, D., & Tobin, K.A. (2007). New outlook for age-related macular degeneration. *Nursing2007, 37*(3), 22-24.

Davis, G. (2006). Anatomy of the eye in relation to common drug therapies. *Nurse Prescribing, 4*(7), 274-278.

Foundation Fighting Blindness. (2008). Retrieved January 2008, from www.blindness.org

Halvorson, P. (2005). The silent thief. *RN, 68*(3), 41-45.

Hodge, W., Horsley, T., Albiani, D., Baryla, J., Belliveau, M., Buhrmann, R., et al. (2007). The consequences of waiting for cataract surgery: A systematic review. *Canadian Medical Association Journal, 176*(9), 1285-1290.

Jarvis, C. (2008). *Physical examination and health assessment* (5th ed.). Philadelphia: Saunders.

Kaiser, P. (2007). Verteporfin photodynamic therapy and anti-angiogenic drugs: Potential for combination therapy in exudative age-related macular degeneration. *Current Medical Research & Opinion, 23*(3), 477-487.

Keeping an eye on abnormalities. (2008). *Nursing2008, 38*(1), 48-49.

Kowing, D., & Kester, E. (2007). Keep an eye out for glaucoma. *The Nurse Practitioner, 32*(7), 18-23.

McCance, K., & Huether, S. (2006). *Pathophysiology: The biologic basis for disease in adults and children* (5th ed.). St. Louis: Mosby.

Meiner, S., & Lueckenotte, A. (Eds.). (2006). *Gerontologic nursing,* (3rd ed.). St. Louis: Mosby.

Nussbaum, R., McInnes, R., & Willard, H. (2007). *Thompson & Thompson: Genetics in medicine* (7th ed.). Philadelphia: Saunders.

Pagana, K., & Pagana, T. (2006). *Mosby's manual of diagnostic and laboratory tests* (3rd ed.). St. Louis: Mosby.

Rushing, J. (2007a). Administering eyedrops. *Nursing2007, 37*(5), 18.

Rushing, J. (2007b). Helping a patient who's visually impaired. *Nursing2007, 37*(8), 29.

Saligan, L., & Yeh, S. (2008). Seeing red: Guiding the management of ocular hyperemia. *The Nurse Practitioner, 33* (6), 14-20.

Schmidt-Luggen, A. (2006). GNP care guidelines: Update on macular degeneration. *Geriatric Nursing, 27*(3), 159.

Sitzman, K. (2006). Promoting eye health: Prevention and detection of cataracts. *American Association of Occupational Health Nurses, 54*(4), 188.

Spires, R. (2006). How you can help when older eyes fail. *RN, 69*(2), 38-43.

*Vaughan, D., Asbury, T., & Riordan-Eva, P. (Eds.). (2004). *General ophthalmology* (16th ed.). New York: McGraw-Hill.

Watkinson, S. (2005). Visual impairment in older people: The nurse's role. *Nursing Standard, 19*(17), 45-52, 54-55.

Whiteside, M., Wallhagen, M., & Pettengill, E. (2006). Sensory impairment in older adults. Part 2. Vision loss. *AJN, 106*(11), 52-61.

Assessment of the Ear and Hearing

50

CHAPTER

Jacquelyn Ann Russek

LEARNING OUTCOMES

For clinical competence and success on the NCLEX Examination, study this chapter with these Learning Outcomes in mind:

Safe and Effective Care Environment

1. Apply principles of infection control when examining an ear with drainage.

Health Promotion and Maintenance

2. Teach all people how to perform ear hygiene safely.
3. Teach all people to use ear protection equipment and strategies.

Psychosocial Integrity

4. Teach patients and family members about what to expect during tests and procedures to assess ear and hearing problems.
5. Provide the opportunity for the patient and family to express their feelings and concerns about a possible change in hearing.

Physiological Integrity

6. Identify people at risk for hearing problems as a result of drug therapy, genetic predisposition, or exposure to environmental hazards.
7. Perform a clinical ear and hearing assessment, including health history and psychosocial assessment.
8. Describe adaptations needed when caring for patients who have age-related changes in the structure of the ear and hearing.
9. Identify 10 common drugs that affect hearing.
10. Demonstrate the correct use of an otoscope.

evolve Go to your Companion CD or Evolve at http://evolve.elsevier.com/Iggy/ for *Self-Assessment Questions for the NCLEX Examination* keyed to these Learning Outcomes.

The ear, along with the brain, is the organ that allows hearing. Hearing is one of the five senses important for communicating with the world. Functional hearing assists in meeting the *human need for sensation and cognition.* It is used to assess surroundings, allow independence, warn of danger, appreciate music, work, play, and interact with other people.

Ear and hearing problems are common among adults of all ages. Assessment of the ear and hearing is an important skill for nurses in any care environment. Therefore an understanding of the anatomy and physiology of the ear is essential. Many ear and hearing problems develop over long periods of time and may be affected by drugs or systemic health problems.

ANATOMY AND PHYSIOLOGY REVIEW

Structure

The ear has three divisions: the external ear, the middle ear, and the inner ear. Each part is important to hearing.

External Ear

The external ear develops in the embryo at the same time as the kidneys and urinary tract. Thus any person with a defect of the external ear should be examined for possible problems of the renal and urinary systems.

The **pinna** is the part of the external ear that is composed of cartilage covered by skin and attached to the head at about a 10-degree angle. It is embedded in the temporal bone on both sides of the head at the level of the eyes. The external ear also includes the **mastoid process,** which is the bony ridge located over the temporal bone behind the pinna. The external ear extends from the pinna through the external ear canal to the **tympanic membrane** (eardrum) (Fig. 50-1). The ear canal is slightly S-shaped and lined with **cerumen** (wax)–producing glands, sebaceous glands, and hair follicles. Cerumen helps protect and lubricate the ear canal. The hair follicles and cerumen protect the eardrum and the middle ear. The distance from the opening of the ear canal to the eardrum in an adult is 1 to $1\frac{1}{2}$ inches (2.5 to 3.75 cm).

Middle Ear

The middle ear begins at the medial or inner side of the eardrum. The eardrum separates the external ear and the middle ear.

The middle ear consists of a compartment called the **epitympanum.** Located in the epitympanum are the top opening of the eustachian tube and three small bones known as the **bony ossicles,** which are the **malleus** (hammer), the **incus** (anvil), and the **stapes** (stirrup) (Fig. 50-2). The bony ossicles are joined loosely, thereby moving with vibrations created when sound waves hit the eardrum.

The eardrum, a thick sheet of tissue, is transparent, opaque, or pearly gray and moves when air is injected into the external canal. The landmarks on the eardrum include the *annulus,* the *pars flaccida,* and the *pars tensa.* These correspond to the parts of the bones of the middle ear that can be seen through the transparent eardrum. The eardrum is attached to the first bony ossicle, the malleus, at the umbo (Fig. 50-3). The umbo is seen through the eardrum membrane as a white dot and is one end of the long process of the malleus. The pars flaccida is that portion of the eardrum above the short process of the malleus. The pars tensa is that portion surrounding the long process of the malleus.

The middle ear is separated from the inner ear by the round window and the oval window. The eustachian tube begins at the floor of the middle ear and extends to the throat. The tube opening in the throat is surrounded by adenoid lym-

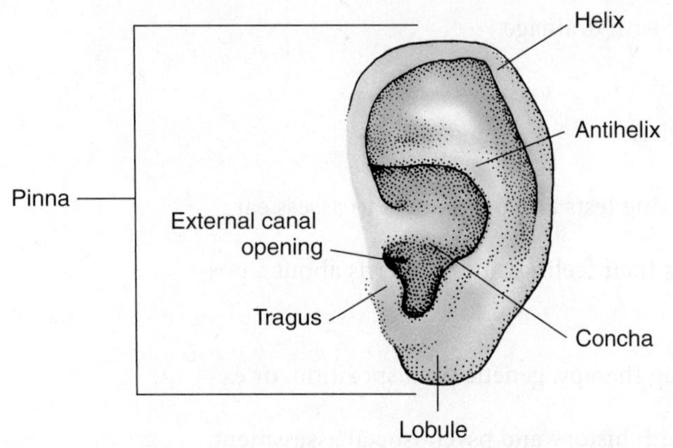
Helix
Antihelix
Pinna
External canal opening
Tragus
Concha
Lobule

Fig. 50-1 • Anatomic features of the external ear.

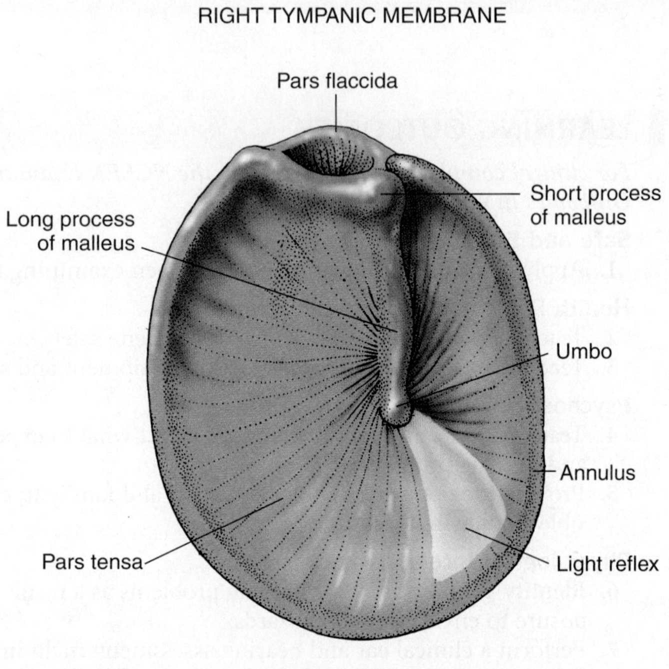
RIGHT TYMPANIC MEMBRANE
Pars flaccida
Short process of malleus
Long process of malleus
Umbo
Annulus
Pars tensa
Light reflex

Fig. 50-3 • Landmarks on the tympanic membrane.

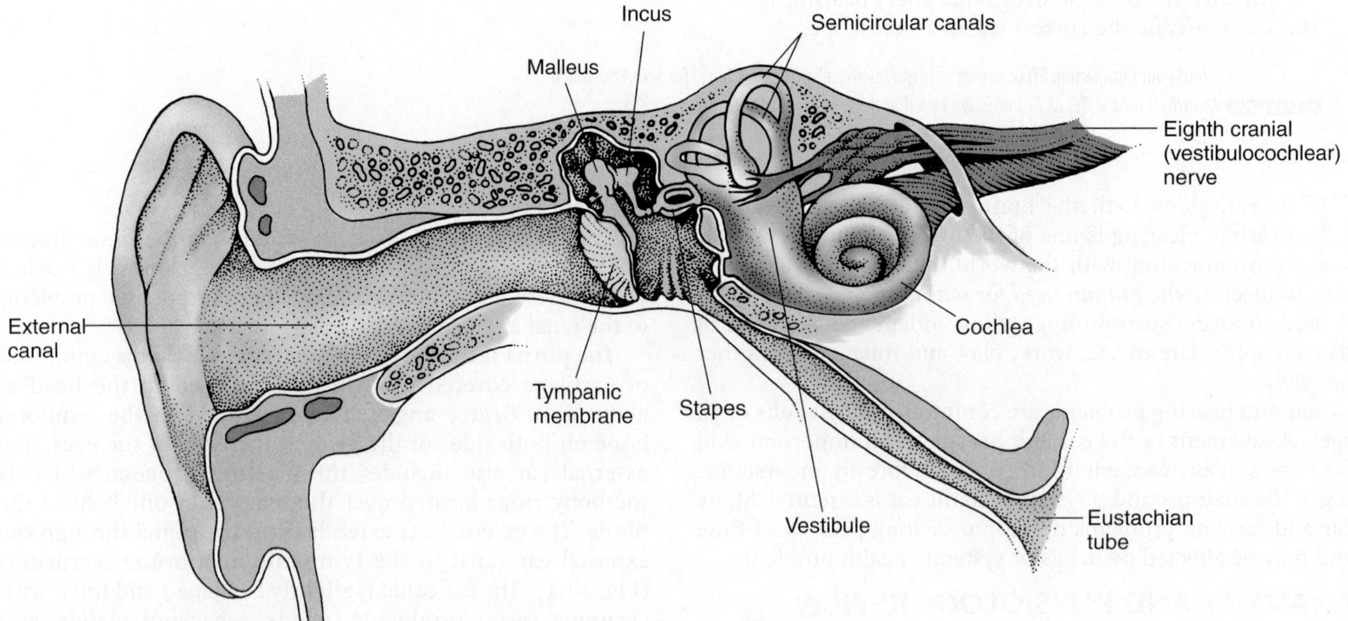
Incus
Semicircular canals
Malleus
Eighth cranial (vestibulocochlear) nerve
External canal
Cochlea
Tympanic membrane
Stapes
Vestibule
Eustachian tube

Fig. 50-2 • Anatomic features of the middle and inner ear.

phatic tissue (Fig. 50-4). The eustachian tube allows the pressure on both sides of the eardrum to equalize. Secretions from the middle ear drain through the tube into the throat.

Inner Ear

The inner ear is on the other side of the oval window and contains the semicircular canals, cochlea, vestibule, and the distal end of the eighth cranial nerve (see Fig. 50-2). The **semicircular canals** are tubes made of cartilage and contain fluid and hair cells. These canals are connected to the sensory nerve fibers of the vestibular portion of the eighth cranial nerve. The fluid and hair cells within the canals help maintain the sense of balance.

The **cochlea,** the spiral organ of hearing, is divided into the scala tympani and the scala vestibuli. The scala media is filled with *endolymph,* and the scala tympani and scala vestibuli are filled with *perilymph.* These fluids protect the cochlea and the semicircular canals by allowing these structures to "float" in the fluids and be cushioned against abrupt head movements.

The **organ of Corti** is the receptor of hearing located on the basilar membrane of the cochlea. The cochlea contains hair cells that detect vibration from sound and stimulate the eighth cranial nerve.

The **vestibule** is a small, oval-shaped, bony chamber between the semicircular canals and the cochlea. It contains the utricle and the sacculus, organs that are important for the sense of balance.

Function

Hearing is the main function of the ear and occurs when sound is delivered through the air to the external ear canal and the temporal bone covering the mastoid air cells. The sound waves strike the mastoid and the movable eardrum, creating vibrations. The eardrum is connected to the first bony ossicle, which allows the sound wave vibrations to be transferred from the eardrum to the malleus, the incus, and the stapes. From the stapes the vibrations are transmitted to the cochlea. Receptors at the cochlea transduce (change) the vibrations into action potentials. The action potentials are conducted to the brain as nerve impulses by the cochlear portion of the eighth cranial (auditory) nerve. The nerve impulses are processed and interpreted as sound by the brain in the auditory cortex of the temporal lobe.

EAR AND HEARING CHANGES ASSOCIATED WITH AGING

Ear and hearing changes related to aging are listed in Chart 50-1, along with implications for care of older patients who have these changes. Some of the ear changes, such as an increase in ear size, are harmless. Other changes to ear structures may pose threats to the hearing ability of older adults.

All older adults should be screened for hearing acuity. Many scales or tools are available to assess hearing loss. However, asking "Do you have a hearing problem now?" may be just as helpful as these scales.

ASSESSMENT METHODS

Patient History

Obtain a thorough history from the patient before performing the physical examination. Hearing assessment begins while observing the patient listening to and answering questions. The patient's posture and appropriateness of responses provide information about hearing acuity. For example, posture changes, such as tilting the head to one side or leaning forward when listening to another person speak, may indicate the presence of a hearing problem. Other indicators of hearing difficulty include frequently asking the speaker to repeat statements or frequently saying "what" or "huh." Notice whether the patient responds to whispered questions and conversa-

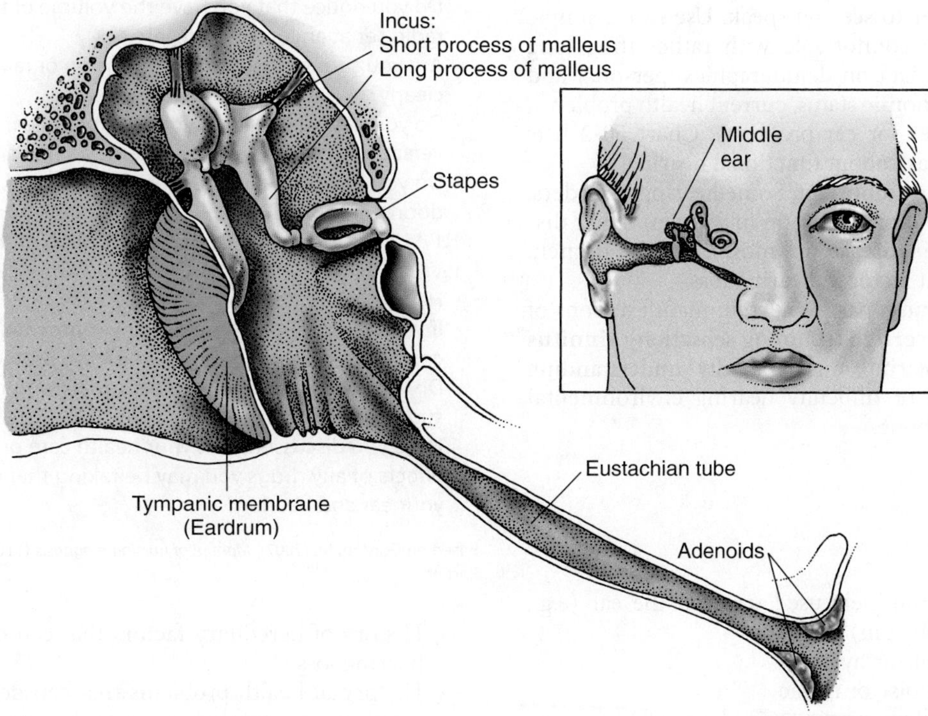
Incus:
Short process of malleus
Long process of malleus
Stapes
Middle ear
Eustachian tube
Tympanic membrane (Eardrum)
Adenoids

Fig. 50-4 • Anatomic features and attached structures of the middle ear.

Chart 50-1 NURSING FOCUS ON THE OLDER ADULT

Age-Related Changes in the Ear and Hearing

Ear or Hearing Change	Nursing Adaptations and Actions
Pinna becomes elongated because of loss of subcutaneous tissues and decreased elasticity.	Reassure the patient that this is normal and does not indicate a problem. When positioning a patient on his or her side, take care not to "fold" the ear under the head.
Hair in the canal becomes coarser and longer, especially in men.	Reassure the patient that this is normal. The patient may require more frequent ear irrigation to keep cerumen from clumping in the hair.
Cerumen is dryer and impacts more easily, reducing hearing function.	Teach the patient to irrigate the ear canal weekly or whenever he or she notices a change in hearing.
Tympanic membrane loses elasticity and may appear dull and retracted.	Do not use this finding as the only indication of otitis media.
Hearing acuity decreases (in some people).	Establish that a hearing deficiency exists, using simple, noninvasive tests such as the voice test and the watch test. If a deficit is present, refer the patient to an ear, nose, and throat specialist to determine what type of hearing loss is present and what can be done to improve hearing. Do not assume all older adults have a hearing loss!!
The ability to hear high-frequency sounds is lost first. Older adults may have particular problems hearing the *f*, *s*, *sh*, and *pa* sounds.	Provide a quiet environment when speaking (close the door to the hallway), and face the patient. If the patient wears glasses, be sure he or she is using them to see your lips and facial expression to enhance speech understanding. Speak slowly and in a deeper voice, and emphasize beginning word sounds. Some patients with a hearing loss that is not corrected may benefit from wearing a stethoscope while listening to you speak.

tions and startles when an unexpected sound occurs in the environment. Also assess whether the patient's responses match the question asked. For example, when you ask the patient, "How old are you?" does the patient respond with an age or does he or she say "No, I don't have a cold?"

During the interview, sit in adequate light and face the patient to allow him or her to see you speak. Use short, simple language the patient is comfortable with rather than long medical terms. Obtain data on demographics, personal and family history, socioeconomic status, current health problems, and the use of remedies for ear problems. Chart 50-2 lists important questions to ask about functional hearing.

The patient's gender is important. Some hearing disorders, such as otosclerosis, are more common in women. Other disorders, such as Ménière's disease, are more common in men. Age is also an important factor in hearing loss.

Personal history includes past or current manifestations of ear pain, ear discharge, **vertigo** (spinning sensation), **tinnitus** (ringing), decreased hearing, and difficulty understanding people when they talk or difficulty hearing environmental noise. Ask the patient about:

- Ear trauma
- Ear surgery
- Past ear infections
- Excessive cerumen
- Ear itch
- Any instruments routinely used to clean the ear (e.g., Q-Tip, match, bobby pin)
- Type and pattern of ear hygiene
- Exposure to loud noise or music
- Air travel (especially in unpressurized aircraft)
- Swimming habits and the use of ear protection when swimming
- History of hereditary factors that can cause progressive hearing loss
- History of health problems that can decrease the blood supply to the ear such as heart disease, hypertension, or diabetes

Chart 50-2 EAR AND HEARING ASSESSMENT

Using Gordon's Functional Health Patterns

COGNITIVE-PERCEPTUAL PATTERN

- Do you have any hearing difficulty?
- Do you use any type of hearing aid?
- Do you notice that you have the volume of the television or radio set at an increased level?
- Are you sitting closer to the television or radio to hear more clearly?
- Do you have difficulty in your ability to hear or follow conversations in a noisy environment, such as a restaurant?
- Do you have difficulty hearing high-pitched sounds like the doorbell?

HEALTH PERCEPTION-HEALTH MANAGEMENT PATTERN

- Have you had your hearing checked?
- If you are or were exposed to environmental noise, have you consistently used appropriate hearing protection?
- Do you avoid cleaning your ear canals with foreign objects such as toothpicks or paper clips?
- Have you discussed with your health care provider the side effects of any drugs you may be taking that might affect your ear and hearing?

Based on Gordon, M. (2007). *Manual of nursing diagnosis* (11th ed.). Boston: Jones & Bartlett.

Chart 50-3 PATIENT AND FAMILY EDUCATION GUIDE

Self–Ear Irrigation for Cerumen Removal

- *Do not attempt to remove ear wax or irrigate the ears if you have ear tubes or if you have blood, pus, or other fluid draining from the ear.*
- Use an ear syringe designed for the purpose of wax removal. These are inexpensive, available at most drug stores, reusable, and can be used by more than one person when cleaned properly between uses.
- The safest type of ear syringe to use is one that has a right-angle or "elbow" in the tip.
- Irrigating your ears in the shower is an easy method.
- Always use tap water that feels just barely warm to you. If you are using a thermometer, keep the water temperature as close as possible to 98° or 99° F. Water that is warmer or colder can make you feel dizzy and nauseated.
- If your ear wax is thick and sticky, you may need to place a few drops of a warm cerumenolytic (commercial eardrops that soften ear wax) into the ear an hour or so before you irrigate the ear. Other substances that can be used for this purpose include baby oil or mineral oil.
- Fill the syringe with the lukewarm tap water.
- If you are using a syringe with an elbow tip, place only the last part of the tip into your ear and aim it toward the roof of your ear canal.
- If you are using a straight-tipped syringe, insert the tip only about one-half to three-fourths inch into your ear canal, aiming toward the roof of the canal.
- Hold your head at a 30-degree angle to the side you are irrigating.
- Use one hand to hold the syringe and the other to push the plunger or squeeze the bulb.
- Apply gentle but firm continuous pressure, allowing the water to flow against the top of the canal.
- *Do not use blasts or bursts of sudden pressure.*
- The ear canal should fill, and water will begin to flow out, bringing ear wax and debris with it.
- If a dental water-pressure irrigator is used, put it on the lowest possible setting.
- This process should not be painful! If pain occurs, decrease the pressure. If pain persists, stop the irrigation.
- Continue the irrigation until at least a cup of solution has washed into and out from your ear canal. (You may have to refill the syringe.)
- Tilting your head at a 90-degree angle to the side should allow most, if not all, of the water to drain out of your ear.
- Repeat the procedure on the other ear.
- If you feel that water is still in the canal, hold a hair dyer on a low setting near the ear.
- Irrigate your ears anywhere from weekly to monthly, depending on how fast your ear wax collects.

- History of vitiligo (a pigment disorder in which there may be a loss of melanin-containing cells [and their protective function] in the inner ear, resulting in hearing loss)
- History of smoking (nicotine may damage sensory cells by increasing the carboxyhemoglobin in the blood and reducing oxygenation of the cochlea)
- History of vitamin B_{12} and folate deficiency (associated with age-related hearing loss)

If the patient uses foreign objects to clean the ear canal (e.g., bobby-pins, Q-tips, toothpicks), take this time to explain the danger in using these objects. They can scrape the skin of the canal, push cerumen up against the eardrum, and even puncture the eardrum. Explain that nothing smaller than the patient's own fingertip should be inserted into the canal. If the patient says that cerumen buildup is a problem, teach him or her to use an ear irrigation syringe and proper solutions to remove it. Chart 50-3 describes techniques to teach patients how to remove cerumen safely.

If the patient uses a hearing aid, assess whether hearing is improved with its use. Obtain the date of the last hearing test, the type of test given, and the results. Ask about problems that may impair hearing such as allergies, upper respiratory infections, hypothyroidism, arteriosclerosis, head trauma, and recent head, facial, or dental surgery. A thorough drug history is important because many drugs are **ototoxic** (damaging to the ear) (Table 50-1).

Ask the patient about his or her occupation and hobbies that involve exposure to loud noise or music. Assess whether he or she uses protective ear devices. Also ask whether any devices are consistently inserted *into* the ear, such ear plugs or earpiece headsets, and for how long each day they are used. Use this opportunity to teach the patient about protecting his or her ears from loud noises by wearing protective ear devices, such as over-the-ear head sets or foam ear inserts, when persistent loud noises are in the environment. Also suggest the use of earplugs when engaging in water sports to prevent ear infections.

Assess the patient's socioeconomic status to determine the availability of health care. Some people might hesitate to have their hearing loss diagnosed because of the fear of needing to wear a hearing aid.

Family History and Genetic Risk

Family history, as well as personal history, is important in determining genetic risk for hearing loss. Although most hearing loss as a result of a genetic mutation is seen in childhood, some genetic problems can lead to progressive hearing loss in adults (Nussbaum et al., 2007). For example, most people with Down syndrome develop hearing loss as adults. People with the genetic disorder osteogenesis imperfecta have bilateral and progressive hearing loss by their 30s.

GENETIC CONSIDERATIONS

One type of hearing loss among adults has a genetic basis with a mutation in gene *GJB2* on chromosome 1. This mutation causes poor production of the protein *connexin-26,* which has a role in function of cochlear hair cells. Other genetic problems slow the metabolism and excretion of drugs, including ototoxic drugs. This allows ototoxic drugs to remain in the body longer, increasing the risk for hearing loss.

TABLE 50-1 Ototoxic Drugs

Drug Type	Drug
Antibiotics	Amikacin Capreomycin Chloramphenicol Dihydrostreptomycin Erythromycin Gentamicin (Garamycin, Cidomycin) Kanamycin Metronidazole (vestibulotoxicity rarely) Neomycin Netilmicin Streptomycin Tobramycin
Diuretics	Acetazolamide (Apo-Acetazolamide🍁, Diamox) Ethacrynic acid (Edecrin) Bumetanide Furosemide (Lasix, Apo-Furosemide🍁, Furoside🍁)
Nonsteroidal anti-inflammatory agents	Ibuprofen (Advil, Nuprin, Motrin) Indomethacin (Indocin) Naproxen (Aleve, Naprosyn, Anaprox) Feldene, Dolobid, Lodine, Relafen, Toradol, Voltaren Salicylates (aspirin, Disalcid, Bufferin, Ecotrin, Trilisate, Ascriptin, Empirin, Excedrin, Fiorinal)
Chemotherapy agents	Actinomycin Bleomycin Cisplatin (Abiplatin, Platinol) Carboplatin Nitrogen mustard (Mustargen) Vincristine
Miscellaneous	Carbamazepine Hydroxychloroquine (Plaquenil) Quinine (Legatrin, Novo-Quinine🍁, Quinamm) Quinidine (Apo-Quinidine🍁, Cardioquin, Quinidex)

Ask the patient:
- Who in your family has hearing problems?
- In those who have hearing problems, are the problems present in men and women equally or are they present more in one gender?
- At what age was hearing loss diagnosed in your relative(s)?
- Are both ears affected?

Current Health Problems

Assess current ear-related problems by asking the patient about any ear "trouble," ear pain, or discharge, including earwax. Ask about any change in hearing, such as **hyperacusis** (the intolerance for sound levels that do not bother other people) or **tinnitus** (ringing in the ears). If a change in hearing is reported, ask whether one or both ears are involved and if the change was sudden or gradual. Also ask about problems with dizziness, sensations of being "off-balance," or **vertigo** (sensation of spinning movement).

NCLEX EXAMINATION CHALLENGE

The nursing assistant tells the nurse that the 80-year-old resident of the LTC facility reports that his ears itch and he wants her to clean them with a Q-tip. What is the nurse's best action?

A. Teach the assistant to use sterile technique to clean the ear canals with cotton-tipped applicators.
B. Advise the assistant that any cleaning of the ear is not a task within his or her scope of practice.
C. Tell the assistant to ask the resident whether both ears are itchy or if only one ear is affected.
D. Instruct the assistant to help the resident to clean his external ear with a soapy washcloth.

evolve For the correct answer, go to http://evolve.elsevier.com/Iggy/.

Physical Assessment

Inspection and palpation are the examination techniques used to assess the ear. Begin the examination by placing the patient in a sitting or supine position. Remove any hearing aids before the examination. After the examination, inspect the hearing aid for cracks, debris, and a proper fit. A complete ear examination is usually performed by a physician, advanced practice nurse, specialty nurse, or physician assistant. The brief assessment of the ear and hearing usually performed by a medical-surgical nurse is described next.

External Ear and Mastoid Assessment

▶ VIDEO CLIP: External Ear

Inspect the entire external ear for shape, location of attachment to the head, and condition, including the condition of the visible external canal. The normal pinna is uniformly shaped without skin tags or deformity. The pinna should be attached to the side of the head at a posterior angle of 10 degrees or less. The normal external canal is dry, clean, free from lesions, and not reddened.

Abnormalities of the pinna include swelling, nodules, and lesions. In chronic gout, collection of uric acid crystals results in hard, painless nodules called **tophi** on the pinna. Other nodules on the pinna might also be from basal cell carcinoma or rheumatoid arthritis. Small, crusted, ulcerated, or indurated lesions on the pinna that fail to heal could be squamous cell carcinoma.

Inspect the mastoid process for redness and swelling, which indicate inflammation. To assess for tenderness, gently tap with one finger over the mastoid process, compress the tragus with one finger, and gently move the pinna forward and backward. Any tenderness suggests an inflammatory process in either the external ear or the mastoid.

Assess for and record these problems:
- Furuncles
- Large amounts of cerumen
- Scaliness
- Redness
- Swelling of or drainage from the ear associated with a foreign object (insects or other substances), trauma, or infection
- Drainage such as blood, cerebrospinal fluid, pus, or serous fluid, and its character

Otoscopic Assessment

The purpose of a brief otoscopic examination is to assess the patency of the external canal, identify lesions or excessive cerumen in the canal, and assess whether the tympanic membrane (eardrum) is intact or inflamed. An instrument called an **otoscope** is used to examine the ear. Many types are available. It consists of a light, a handle, a magnifying lens, and a pressure bulb for injecting air into the external canal to test mobility of the eardrum (Fig. 50-5). Specula of various diameters attach to the head of the otoscope. Select the largest speculum that most comfortably fits the patient's external canal. *Do not examine the ears of a confused patient with an otoscope.*

If the patient has pain during the external ear examination, cautiously attempt an otoscopic examination. The speculum will cause extreme pain if it comes in contact with inflamed tissue in the external canal.

When performing an otoscopic examination, tilt the patient's head slightly away and hold the otoscope upside down, like a large pen (Fig. 50-6). This position permits your hand to lie against the patient's head for support. If the patient moves, both your hand and the otoscope also move, preventing damage to the external canal or eardrum. Hold the otoscope in your dominant hand, and gently pull the pinna up and back with your nondominant hand to straighten the canal. View the ear canal while you slowly insert the speculum. *To avoid perforating the eardrum, observe the ear canal through the otoscope as you insert the speculum into the external canal. Never blindly insert the speculum into the external canal because of the risk of perforating the eardrum.* Use caution to avoid the pain associated with jamming the speculum into the walls of the external canal.

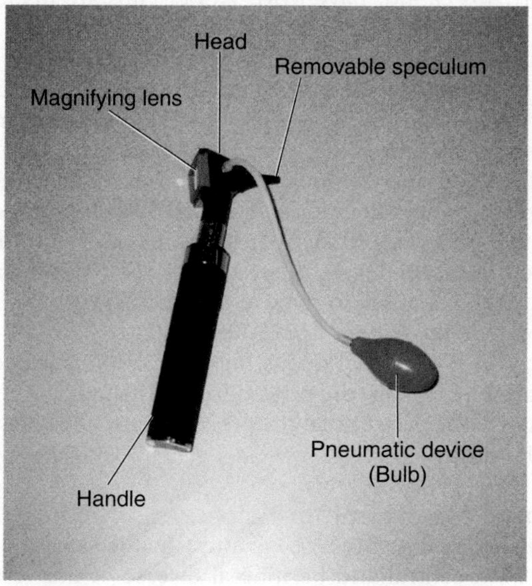
Head
Removable speculum
Magnifying lens
Pneumatic device
(Bulb)
Handle

Fig. 50-5 • Functional components of an otoscope.

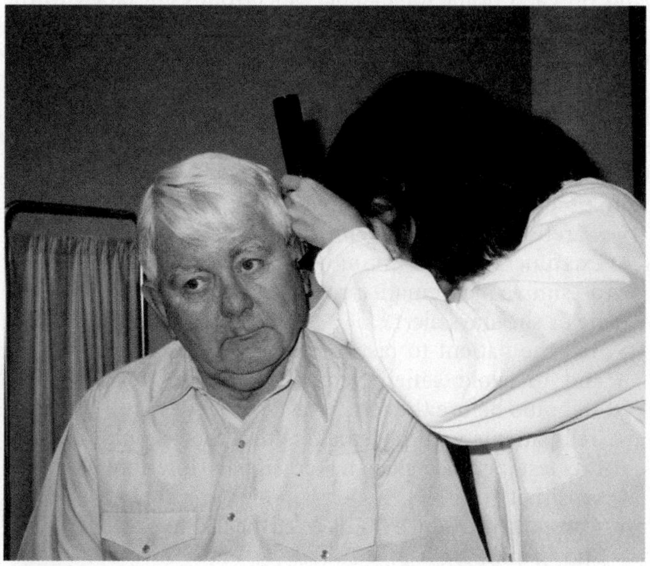

Fig. 50-6 • Proper technique for an otoscopic examination.

VIDEO CLIP: Ear Canal

After the otoscope is comfortably introduced in the external canal, assess for lesions and the amount and consistency of cerumen and hair. The normal external canal is skin colored, intact, and without lesions. It contains various amounts of soft cerumen and small, fine hairs. Assess the eardrum for intactness and color. *The normal eardrum is always intact.* The eardrum is shiny, transparent, and opaque or pearly gray and without lesions. Redness is seen in otitis media. Reflection of the otoscope's light from the normal eardrum is the **light reflex,** and it appears as a clearly outlined triangle of light.

CULTURAL AWARENESS

Cerumen is generally moist and tan or brown in Euro-American patients and African-American patients. It is dry and light brown to gray in Asians and American Indians. The color of the lining of the external ear canal varies with the patient's skin tone. These variations should not be mistaken for indications of problems. Patients with more moist earwax may form cerumen impactions more easily than do patients with drier, flaky earwax and require more frequent ear irrigations.

Auditory Assessment

After assessing the external ear and the canals of both ears, briefly assess the patient's hearing acuity. Several rapid and simple tests for hearing can be performed at the patient's bedside. Although these tests do not determine the true extent or type of hearing loss, they can indicate the patient's functional hearing ability.

The *voice test* for hearing is a simple hearing acuity test that is conducted by asking the patient to block one external ear canal while standing 1 to 2 feet (30 to 60 cm) away. Quietly whisper a statement, and then ask the patient to repeat it. Test each ear separately. If the patient does not respond correctly, use a louder whisper. If you suspect the patient is lip-reading, use your hand to block the view of your mouth, or stand behind him or her while whispering.

The *watch test* for hearing is the use of a ticking watch to test acuity for high-frequency sounds. Hold a ticking watch about 5 inches (12.7 cm) from each ear, and ask whether the ticking is heard. The patient with normal hearing should be able to hear it. If a watch that ticks cannot be found, test hearing by clicking the fingernails of your thumb and forefinger together about 12 inches from the patient's ear or just behind his or her head. More complex assessments of hearing, performed by physicians, advanced practice nurses, specialty nurses, and physician assistants can determine the type and extent of hearing loss.

Sound is transmitted by air conduction and bone conduction. Air conduction of sound is normally more sensitive than bone conduction. If hearing acuity is decreased, the hearing loss is categorized as:

- **Conductive hearing loss,** which results from physical obstruction of sound wave transmission such as a foreign body in the external canal, a retracted or bulging tympanic membrane, or fused bony ossicles.
- **Sensorineural hearing loss,** which results from a defect in the cochlea, the eighth cranial nerve, or the brain itself. Exposure to loud noise and music may cause this type of hearing loss as a result of damage to the cochlear hair cells.
- **Mixed conductive-sensorineural hearing loss,** a profound hearing loss resulting from both conductive and sensorineural hearing loss.

Each auditory function test determines the degree of hearing loss and differentiates the type of loss.

Audioscopy testing involves the use of a handheld device to generate tones of varying intensities to test hearing. Hearing can be measured at a 40-decibel (dB) intensity at frequencies of 500, 1000, 2000, and 4000 cycles per second (cps), or hertz (Hz). The audioscope is larger than a standard otoscope and is easily used to assess hearing.

Tuning fork tests for hearing acuity are the Weber and Rinne tests. These tests are useful, although limited, in distinguishing between conductive and sensorineural hearing losses. The frequency range of the tuning fork used for these tests corresponds to that of normal speech.

The Weber tuning fork test is performed by placing a vibrating tuning fork on the middle of the patient's head and asking him or her to indicate in which ear the sound is louder. The normal test result is sound heard equally in both ears. The term *lateralization* is used if the sound is louder in one ear. For example, lateralization to the right means that the sound is heard loudest in the right ear.

The Rinne tuning fork test compares hearing by air conduction with hearing by bone conduction. Sound is normally heard two to three times longer by air conduction than by bone conduction. The Rinne tuning fork test is performed by placing the vibrating tuning fork stem on the mastoid process (bone conduction) and asking the patient to indicate when the sound is no longer heard. When the patient no longer hears the sound, the fork is quickly brought in front of the pinna (air conduction) without touching the patient. He or she should then indicate when this sound is no longer heard. The patient normally continues to hear the sound two to three times longer in front of the pinna (air conduction) after not hearing it with the tuning fork touching the mastoid process (bone conduction).

Psychosocial Assessment

The patient may become irritable, frustrated, and depressed by an inability to hear and respond appropriately. The inability to hear often isolates the patient from the world. Depression may result from the sensory isolation of hearing loss. Be sensitive to the patient, and conduct the interview at a pace appropriate for that person.

Ask about social and work relationships to determine whether the patient is isolated because of hearing problems. In addition, encourage the patient to express feelings related to hearing loss and discuss any changes in daily living activities that have been made as a result of a change in hearing. Also obtain information from family members, especially if the patient does not acknowledge having a hearing problem. Throughout the assessment, remain patient and empathetic.

Diagnostic Assessment

Laboratory Assessment

Laboratory tests generally are not of value in determining hearing acuity. For an external ear infection, microbial culture and antibiotic sensitivity tests can determine the causative organism and the most appropriate antibiotic.

Imaging Assessment

Computed tomography (CT), with or without contrast enhancement, shows the structures of the ear in great detail by multiple x-ray scans of the head. These scans are then averaged by a computer. CT is especially helpful in diagnosing acoustic tumors.

Magnetic resonance imaging (MRI) is a noninvasive, nonradioactive diagnostic tool that uses a computer to generate images. Because of its superior contrast resolution, no bony artifacts can obscure tissue. Therefore MRI has great sensitivity to soft-tissue changes. Patients with older internal metal vascular clips cannot have MRI. Newer clips are made from titanium and are not a contraindication for MRI.

Other Diagnostic Assessment for Hearing

Auditory brainstem-evoked response (ABR) assesses hearing in patients who are unable to indicate or are unreliable in indicating their recognition of sound stimuli during standard hearing tests, which require cognition. This test helps diagnose both conductive and sensorineural hearing losses. Electrodes are placed on the scalp during the test. After the test, the patient's hair should be cleansed to remove the electrode gel.

To prepare the patient for ABR:

- Tell the patient that no fasting or sedation is needed.
- Carefully explain the procedure and its purpose.
- Inform the patient that the procedure usually takes about 30 minutes.

Diagnostic Assessment for Balance

Electronystagmography (ENG) is a test that is sensitive in detecting both central and peripheral disease of the vestibular system in the ear. The ENG detects and records **nystagmus** (involuntary eye movements) because the eyes and ears depend on each other for balance. Electrodes are taped to the skin near the eyes, and one or more procedures (caloric testing, changing gaze position, or changing head position) are performed to stimulate nystagmus. Failure of nystagmus to occur with cerebral stimulation suggests an abnormality in the vestibulocochlear apparatus, the cerebral cortex, the auditory nerve, or the brainstem.

To prepare the patient for ENG:

- Carefully explain the procedure and its purpose. The examiners will be asking the patient to name names or do simple mathematic problems during the test to ensure he or she stays alert.
- Tell the patient to fast for several hours before the test and to avoid caffeine-containing beverages for 24 to 48 hours before the test.
- Tell patients with pacemakers that they should not have the test because pacemaker signals interfere with the sensitivity of ENG.
- Carefully introduce fluids after the test to prevent nausea and vomiting.

Caloric testing is performed to evaluate the vestibular (inner ear) portion of the auditory nerve. Water warmer or cooler than body temperature is infused into the ear. A normal response is the onset of vertigo and nystagmus within 20 to 30 seconds. To prepare the patient for caloric testing:

- Carefully explain the procedure and its purpose.
- Tell the patient to fast for several hours before the test.
- Tell the patient that the affected side will be tested first.
- Explain that he or she will be on bedrest after the procedure with careful introduction of fluids to prevent nausea and vomiting.

Dix-Hallpike test for vertigo is performed by assisting the patient to a sitting position on an examination table. Stand to the side of the patient, and quickly reposition him or her from sitting to supine with the head extending beyond the end of the table. This change of position is done first to one side and then to the other side. A patient with benign positional vertigo will have a burst of nystagmus after a delay of 5 to 10 seconds.

To prepare the patient for the Dix-Hallpike test:

- Carefully explain the procedure and its purpose.
- Tell him or her to keep the eyes open and try not to blink.
- Explain that double vision may occur during the test.

Audiometry

Audiometry is the measurement of hearing acuity. It is usually performed by audiologists, audiology technicians, or nurses with special training. **Frequency** is the highness or lowness of tones (expressed in hertz). The greater the number of vibrations per second, the higher is the frequency (pitch) of the sound. The fewer the number of vibrations per second, the lower is the frequency (pitch).

Intensity of sound is expressed in decibels (dB). **Threshold** is the lowest level of intensity at which pure tones and speech are heard by a patient about 50% of the time.

The lowest intensity at which a young, normal ear can detect sound about 50% of the time is 0 dB. Sound at 110 dB is so intense (loud) that it is painful for most people with normal hearing. Conversational speech is around 60 dB, and a soft whisper is around 20 dB (Table 50-2). A hearing loss of 45 to 50 dB renders the person unable to hear speech without a hearing aid. A person with a hearing loss of 90 dB may not be able to hear speech even with a hearing aid.

TABLE 50-2 Decibel Intensity and Safe Exposure Time for Common Sounds

Sound	Decibel Intensity (dB)	Safe Exposure Time*
Threshold of hearing	0	
Whispering	20	
Average residence or office	40	
Conversational speech	60	
Car traffic	70	>8 hr
Motorcycle	90	8 hr
Chain saw	100	2 hr
Rock concert, front row	120	3 min
Jet engine	140	Immediate danger
Rocket launching pad	180	Immediate danger

*For every 5-dB increase in intensity, the safe exposure time is cut in half.

Pure tones are generated by an **audiometer** to determine hearing acuity. The two types of audiometry are pure-tone audiometry and speech audiometry.

Pure-Tone Audiometry

Pure-tone audiometry generates tones with an audiometer that are presented to the patient at frequencies for hearing speech, music, and other common sounds. It can be performed by air-conduction testing or bone-conduction testing. The results of pure-tone audiometry are graphed on an audiogram. For some patients, the hearing of one ear is "masked" while the hearing of the other ear is tested.

Pure-tone air-conduction testing determines whether a patient hears normally or has a hearing loss. It is designed to test air-conduction hearing sensitivity (through earphones) at frequencies ranging from 125 to 8000 Hz. Thresholds are usually confined to the frequencies of 250, 500, 1000, 2000, 4000, and 8000 Hz. The intensities for pure tones generally range from 10 to 110 dB.

The patient sits in a sound-isolated room in which background noise does not exceed American National Standards Institute noise standards. Earphones are placed over his or her ears and tones of varying frequencies and intensities are delivered through the earphones, testing one ear at a time. The patient presses a button to indicate when he or she hears a tone and releases the button to indicate that the tone is no longer heard. No follow-up care is needed.

Pure-tone bone-conduction testing determines whether the hearing loss detected by air-conduction testing is due to conductive or sensorineural factors or to a combination of the two. It is used only when the results of air-conduction testing are abnormal. Testing is similar to air-conduction testing except that a bone-conduction vibrator, placed firmly behind the pinna on the mastoid process, is used instead of earphones. No special follow-up care is needed.

Interpretation of audiometric evaluation determines whether the patient's hearing is within normal limits or, with a hearing impairment, whether the hearing loss is conductive, sensorineural, or mixed. The type of loss can be determined by an experienced clinician by examining the shape of the audiogram after completion of pure-tone air-conduction and bone-conduction audiometry.

Speech Audiometry

In speech audiometry, the patient's ability to hear spoken words is measured through a microphone connected to an audiometer. The two components of speech audiometry are the speech reception threshold and speech discrimination.

Speech reception threshold is the minimum loudness at which a patient can repeat simple words. In testing this threshold, try to determine how intense (or loud) a simple speech stimulus must be before the patient can hear it well enough to repeat it correctly. In one common test, lists of two-syllable words called **spondee** are used (i.e., words in which there is generally equal stress on each syllable, such as *airplane, railroad,* and *cowboy*).

The speech reception threshold measured by the audiometer is the hearing level at which the patient can repeat simple words correctly 50% of the time. The test is conducted in a manner similar to the pure-tone tests.

Speech discrimination testing determines the patient's ability to discriminate among similar sounds or among words that contain similar sounds. The ability to understand speech is the most important measurable aspect of human hearing. Speech discrimination testing assesses understanding of speech. A hearing loss may decrease sensitivity to sound and impair understanding of what is being said.

A standard format contains lists of 25 to 50 **monosyllabic** (one-syllable) words, such as *carve, day, toe,* and *ran,* phonemically balanced (designed to include the phonemes of American English in the proper proportion) and with equal word difficulty between lists. The lists are presented to the patient through earphones at a selected loudness level, generally about 30 to 40 dB above the speech reception threshold, or at the patient's most comfortable listening level. A percentage score is derived from the number of words repeated correctly.

Tympanometry

Tympanometry assesses mobility of the eardrum and structures of the middle ear by systematically changing air pressure in the external auditory canal. The progression or resolution of serous otitis and otitis media can be accurately monitored with this procedure.

This test is helpful in distinguishing middle-ear pathologic conditions, such as otosclerosis, ossicular disarticulation, otitis media, and perforation of the eardrum. It is also useful for assessing patency of the eustachian tube and for checking recovery of middle-ear function after surgery.

DECISION-MAKING CHALLENGE
Coordination of Care

A 34-year-old man is seen in the clinic for hearing loss in the left ear and intermittent dizziness. He tells you that he smokes two packs of cigarettes a day, that he is taking no drugs, and that cleaning his ear with a Q-tip does not help his hearing. He is scheduled for a head CT scan and caloric testing tomorrow. He asks whether these tests will be painful and whether he can drive himself to and from the clinic.

1. What is the relationship between cigarette smoking and hearing loss?
2. How will you respond to his questions?
3. What are the teaching priorities for this patient?

evolve For suggested answer guidelines, go to http://evolve.elsevier.com/Iggy/.

HUMAN NEEDS ASSESSMENT REVIEW

What should you expect to NOTICE in a patient with adequate sensation related to the ear and hearing?

- Ears are symmetric on the face on a line about even with the corners of the eyes, and with the tops of the ears rotated slightly toward back.
- Outer ear (pinna) has no open areas, scales, or bumps.
- No drainage from the ear canal.
- Does not tilt one side of the head or lean forward when listening to another person speak.
- Startles when a loud or unexpected sound occurs in the environment.
- Responds appropriately to questions.
- Does not consistently ask a speaker to repeat himself or herself; does not say "what?" or "huh?" frequently.
- Engages in conversation, as appropriate (responds to greetings), with other people in the immediate environment.
- Responds appropriately to whispered questions and conversations, even when the speaker is not facing the patient.

GET READY FOR THE NCLEX EXAMINATION!

Key Points

Review these Key Points for each NCLEX Examination Client Needs Category.

Safe and Effective Care Environment

- Use a separate speculum cover for each ear when conducting an otoscopic examination.
- Slowly and gently introduce the otoscopic speculum into the external ear canal during assessment.
- Use Standard Precautions with any patient who has drainage from the ear canal.
- Do not perform an otoscopic examination on a confused patient.
- Use the suggestions presented in "Patient History" section to enhance communication with a patient who has a hearing impairment.

Health Promotion and Maintenance

- Teach patients the proper way to clean the pinna and external ear canal.
- Identify patients at risk for hearing impairment as a result of work environment or leisure activities.
- Encourage all patients, even if they already have a hearing impairment, to use ear protection in loud environment.
- Inform all patients who smoke that smoking increases the risk for development of hearing problems.

Psychosocial Integrity

- Pace your interview to match the learning needs and style of the individual patient.
- Allow the patient the opportunity to express fear or anxiety about a change in hearing status.
- Explain all diagnostic procedures, restrictions, and follow-up care to the patient scheduled for tests.

Physiological Integrity

- Ask the patient about hearing problems in any other members of the family, because many hearing problems have a genetic component.
- Ask the patient whether any ototoxic drugs have ever been used (see Table 50-1).

Additional Study Resources

Go to your Companion CD or Evolve at http://evolve.elsevier.com/Iggy/ for *Self-Assessment Questions for the NCLEX Examination.*

evolve Go to Evolve at http://evolve.elsevier.com/Iggy/ for *Prioritization and Delegation Questions for the NCLEX Examination.*

SELECTED BIBLIOGRAPHY

Asterisk indicates a classic or definitive work on this subject.

Berry, J., & Stewart, A. (2006). Communicating with the deaf during the health examination visit. *The Journal for Nurse Practitioners—JNP, 2*(8), 509-515.

Bess, F.H., & Humes, L.E. (2007). *Audiology: The fundamentals* (4th ed.). Baltimore: Lippincott Williams & Wilkins.

Boys Town National Research Hospital. Retrieved August 2007, from www.boystownhospital.org/Hearing/index.asp.

Brender, E. (2006). Audiometry. *Journal of the American Medical Association, 295*(4), 460.

Centers for Disease Control and Prevention. (2004). *Developmental disabilities*. Retrieved September 4, 2007, from www.cdc.gov/ncbddd/dd/ddhi.htm.

Clark, S.E., Wantz, M.S., & Brey, R.A. (2005). Developing empathy for hearing-impaired students: Can you hear what I hear? *Journal of School Health, 75*(2), 72-73.

Fields, R. (2007). Food, spices double as folk cures. *Borderlands: An El Paso Community College Local History Project*. Retrieved September 4, 2007, from www.epcc.edu/ftp/Homes/monicaw/borderlands/09_food.htm.

Gordon, M. (2007). *Manual of nursing diagnosis* (11th ed.). Boston: Jones & Bartlett.

Hain, T.C. (2003). *Ototoxic medications*. Retrieved September 4, 2007, from www.tchain.com/otoneurology/disorders/bilat/ototoxins.html.

Harkin, H. (2005). A nurse-led ear care clinic: Sharing knowledge and improving patient care. *British Journal of Nursing, 14*(5), 250-254.

Jarvis, C. (2008). *Physical examination and health assessment* (5th ed.). Philadelphia: Saunders.

*Lusk, S.L. (1997). Noise exposures: Effects on hearing and prevention of noise induced hearing loss. *AAOHN Journal, 45*(8), 397-405, 409-410.

McCance, K., & Huether, S. (2006). *Pathophysiology: The biologic basis for disease in adults and children* (5th ed.). St. Louis: Mosby.

Nussbaum, R., McInnes, R., & Willard, H. (2007). *Thompson & Thompson: Genetics in medicine* (7th ed.). Philadelphia: Saunders.

Pagana, K., & Pagana, T. (2006). *Mosby's manual of diagnostic and laboratory tests* (3rd ed.). St. Louis: Mosby.

*Ventry, I., & Selsnick, S. (1983). Identification of elderly people with hearing problems. *American Speech-Language Hearing Association*, July, 37-42.

Vestibular Disorders Association. (2007). *Diagnostic tests for vestibular disorders*. Retrieved September 2007, from www.vestibular.org/vestibular-disorders/diagnostic-tests.php.

51 CHAPTER

Care of Patients with Ear and Hearing Problems

Jacquelyn Ann Russek

LEARNING OUTCOMES

For clinical competence and success on the NCLEX Examination, study this chapter with these Learning Outcomes in mind:

Safe and Effective Care Environment

1. Apply principles of infection control when examining an ear with drainage.
2. Implement precautions to prevent falls in patients experiencing vertigo or dizziness.
3. Correctly instill eardrops.

Health Promotion and Maintenance

4. Teach patients using hearing aids how to use and care for them properly.

Psychosocial Integrity

5. Use effective communication when teaching patients and family members about what to expect during tests and procedures to assess ear and hearing problems.
6. Provide the opportunity for the patient and family to express their feelings and concerns about a change in hearing.
7. Refer hearing-impaired patients and families to local and Internet-based support services.

Physiological Integrity

8. Compare the clinical manifestations and interventions for external otitis with those of otitis media.
9. Safely remove impacted cerumen from the ear canal of an older patient.
10. Coordinate the care of the patient with Ménière's disease.
11. Prioritize nursing care needs for the patient after tympanoplasty.
12. Prioritize educational needs for the patient after stapedectomy.
13. Identify an appropriate method for communicating with a patient who has recently become hearing impaired.

Go to your Companion CD or Evolve at http://evolve.elsevier.com/Iggy/ for *Self-Assessment Questions for the NCLEX Examination* keyed to these Learning Outcomes.

The ears are important for the sense of hearing and for balance. They play an important role in daily functioning. Ear disorders can cause many problems ranging from hearing difficulty to problems of balance and functional ability. *Hearing problems reduce the ability of the patient to meet the human need for sensation and cognition.* They can lead to confusion, mistrust, social isolation, and the inability to give and receive accurate information. Disorders of the ear and of hearing are often easily treated with proper diagnosis. However, early recognition and intervention are necessary to prevent additional damage and to promote a maximum level of wellness.

CONDITIONS AFFECTING THE EXTERNAL EAR

The external ear is the outermost part of the ear structures and is subject to outside factors that can cause problems. Disorders of the external ear include congenital malformation (birth defects), trauma, and infectious or noninfectious lesions of the pinna, auricle, or auditory canal. Ear structures (external, middle, and inner ear) develop at different times during fetal life. Thus the presence of birth defects in one area does not necessarily mean that other areas also will be affected. Abnormalities of the external ear range from crumpling or falling forward of the pinna to complete absence (**atresia**) of the auditory canal. In addition, trauma can damage or destroy the auricle and external canal. Surgical reconstruction can re-form the pinna with skin grafts and plastic prostheses. Trauma to the auricle resulting in a hematoma requires the removal of blood via needle aspiration to prevent calcification and hardening, which is often referred to as a **cauliflower** or **boxer's ear.**

Benign cysts or polyps of the auricle or external canal are surgically removed if they block the canal and affect hearing. Cancer cells, usually basal cell carcinoma, can also be found on the pinna. In general, treatment consists of simple excision. As the lesion becomes larger, its location near the skull and facial nerve makes treatment more difficult.

EXTERNAL OTITIS

Pathophysiology

External otitis is a painful condition caused when irritating or infective agents come into contact with the skin of the external ear. The result to the external ear canal or the auricle is either an allergic response or inflammation with or without infection. Affected skin becomes red, swollen, and tender to touch or movement. Swelling of the ear canal can lead to hearing loss due to canal obstruction. Allergic external otitis is commonly caused by contact with cosmetics, hair sprays, earphones, earrings, or hearing aids. The most common infectious organisms, usually bacterial or fungal, are *Pseudomonas aeruginosa, Streptococcus, Staphylococcus,* and *Aspergillus.*

External otitis occurs more often in hot, humid environments, especially in the summer, and is commonly referred to as **swimmer's ear** because of the high incidence in people involved in water sports. In addition, patients who have traumatized their external ear canal with sharp or small objects (e.g., hairpins, cotton-tipped applicators) or with headphones are more susceptible to external otitis.

Necrotizing or *malignant otitis* is the most virulent form of external otitis. Organisms spread beyond the external ear canal into the ear and skull. The high mortality rate seen with malignant external otitis results from complications such as meningitis, brain abscess, and destruction of cranial nerve VII.

Patient-Centered Collaborative Care

Manifestations of external otitis include many problems, ranging from mild itching to pain with movement of the pinna or tragus. Patients have pain with movement of the pinna and tragus or when upward pressure is applied to the external canal. They report feeling as if the ear is plugged and hearing is reduced.

Use caution during otoscopic examination to avoid pressing on the walls of the external canal, which causes pain. Drainage from the ear is often greenish white. To prevent cross-contamination, dispose of the otoscope tip and wash your hands before examining the opposite ear. Hearing loss in the affected ear can be severe when inflammation obstructs the ear canal and prevents sounds from reaching the eardrum **(tympanic membrane).**

Treatment focuses on reducing inflammation, edema, and pain. Nursing priorities include comfort measures, such as the application of heat to the ear for 20 minutes three times a day. This can be accomplished by using towels warmed with water and then wrapped in a plastic bag or by using a heating pad placed on a low setting. Teach the patient that bedrest limits head movements, thereby reducing pain.

Topical antibiotic and steroid therapies are most effective in decreasing inflammation and pain (Osguthorpe & Nielsen, 2006). Review best practices for instilling eardrops with the patient, as shown in Chart 51-1. Observe the patient self-administer the eardrops to make sure that he or she uses proper technique. If edema obstructs the external canal, an earwick is inserted past the blockage, with medicated drops applied to the outside end (Fig. 51-1). A long piece of gauze dressing serves as an earwick, which the health care provider inserts using forceps to push carefully through the blocked external auditory canal to the eardrum. The earwick may be removed when eardrops can flow freely into the canal. Coordinate with all members of the health care team to ensure thorough handwashing whenever the infected ear is touched. Oral or IV antibiotics are used in severe cases, especially when cellulitis is present or the lymph nodes in the area are enlarged.

Analgesics, including opioids, may be needed for pain relief during the initial days of treatment. Acetylsalicylic acid (aspirin, Entrophen🍁), ibuprofen (Advil), or acetaminophen (Tylenol, Abenol🍁) may relieve less-severe pain.

After the inflammation has subsided, diluted alcohol may be dropped into the ear to keep it clean and dry and to prevent recurrence. Teach the patient not to use cotton-tipped applicators to dry the ears, because this use could damage the canal and increase the risk for infection or inflammation. Teach him

Chart 51-1 BEST PRACTICE FOR PATIENT SAFETY & QUALITY CARE

Instillation of Eardrops

- Gather the solutions to be administered.
- Check the labels to ensure correct dosage and time.
- Wear gloves to remove and discard any ear packing.
- Wash your hands.
- Perform a gentle otoscopic examination to determine whether the eardrum is intact.
- Irrigate the ear if the eardrum is intact.
- Place the bottle of eardrops (with the top on tightly) in a bowl of warm water for 5 minutes.
- Tilt the patient's head in the opposite direction of the affected ear, and place the drops in the ear.
- With his or head tilted, ask the patient to gently move the head back and forth five times.
- Insert a cotton ball into the opening of the ear canal to act as packing.
- Wash your hands again.

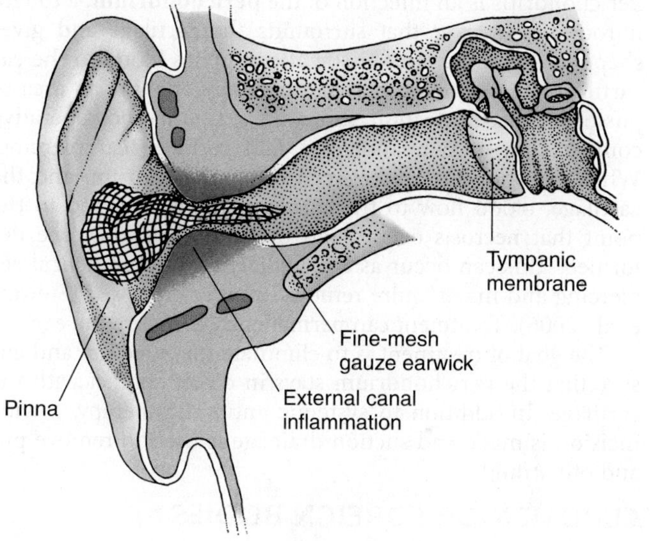
Tympanic membrane
Fine-mesh gauze earwick
Pinna
External canal inflammation

Fig. 51-1 • Earwick for instillation of antibiotics into the external canal. When edema occludes the external auditory canal, it is difficult for antibiotic solutions to enter the canal adequately. An earwick is placed through the meatus. Solutions placed on the external portion of the earwick are absorbed through the canal.

or her to use preventive measures for minimizing ear canal moisture, trauma, or exposure to materials that lead to local irritation or contact dermatitis. Recommend the use of ear plugs when engaging in water sports to those patients with recurrent episodes of external otitis.

FURUNCLE

A **furuncle** is a localized external otitis caused by bacterial infection, usually *Staphylococcus*, of a hair follicle. Most furuncles occur on the outer half of the external canal.

The manifestations of a furuncle include intense local pain to light touch. The area is swollen and red, with tight skin covering the area, possibly with a purulent head. No drainage is seen unless the furuncle has ruptured. Hearing is impaired if the lesion blocks the canal.

Treatment consists of local and systemic antibiotics and local heat application. An earwick may be used with one-half strength Burow's solution to relieve pain. The furuncle may need to be incised and drained if it does not resolve with the use of antibiotics.

PERICHONDRITIS

Perichondritis is an infection of the **perichondrium,** a tough, fibrous tissue layer that surrounds the cartilage and gives shape to the pinna. This tissue also supplies blood to the ear cartilage. The infection can be caused by opening an area of pus or localized infection, insect bites, trauma, postoperative complication of tympanoplasty, and cartilage ear piercing. When infection occurs between the perichondrium and the cartilage, blood flow to the cartilage can be reduced to the point that necrosis occurs and the pinna may become deformed. This can occur as a complication of high helical ear piercing and may require removal of necrotic tissue (Stewart et al., 2006). Treatment can permanently disfigure the ear.

The goal of treatment is to eliminate the infection and ensure that the perichondrium stays in direct contact with the cartilage. In addition to systemic antibiotic therapy, a wide incision is made and suction drainage is used to remove pus and other fluid.

CERUMEN OR FOREIGN BODIES

Pathophysiology

Cerumen (wax) is the most common cause of an impacted canal. A canal can also become impacted as a result of foreign bodies that can enter or be placed in the external ear canal, such as vegetables, beads, pencil erasers, and insects. Although uncomfortable, cerumen or foreign bodies are rarely true emergencies and can be carefully removed by a health care professional. Cerumen impaction in the older adult is common, and often, removal of the cerumen from older adults improves hearing (Walden, 2006). Removal may also improve mental status.

Patient-Centered Collaborative Care

Patients with a cerumen impaction or a foreign body in the ear may experience a sensation of fullness in the ear, with or without hearing loss, and may have ear pain, itching, dizziness, or bleeding from the ear. The object may be visible with direct inspection.

When the occluding material is cerumen, treatment options include watchful waiting, manual removal, and the use of ceruminolytic agents followed by irrigation. The canal can be irrigated with a mixture of water and hydrogen peroxide at body temperature (Fig. 51-2), following best practices for proper irrigation (Chart 51-2). Removal of a cerumen obstruction by irrigation is a slow process and may take more than one sitting. When it is the cause of hearing loss, cerumen removal may improve hearing. Between 50 and 70 ml of solution is the maximum amount that the patient with an impaction usually can tolerate at one sitting. *Do not irrigate an ear with an eardrum perforation or otitis media, because this may spread the infection to the inner ear.*

If the cerumen is thick and dry or cannot be removed easily, the health care professional may prescribe a ceruminolytic product such as Cerumenex to soften the wax before trying to remove it. Another way to soften cerumen is to add 3 drops of glycerin or mineral oil to the ear at bedtime and 3 drops of hydrogen peroxide twice a day. After several days of this treatment, the cerumen is more easily removed by irrigation. In some cases, a small curette or cerumen spoon may be used to scoop out the wax. Only trained health care professionals should use this method, because damage to the canal or the eardrum is likely with improper technique.

Discourage the use of cotton swabs and ear candles (hollow tubes coated in wax inserted into the ear and then lighted at the far end) to clean the ears or remove cerumen. Chart 50-3 in Chapter 50 describes steps to teach patients regarding ear hygiene and self–ear irrigation. Refer to Chart 51-3 for nursing care considerations of older adult patients with cerumen impaction.

Irrigation is not used when the foreign object is vegetable matter, because this material expands when wet, making the impaction worse. The object needs to be physically removed by an experienced health care professional.

Insects are killed before removal unless they can be coaxed out by a flashlight or a humming noise. Lidocaine, a numbing agent, can be placed in the ear canal for immediate pain relief. Mineral oil or diluted alcohol instilled into the ear can suffocate the insect, which is then removed with ear forceps.

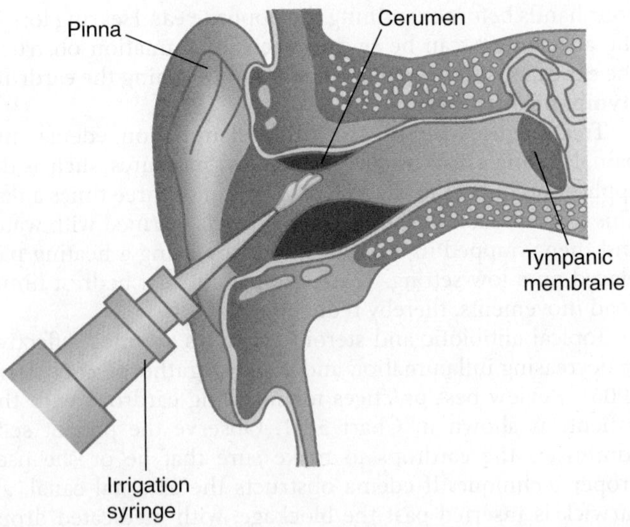
Pinna
Cerumen
Tympanic membrane
Irrigation syringe

Fig. 51-2 • Irrigation of the external canal. Cerumen and debris can be removed from the ear by irrigation with warm water. The stream of water is aimed above or below the impaction to allow back-pressure to push it out rather than further down the canal.

Chart 51-2 BEST PRACTICE FOR PATIENT SAFETY & QUALITY CARE

Ear Irrigation

- Wash your hands.
- Use an otoscope to check the location of the impacted cerumen; ascertain that the eardrum is intact and that the patient does not have otitis media.
- Gather the proper equipment: basin, syringe, otoscope, towel.
- Warm tap water (or other prescribed solution) to body temperature.
- Fill a syringe with the warmed irrigating solution.
- Place a towel around the patient's neck.
- Place a basin under the ear to be irrigated.
- Place the tip of the syringe at an angle so that the fluid pushes on one side of and not directly on the impaction (this helps loosen the impaction instead of forcing it further into the canal).
- Apply gentle but firm continuous pressure, allowing the water to flow against the top of the canal.
- *Do not use blasts or bursts of sudden pressure.*
- If pain occurs, decrease the pressure. If pain persists, stop the irrigation.
- Watch the fluid return for signs of cerumen plug removal.
- Continue to irrigate the ear with about 70 mL of fluid.
- If the cerumen does not drain out, wait 10 minutes and repeat the irrigation procedure.
- Monitor the patient for signs of nausea.
- If the patient becomes nauseated, stop the procedure.
- If the cerumen cannot be removed by irrigation, place (or the patient may place) mineral oil into the ear three times a day for 2 days to soften dry, impacted cerumen, after which irrigation may be repeated.
- After completion of the irrigation, have the patient turn his or her head to the side just irrigated to drain any remaining irrigation fluid.
- Wash your hands.

Chart 51-3 NURSING FOCUS ON THE OLDER ADULT

Cerumen Impaction

- Assess the hearing of all older patients using simple voice tests (see Chapter 50).
- Perform a gentle otoscopic inspection of the external canal and eardrum of any older patient who has a problem with hearing acuity, especially the patient who wears a hearing aid.
- Use ear irrigation to remove any impacted cerumen.
- Make certain that the irrigating fluid is about 98° F (37° C) to reduce the chance of stimulating the vestibular sense.
- Use no more than 5 to 10 mL of irrigating fluid at a time.
- If nausea, vomiting, or dizziness develops, stop the irrigation immediately.
- Teach the patient how to irrigate his or her own ears.
- Obtain a return demonstration of ear irrigation from the patient, observing for specific areas in which the patient may need assistance.
- Encourage the patient to wash the external ears daily using a soapy, wet washcloth over the index finger (best done in the shower or while washing the hair).

If the patient has local irritation, an antibiotic or steroid ointment may be applied to prevent infection and reduce local irritation. Hearing acuity is tested if hearing loss is not resolved by removal of the object.

In rare cases, surgical removal of the foreign object is required. The object is removed through the ear canal (transcanal route) using a wire bent at a 90-degree angle. The wire is looped around the object, and the object is pulled out. Because this procedure is painful, general anesthesia is needed.

CONDITIONS AFFECTING THE MIDDLE EAR

OTITIS MEDIA

Pathophysiology

The three most common forms of otitis media are acute otitis media, chronic otitis media, and serous otitis media. Each type affects the middle ear but has slightly different causes, incidences, and pathologic changes. If otitis progresses or remains untreated, permanent conductive hearing loss may occur. Otitis media is less common in adults than in children.

Acute otitis media and chronic otitis media, also known as *suppurant* or *purulent otitis media,* are similar. An infecting agent introduced into the middle ear causes inflammation of the mucosa, leading to swelling and irritation of the small bones (ossicles) within the middle ear. A purulent inflammatory exudate follows. Acute disease has a sudden onset and lasts 3 weeks or less. Chronic otitis media often follows repeated acute episodes, has a longer duration, and causes greater middle-ear injury. Therapy for complications associated with chronic otitis media, unlike that of acute otitis media, usually involves surgical intervention.

The eustachian tube and mastoid, connected to the middle ear by a sheet of cells, are also affected by the infection. If the eardrum membrane perforates and infective materials spill into the external ear, external otitis develops that thickens and scars the middle ear if left untreated. Necrosis of the ossicles destroys middle-ear structures and causes hearing loss.

Patient-Centered Collaborative Care

Assessment

The patient with acute or chronic otitis media has ear pain with or without movement of the external ear. Pain with chronic otitis media is much less severe than that occurring with acute otitis media. As the pressure in the middle ear increases, there is a sensation of fullness in the ear. Hearing is reduced and distorted. The patient may notice a sticking or cracking sound in the ear on yawning or swallowing or may have tinnitus in the form of a low hum or a low-pitched sound. Conductive hearing loss may occur as sound wave transmission is obstructed. Headaches are common, and systemic symptoms such as malaise, fever, nausea, and vomiting can occur. As the pressure on the middle ear pushes against the inner ear, the patient may have dizziness or vertigo.

Otoscopic examination findings vary, depending on the stage of the condition. The eardrum is initially retracted, which allows landmarks of the ear to be seen clearly. At this early stage, the patient has only vague ear discomfort. As the condition progresses, the eardrum's blood vessels dilate and appear red (Fig. 51-3). In the third stage, the eardrum becomes red, thickened, and bulging, with loss of landmarks. Decreased eardrum mobility is evident on inspection with a pneumatic otoscope. Pus may be seen behind the membrane.

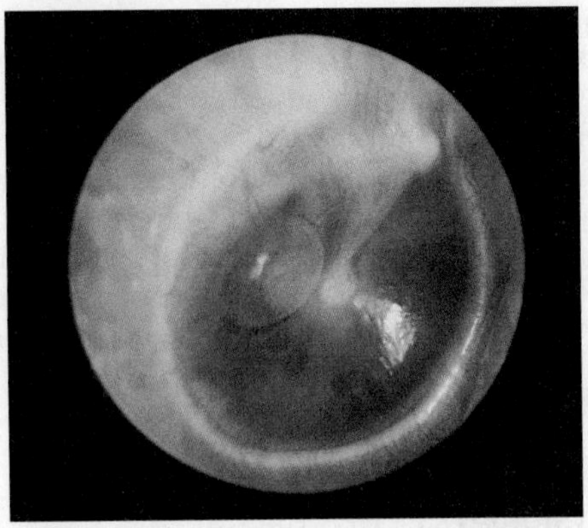

Fig. 51-3 • Otoscopic view of otitis media.

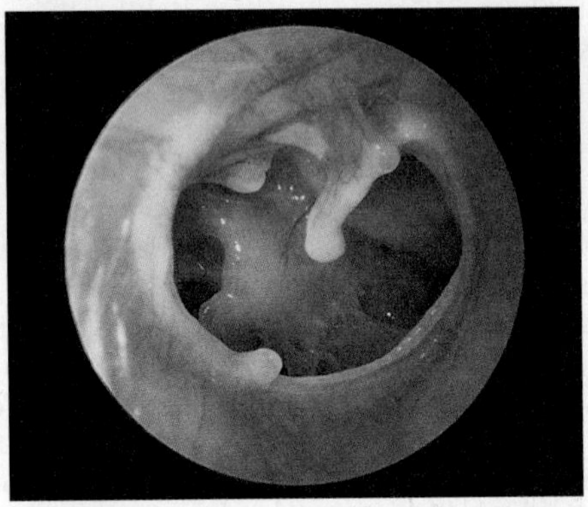

Fig. 51-4 • Otoscopic view of a perforated tympanic membrane.

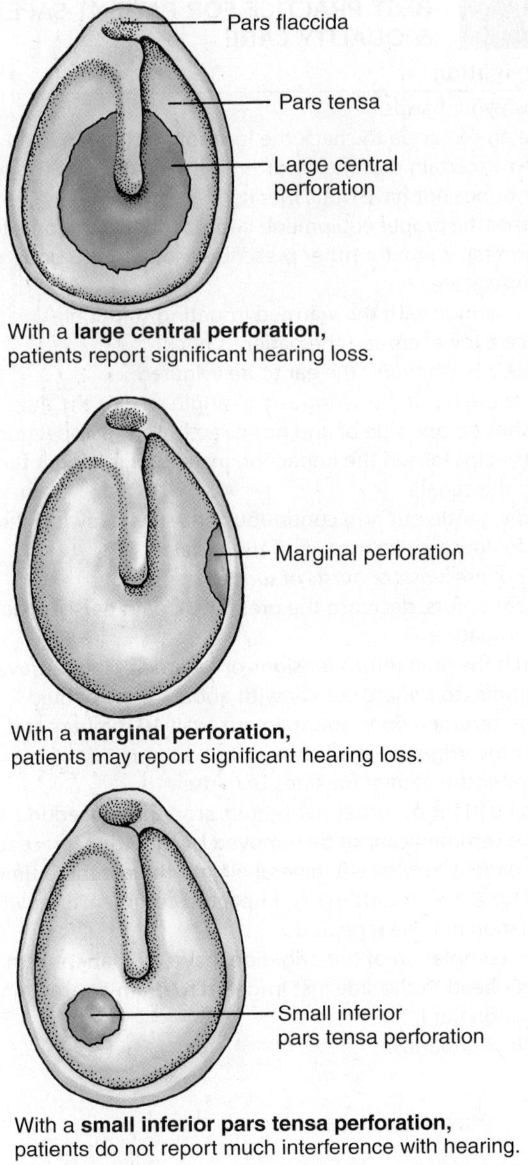
Pars flaccida
Pars tensa
Large central perforation
With a **large central perforation,** patients report significant hearing loss.
Marginal perforation
With a **marginal perforation,** patients may report significant hearing loss.
Small inferior pars tensa perforation
With a **small inferior pars tensa perforation,** patients do not report much interference with hearing.

Fig. 51-5 • Perforations of the tympanic membrane. Central perforations heal more quickly than marginal perforations. Marginal perforations that do not heal allow cholesteatoma formation.

If the condition progresses, the eardrum spontaneously **perforates** (breaks open) and pus or blood drains from the ear (Fig. 51-4). This discharge may be pulsating when viewed through the otoscope. When the membrane ruptures, the patient notices a marked decrease in pain as the pressure on middle-ear structures is relieved (Fig. 51-5). Eardrum perforations from any cause may heal if the underlying problem is controlled. Initially, the eardrum membrane appears thinner over the healed perforation. A simple central perforation does not interfere with hearing unless the small bones of the middle ear are damaged or the perforation is large. However, repeated perforations with extensive scarring can cause hearing loss.

Cultures of drainage after a perforation from uncontrolled otitis media may reveal the infecting agent. Cultures are taken only when previous treatment is ineffective. When the eardrum is not perforated, a needle aspiration or myringotomy draws fluid for culture.

Interventions

Nonsurgical Management

Treatment can be as simple as putting the patient in a quiet environment. Bedrest limits head movements that intensify the pain. Heat may be applied by using a heating pad adjusted to a low setting. Application of cold may occasionally relieve pain.

Systemic antibiotic therapy decreases pain by reducing inflammation. Topical antibiotics are not used to treat otitis media. Teach the patient to complete the antibiotic therapy as prescribed and to not stop taking the drug when manifestations are no longer present. Stopping the drug early may result in infection recurrence and contributes to antibiotic resistance. Analgesics such as aspirin, ibuprofen (Advil), and acetaminophen (Tylenol, Abenol♣) relieve pain and reduce fever, helping the patient feel better. When pain is severe, opioid analgesics such as codeine and meperidine hydrochloride (Demerol) also may be used.

Antihistamines and decongestants are prescribed to decrease mucus production and to decrease fluid in the middle ear. The body can then reabsorb the fluid, reducing pressure and pain.

Surgical Management

If the pain persists after antibiotic therapy and the eardrum continues to bulge, a **myringotomy** (surgical opening of the pars tensa of the eardrum) is performed. This procedure drains middle-ear fluids and immediately relieves pain.

Preoperative care includes reassuring the patient that the myringotomy will relieve pain and is usually performed without anesthesia. Many people are concerned about a perforation and its effect on hearing. To relieve some of this anxiety, discuss the reasons for the procedure and encourage the patient to use techniques such as deep breathing before and dur-

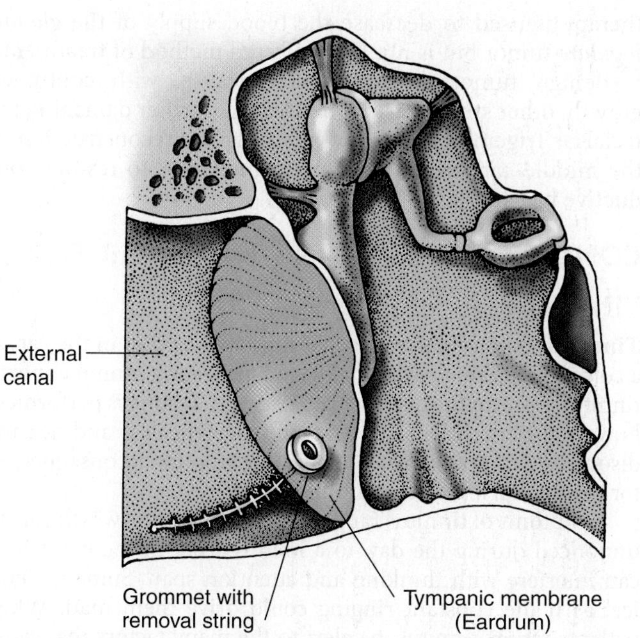
External canal
Grommet with removal string
Tympanic membrane (Eardrum)

Fig. 51-6 • Grommet through the tympanic membrane. A small grommet is placed through the tympanic membrane away from the margins, which allows prolonged drainage of fluids from the middle ear. The grommet can be removed later and the tympanic membrane allowed to heal naturally or patched with a small piece of homogenous tissue.

ing the procedure. Systemic antibiotic therapy continues before and after this procedure. Clean the external canal with a bacteriostatic solution such as povidone-iodine (Betadine) before the myringotomy.

The operative procedure is a small surgical incision. It usually is performed in an office or clinic setting and heals rapidly. Another approach is the removal of fluid from the middle ear with a needle. For relief of pressure caused by serous otitis media and for those patients who have repeated episodes of otitis media, a small **grommet** (polyethylene tube) may be surgically placed through the eardrum to allow continuous drainage of middle-ear fluids (Fig. 51-6).

Postoperative care priorities include teaching the patient to keep the external ear and canal free of other substances while the incision is healing. Instruct him or her to keep the head dry by not washing the hair or showering for several days. Other instructions after surgery are listed in Chart 51-4.

DECISION-MAKING CHALLENGE
Coordination of Care

A 23-year-old woman is being treated for chronic otitis media in the right ear. She rates her pain as 8 on a scale of 1 to 10. She also has decreased hearing in the affected ear and a sensation of fullness. Although she is prescribed an oral antibiotic, she tells you that she does not want to get the prescription filled and asks if she can be treated with eardrops.

1. What are potential problems associated with untreated otitis media?
2. How can pain associated with otitis media be controlled?
3. How would you answer the patient's question regarding treatment with eardrops?

evolve For suggested answer guidelines, go to http://evolve.elsevier.com/Iggy/.

Chart 51-4 PATIENT AND FAMILY EDUCATION GUIDE
Recovery from Ear Surgery

- Avoid straining when you have a bowel movement.
- Do not drink through a straw for 2 to 3 weeks.
- Avoid air travel for 2 to 3 weeks.
- Avoid excessive coughing for 2 to 3 weeks.
- Stay away from people with colds.
- If you need to blow your nose, blow gently, one side at a time, with your mouth open.
- Avoid getting your head wet, washing your hair, and showering for 1 week.
- Keep your ear dry for 6 weeks by placing a ball of cotton coated with petroleum jelly (e.g., Vaseline) in your ear. Change the cotton ball daily.
- Avoid rapidly moving the head, bouncing, and bending over for 3 weeks.
- Change your ear dressing every 24 hours as directed.
- Report excessive drainage immediately to your physician.

MASTOIDITIS
Pathophysiology

The lining of the middle ear is continuous with the lining of the mastoid air cells, which are embedded in the temporal bone. **Mastoiditis** is an infection of the mastoid air cells caused by untreated or inadequately treated otitis media. This infection can be acute or chronic. Antibiotic therapy is aimed at treating the middle-ear infection before it progresses to mastoiditis.

Patient-Centered Collaborative Care

The manifestations of mastoiditis include swelling behind the ear and pain with minimal movement of the tragus, the pinna, or the head. Pain is not relieved by myringotomy. **Cellulitis** (infection spreading sideways through the tissues of the skin) develops on the skin or external scalp over the mastoid process. The ear is pushed sideways and down. Otoscopic examination shows a red, dull, thick, immobile eardrum with or without perforation. Lymph nodes behind the ear are tender and enlarged. Patients may have low-grade fever, malaise, ear drainage, and loss of appetite. Hearing loss occurs, and computed tomography (CT) scans show fluid in the air cells of the mastoid process.

Interventions focus on halting the infection before it spreads to other structures. IV antibiotics are used to prevent the spread of infection. These drugs have limited use in actual mastoiditis treatment because they do not easily penetrate the infected bony structure of the mastoid. Cultures of the ear drainage determine which antibiotics should be most effective.

Surgical removal of the infected tissue is needed if the infection does not respond to antibiotic therapy within a few days. A simple or modified radical mastoidectomy with tympanoplasty is the most common treatment. All infected tissue must be removed so that the infection does not spread to other structures. A tympanoplasty is then performed to reconstruct the ossicles and the eardrum to restore hearing. Patient preparation, the operative procedure, and follow-up care for tympanoplasty are discussed on pp. 1132 and 1133.

Complications occur when infective material is not removed completely or when other structures are contaminated. Complications include damage to cranial nerves VI and VII, decreasing the patient's ability to look sideways (cranial nerve VI) and causing a drooping of the mouth on the affected side (cranial nerve VII). Other complications include vertigo, meningitis, brain abscess, chronic purulent otitis media, and wound infection.

TRAUMA

Pathophysiology

Trauma and damage may occur to the eardrum and ossicles by infection, by direct damage, or through rapid changes in the middle-ear cavity pressure. Foreign objects placed in the external canal exert pressure on the eardrum and cause perforation. If the objects continue through the canal, the bones of the stapes, incus, and malleus may be damaged. Blunt injury to the skull and ears can also damage middle-ear structures through fractures extending to the middle ear. Slapping of the external ear increases the pressure in the ear canal, tearing the eardrum when the pressure is great enough. The eardrum has a limited stretching ability and gives way under high pressure. Excessive nose blowing and rapid changes of pressure that occur with nonpressurized air flight **(barotrauma)** can cause an increase in pressure within the middle ear. High pressure damages the ossicles and can perforate the eardrum.

Patient-Centered Collaborative Care

Most eardrum perforations heal within a week or two without treatment. Repeated perforations, especially from chronic otitis media, heal more slowly, with scarring. Depending on the amount of damage to the ossicles, hearing may or may not return. Hearing aids can improve hearing in this type of hearing loss. Surgical reconstruction of the ossicles and eardrum through a tympanoplasty or a myringoplasty may also improve hearing. (See later discussion of nursing care on p. 1133 in the Tympanoplasty section.)

Nursing care priorities focus on teaching about preventive measures to avoid trauma. Caution patients to avoid inserting objects into the external canal and to follow the steps in Chart 50-3 in Chapter 50 for ear hygiene. Stress the importance of using ear protectors when blunt trauma is likely, especially in sports such as boxing.

NEOPLASMS

Tumors of the middle ear are rare. The most common type of tumor is the *glomus jugulare,* a highly vascular benign lesion arising from the jugular vein. Cancerous ear tumors include adenocarcinoma, adenoid cystic carcinoma, and mucoepidermoid carcinoma. The growth of any lesion within the middle-ear area disrupts conductive hearing, erodes the ossicles, and may spread to the inner ear and nearby cranial nerves.

Patients have progressive hearing loss and tinnitus. Infection and pain rarely occur with *glomus jugulare* tumors. Otoscopic examination shows bulging of the eardrum or a mass extending to the external ear canal. The many blood vessels of the *glomus jugulare* tumor give it a reddish color and a visible pulsation when seen through the eardrum.

Diagnosis is made by physical examination, tomography, and angiography. Tumors are removed by surgery, which often destroys hearing in the affected ear. If all of the edges of the tumor can be seen clearly through the eardrum, surgery is performed through the ear canal to remove the tumor. When the tumor edges extend past the eardrum, more testing is needed to determine the extent of involvement. Radiation therapy is used to decrease the blood supply of the *glomus jugulare* tumor but is not the preferred method of treatment.

Benign tumors are removed because, with continued growth, other structures can be affected, further damaging the facial or trigeminal nerve. When possible, reconstruction of the middle-ear structures is performed later to restore conductive hearing.

CONDITIONS AFFECTING THE INNER EAR

TINNITUS

Tinnitus (continuous ringing or noise perception in the ear) is a common hearing problem. Diagnostic testing cannot confirm tinnitus, nor can the disorder be observed. Testing is performed, however, to assess hearing and rule out other ear and hearing disorders. Tinnitus can have disturbing emotional consequences for the person afflicted with this disorder.

Symptoms of tinnitus range from mild ringing, which can go unnoticed during the day, to a loud roaring in the ear, which can interfere with thinking and attention span. Some patients feel as if the constant ringing could drive them mad. When patients report tinnitus, be alert to the many factors that cause tinnitus: presbycusis, **otosclerosis** (irregular bone growth around ossicles), Ménière's disease, certain drugs, exposure to loud noise, and other inner-ear problems (Daughtery, 2007).

The exact course of the problem and its treatment vary with the underlying cause (Henry et al., 2005). When no cause can be found or the disorder is untreatable, therapy focuses on ways to mask the tinnitus with background sound, noisemakers, and music during sleeping hours. Ear mold hearing aids can amplify sounds to drown out the tinnitus during the day. The American Tinnitus Association assists patients in coping with tinnitus when other therapy is unsuccessful. Refer patients with tinnitus to local and online support groups to help cope with this problem (Table 51-1).

VERTIGO AND DIZZINESS

Vertigo and dizziness are common manifestations of many ear disorders. Dizziness is a disturbed sense of a person's relationship to space. Patients vary greatly in defining dizziness. Vertigo is often used interchangeably with dizziness, but the definition, as well as the cause, is somewhat different. True **vertigo** is a real sense of whirling or turning in space.

The visual system, the vestibular system (cochlea, semicircular canals), and the proprioceptive system (muscles and nerve endings) combine to give input to the brain about balance. Problems in any of these areas lead to a disturbed sense of balance and motion. Factors affecting the ear that cause vertigo include Ménière's disease, labyrinthitis, acoustic neuromas, motion sickness, and drug or alcohol ingestion.

Manifestations of vertigo include nausea, vomiting, falling, nystagmus, hearing loss, and tinnitus. Until the cause of the vertigo can be treated, each manifestation is treated. Teach patients these strategies to reduce manifestations:

- Restrict head motions, and move more slowly.
- Maintain adequate hydration, especially after vomiting.
- Take drugs that reduce the vertigo effects, such as dimenhydrinate (Dramamine, Gravol♣), diazepam (Valium, Apo-Diazepam♣), and scopolamine (Transderm Scop, Transderm-V♣).

Many patients are dissatisfied with treatment because side effects of the drugs, especially drowsiness, can be worse than

TABLE 51-1 Resource Agencies for Ear and Hearing Impairment

House Ear Institute 2100 West Third Street, Fifth Floor Los Angeles, CA 90057 Voice: (800) 388-8612 Fax: (213) 483-8789 www.houseearclinic.com E-mail: info@hei.org	**American Speech-Language-Hearing Association** 2200 Research Boulevard Rockville, MD 20850-3289 Voice: (800) 638-8255 Fax: (301) 296-8580 www.asha.org
Laurent Clerc National Deaf Education Center Gallaudet University 800 Florida Avenue NE Washington, DC 20002 Voice/TTY: (202) 651-5051	**Hearing Loss Association of America** 7910 Woodmont Avenue, Suite 1200 Bethesda, MD 20814 Voice/TTY: (301) 657-2248 Fax: (301) 657-2248 www.shhh.org
American Academy of Otolaryngology/Head and Neck Surgery One Prince Street Alexandria, VA 22314-3357 Voice/TTY: (703) 836-4444 www.entnet.org	**American Tinnitus Association** P.O. Box 5 Portland, OR 97207-0005 Voice: (800) 634-8978 www.ata.org

the vertigo. Teach patients to maintain a safe, uncluttered environment to prevent accidents during periods of vertigo and to use a cane or walker to maintain balance. Also instruct them to not drive or operate machinery when taking these drugs.

LABYRINTHITIS

Labyrinthitis is an infection of the labyrinth, which may occur as a complication of acute or chronic otitis media. Infection results from an erosion of the bony capsule, allowing organisms to invade the inner ear. Labyrinthitis often results from the growth of a **cholesteatoma** (benign overgrowth of squamous cell epithelium) from the middle ear into the semicircular canal. It may follow middle-ear or inner-ear surgery when infection is present. Labyrinthitis may be part of an upper respiratory infection or mononucleosis.

Manifestations include hearing loss, tinnitus, nystagmus to the affected side, and vertigo with nausea and vomiting. **Meningitis** (infection of the brain covering) is a common complication of labyrinthitis.

Treatment of the disease includes the use of systemic antibiotics. Teach the patient to complete the antibiotic therapy as prescribed and to not stop taking the drug when manifestations are no longer present. Stopping the drug early may result in infection recurrence and contributes to antibiotic resistance. Advise patients to stay in bed in a darkened room until manifestations are reduced. Antiemetics and antivertiginous drugs, such as dimenhydrinate (Dramamine, Gravol🍁), relieve symptoms.

The patient also needs psychosocial support. Hearing loss on the affected side may be permanent, although vertigo subsides as the inflammation resolves. Persistent balance problems may improve with gait training and physical therapy.

MÉNIÈRE'S DISEASE

Pathophysiology

Ménière's disease has three features: tinnitus, one-sided sensorineural hearing loss, and vertigo, occurring in attacks that can last for several days. Patients are almost totally incapacitated during an attack, and full recovery often takes several days.

The pathology of Ménière's disease is an excess of endolymphatic fluid that distorts the entire inner-canal system. This distortion decreases hearing from dilation of the cochlear duct, causes vertigo because of damage to the vestibular system, and stimulates tinnitus. At first, hearing loss is reversible, but repeated damage to the cochlea from increased fluid pressure leads to permanent hearing loss.

The exact cause of Ménière's disease is unknown, but it often occurs with infections, allergic reactions, and fluid imbalances. Long-term stress may also have a role in the disease.

Patient-Centered Collaborative Care

Assessment

Ménière's disease usually first occurs in people between the ages of 20 and 50 years. The disease is more common in men and in white people. Times of severe, debilitating attacks alternate with symptom-free periods. Patients often have certain manifestations before an attack of vertigo, such as headaches, increasing tinnitus, and a feeling of fullness in the affected ear. Manifestations are usually only on one side.

Patients describe the tinnitus as a continuous, low-pitched roar or a humming sound, which worsens just before and during a severe attack. Hearing loss occurs first with the low-frequency tones but worsens to include all levels after repeated episodes. In the early stages of Ménière's disease, hearing is normal or nearly normal between episodes, but permanent hearing loss develops as the attacks increase.

Patients describe the vertigo as periods of whirling, which might even cause them to fall. The vertigo is so intense that even while lying down, the patient often holds the bed or ground to prevent the whirling sensation. Severe vertigo usually lasts 3 to 4 hours, but the patient may feel dizzy long after the attack. Nausea and vomiting are common. Other manifestations include rapid eye movements **(nystagmus)** and severe headaches.

Common Nursing Diagnoses and Collaborative Problems

Nursing diagnoses that may apply to patients with Ménière's disease include:

- Anxiety related to loss of control
- Risk for Injury related to loss of balance

- Powerlessness related to loss of control
- Activity Intolerance related to perception of dizziness
- Risk for Deficient Fluid Volume related to nausea and vomiting
- Fear related to potential of hearing loss

Interventions

Nonsurgical Management

Teach patients to move the head slowly to prevent worsening of the vertigo. Nutrition and lifestyle changes can reduce the amount of endolymphatic fluid. Advise patients to stop smoking because of the blood vessel constricting effects.

Nutrition therapy with a hydrops diet aims to stabilize body fluid levels to prevent excess endolymph accumulation. The basic structure of this diet involves:

- Distributing food and fluid intake evenly throughout the day and from day to day
- Avoiding foods or fluids that have a high salt content
- Drinking adequate amounts of fluids (low in sugar) daily
- Avoiding caffeine-containing fluids and foods
- Limiting alcohol intake to one glass of beer or wine each day
- Avoiding foods containing monosodium glutamate (MSG)

Coordinate with a nutritionist for more detailed information about hydrops nutrition therapy for control of Ménière's manifestations.

Drug therapy aims to control the vertigo and vomiting and restore normal balance. Mild diuretics are prescribed to decrease endolymph volume. However, there is insufficient evidence of the effect of diuretics on vertigo, hearing loss, tinnitus, or aural fullness in clearly defined Ménière's disease (Thirlwall & Kundu, 2006). Nicotinic acid has been found to be useful because of its vasodilatory effect. Antihistamines such as diphenhydramine hydrochloride (Benadryl, Allerdryl🍁) and dimenhydrinate (Dramamine, Gravol🍁) help reduce the severity of or stop an acute attack. Antiemetics such as chlorpromazine hydrochloride (Thorazine, Novo-Chlorpromazine🍁), droperidol (Inapsine), and trimethobenzamide hydrochloride (Arrestin, Tigan) help control the nausea and vomiting. Diazepam (Valium, Apo-Diazepam🍁) calms the patient; controls vertigo, nausea, and vomiting; and allows the patient to rest quietly during an attack. Intratympanic therapy with gentamycin and steroids is another method for controlling manifestations. However, some or all hearing is lost in the ear receiving gentamicin.

Another nonsurgical treatment is the Meniett device. This device applies low-pressure micropulses to the inner ear for 5 minutes three times daily. This action is believed to displace fluid from the inner ear and thus relieve manifestations. Placement of a tympanostomy tube in the eardrum of the affected ear is needed to use this therapy. Long-term success in control of vertigo is over 80% (Gates et al., 2006). Although hearing loss is not improved, Meniett device usage does not adversely affect balance, as do most forms of surgical therapy for Ménière's disease. (See the Evidence-Based Practice box below.)

Surgical Management

Surgical treatment of Ménière's disease is a last resort because the hearing in the affected ear is often lost from the procedure. When medical therapy is ineffective and the patient's hearing level has decreased significantly, surgery is performed. The

EVIDENCE-BASED PRACTICE

Self-administered treatment effective in reducing vertigo

Gates, G., Verrall, A., Green, J.D., Tucci, D.L., & Telian, S.A. (2006). Meniett clinical trial: Long-term follow-up. *Archives of Otolaryngology—Head & Neck Surgery, 132*(12), 1311-1316.

Severe vertigo is a distressing manifestation of Ménière's disease resulting in increased sick-day usage and reduced quality of life. Although medical therapy has reduced these side effects in many people, a large percentage of patients with Ménière's disease still suffer from severe vertigo, nausea, and vomiting. In a large, multi-center, randomized, controlled clinical trial, a new device, the Meniett low-intensity alternating-pressure generator, has been shown to significantly reduce vertigo in patients suffering from Ménière's disease in the short term. Self-application of low-intensity alternating pressure involved connecting the device to a polyethylene grommet placed in the eardrum of the affected ear. The device, used three times daily for 5 minutes each time, displaces fluid from the inner ear and thus prevents or relieves manifestations. Results of the initial randomized, controlled clinical trial indicated that about 70% of those patients using the device for 4 months had fewer episodes of vertigo and had fewer sick-day absences from work.

The follow-up study sought to determine whether the effect was maintained long term and what effect the treatment might have had on hearing. Sixty-one subjects who self-administered the treatment were followed for 2 years. The results indicated that about two thirds of the subjects continued to have significant relief from vertigo with fewer sick-day work absences. The treatment was most effective for those patients who did not have a good response with antivertiginous drugs alone. This study showed neither a positive nor a negative effect of the treatment on hearing.

Level of Evidence—1. The study is a follow-up of a multi-site, randomized, controlled clinical trial.

Commentary: Implications for Practice and Research. This nonsurgical approach appears to be effective for many people with Ménière's disease without sacrificing the remaining sense of hearing in the affected ear. It does rely on the patient's adherence to the self-administration treatment schedule, which may assist in increasing the patient's sense of control in management of the disease. Thus nurse promotion and reinforcement of patient education for this treatment may be key in its success. Research studies are needed to develop effective patient education materials and to determine what personal factors may contribute to or predict adherence to the treatment plan.

choice of the surgical procedure depends on the degree of useful hearing, the severity of the spells, and the condition of the opposite ear. The most radical procedure involves resection of the vestibular nerve or total removal of the labyrinth **(labyrinthectomy),** performed through the ear canal. The footplate of the stapes is moved aside, and the labyrinth is removed through the oval window.

Another procedure performed early in the course of the disease is endolymphatic decompression with drainage and a shunt. The effectiveness of this procedure for control of the disease manifestations varies. The endolymphatic sac is drained, and a small tube is inserted to improve fluid drainage. Some patients report relief of vertigo with retention of their hearing. If an endolymphatic decompression has been performed, movement of the vestibular structures of the inner ear causes vertigo early after surgery. Reassure the patient that the vertigo is temporary as a result of the surgical procedure, not the disease.

NCLEX EXAMINATION CHALLENGE

Which is the priority nursing diagnosis for a client with Ménière's disease during an attack?

A. Fear
B. Risk for Injury
C. Powerlessness
D. Risk for Deficient Fluid Volume

evolve For the correct answer, go to http://evolve.elsevier.com/Iggy/.

ACOUSTIC NEUROMA

An **acoustic neuroma** is a benign tumor of cranial nerve VIII. The tumor often damages other structures as it grows. Depending on the size and exact location of the tumor, damage to hearing, facial movements, and sensation can occur (McCance & Huether, 2006). An acoustic neuroma can cause many neurologic manifestations as the tumor enlarges in the brain.

Manifestations begin with tinnitus and progress to gradual sensorineural hearing loss in most patients. Later, patients have constant mild vertigo. As the tumor enlarges, nearby cranial nerves are damaged.

Acoustic neuromas are diagnosed with computed tomography (CT) scanning and magnetic resonance imaging (MRI). Audiograms show sensorineural hearing loss. Cerebrospinal fluid assays show increased pressure and protein.

Surgical removal via a craniotomy is performed, and the remaining hearing is lost. Extreme care is taken to preserve the function of the facial nerve (cranial nerve VII). Care after craniotomy is discussed in Chapter 47. Acoustic neuromas rarely recur after surgical removal.

HEARING LOSS

Pathophysiology

Hearing loss is one of the most common handicaps in North America. It may be conductive, sensorineural, or a combination of the two (Fig. 51-7). *Conductive hearing* loss occurs when sound waves are blocked from contact with inner-ear nerve fibers because of external-ear or middle-ear disorders. If the inner-ear sensory nerve fibers that lead to the cerebral cortex are damaged, the hearing loss is termed *sensorineural.* Combined hearing loss is known as *mixed conductive-sensorineural.*

The differences in conductive and sensorineural hearing loss are listed in Table 51-2. Disorders that cause conductive hearing loss are often corrected with no or minimal permanent damage. Sensorineural hearing loss is often permanent, and measures must be taken to prevent further damage or to amplify sounds as a means to improve hearing.

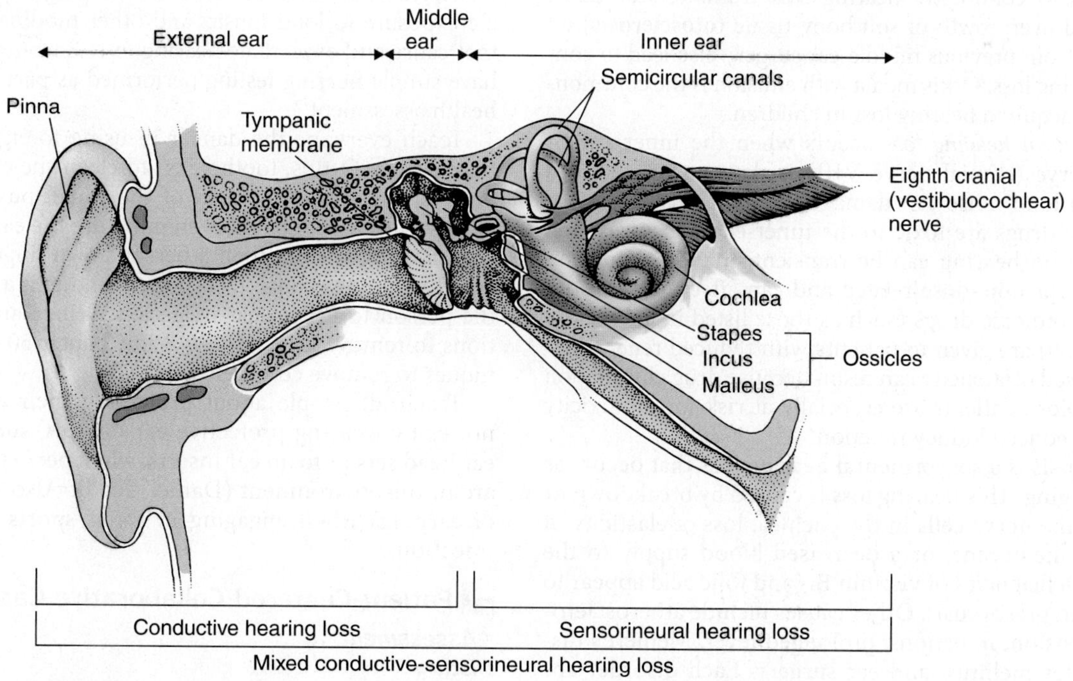
External ear
Middle ear
Inner ear
Semicircular canals
Pinna
Tympanic membrane
Eighth cranial (vestibulocochlear) nerve
Cochlea
Stapes
Incus
Malleus
Ossicles
Conductive hearing loss
Sensorineural hearing loss
Mixed conductive-sensorineural hearing loss

Fig. 51-7 • Anatomy of hearing loss. Hearing loss can be divided into three types: (1) conductive (difficulty in the external or the middle ear); (2) sensorineural (difficulty in the inner ear or the acoustic nerve); and (3) mixed conductive-sensorineural (a combination of the two).

TABLE 51-2 Differential Features of Conductive and Sensorineural Hearing Loss

Conductive Hearing Loss	Sensorineural Hearing Loss
CAUSES	
Cerumen	Prolonged exposure to noise
Foreign body	Presbycusis
Perforation of the tympanic membrane	Ototoxic substance
Edema	Ménière's disease
Infection of the external ear or middle ear	Acoustic neuroma
Tumor	Diabetes mellitus
Otosclerosis	Labyrinthitis
	Infection
	Myxedema
ASSESSMENT FINDINGS	
Evidence of obstruction with otoscope	Normal appearance of external canal and tympanic membrane
Abnormality in tympanic membrane	Tinnitus common
Speaking softly	Occasional dizziness
Hearing best in a noisy environment	Speaking loudly
	Hearing poorly in loud environment
Rinne test: air conduction greater than bone conduction	Rinne test: air conduction less than bone conduction
Weber test: lateralization to affected ear	Weber test: lateralization to unaffected ear

Etiology and Genetic Risk

Conductive hearing loss can be caused by any inflammation or obstruction of the external or middle ear by cerumen or foreign objects. Changes in the eardrum such as bulging, retraction, and perforations may indicate damage to middle-ear structures, which leads to conductive hearing loss. Tumors, scar tissue buildup, and overgrowth of soft bony tissue **(otosclerosis)** on the ossicles from previous middle-ear surgery also lead to conductive hearing loss. Otitis media with effusion is the commonest cause of acquired hearing loss in children.

Sensorineural hearing loss occurs when the inner ear or auditory nerve (cranial nerve VIII) is damaged. Prolonged exposure to loud noise can damage the hair cells of the cochlea. Many drugs are toxic to the inner-ear structures, and their effects on hearing can be transient or permanent and dose related or non–dose related and can affect one or both ears. When ototoxic drugs (such as those listed in Table 50-1 in Chapter 50) are given to patients with reduced renal function, increased ototoxicity can result because drug elimination is slower. Older patients are especially at risk for ototoxicity because of reduced kidney function.

Presbycusis is a sensorineural hearing loss that occurs as a result of aging. This hearing loss is caused by breakdown or atrophy of the nerve cells in the cochlea, loss of elasticity of the basilar membrane, or a decreased blood supply to the inner ear. Deficiencies of vitamin B_{12} and folic acid appear to play a role in presbycusis. Other causes include atherosclerosis, hypertension, infections, prolonged fever, Ménière's disease, diabetes mellitus, and ear surgery. Each disorder appears to speed up degenerative changes of the cochlea. Trauma to the ear or the head also contributes to sensorineural hearing loss.

GENETIC CONSIDERATIONS

In some cases, hearing loss in adults can have a genetic origin. Some syndromes in which a single gene mutation results in many abnormal manifestations also increase the risk for progressive hearing loss in adults. Two such syndromes are Usher's syndrome and Alport's syndrome (Nussbaum et al., 2007). Usher's syndrome, in addition to hearing loss, occurs with blindness as a result of retinitis pigmentosa. This syndrome has an autosomal recessive pattern of inheritance. Alport's syndrome, which causes abnormal renal function in addition to hearing loss, has many forms and many patterns of inheritance. One type of adult-onset hearing loss that does not have any other physical problems is associated with a mutation in the *GJB2* gene on chromosome 1 (Online Mendelian Inheritance in Man [OMIM], 2007). This problem has an autosomal dominant pattern of inheritance.

Incidence/Prevalence

Because hearing loss may be gradual and affect only some aspects of hearing, many adults are unaware that their hearing is impaired. The actual incidence of hearing loss is not known, although about one third of people ages 65 to 75 years have a hearing loss. As many as half of people older than 85 years have some degree of hearing loss (National Institute on Deafness and Other Communication Disorders, 2007).

Health Promotion and Maintenance

For most people, hearing is an important factor in social interactions and to gain knowledge. *Good hearing contributes to meeting the human need for sensation and cognition.* With special care to the ears, hearing can be preserved at maximum levels. Address barriers to the use of hearing protection, deliberate exposure to loud music, and other modifiable risk factors that cause and exacerbate hearing loss. Encourage everyone to have simple hearing testing performed as part of their annual health assessment.

Teach everyone the danger in using foreign objects (e.g., bobby-pins, Q-tips, toothpicks) to clean the ear canal. These objects can scrape the skin of the canal, push cerumen up against the eardrum, and even puncture the eardrum. Explain that nothing smaller than a person's own fingertip should be inserted into the canal. If cerumen buildup is a problem, teach the person to use an ear irrigation syringe and proper solutions to remove it. (Chart 50-3 in Chapter 50 describes techniques to remove cerumen safely.)

Teach all people about protecting their ears from loud noises by wearing protective ear devices, such as over-the-ear head sets or foam ear inserts, when persistent loud noises are in the environment (Daniel, 2007). Also suggest the use of earplugs when engaging in water sports to prevent ear infections.

Patient-Centered Collaborative Care

evolve ONLINE PHARM REVIEW

Assessment

History

Ask patients how long they have noticed a difference in their hearing and whether the changes occurred suddenly or gradually. Age is an important factor, because some ear and hearing changes occur with advanced age. Chronic otitis media occurs more often in the older adult. Ask about occupational exposure to loud or continuous noises, as well as current or previous use of ototoxic drugs. Also ask about any history of external-ear or middle-ear infection and whether eardrum perforation occurred with the infection. Ask patients about any direct trauma to the ears. Because some types of hearing loss have a genetic predisposition, ask whether any family members are hearing impaired.

When pain occurs with acute-onset hearing loss, ask about recent upper respiratory infection and allergies affecting the nose and sinuses.

Physical Assessment/Clinical Manifestations

Chart 51-5 lists focused assessment techniques for patients with suspected hearing loss. Hearing loss may be sudden or gradual and often affects both ears. The ability to hear high-frequency soft, consonants—especially *s, sh, f, th,* and *ch* sounds—is lost first. Patients often state that they have no problem with hearing but cannot understand specific words. They might think that the speaker is mumbling. They often have continuous tinnitus in both ears. Vertigo may be present, depending on the extent of inner-ear involvement.

Tuning fork tests help diagnose hearing loss (see Chapter 50). With the Weber test, the patient can usually hear sounds well in the ear with a conductive hearing loss because of bone conduction. With the Rinne test, the patient reports that sound transmitted by bone conduction is louder and more sustained than that transmitted by air conduction.

Otoscopic examination is performed to assess the external ear canal, the eardrum, and structures of the middle ear that can be seen through the eardrum (see Chapter 50). Findings from examination vary, depending on the cause of the hearing loss.

Chart 51-5 FOCUSED ASSESSMENT

The Patient with Suspected Hearing Loss

Assess whether the patient has any of these ear problems:
- Pain
- Feeling of fullness or congestion
- Dizziness or vertigo
- Tinnitus
- Difficulty understanding conversations, especially in a noisy room
- Difficulty hearing sounds
- The need to strain to hear
- The need to turn the head to favor one ear or the need to lean forward to hear

Assess visible ear structures, particularly the external canal and tympanic membrane:
- Position and size of the pinna
- Patency of the external canal; presence of cerumen or foreign bodies, edema, or inflammation
- Condition of the tympanic membrane: intact, edema, fluid, inflammation

Assess functional ability, including:
- Frequency of asking people to repeat statements
- Withdrawal from social interactions or large groups
- Shouting in conversation
- Failing to respond when not looking in the direction of the sound
- Answering questions incorrectly

Obstruction of the external ear canal can result in hearing loss. Inspect the canal, looking for:
- Whether the canal is open
- The amount and character of cerumen present
- The integrity of the skin lining the canal
- The presence of redness, exudates, lesions, or foreign objects

Middle-ear infections can also reduce hearing. In infection or inflammation, the eardrum appears red, thickened, and bulging, with a loss of landmarks. Loss of eardrum mobility is seen with inspection through a pneumatic otoscope. Document the presence of any scars or perforations on the eardrum. With close observation, exudate may be seen behind the membrane.

Psychosocial Assessment

For people with a hearing loss, communication can become a struggle, and they may isolate themselves because of the difficulty in talking and listening. Social isolation can lead to depression, fear, and despair. Be sensitive to emotional changes that may be related to reduced hearing and a decline in conversational skills. Encourage the patient and family to express their feelings and concerns about an actual or potential hearing loss.

Laboratory Assessment

No laboratory test diagnoses hearing loss. However, some laboratory findings can indicate problems that affect hearing.

White blood cell counts are elevated in the patient with acute or chronic otitis media. Microbial culture and antibiotic sensitivity tests can determine the causative organism and the most appropriate drug therapy when infection causes hearing loss.

The patient with hearing loss from peripheral neuropathy may have other systemic diseases, including human immune deficiency virus (HIV) disease or poorly controlled diabetes mellitus. The blood glucose level may be elevated, and the blood may be positive for serum acetone. Patients undergoing chemotherapy or interferon therapy for cancer are at risk for hearing loss from neuropathy.

Imaging Assessment

Imaging assessment can determine non-auditory problems affecting hearing ability. Some hearing problems can be diagnosed using imaging techniques. Skull x-rays are used to determine bony involvement in otitis media and the location of otosclerotic lesions, and CT and MRI are used to determine soft-tissue involvement and the presence and location of tumors.

Other Diagnostic Assessment

Audiometry can help determine the extent and type of hearing loss. An audiogram shows whether hearing loss is only conductive or whether it has a sensorineural component. This is important in determining possible causes of the hearing loss and in planning interventions.

Analysis

Common Nursing Diagnoses and Collaborative Problems

Priority nursing diagnoses for patients with any degree of hearing impairment are:

1. Disturbed Sensory Perception (Auditory) related to obstruction, infection, damage to the middle ear, or damage to the auditory nerve
2. Impaired Verbal Communication related to reduced sensory perception (auditory)

Additional Nursing Diagnoses and Collaborative Problems

In addition to the common nursing diagnoses, patients with hearing loss or impairment may have one or more of these:

- Deficient Knowledge related to treatment and prevention
- Activity Intolerance related to pain
- Social Isolation related to pain and decreased hearing
- Risk for Injury related to altered auditory perception and infection
- Acute Pain related to an inflammatory process and fluid in the middle ear
- Impaired Physical Mobility related to vertigo

Planning and Implementation

Disturbed Sensory Perception (Auditory)

NOC **Planning: Expected Outcomes.** The patient with hearing loss or impairment is expected to either have an increase in auditory sensory perception to a functional level or maintain existing levels of hearing. Indicators include:

- Mild to no loss of high pitch tones
- Mild to no loss of ability to distinguish conversation from background environmental noise
- Turning to sound
- Maintaining auditory discrimination of discrete sounds

Interventions. Interventions aim at identifying the problem, halting the pathologic processes, and improving auditory perception. Nursing care priorities focus on teaching the patient in the use and care of an appropriate assistive device, providing support to the patient and family who are working to maintain or increase communication, and assisting patients to find local and Internet-based support services.

Nonsurgical Management. Interventions include early detection of hearing impairment, use of drug therapy and comfort measures, and use of assistive devices to amplify or augment the patient's auditory perception.

Early detection helps correct the problem causing the hearing loss. When hearing loss is gradual, the patient can compensate. Assess for indications of hearing loss, as listed in Chart 51-5.

Drug therapy is aimed at either correcting the underlying pathologic change or reducing the side effects of problems occurring with hearing loss. Topical antibiotics are given to patients with external otitis. Systemic antibiotics are needed when patients have other ear infections. Teach the patient receiving antibiotic therapy the importance of taking the drug or drugs exactly as prescribed and completing the entire course. Caution him or her to not stop the drug just because manifestations have improved. By treating the infection, antibiotics reduce local edema and improve hearing. When pain occurs with hearing disorders, analgesics are used, depending on the location and type of pain. Many ear disorders disturb equilibrium, causing vertigo and dizziness with nausea and vomiting. Antiemetic, antihistamine, antivertiginous, and benzodiazepine drugs can help correct nausea, vertigo, and dizziness.

Assistive devices are useful for patients with permanent, progressive hearing loss. Portable amplifiers can be used while watching television to avoid increasing the volume and disturbing others. Telephone amplifiers increase telephone volume, allowing the caller to speak in a normal voice. Flashing lights activated by the ringing telephone or a doorbell alert patients visually. In some cases, patients may have a specially trained dog to help them be aware of sounds (ringing telephones or doorbells, cries of other people, and potential dangers) in much the same way that a seeing eye dog assists a blind person. Provide information about agencies that can assist the hearing-impaired person.

Small, portable audio amplifiers can assist you in communicating with patients with hearing loss but who have chosen not to use a hearing aid. The use of audio amplifiers or allowing patients to use a stethoscope for listening helps you communicate with anyone who requires additional volume to hear speech.

A hearing aid is a miniature electronic amplifier that is usually used for patients with conductive hearing loss. Hearing aids are less effective for sensorineural hearing loss and may make hearing worse by amplifying background noise. The amplifier can be worn in one or both ears. Some hearing-impaired patients refuse to use hearing aids, believing that other people will think they are old. Most common hearing aids are small. Some are attached to a person's glasses and are visible to other people. Another type fits into the ear and is less noticeable. Newer devices fit completely in the canal with only a fine, clear, filament visible at all. The cost of smaller hearing aids is greater than the cost of larger ones. Local agencies offer special classes for the hearing impaired that help the users benefit from this device.

Offer some special tips to help the patient adjust to the hearing aid. Hearing with a hearing aid can be different from natural hearing. Teach the patient to start using the hearing aid slowly, at first wearing it only at home and only during part of the day. Listening to television and the radio and reading aloud can help the patient get used to new sounds. The tone or volume of the hearing aid can be adjusted. The most important and difficult aspect of a hearing aid is the amplification of background noise, as well as voices. The patient must learn to concentrate and filter out background noises.

Teach the patient how to care for the hearing aid (Chart 51-6). Hearing aids are delicate devices that should be handled only by people who know how to care for them properly. The cost of the aids varies greatly but is a significant investment.

Cochlear implantation may help patients with sensorineural hearing loss. Although a superficial surgical procedure is needed to implant the device, the procedure does not enter the inner ear and thus is not considered a surgical correction for hearing impairment. A small computer converts sound waves into electronic impulses. Electrodes are placed near the internal ear, with the computer attached to the external ear. The electronic impulses then directly stimulate nerve fibers. Some patients have a 50% return of their hearing with this method.

Surgical Management. Many surgical interventions are available for patients with specific disorders leading to hearing loss.

Tympanoplasty. Tympanoplasty reconstructs the middle ear to improve conductive hearing loss. The procedures vary from simple reconstruction of the eardrum **(myringoplasty)** to replacement of the ossicles within the middle ear. A type I tympanoplasty is used for a myringoplasty; a type II tympanoplasty is used in cases of greater damage, and it provides more extensive reconstruction (Fig. 51-8).

Preoperative care. The patient requires specific instructions before surgery. Systemic antibiotics reduce the risk for infection. Before surgery, irrigate the ear with a solution of equal parts of vinegar and sterile water to restore normal ear pH.

Teach the patient to follow other measures to decrease the risks for infection, such as avoiding people with upper respiratory infections, getting adequate rest, eating a balanced diet, and drinking adequate amounts of fluid.

Assure the patient that hearing loss immediately after surgery is normal because of canal packing and that hearing will improve when the packing is removed. Explain the importance of deep breathing and coughing after surgery, but stress that forceful coughing increases middle-ear pressure and must be avoided.

Chart 51-6 PATIENT AND FAMILY EDUCATION GUIDE

Hearing Aid Care

- Keep the hearing aid dry.
- Clean the ear mold with mild soap and water while avoiding excessive wetting.
- Clean debris from the hole in the middle of the part that goes into your ear with a toothpick or a pipe cleaner.
- Turn off the hearing aid and remove the battery when not in use.
- Check and replace the battery frequently.
- Keep extra batteries on hand.
- Keep the hearing aid in a safe place.
- Avoid dropping the hearing aid or exposing it to temperature extremes.
- Adjust the volume to the lowest setting that allows you to hear, to prevent feedback squeaking.
- Avoid using hair spray, cosmetics, oils, or other hair and face products that might come into contact with the receiver.
- If the hearing aid does not work:
  - Change the battery.
  - Check the connection between the ear mold and the receiver.
  - Check the on/off switch.
  - Clean the sound hole.
  - Adjust the volume.
  - Take the hearing aid to an authorized service center for repair.

Operative procedures. Surgery is performed only when the middle ear is free of infection and if the condition of the eustachian tube does not promote continued infection. If an infection is present, the graft is more likely to become infected and not heal. Surgery of the eardrum and ossicles requires the use of a microscope and is a delicate procedure. Local anesthesia can be used, although general anesthesia is often used to prevent the patient from moving.

The surgeon can repair the eardrum with many materials, including muscle fascia, a skin graft, and venous tissue. If the ossicles are damaged, more extensive surgery is needed for repair or replacement. The ossicles can be reached in several ways—through the ear canal, with an endaural incision, or by an incision behind the ear with a mastoidectomy (Fig. 51-9).

The surgeon removes diseased tissue and cleans the middle-ear cavity. The ossicles are assessed for damage and the extent of needed repair or replacement. The patient's cartilage or bone, cadaver ossicles, stainless steel wire, or special polymers (Teflon) are used to repair or replace the ossicles.

Postoperative care. An antiseptic-soaked gauze, such as iodoform gauze (NU GAUZE), is packed in the ear canal. If a skin incision is used, a dressing is placed over it. Keep the dressing clean and dry, using sterile technique for changes. Keep the patient flat, with the head turned to the side and the operative ear facing up for at least 12 hours after surgery. Give prescribed antibiotics to prevent infection.

Patients often report hearing improvement after removal of the canal packing. Until that time, communicate as with a hearing-impaired patient, directing conversation to the unaffected ear. Instruct the patient in care and activity restrictions (see Chart 51-4).

Stapedectomy. A partial or complete stapedectomy with a prosthesis corrects hearing loss. This procedure is most effective for patients with hearing loss related to otosclerosis. The average age for patients undergoing primary stapes surgery is increasing. Regardless of age, short-term and long-term hearing results after primary stapes surgery are good. However, a small percentage of patients redevelop conductive hearing loss after undergoing stapes surgery and desire revision surgery to correct this hearing loss. With modern otologic equipment,

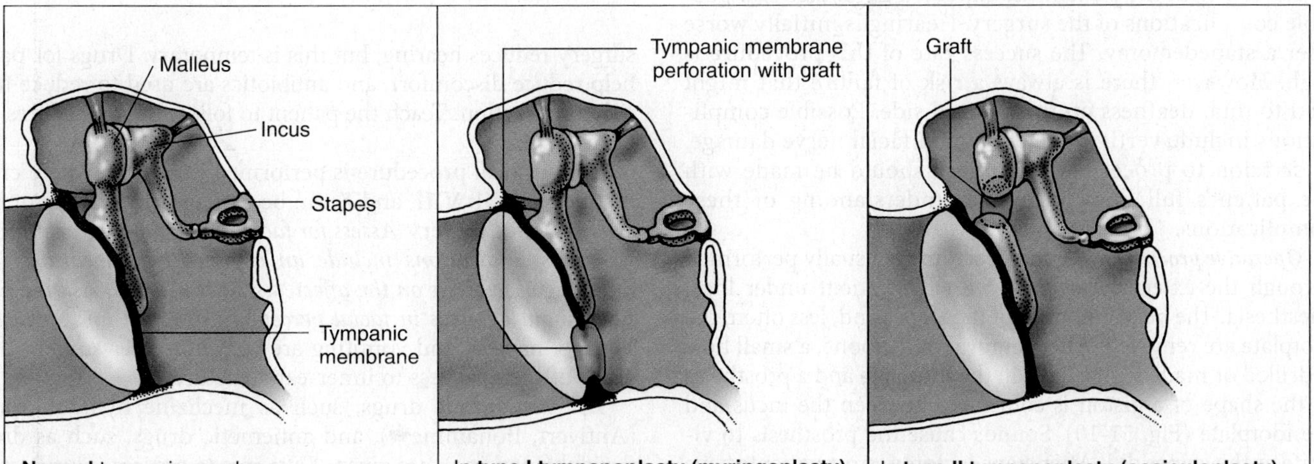
Malleus
Incus
Stapes
Tympanic membrane
Tympanic membrane perforation with graft
Graft

Normal tympanic membrane and ossicles.

In **type I tympanoplasty (myringoplasty)**, a graft is placed over a perforation in the tympanic membrane; other middle ear structures are normal.

In **type II tympanoplasty (ossiculoplasty)**, the malleus, which has become disconnected from the tympanic membrane, is grafted to reconnect the structures.

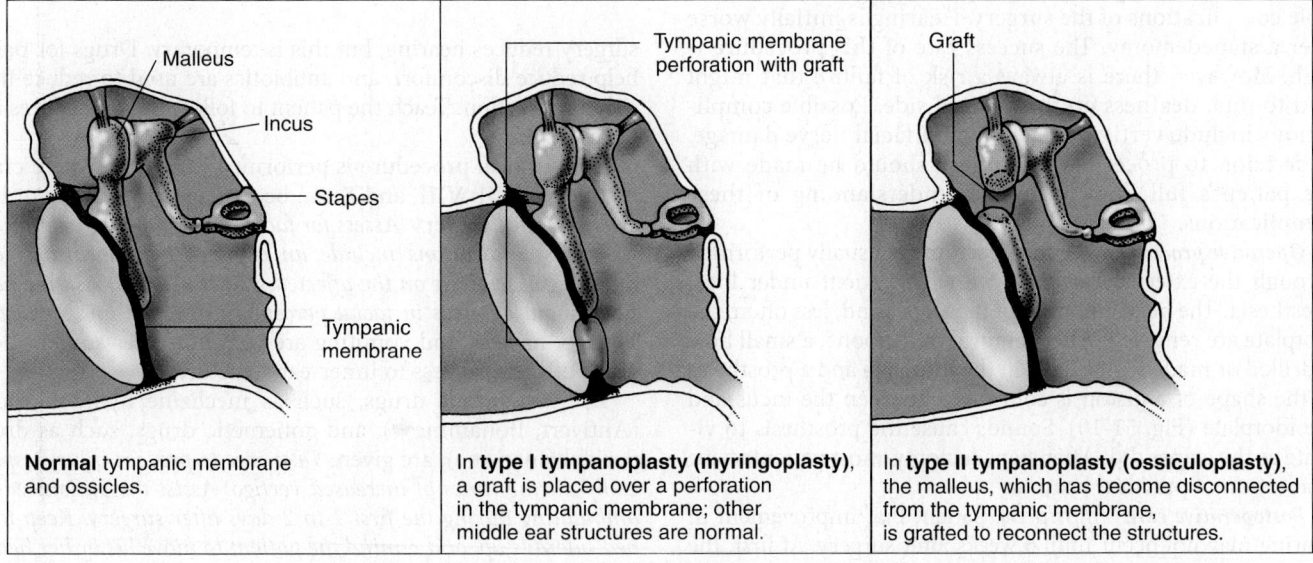

Fig. 51-8 • A normal tympanic membrane and two types of tympanoplasties.

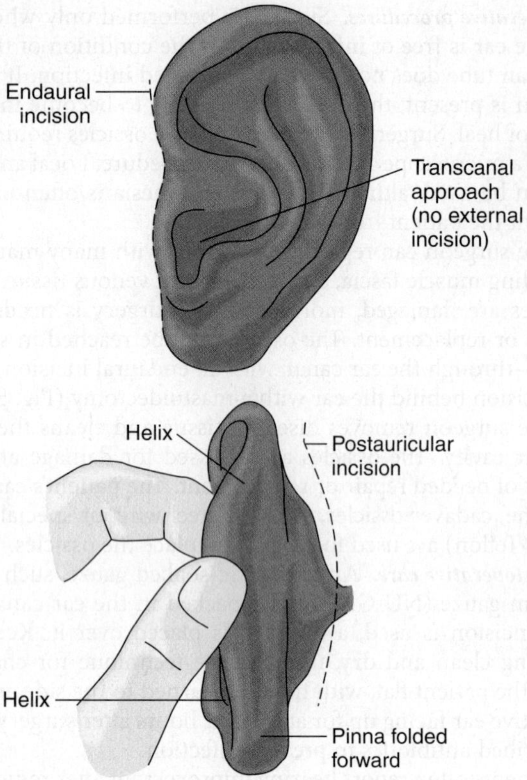
Endaural incision
Transcanal approach (no external incision)
Helix
Postauricular incision
Helix
Pinna folded forward

Fig. 51-9 • Surgical approaches for the ear. The endaural approach is used when the external canal is too small to use for a transcanal approach. The postauricular approach is used for more extensive repair of the middle-ear and inner-ear structures.

including the laser, most patients undergoing revision stapedectomy obtain significant improvement in hearing, regardless of age.

Preoperative care. To prevent infection, the patient must be free from external otitis at surgery. Teach the patient to follow measures that prevent middle-ear or external-ear infections (Chart 51-7).

Review with the patient the expected outcomes and possible complications of the surgery. Hearing is initially worse after a stapedectomy. The success rate of this procedure is high. However, there is always a risk of failure that might lead to total deafness on the affected side. Possible complications include vertigo, infection, and facial nerve damage. A decision to proceed with surgery should be made with the patient's full knowledge and understanding of these complications.

Operative procedures. A stapedectomy is usually performed through the external ear canal with the patient under local anesthesia. The head and neck of the stapes and, less often, the footplate are removed. After removal of the bone, a small hole is drilled or made with a laser in the footplate and a prosthesis in the shape of a piston is connected between the incus and the footplate (Fig. 51-10). Sounds cause the prosthesis to vibrate as the stapes did. After stapedectomy, most patients have restoration of practical hearing.

Postoperative care. Inform the patient that improvement in hearing may not occur until 6 weeks after surgery. At first, the ear packing interferes with hearing. Swelling in the ear after surgery reduces hearing, but this is temporary. Drugs for pain help reduce discomfort, and antibiotics are used to reduce the risk for infection. Teach the patient to follow the procedures in Chart 51-4.

Chart 51-7 PATIENT AND FAMILY EDUCATION GUIDE

Prevention of Ear Infection or Trauma

- Do not use small objects, such as cotton-tipped applicators, matches, toothpicks, or hairpins, to clean your external ear canal.
- Wash your external ear and canal daily in the shower or while washing your hair.
- Blow your nose gently.
- Do not occlude one nostril while blowing your nose.
- Sneeze with your mouth open.
- Wear sound protection around loud or continuous noises.
- Avoid activities with high risk for head or ear trauma, such as wrestling, boxing, motorcycle riding, and skateboarding; wear head and ear protection when engaging in these activities.
- Keep the volume on head receivers at the lowest setting that allows you to hear.
- Frequently clean objects that come into contact with your ear (e.g., headphones, telephone receivers).
- Avoid environmental conditions with rapid changes in air pressure.

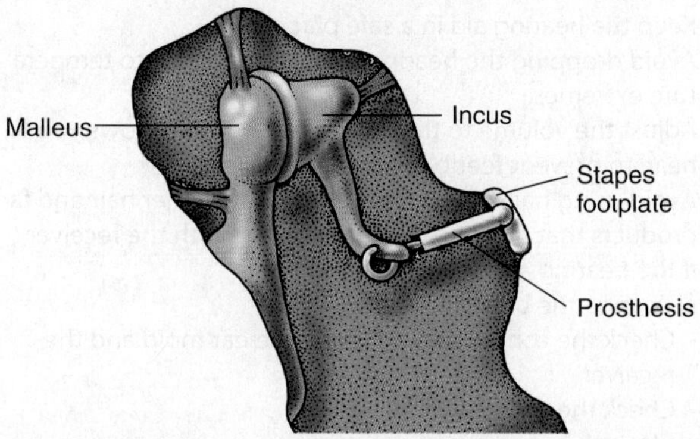
Malleus
Incus
Stapes footplate
Prosthesis

Fig. 51-10 • Prosthesis used with stapedectomy. The stapes is removed, leaving the footplate. After a hole is made in the footplate, a metal or plastic prosthesis is connected to the incus and inserted through the hole to act as a vibration device, much as the stapes worked before the development of otosclerosis.

The surgical procedure is performed in an area where cranial nerves VII, VIII, and X can be damaged by trauma or by swelling after surgery. *Assess for facial nerve damage or muscle weakness. Indications include an asymmetric appearance or drooping of features on the affected side of the face. Ask the patient about changes in facial perception of touch and in taste.* Vertigo, nausea, and vomiting are common after surgery because of the nearness to inner-ear structures.

Antivertiginous drugs, such as meclizine hydrochloride (Antivert, Bonamine♣), and antiemetic drugs, such as droperidol (Inapsine), are given. *Take care to prevent injury, especially during times of increased vertigo. Assist the patient with ambulating during the first 1 to 2 days after surgery. Keep top bed siderails up, and remind the patient to move his or her head slowly when changing position to avoid vertigo.*

Chart 51-8 **BEST PRACTICE FOR PATIENT SAFETY & QUALITY CARE**

Communicating with a Hearing-Impaired Patient

- Position yourself directly in front of the patient.
- Make sure that the room is well lighted.
- Get the patient's attention before you begin to speak.
- Move closer to the better-hearing ear.
- Speak clearly and slowly.
- Do not shout (shouting raises the frequency of the sound and often makes understanding more difficult).
- Keep hands and other objects away from your mouth when talking to the patient.
- Attempt to have conversations in a quiet room with minimal distractions.
- Have the patient repeat your statements rather than just indicating assent.
- Rephrase sentences and repeat information to aid in understanding.
- Use appropriate hand motions.
- Write messages on paper if the patient is able to read.

Impaired Verbal Communication

NOC **Planning: Expected Outcomes.** The patient with hearing loss or impairment is expected to become proficient in hearing compensation behaviors to maintain or improve expressive and receptive communication. Indicators include that the patient consistently demonstrate these behaviors:

- Using hearing assistive devices
- Caring for external hearing assistive devices
- Using sign language, lip-reading, or closed captioning (for television viewing)
- Accurately interpreting messages received
- Using nonverbal language
- Exchanging messages accurately with others

Interventions. Nursing priorities focus on facilitating communication and reducing anxiety.

Use best practices for communicating with a hearing-impaired patient that are listed in Chart 51-8. Do not shout to the patient, because the sound may be projected at a higher frequency, making him or her less able to understand. The most obvious means of communicating with a hearing-impaired person is by the written word (if he or she is able to see, read, and write) or with pictures of familiar phrases and objects. Many television programs are now closed captioned (subtitled).

Assistive Devices. Assistive devices, described on p. 1132, can greatly increase communication for the patient with a hearing impairment.

Lip-Reading. Lip-reading and sign language can also enhance communication. In lip-reading classes, patients are taught the special cues to look for when lip-reading and how to understand body language. However, the best lip-reader still misses more than half of what is being said. Because hearing is assisted by even minimal lip-reading, urge patients to wear their eyeglasses when talking with someone to see lip movement.

Sign Language. For patients with more severe hearing loss, special languages have been developed, including American Sign Language (ASL). Such languages combine speech with hand movements that signify letters, words, and phrases. These languages take time and effort to learn, and many people cannot learn them, just as many people cannot learn foreign languages. However, as the hearing-impaired person becomes less able to function, motivation to learn may increase.

Managing Anxiety. A major source of anxiety is the possibility of permanent hearing loss. Provide honest and accurate information about the likelihood of hearing returning. When the hearing impairment is likely to be permanent or become more profound, reassure patients that communication and social interaction can be maintained.

To reduce anxiety and prevent social isolation, patients use remaining resources to make social contact satisfying. The most obvious way to decrease social isolation is by improving communication (as previously described). Ask about past or present diversional activities to identify the patient's most satisfying activities and social interactions and determine the amount of effort necessary to continue them. Activities can be altered to improve patient satisfaction. Someone accustomed to large gatherings might choose smaller groups instead. A quiet evening meal at home with friends might substitute for dinner in a noisy restaurant.

Community-Based Care

Lengthy hospitalization is rare for most patients with ear and hearing disorders. If surgical repair is needed and the procedure is completed without complications, the procedure may be completed in an ambulatory setting, or the hospital stay is usually only 1 day.

Home Care Management

Patients who have persistent vertigo, either with the disorder or as a side effect of surgery, remain in danger of falling. Assess the home for potential hazards and to determine whether family members or significant others are available to assist with meal preparation and other ADLs. A nurse case manager can coordinate with the home care nurse to assist patients and their families in determining the best ways to maintain adequate self-care abilities, maintain a safe environment, decide about assistance needs, and provide needed care.

Health Teaching

Give patients written instructions about how to take drugs and when to return for follow-up care. If the patient cannot read, give these instructions to a family member who may assist with care. Teach patients how to instill eardrops (see Chart 51-1) and irrigate the ears (see Chart 51-2), and obtain a return demonstration.

To promote health and prevent infections after surgery, instruct patients to follow the suggestions in Chart 51-7. For patients who use a hearing aid, teach them how to use it effectively.

Health Care Resources

If patients do not have family or friends to help during the time before surgery, a referral to a home care agency is needed. Help with meal preparation, cleaning, and personal hygiene can be arranged by the hospital discharge planners.

Follow-up hearing tests are scheduled for patients when the lesions are well healed, in about 6 to 8 weeks. Audiograms done before and after treatment are compared, and evaluation for further intervention to improve hearing begins. A complication of an unsuccessful surgery is continued disability or complete loss of hearing in the affected ear. Surgery is performed on the ear with the greatest hearing loss. If the surgery does not improve hearing, patients must decide to either attempt surgical correction of the other ear or continue to use an amplification device. When the underlying disorder causing the hearing impairment is progressive, this decision is difficult. Support patients by listening to their concerns and giving additional information when needed.

Costs to the person with a hearing impairment can be extensive. Information and support can come from several organizations that publish informative articles to help patients reduce hearing loss (Table 51-1). Many public and private agencies offer hearing evaluations, as well as supply information and counseling for patients with hearing disorders.

Evaluation: Outcomes

Evaluate the care of the patient with hearing loss or hearing impairment on the basis of the identified nursing diagnoses and collaborative problems. The expected outcomes include that the patient will:

- Have at least partial improvement of hearing
- Have reduced anxiety
- Use appropriate hearing compensation behaviors
- Be able to communicate effectively with family, friends, co-workers, and health care professionals

Specific indicators for these outcomes are listed for each nursing diagnosis under the Planning and Implementation section (see earlier).

DECISION-MAKING CHALLENGE
Coordination of Care

An 88-year-old woman with hearing loss and episodes of vertigo is a resident of an assisted-living facility. Her daughter is present and states that her mother recently cleaned her hearing aid and had the battery replaced. During your interaction with the patient, you notice she appears to have no difficulty understanding you. She is taking an antivertiginous drug (meclizine hydrochloride) and an antiemetic drug (droperidol [Inapsine]).

1. What are indicators that the patient does not have impaired communication?
2. What should you consider with regard to safety for this patient?

evolve For suggested answer guidelines, go to http://evolve.elsevier.com/Iggy/.

HUMAN NEEDS NURSING CARE REVIEW

What might you NOTICE if the patient is experiencing reduced sensation as a result of hearing problems?

- Person tilts one side of his or her head or leans forward to listen when another person speaks.
- Person watches the lips of a speaker closely.
- Person does not startle when a loud or unexpected sound occurs in the environment.
- Person frequently asks the speaker to repeat statements or questions.
- Person does not verbally interact with those around him or her.
- When a sentence is whispered to the person, he or she does not accurately repeat it back to the speaker.
- Person responds inappropriately to questions. For example, if asked "Is the room too cold?", the patient may respond "No, I don't feel old."

How should you RESPOND to a patient experiencing reduced sensation as a result of hearing problems?

- Reduce the background sound when speaking to the person (close the door to the hall, use a private area, turn off televisions and radios).
- Speak slowly, distinctly, and with a deeper tone.
- Face the patient while speaking.
- Ensure that all members of the health care team are aware of the patient's impairment and use an appropriate method to communicate with the patient.
- Determine whether the patient can communicate by sign language.
- Use a certified medical interpreter when taking a history from, explaining procedures to, or teaching the patient who has a hearing impairment.

GET READY FOR THE NCLEX EXAMINATION!

Key Points

Review these Key Points for each NCLEX Examination Client Needs Category.

Safe and Effective Care Environment

- Use Contact Precautions with any patient who has drainage from the ear canal.
- Avoid performing an otoscopic examination on a confused or uncooperative patient.
- Use the suggestions presented in the History section to enhance communication with a patient who has a hearing impairment.
- Protect the patient with vertigo or dizziness from injury, and assist with ambulation.

Health Promotion and Maintenance

- Teach patients the proper way to clean the pinna and external ear canal.
- Encourage all patients, even if they already have a hearing impairment, to use ear protection in a loud environment.
- Teach patients how to properly care for their hearing aids.
- Instruct patients to avoid closing off one naris when blowing the nose.
- Tell patients who engage in water sports and who are at risk for external otitis either to wear earplugs when in the water or to rinse the ear canal with drops of dilute alcohol after any immersion of the head in water.
- Teach proper ear hygiene for cleaning cerumen from the external canal.

- Urge everyone to avoid exposure to loud noises for extended periods without proper OSHA-approved ear protection.

Psychosocial Integrity

- Encourage the patient and family the opportunity to express their feelings and concerns regarding a change in hearing status.
- Refer patients newly diagnosed with hearing impairment or any chronic ear problem to appropriate local resources and support groups.
- Explain all diagnostic therapeutic procedures, restrictions, and follow-up care to the patient and family.
- Teach family members ways to communicate with a hearing-impaired patient with and without a hearing aid.

Physiological Integrity

- Ask the patient about hearing problems in any other members of the family, because many hearing problems have a genetic component.
- Check the hearing of any patient receiving an ototoxic drug (Table 50-1 in Chapter 50) for more than 5 days.
- Teach patients the proper technique to use for self-instillation of eardrops and ear irrigation.
- Stress the importance of completing an antibiotic regimen when an ear infection is present.
- Follow the guidelines in Chart 51-2 when irrigating the ear canal.
- Avoid ear canal irrigation if the eardrum is perforated or if the canal contains vegetative matter.

Additional Study Resources

Go to your Companion CD or Evolve at http://evolve.elsevier.com/Iggy/ for *Self-Assessment Questions for the NCLEX Examination.*

evolve Go to Evolve at http://evolve.elsevier.com/Iggy/ for *Prioritization and Delegation Questions for the NCLEX Examination.*

SELECTED BIBLIOGRAPHY

Asterisk indicates a classic or definitive work on this subject.

Berry, J., & Stewart, A. (2006). Communicating with the deaf during the health examination visit. *The Journal for Nurse Practitioners, 2*(8), 509-515.

Daniel, E. (2007). Noise and hearing loss: A review. *Journal of School Health, 77*(5), 225-231.

Daugherty, J. (2007). The latest buzz on tinnitus. *The Nurse Practitioner, 32*(10), 42-47.

Gates, G.A., Verrall, A., Green, J.D. Jr., Tucci, D.L., & Telian, S.A. (2006). Meniett clinical trial: Long-term follow-up. *Archives of Otolaryngology—Head & Neck Surgery, 132*(12), 1311-1316.

Ghossaini, S.N., & Wazen, J.J. (2006). An update on the surgical treatment of Ménière's diseases. *Journal of the American Academy of Audiology, 17*(1), 38-44.

Harkin, H. (2005). A nurse-led ear care clinic: Sharing knowledge and improving patient care. *British Journal of Nursing, 14*(5), 250-254.

Henry, J., Dennis, K., & Schechter, M. (2005). General review of tinnitus: Prevalence, mechanisms, effects, and management. *Journal of Speech, Language, and Hearing Research, 48*(5), 1204-1235.

Jenkins, A. (2006). Deafening silence. *Nursing Standard, 20*(24), 30-31.

Keats, B., Berlin, C., & Gregory, P. (2006). Epidemiology of genetic hearing loss. *Seminars in Hearing, 27*(3), 136-147.

*Lucas, L., & Matthews-Flint, L. (2001). Sound advice about hearing aids. *Nursing2001, 31*(2), 59-61.

McAleer, M. (2006). Communicating effectively with deaf patients. *Nursing Standard, 20*(19), 51-54.

McCance, K., & Huether, S. (2006). *Pathophysiology: The biologic basis for disease in adults and children* (5th ed.). St. Louis: Mosby.

McCarter, D.F., Courtney, A.U., & Pollart, S.M. (2007). Cerumen impaction. *American Family Physician, 75*(10), 1523-1528.

Meiner, S., & Lueckenotte, A. (Eds.). (2006). *Gerontologic nursing* (3rd ed.). St. Louis: Mosby.

Mills, J., Konrad-Martin, D., Leek, M., & Hood, L. (2006). Roundtable discussion: Pathophysiology of the aging auditory system. *Seminars in Hearing, 27*(4), 237-242.

Mills, J., Schmiedt, R., Schulte, B., & Dubno, J. (2006). Age-related hearing loss: A loss of voltage, not hair cells. *Seminars in Hearing, 27*(4), 228-236.

National Institute on Deafness and Other Communication Disorders. *Presbycusis.* NIH Publication No. 97-4235. Retrieved September 4, 2007, from www.nidcd.nih.gov/health/hearing/presbycusis.asp.

Neno, R. (2006). Holistic ear care: Cerumen removal techniques. *Journal of Community Nursing, 20*(9), 26, 28, 30-31.

Nussbaum, R., McInnes, R., & Willard, H. (2007). *Thompson & Thompson: Genetics in medicine* (7th ed.). Philadelphia: Saunders.

Online Mendelian Inheritance in Man, OMIM (TM). (2007). McKusick-Nathans Institute for Genetic Medicine, Johns Hopkins University (Baltimore, MD) and National Center for Biotechnology Information, National Library of Medicine (Bethesda, MD). www.ncbi.nlm.nih.gov/omim/

Osguthorpe, J.D., & Nielsen, D.R. (2006). Otitis externa: Review and clinical update. *American Family Physician, 74*(9), 1510-1516.

Pagana, K., & Pagana, T. (2006). *Mosby's manual of diagnostic and laboratory tests* (3rd ed.). St. Louis: Mosby.

Pullen, R. (2006). Spin control: Caring for a patient with inner ear disease. *Nursing2006, 36*(5), 48-51.

Rosenfeld, R.M., Brown, L., Cannon, C.R., Dolor, R.J., Ganiats, T.G., Hannley, M., et al. (2006). Clinical practice guideline: Acute otitis externa. *Otolaryngology—Head and Neck Surgery, 134*(Suppl. 4), S4-S23.

Smith, J.A., & Danner, C.J. (2006). Complications of chronic otitis media and cholesteatoma. *Otolaryngology Clinics of North America, 39*(6), 1237-1255.

Smy, J. (2005). Hearing aid. *Nursing Times, 101*(11), 24-25.

Souza, P. (2006). Selecting and adjusting amplification for older listeners. *Seminars in Hearing, 27*(4), 303-310.

Stewart, G.M., Thorp, A., & Brown, L. (2006). Perichondritis: A complication of high ear piercing. *Pediatric Emergency Care, 22*(12), 804-806.

Thirlwall, A.S., & Kundu, S. (2006). Diuretics for Ménière's disease or syndrome. *Cochrane Database of Systematic Reviews, 19*(3), CD003599.

Tinnitus. (2006). *Nursing Times 102*(12), 27.

Walden, T. (2006). Evaluating and treating hearing loss in the older patient: Clinical case studies. *Seminars in Hearing, 27*(4), 311-319.

XII

UNIT

Problems of Mobility

Management of Patients with Problems of the Musculoskeletal System

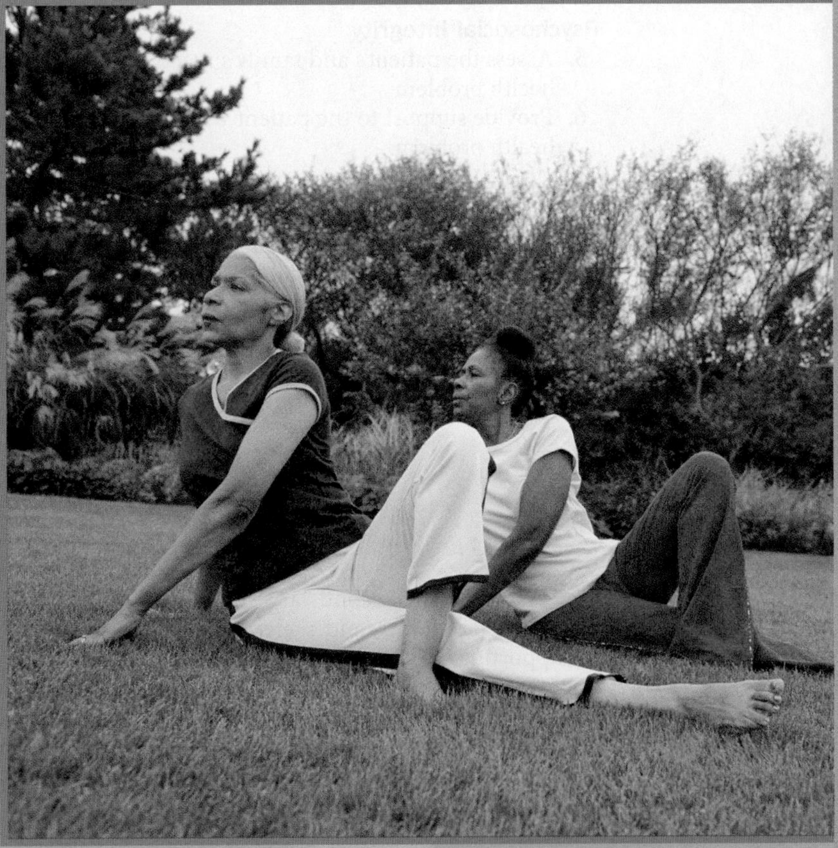

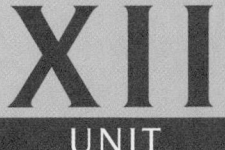

52 CHAPTER

Assessment of the Musculoskeletal System

Cathy A. Murray

LEARNING OUTCOMES

For clinical competence and success on the NCLEX Examination, study this chapter with these Learning Outcomes in mind:

Safe and Effective Care Environment

1. Collaborate with the physical and occupational therapists to perform a complete musculoskeletal assessment, including functional status, as needed.
2. Assess patients regarding iodine allergy before imaging assessments.

Health Promotion and Maintenance

3. Explain the use of laboratory testing for a patient with a musculoskeletal health problem.
4. Educate the patient and family about diagnostic procedures.

Psychosocial Integrity

5. Assess the patient's and family's reaction to change in body image caused by a major musculoskeletal health problem.
6. Provide support to the patient with unexpected altered body image caused by a musculoskeletal health problem.

Physiological Integrity

7. Recall the anatomy and physiology of the musculoskeletal system.
8. Explain how physiologic aging changes of the musculoskeletal system affect care of older adults.
9. Conduct a musculoskeletal history using Gordon's Functional Health Patterns.
10. Assess patients for mobility, gait, motor skills, pain, and the use of assistive devices.
11. Interpret assessment findings in a patient with a musculoskeletal health problem.

evolve Go to your Companion CD or Evolve at http://evolve.elsevier.com/Iggy/ for *Self-Assessment Questions for the NCLEX Examination* keyed to these Learning Outcomes.

The musculoskeletal system is the second largest body system. It includes the bones, joints, and skeletal muscles, as well as the supporting structures needed to move them. *Mobility* (movement) is a basic human need that is essential for performing ADLs. When a patient cannot move to perform ADLs or other daily routines, self-esteem and a sense of self-worth can be diminished.

Disease, surgery, and trauma can affect one or more parts of the musculoskeletal system, often leading to decreased mobility. When mobility is impaired for a long time, other body systems can be affected. For example, prolonged immobility can lead to skin breakdown, constipation, and thrombus formation. If nerves are damaged by trauma or disease, patients may also have problems with *sensation.*

ANATOMY AND PHYSIOLOGY REVIEW

Skeletal System

The skeletal system consists of 206 bones and multiple joints. The growth and development of these structures occur during childhood and adolescence and are not discussed in this text. Common physical skeletal differences among ethnic groups are listed in Table 52-1.

Bones

Types and Structure

Bone can be classified in two ways—by shape and by structure. *Long bones,* such as the femur, are cylindric with rounded ends and often bear weight. *Short bones,* such as the phalanges, are small and bear little or no weight. *Flat bones,* such as

TABLE 52-1 Musculoskeletal Differences in Selected Groups

Group	Musculoskeletal Differences
African Americans	Greater bone density than Europeans, Asians, and Hispanics. Accounts for decreased incidence of osteoporosis.
Amish	Greater incidence of dwarfism than in other populations.
Chinese Americans	Bones are shorter and smaller with less bone density. Increased incidence of osteoporosis.
Egyptian Americans	Shorter in stature than European and African Americans.
Filipino/Vietnamese	Short in stature, adult height about 5 feet.
Irish Americans	Taller and broader than other European Americans. Less bone density than African Americans.
Navajo Native Americans	Taller and thinner than other Native Americans.

Information from Dillon, P.M. (2007). *Nursing health assessment: A critical thinking case studies approach* (2nd ed.). Philadelphia: Davis.

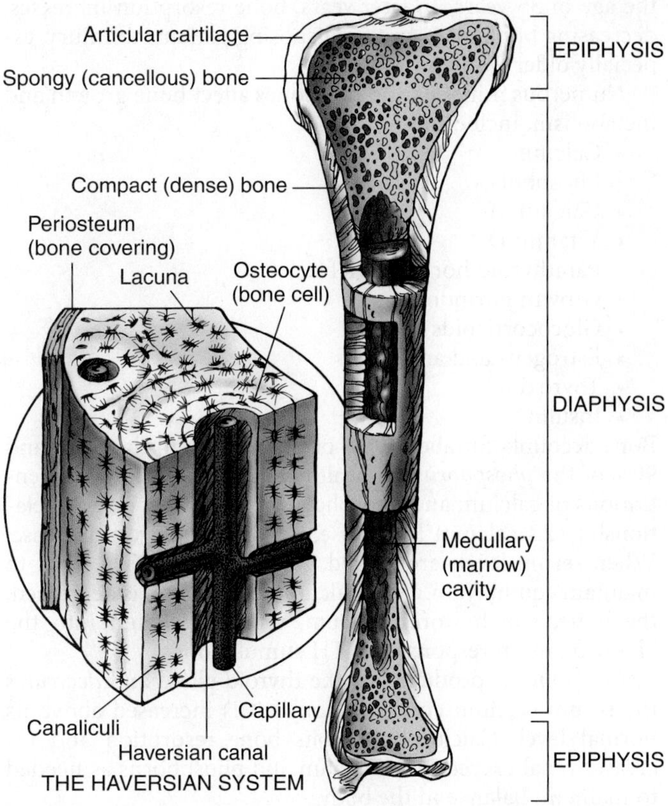
Articular cartilage
Spongy (cancellous) bone
EPIPHYSIS
Compact (dense) bone
Periosteum
(bone covering)
Lacuna
Osteocyte
(bone cell)
DIAPHYSIS
Medullary
(marrow)
cavity
Capillary
Canaliculi
Haversian canal
THE HAVERSIAN SYSTEM
EPIPHYSIS

Fig. 52-1 • The structure of a typical long bone. The cortex, or outer layer, is composed of dense, compact tissue. The microscopic structure of this compact cortical tissue is the haversian system.

the scapula, protect vital organs and often contain blood-forming cells. Bones that have unique shapes are known as *irregular bones.* The carpal bones in the wrist and the small bones in the inner ear are examples of irregular bones. The *sesamoid bone* is the least common type and develops within a tendon; the patella is a typical example.

The second way bone is classified is by *structure* or composition. As shown in Fig. 52-1, the outer layer of bone, or **cortex,** is composed of dense, compact bone tissue. The inner layer, in the medulla, contains spongy, cancellous tissue. Almost every bone has both tissue types but in varying quantities. The long bone typically has a shaft, or **diaphysis,** and two knoblike ends, or **epiphyses.**

The structural unit of the cortical, compact bone is the haversian system, which is detailed in Fig. 52-1. The haversian system is a complex canal network containing microscopic blood vessels that supply nutrients and oxygen to bone, as well as lacunae, which are small cavities that house **osteocytes** (bone cells). The canals run vertically within the hard, cortical bone tissue.

The softer, **cancellous** tissue contains large spaces, or trabeculae, which are filled with red and yellow marrow. **Hematopoiesis** (production of blood cells) occurs in the red marrow. The yellow marrow contains fat cells, which can be dislodged and enter the bloodstream to cause fat embolism syndrome (FES), a life-threatening complication. Volkmann's canals connect bone marrow vessels with the haversian system and periosteum, the outermost covering of the bone. In the deepest layer of the periosteum are osteogenic cells, which later differentiate into **osteoblasts** (bone-forming cells) and **osteoclasts** (bone-destroying cells).

Bone also contains a **matrix,** or *osteoid,* consisting chiefly of collagen, mucopolysaccharides, and lipids. Deposits of inorganic calcium salts (carbonate and phosphate) in the matrix provide the hardness of bone.

Bone is a very vascular tissue. Its estimated total blood flow is between 200 and 400 mL/min. Each bone has a main nutrient artery, which enters near the middle of the shaft and branches into ascending and descending vessels. These vessels supply the cortex, the marrow, and the haversian system. Very few nerve fibers are connected to bone. Sympathetic nerve fibers control dilation of blood vessels. Sensory nerve fibers transmit pain signals experienced by patients who have primary lesions of the bone, like bone tumors.

Function

The skeletal system:

- Provides a framework for the body and allows the body to be weight bearing, or upright
- Supports the surrounding tissues (e.g., muscle and tendons)
- Assists in movement through muscle attachment and joint formation
- Protects vital organs, such as the heart and lungs
- Manufactures blood cells in red bone marrow
- Provides storage for mineral salts (e.g., calcium and phosphorus)

After puberty, bone reaches its maturity and maximal growth. Bone is a dynamic tissue. It undergoes a continuous process of formation and **resorption,** or destruction, at equal rates until the age of 35 years. In later years, bone resorption increases, decreasing bone mass and predisposing patients to injury, especially older women.

Numerous minerals and hormones affect bone growth and metabolism, including:

- Calcium
- Phosphorus
- Calcitonin
- Vitamin D
- Parathyroid hormone (PTH)
- Growth hormone
- Glucocorticoids
- Estrogens and androgens
- Thyroxine
- Insulin

Bone accounts for about 99% of the *calcium* in the body and 90% of the *phosphorus*. In healthy adults, the serum concentrations of calcium and phosphorus maintain an inverse relationship. As calcium levels rise, phosphorus levels decrease. When serum levels are altered, calcitonin and PTH work to maintain equilibrium. If the calcium in the blood is decreased, the bone, which stores calcium, releases calcium into the bloodstream in response to PTH stimulation.

Calcitonin is produced by the thyroid gland and *decreases* the serum calcium concentration if it is increased above its normal level. Calcitonin inhibits bone resorption and increases renal excretion of calcium and phosphorus as needed to maintain balance in the body.

Vitamin D and its metabolites are produced in the body and transported in the blood to promote the absorption of calcium and phosphorus from the small intestine. They also seem to enhance PTH activity to release calcium from the bone. A decrease in the body's vitamin D level can result in osteomalacia (softening of bone) in the adult. Vitamin D metabolism and osteomalacia are described in Chapter 53.

When serum calcium levels are lowered, *parathyroid hormone* (PTH, or parathormone) secretion increases and stimulates bone to promote osteoclastic activity and *release* calcium to the blood. PTH reduces the renal excretion of calcium and facilitates its absorption from the intestine. If serum calcium levels increase, PTH secretion diminishes to preserve the bone calcium supply. This process is an example of the feedback loop system of the endocrine system.

Growth hormone secreted by the anterior lobe of the pituitary gland is responsible for increasing bone length and determining the amount of bone matrix formed before puberty. During childhood, an increased secretion results in gigantism, and a decreased secretion results in dwarfism. In the adult, an increase causes acromegaly, which is characterized by bone and soft-tissue deformities (see Chapter 65).

Adrenal glucocorticoids regulate protein metabolism, either increasing or decreasing catabolism to reduce or intensify the organic matrix of bone. They also aid in regulating intestinal calcium and phosphorus absorption.

Estrogens stimulate osteoblastic (bone-building) activity and inhibit PTH. When estrogen levels decline at menopause, women are susceptible to low serum calcium levels with increased bone loss (osteoporosis). Androgens, such as testosterone in men, promote anabolism (body tissue building) and increase bone mass.

Thyroxine is one of the principal hormones secreted by the thyroid gland. Its primary function is to increase the rate of protein synthesis in all types of tissue, including bone. *Insulin* works together with growth hormone to build and maintain healthy bone tissue.

Joints

A **joint** is a space in which two or more bones come together. This is also referred to as *articulation* of the joint. The major function of a joint is to provide movement and flexibility in the body.

There are three types of joints in the body:

- Synarthrodial, or completely immovable, joints (e.g., in the cranium)
- Amphiarthrodial, or slightly movable, joints (e.g., in the pelvis)
- Diarthrodial (synovial), or freely movable, joints (e.g., the elbow and knee)

Although any of these joints can be affected by disease or injury, the synovial joints are most commonly involved.

The diarthrodial, or synovial, joint is the most common type of joint in the body. **Synovial joints** are the only type lined with synovium, a membrane that secretes synovial fluid for lubrication and shock absorption. As shown in Fig. 52-2, the synovium lines the internal portion of the joint capsule but does not normally extend onto the surface of the cartilage at the spongy bone ends. Articular cartilage consists of a collagen fiber matrix impregnated with a complex ground substance. Patients with inflammatory types of arthritis often have synovitis (synovial inflammation) and breakdown of the cartilage. **Bursae,** small sacs lined with synovial membrane, are located at joints and bony prominences to prevent friction between bone and structures adjacent to bone. These structures can also become inflamed, causing bursitis.

Synovial joints are described by their anatomic structures. *Ball-and-socket* joints (shoulder, hip) permit movement in any direction. *Hinge* joints (elbow) allow motion in one plane,

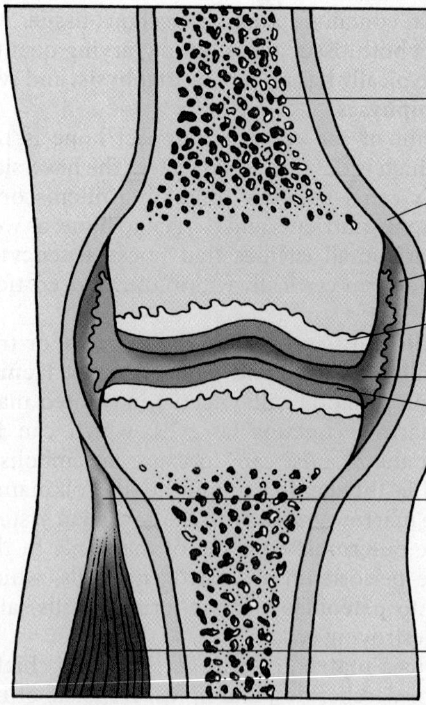
Bone
Joint capsule
Synovium
Subchondral bone plate
Joint cavity
Articular cartilage
Tendon
Muscle

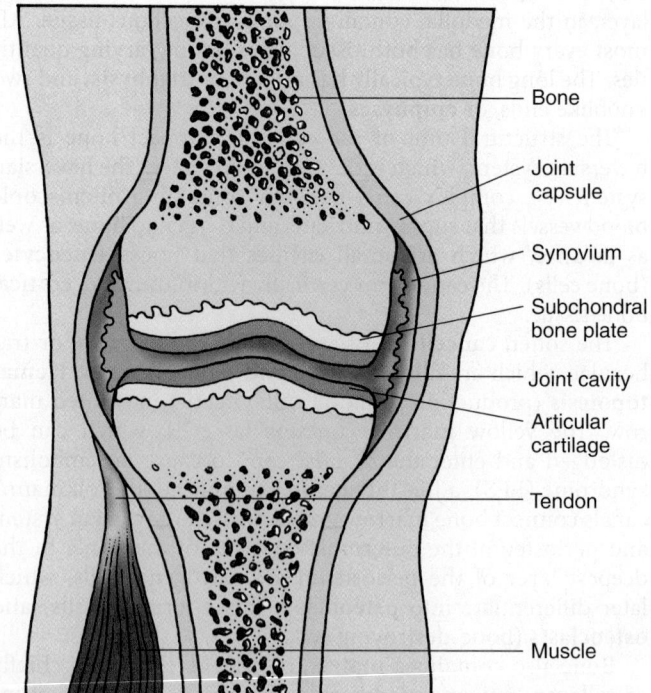

Fig. 52-2 • The structure of a synovial joint. Synovium lines the joint capsule but does not extend into the articular cartilage.

flexion, and extension. The knee is often classified as a hinge joint, but it rotates slightly, as well as flexes and extends. It is best described as a *condylar* type of synovial joint. The gliding movement of the wrist is characteristic of the *biaxial* joint. *Pivot* joints permit rotation only, as in the radioulnar area.

Muscular System

There are three types of muscle in the body: smooth muscle, cardiac muscle, and skeletal muscle. Smooth, or non-striated, involuntary muscle is responsible for contractions of organs and blood vessels and is controlled by the autonomic nervous system. Cardiac muscle, or striated, involuntary muscle, is also controlled by the autonomic nervous system. The smooth and cardiac muscles are discussed with the body systems to which they belong in the assessment chapters.

In contrast to smooth and cardiac muscle, skeletal muscle is striated, voluntary muscle controlled by the central and peripheral nervous systems. The junction of a peripheral motor nerve and the muscle cells that it supplies is sometimes referred to as a **motor end plate.** Muscle fibers are held in place by connective tissue in bundles, or fasciculi. The entire muscle is surrounded by dense, fibrous tissue, or fascia, which contains the muscle's blood, lymph, and nerve supply.

The main function of skeletal muscle is *movement* of the body and its parts. When bones, joints, and supporting structures are adversely affected by injury or disease, the adjacent muscle tissue is often involved, limiting mobility. During the aging process, muscle fibers decrease in size and number, even in well-conditioned adults. Atrophy results when muscles are not regularly exercised, and they deteriorate from disuse.

Supporting structures for the muscular system are very susceptible to injury. They include **tendons** (bands of tough, fibrous tissue that attach muscles to bones) and **ligaments,** which attach bones to other bones at joints.

MUSCULOSKELETAL CHANGES ASSOCIATED WITH AGING

Osteopenia, or decreased bone density (bone loss), occurs as one ages. Many older adults, especially white, thin women, have severe osteopenia, a disease called *osteoporosis.* This condition causes postural and gait changes and predisposes the person to fractures. Chapter 53 discusses this health problem in detail.

Synovial joint cartilage can become less elastic and compressible as a person ages. As a result of these cartilage changes and continued use of joints, the joint cartilage becomes damaged, leading to osteoarthritis (OA). Genetic defects in cartilage may also contribute to joint disease. The most common joints affected are the weight-bearing joints of the hip, knee, and cervical and lumbar spine, but joints in the shoulder and upper extremity, feet, and hands can be affected. Refer to Chapter 20 for a complete discussion of OA.

As one ages, muscle tissue atrophies. Increased activity and exercise can slow the progression of atrophy and restore muscle strength. Musculoskeletal changes cause decreased coordination, loss of muscle strength, gait changes, and a risk for falls with injury. (See Chapter 3 for discussion on fall prevention.) Chart 52-1 lists the major anatomic and physiologic changes and implications for nursing care.

ASSESSMENT METHODS

Patient History

In the assessment of a patient with an actual or potential musculoskeletal problem, a detailed and accurate history is helpful in identifying diagnoses and nursing interventions (Chart 52-2). The history reveals information about the patient that can direct the physical assessment.

Accidents, illnesses, lifestyle, and drugs may contribute to a patient's current problem. Young men are at the greatest risk for trauma related to motor vehicle crashes. Older adults are at the greatest risk for falls that result in fractures and soft-tissue injury. When taking a personal health history, question the patient about any traumatic injuries and sports activities, no matter when they occurred. An injury to the lumbar spine 30 years ago may have caused a patient's current low back pain. A motor vehicle crash or sports injury can cause osteoarthritis years after the event.

Previous or current illness or disease may affect musculoskeletal status. For example, a patient with diabetes who is treated for a foot ulcer is at high risk for acute or chronic osteomyelitis (bone infection). In addition, diabetes slows the healing process. Ask the patient about any previous hospital-

Chart 52-1 NURSING FOCUS ON THE OLDER ADULT

Changes in the Musculoskeletal System Related to Aging

Physiologic Change	Nursing Interventions	Rationales
Decreased bone density	Teach safety tips to prevent falls. Reinforce need to exercise, especially weight-bearing exercise.	Porous bones are more likely to fracture. Exercise slows bone loss.
Increased bone prominence	Prevent pressure on bone prominences.	There is less soft tissue to prevent skin breakdown.
Kyphotic posture: widened gait, shift in the center of gravity	Teach proper body mechanics; instruct the patient to sit in supportive chairs with arms.	Correction of posture problems prevents further deformity; the patient should have support for bony structures.
Cartilage degeneration	Provide moist heat, such as a shower or warm, moist compresses.	Moist heat increases blood flow to the area.
Decreased range of motion (ROM)	Assess the patient's ability to perform ADLs and mobility.	The patient may need assistance with self-care skills.
Muscle atrophy, decreased strength	Teach isometric exercises.	Exercises increase muscle strength.
Slowed movement	Do not rush the patient; be patient.	The patient may become frustrated if hurried.

Chart 52-2 MUSCULOSKELETAL ASSESSMENT
Using Gordon's Functional Health Patterns

ACTIVITY-EXERCISE PATTERN
- Do you have sufficient energy for desired/required activities?
- What is your exercise pattern? Type of exercise? Regularity?
- What spare time (leisure) activities do you engage in?
- What is your perceived ability for (code for level according to key below):

Feeding?	Level 0: Full self-care
Bathing?	Level I: Requires use of equipment or device
Toileting?	
Bed mobility?	Level II: Requires assistance of or supervision by another person
Dressing?	
Grooming?	Level III: Requires assistance of or supervision by another person and equipment or device
General mobility?	
Cooking?	
Home maintenance?	Level IV: Is dependent and does not participate
Shopping?	

COGNITIVE-PERCEPTUAL PATTERN
- Do you experience any discomfort?
- Do you have pain? If so, how do you manage it?
- What is the easiest way for you to learn things?
- Do you have any difficulty learning?

Based on Gordon, M. (2007). *Manual of nursing diagnosis* (11th ed.). Boston: Jones & Bartlett.

izations and illnesses or complications. Inquire about his or her ability to perform ADLs independently or if assistive/adaptive devices are used.

Current lifestyle also contributes to musculoskeletal health. Weight-bearing activities such as walking can reduce risk factors for osteoporosis and maintain muscle strength. High-impact sports, such as excessive jogging or running, can cause musculoskeletal injury to soft tissues and bone. Tobacco use slows the healing of musculoskeletal injuries. Excessive alcohol intake can decrease vitamins and nutrients the person needs for bone and muscle tissue growth.

When assessing a patient with a possible musculoskeletal alteration, inquire about occupation or work life. A person's occupation can cause or contribute to an injury. For instance, fractures are not uncommon in patients whose jobs require manual labor, such as housekeepers, mechanics, and industrial workers. Certain occupations, such as computer-related jobs, may predispose a person to carpal tunnel syndrome (entrapment of the median nerve in the wrist) or neck pain. Construction workers and health care workers may experience back injury from prolonged standing and excessive lifting. Amateur and professional athletes often experience acute musculoskeletal injuries (e.g., joint dislocations and fractures) and chronic disorders (e.g., joint cartilage trauma), which can lead to osteoarthritis.

Ask about allergies, particularly allergy to dairy products, and previous and current use of drugs—prescribed, over-the-counter, and illicit. Allergy to dairy products could cause decreased calcium intake. Some drugs, such as steroids, can negatively affect calcium metabolism and promote bone loss. Other drugs may be taken to relieve musculoskeletal pain. Inquire about herbs, vitamin and mineral supplements, or biologic compounds that may be used for arthritis and other musculoskeletal problems, such as glucosamine and chondroitin. Complementary and alternative therapies are commonly used by patients with various types of arthritis and **arthralgias** (joint aching).

Nutrition History

A brief review of the patient's nutrition history helps determine any risks of inadequate nutrient intake. For example, most people, especially women, do not get enough calcium in their diet. Determine if the patient has had a significant weight gain or loss.

Ask the patient to recall a typical day of food intake to help identify deficiencies and excesses in the diet. Lactose intolerance is a common problem that can cause inadequate calcium intake. People who cannot afford to buy food are especially at risk for undernutrition. Some older adults and others are not financially able to buy the proper foods for adequate nutrition.

Inadequate protein or insufficient vitamin C or D in the diet slows bone and tissue healing. Obesity places excess stress and strain on bones and joints, with resulting fractures and trauma to joint cartilage. In addition, obesity inhibits mobility in patients with musculoskeletal problems, which predisposes them to complications such as respiratory and circulatory problems. People with eating disorders such as anorexia nervosa and bulimia nervosa are also at risk for osteoporosis related to decreased intake of calcium and vitamin D.

Family History and Genetic Risk

Obtaining a family history assists in identifying disorders that have a familial or genetic tendency. Osteoporosis (age-related bone loss) and gout, for instance, often occur in several generations of a family. Osteogenic sarcoma, a type of bone cancer, may be genetically influenced by *TP53* gene mutation (Nussbaum et al., 2007). Positive family history of these types of disorders can increase risks to the patient. Chapters 20 and 53 provide a more complete description of musculoskeletal problems that have strong genetic links.

Current Health Problems

The most common reports of persons with a musculoskeletal problem are pain and weakness, either of which can impair mobility. Collect data pertinent to the patient's presenting health problem as follows:
- Date and time of onset
- Factors that cause or exacerbate (worsen) the problem
- Course of the problem (e.g., intermittent or continuous)
- Clinical manifestations (as expressed by the patient) and the pattern of their occurrence
- Measures that improve clinical manifestations (e.g., heat, ice)

Assessment of pain can present many challenges. Pain can be related to bone, muscle, or joint problems. *Pain* may be described as acute or chronic, depending on the onset and duration. Pain with movement could indicate a fracture and/or muscle or joint injury. Assess the intensity of pain by using a pain scale and asking the patient to rate the level of pain he or she is experiencing. Quality of pain may be described as dull, burning, aching, or stabbing. Determine the location of pain and areas to which the pain may radiate. With any pain assessment, it is always best if the patient describes the pain in his or her own words and points to its location, if possible.

Weakness may be related to individual muscles or muscle groups. Determine if weakness occurs in proximal or distal

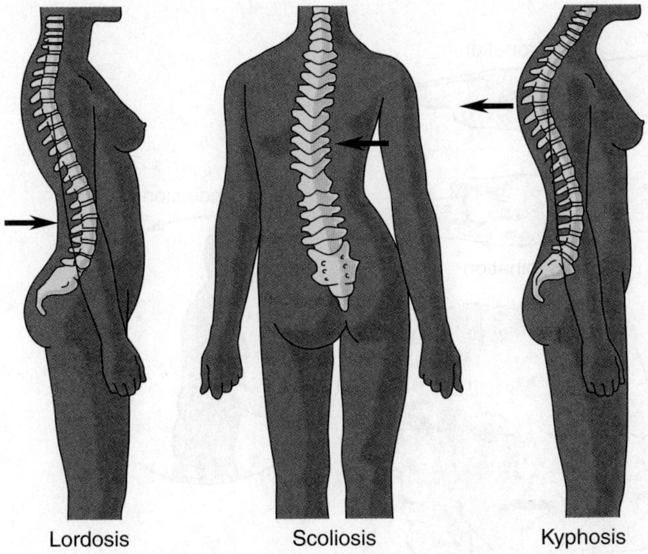
Lordosis
Scoliosis
Kyphosis

Fig. 52-3 • Common spinal deformities.

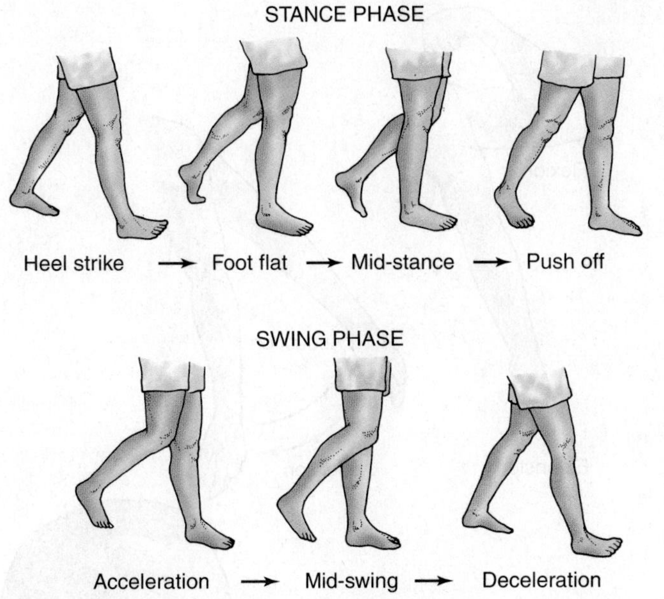
STANCE PHASE
Heel strike
Foot flat
Mid-stance
Push off
SWING PHASE
Acceleration
Mid-swing
Deceleration

Fig. 52-4 • The phases of gait.

muscles or muscle groups. Proximal weakness may indicate **myopathy** (a problem in muscle tissue), whereas distal weakness may indicate **neuropathy** (a problem in nerve tissue). Muscle weakness in the lower extremities may increase the risk for falls and injury. Weakness in the upper extremities may interfere with ADLs.

Assessment of the Skeletal System

Although bones, joints, and muscles are usually assessed simultaneously in a head-to-toe approach, each subsystem is described separately for emphasis and understanding. For physical assessment of the musculoskeletal system, use inspection, palpation, and range of motion (ROM). A general assessment is described in this chapter. More specific assessment techniques are discussed in the musculoskeletal problem chapters in this unit.

General Inspection

Observe the patient's posture, gait, and general mobility for gross deformities and impairment. Note unusual findings, and coordinate with the physical or occupational therapist for an in-depth physical assessment.

Posture and Gait

Posture includes the person's body build and alignment when standing and walking. Assess the curvature of the spine and the length, shape, and symmetry of extremities. Fig. 52-3 illustrates some common spinal deformities. Inspect muscle mass for size and symmetry.

VIDEO CLIP: Gait ▶

Most patients with musculoskeletal problems eventually have a problem with *gait.* The two phases of normal, automatic gait are the stance phase and the swing phase (Fig. 52-4).

The nurse or therapist evaluates the patient's balance, steadiness, and ease and length of stride. Any limp or other asymmetric leg movement or deformity is noted. An abnormality in the stance phase of gait is called an **antalgic** gait. When part of one leg is painful, the patient shortens the stance phase on the affected side. An abnormality in the swing phase is called a **lurch.** This abnormal gait occurs when the muscles in the buttocks and/or legs are too weak to allow the person to change weight from one foot to the other. In this case, the shoulders are moved either side-to-side or front-to-back for help in shifting the weight from one leg to the other. Some patients, such as those with chronic hip pain and muscle atrophy from arthritic disorders, have a combination of an antalgic gait and lurch.

Mobility and Functional Assessment

In collaboration with the physical or occupational therapist, assess the patient's need for ambulatory devices, such as canes and walkers, during transfer from bed to chair and while walking and climbing stairs. Observe his or her ability to perform ADLs, such as dressing and bathing (see Chart 52-2). Pain and deformity may limit physical mobility and function. Coordinate with the physical and occupational therapists to assess the patient's functional status. A complete discussion of functional assessment is found in Chapter 8.

Assess major bones, joints, and muscles by inspection, palpation, and determination of ROM. Pay special attention to areas that are affected or may be affected, according to the patient's history or current problem.

A **goniometer** is a tool that may be used by rehabilitation therapists or nurses to provide an exact measurement of flexion and extension or joint ROM. Active range of motion (AROM) can be evaluated by asking the patient to move each joint through the ROM himself or herself. If the patient cannot actively move a joint through range of motion, ask him or her to relax the muscles in the extremity. Hold the part with one hand above and one hand below the joint to be evaluated and allow passive range of motion (PROM) to evaluate joint mobility. Movements shown in Fig. 52-5 may be used to evaluate active and passive ROM. Circumduction is a movement that can also be evaluated in the shoulder by having the patient move the arm in circles from the shoulder joint. As long as the patient can function to meet personal needs, a limitation in ROM may not be significant. For each anatomic location, observe the skin for color, elasticity, and lesions that may relate to musculoskeletal dysfunction. For instance, redness or warmth may indicate an inflammatory process and/or pressure injury to skin.

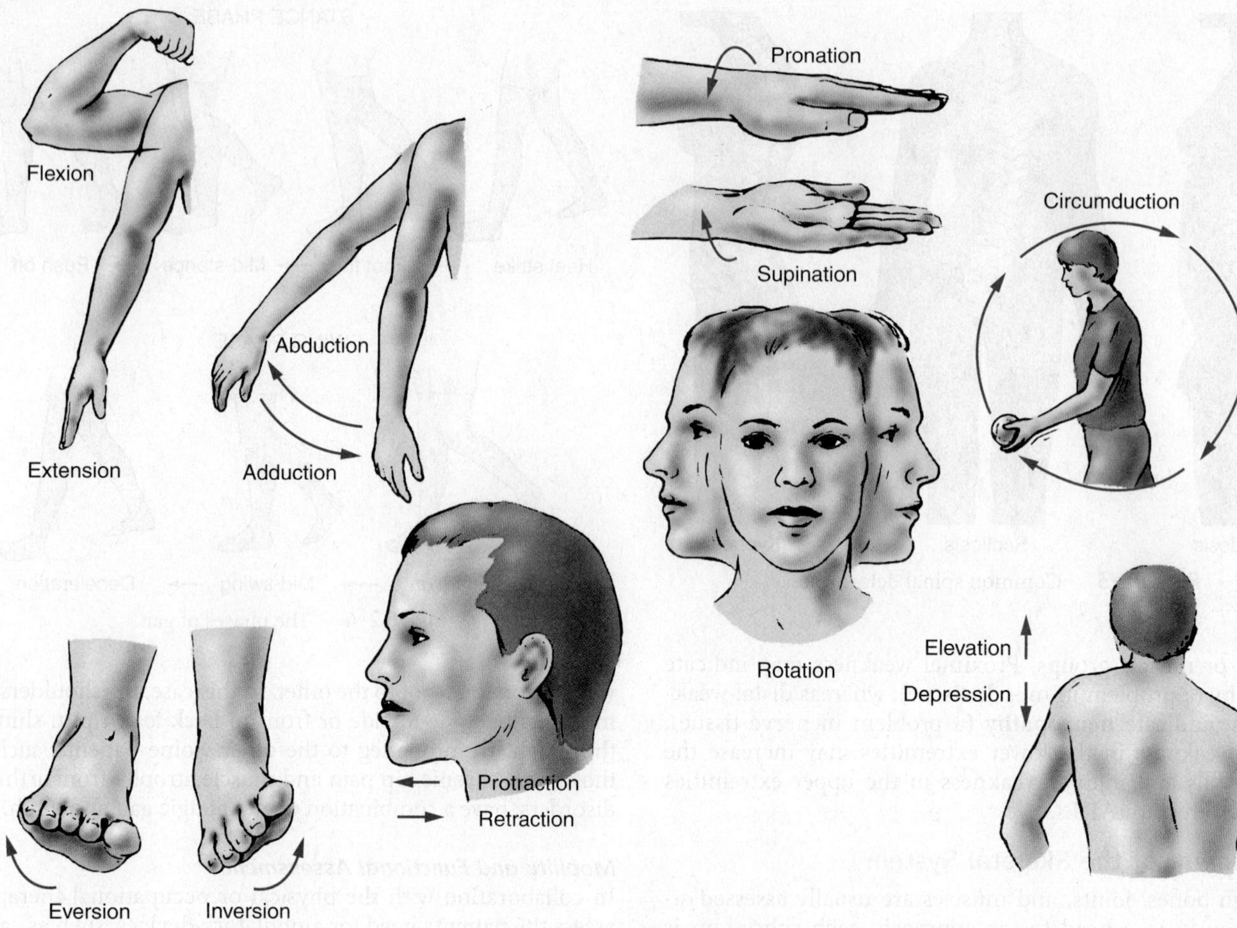
Flexion
Extension
Abduction
Adduction
Pronation
Supination
Circumduction
Rotation
Elevation
Depression
Protraction
Retraction
Eversion
Inversion

Fig. 52-5 • Movements of the skeletal muscles.

Specific Assessments

If the patient has pain or weakness in the *face* or *neck*, inspect and palpate this area for tenderness and masses. Ask the patient to open his or her mouth while palpating the temporomandibular joints (TMJs). Common abnormal findings are tenderness or pain, **crepitus** (a grating sound), and a spongy swelling caused by excess synovium and fluid.

Inspect and palpate each vertebra of the spine in the neck. Proceed cautiously and gently if pain is present. Clinical findings may include malalignment; tenderness; or inability to flex, extend, and rotate the neck as expected. Muscle and nerve pain often accompany neck pain if spinal nerves are involved.

The thoracic *spine,* lumbar spine, and sacral spine are evaluated in the same manner as the neck. Spinal alignment problems are common (see Fig. 52-3). Place both hands over the posterior iliac crests with the thumbs over the lumbosacral area. Apply pressure with the thumbs along the lumbosacral spine to elicit tenderness. Many patients do not have discomfort until the area is palpated. **Lordosis** is a common finding in adults who have abdominal obesity. During screening for **scoliosis,** ask the patient to flex forward from the hips and inspect for a lateral curve in the spine.

If the extremities are affected by a musculoskeletal problem, assess arms or legs at the same time for side-to-side comparisons. For example, inspect and palpate both shoulders for size, swelling, deformity, poor alignment, tenderness or pain, and mobility. A shoulder injury may prevent the patient from combing his or her hair with the affected arm, but severe arthritis may inhibit movement in both arms. Assess the elbows and wrists in a similar way.

Because the hand has multiple joints in a single digit, assessment of hand function is perhaps the most critical part of the examination. If the hands are affected, inspect and palpate the metacarpophalangeal (MCP), proximal interphalangeal (PIP), and distal interphalangeal (DIP) joints. The same digits are compared on the right and left hands (Fig. 52-6). Determine the range of motion (ROM) for each joint by observing active movement. If movement is not possible, evaluate passive motion. For a quick and easy assessment of ROM, ask the patient to make a fist and then appose each finger to the thumb. If he or she can perform these maneuvers, ROM of the hand is not seriously restricted.

Evaluation of the hip joint relies primarily on determination of its degree of mobility, because the joint is deep and difficult to inspect or palpate. The patient with hip pain usually experiences it in the *groin* or has pain that radiates to the knee. The knee is readily accessible for physical assessment, particularly when the patient is sitting and the knee is flexed. Fluid accumulation, or **effusion,** is easily detected in the knee joint. Limitations in movement with accompanying pain are common findings. The knees may be poorly aligned, as in **genu valgum** ("knock-knee") or **genu varum** ("bowlegged") deformities.

The ankles and feet are often neglected in the physical examination. However, they contain multiple bones and joints

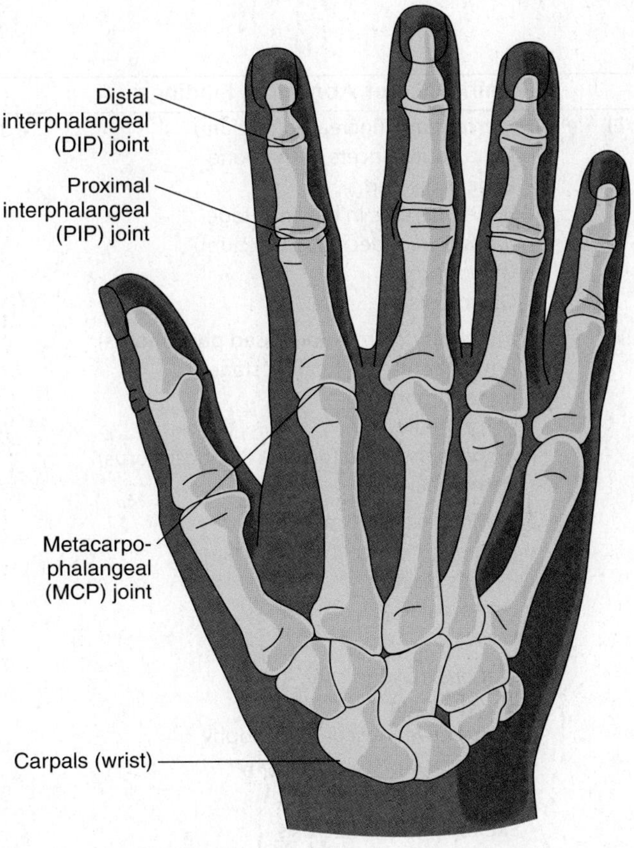

Distal interphalangeal (DIP) joint
Proximal interphalangeal (PIP) joint
Metacarpo-phalangeal (MCP) joint
Carpals (wrist)

Fig. 52-6 • The small joints of the hand.

that can be affected by disease and injury. Observe and palpate each joint and test for ROM if feet are affected by musculoskeletal problems.

Neurovascular Assessment

While completing a physical assessment of the musculoskeletal system, perform an assessment of peripheral vascular and nerve integrity. Beginning with the injured side, always compare one extremity with the other. *Palpation of pulses in the extremities below the level of injury and assessment of sensation, movement, color, temperature, and pain in the injured part give a complete* ***neurovascular assessment.*** If pulses are not palpable, a Doppler should be used to find pulses in the extremities. See Chart 54-3 in Chapter 54 for more details about neurovascular assessment.

Assessment of the Muscular System

During the skeletal assessment, notice the size, shape, tone, and strength of major skeletal muscles. The circumference of each muscle may be measured and compared symmetrically for an estimation of muscle mass if abnormalities are observed.

VIDEO CLIP: Muscular Development and Strength

Ask the patient to demonstrate muscle strength. Apply resistance by holding the extremity and asking the patient to move against resistance. As an option, place your hands on the patient's upper arms and ask the patient to try to raise the arms. Although movement against resistance is not easily quantified, several scales used by nurses and therapists are available for grading the patient's strength. A commonly used scale is shown in Table 52-2.

TABLE 52-2 Lovett's Scale for Grading Muscle Strength

Rating	Description
5	Normal: ROM unimpaired against gravity with full resistance
4	Good: can complete ROM against gravity with some resistance
3	Fair: can complete ROM against gravity
2	Poor: can complete ROM with gravity eliminated
1	Trace: no joint motion and slight evidence of muscle contractility
0	Zero: no evidence of muscle contractility

ROM, Range of motion.

Psychosocial Assessment

The data from the history and physical assessment provide clues for anticipating psychosocial problems. For instance, prolonged absence from employment or permanent disability may cause job or career loss. Further stress may be experienced if chronic pain continues and the patient cannot cope with numerous stressors. Anxiety and depression are common when patients have chronic pain. Deformities resulting from musculoskeletal disease or injury, such as an amputation, can affect a person's body image and self-concept. Help the patient identify support systems and coping mechanisms that may be useful if the patient has long-term musculoskeletal health problems. Encourage the patient to verbalize feelings related to loss and body image changes. Refer the patient for psychological or spiritual counseling if needed and if it is culturally appropriate.

Diagnostic Assessment

Laboratory Assessment

Chart 52-3 lists the common laboratory tests used in assessing patients with musculoskeletal disorders. There is no special patient preparation or follow-up care for any of these tests. Teach the patient about the purpose of the test and the procedure that can be expected. Additional tests performed for patients with connective tissue diseases, such as rheumatoid arthritis, are described in Chapter 20.

Disorders of bone and the parathyroid gland are often reflected in an alteration of the serum calcium or phosphorus level. Therefore these electrolytes, especially calcium, are monitored.

Alkaline phosphatase (ALP) is an enzyme normally present in blood. The concentration of ALP increases with bone or liver damage. In metabolic bone disease and bone cancer, the enzyme concentration rises in proportion to the osteoblastic activity, which indicates bone formation. The level of ALP is normally slightly increased in older adults.

The major *muscle enzymes* affected in skeletal muscle disease or injuries are:

- Creatine kinase (CK-MM)
- Aspartate aminotransferase (AST)
- Aldolase (ALD)
- Lactic dehydrogenase (LDH)

As a result of damage, the muscle tissue releases additional amounts of these enzymes, which increases serum levels.

The serum CK level begins to rise 2 to 4 hours after muscle injury and is elevated early in muscle disease, such as muscu-

Chart 52-3 LABORATORY PROFILE

Musculoskeletal Assessment

Test	Normal Range for Adults	Significance of Abnormal Findings
Serum calcium	9.0-10.5 mg/dL (2.25-2.75 mmol/L) *Older adults:* decreased	*Hypercalcemia* (increased calcium) • Metastatic cancers of the bone • Paget's disease • Bone fractures in healing stage *Hypocalcemia* (decreased calcium) • Osteoporosis • Osteomalacia
Serum phosphorus	3.0-4.5 mg/dL (0.97-1.45 mmol/L) *Older adults:* decreased	*Hyperphosphatemia* (increased phosphorus) • Bone fractures in healing stage • Bone tumors • Acromegaly *Hypophosphatemia* (decreased phosphorus) • Osteomalacia
Alkaline phosphatase (ALP)	30-120 units/L *Older adults:* slightly increased	*Elevations* may indicate: • Metastatic cancers of the bone • Paget's disease • Osteomalacia
Serum muscle enzymes		
Creatine kinase (CK)	Total CK: *Men:* 55-170 units/L *Women:* 30-135 units/L	*Elevations* may indicate: • Muscle trauma • Progressive muscular dystrophy • Effects of electromyography
Lactate dehydrogenase (LDH)	Total LDH: 100-190 units/L *LDH_1:* 17%-27% *LDH_2:* 27%-37% *LDH_3:* 18%-25% *LDH_4:* 3%-8% *LDH_5:* 0% to 5%	*Elevations* may indicate: • Skeletal muscle necrosis • Extensive cancer • Progressive muscular dystrophy
Aspartate aminotransferase (AST)	0-35 units/L *Older adults:* increased	*Elevations* may indicate: • Skeletal muscle trauma • Progressive muscular dystrophy
Aldolase (ALD)	3.0-8.2 units/Dl	*Elevations* may indicate: • Polymyositis and dermatomyositis • Muscular dystrophy

lar dystrophy. The CK molecule has two subunits: M (muscle) and B (brain). Three isoenzymes have been identified. Skeletal muscle CK (CK-MM, or CK_3) is the only isoenzyme that rises in concentration with damage to skeletal muscle.

AST is moderately elevated (three to five times normal) in certain muscle diseases, such as muscular dystrophy. The levels of the isoenzymes aldolase A (ALD-A) and LDH_5 also increase in patients with these disorders.

Imaging Assessment

The skeleton is very visible on *standard x-rays.* Anteroposterior and lateral projections are the initial screening views used most often. Other approaches, such as oblique or stress views, depend on the part of the skeleton to be evaluated and the necessity of the x-ray.

Bone density, alignment, swelling, and intactness can be seen on x-ray. The conditions of joints can be determined, including the size of the joint space, the smoothness of articular cartilage, and synovial swelling. Soft-tissue involvement may be evident but not clearly differentiated.

Inform the patient that the x-ray table is hard and cold, and instruct him or her to remain still during the filming process. Coordinate with the radiology department or clinic to keep older adults and those at risk for hypothermia as warm as possible (e.g., by using blankets).

Whereas standard x-rays superimpose one structure on another, **tomography** produces planes, or slices, for focus and blurs the images of other structures. This procedure is helpful in detailing the musculoskeletal system, because the many close structures make visualization difficult.

Xeroradiography highlights the contrast between structures. Margins and edges can be clearly seen (edge enhancement). Disadvantages of xeroradiography are the higher radiation dose to the patient and inability of the test to determine tissue densities.

Myelography involves the injection of contrast medium into the subarachnoid space of the spine, usually by spinal puncture. The vertebral column, intervertebral disks, spinal nerve roots, and blood vessels can be visualized. Although this test is still performed, it is far less popular. Computed tomography (CT) and magnetic resonance imaging (MRI) have often replaced such invasive and potentially painful and risky diagnostic techniques. The post-test care is similar to that for lumbar puncture, except that the patient is usually placed with the head of the bed elevated 30 to 50 degrees to prevent the contrast medium from getting into the brain (see Chapter 43).

An **arthrogram** is an x-ray study of a joint after contrast medium (air or solution) has been injected to enhance its visualization. Double-contrast arthrography, which uses both air and contrast, may be performed when a traumatic injury is suspected. The physician can often determine bone chips, torn ligaments, or other loose bodies within the joint. This test is not used commonly because of newer advances in diagnostic imaging. Most joints are now studied by MRI.

Computed tomography (CT) has gained wide acceptance for detecting musculoskeletal problems, particularly those of the vertebral column and joints. The scanned images can be used to create additional images from other angles or to create three-dimensional images and view complex structures from any position. The nurse or radiology technologist should ask the patient about iodine-based contrast allergies.

Nuclear Scans

The **bone scan** is a radionuclide test in which radioactive material is injected for viewing the entire skeleton. It may be used primarily to detect tumors, arthritis, osteomyelitis, osteoporosis, vertebral compression fractures, and unexplained bone pain. Bone scans are used less commonly today as more sophisticated MRI equipment becomes more available. However, it may be very useful for detecting hairline fractures in patients with unexplained bone pain and diffuse metastatic bone disease.

The **gallium** and **thallium scans** are similar to the bone scan but are more specific and sensitive in detecting bone problems. Gallium citrate (^{67}Ga) is the radioisotope most commonly used. This substance also migrates to brain, liver, and breast tissue and therefore is used in examination of these structures when disease is suspected.

For patients with osteosarcoma, thallium (^{201}Tl) is better than gallium or technetium for diagnosing the extent of the disease. Thallium has traditionally been used for the diagnosis of myocardial infarctions but can be used for additional evaluation of cancers of the bone.

Because bone takes up gallium slowly, the nuclear medicine physician or technician administers the isotope 4 to 6 hours before scanning. Other tests that require contrast media or other isotopes cannot be given during this time.

Instruct the patient that the radioactive material poses no threat because it readily deteriorates in the body. Because gallium is excreted through the intestinal tract, it tends to collect in feces after the scanning procedure.

Depending on the tissue to be examined, the patient is taken to the nuclear medicine department 4 to 6 hours after injection. The procedure takes 30 to 60 minutes, during which time the patient must lie still for accurate test results to be achieved. The scan may be repeated at 24, 48, and/or 72 hours. Mild sedation may be necessary to facilitate relaxation and cooperation during the procedure for confused older adults or those in severe pain.

No special care is required after the test. The radioisotope is excreted in stool and urine, but no precautions are taken in handling the excreta. Remind the patient to push fluids to facilitate urinary excretion.

Magnetic Resonance Imaging

Magnetic resonance imaging (MRI), with or without the use of contrast media, is commonly used to diagnose musculoskeletal disorders. It is more accurate than computed tomography (CT) and myelography for many spinal and knee problems. MRI is most appropriate for joints, soft tissue, and bony tumors that involve soft tissue. CT is still the test of choice for injuries or pathology that involves only bone.

The image is produced through the interaction of magnetic fields, radio waves, and atomic nuclei showing hydrogen density. Simply put, the radio waves "bounce" off the body tissues being examined. Because each tissue has its own density, the computer image clearly distinguishes normal and abnormal tissues. For some tissues, the cross-sectional image is better than that produced by radiography or CT. The lack of hydrogen ions in cortical bone makes it easily distinguishable from soft tissues. The test is particularly useful in identifying problems with muscles, tendons, and ligaments.

Ensure that the patient removes all metal objects and checks for clothing zippers and metal fasteners. Although joint implants made of titanium or stainless steel are safe, pacemakers, stents, and surgical clips usually are not. Chart 52-4 lists questions that the nurse or technician should consider in preparing the patient for MRI. Open MRIs prevent the claustrophobia that occurs with the older, encased machines.

Ultrasonography

Sound waves produce an image of the tissue in ultrasonography. An ultrasound procedure may be used to view:

- Soft-tissue disorders, such as masses and fluid accumulation
- Traumatic joint injuries
- Osteomyelitis
- Surgical hardware placement

A jelly-like substance applied to the skin over the site to be examined promotes the movement of a metal probe. No special preparation or post-test care is necessary. A quantitative ultrasound (QUS) may be done for determining fractures or bone density.

Other Diagnostic Assessment

Biopsies

In a *bone biopsy,* the physician extracts a specimen of the bone tissue for microscopic examination. This invasive test may confirm the presence of infection or neoplasm, but it is not commonly done today. One of two techniques may be used to retrieve the specimen: needle (closed) biopsy or incisional

Chart 52-4 BEST PRACTICE FOR PATIENT SAFETY & QUALITY CARE

The Patient Preparing for Magnetic Resonance Imaging

- Is the patient pregnant?
- Does the patient have ferromagnetic fragments or implants, such as an older-style aneurysm clip?
- Does the patient have a pacemaker, stent, or electronic implant?
- Can the patient lie still in the supine position for 45 to 60 minutes (may require sedation)?
- Does the patient need life support equipment available?
- Can the patient communicate clearly and understand verbal communication?
- Did the patient get any tattoo *more than* 20 years ago? (If so, metal particles may be in the ink.)
- Is the patient claustrophobic? (Ask this question for closed MRI scanners; open MRIs do not cause claustrophobia.)

(open) biopsy. It is important to watch for bleeding from the puncture site and for tenderness, redness, or warmth that could indicate infection. Mild analgesics may be used.

Muscle biopsy is done for the diagnosis of atrophy (as in muscular dystrophy) and inflammation (as in polymyositis). The procedure and care for patients undergoing muscle biopsy are the same as those for patients undergoing bone biopsy.

Electromyography

Electromyography (EMG) is used to evaluate diffuse or localized muscle weakness. EMG is usually accompanied by nerve conduction studies for determining the electrical potential generated in an individual muscle. EMG helps in the diagnosis of neuromuscular, lower motor neuron, and peripheral nerve disorders. This test is contraindicated for patients undergoing anticoagulant therapy.

Inform the patient that EMG may cause temporary discomfort, especially when the patient is subjected to episodes of electrical current. For selected patients, mild sedation is prescribed. The physician may also prescribe a temporary discontinuation of skeletal muscle relaxants several days before the procedure to prevent drugs from affecting the test results.

The test may be performed at the bedside or in an EMG laboratory. When both EMG and nerve conduction studies are done, nerve conduction is usually tested first. Flat electrodes are placed along the nerve to be evaluated, and low electrical currents are passed through the electrodes to the nerve and muscle innervated. If nerve conduction occurs, the muscle contracts.

For testing muscle potential, multiple small needle electrodes are inserted. The patient is asked to perform activities for measurement of muscle potential during minimal and maximal contraction. The degree of nerve and muscle activity is recorded for later interpretation.

A few medical complications are associated with EMG. The nurse provides comfort measures and inspects the needle sites for hematoma formation. The application of ice can prevent this complication. The patient may also report increased pain and anxiety after the test.

Arthroscopy

The **arthroscopy** may be used as a diagnostic test or a surgical procedure. An arthroscope is a fiberoptic tube inserted into a joint for direct visualization of the ligaments, menisci, and articular surfaces of the joint. The knee and shoulder are most commonly evaluated. In addition, synovial biopsy and surgery to repair traumatic injury can be done through the arthroscope as an ambulatory care procedure.

Patient Preparation. Because the knee is most commonly "scoped," the care described for the patient undergoing arthroscopy relates to that joint. Arthroscopy is performed on an ambulatory basis or as same-day surgery. The patient must be able to flex the knee. Those who cannot flex the knee at least 40 degrees or who have an infected knee are not candidates for the procedure. If the patient cannot flex the knee, the arthroscope cannot be inserted into the joint space to allow visualization. Joint infection may worsen from the mechanical trauma of arthroscope insertion.

If the procedure is done for surgical repair, the patient may have a physical therapy consultation before arthroscopy to learn the leg exercises that are necessary after the test. Straight-leg raises (SLRs) and quadriceps setting exercises (isometrics with the leg extended) are practiced in sets of 10 each. ROM exercises are also taught but may not be allowed immediately after arthroscopic surgery. The nurse in the surgeon's office or at the surgical center can teach these exercises or reinforce the information provided by the physical therapist. The nurse also reinforces the explanation of the procedure and post-test care and ensures that the patient has signed an informed consent.

Procedure. The patient is usually given local, light general, or epidural anesthesia, depending on the purpose of the procedure. In some settings, a large pneumatic tourniquet is used around the thigh to minimize bleeding during the procedure. Drugs that promote vasoconstriction for control of bleeding may be used alone or in conjunction with the tourniquet.

The knee is flexed to at least 40 degrees and is irrigated. As shown in Fig. 52-7, the arthroscope is inserted through a small incision less than ¼ inch (0.6 cm) long. Multiple incisions may be required to allow inspection at a variety of angles. After the procedure, a dressing may be applied, depending on the amount of manipulation during the test or surgery.

Follow-up Care. *The priority for postprocedure care is to evaluate the neurovascular status of the patient's affected limb every hour or according to agency or surgeon protocol. Monitor and document distal pulses, warmth, color, capillary refill, pain, movement, and sensation of the affected extremity.*

Encourage the patient to perform exercises as taught before the procedure, if appropriate. For the mild discomfort experienced after the diagnostic arthroscopy, the physician prescribes a mild analgesic, such as acetaminophen (Tylenol, Ace-Tabs♣). If postoperative, the patient may have short-term activity restrictions, depending on the musculoskeletal problem. Ice is often used for 24 hours, and the extremity should be elevated for 12 to 24 hours. When arthroscopic surgery is performed, the health care provider usually prescribes an opioid-analgesic combination, such as oxycodone and acetaminophen (Percocet, Tylox).

Although complications are not common, monitor and teach the patient to observe for:

- Swelling
- Increased joint pain attributable to mechanical injury
- Thrombophlebitis
- Infection

Severe joint or limb pain after discharge may indicate a possible complication. Teach the patient to contact the physician

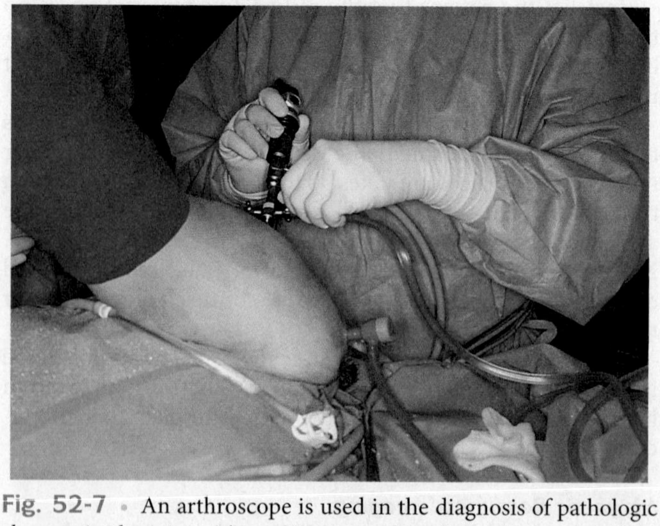

Fig. 52-7 • An arthroscope is used in the diagnosis of pathologic changes in the joints. This patient is undergoing arthroscopy of the shoulder.

immediately. The surgeon usually sees the patient about 1 week after the procedure to check for complications.

NCLEX EXAMINATION CHALLENGE

A client is admitted to the PACU after an arthroscopic procedure to repair a torn knee ligament. Which of these nursing activities can be delegated to the nursing assistant?

A. Teaching the client how to perform his postoperative leg exercises
B. Observing the surgical dressing for bloody drainage
C. Taking the client's temperature, pulse, and respiratory rate
D. Explaining the client's status to his life partner

evolve For the correct answer, go to http://evolve.elsevier.com/Iggy/.

HUMAN NEEDS ASSESSMENT REVIEW

What should you NOTICE in a patient with adequate mobility and sensation related to the musculoskeletal system?

Physical Assessment

- No gross deformities or impairments in posture or gait
- Adequate size, strength, and symmetry of muscle for age
- Can perform ADLs independently
- Can perform other routine daily activities independently
- Can ambulate with or without assistive devices
- No pain or tenderness on palpation or passive range-of-motion (ROM) of joints
- Active ROM of joints within normal limits for age
- No crepitus when moving joints
- No swelling of joints or extremities
- Equal size and alignment of extremities
- Equal sensation in extremities

Diagnostic Assessment

- Muscle enzymes (e.g., CK-MM, ALD) within normal limits for age
- Bone density adequate for age and gender
- Joint changes within normal limits for age

GET READY FOR THE NCLEX EXAMINATION!

Key Points

Review these Key Points for each NCLEX Examination Client Needs Category.

Safe and Effective Care Environment

- Collaborate with the physical and/or occupational therapist to perform a complete musculoskeletal assessment if indicated.
- Ask the patient about allergy to iodine-based contrast media before diagnostic testing such as CT scans.

Health Promotion and Maintenance

- Teach the patient that mild discomfort can be expected during electromyography, a test to assess the electrical potential of muscles and their innervation.
- Instruct the patient to report swelling, infection, and increased pain after an arthroscopy.
- Ask the patient questions to ensure safety before an MRI (see Chart 52-4).

Psychosocial Integrity

- Assess the patient's support systems and coping mechanisms when musculoskeletal trauma or disease affects his or her body image.
- Ask about the patient's occupation, because heavy, manual labor may cause back injury and other musculoskeletal trauma.

Physiological Integrity

- Assess the patient's pain intensity, quality, duration, and location.
- Assess the patient's mobility, including gait, posture, and muscle strength.
- Assess for musculoskeletal changes associated with aging (see Chart 52-1).
- Interpret the patient's laboratory values that are related to musculoskeletal disease (see Chart 52-3).
- Evaluate the neurovascular status of the patient's affected extremity after an arthroscopic procedure as the *priority for care*.

Additional Study Resources

Go to your Companion CD or Evolve at http://evolve.elsevier.com/Iggy/ for *Self-Assessment Questions for the NCLEX Examination.*

evolve Go to Evolve at http://evolve.elsevier.com/Iggy/ for *Prioritization and Delegation Questions for the NCLEX Examination.*

SELECTED BIBLIOGRAPHY

Asterisk indicates a classic or definitive work on this subject.

Dillon, P.M. (2007). *Nursing health assessment: A critical thinking case studies approach* (2nd ed.). Philadelphia: Davis.

Gordon, M. (2007). *Manual of nursing diagnosis* (11th ed.). Boston: Jones & Bartlett.

*Maher, A.B. (2002). Assessment of the musculoskeletal system. In A.B. Maher, S.W. Salmond, & T.A. Pellino (Eds.), *Orthopaedic nursing* (3rd ed.). Philadelphia: Saunders.

*Mangini, M. (1998). Physical assessment of the musculoskeletal system. *Nursing Clinics of North America, 33*(4), 643-652.

*Martsolf, D.S. (1999). Cultural aspects of orthopaedic nursing. *Orthopaedic Nursing, 18*(2), 65-71.

*Mosher, C.M. (2004). *An introduction to orthopaedic nursing.* (3rd ed.). Chicago, IL: National Association of Orthopaedic Nurses.

Nussbaum, R.L., McInnes, R.R., & Willard, H.F. (2007). *Thompson & Thompson genetics in medicine* (7th ed.). Philadelphia: Elsevier.

*O'Hanlon-Nichols, T. (1998). Basic assessment series: A review of the adult musculoskeletal system. *AJN, 98*(6), 48-52.

Pagana, K.D., & Pagana, T.J. (2006). *Mosby's diagnostic and laboratory test reference* (3rd ed.). St. Louis: Mosby.

Schoen, D.C. (2007). Pain in the orthopaedic patient. *Orthopaedic Nursing, 26*(2), 140-144.

Taggart, H.M. (2006). *Core curriculum for orthopaedic nursing* (5th ed.). Boston: Pearson.

53

CHAPTER

Care of Patients with Musculoskeletal Problems

Cathy A. Murray

LEARNING OUTCOMES

For clinical competence and success on the NCLEX Examination, study this chapter with these Learning Outcomes in mind:

Safe and Effective Care Environment

1. Coordinate with health care team members when planning and providing care for patients with musculoskeletal problems.
2. Teach the patient and family about home safety when the patient has a metabolic bone problem such as osteoporosis.
3. Identify community resources for patients with musculoskeletal problems that impair mobility.
4. Review collaborative management options for bone cancer for the patient and family.
5. Apply principles of infection control for patients with osteomyelitis, including Contact Precautions if needed.

Health Promotion and Maintenance

6. Develop a teaching plan for all age-groups about ways to decrease the risk for osteoporosis.
7. Perform health risk assessments for people at risk for osteoporosis and osteomalacia.
8. Assess the genetic risk for patients who have parents with muscular dystrophy.
9. Refer patients with genetic-associated diseases for genetic counseling and testing.

Psychosocial Integrity

10. Assess the patient's and family's responses to a bone cancer diagnosis and treatment options.
11. Evaluate patient and family coping strategies and fears related to grief and loss before and after bone cancer surgery.

Physiological Integrity

12. Educate the patient and family about common drugs used for bone diseases, such as calcium and bisphosphonates.
13. Compare and contrast osteoporosis and osteomalacia.
14. Identify key features of Paget's disease of the bone.
15. Differentiate acute and chronic osteomyelitis.
16. Prioritize care for patients with osteomyelitis.
17. Analyze assessment data to determine priority nursing diagnoses and collaborative problems for the patient with bone cancer.
18. Describe common disorders of the foot, including hallux valgus and plantar fasciitis, that can affect mobility.
19. Explain the role of the nurse when caring for an adult patient with muscular dystrophy.

Go to your Companion CD or Evolve at http://evolve.elsevier.com/Iggy/ for *Self-Assessment Questions for the NCLEX Examination* keyed to these Learning Outcomes.

Musculoskeletal disorders include metabolic bone diseases, such as osteoporosis and Paget's disease, bone tumors and lesions, and a variety of deformities and syndromes. Older adults are at the greatest risk for most of these problems. However, the incidence of bone cancer is increasing in both the younger and older population. Primary bone cancer is most often found in adolescents and young adults. As technologic advances occur and patients survive longer with primary cancers, metastatic lesions have become more prevalent among older adults. Almost all musculoskeletal health problems can cause the patient to have difficulty meeting the human need of *mobility.* This chapter focuses on selected disorders not covered in Chapter 20 on arthritis and other connective tissue diseases.

METABOLIC BONE DISEASES

OSTEOPOROSIS

Pathophysiology

Osteoporosis is a chronic metabolic disease in which bone loss causes decreased density and possible fracture. It is often referred to as a "silent disease" because the first sign of osteoporosis in most people follows some kind of a fracture. The hip, spine, and wrist are most often at risk, although any bone can fracture (National Osteoporosis Foundation, 2007a).

Bone is a dynamic tissue that is constantly undergoing changes in a process referred to as **bone remodeling.** Osteoporosis and **osteopenia** (low bone mass) occur when osteoclastic (bone resorption) activity is greater than osteoblastic (bone building) activity. The result is a decreased **bone mineral density (BMD).** BMD determines bone strength and peaks between 25 and 30 years of age. Before and during the peak years, osteoclastic activity and osteoblastic activity work at the same rate. After the peak years, bone resorption activity exceeds bone-building activity, and bone density decreases. BMD decreases most rapidly in postmenopausal women as serum estrogen levels diminish. Although estrogen does not build bone, it helps prevent bone loss. **Trabecular,** or **cancellous** (spongy), bone is lost first, followed by loss of **cortical** (compact) bone. This results in thin, fragile bone tissue that is at risk for fracture (National Osteoporosis Foundation, 2007b).

Standards for the diagnosis of osteoporosis are based on BMD testing that provides a T-score for the patient. A T-score represents the number of standard deviations above or below the average BMD for young, healthy adults. *Osteopenia is present when the T-score is at −1 and above −2.5. Osteoporosis is diagnosed in a person who has a T-score at or lower than −2.5.* Medicare reimburses for BMD testing every 2 years in people age 65 years and older who (National Osteoporosis Foundation, 2007c):

- Are estrogen deficient
- Receive long-term steroid therapy
- Have hyperparathyroidism
- Are being monitored while on osteoporosis drug therapy

The exact pathophysiology of osteoporosis is unclear, but two broad theories of disease development have been advocated. First, osteoporosis may result from increased osteoclastic (bone resorption) activity and decreased osteoblastic (bone building) activity related to changes in hormone levels or other disease processes. This theory has resulted in treatment directed toward measures to prevent rapid bone resorption. The second theory is that osteoblasts, or bone-forming cells, may have a shortened life span or may be less efficient in the patient with osteoporosis.

Osteoporosis can be classified as generalized or regional. *Generalized* osteoporosis involves many structures in the skeleton and is further divided into two categories, primary and secondary. *Primary* osteoporosis is more common and occurs in postmenopausal women and in men in their seventh or eighth decade of life. Even though men do not experience the rapid bone loss that postmenopausal women have, they do have decreasing levels of testosterone (which builds bone) and altered ability to absorb calcium. This results in a slower loss of bone mass in men, especially those older than 75 years. *Secondary* osteoporosis may result from other medical conditions, such as hyperparathyroidism; long-term drug therapy, such as with corticosteroids; or prolonged immobility, such as that seen with spinal cord injury (Table 53-1). Treatment of the secondary type is directed toward the cause of the osteoporosis when possible.

Regional osteoporosis, an example of secondary disease, occurs when a limb is immobilized related to a fracture, injury, or paralysis. Immobility for longer than 8 to 12 weeks can result in this type of osteoporosis. Bone loss also occurs when people spend prolonged time in a gravity-free or weightless environment (e.g., astronauts). The United States and other countries are studying this problem during trips into space.

Etiology and Genetic Risk

Primary osteoporosis is probably caused by a combination of risk factors and genetic changes (Chart 53-1). Peak bone mass is achieved by about 30 years of age in most women. *Building strong*

TABLE 53-1 Causes of Secondary Osteoporosis

DISEASES/CONDITIONS
- Diabetes mellitus
- Hyperthyroidism
- Hyperparathyroidism
- Cushing's syndrome
- Growth hormone deficiency
- Metabolic acidosis
- Female hypogonadism
- Paget's disease
- Osteogenesis imperfecta
- Rheumatoid arthritis
- Prolonged immobilization
- Bone cancer
- Cirrhosis
- HIV/AIDS
- Chronic airway limitation

DRUGS (CHRONIC USE)
- Corticosteroids
- Heparin
- Anticonvulsants (phenobarbital, phenytoin)
- Ethanol (alcohol)
- Drugs that induce hypogonadism (decreased levels of sex hormones)
- High levels of thyroid hormone
- Cytotoxic agents
- Immunosuppressants
- Loop diuretics

AIDS, Acquired immune deficiency syndrome; *HIV,* human immune deficiency virus.

Chart 53-1 BEST PRACTICE FOR PATIENT SAFETY & QUALITY CARE

Assessing Risk Factors for Primary Osteoporosis

Assess for:
- Age 65 years and older in all women
- Age 75 years and older in men
- Family history of osteoporosis
- History of low-trauma fracture after age 50 years
- Caucasian or Asian ethnicity
- Low body weight, thin build
- Chronic low calcium intake
- Estrogen or androgen deficiency
- Women with other risk factors
- Smoking history
- High alcohol intake
- Lack of physical exercise or prolonged immobility

bone as a young person may be the best defense against osteoporosis in later adulthood (National Osteoporosis Foundation, 2007a). Young women need to be aware of appropriate health and lifestyle practices that can prevent this potentially disabling disease.

Primary osteoporosis most often occurs in women after menopause as a result of decreased estrogen levels. Women lose about 2% of their bone mass every year in the first 5 years after natural or surgical (ovary removal) menopause. For women of any age who do not take estrogen replacement, the risk for osteoporosis increases.

In addition, body build seems to influence who gets the disease. Osteoporosis occurs more often in thin, lean-built European-American and Asian women, particularly those who do not exercise regularly. Obese women can store estrogen in their tissues for use as necessary to maintain a normal level of serum calcium. Weight-bearing exercise reduces bone resorption (loss) and stimulates bone formation. Prolonged immobility produces rapid bone loss.

The relationship of osteoporosis to nutrition is well established. For example, excessive caffeine in the diet can cause calcium loss in the urine. A diet lacking enough calcium and vitamin D stimulates the parathyroid gland to produce parathyroid hormone (PTH). PTH triggers the release of calcium from the bony matrix. Activated vitamin D is needed for calcium uptake in the body. Malabsorption of nutrients in the GI tract also contributes to low serum calcium levels. Institutionalized or homebound patients who are not exposed to sunlight may be at a higher risk because they do not receive adequate vitamin D for the metabolism of calcium.

Calcium loss occurs at a more rapid rate when phosphorus intake is high. (Chapter 13 describes the normal relationship between calcium and phosphorus in the body.) People who drink large amounts of carbonated beverages each day (over 40 ounces) are at high risk for calcium loss and subsequent osteoporosis, regardless of age or gender.

Protein deficiency may also reduce bone density. Because 50% of serum calcium is protein bound, protein is needed to use calcium. However, excessive protein intake may increase calcium loss in the urine. For instance, people who are on high-protein, low-carbohydrate diets, like the Atkins diet, may consume too much protein to replace other food not allowed. Dietary protein intake in healthy adults is recommended at 0.8 grams per kilogram of body weight. Protein is needed for bone healing when a fracture occurs.

Excessive alcohol and tobacco use are other risk factors for osteoporosis. Although the exact mechanisms are not known, these substances promote acidosis, which in turn increases bone loss. Alcohol also has a direct toxic effect on bone tissue, resulting in decreased bone formation and increased bone resorption. For those people who have excessive alcohol intake, alcohol calories decrease hunger and the need to take in adequate amounts of nutrients.

Osteoporosis also occurs in young adults who participate in excessive exercise or weight-loss dieting or in those who have eating disorders, such as anorexia nervosa or bulimia nervosa. Young females with these risk factors have a low body weight and absent menstruation, which contribute to the development of osteoporosis. Dancers, gymnasts, and other athletes may overtrain without sufficient caloric intake, which also results in severe weight loss. Young girls and women may have an obsession with being slim. Particular attention must be paid to bone health for these groups.

GENETIC CONSIDERATIONS

The genetic and immune factors that cause osteoporosis are very complex and unclear. Family history often reveals that the patient's mother had the disease. Many genetic changes have been identified as possible causative factors, but there is no agreement about which ones are most important or constant in all patients. For example, changes in the vitamin D receptor (VDR) gene and calcitonin receptor (CTR) gene have been found in some patients with the disease. Receptors are essential for the uptake and use of these substances by the cells.

The bone morphogenetic protein-2 (BMP-2) gene has a key role in bone formation and maintenance. Some osteoporotic patients who have had fractures have changes in their BMP-2 gene. Alterations in growth hormone-1 (GH-1) have been discovered in petite Asian-American women, those who are likely to have osteoporosis (Lui et al., 2006).

Hormones, tumor necrosis factor (TNF), interleukins, and other substances in the body help control osteoclasts in a very complex pathway. The recent identification of the importance of the cytokine receptor activator of nuclear factor kappa-B ligand (RANKL), its receptor RANK, and its decoy receptor osteoprotegerin (OPG) has helped researchers understand more about the activity of osteoclasts in metabolic bone disease. Disruptions in the RANKL, RANK, and OPG system can lead to increased osteoclast activity in which bone is rapidly broken down (McCance & Huether, 2006).

Incidence/Prevalence

Osteoporosis is a major health problem in the United States and many other countries. Iacono (2007) stated that the disease is a national public health priority. The estimated cost for osteoporosis-related health care alone in the United States is more than $18 billion each year in 2002 dollars with continual cost increases each year (National Osteoporosis Foundation, 2007a).

Osteoporosis is a potential health problem for more than 44 million Americans. About 10 million persons in the United States have the disease, and about 34 million persons 50 years of age and older experience osteopenia and are at risk for development of osteoporosis. Women remain the largest group affected by osteoporosis (8 million). Two million men (especially those older than 75 years) also have the disease. People of all ethnic backgrounds are at some risk (National Osteoporosis Foundation, 2007a), but white, thin women are likely to get primary osteoporosis at an earlier age.

CULTURAL AWARENESS

Although there is some advantage of increased bone density in dark-skinned women, lifestyle and health beliefs about prevention may put all women at an equal risk for osteoporosis. Dietary preferences or the ability to afford high-nutrient food may influence the woman's rate of bone loss. For example, many blacks have lactose intolerance and cannot drink milk or eat other dairy-based foods. Milk and cheese are good sources of protein, a nutrient needed to bind calcium for use by the body.

Osteoporosis results in more than 1.5 million fractures each year. Of these, 300,000 are hip fractures, 700,000 are vertebral fractures, and 250,000 are wrist fractures (National Osteoporosis Foundation, 2007a). A woman who experiences a hip fracture has a four times greater risk for a second fracture. Fractures as a result of osteoporosis can decrease a patient's *mobility* and quality of life. The mortality rate for older patients with hip fractures is very high, especially within the first 6 months, and the debilitating effects can be devastating

Health Promotion and Maintenance

A study by Giangregorio et al. (2007) found that health care professionals, including nurses, who worked with older patients could not identify ways to prevent osteoporosis. (See the Evidence-Based Practice box below). Nurses can play a vital role in patient education to prevent and manage osteoporosis. *Teaching should begin with young women who begin to lose bone after 30 years of age.*

The focus of osteoporosis prevention is to decrease modifiable risk factors. For example, teach patients who do not include enough dietary calcium which foods should be included, such as dairy products and dark green, leafy vegetables. Teach them to read food labels for sources of calcium content. Explain the importance of sun exposure (but not so much as to get sunburned) or adequate vitamin D in the diet. Teach the need to limit the amount of carbonated beverages consumed each day. People who have sedentary lifestyles should be taught about the importance of exercise and what types of exercise builds bone tissue. Weight-bearing exercises are preferred. Teach people to avoid activities that cause jarring, such as horseback riding, to prevent potential vertebral bone damage.

Patient-Centered Collaborative Care

Assessment

A complete health history with assessment of risk factors is important in the prevention, early detection, and treatment of osteoporosis. Patients who have risk factors for osteoporosis are at increased risk for fractures when falls occur. Include a fall risk assessment in the health history, especially for older adults. Assess for fall risk factors, including:

- Delirium
- Dementia
- Immobility
- Muscular weakness
- History of falls
- Visual or hearing deficits
- Current drugs

The Joint Commission's 2007 National Patient Safety Goals (NPSG) document includes a goal to reduce the risk for harm to patients resulting from falls. *Persons with osteoporosis are at an increased risk for fracture if a fall occurs. Implement evidence-based fall reduction strategies when caring for patients with osteoporosis* (The Joint Commission, 2007). Chapter 3 discusses falls in older adults in more detail.

Physical Assessment/Clinical Manifestations

When performing a musculoskeletal assessment, inspect and palpate the vertebral column. The classic "dowager's hump," or kyphosis of the dorsal spine, is usually present (Fig. 53-1). The patient often states that he or she has gotten shorter, perhaps as much as 2 to 3 inches (5 to 7.5 cm) within the previous 20 years. Take or delegate height and weight measurements, and compare with previous measurements if they are available.

The patient may have back pain, which often occurs after lifting, bending, or stooping. The pain may be sharp and acute

EVIDENCE-BASED PRACTICE

Do health care professionals know strategies for prevention of osteoporosis?

Giangregorio, L., Fisher, P., Papaioannou, A, & Adachi, J.D. (2007). Osteoporosis knowledge and information needs in healthcare professionals caring for patients with fragility fractures. *Orthopaedic Nursing, 26*(1), 27-35.

This study explored the knowledge of health care professionals who care for older adult patients who experience fractures of the hip, spine, and wrist. One hundred and twenty-nine persons participated in the study with 90% of those being female. Participants were from fracture clinics and orthopedic and rehabilitation units. Sixty-three of the study participants were nurses. The Osteoporosis Knowledge Questionnaire (OKQ) was administered to each of the participants. The OKQ is a multiple-choice questionnaire designed to assess knowledge of osteoporosis and preventive measures. The responses of the participants to the questionnaire demonstrated that there are gaps in knowledge among health care professionals. Those gaps include the prevalence of osteoporosis, the recommended daily intake of calcium and vitamin D, taking calcium in divided doses with meals, and the use of bisphosphonates to treat osteoporosis. Most study participants did not know that bone loss begins in the third decade. Study participants did, however, know the definition of osteoporosis and the facts that treatments are available and that dairy products are good sources of calcium.

Level of Evidence—6. Study sample is small and not randomized.

Commentary: Implications for Practice and Research. The participants represented a small, convenience sample. However, the results compared to previous results on the OKQ among nurses and nursing students. This group represented professionals who work specifically with persons with or at risk for fracture and one would expect increased knowledge of osteoporosis. Health care professionals who work directly with persons who have a fracture or are at risk for fracture must be knowledgeable in all aspects of prevention and treatment. These gaps in knowledge require education. The interdisciplinary team who has the expert knowledge can play an important role in the prevention of fractures and early treatment of osteoporosis.

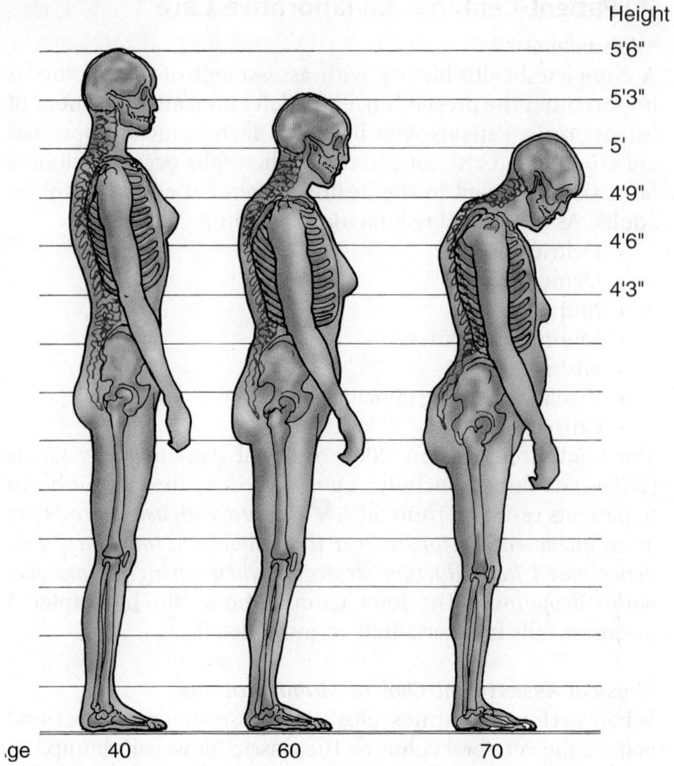
Height
5'6"
5'3"
5'
4'9"
4'6"
4'3"
ge
40
60
70

Fig. 53-1 • A normal spine at age 40 years and osteoporotic changes at ages 60 and 70 years. These changes can cause a loss of as much as 6 inches in height and can result in the so-called dowager's hump *(far right)* in the upper thoracic vertebrae.

in onset. Pain is worse with activity and is relieved by rest. Palpation of the vertebrae, particularly the lower thoracic and lumbar vertebrae, can increase the patient's discomfort. Therefore palpation should be gentle.

Back pain accompanied by tenderness and voluntary restriction of spinal movement suggests one or more compression vertebral fractures, the most common type of osteoporotic fracture. Movement restriction and spinal deformity may result in constipation, abdominal distention, reflux esophagitis, and respiratory compromise in severe cases. The most likely area for spinal fracture is between T8 and L3. This problem is discussed in more detail in Chapter 54.

Fractures are also common in the distal end of the radius (wrist) and the upper third of the femur (hip). Ask the patient to locate all areas that are painful, and observe for signs and symptoms of fractures, such as swelling and malalignment.

Psychosocial Assessment

Women associate osteoporosis with menopause, getting older, and becoming less independent. The disease can result in suffering, deformity, and disability that can affect the patient's well-being and life satisfaction. The quality of life may be further impacted by pain, insomnia, depression, and **fallophobia** (fear of falling).

Assess the patient's concept of body image, especially if he or she is severely kyphotic. For example, the patient may have difficulty finding clothes that fit properly. Social interactions may be avoided because of a change in appearance or the physical limitations of being unable to sit in chairs in restaurants, movie theaters, and other places. Changes in sexuality may occur as a result of poor self-esteem or the discomfort caused by positioning during intercourse.

Because osteoporosis poses a risk for fractures, teach the patient to be extremely cautious about activities. As a result, the threat of fracture can create anxiety and fear and result in further limitation of social or physical activities. Assess for these feelings to assist in treatment decisions and health teaching. For example, the patient may not exercise as prescribed for fear that a fracture will occur.

Laboratory Assessment

There are no definitive laboratory tests that confirm a diagnosis of primary osteoporosis, although a number of *biochemical markers* can provide information about bone resorption and formation activity. These biochemical markers are sensitive to bone changes and can be used to monitor effectiveness of treatment for osteoporosis. *Bone-specific alkaline phosphatase (BSAP)* is found in the cell membrane of the osteoblast and indicates bone formation status. *Osteocalcin* is a protein substance in bone and increases during bone resorption activity. Pyridinium (PYD) cross-links are released into circulation during bone resorption. *N-teleopeptide (NTX)* and *C-teleopeptide (CTX)* are proteins released when bone is broken down. Some laboratories require a 24-hour urine collection for testing, whereas others use a double-voided specimen. Some markers, like NTX and CTX, can also be measured in the blood using immunoassay techniques. Increased levels of any of these markers indicate a risk for osteoporosis. Increased levels are found in patients with osteoporosis, Paget's disease, and bone tumors (Pagana & Pagana, 2006).

A battery of tests can be performed to rule out secondary osteoporosis or other metabolic bone diseases, such as osteomalacia and Paget's disease. These include measurements of serum calcium, vitamin D, and phosphorus. Urinary calcium levels may also be assessed. Serum protein measurements and thyroid function tests are done to check for hyperthyroidism.

Imaging Assessment

Conventional x-rays of the spine and long bones show decreased bone density but only after a 25% to 40% bone loss has occurred. Fractures can also be seen on x-ray.

The most commonly used screening and diagnostic tool for measuring bone mineral density (BMD) is **dual x-ray absorptiometry (DXA).** The spine and hip are most often assessed. Many physicians recommend that women in their 40s have a baseline DXA scan so that later bone changes can be detected and compared. DXA is a painless scan that emits less radiation than a chest x-ray. *It is the best tool currently available for a definite diagnosis of osteoporosis.* The patient stays dressed but is asked to remove any metallic objects such as belt buckles, coins, keys, or jewelry that might interfere with the test. The results are displayed on a computer graph, and a T-score is calculated. No special follow-up care for the test is required. However, the patient needs to discuss the results with the physician for any decisions about possible preventive or management interventions.

Quantitative computed tomography (QCT) can also measure bone density. This procedure analyzes trabecular and cortical bone separately and is especially sensitive to changes in the vertebral column. The test is more expensive than the DXA scan and exposes the patient to more radiation (Raisz, 2005).

Quantitative ultrasound (QUS) of the heel is an effective and low-cost screening tool that can detect osteoporosis and predict risk for hip fracture. The test requires no special preparation, is quick, and has no radiation exposure or specific follow-up care (Pagana & Pagana, 2006).

Common Nursing Diagnoses and Collaborative Problems

The most common nursing diagnoses and collaborative problems that apply to patients with diagnosed osteoporosis include:

- Risk for Falls related to being female 65 years of age or older and environmental hazards
- Impaired Physical Mobility related to decreased muscle strength, pain, and musculoskeletal impairment
- Acute Pain and/or Chronic Pain related to effects of acute physical illness (fracture) or chronic disability
- Potential for Fractures related to weak, porous bone

Interventions

Because the patient is predisposed to fractures, nutritional therapy, exercise, lifestyle changes, and drug therapy are used to slow bone resorption and form new bony tissue. Patient education can help prevent osteoporosis or slow the progress. These measures help reduce the chance of fractures and their complications. The role of drug therapy has increased over the past decade and helps prevent fractures related to osteoporosis. Drug therapy should begin when the BMD T-score for the hip is below −2.0 with no other risk factors or when the T-score is below −1.5 with one or more risk factors or previous fracture.

Nutrition Therapy

The nutritional considerations for the treatment of a patient with a diagnosis of osteoporosis are the same as those for preventing the disease. Adequate amounts of protein, magnesium, vitamin K, and trace minerals are needed for bone formation. Calcium and vitamin D intake should be increased. Teach patients to avoid excessive alcohol and caffeine consumption. For the patient who has sustained a fracture, adequate intake of protein, vitamin C, and iron is important to promote bone healing. People who are lactose intolerant can choose a variety of soy and rice products that are fortified with calcium and vitamin D. In addition, calcium and vitamin D are added to many fruit juices, bread, and cereal products.

A variety of nutrients are needed to maintain bone health. *The promotion of a single nutrient will not prevent or treat osteoporosis.* A nutritional plan that emphasizes fruits and vegetables, low-fat dairy and protein sources, increased fiber, and moderation in alcohol and caffeine intake is most beneficial to maintaining bone health (Whiting & Vatanparast, 2005). Coordinate health teaching and nutrition planning with the nutritionist.

Exercise

Exercise is important in the prevention and management of osteoporosis. It also plays a vital role in pain management, cardiovascular function, and an improved sense of well-being.

In collaboration with the health care provider, the physical therapist may prescribe exercises for strengthening the abdominal and back muscles for those at risk for vertebral fractures. These exercises improve posture and support for the spine. Abdominal muscle tightening, deep breathing, and pectoral stretching are stressed to increase lung capacity. Exercises for the extremity muscles include muscle tightening, resistive, and range-of-motion (ROM) exercises. Encourage active ROM exercises, which improve joint mobility and increase muscle tone, as well as prescribed exercise activities. Swimming provides overall muscle exercise.

In addition to exercises for muscle strengthening, a general weight-bearing exercise program should be implemented. *Walking for 30 minutes three to five times a week is the single most effective exercise for osteoporosis prevention.* Teach the patient that certain high-impact recreational activities, such as running, bowling, and horseback riding, may cause vertebral compression fractures and should be avoided.

Other Lifestyle Changes

In addition to nutrition and exercise, other lifestyle changes should be made. Teach the patient to avoid tobacco in any form, especially cigarette smoking. The patient must be careful to prevent falls and other activities that can cause a fracture. Teach the patient about the importance of having a hazard-free environment, including avoiding scatter rugs, cluttered rooms, and wet floor areas.

Hospitals and long-term care facilities have risk management programs to assess for the risk for falls. For those patients at high risk, communicate this information to other members of the health care team, using colored armbands, tags placed above the head of the bed, or notations made on grease boards in patient rooms. Chapter 3 discusses fall prevention in health care agencies and at home in more detail.

Drug Therapy

The health care provider may prescribe calcium and vitamin D supplements, estrogen or hormone therapy, bisphosphonates, selective estrogen receptor modulators (SERMs), calcitonin, or a combination of several drugs to treat, as well as prevent, osteoporosis (Chart 53-2). Estrogen and combination hormone therapy are the least expensive of the drugs used for osteoporosis, but they increase health risks for women.

Estrogen and Hormone Therapy. Estrogen replacement therapy (ERT) and hormone replacement therapy (estrogen and progesterone) (HRT) have previously been used as primary *prevention* strategies for reducing bone loss in the postmenopausal woman. However, recent studies by the Women's Health Initiative (WHI) demonstrated that long-term effects of ERT/HRT may increase a woman's risk for cardiovascular disease, breast cancer, and venous thromboembolism (VTE). Although treatment using ERT/HRT can reduce the risk for vertebral and hip fractures, the use of estrogen or hormone therapy should be used in a low dose for a short duration of treatment. *Hormones should not be used only for prevention of osteoporosis.* Other approved drugs for treatment or prevention should be considered, and benefits of drug therapy must outweigh the risks to the patient (Woman's Health Initiative, 2005).

Parathyroid Hormone. Parathyroid hormone agent, teriparatide (rDNA origin), under the brand name *Forteo,* is a bone-building agent approved for *treatment* of osteoporosis in postmenopausal women with high risk for fracture. Teach patients to self-administer Forteo as a daily subcutaneous injection. This drug stimulates new bone formation, thus in-

Chart 53-2 COMMON EXAMPLES OF DRUG THERAPY

Osteoporosis

Drug and Usual Dosage	Purpose of Drug	Nursing Interventions	Rationales
Calcium (e.g., Os-Cal, Caltrate-600, Citracal) 1-1.5 g in divided doses orally	Increases calcium intake	Give a third of daily dose at bedtime. Push fluids.	Calcium is most readily utilized by the body when the patient is fasting and immobile. Increased fluid intake aids in preventing the formation of calcium-based urinary stones.
		Assess for a history of urinary stones.	Calcium supplements are not given to patients who are susceptible to urinary stone formation.
		Monitor serum calcium level.	Hypercalcemia, or calcium excess, is a side effect of calcium supplementation.
		Monitor urinary calcium level (no more than 4 mg/kg in 24 hr).	The kidneys attempt to excrete excess calcium.
		Observe for signs of hypercalcemia.	Hypercalcemia can result in urinary stones, cardiac dysrhythmias, and an increase or decrease in skeletal muscle tone.
Estrogen or estrogen/progesterone (e.g., Premarin, Prempro) 0.425-1.25 mg orally for 25 days/mo 0.625 mg conjugated estrogens/2.5 mg medroxyprogesterone acetate (Prempro) (dose may be lower) Use ERT/HRT for short-term after menopause.	Prevents bone loss and increases bone density	Assess for history of tumors, hypertension, thromboembolytic disease, or liver or gallbladder disease.	Estrogen therapy is withheld from patients with susceptibility to an exacerbation of one or more of these problems.
		Teach the importance of gynecologic examinations every 6 months.	Endometrial and breast cancer can result from estrogen therapy.
		Teach breast self-examination.	Patients can detect potentially malignant lesions early so that treatment can begin immediately.
		Observe for vaginal bleeding.	Vaginal bleeding is a side effect of estrogen therapy and a sign of possible endometrial cancer.
		Monitor blood pressure.	Hypertension and other cardiovascular complications may result from combined estrogen-progesterone therapy.
		Observe for venous thromboembolism (VTE).	VTE is a complication of combined estrogen-progesterone therapy.
		Monitor serum liver enzyme and cholesterol levels.	An elevation of liver enzyme levels may be indicative of liver involvement resulting from estrogen. An elevated cholesterol level can result in hypertension and thrombus formation.
BISPHOSPHONATES			
Alendronate (Fosamax) or (Fosamax plus D) **For Prevention:** 5 mg orally daily or 35 mg orally weekly **For Treatment:** 10 mg orally daily or 70 mg orally weekly **Med Error Alert!** Do not confuse Fosamax with Flomax, a selective alpha-adrenergic blocker used for benign prostatic hyperplasia (BPH).	Prevents bone loss and increases bone density	Take on an empty stomach, first thing in the morning with a full glass of water. Take 30 minutes before food, drink, or other drugs. Remain upright, sitting or standing, for 30 minutes after administration.	Difficulty swallowing, esophagitis, esophageal ulcers, and gastric ulcers can result from alendronate therapy. There have been a few reports of osteonecrosis of the jaw and visual disturbances. Any of these should be reported to a health care provider as soon as possible.
Risedronate (Actonel) or (Actonel with Calcium) 5 mg orally daily or 35 mg orally every week preferred)	Same as for alendronate	Follow interventions for alendronate.	Same as for alendronate.
		Observe for CNS side/adverse effects, such as drowsiness, anxiety, agitation.	Drug can cause CNS effects that may not be tolerated.

Chart 53-2 COMMON EXAMPLES OF DRUG THERAPY
Osteoporosis—cont'd

Drug and Usual Dosage	Purpose of Drug	Nursing Interventions	Rationales
BISPHOSPHONATES—cont'd			
Ibandronate sodium (Boniva) 150 mg orally once every month or 3.375 mg IV every 3 months	Same as for alendronate	Take on the same day each month. Take on an empty stomach, first thing in the morning with a full glass of water. Take 60 minutes before food, drink, or other drugs. Remain upright for 1 hour after administration.	Same as for alendronate.
SELECTIVE ESTROGEN RECEPTOR MODULATORS (SERMs)			
Raloxifene (Evista) 60 mg orally daily	Prevents bone loss and increases bone density	Teach patient signs and symptoms of VTE.	Raloxifene can cause increased risk for VTE, especially in the first 4 months of therapy.
Med Error Alert! Do not confuse Evista with Avinza, an extended-release morphine capsule!		Monitor liver function tests (LFTs) in collaboration with health care provider.	Raloxifene can cause increased LFTs or worsen hepatic disease (should not be given to patient who has liver disease).
OTHER AGENTS			
Calcitonin (e.g., Calcimar [salmon], Cibacalcin [human], Miacalcin [salmon; nasal spray]) 100 international units subcutaneously every day or 200 international units intranasally every day	Prevents bone loss and increases bone density	Rotate injection sites for parenteral administration.	Injection sites become irritated and reddened.
		Alternate nares when using intranasal spray.	Can cause rhinitis or epistaxis.
		Monitor for flushing, headache, nausea, and vomiting.	These are common side effects of calcitonin.
		Monitor renal function and calcium and vitamin D levels.	Toxicity from calcitonin can cause renal problems.

CNS, Central nervous system; *ERT,* estrogen replacement therapy; *HRT,* hormone replacement therapy.

creasing BMD. Reduced risk for fracture in the spine, hip, and wrist has been reported in women, and reduced risk for hip fracture has been reported in men. Patients may experience dizziness or leg cramping as side effects of Forteo (National Osteoporosis Foundation, 2007d). Teach the patient to lie down if these problems occur and notify the health care provider as soon as possible.

Calcium and Vitamin D. Intake of *calcium* alone is not a treatment for osteoporosis, but calcium is an important part of a *prevention* program to promote bone health. Most people cannot or do not have enough calcium in their diet, and therefore calcium supplements are needed. Calcium carbonate, found in over-the-counter (OTC) drugs such as Os-Cal, is one of the most cost-effective supplement formulas. Calcium citrate, available OTC as Citracal, is often recommended for those who have gastric upset when taking a calcium supplement. Teach patients to take calcium supplements with food and 6 to 8 ounces of water, although Citracal can be taken anytime. It is best to divide the daily dose, with at least one third of the daily dose being taken in the evening. Teach women to start taking supplements in young adulthood to assist in maintaining peak bone mass. Some drugs contain both calcium and vitamin D, such as Os-Cal Ultra.

Remind patients to take these supplements under the supervision of a health care provider. **Hypercalcemia** (excess serum calcium) can cause serious damage to the urinary system and other body systems. The amount of calcium prescribed is affected by the addition of HRT and the presence of risk factors for osteoporosis. Chapter 13 describes the clinical manifestations of hypercalcemia.

Vitamin D supplementation may also be necessary for institutionalized or homebound patients or for those who do not meet daily requirements. An adequate level of vitamin D is needed for optimal calcium absorption in the intestines. The prescribed dosage is usually 400 to 800 international units/day, depending on the patient's needs. Higher doses can produce toxic effects, such as hypercalcemia and hyperphosphatemia.

Bisphosphonates. Bisphosphonates (BPs) slow bone resorption by binding with crystal elements in bone, especially spongy, trabecular bone tissue. They are the most common drugs used for osteoporosis, but some are also approved for Paget's disease and hypercalcemia related to cancer. Three BPs—alendronate (Fosamax), ibandronate (Boniva), and risedronate (Actonel)—are commonly used for the *prevention and treatment* of osteoporosis in postmenopausal women and hypercalcemia associated with cancer. All three drugs are available as oral preparations, with ibandronate (Boniva) also available as an IV preparation. They are also approved for use in the prevention and treatment of osteoporosis in men.

Oral BPs are commonly associated with a serious problem called **esophagitis** (inflammation of the esophagus). Esophageal ulcers have also been reported with the use of BPs, especially when the tablet is not completely swallowed. Teach patients to take the drug early in the morning with 8 ounces of water and wait 30 minutes in an upright position before eating. If chest discomfort occurs, a symptom of esophageal irritation, instruct patients to discontinue the drug and contact their health care provider. Patients with poor renal function, hypocalcemia, or gastroesophageal reflux disease (GERD) should not take BPs.

The most recent additions to the bisphosphonates are IV pamidronate (Aredia) and IV zoledronic acid (Reclast). These drugs are used when oral BPs are not effective. Aredia is given every 3 to 6 months, and Reclast is needed only once a year. Both drugs have been linked to a complication called jaw **osteonecrosis** (jaw bone death), especially in cancer patients. At this time, the incidence of this serious problem is low but can be a complication of this therapy. More research is needed to determine the relationship of BPs to jaw osteonecrosis. *Teach the patient to have an oral assessment and preventive dentistry before beginning bisphosphonate therapy.* Instruct the patient to inform any dentist who is planning invasive treatment, such as a tooth extraction or implant, that he or she is taking a BP.

Selective Estrogen Receptor Modulators. The selective estrogen receptor modulators (SERMs) are a class of drugs designed to mimic estrogen in some parts of the body while blocking its effect elsewhere. Raloxifene (Evista) is currently the only approved drug in this class and is used for *prevention and treatment* of osteoporosis in postmenopausal women. Raloxifene increases BMD, reduces bone resorption, and reduces the incidence of osteoporotic vertebral fractures. The drug should not be given to women who have a history of thromboembolism.

Other Agents. *Calcitonin* is a thyroid hormone that inhibits osteoclastic activity, thus decreasing bone loss. It is used for the *treatment* of osteoporosis, Paget's disease, and hypercalcemia associated with cancer. The drug also has an analgesic effect after vertebral fracture, thereby promoting early recovery.

Calcitonin (derived from salmon) can be given subcutaneously or intranasally (Miacalcin). The nasal route is preferred because it improves drug adherence, decreases side effects, and is convenient. However, the effect of salmon calcitonin may decrease after use for 2 or more years. Patients may require a holiday from this treatment to maintain effectiveness. Teach the patient to alternate nares to prevent mucosal irritation, a common side effect. The drug must be refrigerated.

Androgens, such as testosterone propionate (Testex, Malogen🍁), have been successful in decreasing bone resorption and increasing bone growth. These drugs may decrease bone resorption in men, particularly in older men. When given to postmenopausal women, however, androgens cause masculine traits and may lead to liver disease.

Surgical Intervention

Vertebroplasty and **kyphoplasty** are minimally invasive procedures used to treat vertebral body compression and fracture found in persons with osteoporosis. **Vertebroplasty** is the injection of bone cement into the vertebral body to reduce a fracture or fill the space created by osteoporosis. **Kyphoplasty** includes the use of a balloon in the vertebral body to contain the bone cement. These procedures greatly reduce pain and increase function in patients with back pain related to osteoporosis. Further discussion of vertebroplasty and kyphoplasty can be found in Chapter 54.

DECISION-MAKING CHALLENGE
Coordination of Care

A 58-year-old patient was told by her gynecologist to have a screening DXA scan. The results show osteopenia in both her hip and spine, even though she is taking a calcium supplement (600 mg) every day. She returns to the office to discuss with you what she can do to prevent osteoporosis.

1. What other assessment data do you need to provide health teaching for this patient?
2. The patient asks you why the calcium supplement did not prevent her from having bone loss. What is your best response?
3. What health teaching do you plan for her?
4. With what members of the health care team might you need to coordinate her care to prevent further bone loss and promote general good health?

evolve For suggested answer guidelines, go to http://evolve.elsevier.com/Iggy/.

Community-Based Care

Patients with osteoporosis are usually managed at home. However, some have fractures that may require hospitalization or medical management in an emergency department (ED) or urgent care setting. In any setting, assess for risk factors of osteoporosis and provide health teaching as appropriate.

The patient with osteoporosis who has one or more fractures may be discharged to the home setting. In some instances, though, the patient is transferred to a long-term care facility for rehabilitation or permanent residence when support systems are not available. Collaborate with case managers or discharge planners to assist in preparing patients and their families for placement in long-term care facilities. Chapter 54 discusses continuing care for patients who have fractures.

The National Osteoporosis Foundation (www.nof.org) in the United States provides information to patients and health care professionals regarding the disease and its treatment. The Osteoporosis Society of Canada (www.osteoporosis.ca) has similar services. Large hospitals often have osteoporosis specialty clinics and support groups for patients with osteoporosis.

OSTEOMALACIA

Pathophysiology

Osteomalacia is loss of bone related to a vitamin D deficiency. It causes softening of the bone caused by inadequate deposits of calcium and phosphorus in the bone matrix. Normal remodeling of the bone is disrupted, and calcification does not occur. Osteomalacia is the adult equivalent of **rickets,** or vitamin D deficiency, in children.

Vitamin D deficiency is the most important factor in development of osteomalacia. In its natural form, vitamin D is activated by the ultraviolet radiation of the sun and obtained from certain foods as a nutritional supplement. In combination with calcium and phosphorus, the vitamin is necessary for bone formation.

Osteomalacia is frequently confused with osteoporosis because of similar characteristics shared by the two disease processes. Table 53-2 shows a comparison and contrast of osteoporosis and osteomalacia.

In addition to primary disease related to lack of sunlight exposure or dietary intake, vitamin D deficiency caused by various health problems may result in osteomalacia (Table 53-3). Malabsorption of vitamin D from the small bowel is a common complication of partial or total gastrectomy and bypass or resection surgery of the small intestine. Disease of the small bowel, such as Crohn's disease, may cause decreased vitamin and mineral absorption.

Liver and pancreatic disorders disrupt vitamin D metabolism and decrease its production. Chronic kidney disease (CKD) interferes with the synthesis of calcitriol, the most active vitamin metabolite. Osteomalacia can also be caused by bone tumors (**oncogenic** or **tumor-induced osteomalacia**).

Conditions that contribute to phosphate depletion (hypophosphatemia) lead to osteomalacia because they stimulate movement from bone and prevent calcium uptake in the bone. Osteomalacia is also an adverse effect of certain drugs, particularly anticonvulsants, barbiturates, and fluoride. The exact mechanism for the drug effects is not known. Genetic deviations in vitamin D or phosphate metabolism may contribute to bone changes seen in osteomalacia.

Osteomalacia is not common in the United States and Western Europe. However, it is more common in less affluent nations and in countries where famine is common. Newcomers from these countries may seek health care in the United States. Older adults are most at risk. This group may have inadequate exposure to sunlight or intake of vitamin D–fortified foods. People who adhere to very restrictive vegan diets without adequate supplement of vitamin D can also be at risk. Assess for the risk for osteomalacia in anyone who has poor nutritional intake related to homelessness, who severely abuses drugs or alcohol, or who is very poor.

TABLE 53-2 Differential Features of Osteoporosis and Osteomalacia

Characteristic	Osteoporosis	Osteomalacia
Definition	Decreased bone mass	Demineralized bone
Pathophysiology	Lack of calcium	Lack of vitamin D
Radiographic findings	Osteopenia, fractures	Pseudofractures, Looser's zones, fractures
Calcium level	Low or normal	Low or normal
Phosphate level	Normal	Low or normal
Parathyroid hormone	Normal	High or normal
Alkaline phosphatase	Normal	High

TABLE 53-3 Causes of Osteomalacia

VITAMIN D DISTURBANCE
- Inadequate production
- Lack of sunlight exposure
- Dietary deficiency
- Abnormal metabolism
- Drug therapy
  - Phenytoin (Dilantin)
  - Fluoride
  - Barbiturates
- Liver disease
- Renal disease
- Inadequate absorption
  - Postgastrectomy
  - Malabsorption syndrome
- Inflammatory bowel disease

KIDNEY DISEASE
- Chronic kidney disease
- Acute tubular disorders
  - Acidosis
  - Hypophosphatemia

FAMILIAL METABOLIC ERROR
- Hypophosphatemia

Health Promotion and Maintenance

To prevent or help treat osteomalacia, teach patients to increase vitamin D through dietary intake, sun exposure, and drug supplements. Instruct the at-risk patient about foods high in vitamin D, such as milk and food that has had it added. Remind patients that cheese and yogurt rarely contain vitamin D although they are rich in calcium. Instruct them to read food labels for nutrient content. Remind patients, especially those who are homebound, about the importance of daily sun exposure (at least 5 minutes each day) for the manufacture of the vitamin.

Some people are lactose intolerant or do not use dairy products related to vegan diets. However, many products are available for people who avoid dairy products. Soy and rice milk, tofu, and soy products are substitutes, but they are expensive. Teach patients to choose those products that are fortified with vitamin D. Other foods rich in the vitamin are eggs, swordfish, chicken, and liver, as well as enriched cereals and bread products. The at-risk patient should also take vitamin D supplements as prescribed by his or her health care provider.

Patient-Centered Collaborative Care

Assessment

Collect important data for the patient with osteomalacia or suspected osteomalacia, including age, ability to be exposed to sunlight, and skin pigmentation. The older adult who has been homebound or chronically institutionalized is at the greatest risk. People who have dark skin and who may consume minimal protein are more at risk than light-skinned people with the same dietary habits. Dark-skinned people tend to avoid the sun and need protein for calcium binding. Take a thorough nutritional history to determine the intake of foods containing vitamin D and calcium. Coordinate the assessment with the nutritionist.

Assessment includes any history of chronic disease processes of the GI tract including inflammatory bowel disease, gastric or intestinal bypass surgery, or any problem that interferes with absorption from the GI tract. A history of renal or liver dysfunction may lead to ineffective metabolism of vitamin D. Drugs such as phenytoin (Dilantin) or fluoride preparations may also interfere with metabolism of vitamin D.

Osteomalacia is easily confused with osteoporosis, and both disorders may occur at the same time (see Table 53-2). In the early stages of osteomalacia, the manifestations are nonspecific. Muscle weakness and bone pain may be misdiagnosed as arthritis or other connective tissue disorder. In some cases, proximal muscle weakness in the shoulder and pelvic girdle area is the only presenting symptom.

Muscle weakness in the lower extremities may cause a waddling and unsteady gait, which contributes to falls and subsequent fractures. Hypophosphatemia leads to an inadequate production of muscle cell adenosine triphosphate, thus resulting in a decrease in muscle cell energy. If hypocalcemia is present, muscle cramping may occur with weakness.

In collaboration with the physical therapist, assess muscle strength and observe the patient's gait. Document concerns about muscle cramps and bone pain. Skeletal discomfort is often vague and generalized. The spine, ribs, pelvis, and lower extremities are most often affected. The patient usually describes the pain as aggravated by activity and worse at night.

Palpate the affected bones for tenderness. Bone tenderness may occur when pressure is applied to the tibia or rib cage. Skeletal malalignment, like long-bone bowing or spinal deformity, may be similar to that seen in osteoporosis. In extreme cases, the pelvis narrows, so vaginal childbirth is difficult. If osteomalacia is untreated, vertebral, rib, and long-bone fractures may occur. The patient may be misdiagnosed as having bone cancer or osteoporosis.

X-rays of bone in patients with osteomalacia reveal a decrease in the cancellous bone and lack of osteoid sharpness. The classic diagnostic finding specific to the disease, however, is the presence of radiolucent bands (Looser's lines or zones). Looser's zones represent stress fractures that have not mineralized. They often appear symmetrically in the medial area of the femoral neck, ribs, and pelvis and may progress to complete fractures with minimal trauma. Bone biopsy of these areas may be needed for complete diagnosis. DXA scan may assist in diagnosis of osteomalacia.

▪ *Interventions*

The major treatment for osteomalacia is vitamin D. The minimum recommended daily allowance (RDA) of vitamin D is 400 international units. Because older adults are at risk for bone demineralization from aging, as well as for osteomalacia, they may need as much as 800 international units daily. Health teaching for patients with osteomalacia is discussed on p. 1161 in the Health Promotion and Maintenance section.

PAGET'S DISEASE OF THE BONE

Pathophysiology

Paget's disease, or **osteitis deformans,** is a chronic metabolic disorder in which bone is excessively broken down (osteoclastic activity) and re-formed (osteoblastic activity). The result is bone that is structurally disorganized, causing bones to be weak with increased risk for bowing of long bones and fractures. Two types of Paget's disease can occur—familial and sporadic.

Three pathophysiologic phases of the disorder have been described: active, mixed, and inactive. In the first phase (the active phase), a rapid increase in osteoclasts (cells that break down bone) causes massive bone destruction and deformity. The osteoclasts of pagetic bone are large and multinuclear, unlike the osteoclasts of normal bone tissue.

In the mixed phase, the osteoblasts (bone-forming cells) react to compensate in forming new bone. The result is bone that is vascular, structurally weak, and deformed. Paget's disease occurs in one bone or in multiple sites. The most common areas of involvement are the vertebrae, femur, skull, clavicle, humerus, and pelvis.

GENETIC CONSIDERATIONS

When the osteoblastic activity exceeds the osteoclastic activity, the inactive phase occurs. The newly formed bone becomes sclerotic and very hard.

It is believed that Paget's disease is caused by a viral respiratory infection that may have been present for many years. Because the disorder is present in identical twins, an autosomal dominant pattern has been suggested. The disease has been noted in up to 30% of people with a positive family history for Paget's disease. Several genetic and immunologic changes have been identified in families with the disease, including mutations in the:

- RANKL/RANK/OPG system, which is needed for osteoclast development and activity (see p. 1154 in the Osteoporosis section)
- Valosin-containing gene of complement binding protein (VCP), an important inflammatory factor
- Sequestosome 1, which helps activate the nuclear factor–kappa B protein complex that is involved in cellular responses to stimuli, such as viruses and bacteria (Daroszewska & Ralston, 2005)

Teach patients the importance of genetics in familial Paget's disease, and refer them to the appropriate genetic counseling resource. Ask the patient if genetic testing is desired.

Paget's disease is second only to osteoporosis as one of the most common bone diseases in the United States, but its occurrence is rapidly declining around the world. The disease is seen more frequently in people age 50 years and older. The risk for developing Paget's disease increases as a person ages, particularly in those 80 years old and older.

Patient-Centered Collaborative Care

▪ *Assessment*

Physical Assessment/Clinical Manifestations

Of all patients with Paget's disease, 80% are asymptomatic, and the disease may be confined to one bone. It may be accidentally discovered during a routine laboratory or x-ray examination. In more severe disease, the manifestations are diverse and potentially fatal (Chart 53-3).

Ask the patient about a history of fracture and current bone pain. Bone pain, usually described as mild to moderate, may cause the patient to seek medical attention. The most

Chart 53-3 KEY FEATURES
Paget's Disease of the Bone

MUSCULOSKELETAL MANIFESTATIONS
- Bone and joint pain (may be in a single bone) that is aching, poorly described, and aggravated by walking
- Low back and sciatic nerve pain
- Bowing of long bones
- Loss of normal spinal curvature
- Enlarged, thick skull
- Pathologic fractures
- Osteogenic sarcoma (bone cancer)

SKIN MANIFESTATIONS
- Flushed, warm skin

OTHER MANIFESTATIONS
- Apathy, lethargy, fatigue
- Hyperparathyroidism
- Gout
- Urinary or renal stones
- Heart failure from fluid overload

common sites for pain are the hip and pelvis. The pain is aching, poorly described, deep, and worsened by pressure and weight bearing. It is most noticeable at night or when the patient is resting. Patients may report redness and warmth at affected sites. These manifestations may be related to increased vascularity and blood flow.

The pain associated with the disorder may result from metabolic bone activity, secondary arthritis, impending fracture, or nerve impingement. Arthritis often occurs at the joints (cartilage) of the affected bones, resulting from bowing in the long bones of the leg. Nerve impingement is particularly common in the lumbosacral area of the vertebral column, presenting as back pain that radiates along one or both legs.

Observe posture, stance, and gait to identify gross bony deformities. Because of the enlargement of the vertebrae, loss of normal spinal curvature, and lower extremity malalignment, the patient may have decreased height. Assess for kyphosis or scoliosis of the spinal column. Note any long-bone bowing in the legs with subsequent varus (bow-leg) deformity. Long bones of the arms may also develop bowing. Flexion contracture in the hip joint is often present. Any of these deformities may be asymmetric. This weakened bone is at risk for fracture from even a minor injury. All of these problems interfere with the patient's *human need for mobility.*

When performing a musculoskeletal assessment in a patient with Paget's disease, pay particular attention to the size and shape of the skull, which is typically soft, thick, and enlarged. Pressure from an enlarged temporal bone may lead to deafness and vertigo (dizziness). Basilar (in the occipital area) complications can compress any of the cranial nerves and result in neurologic problems. Assess the patient for changes in vision, swallowing, and speech. Platybasia, or basilar invagination, causes brainstem (vital sign center) damage that threatens life. In some cases, the bony enlargement of the skull blocks cerebrospinal fluid (CSF), resulting in hydrocephalus.

Pathologic fractures may be the presenting clinical manifestation of the disorder. The femur and the tibia are most often affected, and fracture of these bones can result from minimal trauma. The fracture line is usually perpendicular to the long axis of the bone, and healing is unpredictable because of abnormal metabolic activity within the bone.

Although rare, bones affected by Paget's disease may develop malignant changes. The most dreaded complication of Paget's disease is cancer, most commonly osteogenic sarcoma. Increased incidence of sarcoma occurs in men in the 70- to 80-year-old group. They appear primarily in the femur, the humerus, and old fracture sites and carry a grave prognosis because of early metastasis to the lung or extensive local invasion. When severe bone pain is present in a patient with Paget's disease, bone cancer is suspected.

Assess the skin for its color and temperature. In people with Paget's disease, the skin is typically flushed and warm because of increased blood flow. In addition, assess the patient's energy level because apathy, lethargy, and fatigue are common.

Other less common manifestations of Paget's disease include hyperparathyroidism and gout. Secondary hyperparathyroidism leads to an increase in serum and urinary calcium levels. In severe cases, serum calcium excess results from prolonged immobilization. Calcium deposits occur in joint spaces or as stones in the urinary tract. **Hyperuricemia** (serum uric acid excess) and gout occur because the increased metabolic activity of bone creates an increase in nucleic acid catabolism. Therefore kidney stones are more common in people with Paget's disease.

In a few cases, increased blood flow causes the heart to work harder to increase cardiac output, resulting in heart failure if not treated. Cardiac complications tend to occur only when more than a third of the skeleton is involved.

Other Diagnostic Assessment

Increases in *serum alkaline phosphatase (ALP)* and urinary hydroxyproline levels are the primary laboratory findings indicating possible Paget's disease. Overactive osteoblasts cause an altered ALP level. ALP can be further evaluated by alkaline phosphatase isoenzymes. The isoenzyme testing can further break ALP into three fractions—liver, bone, and intestinal. Elevated bone isoenzymes can help in a more definitive diagnosis of Paget's disease. Serum isoenzyme levels of bone ALP are used to monitor effectiveness of treatment (Pagana & Pagana, 2006).

The 24-hour *urinary hydroxyproline* level reflects bone collagen turnover and indicates the degree of disease severity. The higher the hydroxyproline, the more severe is the disease.

The *calcium* levels in blood and urine may be low, normal, or elevated. The immobilized patient is more likely to have an increase in calcium levels as a result of calcium moving from bone into the blood.

Paget's disease often causes an elevated *uric acid* because nucleic acid from overactive bone metabolism increases. This finding may be misinterpreted as primary gout.

X-rays are also used to diagnose Paget's disease. They reveal characteristic changes including the presence of osteolytic lesions and enlarged bones with radiolucent, or punched-out, appearance. Decrease in joint space may be seen with arthritic changes in joints. Malalignment deformities, fractures, and secondary arthritic changes may be present.

Radionuclide bone scan may be most sensitive in detecting Paget's disease. A radiolabeled bisphosphonate is injected IV and shows pagetic bone in areas of high bone turnover activity. This test can determine the extent of Paget's disease in the skeleton. Computed tomography (CT) is useful in the detection of cancerous tumors, changes in the skull, and spinal cord or nerve compression. Magnetic resonance imaging (MRI) may also be used for the same purpose as the CT scan.

Interventions

Nonsurgical or surgical management may be necessary to reduce pain and promote *mobility.* Nonsurgical interventions are used first.

Nonsurgical Management

The primary intervention for Paget's disease is drug therapy. Potent prescription drugs are used to treat Paget's disease. In addition, simple analgesics such as OTC NSAIDs can be used to control pain.

The purpose of *drug therapy* in Paget's disease is to relieve pain and to decrease bone resorption. Management of mild to moderate pain may include the use of aspirin or NSAIDs, such as ibuprofen (Motrin, Apo-Ibuprofen♣). When the calcium level is more than twice the normal value and the disease is widespread, the health care provider usually prescribes more potent drugs, such as selected bisphosphonates. Treatment with these agents for Paget's disease requires dosages and duration of therapy different from those for osteoporosis. Chart 53-2 includes information about some of these commonly used drugs.

Oral bisphosphonates are a first-line treatment choice for Paget's disease. Currently, six bisphosphonates are approved for use in the United States for treatment of Paget's disease. Alendronate (Fosamax) and risedronate (Actonel) are most commonly used. Etidronate (Didronel) and tiludronate (Skelid) are prescribed less often. These four drugs are oral preparations and require the same nursing considerations during administration as described in osteoporosis use. Two newer drugs have been approved for the treatment of Paget's disease when the oral agents are not effective. Pamidronate (Aredia) and zoledronic acid (Reclast) are administered IV. Aredia is given once every 3 months, and Reclast is given once a year as a single IV dose. These drugs are highly effective. To reduce the risk for hypocalcemia, patients should receive 1500 mg of calcium daily in divided doses and 800 international units of vitamin D daily for at least 2 weeks after zoledronic acid infusion. Chart 53-2 provides additional information about caring for patients receiving bisphosphonates.

Calcitonin is a hormone that seems to reduce bone resorption and, subsequently, relieve pain. The drug often causes a dramatic decrease in the alkaline phosphatase level in a few weeks. Calcitonin is approved for subcutaneous administration in treating Paget's disease because the nasal spray has shown to be ineffective. It binds to osteoclast receptors, therefore slowing bone breakdown. The drug may be used for those patients who do not tolerate bisphosphonates. Side effects of calcitonin include nausea, flushing, and skin rash. Skin testing may be done before administration of the first dose.

In rare instances, patients may not respond to treatment with bisphosphonates or calcitonin and require more aggressive treatment, especially if neurologic symptoms or severe hypercalcemia occur. Plicamycin (Mithracin) is a potent chemotherapeutic agent with many side effects. It is reserved for patients with severe disease and neurologic compromise or marked hypercalcemia. Plicamycin is thought to block the effects of parathyroid hormone on osteoclasts. Observe for signs of toxicity to the liver, GI tract, and kidneys. Monitor liver and kidney function studies and intake and output daily. Electrolyte imbalance can occur. Because plicamycin also suppresses platelets, daily platelet counts and bleeding precautions are taken. When liver enzyme levels become extremely high, drug therapy is interrupted temporarily.

In addition to administering drugs, implement physical measures to reduce pain and increase *mobility.* These measures may include application of heat and gentle massage. An exercise program may be started with the help of a physical therapist. Exercise may be difficult because of pain and danger of fracture. Non-impact exercise should be used, but the patient may benefit from strengthening and weight-bearing exercises. In collaboration with the physical therapist, teach the patient about ROM and gentle stretching. Additional interventions for pain relief, such as relaxation techniques, are discussed in Chapter 5.

Measures to promote bone health are also important and include a diet rich in calcium and vitamin D. Nutrition therapy for bone health is described on p. 1157 in the discussion of interventions in the Osteoporosis section.

Provide the patient with information to contact the U.S. local chapter of the Paget Disease Foundation (www.paget.org) and the Arthritis Foundation (www.arthritis.org). The Arthritis Society in Canada (www.arthritis.ca) is also an excellent service. These resources provide information and support for the patient and family or significant others. Nutritional instruction should be similar to information given to the patient with osteoporosis.

Surgical Management

When a patient with Paget's disease has secondary arthritis and pain relief is not achieved, he or she may undergo a tibial osteotomy or partial or total joint replacement (see Chapter 20). Surgical decompression and stabilization of the spine may be used to retain function, decrease pain, and reduce potential cardiac and respiratory complications.

NCLEX EXAMINATION CHALLENGE

A client is placed on risedronate (Actonel) 35 mg for management of Paget's disease of the bone. Which statement by the client indicates a need for further health teaching?

A. "I have to take this pill faithfully every week."
B. "I am taking this pill to prevent more bone loss."
C. "I need to see my dentist before I start this drug."
D. "I am going to take this pill with food in the morning."

evolve For the correct answer, go to http://evolve.elsevier.com/Iggy/.

OSTEOMYELITIS

Infection in bony tissue can be a severe and difficult-to-treat problem. Bone infection can result in chronic recurrence of infection, loss of function and mobility, amputation, and even death.

Pathophysiology

Bacteria, viruses, or fungi can cause infection in bone known as **osteomyelitis.** Invasion by one or more pathogenic microorganisms stimulates the inflammatory response in bone tissue. The inflammation produces an increased vascular leak and edema, often involving the surrounding soft tissues. Once inflammation is established, the vessels in the area become thrombosed and release exudate (pus) into bony tissue. Isch-

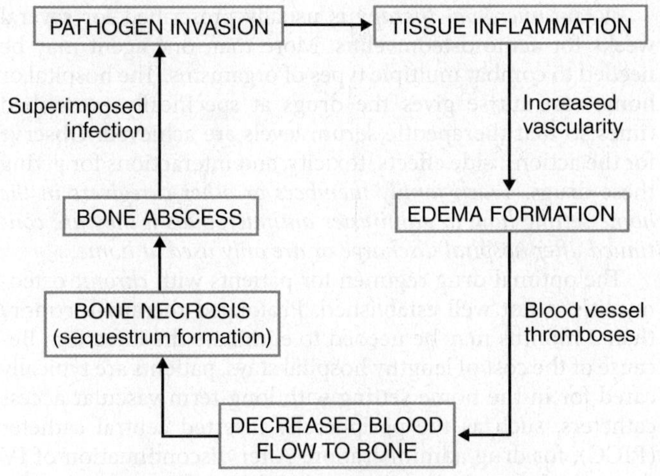
PATHOGEN INVASION
TISSUE INFLAMMATION
Superimposed infection
Increased vascularity
BONE ABSCESS
EDEMA FORMATION
BONE NECROSIS (sequestrum formation)
Blood vessel thromboses
DECREASED BLOOD FLOW TO BONE

Fig. 53-2 • Infection cycle of osteomyelitis.

emia of bone tissue follows and results in necrotic bone. This area of necrotic bone separates from surrounding bone tissue, and **sequestrum** is formed. The presence of sequestrum prevents bone healing and causes superimposed infection, often in the form of bone abscess. As shown in Fig. 53-2, the cycle repeats itself as the new infection leads to further inflammation, vessel thromboses, and necrosis.

Osteomyelitis is categorized as **exogenous,** in which infectious organisms enter from outside the body as in an open fracture, or **endogenous,** in which organisms are carried by the bloodstream from other areas of infection in the body. Endogenous osteomyelitis may also be referred to as **hematogenous** osteomyelitis. A third category is **contiguous,** in which bone infection results from skin infection of adjacent tissues. Osteomyelitis can be further divided into two major types: acute osteomyelitis and chronic osteomyelitis.

Etiology

Each type of bone infection has its own causative factors. Pathogenic microbes favor bone that has a rich blood supply and a marrow cavity. **Acute hematogenous infection** results from bacteremia, underlying disease, or nonpenetrating trauma. Urinary tract infections, particularly in older men, tend to spread to the lower vertebrae. Long-term IV catheters (e.g., Hickman catheters) can be primary sources of infection. Patients undergoing long-term hemodialysis and IV drug abusers are also at risk for osteomyelitis. *Salmonella* infections of the GI tract may spread to bone. Patients with sickle cell disease and other hemoglobinopathies often have multiple episodes of salmonellosis, which can cause bone infection.

Poor dental hygiene and periodontal (gum) infection can be a causative factor in **contiguous** osteomyelitis in facial bones. Minimal nonpenetrating trauma can cause hemorrhages or small-vessel occlusions, leading to bone necrosis. Regardless of the source of infection, many infections are caused by *Staphylococcus aureus.* Treatment of infection may be complicated further by the presence of methicillin-resistant *Staphylococcus aureus* (MRSA) or other drug-resistant microorganism, which is becoming very common in hospitalized and other institutionalized patients. One of the major outcomes in health care settings today is to reduce the number of MRSA infections from any source.

> **CONSIDERATIONS FOR OLDER ADULTS**
>
> Malignant external otitis media involving the base of the skull is sometimes seen in older adults with diabetes. The most common cause of contiguous spread in older adults, however, is found in those who have slow-healing foot ulcers. Multiple organisms tend to be responsible for the resulting osteomyelitis.

In contrast, penetrating trauma leads to acute osteomyelitis by direct inoculation. A soft-tissue infection may be present as well. Animal bites, puncture wounds, and bone surgery can result in bone infection. The most common offending organism is *Pseudomonas aeruginosa,* but other gram-negative bacteria may be found.

If bone infection is misdiagnosed or inadequately treated, **chronic osteomyelitis** may develop. Inadequate care management results when the treatment period is too short or when the treatment is delayed or inappropriate. About half of cases of chronic osteomyelitis are caused by gram-negative bacteria. Although bacteria are the most common causes of osteomyelitis, viruses and fungal organisms also may cause infection.

Incidence/Prevalence

Hematogenous osteomyelitis is the most common type of osteomyelitis. It occurs more often in children but is becoming increasingly common in adults, particularly older adults. Acute infection is more common in children. Chronic infection is more common in adults. Men have osteomyelitis more often than women, related to a higher incidence of blunt or penetrating trauma. Conditions such as malnutrition, alcoholism, diabetes, kidney or liver disease, and immune-suppressing disorders increase the risk and complicate effective treatment. Bone tissues in the vertebrae and long bones are common sites of infection. The adult with a compromised blood supply is at greatest risk for chronic infection. Advanced age and concurrent disease may prolong the course of the infection for as long as a year or more.

Patient-Centered Collaborative Care

Assessment

Bone pain, with or without other manifestations, is a common concern of patients with bone infection. The pain is described as a constant, localized, pulsating sensation that worsens with movement.

The patient with *acute* osteomyelitis has fever, usually with temperature greater than 101° F (38° C). *Older adults may not have an extreme temperature elevation because of lower core body temperature and compromised immune system that occur with normal aging.* The area around the infected bone swells and is tender when palpated. Erythema (redness) and heat may also be present. When vascular compromise is severe, patients may not feel discomfort because of nerve damage from lack of blood supply.

When vascular insufficiency is suspected, assess circulation in the distal extremities. Ulcerations may be present on the feet or hands, indicating inadequate healing ability as a result of poor circulation.

Fever, swelling, and erythema are less common in those with *chronic* osteomyelitis. Ulceration resulting in sinus tract formation, localized pain, and drainage is more characteristic of chronic infection (Chart 53-4).

Chart 53-4 KEY FEATURES

Acute and Chronic Osteomyelitis

ACUTE OSTEOMYELITIS
- Fever; temperature usually above 101° F (38° C)
- Swelling around the affected area
- Erythema of the affected area
- Tenderness of the affected area
- Bone pain that is constant, localized, and pulsating; intensifies with movement

CHRONIC OSTEOMYELITIS
- Ulceration of the skin
- Sinus tract formation
- Localized pain
- Drainage from the affected area

The patient with osteomyelitis usually has an elevated white blood cell (leukocyte) count, which may be double the normal value. In chronic infection, normal values or slight elevations may be seen.

The erythrocyte sedimentation rate (ESR) may be normal early in the course of the disease but rises as the condition progresses. It may remain elevated for as long as 3 months after drug therapy is discontinued.

If bacteremia is present, a potentially life-threatening complication that could lead to septic shock, a blood culture identifies the offending organisms to determine which antibiotics should be used in treatment. Both aerobic and anaerobic blood cultures should be collected before therapy is started.

Although bone changes cannot be detected early with standard x-rays, changes in blood flow can be seen early in the course of the disease by radionuclide scanning. A bone scan, using technetium or gallium, is extremely helpful in the diagnosis of osteomyelitis and identifies most cases. In some cases, MRI may be more sensitive than traditional bone scanning in the diagnosis of osteomyelitis.

Common Nursing Diagnoses and Collaborative Problems

Nursing diagnoses and collaborative problems that may apply to patients with osteomyelitis include:

- Acute Pain or Chronic Pain related to inflammation
- Hyperthermia related to pathogenic invasion of the bone
- Ineffective Tissue Perfusion (Peripheral) related to tissue swelling
- Potential for Sepsis and Septic Shock

Interventions

The specific treatment protocol depends on the type and number of microbes present in the infected tissue. If other measures fail to resolve the infectious process, surgical management may be needed.

Nonsurgical Management

To reverse *acute* osteomyelitis, the health care provider starts antimicrobial (e.g., antibiotic) therapy as soon as possible. In the presence of copious wound drainage, Contact Precautions are used to prevent the spread of the offending organism to other patients and health care personnel. Teach patients, visitors, and staff members how to use these precautions. (See Chapter 25 for a discussion of Contact Precautions.)

IV antimicrobial therapy is usually prescribed for several weeks for acute osteomyelitis. More than one agent may be needed to combat multiple types of organisms. The hospital or home care nurse gives the drugs at specifically prescribed times so that therapeutic serum levels are achieved. Observe for the actions, side effects, toxicity, and interactions for giving these drugs. *Teach family members or other caregivers in the home setting how to administer antimicrobials if they are continued after hospital discharge or are only used at home.*

The optimal drug regimen for patients with *chronic* osteomyelitis is not well established. Prolonged therapy for more than 3 months may be needed to eliminate the infection. Because of the cost of lengthy hospital stays, patients are typically cared for in the home setting with long-term vascular access catheters, such as the peripherally inserted central catheter (PICC), for drug administration. After discontinuation of IV drugs, oral therapy may be needed for weeks or months. Patients and families must understand the complications of inadequate treatment or failure to follow up with health care providers. Teach them that drug therapy must be continued over a long period to be effective. *Even when symptoms of the disease appear to be improved, the full course of IV and oral antimicrobials must be completed.*

In addition to systemic drug therapy, the wound may be irrigated, either continuously or intermittently, with one or more antibiotic solutions. Use sterile technique at all times. A medical technique in which beads made of bone cement are impregnated with an antibiotic and packed into the wound can provide direct contact of the antibiotic with the offending organism.

Drugs are also needed to control pain. Patients experience acute and chronic pain and must receive a regimen of drug therapy for control. Chapter 5 describes pharmacologic and nonpharmacologic interventions for both acute and chronic pain.

If an open wound or ulcer is present in the hospital or long-term care setting, the patient's treatment usually includes Standard Precautions for limited infections in which the wound is not draining but is covered. This practice may vary according to health care agency policy. Contact Precautions are reserved for more severe infections, particularly when the purulent material cannot be adequately contained by a dressing. Cover the open area and use clean technique when dressings are changed to prevent further contamination. The previous clinical practice was to use strict aseptic technique, but most agencies are now using clean technique for contaminated ("dirty") wounds. Wounds may be managed through the window of a cast, which must remain dry during dressing or irrigation procedures. Teach patients and families how to continue clean dressing procedures at home.

A treatment to increase tissue perfusion for patients with chronic, unremitting osteomyelitis is the use of a hyperbaric chamber or portable device to administer hyperbaric oxygen (HBO) therapy. These devices are usually available in large tertiary care centers and may not be accessible to all patients who might benefit from them. With HBO therapy, the affected area is exposed to a high concentration of oxygen that diffuses into the tissues to promote healing. In conjunction with high-dose drug therapy and surgical débridement, HBO has proved very useful in treating a number of anaerobic infections. Other wound management therapies are described in Chapter 27.

Surgical Management

Antimicrobial therapy alone may not meet the desired outcome of treatment. Surgical techniques may be used to minimize the disfigurement that can be a devastating result of severe osteomyelitis. Surgery is reserved for patients with chronic osteomyelitis.

Because bone cannot heal in the presence of necrotic tissue, a *sequestrectomy* may be performed to débride the necrotic bone and allow revascularization of tissue. The excision of dead and infected bone often results in a sizable cavity, or bone defect. The use of bone *grafts* to repair bone defects is also widely used.

When infected bone is extensively resected, reconstruction with *microvascular bone transfers* may be done. This procedure is reserved for larger skeletal defects. The most common donor sites are the patient's fibula and iliac crest. The bone graft may have an attached muscle or skin flap, if necessary. The steps of the procedure are similar to those of bone grafting in that débridement of dead or necrotic bone is done before bone transfer.

Nursing care of the patient after surgery is similar to that for any postoperative patient (see Chapter 18). However, the important difference is that neurovascular (NV) assessments must be done frequently because the patient experiences increased swelling after the surgical procedure. Elevate the affected extremity to increase venous return and thus control swelling. Assess and document the patient's NV status, including:

- Pain
- Movement
- Sensation
- Warmth
- Temperature
- Distal pulses
- Capillary refill (not as reliable as the above indicators)

*Check for signs of neurovascular compromise, including **p**ain that cannot be controlled, **p**aresis or **p**aralysis (weakness or inability to move), **p**aresthesias (abnormal, tingling sensation), **p**allor, and **p**ulselessness. If any of these findings occur, report them immediately to the surgeon.*

If the bony defect is small, a *muscle flap* may be the only surgery required. Local muscle flaps are used in the treatment of chronic osteomyelitis when soft tissue does not fill the dead space, or cavity, resulting from bone débridement. The flap provides wound coverage and enhances blood flow to promote healing. A split-thickness skin graft is often applied several days after the muscle flap.

When the previously described surgical procedures are not appropriate or successful and as a last resort, the affected limb may need to be amputated. The physical and psychological care for a patient who has undergone an amputation is discussed in Chapter 54.

For all of the surgical procedures and their recovery phases, long-term antimicrobial treatment is necessary. The preoperative and postoperative nursing care is similar to that for repair of musculoskeletal trauma and is also discussed in Chapter 54.

BENIGN BONE TUMORS

Pathophysiology

Benign (noncancerous) bone tumors are often asymptomatic and may be discovered on routine x-ray examination or as the cause of pathologic fractures. The cause of benign bone tumors is not known. Tumors may arise from several types of tissue. The major classifications include **chondrogenic** tumors (from cartilage), **osteogenic** tumors (from bone), and **fibrogenic** tumors (from fibrous tissue and found most often in children). Although many specific benign tumors have been identified, only the common ones are described here.

The most common benign bone tumor is the *osteochondroma*. Although its onset is usually in childhood, the tumor grows until skeletal maturity and may not be diagnosed until adulthood. The tumor may be a single growth or multiple growths and can occur in any bone. The femur and the tibia are most often involved.

The *chondroma,* or endochondroma, is a lesion of mature hyaline cartilage affecting primarily the hands and the feet. The ribs, sternum, spine, and long bones may also be involved. Chondromas are slow growing and often cause pathologic fractures after minor injury. They are found in people of all ages, occur in both men and women, and can affect any bone.

The origin of the *giant cell tumor* remains uncertain. This lesion is aggressive and can be extensive and may involve surrounding soft tissue. Although classified as benign, giant cell tumors can metastasize (spread) to the lung. Unlike most other benign bone tumors, giant cell tumors affect women older than 20 years. The peak incidence occurs in patients in their 30s.

Patient-Centered Collaborative Care

Assess for pain, the most common manifestation of benign bone tumors. Pain can range from mild to moderate. It can be caused by direct tumor invasion into soft tissue, compressing peripheral nerves, or by a resulting pathologic fracture.

In addition to assessing the patient's pain, observe and palpate the suspected involved area. When the tumor affects the lower extremities or the small bones of the hands and feet, local swelling may be detected as the tumor enlarges. In some cases, muscle atrophy or muscle spasm may be present. Carefully palpate the bone and muscle to detect these changes and elicit tenderness.

Routine x-rays and tomography are used to find bone tumors. Tumors are characterized by sharp margins, intact cortices, and smooth, uniform periosteal bone.

CT is less useful except in complex anatomic areas, such as the spinal column and sacrum. The test is helpful in evaluating the extent of soft-tissue involvement. MRI may be especially helpful in viewing problems of the spinal column.

The health care provider uses drug therapy and surgery in combination when possible. Non-drug pain relief measures are also used. Depending on the patient's preference and tolerance, measures such as heat or cold may help relieve pain.

In addition to prescribing analgesics to reduce pain, the health care provider usually prescribes one or more NSAIDs to inhibit prostaglandin synthesis that increases pain and inflammation. Give these drugs after meals or with food to reduce GI side effects.

The most common surgical procedure used for benign bone tumors is removal. If the tumor is small, surgery may not be needed. When the tumor is very extensive, as in a giant cell tumor, it is removed with care to restore or maintain the function of the adjacent joint, most often the knee. In some cases, the knee is replaced with a prosthetic device and, less often, is fused **(arthrodesis).** Bone grafting may be needed. The collaborative care for patients undergoing these surgical procedures is discussed in Chapter 20.

BONE CANCER

Cancerous bone tumors may be primary or secondary (those that originate in other tissues and metastasize to bone). *Primary tumors* occur most often in people between 10 and 30 years of age and make up a small percentage of bone cancers. As for other forms of cancer, the exact cause of bone cancer is unknown. *Metastatic lesions* most often occur in the older age-group and account for most bone cancers.

Previous radiation therapy in the anatomic area is a big risk factor. For example, bone cancer of the ribs in the path of radiation for breast cancer is fairly common.

Pathophysiology

Osteosarcoma, or osteogenic sarcoma, is the most common type of *primary* malignant bone tumor. More than 50% of cases occur in the distal femur, followed in decreasing order of occurrence by the proximal tibia and humerus.

The tumor is relatively large, causing acute pain and swelling. The involved area is usually warm because the blood flow to the site increases. The center of the tumor is sclerotic from increased osteoblastic activity. The periphery is soft, extending through the bone cortex in the classic sunburst appearance associated with the neoplasm. An inward spread into the medullary canal is also common.

Osteosarcoma typically **metastasizes** (spreads) to the periphery of the lung within 2 years of treatment. Metastasis usually results in death.

Osteosarcoma occurs twice as often in males as in females between ages 10 and 30 years and in older patients with Paget's disease. Patients who have received radiation for other forms of cancer or who have benign lesions are also at high risk.

Although *Ewing's sarcoma* is not as common as other tumors, it is the most malignant. Like other primary tumors, it causes pain and swelling. In addition, systemic manifestations, particularly low-grade fever, leukocytosis, and anemia, characterize the lesions. The pelvis and the lower extremity are most often affected. Pelvic involvement is a poor prognostic sign. It often extends into soft tissue. Death results from metastasis to the lungs and other bones. Although the tumor can be seen in patients of any age, it usually occurs in children and young adults in their 20s. Men are affected more often than women.

In contrast to the patient with osteosarcoma, the patient with *chondrosarcoma* experiences dull pain and swelling for a long period. The tumor typically affects the pelvis and proximal femur near the diaphysis. Arising from cartilaginous tissue, it destroys bone and often calcifies. The patient with this type of tumor has a better prognosis than one with osteogenic sarcoma. Chondrosarcoma occurs in middle-aged and older people, with a slight predominance in men.

Arising from fibrous tissue, *fibrosarcomas* can be divided into subtypes, of which malignant fibrous histiocytoma (MFH) is the most malignant. Usually, the clinical presentation of MFH is gradual, without specific symptoms. Local tenderness, with or without a palpable mass, occurs in the long bones of the lower extremity. As with other bone cancers, the lesion can metastasize to the lungs. Although MFH affects people of all ages, it typically occurs in middle-aged men but is not common.

Primary tumors of the prostate, breast, kidney, thyroid, and lung are called *bone-seeking* cancers because they spread to the bone more often than other primary tumors. The vertebrae, pelvis, femur, and ribs are the bone sites commonly affected. Simply stated, primary tumor cells, or seeds, are carried to bone through the bloodstream. *Pathologic fractures caused by metastatic bone are a major concern in patient care management.* The most commonly affected areas for fracture are the acetabulum and the proximal femur.

Metastatic bone tumors greatly outnumber primary bone tumors. They affect primarily people older than 40 years. In patients with a history of cancer and local pain, bone metastasis is suspected.

Patient-Centered Collaborative Care

evolve ONLINE PHARM REVIEW

Assessment

The data collected for the patient suspected of having a malignant bone tumor are similar to the data needed for the patient with a benign growth. In addition, ask whether the patient has had previous radiation therapy for cancer and determine the status of the patient's general health.

The clinical manifestations seen in the patient with primary bone cancer or metastatic disease vary, depending on the specific type of lesion. Usually, the patient has a group of nonspecific concerns, including pain, local swelling, and a tender, palpable mass. Marked disability and impaired mobility may occur in those with advanced metastatic bone disease.

In a patient with Ewing's sarcoma, a low-grade fever may occur because of the systemic features of the neoplasm. For this reason, it is often confused with osteomyelitis. Fatigue and pallor resulting from anemia are also common.

In performing a musculoskeletal assessment, inspect the involved area and palpate the mass for size and tenderness. In collaboration with the physical and occupational therapists, assess the patient's ability to perform mobility tasks and ADLs.

Patients with malignant bone tumors may be young adults whose productive lives are just beginning. They need strong support systems to help cope with the diagnosis and its treatment. Family, significant others, and health care professionals are major components of the needed support. Determine what systems or resources are available.

Patients often experience a loss of control over their lives when a diagnosis of cancer is made. As a result, they become anxious and fearful about the outcome of their illness. Coping with the diagnosis becomes a challenge. As patients progress through the grieving process, there may be initial denial. Identify the anxiety level, and assess the stage or stages of the grieving process. Explore any maladaptive behavior, indicating ineffective coping mechanisms. Chapter 24 further describes the psychosocial assessment for patients with cancer.

The patient with a malignant bone tumor typically shows elevated serum alkaline phosphatase (ALP) levels, indicating the body's attempt to form new bone by increasing osteoblastic activity. The patient with Ewing's sarcoma or metastatic bone cancer often has anemia. In addition, leukocytosis is common with Ewing's sarcoma. The progression of Ewing's sarcoma may be evaluated by elevated serum lactate dehydrogenase (LDH) levels.

In some patients with bone metastasis from the breast, kidney, or lung, the serum calcium level is elevated. Massive bone destruction stimulates release of the mineral into the bloodstream. In patients with Ewing's sarcoma and bone metastasis, the erythrocyte sedimentation rate (ESR) may be elevated because of secondary tissue inflammation.

As with benign bone tumors, routine x-rays and CT reveal malignant lesions. Although each tumor type has its own characteristic radiographic pattern, certain findings are common to all. Cancerous tumors typically show poor demonstration of bone margins, bone destruction, irregular periosteal new bone, and breakthrough of the cortical layer.

Metastatic lesions may increase or decrease bone density, depending on the amount of osteoblastic and osteoclastic activity. CT is helpful in determining the extent of soft-tissue damage. The patient may have an MRI for difficult-to-visualize areas such as the vertebrae.

In some cases, a needle bone biopsy may be performed, usually under fluoroscopy to guide the surgeon. Needle biopsy is an outpatient procedure with rare complications. After biopsy, the cancer is staged for size and degree of spread. One popular method is the TNM staging system, based on tumor size and number (T), the presence of cancer cells in lymph nodes (N), and metastasis (spread) to distant sites (M).

Another staging method is to correlate the tumor grade (high or low), tumor site (intracompartmental or extracompartmental), and presence of metastatic disease (positive or negative). Staging guides the health care team in their decision regarding patient-centered collaborative care.

Analysis

Common Nursing Diagnoses and Collaborative Problems

Priority nursing diagnoses for patients with malignant bone tumors are:

- Acute Pain and Chronic Pain related to physical injury (direct tumor invasion into soft tissue)
- Grieving related to a change in body image or impending death

A possible collaborative problem is Potential for Pathologic Fractures.

Additional Nursing Diagnoses and Collaborative Problems

In addition to the common nursing diagnoses and collaborative problems, patients with malignant bone tumors may have one or more of these:

- Fear and Anxiety related to the medical diagnosis, possible disfiguring surgery, or impending death
- Ineffective Coping related to inadequate level of confidence in ability to cope
- Compromised Family Coping related to prolonged disease
- Dysfunctional Grieving related to actual loss
- Impaired Physical Mobility related to pain and musculoskeletal impairment
- Imbalanced Nutrition: Less Than Body Requirements related to an increased metabolic process
- Disturbed Sleep Pattern related to pain
- Self-Care Deficit (Total) related to impaired physical mobility and weakness
- Ineffective Role Performance related to a temporary or permanent inability to maintain the family or community role
- Spiritual Distress related to fear of death
- Potential for Pathologic Fractures

Planning and Implementation

Acute Pain; Chronic Pain

NOC **Planning: Expected Outcomes.** If possible, the patient with bone cancer is expected to take personal actions to control pain. Indicators include that the patient will consistently demonstrate the ability to:

- Recognize pain onset
- Use preventive measures
- Use analgesics appropriately
- Use nonanalgesic relief measures
- Report pain control

If patients cannot take actions to control their pain, the nurse collaborates with the health care team to ensure pain management and pain control.

Interventions. Because the pain is often due to direct primary tumor invasion, treatment is aimed at reducing the size of or removing the tumor. The expected outcome of treating metastatic bone tumors is palliative rather than curative. Palliative therapies may prevent further bone destruction and improve patient function. A combination of nonsurgical and surgical management is used. Members of the interdisciplinary health care team collaborate to plan the best approach for positive patient outcomes.

Nonsurgical Management. In addition to analgesics for local pain relief, chemotherapeutic agents and radiation therapy are often administered to shrink the tumor. In patients with spinal involvement, bracing and immobilization with cervical traction may reduce back pain. Interventional radiology techniques are used to decrease vertebral pain and treat compression fractures.

Drug therapy. The physician may prescribe *chemotherapy* to be given alone or in combination with radiation or surgery. Certain proliferating tumors, such as Ewing's sarcoma, are sensitive to cytotoxic drugs. Others, such as chondrosarcomas, are often totally drug resistant. Chemotherapy seems to work best for small, metastatic tumors and may be administered before or after surgery. In most cases, the physician prescribes a combination of agents. At present, there is no universally accepted protocol of chemotherapeutic agents. The drugs selected are determined in part by the primary source of the cancer in metastatic disease. For example, when metastasis occurs from breast cancer, estrogen and progesterone blockers may be used. Chapter 24 describes the general nursing care of patients who receive chemotherapy. Remember that all chemotherapeutic agents are categorized as high-alert medications (www.ismp.org).

Other drugs are given for specific metastatic cancers, depending on the location of the primary site. For example, biologic agents, such as cytokines, are given to stimulate the immune system to recognize and destroy cancer cells, especially in patients with renal cancer. Zoledronic acid (Zometa) and pamidronate (Aredia) are two of the newer IV bisphosphonates that are approved for bone metastasis from the breast, lung, and prostate. These drugs help protect bones and prevent fractures. Both drugs are given by IV infusion and place patients at risk for flu-like symptoms, hypokalemia, hypomagnesemia, and hypophosphatemia. Inform patients that osteonecrosis of the jaw may also occur, especially in those who have invasive dental procedures (Aschenbrenner, 2005). Patients who are receiving Reclast should not take Zometa because they are essentially the same drug. Monitor associated laboratory tests, such as renal function and electrolytes, because these drugs can be toxic to the kidneys.

Radiation therapy. Radiation, either brachytherapy or external radiation, is used for selected types of malignant tumors. For patients with Ewing's sarcoma and early osteosarcoma, radiation may be the treatment of choice in reducing tumor size and thus pain.

For patients with metastatic disease, radiation is given primarily for palliation. The therapy is directed toward the painful sites to provide a more comfortable life span. One or more treatments are given, depending on the extent of disease. With precise planning, radiation therapy can be used with minimal complications. The general nursing care for patients receiving radiation therapy is described in Chapter 24.

Interventional radiology. Interventional radiologists can perform several noninvasive procedures to help relieve pain in the patient with metastasis to the spinal column. Two types of *thermal ablation techniques, radiofrequency ablation (RFA)* and cryoablation, can be done under moderate sedation or general anesthesia. RFA kills the targeted tissue with heat using a small needle inserted into the tumor. Most patients have pain relief or control after this ambulatory care procedure. *Cryoablation* is similar to RFA, but the radiologist uses an extremely cold gas through a probe into the tumor. Although this procedure has been available for years, newer surgical equipment allows a small incision, and the patient can return to usual daily activities in a day or two.

The radiologist may also perform a *vertebroplasty* if the patient with spinal metastasis has pathologic compression fractures. After making a small incision, bone cement is injected through a needle into the fractured area. The cement hardens within 15 minutes. Like thermal ablation, this procedure is done in an ambulatory care setting and the patient is placed under moderate sedation (Lavelle et al., 2007).

Surgical Management. Primary bone tumors are usually reduced or removed with surgery and often combined with radiation or chemotherapy.

Preoperative care. In addition to the nature, progression, and extent of the tumor, the patient's age and general health state are considered. Chemotherapy may be administered preoperatively.

As for any patient preparing for cancer surgery, the patient with bone cancer needs psychological support from the nurse and other members of the health care team. Assess the level of the patient's and family's understanding about the surgery and related treatments. As an advocate, encourage the patient and family to discuss concerns and questions and provide information regarding hospital routines and procedures. Spiritual support is important to some patients. They may prefer to contact clergy or spiritual leader or talk with the clergy affiliated with the hospital. Assist in arranging for spiritual assistance if requested.

Anticipate postoperative needs as much as possible before the patient undergoes surgery. Remind the patient what to expect postoperatively and how to help ensure adequate recovery.

Operative procedures. Wide or radical resection procedures are used for patients with bone sarcomas to salvage the affected limb. Wide excision is removal of the lesion surrounded by an intact cuff of normal tissue and leads to cure of low-grade tumors only. A radical resection includes removal of the lesion, the entire muscle, bone, and other tissues directly involved. It is the procedure used for high-grade tumors.

Large bone defects that result from tumor removal may require either:

- Total joint replacements with prosthetic implants, either whole or partial
- Custom metallic implants
- Allografts from the iliac crest, rib, or fibula

As an alternative to total replacement, an allograft may be implanted with internal fixation for those patients who do not have metastases. This is a common procedure for sarcomas of the proximal femur. Allograft procedures for the knee are also performed, particularly in young adults. Preoperative chemotherapy is given to enhance the likelihood of success. **Allografts** with adjacent tendons and ligaments are harvested from cadavers and can be frozen or freeze-dried for a prolonged period. The graft is fixed with a series of bolts, screws, or plates.

Although not commonly done, patients with metastatic disease, intractable (not reversible) pain can be surgically treated with percutaneous **cordotomy** (cutting of the spinal nerve roots). **Cryosurgery** (cold application) may reduce pain and tumor size.

Postoperative care. The surgical incision for a limb salvage procedure is often extensive. A pressure dressing with wound suction is typically maintained for several days. The patient who has undergone a limb salvage procedure has some degree of impaired physical mobility and a self-care deficit. The nature and extent of the alterations depend on the location and extent of the surgery. *For patients who have allografts, observe for signs of hemorrhage, infection, or fracture. Report these changes to the surgeon immediately.*

Muscle strengthening and range-of-motion (ROM) exercises begin immediately postoperatively and continue for at least a year. After upper extremity surgery, the patient can engage in active-assistive exercises by using the opposite hand to help achieve motions such as forward flexion and abduction of the shoulder. Continuous passive motion (CPM) using a CPM machine may be initiated as early as the first postoperative day for either upper extremity or lower extremity procedures.

After lower extremity surgery, the emphasis is on strengthening the quadriceps muscles by using passive and active motion when possible. Maintaining muscle tone is an important prerequisite to weight bearing, which progresses from toe touch or partial weight bearing to full weight bearing by 3 months postoperatively. Coordinate the patient's plan of care for ambulation and muscle strengthening with the physical therapist.

The patient who has had a bone graft may have a cast or other supportive device for several months. Weight bearing is prohibited until there is evidence that the graft is incorporated into the adjacent bone tissue.

During the recovery phase, the patient may also need assistance with ADLs, particularly if the surgery involves the upper extremity. Assist if needed, but at the same time encourage the patient to do as much as possible unaided. Some patients need assistive/adaptive devices for a short period while they are healing. Coordinate the patient's plan of care for promoting independence in ADLs with the occupational therapist.

Surrounding tissues, including nerves and blood vessels, may be removed during surgery. Vascular grafting is common, but the lost nerve(s) is (are) usually not replaced. Assess the neurovascular status of the affected extremity and hand or foot every 1 to 2 hours immediately after surgery. Splinting or casting of the limb may also cause neurovascular (NV) compromise and needs to be checked for proper placement. Assess for NV compromise as described on p. 1167 under Surgical Management of Osteomyelitis.

Pelvic lesions, although not common, may also be surgically removed. Reconstruction generally entails bone fusion with muscle and nerve preservation. A hip spica cast or other device may be necessary until the graft has been incorporated. The patient may need a cane, crutches, or walker for ambulation.

The major complications of reconstructive surgery, such as a joint replacement, are superficial and deep wound infection, dislocation or loosening of the implants, and rapid neurovascular compromise. Report an increase in pain or temperature or a rapid deterioration in circulation to the surgeon promptly. Chapter 20 discusses postoperative care of patients having total joint replacements.

In addition to needing emotional support to cope with physical disabilities, the patient may need help coping with the surgery and its effects. Help identify available support systems as soon as possible.

Grieving

NOC **Planning: Expected Outcomes.** The patient with bone cancer is expected to adjust to actual or impending loss. Indicators include that the patient will have the ability to:

- Resolve feelings about loss
- Verbalize reality of loss
- Discuss unresolved conflicts
- Seek social support
- Progress through stages of grief

Interventions. As a result of most of the surgical procedures, the patient experiences an altered body image. Suggest ways to minimize cosmetic changes. For example, a lowered shoulder can be covered by a custom-made pad worn under clothing. The patient can cover lower extremity defects with pants.

The nurse's most important role is to be an active listener and to encourage the patient and family or significant others to verbalize their feelings. Counselors and members of the clergy or spiritual leaders may provide additional assistance in promoting acceptance of the diagnosis, treatment, or, possibly, impending death. Chapter 9 provides information about loss, death, and dying.

Regardless of the prognosis, a diagnosis of bone cancer is a major stressor that causes the patient and family or significant others to grieve. Help the patient and others cope with the loss and resolve the grief (Chart 53-5). Although patients are asked on admission to a health care agency if they want advance directives, they may have chosen not to have them. If a patient has terminal metastatic bone cancer, though, ask if he or she would like to complete advance directives, like a living will. If the patient already has written advance directives, be sure that a copy is on the medical record and has been given to the health care provider.

Advocate for the patient and the family to promote the physician-patient relationship. For instance, the patient may not completely understand the medical or surgical treatment plan but may hesitate to question the physician. The nurse's intervention can increase communication, which is essential in successful management of the patient with cancer.

Community-Based Care

After medical treatment for a primary malignant tumor, the patient is usually managed at home with follow-up care. The patient with metastatic disease may remain in the home or, when home support is not available, may be admitted to a long-term care facility for extended or hospice care. Coordinate the patient's discharge plan and continuity of care with

Chart 53-5 NIC INTERVENTION ACTIVITIES

The Patient with Bone Cancer (Psychosocial Care)

Grief Work Facilitation: *Assistance with the resolution of a significant loss.*

- Identify the loss.
- Assist the patient to identify the nature of the attachment to the lost object or person.
- Assist the patient to identify the initial reaction to the loss.
- Encourage expression of feelings about the loss.
- Instruct in phases of the grieving process, as appropriate.
- Support progression through personal grieving stages.
- Include significant others in discussion and decisions, as appropriate.
- Assist patient to identify personal coping strategies.
- Communicate acceptance of discussing loss.
- Identify sources of community support.
- Reinforce progress made in the grieving process.
- Assist in identifying modifications needed in lifestyle.

Body Image Enhancement: *Improving a patient's conscious and unconscious perceptions and attitudes toward his or her body.*

- Assist patient to discuss changes caused by illness or surgery, as appropriate.
- Help patient determine the extent of actual changes in the body or its level of functioning.
- Assist patient to determine the influence of a peer group on the patient's perception of present body image.
- Identify the effects of the patient's culture, religion, gender, and age in terms of body image.
- Monitor whether patient can look at the changed body part.
- Determine if a change in body image has contributed to increased social isolation.
- Assist patient to identify actions that will enhance appearance.
- Identify support groups available to patient.

NIC intervention activities selected from Bulechek, G.M., Butcher, H.K., & McCloskey Dochterman, J. (Eds.). (2008). *Nursing interventions classification (NIC)* (5th ed.). St. Louis: Mosby. No part of this work is to be altered without prior written permission from the Publisher.

the case manager and other health care team members, depending on the patient's needs.

Home Care Management

In collaboration with the occupational therapist, evaluate the patient's home environment for structural barriers that may hinder mobility. The patient may be discharged with a cast, walker, crutches, or a wheelchair.

Accessibility to eating and toileting facilities is essential to promote ADL independence. Because the patient with metastatic disease is susceptible to pathologic fractures, potential hazards that may contribute to falls or injury should be removed.

Health Teaching

For the patient receiving intermittent chemotherapy or radiation on an ambulatory basis, emphasize the importance of keeping appointments. Review the expected side and toxic effects of the drugs with the patient and family. Teach how to treat less serious side effects and when to contact the health care provider. If the drugs are administered at home via long-term IV catheter, explain and demonstrate the care involved with daily dressing changes and potential catheter complications. Chapter 15 describes the health teaching required for a patient receiving infusion therapy at home.

If the patient has undergone surgery, he or she has a wound and limited *mobility*. Teach the patient, family, and/or significant others how to care for the wound. Help the patient learn how to perform ADLs and mobility activities independently for self-management. Coordinate with the physical and occupational therapists to assist in ADL teaching, and provide or recommend assistive and adaptive devices, if necessary. The physical therapist also teaches the proper use of ambulatory aids, such as crutches, and exercises.

Pain management can be a major problem, particularly for the patient with metastatic bone disease. Discuss the various options for pain relief, including relaxation and music therapy. Emphasize the importance of those techniques that worked during hospitalization.

The patient with bone cancer may fear that the malignancy will return. Acknowledge this fear, but reinforce confidence in the health care team and medical treatment chosen.

Mutually establish realistic outcomes regarding returning to work and participating in recreational activities. Encourage the patient to resume a functional lifestyle, but caution that it should be gradual. Certain activities, such as participating in sports, may be prohibited.

Help the patient with advanced metastatic bone disease prepare for death. The nurse and other support personnel assist the patient through the stages of death and dying. Identify resources that can help the patient write a will, visit with distant family members, or do whatever he or she thinks is needed for a peaceful death. In the later stages of the disease, hospice care may be an option (see Chapter 9). Nurses working in this area of care can be most helpful in managing end-of-life care.

Health Care Resources

In addition to family and significant others, cancer support groups are helpful to the patient with bone cancer. Some organizations, such as *I Can Cope,* provide information and emotional support. Others, such as *CanSurmount,* are geared more toward patient and family education. The American Cancer Society (www.cancer.org) and the Canadian Cancer Society (www.cancer.ca) can also provide education and resources for patients and families.

The hospital staff nurse, discharge planner, or case manager also ensures that follow-up care, including nursing care and physical or occupational therapy, is available in the home. The patient with terminal cancer may choose to become part of a hospice program.

Evaluation: Outcomes

Evaluate the care of the patient with a malignant bone tumor on the basis of the identified nursing diagnoses and collaborative problems. The expected outcomes may include that the patient will:

- Demonstrate ability to control pain
- Adjust to actual or impending loss
- Experience positive perception of own appearance and body function

Specific indicators for these outcomes are listed for each nursing diagnosis under the Planning and Implementation section (see earlier).

NCLEX EXAMINATION CHALLENGE

What is the priority nursing diagnosis for the older adult diagnosed with bone cancer that has metastasized from the lungs?

A. Risk for Injury related to weakness and drug therapy
B. Altered Self-Esteem related to fear of death and dying
C. Impaired Physical Mobility related to weakness and fatigue
D. Chronic Pain related to tumor invasion and nerve involvement

evolve For the correct answer, go to http://evolve.elsevier.com/Iggy/.

DISORDERS OF THE HAND

DUPUYTREN'S CONTRACTURE

Dupuytren's contracture, or deformity, is a slowly progressive thickening of the palmar fascia, resulting in flexion contracture of the fourth (ring) and fifth (little) fingers of the hand. The third or middle finger is occasionally affected. Although Dupuytren's contracture is a common problem, the cause is unknown. It usually occurs in older Euro-American men, tends to occur in families, and can be bilateral.

When function becomes impaired, surgical release is required. A partial or selective fasciectomy (cutting of fascia) is performed. After removal of the surgical dressing, a splint may be used. Nursing care is similar to that for the patient with carpal tunnel repair (see Chapter 54).

GANGLION

A **ganglion** is a round, benign cyst, often found on a wrist or foot joint or tendon. The synovium surrounding the tendon degenerates, allowing the tendon sheath tissue to become weak and distended. Ganglia are painless on palpation, but they can cause joint discomfort after prolonged joint use or minor trauma or strain. The lesion can rapidly disappear and then recur. Ganglia are most likely to develop in people between 15 and 50 years of age. With local or regional anesthesia in a physician's office or clinic, the fluid within the cyst can be aspirated through a small needle. A cortisone injection may follow. If the cyst is very large, it is removed using a small incision. Patients should avoid strenuous activity for 48 hours after surgery and report any signs of inflammation to their physician.

DISORDERS OF THE FOOT

FOOT DEFORMITIES

The **hallux valgus** deformity is a common foot problem in which the great toe drifts laterally at the first metatarsophalangeal (MTP) joint (Fig. 53-3). The first metatarsal head becomes enlarged, resulting in a **bunion.** As the deviation worsens, the bony enlargement causes pain, particularly when shoes are worn. Women are affected more often than men. Hallux valgus often occurs as a result of poorly fitted shoes, in particular, those with narrow toes and high heels. Other causes include osteoarthritis, rheumatoid arthritis, and family history.

The surgical procedure, a simple **bunionectomy,** involves removal of the bony overgrowth and bursa. When other toe deformities accompany the condition or if the bony overgrowth is large, several **osteotomies,** or bone resections, may be performed. Fusions may also be performed. Screws or wires are often inserted to stabilize the bones in the great toe and first metatarsal during the healing process. If both feet are affected, one foot is usually treated at a time. Surgery usually is performed as a same-day procedure.

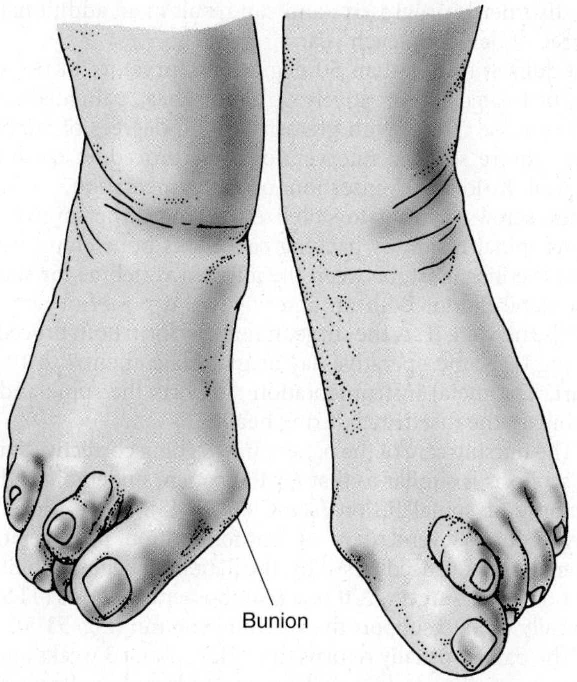
Bunion

Fig. 53-3 • Appearance of hallux valgus with a bunion.

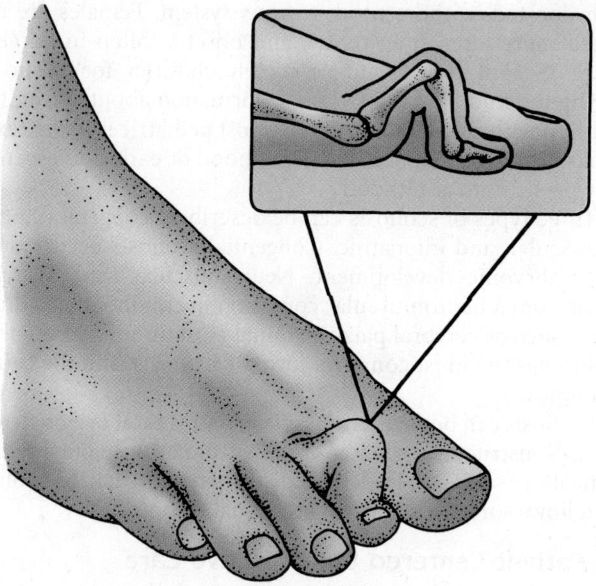

Fig. 53-4 • Hammertoe of the second metatarsophalangeal joint.

Most patients are allowed partial weight bearing while wearing an orthopedic boot or shoe. Walking is difficult because the feet bear body weight. The healing time after surgery may be more than 6 to 12 weeks because the feet receive less blood flow than other parts of the body because of their distance from the heart.

Often patients have hammertoes and hallux valgus deformities at the same time. As shown in Fig. 53-4, a **hammertoe** is the dorsiflexion of any MTP joint with plantar flexion of the proximal interphalangeal (PIP) joint next to it. The second toe is most often affected. As the deformity worsens, uncomfortable corns may develop on the dorsal side of the toe and calluses may appear on the plantar surface. Patients are uncomfortable when wearing shoes and walking.

Hammertoe may be treated by surgical correction of the deformity with **osteotomies** (bone resections) and the insertion of wires or screws for fixation. The postoperative course is similar to that for the patient with hallux valgus repair. The patient uses crutches until full weight bearing is allowed several weeks after surgery.

MORTON'S NEUROMA

In the patient with **Morton's neuroma,** or plantar digital neuritis, a small tumor grows in a digital nerve of the foot. The patient usually describes the pain as an acute, burning sensation in the web space. The pain involves the entire surface of the third and fourth toes. Management involves surgical removal of the neuroma and application of a pressure dressing. Ambulation is usually permitted immediately after surgery.

PLANTAR FASCIITIS

Plantar fasciitis is an inflammation of the plantar fascia, which is located in the area of the arch of the foot. It is often seen in middle-aged and older adults, as well as in athletes, especially runners. In ambulatory care settings, plantar fasciitis accounts for 10% of running injuries. Obesity is also a contributing factor.

Patients report severe pain in the arch of the foot, especially when getting out of bed. The pain is worsened with weight bearing. Although most patients have unilateral plantar fasciitis, the problem can affect both feet.

Most patients respond to conservative management, which includes rest, ice, stretching exercises, strapping of the foot to maintain the arch, shoes with good support, and orthotics. NSAIDs or steroids may be needed to control pain and inflammation. If conservative measures are unsuccessful, endoscopic surgery to remove the inflamed tissue may be required.

Teach the patient about the importance of adhering to the treatment plan and coordinating care with the physical therapist for instruction in exercise.

OTHER PROBLEMS OF THE FOOT

Table 53-4 lists other common foot problems and how they are managed. Although patients are usually not hospitalized for these conditions, the nurse may recognize a foot disorder and alert the physician. Even small deformities or other foot deformities can be very annoying and painful for the patient and may hinder ambulation, as well as interfere with ADLs.

SCOLIOSIS

Pathophysiology

Scoliosis occurs when the vertebrae rotate and begin to compress. The spinal column begins to move into a lateral curve, most commonly in the right lateral thoracic area (see Fig. 52-3 in Chapter 52). As the degree of curvature increases, damage to the vertebral bodies results. The degree of the curvature increases during periods of growth, such as in adolescence. Curvature of greater than 50 degrees results in an unstable spine, and curvature of greater than 60 degrees in the thoracic spine results in compromise of cardiopulmonary function.

The exact cause of scoliosis is not well understood. The process may result from some problem in the balance mechanism located in the central nervous system. Females are affected more often than males, and onset is often in adolescence. School health nurses screen children for scoliosis during the middle school years. Information about caring for children with scoliosis is found in most pediatric nursing textbooks. Scoliosis that occurs in childhood or early adolescence may persist into adulthood.

Three types of scoliosis can be described: congenital, neuromuscular, and idiopathic. Congenital scoliosis occurs during embryonic development. Neuromuscular scoliosis can result from a neuromuscular condition in childhood or adulthood, such as cerebral palsy or spinal cord tumors. Idiopathic scoliosis is the most common form of scoliosis, and the cause is unknown.

Scoliosis can be further classified as structural or nonstructural. Nonstructural scoliosis results from a cause outside the spine itself, such as a leg length discrepancy. Structural scoliosis follows some deviation of the spinal column.

Patient-Centered Collaborative Care

A complete history of the patient with spinal deformity should include onset of problem, in adolescence or adulthood, and what treatments may have been used in the past. Patients who had surgery for scoliosis during adolescence are returning with progressive, debilitating back pain from degenerative disk disease below the level of vertebral fusion. A loss of lumbar curvature, or **lordosis,** described as "flat back" syndrome, may also be present. Complete a thorough pain assessment for patients reporting back pain.

Observe the patient from the front and back, while standing and during forward flexion from the hips. Physical examination usually reveals asymmetry of hip and shoulder height, prominence of the thoracic ribs and scapula on one side, and visible curve in the spinal column. Observation from the side may reveal kyphosis of the thoracic spine. Assess for leg length differences as well.

Methods of managing adult scoliosis differ from those used for children. The adult spinal column is less flexible and therefore less likely to respond to exercises, weight reduction, bracing, and casting for correction of the deformity. In the adult, the disorder is progressive and can result in an additional one degree of deviation each year.

Adults with less than 50 degrees of curvature of the spine may be treated conservatively with moist heat, pain medication, and exercise. Those with greater than 50 degrees of curvature may require surgical intervention. The procedure consists of surgical fusion and insertion of instrumentation, including plates, screws, or rods to stabilize the spine. The surgeon performs spinal fusion by packing cancellous bone chips, usually from the iliac crest, between the affected vertebrae for support and stabilization. Both an anterior and a posterior approach may be needed. If so, the surgeon may perform both procedures during the same operative day or may stage them 7 to 10 days apart. The metal instrumentation supports the spine and immobilizes the fused area during healing.

The nursing care of the patient undergoing corrective surgery for scoliosis is similar to that for the patient undergoing a laminectomy or spinal fusion (see Chapter 45). Some procedures may require several days of immobilization postoperatively, whereas other procedures allow the patient to begin mobility the next day after surgery. A thoracolumbosacral orthosis (TLSO) is typically used to support the vertebral column (Fig. 53-5).

The patient usually returns to work in about 3 weeks and can resume activities such as swimming and bicycling. Recreational sports, such as tennis, may be resumed in 6 weeks for some patients. Other surgical procedures may prevent the patient from performing these activities until 3 to 6 months postoperatively.

Refer patients and their families to the National Scoliosis Foundation (www.scoliosis.org) for information and support services.

PROGRESSIVE MUSCULAR DYSTROPHIES

Many types of **muscular dystrophy (MD)** have been categorized as slowly progressive or rapidly progressive. The slowly progressive types are most commonly seen in adults. Most

TABLE 53-4 Treatment of Common Foot Problems

Description/Cause	Treatment
CORN	
Induration and thickening of the skin caused by friction and pressure; painful conical mass	Surgical removal by podiatrist
CALLUS	
Flat, poorly defined mass on the sole over a bony prominence caused by pressure	Padding and lanolin creams; overall good skin hygiene
INGROWN NAIL	
Nail sliver penetration of the skin, causing inflammation	Removal of sliver by podiatrist; warm soaks; antibiotic ointment
HYPERTROPHIC UNGUAL LABIUM	
Chronic hypertrophy of nail lip caused by improper nail trimming; results from untreated ingrown nail	Surgical removal of necrotic nail and skin; treatment of secondary infection

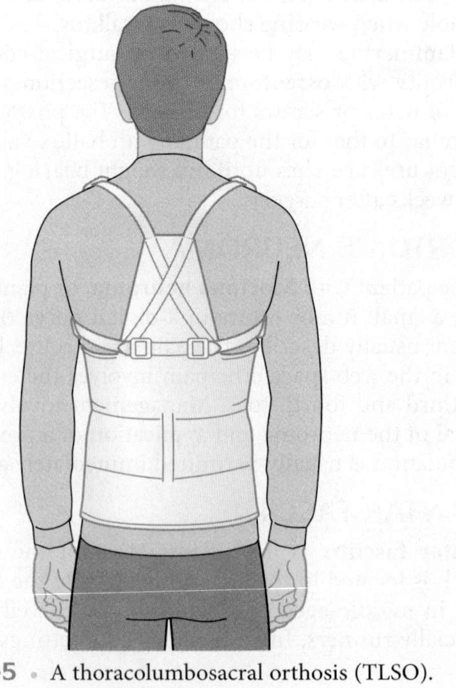

Fig. 53-5 • A thoracolumbosacral orthosis (TLSO).

pediatric nursing books describe the care for patients with MD in detail. Four forms of MD are often seen in adults. Each type has its own distinct characteristics and causes, but all are progressive (Table 53-5).

The exact pathophysiologic mechanisms are unknown, but several causes are possible. These include:

- Poor blood flow to muscle resulting in reduced tissue oxygenation
- Disturbance in nerve-muscle interaction
- Loss of cell membrane integrity as a result of increased enzyme activity

GENETIC CONSIDERATIONS

The major pathologic change that occurs in most types of MD is the production or faulty action of a muscle protein called **dystrophin.** The purpose of this protein is to maintain muscle integrity by sending signals to coordinate smooth, synchronous muscle fiber contraction. The coding of this protein is by a large gene that has many parts located on the X chromosome. Different mutations of the gene where dystrophin is located determine the degree of muscle weakness. Because this protein connects with other substances for final muscle action, genetic mutations of these other substances can make dystrophin fail to work properly.

The most common forms of MD are Duchenne MD (DMD) and Becker MD (BMD). Both are X-linked recessive disorders. Women who are *carriers* (able to pass on the gene without having the disorder) have a 50% chance of passing the MD gene to their daughters, who are then carriers, and to their sons, who then have the disease. These types of MD, then, affect only males. In DMD, most patients die very young and therefore do not have children. In BMD, the patient lives longer and may have children. None of these men's sons will have the disease, but their daughters will be carriers (Nussbaum et al., 2007). Refer carriers for genetic testing and counseling.

Regardless of the type of MD, the primary problem is progressive muscle weakness. The major cause of death is respiratory failure caused by profound respiratory muscle weakness. Cardiac failure also occurs because dystrophin activity is needed for cardiac muscle contraction and maintenance.

Diagnosis of MD is often difficult because the clinical manifestations are similar to those of other muscular disorders. Muscle biopsy often confirms the diagnosis. Muscle weakness and trophic changes are characteristic of all types of MD. Serum muscle enzyme values, such as aldolase and creatine kinase, may be elevated, and electromyographic (EMG) findings are often abnormal.

Collaborative care of the patient with MD is supportive and involves the entire health care team. Physical and occupational therapy help the patient maintain as much function, *mobility,* and independence as possible. Refer the patient and family to the local chapter of the Muscular Dystrophy Association (www.mda.org) for support services and information.

Major organ or body system involvement is medically managed, but the life span is often shortened from these manifestations of the disease. With the exception of steroids, no drug has been found to slow the progression of the disorder, although immunosuppressive agents, anabolic steroids, and growth factors have been tried.

An experimental treatment, myoblast transfer therapy (MTT), has been supported by the Food and Drug Administration (FDA). MTT involves injections of healthy muscle cells (myoblasts) taken from a donor and multiplied in a laboratory. The cells are then given to the patient with MD, where they theoretically fuse with each other and the recipient's unhealthy muscle cells. Gene therapy may also be an option for curing MD in the future.

Nursing interventions focus on making the patient as comfortable as possible and reinforcing techniques and exercises taught in the physical therapy program. The nurse's role in caring for a patient with cardiac or other organ involvement is the same as for any patient with dysfunction of these systems.

TABLE 53-5 Differential Features of Common Muscular Dystrophies Seen in Adults

Onset	Genetic Link	Clinical Manifestations	Progression
BECKER (BENIGN X-LINKED) DYSTROPHY			
5-25 yr	Sex-linked recessive; expression in males	Wasting of pelvic and shoulder muscles; normal cardiac and mental function	Gradual progression; inability to walk 25 yr after onset; usually normal life span
LIMB-GIRDLE DYSTROPHY			
Usually 20s or 30s	Usually autosomal dominant; expression in either gender	Upper extremity and neck muscles and lower extremity and hip muscle weakness	Extremely variable; severe disability within 10-20 yr after onset; life span shortened by 10-20 yr
FACIOSCAPULOHUMERAL (LANDOUZY-DEJERINE) DYSTROPHY			
Usually in 20s	Autosomal dominant; expression in either gender	Facial and shoulder girdle muscle involvement	Usually benign; normal life span
MYOTONIC (STEINERT) DYSTROPHY			
Birth to 40s	Autosomal dominant; expression in either gender	Muscle atrophy with multiple organ involvement (e.g., heart, lungs, smooth muscle, and endocrine system)	Usually gradual if onset in adulthood

HUMAN NEEDS NURSING CARE REVIEW

What might you NOTICE if the patient has impaired mobility as a result of chronic musculoskeletal disorders?

- Spinal deformity (e.g., kyphosis, lateral deviation)
- Bone malalignment (e.g., leg bowing)
- Muscle weakness
- Bone swelling or deformity
- Joint inflammation
- Flushed skin (Paget's disease)
- Fever (bone infection)
- Report of pain
- Report of weight loss

What should you INTERPRET and how should you RESPOND to a patient with impaired mobility as a result of chronic musculoskeletal disorders?

Perform and interpret focused physical assessment findings, including:

- Ability to ambulate (with or without assistive device)
- ADLs ability
- Body weight
- Pain intensity and quality
- Neurovascular assessment findings
- Ability to cope with decreased mobility

Respond:

- Provide pain control interventions, including drugs and nonpharmacologic measures (e.g., music therapy).
- Collaborate with members of the health care team, including PT, OT, nutritionist, as needed.
- Teach about drugs that may be needed for long-term use, including side and toxic effects.
- Explain about the need for adequate calcium and vitamin D for healthy bones and bone healing.
- Assist with ADLs and ambulation as needed, but encourage independence when possible.
- Implement measures to prevent patient falls in the inpatient and home setting.
- Encourage the patient to discuss feelings related to disorders causing impaired mobility.
- Refer patients to appropriate community resources, such as the National Osteoporosis Foundation.

On what should you REFLECT?

- Monitor the patient's response to pain control interventions.
- Monitor the patient for falls.
- Evaluate the patient's knowledge of nutrition and drug therapy.
- Evaluate the patient's coping ability related to disease diagnosis and treatment.
- Think about what else you might do to promote mobility.
- Decide whether you need to provide alternative interventions or additional health teaching.

GET READY FOR THE NCLEX EXAMINATION!

Key Points

Review these Key Points for each NCLEX Examination Client Needs Category.

Safe and Effective Care Environment

- Coordinate with health care team members when assessing patients with osteoporosis for risk for falls.
- In coordination with the physical and occupational therapists, educate the patient and family on home safety when the patient has a metabolic bone disease, such as osteoporosis.
- Use appropriate infection control practices when caring for patients with an open wound associated with osteomyelitis.
- Review treatment options that have been discussed with the patient who has bone cancer.
- Refer patients with musculoskeletal problems to appropriate community resources, such as the Paget's Disease Foundation and the National Osteoporosis Foundation.
- For patients who have surgery for bone cancer, report postoperative manifestations of infection, dislocation, or neurovascular compromise to the surgeon promptly.
- Refer to The Joint Commission for information about 2007 National Patient Safety Goals related to fall injury prevention.

Health Promotion and Maintenance

- Teach patients at risk for osteoporosis to minimize risk factors, such as stopping smoking, decreasing alcohol intake, exercising regularly, and increasing dietary calcium.
- Remind patients at risk for osteoporosis to have screening tests, such as the DXA scan.
- Instruct older adults to have at least 5 to 10 minutes of sun per week and to eat vitamin D–fortified foods to prevent osteomalacia.
- Refer patients with genetic-associated disease for genetic testing and counseling.
- Assess the genetic risk for patients who have parents with muscular dystrophy.

Psychosocial Integrity

- Assist patients with osteoporosis to overcome fear of falling, or fallophobia, which prevents them from socializing or going outside their homes. Collaborate with the physical therapist to determine whether ambulatory devices such as canes are indicated.
- Help patients with bone cancer cope with their illness as described in Chart 53-5.

Physiological Integrity

- Remind patients taking bisphosphonates (BPs) to take them early in the morning, at least 30 minutes before breakfast, with a full glass of water and to remain sitting upright during that time to prevent esophagitis, a common complication of BP therapy.
- Most patients are unaware that they have osteoporosis until they experience a fracture, the most common complication of the disease.
- Osteomalacia, caused by a deficiency in vitamin D, can be caused by the factors listed in Table 53-3.

- Remember that severe chronic pain is a priority for patients with metastatic bone disease.
- Assess for key features of Paget's disease as summarized in Chart 53-3.
- Remember that bone tumors can be benign or malignant.
- Be aware that even minor hand and foot problems can be very painful. Common foot problems are described in Table 53-4.
- In collaboration with the health care team, provide supportive care for the patient with muscular dystrophy.
- Recognize that most major types of muscular dystrophy are genetic and manifest usually in childhood. Care is supportive.

Additional Study Resources

Go to your Companion CD or Evolve at http://evolve.elsevier.com/Iggy/ for *Self-Assessment Questions for the NCLEX Examination.*

evolve Go to Evolve at http://evolve.elsevier.com/Iggy/ for *Prioritization and Delegation Questions for the NCLEX Examination.*

SELECTED BIBLIOGRAPHY

Asterisk indicates a classic or definitive work on this subject.

Aschenbrenner, D.S. (2005). Drug watch—New warnings and safety concerns: Medications and adverse effects. *AJN, 105*(1), 29.

Berg, E.E. (2006). Osteogenic sarcoma. *Orthopaedic Nursing, 25*(5), 348-349.

Childs, S.G. (2005). Dupuytren's disease. *Orthopaedic Nursing, 24*(2), 160-165.

Daroszewska, A., & Ralston, S.H. (2005). Genetics of Paget's disease of the bone. *Clinical Science (London), 109*(3), 257-263.

Estok, P.J., Sedlak, C.A., Doheny, M.O., & Hall, R. (2007). Structural model for osteoporosis preventing behavior in postmenopausal women. *Nursing Research, 56*(7), 148-158.

Geier, K.A. (2006). Metabolic bone conditions. In Taggart, H.M. (Ed.), *Core curriculum for orthopaedic nursing* (pp. 375-397). Boston: Pearson.

Giangregorio, L., Fisher, P., Papaioannou, A., & Adachi, J.D. (2007). Osteoporosis knowledge and information needs in healthcare professionals caring for patients with fragility fractures. *Orthopaedic Nursing, 26*(1), 27-35.

Holcomb, S.S. (2006). Osteoporosis. *Nursing2006, 36*(4), 48-49.

Houghton, D. (2006). Using antibiotics effectively in acute-care patients. *American Nurse Today, 1*(3), 31-35.

Hurwitz, S. (2006). Evaluating bunions, offering relief. *The Journal of Musculoskeletal Medicine, 32*(1), 50-56.

Iacono, M.V. (2007). Osteoporosis: A national public health priority. *Journal of Perianesthesia Nursing, 22*(3), 175-193.

Kessenich, C.R. (2006). Osteoporosis: New options for pain relief. *Nurse Practitioner, 31*(2), 44-47.

Lavelle, W., Carl, A., Lavelle, E.D., & Khaleel, M.A. (2007). Vertebroplasty and kyphoplasty. *Medical Clinics of North America, 91*(2), 299-314.

Lehne, R.A. (2006). *Pharmacology for nursing care.* Philadelphia: Saunders.

Lui, Y-J, Shen, H., Xiao, P., Xiong, D-H., Li, L.H., Recker, R.R., et al. (2006). Molecular genetic studies of gene identification for osteoporosis: A 2004 update. *Journal of Bone and Mineral Research, 21*(10), 1511-1535.

McCance, K.L., & Huether, S.E. (Eds.). (2006). *Pathophysiology: The biologic basis for disease in adults and children.* (5th ed.). St. Louis: Mosby.

National Osteoporosis Foundation. (2007a). *Fast facts.* Retrieved April 15, 2007, from www.nof.org/osteoporosis/disease facts.htm.

National Osteoporosis Foundation. (2007b). *Physician's guide: Basic pathophysiology.* Retrieved April 15, 2007, from www.nof.org/physguide/basic_pathophysiololgy.htm.

National Osteoporosis Foundation. (2007c). *Physicians guide: Diagnosis.* Retrieved April 15, 2007, from www.nof.org/physguid/diagnosis.htm.

National Osteoporosis Foundation. (2007d). *Physicians guide: Pharmacological options.* Retrieved April 15, 2007, from www.nof.org/physguide/pharmacologic.htm.

*Nivens, A.S. (2004). Paget's disease: A case in point. *Orthopaedic Nursing, 23*(6), 355-363.

Nussbaum, R., McInnes, R., & Willard, H. (2007). *Thompson & Thompson: Genetics in medicine* (7th ed.). Philadelphia: Saunders.

Olson, A.F. (2007). Osteoporosis detection: Is BMD testing the future? *The Nurse Practitioner, 32*(6), 20-28.

Pagana, K.D., & Pagana, T.J. (2006). *Mosby's manual of diagnostic and laboratory tests* (3rd ed.). St. Louis: Mosby.

Peer, K.S., & Newsham, K.R. (2005). A case study on osteoporosis in a male athlete. *Orthopaedic Nursing, 24*(3), 193-199.

Raisz, L.G. (2005). Screening for osteoporosis. *New England Journal of Medicine, 353*(2), 164-171.

Sadler, C., & Huff, M. (2007). African-American women: Health beliefs, lifestyle, and osteoporosis. *Orthopaedic Nursing, 26*(2), 96-101.

Schoen, D.C. (2006). Bone neoplasms. *Orthopaedic Nursing, 25*(6), 427-430.

Sedlak, C.A., Doheny, M.O., & Estok, P.J. (2000). Osteoporosis in older men: Knowledge and health beliefs. *Orthopaedic Nursing, 19*(3), 38-46.

Sedlak, C.A., Doheny, M.O., Estok, P.J., & Zeller, R.A. (2005). Tailored interventions to enhance osteoporosis prevention in women. *Orthopaedic Nursing, 24*(4), 270-275.

The Joint Commission. (2007). *2007 National patient safety goals.* Retrieved April 15, 2007, from www.jointcommision.org/PatientSafety/NationalPatientSafetyGoals/07_npsg_facts.htm.

The Paget Foundation. (2007a). *A health professional's guide to the management of Paget's disease.* Retrieved April 15, 2007, from http://paget.org/Information/FactSheet/mgmt_of_pdisbone.html.

The Paget Foundation. (2007b). *A nurse's guide for assessment and management of patients diagnosed with Paget's disease of the bone.* Retrieved April 15, 2007, from http://paget.org/Information/Factsheet/nurses_guide.html.

*Thornton, M.J., Sedlak, C.A., & Doheny, M.O. (2004). Height change and bone mineral density revisited. *Orthopaedic Nursing, 23*(5), 315-320.

Whiting, S.J., & Vatanparast, H. (2005). Nutritional interventions in osteoporosis. *Geriatrics and Aging, 8*(9), 14-20.

Woman's Health Initiative. (2005). *Findings from the WHI postmenopausal hormone therapy trials.* Retrieved April 18, 2007, from www.nhlbi.nih.gov/whi/index.html.

54
CHAPTER

Care of Patients with Musculoskeletal Trauma

Cathy A. Murray

LEARNING OUTCOMES

For clinical competence and success on the NCLEX Examination, study this chapter with these Learning Outcomes in mind:

Safe and Effective Care Environment

1. Collaborate with the health care team when providing care for patients with fractures.
2. Collaborate with the health care team when providing care for patients with amputations.
3. Identify community resources about amputations for patients and their families.
4. Assess patients with musculoskeletal trauma to prioritize interventions for their care.
5. Apply principles of infection control when caring for a patient with a compound fracture.

Health Promotion and Maintenance

6. Teach the public about ways to prevent fractures and other musculoskeletal injuries.
7. Provide discharge teaching for patients with fractures or amputations.
8. Provide care that meets the special needs of older adults with hip fractures, including interventions to increase mobility.

Psychosocial Integrity

9. Assess the patient's and family's reaction to changes in body image resulting from amputation.
10. Assist patients in coping with loss of a body part.

Physiological Integrity

11. Compare and contrast common types of fractures.
12. Describe the usual healing process for bone.
13. Explain the typical clinical manifestations that are seen in patients with fractures.
14. Maintain casts for patients with fractures.
15. Maintain traction and external fixation for patients with fractures.
16. Provide pain management for patients with musculoskeletal trauma.
17. Identify the risk for complications from fractures, and take measures to help prevent them.
18. Perform focused musculoskeletal and neurovascular assessment for patients with musculoskeletal trauma.
19. Provide postoperative care, including health teaching, after fracture repair.
20. Provide emergency care for people who have a traumatic amputation.
21. Provide postoperative care, including health teaching, after an elective amputation.
22. Identify common causes of amputations.
23. Incorporate complementary and alternative therapies into the plan of care for patients with phantom limb pain.
24. Describe the collaborative management for the patient with complex regional pain syndrome.
25. Provide care for patients with common types of sports-related injuries.

Go to your Companion CD or Evolve at http://evolve.elsevier.com/Iggy/ for *Self-Assessment Questions for the NCLEX Examination* keyed to these Learning Outcomes.

Musculoskeletal trauma accounts for about two thirds of all injuries and is one of the primary causes of disability in the United States. It ranges from simple muscle strain to multiple bone fractures with severe soft-tissue damage.

Fractures and other musculoskeletal trauma impair a patient's *mobility* in varying degrees depending on the severity and extent of the injury. These injuries also affect *sensation* because of pressure on nerve endings from edema. In some cases, peripheral nerves are directly damaged as a result of musculoskeletal injury.

Musculoskeletal injury is a correctable event with specific known risks. An important role in nursing is educating the public about how to prevent musculoskeletal trauma and other types of injury.

FRACTURES

Pathophysiology

A **fracture** is a break or disruption in the continuity of a bone that often affects the *human needs for mobility and sensation.* It can occur anywhere in the body and at any age. All fractures have the same basic pathophysiologic mechanism and require similar patient-centered collaborative care, regardless of fracture type or location.

Classification of Fractures

A fracture is classified by the extent of the break:

- *Complete fracture.* The break is across the entire width of the bone in such a way that the bone is divided into two distinct sections.
- *Incomplete fracture.* The fracture does not divide the bone into two portions because the break is through only part of the bone.

A fracture is described by the extent of associated soft-tissue damage as **open** (or **compound**) or **closed** (or **simple**). The skin surface over the broken bone is disrupted in a *compound* fracture, which causes an external wound. These fractures are often graded to define the extent of tissue damage. Grade I is the least severe injury, and skin damage is minimal. In grade II, an open fracture is accompanied by skin and muscle contusions. The most severe injury is grade III, in which there is damage to skin, muscle, nerve tissue, and blood vessels. A *simple* fracture does not extend through the skin and therefore has no visible wound.

Fig. 54-1 shows common types of fractures. In addition to being identified by type, fractures are described by their cause. A **pathologic (spontaneous) fracture** occurs after minimal trauma to a bone that has been weakened by disease. For example, a patient with bone cancer or osteoporosis can easily have a pathologic fracture. A **fatigue (stress) fracture** results from excessive strain and stress on the bone. This problem is

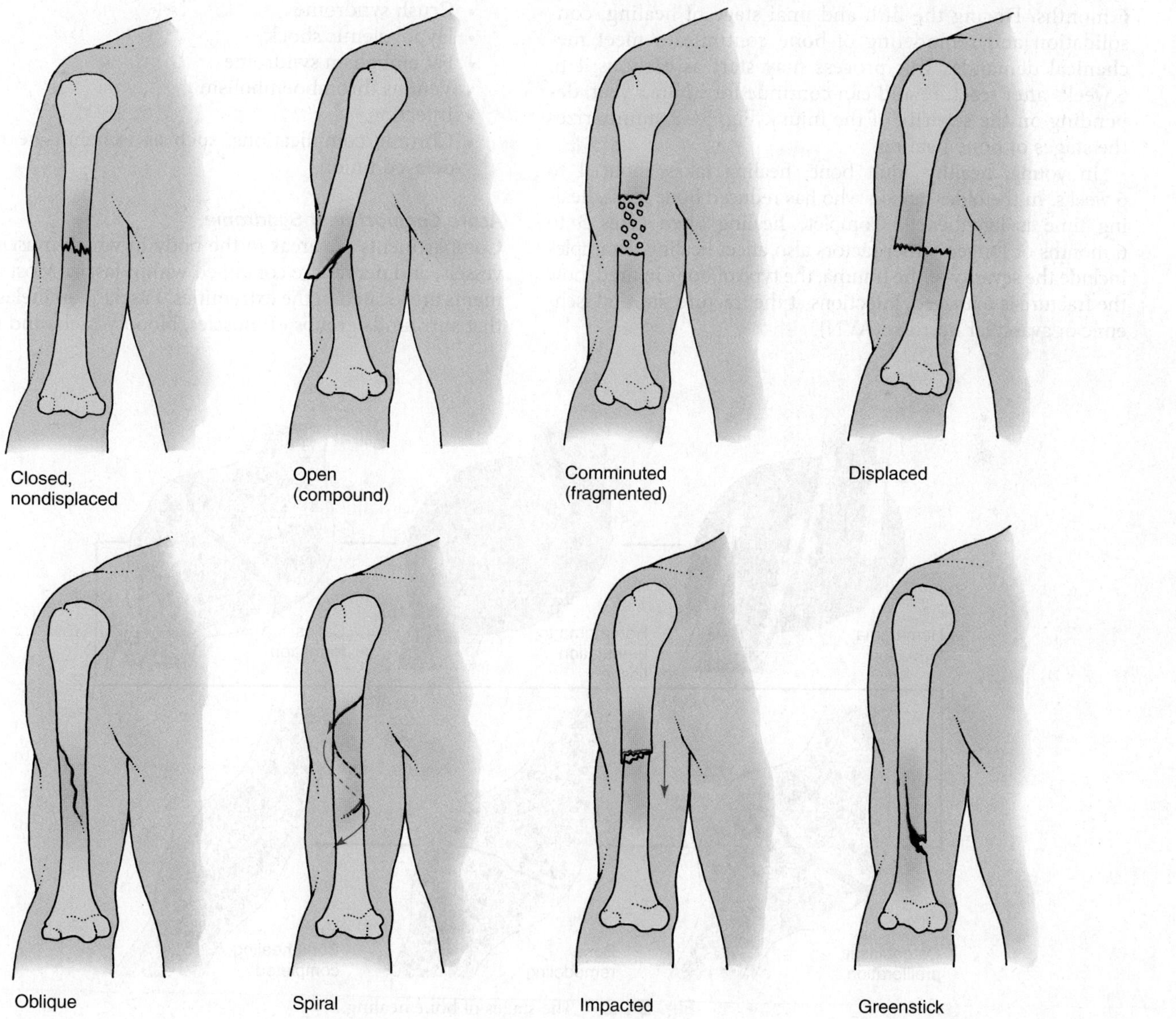
Closed, nondisplaced
Open (compound)
Comminuted (fragmented)
Displaced
Oblique
Spiral
Impacted
Greenstick

Fig. 54-1 • Common types of fractures.

commonly seen in recreational and professional athletes. **Compression fractures** are produced by a loading force applied to the long axis of cancellous bone. They commonly occur in the vertebrae of patients with osteoporosis and are extremely painful.

Stages of Bone Healing

When a bone is fractured, the body immediately begins the healing process to repair the injury and restore the body's equilibrium. Fractures heal in five stages that are a continuous process and not single stages. In stage one, within 24 to 72 hours after the injury, a hematoma forms at the site of the fracture because bone is extremely vascular. Stage two occurs in 3 days to 2 weeks when granulation tissue begins to invade the hematoma. This then prompts the formation of fibrocartilage, providing the foundation for bone healing. Stage three of bone healing occurs as a result of vascular and cellular proliferation. The fracture site is surrounded by new vascular tissue known as a *callus* (within 2 to 6 weeks). **Callus** formation is the beginning of a nonbony union. As healing continues in stage four, the callus is gradually resorbed and transformed into bone. This stage may take 3 weeks to 6 months. During the fifth and final stage of healing, consolidation and remodeling of bone continue to meet mechanical demands. This process may start as early as 4 to 6 weeks after fracture and can continue for up to 1 year, depending on the severity of the injury. Fig. 54-2 summarizes the stages of bone healing.

In young, healthy adult bone, healing takes about 4 to 6 weeks. In the older person who has reduced bone mass, healing time is lengthened. Complete healing often takes 3 to 6 months or longer. Other factors also affect healing. Examples include the severity of the trauma, the type of bone injured, how the fracture is managed, infections at the fracture site, and ischemic or avascular necrosis (AVN).

CONSIDERATIONS FOR OLDER ADULTS

Bone healing can be affected by the aging process. Bone formation and strength rely on adequate nutrition. Calcium, phosphorus, vitamin D, and protein are necessary for the production of new bone (see Chapter 53). For women, the loss of estrogen after menopause decreases the body's ability to form new bone tissue. Chronic diseases can also affect the rate at which bone heals. For instance, peripheral vascular diseases, such as arteriosclerosis, reduce arterial circulation to bone. Thus the bone receives less oxygen and fewer nutrients, both of which are needed for repair.

Complications of Fractures

Regardless of the type or location of the fracture, several limb- and life-threatening complications can result from the injury. Clinical manifestations of beginning complications must be treated early to prevent serious consequences. In some cases, careful monitoring and assessment can prevent these complications:

- Acute compartment syndrome
- Crush syndrome
- Hypovolemic shock
- Fat embolism syndrome
- Venous thromboembolism
- Infection
- Chronic complications, such as ischemic necrosis and delayed union

Acute Compartment Syndrome

Compartments are areas in the body in which muscles, blood vessels, and nerves are contained within fascia. Most compartments are located in the extremities. **Fascia** is an inelastic tissue that surrounds groups of muscles, blood vessels, and nerves in

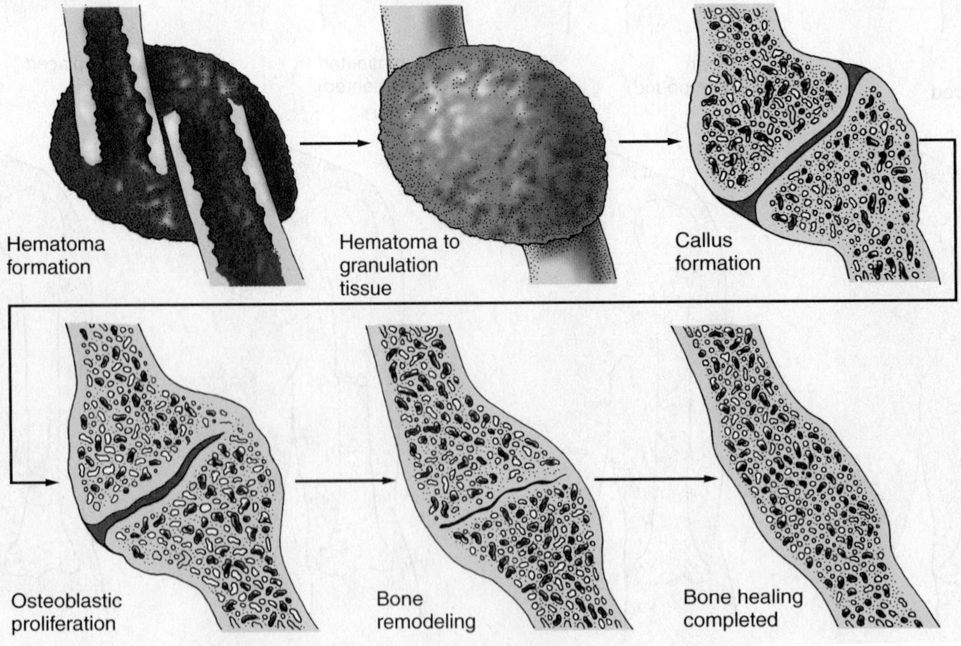

Hematoma formation
Hematoma to granulation tissue
Callus formation
Osteoblastic proliferation
Bone remodeling
Bone healing completed

Fig. 54-2 • The stages of bone healing.

the body. **Acute compartment syndrome (ACS)** is a serious condition in which increased pressure within one or more compartments reduces circulation to the area. The most common sites for this problem in patients with musculoskeletal trauma are the compartments in the lower leg and forearm.

The pathophysiologic changes of increased compartment pressure are sometimes referred to as the *ischemia-edema cycle*. Capillaries within the muscle dilate, which raises capillary pressure. Capillaries then become more permeable because of the release of histamine by the ischemic muscle tissue. As a result, plasma proteins leak into the interstitial fluid space and edema occurs. Edema increases pressure on nerve endings and causes pain. Blood flow to the area is reduced, and further ischemia results. Sensory deficits or paresthesia generally appear before changes in vascular or motor signs. The color of the tissue pales, and pulses begin to weaken but rarely disappear. The affected area is usually palpably tense, and pain occurs with passive motion of the extremity. If the condition is not treated, cyanosis, tingling, numbness, paresis, and severe pain occur. Chart 54-1 summarizes the sequence of pathophysiologic events in compartment syndrome and the associated clinical assessment findings.

The pressure to the compartment can be from an external or internal source. Tight, bulky dressings and casts are examples of *external* pressure. Blood or fluid accumulation in the compartment is a common source of *internal* pressure. The injury or trauma causing the problem is above the compartment involved, which decreases blood flow to the more distal area of injury. ACS is not limited to patients with musculoskeletal problems. It can also occur in those with severe burns, extensive insect bites or snakebites, or massive infiltration of IV fluids. In these situations, edema increases internal pressure in one or more compartments.

Chart 54-1 KEY FEATURES

Compartment Syndrome

Physiologic Change	Clinical Findings
Increased compartment pressure	No change
Increased capillary permeability	Edema
Release of histamine	Increased edema
Increased blood flow to area	Pulses present
	Pink tissue
Pressure on nerve endings	Pain
Increased tissue pressure	Referred pain to compartment
Decreased tissue perfusion	Increased edema
Decreased oxygen to tissues	Pallor
Increased production of lactic acid	Unequal pulses
	Flexed posture
Anaerobic metabolism	Cyanosis
Vasodilation	Increased edema
Increased blood flow	Tense muscle swelling
Increased tissue pressure	Tingling
	Numbness
Increased edema	Paresthesia
Muscle ischemia	Severe pain unrelieved by drugs
Tissue necrosis	Paresis/paralysis

Monitor for early signs of ACS. Assess for the "six Ps" including pain, pressure, paralysis, paresthesia, pallor, and pulselessness (Harvey, 2006). Pain is increased even with passive motion and may seem out of proportion to the degree of injury. Numbness and tingling or paresthesias may be the first signs of a problem. The affected extremity is pale and cool as a result of decreased *arterial* perfusion to the affected area. Capillary refill is an important assessment of perfusion but may not be reliable in an older adult because of arterial insufficiency. *Losses of function and decreased pulses or pulselessness are late signs of ACS.*

Emergency Care: Acute Compartment Syndrome. *Fortunately, ACS is not common, but it creates an emergency situation when it does occur. Within 4 to 6 hours after the onset of compartment syndrome, neurovascular and muscle damage are irreversible. The limb can become useless in 24 to 48 hours.*

In a few cases, compartment pressure may be monitored on a one-time basis with a handheld device with a digital display, or pressure can be monitored continuously. Monitoring is recommended for comatose or unresponsive high-risk patients.

If ACS is verified, the surgeon may perform a **fasciotomy,** or opening in the fascia, by making an incision through the skin and subcutaneous tissues into the fascia of the affected compartment. This procedure relieves the pressure and restores circulation to the affected area. No consensus exists on what pressure requires fasciotomy (normal is 0 to 8 mm Hg). Compartment pressures must be considered in relation to the patient's hemodynamic status. After fasciotomy, the open wound is packed and dressed daily or more often until secondary closure occurs, usually in 4 to 5 days depending on the patient's healing ability. At that time, the surgeon usually débrides the wound and may apply a skin graft to promote healing.

Complications of Acute Compartment Syndrome. Problems resulting from compartment syndrome include infection, persistent motor weakness in the affected extremity, contracture, and myoglobinuric renal failure. In extreme cases, amputation becomes necessary.

Infection from the necrotic tissue may become severe enough that amputation of the limb is needed. *Motor weakness* from injured nerves is not reversible, and the patient may require an orthotic device for assistance in mobility. Volkmann's *contractures* of the forearm, which can begin within 12 hours of the pressure increase, result from shortening of the ischemic muscle and from nerve involvement.

Myoglobinuric renal failure from muscle breakdown is a potentially fatal complication of compartment syndrome. It occurs when large or multiple compartments are involved. Injured muscle tissues release myoglobulin (muscle protein) into the circulation, where it can clog the renal tubules and cause acute renal failure. Although the exact pathophysiologic mechanisms are unknown, it is suspected that myoglobulin has a direct toxic effect on the kidney. Damaged muscle cells also release potassium, which cannot be excreted because of the renal failure. The resulting hyperkalemia may cause dysrhythmias and cardiac arrest.

Early recognition of the signs and symptoms of ACS can prevent loss of function or loss of a limb. Identify patients who may be at risk, and monitor them closely. ACS can begin in 6 to 8 hours after an injury or take up to 2 days to appear. If it is suspected, notify the health care provider immediately, and if possible, implement interventions to relieve the pressure. For example, for the patient with tight, bulky dressings, loosen the bandage or tape. If the patient has a cast, follow agency protocol about who may cut the cast.

Crush Syndrome

Crush syndrome (CS) occurs from an external crush injury that compresses one or more compartments in the leg, arm, or pelvis. It is a potentially life-threatening, systemic complication that results from hemorrhage and edema after a severe fracture injury. As muscle becomes ischemic and necrotic from pressure within the compartment, myoglobin is released into circulation, where it can occlude the distal renal tubules and result in kidney failure.

Specific causes of CS include:
- Twisting-type injuries
- Natural disasters, such as earthquakes
- Work-related injuries, such as being trapped under heavy equipment such as a car
- Drug or alcohol overdose, when one or more limbs may be compressed by body weight for a prolonged time
- Older adults who fall are unable to get up and lie for a prolonged time

Regardless of the cause, CS is indicated by:
- Acute compartment syndrome
- Hypovolemia (decreased circulating blood volume)
- Hyperkalemia (increased serum potassium)
- **Rhabdomyolysis** (myoglobulin release from skeletal muscle into the bloodstream)
- Acute tubular necrosis (ATN) resulting from hypovolemia and rhabdomyolysis
- Dark brown urine
- Muscle weakness and pain

Assess for signs and symptoms of hypovolemia, hyperkalemia, and compartment syndrome. Management focuses on preventing acute tubular necrosis from myoglobin release and cardiac dysrhythmias related to hyperkalemia. Adequate IV fluids, diuretics, and low-dose dopamine to increase renal perfusion may be prescribed. A urine output of 100 to 200 mL/hr is the desired outcome. Kayexalate may reduce serum potassium adequately, but hemodialysis may be required if potassium levels remain high or kidney failure occurs.

Hypovolemic Shock

Bone is very vascular. Therefore there is a risk for bleeding with bone injury. In addition, trauma can cut nearby arteries and cause hemorrhage, resulting in rapidly developing hypovolemic shock. (The pathophysiology of hypovolemic shock is described in Chapter 39.)

Fat Embolism Syndrome

Fat embolism syndrome (FES) is another serious complication in which fat globules are released from the yellow bone marrow into the bloodstream within 12 to 48 hours after an injury or other illness. These globules clog small blood vessels that supply vital organs, most commonly the lungs, and impair organ perfusion. FES usually results from long bone fractures or fracture repair but occasionally is seen in patients who have a total joint replacement. It may also occur, although less often, in those with pancreatitis, osteomyelitis, blunt trauma, or sickle cell anemia.

The problem can occur at any age or in either gender, but young men between ages 20 and 40 years and older adults between ages 70 and 80 years are at the greatest risk. Patients with fractured hips have the highest risk, but FES is also common in those with fractures of the pelvis.

The earliest manifestation of FES is altered mental status, which is caused by a low arterial oxygen level. Assess for decreased level of consciousness (LOC), such as drowsiness and sleepiness. Monitor the patient for anxiety, respiratory distress, tachycardia, tachypnea, fever, and hemoptysis (bloody sputum). **Petechiae,** a macular, measles-like rash, may appear over the neck, upper arms, or chest and abdomen. This rash is a classic manifestation but can be a late sign.

Monitor laboratory findings, which include:
- Increased erythrocyte sedimentation rate (ESR)
- Decreased serum calcium levels
- Decreased red blood cell and platelet counts
- Increased serum lipase level

These changes in blood values are poorly understood, but they aid in diagnosis of the condition.

FES can result in respiratory failure or death, often from pulmonary edema. When the lungs are affected, the complication may be misdiagnosed as a pulmonary embolism from a blood clot (Chart 54-2). Care of the patient is supportive and

Chart 54-2 KEY FEATURES

Pulmonary Emboli: Fat Embolism Versus Blood Clot Embolism

Fat Embolism	Blood Clot Embolism
DEFINITION	
Obstruction of the pulmonary vascular bed by fat globules	Obstruction of the pulmonary artery by a blood clot or clots
ORIGIN	
95% from fractures of the long bones; occurs usually within 48 hr	85% from deep vein thrombosis in the legs or pelvis; can occur anytime
ASSESSMENT FINDINGS	
Altered mental status (earliest sign) Increased respirations, pulse, temperature Chest pain Dyspnea Crackles Decreased Sao_2 Petechiae (50%-60%) Retinal hemorrhage (not common) Mild thrombocytopenia	Same as for fat embolism, except no petechiae
TREATMENT	
Bedrest Gentle handling Oxygen Hydration (IV fluids) Possibly steroid therapy Fracture immobilization	Preventive measures (e.g., leg exercises, antiembolism stockings, SCDs) Bedrest Oxygen Possibly mechanical ventilation Anticoagulants Thrombolytics Possible surgery: pulmonary embolectomy, vena cava umbrella

Sao_2, Arterial oxygen saturation; *SCD*, sequential compression device.

similar to that for those with pulmonary emboli. Prevention of motion at the fracture site and early immobilization can reduce risk for fat embolism.

Venous Thromboembolism

Venous thromboembolism (VTE) includes deep vein thrombosis (DVT) and its major complication, pulmonary embolism (PE). *It is the most common complication of lower extremity surgery or trauma and the most often fatal complication of musculoskeletal surgery.* Factors that make patients with fractures most likely to develop VTE include:

- Cancer or chemotherapy
- Surgical procedure longer than 30 minutes
- History of smoking
- Obesity
- Heart disease
- Prolonged immobility
- Oral contraceptives or hormones
- History of VTE complications
- Older adults (especially with hip fractures)

A discussion of the prevention, assessment, and management of VTE is found in Chapter 38.

Infection

Whenever there is trauma to tissues, the body's defense system is disrupted. Wound infections are the most common type of infection resulting from orthopedic trauma. They range from superficial skin infections to deep wound abscesses. Infection can also be caused by implanted hardware used to repair a fracture surgically, such as pins, plates, or rods. Clostridial infections can result in gas gangrene or tetanus and can prevent the bone from healing properly.

Bone infection, or **osteomyelitis,** is most common with open fractures in which skin integrity is lost and after surgical repair of a fracture. For patients experiencing this type of trauma, the risk for hospital-acquired infections is increased. These infections are common and many are from multiple-drug resistant organisms, such as methicillin-resistant *Staphylococcus aureus* (MRSA) (Okike & Bhattacharyya, 2006). Reducing MRSA infections is a primary outcome for all health care agencies (www.ihi.org). Chapter 25 discusses the prevention, assessment, and management of infection.

Chronic Complications

Ischemic necrosis and delayed bone healing are later complications of musculoskeletal trauma. *Ischemic necrosis* is sometimes referred to as **aseptic** or **avascular necrosis (AVN)** or **osteonecrosis.** Blood supply to the bone is disrupted, leading to the death of bone tissue. This problem is most often a complication of hip fractures or any fracture in which there is displacement of bone. Surgical repair of fractures also can cause necrosis because the hardware can interfere with circulation. Patients on long-term corticosteroid therapy, such as prednisone, are also at high risk for ischemic necrosis.

Delayed union is a fracture that has not healed within 6 months of injury. Some fractures never achieve union; that is, they never completely heal *(nonunion).* Others heal incorrectly *(malunion).* These problems are most common in patients with tibial fractures, fractures that involve many treatment techniques (e.g., cast, traction), and pathologic fractures. Union may also be delayed or not achieved in the older patient. If bone does not heal, he or she typically has chronic pain and immobility from deformity.

Etiology and Genetic Risk

The primary cause of a fracture is trauma from a motor vehicle crash or fall, especially in older adults. The trauma may be a direct blow to the bone or an indirect force from muscle contractions or pulling forces on the bone. Sports, vigorous exercise, and malnutrition are contributing factors. Bone diseases, such as osteoporosis, increase the risk for a fracture in older adults (see Chapter 53). Genetic factors that increase risk for fracture are discussed with the specific health problems throughout this text.

Incidence/Prevalence

The incidence of fractures depends on the location of the injury. Rib fractures are the most common type in the adult population. Femoral shaft fractures occur most often in young and middle-aged adults. The incidence of proximal femur (hip) fractures is highest in older adults. Humeral fractures are common in adults; the older the person, usually the more proximal is the fracture. Wrist (Colles') fractures are typically seen in middle and late adulthood.

Health Promotion and Maintenance

Airbags and seat belts have decreased the number of severe injuries and deaths, but they have increased the number of leg and ankle fractures, especially in older adults. Encourage people to use seat belts, and support legislation for improved vehicle design and re-evaluation of the federal standards for motor vehicle safety. Health teaching should also focus on other risks for musculoskeletal injury, including:

- Osteoporosis screening and education
- Fall prevention
- Home safety assessment and modification, if needed
- Dangers of drinking and driving
- Drug safety (prescribed, over-the-counter, and illicit)
- Older adults and driving
- Helmet use when riding bicycles, motorcycles, ATVs, and skateboards

These educational interventions are discussed throughout this book and in other texts.

Patient-Centered Collaborative Care evolve ONLINE PHARM REVIEW

Assessment

History

If the patient is in severe pain, delay the interview until he or she is more comfortable. Then, ask about the cause of the fracture, which helps in developing an individualized plan of care. Some type of force, such as incisional, crush, acceleration or deceleration, and shearing and friction, leads to most musculoskeletal injuries. As a result, several body systems are often affected.

Incisional injuries, as from a knife wound, and *crush* injuries cause hemorrhage and decrease blood flow to major organs. *Acceleration or deceleration* injuries cause direct trauma to the spleen, brain, and kidneys when these organs are moved from their fixed locations in the body. *Shearing and friction* damage the skin and cause a high level of wound contamination.

Asking about the events leading to the injury helps identify which forces have been experienced and therefore which body systems or parts of the body to assess. For example, a forward fall often results in Colles' fracture of the wrist because the person tries to catch himself or herself with an outstretched hand. Knowing the mechanism of injury also helps determine whether other types of injury, such as head and spinal cord injury, might be present.

A drug history, including substance abuse, is important regardless of the patient's age. For example, a young adult may have had an excessive amount of alcohol, which contributed to a motor vehicle crash or to a fall at the work site. Many older adults also consume alcohol and an assortment of prescribed and over-the-counter drugs, which can cause dizziness and loss of balance.

A medical history may identify possible causes of the fracture and gives clues as to how long it will take for the bone to heal. Certain diseases such as bone cancer and Paget's disease cause pathologic fractures that often do not achieve total healing or union.

Ask about the patient's occupation and recreational activities. Some occupations are more hazardous than others. For instance, construction work is potentially more physically dangerous than office work. Certain hobbies and recreational activities are also extremely hazardous, such as skiing. Contact sports, such as football and ice hockey, often result in musculoskeletal injuries, including fractures. Other activities do not have such an obvious potential for injury but can cause fractures nonetheless. For instance, daily jogging or running can lead to fatigue fractures. Because inadequate nutrition contributes to fractures and can interfere with bone healing, conduct a nutritional screening. If the patient has nutrition deficits, collaborate with the nutritionist to take a complete history and nutritional assessment.

Physical Assessment/Clinical Manifestations

The patient with a fracture often has trauma to other body systems. Consequently, assess all major body systems *first* for life-threatening complications, including head, chest, and abdominal injuries. The assessment of these areas is described elsewhere in this text.

When inspecting the site of a possible fracture, look for a change in bone alignment. The bone may appear deformed, or a limb may be internally or externally rotated. Observe for extremity shortening or a change in bone shape. Ask the patient to gently move the involved body part or area distal to (below) the injury. *If pain occurs, stop the movement immediately.* When the affected part is moved, assess for crepitus—a grating sound created by bone fragments. Range of motion (ROM) is typically decreased.

If the skin is intact (closed fracture), the area over the fracture may be **ecchymotic** (bruised) from bleeding into the underlying soft tissues. **Subcutaneous emphysema,** the appearance of bubbles under the skin because of air trapping, is not uncommon but is usually seen later.

Swelling at the fracture site is rapid and can result in marked neurovascular compromise. *Perform a thorough neurovascular assessment, and compare extremities. Assess skin color and temperature, sensation, mobility, pain, and pulses distal to the fracture site. If the fracture involves an extremity, check the nails for capillary refill by applying pressure to the nail and observing for the speed of blood return. If nails are brittle or thick, assess the skin next to the nail. Checking for capillary refill is not as reliable as other indicators of perfusion.* Chart 54-3 describes the proce-

Chart 54-3 BEST PRACTICE FOR PATIENT SAFETY & QUALITY CARE

Assessment of Neurovascular Status in Patients with Musculoskeletal Injury

Assessment Technique	Normal Findings
SKIN COLOR	
Inspect the area distal to the injury.	No change in pigmentation compared with other parts of the body.
SKIN TEMPERATURE	
Palpate the area distal to the injury (the dorsum of the hands is most sensitive to temperature).	The skin is warm.
MOVEMENT	
Ask the patient to move the affected area or the area distal to the injury (active motion).	The patient can move without discomfort.
Move the area distal to the injury (passive motion).	No difference in comfort compared with active movement.
SENSATION	
Ask the patient if numbness or tingling is present (paresthesia).	No numbness or tingling.
Palpate with a paper clip (especially the web space between the first and second toes or the web space between the thumb and forefinger).	No difference in sensation in the affected and unaffected extremities. (Loss of sensation in these areas indicates peroneal nerve or median nerve damage.)
PULSES	
Palpate the pulses distal to the injury.	Pulses are strong and easily palpated; no difference in the affected and unaffected extremities.
CAPILLARY REFILL (LEAST RELIABLE)	
Press the nail beds distal to the injury until blanching occurs (or the skin near the nail if nails are thick and brittle).	Blood returns (return to usual color) within 3 sec (5 sec for older patients).
PAIN	
Ask the patient about the location, nature, and frequency of the pain.	Pain is usually localized and is often described as stabbing or throbbing. (Pain out of proportion to the injury and unrelieved by analgesics might indicate compartment syndrome.)

dure for a neurovascular assessment, which evaluates circulation, **m**ovement, and sensation (CMS function).

For an open fracture, determine the degree of soft-tissue damage and the amount of bleeding. *The area may be lightly palpated for tenderness, but wear a sterile glove if the skin is broken.*

Patients often report moderate to severe pain at the site of the fracture or in an adjacent or distal area. *For example, those with a fractured hip may have groin pain or pain referred to the back of the knee.* Pain is usually due to muscle spasm and edema, which result from the fracture. In patients with one or more fractured ribs, severe pain occurs when deep breaths are taken. Assess respiratory status, which may be severely compromised from pain or pneumothorax (air in the pleural cavity).

For fractures of the shoulder and upper arm, the physical assessment is best done with the patient in a sitting or standing position, if possible, so that shoulder drooping or other abnormal positioning can be seen. Support the affected arm and flex the elbow to promote comfort during the assessment. For more distal areas of the arm, perform the assessment with the patient in a supine position so that the extremity can be elevated to reduce swelling.

Place the patient in a supine position for assessment of the legs and pelvis. A patient with an impacted hip fracture may be able to walk for a short time after injury, although this is not recommended.

Some fractures can cause internal organ damage resulting in hemorrhage. When a pelvic fracture is suspected, assess vital signs, skin color, and the level of consciousness for indications of possible hypovolemic shock. Check the urine for blood, which indicates damage to the urinary system, often the bladder. If the patient cannot void, suspect that the bladder or urethra has been damaged.

DECISION-MAKING CHALLENGE
Coordination of Care

A 30-year-old man arrives at the emergency department via ambulance. He was the driver of a motorcycle involved in a collision with an SUV. Paramedics report that the patient was hit from the side. The bike fell on him, and he was trapped underneath the vehicle. Initial reports from the ambulance en route describe a person in shock with a mangled left leg below the knee and a left wrist fracture. The patient was wearing a helmet at the time of the crash.

1. What information given above is helpful in predicting other injuries this patient may have?
2. What are the priority assessments you should perform when he arrives at the hospital?
3. With what aspects of care for this patient can you ask the emergency department technician to assist? With what other members of the health care team should you collaborate?
4. What initial assessments of the injured leg should you perform?

evolve For suggested answer guidelines, go to http://evolve.elsevier.com/Iggy/.

Psychosocial Assessment

The psychosocial status of a patient with a fracture depends on the extent of the injury and other complications. Hospitalization is not required for a single, uncomplicated fracture, and the patient returns to usual daily activities within a few days.

In contrast, a patient suffering multiple traumas may be hospitalized for weeks and may undergo many surgical procedures, treatments, and prolonged rehabilitation. These disruptions in lifestyle can create a high level of stress.

The stresses that result from a chronic condition affect relationships between the patient and family members or friends. Assess their feelings, and ask about how they coped with previously experienced stressful events. Body image and sexuality may be altered by deformity, treatment modalities for fracture repair, or long-term immobilization.

Laboratory Assessment

No special laboratory tests are available for assessment of fractures. Hemoglobin and hematocrit levels may often be low because of bleeding caused by the injury. If extensive soft-tissue damage is present, the erythrocyte sedimentation rate (ESR) may be elevated, which indicates the expected inflammatory response. If this value increases during fracture healing, the patient may have a bone infection. During the healing stages, serum calcium and phosphorus levels are often increased as the bone releases these elements into the blood.

Imaging Assessment

The health care provider requests standard x-rays and tomograms to confirm a diagnosis of fracture. These reveal the bone disruption, malalignment, or deformity. If the x-ray film does not show a fracture but the patient is symptomatic, the x-ray is usually repeated with additional views.

The computed tomography (CT) scan is useful in detecting fractures of complex structures, such as the hip and pelvis. It also identifies compression fractures of the spine. Magnetic resonance imaging (MRI) is useful in determining the amount of soft-tissue damage that may have occurred with the fracture. It is also very helpful in visualizing AVN.

▪ *Analysis*

Common Nursing Diagnoses and Collaborative Problems

The priority nursing diagnoses for patients with fractures are:

1. Risk for Peripheral Neurovascular Dysfunction related to fractures (bone and soft-tissue trauma)
2. Acute Pain related to biologic injury (bone disruption, soft-tissue damage, muscle spasm, and edema)
3. Risk for Infection related to trauma
4. Impaired Physical Mobility related to pain
5. Imbalanced Nutrition: Less Than Body Requirements related to additional metabolic need for healing of bone and soft tissues

Additional Nursing Diagnoses and Collaborative Problems

In addition to the common nursing diagnoses, patients with fractures may have one or more of these diagnoses:

- Activity Intolerance related to pain and impaired mobility
- Constipation related to opioids and prolonged immobility (particularly in older adults)
- Ineffective Coping related to prolonged immobility, hospitalization, or lifestyle changes
- Compromised Family Coping related to prolonged hospitalization or lifestyle changes
- Self-Care Deficit related to pain and immobility
- Disturbed Body Image related to deformity and/or treatment modality
- Sexual Dysfunction related to pain and immobility
- Sleep Deprivation related to chronic pain or prolonged hospitalization

- Fear related to possible nursing home placement or death (particularly in older adults)
- Impaired Skin Integrity and Impaired Tissue Integrity related to bone injury and immobility

The collaborative problems that may apply for patients with *severe* fractures include:

- Potential for Acute Compartment Syndrome
- Potential for Hypovolemic Shock
- Potential for Fat Embolism Syndrome
- Potential for Venous Thromboembolism
- Potential for Ischemic Necrosis
- Potential for Delayed Healing, Malunion, or Nonunion

Planning and Implementation

Risk for Peripheral Neurovascular Dysfunction

NOC **Planning: Expected Outcomes.** The patient with a fracture is expected to have adequate blood flow through the small vessels of the extremities to maintain tissue function. Indicators include that the patient will have normal:

- Capillary refill
- Sensation
- Skin color
- Muscle function
- Extremity skin color
- Pedal pulses

Interventions. A fracture can happen anywhere and may be accompanied by multiple injuries to vital organs. Collaborative management of the patient depends on the severity and extent of the injury and the number of fractures the patient has.

Emergency Care: Fracture. *For any patient who experiences trauma in the community, first call 911 and assess for airway, breathing, and circulation (ABCs, or primary survey). Then provide lifesaving care if needed before being concerned about the fracture.*

After a head-to-toe assessment (secondary survey), assess the fracture injury (Chart 54-4). If the person is clothed, cut away clothing from the fracture site, and remove any jewelry from the affected extremity. Control bleeding by direct pressure on the area and digital pressure over the artery above the fracture. At the same time, to prevent shock, place the patient in a supine position and keep him or her warm.

In collaboration with the 911 emergency team:

- Inspect the fracture site for intactness of skin, swelling, and deformity (e.g., shortening and rotation)
- Palpate the area *lightly* to determine temperature (coolness), decreased sensation, and blanching
- Assess distal pulses by comparing affected and unaffected extremities, if applicable
- Assess for motor function by asking the patient to move an area below the fracture. For example, if a femur fracture is suspected, ask him or her to move the ankle and foot on the affected side; the upper portion of the leg should remain still.

To prevent further damage, reduce pain, and increase circulation, the emergency team immobilizes the area of the fracture by splinting. Any object or device that extends to the joints above and below the fracture to immobilize it can be used as a **splint.** Sterile gauze is placed loosely over open areas to prevent further contamination of the wound. Neurovascular assessment is rechecked after splinting.

In the emergency department, physician's office, or urgent care center, fracture management begins with reduction and immobilization of the fracture:

- Reduction, or realignment of the bone ends, for proper healing, is accomplished by a closed method (e.g., cast) or an open (surgical) procedure.
- Immobilization is achieved by the use of bandages, casts, traction, internal fixation, or external fixation.

The health care provider selects the treatment method on the basis of the type, location, and extent of the fracture. These interventions prevent further injury and reduce discomfort.

Nonsurgical Management. Nonsurgical management includes closed reduction and immobilization with a bandage, splint, cast, or traction. *For each modality, the primary nursing concern is assessment and prevention of neurovascular dysfunction or compromise* (Chart 54-5). Assess the patient's neuro-

Chart 54-4 BEST PRACTICE FOR PATIENT SAFETY & QUALITY CARE

Emergency Care of the Patient with an Extremity Fracture

EMERGENCY CARE

1. Assess the patient's airway, breathing, and circulation and perform a quick head-to-toe assessment.
2. Remove the patient's clothing (cut if necessary) to inspect the affected area while supporting the area above and below the injury. Do not remove shoes because this can cause increased trauma.
3. Remove jewelry on the affected extremity in case of swelling.
5. Apply direct pressure on the area if there is bleeding and pressure over the proximal artery nearest the fracture.
5. Keep the patient warm and in a supine position.
6. Check the neurovascular status of the area distal to the extremity: temperature, color, sensation, movement, and capillary refill. Compare affected and unaffected limbs.
7. Immobilize the extremity by splinting; include joints above and below the fracture site. Recheck circulation after splinting.
8. Cover any open areas with a dressing (preferably sterile).

Chart 54-5 NIC INTERVENTION ACTIVITIES

The Patient at Risk for Peripheral Neurovascular Dysfunction

Circulatory Care (Arterial Insufficiency/Venous Insufficiency): *Promotion of arterial and venous circulation*

- Perform a comprehensive appraisal of peripheral circulations (e.g., check peripheral pulses, edema, capillary refill, color, and temperature).
- Monitor degree of discomfort or pain.
- Protect the extremity from injury.
- Place extremity in a dependent position, as appropriate.

Peripheral Sensation Management: *Prevention or minimization of injury or discomfort in the patient with altered sensation*

- Monitor for paresthesia: numbness, tingling, hyperesthesia, and hypoesthesia.
- Monitor fit of bracing devices, prostheses, shoes, and clothing.
- Administer analgesics, as necessary.
- Discuss or identify causes of abnormal sensations or sensation changes.

NIC intervention activities selected from Bulechek, G.M., Butcher, H.K., & McCloskey Dochterman, J. (Eds.). (2008). *Nursing interventions classification (NIC)* (5th ed.). St. Louis: Mosby.

vascular status every hour for the first 24 hours and every 1 to 4 hours thereafter, depending on the injury (see Chart 54-3). The patient usually reports discomfort that is unrelieved by analgesics if the bandage, splint, or cast is too tight. Elevate the fractured extremity higher than the heart, and apply ice for the first 24 to 48 hours as needed to reduce edema.

Closed reduction. Closed reduction is the most common nonsurgical method for managing a simple fracture. While applying a manual pull, or traction, on the bone, the health care provider moves the bone ends so that they realign. Anesthesia or analgesia is typically used during this procedure to decrease pain. An x-ray shows that the bone ends are approximated (aligned) before the bone is immobilized.

Bandages and splints. For certain areas of the body, such as the scapula (shoulder) and clavicle (collarbone), an elastic bandage or commercial immobilizer may be used to keep the bone in place during healing. Because upper extremity bones do not bear weight, splints may be sufficient to keep bone fragments in place for a closed fracture. Fig. 54-3 shows a wrist splint for fracture immobilization. Thermoplastic, a durable, flexible material for splinting, allows custom fitting to the patient's body part.

Casts. For more complex fractures or fractures of the lower extremity, the physician or orthopedic technician applies a cast to hold bone fragments in place after reduction. A **cast** is a rigid device that immobilizes the affected body part while allowing other body parts to move. It also allows early mobility and reduces pain. Although its most common use is for fractures, a cast may be applied for correction of deformities (e.g., clubfoot) or for prevention of deformities (e.g., those seen in some patients with rheumatoid arthritis).

Several types of materials are used to make casts. The traditional plaster-of-Paris cast requires application of a well-fitted stockinette under the material. If the stockinette is too tight, it may impair circulation. If it is too loose, wrinkles can lead to the development of pressure ulcers. Padding is applied over the stockinette, followed by wet plaster rolls wrapped around the extremity or other body part. The cast feels hot because an immediate chemical reaction occurs, but it soon becomes damp and cool. This type of cast takes 24 to 72 hours to dry, depending on the size and location of the cast. A wet cast feels cold, smells musty, and is grayish. The cast is dry when it feels hard and firm, is odorless, and has a shiny white appearance.

On occasion, the plaster cast may have rough edges, which can crumble and cause skin irritation. *Petaling* the cast resolves this problem if the underlying stockinette does not cover the edges of the cast. Small strips of tape are placed over the rough edges to protect the skin. If the skin under the cast is open, the health care provider, orthopedic technician, or specially trained nurse cuts a window into the cast so that the wound can be observed and cared for. The piece of cast removed to make the window must be retained and replaced after wound care to prevent localized edema in the area. This is most important when a window is cut from a cast on an extremity. Tape or elastic bandage wrap may be used to keep the "window" in place. A window is also an access for taking pulses, removing wound drains, or preventing abdominal distention when the patient is in a body or spica cast.

If the cast is too tight, it may be cut with a cast cutter to relieve pressure or allow tissue swelling. The health care provider may choose to bivalve the cast (i.e., cut it lengthwise into two equal pieces) if bone healing is almost complete. Either half of the cast can be removed for inspection or for provision of care. The two halves are then held in place by an elastic bandage wrap.

Synthetic materials for casts include fiberglass and polyester-cotton knit (Fig. 54-4). These materials are lighter than plaster and require minimal drying time. Fiberglass casts are dry in 10 to 15 minutes and can bear weight 30 minutes after application. Polyester-cotton knit casts take 7 minutes to dry and can withstand weight bearing in about 20 minutes. Some health care providers use synthetic casts for upper extremities and plaster-of-Paris casts for lower extremities because plaster casts can bear more weight for a longer time. However, synthetic casts are used much more commonly overall.

Casts can be generally divided into four main groups: arm casts, leg casts, cast braces, and body or spica casts. Table 54-1 describes specific casts that are used for various parts of the body.

When a patient is in bed with an *arm cast,* teach him or her to elevate the arm above the heart to reduce swelling. The hand should be higher than the elbow. Ice may be prescribed for the first 24 to 48 hours. When the patient is out of bed, the arm is supported with a sling placed around the neck to alleviate fatigue caused by the weight of the cast. The sling should distribute the weight over a large area of the shoulders and trunk, not just the neck. Some health care providers prefer that the patient not use a sling after the first few days in an arm cast, particularly a short-arm cast. This encourages normal movement of the mobile joints and enhances bone healing.

A *leg cast* allows mobility and requires the patient to use ambulatory aids such as crutches. A cast shoe, sandal, or boot

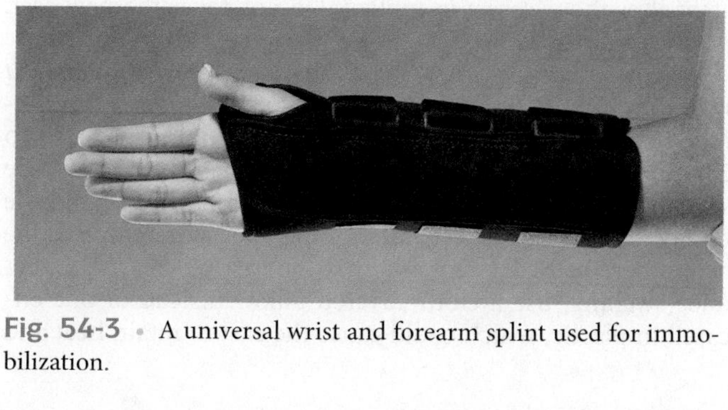

Fig. 54-3 • A universal wrist and forearm splint used for immobilization.

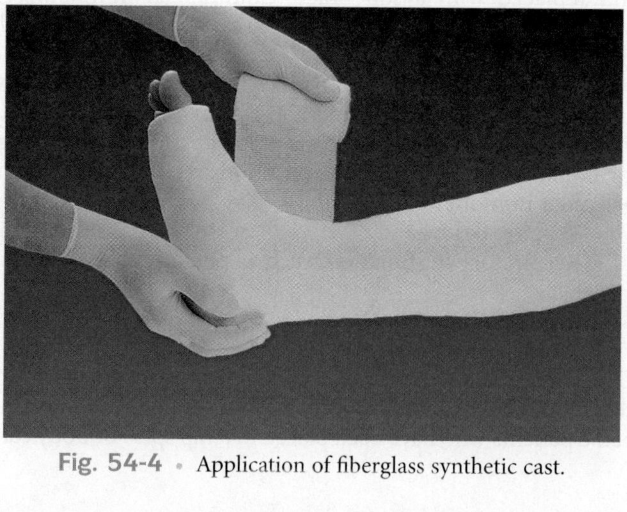

Fig. 54-4 • Application of fiberglass synthetic cast.

TABLE 54-1 Types of Casts Used for Musculoskeletal Trauma

Type and Characteristics of Cast	Use
UPPER EXTREMITY CASTS	
Short-arm cast (SAC) (extends from below the elbow to and including part of the hand)	Stable fractures of the wrist (metacarpals, carpals, or distal radius)
Long-arm cast (LAC) (includes the upper arm to and including part of the hand)	Unstable fractures of the wrist, distal humerus, radius, or ulna
Hanging-arm cast (same as LAC but heavier, with added loop at the mid-forearm)	Fractures of the humerus that cannot be aligned by LAC (light traction is possible while the patient is in bed or by an attached strap that extends around the neck)
Thumb spica (gauntlet) cast (similar to SAC with the thumb casted in abduction)	Fractures of the thumb
Shoulder spica cast (the shoulder is casted in abduction with the elbow flexed)	Unstable fractures of the shoulder girdle or humerus; dislocations of the shoulder
LOWER EXTREMITY CASTS	
Short-leg cast (SLC) (from below the knee to the base of the toes)	Fractures of the ankle, metatarsals, or foot
Long-leg cast (LLC) (from the mid-upper thigh to the base of the toes)	Unstable fractures of the tibia, fibula, or ankle
Walking cast (a walking device on the bottom of SLC or LLC)	Same as for SLC or LLC
Leg cylinder (similar to SLC, but the ankle and foot are not casted)	Stable fractures of the tibia, fibula, or knee
Long-leg cylinder (similar to LLC, but the ankle and foot are not casted)	Stable fractures of the distal femur, proximal tibia, or knee
CAST BRACES (OR BRACE CASTS)	
Patellar weight-bearing cast (similar to SLC or leg cylinder)	Mid-shaft or distal shaft fractures of the femur
External polycentric knee hinge cast (a hinge connects the lower and upper leg and allows 90 degrees of knee flexion)	Same as for the patellar weight-bearing cast
BODY CASTS	
Hip spica (extends from below the nipple line down the affected leg [single], down the leg and half of the unaffected leg [1 1/2], or down both legs [double])	Dislocation of the hip; pelvic or hip injuries
Risser cast (the body jacket extends from the shoulders to beyond the iliac crests and hips, with a large opening over the anterior chest)	Scoliosis; thoracic spinal fractures
Halo cast (the body jacket contains a halo brace)	Fractures of the cervical spine

that attaches to the foot or a rubber walking pad attached to the sole of the cast assists in ambulation (if weight bearing is allowed) and helps prevent damage to the cast. Teach the patient to elevate the affected leg on several pillows to reduce swelling, and apply ice for the first 24 hours or as prescribed.

A *cast brace* allows the patient to bend unaffected joints while the fracture is healing. The fracture must show signs of healing and little tissue edema before this cast is applied. Two cylindric casts are made and connected by a hinge to allow joint movement. As healing occurs, the casts may be removed and replaced with a soft brace. Commercial immobilizers, which serve the same function as a cast brace, are available and are often used instead.

A *body cast* encircles the trunk of the body. A **spica cast** encases a portion of the trunk and one or two extremities. A patient with either of these casts presents a special challenge for nursing care. Potential complications related to severe impairment in mobility include:

- Skin breakdown
- Respiratory dysfunction, such as pneumonia and atelectasis
- Constipation
- Joint contractures

Cast syndrome (superior mesenteric artery syndrome), an uncommon but serious complication, is most often seen in orthopedic patients who have been placed in a hip spica or body cast. Partial or complete upper intestinal obstruction results in classic symptoms: abdominal distention, epigastric pain, nausea, and vomiting. The vomiting often occurs after meals, and patients may have normal bowel sounds. Partial obstruction occurs initially from compression of the third portion of the duodenum between the superior mesenteric artery and the aorta. This can progress to complete obstruction from duodenal edema caused by continued vomiting and distention. Placing a window in the abdominal portion of the cast or bivalving the cast may be sufficient to prevent or relieve pressure on the duodenum. Management of intestinal obstruction is the same as for any patient with this complication.

Cast care. Before the cast is applied, explain the purpose of the cast and the procedure for its application. With a plaster cast, warn the patient about the heat that will be felt immediately after the wet cast is applied. Do not cover the new cast. Allow for air-drying.

When moving a patient with a wet plaster cast, handle it with the palms of the hands to prevent indentations and resulting areas of pressure on the skin. Turn him or her every 1 to 2 hours to allow air to circulate and dry all parts of the cast. Be sure to remind unlicensed assistive personnel (UAP) and the family that the cast is wet and requires special handling. If the health care provider requests that the cast be elevated to reduce swelling, use a cloth-covered pillow instead of one encased in plastic, which could cause the cast to retain heat and prevent drying. Elevation of the casted extremity reduces edema but may impair arterial circulation to the affected limb. Therefore neurovascular assessment of the limb distal to (below) the cast is very important.

For preventing contamination by urine or feces, the perineal area of a dry long-leg or body cast may be covered in plastic. Fracture pans are preferred over traditional bedpans because they are smaller and more comfortable. Remind UAP to take care to prevent spillage onto the cast.

Check to ensure that the cast is not too tight, and frequently monitor neurovascular status, usually every hour for the first 24 hours after application if the patient is hospitalized. You should be able to insert a finger between the cast and the skin. Ice may be applied for the first 24 to 36 hours to reduce swelling and inflammation.

Once the plaster cast is dry, inspect it at least once every 8 hours for drainage, cracking, crumbling, alignment, and fit. Plaster casts act like sponges and absorb drainage, whereas synthetic casts act like a wick pulling drainage away from the drainage site. Padding can also absorb wound drainage. Document in the medical record drainage on any cast. However, sources disagree on whether drainage should be circled on the cast because it may increase anxiety and is not a reliable indicator of drainage amount. *Immediately report to the health care provider any sudden increases in the amount of drainage or change in the integrity of the cast.* After swelling decreases, it is not uncommon for the cast to become too loose and need replacement. If the patient is not admitted to the hospital, provide instructions regarding cast care.

Cast complications. During hospitalization, assess for other complications resulting from casting that can be serious and life threatening, such as infection, circulation impairment, and peripheral nerve damage. If the patient returns home after cast application, teach him or her how to monitor for these complications and when to notify the health care provider.

Infection most often results from the breakdown of skin under the cast (pressure necrosis). If pressure necrosis occurs, the patient typically reports a very painful "hot spot" under the cast and the cast may feel warmer in the affected area. Teach the patient or family to smell the area for mustiness or an unpleasant odor that would indicate infected material. If the infection progresses, a fever may develop.

Circulation impairment and *peripheral nerve damage* can result from tightness of the cast. Teach the patient to assess for circulation at least daily, including the ability to move the area distal to the extremity, numbness, and increased pain.

The patient with a cast may be immobilized for a prolonged period, depending on the extent of the fracture and the type of cast. Assess for complications of immobility, such as skin breakdown, pneumonia, atelectasis, thromboembolism, and constipation. Before the cast is removed, inform the patient that the cast cutter will not injure the skin but that heat may be felt during the procedure.

Because of prolonged immobilization, a joint may become contracted, usually in a fixed state of flexion. Osteoarthritis and osteoporosis may develop from lack of weight bearing. Muscle can also atrophy from lack of exercise during prolonged immobilization of the affected body part, usually an extremity.

Traction. Traction is the application of a pulling force to a part of the body to provide reduction, alignment, and rest. It is also used to decrease muscle spasm (thus relieving pain) and prevent or correct deformity and tissue damage. A patient in traction is usually hospitalized, but in some cases, home care is possible even for skeletal traction.

Mechanical traction can be either:

- Continuous, as in fracture treatment
- Intermittent, for relief of muscle spasm in other types of musculoskeletal/neurologic trauma, such as cervical nerve root compression

Traction may also be classified as running traction or balanced suspension. In *running* traction, the pulling force is in one direction and the patient's body acts as countertraction. Moving the body or bed position can alter the countertraction force. *Balanced suspension* provides the countertraction so that the pulling force of the traction is not altered when the bed or patient is moved. This allows for increased movement and facilitates care.

Traction is typically one of five types: skin traction, skeletal traction, plaster traction, brace traction, or circumferential traction. *Skin traction* involves the use of a Velcro boot (Buck's traction) (Fig. 54-5), belt, or halter, which is usually secured around the affected leg. The primary purpose of skin traction is to decrease painful muscle spasms that accompany fractures. The weight is used as a pulling force and is limited to 5 to 10 pounds (2.3 to 4.5 kg) to prevent injury to the skin.

In *skeletal traction,* pins, wires, tongs (e.g., Crutchfield), or screws are surgically inserted directly into bone. These allow the use of longer traction time and heavier weights—usually 15 to 30 pounds (6.8 to 13.6 kg). Skeletal traction aids in bone realignment. Pin site care is an important part of nursing management to prevent infection.

Plaster traction combines skeletal traction and a plaster cast. A *brace traction* device exerts a pull for correction of alignment deformities. *Circumferential traction* uses a belt around the body, such as pelvic traction for low back problems. Table 54-2 describes commonly used types of traction for various parts of the body.

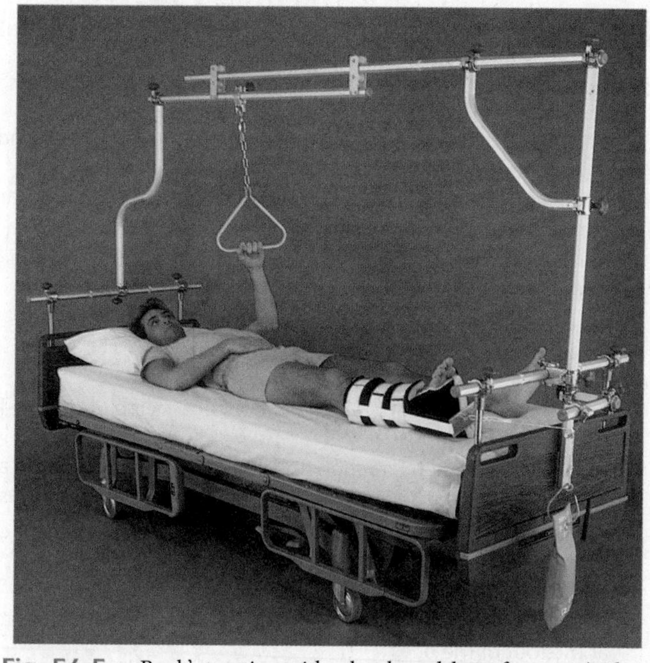

Fig. 54-5 • Buck's traction with a hook-and-loop fastener (Velcro) boot, commonly used for hip fractures.

The nurse may set up or assist in the setup of traction if specially educated. In larger or specialty hospitals or units, orthopedic technicians or physician's assistants often set up traction. Once traction is applied, maintain the correct balance between traction pull and countertraction force. *Weights usually are not removed without a prescription. They should not be lifted manually or allowed to rest on the floor. Weights should be freely hanging at all times. Teach this important point to UAP on the unit, to other personnel such as those in the radiology department, and visitors.*

Inspect the skin at least every 8 hours for signs of irritation or inflammation. When possible, remove the belt or boot that is used for skin traction every 8 hours to inspect under the device.

Check traction equipment frequently to ensure its proper functioning. Inspect all ropes, knots, and pulleys at least every 8 to 12 hours for loosening, fraying, and positioning. Check the weight for consistency with the health care provider's prescription. Sometimes one of the weights is accidentally removed by a staff member or visitor who bumps into it. Replace the weights if they are not correct, and notify the health care provider or orthopedic technician.

If the patient reports severe pain from muscle spasm, the weights may be too heavy or the patient may need realignment. Report the pain to the health care provider if body realignment fails to reduce the discomfort. Assess neurovascular status of the affected body part to detect circulatory compromise and tissue damage. The circulation is usually monitored every hour for the first 24 hours after traction is applied and every 4 hours thereafter.

NCLEX EXAMINATION CHALLENGE

A client is transferred from the operating suite with an external fixator for a compound tibial fracture that has been débrided. He is receiving IV antibiotic therapy and morphine by a PCA pump. Which nursing action is the most important for this client?

A. Monitoring for signs of inflammation and infection
B. Performing frequent neurovascular assessments
C. Teaching the client how to do leg exercises
D. Keeping the affected leg elevated on a pillow

evolve For the correct answer, go to http://evolve.elsevier.com/Iggy/.

Surgical Management. For some types of fractures, closed reduction is not appropriate or sufficient. Surgical intervention may be needed to realign the bone for the healing process.

Preoperative care. For stabilizing the fracture, the patient may be placed in traction before surgery. This procedure is typical for managing a fractured hip when Buck's traction is used (see Fig. 54-5). Teach the patient and family what to expect during and after the surgery. The preoperative care for a patient undergoing musculoskeletal surgery is similar to that for anyone having surgery with general or epidural anesthesia. (See Chapter 16 for a thorough discussion of preoperative nursing care.)

Operative procedures. Open reduction with internal fixation (ORIF) is one of the most common methods of reducing and immobilizing a fracture. External fixation with closed reduction is used when patients have soft tissue injury (open fracture). Although nurses do not decide which surgical technique is used, understanding the procedures enhances patient teaching and care.

Because ORIF permits early mobilization, it is often the preferred surgical method for an older adult who is susceptible to the complications of immobility. **Open reduction** allows the surgeon to directly view the fracture site. **Internal fixation** uses metal pins, screws, rods, plates, or prostheses to immobilize the fracture during healing. The surgeon makes an incision to gain access to the broken bone and implants one or more devices into bone tissue.

After the bone achieves union, the metal hardware may be removed, depending on the location and type of fracture. Hardware is removed most frequently in ankle fractures, depending on the severity of the injury. Specific types of internal

TABLE 54-2 Types of Traction Used for Musculoskeletal Trauma

Type and Characteristics of Traction	Use
UPPER EXTREMITY TRACTION	
Sidearm skin or skeletal traction (the forearm is flexed and extended 90 degrees from the upper part of the body)	Fractures of the humerus with or without involvement of the shoulder and clavicle
Overhead or 90-90 traction, skin or skeletal (the elbow is flexed and the arm is at a right angle to the body over the upper chest)	Same as above (depends on the physician's preference)
Plaster traction (pins inserted through the bone are fixed in the cast)	Fractures of the wrist
LOWER EXTREMITY TRACTION	
Buck's extension traction (skin) (the affected leg is in extension)	Fractures of the hip or femur preoperatively Prevention of hip flexion contractures Hip dislocation
Russell's traction (similar to Buck's traction, but a sling under the knee suspends the leg)	Fractures of the hip or end of the femur
Balanced skin or skeletal traction (the limb is usually elevated in a Thomas splint with Pearson's attachment, or a Böhler-Braun splint is used)	Fractures of the femur or pelvis (acetabulum)
SPINAL COLUMN AND PELVIC TRACTION	
Cervical halter (a strap under the chin)	Cervical muscle spasms, strain/sprain, or arthritis
Cervical skeletal (e.g., halo brace, Crutchfield tongs)	Cervical fractures of the spine; muscle spasms
Pelvic belt (a strap around the hips at the iliac crests is attached to weights at the foot of the bed)	Pain, strain, sprain, or muscle spasms in the lower back
Pelvic sling (a wide strap around the hips is attached to an overhead bar to keep the pelvis off the bed)	Pelvic fractures; other pelvic injuries

fixation devices are discussed later in the Fractures of Specific Sites section.

An alternative modality for the management of fractures is the external fixation apparatus, as shown in Fig. 54-6. **External fixation** is a system in which pins or wires are inserted through the skin and affected bone and then connected to a rigid external frame. The system may be used for upper or lower extremity fractures or for fractures of the pelvis. After a fixator is removed, the patient may be placed in a cast until healing is complete.

External fixation has several advantages over other surgical techniques:

- There is minimal blood loss in comparison with internal fixation.
- The device allows early ambulation and exercise of the affected body part while relieving pain.
- The device maintains alignment in closed fractures that will not maintain position in a cast and stabilizes comminuted fractures that require bone grafting.

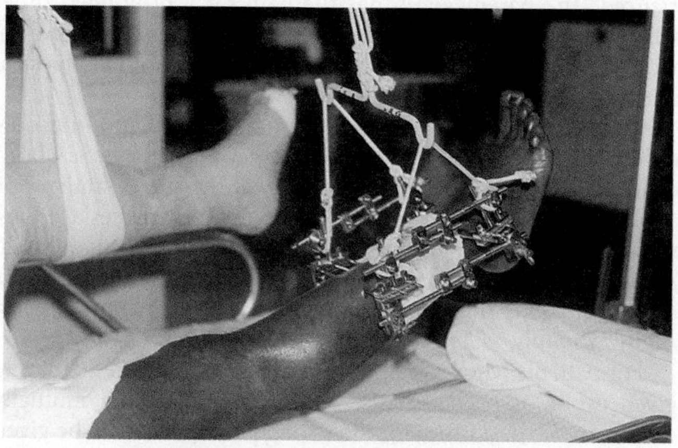

Fig. 54-6 • The Hex-Fix external fixations system for tibia-fibula fractures.

In open fractures, in which skin and tissue trauma accompany the fracture, the device permits easy access to the wound while the bone heals. This method is often preferred over the use of a window in a cast for wound care.

A disadvantage of external fixation is an increased risk for pin site infection. Pin site infections can lead to osteomyelitis, which is serious and difficult to treat (see Chapter 53).

Postoperative care. For patients with an **external fixator,** pay particular attention to the pin sites for signs of inflammation or infection. In the first 48 to 72 hours, *clear* fluid drainage or weeping is expected. Although no standardized method or evidence-based protocol for pin care has been established, recommendations have been made based on the evidence available regarding pin site care. (See the Evidence-Based Practice box below.) Because the pins go through the skin and into bone, the risk for infection is high. Monitor the pin sites at least every 8 to 12 hours for drainage, color, odor, and severe redness, which indicate inflammation and possible infection. Follow agency policy for how to clean the pin site areas, and ensure that it follows the evidence-based guidelines from the National Association of Orthopaedic Nurses (www.naon.org) (Holmes & Brown, 2005).

The patient with an external fixator may have a disturbed body image. The frame may be large and bulky, and the affected area may have massive tissue damage with dressings. Be sensitive to this possibility in planning care. Teach about alterations to clothing that may be required while the fixator is in place.

The Ilizarov technique of circular external fixation is sometimes used to treat new fractures (closed, comminuted fractures and open fractures with bone loss), as well as malunion or nonunion of fractures. It may also be used to treat congenital bone deformities, especially in children.

EVIDENCE-BASED PRACTICE

Improving patient outcomes with pin site care

Holmes, S.B., & Brown, S.J. (2005). Skeletal pin site care: National Association of Orthopaedic Nurses' guidelines for orthopaedic nursing. *Orthopaedic Nursing, 24*(2), 99-107.

This study examined the current literature available concerning methods of pin site care. The purposes of the study were to find as much objective evidence as possible from the studies available regarding pin site care and to describe the level of evidence for recommendations. After systematic review of the literature, the opinions of an expert panel offered four recommendations for skeletal pin site care:

- Pins located in areas of considerable soft tissue should be considered at greater risk for infection.
- After the first 48 to 72 hours, when drainage is the heaviest, pin site care can be done daily or weekly for sites where the pin is very stable in the bone.
- Chlorhexidine 2 mg/mL solution may be the most effective cleansing solution for pin site care.
- Patients and families must be taught pin site care before discharge from the hospital. They should demonstrate the pin site care and be given written instructions for pin site care at home.

Level of Evidence—4. This study is an example of a well-conducted systematic review of literature including randomized control studies and retrospective and prospective case studies from which guidelines were established.

Commentary: Implications for Practice and Research. Only seven studies in the past 10 years were found. Two of those were randomized control studies and the remaining five were prospective or retrospective studies for a total of over 1000 pin sites examined. For many of the considerations in pin site care, there were not enough studies to make a recommendation.

Nurses play an important role in prevention of problems of infection at pin sites. Monitoring pin sites and using the above recommendations can help reduce infection. Teaching patients and families the importance of monitoring and care to pin sites can reduce pin site infection.

The circular external fixation device is used to gently pull apart the cortex of the bone and stimulate new bone growth. Unlike the traditional fixator, the Ilizarov external fixator promotes rotation, angulation, lengthening, or widening of bone to correct bony defects and allows for healing of any soft-tissue defect. The nursing care associated with this device is similar to the care of the patient with other external fixation systems with one major exception. If the device is being used for filling bone gaps using bone transport or distraction, teach the patient how to manually turn the four-sided nuts (also called *clickers*) up to four times a day. Daily distraction rates vary, but 1 mm daily is common. Screening and teaching are particularly important because the patient adjusts and cares for the apparatus over a long period of up to 6 months to 1 year. Pain control is a priority outcome for patients using this device.

The postoperative care for a patient undergoing ORIF or external fixation is similar to that provided for any patient undergoing surgery (see Chapter 18). Because bone is a vascular, dynamic body tissue, the patient is at risk for complications specific to fractures and musculoskeletal surgery. Interventions for preventing and detecting these problems (e.g., fat embolism, venous thromboembolism) were discussed on p. 1180 in the Complications of Fractures section. Additional information about postoperative care is found beginning on p. 1195 in the Fractures of Specific Sites section.

Procedures for Nonunion. Some management techniques are not successful because the bone does not heal. Several additional options are available to the physician to promote bone union, such as electrical bone stimulation, bone grafting, and ultrasound fracture treatment.

For selected patients, *electrical bone stimulation* may be successful. This procedure is based on research showing that bone has electrical properties that are used in healing. The exact mechanism of action is unknown. Several types of devices have been developed. A noninvasive **electrical bone stimulation** system uses magnetic coils applied on the skin or over a cast to deliver a pulsed magnetic field. There are no known risks with this system, although patients with pacemakers cannot use this device on an arm. Implanted direct-current stimulators are placed directly in the fracture site and have no external apparatus. Both systems require about 6 months of treatment, and weight bearing is at the discretion of the health care provider.

Another method of treating nonunion is *bone grafting.* A bone graft may also replace diseased bone or increase bone tissue for joint replacement. In most cases, chips of bone are taken from the iliac crest or other site and are packed or wired between the bone ends to facilitate union. Allografts from cadavers may also be used. These grafts are frozen or freeze-dried and stored under sterile conditions in a bone bank.

Bone banking from living donors is becoming increasingly popular. If qualified, patients undergoing total hip replacement may donate their femoral heads to the bank for later use as bone grafts for others. Careful screening ensures that the bone is healthy and that the donor has no communicable disease. The bone cannot be donated without written consent.

One of the newest modalities for fracture healing is **low-intensity pulsed ultrasound** (Exogen therapy). Used for slow-healing fractures or for new fractures as an alternative to surgery, ultrasound treatment has had excellent results. The patient applies the treatment for about 20 minutes each day. It has no contraindications or adverse effects.

Acute Pain

NOC **Planning: Expected Outcomes.** The patient with a fracture is expected to take personal actions to control pain. Indicators include that he or she will consistently demonstrate the ability to:

- Use preventive measures
- Use nonanalgesic relief measures
- Use analgesic relief measures appropriately
- Report changes in pain symptoms or sites to health care professional
- Report uncontrollable pain symptoms to health care professional
- Report that pain is controlled

Interventions. The nonsurgical or surgical management of fractures through reduction and immobilization helps reduce pain and prevents neurovascular injury. However, the patient often requires drug therapy and other pain-relief measures.

Drug Therapy. *Musculoskeletal pain related to soft-tissue damage, bone disruption, muscle spasm, and peripheral nerve damage is one of the most severe types of pain that can be experienced.* The patient often has the pain for a prolonged time, which makes pain management difficult. The health care provider commonly prescribes opioid and non-opioid analgesics, anti-inflammatory drugs, and muscle relaxants.

For patients with chronic, severe pain, opioid and non-opioid drugs are alternated or given together to manage pain both centrally in the brain and peripherally at the site of injury. For severe or multiple fractures, patient-controlled analgesia (PCA) with morphine, meperidine (Demerol), or other drug is used. *Meperidine should never be used for older adults because it has toxic metabolites that can cause seizures and other complications. Many hospitals no longer use this drug for patients of any age.*

For patients who have less severe injury, the analgesic may be given on an as-needed basis. The nurse and patient mutually decide on the best times for the strong pain relievers to be given (e.g., before a complex dressing change, before physical therapy, and at bedtime). Assess the effectiveness of the analgesic and its side effects. Constipation is a common side effect of opioid therapy, especially for older adults. Assess for frequency of bowel movements, and administer stool softeners as requested by the health care provider. Encourage fluids and activity as tolerated. Chapter 5 discusses the various methods of pain management, including epidural analgesia and patient-controlled analgesia.

Complementary and Alternative Therapies. With chronic, severe pain, the patient cannot depend solely on drugs for relief. Recommend temporary pain-relief measures, such as ice or heat, depending on the cause of the pain. If swelling causes pressure on the affected area, ice and elevation of the affected body part may be appropriate. Teach the patient to plan activities that allow for rest and quiet periods. Some patients like soft music playing while resting. Muscle spasms are best relieved by application of heat and massage. Other physical measures include a warm, soothing bath, a back rub, and the use of therapeutic touch.

If these measures are not effective in reducing pain, distraction, imagery, or music therapy may be used as an alternative. Teach the patient relaxation techniques, such as deep breathing, for use during periods of severe pain. Chapters 2 and 5 discuss these techniques in detail.

Risk for Infection

NOC **Planning: Expected Outcomes.** The patient with a fracture is expected to be free of a wound or bone infection. Indicators include that the patient will not have:

- Foul-smelling discharge
- Purulent drainage
- Fever
- Lethargy
- Wound-site culture colonization (if wound present)
- White blood cell (WBC) elevation (if systemic infection)

Interventions. When caring for a patient with an open fracture, use clean or aseptic technique for dressing changes and wound irrigations. Check agency policy for specific protocols. *Immediately notify the health care provider if you observe inflammation and purulent drainage.* Other infections, such as pneumonia and urinary tract infection, may occur days after the fracture. Monitor the patient's vital signs every 4 to 8 hours because increases in temperature and pulse often indicate systemic infection. *Older adults may not have a temperature elevation even in the presence of severe infection.*

For most patients with an open fracture, the health care provider prescribes one or more broad-spectrum antibiotics prophylactically and performs surgical wound débridement as soon as possible after the injury. First-generation cephalosporins, clindamycin (Cleocin), and ciprofloxacin (Cipro) are commonly used. In addition to systemic antibiotics, local antibiotic therapy through wound irrigation is commonly prescribed, especially during débridement. Antibiotic beads (e.g., tobramycin [Nebcin]) mixed with bone cement can be used during surgery (Okike & Bhattacharyya, 2006).

A newer wound therapy is the vacuum-assisted closure (VAC) system as a method of increasing the rate of wound healing for open fractures. This device allows quicker wound closure, which decreases the risk for infection.

When the bone is surgically repaired, hardware and/or bone grafts have typically been implanted. However, they are limited in their use. The U.S. Food and Drug Administration (FDA) approved the use of recombinant human bone morphogenetic protein-2 (rhBMP-2) for tibial and spinal fractures. The evidence suggests that this implanted genetically engineered substance increases wound healing, decreases hardware failure, and decreases the risk for infection (Okike & Bhattacharyya, 2006).

Impaired Physical Mobility

NOC **Planning: Expected Outcomes.** The patient with a fracture is expected to be free of complications associated with impaired mobility. Indicators include that the patient will not have:

- Pressure ulcers
- Constipation
- Urinary retention
- Contracted joints
- Pneumonia
- Venous thromboembolism (VTE)

The patient is also expected to move purposefully in his or her own environment independently with or without an ambulatory device. Indicators include that the patient will have:

- Balance
- Coordination
- Muscle movement
- Transfer ability
- Ambulation ability (with or without ambulatory aids)

Interventions. The interventions necessary for this diagnosis can be grouped into two types: those that help prevent complications of impaired mobility and those that help increase mobility.

Prevention of Complications. The nurse plays a vital role in preventing and assessing for complications in immobilized patients with fractures. Additional information about nursing care for preventing problems associated with immobility is found in Chapter 8.

Promotion of Mobility. The use of crutches or a walker increases mobility and assists in ambulation. The patient may progress to use of a cane.

Crutches are the most commonly used ambulatory aid for many types of musculoskeletal trauma (e.g., fractures, sprains, amputations). In most agencies, the physical therapist fits the patient for crutches and teaches him or her how to ambulate with them on flat surfaces and stairs. Reinforce the instructions, and evaluate whether the patient is using the crutches correctly. In emergency department and ambulatory settings, nurses routinely teach how to use crutches.

Walking with crutches requires strong arm muscles, balance, and coordination. For this reason, crutches are not often used for older adults. Walkers and canes are preferred. The therapist pads the tips and axillary bars of the crutches. Padding prevents the tips from slipping and the bars from damaging the axillae. To prevent pressure on the axillary nerve, there should be two to three finger breadths between the axilla and the top of the crutch when the crutch tip is at least 6 inches (15 cm) diagonally in front of the foot. The crutch is adjusted so that the elbow is flexed no more than 30 degrees when the palm is on the handle (Fig. 54-7).

There are several types of gaits for walking with crutches. The most common one for musculoskeletal injury is the three-point gait, which allows little weight bearing on the affected leg. The procedure for these gaits is discussed in fundamentals of nursing books.

A *walker* is most often used by the older patient who needs additional support for balance. The physical therapist assesses

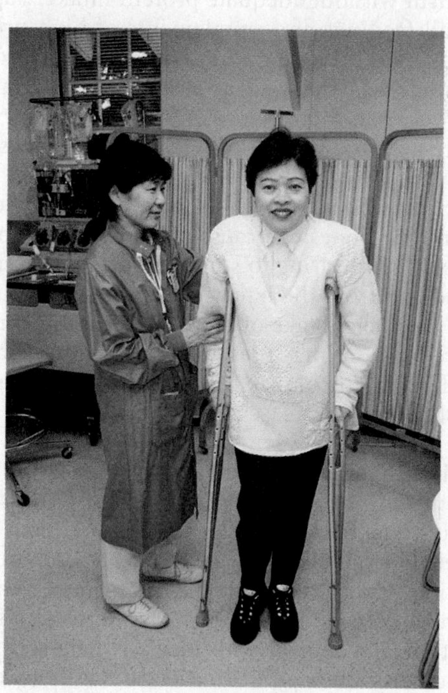

Fig. 54-7 • Assisting the patient with crutch walking. Note how the therapist guards the patient and how the patient's elbows are at no more than 30 degrees of flexion.

the strength of the upper extremities and the unaffected leg. Strength is improved with exercise as needed.

A *cane* is sometimes used if the patient needs only minimal support for an affected leg. The straight cane offers the least support. A hemi-cane or quad-cane provides a broader base for the cane and therefore more support. The cane is placed on the *unaffected* side and should create no more than 30 degrees of flexion of the elbow. The top of the cane should be parallel to the greater trochanter of the femur or stylus of the wrist. Chapter 8 describes these ambulatory devices in more detail.

Imbalanced Nutrition: Less Than Body Requirements

NOC **Planning: Expected Outcomes.** The patient with a fracture is expected to maintain an adequate dietary intake to meet metabolic needs. Indicators include that the patient will have normal:

- Nutrient intake
- Fluid intake
- Serum prealbumin
- Hematocrit and hemoglobin

Interventions. Collaborate with the nutritionist to assess the patient's food likes and dislikes, and plan meals that are both appealing and nutritional. For promotion of bone and tissue healing, the patient needs a high-protein, high-calorie diet. Supplements of vitamins B and C are also required for tissue nutrition. Some patients are immobilized for extended periods. Thus they are predisposed to hypocalcemia, which results in loss of calcium from bone and bone fragility. Teach the patient and family to increase the intake of foods high in calcium, particularly milk and milk products if tolerated. For those who cannot tolerate dairy products or are vegan, calcium-fortified and vitamin D–fortified soy or rice milk and tofu products may be used.

A negative nitrogen balance can develop 7 to 10 days after injury in an immobilized patient because of an increase in catabolism without adequate protein intake. Suggest frequent small feedings and supplements of high-protein nutritional drinks. Milk shakes are an excellent protein and calorie supplement, as well as a source of calcium. If the patient is vegan, is lactose intolerant, or has dairy allergies, collaborate with the nutritionist about non-dairy sources of protein.

For patients who have lower extremity fractures, less weight bearing on long bones can cause anemia. The red bone marrow needs weight bearing to stimulate red blood cell production. Blood loss from the injury or surgery contributes to the anemia. Encourage intake of foods high in iron content. The health care provider may prescribe a daily multivitamin with iron supplement. Encourage the patient to take these supplements with food to decrease possible nausea.

Community-Based Care

The patient with an *uncomplicated* fracture is usually discharged to home from the emergency department or urgent care center. Older adults with hip or other fractures or patients with multiple traumas are hospitalized and then transferred to home, a rehabilitation setting, or a long-term care facility for rehabilitation. Collaborate with the case manager or the discharge planner in the hospital to ensure continuity of care. Be sure to communicate the plan of care to the health care agency receiving the patient.

Home Care Management

If the patient is discharged to home, the nurse, therapist, or case manager (CM) assesses the home environment for structural barriers to mobility, such as stairs. Be sure that the patient has easy access to the bathroom. Ask about scatter rugs, waxed floors, and walkway areas that could increase the risk for falls. If the patient needs to use a wheelchair or ambulatory aid, make sure that he or she can use it safely and that there is room in the house to ambulate with these devices. The physical therapist teaches how to use stairs, but older adults may experience difficulty performing this task. A home health care nurse may make one or two visits to check that the home is safe and that the patient and family are able to follow the interdisciplinary plan of care.

Health Teaching

The patient with a fracture may be discharged from the hospital, emergency department, office, or clinic with a bandage, splint, cast, or external fixator. Provide verbal and written instructions on the care of these devices. Chart 54-6 describes care of the affected extremity after removal of the cast.

The patient may also need to continue wound care at home. Instruct the patient and family about how to assess and dress the wound to promote healing and prevent infection. Teach them how to recognize complications (see the Complications of Fractures section, p. 1180 and when and where to seek professional health care if complications occur. Additional educational needs depend on the type of fracture and fracture repair.

Health Care Resources

In collaboration with the case manager, arrange for follow-up care at home. For example, professional counseling for depression may need to continue after discharge from the hospital. A social worker may need to help the patient apply for funds to pay medical bills. If there is severe bone and tissue damage, be realistic and help the patient and family understand the long-term nature of the recovery period. Multiple treatment techniques and surgical procedures required for complications can be mentally and emotionally draining for the patient and family. A vocational counselor may be needed to help the patient find a different type of job, depending on the extent of the fracture.

An older or incapacitated patient may need assistance with ADLs, which can be provided by home care aides if family or other caregiver is not available. In collaboration with the case manager, anticipate the patient's needs and arrange for these services.

Chart 54-6 PATIENT AND FAMILY EDUCATION GUIDE

Care of the Extremity After Cast Removal

- Remove scaly, dead skin carefully by soaking; do not scrub.
- Move the extremity carefully. Expect discomfort, weakness, and decreased range of motion.
- Support the extremity with pillows or your orthotic device until strength and movement return.
- Exercise slowly as instructed by your physical therapist.
- Wear support stockings or elastic bandages to prevent swelling (for lower extremity).

Evaluation: Outcomes

Evaluate the care of the patient with one or more fractures based on the identified nursing diagnoses and collaborative problems. The expected outcomes include that the patient:

- Has adequate blood flow through the small vessels to maintain tissue perfusion
- Takes personal actions to control pain
- Is free of infection
- Is free of physiologic consequences of impaired mobility
- Moves purposefully and independently in his or her own environment with or without an assistive device
- Meets nutritional needs for healing

Specific indicators for these outcomes are listed for each nursing diagnosis in the Planning and Implementation section (see earlier).

FRACTURES OF SPECIFIC SITES

Upper Extremity Fractures

In addition to the general care discussed in the previous section, management of upper extremity fractures includes specific interventions related to the location and nature of the injury. Unless multiple fractures or massive soft tissue damage occurs, upper extremity fractures do not usually require hospitalization. However, they often take many months to heal. In some cases, patients may not regain complete function for up to a year, even after extensive rehabilitation in occupational therapy. Assess neurovascular status in the affected arm and hand before and after fracture treatment. Monitor for numbness and tingling distal to (below) the injury, which may indicate peripheral nerve damage.

Fractures of the *clavicle* typically result from a fall on an outstretched hand, a fall on the shoulder, or a direct blow to the upper chest and shoulder area. Most clavicular fractures are self-healing. A splint or bandage is used for immobilization. Complicated open fractures, although uncommon, may require open reduction with internal fixation (ORIF) by pins, wires, or screws.

Scapular fractures are not common and are usually caused by direct impact to the area. Serious internal trauma, including pneumothorax, pulmonary contusion, and fractured ribs, can accompany these fractures. The shoulder is kept in position with a commercial immobilizer until the fracture heals, usually in 2 to 4 weeks. Intra-articular neck and glenoid fractures may require surgical intervention with plate and screw fixation.

Fractures of the *proximal humerus,* particularly impacted or displaced fractures, are common in the older adult. As persons age, fractures of the humerus occur more frequently in the area closer to the shoulder joint. This makes treatment more difficult in the older adult. An impacted injury is usually treated with a sling or other device for immobilization. A displaced fracture often requires ORIF with pins or a prosthesis.

Humeral shaft fractures are generally corrected by closed reduction and a hanging-arm cast or splint. If necessary, the fracture is repaired surgically (with an intramedullary rod or metal plate and screws) or with external fixation. Nonunion of the bone and radial nerve palsy are frequent complications of this fracture. Bone grafting helps promote union. Prolonged splinting is necessary while the radial nerve regenerates.

A direct blow to the condyles of the distal humerus can cause either or both condyles to fracture, usually in a T- or Y-shaped configuration. The most serious complication is damage to the brachial or median nerve. Condylar fracture is usually treated by ORIF with a series of screws, although skeletal traction and casting can be used.

Fractures of the *elbow (olecranon)* are common in adults and typically result from a fall on the elbow. Many are successfully treated by closed reduction and application of a cast. ORIF is performed for displaced fractures, and a splint is worn during the healing phase.

Forearm fractures of the ulna without accompanying injury to the radius are rare. As with other fractures of long bones, closed reduction with casting may be the appropriate treatment. If the fracture is displaced, ORIF with intramedullary rods or plates and screws is required.

One or more of the bones in the *wrist and hand* can break, but the most common fracture is of the carpal scaphoid bone in young adult men. This is also one of the most misdiagnosed fractures because it is poorly visualized on an x-ray film. Closed reduction and casting for 6 to 12 weeks is the treatment of choice. If the bone does not heal, ORIF with bone grafting is performed.

A *Colles'* (wrist) fracture is common in older adults, particularly women with osteoporosis. A Colles' fracture occurs in the last inch of the distal radius and often is the result of a fall on an outstretched hand. These fractures can usually be treated by splinting or casting for 6 to 8 weeks.

Fractures of the *metacarpals* and *phalanges (fingers)* are usually not displaced, which makes their treatment less difficult than that of other fractures. Metacarpal fractures are immobilized for 3 to 4 weeks. Phalangeal fractures are immobilized in finger splints for 10 to 14 days.

Lower Extremity Fractures

Fractures of the Hip

Hip fracture is the most common injury in older adults and one of the most frequently seen injuries in any health care setting or community. It has a high mortality rate as a result of multiple complications related to surgery and prolonged immobility. Osteoporosis is the biggest risk factor for hip fractures (see Chapter 53). This disease weakens the upper femur (hip), breaks, and then causes the person to fall. The number of people with hip fracture is expected to continue to increase as the population ages, and the associated health care costs will be tremendous.

CONSIDERATIONS FOR OLDER ADULTS

Teach older adults about the risk factors for hip fracture including physiologic aging changes, disease processes, drug therapy, and environmental hazards. Physiologic changes include sensory changes such as visual acuity and diminished hearing; changes in gait, balance, and muscle strength; and joint stiffness. Disease processes like osteoporosis, foot disorders, and changes in cardiac function increase the risk for hip fracture. Drugs, such as diuretics, antihypertensives, antidepressants, sedatives, opioids, and alcohol are factors that increase the risks for falling in older adults. Use of three or more drugs at the same time drastically increases the risk for falls. Throw rugs, loose carpeting, inadequate lighting, uneven walking surfaces or steps, and pets are environmental hazards that also cause falls.

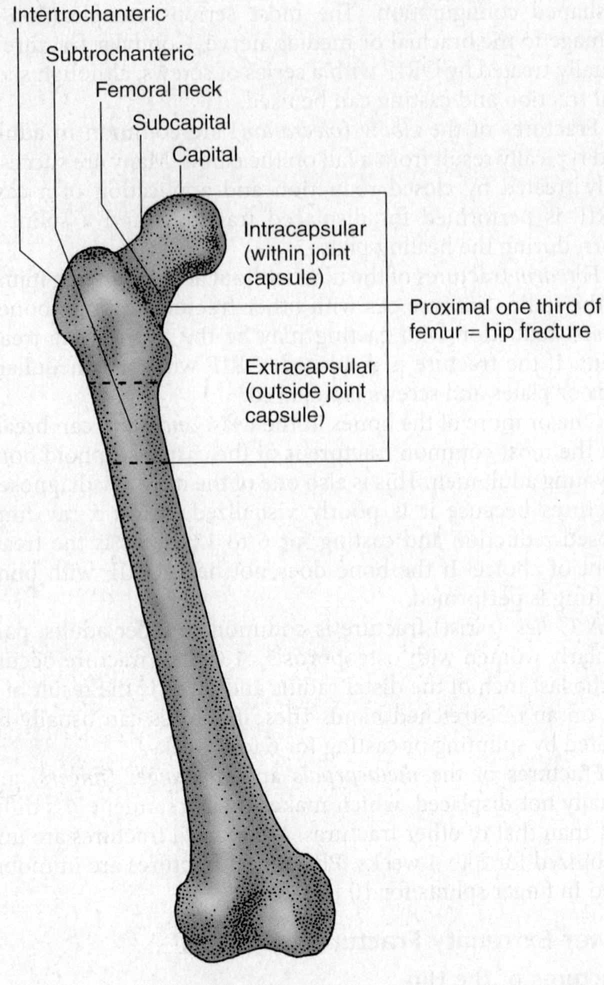
Intertrochanteric
Subtrochanteric
Femoral neck
Subcapital
Capital
Intracapsular (within joint capsule)
Proximal one third of femur = hip fracture
Extracapsular (outside joint capsule)

Fig. 54-8 • Types of hip fractures.

The older adult with hip fracture usually reports groin pain or pain behind the knee on the affected side. In some cases, the patient has pain in the lower back or has no pain at all. However, the patient is not able to stand. X-ray or other imaging assessment confirms the diagnosis. Hip fractures include those involving the upper third of the femur and are classified as **intracapsular** (within the joint capsule) or **extracapsular** (outside the joint capsule). These types are further divided according to fracture location (Fig. 54-8). In the area of the femoral neck there is concern with disruption of the blood supply to the head of the femur, which can result in ischemic or avascular necrosis (AVN) of the femoral head. AVN causes death and necrosis of bone tissue and results in pain and decreased mobility. This problem is most likely in patients with displaced fractures. Prompt surgical repair can prevent this complication and decrease pain.

The treatment of choice is surgical repair, when possible, to allow the older patient to be out of bed and ambulatory. Buck's traction may be applied before surgery to help decrease pain associated with muscle spasm. Depending on the exact location of the fracture, open reduction with internal fixation (ORIF) may include an intramedullary rod, pins, prostheses (for femoral head or neck fractures), or a compression screw.

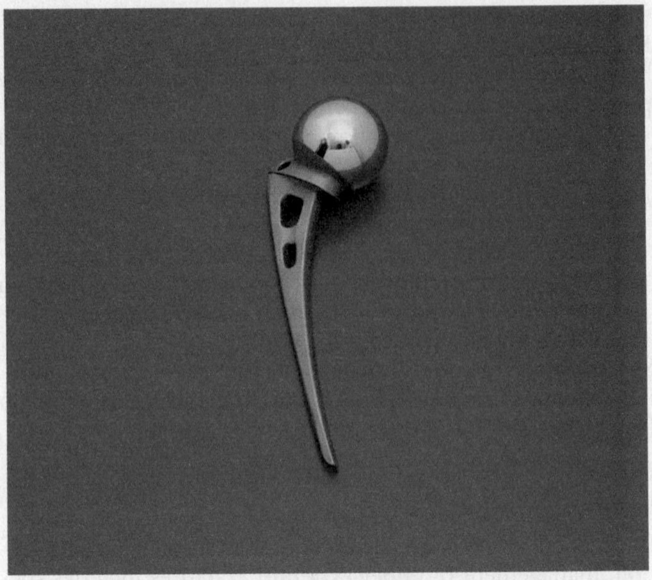

Fig. 54-9 • The Moore prosthesis, which is used for hip fractures.

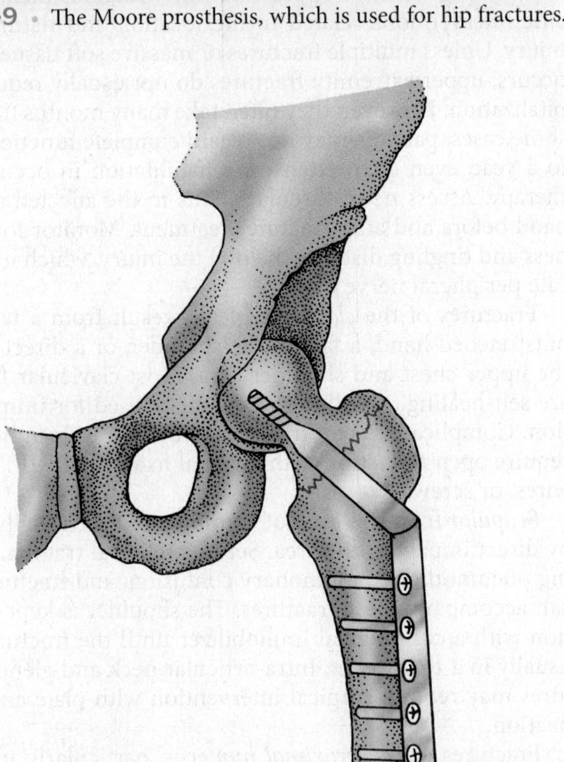

Fig. 54-10 • A compression hip screw used for open reduction with internal fixation (ORIF) of the hip.

Epidural or general anesthesia is used. Figs. 54-9 and 54-10 illustrate examples of these devices. Occasionally a patient will be so debilitated that surgery cannot be done. In these cases, nonsurgical options are Buck's traction, pain management, and bedrest to allow natural fracture healing (Altizer, 2005; Watters & Moran, 2006).

Patients usually receive PCA morphine or other opioid or epidural analgesia after surgery. Chapter 5 discusses the nursing care associated with these pain management modalities in detail. The patient begins ambulating with assistance the day after surgery to prevent complications associated with immobility (e.g., pressure ulcers, atelectasis, venous thromboembo-

EVIDENCE-BASED PRACTICE

What are the major factors that influence functional status after hip surgery?

Folden, S., & Tappen, R. (2007). Factors influencing function and recovery following hip repair surgery. *Orthopaedic Nursing, 26*(4), 234-241.

The purpose of this small descriptive study was to determine which factors predicted the functional ability of patients who had hip repair surgery by 3 months after hospital discharge. Previous studies had suggested many contributing factors, including age, balance, cognitive ability, gender, fatigue, pain, and complications from surgery. Functional status before surgery had also been found to be a factor.

A convenience sample of 73 men and women was evaluated by self-report in an inpatient rehabilitation setting after hospital discharge and again in 3 months. Balance and cognitive ability before surgery were the best predictors of recovery and return to baseline functional status. Fatigue also played a role. Men reported higher functional levels than women and were more likely to return to their presurgical activities. The authors concluded that gender did influence recovery from hip repair surgery.

Level of Evidence—6. This research was a small descriptive study using a convenience sample.

Commentary: Implications for Practice and Research. Although this study was descriptive, it confirmed previous findings of other researchers about which factors predict return to functional ability among patients having hip repair. Physicians can use this information in making decisions about who are the best candidates for surgery. Nurses and rehabilitation therapists can use these findings to plan interventions to improve balance and reduce fatigue as patients recover from surgery during their rehabilitation period.

lism). Early movement and ambulation also decrease the chance of infection and increase surgical site healing.

Patients who have an ORIF are at risk for hip dislocation or subluxation. Be sure to prevent hip adduction and rotation to keep the operative leg in proper alignment. Regular pillows or abduction devices can be used for patients who are confused or restless. If straps are used to hold the device in place, check the skin for signs of pressure. Perform neurovascular assessments to ensure that the device is not interfering with arterial circulation or peripheral nerve conduction.

Special considerations for the patient having a hip repair also include careful inspection of skin including areas of pressure, especially the heels. Use of Buck's traction and periods of bedrest before surgical intervention can increase the risk for pressure injury in this area within 24 hours. *Be sure that the patient's heels are up off the bed at all times. Inspect the heels and other high-risk bony prominence areas every 8 to 12 hours. Delegate turning and repositioning every 1 to 2 hours to unlicensed assistive personnel (UAP), and supervise this nursing activity.* Other measures to decrease the risk for pressure ulcers are described elsewhere in this text and in fundamentals textbooks.

Other nursing and interdisciplinary care is similar to that described for fracture in other sites. Specific interventions are similar to those for total hip replacement (see Chapter 20).

Many patients recover fully from hip fracture repair and regain their functional ability. However, some patients are not able to return to their pre-fracture ADLs and mobility level. These patients usually do not return to their homes and are placed in long-term care facilities. Folden and Tappen (2007) conducted a small descriptive study that identified predictors for patients who are likely to fully recover. They found that balance and cognitive ability were the best predictors (see the Evidence-Based Practice box above).

Other Fractures of the Lower Extremity

Other fractures of the lower extremity may or may not require hospitalization. However, if the patient has severe or multiple fractures, especially with soft tissue damage, hospital admission is usually required. Patients who have surgery to repair their injury may also be hospitalized. Coordinate care with the physical therapist regarding mobility transfers, positioning, and ambulation. Collaborate with the case manager regarding placement after discharge. Most patients go home unless there is no support system or additional rehabilitation is needed. Health teaching and ensuring continuity of care are essential.

Fractures of the *lower two thirds of the femur* usually result from trauma often from a motor vehicle crash. A femur fracture is seldom immobilized by casting because the powerful muscles of the thigh become spastic, which causes displacement of bone ends. Extensive hemorrhage can occur with femur fracture.

Surgical treatment is ORIF with nails, rods, or a compression screw. In a few cases in which extensive bone fragmentation or severe tissue trauma is found, external fixation may be employed. Healing time for a femur fracture may be 6 months or longer. Skeletal traction, followed by a full-leg brace or cast, may be used in nonsurgical treatment.

Like most other fractures, *patellar* (knee cap) fractures result from direct impact. The surgeon typically repairs the fracture by closed reduction and casting or internal fixation with screws. A knee immobilizer is used so that the fracture can heal properly.

Trauma to the lower leg most often causes fractures of both the *tibia* and the *fibula*, particularly the lower third, and is often referred to as a "tib-fib" fracture. The major treatment techniques are closed reduction with casting, internal fixation, and external fixation. If closed reduction is used, the patient wears a cast for at least 8 to 10 weeks. Because of poor blood supply to parts of the tibia and fibula, delayed union is not unusual with this type of fracture. Internal fixation with nails or a plate and screws, followed by a long-leg cast for 4 to 6 weeks, is another option. When the fractures cause extensive skin and soft-tissue damage, the initial treatment may be external fixation, often for 6 to 10 weeks, usually followed by application of a cast until the fracture is completely healed. The patient uses ambulatory aids, usually crutches.

Ankle fractures are described by their anatomic place of injury. For example, a bimalleolar (Pott's) fracture involves the medial malleolus of the tibia and the lateral malleolus of the fibula. Because of the instability of the ankle joint, the fracture can result from supination and eversion, pronation and abduction, or pronation and eversion. These forces generally create spiral, transverse, or oblique breaks, which are often difficult to treat and present problems in healing. A combination of closed and open techniques may be used, depending on the severity and extent of the fracture. An arthrodesis (fusion) may be needed if the bone does not heal.

Treatment of fractures of the foot or phalanges (toes) is similar to that of other fractures, with either closed or open reduction. Phalangeal fractures are more painful than but not as serious as most other types of fractures. Crutches are used for ambulation.

Fractures of the Chest and Pelvis

Chest trauma may cause fractures of the ribs or sternum. The most commonly fractured ribs are numbers 4 through 8. *The major concern with rib and sternal fractures is the potential for puncture of the lungs, heart, or arteries by bone fragments or ends. Assess airway, breathing, and circulation status **first** for any patient having chest trauma.* Fractures of the lower ribs may damage underlying organs, such as the liver, spleen, or kidneys. These fractures tend to heal on their own without surgical intervention. Patients are often uncomfortable during the healing process and require analgesia. They also have a high risk for pneumonia because of shallow breathing caused by pain on inspiration. Encourage them to breathe normally if possible.

Because the pelvis is very vascular and is close to major organs and blood vessels, associated internal damage is the major focus in fracture management. After head injuries, pelvic fractures are the second most common cause of death from trauma. In young adults, pelvic fractures typically result from motor vehicle crashes or falls from buildings. Falls are the most common cause in older adults. The major concern related to pelvic injury is venous oozing or arterial bleeding. Loss of blood volume leads to hypovolemic shock.

Assess for internal abdominal trauma by checking for blood in the urine and stool and by monitoring the abdomen for the development of rigidity or swelling. The trauma team may use peritoneal lavage, computed tomography (CT) scanning, or ultrasound for assessment of hemorrhage. Ultrasound is noninvasive, rapid, reliable, and cost effective and can be done at the bedside.

There are many classification systems for pelvic fractures. A system that is particularly useful divides fractures of the pelvis into two broad categories: non–weight-bearing fractures and weight-bearing fractures.

When a *non–weight-bearing* part of the pelvis is fractured, such as one of the pubic rami or the iliac crest, treatment can be as minimal as bedrest on a firm mattress or bed board. This type of fracture can be quite painful, and the patient may need stool softeners to facilitate bowel movements because of hesitancy to move. Well-stabilized fractures usually heal in 2 months.

A *weight-bearing* fracture, such as multiple fractures of the pelvic ring creating instability or a fractured acetabulum, necessitates external fixation or open reduction with internal fixation (ORIF) or both. Progression to weight bearing depends on the stability of the fracture after fixation. Some patients can fully bear weight within days of surgery, whereas others managed with traction may not be able to bear weight for as long as 12 weeks.

Compression Fractures of the Spine

Most vertebral fractures are associated with osteoporosis, metastatic bone cancer, and multiple myeloma. Compression fractures result when trabecular or cancellous bone within the vertebra becomes weakened and causes the vertebral body to collapse. The patient has severe pain, deformity (kyphosis), and occasional neurologic compromise. As discussed in the Osteoporosis section of Chapter 53, the patient's quality of life is reduced by the impact of this problem.

Nonsurgical management includes bedrest, analgesics, nerve blocks, and physical therapy to maintain muscle strength. Vertebral compression fractures (VCFs) that remain painful and impair mobility may be surgically treated with **vertebroplasty** or kyphoplasty. These procedures are minimally invasive techniques in which bone cement is injected through the skin (percutaneously) directly into the fracture site to provide stability and immediate pain relief. **Kyphoplasty** includes the additional step of inserting a small balloon into the fracture site and inflating it to contain the cement and to restore height to the vertebra. This procedure is preferred because it reduces the complication of leaking of bone cement outside the vertebral body and it may restore height to decrease kyphosis (Gross, 2006).

Minimally invasive surgeries can be done in an operating or interventional radiology suite by a surgeon or interven-

Chart 54-7 BEST PRACTICE FOR PATIENT SAFETY & QUALITY CARE

Nursing Care for Patients Having Vertebroplasty or Kyphoplasty

Provide *preoperative care* including:
- Check the patient's coagulation laboratory test results; platelet count should be more than 100,000/mm^3.
- Make sure that all anticoagulant drugs were discontinued as requested by the physician.
- Assess and document the patient's neurologic status, especially extremity movement and sensation.
- Assess the patient's pain level.
- Assess the patient's ability to lie prone for at least 1 hour.
- Establish an IV line, and take vital signs.

Provide *postoperative care* including:
- Place the patient in a flat supine position for 1 to 2 hours or as requested by the physician.
- Monitor and record vital signs and frequent neurologic assessments; report any change immediately to the physician.
- Apply an ice pack to the puncture site if needed to relieve pain.
- Assess the patient's pain level, and compare it with the preoperative level; give mild analgesic as needed.
- Monitor for complications such as bleeding at the puncture site or shortness of breath; report these findings immediately if they occur.
- Assist the patient with ambulation.

Before discharge, teach the patient and family to:
- Avoid driving or operating machinery for the first 24 hours because of drugs used during the procedure.
- Monitor the puncture site for signs of infection, such as redness, pain, swelling, or drainage.
- Keep the dressing dry, and remove it the next day.
- Begin usual activities, including walking the next day; slowly increase activity level over the next few days.

tional radiologist. They can be done with moderate sedation or general anesthesia. IV ketorolac (Toradol) may be given before the procedure to reduce inflammation at the injection site. Large-bore needles are placed into the fracture site using fluoroscopy or computed tomography guidance. Then the deflated balloon is inserted through the needles and inflated in the fracture site, and the cement is injected (Kessenich, 2006; Lemke, 2005).

Patients may have the procedures in an ambulatory care setting and return home after 2 to 4 hours or be admitted to the hospital for an overnight stay. Chart 54-7 describes the preoperative and postoperative care for percutaneous interventions for VCFs.

Before discharge, teach the patient to report any signs or symptoms of infection from puncture sites. Remind him or her to not soak in a bath for 1 week, use analgesics as needed, resume activity, and contact the health care provider for questions or concerns.

Fractures at Other Sites

Because the skull and vertebral column protect the brain and spinal cord, these fractures are described in Chapters 45 and 47. Fractures of the mandible or nose and other facial trauma are also discussed elsewhere in the text.

AMPUTATIONS

An **amputation** is the removal of a part of the body. Advances in microvascular surgical procedures, better use of antibiotic therapy, and improved surgical techniques for traumatic injury and bone cancer all help reduce the numbers of amputation. The psychosocial aspects of the procedure are often more devastating than the physical impairments that result. The loss is complete and permanent and causes a change in body image and often in self-esteem. Collaborate with members of the health care team, including prosthetists, rehabilitation therapists, psychologists, case managers, and physiatrists (rehabilitation physicians), when providing care to the patient who has an amputation.

Pathophysiology

Types of Amputation

Amputations may be elective or traumatic. Most are *elective* and are related to complications of peripheral vascular disease and arteriosclerosis. These complications result in ischemia in distal areas of the *lower extremity*. Diabetes mellitus is often an underlying cause. Amputation is considered only after other interventions have not restored circulation to the lower extremity, sometimes referred to as *limb salvage procedures* (e.g., percutaneous transluminal angioplasty [PTA]). These procedures are discussed elsewhere in this text.

Traumatic amputations most often result from accidents and are the primary cause of *upper extremity* amputation. A person may be cleaning lawn mower blades or a snow blower without disconnecting the machine. A motor vehicle or industrial machine accident may also cause an amputation. Traumatic amputations also increase during war as a result of mines and bombs (e.g., Iraq), most often affecting one or both legs. Thousands of veterans of war in the United States are amputees and have had to adjust to major changes in their lifestyles.

Injury that causes severe crushing of tissues or significant blood vessel damage usually results in amputation to preserve function of the residual limb. The ability to salvage limbs injured related to trauma, however, is increasing. Some body parts that are severed can be reattached or replanted.

Levels of Amputation

Lower extremity (LE) amputations are performed much more frequently than upper extremity amputations. Five types of lower extremity amputations may be performed (Fig. 54-11).

The loss of any or all of the small toes presents a minor disability. Loss of the great toe is significant because it affects balance, gait, and "push off" ability during walking. Midfoot amputations (e.g., the Lisfranc and the Chopart amputations) and the Syme amputation are common procedures for peripheral vascular disease. In the Syme amputation, most of the foot is removed but the ankle remains. The advantage of this surgery over traditional amputations below the knee is that weight bearing can occur without the use of a prosthesis and with reduced pain.

An intense effort is made to preserve knee joints with below-the-knee amputation (BKA). When the cause for the amputation extends beyond the knee, above-knee or higher amputations are performed. Hip disarticulation, or removal of the hip joint, and hemipelvectomy (removal of half of the pelvis with the leg) are more common in younger patients than in older ones who cannot easily handle the cumbersome prostheses required for ambulation. The higher the level of amputation, the more energy is required for mobility. These higher-level procedures are typically done for cancer of the bone, osteomyelitis, or trauma.

Fewer than 10% of all amputations are upper extremity (UE) amputations. An amputation of any part of the upper extremity is generally more incapacitating than one of the leg. The arms and hands are necessary for ADLs such as feeding, bathing, dressing, and driving a car. In the upper extremity, as

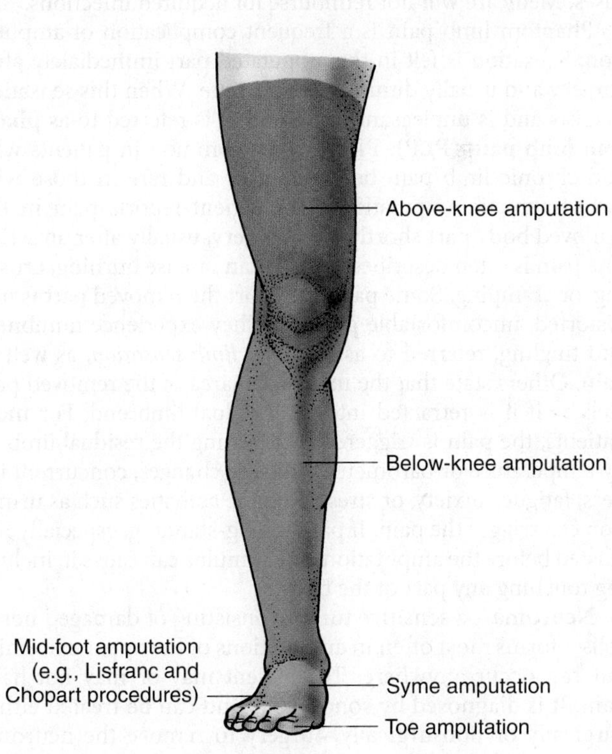
Above-knee amputation
Below-knee amputation
Mid-foot amputation (e.g., Lisfranc and Chopart procedures)
Syme amputation
Toe amputation

Fig. 54-11 • Common levels of lower extremity amputation.

much length as possible is saved to maintain function. Early replacement with a prosthetic device is vital for the patient with this type of amputation.

CULTURAL AWARENESS

The incidence of lower extremity amputations is greater in black and Hispanic populations because the incidence of major diseases leading to amputation, such as diabetes and arteriosclerosis, is greater in these populations. Limited access to health care for these minority groups may also play a major role in limb loss. Language barriers may also be an obstacle to seeking health care providers.

Complications of Amputation

The most common complications of elective or traumatic amputations are:

- Hemorrhage
- Infection
- Phantom limb pain
- Neuroma
- Flexion contractures

When a person loses part or all of an extremity either by surgery or by trauma, major blood vessels are severed, which causes *bleeding.* If the bleeding is uncontrolled, the patient is at risk for hypovolemic shock and possibly death.

As with any surgical procedure or trauma, *infection* can occur in the wound or the bone (osteomyelitis). The older adult who is malnourished and confused is at the greatest risk because excreta may soil the wound or he or she may remove the dressing and pick at the incision. Preventing infection is a major emphasis in hospitals and other health care settings. In some cases, Medicare will not reimburse for acquired infections.

Phantom limb pain is a frequent complication of amputation. Sensation is felt in the amputated part immediately after surgery and usually diminishes over time. When this sensation persists and is unpleasant or painful, it is referred to as **phantom limb pain (PLP).** PLP is more common in patients who had chronic limb pain before surgery and rare in those who have traumatic amputations. The patient reports pain in the removed body part shortly after surgery, usually after an AKA. The pain is often described as either an intense burning, crushing, or cramping. Some patients report the removed part is in a distorted, uncomfortable position. They experience numbness and tingling, referred to as *phantom limb sensation,* as well as pain. Others state that the most distal area of the removed part feels as if it is retracted into the residual limb end. For most patients, the pain is triggered by touching the residual limb or by temperature or barometric pressure changes, concurrent illness, fatigue, anxiety, or stress. Routine activities such as urination can trigger the pain. If pain is long-standing, especially if it existed before the amputation, any stimulus can cause it, including touching any part of the body.

Neuroma—a sensitive tumor consisting of damaged nerve cells—forms most often in amputations of the upper extremity but can occur anywhere. The patient may or may not have pain. It is diagnosed by sonography and can be treated either surgically or nonsurgically. Surgery to remove the neuroma may be performed, but it often regrows and is more painful than before the surgery. Nonsurgical modalities include nerve blocks (e.g., with phenol), steroid injections, and cognitive therapies such as hypnosis.

Flexion contractures of the hip or knee are seen in patients with amputations of the lower extremity. This complication must be avoided so that the patient can ambulate with a prosthetic device. Proper positioning and active range-of-motion exercises help prevent this complication.

Health Promotion and Maintenance

The typical patient undergoing elective amputation is a middle-aged or older man with diabetes and a lengthy history of smoking. He most likely has not cared for his feet properly, which has resulted in a nonhealing, infected foot ulcer and possibly gangrene. Therefore adherence with the disease management plan may help prevent the need for later amputation. Lifestyle habits like maintaining a healthy weight, regular exercise, and avoiding smoking can help prevent chronic diseases like diabetes.

The second largest group with amputations are young men who have motorcycle or other vehicular crashes or who are injured by industrial equipment or by combat or accidents in war. These men may either experience a traumatic amputation or undergo a surgical amputation because of a severe crushing injury and massive soft-tissue damage. Teach young male adults the importance of taking safety precautions to prevent injury at work and to avoid speeding or driving while drinking alcohol. An increasing number of young women also tend to speed and drive while drinking, which endangers themselves and others around them.

Patient-Centered Collaborative Care

Assessment

Physical Assessment/Clinical Manifestations

Assess neurovascular status in the affected extremity that will be amputated. When the patient has peripheral vascular disease, also check circulation in other parts of the body. Assess skin color, temperature, sensation, and pulses in both affected and unaffected extremities. Capillary refill can be difficult to determine in the older adult related to thickened and opaque nails. In this situation, the skin near the nail bed can be used (see Chart 54-3). Capillary refill may not be as reliable as other indicators. Observe and document any discoloration of the skin, edema, ulcerations, presence of necrosis, and hair distribution on the affected extremity before surgery.

Psychosocial Assessment

People react differently to the loss of a body part. Be aware that an amputation of a portion of one finger, especially the thumb, can be traumatic to the patient. The thumb is needed for hand activities. Therefore the loss must not be underestimated. Patients undergoing amputation face a complete, permanent loss. Evaluate their psychological preparation for a planned amputation, and expect them to go through the grieving process. Adjustment to a traumatic, unexpected amputation is often more difficult than accepting a planned one. The young patient may be bitter, hostile, and depressed. In addition to loss of a body part, the patient may lose a job, the ability to participate in favorite recreational activities, or a social relationship if other people cannot accept the body change.

The patient has an altered self-concept. The physical alteration that results from an amputation affects body image and self-esteem. For example, a patient may think that an intimate relationship with a partner is no longer possible. An older adult may feel a loss of independence. Assess the patient's feelings about himself or herself to identify areas in which he or she needs emotional support. Refer the patient to the certified hospital chaplain, other spiritual leader, or social worker if he or she is hospitalized. Counseling resources are also available in the community.

Attempt to determine the patient's willingness and motivation to withstand prolonged rehabilitation after the amputation. Asking questions about how he or she has dealt with previous life crises can provide clues. Adjustment to the amputation and rehabilitation is less difficult if the patient is willing to make needed changes.

In addition to assessing the patient's psychosocial status, assess the family's reaction to the surgery or trauma. Their response usually correlates directly with the patient's progress during recovery and rehabilitation. Expect the family to grieve for the loss, and they must be allowed to adjust to the change.

Assess the patient's and family's coping abilities, and help them identify personal strengths and weaknesses. Assess the patient's religious, spiritual, and cultural beliefs. Certain groups require that the amputated body part be stored for later burial with the rest of the body or be buried immediately. Other cultural customs and rituals may apply depending on the group with which the patient associates.

Diagnostic Assessment

The surgeon determines which tests are performed to assess for viability of the limb based on blood flow. A large number of noninvasive techniques are available for this evaluation. For complete accuracy, the health care provider does not rely on any single test.

One procedure is measurement of segmental limb blood pressures, which can also be used by the nurse at the bedside. In this test, an **ankle-brachial index (ABI)** is calculated by dividing ankle systolic pressure by brachial systolic pressure. A normal ABI is 1 or higher.

Blood flow in an extremity can also be assessed by other noninvasive tests, including Doppler ultrasonography or laser Doppler flowmetry and transcutaneous oxygen pressure ($TcPO_2$). The ultrasonography and laser Doppler measure the speed of blood flow in the limb. The $TcPO_2$ measures oxygen pressure to indicate blood flow in the limb and has proved reliable for predicting healing.

Interventions

Emergency Care: Traumatic Amputation

For a person who has a traumatic amputation in the community, first call 911. Assess the patient for airway or breathing problems. Examine the amputation site and apply direct pressure with layers of dry gauze or other cloth, using clean gloves if available. Many nurses carry gloves and first aid kits for this type of emergency. Elevate the extremity above the patient's heart to decrease the bleeding. Do not remove the dressing to prevent dislodging the clot.

The fingers are the most likely part to be amputated and replanted. The current recommendation for prehospital care is to wrap the completely severed finger in a dry sterile gauze (if available) or clean cloth. Put the finger in a watertight, sealed plastic bag. *Place the bag in ice water, never directly on ice, at 1 part ice and 3 parts water* (Laskowski-Jones, 2006). Avoid contact between the finger and the water to prevent tissue damage. Do not remove any semidetached parts of the digit. Be sure that the part goes with the patient to the hospital.

Patients undergoing amputation today are not confined to a wheelchair. Advancements in the design of prosthetics have enabled them to become independent in ambulation and ADLs. Therefore complications from extended bedrest are not common, even for older adults.

Assessment of Tissue Perfusion

The nurse's primary focus is to monitor for signs indicating that there is sufficient tissue perfusion but no hemorrhage. The skin flap at the end of the residual limb should be pink in a light-skinned person and not discolored (lighter or darker than other skin pigmentation) in a dark-skinned patient. The area should be warm but not hot. Assess the closest proximal pulse for strength, and compare it with that in the other extremity. If the patient has bilateral vascular disease, however, comparison of limbs is not an accurate way of measuring blood flow.

Management of Pain

Phantom limb pain (PLP) must be distinguished from residual limb pain (RLP) because they are managed differently. Some patients have both types of pain at the same time. *If the patient reports PLP, recognize that the pain is real and should be managed promptly and completely! It is not therapeutic to remind the patient that the limb cannot be hurting because it is missing. To prevent increased pain, handle the residual limb carefully when assessing the site or changing the dressing.*

Opioid analgesics are not as effective for PLP as they are for residual limb pain. IV infusions of calcitonin (Miacalcin, Calcimar) during the week after amputation can reduce phantom limb pain. The health care provider prescribes other drugs on the basis of the type of PLP the patient experiences. For instance, beta-blocking agents such as propranolol (Inderal, Apo-Propranolol♣, Detensol♣) are used for constant, dull, burning pain. Antiepileptic drugs such as carbamazepine (Tegretol) and gabapentin (Neurontin) may be used for knifelike or sharp burning pain. Antispasmodics such as baclofen (Lioresal) may be prescribed for muscle spasms or cramping.

Complementary and Alternative Therapies

Many treatments for PLP have been used worldwide, including:

- Ultrasound therapy
- Massage
- Exercises
- Biofeedback
- Distraction therapy
- Hypnosis
- Psychotherapy

Most of these modalities are described in Chapters 2 or 5. Assess the patient's willingness to use any of these therapies. Incorporate them into the plan of care if agreeable with the patient by collaborating with specialists who are trained to perform them. For example, physical therapists often use massage, exercises, TENS, and ultrasound therapy for pain control. Collaborate with the certified hospital chaplain to provide emotional support or a psychologist to provide therapy.

Prevention of Infection

The surgeon typically prescribes broad-spectrum prophylactic antibiotics before elective surgery or immediately before surgery. These may be continued in patients with traumatic amputations or those who have open wounds on the residual limb. The initial pressure dressing and drains are usually removed by the surgeon 48 to 72 hours after surgery. Inspect the wound site for signs of inflammation (e.g., redness and swelling), and monitor for wound healing. Record the appearance, amount, and odor of drainage, if present. Change the soft dressing every day until the sutures or staples are removed. Dressings usually include an elastic bandage wrapped firmly around the residual limb after application of a sterile gauze dressing over the incision.

Promotion of Mobility

Collaborate with the physical therapist to begin exercises as soon as possible after surgery. If the amputation is planned, the therapist may work with the patient before surgery to start muscle-strengthening exercises and evaluate the need for ambulatory aids, such as crutches. If the patient can practice with these devices before surgery, learning how to ambulate after surgery is much easier.

For patients with AKAs or BKAs, teach range-of-motion (ROM) exercises for prevention of flexion contractures, particularly of the hip and knee. A trapeze and an overhead frame, as shown in Fig. 54-12, aid in strengthening the arms and allow the patient to move independently in bed.

A firm mattress is essential for preventing contractures with a leg amputation. Assist the patient into a prone position every 3 to 4 hours for 20- to 30-minute periods if tolerated and not contraindicated. This position may be uncomfortable initially, but it is necessary to prevent hip flexion contractures. Instruct the patient to pull the residual limb close to the other leg and contract the gluteal muscles of the buttocks. For BKAs, also teach how to push the residual limb down toward the bed while supporting it on a pillow. After the sutures are removed, the physical therapist may begin resistive exercises with a "sling-and-spring" apparatus, which can also be used at home.

Elevation of a lower-leg residual limb on a pillow while the patient is in a supine position is controversial. Some practitioners advocate avoiding this procedure at all times because it promotes hip or knee flexion contracture. Others allow elevation for the first 24 to 48 hours to reduce swelling and subsequent discomfort. Inspect the residual limb daily to ensure that it lies completely flat on the bed.

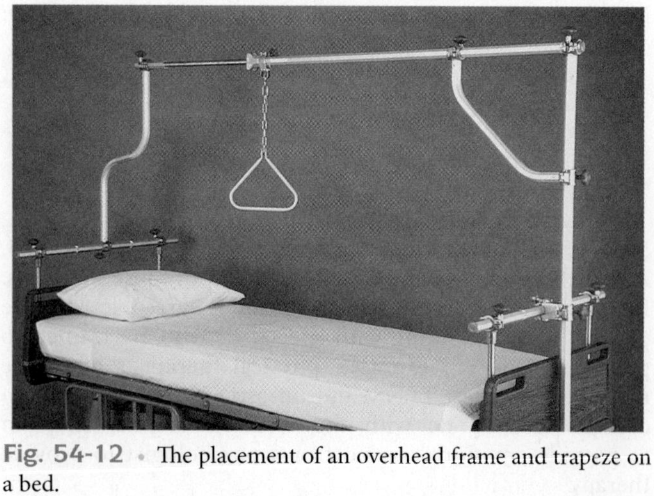

Fig. 54-12 • The placement of an overhead frame and trapeze on a bed.

NCLEX EXAMINATION CHALLENGE

A 78-year-old client has had a left below-the-knee amputation for diabetic peripheral vascular disease. He states that he feels severe burning in his left foot. What is the nurse's best response?

A. "That feeling will go away in a few days; everyone has it."
B. "That foot was amputated so you can't really feel it."
C. "Sometimes the pain medicine makes you feel like that."
D. "On a scale of 1 to 10, what is your pain level now?"

evolve For the correct answer, go to http://evolve.elsevier.com/Iggy/.

Preparation for Prostheses

Before an elective amputation, the patient often sees a certified prosthetist-orthotist (CPO) so that planning can begin for the postoperative period. Arrangements for replacing an arm part are especially important so that the patient can provide self-management. Some patients are fitted with a temporary prosthesis at the time of surgery. Others, particularly older patients with vascular disease, are fitted after the residual limb has healed.

The patient being fitted for a leg prosthesis should bring a sturdy pair of shoes to the fitting. The prosthesis will be adjusted to that heel height.

Several devices help shape and shrink the residual limb in preparation for the prosthesis. Rigid, removable dressings are preferred because they decrease edema, protect and shape the limb, and allow easy access to the wound for inspection. The Jobst air splint, a plastic inflatable device, is sometimes used for this purpose. This device is usually inflated to 20 mm Hg for 22 of every 24 hours. One of its disadvantages is air leakage and loss of compression. Wrapping with elastic bandages can also be effective in reducing edema, shrinking the limb, and holding the wound dressing in place.

For wrapping to be effective, reapply the bandages every 4 to 6 hours or more often if they become loose. *Figure-eight wrapping prevents restriction of blood flow. Decrease the tightness of the bandages while wrapping in a distal-to-proximal direction.* After wrapping, anchor the bandages to the highest joint, such as above the knee for BKAs (Fig. 54-13).

The design of and materials for prostheses have improved dramatically over the years. Computer-assisted design and manufacturing (CAD-CAM) is used for a custom fit. One of the most important developments in lower extremity prosthetics is the ankle-foot prosthesis, such as the Flex-Foot for more active amputees.

Promotion of Body Image and Lifestyle Adaptation

The patient often experiences feelings of inadequacy as a result of losing a body part, especially the older adult who was in poor health before surgery. If possible, arrange for him or her to meet with a rehabilitated amputee who is about the same age as the patient.

Use of the word *stump* for referring to the remaining portion of the limb (residual limb) continues to be controversial. Patients have reported feeling as if they were part of a tree when the term was used. However, some rehabilitation specialists who routinely work with amputees believe the term is appropriate because it forces the patient to realize what has

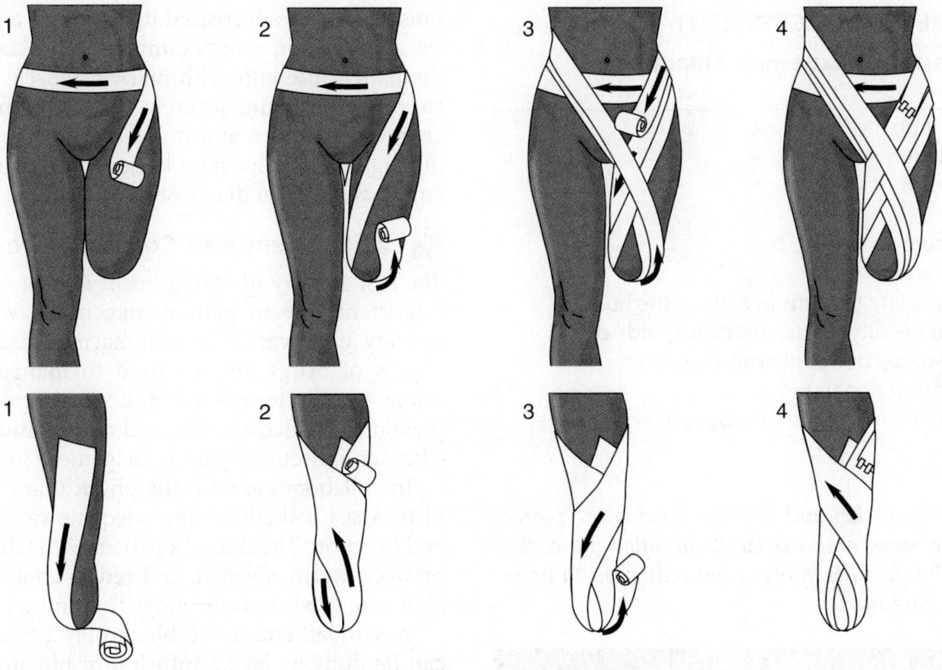
1
2
3
4
1
2
3
4

Fig. 54-13 • A common method of wrapping an amputation stump. *Top,* Wrapping for above-knee amputation. *Bottom,* Wrapping for below-knee amputation.

happened and promotes adjustment to the amputation. Assess the patient to determine what term seems less offensive.

Assess the patient's verbal and nonverbal references to the affected area. Some patients behave euphorically (extremely happy) and seem to have accepted the loss. *Do not jump to the conclusion that acceptance has occurred.* Ask the patient to describe his or her feelings about changes in body image and self-esteem. He or she may verbalize acceptance but refuse to look at the area during a dressing change. This inconsistent behavior is not unusual and should be documented and shared with other health care team members.

A patient who seems to adjust to the amputation during hospitalization may realize that it is difficult to cope with the loss after discharge from the hospital. Teach the patient and family about available resources and support from organizations such as the Amputee Coalition of America (ACA) (www.amputee-coalition.org) and the National Amputation Foundation (NAF) (www.nationalamputation.org). The NAF was originally started for veterans but has since expanded to offer services to civilians.

With advancements in prostheses and surgical techniques, most patients can return to their jobs and other activities. Professional athletes who use prostheses are often quite successful in sports. Patients with amputations ski, hike, golf, bowl, and participate in other physically demanding activities. Many amputees participate actively in organized and recreational sports.

If a job or career change is necessary, collaborate with a social worker or vocational rehabilitation specialist to evaluate the patient's skills. A supportive family or significant other is important for the adjustment to this change. The patient may also think that an intimate relationship is no longer possible because of physical changes. Discuss sexuality issues with the patient and his or her partner as needed. Professional assistance from a sex therapist, intimacy coach, or psychologist may be needed.

Help the patient and family set realistic desired outcomes and take one day at a time. Help them recognize personal strengths. If the outcomes are not realistic, frustration and disappointment may decrease motivation during rehabilitation. Basic principles of rehabilitation are discussed in Chapter 8.

Community-Based Care

The patient is discharged directly to home or to a skilled facility or rehabilitation facility, depending on the extent of the amputation. When rehabilitation is not feasible as in the debilitated or demented older adult, he or she may be discharged to a long-term care facility. Coordinate this transfer with the case manager or discharge planner to ensure continuity of care.

At home, the patient with a leg amputation needs to have enough room to use a wheelchair if the prosthesis is not yet available. He or she must be able to use toileting facilities and have access to areas necessary for self-management, such as the kitchen. Structural home modifications may be required before the patient goes home.

After the sutures or staples are removed, the patient begins residual limb care. A home care nurse may be needed to teach the patient and/or family how to care for the limb and the prosthesis if it is available (Chart 54-8). The limb should be rewrapped three times a day with an elastic bandage applied in a figure-eight manner (see Fig. 54-13). For many patients, a shrinker stocking or sock is easier to apply. After the limb is healed, it is cleaned each day with the rest of the body during bathing with soap and water. Teach the patient and/or family to inspect it every day for signs of inflammation or skin breakdown.

Collaborate with the prosthetist to teach about prosthesis care to ensure its reliability and proper function. These devices are custom made, taking into account the patient's level of amputation, lifestyle, and occupation. Proper teaching regarding

Chart 54-8 HOME CARE ASSESSMENT

The Patient with a Lower Extremity Amputation in the Home

Assess the residual limb for:
- Adequate circulation
- Infection
- Healing
- Flexion contracture
- Dressing/elastic wrap

Assess the patient's ability to perform ADLs in the home.
Evaluate the patient's ability to use ambulatory aids and to care for the prosthetic device (if available).
Assess the patient's nutritional status.
Assess the patient's ability to cope with body image change.

correct cleansing of the socket and inserts, wearing the correct liners, assessing shoe wear, and a schedule of follow-up care is essential before discharge. This information may need to be reviewed by the home care nurse.

DECISION-MAKING CHALLENGE

Coordination of Care

Two days ago a young woman had closed reduction and external fixation for a severely comminuted right ankle and crushed foot. Today she becomes febrile and has an elevated white blood cell count and a decreased hematocrit level. She returns to the operating suite for débridement and exploration where the surgeon finds extensive tissue loss and damage. After this surgery, he recommends an amputation of the foot.

1. What teaching will the patient and family require in preparation for the amputation?
2. What psychosocial assessment and interventions will this patient need? (Consider what health care team members will be needed.)
3. What will you tell her about changes in her lifestyle after the surgery?
4. What community referrals or resources might assist this patient and family with this adjustment?

evolve For suggested answer guidelines, go to http://evolve.elsevier.com/Iggy/.

COMPLEX REGIONAL PAIN SYNDROME

Pathophysiology

Complex regional pain syndrome (CRPS), formerly called **reflex sympathetic dystrophy (RSD),** is a poorly understood dysfunction of the central and peripheral nervous systems. It most often results from traumatic musculoskeletal injury and commonly occurs in the feet and hands. In some cases, specific nerve injuries are present, but in others, no injury can be identified. Typical symptoms include dramatic changes in color and temperature of skin over the affected extremity, intense burning pain, sensitive skin, excessive sweating, and edema.

The most common symptom includes continuous, intense pain out of proportion to the tissue injury that gets progressively worse over time instead of better. The syndrome tends to progress through three classic stages. In stage 1, which lasts 1 to 3 months, the patient reports locally severe, burning pain; edema; vasospasm; and muscle spasm. Over the next 3 months, or stage 2, he or she has more severe, burning pain; edema; muscle atrophy; decreased hair growth; and spotty osteoporosis, as shown on x-ray examination. In stage 3, the final stage, the patient presents with marked muscle atrophy; intractable (unrelenting) pain; severely limited mobility of the affected area; contractures; and marked, diffuse osteoporosis. Timing of diagnosis is important because the syndrome is more difficult to treat when diagnosed in the later stages.

Patient-Centered Collaborative Care

The first priority of management is pain relief. Nurses play an important role in pain management, which includes drug therapy and a variety of nonpharmacologic modalities. Many classes of drugs may be used to manage the intense pain. These include topical analgesics, antiepileptic drugs, antidepressants, corticosteroids, and opioid and non-opioid agents. Chapter 5 discusses pain management in detail.

In collaboration with the physical and occupational therapists, assist in maintaining adequate range of motion (ROM) and function. The skin of a patient with CRPS tends to alternate between warm, swollen, and red to cool, clammy, and bluish. Skin care needs to be gentle with minimal stimulation.

A sympathetic nerve block may be used. This procedure can be done by an IV infusion of phentolamine, a drug that blocks sympathetic receptors, or by injecting anesthetic next to the spine to block sympathetic nerves.

Minimally invasive surgical **sympathectomy,** or cutting of the sympathetic nerve branches via endoscopy through a small axillary incision, may be required. Topical skin adhesive is used to close the very small incision. The patient is discharged to home a few hours later with a follow-up examination the next day with the health care provider. Usual activities can resume a few days later.

Assist the patient in coping with CRPS because it often has a profound psychological effect. A referral for psychological counseling may be indicated. The Reflex Sympathetic Dystrophy Syndrome Association (RSDSA) (www.rsds.org) is available to help patients and their families organize or locate support groups and other resources.

SPORTS-RELATED INJURIES

In addition to the bone and muscle problems already discussed, trauma can cause cartilage, ligament, and tendon injury. Many musculoskeletal injuries are the result of playing sports (professional and recreational) or doing other strenuous physical activities. The popularity of all-terrain vehicles (ATVs) and skateboarding has increased injuries in younger patients. Sports injuries have become so common that large metropolitan hospitals have sports medicine clinics and physicians who specialize in this field.

Although the specific types of injury are numerous, this chapter includes only the most common ones seen in a hospital or ambulatory care setting. The principles of injury to one part of the body are similar to those of other sports injuries. For example, a tendon rupture in a knee is cared for in the same manner as a tendon rupture in the wrist. Chart 54-9 lists general emergency measures for sports-related injuries. All patients require frequent neurovascular monitoring.

Because the knee is most often injured, it is discussed as a typical example of other areas of the body. Trauma to the knee results in **internal derangement,** a broad term for disturbances of an injured knee joint. When surgery is required to resolve the problem, most surgeons prefer to perform the

Chart 54-9 BEST PRACTICE FOR PATIENT SAFETY & QUALITY CARE

Emergency Care of Patients with Sports-Related Injuries

EMERGENCY CARE

- Do not move the victim until spinal cord injury is ascertained (see Chapter 45 for assessment of spinal cord injury).
- Immobilize the injured part, and immobilize the joint above and below the injury by applying a splint.
- Apply ice intermittently for the first 24 to 48 hours (heat may be used thereafter).
- Elevate the affected limb to decrease swelling.
- Always assume the area is fractured until x-ray studies are done.
- Assess neurovascular status in the area distal to the injury.

procedure through an arthroscope when possible. A description of arthroscopy is presented in Chapter 53.

KNEE INJURIES: PATELLOFEMORAL PAIN SYNDROME

Patellofemoral pain syndrome (PFPS) is the most common diagnosis in patients who have knee pain. It occurs most often in people who are runners or who overuse their knee joints. For that reason, it is sometimes referred to as "runner's knee." Patients with this problem describe pain as being behind or around their patella (knee cap) in one or both knees. Swelling is not common although stiffness may be present, especially when the knee is flexed (Dixit et al., 2007).

Management usually involves rest, physical therapy, bracing or splinting, and mild analgesics. For patients who have pain lasting for more than 12 months, arthroscopic surgery is performed.

KNEE INJURIES: MENISCUS

Pathophysiology

There are two semilunar cartilaginous structures, or menisci, in the knee joint: the medial meniscus and the lateral meniscus. These pads act as shock absorbers, but they can tear. Tearing is usually a result of twisting the leg when the knee is flexed and the foot is placed firmly on the ground. The medial meniscus is much more likely to tear than the lateral meniscus because it is less mobile. Internal rotation causes a tear in the medial meniscus. External rotation causes a tear in the lateral meniscus.

Tears can be anterior or posterior, longitudinal or transverse. In the medial meniscus, a longitudinal tear, or "bucket handle" injury, often causes the knee to lock (i.e., the torn cartilage jams between the femur and the tibia and prevents extension of the knee). Surgery is often required for this type of injury. In transverse tears, the knee does not lock and surgery may not be required.

Patient-Centered Collaborative Care

The patient with a torn meniscus typically has pain, swelling, and tenderness in the knee. A clicking or snapping sound can often be heard when the knee is moved.

A common diagnostic technique is the **McMurray test.** The examiner flexes and rotates the knee and then presses on the medial aspect while slowly extending the leg. The test result is positive if clicking is palpated or heard. A negative finding, however, does not rule out a tear.

For a locked knee, the treatment may be manipulation followed by splinting or casting for 3 to 6 weeks. If the problem recurs, a partial or total **meniscectomy** is performed. An *open* meniscectomy requires a surgical incision for removal of all or part of the meniscus and is rarely performed. Most surgeons prefer to remove only the affected portion during a *closed* meniscectomy, which can be done through an arthroscope as a same-day surgical procedure. As described in Chapter 53, an arthroscope is a metal tubular instrument used for examination or surgery of joints. One or more small incisions (less than $\frac{1}{4}$ inch [0.6 cm] long) are made in the knee for insertion of the arthroscope. The surgeon threads a cutting device through the arthroscope for removal of the torn cartilage while the knee is irrigated. The surgeon may use a laser during the procedure, depending on the type and severity of the injury. A bulky pressure dressing is applied after the procedure, and the affected leg is wrapped in elastic bandages.

As for any postoperative patient, check the surgical dressing for bleeding and monitor vital signs after the patient is admitted to the same-day surgical unit. Perform neurovascular checks as outlined in Chart 54-3, usually every hour for the first few hours and then every 4 hours. Teach the patient and family what signs and symptoms to watch for after surgery and when to notify the health care provider.

The patient begins exercises immediately after surgery to strengthen the leg, prevent venous thromboembolism, and reduce swelling. Quadriceps setting, in which the patient straightens the leg while pushing the knee against the bed, is done in sets of 10 or more. Straight-leg raises are also performed. Range-of-motion (ROM) exercises are usually not started for several days.

To prevent bending the affected knee, the physician may request a knee immobilizer, such as the one shown in Fig. 54-14. Elevate the leg on one or two pillows according to the physician's preference, and apply ice to reduce postoperative swelling. Full weight bearing is restricted for several weeks, depending on the amount of cartilage removed. The patient is

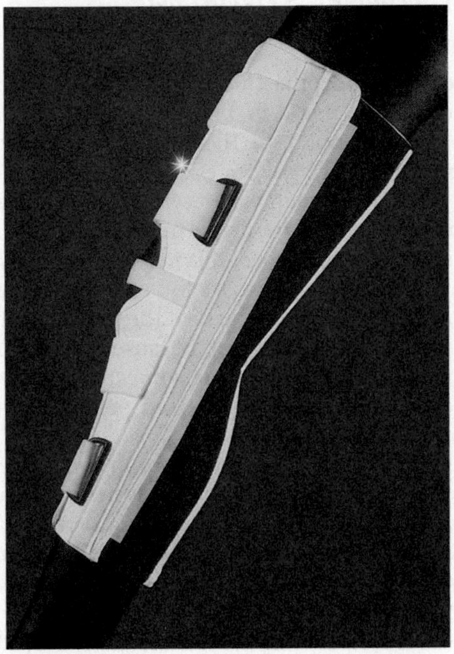

Fig. 54-14 • A knee immobilizer.

usually discharged from the hospital with crutches in less than 23 hours.

KNEE INJURIES: LIGAMENTS

The cruciate and collateral ligaments in the knee are predisposed to injury, often from sports or vehicular crashes. The anterior cruciate ligament (ACL) is the most commonly torn ligament in the knee. Athletes often get these injuries during skiing, skating, or gymnastics. Women have ACL tears more often than men, possibly related to hormonal influences, biomechanical factors, and anatomic differences. Proper athletic shoes and learning how to land when jumping can help prevent this injury (Rodenberg et al., 2006).

When the ACL is torn, the patient feels a snap and the knee gives way because of ACL laxity. Within hours, the knee is swollen, stiff, and painful. Examination by the health care provider shows positive ligament laxity. The diagnosis of an ACL tear is best confirmed by magnetic resonance imaging (MRI) (Rodenberg et al., 2006).

Treatment may be nonsurgical or surgical, depending on the severity of the injury and the activity of the patient. Exercises, bracing, and limits on activities while the ligament heals may be sufficient. If medical management is not effective or the tear is severe, surgery may be needed.

The surgeon repairs the tear by reattaching the torn portions of the ligament through arthroscopy. The leg is placed in a brace or immobilizer. If the ligament cannot be repaired, reconstructive surgery may be performed with autologous grafts. A ligament from another part of the body is used to replace the torn knee ligament. Another option is artificial knee implants such as the GORE-TEX ligament.

Complete healing of knee ligaments after surgery can take 6 to 9 months or longer. These patients may use a continuous passive motion (CPM) machine at home. Teach the patient how to use and care for the machine. CPM use is discussed with the postoperative care of the total knee patient in Chapter 20.

OTHER INJURIES

CARPAL TUNNEL SYNDROME

Pathophysiology

Carpal tunnel syndrome (CTS) is a common condition in which the median nerve in the wrist becomes compressed, causing pain and numbness. The carpal tunnel is a rigid canal that lies between the carpal bones and a fibrous tissue sheet. A group of tendons surrounds the synovium and shares space with the median nerve in the carpal tunnel. When the synovium becomes swollen or thickened, this nerve is compressed.

The median nerve supplies motor, sensory, and autonomic function for the first three fingers of the hand and the palmar aspect of the fourth (ring) finger. Because the median nerve is close to other structures, wrist flexion causes nerve impingement, and extension causes increased pressure in the lower portion of the carpal tunnel.

CTS usually presents as a chronic problem. Acute cases are rare. Excessive hand exercise, edema or hemorrhage into the carpal tunnel, or thrombosis of the median artery can lead to acute CTS. *Patients with hand burns or a Colles' fracture of the wrist are particularly at risk for this problem.* In most cases, the cause may not result in nerve deficit for years.

CTS is a common complication of certain metabolic and connective tissue diseases. For example, **synovitis** (inflammation of the synovium) occurs in patients with rheumatoid arthritis (RA). The hypertrophied synovium compresses the median nerve. In other chronic disorders such as diabetes mellitus, inadequate blood supply can cause median nerve neuropathy or dysfunction, resulting in CTS.

CTS is the most *common* type of **repetitive stress injury (RSI).** RSIs are the fastest growing type of occupational injury. People whose jobs require repetitive hand activities such as pinching or grasping during wrist flexion (e.g., factory workers, computer operators, jackhammer operators) are predisposed to CTS. It can also result from overuse in sports activities such as golf, tennis, or racquetball.

In a few cases, CTS may be a familial or congenital problem that manifests in adulthood. Space-occupying growths such as ganglia, tophi, and lipomas can also result in nerve compression.

Women, especially those over age 50 years, are much more likely than men to experience CTS, most likely due to the higher prevalence of diseases such as RA in women. The problem most often affects the dominant hand but can occur in both hands simultaneously. CTS is beginning to be found in children and adolescents as a result of the increased use of computers in everyday life.

Health Promotion and Maintenance

Most businesses recognize the hazards of repetitive motion as a primary cause of occupational injury and disability. Both men and women in the labor force are experiencing increasing numbers of RSIs. Occupational health nurses have played an important role in ergonomic assessments and in the development of ergonomically designed furniture and various aids to decrease CTS and other musculoskeletal injuries.

U.S federal and state legislation has been passed to ensure that all businesses, including health care organizations (HCOs), provide *ergonomically appropriate workstations* for their employees (www.osha.gov). The Joint Commission also requires that hospitals and other HCOs provide a safe work environment for all staff. In Canada, each country requires the work setting to have joint health and safety committees in which employees are actively involved in setting safety standards (www.ccohs.ca). Chart 54-10 lists best practices for preventing CTS in the health care setting.

Patient-Centered Collaborative Care

Assessment

A medical diagnosis is often made on the basis of the patient's history and report of hand pain and numbness and without further assessment. Ask about the nature, intensity, and location of the pain. Patients often state that the pain is worse at night as a result of flexion or direct pressure during sleep. The pain may radiate to the arm, shoulder and neck, or chest.

In addition to reports of numbness, patients with carpal tunnel syndrome (CTS) may also have **paresthesia** (painful tingling). *Sensory* changes usually occur weeks or months before *motor* manifestations.

The health care provider performs several tests for abnormal sensory findings. Phalen's wrist test, sometimes called **Phalen's maneuver,** produces paresthesia in the median nerve distribution (palmar side of the thumb, index, and middle finger, and half of the ring finger) within 60 seconds. The patient is asked to relax the wrist into flexion or to place

Chart 54-10 **BEST PRACTICE FOR PATIENT SAFETY & QUALITY CARE**

Health Promotion Activities to Prevent Carpal Tunnel Syndrome in Health Care Organizations

- Become familiar with federal and state laws regarding workplace requirements to prevent repetitive stress injuries such as carpal tunnel syndrome (CTS) (www.osha.gov; www.cchos.ca).
- When using equipment or computer workstations that can contribute to developing CTS, assess that they are ergonomically appropriate, including:
  - Specially designed wrist rest devices
  - Geometrically designed computer keyboards
  - Chair height that allows good posture
- Take regular short breaks away from activities that cause repetitive stress, such as computers.
- Stretch fingers and wrists frequently during work hours.
- Stay as relaxed as possible when using equipment that causes repetitive stress.

the back of the hands together and flex both wrists at the same time. The Phalen's test is positive in most patients with CTS.

The same sensation can be created by tapping lightly over the area of the median nerve in the wrist **(Tinel's sign).** If the test is unsuccessful, a blood pressure cuff can be placed on the upper arm and inflated to the patient's systolic pressure (tourniquet). This often causes pain and tingling.

Motor changes begin with a weak pinch, clumsiness, and difficulty with fine movements. These changes progress to muscle weakness and wasting, which can impair self-management. If desired, test for pinching ability and ask the patient to perform a fine-movement task, such as threading a needle. Strenuous hand activity worsens the pain and numbness.

In addition to inspecting for muscle atrophy and task performance, observe the wrist for swelling. Gently palpate the area and note any unusual findings. Autonomic changes may be evidenced by skin discoloration, nail changes (e.g., brittleness), and increased or decreased hand sweating.

When a definitive diagnosis is uncertain, the health care provider may request routine x-rays, electromyography (EMG) and nerve conduction studies (NCS), magnetic resonance imaging (MRI), and/or ultrasonography. NCS testing reveals nerve dysfunction before muscle atrophy is observed. An ultrasound scan or MRI may be done to view the cause of the problem. The most common finding is an enlarged median nerve within the carpal tunnel.

▪ *Interventions*

The health care provider uses conservative measures before surgical intervention. However, CTS can recur with either type of treatment.

Nonsurgical Management. Aggressive drug therapy and immobilization of the wrist are the major components of nonsurgical management. Teach the patient the importance of these modalities in the hope of preventing surgical intervention.

Nonsteroidal anti-inflammatory drugs (NSAIDs) are the most commonly prescribed drugs for the relief of pain and inflammation, if present. In addition to or instead of systemic medications, the physician may inject corticosteroids directly into the carpal tunnel. If the patient responds to the injection, several additional weekly or monthly injections are given. Teach him or her to take NSAIDs with or after meals to reduce gastric irritation.

A splint may be used to immobilize the wrist during the day, during the night, or both. Many patients experience temporary relief with splinting. The occupational therapist places the wrist in the neutral position or in slight extension.

Surgical Management. Surgery is necessary in about half of patients with CTS. Surgery can relieve the pressure on the median nerve by providing nerve decompression. Major surgical complications are rare following CTS surgery. In some cases, however, CTS recurs months to years after surgery.

The nurse in the physician's office or same-day surgical center reinforces the teaching provided by the surgeon regarding the nature of the surgery. Postoperative care is reviewed so the patient knows what to expect. Chapter 16 describes general preoperative care in detail.

Whatever the cause of nerve compression, the surgeon removes it either by cutting or by the newer laser technique. The two most common surgeries are the open carpal tunnel release (OCTR) and the newer endoscopic carpal tunnel release (ECTR). When CTS is a complication of rheumatoid arthritis, a **synovectomy** (removal of excess synovium) through a small inner-wrist incision may resolve the problem. Removal of a space-occupying growth, if present, also decompresses the nerve.

ECTR is a common alternative to OCTR. The surgeon makes a very small incision (less than ½ inch [1.2 cm]) through which the endoscope is inserted. The surgeon then uses special instruments, which may include a laser, to free the trapped median nerve. Although ECTR is less invasive and costs less than the open procedure, the patient may have a longer period of postoperative pain and numbness compared with recovery from OCTR.

After surgery, monitor vital signs and check the dressing carefully for drainage and tightness. If ECTR has been performed, the dressing is very small. The surgeon may require that the patient's affected hand and arm be elevated above heart level for several days to reduce postoperative swelling. Check the neurovascular status of the fingers every hour during the immediate postoperative period, and encourage the patient to move them frequently. Offer pain medication and assure him or her that a prescription for analgesics will be provided before discharge.

Hand movements, including lifting heavy objects, may be restricted for 4 to 6 weeks after surgery. The patient can expect weakness and discomfort for weeks or perhaps months. Teach him or her to report any changes in neurovascular status, including increased pain and numbness, to the surgeon's office immediately.

Remind the patient and family that the surgical procedure might not be a cure. For instance, synovitis may recur with rheumatoid arthritis and may recompress the median nerve. Multiple surgeries and other treatments are common with CTS.

The patient may need assistance with self-management activities during recovery. Ensure that assistance in the home is available before discharge; this is usually provided by the family or significant others.

TENDON RUPTURE AND JOINT DISLOCATION

Other injuries can affect any synovial joint. The nursing management of each of these is similar to the collaborative care previously discussed for knee injuries. Cast care is discussed on p. 1188 in the Fractures section. *Rupture of the Achilles tendon* is common in adults who participate in strenuous sports. In the older adult, quadriceps tendon rupture may occur from a fall down several steps. For severe damage, the tendon is surgically repaired and the leg is immobilized in a cast or brace for 6 to 8 weeks. If the tendon is beyond repair, a **tendon transplant** (also known as *tendon reconstruction*) is performed. A tendon is removed from one part of the body and transplanted to the affected area, or a cadaver donor is used.

Dislocation of a joint occurs when the ends of two or more bones are moved away from each other. If the dislocation is not complete, the joint is partially dislocated, or **subluxed.** It can occur in any diarthrodial (synovial) joint but is most common in the shoulder, hip, knee, and fingers. This injury is usually the result of trauma but can be congenital or pathologic and can result from joint disease, such as arthritis.

The typical manifestations of dislocation are:

- Pain
- Immobility
- Alteration in contour of the joint
- Deviation in length of the extremity
- Rotation of the extremity

The health care provider performs a closed reduction of the joint and moves the joint surfaces back into their normal anatomic position. The patient requires light anesthetic or moderate sedation. The joint is immobilized by a cast, splint, brace, or immobilizer until healing occurs.

Recurrent dislocations are common in the knee and shoulder. For this problem, the joint may be fixed with wires or other device to prevent further displacement. A cast, splint, or traction is applied for 3 to 6 weeks.

STRAINS AND SPRAINS

A **strain** is excessive stretching of a muscle or tendon when it is weak or unstable. Strains are sometimes referred to as *muscle pulls.* Falls, lifting of a heavy item, and exercise often cause this injury.

Strains are classified according to their severity:

- A first-degree (mild) strain causes mild inflammation but little bleeding. Swelling, ecchymosis (bruising), and tenderness are usually present.
- A second-degree (moderate) strain involves tearing of the muscle or tendon fibers without complete disruption. Muscle function may be impaired.
- A third-degree (severe) strain involves a ruptured muscle or tendon with separation of muscle from muscle, tendon from muscle, or tendon from bone. Severe pain and disability result from severe strains.

Management usually involves cold and heat applications, exercise, and activity limitations. The health care provider may prescribe anti-inflammatory drugs to decrease inflammation and pain. Muscle relaxants may also be used. In third-degree strains, surgical repair of the ruptured muscle or tendon may be needed.

A **sprain** is excessive stretching of a ligament. Twisting motions from a fall or sports activity typically cause the injury. Sprains are also classified according to severity:

- A first-degree (mild) sprain involves tearing of a few fibers of a ligament. Function of the joint is not impaired.
- In a second-degree (moderate) sprain, more fibers are torn but the joint remains stable.
- A third-degree (severe) sprain causes marked instability of the joint.

Pain and swelling result from ligament injuries. The treatment for *mild (first-degree)* sprains includes:

- Rest
- Use of ice for the first 24 to 48 hours
- Application of a compression bandage for a few days to reduce swelling and provide joint support
- Elevation

Second-degree sprains require immobilization, such as elastic bandage and an air stirrup ankle brace or splint, and partial weight bearing while the tear heals. For severe ligament damage (*third-degree* sprain), immobilization for 4 to 6 weeks is necessary. Arthroscopic surgery may be done, particularly for chronic joint instability.

ROTATOR CUFF INJURIES

The musculotendinous, or rotator, cuff of the shoulder functions to stabilize the head of the humerus in the glenoid cavity during shoulder abduction. Young adults usually sustain a tear of the cuff by substantial trauma, such as may occur during a fall, while throwing a ball, or with heavy lifting. Older adults tend to have small tears related to aging, repetitive motions, or falls.

The patient with a torn rotator cuff has shoulder pain and cannot easily abduct the arm at the shoulder. When the arm is abducted, he or she usually drops the arm because abduction cannot be maintained (drop arm test).

The health care provider usually treats the patient conservatively with NSAIDs, physical therapy, sling or immobilizer support, and ice and/or heat applications while the tear heals.

For patients who do not respond to conservative treatment or for those who have a complete tear, the surgeon repairs the cuff. After surgery, the affected arm is usually immobilized for several weeks. Pendulum exercises are started on the third or fourth postoperative day and progress to active exercises in about 2 weeks. If the surgery is extensive, the patient's arm may be immobilized for a longer time before exercises begin. Patients then begin outpatient rehabilitation in the occupational therapy department. Teach them that they may not have full function for several months.

HUMAN NEEDS NURSING CARE REVIEW

What might you NOTICE if the patient has impaired mobility and sensation as a result of acute musculoskeletal trauma?

- Extremity swelling, bleeding, bruising, shortening, malalignment, and/or rotation
- Report of severe pain
- Break in skin integrity
- Report of decreased or unusual sensation in extremity
- Inability or decreased ability to move extremity
- Difficulty breathing (rib trauma)
- Severe kyphosis (compression fractures)

What should you INTERPRET and how should you RESPOND to a patient with impaired mobility and sensation as a result of acute musculoskeletal trauma?

Perform and interpret focused physical assessment findings, including:

- ABC (airway, breathing, circulation) ability
- Pain intensity and quality
- Vital signs
- Neurovascular assessment ("circ check")

Respond:

- First, establish ABCs if problem exists.
- If skin is not intact, cover wound with dry, sterile dressing, if available; use clean cloth as an option. Apply pressure to proximal pulse if patient is bleeding; for traumatic intervention, apply direct pressure to the residual body part.
- Implement measures to prevent hypovolemic shock if patient is bleeding, including lying patient flat, keeping him or her warm, and elevating the bleeding part.
- Splint the extremity (in community setting) to prevent movement and further damage.
- If in hospital setting, assist health care provider in splinting.
- Provide pain control interventions by drug therapy as soon as possible.
- Provide emotional assurance for the patient by being present and comforting.

On what should you REFLECT?

- Monitor the patient's response to pain control interventions.
- Think about what else you could do to prevent complications.
- Determine what health teaching will be needed, depending on the treatment that is provided (e.g., surgery, cast).

GET READY FOR THE NCLEX EXAMINATION!

Key Points

Review these Key Points for each NCLEX Examination Client Needs Category.

Safe and Effective Care Environment

- Collaborate with physical and occupational therapists for care of patients with extremity fractures.
- Collaborate with the prosthetist, physical and occupational therapists, psychologist, and sex therapist or intimacy coach for care of patients with amputations.
- Several community organizations, such as the Amputee Coalition of America, are available to help patients and their families cope with the loss of a body part.
- Use strict aseptic technique when caring for wounds in patients with compound fractures to help prevent infection; give antibiotic therapy as prescribed.
- Assess the risk for and implement interventions to prevent complications of immobility in patients having musculoskeletal injury or surgery (e.g., pressure ulcers, venous thromboembolism [VTE]).

Health Promotion and Maintenance

- Teach patients and their family members and significant others how to care for casts or traction at home.
- Reinforce teaching for ambulating with crutches, walkers, or canes.
- Provide special care for older adults with hip fractures, including preventing heel pressure ulcers and promoting early ambulation to prevent complications of immobility.
- Teach exercises to patients with leg amputation to prevent hip flexion contractures.

Psychosocial Integrity

- Be aware that patients with severe musculoskeletal trauma may have a prolonged hospitalization and recovery period.
- For patients with severe trauma or amputation, assess coping skills and encourage verbalization.
- Recognize that the patient having an amputation may need to adjust to an altered lifestyle; however, new custom prosthetics improve mobility.
- Help the patient with an amputation or other musculoskeletal trauma and family to set realistic expected outcomes and take one day at a time.

Continued

Physiological Integrity

- Be aware that open fractures cause a higher risk for infection than do closed fractures.
- Assess patients with fractures for complications, such as VTE, infection, and acute compartment syndrome.
- Recognize that fat embolism syndrome is different from pulmonary (blood clot) embolism as outlined in Chart 54-2.
- Provide emergency care of the patient with a fracture as described in Chart 54-4.
- Identify the patient at risk for acute compartment syndrome; loosen bandages or request that the patient's cast be cut if neurovascular compromise is noted.
- As a priority, assess neurovascular status frequently in patients with musculoskeletal injury, traction, or cast as described in Chart 54-3.
- Provide appropriate cast care, depending on the type of cast (plaster or synthetic); check for pressure necrosis under the cast by feeling for heat, assessing the patient's pain level, and smelling the cast for an unpleasant odor.
- Provide pin care for patients with skeletal traction or external fixation; assess for manifestations of infection at the pin sites.
- Provide postoperative care for the patient having a fracture repair, including promoting mobility and monitoring for complications of immobility.
- Provide care for patients having a vertebroplasty or kyphoplasty as described in Chart 54-7.
- Observe for hemorrhage and infection in the patient having an amputation.
- Postoperatively, assess for and promptly manage phantom limb pain in the patient who has an amputation; collaborate with specialists to incorporate complementary and alternative therapies into the patient's plan of care.
- Provide emergency care for patients with a sports-related injury as outlined in Chart 54-9.

Additional Study Resources

Go to your Companion CD or Evolve at http://evolve.elsevier.com/Iggy/ for *Self-Assessment Questions for the NCLEX Examination.*

evolve Go to Evolve at http://evolve.elsevier.com/Iggy/ for *Prioritization and Delegation Questions for the NCLEX Examination.*

SELECTED BIBLIOGRAPHY

Asterisk indicates a classic or definitive work on this subject.

*Altizer, L. (2004). Compartment syndrome. *Orthopaedic Nursing, 23*(6), 391-396.

Altizer, L. (2005). Hip fractures. *Orthopaedic Nursing, 24*(4), 283-294.

Bongiovanni, M.S., Bradley, S.L., & Kelley, D.M. (2005). Orthopedic trauma. *Critical Care Nursing Quarterly, 28*(1), 60-71.

Centers for Disease Control and Prevention. *Health data for all ages.* Retrieved March 1, 2008, from http://cdc.gov/nchs/health_data_for_all_ages.htm.

Childs, S.G. (2005). Rhabdomyolysis. *Orthopaedic Nursing, 24*(6), 443-447.

Colyar, M. (2006). Reduction of a joint dislocation. *Advance for Nurse Practitioners.* Retrieved March 1, 2008, from www.advanceweb.com.

Day, M.W. (2008). Fracture in the field. *Nursing2008, 38*(6), 72.

Dillon, P.A. (Ed.). (2007). *Nursing health assessment: A critical thinking approach* (2nd ed.). Philadelphia: Davis.

Dixit, S., Difiori, J.P., Burton, M., & Mines, B. (2007). Management of patellofemoral pain syndrome. *American Family Physician, 75*(2), 194-202.

Folden, S., & Tappen, R. (2007). Factors influencing function and recovery following hip repair surgery. *Orthopaedic Nursing, 26*(4), 234-241.

Gross, K.A. (2006). Solid advice on managing vertebral compression fractures. *Nursing2006, 36*(12), 64hn1-3.

Hall, D. (2007). Detect compartment syndrome in time. *American Nurse, 2*(7), 42-43.

Harvey, C. (2006). Complications. *Orthopaedic Nursing, 25*(6), 410-414.

*Holmes, S.B., & Brown, S.J. (2005). Skeletal pin site care: National Association of Orthopaedic Nurses guidelines for orthopaedic nursing. *Orthopaedic Nursing, 24*(2), 99-107.

Huang, T.T., & Liang, S.H. (2005). A randomized clinical trial of the effectiveness of a discharge planning intervention in hospitalized elders with hip fracture due to falling. *Care of Older People, 14,* 1193-1201.

Kessenich, C.R. (2006). Osteoporosis: New options for pain relief. *The Nurse Practitioner, 31*(2), 44-47.

Laskowski-Jones, L. (2006). First aid for amputation. *Nursing2006, 36*(4), 50-52.

Lemke, D.M. (2005). Vertebroplasty and kyphoplasty for treatment of painful osteoporotic compression fractures. *Journal of the American Academy of Nurse Practitioners, 17*(7), 268-276.

*Mosher, C.M. (Ed.). (2004). *An introduction to orthopaedic nursing* (3rd ed.). Chicago: National Association of Orthopaedic Nurses.

National Institute of Neurological Disorders and Stroke. *Complex regional pain syndrome fact sheet.* Retrieved March 1, 2008, from www.ninds.nih.gov/disorders/reflex_sympathetic_dystrophy/detail.htm.

O'Brien, M.S., & DeHoratius, R.J. (2007). Managing the musculoskeletal complications of diabetes mellitus. *The Journal of Musculoskeletal Medicine, 24*(1), 9-18.

Okike, K., & Bhattacharyya, T. (2006). Trends in the management of open fractures. *The Journal of Bone and Joint Surgery, 88A*(12), 2739-2748.

Olsson, L.E., Karlsson, J., & Ekman, I. (2007). Effects of nursing interventions within an integrated care pathway for patients with hip fracture. *Journal of Advanced Nursing, 58*(2), 116-125.

Pagana, K.D., & Pagana, T.J. (2006). *Mosby's manual of diagnostic and laboratory tests* (3rd ed.). St. Louis: Mosby.

Rodenberg, R.E., Cayce K. IV, & Hall, S. (2006). Your guide to a dreaded injury: The ACL tear. *Contemporary Pediatrics, 23*(7), 26-29.

Schoen, D.C. (2005a). The mystery of ankle problems. *Orthopaedic Nursing, 24*(2), 166-169.

Schoen, D.C. (2005b). Injuries of the wrist. *Orthopaedic Nursing, 24*(4), 304-307.

Summerfield, D.L. (2006). Decreasing the incidence of deep vein thrombosis through the use of prophylaxis. *AORN Journal, 84*(4), 642-645.

Sweeney, J., & Ardisson, M. (2006). What's a fat embolism? *Nursing2006, 36*(11), 22.

Taggart, H. (Ed.). (2006). *Core curriculum for orthopaedic nursing* (5th ed.). Boston: Pearson.

Titler, M., Dochterman, J., Taikyoung, K., Kanak, M., Shever, L., Picone, D.M., et al. (2007). Cost of care for seniors hospitalized for hip fracture and related procedures. *Nursing Outlook, 55*(1), 5-14.

Turkoski, B.B. (2005). Fighting infection: An ongoing challenge, Part 1. *Orthopaedic Nursing, 24*(1), 40-48.

Van Horn, E. (2005). An exploration of recurrent injury prevention in patients with trauma. *Orthopaedic Nursing, 24*(4), 249-258.

Watters, C.L., & Moran, W.P. (2006). Hip fractures: A joint effort. *Orthopaedic Nursing, 25*(3), 157-165.

Williams, A., & Jester, R. (2005). Delayed surgical fixation of fractured hips in older people: Impact on mortality. *Journal of Advanced Nursing, 52*(1), 63-69.

HUMAN NEEDS OVERVIEW

Nutrition, Metabolism, and Bowel Elimination

Why do we eat, and how are nutrition, metabolism, and bowel elimination related? Within the human body, as in all living systems, energy is required to perform any function. The word *metabolism* means to change or transform. Humans transform the energy stored within food into the types of energy needed to make the body work.

As shown in Fig. 1, *nutrition* involves ingesting many types of foods that contain proteins, carbohydrates, fats, vitamins, and minerals. Once inside the GI tract, the processes of digestion break down food into its basic elements, which then are absorbed into the blood and delivered to cells. Through metabolism, cells convert these basic elements into chemical energy, mostly adenosine triphosphate (ATP). Different cells then use metabolism to further transform ATP into heat energy, mechanical energy, chemical energy, and electrical energy. The transformation of chemical energy into other types of energy within the human body is *irreversible.* It is lost from the body in the form of heat and work. Thus bringing food into the body on a daily basis is important in meeting the human needs of nutrition and metabolism.

Heat energy helps maintain the core body temperature at or near 98.6° F—the ideal temperature for important physiologic reactions. When environmental temperatures are low, more food is needed to maintain body temperature. When environmental temperatures are high, less food is needed to maintain body temperature. Therefore, in general, more calories need to be consumed per day in the winter than in the summer.

Mechanical energy is used for cell and tissue movement, cell shape changes, and whole body movement. *Electrical energy* generates the action potentials that allow nerves to transmit impulses and muscles to contract. *Chemical energy* is used to drive every chemical reaction in the body. As long as it remains alive, the body continuously needs to change food into these different energies.

Bowel elimination is the way the body rids itself of those food components that cannot be absorbed into the blood and converted into energy, such as fiber and cellulose. If these components remained in the GI tract, they would soon fill it to the point that no nutrients could be ingested.

Consider Fig. 1 as representing the entire nutrition, metabolism, and bowel elimination of a person throughout his or her lifetime. The energy ingested in the form of food exactly matches the energy transformed by metabolism and is used for all the different types of internal and external "work" of the body. When this ideal situation exists, the person always has the right amount of nutrients and neither stores excess nutrients nor breaks down body tissues to use for energy.

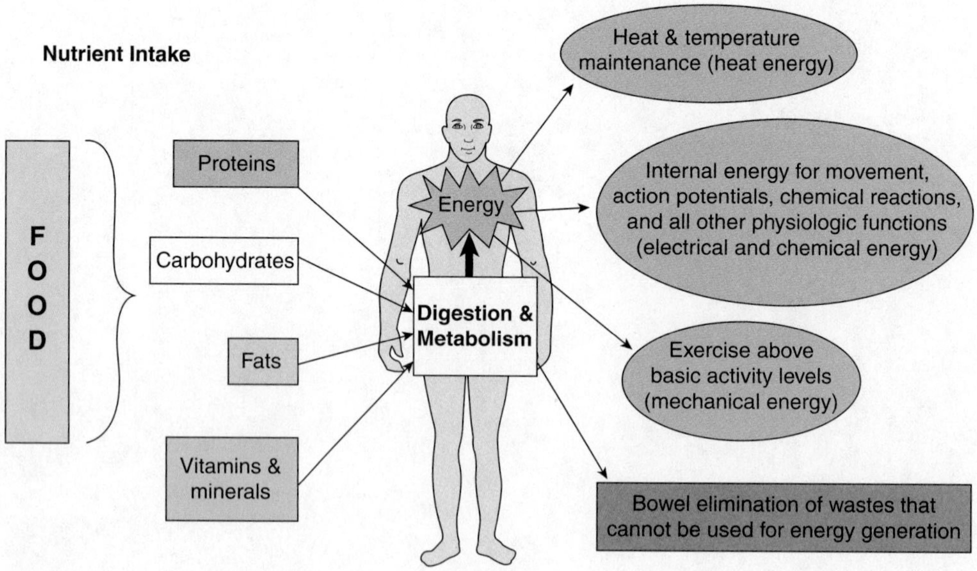

Nutrient Intake
FOOD
Proteins
Carbohydrates
Fats
Vitamins & minerals
Energy
Digestion & Metabolism
Heat & temperature maintenance (heat energy)
Internal energy for movement, action potentials, chemical reactions, and all other physiologic functions (electrical and chemical energy)
Exercise above basic activity levels (mechanical energy)
Bowel elimination of wastes that cannot be used for energy generation

Fig. 1

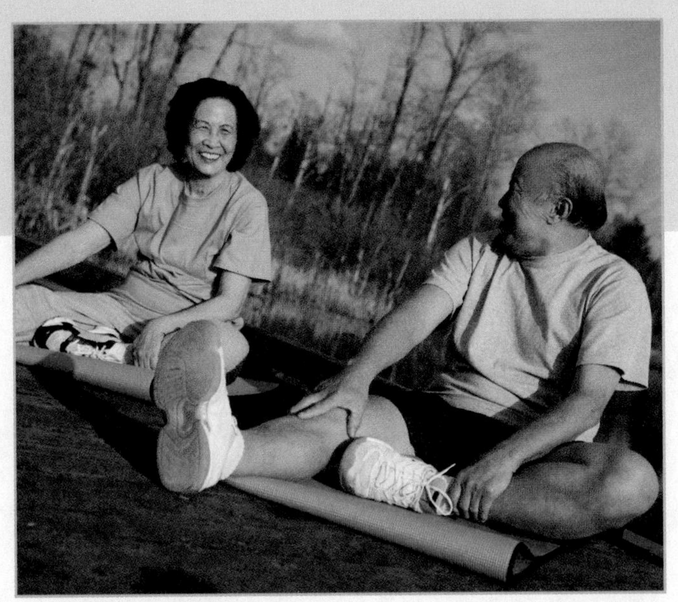

In Fig. 2, the person is not ingesting enough nutrients to meet metabolic energy needs. As a result, the different types of work are less efficient and the person metabolizes his or her own body tissues to provide needed energy. If this situation continues, it will lead to death.

In Fig. 3, the person is ingesting more nutrients than are needed to meet energy needs. As a result, these extra energy compounds are converted first into glycogen and eventually into fat. Although fat represents stored energy, excessive fat can harm the body. In addition, when food is ingested to excess, metabolism and work energies are not increased. Only heat and bowel elimination increase.

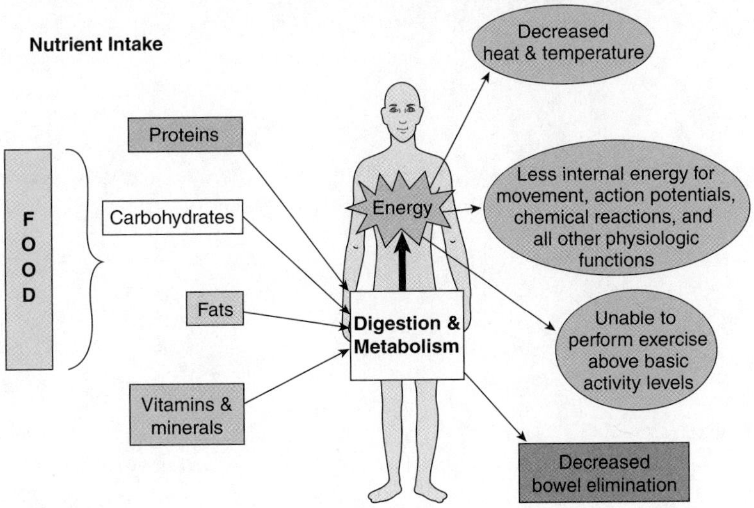
Nutrient Intake
FOOD
Proteins
Carbohydrates
Fats
Vitamins & minerals
Energy
Digestion & Metabolism
Decreased heat & temperature
Less internal energy for movement, action potentials, chemical reactions, and all other physiologic functions
Unable to perform exercise above basic activity levels
Decreased bowel elimination

Fig. 2

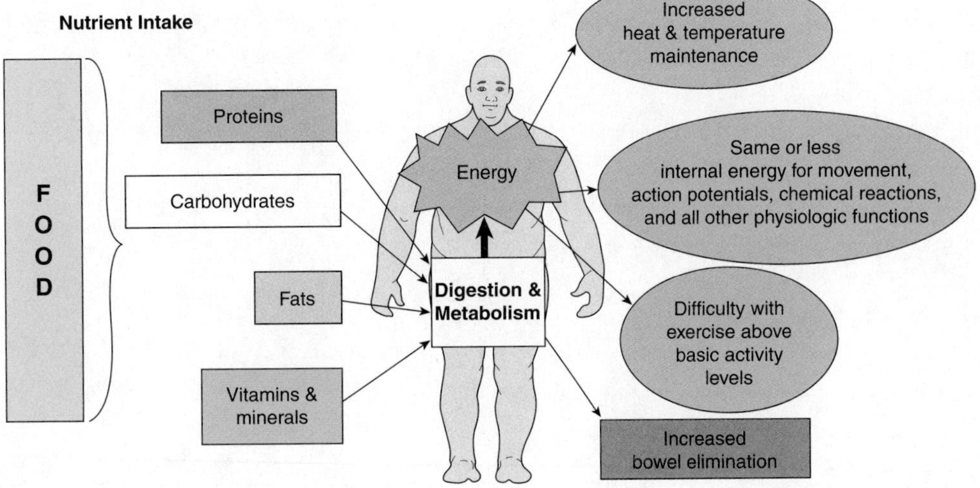
Nutrient Intake
FOOD
Proteins
Carbohydrates
Fats
Vitamins & minerals
Energy
Digestion & Metabolism
Increased heat & temperature maintenance
Same or less internal energy for movement, action potentials, chemical reactions, and all other physiologic functions
Difficulty with exercise above basic activity levels
Increased bowel elimination

Fig. 3

XIII

UNIT

Problems of Digestion, Nutrition, and Elimination

Management of Patients with Problems of the Gastrointestinal System

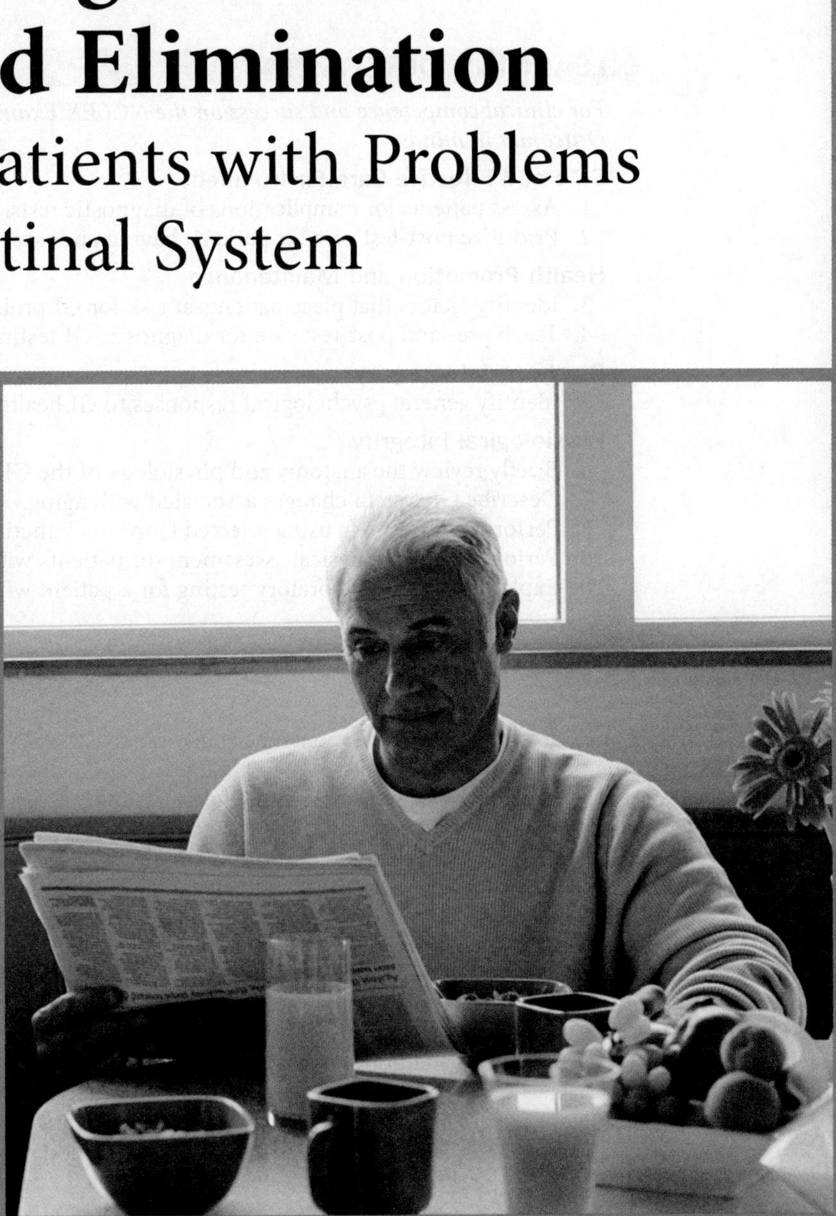

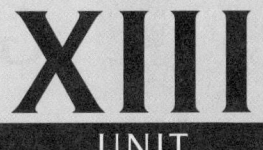

55 CHAPTER

Assessment of the Gastrointestinal System

Karrie K. Dietzen

LEARNING OUTCOMES

For clinical competence and success on the NCLEX Examination, study this chapter with these Learning Outcomes in mind:

Safe and Effective Care Environment

1. Assess patients for complications of diagnostic tests.
2. Prioritize post-test care for patients having endoscopic procedures.

Health Promotion and Maintenance

3. Identify factors that place patients at risk for GI problems.
4. Teach pre- and post-test care for diagnostic GI testing to patients and families.

Psychosocial Integrity

5. Identify general psychological responses to GI health problems.

Physiological Integrity

6. Briefly review the anatomy and physiology of the GI system.
7. Describe GI system changes associated with aging.
8. Perform a GI history using selected Gordon's Functional Health Patterns.
9. Perform focused physical assessment for patients with suspected or actual GI health problems.
10. Explain the use of laboratory testing for a patient with a GI health problem.

evolve Go to your Companion CD or Evolve at http://evolve.elsevier.com/Iggy/ for *Self-Assessment Questions for the NCLEX Examination* keyed to these Learning Outcomes.

The GI system includes the GI tract (alimentary canal), consisting of the mouth, esophagus, stomach, small and large intestines, and rectum. The salivary glands, liver, gallbladder, and pancreas secrete substances into this tract to form the GI system (Fig. 55-1). The main function of the GI tract, with the aid of organs such as the pancreas and the liver, is the *digestion* of food to meet the body's *nutritional* needs and the *elimination* of waste resulting from digestion. Adequate nutrition is required for proper functioning of the body's organs and other cells (see the Human Needs Overview). The GI tract is susceptible to many health problems, including structural or mechanical alterations, impaired motility, infection, and cancer.

ANATOMY AND PHYSIOLOGY REVIEW

Overview of the Gastrointestinal System

ANIMATION: Digestion

Structure

The GI tract is a hollow muscular tube surrounded by four tissue layers. The **lumen,** or inner wall, of the GI tract consists of four layers: mucosa, submucosa, muscularis, and serosa. The *mucosa,* the innermost layer, includes a thin layer of smooth muscle and specialized exocrine gland cells. It is surrounded by the submucosa, which is made up of connective tissue. The *submucosa* layer is surrounded by the muscularis. The *muscularis* is composed of both circular and longitudinal smooth muscles, which work to keep contents moving through the tract. The outermost layer, the *serosa,* is composed of connective tissue. Although the GI tract is continuous from the mouth to the anus, it is divided into specialized regions. The mouth, pharynx, esophagus, stomach, and small and large intestines each perform a specific function. In addition, the secretions of the salivary, gastric, and intestinal glands; liver; and pancreas empty into the GI tract to aid digestion.

Function

The functions of the GI tract include secretion, digestion, absorption, motility, and elimination. Food and fluids are ingested, swallowed, and propelled along the lumen of the GI tract to the anus for elimination. The smooth muscles contract to move food from the mouth to the anus. Before food can be absorbed, it must be broken down to a liquid, called **chyme. Digestion** is the mechanical and chemical process in which complex foodstuffs are broken down into simpler forms that can be used by the body. During digestion, the stomach secretes hydrochloric acid, the liver secretes bile, and digestive enzymes

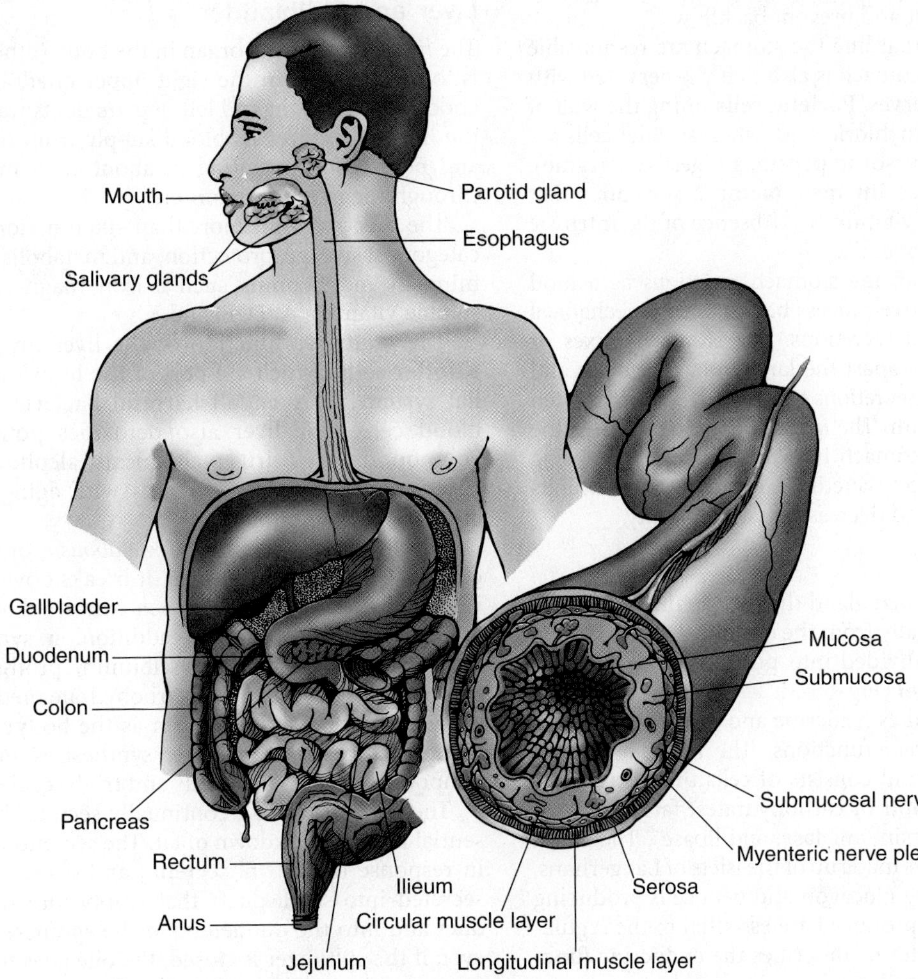
Mouth
Parotid gland
Esophagus
Salivary glands
Gallbladder
Duodenum
Colon
Pancreas
Rectum
Anus
Jejunum
Ilieum
Circular muscle layer
Longitudinal muscle layer
Serosa
Myenteric nerve plexus
Submucosal nerve plexus
Submucosa
Mucosa

Fig. 55-1 • The gastrointestinal system (GI tract) can be thought of as a tube (with necessary structures) extending from the mouth to the anus for a 25-foot length. The structure of this tube *(shown enlarged)* is basically the same throughout its length.

are released from accessory organs, aiding in food breakdown. After the digestive process is complete, absorption takes place. **Absorption** is carried out as the nutrients produced by digestion move from the lumen of the GI tract into the body's circulatory system for uptake by individual cells.

Oral Cavity

The oral cavity (mouth) includes the buccal mucosa, lips, tongue, hard palate, soft palate, teeth, and salivary glands. The buccal mucosa is the mucous membrane lining the inside of the mouth. The tongue is involved in speech, taste, and **mastication** (chewing). Small projections called *papillae* cover the tongue and provide a roughened surface, permitting the movement of food in the mouth during chewing. The hard palate and the soft palate together form the roof of the mouth.

Adults have 32 permanent teeth: 16 each in upper and lower arches. The different types of teeth function to prepare food for digestion by cutting, tearing, crushing, or grinding the food. Swallowing begins after food is taken into the mouth and chewed. Saliva is secreted in response to the presence of food in the mouth and begins to soften the food. Saliva contains mucin and an enzyme called *salivary amylase* (also known as *ptyalin*), which begins the breakdown of carbohydrates.

Esophagus

The esophagus is a muscular canal that extends from the pharynx to the stomach (throat) and passes through the center of the diaphragm. Its primary function is to move food and fluids from the pharynx to the stomach. At the upper end of the esophagus is a sphincter referred to as the **upper esophageal sphincter (UES).** When at rest, the UES is closed to prevent air into the esophagus during respiration. The portion of the esophagus just above the gastroesophageal (GE) junction is referred to as the **lower esophageal sphincter (LES).** When at rest, the LES is normally closed to prevent reflux of gastric contents into the esophagus. If the LES does not work properly, gastroesophageal reflux disease (GERD) can develop (see Chapter 57).

Stomach

The stomach is located in the midline and left upper quadrant (LUQ) of the abdomen and has four anatomic regions. The *cardia* is the narrow portion of the stomach that is below the gastroesophageal (GE) junction. The *fundus* is the area nearest to the cardia. The main area of the stomach is referred to as the *body* or *corpus*. The *antrum* (pylorus) is the distal (lower) portion of the stomach and is separated from the duodenum by the pyloric sphincter. Both ends of the stomach are guarded by sphincters (cardiac and pyloric), which aid in the transport of food through the GI tract and prevent backflow.

Smooth muscle cells that line the stomach are responsible for gastric motility. The stomach is also richly innervated with intrinsic and extrinsic nerves. **Parietal cells** lining the wall of the stomach secrete hydrochloric acid, whereas chief cells secrete pepsinogen (a precursor to pepsin, a digestive enzyme). Parietal cells also produce **intrinsic factor,** a substance that aids in the absorption of vitamin B_{12}. Absence of the intrinsic factor causes pernicious anemia.

After ingestion of food, the stomach functions as a food reservoir where the digestive process begins, using mechanical movements and chemical secretions. The stomach mixes or churns the food, breaking apart the large food molecules and mixing them with gastric secretions to form chyme, which then empties into the duodenum. The *intestinal phase* begins as the chyme passes from the stomach into the duodenum, causing distention. It is assisted by secretin, a hormone that inhibits further acid production and decreases gastric motility.

Pancreas

The pancreas is a fish-shaped gland that lies behind the stomach and extends horizontally from the duodenal C-loop to the spleen. The pancreas is divided into portions known as the *head,* the *body,* and the *tail* (Fig. 55-2).

Two major cellular bodies (exocrine and endocrine) within the pancreas have separate functions. The *exocrine* part is about 80% of the organ and consists of cells that secrete enzymes needed for digestion of carbohydrates, fats, and proteins (trypsin, chymotrypsin, amylase, and lipase). The *endocrine* part of the pancreas is made up of the islets of Langerhans, with alpha cells producing glucagon and beta cells producing insulin. These hormones produced are essential in the regulation of *metabolism.* Chapter 67 describes the endocrine function of the pancreas in detail.

Liver and Gallbladder

The *liver* is the largest organ in the body (other than skin) and is located mainly in the right upper quadrant (RUQ) of the abdomen. The right and left hepatic ducts transport bile from the liver. It receives its blood supply from the hepatic artery and portal vein, resulting in about 1500 mL of blood flow through the liver every minute.

The *liver* performs more than 400 functions in three major categories: storage, protection, and metabolism. It *stores* many minerals and vitamins, such as iron, magnesium, and the fat-soluble vitamins A, D, E, and K.

The *protective* function of the liver involves phagocytic **Kupffer cells,** which are part of the body's reticuloendothelial system. They engulf harmful bacteria and anemic red blood cells. The liver also detoxifies potentially harmful compounds (e.g., drugs, chemicals, alcohol). Therefore the risk for drug toxicity increases with aging because of decreased liver function.

The liver functions in the *metabolism* of proteins considered vital for human survival. It breaks down amino acids to remove ammonia, which is then converted to urea and is excreted via the kidneys. In addition, it synthesizes several plasma proteins, including albumin, prothrombin, and fibrinogen. The liver's role in carbohydrate metabolism involves storing and releasing glycogen as the body's energy requirements change. The organ also synthesizes, breaks down, and temporarily stores fatty acids and triglycerides.

The liver forms and continually secretes bile, which is essential for the breakdown of fat. The secretion of bile increases in response to gastrin, secretin, and cholecystokinin. Bile is secreted into small ducts that empty into the common bile duct and into the duodenum at the sphincter of Oddi. However, if the sphincter is closed, the bile goes to the gallbladder for storage.

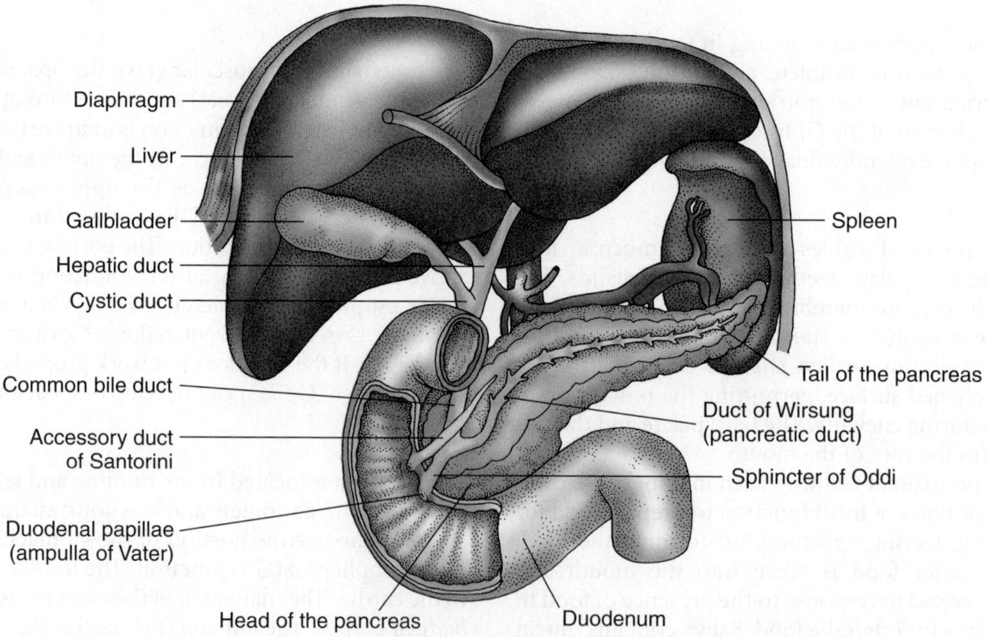

Diaphragm
Liver
Gallbladder
Hepatic duct
Cystic duct
Common bile duct
Accessory duct of Santorini
Duodenal papillae (ampulla of Vater)
Head of the pancreas
Duodenum
Sphincter of Oddi
Duct of Wirsung (pancreatic duct)
Tail of the pancreas
Spleen

Fig. 55-2 • The anatomy of the pancreas, the liver, and the gallbladder.

The *gallbladder* is a pear-shaped, bulbous sac that is located underneath the liver. It is drained by the cystic duct, which joins with the hepatic duct from the liver to form the common bile duct (CBD). The gallbladder collects, concentrates, and stores the bile that has come from the liver. It releases the bile into the duodenum via the CBD when fat is present.

Small Intestine

The small intestine is the longest and most convoluted portion of the digestive tract, measuring 16 to 19 feet (5 to 6 m) in length in an adult. It is composed of three different regions: duodenum, jejunum, and ileum. The *duodenum* is the first 12 inches (30 cm) of the small intestine and is attached to the distal end of the pylorus. The common bile duct and pancreatic duct join to form the ampulla of Vater, emptying into the duodenum at the duodenal papilla. This papillary opening is surrounded by muscle known as the **sphincter of Oddi.** The 8-foot (2.5-m) portion of the small intestine that follows the sphincter of Oddi is the *jejunum.* The last 8 to 12 feet (2.5 to 4 m) of the small intestine is called the *ileum.* The ileocecal valve separates the entrance of the ileum from the cecum of the large intestine.

The inner surface of the small intestine has a velvety appearance because of numerous mucous membrane finger-like projections. These projections are called *intestinal villi.* In addition to the intestinal villi, the small intestine has circular folds of mucosa and submucosa, which increase the surface area for digestion and absorption.

The small intestine has three main *functions:* movement (mixing and peristalsis), digestion, and absorption. Because the intestinal villi increase the surface area of the small intestine, it is the major organ of absorption of the digestive system. The small intestine mixes and transports the chyme to mix with many digestive enzymes. It takes an average of 3 to 10 hours for the contents to be passed by peristalsis through the small intestine. Intestinal enzymes aid in the digestion of proteins, carbohydrates, and lipids.

Large Intestine

The large intestine extends about 5 to 6 feet in length from the ileocecal valve to the anus and is lined with columnar epithelium that has absorptive and mucous cells. It begins with the *cecum,* a dilated, pouchlike structure that is inferior to the ileocecal opening. At the base of the cecum is the vermiform appendix, which has no known digestive function. The large intestine then extends upward from the cecum as the colon. The colon consists of four divisions: ascending colon, transverse colon, descending colon, and sigmoid colon. The sigmoid colon empties into the rectum.

Following the sigmoid colon, the large intestine bends downward to form the rectum. The last 1 to 1½ inches (3 to 4 cm) of the large intestine is called the *anal canal,* which opens to the exterior of the body through the anus. Sphincter muscles surround the anal canal.

The large intestine's *functions* are movement, absorption, and elimination. Movement in the large intestine consists mainly of segmental contractions, like those in the small intestine, to allow enough time for the absorption of water and electrolytes. In addition, peristaltic contractions are triggered by colonic distention to move the contents toward the rectum, where the material is stored until the urge to defecate occurs. Absorption of water and some electrolytes occurs in the large intestine to reduce the fluid volume of the chyme. This process creates a more solid material, the feces, for elimination.

GASTROINTESTINAL CHANGES ASSOCIATED WITH AGING

Physiologic changes occur as people age, especially when they become 65 years of age or older. Changes in digestion and elimination that can affect nutrition are common. For example, decreased gastric HCl can lead to decreased absorption of essential minerals like iron. Chart 55-1 lists common GI changes and nursing implications when caring for older adults.

ASSESSMENT METHODS

Patient History

One tool for assessing GI function is the nutritional-metabolic and elimination pattern assessment found in Gordon's Functional Health Patterns (Chart 55-2). Ask questions about changes in appetite, weight, and stool. The purpose of the health history is to determine the events related to the current health problem.

Collect data about the patient's age, gender, and culture. This information can be helpful in assessing who is likely to have particular GI system disorders. For instance, older adults are more at risk for stomach cancer than are younger adults. Younger adults are more at risk for inflammatory bowel disease (IBD). People of Jewish descent tend to have more IBD than other groups have.

Question the patient about previous GI disorders or abdominal surgeries. Ask about prescription medications being taken, including how much, when the drugs are administered, and why they have been prescribed. Inquire if the patient takes over-the-counter (OTC) drugs, herbs, and/or supplements. In particular, ask whether aspirin, NSAIDs (e.g., ibuprofen), laxatives, herbal preparations, or enemas are routinely taken. Large amounts of aspirin or NSAIDs can predispose the patient to peptic ulcer disease and GI bleeding. Long-term use of laxatives or enemas can cause dependence and result in constipation and electrolyte imbalance. Some herbal preparations, especially ayurvedic herbs, can affect appetite, absorption, and elimination. Determine if the patient smokes or has ever smoked cigarettes, cigars, or pipes. Smoking is a major risk factor for most GI cancers. Chewing tobacco is a major cause of oral cancer.

Finally, investigate the patient's travel history. Ask whether he or she has traveled outside of the country recently. This information may provide clues about the cause of symptoms like diarrhea.

Nutrition History

A nutrition history is important when assessing GI system function. Many conditions manifest themselves as a result of alterations in intake and absorption of nutrients. The purpose of a nutritional assessment is to gather information about how well the patient's nutritional needs are being met. Inquire about any special diet and whether there are any known food allergies. Ask the patient to describe the usual foods that are eaten daily and the times that meals are taken.

Chart 55-1 NURSING FOCUS ON THE OLDER ADULT

Changes in the Gastrointestinal System Related to Aging

Physiologic Change	Disorders Related to Change	Nursing Interventions	Rationales
STOMACH			
Atrophy of the gastric mucosa is characterized by a decrease in the ratio of gastrin-secreting cells to somatostatin-secreting cells. This change leads to decreased hydrochloric acid levels (hypochlorhydria).	Decreased hydrochloric acid levels lead to decreased absorption of iron and vitamin B_{12} and to proliferation of bacteria. Atrophic gastritis occurs as a consequence of bacterial overgrowth.	Encourage bland foods high in vitamins and iron. Assess for epigastric pain.	Bland foods help prevent gastritis. Assessment helps detect gastritis.
LARGE INTESTINE			
Peristalsis decreases, and nerve impulses are dulled.	Decreased sensation to defecate can result in postponement of bowel movements, which leads to constipation and impaction.	Encourage a high-fiber diet and 1500 mL of fluid intake daily (if not contraindicated). Encourage as much activity as tolerated.	These interventions increase the sensation of needing to defecate.
PANCREAS			
Distention and dilation of pancreatic ducts change. Calcification of pancreatic vessels occurs with a decrease in lipase production.	Decreased lipase level results in decreased fat absorption and digestion. Steatorrhea, or excess fat in the feces, occurs because of decreased fat digestion.	Encourage small, frequent feedings. Assess for diarrhea.	Small, frequent feedings help prevent steatorrhea. Diarrhea may be steatorrhea. Excessive diarrhea can lead to dehydration.
LIVER			
A decrease in the number and size of hepatic cells leads to decreased liver weight and mass. This change and an increase in fibrous tissue lead to decreased protein synthesis and changes in liver enzymes. Enzyme activity and cholesterol synthesis are diminished.	Decreased enzyme activity depresses drug metabolism, which leads to accumulation of drugs—possibly to toxic levels.	Assess for adverse effects of all drugs.	Assessment can help detect drug toxicity.

Chart 55-2 GASTROINTESTINAL ASSESSMENT

Using Gordon's Functional Health Patterns

NUTRITIONAL-METABOLIC PATTERN

- What is your typical daily food intake? Describe a day's meals, snacks, and vitamins.
- How much salt do you typically add to your food? Do you use salt substitutes?
- How is your appetite? Any recent change?
- Do you have any difficulty chewing or swallowing?
- Do you wear dentures? How well do they fit?
- Do you ever experience indigestion or "heartburn"? How often? What seems to cause it? What helps it?
- Do you have pain, diarrhea, gas, or any other problems? Do any specific foods cause this for you?
- What is your typical daily fluid intake? What types of fluids (water, juices, soft drinks, coffee, tea)? How much?
- Have you had any recent change in your weight? Weight gain? Weight loss? How much?
- Have you noticed a change in the tightness of your rings or shoes? Tighter? Looser?
- Have you noticed any difference in the size of your abdomen?

ELIMINATION PATTERN

- What is your usual bowel elimination pattern? Frequency? Character? Discomfort? Laxatives?
- Do you have any pain or bleeding associated with bowel movements?
- Have you experienced any changes in your usual bowel pattern?
- When was your last rectal examination?
- Have you ever had an endoscopy or a colonoscopy?
- What is your usual urinary elimination pattern? Frequency? Amount? Color? Odor? Control?
- Have you noticed a change in the amount of urine?

Based on Gordon, M. (2007). *Manual of nursing diagnosis* (11th ed.). Boston: Jones & Bartlett.

CULTURAL AWARENESS

Cultural and religious patterns are important in obtaining a complete nutritional history. Ask if certain foods pose a problem for the patient. For example, the spices or hot pepper used in cooking in many cultures can aggravate or precipitate GI tract symptoms such as indigestion. Note religious patterns such as fasting or abstinence.

About 80% to 90% of black people are lactose intolerant. A much smaller percentage of white people also have this problem. Lactose intolerance causes bloating, cramping, and diarrhea as a result of lack of the enzyme *lactase*. Lactase is needed to convert lactose in milk and other dairy products to glucose and galactose.

Health problems can also affect nutritional intake, so explore any changes that have occurred in eating habits as a result of illness. **Anorexia** (loss of appetite for food) can occur with GI disease. Assess changes in taste and any difficulty or pain with swallowing (dysphagia) that could be associated with esophageal disorders. Also ask if abdominal pain or discomfort occurs with eating and whether the patient has experienced any nausea, vomiting, or **dyspepsia** (indigestion or heartburn). Unknown food allergies often cause these symptoms. Inquire about any unintentional weight loss, because some cancers of the GI tract may present in this manner. Assess for alcohol and caffeine consumption because both substances are associated with many GI disorders, such as gastritis and peptic ulcer disease.

The patient's socioeconomic status may have a profound impact on his or her nutritional status. For example, people who have limited budgets, such as some older adults or the unemployed, may not be able to purchase foods required for a balanced diet. In addition, they may substitute less expensive, and perhaps less effective, OTC medications or herbs for prescription drugs. Necessary medical care may be delayed, and patients may not seek health care until conditions are well advanced.

Family History and Genetic Risk

Ask about a family history of GI disorders. Some GI health problems have a genetic predisposition. For example, familial adenomatous polyposis (FAP) is an inherited autosomal dominant disorder that predisposes the patient to colon cancer. Specific genetic risks are discussed with the GI problems in later chapters.

Current Health Problems

Because GI clinical manifestations are often vague and difficult for the patient to describe, it is important to obtain a chronologic account of the current problem, symptoms, and any treatments taken. Furthermore, ask about the location, quality, quantity, timing (onset, duration), and factors that may aggravate or alleviate each symptom (see Chart 55-2).

For example, a change in bowel habits is a common assessment finding. Obtain this information from the patient:

- Pattern of bowel movements
- Color and consistency of the feces
- Occurrence of diarrhea or constipation
- Effective action taken to relieve diarrhea or constipation
- Presence of frank blood or tarry stools
- Presence of abdominal distention or gas

An unintentional weight gain or loss is another symptom that needs further investigation. Assess the patient's:

- Normal weight
- Weight gain or loss
- Period of time for weight change
- Changes in appetite or oral intake

Pain is a common concern of patients with GI tract disorders. The mnemonic **PQRST** may be helpful in organizing the current problem assessment (Jarvis, 2008):

P: Precipitating or palliative. What brings it on? What makes it better? Worse? When did you first notice it?

Q: Quality or quantity. How does it look, feel, or sound? How intense/severe is it?

R: Region or radiation. Where is it? Does it spread anywhere?

S: Severity scale. How bad is it (on a scale of 1 to 10)? Is it getting better, worse, or staying the same?

T: Timing. Onset—Exactly when did it first occur? Duration—How long did it last?
Frequency—How often does it occur?

Abdominal pain is often vague and difficult to evaluate. Ask the patient to describe the type of pain, such as burning, gnawing, or stabbing. The location of the pain can be determined by asking him or her to point to the involved site. Ask about the relationship of food intake to the onset or worsening of pain. For example, a high-fat meal often causes gallbladder pain.

Changes in the skin may result from several GI tract disorders, such as liver and biliary system obstruction. Ask about whether these clinical manifestations have occurred, or assess whether they are present:

- Skin discolorations or rashes
- Itching
- **Jaundice** (yellowing of skin caused by bilirubin pigments)
- Increased bruising
- Increased tendency to bleed

Physical Assessment

Physical assessment involves a comprehensive examination of the patient's nutritional status, mouth, and abdomen. Nutritional assessment is discussed in detail in Chapter 63. Oral assessment is described in Chapter 56.

In preparation for examination of the *abdomen,* ask the patient to empty his or her bladder and then to lie in a supine position with knees bent, keeping the arms at the sides to prevent tensing of the abdominal muscles.

The abdominal examination usually begins at the patient's right side and proceeds in a systematic fashion (Fig. 55-3):

- Right upper quadrant (RUQ)
- Left upper quadrant (LUQ)
- Left lower quadrant (LLQ)
- Right lower quadrant (RLQ)

Table 55-1 lists the organs that lie in each of these areas.

If areas of pain or discomfort are noted from the history, this area is examined last in the examination sequence. This sequence should prevent the patient from tensing abdominal muscles because of the pain, which would make the examination difficult. Examine any area of tenderness cautiously, and instruct the patient to state whether it is too painful. Observe his or her face for signs of distress or pain.

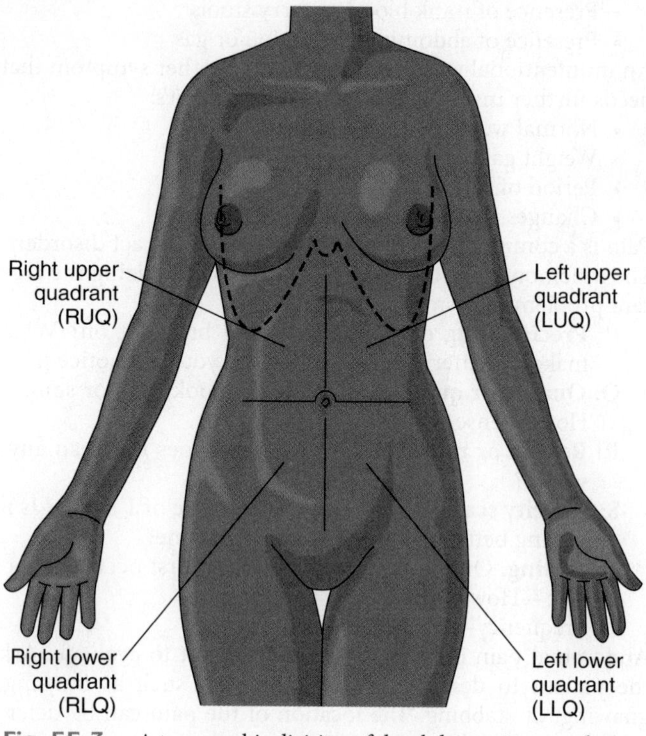
Right upper quadrant (RUQ)
Left upper quadrant (LUQ)
Right lower quadrant (RLQ)
Left lower quadrant (LLQ)

Fig. 55-3 • A topographic division of the abdomen into quadrants.

TABLE 55-1 Location of Body Structures in Each Abdominal Quadrant

RIGHT UPPER QUADRANT (RUQ)
- Most of the liver
- Gallbladder
- Duodenum
- Head of the pancreas
- Hepatic flexure of the colon
- Part of the ascending and transverse colon

LEFT UPPER QUADRANT (LUQ)
- Left lobe of the liver
- Stomach
- Spleen
- Body and tail of the pancreas
- Splenic flexure of the colon
- Part of the transverse and descending colon

LEFT LOWER QUADRANT (LLQ)
- Part of the descending colon
- Sigmoid colon
- Left ureter
- Left ovary and fallopian tube
- Left spermatic cord

RIGHT LOWER QUADRANT (RLQ)
- Cecum
- Appendix
- Right ureter
- Right ovary and fallopian tube
- Right spermatic cord

MIDLINE
- Abdominal aorta
- Uterus (if enlarged)
- Bladder (if distended)

The abdomen is assessed by using the four techniques of examination, but in a sequence different from that used for other body systems: inspection, auscultation, percussion, and then palpation. This sequence is preferred so that palpation and percussion do not increase intestinal activity and bowel sounds. As a nurse generalist, perform inspection, auscultation, and light palpation. Percussion and deep palpation may be done by health care providers or specialty nurses. Advanced practice nurses (APNs) such as nurse practitioners are also qualified for these more difficult skills. If appendicitis or an abdominal aneurysm is suspected, palpation is not done.

Inspection

Inspect the skin, and note any of these findings:
- Overall symmetry of the abdomen
- Presence of discolorations or scarring
- Abdominal distention
- Bulging flanks
- Taut, glistening skin

Observe the shape of the abdomen by observing its contour and symmetry. The contour of the abdomen can be rounded, flat, concave, or distended. It is best determined when standing at the side of the bed or treatment table and looking down on the abdomen. View the abdomen at eye level from the side. Note whether the contour is symmetric or asymmetric. Asymmetry of the abdomen can indicate problems affecting the underlying body structures (see Table 55-1). Note the shape and position of the umbilicus for any deviations. The presence of ecchymosis around the umbilicus **(Cullen's sign)** is an indication of intra-abdominal bleeding.

Finally, observe the patient's abdominal movements, including the normal rising and falling with inspiration and expiration, and note any distress during movement. Occasionally, pulsations may be visible, particularly in the area of the abdominal aorta. *If a bulging, pulsating mass is present, do not touch the area because the patient may have an abdominal aortic aneurysm, a life-threatening problem. Notify the health care provider of this finding immediately!* Peristaltic movements are rarely seen unless the patient is thin and has increased peristalsis. *If these movements are observed, note the quadrant of origin and the direction of peristaltic flow. Report this finding to the health care provider because it may indicate an intestinal obstruction.*

Auscultation

Auscultation of the abdomen is performed with the diaphragm of the stethoscope because bowel sounds are usually high pitched. Place the stethoscope lightly on the abdominal wall while listening for bowel sounds in all four quadrants, beginning in the RLQ at the ileocecal valve area.

▼ VIDEO CLIP: Abdomen, Bowel Sounds

Bowel sounds are created as air and fluid move through the GI tract. They are normally heard as relatively high-pitched, irregular gurgles every 5 to 15 seconds, with a normal frequency range of 5 to 30 per minute. Bowel sounds are characterized as normal, hypoactive, or hyperactive. They are diminished or absent after abdominal surgery or in the patient with peritonitis or paralytic ileus.

For many years, nurses have been taught to count the number of bowel sounds in each quadrant as part of routine and postoperative abdominal assessment to assess for peristalsis. However, recent evidence has shown that the best, most reliable method for assessing the return of peristalsis after abdominal surgery is to ask the patient if he or she has passed flatus within the past 8 hours or a stool within the past 12 to 24 hours (Madsen et al., 2005).

Increased bowel sounds, especially loud, gurgling sounds, result from increased motility of the bowel **(borborygmus).** These sounds are usually heard in the patient with diarrhea or gastroenteritis or above a complete intestinal obstruction.

When auscultating the abdomen, also listen for vascular sounds or **bruits** ("swooshing" sounds) over the abdominal aorta, the renal arteries, and the iliac arteries. A bruit heard over the aorta usually indicates the presence of an aneurysm. *If this sound is heard, do not percuss or palpate the abdomen. Notify the health care provider of your findings!*

VIDEO CLIP: Percussion, Abdomen

Percussion

Percussion may be used by APNs and other health care providers to determine the size of solid organs; to detect the presence of masses, fluid, and air; and to estimate the size of the liver and spleen. The **percussion notes** normally heard in the abdomen are termed **tympanic** (the high-pitched, loud, musical sound of an air-filled intestine) or **dull** (the medium-pitched, softer, thudlike sound over a solid organ, such as the liver).

VIDEO CLIP: Percussion, Liver, Spleen

The liver and spleen can be percussed. An enlarged liver is called **hepatomegaly.** Dullness heard in the left anterior axillary line indicates enlargement of the spleen **(splenomegaly).** Mild to moderate splenomegaly can be detected before the spleen becomes palpable.

Palpation

The purpose of palpation is to determine the size and location of abdominal organs and to assess for the presence of masses or tenderness. Palpation of the abdomen consists of two types: light palpation and deep palpation. Only physicians and APNs, such as clinical nurse specialists and nurse practitioners, should perform deep palpation. Deep palpation is used to further determine the size and shape of abdominal organs and masses.

VIDEO CLIP: Palpation of Abdomen

The technique of *light palpation* is used to detect large masses and areas of tenderness. Place the first four fingers of the palpating hand close together and then place them lightly on the abdomen and proceed smoothly and systematically from quadrant to quadrant. Depress the abdomen to a depth of $\frac{1}{2}$ to 1 inch (1.25 to 2.5 cm). Proceed with a rotational movement of the palpating hand. Note any areas of tenderness or guarding because these areas will be examined last and cautiously during deep palpation. While performing light palpation, notice signs of rigidity, which, unlike voluntary guarding, is a sign of peritoneal inflammation. Areas of pain should be evaluated for rebound tenderness **(Blumberg's sign).** With fingers placed at a 90-degree angle in relation to the abdomen, the examiner pushes slowly and deeply, releasing quickly. Pain felt on release is a positive sign for rebound tenderness and should be reported to the health care provider.

NCLEX EXAMINATION CHALLENGE

A client is admitted with multiple diarrheal stools, fever, and dehydration. Which assessment finding should be reported immediately to the health care provider?

A. Oral temperature of 100° F
B. Increased bowel sounds in all quadrants
C. Dry, flaky skin that easily tents
D. Mid-abdominal pulsating mass

evolve For the correct answer, go to http://evolve.elsevier.com/Iggy/.

Psychosocial Assessment

Psychosocial assessment focuses on how the GI health problem affects the patient's life and lifestyle. Remember that patients are often reluctant to discuss elimination problems, which may be very personal and embarrassing. The interview focus is on whether usual activities have been interrupted or disturbed, including employment. Question the patient about recent stressful events. Emotional stress has been associated with the development or exacerbation (flare-up) of irritable bowel syndrome (IBS) and other GI disorders. If the patient is diagnosed with cancer, he or she is expected to experience the phases of the grieving process. Patients may be depressed, angry, or in denial. More specific psychosocial assessments are included in later GI chapters as part of each disease discussion.

Diagnostic Assessment

Laboratory Assessment

To make an accurate assessment of the many possible causes of GI system abnormalities, laboratory testing of blood, urine, and stool specimens may be performed.

Blood Tests

A *complete blood count (CBC)* aids in the diagnosis of anemia and infection. It also detects changes in the blood's formed elements. *In adults, GI bleeding is the most frequent cause of anemia. It is associated with cancer, peptic ulcer disease, and inflammatory bowel disease.*

Because the liver is the main site of all proteins involved in coagulation, prothrombin time (PT) is useful in evaluating the levels of these clotting factors. *PT* measures the rate at which prothrombin is converted to thrombin, a process that depends on Vitamin K–associated clotting factors. Severe acute or chronic liver damage leads to a prolonged PT secondary to impaired synthesis of clotting proteins.

Many *electrolytes* are altered in GI tract dysfunction. For example, calcium is absorbed in the GI tract and may be measured to detect malabsorption. Excessive vomiting or diarrhea causes sodium or potassium depletion, thus requiring replacement.

Assays of serum enzymes are important in the evaluation of liver damage. **Aspartate aminotransferase (AST)** and **alanine aminotransferase (ALT)** are two enzymes found in the liver and other organs. These enzymes are elevated in most liver disorders, but they are highest in conditions that cause necrosis, such as severe viral hepatitis and cirrhosis.

Elevations in serum *amylase* and *lipase* may indicate acute pancreatitis. In this disease, serum amylase levels begin to elevate within 24 hours of onset and remain elevated for up to 5 days. Serum amylase and lipase are not elevated when *extensive* pancreatic necrosis is present because there are few pancreatic cells manufacturing the enzymes.

Bilirubin is the primary pigment in bile, which is normally conjugated and excreted by the liver and biliary system. It is measured as total serum bilirubin, conjugated (direct) bilirubin, and unconjugated (indirect) bilirubin. These measurements are important in the evaluation of jaundice and in the evaluation of liver and biliary tract functioning. Elevations in direct and indirect bilirubin levels can indicate impaired secretion.

Chart 55-3 LABORATORY PROFILE

Gastrointestinal Assessment

Test (Serum)	Normal Range for Adults	Significance of Abnormal Findings
Calcium (total)	9.0-10.5 mg/dL (values decrease in older adults)	*Decreased* values indicate possible: Malabsorption Renal failure Acute pancreatitis
Potassium	3.5-5.0 mEq/L or 3.5-5.0 mmol/L	*Decreased* values indicate possible: Vomiting Gastric suctioning Diarrhea Drainage from intestinal fistulas
Albumin	3.5-5.0 g/dL	*Decreased* values indicate possible: Hepatic disease
Alanine aminotransferase (ALT)	3-35 international units/L or 8-20 units/L (SI units)	*Increased* values indicate possible: Liver disease Hepatitis Cirrhosis
Aspartate aminotransferase (AST)	5-40 units/L	*Increased* values indicate possible: Liver disease Hepatitis Cirrhosis
Alkaline phosphatase	30-85 international units/L or 42-128 units/L (SI units)	*Increased* values indicate possible: Hepatic disease Biliary obstruction
Bilirubin (total)	0.1-1.0 mg/dL	*Increased* values indicate possible: Hemolysis Biliary obstruction Hepatic damage
Conjugated (direct) bilirubin	0.1-0.3 mg/dL	*Increased* values indicate possible: Biliary obstruction
Unconjugated (indirect) bilirubin	0.2-0.8 mg/dL	*Increased* values indicate possible: Hemolysis Hepatic damage
Ammonia	15-110 mg/dL	*Increased* values indicate possible: Hepatic disease such as cirrhosis
Xylose absorption	*5-g dose in 2 hr:* >20 mg/dL or >1.3 mmol/L *25-g dose in 2 hr:* >25 mg/dL or >1.7 mmol/L	*Decreased* values in blood and urine indicate possible: Malabsorption in the small intestine
Serum amylase	56-90 international units/L or 25-125 units/L (SI units)	*Increased* values indicate possible: Acute pancreatitis
Serum lipase	0-110 units/L	*Increased* values indicate possible: Acute pancreatitis

The serum level of *ammonia* may also be measured to evaluate hepatic function. Ammonia is normally used to rebuild amino acids or is converted to urea for excretion. Elevated levels are seen in conditions that cause severe hepatocellular injury, such as cirrhosis of the liver or fulminant hepatitis (Pagana & Pagana, 2006).

Two primary *oncofetal antigens—CA19-9* and *CEA*—are evaluated to diagnose, monitor the success of cancer therapy, and assess for the recurrence of cancer in the GI tract. These antigens may also be increased in benign GI conditions. Chart 55-3 lists blood tests commonly used by the health care provider in the diagnosis of GI disorders.

Urine Tests

The presence of *amylase* can be detected in the urine. In acute pancreatitis, renal clearance of amylase is increased. Amylase levels in the urine remain high even after serum levels return to normal. This becomes an important finding in patients who are symptomatic for 3 days or longer (Pagana & Pagana, 2006).

Urine *urobilinogen* is a form of bilirubin that is converted by the intestinal flora and excreted in the urine. Its measurement is useful in the evaluation of hepatic and biliary obstruction because the presence of bilirubin in the urine often occurs before jaundice is seen.

Chart 55-3 LABORATORY PROFILE

Gastrointestinal Assessment—cont'd

Test (Serum)	Normal Range for Adults	Significance of Abnormal Findings
Cholesterol	<200 mg/dL	*Increased* values indicate possible: Pancreatitis Biliary obstruction *Decreased* values indicate possible: Liver cell damage
Carbohydrate antigen 19-9 (CA19-9)	<37 units/mL	*Increased* values indicate possible: Cancer of the pancreas, stomach, colon Acute pancreatitis Inflammatory bowel disease
Carcinoembryonic antigen (CEA)	*Nonsmoker:* <2.5 ng/mL *Smoker:* up to 5 ng/mL	*Increased* values indicate possible: Colorectal, stomach, pancreatic cancer Ulcerative colitis Crohn's disease Hepatitis Cirrhosis

SI, International System of Units.

EVIDENCE-BASED PRACTICE

Are patients more compliant if they use an alternate method for stool collection for a FOBT?

Greenwald, B. (2006). A pilot study evaluating two alternate methods of stool collection for the fecal occult blood test. *MEDSURG Nursing, 15*(2), 89-94.

An annual fecal occult blood test (FOBT) is one of the five American Cancer Society screening recommendations for colorectal cancer. Yet, patients have a poor return rate for submitting the required stool samples on the test cards. Many people find stool collection unpleasant. This small pilot study used a convenience sample to determine which of two stool collection methods the subjects preferred: the wooden stick method or the tissue smear method. Using both methods, the return rate of the test cards was 94%, far better than the national average of less than one-half. The authors concluded that if patients have a choice of stool collection method, they would be more likely to complete the test.

Level of Evidence—6. The study was descriptive using a small convenience sample.

Commentary: Implications for Practice and Research. Although this pilot study used a small convenience sample, it suggests that patients would be more compliant in having this important cancer screening test if they had a choice of which stool collection method to use. Nurses can teach patients about these alternate methods and allow them to select the method that they prefer. Additional research is needed to validate these findings that would, it is hoped, help get more people screened for colorectal cancer.

Stool Tests

Stool studies are done to evaluate the function and integrity of the GI tract. The **fecal occult blood test (FOBT)** measures the presence of blood in the stool from GI bleeding, often from colorectal disease. As one option to detect colorectal cancer, the 2005 American Cancer Society Screening Guidelines recommend yearly FOBT using the take-home, multi-sample method rather than having the test done during a digital rectal examination (www.cancer.org). Collecting three samples from three separate bowel movements, the patient applies a small amount of stool with a stick to small cards that are labeled. Although not invasive, the patient return rate of the cards used for testing is low. In her small pilot study, Greenwald (2006) found that the return rate increased when patients had a choice of how to collect the specimen. (See the Evidence-Based Practice above.)

Two methods for testing occult blood in the stool are available: the traditional FOBT and the newer FIT (fecal immunochemical test). The traditionally used FOBT (e.g., Hemoccult II) requires an active component of guaiac and is, therefore, more likely than the FIT (e.g., HemeSelect or InSure) to yield false-positive results. In addition, patients having the guaiac-based test must avoid certain foods before the test, including raw fruits and vegetables and red meat. Vitamin C–rich foods, juices, and tablets must also be avoided. Anticoagulants, such as warfarin (Coumadin), and NSAIDs have to be discontinued for 7 days before testing begins. Patient compliance is likely to be higher with the FIT method because drugs and food do not interfere with the test results (Heseltine, 2007).

Stool samples may also be collected to test for *ova and parasites* to aid in the diagnosis of parasitic infection. They may also be tested for *fecal fats* when **steatorrhea** (fatty stools) or malabsorption is suspected. Fat is normally absorbed in the small intestine in the presence of biliary and pancreatic secretions. In malabsorption, fat is abnormally excreted in the stool.

Another common stool test is for the presence of a bacterial infection called ***Clostridium difficile.*** This test is indicated for patients who have been on antibiotic therapy. Prolonged antibiotic therapy, especially in older adults, depresses the natural intestinal flora, causing an overgrowth of *C. difficile.* The bacterium releases a toxin that causes colonic epithelium necrosis resulting in severe diarrhea that can be transmitted from person to person.

Imaging Assessment

Radiographic examinations and similar diagnostic procedures are useful in detecting structural and functional disorders of the GI system. Teach the patient how to prepare for the examination, provide an explanation of the procedure, and teach the required postprocedure care.

A *plain film of the abdomen* may be the first x-ray study that the health care provider requests when diagnosing a GI problem. This film can reveal abnormalities such as masses, tumors, and strictures or obstructions to normal movement. Patterns of bowel gas appear light on the abdominal film and can be useful in detecting an obstruction (ileus). No preparation is required except to wear a hospital gown and remove any jewelry or belts, which may interfere with the film.

When abdominal pain is severe or when bowel perforation is suspected, an *acute abdomen series* may be requested. This procedure consists of a chest x-ray, supine abdomen film, and an upright abdomen film. The chest x-ray may reveal a hiatal hernia, and an upright abdomen film may show air in the peritoneum from a bowel perforation. Today CT and MRI scans or ultrasound scans are often used instead of abdominal x-rays.

An **upper GI radiographic series** is an x-ray visualization from the mouth to the duodenojejunal junction. It is used to detect disorders of structure or function of the esophagus (barium swallow), stomach, or duodenum. An extension of the upper GI series, the *small bowel follow-through* (SBFT), continues tracing the barium through the small intestine—up to and including the ileocecal junction—to detect disorders of the jejunum or ileum. These tests are not performed as commonly today because endoscopy procedures allow for direct visualization of the internal GI tract.

Remind the patient to withhold foods and liquids for 8 hours before the test. If possible, opioid analgesics and anticholinergic medications are withheld for 24 hours before the test because they decrease intestinal tract motility. Instruct the patient about the barium preparation and the need to drink about 16 ounces of the barium. The radiology nurse or technician explains that a rotating examination table will be used to assist the patient in assuming the vertical, supine, prone, and lateral positions required for this test.

The initial procedure takes about 30 minutes. Fluoroscopy is used to trace the barium through the esophagus and stomach. The patient stands against the x-ray table for this part of the test. The table then moves to a lying position for more views of the stomach and duodenum. The patient then drinks more barium as quickly as possible while x-rays are taken. To attempt to make him or her as comfortable as possible, a pillow for the head and a sheet to prevent chilling are supplied whenever possible. The position changes help coat the mucosa and identify gastroesophageal reflux and hiatal hernia.

If a small bowel radiographic series is included, the patient drinks additional barium and more x-rays are taken at specific intervals. This series can take several hours, depending on how long it takes the barium to reach the cecum.

After either of these series, teach the patient to drink plenty of fluids to help eliminate the barium. A mild laxative or stool softener may be given to assist in its elimination. The radiology nurse or technician instructs the patient that stools may be chalky white for 24 to 72 hours as barium is excreted. When all barium is passed, brown stools return. If the patient is at home, he or she is instructed to report abdominal fullness, pain, or a delay in return to brown stools.

A **barium enema** examination, also known as a **lower GI series,** is an x-ray of the large intestine. This test is not as commonly used today because the colonoscopy can provide a direct view of the colon. Patient preparation is similar to that for colonoscopy. After the study is completed, the patient expels the barium. The radiology nurse or technician teaches the patient to drink plenty of fluids to assist in eliminating the barium. A laxative is given to help remove the barium from the intestinal tract. Stools are chalky white for about 24 to 72 hours, until all barium is passed.

Percutaneous transhepatic cholangiography (PTC) is an x-ray of the biliary duct system using an iodinated dye instilled via a percutaneous needle inserted through the liver into the intrahepatic ducts. This procedure may be performed when a patient has jaundice or persistent upper abdominal pain, even after cholecystectomy, but is rarely done as a diagnostic procedure today. Better information about dilated biliary ducts can be obtained using ultrasound scans and endoscopic retrograde cholangiopancreatography (ERCP) (discussed on p. 1227).

Computed tomography (CT), also referred to as a *CT scan,* provides a noninvasive cross-sectional x-ray view that can detect tissue densities and abnormalities in the abdomen, including the liver, pancreas, spleen, and biliary tract. It may be performed with or without contrast media.

For the CT scan, the patient is told that he or she will need to lie still in a rather enclosed space of the machine. He or she must remove all jewelry and metal. If contrast medium is to be used, ask about allergies to seafood and iodine. The patient is NPO for at least 4 hours before the test if a contrast medium is to be used. IV access will be required for injection of the contrast medium. Advise the patient that he or she may feel warm and flushed on injection. The patient who is mildly claustrophobic may require a mild sedative to tolerate the study. The radiologic technician instructs the patient to lie still and to hold his or her breath when asked to take a series of images. The test takes about 30 minutes.

Like other parts of the body, the abdomen and its organs may also be evaluated by *magnetic resonance imaging (MRI).* For many patients with abdominal symptoms, this may be the first diagnostic test requested by the health care provider.

Other Diagnostic Assessment

Endoscopy

Endoscopy is direct visualization of the GI tract using a flexible fiberoptic endoscope. It is commonly requested to evaluate bleeding, ulceration, inflammation, tumors, and cancer of the esophagus, stomach, biliary system, or bowel. Obtaining specimens for biopsy and cell studies (e.g., *H. pylori)* is also possible through the endoscope. There are several types of endoscopic examinations. The patient must sign an informed consent form before having these invasive studies.

Esophagogastroduodenoscopy. Esophagogastroduodenoscopy (EGD) is a visual examination of the esophagus, stomach, and duodenum. This procedure has significantly reduced the number of upper GI series that are done. If GI bleeding is found during an EGD, the physician can inject a sclerotherapy agent into the affected area to stop the bleeding. If the patient has an esophageal stricture, it can be dilated during an EGD.

Teach the patient preparing for an upper GI endoscopic examination to remain NPO for 6 to 8 hours before the procedure. Usual drug therapy for hypertension or other diseases may be taken the morning of the test. However, diabetic patients should consult their health care provider for special instructions. Patients are also usually asked to avoid anticoagulants, aspirin, or NSAIDs for several days before the test unless it is absolutely necessary. Tell the patient that a flexible tube will be passed down the esophagus while he or she is under moderate sedation. Midazolam hydrochloride (Versed) and fentanyl (Fentanyl, Sublimaze) are commonly used drugs for sedation. Atropine may be administered to dry secretions. In addition, a local anesthetic is sprayed to inactivate the gag reflex and facilitate passage of the tube. Explain that this anesthetic will depress the gag reflex and that swallowing will be difficult. If the patient has dentures, they are removed.

After the drugs are given, the patient is placed in the left lateral decubitus (Sims', or left side-lying) position with a towel or basin at the mouth for secretions. A bite block is inserted to prevent biting down on the endoscope and to protect the teeth. The physician passes the tube through the mouth and into the esophagus (Fig. 55-4). The procedure takes about 20 to 30 minutes.

After the test, the endoscopy nurse or technician checks vital signs frequently (usually every 30 minutes) until the sedation wears off. The siderails of the bed are raised during this time. The patient remains NPO until the gag reflex returns (usually in 1 to 2 hours). *The priority for care is to prevent aspiration. Do not offer fluids or food by mouth until the gag reflex is intact! Monitor for signs of perforation, such as pain, bleeding, or fever*. Teach the patient to not drive for at least 12 hours after the procedure because of sedation. Remind him or her that a hoarse voice or sore throat may persist for several days after the test. Throat lozenges can be used to relieve throat discomfort.

Endoscopic Retrograde Cholangiopancreatography. Endoscopic retrograde cholangiopancreatography (ERCP) includes visual and radiographic examination of the liver, gall-

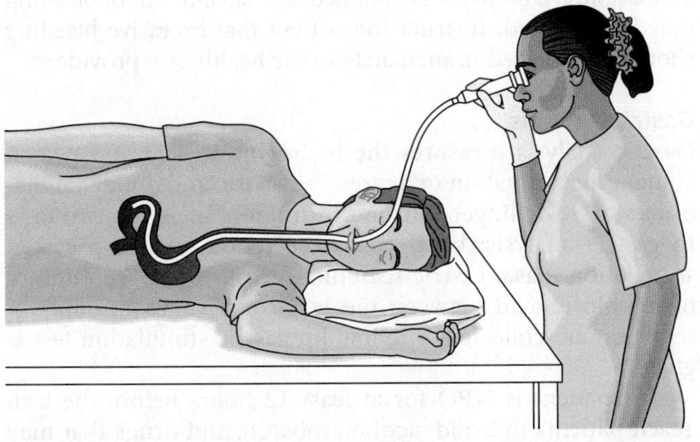

Fig. 55-4 • Esophagogastroduodenoscopy allows visualization of the esophagus, the stomach, and the duodenum. If the esophagus is the focus of the examination, the procedure is called *esophagoscopy*. If the stomach is the focus, the procedure is called *gastroscopy*.

bladder, bile ducts, and pancreas to identify the cause and location of obstruction. After the cannula is inserted into the common bile duct, a radiopaque dye is inserted and then several x-ray images are obtained. The physician may perform a **papillotomy** (a small incision in the sphincter around the ampulla of Vater) to remove gallstones. If a biliary duct stricture is found, plastic or metal stents may be inserted to keep the ducts open. Biopsies of tissue are also frequently taken during this test.

The patient prepares for this test in the same manner as for an EGD, including being NPO for 6 to 8 hours before the test. The patient requires IV access for moderate sedation drugs. Ask about prior exposure to x-ray dye and any sensitivities or allergies. If the patient has dentures, they are removed.

The endoscopic portion of an ERCP is similar to that of an EGD, except that the endoscope is advanced farther to the duodenum and into the biliary tract. Once the cannula is in the common duct, contrast medium is injected and x-rays are taken to view the biliary tract. A tilt table assists in distributing the contrast medium to all areas to be assessed. The patient is placed in a left lateral position for viewing the common bile duct. Once the cannula is placed, he or she is put in a prone position. After examination of the biliary tree, the cannula is directed into the pancreatic duct for examination. The ERCP lasts from 30 minutes to 2 hours depending on the treatment that may be done.

After the test, assess vital signs frequently, usually every 15 minutes, until the patient is stable. *To prevent aspiration, check to ensure that the gag reflex has returned before offering fluids or food. Teach the patient and family to monitor for severe postprocedure complications at home, including cholangitis (gallbladder inflammation), perforation, sepsis, and pancreatitis. The patient has severe pain if any of these complications occur. Fever is present in sepsis. These problems do not occur immediately after the procedure but may take several hours to 2 days to develop.* Colicky abdominal pain can result from air instilled during the procedure. Instruct the patient to report abdominal pain, fever, nausea, or vomiting that fails to resolve after returning home. Be sure that the patient has someone to drive him or her home if the test was done on an ambulatory basis.

Small Bowel Capsule Endoscopy. Small bowel endoscopy, or **enteroscopy,** provides a view of the small intestine. Capsule video endoscopy (M2A) is a small bowel enteroscopy that visualizes the entire small bowel, including the distal ileum. It is used to evaluate and locate the source of GI bleeding. Before the development of the M2A Capsule Endoscope, viewing the small intestine was inadequate. The capsule battery lasts around 8 hours so it is not used to view the colon.

Prepare the patient by explaining the procedure, the purpose, and what to expect during the testing. The patient must fast (water only) for 8 to 10 hours before the test and be NPO for the first 2 hours of the testing.

At the time of the procedure, the patient's abdomen is marked for the location of the sensors, and the eight-lead sensors (Sensor Array) are applied. The patient wears an abdominal belt that houses a data recorder to capture the transmitted images. After the capsule is taken with a glass of water, the patient may return to normal activity for the remainder of the study. He or she can resume a normal diet 4 hours after swallowing the capsule. At the end of the procedure, the patient returns to the facility with the capsule equipment for downloading to a central computer. The procedure lasts about 8 hours.

Because the M2A Capsule Endoscope is a single-use device that moves through the GI tract by peristalsis and is excreted naturally, explain to the patient the capsule will be seen in the stool. No other follow-up is necessary.

Colonoscopy. **Colonoscopy** is an endoscopic examination of the entire large bowel. *The 2005 American Cancer Society Colorectal Cancer Screening Guidelines recommend that beginning at age 50, all men and women should have a colonoscopy every 10 years or chose another equally effective recommended screening option (www.cancer.org).* Those at high risk for cancer (e.g., family history) should have the test more often. The physician may also obtain tissue biopsy specimens or remove polyps through the colonoscope. A colonoscopy can evaluate the cause of chronic diarrhea or locate the source of GI bleeding. A sclerotherapy drug may be injected at the site of any bleeding. An alternative to this invasive procedure is the *virtual colonoscopy,* which is not invasive and uses a CT scanner to view the colon.

Patient Preparation. Teach the patient to stay on a clear liquid diet for 12 to 24 hours before a colonoscopy. He or she should be NPO (except water) 6 to 8 hours before the procedure. Remind patients to avoid aspirin and NSAIDs for several days before the procedure. Anticoagulants may also be withheld, depending on their necessity and the physician's preference. Diabetic patients should check with their health care provider about drug therapy requirements on the day of the test because they are NPO.

The patient drinks an oral liquid preparation for cleaning the bowel (e.g., sodium phosphate [Phospho-Soda]) the evening before the examination and may repeat that procedure the morning of the study. Some physicians prescribe a large amount of Go-Lytely to cleanse the bowel the day before. The solutions should be chilled to improve their taste. Remind the patient to drink them quickly to prevent nausea. These solutions produce a watery diarrhea that begins in about 1 hour. In some cases, the patient may require laxatives, suppositories (e.g., bisacodyl [Dulcolax]), or one or more small-volume cleansing enemas (e.g., Fleets).

Procedure. IV access is necessary for the administration of moderate sedation. The physician prescribes drugs to aid in relaxation, usually IV midazolam hydrochloride (Versed) and/or an opiate. Initially, the patient is placed on the left side with the knees drawn up while the endoscope is passed into the rectum to the cecum. Air may be instilled for better visualization. The entire procedure lasts about 30 to 60 minutes. Atropine sulfate is kept available in case of bradycardia resulting from vasovagal response.

Follow-up Care. Check vital signs every 15 minutes until the patient is stable. Keep the siderails up until the patient is fully alert. Observe for signs of perforation (causes severe pain) and hemorrhage, such as a rapid drop in blood pressure. Reassure the patient that a feeling of fullness, cramping, and passage of flatus are expected for several hours after the test. If a polypectomy or tissue biopsy was performed, there may be a *small* amount of blood in the first stool after the colonoscopy. *However, report excessive bleeding or severe pain to the health care provider immediately* (Chart 55-4). As with other endoscopic procedures, the patient will need someone to provide transportation home. Remind the patient to avoid driving for 12 hours after the procedure because of the effects of sedation.

NCLEX EXAMINATION CHALLENGE

What is the priority for nursing care for a client who just had an esophagogastroduodenoscopy (EGD)?

A. Monitor for return of the gag reflex.
B. Take vital signs every 15 minutes.
C. Assess bowel sounds in all quadrants.
D. Ask about passage of flatus or stool.

evolve For the correct answer, go to http://evolve.elsevier.com/Iggy/.

Virtual Colonoscopy. A noninvasive imaging procedure to obtain multi-dimensional views of the entire colon is the *CT colonography,* most popularly known as the **virtual colonoscopy.** The bowel preparation and dietary restrictions are similar to those for traditional colonoscopy. However, if a polyp is detected during a virtual colonoscopy or bleeding is found, the patient must have a follow-up invasive colonoscopy for treatment. Therefore the advantage of the traditional colonoscopy is that both diagnostic testing and minor surgical procedures can be done at the same time.

Sigmoidoscopy. Proctosigmoidoscopy, often referred to as a *sigmoidoscopy,* is an endoscopic examination of the rectum and sigmoid colon using a flexible scope. The purpose of this test is to screen for colon cancer, investigate the source of GI bleeding, or diagnose or monitor inflammatory bowel disease. If sigmoidoscopy is used as an alternative to colonoscopy for colorectal cancer screening, it is recommended that screening begin at 50 years of age and should be done every 5 years thereafter (www.cancer.org). Patients at high risk for cancer may require more frequent screening.

The patient should have a clear liquid diet for at least 24 hours before the test. A cleansing enema or sodium biphosphate (Fleet's) enema is usually required the morning of the procedure. A laxative may also be prescribed the evening before the test.

The patient is placed on the left side in the knee-chest position. No moderate sedation is required. The endoscope is lubricated and inserted into the anus to the required depth for viewing. Tissue biopsy may be performed during this procedure, but the patient cannot feel it. The examination usually lasts about 30 minutes.

Inform the patient that mild gas pain and flatulence may be experienced from air instilled into the rectum during the examination. If a biopsy was obtained, a small amount of bleeding may be observed. Instruct the patient that excessive bleeding should be reported immediately to the health care provider.

Gastric Analysis

Gastric analysis measures the hydrochloric acid and pepsin content for evaluation of aggressive gastric and duodenal disorders (e.g., Zollinger-Ellison syndrome). There are two tests in gastric analysis: basal gastric secretion and gastric acid stimulation. Basal gastric secretion measures the secretion of hydrochloric acid between meals. If only small amounts of secretion are collected, a follow-up gastric stimulation test is given.

The patient is NPO for at least 12 hours before the test. Teach patients to avoid alcohol, tobacco, and drugs that may affect gastric secretion for 24 hours before the study. A nasogastric (NG) tube is inserted, and gastric residual contents are aspirated and discarded.

The NG tube is attached to suctioning equipment for collecting the contents at 15-minute intervals for 1 hour. Samples are collected and labeled with basal acid output (BAO), time, and volume of each specimen.

For the gastric acid stimulation test, the NG tube is left in place and a drug that stimulates gastric acid secretion (e.g., pentagastrin or betazole dihydrochloride [Histalog]) is given. Fifteen minutes after injection of the drug, specimens are again collected at 15-minute intervals for 1 hour. Samples are collected and labeled with maximal acid output (MAO), time, and volume of each specimen. Depressed levels of gastric secretion suggest the presence of gastric cancer. Increased levels of gastric secretion indicate Zollinger-Ellison syndrome and duodenal ulcers (see Chapter 58).

After the test is completed, the NG tube is removed and the patient can resume normal eating patterns. No other follow-up is necessary.

Ultrasonography

Ultrasonography (US) is a technique in which high-frequency, inaudible vibratory sound waves are passed through the body via a transducer. The echoes of the sound waves created are then recorded and converted into images for analysis. US is commonly used to view soft tissues, such as the liver, the spleen, the pancreas, the gallbladder, and the biliary system. The advantages of this test are that it is painless and noninvasive and requires no radiation.

The patient may be fasting, depending on the abdominal organs to be examined. Inform the patient that it will be necessary to lie still during the study. He or she is instructed to drink 1 to 2 L of fluid just before the test, because a full bladder is necessary for accurate visualization.

The patient is placed in a prone or supine position. The technician applies insulating gel to the end of the transducer and on the area of the abdomen under study. This gel allows airtight contact of the transducer with the skin. The technician moves the transducer back and forth over the skin until the desired images are obtained. The study takes about 15 to 30 minutes. No follow-up care is necessary.

Endoscopic Ultrasonography

Endoscopic ultrasonography (EUS) provides images of the GI wall and high-resolution images of the digestive organs. The ultrasonography is performed through the endoscope. This procedure is useful in diagnosing the presence of lymph node tumors, mucosal tumors, and tumors of the pancreas, stomach, and rectum. The patient preparation and follow-up care are similar to the preparation and follow-up care for both endoscopy and ultrasonography.

Liver-Spleen Scan

A liver-spleen scan uses IV injection of a radioactive material that is taken up primarily by the liver and secondarily by the spleen. The scan evaluates the liver and the spleen for tumors or abscesses, organ size and location, and blood flow.

Teach the patient about the need to lie still during the scanning. Assure the patient that the injection has only small amounts of radioactivity and is not dangerous. Ask female patients of childbearing age if they may be pregnant or are currently breastfeeding. The radionuclide can be found in breast milk, and radiation from x-rays or scans should be avoided in pregnancy.

The technician or the physician gives the radioactive injection through an IV line, and a wait of about 15 minutes is necessary for uptake. The patient is placed in many different positions while the scanning takes place. Tell the patient that the radionuclide is eliminated from the body through the urine in 24 hours. Careful handwashing after toileting decreases the exposure to any radiation present in the urine.

Chart 55-4 BEST PRACTICE FOR PATIENT SAFETY & QUALITY CARE

Care of the Patient After a Colonoscopy

- Do not allow the patient to take anything by mouth until sedation wears off and he or she is alert.
- Take vital signs every 15 to 30 minutes until the patient is alert.
- Keep the siderails up until the patient is alert.
- Assess for rectal bleeding or severe pain.
- Remind the patient that fullness and mild abdominal cramping are expected for several hours.
- Assess for manifestations of bowel perforation, including *severe* abdominal pain and guarding. Fever may occur later.
- Assess for manifestations of hypovolemic shock, including dizziness, light-headedness, decreased blood pressure, tachycardia, pallor, and altered mental status (may be the first sign).
- If the procedure is performed in an ambulatory care setting, arrange for another person to drive the patient home.

HUMAN NEEDS ASSESSMENT REVIEW

What should you NOTICE in a patient with adequate digestion and elimination related to the GI system?

Physical Assessment

- No nausea or vomiting
- Sufficient appetite
- No intentional weight loss
- No dyspepsia (indigestion)
- No jaundice
- Abdomen soft and not tender
- Normoactive bowel sounds present is all quadrants
- No change in bowel habits
- No abdominal pain
- Normal brown, formed stool
- No frequent diarrhea or constipation

Diagnostic Assessment

- No occult blood in stool
- Normal liver enzymes, such as ALT
- Normal bilirubin levels
- Serum and urine amylase within normal limits
- Serum ammonia level within normal limit
- Serum albumin within normal limit
- Electrolytes within normal limits

GET READY FOR THE NCLEX EXAMINATION!

Key Points

Review these Key Points for each NCLEX Examination Client Needs Category.

Safe and Effective Care Environment

- Remember that the priority for care is to check for the return of the gag reflex after an upper endoscopic procedure before offering fluids or food; aspiration may occur if the gag reflex is not intact.
- Monitor vital signs carefully for the patient having any endoscopic procedure and moderate sedation.
- Assess patients who have endoscopies for bleeding, fever, and severe pain.

Health Promotion and Maintenance

- Teach patients to limit caffeine and alcohol in their diets to reduce risk for GI health problems.
- If an endoscopic procedure on an ambulatory basis is scheduled, remind the patient to have someone available to drive him or her home because of the effects of moderate sedation.
- Teach patients having invasive colon diagnostic procedures to follow instructions carefully for the bowel preparation before testing; the bowel must be clear to allow visualization of the colon.
- Instruct the patient to drink plenty of fluids and take a laxative as prescribed to eliminate barium if used during diagnostic testing.

Psychosocial Integrity

- Recognize that most patients are hesitant to openly talk about their elimination patterns because it is embarrassing.
- Remember that problems of digestion, nutrition, and elimination can markedly affect lifestyle.

Physiological Integrity

- Perform a focused abdominal assessment using inspection, auscultation, and light palpation.
- Do not palpate or auscultate any abdominal pulsating mass because it could be a life-threatening aortic aneurysm.
- Assess and report any major complications of GI testing to the health care provider.
- Review laboratory results, and report abnormal findings to the health care provider.

Additional Study Resources

Go to your Companion CD or Evolve at http://evolve.elsevier.com/Iggy/ for *Self-Assessment Questions for the NCLEX Examination.*

evolve Go to Evolve at http://evolve.elsevier.com/Iggy/ for *Prioritization and Delegation Questions for the NCLEX Examination.*

SELECTED BIBLIOGRAPHY

Asterisk indicates a classic or definitive work on this subject.

*Donley, K.M. (2003). Surfing an acidic wave: pH monitoring technologies swim in sea of innovation. *EndoNurse, 3*(1), 22-24.

*Dykes, C.M. (2001). Virtual colonoscopy: A new approach for colorectal cancer screening. *Gastroenterology Nursing, 24*(1), 5-11.

*Given Imaging. (2002). M2A Capsule Endoscopy: Given diagnostic system. Available from Given Imaging, Inc., Oakbrook Technology Center, 5555 Oakbrook Parkway, #355, Norcross, GA 30093.

Gordon, M. (2007). *Manual of nursing diagnosis* (11th ed.). Boston: Jones & Bartlett.

Greenwald, B. (2006). A pilot study evaluating two alternate methods of stool collection for the fecal occult blood test. *MEDSURG Nursing, 15*(2), 89-94.

Heseltine, P. (2007). Fecal immunochemical test. *Clinical Laboratory News,* January. Retrieved March 24, 2008, from www.aacc.org.

Jarvis, C. (2008). *Physical examination and health assessment* (5th ed.). Philadelphia: Saunders.

Madsen, D., Sebolt, T., Cullen, L., Folkedahl, B., Mueller, T., Richardson, C., et al. (2005). Listening to bowel sounds: An evidence-based practice project. *AJN, 105*(12), 40-48.

McCance, K.L., & Huether, S.E. (2006). (Eds.). *Pathophysiology: The biologic basis for disease in adults & children* (5th ed.). St. Louis: Mosby.

National Institutes of Health. (2007). *National digestive disease information clearinghouse publications.* Retrieved March 24, 2008, from www.nih.gov.

Pagana, K.D., & Pagana, T.J. (2006). *Mosby's manual of diagnostic and laboratory tests* (3rd ed.). St. Louis: Mosby.

*Price, A.S. (2003). Primary and secondary prevention of colorectal cancer. *Gastroenterology Nursing, 26*(2), 73-81.

Skidmore-Roth, L. (2007). *Mosby's nursing drug reference.* St. Louis: Mosby.

*Society of Gastroenterology Nurses and Associates. (2003). *Gastroenterology nursing: A core curriculum* (3rd ed.). Chicago: Author.

*Yu, M. (2002). M2A Capsule Endoscopy: A breakthrough diagnostic tool for small intestine imaging. *Gastroenterology Nursing, 25*(1), 24-27.

56
CHAPTER

Care of Patients with Oral Cavity Problems

Karrie K. Dietzen

LEARNING OUTCOMES

For clinical competence and success on the NCLEX Examination, study this chapter with these Learning Outcomes in mind:

Safe and Effective Care Environment

1. Prioritize postoperative care for patients undergoing surgery for oral cancer to promote nutrition.
2. Plan continuity of care between the hospital and community-based agencies for patients having oral surgery.
3. Identify appropriate community resources for patients with oral cavity health problems.

Health Promotion and Maintenance

4. Teach patients ways to prevent oral cancer and maintain good oral health.
5. Develop a teaching plan for patients who have stomatitis to promote digestion and nutrition.
6. Develop a teaching plan for community-based care of patients with oral cancer.

Psychosocial Integrity

7. Assess the patient's response to an oral cancer diagnosis.
8. Refer patients with oral cancer to appropriate support groups.
9. Assist the patient with oral cancer to identify coping mechanisms and support systems.

Physiological Integrity

10. Plan care for patients who have disorders of the salivary glands.
11. Use best practice for teaching or providing oral care for patients.

Go to your Companion CD or Evolve at http://evolve.elsevier.com/Iggy/ for *Self-Assessment Questions for the NCLEX Examination* keyed to these Learning Outcomes.

The oral cavity, or mouth, is where *digestion* of food begins. The teeth tear, grind, and crush food into small particles to promote swallowing. The enzymes in saliva begin the breakdown of carbohydrates. If a person cannot take food or fluid into the mouth, cannot chew food, or cannot swallow, the basic *human need for nutrition* may not be met using the GI tract. Adequate intake of fluids and nutrients into the body is vital to promote function of every body organ and system.

The pharynx (throat) is located just behind the mouth and has a role in *digestion* and oxygenation. Inhaled air passes through the nose, into the pharynx, and down into the trachea. A blockage of the posterior oral cavity, for example, by a tumor, can interfere with oxygenation, another basic human need. Oxygenation and tissue perfusion are discussed in detail in Chapter 29.

Oral cavity disorders, then, can severely affect *nutrition* and oxygenation, as well as speech, body image, and self-esteem. Although there are many oral health problems, this chapter discusses the most common disorders. Nurses play an important role in maintaining and restoring oral health through nursing interventions and patient and family education. Chart 56-1 lists ways to help maintain a healthy oral cavity.

STOMATITIS

Pathophysiology

Painful single or multiple ulcerations (canker sores) that appear as inflammation and erosion of the protective lining of the mouth are called **stomatitis.** The sores cause pain, and open areas make the person at risk for bleeding and infection. Mild erythema (redness) may respond to topical treatments. Extensive stomatitis may require treatment with opioid analgesics. Stomatitis is classified according to the cause of the inflammation. *Primary stomatitis,* the most common type, includes **aphthous** (noninfectious) **stomatitis,** herpes simplex stomatitis, and traumatic ulcers. *Secondary stomatitis* generally results from infection by opportunistic viruses, fungi, or bacteria in patients who are immunocompromised. It can also

Chart 56-1 **PATIENT AND FAMILY EDUCATION GUIDE**

Maintaining a Healthy Oral Cavity

- Perform self-examination of your mouth every month; report any unusual finding.
- Be sure to eat a balanced diet.
- Brush and floss your teeth every day. Set a routine, and keep to it.
- Manage your stress as much as possible; learn how to maintain your emotional health.
- Avoid contact with agents that may cause inflammation of the mouth, such as mouthwashes that contain alcohol.
- If possible, avoid drugs that may cause inflammation of the mouth or reduce the flow of saliva.
- Be aware of any changes in the occlusion of your teeth, mouth pain, or swelling; seek medical attention promptly.
- See your dentist regularly; have problems attended to promptly.
- If you wear dentures, make sure they are in good repair and fit properly.

result from drugs, such as chemotherapy. (See Chapter 24 for discussion of chemotherapy-induced stomatitis.)

A common type of secondary stomatitis is caused by *Candida albicans. Candida* is sometimes present in small amounts in the mouth, especially in older adults. Long-term antibiotic therapy destroys other normal flora and allows the *Candida* to overgrow. The result can be **candidiasis,** also called *moniliasis,* a fungal infection that is very painful. Candidiasis is also common in those undergoing immunosuppressive therapy, such as chemotherapy, radiation, and steroids.

CONSIDERATIONS FOR OLDER ADULTS

Older adults are especially at high risk for candidiasis because aging causes a decrease in immune function. The risk increases for patients who are diabetic, malnourished, or under emotional stress. Those who wear dentures may use soft denture liners that provide comfort but can also be colonized by *C. albicans,* contributing to denture stomatitis. In addition, several studies have found that older adults, especially those in residential or long-term care with dementia, often have poor oral hygiene, which contributes to mouth infections (Chalmers & Pearson, 2005; Gil-Montoya et al., 2006). Chalmers and Pearson recommended that these residents be routinely screened for oral health needs. (See the Evidence-Based Practice box below.)

In addition, the mouth is susceptible to the effects of human immune deficiency virus (HIV) disease. Other systemic diseases that can cause stomatitis include chronic kidney disease and inflammatory bowel disease. Poor oral health is a risk factor for certain infections, such as ventilator-associated pneumonia (Munro et al., 2006).

Stomatitis can result from infection, allergy, vitamin deficiency, systemic disease, and irritants, such as tobacco and alcohol. Infectious agents, such as bacteria and viruses, may have a role in the development of recurrent stomatitis.

Certain foods may trigger allergic responses that cause aphthous ulcers. Foods such as coffee, potatoes, cheese, nuts, citrus fruits, and gluten may be causative factors. In some cases, strict diets have resulted in the improvement of ulcers. Deficiencies in complex B vitamins, folate, zinc, and iron associated with malnutrition can contribute to the formation of recurrent stomatitis.

EVIDENCE-BASED PRACTICE

What are best practices when providing oral hygiene to long-term care residents with dementia?

Chalmers, J., & Pearson, A. (2005). Oral hygiene care for residents with dementia: A literature review. *Journal of Advanced Nursing, 52*(4), 410-419.

Regular oral hygiene for older adults with cognitive impairment is challenging. The researchers conducted a systematic review of 306 articles to determine recommendations for oral care in older adults, especially those in residential facilities (residents).

The study findings confirmed that oral hygiene in older residents with dementia is poor. Contributing factors included swallowing and nutritional problems, the use of multiple drugs, functional dependence, inadequate use of dental care, and lack of oral care assistance. One comprehensive, reliable, and valid oral health screening tool for the study population was found. Recommendations for oral care included oral assessment screening by staff and referral to a dentist to prevent oral diseases and promote resident comfort.

Level of Evidence—5. The study was a systematic review of descriptive and qualitative studies.

Commentary: Implications for Practice and Research. The findings of this research clearly indicate that nurses who work in long-term care facilities with older adults, especially those with dementia, should include oral health screening as part of physical assessment. Although only one reliable and valid tool was located, nurses can use their knowledge of oral health to determine the person's needs. When abnormal findings are found during the assessment, nurses should refer the resident for further dental screening and care.

In addition, nurses are responsible for delegating and supervising selected nursing activities, such as oral hygiene, to unlicensed assistive personnel. Nurses should follow up with staff to ensure that residents receive routine mouth care. It is also important to collaborate with the nutritionist about the patient's dietary needs. The speech-language pathologist can also be helpful by conducting swallowing studies and making suggestions for dietary modifications if needed.

This study examined a fundamental patient health care need that is not being met with all populations. However, further research is needed to develop and validate oral assessment tools, determine the most appropriate oral care products (e.g., an electric toothbrush), and develop staff education programs. Nurses can positively affect patient outcomes to help promote comfort and prevent disease.

Patient-Centered Collaborative Care

Assessment

When performing an oral assessment, ask about a history of recent infections, nutritional changes, oral hygiene habits, oral trauma, or stress. A drug history should also be collected, including over-the-counter (OTC) drugs and herbal supplements. Document the course of the current outbreak, and determine if stomatitis has occurred frequently. Ask the patient if the lesions interfere with swallowing or eating.

The symptoms of stomatitis range in severity from a dry, painful mouth to open ulcerations, predisposing the patient to infection. These ulcerations can alter *nutritional* status because of difficulty with eating or swallowing. When they are severe, stomatitis and edema have the potential to obstruct the airway.

In oral candidiasis, a type of yeast infection, white plaque-like lesions appear on the tongue, palate, pharynx (throat), and buccal mucosa (inside the cheeks) (Fig. 56-1). When these patches are wiped away, the underlying surface is red and sore. Patients may report pain, but others describe the lesions as dry or hot.

While examining the mouth, wear nonsterile gloves. Use adequate lighting, including a flashlight or penlight and tongue blade. Assess the mouth for lesions, coating, and cracking. Document characteristics of the lesions in terms of location, size, shape, odor, color, and drainage.

If lesions are seen along the pharynx and the patient reports **dysphagia** (pain on swallowing), suspect that the lesions might extend down the esophagus. Additional swallowing studies may be required.

The physical assessment should also include palpating the cervical and submandibular lymph nodes for swelling. Advanced practice nurses usually perform this part of the examination.

Interventions

Interventions for stomatitis are aimed toward health promotion through careful *oral hygiene* and food selection. When providing mouth care for the patient, remind unlicensed assistive personnel (UAP) to use a soft-bristled toothbrush or disposable foam swabs to stimulate gums and clean the oral cavity. Teach the patient to rinse the mouth every 2 to 3 hours with a sodium bicarbonate solution or warm saline solution (may be mixed with hydrogen peroxide). He or she should avoid most commercial mouthwashes because they have high alcohol content, causing a burning sensation in irritated or ulcerated areas. Teach the patient to check the labels for alcohol content. Frequent, gentle mouth care promotes débridement of ulcerated lesions and can prevent super-infections. Chart 56-2 lists measures for special oral care.

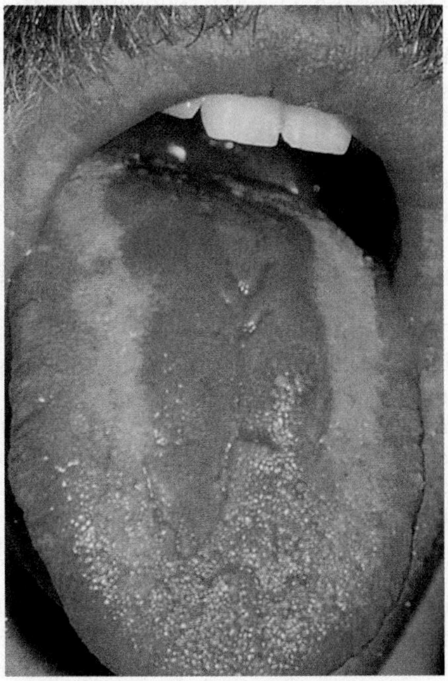

Fig. 56-1 • Oral candidiasis.

Drug therapy used for stomatitis includes antimicrobials, immune modulators, and symptomatic topicals. Complementary and alternative therapies may also be tried.

Antimicrobials, including antibiotics, antivirals, and antifungals, may be necessary for control of infection. Tetracycline syrup (swish/swallow) 250 mg/10 mL four times daily for 10 days may be prescribed, especially for recurrent aphthous ulcers (RAUs). The patient rinses for 2 minutes and swallows the syrup, thus obtaining both topical and systemic therapy. Minocycline swish/swallow and chlorhexidine mouthwashes may also be used.

A regimen of IV acyclovir (Zovirax) is prescribed for immunocompromised patients who contract herpes simplex stomatitis. Acyclovir is typically administered to those with normal kidney function at a dose of 5 mg/kg, infused at a constant rate over a 1-hour period every 8 hours for 7 days. Patients with healthy immune systems may be given acyclovir in oral or topical form.

For fungal infections, nystatin (Mycostatin) oral suspension 600,000 units four times daily for 7 to 10 days is the drug most often used. The patient swishes and swallows the topical preparation. Ice pop troches (lozenges) of the antifungal preparation allow the drug to slowly dissolve, and the cold provides an analgesic effect. Topical triamcinolone in benzocaine (Kenalog in Orabase) and oral dexamethasone elixir used as a swish/expectorate preparation are commonly used for stomatitis, especially RAU.

Immune modulating agents that may be prescribed include:

- Oral levamisole
- Topical amlexanox (Aphthasol)

Chart 56-2 BEST PRACTICE FOR PATIENT SAFETY & QUALITY CARE

Care of the Patient with Problems of the Oral Cavity

- Remove dentures if the patient has severe stomatitis or oral pain.
- Encourage the patient to perform oral hygiene or provide it after each meal and as often as needed.
- Increase mouth care to every 2 hours or more often if stomatitis is not controlled.
- Use a soft toothbrush or gauze for oral care.
- Encourage frequent rinsing of the mouth with warm saline or sodium bicarbonate (baking soda) solution, or a combination of these solutions.
- Teach the patient to avoid commercial mouthwashes and lemon-glycerin swabs.
- Assist the patient in selecting soft, bland, and nonacidic foods.
- Apply topical analgesics or anesthetics as prescribed by the health care provider, and monitor their effectiveness.

- Topical granulocyte-macrophage colony-stimulating factor (GM-CSF)
- Thalidomide

The exact mechanism for how these drugs work is not clear. However, they may inhibit release of mediators that contribute to the inflammation seen in patients with RAU.

Other drugs can be used to control pain, such as OTC benzocaine anesthetics (e.g., Orabase, Anbesol) and camphor phenol (Campho-Phenique). Fifteen mL of 2% viscous lidocaine every 3 hours (maximum of 8 doses per day) can be used as a gargle or mouthwash.

Dietary changes may also help decrease pain. Teach patients to avoid hard, spicy, salty, and acidic foods or fluids that can further irritate the ulcers. Include foods high in protein and vitamin C to promote healing, including scrambled eggs, bananas, custards, puddings, and ice cream, unless the patient has lactose intolerance.

NCLEX EXAMINATION CHALLENGE

An older adult with advanced dementia has been on antibiotic therapy for several days. The nurse notices that she has not been eating as well as usual. What actions should the nurse take? (Select all that apply.)

A. Coordinate with the nutritionist to change her diet.
B. Ask the family to bring in food that she likes from home.
C. Assess the client's mouth for any lesions or swelling.
D. Ask the client why she is not eating well.
E. Take the client's weight to compare with previous weights.
F. Ask the physician to discontinue the client's antibiotic.

evolve For the correct answer, go to http://evolve.elsevier.com/Iggy/.

ORAL TUMORS

Oral cavity tumors can be benign, precancerous, or cancerous. Whether benign or malignant, tumors of the mouth affect many daily functions, including swallowing, chewing, and speaking. Pain accompanying the tumor can also limit daily activities and self-care. Oral tumors affect body image, especially if treatment involves removal of the tongue or part of the mandible (jaw) or requires a tracheostomy.

PREMALIGNANT LESIONS

Leukoplakia

Leukoplakia presents as slowly developing changes in the oral mucous membranes causing thickened, white, firmly attached patches. These patches appear slightly raised and sharply rounded. Most of these lesions are benign. However, a small percentage of them become cancerous. Although leukoplakia can be found anywhere on the oral mucosa, lesions on the lips or tongue are more likely to progress to cancer.

Leukoplakia results from mechanical factors that cause long-term oral mucous membrane irritation, such as poorly fitting dentures, chronic cheek nibbling, or broken or poorly repaired teeth. In addition, oral hairy leukoplakia can be found in patients with HIV infection. Tobacco products, especially chewing tobacco and pipes, have also been implicated in the development of leukoplakia, sometimes referred to as "smoker's patch." Oral leukoplakia can be confused with oral candidal infection. However, unlike candidal infection, leukoplakia cannot be removed by scraping.

Leukoplakia is the most common oral lesion among adults. Oral hairy leukoplakia is an early manifestation of HIV disease and is highly correlated with progression from HIV infection to acquired immune deficiency syndrome (AIDS). Leukoplakia not associated with HIV disease is more often seen in people older than 40 years. Men have twice the incidence of leukoplakia that women have, but this ratio is changing because increasing numbers of women are smoking.

Erythroplakia

Erythroplakia presents as a red, velvety mucosal lesion on the surface of the oral mucosa. There are more malignant changes in erythroplakia than in leukoplakia. As such, these lesions should be regarded with suspicion and analyzed by biopsy. Erythroplakia is most commonly found on the floor of the mouth, tongue, palate, and mandibular mucosa. It can be difficult to distinguish from inflammatory or immune reactions.

ORAL CANCER

In the past decade, dentists and physicians have begun systematically screening their patients for oral cancer. Oral assessment has become a part of the routine dental examination. People should visit a dentist at least once or twice a year for professional dental hygiene and oral cancer screening, which includes inspecting and palpating the mouth for lesions.

Prevention strategies for oral cancer include minimizing sun and tanning bed exposure, tobacco cessation, and decreasing alcohol intake. Most dentists now use digital technology instead of x-rays when performing the annual or bi-annual dental examination. Excessive, prolonged radiation from x-rays has been associated with head and neck cancer (Oral Cancer Foundation, 2007b). Teach patients to follow the guidelines in Chart 56-1 to maintain oral health.

A new mouth rinse has been developed that could diagnose many cases of oral cancer in its early stages. The rinse works by identifying CD44, a protein tumor biomarker on the surface of healthy tissue that increases with oral cancer. This simple, noninvasive test could save thousands of patients whose lives are now shortened because they were diagnosed in the advanced stage of the disease (Oral Cancer Foundation, 2007a).

Pathophysiology

Squamous Cell Carcinoma

More than 90% of oral cancers are squamous cell carcinomas that begin on the surface of the epithelium. Over a period of many years, premalignant (or dysplastic) changes begin. Cells begin to vary in size and shape. Alterations in the thickness of the lining of the epithelium develop, resulting in atrophy. These tumors usually grow slowly, and the lesions may be large before the onset of symptoms unless ulceration is present. *Mucosal erythroplasia is the earliest sign of oral carcinoma. Oral lesions that appear as red, raised, eroded areas are suspicious for cancer. A lesion that does not heal within 2 weeks or a lump or thickening in the cheek is a symptom that warrants further assessment* (Oral Cancer Foundation, 2007b).

Squamous cell cancer can be found on the lips, tongue, buccal mucosa, and oropharynx. The major risk factors in its development are increasing age, tobacco use, and alcohol use. Most oral cancers occur in people older than 40 years. Tobacco use in any form (e.g., smoking or chewing tobacco) can increase the risk for cancer. A person who frequently consumes alcohol and uses tobacco in any form is at the highest risk. Genetic changes in patients with oral cancer have been found, especially the mutation of the *TP53* gene.

An increased rate of oral cancer is found in people with occupations such as textile workers, plumbers, and coal and metal workers. Additional factors, such as sun exposure, poor nutritional habits, poor oral hygiene, and infection with the human papillomavirus (HPV16) may also contribute to oral cancer (Oral Cancer Foundation, 2007b). People with **periodontal** (gum) **disease** in which mandibular (jaw) bone loss has occurred are especially at risk for cancer of the mouth.

Mouth cancers account for about 3% of all cancers in men and 2% of all cancers in women in the United States. Over 34,000 new cases are diagnosed each year, with almost 8000 deaths (Oral Cancer Foundation, 2007b). Most cancers occur in middle-aged and older people, although in recent years, younger adults have been affected, probably as a result of sun exposure.

Basal Cell Carcinoma

Basal cell carcinoma of the mouth occurs primarily on the lips. The lesion is asymptomatic and resembles a raised scab. With time, it evolves into a characteristic ulcer with a raised, pearly border. Basal cell carcinomas do not metastasize (spread) but can aggressively involve the skin of the face. The major risk factor for this type of cancer is excessive sunlight exposure.

Basal cell carcinoma occurs as a result of the failure of basal cells to mature into keratinocytes. It is the second most common type of oral cancer, but it is much less common than squamous cell carcinoma.

Kaposi's Sarcoma

Kaposi's sarcoma is a malignant lesion in blood vessels. It is usually painless and appears as a raised, purple nodule or plaque. In the mouth, the hard palate is the most common site of Kaposi's sarcoma, but it can be found also on the gums, tongue, or tonsils. It is most often associated with AIDS. (See Chapter 21 for a complete discussion of Kaposi's sarcoma.)

Patient-Centered Collaborative Care evolve ONLINE PHARM REVIEW

Assessment

Begin by assessing the patient's routine oral hygiene regimen and use of dentures or oral appliances, which might add to discomfort or mechanically irritate the mucosa. Ask about oral bleeding, which might indicate an ulcerative lesion. Determine the patient's past and current appetite and nutritional state, including difficulty with chewing or swallowing. A continuing trend of weight loss may be related to metastasis, heavy alcohol intake, difficulty in eating or chewing, or an underlying health problem.

An examination of the oral cavity requires adequate lighting. Thoroughly inspect the oral cavity for any lesions, evidence of pain, or restriction of movement. Using a tongue blade, examine all areas of the mouth. Carefully note any change in speech caused by tongue movement. Notice any change in voice or swallowing, and assess for thick or absent saliva. After inspection, the advanced practice nurse or specialty nurse uses bimanual palpation of any visible nodules to determine size and fixation. The cervical lymph nodes should also be palpated (Fig. 56-2).

The functioning and appearance of the mouth are strongly linked with body image and quality of life. Therefore it is important to assess the impact of oral lesions on the patient's self-concept. In addition, assess for any educational or cultural needs that might affect health teaching or treatment. Evaluate the patient's support system and past coping mechanisms.

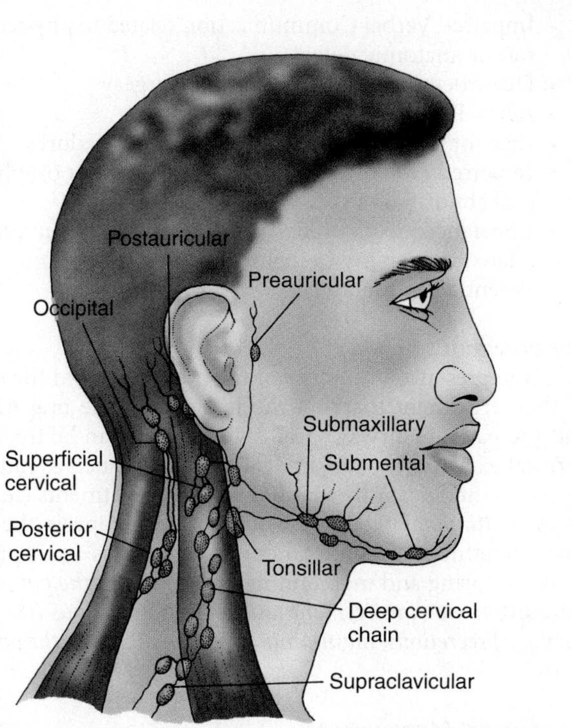
Postauricular
Preauricular
Occipital
Submaxillary
Superficial cervical
Submental
Posterior cervical
Tonsillar
Deep cervical chain
Supraclavicular

Fig. 56-2 • The lymph nodes of the cervical region.

Oral CDx brushing of a lesion is helpful in determining whether it is precancerous. This procedure is usually performed by a dentist during a routine dental examination (Oral Cancer Foundation, 2007a). However, biopsy is the definitive method for diagnosis of oral cancer. The physician obtains a needle biopsy specimen of the abnormal tissue to assess for malignant or premalignant changes. Incisional biopsies may also be performed. An intraoral biopsy can be done under local anesthesia. In very small lesions, an excisional biopsy can permit complete tumor removal. Magnetic resonance imaging (MRI) is useful in detecting perineural involvement and in evaluating thickness in cancers of the tongue. Both computed tomography (CT) and MRI can be used to determine spread to the liver or lungs if further staging of the disease is warranted.

An aqueous solution of toluidine blue 1% can be applied to oral lesions to determine if they are malignant. This preparation stains malignant lesions, leaving normal tissue unaffected. However, a lesion that is the result of an inflammatory process may also absorb the stain, leading to a false-positive result. Although a biopsy is still needed to confirm a cancer diagnosis, toluidine blue may be useful for screening high-risk patients.

Common Nursing Diagnoses and Collaborative Problems

Based on the nursing assessment, nursing diagnoses and collaborative problems that may apply to patients with oral cancer, depending on the extent of the disease, include:

- Risk for Ineffective Airway Clearance related to obstructed airway by the tumor, edema, or secretions
- Impaired Oral Mucous Membrane related to pathologic conditions from the tumor

- Impaired Verbal Communication related to physical barrier or anatomic defect
- Disturbed Body Image related to surgery
- Acute Pain related to physical injury
- Risk for Infection related to invasive procedures
- Impaired Swallowing related to oral cavity or oropharyngeal abnormalities
- Imbalanced Nutrition: Less Than Body Requirements related to inability to ingest food
- Potential for Metastasis

Interventions

Both the presence of tumors of the oral cavity and the effects of their treatment threaten the integrity of the oral mucosa and the patient's airway. Oral cavity lesions can be treated by surgical excision, by nonsurgical treatments such as radiation or chemotherapy, or by a combination of treatments (referred to as *multimodal therapy*). Multimodal therapy is the most costly treatment option. Nursing interventions focus primarily on restoring and maintaining oral health. *If the patient has extensive tumor involvement and copious, tenacious (thick and "stringy") secretions, maintaining an open airway is the primary focus.*

Nonsurgical Management

If needed, implement interventions to *manage the patient's airway* by increasing air exchange, removing secretions, and preventing aspiration (Chart 56-3). Assess for dyspnea resulting from the tumor obstruction or from excessive secretions. Assess the quality, rate, and depth of respirations. Auscultate the lungs for adventitious sounds, such as wheezes caused by aspiration. Listen for stridor caused by partial airway obstruction. Promote deep breathing to help produce an effective cough to mobilize the patient's secretions as described in Chart 56-3.

To increase air exchange, place the patient in a semi-Fowler's or high Fowler's position. Encourage fluids to help liquefy secretions. Chest physiotherapy also increases air exchange as well as promotes effective coughing. If available, collaborate with the respiratory therapist about performing this procedure. If needed, use oral suction equipment with a dental tip or a tonsil tip (Yankauer catheter) to remove secretions that obstruct the airway. Teach the patient and family to use the catheters as needed.

If edema occurs with oral cavity lesions, the patient may receive steroids to reduce inflammation. Antibiotics may be prescribed if infection is present because it can increase inflammation and edema. A cool mist supplied by a face tent may assist with oxygen transport and control of edema.

Aspiration precautions prevent or reduce the risk factors for aspiration. Assess the patient's level of consciousness (LOC), gag reflex, and ability to swallow. To prevent aspiration, place the patient sitting upright at 90 degrees (high Fowler's position). *As a precaution, keep suction equipment nearby. For patients at high risk, assess the gag reflex before giving any fluids. Remind UAP and visitors to feed patients at risk for aspiration in small amounts.* Thickened liquids can be used as an aid to prevent aspiration.

It is important to work with the patient to *establish an oral hygiene routine.* Ideally, oral hygiene is performed every 2 hours for ulcerated lesions, infection, or in the immediate postoperative period. Modifications might be needed because of oral discomfort, bleeding, or edema. Oral care with a soft-bristled toothbrush is preferred. If the platelet count falls below 40,000/mm^3, switch the patient to an ultrasoft "chemobrush." The use of "toothettes" or a disposable foam brush is discouraged because these products may not adequately control bacteremia-promoting plaque. Lubricant can be applied to moisten the lips and oral mucosa as needed.

Chart 56-3 NIC INTERVENTION ACTIVITIES

The Patient with Oral Cancer

Airway Management: *Facilitation of patency of air passages*
- Position patient to maximize ventilation potential.
- Remove secretions by encouraging coughing or by suctioning.
- Instruct how to cough effectively.
- Auscultate breath sounds, noting areas of decreased or absent ventilation and presence of adventitious sounds.
- Administer humidified air or oxygen, as appropriate.
- Position to alleviate dyspnea.
- Monitor respiratory and oxygenation status, as appropriate.

Cough Enhancement: *Promotion of deep inhalation by the patient with subsequent generation of high intrathoracic pressures and compression of underlying lung parenchyma for the forceful expulsion of air*
- Assist patient to a sitting position with the head slightly flexed, shoulders relaxed, and knees flexed.
- Encourage patient to take several deep breaths.
- Encourage patient to take a deep breath, hold it for 2 seconds, and cough two or three times in succession.
- Instruct patient to inhale deeply, bend forward slightly, and perform three or four huffs (against an open glottis).
- Instruct patient to inhale deeply several times, to exhale slowly, and to cough at the end of exhalation.
- Instruct patient to follow coughing with several maximal inhalation breaths.
- Promote systemic fluid hydration, as appropriate.

Aspiration Precautions: *Prevention or minimization of risk factors in the patient at risk for aspiration*
- Monitor level of consciousness, cough reflex, gag reflex, and swallowing ability.
- Monitor pulmonary status.
- Maintain an airway.
- Position upright 90 degrees or as far as possible.
- Feed in small amounts.
- Avoid liquids or use thickening agent.
- Offer foods or liquids that can be formed into a bolus before swallowing.
- Cut food into small pieces.
- Request medication in elixir form.
- Break or crush pills (if appropriate) before administration.
- Keep head of bed elevated 30 to 45 minutes after eating.

NIC intervention activities selected from Bulechek, G.M., Butcher, H.K., & McCloskey Dochterman, J. (Eds.). (2008). *Nursing interventions classification (NIC)* (5th ed.). St. Louis: Mosby.

Teach patients and their families to avoid using commercial mouthwashes and lemon-glycerin swabs. Commercial mouthwashes contain alcohol, and lemon-glycerin swabs are acidic. These substances can cause a burning sensation and contribute to dry oral mucous membranes. Encourage frequent rinsing of the mouth with sodium bicarbonate solution or warm saline (see also Chart 56-2). Follow hospital or health care provider protocol if available.

Radiation therapy has been used alone, as well as with surgery and chemotherapy, for oral cancer. The purpose of radiation therapy is tumor reduction while preserving the patient's function and appearance. There are several ways to apply radiotherapy. In collaboration with the patient, the oncologist or other qualified physician chooses the best mode on the basis of the tumor site and staging.

Radiation therapy for oral cancers can be given by external beam or interstitial implantation. *External-beam* radiation passes through the skin or mucous membrane to the tumor site. Typically, treatments are given as five daily treatments per week over a 6- to 9-week period. Special precautions are taken to minimize the dose of radiation to the brain or spinal cord. Another option is the implantation of radioactive substances (*interstitial radiation* therapy or brachytherapy) either to boost the dosage or to deliver a radiation dose close to the tumor bed. This form of implant therapy can be curative in early-stage lesions in the floor of the mouth or anterior tongue. It may also add a boost of radiation to a tumor that received external-beam radiation.

Interstitial radiation is used for smaller lesions that do not infiltrate surrounding tissues. Radioactive materials can be:

- Seeds, which are permanently implanted into the tissue (usually for tumors that cannot be completely excised or in neck nodes)
- Needles or wires, which are removed at the end of therapy
- Radiation catheters or holders, which are loaded with radioactive materials
- A "mold" of radioactive material placed directly over the lesion for a specific time

With the exception of radioactive seeds, which have a low level of emission, patients receiving interstitial radiation are usually hospitalized for the duration of treatment. Place patients on radiation transmission precautions while the materials are active or in place. A tracheostomy may be required with interstitial implants because of edema and increased oral secretions. (See Chapter 24 for general nursing care of patients undergoing radiation therapy.)

The patient may receive one or more types of *drug therapy*. The advantages of drug therapy instead of or as an adjunct to surgery or radiation for cancer of the oral cavity continue to be evaluated.

Teach the patient undergoing chemotherapy and family about the side effects of the drugs, which vary with each drug. Give antiemetics as prescribed, and provide other comfort measures as needed. (See Chapter 24 for general care of patients receiving chemotherapy.)

One of the most recent advances in the use of drugs for oral cancer is targeted therapy. Hormone-like substances known as *growth factors (GFs)* occur in the body's cells. Oral tumor cells, along with other types of cancers, grow quickly because they have more GF receptors than normal healthy tissue. One of these GFs is called *epidermal growth factor (EGF)*, which has been associated with oral cancers. New drugs that can target and block EGF receptors (EGF-R) are being tested, and more than a dozen have been approved, including cetuximab (Erbitux) and erlotinib (Tarceva). Chapter 24 describes targeted molecular therapy.

Surgical Management

The physician can often remove small, noninvasive lesions of the oral cavity in an ambulatory setting with local anesthesia. The surgical defect is usually small enough to be closed by sutures. These smaller lesions may also be responsive to carbon dioxide laser therapy or **cryotherapy** (extreme cold application), as well as photodynamic therapy. These procedures can be performed as an ambulatory care procedure in a surgical center (but may require general anesthesia).

Small oral cancers are equally responsive to radiation or photodynamic therapy and to surgery. More invasive lesions (stages III and IV) require more extensive surgical excision and result in a greater loss of function and disfigurement. Not all lesions can be excised by the peroral approach (through the mouth). The goal of surgical resection is removal of the tumor with a surgical margin that is free of cancer cells.

Preoperative Care. Before excision of a lesion in the oral cavity, assess and document the patient's level of understanding of the disease process, the rationale for the surgery, and the planned intervention. Problems associated with cancer therapy can be reduced or optimally managed with patient preparation and instruction. Reinforce information as needed. Include family members or other caregivers in the health teaching unless culturally inappropriate.

For small, local excisions, postoperative restrictions include a liquid diet for a day and then advancing as tolerated. There are no activity limitations, and postoperative analgesics are prescribed.

Instructions for the patient undergoing large surgical resections may include but are not limited to these expectations after surgery:

- Placement of a temporary tracheostomy, oxygen therapy, and suctioning
- Temporary loss of speech because of the tracheostomy
- Frequent monitoring of postoperative vital signs
- NPO status until intraoral suture lines are healed
- Need to have IV lines in place for drug delivery and hydration
- Postoperative drug therapy and activity (out of bed on the first postoperative day)
- Possibility of surgical drains

Because communication is interrupted, assess the patient's ability to read and write. In coordination with the patient, select the method of communication to use after surgery with staff and family members (e.g., Magic Slate, computer, picture board, or pad and pencil). Urge the patient to practice the chosen method before surgery to reduce frustration after surgery.

Operative Procedures. Three factors influence the extent of surgery performed for oral cancers: the size and location of the tumor, tumor invasion into the bone, and whether there has been metastasis (cancer spread) to neck lymph nodes. Small, noninvasive tumors can be excised perioraly (inside the mouth). Otherwise, an external approach may be used. The most extensive oral operations are composite resections, which combine partial or total **glossectomy** (tongue removal) and partial **mandibulectomy** (jaw removal). In the *commando* (co-mandible) *procedure,* the surgeon removes a segment of the mandible with the oral lesion and performs a radical neck dissection (see Chapter 31).

Metastasis to cervical lymph nodes usually indicates a poor prognosis for patients with cancer of the oral cavity. In those with cervical node metastasis, a neck dissection may also be performed. A radical neck dissection usually involves the removal of all cervical lymph nodes on the affected side, along with cranial nerve XI, the internal jugular vein, and the sternocleidomastoid (front neck) muscle. Modified and selective neck dissections may be done in patients with minimal lymph node involvement.

Postoperative Care. The patient may have a temporary or permanent tracheostomy, requiring intensive nursing care to promote airway clearance. In addition, care must be taken to protect the surgical incision site from mechanical damage and infection (see Chapter 31). Nursing interventions to relieve pain or discomfort and promote nutrition are also important. Older adults are a special risk for surgery and need to be monitored very carefully (Chart 56-4).

After extensive excision or resection, the most important nursing intervention is maintaining the patient's airway. The patient may not recall on awakening from anesthesia that a tracheostomy tube is in place and may initially panic because of the inability to speak. Remind the patient why he or she cannot speak, and provide reassurance that the vocal cords are intact (unless a total laryngectomy has been performed, in which case the loss of voice is permanent). Ensure that the predetermined method of communication is available for the patient, family members, and staff.

When the patient has an adequate airway and can effectively clear secretions by coughing, the tracheostomy tube may be removed. When the tube is removed, an airtight dressing is placed over the site and the tracheostomy incision heals without the need for sutures.

Patients who have undergone extensive resection may have slurred speech or difficulty in speaking as a result of nerve damage or tongue removal. Collaborate with the speech-language pathologist if speech is altered.

Protect the incision site to avoid infection. It is important to provide gentle mouth care for cleaning away thick secretions and stimulating the flow of saliva. The delivery of oral care depends on the nature and extent of the surgical procedure. Oral care should be provided at least every 4 hours in the early postoperative phase. The presence of unusual odors from the mouth can indicate infection. In the early postoperative phase, care must be taken to avoid disruption of the suture line during oral hygiene.

Chart 56-4 FOCUSED ASSESSMENT

The Postoperative Older Adult with Oral Cancer

- Assess the mouth and surrounding tissues for candidiasis, mucositis, and pain; assess for loss of appetite and taste.
- Monitor the patient's weight.
- Monitor nutritional and fluid intake.
- Assess for difficulty in eating or speech.
- Assess pain status and measures used to control pain.
- Monitor the patient's response to medications.
- Identify psychosocial problems, such as depression, anxiety, and fear.

Elevate the head of the bed to at least 30 degrees to assist in decreasing edema by gravity. If skin grafting was done, inspect the donor site (generally on the anterior thigh) every 8 hours for bleeding or signs of infection. (See Chapter 31 for specific nursing care of the patient with a radical neck dissection.)

To provide optimal *pain relief* in the postoperative period, rely on subjective and objective data to assess the need for analgesics and the effectiveness of the drugs given. The outcome of drug therapy during this period is relief of pain while allowing the patient to function at an optimal level. Those who have undergone surgery for oral cancer describe their pain as throbbing or pounding. IV morphine is usually the initial pain medication given. Tylox or Percocet (Percodan plus acetaminophen) may be used for systemic relief of moderate pain.

Patients who have undergone extensive resections of the oral cavity remain on NPO status for several days. This time allows healing in the oral cavity before food contacts the incision. Nasogastric feeding or total parenteral nutrition may be needed until oral nutrition can begin (see Chapter 63).

When oral fluid intake is started, assess for and document difficulty in swallowing, aspiration, or leakage of saliva or fluids from the suture line. Nursing care should also include monitoring weight and hydration. Nutritional supplementation may be used to improve the patient's quality of life. Patients who have weight loss or who are having difficulty maintaining hydration may be candidates for the surgical placement of a gastrostomy tube. Coordinate dietary care with the nutritionist.

Encourage the patient to perform swallowing exercises. Collaborate with the speech-language pathologist to assist with swallowing techniques. Thickened fluids may be needed to prevent aspiration. A swallowing impairment may be temporary or permanent.

Community-Based Care

Continuing care for the patient with an oral tumor depends on the severity of the tumor, its treatment, and available support systems. Most patients are maintained at home during follow-up care. Ongoing nutritional management remains a vital part of the treatment plan. In addition, the patient and family may benefit from a community-based support group for cancer victims.

Home Care Management

If radiation therapy is part of the patient's treatment plan, home care considerations include health teaching and management strategies. Complications due to radiation to the head or neck can be acute or delayed. Acute effects include treatment-related mucositis, stomatitis, and alterations in taste. Long-term effects such as **xerostomia** (excessive mouth dryness) and dental decay require ongoing oral care, the use of saliva substitutes, and follow-up dental visits. Although ongoing dental care is important, the possible adverse effects that radiation has on bone make elective oral surgical procedures, such as tooth extraction, impossible in the area of the radiation. Fatigue is a common side effect of radiation and chemotherapy.

The patient whose tracheostomy tube has been removed is often taking a soft diet by mouth before discharge. Occasionally, however, patients are discharged from the hospital while still requiring tracheostomy suction, oral suction, and nasogastric feedings. Suction equipment, nutritional supplies, and nursing care can be provided by home care companies. (See Chapter 63 for home care preparation for the patient receiving home parenteral nutrition and Chapter 31 for home care preparation for the patient with a tracheostomy.)

Health Teaching

Teach the patient and family about drug therapy, nutritional therapies, any treatments (e.g., tracheostomy care, suture line care, dressing changes), and early symptoms of infection before hospital discharge. Alterations in taste and dysphagia make maintaining adequate nutrition a challenge for the oral cancer patient. Alterations in taste occur when the taste buds are included in the radiation treatment field. Taste sensation may begin to return several weeks after the completion of treatment. Sometimes the loss of taste is permanent.

Changes in taste include dislike of meat, such as beef or pork, and metallic tastes in the mouth. Teach patients to add seasonings to foods, to use gravies or sauces to make foods more palatable, and to use high-protein foods such as cheeses, milk, eggs, puddings, and legumes in place of meat. Instruct patients with dysphagia in swallowing exercises. Recommend thickened liquids because thin liquids, such as water, are difficult to control during swallowing. Collaborate with the nutritionist to teach the family how to assess the nutritional intake of the patient who is just beginning to eat. Liquid dietary supplements are usually recommended at this time. If bleeding or stomatitis is present, a diet of soft foods is recommended to prevent further injury to the mucous membranes.

Teach the patient or family members to inspect the oral cavity daily for areas of redness, indicating the onset of stomatitis. Meticulous oral hygiene should be continued at home, especially with adjuvant chemotherapy or radiation. Reinforce the oral hygiene routine, emphasizing the need for frequent mouth rinsing to reduce the number of microorganisms and to maintain adequate hydration. The patient should use a chemobrush, rinse the chemobrush with hydrogen peroxide and water or with a diluted bleach solution after each use, and change chemobrushes weekly. The brush may also be cleaned in a dishwasher.

Saliva production is greatly reduced as a consequence of radiation. The resulting xerostomia causes the inability to eat dry foods and may be permanent. Teach the patient regarding the use of saliva substitutes.

Skin reactions are also a common side effect of radiation. Instruct the patient to avoid sun exposure, to avoid perfumed lotions or powders, and to cleanse the face or neck area with a gentle nondeodorant soap. Teach male patients to use an electric razor for shaving and to avoid alcohol-based aftershave lotions to prevent further skin irritation.

Health Care Resources

Patients who have undergone composite resection often require community services because they have both physical and psychosocial needs. Depression related to a change in body image is common. Excision of a portion of the jaw can leave a facial defect that may be difficult to hide. A social worker or other health care professional may be needed for patient and family counseling. Those who have undergone a total glossectomy may be able to speak with special training and the use of an intraoral prosthesis created by a maxillofacial prosthodontist. The prosthesis is similar to dentures.

A case manager provides assistance in obtaining special equipment or nutritional resources required by the patient at home. He or she assesses the patient's financial needs and makes referrals to government, community, and religious organizations as needed. Refer the patient to the American Cancer Society (ACS) (www.cancer.org) or the Oral Cancer Foundation (www.oralcancerfoundation.org) for local support groups and resources, including additional information. The ACS often supplies dressing supplies and transportation to and from follow-up visits or medical treatments.

DECISION-MAKING CHALLENGE
Coordination of Care

You are assigned to visit a middle-aged adult who recently had a partial glossectomy to remove a cancerous tumor. He was formerly a professional baseball player who used chewing tobacco for many years. The patient is receiving parenteral nutrition, and he reports being hungry all the time. He is on Humulin R insulin for his diabetes, which has been uncontrolled since he had his surgery. The patient is very angry and depressed and states to his wife that he "can't live like this." She is concerned that he will try to commit suicide unless his health improves.

1. How should you respond to the patient's wife at this time?
2. What other health care professionals need to be included in managing this patient?
3. How will you coordinate his care with members of the health care team?
4. What other priorities for care do you have for the patient during this home visit?

evolve For suggested answer guidelines, go to http://evolve.elsevier.com/Iggy/.

DISORDERS OF THE SALIVARY GLANDS

ACUTE SIALADENITIS

Pathophysiology

Acute sialadenitis, the inflammation of a salivary gland, can be caused by infectious agents, irradiation, or immunologic disorders. Salivary gland inflammation can have a bacterial or viral cause, such as infection with cytomegalovirus (CMV). The most common bacterial organisms are *Staphylococcus aureus, Staphylococcus pyogenes, Streptococcus pneumoniae,* and *Escherichia coli.* This disorder most commonly affects the parotid or submandibular gland in adults.

A decrease in the production of saliva (as in dehydrated or debilitated patients or in those who are on NPO status postoperatively for an extended time) can lead to acute sialadenitis. The bacteria or viruses enter the gland through the ductal opening in the mouth. Systemic drugs, such as phenothiazines and the tetracyclines, can also trigger an episode of acute sialadenitis. Untreated infections of the salivary glands can evolve into abscesses, which can rupture and spread infection into the tissues of the neck and the mediastinum.

Patients who receive radiation for the treatment of cancers of the head and neck or thyroid may develop decreased salivary flow, predisposing them to acute or persistent sialadenitis. The effect of radiation on the salivary glands is rapid and dose related. Immunologic disorders such as HIV infection can cause enlargement of the parotid gland that result from secondary infection. Sjögren's syndrome, an autoimmune disorder, is characterized by chronic salivary gland enlargement and inflammation (see Chapter 20).

Patient-Centered Collaborative Care

During the initial interview, assess for any predisposing factors for sialadenitis, such as ionizing radiation to the head or neck area. Collect a thorough drug history, and ask about systemic illnesses, such as HIV infection.

Dehydration can be assessed by examining the oral membrane and the skin for turgor. Other assessment findings include pain and swelling of the face over the affected gland. Assess facial function because its branches lie close to the salivary glands. Fever and general malaise also occur, and purulent drainage can often be massaged from the affected duct in the oral cavity.

Collaborative care includes the administration of IV fluids and measures such as these to treat the underlying cause and increase the flow of saliva:

- Hydration
- Application of warm compresses
- Massage of the gland
- Use of a saliva substitute
- Use of **sialagogues** (substances that stimulate the flow of saliva)

Sialagogues include lemon slices and fruit- or citrus-flavored candy. Massage is accomplished by milking the edematous gland with the fingertips toward the ductal opening. Elevation of the head of the bed promotes gravity drainage of the edematous gland.

Acute sialadenitis is best prevented by adherence to routine oral hygiene. This practice prevents infections from ascending to the salivary glands from the mouth.

POSTIRRADIATION SIALADENITIS

The salivary glands are sensitive to ionizing radiation, such as from radiation therapy or radioactive iodine treatment of thyroid cancers. Exposure of the glands to radiation produces **xerostomia** (very dry mouth caused by a severe reduction in the flow of saliva) within 24 hours. Radiation to the salivary glands can also produce pain and edema, which generally abate after several days.

Xerostomia may be temporary or permanent, depending on the dose of radiation and the percentage of total salivary gland tissue irradiated. Little can be done to relieve the patient's dry mouth during the course of radiation therapy. Frequent sips of water and frequent mouth care, especially before meals, are the most effective interventions. After the course of radiation therapy has been completed, saliva substitutes may provide moisture for 2 to 4 hours at a time. Over-the-counter solutions are available, or solutions may be mixed with methylcellulose (Cologel), glycerin, and saline.

SALIVARY GLAND TUMORS

Of all oral tumors, those of the salivary glands are relatively rare. Initially, malignant tumors present as slow-growing, painless masses. Involvement of the facial nerve results in facial weakness or paralysis (partial or total) on the affected side.

Collect information about any prior radiation exposure because radiation to the head and neck areas is associated with the occurrence of salivary gland tumors. Salivary gland tumors present as localized, firm masses. Large tumors may cause facial nerve paralysis. Submandibular and minor salivary gland tumors may be tender or painful. Tumor invasion of the hypoglossal nerve causes impaired movement of the tongue, and a loss of sensation can follow. *Pay particular attention to assessment of the facial nerve because of its proximity to the salivary glands.* Assess the patient's ability to:

- Wrinkle the brow
- Raise the eyebrows
- Squeeze the eyes shut
- Wrinkle the nose
- Pucker the lips
- Puff out the cheeks
- Grimace or smile

The treatment of choice for both benign and malignant tumors of the salivary glands is surgical excision. However, radiation therapy is often used for salivary gland cancers that are large, have recurred, show evidence of residual disease after excision, or are highly malignant.

Patients who have undergone **parotidectomy** (surgical removal of the parotid glands) or submandibular gland surgery are at risk for weakness or loss of function of the facial nerve because the nerve courses directly through the gland. Facial nerve repair with grafting can be done at the time of surgery. A combination of surgery followed by radiation is common for advanced disease. Care for patients after parotidectomy is similar to that required for those having oral cancer surgery, described on p. 1238.

HUMAN NEEDS NURSING CARE REVIEW

What might you NOTICE if the patient has inadequate digestion and oxygenation as a result of oral cavity problems?

- Dysphagia (difficulty swallowing)
- Dyspnea
- Stridor or wheezes
- Changes in speech or voice
- Copious, thickened oral secretions
- Excessive coughing during meals

What should you INTERPRET and how should you RESPOND to a patient experiencing inadequate digestion and oxygenation as a result of oral cavity problems?

Perform and interpret focused physical assessment findings, including:

- Breath sounds
- Oxygen saturation by pulse oximetry
- Ability to cough and clear the airway
- Ability to manage excessive oral secretions
- Ability to chew food and swallow

Respond:

- Place the patient with the head elevated to at least 30 degrees.
- Apply oxygen as needed.
- Suction the oral cavity as needed.
- Encourage deep breathing and coughing every 2 hours.
- Increase fluids to liquefy secretions, depending on swallowing ability.
- Notify the respiratory therapist or Rapid Response Team if interventions are not successful in restoring oxygenation.

On what should you REFLECT?

- Observe patient for evidence of increased oxygenation, including increased ease of breathing.
- Observe patient for evidence of increased ability to swallow.
- Observe patient for evidence of increased ability to manage oral secretions.
- Consider follow-up interventions to manage patient, including coordinating care with nutritionist and speech-language pathologist.
- Think about what else you might do to promote digestion and nutrition.

GET READY FOR THE NCLEX EXAMINATION!

Key Points

Review these Key Points for each NCLEX Examination Client Needs Category.

Safe and Effective Care Environment

- Be aware that airway management is the priority for care for patients having surgery for oral cancer.
- Place patients having oral cancer surgery in a high-Fowler's, sitting position to facilitate breathing and prevent aspiration.
- Be sure to assess for swallowing ability by checking the gag reflex before offering liquids or food to the patient who has had oral cancer surgery to prevent aspiration.
- Plan continuity of care to meet patients' needs when they are transferred from the hospital to community-based agencies.
- Assist the patient and family in identifying and using coping mechanisms to deal with possible changes in body image and altered self-esteem.

Health Promotion and Maintenance

- Teach patients to seek medical or dental attention for oral lesions that do not heal; these lesions could be oral carcinomas.
- Remind patients to visit their dentist regularly for dental hygiene and oral examination.
- Follow the best practice recommendations for maintaining oral health as listed in Chart 56-1.
- Instruct patients to avoid harsh commercial mouthwashes if they have oral lesions.
- Teach patients to avoid tobacco, alcohol, and sun exposure to decrease their chance of having oral cancer.
- Instruct patients with acute sialadenitis to use sialagogues to stimulate saliva, such as citrus foods or candies.

Psychosocial Integrity

- Recognize that patients with stomatitis are often unable to eat or swallow without discomfort.
- Be aware that those who have had surgery for oral cancer may have difficulty coping with the disease.
- Remember that patients having oral cancer may have an impaired body image because of their reconstructive surgery.
- Refer patients with oral cancer to support groups, such as those available through the American Cancer Society.

Physiological Integrity

- Remember that stomatitis usually manifests as painful single or multiple ulcerations within the mouth.
- Recognize that stomatitis can be caused by a variety of organisms; *Candida* infections are very common in patients who receive antibiotic therapy and in those who are immunocompromised.
- Provide gentle oral care for patients with oral lesions, including chemobrushes and warm saline or sodium bicarbonate.
- Be aware that patients with stomatitis receive antimicrobials, anti-inflammatory agents, immune modulators, and topical agents for relief of symptoms, including pain.
- Differentiate leukoplakia and erythroplakia: leukoplakia presents as thin, white patches, and erythroplakia presents as red, velvety lesions.
- Be aware that patients with oral cancer may have chemotherapy, radiation, surgery, or a combination of these treatment methods.
- Provide care for patients having cancer surgery as summarized in Chart 56-3.
- Be aware that sialadenitis can occur as result of radiation therapy.
- For patients with salivary gland tumors, assess for facial nerve involvement.
- Remember that a parotidectomy involves the removal of the salivary glands; postoperative care is similar to that for patients who have oral cancer surgery.

Additional Study Resources

Go to your Companion CD or Evolve at http://evolve.elsevier.com/Iggy/ for *Self-Assessment Questions for the NCLEX Examination.*

evolve Go to Evolve at http://evolve.elsevier.com/Iggy/ for *Prioritization and Delegation Questions for the NCLEX Examination.*

SELECTED BIBLIOGRAPHY

Asterisk indicates a classic or definitive work on this subject.

Bailey, R., Gueldner, S., Ledikwe, J., & Smiciklas-Wright, H. (2005). The oral health of older adults: An interdisciplinary approach. *Journal of Gerontological Nursing, 31*(7), 11-17.

Chalmers, J., & Pearson, A. (2005). Oral hygiene care for residents with dementia: A literature review. *Journal of Advanced Nursing, 52*(4), 410-419.

*Chia-Hui Chen, C. (2003). The Geriatric Oral Health Assessment Index (GOHAI). *Try this: Best practices in nursing for older adults, 14*(6), 5-6.

*Fitzpatrick, J. (2000). Oral health needs of dependent older people: Responsibilities of nurses and care staff. *Journal of Advanced Nursing, 32*, 1325-1332.

*Freer, S.K. (2000). Use of an oral assessment tool to improve practice. *Professional Nurse, 15*(10), 635-639.

Gil-Montoya, J.A., de Mello, A.L., Cardenas, C.B., & Lopez, I.G. (2006). Oral health protocol for the dependent institutionalized elderly. *Geriatric Nursing, 27*(2), 95-101.

Huff, M., Kinion, E., Kendra, M.A., & Klecan, T. (2006). Self-esteem: A hidden concern in oral health. *Journal of Community Health, 23*(4), 245-255.

Jarvis, C. (2008). *Physical examination and health assessment* (5th ed.). Philadelphia: Saunders.

Luggen, A.S. (2005). Gerontologic nurse practitioner guidelines: Oral health of older adults—Problems and management. *Geriatric Nursing, 26*(6), 356-357.

McCance, K.L., & Huether, S.E. (2006). *Pathophysiology: The biologic basis for disease in adults & children* (5th ed.). St. Louis: Mosby.

*Miller, M., & Kearney, N. (2001). Oral care for patients with cancer: A review of the literature. *Cancer Nursing, 24*(4), 241-254.

Munro, C.L., Grap, M.J., Elswick, R.K. Jr., McKinney, J., Sessler, C.N., & Hummel, R.S. III. (2006). Oral health status and development of ventilator-associated pneumonia: A descriptive study. *American Journal of Critical Care, 15*(5), 453-460.

*Neville, B.W., & Day, T.A. (2002). Oral cancer and precancerous lesions. *CA: A Cancer Journal for Clinicians, 52*(4), 195-215.

Oral Cancer Foundation. (2007a). *New diagnostic technologies offer non-invasive method.* Retrieved September 2007, from www.oralcancerfoundation.org.

Oral Cancer Foundation. (2007b). *Oral cancer facts.* Retrieved May 2007, from www.oralcancerfoundation.org.

*Pearson, L. (1996). A comparison of the ability of foam swabs and toothbrushes to remove dental plaque: Implications for nursing practice. *Journal of Advanced Nursing, 23*, 62-69.

*Robins-Sadler, G., Stoudt, A., Fullerton, J.T., Oberle-Edwards, L.K., Nguyen, Q., & Epstein, J.B. (2003). Managing the oral sequelae of cancer therapy. *MedSurg Nursing, 12*(1), 28-36.

Touger-Decker, R., Mobley, C.C.; American Dietetic Association. (2007). Position of the American Dietetic Association: Oral health and nutrition. *Journal of the American Dietetic Association, 107*(8), 1418-1428.

*Walton, J.C., Miller, J., & Tordecilla, L. (2001). Elder oral assessment and care. *MedSurg Nursing, 10*(1), 37-44.

57

CHAPTER

Care of Patients with Esophageal Problems

Donna D. Ignatavicius

LEARNING OUTCOMES

For clinical competence and success on the NCLEX Examination, study this chapter with these Learning Outcomes in mind:

Safe and Effective Care Environment

1. Collaborate with the health care team when providing care to patients with esophageal health problems that impair swallowing or limit nutrition.

Health Promotion and Maintenance

2. Teach the patient and family about lifestyle changes to decrease gastroesophageal reflux disease (GERD) and the discomfort of hiatal hernias.
3. Teach the patient and family about postoperative care after esophageal surgery.

Psychosocial Integrity

4. Provide psychosocial support to patients and their families through diagnosis and treatment of esophageal cancer.

Physiological Integrity

5. Evaluate the impact of esophageal cancer on the patient's nutritional status, including the risk for aspiration.
6. Perform focused assessments for patients with esophageal health problems.
7. Apply knowledge of pathophysiology to monitor for complications of esophageal surgical procedures.
8. Teach patients with GERD about drug therapy.
9. Plan community-based care for patients diagnosed with esophageal cancer.

Go to your Companion CD or Evolve at http://evolve.elsevier.com/Iggy/ for *Self-Assessment Questions for the NCLEX Examination* keyed to these Learning Outcomes.

The esophagus moves partially digested food from the mouth to the stomach. If food cannot reach the stomach, the patient cannot meet the *human need for nutrition.* Nutrients in food are necessary for normal body cell function. Common problems of the esophagus that can interfere with *digestion* and *nutrition* are caused by inflammation, structural defects or obstruction, and cancer. Collaborative management requires dietary and lifestyle changes, as well as medical and surgical therapies.

GASTROESOPHAGEAL REFLUX DISEASE

Pathophysiology

Gastroesophageal reflux disease (GERD) is the most common upper GI disorder in the United States. It occurs most often in middle-aged and older adults but can affect people of any age. **GERD** occurs as a result of **reflux** (backward flow) of GI contents into the esophagus. Reflux produces symptoms by exposing the esophageal mucosa to the irritating effects of gastric or duodenal contents, resulting in inflammation. A person with acute symptoms of inflammation is often described as having **reflux esophagitis,** which may be mild or severe (McCance & Huether, 2006).

The reflux of gastric contents into the esophagus is normally prevented by the presence of two high-pressure areas that remain contracted at rest. A 1.2-inch (3-cm) segment at the proximal end of the esophagus is called the *upper esophageal sphincter (UES).* Another 0.8- to 1.6-inch (2- to 4-cm) portion at the gastroesophageal junction (near the cardiac sphincter) is called the **lower esophageal sphincter (LES).** The function of the LES is supported by its anatomic placement in the abdomen, where the surrounding pressure is significantly higher than in the low-pressure thorax. Sphincter function is also supported by the acute angle (angle of His) that is formed as the esophagus enters the stomach.

The most common cause of GERD is excessive relaxation of the LES, which allows the reflux of gastric contents into the esophagus and exposure of the esophageal mucosa to acidic gastric contents. Nighttime reflux tends to cause prolonged exposure of the esophagus to acid because the supine position decreases peristalsis and the benefit of gravity. Although controversial, *Helicobacter pylori* may contribute to reflux as well (McCance & Huether, 2006).

A person having reflux may be asymptomatic and not aware that reflux is occurring. However, the esophagus has only limited resistance to the damaging effects of the acidic GI contents. The pH of acid secreted by the stomach ranges from 1.5 to 2.0, whereas the pH of the distal esophagus is normally neutral (6.0 to 7.0).

Refluxed material is returned to the stomach by a combination of gravity, saliva, and peristalsis. An inflamed esophagus cannot eliminate the refluxed material as quickly as a healthy one, and therefore the length of exposure increases with each reflux episode. Hyperemia (increased blood flow) and erosion (ulceration) occur in the esophagus in response to the chronic inflammation. Gastric acid and pepsin injure tissue. Minor capillary bleeding often occurs with the erosion, but hemorrhage is rare.

During the process of healing, the body may substitute **Barrett's epithelium** (columnar epithelium) for the normal squamous cell epithelium of the lower esophagus. Although this new tissue is more resistant to acid and therefore supports esophageal healing, it is considered premalignant. It is associated with an increased risk for cancer in patients with prolonged GERD. The fibrosis and scarring that accompany the healing process can produce **esophageal stricture** (narrowing of the esophageal opening). The stricture leads to progressive difficulty in swallowing. Uncontrolled esophageal reflux also creates a risk for other serious complications, such as hemorrhage and aspiration pneumonia. GERD may be one of the causes of adult-onset asthma, laryngitis, and dental decay. It has also been associated with cardiac disease.

Gastric distention caused by eating very large meals or delayed gastric emptying predisposes the patient to reflux. A number of individual factors, including certain foods and drugs, influence the function of the LES (Table 57-1). Smoking and alcohol also weaken the tone of the LES.

Patients who have a nasogastric tube also have decreased esophageal sphincter function. The tube keeps the cardiac sphincter open and allows acidic contents from the stomach to enter the esophagus. Other factors that increase intra-abdominal and intragastric pressure (e.g., pregnancy, wearing tight belts or girdles, bending over, ascites) overcome the gastroesophageal pressure gradient maintained by the LES and allow reflux to occur. Many patients with obstructive sleep apnea report frequent episodes of GERD (Tawk et al., 2006). People with hiatal hernias often have reflux because the upper portion of the stomach protrudes through the diaphragm into the thorax to allow acid to reach the esophagus (see later discussion of hiatal hernia).

Recent research has also associated body weight with GERD. Overweight and obese patients are at an increased risk for the disease (Jacobson et al., 2006). Increased weight increases intra-abdominal pressure, which contributes to reflux of stomach contents into the esophagus.

Patient-Centered Collaborative Care

Assessment

Ask the patient about a history of heartburn or atypical chest pain associated with the reflux of GI contents. Ask whether he or she has been newly diagnosed with asthma or has experienced morning hoarseness or pneumonia. These symptoms are suggestive of severe reflux reaching the pharynx or mouth or pulmonary aspiration.

Physical Assessment/Clinical Manifestations

The clinical manifestations of reflux vary in severity, depending on the patient (Chart 57-1). **Dyspepsia,** *also known as "heartburn," is the main symptom of GERD.* The pain is described as a substernal burning sensation that tends to move up and down the chest in a wavelike fashion. Because heartburn might not be viewed as a serious concern, patients may delay seeking treatment. If the heartburn is severe, the pain may radiate to the neck or jaw or may be referred to the back. The pain typically worsens when the patient bends over, strains, or lies down. Patients may come to the emergency department (ED) fearing that they are having a myocardial infarction ("heart attack").

With severe GERD, the pain occurs after each meal and lasts for 20 minutes to 2 hours. Patients usually obtain prompt relief by drinking fluids, taking antacids, or maintaining an upright posture.

Regurgitation (backward flow into the throat) of food particles or fluids is common. The patient feels warm fluid traveling up the throat without nausea. If the fluid reaches the level of the pharynx, he or she notes a sour or bitter taste in the mouth. This problem can even occur in an upright position. The danger of aspiration is increased if regurgitation occurs when the patient is lying down.

TABLE 57-1 Factors Contributing to Decreased Lower Esophageal Sphincter Pressure

- Fatty foods
- Caffeinated beverages, such as coffee, tea, and cola
- Chocolate
- Citrus fruits
- Tomatoes and tomato products
- Smoking and use of other tobacco products
- Calcium channel blockers
- Nitrates
- Peppermint, spearmint
- Alcohol
- Anticholinergic drugs
- High levels of estrogen and progesterone
- Nasogastric tube placement

Chart 57-1 KEY FEATURES

Gastroesophageal Reflux Disease

- Dyspepsia (heartburn)
- Regurgitation (may lead to aspiration or bronchitis)
- Coughing, hoarseness, or wheezing at night
- Water brash (hypersalivation)
- Dysphagia
- Odynophagia (painful swallowing)
- Epigastric pain
- Belching
- Flatulence
- Nausea
- Pyrosis (retrosternal burning)
- Globus (feeling of something in back of throat)
- Pharyngitis
- Dental caries (severe cases)

Eructation (belching), **flatulence** (gas), and bloating after eating are other common manifestations. Nausea and vomiting rarely occur, and unplanned weight loss is not common.

Assess for crackles in the lung, which can be an indication of associated aspiration. Assess the patient for coughing, hoarseness, or wheezing at night. Bronchitis may occur in those who have long-term regurgitation.

A reflex salivary hypersecretion known as **water brash** occurs in response to reflux. Water brash is different from regurgitation. The patient reports a sensation of fluid in the throat, but unlike with regurgitation, there is no bitter or sour taste.

Chronic GERD can cause **dysphagia** (difficulty swallowing). Dysphagia usually indicates a narrowing of the esophagus because of stricture or inflammation. Assess the patient for:

- The degree of dysphagia
- Whether dysphagia occurs when ingesting solids, liquids, or both
- Whether dysphagia is intermittent or occurs with each swallowing effort

Odynophagia (painful swallowing) can also occur with chronic GERD, but it is rare in people with uncomplicated reflux disease. Severe and long-lasting chest pain may be present if spasms occurring in the esophagus cause the muscle to contract with excess force. The resulting pain can be agonizing and may last for hours.

Other manifestations include chronic cough that occurs mostly at night or when the patient is lying down, asthma, and atypical chest pain. Cough and symptoms of asthma occur when refluxed acid is spilled over into the tracheobronchial tree. *Atypical chest pain* is thought to be caused by stimulation of pain receptors in the esophageal wall and by esophageal spasm. This type of chest pain can mimic angina and needs to be carefully distinguished from cardiac pain.

Diagnostic Assessment

The most accurate method of diagnosing GERD is *24-hour ambulatory esophageal pH monitoring.* This test involves placing a small catheter through the nose into the distal esophagus. The patient is asked to keep a diary of activities and symptoms, and the pH is continuously monitored and recorded. Ambulatory pH monitoring is especially useful in diagnosing patients with atypical symptoms. A wireless monitoring device may be used to promote patient comfort (Lawrence & Taylor, 2007).

Esophagogastroduodenoscopy (EGD) is useful in diagnosing or evaluating reflux esophagitis or in monitoring complications such as Barrett's esophagus. This test requires the use of moderate sedation during the procedure, and patients must have someone accompany them home after recovery. During the procedure, tissue samples can be obtained for biopsy and strictures can be dilated (see Chapter 55).

Although not as common, *esophageal manometry,* or motility testing, may be performed when the diagnosis is uncertain. Water-filled catheters are inserted in the patient's nose or mouth and slowly withdrawn while measurements of LES pressure and peristalsis are recorded. When used alone, manometry is not sensitive or specific enough to establish a diagnosis of GERD.

Common Nursing Diagnoses and Collaborative Problems

Nursing diagnoses that may apply to patients with GERD include:

- Acute Pain and Chronic Pain related to physical (esophageal irritation) injury
- Risk for Aspiration related to inadequate LES function
- Impaired Swallowing related to stricture or inflammation

Interventions

Nonsurgical Management

The purpose of treatment for GERD is the relief of symptoms, treatment of esophagitis, and prevention of complications such as strictures or Barrett's esophagus. For most patients, GERD can be controlled by nutrition therapy, lifestyle changes, and drug therapy. *The most important role of the nurse is patient and family education. Teach the patient that GERD is a chronic disorder that requires ongoing management.*

Nonpharmacologic Interventions. *Nutrition therapy* is used to relieve symptoms in patients with relatively mild GERD. In collaboration with the nutritionist, ask about the patient's basic meal patterns and food preferences. Coordinate with the nutritionist, patient, and family about how to adapt to changes in eating that may decrease reflux symptoms.

Teach the patient to limit or eliminate foods that decrease LES pressure, such as chocolate, alcohol, fatty foods (especially fried), caffeine, and carbonated beverages. The patient should also restrict spicy and acidic foods (e.g., orange juice, tomatoes) until esophageal healing can occur, because these foods irritate the inflamed tissue and cause heartburn. Peppermint may also aggravate symptoms.

Large meals increase the volume of and pressure in the stomach and delay gastric emptying. Therefore remind the patient to eat four to six small meals each day rather than three large ones. Encourage patients to eat no food for at least 3 hours before going to bed. Reflux episodes are most damaging at night. Patients may have the most difficulty restricting evening snacks. Advise the patient to eat slowly and chew thoroughly to facilitate digestion and prevent eructation (belching).

The control of GERD involves *lifestyle changes* to promote health and control reflux (Chart 57-2). Teach the patient to elevate the head by 6 to 12 inches for sleep to prevent nighttime reflux. This can be done by placing blocks under the head of the bed or by using a large, wedge-style pillow instead of a standard pillow.

Teach the patient to sleep in the right side-lying position to decrease the effects of nighttime episodes of reflux. Nighttime

Chart 57-2 PATIENT AND FAMILY EDUCATION GUIDE

Health Promotion Modifications to Control Reflux

- Eat four to six small meals a day.
- Limit or eliminate fatty foods, coffee, tea, cola, and chocolate.
- Reduce or eliminate from your diet any food or spice that increases gastric acid and causes pain.
- Limit or eliminate alcohol and tobacco.
- Do not snack in the evening, and take no food for 2 to 3 hours before you go to bed.
- Eat slowly and chew your food thoroughly to reduce belching.
- Remain upright for 1 to 2 hours after meals, if possible.
- Elevate the head of your bed 6 to 12 inches using wooden blocks or a foam wedge. Never sleep flat in bed.
- If you are overweight, lose weight.
- Do not wear constrictive clothing.
- Avoid heavy lifting, straining, and working in a bent-over position.
- Chew "chewable" antacids thoroughly, and follow with a glass of water.

Chart 57-3 COMMON EXAMPLES OF DRUG THERAPY
Gastroesophageal Reflux Disease (GERD)

Drug/Usual Dosage	Purpose for Drug	Nursing Interventions	Rationales
ANTACIDS			
Aluminum or magnesium salts (Mylanta, Maalox) 30 mL orally between meals and as needed (PRN) throughout the day and at bedtime (Also see Chart 58-3 in Chapter 58)	Increases pH of gastric contents by deactivating pepsin	Give 1 hr before meals, 2-3 hr after meals, and at bedtime.	These drugs work best if the stomach is empty. If given after meals, hydrogen ion load is high in food.
		Observe the patient for constipation or diarrhea.	Aluminum products produce constipation, and magnesium products induce diarrhea.
		Suggest the use of combination mixtures or alternating use of aluminum and magnesium products.	Balancing their effects is important for patient adherence.
Gaviscon, antacid plus alginic acid, 1 tablet or 10-20 mL orally throughout the day and at bedtime	Buffers acid in stomach	Give after meals and at bedtime.	Alginic acid forms a viscous foam that floats on top of the gastric contents, impeding reflux or buffering its effects when it occurs.
HISTAMINE RECEPTOR ANTAGONISTS			
Cimetidine (Tagamet, Peptol) 300 mg orally four times daily or 900-1200 mg orally at bedtime	Decreases gastric acid production (short-acting)	Observe the patient for side effects; fatigue, headache, and diarrhea are common. Instruct patient about potential toxicity with some medications.	Tagamet causes interactions with common medications and *is not used as often as other drugs in this class.*
Ranitidine (Zantac) 150 mg orally twice daily Famotidine (Pepcid) 40 mg orally daily or 20 mg orally twice daily **Med Error Alert!** Do not confuse Zantac with Zytec!		Administer with meals and at bedtime.	Ranitidine and famotidine are more potent, longer-acting drugs but produce fewer side effects.
Nizatidine (Axid) 150 mg orally twice daily		Use cautiously and in reduced dosages in patients with renal disease.	Patients need an adequate creatinine clearance to prevent drug toxicity.
		Observe for dysrhythmias.	Dysrhythmias are common adverse effects of the drug.
		Do not mix with tomato-based, mixed-vegetable juices; apple juice is the preferred choice.	Nizatidine may be less potent when mixed with tomato-based, mixed-vegetable juices.

reflux is extremely common, and infrequent swallowing in combination with a supine position impairs esophageal clearance. Smoking and alcohol cause decreased LES pressure. Explore the possibility and methods for smoking cessation, and make appropriate referrals. Ask the patient about his or her use of alcoholic beverages. If appropriate, assist the patient in finding alcohol cessation programs.

For the obese patient, collaborate with the nutritionist to examine approaches to weight reduction. Decreasing intra-abdominal pressure often reduces reflux symptoms. Teach the patient to avoid wearing constrictive clothing, lifting heavy objects or straining, and working in a bent-over or stooped position. Emphasize that these general adaptations are an essential and effective part of disease management and can produce prompt results in uncomplicated cases.

Obese patients often have obstructive sleep apnea, as well as GERD. Those who receive continuous positive airway pressure (CPAP) treatment report improved sleeping and decreased episodes of reflux at night (Tawk et al., 2006). See Chapter 31 for a discussion of CPAP.

Drug Therapy. Some drugs lower LES pressure and cause reflux, such as oral contraceptives, anticholinergic agents, sedatives, NSAIDs (e.g., ibuprofen), nitrates, and calcium channel blockers. The possibility of eliminating those drugs causing reflux should be explored with the health care provider.

Drug therapy for GERD management includes three major types—antacids, histamine blockers, and proton pump inhibitors. These drugs have one or more of these functions (Chart 57-3):

- Inhibit gastric acid secretion
- Accelerate gastric emptying
- Protect the gastric mucosa

In uncomplicated cases of GERD, *antacids* may be effective for *occasional* episodes of heartburn. Antacids act by elevat-

Chart 57-3 COMMON EXAMPLES OF DRUG THERAPY

Gastroesophageal Reflux Disease (GERD)—cont'd

Drug/Usual Dosage	Purpose for Drug	Nursing Interventions	Rationales
PROKINETIC DRUGS			
Metoclopramide (Reglan) 10 mg orally three or four times daily	Increases gastric emptying	Instruct the patient to take the drug before meals.	This drug increases the rate of gastric emptying.
		Teach the patient to report any neurologic or psychotropic side effects, such as restlessness, anxiety, ataxia, or hallucinations.	Long-term drug use produces adverse effects in up to one third of patients. *Therefore this drug is not commonly used.*
PROTON PUMP INHIBITORS			
Omeprazole (Prilosec, Losec🍁) 20-30 mg orally daily	Decreases gastric acid production (long-acting)	Instruct the patient to take the drug before meals.	Gastric acid suppression is greater than 90%. Action is prolonged, but GI effects are severe in some patients.
		Observe the patient for typical side effects: abdominal cramping, diarrhea, headache.	
Lansoprazole (Prevacid) 15 mg orally daily for gastroesophageal reflux disease (GERD); up to 60 mg orally for GI ulcers or Zollinger-Ellison syndrome		Instruct the patient to take the drug before meals.	Same as omeprazole.
		For the patient who has difficulty swallowing or has a nasogastric tube, open the capsule and mix granules in apple juice (or applesauce if not tube fed).	The drug is safe to administer by opening (not crushing) the capsule.
Rabeprazole (Aciphex) 60 mg orally daily (may increase to 120 mg in two divided doses)		Do not crush, break, or chew delayed-release tablets.	This form of the drug is released into the body slowly throughout the day.
Med Error Alert! Do not confuse Aciphex with Aricept!		Teach patient to wear sunscreen.	The drug predisposes the patient to burns.
Pantoprazole (Protonix, Protonix IV) 40 mg orally daily or 40 mg IV daily for 7-10 days given in 15-min or 2-min infusions		Do not crush, break, or chew delayed-release tablets.	This form of the drug is released slowly into the body throughout the day.
		Do not give Protonix IV with other IV drugs.	Protonix IV is not compatible with most other IV drugs.
Esomeprazole (Nexium) 20-40 mg orally daily; 20-40 mg IV daily for 7-10 days given between 10 and 30 min (do not run less than 3 minutes)		Do not administer with digoxin, rabeprazole, or iron salts.	This drug may alter the effect and absorption of these agents.
		Do not crush, break, or chew this delayed-release oral drug.	The oral form of the drug is released slowly through the day.
		Do not give IV Nexium with other IV drugs.	IV Nexium is not compatible with most other drugs.

ing the pH level of the gastric contents, thereby deactivating pepsin. They are not helpful in controlling frequent symptoms because their length of action is too short and their nighttime effectiveness is minimal. These drugs also *increase* LES pressure and therefore are not given for long-term use.

Antacids containing aluminum hydroxide or magnesium hydroxide may be used. Maalox and Mylanta consist of a combination of these two agents. Patients often tolerate them better because they produce fewer side effects, such as constipation and diarrhea. Teach the patient to take the antacid 1 hour before and 2 to 3 hours after each meal. Some antacids are prepared as double-strength (DS) suspensions or tablets. The advantage of DS preparations is that a smaller amount of the drug is required. For example, 30 mL of regular Mylanta equals 15 mL of Mylanta-II (DS preparation).

Gaviscon, a combination of aluminum hydroxide and magnesium carbonate, is often a very effective drug for GERD. It forms a thick foam that floats on top of the gastric contents and theoretically decreases the incidence of reflux. If reflux occurs, the foam enters the esophagus first and buffers the acid in the refluxed material. Remind the patient to take this drug when food is in the stomach.

Histamine receptor antagonists, commonly called *histamine blockers,* such as famotidine (Pepcid), ranitidine (Zantac), and nizatidine (Axid), decrease acid. With low-dose forms of these drugs available over the counter (OTC) and widely advertised for heartburn, many patients self-medicate before seeking professional assistance from their health care provider. When patients who have self-medicated with OTC preparations have uncontrolled symptoms, the health care provider usually prescribes a *higher* dose.

Cimetidine (Tagamet) is not used as often as the longer-acting preparations because it interferes with the action of other drugs. Ranitidine and the other preparations are longer acting, and less-frequent dosing is necessary. They also appear to produce fewer side effects and may be safe for long-term use. Although these drugs do not affect the occurrence of reflux directly, they do reduce gastric acid secretion, improve symptoms, and promote healing of inflamed esophageal tissue.

Proton pump inhibitors (PPIs), such as omeprazole (Prilosec), lansoprazole (Prevacid), rabeprazole (Aciphex), pantoprazole (Protonix), and esomeprazole (Nexium), are the *main* treatment for more severe GERD. These agents provide effective, long-acting inhibition of gastric acid secretion by affecting the proton pump of the gastric parietal cell. PPIs reduce gastric acid secretion and can be given in a single daily dose. If once-a-day dosing fails to control symptoms, twice-daily dosing may be used. Several PPIs may be administered in IV form for short-term use. PPIs promote rapid tissue healing, but recurrence is common when the drug is stopped. Long-term use may mask reflux symptoms, and stopping the drug determines if reflux has been resolved. Long-term use may also cause community-acquired pneumonia and GI infections (U.S. Department of Health and Human Services, 2005).

Recent research has also found that long-term use of proton pump inhibitors may increase the risk for hip fracture, especially in older adults. PPIs can interfere with calcium absorption and protein digestion and therefore reduce available calcium to bone tissue (Yang et al., 2006). Decreased calcium makes bones more brittle and likely to fracture, especially as people age.

Although used less commonly, *prokinetic drugs* (e.g., metoclopramide [Reglan]) may be given to increase gastric emptying and improve lower esophageal sphincter (LES) pressure. They do not affect gastric acid secretion or directly heal esophageal tissue. Their use is associated with a high incidence of neurologic and psychotropic side effects such as ataxia, tardive dyskinesia (involuntary muscle movements), and hallucinations. Therefore long-term drug use is not recommended.

NCLEX EXAMINATION CHALLENGE

A client with gastroesophageal reflux disease (GERD) is newly diagnosed by the nurse practitioner. Which of these statements by the client indicates a need for further teaching?

A. "I need to lose some weight and stop smoking cigarettes."
B. "I should avoid tight pants and bending over too much."
C. "I have to give up my fried, spicy, and fatty foods."
D. "I am going to eat three balanced meals every day."

evolve For the correct answer, go to http://evolve.elsevier.com/Iggy/.

Endoscopic Therapies. In the past decade, several noninvasive endoscopic procedures have been approved for severe GERD. Two of the new techniques still used are the Stretta procedure and endoluminal gastroplication using the Bard EndoCinch Suturing System (BESS). These nonsurgical methods are becoming more popular and may replace surgery for GERD when other measures are not effective.

In the Stretta procedure, the physician applies radiofrequency (RF) energy through the endoscope using needles placed near the gastroesophageal junction. The RF energy decreases vagus nerve activity, thus reducing discomfort for the patient.

In the gastroplication procedure, the physician tightens the LES through the endoscope using sutures near the sphincter. Chart 57-4 outlines discharge instructions for endoscopic therapies.

The advantages of endoscopic therapies compared with surgery include:

- Use of light or moderate sedation (rather than general anesthesia)
- Ambulatory care procedure (rather than an inpatient stay)
- Short procedure (45 minutes versus several hours)
- 1 to 2 days absence from work (rather than 2 to 3 weeks)
- No antibiotics and lower complication rate, including fewer deaths

Surgical Management

A very small percentage of patients with GERD require anti-reflux surgery. It is usually indicated for otherwise healthy patients who have failed to respond to medical treatment or have developed complications related to GERD. Various surgical procedures may be used through conventional open techniques or laparoscope.

Laparoscopic Nissen fundoplication (LNF) is a minimally invasive surgery (MIS) and is the gold standard for surgical management. A discussion of this procedure can be found in the next section (Hiatal Hernia) in the Surgical Management discussion. Patients who have surgery are encouraged to continue following the basic anti-reflux regimen of antacids and nutritional therapy because the rate of recurrence is high.

Chart 57-4 PATIENT AND FAMILY EDUCATION GUIDE

Postoperative Instructions for Patients Having Endoscopic Therapies for Gastroesophageal Reflux Disease (e.g., Stretta Procedure)

- Remain on clear liquids for 24 hours after the procedure.
- After the first day, consume a soft diet, such as custard, pureed vegetables, mashed potatoes, and applesauce.
- Avoid nonsteroidal anti-inflammatory drugs and aspirin for 10 days.
- Continue drug therapy as prescribed, usually proton pump inhibitors.
- Use liquid medications whenever possible.
- Do not allow nasogastric tubes for at least 1 month because the esophagus could be perforated.
- Contact the health care provider immediately if these problems occur:
  - Chest or abdominal pain
  - Bleeding
  - Dysphagia
  - Shortness of breath
  - Nausea or vomiting

HIATAL HERNIA

Hiatal hernias, also called *diaphragmatic hernias,* involve the protrusion of the stomach through the esophageal hiatus of the diaphragm into the chest. The esophageal hiatus is the opening in the diaphragm through which the esophagus passes from the thorax to the abdomen. Most patients with hiatal hernias are asymptomatic, but some may have daily symptoms similar to those with GERD (McCance & Huether, 2006).

Pathophysiology

The two major types of hiatal hernias are sliding hernias and paraesophageal (rolling) hernias. *Sliding hernias* are the most common type. The esophagogastric junction and a portion of the fundus of the stomach slide upward through the esophageal hiatus into the chest, usually as a result of weakening of the diaphragm (Fig. 57-1). The hernia generally moves freely and slides into and out of the chest during changes in position or intra-abdominal pressure. Although **volvulus** (twisting) and obstruction do occur rarely, the major concern for a sliding hernia is the development of esophageal reflux and its complications (see Gastroesophageal Reflux Disease section earlier in this chapter). The development of reflux is related to chronic exposure of the lower esophageal sphincter (LES) to the low pressure of the thorax, which significantly reduces the effectiveness of the LES. Symptoms associated with decreased LES pressure are worsened by positions that favor reflux, such as bending or lying supine. Coughing, obesity, and ascites also increase reflux symptoms (McCance & Huether, 2006).

With *rolling hernias,* also known as *paraesophageal hernias,* the gastroesophageal junction remains in its normal intra-abdominal location but the fundus (and possibly portions of the stomach's greater curvature) rolls through the esophageal hiatus and into the chest beside the esophagus (see Fig. 57-1). The herniated portion of the stomach may be small or quite large. In rare cases, the stomach completely inverts into the chest. Reflux is not usually present because the LES remains anchored below the diaphragm. However, the risks for **volvulus** (twisting), obstruction (blockage), and strangulation (stricture) are high. The development of iron deficiency anemia is common because slow bleeding from venous obstruction causes the gastric mucosa to become engorged and ooze. Significant bleeding or hemorrhage is rare.

Rolling hernias are thought to develop from an anatomic defect occurring when the stomach is not properly anchored below the diaphragm rather than from muscle weakness. They can also be caused by previous esophageal surgeries, including sliding hernia repair.

Patient-Centered Collaborative Care

Assessment

Ask the patient if he or she has heartburn, regurgitation (backward flow of food into the throat), pain, dysphagia (difficulty swallowing), and eructation (belching). Assess general physical appearance and nutritional status. Note the location, onset, duration, quality, and factors that relieve pain or make it worse. The primary symptoms of sliding hiatal hernias are associated with reflux. Auscultate the lungs because pulmonary symptoms similar to asthma may be triggered by episodes of aspiration, particularly at night. A detailed history is crucial in attempting to differentiate angina from noncardiac chest pain caused by reflux. Symptoms resulting from hiatal hernia typically worsen after a meal or when the patient is in a supine position (Chart 57-5).

In those with rolling hernias, assess for symptoms related to the stretching or displacement of thoracic contents by the hernia. Patients may report a feeling of fullness after eating or have breathlessness or a feeling of suffocation if the hernia interferes with breathing. Some may experience chest pain associated with reflux that mimics angina.

The *barium swallow study with fluoroscopy* is the most specific diagnostic test for identifying hiatal hernia. Rolling hernias are usually clearly visible, and sliding hernias can often be observed when the patient moves through a series of positions that increase intra-abdominal pressure. To visualize sliding hernias, an esophagogastroduodenoscopy (EGD) may be performed to view both the esophagus and gastric lining (see Chapter 55).

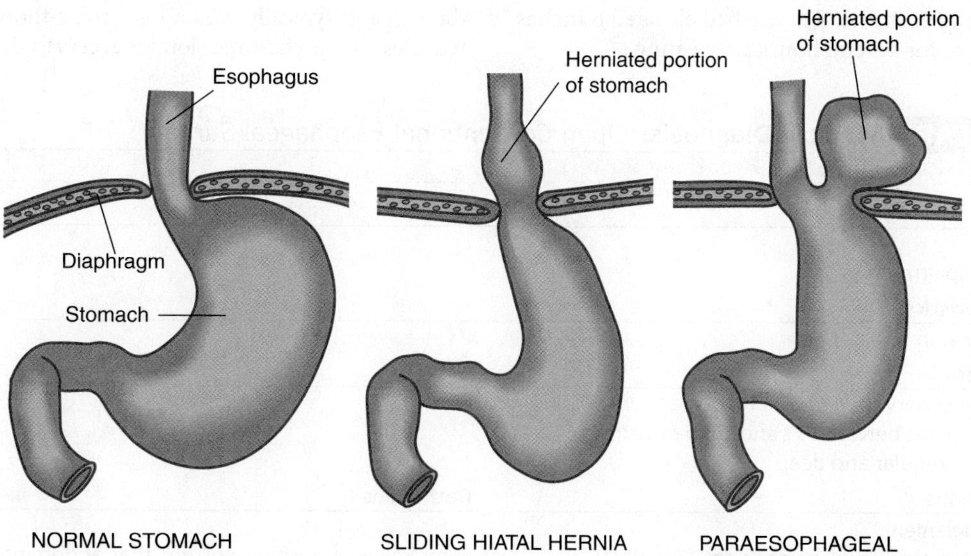
Esophagus
Diaphragm
Stomach
Herniated portion of stomach
Herniated portion of stomach
NORMAL STOMACH
SLIDING HIATAL HERNIA
PARAESOPHAGEAL (ROLLING) HIATAL HERNIA

Fig. 57-1 • A comparison of the normal stomach and sliding and paraesophageal (rolling) hiatal hernias.

Chart 57-5 KEY FEATURES

Hiatal Hernias

SLIDING HIATAL HERNIAS
- Heartburn
- Regurgitation
- Chest pain
- Dysphagia
- Belching

PARAESOPHAGEAL HERNIAS
- Feeling of fullness after eating
- Breathlessness after eating
- Feeling of suffocation
- Chest pain that mimics angina
- Worsening of manifestations in a recumbent position

Interventions

Patients with hiatal hernias may be managed either medically or surgically. Collaborative care is based on the severity of symptoms and the risk for serious complications. Sliding hiatal hernias are most commonly treated medically. Large rolling hernias can become strangulated or obstructed. Therefore early surgical repair is preferred.

Nonsurgical Management

The collaborative interventions for patients with hiatal hernia are similar to those for GERD and include drug therapy, nutrition therapy, and lifestyle changes. The health care provider typically prescribes antacids and histamine receptor antagonists, such as ranitidine (Zantac), in an attempt to control reflux and its symptoms. Nutrition therapy is also important and follows the guidelines discussed earlier for GERD (p. 1245).

The most important role of the nurse in caring for a patient with a hiatal hernia is health teaching. Encourage the patient to avoid eating in the late evening and to avoid foods associated with reflux. In collaboration with the nutritionist, teach the patient and family to follow a restricted diet and exercise to reduce body weight if the patient is overweight. Obesity increases intra-abdominal pressure and worsens both the hernia and the symptoms of reflux. Teach about positioning, including:
- Sleep at night with the head of the bed elevated 6 inches
- Remain upright for several hours after eating
- Avoid straining or excessive vigorous exercise
- Refrain from wearing clothing that is tight or constrictive around the abdomen

Surgical Management

Surgery may be required when the risk for complications is high or when damage from chronic reflux becomes severe.

Preoperative Care. If the surgery is not urgent, the surgeon instructs patients who are overweight to lose weight before surgery. They are also advised to quit or significantly reduce smoking. As part of preoperative teaching, reinforce the surgeon's instructions and prepare the patient for what to expect after surgery.

Laparoscopic Nissen fundoplication (LNF) is the minimally invasive surgery commonly used for hiatal hernia repair. Complications after LNF occur less frequently compared with those seen in patients having the more traditional open surgical approach.

A small percentage of patients are not candidates for LNF and therefore require a conventional open fundoplication. Teach patients having this procedure what to expect after surgery. For example, for the trans-thoracic surgical approach, teach the patient about chest tubes. Inform the patient that a nasogastric tube will be inserted during surgery and will remain in place for several days. Oral intake is started gradually with clear liquids after peristalsis is re-established or to stimulate peristalsis. Instruct the patient how to deep breathe and use the incentive spirometer. These measures are essential to prevent postoperative respiratory complications. The high incision makes deep breathing extremely painful. Teach the patient about postoperative pain, and assure him or her that adequate postoperative analgesic will be given promptly. Pain levels must be continuously monitored.

Operative Procedures. Although several hiatal hernia repair procedures are used, each involves reinforcement of the lower esophageal sphincter (LES) by fundoplication. The surgeon wraps a portion of the stomach fundus around the distal esophagus to anchor it and reinforce the LES (Fig. 57-2). In laparoscopic surgery, the repair is performed through several ½-inch incisions in the abdomen. For the conventional open procedure, the surgeon typically uses a high trans-thoracic approach that requires a large chest incision for access to the surgical area.

PLAN OF CARE Medical Diagnosis: Open Conventional Esophageal Surgery

NURSING DIAGNOSIS NO. 1: Ineffective Breathing Pattern	
Related Factors	
Pain Musculoskeletal impairment	
Defining Characteristics	
Altered chest excursion	
Expected Outcomes	
No verbal report or observation of dyspnea Respiratory rate remains between 11 and 22 breaths/min Respirations remain regular and deep	
Nursing Interventions	**Rationales**
NIC Airway Management	
DPlace the patient in semi-Fowler's position, if possible.	Semi-Fowler's position ensures that abdominal contents do not press against the diaphragm and restrict chest expansion.
Encourage the patient to cough frequently, or suction the patient as necessary.	Coughing or suction will rid the airway of secretions.

DIndicates nursing activities that can be delegated to unlicensed assistive personnel at the discretion of the nurse.

PLAN OF CARE Medical Diagnosis: Open Conventional Esophageal Surgery—cont'd

NURSING DIAGNOSIS NO. 1: **Ineffective Breathing Pattern—cont'd**

D Encourage the patient to take slow, deep breaths; to turn; and to cough.	Effective aeration and coughing will help rid the body of secretions. Frequent position changes will prevent secretions from pooling in one area.
D Assist the patient with an incentive spirometer, as appropriate.	Incentive spirometry encourages the patient to deep breathe.
Regulate fluid intake to optimize fluid balance.	Fluids will help keep lung secretions thin and easier to cough out of the airways.
NIC Respiratory Monitoring	
D Monitor the rate, rhythm, depth, and effort of respirations.	Changes in respiratory rate, rhythm, depth, or effort may signal a descent into respiratory failure.
Note chest movement, watching for symmetry, the use of accessory muscles, and supraclavicular and intercostal muscle retractions.	The use of accessory muscles indicates an increased respiratory effort.
Auscultate breath sounds, noting areas of decreased/absent ventilation and the presence of adventitious sounds.	Absent breath sounds or adventitious breath sounds indicate poor gas exchange or poor movement of air through the airways.
Note changes in Sao_2, Svo_2, end tidal CO_2, and arterial blood gas (ABG) values, as appropriate.	These tests indicate the effectiveness of gas exchange or gas transport.
Monitor the patient's respiratory secretions.	Changes in the color, consistency, or odor of the secretions may indicate infection.
Other Interventions	
Provide pain relief.	Deep breathing and coughing cause diaphragmatic movement and may increase pain.
Continuing Care Considerations	
Teach the patient relaxation techniques.	Stress management and relaxation techniques help control the anxiety resulting from hypoxia.
Encourage the patient to engage in regular physical exercise.	Cardiopulmonary efficiency and endurance improve with exercise.
Encourage the patient to enroll in a smoking cessation program, as indicated.	Smoking damages the airways and alveoli.

NURSING DIAGNOSIS NO. 2: **Imbalanced Nutrition: Less Than Body Requirements**

Related Factors

Inability to ingest or digest food or absorb nutrients due to biologic factors: Surgery

Defining Characteristics

Pain: Abdominal with or without pathology
Perceived inability to ingest food

Expected Outcomes

Has bowel sounds that remain at 3 to 5 per quadrant per minute
Denies abdominal pain
No verbal report or observation of diarrhea
Weight remains within ±5 pounds of desired weight

Nursing Interventions	Rationales
Determine, in collaboration with a nutritionist as appropriate, the number of calories and type of nutrients needed to meet nutrition requirements.	Individual patient needs for nutrients and calories should be the basis for a sound nutritional plan.
Provide foods appropriate for the patient—blenderized or commercial formula via nasogastric, gastrostomy, or jejunostomy tube, or total parental nutrition—as prescribed by physician.	Nutrition therapy and type of surgery dictate the type and form of foods that may be offered to the patient.
D Create a pleasant and relaxing environment at mealtime.	A pleasant and relaxing environment at mealtime improves digestion.
Other Interventions	
Teach the patient and family about high-calorie, high-protein meal planning, as appropriate.	Meal planning that considers the patient's and family's budget and other resources increases the likelihood that appropriate meals will be prepared.
Administer drugs such as simethicone (crushed and dissolved in water) as prescribed.	Simethicone may alleviate or eliminate painful GI gas.
Teach the patient to consciously relax before and after meals.	Patients may have the habit of aerophagia to clear acid reflux. The excess air may be extremely uncomfortable.

Continued

PLAN OF CARE Medical Diagnosis: Open Conventional Esophageal Surgery—cont'd

NURSING DIAGNOSIS NO. 2: **Imbalanced Nutrition: Less Than Body Requirements—cont'd**

Teach the patient and family about nutritional supplements, as appropriate.	Additional vitamins and minerals, calories, dietary fiber, or other nutritional components may need to be added to the diet of patients who are unable to eat a nutritionally adequate diet.
Teach the patient and family about preventing constipation.	Patients on low-fiber diets may need additional fluids and supplemental fiber to maintain bowel regularity.
Continuing Care Considerations	
Encourage the patient and family to use the home nutritional therapy team.	The home nutritional therapy team is able to monitor and adjust the nutritional plan of care to maximize the patient's nutritional status.

NURSING DIAGNOSIS NO. 3: **Acute Pain**

Related Factors

Injury agents (biologic, chemical, physical, psychological): Surgery

Defining Characteristics

Verbal or coded report of pain
Observed evidence of pain

Expected Outcomes

Denies experiencing pain greater than a 5 on a 0-to-10 pain scale
No verbal report or observation of guarding or protective gestures
No verbal report or observation of an alteration in sleep patterns
No verbal report or observation of facial mask of pain
No verbal report or observation of an alteration in activity level

Nursing Interventions	Rationales
NIC Pain Management	
Perform a comprehensive pain assessment that includes location, characteristics, onset/ duration, frequency, quality, intensity or severity of pain, and precipitating factors.	A plan for pain management must be based on the patient's unique responses to pain.
Consider the cultural influences on the pain response.	Cultural stereotypes may lead to an inaccurate assessment of pain.
Select and implement a variety of measures to facilitate pain relief, as appropriate.	Pharmacologic, nonpharmacologic, and interpersonal strategies may provide pain relief depending on the patient's unique responses to the therapeutic interventions.
Use pain control measures before pain becomes severe.	Medicating the patient in a timely manner prevents pain from reaching acutely unpleasant levels.
Teach the use of nonpharmacologic techniques before, after, and if possible, during painful activities; before pain occurs or increases; and along with other pain-relief measures.	Nonpharmacologic techniques help the patient establish a sense of control over his or her pain experience.
NIC Analgesic Administration	
Choose the IV rather than the IM route for frequent pain medication injections, when possible.	The IV route avoids tissue trauma and the unpredictable absorption of medication.
D Institute safety precautions for patients who are receiving opioid analgesics, as appropriate.	Opioid analgesics may impair the patient's judgment and/or coordination.
Document the patient's response to the analgesic and any untoward effects.	Documentation provides the health care team with the information needed to accurately evaluate the patient's response to the analgesic regimen.
Implement actions to decrease the untoward effects of analgesics.	Actions taken to prevent the predictable but unwanted effects of narcotic analgesics (e.g., constipation) increase patient comfort.
Instruct the patient to request PRN pain medication before the pain is severe.	Pain may be managed with lower doses of analgesics and fewer untoward effects if PRN drugs are used before pain becomes severe.
NIC Patient-Controlled Analgesia (PCA) Administration	
Consult with the patient, family members, and physician to adjust lockout interval, basal rate, and demand dosage.	The patient's response to the analgesic will determine the PCA settings.
Teach the patient and family to monitor pain intensity, quality, and duration.	This information will help the patient and family determine when to administer a bolus dose of analgesic, if appropriate, or when to request an increase in basal rate of the analgesic.

D Indicates nursing activities that can be delegated to unlicensed assistive personnel at the discretion of the nurse.

PLAN OF CARE Medical Diagnosis: Open Conventional Esophageal Surgery—cont'd

NURSING DIAGNOSIS NO. 3: Acute Pain—cont'd

Teach the patient and family members to monitor respiratory rate and blood pressure.	This information will help the health care team adjust the analgesic doses to the patient's responses and decrease the untoward effects.
Teach the patient and family how to use the PCA device.	The PCA device will not be used if the patient and/or family do not know how to use or are afraid of the device.
NIC Environmental Management: Comfort	
DFacilitate hygiene measures to keep the patient comfortable.	Hygiene measures may improve the patient's overall sense of well-being.
DPosition the patient to facilitate comfort.	The nurse or UAP may decrease sources of discomfort by using principles of body alignment, supporting with pillows, supporting joints during movement, splinting over incisions, and immobilizing painful body parts.
Other Interventions	
Refer the patient to the Pain Advisory Committee.	The Pain Advisory Committee is a multidisciplinary committee with wide expertise in pain-relief interventions.
Consider the use of complementary and alternative therapies such as yoga, meditation, spirituality, and/or religion.	The experience of meditation and prayer and the reflection on meaning may help the patient relax, thereby easing the muscle tension that contributes to pain sensation.
Consider the use of complementary and alternative therapies such as imagery, aromatherapy, music, touch, and laughter/humor.	Cognitive and behavioral strategies may be used as adjuncts to or in place of pharmacologic or surgical interventions for chronic pain. Each therapy has a different mode of action that may or may not benefit the patient.
Consider using other cutaneous skin stimulation techniques such as massage and/or vibration to complement pain management strategies.	Massage may cause muscle relaxation, which decreases pain signals; vibration interrupts pain signal transmission to decrease pain perception.
Continuing Care Considerations	
Refer the patient to an advanced practice nurse pain specialist, social worker, home care nurse, and/or psychologist, as appropriate.	Health care team members are able to provide continuing support to the patient who is facing chronic pain.

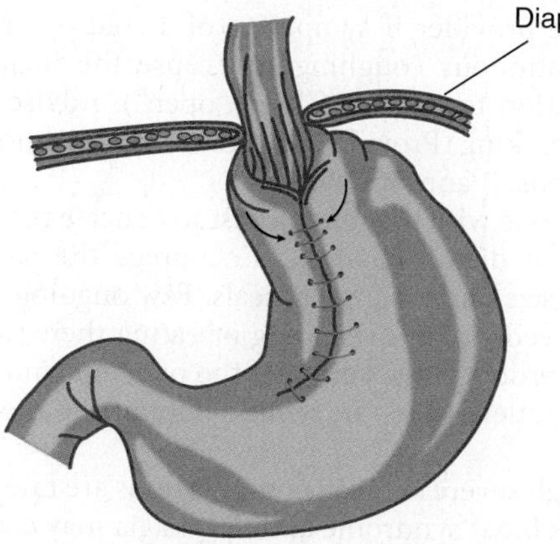
Diaphragm

Fig. 57-2 • Open surgical approach for Nissen fundoplication for gastroesophageal reflux disease or hiatal hernia repair.

Postoperative Care. Patients having the *LNF procedure* are at risk for bleeding and infection, although these problems are not common. *The nursing care priority is to observe for these complications and provide health teaching as described in Chart 57-6.*

Postoperative care after *conventional open repair* closely follows that required after any esophageal surgery (see the Plan of Care on pp. 1250 to 1253). Complications after open surgery are more common and potentially serious. Carefully assess for complications of open fundoplication surgery, described next, and report any complications to the health care provider (Chart 57-7).

Chart 57-6 PATIENT AND FAMILY EDUCATION GUIDE

Postoperative Instructions for Patients Having Laparoscopic Nissen Fundoplication (LNF)

- Stay on a soft diet for about a week, including mashed potatoes, puddings, custard, and milkshakes; avoid carbonated beverages, tough foods, and raw vegetables that are difficult to swallow.
- Remain on antireflux medications as prescribed for at least a month.
- Do not drive for a week after surgery; do not drive if taking opioid pain medication.
- Walk every day, but do not do any heavy lifting.
- Remove gauze dressings 2 days after surgery, and shower; do not remove Steri-Strips until 10 days after surgery.
- Wash incisions with soap and water, rinse well, and pat dry; report any redness or drainage from the incisions to your surgeon.
- Report fever above 101° F (38.3° C), nausea, vomiting, or uncontrollable bloating or pain. For patients over 65 years, report elevations above 100° F (37° C).
- Schedule an appointment for follow-up with your surgeon in 3 to 4 weeks.

The primary focus of care after conventional surgery is the prevention of respiratory complications. Elevate the head of the patient's bed at least 30 degrees to lower the diaphragm and promote lung expansion. Assist the patient out of bed, and begin ambulation as soon as possible. Be sure to support the

Chart 57-7 **BEST PRACTICE FOR PATIENT SAFETY & QUALITY CARE**

Assessment of Postoperative Complications Related to Fundoplication Procedures

Complication	Assessment Findings
Temporary dysphagia	The patient has difficulty swallowing when oral feeding begins.
Gas bloat syndrome	The patient has difficulty belching to relieve distention.
Atelectasis, pneumonia	The patient experiences dyspnea, chest pain, or fever.
Obstructed nasogastric tube	The patient experiences nausea, vomiting, or abdominal distention. The nasogastric tube does not drain.

incision during coughing to reduce pain and to prevent excessive strain on the suture line, especially with obese patients.

Incentive spirometry and deep breathing are routinely used after surgery to maintain patency of the airways and lung expansion. Adequate pain control with analgesics is essential for postoperative deep breathing and coughing. Patients with a smoking history or chronic airway limitation (e.g., chronic obstructive pulmonary disease, asthma) require more aggressive management by the respiratory therapist to prevent atelectasis and pneumonia. Patients with large hiatal hernias are at the highest risk for developing respiratory complications.

The patient having the conventional surgery usually has a large-bore (diameter) nasogastric (NG) tube to prevent the fundoplication wrap from becoming too tight around the esophagus. Initially the NG drainage should be dark brown with old blood but should become normal yellowish green within the first 8 hours after surgery. Check the NG tube every 4 to 8 hours for proper placement in the stomach. The tube should be properly anchored so it is not displaced, because re-insertion could perforate the fundoplication. Follow the surgeon's requests for care of the patient with an NG tube.

Frequent assessment of the patency of the tube is essential to keep the stomach decompressed. This prevents retching or vomiting, which can strain or rupture the stomach sutures. The NG tube is irritating. Therefore provide frequent oral hygiene to increase comfort. Assess the patient's hydration status regularly, including accurate measures of intake and output. Adequate fluid replacement helps thin respiratory secretions.

After open fundoplication, the patient may begin clear fluids when peristalsis is re-established or in an effort to stimulate peristalsis. Some surgeons create a temporary gastrostomy for feeding to allow for undisturbed healing of the repair. The patient gradually progresses to a near-normal diet during the first 4 to 6 weeks. Some foods, especially caffeinated or carbonated beverages and alcohol, are either restricted or eliminated. The food storage area of the stomach is reduced by the surgery, and meals need to be both smaller and more frequent.

Carefully supervise the first oral feedings because temporary dysphagia is common. Continuous dysphagia usually indicates that the fundoplication is too tight, and dilation may be required.

Another common complication of this surgery is the **gas bloat syndrome,** in which patients are unable to voluntarily eructate (belch). The syndrome is usually temporary but may persist, even in those who have the laparoscopic approach. Teach the patient to avoid drinking carbonated beverages and to avoid eating gas-producing foods (especially high-fat foods), chewing gum, and drinking with a straw.

Other patients have **aerophagia** (air swallowing) from attempting to reverse or clear acid reflux. Teach them to relax consciously before and after meals, to eat and drink slowly, and to chew all food thoroughly. Air in the stomach that cannot be removed by belching can be extremely uncomfortable. Frequent position changes and ambulation are often effective interventions for eliminating air from the GI tract. If gas pain is still present, patients are taught to take simethicone, 80 mg four times daily as needed. Be sure to remind the patient to crush and dissolve the medication in water before taking.

Community-Based Care

Patients undergoing one of the open surgical repairs require activity restrictions during the 3- to 6-week postoperative recovery period. For laparoscopic surgery, activity is typically restricted for a shorter time and the patient can return to his or her usual lifestyle more quickly, usually in a few days to a week.

For long-term management, teach the patient and family about appropriate nutritional modifications. The use of stool softeners or bulk laxatives is recommended for the first postoperative weeks until healing is complete. Instruct the patient to avoid straining and to prevent constipation. Teach him or her to inspect the healing incision daily and to notify the health care provider if swelling, redness, tenderness, discharge, or fever occurs. Advise the patient to avoid contact with people with respiratory infections and to contact the health care provider if symptoms of a cold or influenza develop. Continuous coughing can cause the incision or the fundoplication to dehisce ("break open"). Advise the patient to avoid smoking. Provide information about smoking cessation methods, if appropriate.

Collaborate with the nutritionist to educate the patient and family about dietary changes. Encourage the patient to decrease the size and timing of meals. Few ongoing diet restrictions are needed, but overeating or eating the wrong types of foods can produce discomfort if the patient cannot belch. Instruct the patient to report reflux symptoms to the health care provider.

Although severe surgical complications are rare, conditions such as gas bloat syndrome and dysphagia may continue. Prepare the patient for these problems and for the potential that reflux may not be completely controlled or may occur again. Although surgery controls the condition, a cure is rare and lifestyle modifications need to be ongoing.

ACHALASIA

Pathophysiology

Achalasia is a rare esophageal motility disorder that results from loss of nerve impulses to the smooth muscle of the esophagus (McCance & Huether, 2006). Its exact cause is unknown. Patients with achalasia have chronic and progressive dysphagia. Over time, peristaltic failure plus muscle spasm can produce a massively dilated esophagus, which slows food passage. Lower esophageal sphincter (LES) pressure increases.

Epigastric pain, a sensation of food sticking in the lower esophagus, and regurgitation of ingested food may occur. If left untreated, progressive disease can result in weight loss. Complications of achalasia include esophageal candidiasis (yeast infection), lower esophageal diverticula, airway obstruction, and aspiration pneumonia.

Patient-Centered Collaborative Care

A barium swallow is the most sensitive test for viewing the esophagus and is likely to show dilation with a persistent beaklike narrowing at the terminal esophagus. A chest x-ray can show a distorted and dilated tubular esophagus, the absence of a gastric air bubble, and occasionally a tubular mediastinal mass next to the aorta. Esophageal manometry typically reveals an increased LES pressure and incomplete sphincter relaxation when the patient swallows. Endoscopy is used to evaluate the appearance of the esophageal mucosa, especially for changes associated with cancer or the presence of candida.

The symptoms associated with achalasia can be treated with a variety of approaches. A combination of nutritional measures, drug therapy, esophageal dilation, and surgery is used.

Drug therapy is given for symptom relief but is not recommended as an alternative to more definitive therapy. Mild cases of achalasia can be managed with calcium channel blockers, such as nifedipine (Procardia), or nitrates (sublingual nitroglycerin) to reduce LES pressure. Achalasia can also be treated with the direct injection of botulinum toxin (Botox) into the LES muscle via endoscopy. Botulinum toxin acts to suppress acetylcholine release. Most patients have improvement after this procedure. However, repeated regular dosing is required, and the long-term effects are unknown.

Teach the patient to experiment with changes in diet because they can often ease the pressure and reflux associated with achalasia. Discuss any food habits he or she has noted that aggravate or relieve the symptoms. Semisoft foods are often better tolerated, as are warm foods and liquids. Eating four to six smaller meals rather than three large meals during the day facilitates the passage of food. Collaborate with the nutritionist for additional suggestions about diet changes and nutritional balance. Nocturnal (nighttime) reflux of foods and liquids from the dilated esophagus can be prevented if the patient sleeps with the head of the bed elevated or in a semisitting position. Advise him or her to experiment with various changes in position while eating because such changes can reduce pressure sensations during meals. Some patients benefit from arching the back while swallowing. Caution the patient to avoid wearing restrictive clothing, which can increase esophageal pressure and regurgitation.

More severe cases of achalasia require dilation of the LES. The traditional treatment involves the passage of progressively larger sizes of esophageal bougies (dilators) using polyurethane balloons on a catheter. The procedure is performed on an ambulatory care basis. Large-diameter metal stents may be used to keep the esophagus open for longer durations.

After the procedure, monitor the patient for complications of bleeding and signs of perforation, such as chest and shoulder pain, elevated temperature, **subcutaneous emphysema** (air under the skin), or **hemoptysis** (coughing up blood). Teach the patient to expectorate ("spit out") rather than swallow any secretions that are produced. Remind the patient to be NPO for 1 hour and to limit oral intake to liquids for 24 hours. The procedure may be repeated in 2 to 3 months if needed. Most patients report improvement in swallowing.

Surgical procedures for achalasia are done to help food move through the esophagus into the stomach. **Esophagomyotomy,** in which the LES is incised, has been used successfully for decades. Open thoracic and abdominal approaches can be used, but laparoscopic or endoscopic surgery has become more common. An antireflux wrap **(fundoplication)** may or may not be part of the procedure.

Conventional esophagomyotomy is a more complex surgical treatment for achalasia. Using an open approach, general anesthesia is required and the patient is hospitalized for several days. A thoracotomy approach permits exposure of the esophagus. The surgeon cuts muscle fibers around the LES to open the sphincter and thereby lessen obstruction to food.

Immediate postoperative care for patients undergoing transthoracic esophagomyotomy includes managing chest tubes and drains, managing the airway, controlling pain, and managing NG feedings. (See Chapter 18 for general postoperative care and Chapter 32 for care of the patient with a thoracotomy.)

Laparoscopic and endoscopic surgery permits a shorter length of stay and fewer complications compared with either open surgical approach. Patients may receive moderate sedation rather than general anesthesia. Teach patients having laparoscopic surgery to report complications, such as bleeding and fever (see Chart 57-6).

ESOPHAGEAL TUMORS

Pathophysiology

Although esophageal tumors can be benign, they are usually malignant (cancerous). Most esophageal cancers arise from the epithelium. Squamous cell carcinomas of the esophagus are located in the upper two thirds of the esophagus. Adenocarcinomas are more commonly found in the distal third and at the gastroesophageal junction and are now the most common type of esophageal cancer (McCance & Huether, 2006). Esophageal tumors grow rapidly because there is no serosal layer to limit their extension. Because the esophageal mucosa is richly supplied with lymph tissue, there is early spread of tumors to lymph nodes. Esophageal tumors can protrude into the esophageal lumen and can cause thickening or invade deeply into surrounding tissue. In rare cases the lesion may be confined to the epithelial layer (in situ). In most cases, the tumor is large and well established on diagnosis. More than half of esophageal cancers **metastasize** (spread throughout the body).

The two primary risk factors associated with the development of squamous cell carcinoma of the esophagus are tobacco use and heavy alcohol intake. The compounds in tobacco smoke may be responsible for the genetic mutations seen in many esophageal tumors. A smoker has two to six times the risk for eventually developing esophageal cancer than does a nonsmoker (American Cancer Society [ACS], 2008). Some alcoholic beverages contain potent carcinogens that may be responsible for the development of esophageal tumors. Smoking and excessive alcohol can act together in causing esophageal cancer. Obesity and malnutrition are also risk factors.

Long-term, untreated *gastroesophageal reflux disease (GERD)* can lead to esophageal adenocarcinoma. For people with Barrett's esophagus, the risk for developing esophageal cancer also greatly increases. Exposure to acid and pepsin leads to the replacement of normal distal squamous mucosa with columnar epithelium as a response to tissue injury, known as **Barrett's esophagus.** This tissue undergoes dysplasia (cell appearance changes) and, ultimately, becomes cancerous. In parts of the world where esophageal cancer is more common, the incidence of squamous cell carcinoma appears to be linked to high levels of nitrosamines (which are found in pickled and fermented foods) and foods high in nitrate. Diets that are chronically deficient in fresh fruits and vegetables have also been implicated in the development of squamous cell carcinoma.

GENETIC CONSIDERATIONS

Certain *genetic factors* may have a role in the development of esophageal cancers. It is thought that these cancers result from mutations in tumor suppressor genes. Tumor suppressor genes are normal genes that control cell growth and division. When this type of gene is mutated and does not work properly, cells are unable to stop growing and dividing and tumors can result. (See Chapter 23 for a more complete discussion.)

Overexpression and mutations of the *Tp53*, *Tp16*, and *Tp17* tumor suppressor genes have been found in people with esophageal cancer (Nussbaum et al., 2007). In addition, the presence of the mutated *Tp53* gene may be an indication of advanced disease, especially in patients with adenocarcinomas.

Overexpression of cyclin D1, a protein that promotes cell growth and division, has also been found in patients with esophageal squamous cell cancers. Cyclins are products of oncogenes, which are normal genes involved in cell division and are controlled by suppressor genes. Prolonged exposure to carcinogens can cause oncogenes to escape the control of suppressor genes, leading to overexpression of cyclins and uncontrolled cell growth (cancer). For example, many patients with esophageal cancer have abused alcohol and tobacco for a long time. These known carcinogens (cancer-causing agents) enhance each other's ability to damage suppressor genes and overexpress the oncogenes that cause esophageal disease. See Chapter 23 for a more detailed discussion of cancer development.

Patient-Centered Collaborative Care

evolve ONLINE PHARM REVIEW

Assessment

History

Assess for risk factors related to the development or symptoms of esophageal cancer, such as racial and cultural background, age, gender, history of alcohol consumption, tobacco use, dietary habits, and other esophageal problems (e.g., dysphagia, reflux). Esophageal cancer (squamous cell) occurs most often in middle-aged and older adults and tends to occur more in black males, although the exact cause for racial differences has not been found (www.cancer.gov). White males are more predisposed to esophageal adenocarcinoma. Ask the patient about consumption of smoked pickled foods, changes in appetite, changes in taste, or weight loss. *Cancer of the esophagus is a silent tumor in its early stages, with few observable signs. By the time the tumor causes symptoms, it usually has spread extensively.*

Physical Assessment/Clinical Manifestations

***Dysphagia** (difficulty swallowing) is the most common symptom of esophageal cancer, but it may not be present until the esophageal opening has gotten much smaller.* Dysphagia is both persistent and progressive when **stricture** (narrowing) occurs. It is initially associated with swallowing solids, particularly meat, and then progresses rapidly over a period of weeks or months to difficulty in swallowing soft foods and liquids. Late in the disease, even saliva can induce choking. Patients usually report a sensation that food is sticking in the throat or in the substernal area. Careful assessment of the dysphagia is an important part of the diagnosis because dysphagia associated with other esophageal disorders is not usually continuous. Weight loss often accompanies dysphagia and can be more than 20 pounds over several months.

Odynophagia (painful swallowing) is reported by many patients as a steady, dull, substernal pain that may radiate. It occurs most often when the patient drinks cold liquids. The presence of severe or persistent pain often indicates tumor invasion of the mediastinal structures. Assess for regurgitation, vomiting, **halitosis** (foul breath), and chronic hiccups, which often accompany advanced disease. In most patients, pulmonary problems develop. Assess for chronic cough, increased secretions, and a history of recent infections. Tumors in the upper esophagus may involve the larynx and thus cause hoarseness. Chart 57-8 summarizes the common clinical manifestations of esophageal tumors.

Psychosocial Assessment

The diagnosis of esophageal cancer causes high patient anxiety. The disease is accompanied by distressing symptoms and is often terminal. The fear of choking can place unusual stress, especially at mealtimes. The loss of pleasure and social aspects of eating may affect relationships with family and friends. Assess the patient's response to the diagnosis and prognosis. Ask about his or her usual coping strengths and resources. Assess the impact of the disease on the patient's usual daily activity routine. Determine the availability of support systems and the potential financial impact of the disease and its treatment. Refer the patient and family members to psychological counseling, pastoral care, and the social worker or case manager as needed. Chapter 9 describes end-of-life care for patients in the terminal stage of the disease.

Diagnostic Assessment

A barium swallow study with fluoroscopy is usually the first diagnostic test requested to evaluate dysphagia. In a barium swallow, the margins of a tumor may be seen. The definitive diagnosis of esophageal cancer is made by *esophageal ultra-*

Chart 57-8 KEY FEATURES

Esophageal Tumors

- Persistent and progressive dysphagia (most common feature)
- Feeling of food sticking in the throat
- Odynophagia (painful swallowing)
- Severe, persistent chest or abdominal pain or discomfort
- Regurgitation
- Chronic cough with increasing secretions
- Hoarseness
- Anorexia
- Nausea and vomiting
- Weight loss (often more than 20 pounds)
- Changes in bowel habits (diarrhea, constipation, bleeding)

sound (EUS) with fine needle aspiration to examine the tumor tissue. An esophagogastroduodenoscopy (EGD) may also be performed to inspect the esophagus and obtain tissue specimens for cell studies and disease staging. A complete cancer staging workup is performed to determine the extent of the disease and plan appropriate therapy.

Positron emission tomography (PET) may identify metastatic disease with more accuracy than a computed tomography (CT) scan. PET can also help evaluate response to chemotherapy to treat the cancer.

Analysis

Common Nursing Diagnoses and Collaborative Problems

A priority nursing diagnosis for patients with esophageal cancer is:

- Imbalanced Nutrition: Less Than Body Requirements related to impaired swallowing

Additional Nursing Diagnoses and Collaborative Problems

In addition to the common nursing diagnosis, the patient with esophageal cancer may develop any of these resulting from the disease and its treatment:

- Risk for Aspiration related to impaired swallowing secondary to esophageal strictures
- Impaired Swallowing related to obstruction by the tumor or the effects of radiotherapy
- Acute Pain or Chronic Pain related to the physical injury (pressure of the tumor mass in the esophagus or mediastinum)
- Ineffective Coping and Compromised Family Coping related to the effects of the disease and to the terminal prognosis
- Anticipatory Grieving related to declining physical status and terminal prognosis
- Spiritual Distress related to impending death

The additional collaborative problem is Potential for Metastasis resulting from the proximity of the esophagus to lymph tissue and other body structures.

Planning and Implementation

Imbalanced Nutrition: Less Than Body Requirements

Planning: Expected Outcomes. The major concern for a patient with esophageal cancer is weight loss secondary to dysphagia. Therefore he or she is expected to maintain adequate nutrient intake and weight.

Interventions. Interventions to maintain or improve nutritional status focus on treatments that remove or shrink the obstructive tumor. Methods to reduce the effects of treatment that can impact nutrition are also a priority. Surgery is the most definitive intervention for esophageal surgery.

Nonsurgical treatment options for cancer of the esophagus that can assist in both disease and nutrition management include:

- Nutrition therapy
- Swallowing therapy
- Chemotherapy
- Radiation therapy
- Chemoradiation
- Targeted therapies
- Photodynamic therapy
- Esophageal dilation
- Endoscopic therapies

Nonsurgical Management. The treatment of esophageal cancer often involves a combination of the therapies just mentioned. Patients with cancer of the esophagus experience many physical problems, and symptom management becomes essential.

The purpose of nutrition therapy is to administer food and fluids to support the patient who is malnourished or at high risk for becoming malnourished. In collaboration with the nutritionist, conduct a thorough dietary assessment to provide information about the patient's nutritional status. The nutritionist determines the caloric needs of the patient to meet daily requirements. Weigh the patient daily, or teach the patient and family to perform this task. Careful positioning is essential for a patient who is experiencing frequent reflux or who has tubes to keep the esophagus patent. Teach the patient to remain upright for several hours after meals and to avoid lying completely flat. Remind UAP and other health care team members to keep the head of the bed elevated to a 30-degree angle or more to prevent reflux.

Semisoft foods and thickened liquids are preferred because they are easier to swallow. Record the amount of food and fluid intake every day to monitor progress in meeting nutritional outcomes. Liquid nutritional supplements (e.g., Boost, Ensure) are used between feedings to increase caloric intake. Ongoing efforts are made to preserve the ability to swallow, but enteral feedings (tube feedings) may be needed temporarily when dysphagia is severe. In patients with complete esophageal obstruction or life-threatening fistulas, the surgeon may create a gastrostomy or jejunostomy for feeding. Encourage the patient and family to meet with the nutritionist for diet teaching and planning. Chapter 63 describes care for patients receiving enteral feeding.

Collaborate with the speech-language pathologist (SLP) to assist the patient with oral exercises to improve swallowing *(swallowing therapy)*. Ask the patient to suck on a lollipop to enhance tongue strength. Teach the patient to reach for food particles on the lips or chin using the tongue. In preparation for swallowing, remind the patient to position the head in forward flexion (chin tuck). Then tell him or her to place food at the back of the mouth. Monitor him or her for sealing of the lips and for tongue movements while eating. Check for pocketing of food in the cheeks after swallowing. *When the patient is eating or drinking, monitor for signs and symptoms of aspiration, such as choking or coughing! Food aspiration can cause airway obstruction, pneumonia, or both, especially in older adults.* In coordination with the SLP, teach family members and caregivers how to feed the patient, if needed. *Teach them how to monitor for aspiration and implement appropriate measures if choking occurs.* Chart 57-9 provides a summary of NIC interventions for swallowing therapy.

The use of *chemotherapy* in the treatment of esophageal cancer has been only moderately effective. It can be given as a primary treatment if the patient is not a candidate for surgery or for palliation (control of symptoms). In most cases, though, chemotherapy is given in combination with radiation therapy to provide the patient the best chance of cure. The rationale for this approach is to shrink the tumor and eliminate any other tumor that may be in the local lymph nodes, improving the odds for a complete surgical resection. The two most commonly used chemotherapeutic agents have traditionally been 5-fluorouracil (5-FU) and a platinum-based agent, such as cisplatin (Platinol), carboplatin (Paraplatin), and oxaliplatin

Chart 57-9 NIC INTERVENTION ACTIVITIES

The Patient with Esophageal Problems

Nutrition Therapy: *Administration of food and fluids to support metabolic processes of a patient who is malnourished or at high risk for becoming malnourished*

- Determine—in collaboration with the dietitian, as appropriate—the number of calories and type of nutrients needed to meet nutrition requirements.
- Assist patient to a sitting position before eating or feeding.
- Encourage patient to select semisoft food, if lack of saliva hinders swallowing.
- Monitor food/fluid ingested and calculate daily caloric intake, as appropriate.
- Determine need for enteral tube feedings.

Swallowing Therapy: *Facilitating swallowing and preventing complications of impaired swallowing*

- Collaborate with speech/language pathologist to instruct patient/family about swallowing exercise regimen.
- Explain rationale of the swallowing regimen to patient/family.
- Provide a lollipop for patient to suck on to enhance tongue strength, if appropriate.
- Assist patient to position head in forward flexion in preparation for swallowing ("chin tuck").
- Assist patient to place food at back of mouth and on unaffected side.
- Monitor for signs and symptoms of aspiration.
- Instruct family/caregiver how to position, feed, and monitor patient.
- Instruct patient/caregiver on emergency measures for choking.

NIC intervention activities selected from Bulechek, G.M., Butcher, H.K., & McCloskey Dochterman, J. (Eds.). (2008). *Nursing interventions classification (NIC)* (5th ed.). St. Louis: Mosby. No part of this work is to be altered without prior written permission from the Publisher.

(Eloxatin). These drugs make the tumor cells more sensitive to the effects of radiation. Other drugs have been tried successfully for treatment of esophageal cancer, including paclitaxel (Taxol), docetaxel (Taxotere), and irinotecan (Camptosar). Because chemotherapeutic drugs affect healthy cells as well as cancer cells, they have many side effects that cause discomfort to the patient. Chapter 24 describes chemotherapy in detail and discusses the role of the nurse in caring for patients receiving these drugs.

Radiation therapy to manage esophageal cancer is only moderately effective and can be used alone or in combination with other treatments. Radiation alone can provide palliation of symptoms by shrinking the tumor. It is contraindicated for patients with tracheoesophageal fistula, mediastinitis, mediastinal hemorrhage, or infiltration of the cancer to the trachea or bronchus. Normal esophageal tissue is very sensitive to the effects of radiation. Although high doses of radiation demonstrate the best results for tumor shrinkage, esophageal stricture or stenosis can result in many patients, which then requires esophageal dilation. Chapter 24 describes radiation methods and the general nursing care for the patient having radiation therapy.

Chemoradiation is a treatment for esophageal cancer that involves the use of chemotherapy at the same time as radiation therapy. One cycle of chemotherapy is given during the first week of radiation and another is delivered during the fifth week of radiation. Additional drug cycles are given after radiation therapy is complete.

The newest addition to the treatment of esophageal cancer is targeted therapies, used in combination with radiation and chemotherapy. Unlike chemotherapy, these therapies interfere with cancer cell growth in a variety of ways with less impact on healthy cells. Many of these drugs focus on proteins that are involved in signaling cells when to grow and divide. A key to success with targeted therapy is that the cancer cells must overexpress the targeted protein. Thus each patient's cancer cells are first examined for the overexpression to determine if targeted therapy is appropriate and which drug to use. A number of agents have been approved for other GI cancers but are still used experimentally for esophageal cancer. For example, cetuximab (Erbitux) is a monoclonal antibody that targets the epithelial growth factor receptor (EGFR) on the surface of cancer cells. EGRF is often overexpressed in esophageal tumors. Other targeted therapies, such as trastuzumab (Herceptin), gefitinib (Iressa), and erlotinib (Tarceva), have also been used. Chapter 24 describes targeted therapies in detail, including nursing implications for patient safety and quality care.

Photodynamic therapy (PDT) was originally used for the treatment of skin cancer but is now used also as a palliative treatment for patients with advanced esophageal cancer who are not candidates for surgery. It may be used also as a cure for patients who have very small, localized tumors. The patient is injected with porfimer sodium (Photofrin), a light-sensitive drug that collects in cancer cells. Two days after the injection, a fiberoptic probe with a light at the tip is threaded into the esophagus through an endoscope. The light activates the Photofrin, destroying only cancer cells. PDT is far less invasive than surgery and is performed on an ambulatory care basis under moderate sedation.

The side effects of Photofrin are rare but include nausea, fever, and constipation. Before the procedure, the patient is given written guidelines concerning photosensitivity measures. Remind the patient to avoid exposure to sunlight for 1 to 3 months. Sunglasses and protective clothing that covers all exposed body areas are essential. The patient may experience chest pain secondary to tissue damage and will require pain relief with opioid analgesics for a short time. Teach the patient to follow a clear liquid diet for 3 to 5 days after the procedure and advance to full liquids as tolerated. Warn the patient that tissue particles may release from the tumor site and be present in the sputum. Chapter 24 describes in detail the health teaching needed to promote patient safety associated with PDT.

Esophageal dilation may be performed as necessary throughout the course of the disease to achieve temporary but immediate relief of dysphagia. It is usually performed on an ambulatory care basis. Dilators are used to tear soft tissue, thereby widening the esophageal lumen (opening). In most cases, malignant tumors can be dilated safely, but perforation remains a significant risk. Large metal stents may be used to keep the esophagus open for longer durations. A stent covered with graft material can be used to seal a perforation. Bacteremia can also occur. To reduce the risk for endocarditis, antibiotics are given. The treatment is repeated as often as needed to preserve the patient's ability to swallow.

When patients are not candidates for surgery or the tumor is too large to remove surgically, laser therapy or electrocoagulation using endoscopy may be performed as a palliative measure. Both of these methods destroy some cancer cells and reduce tumor size to improve swallowing. The procedures are done in ambulatory care settings or same-day surgery centers using moderate sedation.

Surgical Management. The purposes of surgical resection vary from palliation to cure. **Esophagectomy** is the removal of all or part of the esophagus. An **esophagogastrostomy** involves the removal of part of the esophagus and proximal stomach. The remaining stomach may be "pulled up" to take the place of the esophagus, or a section of the jejunum or colon may be placed as a conduit. Conventional open surgical techniques are lengthy and are associated with many complications or death. Fistula formation between the trachea and esophagus, abscess, and respiratory complications are common.

For patients with early-stage cancer, a laparoscopic-assisted **minimally invasive esophagectomy (MIE)** may be performed. However, most patients require the conventional open surgery because of tumor size and metastasis by the time they are diagnosed with the disease.

Preoperative care. Preoperative preparation for patients undergoing esophagectomy or esophagogastrostomy can be quite extensive, especially before conventional techniques. Advise the patient to stop smoking 2 to 4 weeks before surgery to enhance pulmonary function. Patient preparation may include 5 days to 2 to 3 weeks of nutritional support to decrease the risk for postoperative complications. Ideally this supplementation is given orally, but many patients require tube feeding or parenteral nutrition. Teach the patient and family to monitor the patient's weight and intake and output. A preoperative dental evaluation may be required to treat dental disease. Teach the patient to use meticulous oral care four times daily to decrease the risk for postoperative infection.

Preoperative nursing care focuses on teaching and on psychological support regarding the surgical procedure and preoperative and postoperative instructions. Teach the patient about:

- The number and sites of all incisions and drains
- The placement of a jejunostomy tube for initial enteral feedings
- The need for chest tubes if the pleural space is entered
- The purpose of the nasogastric tube
- The need for IV infusion

Instruct the patient about routines for turning, coughing, deep breathing, and chest physiotherapy. Emphasize the crucial nature of postoperative respiratory care. If colon interposition (resecting a piece of colon and creating an esophagus) is planned, the patient also has a complete bowel preparation with laxatives before surgery.

The patient facing a serious illness and extensive surgery can be expected to have feelings of grief and anxiety. Encourage the patient to talk about personal feelings and fears, and involve the family or significant others in all preoperative teaching and discussions. A social worker or case manager can be extremely helpful in providing continuity of care and support to the entire family.

Operative procedures. In the MIE procedure, the surgeon makes four or five small incisions in the chest and abdomen using a video-assisted thoracoscope and laparoscope. The lower esophagus and gastric fundus are removed. The remaining portion of the esophagus is then anastomosed (reconnected) to the stomach.

For most patients, the surgeon performs an open subtotal or total esophagectomy because tumors are often large and involve distant lymph nodes. For a subtotal (partial) removal, the diseased portion of the esophagus is removed and the cervical portion is anastomosed (connected) to the stomach. The cervical portion of the stomach is then brought up into the thorax through the esophageal hiatus (Fig. 57-3). A **pyloromyotomy** is done by cutting and suturing the pylorus. Finally, a jejunostomy tube may be placed for postoperative enteral feeding.

For patients with early-stage tumors of the lower third of the esophagus, a transhiatal esophagectomy is the preferred surgical approach. The surgery is performed through an upper midline cervical incision. With this approach, the pleural space is not entered, reducing respiratory complications. For patients with tumors in the upper esophagus, a radical neck dissection and laryngectomy may also be needed if the disease has spread to the larynx. Chapter 31 discusses the care of patients having these procedures.

The surgeon may perform a **colon interposition** when the tumor involves the stomach or the stomach is otherwise un-

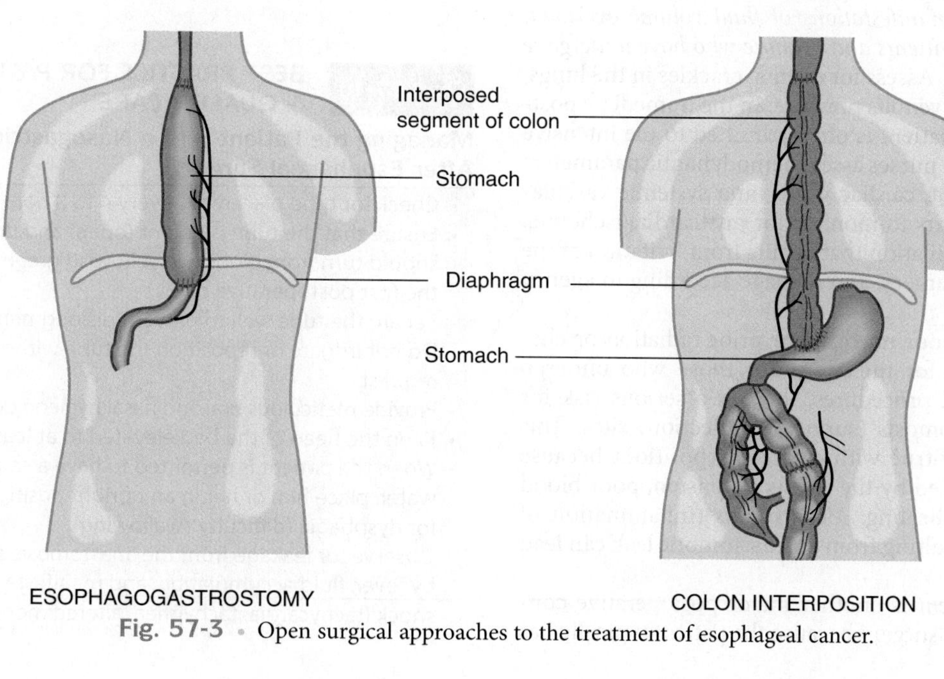
Interposed
segment of colon
Stomach
Diaphragm
Stomach
ESOPHAGOGASTROSTOMY
COLON INTERPOSITION

Fig. 57-3 • Open surgical approaches to the treatment of esophageal cancer.

suitable for anastomosis. A section of right or left colon is removed and brought up into the thorax to substitute for the esophagus (see Fig. 57-3).

Postoperative care. The patient requires intensive postoperative care and is at risk for multiple serious complications. The Plan of Care on pp. 1250 to 1253 outlines common nursing interventions for patients having open esophageal surgery. The patient having an MIE has the same risk for postoperative complications as one having the open procedure. The advantages of MIE, though, include:

- Less blood loss during surgery; fewer blood transfusions
- Decreased healing and recovery time
- Decreased trauma to the body
- No large incisions
- Less postoperative pain
- Shorter hospital stay (5 to 7 days rather than 7 to 10 days)

Respiratory care is the highest postoperative priority for patients having an esophagectomy. For those who had traditional surgery, intubation with mechanical ventilation is needed for at least the first 16 to 24 hours. Pulmonary complications include atelectasis and pneumonia. The risk for postoperative pulmonary complications is increased in the patient who has received preoperative radiation. Once the patient is extubated, begin deep breathing, turning, and coughing every 1 to 2 hours. Collaborate with the respiratory therapist, if available, to begin chest physiotherapy, usually every 2 to 4 hours. Assess the patient for decreased breath sounds and shortness of breath every 1 to 2 hours. Incisional support and adequate analgesia are essential for effective coughing and should be provided regularly if the patient's vital signs remain stable. Pain is often severe and constant as a result of cutting into chest muscle.

Remind nursing and other staff to keep the patient in a semi-Fowler's or high Fowler's position to support ventilation and prevent reflux. The health care provider prescribes prophylactic antibiotics and supplemental oxygen. *Ensure the patency of the chest tube drainage system, and monitor for changes in the volume or color of the drainage.*

Cardiovascular complications, particularly hypotension during surgery, can occur as a result of pressure placed on the posterior heart and usually respond well to IV fluid administration. *Monitor for manifestations of fluid volume overload, particularly in older patients and in those who have undergone lymph node dissection.* Assess for edema, crackles in the lungs, and increased jugular venous pressure. In the immediate postoperative phase, the patient is often admitted to the intensive care unit. Critical care nurses assess hemodynamic parameters such as cardiac output, cardiac index, and systemic vascular resistance every 2 hours to monitor for myocardial ischemia. Observe for atrial fibrillation that results from irritation of the vagus nerve during surgery, and manage according to agency protocol.

The patient with poor nutrition or prior radiation or chemotherapy is at risk for infection. For those who undergo more radical surgical procedures, there is a serious risk for leakage at the anastomosis (surgical connection) sites. This situation is especially true with colon interpositions because several sites are stressed by the effects of tension, poor blood supply, and delayed healing. *Mediastinitis* (inflammation of the mediastinum) resulting from an anastomotic leak can lead to fatal sepsis.

Wound management is another major postoperative concern for conventional surgery because the patient typically has multiple incisions and drains. *Provide direct support to the incision during turning and coughing to prevent dehiscence.* Wound infection can occur 4 to 5 days after surgery. Leakage from the site of anastomosis is a dreaded complication that can appear 2 to 10 days after surgery. If an anastomotic leak occurs, all oral intake is discontinued and is not resumed until the site of the leak has healed. Nutrition may be given through the jejunostomy tube during the healing process. *Carefully assess for fever, fluid accumulation, general signs of inflammation, and symptoms of early shock (e.g., tachycardia, tachypnea). Report any of these findings to the surgeon immediately!*

A nasogastric (NG) tube is placed intraoperatively to decompress the stomach to prevent tension on the suture line. Monitor the NG tube for patency, and carefully secure the tube to prevent dislodgment, which can disrupt the sutures at the anastomosis. *Do not irrigate or reposition the NG tube in patients who have undergone esophageal surgery unless requested by the surgeon!* The initial nasogastric drainage is bloody but should change to a greenish yellow color by the end of the first postoperative day. The continued presence of blood may indicate internal bleeding at the suture line. Provide oral hygiene for the patient every 2 to 4 hours while the tube is in place, or delegate and supervise this activity (Chart 57-10).

The nutritional management of the patient who has undergone an esophageal surgery is an early postoperative concern. After conventional surgery, on the second postoperative day, initial feedings usually begin through the jejunostomy tube (J tube). The feedings are slowly increased over the next several days. Feeding by this method can be discontinued once the patient is taking adequate oral nutrition. However, some patients may require J-tube feedings for about 1 month if small amounts are aspirated.

Before beginning oral feedings, a cine-esophagram study is performed to detect any anastomotic leaks, strictures, or signs of aspiration. If no leaks are seen, a liquid diet is started. If liquids are well tolerated, the patient's diet is advanced to include semisolid foods and then solid foods.

Place the patient in an upright position, and supervise all initial swallowing efforts. The food storage area of the stomach has been radically decreased, and gravity is the only defense

Chart 57-10 **BEST PRACTICE FOR PATIENT SAFETY & QUALITY CARE**

Managing the Patient with a Nasogastric Tube After Esophageal Surgery

- Check for tube placement every 4 to 8 hours.
- Ensure that the tube is patent (open) and draining; drainage should turn from bloody to yellowish green by the end of the first postoperative day.
- Secure the tube well to prevent dislodgment.
- Do not irrigate or reposition the tube without a physician's request.
- Provide meticulous oral and nasal hygiene every 2 to 4 hours.
- Keep the head of the bed elevated to at least 30 degrees.
- When the patient is permitted to have a small amount of water, place him or her in an upright position and observe for dysphagia (difficulty swallowing).
- Observe for leakage from the anastomosis site, as indicated by fever, fluid accumulation, and manifestations of early shock (tachycardia, tachypnea, altered mental status).

against reflux. *Teach the patient and/or family the importance of eating six to eight small meals per day. Fluids should be taken between, rather than with, meals to prevent diarrhea.* Diarrhea can occur 20 minutes to 2 hours after eating and can be managed with loperamide (Imodium) before meals. The diarrhea is thought to be the result of **vagotomy syndrome,** which develops as a result of interrupted vagal fibers to the abdominal organs during surgery.

DECISION-MAKING CHALLENGE
Coordination of Care

A 63-year-old patient had esophageal surgery yesterday and is admitted to your unit from the ICU. He has two chest tubes, a jejunostomy tube, and IV therapy to maintain fluid and electrolyte balance. The patient is also a type II diabetic who was being controlled before surgery by oral antidiabetic agents and nutrition therapy. His FBS this morning was 285 mg/dL. He also has a history of hypertension and mild COPD. When you conduct your assessment, you note that he has diminished breath sounds in both lower lobes. His respirations are 26 and shallow. He is not dyspneic, and his color is good.

1. What are your priorities for this patient's care this evening?
2. Based on his respiratory assessment, what action should you take first?
3. With what members of the health care team will you collaborate to achieve this patient's expected outcomes?
4. Why does this patient have a jejunostomy rather than a gastrostomy?
5. Why do you think this patient's FBS is elevated at this time?

evolve For suggested answer guidelines, go to http://evolve.elsevier.com/Iggy/.

Community-Based Care

Patients with esophageal cancer have many challenges to face once they are discharged home. The combination treatment regimens cause long-lasting side effects, such as fatigue and weakness. These complex treatments also require the patient and family to be knowledgeable about symptom management and to know when to report concerns to the health care provider.

Home Care Management

Once the patient is discharged to home, ongoing respiratory care remains a priority. Give the patient and family instructions for ambulation and incentive spirometer use. Encourage the patient to be as active as possible and to avoid excessive bedrest because this can lead to complications of immobility. Teach the family to protect the patient from infection and to contact the health care provider immediately if signs of respiratory infection develop. Patients should stay away from people with infections and avoid large crowds.

Health Teaching

Remind the patient and family to wash their hands frequently, and teach them to inspect the incisions daily for redness, tenderness, swelling, odor, and discharge because proper wound healing is still a concern at the time of discharge. Instruct them to report a temperature greater than 101° F (38.3° C), or 100° F (37° C) for older adults. Prepare written instructions about the signs of anastomosis leakage. *Teach the patient or family to immediately report to the health care provider the presence of fever and a swollen, painful neck incision.*

Nutritional support also remains a concern. Encourage the patient to continue increasing oral feedings as tolerated. Remind him or her to eat small, frequent meals containing high-calorie, high-protein foods that are soft and easily swallowed. Teach the value of using supplemental eggnogs and milkshakes between meals, and instruct the patient to eat slowly. Lactose-free products should be used if the patient cannot tolerate dairy foods. Patients who have undergone esophageal resection can lose up to 10% of their body weight. Teach the patient to monitor his or her weight at home and to report a weight loss of 5 pounds or more in 1 month. If sufficient oral intake is not possible, the family may need instruction about tube feedings or parenteral nutrition at home.

Emphasize the importance of remaining upright after meals. Dysphagia or odynophagia may recur because of stricture, reflux, or cancer recurrence. These symptoms should be promptly reported to the health care provider. Despite radical surgery, the patient with cancer of the esophagus often still has a terminal illness and a relatively short life expectancy. Emphasis is placed on maximizing quality of life. Realistic planning is important as the patient's condition eventually worsens, and the patient and family are assisted to plan for the future together. Assist family members in exploring formal and informal sources of support. Help the family or significant others arrange for hospice care when it is needed. Chapter 9 describes end-of-life care, including hospice.

Health Care Resources

Referrals to community or home care organizations assist the family in providing care in the home. The patient may need transportation to the radiation treatment center five times per week for up to 6 weeks. Oncology nursing care may be needed to monitor and evaluate the patient who is receiving chemotherapy at home through venous access devices or portable infusion pumps. Inform the patient and family about the services available through the American Cancer Society (www.cancer.org), including support groups and transportation. Familiarize the family with area hospice services for future planning. Coordinate resource referrals with the case manager or home care agency.

▪ *Evaluation: Expected Outcomes*

Evaluate the care of the patient with esophageal cancer on the basis of the identified nursing diagnoses. The major expected outcome is that the patient will be able to consume adequate nutrition and maintain a stable weight. Other outcomes for postoperative esophageal surgical patients are outlined in the Plan of Care on pp. 1250 to 1253. Specific indicators for this outcome are listed for the nursing diagnosis under the Planning and Implementation section (see earlier).

ESOPHAGEAL DIVERTICULA

Diverticula are sacs resulting from the herniation of esophageal mucosa and submucosa into surrounding tissue. They may develop anywhere along the length of the esophagus. No environmental risk factors are known to be involved in their development. The incomplete or late opening of swallowing muscles can cause high pressure in the hypopharynx and lead to *Zenker's diverticula,* the most common form. This type occurs most often in older adults. Patients report dysphagia (difficulty swallowing), regurgitation (reflux), nocturnal cough, and halitosis (bad breath). They can also be at risk for perforation because the mucosa is without the protection of the normal esophageal muscle layer.

Esophageal diverticula are diagnosed most often by esophagogastroduodenoscopy (EGD). This procedure must be performed with strict care because of the risk for perforation. Nutrition therapy and positioning are the major interventions for controlling symptoms related to diverticula. Collaborate with the nutritionist to assist the patient in exploring variations in the size and frequency of meals and in food texture and consistency. Semisoft foods and smaller meals are often best tolerated and may reduce or relieve the symptoms of pressure and reflux. Nocturnal reflux associated with diverticula is managed by teaching the patient to sleep with the head of the bed elevated and to avoid the supine position for at least 2 hours after eating. Advise the patient to avoid vigorous exercise after meals. Teach him or her to avoid restrictive clothing and frequent stooping or bending.

Surgical management is aimed at removing the diverticula. Postoperatively the patient is NPO for several days to promote healing. During that period, the patient receives IV fluids for hydration, tube feedings, and then oral fluid and food. Provide pain-relief measures, and monitor for complications such as bleeding or perforation. *A nasogastric (NG) tube is placed during surgery for decompression and is not irrigated or repositioned unless specifically requested by the surgeon.*

Community-based care includes teaching the patient and family about:

- Nutritional therapy
- Positioning guidelines to prevent reflux
- Warning signs of complications, such as bleeding or infection

ESOPHAGEAL TRAUMA

Trauma to the esophagus can result from blunt injuries, chemical burns, surgery or endoscopy, or the stress of continuous severe vomiting (Table 57-2). Trauma may affect the esophagus directly, impairing swallowing and nutrition, or it may create problems in related structures such as the lungs or mediastinum. The incidence of most forms of esophageal trauma is low in adults. When excessive force is exerted on the esophageal mucosa, it may perforate or rupture, allowing the caustic acid secretions to enter the mediastinal cavity. These tears are associated with a high mortality rate related to shock, respiratory impairment, or sepsis.

TABLE 57-2 Common Causes of Esophageal Perforation

- Straining
- Seizures
- Trauma
- Foreign objects
- Instrument or tubes
- Chemical injury
- Complications of esophageal surgery
- Ulcers

Chemical injury is usually a result of the accidental or intentional ingestion of caustic substances. The damage to the mouth and esophagus is rapid and severe. Acid burns tend to affect the superficial mucosal lining, whereas alkaline substances cause deeper penetrating injuries. Strong alkalis can cause full perforation of the esophagus within 1 minute. Additional problems may include aspiration pneumonia and hemorrhage. Esophageal strictures may develop as scar tissue forms.

Patients with esophageal trauma are initially evaluated and treated in the emergency department. Assessment focuses on the nature of the injury and the circumstances surrounding it. *Assess for airway patency, breathing, chest pain, dysphagia, vomiting, and bleeding as the priority for patient care.* If the risk for extending the damage is not excessive, an x-ray or endoscopic study may be requested to evaluate tears or perforation. A CT scan of the chest can be done to assess for the presence of mediastinal air.

After the injury, keep the patient NPO to prevent further leakage of esophageal secretions. Esophageal and gastric suction can be used for drainage and to rest the esophagus. Esophageal rest is maintained for more than a week after injury to allow for initial healing of the mucosa. Total parenteral nutrition (TPN) is prescribed to provide calories and protein for wound healing while the patient is not eating.

To prevent sepsis, the health care provider prescribes broad-spectrum antibiotics. High-dose corticosteroids may be administered to suppress inflammation and prevent strictures (esophageal narrowing). In addition, opioid and non-opioid analgesics are prescribed for pain management. When caustic burns involve the mouth, topical agents such as topical lidocaine (Viscous Xylocaine) may be used for topical analgesia and local anti-inflammatory action.

If nonsurgical management is not effective in healing traumatized esophageal tissue, the patient may need surgery to remove the damaged tissue. Those with severe injuries may require resection of part of the esophagus with a gastric pull-through and repositioning or replacement by a bowel segment.

HUMAN NEEDS NURSING CARE REVIEW

What might you NOTICE if the patient has inadequate digestion and nutrition as a result of chronic esophageal problems?

- Dysphagia (difficulty swallowing)
- Odynophagia (painful swallowing)
- Dyspepsia (indigestion or "heartburn")
- Regurgitation (reflux)
- Eructation (belching)
- Chronic cough
- Choking
- Halitosis (foul breath)
- Weight loss

What should you INTERPRET and how should you RESPOND to a patient experiencing inadequate digestion and nutrition as a result of chronic esophageal problems?

Perform and interpret focused physical findings, including:

- Assess ability to chew and swallow food.
- Assess chest pain (dyspepsia) for quality, location, and intensity.
- Assess body weight change.

- Auscultate lungs.
- Assess readiness to learn.

Respond:

- Provide semi-solid or thickened liquids if solid foods cannot be swallowed comfortably.
- Collaborate with nutritionist and occupational therapist (OT) for swallowing evaluation and training.
- Monitor for aspiration of secretions or food.
- Teach lifestyle changes, such as foods to avoid, smoking and alcohol cessation, weight reduction (if obese), and importance of drug therapy to control symptoms.
- Monitor weight.
- Monitor for increased dysphagia.

On what should you REFLECT?

- Evaluate for rapid weight changes (decrease if obese, and increase if severe weight loss has occurred).
- Monitor for manifestations of aspiration.
- Observe patient for improvement in GI symptoms.
- Evaluate effectiveness of health teaching.
- Think about what else you might do to promote digestion and nutrition.

GET READY FOR THE NCLEX EXAMINATION!

Key Points

Review these Key Points for each NCLEX Examination Client Needs Category.

Safe and Effective Care Environment

- Consult with the nutritionist, patient, and family regarding nutritional restrictions for patients with GERD.
- Collaborate with the health care team for the patient with impaired swallowing and/or limited nutrition.
- Teach the patient and family to recognize the symptoms of dysphagia.
- Remain with the dysphasic patient during meals to prevent or assist with choking episodes.

Health Promotion and Maintenance

- Teach the patient oral exercises aimed at improving swallowing.
- Stress the importance of recognizing and controlling reflux through nutrition therapy and medications to avoid further esophageal damage that could lead to Barrett's esophagus.
- Teach the patient to elevate the head of the bed by 6 inches for sleep to prevent nighttime reflux.
- Instruct the patient to sleep in the right side-lying position to minimize the effects of nighttime episodes of reflux.
- Teach the patient with esophageal cancer to monitor his or her body weight and to notify the health care provider for a loss of 5 pounds or greater within 1 month.
- Teach the patient to avoid alcoholic beverages, smoking, and other substances as listed in Chart 57-2 because they lead to increased gastroesophageal reflux.
- Teach the patient to prevent gas bloat syndrome by avoiding drinking carbonated beverages, eating gas-producing foods, chewing gum, and drinking with a straw.
- Review postprocedure instructions for patients having endoscopic therapies for GERD as outlined in Chart 57-4.

Psychosocial Integrity

- Allow the patient the opportunity to express fear or anxiety regarding the diagnosis of esophageal cancer and related treatment regimen of surgery, chemotherapy, and radiation.
- Explain all procedures, restrictions, drug therapy, and follow-up care to the patient and family.
- Refer the patient or family members to psychological counseling, hospice, pastoral care, and the case manager as needed.

Physiological Integrity

- For patients with GERD, teach the importance of strict adherence to antireflux agents in preventing esophageal damage (see Chart 57-3).
- Be aware that laparoscopic Nissen fundoplication (LNF) is the most common surgical procedure for patients with GERD and hiatal hernia; LNF may also be performed for those with achalasia.
- Recall that achalasia is an esophageal motility disorder caused by esophageal denervation, which can lead to severe complications, such as carcinoma and aspiration pneumonia.
- Assess for complications and provide postoperative care for patients having the LNF procedure as described in Charts 57-6 and 57-7.
- Teach the patient having open conventional esophageal surgery about incisions, drains, and jejunostomy tube placement before he or she undergoes surgery for esophageal cancer.
- For the patient with a nasogastric (NG) tube, check the NG tube every 4 to 8 hours for proper placement and anchorage; follow guidelines as outlined in Chart 57-10.
- Assess the patient after esophageal surgery for pulmonary and cardiac complications of surgery, and report changes to the health care provider.
- Assess patients for key features of esophageal tumors as listed in Chart 57-8.
- Provide care for patients with open conventional esophageal surgery as discussed in the Plan of Care.

Additional Study Resources

Go to your Companion CD or Evolve at http://evolve.elsevier.com/Iggy/ for *Self-Assessment Questions for the NCLEX Examination.*

Go to Evolve at http://evolve.elsevier.com/Iggy/ for *Prioritization and Delegation Questions for the NCLEX Examination.*

SELECTED BIBLIOGRAPHY

Asterisk indicates a classic or definitive work on this subject.

American Cancer Society. (2008). *Cancer facts and figures 2008.* Retrieved July 30, 2008, from www.cancer.org.

Andreassen, S., Randers, I., Näslund, E., Stockeld, D., & Mattiasson, A.C. (2006). Patients' experiences of living with oesophageal cancer. *Journal of Clinical Nursing, 15*(6), 685-695.

*Brooks-Brunn, J.A. (2000). Esophageal cancer: An overview. *MEDSURG Nursing, 9*(5), 248-254.

Bulechek, G.M., Butcher, H.K., & McCloskey Dochterman, J. (2008). *Nursing interventions classification* (5th ed.). St. Louis: Mosby.

Edmondson, D., & Schiech, L. (2008). Esophageal cancer: A tough pill to swallow. *Nursing2008, 38*(4), 44-51.

*Fennerty, B., et al. (2002). New paradigms for the treatment of acid-related reflux disorders. *Patient Care for the Nurse Practitioner, Special Edition,* Fall, 3-12.

*Hemminger, L.L., & Wolfsen, H.C. (2002). Photodynamic therapy for Barrett's esophagus and high-grade dysplasia: Results of a patient satisfaction survey. *Gastrointestinal Nursing, 25*(4), 139-141.

How to swallow: Understanding dysphagia. *Nursing2008, 38*(3), 45-47.

*Hubbard, P.M. (2002). Update on gastroesophageal reflux disease. *The American Journal for Nurse Practitioners, 6*(2), 9-18.

Jacobson, B.C., Somers, S.C., Fuchs, C.S., Kelly, C.P., & Camargo, C.A. Jr. (2006). Body-mass index and symptoms of gastrointestinal reflux in women. *New England Journal of Medicine, 354*(22), 2340-2348.

Lawrence, B.L., & Taylor, D. (2007). Esophageal pH monitoring goes wireless. *Nursing2007, 37*(10), 26-27.

Ludwig, C. (2005). Gastrointestinal tract. *MEDSURG Nursing, 14*(6), 378.

McCance, K.L., & Huether, S.E. (2006). *The biologic basis for disease in adults and children* (5th ed.). St. Louis: Mosby.

*McCormick, D.G. (2004). Stretta procedure for the treatment of gastroesophageal reflux disease. *Gastroenterology Nursing, 27*(1), 22-28.

*Nilsson, G., Larsson, S., Johnsson, F., & Saveman, B.I. (2002). Patient's experience of illness, operation and outcome with reference to gastroesophageal reflux disease. *Journal of Advanced Nursing, 40*(3), 307-315.

Nussbaum, R.L., McInnes, R.R., & Willard, H.F. (2007). *Thompson and Thompson's genetics in medicine.* Philadelphia: Saunders.

Phan, M., Dyke, S., Whittaker, M.A., Simmerman, A., Abrams, S., Panjehpour, M., et al. (2005). An educational tool for photodynamic therapy of Barrett esophagus with high-grade dysplasia: From screening through follow-up. *Gastroenterology Nursing, 28*(5), 413-421.

Popat, S., Lopez, J., Chan, S., Waters, J., Cominos, M., Rutter, D., et al. (2006). Palliative treatments for patients with inoperable gastrointestinal cancers. *International Journal of Palliative Nursing, 12*(7), 306-317.

*Rockey, A.D. (2002). What you need to know about Barrett's esophagus. *Gastroenterology Nursing, 25*(6), 237-240.

*Sweed, M.R., Schiech, L., Barsevick, A., Babb, J.S., & Goldberg, M. (2002). Quality of life after esophagectomy for cancer. *Oncology Nursing Forum, 29*(7), 1127-1131.

Tawk, M., Goodrich, S., Kinasewitz, G., & Orr, W. (2006). The effect of 1 week of continuous positive airway pressure treatment in obstructive sleep apnea patients with concomitant gastroesophageal reflux. *Chest, 130*(4), 1003-1008.

U.S. Department of Health and Human Services, Agency for Healthcare Research and Quality. (2005). *Comparative analysis of management strategies for gastrointestinal reflux disease.* Rockville, MD: Author.

Yang, Y.X., Lewis, J.D., Epstein, S., & Metz, D.C. (2006). Long-term proton pump inhibitor therapy and the risk of hip fracture. *Journal of the American Medical Association, 296*(24), 2947-2953.

Care of Patients with Stomach Disorders

58

CHAPTER

Donna D. Ignatavicius

LEARNING OUTCOMES

For clinical competence and success on the NCLEX Examination, study this chapter with these Learning Outcomes in mind:

Safe and Effective Care Environment

1. Collaborate with members of the health care team when caring for patients with stomach disorders.
2. Plan individualized care for the patient having gastric surgery.
3. Identify community resources for patients with gastric disorders.

Health Promotion and Maintenance

4. Identify risk factors for gastritis and peptic ulcer disease (PUD).
5. Teach patients about complementary and alternative therapies that have been used to help manage gastritis and PUD.
6. Teach patients ways to promote GI health and prevent gastritis.

Psychosocial Integrity

7. Identify the need for end-of-life care for patients with advanced gastric cancer.

Physiological Integrity

8. Compare etiologies and assessment findings of acute and chronic gastritis.
9. Compare and contrast assessment findings associated with gastric and duodenal ulcers.
10. Identify the most common medical complications that can result from PUD.
11. Teach patients about the purpose and adverse effects of drug therapy for gastritis and PUD.
12. Monitor patients with PUD and gastric cancer for signs of upper GI bleeding.
13. Prioritize interventions for patients with upper GI bleeding.
14. Explain the purpose and procedure for gastric lavage.
15. Evaluate the impact of gastric disorders on the nutrition status of the patient.
16. Provide preoperative and postoperative care for the patient undergoing gastric surgery.
17. Explain Zollinger-Ellison syndrome and its associated clinical manifestations.
18. Identify risk factors for gastric cancer.

Go to your Companion CD or Evolve at http://evolve.elsevier.com/Iggy/ for *Self-Assessment Questions for the NCLEX Examination* keyed to these Learning Outcomes.

Although only a few diseases affect the stomach, they can be very serious and in some cases life threatening. The most common disorders include gastritis, peptic ulcer disease, and gastric cancer. Each of these health problems can result in impaired or altered *digestion* and *nutrition*. The stomach is part of the upper GI system that is responsible for a large part of the digestive process. Collaborative management of patients with stomach disorders often includes therapies to meet the *human need for nutrition.*

GASTRITIS

Gastritis is the inflammation of gastric mucosa (stomach lining). It can be scattered or localized and can be classified according to cause, cellular changes, or distribution of the lesions. Gastritis can be erosive (causing ulcers) or nonerosive. Although the mucosal changes that result from *acute* gastritis typically heal after several months, this is not true for *chronic* gastritis.

Pathophysiology

Prostaglandins provide a protective mucosal barrier that prevents the stomach from digesting itself by a process called acid **autodigestion.** If there is a break in the protective barrier, mucosal injury occurs. The resulting injury is worsened by histamine release and vagus nerve stimulation. Hydrochloric acid can then diffuse back into the mucosa and injure small vessels. This back-diffusion causes edema, hemorrhage, and erosion of the stomach's lining. The pathologic changes of gastritis include vascular congestion, edema, acute inflammatory cell infiltration, and degenerative changes in the superficial epithelium of the stomach lining.

Types of Gastritis

Inflammation of the gastric mucosa or submucosa after exposure to local irritants or other cause can result in **acute gastritis.** The early pathologic manifestation of gastritis is a thickened, reddened mucous membrane with prominent **rugae,** or folds. Various degrees of mucosal necrosis and inflammatory reaction occur in acute disease. The diagnosis cannot be based solely on clinical symptoms. Complete regeneration and healing usually occur within a few days. If the stomach muscle is not involved, complete recovery usually occurs with no residual evidence of gastric inflammatory reaction. If the muscle is affected, hemorrhage may occur during an episode of acute gastritis.

Chronic gastritis appears as a patchy, diffuse (spread out) inflammation of the mucosal lining of the stomach. As the disease progresses, the walls and lining of the stomach thin and atrophy. With progressive gastric atrophy from chronic mucosal injury, the function of the parietal (acid-secreting) cells decreases and the source of intrinsic factor is lost. The intrinsic factor is critical for absorption of vitamin B_{12}. When body stores of vitamin B_{12} are eventually depleted, **pernicious anemia** results. The amount and concentration of acid in stomach secretions gradually decrease until the secretions consist of only mucus and water.

Chronic gastritis is associated with an increased risk for gastric cancer. The persistent inflammation extends deep into the mucosa, causing destruction of the gastric glands and cellular changes. Chronic gastritis may be categorized as type A, type B, or atrophic.

Type A (nonerosive) chronic gastritis refers to an inflammation of the glands, as well as the fundus and body of the stomach. Type B chronic gastritis usually affects the glands of the antrum but may involve the entire stomach. In atrophic chronic gastritis, diffuse inflammation and destruction of deeply located glands accompany the condition. Chronic atrophic gastritis affects all layers of the stomach, thus decreasing the number of cells. The muscle thickens, and inflammation is present. Chronic atrophic gastritis is characterized by total loss of fundal glands, minimal inflammation, thinning of the gastric mucosa, and intestinal metaplasia (abnormal tissue development). These cellular changes can lead to peptic ulcer disease (PUD) and gastric cancer.

Etiology and Genetic Risk

Acute Gastritis

The onset of infection with Helicobacter pylori can result in acute gastritis. H. pylori is a gram-negative, spiral-shaped bacterium that penetrates the mucosal gel layer of the gastric epithelium. Although it is uncommon, other forms of bacterial gastritis from organisms such as staphylococci, streptococci, *Escherichia coli,* or salmonella can cause life-threatening problems such as sepsis and extensive tissue necrosis (death). Other infectious causes of acute gastritis can be found in patients with immunosuppressive disorders. In those with acquired immune deficiency syndrome (AIDS), for example, gastric erosions may be present with herpes simplex and cytomegalovirus (CMV) infection.

Long-term NSAID use creates a high risk for acute gastritis. NSAIDs inhibit prostaglandin production in the mucosal barrier. Other risk factors include alcohol, caffeine, and corticosteroids. Acute gastritis is also caused by local irritation from radiation therapy and accidental or intentional ingestion of corrosive substances, including acids or alkalis (e.g., lye and drain cleaners). Emotional stress and acute anxiety may also cause gastritis.

Chronic Gastritis

Type A gastritis has been associated with the presence of antibodies to parietal cells and intrinsic factor. Therefore an autoimmune cause for this type of gastritis is likely. Parietal cell antibodies have been found in most patients with pernicious anemia and in more than one half of those with type A gastritis. A genetic link to this disease, with an autosomal dominant pattern of inheritance, has been found in the relatives of patients with pernicious anemia (McCance & Huether, 2006).

The most common form of the disease is **type B gastritis,** caused by *H. pylori* infection. A direct correlation exists between the number of organisms and the degree of cellular abnormality present. The host response to the *H. pylori* infection is activation of lymphocytes and neutrophils. Release of inflammatory cytokines, such as interleukin (IL)-1, IL-8, and tumor necrosis factor (TNF)–alpha, damage the gastric mucosa (McCance & Huether, 2006).

Chronic local irritation and toxic effects caused by alcohol ingestion, radiation therapy, and smoking have been linked to chronic gastritis. Surgical procedures that involve the pyloric sphincter, such as a pyloroplasty, can lead to gastritis by causing reflux of alkaline secretions into the stomach. Other systemic disorders such as Crohn's disease, graft-versus-host disease, and uremia can also precipitate the development of chronic gastritis.

Atrophic gastritis is a type of chronic gastritis that is seen most often in older adults. It can occur after exposure to toxic substances in the workplace (e.g., benzene, lead, nickel) or *H. pylori* infection, or it can be related to autoimmune factors.

Health Promotion and Maintenance

Gastritis is a very common health problem in the United States. Yet, a balanced diet, regular exercise, and stress reduction techniques can help prevent it (Chart 58-1). A balanced diet includes following the recommendations of the U.S. Department of Agriculture (USDA) and limiting intake of foods

Chart 58-1 PATIENT AND FAMILY EDUCATION GUIDE

Gastritis Prevention

- Eat a well-balanced diet.
- Avoid drinking excessive amounts of alcoholic beverages.
- Use caution in taking large doses of aspirin, other NSAIDs (e.g., ibuprofen), and corticosteroids.
- Avoid excessive intake of caffeine-containing beverages, especially coffee and tea.
- Be sure that foods and water are safe to avoid contamination.
- Manage stress levels using complementary and alternative therapies, such as relaxation and meditation techniques.
- Stop smoking.
- Protect yourself against exposure to toxic substances in the workplace, such as lead and nickel.
- Seek medical treatment if you are experiencing symptoms of esophageal reflux (see Chapter 57).

and spices that can cause gastric distress such as caffeine, chocolate, mustard, pepper, and other strong or hot spices. Alcohol and tobacco consumption should also be avoided. Regular exercise maintains peristalsis, which helps prevent gastric contents from irritating the gastric mucosa. Stress reduction techniques can include aerobic exercise, meditation, reading, and/or yoga depending on individual preferences. Psychotherapy may also be considered.

Excessive use of aspirin and other NSAIDs should also be avoided. If a family member has *H. pylori* infection or has had it in the past, patient testing should be considered. This test can diagnose the bacteria before they cause gastritis.

Patient-Centered Collaborative Care

Assessment

Physical Assessment/Clinical Manifestations

Symptoms of *acute* gastritis range from mild to severe. The patient may report epigastric discomfort, anorexia, cramping, nausea, and vomiting (Chart 58-2). Assess for abdominal tenderness and bloating, **hematemesis** (vomiting blood), or **melena** (traces of blood in the stool). Symptoms last only a few hours or days and vary with the cause. Aspirin/NSAID–related gastritis may result in **dyspepsia** (heartburn). Gastritis or food poisoning caused by endotoxins, such as staphylococcal endotoxin, has an abrupt onset. Severe nausea and vomiting often occur within 5 hours of ingestion of the contaminated food. *In some cases, gastric hemorrhage is the presenting symptom, which is a life-threatening emergency.*

Chronic gastritis causes few symptoms unless ulceration occurs. Patients may report nausea, vomiting, or upper abdominal discomfort. Periodic epigastric pain may occur after a meal. Some patients have anorexia (see Chart 58-2).

Laboratory Assessment

Several tests are available to detect *H. pylori* if gastritis or an ulcer is suspected. One of the most common methods is a blood test to detect *IgG or IgM anti–H. pylori antibodies.* The IgG antibodies become elevated 2 months after infection and stay elevated until over a year after treatment. The IgM antibodies become elevated 3 to 4 weeks after infection and disappear 3 months after treatment. Another blood test that can be performed in a health care provider's office by a finger stick is immune testing using an *enzyme-linked immunosorbent assay (ELISA)* and *immune chromatography (IMC)* (Pagana & Pagana, 2006).

Chart 58-2 KEY FEATURES

Gastritis

ACUTE GASTRITIS
- Rapid onset of epigastric pain or discomfort
- Nausea and vomiting
- Hematemesis (vomiting blood)
- Gastric hemorrhage
- Dyspepsia (heartburn)
- Anorexia

CHRONIC GASTRITIS
- Vague report of epigastric pain that is relieved by food
- Anorexia
- Nausea or vomiting
- Intolerance of fatty and spicy foods
- Pernicious anemia

Other noninvasive ways to test for *H. pylori* include breath and stool analyses. The *C13 urea breath test* is very accurate and can be used in a health care provider's office or other ambulatory care setting. After being NPO since midnight, the patient drinks a radioactive carbon urea solution. If *H. pylori* are present, they break down urea to carbon dioxide, which is then eliminated by the lungs. The patient's expired air is measured for the amount of carbon dioxide to determine the presence of the bacteria. *Stool testing (HpSA)* is done less commonly because the bacteria do not survive in stool. However, ELISA testing can detect the *H. pylori* antigen in a fresh stool sample (Pagana & Pagana, 2006).

Other Diagnostic Assessment

Esophagogastroduodenoscopy (EGD) via an endoscope with biopsy is the gold standard for diagnosing gastritis. The physician takes a biopsy to establish a definitive diagnosis of the type of gastritis. If lesions are patchy and diffuse, biopsy of several suspicious areas may be necessary to avoid misdiagnosis. A *cytologic examination* of the biopsy specimen is performed to confirm or rule out gastric cancer. Tissue samples can also be taken to detect *H. pylori* using *rapid urease testing.* As the name implies, this test provides quick results unlike the more traditional tissue culture that takes several weeks to determine if the bacteria are present. The results of these tests are not reliable if the patient has not discontinued his or her medications for gastritis, including antacids, for at least a week.

Common Nursing Diagnoses and Collaborative Problems

Nursing diagnoses and collaborative problems that may apply to patients with gastritis include:
- Acute Pain or Chronic Pain related to physical injury (inflammation)
- Nausea and/or vomiting related to gastric irritation
- Deficient Knowledge related to unfamiliarity with information resources
- Potential for Hemorrhage or Perforation

Interventions

Patients with gastritis are not often seen in the acute care setting unless they have an exacerbation ("flare up") of acute or chronic gastritis that results in fluid and electrolyte imbalance or bleeding. Collaborative care is directed toward supportive care for relieving the symptoms and removing or reducing the cause of discomfort.

Acute gastritis is treated symptomatically and supportively because the healing process is spontaneous, usually occurring within a few days. When the cause is removed, pain and discomfort usually subside. If bleeding is severe, a blood transfusion may be necessary. Fluid replacement is prescribed for patients with severe fluid loss. Surgery, such as partial gastrectomy, pyloroplasty, and/or vagotomy, may be needed for patients with major bleeding or ulceration. Treatment of *chronic* gastritis varies with the cause. The approach to management includes the elimination of causative agents, treatment of any underlying disease (e.g., uremia, Crohn's disease), avoidance of toxic substances (e.g., alcohol, tobacco), and health teaching.

Nonsurgical Management

Eliminating the causative factors, such as *H. pylori* infection if present, is the primary treatment approach. Drugs and nutritional therapy are also used. In the *acute* phase, the health care team also provides interventions to relieve pain and discomfort. Drugs that block and buffer gastric acid secretions to relieve pain are usually prescribed.

H_2-receptor antagonists, such as ranitidine (Zantac), famotidine (Pepcid), and nizatidine (Axid), are typically used to block gastric secretions. Sucralfate (Carafate, Sulcrate♣), a *mucosal barrier fortifier,* may also be prescribed. *Antacids* used as buffering agents include aluminum hydroxide combined with magnesium hydroxide (Maalox) and aluminum hydroxide combined with simethicone and magnesium hydroxide (Mylanta). Antisecretory agents **(proton pump inhibitors [PPIs])** such as omeprazole (Prilosec) or esomeprazole may also be used to suppress gastric acid secretion (Chart 58-3). Teach the patient to monitor for symptom relief and side effects of these drugs and to notify the health care provider of any adverse effects or worsening of gastric distress. The dose, frequency, or type of drug may need to be changed if symptoms of gastric irritation appear or persist. *Teach patients not to take additional over-the-counter (OTC) drugs such as Pepcid AC if they are taking similar prescribed drugs.*

Patients with *chronic* gastritis may require vitamin B_{12} for prevention or treatment of pernicious anemia. If *H. pylori* are found, the health care provider treats the infection. Current practice for infection treatment is described on p. *** in the discussion of Drug Therapy in the Peptic Ulcer Disease section.

The nurse, health care provider, or pharmacist teaches patients to avoid drugs and other irritants that are associated with gastritis episodes. These drugs include chemotherapeutic agents, corticosteroids, erythromycin (E-Mycin, Erythromid♣), and NSAIDs, such as aspirin, naproxen (Naprosyn), and ibuprofen (Motrin, Advil, Amersol♣, Novo-Profen♣). NSAIDs are also available as OTC drugs and should not be used. Teach patients to read all OTC drug labels because many preparations contain aspirin or other NSAID. Additional information about these drugs can be found on p. 1274 in the discussion of Drug Therapy in the Peptic Ulcer Disease section.

Instruct the patient to limit intake of any foods and spices that cause distress, such as those that contain caffeine or high acid content (e.g., tomato products, citrus juices) or those that are heavily seasoned with strong or hot spices. Bell peppers and onions are also commonly irritating foods. Most patients seem to progress better with a bland, non-spicy diet and smaller, more frequent meals. Alcohol and tobacco should also be avoided.

Chart 58-3 COMMON EXAMPLES OF DRUG THERAPY

Peptic Ulcer Disease

Drug and Usual Dosage	Purpose of Drug	Nursing Interventions	Rationales
ANTACIDS			
Magnesium hydroxide with aluminum hydroxide (Maalox, Mylanta) 50-80 mEq 1 hr and 3 hr after meals and at bedtime	Increases pH of gastric contents by deactivating pepsin	Give 2 hr after meals and at bedtime.	Hydrogen ion load is high after ingestion of foods.
		Use liquid rather than tablets.	Suspensions are more effective than chewable tablets.
		Do not give other drugs within 1-2 hr of antacids.	Antacids interfere with absorption of other drugs.
		Assess patients for a history of renal disease.	Hypermagnesemia may result. These antacids have a high sodium content. These antacids contain magnesium, which cannot be excreted by poorly functioning kidneys, thus causing toxicity.
		Assess the patient for a history of heart failure.	Inadequate renal perfusion from heart failure decreases the ability of the kidneys to excrete magnesium, thus causing toxicity.
		Observe the patient for the side effect of diarrhea.	Magnesium often causes diarrhea.
Aluminum hydroxide (Amphojel) 50-80 mEq 1 hr and 3 hr after meals and at bedtime		Give 1 hr after meals and at bedtime.	Hydrogen ion load is high after ingestion of food.
		Use liquid rather than tablets if palatable.	Suspensions are more effective than chewable tablets.
		Do not give other drugs within 1-2 hr of antacids.	Antacids interfere with absorption of other drugs.
		Observe patients for the side effect of constipation. If constipation occurs, consider alternating with magnesium antacid.	Aluminum causes constipation, and magnesium has a laxative effect.
		Use for patients with renal failure.	Aluminum binds with phosphates in the GI tract. This antacid does not contain magnesium.

Chart 58-3 COMMON EXAMPLES OF DRUG THERAPY

Peptic Ulcer Disease—cont'd

Drug and Usual Dosage	Purpose of Drug	Nursing Interventions	Rationales
H_2 ANTAGONISTS			
Ranitidine (Zantac) 150 mg orally twice daily or 300 mg orally at bedtime; 50 mg IV every 6 hr or 8 mg/hr IV (continuous) Famotidine (Pepcid) 40 mg orally once daily or in two divided doses; 20 mg IV every 12 hr Nizatidine (Axid) 150 mg orally twice daily or 300 mg at bedtime	Decreases gastric acid secretions by blocking histamine receptors in parietal cells	Give single dose at bedtime for treatment of GI ulcers. **Note:** IV ranitidine may also be given to prevent surgical stress ulcers. **Note:** IV famotidine may also be given to prevent surgical stress ulcers.	Bedtime administration suppresses nocturnal acid production.
MUCOSAL BARRIER FORTIFIERS			
Sucralfate (Carafate, Sulcrate🍁) 1 g orally four times daily or 2 g twice daily	Binds with bile acids and pepsin to protect stomach mucosa	Give 1 hr before and 2 hr after meals, and at bedtime. Do not give within 30 min of giving antacids or other drugs.	Food may interfere with drug's adherence to mucosa. Antacids may interfere with effect.
PROTON PUMP INHIBITORS			
Omeprazole (Prilosec, Losec🍁) 20 mg orally twice daily or 40 mg at bedtime	To suppress H,K–ATPase enzyme system of gastric acid secretion	Have patients take capsule whole; do not crush. Give single dose at bedtime for ulcer disease.	Delayed-release capsules allow absorption after granules leave the stomach. Bedtime administration suppresses nocturnal acid production.
Lansoprazole (Prevacid) 15 or 30 mg orally at bedtime		Give single dose at bedtime for ulcer disease; do not crush.	Bedtime administration suppresses nocturnal acid production.
Rabeprazole (Aciphex) 20 mg orally once daily **Med Error Alert!** Do not confuse Aciphex with Aricept!		Take after the morning meal. Do not crush capsule.	Drug promotes healing and symptom relief of duodenal ulcers. Drug is a sustained-release capsule.
Pantoprazole (Protonix) 40 mg orally or IV daily for 7-10 days		Do not crush. IV form must be given with filter and in a separate line. Do not give Protonix IV with other IV drugs.	Drug is enteric-coated. Given IV, drug precipitates easily. The IV form is not compatible with most other drugs.
Esomeprazole (Nexium) 20 or 40 mg orally daily (or IV daily for 7-10 days)		Give 1 hr before meals. Assess for hepatic impairment. Do not give Nexium IV with other IV drugs.	Food decreases absorption. Patients with severe hepatic problems need a low dose. The IV form is not compatible with most other drugs.
PROSTAGLANDIN ANALOGUES			
Misoprostol (Cytotec) 200 mcg orally four times daily	To decrease gastric secretions and enhance resistance to mucosal injury when patient is taking NSAIDs	Take with food. Avoid magnesium-containing antacids.	Drug protects against NSAID-induced ulcers. Both misoprostol and magnesium-containing antacids can cause diarrhea.
ANTIMICROBIALS			
Clarithromycin (Biaxin) 500 mg orally three times daily Amoxicillin (Amoxil) 1 g orally twice daily Tetracycline 500 mg orally four times daily Metronidazole (Flagyl) 250 mg orally three times daily and at bedtime	To treat *Helicobacter pylori*	Antimicrobials should be given as part of therapy to eradicate *H. pylori* infection. The selection of the specific drug depends on its effectiveness, side effects, and drug interactions.	*H. pylori* is a gram-negative bacterium implicated in the development of peptic ulcer disease (PUD).

TABLE 58-1 Commonly Used Complementary and Alternative Therapies for Gastritis and Peptic Ulcer Disease (PUD)

HERBS AND VITAMINS	
• Gamma-linolenic acid (GLA)	• Cranberry
• Probiotics	• Dandelion
• Vitamin B_{12}	• Ginger
• Bromelain	• Green tea
• Vitamin A	• Licorice
• Vitamin C	• Slippery elm
• Astragalus	• Tumeric
• Barberry	• Yarrow
• Chamomile	
HOMEOPATHY	
• *Pulsatilla*	• *Carbo vegetabilis*
• *Ipecacuanha*	• *Nux vomica*

Assist the patient with various techniques that reduce stress and discomfort, such as progressive relaxation, cutaneous stimulation, guided imagery, and distraction. Other complementary and alternative therapies that have been used are listed in Table 58-1. Chapter 2 describes these therapies in detail.

Surgical Management

Partial gastrectomy, pyloroplasty, vagotomy, or even total gastrectomy may be needed in rare cases for patients who have major bleeding caused by severe erosive gastritis. Such surgery is necessary only if more conservative measures have not controlled the bleeding. Surgical interventions are on p. 1278 in the discussion of Surgical Management in the Peptic Ulcer Disease section.

PEPTIC ULCER DISEASE

A **peptic ulcer** is a mucosal lesion of the stomach or duodenum. **Peptic ulcer disease (PUD)** results when mucosal defenses become impaired and no longer protect the epithelium from the effects of acid and pepsin.

Pathophysiology

Types of Ulcers

Three types of ulcers are commonly seen: gastric ulcers, duodenal ulcers, and stress ulcers. Acid, pepsin, and *H. pylori* infection play an important role in the development of *gastric ulcers.* The gastric mucosal barrier overlies the epithelium. The secretion of mucus and bicarbonate provides a first line of defense in maintaining a near-normal pH on the gastric epithelium and protects the mucosal barrier against acid. Gastromucosal prostaglandins increase the barrier's resistance to ulceration. The integrity of the barrier is enhanced by the rich blood supply of the mucosa of the stomach and duodenum.

When a break in the mucosal barrier occurs, hydrochloric acid injures the epithelium. Gastric ulcers may then result from back-diffusion of acid or dysfunction of the pyloric sphincter (Fig. 58-1). Without normal functioning of the pyloric sphincter, bile refluxes (backs up) into the stomach. This reflux of bile acids may break the integrity of the mucosal barrier and produce hydrogen ion back-diffusion, which leads to mucosal inflammation. Toxic agents and bile then destroy the membrane of the gastric mucosa.

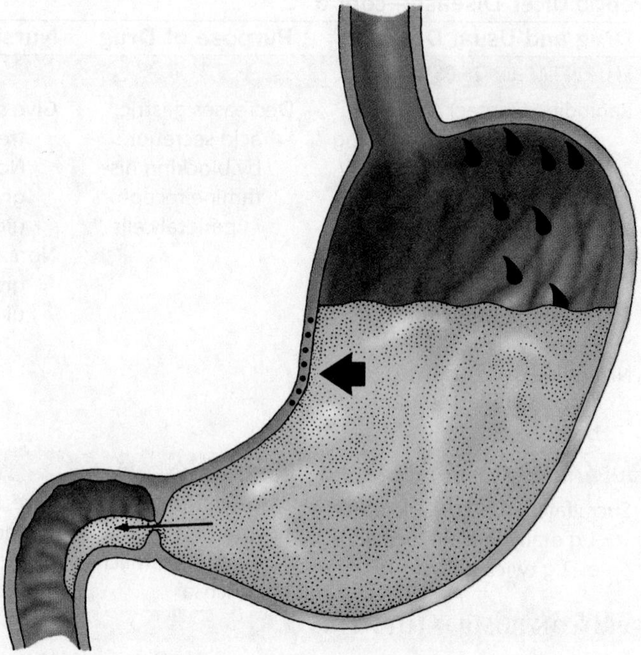

Conditions favoring the development of **gastric ulcers** are normal gastric acid secretion and delayed stomach emptying with *increased diffusion of gastric acid back into the stomach tissues.*

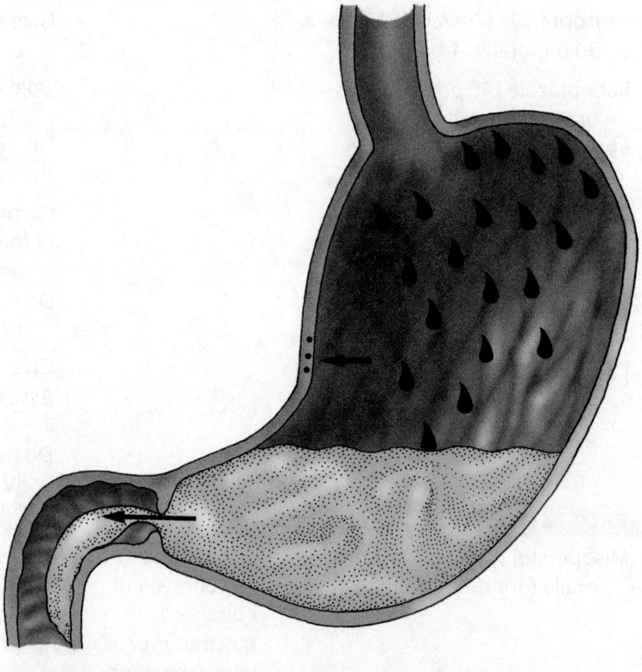

Conditions favoring the development of **duodenal ulcers** are normal diffusion of acid back into stomach tissues with *increased secretion of gastric acid* and *increased stomach emptying.*

Fig. 58-1 • The pathophysiology of peptic ulcer.

Gastric emptying is often delayed in patients with gastric ulceration. This causes regurgitation of duodenal contents, which worsens the gastric mucosal injury. Decreased blood flow to the gastric mucosa may also alter the defense barrier and thereby allow ulceration to occur. Gastric ulcers are deep

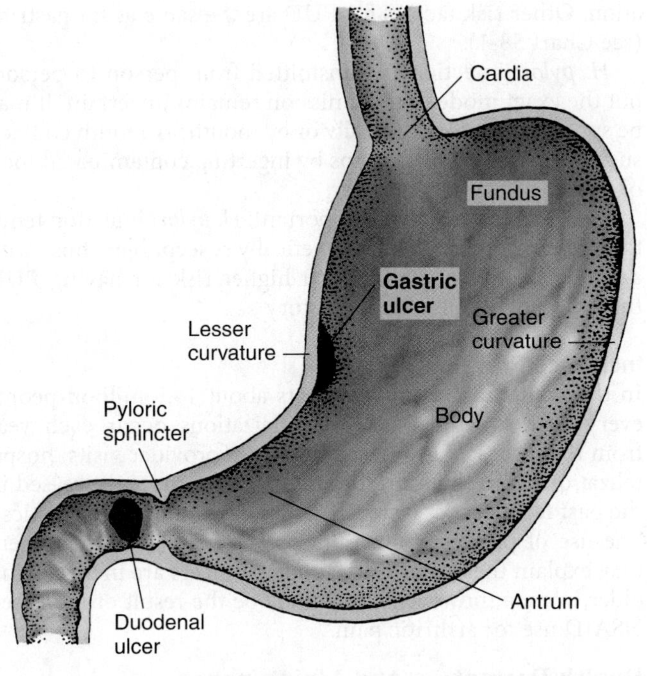
Cardia
Fundus
Gastric ulcer
Lesser curvature
Greater curvature
Pyloric sphincter
Body
Antrum
Duodenal ulcer

Fig. 58-2 • The most common sites for peptic ulcers.

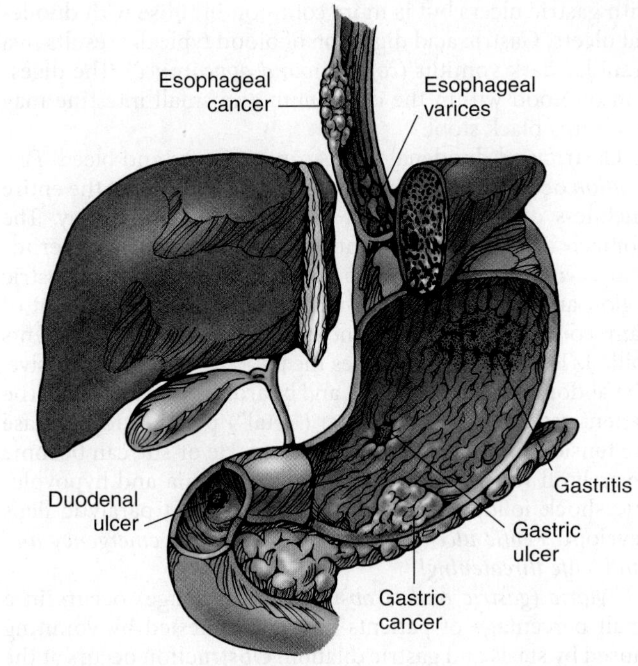
Esophageal cancer
Esophageal varices
Gastritis
Duodenal ulcer
Gastric ulcer
Gastric cancer

Fig. 58-3 • Common causes of upper GI bleeding.

Chart 58-4 KEY FEATURES

Upper GI Bleeding

- Bright red or coffee-ground vomitus (hematemesis)
- Tarry stools or frank (bright red) blood in stools
- Melena (occult blood) (especially in older adults)
- Decreased blood pressure
- Increased weak and thready pulse
- Decreased hemoglobin and hematocrit
- Vertigo
- Acute confusion (in older adults)
- Dizziness
- Syncope

and penetrating, and they usually occur on the lesser curvature of the stomach, near the pylorus (Fig. 58-2).

Most *duodenal ulcers* occur in the upper portion of the duodenum. They are deep, sharply demarcated lesions that penetrate through the mucosa and submucosa into the muscularis propria (muscle layer). The floor of the ulcer consists of a necrotic area residing on granulation tissue and surrounded by areas of fibrosis.

The main feature of a duodenal ulcer is high gastric acid secretion, although a wide range of secretory levels is found. In patients with duodenal ulcers, pH levels are low (excess acid) in the duodenum for long periods. Protein-rich meals, calcium, and vagus nerve excitation stimulate acid secretion. Combined with hypersecretion, a rapid emptying of food from the stomach reduces the buffering effect of food and delivers a large acid bolus to the duodenum (see Fig. 58-1). Inhibitory secretory mechanisms and pancreatic secretion may be insufficient to control the acid load.

Many patients with duodenal ulcer disease have confirmed *H. pylori* infection. These bacteria produce substances that damage the mucosa. Urease produced by *H. pylori* breaks down urea into ammonia. Hydrogen ions are then released in response to the presence of ammonia and contribute further to mucosal damage.

Stress ulcers are acute gastric mucosal lesions occurring after an acute medical crisis or trauma, such as head injury and sepsis. In the patient who is NPO for major surgery, gastritis may lead to **stress ulcers,** which are multiple shallow erosions of the stomach and occasionally the proximal duodenum. Patients who are critically ill, especially those with extensive burns **(Curling's ulcer),** sepsis (ischemic ulcer), or increased intracranial pressure **(Cushing's ulcer),** are also susceptible to these ulcers. To prevent these erosions, drug therapy is prescribed, such as IV famotidine (Pepcid) or pantoprazole (Protonix).

Bleeding caused by gastric erosion is the main manifestation of acute stress ulcers. Multifocal lesions associated with stress ulcers occur in the stomach and proximal duodenum. These lesions begin as areas of ischemia and evolve into erosions and ulcerations that may progress to massive hemorrhage. Little is known of the exact etiology of stress ulcers. However, in the presence of elevated levels of hydrochloric acid, ischemic areas can progress to erosive gastritis and subsequent ulcerations. Stress ulcers are associated with lengthened hospital stay and increased mortality rates.

Complications of Ulcers

The most common complications of PUD are hemorrhage, perforation, pyloric obstruction, and intractable disease. *Hemorrhage is the most serious complication* (Fig. 58-3). It tends to occur more often in patients with *gastric* ulcers and in older adults. Many patients have a second episode of bleeding if underlying infection with *H. pylori* remains untreated or if therapy does not include an H_2 antagonist. With massive bleeding, the patient vomits bright red or coffee-ground blood **(hematemesis).** Hematemesis usually indicates bleeding at or above the duodenojejunal junction (upper GI bleeding) (Chart 58-4).

Minimal bleeding from ulcers is manifested by occult blood in a tarry stool **(melena).** Melena may occur in patients

▶ ANIMATION: Bleeding Ulcer, Pathophysiology

with gastric ulcers but is more common in those with duodenal ulcers. Gastric acid digestion of blood typically results in a granular dark vomitus *(coffee-ground appearance).* The digestion of blood within the duodenum and small intestine may result in a black stool.

Gastric and duodenal ulcers can perforate and bleed. *Perforation* occurs when the ulcer becomes so deep that the entire thickness of the stomach or duodenum is worn away. The stomach or duodenal contents can then leak into the peritoneal cavity. Sudden, sharp pain begins in the midepigastric region and spreads over the entire abdomen. The amount of pain correlates with the amount and type of GI contents spilled. The classic pain causes the patient to be apprehensive. The abdomen is tender, rigid, and boardlike **(peritonitis).** The patient assumes the knee-chest ("fetal") position to decrease the tension on the abdominal muscles. He or she can become severely ill within hours. Bacterial septicemia and hypovolemic shock follow. Peristalsis diminishes, and paralytic ileus develops. *Peptic ulcer perforation is a surgical emergency and can be life threatening!*

Pyloric (gastric outlet) obstruction (blockage) occurs in a small percentage of patients and is manifested by vomiting caused by stasis and gastric dilation. Obstruction occurs at the pylorus (the gastric outlet) and is caused by scarring, edema, inflammation, or a combination of these factors.

Symptoms of obstruction include abdominal bloating, nausea, and vomiting. When vomiting persists, the patient may have hypochloremic (metabolic) alkalosis from loss of large quantities of acid gastric juice (hydrogen and chloride ions) in the vomitus. Hypokalemia may also result from the vomiting or metabolic alkalosis.

Many patients with ulcers have a single episode with no recurrence. However, *intractability* may develop from complications of ulcers, excessive stressors in the patient's life, or an inability to adhere to long-term therapy. He or she no longer responds to conservative management, or recurrences of symptoms interfere with ADLs. In general, the patient continues to have recurrent pain and discomfort despite treatment. Those who fail to respond to traditional treatments or who have a relapse after discontinuation of therapy are referred to a gastroenterologist.

Etiology and Genetic Risk

Peptic ulcer development is associated primarily with NSAID use and bacterial infection with *H. pylori.* NSAIDs (e.g., aspirin, ibuprofen) break down the mucosal barrier and disrupt the mucosal protection mediated systemically by cyclooxygenase (COX) inhibition. COX-2 inhibitors (celecoxib [Celebrex]) are less likely to cause mucosal damage but place patients at high risk for cardiovascular events, such as myocardial infarction. In addition, NSAIDs cause decreased endogenous prostaglandins, resulting in local gastric mucosal injury. GI complications from NSAID use can occur at any time, even after long-term uncomplicated use. NSAID-related ulcers are difficult to treat, even with long-term therapy, because these ulcers have a high rate of recurrence.

Certain substances may contribute to gastroduodenal ulceration by altering gastric secretion, producing localized damage to mucosa and interfering with the healing process. For example, theophylline (Theo-Dur) and caffeine stimulate hydrochloric acid production. The use of corticosteroids is also associated with an increased incidence of peptic ulceration. Other risk factors for PUD are the same as for gastritis (see Chart 58-1).

H. pylori infection is transmitted from person to person, but the exact mode of transmission remains uncertain. It may be spread either fecally–orally or by mouth-to-mouth contact, such as by kissing or perhaps by ingesting contaminated food or water.

Genetic factors may be important. *H. pylori* infection tends to occur in people who are genetically susceptible. Those with a family history of PUD are at higher risk for having PUD than those without a family history.

Incidence/Prevalence

In the United States, PUD affects about 14.5 million people every year. Over 400,000 hospitalizations occur each year from the disease. However, health care provider visits, hospitalizations, and the mortality rate for PUD have decreased in the past few decades (www.digestive.niddk.nih.gov/statistics). The use of proton pump inhibitors and *H. pylori* treatment may explain these declines. Duodenal ulcers are increasing in older women, however, which may be the result of increased NSAID use for arthritic pain.

Health Promotion and Maintenance

Health promotion and illness prevention practices are the same as for gastritis (see Chart 58-1). For critically ill patients, health care providers prescribe drug therapy to prevent stress ulcers. In addition, health care providers may consider starting a patient on enteral nutrition. Enteral nutrition may have a beneficial effect on the stomach mucosa because the products are alkaline.

NCLEX EXAMINATION CHALLENGE

A client with a recent diagnosis of early peptic ulcer disease needs health teaching about nutrition therapy. Which foods should the nurse teach the client to avoid? (Select all that apply.)

A. Red chili peppers
B. Orange juice
C. Green beans
D. Fried chicken
E. Bananas
F. Onions
G. Garlic bread

evolve For the correct answer, go to http://evolve.elsevier.com/Iggy/.

Patient-Centered Collaborative Care

evolve ONLINE PHARM REVIEW

▪ Assessment

History

Collect data related to the causes and risk factors for gastritis and peptic ulcer disease (PUD). Question the patient about factors that can influence the development of PUD, including alcohol intake and tobacco use. Note if certain foods such as tomatoes or caffeinated beverages precipitate or worsen symptoms. Information regarding actual or perceived daily stressors should also be obtained.

A history of current or past medical conditions focuses on GI problems, particularly any history of diagnosis or treatment for *H. pylori* infection. Review all prescription and OTC drugs that the patient is taking. Specifically inquire whether the patient is taking corticosteroids, chemotherapy, aspirin, or other NSAIDs.

Also ask whether he or she has ever undergone radiation treatments. Assess whether the patient has had any GI surgeries, especially a partial gastrectomy, which can cause chronic gastritis.

A history of GI upset, pain and its relationship to eating and sleep patterns, and actions taken to relieve pain are also important. Inquire about any changes in the character of the pain because this may signal the development of complications. For example, if pain that was once intermittent and relieved by food and antacids becomes constant and radiates to the back or upper quadrant, the patient may have ulcer perforation. However, many people with active duodenal or gastric ulcers report having no ulcer symptoms.

Physical Assessment/Clinical Manifestations

Physical assessment findings may reveal epigastric tenderness, usually located at the midline between the umbilicus and the xiphoid process. *If perforation into the peritoneal cavity is present, the patient has a rigid, boardlike abdomen accompanied by rebound tenderness.* Initially, auscultation of the abdomen may reveal hyperactive bowel sounds, but these may diminish with progression of the disorder.

Dyspepsia *(indigestion), which is discomfort in the epigastrium or upper abdomen, is the most commonly reported symptom associated with PUD.* It is typically described as sharp, burning, or gnawing. Some patients may perceive discomfort as a sensation of abdominal pressure or of fullness or hunger. Specific differences between gastric and duodenal ulcers are listed in Table 58-2.

Gastric ulcer pain often occurs in the upper epigastrium with localization to the left of the midline and is aggravated by food. *Duodenal* ulcer pain is usually located to the right of the epigastrium. The pain associated with a duodenal ulcer occurs 90 minutes to 3 hours *after* eating and often awakens the patient at night. Pain may also be exacerbated (made worse) by certain foods (e.g., tomatoes, hot spices, fried foods, onions, alcohol, caffeine drinks) and certain drugs (e.g., aspirin, other NSAIDs, corticosteroids). Perform a comprehensive pain assessment that includes:

- Location
- Characteristics
- Onset/duration
- Frequency
- Quality
- Severity
- All precipitating and alleviating factors

Vomiting may be a symptom accompanying ulcer disease, most commonly with pyloric sphincter dysfunction. It results from gastric stasis associated with pyloric obstruction. Appetite is generally maintained in patients with a peptic ulcer unless pyloric obstruction is present.

To assess for fluid volume deficit that occurs from bleeding, take orthostatic vital signs of all patients suspected of having PUD. Orthostatic changes are present if there is a decrease of more than 20 mm Hg in systolic blood pressure, a decrease of 10 mm Hg in diastolic blood pressure, and/or an increase in pulse when the patient rises from a lying to an erect (sitting or, if possible, standing) position. Also assess for dizziness, especially when the patient is upright, because this is a symptom of fluid volume deficit. This symptom is most common in older adults.

Psychosocial Assessment

Assess the impact of ulcer disease on the patient's lifestyle, occupation, family, and social and leisure activities. Evaluate the impact that lifestyle changes will have on the patient and family. This assessment may reveal information about the patient's ability to adhere to the prescribed treatment regimen and to obtain the needed social support to alter his or her lifestyle.

Laboratory Assessment

Hemoglobin and hematocrit values may be low, indicating bleeding. The stool specimen may be positive for occult (not seen) blood if bleeding is present. Testing methods for *H. pylori* are described on p. 1267 in the discussion of Laboratory Assessment in the Gastritis section.

Imaging Assessment

In the past, upper GI series with barium follow-through were the typical tests for diagnosing peptic ulcers. However, these procedures are not the most reliable ways to visualize any le-

TABLE 58-2 Differential Features of Gastric and Duodenal Ulcers

Feature	Gastric Ulcer	Duodenal Ulcer
Age	Usually 50 yr or older	Usually 50 yr or older
Gender	Male/female ratio of 1.1:1	Male/female ratio of 1:1
Blood group	No differentiation	Most often type O
General nourishment	May be malnourished	Usually well nourished
Stomach acid production	Normal secretion or hyposecretion	Hypersecretion
Occurrence	Mucosa exposed to acid-pepsin secretion	Mucosa exposed to acid-pepsin secretion
Clinical course	Healing and recurrence	Healing and recurrence
Pain	Occurs 30-60 min after a meal; at night: rarely	Occurs $1^1/_2$-3 hr after a meal; at night: often awakens patient between 1 and 2 AM
	Worsened by ingestion of food	Relieved by ingestion of food
Response to treatment	Healing with appropriate therapy	Healing with appropriate therapy
Hemorrhage	Hematemesis more common than melena	Melena more common than hematemesis
Malignant change	Perhaps in less than 10%	Rare
Recurrence	Tends to heal and recurs often in the same location	60% recur within 1 yr; 90% recur within 2 yr
Surrounding mucosa	Atrophic gastritis	No gastritis

sions. If perforation is suspected, the health care provider may request a chest and abdomen x-ray series.

Other Diagnostic Assessment

The major diagnostic test for PUD is esophagogastroduodenoscopy (EGD), which is the most accurate means of establishing a diagnosis. Direct visualization of the ulcer crater by EGD allows the health care provider to take specimens for *H. pylori* testing and for biopsy and cytologic studies for ruling out gastric cancer. EGD may be repeated at 4- to 6-week intervals while the health care provider evaluates the progress of healing in response to therapy. Chapter 55 describes this test in more detail.

Analysis

Common Nursing Diagnoses and Collaborative Problems

The priority nursing diagnosis for patients with peptic ulcer disease (PUD) is Acute Pain or Chronic Pain related to physical (gastric and/or duodenal mucosal) injury.

The most important collaborative problem is Potential for Gastrointestinal (GI) Bleeding.

Additional Nursing Diagnoses and Collaborative Problems

In addition to the common nursing diagnosis and collaborative problem, patients with PUD may have these diagnoses:

- Deficient Knowledge related to management of PUD
- Imbalanced Nutrition: Less Than Body Requirements related to anorexia, nausea, or diet constraints
- Disturbed Sleep Pattern related to discomfort
- Risk for Falls related to orthostatic hypotension
- Fatigue related to loss of blood and chronic illness
- Nausea and/or Vomiting related to GI irritation
- Ineffective Health Maintenance related to lack of knowledge regarding health practices to prevent ulcer formation
- Fear related to threat to well-being or potential death

Possible collaborative problems include:

- Potential for Shock
- Potential for Metabolic Alkalosis

Planning and Implementation

Acute Pain; Chronic Pain

NOC **Planning: Expected Outcomes.** PUD causes significant discomfort that impacts many aspects of daily living. The patient with this disease is expected to:

- Report that pain is controlled.
- Use available resources to manage pain.
- Use previous pain-relief measures.
- Report uncontrolled symptoms to health care professionals.

Interventions. Interventions to manage pain related to PUD include specific ulcer therapy and nutrition changes. One of the primary purposes for drug therapy is to reduce or eliminate pain by eliminating *H. pylori* infection and promoting healing of gastric mucosa.

Teach the patient to eliminate irritants that can precipitate or increase pain from ulcer disease. Measures to promote adequate rest and sleep may be necessary because ulcer pain can cause the patient to awaken.

Drug Therapy. The primary purposes of drug therapy in the treatment of PUD are to (1) provide pain relief, (2) eliminate *H. pylori* infection, (3) heal ulcerations, and (4) prevent recurrence. Several different regimens can be used. In selecting a therapeutic drug regimen, the health care provider must consider the efficacy of the treatment, the anticipated side effects, the ability of the patient to adhere to the regimen, and the cost of the treatment.

Although numerous drugs have been evaluated for the treatment of *H. pylori* infection, no single agent has been used successfully against the organism. A common drug regimen for *H. pylori* infection is triple therapy, which includes a proton pump inhibitor (PPI) such as lansoprazole (Prevacid) plus two antibiotics such as metronidazole (Flagyl, Novonidazol♣) and tetracycline (Ala-Tet, Panmycin, Nu-Tetra♣) or clarithromycin (Biaxin, Biaxin XL) and amoxicillin (Amoxil, Amoxi♣) for 7 to 14 days. Bismuth subsalicylates such as Pepto-Bismol are used less commonly today to treat these bacteria.

Hyposecretory drugs reduce gastric acid secretions and are therefore used for both PUD and gastritis management. These drugs include proton pump inhibitors, H_2-receptor antagonists, and prostaglandin analogues (see Chart 58-3).

Proton pump inhibitors (PPIs) are the drug class of choice for treating patients with acid-related disorders. Omeprazole (Prilosec), lansoprazole (Prevacid), rabeprazole (Aciphex), pantoprazole (Protonix), and esomeprazole magnesium (Nexium) suppress the H,K–ATPase enzyme system of gastric acid production. Omeprazole, lansoprazole, and esomeprazole are each available as delayed-release capsules designed to release their contents after they pass through the stomach. Omeprazole and lansoprazole may be dissolved in a sodium bicarbonate solution and given through any feeding tube. Bicarbonate protects the dissolved omeprazole and lansoprazole granules in gastric acid. Therefore the drugs are still absorbed correctly. These capsules can also be opened. The enteric-coated capsules can be put in apple juice or orange juice and given through a large-bore feeding tube. Rabeprazole (Aciphex) and pantoprazole (Protonix) are enteric-coated tablets that quickly dissolve after the tablet has moved through the stomach and should not be crushed before giving them. Pantoprazole (Protonix) is also available in an IV form, which may be helpful for patients who are NPO.

H_2-receptor antagonists are drugs that block histamine-stimulated gastric secretions. These drugs may also be used for indigestion and gastritis. Lower-dose forms are available in over-the-counter (OTC) products. H_2-receptor antagonists block the action of the H_2 receptors of the parietal cells, thus inhibiting gastric acid secretion. The most common drugs are ranitidine (Zantac), famotidine (Pepcid), and nizatidine (Axid). These drugs are typically administered in a single dose at bedtime and are used for 4 to 6 weeks in combination with other therapy.

Prostaglandins are naturally abundant in the GI tract. *Prostaglandin analogues* are effective in the treatment of duodenal ulcers. They reduce gastric acid secretion and enhance gastric mucosal resistance to tissue injury. Misoprostol (Cytotec), the most commonly used drug in this category, *helps prevent* NSAID-induced ulcers. Some NSAIDs are being manufactured in combination with misoprostol. A significant adverse effect of this drug is uterine contraction. Therefore its use is contraindicated in pregnant women. Teach women that the drug makes menstrual cramps worse.

Antacids buffer gastric acid and prevent the formation of pepsin. They have demonstrated effectiveness in accelerating the healing of duodenal ulcers. Liquid suspensions are the most therapeutic form, but tablets may be more convenient and enhance adherence. The most widely used preparations are mixtures of aluminum hydroxide and magnesium hydroxide. This combination overcomes the unpleasant GI side effects of either of these preparations when used alone. Mylanta and Maalox are examples of this type of combination antacid formulation. The aluminum and magnesium hydroxide combination products neutralize well at small doses. These products must be administered cautiously to patients with renal impairment because elimination is reduced and excessive amounts are retained in the body.

Teach the patient that to achieve a therapeutic effect, sufficient antacid must be ingested to neutralize the hourly production of acid. For optimal effect, take antacids about 2 hours after meals to reduce the hydrogen ion load in the duodenum. Antacids may be effective from 30 minutes to 3 hours after ingestion. If taken on an empty stomach, they are quickly evacuated. Thus the neutralizing effect is reduced. Calcium carbonate (Tums) is a potent antacid, but it triggers gastrin release, causing a rebound acid secretion. Therefore its use in acid inhibition is not recommended.

Antacids can interact with certain drugs such as phenytoin (Dilantin), tetracycline (Ala-Tet, Nu-Tetra🍁), and ketoconazole (Nizoral) and interfere with their effectiveness. Ask what other drugs the patient is using before a specific antacid is prescribed. Other drugs are given 1 to 2 hours before or after the antacid. Inform the patient that flavored antacids, especially wintergreen, should be avoided. The flavoring increases the emptying time of the stomach. Thus the desired effect of the antacid is negated.

Teach the patient with past or present heart failure to avoid antacids with high sodium content, such as aluminum hydroxide, magnesium hydroxide, sodium bicarbonate, and simethicone combination products (Gelusil and Mylanta). Magaldrate (Riopan) has the lowest sodium concentration.

Sucralfate (Carafate) is a *mucosal barrier fortifier* (protector) that forms complexes with proteins at the base of a peptic ulcer. This protective coat prevents further digestive action of both acid and pepsin. Sucralfate does not inhibit acid secretion. Rather, it binds bile acids and pepsins, reducing injury from these substances. The drug may be used in conjunction with H_2-receptor antagonists and antacids but should not be administered within 1 hour of the antacid. Sucralfate is given on an empty stomach 1 hour before each meal and at bedtime. The main side effect of this drug is constipation.

Nutrition Therapy. The value of nutrition in the management of ulcer disease is controversial. There is no evidence that dietary restriction reduces gastric acid secretion or promotes tissue healing, although a bland diet may assist in relieving symptoms. Food itself acts as an antacid by neutralizing gastric acid for 30 to 60 minutes. An increased rate of gastric acid secretion, called *rebound,* may follow. If nutrition therapy is used, it may be directed toward neutralizing acid and reducing hypermotility, which may alleviate symptoms.

Teach the patient to avoid substances that increase gastric acid secretion. This includes caffeine-containing beverages (coffee, tea, cola). Both caffeinated and decaffeinated coffees should be avoided, because coffee contains peptides that stimulate gastrin release.

In collaboration with the nutritionist, teach the patient to exclude any foods that cause discomfort. A bland, nonirritating diet is recommended during the acute symptomatic phase. Bedtime snacks are avoided because they may stimulate gastric acid secretion. Eating six smaller daily meals may help, but this regimen is no longer a regular part of therapy. No evidence supports the theory that eating six daily meals promotes healing of the ulcer. This practice may actually stimulate gastric acid secretion. Patients should avoid alcohol and tobacco because of their stimulatory effects on gastric acid secretion.

Complementary and Alternative Therapies. Teach patients about complementary and alternative therapies that can reduce stress, including hypnosis and imagery. For example, the use of yoga and meditation techniques has demonstrated a beneficial effect on anxiety disorders. Many have suggested that GI disorders result from the dysfunction of both the GI tract itself and the brain. This means that emotional stress is thought to worsen GI disorders such as peptic ulcer disease. Yoga is thought to alter the activities of the central and autonomic nervous systems.

Many herbs, such as powders of slippery elm and marshmallow root, quercetin, and licorice, are used commonly by patients with gastritis and PUD. These herbs are thought to heal inflamed tissue and increase blood flow to the gastric mucosa. Other substances include zinc, vitamin C, essential fatty acids, acidophilus, vitamins E and A, and glutamine. All of these substances enhance healing. Table 58-1 provides a more complete list of therapies that have been used. Many of them have been scientifically supported in animal studies. Additional research using humans is being conducted.

Potential for Gastrointestinal Bleeding

Planning: Expected Outcomes. Fluid volume loss secondary to the development of complications is a risk associated with PUD. Blood loss due to hemorrhage results in high morbidity and mortality. Fluid volume loss secondary to vomiting can lead to dehydration and electrolyte imbalances. The patient with peptic ulcer disease (PUD) is expected to maintain vascular, cellular, and intracellular perfusion. Indicators include that the patient will:

- Have intact mental status
- Have stable blood pressure
- Have warm, dry skin
- Void at least 30 mL/hr of urine per hour

Interventions. Monitoring and early recognition of complications are critical to the successful management of PUD. Interventions aimed at managing complications associated with PUD include prevention and/or management of bleeding, perforation, and gastric outlet obstruction. In some cases, surgical treatment of complications becomes necessary.

Nonsurgical Management. Because prevention or early detection of complications is needed to obtain a positive clinical outcome, monitor the patient carefully and immediately report changes to the health care provider. The type of nonsurgical intervention selected will depend on the type and severity of the complication.

Emergency: upper GI bleeding. *The patient who is actively bleeding has a life-threatening emergency. He or she needs supportive therapy to prevent hypovolemic shock and possible death. The first priority for care is to maintain airway, breathing, and circulation (ABCs).* Provide oxygen and other ventilatory support as needed. Start two large-bore IV lines for replacing fluids and blood. Monitor vital signs, hematocrit, and oxygen saturation (Chart 58-5).

The purpose of managing hypovolemia is to expand intravascular fluid in a patient who is volume depleted. Carefully

Chart 58-5 NIC INTERVENTION ACTIVITIES

The Patient with Peptic Ulcer Disease

Hypovolemia Management: *Expansion of intravascular fluid volume in a patient who is volume depleted*

- Monitor vital signs, as appropriate.
- Monitor fluid status, including intake and output, as appropriate.
- Monitor for fluid loss (e.g., bleeding, vomiting, diarrhea, perspiration, and tachypnea).
- Arrange availability of blood products for transfusion, if necessary.
- Administer blood products (e.g., platelets and fresh frozen plasma), as appropriate.
- Monitor for blood reaction, if appropriate.

Bleeding Reduction: *Gastrointestinal: Limitation of the amount of blood loss from the upper and lower gastrointestinal tract and related complications*

- Monitor for signs and symptoms of persistent bleeding (e.g., check all secretions for frank or occult blood).
- Hematest all excretions and observe for blood loss in emesis, sputum, feces, urine, NG tube drainage, and wound drainage, as appropriate.
- Document color, amount, and character of stools.
- Monitor coagulation studies and complete blood count (CBC) with WBC differential.
- Insert nasogastric tube to suction and monitor secretions, if appropriate.
- Perform nasogastric lavage, as appropriate.
- Avoid extremes in gastric pH level by administration of appropriate medication (e.g., histamine-blocking agent).
- Instruct the patient and/or family on the need for blood replacement, as appropriate.
- Instruct the patient and/or family to avoid the use of anti-inflammatory medications (e.g., aspirin and ibuprofen).

NIC intervention activities selected from Bulechek, G.M., Butcher, H.K., & McCloskey Dochterman, J. (Eds.). (2008). *Nursing interventions classification (NIC)* (5th ed.). St. Louis: Mosby. No part of this work is to be altered without prior written permission from the Publisher.
WBC, White blood cell.

monitor the patient's fluid status, including intake and output. *Fluid replacement in older adults should be closely monitored to prevent fluid overload.* Serum electrolytes are also assessed because depletions from vomiting or nasogastric suctioning must be replaced. Volume replacement with isotonic solutions (e.g., 0.9% normal saline solution, lactated Ringer's solution) should be started immediately. The health care provider may prescribe blood products such as packed red blood cells to expand volume and correct a low complete blood count (CBC). For patients with active bleeding, fresh frozen plasma may be given if the prothrombin time is 1.5 times higher than the midrange control value.

Monitor the patient's hematocrit, hemoglobin, and coagulation studies for changes from the baseline measurements. With mild bleeding (less than 500 mL), slight feelings of weakness and mild perspiration may be present. When blood loss exceeds 1 L/24 hr, manifestations of shock may occur, such as hypotension, chills, palpitations, diaphoresis, and a weak, thready pulse.

A combination of several different treatments, including nasogastric (NG) tube placement and lavage, endoscopic therapy, and acid suppression, can be used to control acute bleeding and prevent rebleeding. If the patient is actively bleeding at home, he or she is usually admitted to the emergency department for GI lavage. If the patient is already a patient in the hospital, lavage can be done at the bedside. After the bleeding has stopped, H_2-receptor antagonists, proton pump inhibitors, and antacids are the primary drugs used.

Nasogastric tube placement and lavage. Upper GI bleeding may require the health care provider or nurse to insert a large-bore nasogastric tube (NGT) to:

- Determine the presence or absence of blood in the stomach
- Assess the rate of bleeding
- Prevent gastric dilation
- Administer lavage

Patients who have upper GI bleeding often have discomfort, nausea, and/or vomiting, which can be worsened by inserting an NGT. Therefore several methods are available to prevent these problems, such as applying lidocaine gel, spray, or nebulized solution before the tube is placed. As another option, IV metoclopramide (Reglan, Maxeran♣) may be given to decrease these symptoms while the tube is inserted (Ozucelik et al., 2005). Some health care providers do not use any of these methods to promote patient comfort, even though they have been shown to be effective.

Once the NGT is placed, proper positioning of the tube is confirmed by x-ray examination. Irrigate the NGT to maintain its patency and prevent obstruction with clotted blood (Chart 58-6).

Gastric lavage requires the insertion of a large-bore NG tube with instillation of a room-temperature solution in volumes of 200 to 300 mL. There is no evidence that sterile saline or water is better than tap water for this procedure. Follow agency protocol for the solution that is required. The solution and blood are repeatedly withdrawn manually until returns are clear or light pink and without clots. Instruct the patient to lie on the left side during this procedure to limit the flow of the lavage solution out of the stomach. The NGT may remain in place for a few days or be removed after lavage.

Endoscopic therapy. Endoscopic therapy via an esophagogastroduodenoscopy (EGD) can assist in achieving homeostasis during an acute bleeding episode. The primary methods of endoscopic therapy are (1) thermal contact using a heater probe or multi-electrocoagulation, (2) injection of the bleeding site with diluted epinephrine, and (3) clipping the bleeding vessel with a mechanical clip. Other methods are also available and are effective in achieving blood clot formation. Thermal contact and injection with epinephrine are most commonly used. Laser therapy is costly and therefore is used less often. Clipping is used mostly when a bleeding vessel is visible. Generally, endoscopic therapy is beneficial for patients with active bleeding. However, ulcers that continue to bleed or continue to rebleed despite endoscopic therapy may require surgical repair. Sometimes endoscopists (physicians) may scope a patient daily during an acute bleed of a peptic ulcer to

Chart 58-6 BEST PRACTICE FOR PATIENT SAFETY & QUALITY CARE

Nasogastric Tubes

1. Inform the patient about the procedure and its potential discomfort.
2. Position the patient with pillows behind the shoulders.
3. Lubricate the tube with a water-soluble lubricant.
4. Measure the length of the tube to be passed:
   a. Measure from the bridge of the nose to the earlobe to the xiphoid process.
   b. Indicate this length with a piece of tape on the tube.

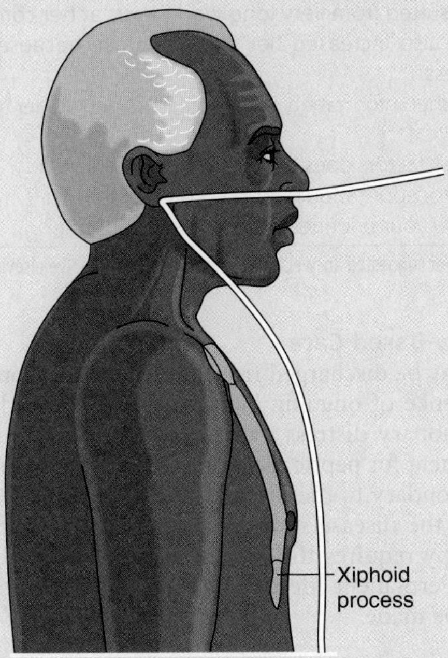
Xiphoid process

5. Determine which nostril is more patent.
6. Encourage the patient to swallow or drink water if the level of consciousness and treatment plan permit.
7. Insert the tube:
   a. Pass the tube gently into the nasopharynx. Ask the patient to swallow repeatedly while the tube is advanced.
   b. If resistance is met, rotate the tube slowly, aiming downward and toward the closer ear.
   c. In the intubated or semiconscious patient, flex the head toward the chest while passing the tube.
8. Withdraw the tube immediately if any change is noted in respiratory status.
9. Test for tube placement by using these techniques:
   a. Obtain a sample of the gastric contents by aspirating with a 50-mL catheter-tipped syringe.
   b. Test the pH of the gastric contents (should be between 1 and 3.5).
   c. Obtain a request for an x-ray study to confirm placement.
10. Connect the tube to suction at low pressure:
    a. The Levin tube is connected to intermittent low suction.
    b. The Salem sump or Anderson tube is connected to continuous low suction.
11. Secure the tube to the patient's nose and to his or her gown:
    a. Tie a slipknot around the tube with a rubber band.
    b. Pin a rubber band to the gown.
12. Check intake and output every 4 hr or more often, as indicated.
13. Observe the patient for nausea, vomiting, abdominal fullness, or distention.
14. If irrigation is indicated, use only a normal saline solution.
15. Observe the patient for alterations in fluid and electrolyte balance.
16. If indicated, instruct the patient about movement that will not dislodge the tube and cause nasal irritation.
17. Remove the tape securing the tube to the nose daily and PRN to clean skin; reapply tape.

assess and possibly re-treat the ulcer if it continues to bleed or begins bleeding again. This regimen may help prevent the patient from having surgery.

Pre-EGD nursing care involves inserting one or two large-bore IV catheters if they are not in place. A large catheter allows the patient to receive IV moderate sedation (e.g., midazolam [Versed] and meperidine [Demerol]) and possibly a blood transfusion. Keep the patient NPO 6 hours before the procedure. This prevents the risk for aspiration and allows the endoscopist to view and treat the ulcer. A patient must sign a consent form before the EGD *after* the physician informs him or her about the procedure. During the EGD, a specialized endoscopy nurse and technician assist the physician with the procedure. Post-EGD nursing care involves checking the vital signs, heart rhythm, and oxygen saturation frequently until they return to baseline. In addition, frequently assess the patient's ability to swallow saliva. The patient's gag reflex may initially be absent after an EGD because of anesthetizing (numbing) the throat with a spray before the procedure. *Do not resume a preprocedure diet until the gag reflex is intact!*

Acid suppression. *Aggressive acid suppression is used to prevent rebleeding.* When acute bleeding is stopped and clot formation has taken place within the ulcer crater, the clot remains in contact with gastric contents. Acid-suppressive agents are used to stabilize the clot by raising the pH level of gastric contents. Several types of drugs are used. H_2-receptor antagonists prevent acid from being produced by parietal cells. Proton pump inhibitors prevent the transport of acid across the parietal cell membrane, whereas antacids buffer acid produced in the stomach.

Octreotide (Sandostatin) may also be given IV and has shown excellent results. It is a synthetic GI hormone (somatostatin analogue) that suppresses gastric acid secretion by decreasing the production of gastrin and other GI substances.

Nonsurgical interventions are also used to prevent peritonitis from GI contents that have entered the peritoneum. *Perforation* is managed by immediately replacing fluid, blood, and electrolytes, administering antibiotics, and keeping the patient NPO. Maintain nasogastric suction to drain gastric secretions and thus prevent further peritoneal spillage. Carefully monitor intake and output and check vital signs at least hourly. Monitor the patient for clinical manifestations of septic shock, such as fever, pain, tachycardia, lethargy, or anxiety.

Pyloric obstruction is caused by edema, spasm, or scar tissue. Symptoms of obstruction related to difficulty in emptying the stomach include feelings of fullness, distention, or nausea after eating, as well as vomiting copious amounts of undigested food.

Treatment of obstruction is directed toward restoring fluid and electrolyte balance and decompressing the dilated stomach. Obstruction related to edema and spasm generally responds to medical therapy. First, the stomach must be decompressed with nasogastric suction. Next, interventions are directed at correcting metabolic alkalosis and dehydration. The NGT is clamped after about 72 hours. Check the patient for retention of gastric contents. If the amount retained is not more than 50 mL in 30 minutes, the health care provider may allow oral fluids. In some cases, surgical intervention may be required to treat PUD.

Surgical Management. Evidence-based guidelines for the treatment of PUD that include *H. pylori* treatment and the development of nonsurgical means of controlling bleeding have led to a decline in the need for surgical intervention. In PUD, surgical intervention may be used to:

- Treat patients who do not respond to medical therapy
- Treat a surgical emergency that develops as a complication of PUD

Two general surgical approaches are available for PUD—minimally invasive surgery and conventional open surgery.

Minimally invasive surgery (MIS) via laparoscopy (a type of endoscope) is occasionally used to remove a chronic gastric ulcer or treat hemorrhage from perforation. Several small incisions allow access to the stomach and duodenum. The patient may have partial stomach removal (subtotal gastrectomy), pyloroplasty (to open the pylorus) and/or a vagotomy (vagus nerve cutting) to control acid secretion (Fig. 58-4). The advantages of MIS over traditional procedures include a shorter hospital stay, fewer complications, less pain, and better, quicker recovery. MIS is discussed in more detail in Chapter 17. Conventional surgery is performed using an open approach. This procedure is discussed on p. 1281 in the discussion of Surgical Management in the Gastric Cancer section.

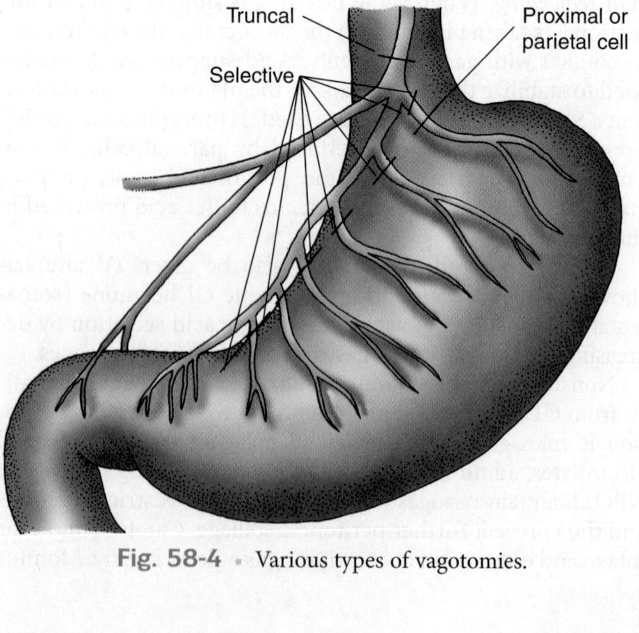
Truncal
Proximal or parietal cell
Selective

Fig. 58-4 • Various types of vagotomies.

DECISION-MAKING CHALLENGE
Critical Rescue

A 46-year-old woman is admitted to the emergency department with severe epigastric pain and hematemesis. She states that she is a newly employed director of the nursing department in a local college. Her husband tells you that she has been under a lot of stress with the new job and has been taking ibuprofen for neck pain that resulted from very long work hours at her computer. The patient has also increased her alcohol intake because of her increased stress.

1. What other information do you need as part of her assessment?
2. What risk factors does she have for her GI bleeding?
3. What procedure should you prepare for and why?
4. What are your priorities for her care at this time?

evolve For suggested answer guidelines, go to http://evolve.elsevier.com/Iggy/.

Community-Based Care

Patients may be discharged from the hospital as long as there is no evidence of ongoing bleeding, orthostatic changes, or cardiopulmonary distress or compromise. Those discharged after treatment for peptic ulcer disease (PUD) and/or complications secondary to the disease must face several challenges to manage the disease successfully. Long-term adherence to drug therapy requires the patient to take several oral drugs each day. Permanent lifestyle alterations in nutrition habits must also be made.

Home Care Management

Most patients are discharged to the home to continue their recovery. Those who have had major surgery or have had complications, such as hemorrhage, may require one or two visits from a home care nurse to assess clinical progress, especially if the patient is an older adult (Chart 58-7).

Health Teaching

The primary focus of home care preparation is patient and family teaching regarding risk factors for the recurrence of PUD. Teach them how to recognize new complications and what to do if they occur, especially abdominal pain; nausea and vomiting; black, tarry stools; and weakness or dizziness.

Instruct the patient and family about risk factors for peptic ulcers. Help them plan ways to make needed lifestyle changes. For postsurgical patients, especially those who have undergone partial stomach removal, a smaller meal may be required. Other postoperative nutrition changes are described on p. 1287 in the discussion of Health Teaching in the Gastric Cancer section.

Teach the patient to avoid any OTC product containing aspirin or other NSAID. Emphasize the importance of adhering to the treatment regimen for eliminating *H. pylori* infection and healing the ulcer. Emphasize the importance of keeping all follow-up appointments. Help the patient identify situations that cause stress, describe feelings during stressful situations, and develop a plan for coping with stressors. Encourage the patient to learn and use relaxation techniques, such as exercise, biofeedback, humor, and imagery. Psychotherapy may be indicated to cope with excessive anxiety or stress.

Chart 58-7 HOME CARE ASSESSMENT

The Patient with Ulcer Disease

Assess gastrointestinal and cardiovascular status, including:
- Vital signs, including orthostatic vital signs
- Skin color
- Presence of abdominal pain (location, severity, character, duration, precipitating factors, and relief measures)
- Character, color, and consistency of stools
- Changes in bowel elimination pattern
- Hemoglobin and hematocrit
- Bowel sounds; palpate for areas of tenderness

Assess nutritional status, including:
- Dietary patterns and habits
- Intake of caffeine and alcohol
- Relationship of food to symptoms

Assess medication history:
- Use of steroids
- Use of NSAIDs
- Use of over-the-counter medications

Assess patient's coping style:
- Recent stressors
- Past coping style

Assess patient's understanding of illness and ability to adhere to the therapeutic regimen:
- Symptoms to report to health care provider
- Expected and side effects of medications
- Food and drug interactions
- Need for smoking cessation

Health Care Resources

Refer the patient and family to the National Digestive Diseases Information Clearinghouse (www.acg.gi.org/patients/gitract/nddic.asp). This group provides information and support to patients who have digestive disorders.

Evaluation: Outcomes

Evaluate the care of the patient with peptic ulcer disease (PUD) on the basis of the identified nursing diagnoses and collaborative problems. The expected outcomes are that the patient:

- Does not have active disease or complications
- Takes personal actions to control pain
- Adheres to the drug regimen and lifestyle changes to prevent recurrence and heal the ulcer

Specific indicators for these outcomes are listed for each nursing diagnosis and collaborative problem under the Planning and Implementation section (see earlier).

ZOLLINGER-ELLISON SYNDROME

Zollinger-Ellison syndrome (ZES) is a rare disease that is manifested by upper GI tract ulceration, increased gastric acid secretion, and one or more duodenal or pancreatic tumors, called **gastrinomas.** About two thirds of these tumors are malignant. Although most grow slowly, a small portion of patients have tumors that develop rapidly and metastasize widely. Metastasis occurs mainly in the liver and regional lymph nodes.

Pathophysiology

ZES is caused by gastrin-secreting tumors that stimulate the acid-secreting cells of the stomach to maximal activity. This large quantity of acid causes GI ulceration. In the early course of the disease, symptoms are similar to those of peptic ulcer disease (PUD). However, these symptoms tend to progress and respond poorly to traditional ulcer therapy. Diarrhea occurs in almost half of patients. It may be associated with large amounts of hydrochloric acid secreted into the proximal duodenum. **Steatorrhea** (an excessive amount of fat in the feces) results from the inactivation of pancreatic lipase secondary to the large concentrations of acid and decreased amounts of bile acids.

In some patients, gastrinoma results from an autosomal dominant disorder called *multiple endocrine neoplasia type 1 (MEN-1) syndrome,* in which there is a mutation in the MEN-1 suppressive gene. Gastrinomas contain multiple hormones, but adrenocorticotropic hormone (ACTH) is most commonly found (McCance & Huether, 2006).

Patient-Centered Collaborative Care

Patients may report PUD symptoms and may have diarrhea and/or steatorrhea. Ask whether any relatives have had ZES. Radiographic and endoscopic findings for ZES are similar to those for PUD. *However, infection with H. pylori is usually absent.* The diagnosis is usually made by radioimmunoassay studies that reveal *increased serum gastrin levels* in conjunction with the clinical features of the disease.

The aim of therapy is to suppress acid secretion to control symptoms. The proton pump inhibitors, such as lansoprazole (Prevacid) and omeprazole (Prilosec, Losec♣), are the drugs of choice to reduce gastric acid secretion and heal the ulcers. High doses of H_2-receptor antagonists such as ranitidine (Zantac) are also effective in reducing gastric acid and providing symptom relief.

The tumor requires complete surgical resection as a curative treatment. In some patients, a radical pancreaticoduodenectomy (Whipple procedure) is performed. Chapter 62 in the discussion of Surgical Management in the Pancreatic Cancer section describes this procedure and nursing care in detail. Patients with aggressive disease can also be treated with chemotherapeutic agents such as 5-fluorouracil, doxorubicin, and streptozocin to reduce tumor size and control symptoms before surgery. Octreotide (Sandostatin) has also been used with success.

GASTRIC CANCER

Most cancers of the stomach are adenocarcinomas. This type of cancer develops in the mucosal cells that form the innermost lining of any portion or all of the stomach. Often there are no symptoms in the early stages, and the disease is advanced when detected.

Pathophysiology

Gastric cancer usually begins in the glands of the stomach mucosa. Atrophic gastritis and intestinal metaplasia (abnormal tissue development) are precancerous conditions. Inadequate acid secretion in patients with atrophic gastritis creates an alkaline environment that allows bacteria, especially *Helicobacter pylori (H. pylori),* to multiply and act on nitrates in food. Nitrates interact with amino acids in the stomach to form carcinogenic nitrosamines. These substances are converted to nitrites, which are a major risk factor for gastric cancer (McCance & Huether, 2006).

Gastric cancers spread by direct extension through the gastric wall and into regional lymphatics, which carry tumor deposits to lymph nodes. Direct invasion of and adherence to adjacent organs (e.g., the liver, pancreas, and transverse colon) may also result. Hematogenous spread via the portal vein to the liver and via the systemic circulation to the lungs and bones is the most common mode of metastasis. Peritoneal seeding of cancer cells from the tumor areas to the omentum, peritoneum, ovary, and pelvic cul-de-sac can also occur.

In people with *advanced* gastric cancer, there is invasion of the muscularis (stomach muscle) or beyond. These lesions are not cured by surgical resection. The overall 5-year survival rate of people with stomach cancer in the United States is poor because most patients have no symptoms until the disease advances.

Etiology and Genetic Risk

Infection with H. pylori is the largest risk factor for gastric cancer because it carries the cytotoxin-associated antigen A (CagA) gene. Patients with pernicious anemia, gastric polyps, chronic atrophic gastritis, and **achlorhydria** (absence of secretion of hydrochloric acid) are two to three times more likely to develop gastric cancer.

The disease also seems to be positively correlated with eating pickled foods, salted fish, salted meat, and nitrates from processed foods, as well as a high consumption of salt. The ingestion of these foods over a long period can lead to atrophic gastritis, a precancerous condition. A low intake of fruits and vegetables is also a risk factor for cancer (McCance & Huether, 2006).

Genetic factors play a role in the development of gastric cancer. Interleukin-1 (IL-1) genotypes are associated with the disease, although the specific genotypes vary when comparing Euro-Americans with Asian Americans. Gastric cancer can also be related to mutations in repair genes *MLH1* and *MSH2*. These genes are generally related to an increased risk for colorectal cancer, specifically hereditary nonpolyposis colon cancer (HNPCC). They also have been related to an increased risk for gastric, ovarian, biliary tract, urinary, and endometrial cancers. This is also inherited in an autosomal dominant process (McCance & Huether, 2006).

Gastric surgery seems to increase the risk for gastric cancer because of the eventual development of atrophic gastritis, which results in changes to the mucosa. Patients with Barrett's esophagus from prolonged or severe gastroesophageal reflux disease (GERD) have an increased risk for cancer in the cardia (at the point where the stomach connects to the esophagus).

Incidence/Prevalence

The National Cancer Institute estimated that in 2008, about 22,000 new cases of gastric cancer were diagnosed in the United States and almost 12,100 people died from the disease. Men appear to have a slightly greater risk than women. Asians and Asian Americans are at an especially high risk because of preferences for salted and smoked fish. Most people with diagnosed stomach cancer are in their 60s and 70s (www.cancer.gov).

Health Promotion and Maintenance

Teach patients with gastritis and/or *H. pylori* infection to follow the treatment regimen to ensure that gastritis heals and *H. pylori* infection is eliminated. *Teach about eating a well-balanced diet and limiting pickled foods, salted foods, and processed foods to help prevent gastric cancer.* Alcohol and tobacco consumption should be avoided, although their role in developing gastric cancer is not known. Patients with a family history of gastric cancer or colon, endometrial, biliary tract, ovarian, or urinary tract cancers should consider genetic counseling to determine whether they are more at risk for these diseases.

Patient-Centered Collaborative Care

Assessment

Question the patient about known risk factors for the development of gastric cancer. Ask about preferred foods, especially pickled, salted, or smoked foods. Ask about tobacco and alcohol use. Inquire whether the patient has ever been diagnosed with or treated for *H. pylori* infection, gastritis, or pernicious anemia. Note whether he or she has a history of gastric surgery or polyps. Also ask whether any of the patient's immediate relatives have gastric cancer.

Although patients with *early* gastric cancer may be asymptomatic, indigestion (heartburn) and abdominal discomfort are the *most* common symptoms (Chart 58-8). These symptoms are often ignored, however, or a change in diet or use of antacids relieves them. As the tumor grows, these symptoms become more severe and do not respond to nutrition changes or antacids. Epigastric or back pain is also an early symptom that may go unrecognized.

In *advanced* gastric cancer, progressive weight loss, nausea, and vomiting can occur. Vomiting represents pronounced dilation, thickening of the stomach wall, or pyloric obstruction. Obstructive symptoms appear earlier with tumors located near the pylorus than with fundic lesions. Patients with advanced disease may have weakness, fatigue, and anemia.

Physical assessment findings in advanced disease may be absent, or a palpable epigastric mass may suggest hepatomegaly (liver enlargement) from metastatic disease. Hard, enlarged lymph nodes in the left supraclavicular chain, left axilla, or umbilicus result from metastasis from gastric cancer.

Chart 58-8 KEY FEATURES

Early Versus Advanced Gastric Cancer

EARLY GASTRIC CANCER*
- Indigestion
- Abdominal discomfort initially relieved with antacids
- Feeling of fullness
- Epigastric, back, or retrosternal pain

ADVANCED GASTRIC CANCER
- Nausea and vomiting
- Obstructive symptoms
- Iron deficiency anemia
- Palpable epigastric mass
- Enlarged lymph nodes
- Weakness and fatigue
- Progressive weight loss
- Signs of distant metastasis
  - Virchow's nodes
  - Blumer's shelf
  - "Sister Mary Joseph nodes"
  - Krukenberg's tumor

***Note:** Many patients with early gastric cancer have no clinical manifestations.

Masses on the right suggest metastasis in the perigastric lymph nodes or liver. Signs of distant metastasis include:

- Virchow's (sentinel or signal) nodes (enlarged supraclavicular lymph nodes, especially on the left)
- Blumer's shelf, resulting from peritoneal seeding that produces a firm mass palpable on rectal or vaginal examination
- "Sister Mary Joseph nodes" (subcutaneous periumbilical deposits)
- Krukenberg's tumor (metastatic ovarian nodules)

In patients with advanced disease, anemia is evidenced by *low hematocrit* and hemoglobin values. Patients may have macrocytic or microcytic anemia associated with decreased iron or vitamin B_{12} absorption. *The stool may be positive for occult blood. Hypoalbuminemia* and *abnormal results of liver tests* (e.g., bilirubin and alkaline phosphatase) occur with advanced disease and with hepatic metastasis. *The level of carcinoembryonic antigen (CEA) is elevated in advanced cancer of the stomach.*

The health care provider uses esophagogastroduodenoscopy (EGD) with biopsy for definitive diagnosis of gastric cancer. The lesion can be viewed directly, and biopsies of all visible lesions can be obtained to determine the presence of cancer cells. During the endoscopy, an endoscopic (endoluminal) ultrasound (EUS) of the gastric mucosa can also be performed. This technology allows the health care provider to evaluate the depth of the tumor and the presence of lymph node involvement that permits more accurate staging of the disease. Computed tomography (CT), positron emission tomography (PET), and magnetic resonance imaging (MRI) scans of the chest, abdomen, and pelvis are used in determining the extent of the disease and planning therapy.

Interventions

Management of gastric cancer includes drug therapy, radiation, and/or surgery. Drug therapy and radiation may be used instead of surgery or as an adjunct before and/or after surgery.

Nonsurgical Management

The treatment of gastric cancer depends highly on the stage of the disease. Radiation and chemotherapy commonly prolong survival of patients with advanced gastric disease.

Combination *chemotherapy* using multiple cycles of cisplatin and epirubicin before and after surgery seems to have the best results (www.cancer.gov/clinicaltrials/results/MAGIC-gastric0706). S-1 chemotherapy, an oral fluoropyrimidine, has had a high success rate as adjuvant therapy in investigational studies but is not yet approved in the United States. Bone marrow suppression, nausea, and vomiting are common side effects. Chapter 24 discusses the general nursing care of patients receiving chemotherapy.

Although gastric cancers are somewhat sensitive to the effects of radiation, the use of this treatment is limited because the disease is often widely spread to other abdominal organs on diagnosis. Organs such as the liver, kidneys, and spinal cord can endure only a limited amount of radiation. Intraoperative radiotherapy (IORT) is not available at many institutions in the United States because special operative suites, equipment, and personnel are required. Radiation may be used for palliative management when surgery is not an option.

The most common side effects of radiation include impaired skin integrity, fatigue, and anorexia. Nausea, vomiting, and diarrhea may occur about 1 week after treatment is initiated and diminish a month or more after treatment ends. (See Chapter 24 for more information on radiation therapy.) The most common potential problems of IORT are hemorrhage and fistula development.

Surgical Management

Surgical resection is the preferred method for treating gastric cancer. The primary surgical procedures for the treatment of gastric cancer are total gastrectomy and subtotal (partial) gastrectomy. In early stages, laparoscopic surgery (minimally invasive surgery [MIS]) plus adjuvant chemotherapy or radiation may be curative. Patients having MIS have less pain, shorter hospital stays, rare postoperative complications, and quicker recovery. However, MIS is seldom performed because very few patients are diagnosed in the early stage of the disease.

Most patients with advanced disease are candidates for palliative surgical treatment. Metastasis in the supraclavicular lymph nodes (Virchow's nodes), inguinal lymph nodes, liver, umbilicus, or perirectal wall indicates that the opportunity for cure by resection has been lost. Palliative resection may significantly improve the quality of life for a patient suffering from obstruction, hemorrhage, or pain.

Preoperative Care. Before conventional open-approach surgery, a nasogastric tube (NGT) is inserted and connected to suction to remove secretions and empty the stomach. This allows surgery to take place without contamination of the peritoneal cavity by gastric secretions. Chart 58-6 describes the procedure for inserting the NGT and nursing care associated with maintenance. The NGT remains in place for a few days *postoperatively* to prevent the accumulation of secretions, which may lead to vomiting or GI distention and pressure on the incision.

Because weight loss is problematic for patients with gastric cancer, nutrition therapy is a vital aspect of preoperative and postoperative management. Preoperatively, compression by the tumor can prevent adequate nutritional intake. To correct malnutrition before surgery, the health care provider may prescribe enteral supplements to the diet and/or total parenteral nutrition (TPN). Vitamin, mineral, iron, and protein supplements are essential to correct nutritional deficits.

Other preoperative nursing measures for the patient undergoing open gastric surgery are the same as those for any patient undergoing abdominal surgery and general anesthesia (see Chapter 16).

Operative Procedures. The surgeon usually removes part or all of the stomach to take out the tumor. When the tumor is located in the mid-portion or distal (lower) portion of the stomach, a subtotal (partial) gastrectomy is typically performed. The omentum, spleen, and relevant nodes are also removed.

For the patient with a resectable growth in the proximal (upper) third of the stomach, a total gastrectomy is performed (Fig. 58-5). In this procedure the surgeon removes the entire stomach along with the lymph nodes and omentum. The surgeon sutures the esophagus to the duodenum or jejunum to reestablish continuity of the GI tract. More radical surgery involving removal of the spleen and distal pancreas is controversial, although the Whipple procedure may be used to prolong life. However, the complications of this drastic surgery are very serious and common. For patients with advanced

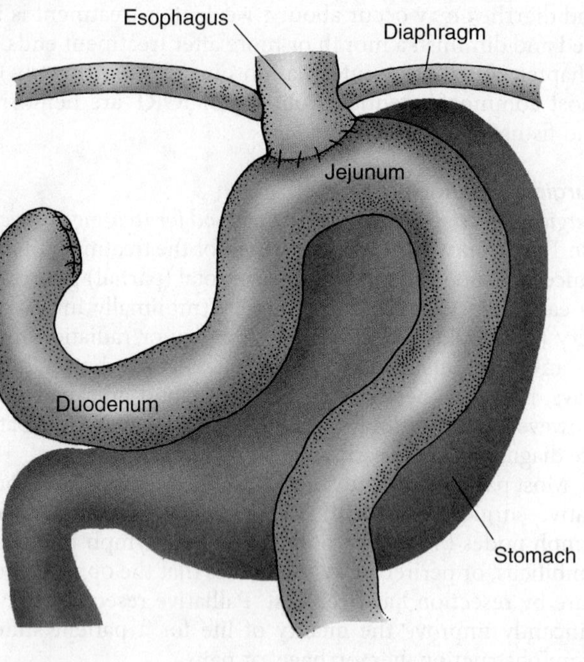
Esophagus
Diaphragm
Jejunum
Duodenum
Stomach

Fig. 58-5 • Total gastrectomy, with anastomosis of the esophagus to the jejunum (esophagojejunostomy), is the principal surgical intervention for extensive gastric cancer.

disease, total gastrectomy is performed only when gastric bleeding or obstruction is present.

Patients with tumors at the gastric outlet who are not candidates for subtotal or total gastrectomy may undergo gastroenterostomy for palliation. The surgeon creates a passage between the body of the stomach and the small bowel, often the duodenum.

Postoperative Care. The postoperative care is similar for all of the open surgical procedures. (See the Plan of Care below and on pages 1283-1285.) Provide the usual postoperative care for patients who have had general anesthesia to prevent atelectasis, paralytic ileus, and wound infection (see Chapter 18). In addition, monitor the patient for the development of complications that are specific to gastric surgery.

Auscultate the lungs for adventitious sounds (crackles or reduced breath sounds), and monitor for the return of bowel sounds. Take vital signs as appropriate to detect signs of infection or bleeding. Aggressive pulmonary exercises and early ambulation can help prevent respiratory complications and deep vein thrombosis. Also inspect the operative site every shift for the presence of redness, swelling, or drainage, which indicates wound infection. Keep the head of the bed elevated to prevent aspiration from reflux.

Assess the NGT for patency, and carefully secure the tube according to agency policy to prevent movement; this action is critical for preventing the retention of gastric secretions. Monitor

PLAN OF CARE Medical Diagnosis: Gastrectomy

NURSING DIAGNOSIS NO. 1: Acute Pain

Related Factors

Injury agents: Surgery

Defining Characteristics

Verbal or coded report of pain
Observed evidence of pain

Expected Outcomes

Denies experiencing pain greater than 5 on a 0-to-10 pain scale
No verbal report or observation of guarding or protective gestures
No verbal report or observation of an alteration in sleep patterns
No verbal report or observation of self-focusing behavior
No verbal report or observation of facial mask of pain
No verbal report or observation of an alteration in activity level

Nursing Interventions	Rationales
NIC Pain Management	
Perform a comprehensive pain assessment that includes location, characteristics, onset/duration, frequency, quality, intensity or severity of pain, and precipitating factors.	A plan for pain management must be based on the patient's unique responses to pain.
D Reduce or eliminate factors that precipitate or increase the pain experience.	Preventing a pain experience is preferred to trying to control or eliminate pain.
Provide information about the pain, such as causes, how long it will last, and anticipated discomforts from procedures.	The patient is better able to monitor his or her own discomfort and to intervene appropriately when informed.
NIC Analgesic Administration	
Choose the IV rather than the IM route for frequent pain medication injections, when possible.	The IV route avoids tissue trauma and the unpredictable absorption of medication.
Administer analgesics around the clock.	Administration around the clock prevents the peaks and troughs of analgesia, especially with severe pain.
D Institute safety precautions for a patient who is receiving opioid analgesics, as appropriate.	Opioid analgesics may impair the patient's judgment and/or coordination.
Document the patient's response to the analgesic and any untoward effects.	Documentation provides the health care team with the information needed to accurately evaluate the patient's response to the analgesic regimen.

D Indicates nursing activities that can be delegated to unlicensed assistive nursing personnel at the discretion of the nurse.

PLAN OF CARE Medical Diagnosis: Gastrectomy—cont'd

NURSING DIAGNOSIS NO. 1: Acute Pain—cont'd

Implement actions to decrease the untoward effects of analgesics.	Actions taken to prevent the predictable but unwanted effects of opioid analgesics (e.g., constipation) increase patient comfort.
Teach about the use of analgesics, strategies to decrease side effects, and expectations for involvement in decisions about pain relief.	Information about analgesics and the expectation for involvement increase the patient's sense of control over his or her pain.
NIC Patient-Controlled Analgesia (PCA) Administration	
Validate that the patient can use a PCA device.	To use a PCA, the patient must be able to communicate, comprehend explanations, and follow directions.
Document the patient's pain, amount and frequency of drug dosing, and response to pain treatment on a pain flow sheet.	Information on the pain flow sheet assists the health care team to adjust the analgesic regimen to the patient's needs.
Teach the patient and family how to use the PCA device.	The device will not be used if the patient and/or family do not know how to use or are afraid of the device.
NIC Environmental Management: Comfort	
D Position the patient to facilitate comfort.	The nurse may decrease sources of discomfort by using principles of body alignment, supporting with pillows, supporting joints during movement, splinting over incisions, and immobilizing painful body parts.
Other Interventions	
Consider the use of alternative therapies such as imagery, aromatherapy, music, touch, and laughter/humor.	Cognitive and behavioral strategies may be used as adjuncts to or in place of pharmacologic or surgical interventions for chronic pain. Each therapy has a different mode of action, which may or may not benefit the patient.

NURSING DIAGNOSIS NO. 2: Ineffective Breathing Pattern

Related Factors

Pain

Defining Characteristics

Altered chest excursion

Depth of breathing: Adult tidal volume 500 mL at rest

Expected Outcomes

No verbal report or observation of dyspnea

Respiratory rate remains between 11 and 22 breaths/min

Has respirations that remain regular and deep

Nursing Interventions	Rationales
NIC Airway Management	
D Place the patient in semi-Fowler's position, if possible.	Semi-Fowler's position ensures that the abdominal contents do not press against the diaphragm and restrict chest expansion.
D Encourage the patient to take slow, deep breaths; to turn; and to cough.	Effective aeration and coughing will help rid the body of secretions. Frequent position changes will prevent secretions from pooling in one area.
D Assist the patient with an incentive spirometer, as appropriate.	Incentive spirometry encourages the patient to deep breathe.
NIC Respiratory Monitoring	
D Monitor the rate, rhythm, depth, and effort of respirations.	Changes in respiratory rate, rhythm, depth, or effort may signal a descent into respiratory failure.
Note chest movement, watching for symmetry, the use of accessory muscles, and supraclavicular and intercostal muscle retractions.	The use of accessory muscles indicates increased respiratory effort.
Auscultate breath sounds, noting areas of decreased/absent ventilation and the presence of adventitious sounds.	Absent or adventitious breath sounds indicate poor gas exchange or poor movement of air through the airways.
Continuing Care Considerations	
D Encourage the patient to engage in regular physical exercise.	Cardiopulmonary efficiency and endurance improve with exercise.
D Encourage the patient to enroll in a smoking cessation program, as indicated.	Smoking damages the airways and alveoli.

NURSING DIAGNOSIS NO. 3: Imbalanced Nutrition: Less Than Body Requirements

Related Factors

Inability to ingest or digest food or absorb nutrients because of biologic, psychological, or economic factors

Continued

PLAN OF CARE Medical Diagnosis: Gastrectomy—cont'd

NURSING DIAGNOSIS NO. 3: Imbalanced Nutrition: Less Than Body Requirements—cont'd

Defining Characteristics

Satiety immediately after ingesting food
Perceived inability to ingest food
Abdomen: Cramping
Pain: Abdominal with or without pathology
Diarrhea

Expected Outcomes

Has bowel sounds that remain at 3 to 5 per quadrant per minute
Denies abdominal pain
No verbal report or observation of diarrhea
Weight remains within ±5 pounds of desired weight

Nursing Interventions	Rationales
NIC Nutrition Management	
Determine, in collaboration with a nutritionist as appropriate, the number of calories and type of nutrients needed to meet nutrition requirements.	Individual patient needs for nutrients and calories should be the basis for a sound dietary plan.
Adjust the diet to the patient's lifestyle, as appropriate.	The dietary division of nutrients, calories, and meals should be adjusted to the patient's lifestyle to increase compliance.
D Provide foods appropriate for the patient—general diet; mechanical soft, blenderized, or commercial formula via a nasogastric or gastrostomy tube; or total parental nutrition—as prescribed by the health care provider.	Nutrition therapy dictates the types and form of foods that may be offered to the patient.
D Create a pleasant, relaxing environment at mealtime.	A pleasant, relaxing environment at mealtime improves digestion.
Other Interventions	
Teach the patient and family about high-calorie, high-protein meal planning as appropriate, as well as refraining from drinking liquids with meals.	Meals must be nutritionally adequate to promote healing and to avoid events such as reflux and dumping syndrome.
Monitor for early signs and symptoms of dumping syndrome—vertigo, tachycardia, syncope, sweating, pallor, palpitations, and the desire to lie down.	Dumping syndrome poses a threat to patient safety.
Teach the patient and family about nutritional supplements, as appropriate.	Additional vitamins and minerals, calories, dietary fiber, or other nutritional components may need to be added to the diet of a patient who is unable to eat a nutritionally adequate diet.
Continuing Care Considerations	
Refer the patient to appropriate community nutritional programs, as needed.	Resources such as Weight Watchers, Overeaters Anonymous, and Take Off Pounds Sensibly provide support to the patient who is attempting to maintain appropriate body weight.

NURSING DIAGNOSIS NO. 4: Risk for Infection

Related Factors

Invasive procedures
Malnutrition
Increased environmental exposure to pathogens
Inadequate primary defenses (broken skin, traumatized tissue, decrease in ciliary action, stasis of body fluids, changes in pH secretions, altered peristalsis)

Expected Outcomes

Denies fatigue
Denies weakness
Denies nausea
Has a blood pressure that remains ±10 mm Hg of baseline
Has a heart rate that remains regular, strong, and between 60 and 100 beats/min
No verbal report or observation of vomiting
Has a body temperature that remains between 97° and 99.6° F (36.1° and 37.5° C)

D Indicates nursing activities that can be delegated to unlicensed assistive nursing personnel at the discretion of the nurse.

PLAN OF CARE Medical Diagnosis: Gastrectomy—cont'd

NURSING DIAGNOSIS NO. 4: Risk for Infection—cont'd	
Nursing Interventions	**Rationales**
NIC Infection Protection	
Monitor for systemic and localized signs and symptoms of infection.	An elevated temperature, pulse, and respirations indicate systemic infection; redness, heat, swelling, and pain indicate local infection.
Monitor absolute granulocyte count, white blood cell (WBC) count, and differential results.	Elevations in these laboratory tests demonstrate the body's response to infection.
Inspect the condition of any surgical incision/wound.	A surgical incision may be slightly reddened and swollen from tissue damage but remain free of the purulent drainage, excess swelling, or excess local pain that indicates infection.
D Maintain asepsis for the patient at risk.	Asepsis will minimize the patient's exposure to pathogenic agents and thus minimize the incidence of infection.
D Encourage coughing and deep breathing, as appropriate.	Coughing and deep breathing clear the lungs of secretions that may encourage the growth of pathogenic microbes.
D Promote sufficient nutritional intake.	Adequate nutrition is essential for the formation of immune system cells and for the repair of damaged body tissues to provide protection against external pathogens.
D Encourage fluid intake, as appropriate.	Adequate fluid intake provides for renal clearance of the toxins produced by pathogens.
D Encourage rest.	Mending tissues require energy. A fatigued patient is stressed and requires greater expenditure of energy to accomplish tasks.
NIC Infection Control	
Administer antibiotic therapy, as appropriate.	Antibiotic therapy should assist the body to destroy pathogens.
Continuing Care Considerations	
Limit numerous visitors, and discourage visits from persons with known infections.	Visitors may provide a needed diversion for the patient, but too many visitors may cause fatigue and bring unwanted exposure to pathogens.
Teach the patient and family about the signs and symptoms of infection and when to report them to the health care provider.	Early intervention to treat infection prevents untoward complications from the infection and its therapy.

the amount of blood draining from the tube. Only a scant amount of blood should be present, and abdominal distention should not develop. If these problems occur, report them immediately to the surgeon. Do not irrigate or reposition the NGT after gastric surgery unless specifically requested!

Decreased patency caused by a clogged NGT can result in *acute gastric dilation* after surgery. This problem is manifested by epigastric pain and a feeling of fullness, hiccups, tachycardia, and hypotension. Irrigation or replacement of the NGT by request of the surgeon can relieve these symptoms.

Dumping syndrome is a term that refers to a group of vasomotor symptoms that occur after eating. This syndrome is believed to occur as a result of the rapid emptying of food contents into the small intestine, which shifts fluid into the gut causing abdominal distention. Observe for *early* manifestations of this syndrome, which typically occurs within 30 minutes of eating. Symptoms include vertigo, tachycardia, syncope, sweating, pallor, palpitations, and the desire to lie down. Report these manifestations to the surgeon and encourage the patient to lie down. Monitor the patient for late symptoms.

Late dumping syndrome, which occurs 90 minutes to 3 hours after eating, is caused by a release of an excessive amount of insulin. The insulin release follows a rapid rise in the blood glucose level that results from the rapid entry of high-carbohydrate food into the jejunum. Observe for manifestations, including dizziness, light-headedness, palpitations, diaphoresis, and confusion.

Dumping syndrome is managed by nutrition changes that include decreasing the amount of food taken at one time and eliminating liquids ingested with meals. In collaboration with the nutritionist, teach the patient to eat a high-protein, high-fat, low- to moderate-carbohydrate diet (Table 58-3). Acarbose may be used to decrease carbohydrate absorption. A somatostatin analogue, octreotide (Sandostatin), 50 mcg subcutaneously 2 to 3 times daily 30 minutes before meals may be prescribed in severe cases. This drug decreases gastric and intestinal hormone secretion and slows stomach and intestinal transit time.

Alkaline reflux gastropathy, also known as *bile reflux gastropathy,* is a complication of gastric surgery in which the pylorus is bypassed or removed. Endoscopic examination reveals regurgitated bile in the stomach and mucosal hyperemia. Symptoms include early satiety (satisfied quickly with little food), abdominal discomfort, and vomiting.

Delayed gastric emptying is often present after gastric surgery and usually resolves within 1 week. Edema at the anastomosis (surgical connection areas) or adhesions (scar tissue) obstructing the distal loop may have mechanical causes. Metabolic causes (e.g., hypokalemia, hypoproteinemia, or hyponatremia) should be considered. The edema is resolved with nasogastric suction, maintenance of fluid and electrolyte balance, and proper nutrition.

Afferent loop syndrome may occur when the duodenal loop is partially obstructed after radical surgery. Pancreatic and biliary secretions fill the intestinal loop, which becomes distended. Painful contractions attempt to propel these secretions from the loop. Teach patients to report abdominal bloating and pain 20 to 60 minutes after eating, often followed by

TABLE 58-3 Diet for Dumping Syndrome

Food Group	Foods Allowed or Encouraged	Foods to Use with Caution	Foods That Must Be Excluded
Soups		Fluids 1 hr before and after meals	Spicy soups
Meat and meat substitutes	8 oz or more per day: fish, poultry, beef, pork, veal, lamb, eggs, cheese, and peanut butter		Spicy meats or meat substitutes
Potato and substitutes	Potato, rice, pasta, starchy vegetables (small amount)		Highly spiced potatoes or substitutes
Bread and cereal	White bread, rolls, muffins, crackers, and cereals (small amount)	Whole-grain bread, rolls, crackers, and cereals	Breads with frosting or jelly, sweet rolls, and coffee cake
Vegetables	Two or more cooked vegetables	Gas-producing vegetables, such as cabbage, onions, broccoli, or raw vegetables	
Fruits	Limit three per day: unsweetened cooked or canned fruits	Unsweetened juice or fruit drinks 30-45 min after meals; fresh fruit	Sweetened fruit or juice
Beverages	Dietetic drinks	Limit to 1 hr after meals; caffeine-containing beverages, such as coffee, tea, and cola; if tolerated, diet carbonated beverages	Milk shakes, malts, and other sweet drinks; regular carbonated beverages and alcohol
Fats	Margarine, oils, shortening, butter, bacon, and salad dressings	Mayonnaise	Any fats with milk products
Desserts	Fruit (see Fruits)	Sugar-free gelatin, pudding, and custard	All sweets, cakes, pies, cookies, candy, ice cream, and sherbet
Seasonings and miscellaneous	Diet jelly, diet syrups, sugar substitutes	Excessive amounts of salt	Excessive amounts of spices, sugar, jelly, honey, syrup, or molasses

GENERAL PRINCIPLES
- Several small meals daily
- Relatively high fat and protein content
- Low roughage
- Relatively low carbohydrate content
- No milk, sweets, or sugars
- Liquid between meals *only*

nausea and vomiting. Treatment consists of surgical correction of the incomplete loop obstruction.

Several problems related to *nutrition* develop as a result of partial removal of the stomach, including deficiencies of vitamin B_{12}, folic acid, and iron; impaired calcium metabolism; and reduced absorption of calcium and vitamin D. These problems are caused by a reduction of intrinsic factor. The decrease results from the resection and from inadequate absorption because of rapid entry of food into the bowel. In the absence of intrinsic factor, clinical manifestations of pernicious anemia may occur. Assess for the development of atrophic glossitis secondary to vitamin B_{12} deficiency. In atrophic glossitis, the tongue takes on a shiny, smooth, and "beefy" appearance. The patient may also have signs of anemia secondary to folic acid and iron deficiency. Monitor the complete blood count (CBC) for signs of megaloblastic anemia and leukopenia (low RBC and WBC levels). These manifestations are corrected by the administration of vitamin B_{12}. The health care provider may also prescribe folic acid or iron preparations.

Community-Based Care

Patients who have undergone total gastrectomy and those who are debilitated with advanced gastric cancer are discharged to home with maximal assistance and support or to a transitional care unit or skilled nursing facility. Patients who have undergone subtotal gastrectomy and are not debilitated may be discharged to home with partial assistance for ADLs. Recurrence of cancer is common, and patients need regular follow-up examinations and imaging assessments. Collaborate with the case manager (CM) to ensure continuity of care and thorough follow-up with diagnostic testing.

Home Care Management

Gastric cancer is a life-threatening illness. Therefore the patient and family members require physical and emotional care. Assess their ability to cope with the disease and the possible need for end-of-life care. The adverse effects of gastric cancer treatment can be debilitating, and patients need to learn symptom management strategies. Hospice programs can help both the patient and the family cope with these physical and emotional needs.

Patients may fear returning home because of their inability for self-management. Enlisting family and health care resources for the patient may ease some of this anxiety. Provide the family with adequate information about community support systems to make the transition to home care easier. If the prognosis is poor, they need continued professional support from case managers, social workers, and/or nurses to cope with death and dying. (See Chapter 9 for a discussion of end-of-life care.)

Health Teaching

Educate the patient and family about any continuing needs, drug therapy, and nutrition therapy. If patients are discharged to home with surgical dressings, teach the patient and family how to change them. Review the manifestations of incisional infection (e.g., fever, redness, and drainage) that they should report to their surgeon.

Patients who will be receiving radiation therapy or chemotherapy require instructions related to the side effects of these treatments. Nausea and vomiting are common side effects of chemotherapy, and instruction in the use of prescribed antiemetics may be needed. (See Chapter 24 for health teaching for patients receiving chemotherapy or radiation therapy.)

In collaboration with the nutritionist, teach the patient and family about the type and quantity of foods that will provide optimal nutritional value. Interventions to minimize dumping syndrome are also emphasized (see Table 58-3). Remind the patient to:

- Eat small, frequent meals
- Avoid drinking liquids with meals
- Avoid foods that cause discomfort
- Eliminate caffeine and alcohol consumption
- Begin a smoking cessation program
- Receive B_{12} injections, as prescribed
- Lie flat after eating for a short time

Health Care Resources

A home care referral provides continued assessment, assistance, and encouragement to the patient and family. A home care nurse can help with care procedures and provide valuable psychological support. Additional referrals to a nutritionist, professional counselor, or clergy/spiritual leader may be necessary. Referral to a hospice agency can be of great assistance for the patient with advanced disease. Hospice care may be delivered in the home or in an institutional setting. Appropriate support groups (e.g., I Can Cope, provided by the American Cancer Society) can be a major resource (www.cancer.org).

HUMAN NEEDS NURSING CARE REVIEW

What might you NOTICE if the patient is experiencing impaired digestion and nutrition as a result of a stomach disorder?

- Report of epigastric pain or indigestion before or after a meal
- Report of inability to tolerate certain foods
- Nausea and/or vomiting (with or without blood)
- Melena or frank blood in stools

What should you INTERPRET and how should you RESPOND to a patient experiencing impaired digestion and nutrition as a result of a stomach disorder?

Perform and interpret physical assessment, including:

- Taking vital signs
- Observing and documenting assessment findings
- Preparing for gastric lavage if hematemesis is present
- Interpreting laboratory values and other diagnostic findings:
  - Presence of *H. pylori*
  - Decreased hemoglobin and hematocrit

Respond by:

- Maintaining airway, breathing, and circulation (ABCs)
- Placing patient in sitting position or on left side to prevent aspiration if vomiting
- Preparing to assist with gastric lavage if hematemesis is present

On what should you REFLECT?

- Think about what else you could do to care for this patient.
- Consider with whom you should collaborate to improve or maintain digestion and nutrition for this patient.
- After patient interventions, monitor for changes in vital signs, hematocrit, and hemoglobin.

GET READY FOR THE NCLEX EXAMINATION!

Key Points

Review these Key Points for each NCLEX Examination Client Needs Category.

Safe and Effective Care Environment

- Provide information about organizations for digestive disorders to receive information and support; refer the patient to the American Cancer Society if gastric cancer is the diagnosis.
- Plan care for the patient having gastric surgery as outlined in the Plan of Care.
- For patients with peptic ulcer disease (PUD), collaborate with the nutritionist to modify food intake.

Health Promotion and Maintenance

- Identify patients at risk for gastritis and PUD, especially older adults who take large amounts of NSAIDs and those with *H. pylori*.
- Teach patients behaviors to prevent PUD, such as avoiding large consumption of caffeine, alcohol, coffee, aspirin, and other NSAIDs. Also teach them to avoid contaminated foods and water and smoking (see Chart 58-1).
- Teach patients the importance of adhering to *H. pylori* treatment to prevent the risk for gastric cancer.
- Teach patients about various complementary and alternative therapies that are currently used for gastritis and PUD.

Psychosocial Integrity

- Allow patients with gastric cancer to express feelings of grief, fear, and anxiety.
- For patients with advanced gastric cancer, identify the need for end-of-life care, including referral to hospice care.

Physiological Integrity

- For patients who have undergone a gastrectomy, collaborate with the nutritionist and instruct the patient regarding diet changes to avoid abdominal distention and dumping syndrome.

- Teach patients with abnormal symptoms, such as abdominal tenderness, abdominal pain that is relieved by food or pain or that becomes worse 3 hours after eating, dyspepsia, melena, and/or distention to consult with their physician immediately for a prompt diagnosis and treatment.
- Teach patients that hematemesis is a medical emergency and that they should go to the emergency department for prompt treatment.
- Teach the proper administration of antacids (one to two after meals). Tell patients that antacids can interfere with the effectiveness of certain drugs, such as phenytoin (Dilantin).
- Teach the proper administration of H_2 antagonists. Explain that they should be given on an empty stomach (see Chart 58-3).
- Teach the proper administration of antisecretory agents, noting that most cannot be crushed because they are sustained-release or enteric-coated tablets.
- Assess patients for clinical manifestations of gastritis.
- Monitor patients with ulcers for any of the signs and symptoms of GI bleeding that are listed in Chart 58-4. Report any of these symptoms if noted to a physician immediately.
- Insert a nasogastric tube (NGT) as outlined in Chart 58-6.
- After an EGD, monitor the patient's vitals signs, heart rhythm, and oxygen saturation frequently until they return to baseline. Assess the gag reflex and ensure that it is intact before giving the patient food to prevent aspiration.
- Observe the patient for signs and symptoms of dumping syndrome after gastric surgery; teach the manifestations and management of this syndrome. Advise the patient to eat six small meals per day and to consume a diet high in protein and fat but low in carbohydrate-rich foods. Liquids should not be taken with meals.

Additional Study Resources

Go to your Companion CD or Evolve at http://evolve.elsevier.com/Iggy/ for *Self-Assessment Questions for the NCLEX Examination.*

evolve Go to Evolve at http://evolve.elsevier.com/Iggy/ for *Prioritization and Delegation Questions for the NCLEX Examination.*

SELECTED BIBLIOGRAPHY

Ables, A.Z., Simon, I., & Melton, E.R. (2007). Update on *Helicobacter pylori* treatment. *American Family Physician, 75*(3), 351-358.

Barba, K., Fitzgerald, P., & Wood, S. (2007). Managing peptic ulcer disease. *Nursing2007, 37*(7), 56hn1-56hn4.

Carlson, D.S., & Pfadt, E. (2004). Perforated peptic ulcer. *Nursing2004, 34*(12), 88.

Cope, D.G., & Reb, A.M. (2006). *An evidence-based approach to the treatment and care of the older adult with cancer.* Pittsburgh, PA: Oncology Nursing Society.

Framp, A. (2006). Diffuse gastric cancer. *Gastroenterology Nursing, 29*(3), 232-238.

Krumberger, J.M. (2005). How to manage an acute upper GI bleed. *RN, 68*(3), 34-40.

McCance, K.L., & Huether, S.E. (2006). *Pathophysiology: The biologic basis for disease in adults and children.* St. Louis: Mosby.

National Digestive Disease Information Clearinghouse. (2008). *H. pylori and peptic ulcer. National Institute of Diabetes and Digestive and Kidney Diseases Home Page.* Retrieved April 2, 2008, from www.niddk.nih.gov./health/digest/pubs/hpylori/hypylori.htm.

National Institute of Diabetes and Digestive and Kidney Diseases. *General information about digestive diseases.* Retrieved April 7, 2008, from www.niddk.nih.gov.

Ozucelik, D.N., Karaca, M.A., & Sivri, B. (2005). Effectiveness of pre-emptive metoclopramide infusion in alleviating pain, discomfort and nausea associated with nasogastric tube insertion: A randomized, double-blind, placebo-controlled trial. *International Journal of Clinical Practice, 59*(12), 1422-1427.

Pagana, K.D., & Pagana, T.J. (2006). *Mosby's manual of diagnostic and laboratory tests.* St. Louis: Mosby.

Ramakrishnan, K., & Salina, R.C. (2007). Peptic ulcer disease. *American Family Physician, 76*(7), 1005-1012.

Rotello, L.C. (2003). Managing critically ill patients at risk for stress ulcers. *CME-Today, 1*(1), 27-30.

Schmidt, E. (2005). Nebulised lidocaine before nasogastric tube insertion reduced patient discomfort but increased risk of nasal bleeding. *Evidence-Based Nursing, 8*(2), 16.

Schuler, A. (2007). Risks versus benefits of long-term proton pump inhibitor therapy in the elderly. *Geriatric Nursing, 28*(4), 225-229.

Snyder, D. (2005). Evidence-based recommendations for older adults with *Helicobacter pylori* or those using nonsteroidal anti-inflammatory drugs. *Gastroenterology Nursing, 28*(4), 309-316.

Care of Patients with Noninflammatory Intestinal Disorders

59
CHAPTER

Lynne Brophy • Donna D. Ignatavicius

LEARNING OUTCOMES

For clinical competence and success on the NCLEX Examination, study this chapter with these Learning Outcomes in mind:

Safe and Effective Care Environment

1. Prioritize nursing care for the patient with abdominal trauma.
2. Identify community-based resources for patients with colorectal cancer (CRC).
3. Collaborate with health care team members to provide care for patients with CRC.

Health Promotion and Maintenance

4. Develop a teaching-learning plan for patients with irritable bowel syndrome (IBS).
5. Teach patients health promotion practices to prevent CRC.
6. Identify risk factors for CRC.
7. Provide health teaching for patients to promote self-management when caring for a colostomy.

Psychosocial Integrity

8. Assess patient and family response to a diagnosis of CRC.

Physiological Integrity

9. Differentiate the most common types of hernias.
10. Develop a plan of care for a patient undergoing a minimally invasive inguinal hernia repair.
11. Interpret assessment findings for patients with CRC.
12. Explain the role of the nurse in managing the patient with CRC.
13. Develop a perioperative plan of care for a patient undergoing a colon resection and colostomy.
14. Explain the differences between small-bowel and large-bowel obstructions.
15. Develop a plan of care for a patient with an intestinal obstruction to promote elimination.
16. Describe the postoperative care for a patient having a hemorrhoid surgical procedure.
17. Explain the pathophysiology of malabsorption syndrome.

Go to your Companion CD or Evolve at http://evolve.elsevier.com/Iggy/ for *Self-Assessment Questions for the NCLEX Examination* keyed to these Learning Outcomes.

Intestinal health problems may be inflammatory or noninflammatory. This chapter describes those disorders that are noninflammatory in origin. Noninflammatory intestinal problems often cause rectal bleeding, changing bowel patterns, and abdominal pain. If not diagnosed and managed early, some intestinal problems can lead to inadequate absorption of vital nutrients and therefore affect the *human need for nutrition* and *elimination.* Fig. 59-1 shows locations and common causes of lower GI bleeding.

IRRITABLE BOWEL SYNDROME

Pathophysiology

Irritable bowel syndrome (IBS) is a functional GI disorder that causes chronic or recurrent diarrhea, constipation, and/or abdominal pain and bloating. It is sometimes referred to as *spastic colon, mucous colon,* or *nervous colon* (Fig. 59-2). The disease exacerbates ("flares up") whenever the patient is exposed to causative agents. No actual pathophysiologic bowel changes occur in IBS.

The disease is believed to be due to impairment in the motor or sensory function of the GI tract. Motility changes, often associated with meals, result in changes in the normal *bowel elimination* pattern to a pattern of diarrhea, constipation, or alternating diarrhea and constipation. Even with these symptoms, the mucosal lining of the bowel remains essentially unchanged. Symptoms of IBS typically begin to appear in young adulthood and continue throughout the patient's life.

No structural or infectious etiology has been identified, so the exact cause is unknown. Physical factors such as diverticular disease, ingestion of coffee or other gastric stimulants,

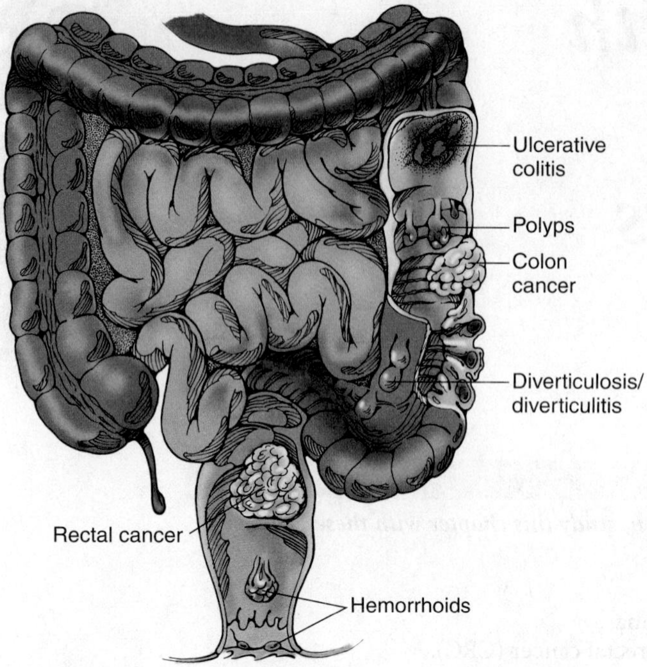
Ulcerative colitis
Polyps
Colon cancer
Diverticulosis/ diverticulitis
Rectal cancer
Hemorrhoids

Fig. 59-1 • Common causes of lower gastrointestinal bleeding.

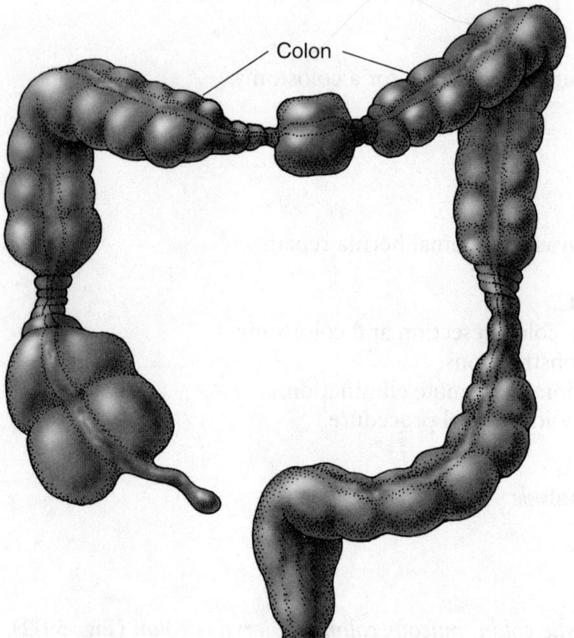
Colon

Fig. 59-2 • Spastic contractions of the colon as they occur with irritable bowel syndrome.

smoking, NSAID intake, increased dietary fat intake, sulfur intake, and milk allergy are being investigated as possible causes (Korzenik, 2005). Researchers are also testing the possibility of increased intestinal permeability exposing the person to antigens or immune deficiency as potential causes. Also, considerable evidence implicates the role of stress and mental or behavioral illness, especially anxiety and depression (Hertig et al., 2007). Many patients diagnosed with IBS meet the criteria for at least one primary psychiatric disorder (Croghan & Heitkemper, 2005). In some cases, the stress may result from a history of sexual or physical abuse. A familial predisposition has also been noted for some patients, and genetically susceptible persons may become ill when environmental factors come into play (Saito et al., 2005).

IBS is the most common digestive disorder seen in clinical practice. It may affect as many as one in five people in the United States, but only a small percentage have serious symptoms. Women are two times more likely to have the disease than men (Lehrer & Lichtenstein, 2007).

Patient-Centered Collaborative Care

Assessment

Ask the patient about a history of weight loss, fatigue, malaise, abdominal pain, changes in the bowel pattern (constipation, diarrhea or an alternating pattern of both) or consistency of stools, and the passage of mucus. Collect information on all drugs the patient is taking because many of them can cause symptoms similar to those of IBS. Ask about the nutrition history, including the use of caffeinated beverages or beverages sweetened with sorbitol or fructose, which can cause bloating or diarrhea.

The course of the illness is specific to the patient. Most patients can identify factors that cause exacerbations, such as diet, stress, or anxiety. There are no changes in the bowel mucosa and therefore no serious health consequences. Food intolerance may be associated with IBS. Dairy products (e.g., lactose intolerance) and grains can contribute to bloating, flatulence, and distention.

The characteristic symptoms known collectively as the **Manning criteria** are typically present:

- Abdominal pain relieved by defecation or falling asleep
- Abdominal pain associated with changes in stool frequency or consistency
- Abdominal distention
- The sensation of incomplete evacuation of stool
- The presence of mucus with stool passage

Bowel function changes progressively and eventually forms the characteristic pattern.

A flare-up of worsening cramps, abdominal pain, and diarrhea or constipation may bring the patient to the health care provider. *The most common symptom of IBS is pain in the left lower quadrant of the abdomen.* Nausea may be associated with mealtime and defecation. The crampy abdominal patterns are accompanied by constipation or diarrhea. The constipated stools are small and hard and are generally followed by several softer stools. The diarrheal stools are soft and watery, and mucus is often present in the stools. Patients with IBS often report belching, gas, anorexia, and bloating.

The patient generally appears well, with a stable weight, and nutritional and fluid levels are within normal ranges. Inspect and auscultate the abdomen. Bowel sounds are generally within normal range and may be somewhat quiet with constipation. On percussion of the abdomen, tympanic sounds may be heard over loops of filled bowel. On light palpation, there may be diffuse (widespread) tenderness, which is generally worse if the sigmoid colon is palpable. Routine laboratory values (including a complete blood count [CBC], serum albumin, erythrocyte sedimentation rate [ESR], and stools for occult blood) are normal in IBS.

Interventions

The patient with IBS is usually cared for in an ambulatory care setting. Interventions include health teaching, drug therapy, and stress management. Some patients use complementary and alternative therapies as well.

Health Teaching

Health promotion focuses on *teaching the patient to avoid problem stimulants.* Educate patients about the chronic nature of the disorder. Assist them to identify and avoid specific foods that they cannot tolerate. These foods may include caffeine, alcohol, egg, wheat products, beverages that contain sorbitol or fructose, and other gastric irritants. Milk and milk products should be avoided if lactose intolerance is suspected. Lactose-free or soy products can be used as a substitute. Patients who are lactose intolerant need to increase intake of calcium-rich, lactose-free foods or take a calcium supplement because they are at high risk for osteoporosis.

Dietary fiber and bulk help produce bulky, soft stools and establish regular bowel habits. The patient should ingest about 30 to 40 g of fiber each day. Eating regular meals, drinking 8 to 10 cups of liquid each day, and chewing food slowly promote normal bowel function. If needed, collaborate with the nutritionist to help the patient and family with meal planning.

Keeping a symptom diary in which the patient records potential triggers and bowel habits for a period of time can assist in identifying new triggers for disease symptoms. Refer patients to the Irritable Bowel Syndrome Association (www.ibsassociation.org) for patient advocacy groups who can provide support and encouragement.

Drug Therapy

Drug therapy is directed at the major symptom of IBS. The health care provider may prescribe bulk-forming or antidiarrheal agents and newer drugs to control symptoms. A 5-HT4 antagonist may be added for women with diarrhea as a predominant symptom of IBS.

For the treatment of constipation-predominant IBS, bulk-forming laxatives, such as psyllium hydrophilic mucilloid (Metamucil), are generally taken at mealtimes with a glass of water. The hydrophilic properties of these drugs help prevent dry, hard, or liquid stools.

Diarrhea-predominant IBS is typically treated with antidiarrheal agents such as loperamide (Imodium). Alosetron (Lotronex), a serotonin (5-HT4) antagonist, is used with caution in women with diarrhea from IBS as a last resort for treatment. Only those who are registered with the manufacturer and agree to report symptoms of colitis or constipation early are allowed to take the drug. Before the patient begins alosetron, take a thorough drug (including herbs) history, both prescribed and over the counter, because it interacts with many drugs in a variety of classes. Teach patients to report constipation, fever, increasing abdominal pain, increasing fatigue, darkened urine, bloody diarrhea, or rectal bleeding as soon as it occurs and stop the drug immediately.

A newer group of drugs called *muscarinic (M3)-receptor antagonists* also inhibit intestinal motility. Some of these agents have been approved for people with overactive bladders but have not yet received U.S. Food and Drug Administration (FDA) approval for IBS. Examples in this group currently undergoing clinical trials are darifenacin (Enablex) and zamifenacin.

For IBS in which pain is the predominant symptom, antidepressants, such as paroxetine (Paxil), have also been successfully used. It is unclear whether their effectiveness is due to the antidepressant or anticholinergic effects of the drugs. If patients have postprandial (after eating) discomfort, they should take these drugs 30 to 45 minutes before mealtime.

Complementary and Alternative Therapies

Hertig et al. (2007) found that GI symptoms associated with IBS are worsened by day-to-day psychological stress, especially in women with anxiety or depression. Therefore strategies that decrease stress may help reduce these symptoms.

Stress management is based on the patient's perceived stressors and available resources. Suggest relaxation techniques and/or hypnotherapy to help the patient decrease GI symptoms.

If the patient is in a stressful work or family situation, personal counseling may be helpful. Make appropriate referrals or assist in making appointments, if necessary. The opportunity to discuss problems and attempt creative problem solving is often helpful. Teach the patient that regular exercise is important for managing stress and promoting regular bowel elimination.

Some patients use other modalities as supplements to their medical treatment plan. Limited evidence from research is available regarding the usefulness and safety of complementary therapies for any inflammatory bowel disease (IBD), including IBS. However, Chinese herbal medicine has been shown to control bowel symptoms (Podovei & Kuo, 2006). Life-threatening side effects of complementary therapies used for IBD have been reported. For this reason, remind patients to discuss the possibly of using complementary therapy with their gastroenterologist before they begin treatment. A few examples of therapies that are used to reduce symptoms and reduce discomfort are:

- Peppermint oil to expel gas and relax spastic intestinal muscles
- Ginger for abdominal discomfort and to expel gas
- Yoga and other relaxation techniques
- Acupuncture
- Artichoke leaf extract (Harmon, 2007)

HERNIATION

Pathophysiology

A **hernia** is a weakness in the abdominal muscle wall through which a segment of the bowel or other abdominal structure protrudes. Hernias can also penetrate through any other defect in the abdominal wall, through the diaphragm, or through other structures in the abdominal cavity.

The most common types of abdominal hernias (Fig. 59-3) are indirect, direct, femoral, umbilical, and incisional.

- An **indirect inguinal hernia** is a sac formed from the peritoneum that contains a portion of the intestine or omentum. The hernia pushes downward at an angle into the inguinal canal. In males, indirect inguinal hernias can become large and often descend into the scrotum.
- **Direct inguinal hernias,** in contrast, pass through a weak point in the abdominal wall.
- **Femoral hernias** protrude through the femoral ring. A plug of fat in the femoral canal enlarges and eventually pulls the peritoneum and often the urinary bladder into the sac.
- **Umbilical hernias** are congenital or acquired. Congenital umbilical hernias appear in infancy. Acquired umbilical hernias directly result from increased intra-abdominal pressure. They are most commonly seen in obese people.
- **Incisional, or ventral, hernias** occur at the site of a previous surgical incision. These hernias result from inadequate healing of the incision, which is usually caused by postoperative wound infections, inadequate nutrition, and obesity.

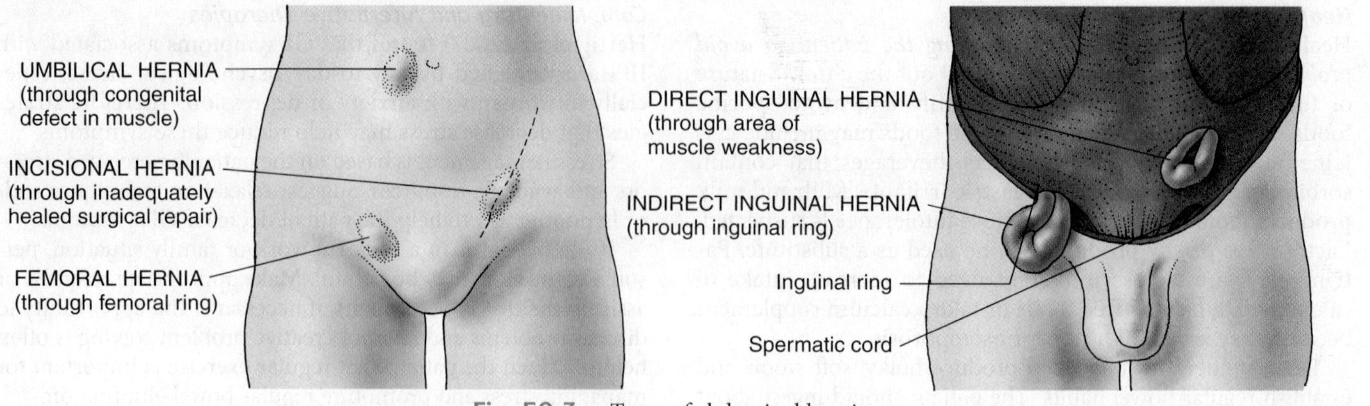
UMBILICAL HERNIA
(through congenital defect in muscle)
INCISIONAL HERNIA
(through inadequately healed surgical repair)
FEMORAL HERNIA
(through femoral ring)
DIRECT INGUINAL HERNIA
(through area of muscle weakness)
INDIRECT INGUINAL HERNIA
(through inguinal ring)
Inguinal ring
Spermatic cord

Fig. 59-3 • Types of abdominal hernia.

Hernias may also be classified as reducible, irreducible (incarcerated), or strangulated. A hernia is **reducible** when the contents of the hernial sac can be placed back into the abdominal cavity by gentle pressure. An **irreducible** (incarcerated) hernia cannot be reduced or placed back into the abdominal cavity. *Any hernia that is not reducible requires immediate surgical evaluation.*

A hernia is **strangulated** when the blood supply to the herniated segment of the bowel is cut off by pressure from the hernial ring (the band of muscle around the hernia). If a hernia is strangulated, there is ischemia and obstruction of the bowel loop. This can lead to necrosis of the bowel and possibly bowel perforation. *Signs of strangulation are abdominal distention, nausea, vomiting, pain, fever, and tachycardia.*

The most important elements in the development of a hernia are congenital or acquired muscle weakness and increased intra-abdominal pressure. The most significant factors contributing to increased intra-abdominal pressure are obesity, pregnancy, and lifting heavy objects.

Indirect inguinal hernias, the most common type, are most common in men because they follow the tract that develops when the testes descend into the scrotum before birth. Direct hernias occur more often in older adults. Femoral and adult umbilical hernias are most common in obese or pregnant women. Incisional hernias can occur in people who have undergone abdominal surgery.

Defects in the muscle wall result from weakened collagen or widened spaces at the inguinal ligament. These muscle weaknesses can be inherited or acquired as part of the aging process. Increases in intra-abdominal pressure as a result of pregnancy, obesity, abdominal distention, ascites, heavy lifting, or coughing can contribute to their occurrence.

Health Promotion and Maintenance

Even though the muscle weakness cannot be prevented, exercises can be performed to strengthen muscles. Obesity is considered a contributing factor because it causes increased intra-abdominal pressure. Weight control helps decrease the likelihood of hernias by decreasing pressure on the abdominal muscles. Heavy lifting and straining also increase intra-abdominal pressure and should be avoided.

Patient-Centered Collaborative Care

Assessment

The patient with a hernia typically comes to the health care provider's office or the emergency department with a report of a "lump" or protrusion felt at the involved site. The development of the hernia may be associated with straining or lifting.

Perform an abdominal assessment inspecting the abdomen when the patient is lying and again when he or she is standing. If the hernia is reducible, it may disappear when the patient is lying flat. The advanced practice nurse or other health care provider asks the patient to strain or perform the Valsalva maneuver and observes for bulging. Auscultate for active bowel sounds. *Absent bowel sounds may indicate obstruction and strangulation, which is a medical emergency!*

To palpate an inguinal hernia, the health care provider gently examines the ring and its contents by inserting a finger in the ring and noting any changes when the patient coughs. *The hernia is never forcibly reduced; that maneuver could cause strangulated intestine to rupture.*

If a male patient suspects a hernia in his groin, the health care provider has him stand for the examination. Using the right hand for the patient's right side and the left hand for the patient's left side, the examiner pushes in the loose scrotal skin with the index finger, following the spermatic cord upward to the external inguinal cord. At this point, the patient is asked to cough, and any palpable herniation is noted.

Interventions

The type of treatment selected depends on patient factors, such as age, as well as the type and severity of the hernia.

Nonsurgical Management

If the patient is not a surgical candidate, often an older adult with multiple health problems, the health care provider may prescribe a truss for an inguinal hernia, most often for men. A **truss** is a pad made with firm material. It is held in place over the hernia with a belt to help keep the abdominal contents from protruding into the hernial sac. If a truss is used, it is applied only after the physician has reduced the hernia if it is not incarcerated. The patient usually applies the truss upon awakening. Teach him to assess the skin under the truss daily and to protect it with a light layer of powder.

Surgical Management

Most hernias are inguinal. Surgical repair of a hernia is the treatment of choice. Surgery is usually performed on an ambulatory care basis for patients who have no pre-existing health conditions that would complicate the operative course. In same-day surgery centers, anesthesia may be regional or general, and the surgery is typically laparoscopic. More extensive surgery, such as a bowel resection or temporary colostomy, may be necessary if strangulation results in a gangrenous section of bowel. Patients undergoing extensive surgery are hospitalized for a longer period.

A **minimally invasive inguinal hernia repair (MIIHR)** through a laparoscope, also called **herniorrhaphy,** is the surgery of choice. An open, conventional herniorrhaphy may be performed when laparoscopy is not appropriate. Patients having minimally invasive surgery (MIS) recover more quickly, have less pain, and develop fewer postoperative complications compared with those having the conventional surgery.

Preoperative Care. In addition to patient education about the procedure, the most important preoperative preparation is to teach the patient to remain NPO for the number of hours before surgery that the surgeon specifies. If same-day surgery is planned, remind the patient to arrange for someone to take him or her home and be available for the rest of the day at home. For patients having an open surgical approach, provide general preoperative care as described in Chapter 16.

Operative Procedures. During an MIIHR, the surgeon makes several small incisions, identifies the defect, and places the intestinal contents back into the abdomen. During a traditional herniorrhaphy, the surgeon makes an abdominal incision to perform this procedure. When a **hernioplasty** is also performed, the surgeon reinforces the weakened outside abdominal muscle wall with a mesh patch.

Postoperative Care. The patient who has had MIIHR is discharged from the surgical center in 3 to 5 hours. Teach him or her to rest for several days before returning to work and a normal routine. Caution patients who are taking opioids for pain management to not drive or operate heavy machinery. Teach them to observe incisions for redness, swelling, heat, drainage, and increased pain and promptly report their occurrence to the surgeon. Remind patients that soreness and discomfort rather than severe, acute pain are common after MIS. Be sure to make a follow-up telephone call on the day after surgery to check on the patient's status.

General postoperative care of patients having an open surgical approach is the same as that described in Chapter 18 *except that they should avoid coughing.* To promote lung expansion, encourage deep breathing and ambulation. With repair of an indirect inguinal hernia, the physician may suggest a scrotal support and ice bags applied to the scrotum to prevent swelling, which often contributes to pain. Elevation of the scrotum with a soft pillow helps prevent and control swelling.

In the immediate postoperative period, the patient having an inguinal hernia repair may experience difficulty voiding. Encourage male patients to stand to allow a more natural position for gravity to facilitate voiding and bladder emptying. Urine output of less than 30 mL per hour should be reported to the surgeon. Techniques to stimulate voiding such as allowing water to run may also be used. A fluid intake of at least 1500 to 2500 mL daily prevents dehydration and maintains urinary function. A "straight" or intermittent catheterization is required if the patient cannot void.

Most patients have uneventful recoveries after an open hernia repair. Surgeons generally allow them to return to their usual activities after surgery, with avoidance of straining and lifting for 8 to 12 weeks while subcutaneous tissues heal and strengthen.

Provide oral instructions and a written list of symptoms to be reported, including fever, chills, wound drainage, redness or separation of the incision, and increasing incisional pain. Teach the patient to keep the wound dry and clean with antibacterial soap and water. Showering is usually permitted in a few days.

NCLEX EXAMINATION CHALLENGE

A postoperative client having a minimally invasive inguinal hernia repair has been given postoperative instructions by the nurse. Which statement by the client indicates a need for further teaching?

A. "I should deep breathe and cough every 2 hours to keep my lungs clear."
B. "I shouldn't lift anything heavy until my surgeon tells me that it's OK."
C. "I need to rest for a few days until I'm strong enough to go back to work."
D. "I'll call the doctor right away if my incisions get red or have drainage."

evolve For the correct answer, go to http://evolve.elsevier.com/Iggy/.

COLORECTAL CANCER

Pathophysiology

Colorectal refers to the colon and rectum, which together make up the large intestine, also known as the *large bowel.* Colorectal cancer (CRC) is cancer of the colon or rectum and is a major health problem worldwide. In the United States, it is one of the most common malignancies.

Most CRCs are **adenocarcinomas,** which are tumors that arise from the glandular epithelial tissue of the colon. They develop as a multi-step process, resulting in a number of molecular changes, such as loss of key tumor suppressor genes and activation of certain oncogenes that alter colonic mucosa cell division. The increased proliferation of the colonic mucosa forms polyps that can transform into malignant tumors. Most CRCs are believed to arise from adenomatous polyps that present as a visible protrusion from the mucosal surface of the bowel.

Tumors occur in different areas of the colon, with about two thirds occurring within the rectosigmoid region. The percentages in Fig. 59-4 indicate an increased incidence of cancer in the proximal sections of the large intestine over the past 30 years.

Colorectal cancer (CRC) can metastasize by direct extension or by spreading through the blood or lymph. The tumor may spread locally into the four layers of the bowel wall and into neighboring organs. It may enlarge into the lumen of the bowel or spread through the lymphatics or the circulatory system. The circulatory system is entered directly from the primary tumor through blood vessels in the bowel or via the lymphatics. The liver is the most frequent site of metastasis from circulatory spread. Metastasis to the lungs, brain, bones, and adrenal glands may also occur. Colon tumors can also spread by peritoneal seeding during surgical resection of the tumor. Seeding may occur when a tumor is excised and cancer cells break off from the tumor into the peritoneal cavity. For this reason, special techniques are used during surgery to decrease this possibility.

Complications related to the increasing growth of the tumor locally or through metastatic spread include bowel obstruction or perforation with resultant peritonitis, abscess formation, and fistula formation to the urinary bladder or the

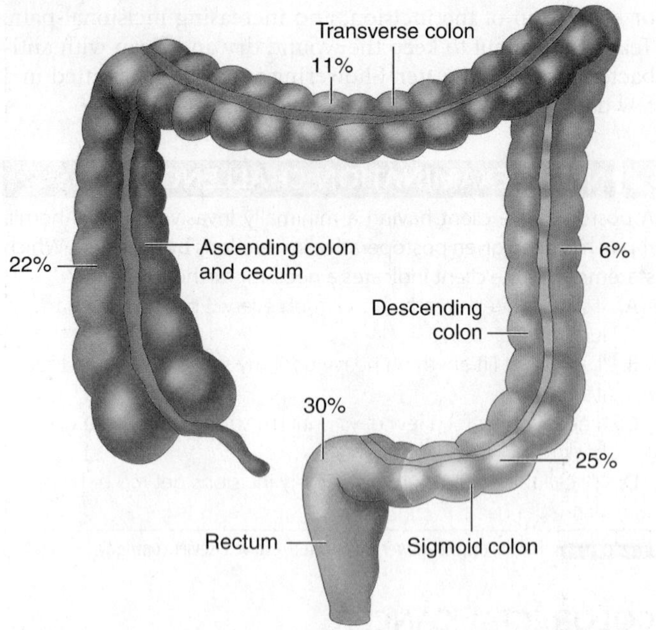
Transverse colon
11%
Ascending colon
and cecum
22%
6%
Descending
colon
30%
25%
Rectum
Sigmoid colon

Fig. 59-4 • The incidence of cancer in relation to colorectal anatomy.

vagina. The tumor may invade neighboring blood vessels and cause frank bleeding. Tumors growing into the bowel lumen can gradually obstruct the intestine and eventually block it completely. Those extending beyond the bowel wall may place pressure on neighboring organs (uterus, urinary bladder, and ureters) and cause symptoms that mask those of the cancer. Chapter 23 discusses cancer pathophysiology in more detail.

Etiology and Genetic Risk

Risk factors for the development of colorectal cancer (CRC) include being older than 50 years, genetic predisposition, personal or family history of cancer, and/or diseases that predispose the patient to cancer such as familial adenomatous polyposis (www.cancer.gov). Research continues to investigate smoking and obesity as risk factors for colorectal cancer.

At least 50% of people in the United States and other Western populations develop either a colorectal tumor or benign polyp by the age of 70 years. About 10% of them eventually develop CRC. Only a small percentage of CRCs are familial and transmitted genetically.

GENETIC CONSIDERATIONS

People with a first-degree relative (sister, sibling, or child) diagnosed with colorectal cancer (CRC) have three to four times the risk for developing the disease. An autosomal dominant inherited genetic disorder known as *familial adenomatous polyposis (FAP)* accounts for 1% of CRCs. FAP is the result of one or more mutations in the adenomatous polyposis coli (APC) gene. In these very young patients, thousands of adenomatous polyps develop over the course of 10 to 15 years and have nearly a 100% chance of becoming malignant. By 20 years of age, most patients require surgical intervention, usually a colectomy with ileostomy or ileoanal pull-through, to prevent cancer. Chemotherapy may also be used for cancer prevention.

Hereditary nonpolyposis colorectal cancer (HNPCC) is another autosomal dominant disorder and accounts for a small percentage of all colorectal cancers. HNPCC is also caused by gene mutations, including *MLH1* and *MLH2*. People with these mutations have an 80% chance of developing CRC at an average of 45 years of age. They also tend to have a higher incidence of endometrial, ovarian, stomach, and ureteral cancers. Genetic testing is available for both of these familial CRC syndromes. Refer patients for genetic counseling and possible testing.

Most CRCs have no known predisposing cause. Age is considered a risk factor in the development of colorectal cancer; most cases are diagnosed in people older than 50 years. Patients who have been diagnosed with and treated for CRC have an increased risk for developing a second primary disease, often at the site of the surgical anastomosis. Those with adenomatous polyps are at an increased risk for developing colorectal cancer. These people need regular follow-up with colonoscopy to detect and remove polyps.

Certain foods *may* place some people at risk for colorectal cancer. These foods also aid in decreasing bowel transit time, which increases the time that the bowel is exposed to **carcinogens** (cancer-causing substances). A high-fat diet, particularly animal fat from red meats, increases bile acid secretion and anaerobic bacteria, which are thought to be carcinogenic within the bowel. Fried and grilled meats and fish are also thought to contain chemicals that are carcinogenic. Diets with large amounts of refined carbohydrates that lack fiber decrease bowel transit time as well.

Inflammatory bowel diseases (IBDs), such as ulcerative colitis and Crohn's disease, pose an increased risk for colorectal cancer, especially if the disease has had a long, severe course.

Incidence/Prevalence

Colorectal cancer (CRC) is the third most common malignancy (after prostate and lung cancer in men and after breast and lung cancer in women), with an estimated 150,000 new cases each year (www.cancer.gov). It is rare before 40 years of age, but incidence increases rapidly with age. The overall incidence is the same in men and women, with cancer of the rectum being more common in men.

Health Promotion and Maintenance

People at risk can take action to decrease their chance of having CRC. For example, those whose family members have had hereditary CRC should be genetically tested for FAP and HNPCC. If gene mutations are present, the person at risk can collaborate with the health care team to decide what prevention or treatment plan to implement.

All people, regardless of risk, should modify their diets to decrease fat, refined carbohydrates, and low-fiber foods. Encourage baked or broiled foods, especially those high in fiber and low in animal fat.

When an adult turns 40 years of age, he or she should discuss with the health care provider about the need for colon cancer screening. The interval depends on level of risk. People of average risk who are older than 50 years, without a family history, should undergo regular CRC screening, including fecal occult blood testing (FOBT) and colonoscopy every 10 years or double-contrast barium enema every 5 years. People who have a personal or family history of the disease should begin screening earlier and more frequently (National Comprehensive Cancer Network, 2008). Teach all patients to follow the American Cancer Society recommendations for CRC screening listed in Chart 59-1.

Aspirin therapy has been extensively researched as a way to prevent CRC. The drug seems to work best with high doses taken for longer than 10 years. Although evidence supports its protective use, GI side effects such as bleeding may cause other major problems (Dube et al., 2007). Dietary calcium supplements have also been studied, but evidence is insufficient to demonstrate its usefulness (Weingarten et al., 2008).

Patient-Centered Collaborative Care evolve ONLINE PHARM REVIEW

Assessment

History

In taking a history, ask the patient about nutritional habits and major risk factors, such as a personal history of breast, ovarian, or endometrial cancer; ulcerative colitis; Crohn's disease; familial polyposis or adenomas; or a family history of CRC. Also assess the patient's participation in age-specific cancer screening guidelines.

Ask whether vomiting and changes in bowel habits, such as diarrhea or constipation, with or without blood in the stool have been noted. The patient may also report fatigue (related to anemias), abdominal fullness, vague abdominal pain, or unintentional weight loss. These symptoms suggest advanced disease.

Physical Assessment/Clinical Manifestations

The clinical manifestations of CRC depend on the location of the tumor. *However, the most common signs are rectal bleeding, anemia, and a change in the stool.* Stools may contain microscopic amounts of blood that are not noticeably visible, or the patient may have mahogany (dark)-colored or bright red stools. Gross blood is not usually detected with tumors of the right side of the colon but is common (but not massive) with tumors of the left side of the colon and the rectum.

Tumors in the transverse and descending colon result in symptoms of obstruction as growth of the tumor blocks the passage of stool. The patient may report "gas pains," cramping, or incomplete evacuation. Tumors in the rectosigmoid colon are associated with **hematochezia** (the passage of red blood via the rectum), straining to pass stools, and narrowing of stools. Patients may report dull pain. Right-sided tumors can grow quite large without disrupting bowel patterns or appearance, because the stool consistency is more liquid in this part of the colon. These tumors ulcerate and bleed intermittently, so stools can contain dark or mahogany-colored blood. A mass may be palpated in the lower right quadrant, and the patient often has anemia secondary to blood loss.

Examination of the abdomen begins with assessment for obvious distention or masses. Visible peristaltic waves accompanied by high-pitched or "tingling" bowel sounds may indicate a partial bowel obstruction from the tumor. Total absence of bowel sounds indicates a complete bowel obstruction. Palpation and percussion are performed by the advanced practice nurse or other health care provider to determine whether the spleen or liver is enlarged or whether masses are present along the colon. The examiner may also perform a digital rectal examination to palpate the rectum and lower sigmoid colon for masses. Fecal occult blood screening should not be done with a specimen from a rectal examination because it is not reliable.

Chart 59-1 BEST PRACTICE FOR PATIENT SAFETY & QUALITY CARE

Screening Recommendations for Men and Women Ages 50 Years and Older at Average Risk for Colorectal Cancer

Procedure: Choice of One of the Following	Interval After Screening Initiated at Age 50 Years	Comments
FOBT and 60 cm colonoscopy (sigmoidoscopy)	Every 5 years	FOBT procedure: two samples from three consecutive bowel movements obtained at home; tested by physician or nurse
OR		
Double-contrast barium enema	Every 5 years	
OR		
Colonoscopy	Every 10 years	

FOBT, Fecal occult blood testing.

Psychosocial Assessment

The psychological consequences associated with a diagnosis of colorectal cancer (CRC) are many. Patients must cope with a diagnosis that instills fear and anxiety about treatment, feelings that life has been disrupted, a need to search for ways to deal with the diagnosis, and concern about family. They also have questions about why colon cancer affected them, as well as concerns about pain, possible disfigurement, and possible death (Houldin & Lewis, 2006). In addition, if the cancer is believed to have a genetic origin, there is anxiety concerning implications for immediate family members.

Laboratory Assessment

Hemoglobin and hematocrit values are usually decreased as a result of the intermittent bleeding associated with the tumor. Colorectal cancer (CRC) that has metastasized to the liver causes liver function tests to be elevated.

A positive test result for occult blood in the stool **(fecal occult blood test [FOBT])** indicates bleeding in the GI tract. These tests can yield false-positive results if certain vitamins or drugs are taken before the test. Remind the patient to avoid aspirin, vitamin C, and red meat for 48 hours before giving a stool specimen. Also assess whether the patient is taking anti-inflammatory drugs (e.g., ibuprofen, corticosteroids, or salicylates). These drugs should be discontinued for a designated period before the test. Two to three separate stool samples should be tested on 3 consecutive days. Negative results do not completely rule out the possibility of CRC.

Carcinoembryonic antigen (CEA), an oncofetal antigen, is elevated in many people with CRC. No relationship exists between the CEA level and the cancer stage. This antigen is not specifically associated with the colorectal cancer, and it may be elevated in the presence of other benign or malignant diseases and in smokers. CEA is often used to monitor the effectiveness of treatment and to identify disease recurrence.

Imaging Assessment

A double-contrast barium enema (air and barium are instilled into the colon) or colonoscopy provides better visualization of polyps and small lesions than a barium enema alone. This test may show an occlusion in the bowel where the tumor is decreasing the size of the lumen.

Computed tomography (CT) or magnetic resonance imaging (MRI) of the chest, abdomen, pelvis, lungs, or liver helps confirm the existence of a mass, the extent of disease, and the location of distant metastases.

Other Diagnostic Assessment

A sigmoidoscopy provides visualization of the lower colon using a fiberoptic scope. Polyps can be visualized, and samples can be taken for biopsy. They are usually removed during the procedure. A colonoscopy provides views of the entire large bowel from the rectum to the ileocecal valve. As with sigmoidoscopy, polyps can be seen and removed, and tissue samples can be taken for biopsy. *Colonoscopy is the definitive test for the diagnosis of colorectal cancer.*

▪ *Analysis*

Common Nursing Diagnoses and Collaborative Problems

The priority nursing diagnosis for patients with colorectal cancer (CRC) is Anticipatory Grieving. The priority collaborative problem is Potential for Metastasis.

Additional Nursing Diagnoses and Collaborative Problems

In addition to the common nursing diagnosis and collaborative problem, patients with colorectal cancer may have:

- Acute Pain or Chronic Pain related to physical injury agents (e.g., tumor obstruction of the intestine with possible pressure on other organs or chronic physical disability)
- Fatigue related to disease state, anemia, and stress
- Disturbed Body Image related to biophysical factors, illness treatment, and/or surgery
- Ineffective Coping related to uncertainty and high degree of threat
- Deficient Knowledge about the disease and its treatment
- Imbalanced Nutrition: Less Than Body Requirements related to inability to digest or absorb food because of biologic factors
- Powerlessness related to illness-related regimen

▪ *Planning and Implementation*

Anticipatory Grieving

NOC **Planning: Expected Outcomes.** A patient faced with a diagnosis of colorectal cancer is expected to adjust to actual or impending loss. Indicators include that he or she will consistently demonstrate the ability to:

- Resolve feelings about loss
- Express spiritual beliefs about death
- Verbalize acceptance of loss
- Report decreased preoccupation with loss
- Report absence of sleep disturbance
- Seek social support
- Progress through stages of grief

Interventions. The patient and family are faced with a possible loss of or alteration in body functions. Medical and surgical interventions for the treatment of colorectal cancer may result in cure, disease control, or palliation. Interventions are designed to assist the patient in planning effective strategies for expressing feelings of grief and developing coping skills.

Observe and identify:

- The patient's and family's current methods of coping
- Effective sources of support used in past crises
- The patient's and family's present perceptions of the health problem
- Signs of anticipatory grief, such as crying, anger, and withdrawal from usual relationships

Encourage the patient to verbalize feelings about the diagnosis, treatment, and anticipated alteration in body functions if a colostomy is planned. (See discussion of Operative Procedures on pp. 1298-1299 in the Surgical Management section.) Sadness, anger, feelings of loss, and depression are normal responses to this change in body function.

If a colostomy is planned, instruct the patient on what to expect about the appearance and care of the colostomy. Postoperatively, encourage him or her to look at and touch the stoma. When the patient is physically able, ask him or her to participate in colostomy care. Participation helps restore the patient's sense of control over his or her lifestyle and thus facilitates improved self-esteem.

NIC ***Grief Work Facilitation.*** The purpose of grief work is to assist the patient with the resolution of a significant loss. Assist in identifying the nature of and reaction to the loss. Encourage the patient to verbalize feelings and identify fears to help move him or her through the appropriate phases of the grief process. Establish a trusting, ongoing relationship with the patient, and provide support through the personal grieving stages.

In collaboration with the social worker or chaplain, and when appropriate, assist the patient in identifying personal coping strategies. Encourage him or her to implement cultural, religious, and social customs associated with the loss, and identify sources of community support. Modifications in lifestyle are needed for patients with CRC. Help the patient and family identify these changes and how best to make them. The chaplain, social worker, or case manager assist in discussions and decisions with them concerning treatment, the prognosis, and end-of-life decisions, as appropriate.

NIC ***Genetic Counseling.*** Refer patients who are at risk for or have familial CRC for genetic counseling. Specially trained nurses can discuss the purposes and goals of genetic testing. Ensure privacy and confidentiality. A review of the family history may provide important information concerning the pattern of colorectal cancer inheritance. To make an informed decision, the patient and family need information about the advantages, risks, and costs of appropriate genetic tests. Monitor the patient's response regarding genetic risk factors. NIC interventions are summarized in Chart 59-2.

Potential for Metastasis

Planning: Expected Outcomes. The patient with colorectal cancer (CRC) is expected to not have the cancer spread to vital organs. Thus the patient's life expectancy will be increased and the quality of life will be improved.

Interventions. Although surgical resection is the primary means used to control the disease, several adjuvant (additional) therapies are used. Adjuvant therapies are administered before or after surgery to effect a cure and to prevent recurrence.

Nonsurgical Management. The type of therapy used is based on the pathologic staging of the disease. The American Joint Committee on Cancer (AJCC) system has begun to replace the older Dukes' staging classification with this description:

- Stage I—Tumor invades up to muscle layer
- Stage II—Tumor invades up to other organs or perforates peritoneum
- Stage III—Any level of tumor invasion and up to 4 regional lymph nodes
- Stage IV—Any level of tumor invasion; many lymph nodes affected with distant metastases

Radiation therapy. The administration of preoperative radiation therapy has not improved overall survival rates for colon cancer, but it has been effective in providing local or regional control of the disease. Postoperative radiation has not demonstrated any consistent improvement in survival or recurrence. However, as a palliative measure, radiation therapy may be used to control pain, hemorrhage, bowel obstruction, or metastasis to the lung in advanced disease. For rectal cancer, unlike colon cancer, radiation therapy is almost always a part of the treatment plan. Reinforce information about the radiation therapy procedure to the patient and family, and monitor for possible side effects (e.g., diarrhea, fatigue). Chapter 24 describes the general care of patients undergoing radiation therapy.

Drug therapy. Adjuvant *chemotherapy* after primary surgery is recommended for patients with stage II or stage III disease to interrupt the DNA production of cells and improve survival. The drugs of choice are IV 5-fluorouracil (5-FU) with leucovorin (LV) (folinic acid), capecitabine (Xeloda), or a combination of drugs referred to as *FOLFOX.* The most frequently used FOLFOX combination is 5-FU, leucovorin, and oxaliplatin (Eloxatin), a platinum analogue. These drugs cannot discriminate between cancer and healthy cells. Therefore common side effects are diarrhea, mucositis, leukopenia, mouth ulcers, and peripheral neuropathy.

If a patient's disease metastasizes, one of the discussed drug regimens may be used in combination with irinotecan (Camptosar) and/or bevacizumab (Avastin). Irinotecan often causes **myelosuppression** (bone marrow suppression) and explosive, immediate diarrhea. For this reason, a dose of atropine is always given just before its administration. Bevacizumab is the first antiangiogenesis drug to be approved for advanced CRC. This type of drug reduces blood flow to the growing tumor cells, thereby depriving them of necessary nutrients needed to grow. It is usually given in combination with other chemotherapeutic agents.

Cetuximab (Erbitux), a monoclonal antibody, may also be given for advanced disease. This drug works by binding to a protein receptor to slow cell growth. Erbitux is usually given in combination with another drug.

Current clinical trials using other monoclonal antibodies and a colorectal tumor vaccine are in progress. In addition, new agents such as fluorinated pyrimidines and oral leucovorin are being tested. The combination of Avastin and Erbitux, as well as new antiangiogenesis drugs, are also being tested. Intrahepatic arterial chemotherapy, often with 5-FU, may be administered to patients with liver metastasis. Patients with CRC also receive drugs for relief of symptoms, such as analgesics and antiemetics.

Surgical Management. Surgical removal of the tumor with margins free of disease is the best method of ensuring removal of CRC. The size of the tumor, its location, the extent of metastasis, the integrity of the bowel, and the condition of the patient determine which surgical procedure is performed for colorectal cancer (Table 59-1). At least 12 regional lymph

Chart 59-2 NIC INTERVENTION ACTIVITIES

The Patient with Noninflammatory Intestinal Disorders

Grief Work Facilitation: *Assistance with the resolution of a significant loss*

- Assist the patient to identify the nature of the attachment to the lost object or person.
- Assist the patient to identify the initial reaction to the loss.
- Encourage expression of feelings about the loss.
- Instruct in phases of the grieving process, as appropriate.
- Support progression through personal grieving stages.
- Include significant others in discussions and decisions, as appropriate.
- Assist patient to identify personal coping strategies.
- Encourage patient to implement cultural, religious, and social customs associated with the loss.
- Identify sources to community support.
- Assist in identifying modifications needed in lifestyle.

Genetic Counseling: *Use of an interactive helping process focusing on assisting a person, family, or group, manifesting or at risk for developing or transmitting a birth defect or genetic condition, to cope*

- Provide privacy and ensure confidentiality.
- Determine the patient's purpose, goals, and agenda for the genetic counseling session.
- Monitor response when patient learns about own genetic risk factors.
- Provide referral to genetic health care specialists, as necessary.

NIC intervention activities selected from Bulechek, G.M., Butcher, H.K., & McCloskey Dochterman, J. (Eds.). (2008). *Nursing interventions classifications (NIC)* (5th ed.). St. Louis: Mosby. No part of this work is to be altered without prior written permission from the Publisher.

TABLE 59-1 Surgical Procedures for Colorectal Cancers in Various Locations

RIGHT-SIDED COLON TUMORS
- Right hemicolectomy for smaller lesions
- Right ascending colostomy or ileostomy for large, widespread lesions
- Cecostomy (opening into the cecum with intubation to decompress the bowel)

LEFT-SIDED COLON TUMORS
- Left hemicolectomy for smaller lesions
- Left descending colostomy for larger lesions

SIGMOID COLON TUMORS
- Sigmoid colectomy for smaller lesions
- Sigmoid colostomy for larger lesions
- Abdominoperineal resection for large, low sigmoid tumors (near the anus) with colostomy (the rectum and the anus are completely removed, leaving a perineal wound)

RECTAL TUMORS
- Resection with anastomosis or pull-through procedure (preserves anal sphincter and normal elimination pattern)
- Colon resection with permanent colostomy
- Abdominoperineal resection with colostomy

TABLE 59-2 Preoperative Assessment by the ET Nurse

KEY POINTS OF PSYCHOSOCIAL ASSESSMENT

- Patient's and family's level of knowledge of disease and ostomy care
- Patient's educational level
- Patient's physical limitations (particularly sensory)
- Support available to patient
- Patient's type of employment
- Patient involvement in activities such as hobbies
- Financial concerns regarding purchase of ostomy supplies

KEY POINTS OF PHYSICAL ASSESSMENT

Before marking, the ET considers:

- Contour of the abdomen in lying, sitting, and standing positions
- Presence of skin folds, creases, bony prominences, and scars
- Need to avoid a prosthesis
- Location of belt line
- Location that is easily visible to the patient
- Possible location in the rectus muscle

Adapted from Pontieri-Lewis, V. (2006). Basics of ostomy care. *MEDSURG Nursing, 15*(4), 199-202.
ET, Enterostomal therapist.

nodes should be removed and examined for presence of cancer. The number of lymph nodes that contain cancer is a strong predictor of prognosis. The most common surgeries performed are **colon resection** (removal of the tumor and regional lymph nodes) with reanastomosis, **colectomy** (colon removal) with *colostomy (temporary or permanent) or ileostomy/ileoanal pull-through,* and **abdominoperineal (AP) resection.** A **colostomy** is the surgical creation of an opening of the colon onto the surface of the abdomen. An AP resection is performed when rectal tumors are present. The surgeon removes the sigmoid colon, rectum, and anus through combined abdominal and perineal incisions.

For patients having a colon resection, minimally invasive surgery (MIS) via laparoscopy is commonly performed today. This procedure results in shorter hospital stays, less pain, fewer complications, and quicker recovery compared with the open conventional surgical approach.

Preoperative care. Reinforce the physician's explanation of the planned surgical procedure. The patient is told as accurately as possible what anatomic and physiologic changes will occur with surgery. The location and number of incision sites and drains are also discussed.

Before evaluating the tumor and colon during surgery, the surgeon may not be able to determine whether a colostomy (or less commonly, an ileostomy) will be necessary. The patient is told that a colostomy is a possibility. If a colostomy is planned, the surgeon consults a certified wound, ostomy, continence nurse (CWOCN) or an enterostomal therapist (ET) (ostomy nurse) to recommend optimal placement of the ostomy. He or she teaches the patient about the rationale and general principles of ostomy care. In many settings, the ET marks the patient's abdomen to indicate a potential ostomy site that will decrease the risk for complications such as interference of the undergarments or a prosthesis with the ostomy appliance. Table 59-2 describes the role of the ET.

The patient who requires low rectal surgery (e.g., AP resection) is faced with the risk for postoperative sexual dysfunction and urinary incontinence after surgery as a result of nerve damage during surgery. The surgeon discusses the risk for these problems with the patient before surgery and allows him or her to verbalize concerns and questions related to this risk. Reinforce teaching about abdominal surgery performed for the patient under general anesthesia, and review the routines for turning and deep breathing (see Chapter 16). Teach the patient about the method of pain management to be used after surgery such as IV patient-controlled analgesia (PCA), epidural analgesia, or other method.

If the bowel is not obstructed or perforated, elective surgery is planned. The patient may be instructed to thoroughly clean the bowel, or "bowel prep," to minimize bacterial growth and prevent complications. Mechanical cleaning is accomplished with laxatives and enemas or with "whole-gut lavage." For whole-gut lavage, the patient may drink large quantities of a sodium sulfate and polyethylene glycol solution (e.g., GoLYTELY). This solution overwhelms the absorptive capacity of the small bowel and clears feces from the colon. However, the use of bowel preps is controversial and some surgeons do not recommend it because of patient discomfort. Infection rates are not different with or without bowel preps.

To reduce the risk for infection, the surgeon may prescribe one dose of oral or IV antibiotics to be given before the surgical incision is made. Teach patients that a nasogastric tube (NGT) may be placed for decompression of the stomach after surgery. A peripheral IV or central venous catheter is also placed for fluid and electrolyte replacement while the patient is NPO after surgery. Patients having minimally invasive surgeries do not need an NGT.

The patient with colorectal cancer faces a serious illness with long-term consequences of the disease and treatment. A case manager or social worker can be very helpful in identifying patient and family needs, as well as ensuring continuity of care and support.

Operative procedures. For the conventional open surgical approach, the surgeon makes a large incision in the abdomen and explores the abdominal cavity to determine whether the tumor can be removed. For a colon resection, the portion of the colon with the tumor is excised and the two open ends of the bowel are irrigated before **anastomosis** (reattachment) of the colon. If an anastomosis is not feasible because of the location of the tumor or the bowel is inflamed, a colostomy is created.

A colostomy may be created in the ascending, transverse, descending, or sigmoid colon (Fig. 59-5). One of several techniques is used to construct a colostomy. A loop **stoma** (surgical opening) is made by bringing a loop of colon to the skin surface, severing and everting the anterior wall, and suturing it to the abdominal wall. Loop colostomies are usually performed in the transverse colon and are usually temporary. An external rod may be used to support the loop until the intestinal tissue adheres to the abdominal wall. Care must be taken to avoid displacing the rod, especially during appliance changes.

An end stoma is often constructed, most often in the descending or sigmoid colon, when a colostomy is intended to be permanent. It may also be done when the surgeon oversews the distal stump of the colon and places it in the abdominal cavity, preserving it for future reattachment. An end stoma is constructed by severing the end of the proximal portion of the bowel and bringing it out through the abdominal wall.

The least common colostomy is the **double-barrel stoma,** which is created by dividing the bowel and bringing both the

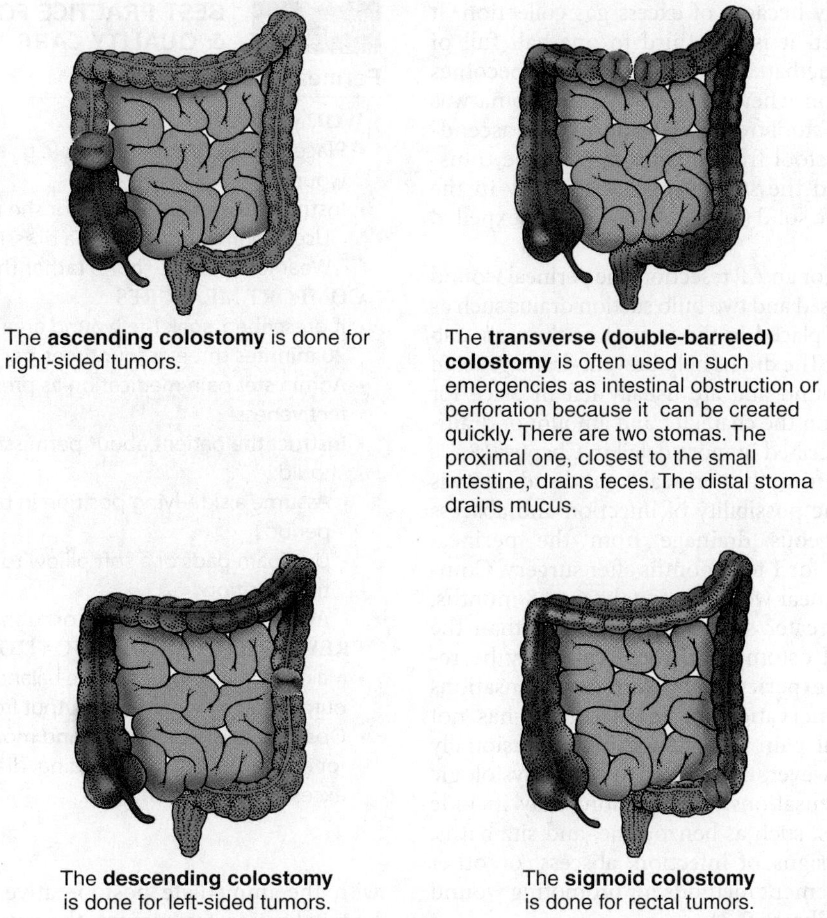
The **ascending colostomy** is done for right-sided tumors.
The **transverse (double-barreled) colostomy** is often used in such emergencies as intestinal obstruction or perforation because it can be created quickly. There are two stomas. The proximal one, closest to the small intestine, drains feces. The distal stoma drains mucus.
The **descending colostomy** is done for left-sided tumors.
The **sigmoid colostomy** is done for rectal tumors.

Fig. 59-5 • Different locations of colostomies in the colon.

proximal and distal portions to the abdominal surface to create two stomas. The proximal stoma (closest to the patient's head) is the functioning stoma and eliminates stool. The distal stoma (farthest from the head) is considered nonfunctioning, although it may secrete some mucus. The distal stoma is sometimes referred to as a *mucous fistula.*

MIS colon resection or total colectomy allows complete tumor removal with an adequate surgical margin and removal of associated lymph nodes. Several small incisions are made, and a miniature video camera is placed within the abdomen to help see the area that is involved. This technique takes longer than the conventional procedure and requires specialized training. However, blood loss is less.

Postoperative care. Patients who have an open colon resection without a colostomy receive care similar to that of those having any abdominal surgery (see Chapter 18). Other patients have surgeries that also require colostomy management. They typically have a nasogastric tube (NGT) after open surgery and receive IV PCA for the first 24 to 36 hours. After NGT removal, the diet is slowly progressed from liquids to solid foods as tolerated. The care of patients with an NGT is found on p. 1304 in the discussion of Interventions in the Intestinal Obstruction section.

By contrast, patients who have laparoscopic (MIS) surgery can progress from liquids to solids more quickly. Because they usually have less pain, they are able to ambulate earlier than those who have the conventional approach. The hospital stay is usually shorter for the patient with MIS—usually 2 to 3 days.

Colostomy management. The patient who has a colostomy may return from surgery with a clear ostomy pouch system in place. A clear pouch allows the health care team to observe the stoma. If no pouch system is in place, a petrolatum gauze dressing is usually placed over the stoma to keep it moist. This is covered with a dry, sterile dressing. In collaboration with the ostomy nurse, place a pouch system as soon as possible. The colostomy pouch system, also called an *appliance,* allows more convenient and acceptable collection of stool than a dressing does.

Assess the color and integrity of the stoma frequently. A healthy stoma should be reddish pink and moist and protrude about $^{3}/_{4}$ inch (2 cm) from the abdominal wall. During the initial postoperative period, the stoma may be slightly edematous. A small amount of bleeding at the stoma is common.

Report any of these problems related to the colostomy to the surgeon:

- Signs of ischemia and necrosis (dark red, purplish, or black color; dry, firm, or flaccid)
- Unusual bleeding
- Mucocutaneous separation (breakdown of the suture line securing the stoma to the abdominal wall)

Also assess the condition of the peristomal skin (skin around the stoma), and frequently check the pouch system for proper fit and signs of leakage. The skin should be intact, smooth, and without redness or excoriation.

The colostomy should start functioning in 2 to 4 days postoperatively. When it begins to function, the pouch may need to be emptied frequently because of excess gas collection. It should be emptied when it is one-third to one-half full of stool. Stool is liquid immediately postoperatively but becomes more solid, depending on where in the colon the stoma was placed. For example, the stool from a colostomy in the ascending colon is liquid, the stool from a colostomy in the transverse colon is pasty, and the stool from a colostomy in the descending colon is more solid (similar to usual stool expelled from the rectum).

Wound management. For an AP resection, the perineal wound is generally surgically closed and two bulb suction drains such as Jackson-Pratt drains are placed in the wound or through stab wounds near the wound. The drains help prevent drainage from collecting within the wound and are usually left in place for several days, depending on the character and amount of drainage. These drains are described in more detail in Chapter 18.

Monitoring drainage from the perineal wound and cavity is important because of the possibility of infection and abscess formation. Serosanguineous drainage from the perineal wound may be observed for 1 to 2 months after surgery. Complete healing of the perineal wound may take 6 to 8 months. This wound can be a greater source of discomfort than the abdominal incision and ostomy, and more care may be required. The patient may experience phantom rectal sensations because sympathetic innervation for rectal control has not been interrupted. Rectal pain and itching may occasionally occur after healing. However, there is no known physiologic explanation for these sensations. Interventions may include use of antipruritic drugs, such as benzocaine, and sitz baths. Continually assess for signs of infection, abscess, or other complications, and implement methods for promoting wound drainage and comfort (Chart 59-3).

DECISION-MAKING CHALLENGE
Coordination of Care

A 59-year-old nurse is admitted to your unit after having urgent surgery for stage IV colorectal cancer. Yesterday she had her first screening colonoscopy at the insistence of her family practice physician. She has been fatigued and anemic for the past year, for which she has taken vitamin and iron supplements. The physician referred her immediately to a surgeon as soon as she was diagnosed with advanced cancer. The surgeon performed a partial colectomy with a right-sided colostomy. She has PCA morphine, an IV antibiotic infusing, an indwelling urinary catheter, oxygen at 3 L/min via nasal cannula, and a large abdominal pressure dressing with two JP drains. When you enter her room, you see her husband and daughter, who are both crying.

1. What is your best response at this time?
2. When you assess the patient, what would you expect to drain from the colostomy?
3. With whom should you collaborate when planning and providing care for this patient and her family?
4. What part of her care could you delegate to an LPN/LVN?

evolve For suggested answer guidelines, go to http://evolve.elsevier.com/Iggy/.

Community-Based Care

Patients undergoing an uncomplicated colon resection by open approach are typically hospitalized for 3 to 5 days or longer, depending on the age of the patient and any complications or concurrent health problems. Collaborate with the case manager to assist patients and their families in coping

Chart 59-3 BEST PRACTICE FOR PATIENT SAFETY & QUALITY CARE

Perineal Wound Care

WOUND CARE
- Place an absorbent dressing (e.g., abdominal pad) over the wound.
- Instruct the patient that he or she may:
  - Use a feminine napkin as a dressing
  - Wear jockey-type shorts rather than boxers

COMFORT MEASURES
- If prescribed, soak the wound area in a sitz bath for 10 to 20 minutes three or four times per day.
- Administer pain medication as prescribed, and assess its effectiveness.
- Instruct the patient about permissible activities. The patient should:
  - Assume a side-lying position in bed; avoid sitting for long periods
  - Use foam pads or a soft pillow to sit on whenever in a sitting position
  - Avoid the use of air rings or rubber donut devices

PREVENTION OF COMPLICATIONS
- Maintain fluid and electrolyte balance by monitoring intake and output and by monitoring output from the perineal wound.
- Observe incision integrity, and monitor wound drains; watch for erythema, edema, bleeding, drainage, unusual odor, and excessive or constant pain.

with the immediate postoperative phase of recovery. After hospitalization for surgery, the patient is usually managed at home. Radiation therapy or chemotherapy is typically done on an ambulatory care basis. For the patient with advanced cancer, hospice care may be an option (see Chapter 9).

Home Care Management

Assess all patients for their ability for self-management within limitations. For those requiring assistance with care, home care visits by nurses or assistive nursing personnel can be provided.

For the patient who has undergone a colostomy, review the home situation to aid the patient in arranging for care. Ostomy products should be kept in an area (preferably the bathroom) where the temperature is neither hot nor cold (skin barriers may become stiff or melt in extreme temperatures) to ensure proper functioning. The home care nurse or ET may serve as a consultant after the patient is discharged home to ensure continuity of care.

No changes are needed in sleeping accommodations. A moisture-proof covering may initially be placed over the bed mattress if patients feel insecure about the pouch system. They may consume their usual diet on discharge.

Health Teaching

Before discharge, teach the patient to avoid lifting heavy objects or straining on defecation to prevent tension on the anastomosis site. If he or she had the open surgical approach, driving should be avoided for 4 to 6 weeks while the incision heals. Patients who have had laparoscopy can usually return to all usual activities in 1 to 2 weeks.

A stool softener may be prescribed to keep stools at a soft consistency for ease of passage. Teach patients to note the frequency, amount, and character of the stools. In addition to this information, teach those with colon resections to watch for and report clinical manifestations of intestinal obstruction and perforation (e.g., cramping, abdominal pain, nausea, vomiting). Advise the patient to avoid gas-producing foods and carbonated beverages. Four to six weeks may be required to establish the effects of certain foods on bowel patterns.

Colostomy Care. Rehabilitation after surgery requires that patients and family members learn how to perform colostomy care. Provide adequate opportunity for patients to learn the psychomotor skills involved in this care before discharge. Plan sufficient practice time for learning how to handle, assemble, and apply all ostomy equipment. Teach patients and families or other caregivers about:

- The normal appearance of the stoma
- Signs and symptoms of complications
- Measurement of the stoma
- The choice, use, care, and application of the appropriate appliance to cover the stoma
- Measures to protect the skin adjacent to the stoma
- Nutrition changes to control gas and odor
- Resumption of normal activities, including work, travel, and sexual intercourse

The appropriate pouch system must be selected and fitted to the stoma. Patients with flat, firm abdomens may use either flexible (bordered with paper tape) or nonflexible (full skin barrier wafer) pouch systems. A firm abdomen with lateral creases or folds requires a flexible system. Patients with deep creases, flabby abdomens, a retracted stoma, or a stoma that is flush or concave to the abdominal surface benefit from a convex appliance with a stoma belt. This type of system presses into the skin around the stoma, causing the stoma to protrude. This protrusion helps tighten the skin and prevents leaks around the stoma opening onto the peristomal skin.

Measurement of the stoma is necessary to determine the correct size of the stomal opening on the appliance. The opening should be large enough not only to cover the peristomal skin but also to avoid stomal trauma. The stoma will shrink within 6 to 8 weeks after surgery. Therefore it needs to be measured at least once weekly during this time and as needed if the patient gains or loses weight. Teach the patient and family caregiver to trace the pattern of the stomal area on the wafer portion of the appliance and to cut an opening about $\frac{1}{8}$- to $\frac{1}{16}$-inch larger than the stomal pattern to ensure that stomal tissue will not be constricted.

Skin preparation may include clipping peristomal hair or shaving the area (moving from the stoma outward) to achieve a smooth surface, prevent unnecessary discomfort when the wafer is removed, and minimize the risk for infected hair follicles. Advise the patient to clean around the stoma with mild soap and water before putting on an appliance. He or she should avoid using moisturizing soaps to clean the area because the lubricants can interfere with adhesion of the appliance. Teach the patient and family to apply a skin sealant (preferably without alcohol) and allow it to dry before application of the appliance (colostomy bag) to facilitate less painful removal of the tape or adhesive. If peristomal skin becomes raw, stoma powder or paste or a combination may also be applied. The paste or other filler cream is also used to fill in crevices and creases to create a flat surface for the faceplate of the colostomy bag. If the patient develops a fungal rash, an antifungal cream or powder should be used.

Control of gas and odor from the colostomy is often an important outcome for patients with new ostomies. Although a leaking or inadequately closed pouch is the usual cause of odor, flatus can also contribute to the odor. Remind the patient that although generally no foods for ostomates are forbidden, certain foods and habits can cause flatus or contribute to odor when the pouch is open. Broccoli, beans, spicy foods, onions, brussels sprouts, cabbage, cauliflower, cucumbers, mushrooms, and peas often cause flatus, as does chewing gum, smoking, drinking beer, and skipping meals. Crackers, toast, and yogurt can help prevent gas. Asparagus, broccoli, cabbage, turnips, eggs, fish, and garlic contribute to odor when the pouch is open. Buttermilk, cranberry juice, parsley, and yogurt will help prevent odor. Charcoal filters, pouch deodorizers, or placement of a breath mint in the pouch will help eliminate odors. The patient should be cautioned to not put aspirin tablets in the pouch because they may cause ulceration of the stoma. Vents that allow release of gas from the ostomy bag through a deodorizing filter are available and may decrease the patient's level of self-consciousness about odor.

The patient with a sigmoid colostomy may benefit from colostomy irrigation to regulate elimination. However, most patients with a sigmoid colostomy can become regulated through diet. An irrigation is similar to an enema but is administered through the stoma rather than the rectum.

In addition to teaching the patient about the clinical manifestations of obstruction and perforation, ask the patient to report any fever or sudden onset of pain or swelling around the stoma. Other home care assessment is listed in Chart 59-4.

Psychosocial Concerns. The diagnosis of cancer can be emotionally immobilizing for the patient and family or significant others, but treatment may be welcomed because it may provide hope for control of the disease. Explore reactions to the illness and perceptions of planned interventions.

The patient's reaction to ostomy surgery may include:

- Fear of not being accepted by others
- Feelings of grief related to disturbance in body image
- Concerns about sexuality

Symms et al. (2008) found in their study of male veterans with intestinal ostomies that problems related to sexual activity and intimacy were their greatest challenge. (See the Evidence-Based Practice box on p. 1302.)

Chart 59-4 HOME CARE ASSESSMENT

The Patient with a Colostomy

Assess gastrointestinal status, including:
- Dietary and fluid intake and habits
- Presence or absence of nausea and vomiting
- Weight gain or loss
- Bowel elimination pattern and characteristics and amount of effluent (stool)
- Bowel sounds

Assess condition of stoma, including:
- Location, size, protrusion, color, and integrity
- Signs of ischemia, such as dull coloring or dark or purplish bruising

Assess peristomal skin for:
- Presence or absence of excoriated skin, leakage underneath drainage system
- Fit of appliance and effectiveness of skin barrier and appliance

Assess patient's and family's coping skills, including:
- Self-care abilities in the home
- Acknowledgment of changes in body image and function
- Sense of loss

EVIDENCE-BASED PRACTICE

What are the sexuality challenges that men with intestinal ostomies have?

Symms, M.R., Rawl, S.M., Grant, M., Wendel, C.S., Coons, S.J., Hickey, S., et al. (2008). Sexual health and quality of life among male veterans with intestinal ostomies. *Clinical Nurse Specialist, 22*(1), 30-40.

The researchers conducted this study of 481 male veterans in three Veterans Administration sites to determine the effect of intestinal ostomies on their sexual health. The design was case-controlled, and both quantitative and qualitative data were collected. The study group was compared with another group who had other surgeries. Quality of life was determined by responses on the modified City of Hope Quality of Life-Ostomy questionnaire.

Compared with sexual activity before surgery, the study group reported more problems with intimacy and sexuality than the control group. They had less sexual activity and more erectile dysfunction than men in the control group. For study group subjects, those who had successful sexual relationships felt less isolation and less trouble adjusting to their ostomies.

Level of Evidence—5. The study used a large sample and a control group for comparison.

Commentary—Implications for Practice and Research. Although the researchers used a convenience sample of one group of men, they had a large sample and obtained both quantitative and qualitative data. Nurses need to include a sexual health assessment in their care of patients with ostomies. They need to be open to discussion about sexual issues and refer patients to other resources, such as intimacy or sexual counselors, as needed. Additional studies should be conducted with non-veterans and include women of various ethnicities.

Allow the patient to verbalize his or her feelings. By teaching how to physically manage the ostomy, help him or her begin to restore self-esteem and improve body image. Inclusion of family and significant others in the rehabilitation process may help maintain relationships and raise self-esteem. Anticipatory instruction includes information on leakage accidents, odor control measures, and adjustments to resuming sexual relationships.

Health Care Resources

Several resources are available to maintain continuity of care in the home environment and provide for patient needs that the nurse is not able to meet. Make referrals to community-based case managers or social workers, who can provide further emotional counseling, aid in managing financial concerns, or arrange for services in the home or long-term care as needed.

Provide information about the United Ostomy Associations of America, Inc. (www.uoaa.org), a self-help group of people who have ostomies. This group has literature such as the organization's publication *(Ostomy Quarterly)* and information about local chapters. The organization conducts a visitor program that sends specially trained visitors (who have an ostomy [ostomate]) to talk with patients. After obtaining consent, make a referral to the visitor program so that the volunteer ostomate can see the patient both preoperatively and postoperatively. A physician's consent for visitation may be necessary.

The local division or unit of the American Cancer Society (ACS) (www.cancer.org) can help provide necessary medical equipment and supplies, home care services, travel accommodations, and other resources for the patient who is having cancer treatment or surgery. Inform the patient and family of the programs available through the local division or unit.

Because of short hospital stays, patients with new ostomies receive much health teaching from nurses working for home care agencies. This resource also helps provide physical care needs, medication management, and emotional support. If the patient has advanced colorectal cancer, a referral for hospice services in the home, nursing home, or other long-term care setting may be appropriate. The home care nurse informs the patient and family about what ostomy supplies are needed and where they can be purchased. Price and location are considered before recommendations are made.

Evaluation: Outcomes

Evaluate the care of the patient with colorectal cancer on the basis of the identified nursing diagnoses and collaborative problems. The expected outcomes are that the patient:

- Adjusts to actual or impending loss
- Is free of complications or metastasis associated with CRC

Specific indicators for these outcomes are listed for each nursing diagnosis and collaborative problem under the Planning and Implementation section (see earlier).

INTESTINAL OBSTRUCTION

Pathophysiology

Intestinal obstructions can be partial or complete and are classified as mechanical or nonmechanical. In **mechanical obstruction,** the bowel is physically blocked by problems outside the intestine (e.g., adhesions), in the bowel wall (e.g., Crohn's disease), or in the intestinal lumen (e.g., tumors). **Nonmechanical obstruction** (also known as **paralytic ileus** or *adynamic ileus*) does not involve a physical obstruction in or outside the intestine. Instead, peristalsis is decreased or absent as a result of neuromuscular disturbance, resulting in a slowing of the movement or a backup of intestinal contents.

Intestinal contents are composed of ingested fluid, food, and saliva; gastric, pancreatic, and biliary secretions; and swallowed air. In both mechanical and nonmechanical obstructions, the intestinal contents accumulate at and above the area of obstruction. Distention results from the intestine's inability to absorb the contents and move them down the intestinal tract. To compensate for the lag, peristalsis increases in an effort to move the intestinal contents forward. This increase stimulates more secretions, which then leads to additional distention. The bowel then becomes edematous, and increased capillary permeability results. Plasma leaking into the peritoneal cavity and fluid trapped in the intestinal lumen decrease the absorption of fluid and electrolytes into the vascular space.

Reduced circulatory blood volume (hypovolemia) and electrolyte imbalances typically occur. Hypovolemia ranges from mild to extreme (hypovolemic shock).

Specific fluid and electrolyte problems result, depending on the part of the intestine that is blocked. An obstruction high in the small intestine causes a loss of gastric hydrochloride, which can lead to *metabolic alkalosis.* Obstruction below the duodenum but above the large bowel results in loss of both acids and bases, so that acid-base imbalance is usually not compromised. Obstruction at the end of the small intestine and lower in the intestinal tract causes loss of alkaline fluids, which can lead to *metabolic acidosis.*

If hypovolemia is severe, renal insufficiency or even death can occur. Bacterial peritonitis with or without actual perforation can also result. Bacteria in the intestinal contents lie stagnant in the obstructed intestine. This is not a problem unless the blood flow to the intestine is compromised. However, with so-called closed-loop obstruction (blockage in two different areas) or a **strangulated obstruction** (obstruction with compromised blood flow), the risk for peritonitis is greatly increased. Bacteria without blood supply can form and release an endotoxin into the peritoneal or systemic circulation and cause septic shock. With a strangulated obstruction, major blood loss into the intestine and the peritoneum can result.

Etiology

Intestinal obstruction is a common and serious disorder caused by a variety of conditions and is associated with significant morbidity. It can occur anywhere in the intestinal tract, although the ileum in the small intestine (the narrowest part of the intestinal tract) is the most common site.

Mechanical obstruction can result from:

- Adhesions (scar tissue from surgeries or pathology)
- Benign or malignant tumor
- Complications of appendicitis
- Hernias
- Fecal impactions (especially in older adults)
- Strictures due to Crohn's disease or previous radiation therapy
- **Intussusception** (telescoping of a segment of the intestine within itself) (Fig. 59-6)
- **Volvulus** (twisting of the intestine) (See Fig. 59-6)
- Fibrosis due to disorders such as endometriosis
- Vascular disorders (e.g., emboli and arteriosclerotic narrowing of mesenteric vessels)

In people age 65 or older, diverticulitis, tumors, and fecal impaction are the most common causes of obstruction.

Paralytic ileus, or nonmechanical obstruction, is most commonly caused by handling of the intestines during abdominal surgery; intestinal function is lost for a few hours to several days. Electrolyte disturbances, especially hypokalemia, predispose the patient to this problem. The ileus can also be a consequence of peritonitis, because leakage of colonic contents causes severe irritation and triggers an inflammatory response. Vascular insufficiency to the bowel, also referred to as *intestinal ischemia,* is another potential cause of an ileus. It results when arterial or venous thrombosis or an embolus decreases blood flow to the mesenteric blood vessels surrounding the intestines, as in heart failure or severe shock. Severe insufficiency of blood supply can result in infarction of surrounding organs (e.g., bowel infarction).

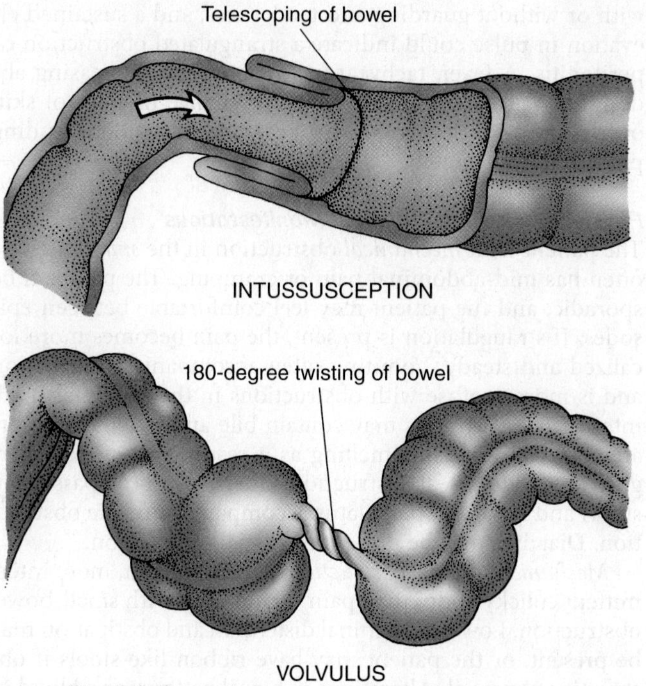
Telescoping of bowel
INTUSSUSCEPTION
180-degree twisting of bowel
VOLVULUS

Fig. 59-6 • Two types of mechanical obstruction.

Incidence/Prevalence

Obstruction of the intestines is the most common reason for surgery of the small intestine. Because bowel obstruction is a result of other disorders, statistics on the incidence of bowel obstruction are not readily available.

Obstruction of the intestines occurs in all age-groups, but the incidence differs with age. In adults, most obstructions occur in the small intestine.

Patient-Centered Collaborative Care

Assessment

History

Collect information about a history of:

- Abdominal surgery
- Radiation therapy
- Inflammatory bowel disease
- Gallstones
- Hernias
- Trauma
- Peritonitis
- Tumors

Question the patient about recent nausea, vomiting, and the color of emesis. Perform a thorough pain assessment with particular attention to the onset, aggravating factors, alleviating factors, and patterns or rhythms of the pain. Severe pain that then stops and changes to tenderness on palpation may indicate perforation and should be reported promptly to the physician. Ask about the passage of flatus and the time, character, and consistency of the last bowel movement. Singultus (hiccups) is common with all types of intestinal obstruction. When an obstruction is suspected, keep the patient NPO and contact the physician promptly for further guidance.

Assess for a family history of colorectal cancer (CRC), and ask about blood in the stool or a change in bowel pattern. Body temperature with uncomplicated obstruction is rarely higher than 100° F (37.8° C). A temperature higher than this, with or without guarding and tenderness, and a sustained elevation in pulse could indicate a strangulated obstruction or peritonitis. A fever, tachycardia, hypotension, increasing abdominal pain, abdominal rigidity, or change in color of skin overlying the abdomen should be reported to the attending physician immediately.

Physical Assessment/Clinical Manifestations

The patient with *mechanical* obstruction in the *small intestine* often has mid-abdominal pain or cramping. The pain can be sporadic, and the patient may feel comfortable between episodes. If strangulation is present, the pain becomes more localized and steady. Vomiting often accompanies obstruction and is more profuse with obstructions in the proximal small intestine. The vomitus may contain bile and mucus or be orange-brown and foul smelling as a result of bacterial overgrowth with low ileal obstruction. **Obstipation** (no passage of stool) and failure to pass flatus accompany complete obstruction. Diarrhea may be present in partial obstruction.

Mechanical colonic obstruction causes a milder, more intermittent colicky abdominal pain than is seen with small-bowel obstruction. Lower abdominal distention and obstipation may be present, or the patient may have ribbon-like stools if obstruction is partial. Alterations in bowel patterns and blood in the stools accompany the obstruction if colorectal cancer or diverticulitis is the cause.

On examination of the abdomen, observe for abdominal distention, which is common in all forms of intestinal obstruction. Peristaltic waves may also be visible. Auscultate for proximal high-pitched bowel sounds **(borborygmi),** which are associated with cramping early in the obstructive process as the intestine tries to push the mechanical obstruction forward. In later stages of mechanical obstruction, bowel sounds are absent, especially distal to the obstruction. Abdominal tenderness and rigidity are usually minimal. The presence of a tense, fluid-filled bowel loop mimicking a palpable abdominal mass may signal a closed-loop, strangulating small-bowel obstruction.

In most types of *nonmechanical* obstruction, the pain is described as a constant, diffuse discomfort. Colicky cramping is not characteristic of this type of obstruction. Pain associated with obstruction caused by vascular insufficiency or infarction is usually severe and constant. On inspection, abdominal distention is typically present. On auscultation of the abdomen, note and document decreased bowel sounds in early obstruction and absent bowel sounds in later stages. Vomiting of gastric contents and bile is frequent, but the vomitus rarely has a foul odor and is rarely profuse. Obstipation may or may not be present. Chart 59-5 compares small-bowel and large-bowel obstructions.

Laboratory Assessment

There is no definitive laboratory test to confirm a diagnosis of mechanical or nonmechanical obstruction. White blood cell (WBC) counts are normal unless there is a strangulated obstruction, in which case there may be leukocytosis (increased WBCs). Hemoglobin, hematocrit, creatinine, and blood urea nitrogen (BUN) values are often elevated, indicating dehydration. Serum sodium, chloride, and potassium concentrations are reduced because of loss of fluid and electrolytes. Elevations in serum amylase levels may be found with strangulating obstructions, which can damage the pancreas.

Patients with high obstruction in the small intestine have arterial blood gas (ABG) values indicative of metabolic alkalosis. Obstruction in the large intestine may show values suggestive of metabolic acidosis. Chapter 14 describes ABGs and these acid-base imbalances in detail.

Chart 59-5 KEY FEATURES

Small-Bowel and Large-Bowel Obstructions

Small-Bowel Obstructions	Large-Bowel Obstructions
Abdominal discomfort or pain possibly accompanied by visible peristaltic waves in upper and middle abdomen	Intermittent lower abdominal cramping
Upper or epigastric abdominal distention	Lower abdominal distention
Nausea and early, profuse vomiting (may contain fecal material)	Minimal or no vomiting
Obstipation	Obstipation or ribbon-like stools
Severe fluid and electrolyte imbalances	No major fluid and electrolyte imbalances
Metabolic alkalosis	Metabolic acidosis (not always present)

Imaging Assessment

The health care provider obtains flat-plate and upright abdominal x-rays and a CT scan as soon as an obstruction is suspected. Distention with fluid and gas in the small intestine with the absence of gas in the colon indicates an obstruction in the small intestine. X-ray findings are often normal when a strangulated obstruction actually exists in the small intestine.

Other Diagnostic Assessment

The diagnostic examination chosen depends on the suspected location of the obstruction. As an initial assessment, the physician may choose to do an abdominal ultrasound to evaluate the potential cause of the obstruction. The physician may perform endoscopy (sigmoidoscopy or colonoscopy) to determine the cause of the obstruction, except when perforation or complete obstruction is suspected.

▪ Interventions

Interventions are aimed at uncovering the cause and relieving the obstruction. Intestinal obstructions can be relieved by nonsurgical or surgical means. If the obstruction is partial and there is no evidence of strangulation, nonsurgical management is the treatment of choice. The patient is placed on NPO status, and decompression of the intestinal tract is initiated along with fluid and electrolyte replacement.

Nonsurgical Management

Paralytic ileus responds well to nonsurgical methods of relieving obstruction. Nonsurgical approaches are also preferred in the treatment of patients with terminal disease associated with bowel obstruction. In addition to being NPO, patients typically have a nasogastric tube (NGT) inserted to decompress the bowel by draining fluid and air. The tube is attached to suction.

ANIMATION: Nasogastric Tube Placement

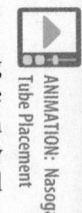

Nasogastric Tubes. Most patients with an obstruction have an NGT unless the obstruction is mild. *A Salem sump tube is*

inserted through the nose and placed into the stomach. It is attached to low continuous suction. This tube has a vent ("pigtail") that prevents the stomach mucosa from being pulled away during suctioning. Levin tubes do not have a vent and therefore should be connected to low intermittent suction. They are used less often than the Salem sump tubes. Chart 58-6 in Chapter 58 describes how to insert an NGT.

At least every 4 hours, assess for proper placement of the tube, tube patency, and output (quality and quantity). Monitor the nasal skin around the tube and opening where the NGT is inserted for irritation. Use a device that secures the tube to the nose to prevent accidental removal. Clean the nose with the same type of skin protectant used for ostomy skin care before applying the NGT securing device. Assess for peristalsis by auscultating for bowel sounds with the suction disconnected (suction masks peristaltic sounds).

Question the patient about the passage of flatus and record flatus and the character of bowel movements daily. Flatus or stool means that peristalsis has returned. Assess for nausea, and ask the patient to report this manifestation.

NG tubes must be monitored for proper functioning. Occasionally, NG tubes move out of optimal drainage position or become plugged. In this case, note a decrease in gastric output or stasis of the tube's contents. Assess the patient for nausea, vomiting, increased abdominal distention, and placement of the tube. If the NG tube is repositioned or replaced, confirmation of proper placement is obtained by x-ray examination before use. After appropriate placement is established, aspirate the contents and irrigate the tube with 30 mL of normal saline every 4 hours or as requested by the health care provider.

Other Nonsurgical Interventions. Most types of nonmechanical obstruction respond to nasogastric decompression in conjunction with medical treatment of the primary disorder. Incomplete mechanical obstruction can sometimes be successfully treated without surgery. Obstruction caused by lower fecal impaction usually resolves after disimpaction and enema administration. Intussusception may respond to hydrostatic pressure changes during a barium enema.

IV fluid replacement and maintenance are indicated for all patients with intestinal obstruction because the patient is NPO and fluids and electrolytes are lost (particularly potassium) through vomiting and nasogastric suction. On the basis of serum electrolytes and blood urea nitrogen (BUN) levels, the health care provider prescribes aggressive fluid replacement with 2 to 4 L of normal saline or lactated Ringer's solution with potassium added. Use care with patients who are susceptible to fluid overload (e.g., older adults with a history of heart or kidney failure). Monitor lung sounds, weight, and intake and output daily. Blood replacement may be indicated in strangulated obstruction because of blood loss into the bowel or peritoneal cavity.

Monitor vital signs and other measures of fluid status (e.g., urine output, skin turgor, mucous membranes) every 2 to 4 hours depending on the severity of the patient's symptoms. In collaboration with the nutritionist, the physician may prescribe total parenteral nutrition (TPN), especially if the patient has had chronic nutritional problems and has been NPO for an extended period. Chapter 63 discusses the nursing care of patients receiving TPN.

The patient with intestinal obstruction is usually thirsty, although older adults have a decreased thirst response as they age. Delegate frequent mouth care to unlicensed assistive personnel (UAP) to help maintain moist mucous membranes. Be sure to supervise this activity. A small amount of ice chips may be allowed if the patient is not having surgery. Follow agency protocol or the physician's request regarding ice chips.

Abdominal distention can cause a great deal of discomfort, especially when it is severe. The colicky, crampy pain that comes and goes with mechanical obstruction and the nausea, vomiting, dry mucous membranes, and thirst contribute to the patient's discomfort. Continually assess the character and location of the pain, and immediately report any pain that significantly increases or changes from a colicky, intermittent type to a constant discomfort. These changes can indicate perforation of the intestine or peritonitis.

Opioid analgesics are normally withheld in the diagnostic workup period so that clinical manifestations of perforation or peritonitis are not masked. Explain to the patient and family the rationale for not giving analgesics. In addition, if analgesics such as morphine are given, they may slow intestinal motility and can cause vomiting. Be alert to this side effect because nausea and vomiting are also signs of NG tube obstruction or worsening bowel obstruction.

Help the patient obtain a position of comfort with frequent position changes to promote increased peristalsis. A semi-Fowler's position helps alleviate the pressure of abdominal distention on the chest. This not only is a good comfort technique but also helps with thoracic excursion and normal breathing patterns.

Discomfort is generally less with nonmechanical obstruction than with mechanical obstruction. With both types of obstruction, discomfort is aggravated by taking in food or fluids.

If strangulation is thought to be likely, the health care provider prescribes IV broad-spectrum antibiotics. In addition, in cases of partial obstruction or paralytic ileus, drugs that enhance gastric motility such as octreotide acetate (Sandostatin) may be used.

Surgical Management

In patients with complete mechanical obstruction and in some cases of incomplete mechanical obstruction, surgical intervention is necessary to relieve the obstruction. A strangulated obstruction is complete, and surgical intervention is always required. An **exploratory laparotomy** (a surgical opening of the abdominal cavity to investigate the cause of the obstruction) is initially performed for many patients with obstruction. More specific surgical procedures depend on the cause of the obstruction.

Preoperative Care. Provide general preoperative teaching for both the patient and family as discussed in Chapter 16. In cases of complete obstruction, the patient may feel too ill to want the information. Reinforce the information with the family or other caregiver. Depending on the cause and severity of the obstruction, as well as the expertise of the surgeon, patients have either minimally invasive surgery (MIS) via laparoscopy or an open conventional approach.

Operative Procedures. In the *open conventional surgical approach,* the surgeon makes a large incision, enters the abdominal cavity, and explores for obstruction and its cause, if possible **(exploratory laparotomy).** If adhesions are found, they are lysed (cut and released). Obstruction caused by a tumor or diverticulitis requires a colon resection with primary anastomosis or a temporary or permanent colostomy. If obstruction is caused by intestinal infarction, an embolectomy, thrombectomy, or resection of the gangrenous small or large bowel may be necessary. In severe cases, a colectomy (removal of the entire colon) may be needed.

For the *MIS* approach, the specially trained surgeon makes several small incisions in the abdomen and places a video camera to view the abdominal contents to determine the extent of the obstruction. A laparoscope (type of endoscope) with a lighted end is inserted along with various surgical instruments to remove the problem. This procedure takes longer than the open approach, but blood loss is less.

Postoperative Care. General postoperative care for the patient undergoing an *exploratory laparotomy* with lysis of adhesions, colon resection, thrombectomy, or embolectomy is similar to that described in Chapter 18. In addition, patients have an NGT in place until peristalsis resumes. A clear liquid diet may be prescribed to encourage peristalsis return. As liquids are started, the NGT can be disconnected from suction and capped for 1 to 2 hours after the patient has taken clear liquids to determine if he or she is able to tolerate them. If the patient vomits after liquids, the suction is resumed. When the patient has return of peristalsis, the NGT is removed slowly by first discontinuing suction and then clamping the tube for a scheduled amount of time. Residual drainage is checked at each stage to assess peristalsis without decompression before removing the tube entirely.

Most patients today have laparoscopic surgery (MIS) for mechanical intestinal obstructions. They usually do *not* have an NGT and can recover more quickly than those with the open surgical approach. The hospital stay for those having MIS to remove tumors, adhesions, and other obstructions may be as short as 2 to 3 days compared with 3 to 5 days or longer for the conventional surgical patients. Recovery is much quicker because there is less pain and fewer postoperative complications among those who had laparoscopic surgery.

NCLEX EXAMINATION CHALLENGE

An older client has a nasogastric tube (NGT) connected to low continuous suction to treat an intestinal obstruction from fecal impaction. The nurse observes that the tube has stopped draining. What is the nurse's best action?

A. Remove the NGT because it is not working.
B. Document the finding, and monitor closely.
C. Notify the health care provider immediately.
D. Irrigate the tube with 30 mL saline.

evolve For the correct answer, go to http://evolve.elsevier.com/Iggy/.

Community-Based Care

All patients with intestinal obstruction are hospitalized for monitoring and treatment. The length of stay varies according to the type of obstruction, the treatment, and the presence of complications. Patients who have complicated obstruction, such as strangulation or incarceration, are at greater risk for peritonitis, sepsis, and shock.

Patients with nonmechanical (adynamic) intestinal obstruction are less likely to require a lengthy hospitalization because of the obstruction alone. Adynamic obstruction generally responds to NG intubation and suction within a few days. However, if the ileus occurs as a complication of an abdominal surgery, the hospital stay could be lengthy.

Chart 59-6 NURSING FOCUS ON THE OLDER ADULT

Preventing Fecal Impaction

- Teach the patient to eat high-fiber foods, including plenty of raw fruits and vegetables and whole-grain products.
- Encourage the patient to drink adequate amounts of fluids, especially water.
- Do not routinely administer a laxative; teach the patient that laxative abuse decreases abdominal muscle tone and contributes to an atonic colon.
- Encourage the patient to exercise regularly, if possible. Walking every day is an excellent exercise for promoting intestinal motility.
- Use natural foods to stimulate peristalsis, such as warm beverages and prune juice.
- Take bulk-forming products, such as Metamucil, to provide fiber.
- Check the patient's stool for amount and frequency; oozing of soft or diarrheal stool often indicates a fecal impaction.
- Have the patient sit on a toilet or bedside commode, rather than on a bedpan, for elimination.

Home Care Management

For the patient who has had an intestinal obstruction, preparation for home care depends on the cause of the obstruction and the treatment required. Those who have resolution of obstruction without surgical intervention are assessed for their knowledge of strategies to avoid recurrent obstruction. For example, if fecal impaction was the cause of the obstruction, assess the patient's ability to carry out a bowel regimen independently (Chart 59-6). For those who have had surgery, evaluate their ability to function at home with the added tasks of incision care and possibly colostomy care.

Health Teaching

Instruct the patient to report any abdominal pain or distention, nausea, or vomiting, with or without constipation, because these symptoms might indicate recurrent obstruction. The patient should be reassured, however, that recurrent paralytic ileus is not common.

Teach the patient who has had surgery about incision care, drug therapy, and activity limitations. Drug therapy consists of an oral opioid analgesic, such as oxycodone hydrochloride with acetaminophen (Tylox, Percocet, Endocet♦), to be taken as needed for incisional discomfort. As with any opioid therapy, scheduled doses of a laxative with a softener (e.g., Docusate with Senna) may be added to prevent constipation and possible recurrent obstruction.

The patient who had curative treatment of the underlying cause most likely requires less support than one who had treatment of obstruction related to a serious disease that will require further management. Encourage the patient to express fears and concerns about the future. Assess the patient's understanding and needs with regard to treatment plans.

Health Care Resources

The need for follow-up appointments depends on the cause of the obstruction and the treatment required. In collaboration with the case manager, make arrangements for a home care nurse if the patient needs help with incision or colostomy care.

ABDOMINAL TRAUMA

Pathophysiology

Abdominal trauma is defined as injury to the structures located between the diaphragm and the pelvis, which occurs when the abdomen is subjected to blunt or penetrating forces. Organs injured may include the large or small bowel, liver, spleen, duodenum, pancreas, kidneys, and urinary bladder.

At least one half of all *blunt abdominal traumas* occur from motor vehicle crashes. Other causes of blunt trauma include falls, aggravated assaults, and contact sports. *Penetrating abdominal trauma* is caused by gunshot wounds, stabbing, or impalement with an object. The liver is the most commonly injured organ in both types of trauma. The spleen is the most commonly injured organ in blunt abdominal trauma. Most penetrating injuries are caused by gunshot wounds (GSWs). *Trauma is the leading cause of death in young adults (younger than 40 years) in the United States.*

Patient-Centered Collaborative Care

Assessment

First, assess any patient experiencing trauma for airway, breathing, and circulation (ABCs). Once these needs are met, focus on the risks of hemorrhage, shock, and peritonitis. Mental status, vital signs, and skin perfusion are *priority* nursing assessments, with skin perfusion being the most reliable clinical guide in assessing hypovolemic shock:

- In a person with mild shock, the skin is pale, cool, and moist.
- With moderate shock, diaphoresis is more marked and urine output ceases.
- With severe shock, changes in mental status are manifested by agitation, disorientation, and recent memory loss.

Assess for abdominal trauma by asking the patient about the presence, location, and quality of pain. Inspect the abdomen, flanks, back, genitalia, and rectum for contusions, abrasions, lacerations, ecchymosis, penetrating injuries, and symmetry. All of the patient's clothes must be removed for this examination.

Inspection of the abdomen may reveal distention. To perform an adequate inspection, turn the patient while maintaining spinal immobilization. *Ecchymosis (bruising) may indicate internal bleeding. Ecchymosis present in the distribution of a lap seat belt should be reported to the health care provider immediately because the bowel or other major organ may be injured.* Ecchymosis around the umbilicus is known as **Cullen's sign.** On either flank, it is known as **Turner's sign** and may indicate retroperitoneal bleeding into the abdominal wall.

Auscultate the abdomen for bowel sounds. Absent or diminished bowel sounds may be caused by the presence of blood, bacteria, or a chemical irritant in the abdominal cavity. Also auscultate for bruits in the abdomen, which could indicate renal artery injury.

During percussion, an abnormal sign associated with abdominal trauma is left flank dullness and resonance over the right flank with the patient lying on the left side. This is known as **Ballance's sign** and is found with a ruptured spleen. Resonance over the normally dull liver is due to free air, which is pathologic. Palpation for lower rib fractures should increase suspicion of liver or spleen injuries. Injury to the spleen is present in many people with left lower rib fractures. Liver injury may be present in those with right lower rib fractures. The presence of **Kehr's sign,** left shoulder pain resulting from diaphragmatic irritation, may be present in splenic injury.

Dullness over hollow organs that normally contain gas such as the stomach and the large and small intestines may indicate the presence of blood or fluid. Light abdominal palpation identifies areas of tenderness, rebound tenderness, guarding, rigidity, and spasm. A palpated mass may be blood or a fluid collection.

The patient without obvious significant bleeding or definite signs of peritoneal irritation undergoes abdominal ultrasound, **diagnostic peritoneal lavage (DPL),** and CT. For DPL, the physician inserts a large-bore catheter into the abdomen and allows fluid to enter the abdominal cavity. If the return drainage from the abdomen is pink or grossly bloody, the health care team prepares for surgery. Abdominal ultrasound or focused abdominal sonography for trauma (FAST) is used to diagnose blunt abdominal trauma and may replace CT and DPL for diagnosis. Patients with hemodynamic instability or peritonitis are candidates for immediate laparotomy.

Interventions

Nonsurgical and surgical interventions are aimed at preserving or restoring hemodynamic stability, preventing or decreasing blood loss, and preventing complications. Patients with abdominal trauma from a vehicle crash often have other injuries such as multiple fractures. *The priority for care is to establish and maintain the ABCs.*

Emergency Care: Abdominal Trauma

Nursing interventions include placement of at least two large-bore IV catheters in the upper extremities. IV catheters are not used in the lower extremities; if the vasculature has been injured, fluid can pool in the abdomen. The health care provider may insert a central venous catheter to assist with rapid fluid volume infusion. IV fluids include saline, crystalloids, and possibly blood. Be sure to type and crossmatch the patient for as many as 4 to 8 units of packed red blood cells.

These laboratory values are monitored:

- Arterial blood gases
- Complete blood count (CBC)
- Serum electrolyte, glucose and amylase, and blood urea nitrogen (BUN) determinations
- Liver function tests
- Coagulation studies

Measuring arterial blood gases may help determine the severity of shock. Hemoglobin and hematocrit values do not initially reflect true blood loss; values can be skewed because of hemoconcentration from volume loss or the dilutional effects of IV fluids. Serial hemoglobin and hematocrit measurements may be more accurate in determining true blood loss. An elevated white blood cell (WBC) count may indicate a ruptured spleen or intestinal injury. Elevated levels of serum transaminases may indicate liver injury. Elevation of serum amylase activity may signal injury to the pancreas or the bowel. All laboratory work is compiled so that values can be compared and subtle changes noted.

Continuous hemodynamic monitoring is begun in the emergency department. Insert an indwelling urinary (Foley) catheter unless there is blood at the urinary meatus. Initially and hourly thereafter, evaluate urine output for bleeding and specific gravity. Laboratory tests indicate the amount of blood and protein in the urine. If there is an open abdominal wound or evisceration, cover it with a sterile dry dressing unless the physician requests otherwise. Unless it is contraindicated, as in the case of a skull fracture, the physician or nurse inserts a nasogastric (NG) tube to identify bleeding and minimize the risk for vomiting and aspiration. Antibiotics are administered as prescribed to reduce the risk for peritonitis.

If the patient with known abdominal trauma has no definite clinical manifestations of active bleeding or organ injury, he or she is admitted to the hospital for observation. Many patients are admitted to the critical care unit. Blunt trauma can cause active, but often not obvious, damage. Assess for abdominal or referred pain and nausea. Every 15 to 30 minutes in the early postinjury period and then hourly, evaluate:

- Mental status
- Vital signs
- Clinical findings, such as vomiting, guarding, rigidity, or rebound tenderness
- Skin temperature
- Bowel sounds
- Urine output
- IV patency

Report any change immediately to the health care provider. It is more important to recognize the high risk for an active abdominal injury and assess for general signs of organ injury (e.g., hemorrhage and peritonitis) than to identify the exact nature of the abdominal injury. Opioid analgesics are given for pain after the physician's initial assessment is complete. Explain to the patient and family the rationale for delaying analgesics.

Intra-abdominal Pressure Monitoring

Some patients are monitored for intra-abdominal pressure (IAP) using a continuous monitoring system. As the name implies, **intra-abdominal pressure** is pressure within the abdominal cavity. The normal IAP in healthy adults is 0 to 5 mm Hg, but obese patients often have a higher normal value. Patients who have uncomplicated abdominal surgery frequently have an increase in IAP but it causes no lasting problems. However, in patients with abdominal injury (especially blunt trauma), IAP may increase to the point that major body organs are damaged.

When IAP becomes higher than the central venous pressure, the inferior vena cava and other abdominal vessels are compressed. This leads to impaired venous return, increased afterload, and decreased preload. The patient is then at risk for deep vein thrombosis and pulmonary embolism (PE). The patient has tachycardia and hypotension. As the IAP increases further (over 20 mm), acidosis and ischemia occur. *If elevated IAP is left untreated, damage to the intestine increases the risk for sepsis, multiple organ dysfunction syndrome (MODS), and death.* Renal, cardiac, and respiratory damage are the most likely to occur, although the central nervous system can be affected, too (www.wsacs.org/consensus.htm).

The health care provider may request continuous or intermittent IAP monitoring in the critical care unit. It is usually done by inserting a urinary catheter and using a stopcock, pressure transducer system, clamp, IV tubing, and bag of saline. *Report any increase in IAP immediately to the physician. A sustained or repeated IAP of 12 mm Hg or higher is considered* ***intra-abdominal hypertension (IAH)*** *or* ***acute compartment syndrome (ACS)*** (Brush, 2007b). Acute IAH has a rapid onset after abdominal trauma (especially blunt trauma) and must be treated immediately using either a nonsurgical (vasopressor drugs and fluids) or surgical approach (fasciotomy). Surgery is risky because it increases the chance of embolic stroke and PE.

Surgical Management

For the patient with severe abdominal trauma, the surgeon performs an *exploratory laparotomy* and repairs abdominal injuries immediately if there are definite signs of peritoneal irritation. These signs include rebound tenderness, significant blood loss, evisceration, or a gunshot wound (GSW) with possible peritoneal involvement. After surgery, many of these patients are admitted to a critical care unit and mechanically ventilated.

Most stab wounds and GSWs require exploratory laparotomy, but as many as 25% are superficial and do not involve the peritoneum. Using local anesthesia, the surgeon explores and cleans superficial penetrating wounds. The patient does not require an exploratory laparotomy.

Patients with multiple trauma stay in the hospital for a prolonged period. Before discharge from the hospital, teach the patient and family the signs and symptoms of abdominal bleeding whether or not surgery has been performed. Instruct them to report abdominal pain, nausea, vomiting, bloody or black stools, fever, weakness, and dizziness.

Hemorrhage can occasionally occur weeks after blunt abdominal trauma, despite medical evaluation or treatment. For the patient who has surgery or exploration of wounds, provide instructions on wound care before discharge from the hospital. Provide additional health teaching as the patient's overall condition requires.

DECISION-MAKING CHALLENGE
Critical Rescue

A 21-year-old woman had a serious car accident last night and has been admitted to the critical care unit with right fractured ribs and a fractured right tibia and lateral malleolus. She also has multiple lacerations and bruises, including some on her abdomen from the seat belt. She is in extreme pain that is not relieved by her PCA morphine. She is very anxious while waiting for her boyfriend to arrive. Her most recent vital signs show that she has an increased heart rate (108) and her blood pressure has decreased (98/58).

1. What are your concerns for the patient at this time? Why?
2. What other assessments should you perform when caring for this patient?
3. What action should you implement as a result of this patient's condition? Why?
4. What are some possible reasons why this patient has anxiety and changes in her vital signs? Think of all the possibilities.

evolve For suggested answer guidelines, go to http://evolve.elsevier.com/Iggy/.

POLYPS

Pathophysiology

Polyps in the intestinal tract are small growths covered with mucosa and attached to the surface of the intestine. Although most are benign, they are significant because some have the potential to become malignant.

Polyps are identified by their tissue type. Although only a very small number of adenomas progress to cancer, almost all colorectal cancers develop from an adenoma. Adenomas are further classified as villous or tubular. Of these, villous adenomas pose a greater cancer risk.

Familial adenomatous polyposis (FAP) and hereditary nonpolyposis colorectal cancer (HNPCC) are inherited syndromes characterized by progressive development of colorectal adenomas. Unless these syndromes are treated, colorectal cancer (CRC) inevitably occurs by the fourth to fifth decade of life. These conditions were discussed on p. 1294 in the Genetic Considerations feature in the Colorectal Cancer section.

Other types of polyps include hyperplastic and hamartomatous polyps. Hyperplastic polyps, which include mucosal and inflammatory varieties, are entirely benign with no malignant potential. Hamartomatous polyps include juvenile and Peutz-Jeghers syndrome polyps. Although both types are generally benign, there are rare reports of malignant changes in juvenile polyps.

In addition to being classified by their tissue type, polyps are described according to their appearance (Fig. 59-7). Pedunculated polyps are stalk-like; a thin stem attaches them to the intestinal wall. They become elongated as peristalsis pulls them into the lumen of the intestine. Polyps attached to the intestinal walls by a broad base are described as sessile. A malignant polyp may be pedunculated or sessile.

Patient-Centered Collaborative Care

Polyps are usually asymptomatic and are discovered during routine colonoscopy screening. However, they can cause gross rectal bleeding, intestinal obstruction, or intussusception (telescoping of the bowel). Biopsy specimens of polyps can be obtained and the entire polyp can be removed (polypectomy) with the use of a snare that fits through the sigmoidoscope or colonoscope. This often eliminates the need for abdominal surgery to remove a suspicious or definitely malignant polyp. The patient with FAP often requires a total colectomy (colon removal) to prevent the development of cancer.

Nursing care focuses on patient education. Instruct the patient about:

- The nature of the polyp
- Clinical manifestations to report to the health care provider
- The need for regular, routine monitoring or screening

If the patient has had a polypectomy, follow-up sigmoidoscopic or colonoscopic examinations are needed because there is an increased risk for developing multiple polyps.

Nursing care of the patient after a polypectomy of the colorectal area includes monitoring for abdominal distention and pain, rectal bleeding, mucopurulent rectal drainage, and fever. A small amount of blood might appear in the stool after a polypectomy, but this should be temporary.

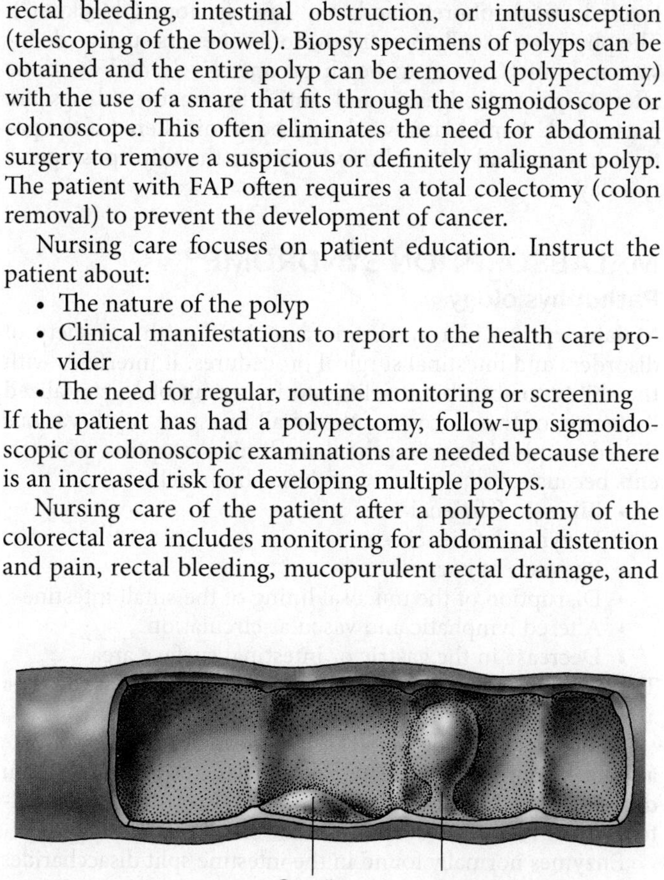

Sessile
Pedunculated

Fig. 59-7 • Pedunculated and sessile polyps. Pedunculated polyps, such as tubular adenomas, are stalk-like. Sessile polyps, such as villous adenomas, are broad based.

HEMORRHOIDS

Pathophysiology

Hemorrhoids are unnaturally swollen or distended veins in the anorectal region. The veins involved in the development of hemorrhoids are part of the normal structure in the anal region. With limited distention, the veins function as a valve overlying the anal sphincter that assists in continence. Increased intra-abdominal pressure causes elevated systemic and portal venous pressure, which is transmitted to the anorectal veins. Arterioles in the anorectal region shunt blood directly to the distended anorectal veins, which increases the pressure. With repeated elevations in pressure from increased intra-abdominal pressure and engorgement from arteriolar shunting of blood, the distended veins eventually separate from the smooth muscle surrounding them. The result is prolapse of the hemorrhoidal vessels.

Hemorrhoids can be internal or external (Fig. 59-8). **Internal hemorrhoids,** which cannot be seen on inspection of the perineal area, lie above the anal sphincter. **External hemorrhoids** lie below the anal sphincter and can be seen on inspection of the anal region. Prolapsed hemorrhoids can become thrombosed or inflamed, or they can bleed.

Hemorrhoids are common and not significant unless they cause pain or bleeding. Caused by increased abdominal pressure, the condition worsens during pregnancy, constipation with straining, obesity, heart failure, prolonged sitting or standing, and strenuous exercise and weight lifting. Decreased fluid intake can also cause hemorrhoids because of the development of hard stool and subsequent constipation. Straining while evacuating stool causes them to enlarge.

Health Promotion and Maintenance

Prevention of constipation is the most important preventive measure. It can be prevented by increasing fiber in the diet, such as eating more whole grains and raw vegetables and fruits.

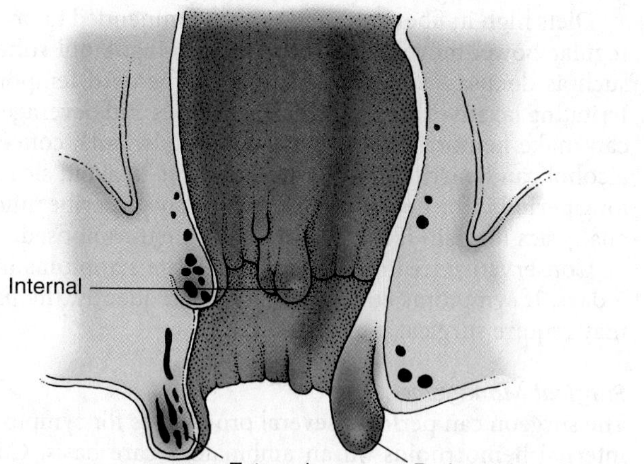

Internal
External
Prolapsed

Fig. 59-8 • Internal, external, and prolapsed hemorrhoids. *Internal hemorrhoids* lie above the anal sphincter and cannot be seen on inspection of the anal area. *External hemorrhoids* lie below the anal sphincter and can be seen on inspection of the anal region. Hemorrhoids that enlarge, fall down, and protrude through the anus are called *prolapsed hemorrhoids*.

Encourage patients to drink plenty of water unless otherwise contraindicated (e.g., kidney disease, heart disease). Remind the patient to avoid straining at stool. Remind him or her to exercise regularly with a gradual buildup in intensity. Maintaining a healthy weight also helps prevent hemorrhoids.

Patient-Centered Collaborative Care

Assessment

The most common symptoms of hemorrhoids are bleeding, swelling, and prolapse (bulging). Blood is characteristically bright red and is present on toilet tissue or streaked in the stool. Pain is a common symptom and is often associated with thrombosis, especially if thrombosis occurs suddenly. Other symptoms include itching and a mucous discharge. Diagnosis is usually made by inspection and digital examination, although anoscopy, proctoscopy, or proctoscopic ultrasonography can be performed.

Interventions

Interventions are typically conservative and are aimed at reducing symptoms with a minimum of discomfort, cost, and time lost from usual activities.

Nonsurgical Management

Local treatment and nutrition therapy are used when symptoms begin. Cold packs applied to the anorectal region for a few minutes at a time beginning with the onset of pain and tepid sitz baths three or four times per day are often enough to relieve discomfort, even if the hemorrhoids are thrombosed.

Topical anesthetics, such as lidocaine (Xylocaine), are useful for severe pain. Dibucaine (Nupercainal) ointment and similar products are available over the counter and may be applied for mild to moderate pain and itching. This ointment should be used only temporarily, however, because it can mask worsening symptoms and delay diagnosis of a severe disorder. If itching or inflammation is present, the health care provider prescribes a steroid preparation, such as hydrocortisone. Cleansing the anal area with moistened cleansing tissues rather than standard toilet tissue helps avoid irritation. The anal area should be cleansed gently by dabbing, rather than by wiping.

Diets high in fiber and fluids are recommended to promote regular bowel movements without straining. Stool softeners, such as docusate sodium (Colace), can be used temporarily. Irritating laxatives are avoided, as are foods and beverages that can make hemorrhoids worse. Spicy foods, nuts, coffee, and alcohol can be irritating. Remind patients to avoid sitting for long periods. The health care provider may prescribe mild oral analgesics for pain if the hemorrhoids are thrombosed.

Conservative treatment should alleviate symptoms in 3 to 5 days. If symptoms continue or recur frequently, the patient may require surgical intervention.

Surgical Management

The surgeon can perform several procedures for symptomatic internal hemorrhoids on an ambulatory care basis. Current recommended therapies include ultrasound coagulation, rubber band ligation, circular stapling, and laser-assisted or simple resection of the hemorrhoids. The type of surgery depends on the degree of prolapse, whether there is thrombosis, and the overall condition of the patient.

The harmonic scalpel is an ultrasonically activated instrument that vibrates to coagulate small and medium-size vessels. In rubber band ligation, a rubber ring is placed around the internal hemorrhoid that constricts blood flow to the hemorrhoid, resulting in shrinking of the hemorrhoid. The rubber band usually causes a feeling of tightness in the area until the rubber band falls off in 2 to 4 days. Complications of these procedures include pain, thrombosis of other hemorrhoids, infection, and abscess formation. Bleeding may occur after the band falls off. If the hemorrhoid is prolapsed, a circular stapling device is used to excise a band of mucosa above the prolapse and restore the hemorrhoidal tissue back into the anal canal.

Hemorrhoidectomy, or resection of the hemorrhoid, tends to cause more pain than the other procedures. Urinary retention can also occur because of rectal spasms and anorectal tenderness. Hemorrhage, which may be internal and not visible or external, is a rare but potential complication.

Teach patients with hemorrhoids about the need to eat high-fiber, high-fluid diets to promote regular bowel patterns before and after surgery. Advise them to avoid stimulant laxatives, which can be habit forming.

For patients who undergo any type of surgical intervention, monitor for bleeding and pain postoperatively and teach them to report these problems to their health care provider. Using moist heat (e.g., sitz baths) three or four times per day can help promote comfort.

Tell the patient that the first postoperative bowel movement may be very painful. Be sure that someone is with or near the patient when this happens. Some patients become light-headed and diaphoretic and may have syncope ("blackout"). The physician usually prescribes stool softeners such as docusate sodium (Colace) to begin preoperatively and continue after surgery. Analgesics and anti-inflammatory drugs are prescribed. A mild laxative should be administered if the patient has not had a bowel movement by the third postoperative day.

MALABSORPTION SYNDROME

Pathophysiology

Malabsorption is a syndrome associated with a variety of disorders and intestinal surgical procedures. It interferes with the ability to absorb nutrients and is a result of a generalized flattening of the mucosa of the small intestine. With various disorders, physiologic mechanisms limit absorption of nutrients because of one or more of these abnormalities:

- Bile salt deficiencies
- Enzyme deficiencies
- Presence of bacteria
- Disruption of the mucosal lining of the small intestine
- Altered lymphatic and vascular circulation
- Decrease in the gastric or intestinal surface area

The nutrient involved in malabsorption depends on the type and location of the abnormality in the intestinal tract.

Deficiencies of bile salts can lead to malabsorption of fats and fat-soluble vitamins. Bile salt deficiencies can result from decreased synthesis of bile in the liver, bile obstruction, or alteration of bile salt absorption in the small intestine.

Enzymes normally found in the intestine split disaccharides (complex sugars) to monosaccharides (simple sugars). Examples of these enzymes are lactase, sucrase, maltase, and isomaltase. Lactase deficiency is the most common disaccharide enzyme deficiency. Without sufficient amounts of this enzyme, the body is not able to break down lactose. Lactase deficiency can be due to genetic inheritance, injury to intestinal mucosa from viral hepatitis, bacterial proliferation in the intestine, or sprue. Deficiencies of the other disaccharide enzymes are rare.

Pancreatic enzymes are also necessary for absorption of vitamin B_{12}. With destruction or obstruction of the pancreas or insufficient pancreatic stimulation, this nutrient is not well absorbed. Chronic pancreatitis, pancreatic carcinoma, resection of the pancreas, and cystic fibrosis can cause these malabsorption problems.

Loops of bowel can accumulate intestinal contents, resulting in bacterial overgrowth, when peristalsis is decreased. Bacteria at these sites break down bile salts, and fewer salts are available for fat absorption. They can also ingest vitamin B_{12}, which contributes to vitamin B_{12} deficiency. This process can occur after a gastrectomy.

Disruption of the mucosal lining of the intestine is responsible for the malabsorption that occurs with celiac (nontropical) sprue, tropical sprue, Crohn's disease, and ulcerative colitis. In celiac (nontropical) sprue, the absorptive surface area in the small intestine is lost; there is malabsorption of most nutrients. Celiac sprue is thought to be due to a genetic immune hypersensitivity response to gluten or its breakdown products or to result from the accumulation of gluten in the diet with peptidase deficiency.

Tropical sprue is caused by an infectious agent that has not been identified but is thought to be bacterial. Mucosal changes occur in a more widespread manner than in celiac sprue. However, the changes are not as severe as in celiac sprue. Tropical sprue results in malabsorption of fat, folic acid, and vitamin B_{12} in later stages of the disease.

The inflammation in Crohn's disease interferes with the surface of cells absorbing bile salts and therefore leads to fat malabsorption. In ulcerative colitis, protein loss may occur.

Obstruction to lymphatic flow in the intestine can lead to loss of plasma proteins along with loss of minerals (e.g., iron, copper, calcium), vitamin B_{12}, folic acid, and lipids. Lymphatic obstruction can be caused by many conditions. Certain cancers such as lymphoma, inflammatory states, radiation enteritis, Crohn's disease, heart failure, and constrictive pericarditis are causes of lymphatic obstruction.

Interference with blood flow to the intestinal mucosa results in malabsorption. With intestinal surgery, there is loss of the surface area needed to facilitate absorption. Resection of the ileum results in vitamin B_{12}, bile salt, and other nutrient deficiencies. Gastric surgery is one of the most common causes of malabsorption and maldigestion. Other conditions associated with poor digestion and malabsorption include small-bowel ischemia and radiation enteritis.

Patient-Centered Collaborative Care

Assessment

Chronic diarrhea is a classic symptom of malabsorption. It occurs as a result of unabsorbed nutrients, which add to the bulk of the stool, and unabsorbed fat. **Steatorrhea** (greater than normal amounts of fat in the feces) is a common sign. It is a result of bile salt deconjugation, nonabsorbed fats, or bacteria in the intestine. Not all patients with malabsorption have diarrhea. Instead, some have an increased stool mass. Other clinical manifestations include:

- Unintentional weight loss
- Bloating and flatus (carbohydrate malabsorption)
- Decreased libido
- Easy bruising (purpura)
- Anemia (with iron and folic acid or vitamin B_{12} deficiencies)
- Bone pain (with calcium and vitamin D deficiencies)
- Edema (caused by hypoproteinemia)

Laboratory studies reveal a decrease in mean corpuscular volume (MCV), mean corpuscular hemoglobin (MCH), and mean corpuscular hemoglobin concentration (MCHC). These decreases indicate hypochromic microcytic anemia resulting from iron deficiency. Increased MCV and variable MCH and MCHC values indicate macrocytic anemia resulting from vitamin B_{12} and folic acid deficiencies. Serum iron levels are low in protein malabsorption because of insufficient gastric acid for use of iron. Serum cholesterol levels may be low from decreased absorption and digestion of fat. Low serum calcium levels may indicate malabsorption of vitamin D and amino acids. Low levels of serum vitamin A (retinol) and carotene, its precursor, indicate a bile salt deficiency and malabsorption of fat. Serum albumin and total protein levels are low if protein is lost. A quantitative fecal fat analysis is elevated in either malabsorption or maldigestion.

A *lactose tolerance test* result that shows less than a 20% rise in the blood glucose level over the fasting blood glucose level indicates lactose intolerance. A monosaccharide test validates or rules out lactase deficiency. The xylose absorption test can reveal low urine and serum D-xylose levels if malabsorption in the small intestine is present, a common finding in celiac sprue. An abnormal D-xylose test can indicate bacterial overgrowth in the small intestine.

The *Schilling test* measures urinary excretion of vitamin B_{12} for diagnosis of pernicious anemia and a variety of other malabsorption syndromes. The *bile acid breath test* assesses the absorption of bile salt. If the patient has bacterial overgrowth, the bile salts will become deconjugated and the carbon dioxide level in the breath will peak earlier than expected.

Biopsy of the small intestine is performed for diagnosis of tropical sprue or celiac sprue. Ultrasonography is used to diagnose pancreatic tumors and tumors in the small intestine that are causing malabsorption. X-rays of the GI tract reveal pancreatic calcifications, tumors, or other abnormalities that cause malabsorption. Barium enema examination shows mucosal changes representative of celiac sprue or other abnormalities. A CT scan may also be done.

Interventions

Interventions for most malabsorption syndromes focus on avoidance of substances that aggravate malabsorption and supplementation of nutrients. Surgical management of the primary disease may be indicated. Drug therapy may also improve or resolve malabsorption.

Nutrition management includes a low-fat diet for patients who have gallbladder disease, severe steatorrhea, or cystic fibrosis. A low-fat diet may or may not be indicated for pancreatic insufficiency because this disorder improves with enzyme replacement. Some clinicians believe that limitation of fat intake is not necessary with enzyme replacement. Dietary intake of fat is actually beneficial to the patient because it has a high number of calories. After a total gastrectomy, a high-protein, high-calorie diet and small, frequent meals are recommended. Lactose-free or lactose-restricted diets are available for patients with lactase deficiency, and gluten-free diets are available for those with celiac sprue.

The physician prescribes nutritional supplements according to the specific deficiency. Common supplements include:

- Water-soluble vitamins, such as folic acid and vitamin B complex
- Fat-soluble vitamins, such as vitamin A, vitamin D, and vitamin K
- Minerals, such as calcium, iron, and magnesium
- Pancreatic enzymes, such as pancrelipase (Pancrease, Viokase)

Antibiotics are used to treat tropical sprue, Whipple's disease, and other disorders involving bacterial overgrowth. Tropical sprue is treated with trimethoprim/sulfamethoxazole (Bactrim, Septra). Bacterial overgrowth can be caused by a variety of disorders but is often treated with tetracycline and metronidazole (Flagyl, Novonidazol♣). Steroids are sometimes given in celiac disease to decrease inflammation.

Drug therapy is used to control the clinical manifestations of malabsorption. Antidiarrheal agents, such as diphenoxylate hydrochloride and atropine sulfate (Lomotil), are often used to control diarrhea and steatorrhea. Anticholinergics, such as dicyclomine hydrochloride (Bentyl, Bentylol♣), may be given before meals to inhibit gastric motility. IV fluids may be necessary to replenish fluid losses associated with diarrhea.

Provide special measures to protect the skin when chronic diarrhea occurs (Chart 59-7). Conduct an ongoing assessment for clinical manifestations of malabsorption, and relate these to activities and dietary intake. For example, patients with steatorrhea are monitored for fluid and electrolyte imbalances and are encouraged to drink electrolyte-rich liquids liberally. Teach them the rationale for dietary, drug, and surgical management of nutritional deficiencies, and evaluate interventions on the basis of changes in or resolution of clinical manifestations.

Chart 59-7 BEST PRACTICE FOR PATIENT SAFETY & QUALITY CARE

Special Skin Care for Patients with Chronic Diarrhea

- Use medicated wipes or premoistened disposable wipes rather than toilet tissue to clean the perineal area.
- Clean the perineal area well with mild soap and warm water after each stool; rinse soap from the area well.
- If the physician allows, provide a sitz bath several times per day.
- Apply a thin coat of vitamin A & D ointment or other medicated protective barrier, such as aloe products, after each stool.
- Keep the patient off the affected buttock area.
- For open areas, cover with thin DuoDerm or Tegaderm occlusive dressing to promote rapid healing.
- Observe for fungal or yeast infections, which appear as dark red rashes with "satellite" lesions. Obtain prescription for medication if this problem occurs.

HUMAN NEEDS NURSING CARE REVIEW

What might you NOTICE if the patient has impaired absorption and inadequate nutrition as a result of noninflammatory intestinal disorders?

- Rectal bleeding
- Report of change in bowel habits
- Diarrhea or report of constipation
- Fatigue
- Vomiting
- Abdominal pain
- Change in bowel sounds (decreased or increased)
- Weight loss

What should you INTERPRET and how should you RESPOND to a patient with impaired absorption and inadequate nutrition as a result of noninflammatory intestinal disorders?

Perform and interpret focused physical assessment findings, including:

- Vital signs
- Complete pain assessment
- Abdominal assessment
- Current weight compared with previous weight

Respond:

- Decrease abdominal pain by sitting patient up.
- Start IV (large-bore) to replace fluids and electrolytes, and give blood transfusion as prescribed.
- Provide rest.
- Provide privacy and dignity.
- Assist with hygiene as needed.
- Insert nasogastric tube and connect to low suction as needed.
- Check laboratory values for hemoglobin and hematocrit.
- Check stool for occult or frank blood.
- Give antidiarrheal drugs if prescribed.
- Record intake and output.
- Assist with ADLs and ambulation as needed.

On what should you REFLECT?

- Continue to monitor for vomiting and diarrhea and for changes in pain.
- Think about what you need to document. Decide when you might need to call the health care provider or Rapid Response Team.
- Determine what health teaching and community resources may be needed for the patient and family.
- Think about what you can do to help prevent complications of the health problem.

GET READY FOR THE NCLEX EXAMINATION!

Key Points

Review these Key Points for each NCLEX Examination Client Needs Category.

Safe and Effective Care Environment

- Refer patients with familial CRC syndromes for genetic counseling and testing.
- Refer ostomy patients to the United Ostomy Associations of America, Inc. and the American Cancer Society for additional information and support groups.
- Consult with the enterostomal therapist (ET) when a patient is scheduled for or has a new colostomy.
- Prioritize care for patients experiencing abdominal trauma: First assess airway, breathing, and circulation (ABCs), and then monitor mental status, vital signs, and skin perfusion to assess for hypovolemic shock.

Health Promotion and Maintenance

- Teach patients with irritable bowel syndrome (IBS) to avoid GI stimulants, such as caffeine, alcohol, and milk and milk products.
- Instruct patients on dietary modifications to decrease the occurrence of colorectal cancer (CRC).
- Teach adults older than 50 years to have routine screening for CRC as listed in Chart 59-1; people with genetic predispositions should have earlier and more frequent screening.
- Teach patients and caregivers how to provide colostomy care, including dietary measures, skin care, and ostomy products.
- Teach people measures for preventing constipation to minimize hemorrhoid occurrence.

Psychosocial Integrity

- Assess effects of IBS on patient lifestyle; recommend stress management techniques.
- Assist the patient with CRC with grief work, as listed in Chart 59-2.
- Be aware that having a colostomy is a life-altering event that severely impacts one's body image; issues related to sexuality and fear of acceptance should be discussed.

Physiological Integrity

- Assess patients with IBS for elimination pattern, abdominal pain, and nausea.
- Be aware that minimally invasive inguinal hernia repair is an ambulatory procedure done via laparoscopy; postoperative management requires health teaching regarding rest for a few days and inspection of incisions for signs of infection.
- Be aware that a strangulated hernia can cause ischemia and bowel obstruction, requiring immediate intervention.
- Monitor patients who have conventional, open herniorrhaphy for ability to void.
- Recognize that surgical procedures for CRC vary depending on tumor location as specified in Table 59-1.
- Keep the peristomal skin clean and dry; observe for leakage around the pouch seal.
- Provide meticulous perineal wound care for patients having an abdominoperineal (AP) resection, as described in Chart 59-3.
- Assess the characteristics of the colostomy stoma, which should be reddish pink and moist; report abnormalities such as ischemia and necrosis (purplish or black) or unusual bleeding to the surgeon.
- Recall that bowel sounds are altered in patients with obstruction; absent bowel sounds imply total obstruction.
- Assess the patient's nasogastric tube for proper placement, patency, and output at least every 4 hours.
- Monitor patients with bowel obstruction for signs and symptoms of fluid, electrolyte, and acid-base imbalances.
- Teach patients having hemorrhoid surgery to take stool softeners before and after surgery to decrease discomfort during defecation.
- Be aware that intestinal polyps are usually benign but can become malignant if not removed.

Additional Study Resources

Go to your Companion CD or Evolve at http://evolve.elsevier.com/Iggy/ for *Self-Assessment Questions for the NCLEX Examination.*

evolve Go to Evolve at http://evolve.elsevier.com/Iggy/ for *Prioritization and Delegation Questions for the NCLEX Examination.*

SELECTED BIBLIOGRAPHY

Asterisk indicates a classic or definitive work on this subject.

American Cancer Society. (2008). *Cancer facts and figures 2008.* Atlanta: Author.

*American College of Gastroenterology Functional Gastrointestinal Disorders Task Force. (2002). Evidence-based position statement on the management of irritable bowel syndrome in North America. *American Journal of Gastroenterology, 97*(Suppl. 11), S1-S5.

*American Gastroenterological Association. (2004). American Gastroenterological Association medical position statement: Diagnosis and treatment of hemorrhoids. *Gastroenterology, 126*(5), 1461-1462.

Brush, K.A. (2007a). Measuring intra-abdominal pressure. *Nursing2007, 37*(7), 42-43.

Brush, K.A. (2007b). The pressure is on. *Nursing2007, 37*(7), 37-40.

Cataldo P., Ellis, C.N., Gregorcyk, S., Hyman, N., Buie, W.D., Church, J., et al. (2005). Practice parameters for the management of hemorrhoids (revised). *Diseases of the Colon and Rectum, 48*(2), 189-194.

Croghan, A., & Heitkemper, M.M. (2005). Recognizing and managing patients with irritable bowel syndrome. *Journal of the American Academy of Nurse Practitioners, 17*(2), 51-59.

Dube, C., Rostom, A., Lewin, G., Tsertsvadze, A., Barrowman, N., Code, C., et al. (2007). The use of aspirin for primary prevention of colorectal cancer: A systematic review prepared for the U.S. Preventive Services Task Force. *Annals of Internal Medicine, 146*(5), 365-375.

Freeman, L.C. (2007). Responding to small-bowel obstruction. *Nursing2007, 37*(5), 56hn1-hn6.

Harmon, H.W. (2007). Treatment options for irritable bowel syndrome. *The Nurse Practitioner, 32*(7), 39-43.

Hertig, V.L., Cain, K.C., Jarrett, M.E., Burr, R.L., & Heitkemper, M.M. (2007). Daily stress and gastrointestinal symptoms in women with irritable bowel syndrome. *Nursing Research, 56*(6), 399-406.

Houldin, A.D., & Lewis, F.M. (2006). Salvaging their normal lives: A qualitative study of patients with recently diagnosed advanced colorectal cancer. *Oncology Nursing Forum, 33*(4), 719-725.

Jemal, A., Siegel, R., Ward, E., Murray, T., Xu, J., & Thun, M.J. (2007). Cancer statistics, 2007. *A Cancer Journal for Clinicians, 57*(1), 43-66.

*Khan, A.N., MacDonald, S., & Howat, J.M.T. (2004). Small bowel obstruction. *eMedicine.* Retrieved April 15, 2008, from www.emedicine.com/radio/topic781.htm.

Korzenik, J.R. (2005). Past and current theories of etiology of IBD: Toothpaste, worms and refrigerators. *Journal of Clinical Gastroenterology, 39*(4 Suppl. 2), S59-S65.

Lehrer, J.K., & Lichtenstein, G.R. (2007). Irritable bowel syndrome. *eMedicine.* Retrieved April 15, 2008, from www.emedicine.com/med/topic1190.htm.

*Levins, T.T. (2000). Using ultrasound to assess blunt abdominal trauma. *Nursing2000, 30*(5), 32cc14-32cc15.

National Comprehensive Cancer Network. (2008). Clinical practice guidelines in oncology. Colorectal cancer screening. Retrieved August 12, 2008, from http://nccn.org/professionals/physician_gls/PDF/colorectal_screening.pdf.

Norton, C.K., Linenfelser, P.I., Cyron, K.E., & Casey, K.A. (2006). Trauma and intraabdominal hypertension. *AJN, 106*(7), 51-55.

Podovei, M., & Kuo, B. (2006). Irritable bowel syndrome: A practical review. *Southern Medical Journal, 99*(11), 1235-1242.

*Pontieri-Lewis, V. (2000). Colorectal cancer: Prevention and screening. *MEDSURG Nursing, 9*(1), 9-13.

Pontieri-Lewis, V. (2006). Basics of ostomy care. *MEDSURG Nursing, 15*(4), 199-202.

Pullen, R.L. (2006). Teaching your patient to irrigate a colostomy. *Nursing2006, 36*(4), 22.

Saito, Y.A., Peterson, G.M., Locke, G.R. III, & Talley, N.J. (2005). The genetics of irritable bowel syndrome. *Clinical Gastroenterology and Hepatology, 3*(11), 1057-1065.

Symms, M.R., Rawl, S.M., Grant, M., Wendel, C.S., Coons, S.J., Hickey, S., et al. (2008). Sexual health and quality of life among male veterans with intestinal ostomies. *Clinical Nurse Specialist, 22*(1), 30-40.

Toth, P.E. (2006). Ostomy care and rehabilitation in colorectal cancer. *Seminars in Oncology Nursing, 22*(3), 174-177.

Viale, P.H., & Sommer, R. (2006). Nursing care of patients receiving chemotherapy for metastatic colorectal cancer: Implications of the treatment continuum concept. *Seminars in Oncology Nursing, 22*(4), 22-35.

Weingarten, M.A., Zalmanovici, A., & Yaphe, J. (2008). Dietary calcium supplementation for preventing colorectal cancer and adenomatous polyps. *Cochrane Database of Systematic Reviews, 23*(1), CD003548.

Wickham, R., & Lassere, Y. (2006). The ABCs of colorectal cancer. *Seminars in Oncology Nursing, 22*(4), 1-8.

Winawer, S., Fletcher, R., Rex, D., Bond, J., Burt, R., Ferrucci, J., et al.; Gastrointestinal Consortium Panel. (2003). Colorectal cancer screening and surveillance: Clinical guidelines and rationale—Update based on new evidence. *Gastroenterology, 124*(2), 544-560.

60

CHAPTER

Care of Patients with Inflammatory Intestinal Disorders

Karen Ruschman

LEARNING OUTCOMES

For clinical competence and success on the NCLEX Examination, study this chapter with these Learning Outcomes in mind:

Safe and Effective Care Environment

1. Collaborate with health care team members to provide care for patients with chronic inflammatory bowel disease (IBD).
2. Identify community resources for patients and families regarding chronic IBD.
3. Apply principles of infection control when caring for patients with infectious intestinal problems.

Health Promotion and Maintenance

4. Apply knowledge of nutrition when assessing weight for patients with chronic IBD.
5. Provide health teaching for patients to promote self-management when caring for ileostomy or other surgical diversion.
6. Discuss ways that helminthes infestation, parasitic infection, and food poisoning can be prevented.

Psychosocial Integrity

7. Identify expected body image changes associated with having an ileostomy or other surgical diversion.
8. Assess patient and family response to chronic IBD.

Physiological Integrity

9. Differentiate common types of acute inflammatory bowel disease.
10. Provide nursing care for the patient who has appendicitis and peritonitis.
11. Discuss the common causes of gastroenteritis.
12. Compare and contrast the pathophysiology and clinical manifestations of ulcerative colitis and Crohn's disease.
13. Explain the purpose of and nursing implications related to drug therapy for patients with IBD.
14. Provide postoperative care for a patient undergoing a colon resection/colectomy and ileostomy.
15. Explain the role of nutrition therapy in managing the patient with diverticular disease.
16. Describe the comfort measures that the nurse can use for the patient with anal disorders.

Go to your Companion CD or Evolve at http://evolve.elsevier.com/Iggy/ for *Self-Assessment Questions for the NCLEX Examination* keyed to these Learning Outcomes.

Inflammatory bowel health problems affect the small intestine, large intestine (colon), or both. Together, these organs are called the *intestinal tract.* Continued digestion of food and absorption of nutrients occur primarily in the small intestine (bowel) to meet the body's needs for energy. Water is reabsorbed in the large intestine to help maintain a fluid balance and promote the passage of waste products. When the intestinal tract and its nearby structures become inflamed, *digestion and nutrition* may be inadequate to meet a patient's needs.

ACUTE INFLAMMATORY BOWEL DISORDERS

Appendicitis, gastroenteritis, and peritonitis are the most common acute inflammatory bowel problems. These disorders are potentially life threatening and can have major systemic complications if not treated promptly.

APPENDICITIS

Pathophysiology

Appendicitis, an acute inflammation of the vermiform appendix, occurs in 5% of the population, peaking among young adults, especially men. It is the most common cause of right lower quadrant (RLQ) pain. The appendix usually extends off the proximal cecum of the colon just below the ileocecal valve. Inflammation occurs when the lumen (opening) of the appendix is obstructed (blocked), leading to infection as bacteria invade the wall of the appendix. The initial obstruction is usually a result of fecaliths (very hard pieces of feces) composed of calcium phosphate–rich mucus and inorganic salts. Less common causes are malignant tumors, worms, or other infections.

When the lumen is blocked, the mucosa secretes fluid, increasing the internal pressure and restricting blood flow, resulting in pain. If the process occurs slowly, an abscess may develop, but a rapid process may result in peritonitis (inflammation of the peritoneum). *All complications of peritonitis are serious. Gangrene can occur within 24 to 36 hours, is life threatening, and is one of the most common indications for emergency surgery. Perforation may develop within 24 hours, but the risk rises rapidly after 48 hours.* Perforation of the appendix also results in peritonitis with a temperature of greater than 101° F (38.3° C) and a rise in pulse rate.

CONSIDERATIONS FOR OLDER ADULTS

Appendicitis is relatively rare at extremes in age. However, perforation is more common in older people, causing a higher mortality rate. The diagnosis of appendicitis is difficult to establish in older adults because symptoms of pain and tenderness may not be as pronounced in this age-group, resulting in treatment delay and an increased risk for perforation, peritonitis, and death.

Recurrent acute appendicitis does sometimes occur, often with complete remission of inflammation between acute attacks. In rare instances, acute appendicitis may be the first manifestation of Crohn's disease.

Patient-Centered Collaborative Care

Assessment

History taking and tracking the sequence of symptoms are important because nausea or vomiting before abdominal pain can indicate gastroenteritis. Abdominal pain followed by nausea and vomiting can indicate appendicitis. Ask about risk factors such as age, familial tendency, and intra-abdominal tumors. Classically, patients with appendicitis have cramplike pain in the epigastric or periumbilical area. Anorexia is a frequent symptom with nausea and vomiting occurring in many cases.

Perform a complete pain assessment. Initially, pain can present anywhere in the abdomen or flank area. As the inflammation and infection progress, the pain becomes more severe and steady and shifts to the RLQ between the anterior iliac crest and the umbilicus. This area is referred to as *McBurney's point* (Fig. 60-1). *Abdominal pain that increases with cough or movement and is relieved by bending the right hip or the knees suggests perforation and peritonitis.* Assess for muscle rigidity and guarding on palpation of the abdomen. The patient may report pain after release of pressure. This is referred to as "rebound" tenderness.

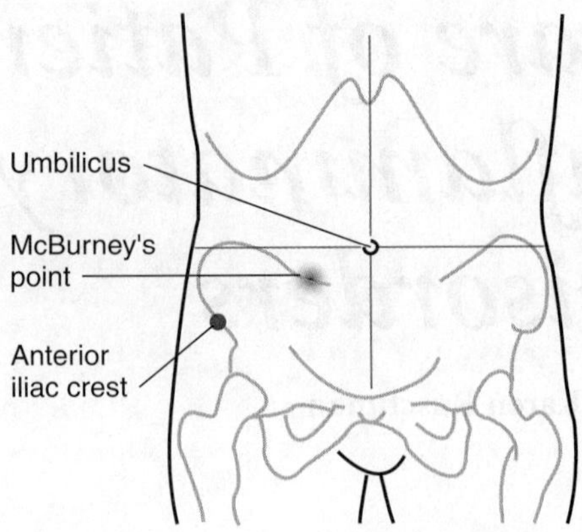
Umbilicus
McBurney's point
Anterior iliac crest

Fig. 60-1 • McBurney's point is located midway between the anterior iliac crest and the umbilicus in the right lower quadrant. This is the classic area for localized tenderness during the later stages of appendicitis.

Laboratory findings do not establish the diagnosis, but often there is a moderate elevation of the white blood cell (WBC) count (leukocytosis) to 10,000 to 18,000/mm^3 with a "shift to the left" (an increased number of immature WBCs). A WBC elevation greater than 20,000/mm^3 may indicate a perforated appendix. An ultrasound study may show the presence of an enlarged appendix. If symptoms are recurrent or prolonged, a computed tomography (CT) scan can be used for diagnosis and may reveal the presence of a fecalith.

Interventions

All patients with suspected or confirmed appendicitis are hospitalized and examined by a surgeon. When the diagnosis is not clear, the health care team observes the patient before surgical exploration.

Nonsurgical Management

Keep the patient with suspected or known appendicitis on NPO to prepare for the possibility of emergency surgery and to avoid making the inflammation worse. Administer IV fluids as prescribed to prevent fluid and electrolyte imbalance and to replace fluid volume. If tolerated, advise the patient to maintain a semi-Fowler's position so that abdominal drainage, if any, can be contained in the lower abdomen.

Once the diagnosis of appendicitis is confirmed and surgery is scheduled, administer opioid analgesics and antibiotics as prescribed. *The patient with suspected appendicitis should not receive laxatives or enemas, which can cause perforation of the appendix. Heat should never be applied to the abdomen because this may increase circulation to the appendix and result in increased inflammation and perforation.*

Surgical Management

Surgery is required as soon as possible. If the diagnosis is not definitive but the patient is at high risk for complications from suspected appendicitis, the surgeon may perform an exploratory laparoscopy or laparotomy to rule out appendicitis. A **laparoscopy** is a minimally invasive surgical (MIS) procedure with several small incisions near the umbilicus through which a small endoscope is placed. A **laparotomy** is an open approach with a larger abdominal incision for complicated or atypical appendicitis or peritonitis.

Preoperative teaching is often limited because the patient is in pain or may be transferred quickly to the operating suite for emergency surgery. The patient is prepared for general anesthesia and surgery, as described in Chapter 16.

An **appendectomy** is the removal of the inflamed appendix by one of the two surgical approaches. Most uncomplicated appendectomy procedures today are done via laparoscopy.

After surgery, care of the patient who has undergone an appendectomy is the same as that required for anyone who has received general anesthesia (see Chapter 18). The patient with an MIS procedure may be discharged on the day of surgery. In a few cases, there is an overnight stay. Most patients recover quickly and can return to usual activities in 2 to 3 weeks or less.

If peritonitis or abscesses are found, wound drains are inserted and a nasogastric tube may be placed to decompress the stomach and prevent abdominal distention. Administer IV antibiotics and opioid analgesics as prescribed. The patient is typically out of bed on the evening of surgery. He or she may be hospitalized for as long as 3 to 5 days and return to normal activity in 4 to 6 weeks.

PERITONITIS

Peritonitis is a life-threatening, acute inflammation of the visceral/parietal peritoneum and endothelial lining of the abdominal cavity. Primary peritonitis is rare and indicates the peritoneum is infected via the bloodstream. This problem is not discussed here.

Pathophysiology

Normally the peritoneal cavity contains about 50 mL of sterile fluid (transudate), which prevents friction in the abdominal cavity during peristalsis. When the peritoneal cavity is contaminated by bacteria, the body first begins an inflammatory reaction walling off a localized area to fight the infection. This local reaction involves vascular dilation and increased capillary permeability, allowing transport of leukocytes and subsequent phagocytosis of the offending organisms. If this walling off process fails, the inflammation spreads and contamination becomes massive, resulting in diffuse (widespread) peritonitis.

Peritonitis is most often caused by contamination of the peritoneal cavity by bacteria or chemicals. Bacteria gain entry into the peritoneum by perforation (from appendicitis, diverticulitis, peptic ulcer disease) or from an external penetrating wound, a gangrenous gallbladder, bowel obstruction, or ascending infection through the genital tract. Less common causes include perforating tumors, leakage or contamination during surgery, and infection by skin pathogens in patients undergoing continuous ambulatory peritoneal dialysis (CAPD). Common bacteria responsible for peritonitis include *Escherichia coli, Streptococcus, Staphylococcus, Pneumococcus,* and *Gonococcus.* Chemical peritonitis results from leakage of bile, pancreatic enzymes, and gastric acid.

When diagnosis and treatment of peritonitis are delayed, blood vessel dilation continues. The body responds to the continuing infectious process by shunting extra blood to the area of inflammation (hyperemia). Fluid is shifted from the extracellular fluid compartment into the peritoneal cavity, connective tissues, and GI tract *("third spacing")*. This shift of fluid can result in a significant decrease in circulatory volume and *hypovolemic shock.* Severely decreased circulatory volume can result in insufficient perfusion of the kidneys, leading to kidney failure with electrolyte imbalance. Assess for clinical manifestations of these life-threatening problems.

Peristalsis slows or *stops* in response to severe peritoneal inflammation, and the lumen of the bowel becomes distended with gas and fluid. Fluid that normally flows to the small bowel and the colon for reabsorption accumulates in the intestine in volumes of 7 to 8 L daily. The toxins or bacteria responsible for the peritonitis can also enter the bloodstream from the peritoneal area and lead to bacteremia or **septicemia** (bacterial invasion of the blood).

Respiratory problems can occur as a result of increased abdominal pressure against the diaphragm from intestinal distention and fluid shifts to the peritoneal cavity. Pain can interfere with respirations at a time when the patient has an increased oxygen demand because of the infectious process.

Patient-Centered Collaborative Care

Assessment

Ask the patient about abdominal pain, and determine the character of the pain (e.g., cramping, sharp, aching), location of the pain, and whether the pain is localized or generalized. Ask about a history of a low-grade fever or recent spikes in temperature.

Physical findings of peritonitis (Chart 60-1) depend on several factors: the stage of the disease, the ability of the body to localize the process by walling off the infection, and whether the inflammation has progressed to generalized peritonitis. The patient most often appears acutely ill, lying still, possibly with the knees flexed. Movement is guarded, and he or she may report and show signs of pain (e.g., facial grimacing) with coughing or movement of any type. During inspection, observe for progressive abdominal distention, often seen when the inflammation markedly reduces intestinal motility. Auscultate for bowel sounds, which usually disappear with progression of the inflammation.

The cardinal signs of peritonitis are abdominal pain and tenderness. In the patient with *localized* peritonitis, the abdomen is tender on palpation in a well-defined area with rebound tender-

Chart 60-1 KEY FEATURES

Peritonitis

- Rigid, boardlike abdomen (classic)
- Abdominal pain (localized, poorly localized, or referred to the shoulder or chest)
- Distended abdomen
- Nausea, anorexia, vomiting
- Diminishing bowel sounds
- Inability to pass flatus or feces
- Rebound tenderness in the abdomen
- High fever
- Tachycardia
- Dehydration from high fever (poor skin turgor)
- Decreased urine output
- Hiccups
- Possible compromise in respiratory status

ness in this area. With *generalized* peritonitis, tenderness is widespread. *Abdominal wall rigidity is a classic finding, sometimes referred to as a "boardlike" abdomen.* The patient may have a high fever because of the infectious process, with tachycardia occurring in response to the fever and decreased circulating blood volume. Assess whether he or she has dry mucous membranes and a low urine output seen with third spacing. Nausea and vomiting may also be present. Hiccups may occur as a result of diaphragmatic irritation.

White blood cell (WBC) counts are often elevated to 20,000/mm^3 with a high neutrophil count. Blood culture studies may be done to determine whether septicemia has occurred and to identify the causative organism to enable appropriate therapy. The health care provider requests laboratory tests to assess fluid and electrolyte balance and renal status, including electrolytes, blood urea nitrogen (BUN), creatinine, hemoglobin, and hematocrit. Oxygen saturation and end-carbon dioxide monitoring may be obtained to assess respiratory function and acid-base balance.

Flat, upright, and decubitus (side) abdominal x-rays can assess for free air or fluid in the abdominal cavity, indicating perforation. The x-rays may also show dilation, edema, and inflammation of the small and large intestines. An abdominal sonogram may be useful in locating the problem.

The physician may perform a diagnostic peritoneal lavage by instilling 1 L of fluid through a peritoneal dialysis catheter. Lavage fluid positive for peritonitis is characterized by more than 500 WBCs/mL of fluid, more than 50,000 red blood cells (RBCs)/mL, or the presence of bacteria on a Gram stain. Bile-stained green fluid may indicate a ruptured gallbladder or perforated intestine.

Interventions

All patients with peritonitis are hospitalized because of the severe nature of the illness. If complications are extensive, they may be admitted to a critical care unit. Nursing interventions focus on the early identification of complications.

Nonsurgical Management

The physician prescribes IV fluids and broad-spectrum antibiotics immediately after establishing the diagnosis of peritonitis. IV fluids are used to replace fluids collected in the peritoneum and bowel. Monitor daily weight and intake and output carefully. A nasogastric tube (NGT) decompresses the stomach and the intestine, and the patient is NPO. Apply oxygen as prescribed and according to the patient's respiratory status. Administer analgesics and monitor pain control as needed. A surgical consultation is requested in case surgery should become necessary.

Surgical Management

Abdominal surgery is the usual treatment for identifying and repairing the cause of the peritonitis. If the patient is so critically ill that surgery would be life threatening, it may be delayed. Surgery focuses on controlling the contamination, removing foreign material from the peritoneal cavity, and draining collected fluid.

Exploratory **laparotomy** (surgical opening into the abdomen) is the usual approach to remove or repair the inflamed or perforated organ (e.g., appendectomy for an inflamed appendix; a colon resection, with or without a colostomy for a perforated diverticulum). Before the abdominal cavity is closed, the surgeon irrigates the peritoneum with antibiotic solutions. Several catheters may be inserted to drain the cavity and provide a route for irrigation after surgery.

The preoperative care is similar to that described in Chapter 16 for patients having general anesthesia. Chapter 18 describes general postoperative care. Multisystem complications can occur with peritonitis.

Maintain the patient in a semi-Fowler's position to promote drainage of peritoneal contents into the lower region of the abdominal cavity. This position also aids in the respiratory effort.

The patient has one or more incisions and drains. Because contamination at the time of surgery slows healing of an incision with edges well approximated (first intention), incisions may be allowed to heal by second or third intention. These wounds require special care involving manual irrigation or packing as prescribed by the surgeon. If the surgeon requests peritoneal irrigation through a drain, *maintain sterile technique during manual irrigation.* Assess whether the patient retains the fluid used for irrigation by comparing the amount of fluid returned with the amount of fluid instilled. Fluid retention could cause abdominal distention or pain.

Loss of fluids from the extracellular space to the peritoneal cavity, NGT suctioning, and NPO status require that the patient receives IV fluid replacement and that intake and output are strictly measured. Fluid rates may be changed frequently based on laboratory values and patient condition. *Therefore monitor the patient's level of consciousness, vital signs, respiratory status (respiratory rate and breath sounds), and intake and output at least hourly immediately after surgery.*

Community-Based Care

The length of hospitalization depends on the extent and severity of the infectious process. Patients who have a localized abscess drained and who respond to antibiotics and IV fluids without multisystem complications are discharged in several days. Others may require mechanical ventilation or hemodialysis with longer hospital stays. Some patients may be transferred to a transitional care unit to complete their antibiotic therapy and recovery. Convalescence is often longer than for other surgeries because of multi-system involvement.

When discharged home, assess the patient's ability for self-management at home with the added task of incision care and a reduced activity tolerance. Provide the patient and family with written and oral instructions to report these problems to the health care provider immediately:

- Unusual or foul-smelling drainage
- Swelling, redness, or warmth or bleeding from the incision site
- A temperature higher than 101° F (38.3° C)
- Abdominal pain
- Signs of wound dehiscence or ileus

Also instruct the patient and family in proper handwashing and dressing change techniques, which include directions to dress each wound separately to avoid cross-contamination.

Review information about antibiotics and analgesics. For patients taking oral opioid analgesics such as oxycodone with acetaminophen (Tylox, Percocet, Endocet♣) for any length of time, a stool softener such as docusate sodium (Colace, Regulex♣) may be prescribed. Older adults are especially at risk for constipation from codeine-based drugs.

Explain nutrition and activity limitations. Nutrition therapy depends on the type of surgery performed and the patient's specific food tolerances at discharge. Tell all patients to refrain from any lifting for *at least* 6 weeks. Other activity limitations are made on an individual basis with the physician's recommendation.

Patients with an incision healing by second or third intention may require dressings, solution, and catheter-tipped syringes to irrigate the wound. A home care nurse may be needed to assess, irrigate, or pack the wound and change the dressing as needed until the patient and family feel comfortable with the procedure. If the patient needs assistance with ADLs, a home care aide or temporary placement in a skilled care facility may be indicated. Collaborate with the case manager to determine the most appropriate setting for seamless continuing care in the community.

GASTROENTERITIS

Pathophysiology

Acute diarrheal illnesses are a significant health problem among adults, especially in less affluent countries. **Gastroenteritis** is an increase in the frequency and water content of stools or vomiting as a result of inflammation of the mucous membranes of the stomach and intestinal tract. It affects mainly the small bowel and can be caused by either viral or bacterial infections, which have similar manifestations. They are considered self-limiting in their course unless complications occur. All organisms implicated in gastroenteritis cause diarrhea. However, the organisms discussed in this section have distinguishing characteristics.

Some clinicians include shigellosis when discussing gastroenteritis. Others consider shigellosis separately as a dysentery type of illness. Dysenteries affect the *large* bowel. Gastroenteritis affects the *small* bowel. Other clinicians classify infectious disease of the intestine as bacterial, viral, or parasitic, without using the term *gastroenteritis*.

Food poisoning is sometimes described in conjunction with gastroenteritis with specific reference to the organism causing the food poisoning. Gastroenteritis, however, differs from food poisoning with regard to transmission in the body, incubation time, and effect on immunity.

The following discussion of gastroenteritis includes the epidemic viral form and the bacterial forms (*Campylobacter, Escherichia coli,* and shigellosis) (Table 60-1). Organisms associated with food poisoning from parasites are discussed on p. 1340 in the Parasitic Infection section.

Infection with viral and bacterial organisms can produce GI illnesses that cause watery diarrhea. These disorders may be caused by noninflammatory, inflammatory, or penetrating mechanisms. Organisms such as enterotoxigenic *E. coli* can release enterotoxin (a noninflammatory toxic substance specific to the intestinal mucosa), which results in diarrhea. *Shigella* or *Campylobacter* can attach itself to mucosal epithelium without penetrating it, resulting in destruction of the intestinal villi and malabsorption. Infections that are caused by bacterial toxins reduce the absorptive capacity of the distal small bowel and proximal colon, resulting in diarrhea. Finally, the organism can penetrate the intestine, causing cellular destruction, necrosis, and a potential for ulceration. Diarrhea occurs often with white blood cells (WBCs) or red blood cells (RBCs) present in the stool.

All of these organisms are transmitted via the oral-fecal route and result in *increased* GI motility, with fluids and electrolytes being secreted into the intestine at rapid rates. Invading organisms more easily attach to the intestinal mucosa if the normal intestinal flora is altered. This can occur in patients who are receiving antibiotics, are malnourished, or are debilitated. Two groups of viruses, the rotaviruses (which usually affect young children) and Norwalk virus, as well as bacterial pathogens, are the most common causes of gastroenteritis. Rotaviruses can also affect older adults in group settings, such as long-term care facilities.

TABLE 60-1 Common Types of Gastroenteritis and Their Characteristics

Type	Characteristics
VIRAL GASTROENTERITIS	
Epidemic viral	Caused by many parvovirus-type organisms Transmitted by the fecal-oral route in food and water Incubation period 10-51 hr Communicable during acute illness
Rotavirus and Norwalk virus	Transmitted by the fecal-oral route and possibly the respiratory route Incubation in 48 hr Rotavirus is most common in infants and young children Norwalk virus affects young children and adults
BACTERIAL GASTROENTERITIS	
Campylobacter enteritis	Transmitted by the fecal-oral route or by contact with infected animals or infants Incubation period 1-10 days Communicable for 2-7 weeks
Escherichia coli diarrhea	Transmitted by fecally contaminated food, water, or fomites
Shigellosis	Transmitted by direct and indirect fecal-oral routes Incubation period 1-7 days Communicable during the acute illness to 4 wk after the illness Humans possibly carriers for months

Types of Gastroenteritis

Viral Gastroenteritis

Norwalk virus infection can occur year-round and affects adults and children. This virus is responsible for one third of all epidemics of viral gastroenteritis in affluent countries and is a common cause of waterborne epidemics of gastroenteritis.

Bacterial Gastroenteritis

The three most common types of bacterial gastroenteritis are *Escherichia coli* diarrhea ("traveler's diarrhea"), *Campylobacter* enteritis (another "traveler's diarrhea"), and *Shigellosis* (bacillary dysentery). The reservoirs of *E. coli* are humans, who are often asymptomatic.

The etiologic feature of *Campylobacter* enteritis is the bacterium *Campylobacter jejuni;* reservoirs are domestic or wild animals and birds. Incubation ranges from 1 to 10 days. The organism is communicable for several days to weeks throughout the course of the infection (usually 2 to 7 weeks).

Shigellosis is caused by infection with *Shigella* bacteria. The incubation period before the illness is 1 to 7 days. The illness can be communicated during the acute phase and for up to 4 weeks after the onset of illness. A person can be a carrier of this illness for months after the acute illness.

Incidence/Prevalence

Acute diarrhea illnesses are the most common cause of morbidity and mortality among children and older adults in Asia, Africa, and Latin America. Gastroenteritis often occurs in epidemic outbreaks.

Diarrhea caused by *E. coli* and *Campylobacter* occur worldwide, commonly in epidemic outbreaks. *E. coli* epidemics are highest in areas of poor sanitation during warm months. Campylobacter incidence is highest during warm months. Shigellosis occurs in every age-group but most frequently in children (younger than 10 years) and older adults because of their depressed immune systems. Outbreaks of shigellosis are common in areas with crowded living conditions.

Patient-Centered Collaborative Care

Assessment

The patient history can provide information related to the potential cause of the illness. Ask about recent travel, especially to tropical regions of Asia, Africa, or Central or South America. Some areas of Mexico may also be the source of gastroenteritis. Newcomers (immigrants) from these countries often have gastroenteritis. Traveler's diarrhea can begin 3 days to 2 weeks after the patient's arrival.

The patient who has gastroenteritis usually looks ill. Nausea and vomiting can occur with all types of gastroenteritis but are usually limited to the first 1 or 2 days. Patients have diarrhea, which varies in consistency and amount with the causative organism.

In patients with epidemic viral gastroenteritis, myalgia (muscle aches), headache, and malaise are often reported. Note any abdominal distention, auscultate for hyperactive bowel sounds, and assess for diffuse tenderness on palpation. However, there should be *no* rebound tenderness, which might indicate peritonitis. Depending on the amount of fluids lost through diarrhea and vomiting, patients may have varying degrees of dehydration manifested by:

- Poor skin turgor
- Dry mucous membranes
- Orthostatic blood pressure changes
- Hypotension
- Oliguria

In some cases, dehydration may be severe, and shock may occur if diarrhea is prolonged. *Dehydration occurs rapidly in older adults and may require hospitalization.*

Diarrhea associated with epidemic viral gastroenteritis is commonly limited to 24 to 48 hours. Infection with the Norwalk virus has a rapid onset of nausea, abdominal cramps, vomiting, and diarrhea. This enteritis is usually mild. *Campylobacter* enteritis is a more severe disease with foul-smelling stools containing blood, which can number 20 to 30 per day for up to 7 days. *E. coli* gastroenteritis may or may not have blood or mucus in the stool. Diarrhea can last for up to 10 days. *Shigella* causes stools to have blood and mucus, which can continue for up to 5 days.

As part of the laboratory assessment, Gram stain of stool is usually done before culture. Cultures positive for the organism are diagnostic. Many WBCs on Gram stain suggest shigellosis. The presence of WBCs and RBCs in the stool indicates *Campylobacter* gastroenteritis.

Interventions

For any type of gastroenteritis, encourage fluid replacement. The amount and route of fluid administration are determined by the patient's hydration status.

Fluid Replacement

Teach patients to drink extra fluids to replace fluid lost through vomiting and diarrhea. Patients may be admitted to the hospital for gastroenteritis if they require IV fluid replacement, or they may stay in the emergency department or urgent care center until they are rehydrated. Commercially prepared rehydration products (e.g., Pedialyte) or IV therapy may prevent hospitalization. Caffeine should be avoided because it increases intestinal mobility and contributes to dehydration.

Obtain a weight, orthostatic blood pressure, and other vital sign measurements at admission. IV fluids such as half-strength normal saline (0.45% sodium chloride) with or without potassium supplements are infused as prescribed. *Potassium is usually needed for patients with excessive diarrhea.* Continue to monitor the patient's vital signs, intake and output, and weight. A rapid gain or loss of 1 kg (2.2 lbs) of body weight is equivalent to the gain or loss of 1 L of fluid. *Use Standard Precautions when handling vomitus and stool.* Advise the patient to alternate periods of rest and activity.

Depending on the type of gastroenteritis, especially if the geographic area is experiencing epidemic infections, the local health department may need to be notified. For example, it is mandatory that every case of shigellosis be reported. In some endemic areas, *Campylobacter* enteritis must be reported.

Drug Therapy

Drugs that suppress intestinal motility, such as anticholinergics and antiemetics, are *not* routinely given for bacterial or viral gastroenteritis. *Use of these drugs can prevent the infecting organisms from being eliminated from the body.* If the health care provider determines that antiperistaltic agents are necessary, an initial dose of loperamide (Imodium) 4 mg can be administered orally, followed by 2 mg after each loose stool, up to 16 mg daily. Bismuth subsalicylate (Pepto-Bismol) 30 mL or two tablets every 30 minutes for a maximum of eight doses can be given to reduce the watery volume of the stool. Diphenoxylate hydrochloride with atropine sulfate (Lomotil, Lomanate) reduces GI motility but is used sparingly because of its habit-forming ability. *The drug should not be used for older adults because it also causes drowsiness and could contribute to falls.*

Treatment with antibiotics may be needed if the gastroenteritis is due to bacterial infection with fever and severe diarrhea. The health care provider may prescribe norfloxacin (Noroxin) 400 mg orally twice daily or ciprofloxacin (Cipro) 500 mg orally twice daily for 3 days or more. If the gastroenteritis is due to shigellosis, anti-infective agents, such as trimethoprim/sulfamethoxazole (Septra DS, Bactrim DS, Roubac🍁), are prescribed.

For relatively short-term diarrhea of 24 to 48 hours' duration, the diagnosis is based primarily on the patient's history and clinical manifestations, not by a stool examination. When diarrhea is severe or persists for long periods, the stool is examined to determine the causative organism and to begin specific treatment. It should be determined whether the diarrhea is caused by *Salmonella* or by parasites because these organisms respond to specific medications (see p. 1339 in the Parasitic Infection section). Diarrhea that continues longer than 10 days, especially if associated with nocturnal diarrhea, is probably *not* due to gastroenteritis.

Skin Care

Frequent stools that are rich in electrolytes and enzymes, as well as frequent wiping and washing of the anal region, can irritate the skin. Teach the patient to avoid toilet paper and harsh soaps. Ideally, he or she can gently clean the area with warm water or absorbent cotton, followed by thorough drying with absorbent cotton. Cream, oil, or gel can be applied to a damp, warm washcloth to remove stool that sticks to open skin. Special prepared skin wipes can also be used. Hydrocortisone cream or protective barrier cream can be applied to the skin between stools. Sitz baths for 10 minutes two or three times daily can also relieve discomfort.

If leakage of stool is a problem, the patient can put absorbent cotton next to the anal orifice and keep it in place with snug underwear. For patients who are incontinent, remind unlicensed assistive personnel (UAP) to keep the perineal and buttock areas clean and dry. The use of incontinent pads at night instead of briefs allows air to circulate to the skin and prevents irritation.

Health Teaching

During the acute phase of the illness, teach the patient and family about the importance of fluid replacement. Teaching the patient and family about reducing the risk for transmission of gastroenteritis is also important (Chart 60-2). Adhere to these precautions for up to 7 weeks after the illness or up to several months if *Shigella* was the offending organism.

INFLAMMATORY BOWEL DISEASE

Although a patient can have idiopathic (unknown cause) inflammatory bowel disease (IBD), the term usually refers to disorders of the GI tract with no known etiology: ulcerative colitis and Crohn's disease. Comparisons and differences are listed in Table 60-2. Viral and bacterial dysenteries can cause symptoms similar to those of IBD, and other problems must be ruled out before a definitive diagnosis is made.

The approach to each patient is individualized. Encourage patients to take control of their incurable but controllable disease by learning about the disease, treatment, drugs, and complications.

Chart 60-2 PATIENT AND FAMILY EDUCATION GUIDE

Preventing Transmission of Gastroenteritis

Advise the patient to:

- Wash hands well for at least 30 seconds with an antibacterial soap, especially after a bowel movement, and maintain good personal hygiene.
- Restrict the use of glasses, dishes, eating utensils, and tubes of toothpaste for their own use. In severe cases, disposable utensils may be wise.
- Maintain clean bathroom facilities to avoid exposure to stool.
- Inform the health care provider if symptoms persist beyond 3 days.
- Do not prepare or handle food that will be consumed by others. If the patient is employed as a food handler, the public health department should be consulted for recommendations about the return to work.

ULCERATIVE COLITIS

Pathophysiology

Ulcerative colitis (UC) creates widespread inflammation of mainly the rectum and rectosigmoid colon but can extend to the entire colon with "backwash ileitis" evident in the terminal ileum when the disease is extensive. Distribution of the disease can remain constant for years. UC is a disease that is associated with periodic remissions and exacerbations (flare-ups).

In mild disease, the intestinal mucosa is hyperemic (has increased blood flow), edematous, and reddened. In more severe inflammation, the lining can bleed and small erosions, or ulcers, occur. Abscesses can form in these ulcerative areas and result in tissue necrosis (cell death). Continued edema and mucosal thickening can lead to a narrowed colon and possibly a partial bowel obstruction. Table 60-3 lists the categories of the severity of UC.

The patient's stool typically contains blood and mucus. Patients report **tenesmus** (an unpleasant and urgent sensation to defecate) and lower abdominal colicky pain relieved with defecation. Malaise, anorexia, and weight loss are common. Anemia occurs less often. Extraintestinal manifestations such as migratory polyarthritis, ankylosing spondylitis, and erythema nodosum are present in some patients. Gallstones are also common. The complications of UC are listed in Table 60-4.

With long-term disease, cellular changes can occur that increase the risk for colon cancer. Damage from inflammatory cytokines (e.g., interleukins [IL-1, IL-6, IL-8) and tumor necrosis factor (TNF)–alpha have cytotoxic effects on the colonic mucosa. Therefore annual colonoscopies are recommended when the patient has longer than a 10-year history of UC involving the entire colon. Primary sclerosing cholangitis (PSC) is a chronic fibrosing inflammation of the intrahepatic/

TABLE 60-2 Differential Features of Ulcerative Colitis and Crohn's Disease

Feature	Ulcerative Colitis	Crohn's Disease
Location	Begins in the rectum and proceeds in a continuous manner toward the cecum	Most often in the terminal ileum, with patchy involvement through all layers of the bowel
Etiology	Unknown	Unknown
Peak incidence at age	15-25 yr and 55-65 yr	15-40 yr
Number of stools	10-20 liquid, bloody stools per day	5-6 soft, loose stools per day, non-bloody
Complications	Hemorrhage Nutritional deficiencies	Fistulas (common) Nutritional deficiencies
Need for surgery	Infrequent	Frequent

extrahepatic bile ducts that can develop into cirrhosis and commonly occurs with UC.

Etiology and Genetic Risk

The exact cause of UC is unknown. A genetic basis of the disease has been proposed because it is often found in families and twins. Immunologic causes, including autoimmune dysfunction, have been explored because of the extraintestinal manifestations of the disease. Epithelial antibodies in the IgG class have been identified in the blood of some patients with UC (McCance & Huether, 2006).

IBD may result from an abnormal response to normal flora present in the intestines. Another possibility is that there may be a defect in intestinal permeability that permits antigens to leak through the mucosa, stimulating an inflammatory response. Psychological factors may result in an exacerbation of the disease. However, little evidence has been found to relate psychological factors to the cause of the disease.

TABLE 60-3 American College of Gastroenterologists Classification of UC Severity

Severity	Stool Frequency	Signs/Symptoms
Mild	<4 stools/day with/without blood	Asymptomatic Laboratory values usually normal
Moderate	>4 stools/day with/without blood	Minimal symptoms Mild abdominal pain Mild intermittent nausea Possible increased C-reactive protein* or ESR†
Severe	>6 bloody stools/day	Fever Tachycardia Anemia Abdominal pain Elevated C-reactive protein* and/or ESR†
Fulminant	>10 bloody stools/day	Increasing symptoms Anemia may require transfusion Colonic distention on x-ray

Adapted from Present, D.H. (2006). *Current and investigational approaches in the management of ulcerative colitis.* Secaucus, NJ: Thomson Professional Postgraduate Services/ Shire Pharmaceuticals, Inc.

*C-reactive protein is a sensitive acute-phase serum marker that is evident in the first 6 hours of an inflammatory process.

†ESR (erythrocyte sedimentation rate) may be helpful but is less sensitive than C-reactive protein.

UC, Ulcerative colitis.

Incidence/Prevalence

The disease occurs at the highest rates in northern Europe and North America. It affects about 2 million people in the United States. A person's risk for the disease is ten times greater if he or she has a first-degree relative (parent, sibling, or child) with the disease. Peak age is between 20 and 40 years old and again at 55 to 65 years old. Women are more often affected than men in their younger years, but men have the disease more often as middle-aged and older adults (www.ccfa.org/info/about/ucp).

People who do not smoke or those who quit smoking are at a *higher* risk for having UC than people who smoke. The reason for this relationship is not known, but nicotine has a positive influence on smooth muscle of the colon.

CULTURAL AWARENESS

Ulcerative colitis is four to five times more common among people of European Jewish or Sephardic origin and commonly affects Euro-American people (www.ccfa/info/about/ucp). The reasons for these ethnic differences are not known.

Patient-Centered Collaborative Care

evolve ONLINE PHARM REVIEW

Assessment

History

Collect data on family history of IBD, previous and current therapy for the illness, and dates and types of surgery. Obtain a nutrition history, including intolerance of milk and milk products and fried, spicy, or hot foods. Ask about usual bowel elimination pattern (color, consistency, character of the stool), abdominal pain, tenesmus, anorexia, and fatigue. Note any

TABLE 60-4 Complications of Ulcerative Colitis and Crohn's Disease

Complication	Description
Hemorrhage/perforation	Lower gastrointestinal bleeding results from erosion of the bowel wall.
Abscess formation	Localized pockets of infection develop in the ulcerated bowel lining.
Toxic megacolon	Paralysis of the colon causes dilation and subsequent colonic ileus, possibly perforation.
Malabsorption	Essential nutrients cannot be absorbed through the diseased intestinal wall, causing anemia and malnutrition (most common in Crohn's disease).
Nonmechanical bowel obstruction	Obstruction results from toxic megacolon or cancer.
Fistulas	In Crohn's disease in which the inflammation is transmural, fistulas can occur anywhere but usually track between the bowel and bladder resulting in pyuria and fecaluria.
Colorectal cancer	Patients with ulcerative colitis with a history longer than 10 years have a high risk for colorectal cancer. This complication accounts for about one third of all deaths related to ulcerative colitis.
Extraintestinal complications	Complications include arthritis, hepatic and biliary disease (especially cholelithiasis), oral and skin lesions, and ocular disorders, such as iritis. The cause is unknown.
Osteoporosis	Osteoporosis occurs especially in patients with Crohn's disease.

relationship between diarrhea, timing of meals, emotional distress, and activity. Inquire about recent (past 2 to 3 month) exposure to antibiotics suggesting *Clostridium difficile* infection. Has the patient traveled to or immigrated from tropical areas? Ask about recent use of NSAIDs that can either present with the initial diagnosis or cause a flare-up of the disease. Ask about any extraintestinal symptoms such as arthritis, mouth sores, vision problems, and skin disorders. Ask if the patient smokes or if symptoms began after smoking cessation.

Physical Assessment/Clinical Manifestations

Symptoms vary with an acuteness of onset. Vital signs are usually within normal limits in mild disease. In more severe cases, the patient may have a low-grade fever (99° to 100° F [37.2° to 37.8° C]). The physical assessment findings are usually nonspecific, and in milder cases the physical examination may be normal. Viral and bacterial infections cause similar symptoms to those of UC.

Note any abdominal distention along the colon. Palpation may reveal areas of increased or localized tenderness. Rebound tenderness may suggest peritonitis. Patients with fever associated with tachycardia may indicate peritonitis, dehydration, and bowel perforation.

Psychosocial Assessment

Many patients are very concerned about the frequency of stools and the presence of blood. *The inability to control the disease symptoms, particularly diarrhea, can be disruptive and stress producing.* Severe illness may limit the patient's activities outside the home with fear of fecal incontinence resulting in feeling "tied to the toilet." Eating may be associated with pain and cramping and an increased frequency of stools. Mealtimes may become unpleasant experiences. Frequent visits to health care providers and close monitoring of the colon mucosa for abnormal cell changes can be anxiety provoking.

Assess the patient's understanding of the illness and its impact on his or her lifestyle. Encourage and support the patient while exploring:

- The relationship of life events to disease exacerbations
- Stress factors that produce symptoms
- Family and social support systems
- Concerns regarding the possible genetic basis and associated cancer risks of the disease
- Internet access for reliable education information

Laboratory Assessment

As a result of chronic blood loss, hematocrit and hemoglobin levels may be low, which indicates anemia and a chronic disease state. *An increased WBC count, platelet count, C-reactive protein, or erythrocyte sedimentation rate (ESR) is consistent with inflammatory disease.* Blood levels of sodium, potassium, and chloride may be *low* as a result of frequent diarrheal stools and malabsorption through the diseased bowel. Hypoalbuminemia (decreased serum albumin) is found in patients with extensive disease from losing protein in the stool.

Other Diagnostic Assessment

A colonoscopy is the most definitive test for diagnosing UC. In some cases, a *computed tomography (CT) scan* may be done to confirm the disease or its complications. *Barium enemas* with air contrast can show differences between UC and Crohn's disease and identify complications, mucosal patterns, and the distribution and depth of disease involvement. In early disease, the barium enema may show incomplete filling as a result of inflammation and fine ulcerations along the bowel contour, which appear deeper in more advanced disease.

DECISION-MAKING CHALLENGE
Coordination of Care

A 43-year-old woman who has 10 to 15 watery loose stools per day since she stopped smoking is admitted to the ED. Bloody mucus is mixed with her stool. She has had no weight loss but has cramping and lower abdominal pain relieved after her bowel movement. Stools for C&S, ova and parasites, and *C. difficile* at her primary care provider's office were negative. She is now admitted for dehydration.

1. What questions should you ask to obtain a thorough history?
2. What other physical assessment should you perform at this time?
3. What other health care team members will likely be involved in this patient's assessment?
4. What laboratory tests will most likely be requested, and what might they show?
5. What interventions will most likely be prescribed to treat this patient's dehydration?

evolve For suggested answer guidelines, go to http://evolve.elsevier.com/Iggy/.

▪ *Analysis*

Common Nursing Diagnoses and Collaborative Problems

The priority nursing diagnoses for patients with ulcerative colitis are:

1. Diarrhea related to inflammation of the bowel mucosa
2. Acute Pain and Chronic Pain related to inflammation and ulceration of the bowel mucosa and skin irritation

The primary collaborative problem is Potential for Lower GI Bleeding with possible anemia.

Additional Nursing Diagnoses and Collaborative Problems

In addition to the common nursing diagnoses and collaborative problem, patients with ulcerative colitis may have:

- Imbalanced Nutrition: Less Than Body Requirements related to inability to absorb food because of biologic factors
- Disturbed Body Image related to biophysical factors and possible surgery
- Activity Intolerance related to generalized weakness
- Risk for Deficient Fluid Volume related to diarrhea
- Potential for colon cancer related to long-term history of UC

▪ *Planning and Implementation*

Diarrhea

Planning: Expected Outcomes. The major concern for a patient with ulcerative colitis is the occurrence of frequent, bloody diarrhea and fecal incontinence from tenesmus (straining). Therefore, with treatment, the patient is expected to have formed stools and a normal elimination pattern with control of bowel movements.

Interventions. Many measures are used to relieve symptoms and to reduce intestinal motility, decrease inflammation, and promote intestinal healing (Chart 60-3). Nonsurgical and surgical management may be needed.

Chart 60-3 NIC INTERVENTION ACTIVITIES

The Patient with Inflammatory Bowel Disease

Diarrhea Management: *Management and alleviation of diarrhea*

- Instruct patient/family members to record color, volume, frequency, and consistency of stools.
- Identify factors (e.g., medications, bacteria, tube feedings) that may cause or contribute to diarrhea.
- Teach the patient to eliminate gas-forming and spicy foods from diet.
- Suggest trial elimination of foods containing lactose.
- Instruct in low-fiber, high-protein, high-calorie diet, as appropriate.
- Teach patient appropriate use of antidiarrheal medications.
- Monitor skin in perianal area for irritation and ulceration.
- Weigh patient regularly.
- Perform actions to rest the bowel (NPO, liquid diet).

Pain Management: *Alleviation of pain or a reduction in pain to a level of comfort that is acceptable to the patient*

- Perform a comprehensive assessment of pain to include location, characteristics, onset/duration, frequency, quality, intensity or severity, and precipitating factors.
- Evaluate, with the patient and the health care team, the effectiveness of past pain control measures that have been used.
- Reduce or eliminate factors that can precipitate or increase the pain experience (e.g., fear, fatigue, monotony, and lack of knowledge).
- Teach the use of nonpharmacologic techniques (e.g., biofeedback, hypnosis, relaxation, guided imagery, music therapy, distraction, activity therapy, acupressure, hot/cold application, and massage) before, after and, if possible, during painful activities; before pain occurs or increases; and along with other pain relief measures.

NIC intervention activities selected from Bulechek, G.M., Butcher, H.K., and McCloskey Dochterman, J. (Eds.). (2008). *Nursing interventions classification (NIC)* (5th ed.). St. Louis: Mosby. No part of this work is to be altered without prior written permission from the Publisher.

Nonsurgical Management. Nonsurgical management includes drug and nutrition therapy. The use of physical and emotional rest is also an important consideration. Teach the patient to record color, volume, frequency, and consistency of stools to determine severity of the problem.

Monitor the skin in the perianal area for irritation and ulceration resulting from loose, frequent stools. Stool cultures may be sent for analysis if diarrhea continues. Teach the patient and family members about the correct use of antidiarrheal drugs. Have the patient weigh himself or herself one or two times per week. If the patient is hospitalized, remind unlicensed assistive personnel to weigh him or her on admission and daily and document all weights.

Drug therapy. Common drug therapy for UC includes aminosalicylates, glucocorticoids, immunomodulators, and antidiarrheal drugs.

The *aminosalicylates* are a class of drug used to treat mild to moderate UC and/or maintain remission after accomplished by other treatments. Four aminosalicylate compounds are available. All deliver 5-aminosalicylic acid (5-ASA) to the affected area. The method of action is unknown but thought to have an anti-inflammatory effect by inhibiting prostaglandins. These agents are effective in 2 to 4 weeks.

Sulfasalazine (Azulfidine, Azulfidine EN-tabs) is metabolized by the intestinal bacteria into 5-ASA, which delivers the beneficial effects of the drug, and sulfapyridine, which is responsible for the side effects (nausea, vomiting, anorexia, folate malabsorption, and headache). With higher doses, rash, hemolytic anemia, hepatitis, male infertility, or agranulocytosis can occur. This drug is in the same family as sulfonamide antibiotics. Therefore assess the patient for an allergy to sulfonamide or other drugs that contain sulfur such as furosemide. The use of a thiazide diuretic is a contraindication for sulfasalazine.

Mesalamine (Asacol, Pentasa, Rowasa) is the generic name for 5-ASA. This drug is better tolerated than sulfasalazine, with side effects of headache and GI upset. Asacol is an enteric-coated drug and is released in the terminal ileum and right side of the colon. Pentasa is a delayed-release drug and is released throughout the small bowel and colon to the rectum. Rowasa is a suppository or enema used nightly to treat left-sided disease. Topical agents (suppository or enema) have minimal systemic absorption and therefore have fewer side effects.

Balsalazide (Colazal) releases 5-ASA and is well tolerated, with headache and abdominal pain as the primary side effects. It is distributed mainly in the colon itself, with little drug effectiveness in the terminal ileum. Table 60-5 lists recommended doses for the 5-ASA drugs.

Glucocorticoids, such as prednisone and budesonide, are corticosteroid therapies prescribed during exacerbations of the disease. Prednisone (Deltasone, Winpred) 40 to 65 mg daily is usually given orally. Once clinical improvement occurs, the corticosteroids are tapered because of the adverse effects that commonly occur with long-term steroid therapy (e.g., hyperglycemia, osteoporosis, peptic ulcer disease, increased risk for infection). For patients with rectal symptoms, topical steroids in the form of small retention enemas may be prescribed. Hydrocortisone rectal foam (Cortifoam) is prescribed as one to two times daily for 2 to 3 weeks and then every other day. Hydrocortisone enemas (Cortenema) are given at bedtime for 21 days, tapered, and discontinued.

Immunomodulators are drugs that alter a person's immune response. They are not thought to be effective in the treatment of ulcerative colitis. However, in combination with steroids, they may offer a synergistic effect to a quicker response, thereby decreasing the amount of steroids needed. For example, cyclosporine used in severely ill patients might avoid an emergent colectomy. Immunosuppressants used with UC (and Crohn's disease) include azathioprine, mercaptopurine, cyclosporine, methotrexate, infliximab, and adalimumab.

To provide symptomatic management of diarrhea, *antidiarrheal drugs* may be prescribed. These drugs are given very cautiously, however, because they can cause colon dilation and toxic megacolon. Common antidiarrheal drugs include diphenoxylate hydrochloride and atropine sulfate (Lomotil) and loperamide (Imodium).

Although not approved as a first-line therapy for ulcerative colitis, *infliximab* (Remicade) may be used for refractory disease or for severe complications, such as **toxic megacolon** (massive dilation of the colon that can lead to peritonitis). Remicade is an immunoglobulin G (IgG) monoclonal antibody that reduces the activity of tumor necrosis factor (TNF) to decrease inflammation. Adalimumab (Humira) is another monoclonal antibody recently approved for refractory cases.

TABLE 60-5 Recommended Doses for 5-ASA Medications

Generic Name	Trade Name	Dosage Available	Recommended Dose
Sulfasalazine	Azulfidine	500 mg tablets	3-4 g daily in divided doses
	Azulfidine En-tabs	250 mg/5 mL liquid	Children >2 yr: 30 mg/kg/day not to exceed 2 g/day
Mesalamine	Asacol	400 mg tablets	800 mg three times daily
	Pentasa	500 mg tablets	1 g four times daily
	Rowasa enemas	4 g/60 mL	At bedtime
	Rowasa suppository	1000 mg/supp	Twice daily or at bedtime
Olsalazine (rarely used)	Dipentum	250 mg tablets	1 g daily in two divided doses
Balsalazide	Colazal	750 mg tablets	3 tablets three times daily

They are used more commonly in management of Crohn's disease. These drugs cause immune suppression and should be used with caution. Teach the patient to report any signs of a beginning infection, including a cold, and to avoid large crowds or others who are sick.

Nutrition therapy. Patients with severe symptoms are kept NPO to ensure bowel rest. The physician may prescribe total parenteral nutrition (TPN) for severely ill and malnourished patients. Chapter 63 describes this therapy in detail. Patients with less severe symptoms may drink elemental formulas such as Vivonex, which are absorbed in the small bowel and reduce bowel stimulation. Those with significant but less severe symptoms may be restricted to a low-fiber (low-residue) diet. Although a fiber-restricted diet remains controversial, teach the patient to limit or omit foods that cause him or her discomfort or diarrhea. Often, lactose-containing foods are poorly tolerated and should be reduced or eliminated. Warn the patient that caffeinated beverages, pepper, alcohol, and smoking are common GI stimulants that could cause discomfort. Smoking and other forms of nicotine have been shown to help heal ulcerative colitis, but this approach is not recommended.

Rest. At the onset of treatment, activity is generally restricted because rest can reduce intestinal activity, provide comfort, and promote healing. Ensure that the patient has easy access to a bedpan, bedside commode, or bathroom in case of urgency or tenesmus.

Complementary and alternative therapies. In addition to nutritional changes, complementary and alternative therapies may be used to supplement traditional management of ulcerative colitis. Examples include herbs, such as flaxseed, selenium, and vitamin C. Biofeedback, hypnosis, yoga, acupuncture, and ayurveda (a combination of diet, yoga, herbs, and breathing exercises) may also be helpful. These therapies have no proven efficacy in randomized double blind studies to date, but some patients find them helpful.

Surgical Management. Some patients with ulcerative colitis require a **colectomy** (surgical colon removal) and ileostomy. Indications for surgery include bowel perforation, toxic megacolon, hemorrhage, dysplastic biopsy results, failure of conventional treatment, and colon cancer.

Preoperative care. General preoperative teaching related to abdominal surgery is described in Chapter 16. When an ileostomy is indicated, provide an in-depth explanation to the patient and family. An **ileostomy** is a procedure in which a loop of the ileum is placed through the abdominal wall **(stoma)** for drainage of fecal material into a pouching system worn on the abdomen. The pouching system consists of a solid skin barrier (wafer) to protect the skin and a fecal collection device (pouch).

The surgeon usually consults with a certified wound, ostomy, continence nurse (CWOCN) or enterostomal therapist (ET) (sometimes called an *ostomy nurse*) before surgery for recommendations on the best location of the stoma. A visit from an **ostomate** (a patient with an ostomy) may be helpful before surgery. Oral or parenteral antibiotics such as neomycin sulfate (Mycifradin) are prescribed as a bowel antiseptic. Cleansing of the bowel with enemas or laxatives may also be needed although the value of preoperative bowel preparation is currently being questioned (Jung et al., 2007).

Operative procedures. Any one of several surgical approaches may be used for the patient with UC. The traditional approach involves a large open incision that cuts through layers of muscle and subcutaneous tissue to create a surgical diversion. The newer minimally invasive surgery (MIS) via laparoscopy for ulcerative colitis involves several small incisions that lead to faster recovery. Patients who are obese, have had previous abdominal surgeries, or have dense scar tissue are not candidates for this technique.

Total proctocolectomy with a permanent ileostomy. Total proctocolectomy (or colectomy) with a permanent ileostomy has traditionally been the standard surgical procedure for patients undergoing a colectomy and involves the removal of the colon, rectum, and anus with surgical closure of the anus (Fig. 60-2, *A*). The surgeon brings the end of the ileum out through the abdominal wall and forms a stoma, or **ostomy.** The stoma (Fig. 60-2, *B*) is usually placed in the right lower quadrant of the abdomen below the belt line. It should not be prolapsed or retract into the abdominal wall. *The stoma should be pinkish to cherry red because it should be receiving an adequate blood supply. If it looks pale, bluish, or dark, report these findings to the health care provider immediately.*

With a permanent ileostomy, initially after surgery the output is a loose, dark green liquid that may contain some blood. Over time, a process called "ileostomy adaptation" occurs. The small intestine begins to perform some of the functions that had previously been done by the colon, including the absorption of increased amounts of sodium and water. Stool volume decreases, becomes thicker (pastelike), and turns yellow-green or yellow-brown. The effluent (fluid material) usually has little odor or a sweet odor. Any foul or unpleasant odor may be a symptom of a problem such as blockage or infection.

The ostomy drains frequently, and the stool is irritating. *The patient must wear a pouch system at all times.* The stool from the small intestine contains many enzymes and bile salts, which can quickly irritate and injure the skin. *Skin care around the stoma is a priority!* A pouch system with a skin barrier (gelatin or pectin) provides sufficient protection for most patients. Other products are also available.

Total colectomy with a continent ileostomy. As an alternative to the traditional ileostomy with an external pouch, the surgeon may create an internal system: a Kock's ileostomy or ileal reservoir referred to as a "continent ileostomy." The surgeon constructs an intra-abdominal pouch or reservoir from the terminal ileum (Fig. 60-3) where stool is stored via a nipple-like valve in the pouch until the patient drains it by using a catheter. Immediately after surgery, an indwelling urinary catheter is placed in the pouch and is connected to low intermittent suction and irrigated as prescribed.

Monitor the character and quality of effluent (drainage). Teach the patient to drain the stoma. Initially the pouch holds only 50 to 75 mL. Over time, the pouch stretches and can hold 500 to 700 mL. When the pouch needs to be emptied, the patient has a sensation of fullness. The patient drains the pouch several times a day and wears a small dressing to keep the stoma moist and protect clothing. This procedure allows for minimal skin irritation. The patient does not need to wear an external pouch. Unfortunately, the need for surgical adjustments and problems with leakage and the development of the ileoanal anastomosis have made this procedure less desirable.

Total colectomy with ileoanal anastomosis. This procedure involves the surgical removal of the colon and the rectum and sutures the ileum into the anal canal or small cuff of rectum. Usually continence is excellent after this procedure, but many patients have some leakage of stool during sleep. Perineal irritation can be a problem. Teach patients who have this surgery to use frequent and careful perineal care.

Ileoanal anastomosis occurs in two stages (Fig. 60-4). First, the surgeon removes the rectal mucosa, performs an abdominal colectomy, constructs the reservoir or pouch to the anal canal, and creates a temporary loop ileostomy. The loop ileostomy allows healing of the internal pouch and all anastomosis sites and allows for an increase in the capacity of the internal reservoir through fluid instillations. After 3 to 4 months, the patient returns to have the loop ileostomy closed. Stool formation resembles that in patients who have undergone a traditional ileostomy.

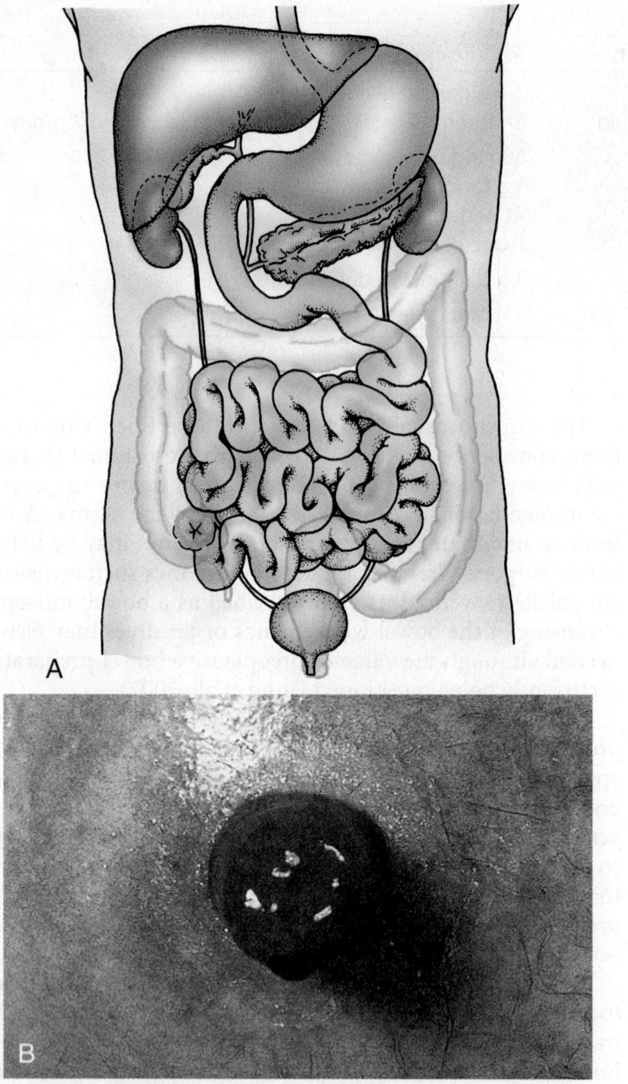
A
B

Fig. 60-2 • **A,** Total proctocolectomy with a permanent ileostomy. This involved removal of the colon, the rectum, and the anus with closure of the anus. Note the missing colon, rectum, and anus with the resultant stoma (**B**) in the right lower quadrant.

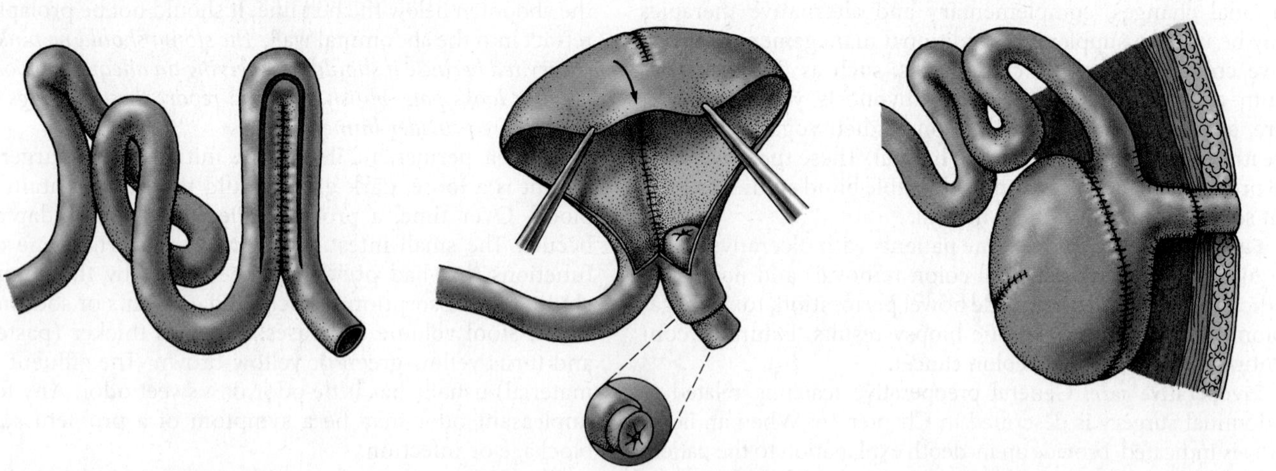

1. A reservoir, in which the patient will retain stool until draining it, is constructed from a loop of ileum folded and sutured together, then cut.
2. A portion of the ileum is intussuscepted to form a nipple valve, and the upper part of the stitched and cut ileum is pulled down and sutured to form a pouch.
3. The nipple valve, which shuts tight against pressure from a filled pouch, is pulled through the stoma and sutured flush with the abdomen.

Fig. 60-3 • The creation of a Kock's (continent) ileostomy.

Ileoanal reservoir. The creation of an ileoanal reservoir, also known as a "J pouch," has become popular for many patients with ulcerative colitis, especially young adults, because it spares the rectal sphincter and eliminates the need for an ostomy. The surgeon removes the colon and sutures the ileum into the rectal stump to form a reservoir. If residual rectal mucosa remains after either an ileoanal anastomosis or a reservoir procedure, proctoscopy is done at on a regular basis to monitor for dysplasia (abnormal cells).

Postoperative care. Provide general postoperative care after surgery, as described in Chapter 18. All patients requiring open approach surgery for ulcerative colitis have a large abdominal incision. At first, most patients are NPO and a nasogastric tube (NGT) is used for suction. The tube is removed in 1 to 2 days as the drainage decreases and fluids and food are slowly introduced. The patient having MIS does not have an NGT.

In collaboration with the ostomy nurse, help the patient adjust and learn the required care. The ileostomy begins to drain within 24 hours after surgery at more than 1 L per day. Be sure that fluids are replaced by adding an additional 500 mL or more each day to prevent dehydration. After about a week of high-volume output, the drainage slows and becomes thicker. During this period, some patients need Lomotil or Imodium. Oral rehydration therapy (ORT) can also be used, including Pedialyte and CeraLyte (Willcutts et al., 2005).

The hospital stay is usually from 4 to 6 days, depending on whether the patient has laparoscopic or open conventional surgery. Patients having MIS have less pain and fewer complications from surgery when compared with other surgical patients.

Surgery for UC may result in altered body image. However, it may be viewed as positive because the patient will have fewer symptoms and feel more comfortable than before the procedure. Patients have to adjust to having an ostomy before they can resume their presurgery activities.

Acute Pain; Chronic Pain

NOC **Planning: Expected Outcomes.** The patient with ulcerative colitis will be able to:

- Use pain prevention measures, such as nutrition changes
- Use non-analgesic relief measures
- Have a decrease in pain to a 2 or 3 on a 1-10 pain intensity scale
- Report changes in pain symptoms to health care professional

Interventions. Pain control requires pharmacologic and nonpharmacologic measures. Physical discomfort can contribute to emotional discomfort. A variety of symptom-reducing interventions and supportive measures is used (see Chart 60-3).

The purpose of pain management is alleviation of pain or a reduction in pain to a level of comfort that is acceptable to the patient. Increases in pain may indicate the development of complications such as peritonitis. Assist the patient in reducing or eliminating factors that can cause or increase the pain experience. For example, he or she may benefit from nutrition changes to decrease abdominal discomfort such as cramping and bloating.

Antidiarrheal drugs such as Imodium or Lomotil are used to control diarrhea, thus reducing the discomfort. However, they must be used with caution and for a short time because toxic megacolon can develop.

Perineal skin can be irritated by contact with loose stools and frequent cleaning. Explain special measures for skin care. Use of medicated wipes is soothing if the rectal area is tender

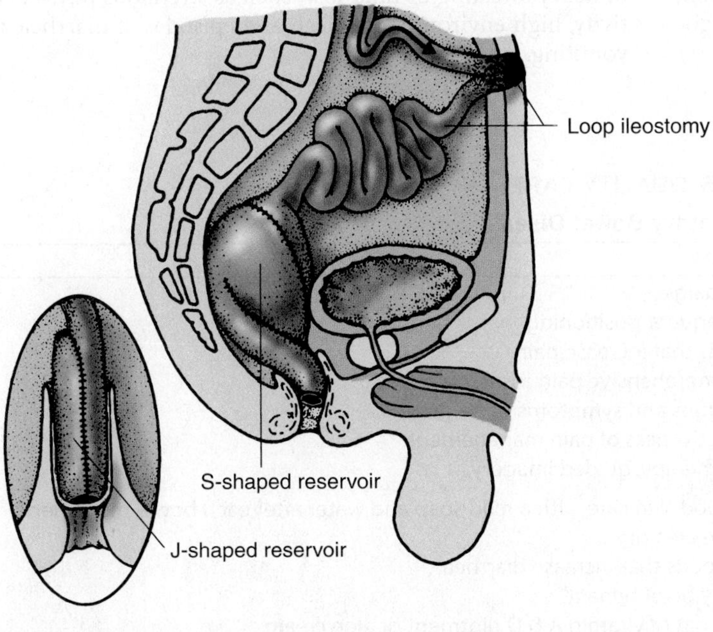
Loop ileostomy
S-shaped reservoir
J-shaped reservoir

Stage 1.
After removal of the colon, a temporary loop ileostomy is created and an ileoanal reservoir is formed. The reservoir is created in an S-shaped reservoir (using three loops of ileum) or a J-shaped reservoir (suturing a portion of ileum to the rectal cuff, with an upward loop).

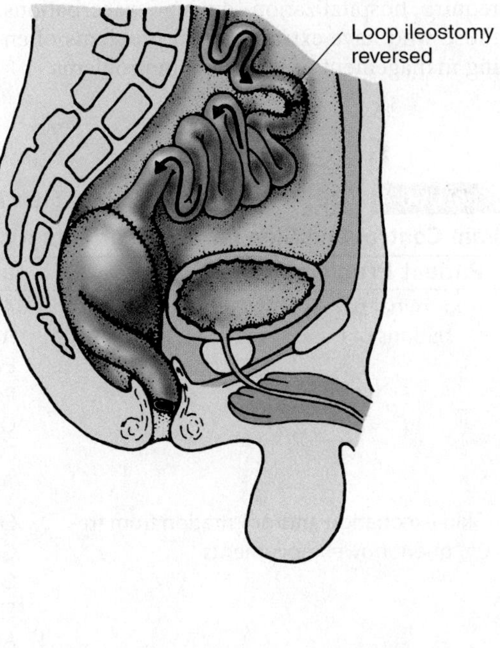
Loop ileostomy reversed

Stage 2.
After the reservoir has had time to heal–usually several months–the temporary loop ileostomy is reversed, and stool is allowed to drain into the reservoir.

Fig. 60-4 • The creation of an ileoanal reservoir.

or sensitive from the use of toilet tissue (Chart 60-4). Various manufacturers of ostomies (Hollister, ConvaTec) produce a three-product system for skin care that may help prevent and heal perineal skin irritation. Such systems include a skin-cleaning solution, a moisturizing and healing cream, and a petroleum jelly–like barrier that prevents contact of moisture and stool with the skin.

Potential for Lower GI Bleeding

Planning: Expected Outcomes. The patient with UC is expected to have a reduction in or cessation of GI bleeding that can occur with the disease. He or she is also expected to remain free of complications of the disease that can cause bleeding, such as perforation.

Interventions. *The primary nursing responsibility is to monitor the patient closely for signs and symptoms of GI bleeding resulting from the disease or its complications.* Monitor stools for blood loss. The blood may be bright red (frank bleeding) or black and tarry **(melena).** Monitor hematocrit, hemoglobin, and electrolyte values, and assess vital signs. Prolonged slow bleeding can lead to anemia. Observe for fever, tachycardia, and signs of fluid volume depletion. Changes in mental status may occur, especially among older adults, and may be the first indication of dehydration or anemia.

If symptoms of GI bleeding begin, notify the health care provider immediately. Blood products may be prescribed for patients with severe anemia. Prepare for the blood transfusion by inserting a large-bore IV catheter if it is not already in place. Chapter 42 outlines nursing actions during blood transfusion.

Community-Based Care

Home Care Management

The patient with ulcerative colitis is managed at home but may require hospitalization during exacerbations. In addition, those who have extraintestinal problems often require ongoing management of joint or skin problems.

Home care management focuses on controlling symptoms and monitoring for complications. Instruct the patient about measures to reduce or control abdominal pain, cramping, and diarrhea. Also teach the patient and family about symptoms that should be reported immediately to the health care provider, such as fever higher than 101° F (38.3° C), tachycardia, palpitations, and an increase in diarrhea, abdominal pain, or nausea/vomiting. Provide written information and contact numbers for the health care provider. For patients returning home or transferring to nursing home or transitional care after surgery, ongoing respiratory care, incision care, ostomy care, and pain management should be continued.

Health Teaching

Teach the patient about the nature of ulcerative colitis, including its acute episodes, remissions, and symptom management. Also stress that even though the cause is unknown, relapses can be resolved with proper health care. Teach the patient taking immunosuppressive drugs to report signs of possible infection, such as sore throat, to the health care provider. Review the drug therapy, when drugs should be taken, and side effects with the patient and family.

There is no special diet for a patient with an ileostomy. However, teach the patient to avoid any foods that cause gas or make the stool thicker. Examples include high-fiber foods like nuts, raw cabbage, corn, celery, apples with peels, and popcorn. The patient needs to learn what foods he or she tolerates best and adjust the diet accordingly.

If he or she has undergone a surgical diversion, collaborate with the ostomy nurse to explain and demonstrate required care so that the patient can self-manage. Also teach the importance of including adequate amounts of salt and water in the diet because the ileostomy increases the loss of these substances. Urge the patient to be cautious in situations that lead to heavy sweating or fluid loss, such as strenuous physical activity, high environmental heat, and episodes of diarrhea and vomiting.

Chart 60-4 BEST PRACTICE FOR PATIENT SAFETY & QUALITY CARE

Pain Control and Skin Care for Patients with Inflammatory Bowel Disease

Patient Problem	Interventions
Abdominal pain (particularly with exacerbations of the disease)	Administer analgesics. Assist with frequent positioning. Evaluate foods that increase pain. Perform a comprehensive pain assessment. Observe for signs and symptoms of peritonitis. Evaluate effectiveness of pain management. Teach music therapy, guided imagery.
Skin excoriation and/or irritation from frequent bowel movements	Encourage good skin care with a mild soap and water after each bowel movement. Gently pat the area dry. Evaluate for foods that increase diarrhea. Sitz baths may be of benefit. Apply a thin coat of vitamin A & D ointment or aloe cream. Use medicated wipes instead of tissue. Ensure good fitting, appropriate ostomy supplies. Antidiarrheal medications may help, but use with caution. Observe for symptoms related to megacolon (fever, leukocytosis, tachycardia, distended abdomen with 3-view abdominal x-ray noting an enlarged colon).

Finding the best ostomy pouching system is a major issue for many patients. An effective system is one that (Willcutts et al., 2005):

- Protects the skin
- Contains the effluent (drainage) and reduces odor, if any
- Remains securely attached to the skin for a dependable period of time

Most patients want an adhesive barrier that will last for 3 to 7 days. The barrier must create a solid seal to prevent the enzymes in the drainage from irritating the skin. Solid barriers are classified as "regular wear" or "extended wear." A person with a high output may want an extended-wear barrier. A special cream can be used to help fill any uneven skin surfaces and provide a consistent seal. Pouches are also individualized by the patient. Large pouches can hold more but are heavy when full. Patients also have to consider the costs of the various systems and how much their insurance (if they have it) will pay for them. Chart 60-5 describes the main areas of ileostomy care.

A patient with an ileostomy may have many concerns about management at home and about sexual and social adjustments. Considering possible sexual issues helps the patient identify and discuss these concerns with the sex partner. For example, a simple change in positioning during intercourse may alleviate apprehension. Social situations may cause anxiety related to decreased self-esteem and a disturbance in body image. Encourage the patient to discuss possible concerns in addressing and resolving these potentially stressful events.

Health Care Resources

If the patient needs assistance with self-management at home, collaborate with the case manager or social worker to arrange the services of a home care aide or nurse. A home care nurse can provide assessment and guidance in integrating ostomy care into the patient's lifestyle. The nurse may also teach about wound care, including the monitoring of wound healing, if needed (Chart 60-6). The patient and family need to know where to purchase ostomy supplies, along with the name, size, and manufacturer's order number.

Identify the local ostomy support group by contacting the United Ostomy Associations of America (www.uoaa.org). The United Ostomy Association of Canada serves the needs of

Chart 60-6 HOME CARE ASSESSMENT
The Patient with Inflammatory Bowel Disease

Assess gastrointestinal function and nutritional status, including:
- Abdominal cramping or pain
- Bowel elimination pattern, specifically frequency, characteristics, and amount of stools and presence or absence of blood in stools
- Food and fluid intake (include relationship of specific foods to cramping and stools)
- Weight gain or loss
- Signs and symptoms of dehydration
- Presence or absence of fever, rectal tenesmus, or urgency
- Bowel sounds
- Condition of perianal skin, including presence or absence of perianal fistula or abscess

Assess patient's and family's coping skills, including:
- Current and ongoing stress level and coping style
- Availability of support system

Assess home environment, including:
- Adequacy and availability of bathroom facilities
- Opportunity for rest and relaxation

Assess ability to self-manage therapeutic regimen, including:
- Drug therapy
- Signs and symptoms to report
- Nutrition therapy
- Availability of community resources
- Importance of follow-up care

Chart 60-5 PATIENT AND FAMILY EDUCATION GUIDE
Ileostomy Care

SKIN PROTECTION
- Use a pectin-based skin barrier to protect your skin from contact with contents from the ostomy.
- Use skin care products, such as skin sealants and ostomy skin creams. If your skin continues to come into contact with ostomy contents, select a product to fill in problem areas and provide an even skin surface.
- Watch your skin for any irritation or redness.

POUCH CARE
- Empty your pouch when it is one-third to one-half full.
- Change the pouch during inactive times, such as before meals, before retiring at night, on waking in the morning, and 2 to 4 hours after eating.
- Change the entire pouch system every 3 to 7 days.

NUTRITION
- Chew food thoroughly.
- Be cautious of high-fiber and high-cellulose foods. You may need to eliminate these from the diet if they cause severe problems (diarrhea, constipation, or blockage). Examples include corn, peanuts, coconut, Chinese vegetables, string beans, tough-fiber meats, shrimp and lobster, rice, bran, and vegetables with skins (tomatoes, corn, and peas).

DRUG THERAPY
- Avoid taking enteric-coated and capsule medications.
- Inform any health care provider who is prescribing medications for you that you have an ostomy. Before having prescriptions filled, inform your pharmacist that you have an ostomy.
- Do not take any laxative or enemas. You should usually have loose stool and should contact a physician if no stool has passed in 6 to 12 hours.

SYMPTOMS TO WATCH FOR
- Report any drastic increase or decrease in drainage to your health care provider.
- If stomal swelling, abdominal cramping, or distention occurs or if ileostomy contents stop draining:
  - Remove the pouch with faceplate.
  - Lie down, assuming a knee-chest position.
  - Begin abdominal massage.
  - Apply moist towels to the abdomen.
  - Drink hot tea.

If none of these maneuvers is effective in resuming ileostomy flow or if abdominal pain is severe, call your health care provider right away.

Canadian patients (www.ostomycanada.ca). A local support group or the Crohn's and Colitis Foundation of America (www.ccfa.org) may be helpful in obtaining supplies and providing education for ostomates. Inform the patient and family of available ostomy ambulatory care clinics and ostomy specialists. If the patient agrees, a visit from an ostomate can be continued after discharge to home.

Evaluation: Outcomes

Evaluate the care of the patient with ulcerative colitis on the basis of the identified nursing diagnoses and collaborative problems. Expected outcomes may include that the patient will:

- Take personal action to control pain
- Self-manage the ileostomy
- Maintain peristomal skin integrity
- Demonstrate behaviors that integrate ostomy care into his or her lifestyle

NCLEX EXAMINATION CHALLENGE

A client who is scheduled for an ileoanal reservoir (J pouch) has received preoperative teaching from the surgeon. Which statement by the client indicates a need for further teaching?

A. "I will be able to have sex with my wife even though we might have to adapt a little."
B. "I'll really need to watch my intake of dairy products because I'm lactose-intolerant."
C. "There are some local support groups I can join that can help me get used to this change."
D. "I'll have to wear a pouch all the time because my stool will be like liquid paste."

evolve For the correct answer, go to http://evolve.elsevier.com/Iggy/.

CROHN'S DISEASE

Pathophysiology

Crohn's disease (CD) is an inflammatory disease of the small intestine (most often), the colon, or both. It can affect the GI tract from the mouth to the anus but most commonly affects the terminal ileum. CD is a slowly progressive, unpredictable, and recurrent disease with involvement of multiple regions of the intestine with normal sections in between (called "skip lesions" on x-rays).

Unlike UC, Crohn's disease presents as transmural inflammation that causes a thickened bowel wall. Strictures and deep ulcerations (cobblestone appearance) also occur, which predispose the patient to developing bowel fistulas. The result is severe diarrhea and malabsorption of vital nutrients. Anemia is common, usually from iron deficiency or malabsorption issues.

The complications associated with Crohn's disease are similar to those of ulcerative colitis (see Table 60-4). Hemorrhage is more common in ulcerative colitis but it can occur in CD as well. Severe malabsorption by the small intestine is more common in patients with CD because UC does not involve the small bowel to any significant extent. *Therefore patients with CD can become very malnourished and debilitated.*

Rarely, cancer of the small bowel and colon develop but usually occurs after the disease has been present for 15 to 20 years. Fistula formation is a common complication of CD but is rare in UC. Fistulas can occur between segments of the intestine or manifest as cutaneous fistulas or perirectal abscesses. They can also extend from the bowel to other organs and body cavities, such as the bladder or vagina (Fig. 60-5). Some patients develop intestinal obstruction, which, at first, is secondary to inflammation and edema. Over time, fibrosis and scar tissue develop and obstruction results from a narrowing of the bowel. Most patients with CD require surgery at some time (Sands, 2006).

Etiology and Genetic Risk

The exact cause of CD is not known, but it seems to include a combination of genetic, immune, and environmental factors. About 10% to 20% of patients have a positive family history for the disease, but no predominant inheritance pattern is present (Nussbaum et al., 2007). The discovery of a mutation in the *NOD2/CARD15* gene on chromosome 16 seems to be associated with some patients who have CD. This gene is found in monocytes that normally recognize and destroy bacteria. In the intestines of some patients with CD, the gene cannot respond to bacterial liposaccharide in the cell wall, which results in an overreaction of the *immune* system. This response leads to uncontrolled inflammation and destruction of intestinal cells.

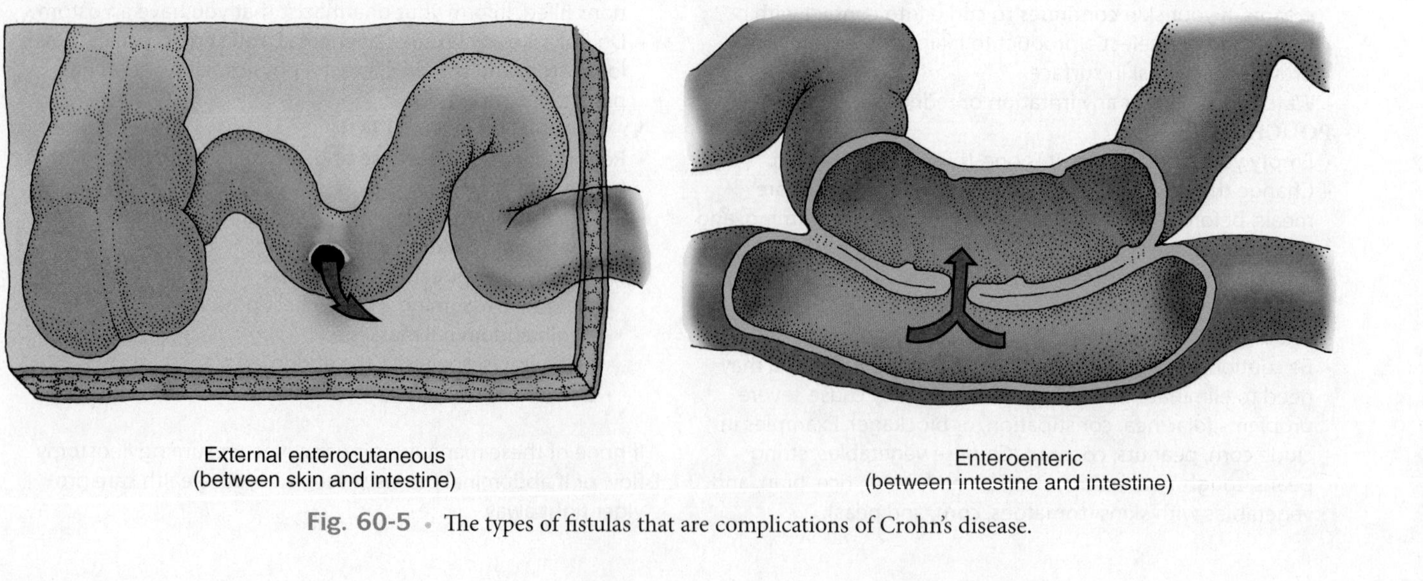
External enterocutaneous
(between skin and intestine)
Enteroenteric
(between intestine and intestine)

Fig. 60-5 • The types of fistulas that are complications of Crohn's disease.

Environmental factors include smoking and bacteria, such as mycobacteria, that are not part of the normal flora (McCance & Huether, 2006). It was once thought that stress and nutrition play a role in the *development* of CD, but these factors have not been proven. However, poor nutrition can worsen the patient's symptoms.

Incidence/Prevalence

More than one million people in the United States have the disease. Most have symptoms and are diagnosed as adolescents or young adults. One in 500 to 1000 people have CD. It is more common in people of Ashkenazi Jewish background than in any other group (Nussbaum et al., 2007).

Patient-Centered Collaborative Care

Assessment

Physical Assessment/Clinical Manifestations

Crohn's disease is made worse by bacterial infection and inflammation. A detailed history is needed to identify manifestations specific to the disease. Ask about recent unintentional weight loss, the frequency and consistency of stools, the presence of blood in the stool, fever, and abdominal pain.

Perform a thorough abdominal examination, assess for manifestations of the disease, and evaluate the patient's nutritional and hydration status. When performing an abdominal assessment, look for findings that are consistent with those in acute appendicitis (e.g., tenderness, guarded movement, a palpable mass in the right lower quadrant).

When inspecting the abdomen, assess for distention, masses, or visible peristalsis. Inspection of the perianal area may reveal ulcerations, fissures, or fistulas. During auscultation, bowel sounds may be decreased or absent with severe inflammation or obstruction. An increase in high-pitched or rushing sounds may be present over areas of narrowed bowel loops. Muscle guarding, masses, rigidity, or tenderness may be noted on palpation.

The clinical presentation of Crohn's disease can vary greatly from person to person. Most patients report diarrhea, abdominal pain, and low-grade fever. Fever is common with fistulas, abscesses, and severe inflammation. If the disease occurs in only the ileum, diarrhea occurs five or six times per day, often with a soft, loose stool. **Steatorrhea** (fatty diarrheal stools) is common. Rarely, stools may contain bright red blood.

Abdominal pain from the inflammatory process is usually constant and often located in the right lower quadrant. The patient also may have pain around the umbilicus before and after bowel movements. If the lower colon is diseased, pain is common in both lower abdominal quadrants.

Most patients with Crohn's disease have *weight loss.* Nutritional problems are the result of increased catabolism from chronic inflammation, anorexia, malabsorption, or self-imposed dietary restrictions. These nutritional problems result in fluid and electrolyte imbalances and protein, iron, vitamin, and mineral deficiencies.

The inflammatory bowel changes decrease the small bowel's ability to absorb nutrients, which may be made worse by surgery and fistulas. Be especially alert for manifestations of peritonitis (discussed earlier in this chapter), bowel obstruction, and nutritional and fluid imbalances. Early detection of a change in the patient's status helps reduce these life-threatening complications.

Psychosocial Assessment

The patient who has Crohn's disease needs a complete psychosocial assessment. The chronic nature of the problem and the troublesome complications can greatly affect patients and their families. Lifestyle changes are necessary to cope with such a disruptive and painful chronic illness. Assess the patient's coping skill, and help identify support systems.

Diagnostic Assessment

The health care provider may request many laboratory studies for patients with Crohn's disease. However, no disease-specific tests are available to confirm the diagnosis except for classic biopsy findings. The results of laboratory tests often indicate the extent and severity of inflammation occurring with the disease.

Anemia is common as a result of slow bleeding and poor nutrition. Serum levels of folic acid and cobalamin (vitamin B_{12} group) are generally low because of malabsorption, further contributing to anemia. Amino acid malabsorption and protein-losing enteropathy may result in *decreased albumin* levels. C-reactive protein and ESR may be elevated to indicate inflammation. White blood cells (WBCs) in the urine may show infection (pyuria), which is caused by ureteral obstruction or an enterovesical (bowel to bladder) fistula. If severe diarrhea or fistula is present, the patient may have electrolyte losses, particularly potassium and magnesium.

X-rays show the narrowing, ulcerations, strictures, and fistulas common with Crohn's disease. An abdominal ultrasound or CT scan may also be performed. In acute illness, these tests may be deferred until the risk for perforation lessens. Biopsies obtained via a colonoscopy may verify the diagnosis.

Interventions

Management of Crohn's disease is similar to that described on p. 1324 in the Nonsurgical Management discussion in the Ulcerative Colitis section.

Nonsurgical Management

Specific interventions vary with the severity of disease and the complications that are present. Drugs used to manage Crohn's disease are similar to those used in the treatment of ulcerative colitis (UC), except that mesalamine is not very effective for CD (see p. 1324 in the Drug Therapy discussion in the Ulcerative Colitis section).

Drug Therapy. In addition to the drugs used for UC, several other drugs may be used for Crohn's disease (CD). Budesonide (Entocort EC) is a delayed-release compound that delivers high local glucocorticoid concentrations to the terminal ileum and right side of the colon for patients with CD. It has little efficacy in UC. Systemic effects are low, but budesonide is tapered slowly if possible.

Although glucocorticoids can be effective, sepsis can result from abscesses or fistulas that may be present. These drugs mask the symptoms of infection. Therefore they must be used with caution. Monitor the patient closely for signs of infection.

Metronidazole (Flagyl, Novonidazole♣) 250 to 500 mg orally three times daily has been helpful in patients with fistulas. Immunosuppressive therapy has been effective in patients with refractory disease or fistulas. Azathioprine (Imuran), an immunosuppressive agent, 50 mg daily for 12 months, may be instituted and then withdrawn. Long-term therapy may be needed in some cases. Methotrexate (MTX) may also be given to suppress immune activity.

Because a defect in the regulation of inflammation may play a role in the development of Crohn's disease, suppression of a cytokine (specifically, tumor necrosis factor) may be useful in decreasing bowel inflammation. Infliximab (Remicade), a monoclonal antibody form of anti–tumor necrosis factor alpha, may be used IV every 8 weeks. The usual dose is 5 mg/kg for treatment of active CD and fistulas. Adalimumab (Humira) is another monoclonal antibody recently approved. Patients who have infections or those with allergies to proteins should not take this drug. Teach the patient to avoid large crowds and anyone who is ill. Remind the patient to report any early signs of infection, including a sore throat or a cold.

Nutrition Therapy. Long-standing nutritional deficits can have severe consequences for the patient with Crohn's disease. Malnutrition can lead to poor fistula and wound healing, loss of lean muscle mass, decreased immune responses, and increased morbidity and mortality. During severe exacerbations of the disease, the patient may be hospitalized to provide bowel rest and nutritional support with total parenteral nutrition (TPN). For less severe exacerbations, an elemental or semi-elemental product such as Vivonex may be prescribed to induce remission. These products are absorbed in the jejunum and therefore permit the distal small intestine and colon to rest. Once remission is achieved, a low-residue diet is usually prescribed. Nutritional supplements, such as Ensure or Sustacal, can be added then to provide nutrients and more calories. Teach the patient to avoid GI stimulants, such as caffeinated beverages and alcohol.

Fistula Management. Fistulas (abnormal tracts between two or more body areas) are common with acute periods of Crohn's disease. They can be between the bowel and bladder (enterovesical), between two segments of bowel (enteroenteral), between the skin and bowel (enterocutaneous), or between the bowel and vagina (enterovaginal) (see Fig. 60-5). The patient with one or more fistulas often has complications such as systemic infections, skin problems, malnutrition, and fluid and electrolyte imbalances. Treatment of the patient with a fistula is complicated and includes nutrition and electrolyte therapy, skin care, and prevention of infection.

Adequate nutrition and fluid and electrolyte balance are priorities in the care of the patient with a fistula. GI secretions are high in volume and rich in electrolytes and enzymes. The patient is at high risk for malnutrition, dehydration, and hypokalemia (decreased serum potassium). Assess for these complications, and collaborate with the health care team to manage them. Monitor urinary output. A decrease indicates possible dehydration, which should be treated immediately by providing additional fluids.

The patient requires at least 3000 calories daily to promote healing of the fistula. If he or she cannot take adequate oral fluids and nutrients, total enteral nutrition (TEN) or TPN may be prescribed (Willcutts et al., 2005). For patients who do not require TEN or TPN, collaborate with the nutritionist to:

- Carefully monitor the patient's tolerance to the prescribed diet.
- Assist the patient in selecting high-calorie, high-protein, high-vitamin, low-fiber meals.
- Offer enteral supplements, such as Ensure and Vivonex.
- Record food intake for accurate calorie counts.

Providing enteral supplements and recording intake may be delegated to unlicensed assistive personnel (UAP) under the supervision of the RN.

Enzymes and bile in the stool contribute to the problem of skin irritation and excoriation. Skin irritation needs to be prevented. This may be accomplished through the use of skin barriers, pouching systems, and insertion of drains (Fig. 60-6). Skin barriers or dressings are used when the fistula drainage in less than 100 mL in 24 hours (Willcutts et al., 2005). A pouch is used for heavily draining fistulas to reduce the risk for skin irritation and measure the **effluent** (drainage). However, they are very challenging because of location and drainage amount. Treatment with an antifungal powder applied to the skin around the fistula is often very helpful.

For some fistulas, pouching may not be possible because of their location. Drainage may need to be managed using regulated wall suction or a vacuum-assisted closure (VAC) device. Continuous low wall suction is attached to a suction catheter in the wound bed of the fistula, not into the fistula tract. These systems are not meant for long-term management.

VAC therapy promotes wound healing by secondary intention as it prepares the wound bed for closure, reduces edema, promotes granulation and perfusion, and removes exudate and infectious material. It should not be used for patients who are at risk for bleeding or only for the purpose of drainage containment.

Collaborate with the wound or ostomy nurse to select the most appropriate wound management for each patient. *Preserving and protecting the skin is the top priority. Wound drainage must never be allowed to be in direct contact with skin without prompt cleaning because intestinal fluid enzymes are caustic. Skin breakdown or fungal infection can cause major discomfort for the patient.*

Patients with fistulas are at high risk for intra-abdominal abscesses and sepsis. Antibiotic therapy is commonly prescribed. Observe for signs of systemic infection or sepsis, such as fever, abdominal pain, or a change in mental status.

Complementary and Alternative Therapies. Other helpful interventions for the patient with CD are those that relax the patient and soothe the GI tract. Such therapies may include naturopathy, herbs (e.g., ginger), acupuncture, hypnotherapy, and ayurveda (a combination of diet, herbs, yoga, breathing exercises). The evidence supporting the use of these substances for CD is lacking, but many patients find them helpful for overall physical and emotional health.

Surgical Management

Surgery for Crohn's disease is usually performed for those patients who have not improved with medical management or those who have complications from the disease. The patient with a fistula may undergo resection of the diseased area. Other indications for surgical treatment include perforation, massive hemorrhage, intestinal obstruction or strictures, abscesses, or cancer.

In some cases, the resection can be performed as minimally invasive surgery (MIS) via laparoscopy, which involves one or more small incisions, less pain, quicker surgical recovery, and quicker return to usual lifestyle. Both small bowel resection (usually the ileum) and ileocecal resection can be done using this procedure.

Stricturoplasty may be performed for bowel strictures related to Crohn's disease. This procedure increases the bowel diameter. Care before and after each of these surgical procedures is similar to care for patients undergoing other types of abdominal surgery (see Chapters 16 and 18.)

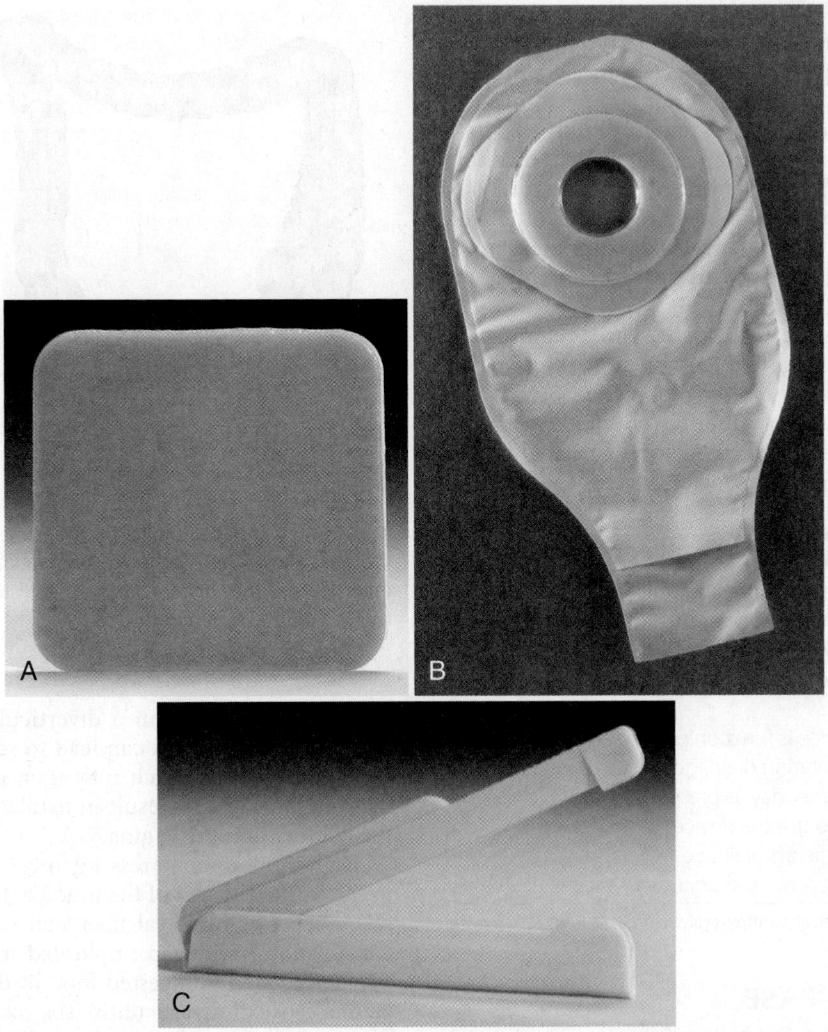
A
B
C

Fig. 60-6 • Skin barriers, such as wafers (**A**) are cut to fit ⅛ inch around the fistula. A drainable pouch (**B**) is applied over the wafer and clamped (**C**) until the pouch is to be emptied. Effluent should drain into the bag and not contact the skin.

Community-Based Care

The discharge care plan for the patient with Crohn's disease is similar to that for the patient with ulcerative colitis (see p. 1328 in the discussion of Community-Based Care in the Ulcerative Colitis section). Collaborate with the case manager and wound nurse to help the patient plan self-management.

Home Care Management

The interventions that were started in the hospital to manage the disease should be continued in the home. Reinforce measures to control the disease and related symptoms and manage nutrition. Supplies for wounds and fistula care may be required. The home should be arranged so that the patient has easy access to the bathroom, as well as privacy to perform fistula care.

Health Teaching

The teaching plan for Crohn's disease is similar to that for the patient with ulcerative colitis. Teach the patient about the usual course of the disease, symptoms of complications, and when to notify the health care provider. Incorporate drug teaching, including purpose, dose, and side effects, into the teaching plan. In addition to other drugs, vitamin supplements, including monthly vitamin B_{12} injections, may be needed because of the inability of the ileum to absorb this nutrient. In collaboration with the nutritionist, instruct the patient to follow a low-residue, high-calorie diet and to avoid foods that cause discomfort, such as milk, gluten, and other GI stimulants like caffeine.

Remind the patient to take rest periods, especially during exacerbations of the disease. If stress appears to increase symptoms of the disease, recommend stress management techniques or counseling. For long-term follow-up, teach the patient about the increased risk for bowel cancer and the importance of having frequent colonoscopies.

If a patient has a fistula, explain and demonstrate fistula care. Provide the opportunity for the patient to practice this care in the hospital. Ideally, he or she should be independent in fistula care before leaving the hospital. However, because of location of the fistula (perirectal or vaginal) or an obese abdomen, assistance may be needed. If this is the case, a family member or a caregiver must learn and practice the care or the case manager (CM) can arrange for home care services.

Health Care Resources

The patient discharged to home after undergoing resection and anastomosis may require visits from a home care nurse to assess the surgical wound and monitor for complications (see Chart 60-6). Assess the patient's and family's ability to monitor the progress of fistula healing and to watch for indications of infection and sepsis. Home care nursing visits may also be appropriate for this purpose. A home care aide or other service might be helpful for the patient who cannot meet nutritional needs or who needs help with grocery shopping and meal preparation.

In collaboration with the CM, assist with obtaining the equipment and supplies for fistula care, such as skin barriers and wound drainage bags. A support group sponsored by the United Ostomy Associations of America (www.uoaa.org) or a local hospital in the community may also be available to help with meeting physical and psychosocial needs.

NCLEX EXAMINATION CHALLENGE

A client is admitted to the skilled nursing unit for long-term management of an enterocutaneous (bowel-to-skin) fistula that is connected to a vacuum-assisted closure (VAC) device. What nursing actions should be implemented when caring for this client? (Select all that apply.)

A. Make sure that the device is functioning properly.
B. Protect the skin from irritating drainage.
C. Use the device every other day as prescribed.
D. Teach the family how to use the device.
E. Measure and record all fistula drainage.
F. Assess the wound for healing, and document.

evolve For the correct answer, go to http://evolve.elsevier.com/Iggy/.

DIVERTICULAR DISEASE

Diverticula are pouchlike herniations of the mucosa through the muscular wall of any portion of the gut but most commonly the colon. **Diverticulosis** is the presence of many abnormal pouchlike herniations (diverticula) in the wall of the intestine. **Diverticulitis** is the inflammation of one or more diverticula.

Pathophysiology

Diverticula can occur in any part of the small or large intestine but usually occur in the sigmoid colon (Fig. 60-7). The muscle of the colon hypertrophies, thickens, and becomes rigid, and herniation of the mucosa and submucosa through the colon wall is seen. Diverticula seem to occur at points of weakness in the intestinal wall, often at areas where blood vessels interrupt the muscle layer. Muscle weakness develops as part of the aging process or as a result of a lack of fiber in the diet.

Without inflammation, diverticula cause few problems. If undigested food or bacteria become trapped in a diverticulum, however, blood supply to that area is reduced. Bacteria invade the diverticulum, resulting in diverticulitis, which then can perforate and develop a local abscess. A perforated diverticulum can progress to an intra-abdominal perforation with peritonitis (inflammation of the peritoneum).

Bleeding from diverticula can range from minor local bleeding to massive hemorrhage. Minor bleeding is often due to inflammation in areas of new blood vessel tissue at the base of the diverticulum. Hemorrhage can result when a blood vessel breaks down within a diverticulum. Inflammation from recurrent diverticulitis can lead to scarring and narrowing of the bowel lumen, which may then result in obstruction. Inflammation can also result in fistulas to other organs, such as the bladder and the vagina.

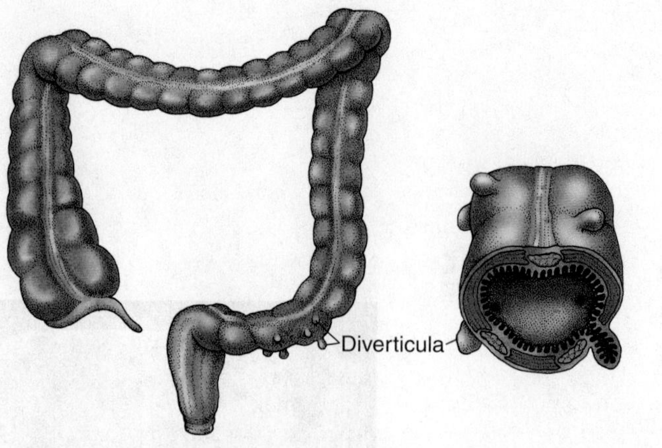
Diverticula

Fig. 60-7 • Several abnormal outpouchings, or herniations, in the wall of the intestine, which are diverticula. These can occur anywhere in the small or large intestine but are found most often in the sigmoid, as shown in this figure. Diverticulitis is the inflammation of a diverticulum that occurs when undigested food or bacteria become trapped in the diverticulum.

High intraluminal pressure forces the formation of a pouch in the weakened area of the mucosa, frequently near blood vessels. Diets low in cereal fiber that cause less bulky stool and constipation have been implicated in the formation of diverticula. Retained undigested food in diverticula is suggested to be one cause of diverticulitis. The retained food reduces blood flow to that area and makes bacterial invasion of the sac easier.

The exact incidence of diverticulosis is unknown, but millions of people are affected by the problem. Diverticulitis is found in one half of adults older than 60 years, with more men than women affected. The cause for this difference is not known. Although diverticulosis is common, only one of five people with this disease has noticeable symptoms.

Patient-Centered Collaborative Care

Assessment

The patient with diverticulosis usually has no symptoms. Unless pain or bleeding develops, the condition may go undiagnosed. Occasionally diverticulosis will cause symptoms. For the patient with uncomplicated diverticulosis, ask about intermittent pain in the left lower quadrant and a history of constipation. If diverticulitis is suspected, ask about a history of low-grade fever, nausea, and abdominal pain. Inquire about recent bowel elimination patterns because constipation may develop as a result of intestinal inflammation. Also ask about any bleeding from the rectum.

On physical examination, uncomplicated *diverticulosis* may produce no clinical manifestations. Occasionally tenderness occurs on abdominal palpation.

The patient with *diverticulitis* may have abdominal pain, most often localized to the left lower quadrant. It is intermittent at first but becomes progressively steady. Occasionally pain may be just above the pubic bone or may occur on one side. Abdominal pain is generalized if peritonitis has occurred. Nausea and vomiting are common. The patient's temperature is elevated, ranging from a low-grade fever to 101° F (38.3° C). Chills may be present. Often an increased heart rate (tachycardia) occurs with fever.

CONSIDERATIONS FOR OLDER ADULTS

The first sign of peritonitis in older adults may be a sudden change in mental status (e.g., acute confusion). For those who have dementia, the confusion worsens. Fever and chills may not be present.

On examination of the abdomen, observe for distention. The patient may report tenderness over the involved area. The colon may be palpable. Localized muscle spasm, guarded movement, and rebound tenderness may be present with peritoneal irritation. If generalized peritonitis is present, profound guarding occurs; rebound tenderness is more widespread; and sepsis, hypotension, or hypovolemic shock can occur. If the perforated diverticulum is close to the rectum, the health care provider may palpate a tender mass during the rectal examination. Blood pressure checks may show orthostatic changes. If bleeding is massive, the patient may have hypotension and dehydration that result in shock.

For the patient with uncomplicated diverticulosis, laboratory studies are not indicated. The patient with diverticulitis, however, has an *elevated white blood cell (WBC) count. Decreased hematocrit and hemoglobin* values are common if chronic or severe bleeding occurs. Stool tests for occult blood, if requested, are sometimes positive. Urinalysis may show a few red blood cells (RBCs) if the left ureter is near a perforated diverticulum.

X-rays of the intestinal tract with barium contrast may show diverticula. An upper GI series shows diverticula of the small intestine, and barium enema shows diverticula of the large intestine. Diverticula are most often diagnosed during routine colonoscopy.

The patient with diverticulitis usually does *not* undergo a barium enema procedure in the acute phase of the illness because of the risk for rupture of the inflamed diverticulum. A barium enema may be completed after the patient has been treated with antibiotics and the inflammation has resolved. A flat-plate film of the abdomen is done to evaluate for free air and fluid indicating perforation. A computed tomography (CT) scan may be performed to diagnose an abscess or thickening of the bowel related to diverticulitis.

Abdominal ultrasonography, a noninvasive test, may also reveal bowel thickening or an abscess. The physician may recommend a colonoscopy 4 to 8 weeks *after the acute phase* of the illness to rule out a tumor in the large intestine, particularly if the patient has rectal bleeding.

▪ Interventions

Patients are managed on an ambulatory care basis if the symptoms are mild. Monitor the patient for any prolonged or increased fever, abdominal pain, or blood in the stool.

The patient with moderate to severe diverticulitis may be hospitalized. Manifestations suggesting the need for admission are a temperature higher than 101° F (38.3° C), persistent and severe abdominal pain for more than 3 days, and/or lower GI bleeding.

Nonsurgical Management

A combination of drug and nutrition therapy with rest to decrease inflammation and improve tissue perfusion is used. Broad-spectrum antimicrobial drugs, such as metronidazole (Flagyl) plus trimethoprim/sulfamethoxazole (Bactrim, Septra), or ciprofloxacin (Cipro) are prescribed. A mild analgesic may be given for pain. Chart 60-7 lists key issues regarding older adults with diverticulitis.

The patient with more severe pain is admitted to the hospital for IV fluids to correct dehydration and IV drug therapy. Anticholinergics may reduce intestinal hypermotility, although they should be avoided for older adults. For patients with moderate to severe diverticulitis, an opioid analgesic, such as meperidine hydrochloride (Demerol) or morphine sulfate, can alleviate pain. *Meperidine is not used for older adults because of its adverse effects. In some agencies, this drug is no longer used for any patient.*

Laxatives and enemas are avoided because they increase intestinal motility. Assess the patient on an ongoing basis for manifestations of fluid and electrolyte imbalance.

Teach the patient to rest during the acute phase of illness. Remind him or her to refrain from lifting, straining, coughing, or bending to avoid an increase in intra-abdominal pressure, which can result in perforation of the diverticulum. Nutrition therapy should be restricted to low fiber or clear liquids based on symptoms.

The patient with more severe symptoms is NPO. A nasogastric tube (NGT) is inserted if nausea, vomiting, or abdominal distention is severe. Infuse IV fluids as prescribed for hydration. In collaboration with the nutritionist, the patient increases dietary intake slowly as symptoms subside. When inflammation has resolved and bowel function returns to normal, a fiber-containing diet is introduced gradually.

Surgical Management

Diverticulitis can result in rupture of the diverticulum with peritonitis, pelvic abscess, bowel obstruction, fistula, persistent fever or pain, or uncontrolled bleeding. The surgeon

Chart 60-7 NURSING FOCUS ON THE OLDER ADULT

Diverticulitis

- Provide antibiotics, analgesics, and anticholinergics as prescribed. Observe older patients carefully for side effects of these drugs, especially confusion (or increased confusion), urinary retention or failure, and orthostatic hypotension.
- Do not give laxatives or enemas. Teach the patient and the family about the importance of avoiding these measures.
- Encourage the patient to rest and to avoid activities that may increase intra-abdominal pressure, such as straining and bending.
- While diverticulitis is active, provide a *low*-fiber diet. When the inflammation resolves, provide a *high*-fiber diet. Teach the patient and family about these diets and when they are appropriate.
- Because older patients do not always experience the typical pain or fever expected, observe carefully for other signs of active disease, such as a sudden change in mental status.
- Perform frequent abdominal assessments to determine distention and tenderness on palpation.
- Check stools for occult or frank bleeding.

performs emergency surgery if peritonitis, bowel obstruction, or pelvic abscess is present. Colon resection, with or without a colostomy, is the most common surgical procedure for patients with diverticular disease. The surgeon removes the portion that is inflamed or diseased and, if possible, creates an anastomosis of the colon to restore patency. Inflammation and infection, however, may prevent an anastomosis. If this is the case, the surgeon may perform a colostomy (see Fig. 60-2, *B* for appearance of a stoma). Some patients may have colostomy closure and anastomosis after the bowel has been allowed to rest for 3 to 6 months.

Preoperative Care. Preparation of the patient for surgery depends on the severity of the condition and whether it is an emergency or is performed a few weeks after the acute stage. The surgeon informs the patient whether a temporary or permanent colostomy might be required.

If the patient is *not* in the acute stage of diverticulitis, a thorough bowel preparation *may* be given consisting of enemas and laxatives daily for 1 to 2 days before surgery. Because of the risk for perforation, however, the surgeon usually does not require an aggressive bowel preparation. If the patient has an acutely inflamed diverticulum or persistent fever and abdominal pain, the bowel preparation is withheld.

The value of preoperative bowel preparation ("bowel prep") for any patient having abdominal surgery is being questioned. For years it was thought that this procedure helped prevent contamination during surgery and sepsis. However, recent studies have shown no difference in clinical outcomes when patients did not have a "bowel prep." Also, this intervention is very uncomfortable and unpleasant for the patient having surgery (Jung et al., 2007).

For patients without acute inflammation, a low-fiber diet may be implemented for several days, followed by a clear-liquid diet for the day or evening before surgery.

Preoperative teaching may include information about the possible need for a colostomy. If a colostomy is a possible outcome, collaborate with the certified wound, ostomy, and continence nurse (CWOCN) or an enterostomal therapist (ET) (ostomy nurse) to describe its function and care.

Operative Procedures. The patient may have one of two surgical approaches: open conventional approach or minimally invasive surgery (MIS) via a laparoscopy. The advantage of MIS is that patients are discharged from the hospital quicker, have less pain after surgery, and have fewer postoperative complications. They are able to resume normal activities much faster than patients having the traditional surgery.

Postoperative Care. The nursing care for patients during the first few days after a colon resection for diverticulitis is the same as that for any patients undergoing abdominal surgery. The patient may have a drain in place at the abdominal incision site for several days. If a colostomy has been performed, the stoma may be covered with a petroleum gauze dressing because the colostomy does not drain for about 2 days or a colostomy bag may be placed over the stoma. If the stoma is visible, monitor for color and integrity. The stoma should be pinkish to cherry red without retraction or prolapse into the abdomen.

The patient is NPO with an NGT until peristalsis returns (about 2 to 3 days). Clear liquids are then introduced *slowly.* Gradually, the diet is advanced to solids, depending on the return of peristalsis and bowel function. Patients who had laparoscopic surgery do not usually have an NGT.

Most patients with a colostomy for diverticulitis have a sigmoid colostomy because the sigmoid colon is the most common site of diverticulitis. Drainage from a sigmoid colostomy at first consists of loose stool, but eventually the stool becomes formed. A tight seal around the stoma is essential to avoid contact of feces with the skin. Colostomy care is detailed in Chapter 59.

Give the patient an opportunity to express feelings about the ostomy. Discuss these feelings with the patient, reinforcing that anger and depression are normal responses. When he or she is physically able, encourage the patient to look at the stoma and touch the pouching system. Collaborate with the ostomy nurse to teach the patient how to self-manage ostomy care.

Community-Based Care

The length of stay for patients hospitalized for diverticulitis ranges from 2 to 4 or more days, depending on the response to treatment and the need for surgery. Discharge plans vary according to the treatment.

Home Care Management

For the patient with diverticulitis who has responded to medical treatment, home care focuses on proper nutrition. Assess the patient's ability to obtain and prepare the recommended high-fiber foods. The patient who has surgical intervention has the added responsibilities of incision care and possibly colostomy care with temporary limitations placed on activities.

Health Teaching

All patients with diverticular disease need education regarding a high-fiber diet. Collaborate with the nutritionist to encourage the patient with *diverticulosis* to eat a diet high in cellulose and hemicellulose types of fiber. These substances can be found in wheat bran, whole-grain breads, and cereals. Teach the patient to eat at least 25 to 35 g of fiber per day. Fresh fruits and vegetables with high-fiber content are added to add bulk to stools.

If not accustomed to eating high-fiber foods, teach the patient to add them to the diet gradually to avoid flatulence and abdominal cramping. If he or she cannot tolerate the recommended fiber requirement, a bulk-forming laxative, such as psyllium hydrophilic mucilloid (Metamucil), can be taken to increase fecal size and consistency. Teach the patient to drink plenty of fluids to help prevent bloating that may occur with a high-fiber diet. Alcohol should be avoided because it irritates the bowel. Foods containing seeds or indigestible material that may block a diverticulum, such as nuts, corn, popcorn, cucumbers, tomatoes, figs, and strawberries, may be eliminated but this is controversial. Some clinicians do *not* believe this is necessary as long as the patient incorporates a high-fiber cereal diet or supplement. Teach the patient that dietary fat intake should not exceed 30% of the total daily caloric intake. Reinforce the teaching performed by the nutritionist.

Teach the patient to avoid all fiber when symptoms of *diverticulitis* are present, because high-fiber foods are then irritating. As it resolves, fiber can gradually be added until progression to a high-fiber diet is once again obtained. The patient who has undergone surgery is usually taking solid food by the time of discharge from the hospital.

The patient who has had abdominal surgery needs oral and written instructions on incision care and the signs and symptoms to report to the health care provider. Provide instructions on colostomy care as needed. Encourage the patient to express concerns about body image. Allow time and address sexual concerns regarding the changed body image.

Instruct the patient with any type of diverticular disease, orally and in writing, about the manifestations of acute diverticulitis, including fever, abdominal pain, and bloody, mahogany, or tarry stools. Advise patients to avoid the use of laxatives (other than bulk-forming types) and enemas. Reassure them that this disorder should not cause problems if a proper diet is followed.

Health Care Resources

In collaboration with the case manager, arrange for a home care nurse, if needed, to assess wound healing and proper functioning of the ostomy and the appliance. If the patient is interested, arrange for a visit from an ostomy volunteer (ostomate) or an ostomy nurse. For information about other community resources, remind the patient to contact the United Ostomy Associations of America (www.uoaa.org).

DECISION-MAKING CHALLENGE
Coordination of Care

A 50-year-old woman had her first screening colonoscopy. She has had no symptoms but her father had colon cancer at age 58 years. His cancer was surgically removed, and he did not require any other treatment. Her father is still alive and well with no recurrence. The patient's colonoscopy showed moderate to severe diverticulosis in the sigmoid colon and mild diverticulitis in the descending colon. She previously had two benign polyps completely removed (one from the cecum and one from the transverse colon). She takes one oral fiber supplement capsule daily, a proton pump inhibitor for GERD, and an ACE inhibitor for hypertension.

1. How would you explain diverticulosis versus diverticulitis to this patient?
2. Is this patient a candidate for antimicrobial therapy? Why or why not?
3. What nutritional modifications and restrictions should she follow and why? (Keep her GERD in mind as well.)
4. What other health teaching does she need? What health care team members might be involved in her care?

evolve For suggested answer guidelines, go to http://evolve.elsevier.com/Iggy/.

ANAL DISORDERS

ANORECTAL ABSCESS

Pathophysiology

Anorectal abscess is a localized area of induration and pus caused by inflammation of the soft tissue near the rectum or anus. It is most often the result of obstruction of the ducts of glands in the anorectal region. Feces, foreign bodies, or trauma can be the cause of the obstruction and stasis, leading to infection that spreads into nearby tissue. Most abscesses begin as a pocket of infection in an anal crypt.

Rectal pain is often the first symptom. There may be no other manifestations at first, but local swelling, redness, and tenderness to touch are present within a few days after the onset of pain. If the abscess becomes chronic, discharge, bleeding, and pruritus (itching) may exist. Fever occurs if larger abscesses are present.

Patient-Centered Collaborative Care

Anorectal abscesses are managed by surgical incision and drainage. The physician can often incise (surgically remove) simple perianal and ischiorectal abscesses using a local anesthetic. For patients with more extensive abscesses, a regional or general anesthetic may be needed. Systemic antibiotics are given only for patients who are immunocompromised, are diabetic, have valvular disease or a prosthetic valve, or are obese. Incision and drainage ("I&D") for these patients is performed after antibiotic therapy.

Nursing interventions are focused on comfort and helping the patient maintain optimal perineal hygiene (Chart 60-8). Encourage the use of warm sitz baths, analgesics, bulk-producing agents, and stool softeners after the surgery until healing occurs. *Stress the importance of good perineal hygiene after all bowel movements and the maintenance of a regular bowel pattern with a high-fiber diet.*

Patients are often embarrassed about having anal problems. Provide privacy and maintain the patient's dignity during the examination and treatment.

ANAL FISSURE

An **anal fissure** is a tear in the anal lining. This common problem can cause much discomfort and disability. Smaller fissures occur with straining to have a stool, such as with diarrhea or constipation. Larger, deeper fissures may occur as a result of another disorder (e.g., Crohn's disease, tuberculosis, leukemia, neoplasm) or from trauma (e.g., from a foreign body, rough anal intercourse, perirectal surgery).

An acute anal fissure is superficial and usually resolves on its own or heals quickly with conservative treatment. Chronic fissures recur, and surgical treatment may be needed. Pain during and after defecation and bright red blood in the stool are the most common symptoms. Other manifestations include pruritus, urinary frequency or retention, dysuria, and **dyspareunia** (painful intercourse).

Chart 60-8 BEST PRACTICE FOR PATIENT SAFETY & QUALITY CARE

Promoting Perineal Comfort

- Keep the perineal area clean with mild soap.
- Pat the perineal area dry instead of rubbing it.
- Provide warm sitz baths, or apply warm compresses to the area.
- If the area is acutely inflamed, apply cold packs.
- Provide a chair cushion for the seated patient. For the older or debilitated patient, monitor the skin carefully to prevent pressure sores.
- Use absorbent pads for drainage, if any, and change them often.
- Use premoistened wipes for cleaning the perineal area after a bowel movement.
- Use witch hazel wipes (e.g., Tucks) to relieve pain.
- Give bulk-forming agents, such as psyllium mucilloid (Metamucil), as prescribed, to reduce pain associated with defecation.
- Apply a topical anesthetic cream to the perineal area, as prescribed.
- Give oral analgesics, as prescribed, for pain relief.
- Do not administer enemas or give potent laxatives.

The diagnosis is made by stretching and inspecting the perianal skin. If the patient is having pain at the time of the examination, diagnostic testing is usually limited to inspection. If he or she is not in severe pain, a digital examination and possibly a sigmoidoscopy are performed. When painless or multiple fissures are present, a colonoscopy may be performed to rule out any inflammatory bowel disorder.

Management of an acute fissure is usually aimed at local pain relief and softening of stools to reduce trauma to the area. Teach the patient to use warm sitz baths, analgesics, and bulk-producing agents (e.g., psyllium hydrophilic mucilloid [Metamucil]) to help minimize the pain from defecation. Topical anti-inflammatory agents (hydrocortisone creams and suppositories) or opiate suppositories (opium and belladonna suppositories) are helpful if spasms are severe.

Explain the pain control measures to the patient. Remind him or her to notify the health care provider if pain is not relieved within a few days. If fissures do not respond to this management within several days to weeks, surgical repair under a local anesthetic may be needed. Teach the patient to report any drainage or bleeding from the rectum to the health care provider.

ANAL FISTULA

An anal fistula, or *fistula in ano,* is an abnormal tract leading from the anal canal to the perianal skin. Most anal fistulas result from anorectal abscesses, which are caused by obstruction of anal glands (see Anorectal Abscess, p. 1337). Fistulas can also occur with tuberculosis, Crohn's disease, or cancer. Intermittent discharge is usually noted over the perianal area.

The patient with an anal fistula has pruritus (itching), purulent discharge, and tenderness or pain that is worsened by bowel movements. A proctoscope may be used to identify the source of symptoms and to locate the fistula. Because fistulas do not heal spontaneously, surgery is necessary. To perform a fistulotomy, the surgeon opens the tissue over the tract and scrapes the base. The incision site then heals by secondary intention. For a fistula higher in the anus, a special surgical technique is used to preserve important sphincters. After surgery, instruct the patient about sitz baths, analgesics, and the use of bulk-producing agents or stool softeners to reduce pain.

PARASITIC INFECTION

Pathophysiology

Parasites can enter and invade the GI tract and cause infections. They commonly enter through the mouth (oral-fecal transmission) from contaminated food or water, oral-anal sexual practices, or contact with feces from a contaminated person. Common parasites that cause infection in humans are *Entamoeba histolytica,* which causes amebiasis (amebic dysentery); *Giardia lamblia,* which causes giardiasis; and *Cryptosporidium. Handwashing is the best way to prevent the spread of parasitic infections.*

Entamoeba histolytica

Humans are the only known hosts for *E. histolytica* (also known as *amebiasis*). This organism occurs in cysts and trophozoites (sporozoan parasites). Trophozoites die rapidly after they leave the body in stool. Cysts, however, can remain alive in the right type of environment for weeks or months. Humans who eliminate cysts are infectious. Flies can spread the cysts, and the problem is more common in areas that use human excrement for fertilizer.

Amebiasis occurs worldwide, but it is most common in tropical areas. Prevalence rates are as high in areas with poor sanitation, crowding, and poor nutrition. Amebiasis causes tens of thousands of deaths annually worldwide. The disease causes less severe symptoms and often goes undiagnosed in temperate climates.

E. histolytica either feeds on bacteria in the intestine or invades and ulcerates the mucosa of the large intestine. The parasite can be limited to the GI tract (intestinal amebiasis), or it can extend outside the intestines (extraintestinal amebiasis). People can have intestinal amebiasis without having any symptoms, or symptoms can range from mild to severe.

Giardia lamblia

G. lamblia is a protozoal parasite that causes superficial invasion, destruction, and inflammation of the mucosa in the small intestine. Like *E. histolytica, G. lamblia* has a trophozoite and cysts form, which is the usual form of transmission. Humans are hosts to this organism, but beavers and dogs may be reservoirs for infection. Giardiasis is a well-recognized problem in travelers, campers, and immunosuppressed patients.

Modes of transmission are similar to those for amebiasis. In the United States, however, giardiasis is much more prevalent and is the most common parasitic infection. Giardiasis affects only the intestinal system, causing acute diarrhea, chronic diarrhea, or malabsorption syndrome. The acute phase usually is self-limiting, lasting days or weeks. The chronic phase can last for years. Diarrhea is usually mild in both forms, but it can be severe. As stools increase in frequency, they become more watery, greasy, frothy, and malodorous with mucus. Weight loss and weakness are also common. Malabsorption can occur with diarrhea that continues for longer than 3 weeks. Manifestations result from malabsorption of fat, protein, vitamin B_{12}, and lactase deficiency.

Cryptosporidium

Cryptosporidium is manifested by diarrhea. This infection occurs most commonly in immunosuppressed patients, particularly those with human immune deficiency virus (HIV). It can also occur in children and older adults from contaminated swimming pools. (See Chapter 21 for a discussion of HIV infection.)

Patient-Centered Collaborative Care

Assessment

A thorough history can help determine potential sources of exposure to parasitic infection. A history of travel to parts of the world where such infections are prevalent increases suspicion for infection with parasites. GI symptoms related to travel may be delayed as long as 1 to 2 weeks after the return home. Immigrants (newcomers) may have the infection upon entering a new country. A nutrition history is especially helpful if several people in a group become ill. Common water supplies or bodies of water may be infected with *Giardia* or *Cryptosporidium.* Trichinosis should be considered if the patient has eaten pork products.

Mild to moderate *E. histolytica* infestation causes the daily passage of several strongly foul-smelling stools, possibly with mucus but without blood, accompanied by abdominal cramping, flatulence (gas), fatigue, and weight loss.

The infected patient usually experiences remissions and recurrences. Severe amebic dysentery is manifested by frequent, more liquid, and foul-smelling stools with mucus *and* blood. Fever up to 104° F (40° C), **tenesmus** (feeling the urge to defecate), generalized abdominal tenderness, and vomiting can also occur. The ulcerations of invading amebiasis that occur in the colon can cause pain, bleeding, and obstruction. Ulcerations can also occur in the rectum, resulting in formed stool with blood. Complications are rare but include appendicitis and bowel perforation.

Extraintestinal amebiasis can occur without symptoms of intestinal infection. The most common form is amebic liver abscess, which causes symptoms of fever, pain, and an enlarged liver. The abscess can rupture, and death can result if the infection and complications are not treated.

The diagnosis of *amebiasis* is made by examining the stool for parasites. Because *E. histolytica* is difficult to detect, serial stool examinations are needed if the disease is suspected. The use of sigmoidoscopy may detect ulcerations in the rectum or colon. Exudate obtained during sigmoidoscopic examination is studied for the parasite. The white blood cell (WBC) count can be as high as 20,000/mm^3 when severe dysentery is present.

The diagnosis of *giardiasis* is also confirmed by the presence of parasites in the stool. Because organisms may not be detected for at least 1 week after symptoms appear, multiple stool samples should be examined.

▪ *Interventions*

Treatment for all types of *amebiasis* involves the use of amebicide drugs. Metronidazole (Flagyl, Novonidazole♣) and diloxanide furoate (Entamide) or diloxanide furoate and tetracycline hydrochloride (Sumycin) followed by chloroquine are commonly prescribed. The patient with severe dysentery requires IV fluids replacement and possibly opiates, such as diphenoxylate hydrochloride and atropine sulfate (Lomotil), to control bowel motility. The patient with extraintestinal amebiasis or severe dehydration is hospitalized, especially the older adult. The patient with asymptomatic, mild, or moderate disease is treated with drug therapy on an ambulatory care basis. Therapy effectiveness is based on the examination of at least three stools at 2- to 3-day intervals, starting 2 to 4 weeks after drug therapy has been completed. *Teach patients the importance of keeping their follow-up appointments and taking all drugs as prescribed.*

Treatment for *giardiasis* is drug therapy. Metronidazole is the drug of choice, 250 mg orally three times daily for 5 days. Tinidazole (Fasigyn) can be used as an alternative. Stools are examined 2 weeks after treatment to assess for drug effectiveness.

Explain modes of transmission and means to avoid the spread of infection and recurrent contact with parasitic organisms. *Inform the patient that the infection can be transmitted to others until amebicides effectively kill the parasites. Teach the patient to:*

- *Avoid contact with stool.*
- *Keep toilet areas clean.*
- *Wash hands meticulously with an antimicrobial soap after bowel movements.*
- *Maintain good personal hygiene by bathing or showering daily.*
- *Avoid stool from dogs and beavers.*

Advise the patient to avoid sexual practices that allow rectal contact until drug therapy is completed. *All household and sexual partners should have stool examinations for parasites.* If the water supply is suspected as the source, a sample is obtained and sent for analysis. Multiple infections are common in households, often as a result of contaminated water supplies. Well water and water from areas with inadequate or no filtration equipment can be sources of contamination.

Infection with *Cryptosporidium* is usually self-limiting in people who have normal immune function. Drug therapy for patients who are immunosuppressed may include paromomycin (Paromycin), an aminoglycoside antibiotic, 500 to 750 mg orally four times daily. Teach patients that this drug can cause dizziness.

HELMINTHIC INFESTATION

Helminths are wormlike animals that are often parasitic and capable of causing infectious disease in humans. There are many species of helminths, which are divided into the general categories of roundworms (nematodes), flukes (trematodes), and tapeworms (cestodes).

Helminths can cause various degrees of GI problems in humans. Most often they enter the human body through the skin or via the oral route with ingestion of contaminated food or water. Some gain access to the body via insects, such as flies and mosquitoes, occurring mostly in tropical areas, and are not discussed here. Flukes (trematodes), which are passed to humans via snail-contaminated water, are also limited to tropical and subtropical areas outside the United States and Canada and are not discussed here. However, travel to or from these areas may result in infestation with flukes.

ROUNDWORMS

Roundworms cause most of the helminthic infections in the United States and worldwide. These infections include enterobiasis, trichinosis, hookworms, and tapeworms.

Enterobiasis

Enterobiasis ("pinworm infection") is caused by *Enterobius vermicularis* and is the most common helminthic infection in the United States. It is transmitted by oral intake of contaminated food or drink. Manifestations of infection include intense perianal pruritus (itching), especially at night; vaginitis; insomnia; and restlessness.

The patient may have vague GI symptoms, such as abdominal pain, nausea, vomiting, and diarrhea. However, many infected people have no symptoms. Diagnosis is made when eggs of the helminths are found on the perianal skin or on cellulose tape that has been applied to the perianal skin.

Treatment of enterobiasis includes meticulous handwashing after defecation and before meals to prevent spread of the worms to others. Drug therapy is indicated for all patients with symptoms and for some who are infected but are not symptomatic. Household members of an infected patient may be treated with drug therapy even if they have no symptoms. Pyrantel pamoate (Antiminth, Combantrin♣) or mebendazole (Vermox) is given orally in one dose, repeated at 2 and 4 weeks.

Infection with pinworms is curable and does not usually lead to complications. However, recurrences are common.

Trichinosis

Trichinosis is caused by roundworms. The incidence in the United States is very low, but many mild or asymptomatic cases go undiagnosed. *Trichinella spiralis,* which lives in the intestine of humans, pigs, bears, and rats, causes trichinosis. *The organism is usually transmitted to people who eat undercooked pork or pork products.* Ingestion of other meats, such as ground beef, can also cause infection if a meat grinder has been used for both beef and pork and the meat is undercooked. After ingestion, the larvae are released by the action of acid and enzymes in the digestive tract. Incubation is 12 hours to 28 days after ingestion. Manifestations range from none to severe; death rarely results.

During the first week after infection, diarrhea results from the invasion of the gut by large numbers of the parasite. Abdominal pain, nausea, and vomiting may follow. During the second week, the larvae begin to invade the muscle, starting a hypersensitivity reaction with fever, edema of the face and around the eyes, and subconjunctival hemorrhage. Occasionally a rash or dyspnea develops. Two to three weeks after infection, symptoms of myositis, myalgia, and muscle weakness develop, particularly in the lower back, neck, jaw, biceps, and muscles controlling eye movement. Vague muscle pain and malaise continue into the recovery phase, which can last several months.

A diagnosis of trichinosis is confirmed by a history of ingestion of raw or undercooked meat. White blood cell (WBC) and eosinophil counts are elevated for 2 weeks after meat is ingested. Biopsy of skeletal muscle shows larvae of the *Trichinella* organism. Worms are rarely seen in feces.

The patient is treated with oral mebendazole (Vermox). During the stage of muscle invasion, hospitalization for high doses of corticosteroids may be required.

Hookworms

Hookworms are also roundworms. They differ from pinworms and *Trichinella* in that they enter the human body through the skin. Hookworm disease is caused by either *Ancylostoma duodenale* or *Necator americanus.*

Hookworms infect a quarter of the world's population, but the disease is rare in areas outside the tropics or in areas with little rain. However, as people travel around the world or enter the United States as newcomers, these diseases may become more common throughout the world. Worms are infective outside the body in warm, moist soil for up to 1 week. Infection occurs when larvae penetrate through the skin. The organism can travel to the lungs via the bloodstream and enter alveoli. Cilia carry the organisms up the respiratory tree to the pharynx and the mouth, where they are swallowed and enter the GI tract. Hookworms probably also enter the GI tract when a person ingests contaminated food.

Early symptoms of hookworm disease include an itchy, red, raised, blister-like inflammation of the skin. Infection in the GI tract may produce no symptoms, or it may cause anorexia, diarrhea, or mild abdominal and epigastric discomfort. Bleeding and anemia may occur when worms suck blood at sites of attachment in the GI tract. If blood loss is severe, the patient may have symptoms of anemia, such as pallor, hair thinning, deformed nails, pica, and shortness of breath.

Diagnosis of hookworm infection is based on the presence of ova (eggs) in the feces. Occult blood is often present in the stool. The patient may also have anemia with low hemoglobin and hematocrit levels or a low serum iron level and high iron-binding capacity. WBC and eosinophil counts are elevated.

All patients with symptoms receive iron therapy and a diet high in protein and vitamins for at least 3 months after anemia is corrected. Pyrantel pamoate (Antiminth) or mebendazole (Vermox) is prescribed for a complete recovery. Severe hookworm disease can cause malabsorption and protein loss, requiring nutritional support in addition to other treatments.

TAPEWORMS

Five types of tapeworms (cestodes) may infect humans: tapeworms found in cattle, fish, dogs, pigs, and rodents. Tapeworm infections generally cause either no symptoms or only occasional GI upset, such as nausea, diarrhea, or abdominal pain. The diagnosis of tapeworm infestation is made by laboratory examination of eggs found in the stool (test of stool for ova and parasites).

Infection by tapeworms occurs when a person eats undercooked beef, raw fish, or other contaminated food or water or accidentally swallows infected lice or fleas from dogs. People can also accidentally eat arthropods, such as cockroaches, in stored foods or cereals.

Treatment is usually with praziquantel (Biltricide) 10 mg/kg except for *Hymenolepis nana* (dwarf tapeworm), in which case the dose is 25 mg/kg in a single dose and may be repeated 1 week later. Beef tapeworm can be treated with albendazole (Albenza) 400 mg daily for 3 days. Niclosamide (Niclocide) (500 mg chewable tablet) is sometimes used for dog tapeworm infestation.

When caring for all patients with helminths, follow Standard Precautions when in contact with any stool. Teach the patient to wash the hands after defecating and before eating. Prevention methods include avoiding eating undercooked beef, fish, or pork and drinking water that might be contaminated. Other prevention strategies include keeping the mouth closed while petting dogs and handwashing after touching any animal. Stored foods should be kept tightly closed to avoid contamination by cockroaches and other insects.

FOOD POISONING

Foodborne illnesses are a common problem in the United States and all other parts of the world and can cause death. The problem results when a person ingests infectious organisms in food. Unlike gastroenteritis, food poisoning is not directly communicable from person to person and incubation periods are shorter. However, like gastroenteritis, it causes diarrhea, nausea, and vomiting. Food poisoning can be differentiated from gastroenteritis by obtaining a thorough history of common food intake in patients who have common symptoms of acute diarrhea, nausea, and vomiting.

Food poisoning is caused by over 250 pathogens. Examples include gram-negative *Salmonella*, *Staphylococcal aureus*, *Escherichia coli*, and botulism. Table 60-6 lists more information about these microbes. All cases of botulism and salmonellosis need to be reported to the local health department. Cases of staphylococcal and *E. coli* food poisoning are reported if epidemic outbreaks occur.

SALMONELLOSIS

Salmonellosis is a bacterial infection caused by the *Salmonella* organism and affects 40,000 people each year in the United States (www.cdc.gov). Salmonella bacteria live in the intestinal tracts of humans and animals. They can be transmitted by the "five Fs": flies, fingers, food, feces, and fomites. Incubation is 8 to 48 hours after the person has ingested the contaminated food or liquid, the most common source. Foods that are most commonly contaminated are eggs, beef, poultry, and green leafy vegetables (e.g., spinach). In 2008 contaminated jalapeno peppers from Mexico caused salmonella infection in hundreds of people in the United States.

Symptoms usually last for 4 to 7 days. Most people have fever, nausea, vomiting, cramping abdominal pain, and foul-smelling diarrhea, which may be bloody (www.cdc.gov./nczved/dfbmd/disease_listing/salmonellosis_gi.html). In some patients, fever is very high.

Salmonellosis is usually self-limiting, but bacteremia that infects the joints or bone may occur later in the disease process. Diagnosis is made by stool culture. Treatment is symptomatic. If bacteremia occurs, antibiotics such as ampicillin or ciprofloxacin (Cipro) are prescribed. Unfortunately, some *Salmonella* bacteria have become resistant to antibiotics because of the use of these drugs in animals. Some patients, especially older adults, are hospitalized with severe diarrhea and dehydration.

Patients may be carriers of the bacterium for up to 1 year. Instruct those with *Salmonella* gastroenteritis and their contacts to wash their hands before meals and after defecating to avoid transmission of the organism.

STAPHYLOCOCCAL INFECTION

Staphylococcus is responsible for 25% of reported food poisoning outbreaks. It is found in meats and dairy products and can be transmitted by carriers of the organism. For staphylococcal food poisoning to occur, there must be contamination of food and a period of time (hours) during which the organisms multiply. This can take place during the slow cooling of food after it is cooked.

Symptoms of staphylococcal food poisoning include an abrupt onset of vomiting, abdominal cramping, and diarrhea. The person usually has symptoms 2 to 4 hours after ingesting the contaminated food. The patient is afebrile but weak.

A diagnosis can be made when stool culture yields 100,000 enterotoxin-producing staphylococci. However, symptoms rarely last more than 24 hours, and people do not always seek medical attention. Antimicrobial drug therapy is not usually indicated unless an agent produces progressive systemic involvement. Parenteral fluids may be needed for dehydration.

ESCHERICHIA COLI INFECTION

E. coli is increasingly becoming associated with food poisoning. Since 1992, a number of outbreaks of *E. coli* food poisoning have occurred in the United States. An estimated 70,000 people are affected each year. Many strains of *E. coli* exist, and not all of them cause harm. However, some cause disease by making a substance called *Shiga toxin.* The bacteria that make these substances are called *Shiga toxin–producing E. coli,* or *STEC* for short. The most commonly identified STEC in the United States is *E. coli* O157:H7 (sometimes just called *O157*). In 2007 prepackaged spinach processed in the United States was contaminated with these bacteria and caused hundreds of people to become ill.

Enterohemorrhagic strains of *E. coli* (EHEC) and STEC can cause serious complications, such as hemorrhagic colitis and hemolytic-uremic syndrome. These problems affect older adults most often.

The symptoms of STEC infections vary, but most people have severe abdominal cramping, vomiting, and diarrhea (often bloody). Treatment of the patient with *E. coli* food poisoning includes IV fluids and supportive therapy, possibly with antidiarrheal agents. Antibiotics are not effective. Chart 60-9 outlines best practices for preventing STEC infections.

BOTULISM

Botulism is a paralytic disease resulting from ingestion of a toxin in food contaminated with *Clostridium botulinum.* Botulism occurs most often with home-canned foods, particularly vegetables, fruits, condiments, and, less commonly, meat and fish. It can also occur in commercially prepared products and with products not adequately heated to destroy toxins before they are eaten.

Incubation is usually 18 to 36 hours. After this time, symptoms occur. Initial symptoms include diplopia (double vision), dysphagia (difficulty swallowing), and dysarthria (slurred speech). Illness may be mild or severe, with paralysis, respiratory failure, and death. Weakness can progress rapidly from the neck to the arms, chest, and legs. Paralytic ileus, severe constipation, and urinary retention can also occur. Nausea,

TABLE 60-6 Common Types of Food Poisoning

STAPHYLOCOCCAL INFECTION
- Caused by contaminated meats and dairy products
- Can be transmitted by human carriers
- Causes abrupt onset of vomiting and diarrhea without fever

***ESCHERICHIA COLI* INFECTION**
- Caused by meat contaminated with animal feces
- Causes abrupt vomiting, diarrhea, abdominal cramping, and fever

BOTULISM
- Commonly associated with improperly canned foods, especially fruits and vegetables
- Nausea, vomiting, diarrhea, and weakness progressing to paralysis
- Diplopia, dysphagia, and dysarthria

SALMONELLOSIS
- Caused by contaminated food or drink but can be transmitted by the fecal-oral route
- Fever, nausea, vomiting, abdominal cramping, and diarrhea lasting for 3 to 5 days

Chart 60-9 PATIENT AND FAMILY EDUCATION GUIDE

Ways to Prevent STEC *(E. coli)* Infections

- Wash your hands *thoroughly* after using the bathroom and after changing diapers and before preparing or eating food.
- Wash your hands after contact with any animals or their environments (e.g., zoo).
- Cook meats thoroughly to at least 160° or 170° internal temperature; use a food thermometer to ensure doneness.
- Avoid raw milk, unpasteurized juices (like fresh apple cider), and unpasteurized dairy products.
- Avoid swallowing water when swimming.
- Prevent cross-contamination during food preparation by washing hands, counters, cutting boards, and utensils after they touch raw meat.

STEC, Shiga toxin–producing *Escherichia coli.*

vomiting, and abdominal pain may occur before or after the onset of paralysis.

The diagnosis is made on the basis of the patient's history and a stool culture of *C. botulinum*. The blood may be positive for toxins.

Treatment with trivalent botulism antitoxin (ABE) is given as soon as the diagnosis is made if the patient is not hypersensitive to it. The physician may lavage the stomach to stop absorption of toxin. All patients are hospitalized to observe for and treat respiratory paralysis. Nothing is given orally until swallowing and respiratory difficulties pass. The physician prescribes IV fluids as needed. If respiratory paralysis occurs, intubation and mechanical ventilation are implemented. If ventilation can be maintained, the patient can survive with no neurologic deficits after the illness.

To prevent botulism, teach patients the importance of discarding cans of food that are punctured or swollen or that have defective seals. Remind them to check for expiration dates and to not use any canned food that has expired. Containers for home-canned foods must be sterilized by boiling for 20 minutes to destroy *C. botulinum* spores before canning.

HUMAN NEEDS NURSING CARE REVIEW

What might you NOTICE if the patient has impaired digestion and inadequate nutrition as a result of inflammatory intestinal problems?

- Report of nausea
- Vomiting
- Report of epigastric or abdominal pain
- Diarrhea (sometimes bloody)
- Elevated temperature
- Weakness

What should you INTERPRET and how should you RESPOND to a patient with impaired digestion and inadequate nutrition as a result of inflammatory intestinal problems?

Perform and interpret focused physical assessment findings, including:

- Vital signs
- Complete pain assessment
- Skin turgor and mucous membrane dryness
- Abdominal assessment
- Current and previous weight
- History of recent food intake
- History of recent travel

Respond:

- Prevent pain and aspiration by sitting patient up.
- Place IV catheter (large-bore) to replace fluids.
- Provide privacy, and assist with hygiene.
- Provide rest.
- Check laboratory values for hemoglobin and hematocrit (anemia).
- Check serum electrolytes (dehydration, hypokalemia).
- Give antidiarrheal drugs if prescribed.
- Record intake and output.
- Assist with ADLs and ambulation as needed.

On what should you REFLECT?

- Continue to monitor for vomiting and diarrhea and changes in pain level.
- Think about what you need to document.
- Decide when you might need to call the health care provider or Rapid Response Team (for hospitalized patients).
- Determine what health teaching and community resources may be needed for this patient and family.
- Think about what you can do to help prevent complications of the health problem.

GET READY FOR THE NCLEX EXAMINATION!

Key Points

Review these Key Points for each NCLEX Examination Client Needs Category.

Safe and Effective Care Environment

- Teach patients to use infection control measures to prevent transmission of gastroenteritis as stated in Chart 60-2.
- Collaborate with a CWOCN or ET nurse for ileostomy teaching and care; collaborate with a case manager when planning for patient discharge.

Health Promotion and Maintenance

- Teach patients with chronic IBD to avoid GI stimulants, such as alcohol and caffeine; each patient's response to foods differs.
- Teach patients how to provide ileostomy care, paying particular attention to skin care; the effluent has a high enzyme content that can easily cause severe skin excoriation (see Charts 60-4 and 60-5).
- Instruct patients with diverticulosis about nutrition modifications, such as avoiding nuts, foods with seeds, and GI stimulants.
- Teach patients with diverticulosis to eat a high-fiber diet; diverticulitis requires a low-fiber diet.

Psychosocial Integrity

- Be aware that all inflammatory bowel diseases (acute and chronic) are very disruptive to one's daily routine; chronic IBD requires a lifetime of modifications.
- Recognize that having an ileostomy impacts the patient's body image and self-esteem; assess for coping strategies that the patient has previously used, and identify personal support systems to assist in coping.

Physiological Integrity

- Assess for the classic clinical manifestations of appendicitis, which include abdominal pain, nausea and vomiting, and abdominal tenderness upon palpation (McBurney's point); some patients also have leukocytosis.

- Assess for the key features of peritonitis as listed in Chart 60-1.
- Assess for signs and symptoms of dehydration in patients who have inflammatory bowel disease.
- Administer antidiarrheal medications, as prescribed, to decrease stools and therefore prevent dehydration in patients with inflammatory bowel diseases.
- Be aware that there are two major types of chronic inflammatory bowel disease (IBD): ulcerative colitis (UC) and Crohn's disease; both have similarities but also have differences (see Table 60-2).
- Recognize that perforation (rupture) of the appendix requires prompt intervention and can result in peritonitis.
- Be alert for GI bleeding in the patient with chronic inflammatory bowel disease (IBD).
- Be aware that patients with Crohn's disease are at high risk for malnutrition as a result of an inability to absorb nutrients via the small intestine.
- Monitor for complications of UC as listed in Table 60-4.
- Provide nursing interventions for patients with IBD as listed in Chart 60-3.
- Administer 5-aminosalicylic acid drugs as prescribed (e.g., Pentasa and Dipentum) to decrease inflammation in patients with UC; most of these same drugs are also used for Crohn's disease management.
- Administer corticosteroids and 6-mercaptopurine, as prescribed, for both UC and Crohn's disease; infliximab (Remicade) is used primarily for Crohn's but may be useful for those with UC in selected cases.
- Observe for GI bleeding in patients with diverticular disease.
- Instruct patients with anorectal disorders to use sitz baths, bulk-forming agents (e.g., Metamucil), and stool softeners to decrease pain.
- Be aware that GI problems, including diarrhea, may also be caused by parasites and helminths.

Additional Study Resources

Go to your Companion CD or Evolve at http://evolve.elsevier.com/Iggy/ for *Self-Assessment Questions for the NCLEX Examination.*

evolve Go to Evolve at http://evolve.elsevier.com/Iggy/ for *Prioritization and Delegation Questions for the NCLEX Examination.*

SELECTED BIBLIOGRAPHY

Asterisk indicates a classic or definitive work on this subject.

Amerine, E., & Keirsey, M. (2006). Managing acute diarrhea. *Nursing2006, 36*(9), 64hn1-hn4.

*Casellas, F., Lopez-Vivancos, J., Badia, X., Vilaseca, J., & Malagelada, J.R. (2000). Impact of surgery for Crohn's disease on health-related quality of life. *American Journal of Gastroenterology, 95*(1), 177-182.

*Dooley, T.P., Curto, E.V., Reddy, S.P., Davis, R.L., Lambert, G.W., Wilborn, T.W., et al. (2004). Regulation of gene expression in inflammatory bowel disease and correlation with IBD drugs: Screening by DNA microassays. *Inflammatory Bowel Diseases, 10*(1), 1-14.

*Goldstein, E.S., Marion, J.F., & Present, D.H. (2004). 6-mercaptopurine is effective in Crohn's disease without concomitant steroids. *Inflammatory Bowel Diseases, 10*(2), 79-84.

Heuer, O.E., Hammerum, A.M., Collignon, P., & Wegener, H.C. (2006). Human health hazard from antimicrobial-resistant enterococci in animals and food. *Clinical Infectious Diseases, 43*(7), 911-916.

*Joachim, G. (2002). An assessment of social support in people with inflammatory bowel disease. *Gastroenterology Nursing, 25*(6), 246-252.

Jung, B., Lannerstad, O., Pahlman, L., Arodell, M., Unosson, M., & Nilsson, E. (2007). Preoperative mechanical preparation of the colon: The patient's experience. *BMC Surgery Journal, 7*(5), 1-8.

*Klonowski, E., & Masoodi, J. (1999). The patient with Crohn's disease. *RN, 62*(3), 32-37.

Lichtenstein, G., Abreu, M., Cohen, R., & Tremaine, W. (2006). American Gastroenterological Association Institute medical position statement on corticosteroids, immunomodulators, and infliximab in inflammatory bowel disease. *Gastroenterology, 130*(3), 935-939.

McCance, K.L., & Huether, S.E. (2006). *Pathophysiology: The biologic basis for disease in adults and children.* St. Louis: Mosby.

*Mikula, C. (1999). Anti-TNF alpha: New therapy for Crohn's disease. *Gastroenterology Nursing, 22*(6), 245-248.

Miller, S., & Alpert, P. (2006). Assessment and differential diagnosis of abdominal pain. *The Nurse Practitioner, 31*(7), 38-47.

Movius, M. (2006). What's causing that gut pain? *RN, 69*(7), 25-29.

Nussbaum, R.L., McInnes, R.R., & Willard, H.F. (2007). *Thompson & Thompson genetics in medicine* (7th ed.). Philadelphia: Saunders.

*Pearson, C. (2004). Inflammatory bowel disease. *Nursing Times, 100*(9), 86-90.

Present, D.H. (2006). Current and investigational approaches in the management of ulcerative colitis. *Thomson Professional Postgraduate Services/Shire Pharmaceuticals, Inc. December* (1-17).

*Rayhorn, N., & Rayhorn, B.S. (2002). Inflammatory bowel disease: Symptoms in the bowel and beyond. *The Nurse Practitioner, 27*(11) 13-16, 23-29.

Rocca, J.D. (2007). Minimizing the perils of appendicitis. *Nursing2007, 37*(1), 64hn1-hn3.

Sands, B.E. (2006). Clinical pearls from ACG 2006: Advances in diagnosis, staging and treatment of Crohn's disease. *Therapeutic Window, LLC CME Certified Newsletter, November,* 1-11.

Snow, M. (2006). Preventing salmonella infection. *Nursing2006, 36*(9), 17.

Willcutts, K., Scarano, K., & Eddins, C.W. (2005). Ostomies and fistulas: A collaborative approach. *Practical Gastroenterology, 29*(11), 63-79.

61 CHAPTER

Care of Patients with Liver Problems

Donna D. Ignatavicius

LEARNING OUTCOMES

For clinical competence and success on the NCLEX Examination, study this chapter with these Learning Outcomes in mind:

Safe and Effective Care Environment

1. Identify community resources for patients with chronic liver disease.
2. Collaborate with health care team members to provide care for patients with liver problems.

Health Promotion and Maintenance

3. Identify risk factors for cirrhosis and hepatitis.
4. Teach patients and families health promotion practices to prevent hepatitis and its spread to others.
5. Teach patients and families health promotion practices to prevent or slow the progress of alcohol-induced cirrhosis.

Psychosocial Integrity

6. Explain the psychosocial needs of patients with hepatitis.
7. Evaluate the psychosocial needs of patients having a liver transplant.

Physiological Integrity

8. Explain the pathophysiology and complications associated with cirrhosis of the liver.
9. Interpret laboratory test findings commonly seen in patients with cirrhosis.
10. Analyze assessment data from patients with cirrhosis to determine priority nursing diagnoses and collaborative problems.
11. Develop a collaborative plan of care for the patient with late-stage cirrhosis.
12. Assess for potentially life-threatening complications of cirrhosis.
13. Identify emergency interventions for the patient with bleeding esophageal varices.
14. Explain the role of the nurse when assisting with a paracentesis procedure.
15. Compare and contrast the transmission of hepatitis viral infections.
16. Explain ways in which each type of hepatitis can be prevented.
17. Assess potentially life-threatening complications of liver trauma.
18. Identify treatment options for patients with cancer of the liver.
19. Describe the common complications that result from liver transplantation.

Go to your Companion CD or Evolve at http://evolve.elsevier.com/Iggy/ for *Self-Assessment Questions for the NCLEX Examination* keyed to these Learning Outcomes.

The liver is the largest and one of the most vital internal organs, performing more than 400 functions and affecting every system in the body. When the liver is diseased or damaged, it cannot provide these activities. As a result, *digestion, nutrition, and metabolism* can be severely affected. Liver diseases range in severity from mild hepatic inflammation to chronic end-stage cirrhosis.

CIRRHOSIS

Cirrhosis is extensive, irreversible scarring of the liver, usually caused by a chronic reaction to hepatic inflammation and necrosis. The disease typically develops slowly and has a progressive, prolonged, destructive course resulting in end-stage liver disease. The most common causes for cirrhosis in the United States are alcoholic liver disease and hepatitis C. Worldwide, hepatitis B and hepatitis D are the leading causes. Without liver transplantation, cirrhosis is usually fatal (Kelso, 2008).

Pathophysiology

Cirrhosis is characterized by widespread fibrotic (scarred) bands of connective tissue that change the liver's normal makeup. Inflammation caused by either toxins or disease results in extensive degeneration and destruction of **hepatocytes** (liver cells). As cirrhosis develops, the tissue becomes nodular. These nodules can block bile ducts and normal blood flow throughout the liver. Impairments in blood and lymph flow result from compression caused by excessive fibrous tissue. In early disease, the liver is usually enlarged, firm, and hard. As the pathologic process continues, the liver shrinks in size, resulting in decreased liver function, which can occur in weeks to years (40% of cirrhotic patients are asymptomatic). This impaired liver function results in elevated serum liver enzymes.

Cirrhosis of the liver can be divided into several types, depending on the cause of the disease:

- Laennec's or alcoholic cirrhosis (caused by chronic alcoholism)
- Postnecrotic cirrhosis (caused by viral hepatitis and certain drugs or chemicals)
- Biliary cirrhosis (also called cholestatic; caused by chronic biliary obstruction, usually from gallbladder disease)
- Cardiac cirrhosis (caused by heart failure as a rare complication)

Complications of Cirrhosis

Common problems and complications associated with hepatic cirrhosis depend on the amount of damage sustained by the liver. In **compensated cirrhosis,** the liver is scarred but can still perform essential functions without causing major symptoms. In **decompensated cirrhosis,** liver function is impaired with obvious manifestations of liver failure.

The loss of hepatic function contributes to the development of metabolic abnormalities. Hepatic cell damage may lead to these common complications:

- Portal hypertension
- Ascites
- Bleeding esophageal varices
- Coagulation defects
- Jaundice
- Portal-systemic encephalopathy (PSE) with hepatic coma
- Hepatorenal syndrome
- Spontaneous bacterial peritonitis

Portal hypertension, a persistent increase in pressure within the portal vein, is a major complication of cirrhosis. It results from increased resistance to or obstruction (blockage) of the flow of blood through the portal vein and its branches. The blood meets resistance to flow and seeks collateral (alternative) venous channels around the high-pressure area.

Blood flow backs into the spleen, causing splenomegaly (spleen enlargement). Veins in the esophagus, stomach, intestines, abdomen, and rectum become dilated. Portal hypertension can result in ascites (abdominal fluid), esophageal varices (distended veins), prominent abdominal veins (caput medusae), and hemorrhoids.

Ascites is the collection of free fluid within the peritoneal cavity caused by increased hydrostatic pressure from portal hypertension. The collection of plasma protein in the peritoneal fluid reduces the amount of circulating plasma protein in the blood. When this decrease is combined with the inability of the liver to produce albumin because of impaired liver cell functioning, the serum colloid osmotic pressure is decreased in the circulatory system. The result is a fluid shift from the vascular system into the abdomen, a form of "third spacing."

Massive ascites may cause renal vasoconstriction, triggering the renin-angiotensin system. This results in sodium and water retention, which increases hydrostatic pressure and the vascular volume, which leads to more ascites.

As a result of portal hypertension, the blood backs up from the liver and enters the esophageal and gastric veins. **Esophageal varices** occur when fragile, thin-walled esophageal veins become distended from increased pressure. The potential for varices to bleed depends on their size; size is determined by direct endoscopic observation. Varices occur most often in the distal esophagus but can also be present in the stomach and rectum.

Bleeding esophageal varices is a life-threatening medical emergency. There can be severe blood loss, resulting in shock from hypovolemia. The bleeding may be either **hematemesis** (vomiting blood) or **melena** (black, tarry stools). Loss of consciousness may occur before any observed bleeding. Variceal bleeding can occur spontaneously with no precipitating factors. However, any activity that increases abdominal pressure may increase the likelihood of a variceal bleed, including heavy lifting or vigorous physical exercise. In addition, chest trauma or dry, hard food in the esophagus can cause bleeding.

Patients with portal hypertension may also have *portal hypertensive gastropathy.* This complication can occur with or without esophageal varices. Slow gastric mucosal bleeding occurs, which may result in chronic slow blood loss, occult-positive stools, and anemia.

In patients with cirrhosis, the production of bile in the liver is decreased. This prevents the absorption of fat-soluble vitamins (e.g., vitamin K). Without vitamin K, clotting factors II, VII, IX, and X are not produced in sufficient quantities and the patient is susceptible to bleeding and easy bruising. These abnormalities are confirmed by coagulation studies.

Splenomegaly (enlarged spleen) results from the backup of blood into the spleen. The enlarged spleen destroys platelets, causing thrombocytopenia (low serum platelet count) and increased risk for bleeding. Thrombocytopenia is often the first clinical sign that a patient has liver dysfunction.

Jaundice (yellowish coloration of the skin) in patients with cirrhosis is caused by one of two mechanisms: hepatocellular disease or intrahepatic obstruction (Table 61-1). Hepatocellular jaundice develops because the liver cells cannot effectively excrete bilirubin. This decreased excretion results in excessive circulating bilirubin levels. Intrahepatic obstructive jaundice results from edema, fibrosis, or scarring of the hepatic bile channels and bile ducts, which interferes with normal bile and bilirubin excretion.

Portal-systemic encephalopathy (PSE) is also known as **hepatic encephalopathy** and **hepatic coma** in the later stages. It is a disorder seen in liver failure and cirrhosis that affects the function of the brain. Patients report sleep disturbance, mood disturbance, mental status changes, and speech problems early as this complication begins (Matthews et al., 2006). Later neurologic symptoms include an altered level of consciousness, impaired thinking processes, and neuromuscular problems. Encephalopathy may be acute and reversible with early intervention.

The exact mechanisms causing hepatic encephalopathy are not clearly understood but probably are the result of the shunting of portal venous blood into the central circulation so that the liver is bypassed. As a result, toxic substances absorbed by the intestine are not broken down or detoxified and may lead to metabolic abnormalities, such as elevated serum ammonia and gamma-aminobutyric acid (GABA) (Kelso,

TABLE 61-1 Laboratory Diagnostic Differentiation of Jaundice

Test	Hepatocellular Jaundice	Obstructive Jaundice	Hemolytic Jaundice
Serum bilirubin			
Indirect (unconjugated)	Increased	Slightly increased	Increased
Direct (conjugated)	Increased	Moderately increased	Normal
Urine bilirubin	Increased	Increased	None
Urobilinogen			
Stool	Normal to decreased	None	Increased
Urine	Normal to increased	None	Increased

TABLE 61-2 Stages of Portal-Systemic Encephalopathy

STAGE I PRODROMAL
- Subtle manifestations that may not be recognized immediately
- Personality changes
- Behavior changes (agitation, belligerence)
- Emotional lability (euphoria, depression)
- Impaired thinking
- Inability to concentrate
- Fatigue, drowsiness
- Slurred or slowed speech
- Sleep pattern disturbances

STAGE II IMPENDING
- Continuing mental changes
- Mental confusion
- Disorientation to time, place, or person
- Asterixis (hand flapping)

STAGE III STUPOROUS
- Progressive deterioration
- Marked mental confusion
- Stuporous, drowsy but arousable
- Abnormal electroencephalogram tracing
- Muscle twitching
- Hyperreflexia
- Asterixis

STAGE IV COMATOSE
- Unresponsiveness, leading to death in most patients progressing to this stage
- Unarousable, obtunded
- Response to painful stimulus
- No asterixis
- Positive Babinski's sign
- Muscle rigidity
- Fetor hepaticus (characteristic liver breath—musty, sweet odor)
- Seizures

2008). Elevated ammonia levels are usually common in patients with hepatic encephalopathy. However, they are not a clear indicator of the presence of encephalopathy. Some patients may have major impairment without high elevations of serum ammonia, and elevations of ammonia can occur without evidence of encephalopathy.

PSE may develop slowly in patients with chronic liver disease and go undetected until the late stages. Symptoms develop rapidly in acute liver dysfunction. Four stages of development have been identified: prodromal, impending, stuporous, and comatose (Table 61-2). The patient's symptoms may gradually progress to coma or fluctuate among the four stages.

Factors that may lead to PSE include:
- High-protein diet
- Infections
- Hypovolemia (deficient fluid volume)
- Hypokalemia (deficient serum potassium)
- Constipation
- GI bleeding (causes a large protein load in the intestines)
- Drugs (e.g., hypnotics, opioids, sedatives, analgesics, diuretics)

PSE may also occur after paracentesis or shunting procedures. The prognosis depends on the severity of the underlying cause, the precipitating factors, and the degree of liver dysfunction.

The development of **hepatorenal syndrome (HRS)** indicates a poor prognosis for the patient with liver failure. It is often the cause of death in these patients. This syndrome is manifested by:
- A sudden decrease in urinary flow (<500 mL/24 hr) (oliguria)
- Elevated blood urea nitrogen and creatinine levels with abnormally decreased urine sodium excretion
- Increased urine osmolarity

HRS often occurs after clinical deterioration from GI bleeding or the onset of PSE. It may also complicate other liver diseases, including acute hepatitis and fulminant liver failure.

Patients with cirrhosis and ascites may develop acute *spontaneous bacterial peritonitis (SBP)*. Those who are particularly susceptible are patients with very advanced liver disease. This may be the result of low concentrations of proteins; proteins normally provide some protection against bacteria.

The bacteria responsible for SBP are typically from the bowel and reach the ascitic fluid after migrating through the bowel wall and transversing the lymphatics. Clinical manifestations vary but may include fever, chills, and abdominal pain and tenderness. However, manifestations can also be minimal with only mild symptoms in the absence of fever. Worsening encephalopathy and increased jaundice may also be present without abdominal symptoms.

The diagnosis of SBP is made when a sample of ascitic fluid is obtained by paracentesis for cell counts and culture. An ascitic fluid leukocyte count of more than 250 polymorphonuclear (PMN) leukocytes can be the basis for treatment.

Etiology

Cirrhosis can occur as a result of many factors and diseases. *Alcohol* has a direct toxic effect on the hepatocytes and causes liver inflammation **(alcoholic hepatitis).** The liver becomes enlarged, with cellular degeneration and infiltration by fat, leukocytes, and lymphocytes. Over time, the inflammatory process decreases and the destructive phase increases. Early scar formation is caused by fibroblast infiltration and collagen formation. Damage to the liver tissue progresses as malnutrition and repeated exposure to the alcohol continue. If alcohol is withheld, the fatty infiltration and inflammation is reversible. If alcohol abuse continues, widespread scar tissue formation and fibrosis infiltrate the liver as a result of cellular necrosis.

The amount of alcohol necessary to cause cirrhosis varies widely from person to person, and there are gender differences. In women, it may take as few as two to three drinks per day over a minimum of 10 years. In men, perhaps six drinks per day over the same time period may be needed to cause disease. Binge drinking can increase risk for hepatitis and fatty liver.

Hepatitis C is now the leading cause of cirrhosis in the United States. It is an infectious bloodborne illness that usually causes chronic disease. Inflammation caused by infection over time leads to progressive scarring of the liver. It usually takes decades for cirrhosis to develop, although alcohol use in combination with hepatitis C may speed the process.

Hepatitis B and hepatitis D are the most common causes of cirrhosis worldwide. Hepatitis B also causes inflammation and low-grade damage over decades that can ultimately lead to cirrhosis. Hepatitis D is another virus that infects the liver but only in people who already have hepatitis B (see discussion of hepatitis on p. 1356). Table 61-3 lists additional causes of liver cirrhosis.

Incidence/Prevalence

The incidence of cirrhosis in the United States is not well known, but about 27,000 die each year. Annual hospital stays are over 400,000 (Kelso, 2008). The disease affects twice as many men as women (www.liverfoundation.org).

Patient-Centered Collaborative Care

evolve ONLINE PHARM REVIEW

Assessment

History

Obtain data from patients with suspected cirrhosis, including age, gender, and employment history, especially history of exposure to chemical toxins or drugs. Keep in mind that all exposures are important regardless of how long ago they occurred. Determine whether there has ever been a needle stick injury. Sexual history and preference may be important in determining an infectious cause for liver disease.

Inquire about whether there is a family history of alcoholism and/or liver disease. Ask the patient to describe his or her alcohol intake, including the amount consumed during a given period. Is there a history of drug use, including oral, IV, and intranasal forms? Is there a history of tattoos? Has the patient been in the military or in prison? Is the patient a health care worker, firefighter, or police officer? For patients previously or currently in an alcohol or drug recovery program, how long have they been sober? This information is sensitive and often difficult for the patient to answer. Be sure to establish why you are asking these questions, and accept answers in a nonjudgmental manner. Provide privacy during the interview. For many people, the behaviors causing the liver disease occurred years before the onset of their current illness and they are regretful and often embarrassed.

Ask the patient about previous medical conditions, such as an episode of jaundice or acute viral hepatitis, biliary tract disorders, viral infections, surgery, blood transfusions, autoimmune disorders, obesity, altered lipid profile, heart failure, respiratory disorders, or liver injury.

Physical Assessment/Clinical Manifestations

Because cirrhosis has a slow onset, many of the *early* manifestations are vague and nonspecific. Assess for:

- Fatigue
- Significant change in weight
- GI symptoms
- Abdominal pain and liver tenderness (both of which may be ignored by the patient)
- Pruritus (itching)

Liver function problems are often found during a routine physical examination or when laboratory tests are completed for an unrelated illness or problem. The patient with *compensated cirrhosis* may be completely unaware that there is a liver problem. The first sign may present before the onset of symptoms when routine laboratory tests, presurgical evaluations, or life and health insurance assessments show abnormalities. These tests could indicate abnormal liver function or thrombocytopenia, requiring a more thorough diagnostic workup.

The development of late signs of *advanced cirrhosis* may cause the patient to seek medical treatment. GI bleeding, jaundice, ascites, and spontaneous bruising indicate poor liver function and complications of cirrhosis.

Thoroughly assess the patient with liver dysfunction or failure because it affects every body system (Fig. 61-1). The clinical picture and course vary from patient to patient depending on the severity of the disease. Assess for:

- Obvious yellowing of the skin (jaundice) and sclerae (icterus)
- Dry skin
- Rashes
- Purpuric lesions, such as **petechiae** (round, pinpoint, red-purple lesions) or **ecchymosis** (large purple, blue, or yellow bruises)
- Warm and bright red palms of the hands (palmar erythema)
- Vascular lesions with a red center and radiating branches, known as **"spider angiomas"** (telangiectases, spider nevi, or vascular spiders), on the nose, cheeks, upper thorax, and shoulders
- Peripheral dependent edema of the extremities and sacrum
- Clubbing of nails
- Fixed flexion of fingers

Abdominal Assessment. Usually *massive* ascites can be detected as a distended abdomen with bulging flanks. The umbilicus may protrude, and dilated abdominal veins (caput medusae) may radiate from the umbilicus. Ascites can cause physical problems. For example, orthopnea and dyspnea from

TABLE 61-3 Common Causes of Cirrhosis

- Alcoholic liver disease
- Viral hepatitis
- Autoimmune hepatitis
- Steatohepatitis (from fatty liver)
- Drugs and chemical toxins
- Gallbladder disease
- Metabolic/genetic causes
- Cardiovascular disease

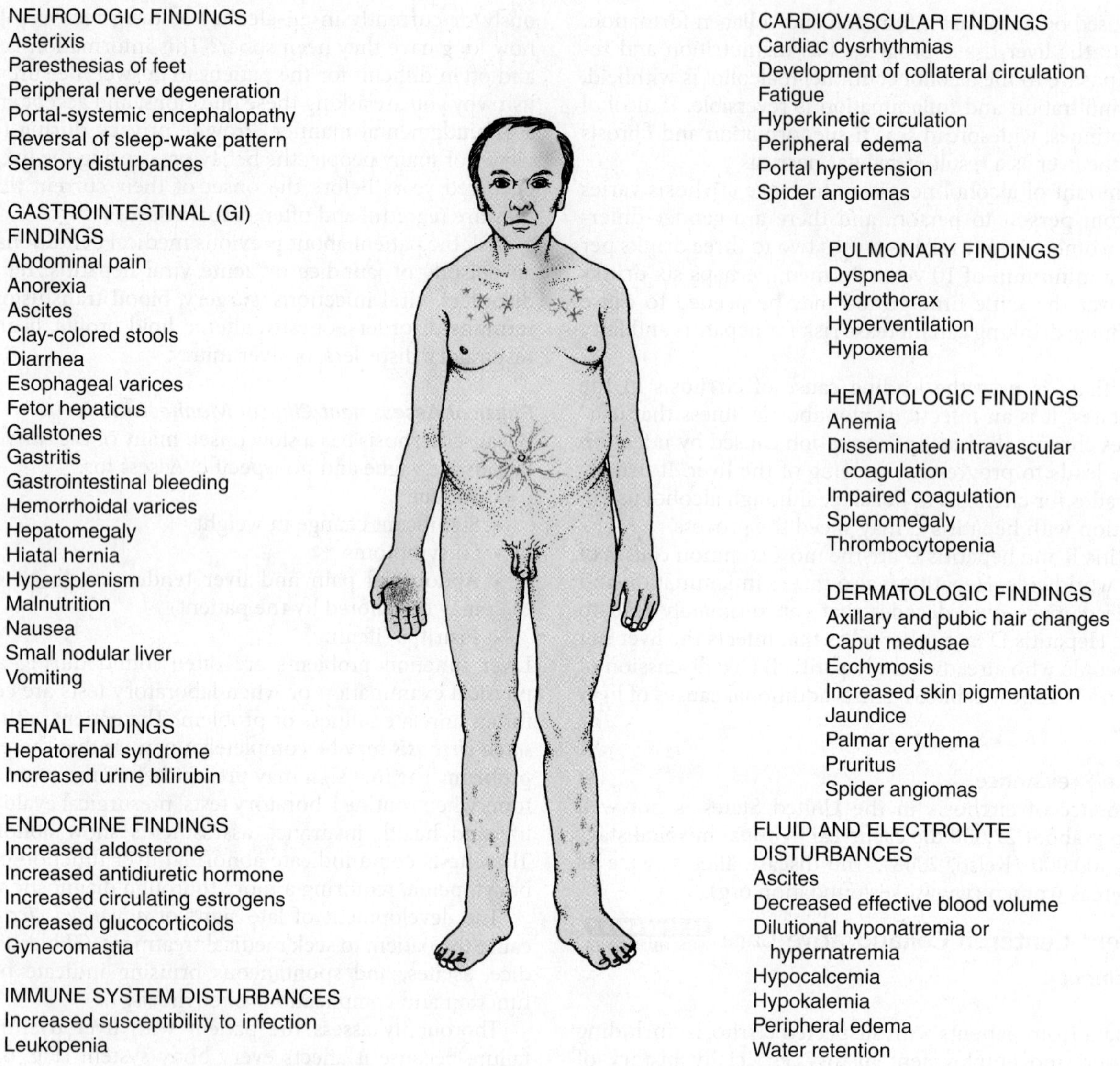
NEUROLOGIC FINDINGS
Asterixis
Paresthesias of feet
Peripheral nerve degeneration
Portal-systemic encephalopathy
Reversal of sleep-wake pattern
Sensory disturbances
GASTROINTESTINAL (GI) FINDINGS
Abdominal pain
Anorexia
Ascites
Clay-colored stools
Diarrhea
Esophageal varices
Fetor hepaticus
Gallstones
Gastritis
Gastrointestinal bleeding
Hemorrhoidal varices
Hepatomegaly
Hiatal hernia
Hypersplenism
Malnutrition
Nausea
Small nodular liver
Vomiting
RENAL FINDINGS
Hepatorenal syndrome
Increased urine bilirubin
ENDOCRINE FINDINGS
Increased aldosterone
Increased antidiuretic hormone
Increased circulating estrogens
Increased glucocorticoids
Gynecomastia
IMMUNE SYSTEM DISTURBANCES
Increased susceptibility to infection
Leukopenia
CARDIOVASCULAR FINDINGS
Cardiac dysrhythmias
Development of collateral circulation
Fatigue
Hyperkinetic circulation
Peripheral edema
Portal hypertension
Spider angiomas
PULMONARY FINDINGS
Dyspnea
Hydrothorax
Hyperventilation
Hypoxemia
HEMATOLOGIC FINDINGS
Anemia
Disseminated intravascular coagulation
Impaired coagulation
Splenomegaly
Thrombocytopenia
DERMATOLOGIC FINDINGS
Axillary and pubic hair changes
Caput medusae
Ecchymosis
Increased skin pigmentation
Jaundice
Palmar erythema
Pruritus
Spider angiomas
FLUID AND ELECTROLYTE DISTURBANCES
Ascites
Decreased effective blood volume
Dilutional hyponatremia or hypernatremia
Hypocalcemia
Hypokalemia
Peripheral edema
Water retention

Fig. 61-1 • The clinical picture of a patient with liver dysfunction. Manifestations vary according to the progression of the disease.

increased abdominal distention can interfere with lung expansion. The patient may have difficulty maintaining an erect body posture, and problems with balance may affect walking. Inspect and palpate for the presence of inguinal or umbilical hernias, which are likely to develop because of increased intra-abdominal pressure.

Minimal ascites is often more difficult to detect, especially in the obese patient. Advanced assessment techniques, such as the percussion test for shifting dullness and the presence of a fluid wave, may be performed by the health care provider.

When performing an assessment of the abdomen, keep in mind that **hepatomegaly** (liver enlargement) occurs in many cases of early cirrhosis. Splenomegaly is common in nonalcoholic causes of cirrhosis. As the liver deteriorates, it may become hard and small. The advanced practice nurse or other health care provider palpates the right upper quadrant for hepatomegaly below the costal (rib cage) border. It may also be assessed by percussing for dullness over the enlarged liver.

Measure the patient's abdominal girth to evaluate the progression of ascites (Fig. 61-2). To measure abdominal girth, the patient lies flat while the nurse or other examiner pulls a tape measure around the largest diameter (usually over the umbilicus) of the abdomen. The girth is measured at the end of exhalation. Mark the abdominal skin and flanks to ensure the same tape measure placement on subsequent readings. *Taking daily weights, however, is the most reliable indicator of fluid retention.*

Other Physical Assessment. Observe vomitus and stool for blood. This may be indicated by frank blood in the excrement or by a positive fecal occult blood test (FOBT) (Hema-Check, Hematest). Gastritis, stomach ulceration, or oozing esophageal varices may be responsible for the blood in the stool.

Note the presence of **fetor hepaticus,** which is the distinctive breath odor of chronic liver disease and portal-systemic encephalopathy (PSE) and is characterized by a fruity or musty odor. Fetor hepaticus results from the inability of the damaged liver to metabolize and detoxify mercaptan, which is produced by bacterial breakdown of methionine, a sulfurous amino acid.

Amenorrhea (no menstrual period) may occur in women, and men may exhibit testicular atrophy, **gynecomastia** (en-

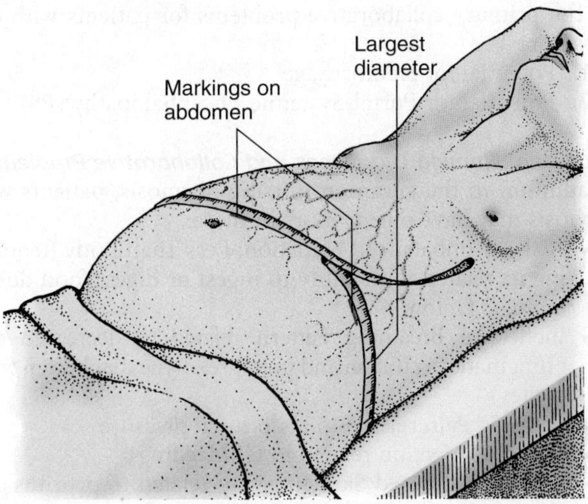
Largest diameter
Markings on abdomen

Fig. 61-2 • How to measure abdominal girth. With the patient supine, bring the tape measure around the patient and take a measurement at the level of the umbilicus. Before removing the tape, mark the abdomen along the sides of the tape on the patient's flanks (sides) and midline to ensure that later measurements are taken in the same place.

larged breasts), and impotence as a result of inactive hormones. Patients with problems of the hematologic system caused by hepatic failure may have bruising and petechiae (small, purplish hemorrhagic spots on the skin).

Continually assess the patient's neurologic function. Subtle changes in mental status and personality often progress to coma, a late complication of PSE. Monitor for **asterixis,** a coarse tremor characterized by rapid, nonrhythmic extensions and flexions in the wrists and fingers.

Psychosocial Assessment

The patient with hepatic cirrhosis may undergo subtle or obvious personality, cognitive, and behavior changes, such as agitation. He or she may experience sleep pattern disturbances or may exhibit signs of emotional lability (fluctuations in emotions), euphoria (a very elevated mood), or depression. A psychosocial assessment identifies needs and helps guide care.

Repeated hospitalizations are common for patients with cirrhosis. It is a life-altering chronic disease, impacting not only the patient but also the immediate and extended family members. There are significant emotional, physical, and financial changes. Substance abuse may continue even as health worsens. It is important, whenever possible, to use resources available to these patients and their families. Collaborate with social workers, substance abuse counselors, and mental health/behavioral health care professionals as needed for patient assessment and management.

Laboratory Assessment

Laboratory study abnormalities are common in patients with liver disease (Table 61-4). Serum levels of aspartate aminotransferase (AST), alanine aminotransferase (ALT), and lactate dehydrogenase (LDH) may be elevated because these enzymes are released into the blood during hepatic inflammation. However, as the liver deteriorates, the hepatocytes may be unable to create an inflammatory response and the AST and ALT may be normal. ALT levels are more specific to the liver because AST can

TABLE 61-4 Assessment of Abnormal Laboratory Findings in Liver Disease

Abnormal Finding	Significance
SERUM ENZYMES	
Elevated serum aspartate aminotransferase (AST)	Hepatic cell destruction, hepatitis (most specific indicator)
Elevated serum alanine aminotransferase (ALT)	Hepatic cell destruction, hepatitis
Elevated lactate dehydrogenase (LDH)	Hepatic cell destruction
Elevated serum alkaline phosphatase	Obstructive jaundice, hepatic metastasis
BILIRUBIN	
Elevated serum total bilirubin	Hepatic cell disease
Elevated serum direct conjugated bilirubin	Hepatitis, liver metastasis
Elevated serum indirect unconjugated bilirubin	Cirrhosis
Elevated urine bilirubin	Hepatocellular obstruction, viral or toxic liver disease
Elevated urine urobilinogen	Hepatic dysfunction
Decreased fecal urobilinogen	Obstructive liver disease
SERUM PROTEINS	
Increased serum total protein	Acute liver disease
Decreased serum total protein	Chronic liver disease
Decreased serum albumin	Severe liver disease
Elevated serum globulin	Immune response to liver disease
OTHER TESTS	
Elevated serum ammonia	Advanced liver disease or portal-systemic encephalopathy (PSE)
Prolonged prothrombin time (PT) or international normalized ratio (INR)	Hepatic cell damage and decreased synthesis of prothrombin

be found in muscle, kidney, brain, and heart. An AST/ALT ratio greater than 2 is usually found in alcoholic liver disease.

Alkaline phosphatase and gamma-glutamyl transpeptidase (GGT) levels are caused by biliary obstruction and therefore may increase in patients with cirrhosis (Kelso, 2008). However, alkaline phosphatase also increases when bone disease is present. Total serum bilirubin levels also rise. Indirect bilirubin levels increase in patients with cirrhosis because of the inability of the failing liver to excrete bilirubin. Therefore bilirubin is present in the urine (urobilinogen) in increased amounts. Fecal urobilinogen concentration is decreased in patients with biliary tract obstruction. These patients have light- or clay-colored stools.

Total serum protein and albumin levels are decreased in patients with severe or chronic liver disease as a result of decreased synthesis by the liver. Prothrombin time/international normalized ratio (PT/INR) is prolonged because the liver decreases the production of prothrombin. The platelet count is low resulting in a characteristic thrombocytopenia of cirrhosis. Anemia may be reflected by decreased red blood cell (RBC), hemoglobin, and hematocrit values. The white blood cell (WBC) count may also be decreased. Ammonia levels are usually elevated in patients with advanced liver disease. Serum creatinine may be elevated in patients with deteriorating kidney function. Dilutional hyponatremia (low serum sodium) is common in patients with ascites.

Imaging Assessment

Plain x-rays of the abdomen may show hepatomegaly, splenomegaly, or massive ascites. A computed tomography (CT) scan may be requested.

Magnetic resonance imaging (MRI) is another test used to diagnose the patient with liver disease. It can reveal mass lesions, giving additional specific information. This information is helpful in determining whether the condition is malignant or benign.

Other Diagnostic Assessment

Ultrasound (US) of the liver is often the first assessment for a person with suspected liver disease to detect ascites, hepatomegaly, and splenomegaly. It can also determine the presence of biliary stones or biliary duct obstruction. Liver US is useful in detecting portal vein thrombosis and evaluating whether the direction of portal blood flow is normal.

Some patients being assessed for liver disease require biopsies to determine the exact pathology and the extent of disease progression. This procedure can be problematic because a large number of patients are at risk for bleeding. Even a **percutaneous** (through the skin) biopsy can pose a significant risk to the patient. To minimize this risk, an interventional radiologist can perform a liver biopsy using a long sheath through a jugular vein that then is threaded into the hepatic vein and liver. A tissue sample is obtained for microscopic evaluation. If a biopsy procedure is not possible, a radioisotope liver scan may be used to identify cirrhosis or other diffuse disease.

The physician may request arteriography if US is not conclusive in finding portal vein thrombosis. To evaluate the portal vein and its branches, a portal venogram may be performed instead by passing a catheter into the liver and into the portal vein. This procedure is described on p. 1354 in the Transjugular Intrahepatic Portal-Systemic Shunt section.

The physician may perform an **esophagogastroduodenoscopy (EGD)** to directly visualize the upper GI tract and to detect the presence of bleeding or oozing esophageal varices, stomach irritation and ulceration, or duodenal ulceration and bleeding. EGD is performed by introducing a flexible fiberoptic endoscope into the mouth, esophagus, and stomach while the patient is under moderate sedation. A camera attached to the scope permits direct visualization of the mucosal lining of the upper GI tract. An **endoscopic retrograde cholangiopancreatography (ERCP)** uses the endoscope to inject contrast material via the sphincter of Oddi to view the biliary tract and allow for stone removals, sphincterotomies, biopsies, and stent placements if required. These procedures are described in more detail in Chapter 55.

▪ *Analysis*

Common Nursing Diagnoses and Collaborative Problems

The most common nursing diagnosis for patients with cirrhosis is Excess Fluid Volume related to edema (portal hypertension).

The primary collaborative problems for patients with cirrhosis are:

1. Potential for Hemorrhage
2. Potential for Portal-Systemic Encephalopathy (PSE)

Additional Nursing Diagnoses and Collaborative Problems

In addition to the common nursing diagnosis, patients with cirrhosis may have one or more of these:

- Risk for Imbalanced Nutrition: Less Than Body Requirements related to inability to ingest or digest food due to biologic factors
- Ineffective Breathing Pattern related to decreased diaphragmatic excursion and pressure on the diaphragm from ascites
- Chronic Pain related to abdominal pressure
- Risk for Infection related to GI bleeding
- Risk for Impaired Skin Integrity related to pruritus and altered nutritional state
- Ineffective Coping related to a chronic and potentially fatal disease
- Sexual Dysfunction related to altered hormonal function and decreased libido
- Disturbed Body Image related to biophysical changes (distended abdomen and skin lesions)

Additional collaborative problems include:

- Potential for Drug Toxicity
- Potential for Hepatorenal Syndrome
- Potential for Hepatopulmonary Syndrome
- Potential for Spontaneous Bacterial Peritonitis
- Potential for Hyponatremia
- Potential for Hypokalemia

▪ *Planning and Implementation*

Excess Fluid Volume

NOC **Planning: Expected Outcomes.** The patient with cirrhosis is expected to have water balance in the intracellular and extracellular compartments of the body. Indicators include that the patient will have:

- Normal blood pressure
- Normal peripheral pulses
- Normal mean arterial pressure
- 24-hour intake and output balance
- Stable body weight
- Normal serum electrolytes
- Normal hematocrit

Interventions. Fluid accumulations are minimal during the early stages of ascites, and therefore interventions are aimed at preventing the accumulation of additional fluid and moving the existing fluid collection. Nonsurgical treatment measures are used to treat ascites. (See the Concept Map for liver failure on p. 1351.)

Nonsurgical Management. Supportive measures to control abdominal ascites include nutrition therapy, drug therapy, paracentesis, and comfort measures. The patient's fluid and electrolyte status is also carefully monitored. If the patient is jaundiced, he or she will likely scratch the skin because the excess bilirubin products cause irritation and pruritus (itching). Teach the patient to use cool rather than warm water on the skin and to not use an excessive amount of soap. Teach unlicensed assistive personnel to use lotion to soothe the skin. Assess for open skins areas from scratching.

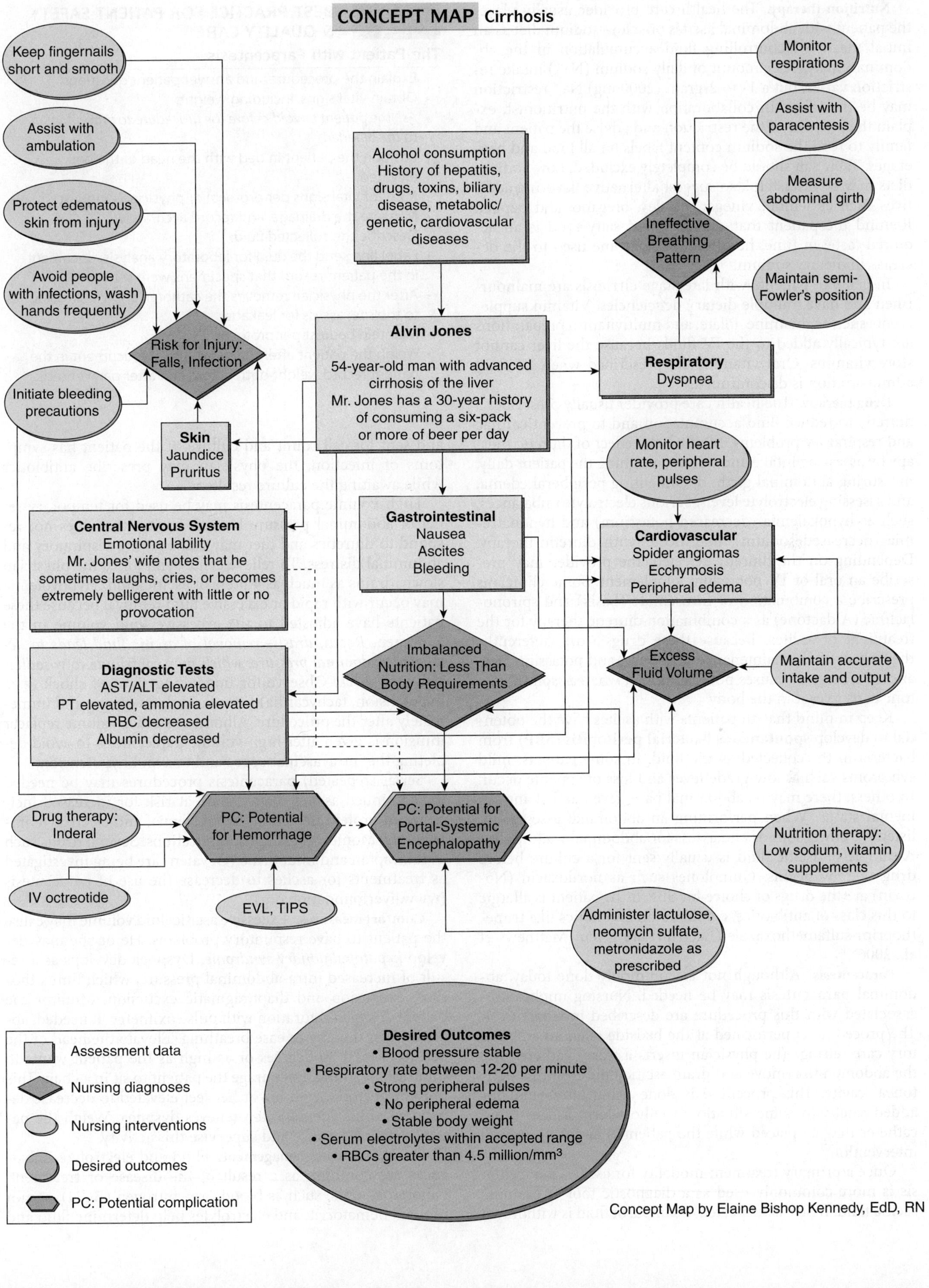
CONCEPT MAP Cirrhosis
Keep fingernails short and smooth
Assist with ambulation
Protect edematous skin from injury
Avoid people with infections, wash hands frequently
Risk for Injury: Falls, Infection
Initiate bleeding precautions
Skin
Jaundice
Pruritus
Alcohol consumption
History of hepatitis, drugs, toxins, biliary disease, metabolic/ genetic, cardiovascular diseases
Alvin Jones
54-year-old man with advanced cirrhosis of the liver
Mr. Jones has a 30-year history of consuming a six-pack or more of beer per day
Monitor respirations
Assist with paracentesis
Measure abdominal girth
Ineffective Breathing Pattern
Maintain semi-Fowler's position
Respiratory
Dyspnea
Monitor heart rate, peripheral pulses
Cardiovascular
Spider angiomas
Ecchymosis
Peripheral edema
Excess Fluid Volume
Maintain accurate intake and output
Gastrointestinal
Nausea
Ascites
Bleeding
Central Nervous System
Emotional lability
Mr. Jones' wife notes that he sometimes laughs, cries, or becomes extremely belligerent with little or no provocation
Diagnostic Tests
AST/ALT elevated
PT elevated, ammonia elevated
RBC decreased
Albumin decreased
Imbalanced Nutrition: Less Than Body Requirements
Drug therapy: Inderal
PC: Potential for Hemorrhage
PC: Potential for Portal-Systemic Encephalopathy
Nutrition therapy: Low sodium, vitamin supplements
IV octreotide
EVL, TIPS
Administer lactulose, neomycin sulfate, metronidazole as prescribed
Assessment data
Nursing diagnoses
Nursing interventions
Desired outcomes
PC: Potential complication
Desired Outcomes
• Blood pressure stable
• Respiratory rate between 12-20 per minute
• Strong peripheral pulses
• No peripheral edema
• Stable body weight
• Serum electrolytes within accepted range
• RBCs greater than 4.5 million/mm3
Concept Map by Elaine Bishop Kennedy, EdD, RN

Nutrition therapy. The health care provider usually places the patient with abdominal ascites on a low-sodium diet as an initial means of controlling fluid accumulation in the abdominal cavity. The amount of daily sodium (Na^+) intake restriction varies, but a 1- to 2-gram (2000 mg) Na^+ restriction may be tried first. In collaboration with the nutritionist, explain the purpose of the restriction and advise the patient and family to read the sodium content labels on all food and beverages. Table salt should be completely excluded. Low-sodium diets may be distasteful, so suggest alternative flavoring additives such as lemon, vinegar, parsley, oregano, and pepper. Remind the patient that seasoned and salty food is an acquired taste; in time, he or she will become used to the decrease in dietary sodium.

In general, patients with late-stage cirrhosis are malnourished and have multiple dietary deficiencies. Vitamin supplements such as thiamine, folate, and multivitamin preparations are typically added to the IV fluids because the liver cannot store vitamins. Oral vitamins are prescribed when IV fluid administration is discontinued.

Drug therapy. The health care provider usually prescribes a diuretic to reduce fluid accumulation and to prevent cardiac and respiratory problems. Monitor the effect of diuretic therapy by assessing intake and output, weighing the patient daily, measuring abdominal girth, documenting peripheral edema, and assessing electrolyte levels. Serious electrolyte imbalances, such as hypokalemia (decreased potassium) and hyponatremia (decreased sodium), may occur with diuretic therapy. Depending on the diuretic selected, the provider may prescribe an oral or IV potassium supplement. Some clinicians prescribe a combination of furosemide (Lasix) and spironolactone (Aldactone) as a combination diuretic therapy for the treatment of ascites. Because these drugs work differently, they are used for maintenance of sodium and potassium balance. Furosemide causes potassium loss, whereas spironolactone conserves it in the body.

Keep in mind that all patients with ascites have the potential to develop **spontaneous bacterial peritonitis (SBP)** from bacteria in the collected ascitic fluid. In some patients, mild symptoms such as low-grade fever and loss of appetite occur. In others, there may be abdominal pain, fever, and change in mental status. When performing an abdominal assessment, listen for bowel sounds and assess for abdominal wall rigidity. A sample of ascitic fluid is usually sent for a culture before drug therapy begins. Quinolones such as norfloxacin (Noroxin) are the drugs of choice for SBP. If the patient is allergic to this class of antibiotics, combination antibiotics like trimethoprim-sulfamethoxazole (Bactrim) are given (Matthews et al., 2006).

Paracentesis. Although not as commonly done today, abdominal **paracentesis** may be needed. Nursing implications associated with this procedure are described in Chart 61-1. The procedure is performed at the bedside or in an ambulatory care setting. The physician inserts a trocar catheter into the abdomen to remove and drain ascitic fluid from the peritoneal cavity. This procedure is done using ultrasound for added safety. In some situations, a short-term ascites drain catheter may be placed while the patient is awaiting surgical intervention.

Once a primary treatment modality for ascites, paracentesis is more commonly used as a diagnostic tool to examine ascitic fluid. If SBP is suspected, a sample of fluid is withdrawn and sent for cell count and culture. If the patient has symptoms of infection, the physician may prescribe antibiotics while awaiting the culture results.

Chart 61-1 BEST PRACTICE FOR PATIENT SAFETY & QUALITY CARE

The Patient with Paracentesis

- Explain the procedure, and answer patient questions.
- Obtain vital signs, including weight.
- *Ask the patient to void before the procedure to prevent injury to the bladder!*
- Position the patient in bed with the head of the bed elevated.
- Monitor vital signs per protocol or physician's request.
- Measure the drainage, and record accurately.
- Describe the collected fluid.
- Label and send the fluid for laboratory analysis; document in the patient record that specimens were sent.
- After the physician removes the catheter, apply a dressing to the site; assess for leakage.
- Maintain bedrest per protocol.
- Weigh the patient after the paracentesis; document in the patient record weight both before and after paracentesis.

High-volume paracentesis may be used for temporary relief of abdominal pressure because ascites that does not respond to diuretics and diet may cause severe respiratory and abdominal distress. To relieve acute symptoms, the physician slowly drains as much as 4 liters of ascitic fluid. Hypovolemia may occur with rapid or excessive fluid removal because these patients have adjusted to the excessive fluid volume in the abdomen. *Rapid, drastic removal of ascitic fluid leads to decreased abdominal pressure, which may contribute to vasodilation and shock.* Observe for impending signs of shock (e.g., hypotension, tachycardia) from fluid shifts during and immediately after the procedure. Albumin or other volume replacer infusion is given after high-volume paracentesis to avoid depleting the intravascular space and to avoid hypotension.

Serial (repeated) paracentesis procedures may be needed for continued ascites. Patients are at risk for increased incidence of protein depletion, hypovolemia, and electrolyte imbalances. Monitor for these complications. Several drugs such as satavaptan and midodrine (Orvaten) are being investigated as treatments for ascites to decrease the use of paracentesis (www.liverfoundation.org).

Comfort measures. Excessive ascitic fluid volume may cause the patient to have respiratory problems. He or she may develop *hepatopulmonary syndrome*. Dyspnea develops as a result of increased intra-abdominal pressure, which limits thoracic expansion and diaphragmatic excursion. Monitor the patient's oxygen saturation with pulse oximetry. If needed, apply oxygen therapy to ease breathing. Elevate the head of the bed to at least 30 degrees or as high as the patient wants to improve breathing. Encourage the patient to sit in a chair. This upright position, with his or her feet elevated to decrease dependent ankle edema, often relieves dyspnea. Weigh the patient daily or delegate and supervise this activity.

NIC **Fluid/electrolyte management.** Fluid and electrolyte imbalances are common as a result of the disease or treatment. Laboratory tests, such as blood urea nitrogen (BUN), serum protein, hematocrit, and electrolytes help determine fluid and

Chart 61-2 NIC INTERVENTION ACTIVITIES

The Patient with Cirrhosis

Fluid/Electrolyte Management: *Regulation and prevention of complications from altered fluid and/or electrolyte levels*

- Obtain laboratory specimens for monitoring of altered fluid and electrolyte levels (e.g., hematocrit, BUN, protein, sodium, and potassium levels), as appropriate.
- Keep an accurate record of intake and output.
- Weigh patient daily, and monitor trends.
- Monitor for signs and symptoms of fluid retention.
- Monitor vital signs, as appropriate.
- Administer prescribed supplemental electrolytes, as appropriate.

Bleeding Precautions: *Reduction of stimuli that may induce bleeding or hemorrhage in at-risk patients*

- Monitor the patient closely for hemorrhage.
- Monitor for signs and symptoms of persistent bleeding (e.g., check all secretions for frank or occult blood).
- Monitor coagulation studies, including prothrombin time (PT), partial thromboplastin time (PTT), fibrinogen, fibrin degradation/split products, and platelet counts, as appropriate.
- Monitor orthostatic vital signs, including blood pressure.
- Use electric razor, instead of straight-edge, for shaving.
- Use soft toothbrush or toothettes for oral care.
- Avoid injections (IV, IM, or subcutaneous), as appropriate.
- Protect the patient from trauma, which may cause bleeding.

Neurologic Monitoring: *Collection and analysis of patient data to prevent or minimize neurologic complications*

- Monitor level of consciousness.
- Monitor level of orientation.
- Monitor recent memory, attention span, past memory, mood, affect, and behaviors.
- Monitor vital signs: temperature, blood pressure, pulse, and respirations.

NIC intervention activities selected from Bulechek, G.M., Butcher, H.K., McCloskey Dochterman, J. (Eds.). (2008). *Nursing interventions classification (NIC)* (5th ed.). St. Louis: Mosby. No part of this work is to be altered without prior written permission from the Publisher.

BUN, Blood urea nitrogen.

electrolyte status. Other nursing intervention activities are listed in Chart 61-2.

Surgical Management. When medical management fails to control ascites, the physician may choose surgical intervention to divert ascites into the venous system by creating a shunt. Older shunts such as portacaval and peritoneovenous shunts to divert fluid away from the diseased liver into the venous system are rarely done today because of serious potential complications. Patients with ascites are poor surgical risks. The transjugular intrahepatic portal-systemic shunt (TIPS) is a nonsurgical procedure that is used to control long-term ascites and to reduce variceal bleeding. This procedure is described in the discussion of Interventions at right in the Potential for Hemorrhage section.

The patient with cirrhosis has many medical problems. An optimal physical state is desired before surgery is performed. Electrolyte imbalances are corrected, and abnormal coagulation is treated with the administration of fresh frozen plasma and vitamin K. Packed red blood cells are made available for transfusion, because these patients have bleeding tendencies.

Provide the usual preoperative and postoperative care for a patient undergoing abdominal surgery (see Chapters 16 and 18). Remain aware that the ascitic fluid is routed into the venous system, resulting in vascular volume expansion and hemodilution. Monitor vital signs carefully and frequently as per surgeon protocol; an increase in blood pressure reflects an increase in vascular volume. Auscultate breath sounds for the presence of crackles, which indicates excessive lung fluid. A diuretic such as furosemide (Lasix) is usually prescribed to rid the body of excessive fluid. Note any abnormal results of coagulation studies (prothrombin time [PT]/INR and partial thromboplastin time [PTT]). Delegate and supervise nursing activities such as weighing the patient, measuring abdominal girth, and recording urine output each shift to determine the effectiveness of the shunting procedure.

Potential for Hemorrhage

Planning: Expected Outcomes. The patient is expected to be free of bleeding episodes. However, if the patient has a hemorrhage, it is expected to be controlled by prompt, evidence-based interdisciplinary interventions.

Interventions. All patients with cirrhosis should be screened for esophageal varices by endoscopy to detect them early *before they bleed.* If patients have varices, they are placed on preventive therapy (Herrine, 2007). If acute bleeding occurs, early interventions are used to manage it. *Because massive esophageal bleeding can cause rapid blood loss, emergency interventions are needed.*

The role of drug therapy is to *prevent* bleeding in patients who have varices. A nonselective beta-blocking agent such as propranolol (Inderal) or nadolol (Corgard) with or without a nitrate is usually prescribed. The patient starts on a low dose that is increased every 3 to 5 days until the heart rate is about 55 beats per minute. By decreasing heart rate and the hepatic venous pressure gradient, the chance of bleeding may be reduced.

If bleeding occurs, the health care team intervenes quickly to control it by providing interventions such as infused vasoactive therapy or endoscopic procedure. After the acute bleeding episode has been controlled, the patient may require a transjugular intrahepatic portal-systemic shunt (TIPS) to decrease portal hypertension, thereby decreasing the risk for further variceal bleeding. The patient is managed in the critical care unit.

Short-term esophagogastric balloon tamponade using a Minnesota or Sengstaken-Blakemore tube is not commonly used today because it is difficult to use, uncomfortable for the patient, and prone to dangerous complications. However, it may be needed if the patient is not able to have an endoscopy or TIPS procedure. Similar to a nasogastric tube, the tube is placed through the nose and into the stomach. An attached balloon is inflated to apply pressure to the bleeding variceal area. Before this tamponade, the patient is usually intubated and placed on a mechanical ventilator to protect the airway (Kelso, 2008). Some patients may need liver transplantation to prevent further bleeding episodes.

Vasoactive Therapy. IV octreotide (Sandostatin), a somatostatin analogue, is the most common drug used in the United States for acute hemorrhage due to esophageal varices. Terlipressin (Lucassin) is used in other countries and is a more effective agent. It is also being tested for the treatment of hepatorenal syndrome. For varices, the purpose of these drugs is to constrict the blood vessels to stop the bleeding episode.

Endoscopic Procedures. Esophageal varices also may be managed with **endoscopic variceal ligation (EVL) (banding).** In some cases, patients who cannot tolerate beta blocker preventive therapy may also have this treatment. This procedure involves the application of small "O" bands around the base of the varices to decrease the blood supply to the varices. The patient is unaware of the bands, and they cause no discomfort.

Endoscopic sclerotherapy (EST), also called injection **sclerotherapy,** may be done to stop bleeding. The varices are injected with a sclerosing agent via a catheter. This procedure is associated with complications such as mucosal ulceration, which could result in further bleeding. Because of the lower potential for treatment-related side effects, EVL is preferred over EST.

Transjugular Intrahepatic Portal-Systemic Shunt. The transjugular intrahepatic portal-systemic shunt (TIPS) is a nonsurgical procedure performed in interventional radiology departments. This procedure is used for patients who have not responded to other modalities for hemorrhage or long-term ascites. If time permits, patients have a Doppler ultrasound to assess vein anatomy and patency. The patient receives heavy IV sedation or moderate general anesthesia for this procedure. The radiologist places a large sheath through the jugular vein. A needle is guided through the sheath and pushed through the liver into the portal vein. A balloon enlarges this tract, and a stent keeps it open. Most patients also have an ultrasound Doppler study of the liver after the TIPS procedure to record the blood flow through the shunt.

Serious complications of TIPS are not common. Patients are discharged in 1 or 2 days and are followed up with ultrasounds for the first year after the shunt is placed. About one third of them need to be re-opened once during the first year as an ambulatory care procedure.

Other Interventions. Depending on the procedure done to control esophageal bleeding, patients may have a nasogastric tube (NGT) inserted to detect any new bleeding episodes. Patients usually receive packed red blood cells, fresh frozen plasma, isotonic saline, and platelets through large-bore IV catheters. Antibiotic therapy should be prescribed because a large number of patients who bleed develop an infection (Garcia-Tsao et al., 2007).

Monitor vital signs every hour and coagulation studies, including prothrombin time (PT), partial thromboplastin time (PTT), platelet count, and international normalized ratio (INR). Chart 61-2 lists additional interventions for patients at risk for bleeding.

A small number of patients with cirrhosis bleed from gastric varices. Interventions for upper GI bleeding are discussed in Chapter 59.

Potential for Portal-Systemic Encephalopathy

Planning: Expected Outcomes. The patient is expected to be managed early to prevent this complication. However, if it occurs, it is expected that the interdisciplinary team will intervene early to prevent further health problems or death.

Interventions. The mechanisms that cause portal-systemic encephalopathy (PSE) are not completely clear, but ammonia probably plays a significant role. The poorly functioning liver cannot convert ammonia and other byproducts of metabolism to a less toxic form. They are carried by the circulatory system to the brain where they affect cerebral function. The aim of PSE management is to halt this process.

Because ammonia is formed in the GI tract by the action of bacteria on protein, nonsurgical treatment measures to decrease ammonia production include nutrition limitations and drug therapy to reduce bacterial breakdown. Collaborate with the nutritionist, pharmacist, and physician to plan and implement these interventions.

Nutrition Therapy. Patients with cirrhosis have increased nutritional requirements—high-carbohydrate, moderate-fat, and high-protein foods. However, the diet is often changed for those who have elevated serum ammonia levels with signs of PSE. Patients should have a moderate amount of protein and fat foods and simple carbohydrates. Previously used protein restrictions are no longer required because patients need protein for healing (Matthews et al., 2006). In collaboration with the nutritionist, be sure to include family members or significant others in nutrition counseling. The patient is often weak and unable to remember complicated guidelines. Brief, simple directions regarding dietary dos and don'ts are recommended. Keep in mind any financial, cultural, or personal preferences when discussing food choices, including the patient's food allergies.

When a patient with cirrhosis has GI bleeding, it can result in the formation of increased amounts of ammonia as intestinal bacteria attempt to metabolize the blood cells. GI bleeding may lead to hepatic coma (stage IV of PSE).

Drug Therapy. Drugs are used sparingly because they are difficult for the failing liver to metabolize. In particular, opioid analgesics, sedatives, and barbiturates should be restricted, especially for the patient with a history of encephalopathy.

Several types of drugs, however, can eliminate or reduce ammonia levels in the body. These include lactulose (e.g., Evalose, Heptalac) or lactilol and nonabsorbable antibiotics.

The health care provider prescribes *lactulose* (or lactitol) to promote the excretion of ammonia in the stool. This drug is a viscous, sticky, sweet-tasting liquid that is given either orally or by NG tube. The purpose is to obtain a laxative effect. Cleansing the bowels rids the intestinal tract of the toxins that contribute to encephalopathy. It works by increasing osmotic pressure to draw fluid into the colon and prevents absorption of ammonia in the colon. The drug may be prescribed to the patient who has manifested signs of PSE, regardless of the stage. The desired effect of the drug is production of two or three soft stools per day and a decrease in patient confusion caused by PSE.

Observe for response to lactulose. The patient may report intestinal bloating and cramping. Serum ammonia levels may be monitored but do not always correlate with symptoms. Hypokalemia and dehydration may result from excessive stools. Remind unlicensed nursing personnel to help the patient with skin care if needed to prevent breakdown caused by excessive stools.

Several *nonabsorbable antibiotics* may be given if lactulose does not help the patient meet the desired outcome or if he or she cannot tolerate the drug. These drugs should not be given together. Older adults can become weak and dehydrated from having multiple stools. Neomycin sulfate (Mycifradin), a broad-spectrum antibiotic, may be given to act as an intestinal antiseptic. It destroys the normal flora in the bowel, diminishing protein breakdown and decreasing the rate of ammonia production. Maintenance doses of neomycin are given orally but may also be administered as a retention enema. Long-term use has the potential for kidney toxicity and therefore is not commonly used. It cannot be used for patients with existing kidney disease.

Metronidazole (Flagyl, Novonidazole♣) is another broad-spectrum antibiotic with similar action to neomycin, but it has less potential for renal toxicity. However, it should also be used for a short period of time and is therefore not commonly used. Rifaximin (Xifaxan) seems to be the most effective and safest for long-term use, but it is not yet FDA approved for PSE. However, many health care providers have used it successfully for their patients.

Frequently assess for changes in level of consciousness and orientation (see Chart 61-2). Check for asterixis (liver flap) and fetor hepaticus (liver breath). These signs suggest worsening encephalopathy.

DECISION-MAKING CHALLENGE

Coordination of Care

A 55-year-old cirrhotic patient is admitted to the general medical unit of the community hospital where you work with new-onset dyspnea, possible pneumonia, and open skin areas and bruises on both arms. During his interview, you find out that he is taking Aldactone, Lactulose, and Corgard. He has had cirrhosis for at least 5 years but continues to drink 12 beers every night. He is self-employed, and his 22-year-old daughter helps him in the office part-time. She tells you that she is very angry that he has continued to drink even though he knows he is supposed to avoid alcohol. At times he has been disoriented and had memory problems.

1. How should you respond to the patient's daughter?
2. What laboratory findings do you expect will be abnormal in view of his diagnosis? Why?
3. What is the priority for this man's care at this time? What interventions should you implement?
4. With what members of the interdisciplinary team should you collaborate to help this patient return home?

evolve For suggested answer guidelines, go to http://evolve.elsevier.com/Iggy/.

Community-Based Care

If the patient with late-stage cirrhosis survives life-threatening complications, he or she is usually discharged to the home or to a long-term care facility after treatment measures have managed the acute medical problems. A home care referral may be needed if the patient is discharged to the home. These chronically ill patients are often readmitted multiple times, and community-based care is aimed at preventing rehospitalization. Some may benefit from hospice care. Collaborate with the case manager (CM) or other discharge planner to coordinate interdisciplinary continuing care.

Home Care Management

In collaboration with the patient, family, and CM, assess physical adaptations needed to prepare the patient's home for recovery. Referrals for physical therapy, nutrition therapy, and transportation for physician and laboratory follow-up may be needed. The patient's rest area needs to be close to a bathroom because diuretic and/or lactulose therapy increases the frequency of urination and stools. If the patient has difficulty reaching the toilet, additional equipment (e.g., bedside commode) is necessary. Special, adult-size incontinence pads or briefs may be helpful if the patient has an altered mental status and has incontinence. If the patient has shortness of breath from massive ascites, elevating the head of the bed and maintaining the patient in a semi-Fowler's to high Fowler's position may help alleviate respiratory distress. Alternatively, a reclining chair with a foot elevator may be used.

Health Teaching

The patient is discharged to the home setting with an individualized teaching plan (Chart 61-3) that includes nutrition therapy, drug therapy, and alcohol abstinence.

In collaboration with the nutritionist and in keeping with the patient's financial, cultural, and personal food preferences, provide information on eating a well-balanced diet. The patient with portal-systemic encephalopathy (PSE) often finds that small, frequent meals are best tolerated. If the patient's nutritional intake or albumin/pre-albumin is decreased after discharge, multivitamin supplements and supplemental liquid feedings (e.g., Ensure, Boost) are usually needed. Teach patients to be careful with vitamins and minerals that can be toxic to the liver, such as megadose vitamin A, excessive iron supplements, and niacin (Matthews et al., 2006). Remind them to check labels for these substances before taking any vitamin supplement.

The patient is often discharged while receiving diuretics. Provide instructions regarding the health care provider's prescription for the diuretic. Teach about side effects of therapy, such as hypokalemia. The patient may need to take a potassium supplement if he or she is taking a diuretic that is not potassium-sparing.

If the patient has had problems with bleeding from gastric ulcers, the provider may prescribe an H_2-receptor antagonist agent or proton pump inhibitor to reduce acid reflux. Patients who have had episodes of spontaneous bacterial peritonitis (SBP) may be on a daily maintenance antibiotic. Because some patients may have alienated relatives over the years because of substance abuse, it may be necessary to help them identify a friend, neighbor, or person in their recovery group for support.

Chart 61-3 PATIENT AND FAMILY EDUCATION GUIDE

Cirrhosis

NUTRITION THERAPY

- Consume a diet that adheres to the guidelines set by your physician, nurse, or nutritionist.
- If you have excessive fluid in your abdomen, follow the low-sodium diet prescribed for you.
- Eat small, frequent meals that are nutritionally well balanced.
- Include in your diet daily supplemental liquids (e.g., Ensure or Ensure Plus) and a multivitamin.

DRUG THERAPY

- Take the diuretics or preventive beta blocker prescribed for you. If you experience muscle weakness, irregular heartbeat, or light-headedness, contact your health care provider right away.
- Take the medication prescribed for you that helps prevent gastrointestinal bleeding.
- Take the lactulose syrup as prescribed to maintain two or three bowel movements every day.
- Do *not* take any other medication (prescribed or over the counter) unless specifically prescribed by your health care provider.

ALCOHOL ABSTINENCE

- Do not consume any alcohol.
- Seek support services for help if needed.

Teach family members about how to recognize signs of PSE and that it is necessary and safe to increase the daily lactulose at the first sign of encephalopathy. The health care provider should also be contacted. Reinforce that constipation, bleeding, and infections may lead to PSE. Remind them that PSE is usually reversible.

Advise the patient to avoid all over-the-counter drugs, especially NSAIDs and hepatic toxic herbs, vitamins, and minerals. Reinforce the need to keep appointments for follow-up medical care. Remind the patient and family to notify the physician immediately if any GI bleeding (overt bleeding or melena) is noted so that re-evaluation can be initiated quickly.

One of the most important aspects of ongoing care is to stress the need to avoid alcohol and illicit drugs (see Chapter 8). By avoiding alcohol and drugs, the patient may:

- Prevent further fibrosis of the liver from scarring
- Allow the liver to heal and regenerate
- Prevent gastric and esophageal irritation
- Reduce the incidence of bleeding
- Prevent other life-threatening complications

Health Care Resources

The patient with chronic cirrhosis may require a home care nurse for several visits after hospital discharge. The home care nurse can monitor the effectiveness of treatment in controlling ascites. The encephalopathic patient may need to be monitored for adherence to drug therapy and alcohol abstinence. Individual and group therapy sessions may be arranged to assist patients in dealing with alcohol abstinence if they are too ill to attend a formal treatment program. If needed, refer the patient and family to self-help groups, such as Alcoholics Anonymous and Al-Anon. The patient may also desire spiritual support. Finances are frequently a problem for the chronically ill patient and family; social support and community services need to be identified. The American Liver Foundation (www.liverfoundation.org) and American Gastroenterological Association (www.gastro.org) are excellent sources for more information about liver disease.

For patients who are not candidates for liver transplantation, address end-of-life issues. Discuss options such as hospice care with patients and their families. Be aware that they will go through a grieving process and will perhaps be in denial or very angry (see Chapter 9).

▪ *Evaluation: Outcomes*

Evaluate the care of the patient with cirrhosis on the basis of the identified nursing diagnoses and collaborative problems. The expected outcomes include that the patient will:

- Have a decrease in or have no ascites
- Have electrolytes within normal limits (WNL)
- Not have hemorrhage or will be managed immediately if bleeding occurs
- Not develop PSE or will be managed immediately if PSE occurs
- Have the highest quality of life possible
- Successfully abstain from alcohol or drugs (if disease is caused by these substances)

Specific indicators for these outcomes are listed for each nursing diagnosis and collaborative problem in the Planning and Implementation section (see earlier).

HEPATITIS

Pathophysiology

Hepatitis is the widespread inflammation of liver cells. *Viral* hepatitis is the most common type and can be either acute or chronic. Less common types of hepatitis are caused by chemicals, drugs, and some herbs. This section discusses hepatitis caused by a virus. **Viral hepatitis** results from an infection caused by one of five major categories of viruses:

- Hepatitis A virus (HAV)
- Hepatitis B virus (HBV)
- Hepatitis C virus (HCV)
- Hepatitis D virus (HDV)
- Hepatitis E virus (HEV)

Some cases of viral hepatitis are not any of these viruses. These patients have non–A-E hepatitis.

Liver injury with inflammation can also develop after exposure to a number of drugs and chemicals by inhalation, ingestion, or parenteral (IV) administration. **Toxic and drug-induced hepatitis** can result from exposure to hepatotoxins (e.g., industrial toxins, alcohol, and drugs). Hepatitis may also occur as a secondary infection during the course of infections with other viruses, such as Epstein-Barr, herpes simplex, varicella-zoster, and cytomegalovirus.

After the liver has been exposed to causative agents (e.g., a virus), it becomes enlarged and congested with inflammatory cells, lymphocytes, and fluid, resulting in right upper quadrant pain and discomfort. As the disease progresses, the liver's normal lobular pattern becomes distorted as a result of widespread inflammation, necrosis, and hepatocellular regeneration. This distortion increases pressure within the portal circulation, interfering with the blood flow into the hepatic lobules. Edema of the liver's bile channels results in obstructive **jaundice** (yellowing of the skin).

Classification of Hepatitis and Etiologies

The five major types of acute viral hepatitis vary by mode of transmission, manner of onset, and incubation periods. Hepatitis cases must be reported to the local public health department, which then notifies the Centers for Disease Control and Prevention (CDC).

Hepatitis A

The causative agent of **hepatitis A,** hepatitis A virus (HAV), is a ribonucleic acid (RNA) virus of the enterovirus family. *It is a hardy virus and survives on human hands.* The virus is resistant to detergents and acids but is destroyed by chlorine (bleach) and a temperature greater than 195° F (Brundage & Fitzpatrick, 2006).

HAV usually has a mild course similar to that of a typical flu-like infection and often goes unrecognized. It is spread via the fecal-oral route by fecal contamination either from person-to-person contact (e.g., oral-anal sexual activity) or by consuming contaminated food or water. Common sources of infection include shellfish caught in contaminated water and food contaminated by food handlers infected with HAV. The incubation period of hepatitis A is usually 15 to 50 days, with a peak of 25 to 30 days (Brundage & Fitzpatrick, 2006). The disease is usually not life threatening, but its course may be more severe in people older than 40 years and those with pre-existing liver disease such as hepatitis C.

TABLE 61-5 Examples of Extrahepatic Manifestations of Hepatitis A

NEUROLOGIC FINDINGS
• Postviral encephalitis
• Guillian-Barré syndrome
• Transverse myelitis
HEMATOLOGIC FINDINGS
• Aplastic anemia
• Autoimmune hemolysis
• Anemia
RENAL FINDINGS
• Acute tubular necrosis (ATN)
• Nephrotic syndrome
GASTROINTESTINAL FINDINGS
• Pancreatitis
• Acalculous cholecystitis
OTHER FINDINGS
• Reactive arthritis
• Cutaneous vasculitis

In a small percentage of HAV cases, severe illness with extrahepatic manifestations can occur (Table 61-5). Advanced age and conditions such as chronic liver disease may cause widespread damage that requires a liver transplant. In some cases, death may occur from HAV.

The incidence of hepatitis A is particularly high in nonaffluent countries in which sanitation is poor. Children are affected the most, and many of them do not have symptoms. Some adults have hepatitis A and do not know it. The course is similar to that of a GI illness, and the disease and recovery are usually uneventful.

Hepatitis B

The **hepatitis B** virus (HBV) is not transmitted like HAV. It is a double-shelled particle containing DNA composed of a core antigen (HBcAg), a surface antigen (HBsAg), and another antigen found within the core (HBeAg) that circulates in the blood. HBV may be spread through these common modes of transmission:

- Unprotected sexual intercourse with an infected partner
- Sharing needles
- Accidental needle sticks or injuries from sharp instruments primarily in health care workers (low incidence)
- Blood transfusions (that have not been screened for the virus, before 1992)
- Hemodialysis
- Maternal-fetal route (more common in Asia)

The clinical course of hepatitis B may be varied. Symptoms usually occur within 25 to 180 days of exposure and include:

- Anorexia, nausea, and vomiting
- Fever
- Fatigue
- Right upper quadrant pain
- Dark urine with light stool
- Joint pain
- Jaundice

Blood tests confirm the disease, although many people with hepatitis B have no symptoms.

Most adults who get hepatitis B recover, clear the virus from their body, and develop immunity. However, a small percentage of people do not develop immunity and become carriers. **Hepatitis carriers** can infect others even though they are not sick and have no obvious signs of hepatitis B. Chronic carriers are at high risk for cirrhosis and liver cancer. Because of the high number of newcomers from endemic areas, the incidence of hepatitis B has increased in the United States.

Hepatitis C

The causative virus of **hepatitis** C (HCV) is an enveloped, single-stranded RNA virus. Transmission is blood to blood. The rate of sexual transmission is very low in a single-couple relationship but increases with multiple sex partners.

HCV is spread most commonly by:

- Illicit IV drug needle sharing (highest incidence)
- Blood, blood products, or organ transplants received before 1992
- Needle stick injury with HCV-contaminated blood (health care workers at high risk)
- Unsanitary tattoo equipment
- Sharing of intranasal cocaine paraphernalia

The disease is **not** transmitted by casual contact or by intimate household contact. However, those infected are advised not to share razors, toothbrushes, or pierced earrings because microscopic blood may be on these items.

The average incubation period is 7 weeks. Acute infection and illness are not common. Most people are completely unaware that they have been infected. They are asymptomatic and not diagnosed until many months or years after the initial exposure when an abnormality is detected during a routine laboratory evaluation or when liver problems occur. Unlike with hepatitis B, most people infected with hepatitis C do not clear the virus and a chronic infection develops.

HCV usually does its damage over decades by causing a chronic inflammation in the liver that eventually causes the liver cells to scar. This scarring may progress to cirrhosis. Alcohol use increases the progression and severity of cirrhosis.

Hepatitis C–induced cirrhosis is the leading indication for liver transplantation in the United States. Unfortunately, the newly transplanted liver often becomes re-infected with the virus.

Hepatitis D

Hepatitis D (delta hepatitis, or HDV) is caused by a defective RNA virus that needs the helper function of HBV. It occurs only with HBV to cause viral replication. This usually develops into chronic HDV. The incubation period is about 14 to 56 days. As with HBV, the disease is transmitted primarily by parenteral routes, especially patients who are IV drug abusers. Having sexual contact with a person with HDV is also a high risk factor.

Hepatitis E

The **hepatitis E** virus (HEV) is a waterborne infection associated with epidemics of hepatitis in the Indian subcontinent, Asia, Africa, the Middle East, Mexico, and Central and South America. Many large outbreaks have occurred after heavy rains and flooding. Like hepatitis A, HEV is caused by fecal contamination of food and water.

In the United States, hepatitis E has been found only in international travelers. It is transmitted via the fecal-oral route, and the clinical course resembles that of hepatitis A. HEV has an incubation period of 15 to 64 days. There is no evidence at this time of a chronic form of HEV. The disease tends to be self-limiting and resolves on its own.

Complications of Hepatitis

Failure of the liver cells to regenerate, with progression of the necrotic process, results in a severe acute and often fatal form of hepatitis known as **fulminant hepatitis.** Hepatitis is considered to be chronic when liver inflammation lasts longer than 6 months. **Chronic hepatitis** usually occurs as a result of hepatitis B or C. Superimposed infection with hepatitis D (HDV) in patients with chronic HBV may also result in chronic hepatitis. Chronic hepatitis can lead to cirrhosis and liver cancer.

Incidence/Prevalence

The incidence of hepatitis A and hepatitis B is declining as a result of CDC recommendations for vaccination. However, hepatitis B and hepatitis C are a concern because of their association with cirrhosis and liver cancer. Although exact numbers are not known, it is estimated that about 200 million people worldwide have the hepatitis C virus (HCV), making this type of hepatitis the most common type (www.cdc.gov). Currently there is no vaccine for HCV. Therefore it is expected that the cases of HCV will rise over the next several decades as a result of increasing illicit drug use. This increase will require a major increase in transplantations and lead to many more deaths.

Health Promotion and Maintenance

Hepatitis vaccines for infants, children, and adolescents have helped decrease the incidence of hepatitis A and hepatitis B. Some adults are also advised to receive these immunizations.

Measures for preventing hepatitis A (HAV) in adults include:

- Proper handwashing, especially after handling shellfish
- Avoiding contaminated food or water (including tap water in countries with high incidence)
- Receiving immune globulin within 14 days if exposed to the virus
- Receiving the HAV vaccine before traveling to areas where the disease is common (e.g., Mexico, Caribbean)
- Receiving the vaccine if living or working in enclosed areas with others, such as college dormitories, correctional institutions, day-care centers, and long-term care facilities

Two HAV vaccines are available—Havrix and Vaqta. Both are made of inactivated hepatitis A virus and are given in the deltoid muscle.

For hepatitis B (HBV) prevention, a vaccine can also provide protection against the disease. Two vaccines, Engerix-B and Recombivax-HB, are available. Twinrix is a combination HAV and HBV vaccine that is also available for adults. Immunization against HBV should be used for:

- People who have unprotected sexual intercourse with more than one partner
- Men having sex with men (MSM)
- People with any chronic liver disease (such as hepatitis C or cirrhosis)
- People who are exposed to blood or body fluids in the workplace, including health care workers, firefighters, and police

Additional measures to prevent viral hepatitis for health care workers and others in contact with infected patients are listed in Charts 61-4 and 61-5.

Patient-Centered Collaborative Care

Assessment

History

Begin by asking the patient whether he or she has had known exposure to a person with hepatitis. For the patient who presents with few or no symptoms of liver disease but has abnormal laboratory tests (e.g., elevated alanine aminotransferase [ALT] or aspartate aminotransferase [AST] level), the history may need to include additional questions regarding risk factors such as:

- Exposure to either inhaled or ingested chemical
- Use of herbal supplement
- Use of any new prescribed medication or over-the-counter (OTC) medication
- Recent ingestion of shellfish
- Exposure to a possibly contaminated water source
- Travel to another country

Chart 61-4 BEST PRACTICE FOR PATIENT SAFETY & QUALITY CARE

Prevention of Viral Hepatitis in Health Care Workers

- Use Standard Precautions to prevent the transmission of disease between patients or between patients and health care staff (see Chapter 25).
- Eliminate needles and other sharp instruments by substituting needleless systems. (Needle sticks are the major source of hepatitis B transmission in health care workers.)
- Take the hepatitis B vaccine (e.g., Recombivax HB), which is given in a series of three injections. This vaccine also prevents hepatitis D by preventing HBV.
- For postexposure prevention of hepatitis A, seek medical attention immediately for immunoglobulin (Ig) administration.
- Report all cases of hepatitis to the local health department.

Chart 61-5 PATIENT AND FAMILY EDUCATION GUIDE

Health Practices to Prevent Viral Hepatitis

- Maintain adequate sanitation and personal hygiene. Wash your hands before eating and after using the toilet.
- Drink water treated by a water purification system.
- If traveling in underdeveloped or nonindustrialized countries, drink only bottled water. Avoid food washed or prepared with tap water, such as raw vegetables, fruits, and soups. Avoid ice.
- Use adequate sanitation practices to prevent the spread of the disease among family members.
- Do not share bed linens, towels, eating utensils, or drinking glasses.
- Do not share needles for injection, body piercing, or tattooing.
- Do not share razors, nail clippers, toothbrushes, or Waterpiks.
- Use a condom during sexual intercourse, or abstain from this activity.
- Cover cuts or sores with bandages.
- If ever infected with hepatitis, never donate blood, body organs, or other body tissue.

- Sexual activities with men, women, or both, and whether it was protected or unprotected
- Illicit drug use, IV or intranasal
- For health care workers, recent needle stick exposure
- Body piercing or tattooing
- Close living accommodations, such as military barracks, correctional institutions, and overcrowded dormitories, long-term facilities, day-care centers, or employment in any such setting
- Blood or blood products or organ transplants received before 1992
- Military service
- Place of birth (United States or other country) and parents' place of birth
- History of alcohol use (how many drinks each day or week)
- Human immune deficiency virus (HIV)

Physical Assessment/Clinical Manifestations

Assess whether the patient has:

- Abdominal pain
- Changes in skin or sclera (icterus)
- **Arthralgia** (joint pain) or **myalgia** (muscle pain)
- Diarrhea/constipation
- Changes in color of urine or stool
- Fever
- Lethargy
- Malaise
- Nausea/vomiting
- Pruritus (itching)

Lightly palpate the right upper abdominal quadrant to assess for liver tenderness. The patient may report right upper quadrant pain with jarring movements. Inspect the skin, sclerae, and mucous membranes for jaundice. He or she may present for medical treatment only after jaundice appears, believing that other vague symptoms are related to an influenza-like syndrome.

Jaundice in hepatitis results from intrahepatic obstruction and is caused by edema of the liver's bile channels. Dark urine and clay-colored stools are often reported by the patient. If possible, obtain a urine and stool specimen for visual inspection and laboratory analysis. The patient may also have skin abrasions from pruritus (itching).

Psychosocial Assessment

Viral hepatitis has various presentations, but for most infected people the initial course is mild with few symptoms. The long-term complications of fibrosis and cirrhosis cause the more serious problem. This is especially true for patients who have chronic HBV and HCV infection.

Emotional problems for affected patients may center on their feeling sick and fatigued. General malaise, inactivity, and vague symptoms contribute to depression. Some patients often feel guilty and are remorseful about decisions made that caused the disease. These feelings are most likely to occur when the source of infection is from drug abuse. Family members may be angry that the patient caused the disease.

Infectious diseases such as hepatitis continue to have a social stigma. The patient may feel embarrassed by the precautions that are imposed in the hospital and continue to be necessary at home. This embarrassment may cause the patient to limit social interactions. Patients may be afraid that they will spread the virus to family and friends.

Family members are sometimes afraid of getting the disease and may distance themselves from the patient. Allow them to verbalize these feelings and explore the reasons for these fears. Educate the patient and family members about modes of transmission and clarify information as needed.

Patients may be unable to return to work for several weeks during the acute phases of illness. The loss of wages and the cost of hospitalization for a patient without insurance coverage may produce great anxiety and financial burden. This situation may last for months or years if hepatitis becomes chronic.

Laboratory Assessment

Hepatitis A, hepatitis B, and hepatitis C are usually confirmed by acute elevations in levels of liver enzymes, indicating liver cellular damage, and by specific serologic markers.

Levels of ALT and AST levels may possibly rise into the thousands in acute or fulminant cases of hepatitis. Alkaline phosphatase levels may be normal or elevated. Serum total bilirubin levels are elevated and are consistent with the clinical appearance of jaundice. Elevated levels of bilirubin are also present in the urine.

The presence of *hepatitis A* is established when hepatitis A virus (HAV) antibodies (anti-HAV) are found in the blood. Ongoing inflammation of the liver by HAV is indicated by the presence of immunoglobulin M (IgM) antibodies, which persist in the blood for 4 to 6 weeks. Previous infection is identified by the presence of immunoglobulin G (IgG) antibodies. These antibodies persist in the serum and provide permanent immunity to HAV.

The presence of the *hepatitis B* virus (HBV) is established when serologic testing confirms the presence of hepatitis B antigen-antibody systems in the blood and a detectable viral count (HBV polymerase chain reaction [PCR] DNA). Antigens located on the surface (shell) of the virus (HBsAg) and IgM antibodies to hepatitis B core antigen (anti-HBc IgM) are the most significant serologic markers. The presence of these markers establishes the diagnosis of hepatitis B. *The patient is infectious as long as HBsAg (hepatitis B surface antigen) is present in the blood.* Persistence of this serologic marker after 6 months or longer indicates a carrier state or chronic hepatitis. HBsAg levels normally decline and disappear after the acute hepatitis B episode. The presence of antibodies to hepatitis B surface antibody (HBsAb) in the blood indicates recovery and immunity to hepatitis B. *People who have been vaccinated against HBV have a positive HBsAb because they also have immunity to the disease.*

Enzyme-linked immunosorbent assay (ELISA) is the initial screening test for patients suspected of being infected with *hepatitis C* virus (HCV). It is also the most commonly used enzyme test for HCV antibodies (anti-HCV). The antibodies can be detected within 4 weeks of the infection (Pagana & Pagana, 2006). A more specific assay called the *recombinant immunoblot assay (RIBA)* has been used as a confirmatory test. These tests show that the patient has been exposed to HCV and has developed the antibody. To identify the actual circulating virus, the HCV PCR RNA test is used. This confirms active virus and can measure the viral load.

The presence of *hepatitis D* virus (HDV) can be confirmed by the identification of intrahepatic delta antigen or, more often, by a rise in the hepatitis D virus antibodies (anti-HDV) titer. This increase can be seen within a few days of infection (Pagana & Pagana, 2006).

Hepatitis E virus (HEV) testing is usually reserved for travelers in whom hepatitis is present but the virus cannot be detected. Hepatitis E antibodies (anti-HEV) are found in people infected with the virus.

Other Diagnostic Assessment

Liver biopsy may be used to confirm the diagnosis of hepatitis and to establish the stage and grade of liver damage. Characteristic changes help the pathologist distinguish among a virus, drug, toxin, fatty liver, iron, and other disease. It is usually performed in an ambulatory care setting as a percutaneous procedure (through the skin) after a local anesthetic is given. If coagulation is abnormal, however, it may be done using either a computed tomography (CT)–guided or transjugular route to reduce the risk for pneumothorax or hemothorax. Ultrasound may also be used.

Interventions

The patient with viral hepatitis can be mildly or acutely ill depending on the severity of the inflammation. Most patients are not hospitalized, although older adults and those with dehydration may be admitted for a short-term stay. The plan of care for all patients with viral hepatitis is based on measures to rest the liver, promote cellular regeneration, and prevent complications, if possible.

During the acute stage of viral hepatitis, interventions are aimed at resting the inflamed liver to promote hepatic cell regeneration. Rest is an essential intervention to reduce the liver's metabolic demands and increase its blood supply. Collaborative care is generally supportive. The patient is usually tired and expresses feelings of general malaise. Complete bedrest is usually not required, but rest periods alternating with periods of activity are indicated and are often enough to promote hepatic healing. Individualize the patient's plan of care and change it as needed to reflect the severity of symptoms, fatigue, and the results of liver function tests and enzyme determinations. Activities such as self-care and ambulating are gradually added to the activity schedule as tolerated.

The diet should be high in carbohydrates and calories with moderate amounts of fat and protein after nausea and anorexia subside. Small, frequent meals are often preferable to three standard meals. Ask the patient about food preferences because favorite foods are tolerated better than randomly selected foods. Encourage the patient to eat foods that are appealing. High-calorie snacks may be needed. Supplemental vitamins are often prescribed.

Drugs of any kind are used sparingly for patients with hepatitis to allow the liver to rest. An antiemetic to relieve nausea may be prescribed. There is no approved drug that is used to treat HAV.

For patients with chronic hepatitis B and hepatitis C, a number of drugs are given, including antiviral and immunomodulating drugs. Antiviral drugs that may be used for HBV include:

- Lamivudine (Epivir-HBV)
- Entecavir (Baraclude)
- Telbivudine (Tyzeka)
- Adefovir dipivoxil (Hepsera)

Teach patients taking these drugs to report any muscle weakness or aching because they can cause myopathy.

Pegylated interferon alpha-2b (PEG-Intron) is given to reduce the replication of the hepatitis B virus in patients with chronic disease and increase immunity. It is now available in a pen injection device. All of the drugs used for HBV can cause renal toxicity.

The current standard of care for hepatitis C is a combination of subcutaneous pegylated interferon alpha once a week and oral ribavirin (Copegus, Rebetol) daily (Patel et al., 2006). Ribavirin should never be given to a pregnant patient. Women of childbearing age must agree to use contraception if they are receiving treatment or if they are sexual partners of patients taking this drug. The length of treatment depends on genotype or strain of hepatitis. There are several different genotypes; most Americans who have hepatitis C are genotype 1. This genotype usually requires 48 weeks of treatment. Genotypes 2 and 3 have a better response rate if the viral load is low and usually need only 24 weeks of treatment. Genotypes 4 and 5 are typically treated for 48 weeks. The desired outcome of treatment is to have a negative HCV PCR RNA level and to sustain a negative level after treatment has ended. The secondary expected outcome is improvement in liver function. Response rates vary, but adults who are young, have a low viral load, and have minimal scarring on liver biopsy have a better chance of clearing the virus and remaining free of hepatitis C after treatment has ended.

NCLEX EXAMINATION CHALLENGE

An older adult is hospitalized with severe dehydration from hepatitis A. What precautions should the nurse use when caring for this client? (Select all that apply.)

A. Gloves
B. Mask
C. Gown
D. Shoe covers
E. Goggles
F. Handwashing

evolve For the correct answer, go to http://evolve.elsevier.com/Iggy/.

Community-Based Care

Home care management varies according to the type of hepatitis and whether the disease is acute or chronic. A primary focus in any case is preventing the spread of the infection. For hepatitis transmitted by the fecal-oral route, careful handwashing and sanitary disposal of feces are important. Standard Precautions are used for hepatitis transmitted percutaneously and permucosally. Education is therefore very important. Collaborate with the certified infection control practitioner and infectious disease specialist if needed in caring for these patients. These experts can also suggest resources for the patient and family.

Teach the patient and the family to use measures to prevent infection transmission (see Chart 61-5). *In addition, instruct the patient to avoid alcohol and to check with the health care provider before taking any medication or vitamin, supplement, or herbal preparation.*

Encourage the patient to increase activity gradually to prevent fatigue. Suggest that he or she eat small, frequent meals of high-carbohydrate foods (Chart 61-6).

FATTY LIVER (STEATOSIS)

Fatty liver is caused by the accumulation of fats in and around the hepatic cells. It may be caused by alcohol abuse or other factors. Nonalcoholic fatty liver disease (NAFLD) and nonal-

Chart 61-6 PATIENT AND FAMILY EDUCATION GUIDE

Viral Hepatitis

- Avoid all medications, including over-the-counter drugs, such as acetaminophen (Tylenol, Exdol♣), unless prescribed by your physician.
- Avoid all alcohol.
- Rest frequently throughout the day, and get adequate sleep at night.
- Eat small, frequent meals with a high-carbohydrate, moderate-fat, and moderate-protein content.
- Avoid sexual intercourse until antibody testing results are negative.
- Follow the guidelines for preventing transmission of the disease (see Chart 61-5).

coholic steatohepatitis (NASH) are types of fatty liver disease. Causes include:

- Diabetes mellitus
- Obesity
- Elevated lipid profile

Fatty infiltration of the liver may result from faulty fat metabolism in the liver and the movement of fatty acids from adipose tissue (fat). Many patients are asymptomatic. The most common and typical finding is an elevated ALT and AST or normal ALT and elevated AST (part of a group of liver function tests [LFTs]).

Magnetic resonance imaging (MRI), ultrasound, and nuclear medicine examinations can be used to confirm excessive fat in the liver. A percutaneous biopsy can provide the same information. Interventions are aimed at removing the underlying cause of the infiltration. Weight loss, glucose control, and aggressive treatment using lipid-lowering agents are recommended. Monitoring LFTs is essential in disease management.

HEPATIC ABSCESS

Although hepatic abscesses are not common, they carry a high mortality (death) rate. Abscesses occur when the liver is invaded by bacteria or protozoa. These organisms destroy the liver tissue, producing a necrotic cavity filled with infective agents, liquefied liver cells and tissue, and leukocytes. The infectious necrotic tissue walls off the abscess from the healthy liver.

A **pyogenic liver abscess** occurs when bacteria invade the liver. Infecting organisms include *Escherichia coli* and *Klebsiella, Enterobacter, Salmonella, Staphylococcus,* and *Enterococcus* species. A pyogenic abscess is generally solitary and confined to the right lobe, but occasionally abscesses are multiple. The usual cause is acute cholangitis, which occurs as a complication of cholelithiasis. Pyogenic liver abscesses may also result from liver trauma, abdominal peritonitis, and sepsis, or an abscess can extend to the liver after pneumonia or bacterial endocarditis. Symptoms are usually sudden.

The protozoan *Entamoeba histolytica* causes an **amebic hepatic abscess,** which may occur after amebic dysentery. These abscesses usually occur in the form of a single abscess in the right hepatic lobe, and the symptoms develop slowly.

Patients with hepatic abscesses are generally quite ill. On occasion, an abscess is not diagnosed until autopsy. Common manifestations include:

- Right upper abdominal pain with a palpable, tender liver
- Anorexia
- Weight loss
- Nausea and vomiting
- Fever and chills
- Weakness and malaise
- Shoulder pain
- Dyspnea
- Pleural pain if the diaphragm is involved

A liver abscess is usually diagnosed by contrast-enhanced CT scan or ultrasound. These abscesses are usually drained under CT or ultrasound guidance. Specimens may be sent for laboratory analysis so that the optimal antibiotic can be selected.

LIVER TRAUMA

The liver is one of the most common organs to be injured in patients with abdominal trauma. Damage or injury should be suspected whenever any upper abdominal or lower chest trauma is sustained. The liver is often injured by steering wheels in vehicular accidents. Common injuries include simple lacerations, multiple lacerations, avulsions (tears), and crush injuries.

The liver is a highly vascular organ and receives almost a third of the body's cardiac output. When hepatic trauma occurs, blood loss can be massive. *Observe for early signs of hemorrhagic shock* (Chart 61-7).

An ultrasound or CT scan of the abdomen is often done to determine the presence of a hematoma (blood clot). A decreased hematocrit may confirm suspected blood loss. Clinical manifestations include right upper quadrant pain with abdominal tenderness, distention, guarding, and rigidity. Abdominal pain exaggerated by deep breathing and referred to the right shoulder may indicate diaphragmatic irritation.

When organ damage is confirmed, a surgeon uses a laparoscope or performs an open exploratory laparotomy to identify and control the source and type of bleeding. Minor surgical interventions, such as suture placement, wound packing, decompression, or a combination of these procedures, are often performed to stop the bleeding. Liver lobe resection is required in some extensive liver injuries. This procedure may be done using laparoscopy.

Patients with hepatic trauma require multiple blood products such as packed red blood cells and fresh frozen plasma, as well as massive volume infusion to maintain adequate hydration. After surgery, the patient is admitted to a critical care unit.

Chart 61-7 KEY FEATURES

Liver Trauma

- Right upper quadrant pain with abdominal tenderness
- Abdominal distention and rigidity
- Guarding of the abdomen
- Increased abdominal pain exaggerated by deep breathing and referred to the right shoulder (Kehr's sign)
- Indicators of hemorrhage and hypovolemic shock:
  - Hypotension
  - Tachycardia
  - Tachypnea
  - Pallor
  - Diaphoresis
  - Cool, clammy skin
  - Confusion or other change in mental state

Monitor the patient for persistent or new bleeding. Closely monitor complete blood count and coagulation studies for trends in changes.

CANCER OF THE LIVER

Pathophysiology

Cancers may be *primary* tumors starting in the liver, or they may be *metastatic* cancers that spread from another organ to the liver. They are most often seen in regions of Asia and the Mediterranean area. Worldwide the disease kills about 1 million people each year, and affects Vietnamese men more than any other group (Pelligrino, 2006). Black and Hispanic populations have twice the rate of the disease as Euro-Americans, and older adults are affected more than other age-groups (www.nci.nih.gov/cancer). In the United States and worldwide, the incidence of liver cancer is increasing because there is an increase in cases of hepatitis C (HCV).

Chronic infection with HBV and HCV frequently lead to cirrhosis, which is a risk factor for developing liver cancer. It is important to remember that cirrhosis from any cause, including alcoholic liver disease, increases the risk for cancer. Other risk factors include:

- Hemochromatosis (hereditary metabolic disease causing iron deposits in the liver)
- Vinyl chloride
- Anabolic steroids
- Smoking
- Androgens or estrogens

Patient-Centered Collaborative Care

Assessment

In the early stage of cancer, most patients are without symptoms. Later in the disease, they report weight loss, anorexia, and weakness. Ask the patient if he or she has or has had recent abdominal pain, the most common concern. It is most often felt in the right upper quadrant before jaundice, bleeding, ascites, and edema develop. Palpation may reveal an enlarged, nodular liver (Pelligrino, 2006).

Elevated serum alpha-fetoprotein (AFP) (a tumor marker for cancers of the liver, testis, and ovary) and increased alkaline phosphatase are also common. Ultrasound (US) and contrast-enhanced CT are both useful in detecting metastasis. If the primary tumor site is not known, a CT- or ultrasound-guided liver biopsy can confirm the diagnosis, although this procedure is risky because of possible bleeding and spread of the cancer cells.

Interventions

Surgical management may be indicated for a small number of patients with a lesion confined to one liver lobe and can be performed through a laparoscope. Liver lobe resection or partial hepatectomy has been successful in achieving survival rates of up to 5 years.

Unfortunately, most patients are not candidates for surgical removal because their tumors are unresectable. The liver cannot tolerate high doses of radiation, so radiation therapy (RT) has not been an option. However, intensity modulated RT with increasing doses has been successful for some patients when used with chemotherapy (Moore, 2007). Other palliative approaches include hepatic artery embolization, ablation techniques, and chemotherapy.

Hepatic artery embolization causes cell death by blocking blood supply to the tumor in the liver. It is performed under moderate sedation by an interventional radiologist who threads a catheter through the femoral artery to inject small particles into the hepatic artery. The patient usually stays overnight in the hospital for observation in case of bleeding. This procedure may be followed by infusing a chemotherapy agent directly into the hepatic artery (chemoembolization) (Pelligrino, 2006).

Common *ablation* procedures include radiofrequency ablation (RFA), percutaneous ethanol injection, and cryotherapy. RFA uses energy waves to heat cancer cells and kill them. It is most often performed as an ambulatory care procedure using a percutaneous laparoscopic approach (Moore, 2007). Ethanol may also be injected directly into the tumor to destroy tumor cells, although this procedure is not as commonly done as RFA. Cryotherapy uses liquid nitrogen to freeze and destroy liver tumors. The general nursing care for patients having these procedures is described in Chapter 24.

Chemotherapy may be administered orally or IV. However, it is not effective in many cases. Examples of drugs used are doxorubicin (Adriamycin), 5-fluorouracil (5-FU), and cisplatin. Sorafenib (Nexavar) is a new kinase inhibitor that has been approved for inoperable liver cancer.

Another drug route is a catheter-directed method directly into the hepatic artery, a procedure called *hepatic arterial infusion (HAI)*. The interventional radiologist places a catheter into the artery that supplies the tumor and injects a mixture of chemotherapy and contrast agent into the tumor. This procedure has the unique effect of depositing chemotherapeutic drugs directly into the tumor without causing major systemic effects. Examples of agents given are fluorodeoxyuridine (FUDR) with or without dexamethasone (the most commonly used), oxaliplatin, mitomycin-C, or irinotecan (Moore, 2007). Chapter 24 describes the general nursing care for patients receiving chemotherapy.

Patients with liver cancer usually need end-of-life care and hospice services. Collaborate with the case manager to help patients and their families find the best community resources that meet their needs. Chapter 9 describes end-of-life care and hospice services in detail. Some patients choose to have their liver removed and wait for a donor liver. Liver transplantation is another method for treating primary liver cancer and offers the best chance of a longer survival.

LIVER TRANSPLANTATION

Liver transplantation has become a common procedure worldwide. The patient with end-stage liver disease or acute liver failure who has not responded to conventional medical or surgical intervention is a potential candidate for liver transplantation. The most common reason for a liver transplant is hepatitis C. It may also be used for the patient with a *primary* liver tumor.

The patient for potential transplantation has extensive physiologic and psychological assessment and evaluation by physicians and transplant coordinators. Alternative treatment should be extensively explored before committing a patient for a liver transplant. Patients who are *not* considered candidates for transplantation are those with:

- Severe cardiovascular instability with advanced cardiac disease
- Severe respiratory disease

- Active alcohol and/or substance abuse
- Metastatic tumors
- Inability to follow instructions regarding drug therapy and self-management

Liver transplantation has become the most effective treatment for patients with an increasing number of acute and chronic liver diseases. Inclusion and exclusion criteria vary among transplantation centers and are continually revised as treatment options change and surgical techniques improve.

Donor livers are obtained primarily from trauma victims who have not had liver damage. They are distributed through a nationwide program—the United Network of Organ Sharing (UNOS). This system distributes donor livers on the basis of regional considerations and patient acuity. Candidates with the highest level of acuity receive highest priority.

The donor liver is transported to the surgery center in a solution that preserves the organ for up to 8 hours. The diseased liver is removed through an incision made in the upper abdomen. The new liver is carefully put in its place and is attached to the patient's blood vessels and bile ducts. The procedure can take many hours to complete and requires a highly specialized team and large volumes of fluid and blood replacement.

Living donors have also been used and are usually close family members or spouse. This is done on a voluntary basis after careful psychological and physiologic preparation and testing. The donor's liver is resected (usually removal of one lobe) and implanted into the recipient after removal of the diseased liver. In both the donor and the recipient, the liver regenerates and grows in size to meet the demands of the body.

Pathophysiology

Although liver transplantations are commonly done, complications can occur. Some problems can be medically managed, whereas others require removal of the transplant. The two most common complications are acute graft rejection and infection.

The success of all transplantations has greatly improved since the introduction many years ago of cyclosporine (cyclosporin A), an immunosuppressant drug. Today, many other anti-rejection drugs are used. (See Chapter 19 for a complete discussion of rejection and preventive drug therapy.)

Clinical manifestations of rejection may include tachycardia, fever, right upper quadrant or flank pain, decreased bile pigment and volume, and increasing jaundice. Laboratory findings include elevated serum bilirubin, rising ALT and AST levels, elevated alkaline phosphatase levels, and increased prothrombin time/international normalized ratio (PT/INR).

Transplant rejection is treated aggressively with immunosuppressive drugs. As with all rejection treatments, the patient is at a greater risk for infection. If therapy is not effective, liver function rapidly deteriorates. Multisystem organ failure, including respiratory and renal involvement, develops along with diffuse coagulopathies and portal-systemic encephalopathy (PSE). The only alternative for treatment is emergency retransplantation.

Infection is another potential threat to the transplanted graft and the patient's survival. Vaccinations and prophylactic antibiotics are helpful in prevention. Immunosuppressant therapy, which must be used to prevent and treat organ rejection, significantly increases the patient's risk for infection. Other risk factors include the presence of multiple tubes and intravascular lines, immobility, and prolonged anesthesia.

In the early post-transplantation period, common infections include pneumonia, wound infections, and urinary tract infections. Opportunistic infections usually develop after the first postoperative month and include cytomegalovirus, mycobacterial infections, and parasitic infections. Latent infections such as tuberculosis and herpes simplex may be reactivated.

The physician prescribes broad-spectrum antibiotics for prophylaxis during and after surgery. Obtain culture specimens from all lines and tubes and collect specimens for culture at predetermined time intervals as dictated by the agency's policy. If an infection is detected, the physician prescribes organism-specific anti-infective agents.

The biliary anastomosis is susceptible to breakdown, obstruction, and infection. If leakage occurs or if the site becomes necrotic or obstructed, an abscess can form or peritonitis, bacteremia, and cirrhosis may develop. Observe for potential complications, which are listed in Table 61-6.

Patient-Centered Collaborative Care

Care of the patient undergoing liver transplantation requires an interdisciplinary team approach. Receiving a transplant has a major psychosocial impact. Transplant complications cause patients to be very anxious. In collaboration with the members of the health care team, assure them and their families that these problems are common and usually successfully treated.

After the patient is identified as a candidate and a donor organ is procured, the actual liver transplantation surgical procedure usually takes 8 hours. The length of the procedure can vary greatly.

In the immediate postoperative period, the patient is managed in the critical care unit and requires aggressive monitoring and care. Assess for signs and symptoms of complications of surgery, and immediately report them to the surgeon (see Table 61-6).

Monitor the patient's temperature frequently per hospital protocol, and report elevations, increased abdominal pain, distention, and rigidity, which are indicators of peritonitis. Nursing assessment also includes monitoring for a change in neurologic status that could indicate encephalopathy from a nonfunctioning liver. Report signs of clotting problems (e.g., bloody oozing from a catheter, petechiae, ecchymosis) to the surgeon immediately because they may indicate impaired function of the transplanted liver.

TABLE 61-6 Assessment and Prevention of Common Postoperative Complications Associated with Liver Transplantation

Assessment	Prevention
ACUTE GRAFT REJECTION	
Occurs from the 4th to 10th postoperative day	Prophylaxis with immunosuppressant agents, such as cyclosporine
Manifested by tachycardia, fever, right upper quadrant (RUQ) or flank pain, diminished bile drainage or change in bile color, or increased jaundice	Early diagnosis to treat with more potent anti-rejection drugs
Laboratory changes: (1) increased levels of serum bilirubin, transaminases, and alkaline phosphatase; (2) prolonged prothrombin time	
INFECTION	
Can occur at any time during recovery	Antibiotic prophylaxis; vaccinations
Frequent cultures of tubes, lines, and drainage	Early diagnosis and treatment with organism-specific anti-infective agents
Manifested by fever or excessive, foul-smelling drainage (urine, wound, or bile); other indicators depend on location and type of infection	
Early removal of invasive lines	
Good handwashing	
HEPATIC COMPLICATIONS (BILE LEAKAGE, ABSCESS FORMATION, HEPATIC THROMBOSIS)	
Manifested by decreased bile drainage, increased RUQ abdominal pain with distention and guarding, nausea or vomiting, increased jaundice, and clay-colored stools	If present, keep T-tube in dependent position and secure to patient; empty frequently, recording quality and quantity of drainage
Laboratory changes: increased levels of serum bilirubin and transaminases	Report manifestations to physician immediately May necessitate surgical intervention
ACUTE RENAL FAILURE	
Caused by hypotension, antibiotics, cyclosporine, acute liver failure, or hypothermia	Monitor all drug levels with nephrotoxic side effects Prevent hypotension
Indicators of hypothermia: shivering, hyperventilation, increased cardiac output, vasoconstriction, and alkalemia	Observe for early signs of renal failure, and report them immediately to the physician
Early indicators of renal failure: changes in urine output, increased blood urea nitrogen (BUN) and creatinine levels, and electrolyte imbalance	

HUMAN NEEDS NURSING CARE REVIEW

What might you NOTICE if the patient is experiencing inadequate digestion, nutrition, and metabolism as a result of impaired liver function?

- Jaundice
- Icterus
- Report of nausea and anorexia
- Vomiting
- Weight loss
- Bruising or bleeding
- Ascites

What should you INTERPRET and how should you RESPOND to a patient experiencing inadequate digestion, nutrition, and metabolism as a result of impaired liver function?

Perform and interpret physical assessment findings, including:

- Assess respiratory status to check for dyspnea or shallow breathing.
- Check level of consciousness and cognition.
- Take vital signs (look for fever or decreased BP) and oxygen saturation.
- Check for blood in the vomitus.
- Perform an abdominal assessment, including measuring girth.
- Check urine for dark color and stool for clay-colored appearance.
- Take current weight, and compare with previous weight.
- Assess skin for open areas.
- Check most recent laboratory values for coagulation studies and LFTs.

Respond by:

- Applying oxygen to assist in ease of breathing
- Keeping head of bed elevated to at least 30 degrees
- Maintaining rest
- Collaborating with nutritionist and pharmacist as needed
- Prioritizing and pacing activities to prevent fatigue
- Monitoring patient closely for complications, such as bleeding; call the rapid response team if bleeding

On what should you REFLECT?

- Monitor the patient for restored digestion and nutrition, such as increased appetite.
- Think about what may have caused the liver problem.
- Consider for what complications the patient is at risk.
- Think about what members of the health care team need to provide care for this patient.

GET READY FOR THE NCLEX EXAMINATION!

Key Points

Review these Key Points for each NCLEX Examination Client Needs Category.

Safe and Effective Care Environment

- Monitor the patient with cirrhosis for bleeding and neurologic changes as described in Chart 61-2.
- When caring for patients with cirrhosis, collaborate with the nutritionist, physician, and pharmacist.
- Refer patients with liver disorders to the American Liver Foundation; refer dying patients to hospice and other community resources as needed.

Health Promotion and Maintenance

- Follow the guidelines listed in Chart 61-4 to prevent viral hepatitis in the workplace.
- Teach patients to take precautions to prevent viral hepatitis in the community as described in Chart 61-5.
- For patients with viral hepatitis, instruct them to follow the guidelines listed in Chart 61-6.

Psychosocial Integrity

- Recognize that patients with cirrhosis have mental and emotional changes due to portal-systemic encephalopathy (PSE).
- Be aware that patients with cirrhosis and/or chronic hepatitis may feel guilty about their disease because of past habits such as drug and alcohol abuse.
- Be aware that family members and friends may fear getting hepatitis from the patient.
- Be aware that patients having liver transplantation have major concerns about the possibility of complications, such as organ rejection.

Physiological Integrity

- Be aware that cirrhosis has many causes in addition to alcohol abuse (see Table 61-3).
- Monitor laboratory values of patients suspected of or diagnosed with cirrhosis of the liver as listed in Tables 61-1 and 61-4.
- Observe for clinical manifestations of portal-systemic encephalopathy (PSE) as listed in Table 61-2.
- Assess for manifestations of cirrhosis as shown in Fig. 61-1.
- Provide care for the patient having a paracentesis as described in Chart 61-1.
- Administer drug therapy to decrease ammonia levels (which cause PSE) in patients with cirrhosis, such as lactulose and nonabsorbable antibiotics.
- Differentiate the five major types of hepatitis: A, B, C, D, and E. HDV occurs only with HBV and is transmitted most commonly by blood and body fluid exposure. Hepatitis A is transmitted via the fecal-oral route. Hepatitis C is the most common type and is also transmitted via blood and body fluids.
- Be aware that patients with chronic viral hepatitis often develop cirrhosis and cancer of the liver.
- Recognize that potent immunomodulators, such as the interferons, and antivirals are being used to treat hepatitis B and hepatitis C.
- Monitor for bleeding in the patient with liver trauma; assume that any abdominal trauma has damaged the liver.
- Observe the patient having a liver transplantation for complications, such as those described in Table 61-6.

Additional Study Resources

Go to your Companion CD or Evolve at http://evolve.elsevier.com/Iggy/ for *Self-Assessment Questions for the NCLEX Examination.*

Go to Evolve at http://evolve.elsevier.com/Iggy/ for *Prioritization and Delegation Questions for the NCLEX Examination.*

SELECTED BIBLIOGRAPHY

Asterisk indicates a classic or definitive work on this subject.

Brundage, S.C., & Fitzpatrick, A.N. (2006). Hepatitis A. *American Family Physician, 73*(12), 2162-2168.

*DeCarlis, L., Giacomoni, A., Pirotta, V., Lauterio, A., Slim, A.O., Sammartino, C., et al. (2003). Surgical treatment of hepatocellular cancer in the era of hepatic transplantation. *Journal of American College of Surgeons, 196*(6), 887-897.

*Dougherty, A.S., & Dreher, H.M. (2001). Hepatitis C: Current treatment strategies for an emerging epidemic. *MEDSURG Nursing, 10*(1), 9-13.

Garcia-Tsao, G., Sanyal, A.J., Grace, N.D., & Carey, W.; Practice Guidelines Committee of the American Association for the Study of Liver Diseases; Practice Parameters Committee of the American College of Gastroenterology. (2007). Prevention and management of gastroesophageal varices and variceal hemorrhage in cirrhosis. *Hepatology, 46*(3), 922-938.

Herrine, S.K. (2007). *Complications of cirrhosis: Clinical insights and implications for practice.* Retrieved April 21, 2008, from www.medscape.com/viewarticle/567230.

Ioannou, G., Doust, J., & Rockey, D.C. (2003). Terlipressin for acute esophageal variceal hemorrhage. *Cochrane Database of Systematic Reviews,* (1), CD002147.

*Iosue, K. (2002). Chronic hepatitis C: Latest treatment options. *The Nurse Practitioner, 27*(4), 32-49.

Kelso, L.A. (2008). Cirrhosis: Caring for patients with end-stage liver failure. *The Nurse Practitioner, 33*(7), 24-30.

Matthews, R.E., McGuire, B.M., & Estrada, C.A. (2006). Outpatient management of cirrhosis: A narrative review. *Southern Medical Association, 90*(6), 600-606.

Moore, S. (2007). Management of hepatic colorectal metastases: A shifting paradigm. *Colorectal Cancer Nursing, 1*(2), 4-7.

*National Institutes of Health Consensus Development Conference Statement. *Management of hepatitis C: 2002.* June 10-12, 2002, Washington, DC: National Institutes of Health.

*Ohata, K., Hamasaki, K., Toriyama, K., Matsumoto, K., Saeki, A., Yanagi, K., et al. (2003). Hepatic steatosis is a risk factor for hepatocellular carcinoma in patients with chronic hepatitis C virus infection. *Cancer, 97*(12), 3036-3043.

Pagana, K., & Pagana, T. (2006). *Mosby's manual of diagnostic and laboratory tests* (3rd ed.). St. Louis: Mosby.

Patel, K., Muir, A.J., & McHutchinson, J.G. (2006). Diagnosis and treatment of chronic hepatitis C infection. *BMJ, 332*(7548), 1013-1017.

Pelligrino, A. (2006). Looking at liver cancer. *Nursing2006, 36*(10), 52-55.

Rushing, J. (2005). Protect your patient during abdominal paracentesis. *Nursing2005, 35*(8), 14.

Schoch, L., & Whiteman, K. (2007). Monitoring liver function. *Nursing2007, 37*(11), 22-23.

62

CHAPTER

Care of Patients with Problems of the Biliary System and Pancreas

Donna D. Ignatavicius • Sarah Pettus

LEARNING OUTCOMES

For clinical competence and success on the NCLEX Examination, study this chapter with these Learning Outcomes in mind:

Safe and Effective Care Environment

1. Prioritize nursing care for the patient with acute pancreatitis.
2. Identify community-based resources for patients with pancreatic disorders.
3. Collaborate with health care team members to provide care for patients with pancreatic disorders.

Health Promotion and Maintenance

4. Identify risk factors for gallbladder disease.
5. Teach patients health promotion practices to prevent gallbladder disease.
6. Teach patients health promotion practices to prevent pancreatitis.

Psychosocial Integrity

7. Describe the psychosocial needs of patients with pancreatic cancer and their families.
8. Assess patient and family response to a diagnosis of pancreatic cancer

Physiological Integrity

9. Identify the common causes of cholecystitis and cholelithiasis.
10. Interpret diagnostic test results associated with gallbladder disease.
11. Interpret laboratory test results associated with acute pancreatitis.
12. Compare postoperative care of patients undergoing a traditional cholecystectomy with that of patients having laparoscopic cholecystectomy.
13. Compare and contrast the pathophysiology of acute and chronic pancreatitis.
14. Interpret common assessment findings associated with acute and chronic pancreatitis.
15. Prioritize nursing care for patients with acute pancreatitis and patients with chronic pancreatitis.
16. Explain the use and precautions associated with enzyme replacement for chronic pancreatitis.
17. Develop a postoperative plan of care for patients having a Whipple procedure.

Go to your Companion CD or Evolve at http://evolve.elsevier.com/Iggy/ for *Self-Assessment Questions for the NCLEX Examination* keyed to these Learning Outcomes.

The biliary system (liver and gallbladder) and pancreas secrete enzymes and other substances that promote food digestion in the stomach and small intestine. When these organs do not work properly, the person has impaired *digestion,* which may result in inadequate *nutrition.* Interdisciplinary management of patients with problems of the biliary system and pancreas includes the need to promote nutrition for normal cellular function. This chapter focuses on problems of the gallbladder and pancreas. Liver disorders were described in Chapter 61.

Because of the close anatomic location of these organs, disorders of the gallbladder and pancreas may extend to other organs if the primary health problem is not treated early. Inflammation is caused by obstruction (blockage) in the biliary system from gallstones, edema, stricture, or tumors. For example, gallstones in the cystic duct cause cholecystitis. Gallstones lodged in the ampulla of Vater block the flow of bile and pancreatic secretions, which can result in pancreatitis.

GALLBLADDER DISORDERS

CHOLECYSTITIS

Pathophysiology

Cholecystitis is an inflammation of the gallbladder that affects many people, most commonly in affluent countries. It may be either acute or chronic, although most patients have the acute type. Over 500,000 surgeries for this health problem are done in the United States each year (Comstock, 2008).

Acute Cholecystitis

Two types of acute cholecystitis can occur: calculous and acalculous cholecystitis. The most common type is **calculous cholecystitis,** in which chemical irritation and inflammation result from gallstones **(cholelithiasis)** that obstruct the cystic duct (most often), gallbladder neck, or common bile duct (Fig. 62-1). When the gallbladder is inflamed, trapped bile is reabsorbed and acts as a chemical irritant to the gallbladder wall; that is, the bile has a toxic effect. Reabsorbed bile, in combination with impaired circulation, edema, and distention of the gallbladder, causes ischemia and infection. The result is tissue sloughing with necrosis and gangrene. The gallbladder wall may eventually perforate (rupture). If the perforation is small and localized, an abscess may form. **Peritonitis,** infection of the peritoneum, may result if the perforation is large.

The exact pathophysiology of gallstone formation is not clearly understood, but abnormal metabolism of cholesterol and bile salts plays an important role in their formation. The gallbladder provides an excellent environment for the production of stones because it only occasionally mixes its normally abundant mucus with its highly viscous, concentrated bile. The constant temperature within the gallbladder also contributes to stone formation by delaying bile emptying, causing biliary stasis.

Gallstones are composed of substances normally found in bile, such as cholesterol, bilirubin, bile salts, calcium, and various proteins. They are classified as either cholesterol stones or pigment stones. Cholesterol calculi form as a result of metabolic imbalances of cholesterol and bile salts. They are the most common type found in people in the United States. Pigmented stones are associated with cirrhosis of the liver (McCance & Huether, 2006).

Bacteria can collect around the stones in the biliary system. Severe bacterial invasion can lead to life-threatening *suppurative* cholangitis when symptoms are not recognized quickly and pus accumulates in the ductal system.

Acalculous cholecystitis (inflammation occurring without gallstones) is typically associated with biliary stasis caused by any condition that affects the regular filling or emptying of the gallbladder. For example, a decrease in blood flow to the gallbladder or anatomic problems such as twisting or kinking of the gallbladder neck or cystic duct can result in pancreatic enzyme reflux into the gallbladder, causing inflammation. Most cases of this type of cholecystitis occur in patients with:

- Sepsis
- Severe trauma or burns
- Long-term total parenteral nutrition
- Multi-system organ failure
- Major surgery (postoperatively)
- Hypovolemia

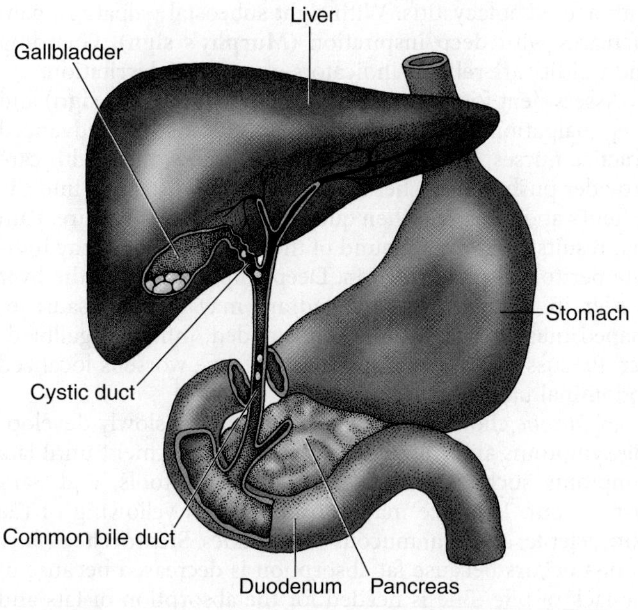
Liver
Gallbladder
Stomach
Cystic duct
Common bile duct
Duodenum
Pancreas

Fig. 62-1 • Gallstones within the gallbladder and obstructing the common bile and cystic ducts.

Chronic Cholecystitis

Chronic cholecystitis results when repeated episodes of cystic duct obstruction cause chronic inflammation. Calculi are almost always present. In chronic cholecystitis, the gallbladder becomes fibrotic and contracted, which results in decreased motility and deficient absorption.

Pancreatitis and cholangitis can occur as chronic complications of cholecystitis. These problems result from the backup of bile throughout the biliary tract. Bile obstruction leads to jaundice.

Jaundice (yellow discoloration of the skin and mucous membranes) and **icterus** (yellow discoloration of the sclerae) can occur in patients with acute cholecystitis but are most commonly seen in those with the *chronic* form of the disease. Obstructed bile flow caused by edema of the ducts or gallstones contributes to *extrahepatic* **obstructive jaundice.** Jaundice in cholecystitis may also be caused by direct liver involvement. Inflammation of the liver's bile channels or bile ducts may cause *intrahepatic* obstructive jaundice, resulting in an increase in circulating levels of bilirubin, the major pigment of bile.

When the concentration of bilirubin in the blood increases, jaundice can occur. In a person with obstructive jaundice, the normal flow of bile into the duodenum is blocked, allowing excessive bile salts to accumulate in the skin. This accumulation of bile salts leads to **pruritus** (itching) or a burning sensation. The bile flow blockage also prevents bilirubin from reaching the large intestine, where it is converted to urobilinogen. Because urobilinogen accounts for the normal brown color of feces, clay-colored stools result. Water-soluble bilirubin is normally excreted by the kidneys in the urine. When an excess of circulating bilirubin occurs, the urine becomes dark and foamy because of the kidneys' effort to clear the bilirubin.

Etiology and Genetic Risk

A familial or genetic tendency appears to play a role in the development of cholelithiasis, but this may be partially related to familial nutrition habits (excessive dietary cholesterol intake) and sedentary lifestyles. Gallstones are seen more frequently in obese patients, probably as a result of impaired fat metabolism or increased cholesterol. Age is also a factor, with people older than 60 years being more likely than younger people to develop stones. Patients with diabetes mellitus are also at increased risk because they usually have higher levels of fatty acids (triglycerides). American Indians and Mexican Americans have a higher incidence of the disease than other groups, which may be due to the higher incidence of diabetes among these populations (McCance & Huether, 2006). Other causes are included in Table 62-1.

TABLE 62-1 Risk Factors for Cholecystitis

- Women
- People older than 60 years
- American Indian, Mexican American, or Caucasian
- Obesity
- Rapid weight loss or prolonged fasting
- Women on hormone replacement therapy (HRT) or older birth control pills
- Family history of gallstones
- Prolonged total parenteral nutrition
- Crohn's disease
- Gastric bypass surgery
- Sickle cell anemia
- Glucose intolerance

WOMEN'S HEALTH CONSIDERATIONS

Women who are between 20 and 60 years of age are twice as likely to develop gallstones as men. Obesity is a major risk factor for gallstone formation, especially in women. Pregnancy tends to worsen gallstone formation. Pregnancy, as well as drugs such as estrogen and birth control pills (especially the older oral contraceptives), alters hormone levels and delays muscular contraction of the gallbladder, decreasing the rate of bile emptying. The incidence of gallstones is higher in women who have had multiple pregnancies. Combinations of causative factors increase the incidence of stone formation, especially in women. Therefore some clinicians refer to the patient most at risk for cholecystitis and gallstones by the four *F*s:

- Female
- Forty
- Fat
- Fertile

Patient-Centered Collaborative Care

Assessment

Physical Assessment/Clinical Manifestations

Patients with acute cholecystitis present with abdominal pain, although clinical manifestations vary in intensity and frequency (Chart 62-1).

Obtain the patient's height, weight, and vital signs, or delegate these activities to unlicensed assistive personnel (UAP). Ask about food preferences, and determine whether excessive fat and cholesterol are part of the diet. Inquire if any foods cause pain. Question whether any GI symptoms occur when fatty food is eaten: **flatulence** (gas), **dyspepsia** (indigestion), **eructation** (belching), anorexia, nausea, vomiting, and abdominal pain or discomfort.

Ask the patient to describe the pain, including its intensity and duration, precipitating factors, and any measures that relieve it. It may be described as indigestion of varying intensity, ranging from a mild, persistent ache to a steady, constant pain in the right upper abdominal quadrant. It may radiate to the right shoulder or scapula. In some cases, the abdominal pain of chronic cholecystitis may be vague and nonspecific. The usual pattern is episodic. Patients often refer to these episodes as "gallbladder attacks."

The severe pain of **biliary colic** is produced by obstruction of the cystic duct of the gallbladder. When a stone is moving through or is lodged within the duct, tissue spasm occurs in an effort to mobilize the stone through the small duct. *This pain may be so severe that it occurs with tachycardia, pallor, diaphoresis, and* ***prostration*** *(extreme exhaustion). Assess the patient for possible shock caused by biliary colic.*

Chart 62-1 KEY FEATURES

Cholecystitis

- Episodic or vague upper abdominal pain or discomfort that can radiate to the right shoulder
- Pain triggered by a high-fat or high-volume meal
- Anorexia
- Nausea and/or vomiting
- Dyspepsia (indigestion)
- Eructation (belching)
- Flatulence (gas)
- Feeling of abdominal fullness
- Rebound tenderness (Blumberg's sign)
- Fever
- Jaundice, clay-colored stools, dark urine, steatorrhea (most common with chronic cholecystitis)

CONSIDERATIONS FOR OLDER ADULTS

Older adults and patients with diabetes mellitus may have atypical manifestations, including the absence of pain and fever. Localized tenderness may be the only presenting sign. The older patient may become acutely confused (delirium) as the first manifestation of gallbladder disease.

Ask patients to describe their daily activity or exercise routines to determine whether they are sedentary. Question whether there is a family history of gallbladder disease. If the patient is female, ask whether she takes hormone replacement therapy (HRT) or birth control pills.

Because of gallbladder tenderness, it is difficult to use abdominal palpation and percussion in assessment of the patient with acute cholecystitis. With right subcostal palpation, pain increases with deep inspiration **(Murphy's sign).** Guarding and rigidity are reliable indicators of peritoneal irritation.

Assessment for rebound tenderness **(Blumberg's sign)** and deep palpation is performed by physicians and advanced practice nurses. To elicit rebound tenderness, the health care provider pushes his or her fingers deeply and steadily into the patient's abdomen and then quickly releases the pressure. Pain that results from the rebound of the palpated tissue may indicate peritoneal inflammation. Deep palpation below the liver border in the right upper quadrant may reveal a sausage-shaped mass, representing the distended, inflamed gallbladder. Percussion over the posterior rib cage worsens localized abdominal pain.

In *chronic* cholecystitis, patients may have slowly developing symptoms and may not seek medical treatment until late symptoms such as jaundice, clay-colored stools, and dark urine occur. Jaundice may also be seen as yellowing of the skin, sclerae, and oral mucous membranes. **Steatorrhea** (fatty stools) occurs because fat absorption is decreased because of the lack of bile. Bile is needed for the absorption of fats and fat-soluble vitamins in the intestine. As with any inflammatory process, the patient may have an elevated temperature of

99° to 102° F (37° to 39° C), tachycardia, and dehydration from fever and vomiting. Older adults become dehydrated much quicker than other age-groups, and they may not present with a fever.

Diagnostic Assessment

No laboratory tests are specific for gallbladder disease. A differential diagnosis must rule out other diseases that may cause similar symptoms, such as peptic ulcer disease and pancreatitis. An increased white blood cell (WBC) count indicates inflammation. Serum levels of alkaline phosphatase, aspartate aminotransferase (AST), and lactate dehydrogenase (LDH) may be elevated, indicating abnormalities in liver function in patients with biliary obstruction, although this is not very common in patients with cholecystitis without gallstones. The direct (conjugated) and indirect (unconjugated) serum bilirubin levels are also elevated. If the pancreas is involved, serum amylase and lipase levels are elevated.

Calcified gallstones are easily viewed on abdominal x-ray. Stones that are not calcified cannot be seen. *Ultrasonography (US) of the right upper quadrant is the best diagnostic test for cholecystitis.* It is safe, accurate, and painless. Acute cholecystitis is seen as edema of the gallbladder wall and pericholecystic fluid. A hepatobiliary scan can be performed to visualize the gallbladder and determine patency of the biliary system.

Interventions

Most patients do not respond to nonsurgical interventions during the acute phase of cholecystitis. Surgery is the treatment of choice.

Nonsurgical Management

Most people with gallstones have no symptoms. Acute pain occurs when gallstones partially or totally obstruct the cystic or common bile duct. Most patients find that they need to avoid fatty foods to prevent further episodes of biliary colic. Withhold food and fluids if nausea and vomiting occur. IV therapy is used for hydration.

Acute biliary pain requires opioid analgesia, such as morphine or hydromorphone (Dilaudid). In the past, meperidine (Demerol) has been the drug of choice because it was thought to cause fewer spasms of the sphincter of Oddi, which blocks bile flow. However, this drug breaks down into a toxic metabolite (normeperidine) and can cause seizures, especially in older adults. All opioids may cause some degree of sphincter spasm (Holcomb, 2007).

Anticholinergic drugs such as dicyclomine (Bentyl, Lomine♣) may be given to relax smooth muscles and decrease ductal tone and spasm. These drugs should not be given to older adults because of adverse drug effects such as constipation, urinary retention, dry mouth, blurred vision, and acute confusion. Ketorolac (Toradol, Acular) may be used for them instead. The health care provider prescribes antiemetics to control nausea and vomiting. IV antibiotic therapy may also be given.

For some patients with small stones or for those who are not good surgical candidates, several other options are available. For example, a treatment that is commonly used for kidney stones is now approved for gallstones—*extracorporeal shock wave lithotripsy (ESWL).* This procedure can be used only for patients who have a normal weight, cholesterol-based stones, and good gallbladder function. The patient lies on a water-filled pad, and shock waves break up the large stones into smaller ones that can be passed through the digestive system. During the procedure, he or she may have pain from the movement of the stones or duct or gallbladder spasms. Oral bile salts may be prescribed after the procedure to help dissolve the remaining fragments.

Another treatment option in people who cannot have surgery is the insertion of a percutaneous transhepatic biliary catheter to open the blocked duct(s) so that bile can flow. Catheters can be placed several ways depending on the condition of the biliary ducts in an internal, external, or internal/external drain. Biliary catheters usually divert bile from the liver into the duodenum to bypass a stricture. When all of the bile enters the duodenum, it is called an *internal* drain. However, in some cases, a patient has an *internal/external* drain in which part of the bile empties into a drainage bag. Patients who need this drain for an extended period may have the external drain capped. If jaundice or leakage around the catheter site occurs, teach the patient to reconnect the catheter to a drainage bag and have a follow-up cholangiogram injection done by an interventional radiologist. An *external* only catheter is connected either temporarily or permanently to a drainage bag. A reduction in bile drainage indicates that the drain is no longer working.

Surgical Management

Cholecystectomy is a surgical removal of the gallbladder. Two procedures are available to the surgeon for performing this surgery: the laparoscopic cholecystectomy and, far less often, the traditional open approach cholecystectomy.

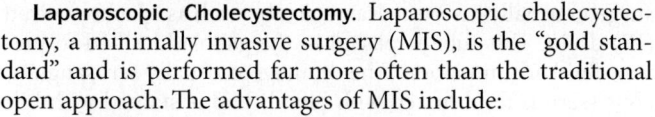

▶ ANIMATION: Laparoscopic Cholecystectomy; Gallbladder Removal

Laparoscopic Cholecystectomy. Laparoscopic cholecystectomy, a minimally invasive surgery (MIS), is the "gold standard" and is performed far more often than the traditional open approach. The advantages of MIS include:

- Complications are not common.
- The death rate is very low.
- Bile duct injuries are rare.
- Patient recovery is quicker.
- Postoperative pain is less severe.

The laparoscopic procedure (often called a "lap chole") is commonly done on an ambulatory care basis in a same-day surgery suite. The surgeon explains the procedure. The nurse answers questions and reinforces the physician's instructions. Reinforce what to expect after surgery, and review pain management, deep-breathing exercises, and incentive spirometry use. There is no special preoperative preparation other than the routine preparation for surgery under general anesthesia described in Chapter 16. An IV antibiotic is usually given immediately before or during surgery.

During the surgery, the surgeon makes a very small midline puncture at the umbilicus. Additional small incisions may be needed. The abdominal cavity is insufflated with 3 to 4 L of carbon dioxide. Gasless laparoscopic cholecystectomy using abdominal wall lifting devices is a more recent innovation in some centers. This technique results in improved pulmonary and cardiac function. A trocar catheter is inserted, through which a laparoscope is introduced. The laparoscope is attached to a video camera, and the abdominal organs are viewed on a monitor. The gallbladder is dissected from the liver bed, and the cystic artery and duct are closed. The surgeon aspirates the bile and crushes any large stones and then extracts the gallbladder through the umbilical port.

Removing the gallbladder with the laparoscopic technique reduces the risk for wound complications. Some patients have pain from carbon dioxide retention in the abdomen. Teach about the importance of early ambulation to promote absorption of the carbon dioxide. Less opioid analgesia is necessary after the laparoscopic procedure than after an open surgical procedure.

The patient is usually discharged from the hospital or surgery center within 1 day, although older and obese patients may stay overnight. Provide postoperative teaching regarding pain management, incision care, and follow-up appointments. After laparoscopic surgery, the patient can return to usual activities much sooner than those having an open cholecystectomy. Most patients are able to resume usual activities within a week.

Traditional Cholecystectomy. Use of the open surgical approach (abdominal laparotomy) has greatly declined during the past 15 years. The patient undergoing this surgery is usually hospitalized for several days after the procedure. Examples of patients who have this type of surgery include those with chronic lung disease or heart failure who cannot tolerate the carbon dioxide that is used in the laparoscopic procedure.

The surgical nurse provides the usual preoperative care and teaching in the operating suite on the day of surgery (see Chapter 16). The surgeon not only removes the gallbladder through a large incision but also may explore the biliary ducts for the presence of stones. If the common bile duct is explored, the surgeon may insert a T-tube drain to ensure patency of the duct, although this is not done as commonly today. Trauma to the common bile duct stimulates inflammation, which can slow bile flow and contribute to bile stasis. In addition, the surgeon usually inserts a drainage tube such as a Jackson-Pratt (JP) drain. This tube is placed in the gallbladder bed to prevent fluid accumulation. The drainage is usually serosanguineous (serous fluid mixed with blood) and is stained with bile in the first 24 hours after surgery. Antibiotic therapy is given to prevent infection.

Patient care for a patient having a traditional open cholecystectomy is similar to the care for any patient having abdominal surgery under general anesthesia as described in Chapter 18. Postoperative incisional pain after a traditional cholecystectomy is controlled with opioids using a patient-controlled analgesia (PCA) pump. Encourage the patient to use coughing and deep-breathing exercises when pain is controlled.

Antiemetics may be necessary for episodes of postoperative nausea and vomiting. Administer the antiemetic early, as prescribed, to prevent retching associated with vomiting and thus decrease pain related to muscle straining.

Provide care for the incision, the surgical drain, and possibly a T-tube. The surgeon typically removes the surgical dressing and drain within 24 hours after surgery. The T-tube, however, may remain in place longer, although it has been associated with many complications. *The priority for caring for the patient with a T-tube is to avoid raising the drainage system above the level of the gallbladder.* Chart 62-2 highlights other important nursing care activities associated with the T-tube system.

The patient is NPO until fully awake postoperatively. Document the patient's level of consciousness, vital signs, and pain level. Assess the surgical incision for signs of infection, such as excessive redness or purulent drainage. Report changes to the surgeon immediately. Begin ambulation as soon as possible to prevent deep vein thrombosis and promote peristalsis.

Chart 62-2 BEST PRACTICE FOR PATIENT SAFETY & QUALITY CARE

Care of the Patient with a T-Tube

- Keep the drainage system below the level of the gallbladder. Maintain the patient in the semi-Fowler's position.
- Assess the amount, color, consistency, and odor of drainage initially every 2 to 4 hours and then every 8 hours after the first 24 hours. In the immediate postoperative period, expect bloody drainage, which changes to green-brown bile. Bile output is about 400+ mL/day with a gradual decrease in amount. Report bile drainage amounts in excess of 1000 mL/day to the physician.
- Report sudden increases in bile output after a normally decreasing output pattern is established.
- Assess for foul odor and purulent drainage, which indicate infection or extensive inflammation. Report changes in drainage to the physician.
- Inspect the skin around the T-tube insertion site for signs of inflammation, including redness, swelling, and erythema, and observe for frank bile leakage. Keep the dressing dry. (Use the hospital's procedure and provide drain care and dressing change per protocol. The site is usually cleaned and the dressing changed daily.)
- *Never irrigate, aspirate, or clamp a T-tube without a physician's request.*
- Assess the drainage system for pulling, kinking, or tangling of tubing, especially when the patient is positioned toward the right side.
- When the patient is allowed to eat, clamp the T-tube for 1 to 2 hours (per physician's protocol) before and after meals. Assess the patient's response to determine tolerance of food.
- Teach patient to observe stools for return of brown color 7 to 10 days postoperatively.

Gradually advance the diet from clear liquids to solid foods as peristalsis returns. Within 1 to 2 days, the patient usually resumes solid foods and is discharged to home. The amount of fat allowed in the patient's diet after a cholecystectomy depends on his or her tolerance of fat. In the early postoperative period, if bile flow is reduced, a low-fat diet may reduce discomfort and prevent nausea. For most patients, a special diet is not required. In collaboration with the nutritionist, advise them to eat nutritious meals and avoid excessive intake of fatty foods, especially fried food, butter, and "fast food." If the patient is obese, recommend a weight-reduction program.

Teach patients that feces will pass more quickly through the colon after surgery. Some patients have diarrhea, which may need to be controlled with a bile acid binder like cholestyramine (Baltimore & Davidson, 2007). Teach them to keep their incision clean and report any changes that may indicate infection. Remind them to report repeat abdominal or epigastric pain with vomiting that may occur several weeks to months after surgery. These symptoms indicate possible **postcholecystectomy syndrome (PCES).**

PCES occurs in fewer than 10% of patients after gallbladder surgery. However, patients who have it are usually discouraged that they have pain after already having surgery to cure it (Comstock, 2008). Causes of PCES are listed in Table 62-2. Management depends on the exact cause but usually involves the use of the endoscopic retrograde cholangiopancreatogra-

TABLE 62-2 Causes of Postcholecystectomy Syndrome

- Pseudocyst
- Common bile duct (CBD) leak
- CBD or pancreatic duct stricture
- Sphincter of Oddi dysfunction
- Retained or new CBD gallstone
- Pancreatic or liver mass
- Primary sclerosing cholangitis
- Diverticular compression

phy (ERCP) to find the cause of the problem and repair it. This procedure and related nursing care are described in Chapter 55. Collaborative care includes pain management, antibiotics, nutrition and hydration therapy (possibly short-term parenteral nutrition), and control of nausea and vomiting.

NCLEX EXAMINATION CHALLENGE

An older client is admitted to the post-anesthesia recovery unit (PACU) after having a laparoscopic cholecystectomy. Which action is the nurse's priority in caring for the client?

A. Assess T-tube drainage and the catheter site for signs of infection.
B. Teach the client to avoid fatty foods for the first 6 weeks after surgery.
C. Manage the pain that is caused by carbon dioxide gas.
D. Remind the client to deep breathe and cough every 2 hours.

evolve For the correct answer, go to http://evolve.elsevier.com/Iggy/.

CANCER OF THE GALLBLADDER

Pathophysiology

Primary cancer of the gallbladder is rare and more common in women than in men. Adenocarcinoma and squamous cell cancer of the gallbladder account for the majority of the cases. The tumor tends to begin in the inner layer (mucosa) of the gallbladder wall. It then grows outward to include the entire gallbladder before it begins to metastasize (spread) to close organs like the liver, small intestine, and pancreas. These rare cancers appear more frequently in patients with pre-existing chronic cholecystitis and cholelithiasis. They also tend to occur more often in American Indians than in any other group, but the reason for this finding is not known (McCance & Huether, 2006).

Patient-Centered Collaborative Care

Assessment

Early symptoms, when present, develop slowly and are similar to those of chronic cholecystitis and cholelithiasis. Assess for characteristic manifestations, which include:

- Anorexia
- Weight loss
- Nausea and vomiting
- Abdominal bloating
- Fever
- General malaise
- Jaundice (in advanced disease)
- Enlargement of the liver and spleen
- Severe abdominal pain (in advanced disease)

A moderately tender, irregularly shaped mass may be palpated. Gallbladder cancer is typically discovered during other procedures for diagnosis of suspected cholecystitis or during cholecystectomy.

The diagnosis of gallbladder cancer is usually made by ultrasonography, but other tests can be done. Some patients have a computed tomography (CT) scan or magnetic resonance cholangiopancreatography (MRCP) in which a contrast medium is injected into the bile ducts. Other more invasive tests, like endoscopic retrograde cholangiopancreatography (ERCP), may also be used. Liver function studies indicate liver involvement. Two serum tests that reveal the presence of cancer cells are carcinoembryonic antigen (CEA) assay and CA 19-9.

Interventions

The prognosis for the patient with cancer of the gallbladder is poor because it is usually diagnosed in late disease due to the lack of specific manifestations. Three treatments are used: surgery, radiation therapy, and chemotherapy. Surgical intervention is either potentially curative (for an early resectable tumor) or palliative (for advanced disease with metastasis). The patient who is diagnosed with early disease has either a simple cholecystectomy (gallbladder removal) or extended cholecystectomy (removal of the gallbladder, surrounding lymph nodes, and a small margin of the liver). For palliative surgery to extend the patient's life or decrease discomfort, radical surgery is done.

Nursing care is similar to that for patients who have a cholecystectomy (see p. 1369) or Whipple procedure (see p. 1382), depending on the extent of disease. These procedures are described elsewhere in this chapter. Teach terminally ill patients and their families about end-of-life care and available hospice services (see Chapter 9).

Radiation therapy and chemotherapy alone are not effective for gallbladder cancer. However, they may be given as adjunctive procedures with surgery or instead of surgery in patients who are not surgical candidates to shrink the tumor. Intensity-modulated radiation therapy that is much more advanced and intense than regular radiation is used. Chemotherapy with 5-fluorourical (5-FU), doxorubicin, and mitomycin has been effective in reducing tumor size in a small percentage of patients (www.cancer.gov). Chapter 24 describes care of the patient receiving radiation and chemotherapy in detail.

Complementary and Alternative Therapies

Like many patients with any cancer, those with gallbladder cancer also use complementary and alternative therapies, such as naturopathic therapies, mind-body therapies, nutrition therapy, and spiritual counseling. Encourage patients to incorporate these modalities into their treatment plan to help decrease anxiety and stress, promote comfort, and increase immune system function. Chapter 2 describes complementary and alternative therapies in more detail.

PANCREATIC DISORDERS

ACUTE PANCREATITIS

Pathophysiology

Acute pancreatitis is a serious and, at times, life-threatening inflammatory process of the pancreas. This process is caused by a premature activation of excessive pancreatic enzymes that destroy ductal tissue and pancreatic cells, resulting in autodigestion and fibrosis of the pancreas. The pathologic changes occur in different degrees. The severity of pancreatitis depends on the extent of inflammation and tissue damage. Pancreatitis can range from mild involvement evidenced by edema and inflammation to **necrotizing hemorrhagic pancreatitis (NHP).** NHP is diffusely bleeding pancreatic tissue with fibrosis and tissue death.

The pancreas is unusual in that it functions as both an exocrine gland and an endocrine gland. The primary *endocrine* disorder is diabetes and is discussed in Chapter 67. The *exocrine* function of the pancreas is responsible for secreting enzymes that assist in the breakdown of starches, proteins, and fats. These enzymes are normally secreted in the inactive form and become activated once they enter the small intestine. Early activation (i.e., activation within the pancreas rather than the intestinal lumen) results in the inflammatory process of pancreatitis. Direct toxic injury to the pancreatic cells and the production and release of pancreatic enzymes (e.g., trypsin, lipase, elastase) result from the obstructive damage. After pancreatic duct obstruction, increased pressure may contribute to ductal rupture allowing spillage of trypsin and other enzymes into the pancreatic parenchymal tissue. Autodigestion of the pancreas occurs as a result (Fig. 62-2). In *acute* pancreatitis, four major pathophysiologic processes occur: lipolysis, proteolysis, necrosis of blood vessels, and inflammation.

The hallmark of pancreatic necrosis is enzymatic fat necrosis of the endocrine and exocrine cells of the pancreas caused by the enzyme *lipase.* Fatty acids are released during this *lipolytic process* and combine with ionized calcium to form a soaplike product. The initial rapid lowering of serum calcium levels is not readily compensated for by the parathyroid gland. Because the body needs ionized calcium and cannot use bound calcium, hypocalcemia occurs.

Proteolysis involves the splitting of proteins by hydrolysis of the peptide bonds, resulting in the formation of smaller polypeptides. Proteolytic activity may lead to thrombosis and gangrene of the pancreas. Pancreatic destruction may be localized and confined to one area or may involve the entire organ.

Elastase is activated by trypsin and causes elastic fibers of the blood vessels and ducts to dissolve. The *necrosis of blood vessels* results in bleeding, ranging from minor bleeding to massive hemorrhage of pancreatic tissue. Another pancreatic enzyme, kallikrein, causes the release of vasoactive peptides, bradykinin, and a plasma kinin known as *kallidin.* These substances contribute to vasodilation and increased vascular permeability, further compounding the hemorrhagic process. This massive destruction of blood vessels by necrosis may lead to generalized hemorrhage with blood escaping into the retroperitoneal tissues. *The patient with hemorrhagic pancreatitis is critically ill, and extensive pancreatic destruction and shock may lead to death. The majority of deaths in patients with acute pancreatitis result from irreversible shock.*

The *inflammatory stage* occurs when leukocytes cluster around the hemorrhagic and necrotic areas of the pancreas. A secondary bacterial process may lead to suppuration (pus formation) of the pancreatic parenchyma or the formation of an abscess. (See discussion of Pancreatic Abscess on p. 1379.) Mild infected lesions may be absorbed. When infected lesions are severe, calcification and fibrosis occur. If the infected fluid becomes walled off by fibrous tissue, a pancreatic pseudocyst is formed. (See discussion of Pancreatic Pseudocyst on p. 1380.)

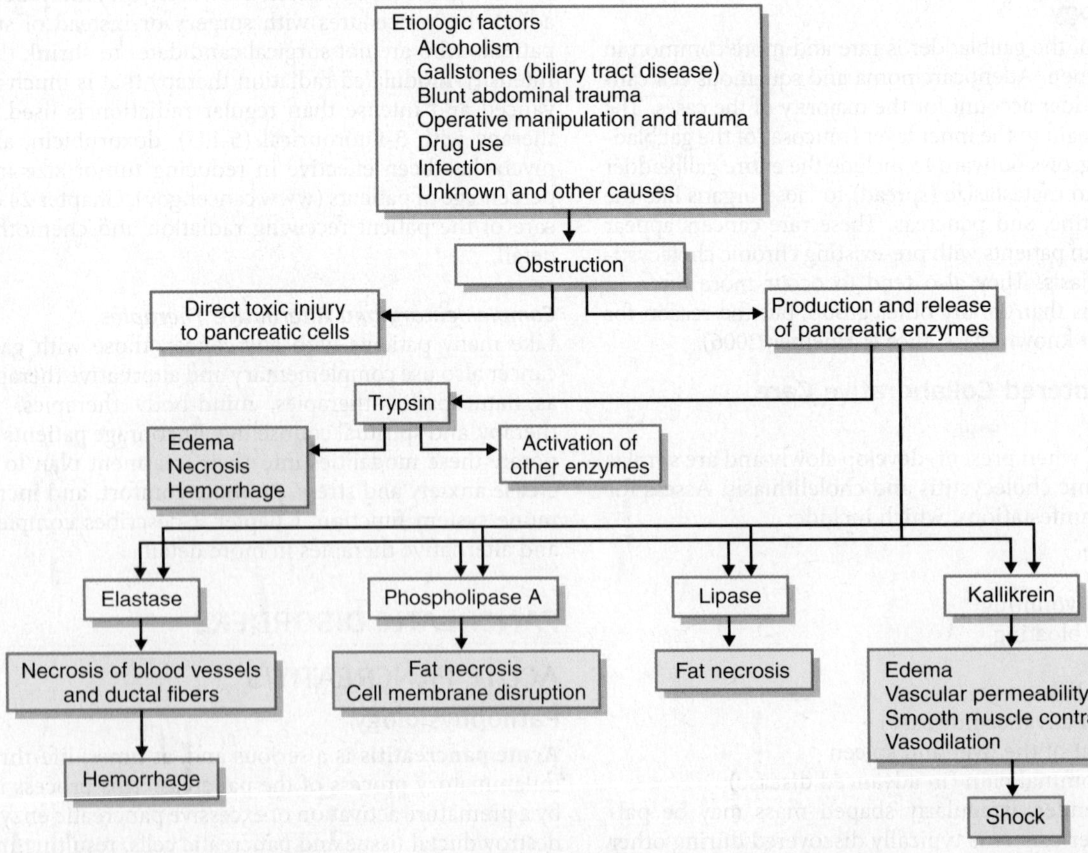
Etiologic factors
Alcoholism
Gallstones (biliary tract disease)
Blunt abdominal trauma
Operative manipulation and trauma
Drug use
Infection
Unknown and other causes
Obstruction
Direct toxic injury to pancreatic cells
Production and release of pancreatic enzymes
Trypsin
Edema
Necrosis
Hemorrhage
Activation of other enzymes
Elastase
Phospholipase A
Lipase
Kallikrein
Necrosis of blood vessels and ductal fibers
Fat necrosis
Cell membrane disruption
Fat necrosis
Edema
Vascular permeability
Smooth muscle contraction
Vasodilation
Hemorrhage
Shock

Fig. 62-2 • The process of autodigestion in acute pancreatitis.

Complications of Acute Pancreatitis

Acute pancreatitis may result in severe, life-threatening complications (Table 62-3). Jaundice occurs from swelling of the head of the pancreas, which slows bile flow through the common bile duct. The bile duct may also be compressed by calculi (stones) or a pancreatic pseudocyst. The resulting total bile flow obstruction causes severe jaundice. Intermittent hyperglycemia occurs from the release of glucagon, as well as the decreased release of insulin due to damage to the pancreatic islet cells. Total destruction of the pancreas may occur, leading to type 1 diabetes.

Left lung pleural effusions frequently develop in the patient with acute pancreatitis. Amylase effusions probably occur when exudate containing pancreatic enzymes passes from the peritoneal cavity into the pleural cavity via the transdiaphragmatic lymph channels. *Atelectasis and pneumonia may occur also, especially in older patients.*

Multi-system organ failure is caused by necrotizing hemorrhagic pancreatitis (NHP). The patient is at risk for acute respiratory distress syndrome (ARDS). This severe form of pulmonary edema is caused by disruption of the alveolar-capillary membrane and is a serious complication of acute pancreatitis. (See Chapter 34 for a discussion of ARDS.) In acute pancreatitis, pulmonary failure accounts for more than half of all deaths that occur in the first week of the disease.

Coagulation defects are another major potential complication and may result in death. Complex physiologic changes in the pancreas cause the release of necrotic tissue and enzymes into the bloodstream, resulting in altered coagulation. Disseminated intravascular coagulation (DIC) involves hypercoagulation of the blood, with consumption of clotting factors and the development of microthrombi.

Shock in acute pancreatitis results from peripheral vasodilation from the released vasoactive substances and the retroperitoneal loss of protein-rich fluid from proteolytic digestion. Hypovolemia may result in decreased renal perfusion and acute renal failure. Paralytic (adynamic) ileus results from peritoneal irritation and seepage of pancreatic enzymes into the abdominal cavity.

Etiology and Genetic Risk

In many cases, the cause of pancreatitis is not known, but many factors can injure the pancreas. The most common causes are excessive alcohol and biliary tract disease, with gallstones accounting for almost half of the cases of obstructive pancreatitis.

TABLE 62-3 Potential Complications of Acute Pancreatitis

- Pancreatic infection (most common cause of death)
- Hypovolemia
- Hemorrhage
- Acute renal failure
- Paralytic ileus
- Hypovolemic or septic shock
- Pleural effusion
- Acute respiratory distress syndrome (ARDS)
- Atelectasis
- Pneumonia
- Multi-organ system failure
- Disseminated intravascular coagulation (DIC)
- Diabetes mellitus

Older adults with pancreatitis typically have biliary obstruction. Acute pancreatitis may occur as a result of trauma from surgical manipulation after biliary tract, pancreatic, gastric, and duodenal procedures, such as cholecystectomy, the Whipple procedure, and partial gastrectomy. The trauma may also occur as a complication of the diagnostic procedure *endoscopic retrograde cholangiopancreatography (ERCP).*

Other causative factors include:

- Trauma: external (blunt trauma) or operative
- Pancreatic obstruction: tumors, cysts, or abscesses; abnormal organ structure
- Metabolic disturbances: hyperlipidemia, hyperparathyroidism, or hypercalcemia
- Renal disturbances: failure or transplantation
- Familial, inherited pancreatitis
- Penetrating gastric or duodenal ulcers, resulting in peritonitis
- Viral infections, such as coxsackievirus B infection
- Toxicities of drugs, including opiates, sulfonamides, thiazides, steroids, and oral contraceptives (The exact mechanism by which these and other drugs cause pancreatitis is unknown.)

Incidence/Prevalence

Pancreatic attacks are especially common during holidays and vacations when alcohol consumption is usually high, especially in men. Women are affected most often after cholelithiasis and biliary tract problems. They are also most at risk for pancreatitis within 2 months after childbirth.

Death occurs in a small percentage of patients with acute pancreatitis, but with early diagnosis and treatment, mortality can be reduced. It occurs at a higher rate in *older adults* and in patients with postoperative pancreatitis. The prognosis for recovery is usually good for pancreatitis associated with biliary tract disease and poor if pancreatitis accompanies alcoholism. Mortality rises when necrosis and hemorrhage occur (Burruss & Holz, 2005).

Health Promotion and Maintenance

In view of the causes of pancreatitis, people who drink alcohol should do so in moderation to prevent alcohol-related health problems such as pancreatitis. Gallbladder disease, especially when triggered by gallstones, should be treated promptly to avoid complications.

To help reduce the incidence of acute pancreatitis in ERCP, several antisecretory agents may be given. The most widely used drugs for this purpose are *somatostatin* and its analogue *octreotide.* These drugs appear to have anti-inflammatory and cytoprotective properties. SecreFlo (injectable *secretin*) has also been used with success. They are most useful during ERCP when measuring pressures of the sphincter of Oddi.

Patient-Centered Collaborative Care

evolve ONLINE PHARM REVIEW

Assessment

History

Most often, the patient reports severe and constant abdominal pain. *Once the pain is controlled, interview him or her to take a history.* Ask whether the abdominal pain occurs when drinking alcohol or eating a high-fat meal. Obtain information about alcohol usage, including the amount of alcohol consumed during what period of time (i.e., years of consumption, how much usually consumed over a particular period). Question the patient about a family or personal history of alcoholism, pancreatitis, or biliary tract disease. Ask whether any abdominal surgical interventions, such as cholecystectomy, or diagnostic procedures, such as ERCP, have been performed recently.

Ask about other medical problems known to cause pancreatitis, including peptic ulcer disease, renal failure, vascular disorders, hyperparathyroidism, and hyperlipidemia. Inquire about recent viral infections. Ask the patient or family member to list all prescription and over-the-counter (OTC) drugs taken recently.

Physical Assessment/Clinical Manifestations

The diagnosis of pancreatitis is made on the basis of the clinical presentation combined with the results of diagnostic studies—both laboratory and imaging assessments. Clinical manifestations of acute pancreatitis vary widely and depend on the severity of the inflammation. Typically, a patient is diagnosed after presenting with severe abdominal pain in the mid-epigastric area or left upper quadrant. Assess the intensity and quality of pain. The patient often states that the pain had a sudden onset and radiates to the back, left flank, or left shoulder. The pain is described as intense, **boring** (feeling that it is going through the body), and continuous and is worsened by lying in the supine position. Often the patient finds relief by assuming the fetal position (with the knees drawn up to the chest and the spine flexed) or by sitting upright and bending forward (Amerine, 2007). He or she may report weight loss resulting from nausea and vomiting. Ask a nursing assistant or technician to weigh the patient.

When performing an abdominal assessment, inspect for:
- Generalized jaundice
- Gray-blue discoloration of the abdomen and periumbilical area **(Cullen's sign)**
- Gray-blue discoloration of the flanks **(Turner's sign),** caused by pancreatic enzyme leakage to cutaneous tissue from the peritoneal cavity

Listen for bowel sounds; absent or decreased bowel sounds usually indicate paralytic (adynamic) ileus. On light palpation, note abdominal tenderness, rigidity, and guarding as a result of peritonitis. A palpable mass may be found if a pancreatic pseudocyst is present. Pancreatic ascites creates a dull sound on percussion.

Monitor and record vital signs frequently to assess for elevated temperature, tachycardia, and decreased blood pressure, or delegate and supervise this activity. Respiratory problems, such as left lung pleural effusions, atelectasis, and pneumonia, are common in patients with acute pancreatitis. Auscultate the lung fields for adventitious sounds or diminished breath sounds, and observe for dyspnea or orthopnea.

Significant changes in vital signs may indicate the life-threatening complication of shock. Hypotension and tachycardia may result from pancreatic hemorrhage, excessive fluid volume shifting, or the toxic effects of abdominal sepsis from enzyme damage. Observe the patient for changes in behavior and level of consciousness (LOC) that may be related to alcohol withdrawal, hypoxia, or impending sepsis with shock.

Psychosocial Assessment

Excessive alcohol intake, particularly in men, is the most frequent cause of acute pancreatitis. Therefore tactfully explore the patient's alcohol intake history. Provide patient privacy and establish a trusting relationship. Discuss the intake of alcohol and the reasons for overindulging. Ask him or her when increased drinking episodes occur, in particular, whether binges occur during holidays, vacations, or weekends or revolve around particular activities, such as television viewing. Question the patient about any recent traumatic or stressful event that may have contributed to increased alcohol consumption, such as the death of a family member or a job loss.

Laboratory Assessment

Diagnostic laboratory abnormalities are typical in patients with acute pancreatitis (Table 62-4). A variety of pancreatic and non-pancreatic disorders can cause increased serum amylase levels. In patients with pancreatitis, *amylase* levels usually increase within 12 to 24 hours and remain elevated for 3 to 4 days. They may be more than three times the normal limit in this disease (Amerine, 2007; Burruss & Holz, 2005). Persistent elevations may be an indicator of pancreatic abscess or pseudocyst.

Lipase is more *specific* in the diagnosis of acute pancreatitis. Serum levels may rise later than amylase and remain elevated for up to 2 weeks. Because these levels stay elevated for such a long time, the health care provider may find this test useful in diagnosing patients who are not examined until several days after the initial onset of symptoms. An increase in lipase and amylase in the urine is also expected.

Trypsin testing is probably the most accurate serum indicator for acute pain but is not widely available. Elastase has not proven to be better than lipase or trypsin in assisting the diagnosis of acute pancreatitis.

If pancreatitis is accompanied by biliary dysfunction (biliary pancreatitis), serum *bilirubin* and *alkaline phosphatase* levels are usually elevated. A sensitive indicator of biliary obstruction in acute pancreatitis is serum *alanine aminotransferase (ALT)*. A threefold or greater rise in concentration indicates that the diagnosis of acute biliary pancreatitis is correct. Elevated *white blood cell (WBC) count and differential, erythrocyte sedimentation rate (ESR),* and serum *glucose* levels are also common in acute pancreatitis. The levels often correlate with disease severity.

TABLE 62-4 Causes of Laboratory Diagnostic Abnormalities in Acute Pancreatitis

Abnormal Finding	Cause
CARDINAL DIAGNOSTIC TESTS	
Increased *serum* amylase	Pancreatic cell injury
Elevated *serum* lipase	Pancreatic cell injury
Elevated *serum* trypsin	Pancreatic cell injury
Elevated *serum* elastase	Pancreatic cell injury
OTHER DIAGNOSTIC TESTS	
Elevated serum glucose	Pancreatic cell injury, resulting in impaired carbohydrate metabolism; decreased insulin release
Decreased serum calcium and magnesium	Fatty acids combined with calcium; seen in fat necrosis
Elevated bilirubin	Hepatobiliary obstructive process
Elevated alanine aminotransferase	Hepatobiliary involvement
Elevated leukocyte count	Inflammatory response

Decreased serum *calcium* and *magnesium* levels are seen with fat necrosis. Calcium levels may fall and remain decreased for 7 to 10 days. Those that consistently remain below 8 mg/dL are associated with a poor prognosis. Other tests include the basal metabolic panel (BMP), complete blood count (CBC), triglycerides, serum total protein, and albumin. The blood urea nitrogen (BUN), serum glucose, and triglycerides are usually elevated. Hemoconcentration is common as a result of third-space fluid loss. Leukocytosis (elevated WBCs) and thrombocytopenia (decreased platelets) are common (Holcomb, 2007). Albumin levels are decreased because cytokines (e.g., tumor necrosis factor [TNF]) released as part of the inflammatory response allow it to move from the bloodstream into the extravascular space. The presence of C-reactive protein suggests pancreatic inflammation and necrosis (Amerine, 2007).

Imaging Assessment

Abdominal ultrasound is the most sensitive test to diagnose causes of pancreatitis like gallstones and can be performed at the bedside. However, it is not helpful in viewing the pancreas because of overlying bowel gas. Therefore *contrast-induced computed tomography (CT)* provides a more reliable image and diagnosis of acute pancreatitis. This noninvasive technique may also be used to rule out pancreatic pseudocyst or ductal calculi.

An abdominal x-ray may also reveal gallstones. A chest x-ray may show elevation of the left side of the diaphragm or pleural effusion.

Analysis

Common Nursing Diagnoses and Collaborative Problems

The priority nursing diagnoses for patients with acute pancreatitis are:

1. Acute Pain related to biologic and injury agents (pancreatic inflammation and enzyme leakage)
2. Imbalanced Nutrition: Less Than Body Requirements related to the inability to ingest food and absorb nutrients

Additional Nursing Diagnoses and Collaborative Problems

In addition to the common nursing diagnoses, patients with acute pancreatitis may have one or more of these nursing diagnoses:

- Nausea related to pancreatic disease
- Risk for Deficient Fluid Volume related to abnormal and normal routines
- Risk for Infection related to necrotic pancreatic tissue
- Ineffective Breathing Pattern related to the complications of pleural effusion or acute respiratory distress syndrome (ARDS)
- Risk for Activity Intolerance related to generalized weakness
- Sleep Deprivation related to pain

The patient with pancreatitis may also have these collaborative problems:

- Potential for Hyperglycemia
- Potential for Hemorrhage
- Potential for Hypovolemic or Septic Shock
- Potential for ARDS
- Potential for Paralytic Ileus
- Potential for Multi-system Organ Failure

Planning and Implementation

Acute Pain

Planning: Expected Outcomes. The patient with acute pancreatitis is expected to state that he or she has a decrease in or absence of abdominal pain, as evidenced by a pain scale measurement.

Interventions. *The priority for patient care is to provide supportive care by relieving symptoms, decrease inflammation, and anticipate or treat complications. As for any patient, continually assess for and support the ABCs (airway, breathing, and circulation). In collaboration with the respiratory therapist, if available, provide oxygen and other respiratory support as needed.* The collaborative care plan depends on the severity of the illness.

Abdominal pain is the most common symptom of pancreatitis. The main focus of nursing care is aimed at controlling pain by interventions that decrease GI tract activity, thus decreasing pancreatic stimulation. Pain assessment to measure the effectiveness of these interventions is an essential part of nursing care.

Nonsurgical Management. *Mild* pancreatitis requires hydration with IV fluids, pain control, and drug therapy. The health care team initially attempts to relieve pain with nonsurgical interventions, which include fasting, drug therapy, and comfort measures. If the patient has a life-threatening complication or requires frequent assessment, he or she is admitted to a critical care unit for invasive hemodynamic monitoring.

Fasting and rest. To rest the pancreas and reduce pancreatic enzyme secretion, withhold food and fluids during the acute period. The health care provider prescribes IV isotonic fluid administration to maintain hydration. IV replacement of calcium and magnesium may also be needed. Measure and document intake and output. Some patients have an indwelling urinary catheter to obtain accurate measurements.

Nasogastric drainage and suction are reserved for more *severely ill* patients who have continuous vomiting or biliary obstruction. Gastric decompression using a nasogastric tube (NGT) prevents gastric juices from flowing into the duodenum. Because paralytic (adynamic) ileus is a common complication of acute pancreatitis, prolonged nasogastric intubation may be necessary. Assess frequently for the return of peristalsis by asking the patient if he or she has passed flatus or had a stool. The return of bowel sounds is not reliable as an indicator of peristalsis return.

Drug therapy. To decrease pain, the primary drug class used is opioid. Other drugs may also be prescribed. Pain management for acute pancreatitis typically begins with the administration of opioids by patient-controlled analgesia (PCA). Drugs such as morphine or hydromorphone (Dilaudid) are typically used because meperidine (Demerol) can cause seizures, especially in older adults. Other options that have been used successfully to manage acute pain include IV or transdermal fentanyl and epidural analgesia.

In mild pancreatitis, the pain usually subsides in 2 to 4 days. However, with severe acute pancreatitis, the abdominal pain and tenderness may persist for up to 2 weeks. The dosages and intervals of drug administration are individualized according to the severity of the disease and the symptoms.

Drugs that relax smooth muscle (spasmolytics) such as papaverine (Pavabid, Cerespan) and nitroglycerin may be used. Anticholinergics such as dicyclomine (Bentyl) help decrease vagal stimulation, motility, and pancreatic flow. *However, these drugs are contraindicated in patients with paralytic ileus.* Histamine receptor antagonists (e.g., ranitidine [Zantac]) and proton pump inhibitors (e.g., omeprazole [Prilosec]) help decrease gastric acid secretion. Drugs such as somatostatin and octreotide are given to decrease pancreatic secretions (Holcomb, 2007). Antibiotics may be used, but they are indicated primarily for patients with acute necrotizing pancreatitis. Common drugs used include cefuroxime (Zinacef), ceftazidime (Ceptaz), and imipenem and cilastatin (Primaxin IV).

Comfort measures. Helping the patient assume a side-lying position (with the legs drawn up to the chest) may decrease the abdominal pain of pancreatitis. Sitting with the knees flexed toward the chest is also helpful.

If the patient is NPO or has an NGT, remind assistive nursing personnel to implement frequent oral hygiene measures to keep mucous membranes moist and free of inflammation or crusting. Because of the drying effect of drugs and the absence of oral fluids, the mouth and oral cavity may be extremely dry, resulting in considerable discomfort and possibly parotitis (inflammation of the parotid [salivary] glands).

Monitor the patient's respiratory status every 8 hours or more often as needed, and provide oxygen to promote comfort in breathing. Respiratory complications such as pleural effusions increase patient discomfort. Fluid overload can be detected by assessing for weight gain, listening for crackles, and observing for dyspnea. Monitor for signs and symptoms of hypocalcemia by assessing for Chvostek's and Trousseau's signs. These tests cause muscle spasms after stimulating the associated nerves. Chapter 13 discusses assessment and interventions for patients with hypocalcemia in more detail.

Lowering the patient's anxiety level may also substantially reduce pain. Explain all procedures and other aspects of patient care thoroughly. Provide reassurance, offer diversional activities such as television, music, and reading material, and encourage visitors to direct attention away from the pain.

Endoscopic retrograde cholangiopancreatography (ERCP). If pancreatitis was caused by gallstones, an ERCP with a **sphincterotomy** (opening of the sphincter of Oddi) may be performed on an urgent or emergent basis. If this procedure is not successful, surgery is required. ERCP is described in detail in Chapter 55.

Surgical Management. Surgical intervention for acute pancreatitis is usually not indicated. However, if an ERCP is not successful in removing gallstones, a laparoscopic cholecystectomy may be performed as described on p. 1369 in the discussion of Surgical Management in the Cholecystitis section.

Complications of pancreatitis, such as pancreatic pseudocyst and abscess, may also require surgical intervention. Laparoscopy (minimally invasive surgery [MIS]) may be done to drain an abscess or pseudocyst. For patients who are high surgical risks, pseudocysts or abscesses can be treated by percutaneous drainage under CT guidance.

Imbalanced Nutrition: Less Than Body Requirements

NOC **Planning: Expected Outcomes.** The patient with acute pancreatitis is expected to have nutrients available to meet metabolic needs. Indicators include that the patient will have normal:

- Nutrient intake
- Fluid intake
- Weight-height ratio
- Hematocrit
- Hydration
- Serum total protein and albumin

Interventions. The patient is maintained on NPO status in the early stages of pancreatitis. Antiemetics for nausea and vomiting are prescribed as needed. Patients who have severe pancreatitis and are unable to eat for 24 to 48 hours after illness onset should begin jejunal tube feeding unless paralytic ileus is present (Holcomb, 2007). Early nutritional intervention enhances immune system functioning and may prevent complications and worsening inflammation. Enteral feeding is preferred over total parenteral nutrition (TPN) because it causes fewer episodes of glucose elevation and other complications associated with TPN. Be sure that the patient is weighed every day. Collaborate with the health care provider, nutritionist, and pharmacist to plan and implement the most appropriate nutritional intervention. Chapter 63 describes interdisciplinary care of patients receiving enteral feeding and TPN.

When food is tolerated during the recovery phase, the health care provider prescribes small, frequent, moderate- to high-carbohydrate, high-protein, low-fat meals. Foods should be bland with little spice. GI stimulants such as caffeine-containing foods (tea, coffee, cola, and chocolate), as well as alcohol, should be avoided. Monitor the patient beginning to resume oral food intake for nausea, vomiting, and diarrhea. *If any of these symptoms occur, notify the health care provider immediately.*

To boost caloric intake, commercial liquid nutritional preparations supplement the diet. The health care provider may also prescribe fat-soluble and other vitamin and mineral replacement supplements. Glutamine, omega-3 fatty acids, fiber, antioxidants, and/or nucleotides may be added to the patient's nutrition plan (Holcomb, 2007).

Community-Based Care

Home Care Management

Home care preparation is individualized for each patient's circumstances. Some patients may be severely weakened from their acute illness and need to confine activity to one floor, limiting stair climbing and other strenuous activities until they regain their strength. Collaborate with the case manager to plan the best place for the patient to recover and resources that may be needed.

Health Teaching

Education needs to be started early in the hospitalization period—as soon as the acute episodes of pain have subsided. Assess the patient's and family's knowledge of the disease.

The desired outcomes for discharge planning and education are to avoid further episodes of pancreatitis and prevent progression to a chronic disease. Instruct the patient to abstain from drinking alcohol to prevent further pain attacks and extension of inflammation and pancreatic insufficiency. Tell the patient that if alcohol is consumed, acute pain will return and further autodigestion of the pancreas may lead to chronic pancreatitis.

Teach the patient to notify the health care provider after discharge to home if acute abdominal pain or biliary tract disease (as evidenced by jaundice, clay-colored stools, or darkened urine) occurs. These signs and symptoms are possible indicators of complications or disease progression.

Health Care Resources

Patients with acute pancreatitis may require several visits by a home care nurse if the hospital course was complicated. In these cases, home care may be needed for wound care and assistance with ADLs. The patient requires medical follow-up with the primary care physician or nurse practitioner to monitor the disease process. For those with alcoholism, provide information about groups such as Alcoholics Anonymous (AA). Family members may attend support groups such as Al-Anon and Alateen.

Evaluation: Outcomes

Evaluate the care of the patient with acute pancreatitis on the basis of the identified nursing diagnoses and collaborative problems. The expected outcomes include that the patient will:

- Have control of abdominal pain, as indicated by self-report
- Have adequate nutrients available to meet metabolic demand

Specific indicators for these outcomes are listed for each nursing diagnosis under the Planning and Implementation section.

DECISION-MAKING CHALLENGE
Coordination of Care

A 72-year-old man is admitted to the critical care unit with acute pancreatitis secondary to alcoholism and a history of gallstones, hypertension, and type 2 diabetes. He has lost 10 pounds (4.5 kg) in the past month and reports severe abdominal pain, fatigue, and weakness. On physical assessment, he has decreased bowel sounds in all quadrants, crackles in the bases of his lungs, and signs of dehydration. Vital signs are: T, 99° F; P, 104; R, 30; and BP, 102/60.

1. What is the priority for this patient's care at this time? Why?
2. What laboratory findings would you expect him to have? Why?
3. With whom should you collaborate to meet the desired outcomes for his care?
4. What community support and health teaching is he going to require when he is discharged?

evolve For suggested answer guidelines, go to http://evolve.elsevier.com/Iggy/.

CHRONIC PANCREATITIS
Pathophysiology

Chronic pancreatitis is a progressive, destructive disease of the pancreas that has remissions and exacerbations ("flare-ups"). Inflammation and fibrosis of the tissue contribute to pancreatic insufficiency and diminished function of the organ. Chronic pancreatitis usually develops after repeated episodes of alcohol-induced acute pancreatitis. It may also be associated with chronic obstruction of the common bile duct. The disease may develop without a known acute disorder. Relief of pain, prevention of recurrence of attacks, prevention of complications, and nutritional support are the principal interventions.

Chronic pancreatitis can be classified into several categories. *Alcoholism* is the primary risk factor for **chronic calcifying pancreatitis (CCP).** In the early stages of the disease, pancreatic secretions precipitate as insoluble proteins that plug the pancreatic ducts and flow of pancreatic juices. As the protein plugs become more widespread, the cellular lining of the ducts changes and ulcerates. This inflammatory process causes fibrosis of the pancreatic tissue. Intraductal calcification and marked pancreatic tissue destruction develop in the late stages. The organ becomes hard and firm as a result of cell atrophy and pancreatic insufficiency.

Chronic obstructive pancreatitis develops from inflammation, spasm, and obstruction of the sphincter of Oddi, often from cholelithiasis (gallstones). Inflammatory and sclerotic lesions occur in the head of the pancreas and around the ducts, causing an obstruction and backflow of pancreatic secretions. (See Complications of Acute Pancreatitis, p. 1373.)

Pancreatic insufficiency in chronic pancreatitis causes loss of *exocrine* function. Most patients with chronic pancreatitis have decreased pancreatic secretions and bicarbonate. Pancreatic enzyme secretion must be greatly reduced to produce steatorrhea resulting from severe malabsorption of fats. These characteristic stools are pale, bulky, and frothy and have an offensive odor. The action of colonic bacteria on unabsorbed lipids and proteins is responsible for the extremely foul odor. On inspection of the stools, the fat content is visible. In severe chronic pancreatitis, stool fat output may be more than 40 g/day.

Fat malabsorption also contributes to weight loss and muscle wasting (a decrease in muscle mass) and leads to general debilitation. Protein malabsorption results in a "starvation" edema of the feet, legs, and hands caused by decreased levels of circulating albumin.

The loss of pancreatic *endocrine* function is responsible for the development of diabetes mellitus in patients with chronic pancreatic insufficiency. (See Chapter 67 for a complete discussion of diabetes mellitus.)

The patient with chronic pancreatitis may have pulmonary complications, such as pleuritic pain, pleural effusions, and pulmonary infiltrates. Pancreatic ascites may decrease diaphragmatic excursion and lung expansion, resulting in impaired ventilation. In the ill patient with chronic pancreatitis, acute respiratory distress syndrome (ARDS) may develop.

Etiology

The cause of chronic calcifying pancreatitis is persistent excessive alcohol intake that results in repeated episodes of acute pancreatitis. The most common cause of chronic obstructive pancreatitis is cholelithiasis and biliary tract disease, which results in persistent inflammation. Other etiologic factors include pancreatic pseudocyst, postoperative ductal scarring, and cancer of the pancreas or duodenum. All of these factors can produce obstruction of the pancreatic duct. Chronic pancreatitis is a risk factor for pancreatic cancer (McCance & Huether, 2006).

Incidence/Prevalence

The leading cause of chronic pancreatitis is alcoholism (McCance & Huether, 2006). Chronic calcifying pancreatitis is found predominantly in men, but the incidence in women is increasing. In women, chronic pancreatitis occurs more commonly among those with biliary tract disease (cholecystitis and cholelithiasis).

Patient-Centered Collaborative Care

Assessment

Clinical manifestations of chronic pancreatitis differ from those of an acute inflammation. However, abdominal pain is the major clinical manifestation (Chart 62-3). The patient typically describes the pain as a continuous burning or gnawing dullness with periods of acute exacerbation (flare-ups). The pain is very intense and relentless. The frequency of acute exacerbations may increase as the pancreatic fibrosis develops.

Perform an abdominal assessment. Abdominal tenderness is less intense in patients with chronic pancreatitis than in those with acute pancreatitis. A mass may be palpated in the left upper quadrant, which may suggest a pancreatic pseudocyst or abscess. Massive pancreatic ascites may be present, producing dullness on abdominal percussion. Because respi-

Chart 62-3 KEY FEATURES

Chronic Pancreatitis

- Intense abdominal pain (major clinical manifestation) that is continuous and burning or gnawing
- Abdominal tenderness
- Ascites
- Possible left upper quadrant mass (if pseudocyst or abscess is present)
- Respiratory compromise manifested by adventitious or diminished breath sounds, dyspnea, or orthopnea
- Steatorrhea; clay-colored stools
- Weight loss
- Jaundice
- Dark urine
- Polyuria, polydipsia, polyphagia (diabetes mellitus)

ratory complications can occur, auscultate the lung fields for adventitious sounds or decreased aeration and observe for dyspnea or orthopnea.

Ask the patient to collect a random stool specimen if able, or ask him or her to describe the stools. The specimen may show **steatorrhea** (foul-smelling fatty stools that may increase in volume as pancreatic insufficiency progresses and lipase production decreases). Assess for unintentional weight loss, muscle wasting, jaundice, dark urine, and the manifestations of diabetes mellitus, such as polyuria (increased urinary output), polydipsia (excessive thirst), and polyphagia (increased appetite).

Diagnosis is based on the patient's clinical manifestations and laboratory and imaging assessment. Endoscopic retrograde cholangiopancreatography (ERCP) is done to visualize the pancreatic and common bile ducts. Imaging studies such as computed tomography (CT) scanning, magnetic resonance imaging (MRI), abdominal ultrasound (US), and endoscopic ultrasound (EUS) are also useful in making the diagnosis. In chronic pancreatitis, laboratory findings include normal or moderately elevated serum amylase and lipase levels. Obstruction of the intrahepatic bile duct can cause elevated serum bilirubin and alkaline phosphatase levels. Intermittent elevations in serum glucose levels are common and can be detected by blood glucose monitoring, both fasting and non-fasting.

▪ *Interventions*

The focus of caring for the patient with chronic pancreatitis is to manage pain, assist in maintaining a sufficient nutritional intake, and prevent recurrence.

Nonsurgical Management

Nonsurgical interventions include primarily drug and nutrition therapy. The major intervention for the pain of chronic pancreatitis is drug therapy. Medicate the patient as prescribed according to the assessment of the intensity of pain. Evaluate the effectiveness of the drug intervention. Opioid analgesia is most frequently used initially, but dependency may occur. Non-opioid analgesics may be tried to relieve pain. (See Chapter 5 for other interventions for chronic pain.)

Pancreatic enzymes are essential dietary supplements (Chart 62-4). These enzymes are given with meals or snacks to aid in digestion and absorption of fat and protein. Drugs such as pancrelipase (Cotazym, Viokase) are prescribed in capsule, tablet, or powder form and contain amylase, lipase, and protease. Teach the patient to take these drugs immediately before or during meals with a glass of water. Enteric-coated tablets should not be broken, crushed, or chewed. Instruct patients who have difficulty swallowing to open capsules and spread the contents over applesauce, mashed fruit, or rice cereal. Enzyme preparations should not be mixed with foods containing proteins, because the enzymatic action dissolves the food into a watery substance. Advise the patient to wipe his or her lips with a wet towel to prevent the skin irritation and breakdown that residual enzymes can cause. Remind the patient to not inhale the enzymatic powder while preparing to take it because it may irritate mucous membranes and cause bronchospasm.

Chart 62-4 PATIENT AND FAMILY EDUCATION GUIDE

Enzyme Replacement for the Patient with Chronic Pancreatitis

- Take pancreatic enzymes before or with meals and snacks with a glass of water.
- Administer enzymes after antacid or H_2 blockers. (Decreased pH inactivates drug.)
- Tell the patient to swallow the tablets without chewing to minimize oral irritation.
- Mix the powder form in applesauce or fruit juice at patient's request.
- Do not mix enzyme preparations in protein-containing foods.
- Have the patient wipe his or her lips after taking enzymes to avoid skin irritation.
- Do not crush enteric-coated preparations.
- Follow up on all scheduled laboratory testing. (Pancrelipase can cause an increase in uric acid levels.)

The dosage of pancreatic enzymes depends on the severity of the malabsorption. Record the number and consistency of stools per day to monitor the effectiveness of enzyme therapy. If pancreatic enzyme treatment is effective, the stools should become less frequent and less fatty.

If the patient has diabetes, the health care provider prescribes insulin or oral hypoglycemic agents for glucose control. Patients maintained on total parenteral nutrition (TPN) are particularly susceptible to elevated glucose levels and may require regular insulin additives to the solution. Closely monitor blood glucose so that hyperglycemia is controlled. Check finger-stick blood glucose or sugar (FSBG or FSBS) levels every 2 to 4 hours.

The health care provider may also prescribe drug therapy to decrease gastric acid. Gastric acid destroys the lipase needed to break down fats. Controlling the acidity of the stomach with H_2 blockers or proton pump inhibitors or neutralizing stomach acid with oral sodium bicarbonate may enhance the effectiveness of the non–enteric-coated enzyme therapy. Subcutaneous octreotide (Sandostatin), a growth hormone similar to somatostatin, is used by some physicians if pain and diarrhea persist.

Protein and fat malabsorption result in significant weight loss and decreased muscle mass in the patient with chronic pancreatitis. Therefore the nutritional interventions for acute pancreatitis are also used for chronic pancreatitis. The patient often limits food intake to avoid increased pain. For this reason, nutrition maintenance is often difficult to achieve. Patients receive either total parenteral nutrition (TPN) or total enteral nutrition (TEN), including vitamin and mineral replacement.

Collaborate with the nutritionist to teach the patient about long-term dietary management. He or she needs an increased number of calories, up to 4000 to 6000 calories/day, to maintain weight. Those high in carbohydrates and protein also assist in the healing process. Foods high in fat are avoided because they cause or increase diarrhea. Teach all patients to avoid alcohol.

Surgical Management

Surgery is not a primary intervention for the treatment of chronic pancreatitis. However, it may be indicated for ongoing abdominal pain, incapacitating relapses of pain, or complications such as abscesses and pseudocysts.

The underlying pathologic changes determine the procedure indicated. Using laparoscopy, the surgeon incises and drains an abscess or pseudocyst. Laparoscopic cholecystectomy or choledochotomy (incision of the common bile duct) may be indicated if biliary tract disease is an underlying cause of pancreatitis. If the pancreatic duct sphincter is fibrotic, the surgeon performs a sphincterotomy (incision of the sphincter) to enlarge it. Endoscopic sphincterotomy may be used for patients who are poor surgical candidates.

In some cases, laparoscopic distal pancreatectomy may be appropriate for resection of the distal pancreas. This procedure is discussed in Surgical Management on p. 1382 in the Pancreatic Cancer section.

In a few cases, pancreas transplantation may be done. However, this procedure is performed most often for patients with severe, uncontrolled diabetes. Chapter 67 discusses pancreas transplantation.

Community-Based Care

Collaborate with the hospital-based case manager (CM) or discharge planner about home care or follow-up in another setting. A community-based CM may continue to follow the patient after hospital discharge. If the patient is discharged to home, the activity area should be limited to one floor until he or she regains strength and can increase activity. Teach patients and families that toilet facilities must be easily accessible because of chronic steatorrhea and frequent defecation. If they are not easily accessible, a bedside commode is obtained for the home.

Because there is no known cure for chronic pancreatitis, patient and family education is aimed at preventing acute episodes of the disease, providing long-term care, and promoting health maintenance (Chart 62-5). Teach the patient to avoid known irritating substances, such as caffeinated beverages (stimulates the GI system) and alcohol. Collaborate with the nutritionist in diet teaching, which focuses on eating bland, low-fat, frequent meals and avoiding rich, fatty foods. Stress the importance of adhering to the nutritional recommendations. Written instructions are essential, with consideration of personal and cultural food preferences.

Remind the patient and family members or significant others of the importance of adhering to pancreatic enzyme replacement. The patient must take the prescribed enzymes with meals and snacks to aid in the digestion of food and promote the absorption of fats and proteins. Teach the patient to take the enzymes before or at the beginning of the meal. Instruct him or her to report any increase in foul-smelling, frothy, fatty stools; abdominal distention; and cramping to the health care provider so that these supplements may be increased as needed. Remind the patient to report any skin breakdown so that therapeutic interventions to promote skin integrity can be started.

The frequency of defecation (whether continent or incontinent) poses challenging skin care problems. Instruct the patient to keep the skin dry and free of the abrasive fatty stools, which damage the skin. The skin should be cleaned thoroughly after each stool and a soothing emollient such as Sween Cream applied. To prevent breakdown and maintain skin integrity, a skin barrier may be needed. Many products on the market such as zinc oxide cream actively repel stool from the skin.

If the patient develops diabetes mellitus as a result of chronic pancreatitis, management of elevated glucose levels after discharge from the hospital may require oral antidiabetic agents or insulin injections. If this is the case, collaborate with the certified diabetic educator (CDE) to provide in-depth teaching concerning diabetes, its signs and symptoms, medical management, drug therapy, nutrition therapy, blood glucose monitoring, and general care.

Chronic illnesses are devastating for families. The high costs of medical insurance, medical treatment, and drug therapy cause serious financial problems. Often the patient with chronic pancreatitis is unable to work. Collaborate with the CM about ways to help the patient with resources for financial help.

The patient may require several home visits by nurses, depending on the severity of the chronic health problems and home maintenance and support needs. The nurse assesses the patient for pain management, adherence to the nutritional plan and alcohol abstinence, the effectiveness of pancreatic enzyme therapy, and psychosocial adaptation to a chronic illness. Refer him or her and the family to a counselor or a self-help group, such as Alcoholics Anonymous (www.aa.org) and Al-Anon (www.al-anon.org), if appropriate.

Chart 62-5 PATIENT AND FAMILY EDUCATION GUIDE

Prevention of Exacerbations of Chronic Pancreatitis

- Avoid things that make your symptoms worse, such as drinking caffeinated beverages.
- Avoid alcohol ingestion; refer to self-help group for assistance.
- Avoid nicotine.
- Eat bland, low-fat, high-protein, moderate-carbohydrate meals; avoid gastric stimulants, such as spices.
- Eat small meals and snacks high in calories.
- Take the pancreatic enzymes that have been prescribed for you with meals.
- Rest frequently; restrict your activity to one floor until you regain your strength.

PANCREATIC ABSCESS

Pancreatic abscesses are the most serious complication of acute necrotizing pancreatitis. If untreated, they are always fatal. After surgery, the recurrence rate is higher than 30%. The abscesses form from collections of purulent liquefaction of the necrotic pancreas.

Pancreatic abscesses occur after severe acute pancreatitis, episodes of chronic pancreatitis, or gallbladder surgery. The development of either a single abscess or multiple abscesses results from extensive inflammatory necrosis of the pancreas that is readily invaded by infectious organisms, such as enteric bacteria and *Candida*. They can erode through the retroperitoneum into the bowel mesentery, the mediastinum, the pleural space, or the pelvis.

Patients with pancreatic abscesses often appear more seriously ill than those with pseudocysts. Clinical manifestations are similar. However, the temperature in patients with abscesses may spike to as high as 104° F (40° C). Blood cultures are helpful in revealing the infective organism. Pleural effusions commonly accompany these abscesses if they enter the pleural space. Ultrasonography and computed tomography (CT) cannot differentiate between pancreatic pseudocysts and abscesses.

Drainage via the percutaneous method or laparoscopy should be performed as soon as possible to prevent sepsis. Antibiotic treatment alone does not resolve the abscess. Death rates remain high even after surgical drainage. Many patients require multiple drainage procedures for repeated abscesses.

PANCREATIC PSEUDOCYST

Pathophysiology

Pancreatic pseudocysts, or false cysts, are so named because, unlike true cysts, they do not have an epithelial lining. They are encapsulated, saclike structures that form on or surround the pancreas. The pseudocyst wall is inflamed, vascular, and fibrotic. It may contain up to several liters of straw-colored or dark-brown viscous fluid, the enzymatic exudate of the pancreas (McCance & Huether, 2006). Risk factors for pseudocysts are acute pancreatitis, abdominal trauma, and chronic pancreatitis.

Patient-Centered Collaborative Care

A pseudocyst can be palpated as an epigastric mass in about half of all cases. The primary presenting symptom is epigastric pain radiating to the back. Other common clinical manifestations include abdominal fullness, nausea, vomiting, and jaundice. Pseudocysts are diagnosed and their growth and resolution monitored by serial pancreatic ultrasonographic examination, CT, or MRI.

Complications of pseudocyst formation include:

- Hemorrhage
- Infection
- Obstruction of the bowel, biliary tract, or splenic vein
- Abscess
- Fistula formation
- Pancreatic ascites

Pseudocysts may spontaneously resolve, or they may rupture and produce hemorrhage. Surgical intervention is necessary if the pseudocyst does not resolve within 6 to 8 weeks or if complications develop. Possible surgeries include:

- Percutaneous drainage using a needle, usually under CT scan guidance
- Endoscopic-assisted drainage using an endoscope to locate the pseudocyst
- Surgical drainage of the pseudocyst into the stomach or jejunum

To provide external drainage, the surgeon inserts a sump drainage tube to remove pancreatic secretions and exudate. Pancreatic fistulas are common after surgery, and skin breakdown from corrosive pancreatic enzymes in patients who have external drainage presents a major nursing care challenge.

INSULINOMA

Insulinoma is the most common type of neuroendocrine pancreatic tumor even though it is rare. As the name implies, these tumors are typically benign tumors of the islets of Langerhans that cause excessive insulin secretion and subsequent hypoglycemia (low serum glucose). Laboratory testing is helpful in most cases for diagnosis. Endoscopic ultrasonography, CT scan, or MRI may be done to locate the tumor.

Management includes removal of the tumor, usually via laparoscopic partial pancreatectomy. Nursing care associated with this surgery is described in the Pancreatic Cancer section, which follows.

PANCREATIC CANCER

Pathophysiology

Cancer of the pancreas is the fourth leading cause of cancer deaths each year in the United States. Over 33,000 people are diagnosed with the disease every year (Halls & Ward-Smith, 2007). It is difficult to diagnose early because the pancreas is hidden and surrounded by other organs. Treatment has limited results, and 5-year survival rates are extremely low (American Cancer Society [ACS], 2008).

Pancreatic tumors usually originate from epithelial cells of the pancreatic ductal system. If the tumor is discovered in the early stages, the tumor cells may be localized within the glandular organ. However, this is highly unlikely. Most often, the tumor is discovered in the late stages of development and may be a well-defined mass or is diffusely spread throughout the pancreas.

The tumor may be a primary cancer, or it may result from metastasis from cancers of the lung, breast, thyroid, kidney, or skin. Primary tumors are generally adenocarcinomas and grow in well-differentiated glandular patterns. They grow rapidly and spread to surrounding organs (stomach, duodenum, gallbladder, and intestine) by direct extension and invasion of lymphatic and vascular systems. This highly metastatic lesion may eventually invade the lung, peritoneum, liver, spleen, and lymph nodes.

Clinical manifestations depend on the site of origin or metastasis. The head of the pancreas is the most common site. The tumors are usually small lesions with poorly defined margins. Jaundice results from tumor compression and obstruction of the common bile duct and from gallbladder dilation, causing the organ to enlarge.

Cancers of the body and tail of the pancreas are usually large and invade the entire tail and body. These tumors may be palpable abdominal masses, especially in the thin patient. Through metastatic spread via the splenic vein, metastasis to the liver may cause **hepatomegaly** (enlargement of the liver up to two to three times its normal size). Cancers of the body and tail spread more extensively than do pancreatic head carcinomas, with invasion of the retroperitoneum, vertebral column, spleen, adrenal glands, colon, or stomach. Regardless of where it originates, it spreads rapidly through the lymphatic and venous systems to other organs.

Venous thromboembolism is a common complication of pancreatic cancer. Necrotic products of the pancreatic tumor are believed to have thromboplastic properties resulting in the blood's hypercoagulable state. In addition, the patient is at high risk because of decreased mobility and extensive surgical manipulation.

The exact cause of pancreatic cancer is unknown. High-risk populations are those in their sixth to eighth decades of life and those with a personal history of smoking.

GENETIC CONSIDERATIONS

A small number of those with pancreatic cancer have an inherited risk. Mutations in certain oncogenes have been identified. Mutations have also been revealed in tumor suppressor genes, such as *p16* and *BRCA2*—the same mutation that makes some women susceptible to breast and ovarian cancer. Genes responsible for hereditary non-polyposis colorectal cancer can also increase a person's risk for pancreatic cancer (ACS, 2008).

Other risk factors associated with the disease include:

- Diabetes mellitus
- Chronic pancreatitis
- Cirrhosis
- High intake of red meat, especially processed meat like bacon
- Long-term exposure to chemicals such as gasoline and pesticides
- Obesity

Patient-Centered Collaborative Care

Assessment

Pancreatic cancer often presents in a slow and vague manner. The presenting symptoms depend somewhat on the location of the tumor. The first sign may be jaundice, which suggests late, advanced disease (Chart 62-6). Jaundice occurs because the gallbladder and liver are commonly involved. As the tumor spreads, the green-gold skin color associated with obstructive jaundice progressively worsens. Ask the patient whether the color of the stool and urine has changed. As a result of the obstructive process, the stool is clay colored and the urine is dark and frothy. Inspect the skin for dryness and scratch marks, indicating pruritus from jaundice caused by bile salt collection. Assess the sclerae for icterus (yellowing) and the mucous membranes for signs of jaundice.

Chart 62-6 KEY FEATURES

Pancreatic Cancer

- Jaundice
- Clay- (light) colored stools
- Dark urine
- Abdominal pain: usually vague, dull, or nonspecific that radiates into the back
- Weight loss
- Anorexia
- Nausea or vomiting
- Glucose intolerance
- Splenomegaly (enlarged spleen)
- Flatulence
- Gastrointestinal bleeding
- Ascites (abdominal fluid)
- Leg or calf pain (from thrombophlebitis)
- Weakness and fatigue

The enlarged gallbladder and liver may be palpable. In advanced cases of pancreatic carcinoma, the tumor may be felt as a firm, fixed mass in the left upper abdominal quadrant or epigastric region.

The most common concern is fatigue, which is described as a diminished energy level and an increased need for rest relative to the level of activity. The patient notices an inability to perform usual physical or intellectual activities.

Question the patient about abdominal pain, which is usually described as a vague, constant dullness in the upper abdomen and nonspecific in nature. Pain also indicates advanced stages of the disease and may be related to eating or activity. Ask whether the patient has pain in other areas of the body. Referred back pain may be caused by pressure on the nerve plexus. Some patients have leg or calf pain with swelling and redness as a result of deep vein thrombosis or thrombophlebitis.

Weigh the patient to determine the extent of weight loss and whether it has occurred rapidly. Ask about food intake and intolerances. Anorexia accompanied by early satiety, nausea, flatulence (gas), and vomiting is common. GI bleeding may develop from esophageal or gastric varices caused by the tumor pressing on the portal vein. A new diagnosis of diabetes is found in some patients.

In addition to the focused history, perform a general abdominal assessment. In particular, observe for distention and swelling, which may be **ascites** (abdominal fluid). Percussion over the ascitic abdomen elicits dullness seen in the advanced stages of the disease process.

No specific blood tests diagnose pancreatic cancer. Serum amylase and lipase levels, as well as alkaline phosphatase and bilirubin levels, are increased. The degree of elevation depends on the acuteness or chronicity of the pancreatic and biliary damage. Elevated carcinoembryonic antigen (CEA) levels occur in most patients with pancreatic cancer. This test may provide early information about the presence of tumor cells. Other tumor markers such as CA 19-9 and CA 242 have been found to be useful serologic tests for monitoring a proven diagnosis and for continuing surveillance for potential spread or recurrence.

Abdominal ultrasound and computed tomography (CT) are the most commonly used imaging techniques for confirming a tumor and can differentiate the tumor from a cyst. The spiral or helical CT scan is preferred over the conventional CT because it can detect tumors less than 1 centimeter by using three-dimensional imaging (Halls & Ward-Smith, 2007). Endoscopic ultrasonography can also be performed to sample tissue for diagnosis and provide information on tumor type and size (Riehl, 2007). Endoscopic retrograde cholangiopancreatography (ERCP) provides the most definitive diagnostic data. An alternative to ERCP is a percutaneous transhepatic biliary cholangiogram with placement of a percutaneous transhepatic biliary drain (PTBD). This drain decompresses the blocked biliary system by draining bile, either internally, externally, or both. Aspiration of pancreatic ascitic fluid by abdominal paracentesis may reveal cancer cells and elevated amylase levels.

Interventions

Management of the patient with pancreatic cancer is geared toward preventing tumor spread and decreasing pain. These measures are not curative, only palliative. The cancers are often metastatic and recur despite treatment.

Nonsurgical Management

As in other types of cancer, chemotherapy or radiation is used to relieve pain by shrinking the tumor. It may be used before, after, or instead of surgery. *Chemotherapy* has had limited success in increasing survival time. In most cases, combining agents has been more successful than single-agent chemotherapy. 5-Fluorouracil (5-FU), a commonly used drug, may be given alone or with gemcitabine (Gemzar) for locally advanced, or unresectable, pancreatic cancers. Gemcitabine may also be given with capecitabine (Xeloda), docetaxel (Taxotere), and/or erlotinib (Tarceva), a targeted agent for unresectable or metastatic tumors. Some patients receive three or four drugs and have had more tumor shrinkage as a result. Observe for adverse drug effects, such as fatigue, rash, anorexia, and diarrhea.

Other targeted therapies being investigated include growth factor inhibitors, anti-angiogenesis factors, and kinase inhibitors (also known as *tyrosine kinase inhibitors*). Kinase inhibitors are a new group of drugs that focus on cancer cells with little or no effect on healthy cells (Van Laethem & Marechal, 2007). Chapter 24 describes general nursing interventions associated with chemotherapy.

To control pain, the patient takes high doses of opioid analgesics (usually morphine) as prescribed and uses other comfort measures before the pain escalates and peaks. Because of the poor prognosis, drug dependency is not a consideration. Chapter 5 describes the care of the patient with chronic cancer pain in detail.

Intensive external beam *radiation* therapy to the pancreas may offer pain relief by shrinking tumor cells, alleviating obstruction, and improving food absorption. It does not improve survival rates. Implantation of radioactive iodine (^{125}I) seeds, in combination with systemic or intra-arterial administration of floxuridine (FUDR), has also been used. The patient may experience discomfort during and after the radiation treatments. Chapter 24 describes radiation therapy in more detail.

For patients experiencing biliary obstruction who are high surgical risks, **biliary stents** placed percutaneously (through the skin) can ensure patency to relieve pain. These stents are devices made of plastic materials that keep the ducts of the biliary system open. Using another approach, self-expandable stents may be inserted endoscopically to relieve obstruction.

Surgical Management

Complete surgical resection of the pancreatic tumor offers the patient with pancreatic cancer the only effective treatment, but it is done only in patients with small tumors. *Partial pancreatectomy* is the preferred surgery for tumors smaller than 3 centimeters in diameter (Halls & Ward-Smith, 2007). Recent technologic advances have expanded the role of **minimally invasive surgery (MIS)** via laparoscopy in the staging, palliation, and removal of pancreatic cancers. The procedure selected depends on the purpose of the surgery and stage of the disease. For example, if the patient has a biliary obstruction, a laparoscopic procedure to relieve the obstruction is performed. This procedure diverts bile drainage into the jejunum.

For larger tumors, the surgeon may perform either a *radical pancreatectomy* or the *Whipple procedure (pancreaticoduodenectomy).* These procedures have traditionally been done using an open surgical approach. Because of new advances in laparoscopic technology using a hand-assist device, this method is beginning to replace the conventional method. Some surgeons are not yet trained in how to perform this technique. Therefore the traditional, open surgical approach remains the most common method of performing these surgeries.

Preoperative Care. The patient with pancreatic cancer may be a poor surgical risk because of malnutrition and debilitation. Specific care depends on the type of surgical approach being used.

Often, in the late stages of pancreatic cancer or before the Whipple procedure, the physician inserts a small catheter into the jejunum **(jejunostomy)** so that enteral feedings may be given. This feeding method is preferred to prevent reflux and to facilitate absorption. Feedings are started in low concentrations and volumes and are gradually increased as tolerated. Provide feedings using a pump to maintain a constant volume, and assess for diarrhea frequency to determine tolerance. Chapter 63 provides additional information about enteral feeding.

For optimal nutrition, TPN may be necessary in addition to tube feedings or as a single measure to provide nutrition. When central venous access is required, a peripherally inserted central catheter (PICC) or other type of IV catheter may be necessary. Meticulous IV line care is an important nursing measure to prevent catheter sepsis. Sterile dressing changes and site observation are extremely important (see Chapter 15). Additional nursing care measures for the patient receiving TPN are given in Chapter 63. Monitor nutrition indicators such as serum prealbumin and albumin.

For the laparoscopic procedure, no bowel preparation is needed. However, either approach requires that the patient have nothing by mouth (NPO) for at least 6 to 8 hours before surgery. Surgeon preference and agency policy determine the preferred protocol for preoperative preparation.

Operative Procedures. The **Whipple procedure (radical pancreaticoduodenectomy)** involves extensive surgical manipulation and is used most often to treat cancer of the head of the pancreas. The procedure entails removal of the proximal head of the pancreas, the duodenum, a portion of the jejunum, the stomach (partial or total **gastrectomy**), and the gallbladder, with anastomosis of the pancreatic duct **(pancreaticojejunostomy),** the common bile duct **(choledochojejunostomy),** and the stomach **(gastrojejunostomy)** to the jejunum (Fig. 62-3). In addition, the surgeon may remove the spleen **(splenectomy).**

Postoperative Care. In addition to routine postoperative care measures, the patient who has undergone an open radical pancreaticoduodenectomy requires intensive nursing care and is usually admitted to a surgical critical care unit. Observe for multiple potential complications of the open Whipple procedure as listed in Table 62-5.

The primary benefit of MIS is the patient's fast postoperative recovery and less pain than with traditional open procedures. The patient having the laparoscopic Whipple surgery or radical pancreatectomy is also less at risk for severe complications. For patients having one of these procedures, observe for and implement preventive measures for these surgical complications:

- Diabetes (Check blood glucose often.)
- Hemorrhage (Monitor pulse, blood pressure, skin color, and mental status [e.g., LOC].)
- Wound infection (Monitor temperature, and assess wounds for redness and induration [hardness].)
- Bowel obstruction (Check bowel sounds and stools.)
- Intra-abdominal abscess (Monitor temperature and patient's report of severe pain.)

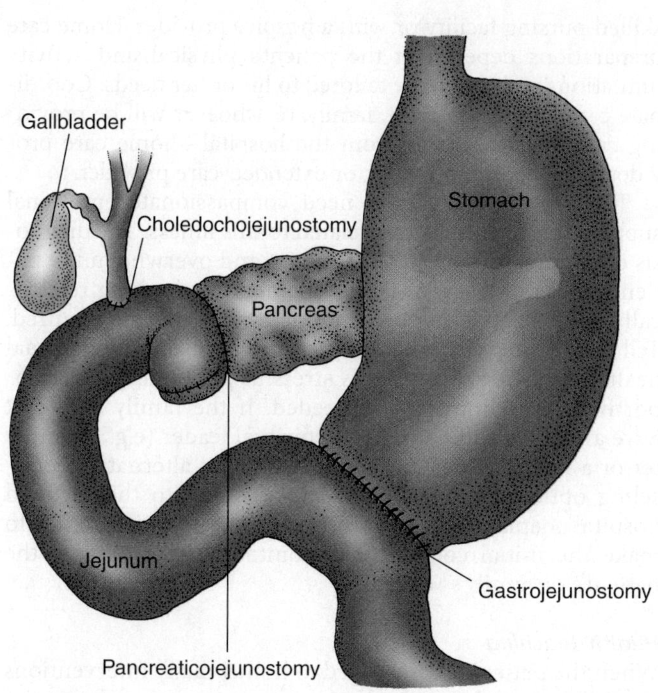
Gallbladder
Choledochojejunostomy
Stomach
Pancreas
Jejunum
Gastrojejunostomy
Pancreaticojejunostomy

Fig. 62-3 • The three anastomoses that constitute the Whipple procedure: choledochojejunostomy, pancreaticojejunostomy, and gastrojejunostomy.

TABLE 62-5 Potential Complications of the Whipple Procedure

CARDIOVASCULAR COMPLICATIONS
- Hemorrhage at anastomosis sites with hypovolemia
- Myocardial infarction
- Heart failure
- Thrombophlebitis

PULMONARY COMPLICATIONS
- Atelectasis
- Pneumonia
- Pulmonary embolism
- Acute respiratory distress syndrome
- Pulmonary edema

GASTROINTESTINAL COMPLICATIONS
- Adynamic (paralytic) ileus
- Gastric retention
- Gastric ulceration
- Bowel obstruction from peritonitis
- Pancreatitis
- Hepatic failure
- Thrombosis to mesentery

WOUND COMPLICATIONS
- Infection
- Dehiscence
- Fistulas: pancreatic, gastric, and biliary

METABOLIC COMPLICATIONS
- Unstable diabetes mellitus
- Renal failure

Immediately after surgery, the patient is NPO and usually has a nasogastric tube (NGT) to decompress the stomach. Monitor GI drainage and tube patency. In open surgical approaches, biliary drainage tubes are placed during surgery to remove drainage and secretions from the area and to prevent stress on the anastomosis sites. Assess the tubes and drainage devices for tension or kinking, and maintain them in a dependent position.

Monitor the drainage for color, consistency, and amount. The drainage should be serosanguineous. The appearance of clear, colorless, bile-tinged drainage or frank blood with an increase in output may indicate disruption or leakage of an anastomosis site. Most of the disruptions of the site occur within 7 to 10 days after surgery. Hemorrhage can occur as an early or late complication.

Place the patient in the semi-Fowler's position to reduce tension on the suture line and anastomosis site as well as to optimize lung expansion. Stress can be decreased by maintaining NGT drainage at a low or high intermittent suction level to keep the remaining stomach (if a partial gastrectomy is done) or the jejunum (if a total gastrectomy is done) free of excessive fluid buildup and pressure. The NGT also reduces stimulation of the remaining pancreatic tissue.

The development of a fistula (an abnormal passageway) is the most common and most serious postoperative complication. Biliary, pancreatic, or gastric fistulas result from partial or total breakdown of an anastomosis site. The secretions that drain from the fistula contain bile, pancreatic enzymes, or gastric secretions, depending on which site is ruptured. *These secretions, particularly pancreatic fluid, are corrosive and irritating to the skin, and internal leakage causes chemical peritonitis.* **Peritonitis** (inflammation and infection of the peritoneum causing boardlike abdominal rigidity) requires treatment with multiple antibiotics. *If you suspect any postoperative complications resulting from MIS or open surgical approaches, call the surgeon immediately and provide assessment findings that support your concerns.*

Because the *open* Whipple procedure is extensive and can take many hours to complete, maintaining fluid and electrolyte balance can be difficult. Patients often have significant intraoperative blood loss and postoperative bleeding. The intestine is exposed to air for long periods, and fluid evaporates. Significant losses of fluid and electrolytes occur from the NGT and other drainage tubes. In addition, these patients may be malnourished and have low serum levels of protein and albumin, which maintain colloid osmotic pressure within the circulating system. Reduction in the serum osmotic pressure makes the patient likely to develop third spacing of body fluids, with fluid moving from the vascular to the interstitial space, resulting in shock. These problems are less likely to occur when MIS is used. Therefore, when possible, the trained surgeon prefers to perform laparoscopic Whipple procedures to shorten operating time and prevent the many complications that can occur.

Closely monitor vital signs for decreased blood pressure and increased heart rate, decreased vascular pressures with a pulmonary artery catheter (Swan-Ganz catheter) (in ICU setting), and decreased urine output to detect early signs of hypovolemia and prevent shock. Be alert for pitting edema of the extremities, dependent edema in the sacrum and back, and an intake that far exceeds output. Maintain sequential compression devices to prevent deep vein thrombosis.

Maintenance of prescribed IV isotonic fluid replacement with colloid replacements is important. Monitor hemoglobin and hematocrit values to assess for blood loss and the need for blood transfusions. Review electrolyte values for decreased serum levels of sodium, potassium, chloride, and calcium. IV fluid concentrations must be altered to correct these electrolyte imbalances. The physician prescribes replacement of electrolytes as needed.

Immediately after the Whipple procedure, the patient may have hyperglycemia or hypoglycemia as a result of stress and surgical manipulation of the pancreas. Most of the endocrine cells (responsible for insulin and glucagon secretion) are located in the body and tail of the pancreas. In some patients, up to half of the gland remains and diabetes does not develop, However, a large number of patients are diabetic before surgery. For patients having a radical pancreatectomy, administer insulin as prescribed, because the entire pancreas is removed. Monitor glucose levels frequently during the early postoperative period, and administer insulin injections as prescribed.

NCLEX EXAMINATION CHALLENGE

A client has had an open Whipple procedure for pancreatic cancer. Which nursing interventions are appropriate for this client in the postoperative period? (Select all that apply.)

A. Maintain IV fluids, and monitor for fluid imbalance.
B. Assess for signs and symptoms of deep vein thrombosis.
C. Connect the nasogastric tube to high intermittent suction.
D. Start pancreatic enzyme replacements as soon as possible.
E. Check finger-stick blood glucose levels regularly.
F. Tell the patient to lie flat to protect the incision.

evolve For the correct answer, go to http://evolve.elsevier.com/Iggy/.

Community-Based Care

The patient with pancreatic cancer is usually followed by a case manager (CM), both in the hospital and in the home or other community-based setting. Collaborate with the CM to ensure that the patient receives cost-effective treatment and that his or her needs are met.

Home Care Management

The stage of progression of pancreatic cancer and available home care resources determine whether the patient can be discharged to home or whether additional care is needed in a skilled nursing facility or with a hospice provider. Home care preparations depend on the patient's physical and activity limitations and should be tailored to his or her needs. Coordinate care with the patient, family, or whoever will be providing care after discharge from the hospital—home care provider, hospice care provider, or extended-care provider.

The patient and family need compassionate emotional support to deal with issues related to this illness. The diagnosis of pancreatic cancer can frighten and overwhelm the patient and family. Assist family members in looking realistically and objectively at the amount of physical care required. Tell family members that their own physical and emotional health are at risk during this stressful period and that supportive counseling may be needed. If the family does not have a religious affiliation or a spiritual leader (e.g., a minister or a rabbi) to provide support, suggest alternative counseling options. Refer patients and families to the certified hospital chaplain if desired. It is appropriate for the nurse to make the initial contact or appointment according to the patient's or family's wishes.

Health Teaching

When the patient is discharged to home, many interventions are palliative and aimed at managing symptoms such as pain. In many cases, the diagnosis of pancreatic cancer is made a few months before death occurs. The patient needs time to adjust to the diagnosis, which is usually made too late for cure or prolonged survival. Help the patient identify what needs to be done to prepare for death, including end-of-life care. For example, he or she may want to write a will or see family members and friends whom he or she has not seen recently. The patient needs to make specific requests for the funeral or memorial service known to family members or others. These actions help prepare for death in a dignified manner. Chapter 9 discusses anticipatory grieving and preparation for death in detail, as well as symptom management during the end-of-life.

Health Care Resources

Regular home care nursing and assistive nursing personnel visits may be scheduled to assist the patient and family by providing physical, psychological, and supportive care. Supply information about local hospice care (see Chapter 9) and cancer support groups.

HUMAN NEEDS NURSING CARE REVIEW

What might you NOTICE if the patient is experiencing inadequate digestion and nutrition as a result of gallbladder and pancreatic disorders?

- Report of intense abdominal pain
- Report of nausea, especially after food
- Report of anorexia
- Vomiting
- Jaundice
- Report of weight loss
- Dark urine
- Clay-colored stools

What should you INTERPRET and how should you RESPOND to a patient experiencing inadequate digestion and nutrition as a result of gallbladder and pancreatic disorders?

Perform and interpret physical assessment, including:

- Take vital signs to assess for hypovolemia and fever.
- Assess respiratory status, including breath sounds.
- Conduct a complete pain assessment if possible.
- Weigh the patient.
- Check laboratory values, especially enzyme levels like amylase and lipase, liver function studies, and CBC. Assess vomitus for quality and amount.

Respond by:

- Keeping the patient's head of the bed elevated and knees flexed
- Providing pain management by comfort measures and analgesia
- Providing oxygen if patient is having dyspnea or adventitious breath sounds
- Reassuring the patient who may be concerned about possible cancer

On what should you REFLECT?

- Observe patient for improvement in signs and symptoms, including pain control.
- Think about what could have caused the health problem.
- Think about what else you could do to help the patient meet desired outcomes.
- Plan health teaching for patient discharge.

GET READY FOR THE NCLEX EXAMINATION!

Key Points

Review these Key Points for each NCLEX Examination Client Needs Category.

Safe and Effective Care Environment

- When caring for a patient with a T-tube, do not place the drainage bag higher than the tube insertion site.
- Recognize that acute pain relief is the first priority for patients with acute pancreatitis.
- Be aware that patients with biliary and pancreatic disorders are at high risk for biliary obstruction, a serious and painful complication.

Health Promotion and Maintenance

- Recognize that obese, middle-aged women are most likely to have gallbladder disease.
- Teach patients to avoid losing weight too quickly and to keep weight under control to help prevent gallbladder disease.
- Instruct patients about ways to prevent exacerbations of chronic pancreatitis as outlined in Chart 62-5.

Psychosocial Integrity

- Provide pain-relief measures for patients with acute pancreatitis to reduce anxiety.
- Refer patients with pancreatitis who use excessive alcohol to community resources such as Alcoholics Anonymous.
- Refer patients with pancreatic cancer for support services such as spiritual leaders and counselors.
- Help prepare the pancreatic cancer patient and family for the death and dying process.

Physiological Integrity

- Be aware that autodigestion of the pancreas causes severe pain in patients with acute pancreatitis (see Fig. 62-2).
- Monitor serum laboratory values, especially amylase and lipase (both elevated), in patients with pancreatitis (see Table 62-4).
- Assess for common clinical manifestations of cholecystitis as listed in Chart 62-1.
- For patients with acute pancreatitis, provide pain management including opioid analgesia.
- Assess for common clinical manifestations of chronic pancreatitis as listed in Chart 62-3.
- Teach patients about enzyme replacement therapy as described in Chart 62-4.
- Assess patients with presenting clinical manifestations of pancreatic cancer as described in Chart 62-6.
- Observe for and implement interventions to prevent life-threatening complications of the Whipple procedure as outlined in Table 62-5.

Additional Study Resources

Go to your Companion CD or Evolve at http://evolve.elsevier.com/Iggy/ for *Self-Assessment Questions for the NCLEX Examination.*

evolve Go to Evolve at http://evolve.elsevier.com/Iggy/ for *Prioritization and Delegation Questions for the NCLEX Examination.*

SELECTED BIBLIOGRAPHY

Asterisk indicates a classic or definitive work on this subject.

American Cancer Society (ACS). (2008). *Cancer facts and figures—2008.* Atlanta: Author.

American College of Gastroenterology. (2006). *Gallstones.* Retrieved April 21, 2008, from www.gi.org/patients/women/gallstones.asp.

Amerine, E. (2007). Get optimum outcomes for acute pancreatitis patients. *The Nurse Practitioner, 32*(6), 44-48.

Baltimore, J.L., & Davidson, J. (2007). Caring for a patient with acute cholecystitis. *Nursing2007, 37*(3), 64hn1-4.

Bellows, C.F., Berger, D.H., & Crass, R.A. (2005). Management of gallstones. *American Family Physician, 72*(4), 637-642.

Burruss, N., & Holz, S. (2005). Understanding acute pancreatitis. *Nursing2005, 35*(3), 32hn1-4.

*Cole, L. (2001). Unraveling the mystery of acute pancreatitis. *Nursing2001, 31*(12), 58-63.

Comstock, D. (2008). Dealing with postcholecystectomy syndrome. *Nursing2008, 38*(4), 17-19.

*Gavaghan, M. (2002). The pancreas: Hermit of the abdomen. *AORN Journal, 75*(6), 1110-1114, 1117, 1119.

*Hale, A.S., Moseley, M.J., & Warner, S.C. (2000). Treating pancreatitis in the acute care setting. *Dimensions of Critical Care Nursing, 19*(4), 15-21.

Halls, B.S., & Ward-Smith, P. (2007). Identifying early symptoms of pancreatic cancer. *Clinical Journal of Oncology Nursing, 11*(2), 245-248.

Holcomb, S.S. (2005). Gallstones. *Nursing2005, 35*(9), 45.

Holcomb, S.S. (2007). Stopping the destruction of acute pancreatitis. *Nursing2007, 37*(6), 43-48.

*Klein, A.P., Brune, K.A., Petersen, G.M., Goggins, M., Tersmette, A.C., Offerhaus, G.J., et al. (2004). Prospective risk of pancreatic cancer in familial pancreatic cancer kindreds. *Cancer Research, 64*(7), 2634-2638.

*Lightner, A.M., Glasgow, R.E., Jordon, T.H., Krassner, A.D., Way, L.W., Mulvihill, S.J., et al. (2004). Pancreatic resection in the elderly. *Journal of the American College of Surgeons, 198*(5), 697-706.

McCance, K.L., & Huether, S.E. (2006). *Pathophysiology: The biologic basis for disease in adults and children* (5th ed.). St. Louis: Mosby.

Pagana, K.D., & Pagana, T.J. (2006). *Mosby's manual of diagnostic and laboratory tests.* St. Louis: Mosby.

*Quillen, S.M. (2001). Identification of pancreatitis in the ambulatory setting. *Gastroenterology Nursing, 24*(1), 20-22.

Riehl, M. (2007). Help your patient cope with pancreatic cancer. *Nursing2007, 37*(4), 54-57.

*Stevens, M., Esler, R., & Asher, G. (2002). Transdermal fentanyl for the management of acute pancreatitis pain. *Applied Nursing Research, 15*(2), 102-110.

Tseng, D., Shappard, B.C., & Hunter, J.G. (2005). New approaches to the minimally invasive treatment of pancreatic cancer. *Cancer Journal, 11*(1), 43-51.

Van Laethem, J.L., & Marechal, R. (2007). Emerging drugs for the treatment of pancreatic cancer. *Expert Opinion on Emerging Drugs, 12*(2), 301-311.

63

CHAPTER

Care of Patients with Malnutrition and Obesity

Donna D. Ignatavicius

LEARNING OUTCOMES

For clinical competence and success on the NCLEX Examination, study this chapter with these Learning Outcomes in mind:

Safe and Effective Care Environment

1. Collaborate with members of the health care team when providing care for patients with malnutrition or obesity.
2. Protect bariatric patients from injury.
3. Delegate and supervise unlicensed assistive personnel (UAP) in assessing and caring for patients with malnutrition.

Health Promotion and Maintenance

4. Provide care that meets the special nutrition needs of older adults.
5. Teach overweight and obese patients the importance of lifestyle changes to promote health.
6. Perform a nutrition screening for all patients to determine if they are at high risk for nutritional health problems.

Psychosocial Integrity

7. Assess patient response to being obese.
8. Incorporate the patient's food preferences when planning nutritional care.

Physiological Integrity

9. Interpret findings of a nutrition screening and assessment.
10. Calculate body mass index (BMI), and interpret findings.
11. Describe the risk factors for malnutrition, especially for older adults.
12. Monitor serum visceral protein levels to indicate change in nutritional status.
13. Provide nutritional supplements as needed to restore or maintain nutrition.
14. Monitor for complications of total enteral nutrition (TEN).
15. Monitor for complications of total parenteral nutrition (TPN).
16. Explain how to maintain enteral tube patency.
17. Intervene to prevent aspiration by checking nasoenteric tube placement.
18. Explain the medical complications associated with obesity.
19. Identify the role of drug therapy in the management of obesity.
20. Prioritize nursing care for patients having bariatric surgery.
21. Develop a discharge teaching plan for patients having bariatric surgery.

Go to your Companion CD or Evolve at http://evolve.elsevier.com/Iggy/ for *Self-Assessment Questions for the NCLEX Examination* keyed to these Learning Outcomes.

Carbohydrates, protein, and fat are nutrients in food that supply the body with energy. In healthy people, most of this energy undergoes digestion and is absorbed from the GI tract. Food energy is used to maintain body temperature, respiration, cardiac output, muscle function, protein synthesis, and the storage and metabolism of food sources. Therefore proper nutrition plays a major role in promoting and maintaining health.

Energy balance refers to the relationship between energy used and energy stored. Weight loss occurs when energy used is more than intake. If food intake is more than energy used, weight is gained. Body proteins are used for energy when calorie intake is insufficient. The body attempts to meet its calorie requirements even if it is at the expense of protein needs.

NUTRITION STANDARDS FOR HEALTH PROMOTION AND MAINTENANCE

The role of nutrition in disease has been a subject of interest for many years. The current focus is on health promotion and the prevention of disease by healthy eating and exercise. In the

TABLE 63-1 Examples of 2005 Dietary Guidelines for Americans

- Consume a variety of nutrient-dense foods and beverages within and among the basic food groups while choosing foods that limit the intake of saturated and *trans* fats, cholesterol, added sugars, salt, and alcohol.
- To maintain body weight in a healthy range, balance calories from foods and beverages with calories expended.
- To prevent gradual weight gain over time, make small decreases in food and beverage calories and increase physical activity.
- Engage in regular physical activity and reduce sedentary activities to promote health, psychological well-being and a healthy body weight.
- Consume a sufficient amount of fruits and vegetables; choose a variety each day.
- Consume 3 or more ounce-equivalents of whole-grain products per day.
- Consume 3 cups per day of fat-free milk or low-fat milk or equivalent milk products.
- Those who drink alcohol may have up to one drink per day for women and up to two drinks per day for men.

Source: U.S. Department of Health and Human Services (DHHS) and the U.S. Department of Agriculture (USDA), 2005. Retrieved June 16, 2008, from *www.healthierus.gov/dietaryguidelines.*

United States, the **Dietary Guidelines for Americans** are revised by the U.S. Department of Agriculture (USDA) and the U.S. Department of Health and Human Services (DHHS) every 5 years. The most recent guidelines (2005) emphasize the need to include preferences of specific racial/ethnic groups, vegetarians, and other populations when selecting foods to maintain a healthful diet that is balanced with moderation and variety (www.health.gov/dietaryguidelines/dga2005/report/html). Examples of some of these guidelines are listed in Table 63-1.

The USDA developed the **Food Guide Pyramid** in 1992 to translate nutrition recommendations into a practical graphic format. A pyramid format was chosen to communicate three key nutrition principles: variety, moderation, and proportion. In 2005, this pyramid was redesigned to help people better understand these principles (Fig. 63-1). MyPyramid also stresses the importance of physical activity to promote health (www.mypyramid.gov).

An increasing number of people are adopting a variety of vegetarian diet patterns for health, environmental, or moral reasons. In general, vegetarians are leaner than those who consume meat. The **lacto-vegetarian** eats milk, cheese, and dairy foods but avoids meat, fish, poultry, and eggs. The **lacto-ovo-vegetarian** includes eggs in his or her diet. The **vegan** eats only foods of plant origin. Some people among these groups eat fish as well. Vegans can develop anemia as a result of vitamin B_{12} deficiency. Therefore they should include a daily source of vitamin B_{12} in their diets, such as a fortified breakfast cereal, fortified soy beverage, or meat substitute. All vegetarians should ensure that they get adequate amounts of calcium, iron, zinc, and vitamins D and B_{12}. Well-planned vegetarian diets can provide adequate nutrition. The **Vegetarian Food Pyramid,** endorsed by many groups, can assist vegetarians with daily food choices (Fig. 63-2).

CULTURAL AWARENESS

A number of other food pyramids have been developed for nutrition preferences of diverse ethnic groups. For example, for people of Hispanic descent, tortillas, beans, and rice *may* be desired over pasta, risotto, and potatoes. *Never assume that a person's racial or ethnic background means that he or she eats only foods associated with his or her primary ethnicity.* Health teaching about nutrition should incorporate any cultural preferences (also see Chapter 4).

Some people have food allergies or intolerances. For instance, lactose intolerance (lactose is found in milk and milk products) is a common problem that occurs in a number of ethnic groups. It is found more often in Mexican Americans and black people as well as in some American Indian groups, Asian Americans, and Ashkenazi Jews. A small percentage of white people, particularly those of Mediterranean descent (e.g., Greek, Italian), are also lactose intolerant. The cause of **lactose intolerance** is an inadequate amount of the lactase enzyme, which converts lactose into absorbable glucose.

Additional pyramids have been developed to reflect the current trend toward specialized diets, such as the "low-carb" Atkins and South Beach diets. The **Atkins Pyramid** emphasizes building the diet on protein sources and vegetables rather than on grains, fruits, and vegetables. Moderate quantities of fruits, dairy products, and nuts are added, and whole grain foods are limited. Refined carbohydrates (e.g., pasta, cakes, white bread) are the least desirable foods for all nutritional plans.

CONSIDERATIONS FOR OLDER ADULTS

The **Food Pyramid for Seniors Over 70** has been developed to guide older adults in food and nutrient selection. The USDA recommends that they drink eight glasses of water a day and eat plenty of fiber to prevent or manage constipation. It also suggests daily calcium and vitamins D and B_{12} supplements.

One of the most recent publications from Health Canada regarding nutrition is the Canada Food Guide. Compared with previous documents, it includes more culturally diverse foods, information on *trans* fats, customized individual recommendations, and exercise guidelines. Several booklets can be purchased to help people select the best foods and nutrients from the new Guide, such as *Eating Well with Canada's Food Guide.* In addition, Canada has published a separate booklet to address the special needs of some of its indigenous people. The *Eating Well with Canada's Food Guide—First Nations, Inuit, and Métis* includes berries, wild plants, and wild game to reflect the values and traditions for aboriginal people living in Canada (www.hc-sc.gc.ca/fn-an/food-guide-aliment/index_e.html).

NUTRITIONAL ASSESSMENT

Malnutrition (also called *undernutrition*) and obesity are common nutritional health problems. These problems lead to deficits that cause many comorbidities and complications, including death.

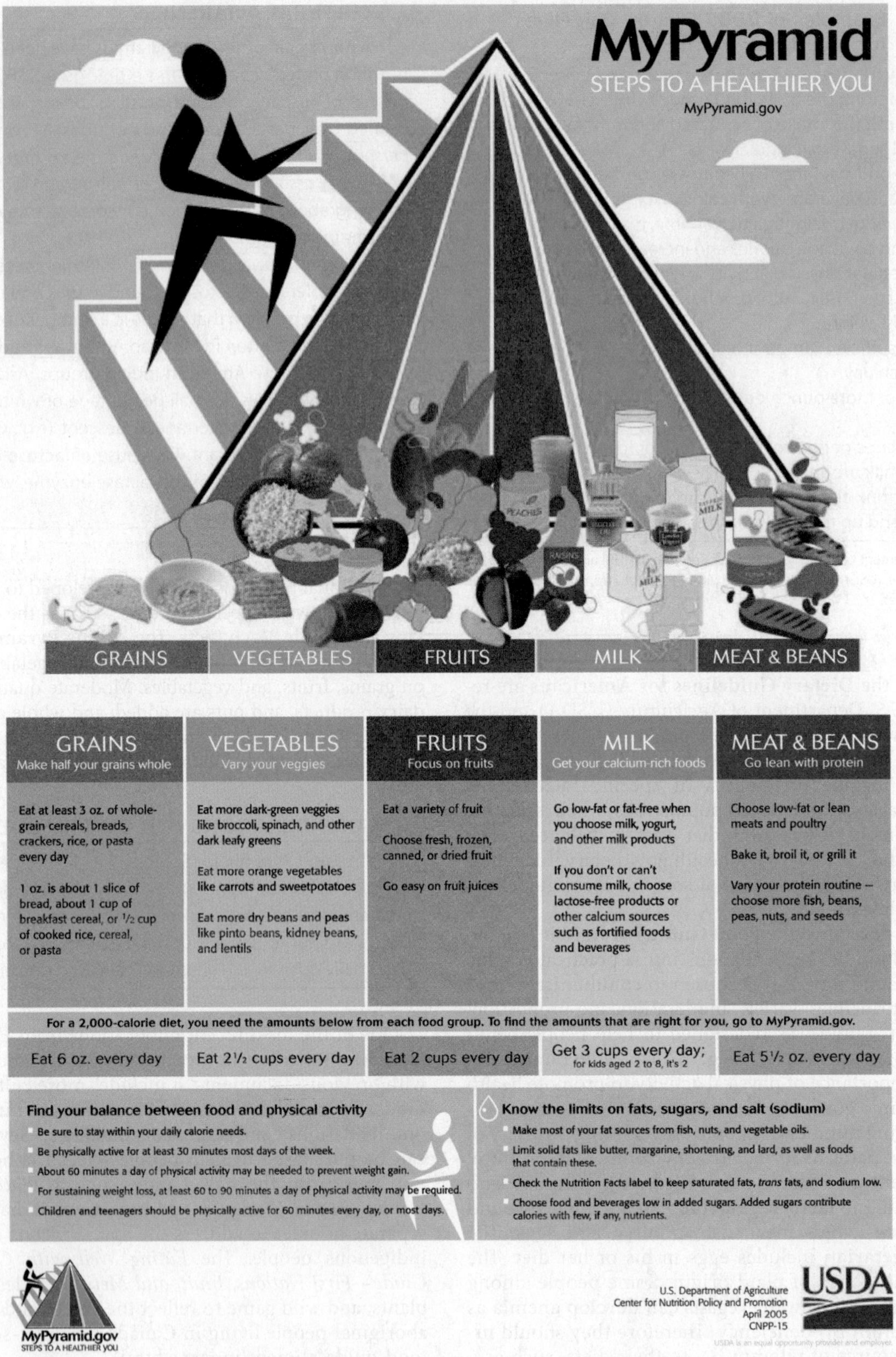
MyPyramid
STEPS TO A HEALTHIER YOU
MyPyramid.gov
GRAINS
VEGETABLES
FRUITS
MILK
MEAT & BEANS
GRAINS
Make half your grains whole
Eat at least 3 oz. of whole-grain cereals, breads, crackers, rice, or pasta every day
1 oz. is about 1 slice of bread, about 1 cup of breakfast cereal, or 1/2 cup of cooked rice, cereal, or pasta
VEGETABLES
Vary your veggies
Eat more dark-green veggies like broccoli, spinach, and other dark leafy greens
Eat more orange vegetables like carrots and sweetpotatoes
Eat more dry beans and peas like pinto beans, kidney beans, and lentils
FRUITS
Focus on fruits
Eat a variety of fruit
Choose fresh, frozen, canned, or dried fruit
Go easy on fruit juices
MILK
Get your calcium-rich foods
Go low-fat or fat-free when you choose milk, yogurt, and other milk products
If you don't or can't consume milk, choose lactose-free products or other calcium sources such as fortified foods and beverages
MEAT & BEANS
Go lean with protein
Choose low-fat or lean meats and poultry
Bake it, broil it, or grill it
Vary your protein routine – choose more fish, beans, peas, nuts, and seeds
For a 2,000-calorie diet, you need the amounts below from each food group. To find the amounts that are right for you, go to MyPyramid.gov.
Eat 6 oz. every day
Eat 2 1/2 cups every day
Eat 2 cups every day
Get 3 cups every day; for kids aged 2 to 8, it's 2
Eat 5 1/2 oz. every day
Find your balance between food and physical activity
Be sure to stay within your daily calorie needs.
Be physically active for at least 30 minutes most days of the week.
About 60 minutes a day of physical activity may be needed to prevent weight gain.
For sustaining weight loss, at least 60 to 90 minutes a day of physical activity may be required.
Children and teenagers should be physically active for 60 minutes every day, or most days.
Know the limits on fats, sugars, and salt (sodium)
Make most of your fat sources from fish, nuts, and vegetable oils.
Limit solid fats like butter, margarine, shortening, and lard, as well as foods that contain these.
Check the Nutrition Facts label to keep saturated fats, trans fats, and sodium low.
Choose food and beverages low in added sugars. Added sugars contribute calories with few, if any, nutrients.
MyPyramid.gov
STEPS TO A HEALTHIER YOU
U.S. Department of Agriculture
Center for Nutrition Policy and Promotion
April 2005
CNPP-15
USDA
USDA is an equal opportunity provider and employer.

Fig. 63-1 • The U.S. Department of Agriculture MyPyramid.

Nutritional status reflects the balance between nutrient requirements and intake. Common factors that affect these requirements include age, gender, disease, infection, and psychological stress. Nutrient intake is influenced by eating behavior, economic factors, emotional stability, disease, drug therapy, and cultural factors.

Evaluation of nutritional status is an important part of total patient assessment and includes:

- Review of the nutritional history
- Food and fluid intake record
- Laboratory data
- Food-drug interactions

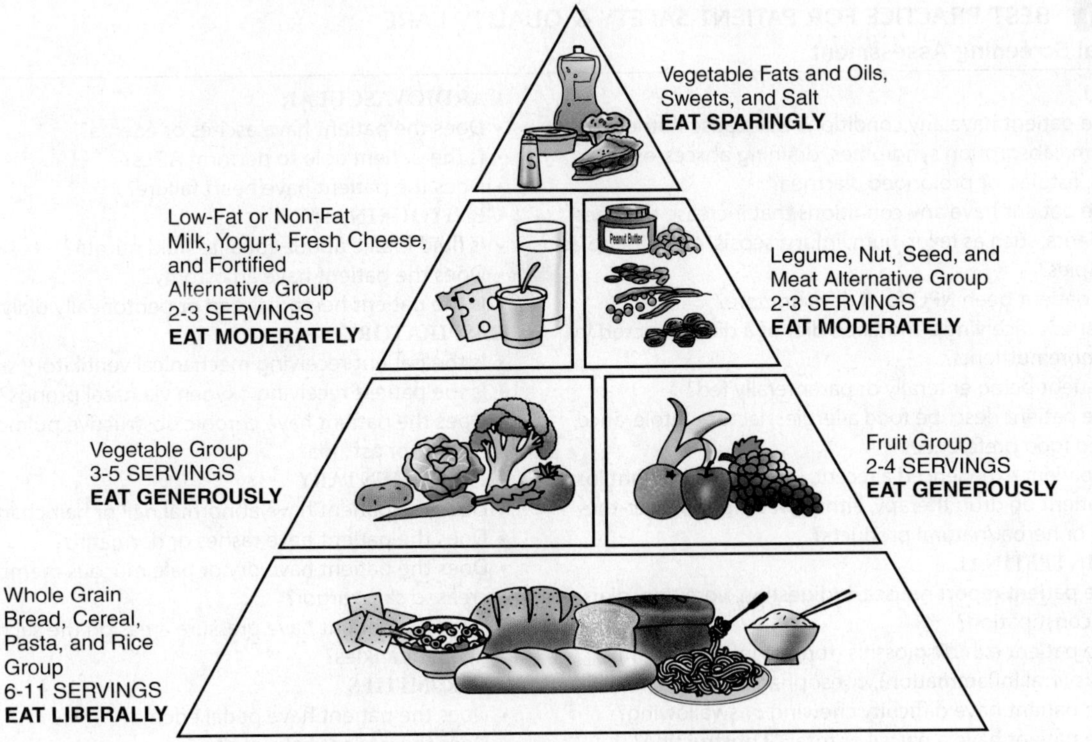
Vegetable Fats and Oils, Sweets, and Salt
EAT SPARINGLY
Low-Fat or Non-Fat Milk, Yogurt, Fresh Cheese, and Fortified Alternative Group
2-3 SERVINGS
EAT MODERATELY
Legume, Nut, Seed, and Meat Alternative Group
2-3 SERVINGS
EAT MODERATELY
Vegetable Group
3-5 SERVINGS
EAT GENEROUSLY
Fruit Group
2-4 SERVINGS
EAT GENEROUSLY
Whole Grain Bread, Cereal, Pasta, and Rice Group
6-11 SERVINGS
EAT LIBERALLY

Fig. 63-2 • Food pyramid for a vegetarian diet.

- Health history and physical assessment
- Anthropometric measurements
- Psychosocial assessment

Monitor the nutritional status of a patient during hospitalization as an important part of your initial assessment. Collaborate with the interdisciplinary health care team to identify patients at risk for nutritional problems.

Initial Nutritional Screening

Not every patient needs a complete nutritional assessment, but it is important to identify those at risk for problems through screening. An initial screening provides an inexpensive, quick way of determining which patients need more extensive nutritional assessment by the health care team. *The Joint Commission Patient Care Standards require that a nutritional screening occur within 24 hours of the patient's hospital admission. If indicated, an in-depth nutritional assessment should be performed.* When patients are in the hospital more than a week, nutritional assessment should be part of the daily plan of care. Unfortunately, this standard is not being consistently met in most hospitals (www.jointcommission.org).

The initial **nutritional screening** includes inspection, measured height and weight, weight history, usual eating habits, ability to chew and swallow, and any recent changes in appetite or food intake. Examples of questions that help identify patients at risk for nutritional problems are part of the history and physical assessment (Chart 63-1).

The Mini Nutritional Assessment (MNA), a two-part tool that has been tested worldwide, provides a reliable, rapid assessment for patients in the community, as well as in any health care setting. The first part asks about food intake, mobility, and body mass index (BMI) (described on p. 1390) and assesses for weight loss, acute illness, and psychological health problems. Part 1 consists of 6 questions and takes about 3 minutes to complete. If the patient scores 11 points or less, the second part of the MNA is completed, for an additional 12 questions. The entire assessment takes less than 15 minutes (Fig. 63-3) (DiMaria-Ghalili & Guenter, 2008).

Anthropometric Measurements

Anthropometric measurements are noninvasive methods of evaluating nutritional status. These measurements include height and weight and assessment of body fat.

Obtain a current *height and weight* to provide a baseline. Be sure to obtain accurate measurements because patients tend to overestimate height and underestimate weight. Measurements taken days or weeks later may indicate an early change in nutritional status. *You may delegate this activity to unlicensed assistive personnel (UAP) under your supervision.*

Patients should be measured and weighed while wearing minimal clothing and no shoes. Determine the height in inches or centimeters using the measuring stick of a weight scale if the patient can stand. He or she should stand erect and look straight ahead, with the heels together and the arms at the sides. For patients who cannot stand or those who cannot stand erect (e.g., some older adults), use a sliding-blade **knee height caliper,** if available. This device uses the distance between the patient's patella and heel to estimate height. It is especially useful for patients who have knee or hip contractures.

UAP weigh ambulatory patients with an upright balance-beam scale. Non-ambulatory patients can be weighed with a movable wheelchair balance-beam scale or a bed scale. *Be sure that the manufacturer calibrates weight scales twice yearly for accurate readings. For daily or sequential weights, obtain the weight at the same time each day, if possible, preferably before breakfast.* Conditions such as congestive heart failure and re-

Chart 63-1 BEST PRACTICE FOR PATIENT SAFETY & QUALITY CARE

Nutritional Screening Assessment

GENERAL
- Does the patient have any conditions that cause nutrient loss, such as malabsorption syndromes, draining abscesses, wounds, fistulas, or prolonged diarrhea?
- Does the patient have any conditions that increase the need for nutrients, such as fever, burn, injury, sepsis, or antineoplastic therapies?
- Has the patient been NPO for 3 days or more?
- Is the patient receiving a modified diet or a diet restricted in one or more nutrients?
- Is the patient being enterally or parenterally fed?
- Does the patient describe food allergies, lactose intolerance, or limited food preferences?
- Has the patient experienced a recent, unexplained weight loss?
- Is the patient on drug therapy, either prescription, over-the-counter, or herbal/natural products?

GASTROINTESTINAL
- Does the patient report nausea, indigestion, vomiting, diarrhea, or constipation?
- Does the patient exhibit glossitis (tongue inflammation), stomatitis (oral inflammation), or esophagitis?
- Does the patient have difficulty chewing or swallowing?
- Does the patient have a partial or total GI obstruction?
- What is the patient's state of dentition?

CARDIOVASCULAR
- Does the patient have ascites or edema?
- Is the patient able to perform ADLs?
- Does the patient have heart failure?

GENITOURINARY
- Is fluid intake about equal to fluid output?
- Does the patient have an ostomy?
- Is the patient hemodialyzed or peritoneally dialyzed?

RESPIRATORY
- Is the patient receiving mechanical ventilatory support?
- Is the patient receiving oxygen via nasal prongs?
- Does the patient have chronic obstructive pulmonary disease (COPD) or asthma?

INTEGUMENTARY
- Does the patient have abnormal nail or hair changes?
- Does the patient have rashes or dermatitis?
- Does the patient have dry or pale mucous membranes or decreased skin turgor?
- Does the patient have pressure areas on the sacrum, hips, heels, or ankles?

EXTREMITIES
- Does the patient have pedal edema?
- Does the patient have cachexia?

Modified with courtesy Ross Products Division, Abbott Laboratories, Columbus, OH.

nal disease cause weight gain; dehydration causes weight loss. *Weight is the most reliable indicator of fluid gain or loss, so accurate weights are essential!*

Normal weights for adult men and women are available from several reference standards, including the 1999 revised Metropolitan Life tables. Some health care professionals prefer these tables because they consider body-build differences by gender and body frame size (www.bcbst.com/MPManual/HW.htm).

Changes in body weight can be expressed by three different formulas:

1. Weight as a percentage of ideal body weight (IBW):

$$\%IBW = \frac{\text{Current weight}}{\text{Ideal body weight}} \times 100$$

2. Current weight as a percentage of usual body weight (UBW):

$$\%UBW = \frac{\text{Current weight}}{\text{Usual body weight}} \times 100$$

3. Change in weight:

$$\text{Weight change} = \frac{\text{Usual weight} - \text{Current weight}}{\text{Usual weight}} \times 100$$

An unintentional weight loss of 10% over a 6-month period at any time significantly affects nutritional status and should be evaluated. Weights may need to be taken daily, several times a week, or weekly for monitoring status and the effectiveness of nutritional support.

In the health care setting, *assessment of body fat* is usually calculated by the nutritionist. For people who participate in a structured exercise program in the community, this assessment is typically performed by a fitness trainer.

The **body mass index (BMI)** is a measure of nutritional status that does not depend on frame size. It indirectly estimates total fat stores within the body by the relationship of weight to height. *Therefore an accurate height is as important as an accurate weight.* The normal BMI is between 18.5 and 24.9.

A simple calculation for estimating BMI can be programmed into handheld computers or calculators using one of these two formulas:

$$\text{BMI} = \frac{\text{Weight (lb)}}{\text{Height (in inches)}^2} \times 703$$

$$\text{BMI} = \frac{\text{Weight (kg)}}{\text{Height (in meters)}^2}$$

BMI can also be determined using a table that is linked with height and weight. The least risk for malnutrition is associated with scores between 18.5 and 25. BMIs above and below these values are associated with increased health risks.

CONSIDERATIONS FOR OLDER ADULTS

Body weight and BMI usually increase throughout adulthood until about 60 years of age. As people get older, they become less hungry and eat less, even if they are healthy. Older adults should have a BMI between 23 and 27 (DiMaria-Ghalili & Amella, 2005).

The average daily energy intake expended by this group tends to be more than the average energy intake. This physiologic change has been called the "anorexia of aging" (Chapman, 2006). Many older adults are underweight, leading to undernutrition and increased risk for illness.

NESTLÉ NUTRITION SERVICES

Nestlé

Mini Nutritional Assessment (MNA)

Last name: First name: Sex: Date:

Age: Weight, kg: Height, cm: I.D. Number:

Complete the screen by filling in the boxes with the appropriate numbers.
Add the numbers for the screen. If score is 11 or less, continue with the assessment to gain a Malnutrition Indicator Score.

Screening

A Has food intake declined over the past 3 months due to loss of appetite, digestive problems, chewing or swallowing difficulties?
0 = severe loss of appetite
1 = moderate loss of appetite
2 = no loss of appetite ☐

B Weight loss during last 3 months
0 = weight loss greater than 3 kg (6.6 lbs)
1 = does not know
2 = weight loss between 1 and 3 kg (2.2 and 6.6 lbs)
3 = no weight loss ☐

C Mobility
0 = bed or chair bound
1 = able to get out of bed/chair but does not go out
2 = goes out ☐

D Has suffered psychological stress or acute disease in the past 3 months
0 = yes 2 = no ☐

E Neuropsychological problems
0 = severe dementia or depression
1 = mild dementia
2 = no psychological problems ☐

F Body Mass Index (BMI) (weight in kg) / (height in m)^2
0 = BMI less than 19
1 = BMI 19 to less than 21
2 = BMI 21 to less than 23
3 = BMI 23 or greater ☐

Screening score (subtotal max. 14 points) ☐☐

12 points or greater Normal – not at risk – no need to complete assessment
11 points or below Possible malnutrition – continue assessment

Assessment

G Lives independently (not in a nursing home or hospital)
0 = no 1 = yes ☐

H Takes more than 3 prescription drugs per day
0 = yes 1 = no ☐

I Pressure sores or skin ulcers
0 = yes 1 = no ☐

J How many full meals does the patient eat daily?
0 = 1 meal
1 = 2 meals
2 = 3 meals ☐

K Selected consumption markers for protein intake
- At least one serving of dairy products (milk, cheese, yogurt) per day? yes ☐ no ☐
- Two or more servings of legumes or eggs per week? yes ☐ no ☐
- Meat, fish or poultry every day yes ☐ no ☐

0.0 = if 0 or 1 yes
0.5 = if 2 yes
1.0 = if 3 yes ☐.☐

L Consumes two or more servings of fruits or vegetables per day?
0 = no 1 = yes ☐

M How much fluid (water, juice, coffee, tea, milk...) is consumed per day?
0.0 = less than 3 cups
0.5 = 3 to 5 cups
1.0 = more than 5 cups ☐.☐

N Mode of feeding
0 = unable to eat without assistance
1 = self-fed with some difficulty
2 = self-fed without any problem ☐

O Self view of nutritional status
0 = views self as being malnourished
1 = is uncertain of nutritional state
2 = views self as having no nutritional problem ☐

P In comparison with other people of the same age, how does the patient consider his/her health status?
0.0 = not as good
0.5 = does not know
1.0 = as good
2.0 = better ☐.☐

Q Mid-arm circumference (MAC) in cm
0.0 = MAC less than 21
0.5 = MAC 21 to 22
1.0 = MAC 22 or greater ☐.☐

R Calf circumference (CC) in cm
0 = CC less than 31 1 = CC 31 or greater ☐

Assessment (max. 16 points) ☐☐.☐

Screening score ☐☐

Total Assessment (max. 30 points) ☐☐.☐

Malnutrition Indicator Score

17 to 23.5 points at risk of malnutrition ☐

Less than 17 points malnourished ☐

Ref.: Guigoz Y, Vellas B and Garry PJ. 1994. Mini Nutritional Assessment: A practical assessment tool for grading the nutritional state of elderly patients. *Facts and Research in Gerontology.* Supplement #2:15-59.
Rubenstein LZ, Harker J, Guigoz Y and Vellas B. Comprehensive Geriatric Assessment (CGA) and the MNA: An Overview of CGA, Nutritional Assessment, and Development of a Shortened Version of the MNA. In: "Mini Nutritional Assessment (MNA): Research and Practice in the Elderly". Vellas B, Garry PJ and Guigoz Y, editors. Nestlé Nutrition Workshop Series. Clinical & Performance Programme, vol. 1. Karger, Bâle, in press.

Fig. 63-3 • The Mini Nutritional Assessment (MNA).

NCLEX EXAMINATION CHALLENGE

An older adult is admitted to the hospital with three pressure ulcers and dehydration. Her height is 5 feet, 2 inches, and she weighs 92 pounds. Her current body mass index (BMI) is _______. (Your answer should be rounded to the nearest tenth.)

evolve For the correct answer, go to http://evolve.elsevier.com/Iggy/.

Skin-fold measurements estimate body fat and can be measured by either the nurse or the nutritionist. The *triceps and subscapular* skin folds are most commonly measured using a special caliper. Both are compared with standard measurements and recorded as percentiles.

The *midarm circumference (MAC) and calf circumference (CC)* can be obtained to measure muscle mass and subcutaneous fat. These measurements are needed if the Mini Nutritional Assessment tool is used. To measure MAC, place a flexible tape around the arm at the midpoint, taking care to hold the tape firmly but gently to avoid compressing the tissue. This measurement is usually recorded in centimeters. The midarm muscle mass (MAMM) measures the amount of muscle in the body and is a sensitive indicator of protein reserves. It can be computed from the MAC and the triceps skin-fold measure. The CC is obtained using a similar procedure on the calf.

MALNUTRITION

Pathophysiology

Protein-energy malnutrition (PEM), also known as **protein-calorie malnutrition (PCM),** may present in three forms: marasmus, kwashiorkor, and marasmic-kwashiorkor. **Marasmus** is generally a calorie malnutrition in which body fat and protein are wasted. Serum proteins are often preserved. **Kwashiorkor** is a lack of protein quantity and quality in the presence of adequate calories. Body weight is more normal, and serum proteins are low. **Marasmic-kwashiorkor** is a combined protein and energy malnutrition. This problem often presents clinically when metabolic stress is imposed on a chronically starved patient. The outcome of unrecognized or untreated PEM is often dysfunction or disability and increased morbidity and mortality.

Malnutrition (also called *undernutrition*) is a multinutrient problem because foods that are good sources of calories and protein are also good sources of other nutrients. In the malnourished patient, protein catabolism exceeds protein intake and synthesis, resulting in negative nitrogen balance, weight loss, decreased muscle mass, and weakness.

The function of the liver, heart, lungs, GI tract, and immune system decreases in the patient with malnutrition. A decrease in serum proteins **(hypoproteinemia)** occurs as protein synthesis in the liver decreases. Vital capacity is also reduced as a result of respiratory muscle atrophy. Cardiac output diminishes. Malabsorption occurs because of atrophy of GI mucosa and the loss of intestinal villi.

Other common complications of severe malnutrition in adults include:

- Leanness and **cachexia** (muscle wasting with prolonged malnutrition)
- Decreased activity tolerance
- Lethargy
- Intolerance to cold
- Edema
- Dry, flaking skin and various types of dermatitis
- Poor wound healing
- Possible death
- Infection, particularly postoperative infection and sepsis

Malnutrition results from inadequate nutrient intake, increased nutrient losses, and increased nutrient requirements. Inadequate nutrient intake can be linked to poverty, lack of education, substance abuse, decreased appetite, and a decline in functional ability to eat independently, particularly in older adults. Infectious diseases, such as tuberculosis and human immune deficiency virus (HIV) infection, can also cause PEM. Diseases that produce diarrhea and infections leading to anorexia result in negative calorie and protein balance. Anorexia then leads to poor food intake. Vomiting causes decreased intestinal absorption with increased nutrient losses. Medical treatments such as chemotherapy can also cause malnutrition. In addition, catabolic processes, such as that caused by prolonged immobility, increase nutrient requirements and metabolic losses.

Inadequate nutrient intake can result also when a person is admitted to the hospital or long-term care facility. For example, decreased staffing may not allow time for patients who need to be fed, especially older adults, who may eat slowly. Many diagnostic tests, surgery, trauma, and unexpected medical complications require a period of NPO or cause **anorexia** (loss of appetite).

CULTURAL AWARENESS

In some cases, malnutrition results when the provided meals are different from what the patient usually eats. Be sure to identify specific food preferences that the patient can eat and enjoy.

CONSIDERATIONS FOR OLDER ADULTS

Older adults in the community or in any health care setting are most at risk for poor nutrition, especially PEM. Risk factors include physiologic changes of aging, environmental factors, and health problems. Chart 63-2 lists some of these major factors. Chapter 3 discusses nutrition for older adults in more detail.

Acute PEM may develop in patients who were adequately nourished before hospitalization but experience starvation while in a catabolic state from infection, stress, or injury. *Chronic* PEM can occur in those who have cancer, end-stage kidney or liver disease, or chronic neurologic disease.

Eating disorders, such as anorexia nervosa and bulimia nervosa seen most often in teens and young adults, also lead to malnutrition. **Anorexia nervosa** is a self-induced starvation resulting from a fear of fatness, even though the patient is underweight. **Bulimia nervosa** is characterized by episodes of binge eating in which the patient ingests a large amount of food in a short time. The binge eating is followed by some form of purging behavior, such as self-induced vomiting or excessive use of laxatives and diuretics. If not treated, death can result from starvation, infection, or suicide. Information about eating disorders can be found in textbooks on mental/behavioral health nursing.

Chart 63-2 NURSING FOCUS ON THE OLDER ADULT

Risk Assessment for Malnutrition

Assess for:
- Decreased appetite
- Weight loss
- Poor-fitting or no dentures/poor dental health
- Poor eyesight
- Dry mouth
- Limited income
- Lack of transportation
- Inability to prepare meals because of functional decline or fatigue
- Loneliness and/or depression
- Chronic constipation (e.g., Alzheimer's disease)
- Decreased meal enjoyment
- Chronic physical illness
- "Failure to thrive" (a combination of three of five symptoms, including weakness, slow walking speed, low physical activity, unintentional weight loss, exhaustion)
- Prescription and OTC drugs (including herbs, vitamins, and minerals)
- Acute or chronic pain

Patient-Centered Collaborative Care evolve ONLINE PHARM REVIEW

Assessment

History

Review the medical history to determine the diagnosis, the possibility of increased metabolic needs or nutritional losses, chronic disease, trauma, recent surgery of the GI tract, drug and alcohol abuse, and recent significant weight loss. Each of these conditions can contribute to malnutrition. For older adults, explore mental status changes and note poor eyesight, diseases affecting major organs, constipation or incontinence, and slowed reactions. Review prescription and over-the-counter (OTC) drugs (including herbal and natural supplements) and physical disabilities (see Chart 63-2).

For patients who live independently in the community, the nurse or occupational therapist may assess their performance of instrumental activities of daily living (IADLs). Functional status can best be evaluated for institutionalized patients by assessing their ADL performance. Poor nutrition is a major contributing factor to decreased functional ability.

In collaboration with the nutritionist, obtain information about the patient's usual daily food intake, eating behaviors, change in appetite, and recent weight changes. If the patient is able to communicate, ask him or her to describe the usual foods eaten daily and the times of meals and snacks. If available, ask the family these questions if the patient cannot communicate. If the patient cannot understand the questions due to language differences, locate an interpreter to assist with communication. The nutritionist can more thoroughly analyze the diet, if necessary, based on your initial nutritional screening.

Ask about changes in eating habits as a result of illness, and document any change in appetite, taste, and weight loss. *A weight loss of 5% or more in 30 days, a weight loss of 10% in 6 months, or a weight that is below ideal may indicate malnutrition.*

Assess for difficulty or pain in chewing or swallowing. *Unrecognized dysphagia is a common problem among nursing home residents and can cause malnutrition, dehydration, and aspiration pneumonia.* Ask the patient whether any foods are avoided and why. Ask UAP to report any choking while the patient eats. Record the occurrence of nausea, vomiting, heartburn, or any other symptoms of discomfort with eating. Finally, ask the patient about dental health problems, including the presence of dentures. Dentures or partial plates that do not fit well interfere with food intake. Dental caries (decay) or missing teeth may also cause discomfort while eating.

Physical Assessment/Clinical Manifestations

Assess for manifestations of various nutrient deficiencies (Table 63-2). Inspect the patient's hair, eyes, oral cavity, nails, and musculoskeletal and neurologic systems. Examine the condition of the skin, including any reddened or open areas. The previously described anthropometric measurements may also be obtained. The nurse or UAP monitor all food and fluid intake and note any mouth pain or difficulty in chewing or swallowing. A 3-day caloric intake may be collected and then calculated by the nutritionist.

Psychosocial Assessment

The psychosocial history provides information about the patient's economic status, occupation, educational level, living and cooking arrangements, and mental status. Determine whether financial resources are adequate for providing the necessary food. If resources are inadequate, the social worker or case manager may refer the patient and family to available community services. Chapter 3 discusses nutrition in older adults in more detail.

Laboratory Assessment

Laboratory tests supply objective data that can support subjective data and identify preclinical deficiencies. However, they must be carefully interpreted with regard to the total patient; an isolated value may yield an inaccurate conclusion.

A low *hemoglobin* level may indicate anemia, recent hemorrhage, or hemodilution caused by fluid retention. Hemoglobin may also be low secondary to conditions such as low serum albumin, infection, catabolism, or chronic disease. High levels may indicate hemoconcentration or dehydration, or they may be secondary to liver disease.

Low *hematocrit* levels may reflect anemia, hemorrhage, excessive fluid, renal disease, or cirrhosis. High hematocrit levels may indicate dehydration or hemoconcentration.

Serum albumin, thyroxine-binding prealbumin, and transferrin are measures of **visceral proteins.** Serum *albumin* reflects nutritional status a few weeks before testing and is not the most sensitive protein study. For example, patients who are dehydrated often have high levels and those with fluid excess have a lowered value. The normal serum albumin level for men and women is 3.5 to 5.0 g/dL (Pagana & Pagana, 2006).

Thyroxine-binding **prealbumin (PAB)** provides a more sensitive indicator of protein deficiency because of its short half-life of 2 days. Depending on the laboratory test used, the normal PAB range is 15 to 36 mg/dL (Pagana & Pagana, 2006). PAB can also assess improvement in nutritional status with

TABLE 63-2 Manifestations of Nutrient Deficiencies

Sign/Symptom	Potential Nutrient Deficiency
HAIR	
Alopecia	Zinc
Easy to remove	Protein
Lackluster hair	Protein
"Corkscrew" hair	Vitamin C
Decreased pigmentation	Protein
EYES	
Xerosis of conjunctiva	Vitamin A
Corneal vascularization	Riboflavin
Keratomalacia	Vitamin A
Bitot's spots	Vitamin A
GASTROINTESTINAL TRACT	
Nausea, vomiting	Pyridoxine
Diarrhea	Zinc, niacin
Stomatitis	Pyridoxine, riboflavin, iron
Cheilosis	Pyridoxine, iron
Glossitis	Pyridoxine, zinc, niacin, folic acid, vitamin B_{12}
Magenta tongue	Riboflavin
Swollen, bleeding gums	Vitamin C
Fissured tongue	Niacin
Hepatomegaly	Protein
SKIN	
Dry and scaling	Vitamin A
Petechiae/ecchymoses	Vitamin C
Follicular hyperkeratosis	Vitamin A
Nasolabial seborrhea	Niacin
SKIN—cont'd	
Bilateral dermatitis	Niacin
Magenta tongue	Vitamin A
Swollen, bleeding gums	Vitamin C
EXTREMITIES	
Subcutaneous fat loss	Calories
Muscle wastage	Calories, protein
Edema	Protein
Osteomalacia, bone pain, rickets	Vitamin D
HEMATOLOGIC	
Anemia	Vitamin B_{12}, iron, folic acid, copper, vitamin E
Leukopenia, neutropenia	Copper
Low prothrombin time, prolonged clotting time	Vitamin K, manganese
NEUROLOGIC	
Disorientation	Niacin, thiamine
Confabulation	Thiamine
Neuropathy	Thiamine, pyridoxine, chromium
Paresthesia	Thiamine, pyridoxine, vitamin B_{12}
CARDIOVASCULAR	
Congestive heart failure, cardiomegaly, tachycardia	Thiamine
Cardiomyopathy	Selenium
Cardiac dysrhythmias	Magnesium

Modified from Ross Products Division, Abbott Laboratories, Columbus, OH.

refeeding; levels can increase by 1 mg/dL daily with adequate nutritional support.

Although not used as commonly, serum **transferrin,** an iron-transport protein, can be measured directly or calculated as an indirect measurement of total iron-binding capacity (TIBC). It has a short half-life of 8 to 10 days and therefore is also a more sensitive indicator of protein status than is albumin.

Cholesterol levels normally range between 160 and 200 mg/dL in adult men and women. Values are typically low with malabsorption, liver disease, pernicious anemia, end-stage cancer, or sepsis. A cholesterol level below 160 mg/dL has been identified as a possible indicator of malnutrition.

Total lymphocyte count (TLC) can be used to assess immune function. Malnutrition suppresses the immune system and leaves the patient more likely to get an infection. When a patient is malnourished, the TLC is usually decreased to below 1500/mm^3.

▪ Analysis

Common Nursing Diagnoses and Collaborative Problems

The most common diagnosis for the patient with malnutrition is Imbalanced Nutrition: Less Than Body Requirements related to inability to ingest or digest food or absorb nutrients because of biologic, psychological, or economic factors.

Additional Nursing Diagnoses and Collaborative Problems

In addition to the common nursing diagnosis, patients with malnutrition may have one or more of these nursing diagnoses:

- Risk for Impaired Skin Integrity related to alterations in nutritional state
- Risk for Infection related to malnutrition
- Risk for Disturbed Body Image related to biophysical changes from weight loss

Patients with prolonged malnutrition are at risk for collaborative problems such as:

- Severe Anemia
- Immunocompromised State
- Multisystem Failure/Death

▪ Planning and Implementation

Imbalanced Nutrition: Less Than Body Requirements

NOC **Planning: Expected Outcomes.** The patient with malnutrition is expected to have nutrients available to meet metabolic needs. Indicators include that he or she will have normal:

Chart 63-3 NIC INTERVENTION ACTIVITIES

The Patient with Malnutrition

Nutrition Management: *Assisting with or providing a balanced dietary intake of foods and fluids*

- Ascertain patient's food preferences.
- Determine, in collaboration with nutritionist as appropriate, number of calories and type of nutrients needed to meet nutrition requirements.
- Encourage increased intake of protein, iron, and vitamin C, as appropriate.
- Encourage calorie intake appropriate for body type and lifestyle.
- Offer snacks (e.g., frequent drinks, fresh fruits/fruit juice), as appropriate.
- Provide patient with high-protein, high-calorie, nutritious finger foods and drinks that can be easily consumed, as appropriate.
- Ensure that the diet includes foods high in fiber content to prevent constipation.
- Monitor and record intake for nutritional content and calories.
- Weigh patient at appropriate intervals.
- Encourage patient to wear properly fitted dentures and/or obtain dental care.
- Determine patient's ability to meet nutritional needs.
- Provide appropriate information about nutritional needs and how to meet them.
- Assist patient in receiving help from appropriate community nutritional programs, as needed.

NIC intervention activities selected from Bulechek, G.M., Butcher, H.K., & McCloskey Dochterman, J. (Eds.). (2008). *Nursing intervention classification (NIC)* (5th ed.). St. Louis: Mosby. No part of this work is to be altered without prior written permission from the Publisher.

- Nutrient intake
- Fluid intake
- Energy
- Weight-height ratio
- Hematocrit and hemoglobin
- Visceral protein levels
- Muscle tone
- Hydration

Interventions. The preferred route for feeding is through the GI tract because it enhances the immune system and is safer, easier, less expensive, and enjoyable for the patient (Chart 63-3).

NIC ***Nutrition Management.*** The nutritionist calculates the nutrients required daily and plans the patient's diet. In collaboration with the health care provider and nutritionist, provide high-calorie, nutrient-rich foods (e.g., milkshakes, cheese). Assess the patient's food likes and dislikes. A feeding schedule of six small meals may be tolerated better than three large ones. A pureed or dental soft diet may be easier for those who have problems chewing or are **edentulous** (toothless).

Malnourished ill patients often need to be encouraged to eat. Instruct UAP who are feeding patients to keep food at the appropriate temperature and to provide mouth care before feeding. Assess for other needs, such as pain management, and provide interventions to make the patient comfortable. Pain can prevent patients from enjoying their meals. Remove bedpans, urinals, and emesis basins from sight. Provide a quiet environment, which is conducive to eating. Soft music may calm those with advanced dementia or delirium.

CONSIDERATIONS FOR OLDER ADULTS

Some patients, especially older adults, may take a long time to eat even small quantities of food because they tend to be less hungry than younger adults. If available, suggest that family members bring in favorite or ethnic foods that the patient might be more likely to eat. Teach them about ways to encourage the patient to increase food intake.

Restorative feeding programs help nursing home residents who need special assistance. These residents often eat in a separate dining area so that time and attention can be given to them. Some nursing homes have designated food and nutrition nursing assistants and/or trained volunteers who are primarily responsible for promoting and maintaining nutrition and hydration. Delegate and supervise these nursing staff during resident mealtime. Chart 63-4 offers additional interventions to increase nutritional intake for older adults in any setting.

If the patient cannot take in enough nutrients in food, fortified **medical nutritional supplements (MNS)** (e.g., Boost, Ensure, Carnation Instant Breakfast) may be given, especially to older adults. Many commercial enteral products are available. For patients with medical diagnoses such as liver and renal disease or diabetes, special products that meet those needs are available.

Nutritional supplements used in acute care, long-term care, and home care are costly. In addition, patients may refuse them and the supplements are then wasted. Bender at al. (2000) found that a more successful alternative to having the MNS given by nursing assistant staff in the nursing home was to have the supplements delivered by nurses during their usual medication passes. In this study, the nurses gave 60 mL or more of the MNS at least four times a day with the residents' medications. As a result, the patients gained weight and had fewer pressure ulcers, thus making the program very cost-effective and providing positive clinical outcomes.

Nutritional supplements are supplied as liquid formulas, powders, soups, coffee, and puddings in a variety of flavors. They come in different degrees of sweetness and are also available as modular supplements that provide single nutrients. Examples of modular supplements are Polycose glucose polymers for carbohydrates and Resource Beneprotein for protein, both available in liquid and powder form. Carbohydrate modulars are useful only if additional calories are needed. Protein modulars are indicated when metabolic stress causes a need for higher protein intake.

The nutritionist may ask the nursing staff to keep a food and fluid intake record for at least 3 consecutive days to help assess the patient's nutritional status. Delegate this activity to UAP under your supervision. UAP also weigh the patient daily, every 3 days, or once a week, depending on the health care setting and severity of malnutrition.

Drug Therapy. Drug therapy may be used for some patients to stimulate appetite. For example, cyproheptadine (Periactin), an antihistamine, may be prescribed for patients who are underweight, especially those with eating disorders. Megestrol acetate (Megace) may be used to increase appetite in those who have cachexia, acquired immune deficiency syndrome (AIDS), or unexplained weight loss. The mechanism for how these drugs work to increase appetite is not well understood.

Multivitamins, zinc, and an iron preparation are often prescribed to treat or prevent anemia. Monitor the patient's hemoglobin and hematocrit levels. Drug therapy can affect nutritional status. For example, iron can cause constipation and zinc can cause nausea and vomiting.

If the patient still does not receive enough nutrition by mouth using the interventions just mentioned, request **specialized nutrition support (SNS).** SNS consists of either total enteral nutrition (TEN) or total parenteral nutrition (TPN).

Total Enteral Nutrition. Patients often cannot meet the desired outcomes of nutritional therapy through their usual oral intake because of increased metabolic demands or a decreased ability to eat. Therefore TEN using enteral tube feeding may be necessary to supplement oral intake or to provide total nutritional support.

Patients likely to receive TEN can be divided into three groups:

- Those who can eat but cannot maintain adequate nutrition by oral intake of food alone
- Those who have permanent neuromuscular impairment and cannot swallow
- Those who do not have permanent neuromuscular impairment but are critically ill and cannot eat because of their condition

Patients in the first group are often older adults or patients receiving cancer treatment who cannot meet their calorie and protein needs. In some cases, this artificial nutrition and hydration may not be desired. For example, some patients have advance directives stating that they do not want to be kept alive by artificial nutrition and hydration if certain conditions exist. *However, legal and ethical questions arise when patients are not able to make their wishes known!*

For many years it was believed that withholding food and fluids would cause discomfort. Terminally or chronically ill patients who do not eat and drink may not suffer. In fact, they may be more comfortable if food and fluids are withheld. *The decision to feed is complex, and there is no clear right or wrong answer. To compound this legal and ethical dilemma, medical complications (e.g., aspiration, pressure ulcers) are common in older adults who are tube-fed.*

Decisions about these dilemmas are aided by the advice of interdisciplinary ethics committees in health care facilities. When clinicians are making decisions about the desirability of tube feedings in these cases, the focus should be on achieving consensus by:

- Reviewing what is known about tube feedings, especially their risks and benefits
- Reviewing the medical facts about the patient
- Investigating any available evidence that would help understand the patient's wishes
- Obtaining the opinions of all stakeholders in the situation
- Delaying any action until consensus is achieved

Those in the second group of patients likely to receive TEN usually have permanent swallowing problems and require some type of feeding tube for delivery of the enteral product on a long-term basis. Examples of conditions that can cause permanent swallowing problems are strokes, severe head trauma, and advanced multiple sclerosis. Patients in the third group receive enteral nutrition for as long as their illness lasts. The feeding is discontinued when the patient's condition improves and he or she can eat again. TEN is contraindicated for patients with diffuse peritonitis, severe pancreatitis, intestinal obstruction, intractable vomiting or diarrhea, and paralytic ileus (Sudakin, 2006).

Many commercially prepared enteral products are available. A therapeutic combination of carbohydrates, fat, vitamins, minerals, and trace elements is available in liquid form. Differences among products allow the nutritionist to select the right formula for each patient. A prescription from the health care provider is required for enteral nutrition, but the nutritionist usually makes the recommendation and computes the amount and type of product needed for each patient.

Chart 63-4 NURSING FOCUS ON THE OLDER ADULT

Promoting Nutritional Intake

- Be sure patient is toileted and receives mouth care before mealtime.
- Be sure that bedpans, urinals, and emesis basins are removed from sight.
- Give analgesics to control pain and/or antiemetics for nausea at least 1 hour before mealtime.
- Remind unlicensed assistive personnel (UAP) to have patient sit in chair, if possible, at mealtime.
- Observe the patient during meals for food intake.
- Ask the patient about food likes and dislikes and ethnic food preferences.
- Encourage self-feeding, or feed the patient slowly; *delegate* this activity to UAP if desired.
- If feeding patient, sit at eye-level if culturally appropriate.
- Create an environment that is conducive to eating and socialization and relaxation, if possible.
- Decrease distractions, such as environmental noise from television, music, or other people.
- Provide adequate, nonglaring lighting.
- Keep patient away from offensive or medicinal odors.
- Keep eye contact with the patient during the meal if culturally appropriate.
- Serve snacks with activities, especially in long-term care settings; *delegate* this activity to UAP if desired.
- Document the percentage of food eaten at each meal and snack; *delegate* this activity to UAP if appropriate.
- Ensure that meals are visually appealing, appetizing, appropriately warm or cold, and properly prepared.
- Do not interrupt patients during mealtimes for nonurgent procedures or rounds.
- Assess for need for supplements between meals and at bedtime.
- Review the patient's drug profile, and discuss with the health care provider the use of drugs that might be suppressing appetite.
- If the patient is depressed, be sure that the depression is treated by the health care provider.

DECISION-MAKING CHALLENGE
Legal/Ethical

An 82-year-old woman has been in the telemetry unit with complications of a total hip replacement. She has been losing weight consistently for the past 5 days and has eaten less than 25% of each meal. She refuses nutritional supplements, stating that "they taste awful." The patient continues to get weaker every day and is starting to become disoriented and confused at night. Her only daughter wants her mother to be tube-fed. The patient has told you on several occasions that she wants to die and doesn't want to be fed through a tube or put on a breathing machine. There are no written advance directives.

1. What will you tell the daughter when she asks you why her mother is not being tube-fed?
2. Is the patient able to make a decision about the possibility of total enteral nutrition?
3. What will you discuss with the physician about this patient's nutritional status?
4. With whom should you collaborate in this situation and why?

evolve For suggested answer guidelines, go to http://evolve.elsevier.com/Iggy/.

Methods of administering total enteral nutrition. TEN is administered as "tube feedings" through one of the available GI tubes, either through a nasoenteric or enterostomal tube. It can be used in the patient's home or any health care setting.

A **nasoenteric tube (NET)** is any feeding tube inserted nasally and then advanced into the GI tract, such as a Keofeed, Enteroflex, or Dobbhoff tube. Commonly used NETs include the **nasogastric (NG) tube** and the smaller (small-bore) **nasoduodenal tube (NDT)** (Fig. 63-4, *A*). A nasojejunal tube (NJT) is also available but is used less often than the other NETs.

The NDTs are used for delivering *short-term* enteral feedings (usually less than 4 weeks) because they are easy to use and are safer for the patient at risk for aspiration *if the tip of the tube is placed below the pyloric sphincter of the stomach and into the duodenum.* Small-bore polyurethane or silicone tubes from 8 to 12 Fr external diameter are preferred. The smaller tubes are more comfortable and are less likely to cause complications such as nasal irritation, sinusitis, tissue erosion, and pulmonary compromise.

Enterostomal feeding tubes are used for patients who need *long-term* enteral feeding. The most common types are gastrostomies and jejunostomies. The surgeon directly accesses the GI tract using various surgical, endoscopic, and laparoscopic techniques.

A **gastrostomy** is a stoma created from the abdominal wall into the stomach, through which a short feeding tube is inserted by the surgeon. It may require a small abdominal incision or may be placed endoscopically. This tube is called a **percutaneous endoscopic gastrostomy (PEG)** or dual-access gastrostomy-jejunostomy (PEG/J) tube. The PEG does not require general anesthesia for placement and is more secure and more durable than traditional gastrostomies. An alternative to either device is the **low-profile gastrostomy device (LPGD)** (Fig. 63-4, *B* and *C*). The LPGD is available with a firm or balloon-style internal bumper or retention disk. An anti-reflux valve keeps GI contents from leaking onto the skin. This device is less irritating to the skin, longer lasting, and more cosmetically pleasing. It also allows greater patient independence. However, skin-level devices do not allow easy access for checking **residuals** (the amount of feeding that remains in the stomach).

Jejunostomies are used less often than gastrostomies. A **jejunostomy** is used for long-term feedings when it is desirable to bypass the stomach, such as with gastric disease, upper GI obstruction, and abnormal gastric or duodenal emptying.

Tube feedings are administered by bolus feeding, continuous feeding, and cyclic feeding. **Bolus feeding** is an intermittent feeding of a specified amount of enteral product at set intervals during a 24-hour period, typically every 4 hours. This method

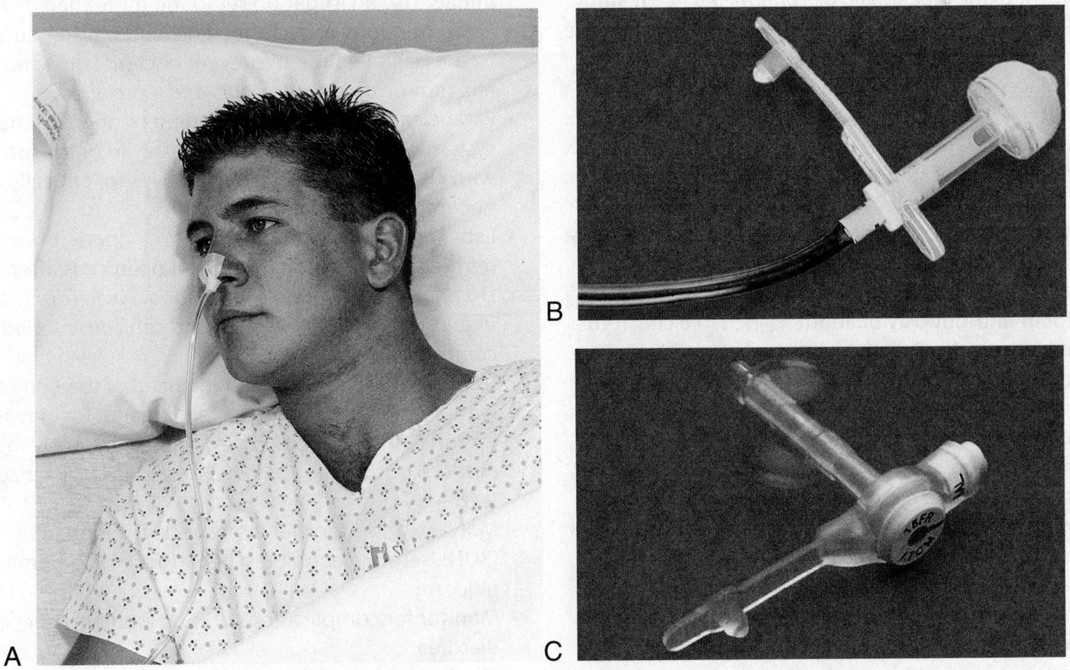
A
B
C

Fig. 63-4 • Feeding tubes used for total enteral nutrition. **A,** Nasoduodenal tube. **B** and **C,** Gastrostomy tubes.

can be accomplished manually or by infusion through a mechanical pump or controller device. Another method of tube feeding is continuous enteral feeding. **Continuous feeding** is similar to IV therapy in that small amounts are continuously infused (by gravity drip or by a pump or controller device) over a specified time. The most commonly seen method, **cyclic feeding,** is the same as continuous feeding except the infusion is stopped for a specified time in each 24-hour period, usually 6 to 10 or more hours ("down time"). Down time typically occurs in the morning to allow bathing, treatments, and other activities.

Infusion rates for cyclic feedings (and to some extent for intermittent bolus feeding) vary with the total amount of solution to be infused, the specific composition of the product, and the response of the patient to the feeding. The health care provider and nutritionist usually decide the type, rate, and method of tube feeding, as well as the amount of additional water ("free water") needed. If the patient can swallow small amounts of food, he or she may also eat orally while the tube is in place.

The nurse is responsible for the care and maintenance of the feeding tube and the enteral feeding. Chart 63-5 lists best practices for the patient receiving TEN.

Complications of total enteral nutrition. The nursing priority for care is preventing, assessing, and managing complications associated with tube feeding. Some complications of therapy result from the type of tube used to administer the feeding, and others result from the enteral product itself. The most common problem is the development of a clogged tube. Use the tips in Chart 63-6 to maintain tube patency.

Patients receiving TEN are at risk for several other complications, including refeeding syndrome, tube misplacement and dislodgement, abdominal distention and nausea/vomiting, and fluid and electrolyte imbalance, often associated with diarrhea. These problems can be prevented if the patient is carefully monitored and complications are detected early.

Chart 63-6 BEST PRACTICE FOR PATIENT SAFETY & QUALITY CARE

Maintaining a Patent Feeding Tube

- Flush the tube with 20 to 30 mL of water (or the amount prescribed by the health care provider or nutritionist):
  - At least every 4 hours during a continuous tube feeding
  - Before and after each intermittent tube feeding
  - Before and after drug administration (use warm water)
  - After checking residual volume
- If the tube becomes clogged, use 30 mL of water for flushing, applying gentle pressure with a 50-mL piston syringe.
- Avoid the use of carbonated beverage, except for existing clogs *when water is not effective.* Do not use cranberry juice.
- Whenever possible, use liquid medications instead of crushed tablets unless liquid forms cause diarrhea; make sure that the drug is compatible with the feeding solution.
- Do not mix drugs with the feeding product before giving. Crush tablets as finely as possible, and dissolve in warm water. *(Check to see which tablets are safe to crush. For example, do not crush slow-acting [SA] or slow-release [SR] drugs.)*
- Consider use of automatic flush feeding pump such as Flexiflo or Kangaroo.

Chart 63-5 BEST PRACTICE FOR PATIENT SAFETY & QUALITY CARE

Tube Feeding Care and Maintenance

- If nasogastric or nasoduodenal feeding is prescribed, use a soft, flexible, small-bore feeding tube (smaller than 12 Fr). *The initial placement of the tube should be confirmed by x-ray study.* Secure the tube with tape or a commercial attachment device after applying a skin protectant; change the tape regularly.
- Check tube placement by x-ray study when the correct position of the tube is in question; *an x-ray study is the only reliable method.* Checking the pH of the aspirant is currently a preferred method for rechecking placement after an x-ray; however, other methods continue to be studied.
- If a gastrostomy or jejunostomy tube is used, assess the insertion site for signs of infection or excoriation (e.g., excessive redness, drainage). Rotate the tube 360 degrees each day, and check for in-and-out play of about 1/4 inch (0.6 cm). If the tube cannot be moved, notify the health care provider immediately because the retention disk may be embedded in the tissue. Cover the site with a dry, sterile dressing, and change the dressing at least once a day.
- Check and record the residual volume every 4 to 6 hours, or per facility policy, by aspirating stomach contents into a syringe. If residual feeding is obtained, check with the health care provider for the appropriate intervention (usually to slow or stop the feeding for a time) or use the American Society of Parenteral and Enteral Nutrition (ASPEN) best practice recommendations.
- Check the feeding pump to ensure proper mechanical operation.
- Ensure that the enteral product is infused at the prescribed rate (mL/hr).
- Change the feeding bag and tubing every 24 to 48 hours; label the bag with the date and time of the change with your initials. Use an irrigation set for no more than 24 hours.
- For continuous or cyclic feeding, add only 4 hours of product to the bag at a time to prevent bacterial growth. *A closed system may be used for 24 hours and is preferred.*
- Wear clean gloves when changing or opening the feeding system or adding product; wipe the lid of the formula can with clean gauze; wear sterile gloves for critically ill or immunocompromised patients.
- Label open cans with date and time opened; cover, and keep refrigerated. Discard any unused open cans after 24 hours.
- *Do not use blue (or any color) food dye in formula because it does not assess aspiration and can cause serious complications.*
- To prevent aspiration, keep the head of the bed elevated at least 30 degrees during the feeding and for at least 1 hour after the feeding for bolus feeding; continuously maintain semi-Fowler's position for patients receiving cyclic or continuous feeding.
- Monitor laboratory values, especially blood urea nitrogen (BUN), serum electrolytes, hematocrit, prealbumin, and glucose.
- Monitor for complications of tube feeding, especially diarrhea.
- Monitor and carefully record the patient's weight and intake and output as requested by the physician or nutritionist.

Refeeding syndrome. **Refeeding syndrome** is a life-threatening metabolic complication that can occur when nutrition is restarted for a patient who is in a *starvation* state. When a patient is starved for nutrition, the body breaks down fat and protein, rather than carbohydrates, for energy. Protein catabolism leads to muscle and cell loss, often in major organs like the heart, liver, and lungs. The body's cells lose valuable electrolytes, including potassium and phosphate, into the plasma. Insulin secretion decreases in response to these changes. When *refeeding* begins, insulin production resumes and the cells take up glucose and electrolytes from the bloodstream, thus depleting serum levels. *This electrolyte shift can cause cardiovascular, respiratory, and neurologic problems, primarily caused by hypophosphatemia (Sudakin, 2006). Observe for clinical manifestations of this electrolyte imbalance, including shallow respirations, weakness, acute confusion, seizures, and increased bleeding tendency. Report and document your findings immediately.* More information on fluid and electrolyte imbalance can be found in Chapters 13 and 14.

Refeeding syndrome can be prevented if patients are carefully assessed and managed for nutritional needs. Interventions to supplement or replace nutrition should be implemented early before the patient is in a starvation state.

Tube misplacement and dislodgement. *A less common but more serious complication is misplacement or dislodgement of the tube, which can cause aspiration and possible death.* Lung intubation occurs in up to 27% of enteral tubes placed in hospitalized patients (Elpern et al., 2007). *Immediately remove any tube that you suspect is dislodged!* The Joint Commission's National Patient Safety Goals requires all health care facilities to establish and implement procedures and systems to prevent patient harm from medical complications.

Several techniques should be used to confirm proper placement to prevent harm and to keep the patient safe. *An x-ray is the most accurate confirmation method and should always be done on* ***initial*** *tube insertion.* After the initial placement is confirmed, check the placement before each intermittent feeding or at least every 4 to 8 hours during feeding. Also check placement before each drug administration.

The traditional auscultatory method for checking tube placement is not reliable, especially for patients with small-bore tubes. In this method, the nurse instills 20 to 30 mL of air into the tube ("insufflation") while listening over the epigastric area (stomach) with a stethoscope. *The resulting whooshing sound does not guarantee correct tube placement!*

Although some patients have respiratory distress if the tube is misplaced into the lungs, some do not. Therefore better methods for patient safety are being researched. Several safer procedures have been recommended for checking tube placement *after the initial placement has been confirmed by x-ray.* These methods include:

- Testing aspirated contents for pH (the most practical and easiest method), bilirubin, trypsin, or pepsin
- Assessing for carbon dioxide using capnometry

Some hospitals and nursing homes support testing the *pH of GI contents* at the bedside. To perform this procedure, aspirate a sample of the GI content, observe its color, and test its pH. When aspirating fluid, wait at least 1 hour after drug administration and then flush the tube with 20 mL of air to clear it. Collect the aspirate, and test it with pH paper. The pH of gastric fluid ranges from 0 to 4.0. If the tube has moved down into the intestines, the pH will be between 7.0 and 8.0. If the tube is in the lungs, the pH will be greater than 6.0 (Metheny et al., 1998). The pH may also be as high as 6 if the patient takes certain drugs, such as H_2 blockers (e.g., ranitidine [Zantac] and famotidine [Pepcid]). Because these drugs affect pH, bilirubin testing may be a more reliable and valid method for predicting tube location.

A newer method that has been researched recently is the use of *capnometry* to determine if carbon dioxide is emitted from the tube (Elpern et al., 2007). A device to measure the presence of the gas is attached to the end of the tube after placement. The test is positive for carbon dioxide if the tube is placed into the lungs, rather than the stomach. *The tube should be immediately removed if the gas is detected.*

If enteral tubes are misplaced or become dislodged, the patient is likely to aspirate. Aspiration pneumonia is a common, life-threatening complication associated with TEN, especially for older adults. Observe for increasing temperature and pulse, as well as for other signs of dehydration such as dry mucous membranes and decreased urinary output. Auscultate lungs every 4 to 8 hours to check for diminishing breath sounds, especially in lower lobes. Patients may become short of breath and report chest discomfort. A chest x-ray confirms this diagnosis, and treatment with antibiotics is started.

Abdominal distention and nausea/vomiting. Abdominal distention, nausea, and vomiting during tube feeding are often caused by overfeeding. To *prevent* overfeeding, check gastric residual volumes every 4 to 6 hours, depending on facility policy and the needs of the patient. The American Society of Parenteral and Enteral Nutrition (ASPEN) recommends holding a feeding if the gastric residual volumes are more than 200 mL on two consecutive assessments (www.nutritioncare.org). In some facilities, feedings are temporarily held if the gastric residual is 150 mL or more. After a period of rest, the feeding can be restarted at a lower flow rate.

A problem with frequent residual assessments is that the formula may clog the tube during aspiration, even if flushed with water. If the patient's residual volumes have been low or zero and he or she has no abdominal distention, nausea, or vomiting, consider discontinuing these assessments, depending on facility policy (Sudakin, 2006).

Fluid and electrolyte imbalances. *Patients receiving enteral nutrition therapy are at an increased risk for fluid imbalances.* They are often older or debilitated and may also have cardiac or renal problems. Fluid imbalances associated with enteral nutrition are usually related to the body's response to increased serum osmolarity, but *fluid overload* from too much tube feeding can also occur.

Osmolarity is the amount or concentration of particles dissolved in solution. This concentration exerts a specific osmotic pressure within the solution. Normal osmolarity of extracellular fluid (ECF) ranges between 270 and 300 mOsm. Enteral feeding products range in osmolarity from isotonic (about 300 mOsm) to extremely hypertonic (600 mOsm). Electrolytes (including sodium) contribute to this hypertonicity, but more of the osmolarity is determined by the concentration of proteins and sugar molecules in the enteral product. Even when the product is isotonic, the ECF can become hyperosmolar unless some hypotonic fluids are also administered to the patient. This situation is most likely to develop in patients who are unconscious, unable to respond to the thirst reflex, on fluid restrictions, or receiving hyperosmotic enteral preparations.

Because increased plasma osmolarity is largely a result of extra glucose and proteins (which tend to remain in the plasma rather than move to interstitial spaces), the plasma osmotic pressure (water-pulling pressure) is increased. In this situation, intracellular and interstitial water move into and expand the plasma volume. This volume expansion results in an increased renal excretion of water (in patients with normal renal function) and leads to osmotic *dehydration.* If patients do *not* have normal renal and cardiac function, expansion of the plasma volume can lead to circulatory overload and pulmonary edema, especially in older adults. Assess for signs and symptoms of circulatory overload, such as peripheral edema, sudden weight gain, crackles, dyspnea, increased blood pressure, and bounding pulse. Collaborate with the nutritionist and health care provider to plan the correct amount of fluid to be provided.

Excessive *diarrhea* may develop when hyperosmolar enteral preparations are delivered quickly. This situation can also lead to *dehydration* through excessive water loss. Collaborate with the health care provider and nutritionist for recommendations to prevent diarrhea. The nutritionist usually changes the feeding to a more iso-osmolar formula. Most of these formulas can be started full strength but slowly at 15 to 20 mL/hr. The rate is gradually increased as the patient tolerates and as the expected nutritional outcome is achieved.

If diarrhea continues, especially if it has a very foul odor, the patient should be evaluated for *Clostridium difficile* or other infectious organisms. Contamination can occur because of repeated and often faulty handling of the feeding solution and system. *Wear clean gloves when changing systems and adding product. Sterile gloves may help prevent infection in critically ill or immunocompromised patients. A closed feeding system is preferred over an open one because the chance of contamination is lessened (see Chart 63-5).* Tubes with ports also minimize contamination by preventing opening the feeding system to administer drugs.

In some cases, diarrhea may be the result of multiple liquid medications, such as elixirs and suspensions that have a very high osmolarity. Examples include acetaminophen (Tylenol), digoxin (Lanoxin), furosemide (Lasix), phenytoin (Dilantin), and potassium chloride. Patients receiving multiple liquid drugs should be evaluated by the health care provider to determine whether their drug regimen can be changed to prevent diarrhea. Diluting these liquids may also be an option.

Depending on the patient's state of health, some electrolyte imbalances can be avoided. This is achieved by the use of enteral preparations containing lower concentrations of the electrolytes that the patient cannot handle well. For example, renal patients with high potassium levels receive a special formula that is used for this imbalance.

The two most common electrolyte imbalances associated with enteral nutrition therapy are hyperkalemia and hyponatremia. Both of these conditions may be related to hyperglycemia-induced hyperosmolarity of the plasma and the resultant osmotic diuresis. Fluid and electrolyte imbalances are discussed in detail in Chapters 13 and 14.

NCLEX EXAMINATION CHALLENGE

A client is being fed through a small-bore nasoduodenal tube with Osmolite. When the nurse attempts to aspirate gastric contents for pH analysis, the client begins to cough and gag. What is the nurse's first action?

A. Flush the tube with 30 mL of warm water until it becomes patent.
B. Remove the tube because it is likely dislodged.
C. Notify the health care provider immediately.
D. Listen to the lungs for adventitious breath sounds.

evolve For the correct answer, go to http://evolve.elsevier.com/Iggy/.

Parenteral Nutrition. When a patient cannot effectively use the GI tract for nutrition, either partial or total parenteral nutrition therapy may maintain or improve his or her nutritional status. This form of IV therapy differs from standard IV therapy in that any or all nutrients (carbohydrates, proteins, fats, vitamins, minerals, and trace elements) can be given. One liter of IV fluid containing 5% dextrose, which is often used as standard therapy, provides only 170 kcal. A hospitalized patient typically receives 3 to 4 L a day, for a total number of calories ranging between 500 and 700 a day. This calorie intake is not sufficient when the patient requires IV therapy for a prolonged period and cannot eat an adequate diet or has increased calorie needs for tissue repair and building.

Partial parenteral nutrition. Partial, or peripheral, parenteral nutrition (PPN) is usually given through a cannula or catheter in a large distal vein of the arm or through a peripherally inserted central catheter (PICC line). (See Chapter 15 for care of patients with PICC lines.) This nutritional alternative is used for some patients who can eat but are not able to take in enough nutrients to meet their needs. The patient must have adequate peripheral vein access and be able to tolerate large volumes of fluid to have PPN. Two types of solutions are commonly used in various combinations for PPN: IV fat (lipid) emulsions (IVFEs) and amino acid–dextrose solutions. IVFEs are usually given using a piggyback method. *For patients receiving fat emulsions, monitor for manifestations of fat overload syndrome, especially in those who are critically ill. These manifestations include fever, increased triglycerides, clotting problems, and multi-system organ failure. Discontinue the IVFE infusion and report any of these changes to the health care provider immediately if this complication is suspected.*

Most IVFEs (20% fat emulsion) are isotonic, but the tonicity of commercially prepared amino acid–dextrose solutions ranges from 300 mOsm to nearly 900 mOsm for PPN. Amino acid–dextrose solutions are considered more stable than IVFEs and therefore additives (e.g., vitamins, minerals, electrolytes, trace elements) tend to be mixed with them. These solutions must be delivered through an in-line filter and are administered by an infusion pump for an accurate and constant delivery rate.

Some PPN products are a *mixture* of lipids (10% or 20% fat emulsion) and an amino acid–dextrose (usually 10%) solution. This mixture of three types of nutrients is referred to as a *3:1, total nutrient admixture (TNA),* or *triple-mix solution.*

Total parenteral nutrition. When the patient requires intensive nutritional support for an extended time, the health care provider prescribes centrally administered **total parenteral nutrition (TPN).** TPN is delivered through access to central veins, usually through a PICC line or the subclavian or internal jugular veins. Central venous catheters and associated nursing care are described in detail in Chapter 15.

Total parenteral nutrition solutions contain higher concentrations of dextrose and proteins, usually in the form of synthetic amino acids or protein hydrolysates (3% to 5%). These solutions are hyperosmotic (three to six times the osmolarity of normal blood). The base solutions are available as commercially prepared solutions. The hospital or community pharmacist adds components (specific electrolytes, minerals, trace elements, and insulin) according to the patient's nutritional needs. This therapy provides needed calories and spares body proteins from catabolism for energy requirements.

The TPN solutions are administered with an infusion pump. The osmolarity of the fluid and the concentrations of the specific components make controlled delivery essential.

Complications of parenteral nutrition. Patients receiving parenteral nutrition fluids are at risk for a wide variety of serious and potentially life-threatening complications. Complications may result from the solutions or from the peripheral or central venous catheter. The following discussion is limited to the complications that involve fluid or electrolyte balance. Complications of IV cannulas and central venous catheters are discussed in Chapter 15, including infection and sepsis.

Fluid imbalances. Patients receiving parenteral nutrition therapy are at high risk for fluid imbalance. Not only is fluid delivered directly into the venous system, but also the extreme hyperosmolarity of the solutions stimulates fluid shifts between body fluid compartments. The hyperosmolarity is caused by their amino acid and dextrose concentrations. Increased dextrose causes hyperglycemia (increased blood glucose). As a result, some of the dextrose moves into the interstitial and intracellular spaces, where it is metabolized. However, dextrose remains in the plasma volume when the solutions are administered too rapidly, without enough insulin coverage, or in the presence of hyponatremia and hypokalemia. The result is a shift of water from the interstitial and intracellular spaces into the plasma. Expansion of the plasma volume together with hyperglycemia can cause osmotic diuresis and lead to serious dehydration and hypovolemic shock. If the patient also has cardiac or renal dysfunction, he or she may develop fluid overload, congestive heart failure, and pulmonary edema. Monitor the infusion rate of the parenteral fluid and give insulin as prescribed.

Monitor for these complications by taking daily weights and by recording accurate intake and output while the patient is receiving parenteral nutrition. Serum glucose and electrolyte values are also monitored (Chart 63-7). Report any major changes or abnormalities to the health care provider and document all assessments and interventions.

Electrolyte imbalances. Patients receiving TPN are at an increased risk for many different electrolyte imbalances, depending on the composition of the solution and whether a fluid imbalance occurs. The health care provider usually requests frequent determinations of serum electrolyte levels to detect these imbalances. The risk for metabolic and electrolyte complications is reduced when the rate of administration is carefully controlled and patients are closely monitored for response to treatment. Potassium and sodium imbalances are common, especially when insulin is also administered as part of the therapy. Calcium imbalances, particularly hypercalcemia, are associated with TPN, although immobility may play more of a role than the actual therapy in developing this imbalance.

Community-Based Care

Malnourished patients can be cared for in a variety of settings, including the acute care hospital, transitional care unit, nursing home, or their own home. Malnutrition is often diagnosed when the patient is admitted to the acute care hospital or shortly after hospitalization if complications such as poor wound healing or sepsis occur. If the patient is severely compromised, he or she may require admission to a traditional nursing home for either transitional or long-term care. If adequate home support is available, he or she may be discharged to home in the care of a family member or other caregiver. Home care nurses may be needed to monitor and direct the care.

Chart 63-7 BEST PRACTICE FOR PATIENT SAFETY & QUALITY CARE

Care and Maintenance of Total Parenteral Nutrition

- Check each bag of total parenteral nutrition (TPN) solution for accuracy by comparing it with the physician's or pharmacist's prescription.
- Monitor the IV pump for accuracy in delivering the prescribed hourly rate.
- If the total parenteral nutrition (TPN) solution is temporarily unavailable, give 10% dextrose/water (D/W) or 20% D/W until the TPN solution can be obtained.
- If the TPN administration is not on time ("behind"), do not attempt to "catch up" by increasing the rate.
- Monitor the patient's weight daily or according to facility protocol.
- Monitor serum electrolytes and glucose daily or per facility protocol. (Some facilities require finger-stick blood sugars [FSBSs] every 4 hours, especially if the patient is receiving insulin. Urine testing for ketones may also be requested.)
- Monitor for complications, including fluid and electrolyte imbalances.
- Monitor and carefully record the patient's intake and output.
- Assess the patient's IV site for signs of infection or infiltration (see Chapter 15).
- Change the IV tubing every 24 hours or per facility protocol.
- Change the dressing around the IV site every 48 to 72 hours or per facility protocol.
- Before administering TPN, have another nurse check the prescription and solution (required by some facilities to prevent patient harm).

Home Care Management

The malnourished patient needs a variety of resources at home to continue aggressive nutrition support. If he or she can consume food by the oral route, the case manager or other discharge planner determines whether financial resources are available for the necessary nutrition supplements. If the hospital provides ambulatory nutrition counseling services, the patient is scheduled for follow-up after discharge for assessment of weight gain.

Health Teaching

The nutritionist instructs the malnourished patient and family about high-calorie, high-protein diet and nutritional supplements. In collaboration with the pharmacist, review specific parenteral solutions with the patient and family or significant others.

Reinforce the importance of adhering to the prescribed diet, and review any drugs the patient may be taking. If using an iron preparation, teach the importance of taking the drug immediately before or during meals. Caution the patient that iron tends to cause constipation. For the older adult already susceptible to constipation, emphasize the importance of measures for prevention, including adequate fiber intake, adequate fluids, and exercise.

Some patients are discharged to home with enteral or parenteral nutrition. Teach the family or other caregiver how to continue these therapies. Remind caregivers to consider the psychosocial aspects of these alternative methods for nutrition. For example, the caregiver can bring the enteral product and napkin to the patient on a decorative tray to make the feeding experience more elegant and "normal." Moving the feeding equipment out of view of the patient when it is not in use is also helpful.

Health Care Resources

The malnourished patient discharged to home on enteral or parenteral nutrition support needs the specialized services of a home nutrition therapy team. This team generally consists of the physician, nurse, nutritionist, pharmacist, and case manager or social worker. Several commercial companies supply these services to patients at home in addition to the feeding supplies and formulas and health teaching.

Evaluation: Outcomes

Evaluate the care of the malnourished patient on the basis of the identified nursing diagnoses and collaborative problems. The primary expected outcome is that he or she has available nutrients to meet the metabolic demands for maintaining weight and total protein. Specific indicators for this outcome are listed for the nursing diagnosis under the Planning: Expected Outcomes section (see earlier).

OBESITY

Pathophysiology

Obesity, like cancer, is not just one disease but instead many conditions with varying causes. The terms *obesity* and *overweight* are often used interchangeably, but they refer to different health problems. **Overweight** is an increase in body weight for height compared with a reference standard, or up to 10% greater than ideal body weight (IBW). However, this weight may not reflect excess body fat. It is possible for well-developed athletes to appear overweight because of increased muscle (lean) mass, in which the proportion of muscle to fat is greater than average.

Obesity refers to an excess amount of body fat when compared with lean body mass. The normal amount of body fat in *men* is between 15% and 20% of body weight. For *women*, the normal amount is 18% to 32%. An obese person weighs at least 20% above the upper limit of the normal range for ideal body weight. **Morbid obesity,** also called *extreme obesity,* refers to a weight that has a severely negative effect on health—usually more than 100% above IBW.

More than one third of the U.S. population are obese, and another third are overweight. About 10% or more of adults are morbidly obese. *This problem is the second leading cause of preventable deaths in the United States, second only to smoking, and has become a national crisis! Obesity across the life span is considered an epidemic in the United States and Canada. Worldwide, it is recognized as a major global health problem, costing billions of dollars for health care and lost productivity.*

The pathophysiology of obesity is very complex. A number of chemicals in the body, including hormones known as *adipokines,* work together to affect appetite and fat metabolism:

- **Leptin:** a hormone released by fat cells and possibly by gastric cells; it also acts on the hypothalamus to control appetite
- **Adiponectin:** an anti-inflammatory and insulin sensitizing hormone
- **Resistin:** a hormone produced by fat cells that creates resistance to insulin activity
- **Inflammatory cytokines:** such as inflammatory interleukins and tumor necrosis factor–alpha
- **Apolipoprotein E:** one of several regulators of lipoprotein metabolism
- **Cholecystokinin:** a hormone that stimulates digestive juices and may work with leptin to increase or decrease appetite

Some adipokines are neuropeptides, including orexins and anorexins, which play a role in body weight. **Orexins** are appetite stimulants; examples are ghrelin secreted by the stomach and peptide YY from the intestines. **Anorexins** decrease appetite and include leptin and insulin (McCance & Huether, 2006). Increased circulating plasma levels of orexins are associated with the development of obesity. However, in some people, high levels of leptin may not be effective in suppressing appetite—a condition known as *leptin resistance.* In this case, overeating and excessive weight gain can result. Hyperleptinemia also stimulates the autonomic nervous system and contributes to blood vessel inflammation and ventricular hypertrophy. These actions may help explain why obese patients are most at risk for hypertension, atherosclerosis, and heart disease (McCance & Huether, 2006). Obesity is also associated with insulin resistance, which predisposes obese patients to type 2 diabetes mellitus (see Chapter 67).

Obesity is determined by weight compared with height, BMI, and waist circumference. To establish the percentage of IBW, the *height and weight* of the patient are compared with the midpoint of the desirable weight using an accepted reference standard. The *body mass index (BMI),* as described previously, is a measure of heaviness and is only an indirect indicator of body fat. It reflects the combined effects of body build, proportions, lean body mass, and body fat. However, BMI has substantial correlations with fat mass for adult men and women and has been validated as a risk factor for cardiovascular disease. A BMI of 25 to 29.9 indicates that a person is overweight. A BMI of 30 or more indicates obesity. *People who are morbidly obese have a BMI of greater than 40 and are at a major risk for life-threatening health problems.*

The distribution of excess body fat rather than the degree of obesity has been used to predict increased health risks. For example, the waist circumference (WC) is a stronger predictor of coronary artery disease (CAD) than is the BMI. A WC greater than 35 inches (89 cm) in women, and a WC greater than 40 inches (102 cm) in men indicate central obesity (Christie et al., 2007). Central obesity is a major risk factor for coronary artery disease (CAD), stroke, type 2 diabetes, some cancers (e.g., colon, breast), sleep apnea, and early death.

The waist-to-hip ratio (WHR) is also a predictor of CAD. This measure differentiates peripheral lower body obesity from central obesity. A WHR of 0.95 or greater in men (0.8 or greater in women) indicates android obesity with excess fat at the waist and abdomen.

Complications of Obesity

The major complications of obesity affect primarily the cardiovascular and respiratory systems. However, excess weight can also cause degeneration of the musculoskeletal system, especially the joints (osteoarthritis). Obese people are also more susceptible to infections and infectious diseases than are

TABLE 63-3 Common Complications of Obesity

- Type 2 diabetes mellitus
- Hypertension
- **Hyperlipidemia** (increased serum lipids)
- Coronary artery disease (CAD)
- Stroke
- Peripheral artery disease (PAD)
- Metabolic syndrome
- Obstructive sleep apnea
- Obesity hypoventilation syndrome
- Depression and other mental health/behavioral health problems
- Urinary incontinence
- **Cholelithiasis** (gallstones)
- Gout
- Chronic back pain
- Early osteoarthritis
- Decreased wound healing

thinner people and tend to heal more slowly. Table 63-3 lists some of the most common complications of obesity.

Etiology and Genetic Risk

The causes of obesity involve complex interrelationships of many environmental, genetic, and behavioral factors. A number of causes of both human and animal obesity have been identified.

One of the most common causes of being overweight or obese is eating *high-fat and high-cholesterol diets.* Obesity is associated with diet when it contains a significant amount of *saturated* fat, which increases low-density lipoproteins (LDL-C). *Trans* fatty acids (TFA), saturated fats, and cholesterol are linked to obesity and CAD (Yantis & Velander, 2007). By contrast, monounsaturated and polyunsaturated fats are healthy fats.

TFA is made when food manufacturers add hydrogen to vegetable oil, a process known as *hydrogenation.* This process increases the food's shelf life and flavor. Large amounts of TFA can be found in vegetable shortening, commercial baked goods, snack foods, and French fries. Food labels in the United States and Canada include amounts of total fat, subtypes of fat, and cholesterol content per serving.

Physical inactivity has been identified as another cause of overweight and obesity. The major barriers to increasing physical activity include a lack of time or decreased mobility associated with prolonged illness. Regular exercise is associated with lower death rates for adults of any age. It also increases lean muscle, decreases body fat, aids in weight control, and enhances psychological well-being. Regular exercise can also decrease the risk for falling in older adults (see Chapter 3).

Another cause of obesity is *drug treatment.* Some prescribed drugs contribute to weight gain when they are taken on a long-term basis. Examples include:

- Corticosteroids
- Estrogens and certain progestins
- Nonsteroidal anti-inflammatory drugs
- Antihypertensives
- Antidepressants and other psychoactive drugs
- Antiepileptic drugs
- Certain oral antidiabetic agents

GENETIC CONSIDERATIONS

Familial and genetic factors seem to play a very important role in obesity. When both parents are overweight, about 80% of their children will be overweight. If neither parent is overweight, fewer than 10% of the children will be overweight. In studies of identical twins, nonidentical twins, and parent-sibling relationships, about 50% of the difference in body fatness is transmitted to children and about 50% of this amount is genetically controlled (McCance & Huether, 2006).

Genetic composition may predispose some people, but not others, to obesity. Leptin, the hormone encoded by the *ob* gene, appears to send a message to the brain that the body has stored enough fat. This message serves as a signal to stop eating. In some obese people, other gene mutations have been identified, including an abnormality of the melanocortin-4 receptor that inhibits appetite in families with a history of obesity.

A small number of obese people have disorders of the neuroendocrine system. Examples include injury to the hypothalamus, Cushing's disease, polycystic ovary failure, hypogonadism, and growth hormone deficiency.

Health Promotion and Maintenance

Obesity is a major public health problem and is associated with many complications, including death. As a result of this increasing problem, the *Healthy People 2010* agenda addresses the need to reduce the proportion of children, adolescents, and adults who are obese. Nurses can help meet this desired outcome through education and role modeling (Table 63-4). In collaboration with the nutritionist, teach the importance of weight management and exercise to improve health. Even a 5% weight loss can drastically decrease the risk for CAD and diabetes.

Patient-Centered Collaborative Care

Assessment

History

In addition to taking a complete history regarding present and past health problems, collect this information about the patient in collaboration with the nutritionist:

- Economic status
- Usual food intake

TABLE 63-4 Meeting *Healthy People 2010* Objectives: Nutrition and Overweight

Objective 19.2: Reduce the proportion of adults who are obese.

- Teach the patient the potential consequences and complications of obesity.
- Teach the patient the importance of eating a healthy diet, including a variety of foods, especially grain products, vegetables, and fruits. The diet should be moderate in salt and sugar and low in fats and cholesterol.
- Remind the patient that foods eaten away from home tend to be higher in fat, cholesterol, and salt and are lower in calcium than foods prepared at home.
- Reinforce the need to engage regularly in moderate physical activity for at least 30 minutes each day.
- Begin education regarding diet and physical activity for children and adolescents, and continue throughout adulthood. (Once an adolescent becomes overweight, he or she is likely to remain overweight.)

- Eating behavior
- Cultural background
- Attitude toward food
- Appetite
- Chronic diseases
- Drugs (prescribed and OTC, including herbal preparations)
- Physical activity/functional ability
- Family history of obesity

A nutritional history usually includes a 24-hour recall of food intake and the frequency with which foods are consumed. The adequacy of the diet can be evaluated by comparing the amount and types of foods consumed daily with the established standards. The nutritionist then provides a more detailed analysis of nutritional intake.

Physical Assessment/Clinical Manifestations

Obtain an accurate height and weight. The nutritionist calculates the percentage of ideal body weight (% IBW) and the body mass index (BMI). He or she may also:

- Measure the waist circumference
- Calculate the waist-hip ratio
- Determine arm and calf circumferences

Examine the skin of the obese patient for reddened or open areas. Lift skin-fold areas, such as pendulous breasts and abdominal aprons **(panniculus),** to observe for *Candida* (yeast) or other infections and lesions. Infection of the panniculus is referred to as **panniculitis.**

Psychosocial Assessment

Obtain a psychosocial history to determine the patient's circumstances and emotional factors that might prevent successful therapy or that might be worsened by therapy. Interview the patient to determine his or her perception of current weight and weight reduction. Some patients do not view weight as a problem, which affects treatment and outcome. Ask the patient questions about their health beliefs related to being overweight, such as:

- What does food mean to you?
- Do you want to lose weight?
- What prevents you from losing weight?
- What do you think will motivate you to lose weight?
- How do you think you might benefit from losing weight?

Many patients report that they have tried multiple diets to lose weight but either the diets have not worked or the weight lost was regained. People who attempt restrictive diets become easy targets for the billion-dollar weight-loss industry, yet 90% to 95% of dieters regain lost weight (May, 2006).

The results of dieting and other efforts can lead to a sense of failure and lowered self-esteem, which often stimulates more overeating (May, 2006). Many overweight and obese people eat in response to environmental and emotional stressors rather than because they are hungry. Ask patients to identify their perceived stressors and what triggers their need for food.

Lifestyle changes are difficult without adequate family and community support. Assess useful coping strategies and support systems that the patient can use during treatment for obesity.

Explore the patient's history to assess:

- Attempts at weight-reduction diets and outcomes
- Effects of obesity on lifestyle
- Effects of obesity on social interactions
- Mental health/behavioral health problems, such as depression
- Effects of obesity on intimate relationships, especially sexuality

Obese men often experience erectile dysfunction (ED), which can cause or worsen depression. Women often experience changes in their menstrual cycles and may have problems getting pregnant.

Interventions

Weight is lost only when energy used is greater than intake. Weight loss may be accomplished by nutritional modification with or without the aid of drugs and in combination with a regular exercise program. Patients who may be candidates for surgical treatment include those who have:

- Repeated failure of nonsurgical interventions
- A BMI equal to or greater than 40
- Weight more than 100% above IBW (i.e., morbidly obese)

Nonsurgical Management

Various nutritional approaches and drug therapy have attempted to help obese patients achieve permanent weight loss.

Diet Programs. Diets for helping people lose weight include fasting, very-low-calorie diets, balanced and unbalanced low-energy diets, and novelty diets.

Short-term fasting programs have not been successful in treating morbidly obese patients, and prolonged fasting does not produce permanent benefits. Most patients regain the weight that was lost by this method. In addition, the risks associated with fasting (e.g., severe ketosis) require close medical supervision.

Very-low-calorie diets generally provide 200 to 800 calories/day. Two types of these diets are the *protein-sparing modified fast* and the *liquid formula diet.* The protein-sparing modified fast provides protein of high biologic value (1.5 g/kg of desirable body weight daily) within a limited number of calories. The diet produces rapid weight loss while preserving lean body mass. The liquid formula diet provides between 33 and 70 g of protein daily.

Both diets require an initial cardiac evaluation, supervision by an interdisciplinary health care team with monitoring by a physician, nutrition counseling by a nutritionist, and supplementation with vitamins and minerals. These diets are only one part of a weight-reduction program. Patients who are on these diets should receive nutrition education, psychological counseling, exercise, and behavior therapy. Comparable weight losses have been achieved with both diets, but again, most patients do not sustain the weight loss and regain the weight.

Nutritionally *balanced diets* generally provide about 1200 calories/day with a conventional distribution of carbohydrate, protein, and fat. Vitamin and mineral supplements may be necessary if energy intakes fall below 1200 calories for women and 1800 calories for men. This diet provides conventional foods that are economical and easy to obtain. Thus the outcome of weight loss is facilitated, and that loss is hopefully maintained. For example, Weight Watchers is an organization that provides education about nutritionally balanced diets based on a point system and weekly group support meetings.

Unbalanced low-energy diets, such as the low-carbohydrate diet (e.g., Atkins or South Beach diet), restrict one or more nutrients. Protein and vegetables are encouraged, but certain carbohydrates and high-fat foods are not. Although they remain controversial in the medical community, these diets are extremely popular. Scientific outcome data have been conflicting.

Novelty diets, such as the grapefruit and Hollywood diet, are often nutritionally *inadequate*. This type of diet implies that a certain food or liquid increases metabolic rate or accelerates the oxidation of body fat. Weight loss is achieved because energy is restricted by food choice, but patients do not sustain weight loss after stopping the diet.

Nutrition Therapy. Nutritional recommendations for each patient should be developed through close interaction among the patient, family, physician, nurse, and nutritionist. The diet should meet the patient's needs, habits, and lifestyle and should be realistic.

The nutritionist develops a diet plan and instructs the patient. At a minimum, the diet should:

- Have a scientific rationale
- Be nutritionally adequate for all nutrients
- Have a low risk-benefit ratio
- Be practical and conducive to long-term success

Calorie estimates are easily calculated. Resting metabolic rate is determined using a gender-specific formula that incorporates the appropriate activity factor. This figure reflects the total calories needed daily for maintaining current weight. To encourage a weight loss of 1 pound (2.2 kg) a week, the nutritionist subtracts 500 calories each day. To encourage a weight loss of 2 pounds (4.4 kg) a week, 1000 calories each day are subtracted. The amount of weight lost varies with the patient's food intake, level of physical activity, and water losses. A reasonable expected outcome of 5% to 10% loss of body weight has been shown to improve glycemic control and reduce cholesterol and blood pressure. These benefits continue if the weight loss is sustained.

Exercise Program. A major intervention to manage obesity is to increase the type and amount of daily exercise to burn calories along with change in eating habits. For most people, adding exercise to a nutritional intervention produces more weight loss than just dieting alone. More of the weight lost is fat, which preserves lean body mass. An increase in exercise can reduce the waist circumference and the waist-hip ratio.

Teach patients that increasing and maintaining physical activity levels are important in maintaining weight loss. Many overweight or obese patients are so unfit that it may take several months of conditioning before they can exercise sufficiently to lose weight.

The physical therapist or exercise physiologist or assistant first obtains a clinical exercise and health history. It is important to determine the patient's current exercise pattern, if any, and exercise habits over a lifetime. Teach about the importance of an exercise component in a weight-loss program. The patient's desire to participate in an exercise program and his or her preferred types of exercise are also identified.

The health care provider may evaluate the patient by an exercise stress test. Not all patients need one, but those with chronic disease may need the results to assist with an individual exercise plan. Patients are counseled about unusual signs and symptoms during exercise (e.g., chest pain) and what to do if they occur. The physical therapist or exercise physiologist first emphasizes the importance of exercising consistently and then stresses its duration, intensity, and frequency.

A minimum-level workout should be developed so that consistency can be achieved. The expected outcome is to maintain a lifetime of increased physical activity. The patient is likely to be less fatigued and discouraged with a low-intensity, short-duration program. Encourage sedentary (physically inactive) patients to increase their activity by walking 30 to 40 minutes at least 5 days each week. The activity may be performed all at once or divided over the course of the day. Remind the patient to exercise only under the supervision of the physician. All members of the interdisciplinary team should encourage and support any increase in physical activity. Structured national programs with support staff, such as Curves, may be helpful for some patients. The staff typically offer diet counseling as well as cardiovascular and muscle-toning activities.

Drug Therapy. A BMI of 30 or a BMI of 27 with comorbidities is one indicator for the use of drug therapy. **Anorectic drugs** suppress appetite, which reduces food intake and, over time, may result in weight loss. The most commonly used drug for the *long-term* treatment of obesity is sibutramine (Meridia). It inhibits the reuptake of serotonin (which enhances satiety [feeling full when eating]) and norepinephrine (which raises the metabolic rate). The usual dosage is 10 mg every day, which may be increased to 15 mg daily after 4 weeks or decreased to 5 mg daily, depending on the patient's response. Adverse effects include dry mouth, constipation, and insomnia.

Orlistat (Xenical) is a different type of long-term use drug that inhibits lipase and leads to partial hydrolysis of triglycerides. Because fats are only partially digested and absorbed, calorie intake is decreased. The usual dosage is 120 mg three times daily. Most patients taking this drug have GI symptoms that include loose stools, abdominal cramps, and nausea. Therefore it should be used with caution and limited to adults between 18 and 75 years of age. Treatment is usually not extended beyond 12 months.

Other sympathomimetic drugs suppress appetite for *short-term* use along with a structured weight-management and exercise program. These drugs act on the central nervous system, including the appetite center of the brain (hypothalamus). Examples include phentermine (Adipex-P), diethylpropion (Tenuate, Tenuate Dospan), and phendimetrazine (Bontril). Patients with hypertension, heart disease, and hyperthyroidism should not take these drugs. Also, any patient taking psychoactive agents should not use these drugs. Side effects include:

- Palpitations
- Diarrhea or constipation
- Restlessness
- Insomnia
- Drug mouth
- Blurred vision (Bontril)
- Change in sex drive or activity
- Anxiety

Behavioral Management. Behavioral management of obesity helps the patient change daily eating habits to lose weight. This ongoing process should produce a change in behavior. Self-monitoring techniques include keeping a record of foods eaten (food diary), exercise patterns, and emotional and situational factors. Stimulus control involves controlling the external cues that promote overeating. Reinforcement techniques are used to self-reward the behavior change. Cognitive restructuring involves modifying negative beliefs by learning positive coping self-statements. Counseling by health care professionals must continue before, during, and after treatment. The 12-step program offered by Overeaters Anonymous (www.oa.org) has helped many people lose weight, especially those who are compulsive eaters.

Complementary and Alternative Therapies. Many complementary and alternative therapies have been tested and used for obesity. These modalities aim to suppress appetite and therefore limit food intake to lose weight:

- Acupuncture
- Acupressure
- Ayurvedic (a combination of holistic approaches)
- Hypnosis

Descriptions of most of these methods can be found in Chapter 2.

Surgical Management

At any weight, some patients seek to improve their appearance by having a variety of cosmetic procedures to reduce the amount of adipose tissue in selected areas of the body. A typical example of this type of surgery is **liposuction,** which can be done in a physician's office. Although the patient's appearance improves, if weight gain continues, the fatty tissue will return. This procedure is not a solution for people who are morbidly obese.

Morbidly obese people who do not respond to traditional interventions may be considered for a major surgical procedure aimed at producing permanent weight loss. Patients with a body mass index (BMI) of 40 or greater or a BMI of 35 or greater along with additional risk factors are considered for surgery. *Surgical intervention is the only method that has a long-term impact on morbid obesity* (Barth & Jenson, 2006).

Bariatrics is a branch of medicine that manages obesity and its related diseases. Surgical procedures include these three types: gastric restrictive, malabsorption, or both. *Restrictive* surgeries decrease the volume capacity of the stomach to limit the amount of food that can be eaten at one time. As the name implies, *malabsorption* procedures interfere with the absorption of food and nutrients from the GI tract.

Every year, more than 100,000 people in the United States have these procedures, and that number is rapidly increasing. The surgeon may use an open conventional approach or minimally invasive surgery (MIS). Most patients have MIS using either laparoscopy or the daVinci Robotic Surgical System. The decision of whether the patient is a candidate for the MIS is based on weight, body build, history of abdominal surgery, and co-existing medical complications. With any surgical approach, patients must agree to modify their lifestyle and follow stringent protocols to lose weight and keep the weight off. After bariatric surgery, many patients no longer have complications of obesity, such as diabetes mellitus, hypertension, depression, or sleep apnea.

Preoperative Care. Preoperative care is similar to that for any patient undergoing abdominal surgery or laparoscopy (see Chapter 16). However, obese patients are at increased surgical risks of pulmonary and thromboembolitic complications, as well as death. Some surgeons require limited weight loss before bariatric surgery to decrease these complications. Patients also have a thorough psychological assessment and testing to detect depression, substance abuse, or other mental health/behavioral health problem that could interfere with their success after surgery. Additional assessments to evaluate cognitive ability, coping skills, development, motivation, expectations, and support systems are also performed. Patients who are not alert and oriented or do not have sufficient strength and mobility are not considered for bariatric surgery. *The primary role of the nurse is to reinforce health teaching in preparation for surgery.* Most bariatric surgical centers provide education sessions for groups of patients who plan to have a bariatric procedure.

Operative Procedures. *Gastric restriction* surgeries allow for normal digestion without the risk for nutritional deficiencies. These procedures include the older *vertical-banded gastroplasty (VBG),* which is seldom done today, and the *laparoscopic adjustable-banded gastroplasty (LABG).* In the LABG procedure, the surgeon places an adjustable band to create a small proximal stomach pouch through a laparoscope (Fig. 63-5, *A*). The band may or may not be inflatable. Restrictive surgeries are the easiest to perform and can be reversed. However, weight lost is often regained after a period of time. By contrast, patients having the malabsorption procedures maintain 60% to 70% of their weight loss even after 20 years.

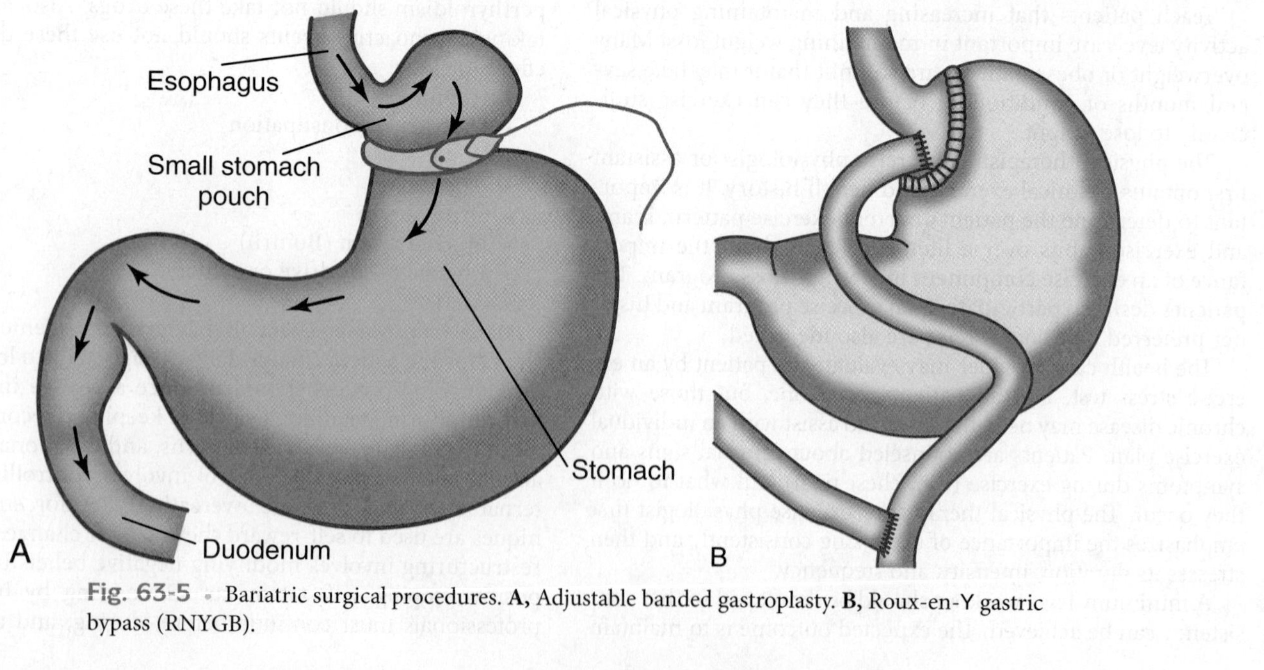
Esophagus
Small stomach pouch
Stomach
A
Duodenum
B

Fig. 63-5 • Bariatric surgical procedures. **A,** Adjustable banded gastroplasty. **B,** Roux-en-Y gastric bypass (RNYGB).

The most common *malabsorption surgery* performed in the United States is the *Roux-en-Y gastric bypass (RGB),* which is often done as a robotic surgical procedure. Other procedures less commonly done are the biliopancreatic diversion (rarely done) and the duodenal switch. All of these procedures result in quicker weight loss, but they are more invasive with a higher risk for postoperative complications. In RGB, most commonly just called a **gastric bypass,** gastric resection is combined with malabsorption surgery. The patient's stomach, duodenum, and part of the jejunum are bypassed so that fewer calories can be absorbed (see Fig. 63-5, *B*).

Postoperative Care. Postoperative care depends on the type of surgery—the open conventional approach or the minimally invasive technique. Although many patients have MIS, they are considered as having major abdominal surgery along with all its risks. However, these patients may require less than 24 hours in the hospital; some may need 1 to 2 days. Patients with open procedures may need several days to recover.

Patients having one of the MIS procedures have less pain, scarring, and blood loss. They typically have a faster recovery time and a faster return to daily activities.

The priority for immediate care of postoperative bariatric surgery patients is airway management. Patients with short and thick necks often have compromised airways and need aggressive respiratory support, possibly mechanical ventilation in the critical care unit. The addition of positive end-expiratory pressure (PEEP) may be helpful in improving oxygenation for these patients (Barth & Jenson, 2006).

All patients experience some degree of pain, but it is usually less severe when MIS is done. Patients may use patient-controlled analgesia (PCA) with morphine for up to the first 24 hours. All patients receive oral opioid analgesic agents as prescribed after the PCA is discontinued. Liquid forms of drug therapy are preferred. Acute pain management is discussed in Chapter 5 in detail.

Care of the bariatric surgical patient is similar to that of any patient having abdominal or laparoscopic surgery. *A major focus is patient and staff safety.* Special bariatric equipment and accommodations, including an extra-wide bed and additional personnel for moving the patient, are needed for both the surgical suite and postoperative care units. Weight-rated beds must be wide enough to allow the patient to turn. Bed rails should not be touching the body because they can cause pressure areas. Pressure between skin folds, as well as tubes and catheters, can also cause skin breakdown. Monitor the skin in these areas, and keep it clean and dry.

Some patients have a nasogastric (NG) tube put in place, especially after open surgical procedures. In gastroplasty procedures, the NG tube drains both the proximal pouch and the distal stomach. Closely monitor the tube for patency. *Never reposition the tube, because its movement can disrupt the suture line!* The NG tube is removed on the second day if the patient is passing flatus. Clear liquids are introduced slowly if the patient can tolerate water, and 1-ounce cups are used for each serving. Pureed foods, juice, and soups thinned with broth, water, or milk are added to the diet 24 to 48 hours after clear liquids are tolerated. Typically, the patient can increase the volume to 1 ounce over 5 minutes or until satisfied, but the diet is limited to liquids or pureed foods for 6 weeks. The patient then progresses to regular food, with an emphasis on nutrient-dense foods. Nausea, vomiting, or discomfort occurs if too much liquid is ingested.

Anastomotic leaks are the most common serious complication and cause of death after gastric bypass surgery. Monitor for manifestations of this life-threatening problem, including increasing back, shoulder, or abdominal pain; restlessness; and unexplained tachycardia and oliguria (scant urine). Report any of these findings to the surgeon immediately!

In addition to the postoperative complications typically associated with abdominal and laparoscopic surgeries, bariatric patients have special needs and risks. Implement these measures to prevent complications:

- Apply an abdominal binder to prevent wound dehiscence.
- Place the patient in semi-Fowler's position or use bi-level or continuous positive airway pressure (Bi-PAP or CPAP) ventilation at night to improve breathing and decrease risk for sleep apnea.
- Monitor oxygen saturation; provide oxygen at 2 L/min as prescribed.
- Apply sequential compression stockings and administer prophylactic anticoagulant (usually heparin) therapy as prescribed to help prevent thromboembolitic complications, including pulmonary embolism (PE).
- Observe skin areas and folds for redness, excoriation, or breakdown to treat these problems early.
- Use absorbent padding between folds to prevent pressure areas and skin breakdown; make sure that tubes and catheters are not causing pressure as well.
- Remove urinary catheter within 24 hours after surgery if possible to prevent urinary tract infection.
- Assist the patient out of bed on the day of surgery; encourage and assist with turning every 2 hours using an appropriate weight-bearing overhead trapeze. Collaborate with the physical or occupational therapist if needed for transfers or ambulation assistive devices, such as walkers.
- Ambulate patient as soon as possible to prevent postoperative complications, such as PE.
- Measure and record abdominal girth daily.
- In collaboration with the nutritionist, provide six small feedings and plenty of fluids to prevent dehydration.
- Observe for signs and symptoms of **dumping syndrome** (caused by food entering the small intestine instead of the stomach) after *gastric bypass,* such as tachycardia, nausea, diarrhea, and abdominal cramping.

DECISION-MAKING CHALLENGE
Critical Rescue

A young adult who had an open gastric bypass is transferred from the post-anesthesia care unit (PACU) to the critical care unit for continued respiratory support. On admission, he is alert and oriented, using paper and pen to communicate. He reports that the PCA is currently keeping him fairly comfortable. His surgical dressing is dry and intact; sequential stockings are in place on his legs. His "sat" is 99%, and he is dozing frequently. Six hours later he uses his call light and writes that he has severe pain in his mid-back and is nauseated. His pulse is 142 and thready, but his blood pressure and temperature have not changed since admission.

1. What further assessment do you need at this time?
2. What action should you take and why?
3. Why is this potential complication life threatening?
4. Could you have taken any action to prevent this complication? Why or why not?

evolve For suggested answer guidelines, go to http://evolve.elsevier.com/Iggy/.

Community-Based Care

Obese patients are cared for in a variety of settings, including the acute care hospital and transitional care unit (particularly after surgery) or in their own home. Obesity is a chronic, lifelong problem. Diets, drug therapy, exercise, and behavior modification can produce short-term weight losses with reasonable safety. However, most patients who do lose weight often regain the weight. Treatment of obesity should focus on the long-term reduction of health risks and medical problems associated with obesity, improving quality of life, and promoting a health-oriented lifestyle. Interdisciplinary team members need to provide a nonjudgmental, supportive atmosphere that encourages the patient to:

- Increase physical activity
- Decrease fat intake and reliance on appetite-reducing drugs
- Establish a normal eating pattern in response to physiologic hunger
- Address psychological problems

Frequent, long-term ambulatory care follow-up coordinated by a case manager is essential for successful treatment.

Teach patients that bowel changes are common after surgery. Constipation is most common after LABG and open gastric bypass surgery. Vitamin and mineral supplements are often needed after surgery, especially vitamin D, B-complex vitamins, iron, and calcium.

The most important features of health teaching for any obese patient and family focus on health-related behavior patterns. In collaboration with the nutritionist, counsel the patient on a healthful eating pattern. The physical therapist or exercise physiologist recommends an appropriate exercise program. A psychologist may recommend cognitive restructuring approaches that help alter dysfunctional eating patterns. For patients who have surgery, additional discharge teaching is needed. Chart 63-8 lists the important areas that should be reviewed.

Bariatric surgery results in a major lifestyle change and a variety of emotions. During weight loss, the patient may become depressed or anxious. Some experience a "hibernation phase" for about a month after surgery because of physical and emotional adjustments. Patients are usually followed closely by the surgeon and nutritionist for several years. Encourage them to keep all appointments and to adhere to the community-based treatment plan to ensure success. Plastic surgery, such as **panniculectomy** (removal of the abdominal apron, or **panniculus**), may be performed after weight is stabilized, usually in about 18 to 24 months.

Provide the patient with a list of available community resources, such as Overeaters Anonymous (www.oa.org) and the American Obesity Association (www.obesity.org). For surgical patients, the American Society for Metabolic and Bariatric Surgery (www.asbs.org) may be helpful.

Chart 63-8 PATIENT AND FAMILY EDUCATION GUIDE

Discharge Teaching for the Patient After Bariatric Surgery

Nutrition: Diet progression, nutrient (including vitamin and mineral) supplements, hydration guidelines

Drug therapy: Analgesics and antiemetic drugs, if needed; drugs for other health problems

Wound care: Clean procedure for open or laparoscopic wounds; cover during shower or bath

Activity level: Restrictions, such as avoiding lifting; activity progression; return to driving and work

Signs and symptoms to report: Fever; excessive nausea or vomiting; epigastric, back, or shoulder pain; red, hot, and/or draining wound(s); pain, redness, or swelling in legs; chest pain; difficulty breathing

Follow-up care: Health care provider office or clinic visits, support groups and other community resources, counseling for patient and family

Continuing education: Nutrition and exercise classes; follow-up visits with nutritionist

HUMAN NEEDS NURSING CARE REVIEW

What might you NOTICE if the patient is experiencing inadequate nutrition as a result of malnutrition or obesity?

Malnutrition

- Weight below ideal body weight or report of unexplained weight loss of 10 pounds in 6 months
- Dry, flaky skin
- Brittle nails and hair
- Leanness
- Activity intolerance
- Report of lethargy or fatigue
- Weakness
- Complications, such as infections, pressure ulcers, poor healing

Obesity

- Weight at least 20% above ideal
- Excessive fat
- Shortness of breath during activity or at rest
- Slowed movement
- Change in gait or limping
- Complications, such as type 2 diabetes mellitus, hypertension, depression

What should you INTERPRET and how should you RESPOND to a patient experiencing inadequate nutrition as a result of malnutrition or obesity?

Perform and interpret assessments, including:

- Take and record height and weight.
- Calculate BMI based on height and weight.
- Check laboratory values for hematocrit and hemoglobin and visceral proteins.
- Take complete medical history to determine associated complications and cause of nutritional problem.
- Assess impact of nutritional status on daily life, including ADLs.
- Assess coping mechanisms, especially for patients who are morbidly obese.

Respond by:

- Teaching patients about their need for a healthy nutritional state

- Teaching patients how to either lose or gain weight, depending on their specific problem (e.g., nutritional supplements for malnutrition; restrictive diet and exercise for obesity)
- Teaching patients to weigh frequently
- Monitoring changes in serum visceral proteins (especially prealbumin) as an indicator of improved nutrition for malnourished patients
- Initiating total enteral or total parenteral nutrition as prescribed for malnutrition
- Informing morbidly obese patients about bariatric surgery options

On what should you REFLECT?

- Monitor patient for indicators of improved nutrition (e.g., increased prealbumins and weights for malnutrition; weight loss and decreased fat for obesity).
- Think about what may have caused these nutritional problems and how they can be prevented.
- Think about what else you can do to improve nutritional health of patients you care for.

GET READY FOR THE NCLEX EXAMINATION!

Key Points

Review these Key Points for each NCLEX Examination Client Needs Category.

Safe and Effective Care Environment

- Ensure that feeding tube placement is verified by x-ray; check placement every 4 to 8 hours by aspirating gastric contents and assessing pH for nasogastric tubes.
- Place patients receiving tube feeding in a semi-Fowler's position at all times to prevent aspiration; check residual contents every 4 hours or as designated per facility policy.
- Use gloves when changing feeding system tubing or adding product; use sterile gloves when working with critically ill or immunocompromised patients.
- Use a feeding pump when the patient receives continuous or cyclic tube feeding.
- Collaborate with the interdisciplinary health care team, especially the nutritionist, health care provider, and case manager, when caring for patients with malnutrition or obesity.
- Be sure that bariatric furniture and equipment are available for the obese patient in the hospital or other health care setting; avoid pressure on skin-fold areas.

Health Promotion and Maintenance

- Perform nutritional screening for all patients to determine if they are at risk (see Charts 63-1 and 63-2).
- For patients receiving enteral or parenteral nutrition at home, teach family members or other caregivers how to provide nutrition while avoiding complications.
- Teach patients who are undernourished to eat high-protein, high-calorie foods and nutritional supplements.
- Instruct obese patients about the importance of health care provider–approved exercise for weight reduction.

Psychosocial Integrity

- Be aware that some obese patients may not view their weight as a problem and are therefore unlikely to be part of a weight-reduction plan.
- Recognize that obesity can cause depression or anxiety, low self-esteem, and a disturbed body image.
- Be aware of legal and ethical issues related to tube-feeding older adults with chronic or terminal illness.

Physiological Integrity

- Review serum prealbumin, hemoglobin, and hematocrit levels to identify patients at nutritional risk.
- Older patients are at increased risk for malnutrition (see Chart 63-2).
- Assess patients with severe malnutrition for common complications, such as edema; lethargy; and dry, flaking skin.
- Implement interventions to promote nutritional intake in older adults as specified in Chart 63-4.
- Provide nursing interventions for managing nutrition as listed in Chart 63-3, including nutritional supplements.
- Provide care for patients receiving total enteral nutrition as described in Charts 63-5 and 63-6.
- Provide care for patients receiving total parenteral nutrition as specified in Chart 63-7.
- Recognize that many people are following low-carbohydrate rather than low-fat diets to lose weight.
- Best practices for maintaining patency of nasoenteric tubes are listed in Chart 63-6.
- Recall that normal body mass index (BMI) for adults should be between 18.5 and 25; older adults should have a BMI between 23 and 27. A BMI of 27 to 30 indicates overweight, over 30 indicates obesity, and 40 and greater indicates morbid obesity.
- Recall that obesity causes early onset of many chronic illnesses, such as osteoarthritis, diabetes mellitus, hypertension, and coronary artery disease. Pulmonary problems, such as obstructive sleep apnea, delayed wound healing, and infections are also common.
- Remember that bariatric surgery includes gastric restriction procedures or gastric bypass; a panniculectomy may be performed to remove skin folds, especially the abdomen, once weight is stabilized.
- Be alert for signs and symptoms of anastomotic leak after bariatric surgery, including severe pain, restlessness, anxiety, and unexplained tachycardia.
- Provide postoperative care for patients having bariatric surgery to prevent complications such as wound dehiscence, respiratory distress, skin breakdown, and thromboembolitic complications, such as pulmonary embolism. Observe for complications, such as dumping syndrome in patients who have a gastric bypass. Tachycardia, nausea, diarrhea, and abdominal cramping are common manifestations of dumping syndrome.
- Provide discharge teaching for patients having bariatric surgery as described in Chart 63-8.

Additional Study Resources

Go to your Companion CD or Evolve at http://evolve.elsevier.com/Iggy/ for *Self-Assessment Questions for the NCLEX Examination.*

Go to Evolve at http://evolve.elsevier.com/Iggy/ for *Prioritization and Delegation Questions for the NCLEX Examination.*

SELECTED BIBLIOGRAPHY

Asterisk indicates a classic or definitive work on this subject.

Arzouman, J., Lacovara, J.E., Blackett, A., McDonald, P.K., Traver, G., & Bartholomeaux, F. Developing a comprehensive bariatric protocol: A template for improving patient care. *MEDSURG Nursing, 15*(1), 21-26.

*Barrow, C.J. (2002). Roux-en-Y gastric bypass for morbid obesity. *AORN Journal, 76*(4), 595-604.

Barth, M.M., & Jenson, C.E. (2006). Postoperative nursing care of gastric bypass patients. *American Journal of Critical Care, 15*(4), 378-388.

*Bender, S., Pusateri, M., Cook, A., Ferguson, M., & Hall, J.C. (2000). Malnutrition: Role of the TwoCal® HN Med Pass Program. *MEDSURG Nursing, 9*(6), 284-296.

*Bowers, S. (2000). All about tubes: Your guide to enteral feeding devices. *Nursing2000, 30*(12), 41-48.

Buchwald, H., Cowan, G., & Pories, W. (2006). *Surgical management of obesity.* Philadelphia: Saunders.

*Cammon, S.A., & Hackshaw, H.S. (2000). Are we starving our patients? *AJN, 100*(5), 43-47.

Chapman, I.M. (2006). Nutritional disorders in the elderly. *Medical Clinics of North America, 90*(5), 887-907.

Christie, C., Meires, J., & Watkins, J.A. (2007). Use your team's might to fight back obesity. *The Nurse Practitioner, 32*(5), 31-36.

*Cowan, D.T., Roberts, J.D., Fitzpatrick, J.M., While, A.E., & Baldwin, J. (2004). Nutritional status of older people in long term care settings: Current status and future directions. *International Journal of Nursing Studies, 41*(3), 225-237.

DiMaria-Ghalili, R.A., & Amella, E. (2005). Nutrition in older adults. *AJN, 105*(3), 40-50.

DiMaria-Ghalili, R.A., & Guenter, P. (2008). The Mini Nutritional Assessment. *AJN, 108*(2), 48-49.

*Edwards, S.J., & Metheny, N.A. (2000). Measurement of gastric residual volume: State of the science. *MEDSURG Nursing, 9*(3), 125-128.

Elpern, E.H., Killeen, K., Talla, E., Perez, G., & Gurka, D. (2007). Capnometry and air insufflation for assessing initial placement of gastric tubes. *American Journal of Critical Care, 16*(6), 544-550.

*Fellows, L.S., Miller, E.H., Frederickson, M., Bly, B., & Felt, P. (2000). Evidence-based practice for enteral feedings: Aspiration prevention strategies, bedside detection, and practice change. *MEDSURG Nursing, 9*(1), 27-32.

*Gallagher, S., & Gates, J.L. (2003). Obesity, panniculitis, panniculectomy, and wound care: Understanding the challenges. *Journal of Wound, Ostomy, and Continence Nursing, 30*(6), 334-341.

Grindel, M.E., & Grindel, C.G. (2006). Nursing care of the person having bariatric surgery. *MEDSURG Nursing, 15*(3), 129-144.

*Guenter, P., & Silkroski, M. (2001). *Tube feeding: Practical guidelines and nursing protocols.* Silver Spring, MD: ASPEN.

Harrington, L. (2006). Postoperative care of patients undergoing bariatric surgery. *MEDSURG Journal, 15*(6), 357-363.

Heddens, C.J. (2007). Body contouring: Shaping the future of patients with an obese past. *American Nurse Today, 2*(3), 46-49.

Jarvis, C. (2008). *Physical examination and health assessment.* (5th ed.). Philadelphia: Saunders.

*Lofgren, I., Herron, K., Zern, T., West, K., Patalay, M., Shachter, N.S., et al. (2004). Waist circumference is a better predictor than body mass index of coronary heart disease risk in overweight premenopausal women. *Journal of Nutrition, 134*(5), 1071-1076.

*Mackie, S.B. (2001). PEGs and ethics. *Gastroenterology Nursing, 24*(3), 138-142.

May, M. (2006). *How to apply a lifestyle approach to counsel overweight patients.* August 2006, 31-40. Retrieved February 16, 2008, from www.patientcareonline.com.

McCance, K.L., & Huether, S.E. (2006). *Pathophysiology: The biologic basis for disease in adults and children.* (5th ed.). St. Louis: Mosby.

*Metheny, N.A., Smith, L., & Stewart, B.J. (2000). Development of a reliable and valid bedside test for bilirubin and utility for improving prediction of feeding tube location. *Nursing Research, 49*(6), 302-309.

*Metheny, N.A., & Stewart, B.J. (2002). Testing feeding tube placement during continuous tube feedings. *Applied Nursing Research, 15*(4), 254-258.

*Metheny, N.A., Wehrle, M.A., Wiersema, L., & Clark, J. (1998). Testing feeding tube placement: Auscultation vs. pH method. *AJN, 98*(5), 37-43.

*Padula, C.A., Kenny, A., Planchon, C., & Lamoureux, C. (2004). Enteral feedings: What the evidence says. *AAJN, 104*(7), 62-64, 66-69.

Pagana, K.D., & Pagana, T.J. (2006). *Mosby's manual of diagnostic and laboratory tests.* (3rd ed.). St. Louis: Mosby.

Palmer, J.L., & Metheney, N.A. (2008). Preventing aspiration in older adults with dysphagia. *AJN, 108*(2), 40-47.

Sudakin, T. (2006). T.E.N. or T.P.N. *Nursing2006, 36*(12), 52-55.

*Yancy, W.S. Jr., Olsen, M.K., Guyton, J.R., Bakst, R.P., & Westman, E.C. (2004). A low-carbohydrate, ketogenic diet versus a low-fat diet to treat obesity and hyperlipidemia: A randomized, controlled trial. *Annals of Internal Medicine, 140*(10), 769-777.

Yantis, M.A., & Velander, R. (2007). Get the skinny on trans-fatty acids. *Nursing2007, 37*(12), 26.

XIV

UNIT

Problems of Regulation and Metabolism

Management of Patients with Problems of the Endocrine System

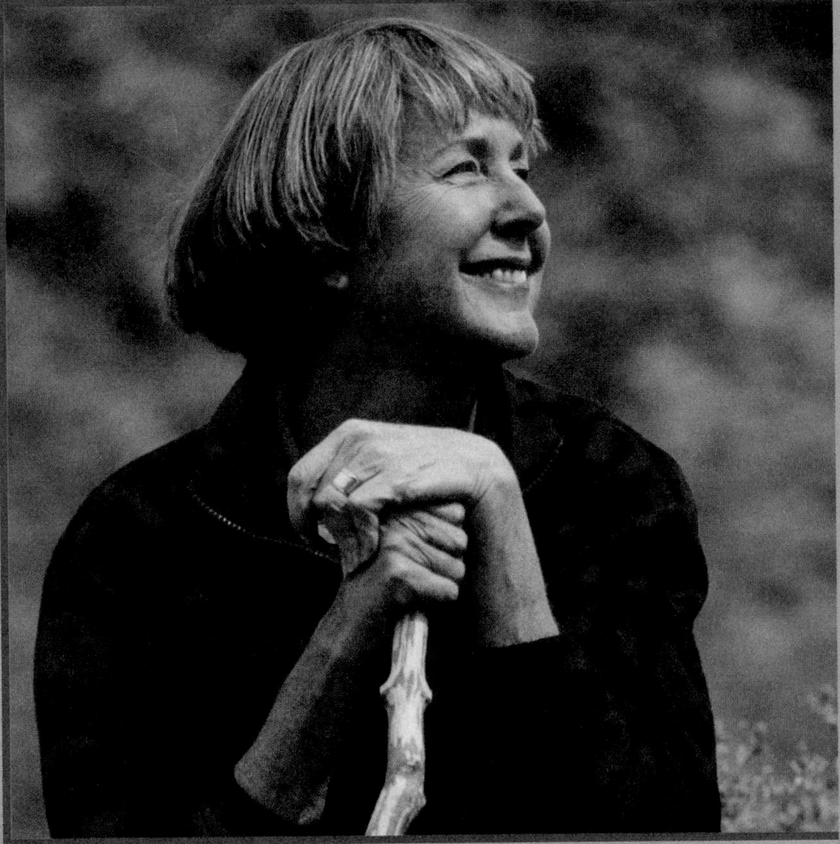

64

CHAPTER

Assessment of the Endocrine System

M. Linda Workman

LEARNING OUTCOMES

For clinical competence and success on the NCLEX Examination, study this chapter with these Learning Outcomes in mind:

Safe and Effective Care Environment

1. Ensure that agency laboratory procedures for collecting and handling specimens for endocrine function studies are followed.

Health Promotion and Maintenance

2. Identify factors that place patients at risk for endocrine health problems.
3. Teach everyone about the dangers of misusing or abusing hormones or steroids.

Psychosocial Integrity

4. Encourage the patient to express feelings or concerns about a change in appearance, sexuality, or fertility.
5. Assess whether the patient has experienced recent changes in behavior or coping responses to stress.
6. Use effective communication when teaching patients and family members about what to expect during tests and procedures to assess for endocrine problems.

Physiological Integrity

7. Describe the relationship between hormones and receptor sites.
8. Explain negative feedback as a control mechanism for hormone secretion.
9. Apply the principles of anatomy and physiology to understand the role of the endocrine system in homeostasis.
10. Identify adaptations in nursing assessment or interventions needed because of age-related changes in endocrine function.
11. Interpret laboratory test findings and clinical manifestations for patients with possible endocrine problems.

evolve Go to your Companion CD or Evolve at http://evolve.elsevier.com/Iggy/ for *Self-Assessment Questions for the NCLEX Examination* keyed to these Learning Outcomes.

The endocrine system is made up of glands in many tissues and organs in a variety of body areas (Fig. 64-1). A key feature of all endocrine glands is the secretion of hormones. **Hormones** are natural chemicals that exert their effects on specific tissues known as **target tissues.** Target tissues are usually located some distance from the endocrine gland, with no direct physical connection between the endocrine gland and its target tissue. For this reason, endocrine glands are called "ductless" glands and must use the blood to transport secreted hormones to the target tissues (Bauer, 2006). Endocrine glands include:

- Hypothalamus (a neuroendocrine gland)
- Pituitary gland
- Adrenal glands
- Thyroid gland
- Islet cells of the pancreas
- Parathyroid glands
- Gonads

The endocrine system works with the nervous system to regulate overall body function, known as **neuroendocrine regulation.** Many interactions must occur between the endocrine system and all other body systems to ensure that each system maintains a constant normal balance **(homeostasis)** in response to environmental changes (Davis, 2007). For example, neuroendocrine control of other body systems keeps the internal body temperature at or near 98.6° F (37° C), even when environmental temperatures are lower or higher. Other neuroendocrine actions help keep the serum sodium level between 136 and 145 mEq/L (mmol/L), regardless of whether a person eats 2 g or 12 g of sodium per day.

Table 64-1 lists the specific hormones secreted by various endocrine glands. Hormones travel through the blood to all

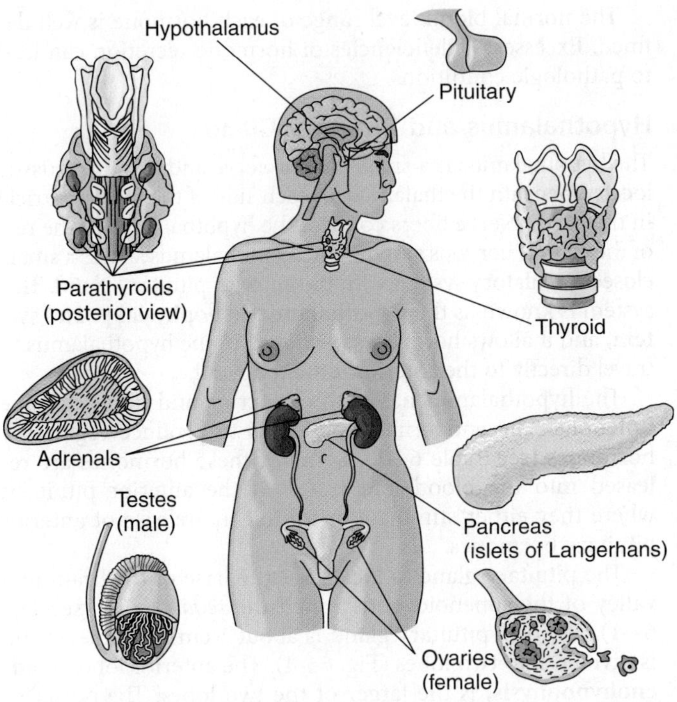
Hypothalamus
Pituitary
Parathyroids
(posterior view)
Thyroid
Adrenals
Testes
(male)
Pancreas
(islets of Langerhans)
Ovaries
(female)

Fig. 64-1 • The endocrine system.

body areas but exert their actions only on target tissues. They recognize their target tissues and exert their actions by binding to receptor sites on or within the target tissue cells. In general, each receptor site type is specific for only one hormone. Hormone-receptor actions work in a "lock and key" manner in that only the correct hormone (key) can bind to and activate the receptor site (lock) (Fig. 64-2). Binding a hormone to its receptor causes the target tissue to change its activity, producing specific responses (McCance & Huether, 2006).

Disorders of the endocrine system are related to either an excess or a deficiency of a specific hormone or to a defect at its receptor site. The onset of these disorders can be either slow and insidious or abrupt and life threatening.

ANATOMY AND PHYSIOLOGY REVIEW

The control of cellular function by any hormone depends on a series of reactions working through negative feedback control mechanisms. Hormone secretion depends on the need of the body for the final action of that hormone. When a body condition starts to move away from the normal range and a specific action or response is needed to correct this change, secretion of the hormone capable of causing the correcting action or response is stimulated until the need (demand) is met. As the correction occurs, hormone secretion decreases (and may halt). This type of control for hormone synthesis is **"negative feedback"** because the hormone causes the *opposite* action of the initial condition change.

An example of a simple negative feedback hormone response is the control of insulin secretion. When blood glucose levels start to rise above normal, the hormone *insulin* is secreted. Insulin increases glucose uptake by the cells, causing a *decrease* in blood glucose levels. Thus the action of insulin (decreasing blood glucose levels) is the opposite of or negative to the condition that stimulated insulin secretion (elevated blood glucose levels).

TABLE 64-1 Principal Hormones of the Endocrine Glands

Gland	Hormones
Hypothalamus	Corticotropin-releasing hormone (CRH)
	Thyrotropin-releasing hormone (TRH)
	Gonadotropin-releasing hormone (GnRH)
	Growth hormone–releasing hormone (GHRH)
	Growth hormone–inhibiting hormone (somatostatin GHIH)
	Prolactin-inhibiting hormone (PIH)
	Melanocyte-inhibiting hormone (MIH)
Anterior pituitary	Thyroid-stimulating hormone (TSH), also known as *thyrotropin*
	Adrenocorticotropic hormone (ACTH, corticotropin)
	Luteinizing hormone (LH), also known as *Leydig cell–stimulating hormone (LCSH)*
	Follicle-stimulating hormone (FSH)
	Prolactin (PRL)
	Growth hormone (GH)
	Melanocyte-stimulating hormone (MSH)
Posterior pituitary	Vasopressin (antidiuretic hormone [ADH])
	Oxytocin
Thyroid	Triiodothyronine (T_3)
	Thyroxine (T_4)
	Calcitonin
Parathyroid	Parathyroid hormone (PTH)
Adrenal cortex	Glucocorticoids (cortisol)
	Mineralocorticoids (aldosterone)
Ovary	Estrogen
	Progesterone
Testes	Testosterone
Pancreas	Insulin
	Glucagon
	Somatostatin

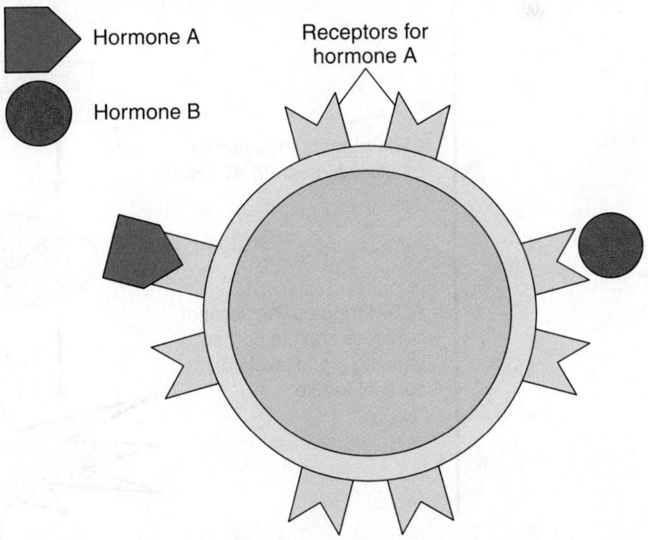
Hormone A
Hormone B
Receptors for
hormone A

Fig. 64-2 • "Lock and Key" hormone-receptor binding. Hormone A fits and binds to receptor sites, causing a change in cell action. Hormone B does not fit or bind to receptor sites; no change in cell action results.

Some hormones that use negative feedback mechanisms have more complex interactions. These interactions involve a series of reactions in which more than one endocrine gland, as well as the final target tissues, is stimulated. In this situation, the first hormone in the series may have another endocrine gland as its target tissue. For this type of mechanism to maintain homeostasis, this series of interactions must occur:

- The central nervous system receives and reacts to various sensory inputs transmitted to the hypothalamus as stimuli.
- The hypothalamus responds to the stimuli with the production and release of either releasing or inhibiting factors, which are transported to the pituitary.
- In the pituitary gland, the releasing or inhibiting factors either stimulate or inhibit the release of specific hormones.
- The anterior pituitary hormones then control the secretion of hormones in other endocrine glands. These glands then secrete hormones into the blood that then act on their target organs or tissues, resulting in a change of at least one function.

One example of this complex control is the interaction of the hypothalamus and the anterior pituitary with the adrenal cortex (Fig. 64-3). Low blood levels of cortisol from the adrenal cortex stimulate the secretion of corticotropic-releasing hormone (CRH) in the hypothalamus. CRH stimulates the anterior pituitary gland to secrete adrenocorticotropic hormone (ACTH). ACTH then triggers the release of cortisol from the adrenal cortex. The rising blood levels of cortisol inhibit CRH release from the hypothalamus. Without CRH, the anterior pituitary gland slows or stops secretion of ACTH. In this way, normal blood levels of cortisol are maintained.

The normal blood level range of each hormone is well defined. Excesses or deficiencies of hormone secretion can lead to pathologic conditions.

Hypothalamus and Pituitary Glands

The hypothalamus is a small area of nerve and glandular tissue located beneath the thalamus on each side of the third ventricle in the brain. Nerve fibers connect the hypothalamus to the rest of the central nervous system. The hypothalamus shares a small, closed circulatory system with the anterior pituitary gland. This system is known as the **hypothalamic-hypophysial portal system,** and it allows hormones produced in the hypothalamus to travel directly to the anterior pituitary gland.

The hypothalamus has both endocrine and nonendocrine functions. The endocrine function is to produce regulatory hormones (see Table 64-1). Some of these hormones are released into the blood and travel to the anterior pituitary, where they either stimulate or inhibit the release of anterior pituitary hormones.

The pituitary gland is located at the base of the brain in a valley of the sphenoid bone called the *sella turcica* (see Fig. 64-1). The oval pituitary gland is about 1 cm in diameter and is divided into two lobes (Fig. 64-4). The anterior lobe, or **adenohypophysis,** is the larger of the two lobes. The posterior lobe, or **neurohypophysis,** stores hormones produced in the hypothalamus. Nerve fibers in the hypophysial stalk, a structure extending from the hypothalamus, connect the hypothalamus to the posterior pituitary.

In response to the releasing hormones of the hypothalamus, the anterior pituitary secretes **tropic hormones,** which are hormones that stimulate other endocrine glands. Other anterior pituitary hormones, such as prolactin, produce their effect directly on final target tissues (Table 64-2).

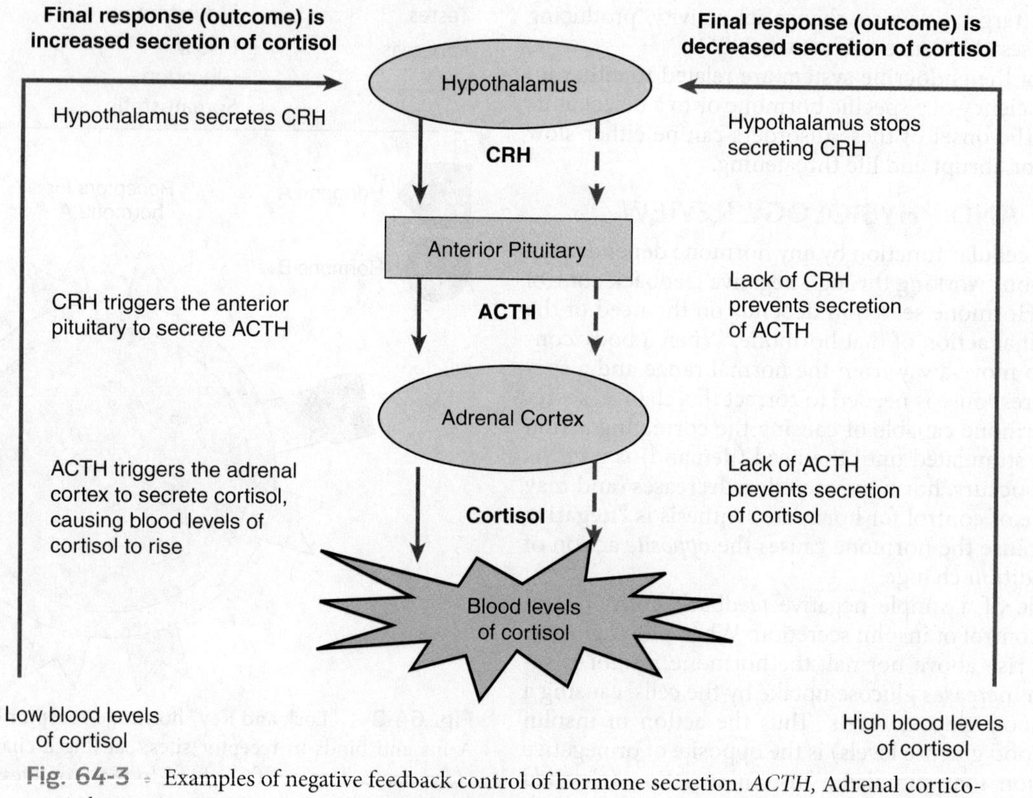

Final response (outcome) is increased secretion of cortisol
Final response (outcome) is decreased secretion of cortisol
Hypothalamus
Hypothalamus secretes CRH
Hypothalamus stops secreting CRH
CRH
Anterior Pituitary
Lack of CRH prevents secretion of ACTH
CRH triggers the anterior pituitary to secrete ACTH
ACTH
Adrenal Cortex
ACTH triggers the adrenal cortex to secrete cortisol, causing blood levels of cortisol to rise
Lack of ACTH prevents secretion of cortisol
Cortisol
Blood levels of cortisol
Low blood levels of cortisol
High blood levels of cortisol

Fig. 64-3 Examples of negative feedback control of hormone secretion. *ACTH,* Adrenal corticotropic hormone; *CRH,* corticotropin-releasing hormone.

The hormones of the posterior pituitary, vasopressin (antidiuretic hormone [ADH]) and oxytocin, are produced in the hypothalamus and sent through the nerve tracts that connect the hypothalamus with the posterior pituitary. These hormones are stored in the nerve endings of the posterior pituitary and are released into the blood when needed.

Other conditions or substances can affect the release of hormones from the pituitary gland. Drugs, diet, lifestyle, and pathologic conditions can increase or decrease pituitary hormone secretion.

Gonads

The **gonads** are the male and female reproductive endocrine glands. Male gonads are the testes, and female gonads are the ovaries. Although these glands are formed before birth and are present at birth, their function does not begin until puberty.

During puberty in the male, the increased secretion of gonadotropins (luteinizing hormone [LH] and follicle-stimulating hormone [FSH]) from the anterior pituitary gland stimulates maturation of the testes, production of testosterone, and maturation of the external genitalia. During puberty in the female, increased secretion of the same gonadotropins stimulates ovarian maturation, estrogen production, ovulation, and maturation of the external genitalia. The function of the testes and ovaries is detailed in Chapter 72.

Adrenal Glands

The adrenal glands are vascular, tent-shaped organs on the top of each kidney (see Fig. 64-1). The adrenal gland has an outer portion **(cortex)** and an inner portion **(medulla);** each area has independent functions. The hormones of the adrenal glands have effects throughout the body.

Adrenal Cortex

The adrenal cortex makes up about 90% of the adrenal gland and has cells divided into three zones or layers (Fig. 64-5). **Mineralocorticoids** are the hormones produced in the zona glomerulosa and help control the body's sodium and potassium content. Glucocorticoids, androgens, and estrogens are

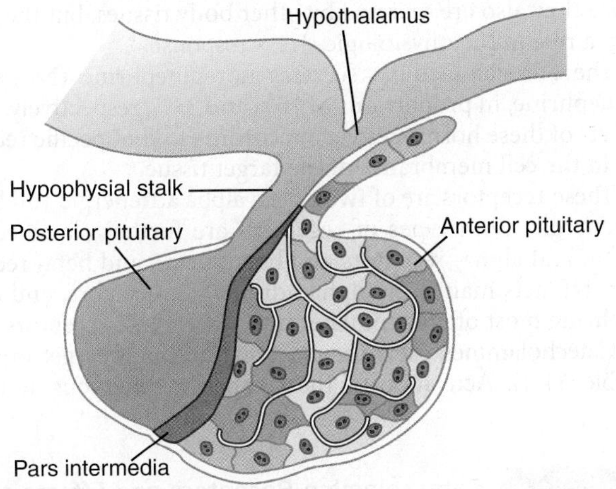
Hypothalamus
Hypophysial stalk
Posterior pituitary
Anterior pituitary
Pars intermedia

Fig. 64-4 • The hypothalamus, anterior pituitary gland, and posterior pituitary gland.

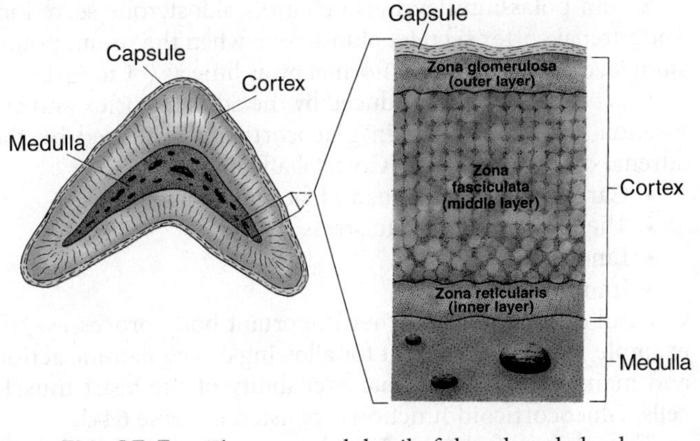
Capsule
Capsule
Cortex
Medulla
Zona glomerulosa (outer layer)
Zona fasciculata (middle layer)
Zona reticularis (inner layer)
Cortex
Medulla

Fig. 65-5 • The structural detail of the adrenal gland.

TABLE 64-2 Pituitary Hormones: Target Tissues and Subsequent Actions

Hormone	Target Tissue	Actions
ANTERIOR PITUITARY		
TSH (thyroid-stimulating hormone or thyrotropin)	Thyroid	Stimulates synthesis and release of thyroid hormone
ACTH (adrenocorticotropic hormone, corticotropin)	Adrenal cortex	Stimulates synthesis and release of corticosteroids and adrenocortical growth
LH (luteinizing hormone or Leydig cell–stimulating hormone)	Ovary Testis	Stimulates ovulation and progesterone secretion Stimulates testosterone secretion
FSH (follicle-stimulating hormone)	Ovary Testis	Stimulates estrogen secretion and follicle maturation Stimulates spermatogenesis
PRL (prolactin)	Mammary glands	Stimulates breast milk production
GH (growth hormone)	Bone and soft tissue	Promotes growth through lipolysis, protein anabolism, and insulin antagonism
MSH (melanocyte-stimulating hormone)	Melanocytes	Promotes pigmentation
POSTERIOR PITUITARY*		
Vasopressin (antidiuretic hormone [ADH])	Kidney	Promotes water reabsorption
Oxytocin	Uterus and mammary glands	Stimulates uterine contractions and ejection of breast milk

*These hormones are synthesized in the hypothalamus and are stored in the posterior pituitary gland. They are transported from the hypothalamus to the posterior pituitary while bound to neurophysins.

produced in the zona fasciculata and zona reticularis. The hormones produced and secreted by the cortex are often called **adrenal steroids** or **corticosteroids.**

Mineralocorticoids are produced and secreted by adrenal cortex to help control body fluids and electrolytes. **Aldosterone,** the chief mineralocorticoid produced by the adrenal cortex, maintains extracellular fluid volume. It promotes sodium and water reabsorption and potassium excretion in the kidney tubules. Aldosterone secretion is regulated by the renin-angiotensin system, serum potassium ion concentration, and adrenocorticotropic hormone (ACTH).

Renin is produced by the juxtaglomerular cells of the renal afferent arterioles. Its release is triggered by a decrease in extracellular fluid volume, which can occur from blood loss, sodium loss, or posture changes. Renin converts renin substrate (formerly called *angiotensinogen*), a plasma protein made in the liver, to angiotensin I. Angiotensin I is converted by a converting enzyme to form angiotensin II, the active form of angiotensin. In turn, angiotensin II stimulates the secretion of aldosterone. Chapters 13 (see Fig. 13-6) and 68 further describe the renin-angiotensin system. Aldosterone causes the kidney to reabsorb sodium and water to bring the plasma volume and osmolarity back to normal.

Serum potassium level also controls aldosterone secretion. The adrenal cortex secretes aldosterone when the serum potassium level increases above normal by as little as 0.1 mEq/L.

Glucocorticoids are produced by the adrenal cortex and are essential for life. The main glucocorticoid produced by the adrenal cortex is **cortisol.** Cortisol affects:

- Carbohydrate, protein, and fat metabolism
- The body's response to stress
- Emotional stability
- Immune function

Cortisol also influences other important body processes. For example, it must be present for allowing catecholamine action and maintaining the normal excitability of the heart muscle cells. Glucocorticoid functions are listed in Table 64-3.

The release of glucocorticoids is regulated directly by the anterior pituitary hormone *ACTH* and indirectly by the hypothalamic corticotropin-releasing hormone *CRH.* The release of CRH and ACTH is affected by the serum level of free cortisol, the normal sleep-wake cycle, and stress.

As described earlier and shown in Fig. 64-3, when blood cortisol levels are low, the hypothalamus secretes CRH, which triggers the pituitary to release ACTH. Then ACTH triggers the adrenal cortex to secrete cortisol. Conversely, adequate or elevated blood levels of cortisol *inhibit* the release of CRH and ACTH. This inhibitory effect is an example of a negative feedback system.

TABLE 64-3 Functions of Glucocorticoid Hormones

- Maintain blood glucose level by increasing hepatic gluconeogenesis and inhibiting peripheral glucose use
- Increase lipolysis, releasing glycerol and free fatty acids
- Increase protein catabolism
- Degrade collagen and connective tissue
- Increase the number of polymorphonuclear leukocytes released from bone marrow
- Exert anti-inflammatory effects that decrease the migration of inflammatory cells to sites of injury
- Maintain behavior and cognitive functions

Glucocorticoid release peaks in the morning and reaches its lowest level 12 hours after each peak. Emotional, chemical, or physical stress increases the release of glucocorticoids.

Sex hormones (androgens and estrogens) are secreted by the adrenal cortex in both genders. Adrenal secretion of these hormones is usually not significant because the **gonads** (ovaries and testes) secrete much larger amounts of estrogens and androgens. In women, however, the adrenal gland is the major source of androgens. Women who have adrenal insufficiency or who have had surgical removal of the adrenals may need a small amount of testosterone replacement.

Adrenal Medulla

The adrenal medulla is actually a sympathetic nerve ganglion that has secretory cells. Stimulation of the sympathetic nervous system results in the release of adrenal medullary hormones, the **catecholamines** (which include epinephrine and norepinephrine). These hormones travel to all areas of the body through the blood and exert their effects on target cells. The adrenal medullary hormones are not essential for life because they also are secreted by other body tissues, but they do play a role in the physiologic stress response.

The adrenal medulla secretes norepinephrine (NE) and epinephrine, in proportions of 15% and 85%, respectively. The effects of these hormones vary according to the specific receptor in the cell membranes of the target tissue.

These receptors are of two types: alpha adrenergic and beta adrenergic. Both types of receptors are further classified as $alpha_1$ and $alpha_2$ receptors and $beta_1$, $beta_2$, and $beta_3$ receptors. NE acts mainly on alpha-adrenergic receptors, and epinephrine most often stimulates beta-adrenergic receptors.

Catecholamines exert their actions on many target organs (Table 64-4). Activation of the sympathetic nervous system,

TABLE 64-4 Catecholamine Receptors and Effects of Adrenal Medullary Hormone Stimulation on Selected Organs and Tissues

Organ or Tissue	Receptors	Effects
Heart	$Beta_1$	Chronotropic action Inotropic action
Blood vessels	Alpha	Vasoconstriction
	$Beta_2$	Vasodilation
Gastrointestinal tract	Alpha	Increased sphincter tone
	Beta	Decreased motility
Kidneys	$Beta_2$	Increased renin release
Bronchioles	$Beta_2$	Relaxation; dilation
Bladder	Alpha	Sphincter contractions
	$Beta_2$	Relaxation of detrusor muscle
Skin	Alpha	Increased sweating
Fat cells	Beta	Increased lipolysis
Liver	Alpha	Increased gluconeogenesis and glycogenolysis
Pancreas	Alpha	Decreased glucagon and insulin release
	Beta	Increased glucagon and insulin release
Eyes	Alpha	Dilation of pupils

which then releases adrenal medullary catecholamines, is an important part of the body's response to stress. Catecholamines are secreted in small amounts at all times to maintain homeostasis. Severe stress triggers increased secretion of these hormones. This sympathetic activation results in the "fight-or-flight" response, a state of heightened physical and emotional awareness.

Thyroid Gland

The thyroid gland is in the anterior neck, directly below the cricoid cartilage (Fig. 64-6). It has two lobes joined by a thin strip of tissue (isthmus) in front of the trachea.

The thyroid gland has a rich blood supply and is composed of follicular and parafollicular cells. Follicular cells produce the thyroid hormones **thyroxine (T_4)** and **triiodothyronine (T_3)**. Parafollicular cells produce and secrete **thyrocalcitonin** (calcitonin [TCT]), which helps regulate serum calcium levels.

Control of metabolism occurs through T_3 and T_4. Both hormones increase metabolism, which causes an increase in oxygen use and heat production in all tissues. The two hormones differ in structure, but their functions are the same. Most circulating T_4 and T_3 are bound to plasma proteins. The proportion of bound hormone is in balance with the free hormone. The free hormone moves into the cell, where it binds to its receptor in the cell nucleus. Once in the cell, T_4 is converted to T_3, the most active thyroid hormone. The conversion of T_4 to T_3 is impaired by stress, starvation, dyes, beta blockers, amiodarone, corticosteroids, and propyl-thiouracil (PTU). Cold temperatures increase the conversion. Table 64-5 lists thyroid hormone functions.

Secretion of T_3 and T_4 is controlled by the hypothalamic-pituitary-thyroid gland axis feedback mechanism. The hypothalamus secretes thyrotropin-releasing hormone (TRH). TRH triggers the anterior pituitary gland to secrete thyroid-stimulating hormone (TSH), which then stimulates the thyroid gland to make and release thyroid hormones. If thyroid hormone levels are high, TSH release is inhibited. If thyroid hormone levels are low, TSH release is increased. This is an example of a negative feedback system. Cold and stress are two factors that cause the hypothalamus to secrete TRH, which then stimulates the anterior pituitary to secrete TSH.

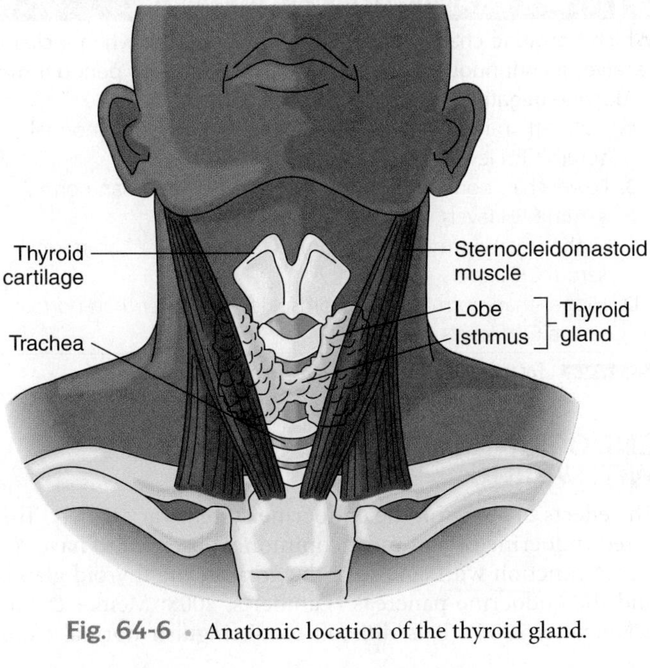
Thyroid cartilage
Trachea
Sternocleidomastoid muscle
Lobe
Isthmus
Thyroid gland
Fig. 64-6 • Anatomic location of the thyroid gland.

TABLE 64-5 Functions of Thyroid Hormones

- Fetal development, particularly neural and skeletal systems
- Control metabolic rate of all cells
- Promote sufficient pituitary secretion of growth hormone and gonadotropins
- Regulate protein, carbohydrate, and fat metabolism
- Exert chronotropic and inotropic cardiac effects
- Increase red blood cell production
- Affect respiratory rate and drive
- Increase bone formation and decrease bone resorption of calcium
- Act as insulin antagonists

Thyroid hormone production involves a series of steps. Dietary intake of protein and iodine is needed to produce thyroid hormones. Iodine is absorbed from the intestinal tract as iodide. The thyroid gland withdraws iodide from the blood and concentrates it. After iodide is in the thyroid, it enters into a series of reactions to form T_4 and T_3. These hormones bind to thyroglobulin and are stored in the follicular cells of the thyroid gland. With stimulation, T_4 and T_3 break off from thyroglobulin and are released into the blood. They enter many cells, bind to the nucleus, and turn on genes important in metabolism. Thus the presence of T_4 and T_3 directly regulates basal metabolic rate (BMR).

Calcium and phosphorus balance occurs through the actions of calcitonin (also called thyrocalcitonin, or TCT). This hormone also is produced in the thyroid gland. Calcitonin lowers serum calcium and serum phosphorus levels by reducing bone resorption (breakdown). Its actions are opposite of parathyroid hormone.

The serum calcium level determines calcitonin secretion. Low serum calcium levels inhibit the release of calcitonin. Elevated serum calcium levels increase its secretion. Other factors that increase calcitonin release are pregnancy, a high-calcium diet, and an increased secretion of gastrin.

Parathyroid Glands

The parathyroid glands consist of four small glands located close to or within the back surface of the thyroid gland (see Fig. 64-1). The chief cells of the parathyroid glands produce and secrete parathyroid hormone (PTH).

Parathyroid hormone regulates calcium and phosphorus metabolism by acting on bone, kidney, and the intestinal tract (Fig. 64-7). Bone is the main storage site of calcium. PTH increases **bone resorption** (bone release of calcium into the blood from bone storage sites), thus increasing serum calcium. In the kidneys, PTH activates vitamin D, which then increases the absorption of calcium and phosphorus from the intestines. In the kidney tubules, PTH allows calcium to be reabsorbed and put back into the blood.

Serum calcium level is the major controlling factor of PTH secretion. Secretion decreases when serum calcium levels are high, and it increases when serum calcium levels are low. Serum phosphorus levels also affect PTH secretion, probably because of the effect on serum calcium levels. PTH and calcitonin work together to maintain a normal level of calcium in the blood and extracellular fluid.

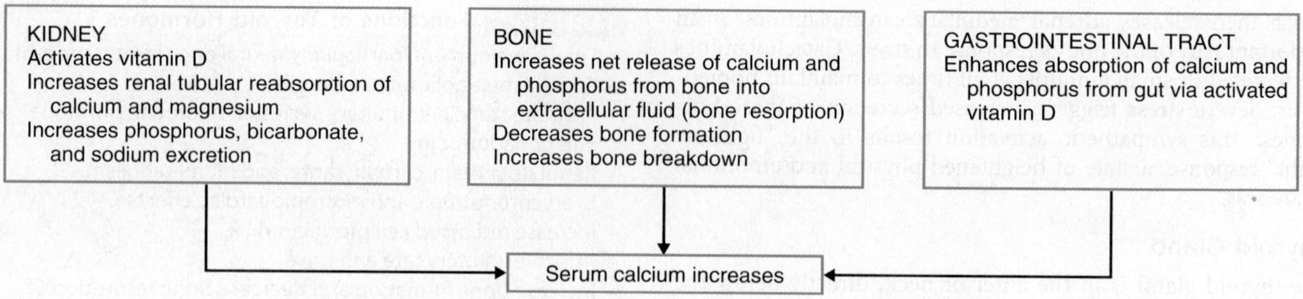
KIDNEY
Activates vitamin D
Increases renal tubular reabsorption of calcium and magnesium
Increases phosphorus, bicarbonate, and sodium excretion
BONE
Increases net release of calcium and phosphorus from bone into extracellular fluid (bone resorption)
Decreases bone formation
Increases bone breakdown
GASTROINTESTINAL TRACT
Enhances absorption of calcium and phosphorus from gut via activated vitamin D
Serum calcium increases

Fig. 64-7 • Effects of parathyroid hormone to maintain calcium balance.

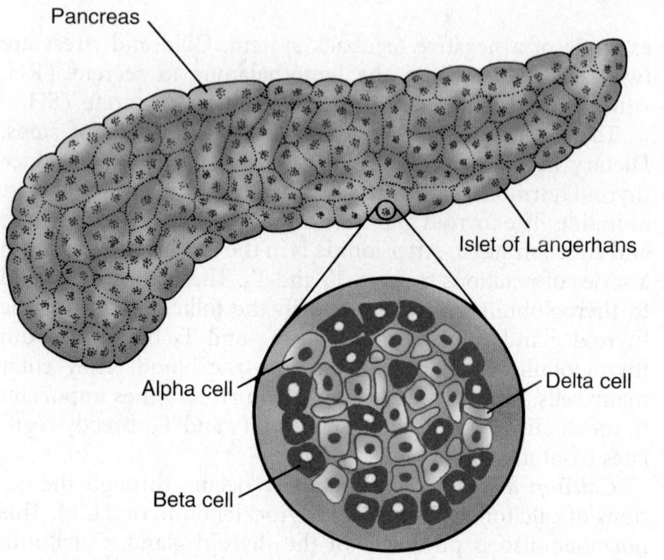
Pancreas
Islet of Langerhans
Alpha cell
Delta cell
Beta cell

Fig. 64-8 • The islets of Langerhans of the pancreas.

Pancreas

The pancreas lies behind the stomach and has endocrine and exocrine functions. The islets of Langerhans areas perform the endocrine functions of the pancreas (Fig. 64-8). About one million islet cells are found throughout the pancreas.

The islets have three distinct cell types: alpha cells, which secrete glucagon; beta cells, which secrete insulin; and delta cells, which secrete somatostatin. Glucagon and insulin affect carbohydrate, protein, and fat metabolism. Somatostatin, which is secreted not only in the pancreas but also in the intestinal tract and the brain, inhibits the release of glucagon and insulin from the pancreas. It also inhibits the release of gastrin, secretin, and other GI peptides.

The exocrine function of the pancreas involves the secretion of digestive enzymes through ducts that empty into the duodenum. The main endocrine function of the pancreas is to regulate blood glucose (sugar) levels.

Glucagon is a hormone that increases blood glucose levels. It is triggered by decreased blood glucose levels and increased blood amino acid levels. Together with epinephrine, growth hormone (GH), and cortisol, glucagon maintains blood glucose levels. In the liver (the main target organ of glucagon), it causes **glycogenolysis** (the conversion of glycogen to glucose). Glucagon also enhances amino acid transport from muscle and promotes **gluconeogenesis** (the conversion of amino acids to glucose). In fat metabolism, glucagon enhances **lipolysis** (fat breakdown) and ketone formation.

TABLE 64-6 Anabolic Effects of Insulin

EFFECTS ON LIVER
• Promotes glycogen synthesis and storage
• Inhibits glycogenolysis, gluconeogenesis, and ketogenesis
• Increases triglyceride synthesis
EFFECTS ON MUSCLE
• Promotes protein synthesis
• Increases amino acid transport
• Promotes glycogenesis
EFFECTS ON FAT
• Increases fatty acid synthesis
• Promotes triglyceride storage
• Decreases lipolysis

Insulin, an **anabolic hormone** (one that stimulates growth), promotes the movement and storage of carbohydrate (CHO), protein, and fat (Table 64-6). Insulin lowers blood glucose levels by enhancing glucose movement across cell membranes and into the cells of many tissues. Basal levels of insulin are secreted continuously to control metabolism. Insulin secretion rises in response to an increase in blood glucose levels. CHO is the main trigger for insulin secretion. More information on insulin is presented in Chapter 67.

NCLEX EXAMINATION CHALLENGE

Which hormone changes should the nurse expect when a client receives a continuous ACTH infusion over a 24-hour period if the endocrine negative feedback loops are normal?

A. Lower-than-normal serum cortisol levels; lower-than-normal serum CRH levels
B. Lower-than-normal serum cortisol levels; higher-than-normal serum CRH levels
C. Higher-than-normal serum cortisol levels; lower–than-normal serum CRH levels
D. Higher-than-normal serum cortisol levels; higher-than-normal serum CRH levels

evolve For the correct answer, go to http://evolve.elsevier.com/Iggy/.

ENDOCRINE CHANGES ASSOCIATED WITH AGING

The effects of aging on the endocrine system vary widely. The three endocrine tissues most commonly observed to have reduced function with aging are the gonads, the thyroid gland, and the endocrine pancreas (Lamberts, 2008; Meiner & Lueckencotte, 2006). It is difficult to distinguish normal from

Chart 64-1 NURSING FOCUS ON THE OLDER ADULT

Changes in the Endocrine System Related to Aging

Changes	Clinical Findings	Nursing Actions/Adaptations
Decreased antidiuretic hormone (ADH) production	Urine is more dilute and may not concentrate when fluid intake is low.	The patient is at greater risk for dehydration as a result of urine loss. Assess the older patient more frequently for dehydration. If fluids are not restricted because of another health problem, teach unlicensed assistive personnel (UAP) to offer fluids at least every 2 hours while awake.
Decreased ovarian production of estrogen	Bone density decreases.	Teach the patient to engage in regular exercise and weight-bearing activity to maintain bone density. Handle the patient carefully to avoid injury from pathologic fractures.
	Skin is thinner, drier, and at greater risk for injury.	Avoid pulling or dragging the patient. Use minimal tape on the skin. Assist patients confined to bed or chairs to change positions at least every 2 hours. Teach patients to use moisturizers on the skin and to avoid agents that promote skin dryness.
	Perineal and vaginal tissues become drier, and the risk for cystitis increases.	Perform or assist the patient to perform perineal care at least twice daily. Unless another health problem requires fluid restriction, encourage all women to drink at least 3 liters of fluids daily. Teach sexually active patients to urinate immediately after sexual intercourse.
Decreased glucose tolerance	Weight becomes greater than ideal along with: • Elevated fasting blood glucose level • Elevated random blood glucose level • Slow wound healing • Frequent yeast infections • Polydipsia • Polyuria	Obtain a family history of obesity and type 2 diabetes. Encourage the patient to engage in regular exercise and to keep body weight within 10 lbs of ideal. Teach patients the clinical manifestations of diabetes, and instruct them to report any of these manifestations to the health care provider. Suggest diabetes testing for any patient with: • Persistent vaginal candidiasis • Failure of a foot or leg skin wound to heal in 2 weeks or less • Increased hunger and thirst • Noticeable decrease in energy level
Decreased general metabolism	Less tolerant of cold. Decreased appetite. Decreased heart rate & blood pressure (BP)	Can be difficult to distinguish from hypothyroidism. Check for additional manifestations of: • Lethargy • Constipation (as a change from usual bowel habits) • Decreased cognition • Slowed speech • Body temperature consistently below 97° F (36° C) • Heart rate below 60 beats/min Teach patient to dress warmly.

abnormal endocrine activity because of these other age-related variables:

- Acute and chronic illnesses
- Alterations in diet, activity, and lean body mass–fat ratio
- Disturbances in sleep patterns
- Decreased metabolic clearance rate of hormones
- Increased use of multiple drugs that may affect hormone function

It is important to consider these factors when assessing the older adult with endocrine dysfunction.

Encourage the older adult patient to participate in regular screening examinations, including fasting and postprandial blood glucose checks, calcium level determinations, and thyroid function testing. Chart 64-1 lists the endocrine changes that occur in the older adult.

ASSESSMENT METHODS

Patient History

Use a systems approach to obtain the history of patients with a possible endocrine problem. This approach can be difficult because of the variety and combination of clinical manifestations. Identify the patient's response to actual or perceived changes, and discuss the potential diagnostic and treatment plan. Chart 64-2 presents some assessment questions based on

Chart 64-2 ENDOCRINE ASSESSMENT

Using Gordon's Functional Health Patterns

NUTRITIONAL-METABOLIC PATTERN

- What is your typical daily food intake? Describe a day's meals, snacks, and vitamins.
- How much salt do you typically add to your food? Do you use salt substitutes?
- How is your appetite?
- Do you have any difficulty chewing or swallowing?
- What is your typical daily fluid intake? What types of fluids (water, juices, soft drinks, coffee, tea)? How much?
- Have you had any recent change in your weight? Weight gain? Weight loss? How much?
- Have you noticed a change in the tightness of your rings or shoes? Tighter? Looser?
- Have you noticed any change in thirst?

ELIMINATION PATTERN

- What is your usual bowel elimination pattern? Frequency? Character? Discomfort? Laxative use?
- What is your usual urinary elimination pattern? Frequency? Amount? Color? Odor? Control?
- Have you noticed a change in the amount of urine?
- Do you have any problem with excessive perspiration?
- Do you have any other type of drainage?

SLEEP-REST PATTERN

- Do you have any difficulty falling asleep when you go to bed?
- Is there a change in the number of hours you sleep per night?
- Do you take any drugs to help you sleep?
- About how many times do you awaken during the night?
- Do you have any difficulty getting back to sleep?
- Are you bothered by nightmares or vivid dreams?
- Do you have difficulty awakening in the morning?
- Do you feel generally rested and ready for daily activities after sleep?
- Do you take scheduled naps or rest periods during the day?
- Do you find yourself falling asleep at work or at home while reading or watching television?
- Have you noticed any difficulty in your ability to concentrate?

SEXUALITY-REPRODUCTIVE PATTERN

- Are you sexually active?
- Are you satisfied with your level of sexual activity?
- Do you participate in sex as often as you would like?
- Do you participate in sex as often as your partner would like?
- Have you noticed a change in your interest in having sex over the past year?

Female:

- At what age did menstruation start?
- How regular are your periods?
- Do you have any pain, cramping, or clotting during your periods?
- Have you ever been pregnant? What was the outcome of the pregnancy(ies)?
- Do you use contraceptives? What type? Have you had any problems with your chosen method of contraception?

ACTIVITY-EXERCISE PATTERN

- Do you feel you have sufficient energy to perform tasks or routines that are required of you?
- Do you feel you have sufficient energy to do what you would like to do?
- Do you exercise? How often? For how long each time? What type(s) of exercise do you perform?
- What activities do you perform in your spare time?
- What is your ability to perform the following tasks?

Feeding _____	Grooming _____
Bathing _____	General Mobility _____
Toileting _____	Cooking _____
Bed Mobility _____	Home Maintenance _____
Dressing _____	Shopping _____

FUNCTIONAL LEVELS CODE

- Level 0: Full self-care
- Level I: Requires use of equipment or device
- Level II: Requires help from another person(s): assistance, supervision, teaching
- Level III: Requires help from another person(s) and equipment or device
- Level IV: Dependent; does not participate in self-care

Based on Gordon, M. (2007). *Manual of nursing diagnosis* (11th ed.). Boston: Jones & Bartlett.

Gordon's Functional Health Patterns. Although endocrine problems can disturb any health pattern, the patterns most commonly affected are nutritional-metabolic, activity, elimination, sleep-rest, and sexuality-reproductive. These data are combined with physical, psychosocial, and laboratory findings for a complete assessment of endocrine function.

The age and gender of the patient provide baseline assessment data. Certain disorders are more common in older than in younger patients, such as diabetes mellitus, loss of ovarian function, and decreased thyroid function.

Manifestations of endocrine disorders can be gender related, such as the sexual effects of hyperpituitarism and hypopituitarism (see Chapter 65). In addition, thyroid problems are much more common in women than in men. Assess the patient for a history of endocrine dysfunction, manifestations that could indicate an endocrine disorder, and hospitalizations. Ask about past and current drugs, such as hydrocortisone, levothyroxine, oral contraceptives, and antihypertensive agents. The use of exogenous hormone drugs, when not needed for hormone replacement, can cause serious dysfunction in many endocrine glands. Use the opportunity to warn patients about the dangers of misusing or abusing hormone-based drugs such as androgens and thyroid hormones.

Because the patient's socioeconomic status is a sensitive issue, explore with the patient whether his or her resources are adequate for a healthy diet, needed drugs, and consistent health care follow-up. It may be appropriate to involve social service and home care agencies at an early stage.

Nutrition History

Nutritional changes or GI tract disturbances may reflect many different endocrine problems. Ask about a history of nausea, vomiting, and abdominal pain. An increase or decrease in food or fluid intake may also indicate specific disorders. For example, diabetes insipidus triggers excessive thirst, and adrenal hypofunction triggers salt craving. Hunger and thirst may also be increased in diabetes mellitus. Rapid changes in weight without diet changes can indicate the onset of a number of endocrine disorders, including diabetes mellitus and thyroid problems.

Dietary deficiencies, especially of protein and iodide-containing foods (saltwater fish and seafood, iodized table salt), may be a cause of an endocrine disorder. Teach the patient about a well-balanced diet that includes at least 60 g of protein daily, less animal fat, and fewer concentrated simple sugars. Teach patients who do not eat saltwater fish on a regular basis to use iodized salt in food preparation.

Family History and Genetic Risk

Ask the patient about any family history of obesity, growth or development difficulties, diabetes mellitus, infertility, or thyroid disorders. These problems may have an autosomal dominant, recessive, or cluster pattern of inheritance.

Current Health Problems

Focus on the patient's reason for seeking health care, asking questions such as:

- Did the symptoms occur gradually, or was the onset sudden?
- Have you been treated for this problem in the past?
- How have the current symptoms affected your activities of daily living?

These types of questions can provide clues to specific endocrine disorders. Also explore changes in energy levels, elimination patterns, sexual and reproductive functions, and physical features.

Energy level changes occur with many endocrine problems, especially thyroid problems (see Chapter 66) and adrenal problems (see Chapter 65). Ask the patient about any change in ability to perform ADLs, and assess his or her current energy level. For instance, has he or she been sleeping longer, or are fatigue and generalized weakness present?

Elimination is also affected by the endocrine system. Identify the patient's past pattern of elimination to determine deviations from the normal routine. Ask about the amount and frequency of urination. Does he or she urinate frequently in large amounts? Does the patient wake during the night to urinate **(nocturia)**, or is pain present with urination **(dysuria)?** Information about the frequency of bowel movements and their consistency and color may provide clues to problems in fluid balance or metabolic rate (i.e., thyroid function).

Sexual and reproductive functions are greatly affected by endocrine disturbances. Ask women about any changes in the menstrual cycle, such as increased flow, duration, and frequency of menses; pain or excessive cramping; or a recent change in the regularity of menses. Ask men whether they have experienced impotence. Question both men and women about a change in libido (sexual desire) or any fertility problems.

Physical appearance changes can reflect an endocrine problem. Discuss any changes that the patient perceives in physical features. Obvious changes are identified during the physical assessment, but patients may be able to describe some of the more subtle changes. Ask about changes in:

- Hair texture and distribution
- Facial contours and eye protrusion
- Voice quality
- Body proportions
- Secondary sexual characteristics

For example, you might ask a man whether he is shaving less often or a woman if she has noticed an increase in facial hair. These changes may be associated with pituitary, thyroid, parathyroid, or adrenal dysfunction.

DECISION-MAKING CHALLENGE
Coordination of Care

The patient is a 27-year-old woman who stopped having menstrual periods 6 months ago. A home pregnancy test indicates she is not pregnant. She is 5′ 2″ tall and weighs 180 lbs. You observe that she has acne and rather heavy facial hair. Her arms and shoulders appear muscular. When you ask her about her diet, she rudely responds that she has been eating only 1200 calories daily and that her weight has increased in the past month.

1. Are there any endocrine glands, based on the patient's age, gender, and manifestations, that do **not** need to be assessed for this patient? Provide a rationale for your answer.
2. What would be an appropriate response to this patient's rude response to your diet question?
3. What specific questions regarding her menstrual cycle should you ask this patient?
4. What other subjective information should you obtain from this patient?

evolve For suggested answer guidelines, go to http://evolve.elsevier.com/Iggy/.

Physical Assessment

Inspection

An endocrine problem can change physical features because of its effect on growth and development, regulation of sex hormone levels, fluid and electrolyte balance, and the body's use of nutrients. Different clinical findings can occur with multiple endocrine disorders or with nonendocrine problems.

Use a head-to-toe approach to inspect the patient. Observe the patient's general appearance, and assess height, weight, fat distribution, and muscle mass in relation to age. It is important to remember that heredity and age rather than a health problem may be responsible for some physical features (e.g., short stature).

When examining the head, focus on abnormalities of facial structure, features, and expression, such as:

- Prominent forehead or jaw
- Round or puffy face
- Dull or flat expression
- Exophthalmos (protruding eyeballs and retracted upper lids)

Check the lower half of the neck for a visible enlargement of the thyroid gland. Normally the thyroid tissue cannot be observed. The isthmus may be noticeable when the patient swallows. Jugular vein distention may be seen on inspection of the neck and can indicate fluid overload.

Skin changes may reflect a specific endocrine dysfunction. Observe skin color, and look for areas of pigment loss (hypopigmentation) or hyperpigmentation. Fungal skin infections, slow wound healing, bruising, and petechiae are often seen in patients with adrenal hyperfunction. Skin infections, foot ulcers, and slow wound healing are common among patients with diabetes mellitus. In secondary hypofunction of the adrenal glands, the skin over the finger joints, elbows, and knees, as well as any scar tissue, may show increased pigmentation due to increased levels of ACTH and melanocyte-stimulating hormone.

Vitiligo (patchy areas of pigment loss with increased pigmentation at the edges) is seen with primary hypofunction of the adrenal glands and is caused by autoimmune destruction of melanocytes in the skin. Areas of pigment loss most often occur on the face, neck, and extremities. Mucous membranes may have large areas of uneven pigmentation. Document the location, color, distribution, and size of skin color changes and lesions.

Inspect the patient's fingernails for malformation, thickness, or brittleness, all of which may suggest thyroid gland problems. Examine the extremities and the base of the spine for edema, which suggests a fluid and electrolyte imbalance.

Inspection of the trunk can show signs of specific endocrine dysfunction. Check for any abnormalities in chest size and symmetry. Truncal obesity and the presence of a "buffalo hump" between the shoulders on the back may indicate adrenocortical excess. Hormonal imbalance may also change secondary sexual characteristics. Inspect the breasts of both men and women for size, symmetry, pigmentation, and discharge. **Striae** (reddish purple "stretch marks") on the breasts or abdomen are often seen with adrenocortical excess.

Assess the patient's hair distribution for indications of endocrine gland dysfunction. Changes can include **hirsutism** (excessive growth of body hair, especially on the face, chest, and the linea alba of the abdomen of women), excessive hair loss, or changes in hair texture.

Examination of the genitalia may reveal a dysfunction in hormone secretion. Observe the size of the scrotum and penis or of the labia and clitoris in relation to standards for the patient's age. The distribution and quantity of pubic hair are often affected in hypogonadism.

Palpation

The thyroid gland and the testes can be examined by palpation. Chapters 72 and 75 discuss examination of the testes. The thyroid gland is palpated for size, symmetry, general shape, and the presence of nodules or other irregularities.

Palpate the thyroid gland by standing either behind or in front of the patient (Fig. 64-9). The posterior approach may be easier. Asking the patient to swallow sips of water during the examination helps the clinician palpate the thyroid gland.

Ask the patient to sit and to lower the chin. Using the posterior approach, place the thumbs of both your hands on the back of the patient's neck, with the fingers curved around to the front of the neck on either side of the trachea. Ask the patient to swallow, and then locate the isthmus of the thyroid as you feel it rising. Identify the anterior surface of the thyroid lobe. To examine the right lobe, proceed in this way:

- Turn the patient's head to the right.
- Displace the thyroid cartilage to the right with the fingers of your left hand.
- Palpate the right lobe with your right hand.
- Reverse this procedure to examine the left lobe.

Auscultation

Auscultate the chest to assess cardiac rate and rhythm. Document this information to use later as a means of assessing treatment effectiveness. Some endocrine problems induce dysrhythmias. Many endocrine disturbances can cause dehydration and volume depletion. Therefore document any difference in the patient's blood pressure and pulse in the lying, standing, or sitting positions (orthostatic vital signs).

If an enlarged thyroid gland is palpated, auscultate the area of enlargement for bruits. Hypertrophy of the thyroid gland causes an increase in vascular flow, which may result in bruits.

Psychosocial Assessment

Information obtained from the history and physical examination may help identify psychosocial problems. Assess the patient's coping skills, support systems, and health-related beliefs. Many endocrine problems can change a patient's behaviors, personality, and psychological responses. Ask the patient whether he or she has noticed a change in how stress is handled, frequency of crying, or degree of patience and anger expression. The patient may not recognize these changes

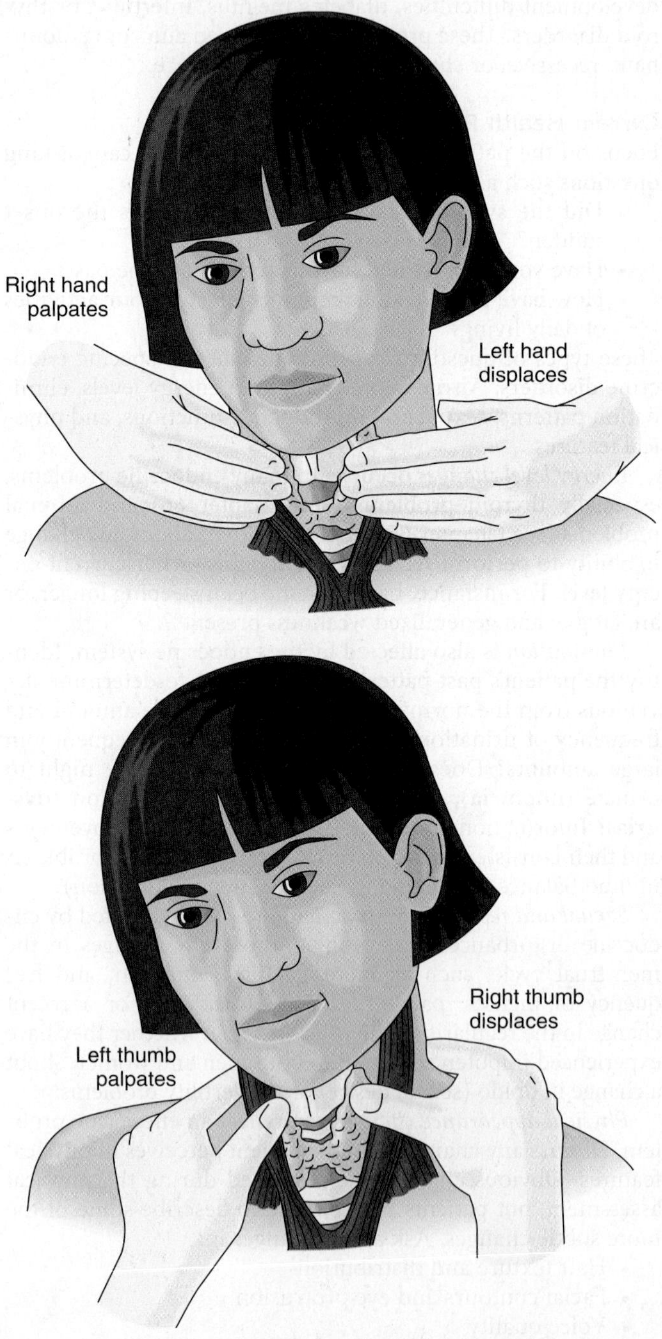
Right hand
palpates
Left hand
displaces
Right thumb
displaces
Left thumb
palpates

Fig. 64-9 • Palpation of the thyroid gland.

in himself or herself. When possible, ask the family about changes in the patient's behaviors or personality.

A number of endocrine disorders affect the patient's perception of self. For example, body features can change significantly in disorders of the pituitary, adrenal, and thyroid glands. Infertility, impotence, and other changes in sexual function may result from endocrine dysfunction. Encourage the patient to express his or her feelings and concerns about a change in appearance or in sexual function. Ask about any difficulty in coping with such changes.

Patients with endocrine problems may require lifelong drugs and follow-up care. Assess their readiness to learn and ability to carry out specific self-management skills. Patients may also face financial difficulties resulting from a prolonged medical regimen or loss of employment. A referral to social service agencies may be needed.

Diagnostic Assessment

Laboratory Assessment

For the patient with possible endocrine dysfunction, laboratory tests are an essential part of the diagnostic process. Body fluids commonly used for these tests include blood, urine, and saliva (Klee, 2008). Regardless of the test requested, check with the agency's laboratory to ensure proper collection and handling of the specimen for accurate results. The specialized testing for specific disorders is described in Chapters 65 to 67. Best practices for the collection of specimens for general endocrine testing are listed in Chart 64-3.

Stimulation/Suppression Tests

Measurement of specific hormone levels does not always distinguish between the normal and the abnormal. The wide normal range for some hormones makes it necessary to trigger responses by stimulation or suppression tests.

For the patient who might have an underactive endocrine gland, a stimulus may be provided to determine whether the gland is capable of normal hormone production. This method is called *stimulation testing.* Measured amounts of selected hormones are given to stimulate the target gland to maximum production. Hormone levels are then measured and compared with expected normal values. Failure of the hormone level to rise with stimulation indicates hypofunction.

Suppression tests are used when hormone levels are high or in the upper range of normal. Failure of suppression of hormone production during testing indicates hyperfunction.

Assays

An assay measures the level of a specific hormone in blood or other body fluid. Some assays are indirect, such as the radioimmunoassay. Other hormone assay methods include immunometric assays, chromatographic assays, and mass spectrometry. An immunometric assay uses a large antibody with a component that "captures" the hormone and a second component that creates a signal when the antibody binds to the hormone (antigen). Chromatographic assays separate molecules in the serum by size, light absorption, and other properties. Each hormone has very specific properties that allow it to separate from other blood substances and form a unique bandwidth. Mass spectrometry methods also allow individual hormones to separate from other serum molecules based on the amount (mass) and charge of individual components. On a graph, these separate hormones each shows as a unique "spike" pattern. Many different hormone concentrations can be analyzed at the same time by this method.

Urine Tests

Hormone levels and the metabolites of specific hormones in the urine are often measured to determine endocrine function. Because many of the endocrine hormones are secreted in a pulsatile fashion, measurement of a specific hormone in a 24-hour urine collection, rather than as a single blood or urine sample, better reflects the overall function of certain glands, such as the adrenal gland. Teach the patient how to collect a 24-hour urine sample (see also Chart 64-3).

Certain hormones require additives in the container at the beginning of the collection. Instruct the patient to not discard

Chart 64-3 BEST PRACTICE FOR PATIENT SAFETY & QUALITY CARE

Endocrine Testing

For blood tests:

- Check your laboratory's method of handling hormone test samples for tube type, timing, drugs to be administered as part of the test, etc. For example, blood samples drawn for catecholamines must be placed on ice and taken to the laboratory immediately.
- Explain the procedure and any restrictions to the patient.
- If you are drawing blood samples from a line, clear the IV line thoroughly. Do not use a double- or triple-lumen line to obtain samples; contamination or dilution from another port is possible.
- Emphasize the importance of taking a drug prescribed for the test on *time.* Tell the patient to set an alarm if the drug is to be taken during the night.

For urine tests:

- Instruct the patient to begin the urine collection (whether for 2, 4, 8, 12, or 24 hours) by first emptying his or her bladder.
- Remind the patient to *not* save the urine specimen that begins the collection. The timing for the urine collection begins *after* this specimen.
- Tell the patient to note the time of the discarded specimen and to plan to collect all urine from this time until the end of the urine collection period.
- To end the collection, instruct the patient to empty his or her bladder at the end of the timed period and *add* that urine to the collection.
- Check with the laboratory to determine any special handling of the urine specimen (e.g., Is a preservative needed? Does the container need to be kept cold?).
- If needed, make sure that the preservative has been added to the collection container at the *beginning* of the collection.
- Tell the patient about any preservative and the need to avoid splashing urine from the container, because some preservatives make the urine caustic.
- If the specimen must be kept cool or cold, instruct the patient to place the container in an inexpensive cooler with ice. The specimen container should not be kept with food or drinks.

the preservative from the container and to use caution when handling it because some solutions are caustic. Remind him or her that this collection is timed for *exactly* 24 hours. Instruct the patient to avoid taking any unnecessary drugs during endocrine testing because some drugs can interfere with the laboratory assays.

Tests for Glucose

Tests for functions of the islet cells of the pancreas are indirect. They measure the *result* of pancreatic islet cell function. Blood glucose values and the oral glucose tolerance test help diagnose diabetes mellitus. The glycosylated hemoglobin (HbA_{1C}) value reveals the *average* blood glucose level over a period of 2 to 3 months. Its primary use is in assessing overall control of glucose level in diabetes mellitus. (See Chapter 67 for a full discussion of diabetes mellitus.)

Imaging Assessment

Anterior, posterior, and lateral skull x-rays may be used to view the sella turcica. Erosion of the sella turcica indicates invasion of the wall from an abnormal growth.

Magnetic resonance imaging (MRI) with contrast is the most sensitive method of imaging the pituitary gland, although computed tomography (CT) scans can also be used to evaluate it. The thyroid, parathyroid glands, ovaries, and testes are evaluated by ultrasound. In addition, CT scans are used to evaluate the adrenal glands, ovaries, and pancreas.

Other Diagnostic Assessment

Needle biopsy is a relatively safe and quick outpatient procedure used to indicate the composition of thyroid nodules. It is used to determine whether surgical intervention is needed.

GET READY FOR THE NCLEX EXAMINATION!

Key Points

Review these Key Points for each NCLEX Examination Client Needs Category.

Safe and Effective Care Environment

- Follow the laboratory's procedures for collecting and handling specimens for endocrine function studies.

Health Promotion and Maintenance

- Teach all patients that abusing or misusing hormones or steroids can have an adverse effect on endocrine function.

Psychosocial Integrity

- Encourage the patient to express his or her feelings and concerns about a change in appearance, sexual function, or fertility as a result of a possible endocrine problem.
- Explain all diagnostic procedures, restrictions, and follow-up care to the patient scheduled for tests.
- Ask family members about changes in the patient's personality or behavior.

Physiological Integrity

- Ask the patient about other family members with endocrine disorders, because some endocrine problems have a genetic component.
- Ask the patient what prescribed and over-the-counter drugs are taken on a regular basis, because some drugs can alter endocrine function.

Additional Study Resources

Go to your Companion CD or Evolve at http://evolve.elsevier.com/Iggy/ for *Self-Assessment Questions for the NCLEX Examination.*

Go to Evolve at http://evolve.elsevier.com/Iggy/ for *Prioritization and Delegation Questions for the NCLEX Examination.*

SELECTED BIBLIOGRAPHY

Bauer, D. (2006). Review of the endocrine system. *MEDSURG Nursing, 14*(5), 335-337.

Davis, G. (2007). Hormonal control and the endocrine system: Achieving homeostasis. *Nurse Prescribing, 4*(11), 446-453.

Gordon, M. (2007). *Manual of nursing diagnosis* (11th ed.). Boston: Jones & Bartlett.

Jarvis, C. (2008). *Physical examination and health assessment* (5th ed.). Philadelphia: Saunders.

Klee, G. (2008). Laboratory techniques for recognition of endocrine disorders. In H. Kronenberg, S. Melmed, K. Polonsky, & P.R. Larsen (Eds.), *Williams' textbook of endocrinology* (11th ed.). Philadelphia: Saunders.

Kronenberg, H., Melmed, S., Polonsky, K., & Larsen, P.R. (Eds.). (2008). *Williams' textbook of endocrinology* (11th ed.). Philadelphia: Saunders.

Lamberts, S. (2008). Endocrinology and aging. In H. Kronenberg, S. Melmed, K. Polonsky, & P.R. Larsen (Eds.), *Williams' textbook of endocrinology* (11th ed.). Philadelphia: Saunders.

McCance, K., & Huether, S. (2006). *Pathophysiology: The biologic basis for disease in adults and children* (5th ed.). St. Louis: Mosby.

Meiner, S., & Lueckenotte, A. (Eds.). (2006). *Gerontologic nursing* (3rd ed.). St. Louis: Mosby.

Nussbaum, R., McInnes, R., & Willard, H. (2007). *Thompson & Thompson: Genetics in medicine* (7th ed.). Philadelphia: Saunders.

Pagana, K., & Pagana, T. (2006). *Mosby's manual of diagnostic and laboratory tests* (3rd ed.). St. Louis: Mosby.

Whitman, K. (2006). ACTH stimulation: Testing the adrenals. *Nursing2006, 36*(7), 24-25.

Care of Patients with Pituitary and Adrenal Gland Problems

65 CHAPTER

M. Linda Workman

LEARNING OUTCOMES

For clinical competence and success on the NCLEX Examination, study this chapter with these Learning Outcomes in mind:

Safe and Effective Care Environment

1. Protect the patient with antidiuretic hormone (ADH) deficiency from dehydration.
2. Use appropriate interventions to prevent injury in the patient who has hypercortisolism.
3. Apply principles of infection control to prevent infection in the patient who is immunosuppressed.
4. Modify the environment to reduce stimulation for the patient with pheochromocytoma.

Health Promotion and Maintenance

5. Teach patients how to avoid increasing intracranial pressure after pituitary surgery.
6. Identify the teaching priorities for the patient taking hormone replacement therapy for pituitary or adrenal hypofunction.
7. Teach patients how to monitor therapy effectiveness for diabetes insipidus or syndrome of inappropriate ADH (SIADH).

Psychosocial Integrity

8. Be accepting of patient behavior.
9. Encourage the patient and family to express their feelings and concerns about a change in endocrine health.
10. Explain all diagnostic and treatment-related procedures to the patient and family.

Physiological Integrity

11. Compare the common clinical manifestations associated with pituitary hypofunction and pituitary hyperfunction.
12. Coordinate nursing care for the patient immediately after a transsphenoidal hypophysectomy.
13. Interpret clinical changes and laboratory data to determine the effectiveness of therapy for diabetes insipidus and for SIADH.
14. Compare the clinical manifestations of Cushing's syndrome and Addison's disease.
15. Identify patients at risk for acute adrenal insufficiency.
16. Prioritize nursing care for the patient with acute adrenal insufficiency.
17. Coordinate nursing care for the patient with Cushing's disease or syndrome.

Go to your Companion CD or Evolve at http://evolve.elsevier.com/Iggy/ for *Self-Assessment Questions for the NCLEX Examination* keyed to these Learning Outcomes.

Pituitary and adrenal gland problems can be caused by or can cause changes in the secretion of one or more other hormones. At times, the correct amount of hormone may be produced but cannot be used because of receptor site failure.

Hormones secreted from the anterior pituitary gland regulate growth, metabolism, pigment changes, and sexual development. These functions are affected when the pituitary gland secretes too much or too little of one or more hormones. The posterior pituitary gland secretes **vasopressin,** also known as *antidiuretic hormone* or *ADH.* Posterior pituitary problems result in fluid and electrolyte imbalances. The adrenal gland produces and secretes hormones that influence homeostasis and are life sustaining. The effects of these endocrine problems occur throughout the body and may induce psychological, as well as physical, changes. Nursing care for the patient with pituitary or adrenal gland disorders includes assessment, patient education, evaluation of patient response to therapy, and providing support.

A complete history and physical examination are performed to detect specific clinical findings. The patient also often undergoes many diagnostic tests and relies on the nurse for specific instructions and explanations. Surgical intervention may be indicated. The patient often needs lifelong hormone replacement therapy, and physical and emotional support are critical.

DISORDERS OF THE ANTERIOR PITUITARY GLAND

The anterior pituitary gland **(adenohypophysis)** controls growth, metabolic activity, and sexual development through the actions of these hormones:

- Growth hormone (GH; somatotropin)
- Thyrotropin (thyroid-stimulating hormone [TSH])
- Corticotropin (adrenocorticotropic hormone [ACTH])
- Follicle-stimulating hormone (FSH)
- Luteinizing hormone (LH)
- Melanocyte-stimulating hormone (MSH)
- Prolactin (PRL)

Disorders of hormones secreted by the anterior pituitary gland can result from problems arising within the anterior pituitary gland itself *(primary pituitary dysfunction)* or from problems in the hypothalamus that change anterior pituitary function *(secondary pituitary dysfunction).* In either case, one or more hormones may be undersecreted *(pituitary hypofunction)* or oversecreted *(pituitary hyperfunction).*

HYPOPITUITARISM

Pathophysiology

A person with hypopituitarism has a deficiency of one or more anterior pituitary hormones, resulting in metabolic problems and sexual dysfunction. If only one hormone is affected, the condition is known as *selective hypopituitarism.* Decreased production of *all* of the anterior pituitary hormones is an extremely rare condition known as **panhypopituitarism.**

More commonly, there is a decrease in the secretion of one hormone and a lesser decrease in the other hormones. Deficiencies of *adrenocorticotropic hormone (ACTH) and thyroid-stimulating hormone (TSH)* are the *most* life threatening because they result in a corresponding decrease in the secretion of vital hormones from the adrenal and thyroid glands. Adrenal gland hypofunction is discussed on p. 1436; hypothyroidism is discussed in Chapter 66.

Deficiency of the **gonadotropins** (luteinizing hormone [LH] and follicle-stimulating hormone [FSH]—hormones that stimulate the ovaries and testes to produce sex hormones) changes sexual function in both men and women. In men, gonadotropin deficiency results in testicular failure, with decreased testosterone production from the Leydig cells and decreased or absent spermatogenesis. Decreased testosterone levels in men cause sterility. In women, gonadotropin deficiency results in ovarian failure, amenorrhea, and infertility.

Growth hormone (GH) deficiency changes tissue growth patterns indirectly. GH itself has little effect on tissues and cells. Rather, the presence of GH stimulates the liver to produce substances known as *somatomedins.* These somatomedins, especially somatomedin C (insulin-like growth factor-1 [IGF-1]), then enhance growth activities in cells and tissues. Somatomedin C is responsible for bone and cartilage growth and maintenance.

GH deficiency may be a result of decreased GH production, failure of the liver to produce somatomedins, or a failure of the cells or tissues to respond to the somatomedins. Deficiency in children leads to short stature and other manifestations of growth retardation. Deficiency in adults does not affect height but does increase the rate of bone destructive activity, leading to thinner, more fragile bones **(osteoporosis)** and an increased risk for fractures.

The cause of hypopituitarism varies. Benign or malignant pituitary tumors can compress and destroy pituitary tissue. Pituitary function can be impaired by severe malnutrition or rapid loss of body fat, such as in people with **anorexia nervosa** (a disorder in which people see themselves as overweight and eat so little that starvation results). Shock or severe hypotension reduces blood flow to the pituitary gland, leading to hypoxia and infarction. Other causes of hypopituitarism include head trauma, brain tumors or infection, radiation or surgery of the head and brain, and acquired immune deficiency syndrome (AIDS) (Melmed & Kleinberg, 2008). Idiopathic hypopituitarism is an isolated hormone deficiency with an unknown cause.

Postpartum hemorrhage is the most common cause of pituitary infarction, which results in decreased hormone secretion. This clinical problem is known as *Sheehan's syndrome.* The pituitary gland normally enlarges during pregnancy, and when hypotension results from hemorrhage, ischemia and necrosis of the gland occur. Usually this condition develops immediately after delivery, although some cases have occurred several years later.

Patient-Centered Collaborative Care

Assessment

Changes in physical appearance and target organ function occur with deficiencies of specific pituitary hormones (Chart 65-1). Gonadotropin (LH and FSH) deficiency results in the loss of or change in secondary sex characteristics in men and women. While assessing the male patient, look for facial and body hair loss. Ask about episodes of impotence and decreased libido (sex drive). Women may report **amenorrhea** (absence of menstrual periods), **dyspareunia** (painful intercourse), **infertility** (difficulty becoming pregnant), and decreased libido. While examining the female patient, check for dry skin, breast atrophy, and a decreased amount or absence of axillary and pubic hair.

Neurologic manifestations of hypopituitarism as a result of tumor growth often first occur as changes in vision. Assess the patient's visual acuity, especially peripheral vision, for changes or loss. Temporal headaches are a common finding. Other manifestations may include **diplopia** (double vision) and ocular muscle paralysis, limiting eye movement.

Laboratory findings vary widely with hypopituitarism. Some pituitary hormone levels may be measured directly. Often, however, the *effects* of the hormones, rather than their actual levels, are assessed. Blood levels of triiodothyronine (T_3) and thyroxine (T_4) from the thyroid, as well as testosterone and estradiol from the gonads, are measured easily. If levels of one or all of these hormones are low or in the low-normal range, further evaluation is necessary. Levels of pituitary gonadotropins (LH and FSH) and TSH are sufficient if function of the target organ is apparent. Function of LH and FSH is assessed by observing for the presence of secondary sexual characteristics. Function of TSH is assessed by measuring circulating levels of thyroid hormones. ACTH levels may be normal or low, and prolactin (PRL) levels are low to high.

Chart 65-1 KEY FEATURES

Pituitary Hypofunction

Deficient Hormone	Clinical Manifestations
ANTERIOR PITUITARY HORMONES	
Growth hormone (GH)	Decreased bone density Pathologic fractures Decreased muscle strength Increased serum cholesterol levels
Gonadotropins (luteinizing hormone [LH], follicle-stimulating hormone [FSH])	Women: • Amenorrhea • Anovulation • Low estrogen levels • Breast atrophy • Loss of bone density • Decreased axillary and pubic hair • Decreased libido Men: • Decreased facial hair • Decreased ejaculate volume • Reduced muscle mass • Loss of bone density • Decreased body hair • Decreased libido • Impotence
Thyroid-stimulating hormone (thyrotropin) (TSH)	Decreased thyroid hormone levels Weight gain Intolerance to cold
Thyroid-stimulating hormone (thyrotropin) (TSH)—cont'd	Scalp alopecia Hirsutism Menstrual abnormalities Decreased libido Slowed cognition Lethargy
Adrenocorticotropic hormone (ACTH)	Decreased serum cortisol levels Pale, sallow complexion Malaise and lethargy Anorexia Postural hypotension Headache Hypoglycemia Hyponatremia Decreased axillary and pubic hair (women)
POSTERIOR PITUITARY HORMONES	
Vasopressin (antidiuretic hormone [ADH])	Diabetes insipidus: • Greatly increased urine output • Low urine specific gravity (<1.005) • Hypovolemia: Hypotension Dehydration • Increased plasma osmolarity • Increased thirst • Output does not decrease when fluid intake decreases

Some tests for pituitary function involve injecting agents that are known to stimulate secretion of specific pituitary hormones and then measuring the response. Such tests are called **stimulation tests.** For example, insulin injection in people with normal pituitary function causes an increased release of GH and ACTH. In people with decreased pituitary function, levels of either of these hormones remain unchanged.

Pituitary problems may cause changes in the sella turcica (the bony nest where the pituitary gland rests) that can be seen with skull x-rays. Changes may include enlargement, erosion, and calcifications as a result of pituitary tumors. Computed tomography (CT) and magnetic resonance imaging (MRI) can more distinctly define bone or soft-tissue lesions. An angiogram may be used to rule out the presence of an aneurysm or other vascular problems in the area before surgery.

Interventions

Management of the adult with hypopituitarism focuses on replacement of deficient hormones. Older patients or those with a chronic disease often require a lower amount of hormone replacement. Men who have gonadotropin deficiency receive sex steroid replacement therapy with androgens (testosterone). The most effective route of androgen replacement is IM, although use of transdermal testosterone patches is increasing. Instruct the patient in self-administration. Therapy begins with high-dose testosterone and is continued until **virilization** (presence of male secondary sex characteristics) is achieved. Maximal effects of treatment include increases in penis size, libido, muscle mass, bone size, and bone strength. Chest, facial, pubic, and axillary hair growth also increases, and the voice deepens. Patients usually report improved self-esteem and body image after therapy is initiated. The dose may then be decreased, but therapy continues throughout life.

Androgen therapy is avoided in men with prostate cancer. Side effects of testosterone therapy include **gynecomastia** (the development of breast tissue in men), acne, baldness, and prostate enlargement.

Achieving fertility in these patients is difficult and requires additional parenteral testosterone therapy and injections of human chorionic gonadotropin (hCG). Teach the patient about the course of additional therapy, and provide emotional support because the outcome of fertility treatment is uncertain.

Women who have gonadotropin deficiency receive hormone replacement with a combination of estrogen and progesterone. The risk for hypertension or thrombosis (formation of blood clots in deep veins) is increased with estrogen therapy, especially among women who smoke. Emphasize measures to reduce risk and the need for regular health visits. For women who wish to become pregnant, clomiphene citrate (Clomid) may be given to induce ovulation. Gonadotropin-releasing hormone (GnRH) and human chorionic gonadotropin (hCG) are used to stimulate ovulation if therapy with clomiphene citrate fails.

Adult patients with GH deficiency may be treated with injections of GH, although this treatment is rare.

HYPERPITUITARISM

Pathophysiology

Hyperpituitarism is hormone oversecretion that occurs with pituitary tumors or hyperplasia (tissue overgrowth). Tumors occur most often in the anterior pituitary cells that produce growth hormone (GH), prolactin (PRL), and adrenocorticotropic hormone (ACTH). Overproduction of PRL also may occur in response to tumors that overproduce GH and ACTH. Hypersecretion of ACTH may occur with increased secretion of melanocyte-stimulating hormone (MSH).

GENETIC CONSIDERATIONS

An uncommon cause of hyperpituitarism is multiple endocrine neoplasia, type 1 (MEN1) in which there is inactivation of the suppressor gene *MENIN* (Melmed & Kleinberg, 2008). This problem has an autosomal dominant inheritance pattern and is usually expressed as a benign tumor that affects the pituitary, parathyroid glands, and pancreas (Quillen, 2006). In pituitary function, MEN1 leads to excessive production of growth hormone and acromegaly. Ask a patient suspected of having acromegaly whether either parent also has this problem or has had a tumor of the pancreas or parathyroid glands.

The most common cause of hyperpituitarism is a pituitary adenoma—a benign tumor of one or more tissues within the anterior pituitary. Adenomas are classified by size, invasiveness, and the hormone secreted. An invasive pituitary adenoma involves a portion or all of the sella turcica. When the sella turcica is not involved, the adenoma is "enclosed."

As an adenoma gets larger and compresses brain tissue, neurologic symptoms, as well as endocrine symptoms, may occur. Such symptoms may include visual changes, headache, and increased intracranial pressure.

Prolactin (PRL)-secreting tumors are the most common type of pituitary adenoma. Excessive PRL inhibits the secretion of gonadotropins and sex hormones in men and women, resulting in galactorrhea (breast milk production), amenorrhea, and infertility.

Overproduction of GH results in gigantism (Fig. 65-1) or acromegaly (Fig. 65-2). The onset of the disease may be gradual with slow progression, and changes may remain unnoticed for years before diagnosis of the disorder. Early detection and treatment are essential to prevent irreversible changes in the soft tissues, such as those of the face, hands, feet, and skin. These changes are, to a certain extent, reversible after treatment, but skeletal changes are permanent.

In the patient with gigantism, the onset of GH hypersecretion occurs *before* puberty, which causes rapid proportional growth in the length of all bones. In the patient with acromegaly, excessive GH secretion occurs *after* closure of the growth plates in bone during puberty and produces increased skeletal thickness, hypertrophy of the skin, and enlargement of many organs, such as the liver and heart (Melmed, 2006).

Bone thinning and bone cell overgrowth occur slowly. Degeneration of joint cartilage and hypertrophy of ligaments, vocal cords, and eustachian tubes are common. Nerve entrapment occurs because of tissue overgrowth and myelin loss in peripheral nerves. Because GH blocks the action of insulin, **hyperglycemia** (elevated blood glucose levels) is also common.

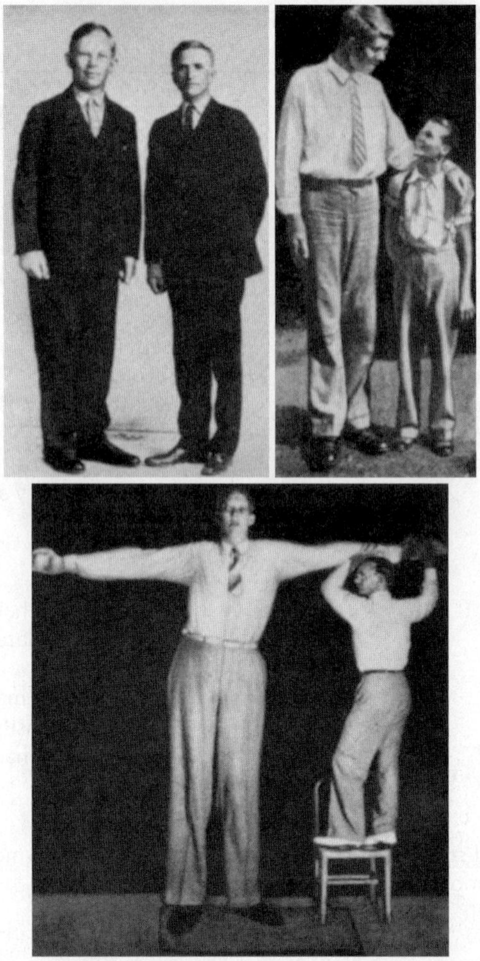

Fig. 65-1 • The clinical features of growth hormone (GH) excess. Robert Wadlow, the "Alton giant," weighed 9 pounds at birth but grew to 30 pounds by the time he was 6 months old. By his first birthday, he had reached 62 pounds. At the time of his death at age 22 from cellulitis of the feet, he was 8 feet, 11 inches tall and weighed 475 pounds.

Excess ACTH overstimulates the adrenal cortex. The result is excessive production of glucocorticoids, mineralocorticoids, and androgens, which leads to the development of Cushing's disease (see Hypercortisolism [Cushing's Syndrome], p. 1439).

Most cases of hyperpituitarism result from hormone-secreting benign tumors (adenomas) arising from one pituitary cell type. Hyperpituitarism can also be caused by hypothalamic problems in which excessive amounts of releasing hormones are produced and then overstimulate the normal pituitary gland.

Patient-Centered Collaborative Care

evolve ONLINE PHARM REVIEW

Assessment

The manifestations of hyperpituitarism vary, depending on which hormone is produced in excess. Obtain data about the patient's age, gender, and family history. Ask the patient about

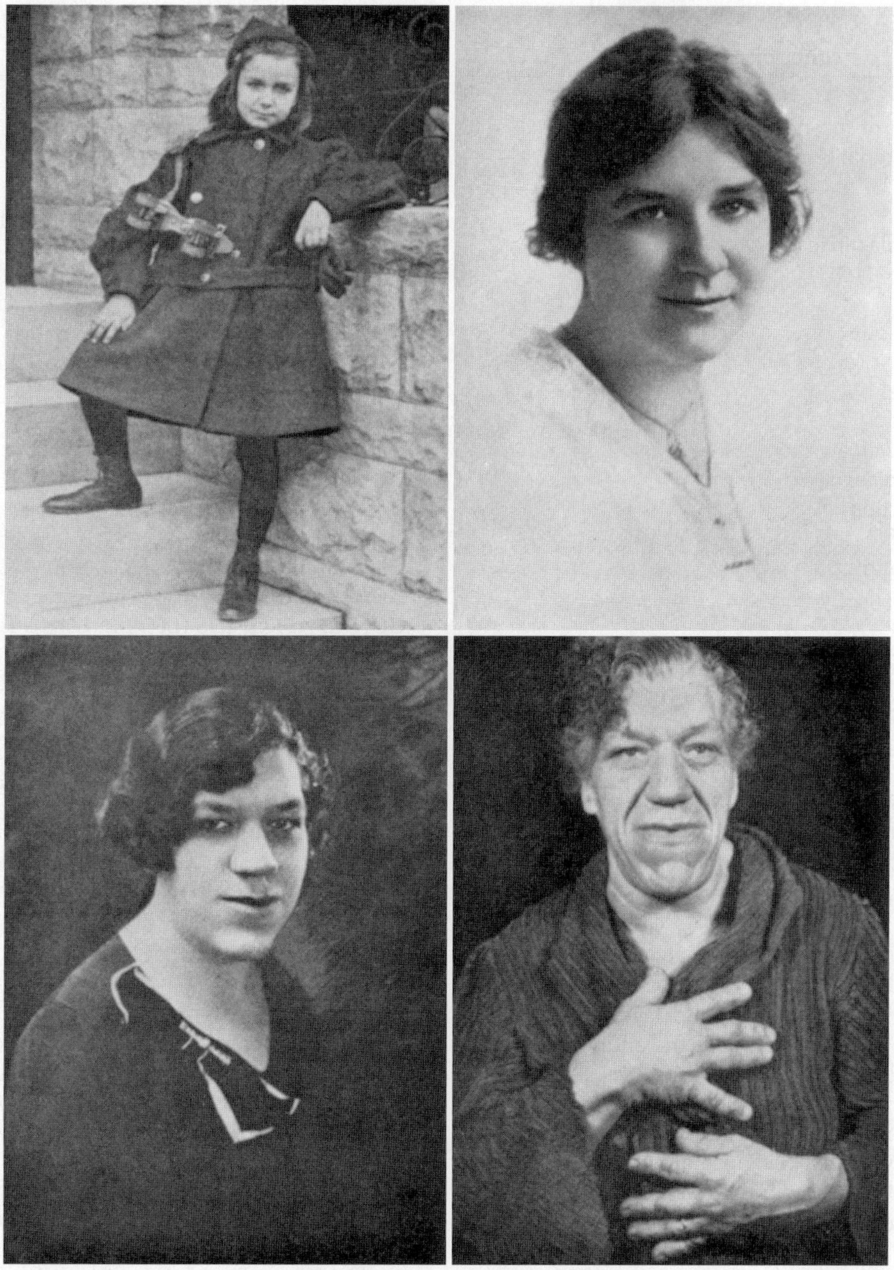

Fig. 65-2 • The progression of acromegaly.

any change in hat, glove, ring, or shoe size. Fatigue and lethargy are common. The patient with high GH levels may have backache and **arthralgias** (joint pain) from bone changes. Ask specifically about headaches and changes in vision.

The patient with hypersecretion of PRL often reports difficulties in sexual functioning. Ask women about menstrual changes (e.g., amenorrhea, irregular menses, and difficulty in becoming pregnant) and about decreased libido or dyspareunia (painful intercourse). Men may report decreased libido and impotence.

Some changes in appearance and target organ function occur with excesses of specific anterior pituitary hormones (Chart 65-2). Initial manifestations of GH hypersecretion are changes in the facial features, including increases in lip and nose sizes and a prominent brow ridge and increases in head, hand, and foot sizes. The patient with hyperpituitarism often seeks health care because of dramatic changes in appearance. Assess the impact of these changes on his or her personal relationships.

In a person with hyperpituitarism, usually only one hormone is produced in excess, because the cell types within the pituitary gland are so discretely organized. The most common hormones produced in excess are PRL, ACTH, and GH. Tumors producing TSH, luteinizing hormone (LH), or follicle-stimulating hormone (FSH) are rare. Elevated levels of any of these hormones warrant evaluation. Elevations of LH and FSH, however, are normal in the postmenopausal woman.

Imaging assessment of the patient with hyperpituitarism is identical to that for a patient with hypopituitarism. Skull x-rays are used to identify abnormalities of the sella turcica. Computed tomography (CT) and magnetic resonance imaging (MRI) can define soft-tissue lesions, and angiography can rule out an aneurysm or vascular malformations.

Chart 65-2 KEY FEATURES

Anterior Pituitary Hyperfunction

PROLACTIN (PRL)
- Hypogonadism (loss of secondary sexual characteristics)
- Decreased gonadotropin levels
- Galactorrhea
- Increased body fat
- Increased serum prolactin levels

GROWTH HORMONE (GH)

ACROMEGALY
- Folding of the scalp skin
- Thickened lips
- Coarse facial features
- Increasing head size
- Protrusion of the lower jaw
- Deepening of the voice
- Tufting of the fingertips
- Enlarged hands and feet
- Joint enlargement and pain
- Kyphosis and backache
- Barrel-shaped chest
- Excessive sweating
- Hyperglycemia
- Airway narrowing, sleep apnea
- Enlarged heart, lungs, and liver

ADRENOCORTICOTROPIC HORMONE (ACTH)

CUSHING'S DISEASE (PITUITARY)
- Elevated plasma cortisol levels
- Weight gain
- Truncal obesity
- "Moon face"
- Extremity muscle wasting
- Loss of bone density
- Hypertension
- Hyperglycemia
- Purple striae
- Acne
- Thin, easily damaged skin
- Hyperpigmentation

THYROTROPIN (THYROID-STIMULATING HORMONE [TSH])
- Elevated plasma TSH levels
- Elevated plasma thyroid hormone levels
- Weight loss
- Tachycardia and dysrhythmias
- Heat intolerance
- Increased GI motility
- Fine tremors

GONADOTROPINS (LUTEINIZING HORMONE [LH], FOLLICLE-STIMULATING HORMONE [FSH])

Men:
- Elevated LH and FSH levels
- Hypogonadism or hypergonadism

Women:
- Normal LH and FSH levels

(The most common clinical manifestations in men and women are related to the physical presence of a tumor rather than to excessive hormone secretion.)

Rather than just measuring the blood level of a specific hormone, some tests measure how well the endocrine gland responds to stimulation changes. Suppression tests help diagnose hyperpituitarism. These tests involve giving agents that induce a suppressed response from the pituitary gland, and they can determine whether the normal negative feedback control mechanisms for hormonal regulation are intact. For example, high blood glucose levels suppress the release of GH. In a suppression test, 100 g of oral glucose or 0.5 g/kg of body weight is given IV. GH levels are measured serially for up to 120 minutes. GH levels that do not fall below 5 ng/mL indicate a positive (abnormal) result.

Common Nursing Diagnoses and Collaborative Problems

Nursing diagnoses that may apply to patients with hyperpituitarism with excesses of prolactin (PRL) and growth hormone (GH) are:

- Disturbed Body Image related to illness or illness treatment
- Sexual Dysfunction related to disease (related to loss of libido, infertility, impotence)
- Acute Pain and Chronic Pain related to compression of tissues by tumor (e.g., discomfort, headache), backache, or arthralgia secondary to the effects of excessive GH levels
- Anxiety related to a threat of or change in health status
- Disturbed Sensory Perception (Visual) related to altered sensory reception, transmission, or integration

Interventions

The goals of therapy for the patient who has hyperpituitarism are to return hormone levels to normal or near normal, reduce or eliminate headache and visual disturbances, prevent complications, and reverse as many of the body changes as possible.

Nonsurgical Management

Encourage the patient to express concerns and fears about his or her altered physical appearance. Help him or her identify personal strengths and positive characteristics, reinforcing each patient's uniqueness and importance. Galactorrhea, gynecomastia, and reduced sexual functioning can disturb body image and personal identity. Reassure the patient that treatment may reverse some of these problems. Encourage the patient to discuss his or her feelings.

Drug therapy may be used alone or in combination with surgery and/or radiation. The most common drugs used are dopamine agonists, including bromocriptine mesylate (Parlodel), cabergoline (Dostinex), and pergolide (Permax) (Melmed & Kleinberg, 2008). These drugs stimulate dopamine receptors in the brain and inhibit the release of many pituitary hormones, most specifically GH and PRL. In most cases, small tumors decrease until the pituitary gland is of normal size. Large pituitary tumors usually decrease to some extent. In patients with acromegaly, bromocriptine reduces GH levels and decreases tumor size, especially when GH levels remain high after surgery or before the full effect of radiation therapy has occurred.

Side effects of bromocriptine include **orthostatic** (postural) hypotension, gastric irritation, nausea, headaches, abdominal cramps, and constipation. Give bromocriptine with a meal or a snack to reduce some of these side effects. Rare but serious side effects include cardiac dysrhythmias, coronary artery spasms, and cerebrospinal fluid leakage. *Teach patients to seek medical care immediately if chest pain, dizziness, or watery nasal discharge occurs.* Treatment starts with a low dose and is gradually increased until the desired level (usually 7.5 mg/day) is reached. *If pregnancy occurs, the drug is stopped immediately.*

Other agents used for acromegaly are the somatostatin analogs, especially octreotide (Sandostatin), and a growth hormone receptor blocker, pegvisomant (Somavert). Octreotide inhibits GH release through negative feedback. Pegvisomant blocks growth hormone (GH) receptor activity and production of insulin-like growth factor (IGF). Although these therapies are effective, a disadvantage is that they must be given as an injection on a daily or weekly schedule. A major side effect is gallbladder disease. Pegvisomant may cause an increase in tumor size.

Radiation therapy is not useful in the immediate management of acute hyperpituitarism. These therapy regimens take a long time to complete, and several years may pass before a therapeutic effect can be seen. Side effects of radiation therapy include hypopituitarism, optic nerve damage, and other eye and vision problems. Use of the gamma knife procedure is increasing the accuracy of radiation therapy.

Surgical Management

Surgical removal of the pituitary gland and tumor (**hypophysectomy**) is the most common treatment for hyperpituitarism.

Preoperative Care. Explain that hypophysectomy decreases hormone levels, relieves headaches, and may reverse changes in sexual functioning. Body changes, organ enlargement, and visual changes are not usually reversible. Explain that because nasal packing is present for 2 to 3 days after surgery, it will be necessary to breathe through the mouth, and a "mustache" dressing ("drip" pad) will be placed under the nose. Instruct the patient not to brush teeth, cough, sneeze, blow the nose, or bend forward after surgery. These activities can open the muscle graft, increase intracranial pressure, and delay healing of the incision.

Operative Procedures. A transsphenoidal hypophysectomy is the most commonly used surgical approach (Fig. 65-3). This procedure is minimally invasive surgery performed with the patient under general anesthesia and in a semi-sitting position. The surgeon makes an incision just above the upper lip and reaches the pituitary gland through the sphenoid sinus. After the gland is removed, a muscle graft is taken, often from the thigh, to support the area and prevent leakage of cerebrospinal fluid (CSF). Nasal packing is inserted after the incision is closed. A mustache dressing is then applied. If the tumor cannot be reached by this approach, a craniotomy may be indicated (see Chapter 47).

Postoperative Care. Monitor the patient's neurologic response, and document any changes in vision, mental status, altered level of consciousness, or decreased strength of the extremities. Observe the patient for complications such as transient diabetes insipidus (discussed on pp. 1432-1433), CSF leakage, infection, and increased intracranial pressure (ICP).

Teach the patient to report any postnasal drip, which might indicate leakage of CSF. Keep the head of the bed elevated after surgery. Assess nasal drainage for quantity, quality, and the presence of glucose (which indicates that the fluid is CSF). A light yellow color at the edge of the clear drainage on the dressing is called the "halo sign" and indicates CSF. If the patient has persistent, severe headaches, CSF fluid may have leaked into the sinus area. Most CSF leaks resolve with bedrest. If the CSF leak persists, the physician may perform a spinal tap to reduce CSF pressure. Surgical intervention is rarely necessary.

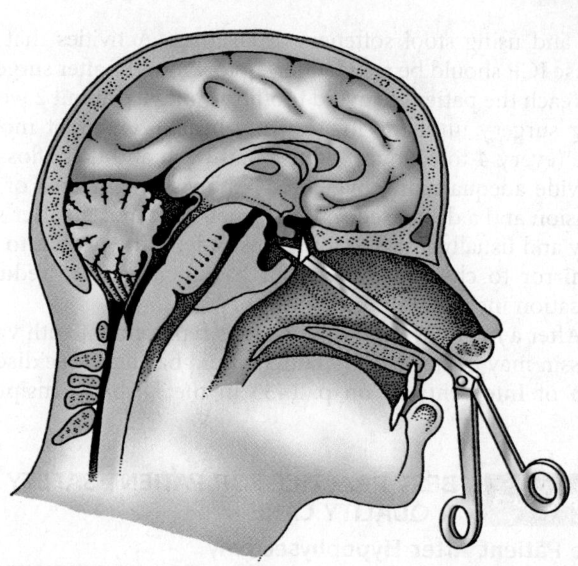

Fig. 65-3 • The transsphenoidal surgical approach to the pituitary gland. Selective adenomectomy leaves normal pituitary tissue undisturbed.

Teach the patient to avoid coughing early after surgery because it increases pressure in the incision area and may lead to a CSF leak. Remind the patient to perform deep-breathing exercises hourly while awake to prevent pulmonary problems. Patients may also have mouth dryness from mouth breathing. Perform frequent oral rinses, and apply a lubricating jelly to dry lips.

Infection can occur after surgery. Specifically assess for manifestations of meningitis, such as headache, fever, and nuchal (neck) rigidity. The surgeon may prescribe antibiotics, analgesics, and antipyretics.

If the entire pituitary gland has been removed, thyroid hormones and glucocorticoid replacement is lifelong. Best practices for care after surgery are listed in Chart 65-3.

After treatment, the patient with hyperpituitarism needs daily self-management regimens and frequent checkups. He or she may also need to develop strategies to reduce stress. The home care nurse performs a focused assessment during any home visit to a patient who has undergone a hypophysectomy (Chart 65-4). Review drug regimens and manifestations of infection and cerebral edema with the family.

After a transsphenoidal hypophysectomy, advise the patient to avoid activities that might interfere with healing. Teach him or her to avoid bending over from the waist to pick up objects or tie shoes because this position increases ICP. Teach the patient to bend the knees and then lower the body to pick up fallen objects. ICP also increases when the patient strains to have a bowel movement. Suggest techniques to prevent constipation, such as eating high-fiber foods, drinking plenty of fluids, and using stool softeners or laxatives. Activities that increase ICP should be avoided for up to 2 months after surgery.

Teach the patient to avoid toothbrushing for about 2 weeks after surgery until the incision has healed. Frequent mouth care (every 4 to 6 hours) with mouthwash and daily flossing provide adequate oral hygiene. Numbness in the area of the incision and a decreased sense of smell are expected after surgery and usually last 3 to 4 months. Advise the patient to use a mirror to check the gums for bleeding, because reduced sensation increases the risk for injury.

After a hypophysectomy, hormone replacement with vasopressin may be needed to maintain fluid balance. (See discussion of Interventions on p. 1433 in the Diabetes Insipidus section.) If the anterior portion of the pituitary gland is removed, instruct the patient in cortisol, thyroid, and gonadal hormone replacement. Teach the patient to report the return of any symptoms of hyperpituitarism immediately to the primary health care provider.

Chart 65-3 BEST PRACTICE FOR PATIENT SAFETY & QUALITY CARE

The Patient After Hypophysectomy

- Monitor the patient's neurologic status hourly for the first 24 hours and then every 4 hours.
- Monitor fluid balance, especially for output greater than intake, because transient diabetes insipidus can occur.
- Encourage the patient to maintain pulmonary hygiene through deep-breathing exercises.
- Instruct the patient to not cough, blow the nose, or sneeze.
- Instruct the patient to use dental floss and oral mouth rinses, because brushing the teeth is not permitted until the incision heals sufficiently.
- Instruct the patient to avoid bending at the waist for any reason, because this position increases intracranial pressure.
- Monitor the nasal drip pad for the type and amount of drainage. The presence of the halo sign may indicate a CSF leak.
- Monitor bowel movements to prevent constipation and subsequent "straining."
- Teach the patient self-administration of the prescribed hormones.

CSF, Cerebrospinal fluid.

DISORDERS OF THE POSTERIOR PITUITARY GLAND

Disorders of the posterior pituitary gland (neurohypophysis) are related to a deficiency or excess of the hormone *vasopressin* (antidiuretic hormone [ADH]) and usually occur independently from anterior pituitary problems (Hanberg, 2005). Diabetes insipidus occurs with ADH deficiency, and the syndrome of inappropriate antidiuretic hormone (SIADH) occurs with ADH excess.

DIABETES INSIPIDUS

Pathophysiology

Diabetes insipidus (DI) is a water metabolism problem caused by an ADH deficiency (either a decrease in ADH synthesis or an inability of the kidneys to respond to ADH). ADH deficiency results in the excretion of large volumes of dilute urine. Without ADH, distal kidney tubules and collecting ducts do not reabsorb water, leading to **polyuria** (excessive water loss through urination) and dehydration.

Dehydration caused by this massive water loss increases plasma osmolarity, which stimulates the osmoreceptors to relay a sensation of thirst to the cerebral cortex. Thirst promotes increased fluid intake and aids in maintaining water homeostasis. *If the thirst mechanism is poor or absent or if the person is unable to obtain water, dehydration becomes more severe and can lead to death. Thus no patient suspected of having DI should be deprived of fluids for more than 4 hours.*

ADH deficiency is classified as nephrogenic, drug-related, primary, or secondary, depending on whether the problem is caused by insufficient production of ADH or an inability of the kidney to respond to the presence of ADH.

Chart 65-4 HOME CARE ASSESSMENT

The Patient Who Has Undergone Transsphenoidal Hypophysectomy for Hyperpituitarism

Assess cardiovascular status:
- Vital signs, including apical pulse, pulse pressure, presence or absence of orthostatic hypotension, and the quality/rhythm of peripheral pulses

Assess cognition and mental status:
- Level of consciousness
- Orientation to time, place, and person
- Accurate reading of a seven-word sentence containing no words longer than three syllables

Assess condition of operative site:
- Observe nasal area for drainage:
  - If present, note color, clarity, and odor
  - Test clear drainage for the presence of glucose

Assess neuromuscular status:
- Reactivity of patellar and biceps reflexes
- Oral temperature
- Handgrip strength
- Steadiness of gait
- Visual fields
- Distant and near visual acuity
- Pupillary responses to light

Assess renal system:
- Observe urine specimen for color, odor, cloudiness, and amount

Ask about:
- Headaches or visual disturbances
- Ease of bowel movements
- 24-hour fluid intake and output
- 24-hour diet recall
- 24-hour activity recall
- Over-the-counter and prescribed drugs taken

Assess patient's understanding of illness and adherence with treatment:
- Signs and symptoms to report to health care provider
- Drug plan (correct timing and dose)

Nephrogenic diabetes insipidus is an inherited disorder. The renal tubules do not respond to the actions of ADH, which results in poor water reabsorption by the kidney. The actual amount of hormone produced is not deficient.

Primary diabetes insipidus is caused by a defect in the hypothalamus or pituitary gland, resulting in a lack of ADH production or release. Secondary diabetes insipidus can result from tumors in or near the hypothalamus or pituitary gland, head trauma, infectious processes, surgical procedures (hypophysectomy), or metastatic tumors. Less often, it is caused by brain hemorrhage, brain disease, or cerebral aneurysm, which reduces ADH production.

Drug-related diabetes insipidus is usually caused by lithium carbonate (Eskalith, Lithobid, Carbolith♣) and demeclocycline (Declomycin). These drugs can interfere with the response of the kidneys to ADH.

Patient-Centered Collaborative Care

Assessment

Most manifestations of DI are related to dehydration (Chart 65-5). The key manifestations are an increase in the frequency of urination and excessive thirst. Ask about a history of any known etiologic factors, such as recent surgery, head trauma, or drug use (e.g., lithium). Although increased fluid intake prevents serious dehydration and volume depletion, the patient who is deprived of fluids or who cannot increase oral fluid intake may develop shock from fluid loss. Manifestations of dehydration, such as poor skin turgor and dry or cracked mucous membranes or skin, may be present. (See Chapter 13 for further discussion of dehydration.)

Water loss produces changes in blood and urine tests. The first step in diagnosis is to measure a 24-hour fluid intake and output. The amount of the patient's food and fluid is not restricted during this measurement. DI is considered if urine output is more than 4 L during this period and is greater than the volume ingested. The amount of urine excreted in 24 hours may vary from 4 to 30 L/day. Urine is dilute with a low specific gravity (less than 1.005) and low osmolarity (50 to 200 mOsm/kg).

Chart 65-5 KEY FEATURES

Diabetes Insipidus

CARDIOVASCULAR MANIFESTATIONS
- Hypotension
- Decreased pulse pressure
- Tachycardia
- Peripheral pulses weak, easily obliterated
- Hemoconcentration:
  - Increased hemoglobin
  - Increased hematocrit
  - Increased BUN

RENAL/URINARY MANIFESTATIONS
- Increased urine output:
  - Dilute, low specific gravity
  - Hypo-osmolar

INTEGUMENTARY MANIFESTATIONS
- Poor turgor
- Dry mucous membranes

NEUROLOGIC MANIFESTATIONS
- Increased sensation of thirst
- Irritability*
- Decreased cognition*
- Hyperthermia*
- Lethargy to coma*
- Ataxia*

*Occurs when access to water is limited and rapid dehydration results.
BUN, Blood urea nitrogen.

Interventions

Medical management is aimed at controlling manifestations with drug therapy (Chart 65-6). If only a partial deficit of ADH is present, effective control can be achieved with oral chlorpropamide (Diabinese, Novo-Propamide♣). This drug increases the action of existing ADH and possibly has a stimulating effect on the production of ADH in the hypothalamus.

When ADH deficiency is severe, ADH is replaced in amounts sufficient to maintain water balance. Desmopressin acetate (DDAVP) is a synthetic form of vasopressin given orally or intranasally in a metered spray and is the drug of choice (Robinson & Verbalis, 2008). The frequency of dosing varies with patient responses. Teach patients that each metered spray delivers 10 mcg, and those with mild DI may need only one or two doses in 24 hours. For the patient with more severe DI, one or two metered doses two or three times daily may be needed. During severe dehydration, ADH may be given IV or IM. Ulceration of the mucous membranes, allergy, a sensation of chest tightness, and pulmonary inhalation of the spray may occur with use of the intranasal preparations. If side effects occur or if the patient has an upper respiratory infection, oral or subcutaneous vasopressin is used.

For the hospitalized patient with DI manifestations, nursing management is aimed at early detection of dehydration and maintaining adequate hydration. Interventions include accurately measuring fluid intake and output, checking urine specific gravity, and recording the patient's weight daily.

Urge the patient to drink fluids in an amount equal to urine output. If fluids are given IV, ensure the patency of the access catheter and accurately monitor the amount infused hourly.

The patient with permanent DI requires lifelong desmopressin or vasopressin therapy. Assess his or her ability to follow instructions and participate in health care. Teach that polyuria and polydipsia are signals for the need for another dose.

Drugs for DI induce water retention and can cause fluid overload and water toxicity (see Chapter 13). *Teach all patients taking these drugs to weigh themselves daily to identify weight gain.* Stress the importance of using the same scale and weighing at the same time of day while wearing a similar amount of clothing. If weight gain or other signs of water toxicity occur (e.g., persistent headache, acute confusion), instruct the patient or family to notify the health care provider. Suggest that the patient should wear a medical alert bracelet identifying the disorder and the drugs.

SYNDROME OF INAPPROPRIATE ANTIDIURETIC HORMONE

Pathophysiology

The **syndrome of inappropriate antidiuretic hormone (SIADH)** is a problem in which vasopressin (antidiuretic hormone [ADH]) is secreted even when plasma osmolarity is low or normal. A decrease in plasma osmolarity normally inhibits ADH production and secretion. SIADH is also known as the

Chart 65-6 COMMON EXAMPLES OF DRUG THERAPY

Diabetes Insipidus

Drug/Dosage	Purpose/Action	Nursing Interventions	Rationales
Desmopressin (DDAVP, Rhinal Tube, Minirin, Stimate) Tablets: 0.1-0.2 mg orally twice daily Nasal spray: 10-20 mcg every 8-12 hr Parenteral: 1-2 mcg IV or subcutaneously every 12 hr **Med Error Alert!** The parenteral form of desmopressin is 10 times stronger than the oral form, and the dosage must be reduced.	The drug is a synthetic type of ADH that serves as a replacement. It binds to kidney receptors and enhances the reabsorption of water, thus reducing urine output.	Teach the patient using the inhaled form of the drug to blow the nose before taking the drug.	Drug is absorbed through the nasal mucosa. Nasal secretions can dilute the drug and inhibit its absorption.
		Teach the patient using the inhaled form to sit upright and hold his or her breath when spraying or using the rhinal tube.	Sitting upright and holding the breath keeps the drug in contact with the nasal mucosa, rather than going down the throat, enhancing drug absorption.
		Warn the patient not to drink more than 3 L of fluids daily while on this drug.	Drug promotes fluid retention and can lead to fluid overload.
		Teach the patient to weigh himself or herself daily and to notify the health care provider if 2 lbs or more is gained in 24 hours.	A rapid increase in weight is an indicator of excessive fluid retention and may require a change in drug dosage.
		Tell the patient to notify the health care provider if he or she experiences a persistent headache or acute confusion.	These are manifestations of water toxicity, which must be treated before seizure activity occurs.
Vasopressin (Pitressin) 5-10 units parenterally two to four times daily	The drug is an exogenous form of ADH that serves as a replacement. It binds to kidney receptors and enhances the reabsorption of water, thus reducing urine output.	For the hospitalized patient, monitor for signs of water intoxication, such as listlessness, drowsiness, confusion, headache, anuria, and weight gain.	Vasopressin-induced water intoxication can also lead to seizures, coma, and death.
		Warn the patient not to drink more than 3 L of fluids daily while on this drug.	Drug promotes fluid retention and can lead to fluid overload.
		Teach the patient to weigh himself or herself daily and to notify the health care provider if 2 lbs or more is gained in 24 hours.	A rapid increase in weight is an indicator of excessive fluid retention and may require a change in drug dosage.
		Tell the patient to notify the health care provider if he or she experiences a persistent headache or acute confusion.	These are manifestations of water toxicity, which must be treated before seizure activity occurs.
Chlorpropamide (Diabinese, Insulase) 250-500 mg orally daily **Med Error Alert!** Do not confuse Diabinese with Diamox, a diuretic.	The drug is an anti-diabetic agent that also has some anti-diuretic activity through an unknown mechanism. It decreases urine output.	Ask whether the patient has any allergies to sulfa-based drugs.	Drug contains sulfa, and a person who is hypersensitive to sulfa drugs is likely to also be hypersensitive to this drug.
		Teach patients the manifestations of hypoglycemia and to always carry candy or concentrated sugar with them.	The main action of the drug is to lower blood glucose levels. When taken by a person whose blood glucose level is normal, hypoglycemia can result.

ADH, Antidiuretic hormone.

Schwartz-Bartter syndrome. It is also discussed in Chapter 24 as a complication of cancer and cancer therapy. SIADH occurs with many pathologic conditions and specific drugs, including selective serotonin reuptake inhibitors (Rottmann, 2007). Table 65-1 lists specific drugs and other common causes of SIADH.

In SIADH, the feedback mechanisms that regulate ADH do not function properly. ADH continues to be released even when plasma is hypo-osmolar. Water is *retained,* which results in dilutional **hyponatremia** (a decreased serum sodium level) and expansion of the extracellular fluid volume. The increase in plasma volume causes an increase in the glomerular filtration rate and inhibits the release of renin and aldosterone. The combined effect is an increased sodium loss in urine, leading to greater hyponatremia.

Patient-Centered Collaborative Care

Assessment

Ask the patient about his or her medical history, which may reveal conditions that occur with the development of SIADH. Information about these conditions should be obtained:

- Recent head trauma
- Cerebrovascular disease
- Tuberculosis or other pulmonary disease
- Cancer
- All past and current drug use

TABLE 65-1 Conditions Causing the Syndrome of Inappropriate Antidiuretic Hormone

MALIGNANCIES
• Small cell carcinoma of the lung
• Pancreatic, duodenal, and GU carcinomas
• Thymoma
• Hodgkin's lymphoma
• Non-Hodgkin's lymphoma
PULMONARY DISORDERS
• Viral and bacterial pneumonia
• Lung abscesses
• Active tuberculosis
• Pneumothorax
• Chronic lung diseases
• Mycoses
• Positive-pressure ventilation
CNS DISORDERS
• Trauma
• Infection
• Tumors (primary or metastatic)
• Strokes
• Porphyria
• Systemic lupus erythematosus
DRUGS
• Exogenous ADH
• Chlorpropamide
• Vincristine
• Cyclophosphamide
• Carbamazepine
• Opioids
• Tricyclic antidepressants
• General anesthetics

ADH, Antidiuretic hormone; *CNS,* central nervous system; *GU,* genitourinary.

The early manifestations of SIADH are related to water retention. GI disturbances, such as loss of appetite, nausea, and vomiting, may occur first. Weigh the patient, and document any recent weight gain. Use this information to monitor responses to therapy. In patients with SIADH, free water (not salt) is retained and dependent edema is not usually present, even though water is retained.

Water retention, hyponatremia, and fluid shifts affect central nervous system function, especially when the serum sodium level drops below 115 mEq/L. The patient may have lethargy, headaches, hostility, disorientation, and a change in level of consciousness. Manifestations can progress from lethargy and headaches to decreased responsiveness, seizures, and coma. Assess deep tendon reflexes, which are usually decreased.

Vital sign changes include tachycardia (caused by the increased fluid volume) and hypothermia (caused by central nervous system disturbance). Chapter 13 presents other findings that occur with hyponatremia.

Water retention changes both plasma and urine osmolarity. Urine volume decreases, and urine osmolarity increases. Plasma volume increases, and plasma osmolarity decreases. Elevated urine sodium levels and specific gravity reflect increased urine concentration. Serum sodium levels are decreased, often as low as 110 mEq/L, because of fluid retention and sodium loss.

Radioimmunoassay of ADH can diagnose SIADH when ADH levels are inappropriately elevated when plasma osmolarity is normal or decreased.

Interventions

Medical interventions for SIADH focus on restricting fluid intake, promoting the excretion of water, replacing any lost sodium, and interfering with the action of ADH. Nursing interventions focus on monitoring response to therapy, preventing complications, teaching the patient and family about fluid restrictions and drug therapy, and preventing injury.

Fluid restriction is essential because fluid intake further dilutes the plasma sodium levels. In some cases, fluid intake may be kept as low as 500 to 600 mL/24 hr. Dilute tube feedings with saline rather than plain water, and use saline to irrigate GI tubes. Mix drugs to be given by GI tube with saline.

Measure intake, output, and daily weights to assess the degree of fluid restriction needed. A weight gain of 2 pounds or more per day or a gradual increase over several days is cause for concern. A 1-kg weight increase is equal to a 1000-mL fluid retention (1 kg = 1 L). The patient is uncomfortable during fluid restriction. Keep mucous membranes moist by offering frequent oral rinsing (remind the patient not to swallow the rinses).

Drug therapy with diuretics may be used to treat SIADH, particularly if heart failure results from fluid overload. Be aware of the diuretic effects on sodium loss. Sodium loss can be potentiated, further contributing to the problems caused by SIADH.

Hypertonic saline (i.e., 3% sodium chloride [3% NaCl]) may be used to treat SIADH when the serum sodium is very low. Give IV saline cautiously because it may add to existing fluid overload and promote heart failure. If the patient needs routine IV fluids, a saline solution rather than a water solution is prescribed.

Demeclocycline (Declomycin) may help treat SIADH. This drug is available only as an oral agent and is a type of antibiotic. One of the common side effects is candidiasis yeast infections from the loss of normal protective bacteria. Check the patient's mouth daily for the presence of white, cheesy material indicating oral yeast. Teach the patient to perform meticulous mouth care at least twice daily, to rinse the toothbrush with a 10% bleach solution daily, and to increase his or her intake of yogurt. The hygiene measures reduce the yeast in the mouth and on the toothbrush. The yogurt replaces protective bacteria suppressed by the antibiotic.

Monitor the patient's response to therapy to prevent the fluid overload from SIADH from becoming worse, leading to pulmonary edema and heart failure. Any patient with SIADH, regardless of age, is at risk for these complications. The older adult or one who has coexisting cardiac problems, kidney problems, pulmonary problems, or liver problems is at greater risk.

Monitor for indicators of increased fluid overload (bounding pulse, increasing neck vein distention, presence of crackles in lungs, increasing peripheral edema, reduced urine output) at least every 2 hours. *Pulmonary edema can occur very quickly and can lead to death.* Notify the health care provider of any change that indicates the fluid overload from SIADH either is not responding to therapy or is becoming worse.

Providing a safe environment is needed when the serum sodium level falls below 120 mmol. Possible neurologic changes and the risk for seizures increase as a result of osmotic fluid shifts into brain tissue. Observe for and document changes in the patient's neurologic status. Assess for subtle changes, such as muscle twitching, before they progress to seizures or coma. Check orientation to time, place, and person every 2 hours because disorientation or confusion may be present. Reduce environmental noise and lighting to prevent overstimulation.

Flow sheets with continuing information about the level of consciousness, motor and sensory neurologic assessments, and laboratory data are helpful in detecting neurologic trends. The frequency of neurologic checks depends on the patient's status. For the patient with SIADH who is hyponatremic but alert, awake, and oriented, neurologic checks every 4 hours are sufficient. For the patient who has had a change in level of consciousness, perform neurologic checks at least every hour. Inspect the environment every shift, making sure that basic safety measures, such as siderails being securely in place, are observed.

DECISION-MAKING CHALLENGE
Critical Rescue

The patient is a 66-year-old man with chronic respiratory fibrosis who has been treated with antibiotics (penicillin [Ampicillin] followed by azithromycin [Zithromax]) for a bacterial pneumonia for the past 3 weeks. He was admitted from the ED because his Spo_2 was 85%. In addition to an antibiotic, he also takes losartan (Cozaar) 50 mg daily, prednisone 10 mg daily, and sertraline (Zoloft). When he gets to the unit, he is slow to answer questions although his answers are correct, and he cannot remember the name of the physician who saw him in the ED. When his blood work comes back, you notice that his serum sodium is 109 mEq/L and his hematocrit is 32%. He is supposed to provide a clean-catch urine specimen but has not urinated since his admission, 3 hours ago.

1. What is the probable source or sources of his mental slowness?
2. What risk factors does he have for SIADH?
3. What other assessment data should you obtain immediately? Provide a rationale for your selection.
4. His admitting prescription reads that he should receive 500 mL of D5% in Ringer's lactate IV over the next 2 hours. What should you do about this prescription?

evolve For suggested answer guidelines, go to http://evolve.elsevier.com/Iggy/.

DISORDERS OF THE ADRENAL GLAND

ADRENAL GLAND HYPOFUNCTION

Pathophysiology

Production of adrenocortical steroids may decrease as a result of inadequate secretion of adrenocorticotropic hormone (ACTH), dysfunction of the hypothalamic-pituitary control mechanism, or direct dysfunction of adrenal gland tissue. Manifestations may develop gradually or occur quickly with stress. In acute adrenocortical insufficiency **(adrenal crisis),** life-threatening manifestations may appear without warning.

Insufficiency of adrenocortical steroids causes problems through the loss of aldosterone and cortisol action. Impaired secretion of cortisol results in decreased **gluconeogenesis** (making glucose from proteins) along with depletion of liver and muscle glycogen, leading to **hypoglycemia** (low blood glucose levels). The glomerular filtration rate and gastric acid production decrease, leading to reduced urea nitrogen excretion, causing anorexia and weight loss.

Reduced aldosterone secretion causes potassium, sodium, and water imbalances. Potassium excretion is decreased, causing hyperkalemia. Sodium and water excretion are increased, causing hyponatremia and hypovolemia. Potassium retention also promotes reabsorption of hydrogen ions, which can lead to acidosis.

Chart 65-7 BEST PRACTICE FOR PATIENT SAFETY & QUALITY CARE

Emergency Care of the Patient with Acute Adrenal Insufficiency

EMERGENCY CARE

HORMONE REPLACEMENT
- Start rapid infusion of normal saline or dextrose 5% in normal saline.
- Initial dose of hydrocortisone sodium succinate (Solu-Cortef) is 100 to 300 mg or dexamethasone 4 to 12 mg as an IV bolus.
- Infuse additional 100 mg of hydrocortisone sodium succinate by continuous IV drip over the next 8 hours.
- Give hydrocortisone 50 mg IM concomitantly every 12 hours.
- Initiate an H_2 histamine blocker (e.g., ranitidine) IV for ulcer prevention.

HYPERKALEMIA MANAGEMENT
- Administer insulin (20 to 50 units) with dextrose (20 to 50 mg) in normal saline to shift potassium into cells.
- Administer potassium binding and excreting resin (e.g., Kayexalate).
- Give loop or thiazide diuretics.
- Avoid potassium-sparing diuretics.
- Initiate potassium restriction.
- Monitor intake and output.
- Monitor heart rate, rhythm, and ECG for manifestations of hyperkalemia (slow heart rate; block; tall, peaked T waves; fibrillation; asystole).

HYPOGLYCEMIA MANAGEMENT
- Administer IV glucose.
- Administer glucagon, as needed.
- Maintain IV access.
- Monitor blood glucose level hourly.

ECG, Electrocardiogram.

Low adrenal androgen levels decrease the body, axillary, and pubic hair, especially in women, because the adrenals produce most of the androgens in females. The severity of symptoms is related to the degree of hormone deficiency.

Acute adrenal insufficiency, or **Addisonian crisis,** is a life-threatening event in which the need for cortisol and aldosterone is greater than the available supply. Often, it occurs in response to a stressful event (e.g., surgery, trauma, severe infection), especially when the adrenal hormone output is already reduced. The problems of acute adrenal insufficiency are the same as those of chronic insufficiency but are more severe. *Unless intervention is initiated promptly, however, sodium levels fall and potassium levels rise rapidly. More severe hypotension results from the blood volume depletion that occurs with the loss of aldosterone.* Best practices for emergency care of patients with acute adrenal insufficiency are listed in Chart 65-7.

Adrenal insufficiency, also known as *Addison's disease,* is classified as primary or secondary. Causes of primary and secondary adrenal insufficiency are listed in Table 65-2. One of the most common causes of secondary adrenal insufficiency is the sudden cessation of long-term, high-dose glucocorticoid therapy. This therapy suppresses production of glucocorticoids through negative feedback by causing atrophy of the adrenal cortex. Glucocorticoid drugs must be withdrawn gradually to allow for pituitary production of ACTH and activation of adrenal cells to produce cortisol.

Patient-Centered Collaborative Care

Assessment

History

When possible, take the history from the patient with possible adrenal insufficiency. If he or she is confused, it may be necessary to ask the family questions about manifestations and factors that cause adrenal hypofunction. Ask about any change in activity level, because lethargy, fatigue, and muscle weakness are often present. Include questions about salt intake because salt craving often occurs with hypofunction.

GI problems, such as anorexia, nausea, vomiting, diarrhea, and abdominal pain, often occur. Ask about weight loss during the past months. Women may have menstrual changes related to weight loss, and men may report impotence.

Ask whether the patient has had radiation to the abdomen or head. Document medical problems (e.g., tuberculosis or previous intracranial surgery) and all past and current drugs, especially steroids, anticoagulants, opioids, or cytotoxic drugs.

Physical Assessment/Clinical Manifestations

The manifestations of adrenal insufficiency vary, and the severity is related to the degree of hormone deficiency (Chart 65-8). In patients with primary insufficiency, plasma ACTH and melanocyte-stimulating hormone (MSH) levels are elevated because of the adrenal-hypothalamic-pituitary feedback system. Elevated MSH levels result in areas of increased pigmentation (Fig. 65-4). In primary autoimmune disease, patchy areas of decreased pigmentation may occur because of destruction of skin melanocytes. Body hair may also be

TABLE 65-2 Causes of Primary and Secondary Adrenal Insufficiency

PRIMARY CAUSES
- Idiopathic (autoimmune) disease*
- Tuberculosis
- Metastatic cancer
- Fungal lesions
- AIDS
- Hemorrhage
- Gram-negative sepsis (Waterhouse-Friderichsen syndrome)
- Adrenalectomy
- Abdominal radiation therapy
- Drugs (mitotane) and toxins

SECONDARY CAUSES
- Pituitary tumors
- Postpartum pituitary necrosis (Sheehan's syndrome)
- Hypophysectomy
- High-dose pituitary radiation
- High-dose whole-brain radiation

*Most common cause.
AIDS, Acquired immune deficiency syndrome.

Chart 65-8 KEY FEATURES
Adrenal Insufficiency

NEUROMUSCULAR MANIFESTATIONS
- Muscle weakness
- Fatigue
- Joint/muscle pain

GASTROINTESTINAL MANIFESTATIONS
- Anorexia
- Nausea, vomiting
- Abdominal pain
- Bowel changes (constipation/diarrhea)
- Weight loss
- Salt craving

INTEGUMENTARY MANIFESTATIONS
- Vitiligo
- Hyperpigmentation

CARDIOVASCULAR MANIFESTATIONS
- Anemia
- Hypotension
- Hyponatremia
- Hyperkalemia
- Hypercalcemia

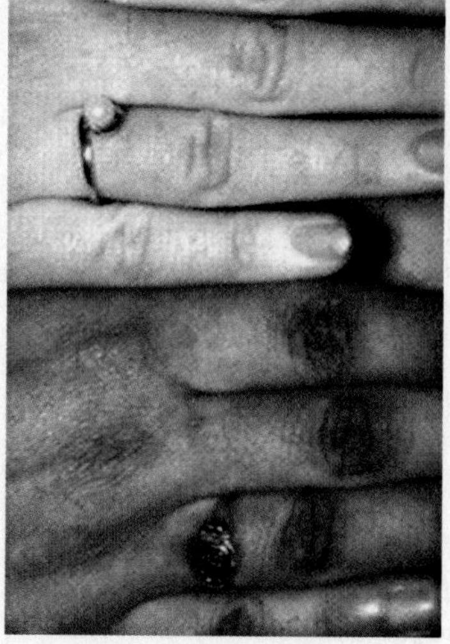

Fig. 65-4 • The increased pigmentation seen in primary adrenocortical insufficiency.

decreased. In secondary disease, there is no change in skin pigmentation.

Assess for manifestations of hypoglycemia (e.g., sweating, headaches, tachycardia, and tremors) and volume depletion (postural hypotension and dehydration). **Hyperkalemia** (elevated blood levels of potassium) can cause dysrhythmias with an irregular heart rate and result in cardiac arrest (Holcomb, 2006).

Psychosocial Assessment

Depending on the degree of imbalance, patients may appear lethargic, depressed, confused, and even psychotic. Observe the patient, and check his or her orientation to person, place, and time. Families may report that the patient has a decreased energy level, experiences wide mood swings, and is forgetful.

Laboratory Assessment

Laboratory findings include low serum cortisol, low fasting blood glucose, low sodium, elevated potassium, and increased blood urea nitrogen (BUN) levels (Chart 65-9). In primary disease, the eosinophil count and ACTH level are elevated. Plasma cortisol levels do not rise during stimulation tests.

Urinary 17-hydroxycorticosteroids are the glucocorticoid metabolites, and 17-ketosteroid levels reflect the adrenal androgen metabolites. Both levels are in the low or low-normal range in adrenal hypofunction.

An ACTH stimulation test is the most definitive test for adrenal insufficiency (Stewart, 2008; Whittman, 2006). A rapid ACTH stimulation test may be performed on an outpatient basis. ACTH 0.25 to 1 mg is given IV, and plasma cortisol levels are obtained at 30-minute and 1-hour intervals. In primary insufficiency, the cortisol response is absent or markedly decreased. In secondary insufficiency, it is increased. When acute adrenal insufficiency is suspected, treatment is started without stimulation testing.

Imaging Assessment

Skull x-rays, CT, MRI, and arteriography may help determine the cause of pituitary problems leading to adrenal insufficiency. CT scans of the adrenal gland may show atrophy of the gland.

NCLEX EXAMINATION CHALLENGE

Which electrolyte values indicate therapy for adrenal insufficiency is effective?

A. Serum sodium 148 mEq/L; serum potassium 7.1 mEq/L
B. Serum sodium 128 mEq/L; serum potassium 3.1 mEq/L
C. Serum sodium 118 mEq/L; serum potassium 6.1 mEq/L
D. Serum sodium 138 mEq/L; serum potassium 4.1 mEq/L

evolve For the correct answer, go to http://evolve.elsevier.com/Iggy/.

▪ Interventions

Nursing interventions aim to promote fluid balance, monitor for fluid deficit, and prevent hypoglycemia (Chart 65-10). Weigh the patient daily, and record intake and output. Assess vital signs every 1 to 4 hours, depending on the patient's condition and the presence of dysrhythmias or postural hypotension. Monitor laboratory values to identify hemoconcentration (e.g., increased hematocrit or BUN). Chapter 13 discusses fluid volume deficit in detail.

Cortisol and aldosterone deficiencies are corrected by replacement therapy. Hydrocortisone corrects glucocorticoid deficiency (Chart 65-11). Therapy replacement regimens vary. Generally, divided doses are given, with two thirds given in the morning and one third in the late afternoon to mimic the normal release of this hormone. Although most patients do well on this regimen, some may not tolerate the dosage or may need more.

An additional mineralocorticoid hormone, such as fludrocortisone (Florinef), may be needed to maintain electrolyte balance (especially sodium and potassium). Dosage adjust-

Chart 65-9 LABORATORY PROFILE
Adrenal Gland Assessment

		SIGNIFICANCE OF ABNORMAL FINDINGS	
Test	**Normal Range for Adults**	**Hypofunction of the Adrenal Gland**	**Hyperfunction of the Adrenal Gland**
Sodium	136-145 mEq/L	Decreased	Increased
Potassium	3.5-5.0 mEq/L	Increased	Decreased
Glucose	70-115 mg/dL *Older adults:* slightly increased	Normal to decreased	Normal to increased
Calcium	9-10.5 mg/dL (total) 4.5-5.6 mg/dL (ionized) *Older adults:* slightly decreased	Increased	Decreased
Bicarbonate	23-30 mEq/L	Increased	Decreased
BUN	10-20 mg/dL *Older adults:* may be slightly higher	Increased	Normal
Cortisol	6 AM to 8 AM: 5-23 mcg/dL or 138-635 SI units (nmol/L) 4 PM to 6 PM: 3-13 mcg/dL or 83-359 SI units (nmol/L)	Decreased	Increased

BUN, Blood urea nitrogen; *SI,* International System of Units.

Chart 65-10 NIC INTERVENTION ACTIVITIES

The Patient with Adrenal Insufficiency

Hypoglycemia Management: *Preventing and treating low blood glucose levels.*

- Determine recognition of hypoglycemia signs and symptoms.
- Monitor blood glucose levels, as indicated.
- Monitor for signs and symptoms of hypoglycemia (e.g., shakiness, tremor, sweating, nervousness, anxiety, irritability, impatience, tachycardia, palpitations, chills, clamminess, light-headedness, pallor, hunger, nausea, headache, tiredness, drowsiness, weakness, warmth, dizziness, faintness, blurred vision, nightmares, crying out in sleep, paresthesias, difficulty concentrating, difficulty speaking, incoordination, behavior change, confusion, coma, seizure).
- Provide simple carbohydrate, as needed.
- Administer glucagon, as indicated.
- Maintain IV access, as appropriate.
- Instruct patient and significant others on signs, symptoms, risk factors, and treatment of hypoglycemia.
- Instruct patient to have simple carbohydrate available at all times.
- Instruct patient to obtain and carry/wear appropriate emergency identification.

NIC intervention activities selected from Bulechek, G.M., Butcher, H.K., & McCloskey Dochterman, J. (Eds.). (2008). *Nursing interventions classification (NIC)* (5th ed.). St. Louis: Mosby.

ment may be needed, especially in hot weather when more sodium is lost because of excessive perspiration. *Salt restriction or diuretic therapy should not be started without considering whether it might lead to an adrenal crisis.*

ADRENAL GLAND HYPERFUNCTION

The adrenal gland may oversecrete just one hormone or all adrenal hormones. Hypersecretion by the adrenal cortex results in hypercortisolism (e.g., **Cushing's disease** or **Cushing's syndrome**), **hyperaldosteronism** (excessive mineralocorticoid production), or excessive androgen production.

Hyperstimulation of the adrenal medulla caused by a tumor **(pheochromocytoma)** results in excessive secretion of catecholamines, of which 80% is epinephrine and the remainder is norepinephrine.

HYPERCORTISOLISM (CUSHING'S DISEASE)

Pathophysiology

Cushing's disease is the exaggerated actions of glucocorticoids, causing widespread problems. The problem is seen as excessive secretion of cortisol from the adrenal cortex. This excess secretion can be a result of a problem in the adrenal cortex itself, a problem in the anterior pituitary gland, or a problem in the hypothalamus. In addition, glucocorticoid therapy can also lead to problems of hypercortisolism.

The presence of excess glucocorticoids, regardless of the cause, affects metabolism and all body systems to some degree. Nitrogen, carbohydrate, and mineral metabolism are

Chart 65-11 COMMON EXAMPLES OF DRUG THERAPY

Hypofunction of the Adrenal Gland

Drug	Usual Dosage	Nursing Interventions	Rationales
Cortisone	25-50 mg orally either once daily in AM or daily in divided doses	Instruct the patient to take the drug with meals or a snack.	GI irritation can occur.
Hydrocortisone (Cortef, Hycort♣)	20-50 mg orally either once daily in AM or daily in divided doses	Instruct the patient to report these signs or symptoms of excessive drug therapy: • Rapid weight gain • Round face • Fluid retention	Cushing's syndrome, which indicates a need for dosage adjustment, can occur.
Prednisone (Winpred♣) **Med Error Alert!** Do not confuse prednisone with prednisolone, another corticosteroid that is 4 to 5 times more potent than prednisone.	5-10 mg orally either once daily in AM or daily in divided doses	Instruct the patient to report illness, such as: • Severe diarrhea • Vomiting • Fever	Other conditions may indicate a need for dosage change. The usual daily dosage may not be adequate during periods of illness or severe stress.
Fludrocortisone (Florinef)	0.05-0.2 mg orally daily	Monitor the patient's blood pressure. Instruct the patient to report weight gain or edema.	Hypertension is a potential side effect. Sodium-related fluid retention is possible.

altered. An increase in total body fat results from slow turnover of plasma fatty acids. This fat is redistributed to produce the typical body pattern of truncal obesity, "buffalo hump," and "moon face" (Fig. 65-5). Increases in the breakdown of tissue protein and an increase in urine nitrogen excretion also occur, resulting in decreased muscle mass, thin skin, and fragile capillaries. The effects on minerals lead to bone density loss.

High levels of corticosteroids kill lymphocytes and shrink organs containing lymphocytes, such as the liver, the spleen, and the lymph nodes. Eosinophils and macrophages are reduced. Although the number of neutrophils may be increased, the reduction of cytokines makes these cells less active. Thus protection of the inflammatory and immune responses is reduced.

In most cases, increased androgen production also occurs and causes acne, **hirsutism** (increased hair growth), and occasionally clitoral hypertrophy. Increased androgen production can also interrupt the normal hormone feedback mechanism for the ovary, decreasing the ovary's production of estrogens and progesterone. **Oligomenorrhea** (scant or infrequent menses) occurs as a result.

Etiology

Cushing's disease or syndrome is a group of clinical problems caused by an excess of cortisol. Table 65-3 lists causes of cortisol excess. When the anterior pituitary gland oversecretes adrenocorticotropic hormone (ACTH), this hormone causes hyperplasia of the adrenal cortex in both adrenal glands and an excess of most hormones secreted by the adrenal cortex. (See Fig. 64-3 in Chapter 64.) This problem is known as **pituitary Cushing's disease** because the tissue causing the problem is the pituitary. When the excess glucocorticoids are caused by a problem in the actual adrenal cortex, usually a benign tumor (adrenal adenoma), the problem is called **adrenal Cushing's disease** and usually occurs in only one adrenal gland. When the excess glucocorticoids are a result of drug therapy for another health problem, the disorder is known as **Cushing's syndrome.**

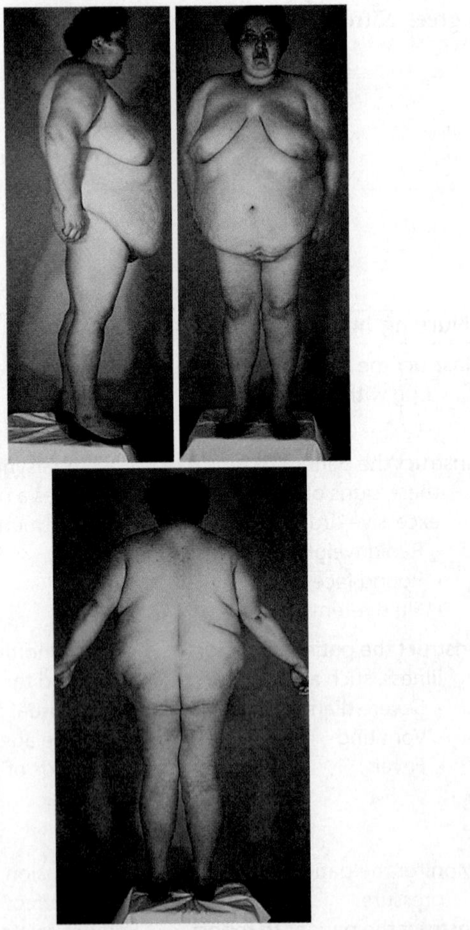

Fig. 65-5 • The typical appearance of a patient with Cushing's disease or syndrome. Note truncal obesity, moon face, buffalo hump, thinner arms and legs, and abdominal striae.

Incidence/Prevalence

The most common cause of Cushing's disease is a pituitary adenoma. Adrenal adenomas account for only about 15% of the disease (Stewart, 2008). Women are more likely than men to develop Cushing's disease. The actual incidence of Cushing's syndrome from chronic use of exogenous corticosteroids is not known. However, because these drugs are commonly used to control serious, chronic inflammatory conditions such as asthma, other respiratory problems, and rheumatoid arthritis, Cushing's syndrome is more common than Cushing's disease and affects both genders equally.

Patient-Centered Collaborative Care

Assessment

History

The first question should be related to the patient's other health problems and drug therapies, because glucocorticoid therapy is a common cause of hypercortisolism. Regardless of cause, the patient with hypercortisolism has many changes because of the widespread effect of excessive cortisol levels. Record age, gender, and usual weight. He or she may report a significant weight gain and an increased appetite. Ask about changes in activity or sleep patterns, fatigue, and muscle weakness. Ask about bone pain or a history of fractures because osteoporosis is common in hypercortisolism. Ask about a history of frequent infections and easy bruising, which sug-

TABLE 65-3 Conditions Causing Increased Cortisol Secretion

ENDOGENOUS SECRETION (CUSHING'S DISEASE)
- Bilateral adrenal hyperplasia*
- Pituitary adenoma increasing the production of ACTH (pituitary Cushing's disease)
- Malignancies: carcinomas of the lung, GI tract, pancreas
- Adrenal adenomas or carcinomas

EXOGENOUS ADMINISTRATION (CUSHING'S SYNDROME)
- Therapeutic use of ACTH or glucocorticoids—most commonly for treatment of:
  - Asthma
  - Autoimmune disorders
  - Organ transplantation
  - Cancer chemotherapy
  - Allergic responses
  - Chronic fibrosis

*Most common cause.
ACTH, Adrenocorticotropic hormone.

gest hypercortisolism. Women may report a cessation of menses. GI problems include ulcer formation from increased hydrochloric acid secretion and decreased production of protective gastric mucus.

Physical Assessment/Clinical Manifestations

The patient with hypercortisolism has specific physical changes, although all body systems are affected (see Fig. 65-5 and Chart 65-12). Observe the patient's general appearance. Changes in fat distribution may result in fat pads on the neck, back, and shoulders ("buffalo hump"); an enlarged trunk with thin arms and legs; and a round face ("moon face"). Other changes include muscle wasting and weakness. Assess and document changes, and use these to prioritize nursing diagnoses and interventions.

Skin changes result from increased blood vessel fragility and include bruises, thin or translucent skin, and wounds that have not healed. Reddish purple **striae** ("stretch marks") are often present on the abdomen, thighs, and upper arms because of the destructive effect of cortisol on collagen.

Excessive cortisol secretion may result in acne and a fine coating of hair over the face and body. In women, look for the presence of hirsutism, clitoral hypertrophy, and male pattern balding related to androgen excess.

Cardiac changes occur as a result of altered water and mineral metabolism. Both sodium and water are reabsorbed and retained, leading to hypervolemia and edema formation. Blood pressure and heart rate are usually elevated.

Musculoskeletal changes occur as a result of nitrogen depletion and mineral loss. Muscle mass decreases. This is most noticeable on the arms and legs, which look too small in proportion to the trunk (see Fig. 65-5). Muscle loss leads to muscle weakness and an increased risk for falls. Bone becomes thinner as a result of mineral loss, and osteoporosis is common. The risk for pathologic fractures greatly increases.

Glucose metabolism is profoundly affected by hypercortisolism. Fasting blood glucose levels are high because the liver is stimulated to convert more glycogen to glucose and the insulin receptors are less sensitive so that blood glucose does not move as easily into the tissues. In addition, muscle mass loss reduces glucose uptake.

Immune changes caused by excess cortisol result in immunosuppression and an increased risk for infection. The excess cortisol reduces the number of circulating lymphocytes, inhibits maturation of macrophages, reduces antibody synthesis, and inhibits production of cytokines and inflammatory chemicals (e.g., histamine). These patients not only are at greater risk for infection but also may not have the expected inflammatory manifestations (fever, purulent exudate, redness in the affected area) when an infection is present.

Psychosocial Assessment

Hypercortisolism can result in emotional lability, and patients often say that they do not feel like themselves anymore. Ask about mood swings, irritability, confusion, or depression. Ask the patient whether he or she has been crying or laughing inappropriately or has had difficulty concentrating. Family members often report these changes in mental or emotional status. The patient may have neurotic or psychotic behavior as a result of high blood cortisol levels. In addition, the hormones stimulate the central nervous system, heightening the awareness of and responses to sensory stimulation. The patient often reports sleep difficulties and fatigue.

Laboratory Assessment

Laboratory tests include blood, salivary, and urine cortisol levels. These are high in patients with hypercortisolism regardless of the origin of the disorder. Plasma ACTH levels vary, depending on the cause of hypercortisolism. In pituitary Cushing's disease, ACTH levels are elevated. In adrenal Cush-

Chart 65-12 KEY FEATURES

Hypercortisolism (Cushing's Disease/Syndrome)

GENERAL APPEARANCE
- Fat redistribution:
  - Moon face
  - Buffalo hump
  - Truncal obesity
- Weight gain

CARDIOVASCULAR MANIFESTATIONS
- Hypertension
- Increased risk for thromboembolic events
- Frequent dependent edema
- Capillary fragility:
  - Bruising
  - Petechiae

MUSCULOSKELETAL MANIFESTATIONS
- Muscle atrophy (most apparent in extremities)
- Osteoporosis (bone density loss)
  - Pathologic fractures
  - Decreased height with vertebral collapse
  - Aseptic necrosis of the femur head
  - Slow or poor healing of bone fractures

SKIN MANIFESTATIONS
- Thinning skin ("paper-like" appearance, especially on the back of the hands)
- Striae
- Increased pigmentation (with ectopic or pituitary production of ACTH)

IMMUNE SYSTEM MANIFESTATIONS
- Increased risk for infection
- Decreased immune function:
  - Decreased circulating lymphocytes
  - Decreased production of immunoglobulins (antibodies)
- Decreased inflammatory responses:
  - Decreased eosinophil count
  - Slight increase in neutrophil count but activity is reduced
- Decreased production of proinflammatory cytokines, histamine, and prostaglandins
- Manifestations of infection/inflammation may be masked

ACTH, Adrenocorticotropic hormone.

ing's disease or when Cushing's syndrome results from chronic steroid use, ACTH levels are very low.

Salivary cortisol levels are becoming increasingly more popular to detect hypercortisolism. This test is very accurate in assessing cortisol levels because cortisol-binding proteins are not present in saliva. Usually, salivary cortisol levels are obtained at midnight (Stewart, 2008). Saliva, not spit, is needed for the assay. Saliva is easily and painlessly collected with the use of a salivary specimen cushion placed in the cheek next to the salivary gland. A normal salivary cortisol level is lower than 2.0 ng/mL. Higher levels indicate hypercortisolism.

Urine is tested to measure levels of free cortisol and the metabolites of cortisol and androgens (17-hydroxycorticosteroids and 17-ketosteroids). In Cushing's disease, levels of urine cortisol, 17-ketosteroids, and 17-hydroxycorticosteroids are all elevated in a 24-hour specimen, as are urine calcium, potassium, and glucose levels.

Dexamethasone suppression testing is another screening tool for hypercortisolism. Suppression testing involves administering set doses of dexamethasone and testing 24-hour urine collections for 17-ketosteroids, 17-hydroxycorticosteroids, creatinine, and urine cortisol. Normally, urinary 17-hydroxycorticosteroid excretion and cortisol levels are suppressed by dexamethasone, and Cushing's disease is ruled out. Suppression testing may take place overnight or over a 3-day period. It may involve low doses or high doses of dexamethasone.

Additional laboratory findings that accompany hypercortisolism include:

- Increased blood glucose level
- Decreased lymphocyte count
- Increased sodium level
- Decreased serum calcium level
- Decreased serum potassium level

Imaging Assessment

Imaging for hypercortisolism includes x-rays, CT scans, MRI, and arteriography. These images can identify lesions of the adrenal or pituitary glands, lung, GI tract, or pancreas.

Analysis

Common Nursing Diagnoses and Collaborative Problems

Priority nursing diagnoses for patients with Cushing's disease or Cushing's syndrome are:

1. Excess Fluid Volume related to excess water and sodium reabsorption
2. Risk for Injury related to skin thinning, poor wound healing, and bone density loss
3. Risk for Infection related to immunosuppression and inadequate primary defenses

A primary collaborative problem is the Potential for Acute Adrenal Insufficiency.

Additional Nursing Diagnoses and Collaborative Problems

- Deficient Knowledge (Illness and Treatment) related to lack of interest in learning and unfamiliarity with information resources
- Sleep Deprivation related to hormone-induced increased sensory stimulation
- Fatigue related to sleep deprivation
- Imbalanced Nutrition: More Than Body Requirements related to excess intake in relation to metabolic need as a result of appetite stimulation by cortisol
- Disturbed Body Image related to illness
- Risk for Falls related to decreased lower extremity strength and impaired balance

Interventions

Goals of treatment for hypercortisolism are the reduction of plasma cortisol levels, removal of tumors, and restoration of normal or acceptable body appearance. When the hypercortisolism is caused by pituitary or adrenal problems, cure is possible. When caused by drug therapy for another health problem, the focus of management is to prevent complications related to hypercortisolism.

Excess Fluid Volume

Planning: Expected Outcomes. The patient with hypercortisolism is expected to achieve and maintain an acceptable fluid balance. Indicators include that these parameters are only mildly compromised or not compromised:

- Blood pressure
- Stable body weight
- Serum electrolytes

Interventions. Interventions for patients with excess fluid (fluid overload) related to hypercortisolism aim to ensure patient safety, restore normal fluid balance, and provide supportive care until the imbalance is resolved. When possible, surgical management is used to reduce cortisol production.

Nonsurgical Management. Patient safety, drug therapy, nutrition therapy, and monitoring are the basis of nonsurgical interventions for hypercortisolism and fluid volume excess.

Patient safety includes preventing fluid overload from becoming worse, leading to pulmonary edema and heart failure. Any patient with fluid overload, regardless of age, is at risk for these complications. The older adult or one who has coexisting cardiac problems, kidney problems, pulmonary problems, or liver problems is at greater risk.

Monitor for indicators of increased fluid overload (increased pulse quality, increasing neck vein distention, presence of crackles in lungs, increasing peripheral edema, reduced urine output) at least every 2 hours. *Pulmonary edema can occur very quickly and can lead to death.* Notify the health care provider of any change that indicates the fluid overload either is not responding to therapy or is becoming worse.

The patient with fluid overload and dependent edema is at risk for skin breakdown. Use a pressure-reducing or pressure-relieving overlay on the mattress. Assess skin pressure areas, especially the coccyx, elbows, hips, and heels, daily for signs of redness or open areas. Because many patients with fluid overload may be receiving oxygen by mask or nasal cannula, check the skin around the mask, nares, ears, and under the elastic band for loss of integrity. Assist the patient to change positions every 2 hours, or ensure that others delegated to perform this intervention are diligent in this action.

Drug therapy involves the use of drugs that interfere with adrenocorticotropic hormone (ACTH) production or adrenal hormone synthesis for temporary relief. Aminoglutethimide (Elipten, Cytadren) and metyrapone (Metopirone) use different pathways to decrease cortisol production. For patients with hypercortisolism from increased ACTH production, cyproheptadine (Periactin) may be used because it interferes with ACTH production. Mitotane (Lysodren) is an adrenal cytotoxic agent used for inoperable adrenal tumors causing hypercortisolism.

Monitor the patient for response to drug therapy, especially weight loss and increased urine output. Observe for manifestations of electrolyte imbalance, especially changes in electrocardiogram (ECG) patterns. Assess laboratory findings, especially sodium and potassium values, every 8 hours or whenever they are drawn.

Nutrition therapy for the patient with hypercortisolism may involve restrictions of both fluid and sodium intake to control fluid volume. Review the patient's serum sodium levels whenever fluid overload is present. Often sodium restriction involves only "no added salt" to ordinary table foods when fluid overload is mild. For more pronounced fluid overload, the patient may be restricted to anywhere from 2 gm/day to 4 gm/day of sodium. When sodium restriction is ongoing, teach the patient and family how to check food labels for sodium content and how to keep a daily record of sodium ingested. Explain to the patient and family the reason for any fluid restriction and the importance of adhering to the prescribed restriction.

Monitoring intake and output, as well as weight, provides information on therapy effectiveness. Ensure that unlicensed assistive personnel (UAP) understand that these measurements need to be accurate, not just estimated, because treatment decisions are based on these findings. In addition to regulating the total amount of fluid ingested in a 24-hour period, schedule fluid offerings throughout the 24 hours. Teach UAP to check urine for color and character and to report these findings. Check the urine specific gravity (a specific gravity below 1.005 may indicate fluid overload). If the patient is receiving IV therapy, infuse the exact amount prescribed.

Fluid retention may not be visible. Remember that rapid weight gain is the best indicator of fluid retention and overload. Metabolism can account for no more than a half pound of weight gain in one day. Each pound of weight gained (after the first half pound) equates to 500 mL of retained water. Weigh the patient at the same time every day (before breakfast), using the same scale. Whenever possible, have the patient wear the same type of clothing for each weigh-in.

Radiation therapy may be used to treat hypercortisolism caused by pituitary adenomas. However, radiation is not always effective and often destroys normal tissue. Observe for any changes in the patient's neurologic status, such as headache, elevated blood pressure or pulse, disorientation, or changes in pupil size or reaction. The patient may have skin dryness, redness, flushing, or alopecia at the radiation site. Review these possible side effects with the patient. Chapter 47 discusses radiation therapy to the head.

Surgical Management. The surgical treatment of adrenocortical hypersecretion depends on the cause of the disease. When adrenal hyperfunction is due to increased pituitary secretion of ACTH, removal of a pituitary adenoma may be attempted. In many instances, a total hypophysectomy (surgical removal of the pituitary gland) is needed. Hypophysectomy is performed via the transsphenoidal or transfrontal craniotomy route. (See earlier discussion of hypophysectomy on p. 1431; see also Chapter 47 for nursing care of patients undergoing a craniotomy.) If hypercortisolism is caused by adrenal tumors, a partial or complete adrenalectomy (removal of the adrenal gland) may be needed.

Preoperative care. Electrolyte imbalances are corrected before surgery. Continue to monitor blood potassium, sodium, and chloride levels. Dysrhythmias from potassium imbalance may occur, and cardiac monitoring is needed. Hyperglycemia is controlled before surgery, and blood glucose levels are monitored.

The patient with hypercortisolism is at risk for complications such as infections and fractures. Prevent infection with handwashing and aseptic technique. Decrease the risk for falls by raising bed upper siderails and encouraging the patient to ask for assistance when getting out of bed. A high-calorie, high-protein diet is prescribed before surgery.

Glucocorticoid preparations are given before surgery. The patient continues to receive glucocorticoids during surgery to prevent adrenal crisis because the removal of the tumor results in a sudden drop in cortisol levels. Before surgery, discuss the care needs for after surgery and the need for long-term drug therapy.

Operative procedures. A unilateral adrenalectomy is performed when one gland is involved. A bilateral adrenalectomy is needed when ectopic ACTH-producing tumors cannot be treated by other means or when both adrenal glands are diseased. Surgery can be abdominal or through the lateral flank. Abdominal surgery causes a higher degree of illness and risk. The flank approach is preferred because the abdominal cavity is not entered and complications are reduced. A laparoscopic adrenalectomy may reduce complications after surgery.

Postoperative care. After an adrenalectomy, the patient is usually sent to a critical care unit. Immediately after surgery, assess the patient every 15 minutes for shock (e.g., hypotension; a rapid, weak pulse; and a decreasing urine output) due to possible insufficient glucocorticoid replacement. Monitor ongoing vital signs and other hemodynamic variables (central venous pressure, pulmonary wedge pressure), intake and output, daily weights, and serum electrolyte levels.

After a bilateral adrenalectomy, patients require lifelong glucocorticoid and mineralcorticoid replacement, starting immediately after surgery. In unilateral adrenalectomy, hormone replacement continues until the remaining adrenal gland increases hormone production. This therapy may be needed for up to 2 years after surgery.

Risk for Injury

The patient who has hypercortisolism is at risk for injury from skin breakdown, bone fractures, and GI bleeding. Prevention of such injuries is a major nursing care focus.

Planning: Expected Outcomes. The patient with hypercortisolism is expected to avoid injury. Indicators include:
- Skin is intact.
- Minimal or no bruising is present.
- Bones are intact.
- Stools, vomitus, and other GI secretions contain no gross or occult blood.

Interventions. Priority nursing interventions for prevention of injury focus on skin assessment and protection, coordinating care to ensure gentle handling, and patient teaching regarding drug therapy for prevention of GI ulcers.

Skin injury is a continuing risk for any patient who has hypercortisolism. Even when surgery has corrected the cortisol excess, the changes induced in the skin and blood vessels are present for weeks to months. Assess the patient's skin for reddened areas, excoriation, breakdown, and edema. If mobility is decreased, turn him or her every 2 hours and pad bony prominences.

Instruct the patient to avoid activities that can result in skin trauma. To reduce tissue injury, teach him or her to use a soft toothbrush and an electric shaver. Instruct patients to keep the skin clean and to dry it thoroughly after washing. Excessive dryness can be prevented by using a moisturizing lotion.

Adhesive tape often causes skin breakdown. Use tape sparingly, and use caution when removing it. After venipuncture or arterial puncture, the patient may have increased bleeding because of blood vessel fragility. Exert pressure over the site for longer than normal to prevent bleeding and bruising.

Pathologic fractures from bone density loss and osteoporosis are possible for months to years after cortisol levels return to normal. Teach the patient about safety issues and dietary needs. He or she is at risk for fractures as a result of minor falls or bumps. When helping the patient to move in bed, use a lift sheet instead of grasping him or her. Remind the patient to call for help when ambulating. Review the use of ambulatory aids (walkers or canes), if needed. Keep rooms free of extraneous objects that might cause a fall. Teach UAP to use a gait belt when ambulating with a patient who has bone density loss.

Coordinate with a nutritionist to counsel the patient about nutrition therapy. A high-calorie diet is prescribed that includes items from all of the major food groups and increased amounts of calcium and vitamin D. Generous amounts of milk, cheese, yogurt, and green leafy and root vegetables add calcium to promote bone density. Advise the patient to avoid caffeine and alcohol, which increase the risk for GI ulcers and may promote bone density loss.

GI bleeding is common with hypercortisolism as a result of systemic changes. Cortisol inhibits production of the thick, gel-like mucus that protects the stomach lining, decreases blood flow to the area, and triggers the release of additional hydrochloric acid. Although surgery reduces the hypercortisolism, the protective mucus and increased blood flow may take days to weeks to return. Interventions aim to reduce gastric irritation, usually through drug therapy to protect the GI mucosa and decrease the secretion of hydrochloric acid.

Antacids buffer stomach acids and protect the GI mucosa. Teach the patient that these drugs should be taken on a regular schedule, rather than on an as-needed basis.

Some agents block the H_2-receptor site in the gastric mucosa. When histamine binds to this receptor site, a series of actions occur that release hydrochloric acid. Drugs that block the H_2-receptor site include cimetidine (Tagamet, Peptol♣, Novo-Cimetine♣), ranitidine (Zantac, Apo-Ranitidine♣), famotidine (Pepcid), and nizatidine (Axid). Omeprazole (Losec♣, Prilosec) and esomeprazole (Nexium) inhibit the gastric proton pump and prevent the formation of hydrochloric acid.

Encourage the patient to reduce or eliminate habits that contribute to gastric irritation, such as consuming alcohol or caffeine, smoking, and fasting. Discuss other prescribed and over-the-counter drugs that he or she may be taking. NSAIDs and drugs that contain aspirin or other salicylates can cause gastritis and intensify GI bleeding.

Risk for Infection

Glucocorticoids reduce both inflammation and the immune responses, increasing the risk for infection. For the patient who is taking glucocorticoid replacement therapy, this is an ongoing risk. For the patient who is recovering from surgery to prevent hypercortisolism, the infection risk continues for weeks after surgery.

Planning: Expected Outcomes. The patient with hypercortisolism is expected to remain free from infection and avoid situations increasing the risk for infection. Indicators include these manifestations and behaviors:

- Absence of fever and foul-smelling or purulent drainage
- Absence of cough, chest pain, and dyspnea
- Absence of urinary frequency, urgency, or pain and burning
- Avoids crowds and large gatherings
- Obtains appropriate vaccinations
- Washes hands frequently

Interventions. A major objective in caring for the patient with hypercortisolism is protection from infection. All personnel must use extreme care during all nursing procedures. Frequent, thorough handwashing is of the utmost importance. Anyone with an upper respiratory tract infection who must enter the patient's room must wear a mask. Observe strict procedures when performing dressing changes or any invasive procedure.

Continually assess the patient for the presence of infection. This task is difficult because manifestations may not be obvious in the patient who is immunosuppressed from hypercortisolism. The development of fever and the formation of pus (both indicators of infection) depend on the presence of white blood cells (WBCs). The immunosuppressed patient may have a severe infection without pus and with only a low fever.

Monitor the patient's daily complete blood count (CBC) with differential WBC count and absolute neutrophil count (ANC). Inspect the mouth during every shift for lesions and mucosa breakdown. Assess the lungs every 8 hours for crackles, wheezes, or reduced breath sounds. Assess all urine for odor and cloudiness. Ask the patient about any urgency, burning, or pain present on urination.

Take vital signs at least every 4 hours to assess for fever. A temperature elevation of even 0.5° F (or 0.5° C) above baseline is significant for a patient who is immunosuppressed and indicates infection until it has been proved otherwise.

Skin care is important for preventing infection because the skin may be the only intact defense. Teach the patient about hygiene, and urge daily bathing. If the patient is immobile, turn him or her every hour and apply skin lubricants.

Perform pulmonary hygiene every 2 to 4 hours. Listen to the lungs for crackles, wheezes, or reduced breath sounds. Urge the patient to cough and deep breathe or to perform sustained maximum inhalations every hour while awake.

Potential for Acute Adrenal Insufficiency

The patient most at risk for acute adrenal insufficiency is the one who has Cushing's syndrome as a result of glucocorticoid drug therapy. The exogenous drug inhibits the feedback control pathway (see Fig. 64-3 in Chapter 64), preventing the hypothalamus from secreting corticotropin-releasing hormone (CRH). The lack of CRH inhibits secretion of ACTH from the anterior pituitary gland. Without normal levels of ACTH, the adrenal glands atrophy and completely stop their own production of any of the corticosteroids. As a result, the patient completely depends on the exogenous drug. If the drug is stopped, even for a day or two, the atrophied adrenal glands cannot produce the glucocorticoids and the patient develops acute adrenal insufficiency, a life-threatening condition. Management of this problem is described on p. 1437.

DECISION-MAKING CHALLENGE
Coordination of Care

The patient is a 70-year-old nursing home resident who has been taking 15 mg of prednisone daily for 15 years to treat a chronic inflammatory problem. She has been a resident of the nursing home for about 6 weeks after falling down her basement steps and breaking her left arm. She has been identified by the staff as a "problem" patient because she has made her roommate cry, has frequent spells of shouting at people intermixed with periods of weeping, and rarely has visitors. She asks for extra food in the evening and at night. Last week, she lost her balance and fell against the doorjamb of the bathroom, resulting in a large bruise on her right hand and arm. When her family visited and asked her about the bruise, she told them that one of the UAP handled her roughly.

1. How should you approach the staff, especially the UAP, about this "problem" patient?
2. What will you tell the family about the bruising?
3. What interventions can you institute to reduce this patient's risk for injury?
4. How can this patient's appetite be managed?

evolve For suggested answer guidelines, go to http://evolve.elsevier.com/Iggy/.

Community-Based Care
Home Care Management

The patient with hypercortisolism usually has muscle weakness and fatigue for some weeks after surgery and remains at risk for falls and other injury. These problems may necessitate one-floor living for a short time, and a home health aide may be needed to assist with hygiene, meal preparation, and maintenance.

Health Teaching

The patient taking exogenous glucocorticoids who is discharged to home remains at continuing risk for fluid volume excess. Teach him or her and the family to monitor weight at home. Verify that the patient understands the relationship between body weight and fluid balance. Suggest that a record of these daily weights be kept to show the health care provider at any checkups. Also, instruct the patient to call the health care provider if he or she gains more than 3 lbs in a week or more than 1 to 2 lbs in a 24-hour period.

Lifelong hormone replacement is needed after bilateral adrenalectomy. Teach the patient and family about adherence with the drug regimen and its side effects (Chart 65-13).

Protecting the patient from infection at home is just as important as it was during hospitalization. Urge him or her to use proper hygiene and to avoid crowds or others with infections. Encourage the patient and all people living in the same home with him or her to have yearly influenza vaccinations. Stress that the patient should immediately notify the physician if he or she has a fever or any other sign of infection. Chart 42-11 in Chapter 42 lists guidelines for patients for infection prevention.

Health Care Resources

Immediately after returning home, the patient may need a support person to stay and provide more attention than could be given by a visiting nurse or home care aide. Contact with the health care team is needed for follow-up and identification of potential problems. The patient taking corticosteroid therapy may have manifestations of adrenal insufficiency if the dosage is inadequate. Suggest that the patient obtain and wear a medical alert bracelet listing the condition and the drug replacement therapy.

Chart 65-13 PATIENT AND FAMILY EDUCATION GUIDE
Cortisol Replacement Therapy

- Take your medication in divided doses—the first dose in the morning and the second dose between 4 and 6 PM.
- Take your medication with meals or snacks.
- Weigh yourself daily.
- Increase your dosage as directed for increased physical stress or severe emotional stress, including surgery, dental work, influenza, fever, pregnancy, and family problems.
- Never skip a dose of medication. If you have persistent vomiting or severe diarrhea and cannot take your medication by mouth for 24 to 36 hours, call your physician. If you cannot reach your physician, go to the nearest emergency department. You may need an injection to take the place of your usual oral medication.
- Always wear your medical alert bracelet or necklace.
- Make regular visits for health care follow-up.
- Learn how to give yourself an intramuscular injection of hydrocortisone.

Evaluation: Outcomes

Evaluate the care of the patient with hypercortisolism on the basis of the identified nursing diagnoses and collaborative problems. The expected outcomes are that the patient should:

- Have an acceptable fluid balance
- Remain free from injury
- Remain free from infection
- Not experience acute adrenal insufficiency

Specific indicators for these outcomes are listed for each nursing diagnosis and collaborative problem under the Planning and Implementation section (see earlier).

HYPERALDOSTERONISM
Pathophysiology

In patients with hyperaldosteronism, increased secretion of aldosterone results in mineralocorticoid excess. Primary hyperaldosteronism (Conn's syndrome) results from excessive secretion of aldosterone from one or both adrenal glands. Usually, this is caused by a benign adrenal tumor (adrenal adenoma). In a person with secondary hyperaldosteronism, the excessive secretion of aldosterone is caused by high levels of angiotensin II that are stimulated by high plasma renin levels. Causes of high renin levels include renal hypoxemia and the use of thiazide diuretics.

Increased aldosterone levels affect the renal tubules and cause sodium retention with potassium and hydrogen ion excretion. Hypernatremia, hypokalemia, and metabolic alkalosis result. Sodium retention increases blood volume, which raises blood pressure and suppresses renin production. The elevated blood pressure may cause strokes and kidney damage. Peripheral edema rarely occurs because of the "renal escape mechanism," in which the kidney decreases sodium reabsorption. However, no compensatory mechanism exists to stop or reverse potassium loss. (See Chapter 13 for discussion of electrolyte imbalances.)

Patient-Centered Collaborative Care

Assessment

Problems from hypokalemia and elevated blood pressure are the most common issues of the patient with hyperaldosteronism. He or she may have headache, fatigue, muscle weakness, **nocturia** (excessive urination at night), and loss of stamina. **Polydipsia** (excessive fluid intake) and **polyuria** (excessive urine output) occur less frequently. **Paresthesias** (sensations of numbness and tingling) may occur if potassium depletion is severe. The patient may have visual changes related to hypertension.

The diagnosis of hyperaldosteronism is made on the basis of laboratory studies, x-rays, and imaging with CT or MRI. Serum potassium levels are decreased, and sodium levels are elevated. Plasma renin levels are low, and aldosterone levels are high. Increased hydrogen ion loss leads to metabolic alkalemia (elevated blood pH). Urine has a low specific gravity and high aldosterone levels.

Interventions

Surgery is the most common treatment for early-stage hyperaldosteronism. One or both adrenal glands may be removed. Surgery is not performed, however, until the patient's potassium levels are normal. Drugs used to increase potassium levels include spironolactone (Aldactone, Spirono, Sincomen♣), a potassium-sparing diuretic and aldosterone antagonist. Potassium supplements may be prescribed to increase potassium levels before surgery. The patient may also benefit from a low-sodium diet before surgery, but sodium restriction is not needed after surgery because aldosterone levels should return to normal.

The patient who has undergone a unilateral adrenalectomy may need temporary glucocorticoid replacement. Replacement is lifelong if both adrenal glands are removed. Glucocorticoids are given before surgery to prevent adrenal crisis. The patient receiving long-term replacement therapy should wear a medical alert bracelet. (See the discussion of adrenalectomy on p. 1443 in the Hypercortisolism [Cushing's syndrome] section for more discussion of care after surgery and patient education.)

When surgery cannot be performed, spironolactone therapy is continued to control hypokalemia and hypertension. *Because spironolactone is a potassium-sparing diuretic, hyperkalemia can occur in patients who have impaired kidney function or excessive potassium intake.* Advise the patient to avoid potassium supplements and foods rich in potassium. Hyponatremia can occur with spironolactone therapy, and the patient may need increased dietary sodium. Instruct the patient to report symptoms of hyponatremia, such as dryness of the mouth, thirst, lethargy, or drowsiness. Teach patients to report any additional side effects of spironolactone therapy, including gynecomastia, diarrhea, drowsiness, headache, rash, **urticaria** (hives), confusion, erectile dysfunction, hirsutism, and amenorrhea.

PHEOCHROMOCYTOMA

Pathophysiology

Pheochromocytoma is a catecholamine-producing tumor that arises in the adrenal medulla. These tumors usually occur as a single lesion in one adrenal gland, although they can be bilateral or in the abdomen. Pheochromocytomas are usually benign, but at least 10% are malignant (Young, 2008).

The tumors produce, store, and release epinephrine and norepinephrine (NE). Excessive epinephrine and NE stimulate adrenergic receptors and can have wide-ranging adverse effects mimicking the action of the sympathetic division of the autonomic nervous system.

The cause is unknown but some pheochromocytomas occur with inherited disorders such as neurofibromatosis and multiple endocrine neoplasia (MEN) syndromes. These tumors are rare and occur slightly more often in women. They can occur at any age but appear most commonly in patients between 40 and 60 years of age.

Patient-Centered Collaborative Care

Assessment

The patient often has intermittent episodes of hypertension or attacks that vary in length from a few minutes to several hours. During these episodes, the patient has severe headaches, palpitations, profuse diaphoresis, flushing, apprehension, or a sense of impending doom. Pain in the chest or abdomen, with nausea and vomiting, can also occur. Increased abdominal pressure, defecation, and vigorous abdominal palpation can provoke a hypertensive crisis. Drugs such as tricyclic antidepressants, droperidol, glucagon, metoclopramide, phenothiazines, and naloxone can induce a hypertensive crisis in the patient with pheochromocytoma. Foods or beverages high in tyramine (e.g., aged cheese, red wine) also induce hypertension. The patient may also report heat intolerance, weight loss, and tremors.

The most common diagnostic test is a 24-hour urine collection for vanillylmandelic acid (VMA) (a product of catecholamine metabolism), metanephrine, and catecholamines, all of which are elevated in the presence of a pheochromocytoma. Other tests that may be conducted when catecholamine levels are not consistent include the clonidine suppression test and, rarely, stimulation testing. MRI or CT scans can precisely locate tumors in the adrenal gland. After diagnosis, CT scans of the chest and abdomen may be used to locate any other tumors.

Interventions

Surgery is the main treatment for a pheochromocytoma. One or both adrenal glands are removed (depending on whether the tumor is bilateral). After surgery, focus on promoting adequate tissue perfusion, nutritional needs, and comfort measures.

Hypertension is the hallmark of the disease and the most common serious complication after surgery (Daub, 2007). Monitor the blood pressure regularly, and place the cuff consistently on the same arm, with the patient in lying and standing positions. Identify stressors that may lead to a hypertensive crisis, and attempt to reduce them. Teach the patient to not smoke, drink caffeine-containing beverages, or change position suddenly. *Do not palpate the abdomen because this action could cause a sudden release of catecholamines and severe hypertension.* Provide a diet rich in calories, vitamins, and minerals.

The patient often benefits from hydration before surgery because decreased blood volume increases the risk for hypotension during and after surgery. Assess the patient's hydration status, and report manifestations of dehydration or fluid overload.

Provide a calm, restful environment for the patient who has a severe headache. Instruct the patient to limit activity. A private, darkened room helps promote rest. If the patient is sleeping, avoid interruptions if possible.

The patient's blood pressure is stabilized with adrenergic blocking agents such as phenoxybenzamine (Dibenzyline) starting several weeks before surgery because of the increased risk for severe hypertension during surgery (Tsegay et al., 2008). The drug dosages are adjusted for 2 to 3 weeks before surgery until blood pressure is controlled and hypertensive attacks do not occur. The blood volume expands, and blood pressure in the supine position returns to normal.

Anesthetic agents and touching of the tumor during surgery can cause a catecholamine release. Short-acting alpha-adrenergic blockers are given by IV bolus or drip for a hypertensive crisis.

Nursing care after surgery is similar to that for the patient who has undergone an adrenalectomy (see Hypercortisolism [Cushing's Syndrome], p. 1443). Closely monitor the patient for hypertension and for hypotension (from the sudden decrease in catecholamine levels) and for hypovolemia. Hemorrhage and shock are possible, and plasma expanders or fluids may be needed. Monitor vital signs, as well as fluid intake and output. If opioids are given, check for their effect on blood pressure.

Tumors may be inoperable because of the patient's other medical conditions. Treatment then is medical, with alpha-adrenergic and beta-adrenergic blocking agents, because the tumors do not respond well to chemotherapy or radiation therapy. For patients who are medically managed, self-measurement of blood pressure with home monitoring equipment is essential. (See Chapter 38 for teaching priorities and community-based care of the patient with chronic hypertension.)

GET READY FOR THE NCLEX EXAMINATION!

Key Points

Review these Key Points for each NCLEX Examination Client Needs Category.

Safe and Effective Care Environment

- Handle all patients with bone density loss carefully, using lift sheets whenever possible.
- Use good handwashing techniques before providing any care to a patient who is immunosuppressed.

Health Promotion and Maintenance

- Instruct patients with adrenal insufficiency to wear a medical alert bracelet and to carry simple carbohydrates with them at all times.
- Teach the patient and family about the clinical manifestations of infection and when to seek medical advice.
- Teach patients who have permanent endocrine hypofunction the proper techniques and timing of hormone replacement therapy.
- Teach patients with diabetes insipidus the proper way to self-administer desmopressin orally or by nasal spray.

Psychosocial Integrity

- Encourage the patient and family to express their feelings and concerns about a change in health status.
- Explain all diagnostic and treatment procedures, restrictions, and follow-up care to the patient scheduled for tests or procedures.
- Allow patients who experience a change in physical appearance to mourn this change.

Physiological Integrity

- Ensure that hormone replacement drugs are given as close to the prescribed times as possible.
- Use Infection Precautions for patients who are immunosuppressed.
- During the immediate period after a transsphenoidal hypophysectomy, teach the patient to avoid activities that increase intracranial pressure (e.g., bending at the waist, straining to have a bowel movement, coughing).
- Measure intake and output accurately on patients who have either diabetes insipidus or syndrome of inappropriate antidiuretic hormone (SIADH).
- Teach the patient with diabetes insipidus the manifestations of dehydration.
- Do not palpate the abdomen of a patient who has a pheochromocytoma.

Additional Study Resources

Go to your Companion CD or Evolve at http://evolve.elsevier.com/Iggy/ for *Self-Assessment Questions for the NCLEX Examination.*

Go to Evolve at http://evolve.elsevier.com/Iggy/ for *Prioritization and Delegation Questions for the NCLEX Examination.*

SELECTED BIBLIOGRAPHY

Bouillon, R. (2006). Acute adrenal insufficiency. *Endocrinology and Metabolism Clinics of North America, 35*(4), 767-775.

Daub, K. (2007). Pheochromocytoma: Challenges in diagnosis and nursing care. *Nursing Clinics of North America, 42*(1), 101-111.

Ezell, J. (2006). What is secondary adrenal insufficiency? *Nursing2006, 36*(5), 12.

Hanberg, A. (2005). Common disorders of the pituitary gland: Hyposecretion versus hypersecretion. *Journal of Infusion Nursing, 28*(1), 36-44.

Holcomb, S. (2005). Confronting Cushing's syndrome. *Nursing2005, 35*(9), 32hn1-32hn6.

Holcomb, S. (2006). Do the clues add up to Addison's disease? *Nursing2006, 36*(3), 64hn1-64hn4.

Johnson, K., & Renn, C. (2006). The hypothalamic-pituitary-adrenal axis in critical illness. *AACN Clinical Issues, 17*(1), 39-49.

McCance, K., & Huether, S. (2006). *Pathophysiology: The biologic basis for disease in adults and children* (5th ed.). St. Louis: Mosby.

Melmed, S. (2006). Medical progress: Acromegaly. *New England Journal of Medicine, 335*(24), 2558-2573.

Melmed, S., & Kleinberg, D. (2008). Anterior pituitary. In H. Kronenberg, S. Melmed, K. Polonsky, & P.R. Larsen (Eds.), *Williams' textbook of endocrinology* (11th ed., pp. 155-261). Philadelphia: Saunders.

Pagana, K., & Pagana, T. (2006). *Mosby's manual of diagnostic and laboratory tests* (3rd ed.). St. Louis: Mosby.

Quillen, T. (2006). Myths & facts about multiple endocrine neoplasia type 1. *Nursing2006, 36*(5), 31.

Robinson, A., & Verbalis, J. (2008). Posterior pituitary. In H. Kronenberg, S. Melmed, K. Polonsky, & P.R. Larsen (Eds.), *Williams' textbook of endocrinology* (11th ed., pp. 263-295). Philadelphia: Saunders.

Rottmann, C. (2007). SSRIs and the syndrome of inappropriate antidiuretic hormone secretion. *AJN, 107*(1), 51-58.

Stewart, P. (2008). The adrenal cortex. In H. Kronenberg, S. Melmed, K. Polonsky, & P.R. Larsen (Eds.), *Williams' textbook of endocrinology* (11th ed., pp. 445-503). Philadelphia: Saunders.

Tsegay, E., Anyango, G., Van Sell, S.L., & Miller-Anderson, M. (2008). Pheochromocytoma: A rare tumor in adults and children. *RN, 71*(6), 31-34.

Whittman, K. (2006). ACTH stimulation: Testing the adrenals. *Nursing2006, 36*(7), 24-25.

Young, W. (2008). Endocrine hypertension. In H. Kronenberg, S. Melmed, K. Polonsky, & P.R. Larsen (Eds.), *Williams' textbook of endocrinology* (11th ed., pp. 505-537). Philadelphia: Saunders.

66

CHAPTER

Care of Patients with Problems of the Thyroid and Parathyroid Glands

M. Linda Workman

LEARNING OUTCOMES

For clinical competence and success on the NCLEX Examination, study this chapter with these Learning Outcomes in mind:

Safe and Effective Care Environment

1. Adjust the environment for the patient with severe hypothyroidism or thyrotoxicosis.
2. Ensure the availability of suction and emergency intubation equipment for anyone who has thyroid or parathyroid surgery.
3. Prevent injury in the patient who has bone density loss or hypocalcemia.

Health Promotion and Maintenance

4. Teach patients taking thyroid hormone inhibitors the correct timing of therapy along with the side effects, adverse effects, and when to seek medical assistance.

Psychosocial Integrity

5. Be accepting of patient behavior.
6. Inform patients and family members that changes in cognition and behavior resulting from thyroid problems are usually temporary.

Physiological Integrity

7. Compare the common clinical manifestations of hyperthyroidism with those of hypothyroidism.
8. Interpret clinical changes and laboratory data to determine the effectiveness of interventions for hyperthyroidism.
9. Coordinate nursing care for the patient during the first 24 hours after thyroid or parathyroid surgery.
10. Identify teaching priorities for the patient taking thyroid hormone replacement therapy.
11. Compare the clinical manifestations of hyperparathyroidism with those of hypoparathyroidism.

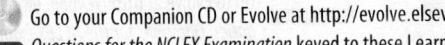

Go to your Companion CD or Evolve at http://evolve.elsevier.com/Iggy/ for *Self-Assessment Questions for the NCLEX Examination* keyed to these Learning Outcomes.

Hormones from the thyroid and parathyroid glands affect overall metabolism, electrolyte balance, and excitable membrane activity. Therefore problems of either thyroid or parathyroid function usually have widespread effects and manifestations. With mild disturbances, the problems are subtle. With more severe disturbances, the problems may be life threatening.

THYROID DISORDERS

HYPERTHYROIDISM

Pathophysiology

Hyperthyroidism is excessive thyroid hormone secretion from the thyroid gland. The manifestations of hyperthyroidism are called **thyrotoxicosis,** regardless of the origin of the thyroid hormones (Davies & Larsen, 2008). (For example, a person who takes a large amount of synthetic thyroid hormones can have thyrotoxicosis but does not have hyperthyroidism.) Thyroid hormones affect metabolism in all body organs. Thus excesses produce many different manifestations. Hyperthyroidism can be temporary or permanent, depending on the cause.

In hyperthyroidism, the normal feedback control over thyroid hormone secretion fails. The excessive thyroid hormones stimulate most body systems, causing hypermetabolism and increased sympathetic nervous system activity (Noble, 2006). Many of the manifestations are caused by the body's response to the demands of hypermetabolism (Chart 66-1).

Thyroid hormones directly stimulate the heart. The resulting increased heart rate and stroke volume cause increased cardiac output, increased systolic blood pressure, and increased blood flow.

Chart 66-1 KEY FEATURES

Hyperthyroidism

SKIN MANIFESTATIONS
- Diaphoresis (excessive sweating)
- Fine, soft, silky hair (body)
- Smooth, warm, moist skin
- Thinning of scalp hair

PULMONARY MANIFESTATIONS
- Shortness of breath with or without exertion
- Rapid, shallow respirations
- Decreased vital capacity

CARDIOVASCULAR MANIFESTATIONS
- Palpitations
- Chest pain
- Increased systolic blood pressure
- Widened pulse pressure
- Tachycardia
- Dysrhythmias

GASTROINTESTINAL MANIFESTATIONS
- Weight loss
- Increased appetite
- Increased stools
- Hypoproteinemia

MUSCULOSKELETAL MANIFESTATIONS
- Muscle weakness
- Muscle wasting

NEUROLOGIC MANIFESTATIONS
- Blurred or double vision
- Eye fatigue
- Corneal ulcers or infections
- Increased tears
- Injected (red) conjunctiva
- Photophobia
- Eyelid retraction, eyelid lag*
- Globe lag*
- Hyperactive deep tendon reflexes
- Tremors
- Insomnia

METABOLIC MANIFESTATIONS
- Increased basal metabolic rate
- Heat intolerance
- Low-grade fever
- Fatigue

PSYCHOLOGICAL/EMOTIONAL MANIFESTATIONS
- Decreased attention span
- Restlessness
- Irritability
- Emotional lability
- Manic behavior

REPRODUCTIVE MANIFESTATIONS
- Amenorrhea
- Decreased menstrual flow
- Increased libido

OTHER MANIFESTATIONS
- Goiter
- Wide-eyed (startled) appearance*
- Decreased total white blood cell count
- Enlarged spleen

*Present in Graves' disease only.

Elevated thyroid hormone levels affect protein, lipid, and carbohydrate metabolism. Protein **synthesis** (buildup) and **degradation** (breakdown) are increased. Breakdown exceeds buildup, causing a net loss of body protein known as a **negative nitrogen balance.** Glucose tolerance is decreased, and the patient has **hyperglycemia** (elevated blood glucose levels). Fat metabolism is increased, and body fat decreases. Although the patient has an increased appetite, food intake does not meet energy demands and the patient loses weight. With prolonged hyperthyroidism, the patient has chronic nutritional deficiency.

Thyroid hormones are produced in response to the stimulation hormones secreted by the hypothalamus and anterior pituitary glands. Thus oversecretion of thyroid hormones changes the secretion of hormones from the hypothalamus and anterior pituitary gland through negative feedback (see Chapter 64). In addition, thyroid hormones have some influence over sex hormone production in both men and women. Women have menstrual problems and decreased fertility. Both men and women with hyperthyroidism have an increased **libido** (sexual urge or interest).

Etiology and Genetic Risk

Hyperthyroidism has many causes, the most common cause of which is **Graves' disease,** also called *toxic diffuse goiter.* The patient with Graves' disease usually has thyrotoxicosis, a **goiter** (enlargement of the thyroid gland), **exophthalmos** (abnormal protrusion of the eyes), and **pretibial myxedema** (dry, waxy swelling of the front surfaces of the lower legs). *Not all patients with a goiter have hyperthyroidism.*

Graves' disease is an autoimmune disorder in which antibodies are made and attach to the thyroid stimulating hormone (TSH) receptor sites on the thyroid tissue. When these antibodies, known as *thyroid-stimulating immunoglobulins (TSIs),* bind to the thyroid gland, the gland increases in size and overproduces thyroid hormones.

Hyperthyroidism caused by multiple thyroid nodules is termed **toxic multinodular goiter.** The nodules may be enlarged thyroid tissues or benign tumors (adenomas). These patients usually have had a goiter for years. The overproduction of thyroid hormones is usually milder than that seen in Graves' disease, and the patient does not have exophthalmos or pretibial edema.

Hyperthyroidism also can be caused by excessive use of thyroid replacement hormones. This type of problem is called **exogenous hyperthyroidism.**

A condition called *thyroid storm* or *thyroid crisis* can occur when hyperthyroidism is untreated or poorly controlled or when the patient is severely stressed. This condition is an extreme state of hyperthyroidism in which all manifestations are more severe and life threatening. It is most common in patients who have Graves' disease (Nayak & Burman, 2006).

GENETIC CONSIDERATIONS

Graves' disease appears to have a strong association with other autoimmune disorders, such as diabetes mellitus, vitiligo, and rheumatoid arthritis. In addition, it often occurs in both members of identical twins, with an inheritance pattern of familial clustering or complex. These facts, together with a higher incidence among women, indicate the predisposition is most likely polygenic (Nussbaum et al., 2007).

Incidence/Prevalence

Hyperthyroidism is a common endocrine disorder. Graves' disease can occur at any age but is diagnosed most often in women between 20 and 40 years of age, affecting women about ten times more often than men (Davies & Larsen, 2008). Toxic multinodular goiter usually occurs after the age of 50 and affects women four times as often as men.

Patient-Centered Collaborative Care

▪ *Assessment*

History

The patient may have noticed many changes and problems because hyperthyroidism affects all body systems, although changes may occur over such a long period that not all patients are aware of them. Record age, gender, and usual weight. The patient may report a recent unplanned weight loss, an increased appetite, and an increase in the number of bowel movements per day.

A hallmark of hyperthyroidism is heat intolerance. The patient may have **diaphoresis** (increased sweating) even when environmental temperatures are comfortable for others. He or she often wears lighter clothing in cold weather. The patient may also report palpitations or chest pain as a result of the cardiovascular effects. Ask about changes in breathing patterns because dyspnea (with or without exertion) is common.

Visual changes may be the earliest problem the patient notices, especially exophthalmos, with Graves' disease (Fig. 66-1). Ask about changes in vision, such as blurring or double vision and tiring of the eyes.

Ask whether he or she has noticed a change in energy level or in the ability to perform ADLs. Fatigue, weakness, and insomnia are common. Family and friends may report that the patient has become irritable or depressed.

Ask women about changes in menses because amenorrhea or a decreased menstrual flow is common. Initially, both men and women may have an increase in libido, but this changes as the patient becomes more fatigued.

Explore the patient's medical history. Previous thyroid surgery or radiation therapy to the neck is important because some people remain hyperthyroid after surgery or are resistant to radiation therapy. Ask about past and current drugs, especially the use of thyroid hormone replacement or antithyroid drugs.

Physical Assessment/Clinical Manifestations

Exophthalmos is common in patients with Graves' disease. The wide-eyed or "startled" look is due to edema in the extraocular muscles and increased fatty tissue behind the eye, which pushes the eyeball forward. Pressure on the optic nerve may impair vision. Swelling and shortening of the muscles may cause problems with focusing. If the eyelid fails to close completely and the eye is unprotected, the eye may become overly dry and develop corneal ulcers or infection. Observe the patient's eyes for excessive tearing and a bloodshot appearance, and ask about sensitivity to light **(photophobia).**

Observe the patient's general appearance. In addition to the exophthalmos of Graves' disease, two other eye problems are common in all types of hyperthyroidism: eyelid retraction (eyelid lag) and globe (eyeball) lag. In eyelid lag, the upper eyelid fails to descend when the patient gazes slowly downward. In globe lag, the upper eyelid pulls back faster than the eyeball when the patient gazes upward. During assessment, ask the patient to look down and then up and document the response.

Observe the size and symmetry of the thyroid gland. Palpate the thyroid gland to assess the presence of a mass or general enlargement. In goiter, a generalized thyroid enlargement, the thyroid gland may increase to four times its normal size (Fig. 66-2). Goiters are common in Graves's disease (Weeks, 2005) and are classified by size (Table 66-1). Bruits (turbulence from increased blood flow) may be heard with a stethoscope. (See Chapter 64 for a discussion of thyroid palpation and auscultation.)

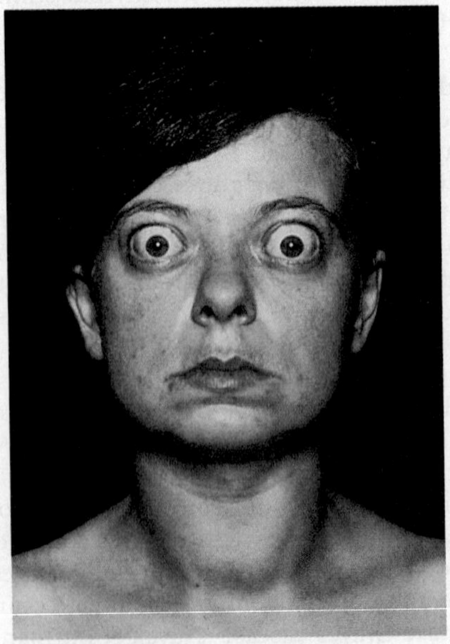

Fig. 66-1 • Exophthalmos.

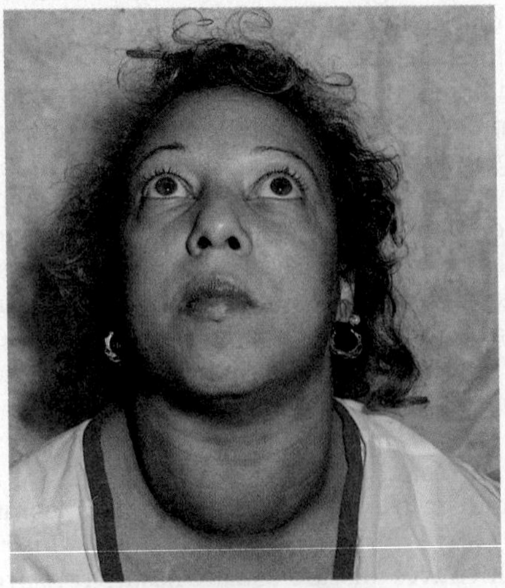

Fig. 66-2 • Goiter.

The cardiac problems of hyperthyroidism include increased systolic blood pressure, tachycardia, and dysrhythmias. Usually the diastolic pressure is decreased, causing a widened pulse pressure.

Inspect the patient's hair and skin. Fine, soft, silky hair and smooth, warm, moist skin are common with hyperthyroidism. The patient may have muscle weakness, hyperactive deep tendon reflexes, or tremors. Observe gross motor movements for tremors, especially of the hands. He or she may appear extremely restless, irritable, and fatigued.

TABLE 66-1 Goiter Classification

Goiter Grade	Description
0	No palpable or visible goiter.
1	Mass is not visible with neck in the normal position. Goiter can be palpated and moves up when the patient swallows.
2	Mass is visible as swelling when the neck is in the normal position. Goiter is easily palpated and is usually asymmetric.

Psychosocial Assessment

The patient with hyperthyroidism often has wide mood swings, irritability, decreased attention span, and manic behavior. Mild to severe hyperactivity often leads to fatigue because of the inability to sleep well. Some patients describe their activity as having two modes—either "full speed ahead" or "completely stopped." Ask the patient whether he or she has been crying or laughing inappropriately or has had difficulty concentrating. Family members often report these changes in mental or emotional status.

Laboratory Assessment

Testing for hyperthyroidism includes measurement of the following blood values: triiodothyronine (T_3), thyroxine (T_4), T_3 resin uptake (T_3RU), and thyroid-stimulating hormone (TSH). Antibodies to TSH (TSH-RAb) are measured to determine the presence of Graves' disease. The most common changes in laboratory tests for Graves' disease and other forms of hyperthyroidism are listed in Chart 66-2.

Other Diagnostic Assessment

Thyroid scan evaluates the position, size, and functioning of the thyroid gland. Radioactive iodine (RAI [^{123}I]) is given by mouth, and the uptake of iodine by the thyroid gland (RAIU) is measured. The half-life of ^{123}I is short, and radiation precau-

Chart 66-2 LABORATORY PROFILE

Thyroid Function

		SIGNIFICANCE OF ABNORMAL FINDINGS	
Test	Normal Range for Adults	Hyperthyroidism	Hypothyroidism
Serum T_3	70-205 ng/dL, or 1.2-3.4 SI units	Increased	Decreased
Serum T_4	4-12 mcg/dL, or 51-154 SI units	Increased	Decreased
Free T_4 index	0.8-2.4 ng/dL, or 10-31 SI units	Increased	Decreased
T_3 resin uptake	24%-34% (varies with different laboratories)	Increased	Decreased
TRH stimulation test	Doubling of baseline TSH 30 min after IV injection of 500 mcg TRH (women have greater response)	Little or no TSH response	Delayed or poor TSH response in secondary hypothyroidism (pituitary failure) Elevated two or more times the normal in primary hypothyroidism (thyroid gland failure)
Thyroid suppression test	N/A	Fails to suppress RAIU or T_4 levels	No change in RAIU or T_4 levels
TSH stimulation test (thyroid stimulation test)	>10% in RAIU or >1.5 mcg/dL	N/A (test differentiates primary from secondary hypothyroidism)	No response in primary hypothyroidism Normal response in secondary hypothyroidism
Thyroid antibodies (antithyroglobulin antibody)	Titer <1:100	High titer of antithyroglobulin antibodies	Increased titers
Thyrotropin receptor antibodies (TSH-RAb)	Titer <130% of basal activity	High titers indicate Graves' disease	No response
TSH	2-10 μU/mL or 2-10 SI units	Low in Graves' disease High in secondary or tertiary hyperthyroidism	High in primary disease Low in secondary or tertiary disease

N/A, Not applicable; *RAIU*, radioactive iodine uptake; *SI*, International System of Units; *T_3*, triiodothyronine; *T_4*, thyroxine; *TRH*, thyrotropin-releasing hormone; *TSH*, thyroid-stimulating hormone.

tions are not needed. Pregnancy, however, should be ruled out before the scan is performed.

Normally the thyroid has an uptake of 5% to 35% of the given dose when measured at 24 hours. RAIU is increased in patients with hyperthyroidism.

Assess whether the patient has undergone procedures or has taken drugs that might affect the results of the scan. Procedures that use iodine-containing dye (e.g., renography) should not be performed for at least 4 weeks before a thyroid scan is done. Any drug that contains iodine should be discontinued for 1 week before the scan.

Ultrasonography of the thyroid gland can determine its size and the general composition of any masses or nodules. This procedure takes about 30 minutes to perform. Reassure the patient that it is painless.

Electrocardiography (ECG) usually shows tachycardia. Other ECG changes with hyperthyroidism include atrial fibrillation, dysrhythmias, and changes in P and T waveforms.

DECISION-MAKING CHALLENGE
Coordination of Care

The patient is a 43-year-old woman who is scheduled to have a hysterectomy later today. During her preadmission testing, her vital signs are T = 100, P = 88 with several "skipped" beats, R = 20, BP = 160/98. She is 5′6″ and weighs 110 lbs. Her current drugs are metoprolol (Toprol) 50 mg orally daily for hypertension and aspirin 81 mg daily. The reason for her surgery is several large fibroid tumors that are causing pain and heavy uterine bleeding. She states that she has no other health problems. When you ask her about her hypertension, she shouts that her blood pressure problem is being managed and that you should focus on her impending surgery. Then she apologizes for her behavior and says that she has not been sleeping well lately, probably because of worrying about the scheduled surgery.

1. What additional physical assessment data should you obtain?
2. Are any of her vital signs of concern before this surgery? If so, which ones and why?
3. What additional assessment questions should you ask?
4. How should you respond to her apology?

evolve For suggested answer guidelines, go to http://evolve.elsevier.com/Iggy/.

Common Nursing Diagnoses and Collaborative Problems

Nursing diagnoses and collaborative problems that may apply to the patient with hyperthyroidism include:

- Imbalanced Nutrition: Less Than Body Requirements related to inadequate intake in relation to metabolic needs
- Hyperthermia related to increased metabolic rate
- Fatigue related to sleep deprivation
- Potential for Hypertension and Cardiac Failure

Interventions

Because Graves' disease is the most common form of hyperthyroidism, the interventions discussed in the following sections include those specific for the problems that occur with Graves' disease. The goals of medical management are to decrease the effect of thyroid hormone on cardiac function and to reduce thyroid hormone secretion. The priorities for nursing care focus on monitoring for complications, reducing stimulation, promoting comfort, and teaching the patient and family about therapeutic drugs and procedures.

Nonsurgical Management

Monitoring includes measuring the patient's apical pulse, BP, and temperature at least every 4 hours. Instruct the patient to report immediately any palpitations, dyspnea, vertigo, or chest pain. Increases in temperature may indicate a rapid worsening of the patient's condition and the onset of "thyroid storm." *Immediately report a temperature increase of even one degree Fahrenheit.* If this task is delegated to UAP, instruct them to report the patient's temperature to you as soon as it has been obtained. If a temperature elevation is reported by UAP, immediately assess the patient's cardiac status. If the patient has a cardiac monitor, check for dysrhythmias.

Reducing stimulation is important because a noisy or stressful environment can increase the manifestations of hyperthyroidism and increase the risk for cardiac complications. Encourage the patient to rest. Keep the environment as quiet as possible by closing the door to his or her room, limiting visitors, and eliminating or postponing nonessential care or treatments.

Promoting comfort can be accomplished through actions such as reducing the room temperature to decrease discomfort caused by heat intolerance. Instruct UAP to ensure the patient always has a fresh pitcher of ice water and to change the bed linen whenever it becomes damp from diaphoresis. Suggest that the patient take a cool shower several times each day. If showering is not possible, cool sponge baths may increase comfort.

Drug therapy with antithyroid drugs is the initial treatment of hyperthyroidism. Chart 66-3 lists teaching priorities for the patient receiving drug therapy for hyperthyroidism. The preferred drugs are the thionamides, which include propylthiouracil (PTU) and methimazole (Tapazole). These drugs block thyroid hormone production by preventing iodide binding in the thyroid gland (see Chart 66-3). In addition, PTU also prevents T_4 from being converted to the more powerful T_3 in the tissues. For this reason, PTU is preferred over methimazole (Davies & Larsen, 2008). However, methimazole doses are lower than PTU doses. The response to these drugs is delayed because the patient may have large amounts of stored thyroid hormones that continue to be released.

Iodine preparations may be used for short-term therapy before surgery. They decrease blood flow through the thyroid gland, reducing the production and release of thyroid hormone. Improvement usually occurs within 2 weeks, but weeks may be needed before metabolism returns to normal. This treatment can result in hypothyroidism, and the patient is monitored closely for the need to adjust the drug regimen.

Lithium also inhibits thyroid hormone release. However, its use is limited because of side effects such as depression, diabetes insipidus, tremors, nausea, and vomiting. Lithium may be used for a patient who cannot tolerate other antithyroid drugs (Nayak & Burman, 2006).

Beta-adrenergic blocking drugs, such as propranolol (Inderal, Detensol🍁) may be used as supportive therapy. These drugs relieve diaphoresis, anxiety, tachycardia, and palpitations but do not inhibit thyroid hormone production. See Chapters 36 and 40 for a discussion of the actions and nursing implications of these agents.

Radioactive iodine (RAI) therapy is not used in pregnant women because ^{131}I crosses the placenta and can damage the fetal thyroid gland. The patient with hyperthyroidism may receive RAI in the form of oral ^{131}I. The dosage depends on the thyroid gland's size and sensitivity to radiation. The thyroid gland picks up the RAI, and some of the cells that produce

Chart 66-3 COMMON EXAMPLES OF DRUG THERAPY*

Hyperthyroidism

Drug/Usual Dosage	Purpose/Action	Nursing Intervention	Rationale
FOR TREATMENT OF MILD TO MODERATE HYPERTHYROIDISM			
Propylthiouracil (PTU, Propyl-Thyracil🍁) Initial dose 100-150 mg orally every 8 hr Maintenance 50-150 mg orally every 8 hr	Reduces manifestations of hyperthyroidism by preventing the new formation of thyroid hormones by inhibiting thyroid binding of iodide and by preventing the conversion of T_4 to T_3 in the tissues.	Teach patient to take the drug every 8 hr.	Taking the drug evenly throughout the day results in better drug action.
		Teach patient to avoid crowds and people who are ill.	Drug reduces blood cell counts and the immune response, increasing the risk for infection.
		Teach patient to report darkening of the urine, a yellow appearance to the skin or whites of the eyes, and an increased tendency to bruise or bleed.	These manifestations may indicate liver toxicity or failure, a possible side effect of the drug.
		Teach patient to check for weight gain, slow heart rate, and cold intolerance.	These indicate hypothyroidism and may require a lower drug dose.
Methimazole (Northyx, Tapazole) Initial dose 5-20 mg orally every 8 hr Maintenance dose 1-4 mg orally every 8 hr	Reduces manifestations of hyperthyroidism by preventing the new formation of thyroid hormones by inhibiting thyroid binding of iodide.	Teach patient to take the drug every 8 hr.	Taking the drug evenly throughout the day results in better drug action.
		Remind women to notify their health care providers if they become pregnant.	This drug causes birth defects and should not be used during pregnancy.
		Teach patient to avoid crowds and people who are ill.	Drug reduces blood cell counts and the immune response, increasing the risk for infection.
		Teach patient to check for weight gain, slow heart rate, and cold intolerance.	These indicate hypothyroidism and may require a lower drug dose.
		Teach patient about the possibility of muscle and joint pain.	Knowing the side effects to expect reduces anxiety.
Lithium carbonate (Eskalith, Lithobid, Lithonate) 300 mg orally every 8 hr	Reduces the manifestations of hyperthyroidism by inhibiting the release of thyroid hormones (temporarily). Used only when the patient cannot take a thionamide.	Teach patient to take the drug every 8 hr.	Taking the drug evenly throughout the day results in better drug action.
		Teach patient to drink at least 3 to 4 quarts of fluids daily.	Drug increases urine output and can cause dehydration.
		Teach patient to check for weight gain, slow heart rate, and cold intolerance.	These indicate hypothyroidism and may require a lower drug dose.
FOR INITIAL TREATMENT OF SEVERE HYPERTHYROIDISM OR THYROTOXICOSIS			
Iodine and iodine-containing agents Lugol's solution Saturated solution of potassium iodide (SSKI) Dosages vary depending on the agent, how the drug is administered, and the severity of the manifestations	The sudden excess of iodine rapidly inhibits thyroid hormone release and dramatically (but temporarily) resolves the cardiac and other manifestations of hyperthyroidism. These agents are not recommended for long-term therapy.	Administer these drugs 1 hour *after* a thionamide has been given.	Initially, the iodine agents can cause an increase in the production of thyroid hormones. Giving a thionamide first prevents this initial increase in thyroid hormone production.
		Check patient for a fever or rash, and ask about a metallic taste, mouth sores, sore throat, or GI distress.	These are manifestations of *iodism*, a toxic effect of the drugs, and may require that the drug be discontinued.

* These drugs are the preferred therapy for hyperthyroidism.

thyroid hormone are destroyed by the local radiation. Because the thyroid gland stores thyroid hormones to some degree, the patient may not have complete symptom relief until 6 to 8 weeks after RAI therapy. Additional drug therapy for hyperthyroidism is still needed during the first few weeks after RAI treatment.

RAI therapy is performed on an outpatient basis. One dose may be sufficient, although some patients need a second or third dose. The radiation dose is low enough that radiation precautions are not needed. Reassure the patient that the radioactivity is quickly eliminated. The degree of thyroid destruction is variable. Some patients become hypothyroid as a result of treatment. This problem may occur within a few weeks, or it may take several years to develop. The patient then needs lifelong thyroid hormone replacement. All patients who have undergone RAI therapy should be monitored regularly for changes in thyroid function.

Surgical Management

Antithyroid drugs and RAI therapy are now the most common treatments for patients with hyperthyroidism. Surgery to remove all or part of the thyroid gland may be needed for patients who have a large goiter causing tracheal or esophageal compression or who do not have a good response to antithyroid drugs. Removal of all **(total thyroidectomy)** or part **(subtotal thyroidectomy)** of the thyroid tissue decreases the production of thyroid hormones. After a total thyroidectomy, patients must take lifelong thyroid hormone replacement.

Preoperative Care. If possible, the patient is treated with drug therapy first to have near-normal thyroid function **(euthyroid)** before thyroid surgery. This state is achieved with antithyroid drugs that decrease the secretion of thyroid hormones. In addition, iodine preparations are used to decrease thyroid size and vascularity, thereby reducing the risk for hemorrhage and the potential for thyroid storm during surgery.

Hypertension, dysrhythmias, and tachycardia must be controlled before surgery. The patient with hyperthyroidism is often not at an optimal weight and may need to follow a high-protein, high-carbohydrate diet for days or weeks before surgery.

Teach the patient to perform coughing and deep-breathing exercises. Stress the importance of supporting the neck when coughing or moving by placing both hands behind the neck. This action reduces the strain on the suture line. Explain that hoarseness may be present for a few days as a result of endotracheal tube placement during surgery.

Patients often fear thyroid surgery, perhaps because the incision is on the neck. Reassure the patient by calmly explaining the surgery and the care after surgery. Remind him or her that a drain as well as a dressing may be in place after surgery. Answer any questions the patient and family have.

Operative Procedures. A thyroidectomy is performed with the patient under general anesthesia. The patient's neck is extended, and the surgeon makes a "collar" incision just above the clavicle. The surgeon attempts to avoid the parathyroid glands and recurrent laryngeal nerves to reduce the risk for complications and injury.

With a subtotal thyroidectomy, the remaining thyroid tissues are sutured to the trachea. With a total thyroidectomy, the entire thyroid gland is removed but the parathyroid glands are left with an intact blood supply to prevent causing hypoparathyroidism.

Postoperative Care. *Monitoring the patient for complications is the most important nursing action after thyroid surgery.* Monitor vital signs every 15 minutes until the patient is stable and then every 30 minutes. Increase or decrease the monitoring of vital signs based on changes in the patient's condition.

Assess the patient's level of discomfort. Use sandbags or pillows to support the head and neck. Place the patient, while he or she is awake, in a semi-Fowler's position. When positioning the patient, decrease tension on the suture line by avoiding neck extension. Give prescribed drugs for pain control as needed.

Humidifying the air promotes easier respiration and thins respiratory secretions. Assist the patient to cough and deep-breathe every 30 minutes to 1 hour. Suction oral and tracheal secretions when necessary.

Thyroid surgery can cause hemorrhage, respiratory distress, parathyroid gland injury (resulting in **hypocalcemia** [low serum calcium levels] and **tetany** [hyperexcitability of nerves and muscles]), damage to the laryngeal nerves, and thyroid storm. Remain alert to the potential for complications, and identify manifestations early.

Hemorrhage is most likely to occur during the first 24 hours after surgery. Inspect the neck dressing and behind the patient's neck for blood. A drain may be present, and a moderate amount of serosanguineous drainage is normal. Hemorrhage may be seen as bleeding at the incision site or as respiratory distress caused by tracheal compression.

Respiratory distress can result from swelling, tetany, or damage to the laryngeal nerve, causing spasms. Laryngeal **stridor** (harsh, high-pitched respiratory sounds) is heard in acute respiratory obstruction. Keep emergency tracheostomy equipment in the patient's room. Check that oxygen and suctioning equipment are nearby and in working order. In some instances, nurses are instructed to remove clips or sutures when medical assistance is not immediately available and swelling at the surgical site is obstructing the airway.

Hypocalcemia and tetany may occur if the parathyroid glands are damaged or their blood supply is impaired during thyroid surgery. These problems result when parathyroid hormone (PTH) levels decrease. Ask the patient hourly about any tingling around the mouth or of the toes and fingers. Assess for muscle twitching as a sign of calcium deficiency. Calcium gluconate or calcium chloride for IV use should be available in an emergency situation. (For information on the later signs of hypocalcemia, see the discussion of postoperative care on p. 1463 in the Hyperparathyroidism section and p. 1463 in the Assessment discussion in the Hypoparathyroidism section. The care of patients with hypocalcemia is discussed also in Chapter 13.)

Laryngeal nerve damage may occur during surgery. This problem results in hoarseness and a weak voice. Assess the patient's voice at 2-hour intervals, and document any changes. Reassure the patient that hoarseness is usually temporary.

Thyroid storm or **thyroid crisis** is a life-threatening event that occurs in patients with uncontrolled hyperthyroidism and occurs most often with Graves' disease (Noble, 2006). Manifestations of crisis develop quickly. It is often triggered by stressors such as trauma, infection, diabetic ketoacidosis, and pregnancy. Other conditions that can lead to thyroid storm include vigorous palpation of the goiter, exposure to iodine, and radioactive iodine (RAI) therapy. Although thyroid storm after surgery is less common because patients receive antithyroid drugs, beta blockers, and iodides before thyroid surgery, it can still occur.

The manifestations of thyroid storm are caused by excessive thyroid hormone release, which dramatically increases metabolic rate. *Key manifestations include fever, tachycardia, and systolic hypertension.* The patient may have GI problems such as abdominal pain, nausea, vomiting, and diarrhea. Often he or she is very anxious and has tremors. As the crisis progresses, the patient may become restless, confused, or psychotic and may have seizures, leading to coma. *Even with treatment, thyroid storm may lead to death.*

Emergency measures to prevent death vary with the intensity and type of specific symptoms. After the cause has been identified, interventions focus on maintaining airway patency, providing adequate ventilation, reducing fever, and stabilizing the hemodynamic status. Chart 66-4 outlines the best practices for emergency management of thyroid storm.

Eye and vision problems of Graves' disease are not corrected by treatment for hyperthyroidism. Treatment of infiltrative ophthalmopathy is symptomatic. Teach the patient with mild symptoms to elevate the head of the bed at night and to use artificial tears. If **photophobia** (sensitivity to light) is present, dark glasses or eye patches are often helpful. For those who cannot close the eyelids completely, recommend gently taping the lids closed with nonallergenic tape at bedtime. These actions prevent irritation and injury. If pressure behind the eye continues and forces the eye forward, blood supply to the eye can be compromised, leading to ischemia and blindness.

In severe cases, short-term steroid therapy is prescribed to reduce swelling and halt the infiltrative process. Prednisone (Deltasone, Winpred♣) is given in high doses (often 120 mg daily) at first and then is tapered down according to the patient's response. Explain the need to reduce the prednisone gradually, and review its side effects with the patient.

Diuretics may be prescribed to decrease edema around the eye. Surgical intervention (orbital decompression) may be needed if loss of sight or damage to the eyeball is possible.

Health teaching includes reviewing with the patient and family the manifestations of hyperthyroidism and instructing the patient to report an increase or recurrence of symptoms.

Chart 66-4 BEST PRACTICE FOR PATIENT SAFETY & QUALITY CARE

Emergency Care of the Patient During Thyroid Storm

EMERGENCY CARE

- Maintain a patent airway and adequate ventilation.
- Give antithyroid drugs as prescribed: propylthiouracil (PTU, Propyl-Thyracil♣), 300 to 900 mg daily; methimazole (Tapazole), up to 60 mg daily.
- Administer sodium iodide solution, 2 g IV daily as prescribed.
- Give propranolol (Inderal, Detensol♣), 1 to 3 mg IV as prescribed. Give slowly over 3 minutes. The patient should be connected to a cardiac monitor, and a central venous pressure catheter should be in place.
- Give glucocorticoids as prescribed: hydrocortisone, 100 to 500 mg IV daily; prednisone, 4 to 60 mg IV daily; or dexamethasone, 2 mg IM every 6 hours.
- Monitor continually for cardiac dysrhythmias.
- Monitor vital signs every 30 minutes.
- Provide comfort measures, including a cooling blanket.
- Give non-salicylate antipyretics as prescribed.
- Correct dehydration with normal saline infusions.
- Apply cooling blanket or ice packs to reduce fever.

Also teach about the manifestations of hypothyroidism (discussed in the next section) and the need for thyroid hormone replacement. Reinforce the need for regular follow-up because hypothyroidism can occur several years after radioactive iodine therapy.

If the patient has had surgery, the surgeon usually removes the sutures on the third or fourth postoperative day. Teach the patient to inspect the incision area and to report redness, tenderness, drainage, or swelling to the surgeon.

The discharged patient may continue to have mood changes as a result of hyperthyroidism. Explain the reason for mood swings to the patient and family, and reassure them that these will decrease with continued treatment.

NCLEX EXAMINATION CHALLENGE

The client who is 12 hours postoperative from a total thyroidectomy has all of the manifestations listed below. For which one should the nurse notify the Rapid Response Team?

A. Inspiratory stridor
B. Blood pressure 180/120
C. Decreased deep tendon reflexes
D. Serosanguineous drainage on dressing

evolve For the correct answer, go to http://evolve.elsevier.com/Iggy/.

HYPOTHYROIDISM

Pathophysiology

The manifestations of hypothyroidism (Chart 66-5) are the result of decreased metabolism from low levels of thyroid hormones. Thyroid cells may fail to produce sufficient levels of thyroid hormones (THs) for several reasons. Sometimes the cells themselves are damaged and no longer function normally. At other times, the thyroid cells are functional but the person does not ingest enough of the substances needed to make thyroid hormones, especially iodide and tyrosine. When the production of thyroid hormones is too low or absent, the blood levels of TH are very low and the patient has a decreased metabolic rate. This lowered metabolism causes the hypothalamus and anterior pituitary gland to make stimulatory hormones, especially thyroid-stimulating hormone (TSH), in an attempt to trigger hormone release from the poorly responsive thyroid gland. The TSH binds to thyroid cells and causes the thyroid gland to enlarge, forming a goiter, although thyroid hormone production does not increase.

Most tissues and organs are affected by the low metabolic rate caused by hypothyroidism. Cellular energy is decreased, and metabolites build up. The metabolites are compounds of proteins and sugars called *glycosaminoglycans.* These compounds build up inside cells, which increases the mucus and water, forms cellular edema, and changes organ texture. The edema is mucinous (called **myxedema**) rather than edema caused by water alone (Fig. 66-3). This edema changes the patient's appearance. Nonpitting edema forms everywhere, especially around the eyes, in the hands and feet, and between the shoulder blades. The tongue thickens and edema forms in the larynx, making the voice husky. General physiologic function is decreased.

Myxedema coma is a rare, serious complication of untreated or poorly treated hypothyroidism. The decreased metabolism causes the heart muscle to become flabby and the chamber size to increase. The result is decreased cardiac output and decreased

Chart 66-5 KEY FEATURES
Hypothyroidism

SKIN MANIFESTATIONS
- Cool, pale or yellowish, dry, coarse, scaly skin
- Thick, brittle nails
- Dry, coarse, brittle hair
- Decreased hair growth, with loss of eyebrow hair
- Poor wound healing

PULMONARY MANIFESTATIONS
- Hypoventilation
- Pleural effusion
- Dyspnea

CARDIOVASCULAR MANIFESTATIONS
- Bradycardia
- Dysrhythmias
- Enlarged heart
- Decreased activity tolerance
- Hypotension

METABOLIC MANIFESTATIONS
- Decreased basal metabolic rate
- Decreased body temperature
- Cold intolerance

MUSCULOSKELETAL MANIFESTATIONS
- Muscle aches and pains
- Delayed contraction and relaxation of muscles

NEUROLOGIC MANIFESTATIONS
- Slowing of intellectual functions
  - Slowness or slurring of speech
  - Impaired memory
  - Inattentiveness
- Lethargy or somnolence
- Confusion
- Hearing loss
- Paresthesia (numbness and tingling) of the extremities
- Decreased tendon reflexes

PSYCHOLOGICAL/EMOTIONAL MANIFESTATIONS
- Apathy
- Depression
- Paranoia
- Withdrawal

GASTROINTESTINAL MANIFESTATIONS
- Anorexia
- Weight gain
- Constipation
- Abdominal distention

REPRODUCTIVE MANIFESTATIONS

WOMEN
- Changes in menses (amenorrhea or prolonged menstrual periods)
- Anovulation
- Decreased libido

MEN
- Decreased libido
- Impotence

OTHER MANIFESTATIONS
- Periorbital edema
- Facial puffiness
- Nonpitting edema of the hands and feet
- Hoarseness
- Goiter (enlarged thyroid gland)
- Thick tongue
- Increased sensitivity to opioids and tranquilizers
- Weakness, fatigue
- Decreased urine output
- Anemia
- Easy bruising
- Iron deficiency
- Folate deficiency
- Vitamin B_{12} deficiency

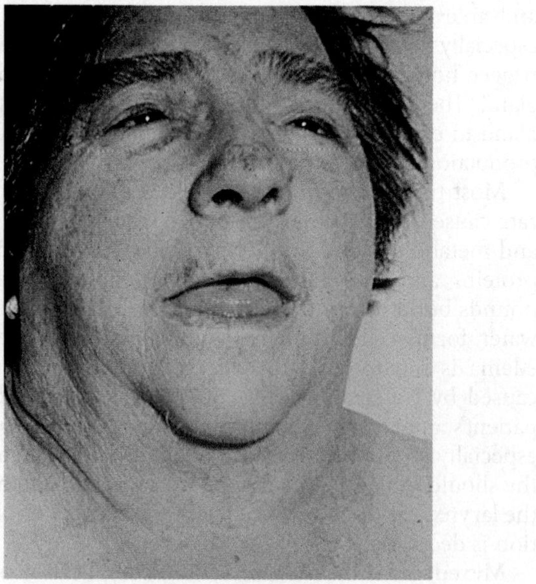

Fig. 66-3 • Myxedema.

perfusion to the brain and other vital organs. The decreased perfusion makes the already slowed cellular metabolism worse, resulting in tissue and organ failure. *The mortality rate for myxedema coma is extremely high, and this condition is considered a life-threatening emergency.* Myxedema coma can be caused by a variety of events, drugs, or conditions.

Etiology

Most cases of hypothyroidism in the United States occur as a result of thyroid surgery and radioactive iodine (RAI) treatment of hyperthyroidism. Worldwide, hypothyroidism is common in areas where the soil and water have little natural iodide, causing endemic goiter. (This problem was common in the midwest region of the United States before iodide was added to table salt and before saltwater fish was widely available.) Hypothyroidism is also caused by a variety of other conditions (Table 66-2).

Incidence/Prevalence

Hypothyroidism occurs most often in women between 30 and 60 years of age. Women are affected 7 to 10 times more often than men (Devdhar et al., 2007). An association exists between the development of hypothyroidism and diabetes mellitus. The incidence increases with age.

TABLE 66-2 Causes of Hypothyroidism

PRIMARY CAUSES
DECREASED THYROID TISSUE
• Surgical removal of the thyroid
• Radiation-induced thyroid destruction
• Autoimmune thyroid destruction
• Congenital thyroid agenesis
• Congenital thyroid hypoplasia
• Congenital thyroid dysgenesis
• Cancer (thyroidal or metastatic)
DECREASED SYNTHESIS OF THYROID HORMONE
• Endemic iodine deficiency
• Excessive exposure to iodine
• Drugs
• Lithium
• Phenylbutazone
• Propylthiouracil
• Sodium or potassium perchlorate
• Aminoglutethimide
SECONDARY CAUSES
INADEQUATE PRODUCTION OF THYROID-STIMULATING HORMONE
• Pituitary tumors, trauma, infections, or infarcts
• Congenital pituitary defects
• Hypothalamic tumors, trauma, infections, or infarcts

Patient-Centered Collaborative Care

evolve ONLINE PHARM REVIEW

Assessment

History

A decrease in thyroid hormones produces many manifestations related to decreased metabolism. However, changes may have occurred slowly, often over weeks or months, and the patient may not have noticed them. Ask him or her to compare activity now with that of a year ago. The patient often reports an increase in time spent sleeping, sometimes up to 14 to 16 hours daily. Generalized weakness, anorexia, muscle aches, and paresthesias may also be present. Constipation is common, as is cold intolerance. Ask whether more blankets at night or sweaters and extra clothing, even in warm weather, have been needed. Some of these changes may be subtle and missed because they are considered part of the aging process (Mauk, 2005).

Both men and women with hypothyroidism may report a decrease in libido. Women may have had difficulty becoming pregnant or have changes in menses (heavy, prolonged bleeding or amenorrhea). Men can have problems with impotence and infertility.

Ask the patient about current or previous use of drugs, such as lithium, amiodarone, aminoglutethimide, sodium or potassium perchlorate, thiocyanates, or cobalt. All these drugs can impair thyroid hormone production. Also determine whether the patient has ever been treated for hyperthyroidism and what specific treatment was used.

Physical Assessment/Clinical Manifestations

Observe the patient's overall appearance. Fig. 66-3 shows the typical appearance of an adult with hypothyroidism. Common changes include coarse features, edema around the eyes and face, a blank expression, and a thick tongue. The patient's overall muscle movement is slow. He or she may not speak clearly and may take a longer time to respond to questions.

Cardiac and respiratory functions are decreased. Heart rate may be below 60 beats per minute, and respiratory rate may be slower than normal. The patient's body temperature is often lower than 97° F.

Weight gain is very common, even when the person is ingesting an appropriate number of calories for size, age, and gender. Weigh the patient, and ask whether the result is the same or different than his or her weight a year ago.

Depending on the cause of hypothyroidism, the patient may have a goiter. However, some types of hypothyroidism do not induce a goiter and some types of hyperthyroidism do. Therefore the presence of a goiter suggests a thyroid problem but does not indicate whether the problem is excessive hormone secretion or too little hormone secretion.

Psychosocial Assessment

Hypothyroidism causes many problems in psychosocial functioning. Depression is the most common reason for seeking medical attention. Family members often bring the patient for the initial evaluation. The patient may be too lethargic, apathetic, or drowsy to recognize changes in his or her condition. Families may report that the patient is withdrawn and has reduced mental function. Assess his or her attention span and memory, both of which can be impaired by hypothyroidism.

Laboratory Assessment

Laboratory findings for hypothyroidism are the opposite of those for hyperthyroidism. Triiodothyronine (T_3) and thyroxine (T_4) serum levels are decreased. TSH levels are high in primary hypothyroidism but can be decreased or near normal in patients with secondary hypothyroidism (see Chart 66-2).

CONSIDERATIONS FOR OLDER ADULTS

Metabolic rate and production of thyroid hormone both decrease with advancing age (Chart 66-6), particularly among people older than 80 years. Until recently, however, data regarding normal levels of T_3 and T_4 were established only for adults between the ages of 20 and 30 years. By such criteria, older people with T_3 and T_4 levels 15% to 20% below "normal levels" (established for a younger population) were considered to have hypothyroidism and therapy with thyroid hormone was initiated. In fact, many of these patients were not truly hypothyroid, and therapy caused pseudohyperthyroidism, stressing many tissues and organs. Daily thyroid hormone therapy decreases the activity of the anterior pituitary gland and the thyroid gland, creating actual hypothyroidism. Health care providers need to assess more than just laboratory data to determine hypothyroidism in the older adult (Holcomb, 2005).

Analysis

Common Nursing Diagnoses and Collaborative Problems

Priority nursing diagnoses for patients with hypothyroidism are:

1. Ineffective Breathing Pattern related to decreased energy, obesity, and fatigue
2. Decreased Cardiac Output related to altered heart rate and rhythm as a result of decreased myocardial metabolism
3. Disturbed Thought Processes related to impaired brain metabolism and edema

Chart 66-6 NURSING FOCUS ON THE OLDER ADULT

Thyroid Problems

Teach the patient these facts about changes in the thyroid gland related to aging:

- The thyroid gland decreases in size with increasing age.
- Thyroid hormone secretion decreases with age, but the hormone level remains stable because cellular clearance of the hormone also decreases with age.
- The basal metabolic rate decreases with age, usually as a result of decreased activity. This decrease changes the body composition from predominantly muscular to predominantly fatty.
- Older patients require lower doses of replacement thyroid hormone. Too large a dose may adversely affect the heart muscle.

The major collaborative problem is the Potential for Myxedema Coma.

Additional Nursing Diagnoses and Collaborative Problems

In addition to the common nursing diagnoses and collaborative problems, patients with hypothyroidism may have one or more of these:

- Imbalanced Nutrition: More Than Body Requirements related to excessive intake in relation to metabolic need
- Hypothermia related to decreased metabolic rate
- Constipation related to decreased motility of the GI tract
- Disturbed Body Image related to illness
- Deficient Knowledge of condition, diagnosis, and treatment related to cognitive limitation

Additional collaborative problems for patients with hypothyroidism are Potential for Paralytic Ileus and Potential for Cardiomyopathy.

Planning and Implementation

Both cardiac and respiratory problems are serious, and their management is a priority. However, the most common cause of death among patients with myxedema coma is respiratory failure.

Ineffective Breathing Pattern

Planning: Expected Outcomes. The patient with hypothyroidism is expected to have not compromised or only mildly compromised respiratory function. Indicators include:

- Maintenance of Spo_2 of at least 90%
- Absence of cyanosis
- Maintenance of cognitive orientation

Interventions. Observe and record the rate and depth of respirations. Measure oxygen saturation by pulse oximetry, and apply oxygen if the patient has hypoxemia. Auscultate the lungs for any problems, such as a decrease in breath sounds. If hypothyroidism is severe, the patient may have such severe respiratory distress that ventilatory support is required. Severe respiratory distress often occurs with myxedema coma.

Sedating a patient with hypothyroidism can make respiratory difficulties worse and is avoided, if possible. When sedation is needed, the dosage is reduced because hypothyroidism increases sensitivity to these drugs. Assess the patient receiving sedation for respiratory adequacy.

Decreased Cardiac Output

Planning: Expected Outcomes. The patient with hypothyroidism is expected to have cardiovascular function that is either not compromised or only mildly compromised. Indicators include that the patient:

- Maintains heart rate above 60 beats/min
- Maintains blood pressure within normal limits for his or her age and general health
- Has no dysrhythmias, peripheral edema, or neck vein distention

Interventions. The patient with hypothyroidism can have decreased blood pressure, bradycardia, and dysrhythmias. Priority nursing actions are focused on monitoring for condition changes and preventing complications. Monitor blood pressure and heart rate and rhythm, and observe closely for signs of shock, such as hypotension, decreasing urine output, and changes in mental status.

If hypothyroidism has been chronic, the patient may have cardiovascular disease. *Instruct the patient to report episodes of chest pain or chest discomfort immediately.*

The patient with hypothyroidism requires lifelong thyroid hormone replacement. Synthetic hormone preparations are usually prescribed. The most common is levothyroxine sodium (Synthroid, T_4, Eltroxin🍁). Therapy is started with low doses and gradually increased over a period of weeks. *The patient with more severe symptoms of hypothyroidism is started on the lowest dose of thyroid hormone replacement.* This caution is especially important when the patient has known cardiac problems. Starting at too high a dose or increasing the dose too rapidly can cause severe hypertension, heart failure, and myocardial infarction (Brent et al., 2008). *Teach patients, as well as the families of patients, who are beginning thyroid replacement hormone therapy to take the drug exactly as prescribed and not to change the dose or schedule without consulting the health care provider.*

Assess the patient for chest pain and dyspnea during initiation of therapy. The final dosage is determined by blood levels of TSH and the patient's physical responses. The dosage and time required for symptom relief vary with each patient. Monitor for and teach the patient and family about the manifestations of hyperthyroidism (see Chart 66-1), which can occur with replacement therapy.

Disturbed Thought Processes

Planning: Expected Outcomes. The patient with hypothyroidism is expected to have not compromised thought processes or compromised only to the extent present before the thyroid problem started. Indicators include that the patient:

- Demonstrates immediate memory
- Communicates clearly and appropriately for age and ability
- Is attentive during conversations

Interventions. Observe for and record the presence and severity of lethargy, drowsiness, memory deficit, poor attention span, and difficulty communicating. These problems should decrease with thyroid hormone treatment, and mental awareness usually returns to the patient's normal level within 2 weeks. Orient the patient to person, place, and time, and explain all procedures slowly and carefully. Provide a safe environment.

Family members may have difficulty coping with the patient's behavior. Encourage them to accept the mood changes and mental slowness as manifestations of the disease. Remind the family that these problems should improve with therapy.

Potential for Myxedema Coma

Any patient with hypothyroidism who has any other health problem or who is newly diagnosed is at risk for myxedema coma. Factors leading to myxedema coma include acute illness, surgery, chemotherapy, discontinuing thyroid replacement therapy, and the use of sedatives or opioids. Problems that often occur with this condition include:

- Coma
- Respiratory failure
- Hypotension
- Hyponatremia
- Hypothermia
- Hypoglycemia

Untreated myxedema coma leads to shock, organ damage, and death. Assess the patient with hypothyroidism at least every 8 hours for changes that indicate increasing severity, especially changes in mental status.

Treatment is instituted quickly according to the patient's manifestations and without waiting for laboratory confirmation. Best practices for emergency care of the patient with myxedema coma are listed in Chart 66-7.

DECISION-MAKING CHALLENGE

Critical Rescue

The adult children of the patient with moderate hypothyroidism, who started treatment last week with levothyroxine, come to her apartment and find her sitting on the couch in her winter coat. When they ask her why she is wearing the coat, she looks at them and asks, "Who are you?" They call the life-squad, and the patient is brought to the ED.

1. What vital sign should you assess first? Provide a rationale for your selection.
2. Should this patient receive oxygen? Why or why not?
3. What IV solution should you be prepared to administer as fluid therapy and why?

evolve For suggested answer guidelines, go to http://evolve.elsevier.com/Iggy/.

Community-Based Care

Hypothyroidism is usually a chronic condition. Patients with hypothyroidism are managed on an outpatient basis and may reside anywhere. Patients in acute care settings, subacute care settings, and rehabilitation centers may have long-standing hypothyroidism in addition to other acute or chronic health problems. Ensure that whoever is responsible for overseeing the patient's daily care is aware of the condition and understands its treatment.

Home Care Management

The patient with hypothyroidism does not usually require changes in the home unless cognition has decreased to the point that he or she poses a danger to himself or herself. Activity intolerance and fatigue may necessitate one-floor living for a short time. If manifestations have not improved before discharge, discuss the need for extra heat or clothing because of cold intolerance. The patient who has a decreased attention span may need help with the drug regimen. Discuss this issue with the family and patient, and develop a plan for drug therapy. One person should be clearly designated as responsible for drug preparation and delivery so that doses are neither missed nor duplicated.

Health Teaching

The most important educational need for the patient with hypothyroidism is about hormone replacement therapy and its side effects. Emphasize the need for lifelong drugs, and review the manifestations of both hyperthyroidism and hypothyroidism. Teach the patient to wear a medical alert bracelet. Teach the patient and family when to seek medical interventions for dosage adjustment and the need for periodic blood tests of hormone levels. Instruct the patient to not take any over-the-counter (OTC) drugs because thyroid hormone preparations interact with many other drugs. Older patients may need additional information about the effects of aging on the thyroid gland (see Chart 66-6).

Advise the patient to eat a well-balanced diet with adequate fiber and fluid intake to prevent constipation. Caution him or her that use of fiber supplements may interfere with the absorption of thyroid hormone. The drug should be taken on an empty stomach. Remind him or her about the importance of adequate rest. Encourage family members to voice their concerns to the health care provider.

Assist the family in understanding that the time required for resolution of hypothyroidism varies. During this time, the patient may continue to have mental dullness or slowness. Teach the family to orient the patient often and to explain everything clearly, simply, and as often as needed.

Teach the patient to monitor himself or herself for therapy effectiveness. The two easiest parameters to check are need for sleep and bowel elimination. When the patient requires more sleep and is constipated, the dose of replacement hormone may need to be increased. When the patient has difficulty getting to sleep and has more bowel movements than normal for him or her, the dose may need to be decreased.

Health Care Resources

Immediately after returning home, the patient may need a support person to stay and provide more attention than could be given by a visiting nurse or home care aide. Contact with the health care team is needed for follow-up and identification of potential problems. The patient taking thyroid drugs may have manifestations of hypothyroidism if the dosage is inadequate or may have manifestations of hyperthyroidism if the dose is too high. The home care nurse performs a focused assessment at every home visit to the patient with thyroid dysfunction (Chart 66-8).

Chart 66-7 BEST PRACTICE FOR PATIENT SAFETY & QUALITY CARE

Emergency Care of the Patient During Myxedema Coma

EMERGENCY CARE

- Maintain a patent airway.
- Replace fluids with IV normal or hypertonic saline.
- Give levothyroxine sodium IV as prescribed.
- Give glucose IV as prescribed.
- Give corticosteroids as prescribed.
- Check the patient's temperature hourly.
- Monitor blood pressure hourly.
- Cover the patient with warm blankets.
- Monitor for changes in mental status.
- Turn every 2 hours.
- Institute Aspiration Precautions.

Chart 66-8 HOME CARE ASSESSMENT

The Patient with Thyroid Dysfunction

Assess cardiovascular status.
- Vital signs, including apical pulse, pulse pressure, presence or absence of orthostatic hypotension, and the quality and rhythm of peripheral pulses
- Presence or absence of peripheral edema
- Weight gain or loss

Assess cognition and mental status.
- Level of consciousness
- Orientation to time, place, and person
- Accurately reading a seven-word sentence containing no words greater than three syllables
- Can the patient count backward from 100 by threes?

Assess condition of skin and mucous membranes.
- Moistness of skin, most reliable on chest and back
- Skin temperature and color

Assess neuromuscular status.
- Reactivity of patellar and biceps reflexes
- Oral temperature
- Handgrip strength
- Steadiness of gait
- Presence or absence of fine tremors in the hand

Ask about:
- Sleep in the past 24 hours
- Patient warm enough or too warm indoors
- 24-hour diet recall
- 24-hour activity recall
- Over-the-counter and prescribed drugs taken
- Last bowel movement

Assess patient's understanding of illness and adherence with treatment.
- Manifestations to report to health care provider
- Drug therapy plan (correct timing and dose)

DECISION-MAKING CHALLENGE

Coordination of Care

The patient with severe hypothyroidism described on p. 1459 is about to be discharged to home.

1. What are the teaching priorities for this patient?
2. Should you include her adult children in the teaching? Why or why not?

evolve For suggested answer guidelines, go to http://evolve.elsevier.com/Iggy/.

Evaluation: Outcomes

Evaluate the care of the patient with hypothyroidism on the basis of the identified nursing diagnoses and collaborative problems. The expected outcomes are that the patient should:

- Maintain normal cardiovascular function
- Maintain adequate respiratory function
- Experience improvement in thought processes

Specific indicators for these outcomes are listed for each nursing diagnosis and collaborative problem in the Planning and Implementation section.

THYROIDITIS

Pathophysiology

Thyroiditis is an inflammation of the thyroid gland. There are three types: acute, subacute, and chronic. Chronic thyroiditis (Hashimoto's disease) is the most common type.

Acute thyroiditis is caused by bacterial invasion of the thyroid gland. Manifestations include pain, neck tenderness, malaise, fever, and dysphagia (difficulty swallowing). It usually resolves with antibiotic therapy.

Subacute or granulomatous thyroiditis results from a viral infection of the thyroid gland after a cold or other upper respiratory infection. Manifestations include fever, chills, dysphagia, and muscle and joint pain. Pain can radiate to the ears and the jaw. The thyroid gland feels hard and enlarged on palpation. Thyroid function can remain normal, although hyperthyroidism or hypothyroidism may develop.

Chronic thyroiditis (Hashimoto's disease) is a common type of hypothyroidism that affects women more often than men, most often patients in their 30s to 50s (Brent et al., 2008). Hashimoto's disease is an autoimmune disorder that is usually triggered by a bacterial or viral infection. The thyroid is invaded by antithyroid antibodies and lymphocytes, causing thyroid tissue destruction. When large amounts of the gland are destroyed, serum thyroid hormone levels are low and secretion of thyroid-stimulating hormone (TSH) is increased.

Patient-Centered Collaborative Care

The manifestations of Hashimoto's disease are dysphagia and painless enlargement of the gland. Diagnosis is based on circulating antithyroid antibodies and needle biopsy of the thyroid gland. Serum thyroid hormone levels, TSH levels, and radioactive iodine uptake (RAIU) vary with disease stage.

The patient is given thyroid hormone to prevent hypothyroidism and to suppress TSH secretion, which decreases the size of the thyroid gland. Surgery (subtotal thyroidectomy) is needed if the goiter does not respond to thyroid hormone, is disfiguring, or compresses other structures.

Nursing interventions focus on promoting comfort and teaching the patient about hypothyroidism, drugs, and surgery. (See Postoperative Care, p. 1454, in the Hyperthyroidism section.)

THYROID CANCER

Pathophysiology

The four distinct types of thyroid cancer are papillary, follicular, medullary, and anaplastic (American Cancer Society, 2008). The initial manifestation of thyroid cancer is a single, painless lump or nodule in the thyroid gland. Additional manifestations depend on the presence and location of **metastasis** (spread of cancer cells).

Papillary carcinoma, the most common type of thyroid cancer, occurs most often in younger women. It is a slow-growing tumor that can be present for years before spreading to nearby lymph nodes. When the tumor is confined to the thyroid gland, the chance for cure is good with a partial or total thyroidectomy.

Follicular carcinoma occurs most often in older patients. The cancer invades blood vessels and spreads to bone and lung tissue. It can adhere to the trachea, neck muscles, great vessels, and skin, resulting in **dyspnea** (difficulty breathing) and **dysphagia** (difficulty swallowing). When the tumor involves the recurrent laryngeal nerves, the patient may have a hoarse voice.

Medullary carcinoma is most common in patients older than 50 years. This tumor often occurs as part of multiple endocrine neoplasia (MEN) type II, a familial endocrine disorder. The tumor usually secretes calcitonin, adrenocorticotropic hormone (ACTH), prostaglandins, and serotonin.

Anaplastic carcinoma is a rapid-growing, aggressive tumor that directly invades nearby structures. Manifestations include stridor (harsh, high-pitched respiratory sounds), hoarseness, and dysphagia.

Patient-Centered Collaborative Care

Radiation therapy is used most often for anaplastic carcinoma because this cancer is usually metastasized (spread) at diagnosis. Surgery is the treatment of choice for papillary, follicular, and medullary carcinomas. A total thyroidectomy is usually performed with a nodal neck dissection if regional lymph nodes are involved. Suppressive doses of thyroid hormone are usually taken for 3 months after surgery. A radioactive iodine uptake (RAIU) study is performed after drugs are withdrawn. If there is RAI uptake, the patient is treated with **ablative** (enough to destroy the tissue) amounts of RAI. If thyroid cancer does not respond to RAI, a course of chemotherapy is initiated.

Usually the patient is hypothyroid after treatment for thyroid cancer. Nursing interventions then focus on teaching the patient about hypothyroidism and its management. (See Patient-Centered Collaborative Care, p. 1457, in the Hypothyroidism section.)

PARATHYROID DISORDERS

HYPERPARATHYROIDISM

Pathophysiology

The parathyroid glands maintain calcium and phosphate balance (Fig. 66-4). Serum calcium level is normally maintained within a narrow range. Phosphate levels vary more widely. Increased levels of parathyroid hormone (PTH) act directly on the kidney, causing increased kidney reabsorption of calcium and increased phosphate excretion. These processes cause **hypercalcemia** (excessive calcium) and **hypophosphatemia** (inadequate phosphate) in the patient with hyperparathyroidism.

In bone, excessive PTH levels increase bone resorption (bone loss of calcium) by decreasing **osteoblastic** (bone production) activity and increasing **osteoclastic** (bone destruction) activity. This process releases calcium and phosphate into the blood and reduces bone density. With chronic calcium excess, as in long-standing hypercalcemia, calcium is deposited in soft tissues.

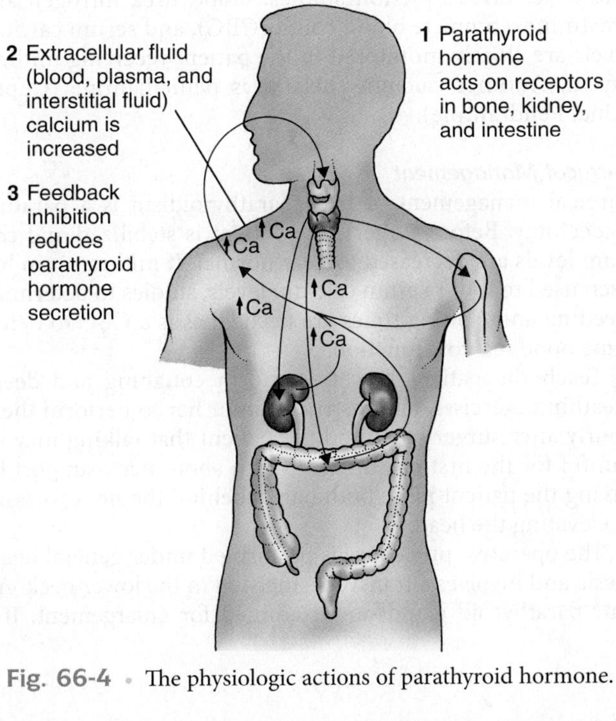
1 Parathyroid hormone acts on receptors in bone, kidney, and intestine
2 Extracellular fluid (blood, plasma, and interstitial fluid) calcium is increased
3 Feedback inhibition reduces parathyroid hormone secretion
Ca
Ca
Ca
Ca
Ca
Ca

Fig. 66-4 • The physiologic actions of parathyroid hormone.

Although the exact triggering mechanisms are unknown, primary hyperparathyroidism results when one or more parathyroid glands do not respond to the normal feedback of serum calcium. The most common cause is a benign tumor in one parathyroid gland. Table 66-3 lists other causes of hyperparathyroidism.

Patient-Centered Collaborative Care

Assessment

Manifestations of hyperparathyroidism may be related either to the effects of excessive PTH or to the effects of the accompanying hypercalcemia.

Ask the patient about any bone fractures, recent weight loss, arthritis, or psychological distress. Determine whether the patient has received radiation treatment to the head or neck. The patient with long-standing disease may have a waxy pallor of the skin and bone deformities in the extremities and back.

High levels of PTH cause **renal calculi** (kidney stones) and deposits of calcium in the soft tissue of the kidney. Bone lesions are due to an increased rate of bone destruction and may result in pathologic fractures, bone cysts, and osteoporosis.

GI manifestations (e.g., anorexia, nausea, vomiting, epigastric pain, constipation, weight loss) are common, particularly when serum calcium levels are high. Elevated serum gastrin levels are caused by hypercalcemia and lead to peptic ulcer disease. Fatigue and lethargy may be present and become more severe as the serum calcium levels increase. When serum calcium levels are greater than 12 mg/dL, the patient may have psychosis with mental confusion, which leads to coma and death if left untreated. (See Chapter 13 for more information about hypercalcemia.)

Serum PTH, calcium, and phosphate levels and urine cyclic adenosine monophosphate (cAMP) are the most commonly used laboratory tests to detect hyperparathyroidism (Chart 66-9). X-rays may show kidney stones, calcium deposits, and bone lesions, such as cysts or fractures. Loss of bone density occurs in the patient with chronic hyperparathyroidism. Other diagnostic tests include arteriography, computed

TABLE 66-3 Causes of Parathyroid Dysfunction

CAUSES OF HYPERPARATHYROIDISM
- Parathyroid adenoma
- Parathyroid carcinoma
- Congenital hyperplasia
- Neck trauma or radiation
- Vitamin D deficiency
- Chronic kidney disease with hypocalcemia
- Parathyroid hormone–secreting carcinomas of the lung, kidney, or GI tract

CAUSES OF HYPOPARATHYROIDISM
- Surgical or radiation-induced thyroid ablation
- Parathyroidectomy
- Congenital dysgenesis
- Idiopathic (autoimmune) hypoparathyroidism
- Hypomagnesemia

Chart 66-9 LABORATORY PROFILE
Parathyroid Function

Test	Normal Range for Adults	SIGNIFICANCE OF ABNORMAL FINDINGS: Hyperparathyroidism	SIGNIFICANCE OF ABNORMAL FINDINGS: Hypoparathyroidism
Serum calcium	Total: 9.0-10.5 mg/dL or 2.25-2.75 SI units Ionized (active): 4.64-5.28 mg/dL or 1.16-1.32 SI units	Increased in primary hyperparathyroidism	Decreased
Serum phosphate	3.0-4.5 mg/dL or 0.97-1.45 SI units *Older adults:* May be slightly lower	Decreased	Increased
Serum parathyroid hormone	C-terminal 50-330 pg/mL	Increased	Decreased

SI, International System of Units.

tomography (CT), venous catheterization of the thyroid veins with sampling of the blood for PTH levels, and ultrasonography. Explain the procedures and care for the patient undergoing diagnostic tests.

NCLEX EXAMINATION CHALLENGE

Which is the priority nursing diagnosis for the client with hyperparathyroidism?

A. Fatigue
B. Constipation
C. Risk for Injury
D. Risk for Acute Confusion

evolve For the correct answer, go to http://evolve.elsevier.com/Iggy/.

■ Interventions

Nonsurgical Management

Diuretic and hydration therapies are used most often for reducing serum calcium levels in patients who are not candidates for surgery. Usually furosemide (Lasix, Uritol♣), a diuretic that increases kidney excretion of calcium, is used together with IV saline in large volumes to promote renal calcium excretion. The priority nursing interventions focus on monitoring and prevention of injury.

Monitor cardiac function and intake and output every 2 to 4 hours during hydration therapy. Continuous cardiac monitoring may be needed. Compare recent ECG tracings with the patient's baseline tracings. Especially look for changes in the T waves and the QT interval, as well as changes in rate and rhythm. Closely monitor serum calcium levels, and immediately report to the health care provider any sudden drop. Sudden drops in calcium levels may cause tingling and numbness in the muscles.

Preventing injury is important because the patient with chronic hyperparathyroidism often has significant bone density loss and is at risk for pathologic fractures. Teach all members of the health care team to handle the patient carefully. Use a lift sheet to reposition the patient rather than pulling him or her. Ensure that the hospitalized patient is accompanied when ambulating to prevent falls.

Drug therapy is used when hydration and furosemide cannot reduce hypercalcemia or if it is necessary to discontinue IV fluids. Other drugs can help reduce the manifestations of hyperparathyroidism, especially those related to hypercalcemia.

Oral phosphates inhibit bone resorption and interfere with calcium absorption. IV phosphates are used only when serum calcium levels must be lowered rapidly. Calcitonin decreases the release of skeletal calcium and increases the kidney excretion of calcium. It is not effective when used alone because of its short duration of action. The therapeutic effects are greatly enhanced if calcitonin is given along with glucocorticoids.

Some drugs, known as *calcium chelators,* lower calcium levels by binding (chelating) calcium, which reduces the levels of free calcium. Mithramycin, a cytotoxic agent, is the most effective and potent calcium chelator used to lower serum calcium levels. In most patients, a single IV dose of 10 to 15 mg/kg of body weight by slow infusion can lower serum calcium levels within 48 hours. However, the toxic effects limit its use to two or three doses. Thrombocytopenia (decreased circulating platelets and an increased tendency to bleed) and kidney and liver toxicity can result after only one dose. Liver function studies, blood urea nitrogen and creatinine, complete blood count (CBC), and serum calcium levels are closely monitored in the patient receiving mithramycin. Another calcium chelator is penicillamine (Cuprimine, Pendramine).

Surgical Management

Surgical management of hyperparathyroidism is a parathyroidectomy. Before surgery, the patient is stabilized and calcium levels are decreased to near normal. If mithramycin has been used to lower serum calcium levels, studies to determine bleeding and clotting times are needed, as is a CBC to determine bone marrow function.

Teach the patient how to perform coughing and deep-breathing exercises, and instruct him or her to perform them hourly after surgery. Remind the patient that talking may be painful for the first day or two. Teach about neck support by having the patient place both hands behind the neck to assist in elevating the head.

The operative procedure is performed under general anesthesia and involves a transverse incision in the lower neck. All four parathyroid glands are examined for enlargement. If a tumor is present on one side but the other side is normal, the surgeon removes the glands containing tumor and leaves the remaining glands on the opposite side intact. If all four glands are diseased, they are all removed.

After surgery, closely observe the patient for respiratory distress, which may occur from compression of the trachea by hemorrhage or swelling of neck tissues. Ensure that emergency equipment, including suction, oxygen, and tracheostomy equipment, is at the bedside. If severe swelling occurs, the surgeon may need to remove clips from the incision to preserve the airway. Monitor vital signs, identify any change in status, and check the neck dressing for abnormal amounts of drainage or bleeding. A small amount (1 to 5 mL) of drainage is normal.

The remaining glands, which may have atrophied as a result of PTH overproduction, require several days to several weeks to return to normal function. A hypocalcemic crisis can occur during this critical period. Usually, the surgeon requests the serum calcium to be assessed frequently after surgery. Check serum calcium levels immediately after surgery and every 4 hours thereafter until calcium levels stabilize. Monitor for manifestations of hypocalcemia, such as tingling and twitching in the extremities and face. Check for Trousseau's and Chvostek's signs, either of which signals potential tetany (see Chapter 13).

The recurrent laryngeal nerve can be damaged. Assess the patient for changes in voice patterns and hoarseness.

When hyperparathyroidism is due to **hyperplasia** (tissue overgrowth), three glands plus half of the fourth gland are usually removed. If all four glands are removed, a small portion of a gland may be implanted in the forearm, where it produces PTH and maintains calcium homeostasis. If all these maneuvers fail, the patient will need lifelong treatment with calcium and vitamin D because the resulting hypoparathyroidism is permanent (see next section).

HYPOPARATHYROIDISM

Pathophysiology

Hypoparathyroidism is a rare endocrine disorder in which parathyroid function is decreased. Problems are directly related to a lack of parathyroid hormone (PTH) secretion or to decreased effectiveness of PTH on target tissue. Whether the problem is a lack of PTH secretion or an ineffectiveness of PTH on tissues, the result is the same: hypocalcemia.

Iatrogenic hypoparathyroidism, the most common form, is caused by the removal of all parathyroid tissue during total thyroidectomy or by deliberate surgical removal of the parathyroid glands.

Idiopathic hypoparathyroidism can occur spontaneously. The exact cause is unknown, but an autoimmune basis is suspected. Hypoparathyroidism may occur with other autoimmune disorders such as adrenal insufficiency, hypothyroidism, diabetes mellitus, pernicious anemia, and vitiligo.

Hypomagnesemia (decreased serum magnesium levels) may also cause hypoparathyroidism. Hypomagnesemia is seen in alcoholics and in patients with malabsorption syndromes, chronic kidney disease, and malnutrition. It causes impairment of PTH secretion and may interfere with the effects of PTH on the bones, the kidneys, and calcium regulation.

Patient-Centered Collaborative Care

Assessment

Ask about any head or neck surgery or radiation therapy because these treatments may cause hypoparathyroidism. Also determine whether the neck has ever sustained a serious injury in a car crash or by strangulation. Assess whether the patient has any manifestations of hypoparathyroidism, which may range from mild tingling and numbness to muscle tetany. Tingling and numbness around the mouth or in the hands and feet reflect mild to moderate hypocalcemia. Severe muscle cramps, spasms of the hands and feet, and seizures (with no loss of consciousness or incontinence) reflect a more severe hypocalcemia. The patient or family may notice mental changes ranging from irritability to psychosis.

The physical assessment may show excessive or inappropriate muscle contractions that cause finger, hand, and elbow flexion. This can signal an impending attack of tetany. Check for Chvostek's sign and Trousseau's sign; positive responses indicate potential tetany (see Chapter 13). Bands or pits may encircle the crowns of the teeth, which indicate a loss of calcium from the teeth with enamel loss.

Diagnostic tests for hypoparathyroidism include electroencephalography (EEG), blood tests, and computed tomography (CT). EEG changes revert to normal with correction of hypocalcemia. Serum calcium, phosphate, magnesium, vitamin D, and urine cyclic adenosine monophosphate (cAMP) levels may be used in the diagnostic workup for hypoparathyroidism (see Chart 66-9). The CT scan can show brain calcifications, which indicate chronic hypocalcemia.

Interventions

Medical management of hypoparathyroidism focuses on correcting hypocalcemia, vitamin D deficiency, and hypomagnesemia. For patients with acute and severe hypocalcemia, IV calcium is given as a 10% solution of calcium chloride or calcium gluconate over 10 to 15 minutes. Acute vitamin D deficiency is treated with calcitriol (Rocaltrol), 0.5 to 2 mg daily. Acute hypomagnesemia is corrected with 50% magnesium sulfate in 2-mL doses (up to 4 g daily) either IM or IV. Long-term oral therapy for hypocalcemia involves the intake of calcium, 0.5 to 2 g daily, in divided doses.

Long-term therapy for vitamin D deficiency is 50,000 to 400,000 units of ergocalciferol daily. The dosage is adjusted to keep the patient's calcium level in the low-normal range (slightly hypocalcemic), enough to prevent symptoms of hypocalcemia. It must also be low enough to prevent increased urine calcium levels, which can lead to stone formation.

Nursing management includes teaching about the drug regimen and interventions to reduce anxiety. Teach the patient to eat foods high in calcium but low in phosphorus. Milk, yogurt, and processed cheeses are avoided because of their high phosphorus content. *Stress that therapy for hypocalcemia is lifelong.* Advise the patient to wear a medical alert bracelet. With adherence to the prescribed drug and diet regimen, the calcium level usually remains high enough to prevent a hypocalcemic crisis.

GET READY FOR THE NCLEX EXAMINATION!

Key Points

Review these Key Points for each NCLEX Examination Client Needs Category.

Safe and Effective Care Environment

- Keep the environment of a patient at risk for thyroid storm cool, dark, and quiet.
- Keep emergency suctioning and tracheostomy equipment in the room of a patient who has had thyroid or parathyroid surgery.
- Use a lift sheet to move or reposition a patient with hypocalcemia.

Health Promotion and Maintenance

- Teach all patients to take antithyroid drugs or thyroid hormone replacement therapy as prescribed.
- Include the person who prepares the patient's meals when teaching about dietary electrolyte restrictions.
- Collaborate with the nutritionist to teach patients about diets that are restricted in calcium or phosphate.

Psychosocial Integrity

- Be accepting of patient behavior.
- Help patients and family members understand that changes in cognition and behavior are usually temporary.
- Encourage the patient who has a permanent change in appearance (e.g., exophthalmia) to mourn the change.

Physiological Integrity

- Monitor the hydration status of patients who have hypercalcemia.
- Teach patients that hormone replacement therapy for hypothyroidism is lifelong.
- Teach patients to use clinical manifestations (e.g., the number of bowel movements per day, the ability to sleep) as indicators of therapy effectiveness and when the dose of thyroid hormone replacement may need to be adjusted.

Additional Study Resources

Go to your Companion CD or Evolve at http://evolve.elsevier.com/Iggy/ for *Self-Assessment Questions for the NCLEX Examination.*

evolve Go to Evolve at http://evolve.elsevier.com/Iggy/ for *Prioritization and Delegation Questions for the NCLEX Examination.*

SELECTED BIBLIOGRAPHY

American Cancer Society. (2008). *Cancer facts and figures 2008*. Report No. 00-300M–No. 5008.08. Atlanta: Author.

Brent, G., Larsen, R.R., & Davies, T. (2008). Hypothyroidism and thyroiditis. In H. Kronenberg, S. Melmed, K. Polonsky, & P.R. Larsen (Eds.), *Williams' textbook of endocrinology* (11th ed., pp. 377-409). Philadelphia: Saunders.

Davies, T., & Larsen, P.R. (2008). Thyrotoxicosis. In H. Kronenberg, S. Melmed, K. Polonsky, & P.R. Larsen (Eds.), *Williams' textbook of endocrinology* (11th ed., pp. 333-375). Philadelphia: Saunders.

Devdhar, M., Ousman, Y., & Burman, K. (2007). Hypothyroidism. *Endocrinology and Metabolism Clinics of North America, 36*(4), 595-615.

Holcomb, S. (2005). Detecting thyroid disease. *Nursing2005, 35*(10), 4-8.

Kronenberg, H., Melmed, S., Polonsky, K., & Larsen, P.R. (Eds.). (2008). *Williams' textbook of endocrinology* (11th ed.). Philadelphia: Saunders.

Mauk, K. (2005). Rooting out hypothyroidism in the elderly. *Nursing2005, 35*(12), 65-66.

McCance, K., & Huether, S. (2006). *Pathophysiology: The biologic basis for disease in adults and children* (5th ed.). St. Louis: Mosby.

Nayak, B., & Burman, K. (2006). Thyrotoxicosis and thyroid storm. *Endocrinology and Metabolism Clinics of North America, 35*(4), 663-686.

Nayak, B., & Hodak, S. (2006). Hyperthyroidism. *Endocrinology and Metabolism Clinics of North America, 35*(4), 617-656.

Noble, K. (2006). Thyroid storm. *Journal of PeriAnesthesia Nursing, 21*(2), 119-125.

Nussbaum, R., McInnes, R., & Willard, H. (2007). *Thompson & Thompson: Genetics in medicine* (7th ed.). Philadelphia: Saunders.

Pagana, K., & Pagana, T. (2006). *Mosby's manual of diagnostic and laboratory tests* (3rd ed.). St. Louis: Mosby.

Porsche, R., & Brenner, Z. (2006). Amiodarone-induced thyroid disfunction. *Critical Care Nurse, 26*(3), 34-41.

Reid, J., & Wheeler, S. (2005). Hyperthyroidism: Diagnosis and treatment. *American Family Physician, 72*(4), 623-630.

Spears. S., Theler, J., & Sorensen, D. (2008). Complications after the surgical treatment of malignant thyroid disease. *Military Medicine, 173*(4), 399-402.

Weeks, B. (2005). Graves' disease: The importance of early diagnosis. *The Nurse Practitioner, 30*(11), 34-45.

Care of Patients with Diabetes Mellitus

67
CHAPTER

Margaret Elaine McLeod

LEARNING OUTCOMES

For clinical competence and success on the NCLEX Examination, study this chapter with these Learning Outcomes in mind:

Safe and Effective Care Environment

1. Administer insulin and other antidiabetic agents in a safe and accurate manner.
2. Apply the principles of infection control in the care of diabetic patients.
3. Individualize teaching methods to ensure the patient's correct understanding of diabetes management.
4. Teach patients and families the safe use of insulin injection equipment and glucose monitoring equipment.
5. Teach diabetic patients with peripheral neuropathy how to avoid injury.

Health Promotion and Maintenance

6. Encourage everyone to prevent type 2 diabetes by achieving and maintaining ideal weight and participating in regular exercise.
7. Teach all patients with diabetes how to self-manage their disease.
8. Teach the patient and family about the manifestations and emergency treatment of hypoglycemia and hyperglycemia.

Psychosocial Integrity

9. Explore with the patient what the diagnosis of diabetes means to him or her.
10. Allow the patient the opportunity to express fear or anxiety regarding the diagnosis of diabetes or the treatment regimen.
11. Explain all procedures, restrictions, drugs, and follow-up care to the patient and family.
12. Refer patients newly diagnosed with diabetes to local resources and support groups.

Physiological Integrity

13. Compare the risk factors, age of onset, manifestations, and pathologic mechanisms of type 1 and type 2 diabetes mellitus.
14. Assess patient risk for type 2 diabetes mellitus.
15. Explain the effects of insulin on carbohydrate, protein, and fat metabolism.
16. Explain how to mix different kinds of insulin together.
17. Evaluate laboratory data to determine whether the patient is using the prescribed dietary, drug, and exercise therapies for diabetes.
18. Explain how to perform foot assessment and foot care for the patient with diabetes.
19. Collaborate with members of the health care team to provide care for patients with diabetic ketoacidosis (DKA).
20. Collaborate with members of the health care team to provide care for patients with hyperglycemic-hyperosmolar state (HHS).

Go to your Companion CD or Evolve at http://evolve.elsevier.com/Iggy/ for *Self-Assessment Questions for the NCLEX Examination* keyed to these Learning Outcomes.

Diabetes mellitus is a common chronic disease requiring lifelong behavioral and lifestyle changes. It is best managed with a collaborative approach to help the patient successfully manage the disease. As part of the team, you will plan, organize, and coordinate care with the various health care team members to provide care and education; and promote the patient's health and well-being.

Diabetes is a major public health problem worldwide. Its complications cause many serious health problems. In the United States, diabetes mellitus (DM) is the leading cause of new cases of blindness, end-stage kidney disease requiring dialysis or transplantation, and foot or leg amputations. Many people have undiagnosed diabetes. Many who are diagnosed have continuous high blood glucose levels. Current evidence shows that **glycemic** (blood glucose) control reduces complications of diabetes. Treatment of hypertension and **hyperlipidemia** (high blood fat levels), which often occur with diabetes, is essential to prevent complications of DM. Thus nursing priorities are aimed at helping the patient with diabetes achieve and maintain lifestyle changes that prevent long-term complications by keeping blood glucose levels and cholesterol levels as close to normal as possible.

Pathophysiology

Classification of Diabetes

For all types of diabetes mellitus (DM), the main feature is chronic **hyperglycemia** (high blood glucose level) resulting from problems with insulin secretion, insulin action, or both. The disease is classified by the underlying problem causing a lack of insulin and the severity of the insulin deficiency. Table 67-1 outlines the types of DM.

The Endocrine Pancreas

The endocrine portion of the pancreas has about 1 million small glands, the islets of Langerhans, scattered through the organ. The islet cells are only a small portion of the gland. Most of the gland has digestive functions. Two types of islet cells are important to glucose control: alpha cells and beta cells. Alpha cells produce glucagon; beta cells produce insulin and amylin. **Glucagon** is a major "counterregulatory" hormone that has actions opposite those of insulin. It causes the release of glucose from cell storage sites whenever blood glucose levels are low. Insulin allows body cells to use and store carbohydrate, fat, and protein.

TABLE 67-1 Classification of Diabetes Mellitus

TYPE 1 DIABETES
- Beta-cell destruction leading to absolute insulin deficiency
- Autoimmune
- Idiopathic

TYPE 2 DIABETES
- Ranges from insulin resistance with relative insulin deficiency to secretory deficit with insulin resistance

OTHER SPECIFIC CONDITIONS RESULTING IN HYPERGLYCEMIA
- Genetic defects of beta-cell function
- Genetic defects in insulin action
- Diseases of the exocrine pancreas: pancreatitis, trauma, neoplasia, cystic fibrosis, hemochromatosis
- Endocrinopathies: acromegaly, Cushing's disease, glucagonoma, pheochromocytoma, hyperthyroidism, aldosteronism
- Drug of chemical-induced conditions (from use of pentamidine, nicotinic acid, glucocorticoids, thyroid hormone, diazoxide, beta-adrenergic agents, thiazides, Dilantin, interferon-alpha, other drugs)
- Infections: congenital rubella, cytomegalovirus
- Uncommon forms of immune-related diabetes
- Other genetic syndromes associated with diabetes: Down syndrome, Klinefelter syndrome, Turner's syndrome, Huntington disease, and others

GESTATIONAL DIABETES MELLITUS (GDM)
- Glucose intolerance with onset or first recognition during pregnancy
- Diagnosis is based on results of a 100-g oral glucose tolerance test during pregnancy

Data from American Association of Diabetes (ADA). (2007). Diagnosis and classification of diabetes mellitus, *Diabetes Care, 30*(Suppl. 1), 42-47.

Insulin Physiology

▶ ANIMATION: Insulin Function

Active insulin is a protein made up of 51 amino acids. Initially, an insulin precursor molecule known as proinsulin is produced. It contains an additional amino acid chain (the C-peptide chain) making the prohormone inactive. Proinsulin is converted in the beta cells into equal amounts of insulin and C-peptide (Fig. 67-1). C-peptide levels are used to measure the rate that beta cells secrete insulin.

The membranes of many cells are impermeable to glucose. Insulin is like a "key" that opens "locked" membranes to glucose, allowing glucose in the blood to move into cells to generate energy. Insulin starts this action by binding to insulin receptors on the cell membranes, which changes membrane permeability to glucose. The liver is the first major organ to be reached by insulin in the blood. In the liver, insulin promotes

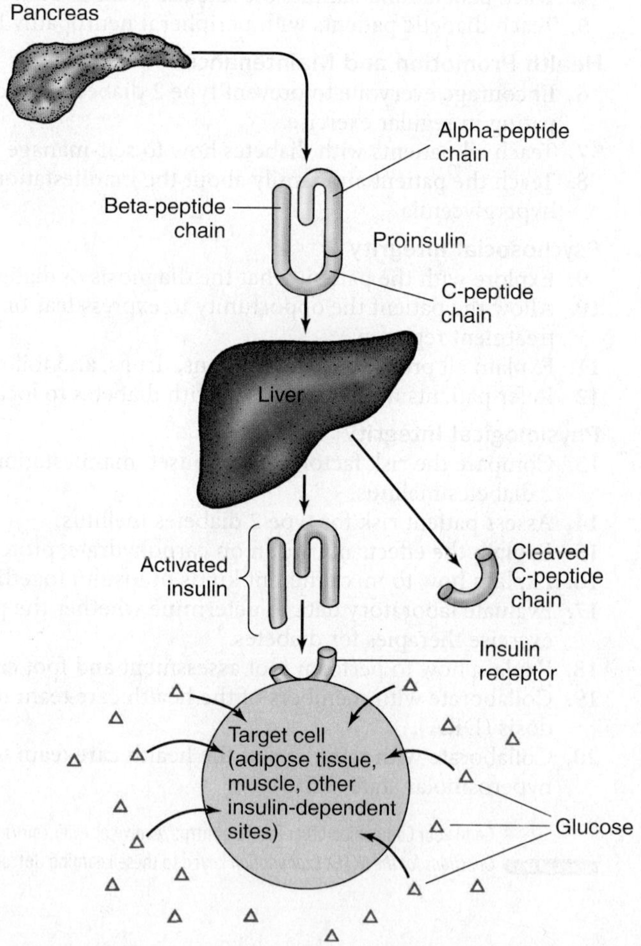
Pancreas
Alpha-peptide chain
Beta-peptide chain
Proinsulin
C-peptide chain
Liver
Activated insulin
Cleaved C-peptide chain
Insulin receptor
Target cell (adipose tissue, muscle, other insulin-dependent sites)
Glucose

Fig. 67-1 • Proinsulin, secreted by and stored in the beta cells of the islets of Langerhans in the pancreas, is transformed by the liver into activated insulin. Insulin attaches to receptors on target cells, where it promotes glucose transport into the cells through the cell membranes.

the production and storage of glycogen **(glycogenesis)** at the same time that it inhibits glycogen breakdown into glucose **(glycogenolysis).** It increases protein and lipid (fat) synthesis and inhibits liver glycogenolysis, **ketogenesis** (conversion of fats to acids), and **gluconeogenesis** (conversion of proteins to glucose). In muscle, insulin promotes protein and glycogen synthesis. In fat cells, it promotes triglyceride storage. Overall, insulin keeps blood glucose levels from becoming too high and helps keep blood lipid levels in the normal range.

The pancreas secretes about 40 to 50 units of insulin daily directly into liver circulation in a two-step manner. It is secreted at low levels during fasting **(basal insulin secretion)** and at increased levels after eating **(prandial).** An early burst of insulin secretion occurs within 10 minutes of eating. This is followed by an increasing release that lasts as long as hyperglycemia is present.

Glucose Homeostasis

Glucose is the main fuel for central nervous system (CNS) cells. Because the brain cannot produce or store much glucose, it needs a continuous supply from circulation to prevent neuronal dysfunction and cell death. Fatty acids can be used as fuel by some cells when glucose is not available. Glucose and free fatty acids are stored inside cells as glycogen in the liver and muscles and as triglyceride in fat cells. Fat, in the form of triglyceride, is the most efficient means of storing energy. Fat has 9 calories of stored energy per gram. Protein and carbohydrate have only 4 calories per gram. During a prolonged fast or after illness or injury, proteins are broken down and some amino acids are converted into glucose.

Several organs and hormones play a role in maintaining glucose homeostasis. During the fasting state, when the stomach is empty, plasma glucose is maintained between 70 and 100 mg/dL (3.9 and 5.6 mmol/L) by a balance between glucose uptake by cells and glucose production by the liver. Liver processes are regulated by glucagon release from pancreatic alpha cells that stimulate glucose production. Insulin is released from pancreatic beta cells to prevent excessive liver glucose output.

Glucose in the blood after a meal is controlled by the emptying rate of the stomach and delivery of nutrients to the small intestine, where they are absorbed into circulation. Incretin hormones (e.g., GLP-1), secreted in response to the presence of food in the stomach, have several actions. They increase insulin secretion, inhibit glucagon secretion, and slow the rate of gastric emptying, thereby preventing hyperglycemia after meals (Kruger et al., 2006).

In type 2 diabetes, hyperglycemia results from excessive liver glucose production and reduced glucose uptake in other cells due to a combination of insulin resistance and deficient insulin secretion. This abnormal glucose homeostasis is most evident at mealtime. During a meal, the rate of gastric emptying for patients with diabetes is faster than normal. Both the rate at which stomach contents reach the intestine and the rate of glucose entry into circulation increase and result in hyperglycemia. The increased rate of gastric emptying is thought due to reduced secretions of amylin and GLP-1 (Kruger et al., 2006).

Counterregulatory hormones increase blood glucose by actions opposite those of insulin when more energy is needed. Glucagon is the main counterregulatory hormone. Other hormones that increase blood glucose levels are epinephrine, norepinephrine, growth hormone, and cortisol. The combined actions of insulin and counterregulatory hormones (discussed in the next section) keep blood glucose levels in the range of 70 to 100 mg/dL (3.9 to 5.6 mmol/L) to support brain functions. When glucose levels fall, insulin secretion stops and glucagon is released. Glucagon causes the release of glucose from the liver. Liver glucose is made through **glycogenolysis,** which is the breakdown of glycogen to glucose, and **gluconeogenesis,** which is the conversion of amino acids into glucose. When liver glucose is unavailable, **lipolysis,** which is the breakdown of fat, and **proteolysis,** which is the breakdown of proteins, provide fuel for energy.

Absence of Insulin

Insulin is needed to move glucose into most body tissues. The lack of insulin in diabetes, from either a lack of production or a problem with insulin use at its cell receptor, prevents some cells from using glucose for energy. Without insulin, the body enters a serious state of breaking down body fat and protein. Levels of counterregulatory hormones increase in an attempt to make glucose from other sources. Table 67-2 outlines the body's response to insufficient insulin.

Without insulin, glucose builds up in the blood, causing **hyperglycemia,** which is high blood glucose levels. Hyperglycemia causes fluid and electrolyte imbalances, leading to the classic symptoms of diabetes: polyuria, polydipsia, and polyphagia.

Polyuria is frequent and excessive urination and results from an osmotic diuresis caused by excess glucose in the urine. As a result of diuresis, sodium, chloride, and potassium are excreted in the urine and water loss is severe. Dehydration results, and **polydipsia,** which is excessive thirst, occurs. Because the cells receive no glucose, cell starvation triggers **polyphagia,** which is excessive eating. Despite eating vast amounts of food, the person remains in starvation until insulin is available to move glucose into the cells.

With insulin deficiency, fats break down, releasing free fatty acids. Conversion of fatty acids to **ketone bodies** (small acids) provides a backup energy source. Because ketone bodies, or "ketones," are abnormal breakdown products of fatty acids, they collect in the blood when insulin is not available. This collection causes metabolic acidosis.

The dehydration that occurs with diabetes leads to **hemoconcentration** (an increased blood concentration), **hypovolemia** (a decreased blood volume), **hyperviscosity** (thick, concentrated blood), **hypoperfusion** (decreased circulation) of tissues, and **hypoxia** (poor tissue oxygenation), especially to the brain. Hypoxic cells do not metabolize glucose efficiently, the Krebs' cycle is blocked, and lactic acid increases, causing

TABLE 67-2 Physiologic Response to Insufficient Insulin

- Decreased glycogenesis (conversion of glucose to glycogen)
- Increased glycogenolysis (conversion of glycogen to glucose)
- Increased gluconeogenesis (formation of glucose from non-carbohydrate sources, such as amino acids and lactate)
- Increased lipolysis (breakdown of triglycerides to glycerol and free fatty acids)
- Increased ketogenesis (formation of ketones from free fatty acids)
- Proteolysis (breakdown of protein with amino acid release in muscles)

more acidosis. Restoring tissue perfusion and oxygenation by giving insulin halts lactic acid production.

The excess acids caused by absence of insulin increase hydrogen ion (H^+) and carbon dioxide (CO_2) levels in the blood, causing metabolic acidosis. These products trigger the respiratory centers of the brain to increase the rate and depth of respiration in an attempt to excrete more carbon dioxide and acid. This type of breathing is known as **Kussmaul respiration.** Acetone is exhaled, giving the breath a "fruity" odor. When the lungs can no longer offset acidosis, the blood pH drops. Arterial blood gas studies show a metabolic acidosis (decreased pH with decreased arterial bicarbonate [HCO_3^-] levels) and compensatory respiratory alkalosis (decreased partial pressure of arterial carbon dioxide [$Paco_2$]).

Insulin lack causes potassium depletion. Because of the increased fluid loss with hyperglycemia, excessive potassium is excreted in the urine, leading to low serum potassium levels. However, high serum potassium levels may occur in acidosis because of the shift of potassium from inside the cells to the blood. Serum potassium levels in diabetes, then, may be low **(hypokalemia),** high **(hyperkalemia),** or normal, depending on hydration, the severity of acidosis, and the patient's response to treatment. Chapter 14 discusses acid-base balance and acidosis in more detail.

Acute Complications of Diabetes

Three glucose-related emergencies can occur in patients with diabetes:

- Diabetic ketoacidosis (DKA) caused by lack of insulin and ketosis
- Hyperglycemic-hyperosmolar state (HHS) caused by insulin deficiency and profound dehydration
- Hypoglycemia from too much insulin or too little glucose

All three problems require emergency treatment and can be fatal if treatment is delayed or incorrect. These problems and their interventions are described later.

Chronic Complications of Diabetes

Diabetes mellitus can lead to health problems and early death because of changes in large blood vessels **(macrovascular)** and small blood vessels **(microvascular)** in tissues and organs. Complications result from poor tissue circulation and cell death. Macrovascular complications, including coronary heart disease, cerebrovascular disease, and peripheral vascular disease, lead to increased early death among those with diabetes. Microvascular complications of blood vessel structure and function lead to **nephropathy** (kidney dysfunction), **neuropathy** (nerve dysfunction), and **retinopathy** (vision problems). Three theories have been used to explain these diabetic vascular complications:

- Chronic hyperglycemia causes irreversible basement membrane thickening and organ damage.
- Glucose toxicity directly or indirectly affects functional cell integrity.
- Chronic ischemia in small blood vessels causes connective tissue hypoxia and microischemia.

Chronic high blood glucose levels are the main cause of microvascular complications and allow premature development of macrovascular complications. These complications in patients with type 2 diabetes seem more related to hypertension, a sedentary lifestyle, high blood lipid levels, and smoking than to hyperglycemia. Obesity is also important for patients with type 2 diabetes. Most patients with type 2 diabetes are obese, and cardiovascular events account for most of their deaths.

Type 2 diabetes often produces no symptoms in its early stages and can remain undiagnosed for years. Many older diabetic patients have no classic signs of high blood glucose levels, and the diagnosis is made when the patient seeks treatment for another illness or for complications of diabetes, such as visual problems. Many patients have reduced vision from retinopathy at the time of diagnosis.

The Diabetes Control and Complications Trial (DCCT), a study involving 29 medical centers and more than 1400 patients with type 1 diabetes, showed that hyperglycemia is a critical factor for long-term diabetic complications. Intensive therapy aiming for blood glucose levels as close to normal as possible delays the onset and progression of retinopathy, nephropathy, neuropathy, and macrovascular disease. Additional studies show that intensive therapy with lowered blood glucose levels delays the onset of retinopathy, nephropathy, and neuropathy in patients with type 2 diabetes. A strong relationship exists between microvascular complications and blood glucose levels. For every percentage point decrease in HbA_{1c}, a 35% reduction in the risk for kidney and eye complications has been shown (ADA, 2003).

Macrovascular Complications

Cardiovascular Disease. Cardiovascular disease (CVD) is the most common complication of diabetes mellitus. Patients with type 1 or type 2 diabetes are at higher risk for MI compared with patients without diabetes. This excess risk affects women to a greater degree than men and is influenced by the patient's ethnic group. More than half of diabetic patients have evidence of CVD at the time of diagnosis.

Myocardial infarction (MI) is the leading cause of death among patients with diabetes. They often have extensive coronary artery disease, diabetic cardiomyopathy, and abnormal blood clotting. Left ventricular dysfunction with cardiac failure and fatal cardiac dysrhythmias are more common in diabetic patients after MI. In the Diabetes Mellitus Insulin-Glucose in Acute MI (DIGAMI) trial, 66% of mortality among patients with diabetes was due to heart failure (Davis et al., 2006).

Diabetic patients often have a higher incidence of traditional cardiovascular risk factors of obesity, hypertension, dyslipidemia (excessive blood levels of cholesterol and other fats), and sedentary lifestyle. Cigarette smoking and a positive family history also increase risk for cardiovascular disease. Renal disease, indicated by **albuminuria** (presence of albumin in the urine), increases the risk for coronary heart disease and mortality from MI. Patients with diabetes tend to have higher levels of C-reactive protein (CRP), an acute-phase inflammatory marker associated with increased risk for future cardiovascular problems and death.

Cardiovascular disease complication rates can be reduced through aggressive management of hyperglycemia, hypertension, and hyperlipidemia. The American Diabetes Association (ADA) recommends that blood pressure (BP) levels be maintained below 130/80 mm Hg and that low-density lipoprotein (LDL) cholesterol be lowered to less than 100 mg/dL (2.60 mmol/L) for patients without manifestations of CVD and to less than 70 mg/dL (1.8 mmol/L) for patients with manifestations of CVD (ADA, 2007b). Diets high in saturated fat raise total cholesterol, and high LDL cholesterol levels increase the incidence of coronary artery disease. The National

Cholesterol Education Panel Guidelines and the ADA recommend reducing intake of saturated and trans-fatty acids to lower the incidence of heart disease (Solano & Goldberg, 2006).

Cerebrovascular Disease. Diabetes damages cerebrovascular (brain) arterial circulation and is a risk factor for stroke. Hypertension, hyperlipidemia, nephropathy, peripheral vascular disease, and alcohol and tobacco abuse, along with diabetes, further increase the risk for stroke (Matz et al., 2006). Diabetes affects stroke outcomes as well. Elevated blood glucose levels at the time of the stroke may lead to greater brain injury and higher mortality.

Microvascular Complications

Eye and Vision Complications. Legal blindness (a corrected visual acuity of 20/200 or less) is 25 times more common in patients with diabetes. Diabetic retinopathy is strongly related to the duration of diabetes. After 20 years of diabetes, nearly all patients with type 1 diabetes have some degree of retinopathy.

The cause and progression of diabetic retinopathy are related to problems that block retinal blood vessels and cause them to leak, leading to retinal hypoxia. Nonproliferative diabetic retinopathy (NPDR) (Fig. 67-2) causes structural problems in retinal vessels, but growth of new blood vessels is not stimulated. There are areas of poor retinal circulation, edema, hard fatty deposits in the eye, and retinal hemorrhages. Microaneurysms are small capillary wall dilations in retinal vessels that form throughout the eye. They leak fluid and blood into the retina, causing retinal edema and hard exudates. Other retinal problems include retinal hemorrhages, optic nerve atrophy from hypoxia, and venous beading. **Venous beading** is the abnormal appearance of retinal veins in which areas of swelling and constriction along a segment of vein resemble links of sausage. It occurs in areas of retinal ischemia and is a predictor of proliferative diabetic retinopathy (PDR). NPDR develops slowly and rarely causes blindness.

Proliferative diabetic retinopathy (PDR) is the growth of new retinal blood vessels, also known as "neovascularization." When retinal blood flow is poor and hypoxia develops, retinal cells secrete a "growth factor" that stimulates formation of new blood vessels in the eye. These new vessels are thin and fragile and bleed easily. They lead to eye hemorrhage and more vision loss (Fig. 67-3). Fibrous tissue bands also develop, causing retinal detachment and permanent vision loss. Chapter 49 discusses treatment of retinal problems.

Retinopathy is linked to fasting blood glucose levels above 129 mg/dL. Hyperglycemia and hypertension increase the rate of retinopathy development in patients with type 1 diabetes. Intensive diabetes management to obtain **near-euglycemic** (near-normal blood glucose) levels reduces the risk for diabetic retinopathy.

Vision loss also occurs from macular degeneration, corneal scarring, and changes in lens shape or clarity. Hyperglycemia may cause blurred vision, even with eyeglasses. Hypoglycemia may cause double vision. Cataracts occur at a younger age and progress faster among patients with diabetes. Open-angle glaucoma also is more common in patients with diabetes. The management of cataracts and glaucoma is the same as for nondiabetic patients (see Chapter 49).

CONSIDERATIONS FOR OLDER ADULTS

The older patient with diabetic retinopathy also has visual changes from aging. As a result, the older diabetic patient's ability to perform self-care may be seriously affected. The patient with retinopathy may have blurred vision, distorted central vision, fluctuating vision, loss of color perception, and mobility problems resulting from loss of depth perception. It is especially important to assess the ability of the patient to perform tasks such as measurement and injection of insulin and blood glucose monitoring to determine if adaptive devices are needed to assist in self-management activities.

Diabetic Neuropathy. Neuropathy is a progressive deterioration of nerves that results in loss of nerve function. It is a common complication of diabetes and often involves all parts of the body. Damage to sensory nerve fibers results in either pain or loss of sensation. Damage to motor nerve fibers results in muscle weakness. Damage to nerve fibers in the autonomic nervous system can cause dysfunction in every part of the body.

Diabetic neuropathy can be focal or diffuse, each with different causes and rates of progression. *Diffuse neuropathies* are

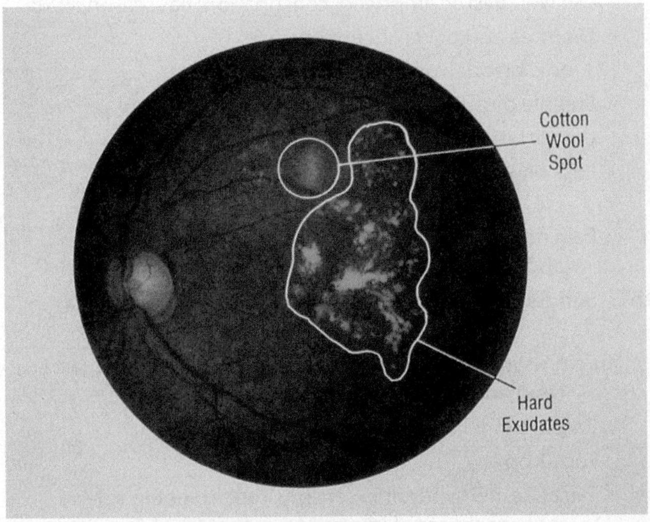
Cotton Wool Spot
Hard Exudates

Fig. 67-2 • Select ophthalmic changes seen in nonproliferative diabetic retinopathy (NPDR).

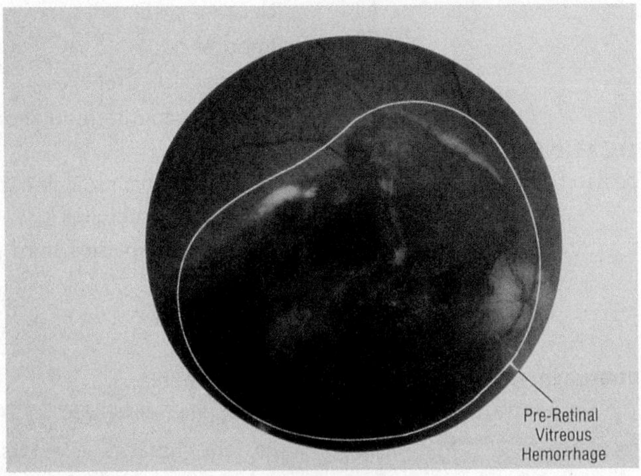
Pre-Retinal Vitreous Hemorrhage

Fig. 67-3 • Ophthalmic hemorrhage that is possible with proliferative diabetic retinopathy.

the most common neuropathies in diabetes and involve widespread nerve function loss. They have a slow onset, affect both sides of the body, involve motor and sensory nerves, progress slowly, are permanent, and include autonomic nerve dysfunction. Late complications include foot ulcers and deformities.

Focal neuropathies affect a single nerve or nerve group. They usually are caused by an acute ischemic event or by the physical trapping of a nerve. Both problems lead to nerve damage or nerve death. Ischemic neuropathies occur when the blood supply to a nerve or group of nerves is disrupted. The symptoms begin suddenly, affect only one side of the body or body area, and are self-limiting. Recovery time varies. Entrapment neuropathies stem from compression of a nerve in a body compartment or between tissues. Symptoms begin gradually and can occur anywhere. They may be bilateral, having a waxing and waning course without spontaneous recovery. An example of focal entrapment neuropathy is carpal tunnel syndrome.

Hyperglycemia leads to neuropathy through blood vessel changes that cause nerve hypoxia. Both the axon and its myelin sheath are damaged by reduced blood flow, resulting in blocked nerve impulse transmission. Excessive glucose is converted to sorbitol, which collects in nerves. The increased sorbitol also impairs motor nerve conduction. Common diabetic neuropathies are listed in Table 67-3. Autonomic nervous system neuropathy leads to problems in cardiovascular, GI, and urinary function. Keeping blood glucose levels in the normal range delays the onset and reduces the severity of diabetic neuropathies.

The cardiovascular problems of **orthostatic** (postural) hypotension and **syncope** (brief loss of consciousness) increase the risk for falls, especially among older adults. In addition, the neuropathy can mask the pain of MI. Common GI symptoms from diabetic neuropathy are **dysphagia** (difficulty swallowing), heartburn, nausea and vomiting, and bowel elimination problems. Diarrhea caused by diabetes is chronic, may be severe, and often occurs at night. Constipation, the most common GI symptom, is intermittent and may alternate with bouts of diarrhea. **Gastroparesis** (delay in gastric emptying) is a cause of hypoglycemia. Loss of nerve input to the bladder results in incomplete emptying, which leads to urinary infection and kidney problems.

Diabetic Nephropathy. **Nephropathy** is a pathologic change in the kidney that reduces kidney function and leads to kidney failure. Diabetes is the leading cause of end-stage kidney disease (ESKD) and kidney failure in the United States. Keeping blood glucose levels in the normal range can delay the onset of nephropathy and, in some cases, may prevent it (ADA, 2007b).

Risk factors for nephropathy include a 10- to 15-year history of diabetes, diabetic retinopathy, poor blood glucose control, uncontrolled hypertension, and genetic predisposition. The earliest clinical sign of nephropathy is **microalbuminuria** (very small amounts of albumin in the urine). Annual testing for microalbuminuria is recommended for patients who have had type 1 diabetes for at least 5 years and in all patients with type 2 diabetes (ADA, 2007b).

TABLE 67-3 Features of Diabetic Neuropathy

	Complication	Manifestation
DIFFUSE NEUROPATHIES		
Distal symmetric polyneuropathy	Sensory alterations	Paresthesias: burning/tingling sensations, starting in toes and moving up legs Dysesthesias: burning, stinging, or stabbing pain Anesthesia: loss of sensation
	Motor alterations in intrinsic muscles of foot	Foot deformities: high arch, claw toes, hammertoes; shift of weight-bearing to metatarsal heads and tips of toes
Autonomic neuropathy	Anhidrosis	Drying, cracking of skin
	Gastroparesis	Delayed gastric emptying, constipation, nausea, anorexia
	Diabetic diarrhea	Diarrhea and bowel incontinence
	Neurogenic bladder	Atonic bladder, urinary retention
	Impotence	Erectile dysfunction
	Loss of cardiac reflexes	Orthostatic hypotension, resting tachycardia
	Defective counterregulation	Loss of warning signs of hypoglycemia
FOCAL NEUROPATHIES		
Focal ischemia	Thoracolumbar radiculopathy with sensory and reflex loss	Pain radiating across back, side, and front of chest or abdomen
	Cranial nerve palsies, third and sixth nerves	Sudden diplopia or ptosis; eye pain
	Amyotrophy	Pain; asymmetric weakness; wasting of iliopsoas, quadriceps, and adductor muscles
Entrapment neuropathies	Median nerve	Carpal tunnel syndrome
	Popliteal nerve/knee	Footdrop
	Posterior tibial nerve at tarsal tunnel	Tarsal tunnel syndrome: sensory impairment in sole of foot; weakness of intrinsic muscles of foot; burning pain and paresthesias at ankle and plantar surface

Chronic high blood glucose levels cause hypertension in kidney blood vessels and excess kidney perfusion. The increased pressure damages the kidney in many ways. The blood vessels become leakier, especially in the glomerulus. This leakiness allows filtration of larger particles (including albumin and other proteins), which then form deposits in the kidney tissue and blood vessels. Deposits narrow the vessels, decreasing kidney oxygenation and leading to kidney cell hypoxia and cell death. These processes worsen over time, with blood vessels in the glomerulus becoming scarred and unable to filter urine from the blood, leading to renal failure.

Kidney damage is also related to hypertension in diabetic patients with cardiovascular disease. Both systolic and diastolic hypertension greatly speed the progression of diabetic nephropathy.

Male Erectile Dysfunction. Erectile dysfunction (ED) is the inability to achieve or maintain a penile erection sufficient for satisfactory sexual performance. ED occurs at a higher rate and an earlier age among men with diabetes as compared with the general population. At least half of men with diabetes have ED. This occurs 10 to 15 years earlier than in the general population and increases with age. It is related to poor blood glucose control, obesity, hypertension, heavy cigarette smoking, and the presence of other chronic vascular complications. Most men with diabetic neuropathy have ED. Chapter 75 discusses erectile function problems in depth.

Etiology and Genetic Risk

Type 1 Diabetes

Type 1 diabetes is an autoimmune disorder in which beta cells are destroyed in a genetically susceptible person (Table 67-4). The immune system fails to recognize normal body cells as "self" and takes destructive actions against them. In type 1 diabetes, immune system cells, mediators, and antibodies attack and destroy insulin-secreting cells in the islets. Although the exact cause of a person's normal cells being attacked by immune system cells is not known, people with certain tissue types are more likely to develop autoimmune diseases, including type 1 diabetes. Specifically, patients who have the tissue types HLA-DR or HLA-DQ are at an increased risk for type 1 diabetes. Certain viral infections, such as mumps, congenital rubella, and coxsackievirus infection, appear to trigger autoimmune destruction of pancreatic beta cells (McCance & Huether, 2006).

Indicators or markers of immune damage to insulin-producing cells (a key feature of type 1 diabetes) are the presence of blood antibodies directed against the beta cells themselves or against substances made by beta cells. Most patients with type 1 diabetes have islet cell antibodies (ICAs), insulin autoantibodies (IAAs), autoantibodies to glutamic acid decarboxylase (GAD), or autoantibodies to tyrosine phosphates (McCance & Huether, 2006). Circulating ICA and IAA may be present before manifestations of type 1 diabetes develop.

GENETIC CONSIDERATIONS

Risk for type 1 diabetes is determined by inheritance of genes coding for the HLA-DR and HLA-DQ tissue types. However, although inheritance of these genes increases the risk, most people with these genes do not develop type 1 diabetes. Development of the disease is an interactive effect of genetic predisposition and exposure to certain environmental factors. The risk for type 1 diabetes in the general population ranges from 1 in 400 to 1 in 1000. The risk greatly increases for those who have at least one parent with diabetes (from 1 in 20 to 1 in 50) (Nussbaum et al., 2007). It is unclear why some genetically susceptible people develop diabetes and others do not.

TABLE 67-4 Differentiation of Type 1 and Type 2 Diabetes

Features	Type 1	Type 2
Former names	Juvenile-onset diabetes Ketosis-prone diabetes Insulin-dependent diabetes mellitus (IDDM)	Adult-onset diabetes Ketosis-resistant diabetes Non–insulin-dependent diabetes mellitus (NIDDM)
Age at onset	Usually younger than 30 yr, occurs at any age	Peaks in 50s; may occur earlier
Symptoms	Abrupt onset, thirst, weight loss	Frequently none; thirst, fatigue, visual blurring, vascular or neural complications
Etiology	Viral infection	Not known
Pathology	Pancreatic beta cell destruction	Insulin resistance Dysfunctional pancreatic beta cell
Antigen patterns	HLA-DR, HLA-DQ	None
Antibodies	ICAs present at diagnosis	None
Endogenous insulin and C-peptide	None	Low, normal, or high
Inheritance	Recessive	Dominant, multifactorial
Nutritional status	Usually nonobese	60% to 80% obese
Insulin	All dependent on insulin	Required for 20% to 30%
Sulfonylurea therapy	None	Effective for most patients
Medical nutrition therapy	Mandatory	Mandatory

ICAs, Islet cell antibodies.

Type 2 Diabetes and Metabolic Syndrome

Type 2 diabetes is a progressive disorder in which the pancreas makes less insulin over time. Patients with type 2 diabetes have **insulin resistance,** which is a reduced ability of most cells to respond to insulin, poor control of liver glucose output, and decreased beta-cell function, eventually leading to beta-cell failure. Most patients with type 2 diabetes are obese. With the increased rate of obesity occurring in younger people, the age of onset for type 2 diabetes is also decreasing. The specific causes of type 2 diabetes are not known. Both insulin resistance and beta-cell failure have many genetic and nongenetic causes. Heredity plays a major role in the development of type 2 diabetes. Offspring of patients with type 2 diabetes have a 15% chance for developing the disease and a 30% risk for having impaired glucose tolerance. Specific gene defects have been identified in certain groups with high incidence rates of type 2 diabetes (Nussbaum, et al., 2007).

Metabolic syndrome, also called **syndrome X,** is the simultaneous presence of metabolic factors known to increase risk for developing type 2 diabetes and cardiovascular disease. Features of the syndrome include:

- Abdominal obesity: waist circumference of 40 inches (100 cm) or more for men, and 35 inches (88 cm) or more for women
- Hyperglycemia: elevated fasting blood glucose level 100 mg/dL or more or on drug treatment for elevated glucose
- Hypertension: systolic BP of 130 mm Hg or more or diastolic BP of 85 mg Hg or more or on drug treatment for hypertension
- Dyslipidemia: triglyceride level 150 mg/dL or more or on drug treatment for elevated triglycerides; high-density lipoprotein (HDL) cholesterol less than 40 mg/dL for men or less than 50 mg/dL for women

Any one of these health problems increases the rate of atherosclerosis and the risk for stroke, coronary heart disease, and early death. Teach patients about the lifestyle changes that can improve health. Reducing weight to within 20% of ideal or body mass index to less than 25 kg/m^2 by modifying diet and exercising more will reduce cardiovascular risk (Appel, 2005). Drug therapy may be required to achieve desired lipid and blood pressure outcomes.

Incidence/Prevalence

Diabetes is the seventh leading cause of death in the United States, where it affects 20.8 million people, or 7% of the population. An additional 6.2 million people are unaware they have the disease (www.diabetes.org).

About 90% of people with diabetes have type 2 diabetes. It is diagnosed most often among middle-aged and older adults, affecting about 9.6% of patients ages 20 to 59 years and 20.9% of patients ages 60 years or older. The prevalence of diabetes is higher for men than for women (www.diabetes.org).

Although type 2 diabetes is a disease of middle-aged and older adults, recent surveys show an increase of the disorder in childhood and adolescence as a result of obesity. Because the prevalence of obesity is rising in North America, diabetes will become even more common. Obesity and a higher-than-normal body mass index (BMI) greatly increase the risk for diabetes.

Health Promotion and Maintenance

The fact that diabetes is a common disorder and causes many preventable but devastating complications makes the disease a major public health problem. Control of diabetes and its complications is a major focus for health promotion activities. No interventions are successful in preventing type 1 diabetes. Health promotion for patients with type 1 diabetes focuses on controlling hyperglycemia to reduce its long-term complications. Teach all patients with diabetes that tight control of blood glucose levels can prevent life-shortening complications. Urge all patients with diabetes to regularly follow-up with their health care provider or endocrinologist, have their eyes and vision tested yearly by an ophthalmologist, and have urine microalbumin levels assessed yearly. Early diagnosis of changes allows adjustments in treatment regimens to be made that slow progression of eye and kidney problems.

Type 2 diabetes can be prevented or delayed by weight loss and increased physical activity. Encourage people to maintain weight within an appropriate range for height and body build. Teach them that strategies to reduce the cardiovascular risk factors of tobacco use, hypertension, and high blood lipid levels also reduce the incidence of type 2 diabetes and its long-term complications.

DECISION-MAKING CHALLENGE
Coordination of Care

You are caring for a 62-year-old woman who has had type 2 diabetes for more than 20 years. She is blind and has renal failure. Her 28-year-old daughter asks you what her own chances are for developing diabetes. The daughter reports that her 38-year-old sister has just been diagnosed with type 2 diabetes. You note that the daughter is 5′ 4″ tall and weighs about 220 lbs. She is a secretary and has a 1-year-old son.

1. What personal questions should you ask the daughter to help determine her risk?
2. Explain the genetics of type 2 diabetes.
3. Does the daughter have any risks for other health problems? If so, what are they?
4. What suggestions do you have for the daughter to reduce her risk for or delay the development of the disease?

evolve For suggested answer guidelines, go to http://evolve.elsevier.com/Iggy/.

CULTURAL AWARENESS

Diabetes is a significant health problem for African Americans, American Indians, and Mexican Americans. The prevalence rates for this disease are 1.6 and 1.9 times higher, respectively, than the rate for white patients (Oldroyd et al., 2005). The increase in obesity and sedentary lifestyles in the U.S. population is the probable cause of this growing problem. The American Diabetes Association (ADA) has identified patients who should be tested for diabetes in Table 67-5.

Racial and ethnic differences affect clinical outcomes for diabetic patients. The prevalence of hypertension in diabetic patients is at least twice the rate of nondiabetic patients, with non-Hispanic whites and African Americans having the highest prevalence. Microvascular complications of the eyes, nerves, and kidneys are more common in African Americans and American Indians with diabetes than in non-Hispanic whites with diabetes. Possible factors for these differences include lack of access to health care, lifestyle issues, mistrust of the health care system, reduced financial resources, and lack of knowledge about the relationship between glucose control and complications.

Patient-Centered Collaborative Care

evolve ONLINE PHARM REVIEW

Assessment

History

Ask questions about risk factors and symptoms related to diabetes. Age is important because type 2 diabetes is more common in older patients, especially among African Americans and Mexican Americans. Ask women how large their children were at birth because many women who develop type 2 diabetes had gestational diabetes or were glucose intolerant during pregnancy. These women often have given birth to infants weighing 9 pounds or more.

Assessing weight and weight change is important because excess weight and obesity are risk factors for type 2 diabetes. The patient with type 1 diabetes often has weight loss with increased appetite during the weeks before diagnosis. For both types of diabetes, patients usually have fatigue, polyuria, and polydipsia. Ask patients about recent major or minor infections. In particular, ask women about frequent vaginal yeast infections. Ask all patients whether they have noticed that small skin injuries become infected more easily or take longer to heal. Also ask whether they have noticed any changes in vision or in their sense of touch.

Laboratory Assessment

Diagnosis of Diabetes. Diabetes can be diagnosed by assessing blood glucose levels. The American Diabetes Association (ADA) defines normal blood glucose values in Chart 67-1. In the absence of hyperglycemia, the diagnosis must be confirmed by any one of three methods. Glycosylated hemoglobin (HbA_{1c}) is not used for the diagnosis of diabetes. ADA criteria for the diagnosis of adult diabetes mellitus are outlined in Table 67-6.

Fasting plasma glucose (FPG) is the preferred test to diagnose diabetes in nonpregnant adults. The patient should have no caloric intake for at least 8 hours (water is permitted). The blood

TABLE 67-5 Indications for Testing for Type 2 Diabetes

Testing for diabetes should be considered in people 45 years of age and older, particularly in those with a BMI greater than 25 kg/m². If normal, it should be repeated at 3-year intervals.

Testing should be considered at a younger age or be carried out more frequently in people who are overweight (BMI >25 kg/m²) and have these additional associated factors:

- Have a first-degree relative with diabetes
- Are habitually physically inactive
- Are members of a high-risk ethnic population (e.g., African American, Hispanic American, American Indian, Asian American, or Pacific Islander)
- Deliver a baby weighing more than 9 pounds or have been diagnosed with GDM
- Are hypertensive (>140/90 mm Hg)
- Have a high-density lipoprotein (HDL) cholesterol level less than 35 mg/dL (0.90 mmol/L) and/or a triglyceride level greater than 250 mg/dL (2.82 mmol/L)
- Have polycystic ovary syndrome
- Have IFG or IGT on previous testing
- Have a history of vascular disease

Data from American Diabetes Association (ADA). (2007). Standard of medical care in diabetes—2007. *Diabetes Care, 30*(Suppl. 1), 4-41.

BMI, Body mass index; *GDM,* gestational diabetes mellitus; *IFG,* impaired fasting glucose; *IGT,* impaired glucose tolerance.

Chart 67-1 LABORATORY PROFILE

Blood Glucose Values

Test	Normal Range for Adults	Significance of Abnormal Results
Fasting blood glucose test	<100 mg/dL (5.6 mmol/L) *Older adults:* Levels rise 1 mg/dL per decade of age	Levels >100 mg/dL (5.6 mmol/L) but <126 mg/dL (7.0 mmol/L) indicate impaired fasting glucose (IFG). Levels >126 mg/dL (7.0 mmol/L) obtained on at least two occasions are diagnostic of diabetes, even in older adults.
Glucose tolerance test (2-hr post-load result)	<140 mg/dL (7.8 mmol/L)	Levels >140 mg/dL (7.8 mmol/L) and <200 mg/dL (11.1 mmol/L) indicate impaired glucose tolerance (IGT). Levels >200 mg/dL (11.1 mmol/L) indicate provisional diagnosis of diabetes.
Glycosylated hemoglobin (hemoglobin A_{1c} [HbA_{1c}]) test	4%-6%	Levels >8% indicate poor diabetic control and need for adherence to regimen or changes in therapy.

Data from American Diabetes Association (ADA). (2007). Diagnosis and classification of diabetes mellitus. *Diabetes Care, 30*(Suppl. 1), 42-47, and the American Diabetes Association (ADA). (2007). Standard of medical care in diabetes. *Diabetes Care, 30*(Suppl. 1), 4-41.

TABLE 67-6 Criteria for the Diagnosis of Type 2 Diabetes

Symptoms of diabetes plus casual blood glucose concentration greater than 200 mg/dL (11.1 mmol/L). *Casual* is defined as any time of day without regard to time since last meal. The classic symptoms of diabetes include polyuria, polydipsia, and unexplained weight loss.

Or

Fasting plasma glucose greater than 126 mg/dL (7.0 mmol/L). *Fasting* is defined as no caloric intake for at least 8 hr.

Or

2-hr plasma glucose greater than 200 mg/dL during an oral glucose tolerance test. The test should be performed using a glucose load containing the equivalent of 75 g glucose dissolved in water.

NOTE: Each test must be confirmed, on a subsequent day, under similar circumstances.

Data from American Diabetes Association (ADA). (2007). Diagnosis and classification of diabetes mellitus. *Diabetes Care, 30*(Suppl. 1), 42-47.

Chart 67-2 PATIENT AND FAMILY EDUCATION GUIDE

Blood Glucose Testing

FASTING BLOOD GLUCOSE

- Do not eat any food or drink any liquid for at least 8 hours.

ORAL GLUCOSE TOLERANCE TEST

- Eat a balanced diet with carbohydrate intake of at least 150 g for a minimum of 3 days while maintaining normal physical activity.
- Carbohydrate restriction, bedrest, acute illness, and certain drugs interfere with the test. Phenytoin (Dilantin), anovulatory drugs, diuretics, nicotinic acid, and glucocorticoids adversely affect results.
- The test is performed in the morning after a 10- to 12-hour fast.
- A fasting blood sample is obtained.
- You will be asked to drink 300 mL (75 g) of a flavored beverage within 5 minutes of the fasting blood sample.
- Blood samples are drawn at 30-minute intervals for 2 hours.
- During the test, you will remain at rest and not be able to smoke or drink liquids.

sample needs to be obtained before insulin or oral antidiabetic agents have been taken. A diagnosis of diabetes is made with two separate test results greater than 126 mg/dL (7 mmol/L) (ADA, 2007a). The guide for patient and family education about blood glucose testing is presented in Chart 67-2.

Oral glucose tolerance testing (OGTT) is the most sensitive test for the diagnosis of diabetes. However, it is not routinely used in the diagnosis of diabetes because the test is inconvenient to patients, costly, and time consuming compared with fasting blood glucose measures. The diagnosis of gestational diabetes mellitus (GDM) is based on the oral glucose tolerance test (75-g, 2-hr test or 100-g, 3-hr test). Before the test, review instructions from Chart 67-2 with the patient. He or she drinks a beverage containing a glucose load, and blood samples are collected at hourly intervals. Two or more of the venous plasma levels must be met or exceeded for a positive diagnosis (ADA, 2007a).

Other blood tests for diabetes can help determine whether a patient has type 1 or type 2 diabetes, although they are not commonly used. Type 1 diabetes is an autoimmune disease with the presence of autoantibodies to proteins. The presence of islet cell antibodies (ICA) is an indicator for type 1 diabetes. Measurement of C-peptide levels indicates beta secretory function of the pancreas. C-peptide levels correlate well with insulin levels and are used to diagnose type 1 diabetes.

Screening for Diabetes. Screening to detect pre-diabetes and diabetes should be considered in patients older than 45 years and those defined as overweight (BMI greater than 25 kg/m^2) (Deatcher, 2008). It is considered also for patients who are younger than 45 years and are overweight if they have additional risk factors for diabetes. Screening for diabetes is done with either fasting plasma glucose test or 2-hour OGTT (75-g glucose load) (ADA, 2007a; ADA, 2007c).

Ongoing Assessment. *Glycosylated hemoglobin assays* are useful because blood glucose permanently attaches to hemoglobin. The higher the blood glucose level is over time, the more glycosylated hemoglobin becomes. Thus glycosylated hemoglobin (HbA_{1c}) is a good indicator of the average blood glucose levels. Measurement of HbA_{1c} shows the average blood glucose level during the previous 120 days—the life span of red blood cells. HbA_{1c} testing is used to assess long-term glycemic control, as well as to predict the risk for complications. *Unlike the fasting blood glucose test, HbA_{1c} test results are not altered by eating habits the day before the test.* This testing is performed at diagnosis and at specific intervals to evaluate the treatment plan. Hemolysis, blood loss, and pregnancy all increase red blood cell turnover and reduce HbA_{1c} levels. Triglycerides and bilirubin interfere with the assay, leading to overestimation of HbA_{1c} levels in patients with hypertriglyceridemia. HbA_{1c} testing is recommended at least twice yearly in patients who are meeting treatment goals and have stable blood glucose control. Quarterly assessment is recommended for patients whose therapy has changed or who are not meeting glycemic goals (ADA, 2007c). Table 67-7 shows the correlation between HbA_{1c} and mean blood glucose levels.

Glycosylated serum proteins and albumin are useful because they become increasingly glycosylated with elevated blood glucose levels in the same way as hemoglobin does. However, because serum proteins and albumin turn over in 14 days, compared with 120 days of red blood cells, these proteins can indicate blood glucose control over a shorter period. These measures are useful when tight control of blood glucose is necessary (e.g., pregnancy) or in short-term follow-up of treatment changes. Available tests are called *glycosylated serum albumin (GSA), glycosylated serum protein (GSP),* and *fructosamine.*

Urine Tests. *Ketone bodies* are a product of fat metabolism. The presence of moderate to high urine ketones (hyperketonuria) indicates a severe lack of insulin. Hyperketonuria in the presence of hyperglycemia is a medical emergency that, when detected early, can be treated with insulin and careful monitoring. Urine testing for ketones should be performed during acute illness or stress, when blood glucose levels consistently exceed 300 mg/dL (16.7 mmol/L), during pregnancy, or when any symptoms of ketoacidosis are present. Ketone testing also is recommended for diabetic patients participating in a weight-loss program. Hyperketonuria without hyperglycemia suggests that weight loss is occurring without disrupting blood glucose control.

Ketone bodies include beta-hydroxybutyric acid, acetoacetic acid, and acetone. They appear in urine in the same proportion as they do in blood but are affected by urine volume and concentration. Ketones are variably reabsorbed by the renal tubules and may be present in urine long after blood levels have returned to normal. For these reasons, urine ketone bodies are not used to evaluate the effectiveness of treatment for ketoacidosis.

TABLE 67-7 Correlation Between HbA_{1c} Level and Mean Plasma Glucose Levels

	MEAN PLASMA GLUCOSE	
HbA_{1c} (%)	mg/dL	mmol/L
6	135	7.5
7	170	9.5
8	205	11.5
9	240	13.5
10	275	15.5
11	310	17.5
12	345	19.5

Data from American Diabetes Association (ADA). (2007). Standards of medical care in diabetes—2007. *Diabetes Care, 30*(Suppl. 1), 4-41.

Tests for kidney function are important because the presence of urine protein without kidney symptoms may indicate microvascular changes in the kidney. Urine albumin excretion rates of 20 to 200 g/min (30 to 300 mg/hr) indicate microalbuminuria. Even minor elevations of albumin are associated with increased mortality.

Once clinical proteinuria has been detected, kidney function (e.g., glomerular filtration rate) is assessed by creatinine clearance tests (see Chapter 68). In patients with nephropathy, a rise in serum creatinine level is related to both poor blood glucose control and hypertension.

Urine glucose testing is an indirect measurement of blood glucose and is much less precise than blood glucose testing. Fluid intake, urine elimination patterns, and certain drugs affect the results. This test may be appropriate for a quick screening but should not be used for monitoring diabetes management.

NCLEX EXAMINATION CHALLENGE

The client with type 2 diabetes admitted for surgery has the following results of today's laboratory testing: FPG = 122 mg/dL; after-meal blood glucose level = 182 mg/dL, and HbA_{1c} = 5.8%. How should these values be interpreted with regard to the client's glucose control?

A. Short-term values elevated, long-term values normal, overall good glucose control
B. Short-term values elevated, long-term values elevated, overall poor glucose control
C. Short-term values normal, long-term values normal, overall good glucose control
D. Short-term values normal, long-term values elevated, overall poor glucose control

evolve For the correct answer, go to http://evolve.elsevier.com/Iggy/.

Analysis

Common Nursing Diagnoses and Collaborative Problems

Priority nursing diagnoses for patients with diabetes are:

1. Risk for Injury related to hyperglycemia
2. Risk for Delayed Surgical Recovery related to endocrine and vascular effects of diabetes
3. Risk for Injury related to sensory alterations (diabetic neuropathy)
4. Chronic Pain related to peripheral nerve dysfunction (diabetic neuropathy)
5. Risk for Injury related to disturbed sensory perception: visual (diabetic retinopathy)
6. Ineffective Tissue Perfusion (Renal) related to impaired transport of oxygen across capillary membranes

Primary collaborative problems are:

1. Potential for Hypoglycemia
2. Potential for Diabetic Ketoacidosis
3. Potential for Hyperglycemic-Hyperosmolar State and Coma

Additional Nursing Diagnoses and Collaborative Problems

In addition to the common nursing diagnoses and collaborative problems, patients with diabetes may have one or more of these:

- Imbalanced Nutrition: More Than Body Requirements related to an imbalance of food intake and physical activity, lack of knowledge, and ineffective coping skills
- Risk for Deficient Fluid Volume related to fluid shifts, failure of regulatory mechanisms, hyperglycemic diuresis, polyuria, vomiting, diarrhea, decreased oral intake, and dehydration
- Impaired Oral Mucous Membrane related to microvascular circulatory changes and uncontrolled blood glucose levels
- Deficient Knowledge about diabetes management related to a lack of familiarity with information resources about disease, diet, exercise, drugs, weight control, and foot care
- Impaired Urinary Elimination and Urinary Retention (with overflow incontinence) related to diabetic neuropathy
- Constipation related to diabetic neuropathy
- Risk for Impaired Skin Integrity related to decreased circulation, increased blood glucose levels, decreased mobility, and decreased sensation
- Risk for Infection related to increased blood glucose levels, decreased tissue perfusion, inadequate primary defenses, and the effects of chronic disease
- Risk for Ineffective Sexuality Pattern (male) related to autonomic neuropathy, decreased circulation, or psychological problems
- Risk for Ineffective Sexuality Pattern (female) related to the stressors of diabetes
- Situational Low Self-Esteem related to an inability to deal with the self-care demands of the diabetic regimen
- Anxiety related to diagnosis of diabetes, potential complications of diabetes, and self-care regimens
- Fear related to diagnosis of diabetes, potential complications of diabetes, and self-care regimens
- Ineffective Coping and Compromised Family Coping related to a chronic disease, a complex self-care regimen, and decreased social support
- Powerlessness related to the complications of diabetes (blindness, amputations, renal failure, and neuropathy)
- Social Isolation related to visual impairment or blindness
- Noncompliance with self-care related to the complexity and duration of the prescribed regimen
- Ineffective Health Maintenance related to insufficient knowledge of diet restriction, weight control, weight maintenance, benefits and risks of exercise, self-monitoring of blood glucose, medications, sick-day care, foot care, hypoglycemia, and available resources

Planning and Implementation

The management of diabetes mellitus is complicated and involves considerable patient involvement and education. The Concept Map on p. 1476 highlights care issues for the patient with type 2 diabetes mellitus.

Risk for Injury Related to Hyperglycemia

NOC **Planning: Expected Outcomes.** The patient with diabetes is expected to manage diabetes mellitus and prevent disease progression by maintaining blood glucose levels in the expected range. Indicators are that the patient consistently demonstrates these behaviors:

- Performs treatment regimen as prescribed
- Follows recommended diet
- Demonstrates correct procedure for blood glucose testing
- Monitors blood glucose
- Treats symptoms of hyperglycemia
- Seeks health care if blood glucose levels fluctuate outside of recommended parameters

CONCEPT MAP Diabetes Mellitus-Type 2

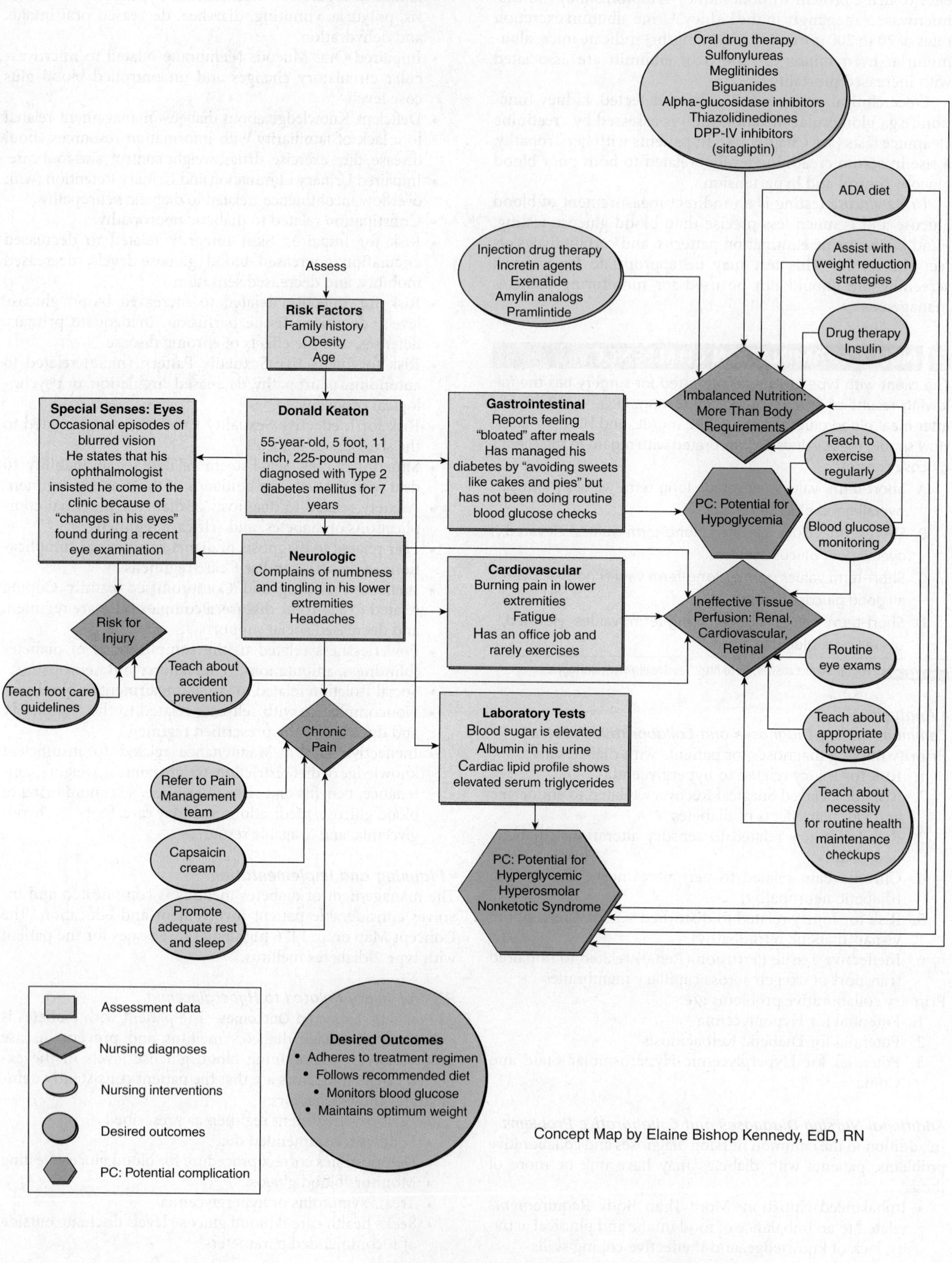
Assess
Risk Factors
Family history
Obesity
Age
Donald Keaton
55-year-old, 5 foot, 11 inch, 225-pound man diagnosed with Type 2 diabetes mellitus for 7 years
Special Senses: Eyes
Occasional episodes of blurred vision
He states that his ophthalmologist insisted he come to the clinic because of "changes in his eyes" found during a recent eye examination
Neurologic
Complains of numbness and tingling in his lower extremities
Headaches
Gastrointestinal
Reports feeling "bloated" after meals
Has managed his diabetes by "avoiding sweets like cakes and pies" but has not been doing routine blood glucose checks
Cardiovascular
Burning pain in lower extremities
Fatigue
Has an office job and rarely exercises
Laboratory Tests
Blood sugar is elevated
Albumin in his urine
Cardiac lipid profile shows elevated serum triglycerides
Oral drug therapy
Sulfonylureas
Meglitinides
Biguanides
Alpha-glucosidase inhibitors
Thiazolidinediones
DPP-IV inhibitors
(sitagliptin)
Injection drug therapy
Incretin agents
Exenatide
Amylin analogs
Pramlintide
ADA diet
Assist with weight reduction strategies
Drug therapy
Insulin
Imbalanced Nutrition: More Than Body Requirements
Teach to exercise regularly
PC: Potential for Hypoglycemia
Blood glucose monitoring
Ineffective Tissue Perfusion: Renal, Cardiovascular, Retinal
Routine eye exams
Teach about appropriate footwear
Teach about necessity for routine health maintenance checkups
PC: Potential for Hyperglycemic Hyperosmolar Nonketotic Syndrome
Risk for Injury
Teach about accident prevention
Teach foot care guidelines
Chronic Pain
Refer to Pain Management team
Capsaicin cream
Promote adequate rest and sleep
Assessment data
Nursing diagnoses
Nursing interventions
Desired outcomes
PC: Potential complication
Desired Outcomes
• Adheres to treatment regimen
• Follows recommended diet
• Monitors blood glucose
• Maintains optimum weight

Concept Map by Elaine Bishop Kennedy, EdD, RN

- Follows recommended activity level
- Uses drugs as prescribed
- Maintains optimum weight

Interventions

Nonsurgical Management. Nonsurgical management of diabetes mellitus involves nutritional interventions, blood glucose monitoring, a planned exercise program, and in some instances, drugs to lower blood glucose levels. The nurse, together with the patient, physician, nutritionist, pharmacist, case manager, and in some cases, physical therapist, plans, coordinates, and delivers care.

The American Diabetes Association (ADA) has proposed these treatment goals for glycosylated hemoglobin (HbA_{1c}) and blood glucose levels (ADA, 2007c):

- HbA_{1c} levels should be maintained at 7% or below.
- The majority of premeal (preprandial) blood glucose levels should be 90 to 130 mg/dL (5.0 to 7.2 mmol/L).
- Blood glucose values at bedtime should be between 100 and 140 mg/dL (5.6 and 7.8 mmol/L).

Drug therapy. Drug therapy is indicated when a patient with type 2 diabetes does not achieve blood glucose control with diet changes, regular exercise, and stress management. Several different categories of drugs are available to lower blood glucose levels.

Oral therapy. Oral agents are prescribed only after dietary control has proven insufficient or if the patient is highly symptomatic.

Sulfonylurea agents are classified as insulin secretagogues and are used for patients with some remaining pancreatic beta-cell function. These drugs stimulate insulin secretion from pancreatic beta cells and increase the number or sensitivity of cell receptor sites for interaction with insulin. The overall effect of sulfonylurea therapy is lowering of fasting plasma glucose levels. These drugs differ in strength, overall effects, metabolism, and risk for complications (Chart 67-3).

Side effects of sulfonylurea agents include weight gain and hypoglycemia. Hypoglycemic episodes are more likely to occur with chlorpropamide (Diabinese, Novo-Propamide🍁)

Text continued on p. 1483

Chart 67-3 COMMON EXAMPLES OF DRUG THERAPY

Diabetes Mellitus: Oral Blood Glucose–Lowering Agents

	Use in Diabetes	Nursing Interventions	Rationales
SULFONYLUREAS			
Acetohexamide (Dymelor) Usual dose: 0.25-1.5 g daily	Increase insulin secretion in the treatment of type 2 diabetes.	Teach patients how to prevent and treat hypoglycemia and hyperglycemia.	Long half-life is associated with increased frequency of hypoglycemia. Older people, people who skip meals, and people who perform intensive exercise are most susceptible.
		Warn patients to avoid drinking alcohol when taking acetohexamide.	Disulfiram-like reaction may occur when alcohol is consumed with acetohexamide. Symptoms include flushing of the face, pulsating headache, sweating, confusion, and slurred speech. Severe reaction can cause death.
Chlorpropamide (Diabinese) Usual dose: 250 mg daily	Increase insulin secretion in the treatment of type 2 diabetes.	Teach patients how to prevent and treat hypoglycemia and hyperglycemia.	Long half-life is associated with increased frequency of hypoglycemia. Older adults, people who skip meals, and people who perform intensive exercise are most susceptible.
		Teach patients to report symptoms of dizziness, nausea, anorexia, mental depression, and/or confusion.	Antidiuretic action of chlorpropamide may result in syndrome of inappropriate ADH secretion manifested as symptoms and signs of water intoxication.
		Caution patients to avoid drinking alcohol when taking acetohexamide.	Alcohol, even in small amounts, can cause disulfiram-like reaction.
Tolazamide (Tolinase) Usual dose: 100-500 mg twice daily	Increase insulin secretion in the treatment of type 2 diabetes.	Administer with meals. Warn patients to avoid drinking alcohol when taking tolazamide.	Severe hypoglycemia, with symptoms resembling neurologic disorders, has occurred in some patients taking tolazamide.

Continued

Chart 67-3 COMMON EXAMPLES OF DRUG THERAPY

Diabetes Mellitus: Oral Blood Glucose–Lowering Agents—cont'd

	Use in Diabetes	Nursing Interventions	Rationales
SULFONYLUREAS—cont'd			
Tolazamide (Tolinase)—cont'd		Teach patients how to prevent and treat hypoglycemia and hyperglycemia.	Debilitated, malnourished, or geriatric patients and those with impaired hepatic and/or renal function should be carefully monitored and the dosage of tolazamide adjusted, since these patients are more prone to development of hypoglycemia.
		Monitor fluid balance. Teach patients to weigh themselves daily and report any weight gain greater than 2 lbs to the health care provider.	Hyponatremia and the syndrome of inappropriate ADH secretion occur in some patients taking tolazamide.
Tolbutamide (Orinase, Mobenol) Usual dose: 750-1000 mg every 12-24 hr	Increase insulin secretion in the treatment of type 2 diabetes.	Teach patients to take the drug in divided doses after meals.	Nausea, epigastric fullness, and heartburn occur frequently with tolbutamide use. Taking tolbutamide with food decreases GI symptoms.
		Teach patients how to prevent and treat hypoglycemia and hyperglycemia.	Long half-life is associated with increased frequency of hypoglycemia. Older adults, people who skip meals, and people who perform intensive exercise are most susceptible.
SECOND-GENERATION SULFONYLUREA AGENTS			
Glipizide (Glucotrol) Usual dose: 2.5-5 mg every 12-24 hr Glucotrol XL (Extended release form) once daily	Increase insulin secretion in the treatment of type 2 diabetes.	Teach patients to take the drug 30 min before meals.	Taking the drug 30 min before a meal achieves the best after-meal blood glucose concentration.
		Teach patients how to prevent and treat hypoglycemia.	Because the drug induces insulin secretion, hypoglycemia is possible.
		Monitor patients with impaired renal function carefully for hypoglycemia.	The drug is eliminated by the renal route. Patients with impaired renal function have higher blood levels of the drug and are a risk for hypoglycemia.
		Instruct patients to swallow the extended-release form of the drug whole and not divided, chewed, or crushed.	Damaging the extended form of the drug causes the rapid release of the entire drug dose and can cause hypoglycemia.
Glyburide (DiaBeta/Micronase) Usual dose: 1.25-20 mg (Glynase PresTabs) Usual dose: 0.75-12 mg (divide doses >6 mg)	Increase insulin secretion in the treatment of type 2 diabetes.	Teach patients to take the drug as a single daily dose with the first main meal of the day.	Glyburide is more likely to produce hypoglycemia than other sulfonylurea agents. The risk for hypoglycemia is increased with the use of other blood glucose–lowering agents or with alcohol.
		Teach patients how to prevent and treat hypoglycemia.	Debilitated, malnourished, or older patients are particularly susceptible to glyburide-induced hypoglycemia. Hypoglycemia is usually, but not always, readily controlled with administration of glucose.

Chart 67-3 COMMON EXAMPLES OF DRUG THERAPY

Diabetes Mellitus: Oral Blood Glucose–Lowering Agents—cont'd

	Use in Diabetes	Nursing Interventions	Rationales
SECOND-GENERATION SULFONYLUREA AGENTS—cont'd			
Glimepiride (Amaryl) Usual dose: 1-4 mg daily	Increase insulin secretion in the treatment of type 2 diabetes.	Teach patients to take the drug as a single daily dose with the first main meal of the day. Teach patients how to prevent and treat hypoglycemia.	Debilitated or malnourished patients or those with impaired kidney or liver function are more sensitive to blood glucose–lowering effects of glimepiride.
MEGLITINIDE ANALOGUES			
Repaglinide (Prandin) Usual dose: 0.5-4 mg daily	Increase insulin secretion in the treatment of type 2 diabetes.	Teach patients to take the drug 1-30 min before meals.	Drug is most effective when administered with or just before eating a meal.
	Short-acting agent used to prevent postmeal blood glucose elevation.	Teach patients to omit the drug when skipping a meal, and instruct them to add a dose if an extra meal is eaten.	Hypoglycemia may occur shortly after dosing when the meal is delayed or omitted.
Nateglinide (Starlix) Usual dose: 60-120 mg before meals	Increase insulin secretion in the treatment of type 2 diabetes.	Teach patients to take the drug 3 times daily, 1-30 min before meals.	Drug is most effective when administered with or just before eating a meal.
	Short-acting agent used to prevent postmeal blood glucose elevation.	Teach patients to omit the drug when skipping a meal, and instruct them to add a dose if an extra meal is eaten.	Hypoglycemia may occur shortly after dosing when the meal is delayed or omitted.
BIGUANIDES			
Metformin (Glucophage) Usual dose: 850 mg twice daily with the morning and evening meals (Glucophage XL) Usual dose: 2.5-5 mg daily before breakfast	Lowers both basal and postmeal blood glucose levels in patients with type 2 diabetes by reducing hepatic glucose production and tissue sensitivity to insulin.	Teach patients to take the drug with food.	Adverse GI side effects such as diarrhea, nausea, vomiting, flatulence, indigestion, and abdominal discomfort are common. Taking the drug with food reduces these effects.
		Monitor liver and renal function before starting metformin and periodically thereafter.	Metformin should be used with caution in older patients since aging is associated with reduced renal function. Metformin is contraindicated in people with serum creatinine in males >1.5 mg/dL (132.6 μmol/L), and in females >1.4 mg/dL (123.8 μmol/L).
		Monitor cardiopulmonary status throughout therapy.	Metformin should not be used in patients with congestive heart failure requiring drug therapy. These patients are at risk for hypoperfusion and hypoxemia, conditions which increase the risk for lactic acidosis.
		Monitor for conditions that increase risk for lactic acidosis.	Metformin is contraindicated in people with risk factors for lactic acidosis: reduced renal function, liver impairment, respiratory insufficiency, severe infection, alcohol abuse.
		Instruct patients taking metformin to report symptoms of lactic acidosis: malaise, unusual muscle pain, respiratory distress, increasing somnolence, and abdominal distress.	Onset of lactic acidosis is subtle and accompanied by nonspecific symptoms.

Continued

Chart 67-3 COMMON EXAMPLES OF DRUG THERAPY
Diabetes Mellitus: Oral Blood Glucose–Lowering Agents—cont'd

	Use in Diabetes	Nursing Interventions	Rationales
BIGUANIDES—cont'd			
Metformin (Glucophage, Glucophage XL)—cont'd		Instruct patients taking metformin to report any illness that causes severe vomiting, diarrhea, or fever.	Precipitating events for lactic acidosis include hypoxemia, dehydration, and sepsis.
		Withhold metformin for 48 hr before use of iodinated contrast materials used in certain radiographic studies.	Iodinated contrast materials can alter renal function and increase the risk for lactic acidosis. Metformin therapy is restarted when renal function has returned to normal.
		Instruct patients taking Glucophage XL that tablets must be swallowed whole and never crushed or chewed.	Damaging the extended form of the drug causes the rapid release of the entire drug dose and can cause hypoglycemia.
ALPHA-GLUCOSIDASE INHIBITORS			
Acarbose (Precose) Usual dose: 50-100 mg three times daily	Used to prevent postmeal blood glucose elevation in the treatment of type 2 diabetes.	Teach patients to take the drug with the first bite of each main meal.	Acarbose must be taken at the beginning of a meal to be fully effective.
		Teach patients the action to take for missed doses of the drug.	Instruct patients to take the missed dose at the next meal and to avoid taking a double dose of drug.
		Monitor for abdominal pain, diarrhea, and flatulence.	GI side effects are very common. Symptoms can be reduced by slow titration of dose.
		Teach patients about dietary habits to decrease GI discomfort.	Avoiding foods that will increase GI discomfort such as rich foods, sauces, beverages including beer and carbonated soft drinks, gas-producing foods such as beans, nuts, bran cereals, broccoli, and cabbage reduce the GI side effects of the drug. Meals and snacks should be low in fat. Drinking plenty of water, especially in the early part of the day, and avoiding overeating also reduce symptoms.
		Monitor kidney function.	Drug may accumulate in patients with renal dysfunction; drug not recommended for patients with serum creatinine >2 mg/dL (176.8 µmol/L).
		Monitor liver function tests. Emphasize the need to report symptoms of unexplained nausea, vomiting, abdominal pain, fatigue, anorexia, or dark urine.	Acarbose is associated with elevation in serum transaminase levels. Doses >150 mg/day associated with increases in ALT (aminotransferase) and AST [SGOT]). ALT should be checked every 3 months for first year and periodically thereafter.

Chart 67-3 COMMON EXAMPLES OF DRUG THERAPY

Diabetes Mellitus: Oral Blood Glucose–Lowering Agents—cont'd

	Use in Diabetes	Nursing Interventions	Rationales
ALPHA-GLUCOSIDASE INHIBITORS—cont'd			
Acarbose (Precose)—cont'd		Instruct patients receiving acarbose to treat hypoglycemia with glucose tablets, glucose gel, or low-fat milk.	Acarbose does not cause hypoglycemia when given alone. Hypoglycemia caused by other agents should be treated with oral dextrose. Sucrose (table sugar or candy bars) will not reverse symptoms of hypoglycemia due to acarbose.
		Teach patients to store drug according to manufacturer's directions.	Remove from wrapper immediately before taking the drug to prevent deterioration of acarbose.
Miglitol (Glyset) Usual dose: 50 mg three times daily	Used to prevent postmeal blood glucose elevation in the treatment of type 2 diabetes.	Instruct patients to take the drug with the first bite of each main meal.	Miglitol must be taken at the beginning of a meal to be fully effective.
		Monitor renal function.	Drug may accumulate in patients with renal dysfunction; drug not recommended for patients with serum creatinine >2 mg/dL.
		Monitor for abdominal pain, diarrhea, and flatulence.	GI side effects are very common. Symptoms can be reduced by slow titration of dose.
		Monitor liver function tests.	Miglitol is associated with elevation in serum transaminase levels.
		Emphasize the need to report symptoms of unexplained nausea, vomiting, abdominal pain, fatigue, anorexia, or dark urine.	These manifestations are associated with reduced liver function.
		Teach patients taking miglitol to treat hypoglycemia with glucose tablets, glucose gel, or low-fat milk.	Miglitol does not cause hypoglycemia when given alone. Hypoglycemia caused by other agents should be treated with oral dextrose. Sucrose (table sugar or candy bars) will not reverse symptoms of hypoglycemia due to acarbose.
THIAZOLIDINEDIONES			
Pioglitazone (Actose) Usual dose: 15 mg or 30 mg once daily without regard to meals Rosiglitazone (Avandia) Usual dose: 8 mg once daily or 4 mg twice daily	Improves tissue sensitivity to insulin in the treatment of type 2 diabetes.	Emphasize the need for liver function tests as recommended. Instruct patients to report symptoms of unexplained nausea, vomiting, abdominal pain, fatigue, anorexia, or dark urine.	Rare cases of liver failure have occurred with pioglitazone. Liver function tests are measured at the start of therapy and at regular intervals thereafter. Not recommended for moderate to severe liver impairment (ALT >2.5 upper limit of normal or active liver disease) or in patients with jaundice.
		Advise women of the need for effective contraception during therapy.	Administration of pioglitazone with certain oral contraceptives may reduce the plasma concentration of the oral contraceptive. Postmenopausal women with insulin resistance may resume ovulation during therapy.
		Monitor weight; assess for edema and shortness of breath.	Fluid retention can lead to weight gain and can cause or exacerbate congestive heart failure.

Continued

Chart 67-3 COMMON EXAMPLES OF DRUG THERAPY

Diabetes Mellitus: Oral Blood Glucose–Lowering Agents—cont'd

	Use in Diabetes	Nursing Interventions	Rationales
THIAZOLIDINEDIONES—cont'd			
Pioglitazone (Actose)—cont'd		Stress importance of continuing therapy even if a response is not evident within 2 weeks.	Full therapeutic response may not be evident for 8-12 weeks after initiation of therapy.
Rosiglitazone (Avandia) Usual dose: 4 mg daily in the morning, or 2 mg twice daily in the morning and evening without regard to food	Improves tissue sensitivity to insulin in the treatment of type 2 diabetes.	Emphasize the need for liver function tests as recommended. Instruct the patient to report symptoms of unexplained nausea, vomiting, abdominal pain, fatigue, anorexia, or dark urine.	Rare cases of liver failure have occurred with rosiglitazone. Liver function tests are measured at the start of therapy and at regular intervals thereafter. Not recommended for moderate to severe liver impairment (ALT >2.5 upper limit of normal or active liver disease) or in patients with jaundice.
		Advise women of the need for effective contraception during therapy.	Administration of rosiglitazone with certain oral contraceptives may reduce the plasma concentration of the oral contraceptive. Postmenopausal women with insulin resistance may resume ovulation during therapy.
		Monitor weight; assess for edema and shortness of breath.	Fluid retention can lead to weight gain and can cause or exacerbate congestive heart failure.
		Stress importance of continuing therapy even if a response is not evident within 2 weeks.	Full therapeutic response may not be evident for 2-3 months after initiation of therapy.
FIXED COMBINATIONS			
Glucovance (glyburide/metformin) 1.25 mg/250 mg 2.5 mg/500 mg 5 mg/500 mg	Metformin added to regimen when blood glucose is inadequately controlled on glyburide therapy alone.	Teach patients how to prevent and treat hypoglycemia.	Hypoglycemia may occur when metformin is given in combination with sulfonylurea agent.
Avandamet (rosiglitazone/metformin) Usual doses: 1 mg/500 mg 2 mg/500 mg 4 mg/500 mg	Rosiglitazone added to regimen when blood glucose is inadequately controlled on metformin therapy alone.	Teach patients how to prevent and treat hypoglycemia.	Hypoglycemia may occur when metformin is given in combination with thiazolidinedione agent.
Metaglip (glipizide/metformin) Usual doses: 2.5 mg/250 mg 2.5 mg/500 mg 5 mg/500 mg	Metformin added to regimen when blood glucose is inadequately controlled on glipizide therapy alone.	Teach patients how to prevent and treat hypoglycemia.	Hypoglycemia may occur when metformin is given in combination with sulfonylurea agent.
Duetact (glimepiride/pioglitazone) Usual doses: 2 mg/30 mg 4 mg/30 mg	Pioglitazone added to regimen when blood glucose is inadequately controlled on glimepiride therapy alone.	Teach patients how to prevent and treat hypoglycemia.	Hypoglycemia may occur when glimepiride is given in combination with thiazolidinedione agent.

Chart 67-3 COMMON EXAMPLES OF DRUG THERAPY
Diabetes Mellitus: Oral Blood Glucose–Lowering Agents—cont'd

	Use in Diabetes	Nursing Interventions	Rationales
FIXED COMBINATIONS—cont'd			
Avandaryl (glimepiride/ rosiglitazone) Usual doses: 1 mg/4 mg 2 mg/4 mg 4 mg/4 mg	Rosiglitazone added to regimen when blood glucose is inadequately controlled on glimepiride therapy alone.	Teach patients how to prevent and treat hypoglycemia.	Hypoglycemia may occur when glimepiride is given in combination with thiazolidinedione agent.
Actoplus Met (pioglitazone/metformin) Usual doses: 15 mg/500 mg 15 mg/850 mg	Pioglitazone added to regimen when blood glucose is inadequately controlled on metformin therapy alone.	Instruct patients in measures to prevent and treat hypoglycemia.	Hypoglycemia may occur when metformin is given in combination with thiazolidinedione agent.

because of its long duration of action. Underweight older patients with cardiovascular, liver, or kidney impairment are more susceptible to hypoglycemia. Many drugs can potentiate or interfere with sulfonylureas (Table 67-8).

First-generation sulfonylurea agents are seldom used but are still available in pharmacies. The Joint Commission 2007 National Patient Safety Goals include improving safety of look-alike/sound alike drugs. Take care to avoid confusing the dosage of acetohexamide (Dymelor) with that of acetazolamide (Diamox), a diuretic used in the treatment of glaucoma, and teach the patient how to avoid this drug error.

Meglitinide analogues are classified as insulin secretagogues and have actions and adverse effects similar to those of sulfonylureas. Repaglinide (Prandin) and Nateglinide (Starlix) lower blood glucose by triggering insulin secretion from pancreatic beta cells. These drugs were designed to increase meal-related insulin secretion. They are rapidly absorbed and have a short duration of action.

Repaglinide (Prandin) is taken before meals, has a rapid onset with a limited duration of action, and is used to treat both fasting and postprandial hyperglycemia. Adverse effects include hypoglycemia, GI disturbances, upper respiratory tract infection, arthralgia or back pain, and headache.

Nateglinide (Starlix) is rapidly absorbed and stimulates insulin secretion within 20 minutes of ingestion. It is taken just before meals to control mealtime hyperglycemia and improves overall glycemic control in patients with type 2 diabetes. The major adverse effect is hypoglycemia. Patients who skip meals should also skip their scheduled dose of Starlix to reduce the risk for hypoglycemia.

Biguanides are antihyperglycemic agents and insulin sensitizers. Metformin (Glucophage) is the major drug in this class. It does not increase insulin secretion. Instead, it decreases liver glucose production, thereby reducing fasting plasma glucose release, and improves insulin receptor sensitivity. The ADA recommends metformin as initial therapy for type 2 diabetes because the drug does not induce weight gain or hypoglycemia, has a relatively low cost, and has few adverse effects. It should not be given to anyone with kidney disease and elevated blood creatinine levels. The drug should be withheld for 48 hours before and after using contrast material and surgical procedures requiring anesthesia.

TABLE 67-8 Drug Interactions with Sulfonylurea Agents

Causes or Worsens Hyperglycemia	Causes or Worsens Hypoglycemia
Adrenalin	Angiotensin-converting agents (captopril [Capoten], enalapril [Vasotec])
Calcium channel blocking agents (diltiazem [Cardizem], nifedipine [Procardia])	Alcohol
Corticosteroids (prednisone)	Allopurinol (Zyloprim)
Diazoxide (Proglycem [oral], Hyperstat [IV])	Analgesics (azapropazone, phenylbutazone, salicylates)
Estrogen (Estrace, Premarin)	Antifungal azoles (fluconazole [Diflucan], ketoconazole [Nizoral], miconazole [Monistat])
Estrogen-progesterone containing oral contraceptives (Brevicon, Depo-Provera, Estrostep)	Beta-adrenergic blocking agents (atenolol, [Tenormin], propranolol [Inderal])
Furosemide (Lasix)	Chloramphenicol (Chloromycetin)
Isoniazid (INH)	Clofibrate (Atromid-S)
Nicotinic acid (Nicolar)	Coumarin anticoagulants (warfarin)
Phenothiazines (chlorpromazine [Thorazine], prochlorperazine [Compazine], trifluoperazine [Stelazine])	Fluoroquinolones (ciprofloxacin [Cipro], gatifloxacin [Tequin], levofloxacin [Levaquin])
Phenytoin (Dilantin)	Heparin
Rifampin (Rifadin)	Histamine H_2 antagonists (cimetidine [Tagamet], ranitidine [Zantac])
Sympathomimetics	Monamine oxidase (MAO) inhibitors (phenelzine [Nardil])
Thiazide diuretics (hydrochlorothiazide [HydroDIURIL], chlorothiazide [Diuril])	NSAIDs (indomethacin [Indocin], ibuprofen [Advil])
	Octreotide (Sandostatin)
	Probenecid (Benemid, Probalan)
	Sulfinpyrazone (Anturane)
	Sulfonamides (trimethoprim/sulfamethoxazole [Bactrim], sulfisoxazole [Gantrisin])
	Tricyclic antidepressants (amitriptyline hydrochloride, desipramine hydrochloride [Norpramin], doxepin hydrochloride [Sinequan])

Data from *AHFS Drug Information*. (2009). Bethesda, MD: American Society of Health-System Pharmacists.

The most common side effects are abdominal discomfort and diarrhea. Metformin can cause lactic acidosis in diabetic patients with renal insufficiency and should not be used in conditions that decrease drug clearance, such as renal insufficiency, liver disease, alcoholism, or severe congestive heart failure or in patients older than 80 years. Hypoxemia, dehydration, and sepsis also increase the risk for lactic acidosis. Symptoms of lactic acidosis can be subtle. Teach the patient to report symptoms of fatigue, unusual muscle pain, difficulty breathing, unusual or unexpected stomach discomfort, dizziness, lightheadedness, or irregular heartbeats to the primary care provider. Instruct patients to take metformin with meals to reduce GI effects. Caution against excessive alcohol intake because alcohol increases the risk for lactic acidosis.

Alpha-glucosidase inhibitors are agents that prevent hyperglycemia by delaying absorption of carbohydrate from the small intestine. These drugs inhibit enzymes in the intestinal tract, reducing the rate of digestion of starches and the absorption of glucose. Acarbose *delays* rather than prevents glucose absorption and does not cause weight loss.

The most common side effects are flatulence, diarrhea, and abdominal discomfort. There are two drugs in this class. Acarbose (Precose) is well tolerated when started at a low dose (25 mg once daily to three times daily with meals) and increased slowly. At higher doses, poor carbohydrate absorption occurs. Miglitol (Glyset) should be taken three times daily with the first bite of each main meal.

These drugs do not cause hypoglycemia unless given with sulfonylureas or insulin. Because alpha-glucosidase inhibitors delay carbohydrate absorption and interfere with the conversion of complex sugars to glucose, many of the standard glucose-based products used to treat hypoglycemia have a slower onset of action. These drugs do not inhibit absorption of glucose or lactose. Teach patients to use oral glucose tablets, glucose gel, or low-fat milk to treat hypoglycemia. Severe hypoglycemia may require glucose infusion or glucagon injection.

Thiazolidinediones (TZDs) are antihyperglycemic agents and insulin sensitizers. They improve insulin sensitivity and reduce liver glucose production. TZDs also improve insulin action in muscle, fat, and liver tissue by stimulating an enzyme receptor that regulates glucose and lipid metabolism (peroxisome proliferator activated receptor). The two drugs in this class are rosiglitazone (Avandia) and pioglitazone (Actos). Although rosiglitazone is available, its use has been associated with an increased risk for heart-related deaths, bone fractures, and macular edema (Ledbetter & Laustsen, 2008). It should be used cautiously in patients who have pre-existing cardiac problems.

All drugs in this class reduce blood lipid levels. Major side effects of TZD treatment are an increase in adipose tissue and fluid retention. Some patients taking these drugs gain weight. Edema, with development of congestive heart failure, is possible but not common. Other side effects of these drugs include infection, headache, peripheral edema, and pain. Patients taking these drugs should have periodic liver function studies because of the potential for liver damage.

Combination agents combine drugs with different mechanisms of action. Glucovance, for example, combines glyburide with metformin. Combining drugs with different mechanisms of action may be highly effective in maintaining desired blood glucose control. Some patients may need a combination of oral agents and insulin to control blood glucose levels.

Drug administration. Drugs are started at the lowest effective dose and increased every 1 to 2 weeks until the patient reaches desired blood glucose control or the maximum dosage. If the maximum dosage does not control blood glucose levels, a second oral agent with a different mechanism of action may be added. Insulin therapy is indicated when blood glucose cannot be controlled after the use of two or three different oral agents.

Antidiabetic drugs are not a substitute for dietary modification and exercise. Teach the patient about the need for continuing dietary restrictions and regular exercise while taking antidiabetic drugs. To avoid adverse drug interactions, teach the patient to consult with the primary care provider or pharmacist before using any over-the-counter drugs.

Drug selection. The choice of oral antidiabetic drug is based on cost, the patient's ability to manage multiple drug doses, age, and response to the drugs. Shorter-acting agents (e.g., glipizide) are preferable in older patients, those with irregular eating schedules, or those with liver, kidney, or cardiac dysfunction, whereas longer-acting agents (e.g., glyburide, glimepiride) with once-a-day dosing are better for adherence. Beta-cell function in type 2 diabetes often declines over time, reducing the effectiveness of some oral agents. The treatment regimen for the patient with type 2 diabetes may eventually require insulin therapy either alone or with oral agents.

Insulin therapy. Insulin therapy is needed for type 1 diabetes and also may be used for type 2 diabetes. The safety of insulin therapy in older patients may be affected by reduced vision, mobility and coordination problems, and decreased memory. There are many types of insulin and regimens, all aimed at achieving normal blood glucose levels.

Types of insulin. Insulin is manufactured using DNA technology to synthesize pure human insulin. Insulin analogues are genetically engineered human insulins in which the structure of the insulin molecule is altered to change the rate of absorption and duration of action within the body. One example is Lispro insulin, a rapid-acting insulin analogue that is created by switching the positions of lysine and proline in one area of the insulin molecule.

Rapid-, short-, intermediate-, and long-acting forms of insulin can be injected separately, and some can be mixed in the same syringe. Insulin is available in 100 units/mL (U-100) and 500 units/mL (U-500). U-500 is used only in rare cases of insulin resistance.

Teach the patient that the insulin types, the injection technique, the site of injection, and the patient response can all affect the absorption, onset, degree, and duration of insulin activity. Reinforce that changing insulins may affect blood glucose control and should be done only under supervision of the health care provider. Table 67-9 outlines the time activity of human insulin.

Insulin regimens. Insulin regimens try to duplicate the normal insulin release pattern from the pancreas. The pancreas produces a constant *(basal)* amount of insulin that balances liver glucose production with glucose use and maintains normal blood glucose levels between meals. The pancreas also produces additional *(prandial)* insulin to prevent blood glucose elevation after meals. The insulin dose required for blood glucose control varies among patients. A usual starting dose is between 0.5 and 1 unit/kg of body weight per day. For multiple-dose regimens or continuous subcutaneous insulin infusion (CSII), basal insulin makes up about 40% to 50% of the

TABLE 67-9 Time Activity of Pharmaceutical Insulin

Preparation	Brand	Onset (hr)	Peak (hr)	Duration (hr)
RAPID-ACTING INSULIN				
Insulin aspart	NovoLog	0.25	1-3	3-5
Insulin glulisine	Apidra	0.3	0.5-1.5	3-4
Human lispro injection	Humalog	0.25	0.5-1.5	5
SHORT-ACTING INSULIN				
Regular human insulin injection	Humulin R Novolin R ReliOn R	0.5 0.5	2-4 2.5-5	5-7 8
Humulin R (Concentrated U-500)	Humulin R (U 500)	1.5	4-12	24
INTERMEDIATE-ACTING INSULIN				
Isophane Insulin NPH injection	Humulin N Novolin N ReliOn N	1.5	4-12	16-24+
Insulin detemir injection	Levemir	1	6-8	5.7-24
70% human insulin isophane suspension/ 30% human insulin injection	Humulin 70/30 Novolin 70/30 ReliOn 70/30	0.5	2-12	24
50% human insulin isophane suspension/ 50% human insulin injection	Humulin 50/50	0.5	3-5	24
70% insulin aspart protamine suspension/ 30% insulin aspart injection	NovoLog Mix 70/30	0.25	1-4	24
75% insulin lispro protamine suspension/ 25% insulin lispro injection	Humalog Mix 75/25	0.25	1-2	24
LONG-ACTING INSULIN				
Insulin glargine injection	Lantus	2-4	None	24

total daily dosage, with the remainder divided into premeal doses of rapid-acting insulin analogues or regular insulin. Basal insulin coverage is provided by NPH insulin or by long-acting insulin analogues, insulin glargine (Lantus) or insulin detemir (Levemir). Because the rate of absorption is slowed by increasing the dosage, adjustments in dosage should be made no more than every 3 to 4 days. Dosage adjustments are based on the results of blood glucose monitoring.

Single daily injection protocols require insulin injection only once daily. This protocol may include one injection of intermediate- or long-acting insulin or a combination of short- and intermediate-acting insulin. Many patients with type 2 diabetes combine once-daily insulin injection with oral agent therapy.

Multiple-component insulin therapy combines short- and intermediate-acting insulin injected twice daily. Two thirds of the daily dose is given before breakfast and one third before the evening meal. Ratios of intermediate-acting and regular insulin are based on results of blood glucose monitoring.

Intensified regimens include a basal dose of intermediate- or long-acting insulin and a bolus dose of short- or rapid-acting insulin designed to bring the next blood glucose value into the target range. Blood glucose elevations above the target range are treated with "correction" doses of short- or rapid-acting insulin. The patient's blood glucose patterns determine insulin dosage. Frequency of blood glucose monitoring is based on the timed action of short- and intermediate- or long-acting insulins and may occur as often as eight times daily. Blood glucose testing 1 to 2 hours after meals and within 10 minutes before the next meal helps determine the adequacy of the bolus dose. The patient determines the effects of basal insulin by monitoring blood glucose levels before breakfast (fasting) and before the evening meal.

Patients on intensified insulin regimens need extensive education to achieve target blood glucose values. They need to know how to adjust insulin doses and understand nutrition therapy to maintain dietary flexibility and target blood glucose values. Patients must also be able to perform accurate blood glucose monitoring so that therapy decisions can be based on accurate data.

Factors influencing insulin absorption. Many factors affect insulin absorption and availability, including injection site; timing, type, or dose of insulin used; and physical activity.

Injection site affects the speed of insulin absorption. Fig. 67-4 shows common insulin injection sites. Absorption is fastest in the abdomen, followed by the deltoid, thigh, and buttocks. Rotating injection sites prevents lipohypertrophy (increased fat deposits in the skin) and lipoatrophy (loss of fatty tissue, leaving an uneven appearance). Rotation *within* one anatomic site is preferred to rotation from one site to another to prevent day-to-day changes in absorption. The abdomen (except for a 2-inch radius around the navel) is the preferred site because it provides the most rapid insulin absorption.

Absorption rate is determined by insulin properties. The longer the duration of action, the more unpredictable is absorption. Larger doses of insulin also prolong the absorption.

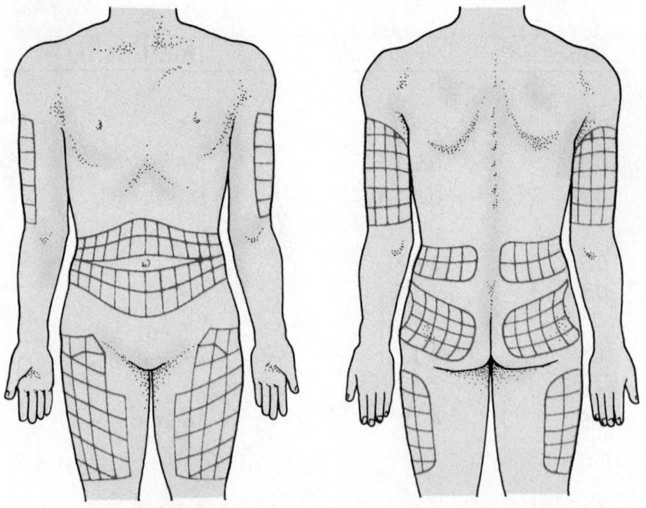
Front
Back
Fig. 67-4 • Common insulin injection sites.

Factors that increase blood flow from the injection site, such as local application of heat, massage of the area, and exercise of the injected area, increase insulin absorption. Scarred sites often become favorite injection sites because they are less sensitive to pain, but these areas usually slow the rate of insulin absorption.

Injection depth changes insulin absorption. Usually, injections are made into the subcutaneous tissue. Most patients lightly grasp a fold of skin and inject at a 90-degree angle. Aspiration for blood is not needed. A thin patient may need to pinch the skin and inject at a 45-degree angle to avoid IM injection. IM injection has a faster absorption and is not used for routine insulin use. Assess the older patient's ability to inject insulin, and arrange for assistance when self-care is no longer possible.

Timing of injection affects blood glucose levels. The interval between premeal injections and eating, known as "lag time," affects blood glucose levels after meals. Insulin lispro, insulin aspart, and insulin glulisine have rapid onsets of action and should be given within 10 minutes before mealtime when blood glucose is in the target range. If hyperglycemia or hypoglycemia is not present, these insulins can be given at any time from 10 minutes before mealtime to just before eating or even immediately after eating. Regular insulin should be given at least 20 to 30 minutes before eating when glucose levels are within the target range. When blood glucose levels are above the target range, the lag time should be increased to permit insulin to begin to have an effect sooner. Rapid-acting insulin analogues can be given 15 minutes before and regular insulin 30 to 60 minutes before eating a meal. When blood glucose levels are below the target range, injection of regular insulin should be delayed until immediately before eating and injection of rapid-acting insulin should be delayed until sometime after eating the meal.

Mixing insulins can change the time of peak action. Mixtures of short- and intermediate-acting insulins produce a more normal blood glucose response in some patients than does a single dose. The patient's response to mixed insulin may differ from the response to the same insulins given separately.

When rapid-acting (Humalog or NovoLog) or short-acting (regular) insulin is mixed with a longer-acting insulin, draw the shorter-acting dose into the syringe first. This action prevents contamination of the shorter-acting insulin vial with the longer-acting insulin. Short-acting and NPH insulins may be used immediately when mixed, or they may be stored. *No other insulin should be mixed with insulin glargine or insulin detemir.* Mixing clouds the solution and makes the onset of action and peak effect time less predictable. Follow American Diabetes Association (ADA) guidelines for mixing insulins (Table 67-10).

TABLE 67-10 American Diabetes Association Guidelines for the Mixing of Insulins

- Patients whose condition is well controlled on a particular mixed-insulin regimen should maintain their standard procedure for preparing insulin doses.
- No other drug or diluent should be mixed with any insulin product unless approved by the prescribing physician.
- Insulin glargine should not be mixed with any other forms of insulin because of the low pH of its diluent.
- Commercially available premixed insulins may be used if the insulin ratio is appropriate to the patient's insulin requirements.
- Currently available NPH and short-acting insulin formulations when mixed may be used immediately or stored for future use.
- Rapid-acting insulin can be mixed with NPH insulin.
- When rapid-acting insulin is mixed with either an intermediate- or long-acting insulin, the mixture should be injected within 15 minutes before a meal.
- Insulin formulations may change; therefore manufacturers should be consulted when their recommendations appear to conflict with the American Diabetes Association guidelines.

Data from American Diabetes Association (ADA). (2004). Insulin administration. *Diabetes Care, 27*(Suppl. 1), 106-109.

Complications of insulin therapy. Hypoglycemia from insulin excess has many causes. Its effects and treatment are discussed on pp. 1506-1509 in the Potential for Hypoglycemia section.

Lipoatrophy is a loss of fat tissue in areas of repeated injection that results from an immune reaction to impurities in insulin. Treatment consists of injection of insulin at the edge of the atrophied area. **Lipohypertrophy** is an increased swelling of fat that occurs at the site of repeated insulin injections. The overlying skin has decreased sensitivity, and the area can become large and unsightly. Treatment consists of rotating the injection site among different body areas. Teach patients who take insulin to rotate injection sites to prevent lipohypertrophy.

Two conditions of fasting hyperglycemia can occur (Fig. 67-5). **Dawn phenomenon** results from a nighttime release of growth hormone that causes blood glucose elevations at about 5 to 6 AM. It is managed by providing more insulin for the overnight period (e.g., giving the evening dose of intermediate-acting insulin at 10 PM). **Somogyi phenomenon** is morning hyperglycemia from the counterregulatory response to nighttime hypoglycemia. It is managed by ensuring adequate dietary intake at bedtime and evaluating the insulin dose and exercise programs to prevent conditions that lead to hypoglycemia. Both problems are diagnosed by blood glucose monitoring during the night. Help identify these problems, and teach the patient and family about management.

Alternative methods of insulin administration. Many methods of insulin delivery are available in addition to traditional subcutaneous injections.

Continuous subcutaneous infusion of a basal dose of insulin (CSII) with increases in insulin at mealtimes is more effective

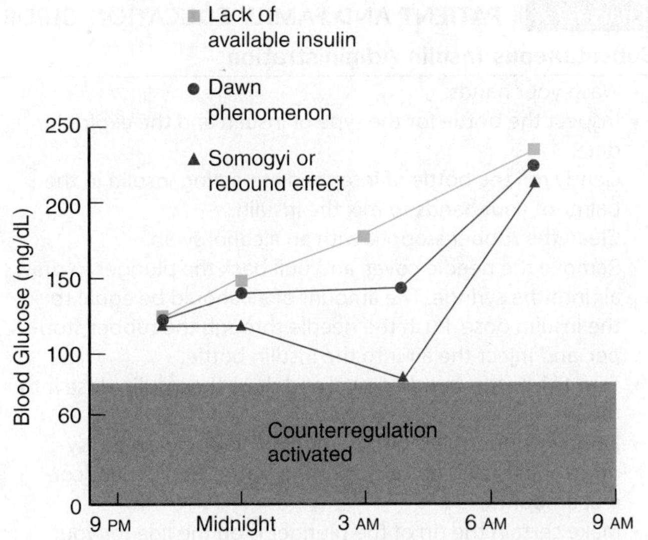
Lack of available insulin
Dawn phenomenon
Somogyi or rebound effect
Blood Glucose (mg/dL)
250
200
150
100
60
0
Counterregulation activated
9 PM
Midnight
3 AM
6 AM
9 AM

Fig. 67-5 • Three blood glucose phenomena in diabetic patients.

in controlling blood glucose levels than a multiple-injection schedule. CSII allows flexibility in meal timing, because if a meal is skipped, the mealtime dose of insulin is not given. It is given by an externally worn pump containing a syringe and reservoir with rapid-acting insulin and is connected to the patient by an infusion set. Teach him or her to adjust the amount of insulin received based on data from blood glucose monitoring. Rapid-acting insulin analogues are used with insulin infusion pumps (Fig. 67-6).

Problems with CSII include skin infections that can occur when the infusion site is not cleaned or the needle is not changed every 2 to 3 days. When the patient is receiving rapid-acting insulin and has normal blood glucose levels, stopping the infusion quickly results in hyperglycemia. CSII may lead to more frequent and more severe ketoacidosis than other methods of insulin delivery because of inexperience in pump use, infection, accidental cessation or obstruction of the infusion, or mechanical pump problems. Stress the importance of testing for ketones when blood glucose levels are greater than 300 mg/dL (16.7 mmol/L).

Patients using CSII need intensive education. Because of the risk for hypoglycemia or hyperglycemia, he or she must be able to operate the pump, adjust the settings, and respond appropriately to alarms. Removing the pump for any length of time can result in hyperglycemia. Provide supplemental insulin schedules for times when the pump is not operational. CSII is more costly than traditional insulin injections, and not all costs are covered by insurance.

Injection devices now include a needleless system and a pen-type injector in addition to traditional insulin syringes. With a needleless device, the needle is replaced by an ultrathin liquid stream of insulin forced through the skin under high pressure. Insulin given by jet injection is absorbed at a faster rate, with a resulting shorter duration of action. Cost is a drawback to this system.

New technology now available includes a system in which the patient's blood is continuously monitored by a skin sensor and the information is transmitted to a pump. The pump then determines the need for insulin, which is injected from the pump through a subcutaneous cannula. Fig. 67-7 shows this type of system. Although expensive and not covered by most

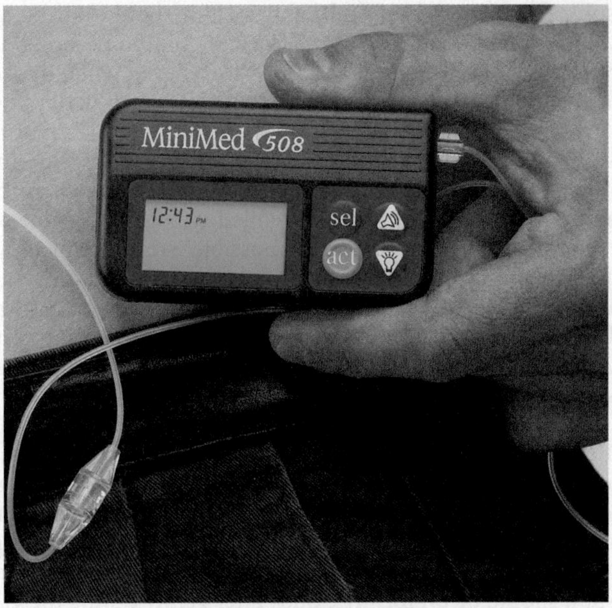
MiniMed 508
12:43 PM
sel
act

Fig. 67-6 • External insulin pump.

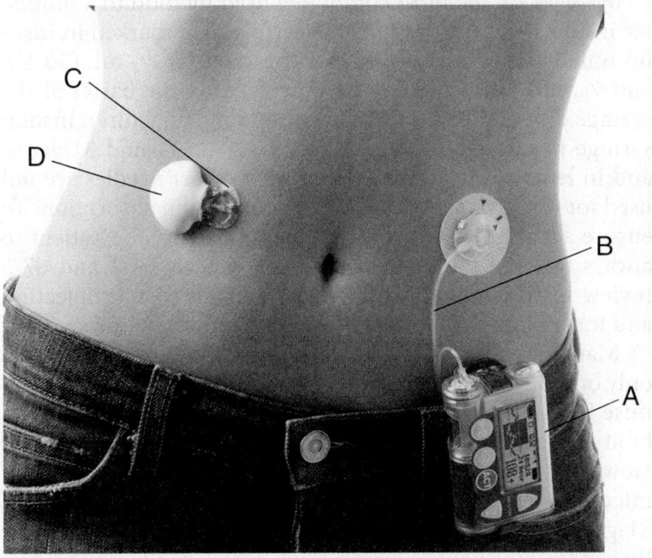
C
D
B
A

Fig. 67-7 • The MiniMed Paradigm® REAL-Time Insulin Pump and Continuous Glucose Monitoring System. **A,** Pump. **B,** Injection cannula. **C,** Glucose sensor. **D,** Data transmitter.

insurance, this system is very convenient for the patient, holding up to a 3-day supply of insulin. Another advantage is that the system can be disconnected easily for activities such as bathing, swimming, or changing clothes.

Patient education: drugs. Provide specific instructions about insulin therapy, new drug therapies, and self-monitoring of blood glucose levels.

Insulin storage varies by use. Teach patients to refrigerate insulin that is not in use to maintain potency, prevent exposure to sunlight, and inhibit bacterial growth. Insulin in use may be kept at room temperature for up to 28 days to reduce irritation at the injection site caused by cold insulin.

To prevent loss of drug potency, teach the patient to avoid exposing insulin to temperatures below 36° F (2.2° C) or above 86° F (30° C), to avoid excessive shaking, and to protect insulin from direct heat and light. Insulin should not be allowed to freeze. Insulin glargine (Lantus) should be stored in a refrigerator (36° to 46° F [2.2° to 7.8° C]) even when in use. Teach patients to discard any unused insulin after 28 days.

Teach patients to always have a spare bottle of each type of insulin used. A slight loss in potency may occur after the bottle has been in use for more than 30 days, even when the expiration date has not passed. Prefilled syringes are stable up to 30 days when refrigerated. If possible, store prefilled syringes in the upright position, with the needle pointing upward, so that insulin particles do not clog it. Teach patients to roll predrawn syringes between the hands before using. The effect of premixing insulins on blood glucose control is assessed by examining blood glucose levels.

Dose preparation is critical for insulin effectiveness and patient safety. Teach patients that the person giving the insulin needs to inspect the insulin before each use for changes (e.g., clumping, frosting, precipitation, or change in clarity or color) that may indicate loss in potency. Rapid-acting, short-acting, and glargine insulins should be clear, and all other types of insulin should be uniformly cloudy after gently rolling the vial between the hands. If potency is questionable, another vial of the same type of insulin should be used.

Syringes are the most commonly used method to administer insulin. The standard insulin syringes are marked in insulin units. They are available in 1-mL (100-U), ½-mL (50-U), and 3/10-mL (30-U) sizes. The unit scale on the barrel of the syringe differs with the syringe size and manufacturer. Insulin syringe needles are measured in 28-, 29-, 30-, and 31-gauge and in lengths of ½-inch and 5/16-inch. Short needles are not used for obese patients because of poor insulin absorption. To ensure accurate insulin measurement, instruct the patient to always buy the same type of syringe. Charts 67-4 and 67-5 review instructions for drawing up a single insulin injection and for mixing regular and NPH insulin in the same syringe.

Manufacturers recommend that disposable needles be used only once. Reuse of an insulin syringe and needle can compromise insulin sterility. Most insulins contain products that inhibit the growth of bacteria commonly found on the skin. However, many diabetic patients are at an increased risk for infection. Another reason to not reuse smaller (30- and 31-gauge) needles is that even with one injection, the needle tip can become bent to form a hook, which can lacerate tissue or break off to leave needle fragments in the skin (Fig. 67-8). Teach the patient to discard the syringe and needle after one use by participating in a community program, such as a drop-off center for household hazardous waste, or in a national disposal program, such as a "sharps" mail-back program. Information on needle disposal can be obtained at www.safeneedledisposal.org.

Pen-type injectors hold small, lightweight, prefilled insulin cartridges. The injectors are easy to carry and make intensive therapy with multiple injections easier. These devices allow greater accuracy than traditional insulin syringes, especially when measuring small doses. Discuss proper storage for prefilled insulin pens or cartridges. More drugs are becoming available in a prefilled syringe or cartridge. Ensure that the product is appropriate to the patient's unique needs. *Pen-type injectors are not designed for independent use by visually impaired patients or by those with cognitive impairment.* Ensure that the patient has received education on its use. Each syringe or cartridge has specific requirements. Patients using the InnoLet (Novo Nordisk) must be able to attach a needle and to perform an air shot of 2 units to ensure that a dose of insulin is administered. The Institute for Safe Medication Practices (ISMP) and the Joint Commission identify insulin as a *High-Alert* drug. The ISMP cautions that digital displays on some

Chart 67-4 PATIENT AND FAMILY EDUCATION GUIDE

Subcutaneous Insulin Administration

- Wash your hands.
- Inspect the bottle for the type of insulin and the expiration date.
- Gently roll the bottle of intermediate-acting insulin in the palms of your hands to mix the insulin.
- Clean the rubber stopper with an alcohol swab.
- Remove the needle cover, and pull back the plunger to draw air into the syringe. The amount of air should be equal to the insulin dose. Push the needle through the rubber stopper, and inject the air into the insulin bottle.
- Turn the bottle upside down, and draw the insulin dose into the syringe.
- Remove air bubbles in the syringe by tapping on the syringe or injecting air back into the bottle. Redraw the correct amount.
- Make certain the tip of the plunger is on the line for your dose of insulin. Magnifiers are available to assist in measuring accurate doses of insulin.
- Remove the needle from the bottle. Recap the needle if the insulin is not to be given immediately.
- Select a site within your injection area that has not been used in the past month.
- Clean your skin with an alcohol swab. Lightly grasp an area of skin, and insert the needle at a 90-degree angle.
- Push the plunger all the way down. This will push the insulin into your body. Release the pinched skin.
- Pull the needle straight out quickly. Do not rub the place where you gave the shot.
- Dispose of the syringe and needle without recapping in a puncture-proof container.

Chart 67-5 PATIENT AND FAMILY EDUCATION GUIDE

How to Mix a Prescribed Dose of 10 Units of Regular Insulin and 20 Units of NPH Insulin

- Wash your hands.
- Inspect the bottle for the type of insulin and the expiration date.
- Gently roll the bottle of intermediate-acting (NPH) insulin in the palms of your hands to mix the insulin.
- Clean the rubber stopper with an alcohol swab.
- Inject 20 units of air into the NPH insulin bottle. The amount of air should be equal to the dose of insulin needed. Always inject air into the intermediate-acting insulin first. Withdraw the needle.
- Inject 10 units of air into the regular insulin bottle. The amount of air is equal to the dose of insulin desired.
- Withdraw 10 units of regular insulin. Be sure that the syringe is free of air bubbles. Always withdraw the shorter-acting insulin first.
- Withdraw 20 units of NPH insulin with the same syringe, being careful not to inject any short-acting insulin into the bottle. (A total of 30 units should be in the syringe.)

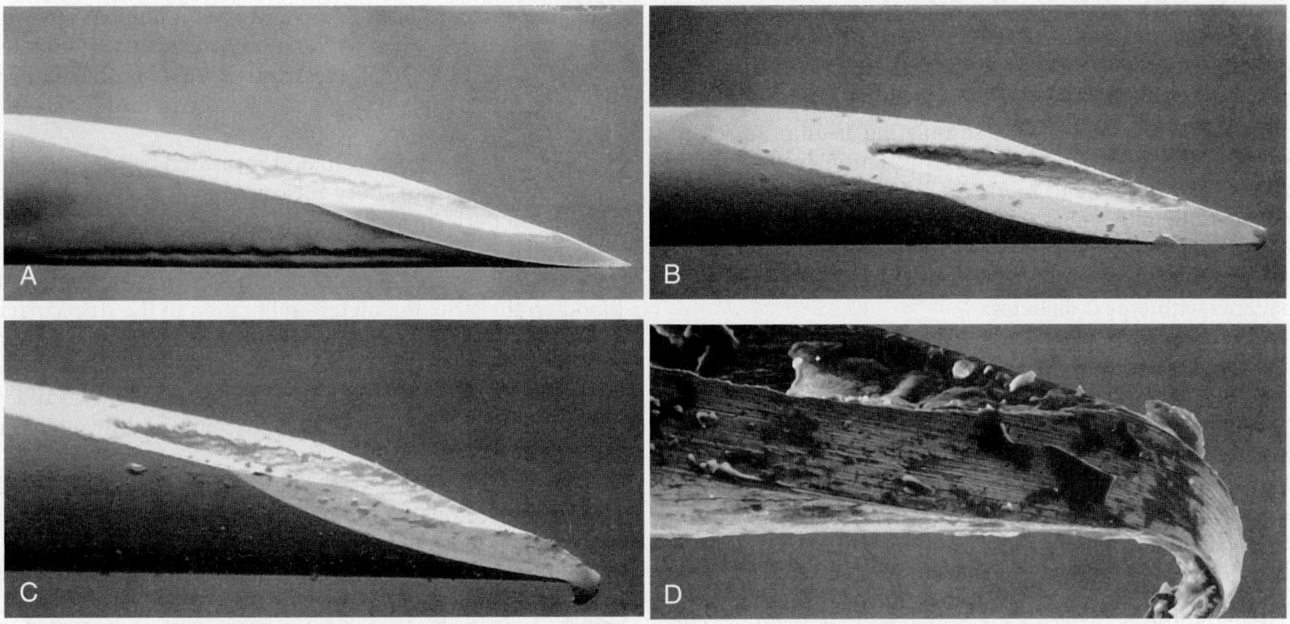
A
B
C
D

Fig. 67-8 • Reuse of insulin needle. **A,** A new needle. **B,** A needle that has been used once. **C,** A needle that has been used twice. **D,** A needle that has been used six times.

of the newer insulin formulations can be misread. If the pen is held upside down, as a left-handed person might do, a dose of 25 units actually appears to be a dose of 52 units.

DECISION-MAKING CHALLENGE
Coordination of Care

A patient with diabetes is admitted to the hospital for treatment of an infection in his foot. He wishes to continue living alone after discharge from the hospital. His current insulin regimen includes 6 units of rapid-acting insulin before each meal and 35 units of long-acting insulin at bedtime.

1. How would you assess this patient's ability to accurately and safely administer insulin?
2. You assess that the patient has difficulty drawing solution into a syringe but can administer insulin accurately. What skills should you evaluate to determine if the patient can safely administer insulin using a preloaded syringe?

evolve For suggested answer guidelines, go to http://evolve.elsevier.com/Iggy/.

Newer drugs. Newer drug therapies for diabetes include amylin analogues, incretin agents, and DDP-IV inhibitors. Extensive patient education is needed to ensure the safety and effectiveness of these drugs.

Amylin analogues are drugs similar to amylin, a naturally occurring hormone produced by beta cells in the pancreas, that works with and is co-secreted with insulin in response to blood glucose elevation. Amylin levels are deficient in patients with type 1 diabetes who are also deficient in insulin. Pramlintide (Symlin), an analogue of amylin, is approved for patients with either type 1 or type 2 diabetes treated with insulin. It is indicated as adjunct therapy for patients who use mealtime insulin delivery and have not achieved desirable glucose control despite optimum insulin therapy (Riddle & Drucker, 2006).

Pramlintide works by three mechanisms: delaying gastric emptying, reducing after-meal blood glucose levels, and by triggering satiety (in the brain), which leads to decreased caloric intake and weight loss. The initial dose of pramlintide is 15 mcg subcutaneously before meals with at least 250 calories or 30 grams of carbohydrate. It can be given up to 4 times per day. Dosage is increased in 15-mcg increments to a target dose of 30 mcg or 60 mcg. Pramlintide alters gastric uptake. Therefore instruct patients to take oral drugs in which rapid onset of action is important (e.g., analgesics) either 1 hour before or 2 hours after eating.

Teach the patient to prepare and self-administer pramlintide. A U-100 syringe is used to administer the drug. However, it is necessary to convert the microgram dosage to insulin syringe unit increments (e.g., 15 mcg is equal to 2.5 units on a U-100 insulin syringe). *Pramlintide and insulin are NOT to be mixed in the same syringe because the pH of the two drugs is not compatible.* Teach the patient to inject pramlintide into a site different from where insulin is injected.

Nausea, vomiting, and anorexia are common side effects of pramlintide therapy. It should not be used for patients with symptomatic gastroparesis. Pramlintide carries a black box warning for insulin-induced severe hypoglycemia. (A **black box warning** is a governmental designation indicating that a drug has at least one serious side effect and must be used with caution.) The hypoglycemic risk is higher in patients with type 1 diabetes and usually occurs within 3 hours of injection. The black box also warns about the risk of hypoglycemia during driving or operating heavy equipment.

Incretin agents are natural "gut" hormones that, in addition to insulin, also lower plasma glucose levels. These agents include glucagon-like-peptide-1 (GLP-1) and glucose-dependent insulinotropic polypeptide (GIP) that are released by the intestine throughout the day in response to food intake. GLP-1 has many effects on the stomach, liver, pancreas, and brain to work together to regulate blood glucose. It lowers glucagon secretion from the pancreas, leading to reduced liver glucose production. It also delays gastric emptying, slows the rate of nutrient absorption into the blood, and reduces food intake, all of which lower blood glucose levels (McKennon & Campbell, 2007).

Patients with type 2 diabetes have a reduced incretin effect, indicating that they have either a decreased level of incretin hormones or a resistance to their effects.

Exenatide (Byetta) is a long-acting analogue of GLP-1. It mimics the actions of GLP-1, stimulating insulin secretion only when blood glucose is high. This action restores "first phase" insulin release and improves blood glucose control by lowering both after-meal and fasting blood glucose levels (McKenna & Campbell, 2007). The drug is approved for use only in combination with a sulfonylurea, metformin, or both in patients with type 2 diabetes.

The main side effect of exenatide is nausea. Most patients taking exenatide lose weight as a result of the anorexic effect of the drug. It stimulates insulin secretion and may cause hypoglycemia when given with sulfonylurea drugs (which also stimulate insulin secretion) but not with metformin alone.

Exenatide is available as a fixed-dose prefilled pen injector delivering either 5 mcg or 10 mcg of exenatide per dose. It is injected subcutaneously in thigh, abdomen, or upper arm within 60 minutes *before* the morning and evening meals. Teach patients not to administer exenatide *after* a meal and to keep the pen injectors refrigerated.

DPP-IV inhibitors work by slowing the inactivation of incretin hormones (McKennon & Campbell, 2007). Sitagliptin (Januvia) increases the body's active incretin hormone levels, reducing both before- and after-meal blood glucose levels. It works only when blood glucose is elevated.

Januvia is approved as single agent for patients with type 2 diabetes unable to manage diabetes with diet and exercise alone and as add-on therapy for those patients with inadequate blood glucose control taking metformin or thiazolidinediones. The recommended dose is 100 mg orally, once daily, with or without food. Its duration of action is 24 hours.

Side effects include stuffy or runny nose, sore throat, upper respiratory infection, and GI effects of abdominal pain, nausea, and diarrhea. Monitor for symptoms of renal insufficiency.

PATIENT EDUCATION: BLOOD GLUCOSE MONITORING. Self-monitoring of blood glucose (SMBG) levels provides information to assess effectiveness of the management plan. SMBG allows patients and providers to evaluate patient response to therapy and assess whether glycemic targets are being reached. Results of SMBG are useful in preventing hypoglycemia and adjusting drug therapy, nutrition therapy, and physical activity. The American Diabetes Association (ADA) recommends SMBG for patients taking insulin or oral therapy. Assessment of blood glucose levels is very important for these situations:

- Symptoms of hypoglycemia/hyperglycemia
- Hypoglycemic unawareness
- Periods of illness
- Before and after exercise
- Gastroparesis
- Adjustment of diabetes medications
- Evaluation of other drug therapies (e.g., steroids)
- Preconception planning
- Pregnancy

Technique for SMBG follows principles that are the same for most self-monitoring systems. The finger is pricked, and a drop of blood is made to flow over a reagent pad on a testing strip. Meters measure blood glucose in one of two ways: using color reflectance or using sensor technology. With reflectance meters, the blood sugar in a drop of blood reacts with an enzyme on the strip and changes the color of the strip. The meter reads the darkness of the strip and gives a number readout of the glucose value. Most of the newer meters use sensor technology to measure small electrical currents produced by the chemical interaction between the glucose in the blood and the chemicals on the strip.

Glucose levels in whole blood measured by SMBG systems vary somewhat from those measured by a clinical laboratory. The overall performance of SMBG systems depends on the accuracy of the specific blood glucose meter, operator proficiency, and test strip quality. Results are influenced by the amount of blood on the strip; the meter's calibration to the strip currently in use; environmental conditions of altitude, temperature, and moisture; and patient-specific conditions of hematocrit level, triglyceride level, and presence of hypotension. The accuracy of SMBG systems decreases at hypoglycemic and hyperglycemic levels.

Most meters display blood glucose results on a screen. For vision-impaired patients, "talking-meters" are available to allow independence in blood glucose monitoring.

Infection control measures are needed for SMBG. Teach the patient to follow Centers for Disease Control and Prevention (CDC) guidelines for infection control during SMBG. The chance of becoming infected from blood glucose monitoring processes is reduced by handwashing before monitoring and by not reusing lancets. *Instruct patients to not share their blood glucose monitoring equipment.* Hepatitis B virus can survive in a dried state for at least 1 week. Infection can be spread by the lancet holder even when the lancet itself has been changed. Small particles of blood can stick to the device and infect multiple users. Regular cleaning of the meter is critical for infection control. Remind health care staff who perform blood glucose testing and family members who help with testing to wear gloves.

Interpretation of results is another area for patient education. Accuracy of blood glucose measurements is reduced by errors in technique or equipment failure. Data obtained from SMBG are evaluated with other measures of blood glucose levels (e.g., glycosylated hemoglobin, or hemoglobin A_{1c} [HbA_{1c}], values) or periodic laboratory blood glucose tests. Even when SMBG is performed correctly, the results are affected by hematocrit values (anemia falsely elevates glucose values; polycythemia falsely depresses them) and may be unreliable in the hypoglycemic or severe hyperglycemic ranges. Accuracy of the meter itself is also an issue. Even when highly trained personnel tested meters under optimal conditions, accuracy and precision varied widely among capillary blood glucose monitoring devices. Teach patients to properly calibrate the machine. Instruct them to recheck the calibration and retest if they obtain a test result that is unusual for them and whenever they are in doubt about test accuracy. Laboratory glucose determinations are more accurate than SMBG.

Frequency of testing varies with the complexity of the drug schedules and the goals of therapy. Patients with unstable blood glucose levels, as well as those using intensive treatment regimens, require frequent monitoring. Those using simple treatment regimens designed to prevent symptomatic hyperglycemia or patients with type 2 diabetes using oral agents need less-frequent testing.

Blood glucose therapy goals are set individually for each patient. The entire health care team works with him or her to reach target blood glucose levels. The American Diabetes Association (ADA) recommends that patients with type 1 diabetes aim for hemoglobin A_{1c} (HbA_{1c}) values less than 7%, premeal glucose levels of 90 to 130 mg/dL (5.0 to 7.2 mmol/L), and postmeal glucose levels less than 180 mg/dL (10.0 mmol/L) (ADA, 2007c).

Accuracy of blood glucose monitors, regardless of type, is usually ensured when the manufacturer's directions are followed. Results are technique-dependent, regardless of whether test strips are read visually or with a meter. Help the patient select a meter based on cost of the meter and strips, ease of use, availability of repair and servicing, and ability to see color. Provide training, explain and demonstrate procedures, assess visual acuity, and check the patient's ability to perform the procedure through a return demonstration. See Table 67-11 for information to help patients determine which blood glucose meter best meets their needs.

Common errors in SMBG involve failing to obtain a sufficient blood drop, poorly storing test strips, using expired strips, and not changing the code number on the meter to match the strip bottle code. Continued retraining of patients performing SMBG helps ensure accurate results because performance accuracy deteriorates over time.

Alternate site testing allows patients to obtain blood from sites other than the fingertip and is available on many meters. However, use caution when interpreting results obtained from alternate sites. These results are not necessarily the same as those from the fingertip when tested at the same time. Comparison studies have shown wide variation between fingertip

TABLE 67-11 Blood Glucose Monitors

Meter	Features	Download to PC	Alternate Site
Freestyle Flash	World's smallest meter for discrete testing. Test does not start until adequate blood sample is present.	Yes	Yes
Freestyle Freedom	Uses colorimetric technology for accuracy.	Yes	Yes
Precision Xtra (for glucose & ketones) Advanced data management system	Simple 2-step testing. Insert strip, add blood, test begins. Test does not start until adequate blood sample is present.	Yes	Yes
Assure 3	Fast, easy-to-use system. Custom design ensures easy handling and fast testing.	No	No
QuickTek	Easy-to-use system with data management capabilities.	Yes	No
Advance Intuition	Large, easy-to-read screen. Fast, simple, two-step testing. Large strips are easy to handle for persons with vision or hand dexterity problems.	No	No
Advance Micro-Draw	Has data management capabilities. 14-day and 30-day averaging. Small sample size with micro-draw test strips.	Yes	No
Assure II	Simple 2-step test. Designed to meet needs of long-term care profession.		
Assure Pro	Designed to meet needs of long-term care profession. Includes safety features such as strip release and "hypo" warnings.		
Ascensia Breeze	Simple-to-use system, no coding, no handling of individual strips. Recommended by the Arthritis Foundation. Disk holds 10 strips.		Yes
Ascensia Contour	Fully automated, requires no coding. Optional premeal and postmeal markers and reminder alarm.	Yes	Yes
Ascensia ELITE			
Ascensia Breeze 2		Yes	Yes
Ascensia ELITE XL			
Prodigy Advance		Yes	Yes
Prodigy Audio		Yes	Yes
Prodigy Autocode		Yes	Yes
Prodigy Duo		Yes	Yes
Prestige IQ	Large, easy-to-read screen.	Yes	No
Sidekick	Smallest testing system available. No coding needed.	No	Yes
TrueTrack Smart System	Easy-to-use system. Simple 2-step test system. Features biosensor technology.	Yes	Yes
OneTouch Basic	Easy to learn and use, large easy-to-read display.	Yes	No
OneTouch SureStep	Easy-to-use meter that is easy to handle and easy to read. Has big screen, big buttons, and big test strip.	Yes	No

Continued

TABLE 67-11 Blood Glucose Monitors—cont'd

Meter	Features	Download to PC	Alternate Site
OneTouch Ultra	Provides separate averages for before-meal and after-meal results. Allows you to link the effects of food to your blood glucose results.	Yes	Yes
OneTouch Ultra 2	Provides before and after meal averages.	Yes	Yes
OneTouch UltraMini	Simple-to-use meter, provides blood glucose value without complicated screens.	No	No
OneTouch UltraSmart	Data management system; collects and organizes glucose data by time of day. Ideal for people who make insulin adjustments.	Yes	Yes
Accu-Chek Active	Apply blood to the test strip either in or out of the meter. Requires 1 microliter blood sample. Results appear in 5 seconds. Stores up to 200 values.	Yes	Yes
Accu-Chek Advantage	Easy-to-use meter. Stores up to 480 values.	Yes	No
Accu-Chek Aviva	Uses Multiclix lancet device (least painful device).	Yes	Yes
Accu-Chek Compact	Preloaded drum of 17 diabetes test strips; no handling of strips. Results appear in 8 seconds. Coding is automatic. Stores up to 100 values.	Yes	Yes
Accu-Chek Compact Plus	Preloaded drum of 17 diabetes test strips for no individual handling of strips. Lancet device can be used attached or detached from the blood glucose meter. Test results appear in 5 seconds. Coding is automatic when test drum is inserted. Stores up to 300 values.	Yes	Yes
Accu-Chek Complete	On-screen data analysis. Stores and analyzes up to 1000 values, plus information on insulin, activity, meals, ketones, A_{1c} values, and event markers.	Yes	No
ReliOn Ultima	Leading industry technology at incredible savings as compared with national brands.	No	No

and alternate sites and are most evident during times when blood glucose levels are rapidly changing. Teach patients that there is a lag time for blood glucose levels between the fingertip and other sites when blood glucose levels are changing rapidly and that the fingertip reading is the only safe choice at those times. *Patients with a history of hypoglycemic unawareness should not test at alternative sites.*

New technology currently approved includes continuous blood glucose monitoring (CGM) devices. These devices measure blood glucose either by continuously measuring glucose in interstitial fluid or by applying electromagnetic radiation through the skin to blood vessels in the body. (See Fig. 67-7.)

A sensor is inserted subcutaneously into the abdomen to measure glucose in interstitial fluid. After a warm-up period of up to 2 hours and a device-specific calibration process, the sensor provides blood glucose readings every 1 to 10 minutes for up to 72 hours. Available CGMs require up to four finger-stick (not alternate site) measurements of blood glucose per day for calibration. CGMs that provide "real-time" readings should not be used to make therapeutic decisions because they are not sufficiently accurate.

Two watchlike devices are available to measure glucose. The GlucoWatch G2 Biographer (GW2B) and Pendra are non-invasive continuous blood glucose monitoring systems worn on the arm, forearm, or wrist that provide real-time blood glucose results. The GW2B sends a tiny electrical current through the skin to measure glucose from interstitial fluid just beneath the skin. It analyzes glucose every 20 minutes for up to 12 hours and is best suited for detecting unsuspected hypoglycemia but has been associated with skin irritation. The Pendra uses radio-wave impedance to measure glucose and can take up to four readings per minute. In addition, it warns patients of high and low glucose levels. The Pendra does not draw fluid from the skin and does not irritate the skin.

Currently available CGMs present problems with accuracy. A major problem is their lack of accuracy for each single data point compared with the accuracy of simultaneous intermittent blood glucose measurements. Depending on activity or eating schedules (and especially during periods of rapid blood glucose fluctuations), equilibration between shifting blood glucose and interstitial fluid glucose level may lag. CGMs are least accurate in the hypoglycemic range. They are expensive, and reimbursement by insurance or other payer organizations has been limited.

Continuous glucose monitoring is meant to supplement, not replace, finger-stick tests. Insulin should be given only after confirming the results of any of the continuous glucose monitoring systems.

Nutrition therapy. Effective self-management of diabetes requires that the meal plan, education, and counseling programs be "patientized" for each patient. A nutritionist should be a member of the treatment team. The nurse, nutritionist, patient, and family work together on all aspects of the meal plan, which must be realistic and as flexible as possible. Plans that consider the patient's cultural background, financial status, and lifestyle are more likely to be successful.

Desired outcomes of nutrition therapy. The ADA (2007b) advocates that nutrition therapy focus on these outcomes:

- Maintaining blood glucose levels in the normal range or as close to normal as is safely possible
- Maintaining a blood lipid profile that reduces the risk for vascular disease
- Achieving blood pressure levels in the normal range or as close to normal as is safely possible
- Preventing or slowing the rate of development of the chronic complications of diabetes by modifying nutrient intake and lifestyle
- Addressing patient nutrition needs taking into account personal and cultural preferences and willingness to change
- Maintaining the pleasure of eating by limiting food choices only when indicated by scientific evidence
- Meeting the nutritional needs of unique times of the life cycle, particularly for pregnant and lactating women and for older adults with diabetes
- Providing self-management training for patients treated with insulin or insulin secretagogues for exercising safely, including the prevention and treatment of hypoglycemia and management of diabetes during acute illness

Principles of nutrition in diabetes. The nutritionist develops a meal plan based on the patient's usual food intake, weight-management goals, and lipid and blood glucose patterns. Day-to-day consistency in the timing and amount of food eaten helps control blood glucose. Patients receiving insulin therapy need to eat at times that are coordinated with the timed action of insulin. Teach patients using intense insulin therapy to adjust premeal insulin to allow for timing and quantity changes in their meal plan.

Protein intake of 15% to 20% of total daily calories is appropriate for diabetic patients with normal kidney function. In patients with microalbuminuria, reduction of protein to 10% of calories (0.8 to 1.0 g/kg) may slow progression of renal failure, and a reduction to not more than 0.8 g/kg body weight in later stages of chronic kidney disease may improve function (ADA, 2007b).

Carbohydrate recommendation for the diabetic patient is a diet containing 45% to 65% of calories from carbohydrate, with a minimum intake of 130 g carbohydrate/day. The diet should include carbohydrate from fruit, vegetables, whole grains, legumes, and low-fat milk. Diets restricting total carbohydrate to less than 130 g/day are not recommended in the management of diabetes (ADA, 2007b).

Food choices that prevent after-meal (postprandial) blood glucose elevation are important in achieving blood glucose control. The amount and types of carbohydrate consumed have the greatest impact on after-meal blood glucose levels.

The percentage of calories from carbohydrates is determined for each patient. Various starches have different blood glucose responses. Place the emphasis on the *total amount* of carbohydrate consumed each day rather than the source of the carbohydrate. Little evidence supports the assumption that sugars are more rapidly absorbed than starches and cause blood glucose values to increase more rapidly.

Dietary fat and cholesterol, especially saturated fatty acids and *trans* fatty acids are restricted to reduce the risk for cardiovascular disease. Current recommendations from the ADA (2007b, 2007c) for patients with diabetes are:

- Limiting saturated fatty intake to less than 7% of total calories
- Minimizing intake of *trans* fat
- Limiting dietary cholesterol to less than 200 mg/day
- Having two or more servings of fish per week (with the exception of commercially fried fish filets) to provide n-3 polyunsaturated fatty acids

Trans fatty acids raise low-density lipoprotein (LDL) cholesterol and lower high-density lipoprotein (HDL) cholesterol, both of which increase the risk for cardiovascular disease. *Trans* fatty acids are found in hard margarine and in foods prepared with or fried in hydrogenated and partly hydrogenated oils. Teach the patient to restrict intake of *trans* fatty acids by limiting the amount of commercially fried foods and bakery goods eaten.

Further dietary fat restrictions for patients with diabetes are determined by a nutritionist on the basis of specific lipid levels. Adults with diabetes should be tested annually for abnormalities of fasting serum cholesterol, triglycerides, high-density lipoprotein (HDL) cholesterol, and calculated low-density lipoprotein (LDL) cholesterol levels (ADA, 2007c).

Fiber improves carbohydrate metabolism and lowers cholesterol levels. Taste and texture, limited food choices, and GI side effects make it difficult to achieve a high-fiber intake. Assist the patient to first reach the goal of 14 g per 1000 calories. The American Heart Association recommends a fiber intake of 25 grams each day. Teach the patient to select a variety of fiber-containing foods such as legumes, fiber-rich cereals (more than 5 g fiber/serving), fruits, vegetables, and whole-grain products because they provide vitamins, minerals, and other substances important for good health.

Teach the patient that adding high-fiber foods to the diet gradually can reduce abdominal cramping, loose stools, and flatulence. An increase in fluid intake should accompany increased fiber intake. The nurse and the patient should pay careful attention to blood glucose levels because hypoglycemia can result when dietary fiber intake increases significantly.

Sweeteners include sucrose and a variety of nonnutritive substances. Dietary sucrose does not increase blood glucose more than equal amounts of other starches. Intake of sucrose and sucrose-containing foods by patients with diabetes does not need to be restricted out of a concern for causing hyperglycemia. Sucrose can be included in the meal plan as long as it is adequately covered with insulin or other glucose-lowering agents.

The use of products to enhance the taste of food while not disturbing blood glucose control is desirable. The Food and Drug Administration (FDA) has approved five nonnutritive sweeteners for use: saccharin, aspartame, acesulfame potassium, neotame, and sucralose.

Alcohol consumption can affect blood glucose levels. Levels are not affected by *moderate* use of alcohol when diabetes is well controlled. Teach diabetic patients that two alcoholic beverages for men and one for women can be ingested with, and in addition to, the usual meal plan. (One alcoholic beverage equals 12 ounces of beer, 5 ounces of wine, or 1½ ounces of distilled spirits.) *Because of the potential for alcohol-induced hypoglycemia, instruct the patient to ingest alcohol only with or shortly after meals.* Alcohol raises plasma triglycerides. Thus reducing or abstaining from alcohol is important for patients with hyperlipidemia. One alcoholic beverage is substituted for two fat exchanges when calculating caloric intake (ADA, 2007b).

Patient education: prescribed nutrition plan. No one meal plan is right for all patients with diabetes. Each patient's nutrition recommendations are based on blood glucose monitoring results, total blood lipid levels, and glycosylated hemoglobin. These tests help determine whether current meal and exercise patterns need adjustment or whether present habits need reinforcement. A specific nutritional prescription is developed for each patient.

Reinforce information provided by the nutritionist. The diabetic patient needs to understand how to adjust food intake during illness, planned exercise, and social occasions (e.g., restaurant meals) when the usual time of eating is delayed. He or she may be unable to follow the prescribed plan because of an inability to see, read, or understand printed materials. Share dietary information with the person who prepares the meals. The nutritionist sees each patient at least yearly to identify changes in lifestyle and make appropriate nutrition therapy changes. Some patients, such as those with weight control problems or low incomes, may need more frequent evaluation and counseling.

Meal-planning strategies. Many meal planning approaches are available. Each approach emphasizes different aspects of nutrition.

Exchange systems are based on three food groups: carbohydrates, meat and meat substitutes, and fat. The exchange list for meal planning assumes that foods with similar nutrient content affect blood glucose levels similarly. Plans based on the exchange system produce predictable blood glucose responses. The patient's prescription identifies how many items from each food group are to be eaten at a meal or snack. Table 67-12 provides an example of the exchange system of nutrition therapy.

Carbohydrate (CHO) counting is a simple approach to meal planning that uses label information of the nutritional content of packaged food items. Because fat and protein have little effect on after-meal blood glucose levels, CHO counting focuses on the nutrient that has the greatest impact on these levels. It uses total grams of carbohydrate, regardless of the food source. The nutritionist determines the number of grams of carbohydrate to be eaten at each meal and snack and helps the patient make appropriate food choices. This method is effective in achieving overall blood glucose control when carbohydrate intake is consistent from day to day.

Patients using intensive insulin or pump therapies can use CHO counting to determine insulin coverage. After the amount of insulin needed to cover the usual meal is determined, insulin may be added or subtracted for changes in carbohydrate intake. An initial formula of 1 unit of rapid-acting insulin for each 15 g of carbohydrate provides flexibility to meal plans. The patient determines the grams of carbohydrate in a specific meal or snack by reading labels or weighing and measuring of each item. The total grams of carbohydrate

TABLE 67-12 Exchange System of Medical Nutrition Therapy

Food Content	Carbohydrate (g)	Protein (g)	Fat (g)	Calories	Example
CARBOHYDRATE					
Breads/grains	15	3	1 or less	80	1 slice bread 1/2 bagel 1/2 hamburger bun 1/2 cup corn 1/2 cup mashed potato
Fruit	15	0	0	60	1 small apple 1/2 medium banana 1/2 grapefruit
Milk					
Skim	12	8	0-3	90	1 cup skim milk (1/2%-1%)
Low-fat	12	8	5	120	1 cup 2% milk
Whole	12	8	5	150	1 cup whole milk
Other carbohydrates	15	Varies	Varies	Varies	Brownie, unfrosted (2-inch square) Fruit juice bar 1 tablespoon jelly, regular
Vegetables	5	2	0	25	Carrots, green beans, spinach, 1/2 cup cooked, 1 cup raw 1 large tomato
MEAT OR MEAT SUBSTITUTE					
Very lean	0	7	0-1	35	1 oz chicken (white meat, skinless), 1 oz fat-free cheese (1 g fat or less)
Lean	0	7	3	55	1 oz lean beef (trimmed rump roast), dark-meat chicken (skinless), or salmon; 1/4 cup cottage cheese (4.5% fat)
Medium-fat	0	7	5	75	1 oz ground beef, pork cutlet, lamb, or dark-meat chicken with skin
FAT					
	0	0	5	45	1 teaspoon butter or margarine, 1 strip bacon

are used to calculate the bolus dose of insulin based on his or her prescribed insulin-to-carbohydrate ratio. See Table 67-13 for an example of carbohydrate counting.

Special considerations for type 1 diabetes include developing insulin regimens that conform to the patient's preferred meal routines, food preferences, and exercise patterns. Patients using rapid-acting insulin by injection or an insulin pump should adjust insulin doses based on the carbohydrate content of the meals and snacks. Insulin-to-carbohydrate ratios are developed and are used to provide mealtime insulin doses. Blood glucose monitoring before and 2 hours after meals determines whether the insulin-to-carbohydrate ratio is correct. For patients who are on fixed insulin regimens and do not adjust premeal insulin dosages, consistency of timing of meals and the amount of CHO eaten at each meal is important to prevent hypoglycemia.

Physical exercise can cause hypoglycemia if insulin is not decreased before activity. For planned exercise, reduction in insulin dosage is the preferred method for hypoglycemia prevention. For unplanned exercise, intake of additional CHO is usually needed. Moderate exercise increases glucose utilization by 2 to 3 mg/kg/min. A 70-kg person would need about 10 to 15 g additional CHO per hour of moderate-intensity physical activity. More CHO is needed for intense activity (ADA, 2007b).

A second goal for patients with type 1 diabetes is to avoid gaining weight. **Hyperinsulinemia** (chronic high blood insulin levels) can occur with intensive treatment schedules and may result in weight gain. These patients may need to manage hyperglycemia by restricting calories rather than increasing insulin. Weight gain can be minimized by following the prescribed meal plan, getting regular exercise, and avoiding overtreatment of hypoglycemia.

Special considerations for type 2 diabetes focus on lifestyle changes. Many patients with type 2 diabetes are overweight and insulin resistant. Nutrition therapy stresses lifestyle changes that reduce calories eaten and increase calories expended through physical activity. Many patients also have abnormal blood fat levels and hypertension (metabolic syndrome), making reductions of saturated fat, cholesterol, and sodium desirable. A moderate caloric restriction (250 to 500 calories less than average daily intake) and an increase in physical activity improve diabetic control and weight control. Decreases of more than 10% of body weight can result in significant improvement in glycosylated hemoglobin (hemoglobin A_{1c}). Decreasing intake of cholesterol-raising fatty acids helps reduce the risk for cardiovascular disease.

When patients with type 2 diabetes need insulin, consistency in timing and carbohydrate content of meals is important. Division of the total daily calories into three meals or into smaller meals and snacks is based on patient preference.

CONSIDERATIONS FOR OLDER ADULTS

Older patients are at increased risk for malnutrition, hypoglycemia, and especially dehydration, a factor in the development of hyperglycemic-hyperosmolar state (HHS). Many factors contribute to malnutrition. Older patients who prepare their own food or have tooth loss or poorly fitting dentures may not eat enough food. Neuropathy with gastric retention or diarrhea compounds poor food intake. Impaired cognition and depression may disrupt self-care. Older patients may have a marginal food supply because of inadequate income, may have poor understanding of meal-planning goals, or may live alone and have reduced incentive to prepare or eat proper meals. They may eat in restaurants or live in situations in which they have little control over meal preparation. Regular visits by home health nurses can assist older patients in following a diabetic meal plan.

A realistic approach to nutrition therapy is essential for the older diabetic patient. Changing the eating habits of 60 to 70 years is very difficult. The nurse, nutritionist, and patient assess the patient's usual eating patterns. Teach the older patient taking antidiabetic drugs about the importance of eating meals and snacks at the same time every day, eating the same amount of food from day to day, and eating all food allowed on the diet.

TABLE 67-13 Carbohydrate Counting

Meal	Food Source	Grams of Carbohydrates	Total	Insulin Dose* (1:15 ratio)
Breakfast	2 slices honey grain bread	32		
	1/4 cup egg substitute	0		
	1/2 cup orange juice	15		
	1 tablespoon lower-fat margarine	0	47	3
Lunch	2 oz tuna, canned in water	0		
	1 hamburger bun	30		
	Fat-free Pringles (#15)	15		
	1 tablespoon reduced-fat mayonnaise	0		
	1 tomato and 1 lettuce slice	0		
	1 medium dill pickle	0		
	Sugar-free pudding made with fat-free milk	15	60	4
Supper	3 oz chicken breast, grilled	0		
	1 small (3 oz) baked potato	15		
	1 cup steamed broccoli	10		
	1 French roll	25		
	1 tablespoon lower-fat margarine	0		
	2 tablespoons reduced-fat sour cream	0		
	1/2 cup canned pineapple (in own juice)	15	65	4

*Insulin dose has been rounded off to the nearest whole unit.

Exercise therapy. Regular exercise is an essential part of diabetic management. It has beneficial effects on carbohydrate metabolism and insulin sensitivity. Programs of increased physical activity and weight loss reduce the incidence of type 2 diabetes in patients with impaired glucose tolerance (Sigal et al., 2006).

Plasma glucose levels remain stable in physically active patients without diabetes because of the balance between glucose use by exercising muscles and glucose production by the liver. Exercise does not result in hyperglycemia or hypoglycemia. The patient with type 1 diabetes cannot make the hormonal changes needed to maintain stable blood glucose levels during exercise. Without an adequate insulin supply, cells cannot use glucose. Low insulin levels trigger release of glucagon and epinephrine (counterregulatory hormones) to increase liver glucose production, further raising blood glucose levels. In the absence of insulin, free fatty acids become the source of energy. Exercise in the patient with uncontrolled diabetes results in further hyperglycemia and the formation of ketone bodies. He or she may have prolonged elevated blood glucose levels after vigorous exercise.

Exercise in the person with diabetes can cause hypoglycemia because of increased muscle glucose uptake and inhibited glucose release from the liver. It can occur during exercise and for up to 24 hours after exercise. Replacement of muscle and liver glycogen stores, along with increased insulin sensitivity after exercise, causes insulin requirements to drop.

Benefits of exercise include better regulation of blood glucose levels and lowering of insulin requirements for patients with type 1 diabetes. Exercise also increases insulin sensitivity, which enhances cell uptake of glucose and promotes weight loss.

Regular exercise decreases the risk for cardiovascular disease. It decreases most blood lipid levels and increases high-density lipoproteins (HDLs). Exercise decreases blood pressure and improves cardiovascular function. Regular vigorous physical activity prevents or delays type 2 diabetes by reducing body weight, insulin resistance, and glucose intolerance.

Exercise in the presence of long-term complications of diabetes often requires some adjustment. Vigorous aerobic or resistance exercise may be contraindicated in the presence of proliferative diabetic retinopathy (PDR) or severe non-PDR (NPDR). Teach the patient with PDR or NPDR to avoid the **Valsalva maneuver** (breath holding while bearing down) and activities that increase blood pressure. Heavy lifting, rapid head motion, or jarring activities can cause vitreous hemorrhage or retinal detachment. Decreased pain sensation in the extremities increases the risk for skin breakdown and infection and for joint destruction. Teach the patient with peripheral neuropathy to engage in non–weight-bearing activities such as swimming, bicycling, or arm exercises. Those with autonomic neuropathy are at increased risk for exercise-induced injury from impaired temperature control, postural hypotension, and impaired thirst with risk for dehydration. Physical activity also can increase urine protein excretion.

Assessment before initiating an exercise program is necessary to ensure patient safety. Advise the patient to have a medical evaluation before starting an exercise program or before participating in activities that will increase the overall level of physical activity. The examination should screen for the presence of complications that may be worsened by the effects of increased physical activity (Zinman et al., 2004).

Regular physical activity increases the risk for both musculoskeletal injury and life-threatening cardiovascular events. The ability of the heart to respond to increasing levels of exercise on a treadmill, as well as the presence of other risk factors, forms the basis of the exercise prescription. A graded exercise test with electrocardiogram (ECG) monitoring should be considered before starting physical activity with increased intensity (more intense than brisk walking) in the previously sedentary patient, as well as in those defined as high risk. High risk is defined by the ADA (Zinman et al., 2004) as:

- Age older than 35 years
- Age older than 25 years and type 2 diabetes of more than 10 year's duration
- Age older than 25 years and type 1 diabetes of more than 15 year's duration
- Presence of any additional risk factors for coronary artery disease
- Presence of microvascular disease (proliferative retinopathy or nephropathy, including microalbuminuria)
- Presence of peripheral vascular disease
- Autonomic neuropathy

For patients who are unable to perform vigorous exercise, exercise tolerance of the heart is tested with cardiac stressor drugs (e.g., coronary vasodilators, dipyridamole thallium scans) (Zinman et al., 2004). Because microalbuminuria and proteinuria are associated with increased risk for cardiovascular disease, an exercise ECG stress test is also recommended for sedentary patients with these conditions before beginning an exercise program.

Guidelines for exercise are based on blood glucose levels and urine ketone levels. The patient checks blood glucose levels before exercise. *Patients with type 1 diabetes should perform vigorous exercise only if blood glucose levels are 80 to 250 mg/dL (4.4 to 13.8 mmol/L) and no ketones are present in the urine.* The absence of urine ketones indicates that enough insulin is available for glucose transport and that exercise should be effective in lowering blood glucose levels. *When urine ketones are present, the patient should **not** exercise.* Ketones indicate that current insulin levels are not adequate and that exercise would elevate blood glucose levels.

The positive benefits of exercise are short term (i.e., triglyceride reduction lasts for up to 72 hours). Systolic blood pressure is reduced for up to 12 hours (Fletcher & Trejo, 2005). Advise the patient to participate in activity according to ADA guidelines. A 5- to 10-minute warm-up period with stretching and low-intensity exercise before exercise prepares the skeletal muscles, heart, and lungs for a progressive increase in exercise intensity. After the activity session, a cool-down should be performed similarly to the warm-up. The cool-down should last 5 to 10 minutes and gradually bring the heart rate down to pre-exercise level.

The American Diabetes Association's Recommendations for Exercise (Sigal et al., 2006) are:

- To improve glycemic control, assist with weight maintenance, and reduce risk for cardiovascular disease, at least 150 min/wk of moderate-intensity aerobic physical activity and/or at least 90 min/wk of vigorous aerobic. The physical activity should occur at least 3 days/wk and with no more than 2 consecutive days without physical activity.
- Performing more than 4 hr/wk of moderate to vigorous aerobic and/or resistance physical activity is associated with greater cardiovascular disease risk reduction compared with lower volumes of activity.

- For long-term maintenance of major weight loss (more than 13.6 kg/30 lb), larger volumes of exercise (7 hr/wk) of moderate or vigorous aerobic physical activity may be helpful.
- Resistance exercise: In the absence of contraindications, patients with type 2 diabetes are urged to perform resistance exercise 3 times a week, targeting all major muscle groups.

Patient education: exercise promotion. Chart 67-6 lists NIC intervention activities for exercise. Instruct the patient to wear shoes with good traction and cushioning and to examine the feet daily and after exercise. Warn him or her to not exercise in extreme heat or cold or during periods of poor blood glucose control. Teach the patient to stay hydrated, especially during and after exercise in a warm environment.

Teach patients not to exercise within 1 hour of insulin injection or at the peak time of insulin action. Exercise can increase absorption of insulin from the injection site, increasing blood insulin levels. The risk for hypoglycemia increases when insulin is injected into an area that is exercised.

Teach patients about the risk for hypoglycemia and its preventive measures. Those taking oral drugs or insulin should monitor blood glucose levels to determine the effects of exercise. Reinforce that snacks containing rapidly absorbable carbohydrate may be eaten before and during exercise to maintain normal blood glucose levels. Extra carbohydrate may be needed for up to 24 hours after exercise to prevent hypoglycemia. The amount of additional carbohydrate is directed by the results of blood glucose monitoring. Teach the patient to decrease insulin dosage before planned exercise as directed.

Advise the nonobese patient who is taking insulin to have a carbohydrate-containing snack before exercise if at least 1 hour has passed since the last food was eaten or if high-intensity exercise is planned. Additional carbohydrate intake is not needed when the blood glucose level exceeds 100 mg/dL (5.6 mmol/L) before exercise and the planned activity is of low intensity and short duration. When vigorous activity of long duration is planned, teach the patient to eat an additional 15 to 30 g of carbohydrate for every 30 to 60 minutes of exercise. Snacks such as fruit, fruit juice, bread products, and whole milk can prevent hypoglycemia. Teach the patient to carry a simple sugar (hard candy) to eat if symptoms of hypoglycemia occur. Also instruct him or her to carry identifying information about having diabetes.

CONSIDERATIONS FOR OLDER ADULTS

With age, the ability of the heart and lungs to deliver oxygen to tissues and organs declines. These changes may be due more to decline in muscle mass than to changes in cardiac output. Aerobic activities are important in maintaining muscle mass. Healthy older adults are able to maintain cardiac output by increasing stroke volume during exercise.

The emphasis for any activity program is on changing sedentary behavior to active behavior at any level. Encourage sedentary older adults to begin with low-intensity physical activity. Start low-intensity activities in short sessions (less than 10 minutes); include warm-up and cool-down components with active stretching. Changes in activity levels should be gradual. Formal evaluation by physical therapy and/or occupational therapy may be needed.

In the absence of retinopathy-related restrictions, strength (resistance) training for major muscles of the legs, arms, stomach, and trunk, performed two or three times weekly, helps preserve muscle mass and minimizes general functional decline. Examples of specific exercise can be found at www.geri.com.

Chart 67-6 NIC INTERVENTION ACTIVITIES

The Diabetic Patient Needing to Increase Physical Activity

Exercise Promotion: *Facilitation of regular physical activity to maintain or advance to a higher level of fitness and health*

- Appraise individual's health beliefs about physical exercise.
- Encourage verbalization of feelings about exercise or need for exercise.
- Assist individual to develop an appropriate exercise program to meet needs.
- Assist individual to set short-term and long-term goals for the exercise program.
- Assist individual to schedule regular periods for the exercise program into weekly routine.
- Include family/caregivers in planning and maintaining the exercise program.
- Inform individual about health beliefs and physiologic effects of exercise.
- Instruct individual about appropriate type of exercise for level of health, in collaboration with physician and/or exercise physiologist.
- Instruct individual about desired frequency, duration, and intensity of the exercise program.
- Instruct individual about conditions warranting cessation of or alteration in the exercise program.
- Instruct individual on proper warm-up and cool-down exercises.
- Instruct individual in techniques to avoid injury while exercising.
- Monitor individual's response to exercise program.
- Provide positive feedback for individual's efforts.

Vital Signs Monitoring: *Collection and analysis of cardiovascular, respiratory, and body temperature data to determine and prevent complications*

- Monitor blood pressure, pulse, temperature, and respiratory status, as appropriate.
- Monitor for and report signs and symptoms of hypothermia and hyperthermia.
- Monitor presence and quality of pulses.
- Monitor cardiac rhythm and rate.
- Monitor respiratory rate and rhythm (e.g., depth and symmetry).
- Monitor for abnormal respiratory patterns (e.g., Cheyne-Stokes, Kussmaul, Biot, apneustic, ataxic, and excessive sighing).
- Monitor skin color, temperature, and moistness.
- Identify possible causes of changes in vital signs.

NIC intervention activities selected from Bulechek, G.M., Butcher, H.K., & McCloskey Dochterman, J. (Eds.). (2008). *Nursing interventions classification (NIC)* (5th ed.). St. Louis: Mosby.

Surgical Management. Surgical interventions for diabetes include transplantation of the pancreas. Successful transplantation improves quality of life by eliminating the need for insulin injections, blood glucose monitoring, and many dietary restrictions. It can eliminate the acute complications related to blood glucose control but is only partially successful in reversing long-term diabetes complications. Pancreatic transplant is successful when the patient no longer needs insulin therapy and all blood measures of glucose are normal.

Transplantation requires lifelong immunosuppressive drugs to prevent graft rejection. These drug regimens have toxic side effects that restrict their use to patients who have serious progressive complications of diabetes. In addition, some anti-rejection drugs have the effect of increasing blood glucose levels. Pancreas-alone transplants are considered for patients with severe metabolic complications, clinical and emotional problems with insulin that are so severe as to be incapacitating, and consistent failure of insulin-based therapy to prevent acute complications.

Pancreas transplantation is considered in diabetic patients with end-stage kidney disease who have had or plan to have a kidney transplant. Normal blood glucose levels after pancreas transplantation improves kidney graft survival. Pancreas graft survival is better when performed at the time of the kidney transplant.

Whole-pancreas transplantation. Improved surgical techniques and newer anti-rejection drugs have improved pancreatic transplantation outcomes. The 1-year survival rate for patients is above 95%, with more than 83% of patients remaining free of insulin injection and diet restrictions after 1 year (ADA, 2006b). The degree of HLA tissue-type matching affects the results.

Pancreatic transplantation is performed in one of three ways: transplant of the pancreas alone (PTA), transplant of the pancreas after kidney transplant (PAK), and simultaneous pancreas and kidney transplant (SPK). SPK is the ideal procedure for diabetic patients with uremia.

Operative procedure. Most pancreatic transplants are from cadaver donors using a total pancreas still attached to the exit of the pancreatic duct. It is placed in the pelvis. The insulin released by the pancreas graft is secreted into the bloodstream. The new pancreas also produces about 800 to 1000 mL of fluid daily, which is diverted to either the bladder or the bowel.

Chronic loss of pancreatic secretions can cause dehydration and electrolyte imbalance, and drainage of these fluids into the urinary bladder causes irritation. When the pancreas is attached to the bladder, the loss of fluid rich in bicarbonate may cause acidosis. Some techniques allow intestinal drainage of pancreatic fluids.

Rejection management. A combination of drugs and antibodies are used to reverse rejection. (See Chapter 19 for a listing of agents used to prevent or treat transplant rejection.) Patients undergoing immunosuppressive therapy first receive drugs to prevent viral, bacterial, and fungal infection because of the risk for opportunistic infections.

In most episodes of rejections, kidney problems occur before pancreatic problems. An increase in serum creatinine indicates rejection of both the transplanted kidney and the pancreas. In patients with bladder drainage of pancreatic hormones, a decrease in the urine amylase level by 25% is an indication to treat rejection. High blood glucose levels are a later marker of rejection and usually indicate irreversible graft failure.

Long-term effects. Long-term immunosuppressive therapy increases the risk for infection, cancer, and atherosclerosis. The transplanted pancreas does not duplicate all the functions of a normal pancreas. When insulin drains into systemic rather than portal (liver) circulation, blood insulin levels rise (hyperinsulinemia) and increase the risk for hypertension and macrovascular disease.

Complications. Complications are common in patients taking long-term immunosuppressive therapy. Monitor laboratory values, fluid and electrolyte status, physical manifestations, and changes in vital signs to identify possible complications. Early removal of IV and intra-arterial lines, use of sterile technique with dressing changes and catheter irrigations, strict handwashing by all health care personnel, and good pulmonary hygiene help prevent infection.

The most serious complication of enteric-drained pancreas transplantation is leaking and intra-abdominal abscess. Observe for and report elevation in temperature, abdominal discomfort, and elevation in white blood cell (WBC) count.

Pancreatitis in the transplanted organ occurs to some degree in all patients after surgery. Report elevations in serum amylase that persist after 48 to 96 hours.

Pancreatic blood vessel thrombosis occurs in about 30% of patients after transplantation. Observe for and report any sudden drop in urine amylase levels, rapid increases in blood glucose, gross **hematuria** (bloody urine), and tenderness or pain in the graft area (iliac fossa).

Bladder-drained pancreas transplantation has a lower rate of intra-abdominal abscess formation. However, drainage of 500 mL of bicarbonate-rich fluid with pancreatic enzymes into the urinary bladder can cause urinary tract infections, cystitis, urethritis, and balanitis. Metabolic acidosis occurs from the loss of large amounts of alkaline pancreatic secretions.

Assess for and document manifestations of rejection. In acute rejection, decreased kidney function is indicated by increased serum creatinine, decreased urine output, hypertension, increased weight, graft tenderness, and fever. Proteinuria is often the first indicator of chronic graft rejection. Check for increased blood amylase, lipase, or glucose; decreased urine amylase; graft tenderness; hyperglycemia; and fever. *It is especially important to assess for signs of infection and start appropriate therapy. Fever can indicate both infection and rejection.*

Monitor for side effects of the anti-rejection drugs. Cyclosporine (Neoral) is toxic to the kidney. Signs of toxicity are elevated creatinine and decreased urine output. Monitor WBC counts daily, because azathioprine (Imuran) can suppress bone marrow function. Prednisone has many side effects, including elevated blood glucose levels. Common side effects of tacrolimus (Prograf) are hypertension, kidney toxicity, neurotoxicity, GI toxicity, and glucose intolerance.

The patient's quality of life improves as a result of freedom from the need for insulin, a less restricted lifestyle, and a return to a normal diet. Stress, however, the potential need for insulin injections to treat hyperglycemia caused by immunosuppressive (anti-rejection) drugs.

Islet cell transplantation. Islet cell transplantation eliminates the need for insulin and protects against the complications of diabetes. Wider use of this procedure is hindered by the limited supply of beta cells available for transplantation and by issues related to rejection. Islet cells from tissue-typed (HLA-matched) cadaver pancreas glands are injected into the portal vein. The new cells lodge in the liver and begin to function, secreting insulin and maintaining near-perfect blood glucose control.

Islet cell transplantation may successfully restore long-term endogenous insulin production and glycemic control in patients with type 1 diabetes and unstable baseline control. Currently, most patients undergoing this procedure eventually have a progressive loss of islet cell function over time. The reasons for this gradual loss of function are not known and make this procedure a long-term but temporary intervention. It is considered an experimental procedure.

Risk for Delayed Surgical Recovery

NOC **Planning: Expected Outcomes.** The patient with diabetes undergoing a surgical procedure is expected to recover completely without complications. Indicators include:

- Wound healing
- Absence of infection
- Maintenance of blood glucose levels within expected range
- Discharge readiness

Interventions. Surgery is a physical and emotional stressor, and the diabetic patient has a higher risk for complications. Anesthesia and surgery cause a stress response with release of counterregulatory hormones that elevate blood glucose. Stress hormones suppress insulin action, increasing the risk for ketoacidosis and metabolic acidosis. Hyperglycemic-hyperosmolar state (HHS) (previously known as *hyperglycemic-hyperosmolar nonketotic syndrome [HHNS]*) is a common complication after major surgery and is associated with increased mortality. Diuresis from hyperglycemia can cause severe dehydration and increase the risk for kidney failure.

Complications of diabetes increase the risk for surgical complications. Diabetics are higher risk for hypertension, ischemic heart disease, cerebrovascular disease, MI, and cardiomyopathy. Heart failure is a serious risk factor and must be improved before surgery. Damage to nerves controlling the heart and blood vessels (autonomic neuropathy) may result in sudden tachycardia, bradycardia, or postural hypotension. The diabetic is at risk for acute renal failure and urinary retention after surgery, especially if he or she has albumin in the urine (indicator of kidney damage). Nerves to the intestinal wall and sphincters can be impaired, leading to delayed gastric emptying and increased reflux of gastric acid and increasing the risk for aspiration on induction of anesthesia. Autonomic neuropathy may cause paralytic ileus after surgery.

Preoperative Care. Patients undergoing major surgery should be admitted to the hospital 2 to 3 days before surgery to optimize blood glucose control. Second-generation sulfonylureas are discontinued 1 day before surgery. Chlorpropamide (Diabinese) is stopped at least 36 hours before surgery. Metformin (Glucophage) is stopped 48 hours before surgery and restarted only after renal function is normal. All other oral drugs are stopped the day of surgery. Patients taking long-acting insulin may need to be switched to intermediate-acting insulin forms 1 to 2 days before surgery.

Preoperative blood glucose levels should be less than 200 mg/dL (11.1 mmol/L) (Hoogwerf, 2006b). Higher levels can cause neutrophil dysfunction and increased infection rates. They also impair wound healing by altering collagen formation, which decreases wound strength.

Plan ahead for pain control after surgery. Pain, a stressor, triggers the release of counterregulatory hormones, increasing blood glucose levels and insulin needs. Opioid analgesics slow GI motility and alter blood glucose levels. The older patient who receives opioids is more at risk for confusion, paralytic ileus, hypoventilation, hypotension, and urinary retention. Patient-controlled analgesia (PCA) systems reduce respiratory complications and confusion. (See Chapter 5 for pain interventions and Chapter 16 for general preoperative care.)

Intraoperative Care. IV infusion of insulin, glucose, and potassium is standard therapy for perioperative management of diabetes. The goal is to keep the glucose level between 120 and 200 mg/dL (6.7 and 11.1 mmol/L) during surgery to prevent hypoglycemia and reduce risks from hyperglycemia. Levels below 200 mg/dL (11.1 mmol/L) reduce the risk for wound infection. Insulin/glucose infusion rates are based on hourly capillary glucose tests. Higher insulin doses may be needed because stress releases glucagon and epinephrine. Patients with diabetes should receive about 5 g of glucose per hour during surgery to prevent hypoglycemia, ketosis, and protein breakdown.

NIC intervention activities for vital sign monitoring are listed in Chart 67-6. Monitor the patient's temperature—it may be lowered deliberately in some surgical procedures and inadvertently in others. Low operating room temperatures and large incisions also lower body temperature. Hypothermia decreases metabolic needs, depresses heart rate and contractility, causes vasoconstriction, and impairs insulin release, resulting in high blood glucose levels. Monitor arterial blood gas values for acidosis.

Postoperative Care. Hyperglycemia is associated with increased mortality and morbidity after surgical procedures. Continuous insulin infusion that maintains blood glucose levels to a target level of 110 mg/dL (6.1 mmol/L) can reduce cardiovascular problems after surgery.

Protocols and computer-based programs are available that determine the insulin infusion rate required to maintain blood glucose levels within a defined target range. Many of these insulin infusion algorithms are implemented by nursing staff. (See the Evidence-Based Practice box on p. 1500.) Continue glucose and insulin infusions as prescribed until the patient is stable and can tolerate oral feedings. Short-term insulin therapy may be needed after surgery for the patient who usually uses oral agents alone. For those receiving insulin therapy, dosage adjustments may be required until the stress of surgery subsides.

Monitoring. Patients with autonomic neuropathy or vascular disease need close monitoring to avoid hypotension or respiratory arrest. Those who take beta blockers for hypertension need close monitoring for hypoglycemia because these drugs mask symptoms of hypoglycemia. Patients with **azotemia** (increased protein or nitrogen waste products in the blood) may have problems with fluid management. Check central venous pressure or pulmonary artery pressure as needed.

Glucose levels are a sensitive marker of counterregulatory hormones, which are often activated before patients become febrile. *When a patient who has had reasonably controlled blood glucose levels in the hospital develops an unexpected rise in blood glucose values, check for wound infection.* Hyperglycemia often occurs before a fever.

Hyperkalemia (high blood potassium level) is common in patients with mild to moderate kidney failure and can lead to cardiac dysrhythmia. In other patients, **hypokalemia** (low blood potassium level) may occur and be made worse by in-

EVIDENCE-BASED PRACTICE

Intensive insulin therapy wins!

Van den Berghe, G., Wilmer, A., Hermans, G., Meerssman, W., Wouters, P.J., Milants, I., et al. (2006). Intensive insulin therapy in the medical ICU. *New England Journal of Medicine, 354*(5), 449-461.

Hyperglycemia is associated with poor outcomes in intensive care units (ICUs). Strict glycemic control has a positive effect on clinical outcomes. Use of an intensive intravenous (IV) insulin infusion protocol to achieve target blood glucose levels of 80 to 100 mg/dL reduces mortality and morbidity in ICUs. However, this degree of control is difficult, in part because nurses are not comfortable with "low-normal" blood glucose levels and lack the experience to effectively manage intensive insulin infusions.

In this study, patients in the ICU for at least 3 days were randomized to one of two groups. One group received intensive insulin therapy by IV infusion for glucose levels exceeding 110 mg/dL, with maintenance values between 80 and 110 mg/dL. The control group received an insulin infusion only for glucose levels greater than 215 mg/dL, with maintenance values between 180 and 200 mg/dL. The dose of insulin was adjusted according to whole blood glucose levels measured at 1-hour to 4-hour intervals. Adjustments were made by nurses in the ICU using approved titration guidelines.

Patients receiving intensive insulin therapy had lower morbidity rates with less new renal injury, earlier weaning from mechanical ventilation, and earlier discharge from the ICU and hospital. Lower mortality rates were noted in those intensively treated patients spending more than 3 days in the ICU.

Level of Evidence—1. (individual randomized controlled trial with narrow confidence interval).

Commentary: Implications for Practice and Research. Hyperglycemia occurs in many critically ill patients. Because controlled trials demonstrate a reduction in both morbidity and mortality as a result of glycemic control, there has been a dramatic shift toward improving glycemic control in the hospital setting. This is accomplished through the use of premeal and basal insulin dosing in general medical and surgical units and IV insulin infusions in intensive care units.

Nurse-implemented intensive insulin protocols are safe and effective in improving glycemic control in critically ill patients. Nurses administer IV insulin according to hospital-approved protocols. Blood glucose levels are monitored every 1 to 4 hours with IV insulin infusion rates adjusted according to blood glucose response and protocol guidelines. The protocol increases the workload of nursing staff. Issues of availability of blood glucose meters and sufficient staff to perform hourly blood glucose testing must be addressed for protocols to be successful. They must be complex enough to achieve strict blood glucose control and practical enough to be easily implemented by ICU nursing staff without the need for physician supervision. Anticipate that the use of intensive insulin protocols will become more widespread as their safety and efficacy are established.

sulin and glucose given during surgery. Monitor the cardiac rhythm and serum potassium values.

Cardiovascular monitoring using serial electrocardiograms (ECGs) is recommended for older diabetic patients, those with long-standing type 1 diabetes, and those with heart disease. Diabetic patients are at higher risk for MI after surgery with a higher mortality rate. Changes in ECG or in potassium level may indicate a silent MI.

Renal monitoring, especially observing fluid balance, helps detect acute kidney failure. Diagnosis of renal impairment may require the use of x-ray studies using dyes, which may be nephrotoxic. Management of infections may require the use of nephrotoxic antibiotics. Ensure adequate hydration when these drugs are used. Check for impending renal failure by assessing fluid and electrolyte status.

Nutritional care. Use of total parenteral nutrition (TPN) in diabetic patients can cause severe metabolic changes. Anticipate that hyperglycemia will occur with TPN therapy. Monitor blood glucose often to determine the need for supplemental short-acting insulin. Insulin can be added to the TPN infusion or given as a separate IV infusion.

Returning to a normal meal plan as soon as possible after surgery promotes healing and metabolic balance. When oral foods are tolerated, make sure the patient takes at least 150 to 200 g of carbohydrate daily to prevent hypoglycemia.

Risk for Injury Related to Sensory Alterations

NOC **Planning: Expected Outcomes.** The patient with diabetes is expected to identify factors that increase the risk for injury, practice proper foot care, and maintain intact skin on the feet. Indicators include that the patient consistently demonstrates these behaviors:

- Follows preventive foot care practices
- Cleanses and inspects the feet daily
- Wears properly fitting shoes
- Avoids walking in bare feet
- Trims toenails properly
- Reports nonhealing breaks in the skin of the feet to the health care provider

Interventions. Patients with diabetes need intensive teaching about foot care. *Foot injury is the most common complication of diabetes leading to hospitalization.* Diabetes is the leading cause of amputation worldwide. The overall risk for amputation is 15 times greater in diabetic patients than in nondiabetic patients. The 5-year mortality rate after leg or foot amputation ranges from 39% to 67%. Risk factors for amputation include long duration of diabetes, poor glucose control, and low levels of high-density lipoprotein (HDL) cholesterol (Driver et al., 2005).

Sensory neuropathy, ischemia, and infection are the leading causes of foot disease among patients with diabetes. Sen-

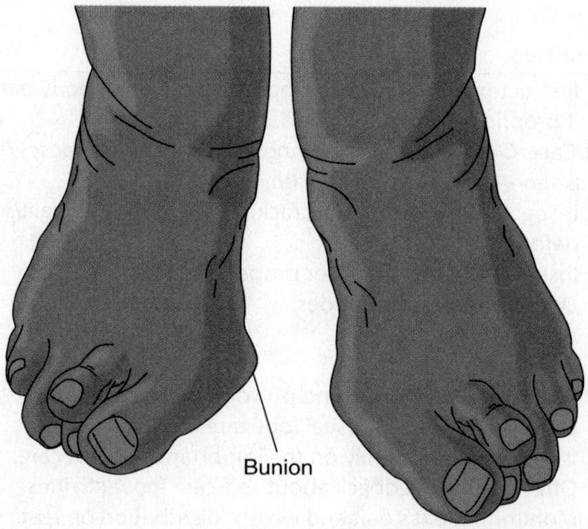
Bunion

Fig. 67-9 • The appearance of hallux valgus with a bunion.

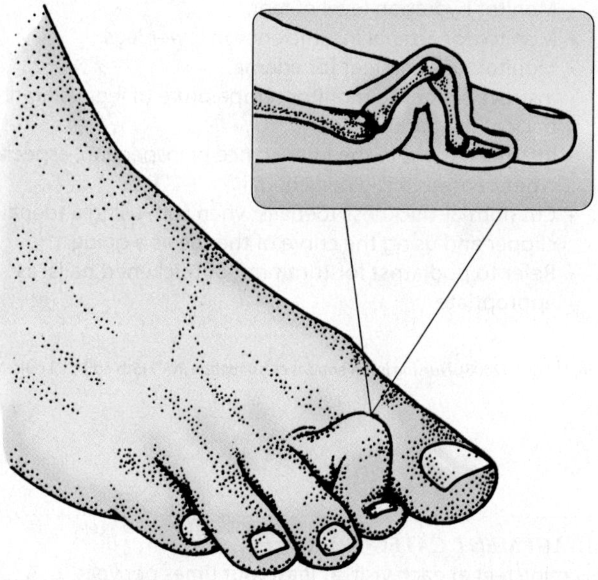

Fig. 67-10 • Hammertoe of the second metatarsophalangeal (MTP) joint.

sory neuropathy occurs in nearly all diabetic foot ulcers. Loss of pain, pressure, and temperature sensation in the foot increases the risk for injury and ulceration. Impaired blood flow to the foot limits wound healing.

Claw toe deformity is common in diabetic neuropathy. Toes are hyperextended, which increases pressure on the metatarsal heads ("ball" of the foot), resulting in ulceration. Thinning or shifting of the fat pad under the metatarsal heads decreases cushioning and increases areas of pressure. These changes predispose the patient to callus formation, ulceration, and infection. Fig. 67-9 shows hallux valgus (turning of the great toe), and Fig. 67-10 shows a hammertoe.

The Charcot foot is a type of diabetic foot deformity. The foot is warm, swollen, and painful. Walking collapses the arch, shortens the foot, and gives the foot a "rocker bottom" shape.

Sensory neuropathy may cause tingling or burning, but more often it produces numbness and reduced sensation. Neuropathy causes loss of normal sweating and skin temperature regulation, resulting in dry, thinning skin. Skin cracks and fissures increase the risk for infection.

Without sensation, the patient does not notice injuries to the foot and does not treat them. Foot injuries can be caused by walking barefoot, wearing ill-fitting shoes, sustaining thermal injuries from hot water (e.g., water bottles, heating pads, baths), or receiving caustic burns from over-the-counter corn treatments. Because the blood supply to the diabetic foot is poor, these injuries can lead to amputation.

Ulcers result from continued pressure. Plantar ulcers (on the sole, usually the ball) are from standing or walking. Those on the top or sides of the foot usually are from shoes. The increased pressure causes calluses. Ulcers usually form over or around the great toe, under the metatarsal heads, and on the tops of claw toes.

Broken skin increases the risk for infection. Skin tends to break in areas of pressure. Infection is common in diabetic foot ulcers and, once present, is difficult to treat. Infection also impairs glucose control, leading to higher blood glucose levels and reduced immune defenses, which further increases the risk for infection.

Prevention of High-Risk Conditions. Neuropathy of the feet and legs can be delayed by keeping blood glucose levels as near normal as possible. Poor blood glucose control increases the risk for neuropathy and amputation (Corbett, 2005). Intensive therapy reduces the risk for peripheral sensory neuropathy by 60%. Encourage smoking cessation to reduce the risk for vascular complications.

The risk for ulcers or amputation increases with duration of diabetes. Other risk factors are male gender; poor glucose control; and cardiovascular, retinal, or renal complications. Foot-related risks include poor gait and stepping mechanics, peripheral neuropathy, increased pressure (callus, erythema, hemorrhage under a callus, limited joint mobility, foot deformities, or severe nail pathology), peripheral vascular disease, and a history of ulcers or amputation.

NIC ***Peripheral Sensation Management.*** The feet should be evaluated closely at least annually. Chart 67-7 lists NIC intervention activities for peripheral sensation management and foot care, and Table 67-14 lists foot risk categories.

Complete a full foot assessment as outlined in Chart 67-8. Sensory examination with Semmes-Weinstein monofilaments is the most practical measure of the risk for foot ulcers. The nylon monofilament is mounted on a holder standardized to exert a 10-g force. There is no agreement on the exact number of sites to test. A person who cannot feel the 10-g pressure at any point is at increased risk for ulcers. To perform the examination:

- Provide a quiet and relaxed setting. Ask the patient to close his or her eyes during the test.
- Test the monofilament on the patient's cheek so he or she knows what to expect.
- Test the sites noted in Fig. 67-11.
- Apply the monofilament at a right angle to the skin surface.
- Apply enough force to bend the filament using a smooth, not jabbing, motion (Fig. 67-12).
- The approach, contact, and removal of the filament at each site should take 1 to 2 seconds.

Chart 67-7 NIC INTERVENTION ACTIVITIES

The Diabetic Patient with Reduced Sensation in the Lower Extremities

Peripheral Sensation Management: *Prevention or minimization of injury or discomfort in the patient with altered sensation*

- Monitor sharp/dull and/or hot/cold discrimination.
- Monitor for paresthesia: numbness, tingling, hyperesthesia, and hypoesthesia.
- Encourage patient to use the unaffected body part to determine temperature of food, liquids, bathwater, and so on.
- Instruct patient or family to monitor position of body parts while bathing, sitting, lying, or changing position.
- Instruct patient or family to examine skin daily for alteration in skin integrity.
- Monitor fit of bracing devices, prostheses, shoes, and clothing.
- Instruct patient or family to use thermometer to test water temperature.
- Encourage use of gloves or other protective clothing over affected body part when body part is in contact with objects that, because of their thermal, textural, or other inherent characteristics, may be potentially hazardous.
- Avoid or carefully monitor use of heat or cold, such as heating pads, hot water bottles, and ice packs.
- Encourage patient to wear well-fitting, low-heeled, soft shoes.
- Check shoes, pockets, and clothing for wrinkles or foreign objects.
- Instruct patient to use timed intervals, rather than presence of discomfort, as a signal to alter position.
- Protect body parts from extreme temperature changes.
- Discuss or identify causes of abnormal sensation or sensation changes.
- Instruct patient to visually monitor position of body parts, if proprioception is impaired.

Foot Care: *Cleansing and inspecting the feet for the purposes of relaxation, cleanliness, and healthy skin*

- Inspect skin for irritation, cracking, lesions, corns, calluses, deformities, or edema.
- Inspect patient's shoes for proper fit.
- Dry carefully between toes.
- Apply lotion.
- Clean nails.
- Apply moisture-absorbing powder, as indicated.
- Discuss with patient usual foot care routine.
- Instruct patient/family on the importance of foot care.
- Offer positive feedback about self-care foot activities.
- Monitor patient's gait and weight distribution on feet.
- Monitor cleanliness and general condition of shoes and stockings.
- Instruct patient to inspect inside of shoes for rough areas.
- Monitor hydration level of feet.
- Monitor for arterial insufficiency in lower legs.
- Monitor legs and feet for edema.
- Instruct patient to monitor temperature of feet using the back of the hand.
- Instruct patient in the importance of inspection, especially when sensation is diminished.
- Cut normal-thickness toenails when soft, using a toenail clipper and using the curve of the toe as a guide.
- Refer to podiatrist for trimming of thickened nails, as appropriate.

NIC intervention activities selected from Bulechek, J.M., Butcher, H.K., & McCloskey Dochterman, J. (Eds.). (2008). *Nursing interventions classification (NIC)* (5th ed.). St. Louis: Mosby.

TABLE 67-14 Foot Risk Categories

RISK CATEGORIES

RISK CATEGORY 0
- Has disease that leads to insensitivity
- Has protective sensation
- Has not had a plantar ulcer

RISK CATEGORY 1
- Does not have protective sensation
- Has not had a plantar ulcer
- Does not have a foot deformity

RISK CATEGORY 2
- Does not have protective sensation
- Has not had a plantar ulcer
- Does have a foot deformity

RISK CATEGORY 3
- Does not have protective sensation
- Has history of plantar ulcer

MANAGEMENT CATEGORIES

MANAGEMENT CATEGORY 0
- Examine feet at each visit, at least four times per year
- Foot clinic visit once a year
- Patient education

MANAGEMENT CATEGORY 1
- Examine feet at each visit, at least four times per year
- Foot clinic visit every 6 months
- Soft insoles
- Patient education

MANAGEMENT CATEGORY 2
- Examine feet at each visit, at least 4 times per year
- Foot clinic visit every 3-4 months
- Custom-molded insoles
- Prescription footwear
- Patient education

MANAGEMENT CATEGORY 3
- Examine feet at each visit, at least four times per year
- Foot clinic visit every 1-2 months
- Custom-molded insoles
- Prescription footwear
- Patient education

From Gillis W. Long Hansen's Disease Center Rehabilitation Branch. (1992). *Foot screening: Care of the foot in diabetes—The Carville approach*. Carville, LA: Department of Health and Human Services.

Chart 67-8 FOCUSED ASSESSMENT

The Diabetic Foot

Assess the patient for risk for diabetic foot problems:
- History of previous ulcer
- History of previous amputation

Assess the foot for abnormal skin and nail conditions:
- Dry, cracked, fissured skin
- Ulcers
- Toenails: thickened, long nails; ingrown nails
- Tinea pedis; onychomycosis (mycotic nails)

Assess the foot for status of circulation:
- Symptoms of claudication
- Presence or absence of dorsalis pedis or posterior tibial pulse
- Prolonged capillary filling time (greater than 25 seconds)
- Presence or absence of hair growth on the top of the foot

Assess the foot for evidence of deformity:
- Calluses, corns
- Prominent metatarsal heads (metatarsal head is easily felt under the skin)
- Toe contractures: clawed toes, hammertoes
- Hallux valgus or bunions
- Charcot foot ("rocker bottom")

Assess the foot for loss of strength:
- Limited ankle joint range of motion
- Limited motion of great toe

Assess the foot for loss of protective sensation:
- Numbness, burning, tingling
- Semmes-Weinstein monofilament testing at 10 points on each foot

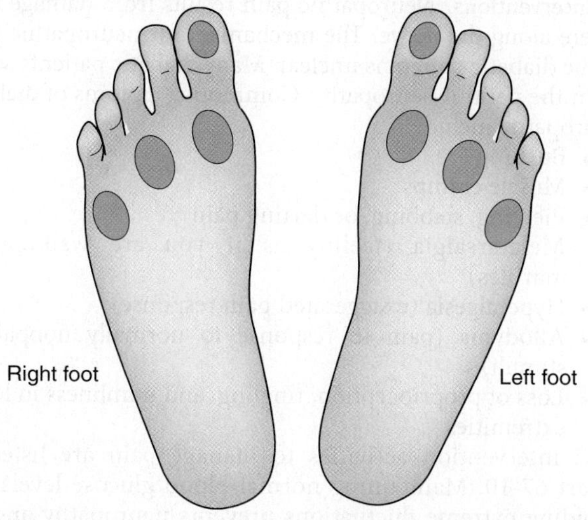
Right foot
Left foot

Fig. 67-11 • Placement sites of monofilaments for testing of protective sensation.

- Apply the filament along the perimeter and **not** on an ulcer site, callus, scar, or necrotic tissue. Do not slide the filament across the skin or make repeated contact at the test site.

Randomize the sequence of applying the filament throughout the examination. Have the patient identify where the filament touched rather than asking "Do you feel this?".

Footwear. All patients with any degree of peripheral neuropathy need to wear protective shoes. They should be fitted by an experienced shoe fitter, such as a certified podiatrist. The shoe should be ½ to ⅝ inch longer than the longest toe. Heels should be less than 2 inches high. Shoes that are too tight damage tissue when worn for 4 hours or longer. Teach the patient to change shoes by midday and again in the evening. Socks or stockings need to fit properly and be appropriate for the planned activity. Socks should feel soft and have no thick seams, creases, or holes. They should pad the foot and absorb excess moisture. Teach patients to avoid tight stockings or those that have constricting bands. Patients with toe deformities should buy custom shoes with high, wide toe boxes and extra depth. Those with severely deformed feet, such as Charcot feet, need specially molded shoes. All new shoes need a long break-in period with frequent inspection for irritation or blistering.

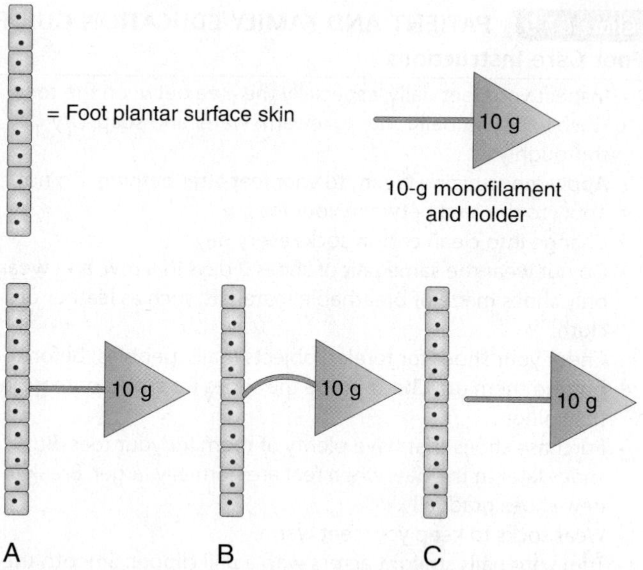
= Foot plantar surface skin
10 g
10-g monofilament and holder
10 g
10 g
10 g
A
B
C

Fig. 67-12 • Correct technique for sensation testing with 10-g monofilament. **A,** Apply monofilament to designated areas of the foot sole (intact skin, see Figure 67-11). **B,** Apply pressure to the filament until either the client states he or she can feel the pressure or until the filament bends (see p. 1501). **C,** Quickly remove the filament without sliding the filament or touching other areas of the foot.

Foot Care. Teach patients about preventive foot care and the need for examination of the feet and legs at each visit to a health care provider. Identify patients with high-risk foot conditions, and teach them about foot care. Explain problems caused by loss of protective sensation, the importance of monitoring the feet daily, proper care of the feet (including nail and skin care), and how to select appropriate footwear. Advise patients with neuropathy to break in new shoes slowly to reduce blisters.

Teach patients to inspect their feet daily. Assess their ability to inspect all areas of the foot and to perform foot care. Teach family members how to inspect and care for the patient's feet if the patient cannot. Chart 67-9 lists foot care instructions.

Wound Care. The standards of care for diabetic ulcers are a moist wound environment, débridement of necrotic tissue, and elimination of pressure (off-loading).

Wound environment is influenced by the dressing. Dressings reduce or prevent infection, allow débridement, reduce wound pain, and stimulate granulation tissue. Many commercial products are available. Antiseptics such as povidone iodine, hydrogen peroxide, and chlorhexidine interfere with wound healing. Dressings that keep the wound moist are essential.

Débridement removes dead tissues that support bacterial growth. Proper débridement is needed to reduce the risk for

Chart 67-9 PATIENT AND FAMILY EDUCATION GUIDE

Foot Care Instructions

- Inspect your feet daily, especially the area between the toes.
- Wash your feet daily with lukewarm water and soap. Dry thoroughly.
- Apply moisturizing cream to your feet after bathing. Do not apply to the area between your toes.
- Change into clean cotton socks every day.
- Do not wear the same pair of shoes 2 days in a row, and wear only shoes made of breathable materials, such as leather or cloth.
- Check your shoes for foreign objects (nails, pebbles) before putting them on. Check inside the shoes for cracks or tears in the lining.
- Purchase shoes that have plenty of room for your toes. Buy shoes later in the day, when feet are normally larger. Break in new shoes gradually.
- Wear socks to keep your feet warm.
- Trim your nails straight across with a nail clipper. Smooth the nails with an emery board.
- See your physician or nurse immediately if you have blisters, sores, or infections. Protect area with a dry, sterile dressing. Do not use adhesive tape to secure dressing.
- Do not treat blisters, sores, or infections with home remedies.
- Do not smoke.
- Do not step into the bathtub without checking the temperature of the water with your wrist or thermometer. Optimal temperature is 95° F (35° C).
- Do not use very hot or cold water. Never use hot water bottles, heating pads, or portable heaters to warm your feet.
- Do not treat corns, blisters, bunions, calluses, or ingrown toenails yourself.
- Do not go barefooted.
- Do not wear sandals with open toes or straps between the toes.
- Do not cross your legs or wear garters or tight stockings that constrict blood flow.
- Do not soak your feet.

infection and to reduce pressure around the wound (Kruse & Edleman, 2006). It is accomplished with surgery, topical débriding agents, and dressings. Mechanical débridement, although helpful, can delay healing by removing newly formed tissue.

Eliminating pressure on an infected area is essential to wound healing. Teach patients with foot ulcers to not wear a shoe on the foot while the ulcer is healing. Those with poor sensation may keep walking on an ulcer because it does not hurt. This results in pressure necrosis that delays healing and increases ulcer size. Pressure is reduced by specialized orthotic devices, custom-molded shoe inserts, or shoe adjustments that redistribute weight.

Total contact casts redistribute pressure over the bottom of the foot (Armstrong et al., 2005). Casting material is molded to the foot and leg so pressure is spread along the entire surface of contact, thereby reducing vertical force. The almost complete elimination of motion of the total-contact cast reduces plantar shear forces. The cast is removed 24 to 48 hours after application and weekly thereafter until the ulcer is healed. *Teach the patient that foot ulcers will recur unless weight is permanently redistributed.*

Growth factors applied to wounds increase healing by stimulating new tissue and enhancing cell growth. This treatment has helped heal foot ulcers present for many months or even years. Because it is costly, this therapy is usually performed in specialized treatment centers.

NCLEX EXAMINATION CHALLENGE

Which specific intervention for complication prevention should the nurse teach the client with diabetes and peripheral neuropathy?

A. "Drink at least 3 L of fluid daily."
B. "Wear a medical alert bracelet."
C. "Never reuse insulin syringes."
D. "Never go barefoot."

evolve For the correct answer, go to http://evolve.elsevier.com/Iggy/.

Chronic Pain

NOC **Planning: Expected Outcomes.** The patient with neuropathic pain is expected to experience relief of pain. Indicators include these consistent behaviors:

- Uses preventive measures
- Uses available resources to increase comfort
- Reports pain controlled

Interventions. Neuropathic pain results from damage anywhere along the nerve. The mechanism for neuropathic pain in the diabetic patient is unclear. Many diabetic patients suffer from the painful neuropathy. Common symptoms of diabetic neuropathy include:

- Burning
- Muscle cramps
- Piercing, stabbing, or darting pain
- Metatarsalgia (feeling as if you are walking on marbles)
- Hyperalgesia (exaggerated pain response)
- Allodynia (pain in response to normally nonpainful stimuli)
- Loss of proprioception, tingling, and numbness in lower extremities

NIC intervention activities to manage pain are listed in Chart 67-10. Maintaining normal blood glucose levels and avoiding extreme fluctuations prevents neuropathy and relieves symptoms of acute nerve dysfunction. Rapid improvement in blood glucose control may actually trigger acute peripheral neuropathy.

Several pharmacologic agents are used to manage neuropathic pain. Anticonvulsants such as gabapentin (Neurontin) is widely used to treat neuropathic symptoms. Tricyclic antidepressants, particularly amitriptyline hydrochloride (Elavil, Levate🍁) and nortriptyline (Pamelor), are also used as first-line therapy for neuropathic pain, especially when pain disturbs sleep and contributes to depression. Smaller doses are needed for analgesia than for antidepressant effects. Duloxetine hydrochloride (Cymbalta), a selective serotonin and norepinephrine

Chart 67-10 NIC INTERVENTION ACTIVITIES

The Diabetic Patient Experiencing Pain

Analgesic Administration: *Use of pharmacologic agents to reduce or eliminate pain*

- Determine pain location, characteristics, quality, and severity before medicating patient.
- Check medical order for drug, dose, and frequency of analgesic prescribed.
- Attend to comfort needs and other activities that assist in relaxation to facilitate response to analgesia.
- Set positive expectations regarding the effectiveness of analgesics to optimize patient response.
- Document response to analgesic and any untoward effects.
- Teach about the use of analgesics, strategies to decrease side effects, and expectations for involvement in decisions about pain relief.

NIC intervention activities selected from Bulechek, G.M., Butcher, H.K., & McCloskey Dochterman, J. (Eds.). (2008). *Nursing interventions classification (NIC)* (5th ed.). St. Louis: Mosby.

reuptake inhibitor (SSNRI), is approved for use in the management of neuropathic pain.

The burning of neuropathy may respond to capsaicin cream 0.075% (Axsain♣, Zostrix-HP). This drug reduces amounts of substance P, which is involved in pain transmission (see Chapter 5). Teach the patient to apply it four times daily for several weeks. Neuropathic pain may worsen for several days after therapy is started before improving.

Unpleasant symptoms are noted with abrupt discontinuation of many of these drugs. Teach the patient about possible side effects of the drug before its initiation, and warn him or her to avoid abrupt discontinuation. A gradual reduction in the dose rather than abrupt cessation is recommended to prevent side effects.

Provide support and practical information on measures to reduce pain. Simple measures such as a bed cradle to lift bed clothes off hypersensitive skin can be beneficial. Assist the diabetic patient to maintain stable glucose control. *All patients with neuropathy are at increased risk for foot ulcers and require more frequent assessment and education in routine foot management.*

Risk for Injury Related to Disturbed Sensory Perception: Visual

Planning: Expected Outcomes. The patient with diabetes is expected to be free of injury related to reduced vision and to maintain current level of vision. Indicators include:

- No further reduction of visual fields
- No double vision

Interventions

Blood Glucose Control. Poor blood glucose control, proteinuria, diastolic hypertension, and long duration of diabetes are risk factors for diabetic retinopathy and vision loss. Surgical intervention for retinal hemorrhage or new retinal blood vessel growth can reduce vision loss.

Besides regular eye examinations to evaluate retinopathy, urge the diabetic patient with impaired vision to have an optometrist or ophthalmologist assess the remaining vision and prescribe appropriate eyewear. A functional vision assessment, performed by a low-vision technician, rehabilitation teacher, or diabetes educator, determines the patient's use of lighting, contrast, non-optical and low-vision devices, large-print options, and central or peripheral vision. Those with macular edema have loss of central vision. This process causes difficulty seeing details, reading printed materials, preparing insulin syringes for injection, and self-monitoring blood glucose (SMBG) levels.

Environmental Management. Not all visually impaired patients need special devices. Adjustments in lighting, contrast, color, distance, type size of printed materials, and eye movement often improve visual abilities. Instruct the patient to supplement overhead fluorescent lighting with an incandescent lamp directed toward the workspace. Placing dark equipment against a white or yellow background (or vice versa) provides contrast to enhance vision. Coding objects such as vials of insulin with bright colors or with felt-tipped markers helps identify the correct bottle. Bringing the blood glucose lancet or insulin syringe close to the eye makes it easier to see. Suggest large type or bold print to ease reading. Teach the patient to use peripheral vision.

Adaptive devices can help the patient self-administer insulin independently. Some syringes may have a magnifier attached to the syringe. Other devices include preset dose gauges (which measure the space between the end of the syringe barrel and the plunger) to help the patient draw up the correct amount of insulin by feeling this distance. The blind patient can accurately measure insulin by using products such as the Count-A-Dose Insulin Measuring Device. This device is designed to be used with the BD Lo-Dose syringe. It holds two insulin vials and has a slot to direct the syringe needle into the vials' rubber stoppers. The patient draws insulin into the syringe by turning a thumb-wheel, which clicks for each unit (clicks can be both heard and felt). When teaching the patient to use an adaptive device, stress:

- Differentiating between bottles of fast-acting and slower-acting insulin by wrapping a rubber band around the fast-acting insulin bottle
- Ensuring proper placement of the device on the syringe
- Holding the insulin bottle upright when measuring insulin
- Avoiding air bubbles in the syringe by pulling a small amount of insulin into the syringe, moving the plunger in and out three times, and measuring insulin on the fourth draw

Design a system to determine how many doses can be drawn from a bottle so the patient does not inject air from an empty bottle instead of insulin.

Specialized adaptive equipment also is available to assist with blood glucose monitoring techniques. Assist the patient to select a blood glucose monitoring device best suited to his or her level of visual impairment. For patients with reliable low vision, monitors with large display screens and easy-to-use features may be used. Some talking blood glucose monitoring systems are available. Add-on voice boxes to provide step-by-step directions can be fitted to some brands of glucose meters. New technology is in development to provide talking meter functions for blood glucose monitoring. Assess the ability of the patient to obtain an adequate blood sample and apply it to the reagent strip. Commercially made blood drop guides can assist with this task.

Ineffective Tissue Perfusion: Renal

NOC **Planning: Expected Outcomes.** The patient with diabetes is expected to maintain a normal urine elimination pattern. Indicators include:

- Urine protein levels within normal limits
- 24-hour intake and output balance
- Blood urea nitrogen (BUN) and serum creatinine within the normal ranges
- Serum electrolytes within the normal ranges

Interventions

Prevention. Tight control of blood glucose levels may slow renal disease in patients with type 1 diabetes. Diabetic kidney disease is more likely to develop in those with poor blood glucose control. Control of hypertension is essential for the reduction of diabetic nephropathy (ADA, 2007c). Both systolic and diastolic hypertension greatly accelerate the progression of diabetic kidney disease.

Stress the need for evaluation of kidney function according to the American Diabetes Association (ADA) Standards of Care. Glomerular filtration rate (GFR) is the best overall measure of kidney function. Serum creatinine should be measured at least annually for an estimation of GFR in all patients with diabetes (ADA, 2007c).

The earliest evidence of nephropathy is the appearance of albumin in the urine. An annual test for microalbumin is performed for patients who have had type 1 diabetes for over 5 years and for all patients with type 2 diabetes starting at diagnosis and during pregnancy. Screening for microalbuminuria is performed by three methods: (1) random, spot urine collection to measure the albumin-creatinine ratio, (2) 24-hour urine collection to measure creatinine clearance, and (3) timed urine collection (e.g., 4 hours or overnight). Timed urine collections are not reliable in patients with neuropathy and incomplete bladder emptying. Random urine albumin/creatinine testing is recommended as the standard measurement of proteinuria in patients with diabetes (ADA, 2007c). Explain the implications of the test, and help the patient collect the specimen if necessary.

Aggressive control of blood glucose and hypertension in patients without microalbuminuria can avoid nephropathy. Once microalbuminuria develops, management is aimed at controlling blood pressure and blood glucose, restricting dietary protein, avoiding nephrotoxic agents, promptly treating urinary tract infections (UTIs), and preventing dehydration.

Control of blood pressure and blood glucose levels requires the patient's participation and effort. Prescribed drugs must be taken according to schedules, and dietary restriction must be maintained. Teach diabetic patients about the roles of blood pressure and blood glucose levels in kidney disease. Help them maintain normal blood glucose levels and blood pressure levels below 130/80 mm Hg. Stress the need for yearly screening for microalbuminuria.

Smoking cessation is important in halting the progression of diabetic kidney disease. Smoking increases the risk for development of microalbuminuria, increases the rate of advancement to overt proteinuria, and accelerates the rate of progression of kidney disease in patients with either type 1 or type 2 diabetes. Teach the patient about the risks of smoking, and refer him or her to appropriate resources for assistance in smoking cessation.

Any UTI can lead to kidney infection and further reduce renal function. Explain the manifestations of UTI. Urge the patient to take antibiotics exactly as prescribed, completing the entire course of treatment. Reinforce the need for follow-up urine cultures to reduce the risk for renal damage. Avoid indwelling urinary catheters when possible.

Drugs can affect renal function either through toxic effects on the kidney or by an acute but reversible reduction in function. The most common nephrotoxic drugs are antifungal agents (amphotericin B) and aminoglycoside antibiotics such as amikacin (Amikin), streptomycin, kanamycin (Kantrex), gentamicin (Garamycin), and tobramycin (Tobrex). Outside the hospital, the leading nephrotoxic agents are NSAIDs such as ibuprofen (Advil) or naproxen (Aleve). To prevent accidental ingestion of nephrotoxic drugs, teach the patient to check with a health care provider before taking over-the-counter drugs or herbal remedies.

Radiocontrast dyes can also affect renal function, especially in patients with preexisting renal insufficiency (Rudnick et al., 2006). Monitor IV hydration before and after contrast is used to prevent contrast-induced nephropathy in diabetic patients.

Drug Therapy. Use of angiotensin-converting enzyme (ACE) inhibitors (ACEIs) or angiotensin-receptor blockers (ARBs) is recommended for all patients with microalbuminuria or advanced stages of nephropathy (Zandi-Nejad & Brenner, 2005). ACE inhibitors reduce the level of albuminuria and the rate of progression of kidney disease. These drugs have not shown to be effective in primary prevention of microalbuminuria. Monitor serum potassium levels for development of hyperkalemia.

Nutrition Therapy. Patients with nephropathy should restrict dietary protein to 0.8 g/kg of body weight per day. Once the glomerular filtration rate (GFR) starts falling, further reducing protein may slow the decline in renal function (ADA, 2007b). Because lifelong dietary restrictions are difficult, provide ongoing teaching to encourage adherence.

NIC ***Fluid Management/Electrolyte Management.*** Fluid and electrolyte management can prevent more loss of kidney function. Avoiding dehydration is important for kidney perfusion and function. Assess fluid balance, and use measures to prevent dehydration. The most common cause of dehydration in patients with diabetes is overuse of diuretics. Teach patients to report edema or symptoms of orthostatic hypotension, and provide ongoing education to promote dietary goals.

Dialysis for patients with diabetes and kidney failure is the same as for patients without diabetes (see Chapter 71). The dosage of insulin needs to be adjusted when dialysis starts.

Potential for Hypoglycemia

Central nervous system (CNS) function depends on a continuous supply of glucose in the blood. The brain cannot make glucose and stores only a few minutes' supply as glycogen. This needed supply is not maintained when blood glucose levels fall below critical levels.

The first defense against falling blood glucose levels in the nondiabetic person is decreased insulin secretion, decreased glucose use, and increased glucose production. Normally, insulin secretion decreases when blood glucose levels drop to about 83 mg/dL (4.5 mmol/L). Counterregulatory hormones are activated at about 67 mg/dL (3.8 mmol/L), a level well above the threshold for symptoms of hypoglycemia. The main counterregulatory hormone is glucagon. Epinephrine also becomes important in diabetic patients who are deficient in glucagon. Both glucagon and epinephrine raise blood glucose levels by stimulating liver glycogen breakdown and conversion of protein to glucose. Epinephrine also limits insulin secretion. Growth hormone and cortisol also are important during prolonged hypoglycemia. Their effects do not become evident until 4 hours after the onset of hypoglycemia.

Type 1 diabetes disrupts the body's response to hypoglycemia, a change that occurs within 1 to 5 years of diagnosis. Regulation of circulating insulin levels is lost because insulin comes from an injection rather than from the pancreas. As blood glucose levels fall, insulin levels do not decrease. Over time, the pancreas loses it ability to secrete glucagon in response to hypoglycemia. After a few more years of type 1 diabetes, the response of epinephrine to falling blood glucose levels is also reduced. It does respond, but it takes a lower blood glucose level to become active. These problems greatly increase the risk for severe hypoglycemia.

A second problem with long-standing type 1 diabetes is *hypoglycemic unawareness* in which patients no longer have the warning symptoms of impending hypoglycemia that should prompt them to take preventive action. This problem occurs most often in diabetic patients who have had type 1 diabetes for 30 years or longer.

Symptoms of hypoglycemia are neuroglycopenic or neurologic. *Neuroglycopenic symptoms* occur when brain glucose *gradually declines* to a low level. *Neurologic symptoms* result from autonomic nervous activity triggered by a *rapid decline* in blood glucose (Table 67-15).

The blood glucose level at which symptoms of hypoglycemia occur varies among patients. Many have symptoms when blood glucose levels are well above 50 mg/dL (2.8 mmol/L), especially if the level dropped rapidly or they are used to chronic hyperglycemia. Thus clinical criteria are used to categorize hypoglycemic severity rather than blood glucose levels. In mild hypoglycemia, the patient remains alert and able to self-manage symptoms. In severe hypoglycemia, neurologic function is so impaired that he or she needs another person's help to increase blood glucose levels.

TABLE 67-15 Symptoms of Hypoglycemia

NEUROGLYCOPENIC SYMPTOMS
- Warmth
- Weakness
- Fatigue
- Difficulty thinking
- Confusion
- Behavior changes
- Emotional lability
- Seizures
- Loss of consciousness
- Brain damage
- Death

NEUROGENIC SYMPTOMS
- Adrenergic
  - Shaky/tremulous
  - Heart pounding
  - Nervous/anxious
- Cholinergic
  - Sweaty
  - Hungry
  - Tingling

Planning: Expected Outcomes. The diabetic patient is expected to have decreased episodes of hypoglycemia and remain oriented to person, place, and time, as indicated by a Glasgow Coma Scale score above 7.

Interventions. A blood glucose level below 70 mg/dL (3.9 mmol/L) alerts you to assess for signs and symptoms of hypoglycemia. (Table 67-15; see also Table 67-16).

NIC ***Hypoglycemia Management.*** NIC activities for hypoglycemia appear in Chart 67-11. Monitor blood glucose levels before giving antidiabetic drugs, before meals, before bedtime, and when the patient is symptomatic. All patients who take insulin, those taking long-acting insulin secretagogues (chlorpropamide, glyburide [glibenclamide]), and those taking long-acting glipizide (Glucotrol XL) are at risk for hypoglycemia. This risk is increased if they are older, have liver or kidney impairment, or are taking drugs that enhance the effects of antidiabetic drugs. Proper patient selection, drug dosage, and instructions are important factors in avoiding severe hypoglycemia. Hypoglycemia may be difficult to recognize in those who take beta-blocking drugs. Symptoms become less intense and less obvious. Manifestations of hypoglycemia in older patients may be mistaken for other conditions (Zammitt & Frier, 2005).

Hypoglycemia occurs when there is an excess of insulin or when the dose of insulin or oral agent is excessive, ill timed, or of the wrong type. Hypoglycemia occurs when meals are missed, when food intake is not increased after exercise, and when food is not eaten in relation to alcohol intake. Sensitivity to insulin is increased with the use of an insulin sensitizer

TABLE 67-16 Differentiation of Hypoglycemia and Hyperglycemia

Feature	Hypoglycemia	Hyperglycemia
Skin	Cool, clammy	Hot, dry*
Dehydration	Absent	Present
Perspiration	Profuse*	Absent
Respirations	No particular or consistent change	Rapid, deep*; Kussmaul type; acetone odor ("fruity" odor) to breath
Mental status	Anxious, nervous,* irritable, mental confusion,* seizures, coma	Varies from alert to stuporous, obtunded, or frank coma
Symptoms	Weakness,* double vision, blurred vision, hunger, tachycardia, palpitations	No specific symptoms for DKA Acidosis; hypercapnia; abdominal cramps, nausea and vomiting Dehydration: decreased neck vein filling, orthostatic hypotension, tachycardia, poor skin turgor
Glucose	<70 mg/dL (3.9 mmol/L)	>250 mg/dL (13.8 mmol/L)
Ketones	Negative	Positive

*Classic symptoms.
DKA, Diabetic ketoacidosis.

Chart 67-11 **NIC INTERVENTION ACTIVITIES**

The Diabetic Patient Experiencing or at Risk for Hypoglycemia

Hypoglycemia Management: *Preventing and treating low blood glucose levels*

- Identify patient at risk for hypoglycemia.
- Monitor blood glucose levels, as indicated.
- Monitor for signs and symptoms of hypoglycemia (e.g., shakiness, tremor, sweating, nervousness, anxiety, irritability, impatience, tachycardia, palpitations, chills, clamminess, light-headedness, pallor, hunger, nausea, headache, tiredness, drowsiness, weakness, warmth, dizziness, faintness, blurred vision, nightmares, crying out in sleep, paresthesias, difficulty concentrating, difficulty speaking, incoordination, behavior change, confusion, coma, seizure).
- Provide simple carbohydrate, as indicated.
- Provide complex carbohydrate and protein, as indicated.
- Administer glucagon, as indicated.
- Contact emergency medical services, as necessary.
- Administer intravenous glucose, as indicated.
- Maintain IV access, as appropriate.
- Maintain patent airway, as necessary.
- Protect from injury, as necessary.
- Review events prior to hypoglycemia to determine probable cause.
- Provide feedback regarding appropriateness of self-management of hypoglycemia.
- Instruct patient and significant others on signs and symptoms, risk factors, and treatment of hypoglycemia.
- Instruct patient to have simple carbohydrates available at all times.
- Instruct patient to obtain and carry/wear appropriate emergency identification.
- Instruct significant others on the use and administration of glucagon, as appropriate.
- Instruct on interaction of diet, insulin/oral agents, and exercise.
- Provide assistance in making self-care decisions to prevent hypoglycemia (e.g., reducing insulin/oral agents and/or increasing food intake for exercise).
- Encourage self-monitoring of blood glucose levels.
- Encourage ongoing telephone contact with diabetes care team for consultation regarding adjustments in treatment regimen.

Chart 67-12 **PATIENT AND FAMILY EDUCATION GUIDE**

Treatment of Hypoglycemia at Home

For *mild* hypoglycemia (hungry, irritable, shaky, weak, headache, fully conscious; blood glucose usually less than 60 mg/dL [3.4 mmol/L]):

- Treat the symptoms of hypoglycemia with 10 to 15 g of carbohydrate. You may use one of the following:
  - Glucose tablets or glucose gel (dosage is printed on the package)
  - $^1/_2$ cup of fruit juice
  - $^1/_2$ cup of regular (nondiet) soft drink
  - 8 ounces of skim milk
  - 6 to 10 hard candies
  - 4 cubes of sugar
  - 4 teaspoons of sugar
  - 6 saltines
  - 3 graham crackers
  - 1 tablespoon of honey or syrup
- Retest blood glucose in 15 minutes.
- Repeat this treatment if symptoms do not resolve.
- Eat a small snack of carbohydrate and protein if your next meal is more than an hour away.

For *moderate* hypoglycemia (cold, clammy skin; pale; rapid pulse; rapid, shallow respirations; marked change in mood; drowsiness; blood glucose usually less than 40 mg/dL [2.2 mmol/L]):

- Treat the symptoms of hypoglycemia with 15 to 30 g of rapidly absorbed carbohydrate.
- Take additional food, such as low-fat milk or cheese, after 10 to 15 minutes.

For *severe* hypoglycemia (unable to swallow; unconsciousness or convulsions; blood glucose usually less than 20 mg/dL [1.0 mmol/L]):

- Treatment administered by family members:
  - Administer 1 mg of glucagon as intramuscular or subcutaneous injection.
  - Administer a second dose in 10 minutes if the person remains unconscious.
  - Notify a primary care provider immediately, and follow instructions.
  - If still unconscious, transport the person to the emergency department.
  - Give a small meal when the person wakes up and is no longer nauseated.

(metformin and thiazolidinedione agents), late after exercise, or after weight loss. Insulin clearance is decreased in kidney failure.

Nutrition Therapy. When the patient is hypoglycemic, start carbohydrate replacement per physician prescription or standing protocols. Ingestion of 15 to 20 g of glucose is the preferred treatment for hypoglycemia. Blood glucose levels begin to fall about 60 minutes after glucose ingestion. If the patient can swallow, give a liquid form of carbohydrate, although any source of carbohydrate can be used to treat hypoglycemia. Specific recommendations are listed in Chart 67-12. The blood glucose level determines the form and amount of glucose used. Fluid is absorbed much more quickly from the GI tract than are solids. Concentrated sweet fluids, such as juice with sugar added or a soft drink, may slow absorption. Blood glucose response correlates better with the glucose content rather than the carbohydrate content of the food. Adding protein to carbohydrate does not improve blood glucose response and does not prevent subsequent hypoglycemia. Adding fat may retard and then prolong the blood glucose response, resulting in post-treatment hyperglycemia. Commercially available products provide predictable glucose absorption.

Drug Therapy. Glucagon given subcutaneously or IM and 50% dextrose given IV is the therapy for diabetic patients who cannot swallow. Glucagon converts liver glycogen to glucose but is not effective in severely starved patients. Take care to prevent aspiration in patients receiving glucagon, because it often causes vomiting. Give 50% dextrose carefully to avoid extravasation because it is hyperosmolar and can damage tissue. The effects of glucagon and dextrose are temporary. After the patient responds and is no longer nauseated, give a simple sugar followed by a small snack or meal. IV glucose is used to maintain mild hyperglycemia. Diazoxide (Proglycem) or octreotide (Sandostatin) may be required to treat sulfonylurea-induced hypoglycemia. Evaluate response by monitoring blood glucose levels for several hours. Symptoms may persist for an hour or more after treatment. A target blood glucose level is 70 to 110 mg/dL (3.9 to 6.2 mmol/L).

Prevention Strategies. Teach the patient how to prevent hypoglycemia. Four common causes of hypoglycemia are (1) excess insulin, (2) deficient intake or absorption of food, (3) exercise, and (4) alcohol intake.

Insulin excess from variable absorption of insulin can cause hypoglycemia even when insulin is injected correctly. This excess also can be caused by lowered insulin resistance, which occurs with termination of pregnancy or resolution of an infection. Increased insulin sensitivity can occur with weight loss or exercise programs. Differences in insulin formulation can result in hypoglycemia. Teach the patient to not change insulin brands without medical supervision.

Deficient food intake from inadequate or incorrectly timed meals can result in hypoglycemia. Changes in gastric absorption sometimes cause hypoglycemia in patients with delayed gastric emptying. This problem is more common in those with diabetes of long duration, is more severe with solid than with liquid meals, and is made worse by illness or poor glucose control. Teach the patient about the importance of regularity in timing and quantity of food eaten.

Exercise usually causes blood glucose levels to fall in a patient with type 1 diabetes. Prolonged exercise increases cellular glucose uptake for several hours after exercise. Teach the patient about blood glucose monitoring and carbohydrate consumption before and during exercise.

Alcohol inhibits liver glucose production and leads to hypoglycemia. It interferes with the counterregulatory response to hypoglycemia and impairs glycogen breakdown, making exercise-induced hypoglycemia more severe. Alcohol is more likely to cause hypoglycemia when the patient does not eat for long periods, when basic nutrition is poor, and when glycogen stores are depleted. Teach him or her to ingest alcohol only with or shortly *after* eating a meal with enough carbohydrate to prevent hypoglycemia. Warn patients to avoid excess alcohol at bedtime to prevent nighttime hypoglycemia.

Patient and Family Education. The cause of hypoglycemia may be subtle. At the onset of menses, a fall in hormone levels decreases insulin needs and contributes to hypoglycemia. When patients switch to a new bottle of insulin, hypoglycemia may occur because the fresh insulin has greater potency. Some patients have hypoglycemia when they change injection sites. Drugs such as propranolol (Inderal, Detensol🍁) or other beta blockers mask warning signs and thus predispose patients to severe hypoglycemia. Some episodes of hypoglycemia occur without an obvious cause, and many are due to the erratic absorption of insulin, a problem for even the most careful patient.

Many patients who have been treated in the emergency department for hypoglycemia do not receive adequate instruction on how to prevent another episode and are at continuing risk (Ginde et al., 2008). Help each patient develop a personal treatment plan for hypoglycemia. Routinely taking 10 to 15 g of carbohydrate results in overtreatment of hypoglycemia in some patients and undertreatment in others. The exact glucose rise from a set amount of carbohydrate varies; however, using the estimate that each 5 g of carbohydrate raises blood glucose about 20 mg/dL is a good starting plan. For example, the patient may be directed to take:

- 20 to 30 g of carbohydrate if the blood glucose level is 50 mg/dL (2.8 mmol/L) or less
- 10 to 15 g of carbohydrate if the blood glucose level is 51 to 70 mg/dL (2.9 to 3.9 mmol/L)

Use blood glucose monitoring results to revise or reinforce this plan.

Recommend that the patient wears a medical alert bracelet, and help him or her obtain one. This bracelet is helpful if the patient becomes hypoglycemic and is unable to provide self-care.

Teach the patient and family about the manifestations of hypoglycemia. Emphasize that delaying a meal for more than 30 minutes raises the risk for hypoglycemia when using some insulin regimens. Instruct him or her to keep a carbohydrate source nearby at all times. Teach the patient and family how to administer glucagon.

Hypoglycemia is a major risk for patients receiving intensive insulin protocols who engage in exercise programs. Explain that nightmares or headaches on days after prolonged or severe exercise occur with hypoglycemia.

Establishing Treatment Plans. Blood glucose monitoring directs hypoglycemia treatment. Treatment continues until blood glucose levels reach and stay in the target range. Once blood glucose control is regained, the specific cause of each hypoglycemic episode should be determined and measures taken to prevent recurrence.

CONSIDERATIONS FOR OLDER ADULTS

Older patients who take antidiabetic drugs are at increased risk for hypoglycemia. Age-related changes in liver and kidney function slow metabolism of these drugs, predisposing to prolonged and recurrent hypoglycemia. Older patients may have a delayed release of epinephrine in response to falling blood glucose levels and are less likely to notice and act on hypoglycemic symptoms. Physical symptoms such as confusion may make the older patient unable to correct hypoglycemia.

Instruct the older diabetic patient and family to check blood glucose values when symptoms such as unsteadiness, lightheadedness, poor concentration, trembling, or sweating occur. Assess eating patterns to make sure he or she is eating sufficient foods at appropriate times. Encourage a patient with a poor appetite to eat a small snack at bedtime to prevent hypoglycemia during the night.

When possible, an antidiabetic drug with low hypoglycemia potential should be selected for older patients. The highest rates of severe and fatal episodes of hypoglycemia are associated with the use of glyburide, and most of these events occurred in patients older than 70 years. Drug regimens that require that meals be eaten on time only increase the potential for hypoglycemic reactions.

Potential for Diabetic Ketoacidosis

Metabolic problems of diabetic ketoacidosis (DKA) are caused by a total or partial lack of insulin combined with the action of counterregulatory hormones (Fig. 67-13). Laboratory diagnosis of DKA is shown in Table 67-17. DKA occurs in patients with type 1 diabetes and most often starts from infection. *Death occurs in up to 10% of these cases even with appropriate treatment.* Mortality is highest for older patients who also have infection, stroke, MI, vascular thrombosis, intestinal obstruction, or pneumonia.

Hormonal changes lead to increased liver and renal glucose production and decreased glucose use in peripheral tissues.

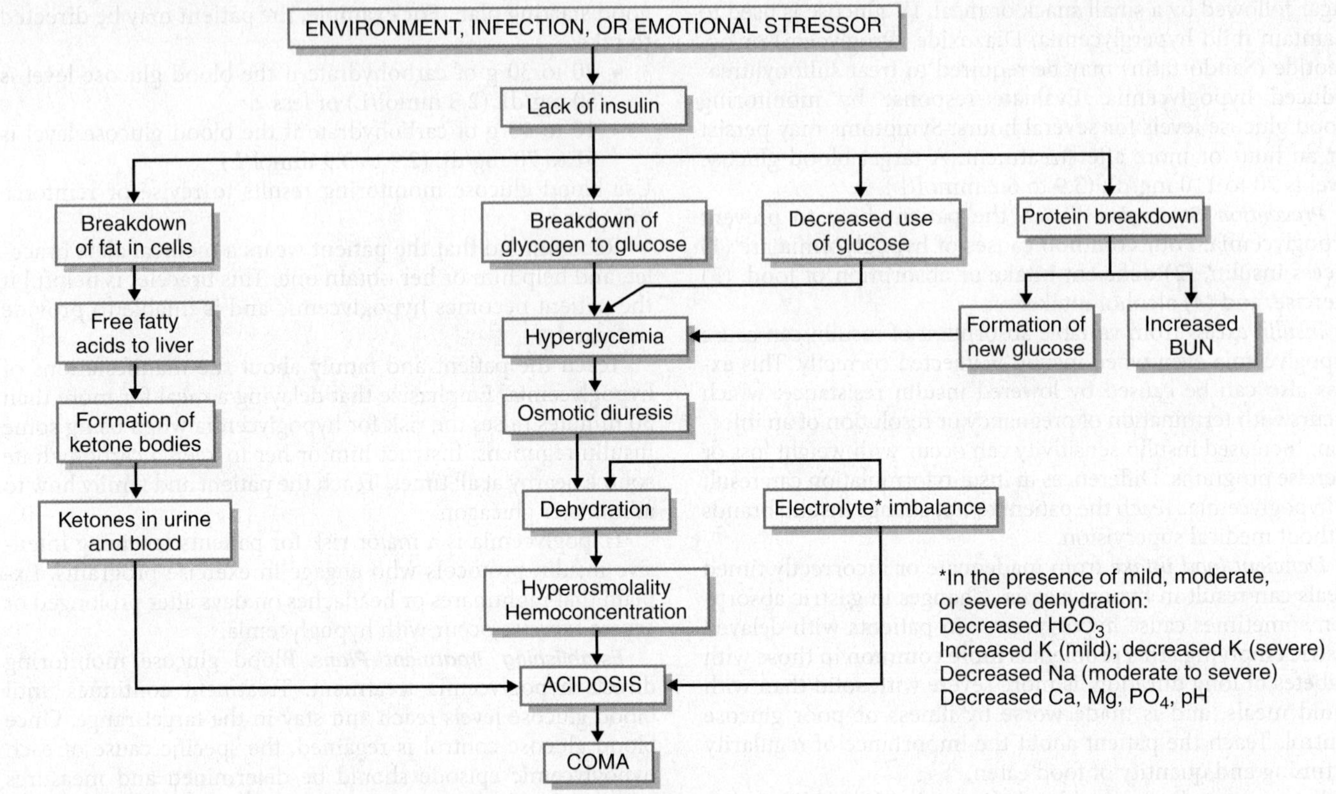
ENVIRONMENT, INFECTION, OR EMOTIONAL STRESSOR
Lack of insulin
Breakdown of fat in cells
Breakdown of glycogen to glucose
Decreased use of glucose
Protein breakdown
Free fatty acids to liver
Hyperglycemia
Formation of new glucose
Increased BUN
Formation of ketone bodies
Osmotic diuresis
Ketones in urine and blood
Dehydration
Electrolyte* imbalance
Hyperosmolality Hemoconcentration
*In the presence of mild, moderate, or severe dehydration:
Decreased HCO_3
Increased K (mild); decreased K (severe)
Decreased Na (moderate to severe)
Decreased Ca, Mg, PO_4, pH
ACIDOSIS
COMA

Fig. 67-13 • The pathophysiologic mechanism of diabetic ketoacidosis.

TABLE 67-17 Differences Between Diabetic Ketoacidosis and Hyperglycemic-Hyperosmolar State

	Diabetic Ketoacidosis (DKA)	Hyperglycemic-Hyperosmolar State (HHS)
Onset	Sudden	Gradual
Precipitating factors	Infection	Infection
	Other stressors	Other stressors
	Inadequate insulin dose	Poor fluid intake
Manifestations	Ketosis: Kussmaul respiration, "fruity" breath, nausea, abdominal pain	Altered central nervous system function with neurologic symptoms
	Dehydration or electrolyte loss: polyuria, polydipsia, weight loss, dry skin, sunken eyes, soft eyeballs, lethargy, coma	Dehydration or electrolyte loss: same as for DKA
LABORATORY FINDINGS		
Serum glucose	>300 mg/dL (16.7 mmol/L)	>600 mg/dL (33.3 mmol/L)
Osmolarity	Variable	>320 mOsm/L
Serum ketones	Positive at 1:2 dilutions	Negative
Serum pH	<7.35	>7.4
Serum HCO_3^-	<15 mEq/L	>20 mEq/L
Serum Na^+	Low, normal, or high	Normal or low
Serum K^+	Normal; elevated with acidosis, low following dehydration	Normal or low
BUN	>20 mg/dL; elevated because of dehydration	Elevated
Creatinine	>1.5 mg/dL; elevated because of dehydration	Elevated
Urine ketones	Positive	Negative

BUN, Blood urea nitrogen; *HCO_3*, bicarbonate.

Increased production of counterregulatory hormones leads to the production of ketoacids with resultant ketonemia and metabolic acidosis.

Hyperglycemia leads to osmotic diuresis with dehydration and electrolyte loss. Classic symptoms of DKA include polyuria, polydipsia, polyphagia, weight loss, vomiting, abdominal pain, dehydration, weakness, altered mental status, shock, and coma. Mental status can vary from total alertness to profound coma. As ketone levels rise, the buffering capacity of the body is exceeded, the pH of the blood decreases, and acidosis occurs. **Kussmaul respirations** (very deep and rapid respirations) cause respiratory alkalosis in an attempt to correct acidosis by exhaling carbon dioxide. Initial serum sodium levels may be low or normal. Initial potassium levels depend on how long DKA lasts before treatment. After therapy starts, serum potassium levels drop quickly.

NOC **Planning: Expected Outcomes.** The patient is expected to have few episodes of hyperglycemia and avoid diabetic ketoacidosis. Indicators include that the patient consistently demonstrates these behaviors:

- Maintains blood glucose levels within the target range
- Adjusts insulin doses to match eating patterns and blood glucose levels during illness
- Describes correct procedure for urine ketone testing
- Describes when to seek help from health care professional

Interventions

Hyperglycemia Management. Monitor for manifestations of DKA (see Table 67-17 and Fig. 67-13). Document and use these findings to determine therapy effectiveness. *First assess the airway, level of consciousness, hydration status, electrolytes, and blood glucose level.* Check the patient's blood pressure, pulse, and respirations every 15 minutes until stable. Record urine output, temperature, and mental status every hour. When a central venous catheter is present, assess central venous pressure every 30 minutes or as prescribed. After treatment starts and these values are stable, monitor and record vital signs every 4 hours. Use blood glucose values to assess therapy and determine when to switch from saline to dextrose-containing solutions.

Fluid and Electrolyte Management. *Closely assess the patient's fluid status.* The kidneys are less able to respond to changes in pH or fluid and electrolyte balance, to concentrate urine, or to regulate blood osmolarity. The risk for kidney failure rises with age. Impaired bicarbonate reabsorption and acid excretion in poorly functioning renal tubules can lead to acidosis. Cardiovascular disease can cause fluid retention. The dehydrated patient's lips and mouth may be dry and the tongue furrowed. Temperature may be elevated. Age-related skin changes, such as loss of elasticity and dryness, make skin turgor an unreliable sign of dehydration in the older patient. In patients with poor renal function and excess fluid volume, assess for edema around the eyes and in the limbs, increasing abdominal girth, increasing blood pressure and pulse volume, jugular venous distention, and orthostatic hypotension. Edema occurs with excess interstitial fluid and often is not apparent until interstitial volume increases by 2 to 3 L. Daily weights are good indicators of fluid status because 1 kg of body weight equals 1 L of fluid.

Check the clinical indicators of fluid imbalance. Fluid overload can cause hypertension, especially in patients with kidney failure. Jugular venous pressure increases with volume overload. Orthostatic hypotension may indicate volume depletion. In that case, jugular venous pulsation may not be visible at a 45-degree angle. In severe volume depletion, the jugular venous pulsation may not be visible even with the patient lying flat.

The first goal of fluid therapy is to restore volume and maintain perfusion to the brain, heart, and kidneys. Infuse 1 L of isotonic saline over 30 to 60 minutes. Usually, a second liter is given in the next hour.

The second goal of fluid therapy, replacing total body fluid losses, is achieved more slowly, usually using 0.45% saline. When blood glucose levels reach 250 mg/dL (13.8 mmol/L), give 5% dextrose in 0.45% saline. This solution prevents hypoglycemia and cerebral edema, which can occur when serum osmolarity declines too rapidly.

During the first 24 hours of treatment, the patient needs enough fluids to replace the actual volume deficit and ongoing losses. This may be as much as 6 to 10 L. Watch for signs of congestive heart failure and pulmonary edema. Central venous pressure may be monitored for older patients and those with myocardial disease. Assess the status of fluid replacement by monitoring blood pressure and urinary intake and output.

Drug Therapy. The outcome of insulin therapy is to lower serum glucose by about 75 to 150 mg/dL/hr. Unless the episode of DKA is mild, regular insulin by continuous IV infusion is the treatment of choice. Effective blood insulin levels are reached quickly when an IV bolus dose is given at the start of the infusion. An initial IV bolus dose of 0.1 unit/kg is followed by an IV drip of 0.1 unit/kg/hr. Continuous insulin infusion is used because of the 4-minute half-life of IV insulin. Subcutaneous insulin is started when the patient can take oral fluids and ketosis has stopped. Assess therapy effectiveness by hourly blood glucose measurements.

Acidosis Management. Regardless of the initial potassium value, there is a large total-body potassium deficit. With insulin therapy, serum potassium levels fall rapidly as potassium shifts into the cells. *Assess for signs of hypokalemia, including fatigue, malaise, confusion, muscle weakness, shallow respirations, abdominal distention or paralytic ileus, hypotension, and weak pulse.* An ECG shows cardiac conduction changes related to potassium. Hypokalemia is a common cause of death in the treatment of DKA. *Before giving IV potassium, make sure the patient produces at least 30 mL/hr of urine.*

Bicarbonate is used only for severe acidosis because it may reverse acidosis too rapidly and lead to severe hypokalemia, which can cause fatal cardiac dysrhythmias. Rapid correction of acidosis can worsen the patient's mental status. Acidosis is corrected with fluid replacement and insulin therapy. Sodium bicarbonate, given by slow IV infusion over several hours, is indicated when the arterial pH is 7.0 or less or the serum bicarbonate level is less than 5 mEq/L (5 mmol/L).

After acid-base disturbances are corrected, efforts are directed toward determining the cause of DKA. Infection is the most common cause (see Table 67-17).

Patient and Family Education: Prevention. Exploring the factors leading to DKA helps in planning specific educational efforts. Teach the patient and family to check blood glucose levels every 4 to 6 hours as long as symptoms such as anorexia, nausea, and vomiting are present and as long as glucose levels exceed 250 mg/dL (13.8 mmol/L). Teach him or her to check urine ketone levels when blood glucose levels exceed 300 mg/dL (16.7 mmol/L).

Teach the patient to reduce the risk for dehydration by maintaining food and fluid intake. Unless another health problem is present that requires fluid restriction, suggest that he or she drink at least 3 L of fluid daily and increase this amount when infection is present. When nausea is present, instruct the patient to take liquids containing both glucose and electrolytes (e.g., soda pop, diluted fruit juice, and sports drinks [Gatorade]). Small amounts of fluid may be tolerated even when vomiting is present. The patient should take 8 to 12 ounces (240 to 360 mL) of calorie-free and caffeine-free liquids every hour while awake.

Liquids containing carbohydrate can be taken if the diabetic patient cannot eat solid food. Ingesting at least 150 g of carbohydrate daily reduces the risk for starvation ketosis. After consulting a primary care provider, urge the patient to take additional rapid-acting (lispro) or short-acting (regular) insulin based on blood glucose levels.

Instruct the patient and family to consult the primary care provider when these problems occur:

- Blood glucose exceeds 250 mg/dL (13.8 mmol/L).
- Ketonuria lasts for more than 24 hours.
- The patient cannot take food or fluids.
- Illness lasts more than 1 to 2 days.

Also instruct them to detect hyperglycemia by monitoring blood glucose whenever the patient is ill. Illness can result in dehydration with DKA, a hyperglycemic-hyperosmolar state, or both. The sooner the patient seeks treatment, the less severe the metabolic alteration. He or she should understand to not omit insulin therapy during illness. Chart 67-13 reviews guidelines for the ill patient.

Potential for Hyperglycemic-Hyperosmolar State (HHS)

Hyperglycemic-hyperosmolar state (HHS), formerly known as *hyperglycemic-hyperosmolar nonketotic syndrome (HHNS),* is a hyperosmolar (increased blood osmolarity) state caused by hyperglycemia. The processes of HHS are outlined in Fig. 67-14. Both HHS and diabetic ketoacidosis (DKA) are caused by hyperglycemia and dehydration. HHS differs from DKA in that ketone levels are low or absent and blood glucose levels are much higher. Blood glucose levels may exceed 600 mg/dL (33.3 mmol/L), and blood osmolality may exceed 320 mOsm/L. Other biochemical problems with HHS also are more severe than those with DKA. Table 67-17 lists the differences between DKA and HHS.

HHS is the end result of a sustained osmotic diuresis. Renal insufficiency in HHS allows for extremely high blood glucose levels. Glucose impairs the concentrating ability of the kidney. Normally, kidneys act as a safety valve to eliminate glucose above levels around 180 mg/dL (10.0 mmol/L). As serum concentrations of glucose exceed the renal threshold, the kidney's capacity to reabsorb glucose is exceeded.

Decreased blood volume, caused by osmotic diuresis, or underlying kidney disease, common in many older patients with diabetes, results in further deterioration of kidney function. The decreased volume further reduces glomerular filtration rate, causing the glucose level to increase. Decreased kidney perfusion associated with hypovolemia further impairs kidney function.

Chart 67-13 PATIENT AND FAMILY EDUCATION GUIDE

Sick-Day Rules

- Notify your health care provider that you are ill.
- Monitor your blood glucose at least every 4 hours.
- Test your urine for ketones when your blood glucose level is greater than 240 mg/dL (13.8 mmol/L).
- Continue to take insulin or oral antidiabetic agents.
- To prevent dehydration, drink 8 to 12 ounces of sugar-free liquids every hour that you are awake.
- Continue to eat meals at regular times.
- If unable to tolerate solid food because of nausea, consume more easily tolerated foods or liquids equal to the carbohydrate content of your usual meal.
- Call your primary care provider for any of these danger signals:
  - Persistent nausea and vomiting
  - Moderate or large ketones
  - Blood glucose elevation after two supplemental doses of insulin
  - High (101.5° F [38.6° C]) temperature or increasing fever; fever for more than 24 hours
- Treat symptoms (e.g., diarrhea, nausea, vomiting, fever) as directed by your primary care provider.
- Get plenty of rest.

CONSIDERATIONS FOR OLDER ADULTS

HHS occurs most often in older patients with type 2 diabetes mellitus, many of whom did not know that they had diabetes. Mortality rates in older patients are as high as 40% to 70%. The onset of HHS is slow and may not be recognized. The older patient often seeks medical attention later and is sicker than the younger patient. HHS does not occur in adequately hydrated patients. Older diabetic patients are at greater risk for dehydration and HHS because of age-related changes in thirst perception and poor urine-concentrating abilities.

Many older adults take diuretics, which contributes to dehydration. Many older adults who are in long-term care settings or who are homebound and depend on others for oral intake do not ingest enough fluids and can more easily become dehydrated. Ensure that older adults with diabetes are weighed every 3 days or at least weekly to monitor trends and detect dehydration early.

Myocardial infarction, sepsis, pancreatitis, stroke, and some drugs (glucocorticoids, diuretics, phenytoin [Dilantin], propranolol [Inderal], and calcium channel blockers) also may cause HHS. Central nervous system (CNS) changes range from confusion to complete coma. Unlike DKA, patients with HHS may have seizures, myoclonic jerking, and reversible paralysis. The degree of neurologic impairment is related to serum osmolarity, with coma occurring once serum osmolarity is greater than 350 mOsm/kg (350 mmol/kg).

The development of HHS rather than DKA is related to residual insulin secretion. In HHS, the patient secretes just enough insulin to prevent ketosis but not enough to prevent hyperglycemia. The hyperglycemia of HHS is more severe than that of DKA, greatly increasing the blood osmolarity and causing profound diuresis. Severe dehydration and electrolyte loss occur, and the patient may lose 15% to 25% of body fluid. When dehydration is severe, glucose is not filtered into the urine, causing even greater hyperglycemia and hyperosmolar-

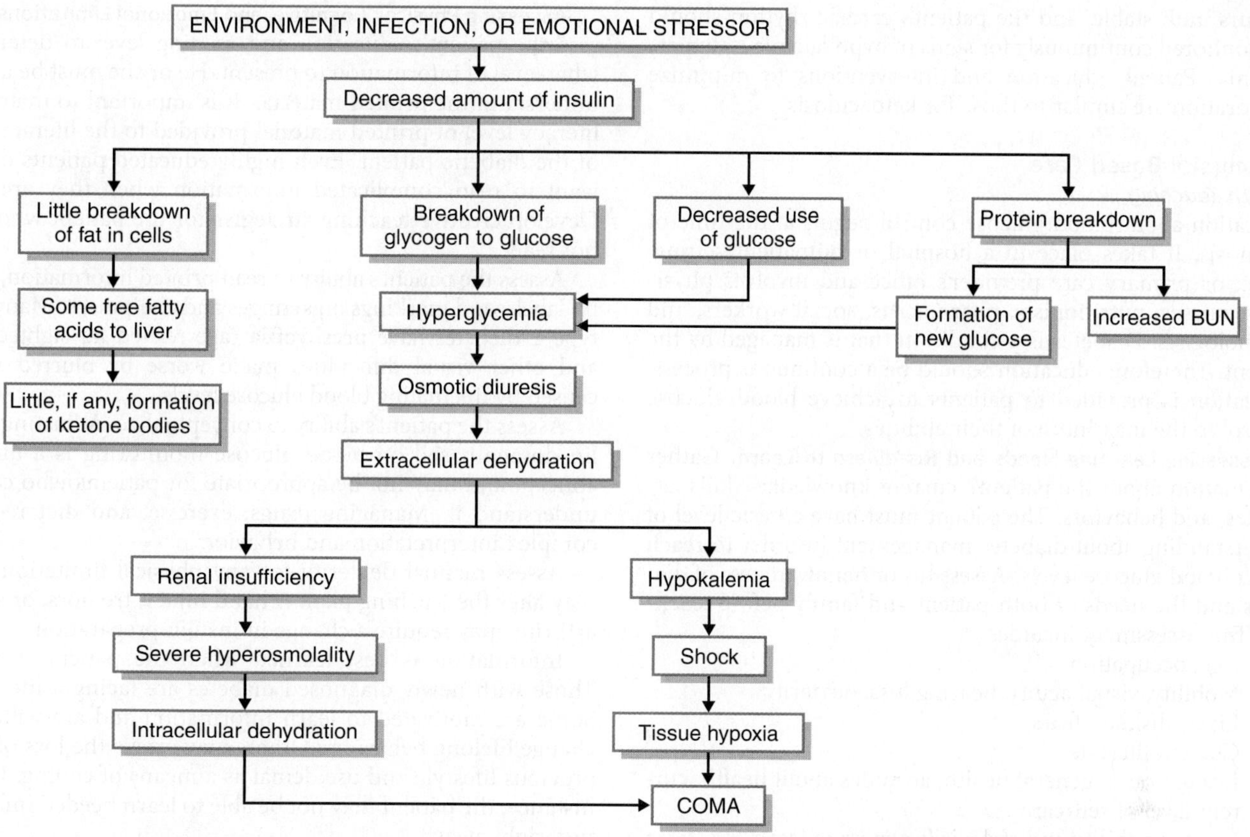
ENVIRONMENT, INFECTION, OR EMOTIONAL STRESSOR
Decreased amount of insulin
Little breakdown of fat in cells
Breakdown of glycogen to glucose
Decreased use of glucose
Protein breakdown
Some free fatty acids to liver
Hyperglycemia
Formation of new glucose
Increased BUN
Little, if any, formation of ketone bodies
Osmotic diuresis
Extracellular dehydration
Renal insufficiency
Hypokalemia
Severe hyperosmolality
Shock
Intracellular dehydration
Tissue hypoxia
COMA

Fig. 67-14 • The pathophysiologic mechanism of hyperglycemic-hyperosmolar state (HHS).

ity. Impairment of the thirst center in the brain occurs, making it impossible for the patient to drink enough fluid to prevent dehydration. This problem is worse in the older adult with diabetes because age-related changes in the thirst center reduce the patient's sensation of thirst.

NOC **Planning: Expected Outcomes.** The diabetic patient is expected to have few episodes of hyperglycemia and avoid HHS. Indicators include that the patient consistently demonstrates these behaviors:

- Maintains blood glucose levels within the target range
- Uses antidiabetic drugs appropriately
- Remains well hydrated
- Describes when to seek help from health care professionals

Interventions

Monitoring. Assess for manifestations of HHS. (See Tables 67-16 and 67-17 for symptoms of hyperglycemia.) Continually assess fluid status.

Fluid Therapy. The goal of therapy is to rehydrate the patient and restore normal blood glucose levels within 36 to 72 hours. The choice of fluid replacement and the rate of infusion are critical in managing HHS. The severity of the CNS problems is related to the level of blood hyperosmolarity and cellular dehydration. Re-establishing fluid balance in brain cells is a difficult and slow process, and many patients do not recover baseline CNS function until hours after blood glucose levels have returned to normal.

The *first* objective for fluid replacement in HHS is to increase blood volume. In shock or severe hypotension, give normal saline. Otherwise, use half-normal saline because it more rapidly corrects the water deficit. Infuse fluids at 1 L/hr until central venous pressure or pulmonary capillary wedge pressure begins to rise or until blood pressure and urine output are adequate. The rate is then reduced to 100 to 200 mL/hr. Half of the estimated water deficit is replaced in the first 12 hours, and the rest is given over the next 36 hours. Body weight, urine output, kidney function, and the presence or absence of pulmonary congestion and jugular venous distention determine the rate of fluid infusion. In patients with congestive heart failure, renal insufficiency, or acute kidney failure, monitor central venous pressure. *Assess the patient hourly for signs of cerebral edema—abrupt changes in mental status, abnormal neurologic signs, and coma. Immediately report changes in the level of consciousness; changes in pupil size, shape, or reaction; or seizures.* Lack of improvement in level of consciousness may indicate inadequate rates of fluid replacement or reduction in plasma osmolarity. Regression after initial improvement may indicate a too-rapid reduction in plasma osmolarity. A slow but steady improvement in CNS function is the best evidence that fluid management is satisfactory.

Continuing Therapy. IV insulin is administered after adequate fluids have been replaced. Stoner (2005) suggests an initial bolus dose of 0.15 unit per kg IV followed by a drip of 0.1 unit per kg per hour until blood glucose levels fall to 250 mg/dL (13.9 mmol/L). A reduction of blood glucose of 50 to 70 mg/dL per hour is a reasonable goal. Monitor the patient closely for indications of hypokalemia. Total body potassium depletion is often unrecognized because the level of potassium in the blood may be normal or high. The serum potassium level may drop quickly when insulin therapy is started. Potassium replacement is initiated once urine output is adequate. Serum electrolytes should be followed every 1 to

2 hours until stable, and the patient's cardiac rhythm should be monitored continuously for signs of hypokalemia or hyperkalemia. Patient education and interventions to minimize dehydration are similar to those for ketoacidosis.

Community-Based Care

Health Teaching

Education about blood glucose control begins at the time of diagnosis. It takes place in a hospital or outpatient setting, clinic, or primary care provider's office and involves physicians, nurses, nutritionists, pharmacists, social workers, and psychologists. Diabetes is a condition that is managed by the patient. Therefore education should be a continuous process. Education is provided to patients to achieve blood glucose control to the maximum of their abilities.

Assessing Learning Needs and Readiness to Learn. Gather information about the patient's current knowledge, skills, attitudes, and behaviors. The patient must have a basic level of understanding about diabetes management in order to reach target blood glucose levels. Assess his or her awareness of diabetes and the needs of both patient and family before teaching. This assessment includes:

- Age, occupation
- Mobility, visual acuity, hearing loss, dexterity
- Likes, dislikes, fears
- Current lifestyle
- Evaluation of general health, attitudes about health, current level of self-care
- Learning ability and style, willingness to learn
- Acceptance of diabetes, current knowledge of diabetes and its treatment
- Psychological status (denial, depression, anxiety)
- Level of alertness and ability to concentrate
- Skills needed, attitudes, goals
- Educational and literacy level
- Ethnic background, cultural and/or religious influences
- Home situation

Adult learners want information that applies directly to them. Find out what concerns the patient most about having diabetes, and ask what he or she wants to learn. Learning is enhanced when it is related to what the learner already knows. Start with what the patient already knows, and build on that base. Because they will be managing their own care after discharge, patients tend to focus on issues most important to them. Treatment measures that need to start soon after diagnosis may be of more interest to the patient than long-term control. Learning is reinforced and retained when it can be applied immediately and repeatedly.

The patient's physical condition dictates the timing of teaching. He or she does not have the energy to learn complex information when blood glucose levels are fluctuating. Explaining that well-controlled blood glucose levels improve the sense of well-being can help the patient accept the therapy plan. Pace your teaching to match the patient's energy level. Use an informal teaching process until he or she feels able to attend a formal class.

Each patient learns in his or her own way. A successful diabetic education program combines several teaching methods. Some patients learn better when they read pamphlets. Others learn better when they watch videos. Learning improves when the equipment is handled, techniques are practiced, success is rewarded, and errors are corrected immediately.

Assessing Physical, Cognitive, and Emotional Limitations. Assess the patient's education and reading level to determine what level of information to present. He or she must be able to understand the printed material. It is important to match the literacy level of printed material provided to the literacy level of the diabetic patient. Even highly educated patients do not want to read complicated information when they are sick. Develop creative teaching strategies for the patient who cannot read.

Assess the patient's ability to read printed information, insulin labels, and markings on syringes and equipment. Many with type 2 diabetes have **presbyopia** (age-related far-sightedness) and other visual difficulties made worse by blurred vision caused by fluctuating blood glucose levels.

Assess the patient's ability to conceptualize. Adjusting insulin dosage based on blood glucose monitoring is a difficult concept and may not be appropriate for patients who cannot understand it. Managing drugs, exercise, and diet requires complex interpretation and behavior.

Assess manual dexterity for any physical limitations that may alter the teaching plan. A hand injury, tremors, or severe arthritis may require a change in insulin preparation.

Information is best learned when the patient is ready. Those with newly diagnosed diabetes are facing a life crisis. Some are motivated to learn information and are willing to change lifelong behaviors. Others may grieve the loss of their previous lifestyle and use denial as a means of coping. In this instance, the patient may not be able to learn needed information right away.

Survival Skills Information. The initial phase of diabetic education involves teaching information necessary for the survival of anyone diagnosed with diabetes. Survival information includes:

- Simple information on pathophysiology of diabetes
- Learning how to prepare and administer insulin or how to take oral medications for diabetes
- Basic diet information
- Monitoring of blood glucose and ketones
- Recognition, treatment, and prevention of hypoglycemia and hyperglycemia
- Sick-day management
- Where to buy diabetic supplies and how to store them
- When and how to notify the primary care provider

A nutritionist provides the initial diet instruction. The patient needs to understand what to eat, how much to eat, and when to eat. Stress the importance of eating on time and the dangers of skipping meals. He or she must know how to maintain food intake during illness. Reinforce dietary instruction, answer questions, and refer questions to the nutritionist or primary care provider as indicated.

After being taught, the patient should be able to identify the drugs needed to control blood glucose levels. If insulin is needed, he or she must be able to prepare and give the dose accurately using sterile technique. The patient must also be able to state when insulin is to be injected, where insulin is injected, and how insulin is stored. Stress the dangers of skipping doses. Carefully review drug interactions, especially with older patients taking oral antidiabetic drugs.

Patients should be able to state their plan for regular physical activity. They must be able to describe the relationship between exercise and blood glucose control and identify situations in which activity should not be performed. Provide guidelines for additional carbohydrate intake to prevent hypoglycemia from excessive exercise.

The diabetic patient also must be able to state the plan for monitoring blood glucose. The person doing the monitoring must be able to do the procedure accurately and understand the results. Explain when blood glucose should be monitored, acceptable ranges, and actions to take when results are out of these ranges. If the patient cannot perform SMBG because of illness, ensure that a resource (e.g., home care agency, health clinic, or primary care provider's office) will be available to do the monitoring.

The most important part of survival level education is to ensure that the patient understands the significance, symptoms, causes, and treatment of hypoglycemia. He or she must be able to state the causes of hypoglycemia and the activities needed to prevent it. The patient must be able to describe appropriate carbohydrates to have available and the need to notify the physician of hypoglycemic episodes. Teach a family member how and when to inject glucagon.

The patient also must understand the significance of hyperglycemia and its relationship to illness. Instruct him or her on actions to take during illness and when to communicate with the primary care provider.

Most of this information is best retained when the patient is ready to learn. Education is a challenge because patients tend to be hospitalized for shorter periods. All diabetic education may be provided in an outpatient setting, where contact with the patient is limited. Important information must be squeezed into the time available. Many patients do not progress in self-management beyond the survival level because of psychological barriers.

In-Depth Education. In-depth education and counseling involve teaching more detailed information related to survival skills as well as learning preventive measures for avoiding long-term complications. Educational sessions with patient and family are needed to "patientize" the diabetes regimen for their needs and abilities. Education is often provided by a team of a physician, nurse educator, nutritionist, social worker, pharmacist, psychologist, case manager, and other health care professionals as needed. It may occur in various outpatient settings.

Besides knowledge gained at the survival level, the patient should be able to discuss the action of insulin in the body and the effects of insulin deficiency. He or she should also be able to explain the effects of diet, drugs, and activity on blood glucose. The patient should be able to relate maintaining normal blood glucose levels to preventing complications. This includes relating changes in glucose level to the possible need for a change in insulin dosage.

The patient must be able to describe the meal plan and explain the adjustments needed to meet diabetic diet requirements. He or she should state how food intake should be altered when eating out or increasing exercise. *The patient must be able to list specific foods to be eaten to prevent and treat hypoglycemia, as well as adjustments to make when ill.* Include in this teaching the family member usually responsible for buying groceries and preparing meals.

The diabetic patient must be able to prepare and give insulin accurately and must be able to discuss the onset, peak, and duration of the insulin used. Review formulas for self-adjustment in insulin (when permitted by the physician), and explain blood glucose monitoring requirements needed to evaluate the effects of additional insulin. If the patient takes an oral diabetic drug, ask him or her to identify the drug and describe its prescribed schedule. The patient must identify over-the-counter drugs with the potential to cause adverse interactions and the need to inform all care providers of the drug regimen.

Review how to perform desired physical activities safely. The patient must state blood glucose levels that are safe for exercise, the frequency of SMBG during exercise, drug adjustments before exercise, food required before exercise, and what food to have available during exercise. He or she should be aware of the risk for injury during exercise and explain the importance of protective footwear.

The goals of in-depth education are to help the diabetic patient solve problems of blood glucose fluctuation through the use of SMBG. He or she should be able to identify practices, such as travel (Chart 67-14), that cause blood glucose to fluctuate and to treat these problems with supplemental insulin, changes in activity, or changes in diet. Ask him or her to demonstrate urine ketone testing and to describe when urine ketones should be measured.

The patient must be able to describe a plan for periodic evaluation of blood glucose control by the primary care provider, as well as periodic dental and eye examinations. He or she must be able to perform foot care, wear properly fitting shoes, and describe hazards related to foot care. The patient must be able to describe ways to reduce specific risk factors, such as cigarette smoking and hypertension.

The patient must state that diabetes is a lifelong disease that requires lifestyle changes, describe the changes being made, and indicate those that need to be made. He or she should be able to identify stress-producing situations and discuss ways to reduce stress.

Psychosocial Preparation

The diagnosis of diabetes may represent a loss of control. All but a few patients lose flexibility. Life becomes ordered, and routines must be followed. Certain events surrounding diabetes are predictable. Taking an insulin injection and not eating for several hours causes hypoglycemia. Poorly controlled diabetes leads to complications and premature death. Tight control of blood glucose levels prevents complications.

The stress of diabetes is in addition to the demands of normal daily life. The patient must be able to integrate the demands of diabetes into daily and recreational schedules while keeping blood glucose stable.

Assist in healthy psychological adaptation to diabetes by providing successful educational experiences. Mastery of blood glucose monitoring helps the patient feel that he or she has control over the disease. Knowing the effects of extra activities, extra food, or extra insulin is helpful in learning to adjust the regimen.

Feeling a sense of control over the condition does much to promote a positive attitude about diabetes. Success in injecting insulin provides concrete evidence that he or she can master the disease. Teach by breaking a task into small, achievable units to ensure mastery. For example, a patient may begin learning how to inject insulin by first obtaining an accurate dose.

Devote as much teaching time as possible to insulin injection and blood glucose monitoring. Patients with newly diagnosed diabetes are often fearful of giving themselves injec-

Chart 67-14 PATIENT AND FAMILY EDUCATION GUIDE

Travel Tips for Diabetic Patients

Before traveling, visit your primary care provider and diabetes educator.

- See your physician to make certain you do not have any other health problems.
- Obtain a letter from your physician (typed on office letterhead) that indicates you have diabetes and lists the drugs you are taking.
- Obtain any needed immunizations or inoculations.
- Obtain prescriptions from your physician for your drugs, including glucagon if you take insulin, and prescriptions for motion sickness, nausea and vomiting, and traveler's diarrhea.
- Develop a plan for changing strengths of insulin if you are traveling to a country that does not carry the type of insulin you use. Learn how to use a U-100 syringe to draw up U-40 insulin.
- Develop a plan for meal and drug adjustment across time zones. Eastbound travel will shorten the day, requiring a reduction in the amount of drug needed. Westbound travel may add an extra meal to the day and require additional drug.
- Obtain a list of foods from your diabetes educator that you can substitute for food served in restaurants or airplanes.

If you are traveling by air, train, or boat, call ahead and request special meals for those with diabetes.

- Plan for delays in eating.
- Eat something every 4 hours.
- Drink a glass of water every 2 hours to prevent dehydration.
- Do not assume that special meals will be available; substitute items you cannot eat with foods you have in your travel kit.

Notify airline and hotel personnel that you have diabetes.

- Always wear medical alert identification and keep your medical alert card in your wallet.

While traveling:

- Check your blood glucose level frequently.
- Do not engage in activities when blood glucose levels are lower than 65 mg/dL.
- Stretch and walk around every 2 hours to help your circulation.
- Check your feet frequently for blisters and sores. You may be doing more walking than usual.
- Take extra shoes with you, and plan to change shoes often when walking more than normal.
- Protect your skin against exposure to the sun. Drug-induced photosensitivity can occur with some oral hypoglycemic agents.

Always have your travel kit with you; do not check your kit along with the rest of your luggage. Include these items in your travel kit:

- Insulin bottles in boxes with prescription labels
- Twice as much drug and twice as many supplies as you think you will need (pack drugs separately from checked luggage)
- Insulin stored in an insulated carrying case that will maintain temperatures according to the manufacturer's directions
- The letter from your physician (typed on office letterhead) that indicates you have diabetes and lists the drugs you are taking
- A supply of fast-acting sugar (e.g., glucose tablets or gel, hard candy, sugar cubes), as well as longer-acting foods (e.g., cheese and crackers, peanut butter and crackers)
- A self-monitoring diary

tions. After this technique has been mastered, they become less anxious and are able to attend to other tasks.

Recognize that not everyone will have a healthy adaptation to diabetes. Major depression affects many patients with diabetes and severely impacts quality of life and all aspects of functioning, including self-management behaviors. Clinical anxiety disorder is another problem common in patients with diabetes. Refer those who have significant problems coping with the day-to-day demands of diabetes to mental health counseling for appropriate treatment.

Home Care Management

Patients with diabetes self-manage their disease. Each day they decide what to eat, whether to exercise, and whether to take prescribed drugs. Maintaining blood glucose control depends on the accuracy of self-management skills. The main role of the health care professional is to provide support and education and to empower the patient to make informed decisions. Self-management education allows patients to identify their problems and provides techniques to help them make decisions, take appropriate actions, and alter these actions as needed.

Provide information about resources. The patient must know whom to contact in case of an emergency. Older adults who live alone need to have daily telephone contact with a friend or neighbor. The patient may also need help shopping and preparing meals. He or she may have limited access to transportation and may not have sufficient supplies of food, particularly in bad weather. Because of the likelihood of visual problems in older patients, they may need assistance in preparing insulin syringes for injection or in monitoring blood glucose. Make referrals to home care or public health agencies as needed. Chart 67-15 identifies areas for assessment during a home or clinic visit.

Health Care Resources

A wide array of diabetic education material is available from drug companies. The American Diabetes Association (ADA) will refer a diabetic patient to specific agencies or resources (phone 800-DIABETES [800-342-2383] in the United States; 800-BANTING [800-226-8464] in Canada). The American Association of Diabetes Educators can refer a diabetic patient to a local certified diabetes educator (phone 800-TEAM-UP-4 [800-832-6874]). Additional resources are listed in the bibliography.

Chart 67-15 FOCUSED ASSESSMENT

The Insulin-Dependent Diabetic Patient During a Home or Clinic Visit

- Assess overall mental status, wakefulness, ability to converse.
- Take vital signs and weight:
  - Fever could indicate infection.
  - Are blood pressure and weight within target range? Why or why not?
- Question patient regarding any change in visual acuity; check current visual acuity.
- Inspect oral mucous membranes, gums, and teeth.
- Question patient about injection areas used; inspect areas being used; assess whether patient is using areas and sites appropriately.
- Inspect skin for intactness, wounds that have not healed, new sores, ulcers, bruises, or burns; assess any previously known wounds for infection, progression of healing.
- Question patient regarding foot care.
- Assess lower extremities and feet for peripheral pulses, lack of or decreased sensation, abnormal sensations, breaks in skin integrity, condition of toes and nails.
- Question patient regarding color and consistency of stools and frequency of bowel movements; assess abdomen for bowel sounds.
- Review patient's home health diary:
  - Is blood glucose within targeted range? Why or why not?
  - Is glucose monitoring being recorded often enough?
  - Is the patient's food intake adequate and appropriate? Why or why not?
  - Is exercise occurring regularly? Why or why not?
- Assess patient's ability to perform self-monitoring of blood glucose.
- Assess patient's procedures for obtaining and storing insulin and syringes, cleaning equipment, disposing of syringes and needles.
- Assess patient's insulin preparation and injection technique.

TABLE 67-18 Outcome Criteria for Diabetic Teaching

Before being discharged to home, the diabetic patient or the significant other should be able to:

- Tell why insulin or an oral hypoglycemic agent is being prescribed.
- Name which insulin or oral hypoglycemic agent is being prescribed, and name the dosage and frequency of administration.
- Discuss the relationship between mealtime and the action of insulin or the oral hypoglycemic agent.
- Discuss plans to follow diabetic diet instructions.
- Prepare and administer insulin accurately.
- Test blood for glucose, or state plans for having blood glucose levels monitored.
- Test urine for ketones, and state when this test should be done.
- Verbalize how to store insulin.
- List symptoms that indicate a hypoglycemic reaction.
- Tell what carbohydrate sources are used to treat hypoglycemic reactions.
- Tell what symptoms indicate hyperglycemia.
- Tell what dietary changes are needed during illness.
- Verbalize when to call the physician or the nurse (frequent episodes of hypoglycemia, symptoms of hyperglycemia).
- Verbalize the procedures for proper foot care.

DECISION-MAKING CHALLENGE

Coordination of Care

The patient was admitted to the hospital for treatment of hyperglycemia and is discharged on a regimen of premeal rapid-acting insulin and long-acting insulin at bedtime.

1. What instruction should you provide to help the patient avoid hypoglycemia?

evolve For suggested answer guidelines, go to http://evolve.elsevier.com/Iggy/.

▪ *Evaluation: Outcomes*

Evaluate the care of the patient with diabetes on the basis of the identified nursing diagnoses and collaborative problems. Outcome success for diabetic education is the ability of the patient to maintain blood glucose levels within their established target range. General outcome criteria are listed below and in Table 67-18. More specific outcomes are listed with each nursing diagnosis and collaborative problem. The expected outcomes include that the patient should:

- Achieve blood glucose control
- Avoid acute and chronic complications of diabetes
- Have a satisfactory and complete postoperative recovery without complications
- Avoid injury
- Experience relief of pain
- Maintain optimal vision
- Maintain a urine elimination pattern in the expected range
- Have an optimal level of mental status functioning
- Have decreased episodes of hypoglycemia
- Have decreased episodes of hyperglycemia

Specific indicators for these outcomes are listed for each nursing diagnosis and collaborative problem under the Planning and Implementation section (see earlier).

GET READY FOR THE NCLEX EXAMINATION!

Key Points

Review these Key Points for each NCLEX Examination Client Needs Category.

Safe and Effective Care Environment

- Use aseptic technique during any invasive procedure when caring for a patient with diabetes.
- Administer antidiabetic drugs and insulin in a safe manner.
- Use good handwashing techniques before providing any care to a patient who has diabetes.
- Wash your hands before and after testing the patient's blood glucose levels.

Health Promotion and Maintenance

- Encourage all patients to maintain weight within an appropriate range.
- Encourage all patients, including patients with diabetes, to participate regularly in exercise or physical activity appropriate to their health status.
- Teach the patient and family about the manifestations of infection and when to seek medical advice.
- Instruct patients with diabetes to wear a medical alert bracelet.
- Instruct patients to not share blood glucose monitoring equipment.
- Reinforce to all patients with diabetes that tight control over blood glucose levels reduces the risk for the vascular complications of diabetes.
- Remind diabetic patients to have yearly eye examinations by an ophthalmologist.
- Teach diabetic patients with peripheral neuropathy to use a bath thermometer to test water for bathing, to avoid walking barefoot, and to inspect their feet daily.

Psychosocial Integrity

- Explore with the patient what the diagnosis of diabetes means to him or her.
- Allow the patient the opportunity to express fear or anxiety regarding the diagnosis of diabetes or the treatment regimen.
- Explain all procedures, restrictions, medications, and follow-up care to the patient and family.
- Pace your education sessions to match the learning needs and style of the patient.
- Use return demonstration strategies when teaching the patient about medication regimen, insulin injection, blood glucose monitoring, and foot assessment.
- Refer patients newly diagnosed with diabetes to local resources and support groups.
- Assess patients' visual acuity and peripheral tactile sensation to determine needed adjustments in teaching self-medication and self-monitoring of blood glucose levels.

Physiological Integrity

- Teach the patient about any drugs to be continued after discharge from the hospital.
- Instruct the patient and family in the manifestations of complications and when to seek assistance.
- Instruct all patients with diabetes to avoid becoming dehydrated and to drink at least 3 L of water each day unless another medical condition requires fluid restriction.
- Instruct patients who are taking sulfonylurea antidiabetic agents, especially chlorpropamide, about an increased risk for hypoglycemic reactions.
- Teach patients who are taking metformin the clinical manifestations of lactic acidosis (fatigue, dizziness, difficulty breathing, stomach discomfort, irregular heartbeat).
- Warn patients to not take over-the-counter drugs with their oral antidiabetic drugs without consulting their primary care provider.
- When mixing different kinds of insulin together, draw the shorter-acting insulin into the syringe before drawing up the longer-acting insulin.
- Never dilute or mix insulin glargine with any other insulin or solution.
- Teach patients to rotate insulin injection areas within one site rather than to other sites, to prevent changes in absorption.
- Avoid injecting insulin within a 2-inch radius of the umbilicus.
- Avoid IM insulin injection.
- Teach patients to administer an accurate dose of insulin using a prefilled or disposable insulin pen.
- Teach patients who experience Somogyi's phenomenon (early morning hyperglycemia) to ensure an adequate dietary intake at bedtime.
- Instruct patients to always carry a glucose source.
- Teach patients who exercise to test urine for ketone bodies if blood glucose levels are greater than 250 mg/dL before engaging in strenuous exercise.
- Instruct patients in foot care as outlined in Chart 67-9.

Additional Study Resources

Go to your Companion CD or Evolve at http://evolve.elsevier.com/Iggy/ for *Self-Assessment Questions for the NCLEX Examination.*

Go to Evolve at http://evolve.elsevier.com/Iggy/ for *Prioritization and Delegation Questions for the NCLEX Examination.*

SELECTED BIBLIOGRAPHY

Asterisk indicates a classic or definitive work on this subject.

*American Diabetes Association (ADA). (2003). Implications of the diabetes control and complications trial. *Diabetes Care, 26*(Suppl. 1), S25-27.

American Diabetes Association (ADA). (2005). ADA Workgroup Report: Defining and reporting hypoglycemia in diabetes: A report of the American Diabetes Association Workgroup on Hypoglycemia. *Diabetes Care, 28*(5), 1245-1249.

American Diabetes Association (ADA). (2006a). Consensus Statement: American College of Endocrinology and American Diabetes Association Consensus Statement on inpatient diabetes and glycemic control: A call to action. *Diabetes Care, 29*(8), 1955-1962.

American Diabetes Association (ADA). (2006b). Pancreas and islet transplantation in type 1 diabetes. *Diabetes Care, 29*(4), 935.

American Diabetes Association (ADA). (2007a). Diagnosis and classification of diabetes mellitus. *Diabetes Care, 30*(Suppl. 1), 42-47.

American Diabetes Association (ADA). (2007b). Nutritional recommendations and interventions for diabetes. *Diabetes Care, 30*(Suppl. 1), 48-65.

American Diabetes Association (ADA). (2007c). Standard of medical care in diabetes—2007. *Diabetes Care, 30*(Suppl. 1), 4-41.

American Diabetes Association (ADA), the North American Association for the Study of Obesity, and the American Society for Clinical Nutrition. (2005). Position Statement: Weight management using life-style modification in the prevention and management of type 2 diabetes: Rationale and strategies. *Clinical Diabetes, 23*(3), 130-136.

Appel, S.J. (2005). Sizing up patients for metabolic syndrome. *Nursing2005, 35*(12), 20-21.

Armstrong, D.G., Lavery, L.A., Wu, S., & Boulton, A.J. (2005). Evaluation of removable and irremovable cast walkers in the healing of diabetic foot wounds. *Diabetes Care, 28*(3), 551-554.

Austin, M.M. (2006). AADE Position Statement: Self-monitoring of blood glucose: Benefits and utilization. *The Diabetes Educator, 32*(6), 835-847.

Baderman, E. (2007). Act fast against severe hypoglycemia. *American Nurse Today, 2*(3), 32.

Boulton, A.J.M. (2005). Management of diabetic peripheral neuropathy. *Clinical Diabetes, 23*(2), 9-15.

Briscoe, V.J., & Davis, S.N. (2006). Hypoglycemia in type 1 and type 2 diabetes: Physiology, pathophysiology and management. *Clinical Diabetes, 24*(3), 115-121.

Brown, J.S., Wessells, H., Chancellor, M.B., Howards, S.S., Stamm, W.E., Stapleton, A.E., et al. (2005). Urologic complications of diabetes. *Diabetes Care, 28*(1), 177-185.

Ceriello, A. (2005). Postprandial hyperglycemia and diabetes complications. *Diabetes, 54*(1), 1-7.

Childs, B. (2006). Pramlintide use in type 1 diabetes resulting in less hypoglycemia. *Diabetes Spectrum, 19*(1), 50-52.

Cohen, A.S., & Ayello, E.A. (2005). Diabetes has taken a toll on your patient's vision: How can you help? *Nursing, 35*(5), 44-47.

Corbett, C.F. (2005). Practical management of patients with peripheral neuropathy. *Diabetes Educator, 31*(4), 523-540.

Cowie, C.C., Rust, K.F., & Byrd-Holt, D.D. (2006). Prevalence of diabetes and impaired fasting glucose in adults in the U.S. population. *Diabetes Care, 29*(6), 1263-1268.

Davis, L.D., Leonard, B., & McGill, J.B. (2006). Achieving optimal control of hypertension in patients with diabetes. *Clinical Advisor, 9*(Suppl. 11), 3-14.

Deatcher, J. (2008). Prediabetes. *AJN, 108*(7), 77-79.

Driver, V.R., Madsen, J., & Goodman, R.A. (2005). Reducing amputation rates in patients with diabetes at a military medical center: The Limb Preservation Service model. *Diabetes Care, 28*(2), 248-253.

Dungan, K., & Buse, J.B. (2005). Glucagon-like peptide 1–based therapies for type 2 diabetes: A focus on exenatide. *Clinical Diabetes, 23*(1), 56-62.

Egede, L.E., & Dagogo-Jack, S. (2005). Epidemiology of type 2 diabetes: Focus on ethnic minorities. *Medical Clinics of North America, 89*(5), 949-975.

Fiorina, P., Venturini, M., Folli, F., Losio, C., Maffi, P., Placidi, C., et al. (2005). Natural history of kidney graft survival, hypertrophy, and vascular function in end-stage renal disease type 1 diabetic kidney-transplanted patients. *Diabetes Care, 28*(6), 1303-1310.

Firdaus, M., Mathew, M.K., & Wright, J. (2006). Health promotion in older adults: The role of lifestyle in the metabolic syndrome. *Geriatrics, 61*(2), 18-25.

Fletcher, G., & Trejo, J.F. (2005). Why and how to prescribe exercise: Overcoming the barriers. *Cleveland Clinic Journal of Medicine, 72*(8), 645-656.

Franz, M. (2006). Medical nutrition therapy for hypertension and albuminuria. *Diabetes Spectrum, 19*(1), 32-38.

Funnell, M. (2008). Standards of care for diabetes: What's new, what's different. *Nursing 2008, 38*(10), 47-49.

Gillespie, K.M. (2006). Type 1 diabetes: Pathogenesis and prevention. *Canadian Medical Association Journal, 175*(2), 165-170.

Ginde, A., Pallin, D., & Camarego, C. (2008). Hospitalization and discharge education of emergency department patients with hypoglycemia. *The Diabetes Educator, 34*(8), 683-691.

Gross, J.L., De Azevedo, M.J., Silveiro, S.P., Canani, L.H., Caramori, M.L., & Zelmanovitz, T. (2005). Diabetic nephropathy: Diagnosis, prevention and treatment. *Diabetes Care, 28*(1), 164-176.

Haas, L. (2007). Functional decline in older adults with diabetes. *AJN, 107*(Suppl. 6), 50-54.

Hall, P.M. (2006). Prevention of progression in diabetic nephropathy. *Diabetes Spectrum, 19*(1), 18-24.

Hood, R., Valentine, V., Mac, S., & Polonsky, W.H. (2006). Use of exenatide in patients with type 2 diabetes. *Diabetes Spectrum, 19*(3), 181-186.

Hoogwerf, B.J. (2006a). Exenatide and pramlintide: New glucose-lowering agents for treating diabetes mellitus. *Cleveland Clinic Journal of Medicine, 73*(5), 477-484.

Hoogwerf, B.J. (2006b). Perioperative management of diabetes mellitus. *Cleveland Clinic Journal of Medicine, 73*(Suppl. 1), 95-99.

Horner, B., & Chase, H.P. (2007). Continuous glucose monitoring. *Practical Diabetology, 29*(1), 30-42.

Jones, M. (2006). Continuous insulin infusion therapy: It's not just for the ICU anymore. *American Nurse Today, 1*(2), 48-51.

King, J. (2006). What is metabolic syndrome? *Nursing, 35*(6), 31.

King, T., & Sole, M.L. (2005). Preventing renal complications from the use of contrast agents: Focus on at-risk patients. *AJN, 105*(11), 72AA.

Kitabchi, A.E., & Nyenwe, E.A. (2006). Hyperglycemic crisis in diabetes mellitus: Diabetic ketoacidosis and hyperglycemic hyperosmolar state. *Endocrinology and Metabolism Clinics of North America, 35*(4), 725-751.

Koski, R. (2006). Practical review of oral antihyperglycemic agents for type 2 diabetes mellitus. *The Diabetes Educator, 32*(6), 869-876.

Kruger, D. (2007). Basal-prandial insulin: When is the right time to initiate treatment? *The Nurse Practitioner, 32*(5), 24-29.

Kruger, D.F., Aronoff, S., & Edleman, S. (2007). Through the looking glass: Current and future perspectives on the role of hormonal interplay in glucose homeostasis. *The Diabetes Educator, 33*(Suppl. 2), 32-48.

Kruger, D.F., Martin, C.L., & Sadler, C.E. (2006). New insights into glucose regulation. *The Diabetes Educator, 32*(2), 221-228.

Kruse, I., & Edleman, S. (2006). Evaluation and treatment of diabetic foot ulcers. *Clinical Diabetes, 24*(2), 91-93.

Kulkarni, K. (2005). Carbohydrate counting: A practical meal-planning option for people with diabetes. *Clinical Diabetes, 23*(3), 120-122.

Lada, P., & Idrees, U. (2005). Toxicity of oral agents used to treat diabetes. *Journal of Pharmacy Practice, 18*(3), 145-156.

Lavery, L.A., Armstrong, D.G., Wunderlich, R.P., Mohler, M.J., Wendel, C.S., & Lipsky, B.A. (2006). Risk factors for foot infections in individuals with diabetes. *Diabetes Care, 29*(6), 1288-1293.

Ledbetter, C., & Laustsen, G. (2008). The truth about rosiglitazone (Avandia). *The Nurse Practitioner, 33*(6), 10-11.

Lidtke, R.H. (2005). How to choose footwear. *Diabetes Self-Management, 22*(4), 33-37.

Mackowiak, L. (2007). Continuous glucose monitoring: Getting started. *Diabetes Self-Management, 24*(2), 15-19.

Matz, K., Keresztes, K., Tatschl, C., Nowotny, M., Dachenhausenm, A., Brainin, M., et al. (2006). Disorders of glucose metabolism in acute stroke patients: An underrecognized problem. *Diabetes Care, 29*(4), 792-797.

McCance, K.L., & Huether, S.E. (2006). (Eds.). *Pathophysiology: The biologic basis for disease in adults & children* (5th ed.) St. Louis: Mosby.

McClellan, W.M. (2005). Epidemiology and risk factors for chronic kidney disease. *The Medical Clinics of North America, 89*(3), 419-445.

McKennon, S.A., & Campbell, R.K. (2007). The physiology of incretin hormones and the basis for DPP-4 inhibitors. *The Diabetes Educator, 33*(1) 55-66.

Meneilly, G.S. (2006). Diabetes in the elderly. *Medical Clinics of North America, 90*(5), 909-923.

Mensing, C., Boucher, J., Cypress, M., Weinger, K., Mulcahy, K., Barta, P., et al. (2007). National standards for diabetes self-management education. *Diabetes Care, 30*(Suppl. 1), 96-103.

Mentes, J. (2006). Oral hydration in older adults: Greater awareness is needed in preventing, recognizing, and treating dehydration. *AJN, 106*(6), 40-49.

Nath, C. (2007). Literacy and diabetes self-management. *AJN, 107*(Suppl. 6), 39-42.

National Institute of Diabetes and Digestive and Kidney Diseases. (2000). *Feet can last a lifetime.* Bethesda: MD. Retrieved April 2007 from www.niddk.nih.gov.

Nugent, B.W. (2005). Hyperosmolar hyperglycemic state. *Emergency Medicine Clinics of North America, 23*(2), 629-648.

Odegard, P.S., Setter, S.M., & Litz, J.L. (2006). Update in pharmacologic treatment of diabetes mellitus: Focus on pramlintide and exenatide. *The Diabetes Educator, 32*(5), 693-712.

Oldroyd, J., Barenrjee, M., Heald, A., & Cruickshank, K. (2005). Diabetes and ethnic minorities. *Postgraduate Medical Journal, 81*(958), 486-490.

Riddle, M.C., & Drucker, D.J. (2006). Emerging therapies mimicking the effects of amylin and glucagon-like peptide 1. *Diabetes Care, 29*(2), 435-449.

Ridge, R. (2007). Boosting insulin safety. *Nursing2007, 37*(2), 14-15.

Roszler, J. (2005). Fast-acting glucose: Why you should always keep some handy. *Diabetes Health, 14*(12), 47-49.

Rudnick, M., Kesselheim, A., & Goldfarb, S. (2006). Contrast-induced nephropathy: How it develops, how to prevent it. *Cleveland Clinic Journal of Medicine, 73*(1), 75-87.

Scemons, D. (2007). Are you up-to-date on diabetes medications? *Nursing2007, 37*(7), 45-49.

Schumann, J. (2005). New recommendations for safe needle disposal. *Diabetes Health, 14*(11), 51.

Seley, J., & Weinger, K. (2007). Executive summary: The state of the science on nursing best practices for diabetes self-management. *AJN, 107*(6), 73-78.

Shapiro, A.M.J., Ricordi, C., Hering, B.J., Auchincloss, H., Lindblad, R., Robertson, R.P., et al. (2006). International trial of the Edmonton protocol for islet transplantation. *New England Journal of Medicine, 355*(13), 1318-1330.

Sigal, R.J., Kenny, G.P., Wasserman, D.H., Castaneda-Sceppa, C., & White, R.D. (2006). Physical activity/exercise and type 2 diabetes: A consensus statement from the American Diabetes Association. *Diabetes Care, 29*(6), 1433-1438.

Sinclair, S.H., Malamut, R., Delvecchio, C., & Li, W. (2005). Diabetic retinopathy: Treating systemic conditions aggressively can save sight. *Cleveland Clinic Journal of Medicine, 72*(2), 447-454.

Solano, M.P., & Goldberg, R.B. (2006). Lipid management in type 2 diabetes. *Clinical Diabetes, 24*(1), 27-32.

Stillman, M. (2006). Clinical approach to patients with neuropathic pain. *Cleveland Clinic Journal of Medicine, 73*(8), 726-739.

Stoner, G.D. (2005). Hyperosmolar hyperglycemic state. *American Family Physician, 71*(9), 1723-1730.

Struck, B.D., & Ross, K.M. (2006). Health promotion in older adults: Prescribing exercise for the frail and home bound. *Geriatrics, 61*(5), 22-27.

Stults, B., & Jones, R.E. (2006). Management of hypertension in diabetes. *Diabetes Spectrum, 19*(1), 25-31.

Tesfaye, S., Chaturvedi, N., Eaton, S.E., Ward, J.D., Manes, C., Ionescu-Tirgoviste, C., et al. (2005). Vascular risk factors and diabetic neuropathy. *New England Journal of Medicine, 352*(4), 341-350.

Thompson, C.L., Dunn, K.C., Menon, M.C., Kearns, L.E., & Braithwaite, S.S. (2005). Hyperglycemia in the hospital. *Diabetes Spectrum, 18*(1), 20-27.

Tomsky, D. (2005). Detection, prevention and treatment of hypoglycemia in the hospital. *Diabetes Spectrum, 18*(1), 39-44.

U.S. Department of Veterans Affairs. (2005a). National PBM Drug Monograph: *Exenatide (Byetta).* VHA Pharmacy Benefits Strategic Healthcare Group and Medical Advisory Panel. Retrieved April 2007, from www.pbm.va.gov/DrugMonograph.aspx.

U.S. Department of Veterans Affairs. (2005b). National PBM Drug Monograph: *Pramlintide (Symlin).* VHA Pharmacy Benefits Strategic Healthcare Group and Medical Advisory Panel. Retrieved April 2007, from www.pbm.va.gov/DrugMonograph.aspx.

U.S. Department of Veterans Affairs. (2006a). National PBM Drug Monograph: *Insulin detemir (Levemir).* VHA Pharmacy Benefits Strategic Healthcare Group and Medical Advisory Panel. Retrieved April 2007, from www.pbm.va.gov/DrugMonograph.aspx.

U.S. Department of Veterans Affairs. (2006b). National PBM Drug Monograph: *Sitagliptin (Januvia).* VHA Pharmacy Benefits Strategic Healthcare Group and Medical Advisory Panel. Retrieved April 2007, from http://www.pbm.va.gov/DrugMonograph.aspx.

Van de Laar, F.A., Lucassen, P.L., Akkermans, R.P., van de Lisdonk, E.H., Rutten, G.E., & van Weel, C. (2005). Alpha-glucosidase inhibitors for patients with type 2 diabetes: Results from a Cochrane systematic review and meta-analysis. *Diabetes Care, 28*(1), 154-163.

Van den Berghe, G., Wilmer, A., Hermans, G., Meerssman, W., Wouters, P.J., Milants, I., et al. (2006). Intensive insulin therapy in the medical ICU. *New England Journal of Medicine, 354*(5), 449-461.

Wamboldt, C., & Kapustin, C. (2006). Evidence-based treatment of diabetic peripheral neuropathy. *The Journal for Nurse Practitioners, 2*(6), 370-378.

Ward, S., & Clark, A. (2006). Improving patient outcomes with intensive insulin therapy. *Clinical Nurse Specialist, 20*(4), 170-174.

Watts, S.A., & Anselmo, J. (2006). Nutrition for diabetes: All in a day's work. *Nursing2006, 35*(6), 46-48.

Weinger, K. (2007). Psychosocial issues and self-care. *AJN, 107*(Suppl. 6), 34-37.

Whiteside, M.M., Wallhagen, M.I., & Pettengill, E. (2006). Sensory impairment in older adults: Part 2. Vision loss. *AJN, 106*(11), 52-61.

Zammitt, N., & Frier, B.M. (2005). Hypoglycemia in type 2 diabetes. *Diabetes Care, 28*(12), 2948-2961.

Zandi-Nejad, K., & Brenner, B.M. (2005). Strategies to retard the progression of chronic kidney disease. *The Medical Clinics of North America, 89*(3), 489-509.

*Zinman, B., Ruderman, N., Campaigne, B., Devlin, J., & Schneider, S. (2004). Physical activity/exercise and diabetes. *Diabetes Care, 27*(Suppl. 1), 58-62.

Zoorob, R., & Smith, V. (2007). How to control the metabolic syndrome. *The Clinical Advisor, 10*(3), 106-109.

HUMAN NEEDS OVERVIEW
Urinary Elimination

The need for urinary elimination is really the need for homeostasis—the ability of the body to maintain its internal environment at a "steady state" and within very narrow ranges of normal, regardless of external changes. The body works best when blood and other extracellular fluids have a serum sodium concentration of 135 to 145 mEq/L (mmol/L) and a serum potassium level of 3.5 to 5.0 mEq/L (mmol/L). Serious health problems and death occur when these electrolytes are much higher or lower than these normal ranges. Keeping the amount of total body water, especially blood volume, within the normal range is also important to proper function and health. When blood volume is too high, hypertension develops and damages vital organs. When blood volume is too low, hypotension can be so severe that vital organs are not perfused with oxygen and become hypoxic. In addition, protein waste products containing nitrogen, such as urea, act as a poison and must be prevented from getting too high. Humans ingest many foods and liquids that contain water, electrolytes, and substances that will be converted to waste products. Without control mechanisms to balance the intake of these substances with their elimination, we would rapidly accumulate too much of everything and die.

As part of the renal/urinary system, the kidneys are responsible for maintaining this balance of what is taken into the body, what is allowed to remain in the body, and what is eliminated from the body. Although some products are eliminated in the stool, there is no discrimination or adjustment in bowel elimination. Urinary elimination, however, allows a person to eat and drink almost anything (except poisons and infectious organisms) in almost any amount without upsetting the homeostatic balance for body water, electrolytes, waste products, and blood pressure. For example, on one day a person may drink 2 L of fluids and eat food that contains 2 g of sodium and 5 g of potassium. The next day this same person may drink 3 L of fluid and eat food that contains 12 g of sodium and 10 g of potassium. Yet because the kidneys selectively adjust to change the amount of each substance that gets eliminated, the blood pressure, serum sodium, and serum potassium levels remain the same and within the normal ranges on both days. A "steady-state" or homeostatic balance of these substances is maintained because the kidneys adjust the output to match the intake (Fig. 1).

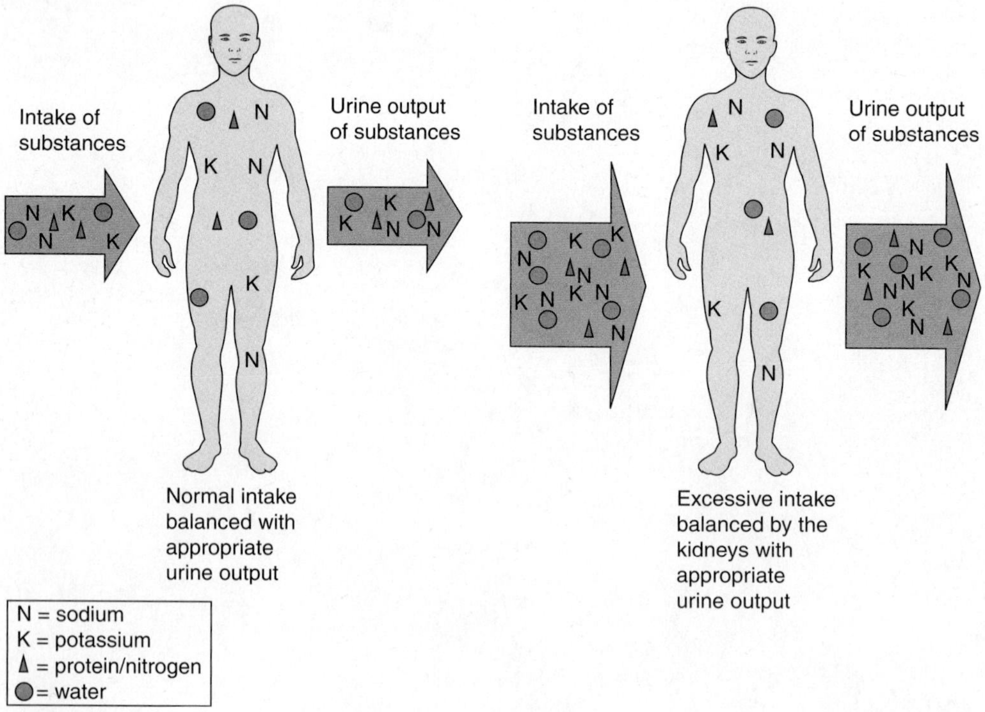
Intake of substances
Urine output of substances
Normal intake balanced with appropriate urine output
Intake of substances
Urine output of substances
Excessive intake balanced by the kidneys with appropriate urine output
N = sodium
K = potassium
= protein/nitrogen
= water

Fig. 1

When kidney function is impaired to any degree as a result of renal/urinary problems, the human need for urinary elimination is not met, and the steady-state homeostasis of water, electrolyte, and waste products is disrupted (Fig. 2). Without intervention, this lack of steady state leads to excesses of body water, electrolytes, and nitrogenous waste products that interfere with normal organ function and can cause death.

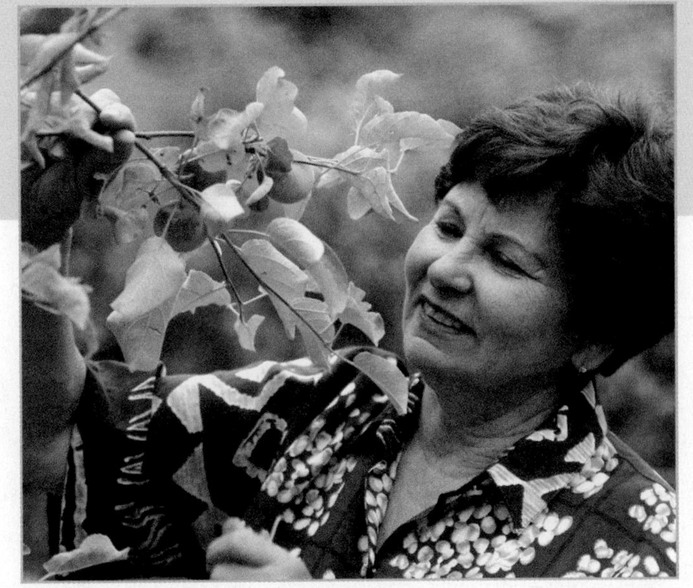

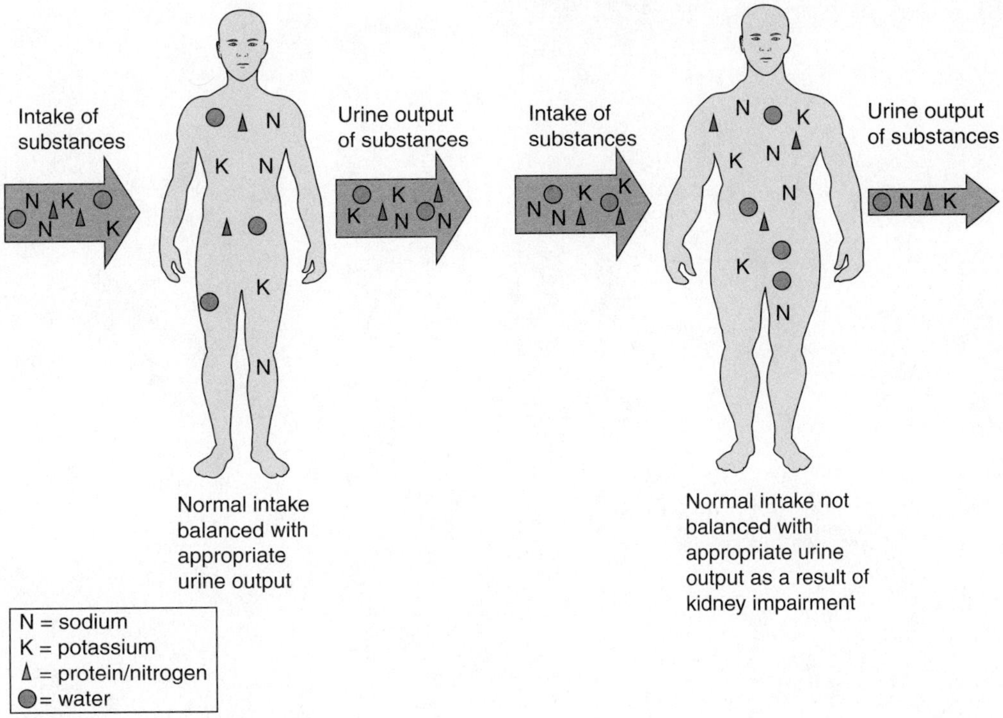

Intake of substances
Urine output of substances
Intake of substances
Urine output of substances
Normal intake balanced with appropriate urine output
Normal intake not balanced with appropriate urine output as a result of kidney impairment
N = sodium
K = potassium
= protein/nitrogen
= water

Fig. 2

XV

UNIT

Problems of Excretion

Management of Patients with Problems of the Renal/Urinary System

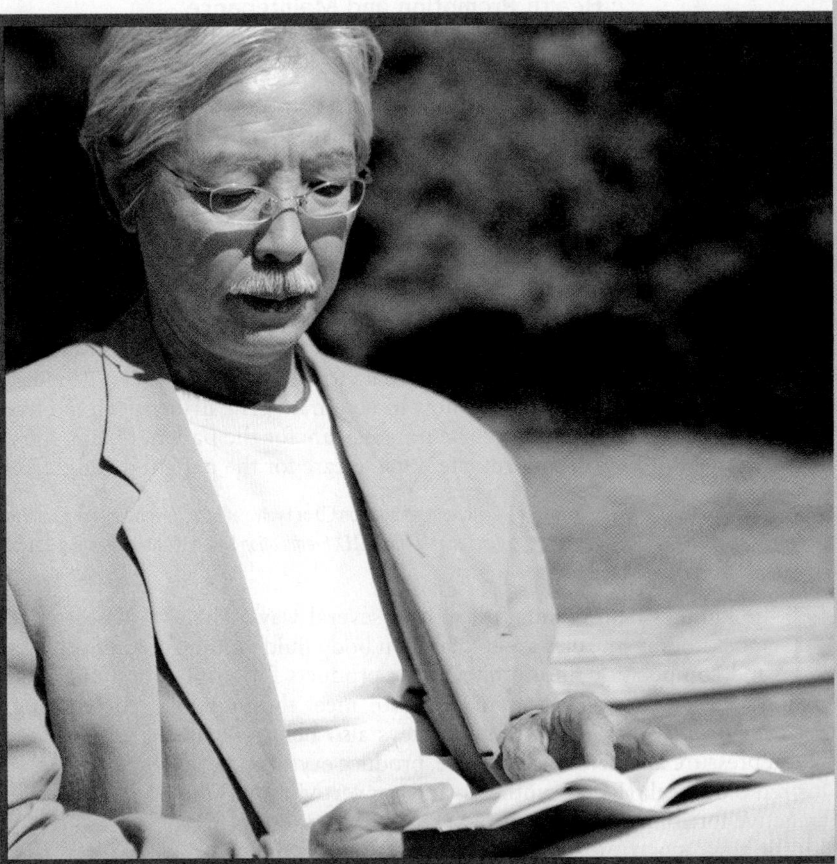

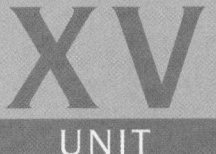

68

CHAPTER

Assessment of the Renal/Urinary System

Chris Winkelman

LEARNING OUTCOMES

For clinical competence and success on the NCLEX Examination, study this chapter with these Learning Outcomes in mind:

Safe and Effective Care Environment

1. Use Standard Precautions when handling urine specimens or examining the patient's genitalia.
2. Determine whether the patient has a risk for an allergic reaction to contrast dyes before testing procedures.
3. Verify that informed consent has been obtained and that the patient has a clear understanding of the potential risks before he or she undergoes invasive procedures to assess renal/urinary function.

Health Promotion and Maintenance

4. Teach all people about the importance of maintaining an adequate oral fluid intake.
5. Teach women the proper method of perineal cleansing.

Psychosocial Integrity

6. Use language the patient is comfortable with during assessment of the renal/urinary system.
7. Encourage the patient to express feelings or concerns about a change in kidney or bladder function.
8. Respect the patient's dignity when performing renal/urinary assessment.
9. Explain all diagnostic procedures, restrictions, and follow-up care to the patient scheduled for tests.

Physiological Integrity

10. Briefly review the anatomy and physiology of the renal/urinary system.
11. Describe age-related changes in the renal/urinary system.
12. Describe the correct techniques to use in physically assessing the renal system.
13. Use laboratory data to distinguish between dehydration and renal impairment.
14. Describe how to obtain a sterile urine specimen from a patient with a Foley catheter.
15. Coordinate nursing care for the patient during the first 24 hours after IV urography.
16. Coordinate nursing care for the patient during the first 24 hours after a renal biopsy.

evolve Go to your Companion CD or Evolve at http://evolve.elsevier.com/Iggy/ for *Self-Assessment Questions for the NCLEX Examination* keyed to these Learning Outcomes.

The kidneys help maintain health in several ways. Their most important roles are to maintain body fluid volume and composition and to filter waste products for elimination. These processes allow the body to meet the *human need for urinary elimination.* The kidneys also help regulate blood pressure and acid-base balance, produce erythropoietin for red blood cell (RBC) synthesis, and convert vitamin D to an active form.

The renal system includes the kidneys and the entire urinary tract. The ureters, bladder, and urethra are the drainage route for the excretion of urine. Structural or functional problems in the kidney or urinary tract may alter fluid, electrolyte, and acid-base balance.

Assessment of the patient at risk for or with actual problems of the renal system begins with a history and physical assessment. Understanding the anatomy, physiology, and diagnostic tests of the renal system helps you in problem-solving about renal function in the clinical setting. It also assists you in teaching the patient about the purpose of procedures and in physically and emotionally preparing the patient for assessment.

ANATOMY AND PHYSIOLOGY REVIEW

Kidneys

Structure

Gross Anatomy

Normally, two kidneys are located behind the peritoneum, not really in the abdominal cavity, one on either side of the spine (Fig. 68-1). The adult kidney is 4 to 5 inches (10 to 13 cm) long, 2 to 3 inches (5 to 7 cm) wide, and about 1 inch (2.5 to

3 cm) thick. It weighs about 8 ounces (250 g). The left kidney is slightly longer and narrower than the right kidney. Larger-than-usual kidneys may indicate renal obstruction or polycystic disease. Smaller-than-usual kidneys may indicate chronic kidney disease.

Several layers of tissue surround the kidney, providing protection and support. On the outer surface of the kidney is a layer of fibrous tissue called the **renal capsule** (Fig. 68-2). This capsule covers most of the kidney except the **hilum,** which is the area where the renal artery and nerve plexus enter and the renal vein and ureter exit. The renal capsule is surrounded by layers of fat and connective tissue.

Lying beneath the renal capsule are the two layers of functional kidney tissue—the cortex and the medulla. The **renal cortex** is the outer tissue layer and is covered by the renal capsule. The **medulla** is the medullary tissue lying below the cortex in the shape of many fans. Each "fan" is called a **pyramid,** and there are 12 to 18 pyramids per kidney. The **renal columns** are cortical tissue that dips down into the interior of the kidney and separate the pyramids.

The tip, or end, of each pyramid is called a **papilla.** The papillae drain urine into the collecting system. A cuplike structure called a **calyx** collects the urine at the end of each papilla. The calices join together to form the **renal pelvis,** which narrows to become the ureter.

The kidneys have a rich blood supply and receive 20% to 25% of the total cardiac output. Renal blood flow per minute varies from about 600 to 1300 mL/min. The blood supply to each kidney comes from the renal artery, which branches from the abdominal aorta. The renal artery divides into progressively smaller arteries, supplying blood to all areas of the renal tissue **(parenchyma)** and the nephrons. The smallest arteries (afferent arterioles) feed the nephrons directly to form urine.

Venous blood from the kidneys starts with the capillaries surrounding each nephron. These capillaries drain into progressively larger veins, with blood eventually returned to the inferior vena cava through the renal vein.

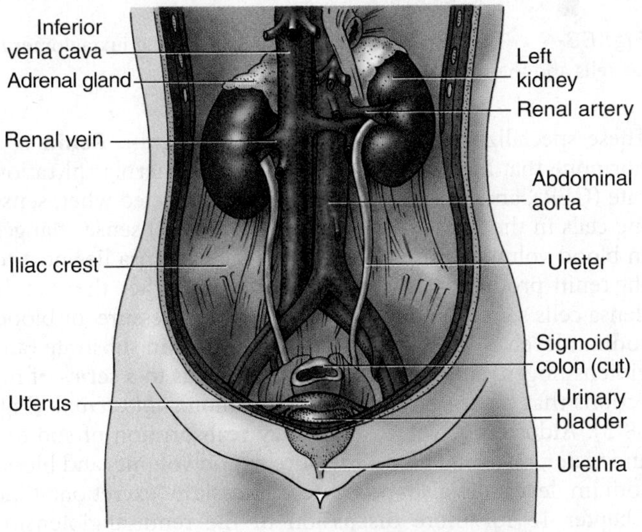
Inferior vena cava
Adrenal gland
Renal vein
Iliac crest
Uterus
Left kidney
Renal artery
Abdominal aorta
Ureter
Sigmoid colon (cut)
Urinary bladder
Urethra

Fig. 68-1 • Anatomic location of organs of the renal/urinary system.

Microscopic Anatomy

The **nephron** is the "working" or functional unit of the kidney, and it is here that urine is actually formed from blood. There are about 1 million nephrons per kidney, and each nephron separately makes urine from blood.

There are two types of nephrons: cortical nephrons and juxtamedullary nephrons. The cortical nephrons are short, with all parts located in the renal cortex. The juxtamedullary nephrons (about 20% of all nephrons) are longer, and their tubes and blood vessels dip deeply into the medulla. The purpose of the juxtamedullary nephrons is to concentrate urine during times of low fluid intake. The ability to concentrate urine allows for continued excretion of body wastes with less fluid loss.

◀ ANIMATION: Nephrons

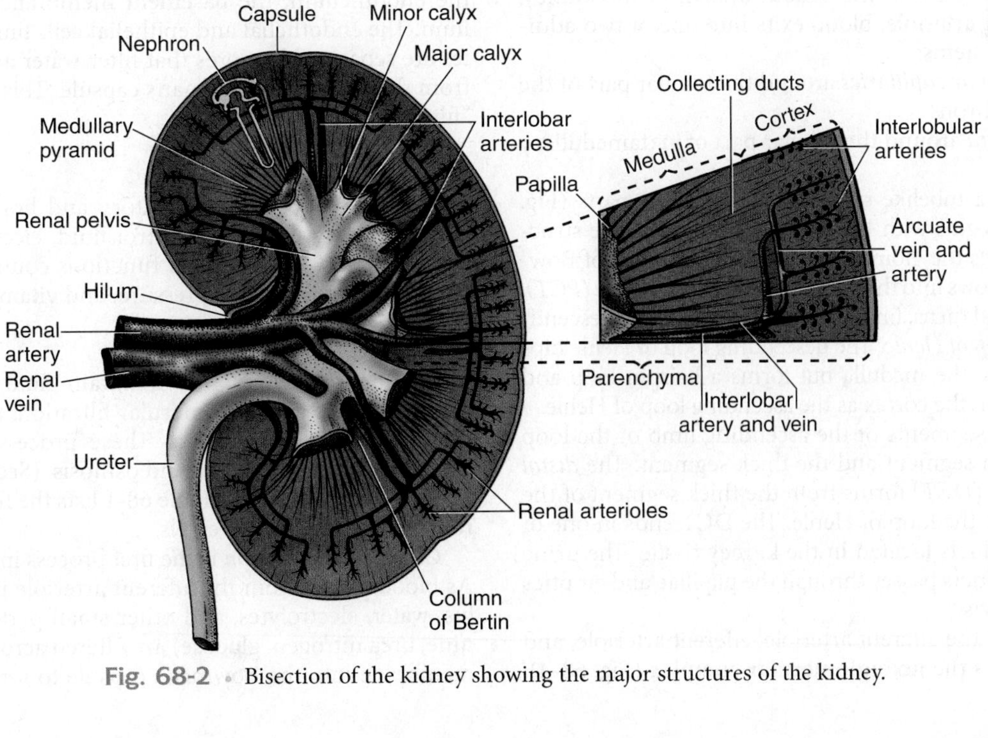
Capsule
Minor calyx
Nephron
Major calyx
Collecting ducts
Medullary pyramid
Interlobar arteries
Cortex
Medulla
Interlobular arteries
Papilla
Renal pelvis
Arcuate vein and artery
Hilum
Renal artery
Renal vein
Parenchyma
Interlobar artery and vein
Ureter
Renal arterioles
Column of Bertin

Fig. 68-2 • Bisection of the kidney showing the major structures of the kidney.

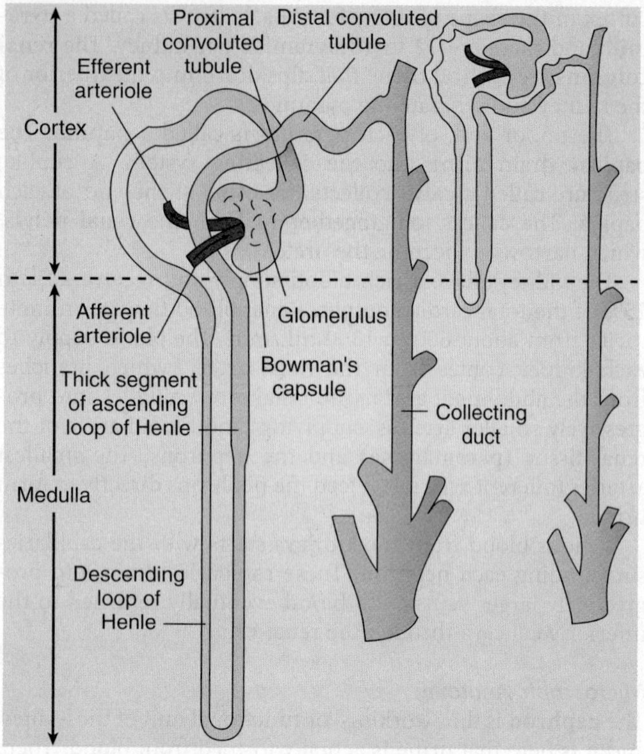
Proximal convoluted tubule
Distal convoluted tubule
Efferent arteriole
Cortex
Afferent arteriole
Glomerulus
Bowman's capsule
Thick segment of ascending loop of Henle
Collecting duct
Medulla
Descending loop of Henle

Fig. 68-3 • Anatomy of the nephron, the functional unit of the kidney. Note that the particular nephron labeled here is a juxtamedullary nephron.

Blood supply to the nephron is delivered through the **afferent arteriole**—the smallest, most distal portion of the renal arterial system. From the afferent arteriole, blood flows into the **glomerulus,** which is a series of specialized capillary loops. It is through these capillaries that water and small particles are filtered from the blood to make urine. The remaining blood leaves the glomerulus through the **efferent arteriole,** which is the first vessel in the venous system of the kidney. From the efferent arteriole, blood exits into one of two additional capillary systems:

- The *peritubular capillaries* around the tubular part of the cortical nephrons
- The *vasa recta* around the tubular part of juxtamedullary nephrons

Each nephron is a tubelike structure with distinct parts (Fig. 68-3). The tube begins with Bowman's capsule, a saclike structure that surrounds the glomerulus. The tubular tissue of Bowman's capsule narrows into the *proximal convoluted tubule (PCT).* The PCT twists and turns, finally straightening into the descending limb of the *loop of Henle.* The descending loop of Henle dips in the direction of the medulla but forms a hairpin loop and comes back up into the cortex as the ascending loop of Henle.

There are two segments of the ascending limb of the loop of Henle: the thin segment and the thick segment. The *distal convoluted tubule (DCT)* forms from the thick segment of the ascending limb of the loop of Henle. The DCT ends in one of many collecting ducts located in the kidney tissue. The urine in the collecting ducts passes through the papillae and empties into the renal pelvis.

Special cells in the afferent arteriole, efferent arteriole, and DCT are known as the **juxtaglomerular complex** (Fig. 68-4).

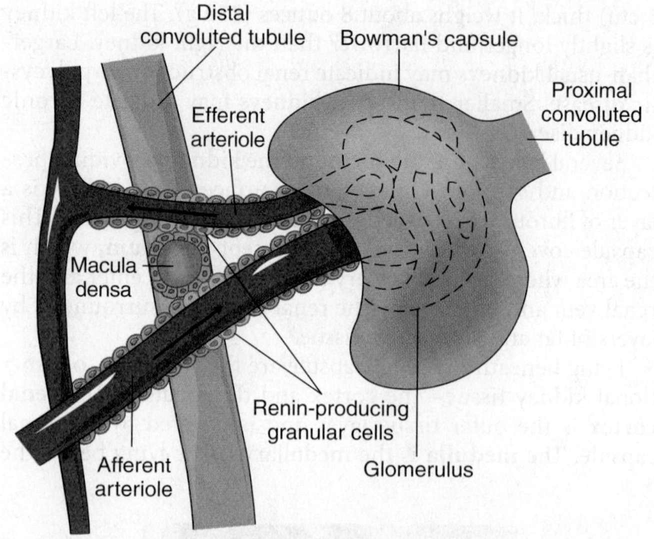
Distal convoluted tubule
Bowman's capsule
Proximal convoluted tubule
Efferent arteriole
Macula densa
Renin-producing granular cells
Afferent arteriole
Glomerulus

Fig. 68-4 • The juxtaglomerular complex showing juxtaglomerular cells and the macula densa.

These specialized cells produce and store renin. **Renin** is a hormone that helps regulate blood flow, glomerular filtration rate (GFR), and blood pressure. Renin is secreted when sensing cells in the DCT (called the *macula densa*) sense changes in blood volume and pressure. The macula densa lies next to the renin-producing cells. Renin is produced when the macula densa cells sense that blood volume, blood pressure, or blood sodium levels is low. Renin then converts renin substrate (angiotensinogen) into angiotensin I. This leads to a series of reactions that cause secretion of the hormone *aldosterone* (Fig. 68-5). Aldosterone increases kidney reabsorption of sodium and water, restoring blood pressure, blood volume, and blood sodium levels. It also promotes potassium excretion. (See Chapter 13 for more discussion of the renin-angiotensin-aldosterone pathway.)

The glomerular capillary wall has three layers (Fig. 68-6): the endothelium, the basement membrane, and the epithelium. The endothelial and epithelial cells lining these capillaries are separated by pores that filter water and small particles from the blood into Bowman's capsule. This fluid is called the "filtrate" or "early urine."

Function

The kidneys have both regulatory and hormonal functions. The regulatory functions control fluid, electrolyte, and acid-base balance. The hormonal functions control red blood cell (RBC) formation, blood pressure, and vitamin D activation.

Regulatory Functions

The kidney processes that maintain fluid, electrolyte, and acid-base balance are glomerular filtration, tubular reabsorption, and tubular secretion. These processes use filtration, diffusion, active transport, and osmosis. (See Chapter 13 for a review of these actions.) Table 68-1 lists the functions of nephron tubules and blood vessels.

◄ ANIMATION: Filtration

Glomerular filtration is the first process in urine formation. As blood passes from the afferent arteriole into the glomerulus, water, electrolytes, and other small particles (e.g., creatinine, urea nitrogen, glucose) are filtered across the glomerular membrane into the Bowman's capsule to form *glomerular fil-*

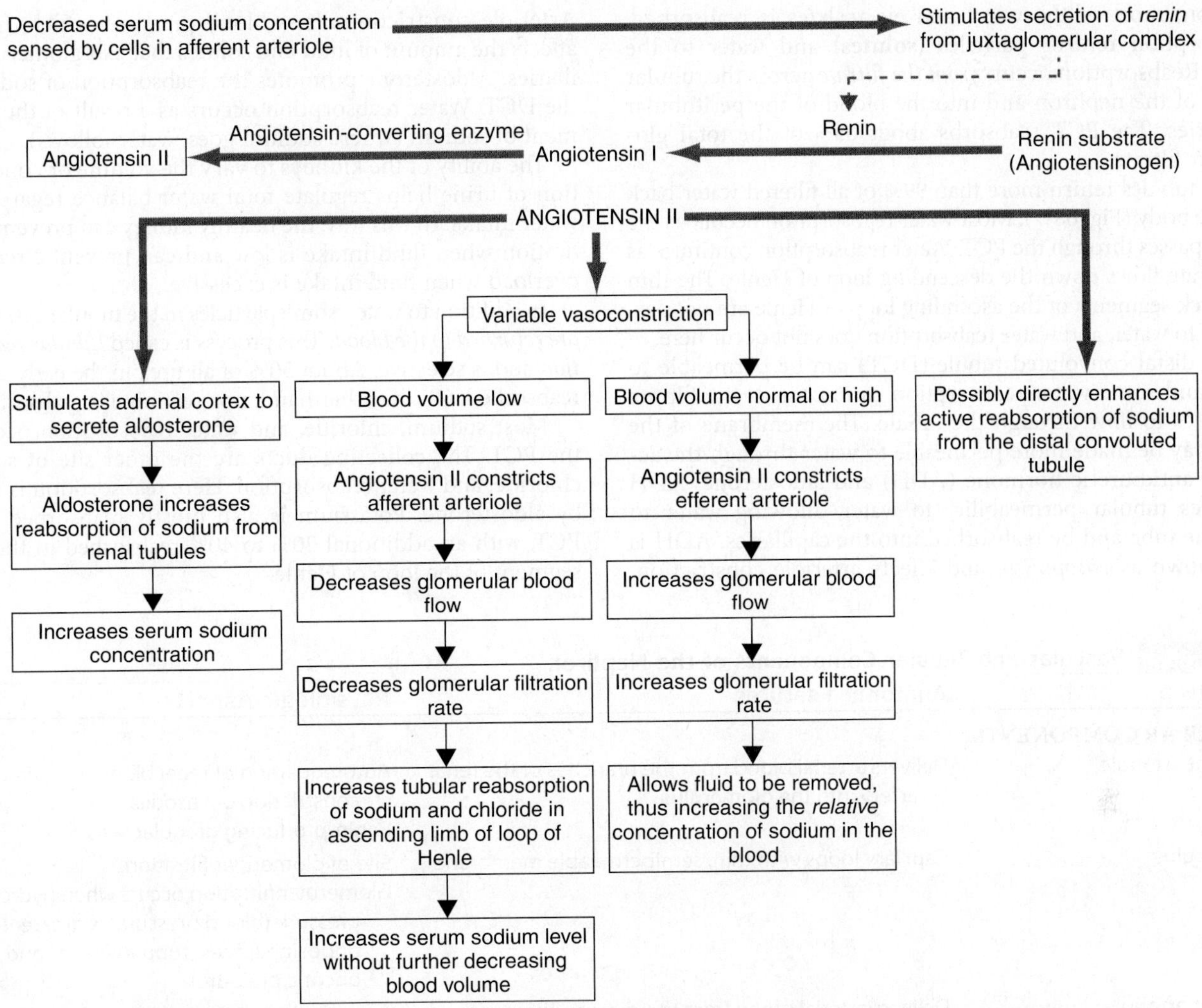
Decreased serum sodium concentration sensed by cells in afferent arteriole
Stimulates secretion of *renin* from juxtaglomerular complex
Renin
Renin substrate (Angiotensinogen)
Angiotensin I
Angiotensin-converting enzyme
Angiotensin II
ANGIOTENSIN II
Variable vasoconstriction
Stimulates adrenal cortex to secrete aldosterone
Aldosterone increases reabsorption of sodium from renal tubules
Increases serum sodium concentration
Blood volume low
Angiotensin II constricts afferent arteriole
Decreases glomerular blood flow
Decreases glomerular filtration rate
Increases tubular reabsorption of sodium and chloride in ascending limb of loop of Henle
Increases serum sodium level without further decreasing blood volume
Blood volume normal or high
Angiotensin II constricts efferent arteriole
Increases glomerular blood flow
Increases glomerular filtration rate
Allows fluid to be removed, thus increasing the *relative* concentration of sodium in the blood
Possibly directly enhances active reabsorption of sodium from the distal convoluted tubule

Fig. 68-5 • The role of aldosterone, renin substrate (angiotensinogen), angiotensin I, and angiotensin II in the renal regulation of water and sodium.

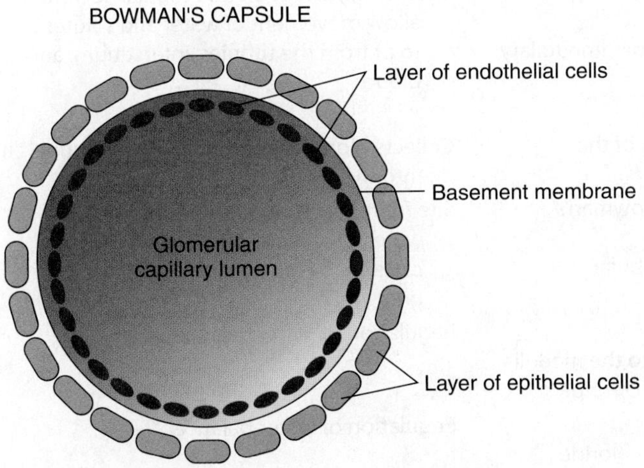
BOWMAN'S CAPSULE
Layer of endothelial cells
Basement membrane
Glomerular capillary lumen
Layer of epithelial cells

Fig. 68-6 • Glomerular capillary wall.

trate. As the filtrate enters the proximal convoluted tubule (PCT), it is called *tubular* filtrate.

Large particles, such as blood cells, albumin, and other proteins, are too large to filter through the glomerular capillary walls. *Therefore these substances are not normally present in the filtrate or in the final urine.*

About 180 L of glomerular filtrate is formed from the blood each day. The rate of filtration is expressed in milliliters per minute. Normal glomerular filtration rate (GFR) averages 125 mL/min. If the entire amount of filtrate were excreted as urine, death would occur quickly from dehydration. Actually, only about 1 to 3 L is excreted each day as urine. The rest is reabsorbed back into the circulatory system.

The GFR is controlled by blood pressure and blood flow. The ability of the kidneys to self-regulate renal blood pressure and renal blood flow keeps GFR constant. GFR is controlled by selectively constricting and dilating the afferent and efferent arterioles. When the afferent arteriole is constricted or the efferent arteriole is dilated, pressure in the glomerular capillaries falls and filtration decreases. When the afferent arteriole is dilated or the efferent arteriole is constricted, pressure in the glomerular capillaries rises and filtration increases. Through this process the kidney can maintain a constant GFR, even when systemic blood pressure changes. When systolic blood pressure drops below about 70 mm Hg, these processes cannot compensate and GFR stops.

Tubular reabsorption is the second process involved in urine formation. This reabsorption of most of the filtrate keeps normal urine output at 1 to 3 L/day and prevents dehydration. As the filtrate passes through the tubular parts of the nephron, most of the water and electrolytes is reabsorbed. Reabsorption returns particles (**solutes**) and water to the blood. Reabsorption occurs *from the filtrate* across the tubular lumen of the nephron and into the blood of the peritubular capillaries. The PCT reabsorbs about 65% of the total glomerular filtrate.

The tubules return more than 99% of all filtered water back into the body (Fig. 68-7). Most water reabsorption occurs as the filtrate passes through the PCT. Water reabsorption continues as the filtrate flows down the descending loop of Henle. The thin and thick segments of the ascending loop of Henle are *not* permeable to water, and water reabsorption does not occur here.

The distal convoluted tubule (DCT) can be permeable to water, and some water reabsorption can occur as the filtrate continues to flow through the tubule. The membrane of the DCT may be made more permeable to water through the action of antidiuretic hormone (ADH) and aldosterone. ADH increases tubular permeability to water, allowing water to leave the tube and be reabsorbed into the capillaries. ADH is also known as *vasopressin* and affects arteriole constriction. Arteriole constriction alters blood pressure, which, in turn, affects the amount of fluid and solutes that exit glomeruli capillaries. Aldosterone promotes the reabsorption of sodium in the DCT. Water reabsorption occurs as a result of the movement of sodium (where sodium goes, water follows).

The ability of the kidneys to vary the volume or concentration of urine helps regulate total water balance regardless of water intake. In this way, the healthy kidney can prevent dehydration when fluid intake is low and can prevent circulatory overload when fluid intake is excessive.

In addition to water, some particles in the tubular filtrate also *are returned to the blood.* This process is called *tubular reabsorption* and is selective. About 50% of all urea in the early urine is reabsorbed. On the other hand, no creatinine is reabsorbed.

Most sodium, chloride, and water reabsorption occurs in the PCT. The collecting ducts are the other site of sodium, chloride, and water reabsorption. Here reabsorption is caused by aldosterone. Potassium is also mostly reabsorbed in the PCT, with an additional 20% to 40% reabsorbed in the thick segment of the loop of Henle.

TABLE 68-1 Vascular and Tubular Components of the Nephron

Structure	Anatomic Features	Physiologic Aspects
VASCULAR COMPONENTS		
Afferent arteriole	Delivers arterial blood from the branches of the renal artery into the glomerulus	Autoregulation of renal blood flow via vasoconstriction or vasodilation Renin-producing granular cells
Glomerulus	Capillary loops with thin, semipermeable membrane	Site of glomerular filtration Glomerular filtration occurs when hydrostatic pressure (blood pressure) is greater than opposing forces (tubular filtrate and oncotic pressure)
Efferent arteriole	Delivers arterial blood from the glomerulus into the peritubular capillaries or the vasa recta	Autoregulation of renal blood flow via vasoconstriction or vasodilation Renin-producing granular cells
Peritubular capillaries (PTCs) and vasa recta (VR)	PTCs: surround tubular components of cortical nephrons VR: surround tubular components of juxtamedullary nephrons	Tubular reabsorption and tubular secretion allow movement of water and solutes to or from the tubules, interstitium, and blood
TUBULAR COMPONENTS		
Bowman's capsule (BC)	Thin membranous sac surrounding $^7/_8$ of the glomerulus	Collects glomerular filtrate (GF) and funnels it into the tubule
Proximal convoluted tubule (PCT)	Evolves from and is continuous with Bowman's capsule Specialized cellular lining facilitates tubular reabsorption	Site for reabsorption of sodium, chloride, water, glucose, amino acids, potassium, calcium, bicarbonate, phosphate, and urea
Loop of Henle	Continues from PCT Juxtamedullary nephrons dip deep into the medulla Permeable to water, urea, and sodium chloride	Regulation of water balance
Descending limb (DL)	Continues from the loop of Henle Permeable to water, urea, and sodium chloride	Regulation of water balance
Ascending limb (AL)	Emerges from DL as it turns and is redirected up toward the renal cortex	Potassium and magnesium reabsorption in the thick segment Thin segment is impermeable to water
Distal convoluted tubule (DCT)	Evolves from AL and twists so the macula densa cells lie adjacent to the juxtaglomerular cells of afferent arteriole	Site of additional water and electrolyte reabsorption, including bicarbonate Potassium and hydrogen secretion
Collecting ducts	Collect formed urine from several tubules and deliver it into the renal pelvis	Receptor sites for antidiuretic hormone regulation of water balance

Bicarbonate, calcium, and phosphate are mostly reabsorbed in the PCT. Bicarbonate reabsorption helps balance acids and maintain a normal blood pH. Blood levels of calcitonin and parathyroid hormone (PTH) (see Chapters 13 and 66) control calcium balance.

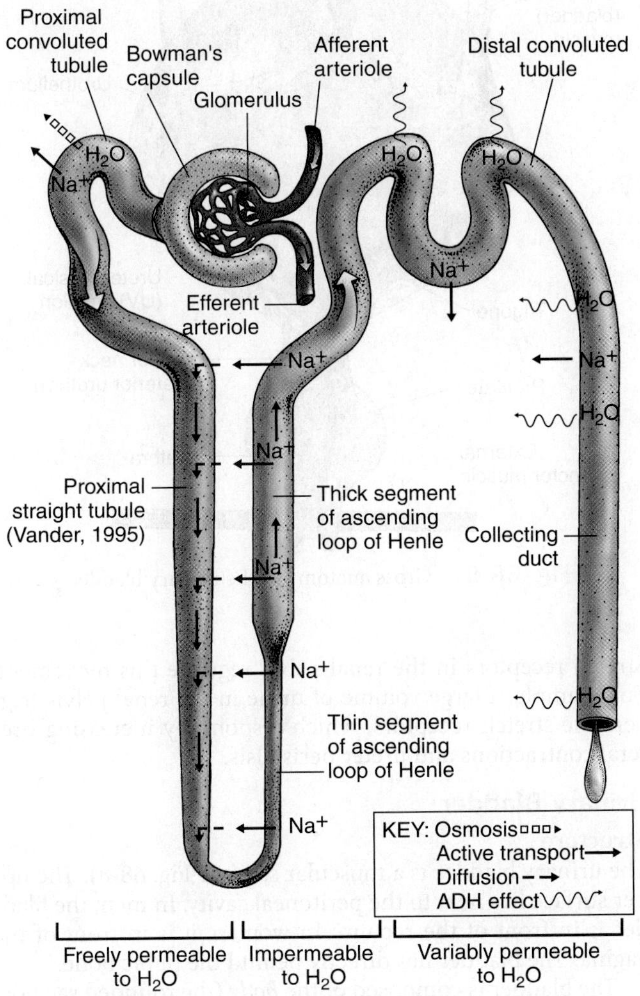
Proximal convoluted tubule
Bowman's capsule
Afferent arteriole
Distal convoluted tubule
Glomerulus
H_2O
Na^+
Efferent arteriole
Proximal straight tubule (Vander, 1995)
Thick segment of ascending loop of Henle
Collecting duct
Thin segment of ascending loop of Henle
KEY: Osmosis
Active transport
Diffusion
ADH effect
Freely permeable to H_2O
Impermeable to H_2O
Variably permeable to H_2O

Fig. 68-7 • Sodium and water reabsorption by the tubules of a cortical nephron.

The kidney reabsorbs some of the glucose filtered from the blood. However, there is a limit to how much glucose the kidney can reabsorb. This limit is called the **renal threshold** for glucose reabsorption or the **transport maximum** for glucose reabsorption. The usual renal threshold for glucose is about 220 mg/dL. This means that at a blood glucose level of 220 mg/dL or less, all glucose is reabsorbed and returned to the blood, with no glucose present in final urine. When blood glucose levels are greater than 220 mg/dL, some glucose stays in the filtrate and is present in the urine. Normally, almost all glucose and any amino acids or proteins are reabsorbed and are not present in the urine. *Thus the presence of these substances in the urine is abnormal and requires further assessment.*

Tubular secretion is the third process involved in urine formation. Like glomerular filtration, it allows substances to move from the blood into the early urine. During tubular secretion, substances move from the peritubular capillaries in reverse, across capillary membranes, and into the cells that line the tubules. From the cells, these substances are moved into the urine and are excreted from the body. Potassium (K^+) and hydrogen ions (H^+) are some of the substances moved in this way to maintain homeostasis of electrolytes and pH.

Hormonal Functions

The kidneys produce renin, prostaglandins, bradykinin, erythropoietin, and activated vitamin D (Table 68-2). Other kidney products, such as the kinins, change renal blood flow and capillary permeability. The kidneys also help break down and excrete insulin.

Renin, as discussed on p. 1528 in the Microscopic Anatomy section, assists in blood pressure control. It is formed and released when there is a decrease in blood flow, blood volume, or blood pressure through the renal arterioles or when too little sodium is present in renal blood. These conditions are detected through the receptors of the juxtaglomerular complex.

Renin release causes the production of *angiotensin II* through a series of steps (see Fig. 68-5). Angiotensin II increases systemic blood pressure through powerful blood vessel constricting effects and triggers the release of aldosterone from the adrenal glands. Aldosterone increases the reabsorption of sodium in the distal tubule of the nephron. Therefore more water is reabsorbed and blood pressure is increased be-

TABLE 68-2 Renal Hormone Production and Hormones Influencing Renal Function

	Site	Action
RENAL HORMONE PRODUCTION		
Renin	Renin-producing granular cells	Raises blood pressure as result of angiotensin (local vasoconstriction) and aldosterone (volume expansion) secretion
Prostaglandins	Renal tissues	Regulate intrarenal blood flow by vasodilation or vasoconstriction
Bradykinins	Juxtaglomerular cells of the arterioles	Increase blood flow (vasodilation) and vascular permeability
Erythropoietin	Renal parenchyma	Stimulates bone marrow to make red blood cells
Activated vitamin D	Renal parenchyma	Promotes absorption of calcium in the GI tract
HORMONES INFLUENCING RENAL FUNCTION		
Antidiuretic hormone (ADH, vasopressin)	Released from posterior pituitary	Makes DCT and CD permeable to water to maximize reabsorption and produce a concentrated urine
Aldosterone	Released from adrenal cortex	Promotes sodium reabsorption and potassium secretion in DCT and CD; water and chloride follow sodium movement
Natriuretic hormones	Cardiac atria, cardiac ventricle, brain	Cause tubular secretion of sodium

CD, Collecting ducts; *DCT,* distal convoluted tubule.

cause of increases in blood volume. When renal blood flow is reduced, this system also regulates pressures in the nephron to prevent fluid loss and maintain circulating blood volume (see also Chapter 13).

Prostaglandins are produced in many tissues, including the kidney. Specific prostaglandins produced in the kidney are prostaglandin E_2 (PGE_2) and prostacyclin (PGI_2). These substances help regulate glomerular filtration, kidney vascular resistance, and renin production. PGE_2 acts on the distal tubule and collecting duct to increase sodium and water excretion.

Bradykinin is release by the kidney in response to the presence of angiotensin II, prostaglandins, and ADH. It is a small hormone that dilates the afferent arteriole and increases capillary membrane permeability to some solutes. These actions maintain kidney blood flow and reabsorption even when other conditions cause systemic blood vessel constriction.

Erythropoietin is produced and released in response to decreased oxygen tension in the renal blood supply. It triggers red blood cell (RBC) production in the bone marrow. When kidney tissue is nonfunctional, erythropoietin production decreases and the person becomes anemic.

Vitamin D activation occurs through a series of steps. Some of these steps take place in the skin when it is exposed to sunlight, and then more processing occurs in the liver. From there, vitamin D is converted to its active form (1,25-dihydroxycholecalciferol) in the kidney. It is needed to absorb calcium in the intestinal tract and to regulate calcium balance.

NCLEX EXAMINATION CHALLENGE

How much glucose is expected to be present in the urine of a client who has a renal threshold for glucose of 220 mg/dL and a blood glucose level of 300 mg/dL?

A. 300 mg/dL
B. 220 mg/dL
C. 80 mg/dL
D. No glucose is present in the urine

evolve For the correct answer, go to http://evolve.elsevier.com/Iggy/.

Ureters

Each kidney has a single ureter—a hollow tube that connects the renal pelvis with the urinary bladder. The ureter is about ½ inch (1.25 cm) in diameter and about 12 to 18 inches (30 to 45 cm) in length. The diameter of the ureter narrows in three areas:

- In the upper third of the ureter, at the point at which the renal pelvis becomes the ureter, is a narrowing known as the **ureteropelvic junction (UPJ)**.
- The ureter also narrows as it bends toward the abdominal wall (aortoiliac bend).
- Each ureter narrows at the point it enters the bladder; this point is called the **ureterovesical junction (UVJ)**.

The ureter tunnels through bladder tissue for a short distance and then opens into the bladder at the trigone (Fig. 68-8).

The ureter has three layers: an inner lining of mucous membrane (urothelium), a middle layer of smooth muscle fibers, and an outer layer of fibrous tissue. The outer layer contains the blood supply. The middle layer of muscle fibers is controlled by several nerve pathways from the lower spinal cord.

Contractions of the smooth muscle in the ureter move urine from the renal pelvis of the kidney to the bladder.

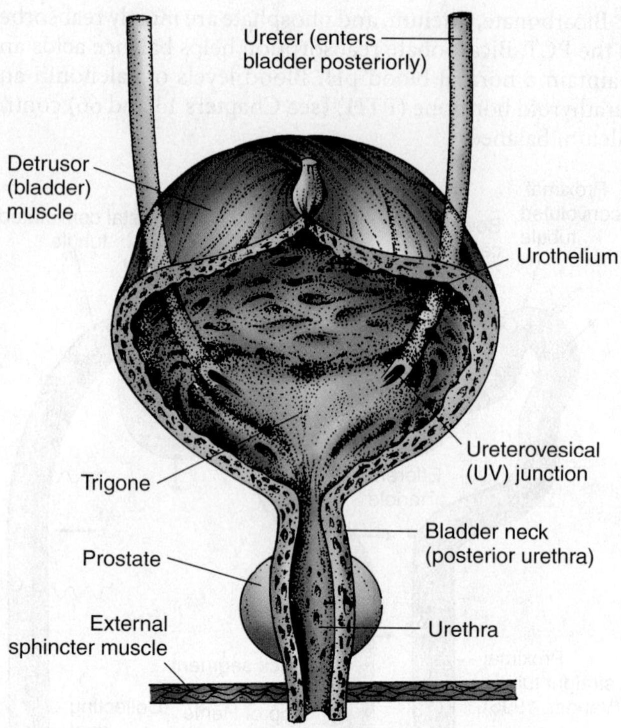
Ureter (enters bladder posteriorly)
Detrusor (bladder) muscle
Urothelium
Ureterovesical (UV) junction
Trigone
Bladder neck (posterior urethra)
Prostate
External sphincter muscle
Urethra

Fig. 68-8 • Gross anatomy of the urinary bladder.

Stretch receptors in the renal pelvis regulate this movement. For example, a large volume of urine in the renal pelvis triggers the stretch receptors, which respond by increasing ureteral contractions and ureter peristalsis.

Urinary Bladder

Structure

The urinary bladder is a muscular sac (see Fig. 68-8). The upper surface lies next to the peritoneal cavity. In men, the bladder is in front of the rectum. In women, it is in front of the vagina. The bladder lies directly behind the pubic bone.

The bladder is composed of the *body* (the rounded sac portion) and the *bladder neck* (posterior urethra), which connects to the bladder body. The bladder has three linings—an inner lining of epithelial cells *(urothelium)*, middle layers of smooth muscle *(detrusor muscle)*, and an outer lining. The *trigone* is an area on the posterior wall between the points of ureteral entry (ureterovesical junctions [UVJs]) and the urethra.

The **internal urethral sphincter** is the smooth detrusor muscle of the bladder neck and elastic tissue. The **external urethral sphincter** is skeletal muscle that surrounds the urethra. In men, the external sphincter surrounds the urethra at the base of the prostate gland. In women, the external sphincter is at the base of the bladder. The pudendal nerve from the spinal cord controls the external sphincter.

Function

The bladder is a temporary urine storage site. The bladder also provides continence and enables voiding. The secretions of the bladder lining resist bacteria.

Continence is the ability to voluntarily control bladder emptying. Bladder continence occurs during bladder filling through the combination of detrusor muscle relaxation, internal sphincter muscle tone, and external sphincter contraction.

As the bladder fills with urine, stretch sensations are transmitted to spinal sacral nerves S2 and S3.

Maintaining continence occurs by the interaction of the nerves that control the muscles of the bladder, bladder neck, urethra, and pelvic floor, as well as by factors that close the urethra. During bladder filling, the sympathetic nervous system fibers prevent detrusor muscle contraction. These control centers are located in the cerebral cortex, the brainstem, and the sacral part of the spinal cord. For urethral closure to be adequate for continence, the mucosal surfaces must be in contact and must be adhesive. Contact depends on the presence and proper function of the involved nerves and muscles. Adhesion depends on the adequate secretion of mucus-like substances.

Micturition (voiding) is a reflex of autonomic control that triggers contraction of the detrusor muscle at the same time as relaxation of the external sphincter and the muscles of the pelvic floor. With detrusor muscle contraction, the UVJ of the ureter closes and the normally round bladder assumes the shape of a funnel. Voiding is a voluntary act as the result of a learned response and is controlled by the cerebral cortex and the brainstem. Contraction of the external sphincter inhibits the micturition reflex and prevents voiding.

Urethra

The urethra is a narrow tube lined with mucous membranes and epithelial cells. Its purpose is to eliminate urine from the bladder. The **urethral meatus,** or opening, is the endpoint of the urethra. In men, the urethra is about 6 to 8 inches (15 to 20 cm) long, with the meatus located at the tip of the penis. The male urethra has three sections:

- The prostatic urethra, which extends from the bladder to the prostate gland
- The membranous urethra, which extends to the wall of the pelvic floor
- The cavernous urethra, which is external and extends through the length of the penis

In women, the urethra is about 1 to 1.5 inches (2.5 to 3.75 cm) long and exits the bladder through the pelvic floor. The meatus lies slightly below the clitoris and directly in front of the vagina and rectum.

RENAL/URINARY SYSTEM CHANGES ASSOCIATED WITH AGING

Renal Changes

Structural and functional changes occur in the kidney as a result of the aging process. These changes often affect health. The kidney loses cortical tissue and gets smaller by 80 years of age. This cortical loss is caused by reduced renal blood flow. The medulla is not affected by aging, and the juxtamedullary nephron functions are preserved. However, the glomerular and tubular linings thicken. Both the number of glomeruli and their surface areas decrease with aging. Tubule length also decreases. These changes reduce the ability of the older adult to filter blood and excrete waste products.

Kidney function also changes with aging (Chart 68-1). Blood flow to the kidney decreases by about 10% per decade as blood vessels thicken. This means that renal blood flow is not as adaptive in older adults compared with younger adults, leaving nephrons more vulnerable to damage during episodes of either hypotension or hypertension.

Glomerular filtration rate (GFR) decreases with age, especially after 45 years of age. By age 65, the GFR is about 65 mL/min (half the rate of a young adult). This decline is more rapid in patients with diabetes, hypertension, or heart failure. As a result, the older patient has a greater risk for fluid overload.

Tubular changes with aging decrease the ability to concentrate urine, resulting in **nocturnal polyuria** (increased urination at night). The regulation of sodium, acids, and bicarbonate remains effective but is less efficient. Along with an age-related impairment in the thirst mechanism, these changes increase the risk for dehydration and **hypernatremia** (increased blood sodium levels) in the older adult (Brenner, 2007). Hormonal changes include a decrease in renin secretion, aldosterone levels, and activation of vitamin D.

Urinary Changes

Changes in the detrusor muscle elasticity lead to decreased bladder capacity and reduced ability to retain urine. The urge to void may cause immediate bladder emptying because the urinary sphincters lose tone and often become weaker with age. In women, weakened muscles shorten the urethra and promote incontinence. In men, an enlarged prostate gland makes starting the urine stream difficult and may cause urinary retention.

CULTURAL AWARENESS

African Americans have more rapid age-related decreases in GFR than do white people (Brenner, 2007). The renal excretion of sodium is less effective in hypertensive African Americans who have high sodium intake, and the kidneys have about 20% less blood flow as a result of anatomic changes in small renal vessels and intrarenal responses to renin (Price et al., 2001; Shulman & Hall, 1991). Thus African American patients are at greater risk for renal failure than are white patients. Yearly health examinations should include urinalysis and checking for the presence of microalbuminuria.

ASSESSMENT METHODS

Patient History

One way to assess renal and urologic function is to use Gordon's Functional Health Patterns (Gordon, 2007). The patterns most related to the renal system are Nutritional/Metabolic and Elimination (Chart 68-2).

Demographic information, such as age, gender, race, and ethnicity, is important to consider as nonmodifiable risk factors in the patient with any renal or urinary problem. A sudden onset of hypertension in patients older than 50 years suggests possible kidney disease. Clinical changes with adult polycystic kidney disease typically occur in patients in their 40s or 50s. In men older than 50 years, altered urine patterns accompany prostate disease.

Anatomic gender differences make some disorders worse or more common. For example, men rarely have urinary tract infections unless there are abnormalities, such as ureteral reflux or prostatic enlargement. Women have a shorter urethra and more commonly develop **cystitis** (bladder infection) because bacteria pass more readily into the bladder.

Ask the patient about any previous renal or urologic problems, including tumors, infections, stones, or urologic surgery. A history of any chronic health problems, especially diabetes mellitus or hypertension, increases the risk for

Chart 68-1 NURSING FOCUS ON THE OLDER ADULT

Changes in the Renal/Urinary System Related to Aging

Physiologic Change	Nursing Interventions	Rationales
Decreased glomerular filtration rate (GFR)	Monitor hydration status.	With aging, the ability of the kidneys to regulate water balance is decreased.
	Ensure adequate fluid intake.	The kidneys are less able to conserve water when necessary.
	Administer potentially nephrotoxic agents or drugs carefully.	Dehydration results in decreased renal blood flow and increases the nephrotoxic potential of many agents. Acute or chronic renal failure may result.
Nocturia	Ensure adequate nighttime lighting and a hazard-free environment.	Nocturia may occur from decreased renal concentrating ability associated with aging.
	Ensure the availability of a toilet, bedpan, or urinal.	The desire to maintain continence prompts people to seek the bathroom. Falls and injuries are common among older patients seeking bathroom facilities.
	Discourage excessive fluid intake for 2-4 hr before the patient retires for the evening.	Excessive fluid intake at night may increase nocturia.
	Evaluate drugs and timing.	Some drugs increase urine output.
Decreased bladder capacity	Encourage the patient to use the toilet, bedpan, or urinal at least every 2 hr.	By emptying the bladder on a regular basis, urinary incontinence from overflow may be avoided.
	Respond as soon as possible to the patient's indication of the need to void.	
Weakened urinary sphincter muscles and shortened urethra in women	Respond as soon as possible to the patient's indication of the need to void.	A quick response may alleviate episodes of urinary stress incontinence.
	Provide thorough perineal care after each voiding.	The shortened urethra increases the potential for bladder infections.
		Good perineal hygiene may prevent skin irritations and urinary tract infection (UTI).
Tendency to retain urine	Observe the patient for urinary retention (e.g., bladder distention) or urinary tract infection (e.g., dysuria, foul odor, confusion).	Urinary stasis may result in a UTI. UTIs may become bloodstream infections, resulting in urosepsis or septic shock.
	Provide privacy, assistance, and voiding stimulants such as warm water over the perineum as needed.	Nursing interventions can help initiate voiding.
	Evaluate drugs for possible contribution to retention.	Anticholinergic drugs promote urinary retention.

Chart 68-2 RENAL/URINARY ASSESSMENT

Using Gordon's Functional Health Patterns

NUTRITIONAL/METABOLIC PATTERN

- What is your typical daily food intake? Describe a day's meals, snacks, and vitamins.
- How much salt do you typically add to your food? Do you use salt substitutes?
- How is your appetite?
- Have you experienced any nausea or vomiting?
- What is your typical daily fluid intake?
- What types of fluids do you drink (water, juices, soft drinks, coffee, tea)?
- How much fluid do you drink each day?
- Have you had any recent change in your weight? Weight gain? Weight loss? How much?
- Have you noticed a change in the tightness of your rings or shoes? Tighter? Looser?
- Have you noticed any skin changes lately? More dry? Less dry? Itchy?

ELIMINATION PATTERN

- What is your usual bowel elimination pattern? Frequency? Character? Discomfort? Laxatives?
- What is your usual urinary elimination pattern? Frequency? Amount? Color? Odor? Control?
- Have you noticed a change in the amount of urine?
- Do you have any problem with excessive perspiration?
- Do you have any other type of drainage?

Based on Gordon, M. (2007). *Manual of nursing diagnosis* (11th ed.). Boston: Jones & Bartlett.

development of renal disease because these disorders damage renal blood vessels.

Ask the patient about chemical exposures at the workplace or with hobbies. Exposure to hydrocarbons (e.g., gasoline, oil), heavy metals (especially mercury and lead), and some gases (e.g., chlorine, toluene) can impair kidney function. Use this opportunity to teach patients who come into contact with chemicals in their workplaces or during leisure time activities to avoid direct skin or mucous membrane contact with these chemicals. Use of heroin, cocaine, methamphetamine, ecstasy, and volatile solvents (inhalants) has also been associated with renal damage.

Specifically ask the patient whether he or she has ever been told about the presence of protein or albumin in the urine. The question "Have you ever been told that your blood pressure is high?" may prompt a response different from the one to the question "Do you have high blood pressure?" Ask women about health problems during pregnancy (e.g., proteinuria, high blood pressure, gestational diabetes, urinary tract infections). Obtain information about:

- Chemical or environmental toxin exposure in occupational or other settings
- Recent travel to geographic regions that pose infectious disease risks
- Recent physical injuries
- Trauma
- Sexual contacts
- A history of altered patterns of urinary elimination

Socioeconomic status may influence health care practices. Prevention, early detection, and treatment of renal or urinary problems may be limited by patients' lack of insurance or access to health care, lack of transportation, and reduced income. These patients may also have difficulty following medical advice, having prescriptions filled, and keeping follow-up appointments.

Educational level may affect health-seeking practices and the patient's understanding of a disease or its symptoms. Recurring urinary tract infections often result from inadequate or incomplete treatment, including lack of follow-up to ensure the infection is cleared. The lack of money to pay for antibiotics or nutritious foods may inhibit or delay recovery.

The patient's health beliefs affect the approach to health and illness. Cultural background or religious affiliation may influence the belief system.

The language used by patients may be different from that used by the health care professional. Anatomic or medical terms may have no meaning for the patient (Table 68-3). When obtaining a history, listen to and explore the terms used by the patient. By using the patient's own terms, you may help him or her provide a more complete description of the problem. This technique may increase the amount of information obtained and decrease the patient's discomfort when discussing bodily functions.

TABLE 68-3 Commonly Used Renal and Urinary Terms

anuria Total urine output of less than 100 mL in 24 hours

azotemia Increased blood urea nitrogen and serum creatinine levels suggestive of renal impairment but without outward symptoms of renal failure

dysuria Discomfort or pain associated with micturition

frequency Feeling the need to void often, usually voiding small amounts of urine each time; may void every hour or even more frequently

hesitancy Difficulty in initiating the flow of urine, even when the bladder has sufficient urine to initiate a void and the sensation of the need to void is present

micturition The act of voiding

nocturia Awakening prematurely from sleep because of the need to empty the bladder

oliguria Decreased urine output; total urine output between 100 and 400 mL in 24 hours

polyuria Increased urine output; total urine output usually greater than 2000 mL in 24 hours

uremia Full-blown manifestations of renal failure; sometimes referred to as the *uremic syndrome,* especially if the cause of the renal failure is unknown

urgency A sudden onset of the feeling of the need to void immediately; may result in incontinence if the patient is unable to locate or get to toileting facilities quickly

Nutrition History

Ask the patient with known or suspected renal or urologic disorders about his or her usual diet and any recent changes in the diet. Note any excessive intake or omission of certain food categories. Ask about food and fluid intake. Assess how much and what types of fluids the patient drinks daily, especially fluids with a high calorie or caffeine content. Use this opportunity to teach the patient the importance of drinking about 3 L of fluid daily (if another medical problem does not require fluid restriction) to prevent dehydration and cystitis. If the patient has followed a diet for weight reduction, the details of the diet plan are important, and collaboration with a nutritionist may be needed. A high-protein intake can result in temporary renal problems. Patients at risk for **calculi** (stone) formation who ingest large amounts of protein or have a poor fluid intake may form new stones.

Ask about any change in appetite or in the ability to discriminate tastes. These symptoms can occur with the build-up of nitrogenous waste products from renal failure. Changes in thirst or fluid intake may also cause changes in urine output. Endocrine disorders may also cause changes in thirst, fluid intake, and urine output (see Chapter 64 for a discussion of endocrine influences on fluid balance).

Medication History

Identify all of the patient's prescription drugs, because many can lead to renal impairment. Ask about the duration of drug use and whether there have been any recent changes in prescribed drugs. Drugs for diabetes mellitus, hypertension, cardiac disorders, hormonal disorders, cancer, arthritis, and psychiatric disorders are potential causes of renal dysfunction. Antibiotics, such as gentamicin (Garamycin, Cidomycin♣), may also cause sudden renal dysfunction.

Explore the past and current use of over-the-counter (OTC) drugs or agents, including dietary supplements, vitamins and minerals, herbal agents, laxatives, analgesics, acetaminophen, and NSAIDs. Many of these agents affect renal function. For example, dietary supplementation with synthetic creatine, used to increase muscle mass, has been associated with compromised renal function. High-dose or long-term use of NSAIDs or acetaminophen can seriously reduce renal function. Some agents are associated with hypertension, hematuria, or proteinuria, which may precede renal dysfunction.

Family History and Genetic Risk

The family history of the patient with a suspected kidney or urologic problem is important because some disorders have a familial inheritance pattern. Ask whether his or her siblings, parents, or grandparents have had renal problems. Past terms used for kidney disease include *Bright's disease, nephritis,* and *nephrosis.* Patients may use these terms to describe kidney disease as it was known by their parents or grandparents years ago. Adult polycystic kidney disease can occur in either gender.

Current Health Problems

The effects of renal failure result in changes in all body systems. Therefore document all of the patient's current health problems. Ask him or her to describe all health concerns, because some renal disorders cause systemic problems or problems in other body systems. Recent upper respiratory problems, achy muscles or joints, chronic fatigue, or GI problems may be related to problems of kidney function.

Assess the kidney and urologic system specifically. Ask the patient about any changes in the appearance (color, odor, clarity) of the urine, pattern of urination, ability to initiate or control voiding, and other unusual symptoms. For example, urine that is reddish, dark brown or black, greenish, or otherwise different from the usual yellowish, straw color usually prompts the patient to seek health care assistance. Urine typically has a mild but distinct odor of ammonia. An increase in the intensity of color, a change in odor quality, or a decrease in urine clarity may suggest infection.

Ask about changes in urination patterns, such as **nocturia** (urination at night), frequency, or an increase or decrease in the amount of urine. The normal urine output for adults is about 1500 to 2000 mL/day, or within 500 mL of the volume of fluid ingested in a day. Ask him or her to consider how closely the urine output is to the volume of fluid ingested. The patient usually does not know the exact amount of urine produced. A bladder diary may provide useful data. Also ask:

- If initiating urine flow is difficult
- If a burning sensation or other discomfort occurs with urination
- If the force of the urine stream is decreased (in men)

Ask about any loss of urinary continence, especially when coughing, sneezing, or laughing. Patients may also report a persistent dribbling of urine.

The onset of pain in the flank, in the lower abdomen or pelvic region, or in the perineal area is often of great concern and usually prompts the patient to seek assistance. Ask about the onset, intensity, and duration of the pain, its location, and its association with any activity or event.

Pain associated with renal or ureteral irritation is often severe and spasmodic. Pain that radiates into the perineal area, groin, scrotum, or labia is described as *renal colic.* This pain occurs with distention or spasm of the ureter, such as in an obstruction or the passing of a stone. Renal colic pain may be intermittent or continuous and may occur with pallor, diaphoresis, and hypotension. These general symptoms occur because of the location of the nerve tracts near or in the kidneys and ureters.

Because the kidneys are close to the GI organs and the nerve pathways are similar, GI manifestations may occur with kidney problems. These renointestinal reflexes often complicate the description of the renal problem.

Uremia is the buildup of nitrogenous waste products in the blood, a result of kidney failure. Manifestations include anorexia, nausea and vomiting, muscle cramps, **pruritus** (itching), fatigue, and lethargy.

Physical Assessment

The physical assessment of the patient with a known or suspected renal or urologic disorder includes general appearance, a review of body systems, and specific structure and functions of the renal/urinary systems.

Assess the general appearance of the patient, and check for a yellowish skin color and the presence of any rashes, bruising, or other discoloration. The skin and tissues may show edema, which with renal disorders may be detected in the **pedal** (foot), **pretibial** (shin), and sacral tissues, and around the eyes. Auscultate the lungs to determine whether fluid is present. Weigh the patient and take his or her blood pressure as a baseline for later comparisons.

Assess the patient's level of consciousness and level of alertness. Record any deficits in concentration, thought processes, or memory. Family members may report subtle changes. Such cognitive changes may be the result of the buildup of waste products when kidney disease is present.

Assessment of the Kidneys, Ureters, and Bladder

Assess the kidneys, ureters, and bladder during an abdominal assessment. Auscultate before percussion and palpation because these activities can enhance bowel sounds and obscure abdominal vascular sounds.

Inspect the abdomen and the flank regions with the patient in both the supine and the sitting positions. Observe the patient for asymmetry (e.g., swelling) or discoloration (e.g., bruising or redness) in the flank region, especially in the area of the costovertebral angle (CVA). The CVA is located between the lower portion of the twelfth rib and the vertebral column.

Listen for a bruit by placing a stethoscope over each renal artery on the midclavicular line. A **bruit** is an audible swishing sound produced when the volume of blood or the diameter of the blood vessel changes. It often occurs with blood flow through a narrowed vessel, as in renal artery stenosis.

Renal palpation is usually performed by a physician or advanced practice nurse. It can help locate masses and areas of tenderness in or around the kidney. Lightly palpate the abdomen in all quadrants. Ask about areas of tenderness or discomfort, and examine nontender areas first. The outline of the bladder may be seen as high as the umbilicus in patients with severe bladder distention. *If tumor or aneurysm is suspected, palpation may harm the patient.*

Because the kidneys are located deep and posterior, palpation is easier in thin patients who have little abdominal musculature. For palpation of the right kidney, the patient is in a supine position while the examiner places one hand under the right flank and the other hand over the abdomen below the lower right part of the rib cage. The lower hand is used to raise the flank, and the upper hand depresses the abdomen as the patient takes a deep breath (Fig. 68-9). The left kidney is deeper and often cannot be palpated. A transplanted kidney is readily palpated in either the lower right or left abdominal quadrant. The kidney should feel smooth, firm, and nontender.

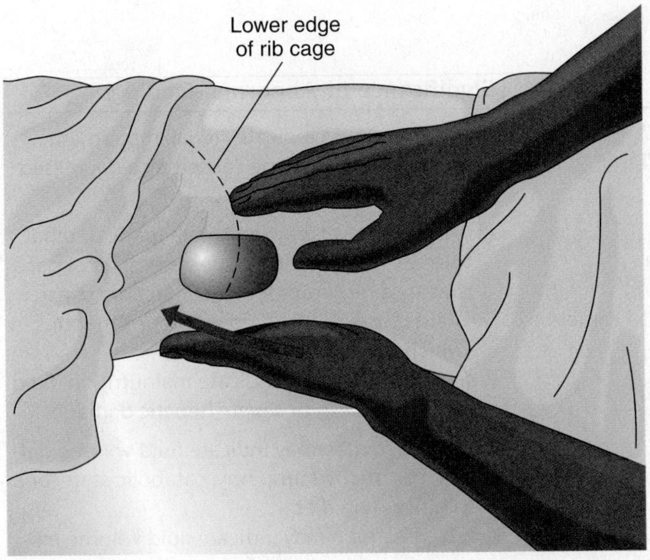
Lower edge
of rib cage

Fig. 68-9 • Advanced technique for palpation of the kidney.

A distended bladder sounds dull when percussed. After gently palpating to determine the outline of the distended bladder, begin percussion on the lower abdomen and continue in the direction of the umbilicus until dull sounds are no longer produced.

If the patient reports flank pain or tenderness, percuss the nontender flank first. Have the patient assume a sitting, side-lying, or supine position, and then form one of your hands into a clenched fist. Place your other hand flat over the CVA of the patient. Then quickly deliver a firm thump to your hand over the CVA area. Costovertebral tenderness often occurs with kidney infection or inflammation. Patients with inflammation or infection in the kidney or nearby structures may describe their pain as severe or as a constant, dull ache.

Assessment of the Urethra

Using a good light source and wearing gloves, inspect the urethra by examining the meatus and the tissues around it. Record any unusual discharge such as blood, mucus, or pus. Inspect the skin and mucous membranes of surrounding tissues. Record the presence of lesions, rashes, or other abnormalities of the penis or scrotum or of the labia or vaginal opening. Urethral irritation is suspected when the patient reports discomfort with urination. Use this opportunity to remind women to clean the perineum by wiping from front to back, never from back to front. Teach them that the front-to-back technique keeps organisms in stool from coming close to the urethra, which could increase the risk for infection.

Women from other cultures may have undergone female circumcision. This procedure alters the anatomic appearance of the vulvar-perineal area and increases the risk for urinary tract infections. It also makes urethral inspection or catheterization difficult. Document any noted anatomic changes and ask the patient to describe her hygiene practices for this area.

Psychosocial Assessment

Concerns about the urologic system may evoke fear, anger, embarrassment, anxiety, guilt, or sadness in the patient. Childhood learning often includes privacy with regard to toilet habits. Urologic disorders may bring up forgotten memories of difficult toilet training and bedwetting or of childhood experiences of exploring one's body. The patient may ignore symptoms or delay seeking health care because of emotional responses or cultural taboos about the urogenital area.

DECISION-MAKING CHALLENGE

Coordination of Care

The patient is a 24-year-old man who arrives with a report of a headache for the past 4 days and nausea and vomiting for the past 3 days. He has never had any serious illness or surgery. He mentions that he has not voided for over 12 hours despite taking in about a liter of fluid over the past 6 hours.

1. What personal or demographic data should you obtain?
2. How would you proceed in gathering physical assessment data?
3. What laboratory or diagnostic testing do you anticipate?

evolve For suggested answer guidelines, go to http://evolve.elsevier.com/Iggy/.

Diagnostic Assessment

Laboratory Assessment

Blood Tests

Serum creatinine is produced when protein or muscle breaks down. Creatinine is filtered by the kidneys and excreted in the urine. Because muscle mass and protein breakdown are usually constant, the serum creatinine level is a good indicator of kidney function. Normal serum creatinine levels vary with age, gender, and body muscle mass. Levels are slightly higher in men than in women (Chart 68-3). In general, men have a larger muscle mass than do women, but there are exceptions. Muscle mass and the amount of creatinine produced decrease with age. Because of decreased rates of creatinine clearance, however, the serum creatinine level remains relatively constant in older adults unless renal disease is present.

No common pathologic condition other than renal disease increases the serum creatinine level. The serum creatinine level does not increase until at least 50% of the renal function is lost, and therefore *any* elevation of serum creatinine values is important.

Blood urea nitrogen (BUN) measures the renal excretion of urea nitrogen, a by-product of protein breakdown in the liver. Urea nitrogen is produced mostly from liver metabolism of food sources of protein. The kidneys filter urea nitrogen from the blood and excrete the waste in urine. BUN levels indicate the extent of renal clearance of this nitrogen waste product.

Other factors influence the BUN level, and an elevation does not always mean renal disease is present (see Chart 68-3). For example, rapid cell destruction from infection, cancer treatment, or steroid therapy may elevate BUN level. In addition, blood is a protein. Blood in the tissues rather than in the blood vessels is reabsorbed as if it were a general protein. Thus reabsorbed blood protein is processed by the liver and increases BUN levels. This means that injured tissues can result in increased BUN levels even when kidney function is normal.

The liver must function properly to produce urea nitrogen. When both liver and kidney dysfunction are present, urea nitrogen levels are actually decreased because the liver failure limits urea production. The BUN level is not always elevated with kidney disease and is not the best indicator of kidney function. However, an elevated BUN level is highly *suggestive* of kidney dysfunction.

Chart 68-3 **LABORATORY PROFILE**

Renal Function Blood Studies

Test	Normal Range for Adults	Significance of Abnormal Findings
Serum creatinine	*Males:* 0.6-1.2 mg/dL (53-106 mmol/L) *Females:* 0.5-1.1 mg/dL (44-97 mmol/L) *Older adults:* may be decreased	An *increased level* indicates renal impairment. A *decreased level* may be caused by a decreased muscle mass.
Blood urea nitrogen (BUN)	10-20 mg/dL (3.6-7.1 mmol/L) *Older adults:* 60-90 yr: 8-23 mg/dL (2.9-8.2 mmol/L) Older than 90 yr: 10-31 mg/dL (3.6-11.1 mmol/L)	An *increased level* may indicate hepatic or renal disease, dehydration or decreased renal perfusion, a high-protein diet, infection, stress, steroid use, GI bleeding, or other situations in which blood is in body tissues. A *decreased level* may indicate malnutrition, fluid volume excess, or severe hepatic damage.
BUN/creatinine ratio	Mass ratio: 12:1 to 20:1 Mole ratio: 48.5:1 to 80.8:1	An *increased ratio* may indicate fluid volume deficit, obstructive uropathy, catabolic state, or a high-protein diet. A *decreased ratio* may indicate fluid volume excess or acute renal tubular acidosis. *No change* in the ratio with increases in both the BUN and creatinine levels indicates renal impairment.

Data from Pagana, K.D., & Pagana, T.J. (2006). *Mosby's manual of diagnostic and laboratory tests* (3rd ed.). St. Louis: Mosby

Blood urea nitrogen to serum creatinine ratio can help determine whether nonrenal factors, such as dehydration or poor renal perfusion, are causing the elevated BUN level rather than kidney damage. When blood volume is deficient (dehydration) or blood pressure is low, the BUN level rises more rapidly than the serum creatinine level. As a result, the ratio of BUN to creatinine is *increased.*

When both the BUN and serum creatinine levels increase at the same rate, the BUN/creatinine ratio remains normal. However, the elevated serum creatinine and BUN levels suggest renal dysfunction that is not related to dehydration or poor perfusion.

Blood osmolarity is a measure of the overall concentration of particles in the blood. The kidneys excrete or reabsorb water to keep blood osmolarity in the range of 285 to 295 mOsm/L. Osmolarity is slightly higher in older adults (285 to 301 mOsm/L). When blood osmolarity is decreased, the release of antidiuretic hormone (ADH) is inhibited. Without ADH, the distal tubule and collecting ducts are *not* permeable to water. As a result, water is *excreted,* not reabsorbed, and blood osmolarity increases. When blood osmolarity increases, ADH is released. ADH increases the permeability of the distal tubule to water. Then water is reabsorbed and blood osmolarity decreases.

Urine Tests

Urinalysis. Urinalysis is a part of any complete physical examination and is especially useful for patients with suspected kidney or urologic disorders (Chart 68-4). Ideally, the urine specimen is collected at the morning's first voiding. Specimens obtained at other times may be too dilute. The specimen may be collected by several techniques (Table 68-4).

Urine color comes from urochrome pigment. Color variations may result from increased levels of urochrome or other pigments, changes in the concentration or dilution of the urine, and the presence of drug metabolites in the urine. Urine smells faintly like ammonia and is normally clear without **turbidity** (cloudiness) or haziness.

Specific gravity of urine is the density of urine compared with water, which has a specific gravity of 1.000. Density is related to the number of particles in a specific volume of urine. The normal specific gravity of urine ranges from 1.005 to about 1.030. In kidney disease, changes in specific gravity do not reflect systemic fluid volume. For example, dilute urine with a low specific gravity may occur in a dehydrated patient who lacks nephron receptors for antidiuretic hormone (ADH).

An *increase* in specific gravity occurs with dehydration, decreased kidney blood flow, or the presence of ADH. (ADH production is normally increased with stress, surgery, anesthetic agents, and certain drugs such as morphine and oral antidiabetic agents.) In these situations, the normal kidney response is to reabsorb water and decrease urine output. As a result, the urine produced is more concentrated.

A *decrease* in specific gravity occurs with increased fluid intake, diuretic drugs, and diabetes insipidus. In these conditions, the normal kidney response is to excrete more water; thus urine output is increased. In kidney disease, the specific gravity decreases because the damaged kidneys reabsorb less water. The specific gravity does not vary with changes in plasma osmolarity (i.e., it becomes fixed).

pH is a measure of urine acidity or alkalinity. A pH value less than 7 is acidic, and a value greater than 7 is alkaline. Many factors influence urine acidity or alkalinity. A diet high in certain fruits and vegetables results in a more alkaline urine. A high-protein diet produces a more acidic urine. The presence of *Escherichia coli* in the urine also results in an acidic urine.

Urine specimens become more alkaline when left standing unrefrigerated for more than 1 hour, when bacteria are present, or when a specimen is left uncovered. Alkaline urine increases cell breakdown; thus the presence of red blood cells may be

Chart 68-4 LABORATORY PROFILE

Urinalysis

Test	Normal Range for Adults	Significance of Abnormal Findings
Color	Pale yellow	*Dark amber* indicates concentrated urine. *Very pale* yellow indicates dilute urine. *Dark red* or brown indicates blood in the urine. Brown also may indicate increased urinary bilirubin level. Red also may indicate the presence of myoglobin. *Other color* changes may result from diet or drugs.
Odor	Specific aroma, similar to ammonia	*Foul smell* indicates possible infection, dehydration, or ingestion of certain foods or drugs.
Turbidity	Clear	*Cloudy urine* indicates infection, sediment, or high levels of urinary protein.
Specific gravity	Usually 1.005-1.030; possible range 1.000-1.040 (after 12-hr fluid restriction, >1.025) *Older adult:* Decreased because of decreased concentrating ability	*Increased* in decreased renal perfusion, inappropriate antidiuretic hormone secretion, or congestive heart failure. *Decreased* in chronic renal insufficiency, diabetes insipidus, malignant hypertension, diuretic administration, and lithium toxicity.
pH	Average: 6; possible range: 4.6-8	*Changes* are caused by diet, the administration of drugs, infection, freshness of the specimen, acid-base imbalance, and altered renal function.
Glucose	<0.5 g/day (<2.78 mmol/L)	*Presence* reflects hyperglycemia or a decrease in the renal threshold for glucose.
Ketones	None	*Presence* reflects incomplete metabolism of fatty acids, as in diabetic ketoacidosis, prolonged fasting, anorexia nervosa.
Protein	0.8 mg/dL	*Increased* amounts may indicate stress, infection, recent strenuous exercise, or glomerular disorders.
Bilirubin (urobilinogen)	None	*Presence* suggests hepatic or biliary disease or obstruction.
Red blood cells (RBCs)	0-2 per high-power field	*Increased* amounts are normal with indwelling or intermittent catheterization or menses but may reflect tumor, stones, trauma, glomerular disorders, cystitis, or bleeding disorders.
White blood cells (WBCs)	*Males:* 0-3 per high-power field *Females:* 0-5 per high-power field	*Increased* amounts may indicate an infectious or inflammatory process anywhere in the renal/urinary tract, renal transplant rejection, fever, or exercise.
Casts	A few or none, composed of RBC, WBC, protein, or tubular cell casts	*Increased* amounts indicate the presence of bacteria or protein, which is seen in severe renal disease and could also indicate urinary calculi.
Crystals	None	*Presence* of normal or abnormal crystals may indicate that the specimen has been allowed to stand.
Bacteria	<1000 colonies/mL	*Increased* amounts indicate the need for urine culture to determine the presence of urinary tract infection.
Parasites	None	*Presence* of *Trichomonas vaginalis* indicates infection, usually of the urethra, prostate, or vagina.
Leukoesterase	None	*Presence* suggests urinary tract infection.
Nitrites	None	*Presence* suggests urinary *Escherichia coli.*

missed on analysis. Ensure that urine specimens are covered and delivered to the laboratory promptly or refrigerated. During acidosis or alkalosis, the kidneys, along with blood buffers and the lungs, normally respond to keep serum pH normal. Chapter 14 discusses acid-base balance and imbalance.

Glucose is filtered by the glomerulus and is reabsorbed in the proximal tubule of the nephron. When the blood glucose level rises above 220 mg/dL, the renal threshold for reabsorption is exceeded and some glucose is present in the urine. Changes in the renal threshold for glucose occur in many patients, such as those with infection or those with long-standing diabetes mellitus. It is possible that their serum glucose level may be high (e.g., greater than 400 mg/dL) and glucose may still not be present in the urine. More often, these patients show glucose in the urine even when blood glucose levels are normal or only slightly elevated.

Ketone bodies are formed from the incomplete metabolism of fatty acids. Three types of ketone bodies are acetone, aceto-

TABLE 68-4 Collection of Urine Specimens

Nursing Interventions	Rationales
VOIDED URINE	
Collect the first specimen voided in the morning.	Urine is more concentrated in the early morning.
Send the specimen to the laboratory as soon as possible.	After urine is collected, cellular breakdown results in more alkaline urine.
Refrigerate the specimen if a delay is unavoidable.	Refrigeration delays the alkalinization of urine. Bacteria are more likely to multiply in an alkaline environment.
CLEAN-CATCH SPECIMEN	
Explain the purpose of the procedure to the patient.	Correct technique is needed to obtain a valid specimen.
Instruct the patient to self-clean before voiding. Instruct the female patient to separate the labia and use the sponges and solution provided to wipe with three strokes over the urethra. The first two wiping strokes are over each side of the urethra; the third wiping stroke is centered over the urethra (from front to back). Instruct the male patient to retract the foreskin of the penis and to similarly clean the urethra, using three wiping strokes with the sponge and solution provided (from the head of the penis downward).	Surface cleaning is necessary to remove secretions or bacteria from the urethral meatus.
Instruct the patient to initiate voiding after cleaning. The patient then stops and resumes voiding into the container. Only 1 ounce (30 mL) is needed; the remainder of the urine may be discarded into the commode.	A midstream collection further removes secretions and bacteria because urine flushes the distal portion of the internal urethra.
Ensure that the patient understands the procedure.	An improperly collected specimen may result in inappropriate or incomplete treatment.
Assist the patient as needed.	The patient's understanding and the nurse's assistance ensure proper collection.
CATHETERIZED SPECIMEN	
For non-indwelling (straight) catheters:	The one-time passage of a urinary catheter may be necessary to obtain an uncontaminated specimen for analysis or to measure the volume of residual urine.
Avoid routine use.	
Follow the facility's procedures for catheterization technique.	These procedures minimize bacterial entry.
For indwelling catheters:	Urine is collected from an indwelling catheter or tubing when patients have catheters for continence or long-term urinary drainage.
Apply a clamp to the drainage tubing, distal to the injection port.	Clamping allows urine to collect in the tubing at the location where the specimen is obtained.
Clean the injection port cap of the catheter drainage tubing with an appropriate antiseptic. Povidone-iodine solution or alcohol is acceptable.	Surface contamination is prevented by following the cleaning procedures.
Attach a sterile 5-mL syringe into the port and aspirate the quantity of urine required.	A minimum of 5 mL is needed for culture and sensitivity (C&S) testing.
Inject the urine sample into a sterile specimen container. Remove the clamp to resume drainage. Properly dispose of the syringe.	A sterile container is used for C&S specimens.
24-HOUR URINE COLLECTION	
Instruct the patient thoroughly.	A 24-hr collection of urine is necessary to quantify or calculate the rate of clearance of a particular substance.
Provide written materials to assist in instruction. Place signs appropriately. Inform all personnel or family caregivers of test in progress.	Instructional materials for patients, signs, and so on remind patients and staff to ensure that the total collection is completed.
Check laboratory or procedure manual on proper technique for maintaining the collection (e.g., on ice, in a refrigerator, or with a preservative).	Proper technique prevents breakdown of elements to be measured.
On initiation of the collection, ask the patient to void, discard the urine, and note the time. If a Foley catheter is in use, empty the tubing and drainage bag at the start time and discard the urine. Collect all urine of the next 24 hr. Twenty-four hours after initiation, ask the patient to empty the bladder and add that urine to the container.	Proper techniques ensure that *all* urine formed within the 24-hr period is collected.
Do not remove urine from the collection container for other specimens.	Urine in the container is not considered a "fresh" specimen and may be mixed with preservative.

acetic acid, and beta-hydroxybutyric acid. *Normally there are no ketones in urine.* Ketone bodies are produced when fat is used instead of glucose for cellular energy. Ketones present in the blood are partially excreted in the urine.

Protein, such as albumin, is not normally present in the urine. Levels greater than 300 mg/24 hr, or 200 mcg/min, are abnormal. Protein molecules are too large to pass through intact glomerular membranes. When glomerular membranes are not intact, protein molecules pass through and are excreted in the urine. Increased membrane permeability is caused by infection, inflammation, or immunologic problems. Some systemic problems cause production of abnormal proteins, such as globulin. These proteins are not detected by routine urinalysis and require electrophoresis or other tests for detection.

A random finding of **proteinuria** (protein in the urine) followed by a series of negative (normal) findings does not imply renal disease. If infection is the cause of the proteinuria, urinalyses after elimination of the infection should be negative for protein. Persistent proteinuria needs further investigation.

Microalbuminuria is the presence of albumin in the urine that is not measurable by a urine dipstick or usual urinalysis procedures. Specialized assays are used to quickly analyze a freshly voided urine specimen for microscopic levels of albumin. The normal microalbumin levels in a freshly voided specimen should range between 2.0 and 20 mg/mmol for men and between 2.8 and 28 mg/mmol for women. Higher levels indicate microalbuminuria and could mean very early kidney disease, especially in patients with diabetes mellitus. In 24-hour urine specimens, levels of 30 to 300 mg/24 hr, or 20 to 200 mcg/min, indicate microalbuminuria.

Leukoesterase is an enzyme found in some white blood cells, especially neutrophils. When the number of these cells increases in the urine or they are broken (lysed), the urine then contains leukoesterase. The presence of leukoesterase and nitrites in the urine is a sensitive screen for assessing urinary tract infections. A normal reading is no leukoesterase in the urine. A positive test (+ sign) indicates increasing leukocytes in the urine.

Nitrites are not usually present in urine. Many types of bacteria, when present in the urine, convert nitrates (normally found in urine) into nitrites. A positive finding indicates urinary tract infection.

Sediment is precipitated particles in the urine. These particles include cells, casts, crystals, and bacteria. Normally, urine contains few, if any, cells. Types of cells abnormally present in the urine include tubular cells (from the tubule of the nephron), epithelial cells (from the lining of the urinary tract), red blood cells (RBCs), and white blood cells (WBCs).

Casts are structures formed around other particles. There may be casts of cells, bacteria, or protein. When cells, bacteria, or proteins are present in the urine, minerals and sticky materials clump around them and form a cast. Casts are described by the type of particle they have surrounded (e.g., RBC cast, WBC cast, tubular epithelial cast) or the stage of cast breakdown. Casts are described as "granular" (coarse or fine) and "waxy."

Urine crystals come from various mineral salts. These minerals may be a result of diet, drugs, or disease. Common salt crystals are formed from calcium, oxalate, urea, phosphate, magnesium, or other substances. Some drugs, such as the sulfates, can also form crystals.

Bacteria in a urine sample multiply quickly, so the specimen must be analyzed promptly. Normally, urine is sterile, but it is easily contaminated by perineal bacteria during collection.

Recent advances in technology and molecular biology are leading to new diagnostic tests using urine, including identification of biomarkers of disease and profiling for specific proteins.

Urine for Culture and Sensitivity. Urine is analyzed for the number and types of organisms present. Manifestations of infection and unexplained bacteria in a urine specimen are indications for urine culture and sensitivity testing. Bacteria from urine are placed in a medium with different antibiotics. In this way we can know which antibiotics are effective in killing the organisms (organisms are "sensitive") and which are not effective (organisms are "resistant"). A clean-catch or catheter-derived specimen is best for culture and sensitivity testing.

Composite Urine Collections. Some urine collections are made for a specified number of hours (e.g., 24 hours) for more precise analysis of one or more substances. These collections are often used to measure urine levels of creatinine or urea nitrogen, sodium, chloride, calcium, catecholamines, or other components (Chart 68-5). For a composite urine specimen, *all* urine within the designated time frame must be collected (see Table 68-4). If other voided or catheterized specimens must be obtained while the collection is in progress, measure and record the amount collected but not added to the timed collection.

The urine collection may need to be refrigerated or stored on ice to prevent changes in the urine during the collection time. Follow the procedure from the laboratory for urine storage. The urine collection must be free from fecal contamination. Menstrual blood and toilet tissue also contaminate the specimen and can invalidate the results.

The collection of urine for a 24-hour period is often more difficult than it seems. With hospitalized patients, the cooperation of staff personnel, the patient, family members, and visitors is essential. Placing signs in the bathroom, instructing the patient and family, and emphasizing the need to save the urine are helpful.

Creatinine Clearance. Creatinine clearance is a calculated measure of glomerular filtration rate. It is the best indication of overall kidney function. The amount of creatinine cleared from the blood (e.g., filtered into the urine) is measured in the total volume of urine excreted in a defined period. A urine specimen for a creatinine clearance test is usually collected for 24 hours, but it can be collected for shorter periods (e.g., 8 or 12 hours). The calculation compares the urine creatinine level with the blood creatinine level, and therefore a blood specimen or creatinine must also be collected.

The laboratory or care provider calculates the creatinine clearance. The patient's age, gender, height, weight, diet, and activity level influence the expected amount of creatinine to be excreted. Thus these factors are considered when interpreting creatinine clearance test results.

The rate of creatinine clearance is expressed as milliliters per minute per square meter of body surface area. The range for normal creatinine clearance is 90 to 139 mL/min/m^2 for men and 80 to 125 mL/min/m^2 for women.

Creatinine clearance values are used to determine the patient's current kidney function. Decreases in the creatinine clearance rate may require reducing drug doses and often signifies the need to further explore the cause of kidney deterioration.

Urine Electrolytes. Urine samples can be analyzed for electrolyte levels (e.g., sodium, chloride). Normally the amount of sodium excreted in the urine is nearly equal to that consumed. Urine sodium levels of less than 10 mEq/L indicate that the tubules are able to conserve (reabsorb) sodium.

Chart 68-5 LABORATORY PROFILE

24-Hour Urine Collections

Component	Normal Range for Adults	Significance of Abnormal Findings
Creatinine	0.8-2 g/24 hr *Males:* 1-2 g/24 hr or 14-26 mg/kg/24 hr (124-230 μmol/kg/24 hr or 7.1-17.7 mmol/24 hr) *Females:* 0.6-1.8 g/24 hr or 11-20 mg/kg/24 hr (97-177 μmol/kg/24 hr or 5.3-15.9 mmol/24 hr) *Older adults:* 10 mg/kg/24 hr (88.4 μmol/kg/24 hr) at 90 yr	*Decreased amounts* indicate a deterioration in renal function caused by renal disease. *Increased amounts* occur with infections, exercise, diabetes mellitus, and meat meals.
Urea nitrogen	12-20 g/24 hr (0.43-0.71 mmol/24 hr)	*Decreased amounts* occur when renal damage or liver disease is present. *Increased amounts commonly result from a high-protein diet, dehydration, trauma, or sepsis.*
Sodium	40-220 mEq/24 hr (40-220 mmol/24 hr)	*Decreased amounts* are seen in hemorrhage, shock, hyperaldosteronism, and prerenal acute renal failure. *Increased amounts* are common with diuretic therapy, excessive salt intake, hypokalemia, and acute tubular necrosis.
Chloride	110-250 mEq/24 hr (110-250 mmol/24 hr) *Older adults:* 95-195 mEq/24 hr (95-195 mmol/24 hr)	*Decreased amounts* are seen in certain renal diseases, malabsorption syndrome, pyloric obstruction, prolonged nasogastric tube drainage, diarrhea, diaphoresis, heart failure, and emphysema. *Increased amounts* are seen with hypokalemia, adrenal insufficiency, and massive diuresis.
Calcium	100-400 mg/24 hr (2.50-7.50 mmol/kg/24 hr)	*Decreased amounts* are often associated with hypocalcemia, hypoparathyroidism, nephrosis, and nephritis. *Increased amounts* are commonly seen with calcium renal stones, hyperparathyroidism, sarcoidosis, certain cancers, immobilization, and hypercalcemia.
Total catecholamines*	<100 mcg/24 hr (<591 mmol/24 hr)	*Increased amounts* occur with pheochromocytoma, neuroblastomas, stress, or strenuous exercise.
Protein	1-14 mg/dL (10-140 mg/L) or 50-80 mg/24 hr at rest	*Increased amounts* indicate glomerular disease, nephrotic syndrome, diabetic nephropathy, urinary tract malignancies, and irritations.

*Epinephrine and norepinephrine only; dopamine is not measured.

Urine Osmolarity. Osmolarity measures the concentration of particles in solution. The particles in urine contributing to osmolarity include electrolytes, glucose, urea, and creatinine. Urine osmolarity can vary from 50 to 1400 mOsm/L, depending on the patient's hydration status and kidney function. With average fluid intake, the range for urine osmolarity is 300 to 900 mOsm/L. Electrolytes, acids, and other wastes of normal metabolism are continually produced. These particles are the solute load that must be excreted in the urine on a regular basis. This is referred to as *obligatory solute excretion.* If the patient loses excessive fluids, the renal response is to save water while excreting wastes by excreting small amounts of highly concentrated urine. Diet, drugs, and activity can change urine osmolarity. Thus urine with an increased osmolarity is concentrated urine with less water and more solutes. Urine with a decreased osmolarity is dilute urine with more water and fewer solutes.

Bedside Sonography/Bladder Scanners

The use of portable ultrasound scanners in the hospital and rehabilitation setting by nurses is a noninvasive method of estimating bladder volume (Fig. 68-10). Bladder scanners are used to screen patients for post-void residual volumes and to determine the need for intermittent catheterization based on the amount of urine in the bladder rather than the time between catheterizations. The scan does not require patient preparation beyond an explanation of what to expect. There is no discomfort with the scan.

Explain why the procedure is being done and what sensations the patient might experience during the procedure. For example, "This test will measure the amount of urine in your bladder. I will place a gel pad just above your pubic area and then place the probe, which is a little bigger and heavier than a stethoscope, on the gel."

Before scanning, select the male or female icon on the bladder scanner. Using the female icon allows the scanner software to subtract the volume of the uterus from any measurement. Use the male icon on all men and on women who have undergone a hysterectomy.

Place an ultrasound gel pad right above the symphysis pubis (pubic bone) or moisten the round dome of the scan head area with 5 mL of conducting gel to improve ultrasound conduction. Use conducting gel on the scanner head for obese

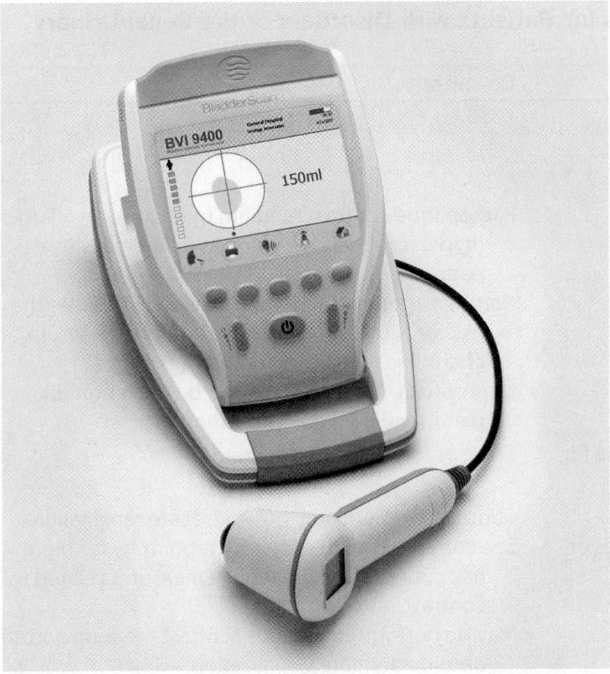
BladderScan
BVI 9400
150ml

Fig. 68-10 • The BladderScan® BVI 9400, a handheld portable bladder scanner.

patients and those with heavy body hair in the area to be scanned. Place the probe midline over the abdomen about 1½ inches (4 cm) above the pubic bone. Aim the scan head so the ultrasound is projected toward the expected location of the bladder, typically toward the patient's coccyx. Press and release the scan button. The scan is complete with the sound of a beep, and a volume is displayed. Two readings are recommended for best accuracy. An aiming icon on the portable bladder scanner indicates whether the bladder image is centered on the crosshairs of the scan head. If the crosshairs on the aiming icon are not centered on the bladder, the measured volume may not be accurate.

DECISION-MAKING CHALLENGE
Coordination of Care

The 24-year-old patient described on p. 1537 has these vital signs and laboratory data: T = 98.4° F; P = 80; R = 16; BP = 138/90; oxygen saturation = 98%; serum sodium = 140; potassium = 4.5; chloride = 101; BUN = 21 mg/dL; creatinine = 8 mg/dL. Urinalysis: 2+ protein; 2+ blood; 1-2 WBCs.

Although he is not taking any prescription drugs, he does take vitamin C regularly and recently increased his dose to 5000 mg daily for 5 days when he had symptoms of a cold about a week before his current symptoms began. He reports that he just finished his undergraduate education and has returned to his parent's house while he looks for employment. He does not believe he has ever had exposure to any environmental hazards.

1. Do any of these data support the possibility of dehydration contributing to acute renal dysfunction?
2. What do the alterations in BUN and creatinine indicate?
3. What independent and collaborative interventions can you anticipate in the care of this patient at this time?

evolve For suggested answer guidelines, go to http://evolve.elsevier.com/Iggy/.

Imaging Assessment

Many imaging procedures are used to diagnose abnormalities within the urinary system (Table 68-5). Explain the procedures thoroughly to the patient, prepare him or her, and provide follow-up care.

Kidney, Ureter, and Bladder X-rays

An x-ray of the kidneys, ureters, and bladder (KUB) is a plain film of the abdomen obtained without any specific patient preparation. The KUB study shows gross anatomic features and obvious stones, strictures, calcifications, or obstructions in the urinary tract. This test identifies the shape, size, and relationship of the organs to other parts of the urinary tract. Other tests are needed to diagnose functional or structural problems.

There is no discomfort or risk from this procedure. Tell the patient that the x-ray will be taken while he or she is in a supine position. No specific follow-up care is needed.

Intravenous Urography

Other names for IV urography include *excretory urography* and (the older term) *IV pyelography (IVP)*.

Patient Preparation. Before urography, assess the patient (Chart 68-6), and explain the need for a bowel preparation. Report allergy information to the physician. Contrast reactions can be minor (nausea and vomiting, urticaria, itching, sneezing), moderate (nephrotoxic effects, congestive heart failure, pulmonary edema), or severe (bronchospasm, anaphylaxis). If the diagnostic test must be performed in a patient with a minor allergy to the contrast dye, drugs such as a steroid (prednisone or methylprednisolone) and an antihistamine (diphenhydramine hydrochloride [Benadryl, Allerdryl🍁]) are prescribed before the procedure to reduce the risk for an allergic response. Explain the rationale for the procedure to the patient.

Some preparations may be needed to ensure that urinary structures are not obscured by bowel contents. Some radiologists recommend a light evening meal or clear liquids and then fasting (NPO status) from midnight on the night before the procedure. Others recommend increased fluid intake to prevent dehydration up until the time of the procedure. Because some patients may vomit as a reaction to the IV contrast, some physicians prefer the patient to remain on NPO status for a few hours before the procedure. Hydration with IV fluids may be prescribed.

A bowel preparation is prescribed to remove fecal contents, fluid, and air from the gut, any of which could obscure part of the outline of the kidneys, ureters, and bladder. Bowel preparation procedures vary but usually include the use of laxatives the day before the procedure. Enemas also may be prescribed, but their use is controversial because some air and fluid can be retained.

CONSIDERATIONS FOR OLDER ADULTS

Bowel preparation procedures increase the risk for dehydration, especially in older adult patients. To help prevent dehydration, contact the testing department and ask that urograms be scheduled early in the day for older patients.

The contrast dye is potentially kidney-damaging (nephrotoxic). The risk for *contrast-induced renal failure* is greatest in patients who are older or dehydrated, who have some renal in-

TABLE 68-5 Common Radiologic and Special Diagnostic Tests for Patients with Disorders of the Renal/Urinary System

Test	Purpose	Comments
Radiography of kidneys, ureters, and bladder (KUB) (plain film of abdomen)	To screen for the presence of two kidneys To measure kidney size To detect gross obstruction	
Excretory urography	To measure kidney size To detect obstruction To assess parenchymal mass	Radiopaque contrast medium may cause an allergic (hypersensitivity) reaction in iodine-sensitive patients. Contrast agent is also hypertonic and increases the risk for acute renal failure in adults with serum creatinine levels greater than 1.5 mg/dL. Nephrotoxic complications can be prevented by parenteral fluid administration.
Nephrotomography	To assess various planes of kidney tissue for cysts, tumors, or calculi	Same as for excretory urogram.
Computed tomography (CT)	To measure kidney size To evaluate contour to assess for masses or obstruction	Contrast medium may provoke acute renal failure. See comments with excretory urography for high-risk patients and preventive measures related to contrast. May be performed without contrast medium and still obtain adequate visualization.
Cystography and cystoscopy	To identify abnormalities of the bladder wall and urethral and ureteral occlusions To treat small obstructions or lesions via fulguration, lithotripsy, or removal with a stone basket	Instrumentation of the urinary tract increases the risk for infection. Monitor for infection for 48-72 hr after the procedure.
Voiding cystourethrography (VCUG)	To outline bladder's contour and detect urinary reflux from vesicourethral junctions	The risk for infection is similar to that in cystography because urinary catheterization is necessary. Monitor for postprocedure infection.
Ultrasonography (US)	To identify the size of the kidneys or obstruction in the kidneys or the lower urinary tract May detect tumors or cysts	Ultrasonography entails minimal risk to the patient. Ultrasonography is a good alternative to excretory urography.
MAG3 study 99m	To assess renal function, structural abnormalities, renal failure, obstruction, and renal calculi	Radioactive material (technetium Tc mertiatide) is used for this test.
Intravenous pyelography (IVP) (fluoroscopy)	To assess renal function, identify anomalies To image renal/urinary calculi (size, location, radiodensity) To screen for renal injury after trauma	Contraindicated during pregnancy (ionizing radiation is a risk to the fetus). Contrast dye can cause renal dysfunction. Colonic cleaning improves quality of image.
Magnetic resonance imaging (MRI)	Staging of cancers, similar to CT	Patient must be able to lie still (motion can interfere with imaging).
Renal scan	Evaluation of renal blood flow Estimation of renal glomerular filtration rate Provides functional information without exposing the patient to iodinated contrast dye	ACE inhibitors should be held for 48 hours before the test. ACE inhibitors may be given during the test, placing the patient at risk for episodes of hypotension. Ensure adequate hydration for best results.

ACE, Angiotensin-converting enzyme.

sufficiency (e.g., serum creatinine levels greater than 1.5 mg/dL), or who are also taking other nephrotoxic drugs. In addition, patients taking metformin are at risk for lactic acidosis when they receive iodinated contrast media (Namasivayam et al., 2006). Metformin should be discontinued at the time of a procedure and for at least 48 hours after the procedure and after renal function has been re-evaluated.

All patients at risk for contrast-induced nephrotoxicity need additional IV fluids before the procedure to maintain hydration and decrease the risk for kidney damage. Acetylcysteine (an antioxidant) may be used to prevent contrast-induced nephrotoxic effects in radiologic procedures, although its benefits have not been proven. Diuretics may be given immediately after the dye is injected to enhance dye excretion in patients who are well hydrated.

Instruct the patient in the preparation procedures for the urogram, and explain the procedure so that he or she knows what to expect (Chart 68-7). Intervene on behalf of

Chart 68-6 **BEST PRACTICE FOR PATIENT SAFETY & QUALITY CARE**

Assessing the Patient About to Undergo a Diagnostic Test or Interventional Procedure Using Contrast Media

Before the procedure:

- Ask the patient if he or she has ever had a reaction to contrast media. (Such a patient has the highest risk for having another reaction.)
- Ask the patient about a history of asthma. (Patients with asthma have been shown to be at greater risk for contrast reactions than the general public. When reactions do occur, they are more likely to be severe.)
- Ask the patient about known hay fever or food or drug allergies, especially to seafood, eggs, milk, or chocolate. (Contrast reactions have been reported to be as high as 15% in these patients.)
- Ask the patients to describe any specific allergic reactions (e.g., hives, facial edema, difficulty breathing, bronchospasm).
- Assess for a history of renal insufficiency and for conditions that have been implicated in increasing the chance of developing renal failure after contrast media (e.g., diabetic nephropathy, class IV heart failure, dehydration, concomitant use of potentially nephrotoxic drugs such as the aminoglycosides or NSAIDs, and cirrhosis).
- Ask the patient if he or she is taking metformin (Glucophage). (Metformin must be discontinued at least 48 hours before any study using contrast media because the life-threatening complication of lactic acidosis, although rare, could occur.)
- Assess hydration status by checking blood pressure, heart and respiratory rates, mucous membranes, skin turgor, and urine concentration.
- Ask the patient when he or she last ate or drank anything.

From Cohan, R.H., & Ellis, J.H. (1997). Iodinated contrast material in uroradiology: Choice of agent and management of complications. *Urologic Clinics of North America, 24*(3), 471-491.

the patient to ensure that questions are answered *before* the procedure.

Procedure. The dye is injected IV with the patient in a supine position. As blood (with the dye) rapidly circulates into the kidney blood vessels and is filtered by the glomeruli, the dye is excreted in the urine. A series of x-rays are taken at various times after injection. Nephrotomograms may be taken at the same time as the urogram. Tomograms take images of different planes of tissue and show any abnormalities present at varying depths. The technologist then asks the patient to empty the bladder and return for a few more x-rays. An outline of the kidneys, ureters, and bladder is visible as urine containing the dye is excreted.

The urogram provides information about:

- The number, size, shape, and location of the kidneys
- The adequacy of filling and the rate of excretion of contrast medium
- The number, size, location, appearance, and patency of the calices, pelves, and ureters
- The size, location, and nature of the urinary bladder

Follow-up Care. After the urogram, monitor the patient for altered renal function and other effects from the dye. Ensure adequate hydration by urging the patient to take oral fluid or by giving IV fluids. Hydration reduces the risk for renal damage. Monitor blood creatinine levels to assess ongoing renal function.

Chart 68-7 **PATIENT AND FAMILY EDUCATION GUIDE**

Excretory Urogram

- The urogram outlines your urinary tract and helps determine any problems there.
- Notify your nurse or physician if you have had any reactions (allergic or otherwise) to any food or drugs, especially shellfish (e.g., shrimp, scallops, crab, lobster) or iodine, or to x-ray "dyes" such as contrast media; if you have a history of asthma; or if you are taking metformin (Glucophage) or Glucovance.
- The day before the test, follow the instructions about changes in your diet and fluid intake to be sure that as much information as possible is gained from the test.
- After you start the bowel preparation, you may need to be close to toileting facilities. The preparation drugs usually work quickly.
- You will be lying on an x-ray table with the x-ray machine above you for most of the procedure.
- A pressure band, similar to a large blood pressure cuff, may be placed around your stomach or abdomen to help obtain better x-rays.
- If you do not already have an IV access site, one will be started to give you the contrast agent.
- After the contrast is injected, you may feel a sense of warmth or heat as it travels throughout your body. You also may have a taste in your mouth that is sometimes described as metallic. These sensations last only a few seconds or minutes.
- When the pressure band is inflated, you may feel some tightness around your abdomen. The sensation is similar to the feeling on your arm when you have your blood pressure taken.
- A series of x-rays will be taken. You may be asked to empty your bladder and return to the table for more films. You also may be asked to have a standing film taken.
- After the test is completed, you are usually able to resume your normal activities and diet.
- You will not notice any change in the color or characteristics of your urine.
- Please do not hesitate to ask your nurse, physician, or x-ray technologist any question, no matter how slight the question may seem to you. It is important that you have as much understanding as possible.

Computed Tomography

Inform the patient that a computed tomography (CT) scan provides three-dimensional information about the kidneys, ureters, bladder, and surrounding tissues. A CT scan is usually performed after other diagnostic procedures and can provide information about tumors, cysts, abscesses, other masses, obstruction, and renal blood vessels.

Some hospitals require patients having abdominal CT scans to be NPO for some period before the scan. For the scan using contrast, extra hydration may be needed before the test, especially if the patient has reduced renal function. Ask about allergy to dyes, and intervene as with IV urography.

The CT scan is performed in a special room, usually in the radiology department. Oral or injected contrast dye is usually given before starting the imaging procedures. Dye use may be omitted in patients at risk for contrast media–

induced acute renal failure, but the images produced are less distinct.

No special follow-up care is needed unless dye was used. In that case, the follow-up care is the same as for IV urography.

Cystography and Cystourethrography

Explain the procedure to the patient. A urinary catheter is temporarily needed to instill contrast dye. The dye is needed to enhance x-ray visibility of the lower urinary tract.

In both cystography and cystourethrography, dye is instilled into the bladder via a urethral catheter. After bladder filling, x-rays are taken from the front, back, and side positions. For the voiding cystourethrogram (VCUG), the patient is requested to void and x-rays are taken during the voiding. A VCUG is obtained to determine whether urine refluxes into the ureter. The cystogram is often used in cases of trauma when urethral or bladder injury is suspected.

Monitor for infection as a result of catheter placement. In this test, the dye is not nephrotoxic because it does not enter the bloodstream and does not reach the kidney. Encourage fluid intake to dilute the urine and reduce the burning sensation from catheter irritation after removal. Also monitor for changes in urine output because pelvic or urethral trauma may be present.

Renography (Kidney Scan)

Explain that a kidney scan is performed to provide general information about renal blood flow. A small amount of radioactive material, a radionuclide, is used. Reassure the patient that there is no danger from the small amount of radioactive material present in the agent. Radionucleotides are not associated with nephrotoxicity.

For a kidney scan, the radionuclide is injected IV. After injection, the agent is absorbed into kidney tissue and gives off low-level radioactive emissions (scintillations). The amount of emission is measured by a scintillation counter. A special camera records the emissions and produces an image. At the same time, the rate and location of the emissions are recorded by computer and information about renal blood flow, or glomerular filtration, is provided.

In some cases, captopril (Capoten), an antihypertensive drug, is given at the start of the procedure to change blood flow in the kidney. This procedure is a "captopril renal scan." The drug can cause severe hypotension during and after the procedure.

When the patient can urinate, urination into a commode does not place anyone at risk from the small amount of radioactive material excreted. If he or she is incontinent, change the bed linens promptly and wear gloves for Standard Precautions. If captopril was used during the procedure, assess the patient's blood pressure frequently. Warn him or her to avoid rapid position changes and about the risk for falling as a result of orthostatic (positional) hypotension.

Ultrasonography

Inform the patient that ultrasonography does not cause discomfort and is without risk. This test usually requires a full bladder. Ask the patient to drink water, if needed, to help fill the bladder. This test applies sound waves to structures of different densities to produce images of the kidneys, ureters, and bladder and surrounding tissues. Ultrasonography allows assessment of kidney size, cortical thickness, and status of the calices. The test can identify obstruction in the urinary tract, tumors, cysts, and other masses without the use of contrast dye.

The patient undergoing renal ultrasound is usually placed in the prone position. Sonographic gel is applied to the skin over the back and flank areas to enhance sound wave conduction. A transducer in contact with and moving across the skin delivers sound waves and measures the echoes. Images of the internal structures are produced. Skin care to remove the gel is all that is needed after ultrasonography.

Renal Arteriography (Angiography)

Renal arteriography allows dye to enter the renal blood vessels and generates images to determine blood vessel size and abnormalities. This test has largely been replaced by other imaging techniques (e.g., nuclear renal scans, ultrasonography, computed tomography) and is seldom used as a stand-alone diagnostic procedure. The most common use of renal arteriography is at the time of a renal angioplasty or other intervention.

Cystoscopy and Cystourethroscopy

Patient Preparation. Cystoscopy and cystourethroscopy are operative procedures and require completion of a preoperative checklist and a signed informed consent statement. The physician provides a complete description of and reasons for the procedure, and the nurse reinforces this information. Cystoscopy may be performed for diagnosis or treatment. This test is used to examine for bladder trauma (cystoscopy) or urethral trauma (cystourethroscopy) and to identify causes of urinary tract obstruction. Cystoscopy may be used to remove bladder tumors or an enlarged prostate gland.

Cystoscopy may be performed under general or local anesthesia with sedation. The patient's age and general health and the expected duration of the procedure are considered in the decision about anesthesia. A light evening meal may be eaten. Usually the patient is NPO after midnight on the night before the cystoscopy. A bowel preparation with laxatives or enemas is performed the evening before the procedure.

Procedure. The cystoscopy is performed in a designated cystoscopic examination room. If the procedure is performed in a surgical suite under general anesthesia, the usual surgical support personnel are present (see Chapter 17). This procedure is often performed in clinics, ambulatory surgery or short-procedure units, or a urologist's office.

Assist the patient onto a table, and after sedation, place him or her in the lithotomy position. After the anesthesia is given and the area cleansed and draped, the urologist inserts a cystoscope through the urethra into the urinary bladder. This examination commonly includes the use of both the cystoscope and the urethroscope.

Follow-up Care. After this procedure with general anesthesia, the patient is returned to a postanesthesia care unit (PACU) or area. If local anesthesia and sedation were used, he or she may be returned directly to the hospital room. Patients undergoing cystoscopic examinations as outpatients are transferred to an area for monitoring before discharge to home. Monitor for airway patency and breathing, changes in vital signs (including temperature), and changes in urine output. Also observe for the complications of bleeding and infection.

A catheter may or may not be present after cystoscopy. The patient without a catheter has urinary frequency as a result of irritation from the procedure. The urine may be pink tinged, but gross bleeding is not expected. Bleeding or the presence of clots may obstruct the catheter and decrease urine output. Monitor urine output, and notify the physician of obvious blood clots or a decreased or absent urine output. Irrigate the Foley catheter with sterile saline, if prescribed. Notify the physician if the patient has a fever (with or without chills) or an elevated white blood cell (WBC) count, which suggests infection. Urge the patient to take oral fluids to increase urine output (which helps prevent clotting) and to reduce the burning sensation on urination.

Retrograde Procedures

Retrograde means going against the normal flow of urine. A retrograde examination of the ureters and pelves (pyelogram), the bladder (cystogram), and the urethra (urethrogram) involves instilling dye into the lower urinary tract. Because the dye is instilled directly to obtain an outline of the structures desired, the dye does not enter the bloodstream. Therefore the patient is not at risk for dye-induced acute renal failure or a systemic allergic response.

The patient is prepared for retrograde procedures (retrograde pyelography, retrograde cystography, and retrograde urethrography) in the same way as for cystoscopy. Retrograde x-rays are obtained during the cystoscopy. After placement of the cystoscope by the urologist, catheters are placed into each ureter and contrast dye is instilled into each ureter and renal pelvis. The catheters are removed by the urologist, and x-rays are taken to outline these structures as the dye is excreted. The procedure identifies obstruction or structural abnormalities.

For patients undergoing retrograde cystoscopy or urethrography, contrast dye is instilled similarly into the bladder or urethra. Cystography and urethrography identify structural problems, such as fistulas, diverticula, and tumors.

After retrograde procedures, monitor the patient for infection caused by placing instruments in the urinary tract. Because these procedures are performed during cystoscopic examination, follow-up care is the same as that for cystoscopy.

Other Diagnostic Assessment

Urodynamic Studies

Urodynamic studies examine the processes of voiding and include:

- Tests of bladder capacity, pressure, and tone
- Studies of urethral pressure and urine flow
- Tests of perineal voluntary muscle function

These tests are often used along with voiding urographic or cystoscopic procedures to evaluate problems with urine flow.

Cystometrography (CMG) can determine how well the bladder wall (detrusor) muscle functions and how sensitive it is to stretching as the bladder fills. This test provides information about bladder capacity, bladder pressure, and voiding reflexes.

Explain the procedure, and inform the patient that a urinary catheter may be needed temporarily during the procedure. Ask the patient to void normally. Record the amount, rate of flow, and time of voiding. Insert a urinary catheter to measure the residual urine volume. The cystometer is attached to the catheter, and fluid is instilled via the catheter into the bladder. The point at which the patient first notes a feeling of the urge to void and the point at which he or she notes a strong urge to void are recorded. Bladder capacity and bladder pressure readings are recorded graphically. The patient is asked to void when the bladder instillation is complete (about 500 mL). The residual urine after voiding is recorded, and the catheter is removed. Electromyography of the perineal muscles may be performed during this examination.

As with any procedure that involves inserting instruments into the urinary tract, monitor for infection. Record the patient's temperature, the character of the urine, and the amount of urine output.

Urethral pressure profile (also called a *urethral pressure profilometry [UPP]*) can provide information about the nature of urinary incontinence or urinary retention.

Explain the procedure, and inform the patient that a urinary catheter may be needed temporarily during the procedure. A special catheter with pressure-sensing capabilities is inserted into the bladder. Variations in the pressure of the smooth muscle of the urethra are recorded as the catheter is slowly withdrawn.

As with any study involving inserting instruments into the urinary tract, monitor the patient for manifestations of infection.

Urine stream testing is used to evaluate pelvic muscle strength and the effectiveness of pelvic muscles in stopping the flow of urine. It is useful in assessing urinary incontinence.

Explain the procedure, and reassure the patient that efforts will be made to ensure privacy. The patient is asked to begin urinating. Three to five seconds after urination begins, the examiner gives the patient a signal to stop urine flow. The length of time required to stop the flow of urine is recorded.

Cleaning the perineal area, as after any voiding, is all that is necessary after the urine stream test.

Electromyography (EMG) of the perineal muscles tests the strength of the muscles used in voiding. This information may help identify methods of improving continence. Inform the patient that some temporary discomfort may accompany placement of the electrodes.

In EMG of the perineal muscles, electrodes are placed in either the rectum or the urethra to measure muscle contraction and relaxation. After the completion of EMG, administer analgesics as prescribed to promote the patient's comfort. Any discomfort is usually mild and of short duration.

Renal Biopsy

Patient Preparation. Explain that a kidney biopsy can help determine a cause of unexplained renal problems and can help direct or change therapy. Most renal biopsies are performed **percutaneously** (through the skin and other tissues) using ultrasound or CT guidance. The patient signs an informed consent. Patients are NPO for 4 to 6 hours before the procedure.

Because of the risk for bleeding after the biopsy, coagulation studies such as platelet count, activated partial thromboplastin time (aPTT), prothrombin time (PT), and bleeding time are performed before surgery. A blood transfusion may be needed to correct anemia before biopsy. Hypertension and uremia increase the risk for bleeding, and antihypertensive drugs or dialysis may be prescribed before a biopsy.

Procedure. In a percutaneous biopsy, the nephrologist or radiologist obtains tissue samples without an incision. Patients receive sedation and are monitored throughout the procedure. The patient is placed in the prone position on the procedure table. The entry site is selected after taking preliminary images. The area is prepped and sterilely draped. A local anesthetic is injected, and the physician then inserts the biopsy device into the tissues toward the kidney. Needle depth and placement are confirmed by ultrasound or CT. While the patient holds his or her breath, the needle is advanced into the renal cortex. Samples are then taken with a spring-loaded coring biopsy needle and sent for pathologic study.

Follow-up Care. After a percutaneous biopsy, the major risk is bleeding from the biopsy site. For 24 hours after the biopsy, monitor the dressing site, vital signs, urine output, hemoglobin level, and hematocrit. Even if the dressing is dry and there is no hematoma, the patient could be bleeding from the site. An internal bleed is not readily visible but is suspected with flank pain, decreasing blood pressure, decreasing urine output, or other signs of hypovolemia or shock.

The patient follows a plan of strict bedrest, lying in a supine position with a back roll for additional support for 2 to 6 hours after the biopsy. The head of the bed may be elevated, and the patient may resume oral intake of food and fluids. After bedrest, the patient may have limited bathroom privileges if there is no evidence of bleeding.

Monitor for hematuria, the most common complication of renal biopsy. Hematuria occurs microscopically in most patients, but 5% to 9% have gross hematuria. This problem usually resolves without treatment in 48 to 72 hours after the biopsy but can persist for 2 to 3 weeks. In rare cases, transfusions and surgery are required. There should be no obvious blood clots in the urine.

The patient may have some local pain after the percutaneous renal biopsy. If aching originates at the biopsy site and begins to radiate to the flank and around the front of the abdomen, bleeding may have started or a hematoma is forming around the kidney. This pattern of discomfort with bleeding occurs because blood in the tissues around the kidney increases pressure on local nerve tracts.

If bleeding occurs, IV fluid, packed red blood cells, or both may be needed to prevent shock. In general, a small amount of bleeding creates enough pressure to compress bleeding sites. This is called a "tamponade effect." If tamponade does not occur and bleeding is extensive, surgery for hemostasis or even nephrectomy may be needed. A hematoma in, on, or around the kidney may become infected, requiring treatment with antibiotics and surgical drainage.

If no bleeding occurs, the patient can resume general activities after 24 hours. Instruct him or her to avoid lifting heavy objects, exercising, or performing other strenuous activities for 1 to 2 weeks after the biopsy procedure. Driving may also be restricted. Refer to Chapter 18 for general postoperative care for the patient undergoing an open renal biopsy.

DECISION-MAKING CHALLENGE

Coordination of Care

A 78-year-old man with hypertension reports worsening symptoms of frequent urination, nocturia, straining to urinate, and a weak stream.

1. What questions can you ask to distinguish between obstructive symptoms associated with benign prostatic hyperplasia (BPH) and irritative symptoms that may indicate an infection?
2. What additional diagnostic testing can you anticipate at this time?
3. What nursing diagnosis do you consider?
4. What educational and psychosocial concerns can you anticipate for this patient?

evolve For suggested answer guidelines, go to http://evolve.elsevier.com/Iggy/.

HUMAN NEEDS ASSESSMENT REVIEW

What should you expect to NOTICE in a patient with adequate urinary elimination?

Vital Signs

- Body temperature is within normal range.
- Blood pressure is within normal range.

Physical Assessment

- Daily urine output is within 500 mL of daily fluid intake.
- Skin texture is normal (no edema or superficial crystals present).
- Skin color is appropriate for race with no excessive yellowing, bruising, or petechiae.
- Urine is clear and some variation of yellow in color.
- Patient voids 300 to 500 mL per voiding.
- Patient does not report pain or burning on urination.
- Patient has no difficulty starting or stopping the stream of urine.
- Patient is continent of urine and can maintain continence without sensation of urgency.

Psychological Assessment

- Patient is alert and oriented.

Laboratory Assessment

- Hematocrit and hemoglobin are within normal limits (no anemia).
- BUN and creatinine are within normal limits.
- Serum electrolytes are within normal ranges.
- Urinalysis shows no bacteria, blood, sediment, or protein.

GET READY FOR THE NCLEX EXAMINATION!

Key Points

Review these Key Points for each NCLEX Examination Client Needs Category.

Safe and Effective Care Environment

- Use sterile technique when inserting a catheter or any other instrument into the urinary system.
- Use Contact Precautions with any patient who has drainage from the genitourinary tract.
- Ask the patient if he or she has ever had an allergic reaction to radiopaque contrast dye, shellfish, or iodine.

Health Promotion and Maintenance

- Teach patients to clean the perineal area after voiding, after having a bowel movement, and after sexual intercourse.

- Urge all patients to maintain an adequate fluid intake (sufficient to dilute urine to a light yellow color). A minimum of 3 L/day may be recommended unless another health problem requires fluid restriction.
- Teach patients who come into contact with chemicals in their workplaces or for leisure time activities to avoid direct skin or mucous membrane contact with these chemicals.

Psychosocial Integrity

- Allow the patient the opportunity to express fear or anxiety about tests of the renal and urinary tract or about a potential change in renal function.
- Assess the patient's level of comfort in discussing issues related to elimination and the urogenital area.
- Explain all diagnostic procedures, restrictions, and follow-up care to the patient scheduled for tests.
- Provide as much privacy as possible for patients undergoing examination or testing of the renal/urinary tract.
- Use language and terminology that the patient can understand during discussions of renal/urinary assessment.

Physiological Integrity

- Ask the patient about renal problems in any other members of the family, because some problems have a genetic component.
- Ask the patient whether any nephrotoxic drugs have ever been used.
- Assess urine output closely after any procedure in which contrast dye is used IV.
- Assess the patient for bleeding or manifestations of infection after any invasive test of renal/urinary function.

Additional Study Resources

Go to your Companion CD or Evolve at http://evolve.elsevier.com/Iggy/ for *Self-Assessment Questions for the NCLEX Examination.*

evolve Go to Evolve at http://evolve.elsevier.com/Iggy/ for *Prioritization and Delegation Questions for the NCLEX Examination.*

SELECTED BIBLIOGRAPHY

Asterisk indicates a classic or definitive work on this subject.

Altschuler, V., & Diaz, L. (2006). Bladder ultrasound. *MEDSURG Nursing, 15*(5), 317-318.

Brenner, B.M., & Levine, S.A. (Eds.). (2007). *Brenner & Rector's the kidney* (8th ed.). Philadelphia: Saunders.

Combest, W., Newton, M., Combest, A., & Kosier, J.H. (2005). Effects of herbal supplements on the kidney. *Urologic Nursing, 25*(5), 381-386, 403.

Gordon, M. (2007). *Manual of nursing diagnosis* (11th ed.). Boston: Jones & Bartlett.

Jarvis, C. (2008). *Physical examination and health assessment* (5th ed.). Philadelphia: Saunders.

*Lancaster, L.E. (Ed.). (2001). *Core curriculum for nephrology nursing* (4th ed.). Pitman, NJ: A.J. Janetti.

Martin, J.L., Williams, K.S., Sutton, A.J., Abrams, K.R., & Assassa, R.P. (2006). Systematic review and meta-analysis of methods of diagnostic assessment for urinary incontinence. *Neurology and Urodynamics, 25*(7), 674-683.

McCance, K., & Huether, S. (2006). *Pathophysiology: The biologic basis for disease in adults and children* (5th ed.). St. Louis: Mosby.

Meiner, S., & Lueckenotte, A. (Eds.). (2006). *Gerontologic nursing* (3rd ed.). St. Louis: Mosby.

Namasivayam, S., Kalra, M.K., Torres, W.E., & Small, W.C. (2006). Adverse reactions to intravenous iodinated contrast media: An update. *Current Problems in Diagnostic Radiology, 35*, 164-169.

Nussbaum, R., McInnes, R., & Willard, H. (2007). *Thompson & Thompson: Genetics in medicine* (7th ed.). Philadelphia: Saunders.

Pagana, K., & Pagana, T. (2006). *Mosby's manual of diagnostic and laboratory tests* (3rd ed.). St. Louis: Mosby.

Price, D.A., Fisher, N.D., Osei, S.Y., Lansang, M.C., & Hollenberg, N.K. (2001). Renal perfusion and function in healthy African Americans. *Kidney International, 59*(3), 1037-1043.

Senese, V. (2006a). Female urethral catheterization. *Urologic Nursing, 26*(4), 314.

Senese, V. (2006b). Male urethral catheterization. *Urologic Nursing, 26*(4), 315.

*Shulman, N.B., & Hall, W.D. (1991). Renal vascular disease in African-Americans and other racial minorities. *Circulation, 83*(4), 1477-1479.

Toughill, E. (2005). Indwelling urinary catheters: Common mechanical and pathogenic problems. *AJN, 105*(5), 35-37.

U.S. Renal Data Systems. (2006). *USRDS 2006 annual data report.* Bethesda, MD: The National Institutes of Health, National Institute of Diabetes and Digestive and Kidney Diseases.

*Vander, A.J., & Navar, L.G. (2003). *Renal physiology* (6th ed.). New York: McGraw-Hill.

Wein, A.J., Kavoussi, L.R., Novick, A.C., Partin, A.W., & Peters, C.A. (2007). *Campbell-Walsh urology* (9th ed.). Philadelphia: Saunders.

Zurakowski, T., Taylor, M., & Bradway, C. (2006). Effective teaching strategies for the older adult with urologic concerns. *Urologic Nursing, 26*(5), 355-360.

69 CHAPTER

Care of Patients with Urinary Problems

Chris Winkelman

LEARNING OUTCOMES

For clinical competence and success on the NCLEX Examination, study this chapter with these Learning Outcomes in mind:

Safe and Effective Care Environment

1. Assess the appropriateness for continuing therapy with indwelling urinary catheters.
2. Use principles of asepsis during catheter insertion.

Health Promotion and Maintenance

3. Encourage everyone to have a daily fluid intake of at least 3 L unless another health problem requires fluid restriction.
4. Teach women hygiene measures to reduce the risk for urinary tract infections.
5. Teach the proper application of pelvic floor exercises to reduce or prevent urinary incontinence.
6. Encourage anyone who comes into contact with chemicals as part of work or hobbies to use appropriate personal protective equipment.

Psychosocial Integrity

7. Use language the patient is comfortable with when discussing urinary and sexual issues.
8. Encourage patients and families to express their feelings and concerns about a change in urinary elimination.
9. Explain to the patient and family what to expect during tests and procedures for urinary problems.
10. Refer patients with long-term urinary problems to appropriate community resources and support groups.

Physiological Integrity

11. Coordinate care to prevent urinary tract infections among hospitalized patients.
12. Compare the pathophysiology and manifestations of stress incontinence, urge incontinence, overflow incontinence, mixed incontinence, and functional incontinence.
13. Coordinate nursing care for the patient who has invasive bladder cancer.

Go to your Companion CD or Evolve at http://evolve.elsevier.com/Iggy/ for *Self-Assessment Questions for the NCLEX Examination* keyed to these Learning Outcomes.

The components of the urinary system are the ureters, bladder, and urethra. Their functions are to store the urine made by the kidney and eliminate it from the body. These actions do not contribute to the homeostatic purposes of the *human need for urinary elimination.* However, when problems in the urinary system interfere with the mechanics of moving urine out of the body, the human need for urinary elimination is not met and homeostasis of fluids, electrolytes, nitrogenous wastes, and blood pressure is disrupted.

Urinary problems affect the storage or elimination of urine. Both acute and chronic urinary problems are common and costly. More than 20 million people in the United States are treated annually for urinary tract infections, cystitis, kidney and ureter stones, or urinary incontinence (U.S. Renal Data Systems, 2006). Although life-threatening complications are rare with urinary problems, patients may have significant functional, physical, and psychosocial changes that reduce quality of life. Nursing interventions are directed toward prevention, detection, and management of urologic disorders.

INFECTIOUS DISORDERS

Infections of the urinary tract and kidneys are common, especially among women. Manifestations of urinary tract infection (UTI) account for more than 7 million health care visits and 1 million hospital admissions annually in the United States (National Kidney and Urologic Diseases Information Clearinghouse, 2007). UTIs are the most common hospital-acquired infection (www.cdc.gov). Total direct and indirect costs for adult urinary tract infections are estimated at $1.6 billion each year (Centers for Disease Control and Prevention [CDC], 2006).

Urinary tract infections are described by their location in the tract. Acute infections in the lower urinary tract include urethritis (urethra), cystitis (bladder), and prostatitis (prostate gland). Acute pyelonephritis is an upper urinary tract (kidney) infection. The site of infection is important to know because site, along with the specific type of bacteria present, determines treatment. Several risk factors are associated with occurrence of UTIs (Table 69-1).

CYSTITIS

Pathophysiology

Cystitis is an inflammation of the bladder. It can be caused by irritation or, more commonly, by infection from bacteria, viruses, fungi, or parasites. Infectious cystitis is the most common of the UTIs. Noninfectious cystitis is caused by irritation from chemicals or radiation. **Interstitial cystitis** is an inflammatory disease that has no known cause.

Infectious agents, most commonly bacteria, move up the urinary tract from the external urethra to the bladder. Less common, spread of infection through the blood and lymph fluid can occur. Once bacteria enter the urinary tract, several factors influence the outcome (Table 69-2).

The presence of bacteria in the urine is **bacteriuria** and can occur with any urologic infection. When bacteriuria is without

TABLE 69-1 Factors Contributing to Urinary Tract Infections

Factor	Mechanism
Obstruction	Incomplete bladder emptying creates a continuous pool of urine in which bacteria can grow, prevents flushing out of bacteria, and allows bacteria to ascend more easily to higher structures. Bacteria have a greater chance of multiplying the longer they remain in residual urine. Overdistention of the bladder damages the mucosa and allows bacteria to invade the bladder wall.
Stones (calculi)	Large stones can obstruct urine flow. The rough surface of a stone irritates mucosal surfaces and creates a spot where bacteria can establish and grow. Bacteria can live within stones and cause reinfection.
Vesicoureteral reflux	Bacteria-laden urine is forced backward from the bladder up into the ureters and kidneys, where pyelonephritis can develop. Reflux of sterile urine can cause kidney scarring, which may promote kidney dysfunction.
Diabetes mellitus	Excess glucose in urine provides a rich medium for bacterial growth. Peripheral neuropathy affects bladder innervation and leads to a flaccid bladder and incomplete bladder emptying.
Characteristics of urine	Alkalotic urine promotes bacterial growth. Concentrated urine promotes bacterial growth.
Gender	Women are susceptible to periurethral colonization with coliform bacteria. Use of diaphragms, frequency of intercourse, and a new partner within the past year are associated with UTI in women. Bladder displacement during pregnancy predisposes women to cystitis and the development of pyelonephritis. A diaphragm or pessary that is too large can obstruct urine flow or traumatize the urethra.
Age	Urinary stasis may be caused by incomplete bladder emptying as a result of an enlarged prostate in men and cystocele and prolapse in women. Neuromuscular conditions that cause incomplete bladder emptying, such as Parkinson disease and strokes, affect older adults more frequently. The use of anticholinergic drugs in older adults contributes to delayed bladder emptying. Fecal incontinence contributes to poor perineal hygiene. Hypoestrogenism in older women adversely affects the cells of the vagina and urethra, making them more susceptible to infections.
Sexual activity	Irritation of the perineum and urethra during intercourse can promote migration of bacteria from the perineal area to the urinary tract in some women. Spermicides can alter vaginal pH, increasing potential numbers of pathogens. Inadequate vaginal lubrication may exacerbate potential urethral irritation. Bacteria may be introduced into the man's urethra during anal intercourse or during vaginal intercourse with a woman who has a bacterial vaginitis.
Recent use of antibiotics	Antibiotics change normal protective flora, providing opportunity for pathogenic bacterial overgrowth and colonization.

TABLE 69-2 Important Factors Influencing the Outcome of Urinary Tract Infection

Facilitating Aspects	Protective Aspects
ANATOMY	
Females: Short length of the urethra and its proximity to the vagina and rectum facilitate colonization of coliform bacteria.	*Males:* Long length of the urethra and its distance from the rectum provide protection from colonization with coliform bacteria.
Males: With age, the prostate enlarges and may obstruct the normal flow of urine, producing stasis.	
PHYSIOLOGY	
Females: Pregnancy predisposes a woman to ureteral reflux and subsequent pyelonephritis; with age, the decline in estrogen facilitates colonization of *Escherichia coli.* In addition, vaginal atrophy can alter urethral competency.	*Females:* Well-estrogenized mucosa in the urethra and trigone may inhibit bacterial colonization and enhance urogenital blood flow.
Males: With age, prostatic secretions lose their antibacterial characteristics and predispose to bacterial proliferation in the urine.	*Males:* Normal prostatic secretions inhibit bacterial growth.
	Both males and females: Mucin is produced by urothelial cells lining the bladder—this helps maintain mucosal integrity and prevent cellular damage; mucin may also prevent bacteria from adhering to urothelial cells.
TRAUMA	
Females: Vaginal penetration with sexual intercourse may traumatize the urethra and bladder base, leading to postcoital (or "honeymoon") cystitis; a vaginal diaphragm that is too large can place pressure on the urethra, causing trauma; vaginal childbirth can cause permanent damage to the urethra.	*Females:* Adequate lubrication, either natural or artificial, with intercourse may prevent any trauma.
Males: Sexually transmitted diseases may cause urethral strictures that obstruct the flow of urine and predispose to urinary stasis.	
Both males and females: Urethral instrumentation (e.g., catheterization) may disturb the urothelial surface and predispose to adherence of bacteria that would ordinarily not be pathogenic.	
INFECTIOUS AGENT	
Some organisms are better able to adhere to host cells and secrete substances that induce inflammation.	A small inoculum (number of microorganisms introduced into the body) is more easily flushed away by the flow of urine.

symptoms of infection, it is called *colonization.* Colonization, asymptomatic bacteriuria, is more common in older adults. This problem does not appear to progress to acute infection or renal insufficiency unless the patient has other pathologic problems, and then it requires treatment.

Etiology and Genetic Risk

UTIs, like other infections, are the result of interactions between a pathogen and the host. Usually, a high bacterial virulence (ability to invade and infect) is needed to overcome normal strong host resistance. However, a compromised host is more likely to become infected even with bacteria that have low virulence. Genetically, invading bacteria with special adhesions are more likely to cause ascending UTIs that start in the urethra or bladder and move up into the ureter and kidney. Patient-specific genetic factors such as blood type and ability to produce bladder surface biofilms that protect bacteria may influence the risk for UTI (Bowen & Hellstrom, 2007).

The most common organisms in infectious cystitis are from the intestinal tract. About 90% of UTIs are caused by *Escherichia coli.* Less common organisms include *Staphylococcus saprophyticus, Klebsiella pneumoniae,* and organisms from the *Proteus* and *Enterobacter* species (Bowen & Hellstrom, 2007).

In most cases, organisms first grow in the perineal area, then move into the urethra as a result of irritation, trauma, or catheterization of the urinary tract, and finally ascend to the bladder. *Catheters are the most common factor placing patients at risk for UTIs in the hospital setting.* Within 48 hours of catheter insertion, bacterial colonization begins. About 50% of patients with indwelling catheters become infected within 1 week of catheter insertion (Toughill, 2005).

How a catheter-related infection occurs varies between genders. Bacteria from a woman's perineal area are more likely to ascend to the bladder by moving along the outside of the catheter. In men, bacteria tend to gain access to the bladder from inside the lumen of the catheter (Toughill, 2005). Any break in the closed urinary drainage system allows bacteria to move through the urinary tract. Best practices to reduce the risk of catheter contamination and catheter-related UTIs are listed in Chart 69-1.

Organisms other than bacteria also can cause cystitis. Fungal infections, such as those caused by *Candida,* can occur during long-term antibiotic therapy, because antibiotics change normal protective flora. Patients who are severely immunosuppressed, are receiving corticosteroids or other immunosuppressive agents, or have diabetes mellitus or acquired immune deficiency syndrome (AIDS) are at higher risk for fungal UTIs.

Viral and parasitic infections are rare and usually are transferred to the urinary tract from an infection at another body site. For example, *Trichomonas,* a parasite found in the vagina, can also be found in the urine. Treatment of the vaginal infection (see Chapter 74) also resolves the UTI.

Noninfectious cystitis may result from chemical exposure, such as to drugs (e.g., cyclophosphamide [Cytoxan, Procytox🍁]), from radiation therapy, and from immunologic responses, as with systemic lupus erythematosus (SLE).

Chart 69-1 BEST PRACTICE FOR PATIENT SAFETY & QUALITY CARE

Minimizing Catheter-Related Infection

- Assess patients daily for those who no longer need indwelling catheters.
- Consider appropriate alternatives to an indwelling catheter.
- Use aseptic routine when handling catheter devices; manipulation can promote an environment favorable to pathogens.
- Select a small-size catheter (14 to 18 Fr with a 5-mL balloon).
- Use strict sterile technique to insert the catheter (in the hospital setting); a break in technique can introduce pathogens into the urinary tract.
- Do not inject more than 10 mL into the balloon.
- Maintain a closed-system irrigation by ensuring that catheter tubing connections are sealed securely; disconnections can introduce pathogens into the urinary tract.
- Avoid routine catheter irrigation.
- Keep urine collection bags below the level of the bladder at all times; elevating the collection bag above the bladder causes reflux of pathogens from the bag into the urinary tract.
- Secure the catheter to the patient's thigh (women) or lower abdomen (men); catheter movement can cause urethral friction and irritation.
- Perform daily catheter care by washing the perineum and proximal portion of the catheter with soap and water and drying gently (removes pathogens and reduces pathogenic population).
- Consider the use of coated catheters for patients requiring indwelling catheters for more than 3 to 5 days. This coating reduces bacterial colonization along the catheter.

Application of antiseptic solutions or antibiotic ointments to the perineal area of catheterized patients has not been demonstrated to have any beneficial effect.

Data from Smith, J. (2003). Indwelling catheter management: From habit to evidence-based practice. *Ostomy and Wound Management, 49*(12), 34-45.

Interstitial cystitis is a rare, chronic inflammation of the entire lower urinary tract (bladder, urethra, and adjacent pelvic muscles) that is not a result of infection. The condition affects women ten times more often than men, and the diagnosis is difficult to make. Manifestations are similar to those of infectious cystitis with more intense urgency and bladder pain. Results from urinalysis and urine culture are negative for infection (Evans & Sant, 2007; Siegel, Sand, & Sasso, 2008).

Although cystitis is not life threatening, infectious cystitis can lead to life-threatening complications, including pyelonephritis and sepsis. The risk for kidney tissue damage followed by kidney failure as a result of bacteria ascending from the bladder to the kidney is controversial. Severe kidney damage is a rare complication unless the patient also has other predisposing factors, such as anatomic abnormalities, pregnancy, obstruction, reflux, calculi, or diabetes mellitus.

The spread of the infection from the urinary tract to the bloodstream is termed **urosepsis.** Sepsis from any source is a systemic infection that can lead to overwhelming organ failure, shock, and death. The most common cause of sepsis in the hospitalized patient is a UTI (www.cdc.gov). Sepsis has a high mortality and prolongs hospital stays (see Chapter 39).

Incidence/Prevalence

The incidence of UTI is second only to that of upper respiratory infections in primary care. Patients who have **frequency** (an urge to urinate frequently in small amounts), **dysuria** (pain or burning with urination), and **urgency** (the feeling that urination will occur immediately) account for more than 5 million health care visits annually. About 50% of these patients will have a confirmed UTI (National Kidney and Urologic Diseases Information Clearinghouse, 2007).

CONSIDERATIONS FOR OLDER ADULTS

The prevalence of UTIs varies with age and gender. Women of any age are more commonly affected with UTIs than are men. In men, the incidence of UTI greatly increases after 73 years of age. In women, the prevalence of UTIs increases from 20% among all women to 50% in those older than 80 years (National Kidney and Urologic Diseases Information Clearinghouse, 2007). Skin and mucous membrane changes from a lack of estrogen appear to account for much of the increased risk in older women. Prostate disease increases risk for UTIs in men.

Health Promotion and Maintenance

Although cystitis is common, in many cases it is preventable. In the health care setting, reducing the use of indwelling urinary catheters is a major prevention strategy. (See the Evidence-Based Practice box on p. 1554.) When catheters must be used, strict attention to sterile technique during insertion can reduce the risk for UTIs as can consistent and adequate perineal and catheter care (see Chart 67-1). Catheters should be removed as early as possible.

Changes in fluid intake patterns, urinary elimination patterns, and hygiene patterns can help prevent or reduce cystitis in the general population. Teach all people to have a minimum fluid intake of 3 L daily unless fluid restriction is needed for another health problem. Encourage people to drink more water rather than sugar-containing drinks. Teach people to avoid urinary stasis by urinating every 3 to 4 hours rather than waiting until the bladder is greatly distended. Encourage everyone either to bathe daily or to thoroughly wash the perineal and urethral areas daily. Other hygiene measures that specifically reduce the risk for cystitis and other UTIs are listed in Chart 69-2.

Patient-Centered Collaborative Care

Assessment

Physical Assessment/Clinical Manifestations

Frequency, urgency, and dysuria are the common manifestations of a urinary tract infection (UTI), but other manifestations may be present (Chart 69-3). Urine may be cloudy, foul smelling, or blood tinged. Ask the patient about risk factors for UTI during the assessment (see Table 69-1). For noninfectious cystitis, the Pelvic Pain and Urgency/Frequency Patient Symptom Scale (PUF) can identify patients with interstitial cystitis.

EVIDENCE-BASED PRACTICE

Take it out, take it out, remove it!

Robinson, S., Allen, L., Barnes, M.R., Berry, T.A., Foster, T.A., Friedrich, L.A., et al. (2007). Development of an evidence-based protocol for reduction on indwelling urinary catheter usage. *MEDSURG Nursing, 16*(3), 157-161.

One large tertiary care center examined its practices for insertion, maintenance, and removal of indwelling urinary catheters and the incidence of urinary tract infections (UTIs) among its patient population. The examination revealed that often catheters were placed in the emergency department automatically with no written prescription and no further evaluation of purpose. Other findings included that 41.5% of patients with indwelling catheters had no appropriate reason for catheter use, only 67% had a physician's prescription for catheter insertion, 64% were not removed until the day of hospital discharge, and 40% had UTI manifestations.

Based on catheter use limitations common in long-term care, a team of nurses implemented a pilot program to change practice regarding indwelling catheter use. The pilot program lasted 2 weeks and included a cohort of 35 patients with indwelling catheters who were similar to a cohort group of 34 patients with catheters on whom information was obtained immediately preceding the implementation of the limited-use protocol. The major intervention was that nurses were asked to evaluate patients with indwelling catheters and to request an order for removal if the use of the catheter did not meet established critical reasons. As a result of this intervention, documentation of catheter insertion and removal greatly increased, the percent of patients with UTI manifestations was reduced to 13%, and only 6% of patients still had catheters in place on day of discharge.

Level of Evidence—4. The study was a well-designed cohort study without randomization.

Commentary: Implications for Practice and Research. In addition to having positive results for a reduction of UTIs, this study pointed out problems with the lack of prescriptions for indwelling catheter insertion and removal, along with the sense of "tradition" rather than proven need for the continued use of indwelling catheters. The dramatic results of this intervention in terms of both reduction of UTIs and reduction in the practice of not removing catheters until day of discharge provide further support for the existing evidence that indwelling catheters are overused and misused. Similar studies with larger samples are needed to continue to provide broader-based support for limiting the use of indwelling catheters. In addition, educating physicians and nurses to think critically about the insertion and maintenance of indwelling catheters is key to the successful outcome of reducing the incidence of hospital-acquired UTIs.

Chart 69-2 PATIENT AND FAMILY EDUCATION GUIDE

Preventing a Urinary Tract Infection

- Drink at least 2 to 3 L of fluid every day.
- Be sure to get enough sleep, rest, and nutrition daily.
- [For women] Clean your perineum (the area between your legs) from front to back.
- [For women] Avoid using or wearing irritating substances, such as bubble bath, nylon underwear, and scented toilet tissue. Wear loose-fitting cotton underwear.
- [For women] Empty your bladder before and after intercourse.
- If you experience burning when you urinate, if you have to urinate frequently, or if you find it difficult to begin urinating, notify your physician or other health care provider right away, especially if you have a chronic medical condition (such as diabetes) or are pregnant.
- Empty your bladder as soon as you feel the urge to urinate.
- Empty your bladder regularly (every 4 hours), even if you do not feel the urge to urinate.
- You may try these home therapies:
  - Cranberry juice (pure), 50 mL daily
  - Apple cider vinegar, 2 tablespoons three times daily in juice
  - Vitamin C, 500 mg daily to acidify the urine
- To prevent recurrent infection:
  - Take your prescribed antibiotic or other drug as directed, even after the symptoms go away.
  - Schedule a follow-up appointment for 10 to 14 days after you finish taking the drug. At your follow-up visit, another urine sample may be taken for analysis or culture.

Before performing the physical assessment, ask the patient to void so that the urine can be examined and the bladder emptied before palpation. Assess vital signs to help rule out sepsis. Inspect the lower abdomen, and palpate the urinary bladder. Distention after voiding indicates incomplete bladder emptying.

Using Standard Precautions, record any lesions around the urethral meatus and vaginal opening. To help differentiate between a vaginal and a urinary tract infection, note whether there is any vaginal discharge (vaginal discharge and irritation are more indicative of vaginal infection). Women often report burning with urination when normal, acidic urine touches labial tissues that are inflamed or ulcerated by vaginal infections or sexually transmitted diseases (STDs). Maintain privacy with drapes during the examination.

The prostate is palpated by rectal examination for size, change in shape or consistency, and tenderness. The physician or advanced practice nurse performs the rectal prostate assessment.

Laboratory Assessment

Laboratory assessment for a UTI is a urinalysis with testing for leukocyte esterase and nitrate. The combination of a positive leukocyte esterase and nitrate is 68% to 88% sensitive in the diagnosis of a UTI (Bowan & Hellstrom, 2007). Although a urinalysis can include a microscopic count of bacteria, white blood cells (WBCs), and red blood cells (RBCs), this additional testing is more expensive, is time consuming, and may not improve diagnostic accuracy. The presence of more than

Chart 69-3 KEY FEATURES

Urinary Tract Infection

COMMON CLINICAL MANIFESTATIONS
- Frequency
- Urgency
- Dysuria
- Hesitancy or difficulty in initiating urine stream
- Low back pain
- Nocturia
- Incontinence
- Hematuria
- Pyuria
- Bacteriuria
- Retention
- Suprapubic tenderness or fullness
- Feeling of incomplete bladder emptying

RARE CLINICAL MANIFESTATIONS
- Fever
- Chills
- Nausea or vomiting
- Malaise
- Flank pain

CLINICAL MANIFESTATIONS THAT MAY OCCUR IN THE OLDER ADULT
- The only symptom may be something as vague as increasing mental confusion or frequent, unexplained falls.
- A sudden onset of incontinence or a worsening of incontinence may be the only symptom of an early UTI.
- Fever, tachycardia, tachypnea, and hypotension, even without any urinary symptoms, may be signs of urosepsis.
- Loss of appetite, nocturia, and dysuria are common symptoms.

UTI, Urinary tract infection.

20 epithelial cells/high power field (hpf) suggests contamination. The presence of 100,000 colonies/mL or the presence of three or more WBCs **(pyuria)** with RBCs **(hematuria)** indicates infection.

A urinalysis is performed on a clean-catch midstream specimen. If the patient cannot produce a clean-catch specimen, you may need to obtain the specimen with a small-diameter (6 Fr) catheter. For a routine urinalysis, 10 mL of urine is needed; smaller quantities are sufficient for culture.

A urine culture confirms the type of organism and the number of colonies. Urine culture is expensive and results take at least 48 hours. It is indicated when the UTI is complicated or does not respond to usual therapy or the diagnosis is uncertain. A UTI is confirmed when more than 10^5 colony-forming units are in the urine from any patient. In patients who also have symptoms of UTI, as few as 10^3 colony-forming units may allow the diagnosis to be made. The presence of many different types of organisms in low colony counts usually indicates that the specimen is contaminated. Sensitivity testing follows culture results when complicating factors are present (e.g., stones or recurrent infection), when the patient is older, or to ensure the appropriate antibiotics are prescribed.

Occasionally the serum WBC count may be elevated, with the differential WBC count showing a "left shift" (see Chapter 19). This shift indicates that the number of immature WBCs is increasing in response to the infection. As a result, the number of bands, or immature WBCs, is elevated. Left shift most often occurs with urosepsis and rarely occurs with uncomplicated cystitis, which is a local rather than a systemic infection.

Other Diagnostic Assessment

The diagnosis of cystitis is based on the history, physical examination, and laboratory data. If urinary retention and obstruction of urine outflow are suspected, urography, abdominal sonography, or computed tomography (CT) may be needed to locate the site of obstruction or the presence of calculi. Voiding cystourethrography (see Chapter 68) is needed when ureteral reflux is suspected.

Cystoscopy (see Chapter 68) may be performed when the patient has recurrent UTIs (more than three or four a year). A urine culture is performed first to ensure no infection is present. If infection is present, the urine is sterilized with antibiotic therapy before the procedure to reduce the risk for sepsis. Cystoscopy identifies abnormalities that increase the risk for cystitis. Such abnormalities include bladder calculi, bladder diverticula, urethral strictures, foreign bodies (e.g., sutures from previous surgery), and **trabeculation** (an abnormal thickening of the bladder wall caused by urinary retention and obstruction). Retrograde pyelography, along with the cystoscopic examination, shows outlines and images of the drainage tract. Areas of obstruction or malformation and the presence of reflux are then identified early.

Cystoscopy is needed to accurately diagnose interstitial cystitis. A urinalysis usually shows WBCs and RBCs but no bacteria. Common findings in interstitial cystitis are a small-capacity bladder, the presence of Hunner's ulcers (a type of bladder lesion), and small hemorrhages after bladder distention.

Common Nursing Diagnoses and Collaborative Problems

Nursing diagnoses and collaborative problems that may apply to patients with cystitis include:
- Acute Pain related to bladder spasms
- Deficient Knowledge (risk factors for cystitis and drug regimen) related to information misinterpretation or unfamiliarity with information resources
- Urge Urinary Incontinence related to irritation of bladder stretch receptors causing spasm (e.g., bladder infection)
- Risk for Impaired Skin Integrity related to moisture from incontinence
- Risk for Sepsis

Interventions

Nonsurgical Management

Drug Therapy. Drugs used to treat bacteriuria and promote patient comfort include urinary antiseptics or antibiotics, analgesics, and antispasmodics. Cure of a UTI depends on the antibiotic levels achieved in the urine (Chart 69-4). Antifungal agents are prescribed for fungal infections. Amphotericin B is most often given in daily bladder instillations, and ketoconazole (Nizoral) is given orally. Antispasmodic drugs decrease bladder spasm and promote complete bladder emptying.

Antibiotic therapy is used for bacterial UTIs (see Chart 69-4). Guidelines indicate that a 3-day course of trimethoprim/sulfamethoxazole or fosfomycin is effective in treating uncomplicated, community-acquired UTIs in women (Bowen & Hellstrom, 2007). Single-dose therapy with long-acting fluoroquinolones is being studied. The shorter courses increase adherence and reduce cost. Longer antibiotic treatment (7 to

Chart 69-4 COMMON EXAMPLES OF DRUG THERAPY

Urinary Tract Infections

Drug/Dosage	Purpose/Action	Nursing Interventions	Rationales
ANTIMICROBIALS			
SULFONAMIDES			
Trimethoprim*/sulfamethoxazole (Bactrim, Bacter-Aid, Septra, Sulfatrim, Sultrex, Roubac♣) 60 mg trimethoprim/800 mg sulfamethoxazole orally every 12 hr	Drug reduces bacteria in the urinary tract by direct killing (trimethoprim) and by inhibiting bacterial reproduction (sulfamethoxazole).	Ask patients about drug allergies, especially to sulfa drugs, before beginning drug therapy.	Allergies to sulfa drugs are common and require changing the drug therapy.
		Teach patients to drink a full glass of water with each dose and to have an overall fluid intake of at least 3 L daily.	Sulfamethoxazole can form crystals that precipitate in the kidney tubules. Fluid intake prevents this complication.
		Teach patients to keep out of the sun or to wear protective clothing outdoors and use a sunscreen.	This drug increases skin sensitivity to the sun and can lead to severe sunburns even in darker-skinned patients.
		Caution patients to complete the drug regimen even if the symptoms improve or disappear sooner.	Not completing the drug regimen can lead to an infection recurrence and to bacterial drug resistance.
QUINOLONES			
Ciprofloxacin (Cipro, ProQuin) 250 mg orally twice daily Gatifloxacin♣ (Tequin, Zymar) 200-400 mg orally or IV once daily **Med Error Alert!** Do not confuse Tequin with Tegretol, an oral anticonvulsant, or with Ticlid, a platelet inhibitor. Levofloxacin (Levaquin) 250 mg orally daily Lomefloxacin (Maxaquin) 250 mg orally daily Norfloxacin (Noroxin) 400 mg orally twice daily **Med Error Alert!** Do not confuse Noroxin with Neurontin, an oral anticonvulsant. Ofloxacin (Floxin) 200 mg orally twice daily Sparfloxacin (Zagam) 200-400 mg orally daily	Drugs from this class reduce bacteria in the urinary tract by direct killing (bactericidal actions) and by inhibiting bacterial reproduction (bacteriostatic actions).	Teach patients taking the extended-release drugs to swallow them whole, not to crush or chew the tablets.	Crushing or chewing the tablet releases all the drug at once, ruining the extended effect.
		Warn patients to not take the drug within 2 hours of taking an antacid.	Many antacids (especially those containing magnesium or aluminum) interfere with drug absorption.
		Teach patients how to take their pulse, to monitor it twice daily while on this drug, and to notify the prescriber if new-onset irregular heartbeats occur.	This class of drugs can induce serious cardiac dysrhythmias.
		Teach patients to keep out of the sun or to wear protective clothing outdoors and use a sunscreen.	Most quinolones increase skin sensitivity to the sun and can lead to severe sunburns even in darker-skinned patients.
		Caution patients to complete the drug regimen even if the symptoms improve or disappear sooner.	Not completing the drug regimen can lead to an infection recurrence and to bacterial drug resistance.
PENICILLINS			
Amoxicillin (Amoxil) 500 mg orally every 12 hr Amoxicillin/clavulanate (Augmentin, Clavulin♣) 500 mg/125 mg orally every 12 hr	Drugs from this class reduce bacteria in the urinary tract by direct killing (bactericidal actions) as a result of interrupting bacterial cell wall synthesis.	Ask patients about drug allergies to penicillin before beginning drug therapy.	Allergies to penicillin are common and require changing the drug therapy.
		Teach patients to take the drug with food.	Taking it with food reduces the risk for GI upset.
		Instruct patients to call the prescriber if severe or watery diarrhea develops.	A complication of penicillin therapy is pseudomembranous colitis, which may require discontinuing the drug.

*Trimethoprim can be given alone to patients with a sulfa allergy.

Chart 69-4 COMMON EXAMPLES OF DRUG THERAPY

Urinary Tract Infections—cont'd

Drug/Dosage	Purpose/Action	Nursing Interventions	Rationales
PENICILLINS—cont'd			
Amoxicillin—cont'd		Suggest that women who take oral contraceptives use an additional method of birth control while taking this drug.	Penicillin appears to reduce the effectiveness of estrogen-containing oral contraceptives.
		Caution patients to complete the drug regimen even if the symptoms improve or disappear sooner.	Not completing the drug regimen can lead to an infection recurrence and to bacterial drug resistance.
CEPHALOSPORINS			
Cefadroxil (Duricef) 1000 mg orally every 12 hr Cefixime (Suprax)	Drugs from this class reduce bacteria in the urinary tract by direct killing (bactericidal actions) as a result of interrupting bacterial cell wall synthesis.	Ask about drug allergies to penicillin or cephalosporins before beginning drug therapy.	Drugs in this class are structurally similar to penicillin. Anyone with allergies to penicillin is likely to be allergic to the cephalosporins.
		Instruct patients to call the prescriber if severe or watery diarrhea develops.	A complication of penicillin therapy is pseudomembranous colitis, which may require discontinuing the drug.
		Caution patients to complete the drug regimen even if the symptoms improve or disappear sooner.	Not completing the drug regimen can lead to an infection recurrence and to bacterial drug resistance.
Fosfomycin (Monurol) 3 g orally as a one-time dose	This drug reduces bacteria in the urinary tract by direct killing (bactericidal actions) as a result of interrupting bacterial cell wall synthesis.	Instruct patients to mix the contents of a package in about $^1/_2$ cup of cold water, stir well, and drink all the liquid.	This oral drug is available as granules that must be dissolved before taking.
		Avoid taking this drug when also taking metoclopramide or any other drug that increases GI motility.	Drugs that increase GI motility reduce the absorption of fosfomycin.
URINARY ANTISEPTICS			
Nitrofurantoin (Furadantin, Macrobid, Macrodantin, Nephronex♣ Urotoin) 100 mg orally every 12 hr	Drugs from this class usually reduce bacteria in the urinary tract by inhibiting bacterial reproduction (bacteriostatic actions).	Teach patients to shake the bottle well before measuring the drug.	Drug is a suspension and requires shaking to ensure homogeneity.
		Suggest that patients obtain a calibrated spoon for liquid drugs and to not use household spoons.	Household spoons are not accurate for measuring drugs.
		Teach patients to drink a full glass of water with each dose and to have an overall fluid intake of at least 3 L daily.	Drug precipitates in the kidney tubules and damages the kidney. Fluid intake prevents this complication.
		Caution patients to complete the drug regimen even if the symptoms improve or disappear sooner.	Not completing the drug regimen can lead to an infection recurrence and to bacterial drug resistance.
BLADDER ANALGESICS			
Phenazopyridine (Azo-Dine, Prodium, Pyridiate, Pyridium, Uristat, Phenazo♣) 200 mg orally 3 times daily, after meals	Drug reduces bladder pain and burning on urination by exerting a topical analgesic or local anesthetic effect on the mucosa of the urinary tract.	Remind patients that this drug will not treat an infection, only the symptoms.	Drug does not have any antibacterial actions.
		Teach patients to take the drug with or immediately after a meal.	Food reduces the risk for GI disturbances.

Continued

Chart 69-4 COMMON EXAMPLES OF DRUG THERAPY

Urinary Tract Infections—cont'd

Drug/Dosage	Purpose/Action	Nursing Interventions	Rationales
BLADDER ANALGESICS—*cont'd*			
Phenazopyridine—cont'd		Warn patients that urine will turn red or orange.	This expected response to the drug may stain clothing or toilets.
ANTISPASMODICS			
Hyoscyamine (Anaspaz, Cystospaz, many others) 0.125 mg-0.25 mg orally, 3 to 4 times daily	Drug relieves bladder spasms by inhibiting nerve stimulation to the bladder muscle.	Teach patients to notify the prescriber if blurred vision or other eye problems, confusion, dizziness or fainting spells, fast heartbeat, fever, or difficulty passing urine occurs.	These are manifestations of drug toxicity.
		Teach patients to wear dark glasses in sunlight or other bright light areas.	Drug dilates the pupil and increases eye sensitivity to light.

21 days) is required for hospitalized patients; those with complicating factors, such as pregnancy, indwelling catheters, or stones; and those with diabetes or immunosuppression.

Long-term antibiotic therapy is used for chronic, recurring infections caused by structural abnormalities or stones. Trimethoprim 100 mg daily may be used for long-term management of the older patient with frequent UTIs. For women who have recurrent UTIs after intercourse, one low-dose tablet of trimethoprim (TMP) (Proloprim, Trimpex) or TMP/sulfamethoxazole (half or single-strength Bactrim, Cotrim, Septra) or nitrofurantoin (Macrodantin, Nephronex🍁, Novofuran🍁) after intercourse is often prescribed. Estrogen used as an intravaginal cream may prevent recurrent UTIs in the postmenopausal woman although this therapy is controversial.

Urinary Elimination Management. The goal is to maintain an optimal urinary elimination pattern. Nursing interventions for the management of cystitis focus on comfort and teaching about therapy and prevention measures.

> **WOMEN'S HEALTH CONSIDERATIONS**
>
> Pregnant women with a bacterial UTI require prompt and aggressive treatment because simple cystitis can lead to acute pyelonephritis during pregnancy. Pyelonephritis in pregnancy can cause preterm labor and adversely affect the fetus.

Nutrition Therapy. The diet should include all food groups and include more calories for the increased metabolism caused by infection. Urge patients to drink enough fluid to maintain diluted urine throughout the day and night unless fluid restriction is needed for another health problem. The daily drinking of 50 mL of concentrated cranberry juice appears to decrease the ability of bacteria to adhere to the epithelial cells lining the urinary tract, decreasing the incidence of symptomatic UTIs in some patients. Cranberry juice must be consumed for 3 to 4 weeks to be effective, and the efficacy of cranberry tablets has not been established (Bowen & Hellstrom, 2007). It is important to note that cranberry juice is an irritant to the bladder with interstitial cystitis and should be avoided by patients with this condition. Avoiding caffeine, carbonated beverages, and tomato products may decrease bladder irritation during cystitis (Janos & Higgins, 2007).

Comfort Measures. A warm sitz bath taken two or three times a day for 20 minutes may provide comfort and some relief of local symptoms. If burning with urination is severe or urinary retention occurs, teach the patient to sit in the sitz bath and urinate into the warm water.

Surgical Management

Surgery for cystitis treats the conditions that increase the risk for recurrent UTIs (e.g., removal of obstructions and repair of vesicoureteral reflux). Procedures may include cystoscopy (see Chapter 68) to identify and remove calculi or obstructions.

Community-Based Care

Assess the patient's level of understanding of the problem. His or her knowledge about factors that promote the development of cystitis determines the type of teaching interventions planned.

Teach the patient how to take prescribed drugs. Stress the need for correct spacing of doses throughout the day and the need to complete all of the prescribed drugs. If the drug will change the color of the urine, as it does with phenazopyridine (Pyridium, Urogesic, Phenazo🍁), inform the patient to expect this change. Offer techniques for remembering the drug schedule, such as the use of a daily calendar or the association of drugs with usual activities (e.g., mealtimes).

Patients may associate symptoms of discomfort with sexual activities and have feelings of guilt and embarrassment. Frank and sensitive discussions with a woman who has recurrences of UTI after sexual intercourse can help her find techniques to handle the problem (see Chart 69-2). Explore with her the factors that contribute to her infections, such as diaphragm use and her general resistance to infection. Remind the patient that vigorous cleaning of the perineum with harsh soaps and vaginal douching may irritate the perineal tissues and increase the risk for UTI. At the patient's request, discuss the problem with her and her partner to help them find ways of maintaining their intimate relationship.

DECISION-MAKING CHALLENGE
Coordination of Care

The patient is a 24-year-old woman with a history of type 1 diabetes mellitus for the past 10 years. She is 2 days postpartum after an emergency C-section. She was 34 weeks pregnant and had difficulties throughout her pregnancy with hypertension. During the delivery, a Foley catheter was inserted to help manage fluid balance. Her Foley catheter was removed last night, and she reported burning during her first void about 4 hours after the Foley was removed. Today with her second void, she continues to describe pain on urination. Her urine is pink-tinged, cloudy, and straw-colored. Current vital signs are: T, 97.8° F; P, 88; R, 12; and BP, 142/88. Morning laboratory test results included a CBC with normal values, including a white blood cell count of 9600. Her basic metabolic panel was normal with a BUN of 13 mg/dL and a creatinine of 1.0 mg/dL.

1. What risk factors are present in this patient related to a urinary tract infection?
2. What other assessment data should you obtain and why?
3. What interventions will you teach her for comfort and treatment of this infection?
4. She asks if this means her kidneys will be harmed; she knows as a diabetic she is already at increased risk for nephropathy. As you respond, what level of language will you use?

evolve For suggested answer guidelines, go to http://evolve.elsevier.com/Iggy/.

URETHRITIS

Pathophysiology

Urethritis is an inflammation of the urethra that causes symptoms similar to urinary tract infection (UTI). In men, manifestations of urethritis are burning or difficulty with urination and a discharge from the urethral meatus. The most common cause of urethritis in men is sexually transmitted diseases (STDs). These include gonorrhea or nonspecific urethritis caused by *Ureaplasma* (a gram-negative bacterium), *Chlamydia* (a sexually transmitted gram-negative bacterium), or *Trichomonas vaginalis* (a protozoan found in both the male and female genital tract).

In women, urethritis causes manifestations similar to those of bacterial cystitis. Urethritis is known by several other terms: *pyuria-dysuria syndrome, frequency-dysuria syndrome, trigonitis syndrome,* and *urethral syndrome.* Urethritis is most common in postmenopausal women and is probably caused by tissue changes related to low estrogen levels.

Patient-Centered Collaborative Care

Ask the patient about a history of STD, painful or difficult urination, discharge from the penis or vagina, and discomfort in the lower abdomen. Urinalysis may show **pyuria** (white blood cells [WBCs] in the urine) without a large number of bacteria. However, results of urethral culture may indicate an STD. In women, the diagnosis may be made by excluding cystitis when urinalysis and urethral culture are negative for bacteria but symptoms persist. In such cases, pelvic examination may reveal tissue changes from low estrogen levels in the vagina. Urethroscopy may show low estrogen changes with inflammation of urethral tissues.

STDs and infection are treated with antibiotic therapy. More information on STDs can be found in Chapter 76.

Postmenopausal women often have improvement in their urethral symptoms with the use of estrogen vaginal cream. Estrogen cream applied locally to the vagina increases the amount of estrogen in the urethra as well, and irritating symptoms are reduced.

NONINFECTIOUS DISORDERS

URETHRAL STRICTURES

Urethral strictures are narrowed areas of the urethra. These problems may be caused by complications of an STD (usually gonorrhea) and by trauma during catheterization, urologic procedures, or childbirth. About one third of urethral strictures have no obvious cause. Strictures occur more often in men than in women. They may be a factor in other urologic problems, such as recurrent UTIs, urinary incontinence, and urinary retention.

The most common symptom of urethral stricture is obstruction of urine flow. Strictures rarely cause pain. Because urine stasis can result when flow is obstructed, the patient with a stricture is at risk for developing a UTI and may have overflow incontinence. **Overflow incontinence** is the involuntary loss of urine when the bladder is overdistended. Assess the patient for these two problems.

A urethral stricture is treated surgically. Dilation of the urethra (using a local anesthetic) is only a temporary measure, not a curative one. Stent placement can be used in some patients. The best chance of long-term cure is with **urethroplasty,** the surgical removal of the affected area with or without grafting to create a larger opening. The recurrence rate after surgery is still high, and most patients need repeated procedures. The urethral stricture location and length are the most important factors affecting choice of interventions and recovery.

URINARY INCONTINENCE

Pathophysiology

Continence is the control over the time and place of urination and is unique to humans and some domestic animals. It is a learned behavior in which a person can suppress the urge to urinate until a socially appropriate location is available (e.g., a toilet). Efficient bladder emptying (i.e., coordination between bladder contraction and urethral relaxation) is needed for continence.

Incontinence is an involuntary loss of urine severe enough to cause social or hygienic problems. It is *not* a normal consequence of aging or childbirth and often is a stigmatizing and an underreported health problem. Many people suffer in silence, are socially isolated, and may be unaware that treatment is available. In addition, the cost of incontinence can be enormous.

Continence occurs when pressure in the urethra is greater than pressure in the bladder. For normal voiding to occur, the urethra must relax and the bladder must contract with enough pressure and duration to empty completely. Voiding should occur in a smooth and coordinated manner under a person's conscious control. Incontinence has several possible causes and can be either temporary or chronic (Table 69-3). Temporary causes usually do not involve a disorder of the urinary tract. The most common forms of adult urinary incontinence are stress incontinence, urge incontinence, overflow incontinence, functional incontinence, and a mixed form.

TABLE 69-3 **Types of Urinary Incontinence**

Type	Definition/Description	Cause	Clinical Manifestations
Stress incontinence	The involuntary loss of urine during activities that increase abdominal and detrusor pressure. Patients cannot tighten the urethra sufficiently to overcome the increased detrusor pressure; leakage of urine results.	Weakening of bladder neck supports; associated with childbirth. Intrinsic sphincter deficiency caused by such congenital conditions as epispadias (abnormal location of the urethra on the dorsum of the penis) or myelomeningocele. Acquired anatomic damage to the urethral sphincter (from repeated incontinence surgeries, prostatectomy, radiation therapy, and trauma).	Urine loss with physical exertion, cough, sneeze, or exercise. Usually only small amounts of urine are lost with each exertion. Normal voiding habits (≤8 times per day, ≤2 or fewer times per night). Postvoid residual usually ≤50 mL. Pelvic examination shows hypermobility of the urethra or bladder neck with Valsalva maneuvers.
Urge incontinence	The involuntary loss of urine associated with a strong desire to urinate. Patients cannot suppress the signal from the bladder muscle to the brain that it is time to urinate.	Unknown.	An abrupt and strong urge to void. May have loss of large amounts of urine with each occurrence.
Detrusor hyperreflexia (reflex incontinence)	The abnormal detrusor contractions result from neurologic abnormalities.	Central nervous system (CNS) lesions from stroke, multiple sclerosis, and parasacral spinal cord lesions. Local irritating factors such as caffeine, medications, or bladder tumor.	Postvoid residual ≤50 mL.
Overflow incontinence	The involuntary loss of urine associated with overdistention of the bladder when the bladder's capacity has reached its maximum. The urethra is obstructed, so it fails to relax sufficiently to allow urine to flow, resulting in incomplete bladder emptying or complete urinary retention, causing overflow incontinence.	Diabetic neuropathy; side effects of medication; after radical pelvic surgery or spinal cord damage; outlet obstruction. Causes external to the mechanism of the urethra: an enlarged prostate (male patients) and large genital prolapse (female patients). When the cause is intrinsic to the urethra, abnormal contraction of the skeletal muscle occurs, causing obstruction. This condition, called *detrusor dyssynergia,* is seen in patients with spinal cord injuries and multiple sclerosis.	Bladder distention, often up to the level of the umbilicus. Constant dribbling of urine.
Mixed incontinence	A combination of stress, urge, and overflow incontinence.	As with each separate disorder.	As with each separate disorder.
Functional incontinence	Leakage of urine caused by factors other than disease of the lower urinary tract.		Quantity and timing of urine leakage vary; patterns are difficult to discern.
Transient causes	Transient causes improve with treatment of the underlying condition.	Loss of cognitive functioning. Loss of awareness that urination is to occur in a socially acceptable place.	Altered mental state, as in delirium, confusion, depression, dementia, sepsis, mental illness, or severe psychological stress.
		Abnormal openings in the urinary tract, such as a fistula or diverticulum.	Urinary drainage noted from areas other than the urinary meatus.
		Drugs, such as sedatives, hypnotics, diuretics, anticholinergics, decongestants, antihypertensives, and calcium channel blockers.	Some drugs cause altered mental state; others cause increased urine production.
		Diabetes insipidus or psychogenic polydipsia.	Increased urine output.
		Inability to get to toileting facilities.	Restraints, restricted mobility.
		Direct bladder pressure or urethral obstruction.	Constipation or fecal impaction.

TABLE 69-3 Types of Urinary Incontinence—cont'd

Type	Definition/Description	Cause	Clinical Manifestations
Permanent causes	Permanent causes are organic but may be improved with treatment.	Cognitive impairment. Traumatic or surgical effects. Those factors contributing to stress incontinence, urge incontinence, and overflow incontinence. Structural or functional defects of the bladder or the sphincters. Injuries or diseases of the spinal cord, brainstem, or cerebral cortex (neurogenic bladder). Congenital defects, including exstrophy of the bladder (bladder turned "inside out") and spina bifida.	Clinical manifestations depend on the cause.

Stress incontinence is the most common type. Its main feature is the loss of small amounts of urine during coughing, sneezing, jogging, or lifting. In the continent person, the urethra can be relaxed and tightened under conscious control because skeletal muscles of the pelvic floor surround it. When a person feels the urge to urinate, the conscious contraction of the urethra can override a bladder contraction if the urethral contraction is strong enough.

Patients who have *stress incontinence* cannot tighten the urethra enough to overcome the increased detrusor pressure. Stress incontinence is common after childbirth, when the pelvic muscles are stretched and weakened. The weakened pelvic floor allows the urethra to move during exertion. If the pelvic muscles are not strengthened, this condition continues. Low estrogen levels after menopause also contribute to stress incontinence. Vaginal, urethral, and pelvic floor muscles become thin and weak without estrogen.

Urge incontinence is the perception of an urgent need to urinate as a result of bladder contractions regardless of the volume of urine in the bladder. When the bladder is full, contraction of the smooth muscle fibers of the bladder detrusor muscle normally signals the brain that it is time to urinate. Continent persons override that signal and relax the detrusor muscle for the time it takes to locate a toilet. Those who suffer from urge incontinence cannot suppress the signal and have a sudden strong urge to void and often leak large amounts of urine at this time. Urge incontinence is also known as an "overactive bladder" or an *unstable bladder.* Overactivity may have no known cause or be the result of abnormal detrusor contractions related to other problems. Such problems include stroke and other neurologic problems, other urinary tract problems, and irritation from concentrated urine or artificial sweeteners, caffeine, alcohol, and citric intake. Drugs, such as diuretics, and nicotine can also irritate the bladder.

Mixed incontinence is the presence of more than one type of incontinence. Often urine loss is related to both stress and urge incontinence. The manifestations mimic more than one subtype. This category is more common in older women.

Overflow incontinence occurs when the detrusor muscle fails to contract and the bladder becomes overdistended. This type of incontinence (also known as "reflex incontinence") occurs when the bladder has reached its maximum capacity and some urine must leak out to prevent bladder rupture. Causes for the underactive (acontractile) bladder may or may not be determined.

The urethra can be obstructed so that it fails to relax enough to allow urine flow. Incomplete bladder emptying or urinary retention due to urethral obstruction results in overflow incontinence.

Functional incontinence is defined as incontinence occurring as a result of factors other than the abnormal function of the bladder and urethra. A common factor is the loss of cognitive function in patients affected by dementia. To maintain continence, a person must be aware that urination needs to occur in a socially acceptable place. Patients with dementia may not have that awareness.

Etiology and Genetic Risk

Incontinence may have temporary or permanent causes. Evaluation of the incontinent patient means considering all possible causes, beginning with those that are temporary and correctable. Surgical and traumatic causes of urinary incontinence are related to procedures or surgery in the lower pelvic structures, areas that contain complex nerve pathways. Radical urologic, prostatic, and gynecologic procedures for treatment of pelvic cancers may result in urinary incontinence. Injury to segments S2 to S4 of the spinal cord may cause incontinence from impairment of normal nerve pathways.

Inappropriate bladder contraction may result from disorders of the brain and nervous system or from bladder irritation due to chronic infection, stones, chemotherapy, or radiation therapy. Failure of bladder contraction occurs with the autonomic neuropathy of diabetes mellitus and syphilis.

CONSIDERATIONS FOR OLDER ADULTS

Many factors contribute to urinary incontinence in older adults (Chart 69-5). An older person may have decreased mobility from many causes. In the hospital or extended-care setting, mobility is limited when the older patient is restrained or placed on bedrest. Vision and hearing impairments may also prevent the patient from locating a call light to notify the nurse or assistive personnel of the need to void. Assess for these factors, and minimize them to prevent urinary incontinence. Getting out of bed to urinate is a common cause of falls among older adults.

Chart 69-5 NURSING FOCUS ON THE OLDER ADULT

Factors Contributing to Urinary Incontinence*

DRUGS

- Central nervous system depressants, such as opioid analgesics, decrease the patient's level of consciousness and the urge to void, and they contribute to constipation.
- Diuretics cause frequent voiding, often of large amounts of urine.
- Multiple drugs can contribute to changes in mental status or mobility, and they can irritate the bladder.
- Anticholinergic drugs or drugs with anticholinergic side effects are especially challenging, because they affect both cognition and the ability to void. Monitor patient responses to these drugs early in treatment.

DISEASE

- Cerebrovascular accidents and other neurologic disorders decrease mobility, sensation, or cognition.
- Arthritis decreases mobility and causes pain.
- Parkinson disease causes muscle rigidity and an inability to initiate movement.

DEPRESSION

- Depression decreases the energy necessary to maintain continence.
- Decreased self-esteem and feelings of self-worth decrease the importance to the patient of maintaining continence.

INADEQUATE RESOURCES

- Patients who have glasses or use a cane, walker, or slippers may be afraid to ambulate.
- Products that help patients manage incontinence are often costly.
- No one may be available to assist the patient to the bathroom or help with incontinence products.

*These factors are in addition to the physiologic changes of aging given in Chapter 3.

Incidence/Prevalence

Incontinence is a major health problem that affects more than 13 million people of all ages in the United States (Agency for Health Care Policy and Research [AHCPR], 2001a). About 85% are women. It is most common in older adults, including 15% to 30% of community-dwelling older people and at least one half of all nursing home residents (AHCPR, 2001a).

In adult patients younger than 65 years, urinary incontinence occurs twice as often in women as in men. Incontinence in women of this age may occur after one or more pregnancies. Men in this age-group rarely experience incontinence unless they have prostate disease or a spinal cord injury.

Patient-Centered Collaborative Care

evolve ONLINE PHARM REVIEW

Assessment

History

Effective screening includes asking patients to respond "always," "sometimes," or "never" to these questions:

- Do you ever leak urine or water when you don't want to?
- Do you ever leak urine or water when you cough, laugh, or exercise?
- Do you ever leak urine or water on the way to the bathroom?
- Do you ever use pads, tissue, or cloth in your underwear to catch urine?

If any answer is always or sometimes, proceed with a focused assessment (AHCPR, 2001b) (Chart 69-6). Incontinence may be underreported because health care professionals do not ask patients about urine loss. *Do not assume that patients will volunteer the information without specifically being asked.*

Physical Assessment/Clinical Manifestations

Assess the abdomen to estimate bladder fullness, to rule out palpable hard stool, and to evaluate bowel sounds. With a physician's request, determine the amount of residual urine

Chart 69-6 FOCUSED ASSESSMENT

The Patient with Urinary Incontinence

Note the presence of risk factors for urinary incontinence:

- Age
- If female, menopausal status
- Neurologic disease:
  - Parkinson disease
  - Dementia
  - Multiple sclerosis
  - Stroke
  - Spinal injury
- Diabetes mellitus
- Childbirth
- Urologic procedures
- Prescribed and over-the-counter drugs
- Bowel patterns
- Stress/anxiety level

Detail the symptoms of urinary incontinence:

- Leakage
- Frequency
- Urgency
- Nocturia
- Sensation of full bladder before leakage

Obtain a 24-hour intake and output record or a voiding diary:

- Time and amount of oral intake and continent voidings
- Time and estimated amount of incontinent leakages
- Activity around the time of leakage

Assess the patient's:

- Mobility
- Self-care ability
- Cognitive ability
- Communication patterns

Assess the environment for barriers to toileting:

- Privacy
- Restrictive clothing
- Access to toilet

Data from Mather, K. (2002). Nursing assistants' perceptions of their ability to provide continence care. *Geriatric Nursing, 23*(2), 76-81; and Agency for Health Care Policy and Research. (2001). *Urinary incontinence in adults: Acute and chronic management. Clinical practice guideline.* AHCPR Publication No. 96-0682. Rockville, MD: Agency for Health Care Policy and Research, Public Health Service, U.S. Department of Health and Human Services; www.ahcpr.gov/clinic/uhistory.html (Clinical Practice Guidelines Online: *Urinary Incontinence Guideline: Real World Examples of Use*).

(urine remaining in the bladder immediately after voiding) by portable ultrasound or catheterizing the patient immediately after voiding. Urinary incontinence is confirmed by evaluating the force and character of the urine stream during voiding. Asking the patient to cough while wearing a perineal pad is useful in evaluating stress incontinence; a wet pad with forceful coughing may indicate stress incontinence. A cystometrogram (see Chapter 68) is used for diagnosis in most cases.

For women, inspect the external genitalia to determine whether there is apparent urethral or uterine prolapse, **cystocele** (herniation of the bladder into the vagina), or rectocele. These conditions occur with pelvic floor muscle weakness. An advanced practice nurse puts on an examination glove and inserts two fingers into the vagina to assess the strength of these muscles. Strength is described as weak, adequate, or strong based on the amount of pressure felt by the nurse as the patient tightens her vaginal muscles. Describe and document the color, consistency, and odor of any secretions from the genitourinary orifices. The urine stream interruption test (see Chapter 68) is another method of determining pelvic muscle strength. For men, inspect the urethral meatus for any discharge.

A digital rectal examination is performed by the physician or advanced practice nurse on both male and female patients. This examination provides information about the integrity of the nerve supply to the bladder. The examiner determines whether there is tactile sensation in the anal area by observing whether the rectal sphincter is relaxed or contracted on digital insertion. Because nerve supply to the bladder is similar to nerve supply to the rectum, the presence of tactile sensation and a rectal sphincter that contracts suggest that the nerve supply to the bladder is intact. The health care provider assesses for prostate enlargement in men as a possible cause of incontinence.

Laboratory Assessment

A urinalysis is useful to rule out infection. This test is the first step in the assessment of incontinent patients of any age. The presence of red blood cells (RBCs), white blood cells (WBCs), leukocyte esterase, or nitrites is an indication for culturing the urine. Any infection is treated before further assessment of incontinence.

Imaging Assessment

Imaging is rarely needed unless surgery is being considered. Urography is the most useful for locating the kidneys and ureters. A voiding cystourethrogram (VCUG) may be performed to assess the size, shape, support, and function of the bladder. Problems identified by this test include obstruction (especially prostate obstruction in men) and post-void residual (PVR). Assessment of PVR also can be made with a portable ultrasonographic bladder scanner.

Other Diagnostic Assessment

Patients who have unusual symptoms, medical complications, or a history of failed incontinence surgery may need urodynamic studies to determine the cause of their incontinence. These studies are not standardized procedures and may consist of any combination of these tests:

- Cystourethroscopy to examine the inside of the bladder and urethra directly
- Cystometrogram (CMG) to measure the pressure inside the bladder as it fills
- Urethral pressure profilometry (UPP) to measure the pressure in the urethra in relation to the bladder pressure during various activities
- Uroflowmetry to measure rate and degree of bladder emptying

Testing may take several hours and more than one visit.

Electromyography (EMG) of the pelvic muscles may be a part of the urodynamic studies. A perineometer is a tampon-shaped instrument inserted into the vagina to measure the strength of pelvic muscle contractions. The graph shows the amplitude of muscle contraction to the patient as a method of biofeedback.

DECISION-MAKING CHALLENGE
Coordination of Care

The patient is a 72-year-old woman who reports new-onset incontinence. She reports three or four episodes of voiding a large amount of urine involuntarily when outside her home. She sensed a full bladder but was unable to find a bathroom quickly. She states, "When I have to go, I really have to go right then." She does not use a diuretic and does not have a history of diabetes. She says she tries to drink very little, especially when she is "out and about" so that she will remain dry. Her only health problem is osteoporosis; she takes vitamin D and calcium supplements. She states that both of her sisters have the same urinary problem.

1. What other questions should you ask?
2. What type or types of incontinence is she most likely to have from the information she has provided thus far?
3. Is this problem likely to be genetic? Why or why not?
4. Which nursing diagnoses would be priority for this patient?

evolve For suggested answer guidelines, go to http://evolve.elsevier.com/Iggy/.

Analysis

Common Nursing Diagnoses and Collaborative Problems

Priority nursing diagnoses for patients with urinary incontinence are:

1. Stress Urinary Incontinence related to weak pelvic muscles and structural supports
2. Urge Urinary Incontinence related to decreased bladder capacity, bladder spasms, diet, and neurologic impairment
3. Reflex Urinary Incontinence related to neurologic impairment
4. Functional Urinary Incontinence related to impaired cognition or neuromuscular limitations
5. Total Urinary Incontinence (Mixed) related to many causes

Additional Nursing Diagnoses and Collaborative Problems

In addition to the common nursing diagnoses, patients with urinary incontinence may have one or more of these:

- Social Isolation related to altered state of wellness or fear of embarrassment
- Risk for Impaired Skin Integrity related to excessive moisture from urinary excretions
- Disturbed Body Image related to odor, need to alter clothing selections, or need to wear protective briefs or supplies
- Risk for Infection related to increased environmental exposure to pathogens from retained or refluxing urine

Planning and Implementation

Several interventions are useful for each type of incontinence. Patient-Centered Collaborative Care uses these interventions, as well as drugs, surgical repair, and nutrition therapy.

Stress Urinary Incontinence

NOC **Planning: Expected Outcomes.** With appropriate therapy, the patient with urinary incontinence is expected to develop urinary continence. Indicators include that the patient rarely or never demonstrates these actions:

- Urine leakage between voidings
- Urine leakage with increased abdominal pressure (e.g., sneezing, laughing, lifting)

Interventions. Initial interventions for patients with stress incontinence include keeping a diary, behavioral interventions, and drugs. Surgery also may be an option if other interventions are not effective. Explain the purpose of a detailed diary in which the patient records times of urine leakage, activities, and foods eaten. The diary is then used by the health care provider to plan and evaluate interventions. Collection devices, absorbent pads, and undergarments may be used during the sometimes lengthy process of assessment and treatment and by those patients who elect not to pursue further interventions.

Nonsurgical Management. Drug therapy and behavioral interventions (primarily diet and exercise) for stress incontinence require the patient's active participation for success. Nursing interventions focus on teaching the patient about the drugs and behavioral strategies and on providing ongoing encouragement, clarification, and support to maximize the effects of all interventions.

Pelvic floor (Kegel) exercise therapy for women with stress incontinence strengthens the muscles of the pelvic floor (circumvaginal muscles). These muscles become strengthened, as any other skeletal muscle does, by frequent, systematic, and repeated contractions.

The most important step in teaching pelvic muscle exercises is to help the patient become aware of which muscle to exercise. During the pelvic examination in women and the rectal examination in men or women, instruct the patient to tighten the pelvic muscles around your fingers. Then provide feedback about the strength of the contraction. Biofeedback devices, such as electromyography (EMG) or perineometers (see discussion on p. 1563 in the Other Diagnostic Assessment section), measure the strength of contraction. Retention of a vaginal weight is also evidence that the patient has identified the proper muscle. The ability to start and stop the urine stream or stop the passage of flatus is evidence that the patient has correctly identified the pelvic muscles.

Instructions for pelvic muscle exercises are given in Chart 69-7. Although improvement may take several months, most patients notice a positive change after 6 weeks. Teach patients to continue the exercises to maintain the improvement.

Nutrition therapy in the form of weight reduction is helpful for obese patients because stress incontinence is made worse by increased abdominal pressure from obesity. Teach the patient to avoid alcohol, nicotine, artificial sweeteners, citrus, and caffeine (bladder irritants). Stress the importance of maintaining an adequate fluid intake, especially water. Refer the patient to the nutritionist as needed.

Drug therapy can be useful for some people with stress incontinence. Because bladder pressure is greater than urethral resistance in patients with stress incontinence, drugs may be used to improve urethral resistance (Chart 69-8).

Estrogen is used to treat postmenopausal women with stress incontinence, although it is not known exactly how this drug helps improve continence. Estrogen may increase the blood flow and tone of the muscles around the vagina and urethra, thus improving the patient's ability to contract those muscles during times of increased intra-abdominal stress.

Vaginal cone therapy involves using a set of five small, cone-shaped weights. They are of equal size but of varying weights and are used together with pelvic muscle exercise. The woman inserts the lightest cone, labeled *1,* into her vagina (Fig. 69-1), with the string to the outside, for a 1-minute test period. If she can hold the first cone in place without its slipping out while she walks around, she proceeds to the second cone, labeled *2,* and repeats the procedure. The patient begins her treatment with the heaviest cone she can comfortably hold in her vagina for the 1-minute test period. Treatment periods are 15 minutes twice a day. When the patient can comfortably hold the cone in her vagina for the 15-minute period, she progresses to the next heaviest weight. Treatment is completed with the cone labeled *5.*

Chart 69-7 PATIENT AND FAMILY EDUCATION GUIDE

Pelvic Muscle Exercises

- The pelvic muscles are composed of a sling of muscles that support your bladder, urethra, and vagina. Like any other muscles in your body, you can make your pelvic muscles stronger by alternately contracting (tightening) and relaxing them in regular exercise periods. By strengthening these muscles, you will be able to stop your urine flow more effectively.
- To identify your pelvic muscles, sit on the toilet with your feet flat on the floor about 12 inches apart. Begin to urinate, and then try to stop the urine flow. Do not strain down, lift your bottom off the seat, or squeeze your legs together. When you start and stop your urine stream, you are using your pelvic muscles.
- To perform pelvic muscle exercises, tighten your pelvic muscles for a slow count of 10 and then relax for a slow count of 10. Do this exercise 15 times while you are lying down, sitting up, and standing (a total of 45 exercises). Repeat—and this time rapidly contracting and relaxing the pelvic muscles 10 times. This should take no more than 10 to 12 minutes for all three positions, or 3 to 4 minutes for each set of 15 exercises.
- Begin with 45 exercises a day in three sets of 15 exercises each. You will notice faster improvement if you can do this twice a day, or a total of 20 minutes each day. Remember to exercise in all three positions so your muscles learn to squeeze effectively despite your position. At first, it is helpful to have a designated time and place to do these exercises because you will have to concentrate to do them correctly. After you have been doing them for several weeks, you will notice improvement in your control of urine. However, many people report that improvement may take as long as 3 months.

Chart 69-8 COMMON EXAMPLES OF DRUG THERAPY
Urinary Incontinence

Drug/Dosage	Purpose/Action	Nursing Interventions	Rationales
Estrogen (Cenestin, Cenestin, Enjuvia, Premarin, C.E.S.🍁) 0.3-1.25 mg orally daily **OR** 2-4 g vaginal cream every other day	This drug reduces incontinence, possibly by improving vaginal and urethral blood flow and tone.	Teach patients to report any unusual vaginal bleeding to their health care provider.	Estrogen increases the risk for endometrial cancer.
		Teach patients to avoid smoking while on this drug and to report any calf pain or swelling.	Estrogen increases the risk for thrombophlebitis, especially among women who smoke.
ANTICHOLINERGICS/ANTISPASMODICS			
Oxybutynin (Ditropan) 5 mg orally 3-4 times daily; (Ditropan XL) 5-10 mg orally daily Tolterodine (Detrol) 2 mg orally twice daily; (Detrol LA) 4 mg orally daily Propantheline (Pro-Banthine, Propanthel🍁) 7.5-30 mg orally 3-4 times daily Dicyclomine (Barmine, Bentyl) 10-40 mg orally 3-4 times daily Trospium (Sanctura) 20 mg orally every 12 hr	These drugs reduce incontinence by causing bladder muscle relaxation and suppressing the urge to void.	Ask whether the patient has glaucoma before starting the drug.	Anticholinergics can increase intraocular pressure and make glaucoma worse.
		Suggest that patients increase fluid intake and use hard candy to moisten the mouth.	Dry mouth is a common side effect of drugs in this category.
		Teach patients to increase fluid intake and the amount of dietary fiber.	Constipation is a common side effect of drugs in this category.
		Teach patients to monitor urine output and to report an output significantly lower than intake to the health care provider.	Drugs in this category can cause urinary retention.
		Instruct patients taking the extended-release forms of these drugs not to chew or crush the tablet/capsule.	Crushing or chewing the tablet releases all the drug at once, ruining the extended effect.
TRICYCLIC ANTIDEPRESSANTS			
Imipramine (Tofranil, Novo-Pramine🍁) 25-100 mg orally 4 times daily Desipramine (Norpramin) 10-25 mg orally 3 times daily Nortriptyline (Pamelor, Aventyl) 10-25 mg orally 3 times daily	Drugs from this class have some anticholinergic actions and also block acetylcholine receptors. Both actions can relieve urinary incontinence.	Warn patients not to take these drugs with any other tricyclic antidepressants or MAO inhibitors.	These drugs prolong the effects of catecholamines (epinephrine and norepinephrine) and lead to hypertensive crisis.
		Teach patients to change positions slowly, especially in the morning.	These drugs cause dizziness and orthostatic hypotension and can increase the risk for falls.
		Teach patients the same interventions as for anticholinergic agents.	These drugs have anticholinergic activity and produce the same side effects.

MAO, Monoamine oxidase.

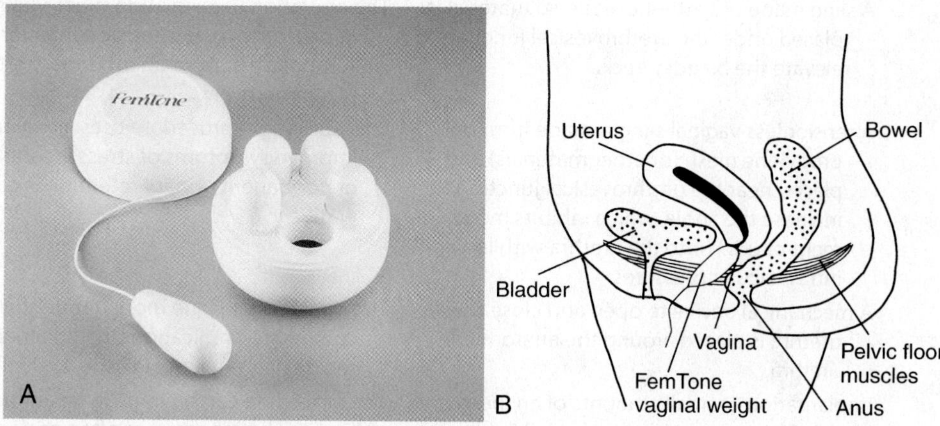
FemTone
A
Uterus
Bowel
Bladder
Vagina
Pelvic floor muscles
FemTone vaginal weight
Anus
B

Fig. 69-1 • **A,** FemTone vaginal weights, or cones. The number on the top of each cone represents increasing weight up to the heaviest cone, a 5. **B,** Diagram showing the correct positioning of a vaginal weight, or cone, in place.

Weighted vaginal cones are helpful in strengthening the pelvic muscles and decreasing stress incontinence but may not help pelvic prolapse. Vaginal cones are available without prescription.

Other interventions for stress incontinence include behavior modification, psychotherapy, and electrical stimulation devices to strengthen urethral contractions. Many intravaginal and intrarectal electrical stimulation devices have been used with varying degrees of success. More research is needed to determine the ideal level of stimulation and methods of reducing discomfort before electrical stimulation becomes a standard treatment for incontinence.

The Reliance insert is like a tiny tampon that the patient inserts into the urethra. After insertion, the patient inflates a tiny balloon, which rests at the bladder neck and prevents the flow of urine. To void, the patient pulls a string to deflate the balloon and removes the device. The applicator is reusable, although the tampon part is disposed of after each void.

Surgical Management. Stress incontinence may be corrected by vaginal, abdominal, or retropubic surgeries. Success rates vary between 50% and 90% for most procedures, but these rates are difficult to evaluate because of the varying definitions of cure. Cure also may vary between short-term and long-term (over 5 years) results. Complications can be significant, with rates ranging from less than 2% for collagen or siloxane injection to 50% for bladder neck suspension.

Preoperative care. Teach the patient about the procedure, and clarify events surrounding the surgery. Extensive urodynamic testing (see Chapter 68) is often performed before surgery, and the need for such thorough assessment should be explained to the patient.

Operative procedures. The procedures used for women include repositioning the urethra and bladder, changing the structure of the involved tissues, or inserting artificial devices to improve function (Table 69-4).

Postoperative care. After surgery, assess for and intervene to prevent or detect complications. For prevention of movement or traction on the bladder neck, secure the urethral catheter with tape or a tube holder. If a suprapubic catheter is used instead of a urethral catheter, monitor the dressing for urine leakage and other drainage. Catheters are usually in place until the patient can urinate easily and has residual urine volume after voiding of less than 50 mL. (See Chapters 16 and 18 for a discussion of general care before and after surgery.)

Urge Urinary Incontinence

NOC **Planning: Expected Outcomes.** The patient with urinary incontinence is expected to use techniques to prevent or man-

TABLE 69-4 Surgical Procedures for Stress Incontinence

Procedure	Purpose	Nursing Considerations
Anterior vaginal repair (colporrhaphy)	Elevates the urethral position and repairs any cystocele.	Because the operation is performed by vaginal incision, it is often done in conjunction with a vaginal hysterectomy. Recovery is usually rapid, and a urethral catheter is in place for 24-48 hr.
Retropubic suspension (Marshall-Marchetti-Krantz or Burch colposuspension)	Elevates the urethral position and provides longer-lasting results.	The operation requires a low abdominal incision and a urethral or suprapubic catheter for several days postoperatively. Recovery takes longer, and urinary retention and detrusor instability are the most frequent complications.
Needle bladder neck suspension (Pereyra or Stamey procedure)	Elevates the urethral position and provides longer-lasting results without a long operative time.	The combined vaginal approach with a needle and a small suprapubic skin incision does not allow direct vision of the operative site; however, the high complication rates may be due to the selection of patients who, because of their medical condition, are not good candidates for longer retropubic procedures.
Pubovaginal sling procedures	A sling made of synthetic or fascial material is placed under the urethrovesical junction to elevate the bladder neck.	The operation uses an abdominal, vaginal, or combined approach to treat intrinsic sphincter deficiencies. Temporary or permanent urinary retention is common postoperatively.
Midurethral sling procedures	A tensionless vaginal sling is made from polypropylene mesh (or other materials) and placed near the urethrovesical junction to increase the angle, which inhibits movement of urine into the urethra with lower intravesicular pressures.	This outpatient procedure uses a vaginal approach to improve symptoms of stress incontinence. Temporary or permanent urinary retention is common postoperatively.
Artificial sphincters	A mechanical device to open and close the urethra is placed around the anatomic urethra.	The operation is done more frequently in men. The most common complications include mechanical failure of the device, erosion of tissue, and infection.
Periurethral injection of collagen or Siloxane	Implantation of small amounts of an inert substance through several small injections provides support around the bladder neck.	The procedure can be done in an ambulatory care setting and can be repeated as often as necessary. Certain compounds may migrate after injection; an allergy test to bovine collagen must be performed before implantation.

age urge incontinence. Indicators include that the patient often or consistently demonstrates these behaviors:

- Responds to urge in a timely manner
- Gets to toilet between urge and passage of urine
- Avoids substances that stimulate the bladder (e.g., caffeine, alcohol)

Interventions. Interventions for patients with urge incontinence or overactive bladder include behavioral interventions and drugs. Surgery is not the recommended treatment of this condition. Collection devices and absorbent pads and undergarments may be used.

Drug Therapy. Because the hypertonic bladder contracts involuntarily in patients with urge incontinence, drugs that relax the smooth muscle and increase the bladder's capacity are prescribed (see Chart 69-8).

The most effective drugs are anticholinergics, such as propantheline (Pro-Banthine, Propanthel♣), and anticholinergics with smooth muscle relaxant properties, such as oxybutynin (Ditropan and Ditropan XL), tolterodine (Detrol and Detrol LA), and dicyclomine hydrochloride (Barmine, Bentyl, Spasmoban♣). This class of drugs has serious side effects and is used along with behavioral interventions. These drugs inhibit the nerve fibers that stimulate bladder contraction. Tricyclic antidepressants with anticholinergic and alpha-adrenergic agonist activity, such as imipramine (Tofranil, Novopramine♣), have been used successfully. The effectiveness of other drugs, such as flavoxate (Urispas) and the antihistamines, NSAIDs, beta-adrenergic agonists, and calcium channel blockers, has yet to be determined.

Nutrition Therapy. Teach the patient to avoid foods that have a direct bladder-stimulating or diuretic effect, such as caffeine and alcohol. Spacing fluids at regular intervals throughout the day (e.g., 120 mL every hour or 240 mL every 2 hours) and limiting fluids after the dinner hour (e.g., only 120 mL at bedtime) help avoid fluid overload on the bladder and allow urine to collect at a steady pace.

Behavioral Interventions. Behavioral interventions for urge incontinence include bladder training, habit training, exercise therapy, and electrical stimulation.

NIC interventions for urinary bladder training and urinary habit training are listed in Chart 69-9. It can be difficult for patients to use these interventions because they involve a great deal of patient participation. Provide ongoing encouragement, clarification, and support to increase the effects of all interventions. Behavioral interventions are often combined with drug therapy for greatest effect.

Bladder training is an education program for the patient that begins with a thorough explanation of the problem of urge incontinence. Instead of the bladder being in control of the patient, the patient learns to control the bladder. For the

Chart 69-9 NIC INTERVENTION ACTIVITIES

The Patient with Urinary Incontinence

Urinary Bladder Training: *Improving bladder function for those with urge incontinence by increasing the bladder's ability to hold urine and the patient's ability to suppress urination*

- Determine ability to recognize urge to void.
- Keep a continence specification record for 3 days to establish voiding pattern.
- Establish interval of initial toileting schedule, based on voiding pattern.
- Establish beginning and ending time for toileting schedule, if not for 24 hours.
- Establish interval for toileting of not less than 1 hour and preferably not less than 2 hours.
- Toilet patient or remind patient to void at prescribed intervals.
- Provide privacy for toileting.
- Use power of suggestion (e.g., running water or flushing toilet) to assist patient to void.
- Avoid leaving patient on toilet for more than 5 minutes.
- Reduce toileting interval by one-half hour if there are more than three incontinence episodes in 24 hours.
- Increase toileting interval by 1 hour if patient has no incontinence episodes for 3 days until optimal 4-hour interval is achieved.
- Teach the patient to consciously hold urine until the scheduled toileting time.
- Discuss daily record of continence with patient to provide reinforcement.

Urinary Habit Training: *Establishing a predictable pattern of bladder emptying to prevent incontinence for persons with limited cognitive ability who have urge, stress, or functional incontinence*

- Keep a continence specification record for 3 days to establish voiding pattern.
- Establish interval of initial toileting schedule, based on voiding pattern and usual routine (e.g., eating, rising, and retiring).
- Establish beginning and ending time for the toileting schedule, if not for 24 hours.
- Establish interval for toileting of preferably not less than 2 hours.
- Assist patient to toilet and prompt to void at prescribed intervals.
- Provide privacy for toileting.
- Use power of suggestion (e.g., running water or flushing toilet) to assist patient to void.
- Avoid leaving patient on toilet for more than 5 minutes.
- Reduce toileting interval by one-half hour if there are more than two incontinence episodes in 24 hours.
- Maintain toileting interval if there are two or less incontinence episodes in 24 hours.
- Increase the toileting interval by one-half hour if patient has no incontinence episodes in 48 hours until optimal 4-hour interval is achieved.
- Discuss daily record of continence with staff to provide reinforcement and encourage compliance with toileting schedule.
- Maintain scheduled toileting to assist in establishing and maintaining voiding habit.
- Give positive feedback or positive reinforcement (e.g., 5 minutes of social conversation) to patient when he or she voids at scheduled toileting times, and make no comment when patient is incontinent.

NIC intervention activities selected from Bulechek, G.M., Butcher, H.K., & McCloskey Dochterman, J. (Eds.). (2008). *Nursing interventions classification (NIC)* (5th ed.). St. Louis: Mosby.

program to succeed, he or she must be alert, aware, and able to resist the urge to urinate.

Start a schedule for voiding, beginning with the longest interval that is comfortable for the patient, even if the interval is only 30 minutes. Instruct the patient to void every 30 minutes and to ignore any urge to urinate between the set intervals. Once he or she is comfortable with the starting schedule, increase the interval by 15 to 30 minutes. Instruct the patient to follow the new schedule until he or she achieves success again. As the interval increases, the bladder gradually tolerates more volume. Teach him or her relaxation and distraction techniques to maximize success in the retraining. Provide positive reinforcement for maintaining the prescribed schedule.

Habit training (scheduled toileting) is a type of bladder training that is successful in reducing incontinence in cognitively impaired patients. To use habit training, caregivers assist the patient in voiding at specific times (e.g., every 2 hours on the even hours). The goal is to get the patient to the toilet before incontinence occurs. There is no effort to increase bladder capacity by gradually lengthening the voiding intervals. This method is undermined when UAP apply absorbent briefs or tell patients to "just wet the bed."

Prompted voiding, a supplement to habit training, attempts to increase the patient's awareness of the need to void and to prompt him or her to ask for toileting assistance. Habit training otherwise relies completely on a time schedule.

Exercise therapy with pelvic muscle exercises for urge incontinence has been helpful and is taught in the same way as for stress incontinence (see Chart 69-7). Improved urethral resistance helps the patient overcome abnormal detrusor contractions long enough to get to the toilet.

Electrical stimulation with either intravaginal or intrarectal electrical stimulation devices is available to treat both urge and stress incontinence.

Reflex Urinary Incontinence

NOC **Planning: Expected Outcomes.** With appropriate intervention, the patient with urinary incontinence is expected to achieve continence. Indicators include that the patient often or consistently demonstrates these behaviors:

- Recognizes the urge to void
- Maintains a predictable pattern of voiding
- Responds to urge in a timely manner
- Empties bladder completely
- Keeps urine volume in the bladder within normal limits, to prevent bladder overdistention

Interventions. Interventions for the patient with reflex (overflow) incontinence caused by obstruction of the bladder outlet may include surgery to relieve the obstruction. The most common surgical procedures are prostate removal (see Chapter 75) and repair of genital prolapse (see Chapter 74). For overflow incontinence related to detrusor muscle weakness, the most effective method of treatment is intermittent catheterization. Behavioral interventions such as bladder compression and intermittent self-catheterization are the main management techniques for this type of incontinence.

Drug Therapy. Drugs are prescribed for short-term management of urinary retention, often after surgery. They are not used in long-term management of overflow incontinence caused by a hypotonic bladder. The most commonly used drug is bethanechol chloride (Urecholine), an agent that increases bladder pressure.

Behavioral Interventions. The most common behavioral interventions are bladder compression and intermittent self-catheterization.

Bladder compression uses techniques that promote bladder emptying and include the Credé method, the Valsalva maneuver, double-voiding, and splinting.

In the Credé method, teach the patient how to press over the bladder area, increasing its pressure, or to trigger nerve stimulation by tugging at pubic hair or massaging the genital area. These techniques manually assist the bladder in emptying. In the Valsalva maneuver, breathing techniques increase chest and abdominal pressure. This increased pressure is then directed toward the bladder during exhalation. With the technique of double-voiding, the patient empties the bladder and then, within a few minutes, attempts a second bladder emptying.

For women who have a large cystocele (prolapse of the bladder into the vagina), a technique called *splinting* both compresses the bladder and moves it into a better position. The woman inserts her fingers into her vagina, gently lifts the cystocele, and begins to urinate.

Intermittent self-catheterization is often used to help patients with long-term problems of incomplete bladder emptying. It is effective and can be learned fairly easily. These points are important in teaching this technique:

- Proper handwashing and cleaning of the catheter reduce the risk for infection.
- A small lumen and good lubrication of the catheter prevent urethral trauma.
- A regular schedule for bladder emptying prevents bladder distention and mucosal trauma.

Patients must be able to understand instructions and have the manual dexterity to manipulate the catheter. Caregivers or family members in the home can also be taught to perform straight catheterization using a clean (rather than sterile) technique with good outcomes.

Functional Urinary Incontinence

NOC **Planning: Expected Outcomes.** The patient with functional urinary incontinence is expected to remain dry. Indicators include that the patient often or consistently demonstrates these behaviors:

- Uses urine containment or collection measures to ensure dryness
- Manages clothing independently

Interventions. Causes of functional (or chronic intractable) incontinence vary greatly. Some are reversible, and others are not. The focus of intervention is treatment of reversible causes. When incontinence is not reversible, urinary habit training (see discussion of habit training at left) is used to establish a predictable pattern of bladder emptying to prevent incontinence. A final strategy focuses on containment of the urine and protection of the patient's skin. Nonsurgical interventions include applied devices, containment, and catheterization.

Applied devices include intravaginal pessaries for women and penile clamps for men. The intravaginal pessary supports the uterus and vagina and helps maintain the correct position of the bladder. (See Chapter 74 for further discussion of pessaries.) The penile clamp is applied around the outside of the penis to compress the urethra and prevent urine leakage.

The dangers of pessaries and penile clamps include damage to the tissues and infection from constant pressure in sensitive areas. Both devices require either that the patient has manual dexterity or that a caregiver applies and removes the device.

Instruct the patient or caregivers in the use of these devices. Male patients may use an external collecting device, such as a condom catheter. Design of an effective external collecting device for women has not been as successful.

Containment is achieved with absorbent pads and briefs designed to collect urine and keep the patient's skin and clothing dry. Many types and sizes of pads are available:

- Shields or liners inserted inside a panty
- Undergarments consisting of full-size pads with waist straps
- Plastic-lined protective underpants with or without elastic legs
- Combination pad and pant systems
- Absorbent bed pads

A major concern with the use of protective pads is the risk that skin breakdown will occur. Materials and costs vary. Some are reusable; others are disposable. The disposal of these products raises ecologic concerns. Avoid use of the word "diaper" when discussing these adult protective pants, however, because of the usual association of diapers with a baby.

Catheterization for control of incontinence may be intermittent or involve an indwelling catheter. Intermittent catheterization is preferred to an indwelling catheter because of the reduced risk for infection. Indwelling urinary catheters should be used temporarily and only when all other interventions have been unsuccessful. A long-term indwelling urinary catheter is appropriate for patients with skin breakdown who need a dry environment for healing, for those who are terminally ill and need comfort, and for those who are critically ill and require careful measurement of urine output.

Total or Mixed Urinary Incontinence

Total or mixed urinary incontinence is a combination of two or more types of involuntary urine loss syndromes. For example, stress incontinence and urge incontinence often occur together in women during and after menopause. For the patient with mixed or total incontinence, combinations of assessment techniques (as discussed under each syndrome) are used. Interventions are also combined to promote continence. The problems and interventions for mixed incontinence are the same as for each specific type of incontinence separately. After identifying the specific types of incontinence an individual patient has, apply the appropriate nursing diagnoses, collaborative problems, interventions, and expected outcomes discussed earlier with each incontinence type.

DECISION-MAKING CHALLENGE
Coordination of Care

Your older patient (described on p. 1563) is diagnosed with mixed stress and urge incontinence. Her environment has no barriers to toileting. Her diet history has little impact on the incontinence, with only infrequent use of caffeine—about twice monthly at a social event. She has been prescribed topical estrogen and bladder training including pelvic muscle exercises. In addition, she is instructed to regularly void to avoid a full bladder.

1. What should you teach her about the effects and side effects of her newly prescribed drug?
2. What approaches are useful to teach her pelvic floor muscle exercises?
3. How can you help evaluate her response to exercise and the prescribed drug to improve continence?

evolve For suggested answer guidelines, go to http://evolve.elsevier.com/Iggy/.

Community-Based Care

Community-based care for the patient with urinary incontinence considers his or her personal, physical, emotional, and social resources. Important personal resources for self-care include mobility, vision, and manual dexterity. When planning care, consider who will be the primary caregiver and what factors may influence the effectiveness of the plan.

Home Care Management

Assess the home environment for barriers that limit access to the bathroom. Eliminate hazards that might slow walking or lead to a fall. These hazards might include small area rugs (throw rugs), tables or chairs with legs that extend into the walking area, slippery waxed or polished floors, and inadequate lighting.

If the patient must climb stairs to reach a bathroom, handrails should be installed and stairs should be kept free of obstacles. Toilet seat extenders may help provide the right level of seating so that maximal abdominal pressure may be applied to encourage voiding. Portable commodes may be obtained for homes in which ambulatory access to toilets is impractical or impossible. Physical and occupational therapists are valuable resources for assisting with home care management.

Health Teaching

Teach the patient and family about the cause of the specific type of incontinence, and discuss available treatment options for its management. The teaching plan addresses the prescribed drugs (purpose, dosage, method and route of administration, and expected and potential side effects). Instruct the patient and family about the importance of weight reduction and dietary modification to help control urinary incontinence.

When external devices or protective pads are needed, describe the possible options, discuss the advantages and disadvantages of each, and help the patient make a selection best for his or her lifestyle and resources. For patients who will use intermittent catheterization or those with artificial urinary sphincters, demonstrate the correct technique to the patient or caregiver. Evaluate return demonstrations for correct technique. Chart 69-10 also addresses teaching.

Psychosocial Preparation

The embarrassment of incontinence can be devastating to a patient's self-esteem, body image, and relationships. The unpredictable nature of incontinence creates anxiety. Patients are often embarrassed to seek help, and even when resources are identified, they may need assistance to feel comfortable in using the resources. Even buying supplies at a local store can be a threat to their privacy.

Accept and acknowledge the personal concerns of the patient and caregiver. Never minimize the concerns or make them seem trivial. Help the patient learn methods of controlling or managing the fear or anxiety. As he or she learns the specifics of the plan that will allow control of urinary incontinence, the confidence to resume social interactions should return.

Health Care Resources

Referral to home care agencies for help with personal care and to continence clinics that specialize in evaluation and treatment may be helpful. In many continence clinics, nurses collaborate with physicians and other health care professionals to evaluate and manage patients. The treatment plan is specific for each patient; supplies and products are custom selected.

Patients may benefit from education and from the support of others who experience similar concerns. The National Association for Continence (NAFC) (www.nafc.org), Access to Continence Care and Treatment (www.wellweb.com/INCONT/acct/contents.htm), and the Wound, Ostomy, and Continence Nurses (www.wocn.org) publish newsletters and educational materials written with simple, easy-to-understand explanations. The American Foundation for Urologic Disease (www.afud.com) provides information on several areas of bladder dysfunction. The Agency for Healthcare Research and Quality (AHRQ) has also published a caregiver guide (AHCPR Publication No. 96-0683) for the public that is available on the Internet or by calling (800) 358-9295 (AHCPR, 2001b). Local hospitals, in collaboration with the NAFC, may conduct local support groups.

NCLEX EXAMINATION CHALLENGE

For which client living in a long-term care facility is habit training the best choice for incontinence management?

A. 56-year-old diabetic who is blind
B. 66-year-old person with Alzheimer's
C. 76-year-old with severe osteoarthritis
D. 86-year-old who has a cystocele

evolve For the correct answer, go to http://evolve.elsevier.com/Iggy/.

Evaluation: Outcomes

Evaluate the care of the patient with urinary incontinence on the basis of the identified nursing diagnoses. The expected outcomes are that the patient will:

- Describe the type of urinary incontinence experienced
- Demonstrate knowledge of proper use of medications and correct procedures for self-catheterization, use of the artificial sphincter, or care of an indwelling urinary catheter
- Demonstrate effective use of the selected exercise or bladder-training program
- Select and use incontinence devices and products
- Have a reduction in the number of incontinence episodes

Specific indicators for these outcomes are listed for each nursing diagnosis under the Planning and Implementation section (see earlier).

UROLITHIASIS

Pathophysiology

Urolithiasis is the presence of calculi (stones) in the urinary tract. Stones often do not cause symptoms until they pass into the lower urinary tract, where they can cause excruciating pain. **Nephrolithiasis** is the formation of stones in the kidney. Formation of stones in the ureter is **ureterolithiasis.**

Urologic stones are caused by many disorders. However, the exact mechanism of stone formation is not entirely understood. Everyone excretes crystals in the urine at some time, but fewer than 10% of people form stones. About 75% of stones contain calcium as one part of the stone complex, which may be calcium oxalate or calcium phosphate. Struvite (15%), uric acid (8%), and cystine (3%) make up the less common stones. Formation of stones seems to involve three conditions:

- Slow urine flow, resulting in supersaturation of the urine with the particular element (e.g., calcium) that first becomes crystallized and later becomes the stone
- Damage to the lining of the urinary tract (e.g., abrasion from crystals)
- Decreased inhibitor substances in the urine that would otherwise prevent supersaturation and crystal aggregation

High urine acidity (as with uric acid and cystine stones) or alkalinity (as with calcium phosphate and struvite stones), as well as drugs (as with triamterene, indinavir, and acetazolamide), contribute to stone formation.

One example of a metabolic problem causing stone formation begins when excessive amounts of calcium are absorbed through the intestinal tract (the most common cause of hypercalciuria). As blood circulates through the kidneys, the excess calcium is filtered into the urine, causing supersaturation of calcium in the urine. If fluid intake is poor, such as when a patient is dehydrated, supersaturation is more likely to occur and the risk for calcium combining with another compound to form a larger molecule increases. Calcium complexes often serve as a center for other deposits, and eventually a stone forms.

Stones that form in the kidney and then pass into the ureter often lodge in areas where the ureter bends or slightly changes shape. When the stone occludes the ureter and blocks the flow of urine, the ureter dilates. Enlargement of the ureter is called **hydroureter.**

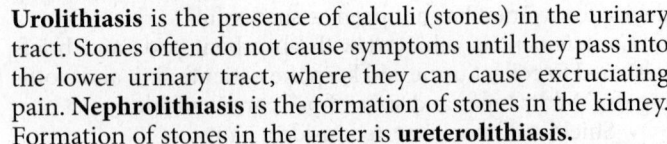

◀ ANIMATION: Renal Stone; Kidney Stone; Nephrolithiasis

Chart 69-10 PATIENT AND FAMILY EDUCATION GUIDE

Urinary Incontinence

- Maintain a normal body weight to reduce the pressure on your bladder.
- Do not try to control your incontinence by limiting your fluid intake. Adequate fluid intake is necessary for kidney function and health maintenance.
- If you have a catheter in your bladder, follow the instructions given to you about maintaining the sterile drainage system.
- If you are discharged with a suprapubic catheter in your bladder, inspect the entry site for the tube daily, clean the skin around the opening gently with warm soap and water, and place a sterile gauze dressing on the skin around the tube. Report any redness, swelling, drainage, or fever to your physician.
- Do not put anything into your vagina, such as tampons, drugs, hygiene products, or exercise weights, until you check with your physician at your 6-week checkup after surgery.
- Do not have sexual intercourse until after your 6-week postoperative checkup.
- Do not lift or carry anything heavier than 5 pounds or participate in any strenuous exercise until your physician gives you postoperative clearance. In some cases, this could be as long as 3 months.
- Avoid exercises, such as running, jogging, step or dance aerobic classes, rowing, cross-country ski or stair-climber machines, and mountain biking. Brisk walking without any additional hand, leg, or body weights is allowed. Swimming is allowed after all drains and catheters have been removed and your incision is completely healed.
- If Kegel exercises are recommended, ask your nurse for specific instructions.

The pain associated with ureteral spasm is excruciating and may cause the patient to go into shock from stimulation of nearby nerves. In addition, **hematuria** (bloody urine) may result from damage to the urothelial lining. If the obstruction is not removed, urinary stasis can cause infection and impair kidney function on the side of the blockage. As the blockage persists, **hydronephrosis** (enlargement of the kidney caused by blockage of urine lower in the tract and filling of the kidney with urine) and permanent kidney damage may develop.

Etiology and Genetic Risk

The cause of urolithiasis is unknown. At least 90% of patients who form stones have a metabolic risk factor. Table 69-5 lists some metabolic defects that commonly cause stone formation.

A diet high in calcium is not believed to cause stones unless a metabolic defect or renal tubular defect already exists. Data suggest that a normal-calcium diet that is relatively low in animal protein, salt, or both may be effective in preventing stone formation. A low-calcium diet does not prevent stone formation (Krieg, 2005). Urinary stasis, urinary retention, immobility, and dehydration all increase the risk for stones to form. Except for the use of the thiazides for calcium oxalate stones, diuretics can cause volume depletion and thus may promote the formation of stones.

GENETIC CONSIDERATIONS

More than 30 genetic variations are associated with the formation of renal stones. Single gene disorders are rare. More commonly, nephrolithiasis is a complex disease, with genetic variation in intestinal calcium absorption, renal calcium transport, or renal phosphate transport all associated with stone formation (Coe et al., 2005). Always ask a patient with a renal stone whether other family members have also had this problem.

Incidence/Prevalence

The incidence of stone disease is high and varies with geographic location, race, and family history. About 12% of adults will have at least one episode of renal stone disease. The incidence is higher in men. However, struvite stones are twice as common in women. Recurrence rates vary depending on the type of treatment. The recurrence rate of untreated calcium oxalate stones is 35% to 50% in 5 to 10 years. A higher recurrence of stones occurs in patients with a family history of stone disease and in those who had their first occurrence by age 25 years.

CULTURAL AWARENESS

The incidence of stone disease is most common in the southeastern United States, Japan, and Western Europe. Calcium stone disease is more common in men than in women and tends to occur in young adults or during early middle adulthood. Kidney stone disease occurs more often in younger adults than older adults and more commonly among white people. For patients in these higher-risk groups, nursing care should include teaching family members, as well as patients, about the manifestations of a stone and interventions to reduce stone formation.

Patient-Centered Collaborative Care

Assessment

Ask the patient about a personal or family history of urologic stones. Obtain a diet history, including fluid intake patterns. If he or she has a history of stone formation, ask about past treatment, whether chemical analysis of the stone was performed, and what preventive measures are followed.

The major manifestation of stones is severe pain, commonly called **renal colic.** Flank pain suggests that the stone is in the kidney or upper ureter. Flank pain that extends toward the abdomen or to the scrotum and testes or the vulva suggests that stones are in the ureters or bladder. Pain is most intense when the stone is moving or when the ureter is obstructed.

Renal colic begins suddenly and is often described as "unbearable." Nausea, vomiting, pallor, and diaphoresis often accompany the pain. A large stationary stone in the kidney (staghorn calculus), however, rarely causes much pain because it is not moving. Frequency and dysuria occur when a stone reaches

TABLE 69-5 Metabolic Defects That Commonly Cause Calculi

Metabolic Deficit	Etiology
Hypercalcemia	
Primary	Absorptive: increased intestinal calcium absorption Renal: decreased renal tubular excretion of calcium
Secondary	Resorptive: hyperparathyroidism, vitamin D intoxication, renal tubular acidosis, prolonged immobilization
Hyperoxaluria	
Primary	Genetic: autosomal recessive trait resulting in high oxalate production
Secondary	Dietary: excess oxalate from foods such as spinach, rhubarb, Swiss chard, cocoa, beets, wheat germ, pecans, peanuts, okra, chocolate, and lime peel
Hyperuricemia	
Primary	Gout is an inherited disorder of purine metabolism (20% of patients with gout have uric acid calculi)
Secondary	Increased production or decreased clearance of purine from myeloproliferative disorders, thiazide diuretics, carcinoma
Struvite	Made of magnesium ammonium phosphate and carbonate apatite; formed by urea splitting by bacteria, most commonly, *Proteus mirabilis;* needs an alkaline urine to form
Cystinuria	Autosomal recessive defect of amino acid metabolism that precipitates insoluble cystine crystals in the urine

the bladder. **Oliguria** (scant urine output) or **anuria** (absence of urine output) suggests obstruction, possibly at the bladder neck or urethra. *Urinary tract obstruction is an emergency and must be treated immediately to preserve kidney function.*

Examine the patient to detect bladder distention. The patient may appear pale, ashen, and diaphoretic and suffer from excruciating pain. Vital signs may be moderately elevated with pain; body temperature and pulse are elevated with infection. Blood pressure may decrease if the severe pain causes shock.

Urinalysis is performed in patients with suspected calculi. Hematuria is a common finding; blood may make the urine appear smoky or rusty. RBCs are usually caused by stone-induced direct trauma on the lining of the ureter, bladder, or urethra. WBCs and bacteria may be present as a result of urinary stasis. Increased turbidity (cloudiness) and odor indicate that infection may also be present. Microscopic examination of the urine may identify crystals from which stones could form. Urinary pH is measured to determine acidity or alkalinity.

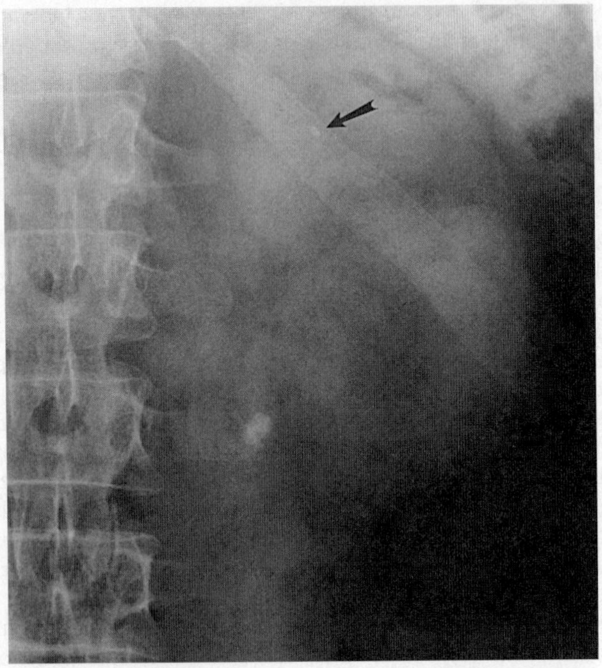

Fig. 69-2 • Urinary stones on x-ray of the kidneys, ureters, and bladder (KUB).

The serum WBC count is elevated with infection. Increases in the serum calcium, serum phosphate, or serum uric acid levels indicate excess minerals are present and may contribute to stone formation.

Stones are easily seen on x-rays of the kidneys, ureters, and bladder (KUB) (Fig. 69-2); IV urograms; or computed tomography (CT). Noncontrast helical CT has the highest sensitivity for the identification of urinary tract stones. These procedures confirm the presence and location of the stones.

IV urography is useful for identifying whether the urinary tract is obstructed. However, because of the risk of acute renal failure induced by contrast dye, other diagnostic tests may be chosen for high-risk patients (older adults and patients with diabetes mellitus, multiple myeloma, or elevated serum creatinine levels).

Renal ultrasonography creates images from sound waves. Structures of varying density are imaged. Solid structures, such as stones, are extremely dense; therefore the images of stones are clear. Small stones are harder to identify and locate. Ultrasound is the main method used to identify hydronephrosis from any cause.

Interventions

Nursing interventions focus on pain management and prevention of infection and urinary obstruction. Most patients can expel the stone without invasive procedures. The most important factors regarding whether a stone will pass on its own are its composition, size, and location. The larger the stone and the higher up in the urinary tract it is, the less likely it is to be passed. Other interventions may be needed when the patient does not pass the stone spontaneously (Fig. 69-3).

Pain Relief Measures

Nonsurgical and surgical approaches are used to assist the patient with a kidney stone achieve an acceptable degree of pain relief.

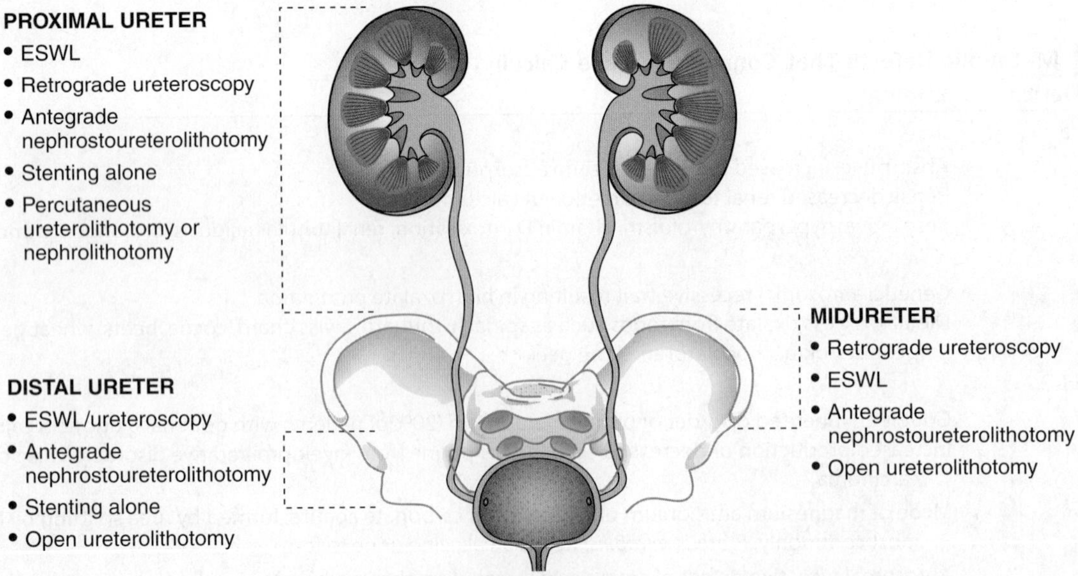
PROXIMAL URETER
• ESWL
• Retrograde ureteroscopy
• Antegrade nephrostoureterolithotomy
• Stenting alone
• Percutaneous ureterolithotomy or nephrolithotomy
MIDURETER
• Retrograde ureteroscopy
• ESWL
• Antegrade nephrostoureterolithotomy
• Open ureterolithotomy
DISTAL URETER
• ESWL/ureteroscopy
• Antegrade nephrostoureterolithotomy
• Stenting alone
• Open ureterolithotomy

Fig. 69-3 • Treatment options for ureteral stones.

Nonsurgical Management. Nonsurgical measures to relieve pain include strategies to enhance stone passing, as well as direct pain management.

Drug therapy is needed most in the first 24 to 36 hours when pain is most severe. Opioid analgesics are often needed to control the severe pain caused by stones in the urinary tract. Opioid agents, such as morphine (Statex🍁), are often given IV for rapid pain relief. NSAIDs such as ketorolac (Toradol) in the acute phase may be quite effective. When NSAIDs are used, the risk for bleeding is increased and the use of extracorporeal shock wave lithotripsy must be delayed.

Control of pain is more effective when drugs are given at regularly scheduled intervals or by a constant delivery system (e.g., skin patch) instead of PRN. Spasmolytic drugs, such as oxybutynin chloride (Ditropan) and propantheline bromide (Pro-Banthine, Propanthel🍁), are important for the relief and control of pain (see Chart 69-8). Give the drugs, and assess the response by asking the patient to rate the discomfort on a pain-rating scale.

Complementary and alternative therapy with relaxation techniques, such as hypnosis and imagery, therapeutic or healing touch, and acupuncture, can relieve pain. Patients often have difficulty finding a comfortable position in which to relax. Thus assisting the patient with positioning can often aid in pain reduction. Breathing techniques, such as those used in childbirth, can also help him or her relax.

Other management techniques include avoiding overhydration and underhydration in the acute phase to help make the passage of a stone less painful. Strain the urine and teach the patient to strain it to monitor for stone passage. Send any stone passed to the laboratory for analysis because preventive therapy is based on stone composition.

Lithotripsy, also known as *extracorporeal shock wave lithotripsy (ESWL),* is the use of sound, laser, or dry shock waves to break the stone into small fragments. The patient receives moderate sedation and lies on a flat table with the lithotriptor aimed at the stone, which is located by fluoroscopy. A local anesthetic cream is applied to the skin site over the stone 45 minutes before the procedure. During the procedure, cardiac rhythm is monitored by electrocardiography (ECG), and the shock waves are delivered in synchrony with the R wave. About 500 to 1500 shock waves are applied in 30 to 45 minutes. Continuous ECG monitoring for dysrhythmia and fluoroscopic observation for stone destruction are maintained.

After lithotripsy, strain the urine to monitor the passage of stone fragments. Bruising may occur on the flank of the affected side after ESWL. Occasionally a stent is placed in the ureter before ESWL to ease passage of the stone fragments. Cystine stones are often resistant to ESWL.

Surgical Management. Minimally invasive surgical and open surgical procedures are used if urinary obstruction occurs or if the stone is too large to be passed.

Minimally Invasive Surgical Procedures. Minimally invasive surgical (MIS) procedures include stenting, retrograde ureteroscopy, and percutaneous ureterolithotomy and nephrolithotomy.

Stenting is performed with a **stent**—a small tube that is placed in the ureter by ureteroscopy. The stent dilates the ureter and enlarges the passageway for the stone or stone fragments. This procedure prevents the passing stone from coming in contact with the ureteral mucosa, thereby reducing pain, bleeding, and infection risk, all of which could block the ureter. A Foley catheter may be placed to facilitate passage of the stone through the urethra.

Retrograde ureteroscopy is an endoscopic procedure. The ureteroscope is passed through the urethra and bladder into the ureter. Once the stone is seen, it is removed using grasping baskets, forceps, or loops. Lithotripsy also can be performed through the ureteroscope. A Foley catheter may be placed to facilitate passage of the stone fragments through the urethra.

Percutaneous ureterolithotomy and nephrolithotomy is the removal of a stone in the ureter or kidney through the skin. The patient lies prone or on the side and receives local or general anesthetic. The physician identifies the ideal entry point with fluoroscopy and then passes a needle into the collecting system of the kidney. Once a tract has been made in the kidney, other equipment, such as an **intracorporeal** (inside the body) ultrasonic or laser lithotriptor, can be used to break up and remove the stone. An endoscope with a special attachment to grasp and extract the stone can be used. Often a nephrostomy tube is left in place at first to prevent the stone fragments from passing through the normal urinary tract.

◀ ANIMATION: Insertion of Foley Catheter

Provide routine nephrostomy tube care and monitor the patient for complications after the procedure. Complications include bleeding at the site or through the tube, pneumothorax, and infection.

Open Surgical Procedures. When other stone removal attempts have failed or when risk of a lasting injury to the ureter or kidney is possible, an open ureterolithotomy (into the ureter), pyelolithotomy (into the kidney pelvis), or nephrolithotomy (into the kidney) procedure may be performed. These procedures are used for a large or impacted stone.

Preoperative care. Prepare the patient for the selected procedure by explaining how, when, and where the procedure will be performed. Describe what he or she can expect to see, hear, and feel before and after the procedure. The patient is given nothing by mouth and also receives a bowel preparation before the procedure. (See Chapter 16 for routine care before surgery.)

Operative procedures. The retroperitoneal area is entered through a large flank incision, as for nephrectomy (see Chapter 70), pyelolithotomy, or nephrolithotomy, and through a lower abdominal incision for ureterolithotomy. The urinary tract is entered surgically, and the stone is removed. Before closure, tubes and drains may be placed (e.g., nephrostomy tube, ureteral stent, Penrose or other wound drainage device, and Foley catheter).

Postoperative care. Follow routine procedures for assessment of the patient who has received anesthesia. (See Chapter 18 for routine care after surgery.) Monitor the amount of bleeding from incisions and in the urine. Maintain adequate fluid intake. Strain the urine to monitor the passage of stone fragments. Teach the patient how to prevent future stones through dietary changes.

Infection Prevention

Control of infections before invasive procedures is critical for the prevention of urosepsis. Interventions include giving appropriate antibiotics, either to eliminate an existing infection or to prevent new infections, and maintaining adequate nutrition and fluid intake. Because infection always occurs with struvite stone formation, the health care team plans for long-term infection prevention.

Drug therapy is the most common intervention. Broad-spectrum antibiotics, such as the aminoglycosides (e.g., gentami-

TABLE 69-6 Dietary Treatment for Renal Stones

Stone Type	Dietary Interventions	Rationales
Calcium oxalate	Avoid oxalate sources, such as spinach, black tea, and rhubarb.	Reduction of urinary oxalate content may help prevent these stones from forming. Urinary pH is not a factor.
	Decrease sodium intake.	High sodium intake reduces renal tubular calcium reabsorption.
Calcium phosphate	Limit intake of foods high in animal protein to 5-7 servings per week and never more than 2 per day.	Reduction of protein intake reduces acidic urine and prevents calcium precipitation.
	Some patients may benefit from a reduced calcium intake (milk, other dairy products).	Reduction of urine calcium concentration may prevent calcium precipitation and crystallization.
	Decrease sodium intake.	High sodium intake reduces renal tubular calcium reabsorption.
Struvite (magnesium ammonium phosphate)	Limit high-phosphate foods, such as dairy products, organ meats, and whole grains.	Reduction of urinary phosphate content may help prevent these stones from forming.
Uric acid (urate)	Decrease intake of purine sources, such as organ meats, poultry, fish, gravies, red wines, and sardines.	Reduction of urinary purine content may help prevent these stones from forming.
Cystine	Limit animal protein intake (as above).	Reduces urinary uric acid.
	Encourage oral fluid intake (500 mL every 4 hours while awake and 750 mL at night).	Increased fluid helps dilute the urine and prevents the cystine crystals from forming.

cin [Garamycin]) and cephalosporins (e.g., cephalexin [Keflex, Novo-Lexin♣]), are first prescribed for infections occurring with stone disease. The broad coverage is effective against gram-negative organisms. After the results of the culture and sensitivity (C&S) studies are obtained, more specific antibiotics may be prescribed. C&S studies are often done 48 hours after the start of antibiotic therapy and again 48 hours after completion of the prescribed course of therapy.

Blood levels of antibiotics may be measured to ensure that adequate levels have been reached. If the desired blood level of these antibiotics is exceeded, toxic effects and kidney damage may result. If the blood level of the antibiotic is not adequate, organisms may not be completely eliminated. Evidence of a new infection (e.g., chills, fever, altered mental status) warrants the collection of a urine sample for repeat C&S tests.

For the patient with struvite stones, periodic and long-term monitoring of the urine for infection is needed. Urine cultures are checked monthly for 3 months and then quarterly for 1 year. Drugs that prevent bacteria from splitting urea, such as acetohydroxamic acid (Lithostat) and hydroxyurea (Hydrea), are often prescribed on a long-term basis for patients with struvite stones. Serum creatinine levels are monitored in patients receiving acetohydroxamic acid. This drug is stopped if creatinine levels are above 2 mg/dL. Review interventions aimed at preventing urinary tract infection (UTI). (See Interventions discussion on pp. 1555 and 1558 in the Cystitis section.)

Nutrition therapy ideally includes adequate calorie intake with a balance of all food groups. Encourage a fluid intake sufficient to dilute urine to a light color throughout the 24-hour day (typically 2 to 3 L/day) unless another health problem requires fluid restriction.

Prevention of Obstruction

Measures to prevent urinary obstruction by stones include a high intake of fluids (3 L/day or more) and careful measures of intake and output. Fluid intake sufficient to provide a diluted urine helps prevent dehydration, promotes the flow of urine, and decreases the chance of crystals forming a stone. Interventions also depend on the type of stone the patient has formed. Drugs, diet modification, and fluid intake are the major strategies used to prevent future stones.

Drug therapy to prevent obstruction depends on what is causing stone formation and the type of stone formed. Teach the patient the reason for the drug, and assess for side effects or adverse drug reactions. Some drugs may need to be avoided because they may contribute to stone formation.

Drugs to treat hypercalciuria (high levels of calcium in the urine) include thiazide diuretics (e.g., chlorothiazide [Diuril] or hydrochlorothiazide [HydroDIURIL, Urozide♣]), orthophosphate, and sodium cellulose phosphate. Thiazide diuretics promote calcium resorption from the renal tubules back into the body, thereby reducing urine calcium loads. Orthophosphates alter calcium-phosphorus metabolism, resulting in decreased urine saturation of calcium oxalate. Sodium cellulose phosphate reduces intestinal absorption of calcium.

For patients with hyperoxaluria (high levels of oxalic acid in the urine), allopurinol (Zyloprim) and vitamin B_6 (pyridoxine) are used.

For patients with chronic gout, allopurinol helps prevent the formation of urate (uric acid) stones. To alkalinize the urine, drugs such as potassium citrate, 50% sodium citrate, and sodium bicarbonate are used. The desired urine pH is 6 to 6.5. Because the normal urine pH averages 5 to 6, the desired values are termed *alkaline*.

For patients with cystinuria (high levels of cystine in the urine), both alpha-mercaptopropionylglycine (AMPG) and captopril (Capoten) lower urine cystine levels. They are used when hydration and urine alkalinization have not been successful.

Nutrition therapy depends on the type of stone formed (Table 69-6). Collaborate with the nutritionist to plan the appropriate diet for the patient.

Chart 69-11 PATIENT AND FAMILY EDUCATION GUIDE

Urinary Calculi

- Finish your entire prescription of antibiotics to ensure that you will not get a urinary tract infection.
- You may resume your usual daily activities.
- Remember to balance regular exercise with sleep and rest.
- You may return to work 2 days to 6 weeks after surgery, depending on the type of intervention, your personal tolerance, and your physician's directives.
- Depending on the type of stone you had, your diet may be restricted to prevent further stone formation.
- Remember to drink at least 3 L of fluid a day to dilute potential stone-forming crystals, prevent dehydration, and promote urine flow.
- Monitor urine pH as directed (possibly up to three times per day).
- Expect bruising after lithotripsy. The bruising may be quite extensive and may take several weeks to resolve.
- Your urine may be bloody for several days after surgery.
- Pain in the region of the kidneys or bladder may signal the beginning of an infection or the formation of another stone. Report any pain, fever, chills, or difficulty with urination immediately to your physician or nurse.
- Keep follow-up appointments to check on infection, and have repeat cultures done.

Other measures can help the patient pass the stone more quickly. Encourage the patient to walk as often as possible. Walking promotes passage of stones and reduces bone calcium resorption. Check the urine pH daily, and strain all urine with filter paper to collect passed stones and fragments.

Health teaching includes the key points listed in Chart 69-11. The patient often has great anxiety and fear that a stone and its pain may recur. In addition to anxiety about the pain, the risk for repeated surgical interventions or permanent and serious kidney damage is of major concern. Psychosocial preparation is enhanced when patients know what to expect and what actions to take if problems develop. Reassure the patient that preventive and health promotion activities help prevent recurrence.

UROTHELIAL CANCER

Pathophysiology

Urothelial cancers are malignant tumors of the urothelium—the lining of transitional cells in the kidney, renal pelvis, ureter, urinary bladder, and urethra. Most urothelial cancers occur in the bladder. Thus the term *bladder cancer* is often used to describe this condition.

In the United States, about 73% of urinary tract cancers are transitional cell carcinomas of the bladder (Jemal et al., 2007). The second most common site of urinary tract cancer is the kidney and renal pelvis. Urothelial cancers are usually low grade, have multiple points of origin **(multifocal),** and are recurrent. Once the cancer spreads beyond the transitional cell layer, it is highly invasive and can spread beyond the bladder. Because of the nature of this cancer, patients may have recurrence up to 10 years after being cancer free (American Cancer Society, 2008).

Tumors confined to the bladder mucosa are treated by simple excision, whereas those that are deeper but not into the muscle layer are treated with excision plus **intravesical** (inside the bladder) chemotherapy. Cancer that has spread deeper into the bladder muscle layer is treated with more extensive surgery, often a **radical cystectomy** (removal of the bladder and surrounding tissue) with urinary diversion. Chemotherapy and radiation therapy are used in addition to surgery. If untreated, the tumor invades surrounding tissues, spreads to distant sites (liver, lung, and bone), and ultimately leads to death.

Exposure to toxins, especially chemicals used in the hairdressing, rubber, paint, electric cable, and textile industries, increases the risk for bladder cancer. The greatest risk factor for bladder cancer is tobacco use. Other risks include *Schistosoma haematobium* (a parasite) infection, excessive use of drugs containing phenacetin, and long-term use of cyclophosphamide (Cytoxan, Procytox🍁).

About 67,160 new cases of bladder cancer are diagnosed each year in the United States and about 13,750 deaths occur each year from the disease (Jemal et al., 2007). This cancer is rare in adults younger than 40 years and is most common after 60 years of age.

Health Promotion and Maintenance

Many people believe that tobacco use is associated with cancers only of organs that come into direct contact with it, such as the lungs. However, many compounds in tobacco enter the bloodstream and affect distant organs, such as the bladder. Therefore encourage everyone who smokes to quit and urge nonsmokers to not start. Just as important, encourage anyone who comes into contact with dry, liquid, or gaseous chemicals to take precautions. Some people work with chemicals and others may come into contact with them while engaging in hobbies, such as photography (developing film) or refinishing furniture. Many chemicals and fumes can enter the body through contact with skin and with mucous membranes in the respiratory tract. Use of personal protective equipment, such as gloves and masks, can reduce this contact. Also encourage anyone who works with chemicals to shower or bathe and change clothing as soon as contact is completed.

Patient-Centered Collaborative Care

Assessment

Physical Assessment/Clinical Manifestations

Ask about the patient's perception of his or her general health. Document the gender and age of the patient. Ask about active and passive exposure to cigarette smoke. To detect exposure to harmful environmental agents, ask the patient to describe his or her occupation or hobbies in detail. Also ask the patient to describe any change in the color, frequency, or amount of urine and any abdominal discomfort.

Observe the overall appearance of the patient, especially skin color and general nutritional status. Inspect, percuss, and palpate the abdomen for asymmetry, tenderness, and bladder distention.

Examine the urine for color and clarity. Blood in the urine may be the first major sign occurring with bladder cancer. It may be gross or microscopic and is usually painless and intermittent. Dysuria, frequency, and urgency are common when infection or obstruction is also present.

Psychosocial Assessment

Assess the patient's emotions, including his or her response to a tentative diagnosis of bladder cancer, and note anxiety, fear, sadness, anger, or guilt. Early manifestations are painless, and many patients ignore the blood in the urine because it is intermittent. They also may be reluctant to seek treatment because they suspect a sexually transmitted disease (STD). As a result, they may have guilt or anger about their own delays in seeking medical attention.

Assess the patient's methods of coping and the degree of support from family members. Social support may provide motivation and improve coping during recovery from treatment.

Diagnostic Assessment

The only significant finding on a routine urinalysis is gross or microscopic hematuria. Cytologic testing on voided urine specimens is not usually helpful. Bladder-wash specimens and bladder biopsies are the most specific tests for cancer.

Cystoscopy with retrograde urography is usually performed to evaluate painless hematuria. A biopsy of a visible bladder tumor can be performed during cystoscopy. This is essential for staging and is usually performed in a day-surgery unit before admission to the hospital for treatment. IV urography may be used when there is blood in the urine. Excretory urography is useful in identifying obstructions, especially where the ureter joins the bladder. Computed tomography (CT) scans show tumor invasion of surrounding tissues. Ultrasonography shows masses but is less valuable for tumor staging. Magnetic resonance imaging (MRI) may help assess deep, invasive tumors.

▪ *Common Nursing Diagnoses and Collaborative Problems*

Nursing diagnoses that may apply to patients with bladder cancer include:

- Fear or Anxiety related to potential diagnosis of a malignant disease
- Disturbed Body Image related to surgery-induced changes in urinary habits or changes in appearance from chemotherapy
- Risk for Infection related to invasive procedures or side effects of systemic chemotherapy
- Risk for Impaired Skin Integrity related to surgical incision or urinary diversion
- Risk for Social Isolation related to altered physical appearance, embarrassment, or odors

▪ *Interventions*

Therapy for the patient with bladder cancer usually begins with surgical removal of the tumor for diagnosis and staging of disease. For tumors extending beyond the mucosa, surgery is followed by intravesical chemotherapy or immunotherapy. High-grade or recurrent tumors are treated with more radical surgery plus intravesical chemotherapy, radiotherapy, or both. Systemic chemotherapy is reserved for patients with distant metastases. (See Chapter 24 for general care of the patient receiving chemotherapy or radiation therapy.)

Nonsurgical Management

Prophylactic immunotherapy with intravesical instillation of bacille Calmette-Guérin (BCG), a compound used to vaccinate against tuberculosis in some countries, is used to prevent tumor recurrence of superficial cancers. This procedure is more effective than single-agent chemotherapy.

Multiagent chemotherapy is successful in prolonging life after distant metastasis has occurred but rarely results in a cure. Radiation therapy is also useful in prolonging life.

Surgical Management

The type of surgery for bladder cancer depends on the type and stage of the cancer and the patient's general health. Complete bladder removal (cystectomy) with additional removal of surrounding muscle and tissue offers the best chance of a cure for large, invasive bladder cancers. Four alternatives are used after cystectomy: ileal conduit; continent pouch; bladder reconstruction, also known as *neobladder;* and ureterosigmoidostomy.

Preoperative Care. Specific patient education depends on the type and extent of the planned surgical procedure. Coordinate education before surgery with the surgeon and enterostomal therapist (ET). Discuss the type of planned urinary diversion and the selection of a site for the stoma. The goal is for the patient to have a positive attitude about body image and a positive self-image. Use educational counseling to ensure understanding about self-care practices, methods of pouching, control of urine drainage, and management of odor.

The site selected for the stoma should be visible and avoid folds of skin, bones, and scar tissue. When possible, the patient's waistline or belt area is avoided. Prepare the patient for the number and type of drains that will be present after surgery. General care before surgery is discussed in Chapter 16.

Operative Procedures. Transurethral resection of the bladder tumor (TURBT) or partial cystectomy is performed for small, early, superficial tumors. In a partial (segmental) cystectomy, a portion of the bladder is removed. This procedure is used when there is only a single isolated bladder tumor.

When the entire bladder must be removed (complete cystectomy), the ureters are diverted into a collecting reservoir. Techniques for urinary diversion are shown in Fig. 69-4. With an ileal conduit, the ureters are surgically placed in the ileum and urine is collected in a pouch on the skin around the stoma. More often, continent reservoirs or "neobladders" are being used. With cutaneous ureterostomy or ureteroureterostomy, the ureter opening is brought out onto the skin. The cutaneous ureterostomies may be located on either side of the abdomen or side by side.

Postoperative Care. After cutaneous ureterostomy, an external pouch covers the ostomy to collect urine. Work with the ET to focus care on the wound, the skin, and urinary drainage. (See Chapters 59 and 60 for ostomy care.)

The patient with a Kock's pouch, a continent reservoir, may have a Penrose drain and a plastic Medena catheter in the stoma. The drain removes lymphatic fluid or other secretions; the catheter ensures urine drainage so that suture lines can heal. The patient with a neobladder will have a drain at first in the event the neobladder requires irrigation. Later, irrigation can be performed with intermittent catheterization. Irrigation is performed to ensure patency. There is no sensation of bladder fullness with a neobladder because sensory nerves are not attached. As a result, the patient will need to learn new cues to void, such as prescribed times or noticing a feeling of neobladder pressure. General care after surgery is discussed in Chapter 18.

Community-Based Care

Health Teaching

Teach the patient and family about drugs, diet and fluid therapy, the use of external pouching systems, and the technique for catheterizing a continent reservoir.

With some procedures, the patient may need electrolyte replacement to prevent long-term deficits. Teach him or her to

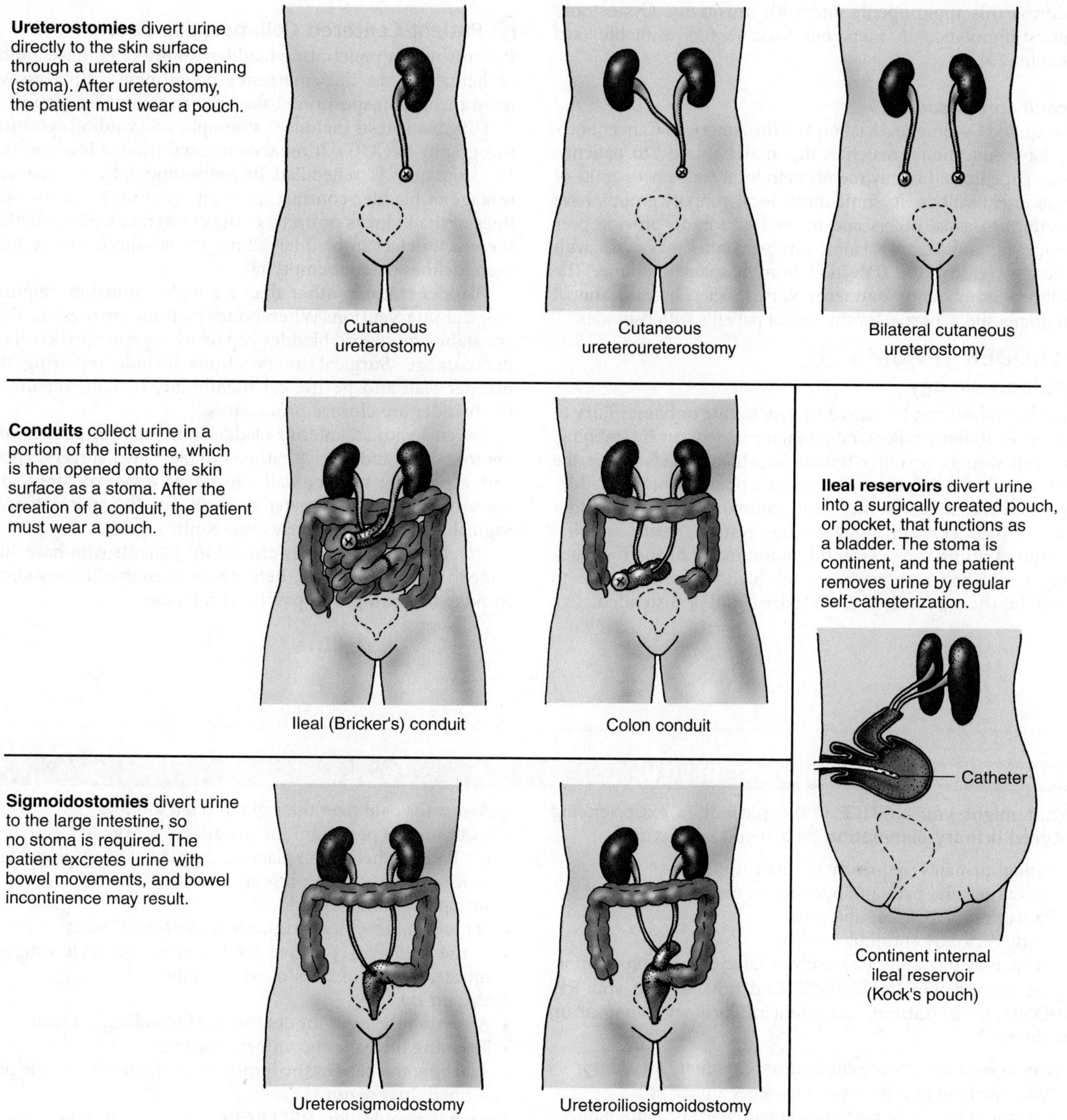
Ureterostomies divert urine directly to the skin surface through a ureteral skin opening (stoma). After ureterostomy, the patient must wear a pouch.
Cutaneous ureterostomy
Cutaneous ureteroureterostomy
Bilateral cutaneous ureterostomy
Conduits collect urine in a portion of the intestine, which is then opened onto the skin surface as a stoma. After the creation of a conduit, the patient must wear a pouch.
Ileal (Bricker's) conduit
Colon conduit
Ileal reservoirs divert urine into a surgically created pouch, or pocket, that functions as a bladder. The stoma is continent, and the patient removes urine by regular self-catheterization.
Catheter
Continent internal ileal reservoir (Kock's pouch)
Sigmoidostomies divert urine to the large intestine, so no stoma is required. The patient excretes urine with bowel movements, and bowel incontinence may result.
Ureterosigmoidostomy
Ureteroiliosigmoidostomy

Fig. 69-4 • Urinary diversion procedures used in the treatment of bladder cancer.

avoid foods that are known to produce gas if the urinary diversion uses the intestinal tract. When intestinal production of gas is excessive, flatus can induce incontinence.

Instruct the patient and family about any changes in self-care activities related to the urinary diversion. In collaboration with the enterostomal therapist, demonstrate external pouch application, local skin care, pouch care, methods of adhesion, and drainage mechanisms. If a Kock's pouch has been created, teach the patient how to use a catheter to drain the pouch. For all instruction, observe at least one return demonstration by the patient or the caregiver. Ideally, the patient assumes responsibility for self-care before discharge.

Assist the patient to prepare for the impact of urinary diversion on self-image, body image, sexual functioning, and self-esteem. Counseling provides information and support to reduce feelings of powerlessness.

Through discussions with the patient about usual social situations, help him or her gain control over new toileting practices. Men with a urinary diversion into the sigmoid colon need to learn the habit of sitting to urinate. For patients of either gender, promote confidence in social situations by encouraging frequent emptying of urinary collection devices before traveling or attending social functions. Resumption of sexual activity is a major concern for many, regardless of age.

Address this topic openly and with sensitivity. Cystectomy causes impotence in men, but treatment is available (see Chapter 75).

Health Care Resources

The United Ostomy Association and the American Cancer Society have educational materials that may be useful to patients. Refer patients and family members to local chapters or units of these organizations. In some areas, local support groups have meetings to assist others and to send visitors to provide peer counseling and support. Home care personnel may assist with follow-up, easing the transition from hospital to home. The Wound, Ostomy, and Continence Nurses Society has educational programs and a journal for the care of patients with ostomies.

BLADDER TRAUMA

Pathophysiology

Bladder trauma can be caused by penetrating or blunt injury to the lower abdomen. Penetrating injury may occur by stabbing, gunshot wound, or other trauma in which objects pierce the abdominal wall. A fractured pelvis with puncture of the bladder by bone fragments is the most common cause of bladder trauma. Bladder trauma may also be a result of sexual assault.

Blunt trauma compresses the abdominal wall and the bladder. A seat belt may compress the bladder hard enough to cause injury, especially if the bladder is full or distended.

Patient-Centered Collaborative Care

Patients with a penetrating bladder wound often have anuria or hematuria. In the emergency department, initial assessment includes inspection of the urinary meatus for blood.

Diagnostic tests include cystography and voiding cystourethrography (VCUG). If renal or ureteral trauma is suspected, IV urography is scheduled before cystography so that any leakage of bladder contrast medium does not mask the outlines of the kidneys or ureters. The cystogram shows whether there is a defect in bladder filling; the voiding cystourethrogram defines bladder emptying.

Bladder trauma, other than a simple contusion, requires surgical intervention. When bone fractures are present, they are stabilized before bladder repair to prevent further bladder damage. Surgical interventions include repairing the bladder wall and peritoneal membrane. Usually, repairs of the bladder are closure procedures.

Patients with an anterior bladder wall injury usually have a Penrose drain and a Foley catheter in place after surgery. Those with a posterior bladder wall injury have a Penrose drain and Foley or suprapubic catheter after surgery. In some instances, vaginal or rectal fistulas may also require repair.

Psychosocial support is critical for patients who have sustained traumatic injuries. Refer them to counseling resources to assist in dealing with psychosocial issues.

HUMAN NEEDS NURSING CARE REVIEW

What might you NOTICE if the patient is experiencing altered urinary elimination as a result of cystitis?

- Patient urinates frequently in small amounts.
- Patient reports pain and burning on urination.
- Patient reports suprapubic pain.
- Urine is cloudy and foul-smelling.
- Urine may be darker or smoky or have obvious blood in it.

What should you INTERPRET and how should you RESPOND to a patient experiencing urinary elimination problems?

Perform and interpret physical assessment, including:

- Ask how long manifestations have been present.
- Ask about low back pain (midline in men) or flank pain.
- Ask whether he or she has had a UTI in the past; how long ago; how it was treated; and if antibiotics were prescribed, whether the drug course was completed.
- Ask about the presence of pregnancy or any chronic health problem, especially diabetes.
- Determine fluid intake and output volumes.
- Assess for bladder distention by palpation or with a bedside bladder scanner (see Chapter 68).
- Assess for pain over the right and left kidneys.
- Examine the perineum for irritation (in women).
- If a Foley catheter is in place, determine why it is in use and how long it has been present.
- Interpret laboratory values:
- Is the complete blood count within normal limits?
- Is the urinalysis positive for bacteria, leukocyte esterase, nitrate, red blood cells, or white blood cells?

Respond by:

- Assessing the need for continuing indwelling catheter
- Teaching the patient comfort measures
- Teaching the patient the importance of completing the prescribed drug regimen

On what should you REFLECT?

- Observe patient for evidence of improved urinary output (see Chapter 68).
- Think about what may have caused this infection in a hospitalized patient (or long-term care resident) and what steps could be taken to prevent a similar episode.
- Think about what patient-teaching focus could help reduce the risk for future UTI.

GET READY FOR THE NCLEX EXAMINATION!

Key Points

Review these Key Points for each NCLEX Examination Client Needs Category.

Safe and Effective Care Environment

- Use sterile technique when inserting a catheter or any other instrument into the urinary system.
- Use Contact Precautions with any patient who has drainage from the genitourinary tract.

Health Promotion and Maintenance

- Teach patients to clean the perineal area after voiding, after having a bowel movement, and after sexual intercourse.
- Encourage all patients to maintain an adequate fluid intake (minimum of 3 L daily unless another health problem requires fluid restriction).
- Instruct women who have stress incontinence the proper way to perform pelvic floor strengthening exercises.
- Teach patients who come into contact with chemicals in their workplaces or with leisure-time activities to avoid direct skin and mucous membrane contact with these chemicals.

Psychosocial Integrity

- Allow the patient the opportunity to express feelings or concerns regarding a potential cancer diagnosis.
- Use a nonjudgmental approach in caring for patients with urinary incontinence.
- Avoid referring to protective pads or pants as "diapers."
- Recognize the need for the patient undergoing cystectomy and urinary diversion to grieve about the body image change.
- Assess the patient's level of comfort in discussing issues related to elimination and the urogenital area.
- Use language and terminology during renal/urinary assessment that the patient is comfortable using.
- Refer patients to community resources and support groups.

Physiological Integrity

- Identify hospitalized patients at risk for bacteruria and urosepsis.
- Report immediately any condition that obstructs urine flow.
- Instruct patients with UTI to complete all prescribed antibiotic therapy even when symptoms of infection are absent.
- Avoid maintaining indwelling catheters long-term in hospitalized patients.
- Teach patients the expected side effects and any adverse reactions to prescribed drugs.
- Assess the patient's manual dexterity and cognitive awareness before teaching a regimen of intermittent self-catheterization.

Additional Study Resources

Go to your Companion CD or Evolve at http://evolve.elsevier.com/Iggy/ for *Self-Assessment Questions for the NCLEX Examination.*

evolve Go to Evolve at http://evolve.elsevier.com/Iggy/ for *Prioritization and Delegation Questions for the NCLEX Examination.*

SELECTED BIBLIOGRAPHY

Asterisk indicates a classic or definitive work on this subject.

*Agency for Health Care Policy and Research (AHCPR). (1996). (Revised 2001a). *Urinary incontinence in adults: Acute and chronic management. Clinical practice guideline.* AHCPR Publication No. 96-0682. Rockville, MD: Agency for Health Care Policy and Research, Public Health Service, U.S. Department of Health and Human Services.

*Agency for Health Care Policy and Research (AHCPR). (1996). (Revised 2001b). *Urinary incontinence in adults: Helping people with incontinence. Clinical practice guideline.* AHCPR Publication No. 96-0683. Rockville, MD: Agency for Health Care Policy and Research, Public Health Service, U.S. Department of Health and Human Services.

Altschuler, V., & Diaz, L. (2006). Bladder ultrasound. *MEDSURG Nursing, 15*(5), 317-318.

American Cancer Society. (2008). *Cancer facts and figures 2008.* Report No. 01-300M–No. 5008.08. Atlanta: Author.

Bowen, A., & Hellstrom, W.J.G. (2007). Urinary tract infections: A primer for clinicians. Retrieved June 15, 2007, from www.Medscape.com.

Bradley, C.S., Rovner, E.S., Morgan, M.A., Berlin, M., Novi, J.M., Shea, J.A., et al. (2005). A new questionnaire for urinary incontinence diagnosis in women: Development and testing. *American Journal of Obstetrics and Gynecology, 192*(1), 66-73.

Centers for Disease Control and Prevention (CDC). (2006). Estimates of nosocomial infections. Retrieved June 15, 2007, from www.cdc.gov/ncidod/dhqp/hai.html.

Coe, F.L., Evan, F., & Worcester, E. (2005). Kidney stone disease. *Journal of Clinical Investigation, 115*(10), 2598-2608.

Colella, J., Kochis, E., Galli, B., & Munver, R. (2005). Urolithiasis/nephrolithiasis: What's it all about? *Urologic Nursing, 25*(6), 427-448, 475.

Dylewski, D.A., Jamison, M.G., Borawski, K.M., Sherman, N.D., Amundsen, C.L., & Webster, G.D. (2007). A statistical comparison of pad numbers versus pad weights in the quantification of urinary incontinence. *Neurourology and Urodynamics, 26*(1), 3-7.

Evans, R.J., & Sant, G.R. (2007). Current diagnosis of interstitial cystitis: An evolving paradigm. *Urology, 69*(Suppl. 4), S82-S84.

Forrest, J.B., & Dell, J.R. (2007). Successful management of interstitial cystitis in clinical practice. *Urology, 69*(4), 82-86.

Gaines, K. (2005). Trospium chloride (Sanctura®): New to the U.S. for overactive bladder. *Urologic Nursing, 25*(1), 64-65, 52.

Hanson, K. (2005). Minimally invasive and surgical management of urinary stones. *Urologic Nursing, 25*(6), 458-464.

Janos, V., & Higgins, L. (2007). Interstitial cystitis. *Advance for Nurse Practitioners, 15*(3), 55-57.

Jemal, A., Siegel, R., Ward, E., Murray, T., Xu, J., & Thun, M.J. (2007). Cancer statistics, 2007. *CA: A Cancer Journal for Clinicians, 57*(1), 43-67.

Karon, S. (2005). A team building approach to bladder retraining: A pilot study. *Urologic Nursing, 25*(4), 269-276.

Kincade, J.E., Dougherty, M.C., Busby-Whitehead, J., Carlson, J.R., Nix, W.B., Kelsey, D.T., et al. (2005). Self-monitoring and pelvic floor muscle exercises to treat urinary incontinence. *Urologic Nursing, 25*(5), 353-363.

Krieg, C. (2005). The role of diet in the prevention of common kidney stones. *Urologic Nursing, 25*(6), 451-456.

Lamm, D., McGee, W., & Hale, K. (2005). Bladder cancer: Current optimal intravesical treatment. *Urologic Nursing, 25*(5), 323-326, 331-332.

Lemmens, D. (2006). Tegress™: A new approach to urethral implants. *Urologic Nursing, 26*(1), 77-79, 52.

Lyons, C.J. (2005). Urethritis. *Clinics in Family Practice, 7*(1), 31-41.

MacDonald, M.F., & Santucci, R.A. (2005). Review and treatment algorithm of open surgical techniques for management of urethral strictures. *Urology, 65*(1), 9-15.

Martin, J.L., Williams, K.S., Sutton, A.J., Abrams, K.R., & Assassa, R.P. (2006). Systematic review and meta-analysis of methods of diagnostic assessment for urinary incontinence. *Neurology and Urodynamics, 25*(7), 674-683.

McCance, K., & Huether, S. (2006). *Pathophysiology: The biologic basis for disease in adults and children* (5th ed.). St. Louis: Mosby.

Meiner, S., & Lueckenotte, A. (Eds.). (2006). *Gerontologic nursing,* (3rd ed.). St. Louis: Mosby.

Milne, J., & Moore, K. (2006). Factors impacting self-care for urinary incontinence. *Urologic Nursing, 26*(1), 41-51.

National Kidney and Urologic Diseases Information Clearinghouse. (2007). Kidney and urologic diseases statistics for the United States, 2004. Retrieved February 2008, from http://kidney.niddk.nih.gov/statistics/.

Nussbaum, R., McInnes, R., & Willard, H. (2007). *Thompson & Thompson: Genetics in medicine* (7th ed.). Philadelphia: Saunders.

Overstreet, D., & Sims, T. (2006). Care of the patient undergoing radical cystectomy with a robotic approach. *Urologic Nursing, 26*(2), 117-123.

Pagana, K., & Pagana, T. (2006). *Mosby's manual of diagnostic and laboratory tests* (3rd ed.). St. Louis: Mosby.

Pelter, M., & Stephens, K. (2008). Evaluation of a device to facilitate female catheterization. *MEDSURG Nursing, 17*(1), 19-25.

Pelvic Pain and Urgency Frequency symptom scale: PUF questionnaire. (2005). Retrieved June 17, 2007, from www.orthoelmiron.com/orthoelmiron/hcptools_puf.html?host=www.orthoelmiron.com.

Robinson, S., Allen, L., Barnes, M.R., Berry, T.A., Foster, T.A., Friedrich, L.A., et al. (2007). Development of an evidence-based protocol for reduction on indwelling urinary catheter usage. *MEDSURG Nursing, 16*(3), 157-161.

Ruff, C. (2005). Risk factors for urinary incontinence in African-American women. *Urologic Nursing, 25*(1), 33-39.

Rushing, J. (2006). Caring for your patient's suprapubic catheter. *Nursing2006, 36*(7), 32.

Saint, S., Kaufman, S.R., Rogers, M.A., Baker, P.D., Boyko, E.J., & Lipsky, B.A. (2006). Risk factors for nosocomial urinary tract–related bacteremia: A case-control study. *American Journal of Infection Control, 34*(7), 401-407.

Senese, V. (2006a). Female urethral catheterization. *Urologic Nursing, 26*(4), 314.

Senese, V. (2006b). Male urethral catheterization. *Urologic Nursing, 26*(4), 315.

Senese, V. (2006c). Suprapubic catheter replacement. *Urologic Nursing, 26*(2), 152.

Siegel, J., Sand, P., & Sasso, K. (2008). Vulvodynia and pelvic pain? Think interstitial cystitis. *The Nurse Practitioner, 33*(10), 41-47.

Smith, P.P., McCrey, R.J., & Appell, R.A. (2006). Current trends in the evaluation and management of female urinary incontinence. *Canadian Medical Association Journal, 175*(10), 607-620.

Specht, J. (2005). 9 myths of incontinence in older adults. *AJN, 105*(6), 58-68.

Toughill, E. (2005). Indwelling urinary catheters: Common mechanical and pathogenic problems. *AJN, 105*(5), 35-37.

U.S. Renal Data Systems. (2006). *USRDS 2006 annual data report.* Bethesda, MD: The National Institutes of Health, National Institute of Diabetes and Digestive and Kidney Diseases.

Wein, A.J., Kavoussi, L.R., Novick, A.C., Partin, A.W., & Peters, C.A. (2007). *Campbell-Walsh urology* (9th ed.). Philadelphia: Saunders.

Weitzel, T. (2008). To cath or not to cath? *Nursing2008, 38*(2), 20-21.

Zarowitz, B., & Ouslander, J. (2006). Management of urinary incontinence in older persons. *Geriatric Nursing, 27*(5), 265-270.

Zurakowski, T., Taylor, M., & Bradway, C. (2006). Effective teaching strategies for the older adult with urologic concerns. *Urologic Nursing, 26*(5), 355-360.

Care of Patients with Renal Disorders

70

CHAPTER

Chris Winkelman

LEARNING OUTCOMES

For clinical competence and success on the NCLEX Examination, study this chapter with these Learning Outcomes in mind:

Health Promotion and Maintenance

1. Encourage patients with diabetes to achieve tight glycemic control.
2. Encourage patients with hypertension to follow their treatment regimens to maintain blood pressure within the target range.
3. Teach patients at risk for urinary tract infection (UTI) to maintain a daily fluid intake of 2 to 3 L unless another health problem requires fluid restriction.
4. Teach patients on antibiotic therapy for a UTI to complete the drug regimen.
5. Teach all people strategies to prevent renal trauma.

Psychosocial Integrity

6. Use language the patient is comfortable with during assessment of the renal/urinary system.
7. Encourage the patient to express feelings or concerns about a change in kidney function.
8. Explain treatment procedures to patients and families.

Physiological Integrity

9. Explain the genetics of autosomal dominant polycystic kidney disease.
10. Use laboratory data and clinical manifestations to determine the effectiveness of therapy for pyelonephritis.
11. Describe the clinical manifestations of hydronephrosis.
12. Explain the relationship between hypertension and renal disease.
13. Coordinate nursing care for the patient with pyelonephritis.
14. Coordinate nursing care for the patient during the first 24 hours after a nephrectomy.

Go to your Companion CD or Evolve at http://evolve.elsevier.com/Iggy/ for *Self-Assessment Questions for the NCLEX Examination* keyed to these Learning Outcomes.

The kidneys are responsible for meeting the *human need for urinary elimination* by filtering wastes and balancing fluids, electrolytes, acids, and bases. Any problem that disrupts kidney function limits the ability to meet that need and has the potential to impair general homeostasis (Fig. 70-1). The kidneys work together with many other organ systems. Thus renal (kidney) disorders affect systemic health and can lead to life-threatening outcomes. Renal disorders are classified as congenital, obstructive, infectious, glomerular, and degenerative. Renal tumors and renal trauma are also described in this chapter. Renal failure is discussed in Chapter 71.

CONGENITAL DISORDERS

POLYCYSTIC KIDNEY DISEASE

Pathophysiology

Polycystic kidney disease (PKD) is an inherited disorder in which fluid-filled cysts develop in the nephrons. In the dominant form, only a few nephrons have cysts until the person reaches his or her 30s. In the recessive form of the disease, nearly 100% of nephrons have cysts from birth. Cysts develop anywhere in the nephron, usually as a result of abnormal kidney cell division.

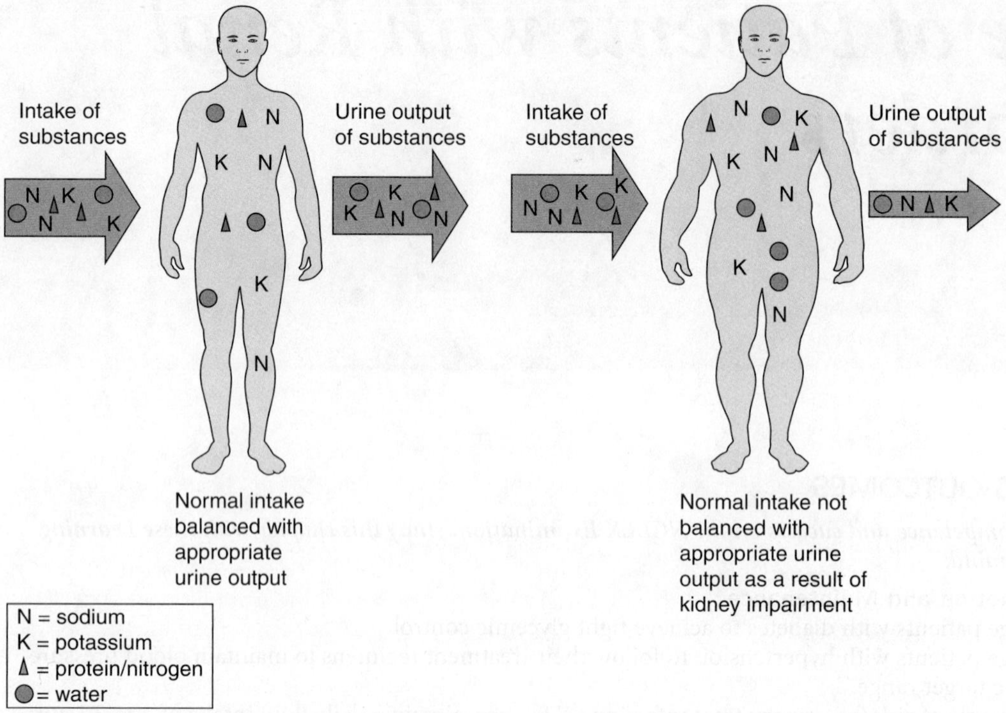
Intake of substances
Urine output of substances
Intake of substances
Urine output of substances
Normal intake balanced with appropriate urine output
Normal intake not balanced with appropriate urine output as a result of kidney impairment
N = sodium
K = potassium
= protein/nitrogen
= water

Fig. 70-1 • Unbalanced body water, electrolytes, and waste products as a result of kidney problems that prevent adjustments in urinary elimination.

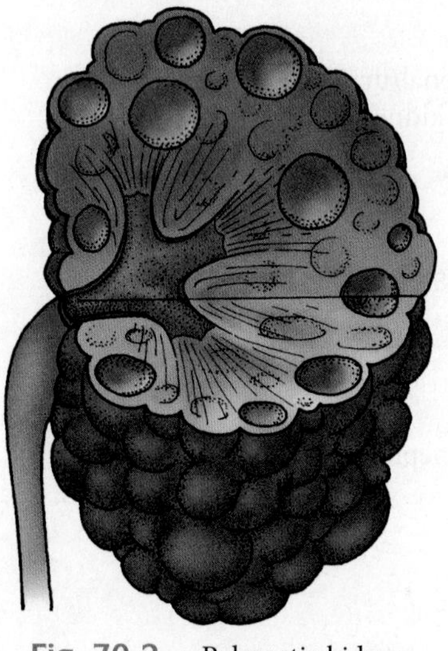

Fig. 70-2 • Polycystic kidney.

Over time, small cysts become much larger (up to a few centimeters in diameter) and more widely distributed. The growing cysts damage the glomerular and tubular membranes. As the cysts fill with fluid and enlarge, the nephron and kidney function become less effective.

The kidney tissue is eventually replaced by nonfunctioning cysts, which look like clusters of grapes (Fig. 70-2). The kidneys become very large. Each cystic kidney may enlarge to two or three times its normal size, becoming as large as a football. Other abdominal organs are displaced, and the patient has discomfort or pain. The fluid-filled cysts are also at increased risk for infection, rupture, and bleeding.

Most patients with PKD have high blood pressure. The cause of hypertension is related to renal ischemia from the enlarging cysts. As the vessels are compressed and renal blood flow decreases, the renin-angiotensin system is activated, raising blood pressure. Control of hypertension is a top priority because proper treatment can disrupt the process that leads to further kidney damage.

Cysts may occur also in other tissues, such as the liver and blood vessels. They may reduce liver function. In addition, the incidence of cerebral *aneurysms* (outpouching and thinning of an artery wall) is higher in patients with PKD. These aneurysms may rupture, causing bleeding and sudden death. For reasons as yet unknown, kidney stones occur in 8% to 36% of the patients with PKD. Heart valve problems (e.g., mitral valve prolapse), left ventricular hypertrophy, and colonic diverticula also are common in patients with PKD.

Etiology and Genetic Risk

PKD has several forms and can be inherited as either an autosomal dominant trait or, less commonly, as an autosomal recessive trait. People who inherit the recessive form of PKD usually die in early childhood. The 5% to 10% incidence of PKD in patients with no family history occurs as a result of a new gene mutation.

GENETIC CONSIDERATIONS

The autosomal dominant form of PKD (ADPKD) is the most common form of polycystic disease. Children of parents who have the autosomal dominant form of PKD have a 50% chance of inheriting the gene that causes the disease. Fig. 70-3 shows a typical pedigree for a family with ADPKD. Presentation of ADPKD can vary for age of onset, manifestations, and illness severity, even within one family. However, it is fully penetrant, meaning that nearly 100% of people who inherit a PKD gene will develop renal cysts by age 30 (Nussbaum et al., 2007). Half of these people develop renal failure by age 50 years. ADPKD-1 is the most common and most severe form of the autosomal dominant disease. ADPKD-2 has a slower rate of cyst formation, so symptoms occur later in life and progression to renal failure and other complications is delayed.

Autosomal recessive PKD is rare, and most people with the disease die in early childhood. It is caused by a different gene mutation than the dominant form. To inherit a recessive gene, both parents must carry a copy of the mutated allele and both mutated alleles must be inherited. Thus each child has a 1-in-4 chance of inheriting autosomal recessive polycystic disease.

There is no way to prevent PKD, although early detection and management of hypertension may slow the progression of kidney damage. Genetic counseling may be useful for adults who have one parent or both parents with PKD. Family history analysis is a simple assessment that can be used to help identify people at risk for PKD (see Fig. 70-3).

Incidence/Prevalence

Polycystic kidney disease (PKD) is a common disorder, affecting 250,000 to 500,000 people in the United States. It is more common in white people than in people of other races. Men and women have an equal chance of inheriting the disease because the gene responsible for PKD is not located on the sex chromosomes (Polycystic Kidney Disease Foundation, 2007).

Patient-Centered Collaborative Care

Assessment

History

Explore the family history of a patient with suspected or actual PKD, and ask whether either parent was known to have PKD or whether there is any family history of kidney disease. The age at which the problem was diagnosed in the parent and any related complications are important to obtain. Ask about constipation, abdominal discomfort, a change in urine color or frequency, high blood pressure, headaches, and a family history of sudden death from a stroke.

Physical Assessment/Clinical Manifestations

Chart 70-1 lists key features of PKD. Pain is often the first manifestation. Inspect the abdomen. A distended abdomen is common as the cystic kidneys swell and push the abdominal contents forward. Polycystic kidneys are easily palpated because of their increased size. Proceed with *gentle* abdominal palpation because the cystic kidneys and nearby tissues may be tender and palpation is uncomfortable.

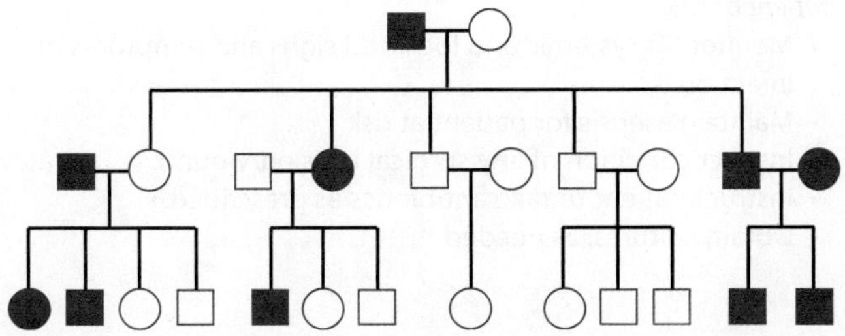

Fig. 70-3 • Three-generation pedigree for autosomal dominant polycystic kidney disease (ADPKD). *Colored-in symbols* indicate family members with ADPKD.

Chart 70-1 KEY FEATURES

Polycystic Kidney Disease

- Abdominal or flank pain
- Hypertension
- Nocturia
- Increased abdominal girth
- Constipation
- Bloody or cloudy urine
- Kidney stones

The patient also may have flank pain as a dull ache or as sharp and intermittent discomfort. Dull, aching pain is caused by increased kidney size with distention or by infection within the cyst. Sharp, intermittent pain occurs when a cyst ruptures or a stone is present. When a cyst ruptures, the patient may have bright-red or cola-colored urine. Infection is suspected if the urine is cloudy or foul smelling or if there is **dysuria** (pain on urination).

Nocturia (the need to urinate excessively at night) is an early manifestation and occurs because of decreased urine concentrating ability. As renal function further declines, the patient has increasing hypertension, edema, and uremic problems such as anorexia, nausea, vomiting, pruritus, and fatigue (see Chapter 71). Because berry aneurysms often occur in patients with PKD, a severe headache with or without neurologic or vision changes deserves particular attention.

Psychosocial Assessment

As an inherited disorder, PKD may cause psychosocial responses. The patient often has seen the effects and problems of the disease in close family members. He or she may have had a parent who died or close relatives who required dialysis or transplantation. While obtaining the family history, listen carefully for spoken and unspoken feelings of anger, resentment, futility, sadness, or anxiety. Such feelings may need further exploration. The focus of the feelings may be one or both parents or the process of diagnosis and treatment. Feelings of guilt and concern for the patient's children may also complicate the issue.

Diagnostic Assessment

Urinalysis shows **proteinuria** (protein in the urine) once the glomeruli are involved. **Hematuria** (blood in the urine) may be gross or microscopic. Bacteria in the urine indicate infection, usually in the cysts. Obtain a urine sample for culture and sensitivity testing when there is evidence of infection. As kidney function declines, serum creatinine and blood urea nitrogen (BUN) levels rise. With decreasing kidney function, creatinine clearance decreases. Changes in kidney handling of sodium may cause either sodium losses or sodium retention.

Diagnostic studies include renal sonography, computed tomography (CT), and magnetic resonance imaging (MRI). Small cysts are detected by sonography, CT, or MRI. Renal sonography shows evidence of PKD, with minimal risk.

Common Nursing Diagnoses and Collaborative Problems

Nursing diagnoses and collaborative problems that may apply to patients with polycystic kidney disease (PKD) include:

- Acute Pain related to cyst rupture or stone formation
- Chronic Pain related to enlarging kidneys compressing abdominal contents
- Constipation related to compression of intestinal tract
- Risk for Infection related to the presence of cysts and decreased renal blood flow
- Potential for Hypertension
- Potential for Stone Formation
- Potential for Renal Failure

Interventions

Chart 70-2 lists some NIC interventions for patients with renal disorders. (See Chapter 69 for information on urinary infections and stone formation. See Chapter 71 for care of the patient with kidney failure.)

Acute Pain; Chronic Pain

Comfort strategies include drug therapy and complementary approaches. A combination may be most effective. NSAIDs are used cautiously because of their tendency to reduce renal blood flow. Aspirin-containing compounds are avoided to reduce the risk for bleeding.

If cyst infection causes discomfort, antibiotics such as trimethoprim/sulfamethoxazole (Bactrim, Septra, Trimpex) or ciprofloxacin (Cipro) are prescribed. (See Chart 69-4 in Chapter 69.) These drugs enter the cyst wall. Monitor the serum creatinine levels because antibiotic therapy can be nephrotoxic. Apply dry heat to the abdomen or flank to promote comfort when renal cysts are infected. When pain is severe, cysts can be reduced by needle aspiration and drainage.

Teach the patient methods of relaxation and comfort using deep breathing, guided imagery, or other strategies. The overall goal is patient self-management. (See Chapter 5 for pain management.)

Constipation

Teach the patient how to prevent constipation by maintaining adequate fluid intake, increasing dietary fiber when fluid intake is more than 2500 mL/24 hr, and exercising regularly. Explain that pressure on the large intestine may occur as the polycystic kidneys increase in size. The patient should know that these recommendations for bowel management might change, particularly if kidney failure also develops. Advise him or her about the use of stool softeners and bulk agents, including the careful use of laxatives, to prevent chronic constipation.

Hypertension and Renal Failure

Blood pressure control is necessary to reduce cardiovascular complications and slow the progression of renal dysfunction. Nursing interventions include education to promote self-management and understanding. When renal impairment results in decreased urine concentration with nocturia and low urine specific gravity, urge the patient to drink at least 2 L of fluid per day to prevent dehydration, which can further reduce renal function. Restricting sodium intake may help control blood pressure. See Chapter 38 for a detailed discussion about the causes and management of hypertension.

Chart 70-2 NIC INTERVENTION ACTIVITIES

The Patient with Renal Problems

Energy Management: *Regulating energy use to treat or prevent fatigue and optimize function*

- Assess patient's physiologic status for deficits resulting in fatigue within the context of age and development.
- Determine patient's/significant other's perceptions of causes of fatigue.
- Encourage verbalization of feelings about limitations.
- Determine what and how much activity is required to build endurance.
- Monitor nutritional intake to ensure adequate energy resources.
- Monitor patient for evidence of excess physical and emotional fatigue.
- Monitor cardiorespiratory response to activity (e.g., tachycardia, other dysrhythmias, dyspnea, diaphoresis, pallor, hemodynamic pressures, and respiratory rate).
- Monitor location and nature of discomfort or pain during movement/activity.
- Promote bedrest/activity limitation (e.g., increase number of rest periods) with protected rest times of choice.
- Encourage alternate rest and activity periods.
- Provide calming diversionary activities to promote relaxation.
- Plan activities for periods when the patient has the most energy.
- Encourage physical activity (e.g., ambulation, performance of activities of daily living) consistent with patient's energy resources).

Fluid Monitoring: *Collection and analysis of patient data to regulate fluid balance*

- Monitor weight.
- Monitor intake and output.
- Monitor serum and urine electrolyte values, as appropriate.
- Monitor serum albumin and total protein levels.
- Monitor serum and urine osmolality levels.
- Keep an accurate record of intake and output.
- Monitor for distended neck veins, crackles in the lungs, peripheral edema, and weight gain.
- Restrict and allocate fluid intake, as appropriate.
- Administer pharmacologic agents to increase urinary output, as appropriate.
- Administer dialysis, as appropriate, noting patient response.

Infection Protection: *Prevention and early detection of infection in a patient at risk*

- Monitor for systemic and localized signs and symptoms of infection.
- Maintain asepsis for patient at risk.
- Inspect condition of any surgical incision/wound.
- Instruct patient to take antibiotics as prescribed.
- Obtain cultures, as needed.

NIC intervention activities selected from Bulechek, G.M., Butcher, H.K., & McCloskey Dochterman, J. (Eds.). (2008). *Nursing interventions classification (NIC)* (5th ed.). St. Louis: Mosby.

Drug therapy for blood pressure control includes antihypertensive agents and diuretics. Antihypertensive agents include angiotensin-converting enzyme (ACE) inhibitors, calcium channel blockers, beta blockers, and vasodilators (see Chapter 38). ACE inhibitors may help control the cell growth aspects of PKD and reduce microalbuminuria. If PKD progresses to chronic kidney disease or end-stage kidney disease, treatment approaches are similar to those in Chapter 71.

Teach the patient and family how to measure and record blood pressure. Help the patient establish a schedule for self-administering drugs, monitoring daily weights, and keeping blood pressure records (Chart 70-3). Explain the potential side effects of the drugs. Make available written materials, such as drug teaching cards and booklets.

A low-sodium diet is often prescribed to control the hypertension that usually occurs with PKD. However, some patients may have salt wasting and should not follow a sodium-restricted diet. As the disease progresses, the protein intake may be limited to slow the development of kidney failure. Assist the patient and family in understanding the diet plan and why it was prescribed. Work closely with the nutritionist to foster the patient's understanding. Also refer the patient for nutritional counseling.

Health Care Resources

The Polycystic Kidney Research Foundation (www.pkdcure.org) and the National Kidney and Urologic Disease division of the National Institute of Health (www.niddk.nih.gov) conduct research and provide education about PKD. Many pamphlets are available; there is a fee for some materials. Chapters of the National Kidney Foundation (NKF) and the American Association of Kidney Patients (AAKP) also have resources for information and support.

OBSTRUCTIVE DISORDERS

HYDRONEPHROSIS, HYDROURETER, AND URETHRAL STRICTURE

Pathophysiology

Hydronephrosis and hydroureter are problems of urine outflow obstruction. Urethral strictures also obstruct urine outflow. Prompt recognition and treatment are crucial to prevent permanent kidney damage.

In **hydronephrosis,** the kidney enlarges as urine collects in the pelvis and kidney tissue. Because the capacity of the renal pelvis is normally 5 to 8 mL, obstruction in the pelvis or at the point where the ureter joins the renal pelvis quickly distends the renal pelvis. Kidney pressure increases as the volume of urine increases. Over time, sometimes in only a matter of hours, the blood vessels and renal tubules can be damaged extensively (Fig. 70-4).

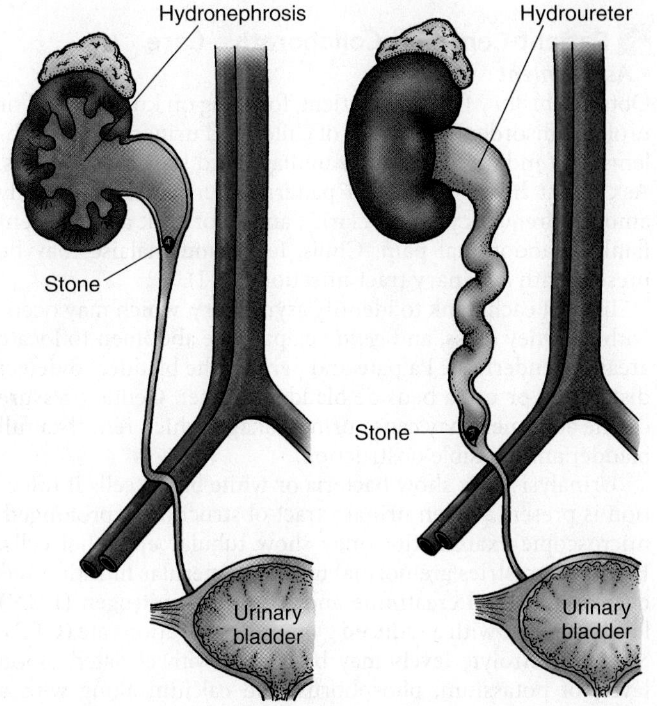
Hydronephrosis
Hydroureter
Stone
Stone
Urinary bladder
Urinary bladder

Fig. 70-4 • Hydronephrosis is caused by obstruction in the upper part of the ureter. Hydroureter is caused by obstruction in the lower part of the ureter.

In patients with **hydroureter** (enlargement of the ureter), the effects are similar but the obstruction is lower in the urinary tract. The ureter is most easily obstructed where the iliac vessels cross or where the ureters enter the bladder. Ureter dilation occurs above the obstruction and enlarges as urine collects (see Fig. 70-4).

In patients with a **urethral stricture,** the obstruction is very low in the urinary tract, causing bladder distention before hydroureter and hydronephrosis. The problems and kidney damage are similar without prompt treatment.

Urinary obstruction causes damage when pressure builds up directly on kidney tissue. Tubular filtrate pressure also increases in the nephron as drainage through the collecting system is impaired. With this added pressure, glomerular filtration decreases or ceases and kidney failure results. Nitrogen waste products (urea, creatinine, and uric acid) and electrolytes (sodium, potassium, chloride, and phosphorus) are retained in the blood, and acid-base balance is impaired.

Causes of hydronephrosis or hydroureter include tumors, stones, trauma, structural defects, and fibrosis. In patients with cancer, obstructed ureters may result from the tumors themselves, pelvic radiation, or surgical treatment. Early treatment of the causes can prevent hydronephrosis and hydroureter and thus prevent permanent kidney damage. The specific time needed to prevent permanent damage depends on the patient's kidney health. Permanent damage can occur in less than 48 hours in some patients and after several weeks in other patients.

Chart 70-3 PATIENT AND FAMILY EDUCATION GUIDE

Polycystic Kidney Disease

- Measure and record your blood pressure daily.
- Take your temperature if you suspect you have a fever.
- Weigh yourself every day at the same time of day and with the same amount of clothing; notify your physician or nurse if you have a sudden weight gain.
- Limit your intake of salt to help control your blood pressure.
- Notify your physician or nurse if your urine is foul smelling or if there is blood in your urine.
- Notify your physician or nurse if you have a headache that does not go away or if you have visual disturbances.
- Monitor bowel movements to prevent constipation.

Patient-Centered Collaborative Care

Assessment

Obtain a history from the patient, focusing on known renal or urologic disorders. A history of childhood urinary tract problems may indicate previously undiagnosed structural defects. Ask about his or her usual pattern of urination, especially amount, frequency, color, clarity, and odor. Ask about recent flank or abdominal pain. Chills, fever, and malaise may be present with a urinary tract infection (UTI).

Inspect each flank to identify asymmetry, which may occur with a kidney mass, and *gently* palpate the abdomen to locate areas of tenderness. Palpate and percuss the bladder to detect distention, or use a bedside bladder scanner. Gentle pressure on the abdomen may cause urine leakage, which reflects a full bladder and possible obstruction.

Urinalysis may show bacteria or white blood cells if infection is present. When urinary tract obstruction is prolonged, microscopic examination may show tubular epithelial cells. Blood chemistries are normal unless glomerular filtration has decreased. Blood creatinine and blood urea nitrogen (BUN) levels increase with a reduced glomerular filtration rate (GFR). Serum electrolyte levels may be altered with elevated blood levels of potassium, phosphorus, and calcium along with a metabolic acidosis (bicarbonate deficit).

IV urography shows ureteral or renal pelvis dilation. Urinary outflow obstruction can be seen with sonography (renal echography) or computed tomography (CT).

Interventions

Urinary retention and potential for infection are the primary problems. (See Fluid Monitoring and Infection Protection in Chart 70-2.) Failure to treat the cause of obstruction leads to infection and renal failure.

Urologic Interventions

If the stricture is caused by a stone, the stone can be located and removed using cystoscopic or retrograde urogram procedures. The urologist uses a cystoscope to guide a stone basket over the stone and removes it through the bladder. After stone removal, a plastic stent is usually left in the ureter for a few weeks to improve urine flow in the area irritated by the stone. The stent is later removed by another cystoscopic procedure.

Radiologic Interventions

When a stricture is causing hydronephrosis and cannot be corrected with urologic procedures, a **nephrostomy** is performed. This procedure diverts urine externally and prevents further damage to the kidney.

Patient Preparation. If possible, the patient is kept NPO for 4 to 6 hours before the procedure. Clotting studies (e.g., international normalized ratio [INR], prothrombin time [PT], and partial thromboplastic time [PTT]) should be normal or corrected. The patient receives moderate sedation for the procedure.

Procedure. The patient is placed in the prone position. The kidney is located under ultrasound or fluoroscopic guidance, and a local anesthetic is given. A needle is placed into the kidney, a soft-tipped guidewire is placed through the needle, and then a catheter is placed over the wire. The catheter tip remains in the renal pelvis, and the external end is connected to a drainage bag. The procedure immediately relieves the pressure in the kidney system and prevents further damage. The nephrostomy tube remains in place until the obstruction is resolved (with or without further intervention).

Follow-up Care. Assess the amount of drainage in the collection bag. The amount of drainage depends on whether a ureteral catheter is also being used (with a separate drainage bag). Patients with ureteral tubes may have all urine pass through to the bladder or may have urine drain into the collection bags. The type of urine drainage expected should be clearly communicated in the chart. If urine is expected to drain into the collection bag, assess the amount of drainage hourly for the first 24 hours. If the amount of drainage decreases and the patient has back pain, the tube may be clogged or dislodged. Notify the physician immediately.

Monitor the nephrostomy site for leaking urine or blood. If either occurs, notify the physician immediately. Urine drainage may be red-tinged for the first 12 to 24 hours after the procedure and should gradually clear. Assess the patient for manifestations of infection, including fever or a change in urine character.

INFECTIOUS DISORDERS: PYELONEPHRITIS

In the healthy person, urine is normally sterile and remains sterile if urine passage is not obstructed in the renal system and urinary tract. When any structural abnormality is present, the risk for damage as a result of infection is greatly increased. **Urinary tract infection (UTI)** is an infection in this normally sterile system. **Pyelonephritis** is a bacterial infection in the kidney and renal pelvis—the *upper* urinary tract. Infections in the *lower* urinary tract are described in Chapter 69.

Pathophysiology

Pyelonephritis is either the presence of active organisms in the kidney or the effects of kidney infections. **Acute pyelonephritis** is the active bacterial infection, whereas **chronic pyelonephritis** results from repeated or continued upper urinary tract infections or the effects of such infections. Chronic pyelonephritis often occurs with a urinary tract defect, obstruction, or, most commonly, when urine refluxes from the bladder back into the ureters. The vesicoureteral junction is the point at which the ureter joins the bladder. **Reflux** is the reverse or upward flow of urine toward the renal pelvis and kidney.

In pyelonephritis, organisms move up from the lower urinary tract into the kidney tissue. Descending infection transmitted by organisms in the blood may occur, but not often. Bacteria trigger the inflammatory response, and local edema results.

Acute pyelonephritis involves acute tissue inflammation, tubular cell necrosis, and possible abscess formation. **Abscesses,** which are pockets of infection with pus, can occur anywhere in the kidney. The infection is scattered within the kidney; healthy tissues can lie next to infected areas. Fibrosis and scar tissue develop from the inflammation. The calices thicken, and scars develop in the interstitial tissue.

Reflux of infected urine from the bladder into the ureters and kidney is responsible for most cases of chronic pyelonephritis. Reflux within the kidney can occur when some papillae in the kidney do not close properly. Inflammation and fibrosis lead to deformity of the renal pelvis and calices. Repeated or continuous infections create additional scar tissue, changing blood vessel, glomerular, and tubular structure.

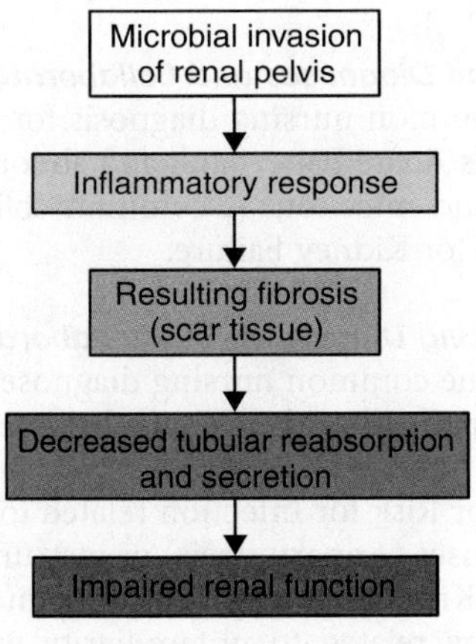
Microbial invasion of renal pelvis
Inflammatory response
Resulting fibrosis (scar tissue)
Decreased tubular reabsorption and secretion
Impaired renal function

Fig. 70-5 • Pathophysiology of pyelonephritis.

As a result, filtration, reabsorption, and secretion are impaired and renal function is reduced (Fig. 70-5).

Etiology and Genetic Risk

Single episodes of *acute pyelonephritis* may result from the entry of bacteria, especially during pregnancy, obstruction, or reflux. *Chronic pyelonephritis* usually occurs with structural deformities or obstruction with reflux. Reflux or obstruction leading to chronic pyelonephritis is often caused by stones or neurogenic impairment of voiding. Reflux is more common in children, who as adults then have scarring with chronic pyelonephritis. Chronic pyelonephritis in adults who did not have reflux as a child usually occurs with spinal cord injury, bladder tumor, prostate enlargement, or urinary tract stones.

Acute or chronic pyelonephritis occurs often in patients who have undergone manipulation of the urinary tract (e.g., placement of a urinary catheter), those with diabetes mellitus or chronic renal stones, or those who overuse analgesics. In those with diabetes mellitus, the reduced bladder tone increases the risk for pyelonephritis. In patients with chronic stone disease, stones may retain organisms, resulting in ongoing infection and kidney scarring. NSAID use can lead to papillary necrosis and reflux.

The most common pyelonephritis-causing organism is *Escherichia coli*. *Enterococcus fecalis* is common in hospitalized patients. Both organisms are in the intestinal tract. Other organisms that cause pyelonephritis in hospitalized patients include *Proteus mirabilis*, *Klebsiella*, and *Pseudomonas aeruginosa*. When the infection is bloodborne, common infecting organisms include *Staphylococcus aureus* and the *Candida* and *Salmonella* species.

Other possible causes of kidney scarring leading to renal function impairment include antibody reactions, cell-mediated immunity against the bacterial antigens, or autoimmune reactions.

Incidence/Prevalence

About 250,000 cases of acute pyelonephritis occur each year, resulting in more than 100,000 hospitalizations (Ramakrishnan & Scheid, 2005). Chronic pyelonephritis is commonly associated with vesicoureteral reflux or other anatomic abnormalities and is more common in women, although exact numbers for incidence and prevalence are not available. After 65 years of age, rates of pyelonephritis for men increase greatly because of the increased incidence of prostatitis.

Patient-Centered Collaborative Care

evolve ONLINE PHARM REVIEW

Assessment

History

Ask about a history of urinary tract infections (UTIs), diabetes mellitus, stone disease, and defects of the genitourinary tract. Determine whether the UTIs occurred with pregnancy, and ask the patient about any previous episodes of pyelonephritis or similar symptoms. Ask about disease or treatment that causes immunosuppression because they can also increase risk for pyelonephritis. Recurrences are common and may lead to a decline of renal function.

Physical Assessment/Clinical Manifestations

Ask about specific manifestations of acute pyelonephritis (Chart 70-4). Chronic pyelonephritis has a less dramatic presentation, with manifestations related to the infection or kidney function. Ask the patient to describe any vague or nonspecific urinary symptoms or abdominal discomfort. Inquire about any history of repeated, low-grade fevers. The patient with chronic pyelonephritis often has bacteriuria that causes no symptoms. Chart 70-5 outlines the renal effects of chronic pyelonephritis.

Inspect the flanks, and gently palpate the costovertebral angle (CVA). Inspect both CVAs for enlargement, asymmetry, edema, or redness, all of which can indicate inflammation. If there is no tenderness to light palpation in either CVA, an advanced practice nurse firmly percusses each area. Tenderness or discomfort may indicate infection or inflammation.

Psychosocial Assessment

The patient with any problem in the genitourinary area may have feelings of anxiety, embarrassment, or guilt. Listen carefully for signs of anxiety or specific fears, and prevent embarrassment during assessment. Feelings of guilt, often associated with sexual habits or practices, may be masked through delay in seeking treatment or through vague, nonspecific responses

Chart 70-4 KEY FEATURES
Acute Pyelonephritis

- Fever
- Chills
- Tachycardia and tachypnea
- Flank, back, or loin pain
- Tender costal vertebral angle (CVA)
- Abdominal, often colicky, discomfort
- Nausea and vomiting
- General malaise or fatigue
- Burning, urgency, or frequency of urination
- Nocturia

Chart 70-5 KEY FEATURES
Chronic Pyelonephritis

- Hypertension
- Inability to conserve sodium
- Decreased urine concentrating ability (nocturia)
- Tendency to develop hyperkalemia and acidosis

to specific or direct questions. Encourage patients to tell their own story in familiar, comfortable language.

Laboratory Assessment
Urinalysis shows a positive leukocyte esterase and nitrite dipstick test and the presence of white blood cells and bacteria. Occasional red blood cells, white blood cell casts, and protein may be present. The urine is cultured to determine whether gram-positive or gram-negative organisms are causing the infection. The urine sample for culture and sensitivity testing, obtained by the clean-catch method, shows the bacterial species and susceptibility or resistance of the specific organism to various antibiotics. In patients with recurrent episodes of pyelonephritis or upper UTIs, more specific testing of bacterial antigens and antibodies may help determine whether the same organism is responsible for the recurrent infections.

Blood cultures are obtained for specific organisms. Other blood tests include the C-reactive protein and erythrocyte sedimentation rate.

Imaging Assessment
An x-ray of the kidneys, ureters, and bladder (KUB) and IV urography are performed to diagnose stones or obstructions. A cystourethrogram is indicated for some patients. These procedures define urinary tract structures and identify any defects. Specific defects to be identified include foreign bodies, such as stones; obstruction to the outflow of urine, such as tumors, structural defects, or prostate enlargement; and urine reflux caused by incompetent bladder-ureter valve closure. (See Chapter 68 for more information on imaging assessment.)

Other Diagnostic Assessment
Other diagnostic tests include examining antibody-coated bacteria in urine, certain enzymes (e.g., lactate dehydrogenase isoenzyme 5), and radionuclide scintillation (e.g., gallium scan). Examining urine for antibody-coated bacteria helps identify patients who may need long-term antibiotic therapy. High-molecular-weight enzymes in urine, such as lactate dehydrogenase isoenzyme 5, are present with any kidney tissue deterioration problem and give trend data. The gallium scan can identify active pyelonephritis or abscesses in or around the kidney.

DECISION-MAKING CHALLENGE
Coordination of Care

The patient is a 31-year-old woman at 24 weeks' gestation with her first pregnancy. She reports new flank and suprapubic pain and dysuria. She states that urgency, nocturia, and frequency are unchanged "but I go a lot since I became pregnant." She says that she has had cystitis a few times in the past but none since she married 1 year ago and that she has had kidney stones twice in the past 7 years. She says, "I usually work the register at the grocery store in the evenings but I had to call in sick yesterday because I was so tired and nauseated." Her vital signs are: T, 102° F; P, 114; R, 22; and BP, 130/90. Her urine is cloudy, amber, and foul smelling, positive for both leukocyte esterase and nitrate, with white blood cells and gram-negative bacteria.

1. What additional assessment data should you obtain?
2. Which manifestations are specific to cystitis, which are specific to pyelonephritis, and which are common to both?
3. What risk factors for pyelonephritis are present for this patient?

evolve For suggested answer guidelines, go to http://evolve.elsevier.com/Iggy/.

■ *Analysis*
Common Nursing Diagnoses and Collaborative Problems
The primary common nursing diagnosis for the patient with pyelonephritis is Acute Pain (flank and abdominal) related to inflammation and infection. A common collaborative problem is Potential for Kidney Failure.

Additional Nursing Diagnoses and Collaborative Problems
In addition to the common nursing diagnoses and collaborative problems, patients with pyelonephritis may have one or more of these:

- Infection or Risk for Infection related to inadequate primary defenses (urinary stasis) or instrumentation
- Deficient Knowledge regarding the medical diagnosis and therapy related to unfamiliarity with information resources
- Activity Intolerance related to fatigue, debilitation, and generalized weakness associated with the infection
- Fear (of Development of Chronic Kidney Disease) related to an inability to control recurrent infections

An additional collaborative problem is:

- Potential for Sepsis and Septic Shock

■ *Planning and Implementation*
Acute Pain
NOC **Planning: Expected Outcomes.** With proper intervention, the patient with pyelonephritis is expected to achieve an acceptable state of comfort. Indicators include that he or she often or consistently demonstrates these behaviors:

- Uses nonanalgesic relief measures
- Uses analgesics appropriately
- Reports pain controlled

Interventions. Interventions may be nonsurgical or surgical. The success of several techniques that crush stones, such as lithotripsy and percutaneous ultrasonic pyelolithotomy (see Chapter 69), has decreased the need for surgery.

Nonsurgical Management. Interventions include the use of drug therapy, nutrition and fluid therapy, and teaching to ensure the patient's understanding of the treatment.

Drug therapy with antibiotics is prescribed to treat the infection. At first, the antibiotics are broad spectrum. After urine and blood culture and sensitivity results are known, more specific antibiotics may be prescribed. Urinary antiseptic drugs (e.g., nitrofurantoin [Macrodantin]) may also be prescribed to provide comfort.

Nutrition therapy involves ensuring that the patient's nutritional intake has adequate calories from all food groups for healing to occur. Fluid intake is recommended at 2 to 3 L/day unless another health problem requires fluid restriction.

Surgical Management. Surgical interventions are used to correct structural problems causing urine reflux or obstruction of urine outflow or to remove the source of infection.

Antibiotics are given, usually IV, to achieve adequate blood levels or sterile blood culture results. Teach the patient the nature and purpose of the proposed surgery, the expected outcome, and how he or she can participate.

The surgical procedures may be one of these: **pyelolithotomy** (stone removal from the kidney), **nephrectomy** (removal of the kidney), ureteral diversion, or reimplantation of ureter to restore proper bladder drainage.

A pyelolithotomy is needed for removal of a large stone in the renal pelvis that blocks urine flow and causes infection. Nephrectomy is a last resort when all other measures to clear the infection have failed. For patients with poor ureter valve closure or dilated ureters, **ureteroplasty** (ureter repair or revision) or ureteral reimplantation (through another site in the bladder wall) preserves kidney function and eliminates infections.

See Chapter 69 for nursing care after surgery for the patient undergoing urologic surgery.

Potential for Kidney Failure

NOC **Planning: Expected Outcomes.** The patient is expected to conserve existing kidney function for as long as possible and have a slow progression of kidney failure once the process of kidney failure begins. Indicators include that he or she consistently demonstrates these behaviors:

- Describes the role of antibiotics and self-administration of drugs
- Explains and offers techniques to ensure adequate nutrition and hydration
- Describes the plan for post-treatment follow-up, including knowledge of recurrent symptoms
- Modifies prescribed regimen as directed by a health care professional

Interventions. Specific antibiotics are prescribed to treat the infection. Stress the importance of completing the drug therapy as directed. Discuss with the patient and family the importance of regular follow-up examinations and completing the recommended diagnostic tests.

Blood pressure control is needed to slow the progression of kidney dysfunction. When impairment decreases urine concentrating ability, encourage the patient to drink at least 2 L of fluid per day to prevent dehydration, which could further reduce kidney function. When dietary protein is restricted, refer the patient to the nutritionist as needed. Other interventions related to the progression of chronic kidney failure are covered in Chapter 71.

Community-Based Care

Pyelonephritis causes fear and anxiety in the patient and family. The severity of the acute process and its potential to develop into a chronic process are frightening. The patient and the family need reassurance that treatment and preventive measures can be successful.

Home Care Management

If no surgery is performed, the patient may need help with self-care, nutrition, and drug management at home. If surgery is performed, he or she may need help with incision care, self-care, and transportation for follow-up appointments.

Health Teaching

After assessing the patient's and family's understanding of pyelonephritis and its therapy, explain:

- Drug regimen (purpose, timing, frequency, duration, and possible side effects)
- The role of nutrition and adequate fluid intake
- The need for a balance between rest and activity, including any limitations after surgery
- The manifestations of disease recurrence
- The use of previously successful coping mechanisms

Advise the patient to complete all prescribed antibiotic regimens and to report any side effects or unusual symptoms to the physician rather than stopping the drugs. Refer the patient and family for nutritional counseling as needed, because many patients have special nutritional requirements, such as those caused by diabetes mellitus or pregnancy.

Health Care Resources

The patient may also briefly need a home health nurse to help with drug or nutrition therapy at home. Housekeeping services may be helpful while he or she is regaining strength.

■ *Evaluation: Outcomes*

Evaluate the care of the patient with pyelonephritis on the basis of the identified nursing diagnoses and collaborative problems. Expected outcomes may include that the patient will:

- Report that pain is controlled
- Be knowledgeable about the disease, its treatment, and interventions to prevent or reduce disease progression

Specific indicators for these outcomes are listed for each nursing diagnosis and collaborative problem under the Planning and Implementation section (see earlier).

DECISION-MAKING CHALLENGE
Coordination of Care

The patient described on p. 1588 is diagnosed with acute pyelonephritis. Because she is pregnant, she is considered a "complicated" presentation of pyelonephritis. A urine culture is obtained along with a Gram stain that shows gram-positive cocci. She is started on ampicillin sulbactam (Unasyn). The perineal examination indicates that her urethral meatus is located abnormally close to her vagina. She will undergo cystography after she recovers from delivery of her child in 6 to 12 months from now. Further testing is deferred because of her pregnancy. Her serum creatinine is normal at 1.0, which indicates adequate renal function, further indicating that additional diagnostic testing can be deferred.

1. Explain whether this patient's acute pyelonephritis is an ascending or a descending infection.
2. How do the findings of the physical examination relate as a cause of her acute pyelonephritis?
3. In addition to adherence to any chronic antiseptic or antibiotic therapy, what could you suggest as measures for this patient to reduce her risk for future episodes of pyelonephritis and cystitis? (You may need to review Chapter 69.)

evolve For suggested answer guidelines, go to http://evolve.elsevier.com/Iggy/.

IMMUNOLOGIC RENAL DISORDERS

Glomerulonephritis (GN) is the third leading cause of end-stage kidney disease (ESKD) (National Kidney and Urologic Diseases Information Clearinghouse [NKUDIC], 2006). Whether the disease starts in the kidney or occurs as the result of other health problems, the glomeruli are usually injured (Table 70-1). For disease that starts in the kidney, a genetic basis and immune

TABLE 70-1 Primary Glomerular Diseases and Syndromes

- Acute glomerulonephritis
- Rapidly progressive glomerulonephritis (RPGN)
- Chronic glomerulonephritis
- Nephrotic syndrome
- Persistent, vague urinary abnormalities with few or no symptoms

problem are common. In addition, systemic diseases and infections can have renal effects and cause glomerular injury (Table 70-2). Conditions that lead to glomerular disease include systemic lupus erythematosus and diabetic nephropathy.

Each type of disease or syndrome has a specific pathophysiology and clinical manifestations. Their *glomerular* effects are caused by injury to the glomeruli and result in proteinuria, hematuria, decreased glomerular filtration rate (GFR), edema, and hypertension. The extent and duration of renal injury, prognosis, and specific cause vary among these syndromes.

Immunologic changes injure the glomeruli, interstitium, or tubules, and the effects may be acute or chronic. Both antibody and cellular immune responses are involved. The resultant renal disorder can be systemic or confined to the kidneys.

Most forms of glomerulonephritis (GN) occur with a collection of immune complexes in the glomeruli (Fig. 70-6). An immune complex is made up of antigens (foreign substances in the body) and antibodies. The antigen can be part of any normal kidney tissue, or it can be dissolved in a body fluid (e.g., blood). Bacteria and viruses are also antigens. Exposure to bacteria, viruses, drugs, or other toxins is believed to be the trigger for glomerular injury.

Antibody reaction with antigens can cause immune complexes to form and become deposited in glomerular tissue. These complexes trigger many inflammatory mediators, such as complement, white blood cells, and blood clotting proteins, which also damage the kidney tissue. Actions that cause tissue injury include damage to cell membranes, local edema, movement of white blood cells to the site of inflammation, and platelet activation.

ACUTE GLOMERULONEPHRITIS

Pathophysiology

An infection often occurs before the renal manifestations of acute glomerulonephritis (GN). The onset of symptoms is about 10 days from the time of infection. Usually, patients recover quickly and completely from acute GN. The term *acute nephritic syndrome* also describes this disorder.

Most causes of acute GN are infectious (Table 70-3) or are related to other systemic diseases (see Table 70-2). The incidence of acute GN is unknown. GN after a systemic streptococcal infection is more common in men.

Patient-Centered Collaborative Care

Assessment

History

Ask about recent infections, particularly of the skin or upper respiratory tract, and about recent travel or other activities with possible exposure to viruses, bacteria, fungi, or parasites.

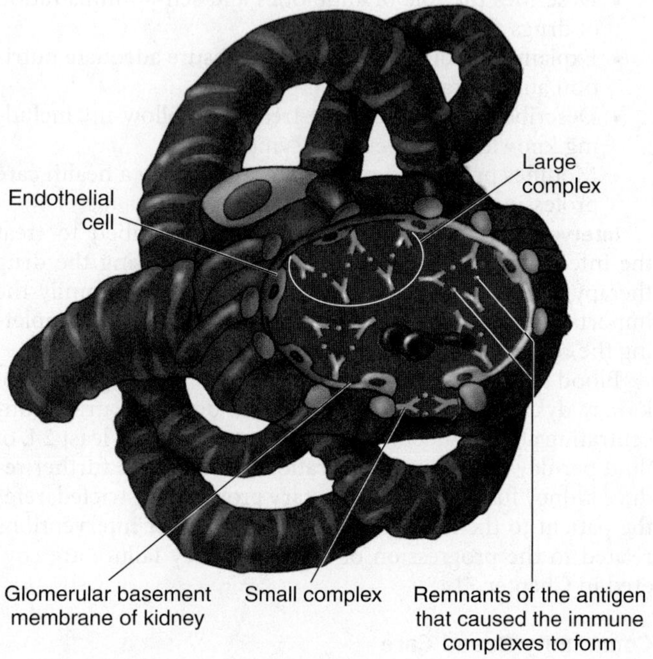
Large complex
Endothelial cell
Glomerular basement membrane of kidney
Small complex
Remnants of the antigen that caused the immune complexes to form

Fig. 70-6 • An immune complex precipitating in the glomerulus of a patient with glomerulonephritis.

TABLE 70-2 Secondary Glomerular Diseases and Syndromes

- Systemic lupus erythematosus (SLE)
- Schönlein-Henoch purpura
- Goodpasture's syndrome
- Systemic necrotizing vasculitis
- Wegener's granulomatosis
- Periarteritis nodosa (also called *polyarteritis nodosa*)
- Amyloidosis
- Diabetic glomerulopathy
- HIV-associated nephropathy
- Alport's syndrome
- Multiple myeloma
- Viral hepatitis B
- Viral hepatitis C
- Cirrhosis
- Sickle-cell disease
- Nonstreptococcal postinfectious acute glomerulonephritis
- Infective endocarditis
- Hemolytic-uremic syndrome
- Thrombotic thrombocytopenic purpura

TABLE 70-3 Infectious Causes of Acute Glomerulonephritis

- Group A beta-hemolytic *Streptococcus*
- Staphylococcal or gram-negative bacteremia or sepsis
- Pneumococcal, *Mycoplasma*, or *Klebsiella* pneumonia
- Syphilis
- Visceral abscesses
- Infective endocarditis
- Hepatitis B
- Infectious mononucleosis
- Measles
- Mumps
- Rocky Mountain spotted fever
- Cytomegalovirus infection
- Histoplasmosis
- Toxoplasmosis
- Varicella
- *Chlamydia psittaci* infection
- Coxsackievirus infection
- Any bacterial, parasitic, fungal, or viral infection (potentially)

Recent illnesses, surgery, or other invasive procedures may suggest infections. Ask about any known systemic diseases, such as systemic lupus erythematosus (SLE), which could cause acute GN.

Physical Assessment/Clinical Manifestations

Inspect the patient's skin for lesions or recent incisions (including body piercings). Assess the face, eyelids, hands, and other areas for edema (present in about 75% of the patients with acute GN). Assess for fluid overload and circulatory congestion (which may accompany the sodium and fluid retention occurring with acute GN). Ask about any difficulty in breathing or shortness of breath. Assess for crackles in the lung fields, an S_3 heart sound (gallop rhythm), and neck vein distention.

Ask about changes in urination pattern and any change in urine color. Microscopic blood in the urine occurs up to 66% of the time, and patients often describe their urine as smoky, reddish brown, rusty, or cola colored. Ask about dysuria or oliguria. Weigh the patient to assess for fluid retention.

Take the patient's blood pressure, and compare it with the baseline blood pressure. Mild to moderate hypertension often occurs with acute GN as a result of sodium and fluid retention. The patient may have fatigue, a lack of energy, anorexia, nausea, and/or vomiting if uremia from kidney failure is present.

CONSIDERATIONS FOR OLDER ADULTS

The less common manifestations of acute GN are more likely to occur in older adults. Circulatory congestion often is present, causing acute GN to be easily confused with congestive heart failure.

Laboratory Assessment

Urinalysis shows red blood cells (hematuria) and protein (proteinuria). An early morning specimen of urine is preferred for urinalysis because the urine is most acidic and formed elements are more intact at that time. Microscopic examination often shows red blood cell casts, as well as casts from other substances. The urine sediment assay is usually positive.

The glomerular filtration rate (GFR), either estimated from a single serum and urine creatinine value or measured by the 24-hour urine test for creatinine clearance, may be decreased to 50 mL/min. Blood urea nitrogen (BUN) levels are usually increased. The older patient may have a greater decline in GFR.

A 24-hour urine collection for total protein assay is obtained. The protein excretion rate for patients with acute GN may be increased from 500 mg to 3 g/24 hr in most patients. Serum albumin levels are decreased because of the protein lost in the urine and because of fluid retention causing dilution.

Specimens from the blood, skin, or throat are obtained for culture, if indicated. Other serologic tests include antistreptolysin-O titers, C3 complement levels, cryoglobulins (immunoglobulin G [IgG]), antinuclear antibodies (ANAs), and circulating immune complexes.

Antistreptolysin-O titers are increased after group A beta-hemolytic *Streptococcus* infections. Complement levels are decreased when the complement system is activated. Type III cryoglobulins may be found during acute illness. ANAs suggest an autoimmune response, and SLE is just one possibility. Circulating immune complexes containing IgG and C3 are often detected.

Other Diagnostic Assessment

A renal biopsy provides a precise diagnosis of the condition, assists in determining the prognosis, and helps outline treatment (see Chapter 68). The specific tissue features are determined by light microscopy, immunofluorescent stains, and electron microscopy to identify cell type, the presence of immunoglobulins, or the type of tissue deposits.

Interventions

Interventions focus on managing infection, preventing complications, and providing appropriate patient education.

Management of infection as a cause of acute GN begins with appropriate antibiotic therapy. Penicillin, erythromycin, or azithromycin is prescribed for GN caused by streptococcal infection. Check the patient's known allergies before giving any drug. To prevent infection spread, antibiotics for people in immediate close contact with the patient also may be prescribed. Stress personal hygiene and basic infection control principles (e.g., handwashing) to prevent spread of the organism. Teach patients the importance of completing the entire course of the prescribed antibiotic.

Prevention of complications is an important nursing intervention. For patients with fluid overload, hypertension, and edema, diuretics and a sodium and water restriction are prescribed. Antihypertensive drugs may be needed to control hypertension (see Chapter 38). The usual fluid allowance is equal to the 24-hour urine output plus 500 to 600 mL. Patients with oliguria usually have increased serum levels of potassium and BUN. Potassium and protein intake may be restricted to prevent hyperkalemia and uremia as a result of the elevated BUN.

Nausea, vomiting, or anorexia indicates that uremia is present. Dialysis is necessary if uremic symptoms or fluid volume excess cannot be controlled (see Chapter 71). **Plasmapheresis** (removal and filtering of the plasma to eliminate antibodies) also may be attempted (see Chapter 42).

To conserve the patient's energy, assist him or her in maintaining a restful environment, balancing activity and rest, and coordinating needed activities. Urge the patient to practice relaxation techniques and to participate in diversional activities to reduce emotional stress.

Patient education includes teaching the patient and family members about the purpose and desired effects of prescribed drugs, the dosage and schedule, and potential adverse side effects. Ensure that they understand dietary or fluid restrictions, including methods of detecting fluid retention. Advise the patient to measure weight and blood pressure daily at the same time each day. Instruct him or her to notify the health care provider of any sudden increase in weight or blood pressure.

If short-term dialysis is required to control fluid volume or uremic symptoms, explain peritoneal or vascular access care and dialysis schedules and routines (also see Chapter 71).

RAPIDLY PROGRESSIVE GLOMERULONEPHRITIS

Rapidly progressive glomerulonephritis (RPGN), a type of acute nephritis, is also called *crescentic glomerulonephritis* because of the presence of crescent-shaped cells in the Bowman's capsule. RPGN develops over several weeks or months and causes loss of kidney function. Patients become quite ill quickly and have manifestations of renal failure (fluid volume excess, hypertension, oliguria, electrolyte imbalances, and uremic symptoms).

The patient may have had previous infection or systemic disease, such as systemic lupus erythematosus (SLE). The renal decline often progresses to end-stage kidney disease (ESKD).

CHRONIC GLOMERULONEPHRITIS

Pathophysiology

Chronic glomerulonephritis, or *chronic nephritic syndrome,* develops over 20 to 30 years or even longer. The exact onset of the disorder is rarely identified. Often the cause of the disease is not known because the kidneys are atrophied and tissue is not available for biopsy or diagnosis. Mild proteinuria and hematuria, hypertension, fatigue, and occasional edema are often the only manifestations.

Although the exact cause is not known, changes in the kidney tissue result from hypertension, infections and inflammation, or poor blood flow to the kidneys. Kidney tissue atrophies, and the number of functional nephrons is greatly reduced. Biopsy in the late stages of atrophy may show glomerular changes, cell loss, protein and collagen deposits, and fibrosis of the kidney tissue. Microscopic examination shows deposits of immune complexes.

The loss of nephrons reduces glomerular filtration. Hypertension and renal arteriole sclerosis are often present. The glomerular damage allows proteins to enter the urine. Chronic glomerulonephritis always leads to kidney failure (see Chapter 71).

Patient-Centered Collaborative Care

▪ Assessment

History

Ask about other health problems, including systemic diseases, renal or urologic disorders, infectious diseases (e.g., streptococcal infections), and recent exposures to infections. Ask about overall health status and whether increasing fatigue and lethargy have occurred.

Identify the patient's pattern of voiding. Ask whether the frequency of voiding has increased or the quantity of urine has decreased. Ask about changes in urine color, odor, or clarity and whether dysuria or incontinence has occurred. Nocturia also is a common symptom.

Assess the patient's general comfort, and ask whether any dyspnea at rest or with exertion has occurred, because fluid overload can occur with decreased urine output. Ask about and observe for changes in mental functioning, such as irritability or an inability to read or to perform job-related functions or other processes requiring concentration. Changes in memory and the ability to concentrate occur as waste products collect in the blood.

Physical Assessment/Clinical Manifestations

Assess for systemic circulatory overload. Auscultate lung fields for crackles, observe the respiratory rate and depth, and measure blood pressure and weight. Auscultate the heart for rate, rhythm, and the presence of an S_3 heart sound. Inspect the neck veins for venous engorgement, and check for edema of the foot and ankle, on the shin, and over the sacrum.

Assess for uremic symptoms, such as slurred speech, ataxia, tremors, or **asterixis** (flapping tremor of the fingers or the inability to maintain a fixed posture with the arms extended and wrists hyperextended). Inspect skin for a yellowish color, texture, bruises, rashes, or eruptions. Ask about itching, and document areas of dryness or any excoriation from scratching.

Diagnostic Assessment

Urine output decreases, but the urine appears normal unless a urinary tract infection (UTI) also is present. Urinalysis shows protein, usually less than 2 g in a 24-hour collection. The specific gravity is fixed at a constant level of dilution (around 1.010). Red blood cells and casts may be in the urine.

The glomerular filtration rate (GFR), measured by creatinine clearance, is low. The serum creatinine level is elevated, usually greater than 6 mg/dL but may be as high as 30 mg/dL or more. The BUN is increased, often as high as 100 to 200 mg/dL.

Decreased kidney function causes abnormal serum electrolyte levels. Sodium retention is common, but dilution of the plasma from excess fluid can result in a falsely normal serum sodium level (135 to 145 mEq/L) or a low sodium level (less than 135 mEq/L). When oliguria develops, potassium is not excreted and hyperkalemia occurs when levels exceed 5.4 mEq/L.

Hyperphosphatemia develops with serum levels greater than 4.7 mg/dL. Serum calcium levels are usually at the lower end of the normal range or are slightly below normal.

Acidosis develops from hydrogen ion retention and loss of bicarbonate. However, there may be a decrease in serum carbon dioxide (CO_2) levels as patients breathe more rapidly to compensate for the acidosis. If respiratory compensation is present, the pH of arterial blood is between 7.35 and 7.45. A pH of less than 7.35 means that the patient's respiratory system is not completely compensating for the acidosis.

The kidneys are abnormally small on x-ray and on IV urography and when measured by sonography or computed tomography (CT).

A renal biopsy is important in the early stages of glomerulonephritis, when protein or blood is first present in the urine. Tissue changes include a variety of cells infiltrating the glomerular tissue, deposits of immune complexes, and blood vessel sclerosis. In advanced disease, when the kidneys are small, renal biopsy usually is not performed.

▪ Interventions

Interventions focus on slowing the progression of the disease and preventing complications. Treatment consists of diet changes, fluid intake sufficient to prevent reduced blood flow volume to the kidneys, and drug therapy to control the problems from uremia. Eventually, the patient requires dialysis or transplantation to prevent death from uremia. (Care for the patient with ESKD requiring dialysis or transplantation is discussed in Chapter 71.)

NEPHROTIC SYNDROME

Pathophysiology

Nephrotic syndrome (NS) is a condition of increased glomerular permeability that allows larger molecules to pass through the membrane into the urine and then be excreted. This process causes massive loss of protein into the urine, edema formation, and decreased plasma albumin levels. Many agents and disorders are possible causes of NS.

The most common cause of glomerular membrane changes is an immune or inflammatory process. Defects in glomerular filtration can also occur as a result of genetic defects of the glomerular filtering system, such as Fabry disease. Altered liver activity may occur with nephrotic syndrome, resulting in increased lipid production and hyperlipidemia.

Patient-Centered Collaborative Care

The main feature of NS is severe proteinuria (more than 3.5 g of protein in 24 hours). Patients also have low serum albumin levels (serum albumin less than 3 g/dL), high serum lipid levels, fats in the urine, edema, and hypertension (Chart 70-6). Renal vein thrombosis often occurs at the same time as NS, either as a cause of the problem or as an effect. NS may progress to ESKD, but this can be prevented with treatment.

Treatment varies depending on what process is causing the disorder (identified by renal biopsy). Immunologic processes may improve with suppressive therapy using steroids and cytotoxic or immunosuppressive agents. Angiotensin-converting enzyme (ACE) inhibitors can decrease protein loss in the urine, and cholesterol-lowering drugs can improve blood lipid levels. Heparin may reduce urine protein and reduce renal insufficiency. Diet changes are often prescribed. If the glomerular filtration rate (GFR) is normal, dietary intake of proteins is needed. If the GFR is decreased, dietary protein intake must be decreased. Mild diuretics and sodium restriction may be needed to control edema and hypertension. Assess the patient's hydration status, because vascular dehydration is common. If the plasma volume is depleted, renal problems worsen. Acute kidney failure may be avoided if good renal blood flow is maintained.

IMMUNOLOGIC INTERSTITIAL AND TUBULOINTERSTITIAL DISORDERS

Problems can arise in the kidney tissues around the nephrons, as well as in the nephron tissues. These interstitial and tubulointerstitial disorders in the kidney are usually caused by immune problems. These kidney changes may be acute or chronic. The acute effects often occur with drugs such as penicillins, cephalosporins, sulfonamides, or NSAIDs. Chronic interstitial nephritis has many causes, including analgesic use, complement activation, cyclosporin use, polycystic kidney disease, autoimmune disorders, multiple myeloma, sickle cell disease, obstructive disorders, and radiation nephritis. Drug-induced problems often occur with a rash or an elevated eosinophil count. Fever is common in interstitial nephritis of unknown cause. Progression to ESKD occurs unless the cause is identified and removed.

DEGENERATIVE DISORDERS

Degenerative disorders that change renal function often occur with a multisystem disorder. Many of these degenerative disorders result from changes in kidney blood vessels.

Chart 70-6 KEY FEATURES

Nephrotic Syndrome

- Massive proteinuria
- Hypoalbuminemia
- Edema
- Lipiduria
- Hyperlipidemia
- Increased coagulation
- Renal insufficiency

NEPHROSCLEROSIS

Pathophysiology

Nephrosclerosis is a problem of thickening in the nephron blood vessels, resulting in narrowing of the vessel lumen. This change decreases renal blood flow, and kidney tissue is chronically hypoxic. Ischemia and fibrosis develop over time.

Nephrosclerosis occurs with all types of hypertension, atherosclerosis, and diabetes mellitus. The more severe the hypertension, the greater is the risk for severe kidney damage. Nephrosclerosis is rarely seen when blood pressure is consistently below 160/110 mm Hg. The changes caused by hypertension may be reversible or may progress to end-stage kidney disease (ESKD) within months or years.

Hypertension is the second leading cause of ESKD. Hypertension is the cause of kidney failure in about 30% of patients requiring renal replacement therapy (e.g., dialysis or transplantation) (Bakris, 2005).

CULTURAL AWARENESS

Hypertension is more common in African Americans, and the risks of ESKD from hypertension are also greater for African Americans (Jamerson, 2005). Between 25 and 45 years of age, the ratio of African Americans to Caucasians at risk for ESKD from hypertension is nearly 20:1. At any health care encounter with an African-American patient, blood pressure should always be assessed. If hypertension is present, treatment and patient education can help reduce the risk for development of ESKD.

Patient-Centered Collaborative Care

Treatment aims to control high blood pressure and reduce albuminuria to preserve kidney function. Although many antihypertensive drugs may lower blood pressure, the patient's response is important in ensuring long-term adherence to the prescribed therapy. Factors that promote adherence include once-a-day dosing, low cost, and minimal side effects.

Lack of knowledge or misinformation about hypertension poses many challenges to health care providers working with patients who have hypertension. When kidney disease occurs, adherence to therapy is even more important for preserving health.

Many drugs can control high blood pressure (see Chapter 38), and more than one agent may be needed for best control. Angiotensin-converting enzyme (ACE) inhibitors are very useful in reducing hypertension and preserving renal function. Diuretics can maintain fluid and electrolyte balance in the presence of renal insufficiency. Hyperkalemia needs to be prevented when potassium-sparing diuretics, alone or in combination, are used to treat hypertensive patients with known kidney disease.

RENOVASCULAR DISEASE

Pathophysiology

Processes affecting the renal arteries may severely narrow the lumen and greatly reduce blood flow to the kidney tissues. Uncorrected renovascular disease, such as renal artery stenosis, atherosclerosis, or thrombosis, causes ischemia and atrophy of kidney tissue (Russell, 2008).

Patients with renovascular disease often have a sudden onset of hypertension, particularly those older than 50 years.

Patients with high blood pressure but with no family history of hypertension also may potentially have renal artery stenosis (RAS). RAS from atherosclerosis or blood vessel hyperplasia is the main cause of renovascular disease. Other causes include thrombosis and renal aneurysms.

Atherosclerotic changes in the renal artery often occur along with sclerosis in the aorta and other major vessels. Changes in the renal artery are often located where the renal artery and aorta meet. Fibrotic changes of the blood vessel wall occur throughout the length of the renal artery.

Patient-Centered Collaborative Care

Assessment

Key features of renovascular disease are listed in Chart 70-7. Hypertension usually first occurs after 40 to 50 years of age, and often the patient does not have a family history of hypertension. Diagnosis is made by magnetic resonance angiography (MRA), renal duplex ultrasonography, radionuclide imaging, renal arteriography, and renal vein renin levels. MRA provides an excellent image of the renal vasculature and kidney anatomy. Radionuclide imaging is a noninvasive way of evaluating renal blood flow and excretory function. Combining radionuclide imaging with ingestion of an ACE inhibitor such as captopril improves the accuracy of the test. A renal arteriogram makes the features of the renal blood vessels visible. The comparison of renal vein renin levels *may* reveal which kidney is producing more renin.

Interventions

Identifying the type of defect, extent of narrowing, and condition of the surrounding blood vessels is critical for treatment choice. The patient's overall health and the size of the atrophied kidney also affect treatment decisions. Many patients with renovascular disease also have cardiovascular disease, and both conditions require treatment.

RAS may be treated by drugs to control high blood pressure and by procedures to restore the renal blood supply. Drugs may control high blood pressure but may not lead to long-term preservation of kidney function. In young and middle-aged adults, a lifetime of treatment with many drugs for high blood pressure may make treatment difficult and the outcomes uncertain.

Balloon angioplasty with or without stent placement to open renal vessels is less risky and requires less time for recovery than does renal artery bypass surgery. Renal artery bypass surgery is a major procedure and requires 2 or more months for recovery. A bypass may be performed for either one or both renal arteries.

Renal angioplasty with metal stent placement is one safe and effective method to repair RAS. After the procedure, the patient usually remains in the ICU for 24 hours to monitor for sudden blood pressure fluctuations as the kidneys adjust to increased blood flow.

Chart 70-7 KEY FEATURES

Renovascular Disease

- Significant, difficult-to-control high blood pressure
- Elevated serum creatinine
- Decreased creatinine clearance

A synthetic blood vessel graft is inserted to redirect blood flow from the abdominal aorta into the renal artery, beyond the area of narrowing. A splenorenal bypass can also restore renal blood flow. The process is similar to other arterial bypass procedures (see Chapter 37).

DIABETIC NEPHROPATHY

Pathophysiology

Diabetes mellitus is the leading cause of end-stage kidney disease (ESKD) among white people in the United States. About 36% of patients requiring dialysis or renal transplantation have diabetes mellitus (NKUDIC, 2006). Diabetic nephropathy occurs with either type 1 or type 2 diabetes mellitus. Severity of diabetic renal disease is related to the extent, duration, and effects of atherosclerosis, hypertension, and neuropathy, which promote loss of bladder tone, urinary stasis, and urinary tract infection.

Patient-Centered Collaborative Care

Diabetic nephropathy is a vascular complication of diabetes. Its first manifestation is persistent albuminuria (as shown by dipstick or a urinary albumin excretion rate above 0.3 g/dL), without evidence of other renal disease. Diabetic kidney disease is progressive (Table 70-4).

Structural and functional changes occur in the kidneys of diabetic patients. Initially, kidney size is slightly increased and glomerular filtration rates (GFRs) are higher than normal. Microlevels of albumin are first detected in the urine. Progressive kidney damage occurs before dipstick procedures can detect protein in the urine. For most patients, proteinuria (albuminuria) indicates the need for follow-up and possibly a renal biopsy for further diagnosis. See Chapter 67 for a detailed discussion of kidney issues in patients with diabetes.

Proteinuria may be mild, moderate, or severe. Diabetic patients are always considered to be at risk for kidney failure. If possible, nephrotoxic agents (e.g., radiopaque contrast media or aminoglycosides) and dehydration are avoided. Patients with worsening renal function may begin to have frequent hypoglycemic episodes and a reduced need for insulin or oral antidiabetic agents. Explain to the patient that the kidneys metabolize and excrete insulin. When renal function is reduced, the insulin is available for a longer time and thus less

TABLE 70-4 The Stages of Progression of Type 1 Diabetic Renal Disease

Stage I, at the time diabetes is diagnosed. Kidney size and glomerular filtration rate are increased. Blood sugar control can reverse the changes.

Stage II, 2 to 3 years after diagnosis. Glomerular and tubular capillary basement membrane changes result in microscopic changes, with loss of filtration surface area and scar formation. Glomerular changes are referred to as *glomerulosclerosis.*

Stage III, 7 to 15 years after diagnosis. Microalbuminuria is present. The glomerular filtration rate (GFR) may still be normal or may be increased.

Stage IV. Albuminuria is detectable by dipstick. GFR is decreased. Blood pressure is increased, and retinopathy is present.

Stage V. GFR decreases at an average rate of 10 mL/min/yr.

NOTE: Progression of renal disease related to type 1 diabetes mellitus can be delayed by maintaining glycemic control with HbA_{1c} levels below 8%.

of it is needed. Unfortunately, many patients believe this means their diabetes is improving. The result is a more rapid progression to ESKD. (See Chapter 67 for specific information on diabetic nephropathy.)

RENAL CELL CARCINOMA

Pathophysiology

Renal cell carcinoma is also known as *adenocarcinoma of the kidney*. As with other cancers, the healthy tissue of the kidney is damaged and replaced by cancer cells.

Systemic effects occurring with this cancer type are called *paraneoplastic syndromes* and include anemia, erythrocytosis, hypercalcemia, liver dysfunction with elevated liver enzymes, hormonal effects, increased sedimentation rate, and hypertension.

Anemia and erythrocytosis may seem confusing. However, most patients with this cancer have *either* anemia or erythrocytosis, not both at the same time. There is some blood loss from hematuria, but the small amount lost does not cause anemia. The cause of the anemia and the erythrocytosis are related to kidney cell production of erythropoietin. At times, the tumor cells produce large amounts of erythropoietin, causing erythrocytosis. Other times, the tumor cells destroy the erythropoietin-producing kidney cells and anemia results. Hypertension may result from increased blood levels of renin.

Parathyroid hormone produced by tumor cells can cause hypercalcemia. Other hormone changes include increased renin levels (causing hypertension) and increased human chorionic gonadotropin (hCG) levels, which decrease libido and change secondary sex features.

Renal cell carcinoma has four distinct cell types. Genetic differences cause a predisposition to develop tumors of each of these types. The most well-known genetic familial syndrome that includes renal cancer is von Hippel-Lindau syndrome. These cancers are highly vascular and may occur with cancers of the pancreas, central nervous system, and adrenal glands.

Renal tumors are classified into four stages (Table 70-5). Complications include metastasis and urinary tract obstruction. The cancer usually spreads to the adrenal gland, liver, lungs, long bones, or the other kidney (Moldawer & Figlin, 2008). When the cancer surrounds a ureter, hydroureter and obstruction may result.

The exact cause of renal cell carcinoma is unknown, but the risk is slightly higher for people who use tobacco or are exposed to lead, phosphate, and cadmium.

TABLE 70-5 Staging Renal Tumors

Stage I. Tumors up to 2.5 cm are situated within the capsule of the kidney. The renal vein, perinephric fat, and adjacent lymph nodes have no tumor.
Stage II. Tumors are larger than 2.5 cm and extend beyond the capsule but are within Gerota's fascia. The renal vein and lymph nodes are not involved.
Stage III. Tumors extend into the renal vein, lymph nodes, or both.
Stage IV. Tumors include invasion of adjacent organs beyond Gerota's fascia or metastasize to distant tissues.

Data from American Cancer Society. (2008). *Cancer facts and figures 2008.* Report No. 00-300M–No. 5008.08. Atlanta: Author.

Renal cancers account for about 51,190 new cases and 12,890 deaths annually in the United States. The 5-year survival rate is 60% in the United States. Renal cell carcinoma occurs most often in patients between 55 and 60 years of age (Jemal et al., 2007).

Patient-Centered Collaborative Care

Assessment

History

Ask the patient about age, known risk factors (e.g., smoking, chemical exposures), weight loss, changes in urine color, abdominal or flank discomfort, and fever. Also ask whether any other family member has ever been diagnosed with cancer of the kidney, bladder, ureter, prostate gland, uterus, or ovary.

Physical Assessment/Clinical Manifestations

Only about 5% to 10% of patients with renal cell cancer have flank pain, obvious blood in the urine, and a kidney mass that can be palpated. Ask about the nature of the flank or abdominal discomfort. Patients often describe the pain as dull and aching. The pain may be more intense if bleeding into the tumor or kidney occurs. Inspect the flank area, checking for asymmetry or an obvious bulge. An abdominal mass may be felt through *gentle* palpation. A renal bruit may be heard on auscultation.

Bloody urine is a *late* common sign. Blood may be visible as bright red flecks or clots, or the urine may appear smoky or cola colored. Without gross hematuria, microscopic examination may or may not reveal red cells.

Inspect the skin for pallor, darkening of the nipples, and, in men, breast enlargement caused by changing hormone levels. Other findings may include muscle wasting, weakness, poor nutritional status, and weight loss. All tend to occur late in the disease.

Diagnostic Assessment

Urinalysis may show red blood cells. Hematologic studies show decreased hemoglobin and hematocrit values, hypercalcemia, increased erythrocyte sedimentation rate, and increased levels of adrenocorticotropic hormone, human chorionic gonadotropin (hCG), cortisol, renin, and parathyroid hormone.

Renal masses may be detected by surgical exploration, IV urogram with nephrograms, or sonography. The mass and surrounding tissues may be outlined by CT with contrast or by MRI. Diagnosis requires a biopsy of the tumor.

Interventions

Interventions focus on controlling the cancer and preventing metastasis.

Nonsurgical Management

Radiofrequency ablation can slow tumor growth. It is a minimally invasive procedure carried out after MRI has precisely located the tumor. The procedure is used most commonly for patients who have only one kidney or who are poor surgical candidates.

Chemotherapy has limited effectiveness against this cancer type. Use of biological response modifiers (BRMs) such as interleukin-2 (IL-2), interferon (INF), and tumor necrosis factor (TNF) has lengthened survival time (see Chapters 19 and 24). Recently, two targeted therapy agents, sorafenib (Nexavar) and temsirolimus (Torisel), were approved as treatment for patients with advanced renal cell carcinoma (Malizzia & Hsu, 2008; Moldawer & Figlin, 2008). Sorafenib, an oral drug taken daily, is a multikinase inhibitor that slows cancer cell division and inhibits blood vessel growth in the tumor. Temsirolimus is a weekly IV infusion and works by inhibiting cell division. Both drugs have increased survival time of patients with advanced cancer.

Surgical Management

Renal cell carcinoma is usually treated surgically by nephrectomy (kidney removal). Renal cell tumors are highly vascular, and blood loss during surgery is a major concern. Before surgery, the arteries supplying the kidney may be occluded (embolized) by radiation to reduce bleeding during nephrectomy.

Preoperative Care. Instruct the patient about surgical routines (see Chapters 16, 17, and 18). Explain the probable site of incision and the presence of dressings, drains, or other equipment after surgery. Reassure the patient about pain relief. Care before surgery may include giving blood and fluids IV to prevent shock.

Operative Procedures. The patient is placed on his or her side with the kidney to be removed uppermost. Usually, the opposite trunk area is flexed to increase exposure of the kidney area. Removal of the eleventh or twelfth rib is needed to provide better access to the kidney. The surgeon removes the entire kidney and all visible tumor, renal artery and vein, and fascia after tying off the ureter. The adrenal gland is left intact. A drain may be placed in the wound before closure.

When a *radical* nephrectomy is performed, local and regional lymph nodes are also removed. The surgical approach may be transthoracic (as discussed in the previous paragraph), lumbar, or through the abdomen, depending on the size and location of the tumor. Radiation therapy may follow a radical nephrectomy.

Postoperative Care. Refer to Chapter 18 for care of the patient after surgery. Nursing priorities are focused on assessing renal function to determine function in the remaining kidney, managing pain, and preventing complications.

Monitoring includes assessing for hemorrhage and adrenal insufficiency. Inspect the patient's abdomen for distention from bleeding. Check the bed linens under the patient, because bleeding may be present. Hemorrhage or adrenal insufficiency causes hypotension, decreased urine output, and an altered level of consciousness.

A decrease in blood pressure is a sign of both hemorrhage and adrenal insufficiency. With hypotension, urine output also decreases immediately. Large water and sodium losses in the urine occur in patients with adrenal insufficiency. As a result, a large urine output is followed by hypotension and oliguria (<400 mL/24 hr or less than 25 mL/hr). IV replacement of fluids and packed red blood cells may be needed.

The second kidney is expected to provide adequate renal function, but this may take days or weeks. Assess urine output hourly for the first 24 hours after surgery (urine output of 30 to 50 mL/hr is acceptable). Output of less than 25 to 30 mL/hr suggests decreased renal blood flow. The hemoglobin level, hematocrit values, and white blood cell count may be measured every 6 to 12 hours for the first day or two after surgery.

Monitor the patient's temperature, pulse rate, and respiratory rate at least every 4 hours. Accurately measure and record fluid intake and output. Weigh the patient daily.

The patient may be in a special care unit for 24 to 48 hours after surgery for monitoring of bleeding and/or adrenal insufficiency. A drain placed near the site of incision removes residual fluid. Because of the discomfort of deep breathing, the patient is at risk for atelectasis. Fever, chills, thick sputum, or decreased breath sounds suggest pneumonia.

Pain management after surgery usually requires opioid analgesics (e.g., hydromorphone [Dilaudid] and morphine [Statex♣]) given parenterally. The incision was made through major muscle groups used with breathing and movement. Liberal use of analgesics is needed for 3 to 5 days to manage the pain after surgery. Oral agents may be tried when the patient is permitted to eat and drink.

Preventing complications focuses on infection and management of adrenal insufficiency. Antibiotics may be prescribed during and after surgery to prevent infection. The need for additional antibiotics is based on evidence of infection. Assess the patient at least every 8 hours for manifestations of systemic infection or local wound infection.

Adrenal insufficiency is possible as a complication of kidney and adrenal gland removal. Although only one adrenal gland may be affected, the remaining gland may not be able to secrete sufficient glucocorticoids immediately after surgery. Steroid replacements may be needed in some patients. Chapter 65 discusses the manifestation of acute adrenal insufficiency in detail, along with specific nursing interventions.

RENAL TRAUMA

Pathophysiology

Trauma to one or both kidneys is always a concern in penetrating wounds or blunt injuries to the back, flank, or abdomen. Blunt trauma to the back, flank, or abdomen accounts for most renal injuries. Injury to the kidney can be minor, major, or pedicle (Fig. 70-7). Anyone can suffer renal trauma. Strategies to prevent trauma are reviewed in Chart 70-8.

Minor injuries include contusions, small lacerations, and tearing of the parenchyma and the calyx (forniceal disruption). With a contusion, one or both kidneys are bruised because of the major impact. Small blood vessels may be damaged, causing some hematuria. Small lacerations may result in small, local hematomas. A small hematoma also may occur at the site of forniceal disruption. Common causes include falls, contact sports, and blows to the back and torso.

Major injuries include lacerations to the cortex, medulla, or branches of the renal artery or vein. Deep tissue injuries may extend throughout the kidney and cause hematomas within or through the capsule. Injuries involving the cortex can cause tissue shattering. The capsule may remain intact or be ruptured.

A major injury often follows penetrating abdominal, flank, or back wounds (e.g., as is seen with gunshot wounds, knife wounds, or motor vehicle crashes). Bleeding is extensive, and surgical exploration is often needed. Because of the hemorrhage, decreased renal blood flow can produce short-term or long-term renin-induced hypertension.

Pedicle injuries are lacerations or breaks in the renal artery or renal vein. Hemorrhage is extensive and rapid, and death may occur unless diagnosis and intervention are prompt.

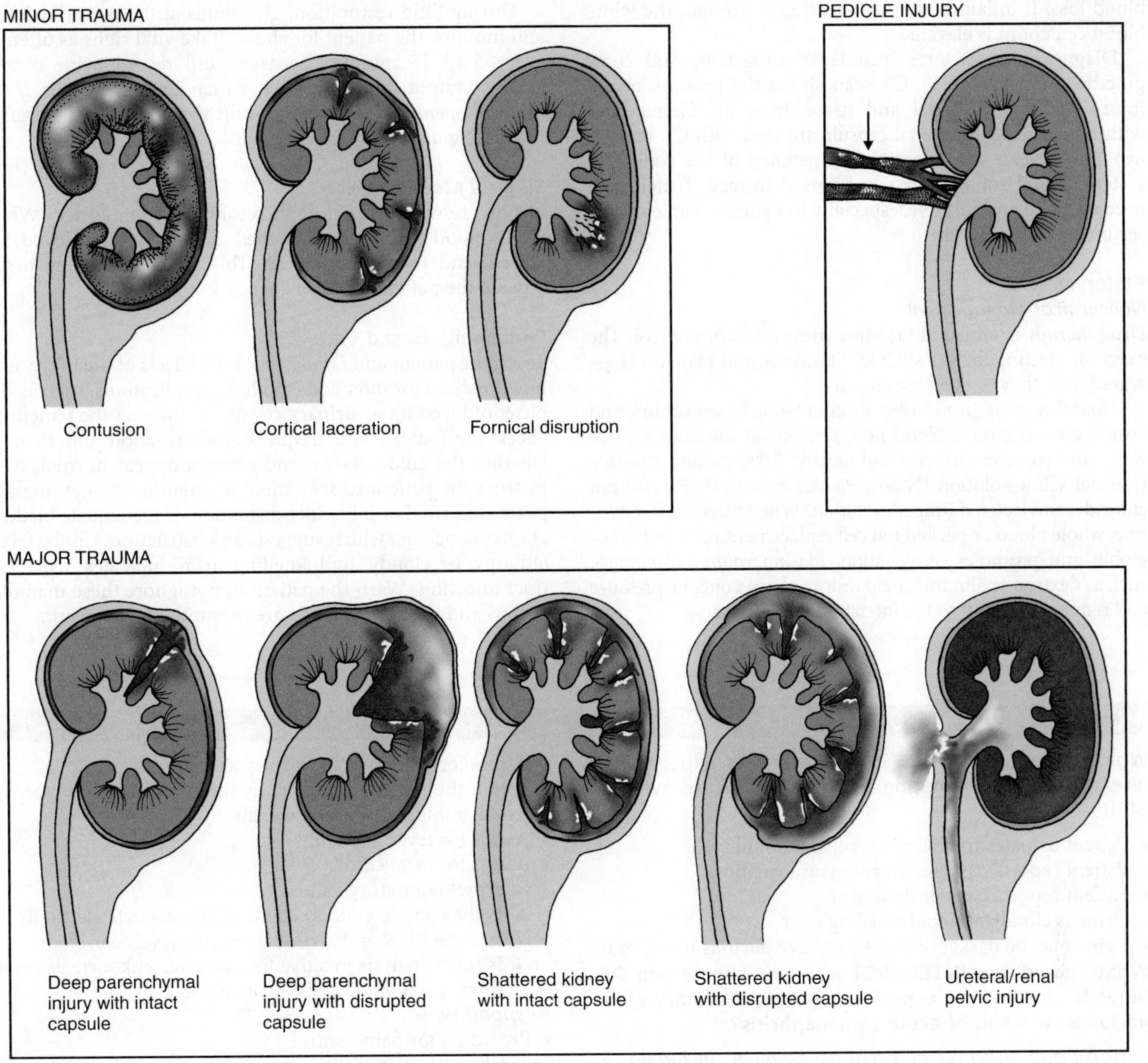
MINOR TRAUMA
Contusion
Cortical laceration
Fornical disruption
PEDICLE INJURY
MAJOR TRAUMA
Deep parenchymal injury with intact capsule
Deep parenchymal injury with disrupted capsule
Shattered kidney with intact capsule
Shattered kidney with disrupted capsule
Ureteral/renal pelvic injury

Fig. 70-7 • Common types and locations of renal trauma.

Chart 70-8 PATIENT AND FAMILY EDUCATION GUIDE

Preventing Renal and Genitourinary Trauma

- Wear a seat belt.
- Practice safe walking habits.
- Use caution when riding bicycles and motorcycles.
- Wear appropriate protective clothing when participating in contact sports.
- Avoid all contact sports and high-risk activities if you have only one kidney.

Patient-Centered Collaborative Care

Assessment

Obtain a history of the patient's usual health and the events involved in the trauma from the patient, a witness, or emergency personnel. Critical information to know is a history of kidney or urologic disease, surgical intervention, or health problems such as diabetes mellitus or hypertension.

Ureteral or renal pelvic injury often causes diffuse abdominal pain, local collections of urine, and infection. Ask the patient about pain in the flank or abdominal pain. Is the pain dull? Sharp? Constant? Intermittent? Made worse by coughing?

Take the patient's blood pressure, apical and peripheral pulses, respiratory rate, and temperature. Inspect both flanks for asymmetry or penetrating injuries of the lower chest or back. Also inspect the abdomen for bruising or penetrating wounds. Percuss the abdomen for distention. Inspect the urethral opening for gross bleeding.

Urinalysis usually shows hemoglobin or red blood cells from renal blood vessel rupture. Microscopic examination may also show red blood cell casts, which suggest tubular damage. Hemoglobin and hematocrit values decrease with blood loss. If inflammation or infection is present, the white blood cell count is elevated.

Diagnostic procedures include IV urography and computed tomography (CT). CT scan shows the location of the injury and blood vessel and tissue integrity. Hematomas within or through the renal capsule are seen with CT scan. A urogram reveals the integrity and patency of the collecting system. Renal sonography can be used instead if there is a need to avoid contrast dye, especially in patients with elevated serum creatinine levels.

Interventions

Nonsurgical Management

Drug therapy is aimed at bleeding prevention or control. The need for clotting factors such as vitamin K and platelets is assessed, and they are given as needed.

Fluid therapy is given to restore circulating blood volume and ensure adequate renal blood flow. *Crystalloid* solutions replace water and some electrolytes and include 0.9% sodium chloride (normal saline solution [NSS]), 5% dextrose in 0.45% sodium chloride, and lactated Ringer's solution. When bleeding is extensive, whole blood or packed red cell replacement restores hemoglobin and promotes oxygenation. *Plasma volume expanders,* such as dextran or albumin, help restore plasma oncotic pressure and reduce fluid shift to the interstitial fluid space.

During fluid restoration, give fluids at the prescribed rate and monitor the patient for shock. Take vital signs as often as every 5 to 15 minutes. Measure and record urine output hourly. Output should be greater than 25 to 30 mL/hr. *If the urethral opening is bleeding, consult with the physician before attempting urinary catheterization.*

Surgical Management

Nephrectomy or partial nephrectomy may be needed. When major blood vessels are torn, the kidney may be removed, repaired, and then reimplanted. This repair of kidney tissue outside the patient is called "bench surgery."

Community-Based Care

Teach the patient and family about the effects of the injury and how to assess for infection or other complications, such as the onset of bleeding or urinary retention. Instruct the patient to check the pattern and frequency of urination and to note whether the color, clarity, and amount appear normal. Also instruct the patient to seek medical attention if anything appears abnormal or if bladder distention or inadequate bladder emptying occurs, which suggests an obstruction. Chills, fever, lethargy, or cloudy, foul-smelling urine indicates a urinary tract infection. Warn the patient to not ignore these manifestations and to seek medical care promptly if they occur.

HUMAN NEEDS NURSING CARE REVIEW

What might you NOTICE if the patient is experiencing altered urinary elimination as a result of acute pyelonephritis?

- Patient urinates frequently in small amounts.
- Patient reports pain and burning on urination.
- Patient reports back or flank pain.
- Urine is cloudy and foul smelling.
- Urine may be darker or smoky or have obvious blood in it.

What should you INTERPRET and how should you RESPOND to a patient experiencing altered urinary elimination as a result of acute pyelonephritis?

Perform and interpret physical assessment, including:

- Ask how long manifestations have been present.
- Ask about low back pain (midline in men) or flank pain.
- Ask whether he or she has had a UTI in the past; how long ago; how it was treated; and if antibiotics were prescribed, whether the drug course was completed.
- Ask about the presence of pregnancy or any chronic health problem, especially diabetes.
- Ask about any nausea or vomiting and its duration.
- Determine fluid intake and output volumes.
- Assess for pain over the right and left kidneys.
- Weigh the patient, and ask whether this weight is more or less than his or her usual weight.
- Assess for fever and chills.
- Assess for tachycardia.
- Interpret laboratory values:
  - Is the complete blood count with leukocyte elevated?
  - Are the BUN and serum creatinine levels elevated?
  - Is the urinalysis positive for bacteria, leukocyte esterase, nitrate, red blood cells, white blood cells?

Respond by:

- Providing for pain control
- Teaching the patient the importance of completing the prescribed antibiotic drug regimen

On what should you REFLECT?

- Observe patient for evidence of improved urinary output (see Chapter 68).
- Think about what may have caused this infection and what steps could be taken to prevent a similar episode.
- Think about what patient teaching focus could help reduce the risk for future pyelonephritis and its complications.

GET READY FOR THE NCLEX EXAMINATION!

Key Points

Review these Key Points for each NCLEX Examination Client Needs Category.

Health Promotion and Maintenance

- Encourage all patients to maintain an adequate fluid intake (minimum of 3 L/day unless another condition requires fluid restriction).
- Encourage patients with diabetes to adhere to regimens for glucose control to prevent hypertension and renal disease.

Psychosocial Integrity

- Allow the patient the opportunity to express fear or anxiety regarding the potential for chronic kidney disease and renal failure.

- Assess the patient's level of comfort in discussing issues related to elimination and the urogenital area.
- Refer patients with polycystic kidney disease to a geneticist or a genetic counselor.
- During renal/urinary assessment, use language and terminology that are comfortable for the patient.
- Refer patients to community resources, support groups, and information organizations such as the National Kidney Foundation and the American Association of Kidney Patients.

Physiological Integrity

- Report immediately any condition that obstructs urine flow.
- Instruct patients with UTI to complete all prescribed antibiotic therapy even when symptoms of infection are absent.
- Check the blood pressure and urine output frequently in patients who have any type of kidney problem.
- Report immediately to the physician any sudden decrease of urine output in a patient with kidney disease or kidney trauma. In general, adult urine output goals are 0.5-1 mL/kg/hr.
- Instruct patients with any type of renal problem to weigh daily and to notify their health care provider if there is a sudden weight gain.
- Teach patients the expected side effects and any adverse reactions to prescribed drugs.
- Teach patients the signs and symptoms of disease recurrence and when to seek medical help.

Additional Study Resources

Go to your Companion CD or Evolve at http://evolve.elsevier.com/Iggy/ for *Self-Assessment Questions for the NCLEX Examination.*

evolve Go to Evolve at http://evolve.elsevier.com/Iggy/ for *Prioritization and Delegation Questions for the NCLEX Examination.*

SELECTED BIBLIOGRAPHY

Asterisk indicates a classic or definitive work on this subject.

American Cancer Society. (2008). *Cancer facts and figures 2008.* Report No. 00-300M–No. 5008.08. Atlanta: Author.

Bakris, G.L. (2005). Protecting renal function in the hypertensive patient: Clinical guidelines. *American Journal of Hypertension, 18*(4 Suppl. 1), 112-119.

Brenner, B.M., & Levine, S.A. (Eds.). (2007). *Brenner & Rector's the kidney* (8th ed.). Philadelphia: Saunders.

Bulechek, G.M., Butcher, H.K., & McCloskey Dochterman, J. (Eds). (2008). *Nursing interventions classification (NIC)* (5th ed.). St. Louis: Mosby.

Combest, W., Newton, M., Combest, A., & Kosier, J.H. (2005). Effects of herbal supplements on the kidney. *Urologic Nursing, 25*(5), 381-386, 403.

Cope, D., & Reb, A. (Eds.). (2006). *An evidence-based approach to the treatment and care of the older adult with cancer.* Pittsburgh: Oncology Nursing Society.

Couser, W.G., & Nangaku, M. (2006). Cellular and molecular biology of membranous nephropathy. *Journal of Nephrology, 19*(6), 699-705.

De Zeeuw, D. (2007). Albuminuria: A target for treatment of type 2 diabetic nephropathy. *Seminars in Nephrology, 27*(2), 172-181.

Galli, B., Munver, R., Sawczuk, I., & Kochis, E. (2005). Laparoscopic radical nephrectomy in renal cell carcinoma. *Urologic Nursing, 25*(2), 83-86, 133.

Garcia, A., & Ngeurue, C.M. (2006). Chronic pyelonephritis. eMedicine. WebMD. Retrieved June 12, 2007, from www.emedicine.com/me/topic2841.htm.

Garcia, J.A., & Rini, B.I. (2007). Recent progress in the management of advanced renal cell carcinoma. *CA: A Cancer Journal for Clinicians, 57*(2), 112-125.

Jamerson, K. (2005). Preventing chronic kidney disease in special populations. *American Journal of Hypertension, 18*(Suppl. 4), 106s-111s.

Jemal, A., Siegel, R., Ward, E., Murray, T., Xu, J., & Thun, M.J. (2007). Cancer statistics, 2007. *CA: A Cancer Journal for Clinicians, 57*(1), 43-67.

Kidney Cancer Association. (2005). Available online at www.curekidneycancer.org/

*Lancaster, L.E. (Ed.). (2001). *Core curriculum for nephrology nursing* (4th ed.). Pitman, NJ: American Association of Nephrology Nurses.

LeHir, M., & Kriz, W. (2007). New insights into structural patterns encountered in glomerulosclerosis. *Current Opinions in Nephrology and Hypertension, 16*(3), 184-191.

Levin, A., Linas, S., Luft, F.C., Chapman, A.B., Textor, S.; ASN HTN Advisory Group. (2007). Controversies in renal artery stenosis: A review by the American Society of Nephrology Advisory Group on Hypertension. *American Journal of Nephrology, 27*(2), 212-220.

Malizzia, L., & Hsu, A. (2008). Temsirolimus, an mTOR inhibitor for treatment of patients with advanced renal cell carcinoma. *Clinical Journal of Oncology Nursing, 12*(4), 639-646.

McCance, K., & Huether, S. (2006). *Pathophysiology: The biologic basis for disease in adults and children* (5th ed.). St. Louis: Mosby.

McCarley, P.B., & Burrows-Hudson, S. (2006). Chronic kidney disease and cardiovascular disease: Using ANNA standards and practice guidelines to improve care. *Nephrology Nursing Journal, 33*(6), 666-674.

Meiner, S., & Lueckenotte, A. (Eds.). (2006). *Gerontologic nursing,* (3rd ed.). St. Louis: Mosby.

Moldawer, N., & Figlin, R. (2008). Renal cell carcinoma: The translation of molecular biology into new treatments, new patient outcomes, and nursing implications. *Oncology Nursing Forum, 35*(4), 699-708.

National Kidney and Urologic Diseases Information Clearinghouse (NKUDIC). (2006). *Kidney and urologic diseases statistics for the United States.* Available online at http://kidney.niddk.nih.gov/kudiseases/pubs/kustats/index.htm

Nussbaum, R., McInnes, R., & Willard, H. (2007). *Thompson & Thompson: Genetics in medicine* (7th ed.). Philadelphia: Saunders.

Pagana, K., & Pagana, T. (2006). *Mosby's manual of diagnostic and laboratory tests* (3rd ed.). St. Louis: Mosby.

Polycystic Kidney Disease Foundation. (2007). Retrieved June 2007, from www.pkdcure.org.

Ramakrishnan, R., & Scheid, D.C. (2005). Diagnosis and management of acute pyelonephritis in adults. *American Family Physician, 71*(5), 933-942.

Rosario, R.F., & Wesson, D.E. (2006). Primary hypertension and nephropathy. *Current Opinion in Nephrology and Hypertension, 15*(2), 130-134.

Russell, S. (2008). Responding to threats to the kidney. *Nursing2008, 38*(2), 36-40.

Schrier, R.W. (2006). Optimal care of autosomal dominant kidney disease. *Nephrology, 11*(2), 124-130.

Shoham, D.A., Vupputuri, S., Diez Roux, A.V., Kaufman, J.S., Coresh, J., Kshirsagar, A.V., et al. (2007). Kidney disease in life-course socioeconomic context: The Atherosclerosis Risk in Communities (ARIC) Study. *American Journal of Kidney Disease, 49*(2), 217-226.

U.S. Renal Data Systems. (2006). *USRDS 2006 annual data report.* Bethesda, MD: The National Institutes of Health, National Institute of Diabetes and Digestive and Kidney Diseases.

Weatherbee, S. (2006). New weapons to snuff out kidney cancer. *Nursing2006, 36*(12), 59-63.

71

CHAPTER

Care of Patients with Acute Renal Failure and Chronic Kidney Disease

Linda A. LaCharity

LEARNING OUTCOMES

For clinical competence and success on the NCLEX Examination, study this chapter with these Learning Outcomes in mind:

Safe and Effective Care Environment

1. Evaluate patient risk for dehydration, shock, and acute renal failure.
2. Collaborate with members of the health care team to reduce patient exposure to nephrotoxins in the acute care setting.
3. Prevent injury in the patient who has bone density loss.
4. Apply principles of infection control to prevent infection in patients receiving immunosuppressive therapy.

Health Promotion and Maintenance

5. Teach everyone to drink fluids to prevent dehydration during hot weather and when engaging in heavy work or exercise.
6. Assess intake and output for anyone at risk for or with hypovolemia.
7. Teach transplant recipients and their families about the importance of adhering to anti-rejection therapy.

Psychosocial Integrity

8. Encourage patients and families to express their feelings and concerns about the risk for death and the disruption of lifestyle as a result of treatment for renal failure.
9. Assess the patient for depression and nonacceptance of his or her diagnosis or treatment plan.
10. Refer patients to community resources and support groups.

Physiological Integrity

11. Compare the pathophysiology and causes of acute renal failure (ARF) with those of chronic kidney disease (CKD).
12. Use laboratory data and clinical assessment to determine the effectiveness of therapy for renal failure.
13. Discuss interventions to prevent ARF.
14. Discuss the mechanisms of peritoneal dialysis (PD) and hemodialysis (HD) as renal replacement therapies.
15. Coordinate nursing care for the patient with severe chronic kidney disease or end-stage kidney disease (ESKD).
16. Plan prevention strategies for the complications of PD.
17. Coordinate nursing care for the patient during the first 24 hours after kidney transplantation.

Go to your Companion CD or Evolve at http://evolve.elsevier.com/Iggy/ for *Self-Assessment Questions for the NCLEX Examination* keyed to these Learning Outcomes.

Renal failure is common in the United States. Acute renal failure (ARF) is most common in the acute care setting, and chronic kidney disease (CKD), which may take years to develop, is more common in the community. Both types of kidney failure cause problems by interfering with the kidney's role in meeting the *human need for urinary elimination* and maintaining homeostasis of fluid volume, blood pressure, electrolytes, wastes, and acid-base balance (see Fig. 70-1 in Chapter 70). These problems can reduce overall physiologic function, shorten life, and decrease quality of life. The incidence of end-stage kidney disease (ESKD) decreased among patients with glomerulonephritis and increased somewhat among those with diabetes mellitus in 2007 (U.S. Renal Data System [USRDS], 2008). Thus overall, the incidence has increased only slightly and is most likely related to the increased use of kidney protective therapy with angiotensin-converting enzyme (ACE) inhibitor and angiotensin II receptor blocker (ARB) drugs, as well as the benefits associated with use of beta-blocker drugs in the

▼ ANIMATION: Renal and Urinary Disorders

treatment of heart failure. The incidence is expected to increase as a result of the aging population and the huge increase in the incidence of type 2 diabetes. The number of treated patients with ESKD has continued to grow, with a 3.4% increase in dialysis patients and a 5.9% increase in kidney transplant patients (USRDS, 2008). Kidney failure has many causes. CKD is most often associated with hypertension (HTN) and diabetes.

As described in Chapter 68, kidney functions include excretion of waste, water and salt balance, acid-base balance, and hormone secretion. When kidney function declines gradually, as occurs most often with CKD, also known as *chronic renal failure (CRF),* 90% to 95% of the nephrons must be destroyed before renal failure is obvious. The patient may have many years of renal insufficiency before the uremia of end-stage kidney disease develops. During this time of decreased renal function, the patient is at increased risk for acute renal failure because of the stress on remaining nephrons.

When renal decline is sudden, the functioning nephrons are overworked and renal failure may develop with the loss of only 50% of functioning nephrons. Acute renal failure and chronic kidney disease are compared in Table 71-1. Acute renal failure affects *many* body systems. Chronic kidney disease affects *every* body system. The problems that occur with renal failure are related to fluid-volume excess, electrolyte and acid-base abnormalities, buildup of nitrogen-based wastes, and loss of kidney hormone function.

When renal function declines to the point that the kidneys can no longer meet the body's homeostatic demands for *urinary elimination,* renal replacement therapy is needed to prevent death from life-threatening consequences.

ACUTE RENAL FAILURE

Pathophysiology

Acute renal failure (ARF) is a rapid decrease in kidney function, leading to the collection of metabolic wastes in the body. ARF can result from conditions that reduce blood flow to the kidneys **(prerenal failure);** damage to the glomeruli, interstitial tissue, or tubules **(intrarenal/intrinsic renal failure);** or obstruction of urine flow **(postrenal failure).** When ARF occurs in patients who already have renal insufficiency, it may lead to **end-stage kidney disease (ESKD)** or it may resolve to nearly the pre-ARF level of renal function. Many factors contribute to renal insults in ARF, but the acute syndrome may be reversible, especially with prompt intervention.

TABLE 71-1 Characteristics of Acute Renal Failure and Chronic Kidney Disease

Characteristic	Acute Renal Failure	Chronic Kidney Disease
Onset	Sudden (hours to days)	Gradual (months to years)
% of nephron involvement	≈50%	90%-95%
Duration	2-4 wks; less than 3 months	Permanent
Prognosis	Good for return of renal function with supportive care; high mortality in some situations	Fatal without a renal replacement therapy such as dialysis or transplantation

The pathologic process of ARF is related to the cause of the sudden decrease in kidney function and to the affected kidney sites(s). Reduced blood flow (poor perfusion), toxins, tubular ischemia, infections, and obstruction have different effects on the renal system. Any of these processes can reduce glomerular filtration rate (GFR), damage nephron cells, and obstruct urine flow in the renal tubules.

With shock or other problems causing an acute reduction in blood flow to the kidney (hypoperfusion), the kidney compensates by constricting renal blood vessels, activating the renin-angiotensin-aldosterone pathway, and releasing antidiuretic hormone (ADH). These responses increase blood volume and improve kidney perfusion. However, these same responses reduce urine volume, resulting in **oliguria** (urine output less than 400 mL/day) and **azotemia** (the retention and build-up of nitrogenous wastes in the blood). Nephron cell injury is more likely to occur from the lack of oxygen (ischemia) related to reduced blood flow (McCance & Huether, 2006). Toxins can cause blood vessel constriction in the kidney, leading to reduced renal blood flow and renal ischemia.

Kidney tissue inflammation caused by infection, drugs, or cancer results in immune-mediated changes in renal tissue. With extensive tubular damage, tubular cells slough and combine with other formed elements (e.g., red blood cell [RBC] casts), which then obstruct tubular lumens and prevent urine outflow. *Obstruction anywhere within the urinary tract may result in reduced urine formation and full or partial obstruction to urine outflow.*

When pressure in the renal tubules (intrarenal pressure) exceeds glomerular pressure, glomerular filtration stops. This problem allows nitrogen-based wastes to collect in the blood, increasing the blood urea nitrogen (BUN) and serum creatinine levels. When the BUN rises faster than the serum creatinine level, the cause is usually related to protein breakdown or volume depletion. When both the BUN and the creatinine levels rise and the ratio between the two remains constant, this indicates kidney failure.

Types of Acute Renal Failure

The types of ARF are described by their causes. These include prerenal azotemia, intrarenal (intrinsic) ARF, and postrenal azotemia. Table 71-2 lists causes of ARF.

Prerenal azotemia is renal failure caused by poor blood flow to the kidneys. The most common problems leading to ARF are hypovolemic shock and heart failure. ARF can be reversed by correcting blood volume, increasing blood pressure, and improving cardiac output. When the reduced blood flow is prolonged, the kidney is severely damaged and intrarenal failure results.

The term *intrarenal ARF* is often shortened to just *ARF* in the clinical setting. Other terms include *acute tubular necrosis (ATN)* and *lower nephron nephrosis.* Infections (bacteria, viral, fungal), drugs (especially aminoglycoside antibiotics and NSAIDs), and invading tumors (e.g., lymphomas, leukemias) can cause acute interstitial nephritis. Other causes of intrarenal ARF include inflammation of the glomeruli (glomerulonephritis) or of the small vessels of the kidneys (vasculitis) or an obstruction of renal blood flow.

Postrenal azotemia develops from obstruction to the outflow of formed urine anywhere within the renal or urinary tract.

TABLE 71-2 Causes of the Three Types of Acute Renal Failure

PRERENAL AZOTEMIA

Any condition decreasing blood flow to the kidneys and leading to ischemia in the nephrons, such as:
- Shock
- Heart failure
- Pulmonary embolism
- Anaphylaxis
- Sepsis
- Pericardial tamponade

INTRARENAL (INTRINSIC)

Actual physical, chemical, hypoxic, or immunologic tissue damage to the kidney, such as:
- Acute interstitial nephritis
- Exposure to nephrotoxins
- Acute glomerular nephritis
- Vasculitis
- Acute tubular necrosis
- Renal artery or vein stenosis
- Renal artery or vein thrombosis
- Formation of crystals or precipitates in the nephron tubules

POSTRENAL AZOTEMIA

Obstruction of the urine collecting system anywhere from the calyces to the urethral meatus (obstruction of the ureter must be bilateral to cause postrenal failure unless only one kidney is functional), such as:
- Ureter, bladder, or urethral cancer
- Kidney, ureter, or bladder stones
- Bladder atony
- Prostatic hyperplasia or cancer
- Urethral stricture
- Cervical cancer

Phases of Acute Renal Failure

When renal function declines, the phases of ARF begin (Table 71-3). Some patients have a *nonoliguric* form of ARF in which urine output remains near normal. The phases of this form of ARF are similar to those listed in Table 71-3 except for the amount of urine excreted. The treatment of these patients is less complicated because renal replacement therapy is rarely needed. Interventions to restore circulating volume, improve cardiac output, or increase blood pressure may prevent progression of the phases when blood flow to the kidneys is poor.

Etiology

Many types of problems can reduce renal function. Severe hypotension from shock or dehydration reduces renal blood flow and can lead to prerenal ARF. Cardiac disease or heart failure also can reduce renal blood flow. The patient may be oliguric or even **anuric** (less than 100 mL/24 hr) if the dehydration or renal blood flow reduction is severe. Conditions causing ARF are listed in Table 71-2.

Incidence/Prevalence

Hospital-acquired ARF occurs in as many as 4% of hospital admissions and 20% of critical care admissions (Sinert & Peacock, 2006). Most ARF episodes are due to acute tubular necrosis (ATN) and worsening of chronic kidney problems. *Volume depletion leading to prerenal azotemia is the most common cause of ARF and is reversible in most cases with prompt intervention.*

For patients who survive the precipitating event, the chance for return of renal function is good. However, complications during the course of ARF can greatly increase the risk for death. Bloodstream infections from contamination through IV lines are the most common complications that lead to death. However, the highest death rate occurs with trauma (70%) and surgery. ARF caused by **nephrotoxic** (kidney dam-

TABLE 71-3 The Phases of Oliguric Acute Renal Failure

Phase	Description	Characteristics
Onset phase	Begins with the precipitating event and continues until oliguria develops. Lasts hours to days.	The gradual accumulation of nitrogenous wastes, such as serum creatinine and BUN, may be noted.
Oliguric phase	Characterized by a urine output of 100-400 mL/24 hr that does not respond to fluid challenges or diuretics. Lasts 1-3 weeks.	Laboratory data include increasing serum creatinine and BUN levels, hyperkalemia, bicarbonate deficit (metabolic acidosis), hyperphosphatemia, hypocalcemia, and hypermagnesemia. Sodium retention occurs, but this is masked by the dilutional effects of water retention. Urinary indices are typically low and fixed; regulation of water balance by the kidneys is impaired, so urine specific gravity and urine osmolarity do not vary as plasma osmolarity changes.
Diuretic phase (high-output phase)	Often has a sudden onset within 2-6 wk after oliguric stage. Urine flow increases rapidly over a period of several days. The diuresis can result in an output of up to 10 L/day of dilute urine.	Electrolyte losses typically precede clearance of nitrogenous wastes. Later in the diuretic phase, the BUN level starts to fall and continues to fall until the level reaches normal limits or reaches a plateau. Normal renal tubular function is re-established during this phase.
Recovery phase (convalescent phase)	In this phase, the patient begins to return to normal levels of activity. Complete recovery may take up to 12 months.	The patient functions at a lower energy level and has less stamina than before the illness. Residual renal insufficiency may be noted through regular monitoring of renal function. Renal function may never return to pre-illness levels, but renal function sufficient for a long and healthy life is likely.

BUN, Blood urea nitrogen.

aging) substances (Table 71-4) has the lowest rates of recovery. The prognosis for ARF caused by obstruction or glomerulonephritis is much better.

Health Promotion and Maintenance

Keep in mind that severe blood volume depletion can lead to renal failure even in people who have no known kidney problems. Urge all people to avoid dehydration by drinking at least 2 to 3 L of fluids daily. This is especially important for athletes or any person who performs strenuous exercise or work and sweats heavily.

Nurses have an essential role in the prevention of acute renal failure (ARF) in hospitalized patients. Always be on the lookout for signs of impending renal impairment through careful physical assessment and close monitoring of laboratory values. Early recognition and correction of problems causing reduced renal blood flow usually restore renal function before tissue damage can occur. Evaluate the patient's fluid status. Accurately measure intake and output and check body weight to identify changes in fluid balance. Assess for manifestations of blood volume depletion, such as decreased urine output, postural hypotension, and tachycardia. Prompt fluid replacement in the prerenal stage can prevent renal tissue damage and renal failure (Venkataraman & Kellum, 2007).

Also monitor laboratory values for any changes that reflect poor kidney function. Decreased urine specific gravity indicates a loss of urine-concentrating ability and is the earliest sign of renal tubular damage. Other laboratory values that are helpful in monitoring renal function include serum creatinine, urine and serum electrolytes, and blood urea nitrogen (BUN).

Be aware of nephrotoxic substances that the patient may ingest or be exposed to (see Table 71-4). Question any prescription for potentially nephrotoxic drugs, and validate the dose before the patient receives the drug. Antibiotics are common drugs that have nephrotoxic side effects. NSAIDs can cause or increase the risk for ARF. Combining two or more nephrotoxic drugs dramatically increases the risk for ARF. If a patient must receive a known nephrotoxic drug, monitor laboratory values, including BUN, creatinine, and drug peak and trough levels, closely for indications of reduced renal function.

TABLE 71-4 Some Potentially Nephrotoxic Substances

DRUGS	Nabumetone
ANTIBIOTICS/ ANTI-INFECTIVES	Naproxen
Amphotericin B	Oxaprozin
Colistimethate	Rofecoxib
Methicillin	Tolmetin
Polymyxin B	***OTHER DRUGS***
Rifampin	Acetaminophen
Sulfonamides	Captopril
Tetracycline hydrochloride	Cyclosporine
Vancomycin	Fluorinate anesthetics
AMINOGLYCOSIDE ANTIBIOTICS	D-Penicillamine
Gentamicin	Phenazopyridine hydrochloride
Kanamycin	Quinine
Neomycin	**OTHER SUBSTANCES**
Netilmicin sulfate	***ORGANIC SOLVENTS***
Tobramycin	Carbon tetrachloride
CHEMOTHERAPY AGENTS	Ethylene glycol
Cisplatin	***NONDRUG CHEMICAL AGENTS***
Cyclophosphamide	Radiographic contrast dye
Methotrexate	Pesticides
NONSTEROIDAL ANTI-INFLAMMATORY DRUGS (NSAIDs)	Fungicides
Celecoxib	Myoglobin (from breakdown of skeletal muscle)
Flurbiprofen	***HEAVY METALS AND IONS***
Ibuprofen	Arsenic
Indomethacin	Bismuth
Ketorolac	Copper sulfate
Meclofenamate	Gold salts
Meloxicam	Lead
	Mercuric chloride

Patient-Centered Collaborative Care

Assessment

History

The accurate diagnosis of ARF, including its type and its cause, depends on a detailed history of potential causes of ARF. Ask the patient about exposure to nephrotoxins, recent surgery or trauma, transfusions, or other factors that might lead to reduced renal blood flow. Obtain a drug history, especially treatment with antibiotics, angiotensin-converting enzyme (ACE) inhibitors, and NSAIDs. Ask about recent imaging procedures requiring injection of a contrast dye. These dyes can cause ARF, especially in older patients with reduced renal reserve. ARF must be differentiated from chronic renal insufficiency (CRI). Ask the patient about diseases that impair renal function, such as diabetes mellitus, long-term hypertension, systemic lupus erythematosus, and other connective tissue diseases.

To identify possible acute glomerulonephritis, ask about acute illnesses such as influenza, colds, gastroenteritis, and sore throats. Ask the patient whether urine color has become darker or appears smoky.

Reversible prerenal azotemia may occur after any episode of acute hypotension, hemorrhage or shock, burns, heart failure, or any problem in which the blood volume is depleted. Extensive bowel preparations, NPO status before surgery, and fluid loss during surgery can cause prerenal azotemia in some patients.

Postrenal ARF is identified by focusing on urinary obstructive problems. Ask the patient about any difficulty in starting the urine stream, changes in the amount or appearance of the urine, narrowing of the urine stream, nocturia, urgency, or symptoms of renal stones. Also ask about any cancer history that may cause urinary obstruction.

Physical Assessment/Clinical Manifestations

The manifestations of ARF are related to the buildup of nitrogenous wastes **(azotemia),** as well as to as the underlying cause (Chart 71-1). Manifestations of *prerenal* azotemia are hypotension, tachycardia, decreased urine output, decreased cardiac output, decreased central venous pressure (CVP), and lethargy. The appearance of a patient with prerenal azotemia is similar to that of a patient with heart failure or dehydration, depending on the cause of the poor renal blood flow.

Intrarenal (intrinsic) ARF usually occurs with damage to the glomeruli, interstitial tissue, or tubules. Manifestations are related to the retention of fluid and nitrogenous wastes. These include **oliguria** (decreased urine output) or **anuria** (absence of urine), edema, hypertension, tachycardia, shortness of breath, distended neck veins, elevated central venous pressure, weight gain, respiratory crackles, anorexia, nausea, vomiting,

Chart 71-1 KEY FEATURES

Acute Renal Failure

PRERENAL AZOTEMIA
- Hypotension
- Tachycardia
- Decreased cardiac output
- Decreased central venous pressure
- Decreased urine output
- Lethargy

INTRARENAL (INTRINSIC) ARF AND POSTRENAL AZOTEMIA
- Renal manifestations:
  - Oliguria or anuria
  - Increased urine specific gravity
- Cardiac manifestations:
  - Hypertension
  - Tachycardia
  - Jugular venous distention
  - Increased central venous pressure
  - ECG changes: tall T waves
- Respiratory manifestations:
  - Shortness of breath
  - Orthopnea
  - Rales or crackles
  - Pulmonary edema
  - Friction rub
- Gastrointestinal manifestations:
  - Anorexia
  - Nausea
  - Vomiting
  - Flank pain
- Neurologic manifestations:
  - Lethargy
  - Headache
  - Tremors
  - Confusion
- General manifestations:
  - Generalized edema
  - Weight gain

ARF, Acute renal failure; *ECG*, electrocardiogram.

and lethargy or changes in levels of consciousness. Manifestations of electrolyte imbalances (particularly elevated potassium levels and low calcium levels), such as electrocardiographic (ECG) changes, may also be present.

In patients with *postrenal* failure, monitor for oliguria or intermittent anuria, symptoms of uremia, and lethargy. Report changes in the urine stream or difficulty starting urination.

Laboratory Assessment

The many changes in laboratory values in the patient with ARF are similar to those occurring in chronic kidney disease (CKD) (Chart 71-2; see also the discussion of Laboratory Assessment on p. 1614 in the Chronic Kidney Disease section). Expect to see rising BUN and serum creatinine and abnormal blood electrolytes values. Patients with ARF, however, usually do *not* have the anemia associated with CKD unless there is hemorrhagic blood loss or unless blood urea levels are high enough to break (lyse) red blood cells.

In the early phases of ARF, urine tests provide important information. Urine sodium levels are often less than 10 to 20 mEq/L in patients with prerenal azotemia. The urine is concentrated, with a specific gravity greater than 1.030. The presence of urine sediment (e.g., red blood cells [RBCs], RBC casts, and tubular cells), myoglobin, or hemoglobin; a urine sodium level lower than 40 mEq/L; and a specific gravity of less than 1.010 or lower indicate intrarenal failure. In postrenal failure, urine sodium levels may be normal (about 40 mEq/L), with a specific gravity of 1.000 to 1.010.

Imaging Assessment

X-rays help determine the cause of ARF. A flat-plate x-ray of the abdomen is used to check the size of the kidneys. Enlarged kidneys, possibly due to obstruction, may result from hydronephrosis. X-rays may show stones obstructing the renal pelvis, ureters, or bladder.

Renal ultrasonography is a noninvasive procedure using high-energy sound waves. It is useful in the diagnosis of urinary tract obstruction. Dilation of the renal calyces and collecting ducts, as well as stones, can be detected. Ultrasonography can show kidney size and the patency of the ureters.

Computed tomography (CT) scans without contrast dye can identify obstruction or tumors. Contrast dyes are usually avoided to prevent further renal damage. A nuclear medicine study called *MAG3* may be used to determine the nature of the renal failure, GFR, or tubular function and its severity. A renal scan can determine whether blood flow to the kidneys is sufficient. Cystoscopy or retrograde pyelography may be needed to identify obstructions of the lower urinary tract.

Other Diagnostic Assessment

Renal biopsy is performed if the cause of ARF is uncertain, an immunologic disease is suspected, or the reversibility of the renal failure needs to be determined after ARF has persisted for an extended period. Prepare the patient before the test, and provide follow-up care. Be aware of all test results, and understand how they might affect the treatment regimen. (See Chapter 68 for a detailed discussion of renal diagnostic tests.)

Common Nursing Diagnoses and Collaborative Problems

Nursing diagnoses and collaborative problems that may apply to patients with acute renal failure include:
- Excess Fluid Volume related to compromised regulatory mechanisms (inability of the kidneys to maintain body fluid balance)
- Potential for Pulmonary Edema
- Potential for Electrolyte Imbalances

Interventions

The patient with ARF may move from the oliguric phase (in which fluid and electrolytes are retained) to the diuretic phase. In the oliguric phase, the plan of care focuses on close monitoring for life-threatening electrolyte changes and nitrogen retention that may require intervention. During the diuretic phase, hypovolemia and electrolyte *loss* are the main problems. The patient in the diuretic phase of ARF needs a plan of care that focuses on fluid and electrolyte *replacement* and monitoring.

These examples of output variation reflect the continually changing nature of ARF and the need for the plan of care to be

Chart 71-2 LABORATORY PROFILE

Renal Failure

Test	Normal Range for Adults	Values in Renal Failure
Serum creatinine	*Male:* 0.6-1.2 mg/dL *Female:* 0.5-1.1 mg/dL *Older adults:* Decreased	**IN CHRONIC KIDNEY DISEASE** May increase by 0.5-1.0 mg/dL every 1-2 yr May be as high as 15-30 mg/dL *before* symptoms of severe CKD are present **IN ACUTE RENAL FAILURE** Gradual increase of 1-2 mg/dL every 24-48 hr May increase 1-6 mg/dL in 1 wk or less
Blood urea nitrogen	10-20 mg/dL *Older adults:* May be slightly increased	**IN CHRONIC KIDNEY DISEASE** May reach 180-200 mg/dL *before* symptoms develop **IN ACUTE RENAL FAILURE** Often increases by 10-20 mg/dL at same pace as serum creatinine level May reach 80-100 mg/dL within 1 wk
Serum sodium	136-145 mEq/L; 136-145 mmol/L (SI units)	Normal, increased, or decreased
Serum potassium	3.5-5.0 mEq/L; 3.5-5.0 mmol/L (SI units)	Increased
Serum phosphorus (phosphate)	3.0-4.5 mg/dL; 0.97-1.45 mmol/L (SI units) *Older adults:* May be slightly decreased	Increased
Serum calcium	Total calcium: 9.0-10.5 mg/dL; 2.25-2.75 mmol/L (SI units) Ionized calcium: 4.5-5.6 mg/dL; 1.05-1.3 mmol/L (SI units) *Older adults:* Slightly decreased	Decreased
Serum magnesium	1.3-2.1 mEq/L; 0.65-1.05 mmol/L (SI units)	Increased
Serum carbon dioxide combining power (bicarbonate)	23-30 mEq/L (venous); 23-30 mmol/L (SI units)	Decreased
Arterial blood pH	7.35-7.45	Decreased (in metabolic acidosis) or normal
Arterial blood bicarbonate (HCO_3^-)	21-28 mEq/L	Decreased
Arterial blood $Paco_2$	35-45 mm Hg	Decreased
Hemoglobin	*Female:* 12-16 g/dL; 7.4-9.9 mmol/L (SI units) *Male:* 14-18 g/dL; 8.7-11.2 mmol/L (SI units) *Older adults:* Slightly decreased	Decreased
Hematocrit	*Female:* 37%-47% *Male:* 42%-52% *Older adults:* May be slightly decreased	Decreased to 20%

SI, International System of Units.

constantly updated to reflect the stages of the disease process. Drug therapy, nutrition therapy, and renal replacement therapy (peritoneal dialysis [PD], hemodialysis [HD], or hemofiltration) are commonly used to manage ARF.

Drug Therapy

Patients with ARF receive many drugs. As kidney function changes, drug dosages are changed. It is important to be knowledgeable about the site of drug metabolism and especially careful when giving drugs. Constantly monitor for possible side effects and interactions of the drugs that the patient with ARF is receiving (Chart 71-3; see also the discussion of drug therapy on pp. 1618-1619 in the Chronic Kidney Disease section). Diuretics may be used to increase urine output.

In patients with prerenal azotemia, fluid challenges and diuretics are often used to promote renal blood flow. In patient without volume excess, 500 to 1000 mL of normal saline may be infused over 1 hour. In prerenal azotemia, the patient responds to the fluid challenge by producing urine soon after the initial bolus. Diuretics such as furosemide (Lasix) also may be prescribed along with a fluid bolus. If oliguric renal failure is diagnosed, the fluid challenges and diuretics are discontinued. Patients often require central venous pressure (CVP) monitoring or measurement of pulmonary arterial pressure by means of a pulmonary artery catheter for accurate evaluation of their hemodynamic status. They also require constant nursing supervision for assessment of the response to fluid and drug therapy. Carefully monitor for signs of possible fluid overload.

Chart 71-3 COMMON EXAMPLES OF DRUG THERAPY

Renal Failure

Drug/Dosage	Action/Purpose	Nursing Interventions	Rationales
CARDIAC GLYCOSIDES			
Digoxin (Digitek, Lanoxicaps, Lanoxin, Novodigoxin♣) 0.125-0.25 mg orally or IV daily or every other day *Older adults:* 0.0625-0.125 mg orally or IV daily or every other day **Med Error Alert!** Watch drug dose; it is very low (0.0625-0.25 mg).	Used when heart failure induces renal failure or makes it worse. Improves ventricular contraction, increasing stroke volume and cardiac output.	Teach patients to take his or her pulse daily before taking the drug and to notify the prescriber if the pulse is below 60.	Drug slows the heart rate and can cause severe bradycardia.
		Instruct patients to notify prescriber if any of these manifestations occur: changes in color vision (more yellow color), blurred vision, eyes sensitive to light, light flashes, or halos around bright lights; changes in behavior, mood, or mental ability; chest pain or palpitations.	These are manifestations of drug toxicity and require the drug be stopped or the dose decreased temporarily.
		Teach patients to not take antacids within 2 hours of taking this drug.	Antacids prevent drug absorption and may delay or inhibit drug effectiveness.
VITAMINS AND MINERALS			
Folic acid (vitamin B_9, Folvite, Novofolacid♣) 0.1 mg orally daily Ferrous sulfate (Feosol, Novoferrosulfa♣) 325 mg orally three or four times daily	When the patient is receiving dialysis, many essential vitamins and minerals are removed from the blood. Replacement is needed to prevent severe deficiencies.	Teach patients to take the drugs after dialysis.	Dialysis removes the drug from the blood.
		Teach patients to take iron supplements (ferrous sulfate) with meals.	Food reduces nausea and abdominal discomfort.
		Teach patients to take stool softeners daily while taking iron supplements.	Oral iron preparations cause constipation, and most patients with renal failure must reduce their fluid intake, further increasing the risk for constipation.
		Remind patients that iron supplements change the color of the stool.	Knowing the expected side effects decreases anxiety when they appear.
SYNTHETIC ERYTHROPOIETIN			
Epoetin Alfa (Epogen, Procrit) 50-100 units/kg subcutaneously or IV three times a week for patients on dialysis Darbepoetin alfa (Aranesp) 0.45 mcg/kg subcutaneously or IV once weekly for patients on dialysis	Drug prevents anemia by stimulating red blood cell growth and maturation in the bone marrow.	Teach patients to report any of these side effects to the prescriber as soon as possible: chest pain, difficulty breathing, high blood pressure, rapid weight gain, seizures, skin rash or hives, swelling of feet or ankles.	Drug can induce serious cardiovascular problems, such as myocardial infarction (MI).
		Reinforce to patients that they must have hemoglobin levels monitored weekly.	Drug can raise hemoglobin and hematocrit levels to the point that blood viscosity increases, raising blood pressure and increasing the risk for MI. Drug dosage is reduced to prevent hemoglobin levels higher than 10 to 12 mg/dL.
PHOSPHATE BINDERS			
Aluminum hydroxide gel (Amphojel, AlternaGEL, Alu-Cap, Nephrox) 500 mg-2 g orally two to four times daily Aluminum carbonate gel (Basaljel) 500 mg-2 g orally two to four times daily	High blood phosphate levels cause hypocalcemia and osteodystrophy. Drugs lower serum phosphate levels by binding phosphorus present in food.	Teach patients to take drugs with meals.	Drug action is to bind phosphate in food, preventing its absorption.
		Remind patients taking digoxin to separate the drugs by at least 2 hours.	These drugs reduce digoxin absorption and effects.
		Teach patients to take stool softeners daily while taking these drugs.	These drugs cause constipation, and most patients with renal failure must reduce their fluid intake, further increasing the risk for constipation.
		Teach patients to report muscle weakness, slow or irregular pulse, or confusion to the prescriber.	These are manifestations of hypophosphatemia, which require dosage adjustment.

Calcium channel blockers may be used to treat ARF resulting from nephrotoxic acute tubular necrosis (ATN). These drugs prevent the movement of calcium into the kidney cells, maintain kidney cell integrity, and improve the glomerular filtration rate (GFR) by improving renal blood flow.

NCLEX EXAMINATION CHALLENGE

The client is a 27-year-old man who received crushing injuries to his legs as a result of a car crash in which he was trapped for 2 hours before being rescued. He is 2 days past the injury and has ATN. For which of his laboratory findings should the nurse immediately notify the Rapid Response Team?

A. Serum sodium 131 mEq/L
B. Serum potassium 6.9 mEq/L
C. Total serum calcium 9.1 mg/dL
D. Hematocrit 35%; hemoglobin 10.2 g/dL

evolve For the correct answer, go to http://evolve.elsevier.com/Iggy/.

Nutrition Therapy

Patients who have ARF often have a high rate of protein breakdown. The exact cause for this state is not known. Increases in metabolism and protein breakdown may be related to the stress of a critical illness, causing an increase in blood levels of catecholamines, cortisol, and glucagon. The rate of protein breakdown correlates with the severity of uremia and azotemia. This state causes the breakdown of muscle for protein, which leads to an increase in azotemia and an even more elevated blood urea nitrogen (BUN) level.

If the patient with ARF has a good dietary intake (see the discussion of Imbalanced Nutrition: Less Than Body Requirements on p. 1615 in the Chronic Kidney Disease section), nutritional support may not be needed. A dietary consult with a nutritionist, who will calculate the patient's caloric needs, may be prescribed. Work with the nutritionist to provide a diet with specified amounts of protein, sodium, and fluids. For the patient who does not require dialysis, 0.6 g/kg of body weight or 40 g/day of protein is usually prescribed. For patients who do require dialysis, the protein level needed will range from 1 to 1.5 g/kg (McCarthy, 2006). The amount of dietary sodium ranges from 60 to 90 mEq. If blood potassium levels are high, dietary potassium is restricted to 60 to 70 mEq. The amount of fluid permitted is generally calculated to be equal to the urine volume plus the insensible loss volume of 500 mL. Assess oral intake every shift to ensure that caloric intake is adequate.

Many patients with ARF are too ill or their appetite is too poor to eat enough food. For these patients, some form of nutritional support (e.g., total parenteral nutrition [TPN] or hyperalimentation) is needed. The desired outcomes of nutritional support in ARF are to provide sufficient nutrients to maintain or improve nutritional status, to preserve lean body mass, to restore or maintain fluid balance, and to preserve renal function.

If TPN is used, the solutions are mixed to meet the patient's specific needs. Because kidney function is unstable in ARF, constantly monitor the serum electrolyte levels to indicate when the TPN solution needs to be changed. IV fat emulsion (Intralipid) infusions can provide a nonprotein source of calories. In uremic patients, fat emulsions are used in place of glucose to avoid the problems of excessive sugars.

Dialysis Therapies

If necessary, hemodialysis (HD) and peritoneal dialysis (PD) may be used for patients with ARF. Indications for dialysis use in ARF include the presence of uremia, persistent high potassium levels, metabolic acidosis, continued fluid volume excess, uremic pericarditis, and encephalopathy.

Immediate vascular access for HD in patients with ARF is made by placement of a dual- or triple-lumen catheter specific for HD. When HD is expected to be used for several weeks, the catheter is usually placed in the subclavian or internal jugular vein. If only one or two HD treatments are needed, as for removal of drugs or toxins, a femoral site may be selected. Longer use of the femoral site is avoided because the patient's mobility is restricted and complications, such as hematomas and infection, are common. Repeatedly accessing the femoral site increases the risk for hematoma formation and makes repeated use of the vein impossible.

The subclavian vein is used, when possible, instead of the femoral site because the catheter can be left in place between dialysis treatments. However, the longer the catheter is left in this place, the greater the chance for infection. The subclavian dialysis catheter (Fig. 71-1) is inserted at the bedside. A physician or nurse practitioner performs the sterile procedure, and then the catheter is covered with a sterile dressing. Monitor

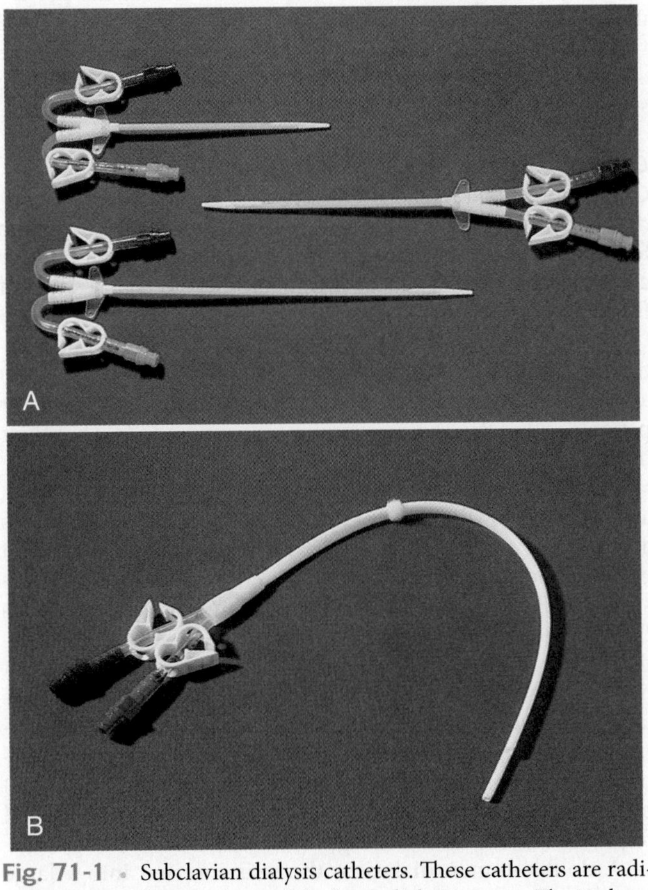
A
B

Fig. 71-1 • Subclavian dialysis catheters. These catheters are radiopaque tubes that can be used for hemodialysis access. The Y-shape tubing allows arterial outflow and venous return through a single catheter. **A,** Mahurkar catheters, made of polyurethane and used for short-term access. **B,** A PermCath catheter, made of silicone and used for long-term access.

for manifestations of procedure complications such as pneumothorax (reduced breath sounds, tracheal deviation away from midline, prominence and poor movement of one side of the chest) or subcutaneous emphysema (crackling and swelling of tissue around the site). Catheter placement is checked by chest x-ray before its use.

If hemodialysis is needed for more than a few days, a long-term dialysis catheter may be used. Most of these catheters are placed in the radiology department using a tunneling technique. The patient receives moderate sedation. Under sonographic or fluoroscopic guidance, the physician makes a small incision where the internal jugular vein passes behind the clavicle. A 6- to 8-cm tunnel is created out from the side of the incision. A long-term hemodialysis catheter is inserted through the tunnel and into the jugular vein. Keeping a segment of the catheter within the subcutaneous tissues before entering the jugular vein reduces the risk for infection.

Hemodialysis catheters have two lumens, one for outflow and one for inflow. This allows the outflow of blood for dialysis to be separated from the dialyzed blood returned through the inflow lumen. A triple-lumen catheter for HD is available. The third lumen is an access for drawing venous blood or giving drugs and fluid without interrupting dialysis.

Peritoneal dialysis (PD) may also be used in the treatment of ARF, although some patients, such as those being mechanically ventilated, may not be able to tolerate the abdominal distention that occurs with PD. PD uses the peritoneum as the dialyzing membrane. The dialysate is infused through a catheter implanted in the peritoneum. A complete discussion of PD is provided the Chronic Kidney Disease section, pp. 1626-1630.

Continuous Renal Replacement Therapy

Continuous renal replacement therapies (CRRTs) are the standard treatment for ARF. Renal replacement therapies in the form of hemofiltration are often better tolerated than HD for critically ill patients because this method avoids rapid shifts of fluids and electrolytes.

Continuous arteriovenous hemofiltration (CAVH) and continuous arteriovenous hemodialysis and filtration (CAVHD) are the renal replacement therapies most commonly used for patients with ARF. These procedures are similar to HD but their use is temporary.

CAVH is used for patients who have fluid volume overload, are resistant to diuretics, and have unstable blood pressures and cardiac output. The use of CAVH requires placement of both arterial and venous catheters and a mean arterial pressure (MAP) of at least 60 mm Hg. (**Mean arterial pressure** is the average arterial pressure of a person and is based on cardiac output and systemic vascular resistance. The typical adult normal MAP is 100 mm Hg.) CAVH continuously removes large amounts of plasma water, wastes, and electrolytes. Electrolytes are replaced through prescribed amounts of IV electrolyte solutions. A major disadvantage of arteriovenous (AV) filtration is the risk for bleeding caused by anticoagulants used to prevent membrane clotting.

A double-lumen dialysis catheter is inserted into a large vein (subclavian, jugular) for CAVHD. A **dialysate** (a solution composed of water, glucose, sodium chloride, potassium, magnesium, calcium, and bicarbonate) delivery system is used to remove waste products in addition to plasma water in patients with limited cardiac output, those with severe hypotension, or those who do not respond to diuretic therapy. These patients cannot tolerate HD, and PD could not remove the large amount of excess fluid.

Continuous venovenous hemofiltration (CVVH) is often used with critically ill patients. CVVH uses only a double-lumen venous catheter for access and is powered by a pump, making the rate of filtration more reliable than methods using mean arterial pressure. The pump increases the risk for an air embolus, but most pumps have alarms that detect air. These systems also require the use of anticoagulants but at lower doses than needed for AV systems. These procedures are used in critical care units, and patients require continuous nursing care.

Posthospital Care

The care for a patient with ARF after discharge from the hospital varies, depending on the status of the disease when the patient is discharged. The course of ARF varies, with recovery lasting up to several months. If the renal failure is resolving, follow-up care may be provided by a nephrologist or by the family physician in consultation with the nephrologist. However, ARF may result in permanent renal damage and the need for chronic dialysis or even transplantation (Bagshaw, 2006b). In these cases, follow-up care is similar to that needed for patients with chronic kidney disease (see Community-Based Care, pp. 1633-1635).

If the ARF is beginning to resolve, the follow-up care may involve many services. Frequent medical visits are necessary, as are scheduled laboratory blood and urine tests to monitor renal function. A nutritionist is needed to modify the patient's diet according to the degree of renal function and ongoing nutritional needs. Teach patients continuing dialysis after discharge to limit foods high in potassium and sodium and to observe protein restrictions. Also teach about any needed fluid intake limitation.

Some patients may need temporary dialysis until their kidneys can eliminate fluid and waste products. The dialysis started while the patient was an inpatient can be continued at an outpatient dialysis center. Teaching about the type of dialysis, how to care for vascular access sites, dietary restrictions, fluid restrictions, and prevention of complications is ongoing throughout the recovery phase. Depending on their level of independence and family support, some patients may also need home care nursing or social work assistance.

DECISION-MAKING CHALLENGE
Coordination of Care

The patient is a 64-year-old man. He visits the primary care provider because of mild lower abdominal pain, decreased urine output, and increased shortness of breath. He is 5 feet, 8 inches tall and weighs 246 pounds. The only drugs he takes are a daily multivitamin, a beta blocker, and occasionally acetaminophen for headache. His past medical history includes kidney stones 1 year ago and mild hypertension over the past 5 years. Physical assessment reveals bilateral crackles in the lung bases. Vital signs are: T, 98.8° F; P, 96/min; R, 28/min; and BP, 148/92.

1. For which type(s) of acute renal failure is he at risk? Why?
2. Do any of his usual drugs increase his risk for ARF? Which one(s) and why?
3. Is there any specific assessment data you could obtain without a prescription to evaluate his risk for acute renal failure? If so, which ones and why?

4. The physician prescribes these interventions:
   - IV placement with a 20-gauge cannula, NS at 20 ml/hr
   - Accurate intake and output
   - Ibuprofen 600 mg orally
   - Furosemide 40 mg IV

In what order (and why) should you perform these interventions?

evolve For suggested answer guidelines, go to http://evolve.elsevier.com/Iggy/.

CHRONIC KIDNEY DISEASE

Pathophysiology

Unlike ARF, chronic kidney disease (CKD) is a progressive, irreversible kidney injury and kidney function does *not* recover. When kidney function is too poor to sustain life, CKD becomes **end-stage kidney disease (ESKD).** Terms used with renal failure include **azotemia** (buildup of nitrogen-based wastes in the blood), **uremia** (azotemia with clinical symptoms [Chart 71-4]), and **uremic syndrome.** ARF and CKD are compared in Table 71-1.

Stages of Chronic Kidney Disease

The kidneys fail in an organized fashion involving five stages based on estimated glomerular filtration rate (GFR) (NIDDK, 2007). Progression toward ESKD in at-risk patients starts with a gradual decrease in GFR (Table 71-5). In the first stage, the person may have a normal GFR (greater than 90 mL/min) with normal kidney function and no obvious kidney disease. However, there may be a *reduced renal reserve* in which reduced kidney function occurs *without* buildup of wastes in the blood because the unaffected nephrons overwork to compensate for the diseased nephrons. Although no manifestations of renal failure are usually present at this stage, if the patient is stressed with infection, fluid overload, or dehydration, renal function at this stage can appear reduced.

In the next stage, *mild CKD,* GFR is reduced, ranging between 60 to 89 mL/min. Kidney nephron damage has occurred and there may be slight elevations of metabolic wastes because not enough healthy nephrons remain to compensate completely for the damaged nephrons. Levels of blood urea nitrogen (BUN), serum creatinine, uric acid, and phosphorus are not sensitive enough to define this stage, however, and reduced GFR is the best measure of CKD. Increased output of dilute urine may occur at this stage of CKD and, if the problem is untreated at this stage, can cause severe dehydration. *Careful management of fluid volume, blood pressure, electrolytes, dietary intake, and other diseases (e.g., heart disease, diabetes) can prevent further damage and slow progression.*

In *moderate CKD,* GRF reduction continues and ranges between 30 to 59 mL/min. Nephron damage has continued and the remaining nephrons cannot manage metabolic wastes, fluid balance, and electrolyte balance. Dietary restrictions of fluids, proteins, and electrolytes are needed.

Over time, patients progress to severe CKD (the fourth stage) and end-stage kidney disease (ESKD, the fifth stage). Excessive amounts of urea and creatinine build up in the blood, and the kidneys cannot maintain homeostasis. Severe fluid, electrolyte, and acid-base imbalances occur (Dinwiddie et al., 2006). Without renal replacement therapy, fatal complications are likely.

Kidney Changes

Kidney failure with greatly reduced glomerular filtration causes many problems, including abnormal urine production, poor water excretion, electrolyte imbalances, and metabolic abnormalities. Because the healthy nephrons become larger and work harder, the kidneys can maintain an effective GFR until about three fourths of kidney function is lost. Homeostasis is maintained until later in the course of kidney failure.

As the disease progresses, the ability to produce dilute urine is reduced, resulting in urine with a fixed osmolarity **(isosthenuria).** As kidney function continues to decline, the BUN increases and urine output decreases. When kidney function declines to this level, the patient is at risk for fluid overload.

Metabolic Changes

Urea and creatinine excretion are disrupted by kidney failure. Creatinine is derived from proteins present in skeletal muscle. The normal rate of creatinine excretion depends on muscle mass, physical activity, and diet. Without major changes in diet or physical activity, the serum creatinine level remains constant. Creatinine is partially excreted by the renal tubules, and a decrease in kidney function leads to a buildup of serum creatinine. Urea is a product of protein metabolism and is excreted by the kidneys. The BUN level normally varies directly with protein intake.

The method for estimating the GFR is the use of a formula that considers the serum creatinine level, age, gender, race, and body size. The most common formula is the Cockcroft-Gault equation, which is described in Chapter 68.

Sodium excretion changes are common. Early in CKD, the patient is at risk for hyponatremia (sodium depletion) because there are fewer healthy nephrons to reabsorb sodium. Thus sodium is lost in the urine. The polyuria often seen in renal failure also causes sodium loss.

Chart 71-4 KEY FEATURES

Uremia

- Metallic taste in the mouth
- Anorexia
- Nausea
- Vomiting
- Muscle cramps
- Itching
- Fatigue and lethargy
- Hiccups
- Edema
- Dyspnea
- Muscle cramps
- Paresthesias

TABLE 71-5 Progression of Chronic Kidney Disease

Stage of Chronic Kidney Disease (CKD)	Estimated Glomerular Filtration Rate
At risk; normal kidney function (early kidney disease may or may not be present)	>90 mL/min
Mild CKD	60-89 mL/min
Moderate CKD	30-59 mL/min
Severe CKD	15-29 mL/min
ESKD	<15 mL/min

In the later stages of CKD, kidney excretion of sodium is reduced as urine production decreases. Then sodium retention and high serum sodium levels (hypernatremia) can occur with only modest increases in dietary sodium intake. This problem leads to severe fluid and electrolyte imbalances (see Chapter 13). Sodium retention causes hypertension and edema.

Even with sodium retention, the serum sodium level may appear normal because plasma water is retained at the same time. If fluid retention occurs at a greater rate than sodium retention, the serum sodium level is falsely low because of dilution (see Chart 71-2).

Potassium excretion occurs mainly through the kidney. Any increase in potassium load during the later stages of CKD can lead to **hyperkalemia** (high serum potassium levels). Normal serum potassium levels of 3.5 to 5 mEq/L are maintained until the 24-hour urine output falls below 500 mL. High potassium levels then develop quickly, reaching 7 to 8 mEq/L or greater. Severe ECG changes result from this elevation, and fatal dysrhythmias can occur. Other factors contribute to high potassium levels in renal failure, including the ingestion of potassium in drugs, failure to restrict potassium in the diet, tissue breakdown, blood transfusions, and bleeding or hemorrhage. (See Chapter 13 for discussion of potassium problems.)

Acid-base balance is affected by CKD. In the early stages, blood pH changes little because the remaining healthy nephrons increase their rate of acid excretion. As more nephrons are lost, acid excretion is reduced and metabolic acidosis results (see Chapter 14).

Many factors lead to acidosis in CKD. First, the kidneys are unable to excrete excessive hydrogen ions (acids). Normally, tubular cells move hydrogen ions into the urine for excretion, but ammonium and bicarbonate are needed for this movement to occur. In patients with renal failure, ammonium production is decreased and reabsorption of bicarbonate does not occur. This process leads to a buildup of hydrogen ions and reduced levels of bicarbonate (base deficit). High potassium levels further reduce renal ammonium production and excretion.

As CKD worsens and acid retention increases, increased respiratory action is needed to keep blood pH normal. The respiratory system adjusts or compensates for the increased blood hydrogen ion levels (decreased pH) by increasing the rate and depth of breathing to excrete carbon dioxide through the lungs. This breathing pattern, called **Kussmaul respiration,** increases with worsening kidney disease. Although hydrogen ions (acids) can leave the body this way, when too much carbon dioxide is "blown off," respiratory alkalosis results. Serum bicarbonate measures the extent of metabolic acidosis (bicarbonate deficit). Patients with CKD usually need alkali replacement to counteract acidosis.

Calcium and phosphorus balance is disrupted by CKD. A complex, balanced normal relationship exists between calcium and phosphate and is influenced by vitamin D (see Chapter 13). The kidney produces a hormone needed to activate vitamin D, which then enhances intestinal absorption of calcium.

In CKD, phosphate retention and a deficiency of active vitamin D disrupt the calcium and phosphate balance. Normally, excessive dietary phosphate is excreted by the kidneys in the urine. Parathyroid hormone (PTH) controls the amount of phosphate in the blood by causing tubular excretion of phosphate when there is an excess. An early effect of CKD is reduced phosphate excretion (Fig. 71-2). As plasma phosphate levels increase **(hyperphosphatemia),** calcium levels decrease **(hypocalcemia).** Chronic low blood calcium levels stimulate the parathyroid glands to release more PTH. Under the influence of additional PTH, calcium is released from storage areas in bones **(bone resorption),** which results in bone density loss. The extra calcium from the bone is needed to balance the excess plasma phosphate level. The problem of low blood calcium levels is made worse with severe CKD because kidney cell damage also reduces production of active vitamin D. Thus less calcium is absorbed through the intestinal tract in the absence of sufficient vitamin D.

The problems in bone metabolism and structure caused by severe CKD–induced low calcium levels and high phosphorus levels are called **renal osteodystrophy.** Bone mineral loss causes bone pain, spinal sclerosis, fractures, bone density loss, osteomalacia, and tooth calcium loss.

Crystals formed from excessive calcium phosphate are known as *metastatic calcifications* and may precipitate in many parts of the body. When the plasma level of the calcium-phosphate product (serum calcium level multiplied by the serum phosphate level) exceeds 70 mg/dL, the crystals may lodge in the kidneys, heart, lungs, major blood vessels, joints, eyes (causing conjunctivitis), and brain. Skin itching increases with calcium-phosphate imbalances and excess PTH release.

Cardiac Changes

Hypertension is common in most patients with CKD. This problem may be either the cause or the result of CKD. In patients who have other causes of hypertension, the increased blood pressure damages the delicate capillaries in the glomerulus and eventually ESKD results.

CKD itself elevates blood pressure by causing fluid and sodium overload and the dysfunction of the renin-angiotensin-

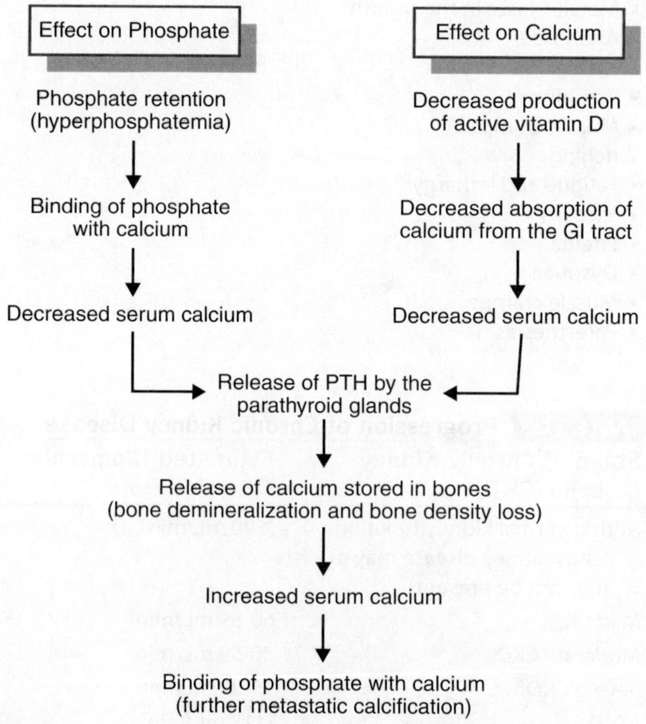
Effect on Phosphate
Effect on Calcium
Phosphate retention (hyperphosphatemia)
Decreased production of active vitamin D
Binding of phosphate with calcium
Decreased absorption of calcium from the GI tract
Decreased serum calcium
Decreased serum calcium
Release of PTH by the parathyroid glands
Release of calcium stored in bones (bone demineralization and bone density loss)
Increased serum calcium
Binding of phosphate with calcium (further metastatic calcification)

Fig. 71-2 • The effects of renal failure on phosphate and calcium balance.

aldosterone system. The retention of sodium and water causes circulatory overload, which elevates blood pressure. The kidneys respond to a decrease in renal blood flow or to low serum sodium levels by trying to improve the renal blood flow. The release of renin triggers the production of more angiotensin and aldosterone. Angiotensin causes blood vessel constriction and increases blood pressure. Aldosterone, a hormone released by the adrenal glands, stimulates kidney tubules to reabsorb sodium and water. These actions increase plasma volume and raise blood pressure. The damaged kidneys do not recognize the increase in blood pressure and continue to produce renin. The result is severe hypertension that is difficult to treat and worsens kidney function. Many patients with CKD also have heart damage and heart enlargement from the long-term hypertension.

Hyperlipidemia occurs in CKD from changes in fat metabolism that increase triglyceride, total cholesterol, and low-density lipoprotein (LDL) levels. These changes increase the patient's risk for coronary artery disease and acute cardiac events. Problems with lipids and atherosclerosis are increased for the patient with CKD and diabetes (Brites et al., 2007).

Heart failure may occur in CKD because it increases the workload on the heart as a result of anemia, hypertension, and fluid overload. Left ventricular enlargement and heart failure are common in end-stage kidney disease (ESKD). Uremia may cause uremic cardiomyopathy, the uremic toxin effect on the myocardium. Heart failure also may occur in these patients because of hypertension and coronary artery disease. Cardiac disease is the leading cause of death in patients with ESKD (USRDS, 2006).

Pericarditis also occurs in patients with CKD. The pericardial sac becomes inflamed by uremic toxins or infection. If it is not treated, this inflammation can lead to pericardial effusion, cardiac tamponade, and death. Manifestations include severe chest pain, an increased pulse rate, a low-grade fever, and a pericardial friction rub that can be heard with a stethoscope placed firmly over the left sternal border. The rub may cause anxiety and pain on deep inspiration that radiates to the left shoulder, neck, and back.

As the pericarditis continues and the pericardial effusion worsens, dysrhythmias may develop. The fluid around the heart makes heart tones softer and harder to hear. Blood pressure decreases, and the patient may be short of breath. If left untreated, pericardial effusion causes cardiac tamponade, an emergency in which pulse pressure decreases and bradycardia results. Treatment of tamponade requires removal of pericardial fluid by placement of a needle, catheter, or drainage tube into the pericardium.

Hematologic Changes

Anemia is a common problem for patients in the later stages of CKD, and it worsens the CKD manifestations. The causes of anemia include a decreased erythropoietin level that decreases red blood cell (RBC) production, decreased RBC survival time resulting from uremia, iron and folic acid deficiencies, and increased bleeding as a result of impaired platelet function.

Gastrointestinal Changes

Uremia affects the entire GI system. The normal flora of the mouth changes with uremia. The mouth contains the enzyme *urease,* which breaks down urea into ammonia. The ammonia generated from this reaction causes **halitosis** (bad breath) and may also cause **stomatitis** (mouth inflammation).

Anorexia, nausea, vomiting, and hiccups are common in patients with uremia. The specific cause of these problems is unknown but may be related to high BUN and creatinine levels, as well as acidosis.

Peptic ulcer disease is also common in patients with uremia. However, the exact cause is unclear. Uremic colitis with watery diarrhea or constipation may also be present in patients with uremia. Ulcers may occur in the stomach or small or large intestine, causing erosion of blood vessels. The blood loss caused by these erosions may lead to hemorrhagic shock from severe GI bleeding.

Etiology and Genetic Risk

The causes of CKD are complex (Table 71-6). More than 100 different disease processes can result in progressive loss of kidney function (see also Chapter 70). Two main causes of

TABLE 71-6 Selected Causes of Chronic Kidney Disease

MORPHOLOGIC

GLOMERULAR DISEASE
- Glomerulonephritis
- Basement membrane disease
- Goodpasture's syndrome
- Intercapillary glomerulosclerosis

TUBULAR DISEASE
- Chronic hypercalcemia
- Chronic potassium depletion
- Fanconi's syndrome
- Heavy metal (lead) poisoning

VASCULAR DISEASE OF THE KIDNEY
- Ischemic disease of the kidney
- Bilateral renal artery stenosis
- Nephrosclerosis
- Hyperparathyroidism

URINARY TRACT DISEASE
- Obstructive uropathy

INHERITED OR GENETIC CONDITIONS
- Hypoplastic kidneys
- Medullary cystic disease
- Polycystic kidney disease

ETIOLOGIC

INFECTION
- Pyelonephritis
- Tuberculosis

SYSTEMIC VASCULAR DISEASE
- Intrarenal renovascular hypertension
- Extrarenal renovascular hypertension

METABOLIC RENAL DISEASE
- Amyloidosis
- Gout (hyperuricemic nephropathy)
- Diabetic nephropathy
- Milk-alkali syndrome
- Sarcoidosis

CONNECTIVE TISSUE DISEASE
- Progressive systemic sclerosis
- Systemic lupus erythematosus
- Polyarteritis

NOTE: List is not all-inclusive.

ESKD are hypertension and diabetes mellitus (USRDS, 2008). In addition, infection and genetic kidney diseases can lead to ESKD (Nussbaum et al., 2007). African-American patients are four times more likely to develop ESKD and seven times more likely to have hypertensive ESKD.

Incidence/Prevalence

The number of patients being treated for CKD is increasing. The 2008 U.S. Renal Data System's annual report stated that more than 340,000 people in the United States are receiving dialysis treatment for ESKD. In 2007, the reported incidence of renal disease (new patients per year requiring renal replacement therapy) was close to 106,000. More than 24% of patients with ESKD die during the first year of treatment. ESKD occurs more often in men than in women (USRDS, 2008). The greatest increase in ESKD is in patients 65 years of age and older. Chart 71-5 addresses the prevention of renal and urinary problems.

Health Promotion and Maintenance

The health-promotion activities to prevent or delay the onset of chronic kidney disease (CKD) focus on controlling the diseases that lead to its development, such as diabetes mellitus and hypertension. Identifying patients who have these disorders at an early stage is critical to CKD prevention. Teach patients to adhere to drug and diet regimens and engage in regular physical activity to prevent the blood vessel changes that lead to kidney damage. Teach patients with diabetes to keep their blood glucose levels within the prescribed range. Teach patients with hypertension that drug therapy is not a cure and must be continued along with lifestyle changes. Urge patients with diabetes or hypertension to have yearly testing for microalbuminuria.

Teach everyone treated for an infection anywhere in the renal/urinary system to take all antibiotics as prescribed. Urge everyone to drink at least 3 L of water daily unless a health problem requires fluid restriction. Caution people who use over-the-counter NSAIDs to avoid abusing these drugs because they reduce renal blood flow and their long-term use reduces kidney function (Schneider et al., 2006). Chart 71-5 is a patient education guide for prevention of renal and urinary problems.

Chart 71-5 PATIENT AND FAMILY EDUCATION GUIDE

Prevention of Renal and Urinary Problems

- Be alert to the general appearance of your urine. Note any changes in its color, clarity, or odor.
- Changes in the frequency or volume of urine passage occur with changes in fluid intake. More frequent or infrequent voiding not associated with changes in fluid intake may signal potential problems.
- Any discomfort or distress with the passage of urine is not normal. Pain, burning, urgency, aching, or difficulty with initiating urine flow or complete bladder emptying is of some concern.
- The kidneys need 1 to 2 quarts of fluid a day to flush out your body wastes. Water is the ideal flushing agent.
- Reduce your intake of soda pop soft drinks.
- Changes in kidney function are often silent for many years. Periodically ask your health care provider to measure your kidney function with a blood test (serum creatinine) and a urinalysis.
- If you have a history of renal disease, diabetes mellitus, hypertension (high blood pressure), or a family history of kidney disease, you should know your serum creatinine level and your 24-hour creatinine clearance. At least one checkup per year that includes laboratory blood and urine testing of kidney function is recommended.
- If you are identified as having decreased kidney function, ask about whether any prescribed drug, diet, diagnostic test, or therapeutic procedure will present a risk to your current kidney function. Check out all nonprescription drugs with your physician or pharmacist before using them.

Patient-Centered Collaborative Care

evolve ONLINE PHARM REVIEW

Assessment

History

When taking a history from a patient with suspected chronic kidney disease (CKD), focus on the manifestations of CKD. Document the patient's age and gender. Accurately measure weight and height, and ask about usual weight and recent weight gain or loss. Weight gain may indicate fluid retention caused by poorly functioning kidneys. Weight loss may be the result of anorexia from high blood urea levels.

Obtain a complete history of known renal or urologic disorders, long-term health problems, drug use, and current health problems. Ask the patient about any existing kidney disease or family history of kidney disease that might indicate a genetic problem. A history of kidney infection or stones may imply past kidney damage. Explore the possibility of long-term health problems because illnesses such as hypertension, diabetes, systemic lupus erythematosus, arthritis, cancer, and tuberculosis can cause decreased kidney function.

Document the use of current and past prescription and over-the-counter drugs because many drugs are nephrotoxic and can cause kidney damage (see Table 71-4).

Examine the patient's dietary habits, and discuss any present GI problems. A change in the taste of foods often occurs with CKD. Patients may report that sweet foods are not as appealing or that meats have a metallic taste. Ask about the presence of nausea, vomiting, anorexia, hiccups, diarrhea, or constipation. These manifestations may be the result of excess wastes that the body cannot excrete because of kidney disease.

Ask about the patient's energy level and any recent injuries or bleeding. Explore changes in his or her daily routine as a possible *result* of fatigue. Weakness, drowsiness, and shortness of breath suggest impending pulmonary edema or neurologic degeneration. Ask about bruising or bleeding, which can be caused by hematologic changes from uremia.

Discuss urine elimination in detail, including frequency of urination, appearance of the urine, and any difficulty starting or controlling urination. These data can help identify urologic problems that may influence existing kidney function.

Physical Assessment/Clinical Manifestations

Chronic kidney disease (CKD) causes changes in many body systems (Chart 71-6). Most manifestations are related to changes in fluid volume, electrolyte and acid-base imbalances, and buildup of nitrogenous wastes.

Neurologic manifestations of CKD and uremic syndrome are numerous (see Chart 71-6) and vary. Observe for problems ranging from lethargy to seizures or coma, which indicate uremic encephalopathy. Assess for sensory changes that appear in a glove and stocking pattern over the hands and feet. Check for weakness in the upper or lower extremities (e.g., uremic neuropathy).

If untreated, encephalopathy progresses to seizures and coma. Dialysis is used to treat CKD when neurologic problems result. The manifestations of encephalopathy resolve with dialysis. However, improvement in neuropathy is limited if it is severe and motor function is impaired.

Cardiovascular manifestations of CKD and uremia result from fluid volume excess, hypertension, heart failure (HF), pericarditis, and potassium-induced dysrhythmias. Assess for signs of reduced sodium and water excretion. Circulatory fluid overload, if untreated, leads to HF, pulmonary edema, peripheral edema, and hypertension.

Assess heart rate and rhythm, listening for extra sounds (particularly an S_3), irregular patterns, or a pericardial friction rub. Unless a hemodialysis (HD) vascular access has been created, measure blood pressure in each arm. Assess the jugular veins for distention, and assess for edema of the feet, shins, and sacrum and around the eyes. Shortness of breath with exertion and at night suggests fluid volume excess.

Respiratory manifestations of CKD also vary (e.g., breath that smells like urine [*uremic fetor* or uremic halitosis], deep sighing, yawning, shortness of breath). Observe the rhythm, rate, and depth of breathing. **Tachypnea** (increased rate of breathing) and **hyperpnea** (increased depth of breathing) occur with metabolic acidosis.

With severe metabolic acidosis, extreme increases in rate and depth of ventilation (Kussmaul respirations) occur. A few patients have pneumonitis, or *uremic lung.* In these patients, assess for thick sputum, reduced coughing, tachypnea, and fever. A pleural friction rub may be heard with a stethoscope. Patients often have pleuritic pain with breathing. Auscultate the lungs for crackles, which indicate fluid volume overload (Pierson, 2006).

Hematologic manifestations of CKD include anemia and abnormal bleeding. Check for indicators of anemia (e.g., fatigue, pallor, lethargy, weakness, shortness of breath, dizziness). Check for abnormal bleeding by observing for bruising,

Chart 71-6 KEY FEATURES
Severe Chronic Kidney Disease

NEUROLOGIC MANIFESTATIONS
- Lethargy and daytime drowsiness
- Inability to concentrate or decreased attention span
- Seizures
- Coma
- Slurred speech
- Asterixis
- Tremors, twitching, or jerky movements
- Myoclonus
- Ataxia (alteration in gait)
- Paresthesias

CARDIOVASCULAR MANIFESTATIONS
- Cardiomyopathy
- Hypertension
- Peripheral edema
- Heart failure
- Uremic pericarditis
- Pericardial effusion
- Pericardial friction rub
- Cardiac tamponade

RESPIRATORY MANIFESTATIONS
- Uremic halitosis
- Tachypnea
- Deep sighing, yawning
- Kussmaul respirations
- Uremic pneumonitis
- Shortness of breath
- Pulmonary edema
- Pleural effusion
- Depressed cough reflex
- Crackles

HEMATOLOGIC MANIFESTATIONS
- Anemia
- Abnormal bleeding and bruising

GASTROINTESTINAL MANIFESTATIONS
- Anorexia
- Nausea
- Vomiting
- Metallic taste in the mouth
- Changes in taste acuity and sensation
- Uremic colitis (diarrhea)
- Constipation
- Uremic gastritis (possible GI bleeding)
- Uremic fetor (breath odor)
- Stomatitis
- Diarrhea

URINARY MANIFESTATIONS
- Polyuria, nocturia (early)
- Oliguria, anuria (later)
- Proteinuria
- Hematuria
- Diluted, strawlike appearance

INTEGUMENTARY MANIFESTATIONS
- Decreased skin turgor
- Yellow-gray pallor
- Dry skin
- Pruritus
- Ecchymosis
- Purpura
- Soft-tissue calcifications
- Uremic frost (late, premorbid)

MUSCULOSKELETAL MANIFESTATIONS
- Muscle weakness and cramping
- Bone pain
- Pathologic fractures
- Renal osteodystrophy

REPRODUCTIVE MANIFESTATIONS
- Decreased fertility
- Infrequent or absent menses
- Decreased libido
- Impotence

GI, Gastrointestinal.

petechiae, purpura, mucous membrane bleeding in the nose or gums, abnormal vaginal bleeding, or intestinal bleeding (black, tarry stools [**melena**]).

GI manifestations of CKD include foul breath and mouth ulceration or inflammation. Document any abdominal pain, cramping, or vomiting. Test all stools for occult blood.

Skeletal manifestations of CKD are related to osteodystrophy from poor absorption of calcium and continuous bone calcium resorption. Adults with osteodystrophy have thin, fragile bones that are at risk for pathologic fractures. These bones break easily with even slight trauma. Vertebrae become more compact and may bend forward, leading to an overall loss of height. Ask about changes in height and any unexplained bone pain. Observe for spinal curvatures and any unusual bumps or protrusions in bone areas that may indicate old fractures. Handle the patient carefully during examination and care.

Urinary manifestations in CKD failure reflect the kidneys' decreasing function. At first, the amount, frequency, and appearance of the urine change. Protein or blood also may be present in the urine.

The amount and composition of the urine change as kidney function decreases. With the onset of mild to moderate CKD, the urine may be more dilute and clearer as tubular reabsorption is reduced. The actual urine output in a patient with CKD varies with the amount of remaining kidney function and glomerular filtration rate (GFR). The patient with severe CKD or ESKD usually has oliguria, but some patients remain able to produce 1 L or more per 24 hours. Daily urine volume usually changes again after dialysis is started.

Skin manifestations of CKD occur as a result of uremia. Pigment is deposited in the skin, causing a yellowish coloration. Some African Americans report a darkening of the skin. The anemia of CKD causes a sallowness, which appears as a faded suntan on lighter-skinned patients.

Skin oils and turgor are decreased in patients with uremia. A distressing problem of uremia is severe **pruritus** (itching). **Uremic frost,** a layer of urea crystals from evaporated sweat, may appear on the face, eyebrows, axilla, and groin of patients with advanced uremic syndrome. Assess for bruises **(ecchymoses),** purple patches **(purpura),** and rashes.

Psychosocial Assessment

Chronic kidney disease and its treatment disrupt many aspects of a patient's life. You are in a unique position to evaluate the patient with newly diagnosed renal failure and to assist with adjustments.

Psychosocial assessment and support are part of the nurse's role from the time that CKD is first diagnosed. Ask about the patient's understanding of the diagnosis and what the treatment regimen means to him or her (e.g., diet, drugs, dialysis). Assess for anxiety and for the coping styles used by the patient or family members. Psychosocial issues affected by CKD include family relations, social activity, work patterns, body image, and sexual activity. The long-term nature of severe CKD and ESKD, the many treatment options, and the uncertainties about the course of the disease and its treatment require ongoing psychosocial assessment.

Laboratory Assessment

Chronic kidney disease causes extreme changes in many laboratory values (see Chart 71-2). Monitor the blood values for creatinine, blood urea nitrogen (BUN), sodium, potassium, calcium, phosphate, bicarbonate, hemoglobin, and hematocrit. Also monitor GFR for trends.

A urinalysis is performed. In the early stages of CKD, urinalysis may show excessive protein, glucose, red blood cells (RBCs), white blood cells (WBCs), and decreased or fixed specific gravity. Urine osmolarity is usually decreased. Glomerular filtration rate (GFR) is calculated based on serum creatinine levels, age, gender, race, and body size. A 24-hour creatinine clearance also may be calculated after blood and urine creatinine levels are collected and quantified but the Cockcroft-Gault estimation is more commonly used. As CKD becomes more severe, the urine output decreases dramatically.

In severe CKD, measurements of the serum creatinine and BUN levels may be used to determine the presence and degree of uremia. Serum creatinine levels may increase gradually over a period of years, reaching levels of 15 to 30 mg/dL or more, depending on the patient's muscle mass. BUN levels are directly related to dietary protein intake. Without protein restriction, BUN levels may rise 10 to 20 times the value of the serum creatinine level. With dietary protein restriction, BUN levels are elevated but less than those of non–protein-restricted patients. Fluid balance also affects BUN. Chapter 68 describes the significance of BUN and creatinine levels, as well as creatinine clearance.

Imaging Assessment

Few x-ray finding are abnormal with CKD. Bone x-rays of the hand can show renal osteodystrophy. With long-term ESKD, the kidneys have shrunk and may be 8 to 9 cm or smaller. This small size results from atrophy and fibrosis. If CKD progresses suddenly, a kidney ultrasound or computed tomography (CT) scan without contrast medium may be used to rule out an obstruction. (See Chapter 68 for a complete description of renal diagnostic tests.)

DECISION-MAKING CHALLENGE
Coordination of Care

The patient is a 27-year-old woman who was diagnosed with type 1 diabetes at the age of 6 years and hypertension at age 21 years. She describes an increase in urine output with clear, dilute-appearing urine. Her skin is pale and dry. She reports palpitations and dizziness when getting out of bed or suddenly rising from her chair. She tells you that she has gained 5 pounds over the past 2 weeks and that when she sits all day, her ankles look swollen.

The drugs she takes include NPH and Regular insulin every morning and evening, hydrochlorothiazide 20 mg once a day, and birth control pills. Vital signs are: T, 98.8° F; P, 94/min and irregular; R, 26/min, and BP, 136/92.

1. What other assessment data should you obtain? What physical manifestations might you find when assessing this patient?
2. What risk factors for the development of CKD are noted in her past medical history? What is the rationale for these risk factors?
3. Why does the patient have an increased urine output at this time?
4. What is the priority nursing diagnosis or collaborative problem for the patient at this time? Provide a rationale for your choice.

evolve For suggested answer guidelines, go to http://evolve.elsevier.com/Iggy/.

Analysis

The patient with CKD has usually had a progressive reduction of renal function and is often hospitalized for adjustment of the treatment plan. The focus of care is to manage symptoms and prevent complications.

Common Nursing Diagnoses and Collaborative Problems

The priority nursing diagnoses for patients with CKD are:

1. Imbalanced Nutrition: Less Than Body Requirements related to inability to ingest or digest food or absorb nutrients as a result of physiologic factors
2. Excess Fluid Volume related to compromised regulatory mechanisms (inability of the kidneys to maintain body fluid balance)
3. Decreased Cardiac Output related to altered stroke volume (reduced) as a result of dysrhythmias and mechanical malfunction (increased preload [excess volume] and increased afterload [increased peripheral vascular resistance])
4. Risk for Infection related to inadequate primary defenses (broken skin), chronic disease, or malnutrition
5. Risk for Injury related to internal biochemical risk factors associated with renal failure (increased susceptibility to bleeding, falls, and fractures)
6. Fatigue related to disease states, altered metabolic energy production, and anemia
7. Anxiety related to threat to or change in health status, economic status, relationships, role function, systems, or self-concept; situational crisis; threat of death; lack of knowledge (diagnostic tests, disease process, treatment); loss of control; or disrupted family life

The primary collaborative problem is Potential for Pulmonary Edema.

Additional Nursing Diagnoses and Collaborative Problems

In addition to the common nursing diagnoses and collaborative problems, patients with CKD may have one or more of these:

- Diarrhea related to chemical or electrolyte imbalances or side effects of drugs
- Constipation related to phosphate-binding drugs
- Impaired Oral Mucous Membrane related to limited fluid intake, malnutrition, and elevated levels of uremic toxins
- Impaired Skin Integrity related to altered chemical balance and uremic toxins
- Social Isolation related to altered state of wellness or alterations in physical appearance
- Interrupted Family Processes related to situational crisis, reduced income, unemployment, or effects of chronic illness
- Sexual Dysfunction related to altered body function, disease process, effects of drugs, depression, or disturbance in body image
- Disturbed Thought Processes related to irritation, central nervous system (CNS) depression, side effects of drugs, sleep deprivation, or clinical depression
- Deficient Knowledge (disease process, care regimen, and follow-up care) related to lack of informational resources and magnitude of the care issues
- Potential for Sepsis
- Potential for Malnutrition
- Potential for Electrolyte Imbalances
- Potential for Metabolic Acidosis

Planning and Implementation

The Concept Map on p. 1616 discusses nursing care issues related to patients who have end-stage kidney disease (ESKD).

Imbalanced Nutrition: Less Than Body Requirements

NOC **Planning: Expected Outcomes.** The patient with CKF is expected to attain and maintain adequate nutrition. Indicators include that the patient should have mild or no deviation from the normal ranges for food intake, weight-to-height ratio, muscle tone, and laboratory values (serum albumin, hematocrit, hemoglobin).

Interventions. The nutritional needs and diet restrictions for the patient with CKD vary according to the degree of remaining kidney function and the type of renal replacement therapy used (Table 71-7).

Nutrition Therapy. The purpose of nutrition therapy is to provide the food and fluids needed to prevent malnutrition. Patients starting hemodialysis (HD) have an increase in protein breakdown and a decrease in intake that result in a loss of lean body mass. NIC nutrition interventions are listed in Chart 71-7.

The patient is referred to a nutritionist for dietary teaching and planning. Work with the nutritionist to teach the patient about diet changes that are needed as a result of CKD. Common changes include control of protein intake; fluid intake limitation; restriction of potassium, sodium, and phosphorus intake; taking vitamin and mineral supplements; and eating enough calories to meet metabolic need.

If adequate calories are not supplied, the body will use muscle protein for energy, which leads to a negative nitrogen balance and malnutrition. The nutritionist determines the number of calories and types of nutrients required to meet body needs.

Protein restriction early in the course of the disease prevents some of the symptoms of CKD and may preserve kidney function. Protein is restricted on the basis of the degree of kidney impairment (reduced GFR) and the severity of the symptoms. Buildup of waste products from protein breakdown is the main cause of uremia. Although lower protein levels are recommended, protein-calorie malnutrition must be avoided in patients receiving hemodialysis (HD). At least 1.5 g of protein per kilogram of body weight per day may be needed for weight gain and improved nutritional status in patients receiving maintenance HD.

The glomerular filtration rate (GFR) is used as an indicator of kidney function and as a guide to safe levels of protein intake. A patient with a severely reduced GFR who is *not* undergoing dialysis is usually permitted 0.55 to 0.60 g of protein per kilogram of body weight (e.g., 40 g of protein daily for a 150-pound [70-kg] adult). If protein is lost in the urine, protein is added to the diet in amounts equal to that lost in the urine. Protein requirements are calculated based on actual body weight (corrected for edema), not ideal body weight.

The patient receiving dialysis needs more protein because some protein is lost through dialysis. While receiving HD, protein requirements are tailored according to the patient's post-dialysis, or "dry," weight. Generally, HD patients are allowed about 1 to 1.5 g of protein/kg/day. Peritoneal dialysis (PD) patients are allowed 1.2 to 1.5 g of protein/kg/day because protein is lost with each exchange. Suggested protein-containing foods are milk, meat, or eggs. If protein intake is

CONCEPT MAP End-Stage Kidney Disease (ESKD)

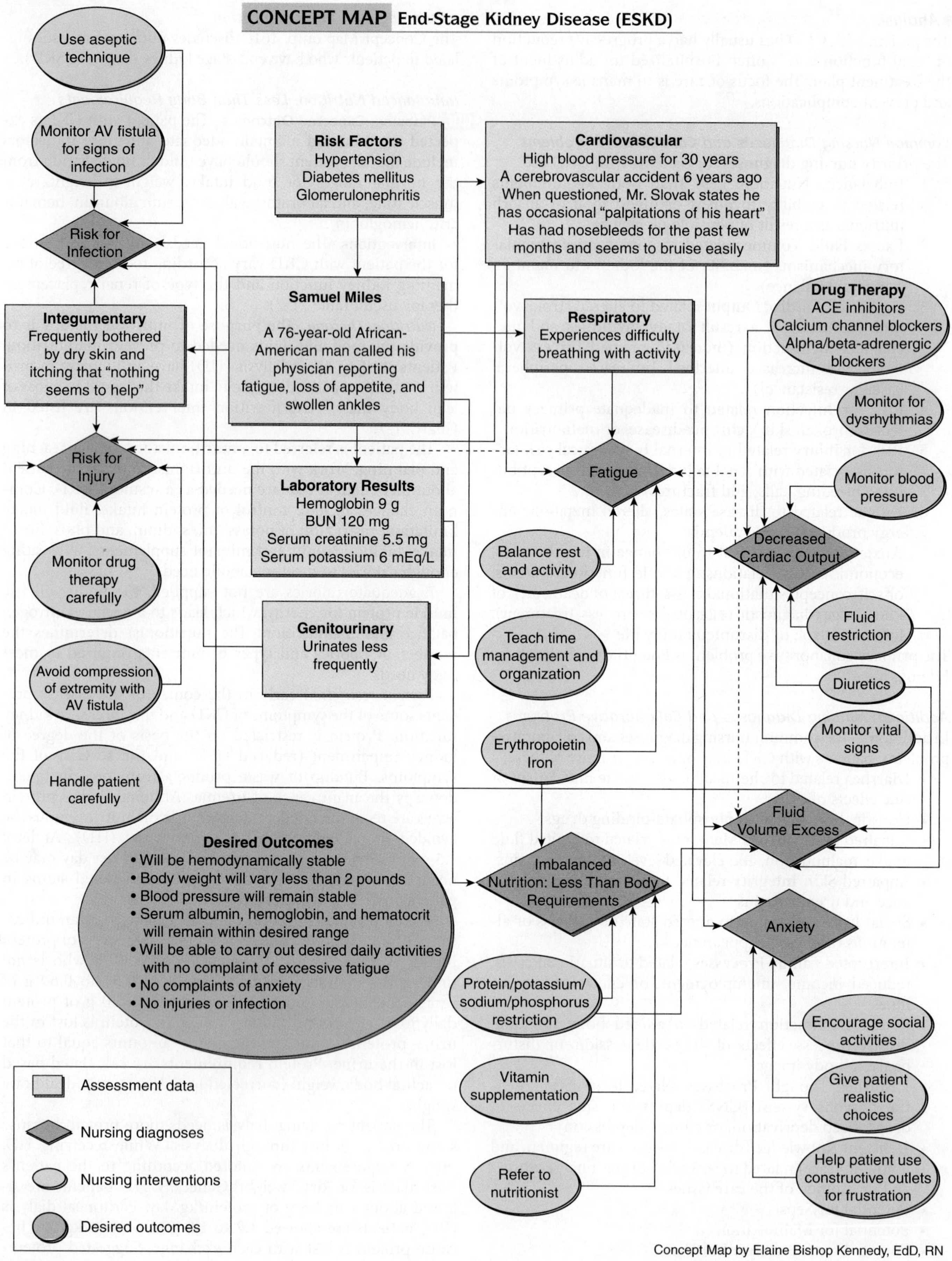
Use aseptic technique
Monitor AV fistula for signs of infection
Risk for Infection
Risk Factors
Hypertension
Diabetes mellitus
Glomerulonephritis
Cardiovascular
High blood pressure for 30 years
A cerebrovascular accident 6 years ago
When questioned, Mr. Slovak states he has occasional "palpitations of his heart"
Has had nosebleeds for the past few months and seems to bruise easily
Samuel Miles
A 76-year-old African-American man called his physician reporting fatigue, loss of appetite, and swollen ankles
Integumentary
Frequently bothered by dry skin and itching that "nothing seems to help"
Respiratory
Experiences difficulty breathing with activity
Drug Therapy
ACE inhibitors
Calcium channel blockers
Alpha/beta-adrenergic blockers
Monitor for dysrhythmias
Risk for Injury
Fatigue
Monitor blood pressure
Laboratory Results
Hemoglobin 9 g
BUN 120 mg
Serum creatinine 5.5 mg
Serum potassium 6 mEq/L
Balance rest and activity
Decreased Cardiac Output
Monitor drug therapy carefully
Fluid restriction
Genitourinary
Urinates less frequently
Teach time management and organization
Avoid compression of extremity with AV fistula
Diuretics
Monitor vital signs
Erythropoietin Iron
Handle patient carefully
Fluid Volume Excess
Desired Outcomes
• Will be hemodynamically stable
• Body weight will vary less than 2 pounds
• Blood pressure will remain stable
• Serum albumin, hemoglobin, and hematocrit will remain within desired range
• Will be able to carry out desired daily activities with no complaint of excessive fatigue
• No complaints of anxiety
• No injuries or infection
Imbalanced Nutrition: Less Than Body Requirements
Anxiety
Protein/potassium/sodium/phosphorus restriction
Encourage social activities
Vitamin supplementation
Give patient realistic choices
Refer to nutritionist
Help patient use constructive outlets for frustration
Assessment data
Nursing diagnoses
Nursing interventions
Desired outcomes

Concept Map by Elaine Bishop Kennedy, EdD, RN

TABLE 71-7 Dietary Restrictions for the Patient with Kidney Failure

Dietary Component	With Chronic Uremia	With Hemodialysis	With Peritoneal Dialysis
Protein	0.55-0.60 g/kg/day	1.0-1.5 g/kg/day	1.2-1.5 g/kg/day
Fluid	Depends on urine output but may be as high as 1500-3000 mL/day	500-700 mL/day plus amount of urine output	Restriction based on fluid weight gain and blood pressure
Potassium	60-70 mEq/day	70 mEq/day	Usually no restriction
Sodium	1-3 g/day	2-4 g/day	Restriction based on fluid weight gain and blood pressure
Phosphorus	700 mg/day	700 mg/day	800 mg/day

Chart 71-7 NIC INTERVENTION ACTIVITIES

The Patient with Chronic Kidney Disease

Nutrition Therapy: *Administration of food and fluids to support metabolic processes of a patient who is malnourished or at high risk for becoming malnourished*

- Complete a nutritional assessment, as appropriate.
- Determine in collaboration with the dietitian, the number of calories and type of nutrients needed to meet nutrition requirements, as appropriate.
- Refer for diet teaching and planning, as needed.
- Instruct patient and family about prescribed diet.
- Provide needed nourishment within limits of prescribed diet.
- Give patient and family written examples of prescribed diet.
- Monitor food/fluid ingested and calculate daily caloric intake, as appropriate.
- Offer herbs and spices as an alternative to salt.
- Monitor lab values, as appropriate.

Fluid Management: *Promotion of fluid balance and prevention of complications resulting from abnormal or undesired fluid levels*

- Maintain accurate intake and output record.
- Monitor hydration status (e.g., moist mucous membranes, adequacy of pulses, and orthostatic blood pressure), as appropriate.
- Monitor for indications of fluid overload/retention (e.g., crackles, elevated CVP or pulmonary capillary wedge pressure, edema, neck vein distention, and ascites), as appropriate.
- Weigh daily and monitor trends.
- Monitor laboratory results relevant to fluid retention (e.g., increased specific gravity, increased BUN, decreased hematocrit, and increased urine osmolality levels).
- Monitor patient's weight change before and after dialysis, if appropriate.
- Assess location and extent of edema, if present.
- Administer prescribed diuretics, as appropriate.
- Distribute the fluid intake over 24 hours, as appropriate.
- Consult physician if signs and symptoms of fluid volume excess persist or worsen.

NIC intervention activities selected from Bulechek, G.M., Butcher, H.K., & McCloskey Dochterman, J. (Eds.). (2008). *Nursing interventions classification (NIC)* (5th ed.). St. Louis: Mosby.

BUN, Blood urea nitrogen; *CVP*, central venous pressure.

not adequate, a negative nitrogen balance develops and causes muscle wasting. BUN and albumin levels are used to monitor the adequacy of protein intake. Decreased serum albumin levels indicate poor protein intake. Excessive protein intake increases BUN levels in patients with CKD.

Sodium restriction is needed in patients with little or no urine output. Both fluid and sodium retention cause edema, hypertension, and heart failure (HF). Most patients with CKD retain sodium; a few cannot conserve sodium.

Estimate fluid and sodium retention status by monitoring the patient's body weight and blood pressure. In uremic patients not receiving dialysis, sodium is limited to 1 to 3 g daily and fluid intake depends on urine output. In patients receiving dialysis, the sodium restriction is 2 to 4 g daily and fluid intake is limited to 500 to 700 mL plus the amount of any urine output. Instruct the patient to not add salt at the table or during cooking. Foods high in sodium (e.g., processed foods, fast foods, potato chips, pretzels, pickles, ham, bacon, sausage) are permitted in moderation. Herbs and spices can be used in place of salt to enhance food flavor.

Potassium restriction may be needed because high blood potassium levels can cause dangerous cardiac dysrhythmias. Monitor the ECG for tall, peaked T waves caused by hyperkalemia. Document serum potassium levels. Instruct the patient with ESKD to limit potassium intake to 60 to 70 mEq/day. Teach him or her to read labels of seasoning agents carefully for sodium and potassium content. Chart 13-8 in Chapter 13 lists common foods that are low in potassium along with common foods that contain high concentrations of potassium and should be avoided. Instruct patients to avoid salt substitutes composed of potassium chloride. Those receiving PD or who are producing urine may not need potassium restriction.

Phosphorus restriction for control of phosphate levels is started early in CKD to avoid osteodystrophy. Monitor serum phosphate levels. Dietary phosphorus restrictions and drugs to assist with phosphate control may be prescribed. Phosphate binders must be taken at mealtimes. Most patients with CKD already restrict their protein intake, and because high-protein foods are also high in phosphorus, this reduces phosphorus intake. Chapter 13 lists foods high in potassium, sodium, and phosphorus.

Vitamin supplementation is needed daily for most patients with CKD. Low-protein diets are also low in vitamins, and water-soluble vitamins are removed from the blood during dialysis. Anemia also is a problem in patients with CKD because of the limited iron content of low-protein diets and decreased kidney production of erythropoietin. Thus supplemental iron is needed. Calcium and vitamin D supplements may be needed, depending on the patient's serum calcium levels and bone status.

Nutritional needs for patients undergoing PD are slightly different from those for patients undergoing HD. Because protein is lost with the dialysate in PD, replacing lost protein is needed. Often 1.2 to 1.5 g of protein per kilogram of body weight per day is recommended. Patients may have anorexia and have difficulty eating enough protein. High-calorie enteral supplements may also be needed. Sodium restriction varies with fluid weight gain and blood pressure. Usually dietary potassium does not need to be restricted because the dialysate is potassium-free. The potassium restriction, if any, is determined by the serum potassium level.

Collaborate with the nutritionist to assess each patient's nutritional needs. Teach the patient and evaluate his or her understanding of and adherence with dietary regimens. Give written examples of the prescribed diet to the patient and family to promote adherence. Help patients adapt the diet to their budget, ethnic background, and food preferences to meet the diet's restrictions.

Excess Fluid Volume

NOC **Planning: Expected Outcomes.** The patient with CKD is expected to achieve and maintain an acceptable fluid balance. Indicators include that the blood pressure, body weight, central venous pressure, and serum electrolytes are only mildly compromised or not compromised.

Interventions. Management of the patient with CKD includes drug therapy, nutrition therapy, fluid restriction, and dialysis. Nutrition therapy is discussed in the Imbalanced Nutrition section, p. 1615, and dialysis is discussed in the Renal Replacement Therapies section, pp. 1620-1630).

The purpose of fluid management is to attain fluid balance and prevent complications of fluid overload (see Chart 71-7). Monitor the patient's intake and output and hydration status. Assess for manifestations of fluid volume excess (e.g., crackles in the bases of the lungs, edema, and distended neck veins).

Drug therapy with diuretics is prescribed for patients with renal insufficiency to treat fluid retention or help control blood pressure. The increased urine output produced from these drugs helps reduce fluid overload in patients who still have some urine output. Diuretics are seldom used in ESKD after dialysis has been initiated because, as kidney function is reduced, these drugs can have harmful side effects on the remaining kidney cells and on the hearing structures.

Assess fluid status by obtaining daily weights and reviewing intake and output. Daily weight gain in these patients indicates fluid retention rather than true body weight gain. Estimate the amount of fluid retained: 1 kg of weight equals about 1 L of fluid retained. Weigh the patient daily at the same time each day, on the same scale, with him or her wearing the same amount of clothing, and after he or she has voided (if the patient is not anuric). Monitor weight for changes before and after dialysis.

Fluid restriction is often needed. The amount of fluid restricted is reviewed in the discussion of sodium restriction on p. 1617. Consider all forms of fluid intake, including oral, IV, and fluid or drugs given through gastric tubes, when calculating fluid intake. Assist the patient in spreading oral fluid intake over a 24-hour period. Monitor his or her response to fluid restriction, and notify the health care provider if manifestations of fluid excess persist or worsen.

Decreased Cardiac Output

NOC **Planning: Expected Outcomes.** The patient with CKD is expected to attain and maintain adequate cardiac output. Indicators include that systolic and diastolic blood pressures, ejection fraction, peripheral pulses, and cognitive status are either only mildly compromised or not compromised.

Interventions. Many patients with long-standing hypertension are at risk for kidney disease and have mild CKD, and some progress to severe CKD and ESKD. *Therefore blood pressure control is essential in preserving kidney function.* To control blood pressure, calcium channel blockers, angiotensin-converting enzyme (ACE) inhibitors, alpha-adrenergic and beta-adrenergic blockers, and vasodilators may be prescribed. ACE inhibitors appear to be the most effective drugs to slow the progression of renal failure. Calcium channel blockers seem to improve the GFR and renal blood flow.

More information on the specific drugs for blood pressure control can be found in Chapter 38. Indications vary depending on the patient, and these drugs are used carefully to avoid complications. Different combinations and doses may be tried until blood pressure control is adequate and side effects are minimized.

Teach the patient and family to measure blood pressure daily. Evaluate their ability to measure and record blood pressure accurately using their own equipment. Recheck measurement accuracy on a regular basis. The patient and family must understand the relationship of blood pressure control to diet and drug therapy. Have the patient or family measure the blood pressure at different times during the day to evaluate control (e.g., in the morning before drugs are taken, after lunch, and at bedtime). Use the results of the measurements to evaluate drug effectiveness and daily BP control. Also teach the patient to weigh daily and to bring records of blood pressure measurements, drug administration times, and weights for discussion with the physician, nurse, or nutritionist.

Assess the patient on an ongoing basis for manifestations of decreased cardiac output, heart failure, and dysrhythmias. These topics are discussed in Chapters 36 through 38.

Risk for Infection

NOC **Planning: Expected Outcomes.** The patient with CKD is expected to remain free of infection. Indicators include that the patient will have only mild or absent fever, lymph node enlargement, positive urine culture, positive dialysis access site culture, or white blood count elevation.

Interventions. Provide meticulous care to any areas where skin integrity has been broken (incisions, site of drains, puncture sites, cracked or excoriated skin, pressure sores), and provide preventive skin care to intact areas. For patients undergoing dialysis, inspect the vascular access site or peritoneal dialysis (PD) catheter insertion site every shift for redness, swelling, pain, and drainage. Monitor vital signs for any manifestation of infection (e.g., fever, tachycardia). Avoid urinary catheterization.

Risk for Injury

NOC **Planning: Expected Outcomes.** The patient with CKD is expected to remain free of injury. Indicators include that the patient should not have any of these problems:

- Fall or experience injury from a fall
- Pathologic fractures
- Bleeding
- Toxic effects of prescribed drugs

Interventions. *Injury prevention strategies* are needed because the patient with long-standing CKD may have brittle, fragile bones that fracture easily and cause little pain. When lifting or moving a patient with fragile bones, use a lift sheet rather than pulling the patient. Observe for normal range of joint motion and for any unusual surface bumps or depressions over bony areas.

Managing drug therapy in patients with CKD is a complex clinical problem. Many over-the-counter drugs contain agents that alter kidney function. Therefore it is important to obtain a detailed drug history. Be aware of the use of each drug, its side effects, and its site of metabolism. Monitor the patient closely for drug-related complications, and ensure that dosages are adjusted as needed.

Certain drugs must be avoided, and the dosages of others must be adjusted according to the degree of remaining renal function. As the patient's renal function decreases, repeated dosage adjustments are necessary. Assess for side effects and signs of drug toxicity, and notify the prescriber as appropriate.

Many drugs are routinely given to patients with renal failure (see Chart 71-3). Know the rationale for these drugs and the indicated nursing interventions. Many patients have cardiac disease and may require cardiac drugs such as digoxin. Patients with severe CKD and ESKD are particularly at risk for digoxin toxicity because the drug is excreted by the kidneys. When caring for patients with CKD who are receiving digoxin, monitor for signs of toxicity, such as nausea, vomiting, anorexia, visual changes, restlessness, headache, fatigue, confusion, **bradycardia** (pulse rate less than 50 to 60 beats/min), and **tachycardia** (pulse rate greater than 100 beats/min). Monitor the serum drug levels to be certain they are in the therapeutic range (0.8-2 ng/mL). Also closely monitor the serum potassium levels of any patient receiving digoxin.

Drugs to control an excessively high phosphate level include phosphate-binding agents. Calcium acetate, calcium carbonate, and aluminum hydroxide are used as phosphate-binding agents in patients with kidney failure. These drugs help prevent renal osteodystrophy and related injuries. Stress the importance of taking these agents and all prescribed drugs.

Hypophosphatemia (low serum phosphorus levels) is a complication of phosphate binding, especially in patients who are not eating adequately but who are continuing to take phosphate-binding drugs. **Hypercalcemia** (excessively high serum calcium levels) also is a possible complication for patients taking calcium-containing compounds to control phosphate excess. In patients taking aluminum-based phosphate binders for prolonged periods, aluminum deposits may cause bone disease or permanent neurologic problems. Monitor the patient for muscle weakness, anorexia, malaise, tremors, or bone pain.

Teach patients with kidney disease to avoid antacids containing magnesium. These patients cannot excrete magnesium and thus should avoid additional intake.

In addition to the drugs used to treat renal failure, the use of certain other drugs requires special attention. These drugs include antibiotics, opioids, antihypertensives, diuretics, insulin, and heparin.

Many antibiotics are safe for patients with CKD, but those excreted by the kidney require dose adjustment. To prevent complications of bloodstream infections from mouth bacteria, prophylactic antibiotic treatment is given to patients with CKD before any dental procedures. The antibiotic used varies with the patient's needs and the physician's preference.

Give opioid analgesics cautiously to patients with severe CKD or ESKD because the effects often last much longer than in those with healthy kidneys. Patients with uremia are very sensitive to the respiratory depressant effects of these drugs. Because opioids are broken down by the liver and not the kidneys, the dosages are often the same regardless of the level of kidney function. Monitor the patient closely after opioids are given, and evaluate his or her reaction to determine whether adjustments are needed.

As CKD progresses, the patient with diabetes often must have insulin doses or oral antidiabetic drug dosages reduced because the failing kidneys do not excrete or metabolize these drugs well. Thus the drugs are effective longer, increasing the risk for low blood glucose levels (hypoglycemia). Monitor blood glucose levels at least four times per day to determine whether a dosage change is needed.

Poor platelet function and capillary fragility in renal failure make anticoagulant therapy risky (Maison et al., 2005). Monitor patients receiving heparin, warfarin, or other anticoagulants every shift for bleeding. See Chapters 41 and 42 for more information on caring for patients at increased risk for bleeding.

Fatigue

NOC **Planning: Expected Outcomes.** The patient with chronic kidney disease (CKD) is expected to conserve energy by balancing activity and rest. Indicators include that the patient will have either only mildly compromised or uncompromised performance of self-care, interest in surroundings, and mental concentration.

Interventions. Some causes of fatigue in the patient with CKD include vitamin deficiency, anemia, and buildup of urea. All patients are given some type of vitamin and mineral supplement because of diet restrictions and vitamin losses from dialysis. Avoid giving these supplements before hemodialysis (HD) treatment because they will be dialyzed out of the body and the patient will receive no benefit.

The anemic patient with CKD is treated with erythropoietin (Epogen, Procrit). The goal of this therapy is to maintain a hematocrit of 30% to 35%. This therapy is effective in triggering bone marrow production of red blood cells if the patient has adequate iron stores. Iron supplements may be needed if patients are iron deficient. Many who receive erythropoietin report improved appetite and sexual function along with decreased fatigue. The increased cell production from this therapy may increase blood pressure. The improved appetite challenges patients in their attempts to maintain protein, potassium, and fluid restrictions and requires additional education.

Anxiety

NOC **Planning: Expected Outcomes.** The patient with CKD is expected to reduce feelings of apprehension and tension. Indicators include that the patient often or consistently demonstrates these behaviors:

- Seeks information to reduce anxiety
- Uses effective coping strategies
- Reports an absence of physical manifestations of anxiety

Interventions. The nurse coordinates a team of health care professionals to support and counsel the patient and family, often over many years of treatment. The nurse has the most contact with the patient with severe CKD and ESKD when the patient is hospitalized or undergoing in-center dialysis treatments. Perform an ongoing assessment of the patient's anxiety level to determine the level of nursing intervention required. Observe his or her behavior for cues indicating anxiety (e.g., anxious facial expressions, clenching of hands, tapping of feet, withdrawn posture, avoidance of eye contact, an increased pulse rate). Evaluate the support systems, such as the involvement of family and friends with the patient's care.

Unfamiliar settings and lack of knowledge about treatments and tests can increase the patient's anxiety level. Explain all procedures, tests, and treatments. Identify the patient's knowledge deficits about kidney function and kidney failure. Provide instruction at a level he or she can understand using a variety of written and video materials.

Provide continuity of care, whenever possible, by using a consistent nurse-patient relationship to decrease anxiety and promote discussions of concerns. As you develop the nurse-patient relationship, encourage the patient to discuss current problems or concerns.

Encourage the patient to ask questions and discuss fears about the diagnosis of severe kidney disease or failure. An open atmosphere that allows for discussion can decrease anxiety level. Facilitate discussions with family members about the prognosis and the impact on the patient's lifestyle.

Potential for Pulmonary Edema

Planning: Expected Outcomes. The patient with CKD is expected to remain free of pulmonary edema by maintaining optimal fluid balance.

Interventions. In the patient with CKD, pulmonary edema can result either from left-sided heart failure or from blood vessel injury. In left-sided heart failure, the heart is unable to eject blood adequately from the left ventricle, leading to an increased pressure in the left atrium and in the pulmonary blood vessels. The increased pressure causes fluid to cross the capillaries into the pulmonary tissue, forming edema. Pulmonary edema can also occur from injury to the pulmonary blood vessels as a result of uremia. This condition causes inflammation and capillary leak. Fluid then leaks into the lung tissue and the alveoli.

Assess the patient for early signs of pulmonary edema, such as restlessness, anxiety, rapid heart rate, shortness of breath, and crackles that begin at the base of the lungs. As pulmonary edema worsens, the level of fluid in the lungs rises. Auscultation reveals increased crackles and decreased air exchange. The patient may have frothy, blood-tinged sputum. As cardiac and pulmonary function decrease further, the patient becomes diaphoretic and cyanotic.

The patient with pulmonary edema usually is admitted to the ICU for aggressive treatment and continuous cardiac monitoring. Place the patient in a high Fowler's position, and give oxygen to improve gas exchange. Drug therapy with renal failure and pulmonary edema is difficult because of potential adverse drug effects on the kidneys. Treatment of pulmonary edema involves giving loop diuretics, such as furosemide (Lasix), IV. Renal impairment increases the risk for ototoxicity with the use of furosemide; thus IV doses are given cautiously. Diuresis usually begins within 5 minutes of giving IV furosemide. Measure urine output every 15 to 30 minutes during the acute episode and every hour thereafter until the patient is stabilized. Monitor vital signs and assess breath sounds at least every 2 hours to evaluate the patient's response to this treatment.

IV morphine sulfate (1 to 2 mg) is often prescribed to reduce myocardial oxygen demand by triggering blood vessel dilation and to provide sedation. Dosage adjustments are needed to achieve the desired response and avoid respiratory depression. Monitor the patient's respiratory rate and blood pressure hourly during this therapy. Other drugs that dilate blood vessels, such as nitroglycerin, also may be given as a continuous infusion to reduce pulmonary pressure. Monitor vital signs at least hourly because this drug combination may cause severe hypotension.

Monitor serum electrolyte levels daily, and report abnormalities to the physician so that imbalances can be corrected quickly. Monitor ECG tracings at least every 2 hours to identify any dysrhythmias. Monitor oxygen saturation levels by pulse oximetry and arterial blood gas values. Adjust the oxygen delivery system to maintain adequate oxygen saturation levels. Monitor the patient for worsening of the condition, manifested as increasing pulmonary edema and hypoxemia. He or she may require temporary intubation and mechanical ventilation to prevent death.

Patients with CKD who have existing cardiac problems, high blood pressure, or chronic fluid retention are at increased risk for developing pulmonary edema. They are less likely to respond quickly to treatment and are more likely to develop problems related to drug therapy. Ultrafiltration may be used with these patients to reduce fluid volume.

Renal Replacement Therapies

Renal replacement therapy is needed when the pathologic changes of stage 4 and stage 5 chronic kidney disease (CKD) are life threatening or pose continuing discomfort to the patient. When he or she can no longer be managed with conservative therapies, such as diet, drugs, and fluid restriction, dialysis is indicated. Transplantation may be discussed at any time.

Hemodialysis

Hemodialysis (HD) is one of several renal replacement therapies used for the treatment of ESKD and kidney failure (Table 71-8). Dialysis removes excess fluids and waste products and restores chemical and electrolyte balance. HD involves passing the patient's blood through an artificial semipermeable membrane to perform the filtering and excretion functions of the kidney.

Patient Selection

Any patient may be considered for HD therapy. Starting this therapy depends on symptoms, not on the glomerular filtration rate (GFR). Dialysis is started immediately for patients who have fluid overload that does not respond to diuretics, pericarditis, uncontrolled hypertension, neurologic problems, and development of bleeding. Most commonly, dialysis is started when uremic manifestations, such as nausea and vomiting, decreased attention span, decreased cognition, worsening anemia, and pruritus, are present.

Many patients survive for years with HD therapy, and others may live only a few months. How long the patient survives using HD therapy depends on his or her age, the cause of renal failure, and the presence of other diseases, such as coronary artery disease, hypertension, or diabetes. General patient selection criteria are:

- Presence of irreversible kidney failure when other therapies are unacceptable or ineffective
- Absence of illnesses that would seriously complicate HD
- Expectation of rehabilitation
- The patient's acceptance of the regimen

TABLE 71-8 A Comparison of Hemodialysis and Peritoneal Dialysis as Renal Replacement Treatment Options

Hemodialysis	Peritoneal Dialysis
ADVANTAGES	
More efficient clearance	Easy access
Short time needed for treatment	Few hemodynamic complications
COMPLICATIONS	
Disequilibrium syndrome	Protein loss
Muscle cramps	Peritonitis
Hemorrhage	Hyperglycemia
Air embolus	Respiratory distress
Hemodynamic changes (hypotension, anemia)	Bowel perforation
Cardiac dysrhythmias	
CONTRAINDICATIONS	
Hemodynamic instability	Extensive peritoneal adhesions
	Peritoneal fibrosis
	Recent abdominal surgery
ACCESS	
Vascular access route	Intra-abdominal catheter
PROCEDURE	
Complex	Simple
Specially trained registered nurses required	Training less complex than for hemodialysis
NURSING IMPLICATIONS	
Vascular access care	Abdominal catheter care
Restrict diet	More flexible diet

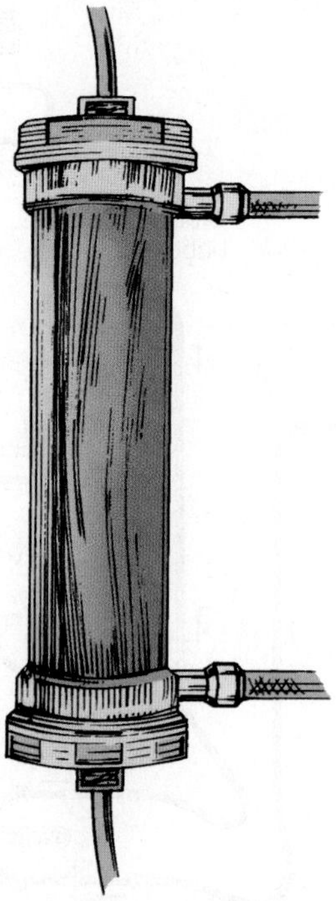

Fig. 71-3 • Artificial kidney (dialyzer) used in hemodialysis.

Dialysis Settings

Patients with CKD may receive HD treatments in many settings, depending on specific needs. Regardless of the setting for therapy, they need ongoing nursing support to maintain this complex and lifesaving treatment.

Patients may be dialyzed in a hospital-based center if they have recently started treatment or have complicated conditions that require close supervision. Stable patients not requiring intense supervision may be dialyzed in a community or freestanding HD center. Select patients may participate in complete or partial self-care in an outpatient center or in in-home HD.

In-home HD is the least disruptive form of therapy and allows the patient to adapt the regimen to his or her lifestyle. Unfortunately, many cannot participate in in-home dialysis because they lack a skilled partner to assist with the therapy and manage the dialysis machine. Some patients and partners find the use of in-home dialysis to be too stressful. In addition, a water treatment system must be installed in the home to provide a safe, clean water supply for the dialysis process.

Procedure

Dialysis works using the passive transfer of toxins by diffusion. **Diffusion** is the movement of molecules from an area of higher concentration to an area of lower concentration. The rate of diffusion during dialysis occurs more rapidly when the membrane pores are large, there is a large surface area of membrane, the temperature of the solutions is higher, and there is a greater difference in the solute concentrations. Molecules that are too large, such as RBCs and most plasma proteins, cannot pass through the membrane.

When HD is started, blood and **dialysate** (dialyzing solution) flow in opposite directions across an enclosed semipermeable membrane. The dialysate contains a balanced mix of electrolytes and water that closely resembles human plasma. On the other side of the membrane is the patient's blood, which contains nitrogen waste products, excess water, and excess electrolytes. During HD, the waste products move from the blood into the dialysate because of the difference in their concentrations **(diffusion).** Excess water is also removed from the blood into the dialysate by osmosis. Electrolytes can move in either direction, as needed, and take some fluid with them. Potassium and sodium typically move out of the plasma into the dialysate. Bicarbonate and calcium generally move from the dialysate into the plasma. This circulating process continues for a preset length of time, restoring water, electrolyte, and acid-base balance and removing wastes. Water volume may be removed from the plasma by applying positive or negative pressure to the system.

The HD system includes a dialyzer, dialysate, vascular access routes, and an HD machine. The artificial kidney, or **dialyzer** (Fig. 71-3), has four parts: a blood compartment, a dialysate compartment, a semipermeable membrane, and an enclosed structure to support the membrane.

Dialysate is made from clear water and chemicals and is free of any waste products or drugs. Bacteria and other organisms are too large to pass through the membrane. Therefore dialysate does not need to be sterile. The water used in dialysate must meet specific standards and usually requires special treatment before mixing the dialysate. The dialysate composition may be altered according to the patient's needs for treatment of electrolyte imbalances. During HD, the dialysate is warmed to 100° F (37.8° C) to increase the rate of diffusion and to prevent hypothermia.

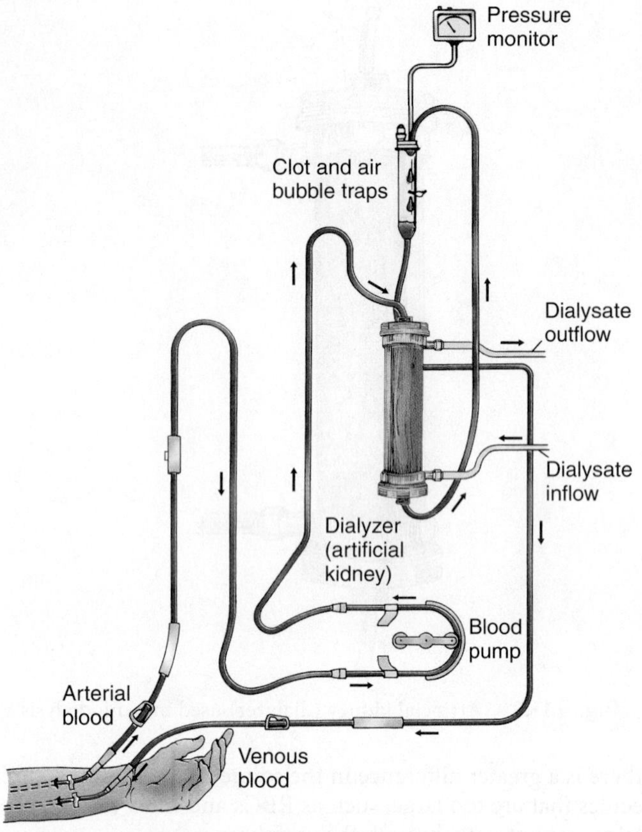
Pressure
monitor
Clot and air
bubble traps
Dialysate
outflow
Dialysate
inflow
Dialyzer
(artificial
kidney)
Blood
pump
Arterial
blood
Venous
blood

Fig. 71-4 • A hemodialysis circuit.

The HD machine has alarm systems to monitor for potential problems, including changes in dialysate temperature, air in the blood tubing, a blood leak in the dialysate compartment, changes in the pressure in either compartment, and changes in composition of the blood or dialysate. If any of these problems are detected, an alarm sounds to protect the patient from life-threatening complications.

All models of HD machines function in a manner similar to that shown in Fig. 71-4. Fig. 71-5 shows one type of HD machine. Fig. 71-6 shows a patient receiving HD. The number and length of treatments depend on the amount of wastes and fluid to be removed, the clearance capacity of the dialyzer, and the blood flow rate to and from the machine. Most patients require about 12 hours per week of total dialysis time. This time is usually divided into three 4-hour treatments. For those with some ongoing urine production, two 5- to 6-hour treatments a week may be adequate. If the patient gains large amounts of fluid weight, a longer treatment time may be needed to remove the fluid without hypotension or severe side effects.

Anticoagulation

To prevent blood clots from forming within the dialyzer or the blood tubing, anticoagulation is needed during HD treatments. Heparin is the most commonly used drug to prevent clots from forming when blood comes in contact with foreign surfaces. Patient response to heparin varies, and the dose is adjusted on the basis of each patient's need. Those receiving erythropoietin may require additional heparin.

Heparin remains active in the body for 4 to 6 hours after dialysis, making the patient at risk for hemorrhage during and immediately after HD treatments. Invasive procedures must be avoided during that time. Monitor him or her closely for any signs of bleeding or hemorrhage. Clotting tendencies can be monitored during HD with a bedside machine (e.g., the HEMOCHRON), by whole-blood clotting times (Lee-White clotting test), or by activated partial thromboplastin times (aPTT) during and after HD. Protamine sulfate is an antidote to heparin and should be available in the dialysis setting.

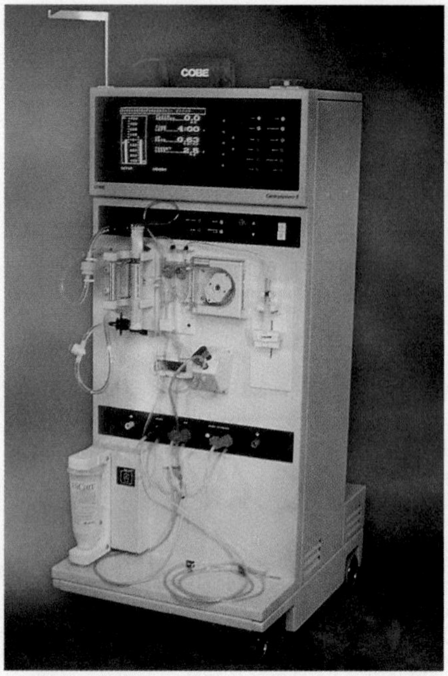

Fig. 71-5 • Hemodialysis machine.

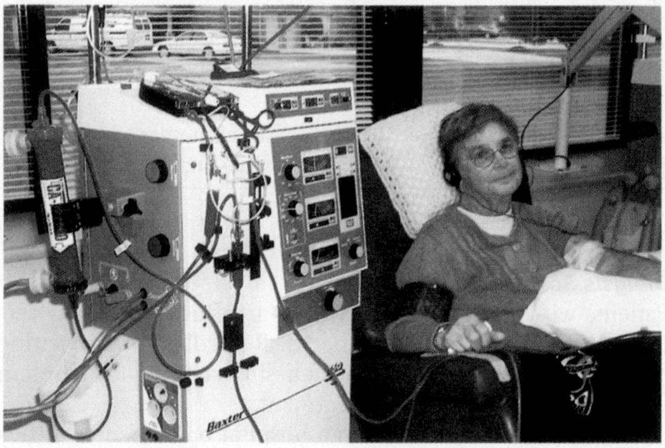

Fig. 71-6 • Patient receiving hemodialysis.

Vascular Access

Vascular access is required for hemodialysis (Table 71-9). The procedure requires the easy availability of a large amount of blood flow: at least 250 to 300 mL/min, usually for a period of 3 to 4 hours. Normal venous cannulation does not provide this rate of blood flow.

Long-term vascular access is internal for most patients having long-term HD (see Table 71-9). The two common choices are an internal arteriovenous (AV) fistula or an AV graft (Fig. 71-7). *AV fistulas* are formed by connecting **(anastomosis)** an artery to a vein. The most commonly used vessels are the radial or

TABLE 71-9 Types of Vascular Access for Hemodialysis

Access Type	Description	Location	Initial Use
PERMANENT			
AV fistula	An internal anastomosis of an artery to a vein	Forearm	2-4 mo or longer
AV graft	Synthetic vessel tubing tunneled beneath the skin, connecting an artery and a vein	Forearm Upper arm Inner thigh	1-2 wk
Dual-lumen hemodialysis catheter	An extended-use catheter, surgically tunneled under the skin with a barrier cuff	Subclavian vein	Immediately postoperatively and after x-ray confirmation of placement
TEMPORARY			
Hemodialysis catheter (dual- or triple-lumen)	A specially designed catheter with two or three lumens Two lumens are for blood outflow and inflow for hemodialysis; a third allows venous access without accessing dialysis lumens	Subclavian, internal jugular, or femoral vein	Immediately after insertion and x-ray confirmation of placement
AV shunt (relatively uncommon)	An external loop of Silastic tubing connecting an artery and a vein Each section of tubing is sutured into a vessel and brought through a skin stab wound	Forearm	Immediately after insertion
Subcutaneous device	An internal device with two metallic access ports and two catheters inserted into large central veins	Subclavian	Immediately after insertion

brachial artery and the cephalic vein of the nondominant arm. Fistulas increase venous blood flow to 250 to 400 mL/min, the amount needed for effective dialysis.

Time is needed after anastomosis for the AV fistula to develop. As the AV fistula "matures," the increased pressure of the arterial blood flow into the vein causes the vessel walls to thicken. This thickening increases their strength and suitability for repeated cannulation. Patients differ in the amount of time needed for the fistula to mature. Some fistulas may not be ready for use for as long as 4 months after the surgery, and a temporary vascular access (AV shunt or HD catheter) is used during this time. Fig. 71-8 shows a mature fistula.

To access a fistula, cannulate it by inserting two needles, one toward the venous blood flow and one toward the arterial blood flow. This procedure allows the HD machine to draw the blood out through the arterial needle and return it through the venous needle.

Arteriovenous grafts are used when the AV fistula does not develop or when complications limit its use. The polytetrafluoroethylene (PTFE) graft is a synthetic material (GORE-TEX). This type of graft is commonly used for older patients using HD. Fig. 71-7, *B* shows a patient's AV graft.

Precautions. Some precautions are needed to ensure the functioning of an internal AV fistula or AV graft. First assess for adequate circulation in the fistula or graft and in the lower portion of the arm. Then check for a bruit or a thrill by auscultation or palpation over the access site. *Repeated compression can result in the loss of the vascular access. Therefore avoid taking the blood pressure or performing venipunctures in the arm with the vascular access. Do not use AV fistula or graft for delivery of IV fluids.* Chart 71-8 lists best practices for care of the patient with an HD access.

Complications. Complications can occur with any type of access. The most common problems are thrombosis or stenosis, infection, aneurysm formation, ischemia, and heart failure.

Thrombosis, or clotting of the AV access, is the most frequent complication. Some patients are at greater risk for clotting than others and may be given anticoagulant drugs. Interventional radiology can treat failing grafts. Most grafts fail because of high-pressure arterial flow entering the venous system. The muscle layers of the veins react to this increased pressure by thickening. The venous thickening reduces or occludes blood flow. Radiologists inject a thrombolytic drug (e.g., tPA) to dissolve the clot. The clot usually dissolves within minutes, and often a stricture is revealed at the point where the graft and the vein connect. The stricture can be treated by balloon angioplasty (Table 71-10).

Most infections of the vascular access are caused by *Staphylococcus aureus* introduced during cannulation. Use sterile technique during cannulation to prevent infection (see Table 71-10).

Aneurysms can form in the fistula and are caused by repeated needle punctures at the same site. Large aneurysms may cause loss of the fistula's function and require surgical repair.

Ischemia occurs in a few patients with vascular access when the fistula decreases arterial blood flow to areas below the fistula. Ischemic symptoms *("steal syndrome")* vary from cold or numb fingers to gangrene. If the collateral circulation is inadequate, the fistula may need to be tied off and a new one created in another area to preserve extremity circulation.

The shunting of blood directly from the arterial system to the venous system, through the fistula, can cause heart failure in patients with a limited cardiac reserve (see Chapter 37). This complication is rare, but if it does occur, the fistula may need to be revised to reduce arterial blood flow.

Temporary Vascular Access. Temporary access with special catheters has replaced the use of the AV shunt for patients

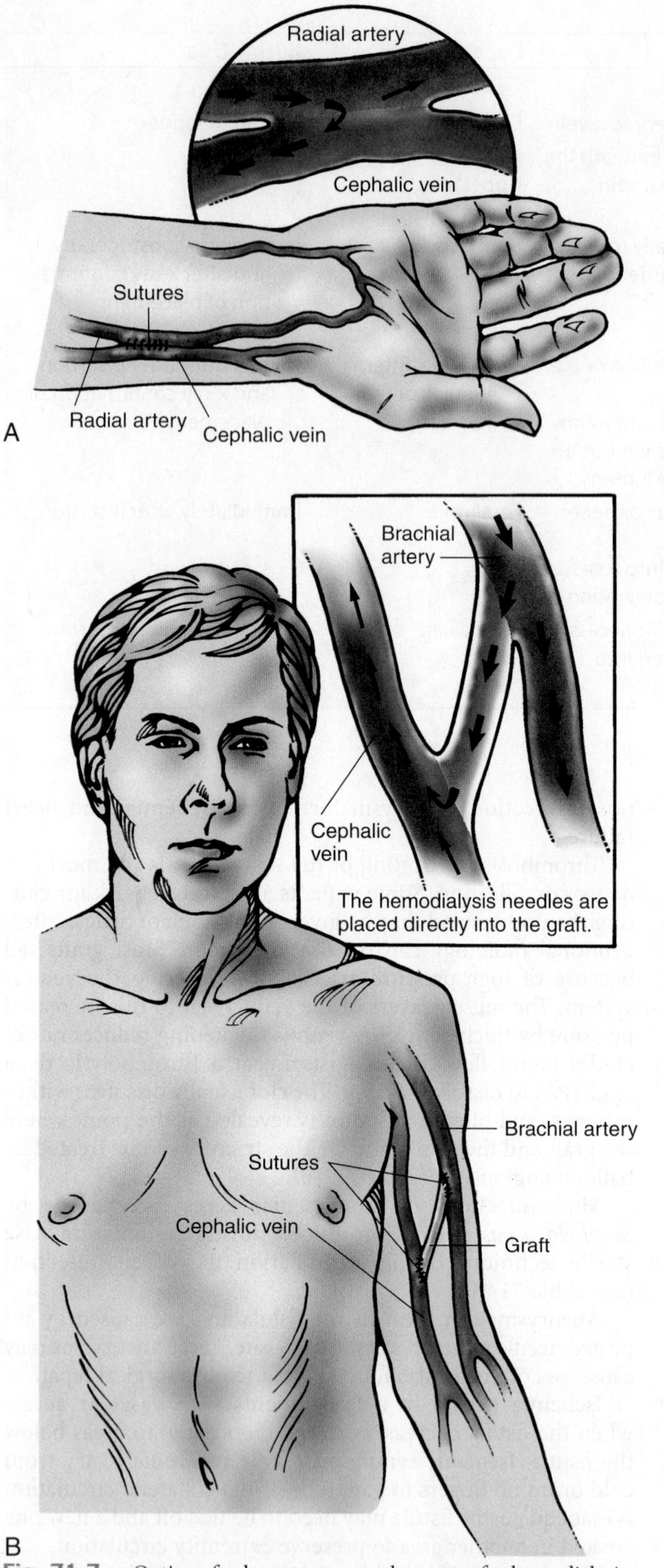
Radial artery
Cephalic vein
Sutures
Radial artery
Cephalic vein
A
Brachial artery
Cephalic vein
The hemodialysis needles are placed directly into the graft.
Brachial artery
Sutures
Cephalic vein
Graft
B

Fig. 71-7 • Options for long-term vascular access for hemodialysis. **A,** A surgically created venous fistula. The increased pressure from the artery forces blood into the vein. This process causes the vein to dilate enough for fistula needles to be placed for hemodialysis. When the vein dilates in this manner, the fistula is said to be "developed" or "mature." **B,** A surgically placed straight vascular graft in the upper arm. The graft creates a shunt between arterial and venous blood.

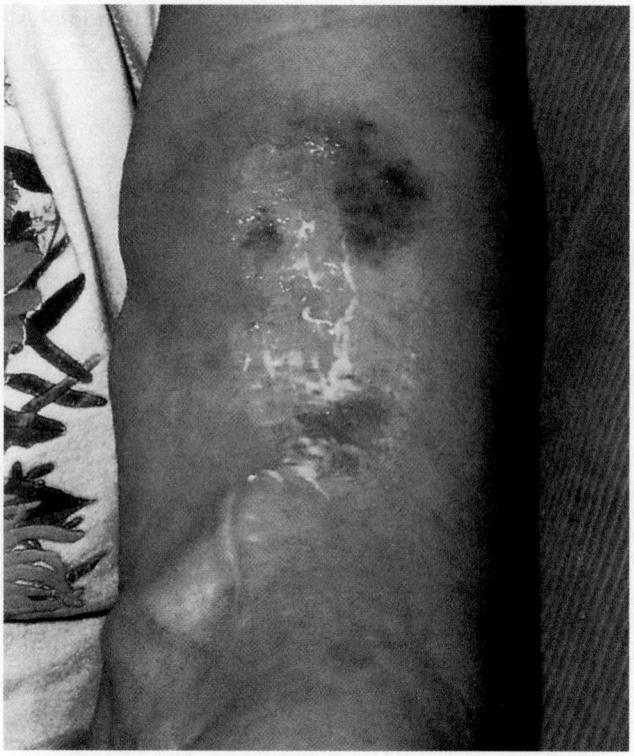

Fig. 71-8 • A mature fistula for hemodialysis access.

Chart 71-8 **BEST PRACTICE FOR PATIENT SAFETY & QUALITY CARE**

Caring for the Patient with an Arteriovenous Fistula, Arteriovenous Graft, or Arteriovenous Shunt

- Do not take blood pressure readings using the extremity in which the vascular access is placed.
- Do not perform venipunctures or start an IV line in the extremity in which the vascular access is placed.
- Palpate for thrills and auscultate for bruits every 4 hours while the patient is awake.
- Assess the patient's distal pulses and circulation.
- Elevate the affected extremity postoperatively.
- Encourage routine range-of-motion exercises.
- Check for bleeding at needle insertion sites or shunt tubing insertion sites. (Keep small clamps handy on the dressing of the AV shunt.)
- Assess for manifestations of infection at needle sites and shunt tubing insertion sites.
- Instruct the patient not to carry heavy objects or anything that compresses the extremity in which the vascular access is placed.
- Instruct the patient not to sleep with his or her body weight on top of the extremity in which the vascular access is placed.

AV, Arteriovenous.

TABLE 71-10 Nursing Interventions for Prevention of Complications in Hemodialysis Vascular Access

Access Type	Bleeding	Infection	Clotting
AV fistula or AV graft	Apply pressure to the needle puncture sites.	Ensure adequate site cleaning before cannulation.	Avoid constrictive devices. Rotate needle insertion sites with each hemodialysis treatment. Assess for thrill and bruit.
AV shunt	Keep clamps available.	Perform exit site care 3 times/wk.	Avoid constrictive devices. Assess for thrill and bruit.
Hemodialysis catheters (temporary and permanent)	Monitor the access site.	Use aseptic technique.	Place a heparin or heparin/saline dwell solution after hemodialysis treatment. Not used between treatments.

AV, Arteriovenous.

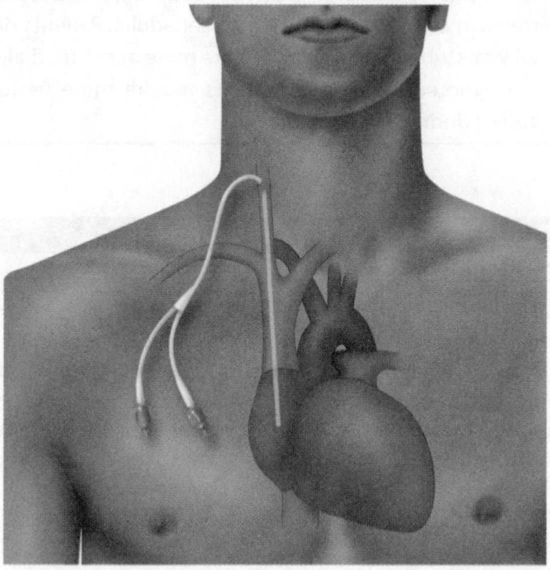

Fig. 71-9 • Temporary subcutaneous hemodialysis access.

requiring immediate HD. A catheter designed for HD may be inserted into the subclavian, internal jugular, or femoral vein. The lumens of these devices are much smaller than the permanent accesses, and more time (4 to 8 hours) is required to complete each dialysis session.

Subcutaneous devices may also be surgically inserted to provide temporary access for HD. Implanted beneath the skin, these devices are composed of two small metallic ports with attached catheters that are inserted into large central veins (Fig. 71-9). The ports of subcutaneous devices have internal mechanisms, which open when needles are inserted and close when needles are removed. Blood from one port flows from the body to the HD machine and returns to the body via the other port. These devices may be ideal for patients awaiting permanent access placement or a kidney transplant.

Hemodialysis Nursing Care

Many drugs are dialyzable (i.e., can be partially removed from the blood during dialysis). Vasoactive drugs can cause hypotension during HD and may also be held until after treatment. Coordinate with the physician to assess the patient's drug regimen and determine which drugs should be held until after HD treatment. Table 71-11 lists common dialyzable and vasoactive drugs that should be given after HD.

TABLE 71-11 Dialyzable and Vasoactive Drugs

DIALYZABLE DRUGS	***MISCELLANEOUS***
AMINOGLYCOSIDES	• Aztreonam
• Amikacin	• Cimetidine
• Gentamycin	• Vitamins
• Tobramycin	**VASOACTIVE DRUGS**
ANTIVIRAL AGENTS	***ANTIDYSRHYTHMICS***
• Acyclovir	• Flecainide
• Ganciclovir	• Lidocaine
PENICILLINS	• Procainamide
• Amoxicillin	• Quinidine
• Ampicillin	***ANTIHYPERTENSIVES***
• Cloxacillin	• Atenolol
• Dicloxacillin	• Captopril
• Mezlocillin	• Diltiazem
• Penicillin G	• Enalapril
• Ticarcillin	• Lisinopril
ANTICONVULSANTS	• Methyldopa
• Ethosuximide	• Nifedipine
• Gabapentin	• Propranolol
• Phenobarbital	• Verapamil
CEPHALOSPORINS	***NARCOTICS***
• Cefaclor	• Codeine
• Cefazolin	• Morphine
• Cefoxitin	***SEDATIVES***
• Ceftizoxime	• Midazolam
• Ceftriaxone	• Phenobarbital
• Cefuroxime	• Propofol
ANTITUBERCULOSIS AGENTS	***VASODILATORS***
• Ethambutol	• Hydralazine
• Isoniazid	• Nitroglycerin
	• Nitroprusside

Post-Dialysis Care

Closely monitor the patient immediately and for several hours after dialysis for any side effects from the treatment. Common problems include hypotension, headache, nausea, malaise, vomiting, dizziness, and muscle cramps.

Obtain vital signs and weight for comparison with predialysis measurements. Blood pressure and weight are expected to be reduced as a result of fluid removal. Hypotension may require rehydration with IV fluids, such as normal saline. The patient's temperature may also be elevated because the dialysis machine warms the blood slightly. If he or she has a fever, sepsis may be present and a blood sample is needed for culture and sensitivity.

The heparin required during hemodialysis (HD) increases the clotting time and thus the risk for excessive bleeding. All invasive procedures must be avoided for 4 to 6 hours after dialysis. Continually monitor the patient for hemorrhage during dialysis and for 1 hour after dialysis (Chart 71-9).

Complications of Hemodialysis

Many fluid-related and infectious complications can occur from HD. The most common complications include disequilibrium syndrome and viral infections.

Dialysis disequilibrium syndrome may develop during HD or after HD has been completed. The cause is thought to be due to the rapid decrease in fluid volume and blood urea nitrogen (BUN) levels during HD. The change in urea levels can cause cerebral edema and increased intracranial pressure. *Neurologic symptoms can result (e.g., headache, nausea, vomiting, restlessness, decreased level of consciousness, seizures, coma, death). Assess for and document these symptoms because early recognition of the syndrome and treatment with anticonvulsants and barbiturates may prevent a life-threatening situation.* The problem may be prevented by starting HD for short periods with low blood flows so that rapid changes in plasma composition are avoided.

Infectious diseases transmitted by blood transfusion are a serious complication of long-term HD. Two of the most serious blood-transmitted infections are hepatitis and human immune deficiency virus (HIV).

Hepatitis infection (B and C) in patients with chronic kidney disease (CKD) has decreased because the use of erythropoietin has reduced the need for blood transfusions to maintain red blood cell counts. Hepatitis is a problem because of the blood access and the risk for contamination during HD. The viruses can be transmitted through the use of contaminated needles or instruments, by entry of contaminated blood through open wounds in the skin or mucous membranes, or through transfusions with contaminated blood. Monitor all patients receiving HD for manifestations of hepatitis (see Chapter 61).

HIV is a bloodborne and body fluid–borne virus that poses some risk for patients undergoing HD. Fortunately, the risks for HIV transmission are reduced by the consistent practice of Standard Precautions (blood and body fluids), routine screening of donated blood for HIV, and decreased need for blood transfusions for patients with CKD and end-stage kidney disease (ESKD). Despite this progress, however, some patients have already been infected with the HIV. Patients who have been undergoing HD or received frequent transfusions during the early 1980s to mid-1980s are at risk for acquired immune deficiency syndrome (AIDS) (see also Chapter 21).

Chart 71-9 BEST PRACTICE FOR PATIENT SAFETY & QUALITY CARE

Caring for the Patient Undergoing Hemodialysis

- Weigh the patient before and after dialysis.
- Know the patient's dry weight.
- Discuss with the physician whether any of the patient's drugs should be withheld until after dialysis.
- Be aware of events that occurred during the dialysis treatment.
- Measure blood pressure, pulse rate, respirations, and temperature.
- Assess for symptoms of orthostatic hypotension.
- Assess the vascular access site.
- Observe for bleeding.
- Assess the patient's level of consciousness.
- Assess for headache, nausea, and vomiting.

CONSIDERATIONS FOR OLDER ADULTS

In 2007, the occurrence of ESKD in patients ages 75 years and older increased to more than 25% of patients beginning ESKD therapy (USRDS, 2008). The overall mean age for new patients is 64.9 years. ESKD incidence caused by diabetes and hypertension continues to grow in older adults. Patients older than 65 years who are receiving HD are more at risk for dialysis-induced hypotension. These patients require more frequent monitoring during and after dialysis.

DECISION-MAKING CHALLENGE

Coordination of Care

A year later, your patient with CKD described on p. 1614 has been diagnosed with ESKD. Her nephrologist has prescribed HD three times a week for 4 to 5 hours, as well as fluid and diet teaching. She has a temporary HD dialysis catheter in place, and the surgeon created an AV fistula 2 weeks ago. The patient tells you that she is concerned about missing so much work and losing her job.

1. What teaching should you provide regarding the diet and fluid needs of this patient?
2. What should you teach the patient regarding care of her temporary and permanent HD sites?
3. What changes, if any, will need to be made in her therapy for diabetes and hypertension?
4. For what complications should you monitor during and immediately after dialysis?

evolve For suggested answer guidelines, go to http://evolve.elsevier.com/Iggy/.

Peritoneal Dialysis

Peritoneal dialysis (PD) allows exchanges of wastes, fluids, and electrolytes to occur in the peritoneal cavity. PD is slower than hemodialysis (HD), however, and more time is needed to achieve the same effect. Advantages and disadvantages are listed in Table 71-12.

Patient Selection

Most patients with chronic kidney disease (CKD) can select either HD or PD. For those who are unstable and those who cannot tolerate anticoagulation, PD is less hazardous than HD. For some patients, vascular access problems may eliminate HD as an option. At times a patient may use PD until a new arteriovenous (AV) fistula matures. PD is also often the treatment of choice for older adults because it offers more flexibility if their status changes frequently.

Peritoneal dialysis *cannot* be performed if peritoneal adhesions are present or if extensive intra-abdominal surgery has been performed. In these cases, the surface area of the peritoneal membrane is not sufficient for adequate dialysis exchange.

Peritoneal membrane fibrosis may occur after repeated infections, which decreases membrane permeability.

Procedure

A siliconized rubber (Silastic) catheter is surgically placed into the abdominal cavity for infusion of dialysate (Fig. 71-10). Usually 1 to 2 L of dialysate is infused by gravity *(fill)* into the peritoneal space over a 10- to 20-minute period, according to the patient's tolerance. The fluid stays *(dwells)* in the cavity for a specified time prescribed by the physician. The fluid then flows out of the body *(drains)* by gravity into a drainage bag. The peritoneal outflow contains the dialysate and the excess water, electrolytes, and nitrogen-based waste products. The dialyzing fluid is called peritoneal *effluent* on outflow. The three phases of the process (infusion, or "fill"; dwell; and outflow, or drain) make up one PD exchange (see Fig. 71-10). The number and frequency of PD exchanges are prescribed by the physician, depending on the patient's manifestations and laboratory data.

TABLE 71-12 Peritoneal Dialysis

Advantages	Disadvantages
Easy to learn	Time-consuming exchanges
Can be done at home	Protein wasting
Ambulatory—no machine needed	Excessive glucose load → hyperlipidemia
When machines are used, they are small	Sterile technique required
Less stressful on the body	Presence of permanent catheter
Hemodynamic tolerance	Weight gain
Continuous process	Peritonitis risk
Better blood pressure control	Peritoneum injury risk
Less dietary and fluid restrictions	Cannot be done if patient has had many abdominal surgeries
Greater freedom in scheduling and traveling	Chronic back pain or development of hernia

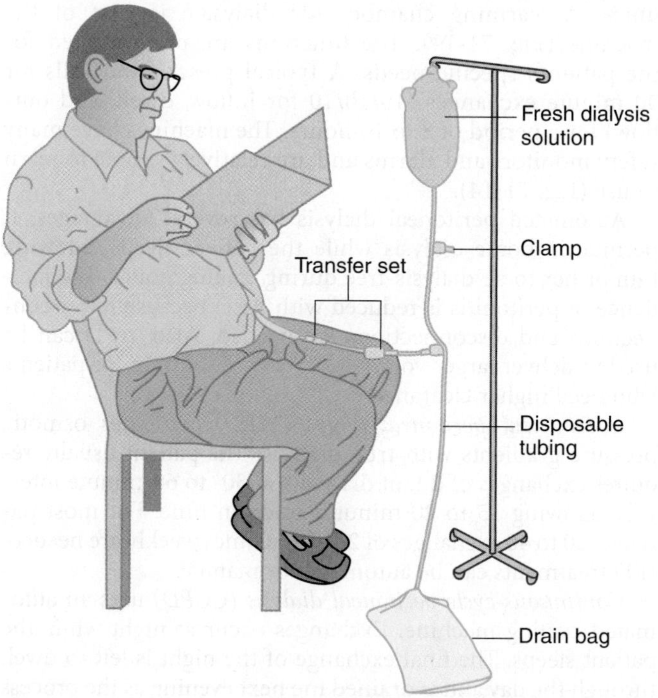
Fresh dialysis solution
Clamp
Transfer set
Disposable tubing
Drain bag

Fig. 71-10 • Peritoneal dialysis exchange for control of fluids, electrolytes, nitrogenous wastes, blood pressure, and acid-base balance.

Process

Peritoneal dialysis occurs through diffusion and osmosis across the semipermeable peritoneal membrane and capillaries. The peritoneal membrane is large and porous. It allows solutes and water to move from an area of higher concentration in the blood to an area of lower concentration in the dialyzing fluid (diffusion) (Fig. 71-11).

The peritoneal cavity is rich in capillaries and is a ready access to the blood supply. The fluid and waste products dialyzed from the patient move through the blood vessel walls, the interstitial tissues, and the peritoneal membrane and are removed when the dialyzing fluid is drained from the body.

The efficiency of PD is affected by many factors, such as decreased peritoneal membrane permeability caused by infection or scarring and reduced capillary blood flow resulting from blood vessel constriction, vascular disease, or decreased perfusion of the peritoneum. Unlike hemodialysis (HD), water removal depends on the concentration of the dialysate. Increasing the glucose concentration of the dialysate makes the solution more hypertonic. The more hypertonic the solution, the greater is the osmotic pressure for water filtration and fluid removal from the patient during an exchange. The dialysate concentration is prescribed on the basis of the patient's fluid status.

Dialysate Additives

Heparin may be added to the dialysate to prevent clotting of the catheter or tubing. Usually intraperitoneal (IP) heparin is needed only after new catheter placement or if peritonitis occurs. IP heparin is not absorbed systemically and does not affect blood clotting.

Other agents that may be given in the dialysate include potassium and antibiotics. Commercially prepared dialysate does not contain potassium. Some patients need potassium added to the dialysate to prevent hypokalemia. Antibiotics may be given by the IP route when peritonitis is present or suspected. Potassium and antibiotics are not mixed in the same dialysate bag because interactions may reduce the antibiotic effect.

Types of Peritoneal Dialysis

Many types of PD are available, including continuous ambulatory PD, multiple-bag continuous ambulatory PD, automated PD, intermittent PD, and continuous-cycle PD. The type selected depends on the patient's ability and lifestyle (Harwood & Leitch, 2006).

Continuous ambulatory peritoneal dialysis (CAPD) is performed by the patient with the infusion of four 2-L exchanges of dialysate into the peritoneal cavity. Each time, the dialysate remains for 4 to 8 hours, and these exchanges occur 7 days a week (Fig. 71-12). During the dwell period, the patient can use a continuous connect system or a disconnect system.

With the continuous *connect* system (straight transfer set), the dialysate bag is attached to the catheter by 48-inch tubing. The empty bag and tubing are folded and worn beneath the clothing until they are used for outflow. After draining, the patient removes the bag and connects a new bag to repeat the process.

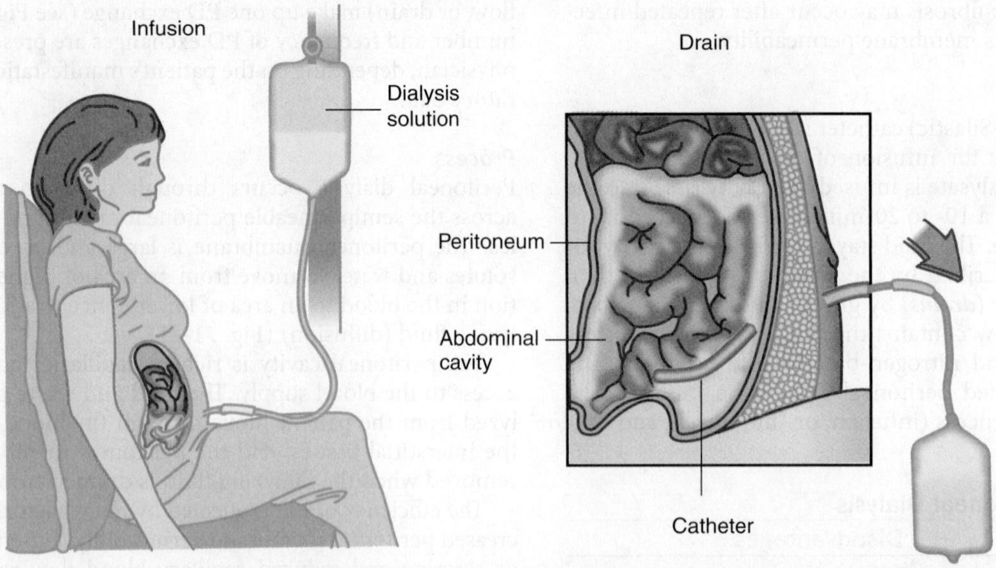
Infusion
Dialysis solution
Peritoneum
Abdominal cavity
Drain
Catheter

Fig. 71-11 • Peritoneal membrane as dialyzing membrane for peritoneal dialysis.

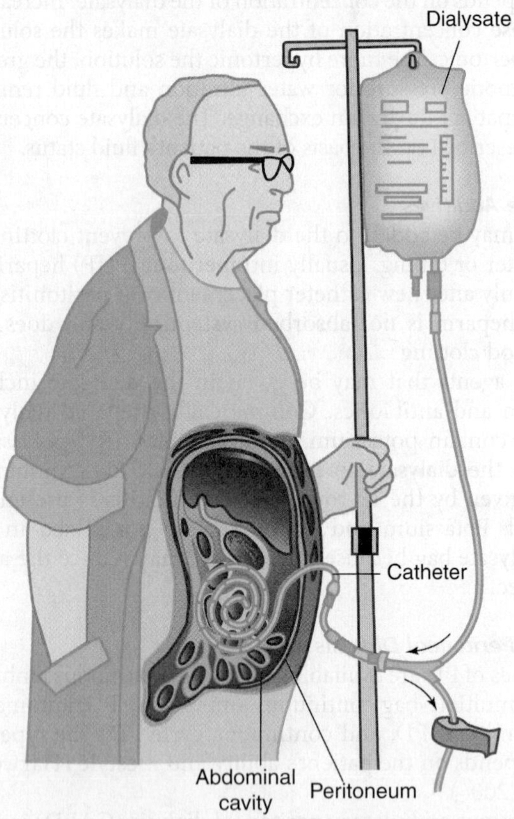
Dialysate
Catheter
Abdominal cavity
Peritoneum

Fig. 71-12 • A patient performing continuous ambulatory peritoneal dialysis (CAPD).

With the *disconnect system* (Y–transfer set), the patient removes the connecting tubing and empty dialysate bag after inflow and attaches a cap to the PD catheter. The disconnect system eliminates the need to wear the tubing and bag but requires opening the system two extra times with each exchange. The extra opening of the system increases the risk for infection.

With CAPD treatment, no machine is necessary and no partner is required. However, it is best for a partner also trained in CAPD to be available as a support for the patient if illness occurs. Devices to assist in the safe, sterile connection of the tubing spike with the dialysate bag are available. These devices are useful for patients with poor vision, limited manual dexterity, or decreased hand and arm strength. CAPD allows constant removal of fluid and wastes and more closely resembles renal function than does HD. Some patients even perform their own exchanges while hospitalized.

Automated peritoneal dialysis (APD) may be used in the acute care setting, the outpatient dialysis center, or the patient's home. APD uses a cycling machine for dialysate inflow, dwell, and outflow according to preset times and volumes. A warming chamber for dialysate is part of the machine (Fig. 71-13). The functions are programmed for the patient's specific needs. A typical prescription calls for 30-minute exchanges (10/10/10 for inflow, dwell, and outflow) for a period of 8 to 10 hours. The machines have many safety monitors and alarms and are relatively simple to learn to use (Fig. 71-14).

Automated peritoneal dialysis has several advantages. It permits in-home dialysis while the patient sleeps, allowing him or her to be dialysis-free during waking hours. The incidence of peritonitis is reduced with APD because fewer connections and disconnections are needed. Also, APD can be used to deliver larger volumes of dialysis solution for patients who need higher clearances.

Intermittent peritoneal dialysis (IPD) combines osmotic pressure gradients with true dialysis. The patient usually requires exchanges of 2 L of dialysate at 30- to 60-minute intervals, allowing 15 to 20 minutes of drain time. For most patients, 30 to 40 exchanges of 2 L three times weekly are needed. IPD treatments can be automated or manual.

Continuous-cycle peritoneal dialysis (CCPD) uses an automated cycling machine. Exchanges occur at night while the patient sleeps. The final exchange of the night is left to dwell through the day and is drained the next evening as the process is repeated. CCPD offers the advantage of 24-hour dialysis, as in CAPD, but the sterile catheter system is opened less often.

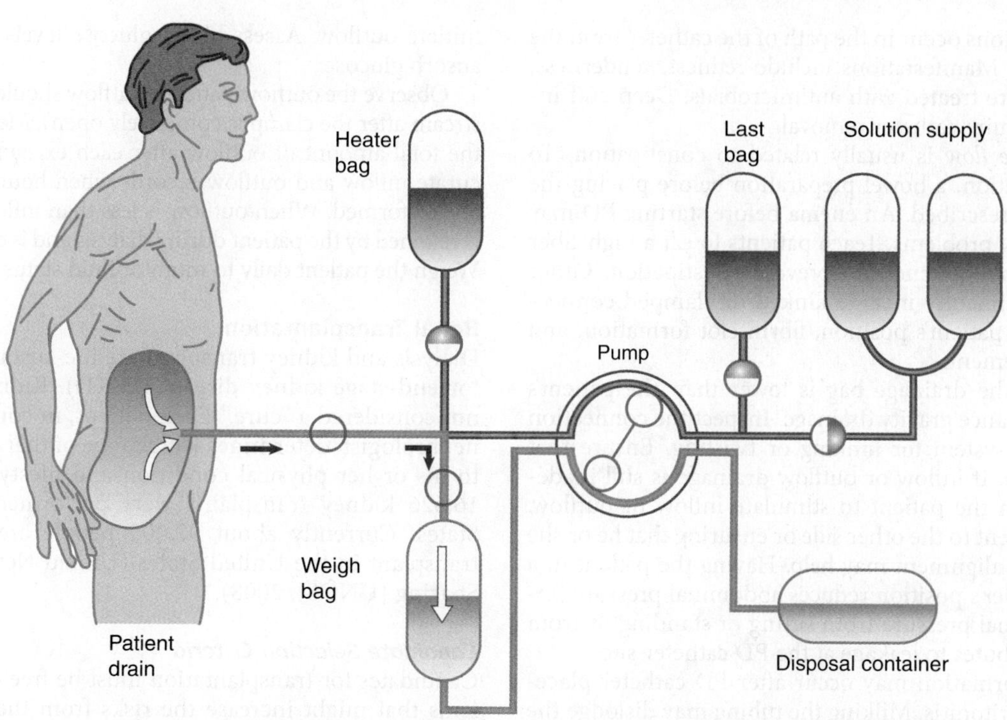
Heater
bag
Last
bag
Solution supply
Pump
Weigh
bag
Patient
drain
Disposal container

Fig. 71-13 • Peritoneal dialysis machine circuit in automated peritoneal dialysis (APD).

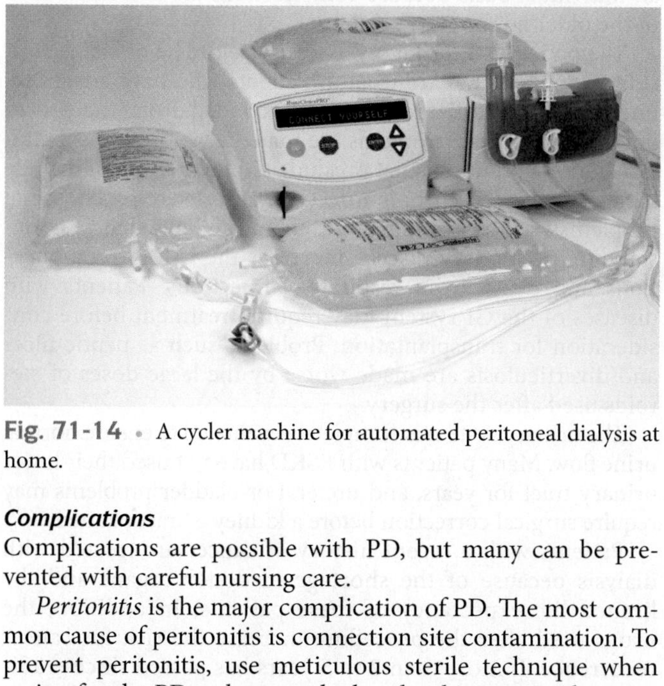
CONNECT YOURSELF

Fig. 71-14 • A cycler machine for automated peritoneal dialysis at home.

Complications

Complications are possible with PD, but many can be prevented with careful nursing care.

Peritonitis is the major complication of PD. The most common cause of peritonitis is connection site contamination. To prevent peritonitis, use meticulous sterile technique when caring for the PD catheter and when hooking up or clamping off dialysate bags (Chart 71-10).

Manifestations of peritonitis include cloudy dialysate outflow (effluent), fever, abdominal tenderness, abdominal pain, general malaise, nausea, and vomiting. Cloudy or opaque effluent is the earliest sign of peritonitis. Examine all effluent for color and clarity to detect peritonitis early. When peritonitis is suspected, send a specimen of the dialysate outflow for culture and sensitivity study, Gram stain, and cell count to identify the infecting organism.

Pain during the inflow of dialysate is common when patients are first started on PD therapy. Usually this pain no longer occurs after a week or two of PD. Cold dialysate increases discomfort. Warm the dialysate bags before instillation by using a heating pad to wrap the bag or by using the warming chamber of the automated cycling machine. *Microwave ovens are **not** recommended for the warming of dialysate.*

Exit site and tunnel infections are serious complications. The exit site from a PD catheter should be clean, dry, and without pain or inflammation. Exit site infections (ESIs) can occur with any type of PD catheter. These infections are difficult to treat and can become chronic. They can lead to peritonitis, catheter failure, and hospitalization. Dialysate leakage and pulling or twisting of the catheter increase the risk for ESIs. A Gram stain and culture should be performed when exit sites have purulent drainage.

Chart 71-10 BEST PRACTICE FOR PATIENT SAFETY & QUALITY CARE

Caring for the Patient with a Peritoneal Dialysis Catheter

- Mask yourself and your patient. Wash your hands.
- Put on sterile gloves. Remove the old dressing. Remove the contaminated gloves.
- Assess the area for signs of infection, such as swelling, redness, or discharge around the catheter site.
- Use aseptic technique:
  - Open the sterile field on a flat surface, and place two precut 4×4–inch gauze pads on the field.
  - Place three cotton swabs soaked in povidone-iodine on the field. Put on sterile gloves.
- Use cotton swabs to clean around the catheter site. Use a circular motion starting from the insertion site and moving away toward the abdomen. Repeat with all three swabs.
- Apply precut gauze pads over the catheter site. Tape only the edges of the gauze pads.

Tunnel infections occur in the path of the catheter from the skin to the cuff. Manifestations include redness, tenderness, and pain. ESIs are treated with antimicrobials. Deep cuff infections may require catheter removal.

Poor dialysate flow is usually related to constipation. To prevent constipation, a bowel preparation before placing the PD catheter is prescribed. An enema before starting PD may also prevent flow problems. Teach patients to eat a high-fiber diet and use stool softeners to prevent constipation. Other causes of flow difficulty include kinked or clamped connection tubing, the patient's position, fibrin clot formation, and catheter displacement.

Ensure that the drainage bag is lower than the patient's abdomen to enhance gravity drainage. Inspect the connection tubing and PD system for kinking or twisting. Ensure that clamps are open. If inflow or outflow drainage is still inadequate, reposition the patient to stimulate inflow or outflow. Turning the patient to the other side or ensuring that he or she is in good body alignment may help. Having the patient in a supine low-Fowler's position reduces abdominal pressure. Increased abdominal pressure from sitting or standing or from coughing contributes to leakage at the PD catheter site.

Fibrin clot formation may occur after PD catheter placement or with peritonitis. Milking the tubing may dislodge the fibrin clot and improve flow. An x-ray is needed to identify PD catheter placement. If displacement has occurred, the physician repositions the PD catheter.

Dialysate leakage is seen as clear fluid coming from the catheter exit site. When dialysis is first started, small volumes of dialysate are used. It may take patients 1 to 2 weeks to tolerate a full 2-L exchange without leakage around the catheter site. Leakage occurs more often in obese or diabetic patients, older adults, and those on long-term steroid therapy. During periods of catheter leak, patients may require hemodialysis (HD) support.

Other complications of PD include bleeding, which is expected when the catheter is first placed, and bowel perforation, which is serious. When PD is first started, the outflow may be bloody or blood tinged. This condition normally clears within a week or two. After PD is well-established, the effluent should be clear and light yellow. Observe for and document any change in the color of the outflow. Brown-colored effluent occurs with a bowel perforation. If the outflow is the same color as urine and has the same glucose level, a bladder perforation is possible. Cloudy or opaque effluent indicates infection.

Nursing Care During Peritoneal Dialysis

In the hospital setting, PD is routinely started and monitored by the nurse. Before the treatment, assess baseline vital signs, including blood pressure, apical and radial pulse rates, temperature, quality of respirations, and breath sounds. Weigh the patient, always on the same scale, before the procedure and at least every 24 hours while receiving treatment. Weight should be checked after a drain and before the next fill to monitor the patient's "dry weight." Baseline laboratory tests, such as electrolyte and glucose levels, are obtained before starting PD and are repeated at least daily during the PD treatment.

Continually monitor the patient during PD. Take and record vital signs every 15 to 30 minutes. Assess for signs of respiratory distress, pain, or discomfort. Check the dressing around the catheter exit site every 30 minutes for wetness during the procedure. Monitor the prescribed dwell time, and initiate outflow. Assess blood glucose levels in patients who absorb glucose.

Observe the outflow pattern (outflow should be a continuous stream after the clamp is completely open). Measure and record the total amount of outflow after each exchange. Maintain accurate inflow and outflow records when hourly PD exchanges are performed. When outflow is less than inflow, the difference is retained by the patient during dialysis and is counted as intake. Weigh the patient daily to monitor fluid status.

Renal Transplantation

Dialysis and kidney transplant are life-sustaining *treatments* for end-stage kidney disease (ESKD). Kidney transplant is not considered a "cure." Each patient, in consultation with a nephrologist, determines which type of therapy is best suited to his or her physical condition and lifestyle. During 2007 16,626 kidney transplants were performed in the United States. Currently about 97,000 people are awaiting renal transplant in the United States (United Network for Organ Sharing [UNOS], 2008).

Candidate Selection Criteria

Candidates for transplantation must be free of medical problems that might increase the risks from the procedure. The usual age range for kidney transplant is 2 to 70 years of age. Patients older than 70 years are considered for transplant on an individual basis because complications are more common in the older adult.

The patient is thoroughly assessed before he or she is considered for a kidney transplant. Patients who have advanced, uncorrectable cardiac disease are excluded from the procedure because these problems are made worse by transplantation. Other conditions that preclude kidney transplant include metastatic cancer, chronic infection, and severe psychosocial problems such as alcoholism or chemical dependency. Long-standing pulmonary disease increases the risk for complications and death from respiratory infections. Patients with diseases of the GI system may require treatment before consideration for transplantation. Problems such as peptic ulcer and diverticulosis are made worse by the large doses of steroids used after the surgery.

The urinary system is completely evaluated to ensure normal urine flow. Many patients with ESKD have not used their lower urinary tract for years, and ureteral or bladder problems may require surgical correction before a kidney is transplanted.

Patients with a recent history of cancer are treated with dialysis because of the shortage of donor organs and the limited life expectancy of these patients. In addition, the drugs used after the procedure increase the risk for cancer recurrence. If more than 2 to 5 years has passed since eradication of the cancer, the patient can be considered for a transplant.

Diabetes mellitus and other endocrine problems cause even greater risks. Patients with these problems can have a renal transplant, but they require intense observation and management to limit complications. Other complicating conditions are considered on an individual basis, depending on the patient's current health status. Renal transplantation can be considered for most patients with ESKD and is the optimal therapy for many people. Most people who have undergone this procedure are satisfied with their quality of life for years after the transplant.

Donors

Kidney donors may be living donors (related or unrelated to the patient), non-heart-beating donors (NHBDs), and cadaveric donors. The available kidneys are matched on the basis of tissue type similarity between the donor and the recipient. Living donors are most often blood relatives, but unrelated donors have been used. NHBDs are persons declared dead by cardiopulmonary criteria. Kidneys from NHBDs are removed (harvested) immediately after death in cases where patients have previously given consent for organ donation. If immediate removal must be delayed, the organ is preserved by infusing a cool preservation solution into the abdominal aorta after death is declared and until surgery can be performed. Cadaveric donors are usually people who suffered irreversible brain injury, usually as a result of trauma. These donors are maintained with mechanical ventilation and must have sufficient renal perfusion for the kidneys to remain viable.

The size of the kidney is seldom a problem in adults. Kidneys transplanted from children become larger to meet adult needs within a few months.

Organs from living *related* donors (LRDs) have the highest rates of renal graft survival (90%). Donors are usually at least 18 years old and are seldom older than 65 years. Physical criteria for donors include:

- Absence of systemic disease and infection
- No history of cancer
- No hypertension or kidney disease
- Adequate renal function as determined by diagnostic studies

In addition, LRDs must express a clear understanding of the surgery and a willingness to give up a kidney. Some transplant centers require a psychiatric evaluation to assess the donor's motivation.

A paired exchange donation can be done when two kidney donor/recipient pairs have blood types that are not compatible within one pair. The two recipients trade donors so that each recipient can receive a kidney with a compatible blood type (Fig. 71-15). Once the evaluations of all donors and recipients are completed, the two kidney transplant operations are scheduled to occur simultaneously (UNOS, 2008).

Because of advances in immunosuppressant therapy and medical management, the United Network of Organ Sharing (UNOS) reported 1-year renal transplant graft survival to be almost 95% for all centers in the United States during 2007 (UNOS, 2008).

Preoperative Care

Many issues related to patient health and the actual transplant procedure must be addressed before surgery. The Clinical Pathway on the Evolve website highlights care needs for the patient undergoing renal transplantation.

Immunologic studies are needed because the major barrier to transplant success after a suitable donor kidney is available is the body's ability to reject "foreign" tissue. This immunologic process can attack the transplanted kidney and destroy it. For immunologic problems to be overcome, in-depth tissue typing is performed on all candidates. These studies include simple blood typing and human leukocyte antigen (HLA) studies, as well as other tests. The HLAs are the main immunologic feature used to match transplant recipients with compatible donors. The more similar the antigens of the donor are to those of the recipient, the more likely the transplant will be successful and rejection will be avoided (see Chapter 19).

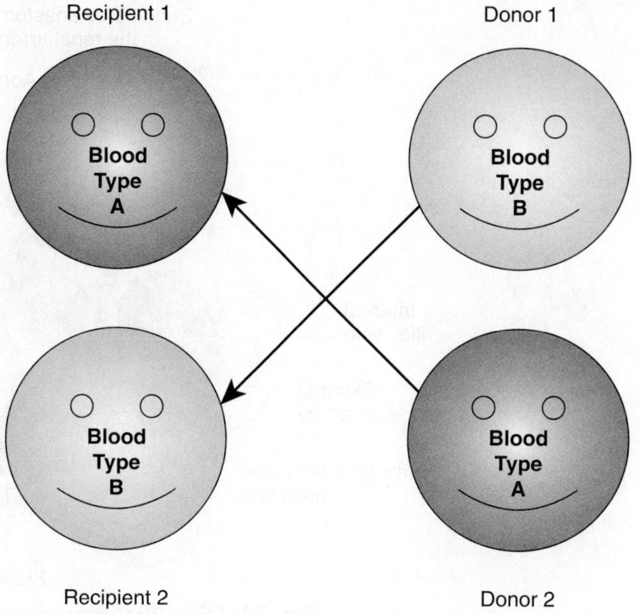
Recipient 1
Donor 1
Blood Type A
Blood Type B
Blood Type B
Blood Type A
Recipient 2
Donor 2

Fig. 71-15 • An example of a paired exchange kidney donation. Donor 1 is related to or acquainted with recipient 1 and has agreed to donate a kidney but is not a blood type or a tissue type match with recipient 1. Donor 1 is compatible with recipient 2 and agrees to donate a kidney to recipient 2 if donor 2 agrees to donate a kidney to recipient 1.

Surgical team members for transplantation include circulating and scrub nurses, clinical nurse specialists, transplant surgeons, anesthesiologists, and nephrologists. Nursing actions before surgery include teaching about the procedure and care after surgery, in-depth patient assessment, coordination of diagnostic tests, and development of treatment plans. See Chapter 16 for more discussion of standard preoperative nursing care.

The patient usually requires dialysis within 24 hours of the surgery. In addition, the recipient often receives a blood transfusion before surgery. Usually blood from the kidney donor is transfused into the recipient. This procedure increases graft survival of organs from living related donors (LRDs).

Operative Procedures

The donor nephrectomy procedure varies depending on whether the donor is a non–heart-beating donor (NHBD), cadaveric donor, or living donor. The NHBD or cadaveric donor nephrectomy is a sterile autopsy in the operating room. All arterial and venous vessels and a long piece of ureter are preserved. After removal, the kidneys are preserved until time for implantation into the recipient. The technique for kidney removal from living donors is a delicate procedure that lasts 3 to 4 hours. A flank incision is used, and care is taken to avoid scarring. Donors usually have more pain after surgery than do recipients. They also need nursing care and support for the psychological adjustment to loss of a body part.

The transplantation surgery usually takes 4 to 5 hours. The transplanted kidney is usually placed in the right or left anterior iliac fossa (Fig. 71-16) instead of the usual anatomic position. This placement allows easier connection of the ureter and the renal artery and vein. It also allows for kidney assess-

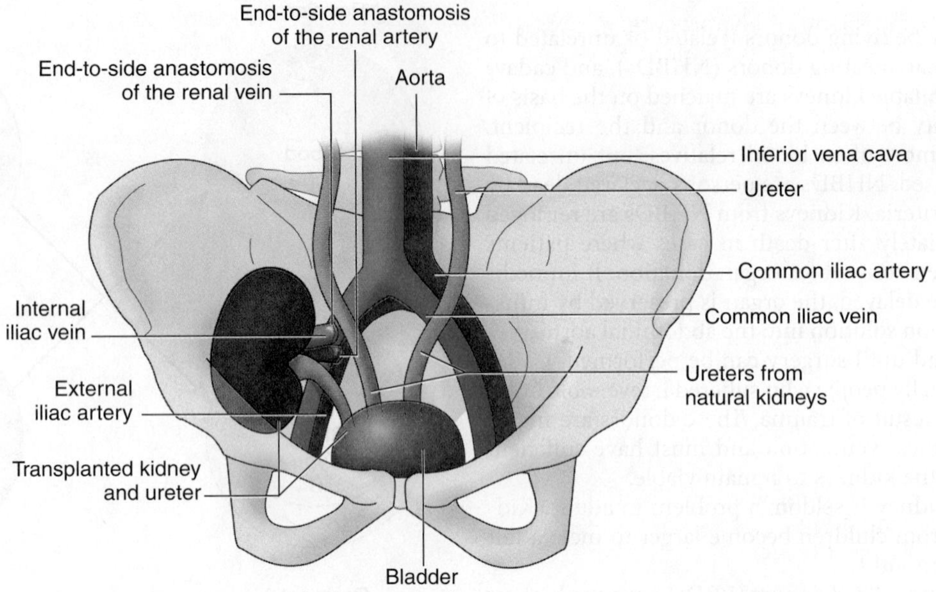
End-to-side anastomosis of the renal artery
End-to-side anastomosis of the renal vein
Aorta
Inferior vena cava
Ureter
Common iliac artery
Common iliac vein
Internal iliac vein
Ureters from natural kidneys
External iliac artery
Transplanted kidney and ureter
Bladder

Fig. 71-16 • Placement of a transplanted kidney in the right iliac fossa.

ment by palpation. The recipient's own failed kidneys are not usually removed unless chronic infection is present in one or both kidneys. After surgery, the patient is taken to the postanesthesia unit and then, when stable, to a designated unit in the transplant center or to a critical care unit.

Postoperative Care

Care of the recipient after surgery requires that nurses be knowledgeable about the expected clinical findings and potential complications. Nursing care includes ongoing physical assessment, especially evaluation of renal function (described below). The transplant recipient requires close attention because the immunosuppressive drug therapy used to prevent tissue rejection impairs healing and increases the risk for infection.

Urologic management is essential to graft success. These patients always have a large-bore indwelling (Foley) catheter for accurate measurements of urine output and decompression of the bladder. Decompression prevents stretch on sutures and ureter attachment sites on the bladder.

Assess urine output at least hourly during the first 48 hours. An abrupt decrease in urine output may indicate complications such as rejection, acute tubular necrosis (ATN), thrombosis, or obstruction. Examine the urine color. The urine is pink or blood-tinged right after surgery and gradually returns to normal over several days to several weeks, depending on renal function. Obtain daily urine specimens for urinalysis, glucose measurement, the presence of acetone, specific gravity measurement, and culture (if needed).

Occasionally, a continuous bladder irrigation is prescribed to decrease blood clot formation, which could increase pressure in the bladder and endanger the graft. Perform routine catheter care, according to agency policy, to reduce catheter contamination. The catheter is removed as soon as possible to avoid infection, usually 3 to 7 days after surgery. After surgery, the function of the transplanted kidney (renal graft) can result in either oliguria or diuresis. Oliguria may occur as a result of ischemia and ATN, rejection, or other complications. To increase urine output, the physician may prescribe diuretics and osmotic agents, such as mannitol. Closely monitor the patient's fluid status because fluid overload can cause hypertension, heart failure, and pulmonary edema. Evaluate his or her fluid status by weighing daily, measuring blood pressure every 2 to 4 hours, and measuring intake and output.

Instead of oliguria, the patient may have diuresis, especially with a kidney from a living related donor (LRD). Carefully monitor intake and output, and observe for serum electrolyte imbalances, such as low potassium and sodium levels. Excessive diuresis may cause hypotension. Prevent this problem, because hypotension reduces blood flow and oxygen to the new kidney, threatening graft survival.

Complications

Many complications are possible after renal transplantation. Early detection and intervention improve the chances of graft survival.

Rejection is the most common and serious complication of transplantation and is the leading cause of graft loss. A reaction occurs between the antigens in the transplanted kidney and the antibodies and cytotoxic T-cells in the recipient's blood. These substances treat the new kidney as a foreign invader and cause tissue destruction, thrombosis, and eventual kidney necrosis.

The three types of rejection are hyperacute, acute, and chronic. Acute rejection is the most common type with kidney transplants. It is treated with increased immunosuppressive therapy and often can be reversible. Rejection is diagnosed by manifestations, a renal scan, and renal biopsy. Table 71-13 lists the features of the three types of rejection. Chapter 19 discusses their causes and treatment.

Acute tubular necrosis (ATN) after surgery can occur as a result of hypoxic damage when transplantation is delayed after kidneys have been harvested. These patients may need dialysis until adequate urine output returns and the blood urea nitrogen (BUN) and creatinine levels normalize. ATN is often difficult to distinguish from acute rejection, and patients need to undergo weekly biopsies to assess the need for further drug therapy if rejection is occurring.

Thrombosis of the major renal blood vessels may occur during the first 2 to 3 days after the transplant. A sudden decrease

TABLE 71-13 A Comparison of Hyperacute, Acute, and Chronic Post-Transplant Rejection

Hyperacute Rejection	Acute Rejection	Chronic Rejection
ONSET		
Within 48 hr after surgery	1 wk to 2 yr postoperatively (most common in first 2 wk)	Occurs gradually during a period of months to years
CLINICAL MANIFESTATIONS		
Increased temperature	Oliguria or anuria	Gradual increase in BUN and serum creatinine levels
Increased blood pressure	Temperature over 100° F (37.8° C)	
Pain at transplant site	Increased blood pressure Enlarged, tender kidney Lethargy Elevated serum creatinine, BUN, potassium levels Fluid retention	Fluid retention Changes in serum electrolyte levels Fatigue
TREATMENT		
Immediate removal of the transplanted kidney	Increased doses of immunosuppressive drugs	Conservative management until dialysis is required

BUN, Blood urea nitrogen.

in urine output may signal impaired perfusion resulting from thrombosis. Ultrasound examination of the kidney may show decreased or absent blood supply. Emergency surgery is required to prevent ischemic damage or graft loss.

Renal artery stenosis may result in hypertension. Other manifestations include a bruit over the artery anastomosis site and decreased renal function. A renal scan can quantify the blood flow to the kidney. The involved artery may be repaired surgically or by balloon angioplasty in the radiology department. The decision to perform a balloon repair is determined by the amount of healing time after the surgery.

Other vascular problems include vascular leakage or thrombosis, both of which require an emergency transplant nephrectomy.

Other complications may involve the surgical wound or urinary tract. Wound problems, such as hematomas, abscesses, and lymphoceles (abnormal lymphatic cysts containing lymph fluid), increase the risk for infection and exert pressure on the new kidney. Infection is a major cause of death in the transplant recipient. Prevention of infection is essential. Strict aseptic technique and handwashing must be rigorously enforced. Transplant recipients may not have the usual manifestations of infection because of the immunosuppressive therapy. Low-grade fevers, mental status changes, and vague reports of discomfort may be the only manifestations before sepsis. Always consider the possibility of infection with any patient after a kidney transplant. Urinary tract complications include ureteral leakage, fistula, or obstruction; stone formation; bladder neck contracture; and graft rupture. Surgical intervention may be required.

Immunosuppressive Drug Therapy

The success of renal transplantation depends on changing the patient's immunologic response so that the new kidney is not rejected as a foreign organ. Immunosuppressive drugs protect the transplanted organ. These drugs include corticosteroids, anti-lymphocyte preparations, monoclonal antibodies, and cyclosporine (Cyclosporin A). Chapter 19 discusses the mechanisms of action for these agents and the associated patient responses. Patients taking these drugs are at an increased risk for death by viral, fungal, bacterial, or protozoal infection.

Teaching patients and families about the importance of adhering to the anti-rejection drug regimen is a critical nursing function. Many patients do not follow the regimen and are at high risk for losing the transplanted kidney. (See the Evidence-Based Practice box on p. 1634.) Work with the patient to identify ways to increase adherence to the drug regimen.

DECISION-MAKING CHALLENGE

Legal/Ethical

The patient is a 58-year-old woman with ESKD from long-standing and uncontrolled hypertension and diabetes. She is scheduled to receive a kidney from her 42-year-old daughter. The daughter, who left home at age 17 when the mother married a man who was abusive toward the daughter, has not been in touch with her mother for more than 25 years. The patient's husband tracked the daughter down because none of this couple's three children have the mother's blood type.

When you meet with the daughter, she is quiet and responds abruptly to direct questions. In response to the question "why are you donating your kidney to your mother?" she responds, "Because my stepfather is giving me $50,000 for doing this." She then admits that she is scared because she is newly married and would like to have a child as soon as possible.

1. Is her concern about a future pregnancy valid? (Consult Chapter 68 and a maternity nursing book.)
2. Are there any other questions you should ask about her decision to donate her kidney?
3. What should you do with the information about the $50,000?

evolve For suggested answer guidelines, go to http://evolve.elsevier.com/Iggy/.

Community-Based Care

Home Care Management

Because of the complex nature of CKD, its progressive course, and many treatment options, a case manager is helpful in planning, coordinating, and evaluating care. As the renal disease progresses, the patient is seen by a physician or nurse practitioner regularly and may be hospitalized often. Together with the nutritionist and social worker, evaluate the home environment and determine equipment needs before discharge. Once the patient is discharged, home care nurses direct care and monitor progress. Chart 71-11 provides a focused assessment guide for the patient after transplantation.

Provide health teaching about the diet in renal disease and the progression of kidney disease. As severe CKD approaches end-stage kidney disease (ESKD), one of these courses of treatment is chosen: hemodialysis (HD), peritoneal dialysis (PD), or transplantation. For each form of treatment, the patient and partner must learn about the procedures and consider his or her personal lifestyle, support systems, and methods of coping. Decision making about treatment type or even whether to pursue treatment is difficult for patients and fami-

EVIDENCE-BASED PRACTICE

Help them try to remember

Russell, C., Conn, V., Ashbaugh, C., Madsen, R., Hayes, K., & Ross. G. (2006). Medication adherence patterns in adult renal transplant recipients. *Research in Nursing & Health, 29*(10), 521-532.

Adherence to immunosuppressive drugs is crucial to survival for patients with transplanted kidneys. Lack of adherence can lead to complications such as rejection, graft loss, return to dialysis, and death. The researchers defined *medication adherence* as the extent to which the patient's medication-taking behavior corresponds with the recommendations of a health care provider.

This study used a prospective, longitudinal, descriptive design to examine the immunosuppressive medication adherence of 44 renal transplant patients. Patients were followed for 6 months at a transplant center, using electronic monitoring. Medication adherence was measured with the medication event monitoring system (MEMS). The MEMS system records data by using a medication bottle cap with microelectronics that record the date and time each time the cap is removed. A MEMS diary was used by patients to document any accidental openings of the caps. Morning and evening doses of immunosuppressant drugs were monitored. Findings of the study indicated 4 adherence patterns:

1. Those who took medications on time
2. Those who took medication on time with late/missed doses
3. Those who rarely took medications on time and who were late with morning and/or evening doses
4. Those who missed doses

Almost 47% of the study participants took both morning and evening drug doses on time (Pattern 1). The author-recommended interventions for this group included continued support and encouragement via oral and written communications. Interventions suggested for Pattern 2 included encouraging the positive efforts toward adherence and exploring the reasons for late or missed doses and then setting strategies to correct late or missed doses (e.g., using an alarm clock for late doses due to oversleeping). Pattern 3 adherence included people who were late taking both morning and evening doses. Suggested interventions for this group included focusing on cues and reminders to help patients take their drugs on time. The 4th pattern included participants who missed both morning and evening doses (N 5 4). Suggested interventions for this group included the use of cues or reminders, as well as further assessment of medication-taking patterns, especially access to medications (e.g., getting medication refills).

Level of Evidence—4. Well-designed cohort study.

Commentary: Implications for Practice and Research. This study contributed to the identification of patterns of poor immunosuppressive drug adherence in renal transplant patients. Identification of poor adherence is essential for treatment of patients at risk for poor post-transplant outcomes and prevention of life-threatening complications. When a pattern of poor adherence is identified, nurses need to work with the patient to identify barriers to adherence and plan strategies to increase adherence. For some patients, this may require a telephone intervention to cue the patient when to take medications.

Chart 71-11 FOCUSED ASSESSMENT

The Patient with Chronic Kidney Disease

Assess cardiovascular and respiratory status, including:
- Vital signs, with special attention to blood pressure
- Presence of S_3 or pericardial friction rub
- Presence of chest pain
- Presence of edema (periorbital, pretibial, sacral)
- Jugular vein distention
- Presence of dyspnea
- Presence of crackles, beginning at the bases and extending upward

Assess nutritional status, including:
- Weight gain or loss
- Presence of anorexia, nausea, or vomiting

Assess renal status, including:
- Amount, frequency, and appearance of urine (in non-anuric patients)
- Presence of bone pain
- Presence of hyperglycemia secondary to diabetes

Assess hematologic status, including:
- Presence of petechiae, purpura, ecchymoses
- Presence of fatigue or shortness of breath

Assess gastrointestinal status, including:
- Presence of stomatitis
- Presence of melena

Assess integumentary status, including:
- Skin integrity
- Presence of pruritus
- Presence of skin discoloration

Assess neurologic status, including:
- Changes in mental status
- Presence of seizure activity
- Presence of sensory changes
- Presence of lower extremity weakness

Assess laboratory data, including:
- BUN
- Serum creatinine
- Creatinine clearance
- CBC
- Electrolytes

Assess psychosocial status, including:
- Presence of anxiety
- Presence of maladaptive behavior

BUN, Blood urea nitrogen; *CBC*, complete blood count.

lies. Provide information and emotional support to assist patients with these decisions.

Teach patients who select hemodialysis (HD) about the dialysis machine and vascular access care. If in-home HD is selected, preparations are needed for the appropriate equipment, including a water treatment system. Regardless of whether the treatment occurs at home or in a center, provide ongoing physical assessment and health teaching to promote independence at home.

The patient receiving PD needs extensive training in the procedure. He or she also needs help obtaining equipment and the many supplies needed. Home care nurses assess patients, monitor vital signs, assess adherence with drug and diet regimens, and monitor for manifestations of peritonitis.

The nurse plays a vital role in the long-term care of the patient with a renal transplant. This patient is usually discharged 3 to 4 weeks after surgery. *Stress that adherence to the prescribed drug therapy is essential for the survival of the kidney.* Facilitate acceptance and understanding of this regimen as a part of daily life. Carefully monitor for signs of graft rejection and for complications, such as infection.

Health Teaching

Instruct patients and family members in all aspects of nutrition therapy, drug therapy, and complications. Teach them to report complications, such as fluid overload and infection. When a patient requires a more advanced form of therapy, such as dialysis or transplantation, focus teaching on the chosen type of intervention.

Hemodialysis (HD) is the most complex form of therapy for the patient and family to understand. Even if patients receive HD in a dialysis center instead of at home, they are expected to have some knowledge of the HD machine. The patient or a family member must be taught to care for the vascular access and to report signs of infection and stenosis. Those who plan to have in-home HD will need a partner. Both the patient and the partner must be taught the entire process of HD and must be able to perform it independently before the patient is discharged.

Peritoneal dialysis (PD) involves extensive health teaching. This instruction can be given to the patient alone or to the patient and a family member if the patient cannot perform the procedure. Emphasize sterile technique because peritonitis is the most common complication of PD. Instruct patients to report any manifestation of peritonitis, especially cloudy effluent and abdominal pain. If peritonitis develops, teach patients how to give themselves antibiotics by the intraperitoneal (IP) route. Stress the importance of completing the antibiotic regimen. Remind patients that repeated episodes of peritonitis can reduce the effectiveness of PD, which may require the transfer to HD.

The patient receiving a kidney transplant also needs extensive health teaching. Provide instruction about drug regimens, home monitoring, immunosuppression, manifestations of rejection, infection, and prescribed changes in the diet and activity level.

Psychosocial Preparation

Provide psychological support for the patient and family. Help the patient adjust to the diagnosis of renal failure and eventually accept the treatment regimens.

Many patients view dialysis as a cure instead of a required lifelong treatment. For many patients, the reduction of uremic symptoms in the first weeks after starting dialysis treatment creates a sense of well-being (the "honeymoon" period). They feel better physically, and their mood may be happy and hopeful. At this time they tend to overlook the discomfort and inconvenience of dialysis. Use this time to begin health care teaching. Stress that, although the uremic symptoms are reduced, they should not expect a complete return to the previous state of well-being.

Many patients become discouraged during the first year of treatment. This mood state may last a few months to a year or longer. The difficulties of incorporating dialysis into daily life are staggering, and patients may become depressed as problems occur. They may struggle with the idea of permanently having to depend on a disruptive therapy. Patients may feel helpless and dependent. Some people retreat into complete or partial denial of the disease and the need for treatment. They may deny the need for dialysis or may not adhere to drug therapy and diet restrictions. Monitor any behaviors that may contribute to nonadherence, and suggest psychiatric referrals. Help the patient and family focus on the positive aspects of the treatments. Continue health care education with patients as active participants and decision makers (Al-Arabi, 2006).

Most patients with CKD eventually enter a phase of acceptance or resignation. The idea of a chronic illness may be devastating for some people, and each person reacts differently. To make this long-term adaptation, the patient must adjust to continuous change. Specific concerns depend on the patient's health and particular treatment method.

After patients have accepted or become resigned to the chronic aspect of their disease, they usually attempt to return to their previous activities. Resuming the previous level of activity, however, may not be possible. Help patients set realistic goals that allow them to lead active, productive lives.

Health Care Resources

Professionals from many disciplines are resources for the patient with renal failure. Home care nurses monitor the patient's status and evaluate maintenance of the prescribed treatment regimen (HD or PD). A patient with advanced renal failure may need a home care aide to help perform ADLs. Social services are often involved because of the complex process of applying for financial aid to pay for the required medical care. A physical therapist may be beneficial in helping improve the patient's functional health. A nutritionist can help the patient and family members understand the special dietary needs. A psychiatric evaluation may be needed if depressive symptoms are present. Clergy and pastoral care specialists offer spiritual support.

Patients with CKD are routinely followed by a physician, usually a nephrologist. Organizations such as the National Kidney Foundation (NKF), the American Kidney Fund, and the National Association of Patients on Hemodialysis and Transplantation (NAPHT) may be helpful to patients and families.

Evaluation: Outcomes

Evaluate the care of the patient with chronic kidney disease (CKD) on the basis of the identified nursing diagnoses and collaborative problems. The expected outcomes are that the patient should:

- Achieve and maintain appropriate fluid volume
- Maintain an adequate nutritional status
- Use effective coping strategies
- Report an absence of physical manifestations of anxiety

Specific indicators for these outcomes are listed for each nursing diagnosis and collaborative problem under the Planning and Implementation section (see earlier).

HUMAN NEEDS NURSING CARE REVIEW

What might you NOTICE if the patient is experiencing altered urinary elimination as a result of acute renal failure?

- Patient urinates infrequently.
- Patient reports back or flank pain.
- Urine may be darker or smoky or have obvious blood in it.

What should you INTERPRET and how should you RESPOND to a patient experiencing altered urinary elimination as a result of acute renal failure?

Perform and interpret physical assessment, including:

- Ask how long manifestations have been present.
- Determine fluid intake and output volumes.
- Weigh the patient, and ask whether this weight is more or less than his or her usual weight.
- Assess for tachycardia.
- Assess for pulmonary congestion.
- Check for presence of generalized or dependent edema.
- Interpret laboratory values:
  - Complete blood count with hemoconcentration
  - BUN and serum creatinine levels elevated
  - Serum potassium level elevated

Respond by:

- Ensuring hemodynamic stability
- Monitoring urine output
- Monitoring for fluid overload

On what should you REFLECT?

- Observe patient for evidence of improved urinary output (see Chapter 68).
- Think about what may have caused this problem and what steps could be taken to prevent a similar episode.
- Consider what changes in the nursing unit environment could reduce the risk for acute renal failure.
- Think about what patient teaching focus could help reduce the risk for future acute renal failure.

GET READY FOR THE NCLEX EXAMINATION!

Key Points

Review these Key Points for each NCLEX Examination Client Needs Category.

Safe and Effective Care Environment

- Use sterile technique when cannulating a vascular access or connecting peritoneal dialysis tubing.
- Handle patients with chronic kidney disease gently to prevent fractures.
- Assess all patients at risk for dehydration or hypovolemia for adequacy of renal perfusion.
- Avoid taking blood pressure measurements or drawing blood from an arm with a vascular access (AV fistula or graft).
- Do not use an AV fistula or graft site to give IV fluids.

Health Promotion and Maintenance

- Encourage patients with chronic kidney disease or kidney failure to follow fluid and dietary restrictions regarding sodium, potassium, and protein.
- Teach patients the expected side effects, any adverse reactions to prescribed drugs, and when to contact the prescriber.
- Teach patients using peritoneal dialysis the manifestations of peritonitis.
- Teach patients on immunosuppressive therapy to assess themselves daily for fever, general malaise, and nausea or vomiting.
- Review with the patient and family the importance of follow-up care and adherence to laboratory testing.

Psychosocial Integrity

- Pace your interview to match the learning needs and style of each patient.
- Allow patients the opportunity to express their feelings and concerns about the risk for death and the disruption of lifestyle as a result of treatment for renal failure.
- Use language and terminology that are comfortable for the patient.
- Assess the patient for depression and nonacceptance of his or her diagnosis or treatment plan.
- Refer patients to community resources and support groups.

Physiological Integrity

- Report immediately any condition that obstructs urine flow.
- Collaborate with the nutritionist to teach patients about needed fluid, sodium, potassium, or dietary protein restriction.
- Teach patients in the early stages of chronic kidney disease the manifestations of dehydration.
- Teach patients in the later stages of chronic kidney disease the manifestations of fluid overload and hyperkalemia.
- Avoid all invasive procedures within 4 to 6 hours after the patient has undergone hemodialysis.
- Use meticulous sterile technique when caring for the peritoneal dialysis catheter and when hooking up or clamping off dialysate bags.

Additional Study Resources

Go to your Companion CD or Evolve at http://evolve.elsevier.com/Iggy/ for *Self-Assessment Questions for the NCLEX Examination.*

Go to Evolve at http://evolve.elsevier.com/Iggy/ for *Prioritization and Delegation Questions for the NCLEX Examination.*

SELECTED BIBLIOGRAPHY

Asterisk indicates a classic or definitive work on this subject.

Al-Arabi, S. (2006). Quality of life: Subjective descriptions of challenges to patients with end-stage renal disease. *Nephrology Nursing Journal, 33*(3), 285-293.

American Association of Kidney Patients. (2007). *Vascular access for hemodialysis.* Retrieved December 2007 from http://kidney.niddk.nih.gov/kudiseases/pubs/vascularaccess/index.htm.

Bagshaw, S.M. (2006a). Epidemiology of renal recovery after acute renal failure. *Current Opinion in Critical Care, 12*(6), 544-550.

Bagshaw, S.M. (2006b). The long-term outcome after acute renal failure. *Current Opinion in Critical Care, 12*(6), 561-566.

Ball, L. (2006). The buttonhole technique for arteriovenous fistula cannulation. *Nephrology Nursing Journal, 33*(3), 299-305.

*Barone, C., Martin-Watson, A., & Barone, G. (2004). The postoperative care of the adult renal transplant recipient. *MEDSURG Nursing, 13*(5), 296-302.

Breiterman-White, R. (2006). C-reactive protein and anemia: Implications for patients on dialysis. *Nephrology Nursing Journal, 33*(5), 555-558.

Brites, F.D., Fernandez, K.M., Verona, J., Malusardi, M.C., Ischoff, P., Beresan, H., et al. (2007). Chronic renal failure in diabetic patients increases lipid risk factors for atherosclerosis. *Diabetes Research and Clinical Practice, 75*(1), 35-41.

Broscious, S., & Castagnola, J. (2006). Chronic kidney disease: Acute manifestations and role of critical care nurses. *Critical Care Nurse, 24*(4), 17-27.

Bulecheck, G.M., Butcher, H.K., & McCloskey Dochterman, J. (2008). *Nursing interventions classification (NIC)* (5th ed.). St. Louis: Mosby.

Burrows-Hudson, S. (2005). Chronic kidney disease: An overview. *AJN, 105*(2), 40-49.

Campoy, S., & Elwell, R. (2005). Pharmacology & CKD. *AJN, 105*(9), 60-71.

Cano, N. (2007). Nutritional supplementation in adult patients on hemodialysis. *Journal of Renal Nutrition, 17*(1), 103-105.

Castner, D. (2008). Kidney dialysis. *Nursing2008, 38*(9), 45.

Castner, D., & Douglas, C. (2005). Now onstage: Chronic kidney disease. *Nursing2006, 35*(12), 58-63.

Centers for Disease Control and Prevention. (2007). Prevalence of chronic kidney disease and associated risk factors—United States 1999-2004. *MMWR Morbidity and Mortality Weekly Report, 56*(8), 161-165.

Deaver, K., & Bennington, L. (2006). Adjusting IV iron and EPO doses in patients on hemodialysis prior to surgery: Can we protect our patients from iron-deficiency anemia? *Nephrology Nursing Journal, 33*(4), 430-437.

Denhaerynck, K., Manhaeve, D., Dobbles, F., Garzoni, D., Nolte, C., & De Geest, S. (2007). Prevalence and consequences of nonadherence to hemodialysis regimens. *American Journal of Critical Care, 16*(3), 222-235.

Dinwiddie, L., Burrows-Hudson, S., & Peacock, E. (2006). Stage 4 chronic kidney disease. *AJN, 106*(9), 40-51.

Dirkes, S., & Hodge, K. (2007). Continuous renal replacement therapy in the adult intensive care unit: History and current trends. *Critical Care Nurse, 27*(2), 61-80.

Harwood, L., & Leitch, R. (2006). Home dialysis therapies. In A. Molzahn & E. Butera (Eds.), *Contemporary nephrology nursing: Principles and practice* (2nd ed., Chapter 26). Pitman, NJ: American Nephrology Nurses Association.

Holcomb, S. (2005). Evaluating chronic kidney disease risk. *The Nurse Practitioner, 30*(4), 12-25.

Katz, A. (2006). What have my kidneys got to do with my sex life? *AJN, 106*(9), 81-83.

Kelman, E., & Watson, D., (2006). Preventing and managing complications of peritoneal dialysis. *Nephrology Nursing Journal, 33*(6), 647-657.

Kohtz, C., & Thompson, M. (2007). Preventing contrast medium–induced nephropathy. *AJN, 107*(9), 40-49.

Kopyt, N. (2007). Management and treatment of chronic kidney disease. *The Nurse Practitioner, 32*(11), 14-23.

Legg, V. (2005). Complications of chronic kidney disease. *AJN, 105*(6), 40-49.

Mahoney, C. (2007). Should patients eat during dialysis? *Nursing2007, 37*(10), 57-58.

Maison, A., Charest, A., & Geerts, W. (2005). Anticoagulant use in patients with chronic renal impairment. *American Journal of Cardiovascular Drugs, 5*(5), 292-305.

McCance, K., & Huether, S. (2006). *Pathophysiology: The biologic basis for disease in adults and children* (5th ed.). St. Louis: Mosby.

McCarthy, M. (2006). Nutrition and transplant: How to help patients on dialysis prepare. *Nephrology Nursing Journal, 33*(5), 570-572.

Medline Plus. (2007). *Acute renal failure, chronic renal failure.* Retrieved December 2007 from www.nlm.nih.gov/medlineplus/ency/encyclopedia_R.htm.

National Kidney and Urologic Diseases Information Clearinghouse. (2007). *Treatment methods for kidney failure: Hemodialysis, peritoneal dialysis, kidney transplantation.* Retrieved December 2007 from http://kidney.niddk.nih.gov/kudiseases/ez.asp.

Nussbaum, R., McInnes, R., & Willard, H. (2007). *Thompson & Thompson: Genetics in medicine* (7th ed.). Philadelphia: Saunders.

Pagana, K., & Pagana, T. (2006). *Mosby's manual of diagnostic and laboratory tests* (3rd ed.). St. Louis: Mosby.

Pearce, J. (2007). Documenting peritoneal dialysis. *Nursing2007, 37*(10), 28.

Pierson, D. (2006). Respiratory considerations in the patient with renal failure. *Respiratory Care, 51*(4), 413-422.

Richard, C. (2006). Self-care management in adults undergoing hemodialysis. *Nephrology Nursing Journal, 33*(4), 387-394.

Russell, C.L., Conn, V.S., Ashbaugh, C., Madsen, R., Hayes, K., & Ross, G. (2006). Medication adherence patterns in adult renal transplant recipients. *Research in Nursing & Health, 29*(10), 521-532.

Sahjian, M., & Frakes, M. (2007). Crush injuries: Pathophysiology and current treatment. *The Nurse Practitioner, 32*(9), 13-18.

Schneider, V., Levesque, L.E., Zhang, B., Hutchinson, T., & Brophy, J.M. (2006). Association of selective and conventional nonsteroidal anti-inflammatory drugs with acute renal failure: A population-based nested case-control analysis. *American Journal of Epidemiology, 164*(9), 881-889.

Sclauzero, P., Casarotto, S., Martingano, M., Morpurgo, F., Rocconi, I., Scala, K., et al. (2006). Improving quality of assistance and outcome in critically ill patients with acute renal failure. *EDTNA/ERCA Journal, 32*(3), 181-185.

Sinert, R., & Peacock, P.R. (2006). *Renal failure, acute.* Retrieved July 9, 2007, from www.emedicine.com/emerg/topic500.htm.

Singh, D., Kaur, R., Chander, V., & Chopra, K. (2006). Antioxidants in the prevention of renal disease. *Journal of Medicinal Food, 9*(4), 443-450.

Thomas-Hawkins, C., & Zazworsky, D. (2005). Self-management of chronic kidney disease. *AJN, 105*(10), 40-48.

Uchino, S. (2006). The epidemiology of acute renal failure in the world. *Current Opinion in Critical Care, 12*(6), 538-543.

United Network for Organ Sharing (UNOS) online. (2008). Website: www.unos.org

U.S. Renal Data System (USRDS). (2008). *USRDS 2007 annual data report.* Bethesda, MD: National Institutes of Health, National Institute of Diabetes and Digestive and Kidney Diseases.

Venkataraman, R., & Kellum, J. (2007). Prevention of acute renal failure. *Chest, 131*(1), 300-308.

Zarifian, A. (2006). Symptom occurrence, symptom distress, and quality of life in renal transplant recipients. *Nephrology Nursing Journal, 33*(6), 609-618.

Zeigler, S. (2007). Prevent dangerous hemodialysis catheter disconnection. *Nursing2007, 37*(3), 70.

HUMAN NEEDS OVERVIEW

Sexuality

Unlike the physiologic human needs introduced in other section openers of this text, *sexuality* is a complex integration of many physiologic, emotional, social, and cultural aspects of well-being. It is closely associated with self-concept, self-esteem, role relationships, sexual response, and reproduction. Sexuality comprises other related human needs, such as belonging, intimacy (e.g., touching, kissing), sharing, and caring. When these needs are met, a person is sexually healthy (Fig. 1).

Sexuality, therefore, is a vital part of one's holistic being from birth to death. During the stages of human development, a person's attitudes, beliefs, and values related to sexuality are influenced and shaped by the environment, including family, friends, and society. For example, cultural beliefs affect the nature of physical sexual pleasure. The media also play a large role in developing views on sexuality. Some societies, such as the United States, tend to value youth and beauty more than aging and wisdom. As a result, people in these societies may feel less physically attractive and desirable for intimacy and belonging as they age.

Various external and internal risk factors can alter or impair sexual health. In many cases they cause physical sexual dysfunction, which then affects emotional needs such as self-esteem (Fig. 2). These factors include:

- Stages of human development
- Physical health problems
- Drugs
- Mental/behavioral health problems

The *stages of human development* typically influence human sexuality, especially when menopause occurs in middle adult-

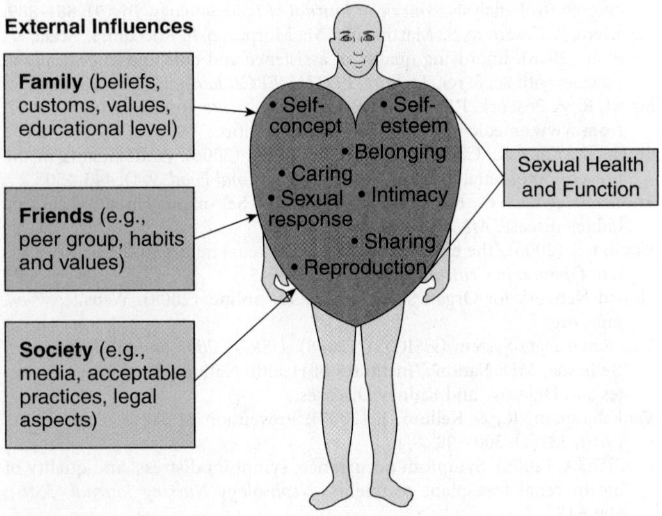

External Influences
Family (beliefs, customs, values, educational level)
Friends (e.g., peer group, habits and values)
Society (e.g., media, acceptable practices, legal aspects)
• Self-concept
• Self-esteem
• Belonging
• Caring
• Sexual response
• Intimacy
• Sharing
• Reproduction
Sexual Health and Function

Fig. 1

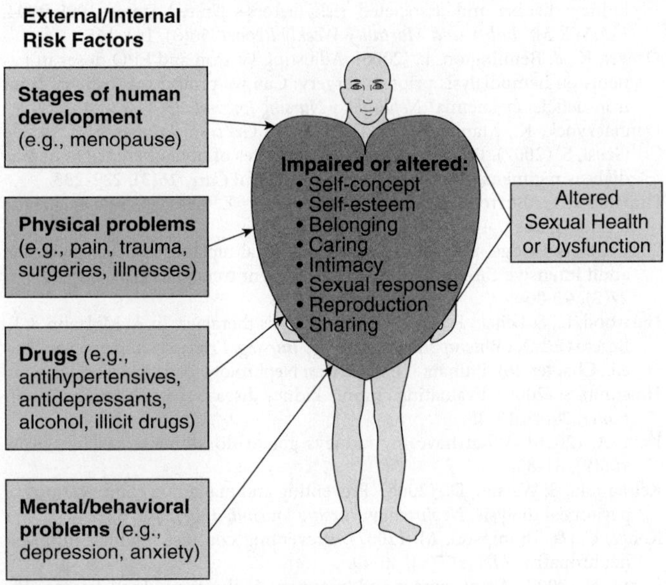

External/Internal Risk Factors
Stages of human development (e.g., menopause)
Physical problems (e.g., pain, trauma, surgeries, illnesses)
Drugs (e.g., antihypertensives, antidepressants, alcohol, illicit drugs)
Mental/behavioral problems (e.g., depression, anxiety)
Impaired or altered:
• Self-concept
• Self-esteem
• Belonging
• Caring
• Intimacy
• Sexual response
• Reproduction
• Sharing
Altered Sexual Health or Dysfunction

Fig. 2

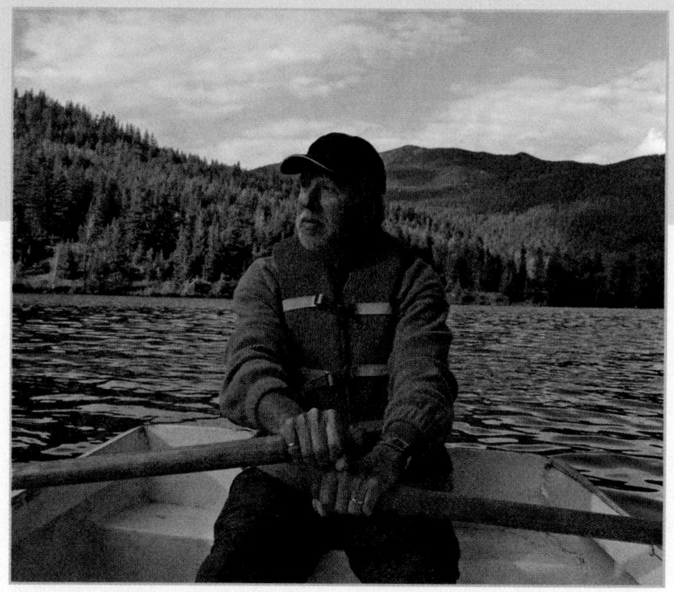

hood. Although each woman's response is different, menopause may result in a decreased libido (desire for sexual contact or intercourse). Relationships with her sexual partner(s) are altered, and interpersonal conflict can occur.

Physical health problems also can negatively affect sexual health. For example, chronic pain may cause decreased physical contact and a lowered self-concept along with chronic fatigue and decreased energy. Sexual dysfunction commonly occurs in people with chronic diseases such as diabetes and hypertension. Reproductive diseases (e.g., sexually transmitted diseases, testicular cancer) and their treatments (e.g., radiation therapy, surgery) can also affect sexuality, both physically and emotionally. Physical trauma such as spinal cord injury may prevent a person from having sexual intercourse.

Certain prescription or recreational *drugs* can cause impotence (inability to have an erection) or infertility. Alcohol and many antihypertensive agents, antidepressants, and illicit drugs interfere with sexual function in men.

Mental/behavioral health problems can also result in altered sexual health. Common examples include depression and severe anxiety states. In some cases, concern about physical performance can lead to sexual dysfunction.

XVI

UNIT

Problems of Reproduction

Management of Patients with Problems of the Reproductive System

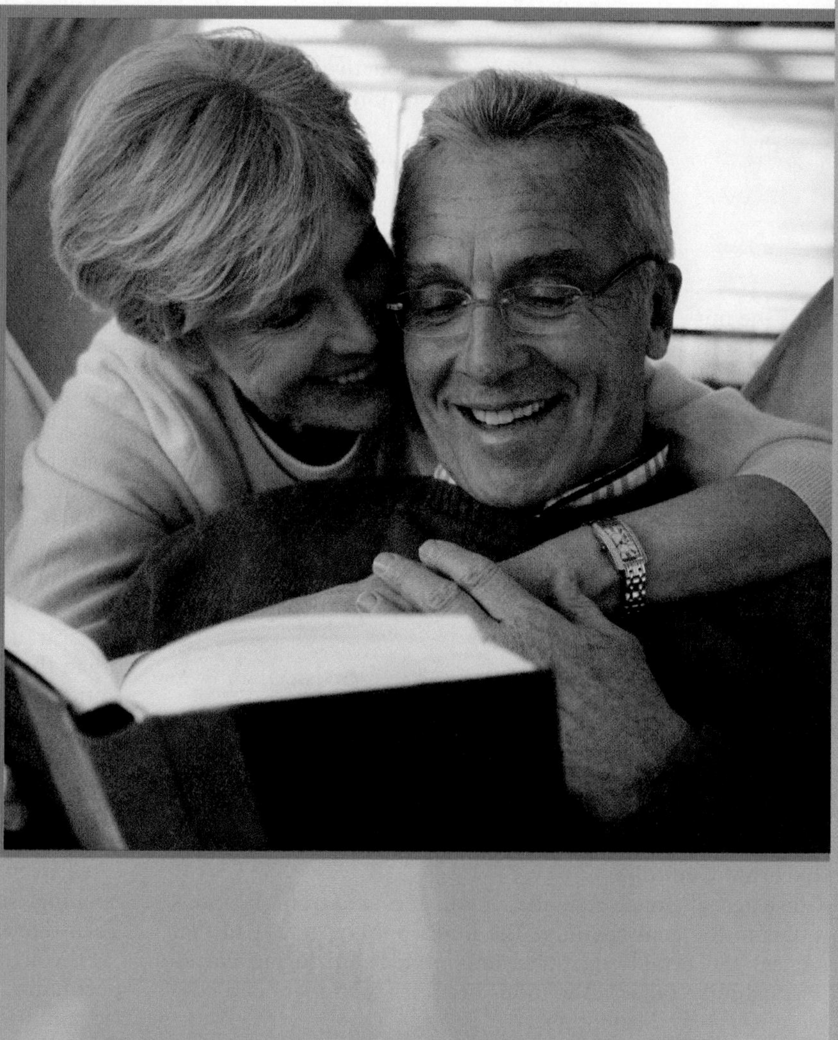

72

CHAPTER

Assessment of the Reproductive System

Deitra Leonard Lowdermilk

LEARNING OUTCOMES

For clinical competence and success on the NCLEX Examination, study this chapter with these Learning Outcomes in mind:

Health Promotion and Maintenance

1. Teach patients about recommended guidelines for selected reproductive screening tests.
2. Teach pre- and post-test care for diagnostic testing for the reproductive system.

Psychosocial Integrity

3. Identify general psychological responses to reproductive health problems.

Physiological Integrity

4. Briefly review the anatomy and physiology of the male and the female reproductive systems.
5. Identify reproductive changes associated with aging.
6. Perform a reproductive history using selected Gordon's Functional Health Patterns.
7. Perform focused physical assessment of the male and the female reproductive systems.
8. Explain the use of laboratory testing for patients with suspected or actual reproductive health problems.
9. Develop a teaching plan for a patient undergoing endoscopic studies for reproductive health problems.

evolve Go to your Companion CD or Evolve at http://evolve.elsevier.com/Iggy/ for *Self-Assessment Questions for the NCLEX Examination* keyed to these Learning Outcomes.

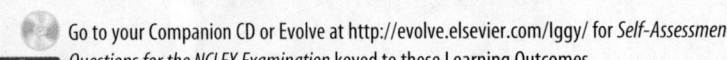

The nurse is often the first health care professional to assess the patient with a reproductive system health problem. These problems usually affect the *human need for sexuality, both its physical and psychosocial aspects,* and are difficult for many people to discuss. Basic assessment of the male and the female reproductive systems should be part of every complete physical assessment. The nurse should be comfortable with his or her sexuality and be nonjudgmental about differences in sexual practices.

This chapter describes basic reproductive system assessment. Refer to a fundamentals or basic nursing text for more information on human sexuality.

ANATOMY AND PHYSIOLOGY REVIEW

Structure and Function of the Female Reproductive System

The female reproductive system is located both outside (external) and inside (internal) the body.

External Genitalia

The external female genitalia, or **vulva,** extend from the mons pubis to the anal opening. The **mons pubis** is a fat pad that covers the symphysis pubis and protects it during **coitus** (sexual intercourse). The mons becomes prominent and covered with hair during puberty.

The **labia majora** are two vertical folds of adipose tissue that extend posteriorly from the mons pubis to the perineum. The size of the labia majora varies depending on the amount of fatty tissue present. The skin over the labia majora is usually darker than the surrounding skin and is highly vascular. It protects inner vulval structures and enhances sexual arousal.

The labia majora surround two thinner, vertical folds of reddish epithelium called the **labia minora.** The labia minora are highly vascular and have a rich nerve supply. Emotional or physical stimulation produces marked swelling and sensitivity. Numerous sebaceous glands in the labia minora lubricate the entrance to the vagina. The **clitoris** is a small, cylindric organ that is composed of erectile tissue with a high concentration of sensory nerve endings. During sexual arousal, the clitoris becomes larger and increases sexual sensation.

The **vestibule** is a longitudinal area between the labia minora, the clitoris, and the vagina that contains Bartholin glands and the openings of the urethra, Skene's glands (paraurethral glands), and vagina. The two Bartholin glands, located deeply toward the back on both sides of the vaginal opening, secrete lubrication fluid during sexual excitement. Their ductal openings are usually not visible.

The area between the vaginal opening and the anus is the **perineum.** The skin of the perineum covers the muscles, fascia, and ligaments that support the pelvic structures.

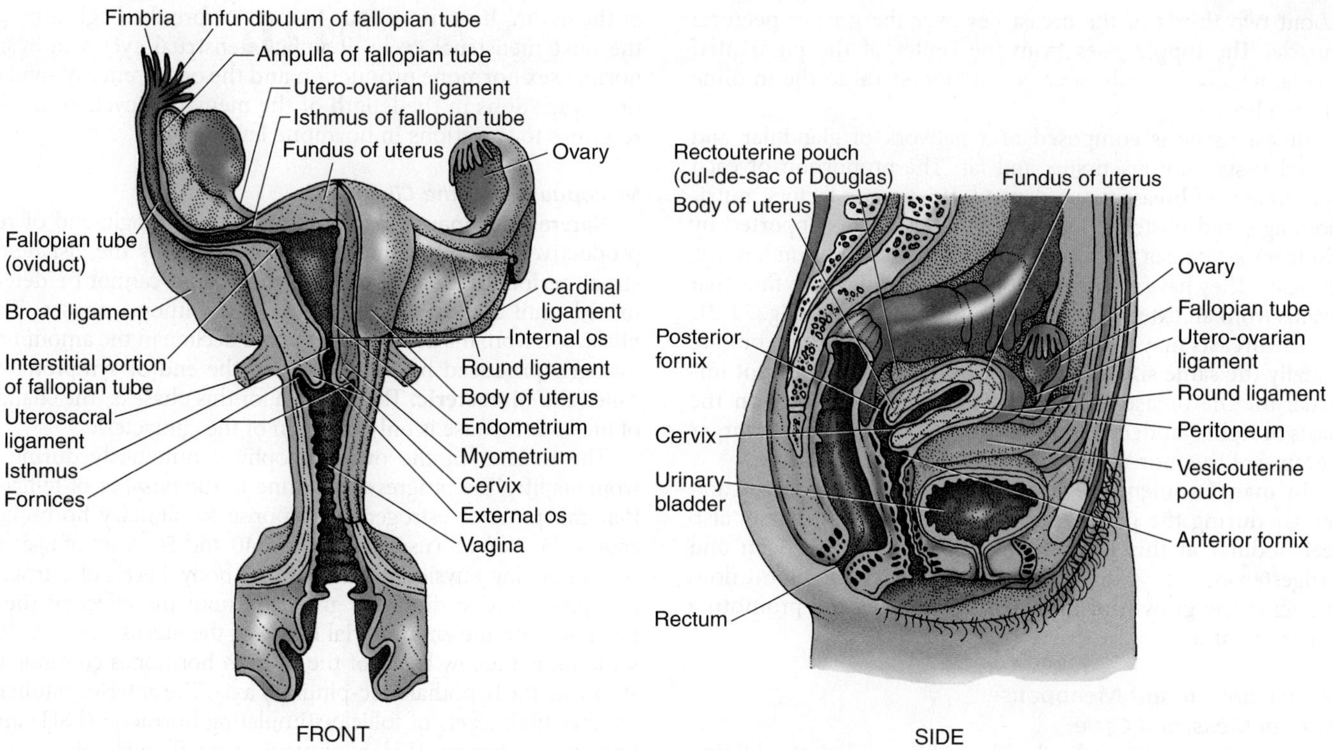
Fimbria
Infundibulum of fallopian tube
Ampulla of fallopian tube
Utero-ovarian ligament
Isthmus of fallopian tube
Fundus of uterus
Ovary
Fallopian tube (oviduct)
Broad ligament
Cardinal ligament
Internal os
Interstitial portion of fallopian tube
Round ligament
Body of uterus
Uterosacral ligament
Endometrium
Myometrium
Isthmus
Cervix
Fornices
External os
Vagina
FRONT
Rectouterine pouch (cul-de-sac of Douglas)
Body of uterus
Fundus of uterus
Ovary
Fallopian tube
Posterior fornix
Utero-ovarian ligament
Round ligament
Cervix
Peritoneum
Urinary bladder
Vesicouterine pouch
Anterior fornix
Rectum
SIDE

Fig. 72-1 • Internal female genitalia.

Internal Genitalia

The internal female genitalia are shown in Fig. 72-1.

Vagina

The **vagina** is a collapsible hollow tube that extends from the vestibule to the uterus. In addition to being the channel for the passage of the menstrual flow, the vagina allows for insertion of the penis during intercourse and passage of the fetus during a vaginal birth. Reduced estrogen levels occurring during menopause cause the vaginal wall to become dry, thinner, and smoother.

The amounts of glycogen and lubricating fluid secreted by the vaginal cells are influenced by ovarian hormones. Döderlein bacilli, the normal vaginal flora, interact with the secretions to produce lactic acid and maintain an acidic pH (3.5 to 5) in the vagina. This acidity helps prevent infection in the vagina.

At the upper end of the vagina, the uterine cervix projects into a cup-shaped vault of thin vaginal tissue. The recessed pockets around the cervix (the fornices) permit palpation of the internal pelvic organs. The posterior area provides access into the peritoneal cavity (through the cul-de-sac of Douglas) for diagnostic or surgical purposes.

Uterus

The uterus (or "womb") is a thick-walled, muscular organ attached to the upper end of the vagina. This inverted pear-shaped organ is located within the true pelvis, between the bladder and the rectum. The uterus is made up of the corpus (body) and the cervix. It responds to hormonal stimulation and prepares to receive, nurture, and, finally, expel the products of conception.

The upper segment of the uterine body, between the insertion sites of the fallopian tubes, is referred to as the *fundus.* Although the uterus is a hollow organ, its walls are in such close proximity in the nonpregnant state that its cavity is merely a slit.

The **cervix** is the lower, narrowed portion of the uterus and extends into the vagina. It is the passage site for sperm to enter the uterus and the passage site for menstrual flow to exit the uterus. The cervix is about 1 inch (2.5 cm) long with a central canal. The upper opening is the internal os, and the lower opening is the external os, which projects into the vagina. The surface of the cervix and the canal are the sites for Papanicolaou (Pap) testing. (See discussion on p. 1652.)

Fallopian Tubes and Ovaries

The **fallopian tubes** (uterine tubes) insert into the fundus of the uterus and extend laterally close to the ovaries. They provide a duct between the ovaries and the uterus for the passage of ova and sperm. In most cases, the ovum is fertilized in these tubes.

The **ovaries** are a pair of almond-shaped organs located near the lateral walls of the upper pelvic cavity. After menopause, they become smaller. These small organs develop and release ova and produce the sex steroid hormones (estrogen, progesterone, androgen, and relaxin). Adequate amounts of these hormones are needed for normal female growth and development and to maintain a pregnancy.

Breasts

The female **breasts** are a pair of mammary glands that develop in response to secretions from the hypothalamus, pituitary gland, and ovaries. The breasts are an accessory of the reproductive system that nourishes the infant after birth. They also are an organ for sexual arousal in the adult.

The breasts are located between the second and sixth ribs, between the edge of the sternum and the midaxillary line.

About two thirds of the breast lies over the greater pectoral muscle. The nipple rises from the center of the pigmented areola, which is usually located slightly lateral to the midline of each breast.

Breast tissue is composed of a network of glandular and ductal tissue, fibrous tissue, and fat. The proportion of each component of breast tissue depends on genetic factors, nutrition, age, and obstetric history. The breasts are supported by Cooper's suspensory ligaments that are attached to underlying muscles. They have abundant blood supply and lymph flow that drains from an extensive network toward the axilla (Fig. 72-2).

The breasts may not develop evenly during puberty but are usually the same size and contour by adulthood. It is not unusual for the breast on the woman's dominant side (on the basis of right-handedness or left-handedness) to appear larger because of the more developed pectoral muscle base.

In many women, the breasts become slightly larger and tender during the premenstrual period. The tissue may also feel nodular at this time. Increasing levels of estrogen and progesterone 3 to 4 days before menses increase blood flow, inducing the growth of the ducts and alveoli and promoting water retention.

Menstruation and Menopause

Normal Menstrual Cycle

Menstruation is the cyclic shedding of the endometrial lining of the uterus. The term **menarche** refers to the female's first menstruation and is one sign of puberty. Most girls begin to menstruate between 10 and 16 years of age.

Cyclic menstruation and reproduction depends on maturation of the hypothalamic-pituitary-ovarian-uterine axis. Normally this cycle is not achieved for the first 1 to 2 years after menarche. The first menstrual cycles are typically anovulatory (without ovulation) and irregular.

The typical menstrual cycle is 28 days, but variation is normal. The first day of the menstrual cycle is the first day of monthly menstrual bleeding. The menstrual flow is referred to as the **menses. Ovulation** is the cyclic maturation of a dominant follicle (the graafian follicle) and the subsequent release of the ovum. It occurs about 14 days before the beginning of the next menstrual cycle. Regular menstrual cycles indicate normal sex hormone production and the occurrence of ovulation. Variations in the length of the menstrual cycle occur in response to variations in hormone levels.

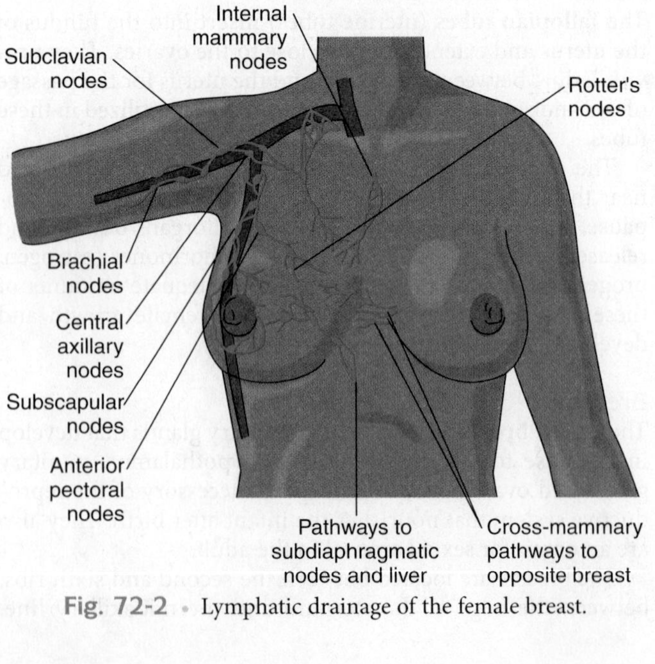
Internal mammary nodes
Subclavian nodes
Rotter's nodes
Brachial nodes
Central axillary nodes
Subscapular nodes
Anterior pectoral nodes
Pathways to subdiaphragmatic nodes and liver
Cross-mammary pathways to opposite breast

Fig. 72-2 • Lymphatic drainage of the female breast.

Menopause and the Climacteric

Natural Menopause. Menopause is the biologic end of reproductive ability, but the term applies to only the last menstrual period. The actual date of menopause cannot be determined until at least 1 year has passed without menses. The phase of a woman's life from the initial decline in the amount of estrogen produced by the ovaries to the end of symptoms is called the **climacteric.** The lay term for this phase is "the change of life." Menopause is only one sign of the climacteric.

The follicles in the ovary atrophy continuously during a woman's life. The progressive decline in the number of follicles that can produce estrogen in response to pituitary hormones causes the woman (usually between 40 and 50 years of age) to begin noticing physical changes in her body. Levels of estrogen and progesterone diminish gradually until the effect of these hormones on the endometrial lining of the uterus stops. At the same time, the low levels of the ovarian hormones continue to stimulate the hypothalamic-pituitary axis. The anterior pituitary secretes high levels of follicle-stimulating hormone (FSH) and luteinizing hormone (LH) after menopause. Blood levels of these hormones are used to confirm the presence of climacteric.

For a time, the inner core of the ovary produces **androgens** (male hormones). In women, most androgens are produced by the adrenal glands. When the ovarian core no longer functions, the adrenal glands are the only source of androgens. The production of androgens is significant, especially after menopause, because they are converted to a form of estrogen (estrone) in body fat. As a result, women with a greater percentage of body fat have higher estrone levels after menopause.

During the climacteric, a woman has irregular menstrual and ovarian cycles. Ovulation often fails to occur. The menstrual flow may be lighter or heavier during these irregular cycles.

Reduced estrogen affects additional body sites such as bone density. The uterus, cervix, ovaries, labia, and clitoris shrink in size. The low estrogen levels cause the vagina to narrow and shorten. The vaginal mucosa becomes thin and dry, which makes intercourse uncomfortable. The muscular support to the pelvis becomes more relaxed. The loss of tone also reduces bladder support, which results in urinary incontinence for many women. Chapter 69 discusses incontinence in more detail.

Bone density is a concern after estrogen production decreases. Estrogen is needed by bone tissue for calcium uptake. It also increases the metabolism of vitamin D, which is needed for the absorption of calcium from the intestines. Bone density declines in patients with decreased calcium uptake. A severe reduction in the amount of bone mass is called **osteoporosis** (see Chapter 53). Thus women are more at risk for bone fractures after menopause.

One of the most common symptoms that occur during the climacteric is the hot flash, which is caused by vasomotor instability. The cause is not clear, but it is thought that surges of FSH and LH cause vasodilation and increased heat production (Fogel, 2007). In addition to physical changes during the climacteric, the woman may also experience emotional changes (including mood changes) and fatigue.

Artificial Menopause. Menopause may occur for reasons other than the natural changes of the climacteric. Artificial menopause is the end of menstruation by some external means, such as an oophorectomy (surgical removal of the ovaries) or radiation to the ovaries. A premenopausal woman who experiences artificial menopause may need estrogen and progesterone therapy. However, the risks and benefits of such therapy need to be understood before making a decision (National Women's Health Information Center, 2006).

Structure and Function of the Male Reproductive System

The male reproductive system also consists of external and internal genitalia.

External Genitalia

The external male genitalia undergo many changes during puberty. The first obvious sign of puberty is enlargement of the scrotum and testes, which typically occurs between 11 and 13½ years of age.

These changes occur from an increase in testosterone production at puberty. The release of gonadotropin-releasing hormone (GnRH) from the hypothalamus stimulates the anterior pituitary to secrete LH (luteinizing hormone) and FSH (follicle-stimulating hormone). As the levels of these hormones increase, the amount of testosterone greatly increases. Other signs of puberty are the growth of axillary hair, lengthening and thickening of the vocal cords, increased sebaceous gland activity, and a general increase in muscle mass and body size.

Testosterone production is fairly constant in the adult male. Only a slight and gradual reduction of testosterone production occurs in the older adult male until he is in his 80s. Low testosterone levels decrease muscle mass, reduce skin elasticity, and lead to postural changes and changes in sexual performance.

The **penis** is an organ for urination and intercourse consisting of the body or shaft and the glans penis (the distal end of the penis). Engorgement of highly vascular, erectile columns with blood during sexual excitement causes the penis to expand and become longer, firm, and erect. The glans is the smooth end of the penis and contains the slitlike opening of the urethral meatus. The urethra is the pathway for the exit of both urine and semen.

The penis is covered by thin skin that is loosely attached to the underlying fascia. The skin allows the penis to enlarge during erections. It is darker than that of the rest of the body, and hair is present only at the base. A continuation of skin covers the glans and folds back on itself to form the prepuce (foreskin). Surgical removal of the foreskin **(circumcision)** for religious or cultural reasons is a common procedure in the United States and other Western countries.

The penis is richly supplied by branches of the sympathetic and parasympathetic nervous systems and by cerebral nerves. Penile erection is under the control of the autonomic nervous system. It can also result from touch and psychogenic mechanisms, such as auditory, visual, or imaginative stimulation. Sympathetic fibers control the rhythmic muscle contractions that lead to the ejaculation of semen.

The **scrotum** is a thin-walled, fibromuscular pouch that is behind the penis and suspended below the pubic bone. This pouch protects the testes, epididymis, and vas deferens in a space that is slightly cooler than inside the abdominal cavity. Normal sperm production and maturation **(spermatogenesis)** require a controlled temperature. The slightly lower temperature, about 6° F (2° C) less than body temperature, is optimal for sperm production and viability.

The scrotal skin is darkly pigmented and contains sweat glands, sebaceous glands, and few hair follicles. It contracts with cold, exercise, tactile stimulation, and sexual excitement.

Internal Genitalia

The internal male genitalia are shown in Fig. 72-3. The major organs are the testes and prostate gland.

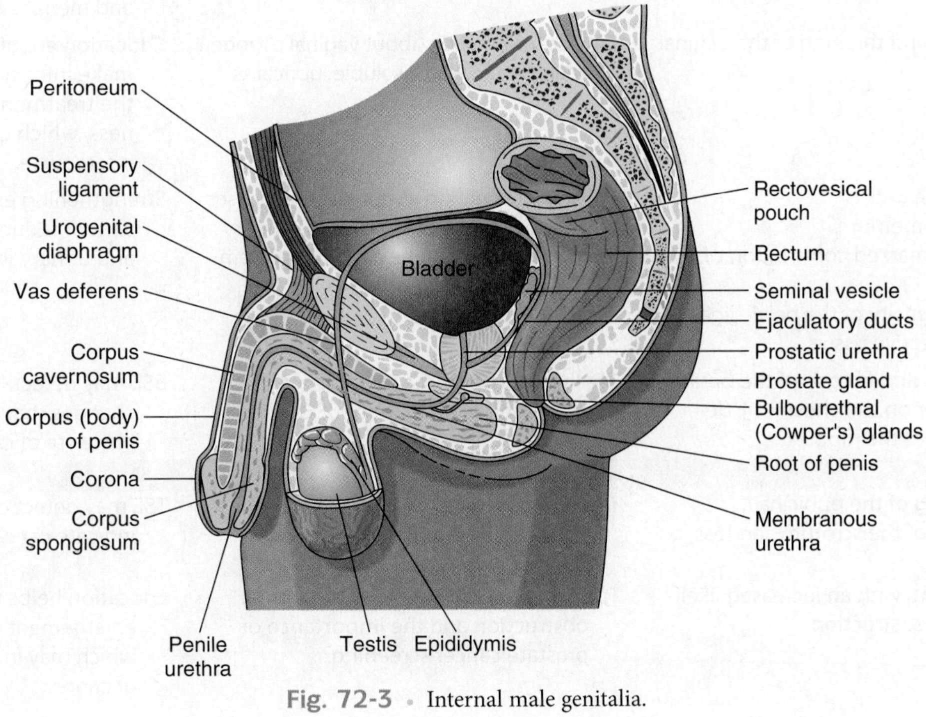
Peritoneum
Suspensory ligament
Urogenital diaphragm
Vas deferens
Corpus cavernosum
Corpus (body) of penis
Corona
Corpus spongiosum
Penile urethra
Testis
Epididymis
Bladder
Rectovesical pouch
Rectum
Seminal vesicle
Ejaculatory ducts
Prostatic urethra
Prostate gland
Bulbourethral (Cowper's) glands
Root of penis
Membranous urethra

Fig. 72-3 • Internal male genitalia.

Testes

The testes are a pair of oval organs in the scrotum that produce sperm and testosterone. Each testis is suspended in the scrotum by the spermatic cord, which provides blood, lymphatic, and nerve supply to the testis. Sympathetic nerve fibers are located on the arteries in the cord, and sympathetic and parasympathetic fibers are on the vas deferens. When the testes are damaged, these autonomic nerve fibers transmit excruciating pain and a sensation of nausea.

The **epididymis** is the first portion of a ductal system that transports sperm from the testes to the urethra and is a site of sperm maturation. The **vas deferens,** or ductus deferens, is a firm, muscular tube that continues from the tail of each epididymis. The end of each vas deferens is a reservoir for sperm and tubular fluids. They merge with ducts from the seminal vesicle to form the ejaculatory ducts at the base of the prostate gland. Sperm from the vas deferens and secretions from the seminal vesicles move through the ejaculatory duct to mix with prostatic fluids in the prostatic urethra.

Prostate Gland

The **prostate gland** is a large accessory gland of the male reproductive system. It secretes a milky alkaline fluid that adds bulk to the semen, enhances sperm movement, and neutralizes acidic vaginal secretions. The prostate gland can be palpated through the rectum and should not project more than ⅜ inch (1 cm) into the rectal lumen.

During **emission,** the first stage of the male orgasm, the prostate gland secretes its fluid at the same time as the vas deferens. The average pH of the combined secretions of semen is about 7.5, whereas secretions from the vagina normally have a pH of 3.5 to 5.

As men age, the prostate gland becomes clinically significant. Men older than 50 years commonly have an enlarged prostate (benign prostatic hyperplasia [BPH]), which can cause problems such as overflow incontinence and nocturia (nighttime urination). Prostate function depends on adequate levels of testosterone. As men age, testosterone production slowly decreases.

Inguinal Area

The inguinal area (groin) is located between the superior iliac spine and the symphysis pubis and is the junction of the lower abdominal wall and thigh. The area is a common site for a **hernia,** which is a loop of bowel that protrudes through a weak spot in the muscles.

◀ VIDEO CLIP: Inguinal Hernia Evaluation

REPRODUCTIVE CHANGES ASSOCIATED WITH AGING

Age affects the function of both the male and the female reproductive systems. After puberty, hormones produced by the gonads (testis and ovary) affect many body systems. Many changes in the reproductive system occur in older adults (Chart 72-1).

Chart 72-1 NURSING FOCUS ON THE OLDER ADULT

Changes in the Reproductive System Related to Aging

Physiologic Change	Nursing Interventions	Rationales
WOMEN		
Graying and thinning of the pubic hair Decreased size of the labia majora and clitoris	Discuss changes with the patient (applies to all structures for both women and men).	Education helps prevent problems with body image (applies to all structures for both women and men).
Drying, smoothing, and thinning of the vaginal walls	Provide information about vaginal estrogen therapy and water-soluble lubricants.	Education enables the patient to make informed decisions about the treatment of vaginal dryness, which can cause painful intercourse.
Decreased size of the uterus Atrophy of the endometrium Decreased size and marked convolution of the ovaries Loss of tone and elasticity of the pelvic ligaments and connective tissue	Provide information about Kegel exercises to strengthen pelvic muscles. Urinary incontinence can be a major problem.	Strengthening exercises may prevent or reduce pelvic relaxation and urinary incontinence.
Increased flabbiness and fibrosis of the breasts, which hang lower on the chest wall; decreased erection of the nipples	Teach or reinforce the importance of breast self-examination (BSE).	BSE may detect lumps or other changes that may indicate the presence of cancer.
MEN		
Graying and thinning of the pubic hair Increased drooping of the scrotum and loss of rugae	Teach or reinforce the importance of testicular self-examination (TSE).	TSE may detect changes that may indicate cancer.
Prostate enlargement, with an increased likelihood of urethral obstruction	Teach the patient the signs of urethral obstruction and the importance of prostate cancer screening.	Education helps the patient detect enlargement or obstruction, which may indicate the presence of cancer.

ASSESSMENT METHODS

Patient History

Use data about the patient's age, gender, and culture to assess the risk for reproductive diseases and to evaluate the reproductive system. The age at which secondary sexual characteristics developed is compared with the typical ranges for males or females.

Assess the patient's health habits, such as diet, sleep, and exercise patterns. Low levels of body fat may be related to ovarian dysfunction. Assess for alcohol, tobacco, and drug use because **libido** (sex drive), sperm production, and **potency** (the ability to have and sustain an erection) can be affected by these substances (Lowdermilk, 2007a).

The patient's personal medical history provides data about his or her general health. Certain childhood illnesses can have an effect on the reproductive system. Women need to be screened for sufficient rubella titers and should be treated, if necessary, to prevent possible **teratogenic** effects (development of birth defects) on their unborn children if they get rubella during the first trimester of pregnancy. Mumps or smallpox in men after puberty may cause **orchitis** (painful inflammation and swelling of the testes) and occasionally leads to testicular atrophy and sterility.

Assess for any major adult illnesses or chronic illnesses that may severely affect reproductive function. Endocrine disorders may affect the hypothalamic-pituitary-gonadal function of men or women. Almost any disease that disturbs a woman's metabolism or nutrition can depress ovarian function and cause **amenorrhea** (absence of menses). Failure of ovulation is associated with a greater risk for endometrial cancer. Patients with diabetes mellitus may experience physiologic changes such as vaginal dryness or impotence. Chronic disorders of the nervous system, respiratory system, or cardiovascular system can alter the sexual response.

Reproductive system dysfunction can also result from irradiation, prolonged use of corticosteroids, external estrogen or testosterone use, and chemotherapy drugs. In addition, past severe infections can alter a person's reproductive ability. For example, pelvic inflammatory disease or a ruptured appendix followed by peritonitis can cause strictures or adhesions in the fallopian tubes and pelvic scarring. **Salpingitis** (uterine tube infection) is usually caused by chlamydial infection and can result in female infertility. Infections or prolonged fever in males may damage sperm production or cause obstruction of the seminal tract, which leads to infertility. Explore the patient's history of illnesses, surgeries, serious injuries, current medications, and allergies. Each of these can affect reproductive structure or function.

Data about sexual activity are important to obtain as part of the history. Heterosexual activity should not be assumed. Lesbian, gay, bisexual, and transsexual (LGBT) issues are often not assessed by health care professionals or shared by the patient. Explore information about sexual practices in a nonjudgmental and sensitive manner. Table 4-3 in Chapter 4 suggests sensitive ways to ask questions about sexual activity.

CULTURAL AWARENESS

Other cultural beliefs and practices influence lifestyle and sexual practices. These beliefs and expectations account for differences in acceptable gender-related identity. A person's attitude and behavior about the meaning and use of genitals begin in early childhood and are modeled on the behavior of significant adults. Religious preferences may be in line with those of a specific culture and strongly affect sexual activity. A person's religious beliefs often influence specific sexual practices, the acceptable number of sexual partners, and contraceptive use. Be sensitive to cultural differences and preferences by being nonjudgmental and showing acceptance.

Nutrition History

A nutrition history is often critical for an accurate interpretation of reproductive system problems. For example, fatigue and low libido may occur with poor diet and anemia. Obesity raises the risk for uterine cancer. High-fat diets may increase the risk for cancer of the breast, ovary, and prostate gland (American Cancer Society [ACS], 2008). Ask the patient to recall his or her dietary intake for a recent 24-hour period to assess quality.

Assess the patient's height, weight, and body mass index. The patient may be hesitant to discuss practices such as bingeing, purging, anorexic behaviors, or excessive exercise. However, these practices may affect the reproductive system. A certain level of body fat and weight is necessary for the onset of menses and the maintenance of regular menstrual cycles. Decreased body fat results in insufficient estrogen levels.

Women have special nutrition needs. Those who use oral contraceptives should have increased sources of folic acid and vitamins B_6, B_{12}, and C. Heavy menstrual bleeding, particularly in women who have intrauterine devices, may require oral iron supplements. Teach all women of any age about their body's need for calcium. Although adequate calcium intake throughout life is optimal, it is especially important during and after menopause. The bone density loss at this time because of reduced estrogen levels predisposes perimenopausal women to osteoporosis and fractures (see Chapter 53).

Family History and Genetic Risk

The family history helps determine the patient's risk for conditions that affect reproductive functioning. A delayed or early development of secondary sex characteristics may be a familial pattern.

The current age and health status of family members are important. Evidence of medical diseases or reproductive problems in family members (e.g., diabetes, endometriosis, reproductive cancer) allows better interpretation of the patient's current symptoms. For example, daughters of women who were given diethylstilbestrol (DES) to control bleeding during pregnancy are at increased risk for infertility and reproductive tract cancer.

Recent advances in genetics have found a hereditary component of many diseases, including those of the reproductive system. For example, about 10% of all cancers have a genetic component but only a small percent of breast cancers are hereditary. Specific *BRCA1* and *BRCA2* gene mutations do increase the overall risk for breast or ovarian cancer (ACS, 2008). Men with first-degree relatives (e.g., father, brother) with prostate cancer are at greater risk for the disease than men in the general population. Testicular cancer can also be familial (ACS, 2008). More information about genetic risks is discussed with specific health problems in later chapters of this unit.

Genitoreproductive History

Obtain genitoreproductive history for both men and women. Chart 72-2 describes assessment data using Gordon's Functional Health Patterns.

Female Patient

Ask the female patient about her menses, including age of menarche, cycle frequency and duration, amount of flow, spotting between periods, **dysmenorrhea** (painful menstrual periods), and premenstrual symptoms. If the patient is of menopausal age, determine the date of her last menstrual period, the presence of climacteric symptoms, and any drugs or complementary and alternative therapies used for these symptoms. Ask all women about the presence of vaginal discharge, a history and treatment of sexually transmitted infections including human immune deficiency virus (HIV), the date and the result of the most recent Papanicolaou (Pap) test, breast self-examination practices, and vulvar self-examination (VSE) practices (Zdanuk, 2007).

Obtain an obstetric history. Women who have never had children have higher rates of ovarian, endometrial, and breast cancer than the rates for women who have had children. If the woman has been pregnant, ask about the outcome of the pregnancies.

An early age at first intercourse and multiple sex partners are associated with an increased risk for cervical cancer. Ask about satisfaction with sexual response, any pain or bleeding with sexual intercourse, and contraceptive use. Religious beliefs or type of sex (oral, anal, and vaginal) may affect the contraceptive practices. Assessment for intimate partner abuse may be included at this point or at another time during the interview for all patients, especially women. Table 72-1 lists suggested questions that you should ask regarding potential abuse.

Male Patient

Ask the male patient about testicular changes and self-examination practices, problems with urination, discharge from the penis, rectal problems, history and treatment of sexually transmitted infections including HIV, and symptoms related to hernias.

Ask about sexual functioning. Reproductive history and contraceptive use, current problems or changes in sexual response, any difficulty with erection or ejaculation, and the use of drugs or treatments direct the physical assessment. The type of sex practiced also allows attention to be focused on the body area involved.

Current Health Problems

If patients seek medical attention for a problem related to the reproductive system, ask additional questions to explore the specific concerns. Most problems are related to pain, bleeding, discharge, and masses (Chart 72-3).

Pain related to reproductive system disorders may be confused with that associated with GI or urinary tract problems. Ask the patient to describe the nature of the pain, including its type, intensity, timing and location, duration, and relationship to menstrual, sexual, urinary, or GI function. Assess the factors that **exacerbate** (worsen) or relieve the pain.

Heavy *bleeding* or a lack of bleeding may concern the patient. Consider the possibility of pregnancy in any sexually active woman with amenorrhea. Any postmenopausal bleeding needs to be evaluated. Ask the patient to describe the amount and character of abnormal vaginal or penile bleeding. Assess whether the bleeding occurs in relation to the menstrual cycle or menopause, intercourse, trauma, or strenuous exercise. Ask about any associated symptoms, such as pain, cramping or abdominal fullness, a change in bowel habits, urinary difficulties, and weight changes. Many factors can cause bleeding, and sites other than the genital tract need to be considered.

Chart 72-2 REPRODUCTIVE ASSESSMENT
Using Gordon's Functional Health Patterns

HEALTH PERCEPTION/HEALTH MANAGEMENT PATTERN

- Has anyone in your family had cancer of the breast or reproductive organs? Who and what type of cancer?
- If you engage in sexual activities, do you practice "safer" sex?
- What do you do to keep healthy—regular health checkups, self-examination (breast, genital [vulvar, testicular]), healthy diet, exercise, use of medications or alternative therapies?

SEXUALITY-REPRODUCTIVE PATTERN

MALE AND FEMALE

- Are you sexually active? Do you find your sexual relationship satisfying? Have there been any changes in your relationship? Are you having any problems in your sexual relationship?
- Do you use contraceptives? If so, do you have any problems with the method of contraception?
- Have you had any sexually transmitted diseases? If yes, when and what type did you have?

FEMALE

- When did you first start menstruating? When was your last menstrual period? Do you have any menstrual problems?
- Have you ever been pregnant? If so, how many times and what were the outcomes?
- Have you had any symptoms of menopause?

MALE

- Do you have any problems with getting and maintaining an erection, or do you have difficulty with ejaculation?
- Have you ever had a hernia or pain in the groin?

SELF-PERCEPTION/SELF-CONCEPT PATTERN

- How would you describe yourself? Do you feel good or not so good about yourself?
- Have you experienced changes in your body appearance or function? If so, are these problematic for you? Have you felt anxious, fearful, or depressed about these changes?

Based on Gordon, M. (2007). *Manual of nursing diagnosis* (11th ed.). Boston: Jones & Bartlett.

TABLE 72-1 Abuse Screening Questions*

1. Are you with a spouse or partner who threatens or physically hurts you?
2. In the past year has anyone hurt, slugged, kicked, or otherwise hurt you?
3. Has your spouse or partner forced you to have sexual activity that made you uncomfortable?
4. Are you afraid of your spouse or partner?

*Never ask questions with partner present.
Source: American College of Obstetricians and Gynecologists. (2006). *Screening tools for domestic violence.* Retrieved February 20, 2007, from www.acog.org.

Chart 72-3 BEST PRACTICE FOR PATIENT SAFETY & QUALITY CARE

Assessing the Patient with Reproductive Health Problems

Patient Concern	Nursing Assessment
Pain	Type and intensity of pain Location and duration of pain Factors that relieve or worsen pain Relationship to menstrual, sexual, urinary, or GI function Medications
Bleeding	Presence or absence of bleeding Character and amount of bleeding Relationship of bleeding to events or other factors (e.g., menstrual cycle) Onset and duration of bleeding Presence of associated symptoms, such as pain
Discharge	Amount and character of discharge Presence of genital lesions, bleeding, itching, or pain Presence of symptoms or discharge in sexual partner
Masses	Location and characteristics of mass Presence of associated symptoms, such as pain Relationship to menstrual cycle

Discharge from either the male or female reproductive tract can cause severe irritation of the surrounding tissues, itching, pain, embarrassment, and anxiety. Ask about the amount, color, consistency, odor, and chronicity of the discharge. Drugs (e.g., antibiotics) and clothing (e.g., tight jeans, synthetic underwear fabric) may cause or worsen genital discharge. Many types of discharge are caused by sexually transmitted infections (see Chapter 76). The body location of these infections depends on the patient's sexual practices. Ask the patient about lesions, bleeding, itching, and pain related to the genitals and orifices used during sexual activity. Also inquire about the presence of symptoms in the sexual partner.

Any reported *masses* in the breasts, testes, or inguinal area need to be evaluated. Some masses change in character or size. The patient can often relate these changes to menstrual cycles, heavy lifting, straining, or trauma. Ask about associated symptoms such as tenderness, heaviness, pain, dimpling, and tender lymph nodes.

Physical Assessment

Assessment of the Female Reproductive System

The medical-surgical nurse usually does not perform a comprehensive female or male reproductive examination. However, perform a focused assessment for specific concerns of the patient. The physician or advanced practice nurse does a more thorough gynecologic assessment as described below. The medical-surgical nurse often assists with the examination.

Inspection of the female genitalia and the pelvic examination are usually performed at the end of a head-to-toe physical assessment. The patient is often more apprehensive about these portions of the examination than about any other part. Pain or lack of privacy during previous pelvic or breast examinations may prevent the patient from relaxing.

Show the patient the equipment to be used, along with three-dimensional models, to demonstrate the assessment procedures. Teach the relaxation and breathing techniques to enhance a sense of control. Inform the patient about what is going to be done and what she may feel as the examination proceeds. If she has pain or exceptional concern during the procedures, the examiner should stop and adjust the assessment plan or techniques. For example, patients who have been sexually abused may become upset during pelvic examinations (Zdanuk, 2007). For some patients, the presence of a support person or having the examination performed by an examiner who is the same gender as the patient may be of benefit.

Other than determining pregnancy or infertility, a pelvic examination is indicated to assess for:

- Menstrual irregularities
- Unexplained abdominal or vaginal pain
- Vaginal discharge, itching, sores, or infection
- Rape trauma or other pelvic injury
- Physical changes in the vagina, cervix, and uterus

Remind the woman not to douche for at least 24 hours before the pelvic examination, because doing so may prevent an accurate evaluation of smears, cultures, and cytologic data (Alexander et al., 2007).

Immediately before the pelvic and breast examinations, ask the patient to empty her bladder and undress completely. Drape the woman adequately to protect modesty throughout the examination. If she is not wearing a gown, a small towel can be placed over the breasts under the larger drape. Remove drapes only over the region being examined, and replace them when that area has been assessed. Drapes that prevent eye contact between the examiner and the patient are dehumanizing and prevent comfort during the examination. Mirrors can be used to facilitate teaching if the patient so desires. The examination is performed in a room that has adequate lighting for body inspection, that is a comfortable temperature, and that ensures privacy.

The physical examination of the reproductive system usually includes the breasts (see Chapter 73). After the breast examination, the examiner generally completes the thoracic and cardiovascular examinations and then inspects, auscultates, and palpates the abdomen. The patient's arms should be at her sides or over her chest to allow better relaxation of the abdominal muscles. During the gynecologic examination, the examiner palpates for symptomatic and asymptomatic abdominopelvic masses. A mass can be of reproductive, intestinal, or urinary tract origin. Careful history-taking combined with the physical examination can usually determine the origin of a mass. Gynecologic masses, such as ovarian masses, may be further differentiated from lesions on the body of the uterus during the bimanual portion of the pelvic examination.

Examination of the External Genitalia

After the abdominal examination, prepare the patient for inspection of the external genitalia and the pelvic examination. Assist the woman into the lithotomy position, and ask her to place her arms at her sides or over her chest. The patient's buttocks extend slightly beyond the edge of the table, and her thighs are abducted. All equipment for the vaginal and speculum examination and cytologic studies is prepared. After thorough handwashing, the examiner wears gloves to protect

▶ VIDEO CLIP: External Genitalia

against possible disease and potential cross-contamination from other patients. The patient is informed that the genitalia will be touched and separated.

The initial inspection and palpation of the external genitalia provide an assessment of age-appropriate development. Hair color and distribution over the symphysis pubis and vulva suggest the woman's age and hormonal functioning. The pubic hair is inspected for the presence of lice or scabies. The skin and mucosa of the vulva are inspected from anterior to posterior for signs of inflammation, infestation, swelling, lesions, and discharge.

The examination of the external female genitalia is an excellent time for teaching about **vulvar self-examination (VSE).** The incidence of precancerous conditions and infectious diseases of the vulva is increasing, especially in young women (ACS, 2008). VSE can easily be taught and can lead to early diagnosis of vulvar conditions, especially cancer (Chart 72-4).

Perineal support and the strength of the vaginal walls may be assessed by asking the woman to squeeze the vaginal opening closed after the examiner has inserted two fingers. The patient is then asked to strain downward while the examiner assesses for urinary incontinence or any bulging of the anterior or posterior vaginal walls that would indicate a cystocele or rectocele, respectively.

VIDEO CLIP: Speculum Examination ▶

Pelvic Examination

After the correct speculum size is selected, it is warmed and lubricated with warm water. No other lubricant should be used if cytologic studies are to be collected because it interferes with specimen analysis. Tell the woman when the speculum is going to be inserted. The examiner's fingers can ease insertion of the speculum by pressing down on the perineal body just inside the vaginal orifice. The woman can also be asked to breathe slowly and to bear down. The closed speculum is inserted, and then the blades are opened.

The cervix is inspected for color, shape, and dilation and for erosions, nodules, masses, discharge, and bleeding. Herpes simplex, syphilis, and cancer can produce characteristic lesions on the cervix. Specimens are obtained from the cervix, endocervix, and vaginal pool for cytologic studies (see Other Laboratory Studies section, p. 1654). After completion of the cervical examination, the speculum is withdrawn. The vaginal tissue is inspected for lesions or inflammation during withdrawal.

Chart 72-4 PATIENT AND FAMILY EDUCATION GUIDE

Vulvar Self-Examination

- Perform a vulvar self-examination monthly between menstrual periods if you are older than 18 years or if you are sexually active.
- Sit in a well-lighted area on a soft surface (bed or carpeted floor).
- Use a handheld mirror to see your external genitalia.
- Examine the area around the vaginal opening from the mons pubis to the perianal area.
- Feel and visually inspect the area.
- Report to your health care provider new nodes, warts, growths of any type, ulcers, sores, blisters, change in skin color, painful areas, areas of itching or inflammation, or any change in vaginal discharge.

VIDEO CLIP: Bimanual Examination ▶

After withdrawing the speculum, the examiner proceeds with the bimanual examination. Using a new glove and lubricant, he or she stands and inserts one or two fingers of one hand into the patient's vagina. The posterior vaginal wall is checked for masses or tenderness. The cervix and fornix around the cervix are identified. The opposite hand is placed on the patient's abdomen—between her umbilicus and symphysis pubis—and pressed downward. The cervix and uterus are lifted with the pelvic hand toward the abdominal hand to trap the uterus for assessment (Fig. 72-4). The size, shape, consistency, location, and mobility of the uterus are assessed. Any tenderness or masses are noted. The ovaries and tubes are examined in the same manner.

The rectovaginal and rectal examination is the last part of the pelvic examination. The glove is changed and lubricated. The gloved middle finger is placed in the rectum and the index finger in the vagina. Insertion of the rectal finger is easier if the patient strains and relaxes the anal sphincter. The procedure for the bimanual examination is repeated. After the examination, any fecal material that remains on the glove may be tested for occult blood.

After the examination, the patient's feet are lowered from the stirrups at the same time to reduce strain on the perineal muscles and lumbosacral ligaments. *Some patients experience orthostatic (postural) hypotension if they sit up too quickly, especially older adults or those with low blood pressure. Evaluate for signs of dizziness before letting her get off the examining table.* Provide supplies, such as perineal wipes and perineal

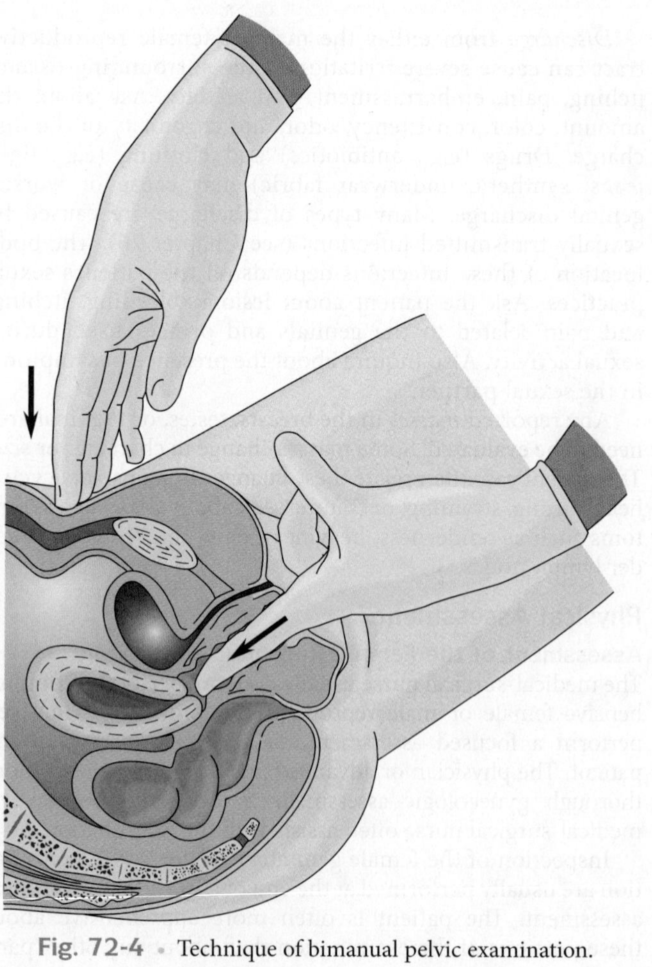

Fig. 72-4 • Technique of bimanual pelvic examination.

napkins or minipads, and allow the patient privacy for dressing. Be available to answer questions and provide support.

Assessment of the Male Reproductive System

Unless a male patient seeks health care for a genital tract problem, the examiner may not inspect and palpate the male genitalia and rectum during physical examinations, depending on the health care setting and the age of the patient. Men are often embarrassed and anxious when the reproductive system is assessed. This concern may be worse when the examiner is a woman. The patient may be concerned about discomfort, the developmental stage of his genitalia, or the likelihood of an erection during the examination. If he does have an erection, the examiner should assure him that this is a normal response to a tactile stimulus (touch) and should continue the examination.

The examination of the male genitalia is a good opportunity to teach about contraceptives, testicular self-examination (TSE), and the need for regular prostate gland examinations. Testicular cancer is one of the most common cancers in young men and can be treated effectively if found early. Prostate cancer is common in older men, and the prognosis is good if diagnosed early. *Although not universally agreed upon, the ACS (2008) recommends annual digital rectal and prostate gland examinations and prostate-specific antigen (PSA) blood tests for men older than 50 years at average risk and for men older than 40 years who are at higher risk (e.g., African-American males and males with a family history).*

As with examinations of other body systems, explain each step of the assessment procedure before it is performed. The patient needs to be reassured that the examiner will stop and change the assessment plan or technique if the patient has pain during the examination. Teach relaxation techniques and provide support during the examination to increase comfort.

VIDEO CLIP: Inspection (Standing)

Examination of the External Genitalia

The patient may be in a lying or a standing position for inspection and palpation of the external genitalia. The examiner sits on a chair in front of the patient. A general observation is made of the secondary sex characteristics. Note the age-appropriateness of the developmental stage, including the pattern of the pubic hair, the descent and size of the testes, and the size of the scrotum and penis. Inspect the pubic hair for the presence of lice or scabies.

Inspect the skin of the penis for intactness. The dorsal vein should be apparent. Note any lesions or ulcers on the penis. A specimen can be scraped for cytologic study if needed. If the patient has not been circumcised, he is asked to retract the foreskin. This should be accomplished easily unless the man has **phimosis** (a tight foreskin that cannot be retracted). Inspect the glans penis for possible inflammation, fungal infection, syphilitic chancres, and cancers. **Smegma,** a white, cheesy secretion from the sebaceous glands in the glans, may accumulate under the foreskin. This secretion is not present in the circumcised male.

The glans is also inspected for placement of the urinary meatus. Positions other than at the distal end of the glans are abnormal. By compressing the glans between the thumb and index finger, the meatus is separated and any discharge present can be determined. Urethral discharge is not normal, and a specimen should be obtained for culture. *The foreskin is replaced if it has been retracted.* The body of the penis is palpated between the thumb and first two fingers; note tenderness, hard areas under the skin, and signs of inflammation.

Inspection of the scrotum and inguinal areas is best accomplished by having the patient hold the penis up and to the side. Document the shape and contour of the scrotum. Normally, the left side of the scrotum is lower than the right because the left testicle has a longer spermatic cord. Both the anterior and posterior surfaces of the scrotum are inspected for lesions, nodules, rashes, pain, and edema. Swelling of the scrotum may indicate a hydrocele (collection of serous fluid in the scrotal sac), infection, or torsion (twisting) of the spermatic cord.

Palpation of the scrotum, testes, epididymis, and spermatic cords is best accomplished in a warm environment so the scrotum hangs low and relaxed. The examiner holds the scrotum gently between the thumb and two fingers and compares the contents of each side of the scrotal pouch. Each testis is inspected for size, shape, symmetry, tenderness, nodules, and consistency.

The normal testis has smooth borders, is somewhat sensitive to light palpation, and feels rubbery. The epididymis can be palpated on the posterior surface of the testis. It is examined for size, shape, and tenderness. In patients with infection of the epididymis, its outline cannot be distinguished. Varicose veins of the spermatic cord (varicocele) feel like a "bag of worms" above the testis.

Any swollen area of the scrotum should be transilluminated. The examining room is darkened for this procedure, and the beam from the penlight is directed through the scrotal swelling from the posterior surface of the scrotum. The light transmits a red glow if the swelling contains serous fluid. Blood and solid tissue do not transmit the light.

The inner thigh can be stroked with a blunt instrument (e.g., the handle of the reflex hammer) to test the **cremasteric reflex.** If this reflex is intact, the testicle and scrotum rise on the stroked side.

Examination of the Rectum and Prostate

The final assessment of the male reproductive system is an examination of the rectum and the prostate gland. This examination can be performed with the patient in a knee-chest position, in a lithotomy position, in a left-lateral-with-knees-flexed position, or standing and leaning over the examining table with the feet turned inward to relax the buttocks. Proper lighting is necessary to view the anus and surrounding tissue. Note and record any lesions, ulcerations, masses, or fissures.

To assess the prostate gland, a rectal examination is performed. The posterior surface of the prostate gland is felt extending less than $\frac{3}{8}$ inch (1 cm) into the rectum. Tell the patient that he may feel an urge to urinate as the prostate is being examined but that he will not do so. The prostate should feel firm (the consistency has been equated to that of a pencil eraser), smooth, and slightly mobile. It should be nontender across its diameter. Any stool on the examiner's glove can be tested for occult blood. However, this practice is controversial because the results may not be reliable.

Psychosocial Assessment

The psychosocial assessment may suggest factors that lead to the patient's health problem. During the social history, ask about sources of support, strengths, and likely reactions to illness or dysfunction.

A patient's personal history or beliefs may negatively influence his or her ability to enjoy a satisfactory sexual life. These factors may include:

- Sexual trauma or abuse inflicted during childhood or adulthood
- Punishment for masturbation
- Psychological trauma
- Cultural influences, such as the idea of female passivity during intercourse
- Concerns about sexual partners or sexual lifestyle
- Use of alcohol or street drugs

Fears may affect the patient's satisfaction with sexuality or body image. He or she may also be concerned about the potential or actual reaction of family members to reproductive health problems (see Chart 72-2).

Diagnostic Assessment

Laboratory Assessment

Papanicolaou Test

The **Papanicolaou test,** or **Pap smear,** is a cytologic study that is effective in detecting precancerous and cancerous cells from the cervix. Health care providers vary in their recommendations for the frequency of routine Pap tests. The American Cancer Society (ACS) advises all women to begin having an annual Pap test within 3 years of becoming sexually active or by 21 years of age. Annual screening is recommended to 30 years of age with the conventional Pap test or every 2 years if a liquid-based test is used. After age 30 and three or more consecutive negative test results, Pap tests may be performed less frequently (i.e., every 2 to 3 years) until 70 years of age. Women older than 70 years who have had normal results for 10 years may discontinue testing (ACS, 2008; U.S. Preventive Services Task Force, 2006). Those who have had a total hysterectomy for benign reasons may need less frequent screening or may not need screening at all (ACS, 2008). However, many clinicians continue to suggest that the test be performed annually during routine physical examinations.

Cytologic examinations can also detect viral, fungal, and parasitic disorders. Examination of cells from the vaginal walls can evaluate the function of steroid hormones.

Patient Preparation. The Pap test should be scheduled between the woman's menstrual periods so that the menstrual flow does not interfere with the test interpretation. The woman should not douche, use vaginal medications or deodorants, or have sexual intercourse for at least 24 hours before the test.

Assist the woman into the lithotomy position. Relaxation techniques, including concentrating on breathing patterns or a visual focal point, may help the apprehensive woman. Explain all steps of the examination to the woman before they are performed.

Procedure. A speculum is inserted into the vagina. Usually, the cervix is visualized and then scraped with one of the various sampling tools available, such as a cytology brush, cotton-tipped applicator, endocervical aspirator, or wooden or plastic spatula. The use of the cytobrush and extended-tip spatula may be the most effective way to collect endocervical cells for analysis.

Two specimens are immediately transferred to glass slides and are either sprayed with or immersed in a fixative solution. If the smear dries on the slide before the fixative is applied, the diagnosis will be inaccurate. The slides are sent to a laboratory for interpretation.

The liquid-based test (e.g., ThinPrep Pap Test) is an improved method of sample preservation. After the sample is obtained, the cells are rinsed into a vial filled with a preserving solution. The vial is sent to the laboratory, where an automated instrument separates the cells from blood and mucus. The thinner layer of cells can then be better visualized under a microscope, which improves the accuracy of the test (Buttin et al., 2006).

Follow-up Care. Provide the woman with a perineal pad, if needed, to protect her clothes from any bleeding from the cervix. The test results may be shared with the woman in person, by telephone, or by letter. Results are not left on answering machines, voice mail, or given to another person without the woman's permission. If a woman's smear has atypical cells, she is urged to have follow-up testing.

DNA Human Papillomavirus

The DNA human papillomavirus (HPV) test can identify 13 high-risk types of HPV associated with the development of cervical cancer. This test can be done at the same time as the Pap test for women older than 30 years and for women of any age who have had an abnormal Pap test result (American College of Obstetricians and Gynecologists [ACOG], 2005). It does not take the place of the Pap test because it tests for the viruses that can cause cell changes in the cervix that, if not treated, could lead to cancer. Cells are collected from the cervix and sent to a laboratory for analysis. Women who have normal Pap test results and no HPV infection are at very low risk for developing cervical cancer. Conversely, women with an abnormal Pap result and a positive HPV test are at higher risk if not treated.

Blood Studies

Serum levels of follicle-stimulating hormone (FSH), luteinizing hormone (LH), and prolactin are helpful in the diagnosis of male and female reproductive tract disorders. No nutrition restrictions are necessary before the test. Serum testing can also detect estrogen, progesterone, and testosterone levels in men and women. Chart 72-5 gives the normal values and the significance of abnormal findings.

Serologic studies detect antigen-antibody reactions that occur in response to foreign organisms. This form of diagnostic testing is helpful only after an infection has become well established. Serologic testing can be used in the evaluation of exposure to organisms causing syphilis, rubella, and herpes simplex virus type 2 (HSV2). Results may be read as nonreactive, weakly reactive, or reactive. A single titer is not as revealing as serial titers, which can detect the rise in antibody reactions as the body continues to fight the infection.

The Venereal Disease Research Laboratory (VDRL) test, the serologic test for syphilis (STS), and the rapid plasma reagin (RPR) test are used to detect, confirm, and monitor cases of syphilis. These tests are recommended for all pregnant women and persons at high risk for syphilis (Centers for Disease Control and Prevention [CDC] et al., 2006). These antigen tests are used to screen for the presence of nonspecific reagin antibodies that appear and increase in titer after infection. They are not totally specific or sensitive for syphilis, but they are economical and highly diagnostic. Some acute and chronic conditions that cause false-positive results include:

- Tuberculosis
- Infectious mononucleosis
- Recent smallpox vaccination
- Rheumatoid arthritis
- Systemic lupus erythematosus

Chart 72-5 LABORATORY PROFILE

Reproductive Assessment

Test	Normal Range for Adults	Significance of Abnormal Findings
SERUM STUDIES		
Follicle-stimulating hormone (FSH) (Follitropin)	*Men:* 1.42-15.4 IU/L *Women:* follicular phase, 1.37-9.9 IU/L; midcycle, 6.17-17.2 IU/L; luteal phase, 1.09-9.2 IU/L; postmenopause, 19.3-100.6 IU/L	Decreased levels indicate possible infertility, anorexia nervosa, neoplasm. Elevations indicate possible Turner's syndrome.
Luteinizing hormone (LH) (Lutropin)	*Men:* 1.24-7.8 IU/L *Women:* follicular phase, 1.68-15 IU/L, midcycle, 21.9-56.6 IU/L; luteal phase, 0.61-16.3 IU/L; postmenopause, 14.2-52.3 IU/L	Decreased levels indicate possible infertility, anovulation. Elevations indicate possible ovarian failure, Turner's syndrome.
Prolactin	*Men:* 0-20 ng/mL *Women:* 0-20 ng/mL *Pregnant women:* 20-400 ng/mL	Elevations indicate possible galactorrhea (breast discharge), pituitary tumor, disease of hypothalamus or pituitary gland, hypothyroidism.
Estradiol	*Men:* 10-50 pg/mL *Women:* follicular phase, 20-350 pg/mL; midcycle, 150-750 pg/mL; luteal phase, 30-450 pg/mL; postmenopause, ≤20 pg/mL	Elevations of estradiol, total estrogens, and estriol in men indicate possible gynecomastia, decreased body hair, increased fat deposits, feminization, testicular tumor; in women, ovarian tumor.
Estriol	*Men and nonpregnant women:* <2.0 ng/dL	Decreased levels or estradiol, total estrogens, and estriol in women indicate possible amenorrhea, climacteric, impending miscarriage, hypothalamic disorders.
Progesterone	*Men:* 10-50 ng/dL *Women:* follicular phase, <50 ng/dL; luteal phase, 300-2500 ng/dL; postmenopausal, <40 ng/dL	Decreased levels in women indicate possible inadequate luteal phase, amenorrhea. Elevations in women indicate possible ovarian luteal cysts. Decreased levels may indicate ovarian neoplasm, ovarian dysfunction.
Testosterone	*Men:* 280-1080 ng/dL *Women:* <70 ng/dL	Increased levels in men indicate possible testicular tumor, hyperthyroidism. Decreased levels in men indicate possible hypogonadism. Elevations in women indicate possible adrenal neoplasm, ovarian neoplasm, polycystic ovary syndrome.
Prostate-specific antigen	*Men:* <4 ng/mL	Increased levels may indicate prostatitis, benign prostatic hypertrophy, prostate cancer.
URINE STUDIES		
Total estrogens	*Men:* 4-25 mcg/24 hr *Women:* 4-60 mcg/24 hr	Elevations indicate possible testicular tumors. Decreased levels indicate possible ovarian dysfunction.
Pregnanediol	*Men:* 0-1.9 mg/24 hr *Women:* follicular phase, <2.6 mg/24 hr; luteal phase, 2.6-10.6 mg/24 hr	Elevations indicate possible luteal ovarian cysts, ovarian neoplasms, adrenal disorders. Decreased levels indicate possible amenorrhea.
17-Ketosteroids	*Men (20-50 yr):* 6-20 mg/24 hr *Women (20-50 yr):* 6-17 mg/24 hr Values decrease with age	Elevations indicate possible Cushing's syndrome, increased androgen or cortisol production, severe stress. Decreased levels indicate possible Addison's disease, hypopituitarism.

Data from Pagana, K.D., & Pagana, T.J. (2006). *Mosby's manual of diagnostic and laboratory tests* (3rd ed.). St. Louis: Mosby.
1 ng, 1 nanogram or 1 billionth of a gram; *1 pg*, 1 picogram or 1 trillionth of a gram; *mcg*, 1 microgram or 1 millionth of a gram.

- Subacute bacterial endocarditis
- Hepatitis
- Recent ingestion of alcohol

Test results vary with the stage of syphilis. The serologic test result is usually positive about 2 weeks after the patient has become infected. If the primary syphilis is treated, the serologic titers almost always return to nonreactive levels within 4 months.

If the VDRL or RPR test is positive, the diagnosis must be confirmed by a more specific test for *Treponema pallidum*, such as the fluorescent treponemal antibody absorption test (FTA-ABS). This expensive and time-consuming test is positive 4 to 6 weeks after infection. Most positive test results for *T. pallidum* remain positive for the rest of the person's life.

HIV testing should be offered to all patients ages 19 to 64 years, especially those with personal risk factors and adolescents who have ever been sexually active (CDC et al., 2006). (See Chapter 21 for further discussion.)

The *prostate-specific antigen (PSA)* test is used to screen for prostate cancer and to monitor the disease after treatment. PSA levels less than 4 ng/mL are normal. Elevated PSA levels, especially above 10 ng/mL, are associated with prostate cancer. Older men, particularly African-American men, often have a higher normal PSA, especially as they age. If combined with a digital rectal examination, almost 90% of all prostate cancers can be detected (Pagana & Pagana, 2006).

The patient should not ejaculate for at least 24 hours before the test to avoid a false-positive result. For the same reason, the blood for the PSA test should be drawn before the digital rectal examination (Pagana & Pagana, 2006).

Other Laboratory Studies

Secretions can be obtained from the vaginal pool at the beginning of a speculum examination. Specimens can also be obtained from the vaginal walls, labia, or vulva during the examination. The specimens are placed on glass slides and are treated with a *wet preparation* ("wet prep") such as saline or potassium hydroxide. The slides are examined under a microscope to confirm or rule out the presence of a pathogen. Table 72-2 lists common types of wet preparations used to diagnose selected vaginal problems.

Cultures identify pathogenic organisms and are used to determine the correct antibiotic therapy. The examiner obtains specimens for culture analysis from any discharge or orifice of the male or female reproductive system. Routine cultures and antibiotic sensitivity studies are performed when a nonspecific bacterial infection is suspected.

The culture to detect Neisseria gonorrhoeae is one of the most important in evaluating the reproductive system. This culture is the only means of confirming a diagnosis of gonorrhea in asymptomatic women. Cervical cultures can be taken after the Pap specimen is obtained. Specimens from men can be taken directly from any penile discharge. Additional specimens from men or women can also be obtained from the urethra, rectum, and throat. The swab is then placed in a culture tube and sent to the laboratory for incubation and analysis.

Cultures to detect *Chlamydia trachomatis* use antigen detection methods. Tissue cultures are the most accurate but are expensive and results take several days. Less expensive and more widely available are a direct immunofluorescent test and an enzyme-linked immunosorbent assay (ELISA) (Pagana & Pagana, 2006). Nucleic acid amplification tests can be used to detect *N. gonorrhoeae and C. trachomatis* in first-voided urine specimens or in specimens collected from the cervix (CDC et al., 2006). Cultures are taken from the cervix in women and from the urethra in men.

TABLE 72-2 Wet Preparations Used for the Diagnosis of Common Vaginal Problems

Wet Preparation	Vaginal Problems
Normal saline	Cervicitis Trichomoniasis Bacterial vaginosis Atrophic vaginitis
Potassium hydroxide (KOH)	Candidiasis *(Candida albicans, Monilia)* Bacterial vaginosis
Gram stain	Mucopurulent cervicitis

NCLEX EXAMINATION CHALLENGE

After completing an assessment of a 50-year-old African-American male, you counsel him about prostate screening. What statement by the client indicates that he understands your teaching?

A. "I'm not at risk for prostate cancer since no male in my family has ever had it."
B. "A PSA level of 4 ng/mL is too high and I might have prostate cancer."
C. "I need a yearly rectal and prostate examination, as well as a PSA screening."
D. "I don't need yearly prostate screening until I am 60 years old because I'm black."

evolve For the correct answer, go to http://evolve.elsevier.com/Iggy/.

Imaging Assessment

General X-rays

A kidney, ureter, and bladder (KUB) x-ray of the abdomen shows these structures and is used in the assessment of disorders of either the male or the female reproductive system. Pelvic masses, calcified tumors or fibroids, dermoid cysts, and metastatic bone changes may be seen. No specific preparation is needed.

Bone scans and chest x-rays may also be included in the workup of the patient with suspected metastatic cancer. They help determine the extent of the cancer spread and obstruction or displacement of the organs. These tests are discussed elsewhere in this text.

Computed Tomography

Computed tomography (CT) scans for reproductive system disorders involve the abdomen and the pelvis. They can detect and evaluate masses and lymphatic enlargement from metastasis. This scan can differentiate solid tissue masses from cystic or hemorrhagic structures.

Hysterosalpingography

A **hysterosalpingogram** is an x-ray of the cervix, uterus, and fallopian tubes and is performed after the injection of a contrast medium. This test is used to evaluate tubal anatomy and patency and uterine problems such as fibroids, tumors, and fistulas. The study should not be attempted for at least 6 weeks after abortion, delivery, or dilation and curettage. Other contraindications include reproductive tract infection and uterine bleeding.

The examination is scheduled in a radiology department 2 to 5 days after the end of the patient's normal menses. The scheduling is important to prevent the accidental flushing of a fertilized ovum from the fallopian tube or the exposure of a fetus to radiation.

The patient is usually instructed to take a laxative the evening before the test, followed by an enema or rectal suppository on the morning of the examination. These procedures reduce the distortion of the x-rays by gas shadows.

On the day of the examination, confirm the date of the patient's last menstrual period and record it in the medical record. Ask about allergies to iodine dye or shellfish. The patient signs a consent form for the procedure. Because discomfort is expected during the examination, premedication with analgesics or NSAIDs may be prescribed. Inform the patient that she may experience some nausea and vomiting, abdominal cramping, or faintness. Provide support and assistance with relaxation techniques.

The patient is placed in the lithotomy position. A speculum is inserted, and the cervix is viewed. Dye is injected through the cervix to fill and highlight the interior of the cervix, uterus, and fallopian tubes. If the fallopian tubes are patent, the contrast material spills into the peritoneal cavity. Usually, only two or three views are obtained to show the path and distribution of the contrast medium.

The patient may experience pelvic pain after the study and should receive analgesic drugs accordingly. She may also have referred pain to the shoulder because of irritation of the phrenic nerve. Provide a perineal pad after the test to prevent the soiling of clothes as the dye drains from the cervix. Instruct the woman to contact her health care provider if bloody discharge continues for 4 days or longer and to report any signs of infection, such as lower quadrant pain, fever, malodorous discharge, or tachycardia.

Mammography

Mammography is an x-ray of the soft tissue of the breast. Mammograms assess differences in the density of breast tissue. They are especially helpful in evaluating poorly defined masses, multiple masses or nodules, nipple changes or discharge, skin changes, and pain. Mammography can detect about 80% to 90% of cancers that are not palpable by physical examination. However, some actual cancers may not appear on mammography or may appear as benign (ACS, 2008).

In young women's breasts, there is little difference in the density between normal glandular tissue and malignant tumors, which makes the mammogram less useful for evaluation of breast masses in these women. For this reason, annual screening mammograms are not recommended for women younger than 40 years (ACS, 2008). In older women, the amount of fatty tissue is higher and the fatty tissue appears lighter than cancers. Cancer and cysts may have the same density. Cysts usually have smooth borders, and cancers often have starburst-shaped margins.

No dietary restrictions are necessary before the mammogram. Remind the patient not to use creams, powders, or deodorant on the breasts or underarm areas before the study because these products can show on the x-ray. If there is any possibility that the patient is pregnant, the test should be rescheduled. Explain the purpose of the examination and its anticipated discomforts. Provide a cover gown and adequate privacy to undress above the waist. The patient also needs support and may need time to express her concerns about the mammogram and the presence of any lumps.

The technician positions the woman next to the x-ray machine with one breast exposed. A film plate and the platform of the machine are placed on opposite sides of the breast to be examined. The technician includes as much breast tissue as possible between the plates. The woman may experience some temporary discomfort when the breast is compressed during the positioning and the test. The test takes about 15 minutes, but the patient is usually asked to wait until the films are developed in case a view needs to be repeated. Some facilities are now using digital imaging rather than films.

The woman should know when to expect the report of the results. Because this is a time when the woman is anxious about the health of her breasts, it is a good opportunity to teach or reinforce the importance of breast self-examination (BSE) and give instructions as needed.

DECISION-MAKING CHALLENGE
Coordination of Care

A 50-year-old Chinese woman comes to the clinic for an employment physical examination. She has difficulty speaking and understanding English, but her son is with her for the appointment. Her history reveals she has never had a Pap test or mammogram.

1. What other information about this patient would be useful?
2. What do you need to include in teaching this patient about the Pap test and mammogram?
3. How could you help her find health care resources in view of her ethnic background?
4. How will you demonstrate cultural appropriateness and sensitivity? (Remember that her son is with her.)

evolve For suggested answer guidelines, go to http://evolve.elsevier.com/Iggy/.

Other Diagnostic Assessment

Ultrasonography

Ultrasonography (US) is a technique that is routinely used to assess problems such as uterine fibroids, ovarian cysts, and pelvic masses. It can be used to monitor the progress of tumor regression after medical treatment. US is also helpful in differentiating solid tumors from cysts in breast examinations. In men, ultrasound can test for varicoceles, scrotal abnormalities, and problems of the ejaculatory ducts and seminal vesicles and the vas deferens (Pagana & Pagana, 2006).

No specific preparations are needed for this study. Women should have a full bladder to help view the uterus and to make the location of other structures more distinct with abdominal ultrasonography. A full bladder is not needed for breast, scrotal, transvaginal, or transrectal scans.

For an abdominal, breast, or scrotal scan, the technician exposes the area and applies oil or gel to the area to be scanned. These substances provide better transmission of sound waves from the transducer through the patient's skin. The transducer is moved in a linear pattern across the area being tested to outline and define soft-tissue masses and to differentiate tumor type, ascites, and encapsulated fluid.

For a *transvaginal* or *transrectal* scan, the transducer is covered with a condom or vinyl glove onto which transmission gel has been placed. The transducer is then inserted into the vagina or rectum as indicated.

The patient may want to watch the viewing screen with a brief explanation of the landmarks and structures seen. There is no special follow-up care for the patient after this procedure except to provide wipes to remove the gel.

Magnetic Resonance Imaging

Magnetic resonance imaging (MRI) uses a magnetic field and radiofrequency energy to scan for pelvic tumors. This scan distinguishes between normal and malignant tissues. MRIs are now being used in the diagnosis of breast cancer in women who have an inherited risk (ACS, 2008). Because of the expense, MRIs are not recommended for general screening.

Endoscopic Studies

Colposcopy

The colposcope allows three-dimensional magnification and intense illumination of epithelium with suspected disease. **Colposcopy** is suited for inspection of the cervical epithelium, vagina, and vulvar epithelium. This procedure can locate the exact site of precancerous and malignant lesions for biopsy.

The woman is placed in the lithotomy position and provided the same support as for a pelvic examination. The patient should not douche or use vaginal preparations for 24 to 48 hours before the test. This nearly painless procedure is better tolerated if it is explained in advance and if the instrument is shown to the patient.

Colposcopy provides accurate site selection for tissue biopsy. Therefore the patient should also be prepared for a biopsy. Materials for cytologic studies and biopsy should be readily available.

The physician locates the cervix or vaginal site through a speculum examination. Lubricants other than water should not be used. Cells in the area may be stained or left unstained to enhance visibility. The physician cleans and moistens the cervix with normal saline. This increases the visibility of vascular patterns and the junction between the columnar epithelium and the squamous epithelium. Acetic acid, 3%, is applied to the cervix to draw moisture from the tissue and to accentuate important features. The physician then uses a colposcope or colpomicroscope to inspect the area in question. A biopsy specimen may also be taken if abnormal cells are seen (Buttin et al., 2006). (See Cervical Biopsy section on p. 1657.)

After the procedure, assist the woman as you would for a pelvic examination, and provide supplies to clean the perineum. Also give her a perineal pad to absorb any dye or discharge. If a biopsy specimen is taken, additional follow-up care is needed.

Laparoscopy

Laparoscopy is a direct examination of the pelvic cavity through an endoscope. This procedure can rule out an ectopic pregnancy, evaluate ovarian disorders and pelvic masses, and aid in the diagnosis of infertility and unexplained pelvic pain. Laparoscopy is also used during surgical procedures such as:

- Tubal sterilization
- Ovarian biopsy
- Cyst aspiration
- Removal of endometriosis tissue
- Lysis of adhesions around the fallopian tubes
- Retrieval of "lost" intrauterine devices

A laparoscopy is used instead of a laparotomy for minor surgical procedures because it uses small incisions, involves less discomfort, and does not require overnight hospitalization.

Patient Preparation. The physician explains the procedure, risks (complications associated with the use of general anesthesia, postoperative shoulder pain, and the rare occurrence of infection or electrical burns), and anticipated discomforts and obtains the patient's consent. The procedure can be performed with either a regional or general anesthetic. Patients should expect mild discomfort from the incision site and may experience referred shoulder pain from phrenic nerve irritation (Lowdermilk, 2007a).

Procedure. The patient is anesthetized and placed in the lithotomy position. A urinary catheter is inserted to drain the bladder. The operating table is placed in a slight Trendelenburg position to cause the intestines to fall away from the pelvis. The cervix is held with a cannula to allow movement of the uterus during laparoscopy (Fig. 72-5). The surgeon inserts a needle below the umbilicus to infuse carbon dioxide into the pelvic cavity, which distends the abdomen and permits better visualization of the organs. After the trocar and cannula are in place in the abdominal cavity, the surgeon removes the trocar and inserts the laparoscope. The surgeon can then visualize the pelvic cavity and reproductive organs. Further instrumentation is possible through one or more small incisions. The laparoscope is removed at the end of the procedure, and the abdomen is deflated. The small incision is closed with absorbable sutures and dressed with an adhesive bandage.

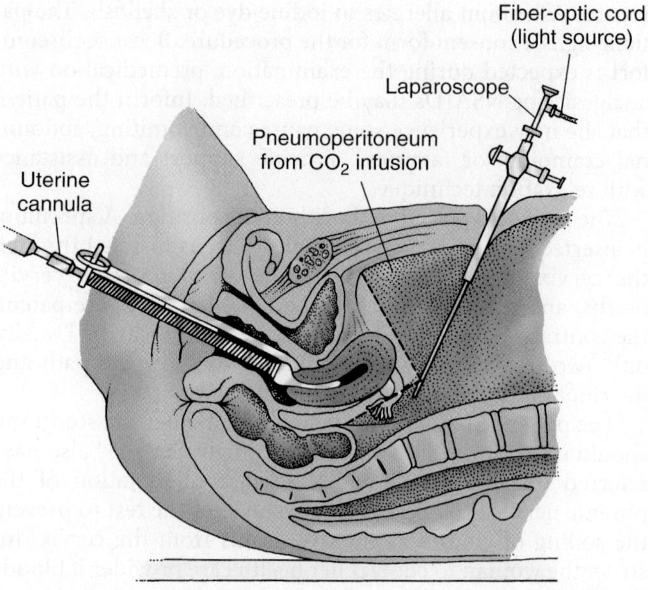
Fiber-optic cord (light source)
Laparoscope
Pneumoperitoneum from CO_2 infusion
Uterine cannula

Fig. 72-5 • Laparoscopy.

Follow-up Care. Care after surgery is similar to that for other patients after general anesthesia. The patient is usually discharged on the day of the procedure. Discomfort from the incision is managed by oral analgesics. The greatest discomfort is due to referred shoulder pain caused by residual gas in the peritoneal cavity. Most of these sensations disappear within 48 hours. Instruct the patient to change the small adhesive bandage as needed and to observe the incision for signs of infection or hematoma. Remind her to avoid strenuous activity for the first week after the procedure.

Hysteroscopy

Hysteroscopy is an endoscopic examination to view the interior of the uterus and the cervical canal. The hysteroscope includes a fiberoptic camera. Aqueous carbon dioxide is the medium used to distend the uterus. Hysteroscopy can be used for the removal of intrauterine devices and as a complement to other diagnostic tests for infertility and unexplained bleeding (Meniru & Hopkins, 2006).

The surgeon informs the patient of all aspects of the procedure and obtains consent. The preparation is the same as for a pelvic examination. The procedure is best performed 5 days after menses have ceased to reduce the possibility of pregnancy. The woman is placed in the lithotomy position and is usually anesthetized with a pericervical or other regional block.

After she is anesthetized, the cervix is dilated. The physician inserts the hysteroscope through the cervix. Because a medium distends the uterus, cells can be pushed through the fallopian tubes and into the pelvic cavity. Therefore hysteroscopy is contraindicated in patients with suspected cervical or endometrial cancer, in those with infection of the reproductive tract, and in pregnant patients.

Care is the same as that after a pelvic examination. Analgesics may be prescribed if the patient has cramping or shoulder pain.

Biopsy Studies

Cervical Biopsy

In a cervical biopsy, cervical tissue is removed for cytologic study. A biopsy is indicated for an identifiable cervical lesion, regardless of the cytologic findings. The health care provider usually performs a biopsy in conjunction with colposcopy as a follow-up to a suspicious Pap test finding. The procedure may be performed in a clinic or office setting.

Several techniques can be used for a cervical biopsy. If a lesion is clearly visible, an endocervical curettage can be performed as an ambulatory care procedure and with little or no anesthetic. **Conization** (removal of a cone-shaped sample of tissue) and loop electrosurgical excision procedures (LEEPs) are usually not done unless the cervical biopsy findings are positive or the results of the colposcopy are unsatisfactory (Lowdermilk, 2007b). Conization can be done as a cold-knife procedure, a laser excision, or an electrosurgical incision.

The biopsy is usually scheduled when the woman is in the early proliferative phase of the menstrual cycle, when the cervix is least vascular. Because a biopsy evaluates potentially cancerous cells, most women are anxious and need time to discuss their feelings and fears. The use of relaxation techniques may assist comfort. Assist the patient into the lithotomy position and prepare her in the same way as for a pelvic examination. Further preparation depends on the type of procedure to be performed.

The physician may anesthetize the patient according to the needs of the chosen procedure. He or she visualizes the cervix and obtains the tissue sample. All specimens are immediately placed into a formalin solution.

The type of anesthetic used for the procedure determines the type of immediate care needed after the procedure. Discharge instructions are listed in Chart 72-6.

Endometrial Biopsy and Aspiration

Both endometrial biopsy and aspiration are used to obtain cells directly from the lining of the uterus to assess for cancer of the endometrium. Biopsy also helps assess menstrual disturbances (especially heavy bleeding) and infertility (corpus luteum dysfunction).

Chart 72-6 PATIENT AND FAMILY EDUCATION GUIDE

The Patient Recovering from Cervical Biopsy

- Do not lift any heavy objects until the site is healed (about 2 weeks).
- Rest for 24 hours after the procedure.
- Report any excessive bleeding (more than that of a normal menstrual period) to your health care provider.
- Report signs of infection (fever, increased pain, foul-smelling drainage) to your health care provider.
- Do not douche, use tampons, or have vaginal intercourse until the site is healed (about 2 weeks).
- Keep the perineum clean and dry by using antiseptic solution rinses (as directed by your health care provider) and changing pads frequently.

When menstrual disturbances are being evaluated, the biopsy is generally done in the immediate premenstrual period to provide an index of progesterone influence and ovulation. A biopsy performed in the second half of the menstrual cycle (about days 21 and 22) evaluates corpus luteum function and the presence or absence of a persistent secretory endometrium. Postmenopausal women may undergo biopsies at any time.

Menstrual data are obtained from the patient and are included on the specimen request for the pathologist. The woman has the same preparation as for a pelvic examination. Advise her that she may experience some cramping when the cervix is dilated. Analgesia before the procedure and relaxation and breathing techniques during the procedure may be helpful.

An endometrial biopsy is usually done as an office procedure with or without anesthesia. After the uterus is measured and the cervix dilated, the physician inserts the curette or intrauterine cannula into the uterus. A portion of the endometrium is withdrawn using either the cuplike end of the curette or with suction equipment. The patient usually has moderate cramping. The specimens are placed into a formalin solution and sent for histologic examination.

Allow the woman to rest on the examining table until the cramping has subsided. Provide a perineal pad and a wipe to clean the perineum. Tell her that spotting may be present for 1 to 2 days but any signs of infection or excessive bleeding should be reported to the physician. Instruct the patient to avoid intercourse or douching until all discharge has ceased. Results of the biopsy are usually available within 72 hours.

Breast Biopsy and Aspiration

One of four different procedures may be used to biopsy breast tissue: needle aspiration, vacuum-assisted biopsy, an advanced breast biopsy instrument (ABBI) method, or surgical biopsy (incisional or excisional). *Aspiration* biopsy is the removal of fluid or tissue from the breast mass through a fine needle or large-bore needle (core-needle biopsy). Another method involves a vacuum-assisted device that is inserted through a small incision to draw multiple samples of tissue. The ABBI device is the newest procedure and is not available in all facilities. Like the surgical excisional biopsy, it can remove the entire lesion without sedating the patient (Carroll, 2006). An incisional biopsy is the surgical removal of some tissue from a breast mass. An excisional biopsy removes the mass itself for histologic (cellular) evaluation.

All breast masses should be evaluated for the possibility of cancer in women or, far less often, in men. Fibrocystic lesions, fibroadenomas, and intraductal papillomas can be differentiated by biopsy. Any discharge from the breasts is examined histologically.

The instructions to the patient depend on the type of biopsy and the type of anesthesia. Explain the procedure. Most biopsies are performed in an ambulatory care setting with or without an anesthetic. The mass is located by palpation of the breast. Aspirated fluid from benign cysts may appear clear to dark green–brown. Bloody fluid suggests cancer. If no fluid is aspirated, the mass is examined by one of the other biopsy methods.

Surgical biopsies are performed as same-day procedures with local or general anesthesia. The specimen undergoes histologic evaluation. If cancer is found, the tissue is sent to the laboratory for estrogen receptor analysis.

Discomfort after surgery is usually mild and is controlled with analgesics or the use of ice or heat, depending on the type and extent of the biopsy. Teach the patient how to assess the area or incision for bleeding and edema. Tell women to wear a properly supportive bra continuously for 1 week after surgery. Numbness around the biopsy site may last 2 to 3 months. Assess the patient's knowledge of breast self-examination, and provide instructions if needed. If cancer is identified, provide emotional support as well as information about follow-up treatment alternatives.

Needle Biopsy of the Prostate

When prostate cancer is suspected, the physician performs a needle aspiration biopsy of the prostate gland for histologic study. This procedure is often performed at the same time as cystoscopy, with the patient under anesthesia. The physician can perform needle biopsies without anesthesia or with the patient under local anesthesia.

Preparation for the procedure depends on the technique used to puncture the gland. Explain about the expected discomforts. Teach the patient about breathing and relaxation techniques for use during the examination. Because the purpose of this procedure is to evaluate prostate cells for cancer, the man needs support and time to discuss his fears. Preparation for a transrectal biopsy involves the use of cleansing enemas. Prophylactic antibiotics are given to reduce the risk for bacterial contamination of the blood or prostate tissue. Local anesthesia is used for transperineal biopsy.

The patent is placed in the same position as for a rectal examination. After injecting a local anesthetic for the transperineal biopsy, the physician places a finger in the rectum to help guide the needle to the prostate. For the transrectal biopsy, the physician places the needle against the examining finger and then inserts it into the rectum to the prostate. From this site, the needle is advanced through the rectal mucosa and into the prostate gland. The aspiration may be repeated several times to obtain a satisfactory specimen.

Although not common, sepsis is a life-threatening complication of transrectal biopsy. Teach the patient to report any manifestations of infection (e.g., fever, low back pain). Prophylactic antibiotics may be prescribed.

HUMAN NEEDS ASSESSMENT REVIEW

What should you expect to see in a patient without reproductive health problems that affect sexuality?

Physical Assessment

- No vaginal bleeding other than usual menstruation
- No unusual vaginal discharge
- No penile bleeding or discharge
- No masses or lesions on internal or external genitalia for men or women
- Reports ability to have intercourse without pain

Psychosocial Assessment

- Reports satisfaction with sexual activity
- Reports satisfaction with body image

Laboratory Assessment

- Sex hormones within normal limits for age
- Prostate-specific antigen within normal limits for age

GET READY FOR THE NCLEX EXAMINATION!

Key Points

Review these Key Points for each NCLEX Examination Client Needs Category.

Health Promotion and Maintenance

- Encourage all women to follow recommended Pap screening guidelines for early detection of precancerous and cancerous cells from the cervix.
- Assess cultural issues when identifying risks for certain reproductive problems and when evaluating health promotion practices.
- Assess and teach all women about breast and vulvar self-examination because these practices can lead to early identification of cancer and other conditions (see Chart 72-4).
- Assess/teach all men about performing testicular or genital self-examinations.
- Explain all diagnostic procedures, restrictions, and follow-up care to the patient scheduled for tests.
- Provide as much privacy as possible for patients undergoing examination or testing of the reproductive system.
- Ask all patients about the use of safer sex practices because sexually transmitted infections can increase the risk for some cancers and infertility, as well as unplanned pregnancy.

Psychosocial Integrity

- Allow the patient the opportunity to express fear or anxiety regarding tests of the reproductive system or regarding a potential change in sexual or reproductive function.
- Assess the patient's level of comfort in discussing issues related to reproduction and sexuality.
- Encourage patients to express feelings of anxiety or discomfort related to genital examinations.

Physiological Integrity

- Urge patients with pain, bleeding, discharge, masses, or changes in reproductive function to seek health care advice.
- Recall that reproductive changes occur with aging, as described in Chart 72-1.
- Selected laboratory tests used for diagnosing reproductive health problems are found in Chart 72-5.
- Teach women to report manifestations of infection to their health care provider after endoscopic procedures and biopsies of the breast, cervix, and endometrium.
- Instruct men to report manifestations of infection to their health care provider after a transrectal biopsy of the prostate.

Additional Study Resources

Go to your Companion CD or Evolve at http://evolve.elsevier.com/Iggy/ for *Self-Assessment Questions for the NCLEX Examination.*

Go to Evolve at http://evolve.elsevier.com/Iggy/ for *Prioritization and Delegation Questions for the NCLEX Examination.*

SELECTED BIBLIOGRAPHY

Asterisk indicates a classic or definitive work on this subject.

Alexander, R., La Rosa, J., Bader, H., & Garfield, S. (2007). *New dimensions in women's health* (4th ed.). Sudbury, MA: Jones & Bartlett.

American Cancer Society (ACS). (2008). *Cancer facts and figures 2008.* Atlanta: Author.

American College of Obstetrics and Gynecology (ACOG). (2005). *Screening tools for domestic violence.* Retrieved February 20, 2007, from www.acog.org.

Buttin, B., Herzog, T., & Mutch, D. (2006). Abnormal cytology and HPV. In M. Curtis, S. Overholtt, & M. Hopkins (Eds.), *Glass' office gynecology* (6th ed., pp. 80-106). Philadelphia: Lippincott Williams & Wilkins.

Carroll, C.M. (2006). Sorting out breast biopsy options. *Nursing2006, 36*(3), 70-71.

Centers for Disease Control and Prevention (CDC), Workowski, K., & Berman, S. (2006). Sexually transmitted diseases treatment guidelines, 2006. *Morbidity & Mortality Weekly Report (MMWR) Recommendations and Reports, 55*(RR-11), 1-94.

*D'Avanzo, C., & Geissler, E. (2003). *Cultural health assessment* (3rd ed.). St. Louis: Mosby.

*Fogel, C. (2007). Reproductive system concerns. In D. Lowdermilk & S. Perry (Eds.), *Maternity and women's health care* (9th ed., pp. 145-173). St. Louis: Mosby.

Hay-Smith, E., & Dumoulin, C. (2007). Pelvic floor muscle training versus no treatment, or inactive control treatments, for urinary incontinence in women. *Cochrane Database of Systematic Reviews, (1),* CD005654.

Lowdermilk, D. (2007a). Infertility. In D. Lowdermilk & S. Perry (Eds.). *Maternity and women's health care* (9th ed., pp. 235-254). St. Louis: Mosby.

Lowdermilk, D. (2007b). Structural disorders and neoplasms of the reproductive system. In D. Lowdermilk & S. Perry (Eds.). *Maternity and women's health care* (9th ed., pp. 276-312). St. Louis: Mosby.

Meniru, G., & Hopkins, M. (2006). Abnormal uterine bleeding. In M. Curtis, S. Overholtt, & M. Hopkins (Eds.), *Glass' office gynecology* (6th ed., pp. 80-106). Philadelphia: Lippincott Williams & Wilkins.

National Women's Health Information Center. (2006). *Menopause and hormone therapy.* Retrieved February 20, 2007, from www.4women.gov/menopause.

Pagana, K., & Pagana, T. (2006). *Mosby's manual of diagnostic and laboratory tests* (3rd ed.). St. Louis: Mosby.

Seidel, H., Ball, J., Dains, J., & Benedict, G. (2006). *Mosby's guide to physical examination* (6th ed.). St Louis: Mosby.

Speroff, L., & Fritz, M. (2005). *Clinical gynecologic endocrinology and infertility* (7th ed.). Philadelphia: Lippincott Williams & Wilkins.

U.S. Preventive Services Task Force. (2006). *The guide to clinical preventive services, 2005. Screening for cervical cancer.* AHRQ Publication No. 05-0570. Rockville, MD: Agency for Healthcare Research and Quality.

Wallace, M.A. (2008). Assessment of sexual health in older adults: Using the PLISSIT model to talk about sex. *AJN, 108*(7), 52-60.

Zdanuk, J. (2007). Assessment and health promotion. In D. Lowdermilk & S. Perry (Eds.), *Maternity and women's health care* (9th ed., pp. 88-124). St. Louis: Mosby.

73 CHAPTER

Care of Patients with Breast Disorders

Mary F. Justice

LEARNING OUTCOMES

For clinical competence and success on the NCLEX Examination, study this chapter with these Learning Outcomes in mind:

Safe and Effective Care Environment

1. Identify community resources for patients with breast cancer.
2. Discuss treatment options for breast cancer with patients and their partners.

Health Promotion and Maintenance

3. Describe the three-pronged approach to early detection of breast masses: mammography, clinical breast examination (CBE), and breast self-examination (BSE).
4. Teach a woman how to do BSE.
5. Explain the options available to a person at high genetic risk for breast cancer.
6. Evaluate patient risk factors for breast cancer.

Psychosocial Integrity

7. Explain the psychosocial aspects related to having breast cancer and undergoing treatments for breast cancer.
8. Discuss sexuality issues with the patient having breast surgery.
9. Assess the patient's acceptance of body image changes that can result from breast cancer surgery.

Physiological Integrity

10. Compare assessment findings associated with benign breast lesions with those of malignant breast lesions.
11. Explain the difference between breast reduction and breast augmentation.
12. Develop a postoperative plan of care for a patient with breast cancer.
13. Describe the role of radiation and drug therapy in the care of patients with breast cancer.
14. Provide information about complementary and alternative therapies.
15. Explain what options are available to a woman considering breast reconstruction.

Go to your Companion CD or Evolve at http://evolve.elsevier.com/Iggy/ for *Self-Assessment Questions for the NCLEX Examination* keyed to these Learning Outcomes.

Breast disorders in women may be benign or cancerous. Breast cancer also affects a small number of men. Women in North America have the highest rate of breast cancer in the world (American Cancer Society [ACS], 2008a). Many symptoms of this disease are the same as those seen in benign disorders, such as a breast lump. Although most lumps are benign, the discovery of a mass in the breast is a frightening experience for the patient and his or her family. The patient may fear cancer, losing a breast, possible treatments, or even losing his or her life.

Western society places a great emphasis on the breast as part of feminine beauty. Any threat to the breast has a significant effect on a woman's self-image and *sexuality.* She may feel unattractive to her partner and worry that their relationship will be negatively affected. She may be embarrassed at how she looks after treatment and refuse to look at herself. Members of the health care team need to be very supportive and acknowledge these feelings and concerns about the woman's perceived inability to meet her *human need for sexuality.* When caring for patients with breast problems, provide privacy and protect their dignity.

BENIGN BREAST DISORDERS

Most breast lumps are benign. Because the incidence of breast disease is related to age, breast disorders are described in an age-related order (Table 73-1).

FIBROADENOMA

Fibroadenomas are the most common benign tumor in women during the reproductive years. However, they also may occur in a few postmenopausal women. A **fibroadenoma** is a mass

TABLE 73-1 Typical Presentation of Benign Breast Disorders

Breast Disorder	Description	Incidence
Fibroadenoma	Most common benign lesion; solid mass of connective tissue that is unattached to the surrounding tissue	During teenage years into the 30s (most commonly)
Fibrocystic breast disease (FBD)	*First stage:* Characterized by premenstrual bilateral fullness and tenderness *Second stage:* Presence of bilateral, multicentric nodules *Third stage:* Presence of microscopic and macroscopic cysts	Late teens and 20s
Ductal ectasia	Hard, irregular mass or masses with nipple discharge, enlarged axillary nodes, redness, and edema; difficult to distinguish from cancer	Women approaching menopause
Intraductal ectasia	Mass in duct that results in nipple discharge; mass is usually not palpable	Women 40 to 55 yr of age

of connective tissue that is unattached to the surrounding breast tissue and is usually discovered by the woman herself or during mammography. Although the immediate fear is that of breast cancer, the risk for it occurring within a fibroadenoma is very small. On clinical examination, the tumors are oval, freely mobile, and rubbery. Their size varies from smaller than 1 cm (0.4 inch) in diameter to as large as 15 cm (6 inches) in diameter.

Fibroadenomas may occur anywhere in the breast. Enlargement is more likely in pregnancy. The health care provider may request a breast ultrasound examination or may perform a needle aspiration to establish whether the lump is cystic or solid. If the lesion is solid, ambulatory care excision using local anesthesia is sometimes the treatment of choice.

FIBROCYSTIC BREAST CONDITION

Pathophysiology

Fibrocystic changes of the breast include a range of changes involving the lobules, ducts, and stromal tissues of the breast. Because these changes affect at least half of women over the life span, they are now referred to as **fibrocystic breast condition (FBC)** rather than fibrocystic disease. This condition most often occurs in premenopausal women between 20 and 50 years of age and is thought to be caused by an imbalance in the normal estrogen-to-progesterone ratio. Typical symptoms include breast pain and tender lumps or areas of thickening in the breasts. The lumps are rubbery, ill defined, and commonly found in the upper outer quadrant of the breast (Hashmi, 2007).

The two main features of FBC are fibrosis and cysts. Areas of fibrosis are made up of fibrous connective tissue and are firm or hard. Cysts are spaces filled with fluid lined by breast glandular cells. Microcysts are small, nonpalpable cysts inside the breast glands. Macrocysts occur when fluid continues to build up. They often enlarge in response to monthly hormonal changes, stretching the surrounding breast tissue and become painful. Macrocysts are easily felt and can reach up to 2 inches across. Symptoms usually resolve after menstruation and then recur before the next menstrual period in a cyclic fashion. Breast ultrasound is used to confirm the presence of a cyst. Fine needle aspiration is used to drain the cyst fluid and reduce pressure and pain. Fluid may return, and more aspirations may be necessary. Older women receiving hormone replacement therapy may develop painful fluid-filled cysts. Having cysts or fibrosis does not increase a woman's chance of developing breast cancer. However, if a lump is very firm or has other features raising the concern about cancer, mammography is indicated. A needle biopsy or a surgical biopsy may be needed to make sure cancer is not present. Biopsy is indicated in these situations:

- No fluid is aspirated.
- The mammogram shows suspicious findings.
- A mass remains palpable after aspiration.
- The aspirated fluid reveals cancer cells.

Symptoms often resolve after menopause when estrogen decreases.

Patient-Centered Collaborative Care

Management of FBC focuses on the symptoms of the condition. Hormones are the main focus of drug therapy. Oral contraceptives can suppress oversecretion of estrogen, and progestins may be used to correct luteal insufficiency. Danazol (Danocrine, Cyclomen🍁) suppresses ovarian function and estrogen stimulation of breast tissue. However, because danazol does not cure FBC and because its side effects are undesirable, it is generally used only in patients with recurrent and severe fibrocystic disease.

Drug therapy may also include the use of vitamins C, E, and B complex. Diuretics may be prescribed to decrease premenstrual breast engorgement. Reduction of dietary fat and caffeine has been suggested, although most studies have questioned the role of caffeine and fat in FBC.

Encourage the patient to continue prescribed drug therapy and monitor the effectiveness of these interventions. Suggest supportive measures such as the use of mild analgesics or limiting salt intake before menses to help decrease swelling. Wearing a supportive bra can reduce pain by decreasing tension on the ligaments, although some women find that not wearing a bra is more comfortable. Local application of ice or heat may provide temporary relief of pain. Teach the patient to perform breast self-examination (BSE) on a regular basis.

DUCTAL ECTASIA

Ductal ectasia is a benign breast problem that is usually seen in women approaching menopause. It occurs when a breast duct dilates and its walls thicken, causing the duct to become blocked. The ducts in the subareolar area are most often affected. These ducts become distended and filled with cellular debris, which activates an inflammatory response. Two manifestations result from these changes:

- A mass develops that feels hard, has irregular borders, and may be tender.
- A greenish brown nipple discharge, enlarged axillary nodes, and redness and edema over the site of the mass are noted.

Ductal ectasia does not affect a woman's breast cancer risk. However, if a mass is present, it may be difficult to distinguish it from breast cancer. Because the risk for breast cancer is increased among women in the menopause age-group, accurate diagnosis is vital. A microscopic examination of the nipple discharge is performed to detect any atypical or malignant cells, and the affected area is excised. Nursing care is directed at reducing the anxiety associated with the threat of breast cancer and at supporting the woman through the diagnostic and treatment procedures. Ductal ectasia may improve without treatment. Warm compresses and antibiotics may be helpful. If symptoms do not improve, the abnormal duct may be surgically removed.

INTRADUCTAL PAPILLOMA

Intraductal papilloma occurs most often in women 40 to 55 years of age. A benign process in the epithelial lining of the duct forms a **papilloma** (pedunculated outgrowth of tissue). As it grows, trauma and erosion within the duct result in a bloody or serous nipple discharge. A mass is rarely palpable.

Diagnosis is aimed first at ruling out breast cancer. Microscopic examination of the nipple discharge and surgical excision of the mass and ductal area are usually indicated.

ISSUES OF LARGE-BREASTED WOMEN

Although Western society emphasizes large breasts as a positive attribute, women with excessive breast tissue often have health problems and discomfort. For instance, a woman with large breasts may have difficulty finding clothes that fit well and in which she feels attractive. The breast size may be out of proportion to the rest of the body, which adds to the problem of finding clothes that fit. Larger bras are expensive and may need to be specially ordered. The woman may have large dents in the shoulders from bra straps. In addition, many large-breasted women develop fungal infections under the breasts, especially in hot weather, because it is difficult to keep this area dry and exposed to air.

Backaches from the added weight are also common. The only alternative for this condition, if well-fitting bras do not help and obesity is not part of the problem, may be breast reduction surgery. The surgeon removes excess breast tissue and then repositions the nipple and remaining skin flaps to produce the best cosmetic effect. This operation is a major surgical procedure and is called a **reduction mammoplasty.**

The decision to have the procedure is usually made after years of living with the discomfort of excessive breast size. Listen to the woman verbalize her feelings, and reinforce information as appropriate. The nursing care after surgery is similar to that for the woman having reconstructive surgery. (See discussion of Breast Reconstruction, p. 1675, in the Surgical Management section.)

ISSUES OF SMALLER-BREASTED WOMEN

Some women choose to have **breast augmentation** surgery to increase or improve the size, shape, or symmetry of their breasts. Most health insurers do not pay for this procedure. Most surgeries involve the implantation of saline-filled or silicon prostheses. Some are constructed from the women's own tissue in much the same way as for reconstruction after mastectomy. *Saline* implants are filled with sterile saline and can be filled with the amount needed to get the shape and firmness the woman wants. If the implant shell leaks, the saline will be safely absorbed by the body. *Silicone* implants are filled with an elastic gel, which can leak into the breast and will not be absorbed. The plastic surgeon reviews the advantages and disadvantages of each implant or natural procedure.

Before surgery, teach the patient to stop smoking (to promote healing), avoid aspirin and other NSAIDs, and avoid herbs that can cause bleeding during the procedure, such as garlic, *Ginkgo biloba,* and ginseng. Tell her that the incisions will be hidden as much as possible, either under the pectoral muscle or directly behind the breast tissue as a submammary placement. One or more wound drains will be inserted during surgery, and she will need to know how to care for those drains at home. Review possible postoperative complications, including infection and prosthesis leakage, which can cause severe pain and possible fever.

After surgery, the patient can be discharged to home the same day or the day after. Someone should stay with her for at least 24 hours after surgery. The incisions may or may not have dressings intact, depending on the surgeon and type of surgery. Remind the patient that for the first few days she should expect soreness in her chest and arms. Her breasts will feel tight and sensitive, and the skin over her breasts may feel warm or may itch. She will have difficulty raising her arms over her head, and she should not lift, push, or pull anything until the surgeon deems it safe. Teach her to also avoid strenuous activity or twisting above her waist. Tell her to walk every few hours to prevent deep vein thrombi. Remind her to expect some swelling for 3 to 4 weeks after surgery.

An important issue for patients who have breast augmentation surgery is breast cancer surveillance. Breast self-examination (BSE) and clinical breast examination (CBE) are easily performed after prostheses are placed. The prosthesis is placed behind the woman's normal breast tissue, actually pushing it forward. Screening mammography, however, is sometimes not as sensitive because the amount of visualized breast tissue is decreased (McCarthy et al., 2007). Magnetic resonance imaging (MRI) or ultrasound may be a better screening option for women with breast augmentation. Women desiring cosmetic breast augmentation should be told about these differences in breast cancer screening.

GYNECOMASTIA

Gynecomastia literally means "female breasts" and is a symptom rather than a disease. It is usually a benign condition of breast enlargement in *men* (Fig. 73-1). However, gynecomastia can be a result of a primary cancer such as lung or testicular cancer. The enlargement is usually bilateral, but enlargement is asymmetric in about 10% of cases. The condition is caused by abnormal growth of the glandular tissue, including the mammary ducts and ductal stroma. In many instances, it is difficult to determine gynecomastia from breast enlargement related to excess adipose tissue. Other causes of gynecomastia include:

- Drugs, such as anti-androgen agents and corticosteroids
- Aging
- Obesity

- Underlying disease causing estrogen excess, such as malnutrition, liver disease, or hyperthyroidism
- Androgen-deficiency states, such as age, chronic kidney disease, or alcoholism

Although gynecomastia is not common, men with abnormal breast findings, especially a breast mass, should be carefully evaluated for breast cancer.

BREAST CANCER

Pathophysiology

Excluding skin cancers, breast cancer is the most commonly diagnosed cancer in women and is second only to lung cancer as a cause of female cancer deaths (ACS, 2008a). Therefore most references in this section are to women with breast cancer. Because of the high incidence of the disease, almost every woman knows of someone with the disease. Thus most women have strong reactions to the threat of breast cancer. These reactions greatly influence health habits, including breast self-examination (BSE) and the patient's readiness to seek care when a suspicious area is discovered. Nurses play a key role in early detection by educating women about screening guidelines, risk factors for breast cancer, and breast self-examination (BSE). Men should also be taught about this disease.

Early detection is the key to effective treatment and survival. The 5-year relative survival rate is lower for women who are diagnosed with an advanced stage of breast cancer. The 5-year survival rate for localized breast cancer is 98%, whereas the rate drops to 81% when the cancer has spread to the regional lymph nodes (ACS, 2008a). Survival drops dramatically when it is metastatic (spread to distant sites).

Cancer of the breast begins as a single transformed cell that grows and multiplies in the epithelial cells lining one or more of the mammary ducts or lobules. It is now identified as a heterogeneous disease in that many forms arise from several different types of cells, which may or may not have hormone receptors (Yang et al., 2007).

There are two broad categories of breast cancer: noninvasive and invasive. About 20% are *noninvasive;* the remaining 80% are invasive. As long as the cancer remains within the duct, it is noninvasive. The cancer is classified as *invasive* when it penetrates the tissue surrounding the duct. Most of these cancers arise from the intermediate ducts.

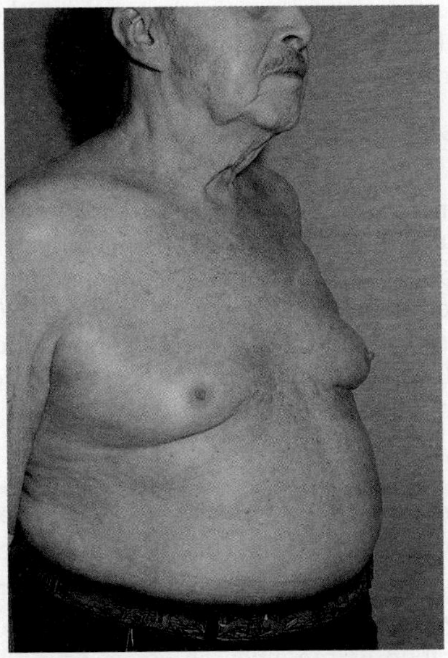

Fig. 73-1 • Gynecomastia.

Noninvasive Breast Cancers

Ductal carcinoma in situ (DCIS) is an early *noninvasive* form of breast cancer. In DCIS, cancer cells are located within the duct and have not invaded the surrounding fatty breast tissue. Because of mammography screening and earlier detection, the number of women with DCIS has increased. If left untreated, it may spread into the breast tissue surrounding the ducts over a period of years. It is then known as *invasive breast cancer. It is important to remember that although DCIS should be treated to prevent it from developing into an invasive breast cancer, it is not harmful at this stage.*

Another type of noninvasive cancer is **lobular carcinoma in situ (LCIS).** This cancer does not show up as a calcified cluster on a mammogram and is therefore most often diagnosed incidentally during a biopsy for another problem. Most of these cancers become invasive and have a high rate of also affecting the contralateral (other) breast. Treatment for LCIS is controversial.

Invasive Breast Cancers

The most common type of invasive breast cancer is **infiltrating ductal carcinoma.** As the name implies, the disease originates in the mammary ducts and grows in the epithelial cells lining these ducts. The rate of growth varies and partially depends on hormonal influences. Once invasive, the cancer grows into the tissue around it in an irregular pattern. For this reason, once the lesion is palpable, it is felt as an irregular, poorly defined mass. As the tumor continues to grow, **fibrosis** (replacement of normal cells with connective tissue and collagen) develops around the cancer. This fibrosis may cause shortening of Cooper's ligaments and the resulting typical skin dimpling that is seen with more advanced disease (Fig. 73-2).

A tumor can also invade the lymphatic channels, blocking skin drainage and causing skin edema, redness, warmth, and an "orange peel" appearance of the skin **(peau d'orange)** as shown in Fig. 73-3. This type of cancer is called *inflammatory breast cancer,* the most malignant of all breast cancers. Invasion of the lymphatic channels carries cancer cells to the lymphatic nodes, including those in the axillary region. For this reason, pathologic examination of the axillary nodes is needed for staging the disease. The cancer eventually replaces the skin

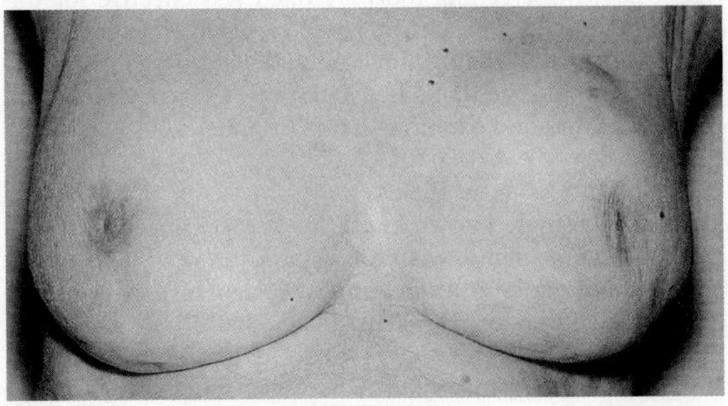

Fig. 73-2 • Skin dimpling on a breast as a result of fibrosis or breast cancer.

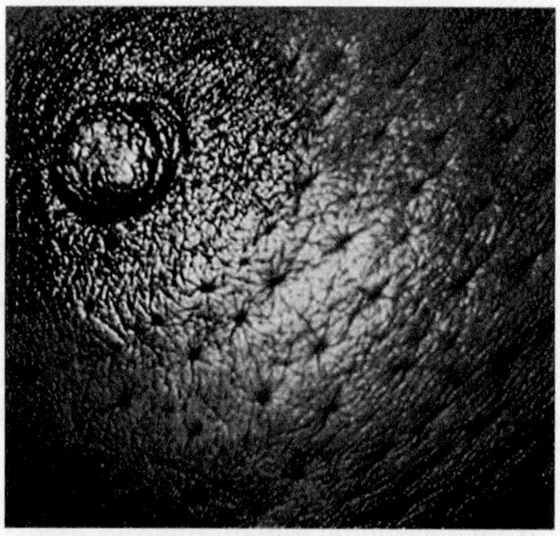

Fig. 73-3 • Breast edema giving the skin an "orange peel" (peau d'orange) appearance.

itself, and the overlying skin ulcerates. Metastasis results from seeding of the cancer cells into the blood and lymph systems, which permits spread of these cells to distant sites. The most common sites of metastatic disease from breast cancer are bone, lungs, brain, and liver.

The course of metastatic breast cancer is related to the site affected and to the function impaired. The processes involved in cancer development are described in Chapter 24.

Breast Cancer in Men

Less than 1% of all cases of breast cancer occur in men. The average age of onset is 60 years. Most cases occur in those with a genetic mutation in either the *BRCA1* or the *BRCA2* gene. (See discussion of genetic risk below.)

Men usually present with a hard, painless, subareolar mass. Gynecomastia may be present. Occasionally the man may have nipple discharge, retraction, erosion, or ulceration. Although nipple discharge is not a common manifestation, most men who present with nipple discharge are diagnosed with breast cancer. The disease is often widespread because it is usually detected at a later stage than in women. However, today survival rates are about the same for men as for women (www.cancer.org). Treatment of breast cancer in men is the same as in women at a similar stage of disease.

Breast Cancer in Young Women

A small number of breast cancers occur in women younger than 40 years (Young Survival Coalition, 2007). Younger women often present with more aggressive or later forms of the disease (ACS, 2008a). Screening tools are often less effective for this group because the breasts are denser. Younger women with breast cancer deal with unique physical and psychosocial aspects of the disease, including infertility after treatment and managing work and parenting issues (Manuel, 2007).

Etiology and Genetic Risk

There is no single known cause for breast cancer. *Being an older woman or man is the primary risk factor, although some people are at higher risk than others.* Family history is also an important risk factor (Nussbaum et al., 2007).

Although most breast cancers occur in women and men with no family history of the disease, having a first-degree relative (mother, sister, or daughter) with breast cancer doubles the risk for the disease. Having two first-degree relatives with breast cancer increases their risk fivefold (ACS, 2008a). This risk is further increased if the relative either had breast cancer in both breasts or was diagnosed before 40 years of age. Family history includes multiple relatives with breast cancer, early age at diagnosis, and in some families, ovarian cancer.

Breast cancer is usually a *sporadic* (not having a definite genetic pattern) rather than an inherited or a familial disorder. Many personal and environmental interactions are related to its development. Known factors that increase risk include exposure to high-dose ionizing radiation to the thorax (especially before 20 years of age), early menarche (before 12 years of age), and late menopause (after 50 years of age). A history of previous breast cancer, **nulliparity** (no pregnancies), and first birth after 30 years of age appear to increase risk. Table 73-2 lists known risk factors for breast cancer development.

GENETIC CONSIDERATIONS

Mutations in several genes, such as *BRCA1* and *BCRA2,* are related to hereditary breast cancer. People who have specific mutations in either one of these genes are at a high risk for developing breast cancer. However, only about 5% of all breast cancers are hereditary. Patients with these mutations have an increased risk for other cancers, including ovarian, renal, and possibly colon cancer. Children of a patient with a *BRCA1* or *BCRA2* germline mutation have a 50% chance of inheriting that mutation (Nussbaum et al., 2007). Ask the patient who has one or more of these risks if he or she wishes to talk with a genetics counselor or other genetics specialist.

Other causative risk factors not as well explained include nutrition and hormone replacement therapy (HRT). Alcohol is clearly linked to an increased risk for breast cancer. Having one or more alcoholic drinks a day increases the risk up to one and a half times (ACS, 2008b). A high-fat diet has not been clearly shown to be a risk factor for breast cancer, although obesity has been found to be a breast cancer risk in all studies (McCance & Huether, 2006). An increase in the risk for breast cancer has been shown in postmenopausal women receiving HRT after 5 or more years of use. HRT that includes the combination of estrogen and progesterone carries the highest increased risk (Reeves et al., 2006). Men who take anti-androgen agents for prostate cancer may also be at risk.

Incidence/Prevalence

In 2008, the projected breast cancer incidence was more than 183,000 women and 2,000 men in the United States. Of these, more than 40,000 women and 400 men are likely to die of the disease. Although these numbers are staggering, the trend is toward earlier diagnosis. In the years between 2001 and 2003, breast cancer incidence rates decreased. Researchers and clinicians think that this decline may be due to the decreased use of HRT after 2002 (Ravdin et al., 2006).

CULTURAL AWARENESS

One of every 8 U.S. women will develop breast cancer by age 70. Euro-American women older than 40 years are at a greater risk than other racial/ethnic groups, but African-American women *younger than 40 years* have breast cancer more often than others in that age-group. African-American women have a higher death

TABLE 73-2 Risk Factors for Breast Cancer

Factors	Comments
HIGH INCREASED RISK (RELATIVE RISK >4.0)	
Female gender	Ninety-nine percent of all breast cancers occur in women.
Age >65 yr	Incidence increases with age and peaks in the sixth decade.
Genetic factors	Inherited mutations of *BRCA1* and/or *BRCA2* increase risk.
Family history	Two or more first-degree relatives with breast cancer at an early age increases risk.
History of a previous breast cancer	The risk for developing a cancer in the opposite breast is 5 times greater than for the average population at risk.
Breast density	Dense breasts contain more glandular and connective tissue.
MODERATE INCREASED RISK (RELATIVE RISK 2.1–4.0)	
Family history	One first-degree relative with breast cancer moderately increases risk.
Biopsy-confirmed atypical hyperplasia	The overactive growth of cells increases risk.
Ionizing radiation	Women who received frequent low-level radiation exposure to the thorax had an increased risk, especially if the exposure occurred during periods of rapid breast formation.
High postmenopausal bone density	High estrogen levels over time both strengthen bone and increase breast cancer risk.
LOW INCREASED RISK (RELATIVE RISK 1.1–2.0)	
Reproductive history Nulliparity First child born after age 30	Childless women have an increased risk, as do women who bear their first child near or after age 30.
Menstrual history Early menstruation or late menopause, or both	The risk for breast cancer rises as the interval between menarche and menopause increases. Women who undergo bilateral oophorectomy before age 35 have only 40% of the risk for breast cancer than do women who undergo natural menopause.
Oral contraceptives	There is a slight increase in breast cancer risk in women taking oral contraceptives.
Hormone replacement therapy (HRT)	Recent and long-term use of hormone replacement therapy slightly increases risk.
Obesity	Postmenopausal obesity (especially increased abdominal fat), increased body mass, insulin resistance, and hyperglycemia have been reported to be associated with an increased risk for breast cancer.
OTHER RISK FACTORS	
Alcohol	The equivalent of two drinks per day may increase risk by 21%.
High socioeconomic status	Breast cancer incidence is greater in women of higher education and socioeconomic background. This relationship is possibly related to lifestyle differences, such as age at first birth.
Jewish heritage	Women of Ashkenazi Jewish heritage have higher incidences of *BRCA1* and *BRCA2* genetic mutations.

Modified from American Cancer Society. *Breast cancer facts & figures 2007-2008*. Atlanta: Author.

rate at any age when compared with other women with the disease (ACS, 2008a). The 5-year survival rate for African Americans is 76% compared with 90% for white people. Research suggests that poverty, less opportunity for education, and inadequate access to screening are related to higher cancer mortality rates in African Americans (ACS, 2008b).

The same factors may apply to American-Indian women. In addition, language barriers may affect their willingness to seek health care. Although they have a low rate of breast cancer, they have one of the poorest 5-year survival rates of all ethnic groups, especially in the southwestern United States. Robinson et al. (2005) found that education about disease prevention, detection, and management was lacking because of communication barriers among Navajo women living in the Four Corners area where Arizona, Utah, Colorado, and New Mexico meet. The authors found that videos and discussion were the most helpful tools in teaching Navajo women about breast cancer.

Like the African-American and American-Indian female population, Latino and Hispanic women have a lower incidence of breast cancer than white women but a higher death rate (ACS, 2008c). The differences in survival rates reflect the stage at which the cancer is diagnosed. Japanese-American women and native Hawaiian women also have a higher-than-average risk for breast cancer (ACS, 2008a). Difference in hormonal levels may help explain some of these variations (Setiawan et al., 2006).

Health Promotion and Maintenance

Early detection by screening for breast masses involves a three-pronged approach: mammography, breast self-examination (BSE), and clinical breast examination (CBE).

Mammography

The American Cancer Society (ACS) has established evidence-based guidelines for breast cancer screening in women. Guidelines have not been recommended for men. However, men at high risk (e.g., known genetic mutations) should be carefully monitored by their health care provider and should perform BSE.

The ACS recommends a baseline screening mammogram (x-ray of the breast) at 40 years of age and yearly screening for asymptomatic, low-risk women beginning at age 40 years (ACS, 2008a). In spite of the importance of mammograms in early breast cancer detection, many women do not get regular screening. Minority women, poor women, and women living in extremely rural areas are especially unlikely to get a mammogram (Paskett, 2006). Barriers to mammography include cost and access. Some women may not be able to afford the cost of a mammogram because they do not have health insurance, and free screening programs may be hard to find. The ability to get a mammogram that is timely and convenient is becoming more difficult for the growing aging population of women (Centers for Disease Control and Prevention [CDC], 2007). One reason is that a number of facilities that offer this test are closing and the prolonged waiting time to have a mammogram can be discouraging.

Breast Self-Examination

Breast self-examination (BSE) is an inexpensive means for detecting breast cancer that has been encouraged by health care providers for decades. The purpose of screening is *early detection, because BSE does not prevent breast cancer.* Detection of breast cancer *before* axillary node invasion increases the chance of survival. The American Cancer Society recommends monthly BSE as a screening option for all women beginning in their 20s. Most women have heard of BSE, but many do not practice it regularly or correctly. This discussion focuses on the female patient, but the BSE procedure is similar for men.

Whether the woman seeks health care because she has found a breast lump, because she needs a routine physical examination, or because she has an unrelated health problem, BSE should be taught. Do not assume that women who practice this examination do so correctly and regularly. Women who are taught BSE on an individual or group basis tend to practice BSE more often, more correctly, and more confidently than do women who learn the technique from pamphlets.

Preparation for Teaching Breast Self-Examination

Before teaching BSE, assess the psychological factors influencing the woman's motivation to practice it. Lack of knowledge about the technique and the benefits of early detection, uneasiness about self-assessment, and lack of confidence in self-assessment may be reasons women fail to perform BSE regularly. Stress that treatment for breast cancer is more successful when the disease is detected earlier. It is also important for the woman to develop confidence in her ability to detect breast changes. A yearly breast examination by a health care provider cannot substitute for BSE.

Emphasize the advantages of early detection, and review risk factors to determine the woman's risk for developing breast cancer. Ask her whether she has ever had a breast problem in the past. Women must believe that there are benefits to practicing BSE and that the barriers to practicing it are minimal.

Discussing the woman's fears, beliefs, and concerns about breast disease and BSE with her is an important step. Discuss the proper timing for BSE. Instruct premenopausal women to examine their breasts 1 week after the menstrual period. At this time, hormonal influence on breast tissue is decreased, so fluid retention and tenderness are reduced. Teach women whose breast tissue is no longer influenced by hormonal fluctuations, such as after a total hysterectomy or menopause, to pick a day each month to do BSE, such as the first day of the month.

Teaching Breast Self-Examination

Ensure that the setting in which you demonstrate BSE is private and comfortable. Ask the woman to undress from the waist up, and provide a gown and sheet. Before teaching breast palpation, ask the woman to demonstrate her own method. If she is unsure or has not performed BSE before, slowly lead her through the examination while explaining the rationale for the technique and answering questions. It is also helpful to point out different findings at this time, especially those that the woman might perceive as abnormal. For example, nodular breast tissue may normally feel lumpy, which may be interpreted as widespread cancer. Placing the woman's hand directly on the involved area and showing her precisely what is normal for her can build self-confidence.

Indicate the *inframammary ridge,* the area of the breast where the skin folds under the breast. This thickened area may be perceived as a lump instead of a normal finding. In thin or small-breasted women, the ribs may be mistaken for masses. Demonstrate how to follow the rib to the sternum to be sure that what she is feeling is bone and not breast tissue. Teach the woman to stand in front of a mirror to inspect the breast for abnormalities. She should raise her arms above her head and press her hands on her hips to emphasize any changes in the shape of the breasts. The breasts are examined in a lying position and while bathing or showering.

Demonstrate the proper amount of pressure needed to palpate the breast tissue and the correct position of the hands. The finger pads, which are more sensitive than the fingertips, are used when palpating the breasts. Teach the woman to press firmly enough to detect the underlying tissue.

Use teaching models of normal and abnormal breasts when teaching BSE. Demonstrate the correct technique of examining the breasts with the arm overhead while lying down instead of having the arm by her side. Showing the difference in the two positions, especially in large-breasted women, reveals the advantage of using the correct method, which spreads the tissue over the chest wall for more effective palpation (Fig. 73-4). Any one of three palpation methods can be used to examine the breast tissue (Fig. 73-5).

Clinical Breast Examination

Clinical breast examination (CBE) is typically performed by advanced practice nurses and physicians. However, nurses in general practice who are skilled in the technique can also perform the procedure. The examination can be done before, after, or during the teaching session. It is recommended that the CBE be part of a periodic health assessment, at least every 3 years for women in their 20s and 30s and every year for asymptomatic women at least 40 years of age (ACS, 2008a). Provide a private and comfortable setting, protect the patient's dignity, and allow time for discussion.

Taking a breast history is vital. Results may be recorded on a breast evaluation form, which is a part of the medical record (Fig. 73-6). This record helps establish the woman's risk for breast disease and the need for follow-up diagnostic tests, such as mammograms, and teaching.

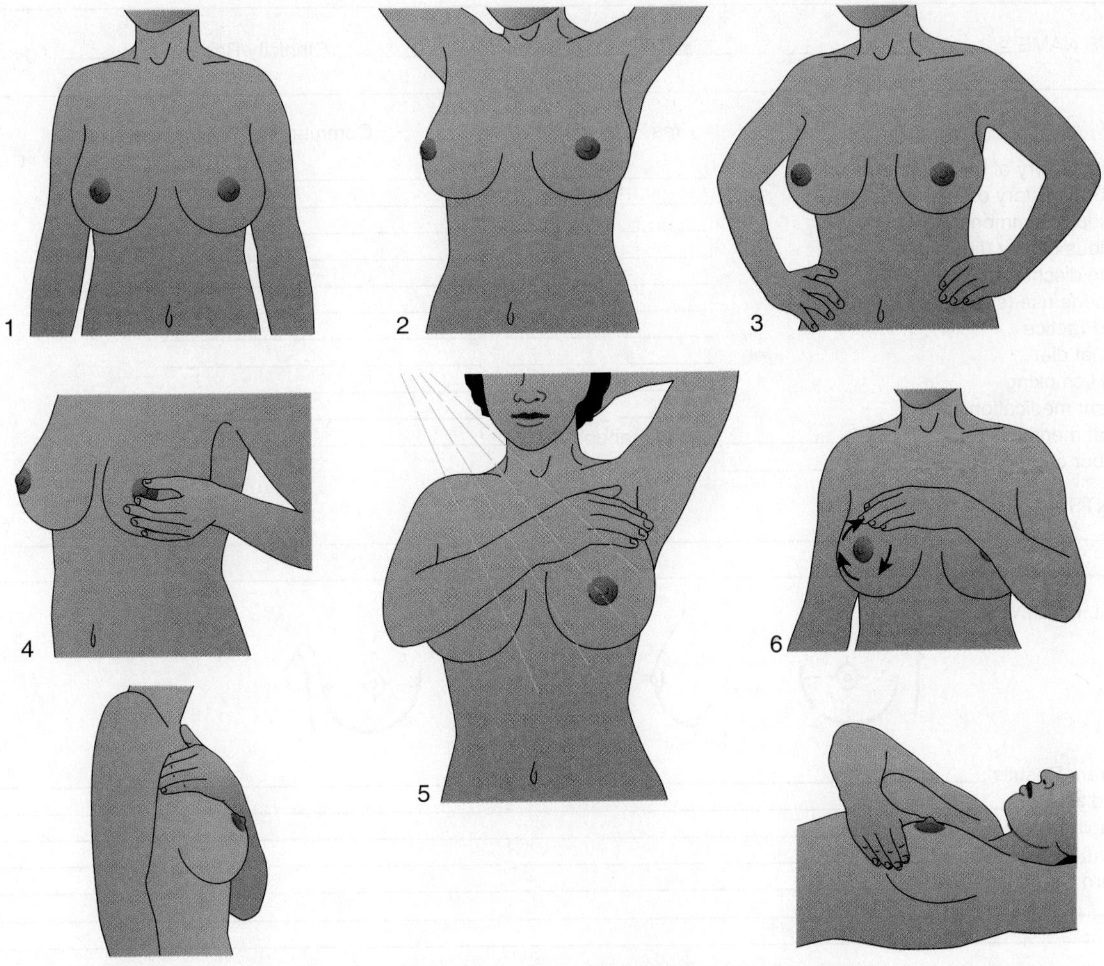
1
2
3
4
5
6

Fig. 73-4 • A woman performing breast self-examination (BSE).

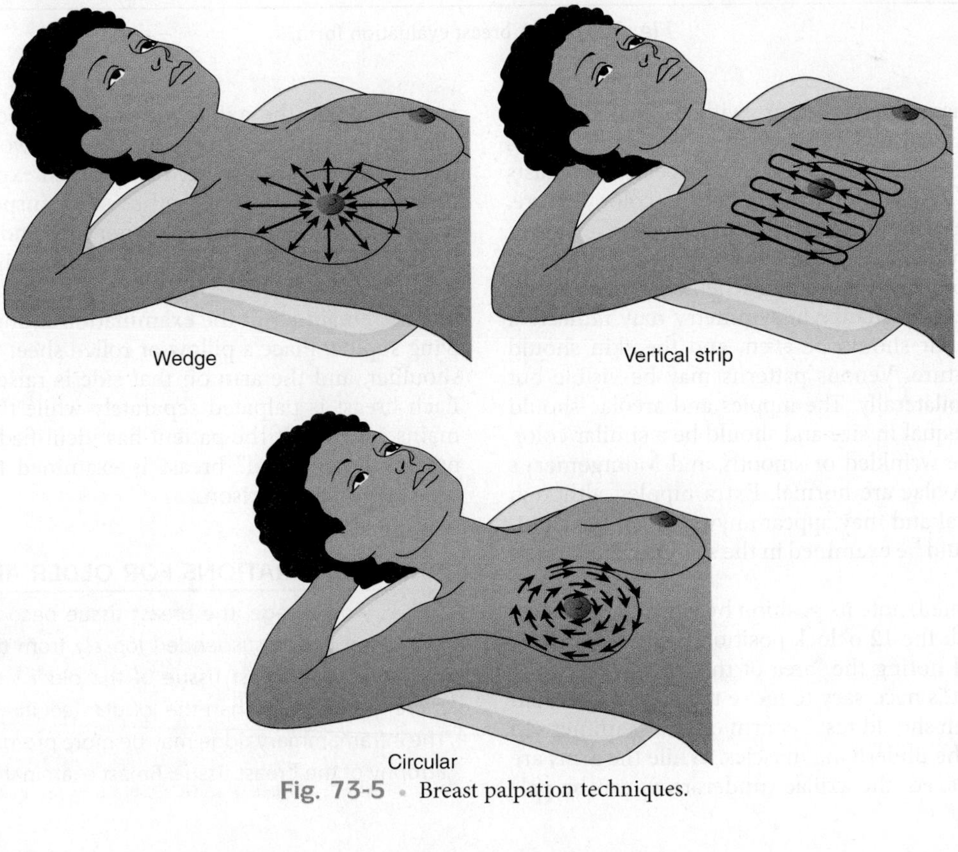
Wedge
Vertical strip
Circular

Fig. 73-5 • Breast palpation techniques.

PATIENT'S NAME ______ Gender ______ Ethnicity/Race ______ Age ______
Weight ______ Ideal Weight ______ Marital Status ______

HISTORY	Yes	No	Comments
Family history of breast cancer	____	____	____
Personal history of breast cancer	____	____	____
Previous mammograms	____	____	____
Previous biopsy (findings)	____	____	____
Nipple discharge	____	____	____
Hormone use (specify)	____	____	____
BSE Practice	____	____	____
High-fat diet	____	____	____
ETOH/smoking	____	____	____
Current medications (list)	____	____	____

Age at menses ______ Age at menopause ______
Number of pregnancies ______

COMMENTS ______

PHYSICAL FINDINGS

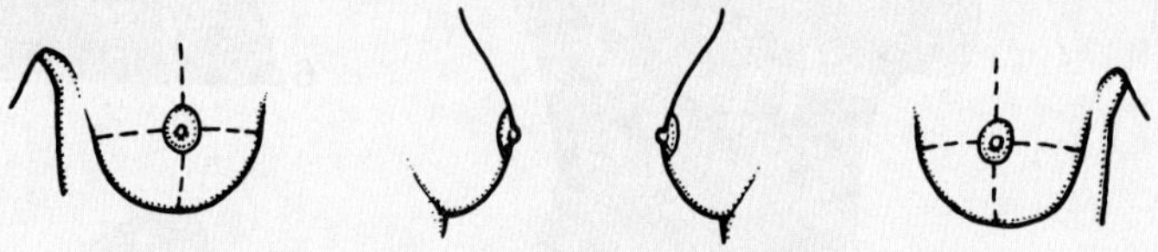

Mammogram Results ______
Ultrasound Results ______
Other Imaging Tests ______
Biopsy/Cytology Results ______
BSE Return Demonstration ______
Plan ______

PATIENT EDUCATION ______

Fig. 73-6 • A breast evaluation form.

VIDEO CLIP: Inspection (Sitting) ▶

The physical assessment begins with inspection. The woman undresses from the waist up and first sits or stands with her hands by her sides. The examiner inspects the breasts for symmetry and size, contour, skin changes (color, texture, and venous patterns), nipple changes, and lesions.

One breast may be larger than the other, and inverted nipples are common. Ask the woman whether these findings are normal for her. Any change in symmetry may indicate a problem. The contour should be even, and the skin should have a smooth texture. Venous patterns may be visible but should be similar bilaterally. The nipples and areolae should be equal or nearly equal in size and should be a similar color. The nipples may be wrinkled or smooth, and Montgomery's tubercles on the areolae are normal. Extra nipples, although rare, are also normal and may appear anywhere on the chest. If present, they should be examined in the same manner as the normal nipples.

If a mass is palpated, note its position by viewing the breast as a clock face (with the 12 o'clock position being toward the woman's head) and noting the "area of the clock" where the mass is located. If it is necessary to move the arms away from the body, the woman should rest her arm on the examiner's to prevent flexion of the underlying muscles. While the arms are by the side and relaxed, the axillae (underarms) can be palpated. Palpate the axilla and the area above and below the clavicle for enlarged lymph nodes. The woman is then asked to raise her arms over her head, which exposes the sides and underneath portions of the breast for inspection. Finally, she is asked to place her hands on her hips and press, thus flexing the pectoral muscles. This action shows skin dimpling, retractions, or masses.

◀ VIDEO CLIP: Inspection (Supine)

The remainder of the examination is done with the patient lying supine. Place a pillow or rolled sheet under the patient's shoulder, and the arm on that side is raised above the head. Each breast is palpated separately while the other breast remains covered. If the patient has identified a problem in one breast, the "normal" breast is examined first to establish a baseline for comparison.

CONSIDERATIONS FOR OLDER ADULTS

As women age, the breast tissue becomes flattened and elongated and is suspended loosely from the chest wall. On palpation, the breast tissue of the older woman has a finer, more granular feel than the lobular feel in a younger woman. The inframammary ridge may be more prominent as a result of atrophy of the breast tissue. Breast examination in older adults may be easier because of tissue atrophy and relaxation of the suspensory ligaments.

Women in nursing homes and other chronic care facilities often do not have clinical breast examinations or perform BSE. Be sure that those who are able learn and perform BSE. Collaborate with the health care provider to ensure that residents have clinical breast examinations.

Fig. 73-5 shows the three breast palpation techniques. The vertical strip method may be the best for ensuring that all breast tissue is examined. Every inch of the breast tissue should be palpated, including the tail of Spence, which extends from the upper outer quadrant of the breast into the axilla. The supraclavicular lymph nodes are palpated for the presence of enlarged nodes by hooking the fingers over the clavicle.

Finally, the nipple is gently compressed to detect the presence of a discharge. If a discharge is produced, note the "area of the clock" where the breast was compressed when the discharge was released. If there is a history of discharge, the woman may be able to express the discharge more successfully than the examiner can and should be asked to do so.

Discovery of a suspicious lesion or discharge during the examination requires referral to a health care provider who specializes in caring for breast disorders. Follow-up usually involves mammography and possibly ultrasound. If there is a dominant mass or high genetic risk, the woman should be referred for biopsy even if the mammogram is negative.

NCLEX EXAMINATION CHALLENGE

A 48-year-old client with a fibrocystic breast condition tells the nurse that she does breast self-examination but is concerned about getting cancer. What is the nurse's best response?

A. "Breast cancer only affects older women after 65 years of age."
B. "I'll make a referral to a genetics counselor as soon as possible."
C. "If you don't feel a lump on your breast, you don't have cancer."
D. "Be sure to have a mammogram and breast exam every year."

evolve For the correct answer, go to http://evolve.elsevier./com/Iggy/.

Options for High-Risk Women

Close surveillance is a prevention option preferred by most *high-risk* women. It is also referred to as "secondary prevention" and is used to detect cancer early in the initial stages. The same combination of breast self-examination (BSE), clinical breast examination (CBE), and mammography is recommended as in the asymptomatic population. The American Cancer Society recommends that high-risk women, such as those with a family history of breast cancer, also have an MRI and a mammogram every year beginning at age 30 (ACS, 2008a).

Prophylactic (preventive) **mastectomy** (surgical breast removal) is another option for reducing the risk for breast cancer. It remains a highly controversial practice. Even though a woman may decide to have a prophylactic mastectomy, there is a small risk that breast cancer will develop in residual breast glandular tissue because no mastectomy reliably removes all mammary tissue. Therefore when prophylactic mastectomy is chosen as an option, careful and regular long-term follow-up is indicated (ACS, 2008c). Prophylactic **oophorectomy** (removal of the ovaries) has been shown to decrease breast cancer risk in woman with genetic mutations of the *BRCA1* and *BRCA2* genes (Wirk, 2005).

Patient-Centered Collaborative Care

evolve ONLINE PHARM REVIEW

Assessment

History

Often, the history is taken after a mass has been discovered but before a diagnosis has been made for the man or woman with breast cancer. For some patients, the history may be obtained at the time they are seen for treatment of an identified cancer. The interview should focus on three major areas: risk factors, the breast mass, and health maintenance practices.

Record age, gender, marital status, weight, and height. Marital status and identifying the patient's primary support person provide information about who should be included in the patient's care, teaching, and support.

CULTURAL AWARENESS

Remember that some cultures do not allow the man to be part of a woman's care or only women are allowed to care for her (e.g., Arab Muslim women). Other cultures are male-predominant, and all decisions about female care are made by the man (e.g., Nigerian women). Chapter 4 describes additional general cultural considerations related to health care.

Ask specific information on personal and family histories of breast cancer. In addition to increasing the woman's own risk, these factors also affect any sisters' or daughters' risk and should be part of later counseling.

Ask about the woman's gynecologic and obstetric history, including:

- Age at menarche
- Age at menopause
- Symptoms of menopause
- Age at first child's birth
- Number of children/pregnancies

Prolonged hormonal stimulation (e.g., early menses, late menopause) increases a woman's risk, as do birth of the first child after 30 years of age and nulliparity (having no children).

A history of the breast mass or lump reveals not only the course of the disease but also information related to health care–seeking practices and health-promoting behaviors. Ask the patient about how, when, and by whom the mass was discovered and the time between discovery and seeking care. If the patient found the mass, ask if it was discovered through breast self-examination (BSE) or by accident? Was it found through a mammogram? The answer to this question reveals the need for discussion and teaching about BSE regardless of whether the mass proves to be cancerous. If there was a delay between discovery and seeing the health care provider, ask what caused the delay. These questions are linked to the psychosocial assessment but also reveal the length of time that the tumor has been present. Ask what procedures have been performed to diagnose the problem. Also, ask patients if they have noticed any other changes in their body within the past year. This information can help determine whether there has been obvious cancer spread. Ask especially about the presence of joint or bone pain.

A brief nutritional history, in which the patient is asked to recall a typical day's menu and alcoholic intake per week, reveals the usual intake of fat and alcohol. These factors may increase the risk for breast cancer.

Ask what prescribed and over-the-counter (OTC) drugs are used, specifically, hormonal supplements such as estrogen and natural or herbal substances that stimulate hormones. Estrogen can be taken orally, intravaginally, or via a transdermal patch. Document the type and form of hormones (birth control pills or patches, supplements) and length of use. Use of estrogen creams intravaginally is common among postmenopausal women and also is a source of estrogen.

Physical Assessment/Clinical Manifestations

Assess for and document specific information about the breast mass (Chart 73-1). Describe the mass in terms of location (using the "face of the clock" method), shape, size, consistency, and whether it is mobile or fixed to the surrounding tissues.

Assess and document any skin change, such as peau d'orange (dimpling, orange peel appearance), redness and warmth, nipple retraction, or ulceration, which can indicate advanced disease. Palpate the axillary and supraclavicular areas thoroughly, and document location of enlargements in the medical record. Evaluate the presence of pain or soreness in the affected breast. Document your assessment findings.

Psychosocial Assessment

The patient with potential or diagnosed breast cancer faces four major issues: (1) the fear of cancer; (2) threats to body image, *sexuality,* and intimacy; (3) decisional conflict related to treatment options; and (4) uncertainty about treatment outcomes and survival.

Assess the patient's need for information. Some people may not be ready for a lot of information at first. Most want to know how advanced the disease is, the likelihood of cure, treatment options and side effects, how treatment will affect their life and self-image, how family or partners will be affected, and home self-care. A previous experience with cancer, especially with other patients with breast cancer, influences the reactions to the disease. Ask patients whether they have known anyone with breast cancer and what types of experiences they have had with breast disease and cancer in general. Explore their feelings about the disease because choices of treatment, recovery, and ability to learn are influenced by these emotions. Assess patients' and families' knowledge of breast cancer, the stage of the disease, and treatment options. Patients' level of education is a significant influencing factor in their treatment choices. Dispel myths or misconceptions by providing current information. Many treatment centers now offer referrals to other breast cancer survivors who have gone through the same treatment. Talking with someone who has been through the experience is particularly helpful in dealing with the emotional aspects of the disease.

Also assess the patient for problems related to *sexuality.* Three critical areas of distress—psychological, physiologic, and relational—contribute to the psychosexual morbidity of these patients. Ask about the frequency of and satisfaction with sexual relations with the partner. Ask about whether and how the breast cancer has changed the intimate relations with, sexual function of, or types of touch by the partner.

Uncertainty is one of the most common experiences reported by women with breast cancer. They have frequent emotional changes and rely on support by family and friends as a coping strategy. Their perspective on life may change as they reflect on their own lives (Shaha et al., 2008).

Evaluate the need for additional resources at this time to help the patient deal with the issues they face. Will extra psychological counseling be needed? Are there financial concerns that need to be discussed with the case manager or social worker? Will the patient's partner, family, or friends support her or him throughout this period? How much support and teaching do they need? When and with whom does the patient expect to hear about the pathology results? Answers to these types of questions help identify expected outcomes for planning patient-centered collaborative care and providing support.

Chart 73-1 BEST PRACTICE FOR PATIENT SAFETY & QUALITY CARE

Assessing a Breast Mass

- Identify the location of the mass by using the "face of the clock" method.
- Describe the shape, size, and consistency of the mass.
- Assess whether the mass is fixed or movable.
- Note any skin changes around the mass, such as dimpling *(peau d'orange),* increased vascularity, nipple retraction, and ulceration.
- Assess the adjacent lymph nodes, both axillary and supraclavicular nodes.
- Ask patients if they experience pain or soreness in the area around the mass.

Laboratory Assessment

The diagnosis of breast cancer relies on pathologic examination of tissue from the breast mass. After the diagnosis of cancer is established, laboratory tests, including pathologic study of the lymph nodes, help detect possible metastases. Elevated liver enzyme levels indicate possible liver metastases, and increased serum calcium and alkaline phosphatase levels suggest bone metastases.

Imaging Assessment

Mammography is a sensitive screening tool for breast cancer. The uniqueness of this test results from its ability to reveal preclinical lesions (masses too small to be palpated manually). Many facilities now use *digital mammography* instead of traditional film mammography. The difference is in the image processing. Digital mammography allows the degree of contrast in the image to be manipulated so that contrast can be increased in dense areas of the breast (Pisano et al., 2005). Greater benefit from digital mammography has been shown in subgroups of women who were premenopausal, younger than 50 years, and had dense breasts (Pisano et al., 2005). A major limitation of digital mammography is that it costs up to 4 times more than film mammography. Patient preparation and the procedure for mammography are discussed in Chapter 72.

Ultrasonography of the breast is an additional diagnostic tool used to clarify findings on mammography. If the mammogram reveals a lesion, ultrasonography is helpful in differentiating a fluid-filled cyst from a solid mass. It also shows the shape of the mass. A newer test, *breast-specific gamma imaging (BSGI),* is available in larger medical centers to aid in the diagnosis when the mammogram is not conclusive. This test requires the patient to be injected with a small amount of tracing agent that concentrates in the tumor area if present. The agent emits x-rays that the imaging system can detect. Like ultrasonography, the results are available the same day and it may prevent unnecessary biopsies.

Other imaging procedures may be used before surgery to rule out metastases. A chest x-ray to screen for lung metastases is routine. Bone, liver, and brain scans and computed tomography (CT) scans of the chest and abdomen can reveal distant metastases.

Magnetic resonance imaging (MRI) may also be helpful in diagnosing breast cancer, especially when the mammogram is inconclusive. The American Cancer Society now recommends that women diagnosed with cancer in one breast have an MRI scan of the other breast to make sure there is no cancer there. Women at a high risk for breast cancer should have an annual MRI screening in addition to the recommended screening guidelines (ACS, 2008a).

Other Diagnostic Assessment

Pathologic examination of the breast tissue, or breast biopsy, is the key to diagnosis of breast cancer. Breast tissue is obtained by one of several types of biopsies (see Chapter 72). Tissue samples are analyzed for estrogen and progesterone receptors. These receptors are cytoplasmic proteins present in breast cancer cells that bind to estrogen and progesterone. In some cancers, when estrogen or progesterone binds to these receptors, the growth rate of the cell increases. Cancer cells that contain estrogen receptors (ER positive) or progesterone receptors (PR positive) have a better prognosis and usually respond to hormonal therapy. More postmenopausal women than premenopausal women are ER positive.

Most women, even those with very small tumors, receive some sort of treatment in addition to surgery for breast cancer. Recent research has focused on predicting the risk for recurrence in women treated for breast cancer so that low-risk women may avoid unnecessary treatments. Gene expression profiling systems, such as Oncotype DX and MammaPrint, can analyze certain patterns of genes in breast cancer tissue. It is hoped that these tests, along with other prognostic factors (size of the tumor, spread to lymph nodes, and hormone receptor status), will be able to predict which women will benefit from adjuvant therapy after surgery (Paik et al., 2006). Clinical trials are underway to assess the clinical benefit of these gene profiling systems. Other research has shown that new classifications of breast cancer, based on its molecular features, may be better able than the current classification system to predict prognosis and response to treatment.

Three breast cancer subtypes have been identified (Yang et al., 2007):

- *Luminal A and Luminal B types:* The luminal types are estrogen receptor positive, low grade, and tend to grow slowly. Luminal A cancers generally have a better prognosis than Luminal B cancers.
- *HER2 type:* This is a type of breast cancer in which the *HER2* or *neu* gene product is overexpressed. Because this gene is part of a family of cell growth factors, the *HER2* type is usually high grade, grows rapidly, and has a poor prognosis. About 25% of breast cancers are *HER2* positive. The targeted therapy *trastuzumab (Herceptin)* has been a successful treatment for this type of breast cancer.
- *Basal type:* This type of breast cancer lacks the estrogen receptors and has normal amounts of *HER2.* The basal type is high grade, grows rapidly, and has a poor prognosis. This type is common in young African-American women and in women with *BRCA* gene mutations (Carey et al., 2006).

The breast biopsy cells should be tested for *HER2* overexpression. The ImmunoHistoChemistry (IHC) test is a protein-based test used to determine the total amount of *HER2* protein receptors on the cell surface. A result of 2+ or 3+ is considered positive for overexpression.

Analysis

Common Nursing Diagnoses and Collaborative Problems

A common nursing diagnosis for patients with breast cancer is Anxiety/Ineffective Coping related to the diagnosis of cancer. A common collaborative problem is Potential for Metastasis.

Additional Nursing Diagnoses and Collaborative Problems

In addition to the common nursing diagnosis and collaborative problem, patients with breast cancer (particularly advanced breast cancer) may have one or more of these nursing diagnoses:

- Anticipatory Grieving related to loss and possible or impending death
- Acute Pain related to tumor compression on nerve endings
- Disturbed Sleep Pattern related to pain and anxiety
- Disturbed Body Image related to illness treatment, surgery, or loss of a body part
- Sexual Dysfunction related to surgery, disease process, or altered body structure

Planning and Implementation

Anxiety; Ineffective Coping

Planning: Expected Outcomes. The patient with breast cancer is expected to report the use of methods to help reduce anxiety and increase coping ability. Indicators include that the patient demonstrates these behaviors:

- Seeks information to reduce anxiety
- Uses and develops new and effective coping strategies
- Maintains social relationships

Interventions. The patient with breast cancer is usually admitted to the health care facility with a definitive diagnosis established through an outpatient biopsy of the mass. The practice of admitting a person with a suspicious lesion and using general anesthesia for a biopsy, frozen section, and possible mastectomy has largely been abandoned. Those who have an interval between the biopsy and treatment, during which they actively participate in the choice of treatment, cope more effectively after surgery, no matter which treatment is chosen.

The anxiety and uncertainty for the patient with breast cancer begins the moment the lump is discovered. These feelings may be related to past experiences and personal associations with the disease. The likelihood that the lesion is or is not cancer is not related to the level of fear. Assess the patient's perceptions of her or his own situation. Allow the patient to ventilate these feelings even if a diagnosis has not been established.

If the mass has been diagnosed as cancer, many people feel a partial sense of relief to be dealing with a known entity. A feeling of shock or disbelief usually occurs. It is difficult to accept a diagnosis of cancer when one feels basically well. Patients and their families or significant others deal in individual ways with the mix of feelings, which include shock, disbelief, and grief. Some may want to read and discuss any available information. Others may want to know as little as possible and resent attempts at teaching. Although some patients may want to talk at length about their concerns, others may want to be alone. Flexibility is the key to nursing care. Adjust your approach to care as the patient's emotional state changes. An integral part of the plan to meet these emotional needs is the use of outside resources. Most health care providers view such groups as the American Cancer Society's Reach to Recovery as a source of support after surgery, but these groups can be suggested in the preoperative phase.

Health care providers working with breast cancer may know other patients willing to make a preoperative visit. For example, the patient who is worried in particular about the side effects of radiation therapy may benefit more from talking to someone who has undergone radiation than from talking to the nurse or health care provider. Be sure to assess his or her preference.

Potential for Metastasis

NOC **Planning: Expected Outcomes.** The patient with breast cancer is expected to remain free of metastases or recurrence of disease, if possible.

Interventions. There are many surgical and nonsurgical options for breast cancer treatment. Because of the various options, the patient with breast cancer often faces difficult decisions. Management of the man with breast cancer is the same as that for a woman.

Although the 5-year survival rate for metastatic breast cancer is only 20%, patients are living longer with metastatic disease than ever before. This is due largely to the use of newer therapeutic agents (Gennari et al., 2005). Once cancer is diagnosed, the extent and location of metastases determine the overall therapeutic strategy. Treatment is tailored specifically to each patient, taking into account other health problems and the patient's ability to tolerate a particular therapy.

Nonsurgical Management. For patients with breast cancer at a stage for which surgery is the main treatment, follow-up with adjuvant radiation, chemotherapy, hormone therapy, or targeted therapy is commonly prescribed. For those who cannot have surgery or whose cancer is too advanced, these therapies are used to promote comfort (palliation). These options are discussed in the Adjuvant Therapy section on p. 1675.

Complementary and alternative therapies. Women with breast cancer must often cope with distressing symptoms related to the disease itself or the side effects of chemotherapy, radiation, and hormonal therapy. Common symptoms associated with these therapies include pain, nausea, hot flashes, anxiety, depression, and fatigue. Physical and emotional symptoms associated with breast cancer may be eased with the use of complementary and alternative medicine (CAM). Between 48% and 66% of breast cancer patients are using some form of CAM (Ernst et al., 2006). Table 73-3 lists the most widely used complementary therapies for specific symptoms associated with breast cancer and its treatments.

Although scientific research on most complementary therapies is relatively new and the studies are small, early results show benefits when they are combined with conventional medicine. For example, acupuncture may help relieve fatigue, hot flashes, nausea, vomiting, and pain. Yoga has been shown to improve physical functioning, reduce fatigue, improve sleep, and improve one's overall quality of life. Meditation helps reduce stress, improve moods, improve quality of sleep, and reduce fatigue. Prayer has been used to cope with many acute and chronic diseases. For example, a study by Morgan et al. (2005) showed that African-American couples obtained strength and increased coping with a breast cancer diagnosis by praying together, walking together, and being together.

TABLE 73-3 Complementary and Alternative Medicine (CAM) for Breast Cancer

Symptom	CAM
PHYSICAL	
Pain	Acupuncture, chiropractic therapy, hypnosis, massage, music, reiki, shiatsu
Nausea/vomiting	Acupuncture, aromatherapy, ginger, hypnosis, progressive muscle relaxation, shiatsu
Fatigue	Acupuncture, massage, meditation, reiki, tai chi, yoga
Hot flashes	Acupuncture, black cohosh, flaxseed
Muscle tension	Aromatherapy, massage, shiatsu
EMOTIONAL	
Anxiety/stress/fear	Aromatherapy, guided imagery, hypnosis, journaling, massage, meditation, music therapy, progressive muscle relaxation, prayer, support groups, tai chi, yoga
Depression	Aromatherapy, yoga, journaling, progressive muscle relaxation

Nutrition and nutritional supplements are used most often for relieving symptoms associated with breast cancer treatment (Lengacher et al., 2006). Current studies are being done on the effect of ginger on chemotherapy-induced nausea; results of previous studies have been mixed (National Center for Complementary and Alternative Medicine, 2007). Although lycopene (a nutrient found in tomatoes) was thought to help protect from breast cancer, results of studies on its value have been contradictory and inconclusive (Wane & Lengacher, 2006). *Encourage patients who are interested in trying CAM therapies to use them after checking with their health care provider regarding their safety.*

There is no proven benefit to using CAM alone as a cure for breast cancer. *Therefore complementary and alternative therapies are not recommended to be used instead of evidence-based treatment for breast cancer* (Ernst et al., 2006). Encourage open communication with patients about conventional therapy options and CAM. Cost may be a factor in decision making, since not all insurances provide coverage for CAMs. Teach the patient that all ingested CAM agents potentially risk interaction with conventional drugs (Itano & Taoka, 2005). Inform the patient that the NIH National Center for Complementary and Alternative Medicine is a very reliable source of information.

Surgical Management. The most common types of breast surgery are shown in Fig. 73-7. Although controversy exists concerning the best treatment for breast cancer, experts agree that the mass itself should be removed to reduce the risk for local recurrence. A large tumor is sometimes treated with chemotherapy, called **neoadjuvant therapy,** to shrink the tumor before it is surgically removed. An advantage of this therapy is that cancers can be removed by lumpectomy rather

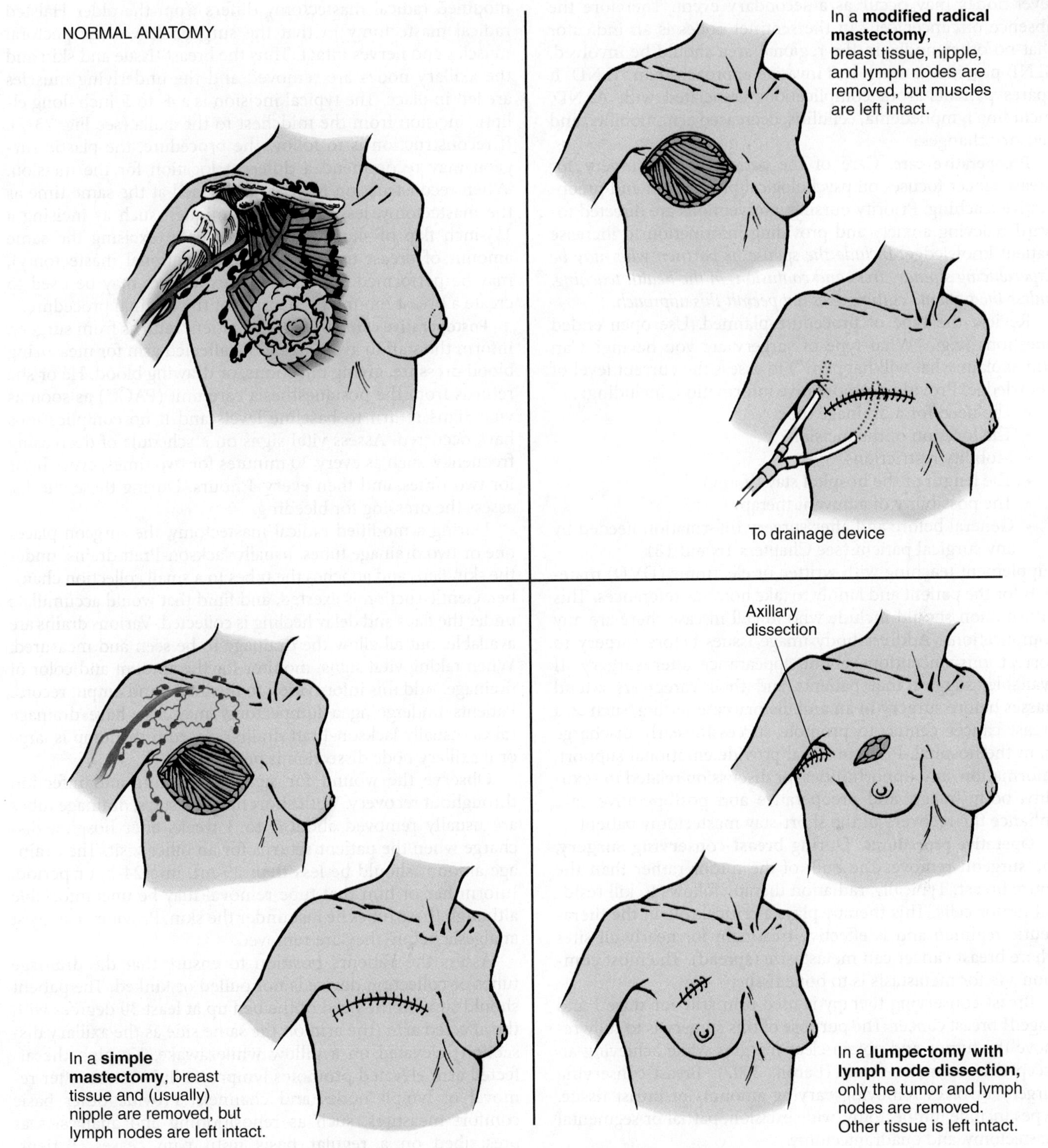

NORMAL ANATOMY
In a **modified radical mastectomy**, breast tissue, nipple, and lymph nodes are removed, but muscles are left intact.
To drainage device
Axillary dissection
In a **simple mastectomy**, breast tissue and (usually) nipple are removed, but lymph nodes are left intact.
In a **lumpectomy with lymph node dissection,** only the tumor and lymph nodes are removed. Other tissue is left intact.

Fig. 73-7 • Surgical management of breast cancer.

than mastectomy. Removal of the axillary lymph nodes for staging purposes may also be recommended. Axillary lymph node dissection (ALND) is usually performed for patients with palpable axillary lymph nodes.

As an alternative to ALND, sentinel lymph node biopsy (SLNB) may be performed. SLNB is an appropriate option for patients with early-stage invasive breast cancer who have a low to moderate risk for lymph node involvement. In this method, the sentinel lymph node is identified during breast surgery by injecting the breast with radioisotope and/or dye that travels via lymphatic pathways to the sentinel lymph node. The nodes that take up the dye (or give off a certain level of radiation picked up by a handheld counter) are removed and examined for the presence of cancer cells. It is believed that if cancer cells have traveled through the lymph channels, the cells will lodge in the sentinel nodes. Travel beyond these nodes to higher level nodes may occur as a secondary event. Therefore the absence of cancer cells in the sentinel nodes is an indicator that no other nodes in the regional area should be involved. SLNB provides a much less invasive approach than ALND. It spares patients from complications associated with ALND, including lymphedema, cellulitis, decreased arm mobility, and sensory changes.

Preoperative care. Care of the patient facing surgery for breast cancer focuses on psychological preparation and preoperative teaching. Priority nursing interventions are directed toward relieving anxiety and providing information to increase patient knowledge. *Include the spouse or partner, who may be experiencing similar stress and confusion, in the health teaching, unless the patient's culture does not permit this approach.*

Review the type of procedure planned. Use open-ended questions (e.g., "What type of surgery are you having? Can you explain what will happen?") to assess the current level of knowledge. Provide postoperative information, including:

- The need for a drainage tube
- The location of the incision
- Mobility restrictions
- The length of the hospital stay (if any)
- The possibility of adjuvant therapy
- General before and after surgery information needed by any surgical patient (see Chapters 16 and 18)

Supplement teaching with written or electronic (DVD) materials for the patient and family to take home as references. This information should include who to call in case there are any complications. Address body image issues before surgery to correct misconceptions about appearance after surgery. If available, suggest that patients and their caregivers attend classes before surgery in an ambulatory care setting, such as a breast cancer center, to promote successful early discharge from the hospital. Programs that provide emotional support, information, and opportunities for discussion related to sexuality, body image, and preoperative and postoperative care enhance the recovery of the short-stay mastectomy patient.

Operative procedures. During **breast-conserving surgery,** the surgeon removes the bulk of the tumor rather than the entire breast. Typically, radiation therapy follows to kill residual tumor cells. This therapy plays a critical role in the therapeutic regimen and is effective treatment for nearly all sites where breast cancer can metastasize (spread). The most common site for metastasis is to bone tissue.

Breast-conserving therapy is used primarily for stage I and stage II breast cancer. The purpose of this surgery is to fully remove the tumor and obtain clear margins while achieving an acceptable cosmetic result (Baron, 2007). Breast-conserving surgery involves removing varying amounts of breast tissue. Types include lumpectomy, wide excision, partial or segmental mastectomy, and quadrantectomy.

Breast-conserving procedures are usually performed in same-day surgical settings. The cosmetic results of these surgeries are good to excellent, and the psychological benefits of avoiding breast removal are significant for patients who choose this option.

The **modified radical mastectomy** does *not* conserve the breast; the affected breast is completely removed. Indications for a modified radical mastectomy include multi-centric disease (tumor is present in different quadrants of the breast), inability to have radiation therapy, presence of a large tumor in a small breast, and patient preference (Baron, 2007). The modified radical mastectomy differs from the older Halsted radical mastectomy in that the surgeon leaves the pectoral muscles and nerves intact. Thus the breast tissue and skin and the axillary nodes are removed and the underlying muscles are left in place. The typical incision is a 4- to 5-inch–long elliptic incision from the midchest to the axilla (see Fig. 73-7). If reconstruction is to follow the procedure, the plastic surgeon may recommend a different location for the incision. When reconstruction is to be performed at the same time as the mastectomy, less invasive techniques, such as incising a 1½-inch flap of skin around the nipple (excising the same amount of breast tissue as with conventional mastectomy), may be performed. Skin flaps or expanders may be used to create a breast mound at the time of the original procedure.

Postoperative care. Before the patient returns from surgery, inform the staff to avoid using the affected arm for measuring blood pressure, giving injections, or drawing blood. He or she returns from the postanesthesia care unit (PACU) as soon as vital signs return to baseline levels and if no complications have occurred. Assess vital signs on a schedule of decreasing frequency, such as every 30 minutes for two times, every hour for two times, and then every 4 hours. During these checks, assess the dressing for bleeding.

During a modified radical mastectomy, the surgeon places one or two drainage tubes, usually Jackson-Pratt drains, under the skin flaps and attaches the tubes to a small collection chamber. Gentle suction is exerted, and fluid that would accumulate under the flaps and delay healing is collected. Various drains are available, but all allow the drainage to be seen and measured. When taking vital signs, monitor for the amount and color of drainage. Add this information to the intake and output record. Patients undergoing a lumpectomy may also have drainage tubes (usually Jackson-Pratt drains) placed if the lump is large or if axillary node dissection is performed.

Observe the wound for signs of swelling and infection throughout recovery. With short hospital stays, drainage tubes are usually removed about 1 to 3 weeks after hospital discharge when the patient returns for an office visit. The drainage amount should be less than 25 mL in a 24-hour period. Inform her or him that tube removal may be uncomfortable although these tubes lie just under the skin. Provide or suggest analgesia before they are removed.

Assess the patient's position to ensure that the drainage tubes or collection device is not pulled or kinked. The patient should sit with the head of the bed up at least 30 degrees with the affected arm (the arm on the same side as the axillary dissection) elevated on a pillow while awake. Keeping the affected arm elevated promotes lymphatic fluid return after removal of lymph nodes and channels. Provide other basic comfort measures, such as repositioning and analgesics as prescribed on a regular basis until pain ceases. Patient-controlled analgesia may be used for some patients for a short time depending on the type of surgery that was performed.

The hospital stay after breast surgery is short, often same-day or just overnight, and recovery is usually not complicated. Because some managed care plans will not authorize an overnight stay in the hospital after a mastectomy, several states have enacted legislation mandating inpatient benefits. The patient who chooses an early discharge should have a home care visit within 24 hours of the discharge.

Ambulation and a regular diet are resumed by the day after surgery. While the patient is walking, the arm on the affected side may need to be supported at first. Gradually, the arm should be allowed to hang straight by the side. Instruct the patient to avoid the hunched-back position with the arm flexed because of the risk for elbow contracture. Beginning exercises that do not stress the incision can usually be started on the first day after surgery. These exercises include squeezing the affected hand around a soft, round object (a ball or rolled washcloth) and flexion/extension of the elbow. The progression to more strenuous exercises depends on the subsequent procedures planned (e.g., reconstruction) and the surgeon's prescription.

As soon as the patient is ambulatory and surgical pain is under control, he or she is discharged to home. Common instructions for exercises after mastectomy are listed in Chart 73-2.

Breast reconstruction. Breast reconstruction after or during mastectomy for women is common with few complications. Patients consult with the plastic surgeon to discuss the type of reconstruction, timing of the procedure, and technique desired. Many of them want breast reconstruction immediately after mastectomy using their own tissue (autogenous reconstruction). Breast reconstruction at the time of mastectomy, both autogenous and prosthetic, may lessen the psychological strain associated with undergoing a mastectomy.

The surgeon should offer the option of breast reconstruction before surgery is performed. If the woman does not choose immediate reconstructive surgery, a temporary prosthesis can be used. Some surgeons allow patients to use a temporary prosthesis in the immediate postoperative period as a part of the postoperative dressing. If this is the case, they return from surgery with a surgical bra and temporary sterile prosthesis in place. Refer them to the American Cancer Society's Reach to Recovery program (www.cancer.org). In this program, a volunteer who has had breast cancer surgery visits the woman at home, offering information on breast forms, clothing, coping with breast cancer, and possible reconstructive options. For this intervention to be as helpful as possible, the volunteer should be about the same age as the patient and have experienced the same surgical procedure.

Evaluate the woman's level of satisfaction with her prosthesis several weeks after surgery. Assess her attitude by asking about future plans for restoring appearance. Although reconstruction is not appropriate for some women and others may not be interested in it, the surgeon should discuss the indications and contraindications, advantages and disadvantages, and typical recovery. If immediate reconstruction is chosen, the surgeon should be aware of this before surgery so that plans can be coordinated with those of the plastic surgeon.

Several procedures are available for restoring the appearance of the breast (Table 73-4). Reconstruction may begin during the original operative procedure or later in one to several stages. Common types of breast reconstruction are (Baron, 2007):

- Breast expanders (saline or gel)
- Autologous reconstruction using the patient's own skin, fat, and muscle

Breast expanders are the most common method of breast reconstruction used today in the United States. A tissue expander is a balloon-like device with a resealable metal port that is placed under the pectoralis muscle. A small amount of normal saline is injected intraoperatively into the expander to partially inflate it. The patient then receives additional weekly saline injections for about 6 to 8 weeks until the expander is fully inflated. When full expansion is achieved, the tissue expander is then exchanged for a permanent implant during outpatient surgery. The permanent implant is filled with either saline or silicone gel. Concerns about silicone gel implants causing autoimmune and connective tissue disease were raised in the early 1990s, and the use of silicone gel implants was restricted to women in Food and Drug Administration (FDA)–approved safety studies. However, an extensive meta-analysis in 1996 found no evidence to support these concerns and the FDA restrictions were lifted (Baron, 2007). Silicone gel has been safely used in the majority of women who choose this type of breast implant.

Autologous reconstruction using the patient's own skin, fat, and muscle is advantageous because the donor site tissue is similar in consistency to the natural breast. Therefore the results more closely resemble a real breast as compared with implant reconstruction (Baron, 2007). Flap donor sites include the latissimus dorsi flap (back muscle); transverse rectus abdominis myocutaneous flap, known as the *TRAM flap* (abdominal muscle); and the gluteal flap (buttock muscle). Reconstruction of the nipple-areola complex is the last stage in the reconstruction of the breast. If necessary, a new nipple may be created with other body tissue, such as from the labia, abdomen, or inner thigh. Nursing care of the woman who has undergone breast reconstruction is outlined in Chart 73-3.

Adjuvant therapy. The decision to follow the original surgical procedure with **adjuvant therapy** (in addition to surgery) for breast cancer is based on:

- The stage of the disease
- The patient's age and menopausal status
- Patient preferences
- Pathologic examination
- Hormone receptor status
- Presence of a known genetic predisposition

Chart 73-2 PATIENT AND FAMILY EDUCATION GUIDE

Postmastectomy Exercises

HAND WALL CLIMBING

- Face the wall, and put the palms of your hands flat against the wall at shoulder level.
- Flex your fingers so that your hands slowly "walk" up the wall.
- Stop when your arms are fully extended.
- Slowly "walk" your hands back down the wall until they return to shoulder level.

PULLEY EXERCISE

- Drape a 6-foot-long rope over a shower curtain rod or over the top of a door. If you use a door for this exercise, have someone put a nail or hook at the top of the door so that the rope does not slip off.
- Grab the ends of the rope, one in each hand, and extend your arms out to your sides until they are straight.
- Keeping your arms straight, pull down with your left arm to raise your right arm as high as you can.
- Pull down with your right arm to raise your left arm as high as you can.

ROPE TURNING

- Tie a rope to the knob of a closed door.
- Hold the other end of the rope and step back from the door until your arm is almost straight out in front of you.
- Swing the rope in a circle. Start with small circles and gradually increase to larger circles as you become more flexible.

TABLE 73-4 Examples of Breast Reconstruction Procedures

Procedure	Description
Implantation	An implant matching the size of the other breast is placed under the muscle on the operative side to create a breast mound. 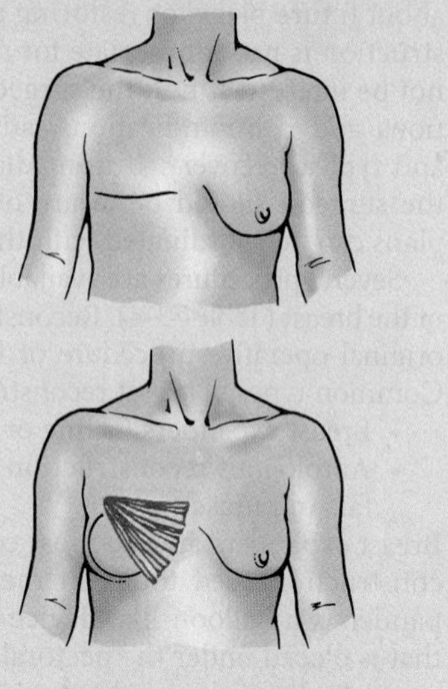
Tissue expansion	A tissue expander is placed under the muscle and gradually expanded with saline to stretch the overlying skin and create a pocket. After several weeks, the tissue expander is exchanged for an implant. 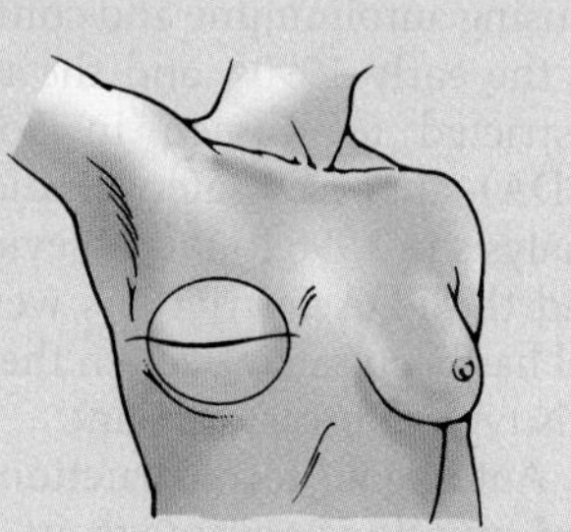
Myocutaneous flaps	A flap of skin, fat, and muscle is transferred from the donor site to the operative area. The flap contains an appropriate amount of fat to match the other breast and is similar in appearance to breast tissue. A blood supply is established by reanastomosis of vessels from the operative area to those with the flap when possible. A new nipple may be created with tissue from areas such as the labia or upper, inner thigh. Nipples can also be created by tattooing. Latissimus dorsi musculocutaneous flap 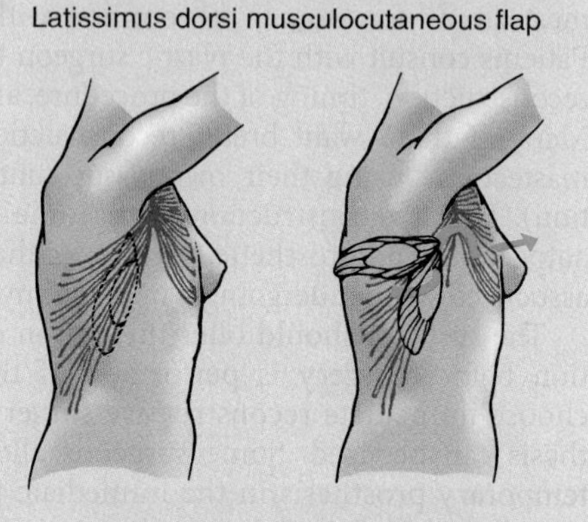 Abdominal myocutaneous flap 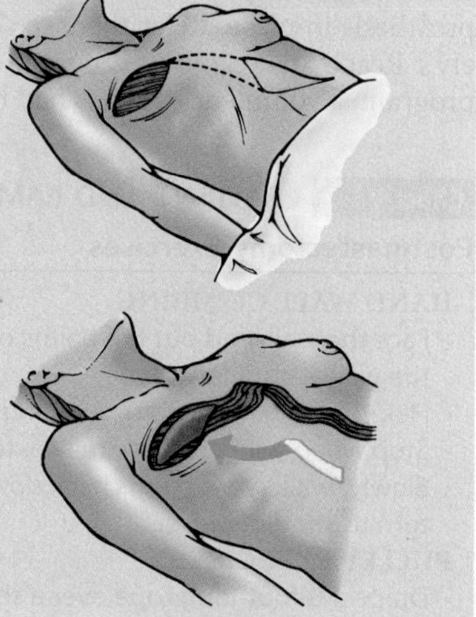

Adjuvant therapy consists of radiation therapy and drug therapy. The purpose of radiation therapy is to reduce the risk for local recurrence of breast cancer. Drug therapy consists of chemotherapy, targeted therapy, and/or hormonal therapy. These drugs destroy breast cancer cells that may be present anywhere in the body. They are typically delivered after surgery for breast cancer, although neoadjuvant chemotherapy may be given to reduce the size of a tumor before surgery. Hormonal therapy is a chemoprevention option for high-risk women with a personal history of breast cancer. The serum level of tumor antigens such as CA 15-3 and CA 27.29 are often monitored during and after therapy to determine the patient's response to therapy for metastatic breast cancer (Pagana & Pagana, 2006).

Radiation therapy. Radiation therapy is administered after breast-conserving surgery to kill breast cancer cells that may remain near the site of the original tumor. This therapy can be delivered to the whole breast or to only part of the breast. Until recently, the traditional method has been whole-breast irradiation delivered by external beam radiation over a period of 5 to 6 weeks. More recently, partial breast irradiation (PBI) has become an option for women with early-stage breast cancer. The types of methods available for delivering partial-breast irradiation include:

- Interstitial brachytherapy, in which several catheters loaded with a radioactive source are inserted at the lumpectomy cavity and surrounding margin, is given over a period of 4 to 5 days.

Chart 73-3 BEST PRACTICE FOR PATIENT SAFETY & QUALITY CARE

Postoperative Care of the Patient After Breast Reconstruction

- Assess the incision and flap for signs of infection (excessive redness, drainage, odor) during dressing changes.
- Assess the incision and flap for signs of poor tissue perfusion (duskiness, decreased capillary refill) during dressing changes.
- Avoid pressure on the flap and suture lines by positioning the patient on her nonoperative side and avoiding tight clothing.
- Monitor and measure drainage in collection devices, such as Jackson-Pratt drains.
- Teach the patient to return to her usual activity level gradually and to avoid heavy lifting.
- Remind the patient to avoid sleeping in the prone position.
- Teach the patient to avoid participation in contact sports or other activities that could cause trauma to the chest.
- Teach the patient to minimize pressure on the breast during sexual activity.
- Remind the patient to refrain from driving until advised by the physician.
- Remind the patient to ask at the 6-week postoperative visit when full activity can be resumed.
- Reassure the patient that optimal appearance may not occur for 3 to 6 months postoperatively.
- If implants have been inserted, teach the proper method of breast massage to enhance expansion and prevent capsule formation (consult with the physician).
- Review the breast self-examination procedure and the need to continue this practice monthly.
- Remind the patient that mammograms should be scheduled at least yearly for the rest of her life.

TABLE 73-5 Drug Therapy for Breast Cancer

Category	Mechanism of Action	Agents
CHEMOTHERAPY		
Anthracyclines	Inhibit DNA synthesis in susceptible cells	Doxorubicin (Adriamycin) (A) Epirubicin (Ellence) (E)
Taxanes	Inhibit microtubule network in rapidly dividing cells	Docetaxel (Taxotere) (D) Paclitaxel (Taxol) (P) Paclitaxel, protein-bound (Abraxane)
Alkylating agents	Interfere with the replication of susceptible cells	Cyclophosphamide (Cytoxan) (C)
Antimetabolites	Inhibit DNA synthesis and cellular replication in rapidly dividing cells	Methotrexate (Mexate) (M) Fluorouracil (5-FU) (F) Capecitabine (Xeloda)
TARGETED THERAPY	Selectively target critical steps in the processes required for tumor growth, viability, or invasion.	Trastuzumab (Herceptin) Bevacizumab (Avastin)
HORMONAL THERAPY		
LH-RH agonists	Block release of LH and FSH, thereby preventing ovarian production of estrogen	Goserelin (Zoladex) Leuprolide (Lupron)
Selective estrogen receptor modulators (SERMs)	Bind to estrogen receptors; have both agonist and antagonist properties (selectively block action of estrogen in the breast but not in other organs)	Tamoxifen (Nolvadex) Raloxifene (Evista)
Aromatase inhibitors	Prevent conversion of adrenal and ovarian androgens to estrogens by inhibiting the aromatase enzyme	Anastrozole (Arimidex) Letrozole (Femara) Exemestane (Aromasin)
Estrogen receptor down-regulators	Induce degradation of estrogen receptor	Fulvestrant (Faslodex)

FSH, Follicle-stimulating hormone; *LH,* luteinizing hormone; *LH-RH,* luteinizing hormone–releasing hormone.

- Balloon brachytherapy, also known as *MammoSite,* involves the use of a single balloon-tipped catheter that is surgically placed near the tumor bed. The catheter is loaded with a radiation source and inflated to conform to the total cavity. Ten total treatments are given, with at least 6 hours between each treatment.
- Intraoperative radiation therapy is the most accelerated form of partial breast irradiation. It utilizes a high single dose of radiation delivered during the lumpectomy surgery.

Nursing care for the patient undergoing radiation therapy involves education and side effect management. Skin changes are a major side effect during this therapy (see Chapter 24). If brachytherapy is planned, instruct patients about the procedure. Assure them that they will be radioactive only while the radiation source is dwelling inside the breast tissue.

Chemotherapy. Chemotherapy for breast cancer is delivered systemically. Its purpose is to kill breast cancer cells that may have left the original tumor and moved to more distant sites. Chemotherapy is usually used for stage II or higher breast cancer, although determination of when it is needed is controversial. As more scientific evidence emerges about the biology of tumors, it is hoped that the need for chemotherapy may be more specifically determined. Chemotherapy may be given before surgery to reduce the size of the tumor. Table 73-5 lists common agents used in breast cancer and their mechanism of action. They are usually delivered in four to six courses of treatment. Combination regimens of chemotherapy have been demonstrated to be more effective than single-agent treatments. A common chemotherapy regimen for breast cancer treatment is Cytoxan, Adriamycin, and 5-FU (CAF), but other combinations may be given. Regimens that contain anthracyclines appear to be more effective than regimens that do not include them. Recently, research has found that *dose-dense* chemotherapy improves survival rates. Using this approach, the patient receives more frequent dosing in shorter intervals. It is a safe method for breast cancer treatments, and the side effects can be managed with newer drugs.

Taxane combinations are commonly used to treat metastatic disease. Some chemotherapy agents are used as a second-line therapy, after another chemotherapy regimen has been used and has stopped working. These agents include protein-bound paclitaxel (Abraxane) and capecitabine (Xeloda).

Targeted therapy. Targeted cancer therapies are drugs that target specific characteristics of cancer cells, such as a protein, an enzyme, or the formation of new blood vessels. The advantage of targeted therapy over traditional chemotherapy is that targeted therapy does not harm normal, healthy cells and therefore it has fewer side effects. The best known targeted therapy for breast cancer is the monoclonal antibody *trastuzumab* (Herceptin). This drug targets the *HER2/neu* gene product in breast cancer cells. Formerly used only in patients with breast cancer metastasis, Herceptin is now used in the standard adjuvant setting as a first-line treatment for *HER2/neu*-positive breast cancers (Plosker & Keam, 2006). Bevacizumab (Avastin) inhibits tumor growth by targeting the growth factor *VEGF* and stopping the formation of new blood vessels that are needed to nourish the tumor.

Hormonal therapy. The purpose of hormonal therapy is to reduce the estrogen available to breast tumors to stop or prevent their growth. *Premenopausal* women whose main estrogen source is the ovaries may benefit from *LH-RH agonists* that inhibit estrogen synthesis. These drugs include leuprolide (Lupron) and goserelin (Zoladex), which suppress the hypothalamus from making luteinizing hormone–releasing hormone (LH-RH). When LH-RH is inhibited, the ovary does not produce estrogen.

Selective estrogen receptor modulators (SERMs) block the effect of estrogen in women who have estrogen receptor (ER)–positive breast cancer. SERMs are also used as chemoprevention in women at high risk for breast cancer and in women with advanced breast cancer. They are generally recommended to be taken for 5 years after breast cancer treatment (Barron et al., 2007). Tamoxifen has been shown to decrease breast cancer recurrence rates by up to 50%. Common side effects of SERMs include hot flashes and weight gain. Rare but serious side effects of these drugs include endometrial cancer and thromboembolytic events.

Aromatase inhibitors (AIs) are used in *postmenopausal* women whose main source of estrogen is the conversion of androgen to estrogen through the action of the enzyme *aromatase.* These drugs inhibit aromatase in this process, thereby reducing estrogen levels. AIs given in addition to tamoxifen have been shown to be more effective than tamoxifen alone in postmenopausal women (Boccardo et al., 2007). A major side effect, not seen with tamoxifen, is loss of bone density. Women taking AIs must be closely monitored for osteoporosis (Justice, 2007). Fulvestrant (Faslodex), a second-line hormonal therapy for postmenopausal women with advanced breast cancer, is used after other hormonal treatments have stopped working.

Nursing care for patients receiving drug therapy. Most chemotherapy for breast cancer is delivered via the IV route through an implantable venous access device. Oncology nurses need to be proficient in the preparation and administration of chemotherapy drugs and knowledgeable about various venous access devices. They must also be able to manage the distressing symptoms associated with side effects of chemotherapy. Chapter 24 discusses general nursing management of alopecia, nausea and vomiting, mucositis, and bone marrow suppression. Fatigue and sleep disturbance are often major concerns as side effects of chemotherapy. In their small study of women in the southwestern United States, Payne et al. (2006) found a relationship between biomarkers, such as melatonin and serotonin, with fatigue, sleep, and depressive symptoms in women with breast cancer. (See the Evidence-Based Practice box below.)

EVIDENCE-BASED PRACTICE

Are biomarkers related to side effects of chemotherapy in women with breast cancer?

Payne, J.K., Piper, B.F., Rabinowitz, I., & Zimmerman, M.B. (2006). Biomarkers, fatigue, sleep, and depressive symptoms in women with breast cancer: A pilot study. *Oncology Nursing Forum, 33*(4), 775-783.

A prospective, correlational, repeated-measures study was done to assess whether selected biomarkers such as melatonin, serotonin, and cortisol were related to patient-reported symptoms associated with chemotherapy. Twenty-two women, 11 who were cancer-free (control group) and 11 who were being treated for stage II breast cancer, were matched by age, ethnicity, and menopausal status. Questionnaires, sleep analysis, and laboratory biomarker analysis were used for all subjects. The results showed that fatigue and depression scores of the cancer group were much higher than those of the control group. Corresponding low serotonin and melatonin quantities were found in the cancer group but not the control group. The authors concluded that interventions studies should be done using this information to help increase sleep and decrease fatigue and depression in women receiving adjuvant chemotherapy. Also, they suggested that selective serotonin reuptake inhibitors and melatonin supplements might be helpful in decreasing these side effects.

Level of Evidence—5. Although this study was small, it used a control group and repeated variable measures.

Commentary: Implications for Research and Practice. The study sample was selected by convenience, but the study group was matched on selected variables with a control group. The authors used multiple measures for correlation, but no causal effects of the biomarkers on the symptoms can be made. A follow-up study using a larger sample and methodology to examine a causal effect would be helpful before intervention studies are undertaken. Nurses should be aware that fatigue is one of the biggest concerns of patients receiving chemotherapy, partially caused by sleep disturbances. Depression also contributes to these symptoms.

Chemotherapy is unpleasant and expensive and can have dangerous short-term and long-term side effects. Since more women are living longer with breast cancer, long-term effects are increasingly emerging. Although targeted therapy is effective with fewer side effects, some side effects are nevertheless life threatening. For example, cardiac toxicity is a risk associated with the use of Herceptin, particularly when it is combined with other chemotherapy. Chemotherapy and ovarian suppression can result in infertility, a devastating effect for women of childbearing age. Hormonal therapy can result in long-term ill effects from bone loss. Discuss patient concerns, provide accurate information, and assist him or her in decision making.

Stem cell transplantation. Autologous or allogeneic stem cell transplantation is an option for patients with a high risk for recurrence or who have advanced disease. **Autologous** bone marrow transplantation (taken from the patient's bone marrow), peripheral blood stem cell transplantation (taken from circulating blood), or **allogeneic** bone marrow transplantation (taken from a healthy donor's bone marrow or peripheral blood) is performed as a means of rescue therapy after very high doses of chemotherapy. The general care of the patient undergoing bone marrow or stem cell transplantation is discussed in Chapter 42.

DECISION-MAKING CHALLENGE

Coordination of Care

A 45-year-old Euro-American woman had a right modified radical mastectomy last night. She is being discharged today with two Jackson-Pratt drainage tubes and a small dry dressing. While you are providing home care teaching for her, she begins to cry and tells you that she thinks her husband is not going to be able to look at her anymore. She feels that he might be tempted to see other women and that their marriage of 20 years may be destroyed. Her daughter is going to drive her home today because he did not want to leave work, where he is a supervisor in a furniture plant.

1. What is your best response to this patient now?
2. What other health care team members of support services may be helpful to her and her husband?
3. What health teaching will you provide?
4. What community resources might you contact for support at home?

evolve For suggested answer guidelines, go to http://evolve.elsevier.com/Iggy/.

Community-Based Care

Home Care Management

In collaboration with the case manager, make the appropriate referrals for care after discharge. Preoperative teaching and arrangements for home care management and referrals (Reach to Recovery, social services, home care) can be started before surgery or other treatment.

The patient who has undergone breast surgery can be discharged to the home setting unless other physical disabilities exist. Some are discharged the day after surgery with Jackson-Pratt or other types of drains in place. Many patients are discharged to home on the day of surgery. Older adults should not be sent home without a family member or friend who can stay with them for 1 to 2 days. These patients may need some assistance at home with drain care, dressings, and ADLs because of pain and impaired range of motion of the affected arm. Summaries of continuing care instructions are given in Charts 73-4 and 73-5.

Teaching patients that activities involving stretching or reaching for heavy objects should be avoided temporarily. This restriction can be discussed with a family member or significant other who can perform these tasks or place the objects within easy reach.

Health Teaching

The teaching plan for the patient after surgery includes:

- Measures to improve body image

Chart 73-4 PATIENT AND FAMILY EDUCATION GUIDE

Recovery from Breast Cancer Surgery

- There may be a dry gauze dressing over the incision when you leave the hospital. You may change this dressing if it becomes soiled.
- A small, dry dressing will be around the site where a drain is placed. Often there is some leakage of fluid around the drain. Check the gauze dressing for drainage, and change it if it becomes soiled. Some leakage is normal, but if the dressing becomes soaked more than once a day, call your health care provider.
- You have been taught how to empty the reservoir from your drain and how to measure the volume of drainage. You should empty the drain twice a day and record the measurements.
- Drains are generally removed when drainage is less than 25 mL in 24 hours.
- Drains are often removed at the same time as the stitches or staples, generally 7 to 10 days after surgery.
- You may take sponge baths or tub baths, making certain that the area of the drain and incision stays dry. You may shower after the stitches, staples, and drains are removed.
- You can begin using your arm for normal activities, such as eating or combing your hair. Exercises involving the wrist, hand, and elbow, such as flexing your fingers, circular wrist motions, and touching your hand to your shoulder, are very good. You can usually resume more strenuous exercises after the drains have been removed.
- You can expect some discomfort or mild pain after surgery, but within 4 to 5 days most women have no need for pain medication or require medication only at bedtime.
- Numbness in the area of the surgery and along the inner side of the arm from the armpit to the elbow occurs in virtually all women. It is the injury to the nerves that causes sensation to the skin in those areas. Women have described sensations of heaviness, pain, tingling, burning, and "pins and needles." Neuropathic pain is sometimes relieved by gabapentin (Neurontin). These sensations change over the months and usually resolve by 1 year.
- Pamphlets on exercises, hand and arm care, and general facts about breast cancer are available from us or from a volunteer visitor. The American Cancer Society has volunteers who have had surgery similar to yours and are available to visit you.

Chart 73-5 HOME CARE ASSESSMENT

Patients Recovering from Breast Cancer Surgery

Assess cardiovascular, respiratory, and urinary status:
- Vital signs
- Lung sounds
- Urine output patterns

Assess for pain and effectiveness of analgesics.

Assess dressing and incision site:
- Excess drainage
- Manifestations of infection
- Wound healing
- Intact staples

Assess drain and site:
- Drainage around drain site and in drain
- Color and amount of drainage
- Manifestations of infection

Review patient's recordings of drainage.

Evaluate patient's ability to care for and empty drain.

Assess status of affected extremity:
- Range of motion
- Ability to perform exercise regimen
- Lymphedema

Assess nutritional status:
- Food and fluid intake
- Presence of nausea and vomiting
- Bowel sounds

Assess functional ability:
- Activities of daily living
- Mobility and ambulation

Assess home environment:
- Safety
- Structural barriers

Assess patient's compliance and knowledge of illness and treatment plan:
- Follow-up appointment with surgeon
- Manifestations to report to health care provider
- Hand and arm care guidelines
- Referral to Reach to Recovery

Assess patient and caregiver coping skills:
- Determine if patient and/or caregiver has looked at incision site.
- Assess their reaction to incision site.

- Information about interpersonal relationships and roles
- Exercises to regain full range of motion
- Measures to prevent infection of the incision
- Measures to avoid lymphedema
- Measures to avoid injury, infection, and swelling of the affected arm
- Care of the incision and drainage device

Teach incisional care to the patient, family, and/or other caregiver. The patient may wear a light dressing to prevent irritation. Explain that no lotions or ointments should be used on the area and that the use of deodorant under the affected arm should be avoided until healing is complete. Although swelling and redness of the scar itself are normal for the first few weeks, swelling, redness, increased heat, and tenderness of the surrounding area indicate infection and should be reported to the surgeon immediately. If a lymph node dissection was performed, instruct the patient to elevate the affected arm on a pillow for at least 30 minutes a day for the first 6 months. Ask the patient to have someone bring a loose-fitting, nonwired bra or camisole for her to try before discharge with a soft, cotton-filled or polyester fiber–filled form supplied by the hospital or by Reach to Recovery. The patient wears this form until the incision is completely healed and the health care provider approves the fitting of a more sophisticated prosthesis, usually 6 to 8 weeks after discharge. Encourage the patient to dress in loose-fitting street clothes at home, not pajamas, to further enhance a positive self-image.

Teach the patient to continue performing the exercises that began in the hospital. Active range-of-motion exercises should begin one week after surgery or when sutures and drains are removed. Emphasize that reaching and stretching exercises should continue only to the point of pain or pulling, never beyond that. ENCORE, a YWCA program, is appropriate for women as early as 3 weeks after surgery and includes exercise to music, exercise in water, and psychological support. Before discharge, the surgeon may prescribe precautions or limitations specific to plans for future procedures, such as reconstruction.

Provide information needed to help the patient avoid infection and subsequent lymphedema of the affected arm after the mastectomy. **Lymphedema** is an abnormal accumulation of protein fluid in the subcutaneous tissue of the affected limb after a mastectomy. Risk factors include injury or infection of the extremity, obesity, presence of extensive axillary disease, and radiation treatment (Baron, 2007). Lymphedema is a commonly overlooked topic in health teaching. Once it develops, it can be very difficult to manage and lifelong measures must be taken to prevent it. Nurses play a vital role in educating patients about this complication. Teach the importance of avoiding having blood pressure measurements taken on, having injections in, or having blood drawn from the arm on the side of the mastectomy. Instruct the patient to wear a mitt when using the oven, wear gloves when gardening, and treat cuts and scrapes appropriately. If lymphedema occurs, early intervention provides the best chance for control. The arm should be elevated when possible and special attention paid to the special precautions. A referral to a lymphedema specialist may be necessary for the patient to be fitted for a compression sleeve and/or glove, to be taught exercises and manual lymph drainage, and to discuss ways to modify daily activities to avoid worsening the problem. Management is directed toward measures that promote drainage of the affected arm. However, prevention is the best cure.

Psychosocial Preparation

Concerns about appearance after surgery are common and are often a threat to the patient's self-concept as a woman. Before breast surgery, the woman and her partner can benefit from an explanation of the expected postoperative appearance. After a modified radical mastectomy, the chest wall is fairly smooth and has a horizontal incision from the axilla to the midchest area. After breast-conserving surgery, scars vary according to the amount of breast tissue removed. Women are sometimes shown pictures of post-mastectomy reconstruction but are disappointed with their own results. Emphasize that scars will fade and edema will lessen with time. Scars may be red and raised at first, but these features lessen in the first few months. After surgery, encourage the woman to look at her incision when she is ready. Do not push her to accept this body image change immediately.

Much of one's body image is a reflection of how others respond. Therefore the response of the patient's family or partner to the surgery is crucial in determining the effect on self-concept. These people may also need the support of the nurse. They may have concerns about their ability to accept the changes and need to discuss these feelings with an objective listener. They may also need help with communicating their feelings, both negative and positive, with their loved one. Involving them in teaching may also help reinforce learning and increase retention.

Discuss sexual concerns before discharge. Young women and men in particular may perceive themselves as less sexually attractive and experience sexual problems after breast cancer surgery (Blakely & King, 2007). Most surgeons recommend avoiding sexual intercourse for 4 to 6 weeks. Patients may prefer to lay a pillow over the surgical site or to wear a bra, camisole, or T-shirt to prevent contact with the surgical site during intercourse. He or she may be embarrassed to discuss the topic of *sexuality.* Be sensitive to possible concerns, and approach the subject first.

For young women, issues related to childbearing may be a concern. Chemotherapy and radiation are considered serious teratogenic (birth defect–causing) agents. Advise sexually active patients receiving chemotherapy or radiotherapy to use birth control during therapy. The method and length of birth control should be discussed with the health care provider.

CONSIDERATIONS FOR OLDER ADULTS

For some older patients, issues such as fear and uncertainty about treatment outcomes, reduced functional status, concurrent chronic diseases, disease recurrence, future well-being and independence, and reduced social resources may be encountered. Older adults who have high physical functioning, emotional and social support, and a positive perception of medical interactions at the time they are diagnosed are likely to have good emotional health during follow-up care (Clough-Gorr et al., 2007).

Health Care Resources

Resources available to the patient after discharge include personal support and community programs. After discharge, the spouse or partner may need help in planning support for home responsibilities. For example, a partner who may be assuming additional duties at home and work may feel stressed. Discussing the need for ongoing emotional support is also beneficial to both the patient and partner. Leaving the hospital and appearing normal do not end the anxiety and fear. Identifying a support person with whom the patient or couple can explore these feelings and discussing the need to ventilate feelings enhance personal and family recovery.

Numerous support and educational resources are available to those diagnosed with breast cancer. There are over two million breast cancer survivors in the United States, and many women and men are active in breast cancer support and advocacy organizations. National breast cancer organizations are accessible online, and many of them have local affiliates. Examples of such organizations are Susan G. Komen for the Cure, the National Breast Cancer Coalition, Y-Me, Sisters Network, Young Survival Coalition, and Pink Ribbon Girls. Also, local support groups can be accessed through the health care provider, the local hospital, home care agencies, or by word of mouth. The American Cancer Society (ACS) (www.cancer.org) is an excellent resource for information and support. The ACS program Reach to Recovery provides a volunteer who visits the patient in the hospital or at home. She brings a personal message of hope, informational materials on breast cancer recovery, and a soft, temporary breast form.

Evaluation: Outcomes

Evaluate the care of the patient with breast cancer on the basis of the identified nursing diagnoses and collaborative problems. The expected outcomes include that he or she will:

- Be able to cope with the diagnosis by being knowledgeable, supported, and actively involved in decision making
- Remain free of metastasis

Specific indicators for these outcomes are listed for each nursing diagnosis and collaborative problem under the Planning and Implementation section (see earlier).

HUMAN NEEDS NURSING CARE REVIEW

What might you NOTICE if a patient is experiencing impaired sexuality as a result of breast cancer or other disorder?

- Breast swelling or lump (with or without pain)
- Discharge from nipple(s)
- Skin dimpling or orange peel appearance
- Asymmetric breast tissue
- Very large or very small breasts
- Skin redness and warmth

What should you INTERPRET and how should you RESPOND to a patient having impaired sexuality as a result of breast cancer or other disorder?

Perform and interpret physical assessment, including:

- Take a thorough patient and family history.
- Examine each breast, comparing sides, and document.
- Assess pain, and document.
- Assess psychosocial reaction to the breast changes.

Respond by:

- Checking recent mammogram test or other imaging assessment results
- Acknowledging patient's concerns about body image and sexuality changes

- Asking the patient about resources for support that have been used in the past for coping with crisis
- Preparing the patient for testing and possible biopsy
- Listening to the patient's concerns in a nonjudgmental manner

On what should you REFLECT?

- Consider what health care resources (team members) the patient and family will need throughout disease management.
- Think about what other community resources the patient and family will need.
- Observe the patient's progress in adapting to body image changes.

GET READY FOR THE NCLEX EXAMINATION!

Key Points

Review these Key Points for each NCLEX Examination Client Needs Category.

Safe and Effective Care Environment

- In collaboration with the health care team, identify community resources for patients with breast cancer, including Reach to Recovery of the American Cancer Society.

Health Promotion and Maintenance

- Identify patients at high risk for breast cancer, especially women with family history of breast cancer, those who have had early menarche, late menopause, or first pregnancy after 30 years of age, or those who are nullipara.
- Reinforce options that women who are high risk for breast cancer have, including close surveillance and prophylactic surgery.
- Teach women how to perform breast self-examination (BSE) as a means of early detection of breast cancer.
- Encourage women to have screening mammography according to recommended guidelines. Baseline screening should begin at 40 years of age and continue yearly. In high-risk women, screening should be started earlier.
- Encourage women to have clinical breast examination (CBE) according to recommended guidelines.

Psychosocial Integrity

- Assess patients' reactions to the diagnosis of breast cancer and the effect of breast cancer treatment on their body image and sexuality.
- Identify resources that facilitate their grief work and coping skills.
- Allow patients opportunities to express feelings of grief, fear, and anxiety.
- Teach women ways to minimize surgical area deformity and enhance body image, such as use of a breast prosthesis or the option of breast reconstruction.
- Address the reactions of family and significant others to the diagnosis of breast cancer; provide support and education.

Physiological Integrity

- Assess benign lumps as mobile and round or oval; assess possible malignant lumps as fixed and irregularly shaped, often in the upper outer breast quadrant.
- A breast reduction is an option for women with very large, heavy breasts to promote comfort.
- A breast augmentation is done for either small breasts or for reconstruction after breast removal.
- After breast cancer surgery, assess vital signs, dressings, drainage tubes, and amount of drainage.
- Notify the health care team that the arm of the surgical mastectomy side should not be used for blood pressures, blood drawing, or injections.
- Assess the return of arm and shoulder mobility after breast surgery and axillary dissection.
- Assess for the presence of lymphedema, and assist the patient to perform therapeutic measures to reduce lymphedema in the affected arm.
- Teach the patient measures to prevent lymphedema after axillary node dissection.
- Observe for and report other complications of breast cancer surgery or breast reconstruction, especially infection and inadequate vascular perfusion.
- After an axillary lymph node dissection, elevate the affected arm on a pillow.
- Radiation and drug therapy are used most often as adjuvant therapy after breast surgery but may be used before surgery to shrink the tumor.

Additional Study Resources

Go to your Companion CD or Evolve at http://evolve.elsevier.com/Iggy/ for *Self-Assessment Questions for the NCLEX Examination.*

Go to Evolve at http://evolve.elsevier.com/Iggy/ for *Prioritization and Delegation Questions for the NCLEX Examination.*

SELECTED BIBLIOGRAPHY

Asterisk indicates a classic or definitive work on this subject.

American Cancer Society (ACS). (2008a). *Breast cancer facts & figures 2007-2008.* Atlanta: Author.

American Cancer Society (ACS). (2008b). *Breast cancer facts & figures for African-Americans 2007-2008.* Atlanta: Author.

American Cancer Society (ACS). (2008c). *Breast cancer facts & figures for Hispanics.* Atlanta: Author.

American Cancer Society (ACS). (2008d). *Detailed guide: Breast cancer.* Retrieved September 18, 2008, from www.cancer.org.

American Cancer Society & National Comprehensive Cancer Network. (2006). *Breast Cancer: Treatment guidelines for patients.* Retrieved May 8, 2008, from www.cancer.org/downloads/CRI/Breast_VIII.pdf.

Antoni, M.H., Wimberly, S.R., Lechner, S.C., Kazi, A., Sifre, T., Urcuyo, K.R., et al. (2006). Reduction of cancer-specific thought intrusions and anxiety symptoms with a stress management intervention among women undergoing treatment for breast cancer. *American Journal of Psychiatry, 163*(10), 1791-1797.

Baron, R. (2007). Surgical management of breast cancer. *Seminars in Oncology Nursing, 23*(1), 10-19.

Barron, T.I., Connolly, R., Bennett, K., Feely, J., & Kennedy, M.J. (2007). Early discontinuation of tamoxifen: A lesson for oncologists. *Cancer, 109*(5), 832-839.

Blakely, M., & King, C. (2007). Research highlights. Young women may experience sexual problems after breast cancer surgery. *Oncology Nursing Forum, 34*(1), 19-20.

Boccardo, F., Rubagotti, A., Aldrighetti, D., Buzzi, F., Cruciani, G., Farris, A., et al. (2007). Switching to an aromatase inhibitor provides mortality benefit in early breast carcinoma. *Cancer, 109*(6), 1060-1067.

Carey, L.A., Perou, C.M., Livasy, C.A., Dressler, L.G., Cowan, D., Conway, K., et al. (2006). Race, breast cancer subtypes, and survival in the Carolina Breast Cancer Study. *Journal of the American Medical Association, 295*(21), 2492-2502.

Centers for Disease Control and Prevention (CDC). (2007). Use of mammograms among women aged >40 years: United States, 2000-2005. *Morbidity and Mortality Weekly Report, 56*(3), 49-51.

Chang, R., et al. (2006). *Complementary medicine: Types of complementary techniques.* Retrieved May 8, 2008, from www.breastcancer.org/comp_med_idx.html.

Clough-Gorr, P., Ganz, P., & Silliman, R. (2007). Older breast cancer survivors: Factors associated with change in emotional well-being. *Journal of Clinical Oncology, 25*(11), 1334-1340.

Doubeni, C.A., Field, T.S., Ulcickas Yood, M., Rolnick, S.J., Quessenberry, C. P., Fouayzi, H., et al. (2006). Patterns and predictors of mammography utilization among breast cancer survivors. *Cancer, 106*(11), 2482-2488.

Ernst, E., Schmidt, K., & Baum, M. (2006). Complementary/alternative therapies for the treatment of breast cancer: A systematic review of randomized clinical trials and a critique of current terminology. *The Breast Journal, 12*(6), 526-530.

Freedman, G.M., Anderson, P., Li, T., Ross, E., Swaby, R., & Goldstein, L. (2006). Identifying breast cancer patients most likely to benefit from aromatase inhibitor therapy after adjuvant radiation and tamoxifen. *Cancer, 107*(11), 2552-2558.

Geiger, A.M., Thwin, S.S., Lash, T.L., Buist, D.S., Prout, M.N., Wei, F., et al. (2007). Recurrences and second primary breast cancer in older women with initial early-stage disease. *Cancer, 109*(5), 966-974.

Gennari, A., Conte, P., Rosso, R., Orlandini, C., & Bruzzi, P. (2005). Survival of metastatic breast carcinoma patients over a 20-year period. *Cancer, 104*(8), 1742-1750.

Guray, M. (2006). Benign breast diseases: Classification, diagnosis, and management. *Oncologist, 11*(5), 435-449.

Hartmann, L.C., Sellers, T.A., Frost, M.H., Lingle, W., Degnim, A.C., Ghosh, K., et al. (2005). Benign breast disease and the risk of breast cancer. *New England Journal of Medicine, 353*(3), 229-237.

Hashmi, T. (2007). Causes of benign breast disease. *General Practitioner, 1*, 25.

Hawkins, R. (2006). Osteoporosis: Cancer survivors are at increased risk for osteoporosis, but how their management differs from that of the general population remains unclear. *Cancer Nursing, 29*(2), 78-82.

Hegel, M.T., Moore, C.P., Collins, E.D., Kearing, S., Gillock, K.L., Riggs, R.L., et al. (2007). Distress, psychiatric syndromes, and impairment of function in women with newly diagnosed breast cancer. *Cancer, 107*(12), 2924-2931.

Howe, H.L., Wu, X., Ries, L.A., Cokkinides, V., Ahmed, F., Jemal, A., et al. (2006). Annual report to the nation on the status of cancer, 1975-2003, featuring cancer among U.S. Hispanic/Latino populations. *Cancer, 107*(8), 1711-1742.

Itano, J., & Taoka, K. (2005). *Core curriculum for oncology nursing* (4th ed.). St. Louis: Mosby.

Jakesz, R., Jonat, W., Gnant, M., Mittlboeck, M., Greil, R., Tausch, C., et al., (2005). Switching of postmenopausal women with endocrine-responsive early breast cancer to anastrozole after 2 years' adjuvant tamoxifen: Combined results of ABCSG trial 8 and ARNO 95 trial. *Lancet, 366*(9484), 455-462.

Justice, M. (2007). New reasons to 'bone up' on osteoporosis. *BCA Bulletin, 12*(1), 2-3.

Keating, N.L., Landrum, M.B., Guadagnoli, E., Winer, E.P., & Ayanian, J.Z. (2006). Factors related to underuse of surveillance mammography among breast cancer survivors. *Journal of Clinical Oncology, 24*(1), 85-94.

Kerlikowske, K. (2007). The mammogram that cried Wolfe. *New England Journal of Medicine, 356*(3), 297-300.

Knobf, M. (2006). Reproductive and hormonal sequelae of chemotherapy in women: Premature menopause and impaired fertility can result, effects that are especially disturbing to young women. *Cancer Nursing, 29*(2), 60-65.

Koren, M.E., & Hertz, J.E. (2007). Older women's breast screening behaviors: What nurses need to know. *MEDSURG Nursing, 16*(2), 80-84.

Krop, I., & Winer, E. (2005). Ovarian suppression for breast cancer: An effective treatment in search of a home. *Journal of Clinical Oncology, 23*(25), 5869-5872.

Lengacher, C., Bennett, M.P., Kip, K.E., Gonzalez, L., Jacobsen, P., & Cox, C.E. (2006). Relief of symptoms, side effects, and psychological distress through use of complementary and alternative medicine in women with breast cancer. *Oncology Nursing Forum, 33*(1), 97-104.

Lester, J. (2007). Breast cancer in 2007: Incidence, risk assessment, and risk reduction strategies. *Clinical Journal of Oncology Nursing, 11*(5), 619-622.

Levine, M., & Whelan, T. (2006). Adjuvant chemotherapy for breast cancer—30 years later. *New England Journal of Medicine, 355*(18), 1920-1922.

Manuel, J. (2007). Younger women's perceptions of coping with breast cancer. *Cancer Nursing, 30*(2), 85-94.

McCance, K.L., & Huether, S.E. (2006). *Pathophysiology: The biologic basis for disease in adults and children* (5th ed.). St. Louis: Mosby.

McCarthy, C.M., Pusic, A.L., Disa, J.J., Cordeiro, P.G., Cody, H.S. III, & Mehrara, B. (2007). Breast cancer in the previously augmented breast. *Plastic and Reconstructive Surgery, 119*(1), 49-58.

Morgan, P.D., Fogel, J., Rose, L., Barnett, K., Mock, V., Davis, B.L., et al. (2005). African American couples merging strengths to successfully cope with breast cancer. *Oncology Nursing Forum, 32*(5), 979-987.

National Center for Complementary and Alternative Medicine, National Institutes of Health. (2007). *Cancer and CAM.* Retrieved May 8, 2008, from http://nccam.nih.gov/health/camcancer/.

Nussbaum, R.L., McInnes, R.R., & Willard, H.F. (2007). *Thompson and Thompson genetics in medicine* (7th ed.). Philadelphia: Saunders.

Pagana, K.D., & Pagana, T.J. (2006). *Mosby's manual of diagnostic and laboratory tests* (3rd ed.). St. Louis: Mosby.

Paik, S., Tang, G., Shak, S., Kim, C., Baker, J., Kim, W., et al. (2006). Gene expression and benefit of chemotherapy in women with node-negative, estrogen receptor–positive breast cancer. *Journal of Clinical Oncology, 24*(23), 3726-3734.

Paskett, E., Tatum, C., Rushing, J., Michielutte, R., Bell, R., Long Foley, K., et al. (2006). Randomized trial of an intervention to improve mammography utilization among a triracial rural population of women. *Journal of the National Cancer Institute, 98*(17), 1226-1237.

Payne, J., Piper, B.F., Rabinowitz, I., & Zimmerman, M.B. (2006). Biomarkers, fatigue, sleep, and depressive symptoms in women with breast cancer: A pilot study. *Oncology Nursing Forum, 33*(4), 775-783.

Pisano, E.D., Gatsonis, C., Hendrick, E., Yaffe, M., Baum, J.K., Acharyya, S., et al., (2005). Diagnostic performance of digital versus film mammography for breast-cancer screening. *New England Journal of Medicine, 353*(17), 1773-1783.

Plosker, G., & Keam, S. (2006). Spotlight on trastuzumab in the management of HER2-positive metastatic and early stage breast cancer. *Biodrugs, 20*(4), 259-262.

Ravdin, P.M., Cronin, K.A., Howlader, N., Berg, C.D., Chlebowski, R.T., Feuer, E.J., et al. (2006). *A sharp decrease in breast cancer incidence in the United States in 2003.* 29th Annual San Antonio Breast Cancer Symposium, Abstract 5. Retrieved May 8, 2008, from www.sabcs.org.

Reeves, G.K., Beral, V., Green, J., Gathani, T., Bull, D.; Million Women Study Collaborators. (2006). Hormonal therapy for menopause and breast-cancer risk by histological type: A cohort study and meta-analysis. *Lancet Oncology, 7*(11), 910-918.

Robinson, F., Sandoval, N., Baldwin, J., & Sanderson, P.R. (2005). Breast cancer education for Native American women: Creating culturally relevant communications. *Clinical Journal of Oncology Nursing, 9*(6), 689-692.

Setiawan, V.W., Haiman, C.A., Stanczyk, F.Z., Le Marchand, L., & Henderson, B.E. (2006). Racial/ethnic differences in postmenopausal endogenous hormones: The multiethnic cohort study. *Cancer Epidemiology Biomarkers & Prevention, 15*(10), 1849-1855.

Shaha, M., Cox, C.L., Talman, K., & Kelly, D. (2008). Uncertainty in breast, prostate, and colorectal cancer: Implications for supportive care. *Journal of Nursing Scholarship, 40*(1), 60-67.

Wane, D., & Lengacher, C.A. (2006). Integrative review of lycopene and breast cancer. *Oncology Nursing Forum, 33*(1), 127-137.

Winer, E.P., Hudis, C., Burstein, H.J., Wolff, A.C., Pritchard, K.I., Ingle, J.N., et al. (2005). American Society of Clinical Oncology technology assessment on the use of aromatase inhibitors as adjuvant therapy for postmenopausal women with hormone receptor–positive breast cancer: Status report 2004. *Journal of Clinical Oncology, 23*(3), 619-629.

Wirk, B. (2005). The role of ovarian ablation in the management of breast cancer. *Breast Journal, 11*(6), 416-424.

Yang, X.R., Sherman, M.E., Rimm, D.L., Lissowska, J., Brinton, L.A., Peplonska, B., et al. (2007). Differences in risk factors for breast cancer molecular subtypes in a population-based study. *Cancer Epidemiology Biomarkers & Prevention, 16*(3), 439-443.

Young Survival Coalition. (2007). *Young women and breast cancer.* Retrieved May 8, 2008, from www.youngsurvival.org/young-women-and-bc.

Ziegler, J., & Citron, M. (2006). Dose-dense adjuvant chemotherapy for breast cancer. *Cancer Nursing, 29*(4), 266-272.

74 CHAPTER

Care of Patients with Gynecologic Problems

Pat Mahaffee Gingrich

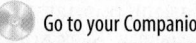

LEARNING OUTCOMES

For clinical competence and success on the NCLEX Examination, study this chapter with these Learning Outcomes in mind:

Safe and Effective Care Environment

1. Identify community resources for patients with gynecologic health problems.
2. Collaborate with members of the health care team when caring for patients with gynecologic cancers.

Health Promotion and Maintenance

3. Identify the risk factors for gynecologic cancers.
4. Describe evidence-based health promotion and maintenance measures to help prevent or early detect gynecologic cancers.

Psychosocial Integrity

5. Explain the psychosocial needs of patients with gynecologic health problems, including their effect on sexuality.
6. Discuss ways to help patients adapt to physical changes, including impaired sexuality, caused by gynecologic problems and their treatment.

Physiological Integrity

7. Compare the pathophysiology, manifestations, and treatments of common menstrual cycle disorders.
8. Describe the mechanisms of action, side effects, and nursing implications of drug therapy for endometriosis.
9. Develop a teaching plan for a patient with a vaginal inflammation or infection.
10. Discuss common assessment findings associated with menopause.
11. Prioritize care after surgery for the woman undergoing an anterior and/or posterior repair.
12. Develop a plan of care for a patient undergoing a hysterectomy.
13. Explain the purpose of radiation and chemotherapy for patients with gynecologic cancers.
14. Provide information about complementary and alternative therapies.
15. Develop a community-based plan of care for patients with gynecologic cancers.

Go to your Companion CD or Evolve at http://evolve.elsevier.com/Iggy/ for *Self-Assessment Questions for the NCLEX Examination* keyed to these Learning Outcomes.

The most common gynecologic manifestations are pain, vaginal discharge, and bleeding. Women are often hesitant to seek medical attention for these problems because of fear of a life-threatening disease diagnosis or concern about privacy and dignity. Be sensitive to the woman's concerns and encourage discussion about menstrual or other reproductive problems. Teach women about their bodies, and help them recognize when professional help should be sought. Teach them how to make informed decisions about treatments. Assess the effects of gynecologic disorders on *sexuality* in any setting. These health problems often impair sexual function and therefore can affect the woman's relationship with her partner. Remember that sexuality affects a woman's sense of being, self-esteem, and body image.

MENSTRUAL CYCLE DISORDERS

PRIMARY DYSMENORRHEA

Pathophysiology

Dysmenorrhea, or painful menstrual flow, is one of the most common gynecologic problems, especially for women in their teens and early 20s. More than half of *all* women report some degree of dysmenorrhea, but only a small percentage are unable to function.

Primary dysmenorrhea occurs after ovulation begins, usually 6 months or more after **menarche** (onset of menstruation). Painful uterine cramping with spasmodic lower abdominal pain begins with the onset of menstrual flow and lasts 12 to 72 hours. The pain often travels to the lower back and thighs.

The cause of primary dysmenorrhea is thought to be increased production and release of uterine prostaglandins, which peak at the onset of menses. Excessive prostaglandin levels cause spasms in the **myometrium** (uterine muscle), which constrict uterine blood flow, resulting in ischemia and pain. Stimulation of other smooth muscles causes GI symptoms, such as nausea, vomiting, diarrhea, and abdominal bloating.

Secondary dysmenorrhea begins with an underlying disease condition. Causes of secondary dysmenorrhea include endometriosis, adhesions, pelvic inflammatory disease (PID), ovarian cysts or tumors, and leiomyomas (fibroids).

Patient-Centered Collaborative Care

Assessment

A thorough history of the patient includes:

- Age at **menarche** (onset of menstruation) and onset of pain
- Characteristics of menstruation and pain
- Obstetric history
- Contraceptive history and preferences
- Risk for sexually transmitted infections
- Previous therapy for dysmenorrhea

To plan care more effectively, assess emotional factors such as each woman's response to dysmenorrhea, her attitudes about menstruation, and the extent to which she believes that dysmenorrhea disrupts her life.

Interventions

NSAIDs such as ibuprofen (Motrin, Actiprofen♣) and naproxen (Naprosyn, Naxen♣) help relieve menstrual pain by inhibiting prostaglandin production. Acetaminophen (Tylenol, Exdol♣) may relieve mild dysmenorrhea. All these drugs can cause GI distress and therefore should be taken with meals or milk if tolerated. Among the newer NSAIDs, valdecoxib (Bextra) is an effective anti-prostaglandin for treatment of dysmenorrhea but questions remain about an association of COX-2 inhibitors with heart disease. Anti-prostaglandins work best if started at the onset of symptoms.

If contraception is desired, ovulation suppression with oral contraceptives may decrease prostaglandin production. Newer regimens of extended or continuous oral contraceptives and depo-medroxyprogesterone (Depo-Provera) provide relief by extending the interval between menses. However, these drugs can cause major side effects. Insertion of the levonorgestrel intrauterine device (Mirena) has demonstrated decreased menstrual pain (Jensen, 2007).

Complementary and Alternative Therapies

Encourage patients to use other measures besides drugs. Continuous low-level heat provided by wearable heat packs applied to the lower abdomen is a cost-effective, non-drug intervention for dysmenorrhea that helps many women. Acupressure, acupuncture, magnet therapy, and relaxation techniques show some evidence for decreasing menstrual pain (Eccles, 2005). Dietary measures to prevent pain for some women include a low-fat vegetarian diet and the use of thiamine, calcium, magnesium, vitamin E, and fish oil supplements (Rapkin, 2005). More clinical research is needed to continue studying these therapies for their usefulness in dysmenorrhea.

PREMENSTRUAL SYNDROME

Pathophysiology

Most ovulating women have some perimenstrual symptoms, but they are usually mild. However, some women have symptoms that disrupt quality of life during the **luteal** (after ovulation) phase of their cycle. These problems are grouped and are called **premenstrual syndrome (PMS)**. During the weeks leading up to menstruation, changes in the levels of the neurotransmitter *serotonin* affect mood. Physical symptoms may be caused by hormonal or fluid shifts. Fortunately, most affected women can be helped with simple lifestyle interventions. Less than 5% of ovulating women experience a more severe and disabling form of PMS, **premenstrual dysphoric disorder (PMDD),** which is included in the *Diagnostic and Statistical Manual of Mental Disorders* (DSM) *IV-TR*.

PMDD occurs most often in women with a history of mental health problems, such as mood or anxiety disorders. It is thought to be caused by low levels of serotonin, gamma-aminobutyric acid, and beta-endorphins, vital neurotransmitters in the body. The risk for PMDD is associated with a genetic variation in *ESR1*, the estrogen receptor alpha gene (Huo et al., 2007).

Premenstrual syndrome is more prevalent in women 20 to 40 years of age. Women are at greater risk for PMS during major life transitions and stresses. Risk factors include smoking, substance abuse, and obesity.

Affective symptoms include depression, angry outbursts, anxiety, irritability, and social withdrawal. Physical discomforts include breast tenderness, edema, headache, bloating, food cravings, insomnia, and fatigue. Decreased **libido** (desire for sex) is also common. Cognitive problems include short-term memory problems, difficulty concentrating, and unclear thinking. Manifestations vary greatly among women and can affect many body systems (Chart 74-1).

Patient-Centered Collaborative Care

Assessment

There is no objective means of diagnosing PMS, although some patterns have been identified. Determining the timing of the symptoms is as critical as noting the type of symptoms. The most effective assessment tool is a menstrual chart. Teach the patient to keep a chart for at least two consecutive menstrual cycles, showing the length of each cycle, the duration of bleeding, and the occurrence of symptoms. True PMS symptoms during the luteal phase are followed by relief with menses and a symptom-free phase of at least 7 days.

When taking a menstrual history, assess to what extent the woman believes her ADLs are disrupted by the symptoms. Offer reassurance that the symptoms are legitimate and that other women have the same problems.

Interventions

Management of PMS focuses on eliminating her unique symptoms. Each woman needs information about her body, especially the menstrual cycle, so that she can begin to understand the physiologic basis of PMS.

Encourage women to express their feelings and discuss their experiences with PMS through support groups. Some groups also encourage significant others to participate because PMS usually affects not only the woman but also her family and friends. Increased family conflict, communication problems with family and friends, and decreased family bond-

Chart 74-1 KEY FEATURES
Premenstrual Syndrome

DERMATOLOGIC MANIFESTATIONS
- Acne
- Urticaria
- Herpes

RESPIRATORY MANIFESTATIONS
- Sinusitis
- Asthma
- Rhinitis
- Colds

UROLOGIC MANIFESTATIONS
- Oliguria
- Cystitis
- Enuresis
- Urethritis

OPHTHALMOLOGIC MANIFESTATIONS
- Conjunctivitis
- Styes
- Glaucoma

NEUROLOGIC MANIFESTATIONS
- Headaches
- Migraine
- Syncope
- Vertigo
- Numbness of hands and feet
- Epilepsy (if susceptible)

METABOLIC MANIFESTATIONS
- Edema
- Breast tenderness

EMOTIONAL OR PSYCHOLOGICAL MANIFESTATIONS
- Depression
- Irritability
- Tension
- Panic attacks
- Change in libido
- Mood swings
- Anxiety

BEHAVIORAL MANIFESTATIONS
- Lowered work performance
- Food cravings
- Alcohol and drug overindulgence
- Confusion
- Sleeplessness
- Lack of coordination
- Suicide
- Lethargy
- Child abuse
- Assaultive behavior

OTHER MANIFESTATIONS
- Allergies
- Hypoglycemia
- Joint pain
- Backache
- Palpitations
- Water retention

ing may occur. Intimate relationships are negatively affected because the woman often loses interest in having sexual intercourse. Other coping strategies for the woman with PMS may include spiritual support.

Teach patients to exercise a minimum of 30 minutes three times a week to boost low perimenstrual endorphin levels. Stress management through adequate rest, meditation, and massage can decrease stress hormones. Many women have sleep disturbances, which increases irritability and mood changes.

Complementary and Alternative Therapies

Nutrition may be useful in managing PMS. Teach patients about how to change their lifestyle to follow healthy eating habits. If hypoglycemia (low blood glucose) occurs, teach the woman to eat six small meals a day and to limit her intake of sugar, red meat, and alcohol. Sugar and red meat tend to contribute to abdominal bloating. Teach patients to avoid alcohol and caffeine to help reduce irritability. Reinforce the need to limit sodium intake if edema occurs. Some women have found that calcium (1200 mg daily) and magnesium (200 to 400 mg daily) supplements help decrease PMS symptoms. Calcium seems to relieve tension, anxiety, and pain; magnesium reduces fluid retention. Clinical evidence supports the use of these minerals (Proctor & Farquhar, 2006). Encourage patients to use these supplements after checking with their health care provider.

Chasteberry (monk's pepper) supplements have shown some promise for reducing PMS discomfort, edema, headache, and mood changes (www.nccam.nih.gov/health/chasteberry). It has been prescribed for women for many years in Europe. The herb is well-tolerated and has no reported drug interactions. Minor side effects include GI distress, dizziness, and dry mouth. In the United States, chasteberry is available as Femaprin (Nature's Way). The usual dosage is 20 to 40 mg per day, but higher doses have been used (Roemheld-Hamm, 2005). Women should not take this herb when pregnant. It should be taken only by women who are using reliable contraception.

Drug Therapy

Hormonal therapy is the first approach for relieving the symptoms associated with PMS. If contraception is desired, *oral contraceptives* can decrease breast pain and bloating. Triphasic pills improve somatic symptoms by decreasing the overall hormone dose, whereas monophasic pills, which do not change dose during the cycle, may help prevent mood swings. Extended and continuous dosing decrease or prevent monthly cyclic fluctuations.

Gonadotropin-releasing hormone (GnRH) agonists such as leuprolide (Lupron Depot) effectively stop ovulation but may cause side effects in some women. Triptorelin (Gonapeptyl Depot) given once each month can be very effective in managing PMS. Teach patients that GnRH agonists can cause menopausal-like side effects, such as hot flashes, headaches, vaginal dryness, and irritability. Long-term use can lead to decreased bone density. Decreased libido is also common when taking these drugs. As an alternative, transdermal estradiol (e.g., Menostar) is available as a patch or gel. Some women use the patch once or twice a week, on a rotating schedule, or all the time depending on its brand. Teach patients how to apply

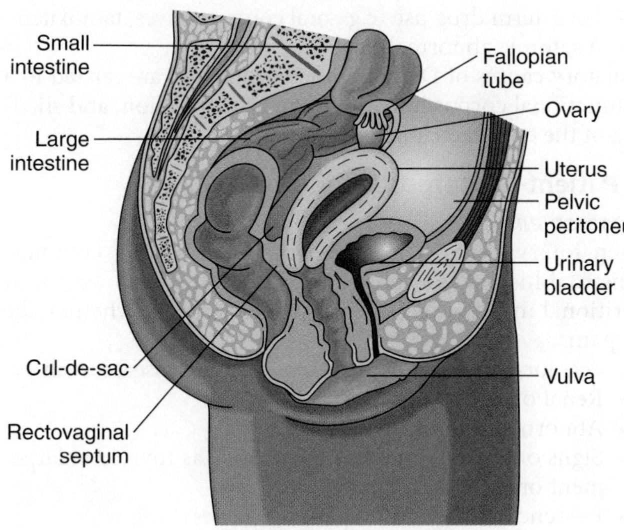
Small intestine
Large intestine
Cul-de-sac
Rectovaginal septum
Fallopian tube
Ovary
Uterus
Pelvic peritoneum
Urinary bladder
Vulva

Fig. 74-1 • Common sites of endometriosis.

the patch or gel for maximum and continuous effectiveness. Side effects associated with GnRH agonists are not common with topical drugs.

Antidepressants, particularly *selective serotonin-reuptake inhibitors (SSRIs)*, are the first-line drugs for PMDD if hormonal therapy is not successful. These drugs may be used for 10 to 14 days before menses begins. A short-term dose decreases the chance of adverse effects. Examples include sertraline (Zoloft), paroxetine (Paxil), and citalopram (Celexa).

ENDOMETRIOSIS

Pathophysiology

Endometriosis is endometrial (inner uterine) tissue implantation *outside* the uterine cavity. The tissue typically appears on the ovaries and the cul-de-sac (posterior rectovaginal wall) and less commonly on other pelvic organs and structures (Fig. 74-1). A "chocolate" cyst is an area of endometriosis on an ovary. The disease affects over 5.5 million women in the United States and Canada (www.endometriosisassn.org).

Endometriosis responds to cyclic hormonal stimulation just as if it were in the uterus. Monthly cyclic bleeding occurs at the **ectopic** (out of place) site of implantation, which irritates and scars the surrounding tissue. Scarring can lead to adhesions, causing infertility (inability to become pregnant). Endometriosis progresses slowly. It regresses during pregnancy and at menopause. Rarely does it become cancerous.

The cause of endometriosis is unknown. One theory is that the endometrial tissue migrates directly through the fallopian tubes during menses. The tissue then implants on pelvic structures or distant organs such as lungs or heart. The formation theory suggests that endometrial tissue develops outside the uterus as a birth defect. Other theories focus on immune, genetic, and environmental factors (e.g., exposure to dioxin, a toxic chemical). Many women with endometriosis have allergies and chemical sensitivities.

The disorder is most often found in women during their reproductive years, but it can affect women into their 80s. The prevalence among infertile women is higher than it is for women who are fertile. It is also common in those whose mothers had endometriosis.

Patient-Centered Collaborative Care

Assessment

Collect a detailed history, including the woman's menstrual history, sexual history, and bleeding characteristics. *Pain is the most common symptom of endometriosis.* The pain usually peaks just before the menstrual flow. It is usually located in the lower abdomen, causing many women to feel a sense of rectal pressure. The degree of pain is not related to the extent of the endometriosis but to the site. Often, women with minimal disease have more severe pain than do women with extensive disease. Other manifestations include **dyspareunia** (painful sexual intercourse), painful defecation, low backache, and infertility. GI disturbances such as nausea and diarrhea are also common. Always ask about current or past physical or sexual abuse.

A pelvic examination may reveal pelvic tenderness, tender nodules in the posterior vagina, and limited movement of the uterus. Psychosocial assessment may reveal anxiety because of uncertainty about the diagnosis. The woman may also have concerns about her self-concept if she is infertile but wants to become pregnant.

Diagnostic studies include tests to rule out pelvic inflammatory disease caused by chlamydia or gonorrhea. Serum cancer antigen CA-125 helps screen for ovarian cancer but also may be positive in women with endometriosis. Transvaginal ultrasound is used to differentiate pelvic masses that might be mistaken for endometriosis. Laparoscopy is still the gold standard diagnostic procedure. Examination of tissue specimens obtained during laparoscopy confirms the diagnosis.

Interventions

Hormonal and surgical management may be used, depending on the symptoms, the extent of disease, and the woman's desire for childbearing. Collaborative care is aimed at:

- Reducing pain
- Restoring sexual function
- Alleviating anxiety related to the disease and the uncertainty of the diagnosis
- Educating the patient about the disease and its treatment
- Alleviating fear related to the possibility of laparoscopy or surgery
- Preventing self-esteem disturbance related to infertility

Nonsurgical Management

Several resources, such as the Endometriosis Association (www.endometriosisassn) and RESOLVE (an organization for infertile couples) (www.resolve.org), offer information on endometriosis that is helpful for patients and caregivers.

Disease management is similar to that of dysmenorrhea: cycle control using hormonal contraceptives for at least 6 months and decreasing prostaglandins via NSAIDs. Other longer-term (6 to 8 months) suppressive hormonal treatments cause pseudo-menopause, which allows the ectopic tissue to atrophy. These suppressive therapies include GnRH agonists (e.g., leuprolide [Lupron Depot]) and androgenic agents (e.g., danazol [Danocrine]). Side effects may include hot flashes and vaginal dryness. In addition, GnRH agonists may cause a decrease in bone density. Androgenic agents may cause acne and hirsutism. Anti-estrogenic aromatase inhibitors can also potentiate cycle suppression (Attar & Bulun, 2006). Endostatins, which block the formation of new blood vessels, have been used to decrease ectopic endometrial growth.

Complementary and Alternative Therapies. Just as with dysmenorrhea, continuous low-level heat using wearable heat packs may provide relief. Relaxation techniques, yoga, massage, and biofeedback may decrease muscle tissue hypoxia and hypertonicity and relieve ischemia by increasing blood flow to the affected areas. Calcium and magnesium may also relieve muscle cramping.

Surgical Management

Surgical management of endometriosis for a woman who wants to remain fertile is the laparoscopic removal of endometrial implants and adhesions in a same-day surgical setting. Chapter 18 describes the general postoperative care for patients having laparoscopic procedures. The surgeon may use a laser to treat endometriosis by vaporizing adhesions and endometrial implants. In women with intractable pain, severing a pelvic nerve may provide relief. Use of the levonorgestrel IUD (Mirena) after surgery can prevent recurrence of painful periods (Abou-Setta et al., 2006). If the patient and partner do not wish to have children, the uterus and ovaries may be removed.

NCLEX EXAMINATION CHALLENGE

A client taking leuprolide is concerned about the drug's side effects. Which statement about preventing side effects should the nurse teach the client?

A. "Eat a diet rich in calcium, and take calcium supplements."
B. "Use massage to decrease tension and stress caused by the drug."
C. "Avoid having sexual intercourse when you have vaginal dryness."
D. "Take cold showers or use ice packs when you have hot flashes."

evolve For the correct answer, go to http://evolve.elsevier.com/Iggy/.

DYSFUNCTIONAL UTERINE BLEEDING

Pathophysiology

Dysfunctional uterine bleeding (DUB) describes bleeding that is excessive in amount (more than 80 mL per cycle) or frequency (more than every 21 days). It is a diagnosis of exclusion, made after ruling out anatomic or systemic conditions such as drug therapy or disease. DUB occurs most often at the beginning or end of a woman's reproductive years—when ovulation is becoming established or when it is becoming irregular at or after menopause.

Normally the menstrual cycle is a series of delicately timed hormonal events regulated by hypothalamic, pituitary, ovarian, and uterine functions. **Menses,** the sloughing of the endometrial lining, is an expected result. DUB occurs when there is a hormonal imbalance. Generally, it happens when the ovaries fail to ovulate. This decreases progesterone production, which is needed to mature the uterine lining and prevent overgrowth. Without progesterone, prolonged estrogen stimulation causes the endometrium to grow past its hormonal support, causing disordered shedding of uterine lining.

Anovulatory DUB during the reproductive years is associated with conditions such as:

- Endocrine disturbances, including type II diabetes and thyroid disease
- Polycystic ovary disease
- Stress
- Obesity or underweight
- Long-term drug use (e.g., oral contraceptives, tamoxifen)
- Anatomic abnormalities

Ovulatory causes of DUB are uncommon and are related to a dysfunctional corpus luteum, irregular maturation, and shedding of the endometrium.

Patient-Centered Collaborative Care

Assessment

When interviewing a woman with DUB, take a complete menstrual history. Ask about illnesses, changes in weight or nutritional intake, exercise, drug ingestion, and whether she has pain.

Assess for symptoms of anemia or systemic disease, such as:

- Renal or hepatic disease
- Abnormal weight
- Signs of hormonal dysfunction, such as thyroid enlargement or male hair pattern
- Evidence of abdominal pain or masses

The health care provider inspects the external genitalia and does a bimanual pelvic examination, Papanicolaou test, and rectal examination to identify infections, lesions, or tenderness.

Transvaginal ultrasound may reveal **leiomyomas** (fibroids) and measure an excessively thick endometrium. *Sonohysterography* uses vaginal ultrasound to visualize the uterus after 5 to 10 mL of sterile saline is infused through the cervix, thus outlining the inner uterine cavity. Direct visualization inside the uterus using a scope through the cervix is called *hysteroscopy.* To evaluate for endometrial cancer, especially in older women, the surgeon usually does an endometrial biopsy by using a thin suction tube through the cervix.

Interventions

Management of the patient often includes nonsurgical and surgical interventions. When nonsurgical treatment is not effective, surgery may be performed.

Nonsurgical Management

As with dysmenorrhea and endometriosis, hormone manipulation is usually the treatment of choice. Estrogen therapy is indicated when bleeding is heavy and acute. Conjugated estrogens (25 mg) are given IV every 4 to 6 hours until bleeding stops or for 24 hours. For nonemergent bleeding, hormonal contraceptives (oral or patch) provide the progestin (artificial progesterone) needed to stabilize the endometrial lining. Progestin-only pills or injectable medroxyprogesterone acetate (Depo-Provera) is preferable for women older than 35 years who smoke or are at risk for thrombophlebitis. The levonorgestrel intrauterine device (IUD) is effective for decreasing dysfunctional bleeding (Lethaby et al., 2005). Women with ovulatory DUB may also benefit from the use of anti-prostaglandin NSAIDs.

Explain the desired effects and the side effects of these drugs, and evaluate the woman's knowledge of the effects, dosage, and schedule. Be sure to remind her to take the drug exactly as prescribed and to not skip a dose or run out of it.

Surgical Management

Dilation and curettage (D&C) is still used as a surgical intervention for DUB, but it is no longer the gold standard. Instead, removal of the built-up uterine lining, called **endometrial ablation,** using a laser, roller ball, or balloon is a safer alternative for women who do not respond to medical management or who do not need a hysterectomy. If leiomyomas are the source of bleeding, they can be removed using a laparoscopic, abdominal, or transcervical hysteroscopic **myomectomy.** A hysterectomy is usually performed only after other treatments have failed. Hysterectomy is discussed later. (See the discussion of Surgical Management on p. 1696 of the Uterine Leiomyoma section.)

MENOPAUSE

Pathophysiology

Menopause is a *normal* biologic event marked for most women by the cessation of menstrual periods (12 months of **amenorrhea** [discontinuation of menses]). Other causes of amenorrhea are listed in Table 74-1. Menopause implies the depletion of *estradiol,* an estrogen hormone produced by the ovaries. Although menopause is a point in time, it is more clinically relevant to look at the months or years surrounding this event. Although the woman no longer has to worry about pregnancy, she may not want to have sex with her partner because of physical symptoms and decreased **libido** (desire for sex).

Women experience menopause as individuals, and care should be taken not to make generalizations. They become menopausal in a variety of ways, including by surgery when the uterus and ovaries are removed and by medical treatment for cancer *(artificial menopause). Natural menopause* is experienced across a wide age range, from as early as the 30s or 40s to as late as the 60s. The average age at which women have their last menstrual period is 51. All women younger than 40 years who have early menopause, regardless of cause, are at higher risk for osteoporosis and related fractures. It is thought that they also may be at higher risk for cardiovascular disease. Most pass through menopause with minimal symptoms. Some women, however, seek care for one or more symptoms related to menopause.

TABLE 74-1 Common Causes of Amenorrhea

PRIMARY
- Congenital anomalies
- Hypothalamic and pituitary disorders, such as delayed puberty
- Systemic disease:
  - Thyroid and adrenal dysfunction
  - Diabetes mellitus
  - Extreme malnutrition
- Ovarian disease
- Malformations of the reproductive tract

SECONDARY
- Pregnancy
- Menopause
- Lactation
- Cervical stenosis
- Polycystic ovary disease
- Pituitary tumor or insufficiency
- Psychogenic stress
- Excessive physical activities
- Medications:
  - Antihypertensive agents
  - Birth control pills
  - Phenothiazines
- Nutritional disorders:
  - Obesity
  - Anorexia nervosa
  - Sudden weight loss
- Ovarian disease, failure, or destruction

Several factors may affect the timing of menopause. These include:
- Autoimmune disease
- Chromosomal abnormalities
- Genetic influence
- Early *menarche* (beginning of menses) (usually means a later menopause)
- Hysterectomy (surgical menopause if ovaries removed)
- Smoking (usually means an earlier menopause)
- Cancer treatment (chemotherapy or radiation)

Patient-Centered Collaborative Care

Assessment

Perimenopause, or "change of life," is the gradual transition to the cessation of spontaneous ovarian function. It is confirmed by laboratory testing of hormone levels (Table 74-2).

Common early features of perimenopause are a change in the woman's usual menstrual periods and the beginning of *vasomotor symptoms,* such as hot flushes (also called *hot flashes*) and night sweats. These symptoms may disturb the woman's usual sleep pattern, which may affect mood, concentration, and memory. Vaginal dryness, **dyspareunia** (painful intercourse), and urogenital atrophy causing stress incontinence can be very distressing and embarrassing for her to discuss with her partner or a health care provider. The woman may not want to be intimate with her partner because it is painful due to vaginal dryness caused by lack of estrogen. Ask the woman about these changes, and reassure her that they are normal during perimenopause. Discuss how perimenopause has affected her sexuality and relationship with her partner(s). Discuss the impact of physical and psychological changes on her relationship with her partner(s) and other family members.

Menstrual irregularity may be the first symptom of menopause. As the transition evolves, most women find that their periods become lighter and farther apart until they finally stop. Some simply stop menstruating without further change. The remaining women experience heavier bleeding, which can be either regularly timed or unpredictable. Abnormal bleeding needs to be evaluated for endometrial cancer, endometrial polyps, or uterine fibroids.

Interventions

In the past decade, there have been many studies about perimenopausal changes and treatment, some of them conflicting and confusing. Before 2002, combined estrogen and progestin *hormone replacement therapy (HRT)* was considered protective against some of the effects of menopause, such as heart

TABLE 74-2 Laboratory Studies That Confirm Menopause

Test	Normal Range	Menopausal Range
Estradiol (serum)	20-750 pg/mL	<20 pg/mL
FSH	1.09-17.2 IU/mL	19.3-100.6 IU/mL
LH	0.61-56.6 IU/mL	14.2-52.3 IU/mL

FSH, Follicle-stimulating hormone; *LH,* luteinizing hormone; *pg,* picograms.

disease and osteoporosis. However, the 2002 Women's Health Initiative reported that HRT was associated with an unexpected *increased* risk for coronary heart disease and breast cancer. It was found that it also did not protect against dementia. Still, some women experience intolerable menopausal symptoms. *To maintain the quality of life for these women, the cautious consensus is to take HRT at the lowest possible dose to relieve symptoms for the shortest period of time.*

Estrogen given alone can cause endometrial cancer, gallbladder disease, and thromboembolic conditions such as deep vein thrombosis and stroke. Finding the right estrogen-progestin combination takes time. Each woman, together with her health care provider, needs to base the decision on whether or not to use HRT on the severity of symptoms and personal risk factors for other health problems.

HRT is available as oral, transdermal, intravaginal, and IM preparations. Transdermal HRT offers a useful alternative route of administration for women who prefer not to take pills, who cannot tolerate oral therapy because of GI side effects such as nausea, or who have abnormal liver function tests.

Atrophic vaginitis (causing vaginal dryness), a common problem with menopause, is best managed by the use of vaginal estrogen therapy (ET) as a ring, tablet, or cream. Teach the patient about this drug including expected outcomes and side effects (Chart 74-2). Vaginal ET can also decrease urinary tract infections in perimenopausal women; however, its effect on urinary incontinence is mixed (Kelley, 2007). The drug is a low enough dose that it is not usually necessary to add progestogen (artificial progesterone) to protect against endometrial cancer. Over-the-counter use of Replens vaginal lubricant can often ease the symptoms of vaginal dryness and irritation that occur with atrophic vaginitis. A water-based lubricant used during intercourse helps reduce vaginal discomfort. Bladder training and pelvic floor exercises (Kegel) may improve stress incontinence.

Symptoms of menopause may be managed using other therapies. For example, for hot flashes, gabapentin and very low doses of antidepressant drugs for a short time may be effective. Preventive therapies are also essential. For instance, many women are on drug therapy to prevent osteoporosis, such as raloxifene (Evista) and alendronate (Fosamax). Expense and convenience of dosing vary widely.

Chart 74-2 PATIENT AND FAMILY EDUCATION GUIDE

Estrogen Replacement Therapy

FOR ALL TYPES OF ESTROGEN REPLACEMENT THERAPY

- Call your health care provider if you have pain in your calves or groin, if you suddenly become short of breath, if you have abnormal vaginal bleeding, if you feel a lump in your breast, if you have a severe headache, or if you feel weak or numb in your arms or legs.
- Use sunscreen if you are in the sun for a prolonged period.
- Keep appointments for checkups.
- If your health care provider has prescribed progesterone to decrease your risk for endometrial cancer, take it as prescribed.

FOR ORAL THERAPY

- Take 1 pill daily for the first 25 days each month.
- If you feel nauseated or have intestinal upset, take your medication with food.

FOR TRANSDERMAL OR SUBDERMAL ADMINISTRATION

- Rotate the sites for the patches or injections to avoid skin irritation.
- Change the patches twice a week or according to your prescribed schedule.

FOR VAGINAL THERAPY

- Use an applicator to insert the suppository or cream as prescribed.
- You may need to wear a minipad to protect your clothing from soiling or staining by the drug.
- Do not use cream as a lubricant for intercourse.

Complementary and Alternative Therapies

Healthy lifestyle habits can reduce the severity and incidence of perimenopausal symptoms. Exercise not only decreases bone loss and prevents chronic hypertension and diabetes but also improves mood and cognitive function. However, increased physical activity may increase hot flashes (Whitcomb et al., 2007). They may be less frequent using mind-based therapies for stress reduction (Carmody et al., 2006) and less severe using acupuncture. Proper nutrition can help manage blood sugar and weight. Supplements of calcium (1200 mg daily) plus vitamin D (400 to 600 IU daily) help prevent fractures. Black cohosh and soy have been popular for menopause symptoms, but randomized controlled trials do *not* support their use (Newton et al., 2006).

VULVOVAGINITIS

Pathophysiology

Vaginal discharge and itching are two problems experienced by most women at some time in their lives. Women can suffer vaginal infections from both sexually and non–sexually transmitted sources. Gonorrhea, syphilis, chlamydia, and herpes simplex virus are sexually transmitted diseases (STDs) discussed in Chapter 76.

Vulvovaginitis is inflammation of the lower genital tract resulting from a disturbance of the balance of hormones and flora in the vagina and vulva. It may be characterized by itching, change in vaginal discharge, odor, or lesions. Possible causes include:

- Fungal (yeast) infections *(Candida albicans)*
- Bacterial vaginosis
- STDs *(Trichomonas vaginalis)*
- Menopausal atrophy
- Changes in the normal flora or pH (from douching)
- Chemical irritant or allergens (vaginal spray, fabric dyes, detergent) or foreign body (tampon)
- Drugs, especially antibiotics
- Immunosuppression from pregnancy, diabetes, or human immune deficiency virus (HIV)

Primary infections that affect the vulva include *herpes genitalis* and *condylomata acuminata* (human papilloma virus, venereal warts) (see Chapter 76). Secondary infections of the vulva are caused by organisms responsible for the many types of vaginitis, including *candidiasis.* Pediculosis pubis (crab lice) and scabies (itch mite) are common parasitic infestations of the skin of the vulva. Other causes of vulvitis include:

- Atrophic vaginitis
- Lichen planus (thickened, leathery skin from scratching)
- Vulvar leukoplakia (postmenopausal atrophy and thickening of vulvar tissues)

- Vulvar cancer
- Urinary incontinence

Some women may have an *itch-scratch-itch cycle,* in which the itching leads to scratching, which causes excoriation that then must heal. As healing takes place, itching occurs again. If the cycle is not interrupted, the chronic scratching may lead to the white, thickened skin of lichen planus. This dry, leathery skin cracks easily, increasing the woman's risk for infection.

Patient-Centered Collaborative Care

Assess for vulvovaginitis by asking questions about the symptoms, assisting with a pelvic examination, and obtaining vaginal smears for laboratory testing. Inquire about symptoms of itching and burning sensation. **Erythema** (redness), edema, and superficial skin ulcers also may be present. Use a nonjudgmental approach and provide reassurance during the assessment because the patient may be embarrassed or afraid to discuss her symptoms. Encourage her to talk about her problem and its effect on her sexual health.

Interventions for vulvovaginitis depend on the causes and the specific vaginal infection. Proper health habits can benefit treatment. Instruct the patient to get enough rest and sleep, observe good dietary habits, exercise regularly, and use good personal hygiene. Teach her about how to manage her infection (Chart 74-3). Chart 74-4 outlines measures to help prevent further infections.

Nursing interventions to relieve itching include applying wet compresses, sitz baths for 30 minutes several times a day, and applying the prescribed topical drugs, such as hydrocortisone and fluorinated corticosteroids. Encourage the removal of any irritant or allergen, such as changing detergents.

Treatment of pediculosis and scabies is used if needed and includes:

- Applying lindane (Kwell, Kwellada) lotion, shampoo, or cream to the affected area as directed
- Cleaning affected clothes, bedding, and towels
- Disinfecting the home environment (lice cannot live for more than 24 hours away from the body)

If the vulvitis is chronic or severe, laser therapy or a "skinning" vulvectomy may be performed (see p. 1707 in the Vulvar Cancer section).

Chart 74-3 PATIENT AND FAMILY EDUCATION GUIDE

Vaginal Infections

- Your risk for getting vaginal infections increases if you have sex with more than one person.
- When you have a vaginal infection, do not have sexual intercourse or at least make sure that your partner wears a condom.
- Sexual partners may need to be treated for infection.
- The only way to identify what infection you have is to be examined by a health care provider and to get the results of laboratory tests.
- Take your medicine as prescribed, not just until your symptoms go away.

Chart 74-4 PATIENT AND FAMILY EDUCATION GUIDE

Prevention of Vulvovaginitis

- Wear cotton underwear.
- Avoid wearing tight clothing, such as pantyhose or tight jeans, because they can cause chafing. You can also get hot and sweaty, which can cause an infection.
- Always wipe front to back after having a bowel movement or urinating.
- During bath or shower, cleanse inner labial mucosa with water, not soap.
- Do not douche or use feminine hygiene sprays.
- If your sexual partner has an infection of the sex organs, do not have intercourse with him or her until he or she has been treated.
- You are more likely to get an infection if you are pregnant, have diabetes, take oral contraceptive drugs, or are menopausal.
- Practice vulvar self-examination monthly.

TOXIC SHOCK SYNDROME

Pathophysiology

Toxic shock syndrome (TSS) was first recognized in 1980 when it was found to be related to menstruation and tampon use. Other conditions associated with TSS include surgical wound infection, nonsurgical infections, and gynecologic surgeries. Use of the diaphragm, cervical cap, and vaginal contraceptive sponge has also been linked to this health problem.

The pathophysiology of TSS is not clearly understood. In menstrually related infection, menstrual blood provides a growth medium for *Staphylococcus aureus* (or, less frequently, *Streptococcus*). Exotoxins produced from the bacteria cross the vaginal mucosa to the bloodstream via microabrasions from tampon insertion or prolonged use.

A small number of TSS cases are fatal. Extensive public education has led to a decreased number of women having the infection.

Patient-Centered Collaborative Care

Within 24 hours of contact with the causative agent, the abrupt onset of a high fever, along with headache, flu-like symptoms, and severe hypotension with fainting, is often present. A sunburn-like rash with broken capillaries in the eyes and skin is another warning sign of TSS. Because not all women have all these manifestations, the criteria established by the Centers for Disease Control and Prevention (CDC) are used to verify cases (Chart 74-5). Educate all women on the prevention of TSS related to the use of tampons, vaginal sponges, and diaphragms (Chart 74-6).

Treatment includes removal of the infection source, such as a tampon; restoring fluid and electrolyte balance; drugs to manage hypotension; and IV antibiotics. Other measures may include transfusions to reverse low platelet counts and corticosteroids to treat skin changes.

UTERINE PROLAPSE

Pathophysiology

The pelvic organs are supported by a sling of muscles and tendons. **Uterine prolapse** (downward displacement) can be caused by neuromuscular damage of childbirth; increased intra-abdominal pressure related to pregnancy, obesity, or physical exertion; or weakening of pelvic support due to decreased estrogen. The stages of uterine prolapse are described by the degree of descent of the uterus (Fig. 74-2) through the pelvic floor.

Whenever the uterus is displaced, other structures such as the bladder, rectum, and small intestine can protrude through

Chart 74-5 KEY FEATURES

Toxic Shock Syndrome

- Fever (temperature >102° F [38.9° C])
- Diffuse rash resembling sunburn
- Peeling of skin—primarily the soles of the feet and the palms of the hands—1 to 2 wk after onset of the illness
- Hypotension (systolic blood pressure <90 mm Hg or orthostatic syncope)
- Involvement of three or more of these:
  - Gastrointestinal system: vomiting, diarrhea at the onset of the syndrome
  - Musculoskeletal system: severe aching or a serum creatinine phosphatase level twice the normal level
  - Respiratory system: acute respiratory distress syndrome (ARDS)
  - Renal/urinary system: decreased urine output, pyuria
  - Cardiovascular system: decreased left ventricular contractility; ischemic changes shown on the electrocardiogram
  - Liver: total bilirubin, aspartate aminotransferase (serum glutamic–oxaloacetic transaminase), and alanine amino-transferase (serum glutamic–pyruvic transaminase) levels elevated; jaundice; disseminated intravascular coagulation (DIC)
  - Hematologic system: platelet levels below normal
  - Central nervous system: disorientation, altered consciousness in the absence of fever or hypertension
  - Mucous membranes: hyperemia of the vaginal walls, the throat, or the conjunctiva of the eye
- Negative results for Rocky Mountain spotted fever, measles, and scarlet fever and for throat, blood, and cerebrospinal fluid cultures
- Positive culture for *Staphylococcus aureus* from blood, urine, or stool

Chart 74-6 PATIENT AND FAMILY EDUCATION GUIDE

Prevention of Toxic Shock Syndrome

TAMPON USE

- Wash your hands before inserting a tampon.
- Do not use a tampon if it is dirty.
- Insert the tampon carefully to avoid injuring the delicate tissue in your vagina.
- Change your tampon every 3 to 6 hours.
- Do not use superabsorbent tampons.
- Use sanitary napkins at night.
- Call your health care provider if you suddenly experience a high temperature, vomiting, or diarrhea.
- Do not use tampons at all if you have had toxic shock syndrome.
- Not using tampons almost guarantees that you will not get toxic shock syndrome.

VAGINAL SPONGE USE

- Wash your hands before inserting a vaginal sponge.
- Use only clean water to wet the sponge.
- Do not use the sponge if it is dirty.
- Do not use the sponge for more than 30 hours at a time.
- Call your health care provider if you have two or more symptoms of toxic shock syndrome.

DIAPHRAGM USE

- Wash your hands and the diaphragm before insertion.
- Remove the diaphragm within 24 hours after intercourse.
- Do not use the diaphragm during your menstrual period.
- After you take out the diaphragm, wash it with mild soap, rinse it, and dry it. Coating the diaphragm with a small amount of cornstarch will absorb any excess water and prevent damage to the latex rubber. Store it in a clean, dry place.

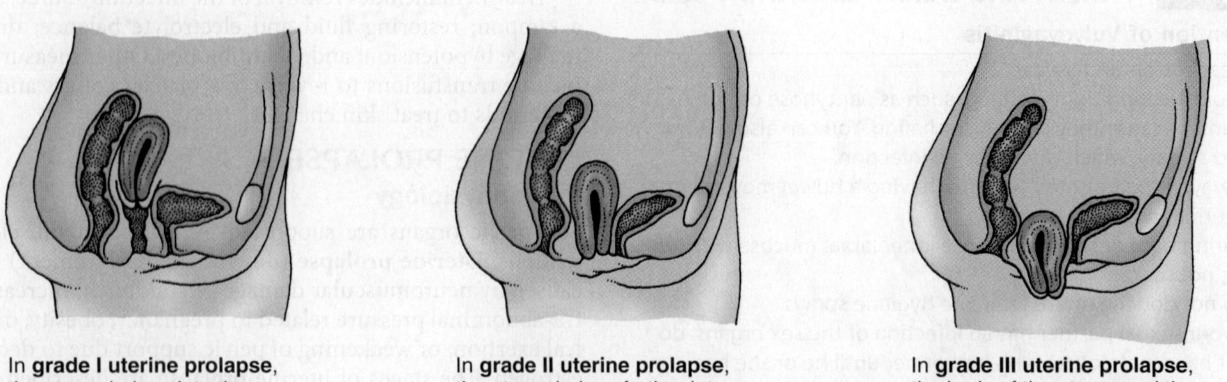

In **grade I uterine prolapse,** the uterus bulges into the vagina, but the cervix does not protrude through the entrance to the vagina.

In **grade II uterine prolapse,** the uterus bulges farther into the vagina, and the cervix protrudes through the entrance to the vagina.

In **grade III uterine prolapse,** the body of the uterus and the cervix protrude through the entrance to the vagina. The vagina is turned inside out.

Fig. 74-2 • Types of uterine prolapse.

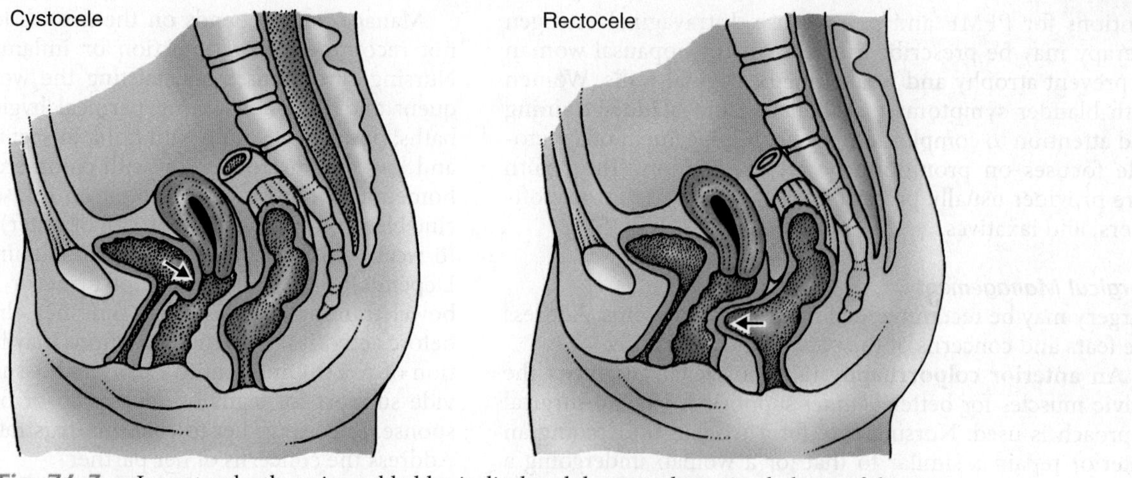
Cystocele
Rectocele

Fig. 74-3 • In cystocele, the urinary bladder is displaced downward, causing bulging of the anterior vaginal wall. In rectocele, the rectum is displaced, causing bulging of the posterior vaginal wall.

Chart 74-7 NIC INTERVENTION ACTIVITIES

The Patient with Weak Pelvic Floor Muscles

Pessary Management: *Placement and monitoring of a vaginal device for treating stress urinary incontinence, uterine retroversion, genital prolapse, or incompetent cervix.*

- Determine ability to perform self-care of pessary.
- Discuss maintenance regimen and cleaning procedures with patient prior to fitting pessary (e.g., fit is trial and error; frequent follow-up visits are required).
- Review manufacturer's directions regarding specific type of pessary.
- Instruct on method for pessary removal, as appropriate.
- Instruct on contraindications for intercourse or douching based on pessary type.
- Instruct to report discomfort; dysuria; changes in color, consistency, or frequency of vaginal discharge.
- Determine therapeutic response to pessary use.

Pelvic Muscle Exercise: *Strengthening and training the levator ani and urogenital muscles through voluntary, repetitive contraction to decrease stress, urge, or mixed types of urinary incontinence.*

- Determine ability to recognize the urge to void.
- Instruct female individual to locate the levator ani and urogenital muscles by placing her finger in the vagina and squeezing.
- Instruct individual to tighten, then relax, the ring of muscle around urethra and anus, as if trying to prevent urination or bowel movement.
- Instruct individual to perform muscle tightening exercises, working up to 300 contractions each day, holding the contraction for 10 seconds each and resting at least 10 seconds between each contraction, per agency protocol.
- Inform individual that it takes 6 to 12 weeks for exercises to be effective.
- Teach individual to monitor response to exercise by attempting to stop urine flow no more often than once a week.
- Provide written instructions describing the intervention and the recommended number of repetitions.

NIC intervention activities selected from Bulechek, G.M., Butcher, H.K., & McCloskey Dochterman, J. (Eds.). (2008). *Nursing interventions classification (NIC)* (5th ed.). St. Louis: Mosby.

the vaginal walls (Fig. 74-3). A **cystocele** is a protrusion of the bladder through the vaginal wall, which can lead to stress incontinence and urinary tract infections. A **rectocele** is a protrusion of the rectum through a weakened vaginal wall.

Patient-Centered Collaborative Care

Assessment

Assessment findings include the patient's feeling as if "something is falling out," dyspareunia (painful intercourse), backache, and a feeling of heaviness or pressure in the pelvis. A pelvic examination may reveal a protrusion of the cervix when the woman is asked to bear down. Listen to her concerns, and note signs of depression.

Ask the patient about manifestations that may indicate that she has a *cystocele.* These signs and symptoms may include:

- Difficulty in emptying the bladder
- Urinary frequency and urgency
- Urinary tract infection
- **Stress urinary incontinence** (loss of urine during activities that increase intra-abdominal pressure, such as laughing, coughing, sneezing, or lifting heavy objects)

A pelvic examination reveals a large bulge of the anterior vaginal wall when the woman is asked to bear down. Diagnostic tests include cystography (to show the presence of bladder herniation), measurement of residual urine by bladder ultrasound, and urine culture and sensitivity testing. Radiographic imaging of urinary anatomy and voiding function is useful in determining the degree of cystocele.

Rectocele assessment usually includes symptoms of constipation, hemorrhoids, fecal impaction, and feelings of rectal or vaginal fullness. A vaginal and rectal examination may show a bulge of the posterior vaginal wall when the woman is asked to bear down.

Interventions

Interventions are based on the degree of prolapse. Conservative treatment is preferred over surgical treatment when possible.

Nonsurgical Management

Teach women to improve pelvic support and tone via pelvic floor muscle exercises (PFME, or Kegel). Space-filling devices such as pessaries or spheres can be worn in the vagina to elevate the uterine prolapse. Chart 74-7 lists NIC interventions for PFME and pessary use. Intravaginal estrogen therapy may be prescribed for the postmenopausal woman to prevent atrophy and weakening of vaginal walls. Women with bladder symptoms may benefit from bladder training and attention to complete emptying. Management of a rectocele focuses on promoting bowel elimination. The health care provider usually prescribes a high-fiber diet, stool softeners, and laxatives.

Surgical Management

Surgery may be recommended for severe symptoms. Address the fears and concerns of the patient and her family.

An **anterior colporrhaphy** (anterior repair) tightens the pelvic muscles for better *bladder* support. A vaginal surgical approach is used. Nursing care for a woman undergoing an anterior repair is similar to that for a woman undergoing a vaginal hysterectomy.

After surgery, instruct the patient to limit her activities. *Teach her to avoid lifting anything heavier than 5 pounds, strenuous exercises, and sexual intercourse for 6 weeks.* For discomfort, tell her to use heat either as a moist heating pad or warm compresses applied to the abdomen. A hot bath may also be helpful. Sutures do not need to be removed because some are absorbable and others will fall out as healing occurs. Tell the woman to notify her health care provider if she has signs of infection, such as fever, persistent pain, or purulent, foul-smelling discharge. Encourage her to keep her follow-up appointment after surgery.

Posterior colporrhaphy (posterior repair) reduces *rectal* bulging. If both a cystocele and a rectocele are present, an *anterior and posterior colporrhaphy (A&P repair)* is performed.

The nursing care after a posterior repair is similar to that after any rectal surgery. After surgery, a low-residue (low-fiber) diet is usually prescribed to decrease bowel movements and allow time for the incision to heal. Instruct the patient to avoid straining when she does have a bowel movement so that she does not put pressure on the suture line. Bowel movements are often painful, and she may need pain medication before having a stool. Provide sitz baths or delegate this activity to unlicensed nursing personnel to relieve the woman's discomfort. Health teaching for the patient undergoing a posterior repair is similar to that for undergoing an anterior repair.

Vaginal hysterectomy may accompany any uterine prolapse repair surgery unless the women wants children or more children. This procedure is described on p. 1696.

FISTULAS

Fistulas are abnormal openings between two adjacent organs or structures. Vaginal fistulas can occur between the vagina and the urethra (urethrovaginal), the vagina and the bladder (vesicovaginal), or the vagina and the rectum (rectovaginal). Traumatic childbirth is the main cause of fistulas, although they can result from complications of surgery, cancer, or radiation therapy for cancer.

Clinical manifestations depend on the location of the fistula. Ask the patient about any:

- Leakage of urine, flatus, or feces into the vagina
- Irritation or excoriation of the vulva and vaginal tissues
- Unpleasant odor (fecal or urine) in the vagina

Women who have fistulas may be embarrassed to seek help until symptoms are severe. They may withdraw from social activities or from relationships with their partners as the symptoms become more difficult to manage.

Management depends on the fistula's location. Surgery is not recommended if infection or inflammation is present. Nursing care focuses on assisting the woman with the frequent and time-consuming perineal hygiene, including sitz baths; perineal cleaning with mild, unscented soap and water; and low-pressure douching with commercial deodorizing or homemade solutions (1 teaspoon [5 mL] of household chlorine bleach to 1 quart [about 1 L] of water). Teach the woman to wear sanitary napkins or disposable undergarments (e.g., Depends) if there is leakage of urine or feces. Bladder and bowel training may help her time her elimination to occur before activities. Other interventions may include the application of A+D Ointment to excoriated tissues. Assess and provide support for signs of depression or other emotional response. Encourage her to voice her frustrations and concerns. Address the concerns of her partner.

If the fistula is repaired surgically, nursing care focuses on preventing infection and avoiding stress on the repaired area (low-residue diet and administration of stool softeners for 2 to 3 weeks after rectovaginal fistula repair). Nursing care and teaching after surgery are similar to the care and teaching of the patient who has a cystocele or rectocele repair.

BENIGN NEOPLASMS

OVARIAN CYST

Functional ovarian cysts can occur in a woman of any age but are rare after menopause. Other cysts and tumors of the ovaries are not related to the menstrual cycle but arise from ovarian tissue. Primary assessment involves pelvic examination and transvaginal ultrasound. Further testing with computerized tomography (CT) or magnetic resonance imaging (MRI) or laparoscopic biopsy to rule out cancer may be indicated. Some ovarian cysts disappear over time, and others cause discomfort for a prolonged period. Laparoscopic surgery to remove the cyst or ovary may be needed.

UTERINE LEIOMYOMA

Pathophysiology

Leiomyomas, also called **fibroids,** are benign, slow-growing solid tumors of the uterine myometrium (muscle layer). They are classified according to their position in the layers of the uterus. The most common types are intramural, submucosal, and subserosal (Fig. 74-4).

Intramural leiomyomas are contained in the uterine wall within the myometrium. *Submucosal* leiomyomas protrude into the cavity of the uterus and can cause bleeding and disrupt pregnancy. *Subserosal* leiomyomas protrude through the outer surface of the uterine wall and may extend to the broad ligament, pressing other organs.

Although most fibroids develop within the uterine wall, a few may appear in the cervix. Pedunculated leiomyomas are attached by a pedicle (stalk) to the outside of the uterus and occasionally break off and attach to other tissues (parasitic fibroids).

Etiology

Although the cause is not known, leiomyomas develop from excessive local growth of smooth muscle cells. This may be a genetic error causing a lack of ability to halt growth. The growth of leiomyomas may be related to stimulation by estro-

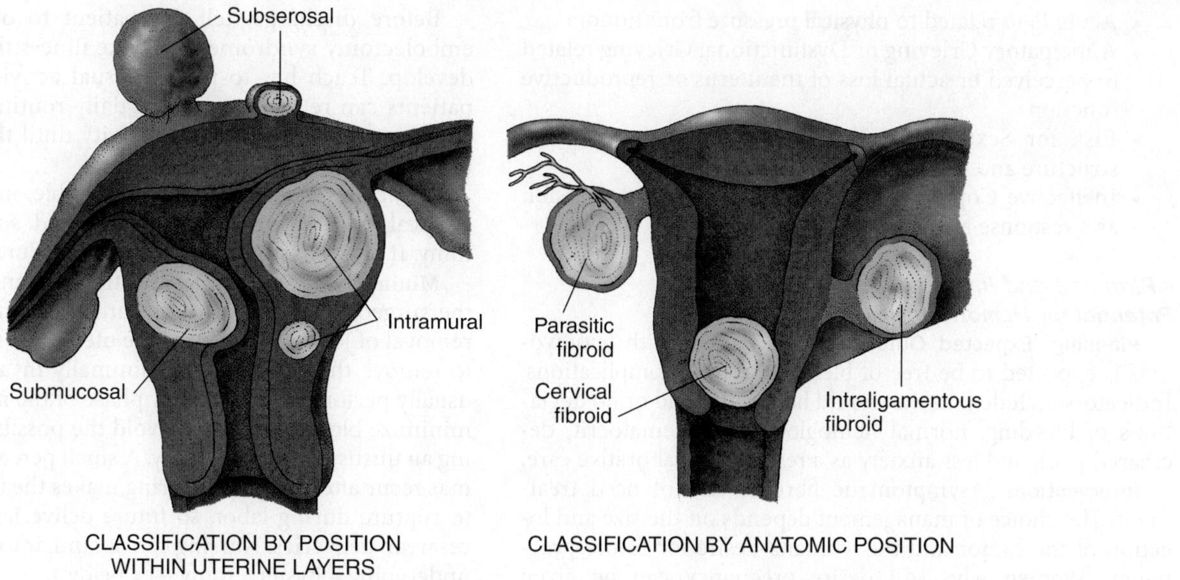
Subserosal
Intramural
Submucosal
CLASSIFICATION BY POSITION WITHIN UTERINE LAYERS
Parasitic fibroid
Cervical fibroid
Intraligamentous fibroid
CLASSIFICATION BY ANATOMIC POSITION

Fig. 74-4 • Classification of uterine leiomyomas.

gen, progesterone, and growth hormone. This explains why fibroids sometimes enlarge during pregnancy and diminish in size after menopause.

Incidence/Prevalence

The incidence of leiomyomas increases as women get older. Many women have asymptomatic fibroids, whereas others have severe symptoms. African-American women have a higher incidence than Euro-American women, but the reason is not known (www.ahrq.gov/reasearch/fibroid). Women who have never been pregnant also are at a high risk.

Patient-Centered Collaborative Care

evolve ONLINE PHARM REVIEW

Assessment

History

Ask the patient if her mother had fibroids. Rapid cellular division in the tumor can outgrow its blood supply, causing degeneration and bleeding. Menstrual bleeding may be increased *(hypermenorrhea)*. The bleeding may occur between menstrual periods *(intermenstrual bleeding)*, or it may be continuous. Any bleeding in the postmenopausal woman should be evaluated.

Physical Assessment/Clinical Manifestations

Women with fibroids do not usually have pain, although acute pain may occur with twisting of the fibroid on its stalk. *The patient often seeks medical attention because of heavy vaginal bleeding.* Ask about how many tampons or menstrual pads she uses a day. The woman may report a feeling of pelvic pressure, constipation, or urinary frequency or retention. These symptoms result when an enlarged fibroid presses on other organs. The patient may notice that her abdomen has increased in size. Assess the woman's abdomen for distention or enlargement. Ask if she has dyspareunia (painful intercourse) and infertility (inability to become pregnant).

Abdominal, vaginal, and rectal examinations usually reveal the presence of a uterine enlargement. Further diagnostic procedures are needed to differentiate benign tumors from cancerous ones.

Psychosocial Assessment

Symptoms may significantly lower the patient's quality of life. A woman who is symptomatic may fear that she has cancer. She may be anxious about abnormal bleeding or her failure to conceive. She may also be concerned if surgery is recommended if she wants to have children or more children. Assess the woman's feelings and concerns about her symptoms and fears of the unknown. If hysterectomy is recommended, explore the significance of the loss of the uterus for the woman and her partner. Discuss sexuality issues with the patient based on your assessment.

Laboratory Assessment

A complete blood count may identify iron deficiency anemia (related to bleeding). A pregnancy test is done to determine whether pregnancy is the cause of the uterine enlargement. An endometrial biopsy may be performed to evaluate for endometrial cancer.

Imaging Assessment

Ultrasound is usually the first choice for imaging. *Transvaginal ultrasound* with saline infusion (saline sonogram) provides a good picture of a submucosal fibroid that may protrude into the uterine cavity. The clinician may then choose to directly view and biopsy a tumor, using *laparoscopy* (for tumors on the outside of the uterus) or hysteroscopy (for tumors accessible inside the uterus). *Magnetic resonance imaging (MRI)* can differentiate between benign and malignant lesions.

Analysis

Common Nursing Diagnoses and Collaborative Problems

The most common collaborative problem for patients with leiomyomas is Potential for Hemorrhage.

Additional Nursing Diagnoses and Collaborative Problems

In addition to the common collaborative problems, patients with leiomyomas may have one or more of these nursing diagnoses:

- Anxiety and Fear related to a threat to or change in health status (uncertain diagnosis; potential surgical treatment)

- Acute Pain related to physical pressure from tumors
- Anticipatory Grieving or Dysfunctional Grieving related to perceived or actual loss of the uterus or reproductive function
- Risk for Sexual Dysfunction related to altered body structure and dyspareunia
- Ineffective Coping related to uncertainty or depression as a response to treatment

Planning and Implementation

Potential for Hemorrhage

Planning: Expected Outcomes. The patient with leiomyomas is expected to be free of bleeding and its complications. Indicators include that she should have only mild or no deviations of bleeding, normal hemoglobin and hematocrit, decreased pain, and less anxiety as a result of collaborative care.

Interventions. Asymptomatic fibroids do not need treatment. The choice of management depends on the size and location of the tumor and the woman's desire for future pregnancy. Women who still desire pregnancy can be given magnetic resonance–guided focused ultrasound surgery or laparoscopic myomectomy to remove the tumor. Uterine artery embolization and hysterectomy are choices for women who no longer desire pregnancy.

Nonsurgical Management. If the woman is menopausal, the fibroids usually shrink and surgery may not be necessary. *Teach the patient who is receiving hormone replacement therapy for menopausal symptoms that the fibroids may continue to grow because of estrogen stimulation.*

If the woman has few symptoms or desires childbearing, the health care provider recommends observation and examination every 4 to 6 months. As with dysmenorrhea and dysfunctional uterine bleeding, mild leiomyoma symptoms can be managed with NSAIDs, extended-cycle hormonal contraception, or levonorgestrel IUD. *Gonadotropin-releasing hormone (GnRH) agonists* such as goserelin (Zoladex) and leuprolide (Lupron Depot) induce artificial menopause. These drugs decrease hormone exposure and give the tumor time to shrink temporarily. This may also be done before surgery.

Magnetic resonance–guided focused ultrasound is a noninvasive, painless technique for women who wish to preserve their fertility. The woman lies prone on an MRI scanner, which provides a three-dimensional image of the pelvis. The technician then guides a focused pulse of ultrasound to heat the tumor to destroy it.

An alternative to surgery for the woman who does not desire pregnancy is **uterine artery embolization** (also called *uterine fibroid embolization [UFE]*) under moderate sedation. The interventional radiologist uses a percutaneous catheter inserted through the femoral artery to inject polyvinyl alcohol pellets into the uterine artery. The resulting blockage starves the tumor of circulation, allowing it (or them) to shrink. The patient stays overnight in the hospital.

After the procedure, the woman may have severe cramping caused by decreased blood flow to the uterus. Cramping continues for 2 to 4 days. Assess her pain level, and provide analgesics as needed. If a vascular closure device is used at the arterial insertion site, raise the head of the bed. Help the patient ambulate in about 2 hours after the procedure. If a closure device was not used, keep her on bedrest with the leg immobilized for 4 hours before ambulating (McDaniel, 2007).

Before discharge, tell the patient to observe for postembolectomy syndrome, a flu-like illness that some women develop. Teach her to resume usual activities slowly. Most patients can return to work or daily routine within a week. She should avoid strenuous activity until the physician recommends it.

Surgical Management. When possible, minimally invasive surgical (MIS) techniques are performed, such as a myomectomy. If not, a hysterectomy is the procedure of choice.

Minimally invasive surgery. If the woman desires children, the surgeon may perform a laparoscopic **myomectomy** (the removal of leiomyomas from the uterus). A laser may be used to remove the tumors. This minimally invasive procedure is usually performed in the early phase of the menstrual cycle to minimize blood loss and to avoid the possibility of interrupting an unsuspected pregnancy. A small percentage of leiomyomas recur after surgery. Scarring makes the uterus more likely to rupture during labor, so future deliveries will be planned cesarean deliveries. Nursing care is similar to that for a woman undergoing a hysterectomy (see below).

In selected cases (e.g., submucous fibroids, menorrhagia), a *transcervical endometrial resection (TCER)* is performed via hysteroscopy. A hysteroscope (endoscope) is inserted into the uterus, and the endometrium is destroyed using diathermy (heat) or radioablation. Potential complications of hysteroscopic surgery include:

- Fluid overload (fluid used to distend the uterine cavity can be absorbed)
- Embolism
- Hemorrhage
- Perforation of the uterus, bowel, or bladder and ureter injury
- Persistent increased menstrual bleeding
- Incomplete suppression of menstruation

Monitor for any indications of these problems, and report signs and symptoms, such as severe pain and heavy bleeding, to the surgeon immediately. Scarring may cause a small risk for complications in future pregnancies.

Hysterectomy. Leiomyomas are the most common reason for hysterectomies. A uterus that has smaller fibroids may be removed via a *total vaginal hysterectomy (TVH).* The surgeon removes the uterus and cervix, sometimes in pieces, through the vagina without an external surgical incision. A *total abdominal hysterectomy (TAH)* is usually performed for leiomyomas larger than the size of a 16-week pregnancy. The uterus and cervix are removed through a horizontal bikini incision (traditional procedure) or by laparoscopic surgery (MIS), which requires several very small umbilical incisions. In both vaginal and abdominal hysterectomies, the surgeon removes the uterus from the five supporting ligaments, which are then attached to the vaginal cuff so that normal depth of the vagina is maintained (Table 74-3).

Preoperative teaching by the health care team begins in the surgeon's office. Explain procedures that routinely take place before surgery, including laboratory tests and expected drugs such as a prophylactic antibiotic. Teach about the need for turning, coughing, and deep-breathing exercises; incentive spirometry; early ambulation; and pain relief (see Chapter 16 for a discussion of general patient care before surgery).

Psychological assessment is essential. Assess the significance of the surgery for the woman and her partner. If it involves loss of the uterus, she may feel a great loss if she wishes to retain her childbearing ability. Many women relate their uterus to self-image and femininity or believe that their sexual function is related to their uterus. Although surgical menopause by hysterectomy can create loss of libido and vaginal changes, teach the patient that vaginal estrogen cream and gentle dilation can help correct that. Reassure her regarding any misperceptions about the effects of hysterectomy, such as association with masculinization and weight gain. Assess the patient's support system. She may fear rejection by her sexual partner. Include the partner in all teaching sessions, unless this practice is not culturally acceptable.

Postoperative care of the woman who has undergone a TAH is similar to that of any patient who has had abdominal surgery (see Chapter 18). Assess (Chart 74-8):

- Vaginal bleeding (there should be less than one saturated perineal pad in 4 hours)
- Abdominal bleeding at the incision site (a small amount is normal)
- Intactness of the incision
- Urine output per urinary catheter for 24 hours or less (for traditional surgery)
- Pain

TABLE 74-3 Common Gynecologic Surgeries

TOTAL HYSTERECTOMY
All the uterus, including the cervix, is removed. The procedure may be vaginal, abdominal, or laparoscopic.

SUBTOTAL HYSTERECTOMY
All the uterus, except the cervix, is removed. This procedure is rarely performed.

BILATERAL SALPINGO-OOPHORECTOMY
Fallopian tubes and ovaries are removed.

PANHYSTERECTOMY
Total abdominal hysterectomy and bilateral salpingo-oophorectomy. The uterus, ovaries, and fallopian tubes are removed abdominally.

RADICAL HYSTERECTOMY
All the uterus is removed abdominally. The lymph nodes, the upper third of the vagina, and the surrounding tissues (parametrium) are also removed.

Specific interventions for a vaginal hysterectomy include:

- Assessment of vaginal bleeding (there should be less than one saturated pad in 4 hours)
- Urinary catheter care
- Perineal care (sitz baths or ice packs)

The surgeon usually removes the abdominal sutures or clips for a traditional TAH at the first postoperative visit. Vaginal sutures are usually absorbed. Monitor for complications associated with hysterectomies, and report them to the health care provider (Table 74-4).

Community-Based Care

The patient with uterine leiomyomas is managed on an ambulatory care basis unless surgery is performed. After discharge, she usually returns to her home.

Home Care Management

Collaborate with the case manager when planning for home care management. The woman is usually discharged to the home setting 1 to 2 days after a traditional TAH, depending on her age and general health. TVH, laparoscopic surgery, or TCER are usually performed as same-day surgery in an ambulatory setting. Teach the patient to limit stair climbing for

TABLE 74-4 Common Postoperative Complications of Traditional Abdominal and Vaginal Hysterectomies

ABDOMINAL HYSTERECTOMY
- Intestinal obstruction (paralytic ileus)
- Thromboembolism
- Atelectasis
- Pneumonia
- Wound dehiscence (especially in obese patients)
- Urinary retention

VAGINAL HYSTERECTOMY
- Hemorrhage
- Urinary tract complications, especially infection or retention
- Wound infection
- Urinary retention

Chart 74-8 FOCUSED ASSESSMENT
The Patient After Total Abdominal Hysterectomy

Assess cardiovascular, respiratory, renal, and gastrointestinal status, including:
- Vital signs
- Heart, lung, and bowel sounds
- Urine output
- Temperature and color of the skin
- Red blood cell, hemoglobin, and hematocrit levels
- Activity tolerance
- Dressing and drains for color and amount of drainage
- Peripads for vaginal bleeding and clots
- Fluid intake (IVs until peristalsis returns and patient is tolerating oral intake)
- Signs of thrombophlebitis

Teach the patient to use these interventions to prevent postoperative complications:
- Cough and deep-breathing exercises
- Incentive spirometry
- Sequential compression devices
- Ambulation
- Avoidance of heavy lifting or strenuous activity

Assess the home care teaching needs of the patient related to the illness and surgery, including:
- Physiologic effects of the surgery
- Signs or symptoms to report
- Side or toxic effects of medications
- Activity limitations related to driving and use of stairs
- Follow-up care
- Postoperative restrictions related to sexual activity, use of tampons, and bathing
- Care of wound and/or drains

Assess the patient's coping skills and reaction to the diagnosis and surgical procedure.

several weeks. If she lives alone and is not permitted to drive for 2 to 6 weeks, she will need to make arrangements for transportation to follow-up visits.

Health Teaching

Teach the woman who has undergone an abdominal hysterectomy about the expected physical changes, any activity restrictions, diet, sexual activity, wound care, complications, and the need for follow-up care. Chart 74-9 lists areas to include for health teaching.

Women who have undergone a hysterectomy need information about possible emotional reactions. Generally, women adjust well to surgery if they have completed childbearing, have interests outside the home, work, have no misconceptions about the effects of hysterectomy, and have support from the family, especially their sexual partner.

Reactions may be different after vaginal and abdominal procedures because women who have undergone a vaginal hysterectomy have no obvious change in body image. Psychological reactions can occur months to years after surgery, particularly if sexual functioning and libido are diminished. Women identified as being at high risk for psychological problems may need long-term follow-up care or referral. They may need to be counseled about signs of depression. Intermittent sadness is normal, but continued feelings of low self-esteem or loss of interest or pleasure in usual activities and pastimes is not normal and should be evaluated. Provide written materials, and focus on the positive aspects of the woman's life to help decrease adverse psychological reactions.

Health Care Resources

Usually no special home equipment is needed for a woman who has undergone a hysterectomy. A home care nurse may be needed to assess and monitor the older adult's progress after surgery if other conditions (e.g., uncontrolled diabetes) are present. Financial assistance may be needed, and referral to the hospital's department of social services or case management department may be indicated if the woman has no insurance coverage. Provide a referral for psychological or sexual counseling if potential problems are identified before discharge.

Evaluation: Outcomes

Evaluate the care of the patient who has undergone surgery for leiomyomas on the basis of the identified nursing diagnoses and collaborative problems. The expected outcomes include that she should:

- Be free of hemorrhage
- Recover from surgery without complications

Specific indicators for these outcomes are listed for each collaborative problem under the Planning and Implementation section (earlier).

DECISION-MAKING CHALLENGE
Coordination of Care

A 77-year-old woman living by herself at home has been having heavy vaginal bleeding for 3 months but is afraid to see a physician. She has become weak and no longer has enough energy to

Chart 74-9 PATIENT AND FAMILY EDUCATION GUIDE
Care After a Total Abdominal Hysterectomy

EXPECTED PHYSICAL CHANGES
- You will no longer have a period, although you may have some vaginal discharge for a few days after you go home.
- It will not be possible for you to become pregnant, and birth control methods are no longer needed.
- If your ovaries were removed, you may have some menopause symptoms such as hot flushes, night sweats, and vaginal dryness.
- It is normal to tire more easily and require more sleep and rest during the first few weeks after surgery (this may last for 2 to 3 months).

ACTIVITY
- Limit stair climbing to fewer than five times per day.
- Take showers rather than tub baths.
- Do not lift anything heavier than 5 lbs.
- Walk indoors for the first week. Then gradually increase walking as exercise, but stop before you become fatigued.
- Avoid the sitting position for any extended period. When you sit, do not cross your legs at the knees.
- Avoid jogging, aerobic exercise, participating in sports, and any strenuous activity for 6 weeks.
- Do not drive for at least 4 weeks or until your surgeon has told you it is alright.

DIET
- Eat a well-balanced diet with extra protein and vitamin C to help heal your tissues.
- Drink at least 3 quarts of fluid, especially water, each day unless you have another health problem (like heart failure or kidney disease) that requires fluid restriction.
- If gas is a problem, avoid foods and beverages that increase gas.

SEXUAL ACTIVITY
- Do not engage in sexual intercourse for 4 to 6 weeks, as prescribed by your surgeon.
- If you had a vaginal "repair" as part of your surgery, the first time you have intercourse you may have some tenderness or pain because the vaginal walls are tighter. Careful intercourse and the use of water-based lubricants can help reduce this discomfort. This discomfort usually goes away with time and stretching of the vagina.

FOLLOW-UP CARE
- If antibiotics are prescribed, take them as directed until all the drugs are gone.
- Make and keep your follow-up appointment(s) with your surgeon.

COMPLICATIONS
- Take your temperature twice each day for the first 2 weeks after surgery.
- Check your incision daily for signs of infection (increasing redness, open areas, drainage that is thick or foul-smelling, incision pain).

REPORT ANY OF THE FOLLOWING TO YOUR SURGEON
- Increased vaginal drainage or change in drainage (bloodier, thicker, foul-smelling)
- Temperature over 100° F
- Pain, tenderness, redness, or swelling in your calves
- Pain or burning on urination

clean her house and prepare meals. Her daughter persuades her to have her problem checked today. The gynecologist suspects uterine fibroids for which she is scheduled to have a vaginal hysterectomy. She also has diabetes mellitus (taking insulin), controlled hypertension, and a history of MI.

1. What preoperative testing might the physician request?
2. What postoperative care will this patient need?
3. With what members of the health care team would you need to collaborate to provide continuity of care after discharge?
4. Do you think she will be able to go home immediately after hospital discharge? Why or why not?

evolve For suggested answer guidelines, go to http://evolve.elsevier.com/Iggy/.

BARTHOLIN CYST

Pathophysiology

Bartholin cyst is a common disorder of the vulva. It results from obstruction of the duct of the Bartholin gland. The secretory function of the gland continues, and the fluid fills the obstructed duct. The main causes of the obstruction are infection, thickened mucus near the ductal opening, or trauma, such as lacerations or episiotomy.

Patient-Centered Collaborative Care

The patient may be asymptomatic if the cyst is small. Ask if she has dyspareunia (painful intercourse) or inadequate genital lubrication. Assess for swelling in the perineal area. A large cyst usually causes constant local pain and may cause difficulty walking or sitting. Physical examination of the vulva reveals a swelling immediately beneath the skin in the posterior portion of the vulva. The cyst may appear brown or bloody, depending on its contents. Usually it is present on only one side and ranges from $^3/_8$ to 4 inches (1 to 10 cm) in size.

If the cyst is draining, a fluid sample is sent to the laboratory for culture (for gonorrhea and aerobic and anaerobic organisms) and sensitivity testing. If the woman is older than 40 years, a biopsy of the cyst is done to identify possible cancer.

If the woman is asymptomatic, no intervention is needed. An abscess usually ruptures spontaneously within 72 hours of forming. Teach the woman with an abscess to take over-the-counter or prescribed analgesics and apply moist heat (sitz baths or hot wet packs) to the vulva. Cultures most often reveal *Escherichia coli* or *Staphylococcus aureus*, for which antibiotics are prescribed.

Simple incision and drainage (I&D) may provide temporary relief. However, cysts tend to recur when the opening of the duct reobstructs. Usually the surgeon establishes a permanent opening for drainage. **Marsupialization** (formation of a pouch that is a new duct opening) is performed using local, regional, or general anesthesia. Discomfort after surgery may be relieved with analgesics and sitz baths. Prophylactic antibiotics may be prescribed.

The Bartholin glands may be totally removed in older women when cancer is suspected or if infections with abscess formation recur. Care after surgery includes:

- Application of ice packs or sitz baths several times a day for comfort and promotion of healing
- Analgesics for pain
- Prophylactic antibiotics
- Assessment of the incision for signs of healing or infection

CERVICAL POLYP

Cervical polyps are *pedunculated* (on stalks) tumors that arise from the mucosa and extend through the opening of the cervical os. They result from a hyperplasia (overgrowth) of the endocervical epithelium in response to hormonal stimulation. Polyps may also be due to inflammation or to localized vascular congestion of the cervical blood vessels. They are the most common benign growth of the cervix and occur most often in women older than 40 years who have had several children.

A woman may be asymptomatic, have premenstrual or postmenstrual bleeding, or have bleeding after intercourse. A speculum examination may reveal a small single polyp or multiple polyps. They are bright red, are soft and fragile, and may bleed when touched.

Polyp removal is a simple office procedure. The base of the polyp is grasped with a clamp, and the polyp is twisted off and sent to the pathology laboratory for evaluation. Cautery usually stops any bleeding at the site of removal. The woman does not feel any pain during the procedure. Instruct her to avoid tampon use, douches, and sexual intercourse for a week or until healing has taken place.

GYNECOLOGIC CANCERS

ENDOMETRIAL (UTERINE) CANCER

Pathophysiology

Endometrial cancer (cancer of the inner uterine lining) is the most common gynecologic malignancy in the United States. Its growth is generally slow, and early symptoms of vaginal bleeding generally lead to prompt evaluation and treatment. As a result, this type of cancer has a good prognosis.

Adenocarcinoma is the most common type, accounting for 80% of all cases. The tumor arises from the glandular part of the endometrium and usually follows endometrial hyperplasia (overgrowth). This usually occurs in younger postmenopausal women. It is strongly associated with conditions causing prolonged exposure to estrogen without the protective effects of progesterone. Risk factors for endometrial cancer are listed in Table 74-5. Although most cases of endometrial cancer do not have a genetic predisposition, it is more common in families who have gene mutations for hereditary nonpolyposis colon cancer (HNPCC) (Nussbaum et al., 2007).

The initial growth of the cancer is within the uterine cavity, followed by extension into the myometrium and the cervix. Metastasis outside the uterus occurs in these ways:

- Through lymphatic spread to the ovaries and parametrial, pelvic, inguinal, and para-aortic lymph nodes
- By blood, to the lungs, liver, or bone
- By transtubal or intra-abdominal spread to the peritoneal cavity

More than 40,000 new cases of endometrial cancer and 7,000 deaths occur annually in the United States. Thus about 1 of every 100 women in the United States has endometrial cancer. The average age at diagnosis is 60 years (American Cancer Society [ACS], 2008).

Patient-Centered Collaborative Care

Assessment

Physical Assessment/Clinical Manifestations

The main symptom of endometrial cancer is postmenopausal bleeding. Ask the patient how many tampons or menstrual pads she uses each day. Some women also have a watery, bloody

TABLE 74-5 Risk Factors for Endometrial Cancer and Cervical Cancer

Endometrial Cancer	Cervical Cancer
Age 50 to 70 yr	Infection with HPV
Family history of endometrial cancer or HNPCC	Multiparity (multiple births)
Diabetes mellitus	Smoking
Hypertension	Younger than 18 yr at first intercourse
Obesity	Multiple sex partners
Uterine polyps	African American
Late menopause	Oral contraceptive use
Nulliparity (no childbirths)	History of STDs
Smoking	Obesity or poor diet
	Family history of cervical cancer
	HIV/AIDS
	Lower socioeconomic status
	Sexual partner had a previous partner who developed cervical cancer
	Intrauterine exposure to DES

AIDS, Acquired immune deficiency syndrome; *DES,* diethylstilbestrol; *HIV,* human immune deficiency virus; *HNPCC,* hereditary nonpolyposis colon cancer; *HPV,* human papillomavirus; *STDs,* sexually transmitted diseases.

vaginal discharge, low back or abdominal pain, and low pelvic pain (caused by pressure of the enlarged uterus). Ask the patient to describe the exact location and intensity of her discomfort. A pelvic examination may reveal the presence of a palpable uterine mass or uterine polyp. The uterus is enlarged if the cancer is advanced.

Diagnostic Assessment

Transvaginal ultrasound and *endometrial biopsy* are the gold standard tests to determine the presence of endometrial thickening and cancer. Saline may be infused during the ultrasound to improve the image of the uterine cavity. The clinician then collects an endometrial biopsy from inside the uterus via a thin, flexible suction curette through the cervix. A dilation and curettage to obtain a tissue sample is seldom done today because an operative suite is needed and because of the risks and cost of the procedure.

Other diagnostic tests to determine the patient's overall health status and the presence of metastasis (cancer spread) include:

- CA-125 tumor marker to rule out ovarian involvement
- Chest x-ray
- Genetic testing for gene causing HNPCC, if there is a family history
- Intravenous pyelography (IVP), or excretory urography, to assess renal function and to assess for renal metastasis
- Barium enema study to assess for intestinal metastasis
- Computed tomography (CT) of the pelvis to identify the spread of the tumor
- Liver and bone scans to assess for distant metastasis

Some women also have a hysteroscopic examination of the uterus and proctosigmoidoscopy depending on the stage of their cancer.

Psychosocial Assessment

Before a diagnosis is made, the woman may deny that the symptoms are related to cancer. During the diagnostic phase, the woman may express fears and concerns about having the disease. After the diagnosis is confirmed, she may express disbelief, anger, depression, anxiety, or withdrawal behaviors. Assess these emotional reactions, and encourage the patient to discuss them. Ask her about how she copes with other stressful events, and assess her support systems.

▪ *Interventions*

Surgical removal of the tumor and lymph nodes and staging are the most important interventions for endometrial cancer. Stage I cancer is confined to the endometrium. Women with early stage I who wish to preserve their fertility may be given a trial of progesterone to reverse the lesion. Stage II involves the cervix. Stage III reaches the vagina or lymph nodes, and stage IV has spread beyond the pelvis.

Surgical Management

For stage I disease, the gynecology oncologist usually removes the uterus, fallopian tubes, and ovaries **(total hysterectomy** and **bilateral salpingectomy/oophorectomy),** as well as peritoneum fluid or washings for cytologic examination. Laparoscopic surgery has fewer complications, shorter hospital stay, and less cost. A radical hysterectomy with bilateral pelvic lymph node dissection and removal of the upper third of the vagina is performed for stage II cancer. Nursing care for a radical hysterectomy is the same as that for a simple hysterectomy except that the woman's hospitalization is usually longer and her convalescence may be extended.

Nonsurgical Management

Nonsurgical interventions (radiation therapy and chemotherapy) are used postoperatively and depend on the surgical staging. An older method was to deliver radiation therapy for 6 weeks before surgery to shrink the tumor and possibly inhibit recurrence. Although this method is still used for some patients, it is not the standard of care based on current evidence.

Radiation Therapy. The oncologist prescribes radiation therapy to be delivered either by external beam or with an internal source for stage II and stage III cancers. Women with stage II disease may use brachytherapy (internal) radiation to prevent recurrence of vaginal cancer and improve survival. Side effects of radiation therapy (RT) are local and include skin lesions, nausea, diarrhea, cystitis, and fistulas. See Chapter 24 for the general nursing care of patients receiving RT.

Intracavitary Radiation (Brachytherapy). The purpose of intracavitary radiation is to prevent disease recurrence. Brachytherapy requires a hospital stay. The radiologist places an applicator within the woman's uterus through the vagina while she is anesthetized. After the correct position of the applicator is confirmed by x-ray, the patient is taken to the hospital room and a radiologist places a radioactive isotope in the applicator, which remains for 1 to 3 days.

Before the procedure, instruct the patient about activities she will need to perform (e.g., deep-breathing and leg exercises) and restrictions during the time the radiation source is in place. While the radioactive implant is in place, the woman is strictly isolated, usually in a private room, because radiation is emitted and can affect other people. The amount of time needed for the therapy depends on the amount of radiation emitted from the source. The radiologist calculates the time needed for a specific dose of radiation. Usually this time ranges from 35 to 60 hours.

Inform the patient that she is restricted to bedrest on her back with the head of the bed flat or slightly elevated. Movement in bed is restricted to prevent dislodgment of the radioactive source. Assess the skin for breakdown over bony pressure points during the activity restriction period.

A urinary catheter is inserted into the bladder before the implant to prevent dislodgment of the implant, which can be caused by a full bladder or attempts to void. Encourage fluid intake to prevent urine stasis and infection. A low-residue diet is prescribed (to prevent bowel movements that might dislodge the implant). The radiologist usually prescribes:

- Antiemetics
- Broad-spectrum antibiotics (to prevent bladder infections)
- Mild sedatives (to help the patient relax)
- Analgesics
- Heparin or Lovenox (to prevent thromboembolism)
- Antidiarrheal medications (to prevent bowel movements)

Chart 74-10 lists the best practices for radiation precautions while caring for the patient with sealed implant radiation sources. *Organize care so that minimal time is spent close to the radiation source!*

External Radiation. External radiation therapy may be used to treat any stage of endometrial cancer in combination with surgery. Depending on the extent of the tumor, the treatment is given on an ambulatory care basis for 4 to 6 weeks. Tissue around the tumor and pelvic wall nodes also are treated. *Teach the patient to monitor for signs of skin breakdown, especially in the perineal area; to avoid sunbathing; and to avoid washing the markings outlining the treatment site.*

Drug Therapy. *Chemotherapy* is used as palliative treatment in advanced (Stage III or IV) and recurrent disease when it has spread to other parts of the body. Usually combinations of three agents are given for chemotherapy. Although the combination can vary, the three most common agents recommended for endometrial cancer are doxorubicin (Adriamycin), cisplatin (Platinol), and paclitaxel (Taxol). Chapter 24 describes chemotherapy and general nursing care during treatment.

Hormone therapy can be used for stage I and stage II cancers that are estrogen dependent and for palliative treatment of stage IV cancer. The hormones commonly prescribed are medroxyprogesterone acetate (Depo-Provera) and megestrol acetate (Megace). Tamoxifen citrate (Nolvadex♣, Tamofen♣), an anti-estrogen, is also used. The progestational agents do not usually cause acute side effects, but nausea and vomiting and hot flushes are associated with tamoxifen.

Complementary and Alternative Therapies. Every woman experiences cancer differently. Many complementary therapies have evidence of benefit in decreasing the side effects of drug therapy and boosting the immune system. Help her make informed, evidence-based decisions. Encourage her to check with her oncologist and/or pharmacist because some alternative therapies can be harmful or interfere with cancer treatment. Current evidence-based information is available about mind-body therapies, healing touch, herbs, vitamins, nutrition, and biologic therapies at the American Cancer Society website (www.cancer.org).

Chart 74-10 BEST PRACTICE FOR PATIENT SAFETY & QUALITY CARE

Care of the Patient with Sealed Implants of Radioactive Sources

- Assign the patient to a private room with a private bath.
- Place a "Caution: Radioactive Material" sign on the door of the patient's room.
- Wear a dosimeter film badge at all times while caring for patients with radioactive implants. The badge offers no protection but measures a person's exposure to radiation. Each badge should be used by only one person.
- Wear a lead shielding apron; always face the radiation source (do not turn your back toward the source).
- Stay as far away from the radiation source as possible.
- Pregnant nurses or those who are trying to become pregnant should not care for these patients; do not allow pregnant women or children younger than 16 years to visit.
- Limit each visitor to one-half hour per day. Be sure visitors are at least 6 feet from the source.
- Never touch the radioactive source with bare hands. In the rare instance that it is dislodged, use a long-handled forceps to retrieve it. Deposit the radioactive source in the lead container kept in the patient's room.
- Save all dressings and bed linens until after the radioactive source is removed. After the source is removed, dispose of dressings and linens in the usual manner. Other equipment can be removed from the room at any time.

Community-Based Care

Home Care Management

The woman with endometrial cancer is managed at home unless surgery is indicated. After surgery, she is usually discharged to her home. Home care after surgery for endometrial cancer is the same as that after a hysterectomy. (See discussion of Hysterectomy on p. 1696 in the Uterine Leiomyoma section.) Patients who are receiving chemotherapy or external radiation therapy are usually treated on an ambulatory care basis. Most women are surprised by the severe fatigue caused by radiation and chemotherapy. Help the patient and her family plan daily activities around trips to the clinic or the health care provider's office. If the tumor recurs and cure is not likely, the woman and her family need to think about hospice care and whether she can be cared for in the home.

Health Teaching

Teach the patient to report vaginal or rectal bleeding, foul-smelling discharge, abdominal pain or distention, and hematuria to the health care provider. These symptoms may be the result of the disease or its treatment.

The high dose of radiation causes sterility, and vaginal shrinkage can occur. Vaginal dilators can be used with water-soluble lubricants for 10 minutes each day until sexual activity resumes (in 10 days to 6 weeks). Reassure the woman that she is not radioactive and that her partner will not "catch" cancer by engaging in sexual intercourse.

Review all prescribed drugs, including the dosage and schedule, effects, and side effects. Emphasize the importance of keeping appointments for follow-up care.

Women need to discuss their concerns about the presence of cancer and the potential for recurrence. Provide emotional support, and create an atmosphere that encourages them to ask questions or express their fears and concerns. Include family members or significant others in discussions when possible.

Reactions to radiation therapy vary. Some women feel radioactive or "unclean" after treatments and may exhibit withdrawal behaviors. Reassure them by correcting any misconceptions. Patients who have chemotherapy may be upset if **alopecia** (hair loss) occurs. Warn them of this possibility before treatment starts. Wigs, scarves, or turbans can be worn until the hair grows back. Many women select these replacements before they lose their hair. Others shave their heads and begin wearing them immediately as the treatment begins. Tell women about these options so that they can make the best decision for them.

Often patients experience emotional crises because of the physical effects of cancer treatments. Radical hysterectomy may be seen as mutilating. Both radiation and chemotherapy have side effects that change physical appearance and body image. Women often may have a grief reaction to these changes. The feelings of loss depend on the visibility of the loss and the loss of function. Help the patient adapt to the body changes. One way to do this is to encourage self-management as soon as her physical condition is stable. Use a calm and accepting attitude.

Death can occur with or without treatment. The patient and family want the woman to pass the 5-year survival mark without a recurrence of disease. If there is a recurrence, they may be hostile and have manifestations of a grief reaction. Encourage patients and their families to discuss their feelings. Refer to support services such as certified hospital chaplains or other spiritual leader, social worker, or counselor. Response to loss and grieving is discussed in Chapter 9.

Health Care Resources

In the United States, local American Cancer Society (www.cancer.org) chapters provide written materials about endometrial cancer and information about local support groups. Each province in Canada also has a division of the Canadian Cancer Society (www.cancer.ca). If the patient is in the terminal stages of cancer, hospice care may be appropriate (see Chapter 9). If nursing care is needed at home, the hospital nurse or case manager makes referrals to a home health care agency. A referral to a social services agency may be needed if the patient cannot meet the financial demands of treatment and long-term follow-up.

CERVICAL CANCER

Pathophysiology

The uterine cervix is covered with squamous cells on the outer cervix and columnar (glandular) cells that line the endocervical canal. Papanicolaou (Pap) tests sample cells from both areas as a screening test for cervical cancer. The squamo-columnar junction is the *transformation zone* where most cell abnormalities occur. The adolescent has more columnar cells exposed on the outer cervix, which may be one reason she is more vulnerable to sexually transmitted diseases, including human immune deficiency virus (HIV). In contrast, in the menopausal woman, the squamo-columnar junction may be higher up in the endocervical canal, making it difficult to sample for a Pap test.

It generally takes years for the cervical cells to transform from normal to premalignant to invasive cancer. Premalignant changes are described on a continuum from atypia (suspicious) to *cervical intraepithelial neoplasia* (*CIN,* also known as *dysplasia,* the earliest premalignant change) to *carcinoma-in-situ (CIS),* which is the most advanced premalignant change.

Once cervical cancer has developed, it is described as preinvasive or invasive. *Preinvasive* cancer is limited to the cervix. *Invasive* cancer has spread to other pelvic structures.

Most cervical cancers arise from the squamous cells on the outside of the cervix. The other cancers arise from the mucus-secreting glandular cells (adenocarcinoma) in the endocervical canal. The disease spreads by direct extension to the vaginal mucosa, lower uterine segment, parametrium, pelvic wall, bladder, and bowel. Metastasis is usually confined to the pelvis, but distant spread can occur through lymphatic spread and the circulation to the liver, lungs, or bones. Table 74-6 shows the staging of cervical cancer.

Etiology

Risk factors for cervical cancer are listed in Table 74-5. Most cases of cervical cancer are caused by certain types of human papillomavirus (HPV). Almost all women will have HPV sometime in their lives, but not all types lead to cancer. HPV is the most common STD in the United States. It stimulates excessive growth in the epithelium, which may present as self-limiting warts, as described in Chapter 76, or may progress to cancer. In most cases, the cells of the cervix return to normal after the immune system attacks the HPV infection. Women who smoke or have HIV infection increase the risk of cervical cancer by impairing the immune system.

Women at the highest risk are those who have a long-standing high-risk HPV strain (Wells, 2008). The high-risk HPV types, especially types 16 and 18, impair the tumor-suppressor gene. The unrestricted tissue growth can spread, becoming invasive and metastatic.

Incidence/Prevalence

Invasive cancer of the cervix is the third most common cancer of the female genital system, after ovarian and uterine cancer. Over 11,000 U.S. women get cervical cancer annually, and about 3,700 women will die of it (ACS, 2008). Although much less common than breast cancer, cervical cancer has a lower 5-year survival rate.

CIN occurs mainly in young women. The peak incidence occurs in patients in their mid-20s. It usually resolves spontaneously within a year. CIS (carcinoma-in-situ) occurs in women about 30 years old, and invasive cancer occurs most commonly in the late 40s. The good news is that the overall U.S. and Canadian death rates for cervical cancer have dropped dramatically in the past two decades because of mass screen-

TABLE 74-6 Clinical Staging of Cervical Cancer*

Stage	Characteristics
I	Carcinoma is strictly confined to cervix (extension to corpus should be disregarded).
II	Carcinoma extends beyond cervix but has not extended to pelvic wall; it involves vagina but not as far as lower third.
III	Carcinoma has extended to pelvic wall; on rectal examination, there is no cancer-free space between tumor and pelvic wall; tumor involves lower third of vagina; all cases with hydronephrosis or nonfunctioning kidney should be included unless they are known to be due to another cause.
IV	Carcinoma has extended beyond true pelvis or has clinically involved mucosa of bladder or rectum.

*An a, b, or c designation at any stage indicates specific degree or depth of spread within that stage.

ing for premalignant and early-stage cancer through the Papanicolaou (Pap) test (also known as a *Pap smear*).

Health Promotion and Maintenance

Girls and young women who receive the currently used HPV vaccine (Gardasil), ideally before onset of intercourse, receive protection against the highest risk HPV types that are responsible for most cervical cancers. Teach them the importance of receiving the vaccine and the need to have the entire series (3 injections over 6 months). Tell the woman that the most frequent side effects are related to local irritation from the injections (e.g., pain, redness). Other common side effects include fever, nausea, dizziness, and diarrhea. Although rare, be sure that women know about long-term adverse effects, such as joint pain, peripheral neuropathy, and blood clots.

The American Cancer Society (ACS) (www.cancer.org) recommends that women have periodic pelvic examinations and Pap tests to screen for cervical cancer early. Teach women that they should begin these screening precautions within 3 years after having sexual intercourse or by the age of 21. Some health care providers, however, recommend the first examination and Pap test by age 18. For conventional Pap testing, *annual* screening is recommended by most experts. If the liquid test is used and the woman has no other risk factors (e.g., weakened immune system, HIV), it may be done *every 2 or 3 years* depending on the health provider's recommendations. The evidence about precise screening frequency remains conflicting (Wells, 2008).

Teach women that if they have a hysterectomy and have no other health risk factors, a Pap test is no longer needed. As women age, the usefulness of testing is also questionable. The ACS recommends that testing be discontinued after 70 years of age unless other risk factors exist that require ongoing screening.

Patient-Centered Collaborative Care

Assessment

Physical Assessment/Clinical Manifestations

The patient who has preinvasive cancer is often asymptomatic. *The classic symptom of invasive cancer is painless, vaginal bleeding.* Ask the patient if she has had or now has bleeding. It may start as spotting between menstrual periods or after sexual intercourse or douching. As the cancer grows, bleeding increases in frequency, duration, and amount and may become continuous.

Ask the woman if she has a watery, blood-tinged vaginal discharge that becomes dark and foul-smelling (occurs as the disease progresses). Leg pain (along the sciatic nerve) or swelling of one leg may be a late symptom or may indicate recurrent disease. Flank pain may be a late symptom of hydronephrosis, indicating advanced cancer pressing on the ureters, backing up the urine into the kidney. Ask the patient if she has had other signs of recurrence or metastasis such as:

- Unexplained weight loss
- **Dysuria** (painful urination)
- Pelvic pain (caused by pressure of the tumor on the bladder or the bowel)
- **Hematuria** (bloody urine)
- Rectal bleeding
- Chest pain
- Coughing

A physical examination may not reveal any abnormalities in early preinvasive cervical cancer. The internal pelvic examination may identify late-stage disease.

Diagnostic Assessment

Diagnostic assessment for cervical cancer begins with a *Pap smear.* Teach the woman not to have this test if she is having her menstrual period. Remind her to avoid these activities at least 48 hours before the test:

- Douching
- Sexual intercourse
- Tampons
- Vaginal creams, jellies, or other drugs

If Pap results are abnormal, an *HPV-typing DNA test* of the cervical sample can determine the presence of one or more high-risk types. The health care provider may perform a colposcopic examination to view the transformation zone. **Colposcopy** is a procedure in which application of a 3% acetic acid solution is applied to the cervix. The cervix is then examined under magnification with a bright filter light that enhances the visualization of the characteristics of dysplasia or cancer. If abnormal tissue is recognized, multiple biopsies of the cervical tissue are performed.

If atypical glandular cells are suspected, the health care provider may perform an *endocervical curettage* (scraping of the endocervix wall) as well. Encourage the patient to relax and breathe deeply during this uncomfortable procedure. Inform her that a small amount of bleeding is expected for up to 2 weeks after the biopsies.

Interventions

Interventions for the woman with cervical cancer are similar to those for endometrial cancer: surgery, which is possibly followed by radiation and chemotherapy for later-stage disease.

Surgical Management

Early stage I management techniques include local cervical ablation therapies of electrosurgical excision, laser therapy, or cryosurgery. Small tumors that are only microinvasive are managed with excisional conization or hysterectomy. Early stage *invasive* cancers are managed with radical surgery and radiation. Advanced inoperable cancers are treated with radiation. Factors that influence the choice of localized treatment versus surgical intervention include patient overall health, desire for future childbearing, tumor size, stage, cancer cell type, degree of lymph node involvement, and patient preference.

Early Surgical Procedures. The **loop electrosurgical excision procedure (LEEP)** is short (10 to 30 minutes) and is performed in a physician's office or in an ambulatory care setting with a local anesthetic injected into the cervix. A thin loop-wire electrode that transmits a painless electrical current is used to cut away affected tissue. LEEP is both a diagnostic procedure and a treatment, because it provides a specimen that can be examined by a pathologist to ensure the lesion was completely removed. Little discomfort is associated with this procedure. Spotting after the procedure is common. Teach patients to adhere for 3 weeks to the restrictions listed in Chart 74-11.

Laser therapy is also an office procedure used for early cancers. A laser beam is directed to the abnormal tissues, where energy from the beam is absorbed by the fluid in the tissues, causing them to vaporize. A small amount of bleeding occurs with the procedure, and the woman may have a slight vaginal discharge. Healing occurs in 6 to 12 weeks. A disadvantage of this procedure is that no specimen is available for study.

Cryotherapy involves freezing of the cancer, causing subsequent necrosis. The procedure is often painless, although some women have slight cramping after the procedure. The patient has a heavy watery discharge for several weeks after the procedure. Instruct her to follow the restrictions in Chart 74-11.

In cases of microinvasive cancer, a *conization* can remove the affected tissue while still preserving fertility. This procedure is done when the lesion cannot be visualized by colposcopic examination. A cone-shaped area of cervix is removed surgically and sent to the laboratory to determine the extent of the cancer. Potential complications from this procedure include hemorrhage and uterine perforation Long-term follow-up care is needed because new cancers can develop.

Chart 74-11 PATIENT AND FAMILY EDUCATION GUIDE

Care After Local Cervical Ablation Therapies

- Refrain from sexual intercourse.
- Do not use tampons.
- Do not douche.
- Take showers rather than tub baths.
- Avoid lifting heavy objects.
- Report any heavy vaginal bleeding, foul-smelling drainage, or fever.

The usual time period for these restrictions is 3 weeks. Your health care provider may prescribe a different (longer or shorter) time frame for you.

Hysterectomy. A simple hysterectomy may be performed as treatment of microinvasive cancer if the woman does not want children or more children. A vaginal approach is commonly used. A radical hysterectomy and bilateral pelvic lymph node dissection are as effective as radiation is for treating cancer that has extended beyond the cervix but not to the pelvic wall. Care for patients undergoing hysterectomy is found in the Uterine Leiomyoma section on p. 1696.

Pelvic Exenteration. One of the most radical surgical procedures, *pelvic exenteration,* is occasionally performed if there is no evidence of tumor outside the pelvis and no lymph node involvement. The three types of exenteration are anterior, posterior, and total (Fig. 74-5). *Anterior* exenteration is the removal of the uterus, cervix, ovaries, fallopian tubes, vagina, bladder, urethra, and pelvic lymph nodes. *Posterior* exenteration is the removal of the uterus, cervix, ovaries, fallopian tubes, descending colon, rectum, and anal canal. *Total* exenteration is a combination of anterior and posterior procedures. When the bladder is removed, urine drains through a urinary diversion (e.g., ileal conduit, Kock ileal urinary pouch). When the colon, rectum, and anal canal are removed, a colostomy is created for passage of feces. The stomas are located on the abdomen—the colostomy on the left and the ileal conduit on the right.

Postoperatively, the patient is admitted to a critical care unit for the first 1 to 2 days because of the high risk for com-

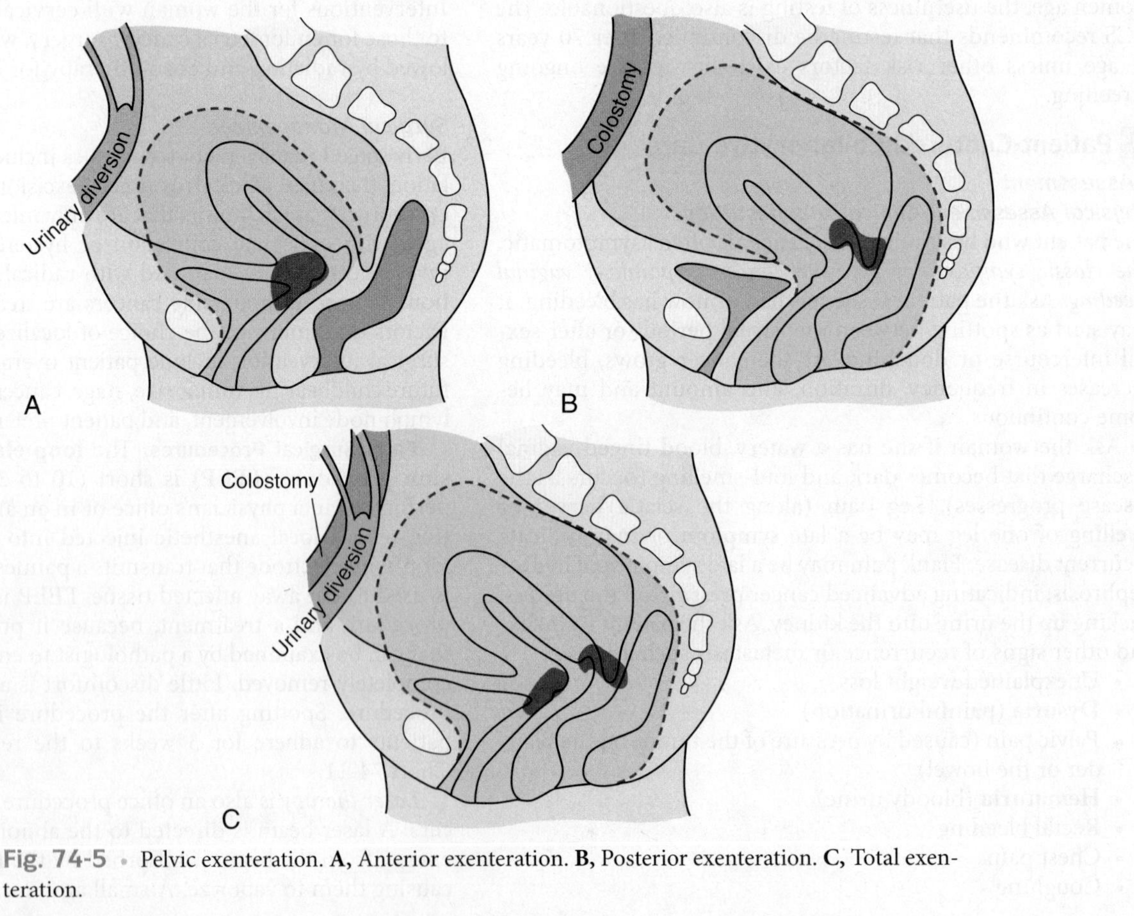
Urinary diversion
A
Colostomy
B
Colostomy
Urinary diversion
C

Fig. 74-5 • Pelvic exenteration. **A,** Anterior exenteration. **B,** Posterior exenteration. **C,** Total exenteration.

plications resulting from this massive surgery. Nursing care of wounds, stomas, and drains is similar to that for any postoperative patient in intensive care. After the surgeon removes the operative dressings, perineal irrigations may be done. Irrigation is usually done with normal saline solution. This is followed by drying of the perineum.

Nonsurgical Management

Radiation therapy is reserved for stage II invasive cervical cancer. For cancer that has extended beyond the cervix but not to the pelvic wall, radiation therapy is as effective as a radical hysterectomy. Intracavitary and external radiation therapies are used in combination, depending on the extent and location of the lesion. Intracavitary implants are usually used after the woman has completed 5 to 6 weeks of external pelvic radiation in combination with chemotherapy. The procedure is similar to that described on p. 1700 for endometrial cancer.

A combination of chemotherapy with cisplatin (Platinol) and radiation may also be used. This treatment modality shows 30% to 50% increased survival times but increased toxicity (anemia, nausea) and cost. Other drugs used alone or in combination include paclitaxel (Taxol), carboplatin, fluorouracil (5-FU), and mitomycin. See Chapter 24 for more information about the general nursing care for the patient on chemotherapy and radiation.

Community-Based Care

Community-based care for the patient after a hysterectomy is described in the discussion of Surgical Management on p. 1697 in the Uterine Leiomyoma section. The woman who has undergone a pelvic exenteration is usually in the hospital for at least 1 week after surgery. She may be discharged to a skilled nursing facility or transitional care unit for continued recovery and care or may be discharged directly to home depending on age and overall health. Physical activities are limited during convalescence. When the patient returns home, she needs personal and household assistance for up to 6 months. Collaborate with the case manager or discharge planner to help arrange for transportation and assistance with meals, self-management, and housework.

Collaborate with the wound and ostomy care nurse to teach the woman who has undergone a pelvic exenteration and her family how to manage her care. A home care nurse can assist with dressing changes and ostomy care and performs assessments for several weeks after discharge to home. The perineal opening may drain mucus for several months to a year, requiring sanitary pads. She will need teaching on nutritional adjustments for the ostomies and information on drug actions, dosages, and side effects.

Until walking is permitted, encourage range-of-motion exercises. Follow-up care is important. Counsel the patient about keeping all follow-up appointments. Provide information about late complications (e.g., infection, bowel obstruction) so that she can seek medical care promptly.

Grieving is common, usually by 3 to 5 days after surgery. At first, she may deny changes by refusing to look at the wound or stoma sites. Later she may become withdrawn or even angry or hostile. She may then move to reality testing by asking questions about her care, watching the nurses do wound care, and becoming actively involved in self-care. The patient needs intensive emotional support if she is to adapt to her altered body image and functions. Monitor for depression, which can persist for years.

Sexual function is different after exenteration (even if an artificial vagina is constructed), and the couple may need counseling about alternatives to intercourse. Even with vaginal reconstruction, the use of vaginal dilators is necessary to achieve desired sexual function. Assess the need for sexual counseling by listening for cues about altered perceptions of body image and anxiety about her sexual partner's response. Refer the patient and her partner as requested to a sexual or intimacy counselor.

OVARIAN CANCER

Pathophysiology

Most ovarian cancers are epithelial tumors that grow on the surface of the ovaries. These tumors grow rapidly, spread quickly, and are often bilateral. Tumor cells spread by direct extension into nearby organs and through blood and lymph circulation to distant sites. Free-floating cancer cells also spread through the abdomen to seed new sites, usually accompanied by ascites (abdominal fluid).

Ovarian cancer seems to be disordered growth in response to excessive exposure to estrogen. This would explain the protective effects of pregnancies and oral contraceptive use, both of which interrupt the monthly estrogen exposure. Table 74-7 lists known and suspected risk factors for ovarian cancer.

Ovarian cancer is the leading cause of death from female reproductive cancers. About 23,000 new cases are diagnosed each year, with 16,000 deaths (ACS, 2008). The incidence increases in women older than 50 years and peaks at 60 to 64 years of age. Family history accounts for a small percentage of cases. These women carry *BCRA1* or *BCRA2* genetic mutations. Of these, some choose to have a bilateral **salpingo-oophorectomy (BSO)** (removal of both ovaries and fallopian tubes). This surgery may reduce the risk for ovarian cancer by more than 90% in these patients (Nussbaum et al., 2007).

Survival rates are low because ovarian cancer is so often not detected until its late stages. The aging of the population makes it important for nurses to teach women to *"think ovarian"* if they have vague abdominal and GI symptoms.

TABLE 74-7 Risk Factors for Ovarian Cancer and Vulvar Cancer

Ovarian Cancer	Vulvar Cancer
Older than 40 years	Older than 40 years
Family history of ovarian or breast cancer or HNPCC	Cervical cancer
Diabetes mellitus	Diabetes mellitus
Nulliparity	Hypertension
Older than 30 years at first pregnancy	Obesity
Breast cancer	Infection with human papillomavirus (especially types 16 and 18)
Colorectal cancer	Cervical cancer
Infertility	Smoking
BRCA1 or *BRCA2* gene mutations	
Early menarche/late menopause	
Endometriosis	
Obesity/high-fat diet	

HNPCC, Hereditary nonpolyposis colon cancer.

Health Promotion and Maintenance

Health promotion measures to help prevent ovarian cancer include maintaining a normal weight and eating a well-balanced diet. Women who have had children, used oral contraception for at least 5 years, and breastfed their children also have less risk for having the disease (Bohnenkamp et al., 2007a).

Patient-Centered Collaborative Care

Assessment

Most women with ovarian cancer have had mild symptoms for several months but may have thought they were due to normal perimenopausal changes or stress. They may report abdominal pain or swelling or have vague GI disturbances such as dyspepsia (indigestion) and gas. Ask the patient if she has had urinary frequency or incontinence, unexpected weight loss, and/or vaginal bleeding.

Complications of advancing metastatic cancer include:

- Pleural effusion
- Ascites
- Lymphedema
- Intestinal obstruction
- Malnutrition

On pelvic examination, an abdominal mass may not be palpable until it reaches a size of 4 to 6 inches (10 to 15 cm). Any enlarged ovary found after menopause should be evaluated as though it were malignant. A Pap smear is of limited value for detecting ovarian cancer.

A cancer antigen test, *CA-125,* measures the presence of damaged endometrial and uterine tissue in the blood. It may be elevated if ovarian cancer is present, but it can also be elevated in patients with endometriosis, fibroids, pelvic inflammatory disease, pregnancy, and even menses. It is not a diagnostic test, but it is useful for monitoring a patient's progress during and after treatment. Transvaginal ultrasonography, chest radiography, and computed tomography (CT) are part of a complete workup to evaluate for metastasis. Complete blood work includes a liver profile if there is ascites.

Diagnosis depends on surgical exploration. Exploratory laparotomy (abdominal surgery) is performed to diagnose and stage ovarian tumors. Ovarian cancer is staged when it is removed. Five-year survival for stage I is 90% but only 10% for stage IV (ACS, 2008).

The woman with ovarian cancer has concerns similar to those described for the patient with endometrial cancer. Because the cancer is often diagnosed in an advanced stage, thoughts of death and dying, menopause, and loss of fertility come as a shock.

Interventions

Nursing care of the patient with ovarian cancer is similar to that for endometrial or cervical cancer. The options for treatment depend on the extent of the cancer and usually include surgery first, followed by chemotherapy. Radiation is used for more widespread cancers.

Surgical Management

Total abdominal hysterectomy (TAH) and bilateral salpingo-oophorectomy (BSO) are the surgical procedures for all stages of ovarian cancer. Surgery confirms disease, allows for surgical staging, and can remove or decrease the size of the tumor. When cancer has spread to other abdominal organs or lymph nodes, the tumors are removed during the surgery. Some women with large tumors may undergo presurgical chemotherapy to shrink the tumors before surgery.

The patient usually has a vertical midline incision instead of a horizontal incision. This incision improves the surgeon's ability to assess disease in the upper abdomen. The oncological surgeon inspects the upper abdomen. Peritoneal washings; frozen sections of the pelvic mass; biopsies of the pelvic organs, diaphragm, peritoneum, and omentum; and lymph nodes are sent to pathology during the surgery.

After surgery, nursing care is similar to that for the patient undergoing a hysterectomy for uterine leiomyomas. The vertical incision is assessed in the same fashion as a horizontal abdominal incision. As for any patient after abdominal surgery, assess vital signs and pain and maintain catheters and drains. Teach her the importance of antiembolism stockings, incentive spirometry, and early ambulation. Monitor for postoperative complications as discussed in Chapter 18. Infections after ovarian cancer surgery commonly affect the respiratory and urinary tract (Bohnenkamp et al., 2007b). Assess vital signs, and monitor the quantity and quality of urine output.

A 1-year "second-look" surgery used to be done routinely to assess and remove any new or residual tumor, but it did not improve outcomes (Martin, 2007). Today the standard of care is periodic CA-125, vaginal ultrasound CT, and chest radiography.

Nonsurgical Management

For all stages of ovarian cancer, cisplatin (Platinol), carboplatin, and taxanes of all types are the most common postoperative *drugs* used for treating ovarian cancer. They may be given IV or intraperitoneally. Intraperitoneal (IP) therapy is described in detail in Chapter 15. The drugs are usually given every 3 to 4 weeks for six cycles in an inpatient or ambulatory care setting. New drugs are being tested that use monoclonal antibodies, hormones, and agents that target cell growth and tumor blood supply.

External *radiation therapy* is used only if the disease is localized. Some areas may be irradiated for palliation in women with advanced disease. The general side effects of chemotherapy and radiation, as well as the associated general nursing care, are discussed in Chapter 24.

Community-Based Care

Patients having surgery usually return to their home. Teach them to avoid tampons, douches, and sexual intercourse for at least 6 weeks. Remind them to keep their follow-up surgical appointment and talk with the health care provider about resuming usual activities. Refer patients and their families to Gilda's Club (www.gildasclub.org) and the National Ovarian Cancer Coalition (NOCC) (www.ovarian.org) for more information and support groups. In Canada, the National Ovarian Cancer Association (www.ovariancanada.org) is available for the same purpose.

For patients with advanced, metastatic disease, collaborate with the case manager, patient, and family for possible referral to hospice. Chapter 9 discusses end-of-life care and hospice in detail. The woman who is faced with the diagnosis of advanced ovarian cancer is usually very anxious about dying. Encourage her to discuss her feelings. Provide realistic assurance, as well as accurate information about treatments. Patients report their most distressing moments in the hospital were when they thought they were not getting adequate information (Carr et al., 2006). Encourage them to use their support systems of family members, friends, and clergy, including the hospital chaplain. Grief counseling is very appropriate. A visit from another woman who has survived a similar disease or referral to a support group may decrease fears. Refer the patient who fears passing the *BRCA1* or *BRCA2* gene to her daughter for genetic counseling and testing.

Ovarian cancer has a high recurrence rate. After recurrence, the cancer is treatable but no longer curable. If this occurs, the patient may deny symptoms at first or express feelings of anger and grief. The family is often fearful of the outcome. Provide encouragement and support during this difficult time, and help the patient and her family work through their grief and prepare for death.

VULVAR CANCER

Pathophysiology

Although vulvar cancer is primarily a disease of older women (average age is 70 years), it has been increasing in women younger than 50 years. In older women, the aging process deteriorates the protective effect of a tumor-suppression gene. In younger women, vulvar cancer may be related to human papillomavirus (HPV). In 2008 the estimated number of vulvar cancer cases in the United States was 3460; the estimated number of U.S. deaths was 870 (www.cancer.gov).

Like other cancers, vulvar cancer has a slow progression from vaginal intraepithelial neoplasia (VIN) to carcinoma-in-situ (CIS) to invasive cancer. It can spread directly to the urethra, the vagina, or the anus and through the lymphatic system to the inguinal, femoral, and deep iliac pelvic nodes.

Other risk factors for vulvar cancer are listed in Table 74-7. Guidelines for the early detection and prevention of vulvar cancer include performing monthly vulvar self-examination with a mirror, having an annual pelvic examination, and practicing "safe sex."

Patient-Centered Collaborative Care

Assessment

Older women may report vulvar irritation or itching. Sometimes they describe a "sore that will not heal." Bleeding is a late symptom. Affected women often have other diseases of aging, such as diabetes and hypertension. Embarrassment may be one reason why older women try to treat themselves and delay seeking medical care, sometimes for years. Younger women may present with a vulvar mass and often report a history of HPV or smoking.

Pelvic examinations usually show multifocal lesions, most often on the labia. The lesions may be white **(leukoplakia)** or red **(erythroplakia),** and the vulvar skin may be very irritated.

A Pap smear and colposcopic examination of the vulva may aid in diagnosis. Toluidine blue stain may be used to stain nuclei in the superficial epithelium, where cells do not normally contain nuclei. Biopsies of the blue areas are easily performed with a dermal punch (a device that removes a disk of tissue). Depending on the site of the lesion, one or more biopsy specimens may be taken. Excisional (removal of entire lesion) biopsies are preferred for smaller lesions.

Prognosis is related to lesion size, contour, cell activity, and whether cancer is present in the lymph nodes. Lesions larger than 2 inches (5 cm) in diameter with infiltrating margins and extensive necrosis are the most likely to recur after surgical resection.

The woman may be anxious or fearful about the diagnosis of cancer. She may fear that her partner(s) will reject her because of the diagnosis, or she may worry about disfigurement related to surgery. Assess the patient's past experiences in coping with stressful situations.

Interventions

Surgery is the major treatment aimed at curing vulvar cancer. Radiation therapy may be used for advanced cancer or for palliation.

If a woman has premalignant vulvar lesions, *laser therapy* may be used. The treatment is usually done on an ambulatory care basis under local, regional, or general anesthesia. Healing occurs over a period of several weeks, usually without scarring.

Vulvectomy is the standard of care for invasive cancer. It may be followed by radiation to prevent recurrence. Chemotherapy is not commonly used, except 5% topical fluorouracil (5-FU) cream for VIN. This treatment should not be used for women who are pregnant or planning a pregnancy. Teach the woman using the cream to wash her hands before and after application. Do not apply the drug to irritated skin. Clean and dry the vulva thoroughly before using the cream.

For some patients, cisplatin (Platinol) is given. However, extensive studies on the use of this drug for vulvar cancer have not been done.

Preoperative Care

Reinforce the information provided by the surgeon about the procedure and care. Photographs of a healed vulvectomy or reconstructed vulva may help reassure the woman about the expected cosmetic outcome. Specific care before a vulvectomy may include an abdominal or perineal shave, enema, and insertion of an indwelling urinary catheter. Other general care before surgery is discussed in Chapter 16.

Operative Procedures

Several surgical procedures are used for the treatment of vulvar cancer. A local wide excision may be used to remove the abnormal area (for CIS). A simple **vulvectomy** (removal of the vulva, the labia majora, the labia minora, and possibly the clitoris) may also be performed for CIS, but this disfiguring surgery is used less often today. Instead, a **skinning vulvectomy**—the removal of superficial vulvar skin (without removal of the clitoris) and replacement of removed skin with split-thickness grafts—is performed (Fig. 74-6). Sexual function and the appearance of the vulva are less affected.

For invasive cancer, a modified radical or **radical vulvectomy** (removal of the entire vulva skin, labia, clitoris, subcutaneous tissues, and possibly inguinal and femoral node dissection) may be performed, depending on node involvement (see Fig. 74-6). Tumors that involve the anus, rectum, rectovaginal septum, or urethra usually require a pelvic exenteration with radical vulvectomy and bilateral groin dissection.

Postoperative Care

After surgery, multiple suction drains (Hemovac or Jackson-Pratt drains) are present in the inguinal or vulvar areas for wound drainage for 7 to 10 days. A pressure-reducing mattress may be placed on the bed to prevent pressure ulcers and increase comfort. A bed cradle may be used to keep linens off

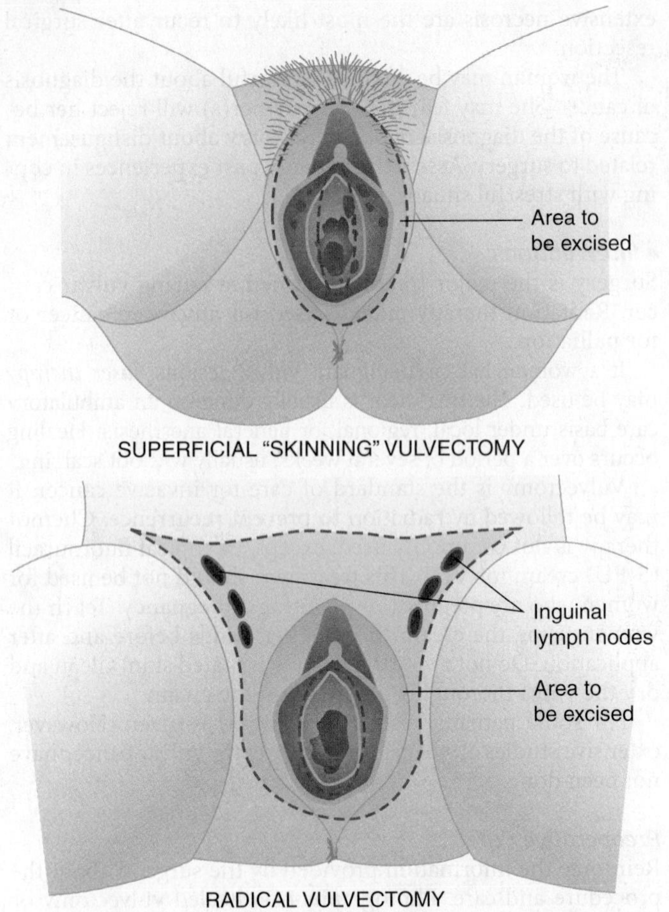
Area to be excised
SUPERFICIAL "SKINNING" VULVECTOMY
Inguinal lymph nodes
Area to be excised
RADICAL VULVECTOMY

Fig. 74-6 • Vulvectomy.

the incision site. The patient usually wears antiembolism stockings or sequential compression devices to prevent thromboembolism and leg edema.

The major focus of nursing care is wound healing and pain relief. Change the dressings over the incision frequently because of the amount of wound drainage and the risk for infection. Wound complications, such as infection and dehiscence, often occur after vulvectomies, and the healing process may take up to 6 months. Meticulous wound care is needed and may involve débridement. Rinse the area with a normal saline solution using a bulb syringe or a Waterpik (on low pressure). Then dry the wound or air-dry it with a hair dryer (using warm air). Wound care is usually done three or four times a day or per agency or surgeon protocol. Provide analgesics before any painful interventions.

Depending on the patient's hygiene and home situation, she may use a sitz bath, tub, or whirlpool bath once or twice a day for wound care. Teach her that the tub should be thoroughly cleaned each time before she uses it. A half-cup of salt may be added to the water. If the patient does not have access to a tub or whirlpool, a squeeze bottle or squirt "gun" can be filled with warm water or a saline solution and poured or squirted over the wound area.

The urinary catheter remains in the bladder for 7 to 10 days to prevent ureteral stenosis and incontinence. After it is removed, the urine stream may be deflected down the leg as a result of edema or even may be uncontrolled. Teach the patient to stand in the shower while voiding if this is a problem. Antiperistaltic drugs are usually given for 7 to 10 days to decrease defecation and the risk for wound infection. Then stool softeners may be given to prevent straining and decrease discomfort related to bowel movements. Teach patients to perform perineal care or sitz baths after voidings or bowel movements to prevent contamination of the incision site.

Women recovering from cancer and disfiguring surgery have similar needs for support, grief counseling, and sexuality as discussed for hysterectomy and pelvic exenteration. In addition, a woman with a radical vulvectomy faces loss of the clitoris and orgasm function. Vaginal dilators may be useful to stretch the remaining vaginal tissues. Discomfort can also be reduced during sexual intercourse by having the couple use water-soluble lubricants or a side-lying position. The couple may need counseling about alternatives to vaginal intercourse. Encourage the woman to express feelings of grief related to her loss of normal sexual function and any fears regarding cancer or recurrence.

VAGINAL CANCER

Pathophysiology

Invasive vaginal cancer is rare. Usually it is an extension of cervical, endometrial, or vulvar cancers. Most vaginal cancers are squamous cell carcinomas that develop in the upper one third of the vagina. They occur most often in women older than 50 years. Most develop after menopause. Risk factors include repeated vaginal injury, such as multiple pregnancies; vaginal trauma; sexually transmitted diseases (STDs), especially syphilis, herpes simplex virus type 2, and papillomavirus infections; and prior radiation.

The spread of vaginal cancer depends on the location of the tumor. Upper vaginal lesions spread in the same manner as cervical cancer, whereas lower lesions spread similarly to vulvar cancer. Because of the rich lymphatic drainage in the vaginal area, metastasis can occur early.

Patient-Centered Collaborative Care

Assessment

Premalignant lesions (vaginal intraepithelial neoplasia) are often asymptomatic. An abnormal Pap smear may be the only indicator of disease. Ask patients about the presence of late symptoms, which include pain, foul-smelling vaginal discharge, painless vaginal bleeding, pruritus, and urinary symptoms from the pressure of the lesion on the bladder.

A pelvic examination may reveal a lesion. Premalignant changes are diagnosed through colposcopic examination and biopsy.

Interventions

Laser therapy may be used to treat vaginal cancer. The health care provider stains the abnormal tissues with an iodine solution to identify the area for treatment. A vaginal discharge may be present for several days after treatment, and healing normally takes a few weeks. Close follow-up is necessary and includes a Pap smear and colposcopic examination every 4 months for 1 year and then every 6 to 12 months. Another treatment option is local wide **excision** (removal of lesion and local surrounding tissue) for localized lesions.

A partial or total **vaginectomy** (vagina removal) is performed for invasive disease. It affects sexual function. Without surgical reconstruction, vaginal intercourse is impossible. The woman and her partner need counseling about alternative activities for achieving sexual satisfaction. Discuss these changes and refer the patient to an intimacy or sexual counselor as soon as possible. A radical hysterectomy or pelvic exenteration may also be performed depending on the extent of the cancer. These procedures were described earlier in this chapter.

Topical chemotherapy with local application of 5-fluorouracil (5-FU) cream to the vagina daily for 1 week is another treatment option. This drug may be irritating to the skin. Zinc oxide ointment application is often recommended to protect the vulvar area. The cream should not be given to women who are pregnant or planning a pregnancy. The treatment is repeated in 3 to 4 weeks, and follow-up is the same as that for laser therapy.

Radiation therapy can be used for all stages of vaginal cancer. Intracavitary radiation therapy (IRT) (brachytherapy) is usually used alone for the treatment of cancer limited to the vaginal wall. External radiation therapy is combined with IRT for cancer that extends beyond the vaginal wall. Complications of radiation therapy include vaginal stenosis, adhesions, and discharge. Women need to use vaginal dilators after treatment and may need follow-up for sexual dysfunction.

FALLOPIAN TUBE CANCER

Pathophysiology

Fallopian tube cancer is the rarest of gynecologic cancers. It occurs in women older than 50 years. Most cases are metastases from ovarian and endometrial cancers.

The cause of squamous cell fallopian tube cancer is unknown. Adenocarcinoma of the fallopian tube may result from pelvic inflammatory disease (PID), chronic salpingitis, and being *BRCA1*-positive. Nulliparity (never experienced childbirth) and infertility (inability to get pregnant) are also risk factors.

Most fallopian tube cancers are serous adenocarcinomas. The spread of this disease is very similar to that of epithelial ovarian cancer. The initial lesion is confined to the lumen of the tube. From there it invades the serosa and spreads to the bowel, omentum, and peritoneum. Lymphatic spread is common.

Patient-Centered Collaborative Care

Women who have fallopian tube cancer often have only a few symptoms. Ask patients if they have the most common manifestations, which include postmenopausal bleeding, increasing abdominal pain, and watery vaginal discharge. Later manifestations include lower abdominal pain or distention and feelings of pressure.

Diagnosis is rare before surgery. Pap smears are abnormal in only a small number of cases. A pelvic mass may be felt on examination in late stages. Vaginal ultrasonography, CT scan, or laparoscopy may be done to confirm a mass.

Treatment of cancer limited to the fallopian tube is a total hysterectomy and bilateral salpingo-oophorectomy (BSO) with **omentectomy** (removal of the connective tissues covering these organs). Care of the patient with fallopian tube cancer is similar to that described for cancer of the ovary. Chemotherapy may be used before surgery in later stages or for recurrence. The lesions respond to paclitaxel (Taxol) and carboplatin (Paraplatin), an alkylating agent. External radiation therapy has been used after surgery for late-stage tumors. Chapter 24 describes the general nursing care for patients receiving chemotherapy and radiation.

HUMAN NEEDS NURSING CARE REVIEW

What might you NOTICE if the patient is experiencing impaired sexuality as a result of gynecologic problems?

- Irregular or abnormal vaginal bleeding
- Vaginal discharge
- Report of perineal itching or burning
- Report of painful intercourse
- Abdominal distention and discomfort
- Report of irritability, anxiety, or depression
- Report of decreased libido

What should you INTERPRET and how should you RESPOND to the patient experiencing impaired sexuality as a result of gynecologic problems?

Perform and interpret physical assessment, including:

- Conducting an abdominal assessment
- Conducting a thorough pain assessment
- Checking for bleeding and amount (number of pads or tampons)
- Listening to patient's concerns about her sexuality

Respond by:

- Helping the patient into a sitting position
- Providing pain-relief measures, such as heat and analgesia
- Referring the patient to a sexual or intimacy counselor (including the patient's partner if desired)

On what should you REFLECT?

- Think about what else you can do to help provide psychosocial support.
- Prepare for complications, such as hemorrhage, if the patient is bleeding.
- Evaluate pain level after interventions.

GET READY FOR THE NCLEX EXAMINATION!

Key Points

Review these Key Points for each NCLEX Examination Client Needs Category.

Safe and Effective Care Environment

- Refer patients with gynecologic problems to appropriate community resources such as the American Cancer Society and the Endometriosis Association.
- Collaborate with the case manager when planning care for patients with gynecologic cancers.

Health Promotion and Maintenance

- Teach women to follow the American Cancer Society's screening guidelines to prevent and early detect for gynecologic cancers.
- Teach all women to have regular Pap tests based on their risk factors.
- Teach women to practice safe sex to prevent infections of the reproductive organs.
- Teach women about risk factors for gynecologic cancers as described in Tables 74-5 and 74-7.
- Teach women how to prevent toxic shock syndrome (TSS) as listed in Chart 74-6.

Psychosocial Integrity

- Reassure women who suffer from premenstrual syndrome (PMS) that their manifestations have a physiologic basis.
- Explain all tests, procedures, and treatments, especially if they cause discomfort during or after the procedures.
- Assess the patient's anxiety before any gynecologic surgery.
- Encourage women who are having procedures that may interfere with fertility to express feelings of fear or grief.
- Encourage women with chronic or serious health problems to consider using support groups or counseling.

Physiological Integrity

- Help patients to be informed enough to make appropriate decisions about whether to use hormone replacement therapy during or after menopause.
- Urge any woman who experiences postmenopausal vaginal bleeding to consult with her gynecologic health care provider as soon as possible.
- Assess for clinical manifestations of TSS as listed in Chart 74-5.
- Teach patients taking danazol for endometriosis about the side effects of the drug (hirsutism, weight gain, decreased breast size, acne).
- Recall laboratory studies for confirming menopause as explained in Table 74-2.
- Teach patients about specific restrictions after local cervical ablation therapy (see Chart 74-11).
- When caring for a patient who has a radioactive implant, use best practices as described in Chart 74-10.
- Teach the patient who is going home after a hysterectomy how to monitor for infection or other complications.
- Instruct patients receiving external beam radiation to the abdomen to gently wash the area; to not apply creams or lotions (unless prescribed by the radiologist); to not wash off marking; to avoid exposing the area to sunlight or temperature extremes; and to wear soft, nonirritating clothing.

Additional Study Resources

Go to your Companion CD or Evolve at http://evolve.elsevier.com/Iggy/ for *Self-Assessment Questions for the NCLEX Examination.*

Go to Evolve at http://evolve.elsevier.com/Iggy/ for *Prioritization and Delegation Questions for the NCLEX Examination.*

SELECTED BIBLIOGRAPHY

Asterisk indicates a classic or definitive work on this subject.

Abou-Setta, A.M., Al-Inany, H.G., & Farquhar, C.M. (2006). Levonorgestrel-releasing intrauterine device (LNG-IUD) for symptomatic endometriosis following surgery. *Cochrane Database of Systematic Reviews, 4,* CD005072.

American Cancer Society (ACS). (2008). *Cancer facts and figures 2008.* Atlanta: Author.

Attar, E., & Bulun, S. (2006). Aromatase inhibitors: The next wave in treatment in endometriosis? *Contemporary Ob/Gyn, Nov 2006,* 82-88.

Ayers, D.M., Lappin, J.E.S., & Liptok, L.M. (2005). Abnormal vaginal bleeding. *Nursing2005, 35*(6), 51.

Bohnenkamp, S., LeBaron, V., & Yoder, L.H. (2007a). The medical-surgical nurse's guide to ovarian cancer: Part I. *MEDSURG Nursing, 16*(4), 259-266.

Bohnenkamp, S., LeBaron, V., & Yoder, L.H. (2007b). The medical-surgical nurse's guide to ovarian cancer: Part II. *MEDSURG Nursing, 16*(5), 323-330.

Carmody, J., Crawford, S., & Churchill, L. (2006). A pilot study on mindfulness-based stress reduction for hot flashes. *Menopause, 13*(5), 760-769.

Carr, E., Brockbank, K., Allen, S., & Strike, P. (2006). Patterns and frequency of anxiety in women undergoing gynaecological surgery. *Journal of Clinical Nursing, 15*(3), 341-352.

Cayir, G., Beji, N.K., & Yalcin, O. (2007). Effectiveness of nursing care after surgery for stress incontinence. *Urological Nursing, 27*(1), 25-33.

Donovan, H., & Ward, S. (2005). Representations of fatigue in women receiving chemotherapy for gynecologic cancers. *Oncology Nursing Forum, 32*(1), 113-116.

Eccles, N.K. (2005). Randomized, double-blinded, placebo-controlled pilot study to investigate the effectiveness of a static magnet to relieve dysmenorrhea. *Journal of Alternative and Complementary Medicine, 11*(4), 681-687.

Edelman, A.B., Gallo, M.F., Jensen, J.T., Nichols, M.D., Schulz, K.F., & Grimes, D.A. (2005). Continuous or extended cycle vs. cyclic use of combined oral contraceptives for contraception. *Cochrane Database of Systematic Reviews, 3,* CD004695.

Farquhar, C.M., Marjoribanks, J., Lethaby, A., Lamberts, Q., Suckling, J.A.; Cochrane Hormone Therapy Study Group. (2005). Long term hormone therapy for perimenopausal and postmenopausal women. *Cochrane Database of Systematic Reviews, 3,* CD004143.

Fitch, M.I., & Turner, F. (2006). Ovarian cancer. *Canadian Nurse, 102*(1), 17-20.

Ford, O., Lethaby, A., Mol, B., & Roberts, H. (2006). Progesterone for premenstrual syndrome. *Cochrane Database of Systematic Reviews, 4,* CD003415.

Gingrich, P.M. (2004). Management and follow-up of abnormal Papanicolaou tests. *Journal of the American Medical Women's Association, 59*(1), 54-60.

Gupta, J.K., Sinha, A.S., Lumsden, M.A., & Hickey, M. (2006). Uterine artery embolization for symptomatic fibroids. *Cochrane Database of Systematic Reviews, 1,* CD005073.

Huo, L., Straub, R.E., Roca, C., Schmidt, P.J., Shi, K., Vakkalanka, R., et al. (2007). Risk for premenstrual dysphoric disorder is associated with genetic variation in ESR1, the estrogen receptor alpha gene. *Biological Psychiatry, 62*(8), 925-933.

Jensen, J.T. (2007). Grand rounds: Don't forget the other benefits of the levonorgestrel IUS. *Contemporary Obstetrics and Gynecology, Jan,* 42-49.

Katz, A. (2007). When sex hurts: Menopause-related dyspareunia. *AJN, 107*(7), 34-37.

Kelley, C. (2007). Estrogen and its effect on vaginal atrophy in postmenopausal women. *Urologic Nursing, 27*(1), 40-45.

Lacey, J.V. Jr., Brinton, L.A., Leitzmann, M., Mouw, T., Hollenbeck, A., Schatzkin, A., et al. (2006). Menopausal hormone therapy and ovarian cancer risk in the National Institutes of Health–AARP Diet and Health Study Cohort. *Journal of the National Cancer Institute, 98*(19), 1397-1405.

Lethaby, A.E., Cooke, I., & Rees, M. (2005). Progesterone or progesterone-releasing intrauterine systems for heavy menstrual bleeding. *Cochrane Database of Systematic Reviews, 4,* CD002126.

Lethaby, A., Hickey, M., & Garry, R. (2005). Endometrial destruction techniques for heavy menstrual bleeding. *Cochrane Database of Systematic Reviews, 4,* CD1501.

Lowdermilk, D.L., & Perry, S.E. (2007). *Maternity and women's health care* (9th ed.). St. Louis: Mosby.

MacDonald, D.J., Sarna, L., Ulman, G.C., Grant, M., & Weitzel, J. (2006). Cancer screening and risk-reducing behaviors of women seeking genetic cancer risk assessment for breast and ovarian cancers. *Oncology Nursing Forum, 33*(2), 27-35.

Martin, V.R. (2005). Straight talk about ovarian cancer. *Nursing2005, 35*(4), 36-42.

Martin, V.R. (2007). Ovarian cancer: An overview of treatment options. *Clinical Journal of Oncology Nursing, 11*(2), 201-207.

McCance, K.L., & Huether, S.E. (2006). *Pathophysiology: The biological basis for disease in adults and children* (5th ed.). St. Louis: Mosby.

McDaniel, C. (2007). Uterine fibroid embolization: The less invasive alternative. *Nursing2007, 37*(7), 26-27.

Newton, K.M., Reed, S.D., LaCroix, A.Z., Grothaus, L.C., Ehrlich, K., & Guiltinan, J. (2006). Treatment of vasomotor symptoms of menopause with black cohosh, multibotanicals, soy, hormone therapy, or placebo: A randomized trial. *Annals of Internal Medicine, 145*(12), 869-879.

Nussbaum, R.L., McInnes, R.R., & Willard, H.F. (2007). *Thompson & Thompson genetics in medicine* (7th ed.). Philadelphia: Saunders.

Proctor, M., & Farquhar, C. (2006). Diagnosis and management of dysmenorrhoae. *British Medical Journal, 332,* 1134-1138 (13 May).

Rapkin, A.J. (2005). New treatment approaches for premenstrual disorders. *American Journal of Managed Care, 11*(Suppl. 16), S480-S491.

Roemheld-Hamm, R. (2005). Chasteberry. *American Family Physician, 72*(5), 821-824.

Sasso, K. (2006). The Copexin Sphere: A new conservative management option for pelvic organ prolapse. *Urologic Nursing, 26*(6), 433-440.

Shan, Y. (2006). Conventional and herbal treatment strategies in the management of endometriosis. *Primary Health Care, 16*(5), 23-26.

Suckling, J., Lethaby, A., & Kennedy, R. (2006). Local oestrogen for vaginal atrophy in postmenopausal women. *Cochrane Database of Systematic Reviews, 4,* CD001500.

Theroux, R. (2005). Factors influencing women's decisions to self-treat vaginal symptoms. *Journal of the American Academy of Nurse Practitioners, 17*(4), 156-162.

Tiffen, J., & Mahon, S.M. (2006b). Cervical cancer: What should we tell women about screening? *Clinical Journal of Oncology Nursing, 10*(4), 527-531.

Tiffen, J.M., & Mahon, S.M. (2006a). Educating women regarding the early detection of endometrial cancer: What is the evidence? *Clinical Journal of Oncology Nursing, 10*(1), 102-104.

Wells, S.F. (2008). Cervical cancer: An overview with suggested practice and policy goals. *MEDSURG Nursing, 17*(1), 43-51.

Whitcomb, B.W., Whiteman, M.K., Langenberg, P., Flaws, J.A., & Romani, W.A. (2007). Physical activity and risk of hot flashes among women in midlife. *Journal of Women's Health, 16*(1), 124-133.

75 CHAPTER

Care of Male Patients with Reproductive Problems

Donna D. Ignatavicius

LEARNING OUTCOMES

For clinical competence and success on the NCLEX Examination, study this chapter with these Learning Outcomes in mind:

Safe and Effective Care Environment

1. Identify community resources for men with reproductive cancers and their partners.
2. Discuss treatment options for prostate cancer with patients, partners, and/or families.
3. Collaborate with health care team members to provide care and discharge planning for patients with male reproductive problems.

Health Promotion and Maintenance

4. Evaluate patient risk factors for male reproductive cancers.
5. Teach men the health promotion practices to prevent or detect early male reproductive cancers.

Psychosocial Integrity

6. Assess the patient's acceptance of body image changes that result from male reproductive surgery.
7. Explain the psychosocial needs of men who have male reproductive problems.

Physiological Integrity

8. Perform a focused physical assessment of the man's reproductive system.
9. Describe the mechanisms of action, side effects, and nursing implications for pharmacologic management of benign prostatic hypertrophy (BPH).
10. Develop a postoperative plan of care for a patient undergoing a transurethral resection of the prostate (TURP) and other newer surgical approaches.
11. Monitor patients' outcomes with continuous bladder irrigation after a TURP.
12. Incorporate complementary and alternative therapies into the patient's plan of care.
13. Provide preoperative teaching for patients having a radical prostatectomy.
14. Educate the patient and family about the role of hormonal therapy in treating prostate cancer.
15. Assess patients for signs and symptoms of adverse effects of radiation therapy for reproductive cancers.
16. Develop a community-based plan of care for a man with prostate cancer.
17. Describe the options for treating erectile dysfunction.
18. Discuss cultural considerations related to male reproductive problems.
19. Develop a plan of care for a patient with testicular cancer, including fertility issues.
20. Compare the assessment and treatment for hydrocele, spermatocele, and varicocele.

Go to your Companion CD or Evolve at http://evolve.elsevier.com/Iggy/ for *Self-Assessment Questions for the NCLEX Examination* keyed to these Learning Outcomes.

Male reproductive problems can range from short-term infections to long-term illnesses that may require end-of-life care. Any health problem that affects the male reproductive system can affect *the human need for sexuality,* either physically or psychologically. For example, some patients have surgeries that damage essential nerves that are needed to have an erection. Others have disorders that psychologically prevent the patient from engaging in his usual sexual activity.

However, male *sexuality* is not limited to intimacy but rather to all aspects of being a man, including relationships with other people of the opposite gender and/or same gender. The role of the nurse and other health care team members is to be open, supportive, and nonjudgmental when caring for men with reproductive problems. Respect the man's privacy at all times.

BENIGN PROSTATIC HYPERTROPHY

Pathophysiology

In a young adult male, the prostatic capsule is thin and attached to the underlying tissue. With aging, the glandular units in the prostate undergo tissue **hyperplasia** (an increase in the number of cells), resulting in prostatic **hypertrophy** (enlargement). High levels of *dihydrotestosterone (DHT),* a testosterone derivative, may accumulate in the prostate and increase cell growth (Ludwig, 2007). Although *benign prostatic hypertrophy* is the more common term used to describe this problem in the clinical setting, **benign prostatic hyperplasia (BPH)** is the most accurate term for the pathologic process.

When the prostate gland enlarges, it extends upward into the bladder and inward, causing *bladder outlet obstruction* (Fig. 75-1). In response, the urinary system is affected in several ways (Fig. 75-2). The detrusor (bladder) muscle then *hypertrophies* (thickens) and *cannot contract* effectively. As a result, the patient has either an increased residual urine (stasis) or acute or chronic urinary retention. Increased residual urine causes **overflow urinary incontinence,** in which the urine "leaks" around the enlarged prostate causing dribbling. Urinary stasis can result in urinary tract infections and bladder calculi (stones).

In a few patients, the prostate becomes very large and the man cannot void (acute retention). In other patients, chronic urinary retention results in a backup of urine and causes a gradual dilation of the ureters **(hydroureter)** and kidneys **(hydronephrosis).** These problems can lead to chronic kidney disease as described in Chapter 71.

GENETIC CONSIDERATIONS

Until recently, BPH was thought to be a single disorder with varying symptoms that resulted from aging. However, researchers have found two types of the problem—a milder form and a more severe form. Men with the severe form of BPH have high levels of a protein made by an androgen-related gene called *JM-27* (Cannon et al., 2007). These patients have more serious bladder damage that can lead to renal involvement. A serum biomarker test to measure the presence and amount of *JM-27* protein is available and being considered for approval by the U.S. Food and Drug Administration (FDA) (Cannon et al., 2007).

Patient-Centered Collaborative Care

Assessment

Physical Assessment/Clinical Manifestations

Ask about the patient's urinary pattern. Assess for frequency, **nocturia** (voiding at night), and other symptoms of bladder outlet obstruction. Together these problems are known as **lower urinary tract symptoms (LUTS).** Other symptoms of LUTS include:

- Difficulty in starting (hesitancy) and continuing urination
- Reduced force and size of the urinary stream
- Sensation of incomplete bladder emptying
- Post-void (after voiding) dribbling

If frequency and nocturia do not occur with restricted urinary flow, the patient may have an infection or other bladder problem. Ask whether the patient has had **hematuria** (blood in the urine) when starting the urine stream or at the end of voiding. BPH is a common cause of hematuria in older men.

Remind the patient to void before the physical examination. Inspect and palpate the abdomen for a distended bladder. The health care provider may percuss the bladder. If the patient has a sense of urgency when gentle pressure is applied, the bladder may be distended. Obese patients are best assessed

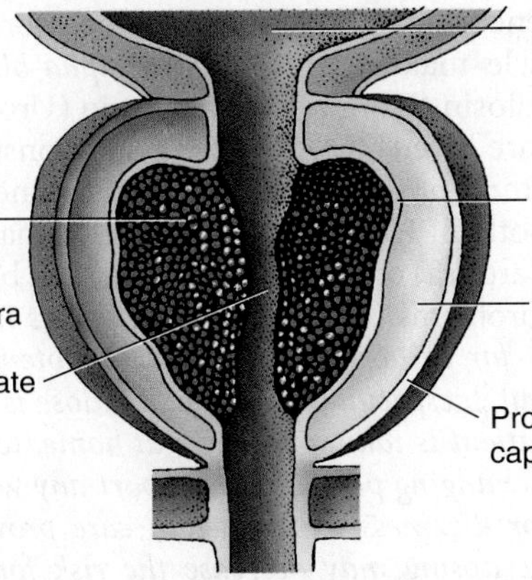

Urinary bladder
BPH tissue
Surgical capsule
Prostatic urethra narrowed by enlarged prostate
True prostate tissue
Prostatic capsule

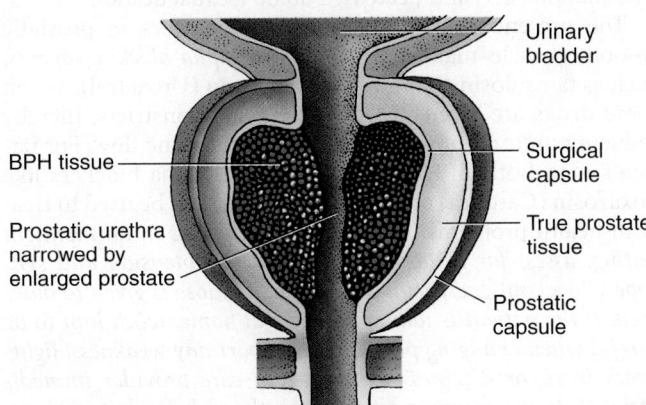

Fig. 75-1 • Benign prostatic hyperplasia (BPH) grows inward, causing narrowing of the urethra.

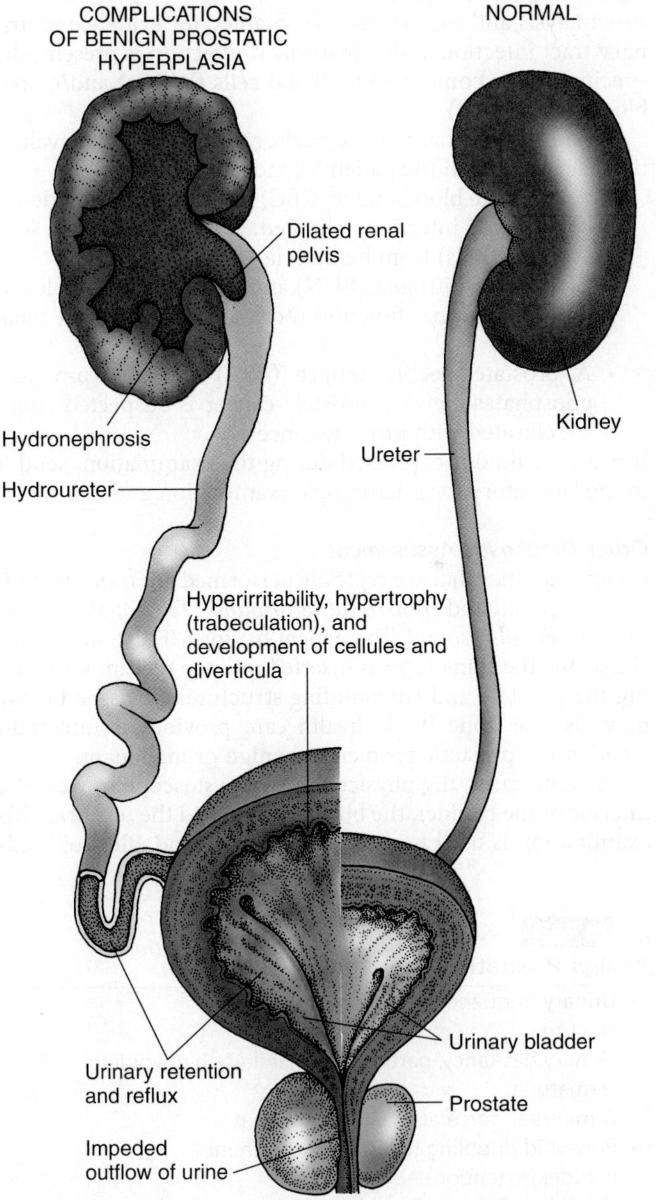

COMPLICATIONS OF BENIGN PROSTATIC HYPERPLASIA
NORMAL
Dilated renal pelvis
Kidney
Hydronephrosis
Ureter
Hydroureter
Hyperirritability, hypertrophy (trabeculation), and development of cellules and diverticula
Urinary bladder
Urinary retention and reflux
Prostate
Impeded outflow of urine

Fig. 75-2 • Potential complications of benign prostatic hyperplasia. The *right side* of the illustration shows a normal male urologic system. The *left side* shows potential complications.

by percussion or bedside ultrasound bladder scanner rather than by inspection or palpation.

Prepare the patient for prostate gland examination. Tell him that he may feel the urge to urinate as the prostate is palpated. Because the prostate is close to the rectal wall, it is easily examined by digital rectal examination (DRE). Help the patient bend over the examination table or assume a side-lying fetal position, whichever is the easiest position for him. The health care provider examines the prostate for size and consistency. BPH presents as a uniform, elastic, nontender enlargement (Chart 75-1), whereas cancer of the prostate gland feels like a stony-hard nodule. Advise the patient that after the prostate gland is palpated, it may be massaged to obtain a fluid sample for examination to rule out **prostatitis** (inflammation of the prostate), a common problem that can occur with BPH.

Laboratory Assessment

A urinalysis and culture may be obtained for evidence of urinary tract infection and hematuria. If infection is present, the specimen may contain white blood cells (WBCs) and/or red blood cells (RBCs).

Blood studies that may be performed at the initial evaluation, depending on the patient's condition, include:

- A complete blood count (CBC) to evaluate any evidence of systemic infection (elevated WBCs) or anemia (decreased RBCs) from hematuria
- Blood urea nitrogen (BUN) and serum creatinine levels to evaluate renal function (both are elevated with renal disease)
- A prostate-specific antigen (PSA) and a serum acid phosphatase level if prostate cancer is suspected (both are elevated with prostate cancer)

If prostatic fluid is expressed during the examination, send it to the laboratory for microscopic examination and culture.

Other Diagnostic Assessment

Imaging studies that are typically performed are *transabdominal ultrasound* and *transrectal ultrasound (TRUS),* also called the *prostate ultrasound.* The patient having a TRUS lies on his side while the transducer is inserted into the rectum for viewing the prostate and surrounding structures. A tissue biopsy may also be done if the health care provider is uncertain whether the prostatic problem is benign or malignant.

In some cases, the physician uses a cystoscope to view the interior of the bladder, the bladder neck, and the urethra. This examination is used to study the presence and effect of bladder neck obstruction. The procedure is usually done in an ambulatory care setting. See Chapter 69 for a detailed description of *cystoscopy* and the nursing care needed for patients having this procedure.

Residual urine may be determined by *bladder ultrasound* immediately after the patient voids. As an alternative, because the patient always voids before cystoscopy, residual urine may be measured at that time. *Urodynamic pressure-flow studies* are the gold standard for diagnosis and grading of bladder outlet obstruction and detrusor muscle function.

Chart 75-1 KEY FEATURES

Benign Prostatic Hypertrophy

- Urinary frequency
- Nocturia
- Urinary hesitancy, particularly on initiation of voiding
- Hematuria
- Diminished force of the urinary stream
- Post-void dribbling (overflow incontinence)
- Bladder distention
- Possible evidence of renal insufficiency, including edema, pallor, and pruritus
- A uniform, elastic, nontender, palpable prostate

Common Nursing Diagnoses and Collaborative Problems

Nursing diagnoses and collaborative problems that may apply to patients with BPH include:

- Urinary Retention related to blockage from the enlarged prostate gland
- Urinary Incontinence related to overdistention of the bladder
- Disturbed Sleep Pattern related to nocturia
- Risk for Infection related to residual urine
- Potential for Renal Insufficiency or Chronic Kidney Disease

Interventions

Drug therapy is a popular option for treating BPH. For patients with acute urinary retention or for those who do not respond or cannot tolerate drug therapy, noninvasive procedures or surgery is the treatment of choice.

Nonsurgical Management

In some cases in which patients are not yet bothered by the symptoms of BPH, "watchful waiting" may be appropriate. During this observation period, the patient is examined every year to determine whether the BPH is causing urinary symptoms. When these symptoms begin, drug therapy is often prescribed.

Drug Therapy. Drugs from two major categories may be used alone or in combination. The health care provider may prescribe a *5-alpha reductase inhibitor (5-ARI),* such as finasteride (Proscar) or dutasteride (Avodart). These drugs lower the level of dihydrotestosterone (DHT). In some men, decreasing the DHT levels can shrink the enlarged prostate and prevent further growth. Remind patients that they may need to take the drug for as long as 6 months before improvement is noticed. Teach them about possible side effects, which include erectile dysfunction (ED) and decreased libido (sexual desire).

The presence of alpha-adrenergic receptors in prostatic smooth muscle makes it respond to *alpha-blocking agents,* such as tamsulosin (Flomax) and alfuzosin (Uroxatral). When these drugs are given, the prostate gland constricts, thereby reducing urethral pressure and improving urine flow. For patients with both BPH and hypertension, alpha blockers like doxazosin (Cardura) or terazosin (Hytrin) can be used to treat both health problems. *If giving alpha blockers in an inpatient setting, assess for orthostatic (postural) hypotension and syncope ("blackout"), especially after the first dose is given to older men. If the patient is taking the drug at home, teach him to be careful when changing position and report any weakness, lightheadedness, or dizziness to the health care provider immediately. Bedtime dosing may decrease the risk for hypotension. Drugs used to treat erection problems (e.g., Viagra) can worsen these side effects.* Teach patients taking a 5-ARI or alpha blocking drug to keep all appointments for follow-up laboratory testing because both drug classes can cause liver dysfunction.

Other drugs, including estrogens and androgens alone or in combination, also have been used less successfully. Therefore these agents are not commonly used today for BPH although hormonal therapy may be given to patients with prostatic cancer. (See Drug Therapy discussion on p. 1723 in the Prostate Cancer section.) Once thought to be contraindicated for BPH, some patients experience relief of annoying urinary symptoms by using antimuscarinic agents like tolterodine (Detrol or Detrol LA). *These drugs should be used with caution in older adults because they can cause constipation, urinary retention, acute confusion, dry mouth, and blurred vision.* Newer drugs for BPH (e.g., Botox) are currently in U.S. clinical research trials.

Complementary and Alternative Therapies. Over 2 million men use herbs and foods to help manage the symptoms of BPH, especially saw palmetto extract (a natural herb) and lycopene (a botanical found in tomatoes). Many men with early to moderate BPH believe these agents have relieved their symptoms and prefer this treatment over prescription drugs or surgery. Studies on the effectiveness of saw palmetto have been contradicting (Bent et al., 2006). Teach patients who want to try these herbs and other natural substances that scientific evidence to prove they are useful is lacking. However, if they choose to take them, remind them to check with their health care provider before taking any over-the-counter natural substance. Some herbs interfere with prescription drugs the patient may be taking for other health problems. Clinical research trials for both agents are continuing.

Other Nonsurgical Measures. Other nonsurgical measures that reduce obstructive symptoms include those that cause the release of prostatic fluid such as frequent sexual intercourse. These measures are helpful for the man whose obstructive symptoms result from an enlarged prostate with a large amount of retained prostatic fluid. Teach the patient to avoid drinking large amounts of fluid in a short time; to avoid alcohol, diuretics, and caffeine; and to void as soon as he feels the urge. These measures are aimed at preventing overdistention of the bladder, which may result in loss of detrusor muscle tone. Teach patients to avoid any drugs that can cause urinary retention, especially anticholinergics, antihistamines, and decongestants. Emphasize the importance of telling any health care provider about the diagnosis of BPH so that these drugs are not prescribed. The Concept Map on p. 1716 presents nursing assessment and care issues related to medical management of the patient with BPH.

If drug therapy or other measures are not helpful in relieving urinary symptoms, several noninvasive techniques are available to destroy excess prostate tissue using a variety of heat methods **(thermotherapy).** These procedures are often done in a physician's office or another ambulatory care setting. Examples include:

- **Transurethral needle ablation (TUNA)** (low radiofrequency energy shrinks the prostate)
- **Transurethral microwave therapy (TUMT)** (high temperatures heat and destroy excess tissue)
- **Interstitial laser coagulation (ILC)** (laser energy coagulates excess tissue)
- **Electrovaporization** (high-frequency electrical current cuts and vaporizes excess tissue)

These procedures have less risk for complications such as intraoperative bleeding and erectile dysfunction when compared with surgery. Patients can return to their usual activities in a day or two. For a small group of men, *prostatic stents* may be placed into the urethra to maintain permanent patency. All of these treatments require local or regional anesthesia and do not require an indwelling urinary catheter.

Surgical Management

For patients who are not candidates for nonsurgical management or do not want to take drugs or have other treatment options, surgery may be performed. The gold standard continues to be a **transurethral resection of the prostate (TURP)** in which the enlarged portion of the prostate is removed through an endoscopic instrument. For a few men, an open prostatectomy (entire prostate removal) may be performed (see discussion of Surgical Management on p. 1721 in the Prostate Cancer section) (Fig. 75-3). Some or all of these criteria indicate the need for surgery:

- Acute urinary retention
- Chronic urinary tract infections secondary to residual urine in the bladder
- Hematuria
- Hydronephrosis

Preoperative Care. When planning surgical interventions, the patient's general physical condition, the size of the prostate gland, and the man's preferences are considered. The patient may have many fears and misconceptions about prostate surgery, such as believing that automatic loss of sexual functioning or permanent incontinence will occur. Assess the patient's anxiety, correct any misconceptions about the surgery, and provide accurate information to him and his family. Regardless of the type of surgery to be performed, provide information about anesthesia (see Chapter 17). The patient may have other medical problems that increase the risk for complications of general anesthesia and may be advised to have regional anesthesia. Epidural or spinal anesthesia are the most common types of anesthesia used for a TURP. Because the patient is awake, it is easier to assess for hyponatremia (low serum sodium), fluid overload, and water intoxication, which can result from large bladder irrigations.

After a TURP, all patients have an indwelling urethral catheter for at least a day. *Be sure that they know that they will feel the urge to void while the catheter is in place.* Tell the patient that he will likely have continuous bladder irrigation (CBI) and traction on the catheter that may cause discomfort. However, reassure him that analgesics will be prescribed to relieve his pain. Explain that it is normal for the urine to be blood-tinged after surgery. Small blood clots and tissue debris may pass while the catheter is in place and immediately after it is removed.

Operative Procedures. The traditional TURP is a "closed" surgery. To perform the procedure, the surgeon inserts a resectoscope (an instrument similar to a cystoscope, but with a cutting and cauterizing loop) through the urethra. The enlarged portion of the prostate gland is then removed in small pieces (prostate chips). A similar procedure is the transurethral incision of the prostate (TUIP), in which small cuts are made into the prostate to relieve pressure on the urethra. This alternate technique is used for smaller prostates. To prevent bleeding and excess clotting, a fibrinolytic inhibitor like tranexamic acid (Cyklokapron) may be used during surgery.

A TURP is safer for the patient who is at high risk for open surgery because a surgical incision is not used. Hospi-

CONCEPT MAP Benign Prostatic Hypertrophy

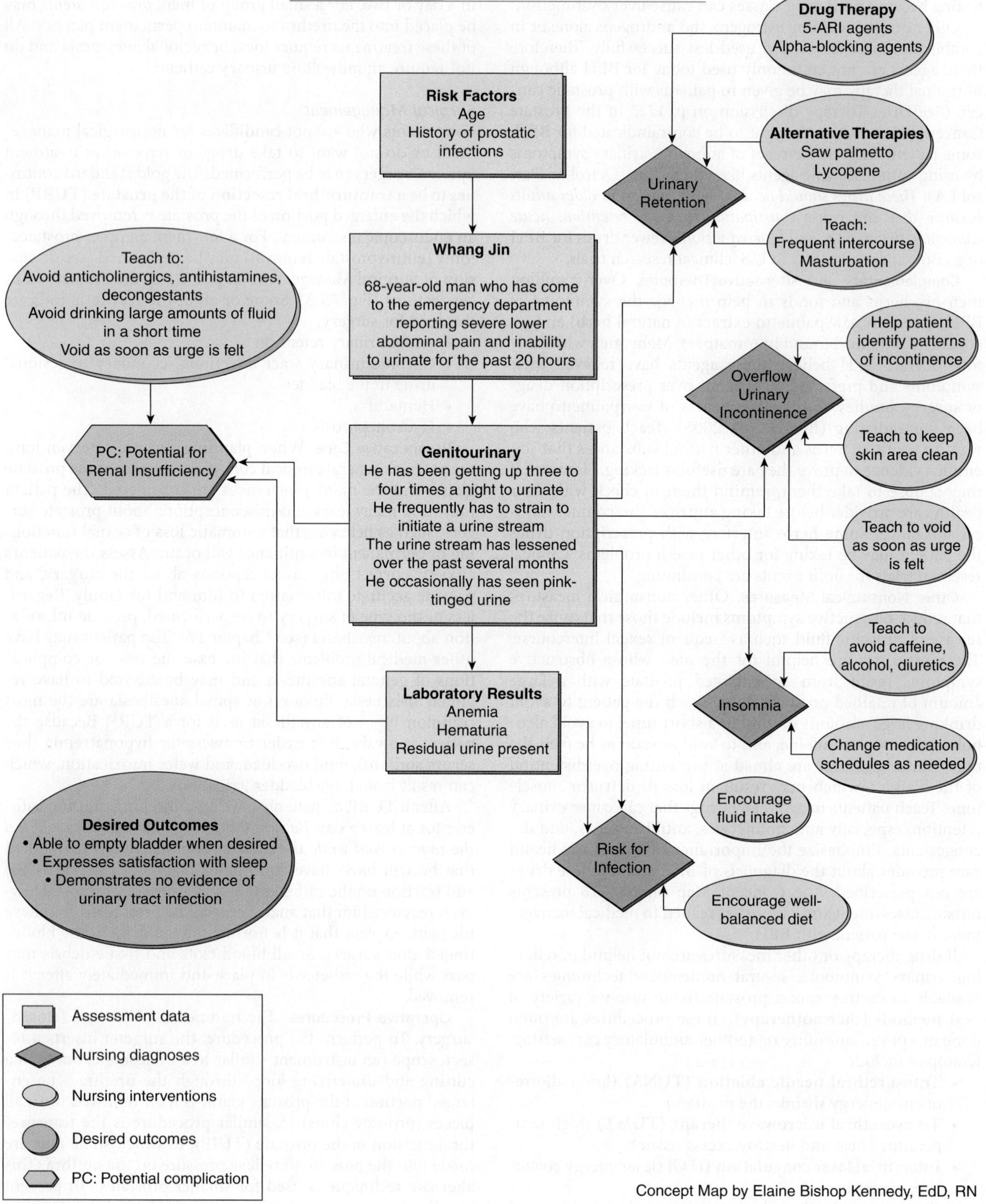
Drug Therapy
5-ARI agents
Alpha-blocking agents
Risk Factors
Age
History of prostatic infections
Alternative Therapies
Saw palmetto
Lycopene
Urinary Retention
Teach:
Frequent intercourse
Masturbation
Teach to:
Avoid anticholinergics, antihistamines, decongestants
Avoid drinking large amounts of fluid in a short time
Void as soon as urge is felt
Whang Jin
68-year-old man who has come to the emergency department reporting severe lower abdominal pain and inability to urinate for the past 20 hours
Help patient identify patterns of incontinence
Overflow Urinary Incontinence
Teach to keep skin area clean
PC: Potential for Renal Insufficiency
Genitourinary
He has been getting up three to four times a night to urinate
He frequently has to strain to initiate a urine stream
The urine stream has lessened over the past several months
He occasionally has seen pink-tinged urine
Teach to void as soon as urge is felt
Teach to avoid caffeine, alcohol, diuretics
Laboratory Results
Anemia
Hematuria
Residual urine present
Insomnia
Change medication schedules as needed
Encourage fluid intake
Desired Outcomes
• Able to empty bladder when desired
• Expresses satisfaction with sleep
• Demonstrates no evidence of urinary tract infection
Risk for Infection
Encourage well-balanced diet
Assessment data
Nursing diagnoses
Nursing interventions
Desired outcomes
PC: Potential complication

Concept Map by Elaine Bishop Kennedy, EdD, RN

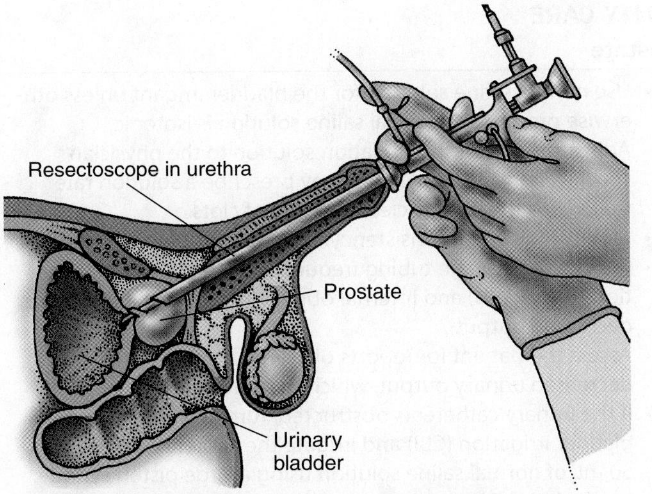
Resectoscope in urethra
Prostate
Urinary bladder

In **transurethral resection of the prostate (TURP),** the surgeon inserts a resectoscope through the urethra and into the bladder and removes pieces of tissue from the prostate gland.

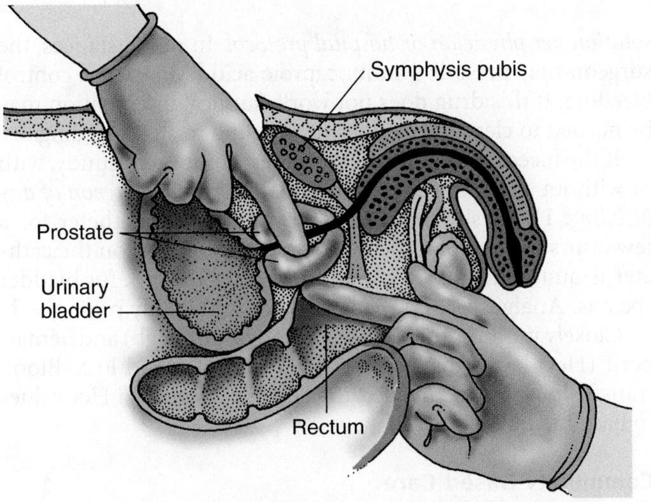
Symphysis pubis
Prostate
Urinary bladder
Rectum

In **retropubic,** or **retrovesical, prostatectomy,** the surgeon removes the BPH tissue directly through an abdominal incision.

Fig. 75-3 • Prostatectomy procedures. *BPH,* Benign prostatic hyperplasia.

talization and recovery are shorter than with any other type of prostate surgery.

The disadvantage of a TURP is that, because only small pieces of the gland are removed, remaining prostate tissue may continue to grow and cause urinary obstruction, requiring additional TURPs. Also, urethral trauma from the resectoscope with resulting urethral strictures is possible.

In many large medical centers, specialists can perform newer surgical treatments. Examples include the *Holmium laser enucleation of the prostate (HOLEP)* and the *transurethral ultrasound-guided laser incision of the prostate (TULIP)* (Ludwig, 2007). These procedures are gaining increased popularity as more urologists learn how to perform them. Men having these newer approaches usually have a urinary catheter for the night after surgery and do not require a CBI unless severe bleeding or clots occur. Therefore they can be done as an ambulatory care or short-stay procedure.

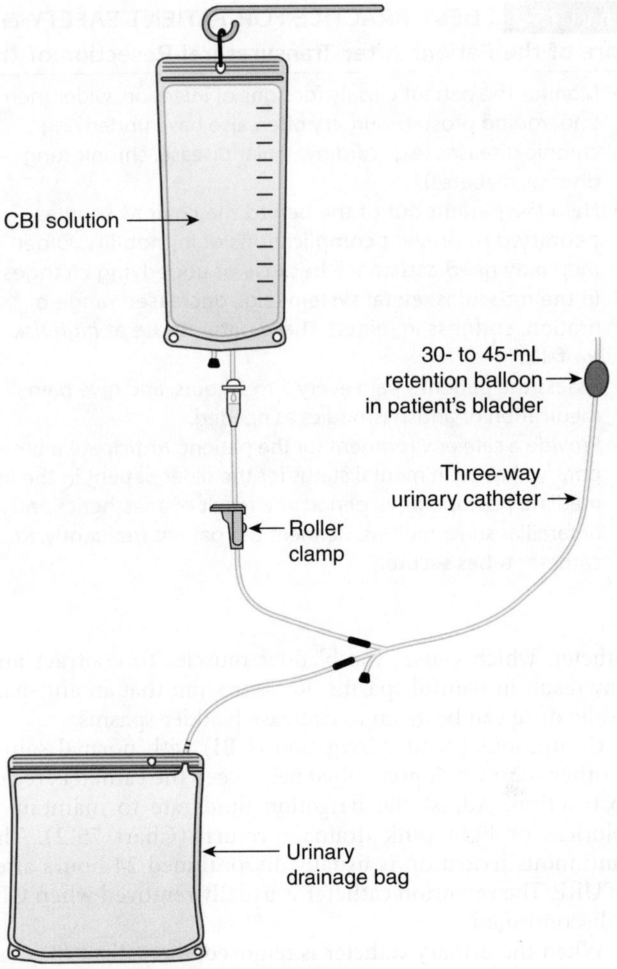
CBI solution
30- to 45-mL retention balloon in patient's bladder
Three-way urinary catheter
Roller clamp
Urinary drainage bag

Fig. 75-4 • Continuous bladder irrigation.

Postoperative Care. After a TURP, the surgeon inserts a three-way urinary catheter with a 30- to 45-mL retention balloon through the urethra into the bladder (Fig. 75-4). The catheter is pulled down into the prostatic fossa to help prevent bleeding. Traction is often applied on the catheter by pulling it taut and taping it to the patient's abdomen or thigh.

If the catheter is taped to the patient's thigh, instruct him to keep his leg straight. The surgeon determines when the traction should be removed; usually it is removed on the first day after surgery.

CONSIDERATIONS FOR OLDER ADULTS

When caring for older men who may become confused after surgery, reorient them frequently and remind them not to pull on the catheter. If the patient is restless or "picks" at tubes, provide a familiar object such as a family picture for him to hold for distraction and a feeling of security. Do not restrain the patient unless all other alternatives have failed.

Remind the patient that because of the retention catheter's large diameter and the pressure of the retention balloon on the internal sphincter of the bladder, he will feel the urge to void continuously. This is a normal sensation, not a surgical complication. Advise the patient not to try to void around the

Chart 75-2 BEST PRACTICE FOR PATIENT SAFETY & QUALITY CARE

Care of the Patient After Transurethral Resection of the Prostate

- Monitor the patient closely for signs of infection. Older men undergoing prostate surgery often also have underlying chronic diseases (e.g., cardiovascular disease, chronic lung disease, diabetes).
- Help the patient out of the bed to the chair as soon as permitted to prevent complications of immobility. Older men may need assistance because of underlying changes in the musculoskeletal system (e.g., decreased range of motion, stiffness in joints). These patients are at *high risk* for falls.
- Assess the patient's pain every 2 to 3 hours, and give pain medication or antispasmodics as needed.
- Provide a safe environment for the patient. Anticipate a temporary change in mental status for the older patient in the immediate postoperative period as a result of anesthetics and unfamiliar surroundings. Reorient the patient frequently. Keep catheter tubes secure.
- Use normal saline solution for the bladder irrigant unless otherwise prescribed. Normal saline solution is isotonic.
- Adjust the rate of the irrigation solution to the physician's specifications. The physician may prescribe a solution rate that keeps the output clear and free of clots.
- Monitor the color, consistency, and amount of urine output.
- Check the drainage tubing frequently for external obstructions (e.g., kinks) and internal obstructions (e.g., blood clots, decreased output).
- Assess the patient for reports of severe bladder spasms with decreased urinary output, which may indicate obstruction.
- If the urinary catheter is obstructed, turn off the continuous bladder irrigation (CBI) and irrigate the catheter with 30 to 50 mL of normal saline solution using a large piston syringe.
- Notify the physician immediately if the obstruction does not resolve by hand irrigation or if the urinary return becomes ketchup-like.

catheter, which causes the bladder muscles to contract and may result in painful spasms. Reassure him that an antispasmodic drug can be given to decrease bladder spasms.

Continuous bladder irrigation (CBI) with normal saline or other solution as prescribed helps keep the catheter free of obstruction. Adjust the irrigation fluid rate to maintain a colorless or light pink drainage return (Chart 75-2). The continuous irrigation is usually discontinued 24 hours after a TURP. The retention catheter is usually removed when CBI is discontinued.

When the urinary catheter is removed, the patient may experience burning on urination and some urinary frequency, dribbling, and leakage. Reassure him that these symptoms are normal and will decrease. The patient may also pass small clots and tissue debris for several days after the TURP. *Instruct him to increase fluid intake to at least 2000 to 2500 mL daily, which helps decrease dysuria and keep the urine clear. An older patient who has renal disease or who is at risk for heart failure may not be able to tolerate this much fluid.* By the time of discharge (usually 1 to 2 days after surgery), he should be voiding 150 to 200 mL of clear yellow urine every 3 to 4 hours. By discharge, pain is minimal and analgesics may not be required.

Observe for other possible but uncommon complications of TURP, such as infection and incontinence. Teach the patient that sexual function should not be affected but that **retrograde ejaculation** is possible. In this case, most of the semen flows backwards into the bladder so only a small amount will be ejaculated from the penis.

Assess for postoperative bleeding. Patients who undergo a TURP or open prostatectomy are at risk for severe bleeding or hemorrhage after surgery. Although rare, bleeding is most likely within the first 24 hours. Bladder spasms or movement may trigger fresh bleeding from previously controlled vessels. This bleeding may be arterial or venous, but venous bleeding is more common.

Monitor the patient's urine output every 2 hours and vital signs every 4 hours. *If the bleeding is arterial, the urinary drainage is bright red or ketchup-like with numerous clots. If arterial bleeding occurs, notify the surgeon immediately and increase the CBI rate or intermittently irrigate the catheter with normal saline solution per physician or hospital protocol.* In rare instances, the surgeon may prescribe aminocaproic acid (Amicar) to control bleeding. If this drug does not work, surgical intervention may be needed to clear the bladder of clots and to stop bleeding.

If the bleeding is *venous,* the urine output is burgundy, with or without any change in vital signs. *Inform the surgeon of any bleeding.* He or she may apply traction on the catheter for a few hours to control it. Be aware that the traction on the catheter is quite uncomfortable and increases the risk for bladder spasms. Analgesics or antispasmodics are usually prescribed.

Closely monitor the patient's hemoglobin (Hgb) and hematocrit (Hct) levels for anemia as a result of blood loss. Blood transfusions may be needed to return the Hgb and Hct values to baseline levels.

Community-Based Care

The patient with benign prostatic hyperplasia (BPH) is typically managed at home. Patients who have surgery are also discharged to their home or other setting from where they were admitted. Some patients, especially those who have had a TURP, may have temporary loss of control of urination or a dribbling of the urine. Reassure the patient that these symptoms are almost always temporary and will resolve. Assist the patient and his family in finding ways to keep his clothing dry until sphincter control returns. Instruct him to contract and relax his sphincter frequently to re-establish urinary control (Kegel exercises). External urinary (condom) catheters are not used except in extreme cases because they may give the patient a false sense of security and delay urinary control.

NCLEX EXAMINATION CHALLENGE

A client had a transurethral resection of the prostate (TURP) this morning. The nurse observes light pink–tinged urine draining from his urinary catheter. What is the nurse's best action?

A. Notify the surgeon as soon as possible.
B. Irrigate the catheter with 30 mL normal saline.
C. Document the assessment in the medical record.
D. Apply additional traction on the catheter.

evolve For the correct answer, go to http://evolve.elsevier.com/Iggy/.

PROSTATE CANCER

Pathophysiology

Prostate cancer is the most common type of cancer in men in the United States. It is the second leading cause of deaths from cancer in men (Wallace & Storms, 2007). Incidence rates have increased rapidly since the introduction of the prostatic-specific antigen serum biomarker to diagnose the disease.

Testosterone and dihydrotestosterone (DHT) are the major androgens (male hormones) in the adult male. Testosterone is produced by the testis and circulates in the blood. DHT is a testosterone derivative in the prostate gland. It binds more easily with androgen receptors than testosterone does. In some patients, the prostate grows very rapidly, leading to noncancerous high-grade prostatic intraepithelial neoplasia (HGPIN). Patients with HGPIN are at a higher risk for developing prostate cancer than men who do not have that growth pattern.

Most prostate tumors are androgen sensitive (McCance & Huether, 2006). More than 95% of them are adenocarcinomas and arise from epithelial cells located in the posterior lobe or outer portion of the gland (Fig. 75-5).

Of all malignancies, prostate cancer is one of the slowest growing, and it metastasizes (spreads) in a predictable pattern. Common sites of metastasis are the nearby lymph nodes, bones, lungs, and liver (McCance & Huether, 2006). The bones of the pelvis, sacrum, and lumbar spine are most often affected.

Etiology and Genetic Risk

Although the cause of prostate cancer remains unclear, several factors influence its development. First, an intact hypothalamic-pituitary-testicular pathway must be present. Men who were castrated before puberty are at little risk for prostate cancer. Second, the advancing age of a man increases his risk for prostate cancer. Men older than 65 years have the greatest risk for the disease.

Other contributing factors may include eating a diet high in animal fat (e.g., red meat), viruses, family history, vitamin D and E deficiencies, and genetic variations. Exposure to environmental toxins, such as arsenic, may also increase the man's risk for prostate cancer (Held-Warmkessel, 2008).

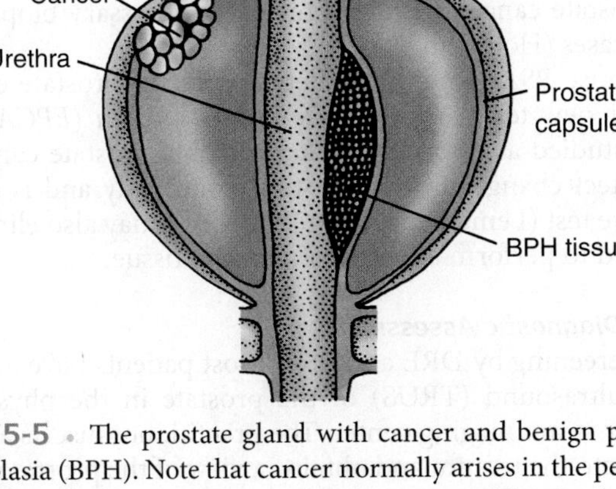
Cancer
Urethra
Prostatic capsule
BPH tissue

Fig. 75-5 • The prostate gland with cancer and benign prostatic hyperplasia (BPH). Note that cancer normally arises in the periphery of the gland, whereas BPH occurs in the center of the gland.

GENETIC CONSIDERATIONS

In the past 10 years, researchers have begun to identify specific genetic alterations that may explain the causes of prostate cancer. For example, the *EphB2* gene is a tumor suppressor gene that is *not* active in some African-American men with prostate cancer who have a family history of the disease. Some men with the most aggressive prostate cancers have *BCRA2* mutations similar to those women who have *BCRA2*-associated breast and ovarian cancers. The androgen receptors are also being researched for their role in the development of prostate cancer (McCance & Huether, 2006).

Incidence/Prevalence

Prostate cancer is common worldwide. It is a cancer of older men and occurs rarely before age 45 years. The National Cancer Institute estimates that almost 187,000 new cases of prostate cancer were diagnosed in 2008 and that over 2 million men are living with the disease (www.cancer.gov). Prostate cancer has a high incidence in less affluent countries and a low incidence in Asian countries. In the United States, it affects African-American men the most and at an earlier age. It is not as common in Asian-American and American-Indian men (www.cancer.gov).

Health Promotion and Maintenance

Teach men about the American Cancer Society's guidelines for prostate cancer screening (Chart 75-3). Beginning at age 50 years, all men should have an annual digital rectal examination (DRE). Men at higher risk for prostate cancer, including African Americans or men who have a first-degree relative with prostate cancer, should start screening at 45 years of age. Men who have multiple first-degree relatives with prostate cancer at an early age should begin screening at age 40 years (www.cancer.org).

Although a family history of prostate cancer cannot be changed, certain nutritional habits can be altered to decrease the risk for the disease. First, teach the patient to eat a healthy, balanced diet. One of the most important changes is to decrease animal fat (e.g., red meat) in the diet. Instead of red meat, teach patients to eat more fish and other foods high in *omega-3 fatty acids* because they are thought to be helpful in preventing cancer. Also instruct them to increase fruits and vegetables, espe-

Chart 75-3 PATIENT AND FAMILY EDUCATION GUIDE

American Cancer Society Prostate Screening and Detection Guidelines (2008)

- An annual digital rectal examination (DRE) and prostate-specific antigen (PSA) test should be offered to:
  - Men beginning at age 50
  - Men who have a life expectancy of at least 10 years
  - African-American men and any man who has a first-degree relative with prostate cancer beginning at age 45
  - Men who have two or more first-degree relatives with prostate cancer beginning at age 40
- DRE should be performed by health care professionals skilled in recognizing subtle prostate abnormalities.
- DRE *and* PSA are needed to detect prostate cancer. An abnormal PSA test result is a value above 4.0 ng/mL.

Data from American Cancer Society, 2008.

cially foods high in *lycopene*, a powerful anticancer antioxidant. Foods high in this substance include tomatoes (raw, cooked, and sauce), watermelons, pink grapefruit, and papaya. Also suggest an increased intake of cruciferous vegetables such as broccoli, cauliflower, cabbage, and kale. These foods may not prevent prostate cancer but have been shown to slow tumor growth (www.prostatecancerfoundation.org).

Other substances that may decrease the risk for getting prostate cancer are selenium, vitamin E, omega-3 oils, and catechin (found in green tea). Exercise may also decrease risk because it lowers lipids, a factor that may increase the likelihood of getting prostate cancer. Too much calcium can increase the risk for the disease (Gray & Sims, 2006).

Tobacco use, especially cigarette smoking, and heavy alcohol consumption increase the growth and improve the prognosis of prostate tumors. Teach patients the importance of not smoking and of drinking alcohol in moderation. These substances also put people at risk for many other diseases (www.prostatecancerfoundation.org).

Patient-Centered Collaborative Care

Assessment

History

Assess the patient's age, race/ethnicity, and family history of prostate cancer. Ask about his nutritional habits, especially focusing on his intake of red meat, fish, and fruits and vegetables. Assess whether the patient has any problems with urination. Take a drug history to determine if he is taking any medication that could affect voiding. The first symptoms that the man may report are related to bladder outlet obstruction, such as difficulty in starting urination, frequent bladder infections, and urinary retention. Ask about urinary frequency, **hematuria** (blood in the urine), and **nocturia** (voiding during the night). Ask if he has had any pain during intercourse, especially when ejaculating. Inquire if the patient has had or currently has any other pain (particularly bone pain), a symptom associated with advanced prostate cancer. Ask him if he has had any recent unexpected weight loss.

Take a sexual history for recent changes in desire or function. Ask about his sexual partner preference, if not known. Also ask about current or previous sexually transmitted diseases, penile discharge, or scrotal pain or swelling.

Physical Assessment/Clinical Manifestations

Most *early* cancers are diagnosed while the patient is having a routine physical examination or is being treated for benign prostatic hypertrophy (BPH). Gross blood in the urine (hematuria) is the most common clinical manifestation of *late* prostate cancer. Assess for pain in the pelvis, spine, hips, or ribs. Complete a thorough pain assessment. Palpate for swollen lymph nodes, especially in the groin areas. Pain and swollen nodes also indicate advanced disease that has spread. Take and record the patient's weight because unexpected weight loss is also common when the disease is advanced.

Prepare the patient for a digital rectal examination (DRE). On rectal examination, a prostate that is found to be stony hard and with palpable irregularities or indurations is suspected to be malignant.

Psychosocial Assessment

A diagnosis of any type of cancer causes fear and anxiety for most people. Some men, particularly African Americans, develop the disease in their 40s and 50s when they are perhaps planning their retirements, putting their children through college, and/or enjoying their middle years. Assess the reaction of the patient to the diagnosis, and observe how his family reacts to the illness. Men may describe their feelings as shock, fear, anger, and "roller coaster" (Wallace & Storms, 2007). Expect that patients will go through the grieving process and may be in denial or depressed. Determine what support systems they have, such as spiritual leaders or community group support, to help them through diagnosis, treatment, and recovery.

One of the biggest concerns for the man may be his ability for sexual function after cancer treatment. Tell him that function will depend on the type of treatment he has. Most surgical techniques used today do not involve cutting the perineal nerves that are needed for an erection. A dry climax may occur if the prostate is removed because it produces most of the fluid in the ejaculate. Refer the patient to his surgeon (urologist), sex therapist, or intimacy counselor if available.

Laboratory Assessment

Prostate-specific antigen (PSA) is a glycoprotein produced by the prostate and, in smaller amounts, by the small intestine, breast, and salivary glands. The normal blood level of PSA in most men is less than 4 ng/mL (National Comprehensive Cancer Network [NCCN], 2007). PSA levels are higher in patients with BPH, prostatitis, and prostate cancer. The levels associated with prostate cancer are usually much higher than those occurring with other prostate tissue problems.

PSA analysis should never be used as a screening test without a digital rectal examination (DRE). Because other prostate problems also increase the PSA level, it is not specifically diagnostic for cancer. In addition, some patients with prostate cancer have PSA levels less than 4 ng/mL. The PSA should be drawn before the DRE because the examination can cause an increase in PSA because of prostate irritation.

The PSA is not elevated in most healthy white men or in men with cancer in other organs. *However, the normal PSA level is slightly higher in older adults and in African Americans.* An elevated PSA level should decrease a few days after a prostatectomy. An increase in the PSA level several weeks after surgery usually indicates that the disease has recurred.

The PSA value measures the total PSA (tPSA) including bound and unbound portions. The PSA bound to alpha$_1$-antichymotrypsin is known as *complexed PSA,* or *cPSA,* that can be measured in the serum. The accepted cPSA level is 2.2-3.4 ng/mL, which is equivalent to a tPSA level of 2.5-4.0 ng/mL. cPSA is more specific and sensitive than tPSA in diagnosing prostate cancer and can prevent unnecessary biopsies in many cases (Holcomb, 2007).

Because PSA is not absolutely specific to prostate cancer, another new test, *early prostate cancer antigen (EPCA-2),* is being studied as a serum marker for only prostate cancer. It can detect changes in the prostate gland early and is a very sensitive test (Leman et al., 2007). EPCA-2 may also eliminate the need to perform a biopsy of prostate tissue.

Other Diagnostic Assessment

After screening by DRE and PSA, most patients have a transrectal ultrasound (TRUS) of the prostate in the physician's office or in an imaging center. The practitioner inserts a small probe into the rectum and obtains a view of the prostate using sound waves. If prostate cancer is suspected, a biopsy is recommended. *Currently, a biopsy is the primary way that this cancer is accurately diagnosed* (NCCN, 2007). A core needle biopsy is the usual method used.

After a *transrectal ultrasound with biopsy,* instruct the patient about possible complications, although rare, including hematuria with clots, signs of infection, and perineal pain. Teach him to report fever, chills, bloody urine, and any difficulty voiding. Advise him to avoid strenuous physical activity and drink plenty of fluids, especially in the first 24 hours after the procedure. Teach him that a small amount of bleeding turning the urine pink is expected during this time.

After prostate cancer is diagnosed, the patient has additional imaging and blood studies to determine the extent of the disease. Common tests include lymph node biopsy, computed tomography (CT) of the pelvis and abdomen, and magnetic resonance imaging (MRI) to assess the status of the pelvic and para-aortic lymph nodes. A radionuclide bone scan may be performed to detect metastatic bone disease. An enlarged liver or abnormal liver function study results indicate possible liver metastases.

Patients with advanced prostate cancer often have *elevated* levels of *serum acid phosphatase.* Most men with bone metastasis have elevated *serum alkaline phosphatase* levels.

Analysis

Common Nursing Diagnoses and Collaborative Problems

A common nursing diagnosis in patients with prostate cancer is Impaired Urinary Elimination related to urinary tract infection caused by bladder outlet obstruction.

Additional Nursing Diagnoses and Collaborative Problems

Additional nursing diagnoses that may apply to patients with prostate cancer include:

- Anxiety and Fear related to a threat to or change in health status and treatment options
- Acute Pain or Chronic Pain related to effects of metastasis, bone pain, and spinal cord compression
- Risk for Sexual Dysfunction related to altered body structure or function (secondary to disease process and treatment)
- Dysfunctional Grieving or Anticipatory Grieving related to loss of a body part or changes in body function

A possible collaborative problem is Potential for Metastasis.

Planning and Implementation

Impaired Urinary Elimination

Planning: Expected Outcomes. The patient with prostate cancer is expected to have normal urinary elimination without hesitancy, urgency, or infection. If the disease is diagnosed and treated early, metastasis may be prevented.

Interventions. As with any cancer, accurate staging and grading of prostate tumors guide treatment planning and monitoring during the course of the disease. Patients are faced with several treatment options. A urologist and oncologist are needed to help them make the best decision. Because prostate cancer is slow growing with late metastasis, older men who are asymptomatic and have other illness may choose observation without immediate active treatment, especially if the cancer is early stage. This option is known as "watchful waiting," or *expectant therapy.* This form of treatment involves initial surveillance with active treatment if the symptoms become bothersome. The average time from diagnosis to start of treatment is up to 10 years. During the watchful waiting period, men are monitored at regular intervals through DRE and PSA testing. Factors that are considered in choosing watchful waiting include potential side effects of treatment (e.g., urinary incontinence, erectile dysfunction), estimated life expectancy, and the risk for increased morbidity and mortality from not seeking active treatment.

Patients who have stage 0 cancer of the prostate who choose watchful waiting require close follow-up by their health care provider. If obstruction occurs, repeated needle biopsies or transurethral resection of the prostate (TURP) should be part of the screening. Hormonal therapy may be given after a period of watchful waiting, but it may also be used later in the disease process.

Active treatment options for the patient with prostate cancer are classified as *local* and *systemic* therapies. Local therapies include surgery and radiation. A variety of drugs are used for systemic therapy. Specific management is based on the extent of the disease and the patient's physical condition. The patient may undergo surgery for a biopsy, staging and removal of the tumor, or palliation to control the spread of disease or relieve distressing symptoms. As with watchful waiting, the health care provider and patient must weigh the benefits of treatment against potential adverse effects such as incontinence and erectile dysfunction (ED).

Surgical Management. Because some localized prostate cancers are resistant to radiation, *surgery is the most common intervention for a cure.* Minimally invasive surgery (MIS) or an open surgical technique for radical prostatectomy (prostate removal) is most often performed. However, a transurethral resection of the prostate (TURP) may be done to promote urination for patients with advanced disease. *It is not used as a curative treatment.* The care of patients having this procedure is described in the discussion of Surgical Management on p. 1715 in the Benign Prostatic Hypertrophy section. A **bilateral orchiectomy** (removal of both testicles) is another palliative surgery that slows the spread of cancer by removing the main source of testosterone. This procedure is described on p. 1729 in the Testicular Cancer section.

Preoperative care. Preoperative care depends on the type of surgery that will be done. The latest advancement in surgical technology for prostate cancer is *laparoscopic radical prostatectomy (LRP).* This minimally invasive surgery may also be done as a robot-assisted procedure (also called the *da Vinci prostatectomy*) (NCCN, 2007). Patients who qualify for LRP must have a PSA less than 10 ng/mL and have no previous hormone therapy or abdominal surgeries. Remind the patient that the advantages of this procedure over open surgery are:

- Decreased hospital stay (1-2 days)
- Minimal bleeding
- Smaller incisions and less scarring
- Less postoperative discomfort
- Decreased time for the urinary catheter
- Fewer complications
- Faster recovery and return to usual activities
- Nerve-sparing advantages

For the patient undergoing an *open* radical prostatectomy, provide preoperative care as for any patient having surgery (see Chapter 16). Both the LRP and open techniques are done as a curative approach.

Operative procedures. For the *LRP procedure,* the urologist makes several small incisions into the abdomen. A laparoscope with a camera on the end is inserted through one of the incisions while other instruments are inserted into the other incisions. The robotic system may be used to control the movement of the instruments by a remote device. The prostate is removed along with nearby lymph nodes.

The *open* radical prostatectomy can be performed via a retropubic or perineal approach, but the retropubic method is done most often to preserve perineal nerves needed for penile erection. The surgeon removes the entire prostate gland along with the prostatic capsule, the cuff at the bladder neck, the seminal vesicles, and the regional lymph nodes. The remaining urethra is connected to the bladder neck. The removal of tissue at the bladder neck allows the seminal fluid to travel upward into the bladder rather than down the urethral tract, resulting in retrograde ejaculations. The patient is sterile and has little ejaculate fluid. After surgery, the patient may experience temporary erectile dysfunction (ED), but normal function usually returns in 3 to 18 months.

Postoperative care. Provide postoperative care of the patient after *open* radical prostatectomy as summarized in Chart 75-4. Nursing interventions include all the typical care for a patient undergoing major surgery. Maintaining hydration, caring for wound drains (open procedure), managing pain, and preventing pulmonary complications are important aspects of nursing care (see Chapter 18).

Assess the patient's pain level, and monitor the effectiveness of pain management with opioids given as patient-controlled analgesia (PCA), a common method of delivery during the first 24 hours after surgery. Administer a stool softener if needed to prevent possible constipation from the drugs. Patients having the minimally invasive surgery have much less pain and fewer complications.

The patient has an indwelling urinary catheter to straight drainage. Monitor intake and output every shift and record, or delegate this activity to and supervise unlicensed assistive personnel (UAP). An antispasmodic may be prescribed to decrease bladder spasm induced by the indwelling urinary catheter. Tell the patient that the catheter will be removed within 7 to 14 days after the LRP procedure, depending on the surgical approach and overall patient condition, if no problems develop. Those with open surgical procedures use the catheter for 7 to 10 days or longer.

Ambulation begins early, usually the night of surgery. Provide assistance in walking the patient when he first gets out of bed. Assess for scrotal or penile swelling from the disrupted pelvic lymph flow. If this occurs, elevate the scrotum and penis and apply ice to the area intermittently (20 minutes on and 20 minutes off) for the first 24 to 48 hours.

Many patients who have the minimally invasive techniques are discharged the day after surgery and can resume usual activities in about a week. Those who have open procedures are discharged in 2 to 3 days, depending on their progress. Teach them that they need about 3 to 5 weeks of rest at home, depending on their age and general physical condition.

Remind patients that common potential long-term complications of open radical prostatectomy are urinary incontinence and erectile dysfunction (ED) (formerly called *impotence*). *Incontinence* may occur because the internal and external sphincters of the bladder lie close to the prostate gland and are often damaged during the surgery. Kegel perineal exercises may reduce the severity of urinary incontinence after radical prostatectomy. Teach the patient to contract and relax the perineal and gluteal muscles in several ways. For one of the exercises, teach him to:

1. Tighten the perineal muscles for 3 to 5 seconds as if to prevent voiding and then relax.
2. Bear down as if having a bowel movement.
3. Relax and repeat the exercise.

Show him how to inhale through pursed lips while tightening the perineal muscles and how to exhale when he relaxes. To regain urinary control, teach the patient to practice holding an object, such as a pencil, in the fold between the buttock and the thigh. He may also sit on the toilet with the knees apart while voiding and start and stop the stream several times.

Difficulty having or maintaining an erection is also possible after radical prostatectomy because of damage to or inflammation of the pudendal nerves. Interventions for erectile dysfunction are discussed on p. 1726.

Nonsurgical Management. Nonsurgical management is usually an adjunct to surgery but may be done as an alternative intervention if the cancer is widespread or the patient's condition or age prevents surgery. Common modalities include radiation therapy, hormonal therapy, and chemotherapy (less often). Several less-common procedures are also available.

Radiation therapy. External or internal radiation therapy may be used in the treatment of prostate cancer. For patients who have severe bone pain from metastasis, systemic therapy may be used in which radioactive substances are given IV (NCCN, 2007). The purposes of radiation therapy are:

- As an alternative curative treatment to surgery for locally contained tumors
- As an adjunct to radical prostatectomy when surgical margins or regional lymph nodes show cancer cells after surgery
- For palliation of the patient's symptoms

Palliative radiation therapy relieves pain caused by bone metastases and may relieve ureteral or bladder outlet obstruction.

External beam radiation therapy (EBRT) comes from a source outside the body. Patients are usually treated 5 days a week for 6 to 9 weeks. Three-dimensional conformal radiation

Chart 75-4 BEST PRACTICE FOR PATIENT SAFETY & QUALITY CARE

Care of the Patient After an Open Radical Prostatectomy

- Encourage the patient to use patient-controlled analgesia (PCA) as needed.
- Help the patient get out of bed into a chair on the night of surgery and ambulate the next day.
- Maintain the sequential compression device until the patient begins to ambulate.
- Monitor the patient for deep vein thrombosis and pulmonary embolus.
- Keep an accurate record of intake and output, including Jackson-Pratt or other drainage device drainage.
- Keep the urinary meatus clean using soap and water.
- Avoid rectal procedures or treatments.
- Teach the patient how to care for the urinary catheter because he will be discharged with the catheter in place.
- Teach the patient how to use a leg bag.
- Emphasize the importance of not straining during bowel movement. Advise the patient to avoid suppositories or enemas.
- Remind the patient about the importance of follow-up appointments with the physician to monitor progress.

therapy (3D-CRT) can more accurately target prostate tissue and can reduce side effects such as damage to the rectum. An advanced type of this radiation called *intensity-modulated radiation therapy* provides very high doses to the prostate. EBRT can also be used to relieve pain from bone metastasis. Teach patients that external beam radiation causes ED in many men well after the treatment is completed.

Other complications from EBRT include *acute radiation cystitis* causing persistent pain and hematuria. Symptoms are usually mild to moderate and subside in 6 weeks after treatment. Drugs to prevent urinary urgency such as tolterodine (Detrol LA) may be prescribed (Gray & Sims, 2006). Teach the patient to avoid caffeine and continue drinking plenty of water and other fluids.

Radiation proctitis (rectal mucosa inflammation) may also develop but is less likely with 3D-CRT. The man reports rectal urgency and cramping and passes mucus and blood. Teach him to report these symptoms to the health care provider. Like cystitis, this problem resolves in 4 to 6 weeks after the treatment stops (Gray & Sims, 2006). If proctitis occurs, teach patients to limit spicy or fatty foods, caffeine, and dairy products.

Internal radiation therapy (brachytherapy) can be delivered by implanting low-dose radiation seeds directly into and around the prostate gland. This treatment includes ultrasonically guided interstitial or radioactive seed implantation. These procedures are done on an ambulatory care basis and are the most cost-effective treatment for early-stage prostate cancer. Reassure the patient that the dose of radiation is low and that he will not pose a hazard to himself or others. Teach him that ED, urinary incontinence, and rectal problems do occur in a small percentage of cases. Fatigue is also common and may last for several months after the treatment stops. Chapter 24 describes general nursing care for patients having radiation therapy.

Drug therapy. Drug therapy may consist of either hormonal therapy (androgen deprivation therapy [ADT]) or chemotherapy. Several vaccines to locate and destroy prostate cancer cells are being studied (Slovin, 2008).

Hormone therapy. Because most prostate tumors are hormone dependent, patients with extensive tumors or those with metastatic disease may be managed by androgen deprivation. Changing the patient's hormone levels may be done in two ways:

- The testosterone influence can be removed by a bilateral orchiectomy (surgery).
- Luteinizing hormone–releasing hormone (LH-RH) agonists or anti-androgens can be given (drugs).

The *LH-RH agonists* currently available in the United States are leuprolide (Lupron), goserelin (Zoladex), and triptorelin (Trelstar) (NCCN, 2007). These drugs first stimulate the pituitary gland to release the luteinizing hormone (LH). After about 3 weeks, the pituitary gland "runs out" of LH, which then reduces testosterone production by the testes. Teach patients taking these drugs that side effects include "hot flashes," erectile dysfunction, and decreased **libido** (desire to have sex). Some men also have **gynecomastia** (breast tenderness and growth). These drugs can also cause osteoporosis. Bisphosphonates like pamidronate (Aredia) are prescribed to prevent bone fractures. They can also be used to slow the damage caused by bone metastasis (NCCN, 2007).

Anti-androgen drugs, also known as androgen deprivation therapy (ADT), work differently in that they block the body's ability to use the available androgens (NCCN, 2007). These drugs are the major treatment for metastatic disease. Examples include flutamide (Eulexin, Euflex♣), bicalutamide (Casodex), and nilutamide (Nilandron). These drugs inhibit tumor progression by blocking the uptake of testicular and adrenal androgens at the prostate tumor site.

Anti-androgens may be used alone or in combination with LH-RH agonists for a total or maximal androgen blockade (hormone ablation). Patients who have this drug combination often have "hot flashes" similar to those experienced by menopausal women, and they can decrease the patient's perceived quality of life. Ask the patient if he has been experiencing this problem. Megestrol acetate may be prescribed for this uncomfortable condition (Lajiness, 2007).

Chemotherapy. Systemic cytotoxic chemotherapy is an option for patients whose cancer has spread and for whom other therapies have not worked. The main agent approved for this use is docetaxel (Taxotere), a drug used also to treat breast cancer. It may be combined with other drugs to reduce the chance that the cancer cells will become resistant to docetaxel. Small cell prostate cancer is rare and is more responsive to chemotherapy than to hormone therapy (NCCN, 2007). Cisplatin (Platinol) and etoposide (VP-16, VePesid) often work for this type of cancer. Clinical trials are testing the effectiveness of many other drugs that may be used for early or late prostate cancer. Chapter 24 describes general nursing care for patients receiving chemotherapy.

Other drugs. Other less commonly used drugs that are available if other drugs have failed or stopped working include high doses of ketoconazole (Nizoral), an antifungal drug that blocks androgen production, and the female hormone *estrogen* (diethylstilbestrol or DES). Teach patients taking ketoconazole that it can cause liver and adrenal problems. Teach them to take the drug on an empty stomach and to avoid drugs such as histamine blockers and antacids, which can interfere with drug absorption (Held-Warmkessel, 2008). Patients are followed closely and have frequent laboratory tests to detect any early organ damage (Liebertz & Fox, 2006). The drug also interacts with many other drugs, including warfarin (Coumadin), phenytoin (Dilantin), and prednisone (Deltasone). Corticosteroids such as prednisone may be given alone as palliation to reduce pain and improve the quality of life (Held-Warmkessel, 2008).

Cryotherapy. Cryotherapy (cryoablation) is a minimally invasive procedure that can be an alternative to radical prostatectomy. This procedure is reserved for patients for whom the cancer is known to be confined to the prostate gland. The patient is placed in the lithotomy position, and a transrectal ultrasound probe is placed in the rectum. The probe helps determine the size of the prostate and the subsequent number of small cryoprobes that are positioned around the prostate gland. Liquid nitrogen freezes the gland and results in prostate cell death. The dead cells are then absorbed gradually by the body (Gray & Sims, 2006).

The main advantage of this procedure is that patients do not have an incision. However, it is associated with a high risk for urinary incontinence and erectile dysfunction (ED). Therefore it is not used commonly at this time. Most patients are able to return to their usual activity level in about 1 week after the procedure.

Complementary and alternative therapies. In addition to increasing foods rich in lycopene and omega-3 fatty acids, many patients with prostate cancer use other foods and supplements

EVIDENCE-BASED PRACTICE

What are the stages that men with prostate cancer go through from diagnosis to recovery?

Wallace, M., & Storms, S. (2007). The needs of men with prostate cancer: Results of a focus group study. *Applied Nursing Research, 20*(4), 181-187.

The purpose of this qualitative study was to identify the psychosocial experiences of men with prostate cancer from diagnosis to surviving the disease. A convenience group of 29 men were interviewed, and demographic questionnaires with open-ended questions were completed by each subject. Most of the volunteers were white and ranged from 49 to 81 years of age. Three distinct stages of emotions were identified: Taking in (the diagnosis), Taking hold (of the experience), and Taking on (survival). The men emphasized that their partners or spouses and family members were very helpful in managing each stage. They also found that finding and talking with other men who had the diagnosis was very helpful. Otherwise they felt that very little patient support was available for them, including patient and partner education. The subjects stated that they wished they had known more about the disease before it affected them so that they would have taken more preventive measures, including regular screening.

Level of Evidence—6. This research was a small qualitative study.

Commentary: Implications for Research and Practice. The study sample was very small and was compiled as a group of volunteers who answered a request to be part of the study. However, the findings of this study are similar to those of studies of women with breast cancer, including the three identified emotional stages. For women having breast surgery, health care agencies often ask the patient if she would like to talk with another woman who has had the procedure. This resource is not usually considered for men having prostate surgery. The men in this study felt that they did not receive adequate health teaching. It is important for urologists to employ nurses or nurse practitioners who can ensure that patients and their partners receive the information they need. Nurses working in the surgical department and other areas of the hospital setting should provide education and support for these patients during treatment.

to slow tumor growth or its spread. Scientific evidence supports soy protein (containing isoflavones) as a useful adjunct to traditional medical therapy for prostate cancer (Hamilton-Reeves et al., 2008; Kumar et al., 2007; Raffoul et al., 2007). Other substances that are used by patients but have not been well researched or are controversial include PC-SPEC (an 8-herb combination used to decrease testosterone and PSA), green tea, and garlic.

Several studies have been done to examine the role of spirituality in patient decision making and recovery. For example, White and Verhoef (2006) found in their qualitative study of 29 men with prostate cancer that spiritual beliefs and practices play an important role in how patients decide which cancer treatment they want. These practices include prayer, meditation, ceremonies, and use of spiritual imagery. In collaboration with the health care team, assess the patient's spiritual beliefs and respect his decision for disease management. Recognize that having prostate cancer may strengthen his link with the spiritual community. While in the hospital setting, ask if the patient wants to talk with his spiritual leader or the certified hospital chaplain.

Community-Based Care

Patient-centered collaborative care of the man with prostate cancer should include his partner, if any. Recognize that he has specific physical and psychosocial needs that should be addressed before hospital discharge and management should continue in the community setting. In their qualitative study of prostate cancer survivors, Wallace and Storms (2007) found that men went through three distinct stages throughout the prostate cancer experience. During each stage, they had varying needs and depended in large part on their partner's support. (See the Evidence-Based Practice box above.)

Patients with prostate cancer may require care in a wide variety of settings: at the hospital, the radiation therapy department, the oncologist's office, or home at any stage of the disease process. Specific interventions depend on which treatment the patient had or if he had a combination of treatments. This section focuses on the needs of those who had a radical prostatectomy.

Home Care Management

Discharge planning and health teaching start early, even before surgery. A patient can better plan home care management when he knows what to expect. Collaborate with the case manager to coordinate the efforts of various health care providers, surgical unit nursing staff, and possibly a home care nurse. Continuity of care is essential when caring for this patient because he may need weeks or months of therapies.

Health Teaching

An important area of teaching for the patient going home after radical prostatectomy is urinary catheter care. An indwelling urinary catheter may be in place for up to 2 weeks, depending on the surgical technique that was used. Teach him and his family how to care for the catheter, use a leg bag, and identify manifestations of infection and other complications. See Chart 75-5 for patient and family education.

Encourage the patient to walk short distances. Lifting is restricted to no more than 15 pounds for up to 6 weeks. Remind him to maintain an upright position and not walk bent or flexed. Vigorous exercise such as running or jumping should be avoided for at least 12 weeks and then gradually introduced.

Teach the patient to not strain to defecate. A stool softener may be prescribed to reduce the need for straining. If an opioid is prescribed for pain management, encourage the patient to drink plenty of water to prevent constipation.

Teach him to shower for the first 2 to 3 weeks rather than soak in a bathtub. Show him how to inspect the incision site daily for signs of infection. Follow-up appointments are scheduled in 1 week for removal of the staples and in 2 to 3 weeks

Chart 75-5 PATIENT AND FAMILY EDUCATION GUIDE

Catheter Care at Home

- Once a day, gently wash the first 6 inches of the catheter starting at the penis and washing outward with mild soap and water.
- Rinse and dry the catheter well.
- If you have not been circumcised, push the foreskin back to clean the catheter site; when finished, push the foreskin forward.
- Change the drainage bag at least once a week:
  - Hold the catheter with one hand and the tubing with the other hand, and twist in opposite directions to disconnect.
  - Place the end of the catheter in a clean container to catch leakage of urine.
  - Remove the rubber cap from the tubing of the leg bag or clean drainage bag.
  - Clean the end of the new tubing with alcohol swabs.
  - Insert the end of the new tubing into the catheter, and twist to connect securely.
- Clean the drainage bag just removed by pouring a solution of one part vinegar to two parts water through the tubing and bag. Rinse well with water, and allow the bag to dry.

for removal of the urinary catheter. PSA blood tests are taken 6 weeks after surgery and then every 4 to 6 months to monitor progress.

Teach the patient about the possibility of developing **Peyronie's disease,** an abnormal bending of the penis during erection that is caused by fibrous plaques (scar tissue) that forms in the penis. Some men have a lump, whereas others have pain but no lump. This rare, non–life-threatening disease occurs most often in middle-aged men after a radical prostatectomy. Teach patients to report his problem to their urologist for possible treatment with penile implants, medication or, less commonly, surgery.

Health Care Resources

Refer the patient and partner to agencies or support groups such as the American Cancer Society's Man to Man program to help cope with prostate cancer. This program provides one-on-one education, personal visits, educational presentations, and the opportunity to engage in open and candid discussions. Another prostate cancer support group is Us TOO International (www.ustoo.com) sponsored by the Prostate Cancer Education and Support Network. This group provides education and support with national and international chapters. Information can also be obtained from the Prostate Cancer Foundation (www.prostatecancerfoundation.org) or the National Prostate Cancer Coalition (www.fightprostatecancer.org). Other personal and community support services such as spiritual leaders or churches and synagogues are also important to many patients.

Many men have erectile dysfunction (ED) for the first 3 to 18 months after a prostatectomy. Refer them to a specialist who can help with this problem. ED is discussed in the next section (Erectile Disfunction). Refer patients with urinary incontinence to a urologist who specializes in this area. Drug therapy and other strategies may be used. Chapter 69 discusses incontinence management in detail.

DECISION-MAKING CHALLENGE

Legal/Ethical

A 61-year-old widower has just been diagnosed with prostate cancer after having a biopsy. He is very upset about the diagnosis, stating that he was planning to get remarried in 6 months. He is very concerned that his fiancée may change her mind about the wedding if she finds out about his cancer. She is 37 years old and has no children from her previous marriage. They have discussed having a baby, and now he does not know if that can still be possible. The urologist has encouraged him to decide on a treatment and begin it soon. The patient is thinking about waiting until after the wedding to deal with his diagnosis but asks you what you think he should do.

1. How should you respond to this patient at this time?
2. What legal/ethical principles are involved in this case?
3. What factors does he need to consider when making his decision?
4. What treatment options does he have given his age and the urologist's suggestion?

evolve For suggested answer guidelines, go to http://evolve.elsevier.com/Iggy/.

ERECTILE DYSFUNCTION

Pathophysiology

Erectile dysfunction (ED), also known as *impotence,* is the inability to achieve or maintain an erection for sexual intercourse. It affects millions of men in the United States. During the past 15 years, there has been a major change in the management of men with ED as a result of increased understanding of the physiology of erectile function and the development of new, effective therapies. There are two classes of ED: organic and functional.

Organic ED is a gradual deterioration of function. The man first notices diminishing firmness and a decrease in frequency of erections. Causes include:

- Inflammation of the prostate, urethra, or seminal vesicles
- Surgical procedures such as prostatectomy
- Pelvic fractures
- Lumbosacral injuries
- Vascular disease, including hypertension
- Chronic neurologic conditions, such as Parkinson disease or multiple sclerosis
- Endocrine disorders, such as diabetes mellitus (a major cause) or thyroid disorders
- Smoking and alcohol consumption
- Drugs, such as antihypertensives
- Poor overall health that prevents sexual intercourse

If the patient has episodes of ED, it usually has a *functional* (psychological) cause. Men with functional ED usually have normal nocturnal (nighttime) and morning erections. Onset is usually sudden and follows a period of high stress.

Patient-Centered Collaborative Care

Assessment

For a man to have an erection, he must have normal innervation and a normal libido (sex drive). Therefore a medical, social, and sexual history and a complete physical examination are needed. The first step is to determine whether the cause is organic. Diagnostic testing is done to rule out possible organic causes.

If test results are negative, the evaluation then focuses on the specific causes that may have been indicated in the medical history. For example, hormone testing is used for patients who have a poor libido, small testicles, or sparse beard growth. Serum levels of *testosterone* and *gonadotropins* such as luteinizing hormone (LH) and follicle-stimulating hormone (FSH) are measured. LH stimulates the Leydig cells in the testicles to produce testosterone.

Duplex Doppler ultrasonography is another test to evaluate ED. It provides information about arterial and venous blood flow to the penis. It can also be used to determine the best treatment for ED. A *nocturnal penile tumescence test* that measures nighttime erections is done in a sleep laboratory. Usually an erection is expected with each rapid eye movement (REM) episode. This study can determine whether ED is caused by an organic or functional problem. If the man has nocturnal erections, the ED is functional. Sex or intimacy counseling is needed in this case, and the patient is referred to a certified sex therapist or other qualified specialist.

Interventions

Current methods of treatment include oral drug therapy, vacuum devices, intracorporal injections, intraurethral applications, and prostheses (implants).

Drug Therapy

First-line oral drugs used to manage ED, phosphodiesterace-5 (PDE-5) inhibitors, work by relaxing the smooth muscles in the corpora cavernosa so blood flow to the penis is increased. The veins exiting the corpora are compressed, limiting outward blood flow and resulting in penile **tumescence** (swelling). Teach patients to take the pill 1 hour before sexual intercourse. For some drugs, such as sildenafil (Viagra) and vardenafil (Levitra), sexual stimulation is needed within ½ to 1 hour to promote the erection. With other drugs, such as tadalafil (Cialis), erection can be stimulated over a longer period. Because the erection occurs more naturally compared with other treatment options, most men and their partners prefer this option.

Instruct patients to abstain from alcohol before sexual intercourse because it may impair the ability to have an erection. Common side effects of these drugs include dyspepsia (heartburn), headaches, facial flushing, and stuffy nose. If more than one pill a day is being taken, leg and back cramps, nausea, and vomiting also may occur. *Teach men who take nitrates to avoid these drugs because the vasodilation effects can cause a profound hypotension and reduce blood flow to vital organs.* For patients who cannot take these drugs or do not respond to them, other methods are available to achieve an erection.

Other Measures

The basic design of a *vacuum constriction device (VCD)* is a cylinder that fits over the penis and sits firmly against the body. Using a pump, a vacuum is created to draw blood into the penis to maintain an erection. A rubber ring (tension band) is placed around the base of the penis to maintain the erection, and the cylinder is removed.

The advantage of this procedure is that the device is easy and safe to use. The disadvantage is its clumsiness and lack of spontaneity. In addition, the man may experience pain from the rubber ring or from pumping the device too quickly. The ring should be removed after an hour, or tissue could be damaged.

Injecting the penis with vasodilating drugs can make the penis erect by engorging it with blood. The most common agents used for this purpose today include (Weeks & Ficorelli, 2006a):

- Alprostadil (Caverject), a synthetic vasodilator identical to prostaglandin E_1 produced in the body
- Paverine, also a vasodilator
- Phentolamine (Regitine), an alpha-1, alpha-2 selective adrenergic receptor antagonist
- A combination of any or all of these drugs

These drugs may be injected into the side of the penis using a 27- or 30-gauge needle. Adverse effects include priapism (prolonged erection), penile scarring, fibrosis, bleeding, bruising at the injection site, pain, infection, and vasovagal responses.

Alprostadil (Muse) is also available as a *transurethral suppository* that is placed in the urethra with an applicator. The drug is absorbed into the corpora, which causes an erection in about 10 minutes; erections last 30 to 60 minutes. Advantages include the simplicity of the procedure and noninvasiveness. Disadvantages are a decrease in spontaneity, syncope, and a burning sensation in the urethra after the application.

Penile implants (prostheses) are used when other modalities fail. Devices include semirigid, flexible, or hydraulic inflatable and multi-component or one-piece instruments. The three-piece inflatable device is the most commonly implanted prosthesis. A reservoir is placed in the scrotum. Tubes carry the fluid into the inflatable pieces that are placed in the penis. To inflate the prosthesis, the man squeezes the pump located in the scrotum. To deflate the prosthesis, a release button is activated. Advantages include the man's ability to control his erections. The major disadvantages include device failure and infection. The device is implanted as an ambulatory surgical procedure. Teach the patient to observe the surgical site for bleeding and infection.

TESTICULAR CANCER

Pathophysiology

Testicular cancer is not very common. However, it is the most common malignancy in men 15 to 34 years of age (www.cancer.org). It strikes young men at a productive time of life and thus has significant economic, social, and psychological impact on the patient and his family and/or partner. Although testicular cancer occurs more often in younger men, middle-aged and older men also may be affected. With early detection by testicular self-examination (TSE) (Chart 75-6) and treatment, testicular cancer can be cured. It can occur in one testicle or both.

Chart 75-6 PATIENT AND FAMILY EDUCATION GUIDE

Testicular Self-Examination

- Examine your testicles monthly immediately after a bath or a shower, when your scrotal skin is relaxed.
- Examine each testicle by gently rolling it between your thumbs and fingers. Testicular tumors tend to appear deep in the center of the testicle.
- Look and feel for any lumps; smooth, rounded masses; or any change in the size, shape, or consistency of the testes.
- Report any lump or swelling to your doctor as soon as possible.

Primary testicular cancers fall into two major groups:

- Germ cell tumors arising from the sperm-producing cells (account for most testicular cancers)
- Non–germ cell tumors arising from the stroma, interstitial, or Leydig cells that produce testosterone (account for a very small percentage of testicular cancers)

Germ Cell Tumors

Testicular germ cell tumors are classified into two broad categories: seminomas and nonseminomas (Table 75-1). The most common type of testicular tumor is *seminoma.* Patients with pure seminomatous tumors have the most favorable prognoses because the tumors are usually localized and metastasize late. They often are diagnosed when they are still confined to the testicles and retroperitoneal lymph nodes. These cancers respond extremely well to radiation therapy. Patients with early-stage seminomas have a 5-year survival rate of 96% with surgery (orchiectomy) and radiation therapy (www.cancer.org).

Nonseminomatous germ cell tumors include three types: embryonal carcinoma, teratoma, and choriocarcinoma (a tumor that is highly malignant and spreads quickly). These tumors are not as sensitive to treatment with radiation therapy. They are treated with surgery or chemotherapy, depending on the extent of the disease at diagnosis.

Non–Germ Cell Tumors

Non–germ cell tumors are classified as either *interstitial cell tumors* or *androblastomas* (testicular adenomas). Most of these tumors do not metastasize. Interstitial cell tumors arise from the Leydig cells, which secrete testosterone into the bloodstream. These tumors secrete an excessive amount of androgenic hormones, which cause young boys with such tumors to undergo early puberty. Androblastomas sometimes secrete estrogen, which accounts for the feminization and **gynecomastia** (breast enlargement) occasionally seen in these men.

The cause of testicular cancer is unknown. The risk for testicular tumors is reported to be higher in males who have an undescended testis **(cryptorchidism).** In males with cryptorchidism, the testicular cancer usually develops in the undescended testis and there is a 25% chance of cancer developing in the normally descended testis. Seminoma is the most common type of testicular cancer associated with cryptorchidism. The undescended testis undergoes gradual involution and degeneration over time, which may contribute to tumor development. It is not known why the normally descended testis is at risk for cancer.

TABLE 75-1 Classification of Testicular Tumors

GERM CELL GERMINAL TUMORS
• Seminoma
• Nonseminoma:
• Embryonal carcinoma
• Teratoma
• Choriocarcinoma
NON–GERM CELL (NONGERMINAL) TUMORS
• Interstitial cell tumor
• Androblastoma

GENETIC CONSIDERATIONS

Men are at a higher risk for testicular cancer if they have a family history of the disease (Hemminki et al., 2008). The incidence is higher among identical twins, brothers, and other close male relatives. A genetic basis is further supported by who gets the disease. Euro-American men are at risk for testicular cancer more than African-American and Asian-American men (McCance & Huether, 2006). The reason for these differences is not known.

Although a history of trauma or infection is common in patients with testicular cancer, neither is a cause of testicular cancer. Testicular trauma or infection can produce changes in the shape, size, or texture of the testes more difficult to determine. The patient with one of these problems should be examined by a health care provider after the acute episode resolves to rule out the presence of a tumor.

Primary testicular cancer is rarely bilateral. Other cancers such as leukemia, lymphoma, and metastatic carcinomas may invade the testes. A man with bilateral testicular tumors is more likely to have metastatic disease to the testes than primary cancer.

Patient-Centered Collaborative Care

evolve ONLINE PHARM REVIEW

Assessment

Physical Assessment/Clinical Manifestations

When taking a history from a patient with a suspected testicular tumor, consider the risk factors. It is important to collect data about age and race because the disease occurs most often in young white males. Assess for other risk factors, including a history or presence of an undescended testis and a family history of testicular cancer.

Ask the patient whether he has noticed a discomfort such as heaviness or aching in the lower abdomen or the scrotum. Determine how long any manifestations have been present.

Assess the patient's family situation. Is the patient sexually active? If so, what is his sexual preference? Does he have children? Does he want children in the future? Depending on the treatment plan chosen, would he be interested in sperm storage in a sperm bank?

If the man has one healthy testis, he can function sexually and may not have any reproductive dysfunction. If he has a retroperitoneal lymph node dissection or chemotherapy, he may become sterile because of treatment effects on the sperm-producing cells or surgical trauma to the sympathetic nervous system resulting in retrograde ejaculations.

The testes, lymph nodes, and abdomen should be thoroughly examined. Patients may feel embarrassed about having this examination. Provide privacy, and explain the procedure to the patient. *Inspect the testicles for swelling or a lump that the patient reports is painless. This is the most common manifestation of testicular cancer.* An advanced practice nurse or other health care provider palpates the testes for lumps and swelling that are not visible (Chart 75-7). The presence of any testicular pain, lymph node swelling, abdominal masses, sudden hydrocele (fluid in the scrotum), or gynecomastia often indicates metastatic disease.

Chart 75-7 FOCUSED ASSESSMENT

A Patient with a Testicular Lump

Obtain a medical history from the patient.
- When was the lump discovered?
- Are there any other symptoms (sensation of heaviness, dragging in testicle, pain, discharge from penis)?
- Is there a history of cryptorchidism?

Assess the genital system. Always wear gloves during the examination of the male genitalia.
- Inspect and palpate the scrotal contents. Have the patient perform a Valsalva maneuver, and palpate for a varicocele.
- Any lump or enlargement that does not transilluminate should be suspected as malignant.

Palpate for any enlarged lymph nodes. Most common lymphadenopathy is in the inguinal or supraclavicular regions.

Assess the abdomen for a possible mass or hepatomegaly.

Psychosocial Assessment

Because testicular cancer and its treatment often lead to sexual dysfunction, pay close attention to the psychosocial aspects of the disease. *Sexuality* is an issue for men of any age, but it may be even more of an issue for younger men. Even if the cancer is detected at an early stage and the patient is cured after surgery, he may be afraid that he will be sexually deficient. He may also think of himself as "less than a whole man." These fears can disrupt the psychosocial and sexual development of young males and can threaten their identity. The patient may be afraid that he will be unable to perform sexually, will no longer be sexually attractive or desirable, and will face rejection. Feelings of sexual inadequacy may be denied, repressed, or displaced, causing increased stress on the man's personal and work relationships.

Assess the man's support systems, including his partner, family members, and friends. Ask him where he feels that he can be supported, such as a religious or spiritual group, community club, or social group. Friends are often very helpful during this difficult time.

Laboratory Assessment

An important diagnostic indicator for testicular cancer is the presence of certain biomarker proteins (tumor markers). These are proteins that normally were produced during embryonic development, and their presence in adults is abnormal. Benign testicular tumors do not elevate the levels of any of these marker proteins.

Common tumor markers for testicular cancer are (www.cancer.gov):
- Alpha-fetoprotein (AFP)
- Beta human chorionic gonadotropin (hCG)
- Lactate dehydrogenase (LDH)

Most patients with nonseminomatous germ cell tumors and teratomas have elevated blood levels of AFP, hCG, or both (Pagana & Pagana, 2006). Patients with a pure seminoma may not have an elevated AFP level, and only a few have a slightly elevated hCG level. This level resolves after orchiectomy. Patients with seminomas have elevated LDH (Pagana & Pagana, 2006).

If a patient has a diagnosis of seminoma and also has an elevated AFP level, the tumor specimen must be re-examined for evidence of a component of nonseminomatous cancer. This step is necessary because the treatments differ for seminomatous and nonseminomatous tumors.

The serum biomarker levels are also used to evaluate responses to therapy for testicular cancer and to document the presence of residual or recurrent disease. With effective treatment, the levels of abnormal markers fall. The persistence of elevated levels of markers after orchiectomy (testicle removal) is evidence that the patient has metastatic disease, even if x-rays and scans do not show a tumor presence. The reappearance of the tumor markers indicates recurrence of the cancer. Therefore marker levels must be monitored regularly during the follow-up of patients treated for testicular cancer.

Serum testosterone levels are increased when the tumor affects the Leydig cells, which produce this hormone. Drugs such as alcohol and antiepileptic drugs can also cause an increase in testosterone (Pagana & Pagana, 2006).

Other Diagnostic Assessment

When a patient has a change in testis size, shape, or texture, *ultrasonography* can determine whether the mass is solid or fluid filled. It also can help differentiate benign masses from malignant ones.

After the diagnosis of testicular cancer, the patient should have a *computed tomography (CT)* scan of the abdomen and the chest to identify small metastatic lesions. *Lymphangiography* shows a view of the body's lymph system to look for spread to other areas.

Magnetic resonance imaging (MRI) is used to detect enlarged lymph nodes and abnormal nodules in certain organs that may indicate metastasis from the testicles. Chest x-rays and bone scans may also be performed if metastasis is suspected.

Common Nursing Diagnoses and Collaborative Problems

Common nursing diagnoses that may apply to the patient with testicular cancer include:
- Risk for Sexual Dysfunction related to altered body structure and function from disease or treatment
- Dysfunctional Grieving or Anticipatory Grieving related to loss of a body part or changes in body function
- Disturbed Body Image related to the diagnosis of cancer and its treatment
- Acute Pain or Chronic Pain related to tumor compression or effects of metastasis
- Anxiety related to threat to health status from the diagnosis of cancer

The primary collaborative problem is Potential for Metastasis.

Interventions

Surgery is the main treatment for testicular cancer. It is often combined with nonsurgical management to prevent metastatic disease (or to alleviate symptoms of metastasis) and to cause tumor regression.

At diagnosis, the incidence of **oligospermia** (low sperm count) and **azoospermia** (absence of living sperm) is common in patients with testicular cancer. This problem is thought to be related to higher testicular temperatures created by cancer cell metabolism. The man may not discover that he has reduced sperm count until he has a sperm count performed before surgery.

Health teaching about reproduction, fertility, and sexuality is started in the pretreatment phase. Review the normal reproductive function, as well as the possible effects of cancer and its treatment on reproductive function. Explore with the patient various reproductive options (e.g., sperm banks, artificial insemination) (Chart 75-8). The sperm bank facility provides comprehensive information on semen collection, storage of semen, the storage contract, costs, and the insemination process.

When preparing the patient for the collection and storage of sperm, assume the role of patient advocate and keep in mind the effect of the cancer diagnosis. The psychological benefit of having stored sperm may be important for the man and may influence his response to treatment. Knowing that the potential for being a father still exists may help the man cope with other fears about his masculinity, such as alopecia or erectile dysfunction (ED).

Suggest that the patient arrange for semen storage as soon as possible after diagnosis. Sperm collection should be completed before he begins radiation therapy or chemotherapy or undergoes a radical lymph node dissection. After radiation therapy or chemotherapy has been started, the patient is at increased risk for producing mutagenic sperm, which may not be viable or may result in fetal abnormalities.

The recommended number of samples to increase the chances of later fertilization is three to six ejaculates, collected 2 to 4 days apart. The process of sperm collection can delay treatment for as long as 1 month, especially if the patient is still recovering from multiple procedures or tests.

The patient's diagnosis and his physical condition may not allow treatment to be postponed, thus making sperm storage impossible. Also, some men may have personal or religious beliefs that do not allow sperm storage. For those who are not candidates for sperm storage in a sperm bank and for those who choose not to bank, discuss other reproductive options such as donor insemination, adoption, or not fathering children.

Surgical Management

The surgeon performs a radical unilateral **orchiectomy** to remove the testicle. Every effort is made to remove the cancerous testis as an intact organ to prevent releasing cancer cells into the surgical site. Depending on the type and stage of the cancer, radical retroperitoneal (abdominal) lymph node dissection may also be done to examine them for cancer cells.

Preoperative Care. Like most patients with cancer, the man with testicular cancer is very apprehensive. Offer support, and reinforce the teaching provided by the surgeon. Teach the patient and his family or partner about what to expect after surgery. Depending on the extent of the lymph node dissection and the need for surgical exploration, the surgeon might make not only a midline incision but also a transthoracic incision or a combination of the two incisions (thoracoabdominal).

Inform the patient and family that traditional open radical retroperitoneal lymph node dissections are long operations, lasting up to 6 or more hours. Tell them that the patient may be cared for in a critical care unit after surgery for close observation.

Operative Procedures. Most patients with seminoma have only one surgery to remove the diseased testicle through the groin (inguinal) for a cure. A frozen section of the tumor is examined to confirm the type and stage of the cancer. A gel-filled silicone prosthesis may be surgically implanted into the scrotum at the time of the orchiectomy or later if the patient desires. Reassure the patient that this procedure does not impair fertility or sexual function. He cosmetically appears to have two testes (reconstructive surgery).

Some men have more advanced disease or tumor types that are more aggressive. These patients require several surgeries to remove both testicles and lymph nodes. Two options are available for the lymph node dissection: a traditional open approach and minimally invasive surgery (MIS) using a laparoscope. To perform the *open* approach, the surgeon removes the retroperitoneal nodes in the iliac and lumbar regions. Because the blood supply and the lymphatic vessels of the testes and kidneys are directly related, an extensive midline incision from the xiphoid process to the pubis is necessary. Removal of the sympathetic ganglia eliminates peristalsis in the vas deferens and contractions of the seminal vesicles. This disruption results in sterility because the man's ejaculate no longer contains sperm. However, having a normal erection and experiencing orgasm usually are not affected.

The MIS procedure involves using a laparoscope through several small "keyhole" incisions through which the nodes are dissected for examination. This technique shortens the time the patient is in the operating suite, minimizes bleeding, and causes less pain after surgery. The patient has fewer postoperative complications and a shorter hospital stay.

Postoperative Care. Because of the length of the *open* surgery, manipulation of the abdominal and retroperitoneal viscera, and the loss of a major part of the lymphatic fluid, nodes, and channels, observe and assess the patient for any of the complications of major abdominal surgery (e.g., paralytic ileus) (see Chapter 18). Intervene for these possible problems:

- Pain from surgical incisions (use ice, analgesics)
- Immobility related to prolonged maintenance of surgical positioning and pain after surgery
- Injuries related to any invasive catheters or tubes

The patient is usually hospitalized for 3 to 4 days after an open radical retroperitoneal lymph node dissection but 1 to 2 days for the MIS procedure. During this time, explain care after discharge.

Nonsurgical Management

Chemotherapy and radiation therapy are indicated for patients at high risk for metastatic disease or those with metastatic disease. Combination *chemotherapy* may be used as adjuvant therapy for nonseminomatous testicular tumors or as primary treatment when there is evidence of metastatic disease. Combination chemotherapy is effective in treating nonseminomatous testicular cancer, particularly if cisplatin (Platinol) is used. The first-line drug combination of choice is cisplatin and etoposide (VePesid, VP-16), with or without

Chart 75-8 PATIENT AND FAMILY EDUCATION GUIDE

Sperm Banking

- You may want to investigate sperm storage in a sperm bank as a way to preserve your sperm for future use.
- No one knows how long sperm can be stored successfully, but pregnancies have resulted from sperm stored for longer than 10 years.
- Check with the sperm bank to see how much it charges to process and store your sperm and to see whether you must pay when the service is provided.
- Investigate whether your health insurance company will reimburse you for sperm collection and storage.

bleomycin (Blenoxane). Treatment is very effective for most patients.

Patients with advanced disease have salvage therapy with ifosfamide (Ifex) and cisplatin *and either* vinblastine (Velban) or paclitaxel (Taxol). The specific combination of drugs and the frequency, cycling, and duration of treatment vary from patient to patient, depending on the extent of the disease and the protocol being followed. Chapter 24 discusses the general nursing care for the patient receiving chemotherapy.

Because most patients live for a long time after having chemotherapy, they are at risk for certain health problems that are associated with these drugs. The best example is the risk for cardiovascular problems associated with cisplatin. These problems include hypertension, hyperlipidemia, Raynaud's phenomenon, and coronary artery disease (Zoltick et al., 2005). Teach patients taking these drugs about the long-term effects for which they should be continually and carefully monitored by their cardiologist or internal medicine specialist.

After orchiectomy (removal of one or both testes), *external beam radiation therapy* is the treatment of choice for men with a pure seminoma. This type of testicular cancer is highly radiosensitive. Before radiation therapy, a staging lymphangiogram is used to determine the treatment fields. An advantage of using radiation therapy instead of radical lymph node dissection is that reproductive function is preserved because surgical dissection of the nerves is avoided.

For the patient undergoing radiation therapy to the retroperitoneal lymph nodes, the remaining testis is shielded with a lead cup to preserve reproductive function. Even with these precautions, he may have a temporary decreased sperm count as a result of radiation scatter. Normally the sperm count returns to the pretreatment level within 24 to 30 months after the radiation treatment is completed. If metastases develop outside the lymphatic system, the man may still be cured with radiation therapy if the area of involvement is limited. If lymphatic involvement is extensive or if the visceral organs are involved, combination chemotherapy is used.

Studies are being conducted to explore whether high-dose chemotherapy with stem cell transplantation may be valuable in treating men with advanced germ cell cancer. In this procedure, the patient's blood-forming stem cells are removed from the blood and preserved by freezing while he receives high-dose chemotherapy. Once the chemotherapy is completed, the stem cells are returned to the patient. This procedure helps prevent the infection and anemia that occur with chemotherapy.

Community-Based Care

After an orchiectomy, the patient is typically hospitalized for 1 to 2 days for rest. This period may need to be extended if he must undergo additional surgery or chemotherapy. Because it may not be known until after the orchiectomy what type of testicular cancer he has or whether he needs additional surgery or treatment, specific discharge planning may need to be delayed until after surgery.

After an *orchiectomy,* unless the patient has a wound complication, he is discharged without a dressing on the inguinal incision. A scrotal support (jock strap) may be needed for several days. He may want to wear a dry dressing to prevent clothing from rubbing on the sutures and causing irritation. Tell him that the sutures will be removed in the physician's office 7 to 10 days after surgery. Patients who also had an *open retroperitoneal lymph node dissection* recover more slowly. They should not lift anything over 15 pounds, should avoid stair climbing, and should not drive a car for several weeks. Be sure that bathroom facilities are on the first floor of the house where he can easily access them.

For the patient who has undergone testicular surgery, emphasize the importance of scheduling a follow-up visit with the surgeon to examine the incision for healing and complications. Instruct him to notify the surgeon if chills, fever, increasing tenderness or pain around the incision, drainage, or dehiscence of the incision occurs. These manifestations may indicate infection for which antibiotics are needed. Instruct the patient who had an orchiectomy that he will be able to resume most of his usual activities within 1 week after discharge, except for lifting heavy objects (objects weighing more than 15 pounds [6.8 kg]) or stair climbing. Remind him to ask his surgeon when strenuous activities may be resumed.

Inform the patient that he may make arrangements to have a silicone prosthesis inserted into the scrotum if one was not inserted during the orchiectomy. Explain the importance of performing monthly testicular self-examination (TSE) on the remaining testis and scheduling follow-up examinations with the physician. The patient who has had testicular cancer should schedule tests for urinary and serum levels of tumor markers and CT or MRI studies as part of his routine follow-up for at least 3 years.

Depending on the pathologic findings and the stage of the cancer, the patient may need further treatment. This information may not be known at the time of discharge. If it is known that the patient needs further surgery, he and his family need information about the future surgery. If it is known that he must undergo radiation therapy or chemotherapy, he needs education about these treatments as soon as possible.

The man who has testicular cancer needs emotional support. If permanent sterility occurs and sperm storage has not been feasible, he may desire counseling about other reproductive options. Refer the patient to agencies or support groups, such as the American Fertility Society (www.theafa.org) or RESOLVE: The National Infertility Association (www.resolve.org) (organizations for infertile couples).

OTHER PROBLEMS AFFECTING THE TESTES AND ADJACENT STRUCTURES

Problems that develop inside the scrotum usually occur as a mass or as scrotal edema. Some problems produce pain, but others do not. Fig. 75-6 shows some of the most common conditions found in men, including hydrocele, spermatocele, varicocele, and scrotal torsion.

HYDROCELE

A hydrocele is a cystic mass, usually filled with straw-colored fluid that forms around the testis (see Fig. 75-6). It results from impaired lymphatic drainage of the scrotum causing a swelling of the tissue surrounding the testes. Unless the swelling becomes large and uncomfortable or begins to impair blood flow to the testis, no treatment is necessary. Hydroceles are usually painless. It is important that the cause of the hydrocele is investigated to rule out a serious condition. The cause may be determined by examination and ultrasound. A small hydrocele may go untreated with no further problems. However, a hydrocele may become very large, which makes clothing uncomfortable and may be cosmetically unacceptable.

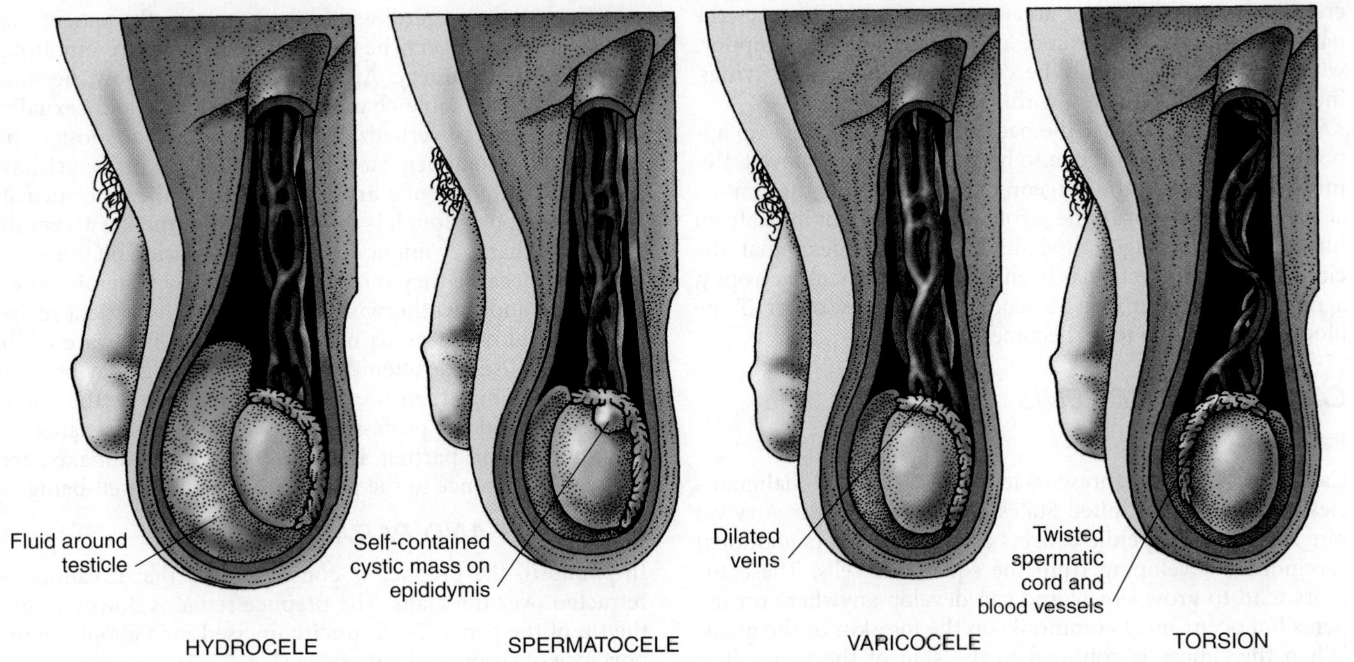
Fluid around testicle
HYDROCELE
Self-contained cystic mass on epididymis
SPERMATOCELE
Dilated veins
VARICOCELE
Twisted spermatic cord and blood vessels
TORSION

Fig. 75-6 • Common problems affecting the testes and adjacent structures.

A hydrocele may be drained via a needle and syringe, or it may be removed surgically in an ambulatory care setting. The patient may or may not have a drain at the incision site. Teach the man that if an incision drain is present, some serosanguineous drainage may be present for the first 24 to 48 hours after surgery. Explain the importance of wearing a scrotal support (jock strap). This device keeps the dressing in place and the scrotum elevated, which helps prevent edema.

The degree of pain experienced after this surgery varies. Assess and observe the patient for pain every 2 to 3 hours immediately after surgery. Moderate incision pain is expected for the first 24 hours after surgery and should markedly decrease within 1 or 2 days. If the pain does not resolve within this time, assess for wound complications, such as infection or bleeding.

Instruct the man to schedule a follow-up visit with the surgeon to have the wound evaluated for healing. Stress the importance of continuing to wear a scrotal support to promote drainage and comfort. The scrotum can remain swollen from residual inflammation and edema for as long as several weeks. Remind the patient to stay off his feet for several days and to limit physical activity for a week. Reassure him that this swelling is normal and eventually subsides.

SPERMATOCELE

A spermatocele is a sperm-containing cyst that develops on the epididymis alongside the testicle (see Fig. 75-6). Trauma, infection, congenital abnormalities, or often for no identifiable reason results in the widening of a portion of the epididymis, creating a small cavity where sperm collects.

Normally, spermatoceles are small and asymptomatic and no interventions are needed. If they become large enough to cause discomfort, a spermatocelectomy is performed. In this simple procedure, the spermatocele is removed through a small scrotal incision. Routinely, no incision drain is used because drainage and swelling are minimal. A few patients have recurrence.

VARICOCELE

A varicocele is a cluster of dilated veins behind and above the testis (see Fig. 75-6). Varicosity of the testicles may result from the increased fluid secondary to damaged or incompetent valves in the testicular veins. The diagnosis is made by scrotal palpation, particularly when the patient performs a Valsalva maneuver, creating additional pressure in the varicose veins. The scrotum feels "wormlike" when palpated. If the varicocele is very small and cannot be palpated, thermography, which detects pockets of heat, or a Doppler, which magnifies the sound of the blood flowing through the veins, is used.

Varicoceles can be either unilateral or bilateral, but most are unilateral. They occur most often on the left side of the scrotum. In many cases, they are asymptomatic and no treatment is required. In a few men, varicoceles are painful and must be removed surgically.

Varicoceles can also cause infertility. It is thought that they increase scrotal temperature from the venous stasis near the testis, altering spermatogenesis. Surgical correction may resolve the infertility. As an alternative, an interventional radiology procedure may be done to embolize the vein that drains the varicocele.

A **varicocelectomy** (surgical removal of the varicocele) is usually performed through an inguinal incision, in which the spermatic veins are ligated in the cord. It can also be performed through an incision near the superior iliac spine, in which the spermatic veins are ligated in the retroperitoneal space. A varicocelectomy may be done on an ambulatory care basis.

Before surgery, explain to the patient that persistent venous congestion of the scrotum is common after this type of surgery because of the changed circulation in the area. To promote drainage of the scrotum, place a rolled towel under the scrotum while he is in bed. Ice may be applied to the scrotum if needed. Any intervention that facilitates drainage and decreases swelling from the area promotes relief. Instruct the patient about the importance of wearing a scrotal support while ambulating. Usually he can resume normal activities, including sexual activities, within a week.

At discharge, instruct the patient to make a follow-up appointment with the surgeon to have the sutures removed. Remind him to notify the surgeon of any increasing discomfort at the incision site or in the scrotum, which might indicate an infection. Increasing scrotal discomfort can mean that the circulation to the testis has been impaired. Testicular atrophy, a rare complication of a varicocelectomy, may occur if the blood supply to the testis becomes insufficient.

CANCER OF THE PENIS

Pathophysiology

Cancer of the penis represents fewer than 1% of all malignancies in men in the United States. The overall 5-year survival rate is 50%. Most penile cancers are epidermoid (squamous) carcinomas developing from the squamous cells. These tumors tend to grow slowly and can develop anywhere on the penis but occur most commonly on the foreskin or the glans. When the cancer is confined to the skin of the penis, it is called *carcinoma in situ (CIS)*. Other types of penile cancers include melanomas, basal cell cancers, and sarcomas.

Circumcision (the surgical removal of the prepuce from the penis) in infancy almost eliminates the possibility of penile cancer in that chronic irritation and inflammation of the glans penis predispose uncircumcised men to penile cancer. Because of the ongoing controversy about neonatal circumcision, teach men and new mothers of boys that strict personal hygiene is an important preventive measure against penile cancer.

Patient-Centered Collaborative Care

Penile cancer usually occurs as a painless, wartlike growth or ulcer on the glans under the **prepuce** (foreskin) and may be mistaken for a venereal wart. It may also appear as a reddened lesion with plaque.

Small lesions involving only the skin may be controlled by excisional biopsy. When the lesion is not curable by excisional biopsy or radiation therapy, a **penectomy** (partial or total removal of the penis) may be required. When the lesion is limited to the glans, a partial penectomy is performed. The distal portion of the corpus cavernosum and the corpus spongiosum is amputated. The urethra is connected to the skin, and a dressing is applied. A retention catheter is in place for 3 to 5 days after surgery until the edema surrounding the urethra subsides. Assess the dressing for drainage, which should be minimal. Check the urinary catheter for patency every 4 hours for the first 24 hours.

A total penectomy is required when the lesion has penetrated the shaft of the penis or when the tumor has recurred after a partial penectomy or radiation therapy. An incision is made from the pubic bone, which encircles the penis and extends into the perineum. The bases of both corpora cavernosa are exposed and excised, and the penis is amputated. An incision drain is placed in the wound before it is sutured. Patients who undergo a total penectomy also have a perineal urethrotomy (connecting the urethra to the skin in the perineum) for urinary drainage.

After a total penectomy, observe the incision dressing every 2 to 4 hours during the first 24 hours. A moderate amount of serosanguineous drainage from the incision drains is expected.

Be aware that regardless of how accepting the patient may appear before surgery, he may experience severe emotional problems after surgery. After a partial penectomy, he must adjust to considerable changes in body image and sexuality. Encourage him to verbalize his feelings about the loss of his penis. After a total penectomy, the patient can no longer have penile-vaginal or penile-anal intercourse and cannot urinate in a standing position. It is difficult for most men to accept the possibility that they might die because of a lesion on the penis, especially because they rarely experience any systemic cancer symptoms and are otherwise healthy. Help the patient realize that removal of his penis may save his life. Be aware of the possibility of suicide attempts because his penis may be more important to him than his life. The nurse may be the one to detect the need for professional psychological assistance for the patient or his partner. Early interventions can make a tremendous difference in the patient's or partner's well-being.

PHIMOSIS AND PARAPHIMOSIS

In *phimosis,* the prepuce is constricted so that it cannot be retracted over the glans. The prepuce remains down, around the tip of the penis. Teach uncircumcised men about the importance of cleaning the prepuce (Fig. 75-7).

In *paraphimosis,* the prepuce has not been returned to its normal position after being retracted and forms a constricting band around the glans. This constricts lymph drainage, causing the penis to swell. Blood flow becomes impeded, and tissue death can occur. *This problem is an emergency requiring immediate treatment. Uncircumcised males are at risk.* Causes include infection, not returning the foreskin to the original position, poor hygiene, vigorous sexual intercourse, and penile piercing. *When caring for a man who is not circumcised, be sure to replace the foreskin over the penis after bathing or catheterizing him to prevent this paraphimosis!*

Phimosis is corrected by **circumcision** (surgical removal of the prepuce or foreskin). This procedure also may be performed for other medical reasons or for aesthetic reasons. Circumcision in the adult male is usually performed in a same-day surgical setting. If the patient has a dressing, instruct him to soak in a warm bath that evening to allow the dressing to loosen. If the dressing falls off before the next day, caution him to not replace it. Explain that the sutures will be absorbed and need not be removed. No residual or side effects result from this surgery, and the patient should be able to re-

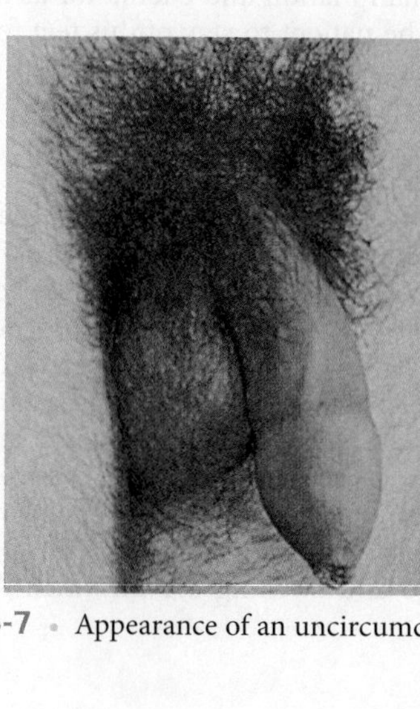

Fig. 75-7 • Appearance of an uncircumcised penis.

sume normal activities within 1 week. Sexual intercourse may be resumed after 1 to 2 weeks when pain has subsided. Advise the man to notify his physician if he has any wound complications, such as swelling at the incision area or drainage, and to schedule a postoperative office visit.

PRIAPISM

Priapism is an uncontrolled, long-maintained erection without sexual desire, which causes the penis to become large, hard, and painful. It affects the two corpora cavernosa. The corpus spongiosum and glans penis are not affected.

Priapism can occur from neural, vascular, or pharmacologic causes, including:

- Thrombosis of the veins of the corpora cavernosa (usually resulting from trauma)
- Leukemia
- Sickle cell disease
- Diabetes mellitus
- Malignancies

Sickle cell disease causes priapism through the collection of erythrocytes within the corporal bodies. Leukemia may cause priapism because the increased number of white blood cells (WBCs) permits persistent engorgement of the corporal bodies. Cancer may also infiltrate the corporal bodies causing persistent engorgement. Priapism can also result from an abnormal neurogenic reflex, psychotropic drugs, antidepressants, antihypertensive drugs, and drugs used to treat erectile dysfunction. Other risk factors include recreational drugs (cocaine, ecstasy, marijuana), overdose of injectable drugs for erectile dysfunction, and prolonged sexual activity.

Priapism is a urologic emergency because the circulation to the penis may be compromised and the patient may not be able to void with an erect penis. The desired outcome for intervention is to improve the venous drainage of the corpora cavernosa. Conservative measures involve prostatic massage, sedation, ice packs, and bedrest. Meperidine (Demerol) is usually given immediately because of its hypotensive effect. Urinary catheterization is required if the man cannot void.

If conservative therapy is unsuccessful, treatment may proceed to aspiration of the corpora cavernosa with a large-bore needle or surgical intervention. The priapism should be resolved within the first 24 to 30 hours to prevent penile ischemia, gangrene, fibrosis, and erectile dysfunction. If a cause is identified, treatment is directed toward that underlying cause.

When caring for the patient with priapism, be sensitive to his emotional needs. He may be uncomfortable and in crisis but at the same time embarrassed by his erection and loss of control. Reassure the patient that it is understood that he is not in control of his erection, and provide him with privacy.

PROSTATITIS

Pathophysiology

Prostatitis is an inflammation of the prostate gland. The four types of prostatitis are acute bacterial (ABP), chronic bacterial (CBP), nonbacterial (NBP)/chronic pelvic pain syndrome (CPPS), and asymptomatic inflammatory prostatitis. Duration of symptoms, presence or absence of WBCs in the urine, and urinary culture results determine the classification.

Bacterial prostatitis often occurs with urethritis or an infection of the lower urinary tract. Organisms may reach the prostate via the bloodstream or the urethra. The most common organisms are *Escherichia coli, Enterobacter, Proteus,* and group D streptococci. Acute bacterial prostatitis may be manifested by fever, chills, **dysuria** (painful urination), urethral discharge, and a boggy, tender prostate. Gentle palpation of the prostate usually results in a urethral discharge, which has WBCs in the prostatic secretions.

Chronic bacterial prostatitis generally occurs in older men and has a less dramatic presentation than acute bacterial prostatitis and without the systemic manifestations. The patient reports experiencing hesitancy, urgency, dysuria, difficulty initiating and terminating the flow of urine, and decreased strength and volume of urine. Also, there may be discomfort in the perineum, scrotum, and penis.

Prostatitis can occur after a viral illness or may be associated with sexually transmitted diseases (STDs), especially in young males. Other causes may be autoimmune disorders, neuromuscular etiologies, allergy-mediated reactions, and psychosexual problems. In many instances, an exact cause of the perineal discomfort cannot be found. The patient reports mild urgency and dysuria. Rectal, perineal, and ejaculatory pain may be present. Decreased libido (sexual desire) may also be present.

Prostatodynia (pelvic floor pain) is a related condition in which manifestations of prostatitis are present but there is no inflammation of the prostate and the urine culture is negative. Also, the patient has low back pain with unilateral testicular pain, narrowed urinary stream with diminished force, and post-void dribbling.

Patient-Centered Collaborative Care

The patient with chronic prostatitis usually reports backache, perineal pain, mild dysuria, and urinary frequency. Hematuria may be present. The prostate may feel irregularly enlarged, firm, and slightly tender when palpated. The patient often has an elevated serum WBC count and prostate-specific antigen (PSA) level.

Complications of prostatitis are **epididymitis** (inflammation of the epididymis) and **cystitis** (inflammation of the bladder). A rare complication is a prostatic abscess. The patient with either acute or chronic bacterial prostatitis is likely to develop urinary tract infections. Sexual functioning may be reduced because of discomfort.

Early diagnosis and treatment of prostatitis with antimicrobials are important. Treatment may last from weeks to many months because there is poor penetration of antibiotics into prostatic tissue. Acute bacterial prostatitis may require hospitalization with aggressive IV antibiotics.

Emphasize the importance of comfort measures, such as sitz baths, muscle relaxants, and NSAIDs. Stool softeners are prescribed to prevent straining and rectal irritation of the prostate during a bowel movement. Alpha blockers such as tamsulosin (Flomax) may be given to promote voiding. Teach patients to avoid alcohol, coffee, tea, and spicy foods that irritate symptoms. Instruct them to avoid over-the-counter cold preparations containing decongestants or antihistamines that may cause urinary retention.

Teach the patient with chronic prostatitis about the long-term nature of the problem. Because prostatitis can cause other urinary tract infections, explain the importance of long-term antibiotic therapy and increasing fluid intake. Remind him to take the prescribed antibiotics on schedule. Because trimethoprim (Bactrim, Septra) diffuses into the prostatic fluid, it is often the antibiotic of choice. Teach the patient about activities that drain the prostate (sexual intercourse, masturbation), which may help in the management of chronic prostatitis. Inform him that prostatitis is not infectious or contagious.

EPIDIDYMITIS

Pathophysiology

Epididymitis is an inflammation of the epididymis and may be a result of an infection or noninfectious source such as trauma. Bacterial infection is the most common cause. The infection may spread from other structures such as the prostate, bladder, or urethra. It can be a complication of an STD, such as gonorrhea or chlamydia. Although not common, epididymitis can also be a complication of long-term use of an indwelling urinary catheter, prostatic surgery, or a cystoscopic examination.

Organisms such as *Staphylococcus* and *E. coli* commonly cause epididymitis. In men younger than 35 years, the major causative organism is *Chlamydia trachomatis,* which is transmitted sexually (see Chapter 76). The infective organism passes upward through the urethra and the ejaculatory duct and then along the vas deferens to the epididymis.

The man with epididymitis usually reports pain along the inguinal canal and along the vas deferens, followed by pain and swelling in the scrotum and the groin. If untreated, the epididymis becomes swollen and painful and fever may be present. Pyuria and bacteriuria may develop with resultant chills and fever. An abscess may form, requiring an **orchiectomy** (removal of one or both testes).

Patient-Centered Collaborative Care

Instruct the patient with epididymitis to remain in bed with his scrotum elevated to prevent traction on the spermatic cord, to facilitate venous drainage, and to relieve pain. The man should wear a scrotal support when ambulating. A smear or culture of the urine or prostate secretions may be obtained to identify the causative organism. Antibiotics appropriate to the specific organism can then be prescribed. These antibiotics are taken until all acute manifestations are gone. If the epididymitis is chlamydial or gonorrheal in origin, the patient's sexual partners are also treated with antibiotics. NSAIDs such as ibuprofen or naproxen (Naprosyn) may be used to decrease inflammation and promote comfort.

The patient may find other comfort measures effective, such as applying cold compresses or ice to the scrotum intermittently and taking sitz baths. Advise him to avoid lifting, straining, or sexual activity until the infection is under control (which may take as long as 4 weeks).

In men with epididymitis, a testicular tumor must always be suspected, especially if the condition does not resolve in a week or two. Ultrasound study is often done to rule out an abscess or tumor. Patients with recurrent or chronic painful conditions may require an **epididymectomy** (excision of the epididymis from the testicle).

ORCHITIS

Orchitis is an acute testicular inflammation resulting from trauma or infection. The infection may be caused by the direct spread of bacteria through the urethra or by an infection elsewhere in the body, such as pneumonia, tuberculosis, gonorrhea, syphilis, or mumps. Usually both the testes and the epididymis are involved (epididymo-orchitis). Risk factors for orchitis include recurrent urinary tract infections, recurrent STDs, congenital abnormalities of the urogenital tract, instrumentation, and chronic indwelling urethral urinary catheter.

Orchitis may be unilateral or bilateral. If it is bilateral, the patient is at increased risk for sterility because of the testicular atrophy and fibrosis that occur during healing.

The manifestations of orchitis are the same as those of epididymitis and include scrotal pain, edema, reports of heavy feelings in the involved testicle(s), dysuria, pain on ejaculation, blood in the semen, and discharge from the penis. In addition, the patient may experience nausea and vomiting and pain radiating to the inguinal canal.

The treatment of orchitis is the same as for epididymitis and includes:

- Bedrest with scrotal elevation
- Application of ice
- Administration of analgesics and antibiotics

Mumps orchitis, which occurs in about 20% of males who have mumps after puberty, is usually bilateral and develops 4 to 6 days after the parotitis. Any adult male who has not had mumps and is exposed to or gets the disease is usually given gamma globulin. Although gamma globulin does not prevent mumps, the clinical course of the disease is likely to be less severe, with fewer complications. However, the outcome is unpredictable and sterility still may result. Childhood vaccination against mumps is an important preventive measure.

HUMAN NEEDS NURSING CARE REVIEW

What might you NOTICE if the patient is experiencing impaired sexuality as a result of male reproductive problems?

- Lump or swelling in prostate or scrotum
- Report of pain in scrotum or during ejaculation
- Report of difficulty voiding (e.g., starting urine stream)
- Hematuria
- Report of dribbling of urine (incontinence)
- Report of inability to have a penile erection
- Report of decreased libido

What should you INTERPRET and how should you RESPOND to a patient experiencing impaired sexuality as a result of male reproductive problems?

Perform and interpret physical assessment, including:

- Conducting a complete pain assessment
- Inspecting and palpating bladder for distention
- Inspecting and palpating scrotum for swelling or masses
- Palpating lymph nodes for swelling, especially in the inguinal areas
- Sending urine sample for urinalysis and culture
- Checking most recent laboratory values for PSA and CBC

Respond by:
- Catheterizing patient if retaining urine
- Providing pain-relief measures, such as ice or medication as prescribed
- Elevating scrotum if swollen
- Arranging for consultation with sex or intimacy therapist, if patient desires

On what should you REFLECT?
- Evaluate patient for need for indwelling urinary catheter.
- Evaluate effectiveness of actions to control pain and swelling.
- Think about what additional resources the patient will need to cope with his problem.

GET READY FOR THE NCLEX EXAMINATION!

Key Points

Review these Key Points for each NCLEX Examination Client Needs Category.

Safe and Effective Care Environment
- Teach patients with prostate cancer about American Cancer Society's Man to Man program and the American Foundation for Urologic Disease's Us TOO program to help men and their partners cope with prostate cancer.
- Use the information listed in Chart 75-5 to teach patients urinary catheter care.
- Have patients report signs of infection when caring for a urinary catheter in the home.
- Teach patients about not lifting more than 15 lb (6.8 kg) after prostate surgery.

Health Promotion and Maintenance
- Teach men at risk for prostate cancer to follow the American Cancer Society's screening guidelines.
- Teach men how to perform testicular self-examination.
- Teach uncircumcised men the importance of keeping the penis clean to prevent penile cancer.

Psychosocial Integrity
- Because most patients with testicular cancer are young adults, assess their reaction to the possible loss of reproductive ability.
- Because of the high incidence of erectile dysfunction after radical prostatectomy, assess the patient's adjustment to these changes in body function.
- Assess the patient's anxiety before prostate surgery, and allow him to express feelings of fear or grief.

Physiological Integrity
- Perform a focused physical assessment for patients reporting lumps or swelling in their genital area; inspect and palpate bladder and scrotum.
- Observe for and report complications after radical prostatectomy.
- Observe for and report bloody urine with clots after TURP; increase continuous irrigation bladder solution or irrigate the bladder per agency or surgeon protocol.
- Maintain traction on the urinary catheter after a TURP.
- Teach patients about drug therapies (5-ARIs and alpha blocking agents) used to treat BPH, including side effects.
- Teach patients to avoid any drugs that can cause urinary retention, especially anticholinergics, antihistamines, and decongestants if BPH is present.
- Remind patients wanting to use complementary and alternative therapies to check with their health care providers before using them.
- Eating a well-balanced diet with plenty of fish and fruits and vegetables may help prevent prostate cancer; eating soy protein with isoflavones has also been shown to be cancer-protective.
- Reinforce the man's option for managing prostate cancer; some procedures and drugs cause erectile dysfunction and incontinence either temporarily or permanently.
- Options for erectile dysfunction (ED) include drug therapy, vacuum assist devices, penile injections, transurethral suppositories, or penile implants.
- Be aware that African-American middle-aged men are the most at risk for prostate cancer; Euro-American young men are the most at risk for testicular cancer.
- Teach patients to report symptoms of radiation cystitis or proctitis to their health care provider as soon as possible; these complications resolve in 4 to 6 weeks after the end of radiation therapy.
- Teach patients and their partners about hormonal therapy used to manage prostate cancer: LH-RH agonists and anti-androgen drugs.

Additional Study Resources

Go to your Companion CD or Evolve at http://evolve.elsevier.com/Iggy/ for *Self-Assessment Questions for the NCLEX Examination.*

Go to Evolve at http://evolve.elsevier.com/Iggy/ for *Prioritization and Delegation Questions for the NCLEX Examination.*

SELECTED BIBLIOGRAPHY

Asterisk indicates a classic or definitive work on this subject.

*Abel, L., Dafoe-Lambie, J., Butler, W.M., & Merrick, G.S. (2003). Treatment outcomes and quality-of-life issues for patients treated with prostate brachytherapy. *Clinical Journal of Oncology Nursing, 7*(1), 48-54.

*Bailey, D.E., Mishel, M.H., Belyea, M., Stewart, J.L., & Mohler, J. (2004). Uncertainty intervention for watchful waiting in prostate cancer. *Cancer Nursing, 27*(5), 339-346.

*Balmer, L., & Greco, K. (2004). Prostate cancer recurrence fear: The prostate-specific antigen bounce. *Clinical Journal of Oncology Nursing, 8*(4), 361-366.

Bent, S., Kane, C., Shinohara, K., Neuhaus, J., Hudes, E.S., Goldberg, H., et al. (2006). Saw palmetto for benign prostatic hyperplasia. *New England Journal of Medicine, 354*(6), 557-566.

Cannon, G.W., Mullins, C., Lucia, M.S., Hayward, S.W., Lin, V., Liu, B.C., et al. (2007). A preliminary study of JM-27: A serum marker that can specifically identify with symptomatic benign prostatic hyperplasia. *Journal of Urology, 177*(2), 610-614.

*Carlson, S. (2004). Prostate disease. *RN, 67*(9), 54-59.

Doyle-Lindrud, S. (2006). Implications of androgen deprivation therapy in patients with prostate cancer: A case study. *Clinical Journal of Oncology Nursing, 10*(5), 565-566.

Doyle-Lindrud, S. (2007). Prostate cancer: A chronic illness. *Clinical Journal of Oncology Nursing, 11*(6), 857-861.

Engstrom, C. (2005). Hot flash experience in men with prostate cancer: A concept analysis. *Oncology Nursing Forum, 32*(5), 1043-1048.

Gray, M., & Sims, T. (2006). Prostate cancer: Prevention and management of localized disease. *The Nurse Practitioner, 31*(9), 15-29.

Hamilton-Reeves, J.M., Rebello, S.A., Thomas, W., Kurzer, M.S., & Slaton, J.W. (2008). Effects of soy protein isolate consumption on prostate cancer biomarkers in men with HGPIN, ASAP, and low-grade prostate cancer. *Nutrition and Cancer, 60*(1), 7-13.

Hawes, S., Malcarne, V., Ko, C., Sadler, G., Banthuia, R., Sherman, S., et al. (2006). Identifying problems faced by spouses and partners of patients with prostate cancer. *Oncology Nursing Forum, 33*(4), 807-814.

Held-Warmkessel, J. (2008). Caring for a patient with metastatic prostate cancer. *Nursing2008, 38*(6), 52-56.

Hemminki, K., Sundquist, J., & Bermejo, J.L. (2008). Familial risks for cancer as the basis for evidence-based clinical referral and counseling. *The Oncologist, 13*(3), 239-247.

Holcomb, S.S. (2007). Prostate cancer screening: An individual decision. *The Nurse Practitioner, 32*(8), 6-8.

Kattan, M.W. (2006). Measuring hot flashes in men treated with hormone ablation therapy: An unmet need. *Urology Nursing, 26*(1), 13-18.

Katz, A. (2006). Erectile dysfunction and its discontents. *AJN, 106*(12), 70-72.

Kumar, N.B., Krischer, J.P., Allen, K., Riccardi, D., Besterman-Dahan, K., Salup, R., et al. (2007). Safety of purified *isoflavones* in men with clinically localized prostate cancer. *Nutrition and Cancer, 59*(2), 169-175.

Lajiness, M.J. (2007). Megestrol acetate for the treatment of hot flashes in men undergoing hormone ablation or orchiectomy. *Urology Nursing, 27*(6), 556-557.

Leman, E.S., Cannon, G.W., Trock, B.J., Sokoll, L.J., Chan, D.W., Mangold, R., et al. (2007). EPCA-2: A highly specific serum marker for prostate cancer. *Urology, 69*(4), 714-720.

Lewis, J., Rosen, R., & Goldstein, I. (2005). Patient education guide: Erectile dysfunction. *Nursing2005, 35*(2), 64.

Liebertz, C., & Fox, P. (2006). Ketoconazole as a secondary hormonal intervention in advanced prostate cancer. *Clinical Journal of Oncology, 10*(3), 361-366.

Ludwig, C.D. (2007). Understanding benign prostatic hyperplasia (BPH). *MEDSURG Nursing, 16*(50), 340-341.

*Maliski, S., Clerkin, B., & Litwin, M. (2004). Describing a nurse case manager intervention to empower low-income men with prostate cancer. *Oncology Nursing Forum, 31*(1), 57-64.

Matthews, P.A. (2007). Hormone ablation therapy: Lightening the load for today's prostate cancer patient. *Urology Nursing, 27*(Suppl.), 3-11.

McCance, K., & Huether, S. (2006). *Pathophysiology: The biologic basis for disease in adults and children* (5th ed.). St. Louis: Mosby.

National Comprehensive Cancer Network (NCCN). (2007). NCCN Clinical Practice Guidelines in Oncology. *Prostate cancer early detection.* Retrieved May 2, 2008, from www.nccn.org/professionals.

Pagana, K.D., & Pagana, T.J. (2006). *Mosby's manual of diagnostic and laboratory tests* (3rd ed.). St. Louis: Mosby.

*Palmer, M.H., Fogarty, L.A., Somerfield, M.R., & Powel, L.L. (2003). Incontinence after prostatectomy: Coping with incontinence after prostate cancer surgery. *Oncology Nursing Forum, 30*(2), 229-238.

Pesquera, M., Yoder, L., & Lynk, M. (2008). Improving cross-cultural awareness and skills to reduce health disparities in cancer. *MEDSURG Nursing, 17*(2), 114-121.

Rackley, J.D., Clark, P.E., & Hall, M.C. (2006). Complementary and alternative medicine for advanced prostate cancer. *Urology Clinics of North America, 33*(2), 237-246.

Raffoul, J.J., Sarker, F.H., & Hillman, G.G. (2007). Radiosensitization of prostate cancer by soy isoflavones. *Current Cancer Drug Targets, 7*(8), 759-765.

Slovin, S.F. (2008). Pitfalls or promise in prostate cancer immunotherapy: Which is winning? *Cancer Journal, 14*(1), 26-34.

*Stevenson, T., & McNeill, J. (2004). Surgical management of testicular cancer. *Clinical Journal of Oncology Nursing, 8*(4), 355-360.

Wallace, M., & Storms, S. (2007). The needs of men with prostate cancer: Results of a focus group study. *Applied Nursing Research, 20*(4), 181-187.

Weeks, B., & Ficorelli, C.T. (2006a). How new drugs help treat erectile dysfunction. *Nursing2006, 36*(1), 18-19.

Weeks, B., & Ficorelli, C.T. (2006b). Treating erectile dysfunction without first-line drugs. *Nursing2006, 36*(3), 26-27.

White, M., & Verhoef, M. (2006). Cancer as part of the journey: The role of spirituality in the decision to decline conventional prostate cancer treatment and to use complementary and alternative medicine. *Integrative Cancer Therapies, 5*(2), 117-122.

Zoltick, B.H., Jacobs, L.A., & Vaughn, D.J. (2005). Cardiovascular risk in testicular cancer survivors treated with chemotherapy: Incidence, significance, and practice implications. *Oncology Nursing Forum, 32*(5), 1005-1012.

Care of Patients with Sexually Transmitted Disease

76

CHAPTER

Shirley E. Van Zandt

LEARNING OUTCOMES

For clinical competence and success on the NCLEX Examination, study this chapter with these Learning Outcomes in mind:

Safe and Effective Care Environment

1. Maintain patient confidentiality and privacy related to sexually transmitted diseases (STDs).
2. Educate patients with STDs and their sexual partners on infection control measures.

Health Promotion and Maintenance

3. Describe the role of expedited partner treatment in reducing STD recurrence.
4. Teach young adults and other at-risk people about risk factors for STDs.
5. Counsel patients and their sexual partners on sexuality issues, such as safe sex practices.

Psychosocial Integrity

6. Assess patients' and their partners' responses to a diagnosis of STD.
7. Respect patients' personal values and beliefs regarding sexual practices.

Physiological Integrity

8. Compare the stages of syphilis.
9. Identify the role of drug therapy in managing patients with STDs.
10. Teach patients how to self-manage their STD, including antibiotic therapy.
11. Describe the assessment findings that are typical in patients with STDs.
12. Develop a collaborative plan of care for a patient with pelvic inflammatory disease (PID).
13. Identify three sexually transmitted vaginal infections.

Go to your Companion CD or Evolve at http://evolve.elsevier.com/Iggy/ for *Self-Assessment Questions for the NCLEX Examination* keyed to these Learning Outcomes.

Sexually transmitted diseases (STDs) are caused by infectious organisms that have been passed from one person to another through intimate contact, usually oral, or vaginal intercourse. Some organisms that cause these diseases are transmitted only through sexual contact. Other organisms are transmitted also by parenteral exposure to infected blood, fecal-oral transmission, intrauterine transmission to the fetus, and perinatal transmission from mother to neonate (Table 76-1). *Sexually transmitted infections (STIs)* is another term that has been used to describe the same group of health problems. This terminology was intended to focus on the management of these infections and to decrease the social stigma of labeling them as diseases. Though used in the literature, STI is the less common terminology. *STD continues to be the most acceptable term by the Centers for Disease Control and Prevention (CDC).*

In spite of improved diagnostic techniques, increased knowledge about organisms that can be sexually transmitted, and changes in sexual attitudes and practices, the number of cases of STDs continues to increase. *Sexual issues are often controversial, and nurses must respect the choices that patients make. Providing confidentiality is essential for patients to receive correct information, make informed decisions, and obtain appropriate care.*

The prevalence of STDs is a major health concern worldwide. Populations at greatest risk for acquiring STDs are pregnant women, adolescents, and men who have sex with men (MSM). External factors such as an increasing population, cultural factors (e.g., early first intercourse), political and economic policies, and international travel and migration affect the prevalence of STDs. It is also affected by changing human physiology patterns such as earlier menarche. Sexual behaviors and access to care play a major role in the risk for acquiring an STD.

TABLE 76-1 Sexually Transmitted Diseases

- Human immune deficiency virus infection
- Chancroid
- Syphilis
- Lymphogranuloma venereum
- Genital herpes simplex virus infection
- Genital warts
- Gonococcal infection
- Chlamydial infection
- Nongonococcal urethritis
- Mucopurulent cervicitis
- Epididymitis
- Pelvic inflammatory disease
- Sexually transmitted enteritis
- Sexually transmitted proctitis
- Trichomoniasis
- Candidal infection
- Bacterial vaginosis
- Viral hepatitis
- Cytomegalovirus infection
- Ectoparasitic infection:
  - Pediculosis pubis
  - Scabies

From Centers for Disease Control and Prevention (CDC). (2006a). 2006 sexually transmitted diseases treatment guidelines. *Morbidity and Mortality Weekly Report, 55* (No. RR-11), 1-94.

WOMEN'S HEALTH CONSIDERATIONS

Because of the very vascular mucous membranes of the vagina, women are more easily infected with STDs than are men and are at greater risk for health problems caused by STDs. Young women who are sexually active with men have an increased risk for contracting a STD for several reasons: (1) increased rates of sexual activity that may be unprotected, (2) a possible lack of previous exposure to infectious agents, and (3) exposure of cervical basal epithelium cells to infections. During adolescence, these cells at the transformation zone of the cervix are rapidly changing (metaplasia) and therefore more exposed to infection (Cox, 2006). Women who identify themselves as lesbians have a decreased risk for STDs, although many of these women also have or have had sex with men.

Some young women may also be at high risk because they:

- Lack knowledge about the risk for disease
- Believe that they are not vulnerable to disease
- Mistakenly believe that oral contraceptives; contraceptive patches, sponges, and foams; and intrauterine devices protect them from STDs, as well as from pregnancy
- Consume large amounts of alcohol, which promotes risky sexual behavior

Postmenopausal women also may be at risk for STDs because many perceive that pregnancy is no longer likely and thus do not use barrier protection. Mucosal tears from vaginal atrophy in postmenopausal women may also place them at risk.

Women have more asymptomatic infections that may delay diagnosis and treatment. This delay increases the likelihood of complications from STDs, including ascending infections that may cause reproductive organ damage and disseminated illness. Embarrassment, denial, or fear about STDs may further delay treatment, increasing the potential for serious complications.

STDs cause complications that can contribute to severe physical and emotional suffering, including infertility, ectopic pregnancy, cancer, and death. Some of the most common complications caused by sexually transmitted organisms are listed in Table 76-2.

Chlamydia, gonorrhea, syphilis, chancroid, human immune deficiency virus (HIV) infection and acquired immune deficiency syndrome (AIDS) are reportable to local health authorities in every state (Centers for Disease Control and Prevention [CDC], 2006b). Other STDs such as genital herpes (GH) may or may not be reported, depending on local legal requirements. Positive results can be reported by clinicians and laboratories. Reports are kept strictly confidential.

Nurses in a variety of community settings are responsible for identifying people at risk for STDs, caring for patients with diagnosed STDs, and preventing further cases through education and case finding. Nurses in secondary and tertiary care settings, such as acute care hospitals, have a responsibility to recognize patients who are at risk for or who have STDs, possibly while being treated for another unrelated health problem. Teach them about self-management and health promotion activities using language that they can understand.

The CDC has recently updated its guidelines for treatment of STDs. These best practice guidelines provide information, treatment standards, and counseling advice to help decrease the spread of these diseases (CDC, 2006a).

INFECTIONS ASSOCIATED WITH ULCERS

SYPHILIS

Pathophysiology

Syphilis is a complex sexually transmitted disease (STD) that can become systemic and cause serious complications, including death. The causative organism is *Treponema pallidum,* a spirochete with a slender, spiral shape that resembles a corkscrew. Nonpathogenic *Treponema* species are found in the mouth, intestinal tract, and genital areas of people and animals. Although the organism can be seen only with a darkfield microscope, several serologic tests may be used to screen for the presence of syphilis antigen or antibody. *T. pallidum* is damaged by dry air or any known disinfectant. The organisms die within hours at temperatures of 105.8° to 107.6° F (41° to 42° C) and are not airborne. *The infection is usually transmitted by sexual contact, but transmission can occur through close body contact and kissing.*

Because of strong U.S. public health efforts between 1990 and 1996, there was a 90% decrease in syphilis cases to an all-time low in 2000. Between 2000 and 2005, an increase occurred, primarily in MSM whose rate increased by 70% during this period (CDC, 2006b).

CULTURAL AWARENESS

In 2005, the incidence of primary and secondary syphilis among women increased, primarily in the black and Hispanic populations, for the first time in over 10 years (CDC, 2006b). African Americans have a 5.4 times greater rate of acquiring syphilis than whites. However, this rate is much lower than it was in previous years because the African-American population has declined. During the same period of time, the Hispanic population has increased. Compared with whites, the 2006 rate

TABLE 76-2 Complications Caused by Sexually Transmitted Organisms

Complication	Causative Organisms
Salpingitis, infertility, and ectopic pregnancy	*Neisseria gonorrhoeae* *Chlamydia trachomatis* *Mycoplasma hominis* *Ureaplasma urealyticum*
Reproductive loss (abortion/miscarriage)	*N. gonorrhoeae* *C. trachomatis* Herpes simplex virus *M. hominis* *U. urealyticum* *Treponema pallidum*
Puerperal infection	*N. gonorrhoeae* *C. trachomatis*
Perinatal infection	Hepatitis B virus Human immune deficiency virus Human papillomavirus *N. gonorrhoeae* *C. trachomatis* Herpes simplex virus *T. pallidum* Cytomegalovirus Group B streptococcus
Cancer of genital area	*C. trachomatis* Herpes simplex virus Human papillomavirus
Male urethritis	*M. hominis* Herpes simplex virus *N. gonorrhoeae* *C. trachomatis* *U. urealyticum*
Vulvovaginitis	Herpes simplex virus *Trichomonas vaginalis* Bacteria causing vaginosis *Candida albicans*
Cervicitis	*N. gonorrhoeae* *C. trachomatis* Herpes simplex virus
Proctitis	*N. gonorrhoeae* *C. trachomatis* Herpes simplex virus *Campylobacter jejuni* *Shigella* species *Entamoeba histolytica*
Hepatitis	*T. pallidum* Hepatitis A, hepatitis B, and hepatitis C viruses
Dermatitis	*Sarcoptes scabiei* *Phthirus pubis*
Genital ulceration or warts	*C. trachomatis* Herpes simplex virus Human papillomavirus *T. pallidum* *Haemophilus ducreyi* *Calymmatobacterium granulomatis*

for Hispanics was almost two times higher (CDC, 2006b). One of the *Healthy People 2010* objectives is to completely eliminate syphilis in the United States (U.S. Department of Health and Human Services [USDHHS], 2007) (Table 76-3).

TABLE 76-3 Meeting *Healthy People 2010* Objectives: Sexually Transmitted Diseases

Objective 25.3: Eliminate sustained domestic transmission of primary and secondary syphilis.

Objective 25.6: Reduce the proportion of females who have ever required treatment for pelvic inflammatory disease.

- Teach sexually active people of all ages to use protection during sexual intercourse.
- Teach people how and when to use condoms.
- Educate people and their partners about the medical complications of STDs and pelvic inflammatory disease (PID).
- Target nonwhite groups for education and screening because these groups have the highest incidence of STDs and PID.
- Target people who are substance abusers for education and screening because they have a high incidence of STDs and PID.
- Participate in health fairs and surveillance programs to screen at-risk groups.
- Develop culturally appropriate education materials.
- Ensure that education materials are written or presented at no greater than a fourth-grade literacy level.

Syphilis progresses through four stages: primary, secondary, latent, and tertiary. The appearance of an ulcer called a **chancre** is the first sign of *primary* syphilis. It develops at the site of entry (inoculation) of the organism from 10 to 90 days after exposure (3 weeks is average). Chancres may be found on any area of the skin or mucous membranes but occur most often on the genitalia, lips, nipples, and hands and in the mouth, anus, and rectum.

During this highly infectious stage, the chancre begins as a small papule. Within 3 to 7 days, it breaks down into its typical appearance: a painless, indurated, smooth, weeping lesion. Regional lymph nodes enlarge, feel firm, and are not painful. Without treatment, the chancre usually disappears within 6 weeks. However, the organism spreads throughout the body and the patient is still infectious.

Secondary syphilis develops 6 weeks to 6 months after the onset of primary syphilis. During this stage, syphilis is a systemic disease because the spirochetes circulate throughout the bloodstream. Common manifestations include:

- Malaise
- Low-grade fever
- Headache
- Muscular aches and pains
- Sore throat
- Generalized rash

These symptoms are often mistaken for those of influenza. The rash involves the palms and soles of the feet. Although it has no typical appearance, the rash tends to change from papules to squamous papules to pustules. Other skin lesions include psoriasis-like rashes (Fig. 76-1), wartlike lesions (condylomata lata), and mucous patches. *These lesions are highly contagious and should not be touched without gloves.* The rash subsides without treatment in 4 to 12 weeks.

After the second stage of syphilis, there is a period of latency. *Early latent* syphilis occurs during the first year after infection, and infectious lesions can recur. *Late latent* syphilis is a disease of more than 1 year's duration after infection. This stage is not infectious except to the fetus of a pregnant woman. Patients with latent syphilis may or may not have reactive serologic test (e.g., Venereal Disease Research Laboratory [VDRL]) findings.

Tertiary, or late, syphilis occurs after a highly variable period, from 4 to 20 years. This stage develops in untreated cases and can mimic almost any pathologic condition because any organ system can be affected. Manifestations of late syphilis include:

- Benign lesions (gummas) of the skin, mucous membranes, and bones
- Cardiovascular syphilis, usually in the form of aortic valvular disease and aortic aneurysms
- Neurosyphilis, causing central nervous system problems (e.g., meningitis, hearing loss, generalized paresis)

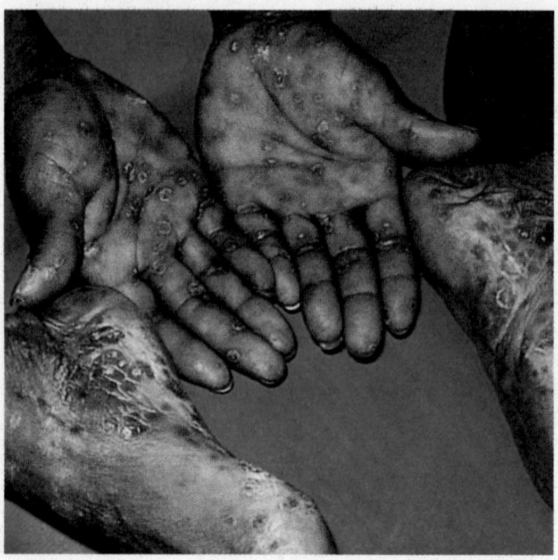

Fig. 76-1 • Palmar and plantar secondary syphilis.

Health Promotion and Maintenance

The most important aspect for prevention of most sexually transmitted diseases (STDs), including syphilis, is education. All people, regardless of age, gender, ethnicity, socioeconomic status, education, or sexual orientation, are susceptible to these diseases. STDs are largely preventable through education that includes safer sex practices. *Do not assume that a person is not sexually active because of his or her age, profession, or religion.* Discuss prevention methods frankly with all patients who are or may become sexually active. *Safer sex practices are those that reduce the risk for nonintact skin or mucous membranes coming in contact with infected body fluids and blood.* Such practices include:

- A latex or polyurethane condom for genital and anal intercourse
- A condom or latex barrier (dental dam) over the genitals or anus during oral-genital or oral-anal sexual contact
- Gloves for finger or hand contact with the vagina or rectum

Abstinence and decreasing the number of sexual partners also decrease the risk for acquiring an STD.

Patient-Centered Collaborative Care

Assessment

Assessment of the patient who has manifestations of syphilis begins with a history to gather information about any lesions or rash. The history should include a risk assessment and sexual history and whether previous testing or treatment for syphilis or other STDs has ever been done (Chart 76-1). Ask

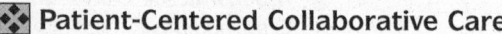

Chart 76-1 FOCUSED ASSESSMENT

The Patient with a Sexually Transmitted Disease

Assess history of present illness:
- Chief concern
- Symptoms by quality and quantity, precipitating and palliative factors
- Any treatments taken (self-prescribed or over-the-counter products)

Assess past medical history:
- Major health problems—including any history of STDs/PID
- Surgeries—obstetric and gynecologic, circumcision

Assess current health status:
- Menstrual history for irregularities
- Sexual history:
  - Type and frequency of sexual activity
  - Number of sexual contacts/partners
  - Sexual orientation
- Contraceptive history
- Medications
- Allergies
- Lifestyle risks—drugs, alcohol, tobacco

Assess preventive health care practices:
- Papanicolaou (Pap) tests
- Regular STD screening
- Use of barrier contraceptives to prevent STDs and pregnancy

Assess physical examination findings:
- Vital signs
- Oropharyngeal findings
- Abdominal findings
- Genital or pelvic findings
- Anorectal findings

Assess laboratory data:
- Urinalysis
- Hematology
- Cervical, urethral, oral, rectal specimens
- Lesion samples for microbiology and virology
- Pregnancy testing

PID, Pelvic inflammatory disease; *STDs*, sexually transmitted diseases.

about allergic reactions to drugs, especially penicillin. A woman may present with inguinal lymph node enlargement, the location that drains the area of the vagina and cervix. She may state a history of sexual contact with a male partner who had an ulcer that she noticed during the encounter. Men usually discover the chancre on the penis or scrotum.

Conduct a physical examination, including inspection and palpation, to identify manifestations of syphilis. *Wear gloves while palpating any lesions because of the highly contagious treponemes that are present.* Women frequently have the chancre on areas that are not easily visible to them, such as the vagina or cervix. Observe for and document rashes of any type because of the variable presentation of secondary syphilis.

After the physical examination, the health care provider obtains a *specimen of the chancre* for examination under a darkfield microscope. Diagnosis of primary or secondary syphilis is confirmed if *T. pallidum* is present. If the first slide is negative, the procedure should be repeated in 3 days, because many conditions can cause a false-negative result.

Blood tests are also used to diagnose syphilis. The usual screening and/or diagnostic nontreponemal tests are the *VDRL* serum test and the more sensitive *rapid plasma reagin (RPR).* These tests are based on an antibody-antigen reaction that determines both the presence and the amount of antibodies produced by the body in response to an infection by *T. pallidum.* They become reactive 2 to 6 weeks after infection. VDRL titers are also used to monitor treatment effectiveness. The antibodies are not specific to *T. pallidum,* and false-positive reactions often occur from such conditions as viral infections, hepatitis, and systemic lupus erythematosus (SLE) (Pagana & Pagana, 2006). HIV testing is also done (Kirkland, 2006).

If a VDRL result is positive, the health care provider requests or the laboratory may automatically perform a more specific test, such as the *fluorescent treponemal antibody absorption (FTA-ABS)* test or the *microhemagglutination assay for T. palladium (MHA-TP),* to confirm the infection. These treponemal tests are more sensitive for all stages of syphilis, although false-positive results may still occur. Patients who have a reactive test will have this positive result for their entire life, even after sufficient treatment. This poses a challenge when receiving a positive result for a patient who denies a history of or does not know he or she had syphilis.

Interventions

Drug Therapy

Benzathine penicillin G given IM as a single 2.4 million units dose is the evidence-based treatment for primary, secondary, and early latent syphilis. Patients in the late latent stage receive the same dose every 7 days for 3 weeks (Kirkland, 2006). Allergic reactions to the antibiotic can occur. Therefore monitor for allergic manifestations (e.g., rash, edema, shortness of breath, chest tightness, anxiety). The patient who has never had penicillin should have a skin test before receiving the injection. Penicillin desensitization is recommended for penicillin-allergic patients. *Keep all patients at the health care agency for at least 30 minutes after they have received the antibiotic so that manifestations of an allergic reaction can be detected and treated.* The most severe reaction is anaphylaxis. Treatment should be available and used immediately if symptoms occur. Chapter 19 describes the management of drug allergies in detail.

After treatment, the CDC recommends follow-up evaluation at 6, 12, and 24 months. Repeat treatment may be needed if the patient does not respond to the initial antibiotic.

The *Jarisch-Herxheimer reaction* may also follow antibiotic therapy for syphilis. This reaction is caused by the rapid release of products from the disruption of the cells of the organism. Symptoms include generalized aches, pain at the injection site, vasodilation, hypotension, and fever. They are usually benign and begin within 2 hours after therapy with a peak at 4 to 8 hours. This reaction may be treated symptomatically with analgesics and antipyretics.

Nursing Management and Health Teaching

Nursing interventions are based on data from the history and physical assessment. Common nursing diagnoses for patients with syphilis and other STDs are listed in Table 76-4.

Reinforce teaching about the cause of infection (sexual transmission); treatment, including side effects; possible complications of untreated or incompletely treated disease; and the need for follow-up care. *Discuss with the patient the importance of partner notification and treatment, including the risk for reinfection if the partner goes untreated. All sexual partners must be prophylactically treated as soon as possible, preferably within 90 days of the syphilis diagnosis.* Inform the patient that the disease will be reported to the local health authority and that all information will be held in strict confidence. Encourage the patient to provide accurate information for this follow-up to ensure that all at-risk partners are treated appropriately. Provide a setting that offers privacy and encourages open discussion. Urge the patient to adhere to the treatment regimen, which includes follow-up visits. Also urge sexual abstinence until the treatment of both the patient and partner(s) is completed.

The emotional responses to syphilis vary and may include feelings of fear, depression, guilt, and anxiety. Patients may experience guilt if they have infected others or anger if they have been infected by a partner. If further psychosocial interventions are needed, encourage the patient to discuss these

TABLE 76-4 Selected Nursing Diagnoses for Patients with Sexually Transmitted Diseases

- Risk for Injury related to the disease process
- Ineffective Coping related to high degree of threat, fear, guilt, or anger
- Noncompliance (treatment and/or partner follow-up) related to cost, significant other, access and convenience of care, cultural influences
- Sexual Dysfunction related to disease process, fear of transmission
- Impaired Skin Integrity related to the presence of genital ulcers, warts, or rash
- Ineffective Health Maintenance related to lack of resources and information about the mode of transmission, disease process, or need for treatment
- Impaired Social Interaction related to self-concept disturbance or social stigma
- Acute Pain related to the physical agent (infection process)
- Anxiety related to threat to health status (possible infertility) as a result of having an STD
- Chronic Low Self-Esteem/Situational Low Self-Esteem related to disturbed body image as a result of having an STD

feelings or refer him or her to other resources such as psychotherapy groups, self-help support groups, or STD clinics.

GENITAL HERPES

Pathophysiology

Genital herpes (GH) is an acute, recurring, incurable viral disease. It is the most common STD in the United States. Two serotypes of herpes simplex virus (HSV) affect the genitalia: type 1 (HSV-1) and type 2 (HSV-2). Most nongenital lesions such as cold sores are caused by HSV-1. Historically, HSV-2 caused most of the genital lesions. However, this distinction is academic because the transmission, symptoms, diagnosis, and treatment are nearly identical for the two types. Either type can produce oral or genital lesions through oral-genital contact with an infected person.

The incubation period is 2 to 20 days, with the average period being 1 week. Many people do not have symptoms during the primary infection. When symptoms do occur, they may be severe during the first infection and occasionally require hospitalization.

Recurrences are not caused by re-infection. Additional episodes are usually less severe and of shorter duration than the primary infection. Some patients have no symptoms at all during recurrence or viral reactivation. *However, there is viral shedding and the patient is infectious.* Long-term complications of GH include the risk for neonatal transmission and an increased risk for acquiring HIV infection.

Fifty million or more people in the United States may have GH (CDC, 2006a). HSV-2 has been thought to cause the majority of the primary episodes of GH, which recurs and sheds asymptomatically more often than HSV-1. Most people with GH have not been diagnosed because they have mild symptoms and shed virus intermittently (CDC, 2006a).

Patient-Centered Collaborative Care

Assessment

The diagnosis of GH is usually based on the patient's history and physical examination (see Chart 76-1). Ask the patient if itching or a tingling sensation was felt in the skin 1 to 2 days before the outbreak. These sensations are usually followed by the appearance of **vesicles** (blisters) in a typical cluster on the penis, scrotum, vulva, vagina, cervix, or perianal region. The blisters rupture spontaneously in a day or two and leave painful erosions that can become extensive. Assess for other symptoms such as headaches, fever, general malaise, and swelling of inguinal lymph nodes. Ask if urination is painful. Patients with urinary retention may need to be catheterized. Lesions resolve within 2 to 6 weeks.

After the lesions heal, the virus remains in a dormant state in the nerve ganglia (specifically, the sacral ganglia). Periodically, the virus may activate and symptoms recur. These recurrences may be triggered by many factors, including stress, fever, sunburn, poor nutrition, menses, and sexual activity. Ask the patient if he or she has had any of these factors recently.

GH is confirmed through a viral culture or serology testing to identify the HSV type. Viral cultures should be done of the lesions and obtained within 48 hours of the first outbreak of the blisters since accuracy decreases as they begin to heal. Fluid from inside the blister is obtained. Polymerase chain reaction (PCR) assays of cerebrospinal fluid (CSF) are done if there is concern of an HSV central nervous system infection.

Type-specific assays can detect antibodies to glycoprotein G for HSV-1 and HSV-2. For example, the POCkit HSV-2 Rapid Test is a point-of-care test with results in 6 minutes. An assay that provides qualitative information is the HerpeSelect 1 and 2 Immunoblot IgG test.

Interventions

The desired outcomes of treatment for HSV-infected patients are to decrease the discomfort from painful ulcerations, promote healing without secondary infection, decrease viral shedding, and prevent infection transmission (Chart 76-2).

Drug Therapy

Antiviral drugs are used to treat GH. *The drugs do not cure the infection but do decrease the severity, promote healing, and decrease the frequency of recurrent outbreaks while they are being used.*

Drug therapy should be offered to anyone with an initial outbreak of GH. Though the initial symptoms may be mild, they may become more severe. Topical therapy is not recommended (Kirkland, 2006). Acyclovir (Zovirax, Avirax♣), famciclovir (Famvir), or valacyclovir (Valtrex) may be prescribed. The main differences in these drugs are cost and frequency of use. Dosage and length of treatment differ for primary outbreaks (lasting 7 to 10 days) and recurrent outbreaks (lasting 5 days). Intermittent or continuous suppressive antiviral therapy is offered to patients to lessen or prevent outbreaks, even for those with infrequent recurrent episodes. Therapy for severe recurrent outbreaks is most beneficial if it is started within 1 day of the appearance of lesions or during the period of itching or tingling before lesions appear.

Patients who have recurrences, either infrequent or frequent (more than six in a year), may benefit from daily sup-

Chart 76-2 BEST PRACTICE FOR PATIENT SAFETY & QUALITY CARE

Care of or Self-Management for the Patient with Genital Herpes

- Administer oral analgesics as prescribed.
- Apply local anesthetic sprays or ointments as prescribed.
- Apply ice packs or warm compresses to the patient's lesions.
- Administer sitz baths three or four times a day.
- Encourage an increase in fluid intake.
- Encourage frequent urination.
- Pour water over the patient's genitalia while voiding, or encourage voiding while the patient is sitting in a tub of water or standing in a shower.
- Catheterize the patient as necessary.
- Encourage genital hygiene, and encourage keeping the skin clean and dry.
- Wash hands thoroughly after contact with lesions, and launder towels that have had direct contact with lesions.
- Wear gloves when applying ointments.
- Advise the patient to avoid sexual activity when lesions are present.
- Advise the patient to use latex or polyurethane condoms during all sexual exposures.
- Instruct the patient in the use, side effects, and risks versus benefits of antiviral agents.

pressive treatment. Suppression reduces recurrences in most patients with frequent outbreaks. However, suppression only reduces but does not prevent viral shedding even when symptoms are absent (CDC, 2006a). Patients receiving continuous therapy should periodically (possibly once a year) be reassessed for recurrences.

IV acyclovir and hospitalization may be indicated for patients with severe HSV infections, such as disseminated disease or encephalitis. These are severe complications of genital herpes.

Nursing Management and Health Teaching

Nursing management includes patient counseling and education about the infection, the potential for recurrent episodes, the correct use and possible side effects of antiviral therapy, and sexual transmission. Discussion about sexual activity is extremely important. *Remind patients to abstain from sexual activity while lesions are present. Urge condom use during all sexual exposures because of the increased risk for HSV transmission.* Viral shedding can occur even when lesions are not present. Teach the patient about how and when to use condoms (Chart 76-3).

Assess the patient's and partner's emotional responses to the diagnosis of genital herpes. Many are initially shocked and need reassurance that they can manage the disease. Infected patients have reported feelings of disbelief, uncleanness, isolation, and loneliness. They have also reported anger at their partners for transmitting the infection or fear of rejection by partners because they have the infection. Help patients cope with the diagnosis by being sensitive and supportive during assessments and interventions. Encourage social support, and refer patients to support groups such as HELP (local support groups of the National Herpes Resource Center [www.healthywomen.org]). Symptomatic care may include oral analgesics, topical anesthetics, sitz baths, and increased oral fluid intake.

Emphasize the risk for neonatal infection to all patients, both male and female. Men and women who have genital herpes need to inform the pregnancy care provider of their history. Infected male partners will be advised to avoid intercourse during pregnancy if the pregnant partner is not infected. This avoids the risk for a new primary infection and outbreak during pregnancy. People who have tested serology positive to HSV-1 or HSV-2 but have never had GH symptoms should be counseled with the same information as those who have symptoms (CDC, 2006a).

INFECTIONS OF THE EPITHELIAL STRUCTURES

CONDYLOMATA ACUMINATA (GENITAL WARTS)

Pathophysiology

Condylomata acuminata (also known as *genital warts*) are caused by certain types of *human papillomavirus (HPV)*, 90% of which are types 6 and 11 or low-risk HPV (Cox, 2006). These types *rarely* result in invasive cancer of the genital tract such as cervical cancer. *However, HPV types 16, 18, 31, 33, and 35, considered high-risk HPV, can be found on the skin of the genitalia and increase the risk for genital cancers, especially cervical cancer.* Infection with several HPV types can occur at the same time. The presence of one strain increases the risk for acquiring a higher-risk strain. Genital warts are the most common viral disease that is sexually transmitted and are often seen with other infections.

HPV infection is thought to be the primary risk factor for development of cervical cancer (Snijders et al., 2006). Sites commonly affected by infection include the urinary meatus, labia, vagina, cervix, penis, scrotum, anus, and perineal area. The incubation period is usually 2 to 3 months.

Chart 76-3 PATIENT AND FAMILY EDUCATION GUIDE

Use of Condoms

- Use latex or polyurethane condoms rather than natural membrane condoms.
- Use a condom with every sexual encounter (including oral, vaginal, and anal).
- Female condoms (Reality)—polyurethane sheaths in the vagina—are effective in preventing transmission of viruses, including HIV.
- Condoms infrequently (2 per 100) break during sexual intercourse, unless used incorrectly.
- Keep condoms (especially latex) in a cool, dry place, out of direct sunlight.
- Do not use condoms that are in damaged packages or that are brittle or discolored.
- Always handle a condom with care to avoid damaging it with fingernails, teeth, or other sharp objects.
- Put condoms on before any genital contact. Hold the condom by the tip and unroll it on the penis. Leave a space at the tip to collect semen.
- If you use a lubricant with condoms, make sure that the lubricant is water based and washes away with water. Oil-based products may damage latex condoms.
- Use of spermicide (nonoxynol-9) with condoms, either lubricated condoms or vaginal application, has *not* been proven to be more or less effective against STDs than use without spermicide. *Spermicide-coated condoms have been associated with* Escherichia coli *urinary tract infections in women. Nonoxynol-9 may increase risk for transmission of HIV during vaginal intercourse and anal intercourse. Its use is discouraged for anal intercourse.*
- If a condom breaks, replace it immediately.
- After ejaculation, withdraw the erect penis carefully, holding the condom at the base of the penis to prevent the condom from slipping off.
- Never use a condom more than once.

Modified from Centers for Disease Control and Prevention (CDC). (2006a). 2006 sexually transmitted diseases treatment guidelines. *Morbidity and Mortality Weekly Report, 55*(RR-11), 4-5.
HIV, Human immune deficiency virus; *STDs,* sexually transmitted diseases.

Patient-Centered Collaborative Care

Assessment

The diagnosis of condylomata acuminata is made by examination of the lesions. They are initially small papillary growths that may grow into large cauliflower-like masses (Fig. 76-2). Multiple warts usually occur in the same area. Bleeding may occur if the wart is disturbed. Warts may heal on their own without treatment.

A Papanicolaou (Pap) test and HPV DNA probe are used to obtain cervical specimens to assess for dysplasia and isolate and diagnose HPV of the cervix. High-risk strains of HPV can be identified and correlated with an abnormal Pap smear finding. High-risk HPV may co-exist with low-risk HPV, the likely cause of the warts. To rule out the presence of other infections, a VDRL test, HIV test, and cultures for chlamydia and gonorrhea infections are done. If a wartlike lesion bleeds easily, appears infected, is atypical, or persists, a specimen for biopsy is obtained to rule out other pathologic problems.

Interventions

The desired outcomes of management are to remove the warts and treat the symptoms. No current therapy eliminates HPV. Therefore recurrences after treatment are likely. It is not known whether removal of visible warts decreases the risk for disease transmission (CDC, 2006a).

Drug Therapy

Patients may apply podofilox (Condylox) 0.5% solution or gel twice daily for 3 days with no treatment for the next 4 days. This regimen should be repeated for four cycles. Another option is imiquimod (Aldara) 5% cream applied topically at bedtime three times a week for up to 16 weeks.

Cryotherapy, podophyllin (Pododerm), and trichloroacetic acid (TCA) or bichloroacetic acid (BCA) are provider-applied treatments. **Cryotherapy** (freezing), usually with liquid nitrogen, can be used every 1 to 2 weeks until lesions are resolved. Podophyllin resin 10% to 25% in a compound of tincture of benzoin can be applied weekly but needs to be washed off 1 to 4 hours after application. TCA/BCA (80% to 90%) can be applied weekly. Extensive warts have been treated with the carbon dioxide laser, intra-lesion interferon injections, and surgical removal.

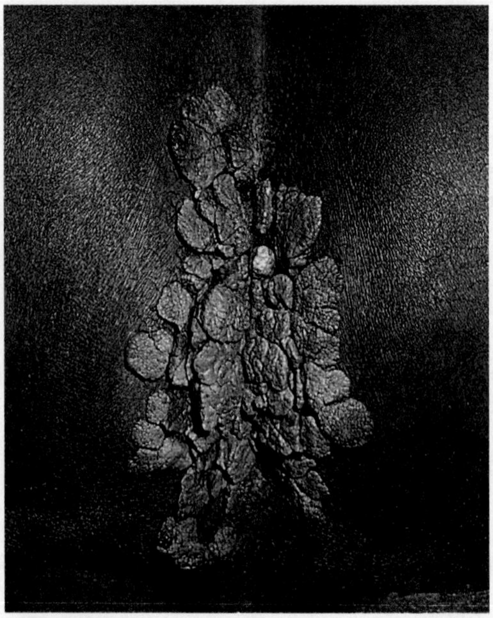

Fig. 76-2 • Perianal condylomata acuminata.

Nursing Management and Health Teaching

The priority for nursing management is patient and sexual partner education about the mode of transmission, incubation period, treatment, and complications, especially the association with cervical cancer. Reinforce instructions about local care of the lesions or patient-applied treatment for self-management. Teach patients that after treatment with cryotherapy, podophyllin, or TCA, they may experience discomfort, bleeding or discharge from the site, or sloughing of parts of warts. Instruct patients to keep the area clean (shower or bath) and dry. Teach them to be alert for any signs or symptoms of infection or side effects of the treatment.

Inform patients that recurrence is likely, especially in the first 3 months, and that repeated treatments may be needed. Urge all patients to have complete STD testing. Condylomata lata (secondary syphilis) can resemble condylomata acuminata. Sexual partners should also be evaluated and offered treatment if warts are present. Teach patients to avoid intimate sexual contact until external lesions are healed. Recommend condoms to help reduce transmission even after warts have been treated (see Chart 76-3). Encourage women to have an annual Pap test. The presence of warts requires HPV testing of the patient and partner.

In 2006, the U.S. Food and Drug Administration (FDA) approved an HPV vaccine that provides almost 100% immunity for HPV types 6 and 11 (low risk) and 16 and 18 (high risk). The vaccine is recommended to be given to all females, ages 9 to 26, as a method for reducing cervical cancer. Controversy has surrounded the vaccine because of legislative efforts in some states to require all girls to receive the drug and because of the long-term adverse effects of the currently used vaccine. Concern has been raised that requiring mandatory vaccination with such a new drug whose efficacy has been established only in clinical trials is premature (CDC, 2007e; Lajiness, 2007; McLemore, 2006).

GONORRHEA

Pathophysiology

Gonorrhea is a sexually transmitted bacterial infection that occurs in both men and women. The causative organism is *Neisseria gonorrhoeae,* a gram-negative intracellular diplococcus. It is transmitted by direct sexual contact with mucosal surfaces (vaginal intercourse, orogenital contact, or anogenital contact).

The first symptoms of gonorrhea may appear 3 to 10 days after sexual contact with an infected person. The disease can be present without symptoms and can be transmitted or progress without warning. In women, ascending spread of the organism can cause pelvic infection **(pelvic inflammatory disease [PID]), endometritis** (endometrial infection), **salpingitis** (fallopian tube infection), and pelvic peritonitis. Rare complications of gonorrhea in adults include arthritis, meningitis, hepatitis, and disseminated infection.

An estimated 600,000 new infections occur each year (CDC, 2006a). The incidence is highest in 15- to 24-year-olds. Fluoroquinolone-resistant *N. gonorrhoeae* has increased and now may represent at least 13% of STD cases. The incidence of gonorrhea may be up to six times greater in men having sex with men (MSM) (CDC, 2007a).

Patient-Centered Collaborative Care

Assessment

A complete history includes reviewing possible symptoms of gonorrhea and taking a sexual history that includes sexual orientation and sites of intercourse. Assess for allergies to antibiotics (see Chart 76-1). Use a nonjudgmental approach to gather more complete information. This approach may decrease the patient's anxiety and fear about having a sexually transmitted disease (STD).

The infection can be asymptomatic in both men and women, but women have asymptomatic, or "silent," infections more often than do men. If symptoms are present, men usually notice dysuria and a penile discharge that can be either profuse yellowish green fluid or scant clear fluid. The urethra is most commonly affected, but infection can extend to the prostate, the seminal vesicles, and the epididymis. Men seek curative treatment sooner, usually because they have symptoms, and thereby avoid some of the serious complications.

Women may report a change in vaginal discharge (yellow, green, profuse, odorous), urinary frequency, or dysuria. The cervix and urethra are the most common sites of infection.

Anal manifestations may include itching and irritation, rectal bleeding or diarrhea, and painful defecation. Assess the mouth for a reddened throat, ulcerated lips, tender gingivae, and blisters in the throat. Fig. 76-3 shows common sites of gonococcal infections.

Inspect for discharge from the urethra, cervix, and rectum. Palpation of the lower abdomen may reveal tenderness. Fever may be present, especially if an ascending or systemic infection has occurred. Gonorrheal infections that have become systemic may develop quickly. Manifestations of disseminated gonococcal infection (DGI) include fever, chills, skin lesions on distal extremities, and joint pain, with or without swelling, heat, or redness.

Clinical symptoms of gonorrhea can resemble those of chlamydia and therefore need to be differentiated. *Molecular testing for N. gonorrhoeae is currently the most widely used standard and preferred over cultures or other tests.* These nucleic acid amplification tests (NAATs) are highly sensitive and specific. Self-collected urine or vaginal swabs can be used to

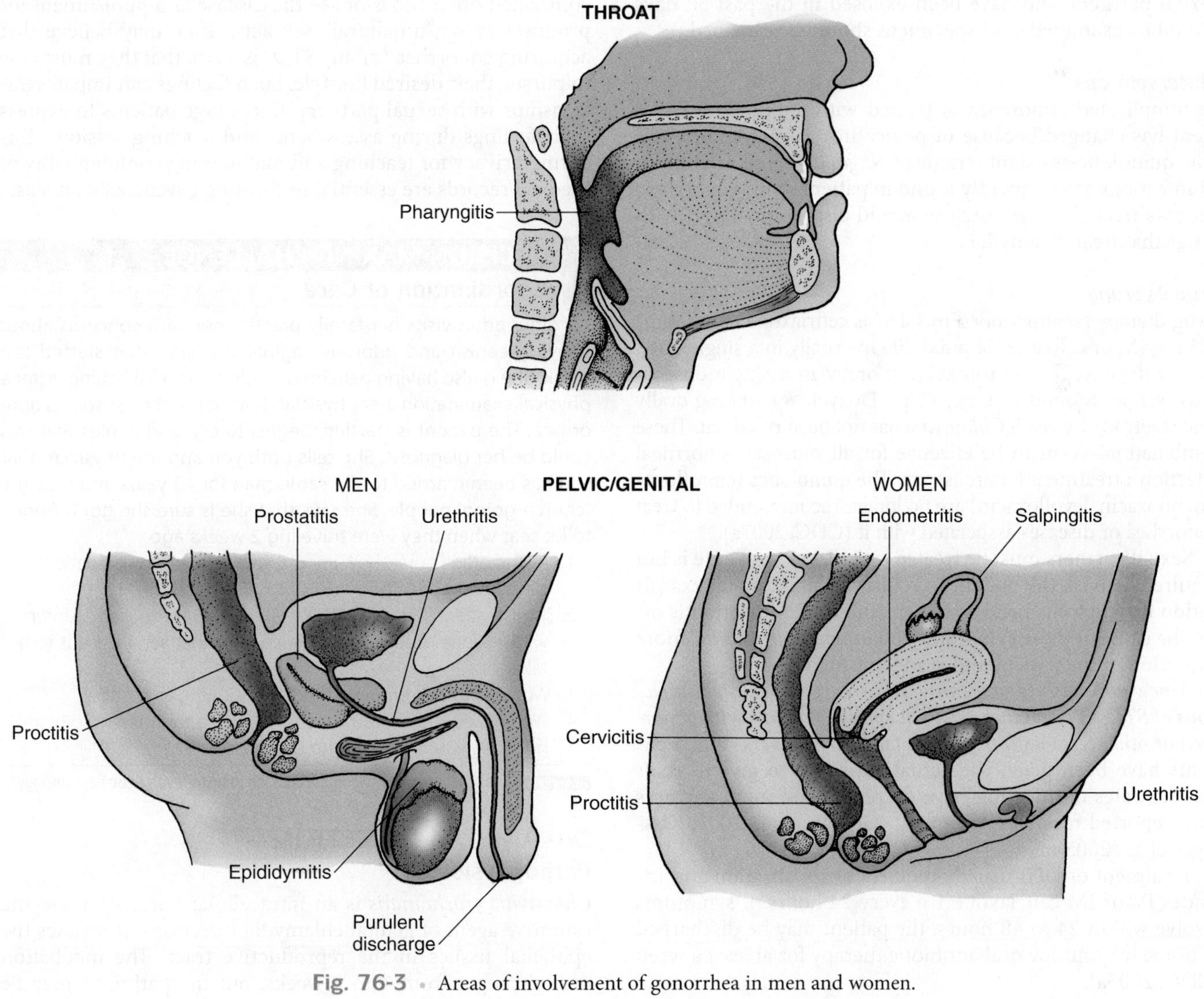
THROAT
Pharyngitis
MEN
PELVIC/GENITAL
WOMEN
Prostatitis
Urethritis
Endometritis
Salpingitis
Proctitis
Cervicitis
Proctitis
Urethritis
Epididymitis
Purulent
discharge

Fig. 76-3 • Areas of involvement of gonorrhea in men and women.

diagnose both gonorrhea and chlamydia infections, allowing for easy screening.

Diagnosis of gonorrhea in men can also be made with smears of the discharge that has been swabbed onto a glass slide, dried, and Gram stained. The presence of gram-negative diplococci is diagnostic for gonococcal urethritis. Gram stains of male urethral discharge if the patient has symptoms are very sensitive and specific for gonorrhea. If the patient has no symptoms, Gram stains are less reliable but allow for immediate diagnosis and early treatment.

Smears do not confirm the diagnosis in women because the female genital tract normally harbors organisms that resemble *N. gonorrhoeae.* Cultures provide a more definitive diagnosis and are the most reliable method of confirming a diagnosis for men and women.

A specimen is obtained from the male urethra or the female cervix and swabbed onto a culture medium. Depending on the patient's history, culture specimens may also be obtained from the throat and rectum. After 24 to 48 hours, the culture is examined for the presence of gram-negative diplococci.

All patients with gonorrhea should be tested for HPV, syphilis, chlamydia, hepatitis B and hepatitis C, and HIV infection because they may have been exposed to these STDs as well. Sexual partners who have been exposed in the past 30 days should be examined, and specimens should be obtained.

Interventions

Uncomplicated gonorrhea is treated with antibiotics. Treatment has changed because of penicillin-resistant strains and now quinolone-resistant strains of *N. gonorrhoeae.* Chlamydial infections are frequently found in patients with gonorrhea. Patients treated for gonorrhea should also be managed with drugs that treat chlamydia.

Drug Therapy

Drug therapy recommended by CDC is ceftriaxone (Rocephin) 125 mg IM or cefixime (Suprax) 400 mg orally in a single dose, *plus* azithromycin (Zithromax) 1 g orally in a single dose *or* doxycycline (Monodox, Doxy-Caps, Doxycin♣) 100 mg orally twice daily for 1 week if *Chlamydia* has not been ruled out. These combinations seem to be effective for all mucosal gonorrheal infections; treatment failure is rare. The quinolones (ciprofloxacin, ofloxacin, levofloxacin) are no longer recommended to treat gonorrhea or diseases associated with it (CDC, 2007a).

Sexual partners must be treated as well. A test of cure is not required. Advise the patient to return for a follow-up examination if symptoms persist after treatment. Re-infection is often the cause of these symptoms and indicates a need for more education of the patient and sexual partner.

A new approach to preventing recurrence or persistent infections of STDs is providing newly diagnosed patients with gonorrhea or other STD with treatment for their partners. When patients have been given the actual antibiotic to give to their partner, rates of infection have decreased and more partners have reported receiving treatment (Golden et al., 2005; Kissinger et al., 2005).

Treatment of DGI usually requires hospitalization and includes IV or IM ceftriaxone 1 g every 24 hours. If symptoms resolve within 24 to 48 hours, the patient may be discharged to home to continue oral antibiotic therapy for at least a week (CDC, 2006a).

Meningitis and endocarditis occur rarely. Hospitalization of patients with these problems is recommended for the initial treatment. Treatment includes IV antibiotic therapy, usually ceftriaxone 1 to 2 g every 12 hours. If meningitis or endocarditis is present, therapy is continued for 10 to 14 days for meningitis and at least 4 weeks for endocarditis. Infectious disease specialists are consulted for management of these infections.

Nursing Management and Health Teaching

Teach the patient about transmission and treatment of gonorrhea. Patients must understand why drugs should be taken for the prescribed time for maximum effectiveness. Discuss the possibility of re-infection, including the risk for pelvic inflammatory disease (PID), and resultant problems such as ectopic pregnancy, infertility, and chronic pelvic pain. Instruct patients to avoid sexual activity until the antibiotic therapy is completed and they no longer have symptoms. Urge men and women to use condoms, especially if abstinence is not possible. Explain that gonorrhea is a reportable disease. All sexual contacts need to be examined and treated for both gonorrhea and *Chlamydia* infection.

When a diagnosis of gonorrhea is made, patients may have feelings of fear or guilt. They may be concerned that they have contracted other STDs or see the disease as a punishment for promiscuity or "unnatural" sex acts. They may believe that acquiring gonorrhea (or any STD) is a risk that they must take to pursue their desired lifestyle. Such feelings can impair relationships with sexual partners. Encourage patients to express their feelings during assessments and teaching sessions. Ensuring privacy for teaching and maintaining confidentiality of medical records are essential in meeting psychosocial needs.

DECISION-MAKING CHALLENGE

Coordination of Care

An older adult visits her family practitioner with concerns about heavy greenish and odorous vaginal drainage that started last week. She is also having pain on urination and anal itching. After a physical examination, her physician tells her that he suspects gonorrhea. The patient is startled, begins to cry, and denies that this could be her diagnosis. She tells both you and the physician that she has been married to the same man for 43 years and they are "church-going" people. She says that she is sure she got it from a toilet seat when they were traveling 2 weeks ago.

1. As the office nurse, how should you respond to this patient based on her reaction?
2. If this patient states that she has not had a sexual encounter with anyone other than her husband, what action needs to be taken?
3. What types of support is this patient going to require?
4. What resources do you have for referring this patient to help her cope with this alarming diagnosis?

evolve For suggested answer guidelines, go to http://evolve.elsevier.com/Iggy/.

CHLAMYDIA INFECTION

Pathophysiology

Chlamydia trachomatis is an intracellular bacterium and the causative agent of genital chlamydia infections. It invades the epithelial tissues in the reproductive tract. The incubation period ranges from 1 to 3 weeks, but the pathogen may be present in the genital tract for months without producing symptoms.

C. trachomatis is now reportable to local health departments in all states. Cases continue to increase yearly, which reflects more sensitive screening tests and increased public health efforts to screen high-risk people. Each year there are an estimated 2.8 million new cases in the United States. African-American women between 16 and 24 years of age are at the highest risk for the disease (CDC, 2006b). The cause for this finding is not known.

The rate of chlamydia in men has increased faster than the rate of increase in women (CDC, 2006b). In women, 20% to 40% of those infected develop pelvic inflammatory disease (PID), discussed later on this page. Some women become infertile.

Patient-Centered Collaborative Care

Assessment

Obtain a complete history including medical, menstrual, and sexual information (see Chart 76-1). In particular, ask about:

- Presence of symptoms, including vaginal or urethral discharge, **dysuria** (painful urination), pelvic pain, irregular bleeding
- Any history of sexually transmitted diseases (STDs)
- Whether sexual partners have had symptoms or a history of STDs

Many women with chlamydial infections are asymptomatic. For men and women, their history may reveal only risk factors associated with *C. trachomatis,* such as new or multiple sexual partners, age younger than 26 years and female, or a male having sex with a male (MSM). As with all interviews concerning sexual behavior, use a nonjudgmental approach and provide privacy and confidentiality.

For men, ask about dysuria, frequent urination, and a mucoid discharge that is more watery and less copious than a gonorrheal discharge. *These manifestations indicate urethritis, the main symptom of chlamydia in men.* Some men have the discharge only in the morning on arising. Complications include epididymitis, prostatitis, infertility, and Reiter's syndrome, a type of connective tissue disease discussed in Chapter 20.

In contrast, many women may have no symptoms. Those with symptoms have a mucopurulent cervicitis with a change in vaginal discharge, easily induced cervical bleeding, urinary frequency, and abdominal discomfort or pain. The vaginal discharge typically becomes yellow and more opaque. Complications of infection with *C. trachomatis* include salpingitis (inflammation of the fallopian tubes), PID, ectopic pregnancy, and infertility. These health problems are discussed in detail in maternal-child textbooks.

Diagnosis is made by sampling cells from the endocervix, urethra, or both. Because chlamydiae can reproduce only inside cells, host cells that harbor the organism (or parts of it) are required in the sample. Absolute diagnosis is made with a tissue culture obtained at the pelvic examination or male urethral examination. Culture for *Chlamydia* has been the gold standard.

However, molecular testing, such as (1) the nucleic acid amplification tests (NAATs), and (2) gene amplification tests (ligand chain reaction [LCR] and polymerase chain reaction [PCR] transcription-mediated amplification), are the newest methods of detecting *Chlamydia* in endocervical samples, urethral swabs, and urine. This less-invasive and self-collected urine testing has been found to be more acceptable and highly sensitive and specific. The increased acceptability of urine testing has resulted in increased identification of asymptomatic people.

All sexually active women 25 years old or younger and all at-risk women older than 25 years should be routinely screened for *Chlamydia* (CDC, 2006b). There is no recommendation for or against screening asymptomatic men, regardless of age or other risk.

Interventions

The treatment of choice for chlamydial infections is azithromycin (Zithromax) 1 g orally in a single dose or doxycycline (Monodox, Doxy-Caps, Doxycin♣) 100 mg orally twice daily for 7 days. The one-dose course, although more expensive, is preferred because of the ease in completing the treatment. Drugs that are prescribed for patients with allergies to these drugs include (CDC, 2006b):

- Erythromycin base (E-Mycin, Eramycin, Erythromid♣) 500 mg orally four times a day for 7 days *or*
- Erythromycin ethylsuccinate (EES, Apo-Erythro♣) 800 mg orally four times a day for 7 days *or*
- Ofloxacin (Floxin) 300 mg orally two times a day for 7 days *or*
- Levofloxacin (Levaquin) 500 mg orally daily for 7 days

Giving the drug while the patient is in the health care agency helps ensure adherence. Sexual partners should be tested and treated. **Expedited partner therapy (EPT),** or patient-delivered partner therapy, shows signs of reducing chlamydia infection rates (CDC, 2006a). Patients are given the drug or a prescription with specific instructions for administration to their partners without direct evaluation by a health care provider (CDC, 2006d).

Patient and partner education is an important nursing intervention. Explain:

- The mode of disease transmission
- The incubation period
- Manifestations, including the possibility of asymptomatic infections
- Treatment of infection with antibiotics
- The need for abstinence from sexual intercourse until the patient and partner(s) have completed treatment (7 days from the start of treatment, including a single-dose regimen)
- No test of cure is required, but all women should be rescreened for re-infection 3 to 12 months after treatment because of the high risk for PID. There is less evidence of the need for re-screening of treated men, but it should be considered
- The need to return for evaluation if symptoms recur or new symptoms develop (most recurrences are re-infections from a new or untreated partner)
- Possible complications of untreated or inadequately treated infection, such as PID, ectopic pregnancy, or infertility

OTHER GYNECOLOGIC CONDITIONS

PELVIC INFLAMMATORY DISEASE

Pathophysiology

Pelvic inflammatory disease (PID) is a complex infectious process in which organisms from the lower genital tract migrate from the endocervix upward through the uterine cavity

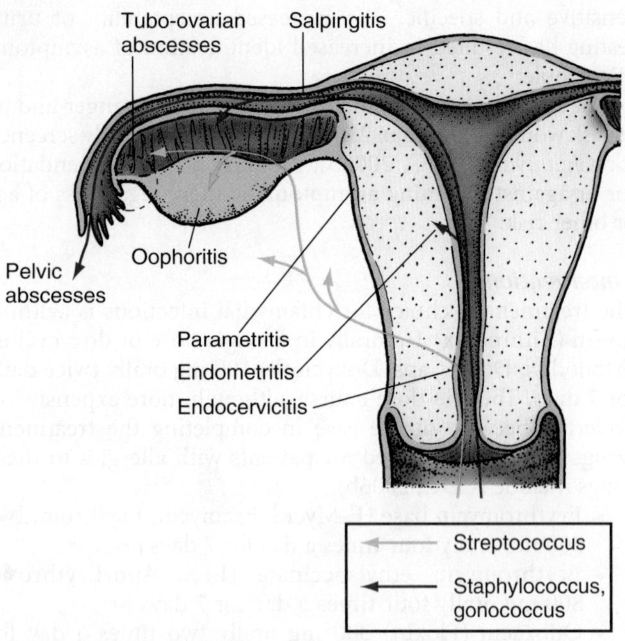
Tubo-ovarian abscesses
Salpingitis
Oophoritis
Pelvic abscesses
Parametritis
Endometritis
Endocervicitis
Streptococcus
Staphylococcus, gonococcus

Fig. 76-4 • The spread of pelvic inflammatory disease.

into the fallopian tubes. The spread of infection to other organs and tissues of the upper genital tract occurs from direct contact with mucosal surfaces or through the fimbriated ends of the tubes to the ovaries, parametrium, and peritoneal cavity (Fig. 76-4). This may involve one or more pelvic structures, including the uterus, fallopian tubes, and adjacent pelvic structures. The most common site is the fallopian tube. Resulting infections include:

- Endometritis (infection of the endometrial cavity)
- Salpingitis (inflammation of the fallopian tubes)
- Oophoritis (ovarian infection)
- Parametritis (infection of the parametrium)
- Peritonitis (infection of the peritoneal cavity)
- Tubal or tubo-ovarian abscess

Many different pathogens are linked to PID. Sexually transmitted organisms are most often responsible, especially *Chlamydia trachomatis* and *Neisseria gonorrhoeae.* Organisms that are part of the vaginal flora can also cause PID. In addition, *Gardnerella vaginalis, Haemophilus influenzae, Staphylococcus, Streptococcus, Escherichia coli,* and other aerobic and anaerobic organisms have been identified in patients with PID. There is increasing evidence that the anaerobes involved in bacterial vaginosis may have a role in the development of PID (CDC, 2006a).

The organisms invade the pelvis from an infection ascending from the vagina or cervix. Infections are spread during sexual intercourse, during childbirth (including the postpartum period), and after abortion. Rarely do they result from transperitoneal spread from a ruptured appendix or intra-abdominal abscess. *Sepsis and death can occur, especially if treatment is delayed or inadequate.*

Many practitioners use the terms *PID* and *salpingitis* as equal terms for acute infections. PID is one of the leading causes of infertility and is related to the increase in the number of ectopic pregnancies reported in the United States. It is an acute syndrome resulting in tenderness in the tubes and ovaries (adnexa) and low, dull abdominal pain. However, many women experience only mild discomfort or menstrual irregularity. Others experience no symptoms at all—so-called "silent" or "subclinical" PID. The diagnosis and treatment of this disease is challenging. Irreversible scarring or stricture, causing sterility, may occur before it is diagnosed.

The incidence of PID is on the rise and is estimated to occur in more than 1 million women annually in the United States (CDC, 2007c). Accurate rates are unavailable because PID is not a reportable disease. The disease may present with mild symptoms and therefore is often underdiagnosed. Estimates suggest that more than 100,000 women become infertile and 150 die from PID each year (CDC, 2007c).

Because of variations in patient manifestations, the diagnosis is difficult because women may have subtle symptoms not typical of the disease. Delay in diagnosis and treatment may add to complications of PID in the upper genital tract. The disease is usually diagnosed on the basis of clinical signs and symptoms. The Centers for Disease Control and Prevention (CDC) has set minimum criteria for diagnosis, but no laboratory or physical examination techniques alone are both sensitive and specific.

Patient-Centered Collaborative Care

evolve ONLINE PHARM REVIEW

Assessment

History

Obtain a complete medical, family, menstrual, obstetric, and sexual history, including a history of previous episodes of pelvic inflammatory disease (PID) or other sexually transmitted diseases (see Chart 76-1). Assess for contraceptive use, a history of reproductive surgery, and other risk factors previously identified. Ask the patient if sexual abuse has occurred. If so, encourage her to discuss what happened and if she was seen by a health care provider.

Many of the same factors that place women at risk for STDs also place them at risk for PID. Risk factors for sexually active women include:

- Age younger than 26 years
- Multiple sexual partners
- Intrauterine device (IUD) in place
- Smoking
- A history of PID
- Chlamydial or gonococcal infection; bacterial vaginosis
- A history of sexually transmitted diseases (STDs)

Physical Assessment/Clinical Manifestations

One of the most frequent symptoms of PID is lower abdominal pain. Conduct a complete pain assessment. Other symptoms include abnormal vaginal bleeding, dysuria (painful urination), an increase or change in vaginal discharge, dyspareunia (painful sexual intercourse), malaise, fever, and chills.

Observe whether the patient has discomfort with movement. Often the patient has a hunched-over gait to protect her abdomen. She may find it difficult to independently get on the examination table or stretcher. Assess for lower abdominal tenderness, possibly with rigidity or rebound tenderness. A pelvic examination by the health care provider may reveal yellow or green cervical discharge and a reddened or **friable** cervix (a cervix that bleeds easily). Criteria for accurate diagnosis of PID are listed in Table 76-5.

Psychosocial Assessment

The woman who has symptoms of PID is usually anxious and fearful of the examination and unknown diagnosis. She may need much reassurance and support during the physical ex-

TABLE 76-5 Diagnostic Criteria for Pelvic Inflammatory Disease

MINIMUM CRITERIA FOR INITIATING EMPIRIC TREATMENT FOR PELVIC INFLAMMATORY DISEASE
- Sexually active woman and at risk for STDs
- Pelvic or lower abdominal pain
- No other cause for illness can be found (appendicitis)

and
- Uterine tenderness *or*
- Adnexal tenderness *or*
- Cervical motion tenderness (chandelier sign)

ADDITIONAL CRITERIA TO INCREASE THE SPECIFICITY OF THE DIAGNOSIS OF PID
- Oral temperature >101° F (>38.3° C)
- Abnormal cervical or vaginal mucopurulent discharge
- Presence of white blood cells on saline microscopy of vaginal secretions
- Elevated erythrocyte sedimentation rate
- Elevated C-reactive protein
- Laboratory documentation of cervical infection with *Neisseria gonorrhoeae* or *Chlamydia trachomatis*

DEFINITIVE CRITERIA FOR DIAGNOSING PID, WARRANTED IN SELECTED CASES
- Histopathologic evidence of endometritis on endometrial biopsy
- Transvaginal sonography or other imaging techniques showing thickened fluid-filled tubes with or without free pelvic fluid or tubo-ovarian complex
- Laparoscopic abnormalities consistent with PID

Modified from Centers for Disease Control and Prevention (CDC). (2006). 2006 sexually transmitted diseases treatment guidelines. *Morbidity and Mortality Weekly Report, 55*(No. RR-11), 57.
PID, Pelvic inflammatory disease.

amination because her abdomen may be very tender or painful. Explain what is taking place to help promote comfort during the examination.

Because PID is often associated with an STD, the woman may feel embarrassed or uncomfortable discussing her symptoms or history. Use a nonjudgmental approach, and encourage the patient to express her feelings and concerns. The patient's ability to follow through with the treatment plan is essential in deciding whether ambulatory care treatment is appropriate.

Laboratory Assessment

The health care provider obtains specimens from the cervix, urethra, and rectum to determine the presence of *N. gonorrhoeae* or *C. trachomatis.* The white blood cell (WBC) count, erythrocyte sedimentation rate (ESR) and C-reactive protein may be elevated but are not specific for PID. A sensitive test that detects human chorionic gonadotropin (hCG) in urine or blood should be performed to determine whether the patient is pregnant. Microscopic examination of vaginal discharge should be done to evaluate for the presence of more than 10 WBCs per high-power field, which correlates with infection. Bacterial vaginosis can be found by observing the diagnostic "clue" cells with microscopic examination of vaginal discharge.

Other Diagnostic Assessment

Abdominal *ultrasonography* may be used to determine the presence of appendicitis and tubo-ovarian abscesses that need to be ruled out when the diagnosis of PID is made. Transvaginal ultrasound and *magnetic resonance imaging (MRI)* are used in some cases to detect tubal wall thickening, fluid-filled tubes, and free pelvic fluid or a tubo-ovarian abscess, all associated with PID. *Endometrial biopsy* also has been used to increase the accuracy of the diagnosis.

Analysis

Common Nursing Diagnoses and Collaborative Problems

The primary collaborative problem for patients with pelvic inflammatory disease (PID) is Infection related to invasion of pelvic organs by pathogens. The common nursing diagnoses for patients with PID are:

1. Acute Pain related to injuring agents (biologic) and the effects of the infectious process
2. Anxiety related to threat to health status and possible infertility as a result of infection

Additional Nursing Diagnoses and Collaborative Problems

In addition to the common nursing diagnoses and collaborative problems, patients with PID may have:

- Ineffective Health Maintenance related to knowledge deficit about risks, prevention, symptoms, treatment, and effects of PID
- Chronic Pain related to chronic presence of organisms that stimulate recurrent PID episodes
- Sexual Dysfunction related to altered body function from the effects of the infectious process
- Situational Low Self-Esteem/Chronic Low Self-Esteem related to disturbed body image or feeling guilty for having PID (associated with sexual transmission)

Planning and Implementation

Infection

Planning: Expected Outcomes. The patient with PID is expected to have her infection resolved. Indicators include that the patient should not have:

- Pain and tenderness of the pelvis
- Fever
- Infectious vaginal discharge

Interventions. Infection control is accomplished with the use of antibiotics, self-management measures, and surgical intervention (rarely).

Infection Control. Uncomplicated PID is usually treated on an ambulatory care basis. The CDC recommends hospitalization for PID if the patient:

- Has appendicitis, ectopic pregnancy, or other surgical emergency that has not been excluded
- Is pregnant
- Does not respond to oral antibiotic therapy
- Is unable to follow or tolerate an outpatient regimen
- Has severe illness, nausea and vomiting, or high fever
- Has a tubo-ovarian abscess

There are no recommendations about whether HIV-infected women should be hospitalized. Assess the ability of high-risk women for self-management at home. The clinical patient's medical condition and availability of support systems are important considerations for home care. If the infection has not responded to treatment, the patient may need to be hospitalized for IV antibiotic therapy and further evaluation.

Drug Therapy. The CDC recommends oral and/or parenteral antibiotics (CDC, 2007b) (Chart 76-4). Treatment lasts for 14 days. If the woman has not responded to oral treatment, she is hospitalized for IV antibiotic therapy and further evalu-

Chart 76-4 COMMON EXAMPLES OF DRUG THERAPY

Acute Pelvic Inflammatory Disease

Drug Dosage	Purpose	Nursing Interventions	Rationales
PARENTERAL TREATMENT (INPATIENT)			
REGIMEN A			
Cefotetan (Cefotan) 2 g IV every 12 hr, which can be changed to oral therapy after 24 hr of clinical improvement *Or* Cefoxitin (Mefoxin) 2 g IV every 6 hr, which can be changed to oral therapy after 24 hr of clinical improvement ***Plus*** Doxycycline (Monodox, Doxy-Caps, Doxycin🍁) 100 mg IV or orally every 12 hr for 14 days (orally is preferred because of the pain associated with infusion) **Med Error Alert!** Do not confuse doxycycline or Doxycin with doxepin, an antidepressant.	Antibiotics are the primary treatment modality for PID. Oral and parenteral treatments appear to have the similar efficacy, especially for mild or moderate PID. Cephalosporins provide coverage for gonococcal infections.	Assess patients for rash, itching, and hypotension.	Assessment detects adverse reactions.
		Assess patients for rash, itching, and hypotension.	Assessment detects adverse reactions.
		Observe the IV site for signs of redness, heat, and tenderness.	Phlebitis can be detected.
		Assess patients for rash, nausea, and diarrhea.	Assessment detects drug side effects.
		Instruct patients about possible photosensitivity and the need for sun protection.	This precaution prevents sunburn by limiting sun exposure.
		Encourage oral fluid intake.	Fluid intake decreases esophageal irritation.
		Instruct patients that it is beneficial to take the drug with food.	Food decreases GI upset.
REGIMEN B			
Clindamycin (Cleocin) 900 mg IV every 8 hr ***Plus*** Gentamicin (Garamycin IV) 2 mg/kg of body weight once IV or IM followed by 1.5 mg/kg every 8 hr IV or IM until there have been signs of clinical improvement for 24 hr	Alternative antibiotic regimens available for allergic patients.	Observe patients for rash and urticaria.	Adverse reactions are detected.
		Observe patients for hypotension, dyspnea, and restlessness.	Anaphylactic reaction is detected.
		Observe patients for severe diarrhea.	This precaution avoids pseudomembranous colitis.
		Observe the IV site for redness, heat, and tenderness.	Phlebitis can be detected.
		Urge oral fluid intake.	Fluid intake prevents irritation to renal tubules.
		Measure fluid intake and output.	Oliguria or anuria can be detected.
		Observe patients for hearing loss, fever, or decreased renal function.	Ototoxicity, nephrotoxicity, and fever are known side effects.
		Draw serum for peak and trough levels.	Serum levels can vary, and the drug has low threshold to toxic level.
ORAL TREATMENT (OUTPATIENT)			
Ceftriaxone 250 mg IM one time only	Oral regimens appear to be as effective as parenteral antibiotics. Fluoroquinolones are no longer used because of resistant isolates of gonorrhea.	Give deep IM injection in the outer upper quadrant of the gluteus maximus.	Local irritation is avoided, and drug absorption is increased.
		Watch for fever, chills, and nausea.	Allergic reactions can be detected.
		Tell patients that the injection may be painful.	Patients are prepared for discomfort related to the inflammatory reaction.
Or			
Cefoxitin 2 g IM in a single dose		Give deep IM injection in the ventral gluteal area.	Local irritation is avoided, and drug absorption is increased.
		Watch for fever, chills, and nausea.	Allergic reactions can be detected.
		Tell patients that the injection may be painful.	Patients are prepared for discomfort related to the inflammatory reaction.

Chart 76-4 COMMON EXAMPLES OF DRUG THERAPY

Acute Pelvic Inflammatory Disease—cont'd

Drug Dosage	Purpose	Nursing Interventions	Rationales
ORAL TREATMENT (OUTPATIENT)—cont'd			
And			
Probenecid (Benemid, Benuryl♣) 1 g orally one time only concurrently **Med Error Alert!** Do not confuse probenecid with Procanbid, a drug used for cardiac dysrhythmias.	Increases level of circulating antibiotics by decreasing renal excretion.	Give with food. Encourage fluid intake (10 glasses per day).	Taking the drug with food avoids GI upset. Fluid intake prevents formation of kidney stones.
Or			
Other parenteral third-generation cephalosporin (e.g., ceftizoxime or cefotaxime)			
ANY OF THE ABOVE ORAL TREATMENT (OUTPATIENT)			
Plus			
Doxycycline (Monodox, Doxy-Caps, Doxycin♣) 100 mg orally twice daily for 14 days	*Chlamydia* is one of the major causes of PID. This drug is highly effective for eradicating it.	See p. 1750 for doxycycline.	See p. 1750 for doxycycline.
With or Without			
Metronidazole (Flagyl, Novonidazol ♣) 500 mg orally twice daily for 14 days	Anaerobes are thought to contribute significantly to the etiology of PID and are eradicated with this medication.	Monitor the serum level if the patient is taking lithium. Avoid alcohol within 24 hr of use.	This drug raises the serum level of lithium. Alcohol causes disulfiram-like effect.

Modified from Centers for Disease Control and Prevention. (2007). *Updated recommended treatment regimens for gonococcal infections and associated conditions—United States, April 2007*. Retrieved online at www.cdc.gov/std/treatment/2006/GonUpdateApril2007.pdf.
PID, Pelvic inflammatory disease.

ation. Inpatient therapy involves a combination of several IV antibiotics until the woman shows signs of improvement (e.g., decreased pelvic tenderness for at least 24 hours). Then oral antibiotics are continued until the course of treatment has lasted 14 days.

Teach women treated as outpatients to rest, abstain from sexual intercourse, and check their temperature twice a day. Teach them to report an increase in temperature to their health care provider. Remind them to be seen by the health care provider within 72 hours from starting the antibiotics and then 1 and 2 weeks from the time of the initial diagnosis.

In a small number of patients, the pain and tenderness may not be relieved by antibiotic therapy. The surgeon may perform a laparoscopy to remove an abscess through one or more sub-umbilical incisions to provide better access to the fallopian tubes. Before surgery, provide information about hospital routines and procedures. After surgery, the care of the woman with PID is similar to that of any patient after laparoscopic abdominal surgery. One difference is that she may have a wound drain for drainage of abscess fluid that may not have been completely removed during surgery. Observe, measure, and record wound drainage every 4 to 8 hours as requested.

Acute Pain

Planning: Expected Outcomes. The patient with PID is expected to have reduced pain and increased comfort as indicated by a 2 or 3 on a pain scale of 1 to 10, with 10 being the worst possible pain.

Interventions. Pain management of PID begins with treatment of the infection. Antibiotic therapy relieves pain by decreasing the inflammation caused by infection. Other pain-relief measures include taking mild analgesics and applying heat to the lower abdomen or back. *Teach the patient to maintain bedrest in a semi-Fowler's position to promote gravity drainage of the infection that may help relieve pain.*

Anxiety

NOC **Planning: Expected Outcomes.** The patient with PID is expected to take actions to reduce anxiety about infertility. Indicators include that the patient will demonstrate:

- Use of effective coping patterns strategies
- Controlled anxiety response
- Use of available social support
- Seeking professional help, as appropriate

Interventions. Infertility is the most common complication of PID. Nursing interventions are aimed at understanding the patient's perspective of the diagnosis and future complications.

If the woman is anxious, provide an atmosphere in which she feels comfortable expressing her feelings and asking questions. Give accurate information about the diagnosis, treatment, and prognosis. Providing information about the advantages of early diagnosis and treatment (to limit damage to organs of the pelvis) and the advances in treatments for infertility may reassure her. Help her assess the emotional support available from family members or significant others. Relaxation techniques may be useful to decrease the anxiety.

Community-Based Care

Collaborate with the case manager before the woman is discharged to home. Teach the patient with PID to have regular follow-up with her health care provider to assess for complications and assess that the infection has resolved. The ongoing role of the nurse is to assess for any continued risk for contracting PID again, signs of persistent or recurrent infection, and education to prevent exposure to and infection with all STDs (e.g., decrease the number of partners, consistently use condoms). Establish an atmosphere of trust that encourages the woman to return frequently, if needed, for education or reassurance.

Home Care Management

Parenteral antibiotic therapy may be given at home, but usually the health care provider changes the treatment regimen to oral antibiotics before hospital discharge.

Health Teaching

Patient teaching focuses on providing information about PID, identifying recurrences (persistent pain, dysmenorrhea, low backache, fever), and urging early and complete self-management to prevent complications. Review information for oral antibiotic therapy (Chart 76-5).

Counsel the patient to contact her sexual partner(s) for examination and treatment. Partners should be treated for gonorrhea and chlamydial infection regardless of their lack of symptoms. Remind the patient about follow-up care, and counsel her about the complications that can occur after an episode of PID. These problems include increased risk for recurrence, ectopic pregnancy, and infertility. Chronic pelvic pain may also develop.

Discuss contraception and the patient's need or desire for it. This discussion includes methods that may decrease the risk for future episodes of PID, such as the use of barrier methods (e.g., condom). Help the patient understand lifestyle factors that increase the risk for recurrent episodes, including sexual intercourse with multiple partners. Douching has also been suggested as a risk behavior for development of PID and/or infection with *Chlamydia* or gonorrhea. However, other researchers have not confirmed that risk factor (Ness et al., 2005).

Chart 76-5 PATIENT AND FAMILY EDUCATION GUIDE

Oral Antibiotic Therapy for Sexually Transmitted Diseases

- Take your medicine for the number of times a day it is prescribed and until it is completed.
- Your sexual partner must be tested and treated if you have a sexually transmitted disease (STD).
- Be sure to return for your follow-up appointment after completing your antibiotic treatment.
- Call if you have any questions or concerns.
- Do not have sex until after you complete your antibiotic therapy. If your partner is being treated, you can go back to having sex together after he or she also completes treatment. This should be 7 days for 1-dose treatment drugs.
- Drink at least 8 to 10 glasses of fluid a day while taking your antibiotics.
- Do not take antacids containing calcium, magnesium, or aluminum, such as Tums, Maalox, or Mylanta, with your antibiotics. They may decrease the effectiveness of the antibiotic.
- Take your antibiotics on an empty stomach unless your health care provider instructs you to take them with food.
- If you are taking oral contraceptives, you should discuss with your health care provider whether the antibiotics will decrease the effectiveness of your pills.

Psychosocial concerns may require teaching and counseling. A patient who has PID may exhibit a variety of feelings (guilt, disgust, anger) about having a condition that may have been transmitted to her sexually. These feelings may affect her relationship with significant others and future sexual relationships. She may also have concerns about future fertility if PID has damaged or scarred the fallopian tubes and other reproductive organs. Provide nonjudgmental emotional support, and allow time for the woman to discuss her feelings.

NCLEX EXAMINATION CHALLENGE

A client with pelvic inflammatory disease is taking antibiotic therapy at home. Which of these statements by the client indicates a need for further health teaching by the nurse?

A. "I have to take all of my antibiotics as prescribed."
B. "I must check my temperature two times a day."
C. "I need to rest as much as possible to help my pain."
D. "If I lie flat on my back, my belly will feel better."

evolve For the correct answer, go to http://evolve.elsevier.com/Iggy/.

Health Care Resources

If infertility is a result of PID, the patient may need referral to a clinic specializing in infertility treatment and counseling. She can also contact support groups for infertile couples, which exist in many local communities.

The costs of antibiotics for care of patients with PID and other STDs may be a concern for those who are uninsured, underinsured, or impoverished. In collaboration with the case manager or social worker, help locate community resources for free or discounted drugs for women who cannot afford them. Ask the patient directly if she has money to pay for the drug therapy, regardless of her apparent financial status.

Evaluation: Outcomes

Evaluate the care of the patient with PID on the basis of the identified nursing diagnoses and collaborative problems. The expected outcomes include that the patient should:

- Show evidence that the infection has resolved
- Report or demonstrate that pain is relieved or reduced and that she feels more comfortable
- Take action to manage anxiety about future infertility

Specific indicators for these outcomes are listed for each nursing diagnosis and collaborative problem under the Planning and Implementation section (see earlier).

VAGINAL INFECTIONS

Vaginal infection associated with sexual activity may produce vaginal discharge or vulvar irritation. The common causes of vaginal infection that can be but are not always sexually transmitted include:

- *Trichomonas vaginalis*
- *Candida,* primarily *C. albicans*
- Bacteria that produce bacterial vaginosis, including *Gardnerella vaginalis, Mycoplasma hominis* and anaerobes including *Prevotella* and *Mobiluncus* species

Men can also get these infections but are not always symptomatic.

Trichomoniasis and candida infections are limited to the vagina. They can be very irritating and bothersome but do not cause any long-term problems. The partner must also be treated for *trichomoniasis* if the infection is to be resolved. *Candidiasis* does not usually require partner treatment. However, if the male partner is symptomatic (irritation of the genital skin), treatment is indicated. It is important to remember that *Candida* is a normal flora on the skin and can easily be relocated to the vagina. Although it can be transmitted sexually, candidiasis occurs among women who are not sexually active. Also, antibiotics that change the normal flora of the vagina contribute to infection.

Bacterial vaginosis (BV) has been implicated in upper genital tract infections. Women undergoing surgery of the upper genital tract should be evaluated and treated if BV is found. Chapter 74 describes the management of each of these infections.

OTHER SEXUALLY TRANSMITTED DISEASES

Less common diseases in the United States that are transmitted by sexual contact are lymphogranuloma venereum, chancroid, and granuloma inguinale. Like syphilis, all of these diseases are associated with ulcers but they are seen most often in less affluent countries. As newcomers migrate into the United States, these STDs may become more common. Ask patients suspected of these infections whether they have traveled out of the United States and whether they had sexual contact with people who live in other countries.

LYMPHOGRANULOMA VENEREUM

Lymphogranuloma venereum (LGV) is the result of genital infection with one of three serotypes of *Chlamydia trachomatis,* which is spread systemically until it localizes in the genital or rectal lymph nodes. The primary lesion at the point of entry is transient, painless, and often not noticed. It usually appears on the penis in men and on the vaginal wall in women. However, sores may also be located in the mouth and rectum.

Lesions vary in form from herpes-like blisters (vesicles), to ulcers, papules, or pustules. Within 1 to 2 weeks after the primary lesion appears, secondary signs of infection appear. Lymphadenopathy (primarily inguinal and femoral) is present, more commonly in men than in women. Swelling from the enlarged lymph nodes occurs on both sides of the inguinal ligament and forms the characteristic "groove sign" of LGV. Other manifestations may include headache, malaise, arthralgia, and anorexia. Most patients seek care at this point.

Complications of the infection include fistulas, rectal strictures, chronic enlarged lymph nodes, and proctitis. Systemic involvement can cause carditis, arthritis, and pneumonia.

The health care provider prescribes doxycycline (Monodox, Doxy-Caps, Doxycin♣) 100 mg orally twice daily or an erythromycin-based drug 500 mg orally four times daily for 21 days. Antibiotic treatment cures the infection and prevents further tissue damage. Infected lymph nodes may be aspirated by needle or incised and drained to prevent ulcer formation. Surgical intervention may be needed for late complications, such as perianal or perirectal strictures and fistulas. Nursing management and patient education are similar to that for syphilis.

Sexual partners should be tested for cervical or urethral chlamydial infection. They should be treated if they had sexual contact during the 60 days before the patient's onset of symptoms.

CHANCROID

Chancroid lesions are painful genital ulcerations caused by infection with *Haemophilus ducreyi,* a gram-negative bacterium. Chancroid ulcers are soft genital lesions. These lesions and inguinal lymphadenopathy without systemic illness are the usual presentation. The infection develops as a result of sexual exposure or self-contamination from a lesion elsewhere on the body. The incubation period for chancroid varies from 3 to 10 days. A tender papule appears at the site of inoculation. This lesion rapidly breaks down to form an irregularly shaped, deep ulcer that has a purulent discharge and bleeds easily.

Complications include inguinal adenitis (ovarian infection), balanitis (penile infection), and urethral fistulas. Chancroids differ from chancres caused by syphilis in that chancroids are soft and painful. Transmission of the disease is through contact with the ulcer or with the discharge from the infected local lymph glands during sexual activity. Uncircumcised men may be at greater risk for infection than circumcised men, and men are more frequently infected than women.

Management consists of azithromycin (Zithromax) 1 g orally in a single dose, ceftriaxone (Rocephin) 250 mg IM in a single dose, ciprofloxacin (Cipro) 500 mg orally twice daily for 3 days, or erythromycin (E-Mycin, Apo-Erythro♣) 500 mg orally four times daily for 7 days. These antibiotics cure the infection, resolve the symptoms, and prevent transmission. Patients should be observed periodically by a health care provider until ulcers heal, usually in 7 days.

GRANULOMA INGUINALE

The causative organism of **granuloma inguinale,** or donovanosis, is *Klebsiella granulomatis.* A nodule appears at the site of inoculation after 1 to 12 weeks. This lesion ulcerates, and others are formed. They are painless and grow together, becoming a spreading ulcer on the genitalia. Left untreated, these lesions can be mutilating. Inguinal lymphadenopathy does not occur; thus the name of this disease may be inappropriate. The ulcerated lesions are very vascular and bleed easily on contact, but they also may appear as necrotic, hypertrophic or sclerotic lesions. As open areas, the ulcerated lesions can become infected with bacteria or other STDs.

Granuloma inguinale is treated with doxycycline 100 mg orally twice daily, azithromycin (Zithromax) 1 g orally once per week, ciprofloxacin (Cipro) 750 mg orally twice daily, erythromycin base (E-Mycin) 500 mg orally four times a day, or trimethoprim/sulfamethoxazole double strength (Bactrim DS, Septra DS) twice daily, all for a minimum of 3 weeks. Treatment needs to continue until all the lesions are completely healed. Relapse can occur within 6 to 18 months, even after successful initial treatment.

HUMAN NEEDS NURSING CARE REVIEW

What might you NOTICE if the patient has altered sexuality as a result of a sexually-transmitted disease (STD)?

- Report of heavy and abnormal vaginal discharge
- Report of urinary frequency or dysuria
- Ulcers, blisters, or warts in the genital area
- Low-grade fever
- Report of malaise
- Report of vaginal, penile, or anal itching or irritation
- Report of abdominal pain (pelvic inflammatory disease [PID])
- Anxious behavior

What should you INTERPRET and how should you RESPOND to a patient with altered sexuality as a result of STD?

Perform and interpret focused physical assessment, including:

- Vital signs
- Pain intensity and quality
- Skin inspection (genital area)

Respond by:

- Reporting and documenting all findings
- Helping patient with abdominal pain into a semi-Fowler's position
- Providing pain-control measures
- Teaching patient about prescribed antibiotic or antiviral therapy
- Teaching patient to avoid sexual intercourse while being treated
- Teaching patient the importance of treating all sexual partners
- Teaching patient and partner(s) about safe sex practices
- Providing support and listening to the patient and partner(s) without judgment

On what should you REFLECT?

- Examine your feelings about patients who make lifestyle choices different from your own.
- Think about what else you could do to help patients meet their physical and emotional needs during this time.
- Determine what other health teaching may be needed for this patient.
- Monitor the patient's response to pain-control interventions.

GET READY FOR THE NCLEX EXAMINATION!

Key Points

Review these Key Points for each NCLEX Examination Client Needs Category.

Safe and Effective Care Environment

- Teach patients to not have sexual intercourse during their treatment for sexually transmitted disease (STD).
- Maintain patient and partner confidentiality and privacy at all times.
- Use gloves when examining the patient's genitalia or skin lesions.

Health Promotion and Maintenance

- Teach the patient about the importance of expedited partner treatment; be sure that all doses of the drug are taken by both the patient and the partner.
- Encourage all patients who are sexually active to use condoms and other precautions during sexual intimacy (see Chart 76-3).
- Urge sexually active people, especially those younger than 25 years or those older than 25 years if at high-risk, to have routine health visits and screenings.

Psychosocial Integrity

- Treat all patients, regardless of diagnosis, with respect.
- Provide as much privacy as possible for patients undergoing examination or testing for STDs.
- Respect the lifestyle choices of all patients regardless of personal feelings.
- Allow the patient the opportunity to express fear or anxiety regarding a diagnosis of STD.
- Refer patients newly diagnosed with an STD to local resources and support groups as needed based on their response.
- Encourage all patients who have an STD to inform their sexual partner(s) of their health status.

Physiological Integrity

- Encourage patients to adhere to their anti-infective drug regimen (see Chart 76-5).
- Teach patients the expected side effects and possible adverse reactions to prescribed drugs.
- Assess patients with STD using the guidelines in Chart 76-1.
- Teach patients about the complications of STD using the information in Table 76-2.
- Be aware that PID is diagnosed based on the criteria in Table 76-5.

Additional Study Resources

Go to your Companion CD or Evolve at http://evolve.elsevier.com/Iggy/ for Self-Assessment Questions for the NCLEX Examination.

evolve *Go to Evolve at http://evolve.elsevier.com/Iggy/ for Prioritization and Delegation Questions for the NCLEX Examination.*

SELECTED BIBLIOGRAPHY

Asterisk indicates a classic or definitive work on this subject.

Apoola, A., & Radcliffe, K. (2004). Antiviral treatment of genital herpes. *International Journal of STD & AIDS, 15*(7), 429-433.

*Ballard, R., & Morse, S. (2003). Chancroid. In S.A. Morse, R. Ballard, K.K. Holmes, & A. Moreland (Eds.), *Atlas of sexually transmitted diseases and AIDS* (3rd ed.). St. Louis: Mosby.

Bartlett, J. (2005). *2005-2006 pocket book of infectious disease therapy.* Philadelphia: Lippincott Williams & Wilkins.

Berman, N.R. (2006) Cervical cancer screening today: The role of HPV DNA testing. *Advance for Nurse Practitioners, 14*(4), 24-29.

*Bowden, F. (2003). Donovanosis. In S.A. Morse, R. Ballard, K.K. Holmes, & A. Moreland (Eds.), *Atlas of sexually transmitted diseases and AIDS* (3rd ed.). St. Louis: Mosby.

Bulechek, G.M., Butcher, H.K., & McCloskey Dochterman, J. (Eds.). (2008). *Nursing interventions classification (NIC)* (5th ed.). St. Louis: Mosby.

Carpenito-Loyet, L. (2007). *Handbook of nursing diagnosis* (12th ed.). Philadelphia: Lippincott Williams & Wilkins.

*Centers for Disease Control and Prevention (CDC). (2004a). Lymphogranuloma venereum among men who have sex with men—Netherlands, 2003-2004. *Morbidity and Mortality Weekly Report, 53*(42), 985-988.

*Centers for Disease Control and Prevention (CDC). (2004b). *STD surveillance 2004: Other STDs—National profile.* Retrieved April 3, 2008, from www.cdc.gov/std/stats04/otherstds.htm.

Centers for Disease Control and Prevention (CDC). (2006a). 2006 sexually transmitted diseases treatment guidelines. *Morbidity and Mortality Weekly Report, 55*(RR-11), 1-94.

Centers for Disease Control and Prevention (CDC). (2006b). *Trends in reportable sexually transmitted diseases in the United States, 2005: National surveillance data for Chlamydia, gonorrhea, and syphilis.* Retrieved April 3, 2008, from www.cdc.gov/std/stats/05pdf/trends-2005.pdf.

Centers for Disease Control and Prevention (CDC). (2006c). *Sexually transmitted disease surveillance 2005.* Atlanta: U.S. Department of Health and Human Services.

Centers for Disease Control and Prevention (CDC). (2006d). *Expedited partner therapy in the management of sexually transmitted diseases.* Atlanta: U.S. Department of Health and Human Services. Retrieved April 3, 2008, from www.cdc.gov/std/treatment/EPTFinalReport2006.pdf.

Centers for Disease Control and Prevention (CDC). (2007a). Update to CDC's sexually transmitted diseases treatment guidelines, 2006: Fluoroquinolones no longer recommended for treatment of gonococcal infections. *Morbidity and Mortality Weekly Report, 56*(14), 332-336.

Centers for Disease Control and Prevention (CDC). (2007b). *Updated recommended treatment regimens for gonococcal infections and associated conditions—United States, April 2007.* Retrieved April 3, 2008, from www.cdc.gov/std/treatment/2006/GonUpdateApril2007.pdf.

Centers for Disease Control and Prevention (CDC). (2007c). *Pelvic inflammatory disease: CDC fact sheet.* Retrieved April 3, 2008, from www.cdc.gov/std/PID/STDFact-PID.htm.

Centers for Disease Control and Prevention (CDC), National Center for HIV/AIDS, Viral Hepatitis, STD, and TB Prevention. (2007d). *Hepatitis.* Retrieved April 3, 2008, from www.cdc.gov/ncidod/diseases/hepatitis/.

Centers for Disease Control and Prevention (CDC). (2007e). Quadrivalent human papilloma virus vaccine: Recommendations of the Advisory Committee on Immunization Practices (ACIP). *Morbidity and Mortality Weekly Report, 56*(RR-2), 1-24.

Chesson, H.W., Blandford, J.M., Gift, T.L., Tao, G., & Irwin, K.L. (2004). The estimated direct medical costs of sexually transmitted diseases among American youth, 2000. *Perspectives on Sexual and Reproductive Health, 36*(1), 11-19.

Cook, R.L., Hutchison, S.L., Ostergaard, L., Braithwaite, R.S., & Ness, R.B. (2005). Systematic review: Noninvasive testing for *Chlamydia trachomatis* and *Neisseria gonorrhoeae. Annals of Internal Medicine, 142*(11), 914-925.

Cottrell, B.H. (2006). Vaginal douching practices of women in eight Florida panhandle counties. *Journal of Obstetric, Gynecologic, and Neonatal Nursing, 35*(1), 24-33.

Cox , J.T. (2006). The development of cervical cancer and its precursors: What is the role of human papillomavirus infection? *Current Opinion in Obstetrics and Gynecology, 18*(Suppl. 1), S5-S13.

Denny-Smith, T., Bairan, A., & Page, M.C. (2006). A survey of female nursing students' knowledge, health beliefs, perceptions of risk, and risk behaviors regarding human papillomavirus and cervical cancer. *Journal of the American Academy of Nurse Practitioners, 18*(2), 62-69.

Dunne, E.F., Unger, E.R., Sternberg, M., McQuillan, G., Swan, D., Patel, S.S., et al. (2007). Prevalence of HPV infection among females in the United States. *Journal of the American Medical Association, 297*(8), 813-819.

Ensor, D. (2005). The significance of herpes simplex for school nurses. *Journal of School Nurses, 21*(1), 10-16.

Golden, M.R., Whittington, W.L., Handsfield, H.H., Hughes, J.P., Stamm, W.E., Hogben, M., et al. (2005). Effect of expedited treatment of sex partners on recurrent or persistent gonorrhea or chlamydial infection. *New England Journal of Medicine, 352*(7), 676-685.

*Hauth, J.C., Goldenberg, R.L., Andrews, W.W., DuBard, M.B., & Copper, R.L. (1995). Reduced incidence of preterm delivery with metronidazole and erythromycin in women with bacterial vaginosis. *New England Journal of Medicine, 333*(26), 1732-1736.

*Hillier, S.L., Nugent, R.P., Eschenbach, D.A., Krohn, M.A., Gibbs, R.S., Martin, D.H., et al. (1995). Association between bacterial vaginosis and preterm delivery of a low birth-weight infant. *New England Journal of Medicine, 333*(26), 1737-1742.

Kirkland, L.G. (2006). New developments in the management of STDs. *Nurse Practitioner, 31*(12), 12-21.

Kissinger, P., Mohammed, H., Richardson-Alston, G., Leichliter, J.S., Taylor, S.N., Martin, D.H., et al. (2005). Patient-delivered partner treatment for male-urethritis: A randomized, controlled trial. *Clinical Infectious Diseases, 41*(5), 623-629.

Lajiness, M.J. (2007). The new vaccine to prevent HPV. *Urologic Nursing, 27*(2), 153-154.

Mabey, D., & Peeling, R.W. (2002). Lymphogranuloma venereum. *Sexually Transmitted Infections, 78*(2), 90-92.

Mashburn, J. (2006). Etiology, diagnosis, and management of vaginitis. *Journal of Midwifery & Women's Health, 51*(6), 423-430.

Mayeaux, E.J. Jr. (2006). Harnessing the power of prevention: Human papillomavirus vaccines. *Current Opinion in Obstetrics and Gynecology, 18*(Suppl. 1), S15-S21.

McLemore, M.R. (2006). Gardasil: Introducing the new human papillomavirus vaccine. *Clinical Journal of Oncology Nursing, 10*(5), 559-560.

*Morse, S.A., Ballard, R., Holmes, K.K., & Moreland, A. (2003). *Atlas of sexually transmitted diseases and AIDS* (3rd ed.). St. Louis: Mosby.

National Digestive Diseases Information Clearinghouse (NDDIC), National Institute of Diabetes and Digestive and Kidney Diseases, National Institutes of Health, U.S. Department of Health and Human Services. (2007). *Chronic hepatitis C: Current disease management.* Retrieved April 3, 2008, from http://digestive.niddk.nih.gov/ddiseases/pubs/chronichepc/.

Ness, R.B., Hillier, S.L., Kip, K.E., Richter, H.E., Soper, D.E., Stamm, C.A., et al. (2005). Douching, pelvic inflammatory disease, and incident gonococcal and chlamydial genital infection in a cohort of high-risk women. *American Journal of Epidemiology, 161*(2), 186-195.

Pagana, K., & Pagana, T. (2006). *Mosby's manual of diagnostic and laboratory tests* (3rd ed.). St. Louis: Mosby.

Peate, I. (2006). Nursing care and the treatment of the patient with human papillomavirus. *British Journal of Nursing, 15*(19), 1063-1069.

*Schacter, J., & Stephens, R. (2003). Infections caused by *Chlamydia trachomatis.* In S.A. Morse, R. Ballard, K.K. Holmes, & A. Moreland (Eds.), *Atlas of sexually transmitted diseases and AIDS* (3rd ed.). St. Louis: Mosby.

Schillinger, J.A., Kissinger, P., Calvet, H., Whittington, W.L., Ransom, R.L., Sternberg, M.R., et al. (2003). Patient-delivered partner treatment with azithromycin to prevent repeated *Chlamydia trachomatis* infection among women: A randomized, controlled trial. *Sexually Transmitted Diseases, 30*(1), 49-56.

Skidmore-Roth, L. (2007). *Mosby's 2007 nursing drug reference.* St. Louis: Mosby.

Snijders, P.J., Steenbergen, R.D., Heideman, D.A., & Meijer, C.J. (2006). HPV-mediated cervical carcinogenesis: Concepts and clinical implications. *Journal of Pathology, 208*(2), 152-164.

Taylor, M.L., Mainous, A.G. III, & Wells, B.J. (2005). Prostate cancer and sexually transmitted diseases: A meta-analysis. *Family Medicine, 37*(7), 506-512.

U.S. Department of Health and Human Services (USDHHS), Office of Disease Prevention and Health Promotion. (2007). *Healthy People 2010.* Retrieved April 3, 2008, from www.healthypeople.gov/Document/HTML/Volume2/25STDs.htm#_Toc489706324.

U.S. Preventive Service Task Force, Agency for Healthcare Research and Quality. (2007). *Guide to clinical preventive services.* Retrieved April 3, 2008, from www.ahrq.gov/clinic/pocketgd.htm.

Weinstock, H., Berman, S., & Cates, W. Jr. (2004). Sexually transmitted diseases among American youth: Incidence and prevalence estimates, 2000. *Perspectives on Sexual and Reproductive Health, 36*(1), 6-10.

Do-Not-Use Abbreviations and Symbols

A

APPENDIX

Symbol or Abbreviation	Intended Meaning	Potential Problem	Preferred Term
μg	Microgram	Mistaken as "mg" (milligrams)	Use "mcg"
ʒ	Dram	Symbol for dram mistaken as "3"	Use the metric system
♍	Minim	Symbol for minim mistaken as "mL"	Use the metric system
@	At	Mistaken as "2"	Use "at"
&	And	Mistaken as "2"	Use "and"
+	Plus or and	Mistaken as "4"	Use "and"
°	Hour	Mistaken as a zero (e.g., q2° seen as "q20")	Use "hr," "h," or "hour"
ī/d	One daily	Mistaken as "tid"	Use "1 daily"
/ (slash mark)	Separates two doses or indicates "per"	Mistaken as the number 1 (e.g., "25 units/ 10 units" misread as "25 units" and "110 units")	Use "per" rather than a slash mark to separate doses
> and <	Greater than and less than	Mistaken as opposite of intended; mistakenly use incorrect symbol; "< 10" mistaken as "40"	Use "greater than" or "less than"
AD, AS, AU	Right ear, left ear, each ear	Mistaken as OD, OS, OU (right eye, left eye, each eye)	Use "right ear," "left ear," or "each ear"
ARA A	vidarabine	Mistaken as cytarabine (ARA C)	Use complete drug name
AZT	zidovudine (Retrovir)	Mistaken as azathioprine or aztreonam	Use complete drug name
BT	Bedtime	Mistaken as "BID" (twice daily)	Use "bedtime"
cc	Cubic centimeters	Mistaken as "u" (units)	Use "mL"
CPZ	Compazine (prochlorperazine)	Mistaken as chlorpromazine	Use complete drug name
D/C	Discharge or discontinue	Premature discontinuation of medications if D/C (intended to mean "discharge") has been misinterpreted as "discontinued" when followed by a list of discharge medications	Use "discharge" and "discontinue"
DPT	Demerol-Phenergan-Thorazine	Mistaken as diphtheria-pertussis-tetanus (vaccine)	Use complete drug name
DTO	Diluted tincture of opium, or deodorized tincture of opium (Paregoric)	Mistaken as tincture of opium	Use complete drug name
HCl	hydrochloric acid or hydrochloride	Mistaken as potassium chloride (the "H" is misinterpreted as "K")	Use complete drug name unless expressed as a salt of a drug
HCT	hydrocortisone	Mistaken as hydrochlorothiazide	Use complete drug name
HCTZ	hydrochlorothiazide	Mistaken as hydrocortisone (seen as HCT250 mg)	Use complete drug name
HS hs	Half-strength At bedtime, hours of sleep	Mistaken as bedtime Mistaken as half-strength	Use "half-strength" or "bedtime"

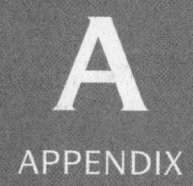

Symbol or Abbreviation	Intended Meaning	Potential Problem	Preferred Term
IJ	Injection	Mistaken as "IV" or "intrajugular"	Use "injection"
IN	Intranasal	Mistaken as "IM" or "IV"	Use "intranasal" or "NAS"
IU	International unit	Mistaken as IV (intravenous) or 10 (ten)	Use "units"
"IV Vanc"	Intravenous vancomycin	Mistaken as Invanz	Use complete drug name
$MgSO_4$	Magnesium sulfate	Mistaken as morphine sulfate	Use complete drug name
MS, MSO_4	Morphine sulfate	Mistaken as magnesium sulfate	Use complete drug name
MTX	methotrexate	Mistaken as mitoxantrone	Use complete drug name
"Nitro" drip	nitroglycerin infusion	Mistaken as sodium nitroprusside infusion	Use complete drug name
"Norflox"	norfloxacin	Mistaken as Norflex	Use complete drug name
OD, OS, OU	Right eye, left eye, each eye	Mistaken as AD, AS, AU (right ear, left ear, each ear)	Use "right eye," "left eye," or "each eye"
o.d. or OD	Once daily	Mistaken as "right eye" (OD-oculus dexter), leading to oral liquid medications administered in the eye	Use "daily"
OJ	Orange juice	Mistaken as OD or OS (right or left eye); drugs meant to be diluted in orange juice may be given in the eye	Use "orange juice"
PCA	procainamide	Mistaken as patient controlled analgesia	Use complete drug name
Per os	By mouth, orally	The "os" can be mistaken as "left eye" (OS-oculus sinister)	Use "PO," "by mouth," or "orally"
PTU	propylthiouracil	Mistaken as mercaptopurine	Use complete drug name
q.d. or QD	Every day	Mistaken as q.i.d., especially if the period after the "q" or the tail of the "q" is misunderstood as an "i"	Use "daily"
qhs	Nightly at bedtime	Mistaken as "qhr" or every hour	Use "nightly"
qn	Nightly or at bedtime	Mistaken as "qh" (every hour)	Use "nightly" or "at bedtime"
q.o.d. or QOD	Every other day	Mistaken as "q.d." (daily) or "q.i.d." (four times daily) if the "o" is poorly written	Use "every other day"
q1d	Daily	Mistaken as q.i.d. (four times daily)	Use "daily"
q6PM, etc.	Every evening at 6 PM	Mistaken as every 6 hours	Use "daily at 6 PM" or "6 PM daily"
SC, SQ, sub q	Subcutaneous	SC mistaken as SL (sublingual); SQ mistaken as "5 every"; the "q" in "sub q" has been mistaken as "every" (e.g., a heparin dose ordered "sub q 2 hours before surgery" misunderstood as every 2 hours before surgery)	Use "subcut" or "subcutaneously"
ss	Sliding scale (insulin) or ½ (apothecary)	Mistaken as "55"	Spell out "sliding scale"; use "one-half" or "½"
SSI	Sliding scale insulin	Mistaken as Strong Solution of Iodine (Lugol's)	Spell out "sliding scale (insulin)"
SSRI	Sliding scale regular insulin	Mistaken as selective-serotonin reuptake inhibitor	Spell out "sliding scale (insulin)"
T3	Tylenol with codeine No. 3	Mistaken as liothyronine	Use complete drug name
TAC	triamcinolone	Mistaken as tetracaine, Adrenalin, cocaine	Use complete drug name
TNK	TNKase	Mistaken as "TPA"	Use complete drug name

Symbol or Abbreviation	Intended Meaning	Potential Problem	Preferred Term
TIW or tiw	3 times a week	Mistaken as "3 times a day" or "twice in a week"	Use "3 times weekly"
U or u	Unit	Mistaken as the number 0 or 4, causing a 10-fold overdose or greater (e.g., 4U seen as "40" or 4u seen as "44"); mistaken as "cc" so dose given in volume instead of units (e.g., 4u seen as "4cc")	Use "unit"
x3d	For three days	Mistaken as "3 doses"	Use "for three days"
$ZnSO_4$	zinc sulfate	Mistaken as morphine sulfate	Use complete drug name
Trailing zero after decimal point (e.g., 1.0 mg)	1 mg	Mistaken as 10 mg if the decimal point is missed	Do not use trailing zeroes for doses expressed in whole numbers
No leading zero before a decimal dose (e.g., .5 mg)	0.5 mg	Mistaken as 5 mg if the decimal point is not seen	Use zero before a decimal point when the dose is less than a whole unit
Drug name and dose run together (especially problematic for drug names that end in "l" such as Inderal40 mg; Tegretol300 mg)	Inderal 40 mg Tegretol 300 mg	Mistaken as Inderal 140 mg Mistaken as Tegretol 1300 mg	Place adequate space between the drug name, dose, and unit of measure
Numerical dose and unit of measure run together (e.g., 10mg, 100mL)	10 mg 100 mL	The "m" is sometimes mistaken as a zero or two zeros, risking a 10- to 100-fold overdose	Place adequate space between the dose and unit of measure
Abbreviations such as mg. or mL., with a period after the abbreviation	mg mL	The period is unnecessary and could be mistaken as the number 1 if written poorly	Use mg, mL, etc. without a terminal period
Large doses without properly placed commas (e.g., 100000 units; 1000000 units)	100,000 units 1,000,000 units	100000 has been mistaken as "10,000" or "1,000,000"; 1000000 has been mistaken as "100,000"	Use commas for dosing units at or above 1,000, or use words such as 100 "thousand" or 1 "million" to improve readability

Data from Institute for Safe Medication Practices (2007). ISMP's list of error-prone abbreviations, symbols, and dose designations (www.ismp.org); and The Joint Commission (2005). The official "do not use" list (www.jointcommission.org).

B

APPENDIX

Communication Quick Reference for Spanish-Speaking Patients

The Body • El Cuerpo (ehl koo-EHR-poh)

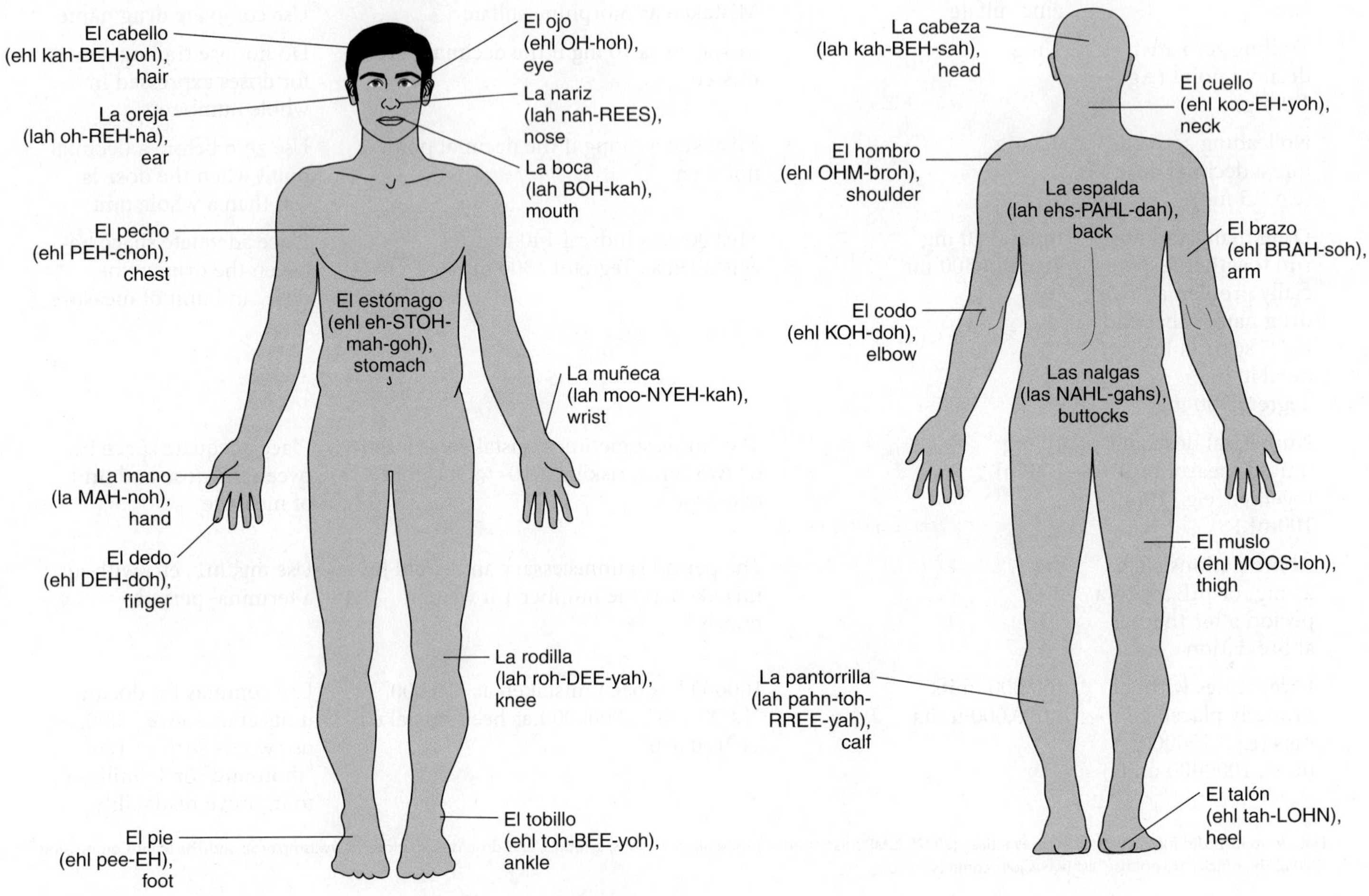

El cabello (ehl kah-BEH-yoh), hair
El ojo (ehl OH-hoh), eye
La oreja (lah oh-REH-ha), ear
La nariz (lah nah-REES), nose
La boca (lah BOH-kah), mouth
El pecho (ehl PEH-choh), chest
El estómago (ehl eh-STOH-mah-goh), stomach
La muñeca (lah moo-NYEH-kah), wrist
La mano (la MAH-noh), hand
El dedo (ehl DEH-doh), finger
La rodilla (lah roh-DEE-yah), knee
El tobillo (ehl toh-BEE-yoh), ankle
El pie (ehl pee-EH), foot
La cabeza (lah kah-BEH-sah), head
El cuello (ehl koo-EH-yoh), neck
El hombro (ehl OHM-broh), shoulder
La espalda (lah ehs-PAHL-dah), back
El brazo (ehl BRAH-soh), arm
El codo (ehl KOH-doh), elbow
Las nalgas (las NAHL-gahs), buttocks
El muslo (ehl MOOS-loh), thigh
La pantorrilla (lah pahn-toh-RREE-yah), calf
El talón (ehl tah-LOHN), heel

Common Instructions to Be Used with the Body Parts

Move the	Mueva	*(mooh-EH-bah)*
Touch the	Toque	*(TOH-keh)*
Point to the	Señale	*(seh-NYAH-leh)*

More Parts of the Body

Armpit	la axila	*(lah ahk-SEE-lah)*
Breasts	los senos	*(lohs SEH-nohs)*
Collarbone	la clavícula	*(lah klah-BEE-koo-lah)*
Diaphragm	el diafragma	*(ehl dee-ah-FRAH-mah)*
Forearm	el antebrazo	*(ehl ahn-teh-BRAH-soh)*
Groin	la ingle	*(lah EEN-gleh)*
Hip	la cadera	*(lah kah-DEH-rah)*

More Parts of the Body—cont'd

Kneecap	la rótula	*(lah ROH-too-lah)*
Nail	la uña	*(lah OO-nyah)*
Pelvis	la pelvis	*(lah PEHL-bees)*
Rectum	el recto	*(ehl REHK-toh)*
Rib	la costilla	*(lah kohs-TEE-yah)*
Spine	la espina dorsal	*(lah ehs-PEE-nah DOHR-sahl)*
Throat	la garganta	*(lah gahr-GAHN-tah)*
Tongue	le lengua	*(lah LEHN-goo-ah)*

Organs

Appendix	el apéndice	*(ehl ah-PEHN-dee-seh)*
Bladder	la vejiga	*(lah beh-HEE-gah)*
Brain	el cerebro	*(ehl seh-REH-broh)*
Colon	el colon	*(ehl KOH-lohn)*
Esophagus	el esófago	*(ehl eh-SOH-fah-goh)*
Gallbladder	la vesícula biliar	*(lah beh-SEE-koo-lah bee-lee-AHR)*
Genitals	los genitales	*(lohs heh-nee-TAH-lehs)*
Heart	el corazón	*(ehl koh-rah-SOHN)*
Kidney	el riñón	*(ehl ree-NYOHN)*
Large intestine	el intestino grueso	*(ehl een-tehs-TEE-noh groo-EH-so)*
Liver	el hígado	*(ehl EE-gah-doh)*
Lungs	los pulmones	*(lohs pool-MOH-nehs)*
Pancreas	el páncreas	*(ehl PAHN-kreh-ahs)*
Small intestine	el intestino delgado	*(ehl een-tehs-TEE-noh dehl-GAH-doh)*
Spleen	el bazo	*(ehl BAH-soh)*
Thyroid gland	la tiroides	*(lah tee-ROH-ee-dehs)*
Tonsils	las amígdalas	*(lahs ah-MEEG-dah-lahs)*
Uterus	el útero	*(ehl OO-teh-roh)*

Essential Phrases

Good morning.	Buenos días.	*Boo-EH-nohs DEE-ahs.*
Good afternoon.	Buenas tardes.	*Boo-EH-nahs TAHR-dehs.*
Good night.	Buenas noches.	*Boo-EH-nahs NOH-chehs.*
Hello.	Hola.	*OH-lah.*
How are you?	¿Cómo está?	*¿KOH-moh ehs-TAH?*
Good (Fine).	Bien.	*Bee-EHN.*
Bad, Better, Worse.	Mal, Mejor, Peor.	*Mahl, Meh-HOHR, Peh-OHR.*
The same.	Igual.	*Ee-GOO-ahl.*
Do you speak English?	¿Habla Inglés?	*¿AH-blah een-GLEHS?*
I don't understand.	No comprendo.	*Noh kom-PREHN-doh.*
Excuse me.	Discúlpeme.	*Dees-KOOL-peh-meh.*
Please speak slowly.	Por favor, hable más lento.	*Pohr fah-VOHR, AH-bleh mahs LEHN-toh.*
Are you in pain?	¿Está adolorido(a)?	*¿Ehs-TAH ah-doh-loh-REE-doh(dah)?*
Yes, No.	Sí, No.	*See, Noh.*
Tell me where it hurts.	Digame donde le duele.	*DEE-gah-meh DOHN-deh leh doo-EH-leh.*
Here, There.	Aquí, Ahi.	*Ah-KEE, Ah-EE.*

Description of Pain

Is your pain...	Tiene un dolor...	*Tee-EH-neh oon doh-LOHR...*
burning?	¿que arde?	*¿keh AHR-deh?*
constant?	¿constante?	*¿kohns-TAHN-teh?*
dull?	¿amortiguado?	*¿ah-MOHR-tee-goo-AH-doh?*
intermittent?	¿intermitente?	*¿een-tehr-mee-TEHN-teh?*
mild?	¿moderado?	*¿moh-deh-RAH-doh?*
severe?	¿muy fuerte?	*¿MOO-ee foo-EHR-teh?*
sharp?	¿agudo?	*¿ah-GOO-doh?*
throbbing?	¿pulsante?	*¿pool-SAHN-teh?*
worse?	¿peor?	*¿peh-OHR?*
Are you allergic to any medication?	¿Es usted alérgico(a) a algun medicamento?	*¿Ehs oos-TEHD ah-LEHR-hee-koh(kah) ah ahl-GOON meh-dee-kah-MEHN-toh?*
I'm here to help you.	Estoy aquí para ayudarle.	*Ehs-TOH-ee ah-KEE pah-rah ah-yoo-DAHR-leh.*
Calm down.	Cálmese.	*KAHL-meh-seh.*
Please.	Por favor.	*Pohr fah-VOHR.*
Thank you.	Gracias.	*GRAH-see-ahs.*
You're welcome.	De nada.	*Deh NAH-dah.*
May I?	¿Puedo?	*¿Poo-EH-doh?*
Who, What, When, Where?	¿Quién, Qué, Cuándo, Dónde?	*¿Kee-EHN, Keh, Koo-AHN-doh, DOHN-deh?*
Zero, One, Two, Three, Four	Cero, Uno, Dos, Tres, Cuatro	*SEH-roh, OO-noh, dohs, trehs, koo-AH-troh*
Five, Six, Seven, Eight, Nine, Ten	Cinco, Seis, Siete, Ocho, Nueve, Diez	*SEEN-koh, SEH-ees, see-EH-teh, OH-choh, noo-EH-beh, dee-EHS*

Preliminary Examination

My name is __, and I am your nurse.	Me llamo __, y soy su enfermera(o).	*Meh YAH-moh ___, ee SOH-ee soo ehn-fehr-MEH-rah(roh).*
I'm going to...	Le voy a...	*Leh VOH-ee ah...*
take your vital signs.	tomar los signos vitales.	*toh-MAHR lohs SEEG-nohs vee-TAH-lehs.*
weigh you.	pesar.	*peh-SAHR.*
take your blood pressure.	tomar la presión.	*toh-MAHR lah preh-see-OHN.*
Extend your arm and relax.	Extienda su brazo y descánselo.	*Ehks-tee-EHN-dah soo BRAH-soh ee dehs-KAHN-seh-loh.*
I'm going to take your...	Le voy a tomar...	*Leh voy ah toh-MAHR...*
pulse.	el pulso.	*ehl POOL-soh.*
temperature.	su temperatura.	*soo tehm-peh-rah-TOO-rah.*
I'm going to count your respirations.	Voy a contar sus respiraciones.	*VOH-ee ah kohn-TAHR soos rehs-pee-rah-see-OH-nehs.*

Obtaining a Blood Sample

I need to draw a blood sample.	Necesito tomar una muestra de la sangre.	*Neh-seh-SEE-toh toh-MAHR OO-nah moo-EHS-trah deh lah SAHN-greh.*
Please give me your arm.	Por favor, déme el brazo.	*Pohr fah-VOHR, DEH-meh ehl BRAH-soh.*
It may cause a little discomfort.	Le puede causar alguna molestia.	*Leh poo-EH-deh kah-OO-sahr ahl-GOO-nah moh-LEHS-tee-ah.*
I am going to put a tourniquet around your arm.	Le voy a poner una liga alrededor del brazo.	*Leh VOH-ee ah poh-NEHR OO-nah LEE-gah ahl-reh-deh-DOHR dehl BRAH-soh.*
I am going to draw blood from this vein.	Voy a sacar la sangre de esta vena.	*VOH-ee ah sah-KAHR lah SAHN-greh deh EHS-tah VEH-nah.*

Obtaining Blood from a Finger Stick

I need to take a few drops of blood from your finger.	Necesito sacar unas gotas de sangre de uno de sus dedos.	*Neh-seh-SEE-toh sah-KAHR OO-nahs GOH-tahs deh SAHN-greh deh OO-noh deh soos DEH-dohs.*

Obtaining a Urine Sample

We also need a urine sample.	También necesitamos una muestra de la orina.	*Tahm-bee-EHN neh-seh-see-TAH-mohs OO-nah moo-EHS-trah deh lah oh-REE-nah.*
It has to be from the middle of the stream.	Tiene que ser de la mitad del chorro.	*Tee-EH-neh keh sehr deh lah mee-TAHD dehl CHOH-rroh.*
Put the urine in this cup.	Ponga la orina en esta tasa.	*POHN-gah lah oh-REE-nah ehn EHS-tah TAH-sah.*

Obtaining a Stool Specimen

I need a sample of your stool.	Necesito una muestra de su excremento.	*Neh-seh-SEE-toh OO-nah moo-EHS-trah deh soo ehks-kreh-MEN-toh.*
Please put a small amount in this cup.	Por favor ponga un poco en esta tasa.	*Pohr fa-VOHR POHN-gah oon POH-koh ehn EHS-tah TAH-sah.*

Obtaining a Sputum Specimen

I need a sample of your sputum.	Necesito una muestra de su esputo.	*Neh-seh-SEE-toh OO-nah moo-EHS-trah deh soo ehs-POO-toh.*
Please spit in this cup.	Por favor, escupa en este vaso.	*Pohr fah-VOHR, ehs-KOO-pah ehn EHS-teh VAH-soh.*

Orders

You need…	Necesita…	*Neh-seh-SEE-tah…*
a bandage.	un vendaje.	*oon behn-DAH-heh.*
a blood transfusion.	una transfusión de sangre.	*OO-nah trahns-foo-see-OHN deh SAHN-greh.*
a cast.	una molde de yeso.	*OO-nah MOHL-deh deh YEH-soh.*
gauze.	la gasa.	*lah GAH-sah.*
intensive care.	cuidado intensivo.	*koo-ee-DAH-doh een-tehn-SEE-boh.*
intravenous fluids.	líquidos intravenosos.	*LEE-kee-dohs een-trah-beh-NOH-sohs.*
an operation.	una operación.	*OO-nah oh-peh-rah-see-OHN.*
physical therapy.	terapia física.	*teh-RAH-pee-ah FEE-see-kah.*
a shot.	una inyección.	*OO-nah een-yehk-see-OHN.*
x-rays.	rayos equis.	*RAH-yohs EH-kees.*
We're going to...	Vamos a...	*VAH-mohs ah...*
change the bandage.	cambiarle el vendaje.	*kahm-bee-AHR-leh ehl behn-DAH-heh.*
give you a bath.	darle un baño.	*DAHR-leh oon BAH-nyoh.*
take out the I.V.	sacarle el tubo intravenoso.	*sah-KAHR-leh ehl TOO-boh een-trah-beh-NOH-soh.*

Description of Tubes

The tube in your...	El tubo en su...	*Ehl TOO-boh ehn soo...*
arm is for I.V. fluids.	brazo es para líquidos intravenosos.	*BRAH-soh ehs PAH-rah LEE-kee-dohs een-trah-beh-NOH-sohs.*
bladder is for urinating.	vejiga es para orinar.	*beh-HEE-gah ehs PAH-rah oh-ree-NAHR.*
stomach is for the food.	estómago es para los alimentos.	*ehs-TOH-mah-goh ehs PAH-rah lohs ah-lee-MEN-tohs.*
throat is for breathing.	garganta es para respirar.	*gahr-GAHN-tah ehs PAH-rah rehs-pee-RAHR.*

Glossary

A

A delta fiber Myelinated fiber found primarily in the skin and muscle; carries rapid, sharp, pricking, or piercing sensations that can generally be localized to a well-defined area; also called "mechanical nociceptor."

abdominoperineal (AP) resection The surgical removal of the sigmoid colon, rectum, and anus through combined abdominal and perineal incisions. This resection is performed when rectal tumors are present.

ablative The process or act of removing.

abscess A localized collection of pus caused by an inflammatory response to bacteria in tissues or organs.

absence seizure A type of generalized seizure consisting of brief periods of loss of consciousness and blank staring, as if day-dreaming. The patient returns to baseline immediately after the seizure. This type is more common in children and tends to run in families. Left untreated, seizures may occur frequently throughout the day, interfering with daily life.

absolute neutrophil count (ANC) The percentage and actual number of mature circulating neutrophils; used to measure a patient's risk for infection. The higher the numbers, the greater the resistance to infection.

absorbable suture A type of suture digested over time by body enzymes.

absorption The uptake from the intestinal lumen of nutrients produced by digestion.

abstinence syndrome Symptoms that occur when a patient who is physically dependent on opioids abruptly ceases using them. Slowly tapering (weaning) the drug dosage lessens or alleviates the physical withdrawal symptoms in a patient who is opioid dependent.

acalculia Difficulty with math calculations; caused by brain injury or disease.

acalculous cholecystitis Inflammation of the gallbladder occurring in the absence of gallstones; typically associated with biliary stasis caused by any condition that affects the regular filling or emptying of the gallbladder.

acceleration-deceleration Forces involved in high-speed crashes or falls from a great height; produce injury by tearing, shearing, and compressing anatomic structures.

acclimatization The process of adapting to a high altitude; involves physiologic changes that help the body compensate for less available oxygen in the atmosphere.

accommodation The process of maintaining a clear visual image when the gaze is shifted from a distant object to a near object. The eye adjusts its focus by changing the curvature of the lens.

achalasia An esophageal motility disorder believed to result from esophageal denervation; involves a failure to relax the smooth muscle fibers of the gastrointestinal tract and characterized by chronic and progressive dysphagia. The term is typically used to refer to failure of the lower esophageal sphincter to relax properly with swallowing and to the replacement of normal peristalsis of the esophagus with abnormal contractions.

achlorhydria The absence of hydrochloric acid from gastric secretions.

acid A substance that releases hydrogen ions when dissolved in water. The strength of an acid is measured by how easily it releases hydrogen ions in solution.

acidosis An acid-base imbalance in which blood pH is below normal.

acinus The structural unit of the lower respiratory tract consisting of a respiratory bronchiole, an alveolar duct, and an alveolar sac.

acorn cardiac support device A polyester mesh jacket that is placed over the ventricles to provide support and avoid overstretching the myocardial muscle in the patient with heart failure; reduces heart muscle hypertrophy and assists with improvement of ejection fraction.

acoustic neuroma A benign tumor of cranial nerve VIII; symptoms include damage to hearing, facial movements, and sensation. The tumor can enlarge into the brain, damaging structures in the cerebellum.

activated protein C An enzyme that helps prevent inappropriate clot formation. It is activated when it binds to healthy endothelial cells of the blood vessels; reduced levels are an indicator of sepsis and septic shock.

active euthanasia Purposeful action that directly causes death; not supported by most professional organizations, including the American Nurses Association.

active immunity Resistance to infection that occurs when the body responds to an invading antigen by making specific antibodies against the antigen. Immunity lasts for years and is natural by infection or artificial by stimulation (e.g., vaccine) of the body's immune defenses.

activities of daily living (ADLs) The activities performed in the course of a normal day, such as bathing, dressing, feeding, and ambulating.

activity therapist A member of the rehabilitation health care team who works to help patients continue or develop hobbies or interests; also called "recreational therapist."

acupoint One of the specific areas for acupressure and acupuncture located on meridians throughout the body.

acupressure A traditional Chinese medicine therapy in which the fingers are used to press certain points on the body to increase the flow of energy and promote the body's self-healing ability.

acupuncture A traditional Chinese medicine therapy in which tiny needles are inserted into the skin and subcutaneous tissues at certain areas of the body to deliver manual vibration or electrical stimulation.

acute Having relatively greater intensity; marked by a sudden onset and short duration.

acute adrenal insufficiency A life-threatening event in which the need for cortisol and aldosterone is greater than the available supply; also called "Addisonian crisis."

acute arterial occlusions The sudden blockage of an artery, typically in the lower extremities, in the patient with chronic peripheral arterial disease.

acute compartment syndrome (ACS) A complication of a fracture characterized by increased pressure within one or more compartments and causing massive compromise of circulation to the area. Compartments are sheaths of inelastic fascia that support and partition muscles, blood vessels, and nerves in the body.

acute coronary syndrome (ACS) A disorder, including unstable angina and myocardial infarction that results from obstruction of the coronary artery by ruptured atherosclerotic plaque and leads to platelet aggregation, thrombus formation, and vasoconstriction.

acute gastritis Inflammation of the gastric mucosa or submucosa after exposure to local irritants. Various degrees of mucosal necrosis and inflammatory reaction occur in acute disease. Complete regeneration and healing usually occur within a few days.

acute hematogenous infection An infection resulting from bacteremia, disease, or nonpenetrating trauma that is disseminated by the blood through the circulation.

acute pain The unpleasant sensory and emotional experience associated with tissue damage that results from acute injury, disease, or surgery.

acute pancreatitis A serious inflammation of the pancreas characterized by a sudden onset of abdominal pain, nausea, and vomiting. It is caused by premature activation of pancreatic enzymes that destroy ductal tissue and pancreatic cells and results in autodigestion and fibrosis of the pancreas.

acute paronychia Inflammation of the skin around the nail, which usually occurs with a torn cuticle or an ingrown toenail.

acute pericarditis An inflammation or alteration of the pericardium, the membranous sac that encloses the heart; may be fibrous, serous, hemorrhagic, purulent, or neoplastic.

acute pyelonephritis Active bacterial infection in the kidney.

acute renal failure A rapid decrease in kidney function that leads to the accumulation of metabolic wastes in the body. It is caused by inadequate kidney perfusion; damage to the glomeruli, interstitial tissue, or tubules; or obstructed urine flow. It can progress to end-stage kidney disease in patients with chronic renal insufficiency.

acute respiratory distress syndrome (ARDS) Respiratory failure marked by hypoxemia that persists even when 100% oxygen is given, as well as decreased pulmonary compliance, dyspnea, noncardiac-associated bilateral pulmonary edema, and dense pulmonary infiltrates on x-ray.

acute sialadenitis Inflammation of a salivary gland; can be caused by infectious agents, irradiation, or immunologic disorders.

adaptive immunity The immunity that a person's body makes (or can receive) as an adaptive response to invasion by organisms or foreign proteins; occurs either naturally or artificially through lymphocyte responses and can be either active or passive.

adaptive mechanism The means of producing compensation; also called "compensatory mechanism."

addiction A primary, chronic neurobiologic disease characterized by impaired control over drug use, compulsive use, continued use despite harm, and craving.

Addisonian crisis Acute adrenal insufficiency; a life-threatening event in which the need for cortisol and aldosterone is greater than the available supply.

additive In pharmacology, a drug that adds an effect, either harmful or beneficial, when given with another drug.

adenocarcinoma Tumors that arise from the glandular epithelial tissue.

adenohypophysis The anterior lobe of the pituitary gland, which makes up about 70% of the gland.

adiponectin An anti-inflammatory and insulin sensitizing hormone.

adipose Fatty.

adjuvant A substance that aids another substance, such as a cancer treatment that uses chemotherapy in addition to surgery.

adjuvant drug Drug used to relieve pain either alone or in combination with an analgesic to enhance the effectiveness of the analgesic.

adjuvant therapy Chemotherapy that is used along with surgery or radiation.

adrenal crisis Acute adrenocortical insufficiency, which can be life threatening.

adrenal Cushing's disease An excess of glucocorticoids caused by a problem in the adrenal cortex, usually a benign tumor (adrenal adenoma). This usually occurs in only one adrenal gland.

adrenal steroid Any of the hormones produced and secreted by the adrenal cortex; also called "corticosteroid."

advance directive A written document prepared by a competent person to specify what, if any, extraordinary actions he or she would want when no longer able to make decisions about personal health care.

adverse drug event (ADE) An unintended harmful reaction to an administered drug.

aerophagia The excessive swallowing of air.

aerosolization Transmission via fine airborne droplets.

aesthetic plastic surgery Plastic surgery that is cosmetic and aims to alter a person's physical appearance.

afferent arteriole The smallest, most distal portion of the renal arterial system that supplies blood to the nephron. From the afferent arteriole, blood flows into the glomerulus, a series of specialized capillary loops.

afferent loop syndrome Chronic partial obstruction of the duodenal loop after partial gastrectomy and gastrojejunostomy, resulting in abdominal bloating and pain after eating; often followed by nausea and vomiting.

afterdrop A continued decrease in core body temperature after a victim is removed from a cold environment; results from equilibration of core and peripheral blood temperature and counter-current cooling of the blood perfusing cold tissue.

afterload The pressure or resistance that the ventricles must overcome to eject blood through the semilunar valves and into the peripheral blood vessels; the amount of resistance is directly related to arterial blood pressure and blood vessel diameter.

agglutination A clumping action that results during the antibody-binding process when antibodies link antigens together to form large and small immune complexes.

aggregation Clumping together.

agnosia A general term for a loss of sensory comprehension; may include an inability to write, comprehend reading material, or use an object correctly.

agraphia Loss of the ability to write; caused by brain injury or disease.

Airborne Precautions Infection control guidelines from the Centers for Disease Control and Prevention; used for patients with infections spread by the airborne transmission route, such as tuberculosis. Negative airflow rooms are required to prevent the airborne spread of microbes.

akinesia Slow or no movement, as seen in a patient with Parkinson disease; also called "bradykinesia."

alanine aminotransferase (ALT) An enzyme found in the liver. Levels of this enzyme are elevated in patients with liver disease, infectious mononucleosis, and other disorders.

albuminuria The presence of albumin in the urine.

alcohol abuse A condition in which a person has problems related to alcohol use but does not have a strong craving for alcohol, loss of control, or physical dependence.

alcoholic hepatitis Liver inflammation caused by the toxic effect of alcohol on hepatocytes. The liver becomes enlarged, with cellular degeneration and infiltration by fat, leukocytes, and lymphocytes.

alcoholism A disease in which a person has a strong need or compulsion to consume alcohol, is unable to quit once he or she begins drinking, experiences a physical dependence, and needs to increase the amount of alcohol to get "high."

aldosterone The chief mineralocorticoid produced by the adrenal cortex. Aldosterone increases kidney reabsorption of sodium and water, thus restoring blood pressure, blood volume, and blood sodium levels. Aldosterone secretion is regulated by the renin-angiotensin system, serum potassium ion concentration, and adrenocorticotropic hormone.

alert Awake and responsive to stimulation.

alexia Problems understanding written language; caused by brain injury or disease.

alkaline reflux gastropathy A complication of gastric surgery in which the pylorus is bypassed or removed. Endoscopic examination reveals regurgitated bile in the stomach and mucosal hyperemia. Symptoms include early satiety, abdominal discomfort, and vomiting; also called "bile reflux gastropathy."

alkalosis An acid-base imbalance in which blood pH is above normal.

allele An alternate form (or variation) of a gene.

allergen A foreign protein that is capable of causing a hypersensitivity response, or allergy, that ranges from uncomfortable (itchy, watery eyes or sneezing) to life threatening (allergic asthma, anaphylaxis, bronchoconstriction, or circulatory collapse); causes a release of natural chemicals, such as histamine, in the body.

allergy An increased or excessive response to the presence of a foreign protein or allergen (antigen) to which the patient has been previously exposed.

allogenic Having cell types that are antigenically distinct; for example, bone marrow transplantation in which the patient receives bone marrow or peripheral blood taken from a healthy donor. Compare with autologous bone marrow transplantation, in which patients receive their own cells, which were collected earlier.

allogenic bone marrow transplantation The transplantation of bone marrow from a sibling.

allogenic transplant Type of bone marrow transplant in which a closely HLA-matched sibling or an unrelated but matched donor provides the stem cells.

allograft A graft of tissue or bone between individuals of the same species but a different genotype; the donor may be a cadaver or a living person, either related or unrelated; also called "homograft."

alopecia Hair loss.

alveolitis Inflammation of the alveoli.

Alzheimer's disease (AD) A chronic, progressive, degenerative disease that accounts for 60% of the dementias occurring in people older than 65 years of age; characterized by loss of memory, judgment, and visuospatial perception and by a change in personality. Over time, the patient becomes increasingly cognitively impaired. Severe physical deterioration takes place, and death occurs as a result of complications of immobility; also called "dementia, Alzheimer type."

amaurosis fugax A transient, brief episode of blindness in one eye.

ambulatory A term that refers to a patient who goes to the hospital or physician's office and returns home on the same day.

ambulatory aid Assistive device such as a cane or a walker.

ambulatory pump Infusion therapy pump generally used with a home care patient to allow a return to his or her usual activities while receiving infusion therapy.

amebic hepatic abscess A liver abscess caused by the protozoan *Entamoeba histolytica;* may occur after amebic dysentery and usually occurs as a single abscess in the right hepatic lobe.

amenorrhea The absence of menstrual periods in women.

amnesia Loss of memory.

amputation The removal of a limb or other appendage of the body.

amyotrophic lateral sclerosis (ALS) A progressive and degenerative disease of the motor system that is characterized by atrophy of the hands, forearms, and legs and results in paralysis and death. There is no known cause, no cure, no specific treatment, no standard pattern of progression, and no method of prevention; also called "Lou Gehrig's disease."

anabolic hormone A hormone that stimulates growth.

anabolic steroids Synthetic substances that mimic the actions of testosterone. Prescribed for people with hormonal difficulties such as delayed puberty or impotence and misused by athletes to increase strength and performance.

anaerobic Lacking adequate oxygen.

anaerobic cellular metabolism Metabolism without oxygen.

anal fissure A painful ulcer at the margin of the anus.

analgesia Pain relief or pain suppression.

analgesia team Team typically consisting of one or more nurses, pharmacists, case managers, and physicians who consult with staff and prescribers on how best to control the patient's pain; also called "multidisciplinary pain team."

anaphylaxis The widespread reaction that occurs in response to contact with a substance to which the person has a severe allergy (antigen); characterized by blood vessel and bronchiolar smooth muscle involvement causing widespread blood vessel dilation, decreased cardiac output, and bronchoconstriction; results in cell damage and the release of large amounts of histamine, severe hypovolemia, vascular collapse, decreased cardiac contraction, and dysrhythmias and causes extreme whole-body hypoxia.

anasarca Generalized edema.

anastomosis Surgical reattachment; also a general term meaning a connection.

anatomic dead space Places in which air flows but the structures are too thick for gas exchange.

androgen Any substance, such as testosterone, that promotes masculinization; male hormones.

anemia A clinical sign of some abnormal condition related to a reduction in one of the following: number of red blood cells, amount of hemoglobin, or hematocrit (percentage of packed red blood cells per deciliter of blood).

anergy The inability to mount an immune response to an antigen.

anesthesia An induced state of partial or total loss of sensation with or without loss of consciousness.

anesthetic Characterized by loss of sensation.
aneuploid An abnormal karyotype with more or fewer than 23 pairs of chromosomes.
aneurysm A permanent localized dilation of an artery (to at least two times its normal diameter) that forms when the middle layer (media) of the artery is weakened, stretching the inner (intima) and outer (adventitia) layers. As the artery widens, tension in the wall increases and further widening occurs, thus enlarging the aneurysm.
aneurysmectomy A surgical procedure performed to excise an aneurysm.
angina pectoris Literally, "strangling of the chest"; a temporary imbalance between the ability of the coronary arteries to supply oxygen and the demand for oxygen by the cardiac muscle. As a result, the patient experiences chest discomfort.
angioedema Diffuse swelling resulting from a vascular reaction in the deep tissues; can occur in a patient having an anaphylactic reaction.
angle-closure glaucoma A form of glaucoma characterized by a narrowed angle and forward displacement of the iris so that movement of the iris against the cornea narrows or closes the chamber angle, obstructing the outflow of aqueous humor. It can have a sudden onset and is an emergency; also called "closed-angle glaucoma," "narrow-angle glaucoma," or "acute glaucoma."
anion Ion that has a negative charge.
anisocoria A difference in the size of the pupils.
ankle-brachial index (ABI) A ratio derived by dividing the ankle blood pressure by the brachial blood pressure; this calculation is used to assess the vascular status of the lower extremities. To obtain the ABI, a blood pressure cuff is applied to the lower extremities just above the malleoli. The systolic pressure is measured by Doppler ultrasound at both the dorsalis pedis and posterior tibial pulses. The higher of these two pressures is then divided by the higher of the two brachial pulses.
ankylosing spondylitis A form of rheumatoid arthritis that affects the vertebral column and causes spinal deformities.
anomia Inability to find words.
anorectal abscess A localized induration and fluctuance that is caused by inflammation of the soft tissue near the rectum or anus and is most often the result of obstruction of the ducts of glands in the anorectal region by feces, foreign bodies, or trauma.
anorectic drugs Drugs that suppress appetite, which reduces food intake and over time may result in weight loss; may be prescribed for obese patients in a comprehensive weight reduction program.
anorexia The loss of appetite for food.
anorexia nervosa An eating disorder of self-induced starvation resulting from a fear of fatness, even though the patient is underweight.
anorexin Neuropeptide that decreases appetite.
anoxic Completely lacking oxygen.
antalgic gait A term that refers to an abnormality in the stance phase of gait. When part of one leg is painful, the person shortens the stance phase on the affected side.
anterior colporrhaphy Surgery for severe symptoms of cystocele in which the pelvic muscles are tightened for better bladder support.
anterior cord syndrome A condition caused by cervical injuries; results from damage to the anterior portion of both the gray and white matter of the spinal cord, usually as a result of decreased blood supply. Motor function and pain and temperature sensation are lost below the level of injury, but the sensations of touch, position, and vibration remain intact.
anterior nares The nostrils or external openings into the nasal cavities.
antibody-mediated immune system The defense response that produces antibodies directed against certain pathogens. The antibodies inactivate the pathogens and protect against future infection from that microorganism.
anticoagulant Something that limits blood clot formation.
antidepressants A group of drugs that help manage clinical depression.
antiepileptic drugs (AEDs) A class of drugs used to control seizures; also called "anticonvulsants."
antigen A foreign protein or allergen that is capable of causing an immune response; protein on the surface of a cell.
antiplatelet agents Drugs that destroy blood platelets.
anuria Complete lack of urine output; usually defined as less than 100 mL/24 hr.
anuric Characterized by anuria (complete lack of urine output).
aortic regurgitation The flow of blood from the aorta back into the left ventricle during diastole; occurs when the aortic valve leaflets do not close properly during diastole and the annulus (the valve ring that attaches to the leaflets) is dilated or deformed.
aortic stenosis Narrowing of the aortic valve orifice and obstruction of left ventricular outflow during systole.
aortic valve The semilunar valve of the heart that separates the left ventricle from the aorta.
aphasia Inability to use or comprehend spoken or written language due to brain injury or disease.
aphonia Inability to produce sound; complete but temporary loss of the voice.
aphthous stomatitis Noninfectious stomatitis.
apical impulse The pulse located at the left fifth intercostal space in the midclavicular line in the mitral area (the apex of the heart); also called the "point of maximal impulse."
aplastic anemia A deficiency of circulating red blood cells because of failure of the bone marrow to produce these cells; usually occurs with leukopenia and thrombocytopenia.
apolipoprotein E One of several regulators of lipoprotein metabolism.
apoptosis Programmed cell death that occurs when deoxyribonucleic acid in the telomere is gone and the chromosomes unravel.
appendectomy Surgical removal of the inflamed appendix.
appendicitis Acute inflammation of the vermiform appendix, which is the blind pouch attached to the cecum of the colon, which is usually located in the right iliac region just below the ileocecal valve.
approximated In a clean laceration or a surgical incision to be closed with sutures or staples, the act of bringing together the wound edges with the skin layers lined up in correct anatomic position so they can be held in place until healing is complete.
apraxia The loss of the ability to carry out a purposeful motor activity.
aqueous humor The clear, watery fluid that is continually produced by the ciliary processes and fills the anterior and posterior chambers of the eye. This fluid drains through the canal of Schlemm into the blood to maintain balanced intraocular pressure (pressure within the eye).

arcus senilis An opaque ring within the outer edge of the cornea caused by fat deposits. Its presence does not affect vision.

areflexic bladder Urinary retention and overflow (dribbling) caused by injuries to the lower motor neuron at the spinal cord level of S2 to S4 (e.g., multiple sclerosis and spinal cord injury below T12). Bladder emptying may be achieved by performing a Valsalva maneuver or tightening the abdominal muscles. The effectiveness of these maneuvers should be ascertained by catheterizing the client for residual urine after voiding. Also called "flaccid bladder."

aromatherapy A complementary therapy that uses essential oils obtained from plants; may be applied in compresses, used in baths, or applied topically to the skin.

arrhythmogenic right ventricular cardiomyopathy (dysplasia) A form of cardiomyopathy that results from the replacement of myocardial tissue with fibrous and fatty tissue.

arterial revascularization The surgical procedure most commonly used to increase arterial blood flow in the affected limb of a patient with peripheral arterial disease.

arterial ulcers A painful complication in the patient with peripheral arterial disease. Typically, the ulcer is small and round, with a "punched out" appearance and well-defined borders. Ulcers develop on the toes (often the great toe), between the toes, or on the upper aspect of the foot. With prolonged occlusion, the toes can become gangrenous.

arteriography Angiography of the arterial vessels; this invasive diagnostic procedure involves fluoroscopy and the use of contrast media and is performed when an arterial obstruction, narrowing, or aneurysm is suspected.

arteriosclerosis A thickening, or hardening, of the arterial wall.

arteriotomy A surgical opening into an artery.

arteriovenous malformation (AVM) An abnormality that occurs during embryonic development, resulting in a tangled mass of malformed, thin-walled, dilated vessels. The congenital absence of a capillary network in these vessels forms an abnormal communication between the arterial and venous systems and increases the risk that the vessels may rupture, causing bleeding into the subarachnoid space or into the intracerebral tissue. In the absence of the capillary network, the thin-walled veins are subjected to arterial pressure.

arteritis Inflammation of arterial walls.

arthralgia Pain in a joint.

arthritis Inflammation of one or more joints.

arthrodesis The surgical fusion of a joint.

arthrogram An x-ray study of a joint after contrast medium (air or solution) has been injected to enhance its visualization.

arthroscopy Examination of the interior of a joint with an arthroscope (a fiberoptic tube).

articulations Joint surfaces.

artifact In the electrocardiogram, interference that is seen on the monitor or rhythm strip and may look like a wandering or fuzzy baseline; can be caused by patient movement, loose or defective electrodes, improper grounding, or faulty equipment.

ascending paralysis Paralysis that begins in the legs and spreads to the arms and upper body.

ascending tracts Groups of nerves that originate in the spinal cord and end in the brain.

ascites The accumulation of free fluid within the peritoneal cavity. Increased hydrostatic pressure from portal hypertension causes this fluid to leak into the peritoneal cavity.

aseptic meningitis A type of meningitis that often occurs after viral illnesses such as measles, herpes simplex, coxsackievirus, and echovirus and is marked by inflammation over the cerebral cortex, white matter, and meninges. The formation of exudate (common in bacterial meningitis) does not occur, and no organisms are obtained from the cerebrospinal fluid. Also called "viral meningitis."

ASKED Model of Cultural Competence created by Dr. Josie Campinha-Bacote that provides a beginning self-assessment tool for cultural competence.

aspartate aminotransferase (AST) An enzyme found in the liver. Levels of this enzyme are elevated in patients with liver disorders and are highest in conditions that cause necrosis, such as severe viral hepatitis.

assistive/adaptive device Any item that enables the patient to perform all or part of an activity independently.

asterixis A coarse tremor characterized by rapid, nonrhythmic extensions and flexions in the wrists and fingers; a motor disturbance seen in portal-systemic encephalopathy; also called a "liver flap" or "flapping tremor."

astigmatism A refractive error caused by unevenly curved surfaces on or in the eye (especially of the cornea) that distort vision.

asynchronous (fixed-rate) pacing mode The mode of temporary cardiac pacing in which the pulse generator does not sense any intrinsic beats of the patient but fires at a fixed rate, regardless of the intrinsic rhythm. Used when the patient is asystolic or profoundly bradycardic, as may occur after open-heart surgery.

ataxia Gait disturbance or loss of balance.

atelectasis Collapse of alveoli.

atherectomy An invasive nonsurgical technique in which a high-speed, rotating metal burr uses fine abrasive bits to scrape plaque from inside an artery while minimizing damage to the vessel surface.

atherosclerosis A type of arteriosclerosis that involves the formation of plaque within the arterial wall; the leading contributor to coronary artery and cerebrovascular disease.

Atkins pyramid A food pyramid based on the Atkins diet that emphasizes building the diet on protein sources and vegetables rather than on grains, fruits, and vegetables, such as in the pyramid approved by the U.S. Department of Agriculture.

atonic (akinetic) seizure A type of generalized seizure characterized by a sudden loss of muscle tone that lasts for seconds and is followed by postictal confusion. These seizures usually cause the patient to fall, which may result in injury.

atresia Congenital absence of a normal body orifice or tubular organ, such as the ear canal.

atrial fibrillation (AF) A cardiac dysrhythmia in which multiple rapid impulses from many atrial foci, at a rate of 350 to 600 times per minute, depolarize the atria in a totally disorganized manner, with no P waves, no atrial contractions, a loss of the atrial kick, and an irregular ventricular response.

atrial flutter A cardiac dysrhythmia that involves rapid atrial depolarization and occurs at a rate of 250 to 350 times per minute.

atrial gallop An abnormal fourth heart sound that occurs as blood enters the ventricles during the active filling phase at the end of ventricular diastole; may be heard in patients with hypertension, anemia, ventricular hypertrophy, myocardial infarction, aortic or pulmonic stenosis, and pulmonary emboli.

atrial overdrive pacing A type of pacing that may be used to terminate symptomatic tachydysrhythmias such as atrial flutter or atrial fibrillation. Overdrive pacing is accomplished by rapidly pacing the atrium to capture the heart and control depolarization and is followed by no pacing in the hope that the sinus node will regain control of the heart.

atrioventricular (AV) block The delay or blockage of supraventricular impulses in the atrioventricular node or intraventricular conduction system; usually classified as first-, second-, or third-degree block. Conduction may be transiently or permanently abnormal.

atrioventricular (AV) junction In the cardiac conduction system, the area consisting of a transitional cell zone, the atrioventricular (AV) node itself, and the bundle of His. The AV node lies just beneath the right atrial endocardium, between the tricuspid valve and the ostium of the coronary sinus.

at-risk drinking Drinking behavior in which five or more alcoholic beverages for men (four or more for women) are consumed.

atrophic gastritis A type of chronic gastritis that is seen most often in older adults. It can occur after exposure to toxic substances in the workplace (e.g., benzene, lead, and nickel) or *Helicobacter pylori* infection, or it can be related to autoimmune factors.

attenuated The quality of making a substance weaker; for example, antigens that are used to make vaccines are specially processed to make them less likely to grow in the body.

atypical angina Angina that manifests itself as indigestion, pain between the shoulders, an aching jaw, or a choking sensation that occurs with exertion. Many women experience atypical angina.

atypical migraine The least common of the three types of migraine headaches, after migraines with aura and migraines without aura; the atypical category includes menstrual and cluster migraines.

audiogram The graphic record of the results of pure-tone audiometry.

audiometer An electronic device that produces pure tones at various frequencies; used in determining hearing acuity.

aura A sensation that signals the onset of a headache or seizure; the patient may experience visual changes, flashing lights, or double vision.

autoamputation of the distal digits A condition in which the tips of the digits fall off spontaneously; can occur in severe cases of Raynaud's phenomenon.

autocontamination The occurrence of infection in which the patient's own normal flora overgrows and penetrates the internal environment.

autodigestion Self-digestion. Specifically, the process of the stomach digesting itself if there is a break in its protective mucosal barrier.

autologous blood transfusion Reinfusing the patient's own blood during surgery.

autologous donation The donation of a patient's own blood before scheduled surgery to eliminate transfusion reactions and reduce the risk of bloodborne disease.

autologous transplant A type of bone marrow transplant in which patients receive their own stem cells, which were collected before high-dose therapy.

autolysis The spontaneous disintegration of tissue by the action of the patient's own cellular enzymes.

automaticity The ability of a cell to initiate an impulse spontaneously and repetitively; in cardiac electrophysiology, the ability of primary pacemaker cells (SA node, AV junction) to generate an electrical impulse.

automatism Behavior of which the patient is not aware and which is not under the patient's control, such as lip smacking or picking at clothes; occurs in some types of seizure disorders.

autonomic dysreflexia A syndrome that affects the patient with an upper spinal cord injury; characterized by severe hypertension and headache, bradycardia, nasal stuffiness, and flushing; caused by a noxious stimulus, usually a distended bladder or constipation. This is a neurologic emergency and must be promptly treated to prevent a hypertensive brain attack.

autonomic nervous system (ANS) The part of the nervous system that is not under conscious control; consists of the sympathetic nervous system and the parasympathetic nervous system.

autoregulation The tendency of an organ or system to maintain blood flow at a fairly constant rate by dilating or constricting arteries in response to changes in blood pressure, carbon dioxide tension, and oxygen tension.

autosome Any of the 22 pairs of human chromosomes containing genes that code for all the structures and regulatory proteins needed for normal function but do not code for the sexual differentiation of a person.

avascular Lacking a blood supply.

avascular necrosis (AVN) The death of bone tissue, usually because the blood supply to the bone is disrupted. It is usually a complication of a hip fracture or any fracture in which there is displacement of bone; also called "osteonecrosis."

axial loading A mechanism of injury that involves vertical compression. An example is a diving accident, in which the blow to the top of the head causes the vertebrae to shatter and pieces of bone enter the spinal canal and damage the cord.

azoospermia The absence of living sperm in the semen.

azotemia An excess of nitrogenous wastes (urea) in the blood.

B

Babinski's sign Dorsiflexion of the great toe and fanning of the other toes, which is an abnormal reflex in response to testing the plantar reflex with a pointed (but not sharp) object; indicates the presence of central nervous system disease. The normal response is plantar flexion of all toes.

bacteremia The presence of bacteria in the bloodstream.

bacteriuria Bacteria in the urine.

bad death A death embodied by pain, not having one's wishes followed at the end of one's life, isolation, abandonment, and constant agonizing about losses associated with death.

Baker's cyst Enlarged popliteal bursa.

balanced analgesia See *multimodal analgesia*.

balanitis circinata Ringlike inflammation of the glans penis.

Ballance's sign During percussion, resonance over the right flank with the patient lying on the left side; this is an abnormal sign associated with abdominal trauma and is found with a ruptured spleen.

ballottement A maneuver to detect fluid in the knee by grasping the medial and lateral aspect of the knee between the thumb and third finger and pushing down on the top surface of the patella with the forefinger. If fluid is present, the patella can be pressed down a distance and rises back up when the forefinger is removed.

banding See *endoscopic variceal ligation.*

barbiturate coma The use of drugs such as pentobarbital sodium or sodium thiopental at dosages to maintain complete unresponsiveness; used for patients whose increased intracranial pressure cannot be controlled by other means. These drugs decrease the metabolic demands of the brain and cerebral blood flow, stabilize cell membranes, decrease the formation of vasogenic edema, and produce a more uniform blood supply. The patient in a barbiturate coma requires mechanical ventilation, sophisticated hemodynamic monitoring, and intracranial pressure monitoring.

bariatrics Branch of medicine that manages obesity and its related diseases.

barium enema See *lower GI series.*

baroreceptor Sensory receptors in the arch of the aorta and at the origin of the internal carotid arteries that are stimulated when the arterial walls are stretched by an increased blood pressure.

barotrauma An injury caused by rapid changes of pressure; usually refers to injury to the eardrum caused by an increase in pressure within the middle ear or to lung damage from excessive pressure.

Barrett's epithelium Columnar epithelium (instead of the normal squamous cell epithelium) that develops in the lower esophagus during the process of healing from gastroesophageal reflux disease. It is considered premalignant and is associated with an increased risk of cancer in patients with prolonged disease.

Barrett's esophagus Ulceration of the lower esophagus caused by exposure to acid and pepsin, leading to the replacement of normal distal squamous mucosa with columnar epithelium as a response to tissue injury.

basal insulin secretion The low levels of insulin that are secreted during fasting.

basal rate A type of regimen for continuous infusion of patient-controlled analgesia that provides more consistent analgesia.

base A substance that binds (reduces) free hydrogen ions in solution. Strong bases bind hydrogen ions easily; weak bases bind less readily.

Bell's palsy Acute paralysis of cranial nerve VII; characterized by a drawing sensation and paralysis of all facial muscles on the affected side. The patient cannot close the eye, wrinkle the forehead, smile, whistle, or grimace. The face appears mask-like and sags; also called "facial paralysis."

beneficence The ethical principle of preventing harm and ensuring the patient's well-being.

benign Altered cell growth that is harmless and does not require intervention.

benign prostatic hyperplasia (BPH) Age-associated enlargement of the prostate gland in men, which may cause bladder compression and can obstruct urinary flow.

benign tumor cells Normal cells growing in the wrong place or at the wrong time.

bereavement Grief and mourning experienced by the survivor before and after a death.

bicaval technique Surgical technique in heart transplantation in which the intact right atrium of the donor heart is preserved by anastomoses at the recipient's superior and inferior vena cavae.

bifurcation The point of division of a single structure into two branches.

bigeminy A type of premature complex that exists when normal complexes and premature complexes occur alternately in a repetitive two-beat pattern, with a pause occurring after each premature complex so that complexes occur in pairs.

bilateral orchiectomy The surgical removal of both testes, typically performed as palliative surgery in patients with prostate cancer. It is not intended to cure the prostate cancer but to arrest its spread by removing testosterone.

bilateral salpingo-oophorectomy (BSO) Surgical removal of both fallopian tubes and both ovaries.

biliary colic Intense pain due to obstruction of the cystic duct of the gallbladder from a stone moving through or lodged within the duct. Tissue spasm occurs in an effort to mobilize the stone through the small duct.

biliary stent A plastic or metal device that is placed percutaneously to keep a duct of the biliary system open in patients experiencing biliary obstruction.

biological response modifiers (BRMs) A class of immunomodulating drugs that attempt to modify the course of disease.

biologically based therapies Therapies that use natural substances for healing, including herbs, foods, vitamins, and minerals.

black box warning A governmental designation indicating that a drug has at least one serious side effect and must be used with caution.

bladder ultrasound Less invasive test to determine postvoiding residual urine volumes for the patient with a reflex (upper motor neuron) or uninhibited bladder; often used to measure residual urine in the bladder of patients with spinal cord injury.

blanch To whiten.

blast effect Injury resulting from impact forces such as that of an exploding bomb.

blast phase cell Immature cell that divides.

blepharitis An inflammation of the eyelid edges.

bloodborne metastasis The release of tumor cells into the blood; the most common cause of cancer spread.

Blumberg's sign Pain felt on abrupt release of steady pressure (rebound tenderness) over the site of abdominal pain.

blunt trauma Injury resulting from impact forces such as those sustained in a motor vehicle collision or a fall.

body mass index (BMI) A measure of nutritional status that does not depend on frame size; indirectly estimates total fat stores within the body by the relationship of weight to height.

bolus feeding A method of tube feeding that involves intermittent feeding of a specified amount of enteral product at specified times during a 24-hour period, typically every 4 hours.

bone mineral density (BMD) The quality of bone that determines bone strength. It peaks between 30 and 35 years of age, when both bone resorption activity and bone-building activity occur at a constant rate. When bone resorption activity exceeds bone-building activity, bone density decreases.

bone remodeling The process of bone tissue constantly undergoing change.

bone resorption Loss of bone density due to demineralization resulting from the release of calcium from storage areas in bones.

bone scan A radionuclide test in which radioactive material is injected for visualization of the entire skeleton; used to detect tumors, arthritis, osteomyelitis, osteoporosis, vertebral compression fractures, and unexplained bone pain.

bony ossicle Small bone; in the ear, the malleus, the incus, and the stapes, which are found in the epitympanum.

borborygmus (borborygmi) Bowel sounds, especially loud gurgling sounds, resulting from hypermotility of the bowel.

boring In pain, the type of intense pain that feels like it is going through the body.

botulism A paralytic disease resulting from ingestion of a toxin in food contaminated with *Clostridium botulinum.* Botulism is associated with home-canned foods, commercially prepared products, and products not adequately heated to destroy toxins. Initial symptoms include diplopia, dysphagia, and dysarthria. Illness may be mild or severe, with paralysis, respiratory failure, and death.

Bouchard's nodes Swelling at the proximal interphalangeal joints in osteoarthritis involving the hands.

bowel training A program for patients with neurologic problems that is designed to include a combination of suppository use and a consistent toileting schedule.

boxer's ear See *cauliflower ear.*

bradycardia Slowness of the heart rate; characterized as a pulse rate less than 50 to 60 beats/min.

bradydysrhythmia An abnormal heart rhythm characterized by a heart rate less than 60 beats/min.

bradykinesia Slow or no movement, as seen in a patient with Parkinson disease; also called "akinesia."

brain abscess A collection of pus that forms in the extradural, subdural, or intracerebral area of the brain as a result of a purulent infection, usually due to bacteria invading the brain directly or indirectly.

brain attack Stroke; disruption in the normal blood supply to the brain, either as an interruption in blood flow (ischemic stroke), or as bleeding within or around the brain (hemorrhagic stroke). A medical emergency that occurs suddenly, a stroke should be treated immediately to prevent neurologic deficit and permanent disability. Formerly called *cerebrovascular accident*, the National Stroke Association now uses the term *brain attack* to describe stroke.

brain herniation syndrome In the patient with untreated increased intracranial pressure, protrusion (herniation) of the brain downward toward the brainstem or laterally from a unilateral lesion within one cerebral hemisphere, causing irreversible brain damage and possibly death.

breast One of a pair of mammary glands that develop in response to secretions from the hypothalamus, pituitary gland, and ovaries. Breasts are an accessory of the reproductive system meant to nourish the infant after birth. They also are organs for sexual arousal in the mature adult.

breast augmentation Cosmetic surgical procedure to enhance the size, shape, or symmetry of the breasts.

breast-conserving surgery Surgical method for breast cancer that removes the bulk of the tumor rather than the entire breast.

Broca's aphasia See *expressive aphasia.*

Broca's area An important speech area of the cerebrum. It is located in the frontal lobe and is composed of neurons responsible for the formation of words, or speech.

bronchoscopy Insertion of a tube in the airway, usually as far as the secondary bronchi, for the purpose of visualizing airway structures and obtaining tissue samples for biopsy or culture.

Brown-Séquard syndrome A condition caused by cervical injuries; generally results from penetrating injuries that cause hemisection of the spinal cord or injuries that affect half of the spinal cord. Motor function, proprioception, vibration, and deep touch sensations are lost on the same side of the body as the lesion (ipsilateral). On the opposite side of the body (contralateral), the sensations of pain, temperature, and light touch are affected.

bruit Swishing sound in the larger arteries (carotid, aortic, femoral, and popliteal) that can be heard with a stethoscope or Doppler probe; may indicate narrowing of the artery and is usually associated with atherosclerotic disease.

bulbar Pertaining to the muscles involved in facial expression, chewing, and speech.

bulimia nervosa An eating disorder that is characterized by episodes of binge eating in which the patient ingests a large amount of food in a short time, followed by purging behavior such as self-induced vomiting or excessive use of laxatives and diuretics.

bunion Hallux valgus deformity of the foot in which lateral deviation of the great toe causes the first metatarsal head to become enlarged.

bunionectomy Surgical removal of the hallux valgus deformity (bunion) of the foot.

bursae The small sacs lined with synovial membrane that are located at joints and bony prominences to prevent friction between bone and structures adjacent to bone.

butterfly rash A dry, scaly, raised rash on the face; the major skin manifestation of systemic lupus erythematosus.

C

C fiber Unmyelinated or poorly myelinated fiber found in muscle, periosteum, and viscera; conducts thermal, chemical, and strong mechanical impulses that produce diffuse, persistent, and dull, burning, or achy sensations.

cachexia Extreme body wasting and malnutrition that develops from an imbalance between food intake and energy use.

calculi An abnormal formation of a mass of mineral salts that can occur in the body; forms in the kidney when excess calcium precipitates out of solution; also called "stones."

calculous cholecystitis Inflammation of the gallbladder usually following and created by obstruction of the cystic duct by a stone (calculus).

callus The loose, fibrous, vascular tissue that forms at the site of a fracture as the first phase of healing and is normally replaced by hard bone as healing continues.

calyx The anatomic term for a cuplike structure.

Canadian Triage Acuity Scale (CTAS) A standardized model for triage in which lists of descriptors are used to establish the triage level.

cancellous The softer tissue inside bones that contains large spaces, or trabeculae, that are filled with red and yellow marrow.

cancer control See *cytoreductive surgery.*

candidiasis An infection caused by the fungus *Candida albicans.*

canthus The place where the upper and lower eyelids meet at the corner of either side of the eye.

capillary closing pressure The amount of pressure needed to occlude skin capillary blood flow.

capillary leak syndrome The response of capillaries to the presence of biologic chemicals (mediators) that change blood vessel integrity and allow fluid to shift from the blood in the vascular space into the interstitial tissues.

Caplan's syndrome The presence of pneumoconiosis and rheumatoid nodules in the lungs; noted primarily in coal miners and asbestos workers.
carboxyhemoglobin Carbon monoxide on oxygen-bending sites of the hemoglobin molecule.
carcinoembryonic antigen (CEA) An oncofetal antigen that may be elevated in 70% of people with colorectal cancer. CEA is not specifically associated with the colorectal cancer and may be elevated in the presence of other benign or malignant diseases and in smokers. CEA is often used to monitor the effectiveness of treatment and to identify disease recurrence.
carcinogen Any substance that changes the activity of the genes in a cell so that the cell becomes a cancer cell.
carcinogenesis Cancer development.
cardiac axis In electrocardiography (ECG), the direction of electrical current flow in the heart. The relationship between the cardiac axis and the lead axis is responsible for the deflections seen on the ECG pattern.
cardiac catheterization The most definitive but most invasive test in the diagnosis of heart disease; involves passing a small catheter into the heart and injecting contrast medium.
cardiac index A calculation of cardiac output requirements to account for differences in body size; determined by dividing the cardiac output by the body surface area.
cardiac output (CO) The volume of blood ejected by the heart each minute; normal range in adults is 4 to 7 L/min.
cardiac rehabilitation The process of actively assisting the patient with cardiac disease to achieve and maintain a productive life while remaining within the limits of the heart's ability to respond to increases in activity and stress. *Phase 1* begins with the acute illness and ends with discharge from the hospital. *Phase 2* begins after discharge and continues through convalescence at home. *Phase 3* refers to long-term conditioning.
cardiac resynchronization therapy (CRT) In patients with some types of heart failure, the use of a permanent pacemaker alone or in combination with an implantable cardioverter-defibrillator to provide biventricular pacing.
cardiac tamponade Compression of the myocardium by fluid that has accumulated around the heart; this compresses the atria and ventricles, prevents them from filling adequately, and reduces cardiac output.
cardiogenic shock Postmyocardial infarction heart failure in which necrosis of more than 40% of the left ventricle has occurred; also called "class IV heart failure."
cardiomegaly Enlarged heart.
cardiomyopathy A subacute or chronic disease of cardiac muscle; classified into three categories based on abnormalities in structure and function dilated, hypertrophic, and restrictive.
cardiopulmonary bypass (CPB) Diversion of the blood from the heart to a bypass machine, where it is heparinized, oxygenated, and returned to the circulation through a cannula placed in the ascending aortic arch or femoral artery to provide oxygenation, circulation, and hypothermia during induced cardiac arrest for coronary artery bypass surgery. This process ensures a motionless operative field and prevents myocardial ischemia.
cardiopulmonary resuscitation (CPR) A procedure that involves forcing air into the lungs of the patient who has stopped breathing, as well as giving chest compressions in the absence of a carotid pulse.
cardioversion A synchronized countershock that may be performed in emergencies for hemodynamically unstable ventricular or supraventricular tachydysrhythmias or electively for stable tachydysrhythmias that are resistant to medical therapies. The shock depolarizes a critical mass of myocardium simultaneously during intrinsic depolarization and is intended to stop the re-entry circuit and allow the sinus node to regain control of the heart.
carina The point at which the trachea branches into the right and left mainstem bronchi.
caring A process, set of actions, and attitude that shows genuine physical and emotional concern for others.
carotid endarterectomy Removal of atherosclerotic plaque from the inner lining of the carotid artery to open the artery enough to re-establish blood flow and decrease risk for brain attack. This surgical procedure prevents progression of brain attack in symptomatic patients with recurrent transient ischemic attacks or carotid stenosis.
carotid sinus massage A method of vagal stimulation of the cardiac conduction system in which the physician massages over one carotid artery for a few seconds and observes for a change in cardiac rhythm. Massaging the carotid sinus causes vagal stimulation, thus slowing sinoatrial and atrioventricular nodal conduction.
carrier (1) A person who harbors an infectious agent without symptoms of active disease; (2) in genetics, a person who has one mutated allele for a recessive genetic disorder. A carrier does not usually have any manifestations of the disorder but can pass the mutated allele to his or her children.
case management The process of assessment, planning, implementation, evaluation, and interaction for patients who have complex health problems and incur a high cost to the health care system. Goals include promoting quality of life, decreasing fragmentation and duplication of care across health care settings, and maintaining cost-effectiveness.
caseation necrosis A type of necrosis in which tissue is turned into a granular mass.
cast A rigid device that immobilizes the affected body part while allowing other body parts to move. It is most commonly used for fractures but may also be applied to correct deformities (e.g., clubfoot) or to prevent deformities (e.g., those seen in some patients with rheumatoid arthritis).
catabolism Any destructive metabolic process by which organisms convert substances into excreted compounds.
catechol *O*-methyltransferase (COMT) inhibitors Enzymes that inactivate dopamine, thereby blocking dopamine activity and increasing the effectiveness of levodopa; a class of drugs prescribed for patients with Parkinson disease.
catecholamines Hormones (dopamine, epinephrine, and norepinephrine) released by the adrenal medulla in response to stimulation of the sympathetic nervous system.
cation Ion that has a positive charge.
cauliflower ear A deformed and hardened auricle caused by trauma and resulting in a hematoma that hardens unless the blood is removed by needle aspiration; also called "boxer's ear."
cell-mediated immunity Microbial resistance that is mediated by the action of specifically sensitized T-lymphocytes.
cellulitis An acute, spreading, edematous inflammation of the deep subcutaneous tissues; usually caused by infection of a wound or burn.

central cord syndrome A condition caused by cervical injuries that involve lesions of the central portion of the spinal cord. Loss of motor function is more pronounced in the upper extremities than in the lower extremities; varying degrees and patterns of sensation remain intact.

central IV therapy IV therapy in which a vascular access device (VAD) is placed in a central blood vessel, such as the superior vena cava.

cerebral angiography (arteriography) Visualization of the cerebral circulation (carotid and vertebral arteries) after injecting a contrast medium into an artery (usually the femoral).

cerebral blood flow (CBF) Useful in evaluating cerebral vasospasm; can be measured in many areas of the brain with the use of radioactive substances.

cerebral perfusion pressure (CPP) The pressure gradient over which the brain is perfused. It is influenced by oxygenation, cerebral blood volume, blood pressure, cerebral edema, and intracranial pressure (ICP) and is determined by subtracting the mean ICP from the mean arterial pressure. A cerebral perfusion pressure above 70 mm Hg is generally accepted as an appropriate goal of therapy.

cerebral salt-wasting (CSW) The primary cause of hyponatremia in the neurosurgical population; characterized by hyponatremia, decreased serum osmolality, and decreased blood volume. It is thought to result from the extrarenal influence of atrial natriuretic factor.

cerumen The wax produced by glands within the external ear canal; helps protect and lubricate the ear canal.

cervical polyp Tumor that arises from the mucosa and extends to the opening of the cervical os. Polyps result from hyperplasia of the endocervical epithelium, inflammation, or an abnormal local response to hormonal stimulation or localized vascular congestion of the cervical blood vessels. Polyps are the most common benign growth of the cervix.

cervix The lower, narrowed portion of the uterus that extends into the vagina. It is the passage site for sperm to enter the uterus and the passage site for menstrual flow to exit the uterus.

chalazion An inflammation of a sebaceous gland in the eyelid.

chancre The ulcer that is the first sign of syphilis. It develops at the site of entry (inoculation) of the organism, usually 3 weeks after exposure. The lesion may be found on any area of the skin or mucous membranes but occurs most often on the genitalia, lips, nipples, and hands and in the oral cavity, anus, and rectum.

chancroid A sexually transmitted disease characterized by painful genital ulcerations and caused by infection with *Haemophilus ducreyi*. Infection develops as a result of sexual exposure or self-contamination from a lesion elsewhere on the body. Incubation period varies from 3 to 10 days. A tender papule appears at the site of inoculation and rapidly breaks down to form an irregularly shaped, deep ulcer that has a purulent discharge and bleeds easily.

chelation A general term referring to a drug or substance that binds or attaches to another substance.

chemoreceptor Specialized sensory receptor in the bifurcation of the carotid arteries and in the aortic arch; sensitive to hypoxemia. When stimulated, the carotid chemoreceptors send impulses along Hering's nerves, and the aortic chemoreceptors send impulses along the vagus nerves to activate a vasoconstrictor response.

chemotaxin Substance secreted by damaged tissues and blood vessels that attracts neutrophils and macrophages so that phagocytosis can occur; also called "leukotaxin."

chemotherapy The treatment of cancer with chemical agents that have systemic effects; used to cure and to increase survival time.

chest tube A drain placed in the pleural space to allow closed-chest drainage, which restores intrapleural pressure and allows re-expansion of the lung after surgery in patients who have undergone thoracotomy (incision of the chest wall).

Cheyne-Stokes respirations Common sign of nearing death in which apnea alternates with periods of rapid breathing.

choked disc See *papilledema*.

cholecystectomy The surgical removal of the gallbladder.

cholecystitis Inflammation of the gallbladder.

cholecystokinin A hormone that stimulates digestive juices and may work with leptin to increase or decrease appetite.

choledochojejunostomy Surgical anastomosis of the common bile duct with the jejunum.

cholelithiasis The presence of gallstones.

cholesteatoma A benign overgrowth of squamous cell epithelium.

cholinergic crisis Overmedication with cholinesterase inhibitors.

cholinesterase inhibitors Drugs that improve cholinergic neurotransmission in the central nervous system by delaying the destruction of acetylcholine by acetylcholinesterase, thus delaying the onset of cognitive decline. These are approved for symptomatic treatment of Alzheimer's disease but do not affect the course of the disease.

chondrogenic Originating from cartilage.

choreiform movement Rapid, jerky movement.

chorioretinitis Inflammation of both the choroid and the retina.

chronic Having a slow onset and symptoms that persist for an extended period.

chronic calcifying pancreatitis (CCP) Alcohol-induced chronic pancreatitis that is characterized by protein precipitates that plug the ducts and lead to ductal obstruction, atrophy, and dilation. The epithelium of the ducts undergoes histologic changes, resulting in metaplasia (cell replacement) and ulceration. This inflammatory process causes fibrosis of the pancreatic tissue.

chronic cancer pain Persistent or recurrent pain that results from cancer or another progressive disease or life-threatening condition.

chronic constrictive pericarditis A fibrous thickening of the pericardium that prevents adequate filling of the ventricles and eventually results in cardiac failure; caused by chronic pericardial inflammation due to tuberculosis, radiation therapy, trauma, kidney failure, or metastatic cancer.

chronic fatigue syndrome (CFS) A chronic illness characterized by severe fatigue for 6 months or longer, usually following flu-like symptoms. At least four of the following criteria are required for diagnosis: sore throat; substantial impairment in short-term memory or concentration; tender lymph nodes; muscle pain; multiple joint pain with redness or swelling; headaches of a new type, pattern, or severity; unrefreshing sleep; and postexertional malaise lasting more than 24 hours.

chronic gastritis A patchy, diffuse inflammation of the mucosal lining of the stomach. Chronic gastritis usually heals without scarring but can progress to hemorrhage and ulcer formation.

chronic health problem A condition that has existed for at least 3 months.

chronic hepatitis Chronic liver inflammation that usually occurs as a result of hepatitis B or C. Superimposed infection with hepatitis D (HDV) in patients with chronic HBV may also result in chronic hepatitis. Can lead to cirrhosis and liver cancer.

chronic noncancer pain Persistent or recurrent pain associated with a tissue injury that has healed or is not associated with cancer, such as arthritis.

chronic obstructive pancreatitis Pancreatitis that develops from inflammation, spasm, and obstruction of the sphincter of Oddi. Inflammatory and sclerotic lesions occur in the head of the pancreas and around the ducts, causing obstruction and backflow of pancreatic secretions.

chronic obstructive pulmonary disease (COPD) Any lung disease characterized by bronchospasm and dyspnea, such as emphysema and chronic bronchitis.

chronic osteomyelitis Bone infection that persists over a long time due to misdiagnosis or inadequate treatment; also called "subchronic osteomyelitis."

chronic pain Pain that persists or recurs for indefinite periods (usually more than 3 months), often involves deep body structures, is poorly localized, and is difficult to describe. Also called "persistent pain."

chronic pancreatitis A progressive, destructive disease of the pancreas characterized by remissions and exacerbations. Inflammation and fibrosis of the tissue contribute to pancreatic insufficiency and diminished function of the organ.

chronic paronychia Inflammation of the skin around the nail that persists for months. People at risk for chronic paronychia are those with frequent exposure to water, such as homemakers, bartenders, and laundry workers.

chronic pyelonephritis A kidney disorder that results from repeated or continued upper urinary tract infections or the effects of such infections.

chronic stable angina (CSA) Type of angina characterized by chest discomfort that occurs with moderate to prolonged exertion and in a pattern that is familiar to the patient.

chyme The transformation of food into a liquid during the digestion process in the gastrointestinal tract.

cilia Hairlike projections from epithelial cells; also, the eyelids or eyelashes.

circle of Willis At the base of the brain, the ring formed by the anterior, middle, and posterior cerebral arteries where they are joined together by small communicating arteries.

circumcision The surgical removal of the prepuce or foreskin of the penis.

circumferential Referring to something that completely surrounds an extremity or the thorax.

cirrhosis Liver disease that is characterized by extensive scarring of the liver and is usually caused by a chronic irreversible reaction to hepatic inflammation and necrosis; disease typically develops insidiously and has a prolonged, destructive course.

classic heat stroke A form of heat stroke in which the body's ability to dissipate heat is significantly impaired; occurs over time as a result of long-term exposure to a hot, humid environment such as a home without air-conditioning in the high heat of the summer.

claudication Pain in the muscles resulting from an inadequate blood supply.

climacteric The phase of a woman's life from the initial decline in the amount of estrogen produced by the ovaries to the end of symptoms. The lay term for this phase is "the change of life."

clinically competent The condition of being legally competent and having decisional capacity.

clitoris A small, cylindric organ of the external female genitalia that is composed of erectile tissue with a high concentration of sensory nerve endings.

clonic Pertaining to a state of alternating muscle stiffness followed by rhythmic jerking motions, as in a tonic-clonic seizure.

clonic seizure A type of generalized seizure lasting several minutes and characterized by muscle contraction and relaxation.

clonus The sudden, brief, jerking contraction of a muscle or muscle group often seen in seizures.

closed fracture A fracture that does not extend through the skin and therefore has no visible wound; also called "simple fracture."

closed head injury A type of traumatic primary brain injury that occurs as the result of blunt trauma; the integrity of the skull is not violated, and damage to brain tissue depends on the degree and mechanisms of injury.

closed reduction A nonsurgical method for managing a simple fracture. While applying a manual pull, or traction, on the bone, the health care provider manipulates the bone ends so they realign.

clubbing Changes in the tissue beds of the fingers and toes, with the base of the nail becoming spongy; results from chronic oxygen deprivation in the tissue beds.

cluster headache A type of oculotemporal or oculofrontal headache marked by unilateral, excruciating, nonthrobbing pain that is felt deep in and around the eye and may radiate to the forehead, temple, cheek, ear, occiput, or neck. Average duration is 10 to 45 minutes. Headaches occur every 8 to 12 hours and up to 24 hours daily at the same time for about 6 to 8 weeks (hence the term *cluster*), followed by remission for 9 months to a year. Cause and mechanism are unknown but have been attributed to vasoreactivity and oxyhemoglobin desaturation.

CO_2 narcosis Loss of sensitivity to high levels of Pa_{CO_2}. For these patients, the stimulus to breathe is a decreased arterial oxygen level.

cochlea The spiral organ of hearing within the inner ear.

cognition The ability of the brain to process, store, retrieve, and manipulate information.

cognitive therapist A member of the rehabilitative health care team, usually a neuropsychologist, who works primarily with patients who have experienced head injuries and have cognitive impairments.

cohorting The practice of grouping patients who are colonized or infected with the same pathogen.

coitus Sexual intercourse.

cold antibody anemia A form of immunohemolytic anemia (in which the immune system attacks a person's own red blood cells for unknown reasons) that occurs with complement protein fixation on immunoglobulin M (IgM). In this condition, the arteries in the hands and feet constrict profoundly in response to cold temperatures or stress.

cold phase A phase after peripheral nerve trauma resulting in complete denervation in which the skin appears cyanotic, mottled, or reddish blue and feels cool compared with the contralateral, unaffected extremity. The cold phase follows the warm phase, which lasts 2 to 3 weeks after injury.

colectomy Surgical removal of part or all of the colon.

collaborative nursing function Activity that is mutually determined by the nurse and the physician or other health care team member or that is directed or prescribed by the health care provider but requires nursing judgment to perform.
collateral circulation Circulation that provides blood to an area with altered tissue perfusion through smaller vessels that develop and compensate for the occluded vessels.
colon interposition A surgical procedure that may be performed in patients with an esophageal tumor when the tumor involves the stomach or the stomach is otherwise unsuitable for anastomosis. In colon interposition, a section of right or left colon is removed and brought up into the thorax to substitute for the esophagus.
colon resection Surgery performed for colorectal cancer in which the tumor and regional lymph nodes are removed.
colonization The presence of microorganisms in the tissues of the host without causing symptomatic disease.
colonoscopy The endoscopic examination of the entire large bowel.
colostomy The surgical creation of an opening between the colon and the surface of the abdomen.
colposcopy Examination of the cervix and vagina using a colposcope, which allows three-dimensional magnification and intense illumination of epithelium with suspected disease. This procedure can locate the exact site of precancerous and malignant lesions for biopsy.
comatose A state of being unconscious and unarousable.
comedones Plural form of *comedo.* Blackheads and whiteheads, the noninflammatory lesions of acne.
command center See *emergency operations center.*
comminuted fracture A type of fracture that involves fragmentation of the bone.
commitment Occurrence in which early embryonic cells start changing into differentiated cells.
communicable The ability of an infection, such as influenza, to be transmitted from person to person.
comorbidity Pre-existing disease state that must be included in patient assessment in regard to how the condition might adversely affect a seemingly unrelated health problem.
compartment syndrome A condition in which increased tissue pressure in a confined anatomic space causes decreased blood flow to the area, leading to hypoxia and pain.
compensated cirrhosis A form of cirrhosis in which the liver has significant scarring but is still able to perform essential functions without causing significant symptoms.
compensatory mechanism The means of producing compensation; also called "adaptive mechanism."
complement activation and fixation Actions triggered by some classes of antibodies that can remove or destroy antigen.
complementary and alternative medicine The broad range of healing philosophies, approaches, and therapies that mainstream Western medicine does not commonly use.
complete spinal cord injury An injury in which the spinal cord has been severed or damaged in a way that eliminates all innervation below the level of the injury.
complex partial seizure A type of partial seizure that occurs in patients with epilepsy, causing loss of consciousness for 1 to 3 minutes. Characteristic behaviors known as automatisms may occur, such as lip smacking or picking at clothes. The patient may experience amnesia after the seizure. Because the area of the brain most often involved is the temporal lobe, complex partial seizures are often called "psychomotor seizures" or "temporal lobe seizures."
complex regional pain syndrome (CRPS) A complex disorder that includes debilitating pain, atrophy, autonomic dysfunction (excessive sweating, vascular changes), and motor impairment (most notably muscle paresis), probably caused by an abnormally hyperactive sympathetic nervous system. This syndrome most often results from traumatic injury and commonly occurs in the feet and hands; formerly called "reflex sympathetic dystrophy (RSD)."
compliance In respiratory physiology, a measure of elasticity within the lung. Also, a patient's fulfillment of a caregiver's prescribed course of treatment.
compound fracture See *open fracture.*
compression fracture A fracture that is produced by a loading force applied to the long axis of cancellous bone. These fractures commonly occur in the vertebrae of patients with osteoporosis.
computed tomography coronary angiography (CTCA) 64-slice diagnostic scan used to diagnose coronary artery disease in symptomatic patients.
computed tomography (CT) scanning Use of a computer to take pictures at many horizontal levels, or slices, of the area being studied. The cross-sectional slices build up three-dimensional pictures; a contrast medium may be used to enhance the image.
concentration gradient Movement across a membrane from an area of higher concentration to an area of lower concentration.
concussion A type of closed head injury that is caused by blunt trauma (e.g., a blow to the head) and is characterized by a brief loss of consciousness.
conductive hearing loss Hearing loss that results from any physical obstruction of sound wave transmission (e.g., a foreign body in the external canal, a retracted or bulging tympanic membrane, or fused bony ossicles).
conductivity The ability of a cell to transmit an electrical stimulus from cell membrane to cell membrane.
congestive heart failure (CHF) Former term for left-sided heart failure. Categorized as either systolic heart failure or diastolic heart failure that may be acute or chronic and mild to severe.
conization The removal of a cone-shaped sample of tissue from the cervix for cytologic study.
conjunctivae The mucous membranes of the eye that line the undersurface of the eyelids (palpebral conjunctiva) and cover the sclera (bulbar conjunctiva).
connective tissue disease (CTD) A group of diseases that are the major focus of rheumatology (the study of rheumatic diseases); most are musculoskeletal disorders.
consensual response In assessing pupillary reaction to light, a slight constriction of the pupil of the eye not being tested when a penlight is brought in from the side of the patient's head and shined into the eye being tested as soon as the patient opens his or her eyes.
consolidation Solidification; lack of air spaces in the lung, such as occurs in pneumonia.
Contact Precautions Infection control guidelines from the Centers for Disease Control and Prevention; used for patients with infections spread by direct contact or contact with items in the patient's environment, such as pediculosis.
contiguous Something in direct contact with, or adjacent to, another area or structure.

continence The ability to voluntarily control emptying the bladder and colon. Continence is a learned behavior whereby a person can suppress the urge to urinate until a socially appropriate location is available.

continuous feeding A method of tube feeding in which small amounts of enteral product are continuously infused (by gravity drip or by a pump or controller device) over a specified time.

contractility The ability of a cell to contract in response to an impulse. In cardiac electrophysiology, the ability of atrial and ventricular muscle cells to shorten their fiber length in response to electrical stimulation, generating sufficient pressure to propel blood forward. Contractility is the mechanical activity of the heart.

contraction The closure of a wound as new collagen replaces damaged tissue, pulling the wound edges inward along the path of least resistance.

contralateral Pertaining to the opposite side.

contrecoup injury Bruising of the brain tissue, with damage occurring on the side opposite the site of impact.

controller A stationary, pole-mounted electronic device that uses a sensor to monitor fluid flow during infusion therapy and to detect flow interruption.

contusion A bruise; when referring to closed head injury, a bruising of brain tissue usually found at the site of impact (coup injury). Compare with "contrecoup injury."

cor pulmonale Right-sided heart failure caused by pulmonary disease.

cordectomy Excision of a vocal cord in surgery for laryngeal cancer.

cordotomy Surgical technique in which the surgeon cuts the pain pathways at the midline portion of the spinal cord, before nerve impulses ascend to the spinothalamic tract. Used to relieve intractable pain in patients with metastatic cancer by interrupting the transmission of pain.

cornea The clear layer that forms the external coat on the front of the eye.

corneal abrasion Scrape or scratch of the cornea that disrupts its integrity.

corneal ulceration Deep disruption of the corneal epithelium that extends into the stromal layer and is caused by bacteria, protozoa, or fungi.

coronary artery bypass graft A surgical procedure in which occluded coronary arteries are bypassed with the patient's own venous or arterial blood vessels or synthetic grafts.

coronary artery calcium score (CAC) A measure of the amount of coronary artery calcification present.

coronary artery disease (CAD) Disease affecting the arteries that provide blood, oxygen, and nutrients to the myocardium; partial or complete blockage of the blood flow through the coronary arteries, causing ischemia and infarction of the myocardium, angina pectoris, and acute coronary syndromes.

coronary artery vasculopathy (CAV) A form of coronary artery disease that presents as diffuse plaque in the arteries of the donor heart in patients who have received a heart transplant.

cortex The outer layer of an organ or body structure.

cortical A term referring to compact bone of the shaft of a bone.

corticosteroids The hormones produced and secreted by the adrenal cortex; also called "adrenal steroids."

cortisol The main glucocorticoid produced by the adrenal cortex.

coryza The common cold, or acute viral rhinitis.

cough assist A technique for assisting the tetraplegic patient to cough. Place his or her hands on either side of the rib cage or upper abdomen below the diaphragm then, as the patient inhales, push upward to help expand the lungs and cough.

craniotomy Surgical incision into the cranium.

creatine kinase (CK) An enzyme specific to cells of the brain, myocardium, and skeletal muscle. Its appearance in the blood indicates tissue necrosis or injury, with levels following a predictable rise and fall during a specified period.

cremasteric reflex Stimulation of the skin on the front and inner side of the thigh retracts the testicle and scrotum on the same side. An intact reflex indicates integrity of the first lumbar nerve segment of the spinal cord.

crepitus (crepitation) A continuous grating sensation caused when irregular cartilage or bone fragments rub together and which may be felt or heard as a joint is put through passive range of motion; also, a crackling sensation that can be felt on a patient's chest, indicating that air is trapped within the tissues.

CREST syndrome In patients with systemic sclerosis, the combination of *c*alcinosis (calcium deposits), *R*aynaud's phenomenon, *e*sophageal dysmotility, *s*clerodactyly (scleroderma of the digits), and *t*elangiectasia (spider-like hemangiomas).

cricothyroidotomy Surgical procedure in which an opening is made between the thyroid cartilage and cricoid cartilage ring and results in a tracheostomy; also called "cricothyrotomy." The procedure is used in an emergency for access to the lower airways.

crises In the patient with sickle cell disease, periodic episodes of extensive cellular sickling that have a sudden onset and can occur as often as weekly or as seldom as once a year.

critical access hospital A small rural facility of 15 or fewer inpatient beds that provides around-the-clock emergency care services 7 days per week. Considered a necessary provider of health care to community residents who are not close to other hospitals in a given region.

critical thinking Purposeful, outcome-directed thinking that is used to make clinical judgments based on scientific evidence rather than on tradition or conjecture (guesswork).

cross-contamination A type of contamination in which organisms from another person or from the environment are transmitted to the patient.

cryoanalgesia The use of cold to achieve permanent ablation of nerve roots.

cryoprecipitate A highly concentrated blood product that is derived from plasma and includes clotting factors VIII and XIII, von Willebrand's factor, and fibrinogen.

cryosurgery Destruction of tissue by applying extreme cold; may reduce pain and tumor size in patients with metastatic cancer.

cryotherapy (1) A way of decreasing muscle pain by "cooling down" the area with a local, short-acting gel or cream, such as after physical therapy; (2) in ophthalmologic surgery, use of a freezing probe to repair retinal detachment.

cryptorchidism Failure of the testes to descend into the scrotum.

Cullen's sign The presence of a bluish discoloration around the umbilicus, which is an indication of intra-abdominal bleeding.

cultural competence The ability of health care provider or organization to understand and respond effectively to the cultural and linguistic needs that patients bring to the health care setting.

cultural diversity The differences among people, which may or may not be visible.

cultural sensitivity The way that one responds to cultural differences.

culture (1) A procedure for identifying a microorganism by cultivating and isolating it in tissue cultures or artificial media; (2) an integrated pattern of human behavior that is learned and transmitted to succeeding generations and includes thought, speech, action, and artifacts.

curandero A folk healer in the Mexican-American medicine system who considers health and health care from a holistic, spiritual perspective rather than the traditional scientific viewpoint.

curative surgery Surgery done to remove all cancer tissue.

Curling's ulcer Acute ulcerative gastroduodenal disease, which may develop within 24 hours of a severe burn injury because of reduced gastrointestinal blood flow and mucosal damage.

Cushing's disease (Cushing's syndrome) Hypercortisolism caused by oversecretion of hormones by the adrenal cortex.

Cushing's triad A classic yet late sign of increased intracranial pressure (ICP) manifested by severe hypertension with a widened pulse pressure and bradycardia. As ICP increases, the pulse becomes thready, irregular, and rapid. Cerebral blood flow increases in response to hypertension.

Cushing's ulcer Acute ulcerative gastroduodenal disease that may develop as a result of increased intracranial pressure.

cutaneous reflexes Superficial reflexes. Usually the plantar and abdominal reflexes are tested.

cuticle A layer of keratin at the nail fold, which attaches the nail plate to the soft tissue of the nail fold.

cyanosis Bluish or darkened discoloration of the skin and mucous membranes; results from an increased amount of deoxygenated hemoglobin.

cyclic feeding A method of tube feeding similar to continuous feeding (see definition of *continuous feeding*) except the infusion is stopped for a specified time in each 24-hour period ("down time"); the down time typically occurs in the morning to allow bathing, treatments, and other activities.

cystectomy (1) Removal of a cysti; (2) surgical removal of the bladder and surrounding tissue.

cystitis Inflammation of the bladder.

cystocele Herniation of the bladder into the vagina.

cytokines Small protein hormones produced by white blood cells.

cytopenia Low blood count.

cytoprotectant Drug that protects specific healthy cells; given to patients to decrease the impact of chemotherapy on normal tissues.

cytoreductive surgery Surgery done to remove part of a tumor while leaving a known amount of gross tumor behind; also called "cancer control."

cytotoxic Having cell-damaging effects.

D

dandruff An accumulation of patchy or diffuse white or gray scales on the surface of the scalp.

dawn phenomenon In the patient with diabetes, a condition of fasting hyperglycemia resulting from a nighttime release of growth hormone that causes blood glucose elevations at about 5 to 6 AM. Providing more insulin for the overnight period helps avoid this condition.

death When illness or trauma overwhelms the compensatory mechanisms of the body and the lungs and heart cease to function.

death rattle Loud, wet respirations caused by secretions in the respiratory tract and oral cavity of a patient who is near death.

débridement The removal of infected tissue from a healing wound.

debriefing After a mass casualty incident or disaster, (1) the provision of sessions for small groups of staff in which teams are brought in to discuss effective coping strategies (critical incident stress debriefing), and (2) the administrative review of staff and system performance during the event to determine opportunities for improvement in the emergency management plan.

debris Dead cells and tissues in a wound.

decerebrate posturing Abnormal posturing and rigidity characterized by extension of the arms and legs, pronation of the arms, plantar flexion, and opisthotonos; usually associated with dysfunction in the brainstem area. Also called "decerebration."

decerebration See *decerebrate posturing.*

decompensated cirrhosis A form of cirrhosis in which liver function is significantly impaired with obvious manifestations of liver failure.

decompressive laminectomy Removal of one or more laminae in the patient with spinal cord injury and compression; allows for cord expansion from edema if more conventional measures fail to prevent neurologic deterioration.

decorticate posturing Abnormal posturing seen in the patient with lesions that interrupt the corticospinal pathways. The arms, wrists, and fingers are flexed with internal rotation and plantar flexion of the legs. Also called "decortication."

decortication See *decorticate posturing.*

deep tendon reflexes Tested as part of the neurologic assessment. An intact reflex arc is indicated when the muscle contracts in response to the tendon being struck with a hammer.

deep vein thrombophlebitis Presence of a thrombus associated with inflammation in the deep veins, usually in the legs. Compared with superficial thrombophlebitis, it presents a greater risk for pulmonary embolism; also called "deep vein thrombosis."

deep vein thrombosis (DVT) Common term for deep vein thrombophlebitis.

defibrillation An asynchronous countershock that depolarizes a critical mass of myocardium simultaneously to stop the re-entry circuit, allowing the sinus node to regain control of the heart.

degradation The process of breaking down.

dehiscence A partial or complete separation of the outer layers of a wound, sometimes described as a "splitting open" of the wound.

dehydration Fluid intake less than what is needed to meet the body's fluid needs.

delayed union Term describing a fracture that has not healed within 6 months of injury.

delirium An acute state of confusion, usually short-term and reversible within 3 weeks. Often seen among older adults in a hospital or other unfamiliar setting.

delirium tremens (DTs) Tremors of the entire body; a symptom of alcohol withdrawal.

demand dose An amount of drug specified by the health care provider that is programmed into a patient-controlled analgesia infusion pump.
dementia A syndrome of slowly progressive cognitive decline with global impairment of intellectual function. The most common type is Alzheimer's disease.
demyelination Destruction of myelin between the nodes of Ranvier; a major pathologic finding in Guillain-Barré syndrome.
demyelinization Occurrence of multiple sclerosis in which the myelin sheath is damaged and its thickness is reduced.
deoxyribonucleic acid (DNA) The basic genetic material required for cell division and growth.
dependence A condition that causes a habitual, compulsive, and uncontrollable urge to use a substance; without the substance, the body experiences severe physiologic, psychological, and emotional disturbances.
depolarization The ability of a cell to respond to a stimulus by initiating an impulse; also called "excitability."
depressant A drug that reduces the activity of the central nervous system, such as a benzodiazepine or barbiturate.
depressed fracture A type of skull fracture in which the bone is pressed inward into the brain tissue.
depression A response to multiple life stresses, a single situation, a primary disorder, or a problem associated with dementia; this response can range from mild, transient feelings of sadness to a severe sense of helplessness and hopelessness.
dermal appendage Collectively, the sweat and oil glands and the hair follicles. The depth of dermal appendages varies from one body area to another.
dermal papillae Fingerlike projections of dermal tissue that anchor the epidermis to the dermis.
dermatomes Specific areas of the skin that receive sensory input from spinal nerves.
dermatomyositis Polymyositis that is accompanied by a rash.
descending tracts Groups of nerves that begin in the brain and end in the spinal cord.
desquamation The shedding or peeling of skin.
diagnostic surgery Surgery done to remove all or part of a suspected lesion for examination and testing; also called "biopsy."
dialysate The solution used in dialysis. It is composed of water, glucose, sodium chloride, potassium, magnesium, calcium, and bicarbonate; dialysate composition may be altered according to the patient's needs for treatment of electrolyte imbalances.
dialyzer The apparatus used to perform hemodialysis. Also known as the artificial kidney, it has four parts: a blood compartment, a dialysate compartment, a semipermeable membrane, and an enclosed structure to support the membrane.
diaphoresis Abnormally profuse sweating.
diaphysis The shaft, or elongated cylindrical portion, between the ends of a long bone.
diastole The phase of the cardiac cycle that consists of relaxation and filling of the atria and ventricles; normally about two thirds of the cardiac cycle.
diastolic blood pressure The amount of pressure/force against the arterial walls during the relaxation phase of the heart.
diastolic heart failure Heart failure that occurs when the left ventricle is unable to relax adequately during diastole, which prevents the ventricle from filling with sufficient blood to ensure adequate cardiac output.
diathermy The use of a high-frequency current to heat body tissues.
Dietary Guidelines for Americans Recommendations made by the USDA and U.S. Department of Health and Human Services to help people maintain nutritional health; updated every 5 years.
diffuse axonal injury (DAI) A type of closed head injury that is usually related to high-speed acceleration/deceleration, as with motor vehicle accidents. There is significant damage to axons in the white matter, and there are lesions in the corpus callosum, midbrain, cerebellum, and upper brainstem. Patients with severe injury may present with immediate coma, and most survivors require long-term care.
diffuse light reflex A description of a light reflex that is spotty or multiple because of a changed eardrum shape from either retraction or bulging.
diffuse scleroderma Skin thickening on the trunk, face, and proximal and distal extremities in patients with systemic sclerosis.
diffusion The spontaneous, free movement of particles (solute) across a permeable membrane down a concentration gradient; that is, from an area of higher concentration to an area of lower concentration.
digitalis toxicity A reaction to therapy with digitalis derivatives (digoxin) that is identified by monitoring serum digoxin and potassium levels (hypokalemia potentiates digitalis toxicity). Signs of toxicity are nonspecific (anorexia, fatigue, changes in mental status). Toxicity may cause dysrhythmia, most commonly premature ventricular contractions.
dilated cardiomyopathy (DCM) A type of cardiomyopathy that involves extensive damage to the myofibrils and interference with myocardial metabolism. There is normal ventricular wall thickness but dilation of both ventricles and impairment of systolic function.
dilation Increase in the diameter of blood vessels.
diplopia Double vision.
direct contact A mode of infection transmission in which microorganisms are transferred directly by physical contact from one person to another.
direct current stimulation (DCS) The placement of an implantable device to promote bone fusion; used as an adjunct for patients for whom spinal fusion may be difficult.
direct inguinal hernia A sac formed from the peritoneum that contains a portion of the intestine and passes through a weak point in the abdominal wall.
direct response Pupil constriction in response to bringing a penlight in from the side of the patient's head and shining the light in the eye being tested as soon as the patient opens his or her eyes.
disabling health problem Any physical or mental health problem that can cause disability.
disaster A mass casualty incident in which the number of casualties exceeds the resource capabilities of a particular community or hospital facility.
disaster triage tag system A system that categorizes triage priority by colored and numbered tags.
discoid lesion Round lesion in patients who have discoid lupus erythematosus; evident when exposed to sunlight or ultraviolet light.
disease-modifying antirheumatic drugs (DMARDs) Drugs prescribed to slow the progression of mild rheumatoid disease before it worsens, such as hydroxychloroquine, sulfasalazine, or minocycline.

disequilibrium A condition in which the hydrostatic pressure is not the same in the two fluid spaces on either side of a permeable membrane.

disinfection A method of infection control in which the level of disease-causing organisms is reduced but the organisms are not killed; adequate when an item is entering a body area that has resident bacteria or normal flora, such as the respiratory tract.

diskitis Disk inflammation.

dislocation of a joint Occurrence of the articulating surfaces of two or more bones moving away from each other.

dissociate The act of separating and releasing ions.

distal protection device (DSP) A device that is placed beyond (distal to) the stenosis during an angioplasty/stenting procedure for the purpose of catching debris that breaks off during the procedure.

divalent cation An ion having two positive charges.

diverticula Sacs resulting from the herniation of the mucosa and submucosa of a tubular organ into surrounding tissue.

diverticulitis The inflammation of one or more diverticula.

diverticulosis The presence of many abnormal pouchlike herniations (diverticula) in the wall of the intestine.

DNA replication The process of making a new copy of an entire strand of DNA.

dopamine agonist A class of drugs that mimic dopamine. Dopamine agonists stimulate dopamine receptors and are typically the most effective during the first 3 to 5 years of use. Prescribed for the patient with Parkinson disease to reduce dyskinesias (problems with movement).

dose (1) In radiation therapy, the amount of radiation absorbed by recipient tissue during radiation therapy as determined by intensity of exposure, duration of exposure, and closeness of the radiation source to the cells; (2) the amount of drug or other substance to be administered at one time.

dose-dense chemotherapy Chemotherapy that uses higher doses more often for aggressive cancer treatment, especially breast cancer.

double-barrel stoma The least common type of colostomy, which is created by dividing the bowel and bringing both the proximal and distal portions to the abdominal surface to create two stomas.

doubling time The amount of time it takes for a tumor to double in size.

Dressler's syndrome Pericarditis, fever, and pericardial and pleural effusions occurring together from 1 to 12 weeks after myocardial infarction.

droplet The small particles produced when a person coughs or sneezes; may be involved in indirect transmission of infection.

Droplet Precautions Infection control guidelines from the Centers for Disease Control and Prevention; used for patients with infections spread by the droplet transmission route, such as influenza.

drug holiday Period of time lasting up to 10 days in which the patient with Parkinson disease receives no drug therapy.

dual x-ray absorptiometry (DXA) A type of radiographic scan that measures bone mineral density in the hip, wrist, or vertebral column; used as a screening and diagnostic tool for diagnosis and for follow-up evaluation of treatment of osteoporosis.

ductal carcinoma in situ (DCIS) An early, noninvasive form of breast cancer in which cancer cells are located within the duct and have not invaded the surrounding fatty breast tissue.

ductal ectasia A benign breast disease caused by dilation and thickening of the collecting ducts in the subareolar area. The ducts become distended and filled with cellular debris, which activates an inflammatory response. It is usually seen in women approaching menopause.

dull A term that describes the medium-pitched, soft, thudlike sound over a solid organ (e.g., liver) that is obtained upon percussion of the abdomen.

dumping syndrome A constellation of vasomotor symptoms that typically occur within 30 minutes after eating; believed to occur as a result of the rapid emptying of gastric contents into the small intestine, which shifts fluid into the gut and causes abdominal distention. Early manifestations include vertigo, tachycardia, syncope, sweating, pallor, and palpitations.

Dupuytren's contracture A slowly progressive contracture of the palmar fascia that results in flexion of the fourth or fifth digit of the hand and occasionally affects the third digit. Although a fairly common problem, the cause is unknown. It usually occurs in older men, tends to occur in families, and can be bilateral.

durable power of attorney (DPOA) for health care A legal document in which a person appoints someone else to make health care decisions in the event he or she becomes incapable of making decisions.

dysarthria Slurred speech.

dysfunctional uterine bleeding (DUB) A nonspecific term to describe bleeding that is excessive or abnormal in amount or frequency without predisposing anatomic or systemic conditions. Such bleeding occurs most often at either end of the span of a woman's reproductive years, when ovulation is becoming established or when it is becoming irregular at menopause.

dyskinesia Difficulty with movement.

dysmenorrhea Painful menstruation.

dysmetria The inability to direct or limit movement.

dyspareunia Painful sexual intercourse.

dyspepsia Indigestion or heartburn following meals.

dysphagia Difficulty in swallowing.

dyspnea Difficulty in breathing or breathlessness.

dyspnea on exertion (DOE) Dyspnea that is associated with activity, such as climbing stairs.

dysrhythmia A disorder of the heartbeat involving a disturbance in cardiac rhythm; irregular heartbeat.

dystrophic Pertaining to or characterized by dystrophy; abnormal.

dystrophin A muscle protein that maintains muscle integrity by sending signals to coordinate smooth, synchronous muscle fiber contraction. Faulty action of this protein causes muscular dystrophy.

dysuria Painful urination.

E

early-onset seizure Seizure that occurs within 7 days of a head injury.

Eaton-Lambert syndrome A form of myasthenia gravis that affects the muscles of the trunk and the pelvic and shoulder girdles; often observed in combination with small cell carcinoma of the lung. Although weakness increases after exertion, there may be a temporary increase in muscle strength during the first few contractions, followed by a rapid decline.

ecchymoses Bruises of the skin resulting from small hemorrhages; these bruises are larger than petechiae.

ecchymotic Pertaining to a bruise.
ECG caliper A measurement tool used in analysis of an electrocardiographic (ECG) rhythm strip.
echocardiography In cardiovascular assessment, the use of ultrasound waves to assess cardiac structure and mobility, particularly of the valves; a noninvasive, risk-free test that is easily performed at the bedside or on an ambulatory care basis.
echolalia Automatic repetition of what another person says.
ectopic Out of place.
ectopic beats Heartbeats generated outside the normal conduction system in the ventricles; a cardiac manifestation of hyperkalemia.
ectropion A turning outward and sagging of the eyelid, which is caused by relaxation of the orbicular muscle.
edema Tissue swelling as a result of the accumulation of excessive fluid in the interstitial spaces.
edentulous Without teeth.
efferent arterioles The extremely small blood vessels that carry the remaining blood out of the glomerulus (once the glomerulus has filtered the blood to make urine) and into one of two additional capillary systems (the peritubular capillaries or the vasa recta).
effluent Drainage.
effusion An accumulation of fluid, such as in a joint (where it may limit movement).
ejection fraction The percentage of blood ejected from the heart during systole.
elastin The major component of the elastic fibers that are scattered among the collagen fibers. Elasticity of the skin depends on both the amount and quality of the elastic fibers.
electrical bone stimulation The use of an electronic device (e.g., magnetic coils applied on the skin or over a cast to deliver a pulsed magnetic field) to promote bone union after a fracture. The exact mechanism of action is unknown, but this procedure is based on research showing that bone has inherent electrical properties that are used in healing.
electrocardiogram (ECG) A graphic recording of the electrical current generated by the heart. The ECG provides information about cardiac dysrhythmias, myocardial ischemia, site and extent of myocardial infarction, cardiac hypertrophy, electrolyte imbalances, and effectiveness of cardiac drugs. It is a routine part of cardiovascular evaluation and is a valuable diagnostic test.
electroencephalography (EEG) A recording of the electrical activity of the cerebral hemispheres; it represents the voltage changes in various areas of the brain as determined by recording the difference between two electrodes.
electrolyte A substance in body fluids that carries an electrical charge; also called an "ion."
electromyography (EMG) A recording of the electrical activity of peripheral nerves by testing muscle activity.
electrophysiologic study (EPS) In cardiovascular assessment, an invasive procedure performed in a catheterization laboratory during which programmed electrical stimulation of the heart is used to induce and evaluate lethal dysrhythmias and conduction abnormalities to permit accurate diagnosis and effective treatment. The study is used in patients who have survived cardiac arrest, have recurrent tachydysrhythmias, or experience unexplained syncopal episodes.
electrovaporization Procedure for treating benign prostatic hyperplasia with high-frequency electrical current to cut and vaporize excess tissue.
emboli (1) Tumor pieces that spread to distant body areas; (2) small blood clots that can enter circulation.
embolic protection device (EPD) A device that is placed beyond the stenosis during an angioplasty/stenting procedure to catch debris that breaks off during the procedure.
embolus The occurrence of inflammation and thickening of the vein wall around a clot (thrombus).
emergence Recovery from anesthesia.
emergency medical technician (EMT) Prehospital care provider who supplies basic life-support interventions such as oxygen, basic wound care, splinting, spinal immobilization, and monitoring of vital signs.
emergency medicine physician A member of the emergency health care team with education and training in the specialty of emergency patient management.
emergency operations center (EOC) A designated location in the HICS system with accessible communication technology; also called the "command center."
emergency preparedness A goal or plan to meet the extraordinary need for hospital beds, staff, drugs, personal protective equipment, supplies, and medical devices such as mechanical ventilators.
Emergency Severity Index (ESI) A standardized model for triage that categorizes both patient acuity and resource utilization into five levels, from most urgent to least urgent.
emergent phase The first phase of a burn injury, beginning at the onset of injury and continuing to about 48 hours.
emergent triage In a three-tiered triage scheme, the category that includes any condition or injury that poses an immediate threat to life or limb, such as crushing chest pain or active hemorrhage.
emetogenic A substance that induces nausea and vomiting.
emission The first stage of the male orgasm in which the prostate gland secretes its fluid at the same time as the vas deferens.
emmetropia The state of perfect refraction of the eye; with the lens at rest, light rays from a distant source are focused into a sharp image on the retina.
emotional abuse The intentional use of threats, humiliation, intimidation, and isolation to another person.
emotional lability Having uncontrollable emotions; for example, the patient laughs and then cries unexpectedly for no apparent reason.
empyema A collection of pus in the pleural space.
encephalitis An inflammation of the brain parenchyma (brain tissue) and meninges that affects the cerebrum, brainstem, and cerebellum; usually caused by a virus.
endogenous Originating inside the body.
endometrial ablation Procedure for dysfunctional uterine bleeding that removes a built-up uterine lining using a laser, roller ball, or balloon.
endometrial cancer Cancer of the inner uterine lining.
endometriosis The abnormal occurrence of endometrial tissue outside the uterine cavity.
endometritis An infection of the endometrium.
endorphins Morphine-like substances in the body that are released when the large-diameter nerve fibers are stimulated. They close the gate and decrease pain transmission.

endoscope A tube that allows viewing and manipulation of internal body areas.

endoscopic retrograde cholangiopancreatography (ERCP) The visual and radiographic examination of the liver, gallbladder, bile ducts, and pancreas by means of an endoscope and the injection of radiopaque dye to identify the cause and location of obstruction.

endoscopic variceal ligation (EVL) The application of small "O" bands around the base of the esophageal varices to cut off their blood supply; also called "banding."

endoscopy The direct visualization of the gastrointestinal tract by means of a flexible fiberoptic endoscope.

endotoxin Any toxic substance that is produced in the cell walls of certain bacteria and released only with cell lysis. Typhoid and meningococcal diseases are caused by endotoxins.

endovascular stent graft The repair of an abdominal aortic aneurysm using a stent made of flexible material; the stent is inserted through a skin incision into the femoral artery by way of a catheter-based system.

endoventricular circular patch cardioplasty In the patient with heart failure, a procedure in which the surgeon removes portions of the cardiac septum and left ventricular wall and grafts a circular patch (synthetic or autologous) into the opening. This procedure provides a more normal shape to the left ventricle to improve hemodynamics.

end-stage kidney disease (ESKD) Acute renal failure combined with chronic renal insufficiency, resulting in the inability of the kidney to excrete waste products normally. The patient may need hemodialysis or a kidney transplant.

energy conservation Strategies to reduce the fatigue associated with chronic and disabling conditions, such as allowing rest periods and setting priorities.

engraftment The successful transplantation of cells in the patient's bone marrow.

enophthalmos Backward displacement of the eyeball into the orbit so that the eye appears sunken.

enteroscopy Visualization of the small intestine.

enterostomal feeding tube A tube used for patients who need long-term enteral feeding; the physician directly accesses the gastrointestinal tract using surgical, endoscopic, and laparoscopic techniques.

entropion The turning inward of the eyelid, causing the eyelashes to rub against the eye.

enucleation The surgical removal of the entire eyeball.

envenomation Venom injection from a snake bite.

epididymectomy Surgical excision of the epididymis from the testicle.

epididymis The cordlike structure along the posterior border of the testis; it is the first portion of a ductal system that transports sperm from the testes to the urethra.

epididymitis Inflammation of the epididymis.

epidural Term for the space between the dura mater and vertebrae; it consists of fat, connective tissue, and blood vessels.

epidural analgesia The instillation of a pain-blocking agent into the epidural space (between the dura mater and the vertebral column).

epidural catheter A transducer or sensor that is placed between the skull and the dura (leaving the dura intact) to monitor intracranial pressure.

epidural hematoma An accumulation of clotted blood resulting from arterial bleeding into the space between the dura and the skull; a neurosurgical emergency.

epidural hemorrhage Arterial bleeding into the space between the dura and the skull.

epiglottis A leaf-shaped, elastic structure that is attached along one edge to the top of the larynx; it closes over the glottis during swallowing to prevent food from entering the trachea and opens during breathing and coughing.

epilepsy A chronic disorder characterized by recurrent, unprovoked seizure activity; may be caused by an abnormality in electrical neuronal activity, an imbalance of neurotransmitters, or a combination of both.

epiphyses The two knoblike ends of a long bone.

epistaxis Nosebleed.

epitympanum The upper portion of the tympanic cavity; a compartment containing the three bony ossicles.

equianalgesic Refers to the dose and route of administration of one drug that produces approximately the same degree of analgesia as the given dose and route of another drug.

equilibrium (1) A state of balance; (2) a condition in which there is no hydrostatic pressure difference between the two fluid spaces on either side of a permeable membrane.

erectile dysfunction (ED) The inability to achieve or maintain a penile erection sufficient for sexual intercourse.

ergonomics An applied science in which the workplace is designed to increase worker comfort (thus reducing injury) while increasing efficiency and productivity.

eructation The act of belching.

erythema Redness of the skin.

erythema migrans A round or oval flat or slightly raised rash.

erythrocyte A red blood cell. Red blood cells are the major cells in the blood and are responsible for tissue oxygenation.

erythroplakia A velvety red mucosal lesion, most often occurring in the oral cavity.

erythroplasia Red, velvety patches on a mucous membrane.

erythropoiesis The selective maturation of stem cells into mature erythrocytes.

eschar The crust of dead tissue that forms from coagulated particles of destroyed dermis in a patient with a full-thickness burn injury.

escharotomy Incision made through tight eschar to relieve pressure and allow normal blood flow and breathing.

esophageal stricture Narrowing of the esophageal opening.

esophageal varices The distention of fragile, thin-walled esophageal veins due to increased pressure; the increased pressure is a result of portal hypertension, in which the blood backs up from the liver and enters the esophageal and gastric vessels that carry it into the systemic circulation.

esophagectomy The surgical removal of all or part of the esophagus.

esophagitis Inflammation of the esophagus.

esophagogastroduodenoscopy (EGD) The visual examination of the esophagus, stomach, and duodenum by means of a fiberoptic endoscope.

esophagogastrostomy The surgical creation of a communication between the stomach and the esophagus; it involves the removal of part of the esophagus and proximal stomach.

esophagomyotomy A surgical procedure in which the lower esophageal sphincter is incised to facilitate the passage of food for patients with achalasia.

essential hypertension Elevated blood pressure that is not caused by a specific disease. The major risk factor is a family history of hypertension; also called "primary hypertension."

ethnopharmacology The study of how ethnicity affects how drugs work in the body, including drug absorption, distribution, metabolism, and excretion.
euploid Having the correct number of chromosome pairs for the species.
eustachian tube Tube that connects the nasopharynx with the middle ear and opens during swallowing to equalize pressure within the middle ear.
euthyroid Having normal thyroid function.
evidence-based practice Care that nurses provide that is based on research and identified standards and considers the patient's preferences and values and the nurse's clinical expertise.
evisceration The total separation of all layers of a wound and the protrusion of internal organs through the open wound.
evoked potentials Tests to measure the electrical signals to the brain generated by hearing, touch, or sight; also called "evoked response."
exacerbate To increase in severity of disease or its symptoms.
exacerbation An increase in severity of a disease; also called "flare-up."
excision Removal of a lesion and local surrounding tissue.
excitability The ability of a cell to respond to a stimulus by initiating an impulse; also called "depolarization." In cardiac electrophysiology, it is the ability of non-pacemaker myocardial cells to respond to an electrical impulse generated from pacemaker cells and to depolarize.
exercise electrocardiography In cardiovascular assessment, a test that assesses cardiovascular response to an increased workload; also called "exercise tolerance" or a "stress test." Exercise electrocardiography helps determine the functional capacity of the heart, screens for coronary artery disease, and identifies dysrhythmias that develop during exercise. It also aids in evaluating the effectiveness of antidysrhythmic drugs.
exertional dyspnea Breathlessness or difficulty breathing that develops during activity or exertion.
exertional heat stroke A form of heat stroke with a sudden onset, typically due to strenuous physical activity in hot, humid conditions. Lack of acclimatization to hot weather and wearing clothing too heavy for the environment are common contributing factors.
exogenous Originating outside the body.
exogenous hyperthyroidism Hyperthyroidism caused by excessive use of thyroid replacement hormones.
exophthalmos Abnormal protrusion of the eyeball (proptosis).
exotoxin Any toxic substance that is produced and released by certain bacteria into the surrounding environment. Botulism, tetanus, and diphtheria are attributed to exotoxins.
expedited partner therapy (EPT) Therapy used to treat chlamydia in which patients are given a drug or prescription with specific instructions for administration to their partners without direct evaluation by a health care provider; also called "patient-delivered partner therapy."
exploratory laparotomy A surgical opening of the abdominal cavity to investigate the cause of an obstruction or peritonitis.
exposure (1) The final component of the primary survey that allows for thorough assessment of the trauma patient; (2) in radiation therapy, the amount of radiation that is delivered to a tissue.
expressed gene When a particular gene has been "turned on."
expression (gene) The selective activation of a particular gene in a specific cell type.
expressive aphasia A type of aphasia resulting from damage in Broca's area of the frontal lobe of the brain. A motor speech problem in which the patient understands what is said but is unable to communicate verbally and has difficulty writing; rote speech and automatic speech, such as responses to a greeting, are often intact. The patient is aware of the deficit and may become frustrated and angry. Also called "Broca's aphasia" or "motor aphasia."
expressivity In genetics, the degree of expression a person has when a specific autosomal dominant gene is present. The gene is always expressed, but some people have more severe results.
external catheter An epidural catheter, a portion of which exits the skin.
external fixation A system in which pins or wires are passed through skin and bone and connected to a rigid external frame to immobilize a fracture during healing.
external hemorrhoid A hemorrhoid that lies below the anal sphincter and can be seen on inspection of the anal region.
external otitis A painful irritation or infection of the skin of the external ear, with resulting allergic response or inflammation. When it occurs in patients who participate in water sports, external otitis is called "swimmer's ear."
external urethral sphincter The sphincter composed of the skeletal muscle that surrounds the urethra.
extracapsular Located outside the joint capsule.
extracellular fluid (ECF) The portion of total body water (about one third) that is in the space outside the cells. This space also includes interstitial fluid, blood, lymph, bone and connective tissue water, and the transcellular fluids.
extracranial-intracranial bypass A surgical procedure in which the surgeon performs a craniotomy and bypasses the blocked artery by making a graft (bypass) from the first artery to the second artery to establish blood flow around the blocked artery and re-establish blood flow to the involved areas.
extramedullary tumor A tumor found within the spinal dura but outside the cord.
extrapulmonary Involving nonpulmonary tissues.
extravasation Escape of fluids or drugs into the subcutaneous tissue; a complication of intravenous infusion.
extrinsic factors In hematology, an event (e.g., trauma) that occurs outside the blood to cause platelet plugs to form.
extubation The removal of an endotracheal tube.
exudate Pus.

F

facial paralysis See *Bell's palsy*.
facilitated diffusion Diffusion across a cell membrane that requires the assistance of a transport system or membrane-altering system; also called "facilitated transport."
facilitated transport See *facilitated diffusion*.
failed back surgery syndrome (FBSS) A combination of organic, psychological, and socioeconomic factors in patients for whom back surgery is not successful. Discouraged by repeated surgical procedures, these patients must continue long-term nonsurgical management of pain, including nerve blocks.
fall An unintentional change in body position that results in the patient's body coming to rest on the floor or ground.
fallophobia In some older adults, the fear of falling and sustaining a serious injury.

fallopian tubes The tubes that insert into the fundus of the uterus, extending laterally close to the ovaries, and provide a duct between the ovaries and uterus for the passage of ova and sperm; also called "uterine tubes."

far point of vision The farthest point at which the eye can see an object.

fascia An inelastic tissue that surrounds groups of muscles, blood vessels, and nerves in the body.

fasciculation Abnormal, involuntary twitching of a muscle.

fasciotomy A surgical procedure in which an incision is made through the skin and subcutaneous tissues into the fascia of the affected compartment to relieve the pressure in and restore circulation to the affected area in the patient with acute compartment syndrome.

fat embolism syndrome (FES) A serious complication, usually resulting from a fracture, in which fat globules are released from the yellow bone marrow into the bloodstream. This syndrome usually occurs within 48 hours of the fracture and can result in respiratory failure or death, often from pulmonary edema.

fatigue (stress) fracture A fracture that results from excessive or repeated strain and stress on a bone.

fecal occult blood test (FOBT) A diagnostic test that measures the presence of blood in the stool from gastrointestinal bleeding; this is a common finding associated with colorectal cancer.

Felty's syndrome The combination of rheumatoid arthritis, hepatosplenomegaly (enlarged liver and spleen), and leukopenia.

femoral hernia A hernia that protrudes through the femoral ring.

fetor hepaticus The distinctive fruity or musty breath odor of chronic liver disease and portal-systemic encephalopathy.

fibrinolysis The breakdown of a clot.

fibrinolytic Drug that targets the fibrin component of the coronary thrombosis; used to dissolve thrombi in the coronary arteries and restore myocardial blood flow; examples include tissue plasminogen activator, anisoylated plasminogen-streptokinase activator complex, and reteplase.

fibroadenoma A solid, slowly enlarging, benign mass of connective tissue that is unattached to the surrounding breast tissue and is typically discovered by the patient herself. The mass is usually round, firm, easily movable, nontender, and clearly delineated from the surrounding tissue.

fibrocystic breast condition (FBC) Physiologic nodularity of the breast that is thought to be caused by an imbalance in the normal estrogen to progesterone ratio. It is the most common breast problem of women between 20 and 30 years of age.

fibrogenic Originating from fibrous tissue.

fibroids See *leiomyomas.*

fibromyalgia syndrome (FMS) A chronic pain syndrome characterized by pain and tenderness at specific sites in the back of the neck, upper chest, trunk, low back, and extremities along with fatigue, sleep disturbances, and headache.

fibrosis Replacement of normal cells with connective tissue and collagen (scar tissue).

filter The movement of fluid from the space with higher hydrostatic pressure through the membrane into the space with lower hydrostatic pressure.

filtration The movement of fluid through a cell or blood vessel membrane because of hydrostatic pressure differences on both sides of the membrane.

financial abuse Mismanagement or misuse of the patient's property or resources.

first intention healing Healing in which the wound can be easily closed and dead space eliminated without granulation, which thus shortens the phases of tissue repair. Inflammation resolves quickly, and connective tissue repair is minimal, resulting in a thin scar.

fistula An abnormal opening between two adjacent organs or structures.

five cardinal manifestations of inflammation Warmth, redness, swelling, pain, and decreased function.

fixed occlusion Wiring the jaws together in the mouth closed position.

flaccid bladder See *areflexic bladder.*

flaccid paralysis Paralysis of a part of the body that is characterized by loss of muscle tone due to hypotonia; may be seen in the patient who has experienced a brain attack.

flail chest Inward movement of the thorax during inspiration, with outward movement during expiration; results from multiple rib fractures caused by blunt chest trauma that leaves a segment of the chest wall loose.

flatulence The presence of an excessive amount of gas in the stomach or intestines.

fluid overload An excess of body fluid. Also called "overhydration."

folliculitis A superficial bacterial infection involving only the upper portion of the hair follicle.

Food Guide Pyramid Food recommendations of the U.S. Department of Agriculture presented in a graphic pyramid design format to communicate the key dietary principles of variety, moderation, and proportionality. In the pyramid design, the diet is built on a base of grains, fruits, and vegetables, with moderate quantities of lean meats, protein sources, and dairy products and limited intake of fats and sweets. In 2005, this pyramid was redesigned into the MyPyramid to help people better understand these principles. MyPyramid also stresses the importance of physical activity to promote health.

Food Pyramid for Seniors Over 70 A food pyramid developed to guide older adults in food and nutrient selection.

forced expiratory volume in the first second (FEV$_1$) Volume of air blown out as hard and fast as possible during the first second of the most forceful exhalation after the greatest full inhalation.

forced vital capacity (FVC) Volume of air exhaled from full inhalation to full exhalation.

forensic nurse examiner Emergency department specialist who is trained to recognize evidence of abuse and to intervene on the patient's behalf and who obtains patient histories, collects forensic evidence, and offers counseling and follow-up care for victims of rape, child abuse, and domestic violence.

fracture A break or disruption in the continuity of a bone.

fremitus Vibration.

frequency (1) The highness or lowness of tones (expressed in hertz). The greater the number of vibrations per second, the higher the frequency (pitch) of the sound; the fewer the number of vibrations per second, the lower the pitch; (2) an urge to urinate frequently in small amounts.

fresh frozen plasma (FFP) Plasma that is frozen immediately after donation so that the clotting factors are preserved.

friable Easily crumbled or damaged.

frostbite A cold injury characterized by the degree of tissue freezing and the resultant damage it produces. Frostbite injuries can be superficial, partial, or full thickness.

frostnip A form of superficial frostbite (typically on the face, fingers, or toes) that produces pain, numbness, and pallor but is easily remedied with the application of warmth and does not induce tissue injury.

full agonist Morphine-like opioid analgesic that binds to mu receptors and blocks the release of substance P, preventing the transmission of pain; the most potent of all analgesics.

Fulmer SPICES A framework that identifies six serious "marker conditions" that can lead to longer hospital stays for patients, higher medical costs, and deaths.

fulminant hepatitis A severe acute and often fatal form of hepatitis caused by failure of the liver cells to regenerate, with progression to necrosis.

fundoplication A procedure in which the fundus of the stomach is wrapped around the lower end of the esophagus to anchor it and reinforce the lower esophageal sphincter; the most common surgical technique for hiatal hernia repair. A laparoscopic Nissen fundoplication is one variation of this type of procedure; a traditional, open surgical approach (using a large abdominal incision) is another variation.

furuncle A localized inflammation of the skin caused by bacterial infection, usually *Staphylococcus,* of a hair follicle; also called "a boil."

G

G_1 phase Phase of cell division in which the cell gets ready for division by taking on extra nutrients, making more energy, growing extra membrane, and increasing the amount of cytoplasm.

G_2 phase Phase of cell division in which the cell makes proteins that will be used in actual cell division and in normal physiologic function after cell division is complete.

gallium scan A test that is similar to the bone scan but uses the radioisotope gallium citrate and is more specific and sensitive in detecting bone problems. This substance also migrates to brain, liver, and breast tissue and therefore is used to examine these structures when disease is suspected.

gamma globulins See *immunoglobulin.*

ganglion A round, cystlike lesion, often overlying a wrist joint or tendon.

gas bloat syndrome A common, usually temporary, complication of fundoplication surgery. In this syndrome, patients are unable to voluntarily eructate (belch).

gastrectomy The surgical removal of part or all of the stomach.

gastric bypass (Roux-en-Y gastric bypass) A type of gastric restriction surgery in which gastric resection is combined with malabsorption surgery. The patient's stomach, duodenum, and part of the jejunum are bypassed so that fewer calories can be absorbed.

gastric lavage Procedure of irrigating the stomach in which a large-bore nasogastric tube is inserted into the stomach and room-temperature solution is instilled in volumes of 200 to 300 mL. The solution and blood are repeatedly withdrawn manually until returns are clear or light pink and without clots.

gastrinoma A non–beta cell islet tumor of the pancreas; the usual cause of Zollinger-Ellison syndrome.

gastritis An inflammation of the gastric mucosa (stomach lining).

gastroenteritis An increase in the frequency and water content of stools or vomiting as a result of inflammation of the mucous membranes of the stomach and intestinal tract. It primarily affects the small bowel and can be of either viral or bacterial origin.

gastroesophageal reflux disease (GERD) An upper gastrointestinal disease caused by the backward flow (reflux) of gastrointestinal contents into the esophagus.

gastrojejunostomy Surgical anastomosis of the stomach to the jejunum.

gastroparesis Delay in gastric emptying.

gastrostomy A stoma created from the abdominal wall into the stomach.

gate control theory A theory to explain the observed relationship between pain and emotion; a gating mechanism occurs in the spinal cord. Nerve fibers (A delta and C fibers) transmit pain impulses from the periphery of the body. The impulses travel to the dorsal horns of the spinal cord, specifically to the *substantia gelatinosa*. The cells of the substantia gelatinosa can inhibit or facilitate the pain impulses transmitted to the trigger cells (T-cells). When T-cell activity is inhibited, the gate is closed and impulses are less likely to be transmitted to the brain. When the gate is opened, pain impulses ascend to the brain.

gel phenomenon In patients with rheumatoid arthritis, morning stiffness that lasts between 45 minutes and several hours after awakening.

gene The deoxyribonucleic acid in the form of chromosomes within the nucleus of each cell that contains the instructions for making all the different proteins any organism makes. Every human cell with a nucleus contains the entire set of human genes.

general anesthesia A reversible loss of consciousness induced by inhibiting neuronal impulses in the central nervous system.

generalized seizure One of the three broad categories of seizure disorders along with partial seizures and unclassified seizures. There are six types: tonic-clonic, tonic, clonic, absence, myoclonic, and atonic (akinetic).

generation time The time it takes one cell to divide into two cells.

genital herpes (GH) An acute, recurring, incurable viral disease of the genitalia caused by the herpes simplex virus and transmitted through contact with an infected person. An outbreak typically is preceded by a tingling sensation of the skin followed by the appearance of vesicles (blisters) on the penis, scrotum, vulva, perineum, vagina, cervix, or perianal region. The blisters rupture spontaneously, leaving painful erosions. After the lesions heal, the virus remains dormant, periodically reactivating with a recurrence of symptoms.

genome The complete set of human genes. Each human cell with a nucleus contains the entire set of human genes. The human genome contains about 35,000 individual genes.

genotype The actual alleles for a genetic trait, not just what can be observed.

genu valgum A deformity in which the knees are abnormally close together and the space between the ankles is increased; also called "knock-knee."

genu varum A deformity in which the knees are abnormally separated and the lower extremities are bowed inward; also called "bowleg."

Geriatric Depression Scale—Short Form A valid and reliable screening tool to help determine if an older patient has clinical depression.
Ghon tubercle A mass of necrotic lung tissue, visible on x-ray, that is the primary lesion of tuberculosis.
Glasgow Coma Scale An objective and widely accepted tool for neurologic assessment and documentation of level of consciousness. It establishes baseline data for eye opening, motor response, and verbal response. The patient is assessed and assigned a numerical score for each of these areas. A score of 15 represents normal neurologic functioning, and a score of 3 represents a deep coma state.
glaucoma A group of ocular diseases resulting in increased intraocular pressure, causing reduced blood flow to the optic nerve and retina and followed by tissue damage.
glomerulus A series of specialized capillary loops that receive blood from the afferent arteriole and then filter water and small particles from the blood to make urine. The remaining blood leaves the glomerulus via the efferent arteriole.
glossectomy The partial or total surgical removal of the tongue.
glossitis A smooth, beefy red tongue.
glottis The opening between the true vocal cords inside the larynx.
glucagon A hormone secreted by the pancreas that increases blood glucose levels. It is a "counterregulatory" hormone that has actions opposite those of insulin. It causes the release of glucose from cell storage sites whenever blood glucose levels are low.
gluconeogenesis The conversion of proteins and amino acids to glucose in the body.
glycemic A term referring to blood glucose.
glycogenesis The production of glycogen in the body.
glycogenolysis The breakdown of glycogen into glucose.
glycoprotein IIa/IIIb inhibitors Drugs that target the platelet component of the thrombus. They are administered intravenously to prevent fibrinogen from attaching to activated platelets at the site of a thrombus and are given to patients with acute coronary syndromes (especially unstable angina and non–Q-wave myocardial infarction). Examples include abciximab, eptifibatide, and tirofiban.
"go bag" See *personal readiness supplies.*
goiter Enlargement of the thyroid gland.
gonadotropins Hormones that stimulate the ovaries and testes to produce sex hormones.
gonads The male and female reproductive endocrine glands. Male gonads are the testes, and female gonads are the ovaries.
goniometer An instrument for measuring angles; also used to refer to a tool used to measure joint range of motion.
good death A death that is free from avoidable distress and suffering for patients, families, and caregivers; in agreement with patients' and families' wishes; and consistent with clinical practice standards.
gout A systemic disease in which urate crystals deposit in the joints and other body tissues, causing inflammation.
gradient A graded difference of hydrostatic pressure in a state of disequilibrium; that is, one fluid space has a higher hydrostatic pressure than the other.
grading System of classifying cellular aspects of a cancer tumor.
granulation The formation of scar tissue for wound healing to occur.
granulocyte Neutrophil that contains a large number of granules.
granuloma Growth that develops in the lungs of patients with sarcoidosis and contains lymphocytes, macrophages, epithelioid cells, and giant cells; scar tissue.
granuloma inguinale An ulcerative disease of the genital area that appears as a painless nodule.
Graves' disease Toxic diffuse goiter characterized by hyperthyroidism, enlargement of the thyroid gland, abnormal protrusion of the eyes, and dry, waxy swelling of the front surfaces of the lower legs.
gray matter In the spinal cord, neuron cell bodies.
grief The emotional feeling related to the perception of loss.
grommet A polyethylene tube that is surgically placed through the tympanic membrane to allow continuous drainage of middle-ear fluids in the patient with otitis media.
ground substance A lubricant composed of protein and sugar groups that surrounds the dermal cells and fibers and contributes to the skin's normal suppleness and turgor.
Guillain-Barré syndrome (GBS) An acute autoimmune disorder characterized by varying degrees of motor weakness and paralysis. It may be referred to by a variety of other names, such as "acute idiopathic polyneuritis" and "polyradiculoneuropathy."
gynecomastia Abnormal enlargement of the breasts in men.

H

H_2-receptor antagonists A group of drugs that inhibit gastric acid secretion by blocking the effects of histamine on parietal cell receptors in the stomach.
halitosis A foul odor of the mouth.
hallucinogens Chemical substances that possess mind-altering or perception-altering properties, such as lysergic acid (LSD), phencyclidine (PCP), and marijuana.
hallux valgus A common deformity of the foot that occurs when the great toe deviates laterally at the metatarsophalangeal joint; sometimes referred to as a *bunion.*
hammertoe The dorsiflexion of any metatarsophalangeal joint with plantar flexion of the adjacent proximal interphalangeal joint. The second toe is most often affected.
hand hygiene Infection control protocol that refers to both handwashing and alcohol-based hand rubs.
handwashing The process of wetting, soaping, lathering, applying friction under running water for at least 15 seconds, rinsing, and drying the hands; an important part of infection control.
health care–associated infections (HAI) Infections that are associated with the provision of health care; for example, microorganisms can enter the body through the genitourinary tract in patients with indwelling urinary catheters.
Healthy People 2010 A program created by the U.S. Department of Health and Human Services (2000) with the goal of eliminating differences in health status among racial and ethnic minorities while continually improving the overall health of all Americans through research, preventive programs, and inclusion of members of minority groups.
heart failure A general term for the inadequacy of the heart to pump blood throughout the body, causing insufficient perfusion of body tissues with vital nutrients and oxygen; also called "pump failure."
heart rate (HR) Term referring to the number of times the ventricles contract each minute.

heart reduction surgery Partial left ventriculectomy; in the patient with heart failure, a surgical procedure to remove a triangle-shaped section of the weakened heart in the left lateral ventricle to reduce the ventricle's diameter and decrease wall tension.

heart transplantation A surgical procedure in which a heart from a donor with a comparable body weight and ABO compatibility is transplanted into a recipient less than 6 hours after procurement. It is the treatment of choice for patients with severe dilated cardiomyopathy and may be considered for patients with restrictive cardiomyopathy.

heat exhaustion A syndrome primarily caused by dehydration from heavy perspiration and inadequate fluid and electrolyte consumption during heat exposure over hours to days; if left untreated, can be a precursor to heat stroke.

heat stroke A true medical emergency in which the victim's heat regulatory mechanisms fail and are unable to compensate for a critical elevation in body temperature; if uncorrected, organ dysfunction and death will ensue.

Heberden's nodes Swelling at the distal interphalangeal joints in osteoarthritis that involves the hands.

helminths Parasitic worms that are capable of causing infectious disease with gastrointestinal symptoms in humans. The three general categories are roundworms (nematodes), flukes (trematodes), and tapeworms (cestodes).

hematemesis The vomiting of blood.

hematochezia The passage of red blood via the rectum.

hematocrit The percentage of packed red blood cells per deciliter of blood.

hematogenous Disseminated by the blood through the circulation.

hematogenous tuberculosis A form of tuberculosis that spreads throughout the body when a large number of organisms enter the blood. Also called "miliary tuberculosis."

hematopoiesis The production of blood cells, which occurs in the red marrow of bones.

hematuria Blood in the urine.

hemianopsia Blindness in half of the visual field of one or both eyes; also called "hemianopia."

hemiarthroplasty Surgical replacement of part of the shoulder joint, typically the humeral component, as an alternative to total shoulder arthroplasty.

hemiparesis Weakness on one side of the body.

hemiplegia Paralysis on one side of the body.

hemoconcentration Elevated plasma levels of hemoglobin, hematocrit, serum osmolarity, glucose, protein, blood urea nitrogen, and electrolytes that occur when only the water is lost and other substances remain.

hemodilution Excessive water in the vascular space.

hemodynamic monitoring An invasive system that directly measures pressures in the heart and great vessels; used in critical care areas to provide quantitative information about vascular capacity, blood volume, pump effectiveness, and tissue perfusion.

hemoglobin A (HbA) Normal adult hemoglobin. The molecule has two alpha chains and two beta chains of amino acids.

hemolytic The characteristic of destroying red blood cells.

hemoptysis Coughing up blood or blood-stained sputum.

hemorrhoid Unnaturally swollen or distended vein in the anorectal region.

hemorrhoidectomy The excision of a hemorrhoid.

heparin-induced thrombocytopenia and thrombosis (HIT) The aggregation of platelets into "white clots" that can cause thrombosis, usually in the form of an acute arterial occlusion; occurs with heparin administration; also called "white clot syndrome."

hepatic coma See *portal-systemic encephalopathy.*

hepatic encephalopathy See *portal-systemic encephalopathy.*

hepatitis The widespread inflammation of liver cells.

hepatitis A Hepatitis that is caused by the hepatitis A virus (HAV) and is characterized by a mild course similar to that of a typical viral syndrome and often goes unrecognized. It is spread via the fecal-oral route by oral ingestion of fecal contaminants. Sources of infection include contaminated water, shellfish caught in contaminated water, and food contaminated by infected food handlers. The virus may also be spread by oral-anal sexual activity. The incubation period is usually 15 to 50 days. The disease is usually not life threatening but may be more severe in people older than 40 years of age. It can also complicate pre-existing liver disease.

hepatitis B A form of hepatitis that is caused by the hepatitis B virus, which is shed in the body fluids of infected people and asymptomatic carriers. It is spread through unprotected sexual intercourse with an infected partner, needle sharing, blood transfusions, and other modes. Symptoms usually occur within 25 to 180 days of exposure and include nausea, fever, fatigue, joint pain, and jaundice. Most adults who get hepatitis B recover, clear the virus from their body, and develop immunity; however, up to 10% of patients with the disease do not develop immunity and become carriers.

hepatitis C Hepatitis that is caused by the hepatitis C virus. Transmission is blood to blood, most commonly by needle sharing or needle stick injury with contaminated blood. The rate of sexual transmission is very low; it is not spread by casual contact and is rarely transmitted from mother to fetus. The average incubation period is 7 weeks. Most people are asymptomatic and are not diagnosed until long after the initial exposure when an abnormality is detected during a routine laboratory evaluation or when symptoms of liver impairment appear. Hepatitis C causes chronic inflammation in the liver that eventually causes the hepatocytes to scar and may progress to cirrhosis.

hepatitis carrier Person who has had hepatitis B but has not developed immunity. Hepatitis carriers can infect others even though they are not sick and demonstrate no obvious signs of disease. Chronic carriers are at high risk for cirrhosis and liver cancer.

hepatitis D The hepatitis D virus (HDV) co-infects with hepatitis B virus (HBV) and needs the presence of HBV for viral replication. HDV can co-infect a patient with HBV or can occur as a superinfection in a patient with chronic HBV. Superinfection usually develops into chronic HDV infection. The incubation period is 14 to 56 days. As with HBV, the disease is transmitted primarily by parenteral routes.

hepatitis E Hepatitis E virus (HEV) was originally identified by its association with waterborne epidemics of hepatitis in the Indian subcontinent. Since then, it has occurred in epidemics in Asia, Africa, the Middle East, Mexico, and Central and South America, typically after heavy rains and flooding. In the United States, hepatitis E has been found only in travelers returning from endemic areas. The virus is transmitted via the fecal-oral route, and the clinical course resembles that of hepatitis A.

HEV has an incubation period of 15 to 64 days. There is no evidence at this time of a chronic form of hepatitis E.

hepatocyte Liver cell.

hepatomegaly Enlargement of the liver.

hepatorenal syndrome (HRS) A state of progressive oliguric renal failure associated with hepatic failure, resulting in functional impairment of kidneys with normal anatomic and morphologic features. It indicates a poor prognosis for the patient with hepatic failure and is often the cause of death in patients with cirrhosis.

herbal preparation Plant used for medicinal purposes.

hernia A weakness in the abdominal muscle wall through which a segment of the bowel or other abdominal structure protrudes.

herniated nucleus pulposus (NHP) The protrusion (herniation) of the pulpy material from the center of a vertebral disk; herniated disks occur most often between the fourth and fifth lumbar vertebrae (L4-5) but may occur at other levels. A herniation in the lumbosacral area can press on the adjacent spinal nerve (usually the sciatic nerve), causing severe burning or stabbing pain into the leg or foot, or it may press on the spinal cord itself, causing leg weakness and bowel and bladder dysfunction. The specific area of pain depends on the level of herniation.

hernioplasty Surgical repair of a hernia in which the surgeon reinforces the weakened outside muscle wall with a mesh patch.

herniorrhaphy The surgical repair of a hernia.

heterotopic ossification Abnormal bony overgrowth, often into muscle; seen as a complication of prolonged immobility in patients with spinal cord injury.

hiatal hernia Protrusion of the stomach through the esophageal hiatus of the diaphragm and into the thorax; also called "diaphragmatic hernia."

high altitude Elevations above 5000 feet, which can produce a range of physiologic consequences in the body.

high altitude pulmonary edema (HAPE) A form of acute mountain sickness often seen with high altitude cerebral edema. Clinical indicators include persistent dry cough, cyanosis of the lips and nail beds, tachycardia and tachypnea at rest, and rales auscultated in one or both lungs. Pink, frothy sputum is a late sign.

highly sensitive C-reactive protein (hsCRP) A serum marker of inflammation and a common and critical component to the development of atherothrombosis.

high-output heart failure Heart failure that occurs when cardiac output remains normal or above normal. It is usually caused by increased metabolic needs or hyperkinetic conditions such as septicemia (fever), anemia, and hyperthyroidism. This type of heart failure is different from left- and right-sided heart failure, which are typically low-output states, and is not as common as other types.

hilum The area of the kidney in which the renal artery and nerve plexus enter and the renal vein and ureter exit. This area is not covered by the renal capsule.

hirsutism Abnormal growth of body hair, especially on the face, chest, and the linea alba of the abdomen of women.

homeopathic medicine Practice of medicine that uses small doses of specially prepared plant extracts and minerals to promote healing.

homeostasis The narrow range of normal conditions (e.g., body temperature, blood electrolyte values, blood pH, blood volume) in the human body; the tendency to maintain a constant balance in normal body states.

homeostatic mechanism A safeguard or control mechanism within the human body that prevents dangerous changes.

homocysteine An essential sulfur-containing amino acid that is produced when dietary protein breaks down; elevated values (greater than 15 mmol/L) may be a risk factor for the development of cardiovascular disease.

homonymous hemianopsia Condition in which there is blindness in the same side of both eyes.

hormone Chemical produced in the body that exerts its effects on specific tissues known as target tissues.

hospice care An interdisciplinary approach to facilitate quality of life and a "good" death for patients near the end of their lives, with care provided in a variety of settings.

Hospital Incident Command System (HICS) An organizational model for disaster management in which roles are formally structured under the hospital or long-term care facility incident commander, with clear lines of authority and accountability for specific resources.

hospital incident commander As defined in a hospital's emergency response plan, the person (either an emergency physician or administrator) who assumes overall leadership for implementing the institutional plan at the onset of a mass casualty incident. The hospital incident commander has a global view of the entire situation, facilitates patient movement through the system, and brings in resources to meet patient needs.

Huber needle A noncoring port access needle used in central IV therapy.

human leukocyte antigen (HLA) Antigen that is present on the surfaces of nearly all body cells as a normal part of the person and acts as an antigen only if it enters another person's body.

humoral immunity A type of immunity provided by antibodies circulating in body fluids.

Huntington disease (HD) A hereditary disorder transmitted as an autosomal dominant trait at the time of conception (formerly called Huntington chorea). Men and women between 35 and 50 years of age are affected; clinical onset is gradual. The two main symptoms are progressive mental status changes (leading to dementia) and choreiform movements (rapid, jerky movements) in the limbs, trunk, and facial muscles.

hydrocephalus The abnormal accumulation of cerebrospinal fluid within the skull.

hydronephrosis Abnormal enlargement of the kidney caused by a blockage of urine lower in the tract and filling of the kidney with urine.

hydrophilic Tending to absorb water readily.

hydrophobic Not readily absorbing water; waterproof.

hydrostatic pressure The force of the weight of water molecules pressing against the confining walls of a space.

hydrotherapy The application of water for treatment of injury or disease.

hydroureter Abnormal distention of the ureters.

hyperacusis An intolerance for sound levels that do not bother other people.

hyperaldosteronism Excessive mineralocorticoid production.

hypercalcemia A total serum calcium level above 10.5 mg/dL or 2.75 mmol/L, which can cause fatigue, anorexia, nausea and vomiting, constipation, polyuria, and serious damage to the urinary system.

hypercapnia Increased arterial carbon dioxide levels.
hypercarbia Increased partial pressure of arterial carbon dioxide ($Paco_2$) levels.
hypercellularity An abnormal number of cells.
hyperemia Increased blood flow to an area.
hyperesthesia Abnormally increased sensation.
hyperextension A mechanism of injury that occurs when a part of the body is suddenly accelerated and then decelerated, causing extreme extension.
hyperflexion A mechanism of injury that occurs when a part of the body is suddenly and forcefully accelerated forward, causing extreme flexion.
hyperglycemia Abnormally high levels of blood glucose.
hyperglycemic-hyperosmolar state (HHS) State of increased blood osmolarity caused by hyperglycemia.
hyperinsulinemia Chronic high blood insulin levels.
hyperkalemia An elevated level of potassium in the blood.
hyperlipidemia An elevation of serum lipid (fat) levels in the blood.
hypermagnesemia A serum magnesium level above 2.1 mEq/L.
hypernatremia An excessive amount of sodium in the blood.
hyperopia An error of refraction that occurs when the eye does not refract light enough, causing images to fall (converge) behind the retina and resulting in poor near vision; also called "farsightedness."
hyperosmotic Describes fluids with osmolarities (solute concentrations) greater than 300 mOsm/L; hyperosmotic fluids have a greater osmotic pressure than do isosmotic fluids and tend to pull water from the isosmotic fluid space into the hyperosmotic fluid space until an osmotic balance occurs. Also called "hypertonic."
hyperphosphatemia A serum phosphorus level above 4.5 mEq/L.
hyperpituitarism Hormone oversecretion that occurs with pituitary tumors or hyperplasia.
hyperplasia Growth that causes tissue to increase in size by increasing the number of cells; abnormal overgrowth of tissue.
hyperpnea An abnormal increase in the depth of respiratory movements.
hypersensitivity An overreaction to a foreign substance.
hypertension A cardiovascular condition pertaining to people who have a systolic blood pressure of 140 mm Hg or higher or a diastolic blood pressure of 90 mm Hg or higher, or who take medication to control blood pressure; approximately 1 out of every 5 Americans have hypertension.
hyperthermia Elevated body temperature; fever.
hyperthyroidism A condition caused by excessive production of thyroid hormone.
hypertonia A condition of excessive muscle tone, which tends to cause fixed positions or contractures of the involved extremities and restricted range of motion of the joints.
hypertonic See *hyperosmotic.*
hypertriglyceridemia Elevated levels (150 mg/dL or above) of triglyceride in the blood.
hypertrophic cardiomyopathy (HCM) A type of cardiomyopathy that involves disarray of the myocardial fibers and asymmetric ventricular hypertrophy; leads to a stiff left ventricle that results in diastolic filling abnormalities.
hypertrophy The enlargement or overgrowth of an organ; tissue increases in size by the enlargement of each cell.
hyperuricemia An excess of uric acid in the blood.
hyperventilation A state of increased rate and depth of breathing.
hyperviscosity Excessively thick or concentrated, as of the blood.
hyperviscous The quality of being thicker than normal.
hypervolemia Increased plasma volume; or fluid excess.
hyphema A hemorrhage in the anterior chamber of the eye that occurs when a force is applied to the eye and breaks the blood vessels.
hypnosis An altered state of consciousness in which a person enters a trance and loses an overall sense of reality.
hypocalcemia A total serum calcium level below 9.0 mg/dL or 2.25 mmol/L.
hypocapnia Decreased arterial carbon dioxide levels.
hypodermoclysis The slow infusion of isotonic fluids into subcutaneous tissue.
hypoesthesia Abnormally decreased sensation.
hypoglycemia Abnormally low levels of glucose in the blood.
hypokalemia A decreased serum potassium level; a common electrolyte imbalance.
hypomagnesemia Decreased serum magnesium levels.
hyponatremia A serum sodium level below 136 mEq/L (mmol/L).
hypo-osmotic Describes fluids with osmolarities of less than 270 mOsm/L. Hypo-osmolar fluids have a lower osmotic pressure than isosmotic fluids, and water tends to be pulled from the hypo-osmotic fluid space into the isosmotic fluid space until an osmotic balance occurs. Also called "hypotonic."
hypoperfusion Decreased blood flow through an organ.
hypophonia Soft voice.
hypophosphatemia Inadequate levels of phosphate in the blood (below 3.0 mEq/L).
hypophysectomy Surgical removal of the pituitary gland.
hypoplasia Reduced production of cells.
hypoproteinemia A decrease in serum proteins.
hyporeflexia A decreased response to deep tendon reflex stimulation.
hyposthenuria The inability to form urine of high specific gravity; loss of urine-concentrating ability.
hypothalamic-hypophysial portal system The small, closed circulatory system that the hypothalamus shares with the anterior pituitary gland, which allows hormones produced in the hypothalamus to travel directly to the anterior pituitary gland.
hypothalamus A structure within the brain; an integral part of autonomic nervous system control (controlling temperature and other functions) that is essential in intellectual function.
hypothermia A core body temperature less than 95° F (35° C).
hypotonia An abnormal condition of inadequate muscle tone, with an inability to maintain balance.
hypotonic See *hypo-osmotic.*
hypoventilation A state in which gas exchange at the alveolar-capillary membrane is inadequate so that too little oxygen reaches the blood and carbon dioxide is retained.
hypovolemia Abnormally decreased volume of circulating fluid in the body; fluid deficit.
hypoxemia (hypoxemic) Decreased blood oxygen levels; hypoxia.
hypoxia (hypoxic) A reduction of oxygen supply to the tissues.
hysterosalpingogram An x-ray of the cervix, uterus, and fallopian tubes that is performed after injection of a contrast medium. This test is used in infertility workups to evaluate

tubal anatomy and patency and uterine problems such as fibroids, tumors, and fistulas.

hysteroscopy Examination of the interior of the uterus and cervical canal using an endoscope.

I

icterus Yellow discoloration of the sclerae.

idiopathic seizure See *unclassified seizure.*

idioventricular rhythm A heart rhythm in which the ventricular nodal cells pace the ventricles at a rate that is usually less than 40 beats/min; also called "ventricular escape rhythm."

ileostomy The surgical creation of an opening into the ileum, usually by bringing the end of the terminal ileum through the abdominal wall and forming a stoma, or ostomy.

imagery In complementary medicine, a mind-body therapy or form of distraction in which the patient is encouraged to visualize or think about some pleasant or desirable feeling, sensation, or event.

immediate memory Short-term or new memory. Test by asking the patient to repeat two or three unrelated words to make sure they were heard; after about 5 minutes, while continuing the examination, ask the patient to repeat the words.

immunity Resistance to infection; usually associated with the presence of antibodies or cells that act on specific microorganisms.

immunocompetence Full immunity, which requires the interaction of the processes of inflammation, antibody-mediated immunity (humoral immunity), and cell-mediated immunity.

immunocompetent Having proper functioning of the body's ability to maintain itself and defend against disease.

immunoglobulin Antibody; also called "gamma globulins."

impedance The pressure that the heart must overcome to open the aortic valve. The amount of impedance depends on aortic compliance and total systemic vascular resistance, a combination of blood viscosity and arteriolar constriction.

impedance cardiography (ICG) A noninvasive monitoring system that measures the total impedance (resistance) to the flow of electricity in the heart and provides measures of thoracic fluid, left ventricular function (cardiac output and cardiac index), preload, afterload, and contractility of the heart.

impermeable Not porous.

implanted port A device used for long-term or frequent infusion therapy; consists of a portal body, a dense septum over a reservoir, and a catheter that is surgically implanted on the upper chest or upper extremity.

inactivation The process of binding an antibody to an antigen to cover the antigen's active site and to make the antigen harmless without destroying it; also called "neutralization."

incisional hernia Protrusion of the intestine at the site of a previous surgical incision resulting from inadequate healing. Most often caused by postoperative wound infections, inadequate nutrition, and obesity.

incomplete spinal cord injury An injury in which the spinal cord has been damaged in a way that allows some function or movement below the level of the injury.

incontinence Involuntary loss of urine severe enough to cause social or hygienic problems.

incus One of the three bony ossicles of the ear; also called the "anvil."

independent living skills See *instrumental activities of daily living (IADLs).*

independent nursing function A nursing function initiated and carried out by the nurse without direction from the health care provider.

indirect contact A mode of infection transmission in which microorganisms are transferred passively from a contaminated inanimate object to a susceptible person.

indirect inguinal hernia A sac formed from the peritoneum that contains a portion of the intestine or omentum. The hernia pushes downward at an angle into the inguinal canal. In males, indirect inguinal hernias can become large and often descend into the scrotum.

indolent Slow-growing.

infarction Necrosis, or cell death.

infective endocarditis A microbial infection (e.g., viruses, bacteria, fungi) involving the endocardium; previously called "bacterial endocarditis."

inferior vena caval interruption Surgical procedure in which the surgeon inserts a filter device percutaneously into the inferior vena cava of a patient with recurrent deep vein thrombosis (to prevent pulmonary emboli) or pulmonary emboli that do not respond to medical treatment. The device is meant to trap emboli in the inferior vena cava before they progress to the lungs. Holes in the device allow blood to pass through, thus not significantly interfering with the return of blood to the heart.

inferior wall myocardial infarction A type of myocardial infarction that occurs in patients with obstruction of the right coronary artery, causing significant damage to the right ventricle.

infertility Difficulty becoming pregnant.

infiltrating ductal carcinoma The most common type of breast cancer; it originates in the mammary ducts and grows in the epithelial cells lining these ducts.

inflammatory cytokines Proteins produced primarily by white blood cells that assist in the inflammatory and immune responses of the body (e.g., tumor necrosis factor, interleukins).

inflow disease Chronic peripheral arterial disease with obstruction at or above the common iliac artery, abdominal aorta, or profunda femoris artery. The patient experiences discomfort in the lower back, buttocks, or thighs after walking a certain distance. The pain usually subsides with rest.

informatics A specialized computer science that is used to manage information and technology.

infrapatellar notch The area directly below the knee.

infratentorial Located below the tentorium of the cerebellum.

infusate A solution that is infused into the body.

infusion therapy The delivery of parenteral medications and fluids through a variety of catheter types and locations using multiple techniques and procedures, such as intravenous and intra-arterial therapy to deliver solutions into the vascular system.

inhalants Breathable chemical vapors that produce psychoactive effects.

initial First or, in phases of shock, early.

initiation In oncology, the first step in carcinogenesis; caused by damage to the genes.

innate-native immunity Also called "natural immunity"; a type of immunity that cannot be developed or transferred from one person to another and is not an adaptive response to exposure or invasion by foreign proteins.

inpatient A patient who is admitted to a hospital.

insensible water loss Water loss from the skin, lungs, and stool that cannot be controlled.
instrumental activities of daily living (IADLs) Special activities performed in the course of a day such as using the telephone, shopping, preparing food, and housekeeping. Also called "independent living skills."
insufflation The practice of injecting gas or air into a cavity before surgery to separate organs and improve visualization.
insulin resistance A reduced ability of most cells to respond to insulin. It is associated with type 2 diabetes.
insulinoma A usually benign tumor of the islets of Langerhans that causes excessive insulin secretion and subsequent hypoglycemia (low serum glucose); the most common type of neuroendocrine pancreatic tumor, even though it is rare.
integrative medicine Practice of medicine that combines therapies from traditional western medicine and complementary and alternative medicine (CAM).
intensity A quality of sound that is expressed in decibels; generally, having a high degree of energy or activity.
intensivist A physician who specializes in critical care.
intention tremor A tremor that occurs when performing an activity.
interbody cage fusion Cagelike spinal device that is implanted into the space where a disk was removed. Bone graft tissue grows into and around the cage and creates a stable spine at that level.
intercostally Located between the ribs.
intermittent claudication A characteristic leg pain experienced by patients with chronic peripheral arterial disease. Typically, patients can walk only a certain distance before a cramping muscle pain forces them to stop. As the disease progresses, the patient can walk only shorter and shorter distances before pain recurs. Ultimately, pain may occur even at rest.
internal derangement A broad term for disturbances of an injured knee joint.
internal fixation The use of metal pins, screws, rods, plates, or prostheses to immobilize a fracture during healing. The surgeon makes an incision (open reduction) to gain access to the broken bone and implants one or more devices.
internal hemorrhoid A hemorrhoid that is located above the anal sphincter and cannot be seen on inspection of the perineal area.
internal urethral sphincter The smooth detrusor muscle that lines the interior of the bladder neck.
interstitial cystitis A bladder inflammation of unknown etiology that occurs predominantly in women and is characterized by urinary frequency and pain on bladder filling.
interstitial fluid A portion of the extracellular fluid that is between cells, sometimes called the "third space."
interstitial laser coagulation (ILC) Procedure for treating benign prostatic hyperplasia that uses laser energy to coagulate excess tissue.
intra-abdominal hypertension (IAH) Condition of sustained or repeated intra-abdominal pressure of 12 mm Hg or higher.
intra-abdominal pressure Pressure contained within the abdominal cavity.
intra-aortic balloon pump (IABP) An intra-aortic counterpulsation device. It may be used as an invasive intervention to improve myocardial perfusion during an acute myocardial infarction, reduce preload and afterload, and facilitate left ventricular ejection. It is also used when patients do not respond to drug therapy with improved tissue perfusion, decreased workload of the heart, and increased cardiac contractility.
intra-arterial thrombolysis Therapy for brain attack that delivers the thrombolic agent directly into the thrombus within 6 hours of the attack's onset.
intracapsular Located within the joint capsule.
intracellular fluid (ICF) The portion of total body water (about two thirds) that is found inside the cells.
intracerebral hemorrhage Bleeding within the brain tissue caused by the tearing of small arteries and veins in the subcortical white matter.
intracorporeal Situated or occurring inside the body.
intractable pain Chronic pain that cannot be managed using standard therapies.
intramedullary tumor Tumor originating within the spinal cord in the central gray matter and anterior commissure. It is often malignant.
intraocular pressure (IOP) Pressure of the fluid within the eye; may be measured by methods that involve direct contact with the eye or by noncontact techniques.
intraoperative During surgery.
intraosseous (IO) therapy Infusion therapy that is delivered to the vascular network in the long bones.
intraperitoneal (IP) therapy The administration of antineoplastic agents into the peritoneal cavity.
intrapulmonary Within the respiratory tract.
intrarenal/intrinsic renal failure Decreased renal function resulting from damage to the glomeruli, interstitial tissue, or tubules. It can contribute to acute renal failure.
intrathecal Referring to the spine.
intrathecal (subarachnoid) analgesia The introduction of a pain-blocking agent into the space between the arachnoid mater and pia mater of the spinal cord (where the cerebrospinal fluid is located).
intravascular ultrasonography (IVUS) In cardiac catheterization, the use of a flexible catheter with a miniature transducer that emits sound waves. Sound waves are reflected off the plaque and the arterial wall, creating an image of the blood vessel; used as an alternative to injecting a medium into the coronary arteries.
intravenous (systemic) thrombolytic therapy The intravenous administration of thrombolytic agents to dissolve a thrombus.
intraventricular catheter (IVC) A small tube that is inserted into the anterior horn of the lateral ventricle of the nondominant cerebral hemisphere to monitor intracranial pressure; can also be used to drain cerebrospinal fluid to decrease pressure and obtain specimens for laboratory analysis.
intravesical Situated inside the bladder.
intrinsic factor A substance normally secreted by the gastric mucosa and needed for intestinal absorption of vitamin B_{12}. A deficiency of intrinsic factor and the resulting failure to absorb vitamin B_{12} leads to pernicious anemia.
intussusception The telescoping of a segment of the intestine within itself.
invasive Pertaining to the ability to penetrate nearby tissue; said of cancers.
invasive temporary pacemaker A cardiac pacing system consisting of an external battery-operated pulse generator and pacing electrodes, or lead wires, that attach to the generator on one end and are in contact with the heart on the other end. Electrical pulses are emitted from the negative terminal of the generator, flow through a lead wire, and stimulate the cardiac

cells to depolarize. The current seeks ground by returning through the other lead wire to the positive terminal of the generator, thus completing a circuitous route.

ion A substance found in body fluids that carries an electrical charge; also called "electrolyte."

ipsilateral Occurring on the same side.

iris The colored portion of the external eye; its center opening is the pupil. Muscles of the iris contract and relax to control pupil size and the amount of light entering the eye.

iritis Inflammation of the iris.

irreducible hernia A hernia that cannot be reduced or placed back into the abdominal cavity; requires immediate surgical evaluation.

irreversible stage The former name for the refractory stage of shock. See *refractory stage.*

irritability An overresponse to stimuli.

irritable bowel syndrome (IBS) A chronic gastrointestinal disorder characterized by chronic or recurrent diarrhea, constipation, and/or abdominal pain and bloating; also called "spastic colon," "mucous colon," or "nervous colon."

ischemia Blockage of blood flow through a blood vessel. Prolonged severe ischemia can cause irreversible damage to tissue.

ischemic Cell dysfunction or death from a lack of oxygen resulting from decreased blood flow in a body part.

ischemic stroke A type of brain attack caused by occlusion of a cerebral artery by either a thrombus or an embolus. About 80% of all brain attacks are ischemic.

Ishihara chart The most commonly used tool for testing color vision. The chart shows numbers composed of dots of one color within a circle of dots of a different color. Each eye is tested separately by asking the patient what numbers he or she sees on the chart; reading the numbers correctly indicates normal color vision.

isoelectric Having equal electric potentials, such as in the heart.

isosmotic Having the same osmotic pressures; also called "isotonic" or "normotonic."

isosthenuria Excretion of urine with the same osmolality as that of plasma; occurs in patients with declining renal function due to chronic renal failure.

isotonic See *isosmotic.*

isotope A different form of a specific element; has a slightly different atomic weight and number of neutrons.

"itch-scratch-itch" cycle A pattern seen in patients with pruritus who try to relieve the itching sensation by scratching the skin, further stimulating the itch receptors and causing the itching sensation to continue.

J

jaundice A syndrome characterized by excessive circulating bilirubin levels. Liver cells cannot effectively excrete bilirubin, and skin and mucous membranes become characterized by a yellow coloration.

jejunostomy The surgical creation of an opening between the jejunum and the surface of the abdominal wall.

joint The place at which two or more bones come together; also referred to as *articulation* of the joint. The primary function is to provide movement and flexibility in the body.

journaling A mind-body therapy in which the patient records the process of life and reflects on it to express feelings, gain new perspectives, and pay attention to what is in the unconscious.

jugular venous distention (JVD) Enlargement of the jugular vein of the neck; caused by an increase in jugular venous pressure.

justice The ethical principle that refers to patient equality.

juxtaglomerular complex Specialized cells that produce and store renin in the afferent arteriole, efferent arteriole, and distal collecting tubule; taken together, the juxtaglomerular cells and the macula densa.

K

karyotype Technique used to make an organized arrangement of all the chromosomes within one cell during the metaphase section of mitosis.

Kehr's sign Pain in the left shoulder resulting from diaphragmatic irritation; may be present in splenic injury.

keratin The protein produced by keratinocytes; makes the outermost skin layer waterproof.

keratoconjunctivitis sicca A condition of the eyes that results from changes in tear composition, lacrimal gland malfunction, or altered tear distribution; also called "dry eye syndrome."

keratoplasty Corneal transplant. The surgical removal of diseased corneal tissue and replacement with tissue from a human donor cornea.

ketogenesis The conversion of fats to acids in the body.

ketone bodies Substances, including acetone, that are produced as by-products of the incomplete metabolism of fatty acids. When insulin is not available (as in uncontrolled diabetes mellitus), they accumulate in the blood and cause metabolic acidosis; also called "ketones."

ketorolac (Toradol) Popular nonsteroidal anti-inflammatory drug prescribed for short-term use in acute pain because it can be given orally, intramuscularly, or by IV push.

knee height caliper Device that uses the distance between the patella and heel to estimate height.

Kupffer cells Phagocytic cells that are part of the body's reticuloendothelial system and are involved in the protective function of the liver. Kupffer cells engulf harmful bacteria and anemic red blood cells.

Kussmaul respiration A type of breathing that occurs when excess acids caused by the absence of insulin increase hydrogen ion and carbon dioxide levels in the blood. This state triggers an increase in the rate and depth of respiration in an attempt to excrete more carbon dioxide and acid.

kwashiorkor Lack of protein quantity and quality in the presence of adequate calories. Body weight is somewhat normal, and serum proteins are low.

kyphoplasty A minimally invasive surgery for managing vertebral fractures in patients with osteoporosis. Bone cement is injected into the fracture site to provide pain relief, and an inflated balloon is used to restore height to the vertebra.

L

labia majora Two vertical folds of adipose tissue that extend posteriorly from the mons pubis to the perineum.

labia minora Two thinner, vertical folds of reddish epithelium that are surrounded by the labia majora.

labyrinthectomy Surgical removal of the labyrinth; used as a radical treatment of Ménière's disease when medical therapy is ineffective and the patient already has significant hearing loss.

labyrinthitis An infection of the labyrinth of the ear; may occur as a complication of acute or chronic otitis media.

laceration A type of wound characterized by tearing or mangling and usually caused by sharp objects and projectiles.
lacrimal gland A small gland that produces tears; located in the upper outer part of each ocular orbit.
lacto-ovo-vegetarian A vegetarian diet pattern in which milk, cheese, eggs, and dairy foods are eaten but meat, fish, and poultry are avoided.
lactose intolerance The inability to convert lactose (found in milk and dairy products) to glucose and galactose in the body.
lacto-vegetarian A vegetarian diet pattern in which milk, cheese, and dairy foods are eaten but meat, fish, poultry, and eggs are avoided.
lacunae Small, deep cavities within the brain that result from occlusion of a small vessel; this leads to infarct and necrosis of the area of the brain supplied by the affected vessel.
laparoscopy A minimally invasive procedure in which the surgeon makes several small incisions near the umbilicus through which a small endoscope is placed to examine the abdomen; direct examination of the pelvic cavity through an endoscope.
laparotomy An open surgical approach in which a large abdominal incision is made.
laryngitis Inflammation of the mucous membranes lining the larynx.
laryngopharynx The area behind the larynx that extends from the base of the tongue to the esophagus. It is the critical dividing point at which solid foods and fluids are separated from air.
larynx The "voice box"; it is composed of several cartilages and is located above the trachea and just below the throat at the base of the tongue; part of the upper respiratory tract.
laser An acronym for <u>l</u>ight <u>a</u>mplification by <u>s</u>timulated <u>e</u>mission of <u>r</u>adiation. As a surgical tool, a laser emits a high-powered beam of light that cuts tissue more cleanly than do scalpel blades. A laser creates intense heat, rapidly clots blood vessels or tissue, and turns target tissue (e.g., a tumor) into vapor.
laser-assisted angioplasty A procedure using heat from a laser probe that is advanced through a cannula to vaporize arteriosclerotic plaque and open the occluded or stenosed artery.
latency period The time between the initiation of a cell and the development of an overt tumor.
late-onset seizure Seizure that occurs initially more than 7 days after a head injury.
latex allergy Reactions to exposure to latex in gloves and other medical products; reactions include rashes, nasal or eye symptoms, and asthma.
latrodectism A syndrome caused by the venom of a black widow spider bite in which neurotransmitter releases from nerve terminals to cause severe abdominal pain, muscle rigidity and spasm, hypertension, and nausea and vomiting.
lead axis In electrocardiography, the imaginary line that joins the positive and negative poles of the lead systems.
left shift An increase in the band cells (immature neutrophils) in the white blood cell differential count; an early indication of infection.
left-sided heart (ventricular) failure Inadequacy of the left ventricle of the heart to pump adequately; results in decreased tissue perfusion from poor cardiac output and pulmonary congestion from increased pressure in the pulmonary vessels; typical causes include hypertensive, coronary artery, or valvular disease involving the mitral or aortic valve. Most heart failure begins with failure of the left ventricle and progresses to failure of both ventricles.
legally competent A person 18 years of age or older, a pregnant or a married minor, a legally emancipated (free) minor who is self-supporting, or a person not declared incompetent by a court of law.
leiomyomas Benign, slow-growing solid tumors of the uterine myometrium (muscle layer). These are the most commonly occurring pelvic tumors; also called "myomas" and "fibroids."
lens The circular, convex structure of the eye that lies behind the iris and in front of the vitreous body. Normally transparent, the lens bends the rays of light entering through the pupil so they focus on the retina. The curve of the lens changes to focus on near or distant objects.
leprosy (Hansen's disease) A chronic, contagious, systemic mycobacterial infection of the peripheral nervous system with skin involvement. The clinical course is either progressive or self-limiting depending on the immunologic status of the host. Although the exact mechanism of infection remains unknown, studies suggest transmission via the airborne route, by insects, or through direct contact with skin lesions.
leptin A hormone that is released by fat cells and possibly by gastric cells; it also acts on the hypothalamus to control appetite.
lethargic A state of drowsiness or sleepiness.
leukemia A type of cancer with uncontrolled production of immature white blood cells in the bone marrow; the bone marrow becomes overcrowded with immature, nonfunctional cells, and the production of normal blood cells is greatly decreased.
leukocyte White blood cell (WBC); this immune system cell protects the body from the effects of invasion by organisms.
leukocytosis An elevated white blood count.
leukopenia A reduction in the number of white blood cells.
leukoplakia White, patchy lesions on a mucous membrane.
level I trauma center According to the American College of Surgeons, a regional resource facility that is capable of "providing leadership and total care for every aspect of injury, from prevention through rehabilitation."
level II trauma center A community facility that is capable of providing care to the vast majority of injured patients but may not be able to meet the resource needs of patients who require very complex injury management.
level III trauma center A critical link to higher capability trauma centers in communities that do not have ready access to Level I or Level II centers; the primary focus is injury stabilization and patient transfer.
level IV trauma center A facility that offers advanced life support care in rural or remote settings that do not have ready access to a higher level trauma center, such as a ski area.
LGBT Acronym for "lesbian, gay, bisexual, and transgender" culture.
libido Sexual desire.
lichenification An abnormal thickening of the skin to a leathery appearance; can occur in patients with chronic dermatitis because of their continual rubbing of the area to relieve itching.
Lichtenberg figures Branching or ferning marks that appear on the skin as a result of a lightning strike; also called "keraunographic markings" or "erythematous arborization."
life review A structured process of reflecting on one's life that is often facilitated by an interviewer.

ligament One of many bands of tissue that attach bones to other bones at joints and serve to support joints.

light reflex The reflection of the otoscope's light off the eardrum in the form of a clearly demarcated triangle of light in the normal ear.

limited scleroderma Thick skin that is limited to sites distal to the elbow and knee but also involves the face and neck.

linear fracture A type of bone fracture involving a simple, clean break in which the impacted area of bone bends inward and the area around it bends outward.

lipid Fat, including cholesterol and triglycerides, that can be measured in the blood.

lipoatrophy The loss or atrophy of subcutaneous fat; in patients with diabetes, the loss of fat tissue in areas of repeated insulin injection.

lipohypertrophy The enlargement or hypertrophy of subcutaneous fat; in patients with diabetes, an increased swelling of fat that occurs at the site of repeated insulin injections.

lipolysis The decomposition or splitting up of fat to provide fuel for energy when liver glucose is unavailable.

liposuction A cosmetic procedure to reduce the amount of adipose tissue in selected areas of the body.

lithotripsy The use of sound, laser, or dry shock wave energy to break a kidney stone into small fragments; also called "extracorporeal shock wave lithotripsy."

living will A legal document that instructs physicians and family members about what life-sustaining treatment is wanted (or not wanted) if the patient becomes unable to make decisions.

lobectomy Surgical removal of an entire lung lobe.

lobular carcinoma in situ (LCIS) A noninvasive form of breast cancer that does not show up as a calcified cluster on a mammogram and is therefore most often diagnosed incidentally during a biopsy for another problem.

local anesthesia Anesthesia that is delivered by applying it to the skin or mucous membranes of the area to be anesthetized or by injecting it directly into the tissue around an incision, wound, or lesion.

localized pain Confined to the site of origin.

lockout interval A specific interval between doses programmed into a patient-controlled analgesia infusion pump. No drug is administered if the patient attempts to access the drug before the interval has elapsed.

locus The specific chromosome location for a gene.

log rolling Turning technique in which the patient turns all at once while his or her back is kept as straight as possible.

long-term nonprogressor (LTNP) A person who has been infected with the human immune deficiency virus for at least 10 years and has remained asymptomatic with CD4+ cell counts within a normal range. About 1% of those infected are long-term nonprogressors.

loop electrosurgical excision procedure (LEEP) Diagnostic procedure/treatment in which a thin loop-wire electrode that transmits a painless electrical current is used to cut away affected cervical cancer tissue.

lordosis The anterior concavity in the curvature of the lumbar and cervical spine when viewed from the side; a common finding in pregnancy and abdominal obesity.

Lou Gehrig's disease See *amyotrophic lateral sclerosis (ALS)*.

low back pain (LBP) Pain in the lumbosacral region of the back caused by muscle strain or spasm, ligament sprain, disk degeneration, or herniation of the nucleus pulposus from the center of the disk. Herniated disks occur most often between the fourth and fifth lumbar vertebrae (L4-5) but may occur at other levels.

lower esophageal sphincter (LES) The portion of the esophagus proximal to the gastroesophageal junction; when at rest, the sphincter is closed to prevent reflux of gastric contents into the esophagus.

lower GI series Radiographic visualization of the large intestine; usually ordered for a patient with a complaint of blood or mucus in the stool or a change in bowel pattern, such as diarrhea or constipation; also called a "barium enema."

lower motor neuron Neurons that carry motor impulses to skeletal muscles. Patients with spinal cord injuries involving lower motor neuron lesions experience muscle wasting due to long-term flaccid paralysis.

lower urinary tract symptom (LUTS) Any of a collection of symptoms seen in benign prostatic hyperplasia, including hesitancy, intermittency, reduced force and size of the urinary stream, a sensation of incomplete bladder emptying, and postvoid dribbling.

low-intensity pulsed ultrasound A method using ultrasonic waves to promote bone union in slow-healing fractures or for new fractures as an alternative to surgery.

low-profile gastrostomy device (LPGD) A gastrostomy device that uses a firm or balloon-style internal bumper or retention disk; an antireflux valve keeps gastric contents from leaking onto the skin.

loxoscelism Systemic effects from the injected toxin of a spider bite.

lumbar puncture The insertion of a spinal needle into the subarachnoid space between the third and fourth (sometimes the fourth and fifth) lumbar vertebrae to withdraw spinal fluid for analysis; also called a "spinal tap."

lumen The inside cavity of a tube or tubular organ, such as a blood vessel or airway.

lung compliance The quality of elasticity of the lungs.

lunula The white crescent-shaped portion of the nail at the lower end of the nail plate.

lurch An abnormality in the swing phase of gait; occurs when the muscles in the buttocks or legs are too weak to allow the person to change weight from one foot to the other.

luteal Pertaining to the post-ovulation phase of the menstrual cycle.

Lyme disease A systemic infectious disease that is caused by the spirochete *Borrelia burgdorferi* and results from the bite of an infected deer tick. Signs and symptoms include a large "bull's-eye" circular rash, malaise, fever, headache, and muscle or joint aches.

lymph Fluid that has moved out of the capillaries and is returned to the systemic circulation.

lymphadenopathy Persistently enlarged lymph nodes.

lymphedema Abnormal accumulation of protein fluid in the subcutaneous tissue of the affected limb after a mastectomy.

lymphoblastic Pertaining to abnormal leukemic cells that come from the lymphoid pathways and develop into lymphocytes.

lymphocytic Pertaining to abnormal leukemic cells that come from the lymphoid pathways.

lymphokine Cytokine produced by T-cells.

lysergic acid (LSD) The prototype major hallucinogenic drug that is odorless and colorless with a slightly bitter taste; also called "acid."

lysis Breakage, for example, of a cell membrane.

lysozyme A component that is present in large quantities in many body secretions and dissolves the cell walls of some bacteria.

M

M phase The phase of cell division in which a single cell splits into two cells (actual mitosis).
macrocytic anemia A form of vitamin B_{12} deficiency anemia characterized by abnormally large precursor cells.
macrovascular Referring to large blood vessels.
macular A term referring to a macula, a discolored spot on the skin that is not raised above the surface.
macular degeneration The deterioration of the macula, the area of central vision.
magnesium (Mg^{2+}) A mineral that forms a cation when dissolved in water.
magnetoencephalography (MEG) A noninvasive imaging technique that measures the magnetic fields produced by electrical activity in the brain via extremely sensitive devices such as superconducting quantum interference devices (SQUIDs).
malabsorption A syndrome associated with a variety of disorders and intestinal surgical procedures and characterized by impaired intestinal absorption of nutrients.
malignant Referring to cancer.
malignant growth Altered cell growth that is serious and, without intervention, leads to death; cancer.
malignant hypertension A severe type of elevated blood pressure that rapidly progresses, with systolic blood pressure greater than 200 mm Hg and diastolic blood pressure greater than 150 mm Hg (greater than 130 mm Hg when there are pre-existing complications).
malignant transformation The process of changing a normal cell into a cancer cell.
malleus The outermost bony ossicle of the ear; also called the "hammer."
malpighian layers The stratified layers of the epithelium that are formed when older keratinocytes are pushed upward.
mammography An x-ray of the soft tissue of the breast.
mandibulectomy Surgical removal of the jaw.
Manning criteria A collective term for the characteristic symptoms of irritable bowel syndrome: abdominal pain relieved by defecation or associated with changes in stool frequency or consistency, abdominal distention, the sensation of incomplete evacuation of stool, and the presence of mucus with stool passage.
marasmic-kwashiorkor A combined protein and energy malnutrition that often presents clinically when metabolic stress is imposed on a chronically starved patient.
marasmus A calorie malnutrition in which body fat and protein are wasted but serum proteins are often preserved.
marsupialization Surgical formation of a pouch that is a new duct opening.
masklike facies Facial expression characterized by wide-open, fixed, staring eyes caused by rigidity of the facial muscles; often seen in patients with Parkinson disease.
mass casualty event A situation affecting the public health that is defined based on the resource availability of a particular community or hospital facility. When the number of casualties exceeds the resource capabilities, a disaster situation is recognized to exist.
massage The use of various strokes and pressure to manipulate soft tissues for therapeutic purposes.
mastication The process of chewing.
mastoid process The bony ridge located over the temporal bone behind the pinna; part of the external ear.
mastoiditis An acute or chronic infection of the mastoid air cells caused by untreated or inadequately treated otitis media.
matrix In referring to bone, the substance of bone consisting chiefly of collagen, mucopolysaccharides, and lipids. Deposits of inorganic calcium salts (carbonate and phosphate) in the matrix provide the hardness of bone.
maze procedure An open chest surgical technique often performed with coronary artery bypass grafting for patients in atrial fibrillation with decompensation.
McMurray test A common diagnostic technique for the patient with a torn meniscus. The examiner flexes and rotates the knee and then presses on the medial aspect while slowly extending the leg. The test result is positive if clicking is palpated or heard; however, a negative finding does not rule out a tear.
mean arterial pressure (MAP) The arterial blood pressure (between 60 and 70 mm Hg) necessary to maintain perfusion of major body organs, such as the kidneys and brain.
mechanical débridement Method of débriding a wound by mechanical entrapment and detachment of dead tissue.
mechanical obstruction The physical obstruction of the bowel by disorders outside the intestine (e.g., adhesions or hernias) or by blockages in the lumen of the intestine (e.g., tumors, inflammation, strictures, or fecal impactions).
mechanical patient lift Electrically operated devices used to lift, transfer, move, and reposition patients.
mechanism of injury (MOI) The manner in which a patient's traumatic event occurred, such as a high-speed motor vehicle crash or gunshot wound.
mediastinal shift A shift of central thoracic structures toward one side; seen on chest x-ray.
mediastinitis Infection of the mediastinum.
medical command physician As defined in a hospital's emergency response plan, the person responsible for determining the number, acuity, and medical resource needs of victims arriving from the incident scene and for organizing the emergency health care team response to injured or ill patients.
medical harm Physician incidents and all errors caused by members of the health care team that lead to patient injury or death.
medical nutritional supplements (MNS) Enteral products taken by patients who cannot consume enough nutrients in their usual diet (e.g., Ensure, Boost).
medication overuse headache See *rebound headache*.
meditation A mind-body therapy using self-directed practices to relax the body and calm the mind.
medulla A general term for the most interior portion of an organ or structure.
melena Blood in the stool, with the appearance of black tarry stools.
memory cell A type of B-lymphocyte that remains sensitized but does not start to produce antibodies until the next exposure to the same antigen.
menarche A female's first menstruation, which is one sign of puberty.
Ménière's disease Tinnitus, one-sided sensorineural hearing loss, and vertigo that is related to overproduction or decreased reabsorption of endolymphatic fluid and causes a distortion of the entire inner canal system.

meninges The immediate protective covering of the brain and the spinal cord.
meningioma A type of benign brain tumor that arises from the coverings of the brain (the meninges) and causes compression and displacement of adjacent brain tissue.
meningitis Inflammation, usually bacterial or viral, of the arachnoid and pia mater of the brain and spinal cord and the cerebrospinal fluid. May be caused by bacteria or viruses; symptoms are the same regardless of the causative organism.
meniscectomy Surgical excision of a meniscus, as in a knee joint.
menopause The end of menstruation and the biologic end of reproductive ability. The term applies only to the last menstrual period. The actual date of menopause cannot be determined until at least 1 year has passed without menses.
menses The monthly flow of blood from the genital tract of women.
menstruation The cyclic shedding of the endometrial lining of the uterus.
metabolic syndrome A collection of related health problems with insulin resistance as a main feature. Other features include obesity, low levels of physical activity, hypertension, high blood levels of cholesterol, and elevated triglyceride levels. Metabolic syndrome increases the risk for coronary heart disease. Also called "Syndrome X."
metastasis The growth and spread of cancer.
metastasize To spread cancer from the main tumor site to many other body sites.
metastatic Referring to disease, such as cancer, that transfers from one organ to another organ or part not directly connected; pertains to additional tumors that form after cancer cells move from the primary location by breaking off from the original group and establishing remote colonies.
methemoglobinemia The conversion of normal hemoglobin to methemoglobin.
microalbuminuria The presence of very small amounts of albumin in the urine that are not measurable by a urine dipstick or usual urinalysis procedures. Specialized assays are used to analyze a freshly voided urine specimen for microscopic levels of albumin.
microcytic Abnormally small in size, such as an abnormally small red blood cell.
microvascular Referring to small blood vessels.
microvascular decompression A surgical procedure to relieve the pain of trigeminal neuralgia by relocating a small artery that compresses the trigeminal nerve as it enters the pons. The surgeon carefully lifts the loop of the artery off the nerve and places a small silicone sponge between the vessel and the nerve.
midline catheter A type of catheter that is 6 to 8 inches long and inserted through the veins of the antecubital fossa; used in therapies lasting from 1 to 4 weeks.
migraine headache An episodic familial disorder manifested by a unilateral, frontotemporal, throbbing pain that is often worse behind one eye or ear. It is often accompanied by a sensitive scalp, anorexia, photophobia, and nausea with or without vomiting. Three categories of migraine headache are migraines with aura, migraines without aura, and atypical migraines.
migratory arthritis In the early stage of rheumatoid arthritis, symptoms that are migrating or involve more joints.
miliary tuberculosis See *hematogenous tuberculosis.*
mineralocorticoids Corticosteroids produced in the zona glomerulosa of the adrenal gland to help control the body's sodium and potassium content.
minimally invasive direct coronary artery bypass (MIDCAB) Surgical procedure that does not require cardiopulmonary bypass and may be used for patients with a lesion of the left anterior descending artery.
minimally invasive esophagectomy (MIE) A laparoscopic surgical procedure to remove part of the esophagus; may be performed in patients with early-stage cancer.
minimally invasive inguinal hernia repair (MIIHR) Surgical repair of an inguinal hernia through a laparoscope, which is the treatment of choice.
minimally invasive surgery (MIS) A general term for any surgery performed using laparoscopic technique.
miosis Constriction of the pupil of the eye.
mitochondria Within the cytoplasm of cells, the sites of production of adenosine triphosphate.
mitosis Cell division.
mitotic index The percentage of actively dividing cells within a tumor.
mitral (bicuspid) valve The atrioventricular valve that separates the left atrium of the heart from the left ventricle.
mitral regurgitation Inability of the mitral valve to close completely during systole, which allows the backflow of blood into the left atrium when the left ventricle contracts; usually due to fibrosis and calcification caused by rheumatic disease. Also called "mitral insufficiency."
mitral stenosis Thickening of the mitral valve due to fibrosis and calcification and usually caused by rheumatic fever. The valve leaflets fuse and become stiff, the chordae tendineae contract, and the valve opening narrows, preventing normal blood flow from the left atrium to the left ventricle. As a result, left atrial pressure rises, the left atrium dilates, pulmonary artery pressures increase, and the right ventricle hypertrophies.
mitral valve prolapse (MVP) Dysfunction of the mitral valve that occurs because the valvular leaflets enlarge and prolapse into the left atrium during systole; usually benign but may progress to pronounced mitral regurgitation.
mixed conductive-sensorineural hearing loss A profound hearing loss that results from a combination of both conductive and sensorineural types of hearing loss.
modifiable risk factor A factor in disease development that can be altered or controlled by the patient. Examples include elevated serum cholesterol levels, cigarette smoking, hypertension, impaired glucose tolerance, obesity, physical inactivity, and stress.
modified radical mastectomy Surgical procedure for breast cancer in which the affected breast is completely removed.
monokine Cytokine made by macrophages, neutrophils, eosinophils, and monocytes.
monosyllabic One-syllable words, such as *day, toe,* and *ran,* used in speech discrimination testing to determine the patient's ability to discriminate among similar sounds or among words that contain similar sounds.
mons pubis The fat pad that covers the symphysis pubis and protects it during sexual intercourse; it becomes prominent and covered with hair during puberty.
morbid obesity A weight that has a severely negative effect on health; usually more than 100% above ideal body weight or a body mass index greater than 40.
morbidity An illness or an abnormal condition or quality.

mortality Death.
Morton's neuroma Plantar digital neuritis, a condition in which a small tumor grows in a digital nerve of the foot. The patient usually describes the pain as an acute, burning sensation in the web space that involves the entire surface of the third and fourth toes.
motor Facilitating movement.
motor aphasia See *expressive aphasia.*
motor cortex Area in the frontal lobe of the brain that controls voluntary movement.
motor end plate The junction of a peripheral motor nerve and the muscle cells that it supplies.
mourning The outward social expression of loss.
mu opioids Drugs that cause side effects that include constipation, nausea and vomiting, urinary retention, pruritus (itching), sedation, and respiratory depression because of their action on the mu receptor, the most important type of opioid receptor.
mucosa The innermost layer of the gastrointestinal tract; consists of a thin layer of smooth muscle and specialized exocrine gland cells.
mucositis Open sores on mucous membranes.
multi-casualty event A disaster event in which a limited number of victims or casualties are involved and can be managed by a hospital using local resources.
multidisciplinary pain team Team typically consisting of one or more nurses, pharmacists, case managers, and physicians who consult with staff and prescribers on how best to control the patient's pain; also called "analgesia team."
multifocal Having multiple points of origin.
multigated blood pool scanning In nuclear cardiology, cardiac blood pool imaging is a noninvasive test to evaluate cardiac motion and calculate ejection fraction by using a computer to synchronize the patient's electrocardiogram with pictures obtained by a gamma-scintillation camera. In multigated blood pool scanning, the computer breaks the time between R waves into fractions of a second, called "gates." The camera records blood flow through the heart during each gate. By analyzing information from multiple gates, the computer can evaluate ventricular wall motion and calculate ejection fraction (percentage of the left ventricular volume that is ejected with each contraction) and ejection velocity.
multimodal analgesia The use of a combination of opioids, nonopioids, and local anesthetics for postoperative pain; also called "balanced analgesia."
multiple organ dysfunction syndrome (MODS) The sequence of inadequate blood flow to body tissues, which deprives cells of oxygen and leads to anaerobic metabolism with acidosis, hyperkalemia, and tissue ischemia; this is followed by dramatic changes in vital organs and leads to the release of toxic metabolites and destructive enzymes.
multiple sclerosis (MS) A chronic autoimmune disease that affects the myelin sheath and conduction pathway of the central nervous system. It is one of the leading causes of neurologic disability in persons 20 to 40 years of age.
murmur Abnormal heart sound that reflects turbulent blood flow through normal or abnormal valves; murmurs are classified according to their timing in the cardiac cycle (systolic or diastolic) and their intensity depending on their level of loudness.
Murphy's sign A sign of gallbladder disease consisting of pain that increases with deep inspiration with right subcostal palpation.
muscle biopsy The extraction of a muscle specimen for the diagnosis of atrophy (as in muscular dystrophy) and inflammation (as in polymyositis).
muscular dystrophy (MD) A group of degenerative myopathies characterized by weakness and atrophy of muscle without nervous system involvement. At least nine types have been clinically identified and can be broadly categorized as slowly progressive or rapidly progressive.
mutation A change in deoxyribonucleic acid that is passed from one generation to another.
myalgia Muscle aches/muscle pain.
myasthenia gravis (MG) A chronic autoimmune disease of the neuromuscular junction. It is characterized by remissions and exacerbations, with fatigue and weakness primarily in the muscles innervated by the cranial nerves and in the skeletal and respiratory muscles. It ranges from mild disturbances of the ocular muscles to a rapidly developing, generalized weakness that may lead to death from respiratory failure.
myasthenic crisis Undermedication with cholinesterase inhibitors.
mydriasis Dilation of the pupil of the eye.
myelin sheath A white, lipid covering of the axon.
myelocytic Pertaining to leukemias in which the abnormal cells come from the myeloid pathways.
myelogenous Pertaining to leukemias in which the abnormal cells come from the myeloid pathways.
myelography Radiography of the spine after injection of contrast medium into the subarachnoid space of the spine; used to visualize the vertebral column, intervertebral disks, spinal nerve roots, and blood vessels.
myelosuppression Suppression of bone marrow activity that causes decreased numbers of blood cells (pancytopenia).
myocardial contractility The force of cardiac contraction independent of preload.
myocardial infarction (MI) Injury and necrosis of myocardial tissue that occurs when the tissue is abruptly and severely deprived of oxygen; usually caused by atherosclerosis of a coronary artery, rupture of the plaque, subsequent thrombosis, and occlusion of blood flow.
myocardial nuclear perfusion imaging (MNPI) The use of radionuclide techniques in which radioactive tracer substances are used to view, record, and evaluate cardiovascular abnormalities; useful for detecting myocardial infarction and decreased myocardial blood flow and for evaluating left ventricular ejection.
myocardium The heart muscle.
myoclonic seizure A type of generalized seizure characterized by a brief jerking or stiffening of the extremities. The contractions last for just a few seconds and may be symmetric or asymmetric.
myofibril sarcomere The basic contractile unit of the myocardial cell.
myoglobin A low–molecular-weight heme protein found in cardiac and skeletal muscle; an early marker of myocardial infarction.
myoglobinuria The release of muscle myoglobulin into the urine.
myoglobinuric renal failure Renal failure that is caused by the release of myoglobulin (muscle protein) from injured muscle

tissues into the circulation. Myoglobulin, which is believed to have a direct toxic effect on the kidney, can occlude the distal convoluted tubule and precipitate acute renal failure.

myomectomy The surgical removal of leiomyomas with preservation of the uterus.

myometrium The thick, middle, muscular layer of the body of the uterus. Contraction of these muscle fibers can expel the products of conception and can constrict the blood vessels to control bleeding after childbirth.

myopathy A problem in muscle tissue.

myopia An error of refraction that occurs when the eye overrefracts or overbends the light and focuses images in front of the retina; this results in normal near vision but poor distance vision; also called "nearsightedness."

myositis Inflammation of a muscle.

myosplint Electrical stimulation of tension splints in the heart to help the ventricle change to a more normal shape in the patient with heart failure; under investigation in Europe and the United States.

myringoplasty Surgical reconstruction of the eardrum.

myringotomy The surgical creation of a hole in the eardrum; performed to drain middle-ear fluids and relieve pain in the patient with otitis media (middle-ear infection).

myxedema Dry, waxy swelling of the skin that is accompanied by nonpitting edema (especially around the eyes, in the hands and feet, and between the shoulder blades) and is associated with primary hypothyroidism.

myxedema coma A rare, serious complication of untreated or poorly treated hypothyroidism in which decreased metabolism causes the heart muscle to become flabby and the chamber size to increase, resulting in decreased cardiac output and decreased perfusion to the brain and other vital organs.

N

nadir In chemotherapy, the period of greatest bone marrow suppression, when the patient's platelet count may be very low.

nasoduodenal tube (NDT) A tube that is inserted through a nostril and into the small intestine.

nasoenteric tube (NET) Any feeding tube that is inserted nasally and then advanced into the gastrointestinal tract.

nasogastric (NG) tube A tube that is inserted through a nostril and into the stomach for liquid feeding or for withdrawing gastric contents.

nasotracheal The route for inserting a tube into the trachea via the nose.

National Patient Safety Goals Goals published by The Joint Commission that require health care organizations to focus on specific priority safety practices.

natural chemical débridement Method of débriding a wound by creating an environment that promotes self-digestion of dead tissues by bacterial enzymes.

naturopathic medicine The practice of medicine that incorporates herbs and nutrition into its health care practice.

near point of vision The closest distance at which the eye can see an object clearly.

near-drowning Recovery after submersion in a liquid medium (usually water).

near-euglycemic A term that refers to near-normal blood glucose levels.

near-syncope Dizziness with an inability to remain in an upright position.

necrosis Cell death, or infarction.

necrotic arachnidism A necrotic wound resulting from a spider bite.

necrotizing hemorrhagic pancreatitis (NHP) Inflammation of the pancreas that is characterized by diffusely bleeding pancreatic tissue with fibrosis and tissue death. This form affects about 20% of patients with pancreatitis.

necrotizing vasculitis A group of diseases whose primary manifestation is inflammation of arterial walls, which causes ischemia in the tissues usually supplied by the involved vessels.

needle thoracostomy A quick, temporary method of chest decompression in which a large-bore needle is used to vent trapped air pending chest tube insertion.

negative deflection In electrocardiography, the flow of electrical current in the heart (cardiac axis) away from the positive pole and toward the negative pole.

negative feedback control mechanism The condition of maintaining a constant output of a system by exerting an inhibitory control on a key step by a product of that system. Used in a series of reactions that control hormone secretion and cellular activity based on responses to correct any movement away from normal function. An example of a simple negative feedback hormone response is the control of insulin secretion in which the action of insulin (decreasing blood glucose levels) is the opposite of the condition that stimulated insulin secretion (elevated blood glucose levels).

negative nitrogen balance A net loss of protein that occurs when the breakdown (degradation) of protein exceeds buildup (synthesis).

neglect In nursing, failure to provide for a patient's basic needs.

neglect syndrome In the patient who has had a brain attack, an unawareness of the existence of the paralyzed side. For example, the patient may believe he or she is sitting up straight when actually he or she is leaning to one side. Another typical example is the patient who washes or dresses only one side of the body.

neoadjuvant therapy Treatment of a cancerous tumor with chemotherapy to shrink the tumor before it is surgically removed.

neoplasia Any new or continued cell growth not needed for normal development or replacement of dead and damaged tissues.

nephrectomy The surgical removal of the kidney.

nephrolithiasis The formation of stones in the kidney.

nephron The "working" unit of the kidney where urine is formed from blood. Each kidney consists of about 1 million nephrons, and each nephron separately makes urine. There are two types of nephrons cortical and juxtamedullary.

nephropathy Pathologic change in the kidney that reduces kidney function and leads to renal failure.

nephrosclerosis Thickening in the nephron blood vessels that results in narrowing of the vessel lumen, with decreased renal blood flow and chronically hypoxic kidney tissue.

nephrostomy The surgical creation of an opening directly into the kidney; performed to divert urine externally and prevent further damage to the kidney when a stricture is causing hydronephrosis and cannot be corrected with urologic procedures.

nephrotic syndrome (NS) A condition of increased glomerular permeability that allows larger molecules to pass through the membrane into the urine and be removed from the blood. This process causes massive loss of protein into the urine, edema formation, and decreased plasma albumin levels.

nephrotoxicity (nephrotoxic) The disruption of kidney function.

neuritic plaques Degenerating nerve terminals found particularly in the hippocampus, an important part of the limbic system, and marked by increased amounts of an abnormal protein called beta amyloid; a characteristic change of the brain found in patients with Alzheimer's disease.

neuroaxial Referring to the epidural or spinal area.

neuroendocrine regulation The regulation of overall body function by the combined actions of the endocrine system and the nervous system.

neurofibrillary tangles Tangled masses of fibrous elements throughout the neurons; a classic finding at autopsy in the brains of patients with Alzheimer's disease.

neurogenic shock Hypotension and bradycardia associated with cervical spinal injuries and caused by a loss of autonomic function. The patient is at greatest risk in the first 24 hours after injury.

neuroglial cells Cells of varying size and shape that provide protection, structure, and nutrition for the neurons.

neurohypophysis The posterior lobe of the pituitary gland that stores hormones produced in the hypothalamus.

neurolysis Permanent nerve destruction.

neuroma A sensitive tumor consisting of nerve cells and nerve fibers.

neuropathic pain A type of chronic noncancer pain that results from a nerve injury. Examples of causes include diabetic neuropathy, postherpetic neuralgia, radiculopathy (spinal nerve damage), and trigeminal neuralgia. Neuropathic pain is described as burning, shooting, stabbing, and the sensation of "pins and needles."

neuropathy A progressive deterioration of nerves that results in loss of nerve function. A common complication of diabetes, it often involves all parts of the body.

neurotransmitter Regulatory chemical that exerts inhibitory (slowing down) or excitatory (speeding up) activity at postsynaptic nerve cell membranes. Acetylcholine, norepinephrine, epinephrine, dopamine, and serotonin are neurotransmitters.

neurovascular assessment Assessment of the neuromuscular system that includes inspection of skin color, temperature, and capillary refill distal to an injury, surgical procedure, or cast. Palpation of pulses in the extremities below level of injury and assessment of sensation, movement, and pain in the injured part give a complete assessment.

neutralization See *inactivation.*

neutropenia Decreased numbers of leukocytes, especially neutrophils, which causes immunosuppression.

neutrophilia Increased number of circulating neutrophils.

nevus A mole; a benign skin growth of the pigment-forming cells.

new-onset angina Cardiac chest pain that occurs for the first time.

nitroglycerin (NTG) A drug prescribed for patients with angina. It increases collateral blood flow, redistributes blood flow toward the subendocardium, and causes dilation of the coronary arteries.

nits Lice eggs.

NMDA (*N*-methyl-D-aspartate) receptor antagonist A group of drugs that block excess amounts of glutamate, which damages nerve cells in the brain; used to treat Alzheimer's disease.

nociceptive pain Pain related to the skin, musculoskeletal structures, or body organs.

nocturia The need to urinate excessively at night. Also called "nocturnal polyuria."

nocturnal polyuria See *nocturia.*

nodule A small node. In the vocal cords, enlarged fibrous tissue caused by infectious processes or overuse of the voice.

nonabsorbable suture Suture that becomes encapsulated in the tissue during the healing process and remains in the tissue unless removed; made of silk, cotton, steel, nylon, polyester, or other synthetic material.

nonadherence In health care, accidental failure by a patient to take medication.

noncompliance In health care, deliberate failure by a patient to take medication.

noninvasive temporary pacing (NTP) Cardiac pacing that is accomplished through the application of two large external electrodes attached to an external pulse generator; used as an emergency measure to provide demand ventricular pacing in a profoundly bradycardic or asystolic patient until invasive pacing can be instituted or the patient's intrinsic rate returns to normal.

nonmechanical obstruction Intestinal obstruction that does not involve a physical obstruction in or outside the intestine. Instead, decreased or absent peristalsis results in a slowing of the movement or a backup of intestinal contents. This is also known as "paralytic ileus" or "adynamic ileus" because it is a result of neuromuscular disturbance.

nonmodifiable risk factor Factor in disease development that cannot be altered or controlled by the patient. Examples include age, gender, family history, and ethnic background.

nonprogressive (compensatory) stage of shock The stage of shock that occurs when kidney and hormonal mechanisms are activated because cardiovascular compensation alone is not enough to maintain mean arterial pressure and supply needed oxygen to the vital organs.

nonsteroidal anti-inflammatory drugs (NSAIDs) Potent anti-inflammatory agents that inhibit the synthesis of prostaglandins, thus decreasing pain and inflammation.

nonsustained ventricular tachycardia (NSVT) Occurrence of three or more successive premature ventricular complexes.

nontunneled percutaneous central catheter A type of catheter, usually 15 to 20 cm long and with dual or triple lumens, that is inserted through the subclavian vein in the upper chest or through the jugular veins in the neck using sterile technique.

nonurgent In a three-tiered triage scheme, the category that includes patients who can generally tolerate waiting several hours for health care services without a significant risk of clinical deterioration, such as those with sprains, strains, or simple fractures.

"normal" adult blood pressure According to 2003 guidelines, blood pressure less than 120 mm Hg systolic *and* less than 80 mm Hg diastolic in adults.

normal flora The microorganisms living in or on the human host without causing disease; the bacteria that are characteristic of each body location. Normal flora often compete with and prevent infection from unfamiliar microorganisms attempting to invade a body site.

normal sinus rhythm (NSR) The rhythm originating from the sinoatrial node (dominant pacemaker), with atrial and ventricular rates of 60 to 100 beats/min and regular atrial and ventricular rhythms.

normotonic See *isosmotic.*

North American pit vipers The Crotalidae, one of two families of indigenous poisonous snakes in North America; named for the characteristic depression between each eye and nostril. They include rattlesnakes, copperheads, and water moccasins and account for most poisonous snakebites in the United States.

nosocomial infection Acquired in an inpatient health care setting; for example, infections that were not present at hospital admission; also called "hospital-acquired infections" and "health care–associated infections."

nothing by mouth (NPO) No eating, drinking (including water), or smoking.

nuchal rigidity Stiff neck, which can be a sign of cerebrospinal fluid leak; nuchal rigidity is not checked until a spinal cord injury has been ruled out.

nucleoside What the four bases in deoxyribonucleic acid (adenine, guanine, cytosine, thymine) become when a five-sided sugar (deoxyribose sugar) attaches to them.

nucleotide The final form of a base that actually gets put into the strand of deoxyribonucleic acid. A nucleoside becomes a complete nucleotide by the attachment of phosphate groups.

nulliparity The condition of never having given birth.

nursing assistant A member of the rehabilitative health care team who assists the registered nurse in the care of patients.

nutritional screening A screening by the health care provider that includes visual inspection, measured height and weight, weight history, usual eating habits, ability to chew and swallow, and any recent changes in appetite or food intake. The screening is a way to determine which patients need more extensive nutritional assessment.

nutritional status Reflects the balance between nutrient requirements and intake.

nutritionist A member of the health care team that ensures patients meet their nutritional needs. Formerly called "dietitian."

nystagmus Involuntary, rapid eye movements.

O

obesity An increase in body weight at least 20% above the upper limit of the normal range for ideal body weight, with an excess amount of body fat; in an adult, a body mass index greater than 30.

obligatory urine output The minimum amount of urine per day needed to dissolve and excrete toxic waste products.

obstipation The inability to pass stool; intractable constipation.

obstructive jaundice Jaundice caused by an impediment to the flow of bile from the liver to the duodenum; may be caused by edema of the ducts or gallstones.

occlusion Blockage.

occlusive stroke A type of brain attack caused by ischemia (interruption in blood flow) in the brain tissue supplied by the affected artery.

Occupational Safety and Health Administration (OSHA) A federal agency that protects workers from injury or illness at their place of employment.

occupational therapist (OT, OTR) A member of the rehabilitation health care team who works to develop the patient's fine motor skills used for activities of daily living and the skills related to coordination and cognitive retraining.

odynophagia Pain on swallowing.

oligomenorrhea Scant or infrequent menses.

oligospermia Low sperm count.

oliguria Decreased excretion of urine in relation to amount of fluid intake; usually defined as urine output less than 400 mL/day.

omentectomy Surgical removal of the connective tissues covering the pelvic organs.

oncogene Proto-oncogene that has been "turned on" and can cause cells to change from normal cells to cancer cells.

oncogenesis Cancer development.

oncogenic osteomalacia Osteomalacia that is caused by malignant tumors of the bone; also called "tumor-induced osteomalacia."

oncovirus Virus that causes cancer.

oophorectomy Surgical removal of the ovary.

open fracture A fracture in which the skin surface over the broken bone is disrupted, causing an external wound; also called "compound fracture."

open head injury A type of traumatic primary brain injury that occurs with a skull fracture or when the skull is pierced by a penetrating object. The integrity of the brain and the dura is violated and there is exposure to outside contaminants, with damage to the underlying vessels, dural sinus, brain, and cranial nerves.

open reduction The reduction of a fracture after surgical incision into the site to allow direct visualization of the fracture. See *internal fixation*.

ophthalmoplegia Paralysis or weakness of the eye muscles.

opioids Any of a group of drugs made from the Asian poppy or produced as a synthetic drug that produces the same effects of the opium plant. The street term for opioids is *narcotics* or *narcs*.

opportunistic infection Infection caused by organisms that are present as part of the normal environment and would be kept in check by normal immune function.

optic disc The point at the inside back of the eye where the optic nerve enters the eyeball. It appears as a creamy pink to white depressed area in the retina and contains only nerve fibers and no photoreceptor cells.

optic fundus The area at the inside back of the eye that can be seen with an ophthalmoscope.

optic nerve The nerve of sight; connects the optic disc to the brain.

orbit The bony socket of the skull that surrounds and protects the eye along with the attached muscles, nerves, vessels, and tear-producing glands.

orchiectomy The surgical removal of one or both testes.

orchitis An acute testicular inflammation resulting from trauma or infection.

orexin Neuropeptide that is an appetite stimulate.

organ of Corti The receptor end-organ of hearing located on the basilar membrane of the cochlea; contains hair cells that detect vibration from sound and stimulate the eighth cranial nerve.

orotracheal The route for inserting a tube into the trachea via the mouth.

orthopnea Shortness of breath that occurs when lying down but is relieved by sitting up.

orthostatic Pertaining to or caused by standing erect.

orthostatic hypotension A decrease in blood pressure (20 mm Hg systolic and/or 10 mm Hg diastolic) that occurs during the first few seconds to minutes after changing from a sitting or lying position to a standing position; also called "postural hypotension."

orthotopic transplantation The most common type of transplantation procedure in which a diseased organ is removed and a donor organ is grafted in its place. For example, during heart transplantation, the surgeon removes the diseased heart and leaves the posterior walls of the patient's atria, which serve as the anchor for the donor heart; anastomoses are made between the recipient and donor atria, aorta, and pulmonary arteries.

osmolality The number of milliosmoles in a kilogram of solution.

osmolarity The number of milliosmoles in a liter of solution.

osmosis The movement of a solvent across a semipermeable membrane (a membrane that allows the solvent, but not the solute, to pass through) from a lesser to a greater concentration.

osteitis deformans A metabolic disorder of bone remodeling, or turnover, in which increased resorption or loss results in bone deposits that are weak, enlarged, and disorganized; also called "Paget's disease."

osteoarthritis Noninflammatory form of arthritis characterized by the progressive deterioration and loss of cartilage in one or more joints; most common form of arthritis.

osteoblast Cell associated with formation of bone.

osteoblastic Referring to bone production activity.

osteoclast Cell associated with destruction or resorption of bone.

osteoclastic Referring to bone destruction.

osteocyte Bone cell.

osteogenic Originating from bone.

osteomalacia Abnormal softening of the bone tissue characterized by inadequate mineralization of osteoid. It is the adult equivalent of rickets (vitamin D deficiency) in children.

osteomyelitis An inflammation of bone tissue caused by pathogenic microorganisms; produces an increased vascularity and edema often involving the surrounding soft tissues.

osteonecrosis See *avascular necrosis.*

osteopenia A condition of low bone mass that occurs when there is a disruption in the bone remodeling process.

osteophyte Bone spur.

osteoporosis A metabolic disease in which bone demineralization results in decreased density and subsequent fractures.

osteotomy Surgical resection of bone.

ostomate A patient with an ostomy.

ostomy The surgical creation of an opening, usually referring to an opening in the abdominal wall; stoma.

otorrhea Ear discharge.

otosclerosis Irregular bone growth around the ossicles.

otoscope An instrument used to examine the ear; consists of a light, a handle, a magnifying lens, and a pneumatic bulb for injecting air into the external canal to test mobility of the eardrum.

ototoxic Having a toxic effect on the inner ear structures.

ototoxicity Disruption of hearing and/or balance.

outflow disease Chronic peripheral arterial disease with obstruction at or below the superficial femoral or popliteal artery. The patient experiences burning or cramping in the calves, ankles, feet, and toes after walking a certain distance; the pain usually subsides with rest.

outpatient A patient who goes to the hospital for treatment and returns home on the same day.

ovaries A pair of almond-shaped organs that are located near the lateral walls of the upper pelvic cavity. They develop and release ova and produce the sex steroid hormones (estrogen, progesterone, androgen, and relaxin).

overflow (urinary) incontinence The involuntary loss of urine when the bladder is overdistended.

overhydration See *fluid overload.*

overweight An increase in body weight for height compared with a reference standard (e.g., the Metropolitan Life height and weight tables) or 10% greater than ideal body weight. However, this weight may not reflect excess body fat, which in an adult is a body mass index of 25 to 30.

ovoid pupil In evaluating pupils for size and reaction to light, the midstage between a normal-sized pupil and a dilated pupil; indicates the development of increased intracranial pressure.

ovulation The cyclic maturation of a dominant follicle (the graafian follicle) in the ovary and the subsequent release of the ovum.

oxygen concentrator A machine that removes nitrogen, water vapor, and hydrocarbons from room air.

oxygen dissociation The transfer of oxygen from hemoglobin to tissues.

P

P wave In the electrocardiogram, the deflection representing atrial depolarization.

pacemaker In the cardiac conduction system, the sinus node.

pack-years The number of packs of cigarettes per day multiplied by the number of years the patient has smoked; used in recording the patient's smoking history.

Paget's disease An alternative name for osteitis deformans, a metabolic disorder of bone remodeling, or turnover, in which increased resorption or loss results in bone deposits that are weak, enlarged, and disorganized.

pain An unpleasant sensory and emotional experience associated with actual or potential tissue damage; the most reliable indication of pain is the patient's self-report.

palliation Relieving symptoms.

palliative care A compassionate and supportive approach to patients and families who are living with life-threatening illnesses; involves a holistic approach that provides relief of symptoms experienced by the dying patient.

palliative surgery Surgery done to make the patient more comfortable.

palpitations A feeling of fluttering in the chest, an unpleasant awareness of the heartbeat, and an irregular heartbeat; may result from a change in heart rate or rhythm or from an increase in the force of heart contractions.

pancreatic abscess A collection of purulent material that results from extensive inflammatory necrosis of the pancreas after infection by organisms such as *Escherichia coli*; the most serious complication of pancreatitis. It is fatal if left untreated.

pancreatic pseudocyst A false cyst, so named because, unlike a true cyst, it does not have an epithelial lining. It is an encapsulated saclike structure that forms on or surrounds the pancreas and develops as a complication of acute or chronic pancreatitis. It may contain up to several liters of straw-colored or dark-brown viscous fluid, the enzymatic exudate of the pancreas.

pancreaticojejunostomy Surgical anastomosis of the pancreatic duct with the jejunum.

pancytopenia A deficiency of all three cell types (red blood cells, white blood cells, and platelets) of the blood.

pandemic A general epidemic spread over a wide geographic area and affecting a large proportion of the population.
panhypopituitarism The decreased production of all anterior pituitary hormones; an extremely rare condition.
panniculectomy The surgical removal of any panniculus, most often the abdominal apron; usually done as a follow-up to bariatric surgery in an obese patient.
panniculitis Infection of the panniculus.
panniculus A layer of membrane; also used to refer to skinfold areas in the obese patient.
pannus Vascular granulation tissue composed of inflammatory cells that forms in a joint space; erodes articular cartilage and eventually destroys bone.
Papanicolaou test (Pap smear) A cytologic study that is effective in detecting precancerous and cancerous cells obtained from the cervix.
papilla The anatomic term for a small, nipple-shaped projection or structure.
papilledema Edema and hyperemia of the optic disc; a sign of increased intracranial pressure found on ophthalmoscopic examination; also called a "choked disc."
papilloma A pedunculated outgrowth of tissue.
papillotomy An incision of a papilla, a small nipple-shaped projection or structure.
papular Referring to a papule, a small, solid elevation of the skin.
paracentesis A procedure in which the physician inserts a trocar catheter into the abdomen to remove and drain ascitic fluid from the peritoneal cavity.
paradoxical blood pressure (paradoxical pulse) An exaggerated decrease in systolic pressure by more than 10 mm Hg during the inspiratory phase of the respiratory cycle (normal is 3 to 10 mm Hg); clinical conditions that may produce a paradoxical blood pressure include pericardial tamponade, constrictive pericarditis, and pulmonary hypertension.
paradoxical chest movement The "sucking inward" of the loose chest area during inspiration and a "puffing out" of the same area during expiration in a patient with a flail chest.
paradoxical splitting Abnormal splitting of the S_2 heart sound heard in patients with severe myocardial depression; causes early closure of the pulmonic valve or a delay in aortic valve closure.
paralysis Absence of movement.
paralytic ileus Absence of peristalsis.
paramedic Prehospital care provider for patients who require care that exceeds basic life support resources. Advanced life support (ALS) may include cardiac monitoring, advanced airway management and intubation, establishing IV access, and administering drugs en route to the emergency department.
paranasal sinuses The air-filled cavities within the bones that surround the nasal passages. Lined with ciliated membrane, the sinuses provide resonance during speech and decrease the weight of the skull.
paraparesis Weakness that involves only the lower extremities, as seen in lower thoracic and lumbosacral injuries or lesions.
paraplegia Paralysis that involves only the lower extremities, as seen in lower thoracic and lumbosacral injuries or lesions.
parathyroid hormone (PTH) A hormone released from the parathyroid glands in response to decreased serum calcium levels.
parenchyma A general term for the functional elements of an organ as differentiated from its framework (stroma).
paresis Weakness.
paresthesia Unusual nerve sensations of touch, such as tingling and burning.
parietal cells Cells lining the wall of the stomach that secrete hydrochloric acid and produce intrinsic factor.
Parkinson disease (PD) A debilitating neurologic disease that affects motor ability and is characterized by four cardinal symptoms: tremor, rigidity, akinesia (slow movement), and postural instability. It is the third most common neurologic disorder of older adults; also called "paralysis agitans."
parotidectomy The surgical removal of the parotid glands.
paroxysmal nocturnal dyspnea (PND) In the patient with heart disease, difficulty breathing that develops after lying down for several hours and causes the patient to awaken abruptly with a feeling of suffocation and panic. Occurs because the heart is unable to compensate for the increased volume when blood from the lower extremities is redistributed to the venous system, which increases venous return to the heart. A diseased heart is ineffective in pumping the additional fluid into the circulatory system, and pulmonary congestion results.
paroxysmal supraventricular tachycardia (PSVT) A form of supraventricular tachycardia that occurs when the rhythm is intermittent, initiated suddenly by a premature complex such as a premature atrial complex, and terminated suddenly with or without intervention.
partial seizure One of the three broad categories of seizure disorders along with generalized seizure and unclassified seizure. Partial seizures are of two types: complex and simple. Partial seizures begin in a part of one cerebral hemisphere; some can evolve into generalized tonic-clonic, tonic, or clonic seizures. They are most often seen in adults and in general are less responsive to medical treatment; also called "focal seizures" or "local seizures."
passive euthanasia See *withdrawing or withholding life-sustaining therapy.*
passive immunity Resistance to infection that is of short duration (days or months) and either natural by transplacental transfer from the mother or artificial by injection of antibodies (e.g., immune globulin).
passive smoking The exposure to secondhand smoke produced by a person smoking cigarettes.
pathogen Any microorganism capable of producing disease.
pathogenicity The ability to cause disease.
pathologic (spontaneous) fracture A fracture that occurs after minimal trauma to a bone that has been weakened by a disease such as bone cancer or osteoporosis.
patient-controlled analgesia A method that allows the patient to control the dosage of opioid analgesia received by using an infusion pump to deliver the desired amount of medication through a conventional IV route.
patients Recipients of care in mutually trusting relationships with nurses and other members of the health care team.
peak expiratory flow (PEF) The fastest airflow rate reached at any time during exhalation.
peau d'orange A dimpled appearance of the skin, resembling an orange peel.
pedal Pertaining to the feet.
pediculosis An infestation by human lice.
pedigree A graph of a family history for a specific trait or health problem over several generations.
pelvic inflammatory disease (PID) Any infection of the pelvis involving the upper genital tract beyond the cervix in women. It occurs when organisms from the lower genital tract migrate

from the endocervix upward through the uterine cavity into the fallopian tubes.

pemphigus vulgaris A rare, chronic blistering disease that can occur anywhere on the skin and is associated with high morbidity and mortality rates. It is caused by an autoimmune disorder that occurs most often during middle and old age.

penectomy Surgical removal of the penis.

penetrance In genetics, how often or how well a gene is expressed when it is present within a population.

penetrating injury See *penetrating trauma.*

penetrating trauma Injuries caused by piercing; classified by the velocity of the vehicle (e.g., knife or bullet) causing the injury. Low-velocity injuries from knife wounds cause damage directly at the site; high-velocity injuries from gunshot wounds cause both direct and indirect damage; also called "penetrating injury."

penis An organ for urination and intercourse. It consists of the body or shaft and the glans penis (the distal end of the penis).

peptic ulcer A mucosal lesion of the stomach or duodenum.

peptic ulcer disease (PUD) The impairment of gastric mucosal defenses so they no longer protect the epithelium from the effects of acid and pepsin.

percussion notes The sounds heard upon striking a part of the body with short, sharp blows; aids diagnosis through a systematic assessment of changes in the sound quality obtained.

percutaneous Performed through the skin.

percutaneous alcohol septal ablation Surgical procedure for hypertrophic cardiomyopathy (HCM) in which alcohol is injected into a target septal branch of the left anterior descending coronary artery to produce a small septal infarction. This procedure also widens the LV outflow tract.

percutaneous electrical nerve stimulation (PENS) See *transcutaneous electrical nerve stimulation (TENS).*

percutaneous endoscopic gastrostomy (PEG) A stoma created from the abdominal wall into the stomach for insertion of a short feeding tube.

percutaneous stereotactic rhizotomy (PSR) Procedure performed under general anesthesia to treat trigeminal neuralgia; a hollow needle is passed through the inside of the patient's cheek into the trigeminal nerve fibers, and a heating current (radiofrequency thermocoagulation) goes through the needle to destroy some of the fibers.

percutaneous transhepatic cholangiography (PTC) The radiographic study of the biliary duct system using an iodinated dye instilled via a percutaneous needle inserted through the liver into the intrahepatic ducts. It may be performed when a patient has jaundice or persistent upper abdominal pain, even after cholecystectomy, but it is rarely performed as a diagnostic procedure.

percutaneous transluminal angioplasty (PTA) A nonsurgical method of improving arterial flow by opening the vessel lumen and creating a smooth inner vessel surface. One or more arteries are dilated with a balloon catheter advanced through a cannula, which is inserted into or above an occluded or stenosed artery.

percutaneously Performed through the skin and other tissues.

perforate To break open or pierce through a part.

pericardial effusion Complication of pericarditis that occurs when the space between the parietal and visceral layers of the pericardium fills with fluid.

pericardial friction rub An abnormal sound that originates from the pericardial sac and occurs with the movements of the heart during the cardiac cycle; usually transient and a sign of inflammation, infection, or infiltration; may be heard in patients with pericarditis resulting from myocardial infarction, cardiac tamponade, or post-thoracotomy.

pericardiectomy Surgical excision of the pericardium (the sac around the heart).

pericardiocentesis Withdrawal of pericardial fluid through a catheter inserted into the pericardial space to relieve the pressure on the heart.

perichondrium A tough, fibrous tissue layer that surrounds the ear cartilage and gives shape to the pinna.

perimenopause Menopause transition; changes in spontaneous ovarian function that precede the last menstrual period and occur gradually. Common features are a change in the woman's usual menstrual periods and the beginning of vasomotor symptoms, such as hot flushes and night sweats.

perineum The area between the vaginal opening and the anus. The skin of the perineum covers the muscles, fascia, and ligaments that support the pelvic structures.

periodontal disease Gum disease in which mandibular bone loss has occurred.

perioperative The operative experience consisting of the preoperative, intraoperative, and postoperative time periods.

peripheral blood stem cells (PBSCs) Stem cells that are collected from peripheral blood for transplantation into the patient.

peripheral IV therapy IV therapy in which a vascular access device (VAD) is placed in a peripheral vein, usually in the arm.

peripheral neuropathy (PN) A general term for inflammation of peripheral nerves; also called "polyneuritis" and "polyneuropathy."

peripheral vascular disease (PVD) Any disorder that alters the natural flow of blood through the arteries and veins of the peripheral circulation.

peritonitis Acute inflammation of the visceral/parietal peritoneum and endothelial lining of the abdominal cavity, or peritoneum.

periungual lesion Skin lesion around the nail bed.

permeable The quality of being porous.

pernicious anemia A form of megaloblastic anemia caused by failure to absorb vitamin B_{12} because of a deficiency of intrinsic factor (normally secreted by the gastric mucosa) needed for intestinal absorption of vitamin B_{12}.

PERRLA An acronym that stands for the phrase "Pupils should be equal in size, round and regular in shape, and react to light and accommodation."

persistent pain See *chronic pain.*

personal emergency preparedness plan An individual plan that outlines specific arrangements in the event of disaster, such as child care, pet care, and older adult care.

personal protective equipment (PPE) Infection control protocol that refers to the use of gloves, isolation gowns, face protection, and respirators with N95 or higher filtration.

personal readiness supplies A preassembled disaster supply kit for the home and/or automobile that contains clothing and basic survival supplies; also called a "go bag."

petechiae Pinpoint red spots on the mucous membranes, palate, conjunctivae, or skin.

pH A measure of the free hydrogen ion level in body fluid.

phagocytosis The process of engulfing, ingesting, killing, and disposing of an invading organism by neutrophils and macrophages; a key process of inflammation.

phantom limb pain (PLP) A frequent complication of amputation in which the patient perceives sensation in the absent (amputated) foot or hand. This sensation usually diminishes over time.

pharmacologic stress echocardiogram A form of echocardiography in which either dobutamine (increases heart's contractility) or adenosine (dilates coronary arteries) is given to the patient; usually used when patients cannot tolerate exercise.

pharynx The throat, which extends from the soft palate to the esophagus and is lined with mucous membrane; part of the upper respiratory tract.

phenotype Any genetic characteristic that can actually be observed or, in some cases, determined by laboratory test.

pheochromocytoma A tumor of the adrenal medulla, which can cause excessive secretion of catecholamines.

pheresis A procedure in which whole blood is withdrawn from the patient, a blood component (such as stem cells) is filtered out, and the plasma is returned to the patient.

phimosis A tight foreskin of the penis, which cannot be retracted.

phlebitis Inflammation of a vein, which can predispose patients to thrombosis.

phlebothrombosis Presence of a thrombus in a vein without inflammation.

phlebotomy Drawing of blood from a vein.

phonation Normal speech.

phonophobia Abnormal sensitivity to sound.

phonophoresis Treatment for back pain in which a topical drug (e.g., lidocaine, hydrocortisone) is applied followed by continuous ultrasound for 10 minutes.

photocoagulation Use of a laser, such as in treatment of retinal detachment.

photophobia Abnormal sensitivity to light.

photopsia The appearance of bright flashes of light due to the onset of retinal detachment.

physiatrist A physician who specializes in rehabilitative medicine.

physical abuse The use of a physical force, such as hitting, burning, pushing, and molesting the patient, that results in bodily injury.

physical dependence The adaptation manifested by a drug class–specific withdrawal syndrome. Manifestations can be produced by abrupt cessation, rapid dose reduction, decreasing blood level of the drug, or administration of an antagonist.

physical therapist (PT, RPT) A member of the rehabilitation health care team who helps the patient achieve mobility and who teaches techniques for performing certain activities of daily living.

piggyback set See *secondary administration set.*

pilonidal cyst A lesion of the sacral area that often has a sinus track extending into deeper tissue structures.

pinna The external ear, which is composed of cartilage covered by skin.

pitting Indentation of the skin; often occurs with edema.

pituitary Cushing's disease Oversecretion of ACTH by the anterior pituitary gland, which causes hyperplasia of the adrenal cortex in both adrenal glands and an excess of most hormones secreted by the adrenal cortex.

placebo Substance or action that produces an effect regardless of its known intrinsic value or specific physical or chemical properties.

placebo effect A patient's favorable response to a placebo.

plantar fasciitis An inflammation of the plantar fascia, which is located in the area of the arch of the foot. It is often seen in athletes, especially runners.

plasma cell A short-lived B-lymphocyte that begins functioning immediately to produce antibodies against sensitizing antigens.

plasmapheresis The separation of plasma from whole blood, after which the blood cells are returned to the patient without the plasma to eliminate antibodies.

pleiotropic Having widespread or numerous effects.

plethoric A flushed appearance of the skin.

pleura The continuous smooth membrane composed of two surfaces that totally enclose the lungs.

pleural effusion Fluid in the pleural space.

pleuritic chest pain A stabbing pain on taking a deep breath.

pleurodesis An inflammation created by instilling a sclerosing agent through a chest tube into the pleural space, which causes the pleura to stick to the chest wall and prevent formation of effusion fluid.

plexus Cluster of nerves.

ploidy The number and appearance of chromosomes; used to describe cancer cells.

pluripotency The unlimited potential of early embryonic cells to mature into any body cell; also called "multipotency" or "totipotency."

pluripotent stem cell The precursor cell involved in the production of red blood cells.

pneumonectomy Removal of an entire lung, including all blood vessels.

pneumothorax Air in the pleural (chest) cavity.

podagra Inflammation of the metatarsophalangeal joint of the great toe.

point of maximal impulse (PMI) See apical impulse.

polyarthralgia Aching around multiple joints.

polycystic kidney disease (PKD) An inherited disorder in which fluid-filled cysts develop in the kidneys.

polycythemia An excess of red blood cells.

polycythemia vera (PV) A disease that involves massive production of red blood cells, leukocytes, and platelets.

polydipsia Excessive intake of water.

polymorphism A variation in form.

polymyalgia rheumatica (PMR) A clinical syndrome characterized by stiffness, weakness, aching of the proximal musculature (the shoulder and pelvic girdles), and systemic manifestations such as low-grade fever, arthralgias and stiffness, fatigue, and weight loss.

polymyositis A diffuse inflammatory disease of skeletal (striated) muscle that causes symmetric weakness and atrophy.

polyp An abnormal outgrowth from a mucous membrane.

polypectomy Surgical removal of a nasal polyp.

polyphagia Excessive eating.

polypharmacy The use of multiple drugs, both prescription and nonprescription.

polyuria Frequent and excessive urination.

pores Openings or spaces.

portal hypertension An abnormal persistent increase in pressure within the portal vein; a major complication of cirrhosis.

portal hypertensive gastropathy A complication that can occur in patients with portal hypertension, with or without esophageal varices. Slow gastric mucosal bleeding may result in chronic slow blood loss, occult positive stools, and anemia.

portal-systemic encephalopathy (PSE) A clinical disorder seen in hepatic failure and cirrhosis; it is manifested by neurologic symptoms and is characterized by an altered level of consciousness, impaired thinking processes, and neuromuscular disturbances; also called "hepatic encephalopathy" and "hepatic coma."

positive deflection In electrocardiography, the flow of electrical current in the heart (cardiac axis) toward the positive pole.

positive inotropic agents Drugs that increase myocardial contractility and are prescribed to improve cardiac output.

positron emission tomography (PET) A diagnostic tool that provides information about the function of the brain, specifically glucose and oxygen metabolism and cerebral blood flow. The patient is injected with the molecule deoxyglucose, which is tagged to an isotope. The isotope emits activity in the form of positrons, which are scanned and converted into a color image by a computer.

postanesthesia care unit (PACU) Recovery room.

postcholecystectomy syndrome (PCES) The occurrence of the clinical manifestations of biliary tract disease following cholecystectomy; caused by residual or recurring calculi, inflammation, or stricture of the common bile duct.

post-concussion syndrome A group of clinical manifestations following a concussion that consist of personality changes, irritability, headaches, dizziness, restlessness, nervousness, insomnia, memory loss, and depression. The prolonged pattern is classified as post-trauma syndrome.

posterior colporrhaphy The surgical procedure to repair a rectocele by strengthening pelvic supports and reducing the bulging.

posterior cord lesion A condition caused by cervical injuries; results from damage to the posterior gray and white matter of the spinal cord. Motor function remains intact, but the patient experiences a loss of vibratory sense, crude touch, and position sensation; this is the opposite of anterior cord syndrome.

posteroanterior Back to front; position for standard chest x-rays.

postherpetic neuralgia Pain that persists after herpes zoster lesions have resolved.

postictal stage Referring to the time immediately after a seizure.

postoperative After surgery.

postpericardiotomy syndrome Symptoms, including pericardial and pleural pain, pericarditis, friction rub, elevated temperature and white blood cell count, and dysrhythmias that occur in patients after cardiac surgery; may occur days to weeks after surgery and seems to be associated with blood that remains in the pericardial sac.

postrenal failure Decrease in renal function related to an obstruction in the flow of urine. It can progress to acute renal failure.

postural (orthostatic) hypotension A decrease of more than 20 mm Hg of systolic pressure or more than 10 mm Hg of diastolic pressure, with a 10% to 20% increase in heart rate; patients may report dizziness or light-headedness when they move from a lying to a sitting or standing position.

post-void residual (PVR) The amount of urine remaining in the bladder within 20 minutes after voiding.

potency The ability to have and sustain an erection.

PQRST A mnemonic (memory device) that may help in the current problem assessment of patients with gastrointestinal tract disorders. The letters represent the following areas P, precipitating or palliative (What brings it on? What makes it better or worse?); Q, quality or quantity (How does it look, feel, or sound?); R, region or radiation (Where is it? Does it spread anywhere?); S, severity scale (How bad is it [on a scale of 1 to 10]? Is it getting better, worse, or staying the same?); T, timing (onset, duration, and frequency).

PR interval In the electrocardiogram, the interval measured from the beginning of the P wave to the end of the PR segment; represents the time required for atrial depolarization as well as impulse delay in the atrioventricular node and travel time to the Purkinje fibers.

PR segment In the electrocardiogram, the isoelectric line from the end of the P wave to the beginning of the QRS complex, when the electrical impulse is traveling through the atrioventricular node, where it is delayed.

prandial insulin secretion The increased levels of insulin that are secreted after eating. Within 10 minutes of eating, an early burst of insulin secretion occurs, which is followed by an increasing insulin release that lasts as long as hyperglycemia is present.

prealbumin (PAB) A protein secreted by the liver that binds thyroxine.

precipitation The formation of large, insoluble, antigen-antibody complexes during the antibody-binding process.

pre-emptive analgesia A technique to decrease postoperative pain and the requirements for analgesia, improve morbidity, and decrease hospital stay by administering local anesthetics, opioids, and nonsteroidal anti-inflammatory drugs in the preoperative, intraoperative, or postoperative period.

prehospital care provider Typically, any of the first caregivers encountered by the patient if he or she is transported to the emergency department by an ambulance or helicopter.

prehypertension A blood pressure category that includes blood pressure readings of 120 to 139 mm Hg systolic or 80 to 89 mm Hg diastolic. Prehypertensive patients are at a higher risk for the development of hypertension.

preictal phase Referring to events that a patient experiences before a seizure, such as the presence of an aura.

preinfarction angina Chest pain that occurs in the days or weeks before a myocardial infarction.

preload The degree of myocardial fiber stretch at the end of diastole and just before contraction; determined by the amount of blood returning to the heart from both the venous system (right heart) and the pulmonary system (left heart).

premature atrial complex (PAC) In the electrocardiogram, an early complex that occurs when atrial tissue becomes irritable. This ectopic focus fires an impulse before the next sinus impulse is due, thus usurping the sinus pacemaker. The premature P wave from the atrial focus is early and has a shape different from that of the P wave generated from the sinus node.

premature complex In the electrocardiogram, an early complex that occurs when a cardiac cell or cell group other than the sinoatrial node becomes irritable and fires an impulse before the next sinus impulse is generated. After the premature complex, there is a pause before the next normal complex, which creates an irregularity in the rhythm.

premature ventricular complex (PVC) In the electrocardiogram, an early ventricular complex is followed by a pause that results from increased irritability of ventricular cells. The QRS complexes may be unifocal or uniform (of the same shape), or multifocal or multiform (of different shapes).

premenstrual dysphoric disorder (PMDD) A more disabling and severe form of premenstrual syndrome.

premenstrual syndrome (PMS) A collection of symptoms that occur in the 2 weeks before menstruation and are followed by relief with menses and a symptom-free phase. Symptoms may include emotional, physical, and cognitive manifestations such as irritability, breast tenderness, and short-term memory problems.

preoperative Before surgery.

prepuce The foreskin of the penis.

prerenal failure Condition that causes inadequate kidney perfusion; can progress to acute renal failure.

presbycusis The loss of hearing, especially for high-pitched sounds; occurs as a result of aging.

presbyopia An age-related impairment of vision characterized by a loss of lens elasticity and the ability of the eye to accommodate. The near point of vision increases, and near objects must be placed farther from the eye to be seen clearly.

presence A type of communication that consists of listening and acknowledging the legitimacy of the patient's and/or family's pain.

pressure ulcer Tissue damage caused when the skin and underlying soft tissue are compressed between a bony prominence and an external surface for an extended period; commonly occurs over the sacrum, hips, and ankles.

pretibial Pertaining to the front of the leg below the knee.

pretibial myxedema Dry, waxy swelling of the front surfaces of the lower legs.

preventive therapy drugs For asthma, drugs that are used every day regardless of symptoms to change airway responsiveness and prevent asthma attacks from occurring.

priapism An abnormal, long-maintained erection without sexual desire, which causes the penis to become large, hard, and painful. It can occur from neural, vascular, or pharmacologic causes.

primary arthroplasty A total hip arthroplasty procedure that has been performed for the first time.

primary gout The most common type of gout; results from one of several inborn errors of purine metabolism.

primary lesions In describing skin disease, the initial reaction to a problem that alters one of the structural components of the skin.

primary open-angle glaucoma (POAG) The most common form of primary glaucoma; characterized by reduced outflow of aqueous humor through the chamber angle. Because the fluid cannot leave the eye at the same rate it is produced, intraocular pressure gradually increases.

primary prevention Strategies used to avoid or delay the actual occurrence of a specific disease.

primary progressive multiple sclerosis A type of multiple sclerosis (MS) that involves a steady and gradual neurologic deterioration without remission of symptoms. Patients with this type of MS are usually between 40 and 60 years of age at onset of the disease and experience progressive disability with no acute attacks.

primary survey Priorities of care addressed in order of immediate threats to life as part of the initial assessment in the emergency department. Survey is based on an "ABC" mnemonic with "D" and "E" added for trauma patients: airway/cervical spine (A), breathing (B), circulation (C), disability (D), and exposure (E).

primary tumor The original tumor, usually identified by the tissue from which it arose (parent tissue), such as in breast cancer or lung cancer.

progressive stage of shock The stage of shock that occurs with a sustained decrease in mean arterial pressure, when compensatory mechanisms are functioning but are no longer delivering sufficient oxygen, even to vital organs.

progressive-relapsing multiple sclerosis A type of multiple sclerosis (MS) that occurs in only 5% of patients with MS. It is characterized by the absence of periods of remission, and the patient's condition does not return to baseline. Progressive, cumulative symptoms, and deterioration occur over several years.

proinsulin A precursor of insulin that includes the alpha and beta chains of the insulin molecule.

projected pain Pain that occurs along a specific nerve or nerves.

proliferative diabetic retinopathy (PDR) A form of retinopathy associated with diabetes mellitus in which a network of fragile new blood vessels develops, leaking blood and protein into surrounding tissue. The new blood vessels are stimulated by retinal hypoxia that results from poor capillary perfusion of the retinal tissues. New blood vessels grow in the retina, onto the iris, and into the back of the vitreous. The vitreous contracts and pulls away from the retina, causing blood vessels to break and bleed into the vitreous.

promoter In oncology, a substance that promotes or enhances growth of the initiated cancer cell; may be a hormone, drug, or chemical.

pronator drift Occurs in a patient with muscle weakness due to cerebral or brainstem reasons. The arm on the weak side tends to fall, or "drift," with the palm pronating (turning inward) after the patient has closed his or her eyes and held the arms perpendicular to the body with the palms up for 15 to 30 seconds; part of the neurologic assessment.

prophylactic mastectomy Highly controversial practice of surgically removing the breast in order to reduce the risk of breast cancer.

prophylactic surgery Surgery done to remove "at-risk" tissue to prevent cancer development.

proportional pulse pressure A measurement of cardiac output that is calculated from blood pressure measurements, as follows: subtract diastolic from systolic blood pressure, and divide the result by systolic blood pressure. A proportional pulse pressure less than 25% indicates severely compromised cardiac output.

proprioception Position sense.

proprioceptive Awareness of body position.

prosopagnosia The inability to recognize oneself and other familiar faces; occurs in patients in the later stages of Alzheimer's disease.

prostaglandins Chemicals that are produced in the cells and cause inflammation and swelling.

prostate gland A large accessory gland of the male reproductive system. It secretes a milky alkaline fluid that adds bulk to the semen, enhances sperm motility, and neutralizes acidic vaginal secretions.

prostatectomy Surgical removal of the prostate.

prostate-specific antigen (PSA) A glycoprotein produced solely by the prostate. The normal blood level of PSA is less than 4 ng/mL; levels are higher in patients with increased prostatic tissue as a result of benign prostatic hyperplasia, prostatic infarction, prostatitis, and prostate cancer. Levels associated with prostate cancer are usually much higher than those occurring with other prostate tissue enlargement.

prostatitis Inflammation of the prostate.

prostatodynia Pain in the prostate with manifestations of prostatitis but no inflammation of the prostate and a negative urine culture.

prostration Extreme exhaustion.

protein-calorie malnutrition (PCM) A disorder of nutrition that may present in three forms marasmus, kwashiorkor, and marasmic-kwashiorkor; also called "protein-energy malnutrition."

protein-energy malnutrition (PEM) See *protein-calorie malnutrition.*

proteinuria The presence of protein in the urine.

proteolysis The breakdown of proteins to provide fuel for energy when liver glucose is unavailable.

proton-pump inhibitor (PPI) A group of drugs that inhibit the proton pump in the stomach to decrease gastric acid production.

pruritus An unpleasant itching sensation.

pseudoaddiction An iatrogenic syndrome created by the undertreatment of pain and characterized by patient behaviors such as anger and escalating demands for more or different medications; results in suspicion and avoidance by staff. Pseudoaddiction can be distinguished from true addiction because the behaviors resolve when pain is effectively treated.

pseudogout A disease that mimics the clinical manifestations of gout; however, the crystals deposited in the joints are calcium pyrophosphate, not sodium urate.

psoriatic arthritis (PsA) A syndrome of inflammatory arthritis associated with psoriasis, the skin condition characterized by a scaly, itchy rash.

psychiatric crisis nurse team An emergency department specialty team whose nurses interact with patients and families in crisis.

psychotropic drugs Antipsychotic and neuroleptic drugs. These are appropriately given to patients with emotional and behavioral health problems (e.g., hallucinations and delusions) that accompany dementia but are sometimes inappropriately used for agitation, combativeness, or restlessness. They are considered chemical restraints because they decrease mobility and patients' ability to care for themselves.

ptosis Drooping of the eyelid.

pulmonary artery occlusive pressure (PAOP) See *pulmonary artery wedge pressure.*

pulmonary artery wedge pressure (PAWP) Measurement of pressure in the left atrium using a balloon-tipped catheter introduced into the pulmonary artery. When the balloon at the catheter tip is inflated, the catheter advances and wedges in a branch of the pulmonary artery. The tip of the catheter is able to sense pressures transmitted from the left atrium, which reflect left ventricular end-diastolic pressure; also called "pulmonary artery occlusive pressure."

pulmonary autograph The relocation of the patient's own pulmonary valve to the aortic position for aortic valve replacement (Ross procedure).

pulmonary embolism (PE) A collection of particulate matter, most commonly a blood clot, that enters venous circulation and lodges in the pulmonary vessels, obstructing pulmonary blood flow and leading to decreased systemic oxygenation, pulmonary tissue hypoxia, and potential death.

pulmonic valve The semilunar valve of the heart that separates the right ventricle from the pulmonary artery.

pulse deficit The difference between the apical and peripheral pulses.

pulse pressure The difference between the systolic and diastolic pressures.

pulse therapy Any therapy given at a high dose for a short duration.

pulsus alternans A type of pulse in which a weak pulse alternates with a strong pulse despite a regular heart rhythm; seen in patients with severely depressed cardiac function.

pump A pole-mounted or portable device that pumps medication or fluid under pressure during infusion therapy.

pump failure See *heart failure.*

punctum The opening through which tears drain; located at the nasal side of the eyelid edges.

pupil The opening through which light enters the eye; located in the center of the iris of the eye.

pure tones Tones generated by an audiometer to determine hearing acuity.

Purkinje cells In the cardiac conduction system, the cells that make up the bundle of His, bundle branches, and terminal Purkinje fibers. These cells are responsible for the rapid conduction of electrical impulses throughout the ventricles, leading to ventricular depolarization and subsequent ventricular muscle contraction.

purpura Purple patches on the skin that may be caused by blood disorders, vascular abnormalities, or trauma.

pyelolithotomy The surgical removal of a stone from the kidney.

pyelonephritis A bacterial infection in the kidney and renal pelvis (the upper urinary tract).

pyloromyotomy An incision through the serosa and muscularis of the pylorus, down to the mucosa; created to prevent gastric motility disturbances in patients who have undergone esophagectomy.

pyogenic liver abscess A liver abscess resulting from bacterial infection by *Escherichia coli* and *Klebsiella, Enterobacter, Salmonella, Staphylococcus,* and *Enterococcus* species. A pyogenic abscess is generally solitary and is confined to the right lobe, but occasionally abscesses are multiple.

pyramid The fan-shaped structures that constitute the medulla of the kidney. Each kidney has 12 to 18 pyramids.

pyuria The presence of white blood cells (pus) in the urine.

Q

QRS complex In the electrocardiogram, the portion consisting of the Q, R, and S waves, representing ventricular depolarization.

QRS duration In the electrocardiogram, the time required for depolarization of both ventricles; measured from the beginning of the QRS complex to the J point (the junction where the QRS complex ends and the ST segment begins).

QT interval In the electrocardiogram, the time from the beginning of the QRS complex to the end of the T wave. It represents the total time required for ventricular depolarization and repolarization.

quadriceps-setting exercise Postoperative leg exercise performed by straightening the legs and pushing the back of the knees into the bed.

quadrigeminy A type of premature complex consisting of a repetitive four-beat pattern; usually occurs as three sequential normal complexes followed by a premature complex and a pause, with the same pattern repeating itself in a four-beat pattern.

quadriparesis Weakness that involves all four extremities; seen with cervical spinal cord injury.

R

Rad Acronym for "radiation absorbed dose."

radiating pain Diffuse, unlocalized pain around the site of origin.

radiation exposure The amount of radiation delivered to a tissue during radiation therapy.

radiation proctitis Rectal mucosa inflammation that results from external beam radiation therapy.

radical vulvectomy The surgical removal of the entire vulva skin, labia, clitoris, subcutaneous tissues, and possibly inguinal and femoral node dissection.

radicular Referring to a nerve root.

radiculopathy Referring to radicular pain; spinal nerve root involvement.

radiofrequency ablation The use of heat to achieve permanent ablation of nerve roots.

radiofrequency catheter ablation An invasive procedure that uses radiofrequency waves to abolish an irritable focus that is causing a supraventricular or ventricular tachydysrhythmia.

Rapid Response Team Team of critical care experts that save lives and decrease the risk for harm by providing care to patients before a respiratory or cardiac arrest occurs. Also called "Medical Emergency Team."

rebound headache Headache that occurs as a side effect of a drug that has relieved an initial migraine headache; also called "medication overuse headache."

recall memory Recent memory, which can be tested during the history taking by asking about items such as the dates of clinic or physician appointments.

receptive aphasia A type of aphasia caused by injury to Wernicke's area in the temporoparietal area of the brain and characterized by an inability to understand the spoken and written word; both reading and writing ability are equally affected. Although the patient can talk, the language is often meaningless, and neologisms (made-up words) are common parts of speech. Also called "Wernicke's aphasia" or "sensory aphasia."

reconstructive plastic surgery Type of plastic surgery that corrects or improves functional defects that have occurred as a result of congenital problems, trauma and scarring, or other types of therapy.

reconstructive surgery Surgery done to increase function, enhance appearance, or both; also called "rehabilitative surgery."

recreational exercise A type of exercise that includes hobbies and sports, with no planned purpose other than relaxation.

recreational therapist A member of the health care team who works to help patients continue or develop hobbies or interests; also called "activity therapist."

red reflex A reflection of light on the retina seen as a red glare during ophthalmoscopic examination. An absent red reflex may indicate a lens opacity or cloudiness of the vitreous.

redirection An intervention to help with communication problems in patients with dementia; consists of attracting the patient's attention before conversing, keeping the environment as free of distractions as possible, and speaking directly to the patient in a distinct manner using clear and short sentences.

reducible hernia A hernia that can be placed back into the abdominal cavity by gentle pressure.

reduction mammoplasty Breast reduction surgery in which the surgeon removes excess breast tissue and then repositions the nipple and remaining skin flaps to produce an optimal cosmetic effect.

Reed-Sternberg cell A specific cancer cell type, found in lymph nodes, that is a marker for Hodgkin's lymphoma.

re-epithelialization In partial-thickness (superficial) wounds involving damage to the epidermis and upper layers of the dermis, a form of healing by means of the production of new skin cells by undamaged epidermal cells in the basal layer of the dermis.

refeeding syndrome Life-threatening metabolic complication that can occur when nutrition is restarted for a patient who is in a starvation state.

referred pain Perceived pain in an area distant from the site of painful stimuli.

reflex arc A closed circuit of spinal and peripheral nerves that requires no control by the brain.

reflex bladder Incontinence characterized by sudden, gushing voids, usually without completely emptying the bladder; caused by neurologic problems affecting the upper motor neuron, such as with spinal cord injuries above the twelfth thoracic vertebra; also called "spastic bladder."

reflex sympathetic dystrophy (RSD) See *complex regional pain syndrome.*

reflux Reverse or backward flow.

reflux esophagitis Damage to the esophageal mucosa, often with erosion and ulceration, in patients with gastroesophageal reflux disease.

refract To cause to bend.

refraction The bending of light rays.

refractory stage The stage of shock that occurs when too much cell death and tissue damage result from too little oxygen reaching the tissues; the vital organs have overwhelming damage, and the body is unable to respond effectively to interventions. Formerly called the "irreversible stage."

regional anesthesia A type of local anesthesia that blocks multiple peripheral nerves in a specific body region.

regurgitation Flowing in the opposite direction from normal, as the occurrence of warm fluid traveling up the throat, unaccompanied by nausea, in the patient with gastroesophageal reflux disease.

rehabilitation The process of learning to live with chronic and disabling conditions by returning the patient to the fullest possible physical, mental, social, vocational, and economic capacity.

rehabilitation case manager Nurse or other health care professional who coordinates health care for patients undergoing rehabilitation in home or acute care settings.

rehabilitation nurse Nurse who coordinates the efforts of health care team members for patients undergoing rehabilitation in the inpatient setting; may be designated as the patient's case manager.

rehabilitative surgery See *reconstructive surgery.*

relapsing-remitting multiple sclerosis A type of multiple sclerosis that occurs in 85% of cases and is characterized by a mild or moderate course, depending on the degree of disability. Relapses develop over 1 to 2 weeks and resolve over 4 to 8 months, after which the patient returns to baseline.

religion The formal expression of spirituality.

relocation stress syndrome Physiologic or psychosocial distress following transfer from one environment to another, such as after admission to a hospital or nursing home; also called "relocation trauma."

reminiscence The process of randomly reflecting on memories of events in one's life.

remote memory Long-term memory of events; can be tested by asking patients about their birth date, schools attended, city of birth, or anything from the past that can be verified.

renal calculi Kidney stones.

renal capsule The layer of fibrous tissue on the outer surface of the kidney, which provides protection and support. The renal capsule itself is surrounded by layers of fat and connective tissue.

renal colic Severe pain associated with distention or spasm of the ureter, such as with an obstruction or the passing of a stone; the pain radiates into the perineal area, groin, scrotum, or labia. Pain may be intermittent or continuous and may be accompanied by pallor, diaphoresis, and hypotension.

renal columns Cortical tissue that dips into the interior of the kidney and separates the pyramids in the medulla; also called "columns of Bertin."

renal cortex The outermost layer of functional kidney tissue lying beneath the renal capsule.

renal osteodystrophy The problems in bone metabolism and structure caused by renal failure–induced hypocalcemia and hyperphosphatemia.

renal pelvis The expansion from the upper end of the ureter into which the calices of the kidney open.

renal threshold The limit to the amount of glucose that the kidney can reabsorb as glucose is filtered from the blood; also called the "transport maximum."

renin A hormone that is produced in the juxtaglomerular complex of the kidney and helps to regulate blood flow, glomerular filtration rate, and blood pressure. Renin is secreted when sensing cells (macula densa) in the distal convoluted tubule sense changes in blood volume and pressure.

repolarization A return to baseline after depolarization.

rescue drugs For asthma, drugs that are used to actually stop an asthma attack once it has started.

reservoir In health care, a source of infectious agents. Animate reservoirs include people, animals, and insects. Inanimate reservoirs include environmental sources and medical equipment. Community reservoirs include sewage, contaminated water, and improperly handled foods.

resistin A hormone produced by fat cells that creates resistance to insulin activity.

resorption In referring to bone, the loss of bone minerals and density; the release of free calcium from bone storage sites directly into the extracellular fluid.

restorative aid A member of the health care team, often with the nursing department, who assists the therapists, especially in the long-term care setting.

restraint Any device (physical restraint) or drug (chemical restraint) that prevents the patient from moving freely.

restrictive cardiomyopathy A form of cardiomyopathy that results restricts the filling of the ventricles; a type of lung disease that prevents good expansion and recoil of the gas exchange unit.

restrictive lung disorder Any lung disorder that prevents good expansion and recoil of the gas exchange unit.

resurfacing Regrowth of new skin cells across the open area of a wound as it heals.

rete pegs The fingers of epidermal tissue that project into the dermis.

reticular activating system (RAS) Special cells throughout the brainstem that constitute the system that controls awareness and alertness.

retina The innermost layer of the eye, made up of sensory receptors that transmit impulses to the optic nerve. It contains blood vessels and two types of photoreceptors called rods and cones. Rods work at low light levels and provide peripheral vision; cones are active at bright light levels and provide color and central vision.

retinal detachment Separation of the retina from the epithelium.

retinal hole A break in the retina; can be caused by trauma or can occur with aging.

retinal tear Jagged and irregularly shaped break in the retina resulting from traction on the retina.

retinitis Inflammation of the retina.

retinopathy Inflammation of the retina; also used as a general term for vision problems.

retrograde Going against the normal direction of flow.

retrograde ejaculation Condition in which semen flows backwards into the bladder so that only a small amount is ejaculated from the penis.

retroviruses The family of viruses that includes the human immune deficiency virus.

reversible ischemic neurologic deficit (RIND) A type of transient focal neurologic dysfunction resulting from a brief interruption in cerebral blood flow; symptoms last longer than 24 hours but less than a week.

revision arthroplasty Surgical replacement of a prosthesis that has loosened and is causing pain.

rhabdomyolysis The breakdown or disintegration of muscle tissue; associated with excretion of myoglobin in the urine.

rheumatic carditis Inflammatory lesions in the heart due to a sensitivity response that develops after an upper respiratory tract infection with group A beta-hemolytic streptococci, which occurs in about 40% of patients with rheumatic fever. Inflammation results in impaired contractile function of the myocardium, thickening of the pericardium, and valvular damage.

rheumatic disease Any disease or condition involving the musculoskeletal system.

rheumatoid arthritis (RA) A chronic, progressive systemic inflammatory autoimmune disease process that primarily affects the synovial joints; one of the most common connective tissue diseases and the most destructive to the joints.

rhinitis An inflammation of the nasal mucosa.

rhinitis medicamentosa Nasal congestion from overuse of nose drops or sprays.

rhinoplasty A surgical reconstruction of the nose done for cosmetic purposes and improvement of airflow.

rhinorrhea Watery drainage from the nose; a "runny" nose.

rhizotomy Surgical technique in which sensory nerve roots are destroyed where they enter the spinal cord; used to interrupt the transmission of pain.

rhytidectomy Plastic surgery to eliminate wrinkles from the facial skin; commonly known as a "face lift."

rickets Vitamin D deficiency in children.

right-sided heart (ventricular) failure The inability of the right ventricle to empty completely, resulting in increased volume and pressure in the systemic veins and systemic venous congestion with peripheral edema.

rigidity Abnormal resistance to passive movement of the extremities, an early sign of Parkinson disease.

rigors Severe chills.

Romberg sign Swaying or falling when the patient is standing with arms at the sides, feet and knees close together, and eyes closed; a test of equilibrium in neurologic assessment.

rotation A mechanism of injury in which the head is turned excessively beyond the normal range.

rubor Dusky red discoloration of the skin.

rugae Folds, as of a mucous membrane.

S

S phase The phase of cell division in which the cell doubles its deoxyribonucleic acid (DNA) content by separating the double strands of DNA and building a new strand complementary to the original strand (DNA synthesis).

S_3 gallop The third heart sound; an early diastolic filling sound that indicates an increase in left ventricular pressure and may be heard on auscultation in patients with heart failure.

salpingitis Infection of the fallopian tube.

sanguineous Having a bloody appearance.

sarcoidosis A granulomatous disorder of unknown cause that can affect any organ but most often involves the lung.

SBAR Acronym for a formal method of communication between two or more members of the health care team. It is used most often when there is an unmet patient need or problem but can also be used to communicate continuing care issues when a patient is discharged from one agency to another. It consists of four steps Situation, Background, Assessment, Recommendation.

scabies A contagious skin disease caused by mite infestations.

sclera The external white layer of the eye.

scleroderma See *systemic sclerosis.*

sclerosing agent An irritant that causes inflammation; often used to relieve pleural effusion.

sclerotherapy The injection of a sclerosing agent via a catheter, usually in an endoscopic procedure, to stop variceal bleeding.

sclerotic Hard, or hardening.

scoliosis An abnormal lateral curve in the spine, which normally should be a straight vertical line.

scotoma Blind spot in the visual field.

scrotum A thin-walled, fibromuscular pouch that lies behind the penis and is suspended below the pubic bone. This pouch protects the testes, epididymis, and vas deferens in a space that is slightly cooler than inside the abdominal cavity.

seborrhea Excessive secretion of sebum, resulting in greasy, itchy scaling.

sebum A mildly bacteriostatic, fat-containing substance produced by the sebaceous glands. Sebum lubricates the skin and reduces water loss from the skin surface.

second intention healing Healing of deep tissue injuries or wounds with tissue loss in which a cavity-like defect requires gradual filling of the dead space with connective tissue, which prolongs the repair process.

secondary administration set A short conduit that is attached to the primary administration set at a Y-injection site and is used to deliver intermittent medications; also called a "piggyback set."

secondary hypertension Elevated blood pressure that is related to a specific disease (e.g., kidney disease) or medication (e.g., estrogen).

secondary lesion Describing skin disease in terms of changes in the appearance of the primary lesion. These changes occur with progression of an underlying disease or in response to a topical or systemic therapeutic intervention.

secondary prevention Early detection of a disease or condition, sometimes before signs and symptoms are evident, to prevent or limit permanent disability or death.

secondary progressive multiple sclerosis A type of multiple sclerosis that begins with a relapsing-remitting course and later becomes steadily progressive. Attacks and partial recoveries may continue to occur.

secondary seizure Non-epileptic seizure that results from an underlying brain lesion, most commonly a tumor or trauma.

secondary survey In the emergency department, a more comprehensive head-to-toe assessment performed to identify other injuries or medical issues that need to be managed or that might impact the course of treatment.

secondary tumor Additional tumor that is established when cancer cells move from the primary location to another area in the body; also called "metastatic tumor."

second-look surgery Surgery done to assess the disease status in patients who have been treated and have no symptoms of remaining cancer tumor.

segmentectomy A lung resection (segmental resection) that includes the bronchus, pulmonary artery and vein, and tissue of the involved lung segment or segments, which are divisions of lobes.

seizure An abnormal, sudden, excessive, uncontrolled electrical discharge of neurons within the brain that may result in an alteration in consciousness, motor or sensory ability, and/or behavior. A single seizure may occur for no known reason; however, seizures may be due to a pathologic condition of the brain, such as a tumor.

self-determination An individual sense of autonomy; capable of making informed decisions about care. Also called "self-management."

self-management See *self-determination.*

self-tolerance In immunology, the ability to recognize self cells versus non-self cells, which is necessary to prevent healthy body cells from being destroyed along with invading cells.

semicircular canals Within the inner ear, tubes made of cartilage that contain fluid and hair cells and are connected to the sensory nerve fibers of the vestibular portion of the eighth cranial nerve. The fluid and hair cells within the canals help maintain the sense of balance.

sensitivity The likelihood that infecting bacterial organisms will be killed or stopped by a particular antibiotic drug. Sensitivity is determined by testing different antibiotics against the organisms. Organisms are "sensitive" if the antibiotic is effective in stopping their growth; organisms are "resistant" if the antibiotic is not effective.

sensorineural hearing loss Hearing loss that results from a defect in the cochlea, the eighth cranial nerve, or the brain itself. Exposure to loud noises and music may cause this type of hearing loss as a result of damage to the cochlear hair cells.

sensory Facilitating sensation.

sensory aphasia See *receptive aphasia.*

sepsis Systemic infection.

septic shock The type of shock that occurs when large amounts of toxins and endotoxins produced by bacteria are released into the blood, causing a whole-body inflammatory reaction.

septicemia Systemic disease associated with sepsis; the presence of pathogens in the blood.

sequestrum A piece of necrotic bone that has separated from surrounding bone tissue; a common complication of osteomyelitis.

serologic testing Laboratory testing that is performed to identify pathogens by detecting antibodies to the organism.

serositis Inflammation of a serous membrane, such as the pleura or peritoneum.

serous Having a serum-like appearance, or yellow color.

serum sickness A type III hypersensitivity reaction that develops first as a skin rash and occurs within 3 to 21 days of the administration of antivenin (Crotalidae) polyvalent. This allergic response is often accompanied by other manifestations such as fever, arthralgias (joint pains), and pruritus (itching).

severe acute respiratory syndrome (SARS) An easily spread respiratory infection first identified in China in November 2002. At first appearing as an atypical pneumonia, it is caused by a new, more virulent form of coronavirus, and there is no known effective treatment.

severe sepsis The progression of sepsis with an amplified inflammatory response.

sex chromosomes The pair of chromosomes containing the genes for sexual differentiation in humans. In males, the sex chromosomes are an X and a Y; in females, the sex chromosomes are two Xs.

sexually transmitted diseases (STDs) Any of a group of diseases caused by infectious organisms that have been passed from one person to another through intimate contact. Some organisms that cause these diseases are transmitted only through sexual contact. Other organisms are transmitted by parenteral exposure to infected blood, fecal-oral transmission, intrauterine transmission to the fetus, and perinatal transmission from mother to neonate.

shift to the left An increased number of immature neutrophils found on a differential count in patients with infections; can be characterized by changes in percentages of different types of leukocytes.

shock The whole-body response to poor tissue oxygenation. Any problem that impairs oxygen delivery to tissues and organs can start the syndrome of shock and lead to a life-threatening emergency.

short peripheral catheter A catheter that consists of a plastic cannula built around a sharp stylet for venipuncture, which extends slightly beyond the cannula and is advanced into the vein.

sialagogue An agent that stimulates the flow of saliva.

simple fracture See *closed fracture.*

simple partial seizure A type of partial seizure in which the patient remains conscious, often reporting an aura (e.g., perception of an offensive smell) before the seizure occurs. Characterized by unilateral movement of an extremity, unusual sensations, and autonomic or psychic symptoms. Autonomic changes include a change in heart rate, skin flushing, and epigastric discomfort.

single-photon emission computed tomography (SPECT) A diagnostic tool using a radiopharmaceutical (agent that enables radioisotopes to cross the blood-brain barrier) that is administered by IV injection, after which the patient is scanned.

sinoatrial (SA) node In the cardiac conduction system, the primary pacemaker of the heart; located close to the epicardial surface of the right atrium near its junction with the superior vena cava. It can spontaneously and rhythmically generate electrical impulses at a rate of 60 to 100 beats/min; also called the "sinus node."

sinus arrhythmia A variant of normal sinus rhythm that results from changes in intrathoracic pressure during breathing; heart rate increases slightly during inspiration and decreases slightly during exhalation. Atrial and ventricular rates are between 60 and 100 beats/min, and atrial and ventricular rhythms are irregular.

sinus bradycardia A cardiac dysrhythmia caused by a decreased rate of sinus node discharge, with a heart rate that is less than 60 beats/min.

sinusitis An inflammation of the mucous membranes of the sinuses.

Sjögren's syndrome In patients with advanced rheumatoid arthritis, the triad of dry eyes, dry mouth, and dry vagina caused by the obstruction of secretory ducts and glands by inflammatory cells and immune complexes.

skin fold measurement Measurement that estimates body fat.

skinning vulvectomy The surgical removal of superficial vulvar skin (without removal of the clitoris) and the replacement of removed skin with split-thickness grafts.

sleep apnea A breathing disruption during sleep that lasts at least 10 seconds and occurs a minimum of 5 times in an hour.

sliding board Alternative transfer technique for a patient who cannot bear weight but who has balance skills.

smart pump An infusion pump with dosage calculation software.

smegma A white, cheesy secretion from the sebaceous glands in the glans; may accumulate under the foreskin of the penis. This secretion is not present in the circumcised male.

social worker Members of the health care team who help patients identify support services and resources and who coordinate transfers to or discharges from the rehabilitation setting.

sodium (Na^+) A mineral that is the major cation in the extracellular fluid and maintains ECF osmolarity.

solubility The degree to which a solute dissolves in water.

solute A particle dissolved or suspended in the water portion (solvent) of body fluids; a solution consists of a solute and a solvent.

Somogyi's phenomenon In the patient with diabetes, morning hyperglycemia from the effective counterregulatory response to nighttime hypoglycemia. Treat by ensuring adequate dietary intake at bedtime and by evaluating the insulin dose and exercise programs to prevent conditions that lead to hypoglycemia.

spastic bladder See *reflex bladder.*

spastic paralysis Paralysis of a part of the body that is characterized by spasticity of muscles due to hypertonia; may be seen in the patient who has experienced a brain attack.

specialized nutritional support (SNS) Total nutritional intake orally or intravenously with commercially prepared products (either total enteral nutrition or total parenteral nutrition).

speech-language pathologist (SLP) A member of the rehabilitation health care team who evaluates and retrains patients with speech, language, or swallowing problems.

spermatogenesis Normal sperm production and maturation.

sphincter of Oddi The sheath of muscle fibers surrounding the papillary opening of the duodenum.

sphincterotomy A procedure for opening a sphincter.

spica cast A type of cast that encases a portion of the trunk and one or two extremities; contrasted with a body cast, which encircles the trunk of the body.

spider angiomas Vascular lesions with a red center and radiating branches; also called "telangiectasias," "spider nevi," or "vascular spiders."

spinal fusion (arthrodesis) A surgical procedure to stabilize the spine after repeated laminectomies have been unsuccessful. Chips of bone are removed (typically from the iliac crest) or are obtained from donor bone; the chips are grafted between the vertebrae for support and to strengthen the back.

spinal shock See *spinal shock syndrome.*

spinal shock syndrome Loss of reflex activity below the level of a spinal lesion; occurs immediately after injury as a result of disruption in the communication pathways between the upper motor neurons and the lower motor neurons; also called "spinal shock."

spinal stenosis Narrowing of the spinal canal; typically seen in people over 60 years of age.

spirituality The connection to self, others, the environment, and a "higher power."

splenectomy Surgical removal of the spleen.

splenomegaly Enlargement of the spleen.

splint Any object or device that extends to the joints above and below a fracture to immobilize it.

splinter hemorrhage Black longitudinal line or small red streak on the distal third of the nail bed; seen in patients with infective endocarditis.

spondee Two-syllable words in which there is generally equal stress on each syllable, such as *airplane, railroad,* and *cowboy;* used in testing speech reception threshold.

spondylolisthesis Condition in which one vertebra slips forward on the one below it, often as a result of spondylolysis. This problem causes pressure on the nerve roots, leading to pain in the lower back and into the buttocks.

spondylolysis A defect in one of the vertebrae; usually found in the lumbar spine.

spontaneous bacterial peritonitis (SBP) Bacterial infection of the abdominal peritoneum caused by ascites; often seen in patients with cirrhosis of the liver.

spore An encapsulated, inactive organism.

sprain Excessive stretching of a ligament.

ST segment In the electrocardiogram, the line (normally isoelectric) representing early ventricular repolarization. It occurs from the J point to the beginning of the T wave.

staging System of classifying clinical aspects of a cancer tumor.

Standard Precautions Infection control guidelines from the Centers for Disease Control and Prevention stating that all body excretions, secretions, and moist membranes and tissues are potentially infectious; combines protective measures from Universal Precautions and Body Substance Isolation.

stapes One of the three bony ossicles of the ear; also called the "stirrup."

stasis dermatitis In patients with venous insufficiency, discoloration of the skin along the ankles, which extends up to the calf.

stasis ulcer In patients with long-term venous insufficiency, ulcer formed as a result of edema or minor injury to the limb; typically occurs over the malleolus.

status epilepticus Prolonged seizures lasting more than 5 minutes or repeated seizures over the course of 30 minutes; a potential complication of all types of seizures.

steatorrhea An excessive amount of fat in the stool.

stem cell An immature, undifferentiated cell produced by the bone marrow.

stent A small tube that is placed in a tubular structure to dilate it; a wirelike device that may be used along with percutaneous transluminal angioplasty to help keep the vessel open.

stereotactic pallidotomy A surgical treatment for the patient with Parkinson disease when drugs are ineffective in symptom management. An electrode is used to create a lesion in a targeted area within the pallidum, with the goal of reducing tremor and rigidity.

stereotyping Assuming that all people in a particular culture have the group's values and beliefs or practice the group's customs.

sterilization A method of infection control in which all living organisms and bacterial spores are destroyed; used on items that invade human tissue where bacteria are not commonly found.

stimulant Any of a group of drugs that excite the cerebral cortex of the brain, producing a variety of behavioral responses and causing an increase in body activity, such as caffeine, nicotine, amphetamines, and methamphetamines.

stimulation test A type of test for pituitary function that involves injecting agents known to stimulate secretion of specific pituitary hormones and then measuring the response.

stoma The surgical creation of an opening; usually refers to an opening in the abdominal wall.

stomatitis Inflammation of the oral mucosa; characterized by painful single or multiple ulcerations that impair the protective lining of the mouth. The ulcerations are commonly referred to as canker sores.

strain Excessive stretching of a muscle or tendon when it is weak or unstable; sometimes referred to as "muscle pulls."

strangulated hernia A tightly constricted hernia that compromises the blood supply to the herniated segment of the bowel as a result of pressure from the hernial ring (the band of muscle around the hernia); leads to ischemia and obstruction of the bowel loop, with necrosis of the bowel and possibly bowel perforation.

strangulated obstruction Intestinal obstruction with compromised blood flow.

stratum corneum The outermost layer of the skin.

stress test See *exercise electrocardiography.*

stress ulcers Multiple shallow erosions of the proximal stomach and occasionally the duodenum.

stress urinary incontinence Loss of urine during activities that increase intra-abdominal pressure, such as laughing, coughing, sneezing, or lifting heavy objects.

striae Reddish purple streaks on the skin, also called "stretch marks."

stricture Narrowing.

stridor A high-pitched crowing sound caused by laryngospasm or edema above or below the glottis; heard during respiration.

stroke Former name for brain attack; see *brain attack.*

stroke volume The amount of blood ejected by the left ventricle during each heartbeat.

stuporous A state of being arousable with only vigorous or painful stimulation.

subarachnoid See *subarachnoid space.*

subarachnoid screw or bolt A hollow device placed into the subarachnoid space for direct measurement of intracranial pressure. It does not allow drainage of cerebrospinal fluid to treat increased pressure, but it is less invasive, which lowers the risk of infection. Compare with "intraventricular catheter."

subarachnoid space Term for the space between the arachnoid mater and pia mater of the spinal cord; also called "subarachnoid."

subcutaneous emphysema The presence of bubbles under the skin because of air trapping; an uncommon late complication of fracture.

subcutaneous nodule Characteristic round, movable, nontender swelling under the skin of the arm or fingers in patients with severe rheumatoid arthritis.

subcutaneous therapy Infusion therapy that is delivered under the skin when patients cannot tolerate oral medications, when intramuscular injections are too painful, or when vascular access is not available.

subdural hematoma (SDH) The collection of clotted blood that typically results from venous bleeding into the space beneath the dura and above the arachnoid.

subdural hemorrhage Venous bleeding into the space beneath the dura and above the arachnoid.

subdural space Term for the space between the dura mater and the middle layer (arachnoid).

subendocardial myocardial infarction An infarction that involves only the subendocardium, the inner layer of the cardiac muscle.

subluxation Partial joint dislocation.

submucous resection (SMR) Surgical procedure to straighten a deviated septum when chronic symptoms or discomfort occur; also called "nasoseptoplasty."

substance abuse The overindulgence of a chemical substance and the resulting dependence that interferes with life's activities.

substance misuse The taking of chemicals for reasons other than their intended action.

substance use The taking of chemicals for pleasure without dependence.

substernally Located below the ribs.

subtotal thyroidectomy The surgical removal of part of the thyroid tissue.

sundowning In patients with Alzheimer's disease, increased confusion at night or when excessively fatigued.

superinfection Reinfection or a second infection of the same type.

suppressed gene A particular gene that has been "turned off."

suprapatellar area The area directly above the knee.

supratentorial Located within the cerebral hemispheres, in the area above the tentorium of the cerebellum; the tentlike fold of dura that surrounds the cerebellar hemisphere and supports the occipital lobe.

supraventricular tachycardia (SVT) A form of tachycardia that involves the rapid stimulation of atrial tissue at a rate of 100 to 280 beats/min. It is most often due to a re-entry mechanism in which one impulse circulates repeatedly throughout the atrial pathway, restimulating the atrial tissue at a rapid rate.

surfactant A fatty protein secreted by type II pneumocytes to reduce surface tension in the alveoli.

surgical débridement Method of débriding a wound by removing thick, adherent wound crust using a scalpel or scissors.

surveillance Term used to describe the tracking of infections by health care agencies.

susceptibility The risk of the host to infection; may be increased by the breakdown of host defenses against pathogens.

swimmer's ear See *external otitis.*

sympathectomy Surgical cutting of the sympathetic nerve branches via endoscopy through a small axillary incision.

sympathetic tone A state of partial blood vessel constriction caused when nerves from the sympathetic division of the autonomic nervous system continuously stimulate vascular smooth muscle.

synapse The area through which impulses are transmitted to their eventual destination.

synchronous (demand) pacing mode The mode of temporary cardiac pacing in which the pacemaker's sensitivity is set to sense the patient's own beats. When the patient's intrinsic rate is above the rate set on the pulse generator, the pacemaker is inhibited from firing. When the patient's rate is below that set on the generator, the pacemaker fires electrical impulses to stimulate depolarization.

syncope Transient loss of consciousness (blackouts), most commonly caused by decreased perfusion to the brain.

syndrome of inappropriate antidiuretic hormone (SIADH) Persistent hyponatremia, hypovolemia, and inappropriately elevated urine osmolality that occurs when vasopressin (antidiuretic hormone) is secreted even when plasma osmolarity is low or normal.

syndrome X See *metabolic syndrome.*

syngeneic transplant Bone marrow transplant in which stem cells are taken from the patient's own identical sibling.

synovectomy The surgical removal of synovium.

synovial joint Type of joint lined with synovium, a membrane that secretes synovial fluid for lubrication and shock absorption.

synovitis Inflammation of synovial membrane.

synthesis The process of building up.

syphilis A complex sexually transmitted disease that can become systemic and cause serious complications and even death. It is caused by the spirochete *Treponema pallidum,* which is found in the mouth, intestinal tract, and genital areas of people and animals. The infection is usually transmitted by sexual contact, but transmission can occur through close body contact and kissing.

syringe pump Pump for infusion therapy that uses a battery-powered piston to push the plunger continuously at a selected mL/hr rate; limited to small-volume continuous or intermittent infusions.

systemic Affecting the body system as a whole.

systemic lupus erythematosus (SLE) A chronic, progressive, inflammatory connective tissue disorder that can cause major body organs and systems to fail; characterized by spontaneous remissions and exacerbations.

systemic sclerosis (SSc) A chronic connective tissue disease characterized by inflammation, fibrosis, and sclerosis of the skin and vital organs; also called "scleroderma" and formerly called "progressive systemic sclerosis."

systemic vascular resistance The resistance to the flow of blood through the body's blood vessels; it increases when vessels construct and decreases when vessels dilate.

systole The phase of the cardiac cycle that consists of the contraction and emptying of the atria and ventricles.

systolic blood pressure The amount of pressure/force generated by the left ventricle to distribute blood into the aorta with each contraction of the heart.

systolic heart failure (systolic ventricular dysfunction) Heart failure that results when the heart is unable to contract forcefully enough during systole to eject adequate amounts of blood into the circulation.

T

T wave In the electrocardiogram, the deflection that follows the ST segment and represents ventricular repolarization.

tachycardia An excessively fast heart rate; characterized as a pulse rate greater than 100 beats/min.

tachydysrhythmia An abnormal heart rhythm with a rate greater than 100 beats/min.

tachypnea An increased rate of breathing.

tactile (vocal) fremitus A vibration of the chest wall produced when the patient speaks; can be palpated on the chest wall.

tai chi A holistic movement therapy derived from a traditional Chinese martial art; has been adapted as a mind-body exercise that integrates body movements, mental concentration, muscle relaxation, and breathing to promote the flow of *qi*, or energy, in the body.

target tissues The tissues that respond specifically to a given hormone.

taut Tightly stretched.

telemetry In electrocardiography (ECG), the use of a battery-powered transmitter system for monitoring an ambulatory patient; allows freedom of movement within a certain radius without losing transmission of the ECG.

telesurgery The use of robotics to perform surgical procedures over long distances.

telomeres The "tips" of the chromosomes.

temporal field blindness A decrease in lateral peripheral vision.

temporary pacing A nonsurgical intervention for cardiac dysrhythmia that provides a timed electrical stimulus to the heart when either the impulse initiation or the intrinsic conduction system of the heart is defective.

tendon Any one of many bands of tough, fibrous tissue that attach muscles to bones.

tendon transplant Removal of a tendon from one part of the body and transplantation into the affected area to replace a ruptured tendon that cannot be repaired surgically.

tenesmus Straining, especially painful straining to defecate.

tension headache A type of headache characterized by neck and shoulder muscle tenderness and bilateral pain at the base of the skull and in the forehead; usually treated with non-opioid analgesics such as acetaminophen, aspirin, and non-steroidal anti-inflammatory drugs.

teratogenic Tending to produce birth defects.

tetany Continuous contractions of muscle groups; hyperexcitability of nerves and muscles.

tetraplegia Another term for quadriplegia (paralysis that involves all four extremities).

thalamotomy An alternative to stereotactic pallidotomy as a surgical treatment for the patient with Parkinson disease; uses thermocoagulation of brain cells to reduce tremor. Usually only unilateral surgery is performed to benefit the side of the body most affected by the disease.

thalamus A structure within the brain; functions as the "central switchboard" for the central nervous system.

thallium scan A test that is similar to the bone scan but uses the radioisotope thallium and is more sensitive in diagnosing the extent of disease in patients with osteosarcoma.

The Joint Commission An organization that offers peer evaluation for accreditation every 3 years for all types of health care agencies that meet their standards. Formerly known as the "Joint Commission for Accreditation of Healthcare Organizations (JCAHO)."

therapeutic exercise A type of exercise that includes carefully planned activities designed to improve muscle strength, muscle tone, and joint range of motion and to reduce pain and improve the patient's psychological health.

thermotherapy Technique for treating benign prostatic hyperplasia that uses a variety of heat methods to destroy excess prostate tissue.

third intention healing Delayed primary closure of a wound with a high risk for infection. The wound is intentionally left open for several days until inflammation has subsided and is then closed by first intention.

thoracentesis The aspiration of pleural fluid or air from the pleural space.

threshold In evaluating hearing, the lowest level of intensity at which pure tones and speech are heard by a patient; in general, the lowest level at which a stimulus is perceived.

thrombectomy Removal of a clot (thrombus) from a blood vessel.

thrombocytopenia A reduction in the number of blood platelets below the level needed for normal coagulation, resulting in an increased tendency to bleed.

thrombophlebitis The presence of a thrombus associated with inflammation; usually occurs in the deep veins of the lower extremities.

thrombosis The formation of a blood clot (thrombus) within a blood vessel.

thrombus A blood clot believed to result from an endothelial injury, venous stasis, or hypercoagulability.

thymoma An encapsulated tumor of the thymus gland.

thyrocalcitonin (TCT) A hormone produced and secreted by the parafollicular cells of the thyroid gland to help regulate serum calcium levels; secreted in response to excess plasma calcium.

thyroid storm (thyroid crisis) A life-threatening event that occurs in patients with uncontrolled hyperthyroidism and is usually caused by Graves' disease. Key manifestations include fever, tachycardia, and systolic hypertension.

thyrotoxicosis The condition caused by excessive amounts of thyroid hormones.

thyroxine (T_4) A hormone that is produced by the follicular cells of the thyroid gland and increases metabolism.

tinnitus A continuous ringing or noise perception in the ears.

titration Adjustment of IV fluid rate on the basis of the patient's urine output plus serum electrolyte values.

TNM (tumor, node, metastasis) System developed by the American Joint Committee on Cancer to describe the anatomic extent of cancers.

toe brachial pressure index (TBPI) Toe systolic pressure divided by brachial (arm) systolic pressure; may be performed instead of or in addition to ankle-brachial index to determine arterial perfusion in the feet and toes.

tolerance A state of adaptation in which exposure to a drug induces changes that result in a decrease in one or more of the drug's effects over time.

tomography An imaging technique that produces planes, or slices, for focus and blurs the images of other structures; different from standard x-rays, which superimpose one structure on another.

tonic Pertaining to a state of stiffening or rigidity of the muscles, particularly of the arms and legs, and immediate loss of consciousness.

tonic seizure A type of generalized seizure characterized by an abrupt increase in muscle tone, loss of consciousness, and loss of autonomic signs; lasts from 30 seconds to several minutes.

tonic-clonic seizure A type of generalized seizure consisting of a tonic phase (characterized by stiffening or rigidity of the muscles and immediate loss of consciousness); this is followed by clonic or rhythmic jerking of the extremities and lasts 2 to 5 minutes. The patient may bite his or her tongue and may become incontinent of urine or feces. Fatigue, confusion, and lethargy may last up to an hour after the seizure.

tophi A collection of uric acid crystals that form hard, irregular, painless nodules on the ears, arms, and fingers of patients with gout.

torsades de pointes A type of ventricular tachycardia that is related to a prolonged QT interval.

total body surface area (TBSA) The total amount of skin surface for one person.

total hysterectomy Removal of the uterus and cervix through the vagina without an external surgical incision.

total joint arthroplasty (TJA) Surgical creation of a joint, or total joint replacement; commonly performed in patients with osteoarthritis. Also called "total joint replacement (TJR)."

total joint replacement (TJR) See *total joint arthroplasty.*

total parenteral nutrition (TPN) Provision of intensive nutritional support for an extended time; delivered to the patient through access to central veins, usually the subclavian or internal jugular veins.

total thyroidectomy The surgical removal of all of the thyroid tissue.

touch discrimination Part of the neurologic examination. The patient closes his or her eyes while the practitioner touches the patient with a finger and asks that the patient point to the area touched.

toxic and drug-induced hepatitis Liver inflammation resulting from exposure to hepatotoxins (e.g., industrial toxins, alcohol, and medications).

toxic epidermal necrolysis (TEN) A rare acute drug reaction of the skin that results in diffuse erythema and blister formation, with mucous membrane involvement and systemic toxicity.

toxic megacolon Acute enlargement of the colon along with fever, leukocytosis, and tachycardia; usually associated with ulcerative colitis.

toxic multinodular goiter Hyperthyroidism caused by multiple thyroid nodules, which may be enlarged thyroid tissues or adenomas, and a goiter that has been present for several years.

toxic shock syndrome (TSS) A severe illness caused by a toxin produced by certain strains of *Staphylococcus aureus*. It was first recognized in 1980 as related to menstruation and tampon use. It is characterized by abrupt onset of a high fever and headache, sore throat, vomiting, diarrhea, generalized rash, and hypotension. The most common manifestations are skin changes (initially a rash that resembles a severe sunburn and changes to a macular erythema similar to a drug-related rash).

toxin Protein molecule released by bacteria that affects host cell at a distant site. Continued multiplication of a pathogen is sometimes accompanied by toxin production.

trabecular Spongy bone; also called "cancellous bone."

trabeculation An abnormal thickening of the bladder wall caused by urinary retention and obstruction.

tracheostomy The (tracheal) stoma, or opening, that results from a tracheotomy.

tracheotomy The surgical incision into the trachea for the purpose of establishing an airway.

traction The application of a pulling force to a part of the body to provide reduction, alignment, and rest.

transcellular fluid Any of the fluids in special body spaces, including cerebrospinal fluid, synovial fluid, peritoneal fluid, and pleural fluid.

transcultural nursing The area of study and practice that focuses on the care, health, and illness patterns of people with similarities and differences in their cultural beliefs, values, and practices; also, care that considers the cultural aspects of the patient.

transcutaneous electrical nerve stimulation (TENS) The use of a battery-operated device to deliver small electrical currents to the skin and underlying tissues for pain management; also called "percutaneous electrical nerve stimulation (PENS)."

transesophageal echocardiography (TEE) A form of echocardiography performed transesophageally (through the esophagus); an ultrasound transducer is placed immediately behind the heart in the esophagus or stomach to examine cardiac structure and function.

transferrin An iron-transport protein that can be measured directly or calculated as an indirect measurement of total iron-binding capacity.

transient ischemic attack (TIA) A brief attack (lasting a few minutes to less than 24 hours) of focal neurologic dysfunction caused by a brief interruption in cerebral blood flow, possibly resulting from cerebral vasospasm or transient systemic arterial hypertension. Repeated attacks may damage brain tissue; multiple attacks indicate significant increased risk for brain attack.

transmitted In genetics, the passage of a gene for a specific trait from one human generation to the next.

transmural myocardial infarction An infarction that involves all three layers of cardiac muscle.

transmyocardial laser revascularization A new surgical procedure for patients with unstable angina and inoperable coronary artery disease with areas of reversible myocardial ischemia. After a single-lung intubation, a left anterior thoracotomy is performed and the heart is visualized. A laser is used to create 20 to 24 long, narrow channels through the left ventricular muscle to the left ventricle. The channels eventually allow oxygenated blood to flow from the left ventricle during diastole to nourish the muscle.

transport maximum See *renal threshold.*

transurethral microwave therapy (TUMT) Procedure for treating benign prostatic hyperplasia using high temperatures to heat and destroy excess tissue.

transurethral needle ablation (TUNA) Procedure for treating benign prostatic hyperplasia using low radiofrequency energy to shrink the prostate.

transurethral resection of the prostate (TURP) The traditional "closed" surgical procedure for removal of the prostate. In this procedure, the surgeon inserts a resectoscope (an instrument similar to a cystoscope, but with a cutting and cauterizing loop) through the urethra. The enlarged portion of the prostate gland is then resected in small pieces.

trauma Bodily injury.

trauma activation criteria Certain injury mechanisms associated with life-threatening consequences that serve as criteria for summoning the trauma team for a rapid and coordinated resuscitation response.

trauma center Specialty care facility that provides competent and timely trauma services to patients depending on its designated level of capability.

trauma nursing Nursing specialty that encompasses the continuum of care from injury prevention and prehospital services to acute care, rehabilitation and, ultimately, community reintegration.

trauma system An organized and integrated approach to trauma care designed to ensure that all critical elements of trauma care delivery are aligned to meet the injured patient's needs.

triage In the emergency department, sorting or classifying patients into priority levels depending on illness or injury severity, with the highest acuity needs receiving the quickest evaluation and treatment.

triage officer In a hospital's emergency response plan, the person who rapidly evaluates each patient who arrives at the hospital. In a large hospital, this person is generally a physician who is assisted by triage nurses; however, a nurse may assume this role when physician resources are limited.

tricuspid valve The atrioventricular valve of the heart; separates the right atrium from the right ventricle.

tricyclic antidepressants Drugs used to treat depression.

trigeminy A type of premature complex consisting of a repetitive three-beat pattern; usually occurs as two sequential normal complexes followed by a premature complex and a pause, with the same pattern repeating itself in triplets.

trigger points In patients with fibromyalgia syndrome, tender areas that can typically be palpated to elicit pain in a predictable, reproducible pattern.

triiodothyronine (T3) A hormone produced by the follicular cells of the thyroid gland.

tropic hormones Hormones secreted by the anterior pituitary gland that stimulate other endocrine glands.

troponin A myocardial muscle protein released into the bloodstream after injury to myocardial muscle. Because it is not found in healthy patients, any rise in values indicates cardiac necrosis or acute myocardial infarction.

truss A device, usually a pad made with firm material, that is held in place over the hernia with a belt to keep the abdominal contents from protruding into the hernial sac.

tube thoracostomy A method of chest decompression performed after needle thoracostomy in which a chest tube is inserted in the fifth intercostal space, just anterior to the midaxillary line, to promote air and fluid drainage.

tumescence The condition of being swollen.

tumor-induced osteomalacia See *oncogenic osteomalacia.*

tunneled central venous catheter A type of catheter used for long-term infusion therapy in which a portion of the catheter lies in a subcutaneous tunnel, separating the points where the catheter enters the vein from where it exits the skin.

turbidity Cloudiness of a solution.

turbinates Three bony projections that protrude into the nasal cavities from the walls of the internal portion of the nose.

turgor The condition of being swollen and congested; indicates the amount of skin elasticity; the normal resiliency of a pinched fold of skin.

Turner's sign Ecchymosis on either flank, which may indicate retroperitoneal bleeding into the abdominal wall.

tympanic A term that describes the high-pitched, loud, musical sound heard over an air-filled intestine; obtained upon percussion of the abdomen.

tympanic membrane The eardrum; a thick, transparent sheet of tissue that provides a barrier between the external ear and the middle ear.

type A gastritis A form of chronic gastritis associated with the presence of antibodies to parietal cells and intrinsic factor. An autoimmune pathogenesis for this type of gastritis has been proposed.

type B gastritis The most common form of chronic gastritis; caused by *Helicobacter pylori* infection; 50% of patients who have gastric ulcers have associated chronic gastritis.

U

U wave In the electrocardiogram, the deflection that follows the T wave and may result from slow repolarization of ventricular Purkinje fibers. When present, it is of the same polarity as the T wave, although generally smaller. Abnormal prominence of the U wave suggests an electrolyte abnormality or other disturbance.

ulcerative colitis (UC) A chronic inflammatory process that affects the mucosal lining of the colon or rectum; one of a group of bowel diseases of unknown etiology characterized by remissions and exacerbations. It can result in loose stools containing blood and mucus, poor absorption of vital nutrients, and thickening of the colon wall.

umbilical hernia Protrusion of the intestine at the umbilicus; can be congenital or acquired. Congenital umbilical hernias appear in infancy. Acquired umbilical hernias directly result from increased intra-abdominal pressure and are most commonly seen in obese people.

unclassified seizure One of the three broad categories of seizure disorders along with partial seizure and generalized seizure. They occur for no known reason, do not fit into the generalized or partial classifications, and account for about half of all seizure activity; also called "idiopathic seizures."

uncus The inner part of the temporal lobe of the brain that can move downward and cause pressure on the brainstem; the vital sign center.

undermining Separation of the skin layers at the wound margins from the underlying granulation tissue.

uninhibited bladder May occur with a neurologic problem that affects the cortical bladder center of the brain (frontal lobe), such as brain attack or brain injury. The patient has little sensorimotor control and cannot wait until he or she is on the commode or bedpan before voiding.

Unna boot A wound dressing constructed of gauze moistened with zinc oxide; used to promote venous return in the ambulatory patient with a stasis ulcer and to form a sterile environment for the ulcer. The boot is applied to the affected limb, from the toes to the knee, after the ulcer has been cleaned with normal saline solution and covered with an elastic wrap. The dressing hardens like a cast.

unroofing Lifting or puncturing of the outer surface of a skin lesion to obtain specimens for bacterial culture.

unstable angina Chest pain or discomfort that occurs at rest or with exertion and causes marked limitation of activity; characterized by an increase in the number of attacks and an increase in the intensity of pain. Pain may last longer than 15 minutes or may be poorly relieved by rest or nitroglycerin.

upper esophageal sphincter (UES) The ringlike band of muscle fibers at the upper end of the esophagus. When at rest, the sphincter is closed to prevent air from entering into the esophagus during respiration.

upper GI (gastrointestinal) radiographic series The radiographic visualization of the gastrointestinal tract from the oral part of the pharynx to the duodenojejunal junction; used to detect disorders of structure or function of the esophagus (barium swallow), stomach, or duodenum.

upper motor neuron Neurons that carry motor impulses from the cerebral cortex to the cerebral nerves. Patients with spinal cord injuries involving upper motor neuron lesions experience muscle spasticity, which can lead to contractures after spinal shock has resolved.

uremia The accumulation of nitrogenous wastes in the blood (azotemia); a result of renal failure, with clinical symptoms including nausea and vomiting.

uremic frost A layer of urea crystals from evaporated sweat; may appear on the face, eyebrows, axilla, and groin in patients with advanced uremic syndrome.

uremic syndrome The systemic clinical and laboratory manifestations of end-stage kidney disease.

ureterolithiasis Formation of stones in the ureter.

ureteropelvic junction (UPJ) The narrow area in the upper third of the ureter at the point at which the renal pelvis becomes the ureter.

ureteroplasty Surgical repair of the ureter.

ureterovesical junction (UVJ) The point at which each ureter becomes narrow as it enters the bladder.

urethral meatus The opening at the endpoint of the urethra.

urethral stricture An obstruction that occurs low in the urinary tract due to decreased diameter of the urethra, causing bladder distention before hydroureter and hydronephrosis.

urethritis An inflammation of the urethra that causes symptoms similar to urinary tract infection.

urethroplasty Surgical treatment of the urethral stricture to remove the affected area with or without grafting to create a larger opening.

urgency The feeling that urination will occur immediately.

urgent triage In a three-tiered triage scheme, the category that includes patients who should be treated quickly but in whom an immediate threat to life does not currently exist, such as those with abdominal pain or displaced fractures or dislocations.

urinary tract infection (UTI) An infection in the normally sterile urinary system. The unobstructed and complete passage of urine from the renal and urinary systems is critical in maintaining a sterile urinary tract. When any structural abnormality is present, the risk for damage as a result of infection is greatly increased.

urolithiasis The presence of calculi (stones) in the urinary tract.

urosepsis The spread of an infection from the urinary tract to the bloodstream, resulting in systemic infection accompanied by fever, chills, hypotension, and altered mental status.

urticaria A transient vascular reaction of the skin marked by the development of wheals (hives).

uterine artery embolization Treatment for leiomyomas in which a radiologist uses a percutaneous catheter inserted through the femoral artery to inject polyvinyl alcohol pellets into the uterine artery. The resulting blockage starves the tumor of circulation, allowing it (or them) to shrink.

uterine prolapse Downward displacement of the uterus into the vagina.

uvea The middle layer of the eye, which consists of the choroid, ciliary body, and iris. The choroid has many blood vessels that supply nutrients to the retina.

uveitis Inflammation of part or all of the uvea.

V

vagal maneuver Nonsurgical management of cardiac dysrhythmias that is intended to induce vagal stimulation of the cardiac conduction system, specifically the sinoatrial and atrioventricular nodes. Vagal maneuvers may be attempted to terminate supraventricular tachydysrhythmia.

vagina The collapsible hollow tube with thin, muscular walls lined by mucous membrane and many blood vessels; extends from the vestibule to the uterus. It is the channel for the passage of menstrual flow, allows reception of the penis during intercourse, and allows passage of the fetus during a vaginal birth.

vaginectomy Surgical removal of part or all of the vagina.

vagotomy syndrome Diarrhea that develops as a result of the interruption of vagal fibers to the abdominal viscera during esophageal surgery.

validation therapy For the patient with moderate or severe Alzheimer's disease, the process of recognizing and acknowledging the patient's feelings and concerns without reinforcing an erroneous belief (e.g., if the patient is looking for his or her deceased mother).

Valsalva maneuver A form of vagal stimulation of the cardiac conduction system in which the health care provider instructs the patient to bear down as if straining to have a bowel movement.

variant (Prinzmetal's) angina A type of angina caused by coronary vasospasm (vessel spasm); usually associated with elevation of the ST segment on an electrocardiogram obtained during anginal attacks.

varicocelectomy The surgical removal of a varicocele (a cluster of dilated veins behind and above the testis).

varicose veins Distended, protruding veins that appear darkened and tortuous; common in patients older than 30 years of age whose occupations require prolonged standing. As the vein wall weakens and dilates, venous pressure increases and the valves become incompetent (defective). The incompetent valves enhance the vessel dilation, and the veins become tortuous and distended.

vas deferens A firm, muscular tube that continues from the tail of each epididymis and is a reservoir for sperm and tubular fluids. They merge with ducts from the seminal vesicle to form the ejaculatory ducts at the base of the prostate gland. Sperm from the vas deferens and secretions from the seminal vesicles are transported through the ejaculatory duct to mix with prostatic fluids in the prostatic urethra. Also called "ductus deferens."

vascular access device A catheter; a plastic tube placed in a blood vessel to deliver fluids and medications.

vasculitis Blood vessel inflammation.

vasoconstriction Decrease in diameter of blood vessels.

vasospasm A sudden and transient constriction of a blood vessel.

Vaughn-Williams classification System used to categorize antidysrhythmic agents according to their effects on the action potential of cardiac cells.

vegan A vegetarian diet pattern in which only foods of plant origin are eaten.

Vegetarian Food Pyramid A food pyramid to assist vegetarians with daily food choices.

venous beading A complication of diabetes; the abnormal appearance of retinal veins in which areas of swelling and constriction along a segment of vein resemble links of sausage. Such bleeding occurs in areas of retinal ischemia and is a predictor of proliferative diabetic retinopathy.

venous duplex ultrasonography A noninvasive test using ultrasonic waves; the preferred diagnostic test for deep vein thrombosis.

venous insufficiency Alteration of venous efficiency by thrombosis or defective valves; caused by prolonged venous hypertension, which stretches the veins and damages the valves, resulting in further venous hypertension, edema and, eventually, venous stasis ulcers, swelling, and cellulitis.

venous thromboembolism (VTE) A term that refers to both deep vein thrombosis and pulmonary embolism; obstruction by a thrombus.

ventilation assistance Process or devices to help the patient breathe easily (e.g., mechanical ventilation assistance).

ventral hernia Protrusion of the intestine at the site of a previous surgical incision resulting from inadequate healing. Most often caused by postoperative wound infections, inadequate nutrition, and obesity.

ventricular asystole The complete absence of any ventricular rhythm. There are no electrical impulses in the ventricles and therefore no ventricular depolarization, no QRS complex, no contraction, no cardiac output, and no pulse, respirations, or blood pressure. The patient is in full cardiac arrest.

ventricular fibrillation (VF) A cardiac dysrhythmia that results from electrical chaos in the ventricles; impulses from many irritable foci fire in a totally disorganized manner so that ventricular contraction cannot occur; there is no cardiac output or pulse and therefore no cerebral, myocardial, or systemic perfusion. This rhythm is rapidly fatal if not successfully terminated within 3 to 5 minutes.

ventricular gallop An abnormal third heart sound that arises from vibrations of the valves and supporting structures and is produced during the rapid passive filling phase of ventricular diastole when blood flows from the atrium to a noncompliant ventricle. In patients older than 35 years of age, it is an early sign of heart failure or ventricular septal defect.

ventricular remodeling (1) Progressive myocyte (myocardial cell) contractile dysfunction over time; results from activation of the renin-angiotensin system caused by reduced blood flow to the kidneys, a common occurrence in low-output states; (2) after a myocardial infarction, permanent changes in the size and shape of the left ventricle due to scar tissue; such remodeling may decrease left ventricular function, cause heart failure, and increase morbidity and mortality.

ventricular tachycardia (VT) An abnormal heart rhythm that occurs with repetitive firing of an irritable ventricular ectopic focus, usually at a rate of 140 to 180 beats/min or more.

ventriculomyomectomy The surgical excision of a portion of the hypertrophied ventricular septum to create a widened outflow tract in patients with obstructive hypertrophic cardiomyopathy.

ventriculostomy The surgical placement of an intraventricular catheter to drain cerebrospinal fluid in patients with increased intracranial pressure and rapidly deteriorating neurologic function.

vertebroplasty A minimally invasive surgery for managing vertebral fractures in patients with osteoporosis. Bone cement is injected directly into the fracture site to provide immediate pain relief.

vertigo A sense of spinning movement that may result from diseases of the inner ear.

vesicant Chemicals that cause tissue damage on direct contact.

vesicant medication A drug that causes tissue damage when extravasated.

vesicle In health care, a small bladder or blister.

vestibule A longitudinal area between the labia minora, the clitoris, and the vagina that contains Bartholin's glands and the openings of the urethra, Skene's glands (paraurethral glands), and vagina.

viral hepatitis Inflammation of the liver that results from an infection caused by one of five major categories of viruses (hepatitis A, B, C, D, or E). Viral hepatitis is the most prevalent type and can be either acute or chronic.

viral load testing Test that measures the presence of human immune deficiency virus genetic material (ribonucleic acid) or other viral proteins in the patient's blood.

viral meningitis A type of meningitis that often occurs after viral illnesses such as measles, herpes simplex, coxsackievirus, and echovirus; it is marked by inflammation over the cerebral cortex, white matter, and meninges. The formation of exudate (common in bacterial meningitis) does not occur, and no organisms are obtained from the cerebrospinal fluid. Also called "aseptic meningitis."

Virchow's triad The occurrence of stasis of blood flow, endothelial injury, or hypercoagulability; often associated with thrombus formation.

viremia The presence of viruses in the blood.

virilization The presence of male secondary sex characteristics.

virtual colonoscopy A noninvasive alternative to the colonoscopy procedure. A scanner is used to view the colon.

virulence A term used to describe the frequency with which a pathogen causes disease (degree of communicability) and its ability to invade and damage a host. Virulence can also indicate the severity of the disease; often used as a synonym for pathogenicity.

visceral protein Proteins such as albumin that circulate in the bloodstream and may be produced by the liver.

viscous Of thick consistency.

vitiligo An abnormality of the skin characterized by patchy areas of pigment loss with increased pigmentation at the edges. It is seen with primary hypofunction of the adrenal glands and is due to autoimmune destruction of melanocytes in the skin.

vitrectomy The surgical removal of the vitreous.

vitreous body The clear, thick gel that fills the vitreous chamber of the eye (the space between the lens and the retina). This gel transmits light and shapes the eye.

vocational counselor A member of the rehabilitative health care team who assists the patient with job placement, training, or further education.

volutrauma Damage to the lung by excess volume delivered to one lung over the other.

volvulus Obstruction of the bowel caused by twisting of the bowel.

vulva The external female genitalia; extends from the mons pubis to the anal opening.

vulvar self-examination (VSE) A method for self-examination of the external female genitalia for early detection of diseases of the vulva.

vulvectomy Surgical removal of the vulva, labia majora, labia minora and, possibly, the clitoris.

vulvovaginitis Inflammation of the lower genital tract resulting from a disturbance of the balance of hormones and flora in the vagina and vulva.

W

warm antibody anemia A form of immunohemolytic anemia (in which the immune system attacks a person's own red blood cells for unknown reasons) that occurs with immunoglobulin G antibody excess and may be triggered by drugs, chemicals, or other autoimmune problems.

warm phase A phase lasting 2 to 3 weeks after peripheral nerve trauma resulting in complete denervation; the extremity is warm, and the skin appears flushed or rosy. The warm phase is gradually superseded by a cold phase.

water brash Reflex salivary hypersecretion that occurs in response to reflux in the patient with gastroesophageal reflux disease.

"wearing off" phenomenon Loss of response over time to a medication.

wedge resection Removal of small, localized areas of disease.

Wernicke's aphasia See *receptive aphasia.*

Wernicke's area An important speech area of the cerebrum. It is located in the temporal lobe and plays a significant role in higher-level brain function. It enables the processing of words into coherent thought and recognition of the idea behind written or printed words (language).

Whipple procedure (radical pancreaticoduodenectomy) A surgical treatment for cancer of the head of the pancreas. The procedure entails removal of the proximal head of the pancreas, the duodenum, a portion of the jejunum, the stomach (partial or total gastrectomy), and the gallbladder, with anastomosis of the pancreatic duct (pancreaticojejunostomy), the common bile duct (choledochojejunostomy), and the stomach (gastrojejunostomy) to the jejunum.

white matter In the spinal cord, myelinated axons that surround the gray matter (neuron cell bodies).

Williams position A position in which the patient lies in the semi-Fowler's position and flexes the knees to relax the muscles of the lower back and relieve pressure on the spinal nerve root. This is typically more comfortable and therapeutic for the patient with low back pain.

withdrawal syndrome Symptoms that occur when a patient who is physically dependent on opioids abruptly stops using them. Slowly tapering (weaning) the drug dosage lessens or alleviates the physical withdrawal symptoms in a patient who is opioid dependent. Also called "abstinence syndrome."

withdrawing or withholding life-sustaining therapy (WWLST) The withdrawal or withholding of one or more therapies that might prolong the life of a person who cannot be cured by the therapy; the withdrawal of therapy does not directly cause death. Formerly called "passive euthanasia."

X

xenograft Tissue transplanted (grafted) from another species; for example, a heart valve transplanted from a pig to a human.

xeroradiography A diagnostic x-ray technique in which images are produced electrically rather than chemically, permitting lower exposure times and radiation energies than those of ordinary x-rays. The images exhibit "edge contrast," which is useful for identifying minute calcifications in the breast.

xerosis Abnormally dry skin.

xerostomia Abnormal dryness of the mouth caused by a severe reduction in the flow of saliva.

x-ray Radiation that is generated by machine.

Z

Zollinger-Ellison syndrome (ZES) The occurrence of upper gastrointestinal tract ulceration, increased gastric acid secretion, and the presence of a non–beta cell islet tumor of the pancreas, called a gastrinoma. Affected people may have more than one gastrinoma.

Illustration Credits

Chapter 1

1-1, From Harkreader, H., & Hogan, M.A. (2004). *Fundamentals of nursing: Caring and clinical judgment* (2nd ed.). Philadelphia: Saunders.

Chapter 2

2-1, From Potter, P.A., & Perry, A.G. (2001). *Fundamentals of nursing* (5th ed.). St. Louis: Mosby; **2-2, 2-3,** from Potter, P.A., & Perry, A.G. (2005). *Fundamentals of nursing* (6th ed.). St. Louis: Mosby.

Chapter 3

3-3, From the Aging Clinical Research Center (ACRC), a joint project of Stanford University and the VA Palo Alto Health Care System, Palo Alto, CA, funded by the National Institute of Aging and the Department of Veterans Affairs.

Chapter 4

4-1, 4-3, From Harkreader, H., Hogan, M.A., & Thobaben, M. (2007). *Fundamentals of nursing: Caring and clinical judgment* (3rd ed.). Philadelphia: Saunders.

Chapter 5

5-2, From Melzack, R. (1975). The McGill Pain Questionnaire: Major properties and scoring methods. *Pain, 1,* 272-281; **5-3,** Simple descriptive pain distress scale, 0-10 numeric pain distress scale, and visual analog scale redrawn from Acute Pain Management Guideline Panel. (1992). *Acute pain management: Operative or medical procedures and trauma. Clinical practice guideline.* AHCPR Publication No. 92-0032. Rockville, MD: Agency for Health Care Policy and Research, Public Health Service, U.S. Department of Health and Human Services. Pain relief visual analog scale redrawn from Fishman, B., Pasternak, S., Wallenstein, S.L., Houde, R.W., Holland, J.C., & Foley, K.M. (1987). The Memorial Pain Assessment Card: A valid instrument for the evaluation of cancer pain. *Cancer, 60*(5), 1151-1158. Percent relief scale redrawn from the Brief Pain Inventory. Pain Research Group, Department of Neurology, University of Wisconsin—Madison; **5-4,** CADD-PCA is a registered trademark of Pharmacia Deltec, St. Paul, MN; **5-5,** courtesy Medtronic, Inc., Columbia Heights, MN.

Chapter 6

6-1, 6-6, 6-13, 6-17, 6-19, Modified from Jorde, L., Carey, J., Bamshad, M., & White, R. (2000). *Medical genetics* (2nd ed.). St. Louis: Mosby; **6-3,** modified from Nussbaum, R., McInnes, R., & Willard, H. (2001). *Thompson & Thompson: Genetics in medicine* (6th ed.). Philadelphia: Saunders; **6-12,** from Nussbaum, R., McInnes, R., & Willard, H. (2001). *Thompson & Thompson: Genetics in medicine* (6th ed.). Philadelphia: Saunders.

Chapter 7

7-2, Used with permission of the American Dental Association, 211 E. Chicago Ave., Chicago, IL 60611.

Chapter 8

8-4, Courtesy Kinetic Concepts, Inc., San Antonio, TX.

Chapter 9

9-1, Copyright 2005 National Hospice and Palliative Care Organization, 2007 Revised. All rights reserved. Reproduction and distribution by an organization or organized group without the written permission of the National Hospice and Palliative Care Organization is expressly forbidden. Visit caringinfo.org for more information.

Chapter 11

11-1, From Auerbach, P.S., Donner, H.J., & Weiss, E.A. (2007). *Wilderness medicine* (5th ed.). St. Louis: Mosby (courtesy Michael Cardwell and Carl Barden Venom Laboratory); **11-2,** from Auerbach, P.S., Donner, H.J., & Weiss, E.A. (2007). *Wilderness medicine* (5th ed.). St. Louis: Mosby (courtesy Sherman Minton, MD); **11-3,** from Auerbach, P.S., Donner, H.J., & Weiss, E.A. (2007). *Wilderness medicine* (5th ed.). St. Louis: Mosby (courtesy Michael Cardwell and Jude McNally); **11-4,** from Auerbach, P.S., Donner, H.J., & Weiss, E.A. (2007). *Wilderness medicine* (5th ed.). St. Louis: Mosby (courtesy Indiana University Medical Center); **11-5,** from Auerbach, P.S., Donner, H.J., & Weiss, E.A. (2007). *Wilderness medicine* (5th ed.). St. Louis: Mosby (courtesy Paul Auerbach, MD); **11-6,** from Auerbach, P.S., Donner, H.J., & Weiss, E.A. (2007). *Wilderness medicine* (5th ed.). St. Louis: Mosby; **11-7,** from Auerbach, P.S., Donner, H.J., & Weiss, E.A. (2007). *Wilderness medicine* (5th ed.). St. Louis: Mosby (courtesy Cameron Bangs, MD).

Chapter 12

12-1, Courtesy Ann Breslin; **12-2,** Courtesy Jeanne McConnell, MSN, RN.

Chapter 13

13-2, 13-7, 13-10, ©1992 by M. Linda Workman. All rights reserved.

Chapter 14

14-1, 14-6, ©1992 by M. Linda Workman. All rights reserved.

Chapter 15

15-2, Courtesy Becton Dickinson Infusion Therapy Systems, Sandy, UT; **15-3,** from Potter, P.A., & Perry, A.G. (2005). *Fundamentals of nursing* (6th ed.). St. Louis: Mosby; **15-4,** courtesy ICU Medical Inc., San Clemente, CA; **15-5,** courtesy HMP-Horizon Medical Products Inc., Manchester, GA; **15-6,** courtesy NowMedical, Chadds Ford, PA; **15-7,** courtesy Venetec International, San Diego, CA; **15-8,** courtesy I.V. House, Hazelwood, MO.

Chapter 16

16-1, 16-5, Courtesy Christiana Care Health Services, Newark, DE; **16-3,** from Perry, A.G., & Potter, P.A. (2006). *Clinical nursing skills and techniques* (6th ed.). St. Louis: Mosby; **16-4,**

A, courtesy The Kendall Healthcare Company, Mansfield, MA; **16-4, B,** courtesy Venodyne, Inc., Norwood, MA; **16-4, C,** courtesy Huntleigh Healthcare, Eatontown, NJ.

Chapter 17

17-1, Courtesy Christiana Care Health Services, Newark, DE; **17-4,** courtesy HGM Medical Laser Systems, Santa Clara, CA; **17-5,** redrawn with permission by Intuitive Surgical, Inc., 2007.

Chapter 18

18-1, Courtesy Forrest General Hospital, Hattiesburg, MS; **18-2,** from Harkreader, H., Hogan, M.A., & Thobaben, M. (2007). *Fundamentals of nursing: Caring and clinical judgment* (3rd ed.). Philadelphia: Saunders; **18-3, C and D,** courtesy CR Bard, Inc., Covington, GA.

Chapter 19

19-3, Modified from Goldman, L., & Ausiello, D. (Eds.). (2008). *Cecil medicine* (23rd ed.). Philadelphia: Saunders.

Chapter 20

20-4, From Damjanov, I. (2006). *Pathophysiology for the health professions* (3rd ed.). Philadelphia: Saunders; **20-5,** courtesy Whitehall Manufacturing, City of Industry, CA; **20-8,** from Goldman L., & Ausiello, D. (2007). *Cecil medicine* (23rd ed.). Philadelphia: Saunders.

Chapter 21

21-1, From Kumar, V., Abbas, A., & Fausto, N. (2005). *Robbins & Cotran pathologic basis of disease* (7th ed.). Philadelphia: Saunders; **21-4,** from McCance, K.L., & Huether, S.E. (2002). *Pathophysiology: The biologic basis for disease in adults and children* (4th ed.). St. Louis: Mosby; **21-5,** data from The Centers for Disease Control and Prevention HIV/AIDS Fact Sheet: *HIV/AIDS among women*. Revised June 2007; **21-6,** data from The Centers for Disease Control and Prevention HIV/AIDS Fact Sheet: *A glance at the HIV/AIDS epidemic*. Revised June 2007.

Chapter 22

22-3, Courtesy Dey, Napa, CA; **22-4,** from Goldstein, B.G., & Goldstein, A.O. (1997). *Practical dermatology* (2nd ed.). St. Louis: Mosby.

Chapter 23

23-7, From American Cancer Society. *Cancer facts and figures 2008*. Atlanta, GA: Author.

Chapter 25

25-1, A, From deWit, S.C. (2008). *Fundamental concepts and skills for nursing* (3rd ed.). Philadelphia: Saunders; **B,** from Elkin, M.C., Perry, A., & Potter, P.A. (2007). *Nursing interventions and clinical skills* (4th ed.). St. Louis: Mosby (courtesy Kimberly-Clark Health Care, Roswell, GA).

Chapter 26

26-14, From Marks, J., & Miller, J. (2006). *Lookingbill and Marks' principles of dermatology* (4th ed.). Philadelphia: Saunders.

Chapter 27

27-2, Modified from Swaim, S.F. (1980). *Surgery of traumatized skin*. Philadelphia: Saunders; **27-4,** from Barbara Braden and Nancy Bergstrom. Copyright 1988. Reprinted with permission; **27-10,** from Lookingbill, D.P., & Marks, J.G. (2000). *Principles of dermatology* (3rd ed.). Philadelphia: Saunders.

Chapter 28

28-1, Modified from Moritz, A.R. (1947). Studies of thermal injuries. II: The relative importance of time and surface temperature in causation of cutaneous burns. *American Journal of Pathology, 23,* 695; **28-14,** courtesy Beiersdorf-Jobst, Inc, Charlotte, NC.

Chapter 29

29-11, From Harkreader, H., Hogan, M.A., & Thobaben, M. (2007). *Fundamentals of nursing: Caring and clinical judgment* (3rd ed.). Philadelphia: Saunders.

Chapter 30

30-3, 30-9, 30-10, From Perry, A.G., & Potter, P.A. (2006). *Clinical nursing skills and techniques* (6th ed.). St. Louis: Mosby; **30-13,** courtesy Mallinckrodt, Inc., Shiley Tracheostomy Products, St. Louis, MO; **30-14,** courtesy J.T. Posey Company, Arcadia, CA; **30-15,** courtesy Dale Medical Products, Inc., Plainville, MA.

Chapter 31

31-1, From Tardy, M.E. (1997). *Rhinoplasty: The art and science*. Philadelphia: Saunders. Used with permission; **31-2, A,** courtesy Invotec International, Jacksonville, FL; **31-5,** courtesy InHealth Technologies, a division of Helix Medical, LLC, Carpinteria, CA.

Chapter 32

32-2, From Jarvis, C. (2008). *Physical examination and health assessment* (5th ed.). Philadelphia: Saunders; **32-9,** modified from Gift, A. (1989). A dyspnea assessment guide. *Critical Care Nurse, 9*(8), 79. Used with permission; **32-10,** from Swartz, M.H. (1998). *Textbook of physical diagnosis: History and examination*. Philadelphia: Saunders; **32-12,** courtesy Axcan Pharma, Mont-Saint-Hilaire, Quebec, Canada; **32-16,** courtesy Atrium Medical Corporation, Hudson, NH.

Chapter 33

33-1, Courtesy Covidien AG, Switzerland; **33-2,** courtesy Uvex Safety, Smithfield, RI.

Chapter 34

34-2, Modified from Gift, A. (1989). A dyspnea assessment guide. *Critical Care Nurse, 9*(8), 79. Used with permission; **34-3, A,** courtesy Sims Porter, Inc.; **34-4,** copyright Dräger Medical AG & Co. KG, Lübeck, Germany. All rights reserved. Not to be reproduced without written permission, not to be saved or copied in any electronic format, not to be transmitted electronically or mechanically by way of photocopying or photographing, in any way, shape or form, whether fully or partially; **34-5,** from McCance, K.L., & Huether, S.E. (2006). *Pathophysiology: The biologic basis for disease in adults and children* (5th ed.). St. Louis: Mosby.

Chapter 36

36-13, courtesy Philips Medical Systems, Andover, MA.

Chapter 37

37-1, From McCance, K.L., & Huether, S.E. (2002). *Pathophysiology: The biologic basis for disease in adults & children* (4th ed.). St. Louis: Mosby; **37-2,** courtesy Abiomed, Inc., Danvers, MA; **37-3, A** and **B,** courtesy Medtronic, Inc., Minneapolis, MN; **C,** courtesy Baxter Healthcare Corporation, Edwards CVS Division, Santa Ana, CA.

Chapter 38

38-7, From Rutherford, R. (2005). *Vascular surgery* (6th ed.). Philadelphia: Saunders; **38-8,** from Forbes, C.D., & Jackson, W.F. (2003). *Color atlas and text of clinical medicine* (3rd ed.). St. Louis: Mosby.

Chapter 40

40-1, From Huether S.E., & McCance, K.L. (2008). *Understanding pathophysiology* (4th ed.). St. Louis: Mosby.

Chapter 44

44-2, A, From Mini-Mental State Examination © 1975, 1998, 2001 by MiniMental, LLC. All rights reserved. Published 2001 by Psychological Assessment Resources, Inc. May not be reproduced in whole or in part in any form or by any means without written permission of Psychological Assessment Resources, Inc., 16204 N. Florida Ave., Lutz, FL 33549, (800) 331-8378 or (813) 968-3003; **B,** from Seidel, H.M., Benedict, G.W., Ball J.W., & Dains, J.E. (1999). *Mosby's guide to physical examination* (4th ed.). St. Louis: Mosby.

Chapter 45

45-6, From Harkreader, H. (2007). *Fundamentals of nursing: Caring and clinical judgment* (3rd ed.). Philadelphia: Saunders.

Chapter 47

47-3, From Seidel, H.M., Ball, J.W., Dains, J.E., & Benedict, G.W. (2006). *Mosby's guide to physical examination* (6th ed.). St. Louis: Mosby; **B,** modified from Stein, Slatt, Stein, 1994.

Chapter 48

48-8, Courtesy the National Society to Prevent Blindness; **48-13,** courtesy Medtronic Ophthalmics, Minneapolis, MN.

Chapter 49

49-4, Courtesy John A. Costin, MD; **49-6,** from Thibodeau G.A., & Patton K.T. (2007). *Anatomy and physiology* (6th ed.). St. Louis: Mosby.

Chapter 50

50-10, 50-11, Courtesy the Cleveland Hearing and Speech Center, Cleveland, OH.

Chapter 52

52-5, Modified from Jarvis, C. (2004). *Physical examination and health assessment* (4th ed.). Philadelphia: Saunders.

Chapter 53

53-5, Courtesy Truform Orthotics and Prosthetics, Cincinnati, OH.

Chapter 54

54-3, 54-4, 54-9, Courtesy Smith & Nephew, Inc., Orthopaedics Divisions, Memphis, TN; **54-5,** from Christensen, B.L., & Kockrow, E.O. (2006). *Adult health nursing* (5th ed.). St. Louis: Mosby; **54-6,** from McCance, K.L., & Huether, S.E. (2006). *Pathophysiology: The biologic basis for disease in adults and children* (5th ed.). St. Louis: Mosby; **54-14,** courtesy Zimmer, Inc., Warsaw, IN.

Chapter 56

56-1, From Friedman-Kien, A.E., & Cockerell, C.J. (1996). *Color atlas of AIDS* (2nd ed.). Philadelphia: Saunders.

Chapter 60

60-2, B, 60-6, Courtesy ConvaTec, a Bristol-Myers Squibb Company, Princeton, NJ.

Chapter 63

63-1, From U.S. Department of Agriculture: Center for Nutrition Policy and Promotion, April 2005, www.MyPyramid.gov; **63-2,** courtesy The Health Connection, Hagerstown, MD; **63-3,** ®Société des Produits Nestlé S.A., Vevey, Switzerland, Trademark Owners; **63-4, A,** from Lilley, L. (2007). *Pharmacology and the nursing process* (5th ed.). St. Louis: Mosby; **B,** courtesy C.R. Bard, Inc., Billerica, MA; **C,** courtesy Ballard Medical Products, Draper, UT.

Chapter 64

64-4, From Guyton, A., & Hall, J. (2006). *Textbook of medical physiology* (11th ed.). Philadelphia: Saunders.

Chapter 65

65-1, A and B, From Fadner, F. (1944). *Biography of Robert Wadlow* (courtesy Bruce Humphries, Publishers). **C,** courtesy C.M. Charles and C.M. MacBryde; **65-2,** from Mendelhoff, A., & Smith, D.E. (Eds.). (1956). Acromegaly, diabetes, hypermetabolism, proteinuria, and heart failure. Clinical Pathological Conference, *American Journal of Medicine, 20,* 133; **65-4,** from Wilson, J.D., Foster, D., Kronenberg, H., & Larsen, P.R. (1998). *Williams textbook of endocrinology* (9th ed.). Philadelphia: Saunders (courtesy Dr. H. Patrick Higgins); **65-5,** from Wenig, B.M., Heffess, C.S., & Adair, C.F. (1997). *Atlas of endocrine pathology.* Philadelphia: Saunders.

Chapter 67

67-6, 67-7, Courtesy MiniMed, Inc., Northridge, CA; **67-8,** courtesy Becton, Dickinson and Company, Franklin Lakes, NJ.

Chapter 68

68-10, Courtesy Verathon Corporation, Bothell, WA.

Chapter 69

69-1, A, Courtesy ConvaTec, A Bristol-Meyers Squibb Company, a Division of E.R. Squibb & Sons, Inc., Princeton, NJ; **B,** from ConvaTec. (1996). *FemTone vaginal weights: A training aid for pelvic floor exercises* (brochure). Princeton, NJ: Author; **69-2,** from Pollack, H.M. (2000). *Clinical urography* (2nd ed.).

Philadelphia: Saunders; **69-3,** modified from Singal, R.K., & Denstedt, J.D. (1997). Contemporary management of ureteral stones. *The Urologic Clinics of North America, 24*(1), 59-70.

Chapter 71

71-1, Courtesy Kendall Company, Bothell, WA; **71-5,** courtesy GAMBRO Healthcare, Stockholm, Sweden; **71-14,** courtesy Baxter International, Inc., Deerfield, IL.

Chapter 73

73-1, From Swartz, M.H. (2006). *Textbook of physical diagnosis: History and examination* (5th ed.). Philadelphia: Saunders; **73-2,** from Mansel, R., & Bundred, N. (1995). *Color atlas of breast disease.* St. Louis: Mosby; **73-3,** from Gallager, H.S., Leis, H.P. Jr., Snyderman, R.K., & Urban, J.A. (1978). *The breast.* St. Louis: Mosby.

Chapter 74

74-5, From Lowdermilk, D., & Perry, S. (2007). *Maternity and women's health care* (9th ed.). St. Louis: Mosby.

Chapter 75

75-7, From Seidel, H.M., Ball, J., Dains, J., & Benedict, G.W. (2006). *Mosby's guide to physical examination* (6th ed.). St. Louis: Mosby.

Chapter 76

76-1, 76-2, From Morse, S., Ballard, R., Holmes, K., & Moreland, A. (2003). *Atlas of sexually transmitted diseases and AIDS* (3rd ed.). St. Louis: Mosby.

Index

A

A delta fiber, 38
AACN; *See* American Association of Colleges of Nursing
Abacavir, 376*c*, 379
Abacavir-lamivudine, 376*c*
Abatacept, 342*c*, 344
ABCD features in skin cancer, 467
ABCDE mnemonic, 136
Abciximab
 for acute myocardial infarction, 859
 for acute peripheral arterial occlusion, 810
 for deep vein thrombosis, 819
 for postoperative graft occlusion, 809
Abdomen
 quadrants of, 1222*f*, 1222*t*
 sickle cell disease and, 895
Abdominal aortic aneurysm, 811, 812
Abdominal assessment, 1221-1223, 1222*f*, 1222*t*
 in abdominal hernia, 1292
 in abdominal trauma, 1307
 in chronic pancreatitis, 1377-1378
 in cirrhosis, 1347-1348
 in Crohn's disease, 1331
 in hematologic disorders, 885-886
 in infective endocarditis, 784
 in spinal cord injury, 994
Abdominal distention
 in abdominal trauma, 1307
 in Crohn's disease, 1331
 in cystic fibrosis, 635
 in diverticulitis, 1335
 in hypokalemia, 188
 in intestinal obstruction, 1302, 1304, 1305
 in tube feeding, 1399
 in ulcerative colitis, 1323
Abdominal girth
 in cirrhosis, 1348, 1349*f*
 in right-sided heart failure, 769
Abdominal hemorrhage in spinal cord injury, 993, 994
Abdominal herniation, 1291-1293, 1292*f*
Abdominal pain
 in acute pancreatitis, 1375-1377
 in appendicitis, 1316
 in black widow spider bite, 148
 in botulism, 1342
 bromocriptine-related, 1431
 in coral snake envenomation, 146
 in Crohn's disease, 1331
 in diverticulitis, 1334-1335
 in dysmenorrhea, 1684-1685
 in *Escherichia coli* infection, 1341
 in food poisoning, 1341
 gastrointestinal assessment of, 1221
 in hookworm infection, 1340
 in hypercalcemia, 194
 in intestinal obstruction, 1304
 in irritable bowel syndrome, 1290
 in pancreatic cancer, 1380
 in pelvic inflammatory disease, 1748
 in peritonitis, 1317-1318
 in sickle cell disease, 895
 in systemic lupus erythematosus, 349
 in ulcerative colitis, 1321
Abdominal radiography
 in cirrhosis, 1350
 in gastrointestinal assessment, 1226
 in intestinal obstruction, 1304
Abdominal surgery, skin preparation for, 256*f*

c indicates charts, *f* indicates illustrations, and *t* indicates tables.

Abdominal thrust maneuver, 597*f*
Abdominal trauma, 1307-1308
 kidney injury in, 1596
 liver injury in, 1361
 pelvic fracture and, 1198
Abdominal ultrasound
 in abdominal trauma, 1307
 in acute pancreatitis, 1375
 in benign prostatic hypertrophy, 1714
 in diverticulitis, 1335
 in liver trauma, 1361
 in pancreatic cancer, 1380
Abdominoperineal resection, 1298
Abducens nerve, 935*t*, 1072
Abduction, 1146*f*
Abenol; *See* Acetaminophen
ABGs; *See* Arterial blood gases
ABI; *See* Ankle-brachial index
AbioCor System, 774, 774*f*
Ablation procedures
 in liver cancer, 1362
 in thyroid cancer, 1461
Abnormal cell, 402*t*, 402-403
Abnormal heart sounds, 718-719, 719*t*
Abnormal spontaneous movement, 933
ABO system, 919
Abortive therapy for migraine headache, 952-953, 953*t*
Above-knee amputation, 1199*f*, 1203*f*
Abrasion, corneal, 1089
Abraxane; *See* Paclitaxel
Abscess
 after pancreatic transplant, 1498
 after renal transplantation, 1633
 anorectal, 1337, 1337*c*
 Bartholin cyst and, 1699
 brain, 1065-1066
 in epididymitis, 1734
 hepatic, 1361
 in inflammatory bowel disease, 1322*t*
 lung, 672
 pancreatic, 1379-1380
 in pelvic inflammatory disease, 1748
 peritonsillar, 657
 in pyelonephritis, 1586
Absence seizure, 956
Absolute granulocyte count, 310
Absolute neutrophil count, 310
Absorbable sutures, 281-282, 282*f*
Absorption, 1217
Absorption atelectasis, 573
Abstinence syndrome, 40
Abuse, elder, 22*c*, 22-23, 977
Abuse screening questions, 1648*t*
AC ventilation, 693
Acalculia, 1034, 1034*c*
Acalculous cholecystitis, 1367
Acanthosis, 597
Acarbose, 1480-1481*c*, 1484
Accelerated graft atherosclerosis, 319
Acceleration injury, 1050*f*, 1050-1051, 1183
Acceleration-deceleration forces, 136
Accessory duct of Santorini, 1218*f*
Accessory muscles of respiration, 556
Accessory nerve, 935*t*
Accessory organs of blood formation, 879
Accidental decannulation, 580
Acclimatization, 155
Accolate; *See* Zafirlukast
Accommodation, 1074
Accutane; *See* Isotretinoin
ACE inhibitors; *See* Angiotensin-converting enzyme inhibitors
ACE unit, 23
Acebutolol, 742*c*
Acetaminophen
 after cataract surgery, 1094
 for fever, 451
 for low back pain, 985
 for migraine headache, 952, 953*t*
 for osteoarthritis, 326
 for pain, 45, 46
 for postoperative pain, 297-299
 for rheumatoid arthritis, 344
 for tension headache, 955
Acetazolamide, 155
Acetoacetic acid, 1474, 1539-1541
Acetohexamide, 1477*c*
Acetone
 diabetes mellitus and, 1467, 1474
 in urine, 1539-1541
Acetylcholine, 930*t*
 Alzheimer's disease and, 970
 myasthenia gravis and, 1016, 1017
 Parkinson disease and, 965
Acetylcysteine, 629
Acetylsalicylic acid
 for pain, 45
 for peripheral arterial disease, 807
 as trigger for asthma, 611
Achalasia, 1254-1255
Achilles reflex, 940*f*
Achilles tendon rupture, 1208
Achlorhydria, 1280
Achromycin; *See* Tetracycline
Acid deficit, 210
Acid-base balance, 199
 postoperative assessment of, 290
 regulatory mechanisms of, 202*c*, 202-204, 203*f*, 203*t*
Acid-base chemistry, 200*f*, 200-201, 201*f*
Acid-base imbalance, 199-212
 acid-base chemistry and, 200*f*, 200-201, 201*f*
 acid-base regulatory mechanisms and, 202*c*, 202-204, 203*f*, 203*t*
 acidosis and, 204-209
  assessment of, 206-209, 207*c*, 208*c*, 208*f*
  in chronic glomerulonephritis, 1592
  in chronic kidney disease, 1610
  in chronic obstructive pulmonary disease, 623
  combined metabolic and respiratory, 206, 208*c*
  in cystic fibrosis, 636
  in hypovolemic shock, 831
  metabolic, 205-206, 209, 209*c*
  in myocardial infarction, 849
  nursing diagnoses in, 209
  pathophysiology of, 204-205, 205*c*, 205*t*
  respiratory, 206, 209
 alkalosis and, 210*f*, 210*t*, 210-211, 211*c*
 body fluid chemistry and, 201*f*, 201-202
 in chronic kidney disease, 1610
 in hypothermia, 153
Acidosis, 204-209
 assessment of, 206-209, 207*c*, 208*c*, 208*f*
 in chronic glomerulonephritis, 1592
 in chronic kidney disease, 1610
 in chronic obstructive pulmonary disease, 623
 combined metabolic and respiratory, 206, 208*c*
 in cystic fibrosis, 636
 in hypovolemic shock, 831
 metabolic, 205-206, 209, 209*c*
  causes of, 205*t*
  in chronic obstructive pulmonary disease, 626-627
Acidosis *(Continued)*
  in diabetes mellitus, 1467
  in intestinal obstruction, 1303
  laboratory assessment of, 208, 208*c*, 208*f*
  in septic shock, 842
 in myocardial infarction, 849
 nursing diagnoses in, 209
 pathophysiology of, 204-205, 205*c*, 205*t*
 respiratory, 206, 209
  causes of, 205*t*
  in chronic obstructive pulmonary disease, 626
  laboratory assessment of, 208*c*, 208*f*, 208-209
Acid(s), 200
 renal formation of, 204
 sources of, 201-202
Acinus, 555, 555*f*
Aciphex; *See* Rabeprazole
ACLS; *See* Advanced cardiac life support
Acne, 515
Acorn cardiac support device, 775
Acoustic neuroma, 1061, 1129
Acquired immunodeficiency syndrome, 363-383
 brain abscess in, 1066
 chronic low self-esteem in, 381-382
 diarrhea in, 380-381
 disturbed thought processes in, 381
 drug therapy for, 375-379, 376-378*c*
 etiology and genetic risk in, 363*f*, 363-366, 364*f*, 365*t*
 health care resources for, 383
 health teaching in, 383, 384*c*
 home care management of, 382, 383*c*
 impaired gas exchange in, 379
 impaired skin integrity in, 381
 incidence and prevalence of, 366*f*, 366-367, 367*f*
 laboratory assessment in, 373-374
 lung abscess in, 672
 nursing diagnoses in, 374-375
 nutritional status and, 380
 pain in, 379-380
 parenteral transmission of, 367-368
 patient history and, 370
 perinatal transmission of, 368
 physical assessment in, 370-373, 371*c*, 372*t*
 psychosocial assessment in, 373
 risk for infection in, 375, 375*c*, 376*c*
 sexual transmission of, 367, 368*c*
 social isolation in, 382
 testing for, 369-370, 370*c*
 transmission and health care workers and, 368-369, 369*c*
Acromegaly, 1428, 1428*f*, 1429*f*
Actemra; *See* Tocilizumab
ACTH; *See* Adrenocorticotropic hormone
Acticin; *See* Permethrin
Actinic keratoses, 509, 510*t*
Actinic lentigo, 465*f*
Activase; *See* Alteplase
Activated partial thromboplastin time
 in leukemia, 904
 peripheral venous access device for blood sample for, 888
 preoperative assessment of, 251*c*
 in pulmonary embolism, 680, 682*c*
Activated protein C, 842, 843-844
Activation of emergency preparedness plans, 161-162
Active assisted range-of-motion exercises, 102*t*
Active euthanasia, 121-122, 122*t*

Active external rewarming methods, 153
Active immunity, 316, 441
Active range of motion, 1145, 1146*f*
Active range-of-motion exercises, 102*t*
Activities of daily living
acquired immunodeficiency syndrome and, 383
after bone cancer surgery, 1170
assessment before rehabilitation, 98-99
dyspnea and, 559, 560*t*
Huntington disease and, 980
peripheral vascular disease and, 810
self-care deficit and, 102
spinal cord injury and, 999
stroke and, 1047
Activity
after hysterectomy, 1698*c*
after total hip arthroplasty, 331-332, 332*f*
asthma and, 621
Braden Scale for pressure ulcer risk and, 487*f*
coronary artery disease and, 852, 854*c*, 871, 871*c*
obesity and, 1403
older adult and, 17, 17*f*
Activity intolerance
in acute coronary syndromes, 860
in chronic obstructive pulmonary disease, 633
in heart failure, 775
Activity therapist, 96
Activity-exercise pattern
in acid-base assessment, 207*c*
in cardiovascular assessment, 711*c*
in endocrine assessment, 1420*c*
in hematologic assessment, 882*c*
in musculoskeletal assessment, 1144*c*
in neurologic assessment, 937*c*
in respiratory assessment, 558*c*
Actonel; *See* Risedronate
Actoplus Met; *See* Pioglitazone-metformin
Actose; *See* Pioglitazone
Acular; *See* Ketorolac
Acupoints, 9
Acupressure, 9
Acupuncture, 57
Acute abdomen series, 1226
Acute adrenal insufficiency
in Cushing's disease, 1444
emergency care in, 1436*c*, 1437
Acute back pain, 984
Acute care nurse practitioner, 3
Acute Care of the Elderly unit, 23
Acute cholecystitis, 1367, 1367*f*
Acute compartment syndrome
in abdominal trauma, 1308
fracture and, 1180-1182, 1181*c*
Acute coronary syndromes, 847-874
activity intolerance in, 860
acute pain in, 856*c*, 856-858, 857-858*c*
chronic stable angina pectoris and, 847-848
coronary artery bypass graft surgery in, 866-870, 867*f*
diagnostic tests in, 855
dysrhythmias in, 861-862
etiology and genetic risk in, 850
health care resources for, 872
health teaching in, 870-872, 871*c*, 872*c*
heart failure in, 862*t*, 862-864, 863-864*c*
history in, 853
home care management in, 870, 870*c*, 871*c*
imaging studies in, 855
incidence and prevalence of, 850
ineffective coping in, 860-861
ineffective tissue perfusion in, 858-860, 859*t*
intervention activities in, 861*c*
laboratory assessment in, 855
nursing diagnoses in, 855-856
pathophysiology of, 848*f*, 848-850, 849*f*
Acute coronary syndromes *(Continued)*
percutaneous transluminal coronary angioplasty in, 865, 865*t*
physical assessment in, 853*c*, 853-855
prevention of, 850-853, 853*t*, 854*c*
psychosocial assessment in, 855
serum markers of myocardial damage in, 719-721
stent in, 865-866, 866*f*
Acute diarrheal illness, 1319*t*, 1319-1321, 1321*c*
Acute gastritis, 1265-1270, 1266-1269*c*, 1270*t*
Acute gastroduodenal ulcer, burn-related, 525
Acute glaucoma, 1095*t*, 1095-1098, 1098*c*
Acute glomerulonephritis, 655, 1590*t*, 1590-1591
Acute gout, 353
Acute hematogenous osteomyelitis, 1165
Acute idiopathic polyneuritis, 1011-1016, 1012*c*, 1012*t*, 1013*t*, 1014*c*, 1015*c*
Acute inflammatory bowel disorders, 1316-1321
appendicitis in, 1316*f*, 1316-1317
gastroenteritis in, 1319*t*, 1319-1321, 1321*c*
peritonitis in, 1317*c*, 1317-1319
Acute leukemia, 902
drug therapy for, 905
thrombocytopenia in, 910, 910*c*
Acute lung injury, 686-689, 687*t*
Acute lymphocytic leukemia, 902
Acute mountain sickness, 154-156, 156*c*
Acute myelogenous leukemia, 902
Acute myocardial infarction, 848-850, 849*f*
in diabetes mellitus, 1468
emergency care in, 856-858, 857-858*c*
home care management after, 870, 870*c*, 871*c*
serum markers of myocardial damage in, 719-721
Acute nephritic syndrome, 1590
Acute normovolemic hemodilution, 921
Acute otitis media, 1123-1125, 1124*f*, 1125*c*, 1125*f*
Acute pain, 36*t*, 36-38, 37*t*
in acute coronary syndromes, 856*c*, 856-858, 857-858*c*
in acute pancreatitis, 1375-1376
in bone cancer, 1169
in burn, 535-536
in cholecystitis, 1369
in fracture, 1192
in pelvic inflammatory disease, 1751-1752
in peptic ulcer disease, 1274-1275
in polycystic kidney disease, 1584
postoperative, 297-299, 297-299*c*
psychosocial assessment of, 44
in pyelonephritis, 1588-1598
in ulcerative colitis, 1327-1328, 1328*c*
Acute pancreatitis, 1371-1377, 1372*f*, 1373*t*, 1374*t*
acute pain in, 1375-1376
community-based care in, 1376-1377
complications of, 1373, 1373*t*
history in, 1373-1374
laboratory assessment in, 1374*t*, 1374-1375
pancreatic abscess and, 1379-1380
pathophysiology of, 1371-1373, 1372*f*
physical assessment in, 1374
Acute paronychia, 474
Acute pericarditis, 785
Acute peripheral arterial occlusion, 810
Acute phase of burn, 537-545
disturbed body image and, 544-545
imbalanced nutrition: less than body requirements in, 543
impaired physical mobility in, 543-544, 544*c*, 544*f*
Acute phase of burn *(Continued)*
nursing diagnoses in, 537-538
physical assessment in, 537, 538*t*
risk for infection in, 540-543, 542-543*c*
wound care management in, 538-540, 539*t*
Acute promyelocytic leukemia, 902
Acute pulmonary edema, 775
Acute pyelonephritis, 1586-1589, 1587*c*, 1587*f*
Acute radiation cystitis, 1723
Acute rehabilitation, 95
after total hip arthroplasty, 332
after total knee arthroplasty, 334
Acute rejection, 319
in liver transplantation, 1363, 1364*t*
in renal transplantation, 1633*t*
Acute renal failure, 1601-1609
after liver transplantation, 1364*t*
chronic kidney disease *versus*, 1601*t*
continuous renal replacement therapy for, 1608
dialysis therapies for, 1607*f*, 1607-1608
drug therapy for, 1605-1607, 1606*c*
health promotion and maintenance in, 1603
history in, 1603
imaging studies in, 1604
incidence and prevalence of, 1602-1603, 1603*t*
laboratory assessment in, 1604, 1605*c*
nursing diagnoses in, 1604
nutrition therapy for, 1607
phases of, 1602, 1602*t*
physical assessment in, 1603-1604, 1604*c*
posthospital care in, 1608
types of, 1601, 1602*t*
Acute respiratory distress syndrome, 686-689, 687*t*
in acute pancreatitis, 1373
burn-related, 537
heart failure in, 767
oxygen toxicity and, 573
in septic shock, 842
ventilation-perfusion mismatch in, 685, 685*t*
Acute respiratory failure, 685*t*, 685-686, 686*f*
Acute respiratory problems, 677-701
acute respiratory distress syndrome in, 686-689, 687*t*
acute respiratory failure in, 685*t*, 685-686, 686*f*
cardiac oxygen delivery impairment in, 678*f*
endotracheal intubation in, 689-692, 690*f*, 691*c*
flail chest in, 698, 698*f*
hemothorax in, 699
mechanical ventilation in, 692*c*, 692-697
extubation in, 697
managing ventilator system in, 695*t*, 695-696
modes of ventilation in, 693
monitoring in, 694-695
preventing complications in, 696
types of ventilators in, 692-693, 693*f*
ventilator controls and settings in, 693-694
weaning from, 696-697, 697*t*
pain assessment in, 43-44
pneumothorax in, 698-699
pulmonary contusion in, 697-698
pulmonary embolism in, 677-684
anxiety and, 682-683
decreased cardiac output in, 682
health care resources for, 683-684, 684*c*
health promotion and maintenance and, 678, 678*c*
health teaching in, 683, 684*c*
history in, 679
Acute respiratory problems *(Continued)*
home care management in, 683
hypoxemia in, 680-682, 680-682*c*
imaging assessment in, 679
laboratory assessment in, 679
nursing diagnoses in, 679-680
pathophysiology of, 677-678
physical assessment in, 679, 679*c*
potential for bleeding in, 683, 683*c*
psychosocial assessment in, 679
total hip arthroplasty and, 330-331
rib fracture in, 698
tension pneumothorax in, 699
tracheobronchial trauma in, 699
Acute sialadenitis, 1239-1240
Acute thyroiditis, 1460
Acute tonsillitis, 657, 657*c*
Acute tubular necrosis, 1601
after abdominal aortic aneurysm resection, 812
after renal transplantation, 1632
Acute viral rhinitis, 654
Acyclovir
for encephalitis, 965
for facial paralysis, 1026
for genital herpes, 1742
for viral skin infection, 503
for viral stomatitis, 1233
Adalimumab
for rheumatoid arthritis, 342*c*, 344
for ulcerative colitis, 1324-1325
Adam's apple, 554, 554*f*
Adaptive devices, 102-103, 103*t*
Adaptive immunity, 316
Adaptive mechanisms
in burn, 525, 526*f*
in heart failure, 765-767, 766*f*
in hypovolemic shock, 833-835
Addiction, 39-40, 80
barbiturates and, 89
cocaine and, 86
opioid analgesics and, 90
Addisonian crisis, 1437
Addison's disease, 1436-1439, 1436-1439*c*, 1437*f*, 1437*t*
Additives in adjuvant analgesics, 54
Add-on device in infusion system, 220-221, 221*f*
Adduction, 1146*f*
Adenine, 64, 64*f*
Adenocarcinoma
cervical, 1702
colorectal, 1293
endometrial, 1699
esophageal, 1255
fallopian tube, 1709
gallbladder, 1371
gastric, 1279
lung, 641
renal, 1595*t*, 1595-1596
Adenocard; *See* Adenosine
Adenohypophysis, 1414, 1426
Adenoids, 553*f*, 554
Adenoma
adrenal, 1440
testicular, 127, 1727*t*
Adenosine, 741, 745*c*
Adenosine triphosphate, 885
ADH; *See* Antidiuretic hormone
Adhesive transparent film dressing, 494-495*t*
Adipex-P; *See* Phentermine
Adipokines, 1402
Adiponectin, 1402
Adipose tissue, 248, 461, 461*f*
Adjuvant analgesics, 45*t*, 54*t*, 54-55
Adjuvant therapy in cancer, 421, 1675-1676
Administration set, 220, 220*c*, 224
Administrative review after mass casualty event, 165
Adrenal adenoma, 1440
Adrenal cortex, 1415*f*, 1415*t*, 1415-1416
Adrenal crisis, 1436
Adrenal Cushing's disease, 1440

Adrenal gland, 1413*f*, 1415*f*, 1415*t*, 1415-1417, 1416*t*, 1436-1447
  Cushing's disease and, 1439-1445
    acute adrenal insufficiency in, 1444
    community-based care in, 1445, 1445*c*
    excess fluid volume in, 1442-1443
    history in, 1440-1441
    imaging studies in, 1442
    laboratory assessment in, 1441-1442
    pathophysiology of, 1439-1440, 1440*f*, 1440*t*
    physical assessment in, 1441, 1441*c*
    psychosocial assessment in, 1441
    risk for infection in, 1444
    risk for injury in, 1443-1444
  hyperaldosteronism and, 1445-1446
  hypofunction of, 1436-1439, 1436-1439*c*, 1437*f*, 1437*t*
  negative feedback mechanism and, 1414, 1414*f*
  pheochromocytoma and, 1446-1447
Adrenal hormones, 1413*t*
Adrenal insufficiency, 1436-1439, 1436-1439*c*, 1437*f*, 1437*t*
  in renal cell carcinoma, 1596
  in septic shock, 843
Adrenal medulla, 1415*f*, 1416*t*, 1416-1417
Adrenal steroids, 1416
Adrenalectomy
  in Cushing's disease, 1443
  in hyperaldosteronism, 1446
Adrenalin; *See* Epinephrine
Adrenocorticotropic hormone, 1415*t*
  deficiency of, 1426, 1427*c*
  glucocorticoid release and, 1416
  overproduction of, 1429, 1430*c*
Adrenocorticotropic hormone stimulation test, 1438
Adriamycin; *See* Doxorubicin
Adrucil; *See* 5-Fluorouracil
Adsorbocarpine; *See* Pilocarpine
Adult health nursing, 2-7
  core competencies and, 3-6
    collaboration with interdisciplinary health care team and, 5
    in emergency nursing, 130-131
    evidence-based practice and, 5-6, 6*t*
    informatics and, 6, 6*f*
    patient-centered care and, 3-5, 4*c*
    quality improvement and, 6
  Institute for Healthcare Improvement and, 3, 3*t*
  national patient safety goals and, 2
Adult respiratory distress syndrome, 686-689, 687*t*
Advance directive, 113, 114*f*
  in heart failure, 778
  intraoperative medical record review and, 278
Advanced cardiac life support
  in cardiac arrest, 756
  in idioventricular rhythms, 747
  in lightning strike, 152
  paramedic and, 127
  training and certification in, 131, 131*t*
  in ventricular asystole, 750
  in ventricular fibrillation, 749
Advanced Disaster Life Support training, 161
Advanced older adult population, 15-16
Adventitious breath sounds, 562-564, 563*t*
Adverse drug events
  dapsone and, 147
  intravenous drug therapy and, 214-215
  older adult and, 19, 19*t*
Advicor; *See* Niacin-lovastatin
Advocate, 5
Adynamic ileus, 1302
AED; *See* Automated external defibrillator
AEDs; *See* Antiepileptic drugs
Aerophagia after esophageal surgery, 1254, 1254*c*
Aerosol inhalation, 91
Aerosol mask, 577, 577*t*
Aerosolization, tuberculosis and, 668
Aesthetic plastic surgery, 513-515, 514*t*
Afferent arteriole, 1528, 1528*f*, 1530*t*
Afferent loop syndrome, 1285-1286
Afferent pathway, 928
African Americans
  age-related glomerular filtration rate changes in, 1533
  beliefs regarding death, dying, and afterlife, 119*t*
  breast cancer in, 1664-1665
  burn assessment and, 532
  cancer development and, 410, 410*t*
  chronic obstructive pulmonary disease and, 622
  coronary artery disease and, 850, 852, 855
  diabetes mellitus and, 1472
  hypertension and, 798, 803, 852, 1593
  lactose intolerance and, 1221
  musculoskeletal differences in, 119*t*
  oxygen saturation in, 556
  sickle cell disease in, 895
  syphilis and, 1738
Africanized bee sting, 149-150
After-drop, 153
Afterlife beliefs, 119*t*
Afterload, 708, 766
Agammaglobulinemia, Bruton's, 385
Age
  breast cancer risk and, 1665*t*
  cancer development and, 409, 409*c*
  cataract formation and, 1092*c*
  coronary artery disease and, 850
  hemoglobin levels and, 882
  hyperkalemia and, 190
  hypokalemia and, 187
  hypovolemic shock and, 833
  risk for infection and, 441*t*
  surgical risk and, 244*t*
  urinary tract infection and, 1551*t*
  vision assessment and, 1076
Age-related macular degeneration, 1100-1101
Agglutination, antigen-antibody interaction and, 314-315, 315*f*
Aggrastat; *See* Tirofiban
Aggregation of platelets, 878
Aging
  changes associated with
    cardiovascular, 709, 710*c*
    ear and hearing, 1111, 1112*c*
    endocrine, 1418-1419, 1419*c*
    fluid balance, 174*c*
    gastrointestinal, 1219, 1220*c*
    hematologic, 881, 882*c*
    immune function, 308*c*
    musculoskeletal, 1143, 1143*c*
    neurologic, 933-935, 936*c*
    renal, 1533, 1534*c*
    reproductive, 1646, 1646*c*
    respiratory, 556, 557*c*
    skin, 462-466, 463-464*c*, 465*f*, 466*f*
    stomach, 1220*c*
    vision, 1074, 1075*c*, 1075*f*
  complications from burn injury and, 529*c*
  drug effects and, 19, 19*t*
  nutritional status and, 16-17
Agitation
  in Alzheimer's disease, 977, 977*t*
  end-of-life care and, 118
  in heat stroke, 142
  in hypovolemic shock, 835
Agnosia
  after stroke, 1034
  in Alzheimer's disease, 971
Agraphia, 1034, 1034*c*
AIDS; *See* Acquired immunodeficiency syndrome
AIDS dementia complex, 373
AIDS wasting syndrome, 373
Air conduction of sound, 1115-1116
Air embolism
  central venous catheter insertion-related, 231*t*
  changing administration set and, 224
Air pollution, chronic obstructive pulmonary disease and, 623
Air warming and humidification in tracheostomy, 583
Airborne precautions, 447*t*, 448
  in tuberculosis, 670
Airborne transmission of infection, 442
  in severe acute respiratory syndrome, 666
  in tuberculosis, 668
Airway, 554-555, 555*f*
  asthma and, 610-621
    drug therapy in, 615-621, 616-618*c*
    exercise and activity in, 621
    health teaching in, 613-615, 615*c*
    history in, 612
    laboratory assessment in, 612
    oxygen therapy in, 621
    pathophysiology of, 610-611, 611*f*
    physical assessment in, 612, 614*f*
    smoking cessation and, 614*c*
    status asthmaticus and, 621
    step system in, 613*c*
    subcutaneous infusion therapy in, 237*t*
    surgical risk and, 246
  inhalation burn of, 529
Airway management
  after discharge from postanesthesia care unit, 289*c*
  in bariatric surgery, 1407
  in burn, 535
  in cervical neck pain surgery, 989, 989*f*
  in chronic obstructive pulmonary disease, 628, 631-632, 632*f*, 633*t*
  in facial trauma, 593
  in Guillain-Barré syndrome, 1014, 1015*c*
  in head and neck cancer, 600-601, 601*f*
  in laryngeal trauma, 596
  in oral cancer, 1236, 1236*c*, 1238, 1238*c*
  in pneumonia, 664
  postoperative, 294
  in spinal cord injury, 993, 995*c*, 997
  trauma nursing and, 136, 137*f*, 138*t*
  in traumatic brain injury, 1954
Airway obstruction
  after extubation, 697
  in burn injury, 529, 529*t*, 535
  in cancer, 417
  in facial trauma, 593
  in head and neck cancer, 599-602, 600*t*, 601*f*, 603*f*
  respiratory acidosis and, 206
  upper, 596, 597*f*
  in vocal cord paralysis, 594
Akarpine; *See* Pilocarpine
Akinesia, 965
Akinetic seizure, 956
AK-Taine; *See* Proxymetacaine
Alafacept, 508
Alanine, 70*f*, 70*t*
Alanine aminotransferase
  in acute pancreatitis, 1374, 1374*t*
  in cirrhosis, 1349, 1349*t*
  in gastrointestinal assessment, 1223, 1224*c*
  in hepatitis, 1359
Al-Anon, 84
Alarm system of ventilator, 695, 695*t*
Albendazole, 1340
Albenza; *See* Albendazole
Albumin, 877
  burn assessment and, 532*c*
  gastrointestinal assessment and, 1224*c*
  rheumatoid arthritis and, 339*c*
  in urine, 1541
Albumin/globulin ratio, 948*t*
Albuminuria, 1468
Albuterol
  for anaphylaxis, 393*c*, 394
  for asthma, 616*c*, 618
  for dyspnea in dying patient, 117
Alcohol
  abuse of, 82-84, 83*t*, 84*c*, 84*t*
  acute pancreatitis and, 1373
  breast cancer risk and, 1665*t*
  coronary artery disease and, 852
  diabetes mellitus and, 1493
  esophageal cancer and, 1255
  folic acid deficiency anemia and, 900
  gout and, 354
  head and neck cancer and, 598
  hematologic assessment and, 884
  hypoglycemia and, 1509
  osteoporosis and, 1154
  prostate cancer and, 1720
Alcohol-based surgical scrub agents, 270, 444
Alcoholic cirrhosis, 1345
Alcoholic hepatitis, 1346-1347
Alcoholics Anonymous, 84
Alcoholism, 82-84, 83*t*, 84*c*, 84*t*
Aldactone; *See* Spironolactone
Aldolase, 1148*c*
Aldosterone, 1416, 1528, 1529*f*
  chronic kidney disease and, 1611
  fluid balance and, 175, 176*f*
  heart failure and, 766
  hypertension and, 797
  hypovolemic shock and, 831
  influence on renal function, 1531*t*
Aldosterone receptor antagonists, 802
Alemtuzumab, 435*t*
Alendronate
  for osteoporosis prevention, 1158*c*, 1160
  for Paget's disease of bone, 1164
Alexia, 1034, 1034*c*
Alfenta; *See* Alfentanil
Alfentanil, 274*t*, 276
Alfuzosin, 1714
ALG; *See* Antithymocyte globulin
Alginate dressing, 494-495*t*
Aliskiren, 802
Alkali burn, 525-526
Alkaline, term, 1574
Alkaline phosphatase, 1147, 1148*c*
  in acute pancreatitis, 1374
  in cirrhosis, 1349, 1349*t*
  in gastrointestinal assessment, 1224*c*
  in Paget's disease of bone, 1163
Alkaline reflux gastropathy, 1285
Alkalosis, 210*f*, 210*t*, 210-211, 211*c*
  combined metabolic and respiratory, 208*c*
  metabolic, 208*c*, 210*t*, 210-211, 211*c*
    in hyperaldosteronism, 1445
    in intestinal obstruction, 1303
  respiratory, 208*c*, 210*f*, 210*t*, 210-211, 211*c*
    acclimatization and, 155
    in diabetes mellitus, 1467
    in heart failure, 769-770
    in high altitude pulmonary edema, 155
Alkeran; *See* Melphalan
Alkylating agents, 422, 422*t*
  for breast cancer, 1677*t*
Allegra; *See* Fexofenadine
Allele, 69, 69*f*
Aller-Chlor; *See* Chlorpheniramine
Allerdryl; *See* Diphenhydramine
Allergen, 388, 388*f*
  rhinitis and, 654
Allergic asthma, 612, 640*c*
Allergic conjunctivitis, 1087
Allergic rhinitis, 388*f*, 388-391, 389*f*, 390*c*, 654
Allergic transfusion reaction, 921
Allergy, 387-398, 388*t*
  to antibiotic therapy, 452*c*
  to antivenom, 146

Allergy *(Continued)*
aromatherapy and, 12
autoimmunity and, 395-397, 396*t*
Goodpasture's syndrome in, 397
Sjögren's syndrome in, 396-397
intraoperative medical record review and, 278
to intravenous therapy, 230*t*
respiratory assessment and, 558
skin problems and, 467
surgical risk and, 246
to targeted therapy, 434
type I: rapid hypersensitivity reactions, 387-394
allergic rhinitis in, 388*f*, 388-391, 389*f*, 390*c*
anaphylaxis in, 391*t*, 391-394, 392*c*, 392*f*, 393*c*
latex allergy in, 394
type II: cytotoxic reactions, 394, 394*f*
type III: immune complex reactions, 394-395, 395*f*
type IV: delayed hypersensitivity reactions, 395
type V: stimulatory reactions, 395
Allergy testing, 389
Allogenic bone marrow transplantation, 907, 907*t*, 909*f*, 1679
Allograft
in bone cancer, 1170
for burn wound, 539
Allopurinol
for gout, 354
for hyperoxaluria, 1574
Aloe vera-coated gloves, 445
Alopecia
aging and, 473
chemotherapy-induced, 424, 428-430, 644, 1702
in induction therapy in acute leukemia, 905
in nutrient deficiencies, 1394*t*
in systemic lupus erythematosus, 350
Alosetron, 1291
Aloxi; *See* Palonosetron
Alpha adrenergic receptors, 1416, 1416*t*
Alpha cell, 1418, 1418*f*, 1466
Alpha$_1$ globulin, 339*c*
Alpha$_2$ globulin, 339*c*
Alpha particles, 418, 418*f*
5-Alpha reductase inhibitors, 1714
Alpha-adrenergic agonists for glaucoma, 1099*c*
Alpha-adrenergic antagonists
for benign prostatic hypertrophy, 1714
for hypertension, 802
Alpha$_1$-antitrypsin deficiency, 623, 623*t*
Alpha-fetoprotein
in liver cancer, 1362
in testicular cancer, 1728
Alphagan; *See* Brimonidine tartrate
Alpha-glucosidase inhibitors, 1480-1481*c*, 1484
Alport's syndrome, 1130
Alprazolam, 55
Alprostadil, 1726
ALS; *See* Amyotrophic lateral sclerosis
ALT; *See* Alanine aminotransferase
Altace; *See* Ramipril
Alteplase
for acute peripheral arterial occlusion, 810
for pulmonary embolism, 680, 681*c*
AlternaGEL; *See* Aluminum hydroxide gel
Alternate site testing in self-monitoring of blood glucose, 1491-1492
Alternative medicine; *See* Complementary and alternative therapies
Alternative sites for infusion, 236-239
arterial therapy and, 236
intraosseous therapy and, 238-239
intraperitoneal infusion and, 236-237
intraspinal infusion and, 237-238
subcutaneous infusion and, 237, 237*t*
Altitude-related illnesses, 154-156, 156*c*
Altretamine, 422*t*
Alu-Cap; *See* Aluminum hydroxide gel
Aluminum carbonate gel, 1606*c*
Aluminum hydroxide
for gastritis, 1268, 1268*c*
for gastroesophageal reflux disease, 1246*c*, 1247
for peptic ulcer disease, 1268*c*
Aluminum hydroxide gel, 1606*c*
Alupent; *See* Metaproterenol
Alveolar duct, 555, 555*f*
Alveolar edema, 524-525
Alveolar sac, 555, 555*f*
Alveolar-arterial gradient, 679
Alveolar-capillary diffusion, 206
Alveolitis
extrinsic allergic, 640*c*
in pulmonary sarcoidosis, 638
Alveolus, 555, 555*f*
Alzheimer's disease, 21, 969-980
caregiver role strain in, 978
chronic confusion in, 974*c*, 974*t*, 974-976, 976*c*
disturbed sleep pattern in, 977-978
health care resources for, 979
health promotion and maintenance in, 970
health teaching in, 978-979
history in, 970-971, 971*t*
home care management of, 978, 978*c*
imaging studies in, 973
laboratory assessment in, 973
nursing diagnoses in, 973-974
pathophysiology of, 969-970
physical assessment in, 971-973, 972*c*, 972*f*
psychosocial assessment in, 973
risk for injury in, 976-977, 977*t*
Alzheimer's Society of Canada, 978
Amantadine
for influenza, 658
for Parkinson disease, 968
Amaryl; *See* Glimepiride
Amaurosis fugax, 1035
Ambulation
after open radical prostatectomy, 1722
after total hip arthroplasty, 330
assistive devices for, 101*f*
burn patient and, 543
in Parkinson disease, 968
preoperative patient education about, 258
reduced vision and, 1107
Ambulatory aids, 100, 100*f*
Ambulatory blood pressure monitoring device, 803
Ambulatory care clinic for heart failure patients, 777
Ambulatory esophageal pH monitoring, 1245
Ambulatory pump, 222
Ambulatory surgery, 244, 444
Amebiasis, 1338-1339
Amebic dysentery, 1339
Amebic encephalitis, 964
Amebic hepatic abscess, 1361
Amenorrhea, 1647
in cirrhosis, 1348
in hypopituitarism, 1426
in menopause, 1689, 1689*t*
American Academy of Otolaryngology/Head and Neck Surgery, 1127*t*
American Association of Colleges of Nursing, 112*t*
American Brain Tumor Association, 1065
American Cancer Society, 417
American College of Cardiology/American Heart Association staging system, 765
American Diabetes Association, 1516
American Heart Association, 765, 872
American Indians, 28
beliefs regarding death, dying, and afterlife, 119*t*
American Indians *(Continued)*
breast cancer and, 1665*t*
coronary artery disease and, 850, 852
diabetes mellitus and, 1472
American Lung Association classification of tuberculosis, 668*t*
American Red Cross, 162
American Sign Language, 1135
American Society of Anesthesiologist physical status system, 271
American Society of Parenteral and Enteral Nutrition, 214
American Speech-Language-Hearing Association, 1127*t*
American Tinnitus Association, 1127*t*
Americans with Disabilities Act, 99
Amersol; *See* Ibuprofen
Amevive; *See* Alafacept
AMI; *See* Acute myocardial infarction
Amicar; *See* Aminocaproic acid
Amidate; *See* Etomidate
Amifostine, 424*t*
Amiloride, 189
Amino acid-dextrose solutions, 1400
Amino acids, 70, 70*f*, 70*t*, 930*t*
Aminocaproic acid, 680
Aminoglutethimide, 1442
Aminoglycoside antibiotics, 1603*t*
Aminophylline
for anaphylaxis, 393*c*, 393-394
for asthma, 620
5-Aminosalicylic acid
after percutaneous transluminal coronary angioplasty, 865
after stent procedure, 866
after stroke, 1043
for coronary artery disease, 858*c*, 859
for pain, 45
for peripheral arterial disease, 807
for prevention of colorectal cancer, 1295
as trigger for asthma, 611
for ulcerative colitis, 1324, 1325*t*
Amiodarone, 743*c*
for atrial fibrillation, 746
for valvular heart disease, 781
Amitriptyline
for diabetic neuropathy, 1504
for fibromyalgia, 358
for irritable bowel syndrome, 1291
for pain, 54, 54*t*
for pain in acquired immunodeficiency syndrome, 380
Amlodipine-atorvastatin, 796
Ammonia
gastrointestinal assessment and, 1224, 1224*c*
hepatic encephalopathy and, 1346
Ammonium, 204
Amnesia
in complex partial seizure, 956
general anesthesia and, 272
in lightning strike, 151
in traumatic brain injury, 1053
Amniotic fluid embolism, 678
Amniotic membrane dressing, 539
Amoxicillin
for inhalation anthrax, 673*c*
for Lyme disease, 356
for peptic ulcer disease, 1269*c*, 1274
for urinary tract infection, 1556*c*
Amoxicillin-clavulanate, 1556*c*
Amoxil; *See* Amoxicillin
Amphetamines, 85-86, 86*f*, 86*t*
Amphiarthrodial joint, 1142
Amphojel; *See* Aluminum hydroxide gel
Amphotericin B
nephrotoxicity of, 1506
for ocular infection, 1086*c*
Ampulla of Vater, 1218*f*
Amputation, 1199-1204
community-based care in, 1203-1204, 1204*c*
diabetic foot and, 1501
levels of, 1199*f*, 1199-1200
Amputation *(Continued)*
lifestyle adaptation and, 1202-1203
mobility after, 1202, 1202*f*
pain in, 1201
pathophysiology of, 1199
physical assessment in, 1200
preparation for prosthesis, 1202, 1203*f*
Amputee Coalition of America, 1203
Amulet, 32, 32*f*
Amylin analogues, 1489
Amyloid beta protein precursor, 973
Amyotrophic lateral sclerosis, 1007*c*, 1007-1008
Amytal abuse, 89
Anabolic hormone, 1418
Anabolic steroid abuse, 91-92
Anaerobic metabolism, 202, 830
Anakinra, 342*c*, 344
Anal canal, 1219
Anal fissure, 1337-1338
Anal fistula, 1338
Analgesia team, 35
Analgesics, 44-55, 45*t*
acetaminophen in, 46
adjuvant, 54*t*, 54-55
for black widow spider bite, 148
for burn pain, 536
for cholecystitis, 1369
for chronic pain in diabetic neuropathy, 1505*c*
in end-of-life care, 49, 116-117
epidural, 52-54, 53*f*
for external otitis, 1121
for frostbite, 154
general anesthesia and, 272, 274*t*
non-opioid, 45
nonsteroidal antiinflammatory drugs in, 45-46
opioid, 46-51, 47*t*, 49-51*t*
for osteoarthritis, 326-327, 327*c*
for otitis media, 1124
for pain in acquired immunodeficiency syndrome, 380
patient-controlled, 51*f*, 51-52
for pit viper envenomation, 145
for postoperative pain, 297-298*c*, 297-299
preemptive, 37
preoperative, 261
for rheumatoid arthritis, 344
routes of administration, 49-51, 50-51*t*
for scorpion sting, 149
side effects of, 48-49, 49*t*
substance abuser and, 82
for traumatic brain injury, 1057
Anaphase of cell cycle, 67*f*
Anaphylaxis, 388, 391*t*, 391-394, 392*c*, 392*f*, 393*c*, 830
antivenom-induced, 146
in bee sting, 149, 150
in intradermal testing for allergy, 390
Anaplasia, 401, 403
Anaplastic thyroid carcinoma, 1461
Anascara, 714
Anaspaz; *See* Hyoscyamine
Anastomosis
bariatric surgery, 1407
in colorectal cancer surgery, 1298
ileoanal, 1326, 1327*f*
in lung transplantation, 637
in Whipple procedure, 1383*f*
Anastrozole, 432
Anatomic dead space, 574
Ancasal; *See* Aspirin
Ancylostoma duodenale, 1340
Androblastoma, 127, 1727*t*
Androgen deprivation therapy, 1723
Androgen(s), 1416
for hormonal manipulation in cancer, 431*t*
menopause and, 1644
for osteoporosis prevention, 1160
Anectine; *See* Succinylcholine

Anemia, 878, 893-898
after total hip arthroplasty, 331
aplastic, 900
bleeding gastrointestinal ulcer or polyp and, 886
chemotherapy-related, 424, 426
in chronic kidney disease, 1611, 1613-1614
in cirrhosis, 1350
in colorectal cancer, 1295
common causes of, 893*t*
community-based care in, 898, 898*c*
in Crohn's disease, 1331
Fanconi's, 900
in folic acid deficiency, 900
in gastric cancer, 1281
in glucose-6-phosphate dehydrogenase deficiency, 898-899
hematologic assessment and, 885
immunohemolytic, 899
iron-deficiency, 899, 899*c*
in leukemia, 902
in myelodysplastic syndromes, 901-902
in renal cell carcinoma, 1595
in sickle cell disease, 894*f*, 894-898, 895*f*, 897*c*, 898*c*
systemic manifestations of, 894*c*
in vitamin B_{12} deficiency, 900
Anergy, 372
Mantoux test and, 669
Aneroid pressure manometer, 583*f*
Anesthesia, 270-277
advantages and disadvantages of various types of, 272*t*
for burn pain, 536
general, 272-275, 273*t*, 274*t*, 275*c*
local or regional, 275-276, 276*f*, 276*t*, 277*f*
moderate sedation and, 276-277
surgical risk and, 246
in total hip replacement, 329
Anesthesia provider, 265
Anesthesia station, 268*f*
Anesthesiologist, 265
Aneuploidy, 68, 403, 407
Aneurysm, 810-814
abdominal aortic, 811, 812
central artery, 810-814, 811*f*
cerebral, 1031-1032, 1033, 1045, 1582
dissecting, 810, 814, 1031
hemorrhagic stroke and, 1031
microaneurysm in diabetic retinopathy, 1469
mycotic, 1031-1032
peripheral artery, 814
ventricular, 758
Aneurysmectomy, 812
Angel dust, 87
Angina, 713*t*, 847-848
atypical, 853
myocardial infarction *versus*, 854*c*
nitroglycerin for, 856
Angioedema, 392, 392*f*
Angiography
in cardiovascular assessment, 722
cerebral, 943, 943*c*, 944*t*
renal, 1546
Angiomax; *See* Bivalirudin
Angiotensin
chronic kidney disease and, 1611
hypertension and, 797
Angiotensin I, 176*t*, 1416, 1529*f*
Angiotensin II, 176*t*, 766, 1416, 1529*f*, 1531
Angiotensin II receptor antagonists
for heart failure, 771-772
for hypertension, 801
for microalbuminuria in diabetes mellitus, 1506
for myocardial infarction, 859-860
Angiotensin-converting enzyme inhibitors
for chronic kidney disease, 1618
for heart failure, 771-772
for hypertension, 801
Angiotensin-converting enzyme inhibitors *(Continued)*
for microalbuminuria in diabetes mellitus, 1506
for myocardial infarction, 859-860
for polycystic kidney disease, 1585
Angiotensinogen, 176*t*, 1416, 1529*f*
Angle-closure glaucoma, 1095*t*, 1095-1098, 1098*c*
Animal-assisted therapy, 10-11
Anion, 183
Anisocoria, 1077
Ankle
arthroplasty of, 335
fracture of, 1197-1198
musculoskeletal assessment of, 1146-1147
positioning for prevention of contracture, 544*c*
Ankle surgery, skin preparation for, 256*f*
Ankle-brachial index
before amputation, 1201
cardiovascular assessment and, 716, 717
in peripheral arterial disease, 806
Ankylosing spondylitis, 355
Annular skin lesion, 471*t*
Annulus, 1110, 1110*f*
Anomia, 971, 975-976
Anorectal abscess, 1337, 1337*c*
Anorectic drugs, 1405
Anorexia
in acute glomerulonephritis, 1591
in acute mountain sickness, 155
in acute renal failure, 1603
in cancer, 415
in chronic kidney disease, 1611
in heat exhaustion, 142
in hookworm infection, 1340
in hypercalcemia, 194
in hyperparathyroidism, 1461
in hypomagnesemia, 196
in hypothyroidism, 1457
in influenza, 658
in leukemia, 904
in lung cancer, 644
in malnutrition, 1392
nutrition history and, 1221
in pancreatic cancer, 1380
in tuberculosis, 669
Anorexia nervosa, 1392, 1426
Anorexins, 1402
Anovulatory dysfunctional uterine bleeding, 1688
Anoxia, 832
ANP; *See* Atrial natriuretic peptide
Antacids
drug interactions with, 1275
for gastritis, 1268, 1268*c*
for gastroesophageal reflux disease, 1246*c*, 1246-1247
for gastrointestinal protection in Cushing's disease, 1444
mechanical ventilation and, 696
for peptic ulcer disease, 1268*c*, 1274-1275
Antalgic gait, 1145
Anterior cerebral artery, 931, 932*f*
stroke and, 1033*c*
Anterior cervical diskectomy and fusion, 990*c*
Anterior chamber, 1071*f*, 1072*f*
hyphema and, 1103
Anterior colporrhaphy, 1694
Anterior communicating artery, 932*f*
Anterior cord syndrome, 992, 992*f*
Anterior cruciate ligament injury, 1206
Anterior exenteration, 1704*f*, 1704-1705
Anterior fornix, 1643*f*
Anterior horn, 932*f*, 933
Anterior inferior cerebellar artery, 932*f*
Anterior myocardial infarction, 862
Anterior nares, 553
Anterior nosebleed, 592*c*
Anterior pectoral nodes, 1644*f*
Anterior pituitary, 1415*f*, 1426-1432
hormones of, 1413*t*, 1415*t*
hyperpituitarism and, 1428*f*, 1428-1432, 1429*f*, 1430*c*, 1431*f*
hypopituitarism and, 1426-1428, 1427*c*
negative feedback mechanism and, 1414, 1414*f*
Anterior segment of eye, 1071*f*, 1072*f*
Anterior spinal artery, 932*f*
Anterior spinocerebellar tract, 932*f*, 932-933
Anterior thoracic landmarks, 561*f*
Anterior tibial artery, 804*f*
Anterior uveitis, 1100
Anterior vaginal repair, 1566*t*
Anterior wall myocardial infarction, 850
Anthracyclines, 1677*t*
Anthraforte; *See* Anthralin
Anthralin, 507
Anthrax, 166*f*, 166-167
in bioterrorism, 454*t*, 455
cutaneous, 503-504
inhalation, 672-673, 673*c*
Anthropometric measurements, 1389-1392
Antiandrogen drugs, 431*t*, 1723
Antianxiety agents
for LSD withdrawal, 87
for pain, 55
preoperative, 261
Antibiotic sensitivity testing, 450
Antibiotic(s), 451
for acne, 515
for acute pancreatitis, 1376
allergic reactions to, 452*c*
antacid interaction with, 1275
antitumor, 421*t*, 422
for brain abscess, 1066
for brown recluse spider bite, 147
for burn infection, 541
for chancroid, 1753
for chlamydial infection, 1747
chronic kidney disease and, 1619
before colorectal cancer surgery, 1298
for corneal infection, 1089
for corneal laceration, 1104
for cutaneous anthrax, 504
for cystitis, 1555-1558, 1556-1558*c*
for diverticulitis, 1335
for empyema, 674
for gastroenteritis, 1320
for gonorrhea, 1746
for granuloma inguinale, 1754
inadequate, 449
for infection, 451
in leukemia, 906
in urolithiasis, 1574
for infective endocarditis, 784-785
for inhalation anthrax, 673*c*
before invasive procedures, 781
for leprosy, 516
for Lyme disease, 356
for lymphogranuloma venereum, 1753
for meningitis, 963
nephrotoxicity of, 1603*t*
for ocular infection, 1086*c*
for osteomyelitis, 1166
for otitis media, 1124
ototoxicity of, 1114*t*
for pelvic inflammatory disease, 1750-1752*c*
for peptic ulcer disease, 1269*c*, 1274
for peritonitis, 1318
for peritonsillar abscess, 657
for pharyngitis, 656-657
for pneumonia, 664-665, 665*t*
for portal-systemic encephalopathy, 1354-1355
for pyelonephritis, 1588
for respiratory infection-related dyspnea in dying patient, 117
for rheumatic carditis, 787
for rhinitis, 654
for septic shock, 843, 843*t*
Antibiotic(s) *(Continued)*
serum sickness and, 395
for sexually transmitted diseases, 1752*c*
for sinusitis, 655
for skin infection, 503
for stomatitis, 1233
for syphilis, 1741
for tonsillitis, 657
for trachoma, 1088
for tropical sprue, 1312
for urinary tract infection, 1556-1557*c*, 1558
Antibody, 316
Antibody test in acquired immunodeficiency syndrome, 373
Antibody-antigen complexes, 314-315, 315*f*
type II cytotoxic reactions and, 394, 394*f*
Antibody-mediated immunity, 313-317, 314*f*, 315*f*
host defense against infection and, 443
immune function changes related to aging and, 308*c*
leukocytes in, 309*t*
macrophages and, 311
white blood cell and, 878, 878*t*
Anticholinergic drugs
for acute pancreatitis, 1375-1376
for asthma, 616*c*, 620
for cholecystitis, 1369
for diverticulitis, 1335
for malabsorption syndrome, 1312
for Parkinson disease, 968
preoperative, 261
for pulmonary secretions in dying patient, 117
for urinary incontinence, 1565*c*, 1567
Anticholinesterases, 1018-1019
Anticlotting forces, 881, 882*f*
Anticoagulation
after stroke, 1043
after total hip arthroplasty, 330-331
after transient ischemic attack, 1030
hematologic assessment and, 884
in hemodialysis, 1622
patient safety and, 819*c*
prevention of injury in patient receiving, 683*c*
for pulmonary embolism, 680, 681*c*, 682*c*
Anticonvulsants
for cluster headache, 954-955
for migraine headache, 953, 953*t*
for multiple sclerosis, 1006
for pain, 54, 54*t*
for pain in acquired immunodeficiency syndrome, 380
for restless legs syndrome, 1024
for seizure in meningitis, 963
for seizure in traumatic brain injury, 1057
for seizures and epilepsy, 957-959, 957-959*c*
for trigeminal neuralgia, 1025
Antidepressants
for Alzheimer's disease, 976
for diabetic neuropathy, 1504
for fibromyalgia, 358
for Guillain-Barré syndrome, 1015
for multiple sclerosis, 1006
for pain, 54*t*, 54-55
for premenstrual dysphoric disorder, 1687
for urinary incontinence, 1565*c*, 1567
Antidiabetic drugs, 1477-1483*c*
Antidiarrheal agents
for irritable bowel syndrome, 1291
for malabsorption syndrome, 1312
for ulcerative colitis, 1324
Antidiuretic hormone, 1415, 1415*t*, 1425, 1530, 1531*t*
changes in older adult, 1419*c*
deficiency of, 1427*c*

Antidiuretic hormone *(Continued)*
diabetes insipidus and, 1432
fluid balance and, 175, 176*f*
hypovolemic shock and, 831
sodium effects on, 184
syndrome of inappropriate antidiuretic hormone secretion and, 435-436, 1433-1436, 1435*t*
Antidysrhythmic drugs, 741-745*c*, 751-753, 752-753*c*
Antiembolism stockings, 258, 822
Antiemetics
for Meniere's disease, 1128
for migraine headache, 952
Antiepileptic drugs
for cluster headache, 954-955
for migraine headache, 953, 953*t*
for multiple sclerosis, 1006
for pain, 54, 54*t*
for pain in acquired immunodeficiency syndrome, 380
for restless legs syndrome, 1024
for seizure in meningitis, 963
for seizure in traumatic brain injury, 1057
for seizures and epilepsy, 957-959, 957-959*c*
for trigeminal neuralgia, 1025
Antiestrogens, 431*t*
Antifungal agents, 451
for corneal infection, 1089
for infection in leukemia, 906
for ocular infection, 1086*c*
for stomatitis, 1233
Antigen, 307
allergy and, 387
leukemia and, 904
oncofetal, 1223, 1224*c*
Antigen-antibody interactions, 313-316, 314*f*, 315*f*
Antiglobulins, 886
Antihelix, 1110*f*
Antihemophilic factor, 881*t*
Antihistamines
for allergic rhinitis, 390
for anaphylaxis, 393, 393*c*
for bee sting, 150
for inflammatory skin disease, 506
for Meniere's disease, 1128
for pruritus, 480
for rhinitis, 654
for tarantula bite, 148
for urticaria, 480
Antihyperlipoproteinemics, 796, 796*t*
Antihypertensive drugs, 801*t*, 801-802
for black widow spider bite, 148
Antiinfective agents, 451
Antiinflammatory drugs
for acquired immunodeficiency syndrome, 380
acute gastritis risk and, 1266
after total hip arthroplasty, 331
for asthma, 617*c*, 618*c*, 620-621
for carpal tunnel syndrome, 1207
for dysmenorrhea, 1685
for endometriosis, 1687
for fibromyalgia, 358
gastrointestinal assessment and, 1219
for gout, 354
heart failure and, 767
hematologic assessment and, 884
for low back pain, 985
for migraine headache, 952, 953*t*
nephrotoxicity of, 1506, 1603*t*
for ocular inflammation, 1086*c*
for osteoarthritis, 326
ototoxicity of, 1114*t*
peptic ulcer disease risk and, 1272
for pericarditis, 786
for postoperative pain, 297-299, 298*c*
for rheumatoid arthritis, 341*c*, 343
Antimetabolites, 421*t*, 422, 1677*t*
Antimicrobial soap, 270
Antiminth; *See* Pyrantel pamoate
Antimitotics, 421*t*, 421-422
Antimyasthenics, 1018-1019
Antineoplastic agents
arterial catheter for, 236
categories of, 421-422*t*, 422
nephrotoxicity of, 1603*t*
Antinuclear antibody
in lupus erythematosus, 347
in rheumatoid arthritis, 339*c*, 339-340
Antiplatelet agents
after percutaneous transluminal coronary angioplasty, 865
after stroke, 1043
for coronary artery disease, 858*c*
for peripheral arterial disease, 807
Antipsychotic drugs, 976
Antipyretics
for fever, 451-452
for rhinitis, 654
Antiseptic handwashing solutions, 444
Antispasmodics, 1558*c*, 1565*c*
Antithrombin III, 882
Antithymocyte globulin, 320, 900
Antithyroglobulin antibody, 1451*c*
Antithyroid drugs, 1452-1454, 1453*c*
Antitumor antibiotics, 421*t*, 422
Antivenom
for black widow spider bite, 148
for coral snake envenomation, 146
for pit viper envenomation, 145
for scorpion sting, 149
Antiviral agents
for corneal infection, 1089
for encephalitis, 965
for facial paralysis, 1026
for genital herpes, 1742-1743
for hepatitis, 1360
for infection in leukemia, 906
for influenza, 658
for stomatitis, 1233
for viral skin infection, 503
Antral irrigation, 655
Antrum of stomach, 1217
Anuria, 1535*t*
in acute renal failure, 1602, 1603
in urolithiasis, 1572
Anus, 1217*f*
abscess of, 1337, 1337*c*
fissure of, 1337-1338
fistula of, 1338
hemorrhoids and, 1309*f*, 1309-1310
Anvil, 1110, 1110*f*
Anxiety
in acute pancreatitis, 1376
in anaphylaxis, 392
in breast cancer, 1671-1672
chest pain and, 713*t*
in chronic kidney disease, 1619-1620
in chronic obstructive pulmonary disease, 633
in coronary artery disease, 855, 860
in head and neck cancer, 604
hearing loss and, 1135
in heart failure, 769
in heat stroke, 142
in hypovolemic shock, 835
massage for, 11, 11*t*
music therapy for, 10
in pelvic inflammatory disease, 1752
postoperative, 293
in premenstrual syndrome, 1685
preoperative, 248, 258-260
in pulmonary embolism, 682-683
relationship with postoperative pain, 249
Anxiolytics
for LSD withdrawal, 87
for pain, 55
preoperative, 261
Anzemet; *See* Dolasetron
Aorta, 705*f*, 706, 706*f*
aging-related changes in, 710*c*
site of inflow and outflow lesions, 804*f*
Aortic arch syndrome, 355
Aortic area, 718*t*
Aortic dissection, 814
Aortic regurgitation, 779*c*, 780
Aortic stenosis, 779*c*, 780
Aortic valve, 705*f*, 706
Aortic valvuloplasty, 781-782
Aortofemoral bypass surgery, 808, 808*f*
Aortoiliac bypass surgery, 808, 808*f*
APAP; *See* Autotitrating positive airway pressure
Aphasia
in Alzheimer's disease, 971, 975-976
in stroke, 1034, 1034*c*
Aphonia in laryngeal trauma, 596
Aphthous stomatitis, 1231
Apical impulse, 717-718, 718*f*
Apidra, 1485*t*
Aplastic anemia, 893*t*, 900
Apo-Acetazolamide; *See* Acetazolamide
Apo-Amitriptyline; *See* Amitriptyline
Apo-ASA; *See* Aspirin
Apocrine sweat gland, 462, 462*f*
Apo-Dipyridamole; *See* Dipyridamole
Apo-Ipravent; *See* Ipratropium
Apokyn; *See* Apomorphine
Apolipoprotein E, 973, 1402
Apo-Lorazepam; *See* Lorazepam
Apomorphine, 967
Apo-Prednisone; *See* Prednisone
Apo-Propranolol; *See* Propranolol
Apoptosis, 66, 400
Apo-Sulfatrim; *See* Trimethoprim-sulfamethoxazole
Apo-Tetra; *See* Tetracycline
Appendectomy, 1317
Appendicitis, 1316*f*, 1316-1317
Appendix, 1219
Approximated wound edges, 481
Apraclonidine, 1099*c*
Apraxia
after stroke, 1034, 1047
in Alzheimer's disease, 971, 975-976
Aprepitant, 429*c*
aPTT; *See* Activated partial thromboplastin time
AquaMEPHYTON; *See* Vitamin K_1
Aqueous humor, 1071, 1072*f*
ara-C; *See* Cytarabine
Arachidonic acid cascade, 312-313
Arachnoid, 929
Aranesp; *See* Darbepoetin alfa
Arava; *See* Leflunomide
Arboviral encephalitis, 964
ARBs; *See* Angiotensin II receptor antagonists
Arcuate artery, 1527*f*
Arcuate vein, 1527*f*
Arcus senilis, 465*f*, 1074, 1075*f*
Ardeparin, 819
ARDS; *See* Acute respiratory distress syndrome
Aredia; *See* Pamidronate
Areflexic bladder, 105, 994
Arformoterol, 629
ARGYLE specimen trap, 663*f*
Aricept; *See* Donepezil
Arimidex; *See* Anastrozole
Arixtra; *See* Fondaparinux
Arizona coral snake envenomation, 145-146, 146*f*
Arm
complications related to intraoperative positioning, 281*c*
intravenous sites in, 216*f*
Arm cast, 1187, 1188*t*
Aromatase inhibitors
for breast cancer, 1677*t*, 1678
for endometriosis, 1687
Aromatherapy
in end-of-life care, 117, 118
in pain management, 12
Arrhythmias; *See* Dysrhythmias
Arrhythmogenic right ventricular cardiomyopathy, 787-790, 788*t*, 789*f*, 790*c*
Arsenic trioxide, 422*t*
Arterial baroreceptor, 797
Arterial blood gases
in acute respiratory distress syndrome, 687
in acute respiratory failure, 685
in asthma, 612
in burn, 532*c*
in cardiovascular assessment, 721
in chronic obstructive pulmonary disease, 626
in Guillain-Barré syndrome, 1013, 1014
in heart failure, 769-770
oxygen toxicity and, 573
in pneumonia, 663
postoperative, 293
in pulmonary embolism, 679
in respiratory assessment, 565*c*
in respiratory disorders, 564
Arterial blood pressure, 728
Arterial catheter, 236
Arterial embolization in infective endocarditis, 784
Arterial partial pressure of carbon dioxide
in burn, 532*c*
normal range for adult, 202*c*
in respiratory assessment, 565*c*
uncompensated acid-base imbalances and, 208*c*
Arterial pulses, 716-717, 717*f*
Arterial puncture, 232*t*
Arterial revascularization, 808
Arterial system, 708-709, 710*c*
Arterial ulcer, 805, 806*c*
Arteriography
in Buerger's disease, 815
in cardiovascular assessment, 722, 722*t*, 723
cerebral, 943, 943*c*, 944*t*
in peripheral arterial disease, 805
renal, 1546
Arteriole, 708
Arteriosclerosis, 793-796, 794*f*, 794*t*, 796*t*
Arteriotomy, 810
Arteriovenous fistula, 1622-1623, 1623*t*, 1624*c*, 1624*f*
Arteriovenous graft, 1623, 1623*t*, 1624*c*, 1625*t*
Arteriovenous malformation, 1032, 1032*f*, 1044*f*, 1044-1045
Arteriovenous shunt, 1623*t*, 1624*c*
Arteritis, 354-355
Arthralgia, 1144
in acquired immunodeficiency syndrome, 380
in ankylosing spondylitis, 355
in growth hormone overproduction, 1429
in hepatitis, 1359
in scleroderma, 351
in serum sickness, 395
Arthritis, 322-361
ankylosing spondylitis and, 355
chronic fatigue syndrome and, 358
disease-associated, 357, 357*t*
fibromyalgia and, 357*f*, 357-358
gouty, 353-354, 354*f*
infectious, 356
lupus erythematosus and, 347-350, 348*c*, 349*f*, 350*c*
Lyme disease and, 356, 356*c*
Marfan syndrome and, 355-356
mixed connective tissue disease and, 358
osteoarthritis and, 323-336
chronic pain in, 326-328, 327*c*
complementary and alternative therapies in, 327-328, 328*c*
health care resources in, 336
health promotion and maintenance in, 324
health teaching in, 336, 336*c*
home care management in, 335-336
imaging assessment in, 325

Arthritis *(Continued)*
impaired physical mobility in, 335, 336*c*
laboratory assessment in, 325
nursing diagnoses in, 325-326
pathophysiology of, 323*f*, 323-324
patient history in, 324
physical assessment in, 324-325, 325*t*
psychosocial assessment in, 325
total elbow arthroplasty in, 335
total hip arthroplasty in, 328-332, 330*c*, 330*t*, 332*c*, 332*f*
total knee arthroplasty in, 333*f*, 333-334, 334*c*
total shoulder arthroplasty in, 334-335
Paget's disease of bone and, 1162-1164, 1163*c*
polymyalgia rheumatica and temporal arteritis and, 355, 355*c*
polymyositis/dermatomyositis and, 354
pseudogout and, 356
psoriatic, 357, 506
Reiter's syndrome and, 355
rheumatoid, 337-347
body image and, 346
complementary and alternative therapies for, 345
diagnostic assessment in, 340
drug therapy for, 340-344, 341-342*c*
fatigue in, 346, 346*c*
gene therapy for, 345
health care resources in, 347
health teaching in, 347
home care management in, 346, 346*f*
laboratory assessment in, 339*c*, 339-340
nonpharmacologic interventions for, 344-345, 345*f*
pathophysiology of, 337, 337*c*
physical assessment in, 337-339, 338*f*
promotion of self-care in, 345-346
psychosocial assessment in, 339
Sjögren's syndrome with, 396
scleroderma and, 351*f*, 351-353, 352*c*
systemic necrotizing vasculitis and, 354-355
Arthritis Foundation, 336, 1164
Arthritis Society in Canada, 1164
Arthrocentesis, 340
Arthrodesis
for back pain, 987
in benign bone tumor, 1167
Arthrogram, 1149
Arthroplasty
elbow, 335
hip, 328-332, 330*c*, 330*t*, 332*c*, 332*f*
knee, 333*f*, 333-334, 334*c*
shoulder, 334-335
Arthropod bites and stings, 146-150, 147*f*, 149*f*, 150*c*
Arthroscopy, 1150*f*, 1150-1151
Articular cartilage, 1141*f*, 1142*f*
osteoarthritis and, 323, 323*f*
Articulation, 1142
Artificial active immunity, 316
Artificial airway
postoperative evaluation of, 287
suctioning of, 583-584, 584*c*
Artificial kidney, 1621, 1621*f*
Artificial menopause, 1645, 1689
Artificial nails
infection control and, 445
preoperative removal of, 260
Artificial passive immunity, 317
Artificial saliva, 396
Artificial skin, 540
Artificial sphincter, 1566*t*
Artificial tears
for keratoconjunctivitis sicca, 1087
for Sjögren's syndrome, 396
Arytenoid cartilage, 554, 554*f*
Asacol; *See* Mesalamine
Asbestosis, 640*c*
Ascabiol; *See* Benzyl benzoate
Ascending colon, 1219, 1294*f*
Ascending colostomy, 1299*f*
Ascending Guillain-Barré syndrome, 1012, 1013*t*
Ascending loop of Henle, 1528*f*, 1530*t*, 1531*f*
Ascending tracts, 931-933
Aschoff bodies, 787
Ascites
abdominal assessment and, 1347-1348
in chronic pancreatitis, 1377-1378
in cirrhosis, 1345, 1350
in pancreatic cancer, 1380
Aseptic meningitis, 961-963, 962*c*, 962*t*, 963*c*
ASKED Model of Cultural Competence, 28, 28*t*
Asmanex; *See* Memetasone
Asparaginase, 422*t*
Aspartate, 930*t*
Aspartate aminotransferase, 1148, 1148*c*
in cholecystitis, 1369
in cirrhosis, 1349, 1349*t*
in gastrointestinal assessment, 1223, 1224*c*
in hepatitis, 1359
Aspergillus in external otitis, 1121
Asphyxiation in drowning, 156
Aspiration
of gastric contents
acute respiratory distress syndrome and, 687
in endoscopic gastrointestinal tests, 1227
in head and neck cancer, 603*c*, 603-604, 604*c*
nasogastric tube and, 291
in oral cancer, 1236, 1236*c*
in vocal cord paralysis, 594, 595
Aspiration biopsy
bone marrow, 889-890, 904
of breast, 1657-1658
endometrial, 1657
Aspiration pneumonia, 665, 1399
Aspirin
after percutaneous transluminal coronary angioplasty, 865
after stent procedure, 866
after stroke, 1043
for coronary artery disease, 858*c*, 859
for pain, 45
for peripheral arterial disease, 807
for prevention of colorectal cancer, 1295
as trigger for asthma, 611
Aspirin-pravastatin, 796
Assay
in endocrine assessment, 1423, 1423*c*
in human immunodeficiency virus infection, 374
in infection assessment, 450
Assist-control ventilation, 693
Assisted coughing
in myasthenia gravis, 1018
in spinal cord injury, 997
Assistive technology, 103
Assistive/adaptive devices, 102-103, 103*t*
for hearing loss, 1132, 1135
Association for Vascular Access, 214
AST; *See* Aspartate aminotransferase
Asterixis
in chronic glomerulonephritis, 1592
in cirrhosis, 1349
Asthma, 610-621
combined ventilatory and oxygenation failure in, 685
drug therapy for, 615-621, 616-618*c*
exercise and activity in, 621
health teaching in, 613-615, 615*c*
history in, 612
laboratory assessment in, 612
Asthma *(Continued)*
occupational, 640*c*
oxygen therapy for, 621
pathophysiology of, 610-611, 611*f*
physical assessment in, 612, 614*f*
smoking cessation and, 614*c*
status asthmaticus and, 621
step system in, 613*c*
subcutaneous infusion therapy in, 237*t*
surgical risk and, 246
Astigmatism, 1073, 1102
Astrocytoma, 1060
Asymmetry of reflexes, 941
Asynchronous pacing mode, 754
Asystole
in hypothermia, 153
in lightning strike, 151
Atarax; *See* Hydroxyzine
Atasol; *See* Acetaminophen
Ataxia
after stroke, 1034
in brain abscess, 1066
in chronic glomerulonephritis, 1592
in high altitude cerebral edema, 155
in multiple sclerosis, 1006
in spinal tumor, 1001
in traumatic brain injury, 1056
Atazanavir, 377*c*, 379
Atelectasis
absorption, 573
in acute pancreatitis, 1373
after brain tumor surgery, 1064
after coronary artery bypass graft, 869
after open conventional esophageal surgery, 1254, 1254*c*
surfactant and, 555
surgical risk and, 246
Atherectomy, 807-808, 865
Atherosclerosis, 793-796, 794*f*, 794*t*, 796*t*
aneurysms and, 811
myocardial infarction and, 849
peripheral arterial disease and, 804
Atherosclerotic plaque, 848, 848*f*
Athlete's foot, 501
Ativan; *See* Lorazepam
Atkins Pyramid, 1387
Atonic seizure, 956
Atopic allergy, 387-394
allergic rhinitis in, 388*f*, 388-391, 389*f*, 390*c*
anaphylaxis in, 391*t*, 391-394, 392*c*, 392*f*, 393*c*
latex allergy in, 394
Atopic asthma, 612
Atopic dermatitis, 505, 505*c*
Atorvastatin, 796, 796*t*
Atovaquone, 379
Atracurium, 274*t*, 535
Atresia of ear, 1120
Atrial dysrhythmias, 740-747
atrial fibrillation in, 745-746, 746*f*
atrial flutter in, 747
drug therapy for, 741-745*c*
premature atrial complexes in, 740
supraventricular tachycardia in, 740-741
Atrial fibrillation, 745-746, 746*f*
in dilated cardiomyopathy, 787
in left-sided heart failure, 769
in mitral regurgitation, 779*c*, 780
in mitral stenosis, 779, 779*c*
Atrial flutter, 747
Atrial gallop, 718-719
Atrial kick, 731, 745
Atrial natriuretic peptide, 175-176
Atrial overdrive pacing, 754
Atrioventricular block, 750
Atrioventricular junctional area, 731, 731*f*
Atrioventricular valves, 705*f*, 706
At-risk drinking, 83
Atrophic gastritis, 1266
Atrophic vaginitis, 1690
Atrophy, 470
in carpal tunnel syndrome, 1207
in myasthenia gravis, 1017
Atropine, 745*c*
preoperative, 261
for sinus bradycardia, 740
for spinal cord injury, 996
Atrovent; *See* Ipratropium
Attenace; *See* Modafinil
Attention, assessment of, 938
Attenuated antigen, 316
Attenuated influenza virus vaccine, 658
Atypical angina, 853, 1245
Atypical migraine, 951
Audio amplifier, 1132
Audiometer, 1117
Audiometry, 1117*t*, 1117-1118, 1131
Audioscopy, 1116
Auditory assessment, 1115-1116
Auditory brainstem-evoked response, 1116
Auditory evoked potentials, 947
Augmentation mammoplasty, 514*t*, 515
Augmentin; *See* Amoxicillin-clavulanate
Aura
in migraine headache, 951, 952*c*
in simple partial seizure, 956
Aureomycin; *See* Chlortetracycline
Auscultation
in abdominal assessment, 1222-1223
for breath sounds, 561-564, 562*f*, 563*t*
in endocrine assessment, 1422
of heart sounds, 718
Autoamputation of distal digits, 352
Autocontamination
burn wound and, 540
in leukemia, 905
Autodigestion, 1265
in acute pancreatitis, 1372, 1372*f*
Autograft for burn wound, 540, 541*f*
Autoimmune disorders, 395-397, 396*t*
ankylosing spondylitis in, 355
chronic fatigue syndrome in, 358
disease-associated arthritis in, 357, 357*t*
fibromyalgia in, 357*f*, 357-358
Goodpasture's syndrome in, 397
gout in, 353-354, 354*f*
Hashimoto's disease in, 1460
infectious arthritis in, 356
lupus erythematosus in, 347-350, 348*c*, 349*f*, 350*c*
Lyme disease in, 356, 356*c*
Marfan syndrome in, 355-356
mixed connective tissue disease in, 358
polymyalgia rheumatica and temporal arteritis in, 355, 355*c*
polymyositis/dermatomyositis in, 354
pseudogout in, 356
psoriasis in, 506-508, 507*f*
psoriatic arthritis in, 357
Reiter's syndrome in, 355
rheumatoid arthritis in, 337-347
body image and, 346
complementary and alternative therapies for, 345
diagnostic assessment in, 340
drug therapy for, 340-344, 341-342*c*
fatigue in, 346, 346*c*
gene therapy for, 345
health care resources in, 347
health teaching in, 347
home care management in, 346, 346*f*
laboratory assessment in, 339*c*, 339-340
nonpharmacologic interventions for, 344-345, 345*f*
pathophysiology of, 337, 337*c*
physical assessment in, 337-339, 338*f*
promotion of self-care in, 345-346
psychosocial assessment in, 339
Sjögren's syndrome with, 396

Autoimmune disorders *(Continued)*
scleroderma in, 351*f*, 351-353, 352*c*
Sjögren's syndrome in, 396-397
systemic necrotizing vasculitis in, 354-355
Autoimmune hemolytic anemia, 893*t*, 899
Autoimmune response, 387
Autoimmune thrombocytopenic purpura, 916
Autoimmunity, 395-396, 396*t*
Autoinoculation, 499
Autologous blood donation, 246, 278, 279*c*, 921
Autologous bone marrow transplantation, 1679
Autologous transplant, 907, 907*t*
Autolysis, 539
Automated external defibrillator, 757, 757*f*
in coronary artery disease, 850
in ventricular fibrillation, 749
Automated peritoneal dialysis, 1628, 1629*f*
Automaticity of heart, 730
Automatisms, 956
Autonomic dysfunction, 1011-1028
cast-related, 1189
chemotherapy-related, 430-431, 431*c*
in facial paralysis, 1026
in Guillain-Barré syndrome, 1011-1016, 1012*c*, 1012*t*, 1013*t*, 1014*c*, 1015*c*
in myasthenia gravis, 1016-1022
community-based care in, 1021*t*, 1021-1022, 1022*c*
electromyography in, 1018
nonsurgical management of, 1018-1020, 1019*t*, 1020*c*
nursing diagnoses in, 1018
pathophysiology of, 1016
physical assessment in, 1-17*c*, 1016-1017
surgical management of, 1020-1021
in Parkinson disease, 966*c*
in peripheral nerve trauma, 1022*f*, 1022-1024, 1023*f*
in restless legs syndrome, 1024
in spinal cord injury, 994
in trigeminal neuralgia, 1025*f*, 1025-1026
Autonomic dysreflexia, 998, 998*c*
Autonomic nervous system, 933
blood pressure and, 708
Autonomic neuropathy, 1470*t*
Autonomy of patient, 5
Autoregulation, vascular, 797
Autosomal dominant pattern of inheritance, 72*t*, 73
Autosomal dominant polycystic kidney disease, 1582-1583, 1583*f*
Autosomal recessive pattern of inheritance, 72*t*, 73*f*, 73-74
Autosome, 68
Autotitrating positive airway pressure, 594
Avandamet; *See* Rosiglitazone-metformin
Avandaryl; *See* Glimepiride-rosiglitazone
Avandia; *See* Rosiglitazone
Avapro; *See* Irbesartan
Avascular burn tissue, 523
Avascular necrosis, fracture-related, 1183
Avastin; *See* Bevacizumab
Avian influenza, 455, 667-668
Avinza; *See* Morphine
Avlosulfon; *See* Dapsone
Avodart; *See* Dutasteride
Avoidance therapy, 390
AVPU mnemonic, 138
Axial images, 1079
Axial loading injury, 991, 991*f*
Axid; *See* Nizatidine
Axilla, positioning for prevention of contracture, 544*c*
Axillary lymph node dissection, 1673
Axillary nerve, 1022*f*
Axillofemoral bypass surgery, 808, 808*f*
Axon, 928, 929*f*
Azacitidine, 435*t*
Azathioprine
for idiopathic pulmonary fibrosis, 639
for immunohemolytic anemia, 899
for psoriasis, 508
for rheumatoid arthritis, 341*c*, 344
for systemic lupus erythematosus, 350
for transplant immunosuppression, 319
Azilect; *See* Rasagiline mesylate
Azithromycin
for chancroid, 1753
for chlamydial infection, 1747
for gonorrhea, 1746
for granuloma inguinale, 1754
for trachoma, 1088
Azo-Dine; *See* Phenazopyridine
Azoospermia, 1728
Azopt; *See* Brinzolamide
Azotemia, 1535*t*
in acute renal failure, 1601, 1603
after pancreas transplantation, 1499
in chronic kidney disease, 1609
Azulfidine; *See* Sulfasalazine

B

Babinski's sign, 940*f*, 940-941
Bacillary dysentery, 1319*t*, 1319-1321, 1321*c*
Bacillus anthracis, 454*t*, 503-504, 672
Bacillus Calmette-Guérin vaccine, 669
Bacitracin; *See* Polymyxin B
Back pain, 983-989
complementary and alternative therapies for, 986
diagnostic assessment in, 985
in growth hormone overproduction, 1429
health care resources for, 989
health teaching in, 988*c*, 988-989
home care management in, 988
in large-breasted woman, 1662
nonsurgical management of, 985-986, 986*c*
in osteoporosis, 1155-1156
pathophysiology of, 984
physical assessment in, 984-985
prevention of, 984, 984*c*
in prostatitis, 1733
surgical management of, 986-988, 987*c*
Backpriming method for infusing intermittent drug, 220*c*
Baclofen
for multiple sclerosis, 1006
for spinal cord injury, 996
for trigeminal neuralgia, 1025
Bacteremia
catheter-acquired, 442
in osteomyelitis, 1166
Bacteria in urine, 1539*t*
Bacterial infection
in acute sialadenitis, 1239-1240
of bladder, 1533, 1551-1559
community-based care in, 1558-1559
drug therapy for, 1555-1558, 1556-1558*c*
laboratory assessment in, 1554-1555
nursing diagnoses in, 1555
nutrition therapy for, 1558
pathophysiology of, 1551-1553, 1552*t*, 1553*c*
physical assessment in, 1553-1554, 1555*c*
prevention of, 1553, 1554*c*
Bacterial infection *(Continued)*
in brain abscess, 1065-1066
chlamydial, 1746-1747
in conjunctivitis, 1087-1088
cutaneous, 499, 500*c*, 501*f*, 502*c*, 503*c*
in cystic fibrosis, 636
in endocarditis, 783-785, 784*c*
in external otitis, 1121*c*, 1121*f*, 1121-1122
in furuncle of ear, 1122
in gastroenteritis, 1319*t*, 1319-1321, 1321*c*
in gonorrhea, 1744-1746, 1745*f*
in HIV-infected patient, 371
in leukemia, 906
in lung abscess, 672
in meningitis, 961*t*, 961-963, 962*c*, 962*t*, 963*c*
in osteomyelitis, 1164-1167, 1165*f*, 1166*c*
in peritonitis, 1317*c*, 1317-1319
in pharyngitis, 655-657, 656*c*, 656*t*
in pneumonia, 659-666
concept map for, 662
health care resources for, 666
health teaching in, 665-666
history in, 660-661
home care management in, 665, 665*c*
imaging assessment in, 663
impaired gas exchange in, 664, 664*c*
ineffective airway clearance in, 664
laboratory assessment in, 663, 663*f*
nursing diagnoses in, 663-664
pathophysiology of, 659, 659*t*
physical assessment in, 661, 663*t*
prevention of, 660, 660*c*
psychosocial assessment in, 661
risk in chronic obstructive pulmonary disease, 633
sepsis in, 664-665, 665*t*
in prostatitis, 1733-1734
in pyelonephritis, 1586-1589, 1587*c*, 1587*f*
in rhinitis, 654
risk in sickle cell disease, 897
septic shock and, 838
in sinusitis, 654-655, 655*c*
skin culture in, 477
in stomatitis, 1231-1234, 1233*c*, 1233*f*
in syphilis, 1738-1742, 1740*f*
in tonsillitis, 657, 657*c*
in toxic shock syndrome, 1691, 1692*c*
in tuberculosis, 668-672
directly observed therapy in, 449
drug therapy for, 670, 671*c*
health care resources for, 672
health teaching in, 670-672
history in, 669
in HIV-infected patient, 372
home care management in, 670
laboratory assessment in, 669
nursing diagnoses in, 669
pathophysiology of, 668, 668*t*
physical assessment in, 669
in vaginosis, 1753
Bacterial overgrowth, 1312
Bacterial transfusion reaction, 921
Bacteriuria, 1551-1552
Bacteroides
in brain abscess, 1065
in sinusitis, 654
Bactrim; *See* Trimethoprim-sulfamethoxazole
Bad death, 112
Bag-valve mask, 136, 137, 137*f*
Baker's cyst, 338
Balance, diagnostic testing of, 1116-1117
Balanced analgesia, 52
Balanced anesthesia, 272, 272*t*
Balanced suspension traction, 1189, 1190*t*
Balanitis circinata, 355
Ballance's sign, 1307
Ball-and-socket joint, 1142
Balloon angioplasty, 1594
Balloon brachytherapy, 1677
Balloon valvuloplasty, 781
Ballottement, 324
Balsalazide, 1324, 1325*t*
Band neutrophil, 310
Bandage
for fracture, 1187, 1187*f*
for stump, 1203*f*
Bandemia, 293, 311
Bar code medication administration system, 215
Barbita; *See* Phenobarbital
Barbiturate coma, 1057
Barbiturate(s)
abuse of, 89
for dying patient, 118
Bard EndoCinch Suturing System, 1248, 1248*c*
Bariatrics, 1046*f*, 1406-1407
Barium enema, 1226
in colorectal cancer, 1296
in diverticulitis, 1335
Barium swallow
in achalasia, 1255
in hiatal hernia, 1249
Bark scorpion, 148-149, 149*f*
Barmine; *See* Dicyclomine
Baroreceptor, 708
aging-related changes in, 710*c*
hypertension and, 797
Barotrauma
mechanical ventilation and, 696
middle ear and, 1126
Barrel chest
in asthma, 612, 614*f*
in chronic obstructive pulmonary disease, 626
Barrett's epithelium, 1244
Barrett's esophagus, 1256
Bartholin cyst, 1699
Basal cell carcinoma
cutaneous, 509, 510*f*, 510*t*
in oral cancer, 1235
Basal ganglia, 929
Basal gastric secretion, 1228-1229
Basal insulin secretion, 1467
Basal metabolic panel, 1375
Basal rate in patient-controlled analgesia regimen, 52
Basal type breast cancer, 1671
Basaljel; *See* Aluminum carbonate gel
Base deficit, 205, 206
Base pair, 64, 64*f*
Basement membrane, burn-related skin changes and, 520, 522*f*
Bases, 200, 201-202
Bases of deoxyribonucleic acid, 64, 64*f*
Basic cardiac life support, 127, 131, 131*t*, 755
Basic disaster life support training, 161
Basilar artery, 932*f*
Basilar skull fracture, 1050
Basilic vein, 216*f*, 217
Basiliximab, 320
Basophil, 311
asthma and, 610
count in respiratory assessment, 565*c*
functions of, 309*t*, 878*t*
Batista procedure, 775
Battle sign, 593
B-cell lymphoma, 914
BCLS; *See* Basic cardiac life support
BCNU; *See* Carmustine
Beau's grooves, 475*t*
Becker muscular dystrophy, 1175, 1175*t*
Beclomethasone, 393*c*
Bed to wheelchair or chair transfer, 100*c*
Bedside bladder scan, 1542-1543, 1543*f*
Bee sting, 149-150, 150*c*
Beef tapeworm, 1340
Behavior
after traumatic brain injury, 1058
in Alzheimer's disease, 971-973, 977, 977*t*

Behavior *(Continued)*
in hypokalemia, 188
premenstrual syndrome and, 1686*c*
Behavioral health, older adult and, 20-22, 21*f*, 22*t*
Behavioral interventions
in obesity, 1405-1406
in reflex urinary incontinence, 1568
in urge urinary incontinence, 1567, 1567*c*
Belching
in cholecystitis, 1368
in gastroesophageal reflux disease, 1245
in hiatal hernia, 1249
Bell's palsy, 1026
Below-knee amputation, 1199, 1199*f*, 1203*f*
Benadryl; *See* Diphenhydramine
Bence-Jones protein, 915
Bench surgery, 1598
Beneficence, 5
Benemid; *See* Probenecid
Benign breast disorders, 1660-1663, 1661*t*
ductal ectasia in, 1661-1662
fibroadenoma in, 1660-1661
fibrocystic breast condition in, 1661
gynecomastia in, 1662-1663, 1663*f*
intraductal papilloma in, 1662
large-breasted woman and, 1662
small-breasted woman and, 1662
Benign cell growth, 399
Benign prostatic hypertrophy, 1712-1718
community-based care in, 1718
concept map for, 1716
drug therapy for, 1714-1715
laboratory assessment in, 1714
nursing diagnoses in, 1714
pathophysiology of, 1712-1713, 1713*f*
physical assessment in, 1713-1714, 1714*c*
prostate cancer and, 1720
surgical management of, 1715-1718, 1717*f*, 1718*c*
Benign tumor
acoustic neuroma, 1129
Bartholin cyst, 1699
of bone, 1167
of brain, 1060*t*, 1060-1061
cervical polyp, 1699
classification by tissue of origin, 405*t*
cutaneous, 508-509, 509*f*
of middle ear, 1126
ovarian, 1694
uterine leiomyoma, 1694-1699, 1695*f*, 1697*c*, 1697*t*, 1698*c*
Benign tumor cell, 402
Benign X-linked dystrophy, 1175*t*
Bentyl; *See* Dicyclomine
Benuryl; *See* Probenecid
Benzathine penicillin G, 1741
Benzocaine-related methemoglobinemia, 568
Benzodiazepines
abuse of, 89
for alcohol withdrawal, 84
for chemotherapy-induced nausea and vomiting, 429*c*
for dying patient, 118
for LSD withdrawal, 87
overdose of, 300*c*
Benzoyl peroxide, 515
Benztropine, 968
Benzyl benzoate, 504
Bereavement, 120
Berylliosis, 640*c*
Beta adrenergic receptors, 1416, 1416*t*
Beta amyloid, 970
Beta cell, 63, 1418, 1418*f*, 1466
Beta globulin, 339*c*
Beta human chorionic gonadotropin, 1728
Beta particles, 418, 418*f*
Beta-adrenergic agonists
for anaphylaxis, 393*c*
for asthma, 615-618
to enhance contractility, 773
Beta-adrenergic blockers
for acute myocardial infarction, 859
for alcohol withdrawal, 84
for coronary artery disease, 857*c*
for glaucoma, 1099*c*
for heart failure, 774
for hypertension, 802
for hyperthyroidism, 1452
for hypertrophic cardiomyopathy, 788
for migraine headache, 953, 953*t*
patient education in, 778*c*
Beta-hydroxybutyric acid, 1474, 1541
Betaloc; *See* Metoprolol
Betamethasone, 1086*c*
Betamol; *See* Timolol
Betapace; *See* Sotalol
Betaxolol hydrochloride, 1099*c*
Betaxon; *See* Levobetaxolol
Bethanechol chloride
for epidural opioid-related urinary retention, 53
for reflex urinary incontinence, 1568
for urinary elimination problems, 106
Betnesol; *See* Betamethasone
Betopic; *See* Betaxolol hydrochloride
Bevacizumab, 435*t*
for brain tumor, 1062
for breast cancer, 1678
for colorectal cancer, 1297
for lung cancer, 645
Bextra; *See* Valdecoxib
Biaxial joint, 1143
Biaxin; *See* Clarithromycin
Bicalutamide, 1723
Bicarbonate, 201, 201*f*
in acid-base control, 202
in acute renal failure, 1605*c*
adrenal gland assessment and, 1438*c*
alkalosis and, 210, 210*f*
chloride shift and, 197
metabolic acidosis and, 206, 208, 208*c*
normal range for adult, 202*c*
in respiratory assessment, 565*c*
uncompensated acid-base imbalances and, 208*c*
Bicaval technique in heart transplantation, 789
Biceps reflex, 940*f*
BiCNU; *See* Carmustine
Bicuspid valve, 706
Bifurcation, 1031
Big block method of heart rate determination, 736, 736*f*
Bigeminy, 738
Biguanides, 1479-1480*c*, 1483-1484
Bilateral adrenalectomy, 1443
Bilateral cutaneous ureterostomy, 1577*f*
Bilateral orchiectomy, 1721
Bilateral salpingectomy/oophorectomy, 1700
Bilateral salpingo-oophorectomy, 1697*t*, 1705, 1706
Bile, 1218
Bile acid breath test, 1311
Bile reflux gastropathy, 1285
Bile salt deficiency, 1311-1312, 1312*c*
Bilevel positive airway pressure, 693
in amyotrophic lateral sclerosis, 1008
in myasthenia gravis, 1018
noninvasive positive-pressure ventilation and, 578
in obstructive sleep apnea, 594
oxygen toxicity and, 573
Bilevel positive airway pressure ventilator, 692-693
Biliary cirrhosis, 1345
Biliary colic, 1368
Biliary disorders, 1366-1385
acute pancreatitis in, 1371-1377, 1372*f*, 1373*t*, 1374*t*
acute pain in, 1375-1376
Biliary disorders *(Continued)*
community-based care in, 1376-1377
complications of, 1373, 1373*t*
history in, 1373-1374
laboratory assessment in, 1374*t*, 1374-1375
pancreatic abscess and, 1379-1380
pathophysiology of, 1371-1373, 1372*f*
physical assessment in, 1374
cholecystitis in, 1366-1371, 1367*f*, 1368*c*, 1368*t*, 1370*c*, 1371*t*
chronic pancreatitis in, 1377-1379, 1378*c*, 1379*c*
gallbladder cancer in, 1371
insulinoma in, 1380
pancreatic abscess in, 1379-1380
pancreatic cancer in, 1380-1384, 1381*c*, 1383*c*, 1383*t*
pancreatic pseudocyst in, 1380
Biliary stent, 1382
Bilirubin
cirrhosis and, 1349, 1349*t*
in gastrointestinal assessment, 1223, 1224*c*
urine, 1539*t*
Biltricide; *See* Praziquantel
Bimanual pelvic examination, 1650, 1650*f*
Bimatoprost, 1099*c*
Biobrane, 540
Biochemical markers for osteoporosis, 1156
Bioclate; *See* Factor VIII cryoprecipitate
Bio-Freeze, 55
Biologic dressing, 494-495*t*
for burn wound, 539*t*, 539-540, 541*f*
Biologic ecology, 31
Biologic heart valves, 782, 782*f*
Biological response modifiers
for cancer, 433*t*, 433-434
for chemotherapy-related anemia, 426
for chemotherapy-related thrombocytopenia, 426-427
for drug-induced immune deficiency, 385
for lung cancer, 645
for rheumatoid arthritis, 342*c*, 343-344
Biologically based therapies, 9*t*, 11-12, 12*t*
Biomarkers
in chemotherapy for breast cancer, 1678
in testicular cancer, 1728
Biomedicine, 8
Biopsy
in bladder cancer, 1576
bone, 1149-1150
bone marrow, 889-890
brain, 1062
breast, 1671
cervical, 1647, 1657, 1657*c*
endometrial, 1700
in head and neck cancer, 598-599
liver, 1360
lung, 569, 644
muscle, 949, 1149-1150
nerve, 949
prostate, 1658, 1720-1721
renal, 1547-1548
in acute glomerulonephritis, 1591
in acute renal failure, 1604
in chronic glomerulonephritis, 1592
in reproductive assessment, 1657*c*, 1657-1658
skin, 477
in discoid lupus erythematosus, 349
in skin cancer, 512
small intestine, 1311
thyroid, 1424
Biosynthetic dressing for burn wound, 540
Bioterrorism, 453-455, 454*t*, 455*t*
Bio-Well; *See* Lindane
BiPAP; *See* Bilevel positive airway pressure
Bipolar limb leads, 732, 733*t*
Bird fancier's lung, 640*c*
Bird flu, 455, 667-668
Birth defects of ear, 1120
Bisacodyl, 107
Bisexual health care, 30*c*, 30-31, 31*t*
Bismuth subsalicylate, 1320
Bisoprolol, 774
Bisphosphonates
for hypercalcemia, 194
for osteoporosis prevention, 1158-1159*c*, 1160
for Paget's disease of bone, 1164
steroid therapy and, 344
Bitemporal hemianopia, 1035, 1035*f*
Bites and stings, 146-150, 147*f*, 149*f*, 150*c*
Bitolterol, 618
Bivalirudin, 818
Biventricular pacing, 746, 774
Black box warning, 1489
Black cohosh, 246*t*
Black eye, 1103
Black lung disease, 640*c*
Black widow spider, 147*f*, 147-148
Blackhead, 515
Bladder, 1527*f*, 1532-1533
cancer of, 409*c*, 1575-1578, 1577*f*
catecholamine receptors and, 1416*t*
female, 1643*f*
infection of, 1533, 1551-1559
community-based care in, 1558-1559
drug therapy for, 1555-1558, 1556-1558*c*
laboratory assessment in, 1554-1555
nursing diagnoses in, 1555
nutrition therapy for, 1558
pathophysiology of, 1551-1553, 1552*t*, 1553*c*
physical assessment in, 1553-1554, 1555*c*
prevention of, 1553, 1554*c*
multiple sclerosis and, 1006
physical assessment of, 1536-1537
trauma to, 1578
Bladder analgesics, 1557-1558*c*
Bladder compression techniques, 1568
Bladder outlet obstruction, 1713, 1713*f*
Bladder scan, 1542-1543, 1543*f*
Bladder training, 105*t*, 105-106, 1047, 1567*c*, 1567-1568
Bladder ultrasound, 105
in benign prostatic hypertrophy, 1714
in spinal cord injury, 998
Blanching of skin
pressure ulcer assessment and, 488
in superficial partial-thickness burn, 522, 522*f*
Blast effect, 136
Blast phase cell, 904
Bleeding
in acute myelogenic leukemia, 910
in chronic kidney disease, 1613-1614
in cirrhosis, 1353*c*, 1353-1354
dysfunctional uterine, 1688-1689
in endometrial cancer, 1699-1700
during hemodialysis, 1625*t*
in hemophilia, 917
in hemorrhoids, 1309, 1310
in idiopathic thrombocytopenic purpura, 916
iron deficiency anemia and, 899
in lower extremity amputation, 1200
nasal fracture and, 591
peritoneal dialysis-related, 1630
postoperative
in bone marrow transplantation, 912*c*
in brain tumor surgery, 1064

Bleeding (Continued)
in coronary artery bypass graft, 868
in glaucoma surgery, 1098
in laryngectomy, 601
in renal biopsy, 1548
in total hip arthroplasty, 330c, 331
in transurethral resection of prostate, 1718
in pulmonary embolism, 683, 683c, 684c
reproductive assessment and, 1648, 1649c
in spinal cord injury, 993
tracheotomy-related, 581
in traumatic brain injury, 1051-1052, 1052f
in uterine leiomyoma, 1695, 1696
in vulvar cancer, 1707
Bleeding precautions, 428c
Bleeding time, 887c, 888
Blenoxane; See Bleomycin
Bleomycin, 421t, 1730
Blepharitis, 1084-1085
Blepharoplasty, 514t
Blind spot, 1071, 1071f
Blindness, 1106c, 1106-1107
after stroke, 1035, 1035f
in diabetes mellitus, 1469
in glaucoma, 1097
preoperative informed consent and, 254
in retinitis pigmentosa, 1102
in trachoma, 1088
Blink reflex, 1072, 1077
Blister
in classification of burn depth, 521t
in frostbite, 154, 154f
in genital herpes, 1742
in pemphigus vulgaris, 516
in toxic epidermal necrolysis, 516
Bloating in gastroesophageal reflux disease, 1245
Blom-Singer Trapdoor prosthesis, 603f
Blood
components of, 877-879, 878f, 878t, 879f
HIV transmission and, 368
viscosity in polycythemia vera, 901
Blood alcohol, 83, 83t
Blood clotting, 879-880, 880f, 881t
anti-clotting forces and, 881, 882f
hypercalcemia and, 194
hypovolemic shock and, 832
Blood coagulation studies, 721
Blood components infusion, 214
Blood culture, 784
Blood disorders, 892-925
hematologic assessment in, 876-891
accessory organs of blood formation and, 879
aging-related changes in hematologic system and, 881, 882c
anti-clotting forces and, 881, 882f
blood clotting and, 879-880, 880f, 881t
blood components and, 877-879, 878f, 878t, 879f
bone marrow and, 876-877, 877f
bone marrow aspiration and biopsy in, 889-890
imaging studies in, 889
laboratory assessment in, 886-889, 887c
patient history in, 882c, 882-885, 883-884t
physical assessment in, 885-886
psychosocial assessment in, 886
hemophilia in, 917
platelet disorders in, 916
red blood cell disorders in, 893-902
anemia in, 893t, 893-898, 894c, 894f, 895f, 897c, 898c
aplastic anemia in, 900
folic acid deficiency anemia in, 900
Blood disorders (Continued)
glucose-6-phosphate dehydrogenase deficiency anemia in, 898-899
immunohemolytic anemia in, 899
iron-deficiency anemia in, 899, 899c
myelodysplastic syndromes in, 901-902
polycythemia vera in, 901, 901c
vitamin B_{12} deficiency anemia in, 900
transfusion therapy for, 917t, 917-921, 918c, 919c, 919t
white blood cell disorders in, 902-916
Hodgkin's lymphoma in, 913t, 913-914
leukemia in, 902-913; See also Leukemia
multiple myeloma in, 915
non-Hodgkin's lymphoma in, 914-915
Blood donation, autologous, 246-247, 278, 279c
Blood flow
acute compartment syndrome and, 1181
before amputation, 1201
in bone, 1141
glomerular filtration rate and, 1529
oxygenation and tissue perfusion and, 827
in portal hypertension, 1345
pulmonary, 556
to site of infection, 839
through heart, 705f, 706
Blood glucose
diabetes mellitus and, 1505
after pancreas transplantation, 1499
diagnosis in, 1474c
hypoglycemia and, 1506-1509, 1507t, 1508c
insulin therapy and, 1485-1486
neuropathy and, 1470
oral blood glucose-lowering agents for, 1477-1483c
retinopathy and, 1469
self-monitoring of, 1490-1492, 1491-1492t
metabolic syndrome and, 853t
preoperative, 1499
septic shock and, 841, 841t, 843
Blood glucose monitor, 1491-1492t
Blood loss
in hemothorax, 699
hypovolemic shock and, 830-831, 831t
Blood osmolarity, 1538
Blood pH, 199
in acute renal failure, 1605c
alkalosis and, 211
Blood pressure, 708
activity intolerance and, 775
after discharge from postanesthesia care unit, 289c
beta-adrenergic blockers and, 774
coronary artery disease and, 854, 854c
dehydration and, 178
glomerular filtration rate and, 1529
in hematologic assessment, 885
hypertension and, 796-804
in acute renal failure, 1603
after coronary artery bypass graft, 868
atherosclerosis and, 794
in black widow spider bite, 148
cardiovascular assessment and, 716
in chronic kidney disease, 1610-1611, 1618
concept map for, 800
coronary artery disease and, 852
diabetes mellitus and, 1468, 1472
in diabetic nephropathy, 1471
diagnostic tests for, 799
drug therapy for, 801t, 801-802
in Guillain-Barré syndrome, 1014
Blood pressure (Continued)
health teaching in, 803-804
heart failure and, 767
heath care resources for, 804
history in, 798
home care management in, 802-803
hypertensive crisis and, 802, 803c
ineffective therapeutic regimen management in, 802, 803c
lifestyle modifications in, 800-801
in nephrosclerosis, 1593
in nephrotic syndrome, 1593
nursing diagnoses in, 799
pathophysiology of, 796-798, 796-798t
peripheral arterial disease and, 807
in pheochromocytoma, 1446
physical assessment in, 798-799, 799f
in polycystic kidney disease, 1584-1585, 1585c
psychosocial assessment in, 799
in renovascular disease, 1593-1594
in scorpion sting, 149
in thyroid storm, 1455
vision changes in, 1075
hyponatremia and, 185
hypovolemic shock and, 833-834
metabolic syndrome and, 853t
normal adult range, 796, 796t
orthostatic hypotension and, 799
alpha blocker-related, 1714-1715
bromocriptine-related, 1431
cardiovascular assessment and, 716
dehydration and, 178
in diabetic neuropathy, 1470
in hypernatremia, 186
in hyponatremia, 185
spinal cord injured patient and, 997
postoperative assessment of, 287
spinal cord injury and, 994
trauma patient and, 136
Blood replacement therapy, 214
Blood sampling
peripheral venous access device for, 888
from peripherally inserted central catheter, 218
before transfusion, 918
Blood tests
in endocrine assessment, 1423, 1423c
in gastrointestinal assessment, 1223-1224
in pulmonary embolism, 682c
in renal assessment, 1537-1538, 1538c
in reproductive assessment, 1652-1654, 1653c
in respiratory assessment, 565c
for syphilis, 1741
Blood thinners, 884
Blood transfusion, 917-921
in aplastic anemia, 900
autologous, 921
in burn, 524
filter in, 221
in hypovolemic shock, 837
indications for, 917t
in leukemia, 911
in myelodysplastic syndromes, 901
older adult and, 919c
pretransfusion responsibilities in, 917-919, 918c
reactions to, 920-921
in septic shock, 844
in sickle cell disease, 897
via peripherally inserted central catheter, 218
Blood urea nitrogen, 1537, 1538c
in acute pancreatitis, 1375
in acute renal failure, 1601, 1605c
in adrenal gland assessment, 1438c
in chronic kidney disease, 1609, 1614
preoperative assessment of, 250c
secondary hypertension in renal disease and, 799
Blood urea nitrogen to serum creatinine ratio, 1538, 1538c
Blood vessels
cancer cell and, 404f
catecholamine receptors and, 1416t
changes resulting from burn injury, 523-524, 524f
cutaneous, 461f
deep partial-thickness burn and, 522-523
of eye, 1072
sympathetic tone of, 827
Blood volume, mean arterial pressure and, 829t
Bloodborne metastasis, 405
Blood-brain barrier, 931
Bloodroot, 246t
Bloodstream infection, central venous catheter-related, 234t
Blumberg's sign, 1223, 1368
Blunt trauma, 136
abdominal, 1307-1308
bladder, 1578
renal, 1596-1598, 1597f
B-lymphocyte
antibody-mediated immunity and, 313-317, 314f, 315f
functions of, 309t, 878t
BMD; See Bone mineral density
BMI; See Body mass index
BNP; See Brain natriuretic peptide
Body cast, 1188, 1188t
Body fluids
burn-related changes in, 524
chemistry of, 201f, 201-202
composition of, 183f
fluid balance and, 174c, 174-175, 175t
particle concentration in, 173-174
pH of, 199
Body image
amputation and, 1201, 1202-1203
bone cancer and, 1171c
burn injury and, 544-545
head and neck cancer and, 604
rheumatoid arthritis and, 346
tracheostomy and, 586
Body mass index
calculation of, 1390
heart disease risk and, 710-711
nutritional screening and, 1389
obesity and, 1402, 1406
Body piercings, 471
Body temperature
after discharge from postanesthesia care unit, 289c
assessment in musculoskeletal trauma, 1184c
burn-related changes in skin and, 520, 520f
coronary artery disease and, 854-855
fever and
in bronchiolitis obliterans organizing pneumonia, 640c
in cholecystitis, 1368-1369
in Crohn's disease, 1331
dehydration and, 179
in food poisoning, 1341
in infection, 450, 451-452, 452c, 452t
in infective endocarditis, 784
in influenza, 658
in inhalation anthrax, 673
in intestinal parasitic infection, 1339
in lung abscess, 672
in meningitis, 961
in pharyngitis, 655, 656c
in pneumonia, 661, 663t
in rheumatic carditis, 787
in rheumatoid arthritis, 338
in scorpion sting, 149
in sepsis, 839
in serum sickness, 395
in severe acute respiratory syndrome, 666

Body temperature (*Continued*)
in systemic lupus erythematosus, 349
in thyroid storm, 1455
in toxic shock syndrome, 1691, 1692*c*
in traumatic brain injury, 1056-1057
in tuberculosis, 669
in ulcerative colitis, 1323
heat exhaustion and, 142
heat stroke and, 142-143, 143*c*
hypothermia and, 152-154
after coronary artery bypass graft, 868
in drowning, 156
postoperative, 288, 299
in spinal cord injury, 994
in syndrome of inappropriate antidiuretic hormone secretion, 1435
trauma patient and, 138
skin role in, 463*t*
Body-based therapies, 9*t*, 11, 11*f*, 11*t*
Boil, 499, 500*c*, 501*f*
Bolus feeding, 1397-1398
Bone, 1140-1142, 1141*f*
cancer of, 1168-1172, 1171*c*
chronic kidney disease and, 1613*c*, 1614
Cushing's disease and, 1441
estrogen changes in older adult and, 1419*c*
fracture of, 1179-1199
acute compartment syndrome and, 1180-1182, 1181*c*
acute pain in, 1192
cast application for, 1187*f*, 1187-1189, 1188*t*
chronic complications of, 1183
classification of, 1179*f*, 1179-1180
crush syndrome and, 1182
emergency care of, 1186, 1186*c*
fat embolism syndrome and, 1182*c*, 1182-1183
health care resources for, 1194
health teaching in, 1194, 1194*c*
hip, 1195-1197, 1196*f*
history in, 1183-1184
home care management in, 1194
hypovolemic shock and, 1182
imaging studies in, 1185
imbalanced nutrition: less than body requirements in, 1194
impaired physical mobility in, 1193*f*, 1193-1194
incidence and prevalence of, 1183
infection and, 1183, 1192-1193
laboratory assessment in, 1185
lower extremity, 1197-1198
mandibular, 593
nasal, 590-591, 591*f*
nursing diagnoses in, 1185-1186
open reduction of, 1190-1192, 1191*f*
osteoporosis-related, 1155
pelvic, 1198
peripheral neurovascular dysfunction and, 1186, 1186*c*
physical assessment in, 1184*c*, 1184-1185
prevention of, 1183
psychosocial assessment in, 1185
rib, 698, 1198
skeletal pin site care in, 1191
stages of bone healing and, 1180, 1180*f*
sternal, 1198
traction for, 1189*f*, 1189-1190, 1190*t*
upper extremity, 1195
venous thromboembolism and, 1183
vertebral, 1198*c*, 1198-1199
growth hormone and, 1415*t*
Bone (*Continued*)
healing of, 1180, 1180*f*
intraosseous therapy and, 238-239
menopause and, 1644
osteomalacia and, 1160-1162, 1161*t*
osteomyelitis and, 1164-1167, 1165*f*, 1166*c*
fracture-related, 1183
halo device-related, 996
intraosseous therapy-related, 239
lower extremity amputation-related, 1200
open fracture-related, 1183
osteonecrosis of
fracture-related, 1183
in osteoarthritis, 328
in systemic lupus erythematosus, 348
osteopenia and, 1143, 1153
osteoporosis and, 1143, 1153-1160
community-based care for, 1160
drug therapy for, 1157-1160, 1158-1159*c*
exercise and, 1157
history in, 1155
hypocalcemia and, 193
imaging studies in, 1156-1157
laboratory assessment in, 1156
lifestyle changes in, 1157
nursing diagnoses in, 1157
nutrition therapy in, 1157
osteomalacia *versus*, 1161, 1161*t*
pathophysiology of, 1153*c*, 1153*t*, 1153-1155
physical assessment in, 1155-1156, 1156*f*
prevention of, 1155
psychosocial assessment in, 1156
surgery for, 1160
overproduction of growth hormone and, 1428
Paget's disease of, 1162-1164, 1163*c*
pathologic fracture of, 1179
in bone cancer, 1168
in chronic kidney disease, 1614
in Cushing's disease, 1444
in hyperparathyroidism, 1462
in Paget's disease of bone, 1163
resorption of
in chronic kidney disease, 1610, 1610*f*
in leukemia, 904
parathyroid hormone and, 1417, 1418*f*
Bone banking, 1192
Bone biopsy, 1149-1150
Bone cyst, 323
Bone graft
in bone cancer, 1170-1171
for nonunion of fracture, 1192
in osteomyelitis, 1167
in spinal fusion, 986
Bone marrow, 876-877, 877*f*
drugs causing suppression of, 883*t*
immune system cells and, 308, 309*f*
Bone marrow aspiration and biopsy, 889-890, 904
Bone marrow harvesting, 907
Bone marrow hypoplasia, 902
Bone marrow suppression, chemotherapy-related, 424-427, 426-428*c*
Bone marrow transplantation
in leukemia, 907*t*, 907-910, 909*f*
in multiple myeloma, 915
Bone mineral density, 1153
Bone morphogenic protein-2, 1154
Bone pain
in multiple myeloma, 915
in osteomalacia, 1162
in osteomyelitis, 1165
in Paget's disease of bone, 1162-1163
Bone remodeling, 1153, 1180, 1180*f*
Bone scan
in musculoskeletal assessment, 1149
in Paget's disease of bone, 1163
in rheumatoid arthritis, 340
Bone spur, 323, 323*f*
Bone tumor
benign, 1167
malignant, 1168-1172, 1171*c*
osteomalacia and, 1161
Boneset, 246*t*
BoneSource, 593
Bone-specific alkaline phosphatase, 1156
Boniva; *See* Ibandronate
Bontril; *See* Phendimetrazine
Bony ossicle, 1110, 1110*f*
ossiculoplasty and, 1134*f*
trauma to, 1126
BOOP; *See* Bronchiolitis obliterans organizing pneumonia
Borborygmus, 1223, 1304
Borrelia burgdorferi, 356
Bortezomib, 435*t*
Bosentan
for primary pulmonary hypertension, 638
for scleroderma, 352
Botulinum toxin, 513
Botulism, 454*t*, 1341*t*, 1341-1342
Bouchard's node, 324
Bowel dysfunction
in chronic and disabling conditions, 106-107, 107*t*
in spinal cord injury, 997-998, 998*c*
in spinal tumor, 1001
Bowel incontinence, 1323
in Alzheimer's disease, 975
in stroke, 1047
Bowel preparation, 254, 1298
in diverticular disease, 1336
for intravenous urography, 1543
Bowel sounds, 1222-1223
in abdominal hernia, 1292
in burn, 531
in colorectal cancer, 1295
in hyperkalemia, 190
in hypokalemia, 188
in intestinal obstruction, 1304
in irritable bowel syndrome, 1290
postoperative assessment of, 290
in viral gastroenteritis, 1320
Bowel training, 107
Bowlegged deformity, 1146
Bowman's capsule, 1528, 1528*f*, 1529*f*, 1530*t*, 1531*f*
Boxer's ear, 1120
Brace casts, 1188*t*
Brace traction, 1189
Brachial node, 1644*f*
Brachial plexus, 281*c*, 1022*f*
Brachial plexus block, 276*f*
Brachial pulse, 717*f*
Brachioradialis reflex, 940*f*
Brachytherapy, 419
in bone cancer, 1169
in endometrial cancer, 1700-1701, 1701*c*
in oral cancer, 1237
in prostate cancer, 1723
Braden Scale for pressure ulcer risk, 486, 487*f*
Bradycardia, 736
in chronic kidney disease, 1619
in hyperkalemia, 190
in hypermagnesemia, 196
in hypothermia, 153
postoperative assessment of, 287-289
sinus, 739*f*, 740
in spinal cord injury, 994, 996
Bradydysrhythmias, 738, 738*c*
prevention of, 759*c*
temporary pacing for, 754-755
Bradykinesia, 965
Bradykinin, 1531*t*, 1532
Brain
abscess of, 1065-1066
herniation in head injury, 1052, 1053*f*
hyponatremia and, 185
pain transmission and, 38, 39*f*
pathophysiologic changes in stroke, 1030
Brain (*Continued*)
in respiratory regulation of acid-base balance, 203, 203*f*
structure and function of, 929-931, 931*f*, 931*t*, 932*f*
traumatic injury of, 1049-1060
brain herniation in, 1052, 1053*f*
closed head injury in, 1050, 1050*f*
community-based care in, 1059-1060
drug therapy for, 1057
fluid and electrolyte management in, 1057
hemorrhage in, 1051-1052, 1052*f*
history in, 1053, 1054*c*
hydrocephalus after, 1052
imaging studies in, 1055
incidence and prevalence of, 1052
increased intracranial pressure in, 1051, 1055-1057
laboratory assessment in, 1055
minor head injury in, 1056*c*
nutrition management in, 1057-1058
in older adult, 1054*c*
open head injury in, 1049-1050
pathophysiology of, 1049, 1049*c*
physical assessment in, 1053-1055
prevention of, 1053
psychosocial assessment in, 1055
sensory, cognitive, and behavioral management in, 1058
surgical management in, 1058, 1059*t*
types of force in, 1050*f*, 1050-1051
Brain attack, 1030-1049
arteriovenous malformation and, 1044*f*, 1044-1045
atrial fibrillation and, 745-746
carotid artery angioplasty with stenting in, 1044
carotid endarterectomy in, 1045
community-based rehabilitation in, 1048
in diabetes mellitus, 1469
diastolic blood pressure and, 797
disturbed sensory perception in, 1047
drug therapy for, 1043-1044
etiology and genetic risk for, 1032, 1033*c*
extracranial-intracranial bypass in, 1045
family history of, 936
health care resources for, 1048-1049
health teaching in, 1048, 1048*f*
history in, 1032-1033
home care management in, 1047-1048
homocysteine and, 795
in idiopathic thrombocytopenic purpura, 916
imaging studies in, 1036
impaired physical mobility in, 1046
impaired swallowing in, 1045
impaired verbal communication in, 1046, 1046*t*
ineffective tissue perfusion in, 1036-1037
in infective endocarditis, 784
intracranial pressure monitoring in, 1037*c*, 1037-1043
laboratory assessment in, 1036
migraine headache and, 952
nursing care plan for, 1038-1043
nursing diagnoses in, 1036
pathophysiologic changes in brain and, 1030
physical assessment in, 1033*c*, 1033*f*, 1033-1035, 1034*c*
prevention of, 1032
psychosocial assessment in, 1035-1036
thrombolytic therapy for, 1037, 1037*c*
types of, 1030*f*, 1030-1032, 1031*t*
unilateral neglect in, 1047
urinary and bowel incontinence in, 1047

Brain biopsy, 949
Brain death, 1056
Brain disorders, 950-982
Alzheimer's disease in, 969-980
caregiver role strain in, 978
chronic confusion in, 974c, 974t, 974-976, 976c
disturbed sleep pattern in, 977-978
health care resources for, 979
health promotion and maintenance in, 970
health teaching in, 978-979
history in, 970-971, 971t
home care management of, 978, 978c
imaging studies in, 973
laboratory assessment in, 973
nursing diagnoses in, 973-974
pathophysiology of, 969-970
physical assessment in, 971-973, 972c, 972f
psychosocial assessment in, 973
risk for injury in, 976-977, 977t
headaches in, 951-955
cluster headache in, 954-955
migraine in, 951-954, 952c, 953t, 954c, 954t
tension headache in, 955
Huntington disease in, 979-980
infections in, 961-965
encephalitis in, 963-965, 964c
meningitis in, 961t, 961-963, 962c, 962t, 963c
Parkinson disease in, 965t, 965-969, 966c, 966f, 967c
seizures and epilepsy in, 955-961
drug therapy for, 957-959, 957-959c
emergency care in, 959-961
management of, 959, 959c, 960c
nursing diagnoses in, 957
pathophysiology of, 955-956
surgical management of, 960-961
Brain herniation syndrome, 1051
Brain natriuretic peptide, 175-176
Brain stem auditory evoked response, 947
Brain tumor, 1060t, 1060-1065, 1061c, 1062f, 1064t
sites of metastasis in, 405t
Brainstem tumor, 1061c
BRCA1 and *BRCA2* gene mutations
in breast cancer, 73, 78, 1647, 1664, 1705
in prostate cancer, 1719
Breakthrough pain, 47-48
Breast, 1660-1683
anatomy of, 1643-1644, 1644f
benign disorders of, 1660-1663, 1661t
ductal ectasia in, 1661-1662
fibroadenoma in, 1660-1661
fibrocystic breast condition in, 1661
gynecomastia in, 1662-1663, 1663f
intraductal papilloma in, 1662
large-breasted woman and, 1662
small-breasted woman and, 1662
biopsy of, 1657-1658, 1671
cancer of; *See* Breast cancer
examination of, 1649
mammography of, 1655
Breast augmentation, 514t, 515, 1662
Breast cancer, 1663-1681
anxiety in, 1671-1672
BRCA1 and *BRCA2* gene mutations and, 73, 78, 1647
breast reconstruction in, 1675, 1676t, 1677c
chemotherapy in, 1677t, 1677-1679
complementary and alternative therapies in, 1672, 1672t
conditions associated with genetic predisposition for, 410t
cultural considerations in, 1664-1665
etiology and genetic risk in, 1664, 1665t
health care resources for, 1681
Breast cancer *(Continued)*
health promotion and maintenance and, 1665-1669
breast self-examination in, 1666, 1667f
clinical breast examination in, 1666-1668, 1667f
mammography in, 1665-1666
options for high-risk women in, 1669
health teaching in, 1679-1680
history in, 1669-1670
home care management in, 1679, 1679c, 1680c
imaging studies in, 1670-1671
incidence and prevalence of, 1664
invasive, 1663f, 1663-1664, 1664f
laboratory assessment in, 1670
in men, 1664
metastasis in, 1672
noninvasive, 1663
nursing diagnoses in, 1671
in older adult, 1668-1669
physical assessment in, 1670, 1670c
psychosocial assessment in, 1670
psychosocial preparation in, 1680-1681
radiation therapy in, 1676-1678, 1677t
sites of metastasis for, 405t
stem cell transplantation in, 1679
subtypes of, 1671
surgical management of, 1672-1675, 1673f, 1675c
in young women, 1664
Breast evaluation form, 1668f
Breast expanders, 1675
Breast reconstruction surgery, 1675, 1676t, 1677c
Breast reduction, 514t
Breast self-examination, 1666, 1667f
Breast-conserving surgery, 1674
Breast-specific gamma imaging, 1670-1671
Breath sounds
auscultation for, 561-564, 562f, 563t
endotracheal tube and, 690
in lung cancer, 643-644
postoperative, 287
in pulmonary embolism, 679
Breathaire; *See* Terbutaline
Breathing
accessory muscles of respiration and, 556
after discharge from postanesthesia care unit, 289c
interventions in trauma nursing, 137, 138t
spinal cord injury and, 993
Breathing exercises, 294
after lung transplantation, 630, 631c
preoperative patient education in, 255, 257c
for urolithiasis, 1573
Breathing pattern
approaching death and, 115c
in burn injury, 535
in chronic obstructive pulmonary disease, 626, 630-631, 631c
in hypothyroidism, 1458
in lung cancer, 643
mechanical ventilation and, 694
in spinal cord injury, 997
in traumatic brain injury, 1054
Brevibloc; *See* Esmolol
Brevitol; *See* Methohexital sodium
Bricker's conduit, 1577f
Bright's disease, 1536
Brimonidine tartrate, 1099c
Brimonidine tartrate-timolol maleate, 1100c
Brinzolamide, 1100c
Brittle nails, 473
BRMs; *See* Biological response modifiers
Broad ligament, 1643f
Broca's aphasia, 1046, 1046t
Broca's area, 930
Bromfenac, 1086c
Bromocriptine
for hyperpituitarism, 1430-1431
for Parkinson disease, 968
Bronchial breath sounds, 562, 563t, 661
Bronchial hygiene, tracheostomy and, 585
Bronchiole, 554-555, 555f, 1416t
Bronchiolitis obliterans organizing pneumonia, 641
Bronchoconstriction in anaphylaxis, 392
Bronchodilators
for asthma, 615-620, 616c, 619c, 619f
for dyspnea in dying patient, 117
Bronchogenic carcinoma, 641
Bronchoscopy
in burn, 535
in lung cancer, 644
in respiratory assessment, 567-568
Bronchospasm
in asthma, 611, 611f
in bee sting, 150
tracheostomy-related, 584
Bronchovesicular breath sounds, 562, 563t
Bronchus, 554, 555f
Brovana; *See* Arformoterol
Broviac catheter, 218
Brown recluse spider, 147, 147f
Brown-Séquard syndrome, 992, 992f
Bruising, 471
in abdominal trauma, 1307
in cirrhosis, 1347
hematologic assessment and, 885
in idiopathic thrombocytopenic purpura, 916
intravenous therapy-related, 228t
in multiple myeloma, 915
in musculoskeletal trauma, 1184
in pit viper envenomation, 144
in uremic syndrome, 1614
Bruit, 717
abdominal, 1223
in abdominal aortic aneurysm, 811
in atherosclerosis, 795
in leukemia, 903
Bruton's agammaglobulinemia, 385
B-type natriuretic peptide, 767, 769
Bubble humidifier, 573, 573f
Buccal mucosa, 1217
squamous cell carcinoma of, 1234-1235
Buck's traction, 1189f, 1190t
Budesonide
for asthma, 620
for Crohn's disease, 1331
for ulcerative colitis, 1324
Buerger's disease, 815
Buffalo hump, 1440, 1440f, 1441
Buffers, 200f, 200-201, 201f
Bulbourethral gland, 1645f
Bulimia nervosa, 1392
Bulk-forming laxatives, 107
Bullae, 469f
in emphysema, 621
Bull's eye lesion, 356
Bumetanide
for hypernatremia, 187
for pulmonary edema, 776
to reduce preload in heart failure, 772
Bumex; *See* Bumetanide
BUN; *See* Blood urea nitrogen
Bundle branch block, 750
Bundle of His, 731, 731f
Bundles for resuscitation in septic shock, 843, 843t
Bunion, 1172-1173, 1173f, 1501f
Bunionectomy, 1172
Bupivacaine
epidural, 52
postoperative, 297
Burch colposuspension, 1566t
Burkholderia cepacia, 636
Burkitt's lymphoma, 914
Burn, 519-549
acute phase of, 537-545
disturbed body image and, 544-545
imbalanced nutrition: less than body requirements in, 543
impaired physical mobility in, 543-544, 544c, 544f
nursing diagnoses in, 537-538
physical assessment in, 537, 538t
risk for infection in, 540-543, 542-543c
wound care management in, 538-540, 539t
classification of, 521t
compensatory responses to, 525, 526f
etiology of, 525-527, 527f
incidence and prevalence of, 527
in lightning strike, 151
pathophysiology of, 520f, 520-525, 522-524f
prevention of, 527-528
rehabilitative phase of, 545-547, 546t
resuscitation/emergent phase of, 528c, 528-537
acute respiratory distress syndrome and, 537
history and, 528, 529c
ineffective breathing pattern and, 535
ineffective tissue perfusion and, 533c, 533t, 533-535, 534f
laboratory assessment in, 531-532, 532c
nursing diagnoses in, 532-533
pain and, 535-536
physical assessment in, 529t, 529-531, 530t, 531f
pulmonary edema and, 536
Burn center referral criteria, 521t
Burn fluid resuscitation formulas, 533t
Burn wound sepsis, 537, 538t
Burr hole, 1058
Bursa, 1142, 1142f
Busulfan, 422t
Busulfex; *See* Busulfan
Butorphanol, 297, 298c
Butterfly rash in systemic lupus erythematosus, 348, 349f
Buttonhook, 103t

C

C cylinder, 579
C fiber, 38
C13 urea breath test, 1267
CA-125 cancer antigen, 1706
Cabergoline, 1430
CABG; *See* Coronary artery bypass graft
Cachexia
in cancer, 415
in malnutrition, 1392
CAD; *See* Coronary artery disease
Caduet; *See* Amlodipine-atorvastatin
Caf[ac]e au lait spot, 73
Caffeine
abuse of, 85
for migraine headache, 952
palpitations and, 747
CAGE alcohol use assessment, 83, 83t
Calan; *See* Verapamil
Calcimar; *See* Calcitonin
Calcipotriene, 507
Calcitonin, 1142
for hypercalcemia, 194
for osteoporosis prevention, 1159c, 1160
for Paget's disease of bone, 1164
Calcium, 191-194
adrenal gland assessment and, 1438c
in body fluids, 183f
bone and, 1142
calcitonin and, 1417
cardiac muscle and, 707
chronic kidney disease and, 1610, 1610f

Calcium (Continued)
in gastrointestinal assessment, 1224c
hypercalcemia and, 193-194, 194t
calcium supplementation-related, 1159
cancer and, 436
cardiovascular assessment and, 721-722
in chronic kidney disease, 1619
in hyperparathyroidism, 1461
in urolithiasis, 1571t
hyperparathyroidism and, 1461
hypocalcemia and, 191-193, 192t, 193f
after parathyroidectomy, 1463
cardiovascular assessment and, 721
in chronic kidney disease, 1610, 1610f
in hyperparathyroidism, 1463
hypomagnesemia and, 196
plasmapheresis-related, 1014c
in thyroidectomy, 1454
imbalance after coronary artery bypass graft, 868
long-term use of proton pump inhibitors and, 1248
normal plasma values for older adult, 184t
osteoporosis and, 1154
Paget's disease of bone and, 1163
parathyroid hormone control of, 1417, 1418f
role in blood coagulation, 881t
serum, 184t
supplementation of
hypercalcemia and, 1159
in hypocalcemia, 193
for osteoporosis prevention, 1158c, 1159-1160
in rheumatoid arthritis, 345
steroid therapy and, 344
twenty-four hour urine collection range and, 1542c
uncompensated acid-base imbalances and, 208, 208c
Calcium carbonate, 1159
Calcium channel blockers
for achalasia, 1255
for acute renal failure, 1607
for atrial fibrillation, 746
for cerebral vasospasm, 1044
for chronic stable angina, 860
for hypertension, 801
for primary pulmonary hypertension, 637
Calcium chelators, 1462
Calcium chloride, 753c
Calcium citrate, 1159
Calcium gluconate, 148
Calcium oxalate stones, 1574t
Calcium phosphate stones, 1574t
Calculous cholecystitis, 1367
Caldwell-Luc procedure, 655
Calf circumference, 1392
Calf pain, 817
Callus, 1174t, 1180, 1180f
CaloMist; *See* Cyanocobalamin
Caloric testing, 1117
Calorie needs
in burn, 525, 543
in chronic pancreatitis, 1379
obesity and, 1405
Calyx, 1527, 1527f
CAM; *See* Complementary and alternative therapies
cAMP; *See* Cyclic adenosine monophosphate
Campath; *See* Alemtuzumab
Campinha-Bacote's ASKED Model for Cultural Competence, 28, 28t
Camptosar; *See* Irinotecan
Campylobacter enteritis, 1319t, 1319-1320
Canada Food Guide, 1387
Canadian Triage Acuity Scale, 132
Canal of Schlemm, 1071f, 1072f
Cancellous bone, 1141, 1141f, 1153
Cancer, 399-439
altered gastrointestinal structure and function in, 415
biological response modifiers for, 433t, 433-434
bladder, 1575-1578, 1577f
bone, 1168-1172, 1171c
breast, 1663-1681
anxiety in, 1671-1672
BRCA1 and *BRCA2* gene mutations and, 73, 78, 1647
breast reconstruction in, 1675, 1676t, 1677c
breast self-examination and, 1666, 1667f
chemotherapy in, 1677t, 1677-1679
clinical breast examination and, 1666-1668, 1667f
complementary and alternative therapies in, 1672, 1672t
conditions associated with genetic predisposition for, 410t
cultural considerations in, 1664-1665
etiology and genetic risk in, 1664, 1665t
health care resources for, 1681
health teaching in, 1679-1680
history in, 1669-1670
home care management in, 1679, 1679c, 1680c
imaging studies in, 1670-1671
incidence and prevalence of, 1664
invasive, 1663f, 1663-1664, 1664f
laboratory assessment in, 1670
mammography and, 1665-1666
in men, 1664
metastasis in, 1672
noninvasive, 1663
nursing diagnoses in, 1671
in older adult, 1668-1669
options for high-risk women in, 1669
physical assessment in, 1670, 1670c
psychosocial assessment in, 1670
psychosocial preparation in, 1680-1681
radiation therapy in, 1676-1678, 1677t
sites of metastasis for, 405t
stem cell transplantation in, 1679
subtypes of, 1671
surgical management of, 1672-1675, 1673f, 1675c
in young women, 1664
cervical, 1700t, 1702t, 1702-1705, 1704c, 1704f
chemotherapy for, 421-431
alopecia in, 428-430
bone marrow suppression in, 424-427, 426-428c
categories of chemotherapeutic drugs in, 421-422t, 422
cognitive function changes in, 430
combination, 422-423
epidural infusion in, 237-238
mucositis in, 428, 429c
nausea and vomiting in, 427-428, 429c
peripheral neuropathy in, 430-431, 431c
side effects of, 423-424, 424c
treatment issues in, 423, 423t, 424c
chronic pain in, 36-37, 37t, 416
colorectal, 1293-1302
anticipatory grieving in, 1296, 1297c
conditions associated with genetic predisposition for, 410t
drug therapy in, 1297
genetic testing for, 76
health care resources for, 1302
health promotion and maintenance in, 1294-1295, 1295c
Cancer (Continued)
health teaching in, 1300-1302, 1301c
hematologic assessment in, 409c
history in, 1295
home management in, 1300
imaging studies in, 1296
inflammatory bowel disease and, 1322t
intestinal obstruction and, 1303
laboratory assessment in, 1295-1296
lower gastrointestinal bleeding in, 1290f
metastasis in, 1296
nursing diagnoses in, 1296
pathophysiology of, 1293-1294, 1294f
physical assessment in, 1295
psychosocial assessment in, 1295
radiation therapy in, 1297
sites of metastasis for, 405t
surgical management of, 1297t, 1297-1300, 1298t, 1299f, 1300c
decreased respiratory function in, 417
development of, 399-413
carcinogenesis and oncogenesis and, 403t, 403-405, 404f, 404t, 405t
classification of, 405t, 405-406, 406f
external factors in, 407-408, 408c, 408t
grading, ploidy, and staging and, 406t, 406-407, 407t
pathophysiology and, 399-403, 400f
personal factors in, 408-411, 409c, 409t, 410t
prevention of, 411t, 411-412
endometrial, 1699-1702, 1700t, 1701c
esophageal, 1255-1261
community-based care in, 1261
history in, 1256
imbalanced nutrition: less than body requirements in, 1257
nonsurgical management of, 1257-1259, 1258c
nursing diagnoses in, 1257
pathophysiology of, 1255-1256
physical assessment in, 1256, 1256c
psychosocial assessment in, 1256
surgical management of, 1259f, 1259-1261, 1260c
fallopian tube, 1709
gallbladder, 1371
gene therapy in, 434
head and neck, 597-606
anxiety in, 604
assessment in, 598t, 598-599
disturbed body image in, 604
health care resources in, 606
health teaching in, 605c, 605-606, 606f
home care management in, 605, 605c
nursing diagnoses in, 599
pathophysiology of, 597-598
psychosocial preparation for, 606
respiratory obstruction in, 599-602, 600t, 601f, 603f
risk for aspiration in, 603c, 603-604, 604c
subcutaneous infusion therapy in, 237t
in HIV-infected patient, 372
Hodgkin's lymphoma, 913t, 913-914
hormonal manipulation in, 431t, 431-432
hypercalcemia in, 436
leukemia, 902-913
conditions associated with genetic predisposition for, 410t
fatigue in, 910-911, 911c
health care resources for, 912
health teaching in, 911-912, 912c
hematologic assessment in, 409c
Cancer (Continued)
hematopoietic stem cell transplantation in, 907t, 907-910, 909f
history in, 903
home care management in, 911, 911c
imaging studies in, 904
laboratory assessment in, 904
nursing diagnoses in, 904
pathophysiology of, 902-903
physical assessment in, 903c, 903-904
psychosocial assessment in, 904
psychosocial preparation in, 912
risk for infection in, 905c, 905-907, 912c
risk for injury in, 910, 910c
liver, 1362
lung, 641-650
hematologic assessment in, 409c
history in, 642-643, 643t
nonsurgical management of, 644-645
palliation in, 650, 650c
pathophysiology of, 641-642
physical assessment in, 643-644
prevention of, 642
psychosocial assessment in, 644
sites of metastasis for, 405t
surgical management of, 645-649, 646f, 647f, 648c
motor and sensory deficits in, 416-417
of nose and sinuses, 592-593
oral cavity, 1234-1239, 1235f, 1236c, 1238c
ovarian, 1705t, 1705-1707
pancreatic, 1380-1384, 1381c, 1383c, 1383t
photodynamic therapy in, 432c, 432-433
prostate, 1719-1725
complementary and alternative therapies in, 1723-1724
cryotherapy in, 1723
drug therapy, 1723
health promotion and maintenance in, 1719c, 1719-1720
health teaching in, 1724-1725, 1725c
heath care resources for, 1725
history in, 1720
home care management in, 1724
impaired urinary elimination in, 1721
laboratory assessment in, 1720
nursing diagnoses in, 1721
pathophysiology of, 1719, 1719f
physical assessment in, 1720
psychosocial assessment in, 1720
radiation therapy in, 1722-1723
surgical management of, 1721-1722, 1722c
radiation therapy for, 418f, 418-420, 419f, 420c
in bladder cancer, 1576
in bone cancer, 1169-1170
in brain tumor, 1062
in breast cancer, 1676-1678, 1677t
in cervical cancer, 1705
in colorectal cancer, 1297
in Cushing's disease, 1443
in endometrial cancer, 1700-1701, 1701c
in esophageal cancer, 1258
in gallbladder cancer, 1371
in gastric cancer, 1281
in head and neck cancer, 599
in lung cancer, 645, 650
in nasopharyngeal cancer, 593
in ocular melanoma, 1106
in oral cancer, 1237
in ovarian cancer, 1706
in pancreatic cancer, 1382
postirradiation sialadenitis and, 1240

Cancer *(Continued)*
in prostate cancer, 1722-1723
in skin cancer, 512
in spinal tumor, 1002
in testicular cancer, 1730
in thyroid cancer, 1461
in vaginal cancer, 1709
reduced immunity and blood-producing functions in, 415
renal cell carcinoma, 1595*t*, 1595-1596
sepsis and disseminated intravascular coagulation in, 435
seven warning signs of, 409*t*
skin, 509-512, 510*f*, 510*t*, 511*c*
spinal cord compression in, 436
stomach, 1279-1287
assessment in, 1280*c*, 1280-1281
chronic gastritis and, 1266
community-based care in, 1286-1287
nonsurgical management of, 1281
pathophysiology of, 1279-1280
postoperative afferent loop syndrome and, 1285-1286
postoperative alkaline reflux gastropathy and, 1285
postoperative dumping syndrome and, 1285, 1286*t*
prevention of, 1280
surgery for, 1281-1285, 1282*f*
upper gastrointestinal bleeding in, 1271*f*
superior vena cava syndrome in, 436*f*, 436-437
surgery in, 417-418
syndrome of inappropriate antidiuretic hormone secretion and, 435-436, 1435*t*
targeted therapy in, 434, 435*t*
testicular, 1726*c*, 1726-1730, 1727*t*, 1728*c*, 1729*c*
thyroid, 1460-1461
tumor lysis syndrome in, 437, 437*f*
vaginal, 1708-1709
vulvar, 1707-1708, 1708*f*
Cancer cell, 403
Cancer control surgery, 417
Candida albicans, 500*c*, 501
in HIV-infected patient, 371
oral, 1232, 1233*f*
urinary tract, 1552, 1587
vaginal, 1753
in vulvovaginitis, 1690-1691, 1691*c*
Cane, 1194
Cane assisted gait training, 101*c*
Canertinib, 435*t*
Canker sore, 1231-1234, 1233*c*, 1233*f*
Canthus, 1072
CAPD; *See* Continuous ambulatory peritoneal dialysis
Capecitabine, 421*t*
for breast cancer, 1678
for colorectal cancer, 1297
for pancreatic cancer, 1382
Capillary
filtration and, 172, 172*f*
osmosis and, 174
Capillary closing pressure, 486
Capillary filling time, 794-795
Capillary fragility test, 888
Capillary leak syndrome, 523-524, 524*f*, 830
Capillary refill
in hypovolemic shock, 835
in musculoskeletal assessment, 1184*c*
Capital hip fracture, 1196*f*
Caplan's syndrome, 339
Capnography, 566
Capnometry, 566, 1399
Capsaicin
after total knee arthroplasty, 333
for osteoarthritis, 327-328
Captopril, 801
Captopril renal scan, 1546
Carafate; *See* Sucralfate
Carbachol, 1099*c*
Carbamazepine, 957*c*
for multiple sclerosis, 1006
for pain in acquired immunodeficiency syndrome, 380
for restless legs syndrome, 1024
for trigeminal neuralgia, 1025
Carbatrol; *See* Carbamazepine
Carbohydrate antigen 19-9, 1225*c*
Carbohydrate counting, 1494-1495, 1495*t*
Carbohydrate(s)
exchange system for, 1494*t*
intake in diabetes mellitus, 1493
metabolism of
carbon dioxide and, 201-202
liver role in, 1218
Carbon dioxide
carbonic acid and, 201
preoperative assessment of, 250*c*
relationship with hydrogen ions, 201
Carbon dioxide narcosis, 573
Carbon dioxide partial pressure
normal range for adult, 202*c*
uncompensated acid-base imbalances and, 208*c*
Carbon monoxide poisoning, 529-530, 530*t*
Carbonic acid, 201, 201*f*
Carbonic anhydrase, 201
Carbonic anhydrase inhibitors, 1100*c*
Carboplatin, 422*t*
for cervical cancer, 1705
for esophageal cancer, 1257
for fallopian tube cancer, 1709
for ovarian cancer, 1706
Carboptic; *See* Carbachol
Carboxyhemoglobin
burn assessment and, 532*c*
smoking and, 246
Carcinoembryonic antigen, 1225*c*
in colorectal cancer, 1295-1296
in pancreatic cancer, 1380
Carcinogen, 403, 404*t*, 1294
Carcinogenesis, 403*t*, 403-405, 404*f*, 404*t*, 405*t*
Carcinoma-in-situ, cervical, 1702
Cardiac arrest
in anaphylaxis, 392
cardiopulmonary resuscitation for, 755
drug therapy for, 752-753*c*
in hypothermia, 153-154
in lightning strike, 151
spinal anesthesia and, 276
in status asthmaticus, 621
ventricular asystole and, 750
ventricular tachycardia and, 748
Cardiac assessment; *See* Cardiovascular assessment
Cardiac axis, 732, 732*f*
Cardiac blood pool imaging, 726
Cardiac care, 751, 751*c*, 861*c*
Cardiac catheterization, 722*t*, 722-724, 723*f*, 855
Cardiac cirrhosis, 1345
Cardiac conduction system, 731, 731*f*
Cardiac cycle, 706-707, 707*f*
Cardiac disease; *See* Heart disease
Cardiac drugs
classification of, 771*t*
to enhance contractility, 773-774
to reduce afterload, 771-772
to reduce preload, 772-773
Cardiac dysrhythmias, 730-763
advanced cardiac life support for, 756
after coronary artery bypass graft, 868
after thoracic aortic aneurysm repair, 813
in anaphylaxis, 392
atrial, 740-747
atrial fibrillation in, 745-746, 746*f*
atrial flutter in, 747
drug therapy for, 741-745*c*
premature atrial complexes in, 740
Cardiac dysrhythmias *(Continued)*
supraventricular tachycardia in, 740-741
atrioventricular blocks in, 750
automatic external defibrillation for, 757, 757*f*
in bee sting, 150
bundle branch blocks in, 750
cardiac conduction system and, 731, 731*f*
in cardiomyopathy, 789
cardiopulmonary resuscitation in, 755-756
cardioversion for, 756
in chronic obstructive pulmonary disease, 623
coronary artery bypass graft for, 758
decreased cardiac output and ineffective tissue perfusion in, 750-751, 751*c*
defibrillation for, 756-757
in digitalis toxicity, 773
drug therapy for, 751-753, 752-753*c*
electrocardiography and, 731-737, 732*f*
complexes, segments, and intervals in, 733-736, 735*f*
continuous electrocardiographic monitoring and, 732-733, 734*f*
determination of heart rate in, 736, 736*f*
heart rhythm analysis in, 736-737
lead systems for, 732, 733*t*
electrophysiologic properties of heart and, 730-731, 731*f*
health teaching in, 758-761, 759-761*c*
home care management in, 758
in hypercalcemia, 194
in hypothermia, 153
junctional, 747
key features of, 738*c*
in Lyme disease, 356
in malignant hyperthermia, 273
normal rhythms and, 737*f*, 737-738
nursing diagnoses in, 750
pacemaker insertion for, 757
radiofrequency catheter ablation for, 757
sinus, 739*f*, 739-740
temporary pacing for, 754-755
terminology in, 738-739
vagal maneuvers for, 753-754
ventricular, 747-750, 748*f*, 749*f*
Cardiac electrophysiology, 730-731, 731*f*
Cardiac enzymes, 720*c*, 720-721
Cardiac glycosides, 1606*c*
Cardiac index, 707
Cardiac markers in myocardial infarction, 855
Cardiac monitoring
in hypercalcemia, 194
in hyperkalemia, 191
in lightning strike, 152
postoperative, 288-289
in brain tumor surgery, 1063
in pancreas transplantation, 1500
Cardiac muscle, 706, 707, 1143
Cardiac output, 707
blood pressure and, 708
in burn, 524, 533*c*, 533*t*, 534*f*, 534-535
in chronic kidney disease, 1618
dysrhythmias and, 750-751, 751*c*
heart failure and, 765-767, 766*f*, 770-775, 771*t*, 774*f*
of heart transplant recipient, 790
hemodynamic monitoring of, 728
in hyponatremia, 185
in hypothermia, 153
hypothyroidism and, 1458
in left-sided heart failure, 769
in pulmonary embolism, 682
in septic shock, 841, 841*t*
in severe sepsis, 840
Cardiac rehabilitation, 860, 861*c*, 870
Cardiac resynchronization therapy, 774
Cardiac sphincter, 1218
Cardiac surgical-critical care unit, 866
Cardiac tamponade
after coronary artery bypass graft, 868-869
in pericarditis, 786
Cardiac valves, 705*f*, 706, 710*c*
Cardinal ligament, 1643*f*
Cardinal positions of gaze, 1078*f*, 1078-1079
Cardiogenic shock, 828, 828*t*
causes of, 830*c*
in coronary artery disease, 862-863
risk factors in older adult, 841*c*
Cardiomegaly, 787
Cardiomyopathy, 787-790, 788*t*, 789*f*, 790*c*
Cardiopulmonary bypass
in coronary artery bypass graft, 867, 867*f*
in hypothermia, 153
Cardiopulmonary resuscitation
advance directive and, 113
in anaphylaxis, 393
in cardiac arrest, 755
in drowning, 157
end-of-life care and, 112
in idioventricular rhythms, 747
in lightning strike, 152
training and certification in, 131, 131*t*
in ventricular asystole, 750
in ventricular fibrillation, 749
Cardioselective beta blockers, 802
Cardiovascular assessment, 704-729
after stroke, 1035
arterial system and, 708-709
in burn, 530, 537
cardiac catheterization in, 722*t*, 722-724, 723*f*
changes associated with aging, 709, 710*c*
echocardiography in, 725
electrocardiography in, 724
electronic-beam computed tomography scan in, 726
electrophysiologic studies in, 724
heart structure and function in, 704-708, 705-707*f*
of heart transplant recipient, 790
in hematologic disorders, 885
hemodynamic monitoring in, 726-728, 727*c*, 727*f*
laboratory assessment in, 719-722, 720*c*
magnetic resonance imaging in, 726
myocardial nuclear perfusion imaging in, 725-726
patient history in, 709-714
current health problems in, 712-714, 713*t*
family history and genetic risk in, 712
functional history in, 714, 714*t*
Gordon's Functional Health Patterns and, 711*c*
nutrition history in, 712
physical assessment in, 714-719
blood pressure and, 716
extremities and, 715, 715*f*
general appearance and, 714
precordium and, 717-719, 718*f*, 719*t*
skin and, 715
venous and arterial pulses and, 716-717, 717*f*
preoperative, 247
psychosocial assessment in, 719
rehabilitation and, 97, 97*t*
in spinal cord injury, 994
stress test in, 724-725
transesophageal echocardiography in, 725
venous system and, 709
Cardiovascular disease, 793-825
acute peripheral arterial occlusion in, 810

Cardiovascular disease *(Continued)*
aneurysms in, 810-814
of central arteries, 810-814, 811*f*
of peripheral arteries, 814
aortic dissection in, 814
arteriosclerosis and atherosclerosis in, 793-796, 794*f*, 794*t*, 796*t*
Buerger's disease in, 815
in diabetes mellitus, 1468-1469
hypertension in, 796-804
cardiovascular assessment and, 716
concept map for, 800
diagnostic tests for, 799
drug therapy for, 801*t*, 801-802
health teaching in, 803-804
heart failure and, 767
heath care resources for, 804
history in, 798
home care management in, 802-803
ineffective therapeutic regimen management in, 802, 803*c*
lifestyle modifications in, 800-801
nursing diagnoses in, 799
pathophysiology of, 796-798, 796-798*t*
physical assessment in, 798-799, 799*f*
psychosocial assessment in, 799
peripheral arterial disease in, 804-810
community-based care in, 809*c*, 809-810, 810*c*
diagnostic tests for, 805-806
drug therapy for, 807
pathophysiology of, 804, 804*f*
physical assessment in, 805, 805*c*, 806*c*
surgical management of, 808*f*, 808-809
peripheral venous disease in, 816-823
phlebitis in, 823
varicose veins in, 822-823
vascular trauma in, 823
venous insufficiency in, 821-822, 822*c*
venous thromboembolism in, 816-821, 817*f*, 819*c*, 821*c*
popliteal entrapment in, 816
Raynaud's phenomenon in, 815-816, 816*f*
subclavian steal in, 815
thoracic outlet syndrome in, 815
Cardiovascular system
acidosis and, 207, 207*c*
adrenal insufficiency and, 1437*c*
age-related surgical risks and, 245*c*
alkalosis and, 210-211, 211*c*
anemia and, 894*c*
cirrhosis and, 1348*f*
complications of surgery and, 287*t*
esophageal surgery and, 1260
preventive procedures and exercises for, 258, 259*f*
Whipple procedure and, 1383*t*
Cushing's disease and, 1441*c*
dehydration and, 178
diabetes insipidus and, 1433*c*
fluid overload and, 182*c*
hypercalcemia and, 194
hyperkalemia and, 190
hypermagnesemia and, 196
hypernatremia and, 186
hyperthyroidism and, 1449*c*
hypocalcemia and, 192
hypokalemia and, 188
hyponatremia and, 185
hypophosphatemia and, 195
hypothyroidism and, 1456*c*
immobility and, 102*t*
infusion therapy and, 235-236
leukemia and, 903, 903*c*
Marfan syndrome and, 356
nutrient deficiencies and, 1394*t*
nutrition screening assessment and, 1390*c*
shock and, 829*c*
sickle cell disease and, 895
Cardioversion, 756
for atrial fibrillation, 746
for atrial flutter, 747
for ventricular tachycardia, 748
Carditis, 356
Cardizem; *See* Diltiazem
Cardura; *See* Doxazosin
Caregiver role of nurse, 4
Caregiver support
in Alzheimer's disease, 978, 978*c*
elder neglect and abuse and, 22*c*
Carina, 554, 555*f*, 689-690, 690*f*
Carmustine, 422*t*
for brain tumor, 1062
for spinal tumor, 1002
Carotid artery
palpation in atherosclerosis, 794-795
rupture after laryngectomy, 601
Carotid artery angioplasty with stenting, 1044
Carotid artery bruit, 717
Carotid endarterectomy, 1045
Carotid pulse, 717*f*
Carotid sinus massage, 754
Carpal tunnel syndrome, 1206-1207
Carpal(s), 1147*f*
Carpentier-Edwards pericardial bioprosthesis, 782*f*
Carrier, 73-74, 441
Carrier testing, 75*t*
Carteolol, 1099*c*
Cartrol; *See* Carteolol
Carvedilol
for acute myocardial infarction, 859
for coronary artery disease, 857*c*
for heart failure, 774
for hypertrophic cardiomyopathy, 789
Case management, 5
in acute respiratory distress syndrome, 689
in emergency nursing, 133-134
Case manager, 5
Caseation necrosis in tuberculosis, 668
Casodex; *See* Bicalutamide
Cast, renal, 1539*t*, 1541
Cast application for fracture, 1187*f*, 1187-1189, 1188*t*
Cast brace, 1188, 1188*t*
Cast syndrome, 1188
Catabolism, burn-related, 525
Catapres; *See* Clonidine
Cataract, 1074, 1091*f*, 1091-1095, 1092*f*, 1092*t*, 1094*f*, 1095*c*
Catechol O-methyltransferases, 968
Catecholamines, 930*t*, 1416-1417
Catheter
arterial, 236
dual-lumen hemodialysis, 1623*t*
epistaxis, 592, 592*f*
in infusion therapy
blood sampling from, 225
confirming tip location of, 222
controlling infusion pressure and, 224
flushing of, 224-225
older adult and, 235, 236*f*
removal of, 225
securing and dressing of, 223*f*, 223-224, 224*f*
preoperative preparation for, 255
subclavian dialysis, 1607*f*, 1607-1608
Catheter embolism in intravenous therapy, 230*t*
Catheter infection, 442
blood sampling and, 225
central venous catheter and, 234*t*
in epidural analgesia, 52
urinary tract, 1552, 1553*c*
Catheterized urine specimen, 1540*t*
Cation, 183
Cauda equina syndrome, 992, 992*f*
Cauliflower ear, 1120
CAVH; *See* Continuous arteriovenous hemofiltration
CAVHD; *See* Continuous arteriovenous hemodialysis and filtration
CCNU; *See* Lomustine
CCP; *See* Chronic calcifying pancreatitis
CD16+ cell, 317
CD4+ T-cell, 363, 363*f*
CD4+ T-cell count, 364, 365*t*, 373
CD8+ T-cell count, 373
CEA; *See* Carcinoembryonic antigen
Cecum, 1219
CeeNU; *See* Lomustine
Cefadroxil, 1557*c*
Cefixime
for gonorrhea, 1746
for urinary tract infection, 1557*c*
Cefotan; *See* Cefotetan
Cefotetan, 1750*c*
Cefoxitin, 1750*c*, 1751*c*
Ceftazidime, 1376
Ceftin; *See* Cefuroxime
Ceftriaxone
for chancroid, 1753
for gonorrhea, 1746
for pelvic inflammatory disease, 1750*c*
Cefuroxime
for acute pancreatitis, 1376
for Lyme disease, 356
Celebrex; *See* Celecoxib
Celecoxib
for heterotopic ossification, 996
for osteoarthritis, 326
for pain, 46
for rheumatoid arthritis, 343
Celexa; *See* Citalopram
Celiac sprue, 1311
Cell
abnormal, 402*t*, 402-403
anatomy of, 63, 63*f*
division of, 65*f*, 65-66, 66*f*
malignant transformation of, 403*t*, 403-405, 404*f*, 405*t*
normal, 400*f*, 400-402, 402*f*
self *versus* non-self and, 307*f*, 307-308, 308*c*, 308*f*
Cell cycle, 65-66, 65-68*f*, 400-401, 401*f*
Cell membrane, 63*f*
fluid and electrolyte balance and, 171-174
diffusion and, 172*f*, 172-173
filtration and, 171*f*, 171-172, 172*f*
lymph and, 174
osmosis and, 173*f*, 173-174
self *versus* non-self and, 307*f*, 307-308, 308*c*, 308*f*
CellCept; *See* Mycophenolate
Cell-mediated immunity, 317-320, 318*f*, 318*t*
host defense against infection and, 443
immune function changes related to aging and, 308*c*
leukocytes in, 309*t*
macrophages and, 311
tuberculosis and, 668
white blood cell and, 878, 878*t*
Cellular immunity, 317
Cellulitis, 499, 500*c*
in mastoiditis, 1125
pressure ulcer and, 489-490
Centers for Disease Control and Prevention transmission-based guidelines, 446*t*, 446-449, 447*t*
Central alpha agonists, 802
Central axillary nodes, 1644*f*
Central chemoreceptor, 708
Central cord syndrome, 992, 992*f*
Central cyanosis, 715
Central herniation, 1052, 1053*f*
Central intravenous therapy, 217-219, 218*f*, 219*f*
blood sampling from central venous catheter and, 225
catheter removal in, 225
complications of
during dwell of catheter, 232-234*t*
insertion-related, 231-232*t*
Central nervous system, 929-933
acidosis and, 207, 207*c*
alkalosis and, 210, 211*c*
brain in, 929-931, 931*f*, 931*t*, 932*f*
hypermagnesemia and, 196
hypomagnesemia and, 196
hypophosphatemia and, 195
lightning strike and, 151
negative feedback mechanism and, 1414
in respiratory regulation of acid-base balance, 203, 203*f*
spinal cord in, 931-933, 932*f*
Central nervous system problems, 950-1010
Alzheimer's disease in, 969-980
caregiver role strain in, 978
chronic confusion in, 974*c*, 974*t*, 974-976, 976*c*
disturbed sleep pattern in, 977-978
health care resources for, 979
health promotion and maintenance in, 970
health teaching in, 978-979
history in, 970-971, 971*t*
home care management of, 978, 978*c*
imaging studies in, 973
laboratory assessment in, 973
nursing diagnoses in, 973-974
pathophysiology of, 969-970
physical assessment in, 971-973, 972*c*, 972*f*
psychosocial assessment in, 973
risk for injury in, 976-977, 977*t*
amyotrophic lateral sclerosis in, 1007*c*, 1007-1008
back pain in, 983-989
complementary and alternative therapies for, 986
diagnostic assessment in, 985
health care resources for, 989
health teaching in, 988*c*, 988-989
home care management in, 988
nonsurgical management of, 985-986, 986*c*
pathophysiology of, 984
physical assessment in, 984-985
prevention of, 984, 984*c*
surgical management of, 986-988, 987*c*
cervical neck pain in, 989*f*, 989-990, 990*c*
headaches in, 951-955
cluster headache in, 954-955
migraine in, 951-954, 952*c*, 953*t*, 954*c*, 954*t*
tension headache in, 955
Huntington disease in, 979-980
infections in, 961-965
encephalitis in, 963-965, 964*c*
meningitis in, 961*t*, 961-963, 962*c*, 962*t*, 963*c*
multiple sclerosis in, 1002-1007, 1003*c*
Parkinson disease in, 965*t*, 965-969, 966*c*, 966*f*, 967*c*
seizures and epilepsy in, 955-961
drug therapy for, 957-959, 957-959*c*
emergency care in, 959-961
management of, 959, 959*c*, 960*c*
nursing diagnoses in, 957
pathophysiology of, 955-956
surgical management of, 960-961
spinal cord injury in, 990-1000
etiology of, 992-993
extent of injury in, 991-992, 992*f*
health care resources for, 1000
health teaching in, 999*c*, 999-1000, 1000*c*
history in, 993
home care management in, 999
imaging studies in, 994-995
impaired adjustment in, 998
impaired elimination in, 997-998, 998*c*

Central nervous system problems *(Continued)*
impaired gas exchange in, 997
ineffective tissue perfusion in, 995*c*, 995-997, 996*f*
laboratory assessment in, 994
mechanisms of injury in, 990-991, 991*f*
nursing diagnoses in, 995
physical assessment in, 993-994, 994*c*
psychosocial assessment in, 994
self-care deficit in, 997
spinal cord tumor in, 1000-1002, 1001*c*
Central obesity, 1402
Central venous catheter
in acute renal failure, 1605
home care of, 911*c*
in hypovolemic shock, 838
risk for infection and, 442
Centrilobular emphysema, 611*f*, 622
Centriole, 63*f*
Centroacinar emphysema, 611*f*
Centromere, 66, 67*f*
Cephalic vein for intravenous access, 216*f*, 217
Cephalosporins
for acute pancreatitis, 1376
for chancroid, 1753
for gonorrhea, 1746
for infection in urolithiasis, 1574
for Lyme disease, 356
for pelvic inflammatory disease, 1750*c*
for urinary tract infection, 1557*c*
Ceptaz; *See* Ceftazidime
Cerebellar abscess, 1066
Cerebellar function
after lightning strike, 151
assessment of, 940
Cerebellar pontine angle tumor, 1061
Cerebellum, 930
Cerebral abscess, 1065-1066
Cerebral aneurysm, 1031-1032, 1033, 1045
in polycystic kidney disease, 1582
Cerebral angiography, 943, 943*c*, 944*t*
Cerebral blood flow evaluation, 946
Cerebral circulation, 932*f*
Cerebral edema
in brain tumor, 1060
high-altitude, 154-156, 156*c*
in traumatic brain injury, 1051
Cerebral function assessment, 289*t*, 289-290
Cerebral hemisphere, 929
Cerebral infarction
in lightning strike, 151
in stroke, 1030
Cerebral perfusion
heart failure and, 767
stroke and, 1036-1037
Cerebral perfusion pressure, 1051
Cerebral salt wasting, 1065
Cerebral tumor, 1060*t*, 1060-1065, 1061*c*, 1062*f*, 1064*t*
Cerebral vasospasm, 1043-1044
Cerebrospinal fluid, 931
hydrocephalus and, 1044
lumbar puncture and, 947-949, 948*t*
traumatic brain injury and, 1049
Cerebrospinal fluid analysis
in encephalitis, 964
in Guillain-Barré syndrome, 1013
in meningitis, 962, 962*t*
in multiple sclerosis, 1004
Cerebrospinal fluid leak
after hypophysectomy, 1431
after lumbar spinal surgery, 987*c*
in nasal fracture, 591
in traumatic brain injury, 1056
Cerebrum, 929-930
Cerebyx; *See* Fosphenytoin
Cerespan; *See* Papaverine
CERT; *See* Community Emergency Response Team
Certican; *See* Everolimus
Certification in emergency nursing, 131, 131*t*
Certified diabetic educator, 1379
Certified in infection control, 444
Certified registered nurse anesthetist, 265, 270-271
Certified registered nurse first assistant, 265
Certified registered nurse infusion, 214
Cerubidine; *See* Daunorubicin
Cerumen, 1109
changes with aging, 1112*c*
cultural considerations and, 1115
impaction of, 1122*f*, 1122-1123, 1123*c*
self-ear irrigation for, 1113*c*
Cervical biopsy, 1647, 1657*c*
Cervical cancer, 1700*t*, 1702*t*, 1702-1705, 1704*c*, 1704*f*
Cervical chordotomy, 58*f*
Cervical culture, 1654
Cervical diskectomy and fusion, 990*c*
Cervical halter, 1190*t*
Cervical intraepithelial neoplasia, 1702
Cervical lymph nodes, 1235*f*
oral cancer metastasis to, 1238
Cervical neck pain, 989*f*, 989-990, 990*c*
Cervical plexus block, 276*f*
Cervical skeletal traction, 1190*t*
Cervical spine
trauma nursing and, 136, 137*f*, 138*t*
trauma to, 990-1000
etiology of, 992-993
extent of injury in, 991-992, 992*f*
health care resources for, 1000
health teaching in, 999*c*, 999-1000, 1000*c*
history in, 993
home care management in, 999
imaging studies in, 994-995
impaired adjustment in, 998
impaired elimination in, 997-998, 998*c*
impaired gas exchange in, 997
ineffective tissue perfusion in, 995*c*, 995-997, 996*f*
laboratory assessment in, 994
in lightning strike, 151
mechanisms of injury in, 990-991, 991*f*
neck injury and, 597
nursing diagnoses in, 995
physical assessment in, 993-994, 994*c*
psychosocial assessment in, 994
self-care deficit in, 997
tumor of, 1001*c*
Cervical tongs, 886
Cervicitis, 1745*f*
Cervix, 1643, 1643*f*
biopsy of, 1647, 1657*c*
cancer of, 1702*t*, 1702-1705, 1704*c*, 1704*f*
colposcopy of, 1656
Pap smear and, 1652
pelvic examination and, 1650, 1650*f*
polyp of, 1699
Cestode infection, 1340
Cetirizine, 390
Cetuximab, 435*t*
for colorectal cancer, 1297
for esophageal cancer, 1258
for oral cancer, 1237
Chalazion, 1087
Chancre, 1739
Chancroid, 1753
Chaplain, 31-32
Charcot foot, 1501
Chart review, preoperative, 260
Chasteberry, 1686
Chelation in myelodysplastic syndromes, 901
Chemical acid-base control mechanisms, 202, 203*t*
Chemical burn, 525-526, 528*c*, 1262
Chemical carcinogenesis, 407-408, 408*t*
Chemical peritonitis, 1317
Chemical responses to heart failure, 767
Chemical restraints, 25
Chemical-induced distributive shock, 830
Chemical-induced leukemia, 902
Chemoprevention of cancer, 411, 411*t*
Chemoreceptor, 708
Chemotaxins, 312
Chemotherapy, 421-431
alopecia in, 428-430
arterial catheter for, 236
for bladder cancer, 1576
for bone cancer, 1169
bone marrow suppression in, 424-427, 426-428*c*
for brain tumor, 1062
for breast cancer, 1677*t*, 1677-1678, 1677-1679
categories of chemotherapeutic drugs in, 421-422*t*, 422
for cervical cancer, 1705
cognitive function changes in, 430
for colorectal cancer, 1297
combination, 422-423
for endometrial cancer, 1701
for esophageal cancer, 1257-1258
for gallbladder cancer, 1371
for gastric cancer, 1281
for head and neck cancer, 599
for liver cancer, 1362
for lung cancer, 644-645
mucositis in, 428, 429*c*
for multiple myeloma, 915
nausea and vomiting in, 427-428, 429*c*
for non-Hodgkin's lymphoma, 914
for oral cancer, 1237
ototoxic, 1114*t*
for ovarian cancer, 1706
for pancreatic cancer, 1382
peripheral neuropathy in, 430-431, 431*c*
for prostate cancer, 1723
for renal cell carcinoma, 1595-1596
side effects of, 423-424, 424*c*
for spinal tumor, 1002
for testicular cancer, 1729-1730
treatment issues in, 423, 423*t*, 424*c*
for vaginal cancer, 1709
Chemotherapy-induced nausea and vomiting, 427-428, 429*c*, 644
Cherry angioma, 466*f*
Chest
physical assessment of, 560-564, 561*f*, 562*f*, 562*t*, 563*t*
positioning for prevention of contracture, 544*c*
Chest decompression, 136
Chest leads, 732, 733*t*
Chest pain
after cardiac catheterization, 724
in aortic stenosis, 779*c*, 780
assessment of, 712-713, 713*t*
in chronic stable angina pectoris, 848
in coronary artery disease, 853*c*, 853-855
in empyema, 674
in hypertrophic cardiomyopathy, 789
in inhalation anthrax, 673
in lung abscess, 672
in lung cancer, 643
management at home, 872*c*
in mitral valve prolapse, 779*c*, 780
in pneumonia, 661, 663*t*
in pulmonary embolism, 679, 679*c*
respiratory assessment and, 559
in tuberculosis, 669
Chest physiotherapy
in burn, 535
in chronic obstructive pulmonary disease, 631, 632*f*
Chest surgery, skin preparation for, 256*f*
Chest trauma, 697-699
Chest tube
in empyema, 674
in lung cancer, 646*f*, 646-648, 647*f*, 648*c*
trauma patient and, 136
Chest wall
of older adult, 557*c*
postoperative assessment of, 287
Chest x-ray
in acute respiratory distress syndrome, 687
in asthma, 612
in cardiovascular assessment, 722
in chronic obstructive pulmonary disease, 627
in empyema, 674
in heart failure, 770
in pneumonia, 663
preoperative, 249
in pulmonary embolism, 679
in pulmonary sarcoidosis, 639
in respiratory problems, 564
in severe acute respiratory syndrome, 666
in valvular heart disease, 781
Cheyne-Stokes respirations, 115
Chills
in influenza, 658
in pneumonia, 661
Chlamydia trachomatis, 1088, 1654
in epididymitis, 1734
in lymphogranuloma venereum, 1753
in pelvic inflammatory disease, 1748
sexually transmitted, 1746-1747
Chlorambucil, 422*t*, 639
Chlordiazepoxide, 84
Chloride
balance and imbalance of, 197
in body fluids, 183*f*
burn-related changes in, 532*c*
cystic fibrosis and, 635
normal plasma values for older adult, 184*t*
preoperative assessment of, 250*c*
serum, 184*t*
tubular reabsorption of, 1530
twenty-four hour urine collection range and, 1542*c*
uncompensated acid-base imbalances and, 208, 208*c*
Chloride shift, 197
Chlorothiazide, 1574
Chlorpheniramine
for allergic rhinitis, 390
for bee sting, 150
Chlorpromazine, 143
Chlorpropamide, 1433, 1434*c*, 1477*c*, 1477-1483
Chlortetracycline, 1086*c*
Chlor-Trimeton; *See* Chlorpheniramine
Chocolate cyst, 1687
Cholecystectomy, 1369-1371, 1370*c*, 1371*t*
Cholecystitis, 1366-1371, 1367*f*, 1368*c*, 1368*t*, 1370*c*, 1371*t*
Cholecystokinin, 1402
Choledochojejunostomy, 1382, 1383*f*
Choledyl; *See* Oxtriphylline
Cholelithiasis, 1367
Cholesteatoma, 1127
Cholesterol
atherosclerosis and, 794, 795-796
cardiovascular assessment and, 720*c*, 721
coronary artery disease and, 850-851, 854*c*
gastrointestinal assessment and, 1225*c*
intake in diabetes mellitus, 1493
malnutrition and, 1394
Cholinergic agents, 1099*c*
Cholinergic antagonists, 616*c*, 620
for acute pancreatitis, 1375-1376
for asthma, 616*c*, 620
for cholecystitis, 1369
for diverticulitis, 1335

Cholinergic antagonists (Continued)
for malabsorption syndrome, 1312
for Parkinson disease, 968
preoperative, 261
for pulmonary secretions in dying patient, 117
for urinary incontinence, 1565c, 1567
Cholinergic crisis, 1017, 1019, 1019t
Cholinergics, 106
Cholinesterase inhibitor drugs, 1018-1019
Cholinesterase inhibitors
for Alzheimer's disease, 976
for Parkinson disease, 968
Chondrogenic tumor, 1167
Chondroitin, 328, 328c
Chondroma, 1167
Chondrosarcoma, 1168
Chopart amputation, 1199f
Chordotomy, 57-58, 58f
Choreiform movements in Huntington disease, 980
Choriocarcinoma, 127, 1727t
Chorioretinitis, 1100
Choroid, 1071f
Choroidal hemorrhage, 1098
Christmas factor, 881t
Chromatid, 63f, 67f
Chromatin, 63f
Chromatographic assay, 1423
Chromosomal analysis, 67-68, 68f
in leukemia, 904
Chromosome, 63f
deoxyribonucleic acid and, 64f, 65
formation of, 66, 67f
function of, 66-67, 67f
Chronic airflow limitation, 610-638
in asthma, 610-621
drug therapy in, 615-621, 616-618c
exercise and activity in, 621
health teaching in, 613-615, 615c
history in, 612
laboratory assessment in, 612
oxygen therapy in, 621
pathophysiology of, 610-611, 611f
physical assessment in, 612, 614f
smoking cessation and, 614c
status asthmaticus and, 621
step system in, 613c
subcutaneous infusion therapy in, 237t
surgical risk and, 246
in chronic obstructive pulmonary disease, 621-635
activity intolerance in, 633
anxiety in, 633
health care resources in, 634, 634c
health teaching in, 634
history in, 624
home care management in, 634
imaging studies, 627
imbalanced nutrition: less than body requirements in, 632-633
impaired gas exchange in, 628-630, 629c
ineffective airway clearance in, 631-632, 632f, 633t
ineffective breathing pattern in, 630-631, 631c
laboratory assessment in, 626-627
nursing diagnoses in, 628
physical assessment in, 624f, 624-626, 626f
pneumonia and respiratory infection risks in, 633
prevention of, 624
psychosocial assessment in, 626
pulmonary function tests in, 627, 627t
in cystic fibrosis, 635-637
in primary pulmonary hypertension, 637-638, 638t
Chronic bacterial prostatitis, 1733
Chronic brain syndrome, 21
Chronic bronchitis, 622
combined ventilatory and oxygenation failure in, 685
pathophysiology of, 611f
surgical risk and, 246
Chronic calcifying pancreatitis, 1377
Chronic cancer pain, 36, 37, 37t
Chronic cholecystitis, 1367
Chronic confusion, 21, 974c, 974t, 974-976, 976c
Chronic constrictive pericarditis, 785
Chronic fatigue and immune dysfunction syndrome, 358
Chronic fatigue syndrome, 358
Chronic gastritis, 1265-1270, 1266-1269c, 1270t
Chronic glomerulonephritis, 1592
Chronic gout, 353, 354f
Chronic health problems
drug reactions in older adult and, 19, 19t
potassium loss in, 188
rehabilitation and, 94-110
constipation and, 106-107, 107t
coping issues in, 107-108
functional assessment and, 98-99
health care resources for, 109
health teaching and, 108-109
home care management and, 108
impaired physical mobility and, 99-101, 100c, 101c, 101f, 102t
impaired skin integrity and, 103-105, 104c
nursing diagnoses and, 99
patient history and, 97
physical assessment and, 97t, 97-98
psychosocial assessment and, 99
rehabilitation team and, 95f, 95-97, 96f, 96t
self-care deficit and, 101-103, 103t
urinary elimination impairment and, 105t, 105-106
vocational assessment and, 99
Chronic hepatitis, 1358
Chronic kidney disease, 1609c, 1609-1635
acute renal failure versus, 1601t
anxiety in, 1619-1620
cardiac changes in, 1610-1611, 1613, 1613c
concept map for, 1616
decreased cardiac output in, 1618
etiology and genetic risk in, 1611t, 1611-1612
excess fluid volume in, 1618
fatigue in, 1619
gastrointestinal changes in, 1611, 1613c, 1614
health care resources for, 1635
health promotion and maintenance in, 1612
health teaching in, 1635
hematologic changes in, 1611, 1613c, 1613-1614
hemodialysis in, 1620-1626, 1621t
anticoagulation in, 1622
complications of, 1626
dialysis settings for, 1621
nursing care in, 1625, 1625t
patient selection for, 1620
post-dialysis care in, 1625-1626, 1626c
procedure of, 1621f, 1621-1622, 1622f
vascular access for, 1622-1625, 1623t, 1624c, 1625f
history in, 1612
home care management in, 1633-1635, 1634c
imaging studies in, 1614
imbalanced nutrition: less than body requirements in, 1615-1618, 1617c, 1617t
incidence and prevalence of, 1612, 1612c
Chronic kidney disease (Continued)
integumentary manifestations in, 1613c, 1614
kidney changes in, 1609
laboratory assessment in, 1614
metabolic changes in, 1609-1610, 1610f
musculoskeletal manifestations in, 1613c, 1614
neurologic manifestations in, 1613c
nursing diagnoses in, 1615
osteomalacia and, 1161
peritoneal dialysis in, 1626-1630, 1627t, 1627-1629f, 1629c
physical assessment in, 1612-1614, 1613c
psychosocial assessment in, 1614
psychosocial preparation in, 1635
pulmonary edema in, 1620
renal transplantation in, 1630-1633, 1631f, 1632f, 1633t
reproductive manifestations in, 1613c
respiratory manifestations in, 1613, 1613c
risk for infection in, 1618
risk for injury in, 1618-1619
sickle cell disease and, 895-896
stages of, 1609, 1609t
Chronic leukemia, 902
Chronic lymphocytic leukemia, 903, 906
Chronic myelogenous leukemia, 902-903
Chronic nephritic syndrome, 1592
Chronic non-cancer pain, 37, 37t
Chronic obstructive pancreatitis, 1377
Chronic obstructive pulmonary disease, 621-635
activity intolerance in, 633
anxiety in, 633
health care resources in, 634, 634c
health teaching in, 634
heart failure in, 767
history in, 624
home care management in, 634
imaging studies, 627
imbalanced nutrition: less than body requirements in, 632-633
impaired gas exchange in, 628-630, 629c
ineffective airway clearance in, 631-632, 632f, 633t
ineffective breathing pattern in, 630-631, 631c
laboratory assessment in, 626-627
nursing diagnoses in, 628
physical assessment in, 624f, 624-626, 626f
pneumonia and respiratory infection risks in, 633
prevention of, 624
psychosocial assessment in, 626
pulmonary function tests in, 627, 627t
Chronic osteomyelitis, 1165
Chronic otitis media, 1123-1125, 1124f, 1125c, 1125f
Chronic pain, 36t, 36-38, 37t
in bone cancer, 1169
in burn, 535-536
in cancer, 416
in connective tissue diseases, 323
in diabetes mellitus, 1504-1505, 1505c
end-of-life care and, 117
epidural opioids for, 53
in fibromyalgia, 357-358
guided imagery for, 56
intractable, 52
invasive techniques for, 57-58, 58f
lightning strike victim and, 151
opioids abuse in, 82
in osteoarthritis, 324, 326-328, 327c
in peptic ulcer disease, 1274-1275
in polycystic kidney disease, 1584
psychosocial assessment of, 44
referral in, 59
in sickle cell disease, 896-897, 897c
Chronic pain (Continued)
subcutaneous infusion therapy in, 237t
in trigeminal neuralgia, 1025
in ulcerative colitis, 1327-1328, 1328c
Chronic pain syndromes, 38t
Chronic pancreatitis, 1377-1379, 1378c, 1379c
Chronic paronychia, 474
Chronic pyelonephritis, 1586-1589, 1587c, 1587f
Chronic rejection of transplant, 319, 1633t
Chronic renal failure; See Chronic kidney disease
Chronic rhinitis, 654
Chronic stable angina, 847-848, 860
Chronic thyroiditis, 1460
Chvostek's sign
in hyperparathyroidism, 1463
in hypocalcemia, 192, 193f
Chylothorax, 231t
Chyme, 1216
Cialis; See Tadalafil
Cibacalcin; See Calcitonin
Cilia, nasal, 553
Ciliary artery, 1072
Ciliary body, 1071f, 1072f
Ciliary processes of eye, 1071f
Ciloxin; See Ciprofloxacin
Cimetidine
for gastroesophageal reflux disease, 1246c, 1248
for gastrointestinal protection in Cushing's disease, 1444
preoperative, 261
CIN; See Chemotherapy-induced nausea and vomiting
Cingulate gyrus herniation, 1053f
Ciprofloxacin
for chancroid, 1753
for cutaneous anthrax, 504
for diverticulitis, 1335
for gastroenteritis, 1320
for granuloma inguinale, 1754
for inhalation anthrax, 673c
for ocular infection, 1086c
for urinary tract infection, 1556c
Circinate skin lesion, 471t
Circle of Willis, 931, 932f
Circulating nurse, 265
Circulation management
in spinal cord injury, 993
in trauma nursing, 137-138, 138t
Circulatory overload
in chronic kidney disease, 1611
from fluid resuscitation in burn, 530
intravenous therapy-related, 230t
transfusion-related, 921
Circumcision, 1645, 1732
Circumduction, 1146f
Circumferential burn wound, 523
Circumferential traction, 1189
Circumflex coronary artery, 706f, 850
Circumscribed skin lesion, 471t
Cirrhosis, 1344-1356
complications of, 1345-1346, 1346t
concept map for, 1351
etiology of, 1346-1347, 1347t
excess fluid volume in, 1350-1353, 1352c, 1353c
health care resources for, 1356
health teaching in, 1355c, 1355-1356
hemorrhage in, 1353-1354
hepatitis C-induced, 1357
history in, 1347
home care management in, 1355
imaging studies in, 1350
laboratory assessment in, 1349t, 1349-1350
nursing diagnoses in, 1350
pathophysiology of, 1344-1345
physical assessment in, 1347-1349, 1348f, 1349f
portal-systemic encephalopathy in, 1354-1355
psychosocial assessment in, 1349

Cisatracurium, 274*t*, 1057
Cisplatin, 422*t*
for cervical cancer, 1705
for esophageal cancer, 1257
for ovarian cancer, 1706
for prostate cancer, 1723
for testicular cancer, 1729-1730
Cistern, 931
Citalopram, 1687
CK; *See* Creatine kinase
CKD; *See* Chronic kidney disease
Cladribine, 421*t*
Clarinex; *See* Desloratadine
Clarithromycin
for leprosy, 516
for peptic ulcer disease, 1269*c*, 1274
Class I antidysrhythmics, 741-742*c*, 751
Class I antigens, 307
Class II antidysrhythmics, 742*c*, 751
Class III antidysrhythmics, 743-744*c*, 751
Class IV antidysrhythmics, 744*c*, 751
Classic heat stroke, 142
Classic migraine, 952*c*
Claudication
in Buerger's disease, 815
in peripheral arterial disease, 805
Clavicle fracture, 1195
Clavulin; *See* Amoxicillin-clavulanate
Claw hand, 281*c*
Claw toe deformity, 1501
Clean-catch urine specimen, 1540*t*
Cleocin; *See* Clindamycin
Click in mitral valve prolapse, 779*c*, 780
Climacteric, 1644-1645
Clindamycin
for inhalation anthrax, 673*c*
for methicillin-resistant *Staphylococcus aureus*, 503*c*
for pelvic inflammatory disease, 1750*c*
Clinical breast examination, 1666-1668, 1667*f*
Clinical staging of cancer, 407
Clinically competent person, 20
Clitoris, 1642
Clofazimine, 516
Clomid; *See* Clomiphene citrate
Clomiphene citrate, 1427-1428
Clonazepam, 957*c*
for multiple sclerosis, 1006
for pain, 55
Clonic seizure, 955-956
Clonidine, 802
Clopidogrel
after percutaneous transluminal coronary angioplasty, 865
after stent procedure, 866
after transient ischemic attack, 1030
for coronary artery disease, 858*c*
for peripheral arterial disease, 807
for pulmonary embolism risk, 678
Clorazepate dipotassium, 957*c*
Closed fracture, 1179, 1179*f*
Closed head injury, 1050, 1050*f*
Closed infusion system, 219
Closed reduction of fracture, 591, 1187*f*, 1187-1190, 1188*t*, 1189*f*, 1190*t*
Closed rhizotomy, 57
Closed-angle glaucoma, 1095*t*, 1095-1098, 1098*c*
Clostridium botulinum, 454*t*, 1341*t*, 1341-1342
Clostridium difficile, 455
enteral nutrition therapy and, 1400
stool test for, 1225-1226
Clotting
after renal transplantation, 1632
during hemodialysis, 1625*t*
hypercalcemia and, 194
peritoneal dialysis-related, 1630
Clotting factors, 880, 881*t*
disorders of, 916-917
Clubbing, 475*t*
cardiovascular assessment and, 715, 715*f*
in chronic obstructive pulmonary disease, 626, 626*f*
Cluster headache, 954-955
Clustered skin lesion, 471*t*
CMG; *See* Cystometrography
CMI; *See* Cell-mediated immunity
Coagulation, 879-880, 880*f*, 881*t*
anti-clotting forces and, 881, 882*f*
hypercalcemia and, 194
Coagulation disorders, 915-917
Coagulation studies, 721
Coagulopathy in pit viper envenomation, 144, 145
Coal miner's disease, 640*c*
Coalesced skin lesion, 471*t*
Coarse crackles, 563*t*
Cobalt-60 radioisotope, 1062, 1062*f*
Cocaine, 86, 1086*c*
Cochlea, 1110*f*
Cochlear implantation, 1132
Codeine, 46
abuse of, 90*t*, 90-91, 91*c*
equianalgesic dose of, 47*t*
for postoperative pain, 297, 298*c*
Co-dominant allele, 69
Codon, 70, 70*t*
Cogentin; *See* Benztropine
Cognitive function
after lightning strike, 151
after stroke, 1034
after traumatic brain injury, 1058
Alzheimer's disease and, 971, 971*t*
assessment of, 98, 938
chemotherapy-related changes in, 430
hypernatremia and, 186
multiple sclerosis and, 1006
older adult and, 935
severe sepsis and, 840
Cognitive stimulation and memory training, 974, 974*c*
Cognitive therapist, 96
Cognitive-behavior measures for pain, 56-57
Cognitive-perceptual pattern
in acid-base assessment, 207*c*
in cardiovascular assessment, 711*c*
in ear and hearing assessment, 1112*c*
in musculoskeletal assessment, 1144*c*
in neurologic assessment, 937*c*
in vision assessment, 1076*c*
Cohorting, 445
Coitus, 1642
Colazal; *See* Balsalazide
Colchicine, 354
Cold antibody anemia, 899
Cold application
for hemorrhoids, 1310
for muscle strain, 1208
for osteoarthritis, 327
for pain, 56
for rheumatoid arthritis, 344
Cold injuries, 152-154, 154*f*
Cold intolerance in hypothyroidism, 1457
Cold phase of peripheral nerve trauma, 1023
Cold spot in thallium scan, 855
Colectomy, 1325-1327, 1326*f*, 1327*f*
Colitis
ulcerative, 1321-1330
Crohn's disease *versus*, 1321*c*
diarrhea in, 1323-1325, 1324*c*
health care resources for, 1329*c*, 1329-1330
health teaching in, 1328-1329, 1329*c*
history in, 1322-1323
home care management in, 1328
laboratory assessment in, 1323
lower gastrointestinal bleeding in, 1290*f*, 1328
malabsorption in, 1311
nursing diagnoses in, 1323
pain in, 1327-1328, 1328*c*
pathophysiology of, 1321-1322, 1322*t*
physical assessment in, 1323
Colitis *(Continued)*
psychosocial assessment in, 1323
surgical management of, 1325-1327, 1326*f*, 1327*f*
uremic, 1611
Collaboration with interdisciplinary health care team, 5
Collaborative nursing functions, 4
Collagen, 461
Collagenase, 539, 542*c*
Collateral circulation, 807
silent myocardial infarction and, 856
Collecting duct, 1527*f*, 1530*t*, 1531*f*
Colles fracture, 1183, 1195, 1206
Colloids, 837
Colon, 1217*f*, 1219
Colon cancer; *See* Colorectal cancer
Colon conduit, 1577*f*
Colon interposition in esophageal cancer, 1259*f*, 1259-1260
Colonization of bacteria, 441, 1552
Colonoscopy, 1228, 1229*c*
in colorectal cancer, 1294-1295, 1296
in ulcerative colitis, 1321, 1323
Colony-stimulating factor, 312
Color vision
assessment of, 1079, 1079*f*
changes with aging, 1075*c*
Colorectal cancer, 1293-1302
anticipatory grieving in, 1296, 1297*c*
conditions associated with genetic predisposition for, 410*t*
drug therapy in, 1297
genetic testing for, 76
health care resources for, 1302
health promotion and maintenance in, 1294-1295, 1295*c*
health teaching in, 1300-1302, 1301*c*
hematologic assessment in, 409*c*
history in, 1295
home management in, 1300
imaging studies in, 1296
inflammatory bowel disease and, 1322*t*
intestinal obstruction and, 1303
laboratory assessment in, 1295-1296
lower gastrointestinal bleeding in, 1290*f*
metastasis in, 1296
nursing diagnoses in, 1296
pathophysiology of, 1293-1294, 1294*f*
physical assessment in, 1295
psychosocial assessment in, 1295
radiation therapy in, 1297
sites of metastasis for, 405*t*
surgical management of, 1297*t*, 1297-1300, 1298*t*, 1299*f*, 1300*c*
Colostomy
in colorectal cancer, 1298-1300, 1299*f*
in diverticulitis, 1336
health care resources for, 1302
home care of, 1301, 1301*c*
Colporrhaphy, 1566*t*, 1694
Colposcopy, 1656
in cervical cancer, 1703
in vulvar cancer, 1707
Colsalide; *See* Colchicine
Coltsfoot, 246*t*
Column of Bertin, 1527*f*
Coma, 938
barbiturate, 1057
in brown recluse spider bite, 147
heat stroke-related, 142
hepatic, 1345-1346, 1346*t*
in high altitude cerebral edema, 155
myxedema, 1459, 1459*c*
in phencyclidine withdrawal, 87
Combantrin; *See* Pyrantel pamoate
Combigan; *See* Brimonidine tartrate-timolol maleate
Combination therapy, 422-423
for breast cancer, 1677-1678
for colorectal cancer, 1297
for diabetes mellitus, 1484
for glaucoma, 1100*c*
Combination therapy *(Continued)*
for idiopathic pulmonary fibrosis, 639
for prostate cancer, 1723
for testicular cancer, 1729-1730
for tuberculosis, 670, 671*c*
Combined metabolic and respiratory acidosis, 206, 208*c*
Combined metabolic and respiratory alkalosis, 208*c*
Combined ventilatory and oxygenation failure, 685
Combivir; *See* Zidovudine-lamivudine
Combustion hazard in oxygen therapy, 572
Comedone, 515
Command center, 162
Commando procedure, 1237-1238
Comminuted fracture, 1179*f*
Comminuted skull fracture, 1050
Commitment of embryonic cell, 402
Common bile duct, 1218*f*, 1219
Common cold, 654
Common femoral artery, 804*f*
Common iliac artery, 804*f*
Common peroneal nerve, 1022*f*
Common variable immune deficiency, 385
Communicable infection, 440
Communicating hydrocephalus, 1052
Communication
after laryngectomy, 606, 606*f*
in emergency care, 128, 130-131
genetic counseling and, 77
Guillain-Barré syndrome and, 1015-1016
hearing loss and, 1135, 1135*c*
with lesbian, gay, bisexual, and transgender patients, 30*c*
mechanical ventilation and, 694-695
medical errors and, 5
myasthenia gravis and, 1020
non-English-speaking patients and, 29, 29*c*
older adult and
Alzheimer's disease and, 875-976, 976*c*
drug errors and, 19-20
with impaired vision, 1098*c*
Parkinson disease and, 968-969
preoperative anxiety and, 259
pulmonary embolism and, 682-683
reduced vision and, 1106, 1106*c*
stroke and, 1046, 1046*t*
tracheostomy and, 586
Community Emergency Response Team, 161
Community-acquired pneumonia, 659, 659*t*
Community-associated methicillin-resistant *Staphylococcus aureus*, 448
Community-based care
in acute pancreatitis, 1376-1377
in Alzheimer's disease, 978
in amputation, 1203-1204, 1204*c*
in aneurysms, 813-814
in back pain, 988*c*, 988-989
in benign prostatic hypertrophy, 1718
in bladder cancer, 1576-1578
in bone cancer, 1171-1172
in brain tumor, 1065
in breast cancer, 1679*c*, 1679-1681, 1680*c*
in burn, 545-546, 546*t*
in cataracts, 1094-1095, 1095*c*
in cervical cancer, 1705
in chronic and disabling diseases, 108-109
in chronic obstructive pulmonary disease, 634, 634*c*
in chronic pancreatitis, 1379, 1379*c*
in cirrhosis, 1355*c*, 1355-1356
in colorectal cancer, 1300-1302, 1301*c*
in coronary artery disease, 870-872, 870-872*c*
in Crohn's disease, 1333-1334

Community-based care (*Continued*)
in Cushing's disease, 1445, 1445*c*
in cystitis, 1558-1559
in deep vein thrombosis, 820-821, 821*c*
in diabetes mellitus, 1514-1517, 1516*c*, 1517*c*
in diverticular disease, 1336-1337
in dysrhythmias, 758-761, 759-761*c*
in endometrial cancer, 1701-1702
in esophageal cancer, 1261
in fracture, 1194
in gastric cancer, 1286-1287
in Guillain-Barré syndrome, 1016
in head and neck cancer, 604-605, 605*c*
in hearing loss, 1135-1136
in heart failure, 776*c*, 776-779, 777*t*, 778*c*
in hepatitis, 1360, 1361*c*
in hypertension, 802-804
in hypothyroidism, 1459
in hypovolemic shock, 838
in infection, 452-453
in infective endocarditis, 785
in intestinal obstruction, 1306, 1306*c*
in leukemia, 911*c*, 911-913, 912*c*
in malnutrition, 1401-1402
in multiple sclerosis, 1006-1007
in myasthenia gravis, 1021*t*, 1021-1022, 1022*c*
in obesity, 1408, 1408*c*
in open conventional esophageal surgery, 1254
in oral cancer, 1238-1239
in osteoarthritis, 335-336, 336*c*
in osteoporosis, 1160
in ovarian cancer, 1706-1707
in oxygen therapy, 578-579, 579*f*
pain management and, 58-59
in pancreatic cancer, 1384
in pelvic inflammatory disease, 1752
in peptic ulcer disease, 1278-1279, 1279*c*
in peripheral arterial disease, 809*c*, 809-810, 810*c*
in peritonitis, 1318-1319
in pneumonia, 665*c*, 665-666
postoperative, 299-301
in pressure ulcer, 498-499, 499*c*
in prostate cancer, 1724*c*, 1724-1725
in pulmonary embolism, 683-684, 684*c*
in pyelonephritis, 1589
in renal transplantation, 1633-1635, 1634*c*
in renal trauma, 1598
in rheumatoid arthritis, 346*f*, 346-347
in scleroderma, 352-353
in septic shock, 844, 844*c*
in sickle cell disease, 897, 898*c*
in spinal cord injury, 998-1000, 999*c*, 1000*c*
in spinal tumor, 1002
in stroke, 1047-1048, 1048*f*
in systemic lupus erythematosus, 350, 350*c*
in testicular cancer, 1730
in tracheostomy, 587
in traumatic brain injury, 1059-1060
in tuberculosis, 670-672
in ulcerative colitis, 1328-1330, 1329*c*
in uterine leiomyomas, 1697*c*, 1697-1698, 1698*c*
in valvular heart disease, 782-783, 783*c*
in venous insufficiency, 822
Comorbidities, emergency care and, 130
Compact bone, 1141, 1141*f*, 1153
Compartment syndrome
in abdominal trauma, 1308
after peripheral arterial disease surgery, 809
in crush syndrome, 1182
fracture and, 1180-1182, 1181*c*
intraosseous therapy-related, 239
Compatibility chart for red blood cell transfusion, 919*t*
Compensated cirrhosis, 1345, 1347
Compensation, 204
Compensatory mechanisms
in burn, 525, 526*f*
in heart failure, 765-767, 766*f*
in hypovolemic shock, 833-835
Compensatory stage of shock, 831-832
Complement activation and fixation, 312, 315-316
Complementary and alternative therapies, 8-14
for allergic rhinitis, 391
for Alzheimer's disease, 976
for benign prostatic hypertrophy, 1715
biologically based therapies in, 11-12, 12*t*
to boost immune function, 425-426
for breast cancer, 1672, 1672*t*
for chemotherapy-induced nausea and vomiting, 428
for coronary artery disease, 851, 871-872
for Crohn's disease, 1332
for dysmenorrhea, 1685
in end-of-life care, 117, 118
for endometrial cancer, 1701
for endometriosis, 1688
energy therapies in, 12-13, 13*f*
for gallbladder cancer, 1371
for gastritis and peptic ulcer disease, 1270*t*
for human immunodeficiency virus infection, 379
implications for nursing, 13
for irritable bowel syndrome, 1291
manipulative and body-based therapies in, 11, 11*f*, 11*t*
for menopause, 1690
mind-body therapies in, 9-11, 10*f*
for multiple sclerosis, 1006
National Center for Complementary and Alternative Medicine, 8, 9*t*
for obesity, 1406
for osteoarthritis, 327-328, 328*c*
for pain, 55
in acquired immunodeficiency syndrome, 380
back, 986
in burn injury, 536
in fracture, 1192
in migraine, 953, 954*t*
phantom limb, 1201
postoperative, 299, 299*c*
in tension headache, 955
for peptic ulcer disease, 1275
for prostate cancer, 1723-1724
to reduce cholesterol levels, 796
for rheumatoid arthritis, 345
for rhinitis, 654
for sickle cell disease, 897
systems of care in, 9
for total knee arthroplasty, 333
for ulcerative colitis, 1325
for urolithiasis, 1573
Complementary base pair, 64*f*, 64-65, 65*f*
Complete blood count
in allergic rhinitis, 389
in Cushing's disease, 1444
in gastrointestinal assessment, 1223
in hematologic assessment, 886
in human immunodeficiency virus infection, 373
in infection assessment, 450
in meningitis, 962
in pharyngitis, 656, 656*c*
in pneumonia, 663
in respiratory assessment, 565*c*
in rheumatoid arthritis, 340
in tonsillitis, 657
Complete cystectomy, 1576
Complete fracture, 1179
Complete heart block, 750
Complete partial seizure, 959*c*
Complete spinal cord injury, 990
Complex inheritance and familial clustering, 72*t*, 74
Complex partial seizure, 956
Complex regional pain syndrome, 1204
Complicated lesion in atherosclerotic coronary artery, 848*f*
Composite resection in head and neck cancer, 602
Composite urine collections, 1541, 1542*c*
Compound fracture, 1179, 1179*f*
Compress for skin infection, 503
Compression bandage
for coral snake envenomation, 146
for pit viper envenomation, 145
Compression fracture, 1180
vertebral, 1156, 1198*c*, 1198-1199
Compression hip screw, 1196*f*
Compression stockings, 821, 822*c*
Computed tomography
in abdominal aortic aneurysm, 812
in abdominal trauma, 1307
in acute renal failure, 1604
in Alzheimer's disease, 973
in bladder cancer, 1576
in bone cancer, 1168
in brain abscess, 1066
in brain tumor, 1061
in chronic pancreatitis, 1378
in cirrhosis, 1350
in colorectal cancer, 1296
in ear assessment, 1116
in endocrine assessment, 1424
in fractures, 1185
in gallbladder cancer, 1371
in gastrointestinal assessment, 1226
in Guillain-Barré syndrome, 1013
in head and neck cancer, 598
in infection assessment, 451
in intestinal obstruction, 1304
in lung cancer, 644
in musculoskeletal assessment, 1149
in neurologic assessment, 943-945, 944*t*
in ocular problems, 1079
in osteoporosis, 1156
in Paget's disease of bone, 1163-1164
in pancreatic cancer, 1380
in penetrating ocular trauma, 1104
in prostate cancer, 1721
renal, 1544*t*, 1545-1546, 1598
in reproductive assessment, 1654
in respiratory assessment, 566
in spinal cord injury, 994-995
in spinal tumor, 1001
in stroke, 1035
in testicular cancer, 1728
in traumatic brain injury, 1056
in urolithiasis, 1572
Computed tomography angiography, 855, 944*t*, 945, 1035
Computer physician order entry, 215
Comtan; *See* Entacapone
COMTs; *See* Catechol O-methyltransferases
Concentration gradient, 172
Concept map
for bacterial pneumonia, 662
for benign prostatic hypertrophy, 1716
for chronic cancer pain, 416
for chronic kidney disease, 1616
for cirrhosis, 1351
for glaucoma, 1096
for hypertension, 800
for hypovolemic shock, 834
for multiple sclerosis, 1005
for pressure ulcer, 492
for respiratory acidosis, 625
for type 2 diabetes mellitus, 1476
Concha, 1110*f*
Concussion, 1050
Conditioning regimen in stem cell transplantation, 908-909, 909*f*
Condom, 1743*c*
safer sex practices and, 367
sexually transmitted diseases and, 368*c*
syphilis prevention and, 1740
Conduction system of heart, 710*c*, 731, 731*f*
Conductive hearing loss, 1116, 1129-1130
anatomy of, 1129*f*
in otitis media, 1123
sensorineural hearing loss *versus*, 1130*t*
Conductivity, 731
Conduit, 1577*f*
Condylar joint, 1143
Condylomata acuminata, 1690, 1743-1744, 1744*f*
Condylox; *See* Podofilox
Cones, 1071
Confusion
in Alzheimer's disease, 974*c*, 974*t*, 974-976, 976*c*
delirium and, 21-22, 22*t*
dementia and, 21, 22*t*
in heat stroke, 142
in high altitude cerebral edema, 155
hospitalized older adult and, 23
in hypomagnesemia, 196
in hypothermia, 153
in hypovolemic shock, 835
in lightning strike, 151
opioid analgesic-related, 49*t*
in pulmonary edema, 775
Confusion Assessment Method, 21, 22*t*
Congenital aneurysm, 1031
Congenital immune deficiencies, 385
Congenital scoliosis, 1174
Congestion, approaching death and, 115*c*
Congestive heart failure; *See* Heart failure
Conivaptan
for fluid overload, 182
for hyponatremia, 186
Conization, 1657, 1704
Conjugated bilirubin
in gastrointestinal assessment, 1224*c*
in jaundice, 1346*t*
Conjunctiva, 1071*f*, 1072
Conjunctival hemorrhage, 1087
Conjunctivitis, 1087-1088
Connective tissue diseases, 322-361
ankylosing spondylitis in, 355
chronic fatigue syndrome in, 358
disease-associated arthritis in, 357, 357*t*
fibromyalgia in, 357*f*, 357-358
gout in, 353-354, 354*f*
infectious arthritis in, 356
lupus erythematosus in, 347-350, 348*c*, 349*f*, 350*c*
Lyme disease in, 356, 356*c*
Marfan syndrome in, 355-356
mixed connective tissue disease in, 358
osteoarthritis in, 323-336
chronic pain in, 326-328, 327*c*
complementary and alternative therapies in, 327-328, 328*c*
health care resources in, 336
health promotion and maintenance in, 324
health teaching in, 336, 336*c*
home care management in, 335-336
imaging assessment in, 325
impaired physical mobility in, 335, 336*c*
laboratory assessment in, 325
nursing diagnoses in, 325-326
pathophysiology of, 323*f*, 323-324
patient history in, 324
physical assessment in, 324-325, 325*t*
psychosocial assessment in, 325

Connective tissue diseases *(Continued)*
total elbow arthroplasty in, 335
total hip arthroplasty in, 328-332, 330*c*, 330*t*, 332*c*, 332*f*
total knee arthroplasty in, 333*f*, 333-334, 334*c*
total shoulder arthroplasty in, 334-335
polymyalgia rheumatica and temporal arteritis in, 355, 355*c*
polymyositis/dermatomyositis in, 354
pseudogout in, 356
psoriatic arthritis in, 357
Reiter's syndrome in, 355
rheumatoid arthritis in, 337-347
body image and, 346
complementary and alternative therapies for, 345
diagnostic assessment in, 340
drug therapy for, 340-344, 341-342*c*
fatigue in, 346, 346*c*
gene therapy for, 345
health care resources in, 347
health teaching in, 347
home care management in, 346, 346*f*
laboratory assessment in, 339*c*, 339-340
nonpharmacologic interventions for, 344-345, 345*f*
pathophysiology of, 337, 337*c*
physical assessment in, 337-339, 338*f*
promotion of self-care in, 345-346
psychosocial assessment in, 339
scleroderma in, 351*f*, 351-353, 352*c*
systemic necrotizing vasculitis in, 354-355
Connexin-26, 1113
Conscious sedation; *see* moderate sedation
Consensual response, 942, 1077
Consent form, 253*f*
Conservation of energy
after lung transplantation, 631
in chronic and disabling conditions, 103
in heart failure, 775
in leukemia, 911
in polycystic kidney disease, 1584*c*
in rheumatoid arthritis, 346, 346*c*
Consolidation in lobar pneumonia, 659
Consolidation therapy in acute leukemia, 905
Constipation
after bariatric surgery, 1408
in botulism, 1341
bromocriptine-related, 1431
in chronic and disabling conditions, 106-107, 107*t*
dying patient and, 118
hemorrhoids and, 1309-1310
in hypercalcemia, 194
in hyperparathyroidism, 1461
in hypokalemia, 188
in hypomagnesemia, 196
in hypothyroidism, 1457
in irritable bowel syndrome, 1289-1290
opioid analgesic-related, 48, 49*t*
in polycystic kidney disease, 1584
postoperative assessment of, 291
spinal cord injury and, 997-998, 998*c*
Contact burn, 525
Contact dermatitis, 505, 505*c*
Contact lenses, 1103
Contact precautions, 447*t*, 448
Contact transmission of infection, 442
Container in infusion system, 219
Contiguous osteomyelitis, 1165
Continence, 1532-1533, 1559
Continent ileostomy, 1326, 1326*f*
Continent internal ileal reservoir, 1576-1577, 1577*f*
Continuous ambulatory peritoneal dialysis, 1627, 1628*f*
Continuous arteriovenous hemodialysis and filtration, 1608
Continuous arteriovenous hemofiltration, 1608
Continuous arteriovenous rewarming, 153
Continuous bladder irrigation, 1717*f*, 1718, 1718*c*
Continuous blood glucose monitoring device, 1492
Continuous electrocardiographic monitoring, 732-733, 734*f*
Continuous feeding, 1398
Continuous passive motion machine
for sports-related knee injury, 1206
in total knee arthroplasty, 333*f*, 333-334, 334*c*
Continuous peripheral nerve blockade, 334
Continuous positive airway pressure, 694
in acute respiratory distress syndrome, 688
in heart failure, 774
noninvasive positive-pressure ventilation and, 578
in obstructive sleep apnea, 594
oxygen toxicity and, 573
Continuous renal replacement therapy, 1608
Continuous subcutaneous infusion of insulin, 1486-1487, 1487*f*
Continuous sutures, 282*f*
Continuous venovenous hemofiltration, 1608
Continuous wet gauze for wound débridement, 493*t*
Continuous-cycle peritoneal dialysis, 1628
Contraceptive diaphragm, toxic shock syndrome and, 1692*c*
Contractility of heart, 731
Contraction, wound healing and, 482*f*, 484
Contracture
Dupuytren's, 1172
positioning for prevention of, 544*c*
spinal cord injured patient and, 997
Contrast agent injection, 943*c*
Contrast-enhanced cardiovascular magnetic resonance, 855
Contrast-induced computed tomography, 1375
Contrast-induced renal failure, 1543-1544
Contrecoup head injury, 1050, 1050*f*
Controlled coughing
after laryngectomy, 601
in chronic obstructive pulmonary disease, 628, 629*c*, 631
preoperative teaching of, 258
Controller of infusion rate, 222
Contusion
in closed head injury, 1050
ocular, 1103
pulmonary, 697-698
renal, 1596-1598, 1597*f*
Conus medullaris, 992, 992*f*
Conventional open esophageal surgery, 1250-1253
Convergence, 1074
Convulsive status epilepticus, 959-960
Cooling measures
in fever treatment, 452
in heat exhaustion, 142
in heat stroke, 142, 143
Coombs' test, 886, 887*c*
Cooper's suspensory ligaments, 1644
Coordination assessment, 940
Copaxone; *See* Glatiramir acetate
Coping
in breast cancer, 1671-1672
in chronic and disabling diseases, 107-108
in coronary artery disease, 860-861, 861*c*
Coping *(Continued)*
in osteoarthritis, 326
in spinal cord injury, 998
Coping/stress tolerance pattern in cardiovascular assessment, 711*c*
Copperhead envenomation, 144*f*, 144-145
Cor pulmonale
in chronic obstructive pulmonary disease, 623, 623*c*
in pulmonary sarcoidosis, 638
Coral snake envenomation, 145-146, 146*f*
Cord blood harvesting, 908
Cordarone; *See* Amiodarone
Cordectomy, 600, 600*t*
Cordotomy, 57-58, 58*f*, 1170
Core body temperature, burn-related changes in, 525
Core competencies, 3-6
collaboration with interdisciplinary health care team and, 5
in emergency nursing, 130-131
evidence-based practice and, 5-6, 6*t*
informatics and, 6, 6*f*
patient-centered care and, 3-5, 4*c*
in peaceful death, 112*t*
quality improvement and, 6
Core rewarming methods, 153
Coreg; *See* Carvedilol
Corgard; *See* Nadolol
Corium, 461, 461*f*
Corlopam; *See* Fenoldopam
Corn, 1174*t*
Cornea, 1071, 1071*f*, 1088-1091
abrasion, ulceration, and infection of, 1089
assessment of, 1077
changes with aging, 1075*c*
keratoconus and opacities of, 1089*f*, 1089-1091, 1090*f*, 1091*t*
laceration of, 1104
transplantation of, 1090, 1090*f*
Corneal light reflex, 1078
Corneal staining, 1079-1080
Corona, 1645*f*
Coronal images, 1079
Coronary arterial system, 705*f*, 706
Coronary arteriography, 722, 722*t*, 723
Coronary artery bypass graft, 866-870, 867*f*
in dysrhythmias, 758
maze procedure and, 746
Coronary artery calcium score, 726
Coronary artery disease, 847-874
activity intolerance in, 860
acute pain in, 856*c*, 856-858, 857-858*c*
chronic stable angina pectoris and, 847-848
coronary artery bypass graft surgery in, 866-870, 867*f*
diagnostic tests in, 855
dysrhythmias in, 730-763, 861-862
advanced cardiac life support for, 756
atrial fibrillation in, 745-746, 746*f*
atrial flutter in, 747
atrioventricular blocks in, 750
automatic external defibrillation for, 757, 757*f*
bundle branch blocks in, 750
cardiac conduction system and, 731, 731*f*
cardiopulmonary resuscitation in, 755-756
cardioversion for, 756
coronary artery bypass graft for, 758
decreased cardiac output and ineffective tissue perfusion in, 750-751, 751*c*
defibrillation for, 756-757
drug therapy for, 741-745*c*, 751-753, 752-753*c*
electrocardiography and, 731-737, 732*f*, 733*t*, 734*f*, 735*f*, 736*f*
Coronary artery disease *(Continued)*
electrophysiologic properties of heart and, 730-731, 731*f*
health teaching in, 758-761, 759-761*c*
home care management in, 758
in hypercalcemia, 194
junctional, 747
key features of, 738*c*
normal rhythms and, 737*f*, 737-738
nursing diagnoses in, 750
pacemaker insertion for, 757
premature atrial complexes in, 740
radiofrequency catheter ablation for, 757
sinus, 739*f*, 739-740
supraventricular tachycardia in, 740-741
temporary pacing for, 754-755
terminology in, 738-739
vagal maneuvers for, 753-754
ventricular, 747-750, 748*f*, 749*f*
etiology and genetic risk in, 850
health care resources for, 872
health teaching in, 870-872, 871*c*, 872*c*
heart failure in, 862*t*, 862-864, 863-864*c*
history in, 709, 853
home care management in, 870, 870*c*, 871*c*
homocysteine and, 795
imaging studies in, 855
incidence and prevalence of, 850
ineffective coping in, 860-861
ineffective tissue perfusion in, 858-860, 859*t*
intervention activities in, 861*c*
laboratory assessment in, 855
nursing diagnoses in, 855-856
obesity and, 1402
pathophysiology of, 848*f*, 848-850, 849*f*
percutaneous transluminal coronary angioplasty in, 865, 865*t*
physical assessment in, 853*c*, 853-855
prevention of, 850-853, 853*t*, 854*c*
psychosocial assessment in, 855
serum markers of myocardial damage in, 719-721
stents in, 865-866, 866*f*
Coronary artery vasculopathy, 790*c*
Coronary heart disease; *See* Coronary artery disease
Coronary sinus, 705*f*
Coronavirus, 666-667
Corpus callosum, 929
Corpus cavernosum, 1645*f*
Corpus of stomach, 1217
Corpus spongiosum, 1645*f*
Cortef; *See* Hydrocortisone
Cortex of bone, 1141
Cortical bone, 1153
Cortical nephron, 1527
Corticosteroids, 1416
for acute respiratory distress syndrome, 688
after lung transplantation, 637
for allergic rhinitis, 390
for anaphylaxis, 393*c*
for asthma, 617*c*, 620
for bee sting, 150
for bronchiolitis obliterans organizing pneumonia, 640*c*
for chemotherapy-induced nausea and vomiting, 429*c*
for Crohn's disease, 1331
drug-induced immune deficiency and, 384
for dyspnea in dying patient, 117
for facial paralysis, 1026
for inflammatory skin disease, 505
for psoriasis, 507
for pulmonary sarcoidosis, 639
for septic shock, 843*t*
for Sjögren's syndrome, 396
for ulcerative colitis, 1324

Corticotropin-releasing hormone, 1416
Cortisol, 1414*f*, 1416
  adrenal gland assessment and, 1438*c*
  glucose homeostasis and, 1467
  hypercortisolism and, 1439-1445
    acute adrenal insufficiency in, 1444
    community-based care in, 1445, 1445*c*
    excess fluid volume in, 1442-1443
    history in, 1440-1441
    imaging studies in, 1442
    laboratory assessment in, 1441-1442
    pathophysiology of, 1439-1440, 1440*f*, 1440*t*
    physical assessment in, 1441, 1441*c*
    psychosocial assessment in, 1441
    risk for infection in, 1444
    risk for injury in, 1443-1444
    secondary hypertension in, 798
Cortisol replacement therapy, 1445*c*
Cortisone, 1439*c*
Corvert; *See* Ibutilde
Coryza, 654
Cosmegen; *See* Dactinomycin
Cosmetic surgery, 243*t*, 545
Costovertebral angle, 1536
Cotazym; *See* Pancrelipase
Cotrim; *See* Trimethoprim-sulfamethoxazole
Cotton gauze dressing, 494-495*t*
Cottonmouth envenomation, 144-145, 145*f*
Cough
  after extubation, 697
  in asthma, 612
  in bronchiolitis obliterans organizing pneumonia, 640*c*
  in empyema, 674
  in esophageal diverticula, 1261
  in gastroesophageal reflux disease, 1245
  in high altitude pulmonary edema, 155
  history in, 559
  in influenza, 658
  in inhalation anthrax, 673
  in laryngitis, 658
  in lung abscess, 672
  in pneumonia, 661, 663*t*
  in severe acute respiratory syndrome, 666
  in tuberculosis, 669
Cough assist
  after laryngectomy, 601
  after peripheral arterial disease surgery, 809
  in chronic obstructive pulmonary disease, 628, 629*c*, 631
  in myasthenia gravis, 1018
  in oral cancer, 1236*c*
  preoperative teaching of, 258
  in spinal cord injury, 997
Coumadin; *See* Warfarin
Counterimmunoelectrophoresis, 962
Counterregulatory hormones, 1467
Coup injury, 1050, 1050*f*
Cowper's gland, 1645*f*
COX-2 inhibitors, 46
Cozaar; *See* Losartan
CPAP; *See* Continuous positive airway pressure
C-peptide, 1474
CPR; *See* Cardiopulmonary resuscitation
Crab lice, 504
Crack cocaine, 86
Crackles
  in acute renal failure, 1603
  in bronchiolitis obliterans organizing pneumonia, 640*c*
  in circulatory overload from fluid resuscitation in burn, 530
  in high altitude pulmonary edema, 155
  in left-sided heart failure, 769, 854
  in pneumonia, 661
  in pulmonary edema, 775
  in pulmonary embolism, 679, 679*c*
Cramping in osteomalacia, 1162
Cranberry juice, 1558
Cranial nerves, 933, 935*t*
  assessment of, 938
  encephalitis and, 964
  eye and, 1072
  Guillain-Barré syndrome and, 1012*c*, 1012-1013
  meningitis and, 963
  stroke and, 1035
  traumatic brain injury and, 1055
  trigeminal neuralgia and, 1025*f*, 1025-1026
Cranial polyneuritis, 1026
Craniofacial disjunction, 593
Craniotomy
  in brain abscess, 1066
  in brain tumor, 1062-1063
  in cerebral aneurysm, 1045
  postoperative complications of, 1064*t*
  in traumatic brain injury, 1058
Crank, 85
C-reactive protein
  in cardiovascular assessment, 721
  in osteoarthritis, 325
  in rheumatoid arthritis, 340
Creatine kinase, 720*c*, 720-721
  in amyotrophic lateral sclerosis, 1007
  in lightning strike, 152
  in musculoskeletal assessment, 1148*c*
Creatine kinase-BB, 720*c*, 721
Creatine kinase-MB, 720*c*, 721, 855
Creatine kinase-MM, 720*c*, 721, 1147-1148
Creatinine
  chronic kidney disease and, 1609
  preoperative assessment of, 250*c*
  twenty-four hour urine collection range and, 1542*c*
Creatinine clearance, 799, 1541
Credé maneuver, 105-106, 1568
Cremasteric reflex, 1651
Crepitus, 561
  in esophageal injury, 597
  musculoskeletal assessment of, 1146
  in osteoarthritis, 324
Crescentic glomerulonephritis, 1591-1592
CREST syndrome, 351
CRH; *See* Corticotropin-releasing hormone
Cricoid cartilage, 554, 554*f*
Cricothyroid membrane, 554, 554*f*
Cricothyroidotomy, 554
  in facial trauma, 593
  in upper airway obstruction, 596
Critical access hospital, 126
Critical incident stress debriefing, 164*c*, 164-165
Critical thinking, 6
Critically ill patient, 677-701, 1029-1068
  acute respiratory distress syndrome and, 686-689, 687*t*
  acute respiratory failure and, 685*t*, 685-686, 686*f*
  arterial blood pressure measurement in, 728
  cardiac oxygen delivery impairment in, 678*f*
  endotracheal intubation in, 689-692, 690*f*, 691*c*
  flail chest and, 698, 698*f*
  hemothorax and, 699
  mechanical ventilation in, 692*c*, 692-697
    extubation in, 697
    managing ventilator system in, 695*t*, 695-696
    modes of ventilation in, 693
    monitoring in, 694-695
    preventing complications in, 696
    types of ventilators in, 692-693, 693*f*
    ventilator controls and settings in, 693-694
    weaning from, 696-697, 697*t*
Critically ill patient *(Continued)*
  pain assessment in, 43-44
  pneumothorax and, 698-699
  pulmonary contusion and, 697-698
  pulmonary embolism and, 677-684
    anxiety and, 682-683
    decreased cardiac output in, 682
    health care resources for, 683-684, 684*c*
    health promotion and maintenance and, 678, 678*c*
    health teaching in, 683, 684*c*
    history in, 679
    home care management in, 683
    hypoxemia in, 680-682, 680-682*c*
    imaging assessment in, 679
    laboratory assessment in, 679
    nursing diagnoses in, 679-680
    pathophysiology of, 677-678
    physical assessment in, 679, 679*c*
    potential for bleeding in, 683, 683*c*
    psychosocial assessment in, 679
    total hip arthroplasty and, 330-331
  rib fracture and, 698
  stroke and, 1030-1049
    arteriovenous malformation and, 1044*f*, 1044-1045
    carotid artery angioplasty with stenting in, 1044
    carotid endarterectomy in, 1045
    community-based rehabilitation in, 1048
    disturbed sensory perception in, 1047
    drug therapy for, 1043-1044
    etiology and genetic risk for, 1032, 1033*c*
    extracranial-intracranial bypass in, 1045
    health care resources for, 1048-1049
    health teaching in, 1048, 1048*f*
    history in, 1032-1033
    home care management in, 1047-1048
    imaging studies in, 1036
    impaired physical mobility in, 1046
    impaired swallowing in, 1045
    impaired verbal communication in, 1046, 1046*t*
    ineffective tissue perfusion in, 1036-1037
    intracranial pressure monitoring in, 1037*c*, 1037-1043
    laboratory assessment in, 1036
    nursing care plan for, 1038-1043
    nursing diagnoses in, 1036
    pathophysiologic changes in brain and, 1030
    physical assessment in, 1033*c*, 1033*f*, 1033-1035, 1034*c*
    prevention of, 1032
    psychosocial assessment in, 1035-1036
    thrombolytic therapy for, 1037, 1037*c*
    types of, 1030*f*, 1030-1032, 1031*t*
    unilateral neglect in, 1047
    urinary and bowel incontinence in, 1047
  tension pneumothorax and, 699
  tracheobronchial trauma and, 699
  transient ischemic attack and, 1030
Crixivan; *See* Indinavir
CRNA; *See* Certified registered nurse anesthetist
CRNFA; *See* Certified registered nurse first assistant
Crohn's disease, 1330*f*, 1330-1334, 1333*f*
  complications of, 1322*t*
  folic acid deficiency anemia in, 900
  malabsorption in, 1311
  pain management in, 1324*c*
  ulcerative colitis *versus*, 1321*c*
Cromolyn sodium, 391
Cross-bridges, 707
Cross-contamination
  burn wound and, 540
  in leukemia, 905
Crossmatching before transfusion, 918
Crotalidae envenomation, 143*f*, 143-146, 144*c*, 144*f*, 145*t*, 146*t*
Cruciate ligament injury, 1206
Crush syndrome, 1182
Crust, 470*f*
Crutches, 1193, 1193*f*
Cryoablation in bone cancer, 1170
Cryoanalgesia for chronic pain, 57
Cryoprecipitate, 917*t*, 920
Cryosurgery
  in bone cancer, 1170
  in skin cancer, 512
Cryotherapy
  in cervical cancer, 1704
  in genital herpes, 1744
  in oral cancer, 1237
  for pain, 55
  in prostate cancer, 1723
  in retinal detachment, 1101
Cryothermia, 272*t*
Cryptococcosis, 371
Cryptococcus neoformans meningitis, 961
Cryptorchidism, 1727
Cryptosporidium, 371, 1338-1339
Crystalloids
  for hypovolemic shock, 837
  for renal trauma, 1598
  for septic shock, 843*t*
Crystals in urine, 1539*t*, 1541
CT; *See* Computed tomography
C-teleopeptide, 1156
CTX; *See* C-teleopeptide
Cul-de-sac of Douglas, 1643*f*
Cullen's sign, 1222
  in abdominal trauma, 1307
  in acute pancreatitis, 1374
Cultural competence, 27-38, 28*f*, 28*t*
Cultural considerations, 27-34
  in beliefs regarding death, dying, and afterlife, 119*t*
  in bone marrow donation, 907
  in breast cancer, 1664-1665, 1669
  in burn assessment, 532
  in cancer, 410, 411*t*
  in cerumen, 1115
  in chronic obstructive pulmonary disease, 622
  in coronary artery disease, 850, 852, 855
  culture and cultural competence and, 27-38, 28*f*, 28*t*
  in cyanosis in dark-skinned patient, 805
  in diabetes mellitus, 1472, 1473*t*
  in emergency nursing, 133, 134
  in food pyramids, 1387
  in glomerular filtration rate, 1533
  health care disparities and, 28
  in hematologic assessment, 885
  in human immunodeficiency virus infection, 366, 366*f*
  in hypertension, 798, 852, 1593
  in lactose intolerance, 192
  in lower extremity amputation, 1200
  in lupus, 348
  in malnutrition, 1392
  in nutritional history, 1221
  in osteoporosis, 1154
  in oxygen saturation, 556
  Purnell's domains of culture and, 29*t*, 29-33
    biologic ecology in, 31
    culture overview and communication in, 29, 29*c*
    family and workplace issues in, 29-30
    health care practices and practitioners in, 32*f*, 32-33, 33*f*
    lesbian, gay, bisexual, and transgender health in, 30*c*, 30-31, 31*t*

Cultural considerations *(Continued)*
nutrition in, 31
spirituality in, 31-32
in renal stones, 1571
in sexual practices, 1647
in skin color, 474-475, 476*f*
in substance abuse, 81
in syphilis, 1738-1739
in ulcerative colitis, 1322
Cultural diversity, 27-28
Cultural sensitivity, 28
Culture, 27-38, 28*f*, 28*t*
Culture and sensitivity
in cystitis, 1555
in reproductive assessment, 1654
Cultured skin for burn wound, 540
Cuprimine; *See* Penicillamine
Curandera, 33
Curandero, 33, 33*f*
Curative surgery, 243*t*, 417
Curettage and electrodesiccation, 512
Curling's ulcer, 525, 1271
Current health problems
in cardiovascular assessment, 712-714, 713*t*
in ear and hearing assessment, 1114
in endocrine assessment, 1421
in hematologic assessment, 884-885
in musculoskeletal assessment, 1144-1145
in neurologic assessment, 936, 937*c*
in renal assessment, 1536
in reproductive assessment, 1648-1649, 1649*c*
in respiratory assessment, 559, 560*t*
in skin disorders, 466*c*, 467
in vision assessment, 1077
Cushing's disease, 1439-1445
acute adrenal insufficiency in, 1444
community-based care in, 1445, 1445*c*
excess fluid volume in, 1442-1443
history in, 1440-1441
imaging studies in, 1442
laboratory assessment in, 1441-1442
pathophysiology of, 1439-1440, 1440*f*, 1440*t*
physical assessment in, 1441, 1441*c*
psychosocial assessment in, 1441
risk for infection in, 1444
risk for injury in, 1443-1444
secondary hypertension in, 798
Cushing's syndrome, 1439, 1440, 1440*t*
Cushing's triad, 1054
Cushing's ulcer, 1271
Customs surrounding food, 31
Cutaneous infection, 499-503, 500*c*
anthrax in, 503-504
bacterial, 499, 501*f*
fungal, 501
pediculosis in, 504
prevention of, 501-502, 502*c*
scabies in, 504
viral, 499-501, 501*f*
Cutaneous reflexes, 940*f*, 940-941
Cutaneous stimulation for pain management, 55
Cutaneous ureterostomy, 1557*f*, 1576
Cutaneous ureteroureterostomy, 1577*f*
Cuticle, 462, 462*f*
CVD; *See* Cardiovascular disease
CVVH; *See* Continuous venovenous hemofiltration
Cyanocobalamin, 900
Cyanosis, 468*t*
in acute respiratory distress syndrome, 687
cardiovascular assessment and, 715
in dark-skinned patient, 805, 885
in high altitude pulmonary edema, 155
in hypovolemic shock, 835
in inhalation anthrax, 673
in lung cancer, 644
in malignant hyperthermia, 273
in patient with dark skin, 475, 476*c*
Cyanosis *(Continued)*
in pulmonary embolism, 679
in Raynaud's phenomenon, 816
in seizure, 959
in septic shock, 842
in severe acute respiratory syndrome, 666
in sickle cell disease, 895
CyberKnife, 1062
Cyclandelate, 816
Cyclic adenosine monophosphate, 615
Cyclic feeding, 1398
Cyclins, 400-401
Cyclobenzaprine, 327
Cyclomen; *See* Danazol
Cyclooxygenase-2 inhibitors, 46
Cyclophosphamide, 422*t*
for aplastic anemia, 900
for bladder cancer, 1575
for idiopathic pulmonary fibrosis, 639
for immunohemolytic anemia, 899
for multiple sclerosis, 1006
for rheumatoid arthritis, 341*c*, 344
for Sjögren's syndrome, 396
Cyclospasmol; *See* Cyclandelate
Cyclosporine, 319
for aplastic anemia, 900
drug-induced immune deficiency and, 384
for lung transplantation, 637
nephrotoxicity of, 1498
for psoriasis, 508
for renal transplantation, 1633
for Sjögren's syndrome, 396
Cymbalta; *See* Duloxetine hydrochloride
Cyproheptadine
for Cushing's disease, 1442
to stimulate appetite, 1395
Cyst, 469*f*, 508
Baker's, 338
Bartholin, 1699
bone, 323
of ear, 1120-1121
in fibrocystic breast condition, 1661
ganglion, 1172
ovarian, 1694
in polycystic kidney disease, 1581-1585, 1582*f*, 1583*f*, 1583-1585*c*
vocal cord, 595
Cystectomy, 1575, 1576
Cystic duct, 1218*f*
Cystic fibrosis, 635-637
Cystine stones, 1574*t*
Cystinuria, 1571*t*, 1574
Cystitis, 1533, 1551-1559
community-based care in, 1558-1559
drug therapy for, 1555-1558, 1556-1558*c*
laboratory assessment in, 1554-1555
nursing diagnoses in, 1555
nutrition therapy for, 1558
pathophysiology of, 1551-1553, 1552*t*, 1553*c*
physical assessment in, 1553-1554, 1555*c*
prevention of, 1553, 1554*c*
prostatitis-related, 1733
Cystocele, 1563, 1568, 1693, 1693*f*
Cystography, 1544*t*, 1546, 1578
Cystometrography, 1547
Cystoscopy, 1544*t*, 1546-1547
in bladder cancer, 1576
in cystitis, 1555
Cystospaz; *See* Hyoscyamine
Cystourethrography, 1546, 1588
Cystourethroscopy, 1546-1547
Cytadren; *See* Aminoglutethimide
Cytarabine, 421*t*
Cytokines, 317-318, 318*f*, 318*t*
as biological response modifiers, 433*t*, 433-434
heart failure and, 767
multiple myeloma and, 915
obesity and, 1402
osteoarthritis and, 323
Cytokines *(Continued)*
septic shock and, 842
systemic inflammatory response and, 839
Cytokinesis, 65*f*, 66
Cytologic examination
in gastritis, 1267
in lung cancer, 644
Cytomegalovirus infection, 372
Cytopenia, 901
Cytoplasm, 63*f*
Cytoprotectants, 424*t*, 425
Cytoreductive surgery in cancer, 417
Cytosar; *See* Cytarabine
Cytosine, 64, 64*f*
Cytotec; *See* Misoprostol
Cytotoxic drugs, 384
Cytotoxic edema in traumatic brain injury, 1051
Cytotoxic effects of chemotherapy, 421
Cytotoxic reactions, 394, 394*f*
Cytotoxic/cytolytic T-cell, 309*t*, 317, 878*t*
Cytoxan; *See* Cyclophosphamide

D

D cylinder, 579
Dacarbazine, 422*t*
Daclizumab, 320
Dactinomycin, 421*t*
DAI; *See* Diffuse axonal injury
Daily-wear contact lenses, 1103
Dalteparin
after total hip arthroplasty, 330
for deep vein thrombosis, 819
Danazol
for endometriosis, 1687
for fibrocystic breast condition, 1661
Dandelion, 246*t*
Dandruff, 473
Danocrine; *See* Danazol
Dantrolene, 273, 1006
Dapsone
for brown recluse spider bite, 147
for leprosy, 516
for *Pneumocystis jiroveci* pneumonia, 379
Darbepoetin alfa
for acute renal failure, 1606*c*
for cancer therapy support, 433*t*
for chemotherapy-related anemia, 426
for leukemia, 911
Darifenacin, 1291
Dark skin assessment, 475-476, 476*c*
Darunavir, 377*c*, 379
Dasatinib, 435*t*
Daunorubicin, 421*t*
Davol; *See* DuPen Silastic catheter
Dawn phenomenon, 1486, 1487*f*
DDAVP; *See* Desmopressin
ddC; *See* Zalcitabine
D-dimer test, 818
ddI; *See* Didanosine
Death, 112
in acute pancreatitis, 1373
in amyotrophic lateral sclerosis, 1007
in botulism, 1341
in brown recluse spider bite, 147
cancer and, 406*f*
in diabetic ketoacidosis, 1510
dyspnea management in, 117-118
in emergency department, 134
in endometrial cancer, 1702
euthanasia and, 121-122, 122*t*
in high altitude cerebral edema, 155
in high altitude pulmonary edema, 155
hyperkalemia and, 190
incidence of, 113
in myxedema coma, 1456, 1459
in pancreatic cancer, 1380
pathophysiology of dying and, 112
patient and family education in, 115*c*
in pelvic inflammatory disease, 1748
Death *(Continued)*
perception of, 111-112, 112*t*
in phencyclidine withdrawal, 87
planning for, 113, 114*f*
postmortem care and, 121, 121*c*, 122*c*
from preventable health care errors, 2
in scorpion sting, 149
in septic shock, 840
in stroke, 1030
in thyroid storm, 1455
ventricular tachycardia and, 748, 749
Death rattle, 117
Débridement
in brown recluse spider bite, 147
in burn, 539
in diabetic foot care, 1503-1504
in facial trauma, 593
in frostbite, 154
in open fracture, 1193
in postoperative wound infection, 296
of pressure ulcer, 491, 493*t*
Debriefing after mass casualty incident, 164*c*, 164-165
Decadron; *See* Dexamethasone
Decannulation, accidental, 580
Deceleration injury, 1050*f*, 1050-1051, 1183
Decerebrate posturing, 942, 942*f*, 1055
Decibel intensity, 1117*t*
Declomycin; *See* Demeclocycline
Decompensated cirrhosis, 1345
Decompressive laminectomy, 996-997
Decongestants
for allergic rhinitis, 390
for rhinitis, 654
for sinusitis, 655
Decorticate posturing, 942, 942*f*, 1055
Dedicated administration set, 220
Deep brain stimulation
for cluster headache, 955
for Parkinson disease, 969
Deep breathing
after laryngectomy, 601
after lumbar spinal surgery, 988
after peripheral arterial disease surgery, 809
in heart failure, 770
preoperative teaching of, 257*c*
for ventilatory support in burn, 535
Deep cervical lymph nodes, 1235*f*
Deep femoral artery, 804*f*
Deep full-thickness burn, 521*t*, 523, 523*f*
Deep partial-thickness burn, 521*t*, 522*f*, 522-523, 523*f*
Deep peroneal nerve, 1022*f*
Deep tendon reflexes
assessment of, 940, 940*f*
hypercalcemia and, 194
hypermagnesemia and, 196
hypernatremia and, 186
spinal cord injury and, 993-994
Deep vein thrombophlebitis, 817
Deep vein thrombosis, 816-821, 817*f*, 819*c*, 821*c*
after stroke, 1046
in lower extremity fracture, 1183
preoperative patient education in, 258, 259*f*
pulmonary embolism and, 678
spinal cord injured patient and, 997
total hip arthroplasty and, 330-331
Deep venous circulation, 709
Defibrillation, 756-757
Degenerative joint disease; *See* Osteoarthritis
Dehiscence, 291*f*, 291-292, 296
Dehydration, 176-181
in acute sialadenitis, 1240
approaching death and, 116
assessment of, 178*c*, 178-179, 179*f*
in cholecystitis, 1369
in diabetes insipidus, 1432
in diabetes mellitus, 1467
in diabetic ketoacidosis, 1512
in enteral nutrition therapy, 1400

Dehydration *(Continued)*
fever and, 452
in heat exhaustion, 142
in high altitude-related illnesses, 155
in hyperglycemic-hyperosmolar state, 1512-1513
in hypothermia, 153
hypovolemic shock and, 832
interventions for, 179-181, 180*c*, 180*t*
nursing diagnoses for, 179
in older adult, 1419*c*
pathophysiology of, 176*t*, 176-177, 177*f*
prevention of, 178
specific gravity of urine and, 1538
thermal airway burn and, 530
Delavirdine, 377*c*, 379
Delayed closure in wound healing, 482*f*
Delayed gastric emptying
in alkaline reflux gastropathy, 1285
in gastric ulcer, 1270-1271
Delayed hypersensitivity reactions, 395
Delayed union, 1183
Delirium
older adult and, 21-22, 22*t*
in Parkinson disease, 968
Delirium tremens, 84
Delta cell, 1418, 1418*f*
Delta-Cortef; *See* Prednisolone
Deltasone; *See* Prednisone
Demadex; *See* Torsemide
Demand dose in patient-controlled analgesia, 52
Demeclocycline, 1435-1436
Dementia, 21, 22*t*
in Alzheimer's disease, 969-980
caregiver role strain in, 978
chronic confusion in, 974*c*, 974*t*, 974-976, 976*c*
disturbed sleep pattern in, 977-978
health care resources for, 979
health promotion and maintenance in, 970
health teaching in, 978-979
history in, 970-971, 971*t*
home care management of, 978, 978*c*
imaging studies in, 973
laboratory assessment in, 973
nursing diagnoses in, 973-974
pathophysiology of, 969-970
physical assessment in, 971-973, 972*c*, 972*f*
psychosocial assessment in, 973
risk for injury in, 976-977, 977*t*
in Huntington disease, 980
oral hygiene in long-term care and, 1232
in Parkinson disease, 967
Demerol; *See* Meperidine
Demographic data in emergency nursing, 124-125
Demyelination
in Guillain-Barré syndrome, 1011-1012
in multiple sclerosis, 1002-1003
Dendrite, 928, 929*f*
Dental problems
methamphetamine use and, 86, 86*f*
older adult and, 17
Dentures, preoperative removal of, 260, 277-278
Deoxyribonucleic acid, 63-68
cell division and, 65*f*, 65-66, 66*f*
chromosomal analysis and, 67-68, 68*f*
chromosome formation and, 66, 67*f*
chromosome function and, 66-67, 67*f*
mutations of, 70-71
protein synthesis and, 70, 70*f*, 70*t*, 71*f*
structure of, 63-65, 64*f*, 65*f*
Depacon; *See* Valproate
Depade; *See* Naltrexone
Depakene; *See* Valproic acid
Depakote; *See* Divalproex
Dependence, 80
cocaine and, 86
opioid analgesics and, 90
DepoDur; *See* Morphine sulfate extended-release liposome
Depolarization, 731
Depo-Provera; *See* Medroxyprogesterone acetate
Deprenyl; *See* Selegiline
Depressants abuse, 81, 81*t*, 88-89
Depressed skull fracture, 1050
Depression
chronic pain and, 37
in coronary artery disease, 855
in Guillain-Barré syndrome, 1015
in heart failure, 769
in hypothyroidism, 1457
lesbian and, 30
in lightning strike, 151
older adult and, 20-21, 21*f*
in premenstrual syndrome, 1685
Dermabrasion, 514*t*
Dermal appendages, 462, 462*f*
burn-related skin changes and, 520, 522*f*
Dermal papilla, 461, 461*f*
Dermatomes, 933, 933*f*
Dermatomyositis, 354
Dermatophytosis, 500*c*, 501
Dermis, 461, 461*f*, 462*f*
burn-related skin changes and, 520, 522*f*
changes related to aging, 464*c*
functions of, 463*t*
Deronil; *See* Dexamethasone
DES; *See* Diethylstilbestrol
Descending colon, 1219
Descending colostomy, 1299*f*
Descending Guillain-Barré syndrome, 1013*t*
Descending loop of Henle, 1528*f*, 1530*t*, 1531*f*
Descending tracts, 933
Descriptive pain distress scale, 43, 43*f*
Desensitization therapy, 391
Desflurane, 274*t*
Desipramine, 1565*c*
Desloratadine, 390
Desmopressin
after brain tumor surgery, 1065
for diabetes insipidus, 1433, 1434*c*
Desquamation, 522
Desyrel; *See* Trazodone
Detached retina, 151, 1101-1102, 1102*b*
Detrol; *See* Tolterodine
Detrusor dyssynergia, 1560*t*
Detrusor hyperreflexia, 1006, 1560*t*
Detrusor muscle, 1532, 1532*f*
aging related changes in, 1533
benign prostatic hypertrophy and, 1713, 1713*f*
Dexair; *See* Dexamethasone
Dexamethasone
for acute mountain sickness, 156
for cerebral edema, 1062
for chemotherapy-induced nausea and vomiting, 429*c*
for dyspnea in dying patient, 117
for high altitude cerebral edema, 156
for ocular infection, 1086*c*
Dexamethasone suppression testing, 1442
Dexotic; *See* Dexamethasone
Dexrazoxane, 424*t*
Dextran, 1598
Dextromethorphan, 55
Dextrose in Ringer's lactate, 180*t*
Dextrose in saline, 180*t*
Dextrose in water, 180*t*
DHE; *See* Dihydroergotamine
DHT; *See* Dihydrotestosterone
DI; *See* Diabetes insipidus
DiaBeta; *See* Glyburide
Diabetes insipidus, 1427*c*, 1432-1433, 1433*c*, 1434*c*
after brain tumor surgery, 1064
after traumatic brain injury, 1057
in brain tumor, 1060
Diabetes mellitus, 1465-1520
absence of insulin in, 1467*t*, 1467-1468
amputation and, 1200
atherosclerosis and, 794
blood glucose control in, 1505
blood glucose monitoring in, 1490-1492, 1491-1492*t*
chronic kidney disease and, 1619
chronic pain in, 1504-1505, 1505*c*
chronic pancreatitis and, 1377, 1379
classification of, 1466, 1466*t*
complications of
acute, 1468
diabetic ketoacidosis in, 1510-1512, 1512*c*
erectile dysfunction in, 1471
heart disease in, 709, 852, 854*c*
hyperglycemic-hyperosmolar state in, 1512*c*, 1512-1514, 1513*f*
hypoglycemia in, 1506-1509, 1507*t*, 1508*c*
macrovascular, 1468-1469
microvascular, 1469, 1469*f*, 1470*t*
nephropathy in, 1470-1471
neuropathy in, 1469-1470, 1470*t*
sensory alterations in, 1500-1501, 1501*f*
urinary tract infection in, 1551*t*
vision changes in, 1075
concept map for, 1476
cultural considerations in, 1472, 1473*t*
cystic fibrosis and, 636
endocrine pancreas and, 1466
etiology and genetic risk in, 1471*t*, 1471-1472
exercise therapy for, 1496-1497, 1497*c*
foot care in, 1501-1503, 1502*c*, 1502*t*, 1503*b*, 1503*f*, 1504*c*
glucose homeostasis and, 1467
health care resources for, 1516
health promotion and maintenance in, 1472
health teaching in, 1514-1515, 1516*c*, 1517*t*
history in, 1473
home care management in, 1516, 1516*c*
hyperglycemia in, 1475-1477
incidence and prevalence of, 1472
ineffective renal tissue perfusion in, 1506
insulin physiology and, 1466*f*, 1466-1467
insulin therapy for, 1484-1489
alternative methods of administration in, 1486-1489, 1487*c*, 1488*b*, 1489*f*
complications of, 1486, 1487*f*
evidence-based practice in, 1500
factors influencing insulin absorption and, 1485-1486, 1486*f*, 1486*t*
insulin regimens in, 1484-1485
types of insulin in, 1484, 1485*t*
laboratory assessment in, 1473*c*, 1473*t*, 1473-1475, 1474*c*, 1474*t*
newer drug therapies for, 1489-1490
nursing diagnoses in, 1475
nutrition therapy for, 1492-1495, 1494*t*, 1495*t*
oral drug therapy for, 1477-1483*c*, 1477-1484, 1483*t*
pancreatic transplantation for, 1498-1500
subcutaneous infusion therapy in, 237*t*
wound care in, 1503-1504
Diabetic ketoacidosis, 1510-1512, 1512*c*
Diabetic nephropathy, 1468, 1470-1471, 1506, 1590, 1594*t*, 1594-1595
Diabetic neuropathy, 1468, 1469-1470, 1470*t*
chronic pain in, 1504-1505, 1505*c*
foot and, 1501-1503, 1502*c*, 1502*t*, 1503*c*, 1503*f*, 1504*c*
Diabetic retinopathy, 1468, 1469
Diabetic ulcer, 806*c*
Diabinese; *See* Chlorpropamide
Diagnostic peritoneal lavage
in abdominal trauma, 1307
in peritonitis, 1318
Diagnostic surgery, 243*t*
Dialysate, 1608, 1621
additives in, 1627
peritoneal dialysis-related leakage of, 1630
Dialysis, 1620-1630
in Goodpasture's syndrome, 397
health teaching in, 1635
hemodialysis in, 1620-1626, 1621*t*
in acute renal failure, 1607*f*, 1607-1608
anticoagulation in, 1622
complications of, 1626
dialysis settings for, 1621
dietary restrictions in, 1617*t*
in hypothermia, 153
nursing care in, 1625, 1625*t*
patient selection for, 1620
post-dialysis care in, 1625-1626, 1626*c*
procedure of, 1621*f*, 1621-1622, 1622*f*
vascular access for, 1622-1625, 1623*t*, 1624*c*, 1625*f*
in hypercalcemia, 194
peritoneal, 1626-1630, 1627*t*, 1627-1629*f*, 1629*c*
in acute renal failure, 1608
dietary restrictions in, 1617*t*, 1618
hemodialysis *versus*, 1621*t*
protein needs in, 1615-1617
Dialysis catheter, 219
Dialysis disequilibrium syndrome, 1626
Dialyzable drugs, 1625*t*
Dialyzer, 1621, 1621*f*
Diamox; *See* Acetazolamide
Diaphoresis
in aortic dissection, 814
in black widow spider bite, 148
in hyperthyroidism, 1450
in inhalation anthrax, 673
in pheochromocytoma, 1446
in urolithiasis, 1571
Diaphragm, 1218*f*
emphysema and, 621, 622*f*
Diaphragmatic breathing
after lung transplantation, 630, 631*c*
preoperative teaching of, 257*c*
Diaphragmatic hernia, 1249*f*, 1249-1254, 1253*c*, 1253*f*, 1254*c*
Diaphysis, 1141, 1141*f*
Diarrhea
in acquired immunodeficiency syndrome, 380-381
in avian influenza, 668
in bee sting, 149
in Crohn's disease, 1331
in enteral nutrition therapy, 1400
in *Escherichia coli* infection, 1341
in food poisoning, 1341
in gastroenteritis, 1319*t*, 1319-1321, 1321*c*
in hookworm infection, 1340
in irritable bowel syndrome, 1289-1290
in malabsorption syndrome, 1311
in malnutrition, 1392
metabolic acidosis and, 209
in scleroderma, 352
skin care in, 1312*c*
in ulcerative colitis, 1323-1325, 1324*c*
Diarthrodial joint, 1142
Diascopy, 477
Diastole, 706
Diastolic blood pressure, 708
heart disease and, 797
hypovolemic shock and, 834
Diastolic heart failure, 765
Diastolic murmur, 719

Diathermy for retinal detachment, 1101
Diazepam, 957*c*
 for alcohol withdrawal, 84
 for anxiety in head and neck cancer, 604
 for black widow spider bite, 148
 for dying patient, 118
 for heat stroke-related seizures, 143
 for moderate sedation, 276
 for multiple sclerosis, 1006
 for status epilepticus, 959, 960
Diazoxide, 1509
Dibenzyline; *See* Phenoxybenzamine
DIC; *See* Disseminated intravascular coagulation
Diclofenac, 1086*c*
Dicyclomine
 for acute pancreatitis, 1375-1376
 for cholecystitis, 1369
 for urinary incontinence, 1565*c*, 1567
Didanosine, 376*c*, 379
Didronel; *See* Etidronate
Diencephalon, 930
Diet
 achalasia and, 1255
 after hysterectomy, 1698*c*
 atherosclerosis and, 795
 chronic kidney disease and, 1615-1618, 1617*c*, 1617*t*
 coronary artery disease and, 851, 854*c*
 diabetic nephropathy and, 1506
 for dumping syndrome, 1286*t*
 dysmenorrhea and, 1685
 edentulous patient and, 1395
 hemorrhoids and, 1310
 hypothyroidism and, 1459
 iron deficiency anemia and, 899
 malabsorption syndrome and, 1311-1312
 Meniere's disease and, 1128
 minimal bacteria, 906
 obesity and, 1403, 1404-1405
 polycystic kidney disease and, 1585
 preoperative restrictions, 254
 to reduce cancer risk, 408*c*
 renal stones and, 1574*t*
 restrictions in hemodialysis, 1617*t*
 urolithiasis and, 1571
Dietary Guidelines for Americans, 1387, 1387*c*
Diethylpropion, 1405
Diethylstilbestrol, 1723
Dietitian; *See* Nutritionist
Differential white blood cell count, 311, 311*t*
 in allergic rhinitis, 389
 in cystitis, 1555
 in infection assessment, 450
 in respiratory assessment, 565*c*
Diffuse axonal injury, 1050
Diffuse interstitial fibrosis, 338, 640*c*
Diffuse neuropathies in diabetes mellitus, 1469-1470, 1470*t*
Diffuse scleroderma, 351
Diffuse skin lesion, 471*t*
Diffusion, 172*f*, 172-173
 hemodialysis and, 1621
Diffusion capacity of carbon monoxide, 567*t*
Diffusion imaging, 945-946
Diffusion test in chronic obstructive pulmonary disease, 627
Diflucan; *See* Fluconazole
Digestion, 1216-1217
Digital clubbing, 475*t*, 626, 626*f*
Digital mammography, 1670
Digital rectal examination
 in benign prostatic hypertrophy, 1714
 in prostate cancer, 1719, 1719*c*, 1720
 in urinary incontinence, 1563
Digitalis toxicity, 773
Digoxin, 744*c*
 for acute renal failure, 1606*c*
 for heart failure, 773
 hypokalemia and, 188
Digoxin, *(Continued)*
 patient education in, 778*c*
 for primary pulmonary hypertension, 638
Dihydroergotamine, 953, 953*t*
Dihydrotestosterone
 benign prostatic hypertrophy and, 1713, 1714
 prostate cancer and, 1719
Dilantin; *See* Phenytoin
Dilated cardiomyopathy, 787-790, 788*t*, 789*f*, 790*c*
Dilation and curettage, 1688
Dilaudid; *See* Hydromorphone
Dilor; *See* Dyphylline
Diloxanide furoate, 1339
Diltiazem, 744*c*
 for atrial fibrillation, 746
 for hypertrophic cardiomyopathy, 788
 for primary pulmonary hypertension, 637
 for supraventricular tachycardia, 741
 for valvular heart disease, 781
Diopter, 1102
Diovan; *See* Valsartan
Diphenhydramine
 for allergic rhinitis, 390
 for anaphylaxis, 392, 393, 393*c*
 for asthma, 610
 for bee sting, 150
 for urticaria, 480
Diphenoxylate hydrochloride with atropine sulfate
 for gastroenteritis, 1320
 for ulcerative colitis, 1324
Dipivefrin hydrochloride, 1099*c*
Diplococcus sinusitis, 654
Diploid number of chromosomes, 66
Diplopia
 after stroke, 1047
 in hypopituitarism, 1426
 in migraine headache, 951
 in multiple sclerosis, 1004, 1006
 in myasthenia gravis, 1016
Diprivan; *See* Propofol
Dipyridamole, 725
Direct commissurotomy, 782
Direct contract transmission of infection, 442
Direct Coombs' test, 886, 887*c*
Direct current stimulation for back pain, 987
Direct inguinal hernia, 1291-1293, 1292*f*
Direct response of pupil, 942
Direct traumatic brain injury, 1049
Directed blood donation, 246-247
Directly observed therapy in tuberculosis, 449
Disability examination in trauma nursing, 138, 138*t*
Disaccharide enzyme deficiency, 1311-1312, 1312*c*
Disaster Medical Assistance Team, 162
Disaster Mortuary Team, 162
Disaster preparedness, 159-168
 case presentation of anthrax exposure and, 166*f*, 166-167
 event resolution and, 164*c*, 164-166
 hospital incident command system and, 162-163, 163*t*
 impact of recent disasters and, 159-160, 160*f*
 mass casualty triage and, 160-161, 161*t*
 notification and activation of emergency plans and, 161-162
 role of nursing in, 163-164, 164*t*
Disaster supply kit, 163, 164*t*
Disaster triage tag system, 161, 161*t*
Discharge instructions, 300
 in anterior cervical diskectomy and fusion, 990*c*
 in bariatric surgery, 1408*c*
 cultural awareness in, 134
 in total hip arthroplasty, 332, 332*c*
Discharge planning, 247
 in rehabilitation, 108
Discoid lesion, 348
Discoid lupus erythematosus, 347-350, 348*c*, 349*f*, 350*c*
Discrimination in health care, 30-31
Disease-associated arthritis, 357, 357*t*
Disease-modifying antirheumatic drugs
 for ankylosing spondylitis, 355
 for rheumatoid arthritis, 340
Disequilibrium, hydrostatic pressure and, 171, 171*f*
Disinfection, 445
Diskectomy, 986
Diskitis, laminectomy-related, 986
Dislocation, 1208
 of hip after open reduction and internal fixation, 1197
 total hip arthroplasty and, 329-330, 330*c*
 total shoulder arthroplasty and, 334
Dislodgement of central venous catheter, 232*t*
Disopyramide, 741*c*
Disorientation
 approaching death and, 115*c*
 in lightning strike, 151
 in pulmonary edema, 775
 in traumatic brain injury, 1058
Displaced fracture, 1179*f*
Disposition of patient
 in emergency care, 133
 trauma nursing and, 138-139
Dissecting aneurysm, 810, 814, 1031
Dissecting hematoma, 810, 814
Disseminated intravascular coagulation
 in acute pancreatitis, 1373
 in cancer, 435
 in pit viper envenomation, 144
 in septic shock, 842
 in severe sepsis, 840
Dissociative drugs, 87-88
Distal convoluted tubule, 1528, 1528*f*, 1530, 1530*t*, 1531*f*
Distal interphalangeal joint
 musculoskeletal assessment of, 1146, 1147*f*
 positioning for prevention of contracture, 544*c*
Distal symmetric polyneuropathy, 1470*t*
Distal/embolic protection device, 1044
Distraction methods
 for chemotherapy, 425
 for pain management, 56
 for preoperative anxiety, 259
Distributive shock, 828, 828*t*
 causes of, 830*c*
 risk factors in older adult, 841*c*
Ditropan; *See* Oxybutynin
Diuretics
 for acute renal failure, 1605
 for chronic kidney disease, 1618, 1620
 for cirrhosis, 1352
 for dyspnea in dying patient, 117
 fluid balance disturbance and, 178
 for fluid overload, 182
 for hypernatremia, 187
 for hyperparathyroidism, 1462
 for hypertension, 801
 for hypokalemia, 189
 hypokalemia and, 188
 ototoxic, 1114*t*
 for primary pulmonary hypertension, 638
 to reduce preload, 772-773
 for syndrome of inappropriate antidiuretic hormone secretion, 1435
Divalent cation, 191
Divalproex, 955, 957*c*
Diverticula, esophageal, 1261-1262
Diverticular disease, 1334*f*, 1334-1337, 1335*c*
Diverticulitis, 1290*f*, 1334*f*, 1334-1337, 1335*c*
Diverticulosis, 1290*f*, 1334*f*, 1334-1337, 1335*c*
Diving reflex, 156
Dix-Hallpike test, 1117
Dizziness, 1126-1127
 after cardiac catheterization, 724
 in aortic dissection, 814
 in Lyme disease, 356
DKA; *See* Diabetic ketoacidosis
DLCO; *See* Diffusion capacity of carbon monoxide
DMARDs; *See* Disease-modifying antirheumatic drugs
DMAT; *See* Disaster Medical Assistance Team
DMORT; *See* Disaster Mortuary Team
DNA; *See* Deoxyribonucleic acid
DNA human papillomavirus test, 1652
DNR order
 advance directive and, 113
 end-of-life care and, 112
 intraoperative medical record review and, 278
Dobutamine
 for cardiac arrest, 753*c*
 to enhance contractility, 773
 for heart failure, 864*c*
 for hypovolemic shock, 837*c*, 838
 for pharmacologic stress echocardiogram, 725
 for pulmonary embolism, 682
Dobutrex; *See* Dobutamine
Docetaxel, 421*t*
 for esophageal cancer, 1258
 for pancreatic cancer, 1382
 for prostate cancer, 1723
Docking proteins, 363, 363*f*
Documentation
 of autologous or directed blood donation, 247
 of extravasation, 423, 424*c*
 of health teaching, 5
 of infusion therapy, 225
 of wound assessment, 488-489
Dofetilide, 744*c*
Dog tapeworm infestation, 1340
Dolasetron, 429*c*
Dolophine; *See* Methadone
Donepezil, 968
Donor, kidney, 1631, 1631*f*
Donovanosis, 1753-1754
Dopamine, 930*t*
 Alzheimer's disease and, 970
 for anaphylaxis, 393*c*
 for cardiac arrest, 752, 752*c*
 for heart failure, 864*c*
 for hypovolemic shock, 837*c*, 838
 methamphetamine and, 85
 Parkinson disease and, 965
Dopamine agonists
 for hyperpituitarism, 1430
 for Parkinson disease, 967
 for restless legs syndrome, 1024
Dopamine receptor antagonists, 968
Doppler flow studies in deep vein thrombosis, 817
Doppler ultrasonography
 in erectile dysfunction, 1726
 transcranial, 949
Dornase alfa, 629
Dorsal rhizotomy, 58*f*
Dorsal venous arch, 216*f*
Dorsalis pedis artery, 804*f*
Dorsalis pedis pulse, 717*f*
Doryx; *See* Doxycycline
Dorzolamide, 1100*c*
Dose-dense chemotherapy, 423
Dostinex; *See* Cabergoline
Double-barrel stoma, 1298-1299, 1299*f*
Double-voiding for reflex urinary incontinence, 1568
Doubling time of tumor, 407
Dovonex; *See* Calcipotriene
Dowager's hump, 1155, 1156*f*

Doxazosin
for benign prostatic hypertrophy, 1714
for hypertension, 802
Doxorubicin, 421*t*
Doxycin; *See* Doxycycline
Doxycycline
for chlamydial infection, 1747
for cutaneous anthrax, 504
for gonorrhea, 1746
for granuloma inguinale, 1754
for inhalation anthrax, 673*c*
for Lyme disease, 356
for lymphogranuloma venereum, 1753
for pelvic inflammatory disease, 1750*c*
DPL; *See* Diagnostic peritoneal lavage
DPP-IV inhibitors, 1490
Drain
in gallstones, 1369
postoperative assessment of, 292, 292*f*
postoperative care of, 295
preoperative preparation for, 255
Dressing
in brain tumor surgery, 1063
for burn wound, 539-540, 541*f*, 549*t*
for intravenous catheter, 223*f*, 223-224, 224*f*
postoperative assessment of, 292
postoperative care and, 294-295, 295*f*
for pressure ulcer, 491-493, 493-495*t*
in rhinoplasty, 591, 591*f*
risk for infection and, 282
for tracheostomy, 585, 585*f*
for venous stasis ulcer, 822
Dressler's syndrome, 785
Drithocreme; *See* Anthralin
Droplet precautions, 447*t*, 448
Droplet transmission of infection, 442
Drotrecogin, 843*t*, 844
Drowning, 156-157
Droxia; *See* Hydroxyurea
DRSP; *See* Drug-resistant *Streptococcus pneumoniae*
Drug abuse, 80-93
alcohol and, 82-84, 83*t*, 84*c*, 84*t*
barbiturates and, 89
commonly abused substances, 81*t*
depressants and, 88-89
effects on lung function, 558
hallucinogens and, 86-88
hospitalized patient and, 81-82
infective endocarditis and, 783-784
inhalants and, 91
nicotine and, 84-85, 85*f*
nurse and, 82
opioids and, 90*t*, 90-91, 91*c*
parenteral transmission of HIV and, 367-368
steroids and, 91-92
stimulants and, 85-86, 86*f*, 86*t*
stress and, 81
Drug errors
intravenous drug therapy and, 215
older adult and, 19-20
patient-controlled analgesia and, 52
Drug eruption, 505*c*
Drug history
in cardiovascular assessment, 711
in musculoskeletal trauma, 1184
in renal assessment, 1535-1536
in skin problems, 466*c*
in vision assessment, 1076, 1076*t*
Drug holiday in Parkinson disease, 968
Drug therapy
for acquired immunodeficiency syndrome, 375-379, 376-378*c*
for acute leukemia, 905
for acute myocardial infarction, 856-858, 857-858*c*, 859
for acute pancreatitis, 1375-1376
for acute renal failure, 1605-1607, 1606*c*
for acute respiratory distress syndrome, 688-689
for alcohol withdrawal, 84
for allergic rhinitis, 390-391
Drug therapy *(Continued)*
for Alzheimer's disease, 976
for asthma, 615-621, 616-618*c*
for atherosclerosis, 796, 796*t*
for atrial dysrhythmias, 741-745*c*
for benign prostatic hypertrophy, 1714-1715
biologic ecology and, 31
for bone cancer, 1169
for brain abscess, 1066
for brain tumor, 1062
for burn patient
for decreased cardiac output, 534
for impaired breathing, 535
for infection, 541, 542-543*c*
for infection prevention, 540-541
for pain, 536
for chronic kidney disease, 1618
for chronic leukemia, 905-906
for chronic obstructive pulmonary disease, 628-629
for chronic pancreatitis, 1378
for cirrhosis, 1352, 1355*c*
for colorectal cancer, 1297
for coronary artery disease, 872, 872*c*
for Crohn's disease, 1331-1332
for Cushing's disease, 1442
for cystitis, 1555-1558, 1556-1558*c*
for deep vein thrombosis, 818-820, 819*c*
for dehydration, 180-181
for diabetes insipidus, 1433, 1434*c*
for diabetes mellitus, 1477-1489
for diabetic ketoacidosis, 1511
for hypoglycemia, 1508-1509
insulin therapy in, 1484-1489, 1485*t*, 1486*f*, 1486*t*, 1487*c*, 1487*f*, 1488*c*, 1489*f*
for microalbuminuria, 1506
newer drugs in, 1489-1490
oral agents in, 1477-1483*c*, 1477-1484, 1483*t*
for dyspnea in dying patient, 117
for dysrhythmias, 751-753, 752-753*c*
effects on lung function, 558
for endometrial cancer, 1701
for erectile dysfunction, 1726
for fibrocystic breast condition, 1661
for fluid overload, 182
for fracture pain, 1192
for gastroenteritis, 1320-1321
for gastroesophageal reflux disease, 1246-1247*c*, 1246-1248
for genital herpes, 1742-1743, 1744
for glaucoma, 1097, 1099-1100*c*
for gonorrhea, 1746
for Goodpasture's syndrome, 397
for gout, 354
for Guillain-Barré syndrome, 1013-1014
for hearing loss, 1132
for heart failure
in acute coronary syndromes, 863-864*c*
classification of, 771*t*
to enhance contractility, 773-774
health teaching in, 777-778, 778*c*
to reduce afterload, 771-772
to reduce preload, 772-773
for Huntington disease, 980
for hypercalcemia, 194
for hyperkalemia, 190
for hypernatremia, 187
for hyperparathyroidism, 1462
for hyperpituitarism, 1430-1431
for hypertension, 801*t*, 801-802
for hyperthyroidism, 1452-1454, 1453*c*
for hypocalcemia, 193
for hypokalemia, 188-189
for hyponatremia, 186
for hypovolemic shock, 837*c*, 837-838
for idiopathic thrombocytopenic purpura, 916
for infection, 451
Drug therapy *(Continued)*
in leukemia, 906
in urolithiasis, 1573-1574
for infective endocarditis, 784-785
for inhalation anthrax, 673, 673*c*
for intestinal parasitic infection, 1339
intravenous, 214-215
for irritable bowel syndrome, 1291
for leukemia, 911
for lung cancer palliation, 650
for malabsorption syndrome, 1312
for malnutrition, 1395-1396
for Meniere's disease, 1128
for meningitis, 963
for migraine headache, 952-953, 953*t*
for multiple sclerosis, 1004-1006
for myasthenia gravis, 1018-1019
for obesity, 1405
for ocular inflammation and infection, 1086*c*
older adult issues in, 18-20, 19*t*, 20*f*
older adult with impaired vision and, 1098*c*
for oral cancer, 1237
for osteoporosis, 1157-1160, 1158-1159*c*
for Paget's disease of bone, 1164
for pain, 44-55, 45*t*
acetaminophen in, 46
acute, 297-298*c*, 297-299
adjuvant analgesics in, 54*t*, 54-55
epidural analgesia in, 52-54, 53*f*
non-opioid analgesics in, 45
nonsteroidal antiinflammatory drugs in, 45-46
opioid analgesics in, 46-51, 47*t*, 49-51*t*
patient-controlled analgesia in, 51*f*, 51-52
postoperative, 297-298*c*, 297-299
for Parkinson disease, 967-968
for pelvic inflammatory disease, 1749-1751, 1750-1751*c*
for peptic ulcer disease, 1268-1269*c*, 1274-1275
for peripheral arterial disease, 807
for portal-systemic encephalopathy, 1354-1355
postoperative, 295-296
in brain tumor surgery, 1063
in ileostomy, 1329*c*
for pain, 297-298*c*, 297-299
in percutaneous transluminal coronary angioplasty, 865
for premenstrual syndrome, 1686-1687
preoperative administration of regularly scheduled drugs and, 254
for pressure ulcer, 493
for prostate cancer, 1723
for pulmonary embolism, 680, 681*c*
for pyelonephritis, 1588
for reflex urinary incontinence, 1568
for renal trauma, 1598
for respiratory acidosis, 209
for restless legs syndrome, 1024
for rheumatoid arthritis, 340-344, 341-342*c*
for rhinitis, 654
for seizures and epilepsy, 957-959, 957-959*c*
for septic shock, 843-844
for sinusitis, 655
for skin cancer, 512
for skin infection, 503, 503*c*
for spinal cord injury, 996, 999-1000
for stomatitis, 1233
for stroke, 1043-1044
for syndrome of inappropriate antidiuretic hormone secretion, 1435-1436
for syphilis, 1741
for systemic lupus erythematosus, 350
for traumatic brain injury, 1057
for tuberculosis, 670, 671*c*
Drug therapy *(Continued)*
for ulcerative colitis, 1324-1325, 1325*t*
for urge urinary incontinence, 1567
for urinary elimination problems, 106
for urinary incontinence, 1564, 1565*c*
for urolithiasis, 1573
via subcutaneous infusion, 237, 237*t*
Drug tolerance, 39-40
alcohol and, 83
opioid analgesics and, 90
Drug-eluting stent, 866
Drug-induced disorders
cataract formation in, 1092*c*
cystitis in, 1552-1553
heart failure in, 767
hepatitis in, 1356
immune deficiencies in, 384
leukemia in, 902
secondary hypertension in, 798
syndrome of inappropriate antidiuretic hormone secretion in, 1435*t*
Drug-related diabetes insipidus, 1433
Drug-resistant *Streptococcus pneumoniae*, 665
Drug(s)
associated with gastritis, 1268
causing anaphylaxis, 391*t*
dialyzable, 1625*t*
hematologic system impairing, 883-884*t*
interference with warfarin, 821*c*
nephrotoxic, 1506, 1603*t*
ototoxic, 1113, 1114*t*
surgical risk and, 244*t*
Dry age-related macular degeneration, 1100-1101
Dry cough
in high altitude pulmonary edema, 155
in laryngitis, 658
in mitral stenosis, 779
in severe acute respiratory syndrome, 666
Dry eyes, 396, 1087
Dry heat injury, 525
Dry mouth
after oral cancer surgery, 1238
in postirradiation sialadenitis, 1240
radiation therapy-related, 420, 599
in Sjögren's syndrome, 396
Dry powder inhaler, 618-619, 619*c*, 619*f*, 620*f*
Dry skin, 465*f*, 471, 480, 480*c*
d4T; *See* Stavudine
DTIC; *See* Dacarbazine
Dual x-ray absorptiometry, 1156
Dual-lumen cuffed tracheostomy tube, 582*f*
Dual-lumen hemodialysis catheter, 1623*t*
DUB; *See* Dysfunctional uterine bleeding
Duchenne muscular dystrophy, 1175, 1175*t*
Duct of Wirsung, 1218*f*
Ductal carcinoma in situ, 1663
Ductal ectasia, 1661*t*, 1661-1662
Ductus deferens, 1646
Duetact; *See* Glimepiride-pioglitazone
Dulcolax; *See* Bisacodyl
Dull percussion sound, 562*t*, 1223
Duloxetine hydrochloride, 1504-1505
Dumping syndrome, 1285, 1286*t*
Duodenal papillae, 1218*f*
Duodenal tumor, 1279
Duodenal ulcer, 1270-1279
complementary and alternative therapies for, 1270*t*
complications of, 1271*c*, 1271*f*, 1271-1272
drug therapy for, 1268-1269*c*
etiology and genetic risk in, 1272
gastrointestinal bleeding in, 1275-1278, 1276*c*, 1277*c*, 1278*f*

Duodenal ulcer *(Continued)*
health care resources for, 1279
health teaching in, 1278
history in, 1272-1273
home care management in, 1278, 1279*c*
imaging studies in, 1273-1274
laboratory assessment in, 1273
nursing diagnoses in, 1274
pain in, 1274-1275
pathophysiology of, 1270*f*, 1270-1271, 1271*f*
physical assessment in, 1273, 1273*t*
prevention of, 1272
psychosocial assessment in, 1273
Duodenum, 1217*f*, 1218*f*, 1219
DuPen Silastic catheter, 53
Dupuytren's contracture, 1172
Dura mater, 929
Durable power of attorney for health care, 113, 114*f*
Duragesic; *See* Fentanyl
Duramorph; *See* Morphine
Duricef; *See* Cefadroxil
Dutasteride, 1714
DVT; *See* Deep vein thrombosis
Dwarf tapeworm, 1340
DXA; *See* Dual x-ray absorptiometry
Dying patient, 111-123
dyspnea management in, 117-118
euthanasia and, 121-122, 122*t*
hospice and palliative care in, 113
incidence of death and, 113
nausea and vomiting management in, 118
pain management in, 116-117
pathophysiology of dying and, 112
patient and family education in, 115*c*
perception of death and, 111-112, 112*t*
physical assessment and, 115*c*, 115-116
planning for, 113, 114*f*
postmortem care and, 121, 121*c*, 122*c*
psychosocial assessment and, 116, 116*c*
psychosocial management in, 119*t*, 119-121, 120*c*, 121*c*
refractory symptoms of distress and, 118
restlessness and agitation management in, 118
seizure management in, 118
weakness management in, 116
Dymelor; *See* Acetohexamide
Dynacin; *See* Minocycline
Dyphylline, 620
Dyrenium; *See* Triamterene
Dysarthria
in amyotrophic lateral sclerosis, 1007*c*
in multiple sclerosis, 1006
in myasthenia gravis, 1020
in Parkinson disease, 966*c*
in stroke, 1046
Dysentery, 1319*t*, 1319-1321, 1321*c*
Dysfunctional uterine bleeding, 1688-1689, 1695
Dyskinesia, 967
Dyslipidemia, 1472
Dysmenorrhea, 1648, 1684-1685
Dysmetria, 1004
Dyspareunia
after vulvectomy, 1708
in anal fissure, 1337
in Bartholin cyst, 1699
in endometriosis, 1687
in hypopituitarism, 1426
in menopause, 1689
Dyspepsia
in cholecystitis, 1368
in gastritis, 1267
in gastroesophageal reflux disease, 1244
nutrition history and, 1221
in peptic ulcer disease, 1273
Dysphagia
in achalasia, 1254-1255
after open conventional esophageal surgery, 1254
in amyotrophic lateral sclerosis, 1007*c*
in diabetic neuropathy, 1470
in esophageal cancer, 1256
in esophageal diverticula, 1261
in follicular thyroid carcinoma, 1460
in gastroesophageal reflux disease, 1245
in Guillain-Barré syndrome, 1015
in hiatal hernia, 1249
in laryngitis, 658
in lung cancer, 644, 650
malnutrition and, 1393
in myasthenia gravis, 1016
in pharyngitis, 655, 656*c*
in scleroderma, 352
in severe acute respiratory syndrome, 666
in stomatitis, 1233
in stroke, 1035
in thyroiditis, 1460
Dyspnea
in acute renal failure, 1603
in acute respiratory failure, 686
after extubation, 697
in amyotrophic lateral sclerosis, 1008
in anaphylaxis, 392
in asthma, 612
in bronchiolitis obliterans organizing pneumonia, 640*c*
cardiovascular assessment and, 713
in chronic obstructive pulmonary disease, 626, 633
in circulatory overload from fluid resuscitation in burn, 530
in cystic fibrosis, 636
in empyema, 674
end-of-life care and, 117-118
in follicular thyroid carcinoma, 1460
in inhalation anthrax, 673
in laryngeal trauma, 596
in left-sided heart failure, 768
in lung cancer, 643
in Lyme disease, 356
nutrition status and, 559
in oral cancer, 1236
patient positioning for, 770
in pneumonia, 661, 663*t*
in primary pulmonary hypertension, 637
in pulmonary embolism, 679, 679*c*
respiratory assessment and, 559, 560*t*
in vocal cord paralysis, 594
Dyspnea assessment tool, 686*f*
Dyspnea on exertion
in aortic regurgitation, 779*c*, 780
in aortic stenosis, 779*c*, 780
cardiovascular assessment and, 713
in hypertrophic cardiomyopathy, 789
in left-sided heart failure, 768
in mitral regurgitation, 779*c*, 780
in mitral stenosis, 779, 779*c*
Dysrhythmias, 730-763
advanced cardiac life support for, 756
after coronary artery bypass graft, 868
after thoracic aortic aneurysm repair, 813
in anaphylaxis, 392
atrial, 740-747
atrial fibrillation in, 745-746, 746*f*
atrial flutter in, 747
drug therapy for, 741-745*c*
premature atrial complexes in, 740
supraventricular tachycardia in, 740-741
atrioventricular blocks in, 750
automatic external defibrillation for, 757, 757*f*
bundle branch blocks in, 750
cardiac conduction system and, 731, 731*f*
in cardiomyopathy, 789
Dysrhythmias *(Continued)*
cardiopulmonary resuscitation in, 755-756
cardioversion for, 756
in chronic obstructive pulmonary disease, 623
coronary artery bypass graft for, 758
in coronary artery disease, 854, 861-862
decreased cardiac output and ineffective tissue perfusion in, 750-751, 751*c*
defibrillation for, 756-757
in digitalis toxicity, 773
drug therapy for, 751-753, 752-753*c*
electrocardiography and, 731-737, 732*f*
complexes, segments, and intervals in, 733-736, 735*f*
continuous electrocardiographic monitoring and, 732-733, 734*f*
determination of heart rate in, 736, 736*f*
heart rhythm analysis in, 736-737
lead systems for, 732, 733*t*
electrophysiologic properties of heart and, 730-731, 731*f*
health teaching in, 758-761, 759-761*c*
home care management in, 758
in hypercalcemia, 194
junctional, 747
key features of, 738*c*
in Lyme disease, 356
in malignant hyperthermia, 273
normal rhythms and, 737*f*, 737-738
nursing diagnoses in, 750
in older adult, 760*c*
pacemaker insertion for, 757
radiofrequency catheter ablation for, 757
sinus, 739*f*, 739-740
temporary pacing for, 754-755
terminology in, 738-739
vagal maneuvers for, 753-754
ventricular, 747-750, 748*f*, 749*f*
Dystrophin, 1175
Dysuria, 1535*t*
in cervical cancer, 1703
in chlamydial infection, 1747
in cystitis, 1553
endocrine system and, 1421
in orchitis, 1734
in polycystic kidney disease, 1583
preoperative assessment of, 247
in prostatitis, 1733
in urolithiasis, 1571-1572

E

E cylinder, 579, 579*f*
Ear, 1109-1137
acoustic neuroma of, 1129
anatomy and physiology of, 1109-1111, 1110*f*, 1111*f*
cerumen impaction and, 1122*f*, 1122-1123, 1123*c*
changes associated with aging, 1111, 1112*c*
external otitis and, 1121*c*, 1121*f*, 1121-1122
furuncle of, 1122
hearing assessment and, 1109-1119
anatomy and physiology review and, 1109-1111, 1110*f*, 1111*f*
audiometry in, 1117*t*, 1117-1118
auditory assessment in, 1115-1116
diagnostic assessment for balance in, 1116-1117
external ear and mastoid inspection in, 1114
imaging assessment in, 1116
otoscopic assessment in, 1115, 1115*f*
patient history in, 1111-1114, 1112*c*, 1113*c*, 1114*t*
psychosocial assessment and, 1116
Ear *(Continued)*
hearing loss and, 1129-1136
health care resources for, 1135-1136
health teaching in, 1135
hearing aid care in, 1132, 1133*c*
history in, 1130-1131
home care management in, 1135
imaging studies in, 1131
impaired verbal communication and, 1135, 1135*c*
nursing diagnoses in, 1131-1132
pathophysiology of, 1129*f*, 1129-1130, 1130*t*
physical assessment in, 1131, 1131*c*
prevention of, 1130
psychosocial assessment in, 1131
surgical management of, 1132-1133, 1133*f*, 1134*c*, 1134*f*
labyrinthitis and, 1127
mastoiditis and, 1125-1126
Meniere's disease and, 1127-1129
middle ear neoplasms and, 1126
otitis media and, 1123-1125, 1124*f*, 1125*c*, 1125*f*
perichondritis and, 1122
pharyngitis and, 656
tinnitus and, 1126, 1127*t*
trauma to, 1126
vertigo and dizziness and, 1126-1127
Eardrops, 1121*c*
Eardrum, 1109, 1110, 1110*f*, 1111*f*
changes with aging, 1112*c*
myringotomy and, 1125, 1125*f*
perforation of
in middle ear trauma, 1126
in otitis media, 1124, 1124*f*
Early ambulation
after total hip arthroplasty, 330
preoperative patient education about, 258
Early dementia, Alzheimer type, 969
Early latent syphilis, 1740
Early prostate cancer antigen, 1720
Early-onset familial Alzheimer's disease, 970
Early-onset seizure in traumatic brain injury, 1057
Earwax, 1109
cultural considerations and, 1115
impaction of, 1122*f*, 1122-1123, 1123*c*
self-ear irrigation for, 1113*c*
Earwick for instillation of antibiotics, 1121*f*
Eating disorders, 1392
Eaton-Lambert syndrome, 1017
EBRT; *See* External beam radiation therapy
Ecchymosis, 471
in abdominal trauma, 1307
in cirrhosis, 1347
hematologic assessment and, 885
in idiopathic thrombocytopenic purpura, 916
intravenous therapy-related, 228*t*
in multiple myeloma, 915
in musculoskeletal trauma, 1184
in pit viper envenomation, 144
in uremic syndrome, 1614
Eccrine sweat gland, 462, 462*f*
ECF; *See* Extracellular fluid
ECG; *See* Electrocardiography
Echinacea, 12*t*
Echocardiography
in cardiovascular assessment, 725
in coronary artery disease, 855
in heart failure, 770
in infective endocarditis, 784
in valvular heart disease, 780
Echolalia, 966*c*
Echothiophate, 1099*c*
Ecotrin; *See* Aspirin
Ecstasy, 88
Ectopic beats
in hyperkalemia, 190
prevention of, 759*c*

Ectopic focus, 738
Ectopic pregnancy, 1739*t*
Ectropion, 1085
Eczema, 505, 505*c*
Edema, 468
in acute compartment syndrome, 1181
in acute osteomyelitis, 1165, 1166*c*
in acute pancreatitis, 1372
in acute renal failure, 1603
after coronary artery bypass graft, 868
in bee sting, 149
in black widow spider bite, 148
in brown recluse spider bite, 147
capillary hydrostatic pressure and, 172
cardiovascular assessment and, 714, 715
cerebral
in brain tumor, 1060
high-altitude, 154-156, 156*c*
in traumatic brain injury, 1051
in classification of burn depth, 521*t*
in coronary artery disease, 854
in deep vein thrombosis, 817, 817*f*
in fracture, 1184
in frostbite, 154, 154*f*
in hemorrhoids, 1310
hydrostatic pressure and, 172
in infection, 839
inflammation and, 312
in nephrotic syndrome, 1593
in oral cancer, 1236
in orchitis, 1734
palpation of, 472*t*
in pit viper envenomation, 144
pitting, 181, 181*f*
pulmonary
after brain tumor surgery, 1064
in black widow spider bite, 148
in burn injury, 536
in chronic kidney disease, 1620
in coronary artery disease, 862
in Cushing's disease, 1442
fluid overload and, 182
in heart failure, 775*c*, 775-776
high-altitude, 154-156, 156*c*
in mitral stenosis, 779
in pit viper envenomation, 144
in scorpion sting, 149
in syndrome of inappropriate antidiuretic hormone secretion, 436, 1436
in thermal airway burn, 530
in renal problems, 1536
in right-sided heart failure, 768, 769
in tarantula bite, 148
in traumatic brain injury, 1051
in venous insufficiency, 821
in vulvovaginitis, 1691
Edentulous patient, nutrition management and, 1395
Efalizumab, 508
Efavirenz, 377*c*, 379
Efferent arteriole, 1528, 1528*f*, 1530*t*, 1531*f*
Efferent pathway, 928
Effusion, 1146
in osteoarthritis, 324
pleural, 561
in acute pancreatitis, 1373
in inhalation anthrax, 673
in lung cancer, 650
in rheumatoid arthritis, 338
Efudex; *See* 5-Fluorouracil
EGD; *See* Esophagogastroduodenoscopy
Ejaculatory duct, 1645*f*
Ejection fraction, 765
ELA-Max cream, 55
Elapidae envenomation, 143*f*, 143-146, 144*c*, 144*f*, 145*t*, 146*t*
Elastase, 1372
Elastic shoelaces, 103*t*
Elastic stockings, 821, 822*c*
Elastin, 461
Elavil; *See* Amitriptyline
Elbow
fracture of, 1195
positioning for prevention of contracture, 544*c*
total elbow arthroplasty and, 335
Elbow surgery, skin preparation for, 256*f*
Eldepryl; *See* Selegiline
Elder neglect and abuse, 22*c*, 22-23, 977
Elderly; *See* Older adult
Elective surgery, 243*t*
Electrical bone stimulation, 1192
Electrical burn, 526, 527*f*, 528*c*
Electrical stimulation
for pain management, 55-56, 56*f*
for pressure ulcer, 495
for urge urinary incontinence, 1568
Electrocardiographic caliper, 736
Electrocardiographic strip, 733, 734*f*
Electrocardiography, 731-737, 732*f*
in burn, 530
in cardiovascular assessment, 724
complexes, segments, and intervals in, 733-736, 735*f*
continuous electrocardiographic monitoring and, 732-733, 734*f*
in coronary artery disease, 855
determination of heart rate in, 736, 736*f*
in heart failure, 770
heart rhythm analysis in, 736-737
in hyperkalemia, 190
in hyperthyroidism, 1452
hypocalcemia and, 192
lead systems for, 732, 733*t*
in lightning strike, 152
in myocardial infarction, 849, 849*f*
in pit viper envenomation, 145
preoperative, 249
in sickle cell disease, 896
in stress test, 724-725
in valvular heart disease, 781
Electrode placement in electrocardiography, 732, 733*t*
Electroencephalography, 946-947, 947*c*
in Alzheimer's disease, 973
in brain abscess, 1066
in neurologic assessment, 946-947, 947*c*
Electrolarynges, 602
Electrolytes, 170-198
acute renal failure and, 1604
after blood transfusion, 919
body fluids and, 174*c*, 174-175, 175*t*
burn-related changes in, 524, 532*c*
calcium and, 191-194
hypercalcemia and, 193-194, 194*t*
hypocalcemia and, 191-193, 192*t*, 193*f*
chloride and, 197
coronary artery bypass graft and, 868
dehydration and, 176-181
assessment of, 178*c*, 178-179, 179*f*
interventions for, 179-181, 180*c*, 180*t*
nursing diagnoses for, 179
pathophysiology of, 176*t*, 176-177, 177*f*
prevention of, 178
diabetic nephropathy and, 1506
fluid overload and, 181*f*, 181-183, 182*c*
gastrointestinal tract dysfunction and, 1223
heart failure and, 769
homeostasis and, 170-171, 171*f*
hormonal regulation of fluid balance and, 175-176, 176*f*
magnesium and, 195-197
hypermagnesemia and, 196-197
hypomagnesemia and, 196, 196*t*
major serum electrolyte concentrations and functions and, 184*t*
normal plasma values of, 184*t*
parenteral nutrition and, 1401, 1401*c*
phosphorus and, 194-195
hyperphosphatemia and, 195
Electrolytes *(Continued)*
hypophosphatemia and, 194-195, 195*c*, 195*t*
physiologic influences on balance of, 171-174
diffusion in, 172*f*, 172-173
filtration in, 171*f*, 171-172, 172*f*
lymph and, 174
osmosis in, 173*f*, 173-174
postoperative assessment of, 290
potassium and, 187*t*, 187-189, 189*c*
hyperkalemia and, 190*t*, 190-191, 191*c*
hypokalemia and, 187*t*, 187-189, 189*c*
preoperative assessment of, 249
refeeding syndrome and, 1399
replacement during mechanical ventilation, 696
sodium and, 183-187
hypernatremia and, 186*t*, 186-187
hyponatremia and, 185*t*, 185-186
urine, 1541
Electromyography, 946, 1150
in amyotrophic lateral sclerosis, 1007
in low back pain, 985
in myasthenia gravis, 1018
of perineal muscles, 1547
in urinary incontinence, 1563
Electronic infusion device, 221-222
Electronic mail, 6
Electronic medical records, 6, 6*f*
Electronic-beam computed tomography scan, 726
Electronystagmography, 1116
Electrophysiologic properties of heart muscle, 706
Electrophysiologic studies
in cardiovascular assessment, 724
in Guillain-Barré syndrome, 1013
Electroretinography, 1082
Electrovaporization for benign prostatic hypertrophy, 1715
Elevation, 1146*f*
Elimination
chronic and disabling diseases and, 105*t*, 105-106
effect of endocrine system on, 1421
prostate cancer and, 1721
spinal cord injury and, 997-998, 998*c*
Elimination pattern
in acid-base assessment, 207*c*
in cardiovascular assessment, 711*c*
in dehydration, 178*c*
in endocrine assessment, 1420*c*
in gastrointestinal assessment, 1220*c*
in renal assessment, 1534*c*
Elimite; *See* Permethrin
Elipten; *See* Aminoglutethimide
ELISA; *See* Enzyme-linked immunosorbent assay
Elixophyllin; *See* Theophylline
Ellence; *See* Epirubicin
Eloxatin; *See* Oxaliplatin
Elspar; *See* Asparaginase
Eltroxin; *See* Levothyroxine sodium
E-mail, 6
EMB; *See* Ethambutol
Embolectomy
in acute peripheral arterial occlusion, 810
in pulmonary embolism, 682
Embolic stroke, 1031, 1031*t*
Embolism
in acute peripheral arterial occlusion, 810
amniotic fluid, 678
fat, 678, 1141
after lumbar spinal surgery, 987*c*
fracture and, 1182*c*, 1182-1183
ischemic stroke and, 1030
in lung cancer, 641
pulmonary, 677-684
anxiety and, 682-683
atrial fibrillation and, 745-746
Embolism *(Continued)*
decreased cardiac output in, 682
fat embolism syndrome *versus*, 1182*c*
fracture-related, 1183
health care resources for, 683-684, 684*c*
health promotion and maintenance and, 678, 678*c*
health teaching in, 683, 684*c*
history in, 679
home care management in, 683
hypoxemia in, 680-682, 680-682*c*
imaging assessment in, 679
laboratory assessment in, 679
nursing diagnoses in, 679-680
pathophysiology of, 677-678
physical assessment in, 679, 679*c*
potential for bleeding in, 683, 683*c*
psychosocial assessment in, 679
spinal cord injured patient and, 997
total hip arthroplasty and, 330-331
in venous thromboembolism, 816-821, 817*f*, 819*c*, 821*c*
fracture and, 1183
homocysteine and, 795
pancreatic cancer and, 1380
total hip arthroplasty and, 329, 330*c*, 330-331
Embolization procedure for arteriovenous malformation, 1044*f*, 1044-1045
Embryonal carcinoma, 127, 1727*t*
Embryonic cell, 401*f*, 401-402, 402*t*
Emcyt; *See* Estramustine
Emend; *See* Aprepitant
Emergence from general anesthesia, 272
Emergency and disaster preparedness, 159-168
case presentation of anthrax exposure and, 166*f*, 166-167
event resolution and, 164*c*, 164-166
hospital incident command system and, 162-163, 163*t*
impact of recent disasters and, 159-160, 160*f*
mass casualty triage and, 160-161, 161*t*
notification and activation of emergency plans and, 161-162
role of nursing in, 163-164, 164*t*
Emergency care, 125-158
in abdominal trauma, 1307-1308
in acute adrenal insufficiency, 1436*c*
in acute cardiac tamponade, 786
in acute compartment syndrome, 1181
in anaphylaxis, 392*c*
in aortic dissection, 814
in autonomic dysreflexia, 998
in benzodiazepine overdose, 300*c*
in burn injury, 528*c*, 528-537
acute respiratory distress syndrome and, 537
compensatory responses and, 525, 526*f*
history and, 528, 529*c*
ineffective breathing pattern and, 535
ineffective tissue perfusion and, 533*c*, 533*t*, 533-535, 534*f*
laboratory assessment in, 531-532, 532*c*
nursing diagnoses in, 532-533
pain and, 535-536
physical assessment in, 529*t*, 529-531, 530*t*, 531*f*
pulmonary edema and, 536
in cholinergic crisis, 1019
emergency nursing concepts in, 126-140
case management in, 133-134
core competencies in, 130-131
death and, 134
emergency department environment and, 126-128, 127*f*, 128*f*

Emergency care (Continued)
mentally ill patient and, 133
patient and family education in, 134
patient disposition and, 133
staff and patient safety considerations in, 128-130, 129c
training and certification in, 131, 131t
triage and, 131t, 131-132
in environmental emergencies, 141-158
altitude-related illnesses in, 154-156, 156c
arthropod bites and stings in, 146-150, 147f, 149f, 150c
cold injuries in, 152-154, 154f
drowning in, 156-157
heat-related illnesses in, 141-143, 142c, 143c
lightning injuries in, 150-152, 151c
snakebite in, 143f, 143-146, 144c, 144f, 145t, 146f
in fracture, 1186, 1186c
in gastrointestinal bleeding, 1275-1276, 1276c
in hypertensive crisis, 802, 803c
in idioventricular rhythms, 747
intubation in, 690
in malignant hyperthermia, 275c
in myasthenic crisis, 1019
in myocardial infarction, 856-858, 856-858c
in myxedema coma, 1459c
in opiate intoxication, overdose, or withdrawal, 91c, 299c
in posterior nasal bleeding, 591-592, 592f
in seizures and epilepsy, 959-961
in sports-related injury, 1205c
in surgical wound evisceration, 296c
in thyroid storm, 1455, 1455c
in traumatic amputation, 1201
in ventricular asystole, 750
in ventricular fibrillation, 749-750
Emergency department, 126-128, 127f, 128f
Emergency medical technician, 127
Emergency medicine physician, 128
Emergency nurse, 128
Emergency nursing specialty certification, 131, 131t
Emergency operations center, 162
Emergency Severity Index, 132
Emergency thrombectomy, 809
Emergent surgery, 243t
Emergent triage categories, 131-132, 132t
Emerging infections, 453-455, 454t, 455t
Emetogenic chemotherapy agents, 645
EMG; See Electromyography
Emission, 1646
EMLA cream, 55
Emmetropia, 1073, 1073f
Emotional abuse, 22
Emotional lability
after stroke, 1035
in premenstrual syndrome, 1686c
Emotional stress
coronary artery disease and, 852
older adult and, 17-18, 18c
substance abuse and, 81
tension headache and, 955
Emotional support
in amputation, 1200-1201
in Guillain-Barré syndrome, 1016
in pancreatic cancer, 1384
in psoriasis, 508
in tracheostomy, 586
Emphysema, 621-622, 622f
combined ventilatory and oxygenation failure in, 685
pathophysiology of, 611f
surgical risk and, 246
Empirin; See Aspirin
Empyema, 673-674
Emtricitabine, 376c, 379
Emtriva; See Emtricitabine
Enablex; See Darifenacin
Enalapril
for hypertension, 801
to reduce afterload in heart failure, 771
Enbrel; See Etanercept
Encephalitis, 963-965, 964c
Encephalopathy, hepatic, 1345-1346, 1346t
Endaural approach in ear surgery, 1134f
Endocarditis, 783-785, 784c
gonorrhea-related, 1746
Endocardium, 705f
Endocervical curettage, 1703
Endocet; See Oxycodone-acetaminophen
Endochondroma, 1167
Endocrine assessment, 1412-1424
aging-related changes in endocrine system and, 1418-1419, 1419c
auscultation in, 1422
in burn, 537
hormones and, 1412-1413, 1413t
imaging studies in, 1424
inspection in, 1421-1422
laboratory assessment in, 1423c, 1423-1424
palpation in, 1422, 1422f
patient history in, 1419-1421, 1420c
psychosocial assessment in, 1422-1423
thyroid needle biopsy in, 1424
Endocrine disorders
adrenal, 1436-1447
Cushing's disease in, 1439-1445, 1440f, 1440t, 1441c, 1445c
hyperaldosteronism in, 1445-1446
hypofunction in, 1436-1439, 1436-1439c, 1437f, 1437t
pheochromocytoma in, 1446-1447
diabetes mellitus in, 1465-1520
absence of insulin in, 1467t, 1467-1468
acute complications of, 1468
amputation and, 1200
atherosclerosis and, 794
blood glucose control in, 1505
blood glucose monitoring in, 1490-1492, 1491-1492t
chronic pain in, 1504-1505, 1505c
chronic pancreatitis and, 1377, 1379
classification of, 1466, 1466t
concept map for, 1476
coronary artery disease and, 852, 854c
cultural considerations in, 1472, 1473t
cystic fibrosis and, 636
diabetic ketoacidosis in, 1510-1512, 1512c
endocrine pancreas and, 1466
erectile dysfunction in, 1471
etiology and genetic risk in, 1471t, 1471-1472
evidence-based practice and, 1500
exercise therapy for, 1496-1497, 1497c
foot care in, 1501-1503, 1502c, 1502t, 1503b, 1503f, 1504c
glucose homeostasis and, 1467
health care resources for, 1516
health promotion and maintenance in, 1472
health teaching in, 1514-1515, 1516c, 1517t
heart disease and, 709
history in, 1473
home care management in, 1516, 1516c
hyperglycemia in, 1475-1477
hyperglycemic-hyperosmolar state in, 1512c, 1512-1514, 1513f
Endocrine disorders (Continued)
hypoglycemia in, 1506-1509, 1507t, 1508c
incidence and prevalence of, 1472
ineffective renal tissue perfusion in, 1506
insulin physiology and, 1466f, 1466-1467
insulin therapy for, 1484-1489, 1485t, 1486f, 1486t, 1487c, 1487f, 1488c, 1489f
laboratory assessment in, 1473c, 1473t, 1473-1475, 1474c, 1474t
macrovascular complications in, 1468-1469
microvascular complications in, 1469, 1469f, 1470t
nephropathy in, 1470-1471
neuropathy in, 1469-1470, 1470t
newer drug therapies for, 1489-1490
nursing diagnoses in, 1475
nutrition therapy for, 1492-1495, 1494t, 1495t
oral drug therapy for, 1477-1483c, 1477-1484, 1483t
pancreatic transplantation for, 1498-1500
sensory alterations in, 1500-1501, 1501f
subcutaneous infusion therapy in, 237t
vision changes in, 1075
wound care in, 1503-1504
in HIV-infected patient, 372t, 372-373
parathyroid, 1461-1463
hyperparathyroidism in, 1461f, 1461t, 1461-1463, 1462c
hypoparathyroidism in, 1463
pituitary, 1426-1436
diabetes insipidus in, 1432-1433, 1433c, 1434c
hyperpituitarism in, 1428f, 1428-1432, 1429f, 1430c, 1431f
hypopituitarism in, 1426-1428, 1427c
syndrome of inappropriate antidiuretic hormone secretion in, 1433-1436, 1435t
tumor in, 1061, 1426, 1428, 1440
thyroid, 1448-1461
cancer in, 1460-1461
hyperthyroidism in, 1448-1455, 1449c, 1450f, 1451c, 1451t, 1453c, 1455c
hypothyroidism in, 1455-1460, 1456c, 1456f, 1459c, 1460c
thyroiditis in, 1460
Endocrine pancreas, 1218, 1418
diabetes mellitus and, 1466
Endocrine paraneoplastic syndromes, 641, 642t
Endocrine system, 1413-1418
adrenal glands in, 1415f, 1415t, 1415-1417, 1416t
blood pressure and, 708
changes associated with aging, 1418-1419, 1419c
cirrhosis and, 1348f
fluid balance and, 174c, 175-176, 176f
gonads in, 1415
hormones and, 1412-1413, 1413f, 1413t
hypothalamus and pituitary gland in, 1414-1415, 1415f, 1415t
pancreas in, 1418, 1418f, 1418t
parathyroid glands in, 1417, 1418f
thyroid gland in, 1417, 1417f, 1417t
Endodan; See Oxycodone-aspirin
End-of-life care, 111-123
dyspnea management in, 117-118
euthanasia and, 121-122, 122t
hospice and palliative care and, 113
incidence of death and, 113
End-of-life care (Continued)
nausea and vomiting management in, 118
pain management and, 116-117
pathophysiology of dying and, 112
patient and family education in, 115c
perception of death and, 111-112, 112t
physical assessment and, 115c, 115-116
planning for death and, 113, 114f
postmortem care and, 121, 121c, 122c
psychosocial assessment and, 116, 116c
psychosocial management in, 119t, 119-121, 120c, 121c
refractory symptoms of distress and, 118
restlessness and agitation management in, 118
seizure management and, 118
weakness management in, 116
Endogenous osteomyelitis, 1165
Endoluminal gastroplication, 1248, 1248c
Endolymph, 1110f
Endometrial ablation in dysfunctional uterine bleeding, 1688-1689
Endometrial biopsy, 1657, 1700
Endometrial cancer, 1699-1702, 1700t, 1701c
Endometriosis, 1687f, 1687-1688
Endometritis
gonorrhea and, 1744, 1745f
pelvic inflammatory disease and, 1748
Endometrium, 1643f
Endoplasmic reticulum, 63f, 70
Endorphins, 38, 930t
Endoscope, 267, 269f
Endoscopic carpal tunnel release, 1207
Endoscopic retrograde cholangiopancreatography, 1227
in acute pancreatitis, 1373, 1376
in chronic pancreatitis, 1378
in cirrhosis, 1350
in gallbladder cancer, 1371
in pancreatic cancer, 1380
Endoscopic ultrasonography, 1229
Endoscopic variceal ligation, 1354
Endoscopic vessel harvesting, 870
Endoscopy
in esophageal varices, 1354
in gastroesophageal reflux disease, 1248, 1248c
in gastrointestinal assessment, 1226-1228, 1227f
in gastrointestinal bleeding, 1276-1277
preparation of surgical suite for, 267-270, 271f
in reproductive assessment, 1656f, 1656-1657
in respiratory assessment, 567-568
in sinus assessment, 655
Endostatins, 1687
Endothelial injury in atherosclerosis, 794, 848f
Endothelin, 767
Endothelin-receptor antagonists
for primary pulmonary hypertension, 637-638
for scleroderma, 352
Endotoxin, 441
Endotracheal intubation, 689-692, 690f, 691c
in advanced cardiac life support, 756
in drowning, 157
postoperative evaluation of, 287
in trauma patient, 136
in upper airway obstruction, 596
Endotracheal tube, 689-690, 690f
extubation of, 697
mechanical ventilation and, 696
securing of, 691c
stabilization of, 690, 691c
T-piece apparatus for, 577, 577t, 578f
verification of placement of, 690

Endovascular repair of abdominal aortic aneurysm, 813
Endovascular stent graft, 813
Endovascular vessel harvesting, 870
Endoventricular circular patch cardioplasty, 775
End-stage kidney disease, 1600-1601
  acute renal failure and, 1601
  chronic kidney disease and, 1609*c*, 1609-1635
    acute renal failure *versus*, 1601*t*
    anxiety in, 1619-1620
    cardiac changes in, 1610-1611, 1613, 1613*c*
    concept map for, 1616
    decreased cardiac output in, 1618
    etiology and genetic risk in, 1611*t*, 1611-1612
    excess fluid volume in, 1618
    fatigue in, 1619
    gastrointestinal changes in, 1611, 1613*c*, 1614
    health care resources for, 1635
    health promotion and maintenance in, 1612
    health teaching in, 1635
    hematologic changes in, 1611, 1613*c*, 1613-1614
    hemodialysis in, 1620-1626; *See also* Hemodialysis
    history in, 1612
    home care management in, 1633-1635, 1634*c*
    imaging studies in, 1614
    imbalanced nutrition: less than body requirements in, 1615-1618, 1617*c*, 1617*t*
    incidence and prevalence of, 1612, 1612*c*
    integumentary manifestations in, 1613*c*, 1614
    kidney changes in, 1609
    laboratory assessment in, 1614
    metabolic changes in, 1609-1610, 1610*f*
    musculoskeletal manifestations in, 1613*c*, 1614
    neurologic manifestations in, 1613*c*
    nursing diagnoses in, 1615
    osteomalacia and, 1161
    peritoneal dialysis in, 1626-1630, 1627*t*, 1627-1629*f*, 1629*c*
    physical assessment in, 1612-1614, 1613*c*
    psychosocial assessment in, 1614
    psychosocial preparation in, 1635
    pulmonary edema in, 1620
    renal transplantation in, 1630-1633, 1631*f*, 1632*f*, 1633*t*
    reproductive manifestations in, 1613*c*
    respiratory manifestations in, 1613, 1613*c*
    risk for infection in, 1618
    risk for injury in, 1618-1619
    sickle cell disease and, 895-896
    stages of, 1609, 1609*t*
  in diabetic nephropathy, 1594-1595
  in immunologic interstitial and tubulointerstitial disorders, 1593
  in nephrosclerosis, 1593
End-tidal carbon dioxide, 566
Enema, preoperative, 254
Energy balance, 1386
Energy conservation
  after lung transplantation, 631
  in chronic and disabling conditions, 103
  in heart failure, 775
  in leukemia, 911
  in polycystic kidney disease, 1584*c*
  in rheumatoid arthritis, 346, 346*c*
Energy therapies, 9*t*, 12-13, 13*f*
Enflurane, 274*t*
Enfuvirtide, 378*c*, 379
ENG; *See* Electronystagmography
Engraftment in bone marrow transplantation, 909-910
Enkephalins, 930*t*
Enophthalmos, 1077
Enoxaparin
  after total hip arthroplasty, 330
  for atrial fibrillation, 746
  for deep vein thrombosis, 819
  for pulmonary embolism, 681*c*
Entacapone, 968
Entamide; *See* Diloxanide furoate
Entamoeba histolytica, 1338-1339
Enteral nutrition, 1396-1400, 1397*f*, 1398*c*
  in acute respiratory distress syndrome, 689
  after laryngectomy, 602
  burn patient and, 543
  during mechanical ventilation, 696
Enterobacter
  in brain abscess, 1065
  in prostatitis, 1733
  in pyogenic liver abscess, 1361
  in urinary tract infection, 1552
Enterobiasis, 1339
Enterococcus
  in pyelonephritis, 1587
  in pyogenic liver abscess, 1361
  vancomycin-resistant, 448
Enterohemorrhagic *Escherichia coli*, 1341, 1341*c*
Enteroscopy, 1227-1228
Enterostomal feeding tube, 1397
Entocort EC; *See* Budesonide
Entrapment neuropathies, 1470*t*
Entropion, 1085, 1085*c*, 1085*f*
Entry inhibitors, 378*c*, 379
Enucleation, 1105, 1105*c*
Envenomation
  bee and wasp, 149-150
  black widow spider, 147*f*, 147-148
  brown recluse spider, 147, 147*f*
  scorpion, 148-149, 149*f*
  snake, 143*f*, 143-146, 144*c*, 144*f*, 145*t*, 146*t*
  tarantula, 148
Environment
  disaster workers and, 161
  protective, 445
    in Alzheimer's disease, 974
    burn patient and, 536, 541
  standard precautions and, 446*t*
Environmental emergencies, 141-158
  altitude-related illnesses in, 154-156, 156*c*
  arthropod bites and stings in, 146-150, 147*f*, 149*f*, 150*c*
  cold injuries in, 152-154, 154*f*
  drowning in, 156-157
  heat-related illnesses in, 141-143, 142*c*, 143*c*
  lightning injuries in, 150-152, 151*c*
  snakebite in, 143*f*, 143-146, 144*c*, 144*f*, 145*t*, 146*f*
Environmental exposure
  cancer development and, 407-408, 408*c*, 408*t*
  risk for infection and, 441, 441*t*
Enzymatic débridement in burn injury, 539
Enzyme-linked immunosorbent assay
  in acquired immunodeficiency syndrome, 373-374
  in gastritis, 1267
  in hepatitis, 1359
Enzymes
  deficiencies in malabsorption syndrome, 1311-1312, 1312*c*
  in deoxyribonucleic acid synthesis, 65-66
Eosinophil, 309*t*, 311, 878*t*
Eotaxin, 610
Ephedra, 246*t*
Ephedrine sulfate, 393*c*
Epicardium, 705*f*
Epidermal growth factor, 1237
Epidermal inclusion cyst, 508
Epidermis, 461, 461*f*, 462*f*
  burn-related skin changes and, 520, 522*f*
  changes related to aging, 463-464*c*
  functions of, 463*t*
Epidermoid lung cancer, 641
Epididymectomy, 1734
Epididymis, 1645*f*, 1646
Epididymitis, 1733, 1734, 1745*f*
Epidural analgesia, 52-54, 53*f*
  in lung transplantation, 630
  postoperative, 297
Epidural anesthesia, 275, 276*t*, 277*f*, 329
Epidural catheter, 1058, 1059*t*
Epidural hematoma, 1051-1052, 1052*f*, 1064
Epidural space, 237, 929
Epidural spinal tumor, 1001
Epidural therapy, 237-238
Epifrin; *See* Epinephrine borate
Epigastric area, 718*t*
Epigastric pain
  in achalasia, 1255
  in hookworm infection, 1340
  in hyperparathyroidism, 1461
Epiglottis, 553*f*, 554, 554*f*
Epiglottitis
  pharyngitis-related, 657
  thermal airway burn and, 530
Epilepsy, 955-961
  drug therapy for, 957-959, 957-959*c*
  emergency care in, 959-961
  management of, 959, 959*c*, 960*c*
  nursing diagnoses in, 957
  pathophysiology of, 955-956
  surgical management of, 960-961
Epimorph; *See* Morphine
Epinal; *See* Epinephrine borate
Epinephrine, 1416
  for anaphylaxis, 393, 393*c*
  for bee sting, 150
  for cardiac arrest, 752, 752*c*
  glucose homeostasis and, 1467
Epinephrine borate, 1099*c*
EpiPen, 150
Epi-Pen, 391, 392*f*
Epiphysis, 1141, 1141*f*
Epirubicin, 421*t*
Epistaxis, 396, 591-592, 592*c*, 592*f*
Epistaxis catheter, 592, 592*f*
Epithalamic nucleus, 931*f*
Epitympanum, 1110
Epivir; *See* Lamivudine
Eplerenone, 802
Epoetin alfa
  for acute renal failure, 1606*c*
  in cancer therapy support, 433*t*
  for chemotherapy-related anemia, 426
  for leukemia, 911
  before total hip arthroplasty, 329
Epogen; *See* Epoetin alfa
Epoprostenol, 638
Eppy/N; *See* Epinephrine borate
Epratuzumab, 435*t*
Eprex; *See* Epoetin alfa
Epstein-Barr virus
  Burkitt's lymphoma and, 914
  cancers associated with, 408*t*
Eptifibatide
  for acute myocardial infarction, 859
  for deep vein thrombosis, 819
  for postoperative graft occlusion, 809
Epzicom; *See* Abacavir-lamivudine
Equianalgesic chart, 46, 47*t*
Equilibrium
  cerebellar assessment and, 940
  hydrostatic pressure and, 171, 171*f*
Erbitux; *See* Cetuximab
Erb's point, 718*t*
ERCP; *See* Endoscopic retrograde cholangiopancreatography
Erectile dysfunction, 1725-1726
  after prostatectomy, 1722, 1725
  in diabetes mellitus, 1471
  obesity and, 1404
Erection, 1647
Ergonomically appropriate workstation, 1206
Ergonomics, 984
Ergotamine preparations, 953, 953*t*
Erlotinib, 435*t*
  for brain tumor, 1062
  for esophageal cancer, 1258
  for lung cancer, 645
  for oral cancer, 1237
  for pancreatic cancer, 1382
Erosion, 470*f*
Eructation
  in cholecystitis, 1368
  in gastroesophageal reflux disease, 1245
  in hiatal hernia, 1249
Erythema, 468*t*
  in acute osteomyelitis, 1165, 1166*c*
  in brown recluse spider bite, 147
  in sunburn, 480
  in toxic epidermal necrolysis, 516
  in vulvovaginitis, 1691
Erythema migrans, 356
Erythrocyte, 877-878, 878*f*
Erythrocyte disorders, 893-902
  anemia in, 878, 893*t*, 893-898, 894*c*, 894*f*, 895*f*, 897*c*, 898*c*
    after total hip arthroplasty, 331
    aplastic, 900
    bleeding gastrointestinal ulcer or polyp and, 886
    chemotherapy-related, 424, 426
    common causes of, 893*t*
    community-based care in, 898, 898*c*
    folic acid deficiency, 900
    glucose-6-phosphate dehydrogenase deficiency, 898-899
    hematologic assessment and, 885
    immunohemolytic, 899
    iron-deficiency, 899, 899*c*
    sickle cell, 894*f*, 894-898, 895*f*, 897*c*, 898*c*
    systemic manifestations of, 894*c*
    vitamin B_{12} deficiency, 900
  myelodysplastic syndromes in, 901-902
  polycythemia vera in, 901, 901*c*
Erythrocyte sedimentation rate
  in acute pancreatitis, 1374
  in brain abscess, 1066
  in infection assessment, 450-451
  in osteoarthritis, 325
  in osteomyelitis, 1166
  in polymyalgia rheumatica, 355
  in rheumatoid arthritis, 339*c*, 340
  in ulcerative colitis, 1323
Erythrocytosis, 1595
Erythrodermic psoriasis, 506
Erythromycin
  for chancroid, 1753
  for chlamydial infection, 1747
  for granuloma inguinale, 1754
  for Lyme disease, 356
  for ocular infection, 1086*c*
  for trachoma, 1088
Erythroplakia, 1234, 1707
Erythroplasia, 597
Erythropoiesis, 878
Erythropoietin, 318*t*, 878
  for acute renal failure, 1606*c*
  for chronic kidney disease, 1619
  for myelodysplastic syndromes, 901
  renal production of, 1531*t*, 1532
Esalen massage, 11
Escape complexes, 738-739
Escape rhythms, 738-739
Eschar, 490
  in brown recluse spider bite, 147
  in classification of burn depth, 521*t*
  in full-thickness burn, 523, 523*f*

Escharotomy, 523, 534*f*, 534-535
Escherichia coli
in acute sialadenitis, 1239-1240
in Bartholin cyst, 1699
in brain abscess, 1065
in epididymitis, 1734
in food poisoning, 1341, 1341*t*
in foodborne infection, 455
in gastroenteritis, 1319*t*, 1319-1329
in pelvic inflammatory disease, 1748
in peritonitis, 1317
in prostatitis, 1733
in pyelonephritis, 1586
in pyogenic liver abscess, 1361
in sepsis, 840
in urinary tract infection, 1552
Escitalopram oxalate, 358
Eskalith; *See* Lithium carbonate
ESKD; *See* End-stage kidney disease
Esmolol, 742*c*
Esomeprazole
for gastritis, 1268
for gastroesophageal reflux disease, 1247*c*, 1248
for gastrointestinal protection in Cushing's disease, 1444
mechanical ventilation and, 696
for peptic ulcer disease, 1269*c*, 1274
Esophageal dilation, 1258
Esophageal manometry, 1245
Esophageal pain, 713*t*
Esophageal pH monitoring, 1245
Esophageal reflux, 352
Esophageal speech, 602
Esophageal varices, 1345, 1353-1354
Esophagectomy, 1259
Esophagitis
bisphosphonate-related, 1160
in scleroderma, 352*c*
Esophagogastric balloon tamponade, 1353
Esophagogastroduodenoscopy, 1226-1227, 1227*f*
in cirrhosis, 1350
in esophageal diverticula, 1262
in gastric cancer, 1281
in gastritis, 1267
in gastroesophageal reflux disease, 1245
in gastrointestinal bleeding, 1276
in peptic ulcer disease, 1274
Esophagogastrostomy, 1259, 1259*f*
Esophagomyotomy, 1255
Esophagoscopy, 1227*f*
Esophagus, 553*f*, 1217, 1217*f*, 1243-1264
achalasia and, 1254-1255
diverticula of, 1261-1262
gastroesophageal reflux disease and, 1243-1248
drug therapy for, 1246-1247*c*, 1246-1248
endoscopic therapies for, 1248, 1248*c*
nonpharmacologic interventions in, 1245*c*, 1245-1246
nursing diagnoses in, 1245
pathophysiology of, 1243-1244, 1244*t*
physical assessment in, 1244*c*, 1244-1245
surgical management of, 1248
hiatal hernia and, 1249*f*, 1249-1254, 1253*c*, 1253*f*, 1254*c*
nursing care plan for open conventional esophageal surgery, 1250-1253
scleroderma and, 352
stricture of, 1244, 1256
trauma to, 597, 1262, 1262*t*
tumor of, 1255-1261, 1271*f*
community-based care in, 1261
history in, 1256
imbalanced nutrition: less than body requirements in, 1257
nonsurgical management of, 1257-1259, 1258*c*
Esophagus *(Continued)*
nursing diagnoses in, 1257
pathophysiology of, 1255-1256
physical assessment in, 1256, 1256*c*
psychosocial assessment in, 1256
surgical management of, 1259*f*, 1259-1261, 1260*c*
ESR; *See* Erythrocyte sedimentation rate
Essential hypertension, 797-798, 798*t*; *See also* Hypertension
Essential oils, 12
Estracyte; *See* Estramustine
Estradiol
menopause and, 1689, 1689*t*
for premenstrual syndrome, 1686
serum levels in reproductive assessment, 1653*c*
Estramustine, 422*t*
Estriol, 1653*c*
Estrogen, 1416
bone and, 1142, 1644
changes in older adult, 1419*c*
Estrogen therapy
for dysfunctional uterine bleeding, 1688
for hormonal manipulation in cancer, 431*t*
in menopause, 1689-1690, 1690*c*
for osteoporosis prevention, 1157, 1158*c*
for urinary incontinence, 1564, 1565*c*
ESWL; *See* Extracorporeal shock wave lithotripsy
Etanercept
for psoriasis, 508
for rheumatoid arthritis, 342*c*, 343
$ETCO_2$; *See* End-tidal carbon dioxide
Ethambutol, 670, 671*c*
Ethical considerations
in end-of-life care, 118
in genetic testing, 75-76
in total enteral nutrition, 1396
Ethical principles, 5
Ethmoid sinus, 553*f*
Ethnicity, 27-28
Ethnopharmacology, 31
Ethosuximide, 957*c*
Ethrane; *See* Enflurane
Ethyol; *See* Amifostine
Etidronate
for hypercalcemia, 194
for Paget's disease of bone, 1164
Etomidate, 274*t*
for bone marrow aspiration, 890
for moderate sedation, 276
Etoposide, 421*t*
for prostate cancer, 1723
for testicular cancer, 1729-1730
Etravirine, 377*c*, 379
Euflex; *See* Flutamide
Eulexin; *See* Flutamide
Euploid number of chromosomes, 68
Euploidy, 401, 406
Eustachian tube, 1110*f*, 1110-1111
opening of, 553*f*
otitis media and, 1123
Euthanasia, 121-122, 122*t*
Euthyroid, 1454
Event resolution in disaster, 164*c*, 164-166
Everolimus, 320
Eversion, 1146*f*
Evidence-based practice, 5-6, 6*t*
activated partial thromboplastin time, 888
ankle-brachial index, 717
biomarkers in chemotherapy for breast cancer, 1678
cataract surgery delay, 1093
community-based rehabilitation for stroke patient, 1048
dietary supplements in prevention of coronary artery disease, 851
distraction intervention for chemotherapy, 425
Evidence-based practice *(Continued)*
early diagnosis of lung cancer, 643
fluid management in acute lung injury, 688
functional status after hip surgery, 1197
heart failure self-care, 777
implanted cardiac devices, 758
indwelling urinary catheter usage, 1554
intensive insulin therapy in intensive care unit, 1500
medication event monitoring system, 1634
Meniett device, 1128
music therapy effect on pain and anxiety, 10
nurse-managed telemonitoring of blood pressure, 803
oral hygiene in dementia patient, 1232
pain assessment in older adult, 44
preoperative denture removal, 278
prevention of osteoporosis, 1155
prevention of ventilator-associated pneumonia, 661
prostate cancer, 1724
relationship between anxiety and postoperative pain, 249
sexual health in men with intestinal ostomies, 1302
skeletal pin site care, 1191
skin self-examination in melanoma, 511
stem cell donation, 908
stool collection for fecal occult blood test, 1225
stressors and coping strategies in osteoarthritis, 326
Evil eye, 32
Evisceration, 291*f*, 291-292, 296, 296*c*
Evista; *See* Raloxifene
EVL; *See* Endoscopic variceal ligation
Evoked potentials, 947
Evoked response, 947
Ewing's sarcoma, 1168
Exacerbation
in chronic pancreatitis, 1379*c*
in multiple sclerosis, 1002
in myasthenia gravis, 1016
in rheumatoid arthritis, 338
in systemic lupus erythematosus, 347
Exacerbation therapy in cystic fibrosis, 636
Exchange system, 1494, 1494*t*
Excisional biopsy, 477, 512
Excisional conization, 1703
Excitability of heart, 730-731
Excretory urography, 1543-1545, 1544*t*, 1545*c*
Exelon; *See* Rivastigmine
Exercise
after amputation, 1202
after bone cancer surgery, 1170
after total hip arthroplasty, 330
asthma and, 621
for back pain, 985-986, 986*c*
in chronic obstructive pulmonary disease, 629-630
coronary artery disease and, 871, 871*c*
in diabetes mellitus, 1496-1497, 1497*c*
in heart failure, 777
hypoglycemia and, 1509
in multiple sclerosis, 1007
for obesity, 1405
older adult and, 17, 17*f*
in osteoarthritis, 335, 336*c*
osteoporosis and, 1157
in Parkinson disease, 968
in peripheral arterial disease, 807
postmastectomy, 1675*c*
in rheumatoid arthritis, 336*c*
for urge urinary incontinence, 1568
Exercise electrocardiography, 724-725
Exercise intolerance
in mitral valve prolapse, 780
older adult and, 557*c*
Exercise tolerance testing, 724-725
in coronary artery disease, 855
in peripheral arterial disease, 806
in respiratory assessment, 567
in valvular heart disease, 780
Exertional dyspnea
in acute mountain sickness, 155
in aortic regurgitation, 779*c*, 780
in aortic stenosis, 779*c*, 780
cardiovascular assessment and, 713
in hypertrophic cardiomyopathy, 789
in left-sided heart failure, 768
in mitral regurgitation, 779*c*, 780
in mitral stenosis, 779, 779*c*
Exertional heat stroke, 142
Exfoliative psoriasis, 506
Exocrine pancreas, 1218, 1418
Exogen therapy, 1192
Exogenous hyperthyroidism, 1449
Exogenous osteomyelitis, 1165
Exophthalmos, 1077, 1449, 1450, 1450*f*
Exotoxin, 441
Expansion breathing, 257*c*
Expedited partner therapy in chlamydial infection, 1747
Exploratory laparotomy
in abdominal trauma, 1308
in appendicitis, 1316-1317
in intestinal obstruction, 1305-1306
in liver trauma, 1361
in peritonitis, 1318
Exposure assessment in trauma nursing, 138, 138*t*
Expressive aphasia, 1046, 1046*t*
Expressivity of gene, 73, 402
Extended shoehorn, 103*t*
Extended-wear contact lenses, 1103
Extension, 1146*f*
Extension exercises for back pain, 986*c*
Extension set, 220
External catheter for epidural analgesia, 53
External clip insertion in deep vein thrombosis, 820
External cooling, 452
External ear, 1109-1110, 1110*f*
benign cyst or polyp of, 1120-1121
cerumen impaction or foreign body in, 1122*f*, 1122-1123, 1123*c*
external otitis and, 1121*c*, 1121*f*, 1121-1122
furuncle of, 1122
inspection of, 1114
instillation of antibiotics and, 1121*f*
irrigation of, 1122, 1122*f*, 1123*c*
perichondritis of, 1122
External fixation, 1191, 1191*f*
External fixator, 1191-1192
External genitalia
female, 1642, 1643*f*, 1649-1650, 1650*c*
male, 1645, 1651
External hemorrhage, 136
External hemorrhoids, 1309, 1309*f*
External iliac artery, 804*f*
External os, 1643*f*
External otitis, 1121*c*, 1121*f*, 1121-1122
External polycentric knee hinge cast, 1188*t*
External urethral sphincter, 1532
External-beam radiation therapy
in bone cancer, 1169
in endometrial cancer, 1701
in oral cancer, 1237
in prostate cancer, 1722-1723
in testicular cancer, 1730
Extracapsular cataract extraction, 1094, 1094*f*
Extracapsular hip fracture, 1196, 1196*f*
Extracellular fluid, 170
bicarbonate buffer in, 202
electrolytes in, 183, 183*f*
impermeability and, 173
osmosis and, 174
overhydration and, 181*f*, 181-183, 182*c*

Extracellular fluid *(Continued)*
potassium in, 187
sodium in, 183-184
transmission of nerve impulse and, 929
Extracorporeal shock wave lithotripsy, 1369, 1573
Extracranial-intracranial bypass, 1045
Extradural analgesia, 52-54, 53*f*
Extradural spinal tumor, 1001
Extrahepatic obstructive jaundice, 1367
Extramedullary spinal tumor, 1001
Extraocular muscles, 1072, 1073*f*, 1073*t*
changes with aging, 1075*c*
function testing of, 1078
Extrapulmonary causes of ventilatory failure, 685, 685*c*
Extrapyramidal system, 933
Extravasation
in chemotherapy, 423, 424*c*
in intravenous therapy, 226*t*
of vesicant medications, 217
Extreme obesity, 1402
Extremities
cardiovascular assessment and, 715
nutrient deficiencies and, 1394*t*
nutrition screening assessment and, 1390*c*
Extrinsic allergic alveolitis, 640*c*
Extrinsic factors, 879, 880*f*
Extubation in mechanical ventilation, 697
Exubera, 1485*t*
Exudate, 490, 490*t*, 961
Exudative macular degeneration, 1101
Exudative retinal detachment, 1101
Eye, 1084-1108
aging of, 1074, 1075*c*, 1075*f*
application of eye patch, 1088*c*
application of ocular compress, 1087*c*
assessment of, 1070-1083
anatomy and physiology review in, 1070-1074, 1071-1074*f*, 1073*t*
changes associated with aging and, 1074, 1075*c*, 1075*f*
corneal staining in, 1079-1080
electroretinography in, 1082
fluorescein angiography in, 1081*c*, 1081-1082
health promotion and maintenance and, 1074-1075, 1076*c*
imaging studies in, 1079
inspection in, 1077
laboratory assessment in, 1079
ophthalmoscopy in, 1080-1081, 1081*f*, 1081*t*
patient history in, 1075-1077, 1076*c*, 1076*t*
psychosocial assessment in, 1079
slit-lamp examination in, 1079, 1080*f*
tonometry in, 1080, 1080*f*
vision testing in, 1077-1079, 1078*f*, 1079*f*
blepharitis and, 1084-1085
cataracts and, 1091*f*, 1091-1095, 1092*f*, 1092*t*, 1094*f*, 1095*c*
catecholamine receptors and, 1416*t*
chalazion and, 1087
conjunctival hemorrhage and, 1087
conjunctivitis and, 1087-1088
contusion of, 1103
corneal abrasion, ulceration, and infection, 1089
drug therapy for inflammation and infection of, 1086*c*
ectropion and, 1085
entropion and, 1085, 1085*c*, 1085*f*
external structures of, 1072, 1072*f*
foreign body in, 1103-1104
function of, 1073*f*, 1073-1074
glaucoma and, 1095*f*, 1095-1098, 1099-1100*c*
hordeolum and, 1085-1087
hyphema and, 1103
Eye *(Continued)*
insertion and removal of ocular prosthesis, 1105*c*
instillation of ophthalmic ointment, 1085*c*
irrigation of, 1104*c*
keratoconjunctivitis sicca and, 1087
keratoconus and corneal opacities and, 1089*f*, 1089-1091, 1090*f*, 1091*t*
laceration of, 1104
layers of eyeball and, 1071, 1071*f*
macular degeneration and, 1100-1101
microvascular complications in diabetes mellitus, 1469, 1469*f*
muscles, nerves, and blood vessels of, 1072, 1073*f*, 1073*t*
nutrient deficiencies and, 1394*t*
ocular melanoma and, 1104-1106
penetrating injury of, 1104
premenstrual syndrome and, 1686*c*
promotion of independent living in patient with impaired vision, 1098*c*
reduced vision and, 1106*c*, 1106-1107
refractive errors and, 1102-1103
refractive structures and media of, 1071-1072, 1072*f*
retinal holes, tears, and detachments, 1101-1102, 1102*f*
retinitis pigmentosa and, 1102
rheumatoid arthritis and, 338
systemic lupus erythematosus and, 350
trachoma and, 1088
traumatic brain injury and, 1055
uveitis and, 1100
vitreous hemorrhage and, 1098-1100
Eye chart, 1077-1078, 1078*f*
Eye contact, 29
Eye donation, 1091
Eye patch, 1088*c*
Eye protection
in Bell's palsy, 1026
myasthenia gravis and, 1020
standard precautions and, 446*t*
Eyedrops, 1076*c*, 1081*c*, 1099-1100*c*
Eyeglasses, 1102-1103
Eyelid, 1072, 1072*f*
blepharitis and, 1084-1085
chalazion and, 1087, 1088*c*
ectropion and, 1085
entropion and, 1085, 1085*c*, 1085*f*
hordeolum and, 1085-1087, 1087*c*
lag in hyperthyroidism, 1450
Eyelid eversion, 465*f*
Ezetimibe, 796
Ezetimibe-simvastatin, 796

F

Face
edema in black widow spider bite, 148
expression in Parkinson disease, 966, 966*f*
musculoskeletal assessment of, 1146
trauma to, 593-594
Face shield, 446*t*
Face tent, 577, 577*t*
Face-lift, 514*t*, 515
Facemask for oxygen delivery, 574-576, 575*t*, 576*f*
Facial nerve
eye and, 1072
functions of, 935*t*
salivary gland tumor and, 1240
Facial paralysis, 356, 1026
Facial sling in Bell's palsy, 1026
Facial x-ray, 566
Facilitated diffusion, 173
Facilitated transport, 173
Facilitating techniques in bladder training, 105-106
Facioscapulohumeral dystrophy, 1175*t*
Factor VIII cryoprecipitate, 917
Failed back surgery syndrome, 988*c*, 988-989
Fainting
in pulmonary embolism, 679
in toxic shock syndrome, 1691
Fall
in emergency department, 129*c*
older adult and, 18, 23-24, 24*c*
prevention of, 180*c*
traumatic brain injury and, 1052, 1053
vertigo and, 1126
Fallophobia, 18, 1156
Fallopian tube, 1643, 1643*f*
cancer of, 1709
False aneurysm, 810
Famciclovir
for genital herpes, 1742
for viral skin infection, 503
Familial adenomatous polyposis, 1294, 1309
Familial hemiplegic migraine, 951
Familial Paget's disease of bone, 1162
Family
coping in Alzheimer's disease, 978
culture and, 29-30
Family history
breast cancer risk and, 1665*t*
in cardiovascular disease, 712
in coronary artery disease, 850
in endocrine assessment, 1421
in gastrointestinal problems, 1221
in hearing problems, 1113-1114
in hematologic assessment, 884
in musculoskeletal disorders, 1144
in neurologic disorders, 936
in ocular problems, 1077
in osteoporosis, 1154
in prostate cancer, 1719
in renal assessment, 1536
in reproductive assessment, 1647
in respiratory assessment, 559
in skin problems, 466*c*, 467
surgical risk and, 244*t*
in testicular cancer, 1726
Family tree, 71-72, 72*f*
Famotidine
for gastritis, 1268
for gastroesophageal reflux disease, 1246*c*, 1247-1248
for peptic ulcer disease, 1269*c*, 1274
Famvir; *See* Famciclovir
Fanconi's anemia, 900
FAP; *See* Familial adenomatous polyposis
Far point of vision, 1074
Farmer's lung, 640*c*
Farsightedness, 1073, 1073*f*, 1102
Fascia, acute compartment syndrome and, 1180-1182, 1181*c*
Fasciculations
in amyotrophic lateral sclerosis, 1007*c*
in black widow spider bite, 148
in hyperkalemia, 190
in hypernatremia, 186
in myasthenia gravis, 1017, 1019*t*
in pit viper envenomation, 144
Fasciculus cuneatus, 932*f*
Fasciculus gracilis, 932*f*
Fasciotomy
in acute compartment syndrome, 1181
in acute peripheral arterial occlusion, 810
in burn patient, 523, 535
FAST; *See* Focused abdominal sonography for trauma
Fasting blood glucose
metabolic syndrome and, 853*t*
preoperative assessment of, 250*c*
Fasting plasma glucose, 1473*t*, 1473-1474
Fat
exchange system for, 1494*t*
intake in diabetes mellitus, 1493
Fat cell
anabolic effects of insulin on, 1418*t*
catecholamine receptors and, 1416*t*
Fat embolism syndrome, 678, 1141
after lumbar spinal surgery, 987*c*
fracture and, 1182*c*, 1182-1183
Fat emulsion, 1400
Fatigue
in anemia, 885
in aortic stenosis, 779*c*, 780
cardiovascular assessment and, 713
in chronic and disabling conditions, 103
in chronic kidney disease, 1619
in cystic fibrosis, 636
end-of-life care and, 116
in heat exhaustion, 142
in high altitude pulmonary edema, 155
in hyperaldosteronism, 1446
in hyperthyroidism, 1450
in influenza, 658
in inhalation anthrax, 673
in leukemia, 903, 910-911, 911*c*
in lightning strike, 151
in lung cancer, 644
in Lyme disease, 356
in mitral regurgitation, 779*c*, 780
in multiple myeloma, 915
in multiple sclerosis, 1003
in myasthenia gravis, 1016
in pancreatic cancer, 1380
in primary pulmonary hypertension, 637
in rheumatoid arthritis, 338, 346, 346*c*
in systemic lupus erythematosus, 349
in tuberculosis, 669
Fatigue fracture, 1179-1180
Fatty liver, 1360-1361
Fatty stools, 1225
in cholecystitis, 1368
in malabsorption syndrome, 1311
Fatty streak, 848*f*
Faucial tonsils, 553*f*, 554
Fc fragment, 314, 315*f*, 388*f*
Fc receptor, 314, 315*f*, 388*f*
Fear of death, 116
Febrile transfusion reaction, 920
Fecal fats, 1225
Fecal immunochemical test, 1225
Fecal impaction, 1306*c*
Fecal incontinence, 1323
in Alzheimer's disease, 975
in stroke, 1047
Fecal occult blood test, 1225, 1295, 1295*c*
Federal Emergency Management Agency, 161
Felbamate, 957*c*
Felbatol; *See* Felbamate
Felt-tip marker inhalation, 91
Felty's syndrome, 339
FEMA; *See* Federal Emergency Management Agency
Female
autoimmune disorders in, 396
blood cell counts and, 882
breast cancer in, 1663-1681
anxiety in, 1671-1672
BRCA1 and *BRCA2* gene mutations and, 73, 78, 1647
breast reconstruction in, 1675, 1676*t*, 1677*c*
breast self-examination and, 1666, 1667*f*
chemotherapy in, 1677*t*, 1677-1679
clinical breast examination and, 1666-1668, 1667*f*
complementary and alternative therapies in, 1672, 1672*t*
conditions associated with genetic predisposition for, 410*t*
cultural considerations in, 1664-1665
etiology and genetic risk in, 1664, 1665*t*
health care resources for, 1681
health teaching in, 1679-1680

Female (Continued)
history in, 1669-1670
home care management in, 1679, 1679c, 1680c
imaging studies in, 1670-1671
incidence and prevalence of, 1664
invasive, 1663f, 1663-1664, 1664f
laboratory assessment in, 1670
mammography and, 1665-1666
in men, 1664
metastasis in, 1672
noninvasive, 1663
nursing diagnoses in, 1671
in older adult, 1668-1669
options for high-risk women in, 1669
physical assessment in, 1670, 1670c
psychosocial assessment in, 1670
psychosocial preparation in, 1680-1681
radiation therapy in, 1676-1678, 1677t
sites of metastasis for, 405t
stem cell transplantation in, 1679
subtypes of, 1671
surgical management of, 1672-1675, 1673f, 1675c
in young women, 1664
cancer incidence and death in, 406f
carpal tunnel syndrome in, 1206-1207
chronic calcium loss in, 192
coronary artery disease in, 709, 712, 850, 853
gallstones in, 1368
gynecologic problems in, 1684-1711
Bartholin cyst in, 1699
cervical cancer in, 1702t, 1702-1705, 1704c, 1704f
cervical polyp in, 1699
dysfunctional uterine bleeding in, 1688-1689
endometrial cancer in, 1699-1702, 1700t, 1701c
endometriosis in, 1687f, 1687-1688
fallopian tube cancer in, 1709
menopause in, 1689t, 1689-1690, 1690c
ovarian cancer in, 1705t, 1705-1707
ovarian cyst in, 1694
premenstrual syndrome in, 1685-1687, 1686c
primary dysmenorrhea in, 1684-1685
toxic shock syndrome in, 1691, 1692c
uterine leiomyoma in, 1694-1699, 1695f, 1697c, 1697t, 1698c
uterine prolapse in, 1691-1694, 1692f, 1693c, 1693f
vaginal cancer in, 1708-1709
vulvar cancer in, 1707-1708, 1708f
vulvovaginitis in, 1690-1691, 1691c
human immunodeficiency virus infection in, 366, 367f
migraine headache in, 951
osteoporosis in, 1143, 1153-1160
community-based care for, 1160
drug therapy for, 1157-1160, 1158-1159c
exercise and, 1157
history in, 1155
hypocalcemia and, 193
imaging studies in, 1156-1157
laboratory assessment in, 1156
lifestyle changes in, 1157
nursing diagnoses in, 1157
nutrition therapy in, 1157
pathophysiology of, 1153c, 1153t, 1153-1155
physical assessment in, 1155-1156, 1156f
prevention of, 1155
psychosocial assessment in, 1156
surgery for, 1160

Female (Continued)
pelvic inflammatory disease in, 1747-1753
acute pain in, 1751-1752
anxiety in, 1752
community-based care in, 1752
drug therapy for, 1749-1751, 1750-1751c
fallopian tube cancer and, 1709
history in, 1748
infection control in, 1749
laboratory assessment in, 1749
Neisseria gonorrhoeae in, 1744
nursing diagnoses in, 1749
pathophysiology of, 1747-1748, 1748f
physical assessment in, 1748, 1749t
psychosocial assessment in, 1748-1749
sexually transmitted diseases in, 1738
sickle cell disease in, 898
smoking and, 556
substance abuse and, 81
total body water of, 175
urinary tract infection during pregnancy, 1558
Female reproductive system
aging related changes in, 1646c
endoscopic studies of, 1656f, 1656-1657
genitoreproductive history and, 1648, 1648c
imaging studies of, 1654-1655
physical assessment of, 1649-1651, 1650c, 1650f
structure and function of, 1642-1645, 1643f, 1644f
Femoral artery aneurysm, 814
Femoral fracture, 1197
Femoral hernia, 1291-1293, 1292f
Femoral neck fracture, 1196f
Femoral nerve, 1022f
Femoral pulse, 717f
Femoral shaft fracture, 1183
Femoral vein, 723f
Fenestrated tracheostomy tube, 582f, 582-583
Fenoldopam
for heart failure, 864c
for hypertensive crisis, 802
Fentanyl, 47-48
abuse of, 90t
for burn pain, 536
epidural, 52, 297
for general anesthesia, 274t
for moderate sedation, 276
for pain in acquired immunodeficiency syndrome, 380
for traumatic brain injury, 1057
Ferritin, 879
Ferrous sulfate, 1606c
Fetal tissue transplantation, 969
Fetor hepaticus, 1348
FEV_1; *See* Forced expiratory volume at 1 second
Fever
in acute osteomyelitis, 1165, 1166c
in bronchiolitis obliterans organizing pneumonia, 640c
in cholecystitis, 1368-1369
in Crohn's disease, 1331
dehydration and, 179
in food poisoning, 1341
in infection, 450, 451-452, 452c, 452t
in infective endocarditis, 784
in influenza, 658
in inhalation anthrax, 673
in intestinal parasitic infection, 1339
in lung abscess, 672
in meningitis, 961
in pharyngitis, 655, 656c
in pneumonia, 661, 663t
in rheumatic carditis, 787
in rheumatoid arthritis, 338
in scorpion sting, 149

Fever (Continued)
in sepsis, 839
in serum sickness, 395
in severe acute respiratory syndrome, 666
in systemic lupus erythematosus, 349
in thyroid storm, 1455
in toxic shock syndrome, 1691, 1692c
in traumatic brain injury, 1056-1057
in tuberculosis, 669
in ulcerative colitis, 1323
Feverfew, 246t
Fexofenadine, 390
FFP; *See* Fresh frozen plasma
Fiber intake in diabetes mellitus, 1493
Fiberglass synthetic cast, 1187, 1187f
Fiberoptic bronchoscopy, 644
Fiberoptic transducer-tipped pressure sensor, 1058, 1059t
Fibrillation
atrial, 745-746, 746f
in dilated cardiomyopathy, 787
in left-sided heart failure, 769
in mitral regurgitation, 779c, 780
in mitral stenosis, 779, 779c
ventricular, 748-750, 749f
in coronary artery disease, 850
in hypothermia, 153
in lightning strike, 151
Fibrin clot, 880
Fibrin degradation products, 887c
Fibrinogen, 877, 881t
Fibrinolysis, 687, 881, 882f
Fibrinolytic therapy, 884
in acute myocardial infarction, 859
prevention of injury in patient receiving, 683c
in pulmonary embolism, 680
in stroke, 1037, 1037c
Fibrin-stabilizing factor, 881t
Fibroadenoma, breast, 1660-1661, 1661t
Fibroblast, 461
Fibroblastic phase of wound healing, 481t
Fibrocystic breast condition, 1661, 1661t
Fibrogenic tumor, 1167
Fibroids, 1688, 1694-1699, 1695f, 1697c, 1697t, 1698c
Fibromyalgia, 357f, 357-358
Fibrosarcoma, 1168
Fibrosis
in fibrocystic breast condition, 1661
in infiltrating ductal carcinoma, 1663, 1663f
in pulmonary sarcoidosis, 638
Fibrositis, 357
Fibrotic lung diseases, 638
Fibrous atherosclerotic plaque, 848f
Fibula fracture, 1191f, 1197
Fiddleback spider, 147, 147f
Field block, 275, 276t
Fifth nerve rhizotomy, 58f
Fight-or-flight response, 1417
Filgrastim, 433t
Filter
in add-on device of infusion system, 220-221
cell membrane as, 171-172
Filtering microsurgery, 1097
Filtration, 171f, 171-172, 172f
FIM; *See* Functional Independence Measure
Finasteride, 1714
Fine crackles, 563t
Fine needle aspiration in fibrocystic breast condition, 1661
Fine rales, 563t
Finger
clubbing of, 475t
cardiovascular assessment and, 715, 715f
in chronic obstructive pulmonary disease, 626, 626f
fracture of, 1195
hand massage and, 11t

Finger (Continued)
positioning for prevention of contracture, 544c
traumatic amputation of, 1201
Fingernail polish, preoperative removal of, 260
Fingernail(s), 462, 462f, 473-475
alterations in color of, 474f, 474t
changes related to aging, 464c, 466f
endocrine assessment and, 1422
variations in shape of, 475t
FiO_2; *See* Fraction of inspired oxygen
Fire hazard in oxygen therapy, 572
First aid
in bee sting, 150
in black widow spider bite, 148
in brown recluse spider bite, 147
in coral snake envenomation, 146
in drowning, 157
in heat stroke, 142
in high altitude-related illnesses, 155
in hypothermia, 153
in lightning strike, 152
in pit viper envenomation, 144-145
First heart sound, 718
First intention healing, 481, 482f
First-degree atrioventricular block, 750
First-degree frostbite, 154
Fissure, 470f
anal, 1337-1338
Fistula
anal, 1338
arteriovenous, 1622-1623, 1623t, 1624c, 1624f, 1625t
in Crohn's disease, 1330, 1330f, 1332, 1333f
in inflammatory bowel disease, 1322t
in lymphogranuloma venereum, 1753
mucous, 1299
tracheoesophageal, 602, 603f
tracheostomy-related, 581t
vaginal, 1694
FIT; *See* Fecal immunochemical test
Five cardinal manifestations of inflammation, 312
Fixed occlusion in jaw fracture, 593
Fixed-rate pacing mode, 754
Flaccid bladder, 105, 105t, 998
Flaccid paralysis
after stroke, 1034, 1046
in coral snake envenomation, 146
in peripheral nerve trauma, 1023
Flagyl; *See* Metronidazole
Flail chest, 698, 698f
Flame burn, 525, 528c
FLAMP; *See* Fludarabine
Flank pain, 1536
in infective endocarditis, 784
in polycystic kidney disease, 1583
in urolithiasis, 1571
Flap
in laryngectomy, 601
for pressure ulcer repair, 495-496, 496f
Flash burn, 526
Flashover phenomenon, 151
Flat back syndrome, 1174
Flat bones, 1140-1141
Flatness, percussion note, 562t
Flatulence
in cholecystitis, 1368
in gastroesophageal reflux disease, 1245
Flavoxate, 1567
Flecainide, 742c
Flexeril; *See* Cyclobenzaprine
Flexion, 1146f
Flexion contracture, 1200
Flexion exercises for back pain, 986c
Floaters, 1100
Flolan; *See* Epoprostenol
Flomax; *See* Tamsulosin
Florinef; *See* Fludrocortisone
Flovent; *See* Fluticasone
Floxin; *See* Ofloxacin
Floxuridine, 421t

Fluconazole, 380
Fludarabine, 421*t*
Fludrocortisone, 1438-1439, 1439*c*
Fluid and electrolyte imbalances, 170-198
after blood transfusion, 919
after coronary artery bypass graft, 868
body fluids and, 174*c*, 174-175, 175*t*
burn-related, 524
calcium and, 191-194
hypercalcemia and, 193-194, 194*t*
hypocalcemia and, 191-193, 192*t*, 193*f*
cardiovascular assessment and, 721-722
chloride and, 197
in cirrhosis, 1348*f*, 1352-1353, 1353*c*
common causes of, 176*t*
in Crohn's disease, 1332
dehydration and, 176-181
assessment of, 178*c*, 178-179, 179*f*
interventions for, 179-181, 180*c*, 180*t*
nursing diagnoses for, 179
pathophysiology of, 176-177, 177*f*
prevention of, 178
in enteral nutrition therapy, 1399-1400
fluid overload and, 181*f*, 181-183, 182*c*
homeostasis and, 170-171, 171*f*
hormonal regulation of fluid balance and, 175-176, 176*f*
magnesium and, 195-197
hypermagnesemia and, 196-197
hypomagnesemia and, 196, 196*t*
major serum electrolyte concentrations and functions and, 184*t*
older adult and, 184*t*
parenteral nutrition and, 1401, 1401*c*
phosphorus and, 194-195
hyperphosphatemia and, 195
hypophosphatemia and, 194-195, 195*c*, 195*t*
physiologic influences on balance and, 171-174
diffusion in, 172*f*, 172-173
filtration in, 171*f*, 171-172, 172*f*
lymph and, 174
osmosis in, 173*f*, 173-174
potassium and, 187*t*, 187-189, 189*c*
hyperkalemia and, 190*t*, 190-191, 191*c*
hypokalemia and, 187*t*, 187-189, 189*c*
sodium and, 183-187
hypernatremia and, 186*t*, 186-187
hyponatremia and, 185*t*, 185-186
traumatic brain injury and, 1057
Fluid balance
body fluids and, 174*c*, 174-175, 175*t*
hormonal regulation of, 175-176, 176*f*
hypertension and, 797
parenteral nutrition and, 1401, 1401*c*
postoperative assessment of, 290
Fluid intake
after oral cancer surgery, 1238
after transurethral resection of prostate, 1718
fluid balance and, 175
in glucose-6-phosphate dehydrogenase deficiency, 898-899
in sickle cell disease, 897
urinary elimination problems and, 106
Fluid management
in acute lung injury, 688
after brain tumor surgery, 1065
in avian influenza, 668
in chronic kidney disease, 1617*c*
in cirrhosis, 1352-1353, 1353*c*
in dehydration, 180, 180*c*
in diabetic ketoacidosis, 1511
in diabetic nephropathy, 1506
in gastroenteritis, 1320
in gastrointestinal bleeding, 1276
in hypercalcemia, 194
in hyperglycemic-hyperosmolar state, 1513
Fluid management *(Continued)*
in intestinal obstruction, 1305
in intestinal parasitic infection, 1339
in polycystic kidney disease, 1584*c*
in renal trauma, 1598
Fluid overload, 181*f*, 181-183, 182*c*
in chronic kidney disease, 1618
in Cushing's disease, 1442
dyspnea in dying patient and, 117
in enteral nutrition therapy, 1399-1400
from fluid resuscitation, 530
in syndrome of inappropriate antidiuretic hormone secretion, 1436
Fluid restriction
in chronic kidney disease, 1617*t*, 1618
in hyponatremia, 186
infusion therapy and, 235-236
in syndrome of inappropriate antidiuretic hormone secretion, 1435
Fluid resuscitation
in acute respiratory distress syndrome, 688-689
in burn, 531, 533*c*, 533*t*, 533-534
in hypovolemic shock, 837
in pulmonary embolism, 682
in septic shock, 843*t*
Fluid retention
cardiovascular assessment and, 714
in Cushing's disease, 1443
fluid overload and, 182-183
mechanical ventilation and, 696
in right-sided heart failure, 768
in syndrome of inappropriate antidiuretic hormone secretion, 1435
Fluid shift in burn injury, 523-524, 524*f*
Fluid volume deficit
after lumbar spinal surgery, 987*c*
in burn, 533*c*, 533*t*, 533-535, 534*f*
isotonic dehydration and, 177
in peptic ulcer disease, 1273, 1275
Fluid volume excess
in chronic kidney disease, 1618
in cirrhosis, 1350-1353, 1352*c*, 1353*c*
in Cushing's disease, 1442-1443
FluidAir Elite bed, 104*f*
Flumadine; *See* Rimantadine
Flumazenil, 299, 300*c*
Flunitrazepam, 89
Fluorescein angiography, 1081*c*, 1081-1082
Fluorescent treponemal antibody absorption test, 948, 1653-1654, 1741
Fluorometholone, 1086*c*
Fluor-Op; *See* Fluorometholone
Fluoroplex; *See* 5-Fluorouracil
5-Fluorouracil, 421*t*
for cervical cancer, 1705
for colorectal cancer, 1297
for esophageal cancer, 1257
for pancreatic cancer, 1382
for vulvar cancer, 1707
Fluothane; *See* Halothane
Flurbiprofen, 1086*c*
Flushing of implanted port, 219
Flutamide, 1723
Fluticasone, 617*c*, 620
Flutter valve mucus clearance device, 632, 633*f*
Foam buildups, 103*t*
Foam dressing, 494-495*t*
FOBT; *See* Fecal occult blood test
Focal ischemia, 1470*t*
Focal neuropathies in diabetes mellitus, 1470, 1470*t*
Focal seizure, 956
Focused abdominal sonography for trauma, 1307
Focused assessment
in acquired immunodeficiency syndrome, 383*c*
after discharge from postanesthesia care unit, 289*c*
Focused assessment *(Continued)*
in chronic kidney disease, 1634*c*
in diabetic foot, 1503*c*
in home visit to type 1 diabetic patient, 1516*c*
in pneumonia, 665*c*
of postoperative older adult with oral cancer, 1238*c*
preoperative, 251*c*
in prevention of infection, 375*c*
in sexually transmitted diseases, 1740*c*
in suspected hearing loss, 1131*c*
in testicular cancer, 1728
in total abdominal hysterectomy, 1697*c*
in urinary incontinence, 1562*c*
Folex; *See* Methotrexate
Foley catheter
for functional urinary incontinence, 1569
home care of, 1725*c*
postoperative monitoring of, 290
preoperative preparation for, 255
in spinal cord injury, 1000
in transurethral resection of prostate, 1715
urinary tract infection and, 1554
Folic acid
for acute renal failure, 1606*c*
deficiency of, 1394*t*
anemia in, 893*t*, 900
presbycusis in, 1130
vitamin B_{12} deficiency and, 900
Folk health beliefs and practices, 32*f*, 32-33, 33*f*
Follicle-stimulating hormone, 1415, 1415*t*, 1645
deficiency of, 1426, 1427*c*
menopause and, 1689*t*
overproduction of, 1430*c*
serum levels in reproductive assessment, 1653*c*
Follicular lymphoma, 914
Follicular thyroid carcinoma, 1460-1461
Folliculitis, 499, 500*c*, 501*f*
Folstein's Mini-Mental State Examination, 971, 972*f*
Fondaparinux, 330
Food
achalasia and, 1255
causing anaphylaxis, 391*t*
colorectal cancer and, 1294
diverticular disease and, 1336
dumping syndrome and, 1286*t*
gastroesophageal reflux disease and, 1244
interference with warfarin, 821*c*
monoamine oxidase inhibitors and, 968
older adult with impaired vision and, 1098*c*
peptic ulcer disease and, 1275
potassium in, 187
rituals and customs surrounding, 31
sodium in, 184
Food and Drug Administration, 12
Food guide pyramid, 1387, 1388*f*
Food poisoning, 1319, 1340-1342, 1341*c*, 1341*t*
Foot
common problems of, 1173, 1174*t*
deformities of, 1172-1173, 1173*f*
diabetic, 1501-1503, 1502*c*, 1502*t*, 1503*b*, 1503*f*, 1504*c*
Morton's neuroma of, 1173
musculoskeletal assessment of, 1146-1147
peripheral vascular disease and, 810*c*
plantar fasciitis of, 1173
popliteal entrapment and, 816
Foot drop, 281*c*
Foot plexus pump, 821
Foot surgery, skin preparation for, 256*f*
Footwear for diabetic patient, 1503
Foradil; *See* Formoterol
Forane; *See* Isoflurane
Forced expiratory volume at 1 second, 567*t*
in asthma, 612
in chronic obstructive pulmonary disease, 627, 627*t*
Forced expiratory volume at 1 second/forced vital capacity ratio, 567*t*
Forced vital capacity, 567*t*
in asthma, 612
in chronic obstructive pulmonary disease, 627, 627*t*
Forearm fracture, 1195
Forearm splint, 1187*f*
Forearm surgery, skin preparation for, 256*f*
Foreign body
in ear, 1113, 1122*f*, 1122-1123, 1123*c*, 1126
ocular, 1103-1104
Forensic nurse examiner, 127
Formoterol, 620
Fornices, 1643*f*
Fosamax; *See* Alendronate
Fosamprenavir, 377*c*, 379
Fosfomycin, 1557*c*
Fosinopril, 771
Fosphenytoin, 958*c*, 959, 960
Fourth-degree frostbite, 154
Fovea centralis, 1071, 1071*f*
Fraction of inspired oxygen, 572, 693, 694
Fracture, 1179-1199
acute compartment syndrome and, 1180-1182, 1181*c*
acute pain in, 1192
cast application for, 1187*f*, 1187-1189, 1188*t*
chronic complications of, 1183
classification of, 1179*f*, 1179-1180
crush syndrome and, 1182
emergency care of, 1186, 1186*c*
fat embolism syndrome and, 1182*c*, 1182-1183
health care resources for, 1194
health teaching in, 1194, 1194*c*
hip, 1195-1197, 1196*f*, 1248
history in, 1183-1184
home care management in, 1194
hypovolemic shock and, 1182
imaging studies in, 1185
imbalanced nutrition: less than body requirements in, 1194
impaired physical mobility in, 1193*f*, 1193-1194
incidence and prevalence of, 1183
infection and, 1183, 1192-1193
laboratory assessment in, 1185
lower extremity, 1197-1198
mandibular, 593
nasal, 590-591, 591*f*
nursing diagnoses in, 1185-1186
open reduction of, 1190-1192, 1191*f*
osteoporosis-related, 1155
pathologic
in bone cancer, 1168
in chronic kidney disease, 1614
in Paget's disease of bone, 1163
pelvic, 1198
peripheral neurovascular dysfunction and, 1186, 1186*c*
physical assessment in, 1184*c*, 1184-1185
prevention of, 1183
psychosocial assessment in, 1185
rib, 698, 1198
skeletal pin site care in, 1191
skull, 1050
stages of bone healing and, 1180, 1180*f*
sternum, 1198
traction for, 1189*f*, 1189-1190, 1190*t*
upper extremity, 1195
venous thromboembolism and, 1183
vertebral, 1198*c*, 1198-1199

Fragmented fracture, 1179*f*
Fragmin; *See* Dalteparin
Frail elderly, 15-16
Frameshift mutation, 71
FRC; *See* Functional residual capacity
Free hydrogen ion level, 201
Free thyroxine index, 1451*c*
Freestyle stentless pig valve, 782*f*
Freezing gait in Parkinson disease, 968
Fremitus, 560
in chronic obstructive pulmonary disease, 626
in lung cancer, 643
Frequency, 1535*t*
in benign prostatic hypertrophy, 1713
in chlamydial infection, 1747
in cystitis, 1553
in prostate cancer, 1720
in prostatitis, 1733
in urolithiasis, 1571-1572
Frequency of sound, 1117
Frequency-dysuria syndrome, 1559
Fresh frozen plasma, 917*t*, 920
Friction
musculoskeletal trauma and, 1183
pressure ulcer and, 485, 485*f*, 487*f*
Frontal lobe, 931*f*, 931*t*
Frontal sinus, 553*f*
Frostbite, 154, 154*f*
Frostnip, 154
Fructosamine, 1474
FSH; *See* Follicle-stimulating hormone
FTA-ABS; *See* Fluorescent treponemal antibody absorption test
FUDR; *See* Floxuridine
Full agonists, 46
Full-disclosure electrocardiogram monitor, 733
Full-thickness burn, 521*t*, 522*f*, 523, 523*f*
Full-thickness skin graft, 495-496, 496*f*
Full-thickness wound
in burn injury, 522*f*, 523, 523*f*
healing of, 483-484
Fulmer SPICES framework, 23
Fulminant hepatitis, 1358
Functional assessment
in mobility disorders, 1145, 1146*f*
in rehabilitation, 98-99
Functional Health Patterns
in acid-base assessment, 207*c*
in cardiovascular assessment, 711*c*
in ear and hearing assessment, 1112*c*
in endocrine assessment, 1420, 1420*c*
in fluid and electrolyte assessment, 178*c*
in gastrointestinal assessment, 1219, 1220*c*
in hematologic assessment, 882*c*
in musculoskeletal assessment, 1144*c*
in neurologic assessment, 937*c*
in renal assessment, 1534*c*
in reproductive assessment, 1658*c*
in respiratory assessment, 558*c*
in vision assessment, 1076*c*
Functional history in cardiovascular assessment, 714, 714*t*
Functional Independence Measure, 98-99
Functional levels code
in endocrine assessment, 1420*c*
in respiratory assessment, 558*c*
Functional magnetic resonance imaging, 945
Functional residual capacity, 567*t*
Functional urinary incontinence, 1560*t*, 1561, 1568-1569
Fundoplication
in achalasia, 1255
in gastroesophageal reflux disease, 1248
in hiatal hernia, 1250-1253, 1253*c*
Fundus
of stomach, 1217
of uterus, 1643, 1643*f*
Fungal infection
in burn wound sepsis, 538*t*
cutaneous, 500*c*, 501
in cystitis, 1552
in external otitis, 1121*c*, 1121*f*, 1121-1122
in HIV-infected patient, 371
in leukemia, 906
in lung abscess, 672
in meningitis, 961
in osteomyelitis, 1164-1167, 1165*f*, 1166*c*
septic shock and, 838
skin culture in, 476-477
in stomatitis, 1231-1234, 1233*c*, 1233*f*
Furacin; *See* Nitrofurazone
Furadantin; *See* Nitrofurantoin
Furosemide
for acute renal failure, 1605
for cirrhosis, 1352
for dyspnea in dying patient, 117
for fluid overload, 182
for high altitude cerebral edema, 156
for hypercalcemia, 194
for hypernatremia, 187
for hyperparathyroidism, 1462
for pulmonary edema, 776, 1620
to reduce preload in heart failure, 772
for traumatic brain injury, 1057
Furuncle, 499, 500*c*, 501*f*, 1122
Fusiform aneurysm, 810
Fusion inhibitors, 378*c*, 379
Fuzeon; *See* Enfuvirtide
FVC; *See* Forced vital capacity

G

G_0 phase of cell cycle, 65, 65*f*, 400-401, 401*f*
G_1 phase of cell cycle, 65*f*, 66, 401, 401*f*
G_2 phase of cell cycle, 65*f*, 66, 401, 401*f*
GABA; *See* Gamma-aminobutyric acid
Gabapentin, 957*c*
for chronic low back pain, 985
for diabetic neuropathy, 1504
for facial paralysis, 1026
for Guillain-Barr[ac]e syndrome, 1015
for pain, 54, 54*t*
for restless legs syndrome, 1024
for seizures after stroke, 1043
for trigeminal neuralgia, 1025
Gabitril; *See* Tiagabine
Gait
cerebellar assessment and, 940
musculoskeletal assessment and, 1145, 1145*f*
in Parkinson disease, 966*c*, 968
Gait training, 100-101, 101*c*, 101*f*, 102*t*
Galantamine, 976
Galiximab, 435*t*
Gallbladder, 1217*f*, 1218*f*, 1218-1219, 1366-1371
cancer of, 1371
cholecystitis and, 1366-1371, 1367*f*, 1368*c*, 1368*t*, 1370*c*, 1371*t*
Gallium scan, 1149
Gallop, 718
in coronary artery disease, 854
in left-sided heart failure, 769
Gallstones, 1366-1371, 1367*f*, 1368*c*, 1368*t*, 1370*c*, 1371*t*
Gamma globulin, 316, 339*c*
Gamma hydroxybutyrate, 89
Gamma knife surgery, 1062, 1062*f*
Gamma rays, 418, 418*f*
Gamma-aminobutyric acid, 930*t*
Huntington disease and, 980
Gamma-linolenic acid, 328
Ganglion, 1172
Gangrene, appendicitis and, 1316
Gantrisin; *See* Sulfisoxazole
Garamycin; *See* Gentamicin
Gardasil, 1703
Gardnerella vaginalis, 1748
Garlic, 12*t*, 246*t*
Gas bloat syndrome, 1254, 1254*c*
Gas exchange impairment
in acquired immunodeficiency syndrome, 379
in chronic obstructive pulmonary disease, 628-630, 629*c*
in heart failure, 770, 771*c*
in pneumonia, 664, 664*c*
postoperative, 294, 295*c*
in spinal cord injury, 997
Gasoline inhalation, 91
Gastrectomy, 1282*f*, 1282-1285, 1382
Gastric acid
chronic pancreatitis and, 1378
duodenal ulcer and, 1271
gastritis and, 1268
gastrointestinal bleeding and, 1277
Zollinger-Ellison syndrome and, 1279
Gastric acid stimulation, 1228-1229
Gastric analysis, 1228-1229
Gastric bypass, 1406*f*, 1407
Gastric cancer, 1279-1287
assessment in, 1280*c*, 1280-1281
chronic gastritis and, 1266
community-based care in, 1286-1287
nonsurgical management of, 1281
pathophysiology of, 1279-1280
postoperative afferent loop syndrome and, 1285-1286
postoperative alkaline reflux gastropathy and, 1285
postoperative dumping syndrome and, 1285, 1286*t*
prevention of, 1280
surgery for, 1281-1285, 1282*f*
upper gastrointestinal bleeding in, 1271*f*
Gastric contents aspiration
acute respiratory distress syndrome and, 687
in endoscopic gastrointestinal tests, 1227
Gastric lavage, 1276
Gastric outlet obstruction, 1272
Gastric restriction surgery, 1406
Gastric ulcer, 1270-1279
complementary and alternative therapies for, 1270*t*
complications of, 1271*c*, 1271*f*, 1271-1272
drug therapy for, 1268-1269*c*
etiology and genetic risk in, 1272
gastrointestinal bleeding in, 1275-1278, 1276*c*, 1277*c*, 1278*f*
health care resources for, 1279
health teaching in, 1278
history in, 1272-1273
home care management in, 1278, 1279*c*
imaging studies in, 1273-1274
laboratory assessment in, 1273
nursing diagnoses in, 1274
pain in, 1274-1275
pathophysiology of, 1270*f*, 1270-1271, 1271*f*
physical assessment in, 1273, 1273*t*
prevention of, 1272
psychosocial assessment in, 1273
Gastrinoma, 1279
Gastrin-secreting tumor, 1279
Gastritis, 1265-1270, 1266-1269*c*, 1270*t*, 1271*f*
Gastroccult; *See* Occult blood test
Gastroenteritis, 1319*t*, 1319-1321, 1321*c*
Gastroesophageal reflux disease, 1243-1248
in cystic fibrosis, 635
drug therapy for, 1246-1247*c*, 1246-1248
endoscopic therapies for, 1248, 1248*c*
esophageal adenocarcinoma and, 1255-1256
laryngitis in, 658
nonpharmacologic interventions for, 1245*c*, 1245-1246
Gastroesophageal reflux disease *(Continued)*
nursing diagnoses in, 1245
pathophysiology of, 1243-1244, 1244*t*
physical assessment in, 1244*c*, 1244-1245
surgical management of, 1248
Gastrointestinal assessment, 1216-1230
anatomy and physiology review and, 1216-1219, 1217*f*, 1218*f*
in burn, 531
colonoscopy in, 1228, 1229*c*
endoscopic retrograde cholangiopancreatography in, 1227
endoscopic ultrasonography in, 1229
esophagogastroduodenoscopy in, 1226-1227, 1227*f*
gastric analysis in, 1228-1229
gastrointestinal changes associated with aging and, 1219, 1220*c*
imaging studies in, 1226
laboratory assessment in, 1223-1226, 1224-1225*c*
liver-spleen scan in, 1229
patient history in, 1219-1221, 1220*c*
physical assessment in, 1221-1223, 1222*f*, 1222*t*
psychosocial assessment in, 1223
rehabilitation and, 97*t*, 97-98
small bowel capsule endoscopy in, 1227-1228
in spinal cord injury, 994
ultrasonography in, 1229
Gastrointestinal bleeding
common causes of, 1290*f*
in Cushing's disease, 1444
in diverticular disease, 1334
gastritis-related, 1267
nonsteroidal antiinflammatory drug-related, 46
in peptic ulcer disease, 1271, 1271*f*, 1275-1278, 1276*c*, 1277*c*, 1278*f*
in ulcerative colitis, 1290*f*, 1328
Gastrointestinal disorders, 1215-1410
biliary, 1366-1385
acute pancreatitis in, 1371-1377, 1372*f*, 1373*t*, 1374*t*
cholecystitis in, 1366-1371, 1367*f*, 1368*c*, 1368*t*, 1370*c*, 1371*t*
chronic pancreatitis in, 1377-1379, 1378*c*, 1379*c*
gallbladder cancer in, 1371
insulinoma in, 1380
pancreatic abscess in, 1379-1380
pancreatic cancer in, 1380-1384, 1381*c*, 1383*c*, 1383*t*
pancreatic pseudocyst in, 1380
esophageal, 1243-1264
achalasia in, 1254-1255
diverticula in, 1261-1262
gastroesophageal reflux disease in, 1243-1248, 1244*t*, 1244-1248*c*
hiatal hernia in, 1249*f*, 1249-1254, 1253*c*, 1253*f*, 1254*c*
nursing care plan for open conventional esophageal surgery and, 1250-1253
trauma and, 1262, 1262*t*
tumor in, 1255-1261, 1256*c*, 1258*c*, 1259*f*, 1260*c*
hepatic, 1344-1365
cirrhosis in, 1344-1356; *See also* Cirrhosis
fatty liver in, 1360-1361
hepatitis in, 1356-1360, 1357*t*, 1358*c*, 1361*c*
liver abscess in, 1361
liver cancer in, 1362
liver transplantation for, 1362-1363, 1364*t*
liver trauma in, 1361*c*, 1361-1362
inflammatory intestinal, 1315-1343
anal fissure in, 1337-1338
anal fistula in, 1338
anorectal abscess in, 1337, 1337*c*

Gastrointestinal disorders *(Continued)*
appendicitis in, 1316*f*, 1316-1317
Crohn's disease in, 1330*f*, 1330-1334, 1333*f*
diverticular disease in, 1334*f*, 1334-1337, 1335*c*
food poisoning in, 1340-1342, 1341*c*, 1341*t*
gastroenteritis in, 1319*t*, 1319-1321, 1321*c*
helminthic infestation in, 1339-1340
parasitic infection in, 1338-1339
peritonitis in, 1317*c*, 1317-1319
ulcerative colitis in, 1321-1330; *See also* Ulcerative colitis
malnutrition and, 1392-1402
community-based care in, 1401-1402
drug therapy for, 1395-1396
history in, 1393
intervention activities for, 1395*c*
laboratory assessment in, 1393-1394
mechanical ventilation and, 696
nursing diagnoses in, 1394
nutrition management in, 1395
older adult and, 16, 1393*c*, 1395, 1396*c*
parenteral nutrition in, 1400-1401, 1401*c*
pathophysiology of, 1392
physical assessment in, 1393, 1394*t*
psychosocial assessment in, 1393
total enteral nutrition in, 1396-1400, 1397*f*, 1398*c*
noninflammatory intestinal, 1289-1314
abdominal herniation in, 1291-1293, 1292*f*
abdominal trauma in, 1307-1308
colorectal cancer in, 1293-1302; *See also* Colorectal cancer
hemorrhoids in, 1309*f*, 1309-1310
intestinal obstruction in, 1302-1306, 1303*f*, 1304*c*, 1306*c*
intestinal polyps in, 1308-1309, 1309*f*
irritable bowel syndrome in, 1289-1291, 1290*f*
malabsorption syndrome in, 1311-1312, 1312*c*
obesity and, 1402-1408
abdominal hernia and, 1292
behavioral management in, 1405-1406
community-based care in, 1408, 1408*c*
complementary and alternative therapies for, 1406
complications of, 1402-1403, 1403*t*
coronary artery disease and, 852, 854*c*
diet programs for, 1404-1405
drug therapy for, 1405
etiology and genetic risk for, 1403
exercise program for, 1405
gastroesophageal reflux disease and, 1246
heart disease risk and, 710-711
history in, 1403-1404
nutrition therapy for, 1405
osteoarthritis and, 323
pathophysiology of, 1402
preoperative assessment of, 248
prevention of, 1403, 1403*t*
psychosocial assessment in, 1404
surgical management of, 1406*f*, 1406-1407
oral cavity, 1231-1242
acute sialadenitis in, 1239-1240
cancer of, 1234-1239, 1235*f*, 1236*c*, 1238*c*
maintenance of healthy mouth and, 1232*c*

Gastrointestinal disorders *(Continued)*
postirradiation sialadenitis in, 1240
premalignant lesions in, 1234
salivary gland tumors in, 1240
stomatitis in, 1231-1234, 1233*c*, 1233*f*
stomach, 1265-1288
gastric cancer in, 1279-1287, 1280*c*, 1282*f*, 1286*t*
gastritis in, 1265-1270, 1266-1269*c*, 1270*t*
peptic ulcer disease in, 1270-1279; *See also* Peptic ulcer disease
Zollinger-Ellison syndrome in, 1279
Gastrointestinal preparation for surgery, 254
Gastrointestinal system
adrenal insufficiency and, 1437*c*
burn-related changes in, 525
cancer effects on, 415
catecholamine receptors and, 1416*t*
chronic kidney disease and, 1611, 1613*c*, 1614
cirrhosis and, 1348*f*
complications of mechanical ventilation and, 696
fluid overload and, 182*c*
hepatitis A and, 1357*t*
hyperkalemia and, 190
hyperparathyroidism and, 1461
hyperthyroidism and, 1449*c*
hypocalcemia and, 193
hypokalemia and, 188
hypomagnesemia and, 196
hyponatremia and, 185
hypothyroidism and, 1456*c*
immobility and, 102*t*
leukemia and, 903*c*, 904
nutrient deficiencies and, 1394*t*
nutrition screening assessment and, 1390*c*
parathyroid hormone and, 1417, 1418*f*
pathogen entry via, 442
postoperative complications of, 287*t*
shock and, 829*c*
Whipple procedure and, 1383*t*
Gastrojejunostomy, 1382, 1383*f*
Gastroparesis, 1470
Gastroplication procedure, 1248, 1248*c*
Gastroscopy, 1227*f*
Gastrostomy, 602, 1397, 1397*f*
Gate control theory of pain, 38, 39*f*
Gatifloxacin, 1556*c*
Gauge size for peripheral catheter, 216*t*
Gaviscon, 1246*c*, 1247
Gay health care, 30*c*, 30-31, 31*t*
Gaze, cardinal positions of, 1078*f*, 1078-1079
G-CSF; *See* Granulocyte colony-stimulating factor
Gefitinib, 435*t*
for brain tumor, 1062
for esophageal cancer, 1258
Gel pad, 103*t*
Gel phenomenon, 338
Gemcitabine, 421*t*, 1382
Gemtuzumab, 435*t*
Gemzar; *See* Gemcitabine
Gender
cancer incidence and death and, 406*f*
carpal tunnel syndrome and, 1206
human immunodeficiency virus infection and, 366, 367*f*
total body water and, 175
urinary tract infection and, 1551*t*, 1552*t*
vision assessment and, 1076
Gene, 62-71
deoxyribonucleic acid and, 63-68
cell division and, 65*f*, 65-66, 66*f*
chromosomal analysis and, 67-68, 68*f*
chromosome formation and, 66, 67*f*
chromosome function and, 66-67, 67*f*
structure of, 63-65, 64*f*, 65*f*

Gene *(Continued)*
expression of, 69-70
protein synthesis and, 70, 70*f*, 70*t*, 71*f*
structure and function of, 68-69, 69*f*
Gene mutation, 70-71
in breast cancer, 73, 78, 1647, 1664, 1705
in Crohn's disease, 1330
in esophageal cancer, 1256
in gastric cancer, 1280
in pancreatic cancer, 1380
in prostate cancer, 1719
Gene products, 70
Gene therapy
in cancer, 434
in heart failure, 774
in rheumatoid arthritis, 345
General anesthesia, 272*t*, 272-275, 273*t*, 274*t*, 275*c*
General appearance
in cardiovascular assessment, 714
in chronic obstructive pulmonary disease, 624
in Cushing's disease, 1441*c*
as indicator of respiratory adequacy, 564
Generalized osteoporosis, 1153
Generalized seizure, 955-956
Generation time of cell, 401
Generic administration set, 220
Genetic biology, 62-71
cell anatomy and, 63*f*
deoxyribonucleic acid and, 63-68
cell division and, 65*f*, 65-66, 66*f*
chromosomal analysis and, 67-68, 68*f*
chromosome formation and, 66, 67*f*
chromosome function and, 66-67, 67*f*
structure of, 63-65, 64*f*, 65*f*
gene expression and, 69-70
gene mutation and, 70-71
gene structure and function and, 68-69, 69*f*
protein synthesis and, 70, 70*f*, 70*t*, 71*f*
Genetic considerations, 62-79
in acute pancreatitis, 1373
in acute respiratory distress syndrome, 687
in allergies, 388-389
in Alzheimer's disease, 970
in asthma, 610
in atherosclerosis, 794
in benign prostatic hypertrophy, 1713
in cancer, 408-411, 409*c*, 409*t*, 410*t*
breast, 1664, 1665*t*
colorectal, 410*t*
esophageal, 1256
leukemia, 902
lung, 642
pancreatic, 1380
prostate, 1719
testicular, 1726
in cardiovascular disease, 712
in cataract, 1091
in cholelithiasis, 1367, 1368*t*
in chronic obstructive pulmonary disease, 623, 623*t*
in coronary artery disease, 850
in Crohn's disease, 1330
in cystic fibrosis, 635-637
in diabetes mellitus, 1471*t*, 1471-1472
in endocrine assessment, 1421
in epilepsy, 956
in gastrointestinal problems, 1221
in hearing loss, 1130
in hearing problems, 1113-1114
in hematologic disorders, 884
in hemophilia, 917
in human immunodeficiency virus infection, 366
in Huntington disease, 979
in hyperpituitarism, 1428
in hyperthyroidism, 1449-1450
in lupus, 348

Genetic considerations *(Continued)*
in malignant hyperthermia, 274
in Marfan syndrome, 356
in multiple sclerosis, 1003
in muscular dystrophy, 1175
in musculoskeletal disorders, 1144
in neurologic disorders, 936
in obesity, 1403
in ocular problems, 1077
in osteoarthritis, 323
in osteoporosis, 1153*c*, 1153-1154
in Paget's disease of bone, 1162
in Parkinson disease, 965
in peptic ulcer disease, 1272
in polycystic kidney disease, 1582-1583, 1583*f*
in primary pulmonary hypertension, 637
in renal problems, 1536
in renal stones, 1571
in reproductive assessment, 1647
in respiratory disorders, 559
in retinitis pigmentosa, 1102
in rheumatoid arthritis, 337
in scleroderma, 351
in septic shock, 840
in sickle cell disease, 894, 895*f*
in skin problems, 467
in stroke, 1032, 1033*c*
in substance abuse, 81
in ulcerative colitis, 1322
Genetic counseling, 75, 76*c*, 77*c*
in colorectal cancer, 1296, 1297*c*
nurse role in, 77-78
Genetic testing, 74-76, 75*t*, 76*c*, 77*c*, 410
Gengraf; *See* Cyclosporine
Genital herpes, 1742*c*, 1742-1743
Genital warts, 1743-1744, 1744*f*
Genitoreproductive history, 1648, 1648*c*
Genitourinary surgery, skin preparation for, 256*f*
Genome, 63
Genomic medicine, 62
Genomics, 62
Genoptic; *See* Gentamicin
Genotype, 69
Gentak Alcomicin; *See* Gentamicin
Gentamar; *See* Gentamicin
Gentamicin
for burn infection, 542*c*
for infection in urolithiasis, 1573-1574
for ocular infection, 1086*c*
for pelvic inflammatory disease, 1750*c*
Genu valgum, 1146
Genu varum, 1146
GERD; *See* Gastroesophageal reflux disease
Geriatric Depression Scale-Short Form, 20, 21*f*
Geriatric patient; *See* Older adult
Germ cell, 63
Germ cell tumor, 1727, 1727*t*
Germline mutation, 70
Gestational diabetes mellitus, 1466*t*
GH; *See* Growth hormone
GHB; *See* Gamma hydroxybutyrate
Ghon tubercle, 668
Giant cell arteritis, 355, 355*c*
Giant cell tumor, 1167
Giardia lamblia, 1338-1339
Gigantism, 1428, 1428*f*, 1429*f*
Ginkgo biloba, 12*t*, 156
Ginseng, 12*t*, 246*t*
GLA; *See* Gamma-linolenic acid
Gland changes related to aging, 464*c*
Glasgow Coma Scale, 941, 941*f*
in spinal cord injury, 993
in traumatic brain injury, 1049, 1055
Glass infusion container, 219
Glatiramir acetate, 1005
Glaucoma, 1095*t*, 1095-1098, 1099-1100*c*
Gleevec; *See* Imatinib mesylate
Glimepiride, 1479*c*
Glimepiride-pioglitazone, 1482*c*

Glimepiride-rosiglitazone, 1483*c*
Glioma, 1060
Glipizide, 1478*c*
Glipizide-metformin, 1482*c*
Global aphasia, 1046, 1046*t*
Globulins, 877
  in rheumatoid arthritis, 339*c*
Glomerular diseases and syndromes, 1589*t*
Glomerular filtrate, 1529
Glomerular filtration, 1528-1529
Glomerular filtration rate, 1529
  in acute glomerulonephritis, 1591
  changes with aging, 1533, 1534*c*
  in chronic glomerulonephritis, 1592
  in chronic kidney disease, 1609, 1609*t*, 1614
  in diabetic nephropathy, 1594*t*, 1594-1595
  guide to safe levels of protein intake, 1615
Glomerulonephritis
  acute, 1590*t*, 1590-1591
  chronic, 1592
  rapidly progressive, 1591-1592
Glomerulus, 1528, 1528*f*, 1530*t*, 1531*f*
Glomus jugulare tumor, 1126
Glossectomy, 1237-1238
Glossitis, 900
Glossopharyngeal nerve, 935*t*
Glottis, 553*f*, 554, 554*f*
Gloving
  standard precautions and, 445, 446*t*
  surgical scrub and, 270, 271*f*
Glucagon, 1418, 1466, 1467
Glucagon-like peptide-1, 1489
Glucocorticoids, 1415-1416, 1416*t*
  bone and, 1142
  for Crohn's disease, 1331
  hypercortisolism and, 1439-1445
    acute adrenal insufficiency in, 1444
    community-based care in, 1445, 1445*c*
    excess fluid volume in, 1442-1443
    history in, 1440-1441
    imaging studies in, 1442
    laboratory assessment in, 1441-1442
    pathophysiology of, 1439-1440, 1440*f*, 1440*t*
    physical assessment in, 1441, 1441*c*
    psychosocial assessment in, 1441
    risk for infection in, 1444
    risk for injury in, 1443-1444
    secondary hypertension in, 798
  for ulcerative colitis, 1324
Gluconeogenesis, 1418, 1436, 1467
Glucophage; *See* Metformin
Glucosamine
  for osteoarthritis, 328, 328*c*
  for pain management in arthritis, 57
Glucose
  adrenal gland assessment and, 1438*c*
  burn assessment and, 532*c*
  in cerebrospinal fluid, 948*t*
  changes in older adult, 1419*c*
  Cushing's disease and, 1441
  diabetes mellitus and, 1466, 1466*f*, 1475
  diffusion across cell membrane, 173
  homeostasis of, 1467
  incomplete breakdown of, 202
  preoperative assessment of, 250*c*
  renal reabsorption of, 1531
  in urine, 1539, 1539*t*
Glucose tests, 1424
Glucose tolerance test, 1473*t*, 1474*c*
Glucose-dependent insulinotropic polypeptide, 1489
Glucose-6-phosphate dehydrogenase anemia, 893*t*
Glucotrol; *See* Glipizide
Glucovance; *See* Glyburide-metformin
GlucoWatch G2 Biographer, 1492
Glue inhalation, 91
Glutamate, 930*t*
  Alzheimer's disease and, 976
  dissociative drugs and, 87
  Huntington disease and, 980
  migraine headache and, 951
Glutamine, 948*t*
Glyburide, 1478*c*
Glyburide-metformin, 1482*c*, 1484
Glycemic control in diabetes mellitus, 1466
Glycerin, 107
Glycine, 70*f*, 70*t*, 930*t*
Glycogenesis, 1467
Glycogenolysis, 1418, 1467
Glycoprotein IIb/IIIa inhibitors
  for acute myocardial infarction, 859
  for postoperative graft occlusion, 809
Glycosaminoglycans, 1455
Glycosylated hemoglobin, 1424, 1473*t*, 1474, 1474*t*
Glycosylated serum albumin, 1474
Glycosylated serum protein, 1474
Glynase PresTabs; *See* Glyburide
Glyset; *See* Miglitol
GM-CSF; *See* Granulocyte-macrophage colony-stimulating factor
Go bag, personal readiness supplies, 163, 164*t*
Goggles, standard precautions and, 446*t*
Goiter, 1449, 1450, 1450*f*, 1451*t*
Gold therapy for rheumatoid arthritis, 344
Goldenseal, 246*t*
Goldmann's applanation tonometer, 1080*f*
Golgi apparatus, 63*f*
Gonadotropin-releasing hormone, 1645
Gonadotropin-releasing hormone agonists
  for endometriosis, 1687
  for premenstrual syndrome, 1686
  for uterine leiomyoma, 1696
Gonadotropins
  deficiency of, 1426, 1427*c*
  overproduction of, 1430*c*
Gonads, 1413*f*, 1415, 1416
Goniometer, 1145
Gonioscopy, 1097
Gonococcal peritonitis, 1317
Gonorrhea, 1744-1746, 1745*f*
Good death, 112, 112*t*
Gordon's Functional Health Patterns
  in acid-base assessment, 207*c*
  in cardiovascular assessment, 711*c*
  in ear and hearing assessment, 1112*c*
  in endocrine assessment, 1420, 1420*c*
  in fluid and electrolyte assessment, 178*c*
  in gastrointestinal assessment, 1219, 1220*c*
  in hematologic assessment, 882*c*
  in musculoskeletal assessment, 1144*c*
  in neurologic assessment, 937*c*
  in renal assessment, 1534*c*
  in reproductive assessment, 1658*c*
  in respiratory assessment, 558*c*
  in vision assessment, 1076*c*
Goserelin
  for breast cancer, 1678
  for prostate cancer, 1723
  for uterine leiomyoma, 1696
Gout, 353-354, 354*f*
  Paget's disease of bone and, 1163
Gouty arthritis, 353-354, 354*f*
Gown
  standard precautions and, 446*t*
  surgical scrub and, 270, 271*f*
Gradient, 171
Grading
  of cancer, 406*t*, 406-407, 407*t*
  of heart murmur, 719*t*
Graft
  arteriovenous, 1623, 1623*t*, 1624*c*, 1624*f*, 1625*t*
  nerve, 1024
  skin
Graft *(Continued)*
    in brown recluse spider bite, 147
    in burn, 539, 540
    for pressure ulcer repair, 495-496
Graft occlusion
  after abdominal aortic aneurysm resection, 812
  in peripheral arterial disease surgery, 809
Graft rejection
  cardiac, 790*c*
  corneal, 1091
Graft-*versus*-host disease
  in bone marrow transplantation, 910
  transfusion-associated, 921
Gram-negative organisms
  in burn wound sepsis, 538*t*
  in infection in leukemia, 905
  in sepsis, 840
Gram-positive organisms
  in burn wound sepsis, 538*t*
  in sepsis, 840
Granisetron, 429*c*
Granulation tissue
  in bone healing, 1180, 1180*f*
  myocardial infarction and, 849
  wound healing and, 482*f*, 483-484, 490
Granulocyte, 310*f*, 310-311, 311*t*
Granulocyte colony-stimulating factor, 310, 318*t*
Granulocyte transfusion, 920
Granulocyte-macrophage colony-stimulating factor, 310, 318*t*
Granuloma in sarcoidosis, 638
Granuloma inguinale, 1753-1754
Granulomatous thyroiditis, 1460
Grapefruit diet, 1405
Grapefruit juice, antihypertensives and, 802
Graves' disease, 395, 1448-1455
  drug therapy for, 1452-1454, 1453*c*
  history in, 1450, 1450*f*
  laboratory assessment in, 1451, 1451*c*
  nursing diagnoses in, 1452
  pathophysiology of, 1448-1450, 1449*c*
  physical assessment in, 1450*f*, 1450-1451, 1451*t*
  psychosocial assessment in, 1451
  surgical management of, 1454-1455, 1455*c*
Gravity, pressure ulcer shearing forces and, 485
Gravity drain, 292, 292*f*
Gray matter
  of brain, 929
  of spinal cord, 931, 932*f*
Graying of hair, 465*f*
Greenfield filter, 820
Greenstick fracture, 1179*f*
Grief, 119
  after burn injury, 545
  bone cancer and, 1171, 1171*c*
  cervical cancer and, 1705
  colorectal cancer and, 1296, 1297*c*
Groin, 1646
Grommet in myringotomy, 1125, 1125*f*
Ground substance, 461
Group A beta-hemolytic *Streptococcus*
  in peritonsillar abscess, 657
  in pharyngitis, 655, 656*t*
Growth factors, 318*t*
  neutrophils and, 310
  oral cancer and, 1237
Growth hormone, 1415*t*
  bone and, 1142
  deficiency of, 1426, 1427*c*
  glucose homeostasis and, 1467
  overproduction of, 1428, 1428*f*, 1429*f*, 1430*c*
Guaifenesin, 629
Guanine, 64, 64*f*
Guided imagery, 9-10, 56
Guillain-Barré syndrome, 1011-1016, 1012*c*, 1012*t*, 1013*t*, 1014*c*, 1015*c*
Gunshot wound
  abdominal, 1307-1308
  to head, 1050
Gurgling, approaching death and, 115*c*
Gusperimus, 320
GVHD; *See* Graft-*versus*-host disease
Gynecologic cancers, 1699-1709
  cervical cancer in, 1702*t*, 1702-1705, 1704*c*, 1704*f*
  endometrial cancer in, 1699-1702, 1700*t*, 1701*c*
  fallopian tube cancer in, 1709
  ovarian cancer in, 1705*t*, 1705-1707
  vaginal cancer in, 1708-1709
  vulvar cancer in, 1707-1708, 1708*f*
Gynecologic problems, 1684-1711
  Bartholin cyst in, 1699
  cervical cancer in, 1702*t*, 1702-1705, 1704*c*, 1704*f*
  cervical polyp in, 1699
  dysfunctional uterine bleeding in, 1688-1689
  endometrial cancer in, 1699-1702, 1700*t*, 1701*c*
  endometriosis in, 1687*f*, 1687-1688
  fallopian tube cancer in, 1709
  menopause in, 1689*t*, 1689-1690, 1690*c*
  ovarian cancer in, 1705*t*, 1705-1707
  ovarian cyst in, 1694
  pelvic inflammatory disease in, 1747-1753
    acute pain in, 1751-1752
    anxiety in, 1752
    community-based care in, 1752
    drug therapy for, 1749-1751, 1750-1751*c*
    fallopian tube cancer and, 1709
    history in, 1748
    infection control in, 1749
    laboratory assessment in, 1749
    Neisseria gonorrhoeae in, 1744
    nursing diagnoses in, 1749
    pathophysiology of, 1747-1748, 1748*f*
    physical assessment in, 1748, 1749*t*
    psychosocial assessment in, 1748-1749
  premenstrual syndrome in, 1685-1687, 1686*c*
  primary dysmenorrhea in, 1684-1685
  toxic shock syndrome in, 1691, 1692*c*
  uterine leiomyoma in, 1694-1699, 1695*f*, 1697*c*, 1697*t*, 1698*c*
  uterine prolapse in, 1691-1694, 1692*f*, 1693*c*, 1693*f*
  vaginal cancer in, 1708-1709
  vulvar cancer in, 1707-1708, 1708*f*
  vulvovaginitis in, 1690-1691, 1691*c*
Gynecologic surgery, skin preparation for, 256*f*
Gynecomastia, 1662-1663, 1663*f*
  androgen therapy-related, 1427
  in cirrhosis, 1348-1349
  hormonal manipulation in cancer and, 432
  LH-RH agonist-related, 1723
  in testicular cancer, 1727

H

H cylinder, 579
HAART; *See* Highly active antiretroviral therapy
Habit training, 1567*c*, 1568
HACE; *See* High-altitude cerebral edema
Haemophilus ducreyi, 1753
Haemophilus influenzae
  in conjunctivitis, 1087
  in meningitis, 961*t*, 961-962
  in pelvic inflammatory disease, 1748
  in sinusitis, 654
  in tonsillitis, 657
Hageman factor, 881*t*
HAI; *See* Healthcare-associated infection

Hair, 461f, 462, 462f
assessment of, 473
changes related to aging, 464c
in ear canal, 1112c
graying of, 465f
hematologic assessment in older adult and, 882c
hyperthyroidism and, 1451
nutrient deficiencies and, 1394t
systemic lupus erythematosus and, 350
Hair follicle, 461f, 462
burn-related skin changes and, 520, 522f
furuncle of ear and, 1122
Hair loss
aging and, 473
chemotherapy-induced, 424, 428-430, 644, 1702
in induction therapy in acute leukemia, 905
in nutrient deficiencies, 1394t
in systemic lupus erythematosus, 350
Haldol; See Haloperidol
Halitosis
in chronic kidney disease, 1611
in esophageal cancer, 1256
in esophageal diverticula, 1261
Hallucinogens abuse, 81, 81t, 86-88
Hallux valgus, 1172-1173, 1173f, 1501f
Halo cast, 1188t
Halo fixator, 996, 996f, 1000c
Halo sign in hypophysectomy, 1431
Haloperidol, 87
Halothane, 274t
Hamartomatous intestinal polyp, 1309
Hammer, 1110, 1110f
Hammertoe deformity, 1173, 1173f, 1501
Hancock II stented pig valve, 782f
Hand
arthroplasty of, 335
carpal tunnel syndrome and, 1206-1207
complications related to intraoperative positioning, 281c
Dupuytren's contracture of, 1172
fracture of, 1195
ganglion of, 1172
intravenous sites in, 216f
musculoskeletal assessment of, 1146, 1147f
rheumatoid arthritis of, 338, 338f
strength assessment of, 939, 939f
Hand hygiene
infection control and, 444, 444c
in severe acute respiratory syndrome, 666
standard precautions and, 446t
Hand massage, 11, 11t
Hand motion acuity, 1078
Hand surgery, skin preparation for, 256f
Hand wall climbing exercise, 1675c
Hand-off communication, 5
in emergency care, 128
postoperative, 286, 286c
Hanging-arm cast, 1188t
Hansen's disease, 516
HAPE; See High-altitude pulmonary edema
Hard contact lenses, 1103
Hard palate, 553f, 1217
Harmonic scalpel, 1310
Hashimoto's disease, 1460
Haversian system, 1141, 1141f
Hawthorn, 246t
Hay fever, 388f, 388-391, 389f, 390c, 654
Hazardous materials training, 160
HBO; See Hyperbaric oxygen therapy
HCTZ; See Hydrochlorothiazide
Head
hematologic assessment and, 885
positioning for prevention of contracture, 544c
Head and neck cancer, 597-606
anxiety in, 604
assessment in, 598t, 598-599
disturbed body image in, 604
health care resources in, 606
health teaching in, 605c, 605-606, 606f
home care management in, 605, 605c
laryngitis in, 658
nursing diagnoses in, 599
pathophysiology of, 597-598
psychosocial preparation for, 606
respiratory obstruction in, 599-602, 600t, 601f, 603f
risk for aspiration in, 603c, 603-604, 604c
subcutaneous infusion therapy in, 237t
Head injury, 1049-1060
brain herniation in, 1052, 1053f
closed head injury in, 1050, 1050f
community-based care in, 1059-1060
drug therapy for, 1057
fluid and electrolyte management in, 1057
hemorrhage in, 1051-1052, 1052f
history in, 1053, 1054c
hydrocephalus after, 1052
imaging studies in, 1055
incidence and prevalence of, 1052
increased intracranial pressure in, 1051, 1055-1057
laboratory assessment in, 1055
minor head injury in, 1056c
nutrition management in, 1057-1058
in older adult, 1054c
open head injury in, 1049-1050
pathophysiology of, 1049, 1049c
physical assessment in, 1053-1055
prevention of, 1053
psychosocial assessment in, 1055
sensory, cognitive, and behavioral management in, 1058
surgical management in, 1058, 1059t
types of force in, 1050f, 1050-1051
Head lice, 504
Head surgery, skin preparation for, 256f
Headache, 951-955
in acute mountain sickness, 155
bromocriptine-related, 1431
in cerebral aneurysm, 1033
cluster, 954-955
in coral snake envenomation, 146
in heat exhaustion, 142
in hyperaldosteronism, 1446
in hypopituitarism, 1426
in influenza, 658
in lightning strike, 151
in meningitis, 961
migraine, 951-954, 952c, 953t, 954c, 954t
in pheochromocytoma, 1446
in pneumonia, 661
in severe acute respiratory syndrome, 666
tension, 955
in toxic shock syndrome, 1691
in viral gastroenteritis, 1320
Healing, 481-484
of bone, 1180, 1180f
classification of burn depth and, 521t
mechanisms of, 482-484, 484f
older adult and, 484
phases of, 481, 481t, 482f, 483t
postoperative assessment of, 291f, 291-292
Healing touch, 12
Health
cultural aspects of, 27-34
culture and cultural competence and, 27-38, 28f, 28t
health care disparities and, 28
Purnell's domains of culture and, 29c, 29t, 29-33, 30c, 31t, 32f, 33f
of surgical team members, 270
Health care
complementary and alternative medicine and, 8-14
biologically based therapies in, 11-12, 12t
energy therapies in, 12-13, 13f
implications for nursing, 13
manipulative and body-based therapies in, 11, 11f, 11t
mind-body therapies in, 9-11, 10f
National Center for Complementary and Alternative Medicine, 8, 9t
systems of care in, 9
cultural aspects of, 27-34
culture and cultural competence and, 27-38, 28f, 28t
health care disparities and, 28
Purnell's domains of culture and, 29c, 29t, 29-33, 30c, 31t, 32f, 33f
older adult issues in, 23-25, 24c
Health care errors, 2-7
core competencies and, 3-6
collaboration with interdisciplinary health care team and, 5
in emergency nursing, 130-131
evidence-based practice and, 5-6, 6t
informatics and, 6, 6f
patient-centered care and, 3-5, 4c
quality improvement and, 6
in emergency department, 129c, 130
Institute for Healthcare Improvement and, 3, 3t
National Patient Safety Goals and, 2
Health care personnel
carpal tunnel syndrome and, 1207c
emergency preparedness roles and responsibilities of, 162-164, 163t, 164t
human immunodeficiency virus infection and, 368-369, 369c
personal protective equipment and, 445, 445f
posttraumatic stress disorder after mass casualty event and, 164c, 164-165
prevention of viral hepatitis in, 1358c
professional core competencies of, 3-6
collaboration with interdisciplinary health care team and, 5
in emergency nursing, 130-131
evidence-based practice and, 5-6, 6t
informatics and, 6, 6f
patient-centered care and, 3-5, 4c
in peaceful death, 112t
quality improvement and, 6
safety in emergency care, 128-130, 129c
surgical team members in, 264-267, 266f, 267f
Health care practices, 32f, 32-33, 33f
Health care practitioner, 32f, 32-33, 33f
Health care resources
for acquired immunodeficiency syndrome, 383
for acute coronary syndromes, 872
for acute pancreatitis, 1376-1377
for Alzheimer's disease, 979
for back pain, 989
for bladder cancer, 1578
for bone cancer, 1172
for breast cancer, 1681
for burns, 546
for cataracts, 1095
for chronic and disabling diseases, 109
for chronic kidney disease, 1635
for chronic obstructive pulmonary disease, 634, 634c
for cirrhosis, 1356
for colorectal cancer, 1302
for Crohn's disease, 1334
for Cushing's disease, 1445
for diabetes mellitus, 1516
for diverticular disease, 1337
Health care resources (Continued)
for endometrial cancer, 1702
for esophageal cancer, 1261
for fracture, 1194
for gastric cancer, 1287
for head and neck cancer, 606
for hearing loss, 1127t, 1135-1136
for heart failure, 778
for hypertension, 804
for hypothyroidism, 1459, 1460c
for infection, 453
for intestinal obstruction, 1306
for leukemia, 912
for malnutrition, 1402
for multiple sclerosis, 1007
for myasthenia gravis, 1022
for oral cancer, 1239
for osteoarthritis, 336
for pain management, 59
for pancreatic cancer, 1384
for pelvic inflammatory disease, 1752
for peptic ulcer disease, 1279
for pneumonia, 666
for polycystic kidney disease, 1585
postoperative care and, 300-301
for pressure ulcer, 498, 499c
for prostate cancer, 1725
for pulmonary embolism, 683-684, 684c
for pyelonephritis, 1589
for rheumatoid arthritis, 347
for spinal cord injury, 1000
for spinal tumor, 1002
for stroke, 1048-1049
for traumatic brain injury, 1060
for tuberculosis, 672
for ulcerative colitis, 1329c, 1329-1330
for urinary incontinence, 1569-1570
for uterine leiomyomas, 1698
for valvular heart disease, 783
Health history; See History
Health perception-health management pattern
in cardiovascular assessment, 711c
in ear and hearing assessment, 1112c
in neurologic assessment, 937c
in reproductive assessment, 1648c
in respiratory assessment, 558c
Health promotion and maintenance
in abdominal hernia, 1292
in acute pancreatitis, 1373
in acute renal failure, 1603
in acute respiratory distress syndrome, 687
in Alzheimer's disease, 970
in amputation, 1200
in anaphylaxis, 391t, 391-392, 392f
in arthropod bite and sting prevention, 150c
in avian influenza, 667
in back pain, 984, 984c
in bladder cancer, 1575
in breast cancer, 1665-1669
breast self-examination in, 1666, 1667f
clinical breast examination in, 1666-1668, 1667f
mammography in, 1665-1666
options for high-risk women in, 1669
in burns, 527-528
in carpal tunnel syndrome, 1206
in cataract prevention, 1091-1092
in cervical cancer, 1703
in chronic kidney disease, 1612
in chronic obstructive pulmonary disease, 624
in cold injury prevention, 152
in colorectal cancer, 1294-1295, 1295c
in coronary artery disease, 850-853, 853t, 854c
in dehydration, 178
in diabetes mellitus, 1472
in drowning prevention, 156
in fractures, 1183

Health promotion and maintenance (Continued)
in gastric cancer, 1280
in gastritis, 1266, 1266c
in hearing loss, 1130
in heat-related illnesses, 141-142, 142c
in hemorrhoids, 1309-1310
in hepatitis, 1358, 1358c
in human immunodeficiency virus infection, 367-370, 368-370c
in hypertension, 798
in hypovolemic shock, 832-833, 833c
in infection prevention and control, 443c, 443-446, 444c, 445f
in influenza, 658
in lightning strike prevention, 151c
in lung cancer, 642
in nutrition, 1386-1387, 1387t, 1388f, 1389f
in osteoarthritis, 324
in osteomalacia, 1161
in osteoporosis, 1155
in osteoporosis-, 1155
in ovarian cancer, 1706
in peptic ulcer disease, 1272
in pressure ulcer prevention, 485c, 485-488, 487f
in prostate cancer, 1719c, 1719-1720
in pulmonary embolism, 678, 678c
in sepsis, 840t, 840-841
in skin cancer prevention, 509-511, 511c
in skin infection prevention, 501-502, 502c
in snakebite prevention, 144c
in stroke, 1032
in syphilis, 1740
in traumatic brain injury, 1053
in urinary tract infections, 1553, 1554c
in venous thromboembolism, 817
in vision, 1074-1075, 1076c
Health teaching
in acquired immunodeficiency syndrome, 383, 384c
in acute coronary syndromes, 870-872, 871c, 872c
in acute glomerulonephritis, 1591
in acute pancreatitis, 1376
in Alzheimer's disease, 978-979
in arthropod bite/sting prevention, 150c
in asthma, 613-615, 615c, 619c
in back pain, 988c, 988-989
in bladder cancer, 1576-1578
in bone cancer, 1171-1172
in breast cancer, 1679-1680
in breast self-examination, 1666, 1667f
in burn, 546
in cataracts, 1094-1095, 1095c
in chemotherapy-related peripheral neuropathy, 431c
in chronic and disabling diseases, 108-109
in chronic kidney disease, 1635
in chronic obstructive pulmonary disease, 634
in cirrhosis, 1355c, 1355-1356
in colorectal cancer, 1300-1302, 1301c
in condom use, 1743c
in condom use to prevent sexually transmitted diseases, 368c
in Crohn's disease, 1333
in Cushing's disease, 1445, 1445c
in death and dying
emotional signs of approaching death and, 116c
occurrence of death and, 121c
signs and symptoms of approaching death and, 115c
in diabetes mellitus, 1514-1515, 1516c, 1517t
diagnostic blood glucose testing and, 1474b
exercise and, 1497, 1497c
foot care and, 1504c
Health teaching (Continued)
hypoglycemia and, 1509
insulin therapy and, 1487-1488
nutrition plans and, 1494t, 1494-1495, 1495t
self-monitoring of blood glucose and, 1490-1492, 1491-1492t
sick-day rules and, 1512c
in dietary habits to reduce cancer risk, 408c
in diverticular disease, 1336-1337
in dry skin, 480c
in dysrhythmias, 758-761, 759-761c
emergency nursing and, 134
in endometrial cancer, 1701-1702
in energy conservation, 346c
in esophageal cancer, 1261
in excretory urogram, 1545c
in fracture, 1194, 1194c
in gastric cancer, 1287
in gastroenteritis, 1321, 1321c
in genital herpes, 1743, 1744
in gonorrhea, 1746
in head and neck cancer, 605c, 605-606, 606f
in hearing aid care, 1133c
in hearing loss, 1135
in heart failure, 776-778, 777t, 778c
in heat-related illness prevention, 142
in hiatal hernia, 1250
in HIV testing, 370c
in hyperkalemia, 191, 191c
in hypertension, 803-804
in hyperthyroidism, 1455
in hypophosphatemia, 195c
in hypothyroidism, 1459
in hysterectomy, 1696
in infection, 453
in infusion therapy, 222
in intestinal obstruction, 1306
in irritable bowel syndrome, 1291
in leukemia, 911-912, 912c
in lifestyles and practices to promote wellness, 16, 16c
in malnutrition, 1401-1402
in multiple sclerosis, 1006-1007
in myasthenia gravis, 1021, 1021t, 1022c
in nonoccupational postexposure prophylaxis to HIV, 368c
nurse role in, 4
older adult and, 4c
in oral cancer, 1239
in osteoarthritis, 336, 336c
in pain management, 58-59
in pancreatic cancer, 1384
in pelvic inflammatory disease, 1752, 1752c
in peptic ulcer disease, 1278
in perioperative respiratory care, 257c
in photodynamic therapy, 432c
in pneumonia, 665-666
in polycystic kidney disease, 1585c
postoperative care and, 300
in postoperative procedures and exercises, 255-258, 256c, 257c, 258f, 259f
in preoperative anxiety, 259
in pressure ulcer, 498
in prevention of ear infection or trauma after ear surgery, 1134c
in prevention of infection, 427c
in prevention of migraine headache, 953-954, 954c
in prevention of pneumonia, 660c
in prevention of renal and urinary problems, 1612c
in prostate cancer, 1724-1725, 1725c
in pulmonary embolism, 683, 684c
in pyelonephritis, 1589
in renal trauma, 1597
in rheumatoid arthritis, 347
in septic shock, 844, 844c
Health teaching (Continued)
in skin protection
during radiation therapy, 420c
in systemic lupus erythematosus, 350c
in snakebite prevention, 144c
in spinal cord injury, 999c, 999-1000, 1000c
in spinal tumor, 1002
in stroke, 1048, 1048f
in supraglottic method of swallowing, 604c
in syphilis, 1741-1742
in total hip arthroplasty, 332c
in traumatic brain injury, 1059-1060
in tuberculosis, 670-672
in ulcerative colitis, 1328-1329, 1329c
in urinary incontinence, 1569, 1570c
in urolithiasis, 1575, 1575c
in uterine leiomyomas, 1687, 1698c
in vaginal infections, 1691c
in valvular heart disease, 783, 783c
Healthcare-associated infection, 442, 443-444
Health-enhancing behaviors of older adult, 16c
Health-protecting behaviors of older adult, 16c
Healthy People 2010 objectives, 28
in blood pressure, 797t
in heart failure, 767, 768t
in nutrition and overweight, 1403t
in sexually transmitted diseases, 1739t
Hearing, 1111
Hearing acuity testing, 1115
Hearing aid, 260, 1132, 1133c
Hearing assessment, 1109-1119
anatomy and physiology review and, 1109-1111, 1110f, 1111f
audiometry in, 1117t, 1117-1118
auditory assessment in, 1115-1116
diagnostic assessment for balance in, 1116-1117
external ear and mastoid inspection in, 1114
imaging assessment in, 1116
otoscopic assessment in, 1115, 1115f
patient history in, 1111-1114, 1112c, 1113c, 1114t
psychosocial assessment and, 1116
Hearing loss, 1129-1136
in acoustic neuroma, 1129
in external otitis, 1121
health care resources for, 1135-1136
health teaching in, 1135
hearing aid care in, 1132, 1133c
history in, 1130-1131
home care management in, 1135
imaging studies in, 1131
impaired verbal communication and, 1135, 1135c
in labyrinthitis, 1127
in Meniere's disease, 1127-1129
nursing diagnoses in, 1131-1132
in otitis media, 1123
pathophysiology of, 1129f, 1129-1130, 1130t
physical assessment in, 1131, 1131c
preoperative informed consent and, 254
prevention of, 1130
psychosocial assessment in, 1131
stapedectomy in, 1133-1134, 1134c, 1134f
tympanoplasty in, 1132-1133, 1133f, 1134c, 1134f
in vertigo, 1126
Hearing Loss Association of America, 1127t
Heart
burn-related changes in, 524
cardiovascular assessment and, 704-729
arterial system and, 708-709
blood pressure and, 716
Heart (Continued)
cardiac catheterization in, 722t, 722-724, 723f
changes associated with aging and, 709, 710c
current health problems in, 712-714, 713t
echocardiography in, 725
electrocardiography in, 724
electronic-beam computed tomography scan in, 726
electrophysiologic studies in, 724
extremities and, 715, 715f
family history and genetic risk in, 712
functional history in, 714, 714t
general appearance and, 714
Gordon's Functional Health Patterns and, 711c
hemodynamic monitoring in, 726-728, 727c, 727f
laboratory assessment in, 719-722, 720c
magnetic resonance imaging in, 726
myocardial nuclear perfusion imaging in, 725-726
nutrition history in, 712
precordium and, 717-719, 718f, 719t
psychosocial assessment and, 719
skin and, 715
stress test in, 724-725
transesophageal echocardiography in, 725
venous and arterial pulses in, 716-717, 717f
venous system and, 709
catecholamine receptors and, 1416t
chronic kidney disease and, 1610-1611, 1613, 1613c
complications of mechanical ventilation and, 696
conduction system of, 731, 731f
Cushing's disease and, 1441
dysrhythmias of, 730-763
advanced cardiac life support for, 756
atrial fibrillation in, 745-746, 746f
atrial flutter in, 747
atrioventricular blocks in, 750
automatic external defibrillation for, 757, 757f
bundle branch blocks in, 750
cardiac conduction system and, 731, 731f
cardiopulmonary resuscitation in, 755-756
cardioversion for, 756
coronary artery bypass graft for, 758
decreased cardiac output and ineffective tissue perfusion in, 750-751, 751c
defibrillation for, 756-757
drug therapy for, 741-745c, 751-753, 752-753c
electrocardiography and, 731-737, 732f, 733t, 734f, 735f, 736f
electrophysiologic properties of heart and, 730-731, 731f
health teaching in, 758-761, 759-761c
home care management in, 758
in hypercalcemia, 194
junctional, 747
key features of, 738c
normal rhythms and, 737f, 737-738
nursing diagnoses in, 750
older adult and, 760c
pacemaker insertion for, 757
premature atrial complexes in, 740
radiofrequency catheter ablation for, 757
sinus, 739f, 739-740

Heart (Continued)
supraventricular tachycardia in, 740-741
temporary pacing for, 754-755
terminology in, 738-739
vagal maneuvers for, 753-754
ventricular, 747-750, 748f, 749f
electrophysiologic properties of, 730-731, 731f
Guillain-Barré syndrome and, 1014
infusion therapy and, 235-236
leukemia and, 903, 903c
Marfan syndrome and, 356
shock and, 829c
structure and function of, 704-708, 705-707f
Heart disease, 764-792, 847-874
acute coronary syndromes in, 847-874
activity intolerance in, 860
acute pain in, 856c, 856-858, 857-858c
chronic stable angina pectoris and, 847-848
coronary artery bypass graft surgery in, 866-870, 867f
diagnostic tests in, 855
dysrhythmias in, 861-862
etiology and genetic risk in, 850
health care resources for, 872
health teaching in, 870-872, 871c, 872c
heart failure in, 862t, 862-864, 863-864c
history in, 853
home care management in, 870, 870c, 871c
imaging studies in, 855
incidence and prevalence of, 850
ineffective coping in, 860-861
ineffective tissue perfusion in, 858-860, 859t
intervention activities in, 861c
laboratory assessment in, 855
nursing diagnoses in, 855-856
pathophysiology of, 848f, 848-850, 849f
percutaneous transluminal coronary angioplasty in, 865, 865t
physical assessment in, 853c, 853-855
prevention of, 850-853, 853t, 854c
psychosocial assessment in, 855
stents in, 865-866, 866f
cardiomyopathy in, 787-790, 788t, 789f, 790c
diastolic blood pressure and, 797
heart failure in, 765-779
in chronic obstructive pulmonary disease, 623, 623c
classification and staging of, 765
compensatory mechanisms in, 765-767, 766f
decreased cardiac output in, 77o0-775, 771t, 774f
diagnostic tests in, 770
etiology of, 767, 767t
health care resources for, 778
health teaching in, 776-778, 777t, 778c
history in, 767-768
home care management in, 776, 776c
imaging assessment in, 770
impaired gas exchange in, 770, 771c
incidence and prevalence of, 767
laboratory assessment in, 769-770
nursing diagnoses in, 770
physical assessment in, 768c, 768-769
potential for pulmonary edema in, 775c, 775-776
psychosocial assessment in, 769
types of, 765
infective endocarditis in, 783-785, 784c
Heart disease (Continued)
pericarditis in, 785-786, 786c
rheumatic carditis in, 787
surgical risk and, 246
valvular, 779c, 779-783, 782f, 783c
Heart failure, 765-779
in acute coronary syndromes, 862t, 862-864, 863-864c
in chronic kidney disease, 1611
in chronic obstructive pulmonary disease, 623, 623c
in circulatory overload from fluid resuscitation, 530
classification and staging of, 765
compensatory mechanisms in, 765-767, 766f
in coronary artery disease, 862t, 862-864, 863-864c
decreased cardiac output in, 77o0-775, 771t, 774f
diagnostic tests in, 770
etiology of, 767, 767t
health care resources for, 778
health teaching in, 776-778, 777t, 778c
history in, 767-768
home care management in, 776, 776c
hypertension and, 767
imaging assessment in, 770
impaired gas exchange in, 770, 771c
incidence and prevalence of, 767
in infective endocarditis, 784
laboratory assessment in, 769-770
nursing diagnoses in, 770
physical assessment in, 768c, 768-769
postmyocardial infarction, 862, 862t
potential for pulmonary edema in, 775c, 775-776
with preserved left ventricular function, 765
psychosocial assessment in, 769
types of, 765
Heart murmur, 718, 719, 719t
in aortic regurgitation, 779c, 780
in aortic stenosis, 779c, 780
in infective endocarditis, 784
in leukemia, 903
in mitral regurgitation, 779c, 780
in mitral stenosis, 779, 779c
Heart rate, 707
in atrial fibrillation, 745, 746f
in atrial flutter, 746f, 747
bradydysrhythmias and tachyrhythmias and, 738, 738c
burn-related changes in, 524
in chronic obstructive pulmonary disease, 626
coronary artery disease and, 854
dehydration and, 178
electrocardiographic determination of, 736, 736f
in heart failure, 766
of heart transplant recipient, 790
hypocalcemia and, 192
in hypothyroidism, 1457
hypovolemic shock and, 833
in idioventricular rhythm, 747
in junctional dysrhythmias, 747
normal sinus rhythm and, 737
in pulmonary embolism, 679
sinus arrhythmia and, 737
in sinus bradycardia, 739f
in sinus tachycardia, 739, 739f
in supraventricular tachycardia, 740
in ventricular tachycardia, 749f
Heart reduction surgery, 775
Heart rhythm
electrocardiographic analysis of, 736-737
in left-sided heart failure, 769
normal sinus rhythm and, 737
sinus arrhythmia and, 737
Heart sounds
abnormal, 718-719, 719t
normal, 718
Heart sounds (Continued)
postoperative assessment of, 287
in pulmonary embolism, 679
Heart transplantation
in cardiomyopathy, 789, 789f
in heart failure, 774
Heart valves, 705f, 706
aging-related changes in, 710c
valvular heart disease and, 779c, 779-783, 782f, 783c
Heartburn
in gastritis, 1267
in gastroesophageal reflux disease, 1244
in hiatal hernia, 1249
Heat application
for back pain, 985
for dysmenorrhea, 1685
for endometriosis, 1688
for muscle strain, 1208
for osteoarthritis, 327
for pain, 56
for rheumatoid arthritis, 344-345, 345f
Heat exhaustion, 142
Heat intolerance in hyperthyroidism, 1450
Heat stroke, 142-143, 143c
Heat-related illnesses, 141-143, 142c, 143c
Heavy metals, 1603t
Heberden's node, 324
Height
nutritional assessment and, 1389-1390
obesity and, 1402
Heimlich maneuver, 597f
Helicobacter pylori
in duodenal ulcer, 1271
in gastric cancer, 1280
in gastritis, 1266
gastroesophageal reflux disease and, 1244
in peptic ulcer disease, 1272
Heliox
for asthma, 621
for cystic fibrosis, 636
Helix, 1110f
Helixate; *See* Factor VIII cryoprecipitate
Helminthic infestation, 1339-1340
Helper/inducer T-cell, 317, 318f
antigen-antibody interactions and, 313
functions of, 309t, 878t
human immunodeficiency virus and, 363, 363f
Hematemesis
in bleeding esophageal varices, 1345
in gastritis, 1267
in peptic ulcer disease, 1271
Hematochezia, 1295
Hematocrit
in acute renal failure, 1605c
in anemia, 893
in burn, 532c
in cardiovascular assessment, 722
in colorectal cancer, 1295
in diverticulitis, 1335
in heart failure, 769
in hematologic assessment, 887c
in hypovolemic shock, 835, 836c
in malnutrition, 1393
in peptic ulcer disease, 1273
preoperative assessment of, 251c
in respiratory assessment, 565c
in sickle cell disease, 896
in ulcerative colitis, 1323
Hematogenous metastasis, 641
Hematogenous osteomyelitis, 1165
Hematogenous tuberculosis, 668
Hematologic assessment, 876-891
aging-related changes in hematologic system and, 881, 882c
anatomy and physiology review and, 876-881
accessory organs of blood formation and, 879
anti-clotting forces and, 881, 882f
Hematologic assessment (Continued)
blood clotting and, 879-880, 880f, 881t
blood components and, 877-879, 878f, 878t, 879f
bone marrow and, 876-877, 877f
bone marrow aspiration and biopsy in, 889-890
in cancer, 409, 409c
in colorectal cancer, 409c
imaging studies in, 889
laboratory assessment in, 886-889, 887c
patient history in, 882c, 882-885, 883-884t
physical assessment in, 885-886
psychosocial assessment in, 886
Hematologic disorders, 892-925
hemophilia in, 917
platelet disorders in, 916
red blood cell disorders in, 893-902
anemia in, 893t, 893-898, 894c, 894f, 895f, 897c, 898c
aplastic anemia in, 900
folic acid deficiency anemia in, 900
glucose-6-phosphate dehydrogenase deficiency anemia in, 898-899
immunohemolytic anemia in, 899
iron-deficiency anemia in, 899, 899c
myelodysplastic syndromes in, 901-902
polycythemia vera in, 901, 901c
vitamin B_{12} deficiency anemia in, 900
transfusion therapy for, 917t, 917-921, 918c, 919c, 919t
white blood cell disorders in, 902-916
Hodgkin's lymphoma in, 913t, 913-914
leukemia in, 902-913; *See also* Leukemia
multiple myeloma in, 915
non-Hodgkin's lymphoma in, 914-915
Hematologic system
aging-related changes in, 881, 882c
chronic kidney disease and, 1611, 1613c, 1613-1614
cirrhosis and, 1348f
drugs impairing, 883-884t
hepatitis A and, 1357t
nutrient deficiencies and, 1394t
role in oxygenation and tissue perfusion, 876f
Hematoma
after renal transplantation, 1633
in bone healing, 1180, 1180f
intravenous therapy-related, 228t
Hematopoiesis, 1141
Hematopoietic stem cell transplantation
in leukemia, 907t, 907-910, 909f
platelet transfusion and, 920
in sickle cell disease, 897
Hematuria
after renal biopsy, 1548
in benign prostatic hypertrophy, 1713
in bladder cancer, 1576
in cervical cancer, 1703
in cystitis, 1555
hematologic assessment and, 885
in pancreatic transplant rejection, 1498
in polycystic kidney disease, 1583
in prostate cancer, 1720
in prostatitis, 1733
in urolithiasis, 1571, 1572
Hemianopsia, 1035, 1035f
Hemiarthroplasty of shoulder, 334
Hemilaryngectomy, 600t
Hemiparesis, 1034
Hemiplegia
after stroke, 1034
in brain abscess, 1066

Hemoconcentration
burn-related changes in, 524
dehydration and, 179
in diabetes mellitus, 1467
Hemodialysis
in acute renal failure, 1607f, 1607-1608
in chronic kidney disease, 1620-1626, 1621t
anticoagulation in, 1622
complications of, 1626
dialysis settings for, 1621
nursing care in, 1625, 1625t
patient selection for, 1620
post-dialysis care in, 1625-1626, 1626c
procedure of, 1621f, 1621-1622, 1622f
vascular access for, 1622-1625, 1623t, 1624c, 1625f
complications of, 1626
dialysis settings for, 1621
dietary restrictions in, 1617t
health teaching in, 1635
in hypothermia, 153
nursing care in, 1625, 1625t
procedure of, 1621f, 1621-1622, 1622f
Hemodialysis catheter, 1623t
Hemodynamic monitoring, 726-728, 727c, 727f, 1307-1308
Hemodynamic regulation in heart failure, 771c, 771t, 771-775, 774f
Hemoglobin
in acid-base control, 202
in acute renal failure, 1605c
in burn, 532c
in cardiovascular assessment, 722
changes with age, 882
in colorectal cancer, 1295
in diverticulitis, 1335
in heart failure, 769
in hematologic assessment, 887c
in hypovolemic shock, 835, 836c
in malnutrition, 1393
in peptic ulcer disease, 1273
preoperative assessment of, 251c
red blood cell production of, 877
sickle cell disease and, 894
in ulcerative colitis, 1323
Hemoglobin A, 894
Hemoglobin A_1c, 1473t, 1474, 1474t
Hemoglobin electrophoresis, 886, 887c
Hemoglobin S, 894
Hemolysis, drugs causing, 883t
Hemolytic anemia
in brown recluse spider bite, 147
in glucose-6-phosphate dehydrogenase deficiency, 898-899
in sickle cell disease, 894
Hemolytic jaundice, 1346t
Hemolytic transfusion reaction, 920-921
Hemophilia, 917
Hemoptysis
after dilation of lower esophageal sphincter, 1255
in laryngeal trauma, 596
in mitral stenosis, 779, 779c
respiratory assessment and, 559
Hemorrhage
in blunt abdominal trauma, 1308
in cirrhosis, 1353c, 1353-1354
conjunctival, 1087
in diverticular disease, 1334
hypovolemic shock and, 832
in inflammatory bowel disease, 1322t
in inhalation anthrax, 672
intracerebral
after brain tumor surgery, 1064
in lightning strike, 151
in traumatic brain injury, 1051-1052, 1052f
in pit viper envenomation, 145
postoperative
in bone marrow transplantation, 912c
in coronary artery bypass graft, 868
Hemorrhage (Continued)
in glaucoma surgery, 1098
in laryngectomy, 601
in renal biopsy, 1548
in thyroidectomy, 1454
in total hip arthroplasty, 330c, 331
in transurethral resection of prostate, 1718
in renal cell carcinoma, 1596
in spinal cord injury, 993
trauma patient and, 136
in uterine leiomyoma, 1696
vitreous, 1098-1100
Hemorrhagic bullae, 144
Hemorrhagic pancreatitis, 1372
Hemorrhagic shock, 1361
Hemorrhagic stroke, 1031t, 1031-1032
Hemorrhoidectomy, 1310
Hemorrhoids, 1290f, 1309f, 1309-1310
Hemostasis, 879-880, 880f, 881t
Hemothorax, 231t, 699
Hemovac drain, 292, 292f, 295
HEPA respirator
in severe acute respiratory syndrome, 666-667
in tuberculosis, 670, 672f
Hepalean; See Heparin
Heparin
after percutaneous transluminal coronary angioplasty, 865
after stroke, 1043
for anticoagulation in hemodialysis, 1622
for atrial fibrillation, 746
basophil production of, 311
for pulmonary embolism, 678, 680, 681c
Heparin-induced thrombocytopenia, 818
Hepatic arterial infusion, 1362
Hepatic artery embolization, 1362
Hepatic coma, 1345-1346, 1346t
Hepatic disorders, 1344-1365
cirrhosis in, 1344-1356
complications of, 1345-1346, 1346t
concept map for, 1351
etiology of, 1346-1347, 1347t
excess fluid volume in, 1350-1353, 1352c, 1353c
health care resources for, 1356
health teaching in, 1355c, 1355-1356
hemorrhage in, 1353-1354
history in, 1347
home care management in, 1355
imaging studies in, 1350
laboratory assessment in, 1349t, 1349-1350
nursing diagnoses in, 1350
pathophysiology of, 1344-1345
physical assessment in, 1347-1349, 1348f, 1349f
portal-systemic encephalopathy in, 1354-1355
psychosocial assessment in, 1349
fatty liver in, 1360-1361
hepatitis in, 1356-1360, 1357t, 1358c, 1361c
liver abscess in, 1361
liver cancer in, 1362
liver transplantation for, 1362-1363, 1364t
liver trauma in, 1361c, 1361-1362
Hepatic duct, 1218f
Hepatic encephalopathy, 1345-1346, 1346t
Hepatic thrombosis after liver transplantation, 1364t
Hepatitis, 1356-1360, 1357t, 1358c, 1361c
Hepatitis A, 1356-1357, 1357t, 1358
Hepatitis A virus antibody, 1359
Hepatitis B, 1357
cancers associated with, 408t
cirrhosis and, 1347
hemodialysis-related, 1626
liver cancer and, 1362
Hepatitis B antigen-antibody system, 1359
Hepatitis B vaccine, 1358
Hepatitis C, 1357
cancers associated with, 408t
cirrhosis and, 1347
hemodialysis-related, 1626
Hepatitis carrier, 1357
Hepatitis D, 1347, 1357
Hepatitis E, 1357-1358
Hepatocellular jaundice, 1346t
Hepatocyte, 1344-1345
Hepatomegaly, 1223
in cirrhosis, 1348
in pancreatic cancer, 1380
in right-sided heart failure, 769
Hepatopulmonary syndrome, 1352
Hepatorenal syndrome, 1346
HER2 type breast cancer, 1671
Herbal preparations, 12, 12t
for gastritis and peptic ulcer disease, 1270t, 1275
for migraine headache, 953, 954t
surgical risk and, 246, 246t
for ulcerative colitis, 1325
Herceptin; See Trastuzumab
Hereditary nonpolyposis colorectal cancer, 76, 1294, 1309
Hernia
abdominal, 1291-1293, 1292f
brain, 1052, 1053f
hiatal, 1249f, 1249-1254, 1253c, 1253f, 1254c
inguinal, 1291-1293, 1292f
umbilical, 1291-1293, 1292f
uncal, 1052, 1053f
Herniated nucleus pulposus, 984, 989, 989f
Hernioplasty, 1293
Herniorrhaphy, 1293
Heroin, 90t, 90-91, 91c
Herpes genitalis, 1690
Herpes simplex virus, 499-501, 501f
in encephalitis, 964
in facial paralysis, 1026
in genital herpes, 1742c, 1742-1743, 1743c
in HIV-infected patient, 372
Herpes zoster, 500c, 501, 501f
HerpeSelect 1 and 2 Immunoblot IgG test, 1742
Herpetic whitlow, 500-501
Hesitancy, 1535t
Heterograft for burn wound, 539
Heterotopic ossification, 994, 996
Heterozygous allele, 69
Hexalen; See Altretamine
Hex-Fix external fixations system, 1191f
HHS; See Hyperglycemic-hyperosmolar state
Hiatal hernia, 1249f, 1249-1254, 1253c, 1253f, 1254c
Hiccups in chronic kidney disease, 1611
Hickman catheter, 218
Hierarchy of evidence, 6t
High-alert drugs, 1043
High-altitude cerebral edema, 154-156, 156c
High-altitude pulmonary edema, 154-156, 156c
High-density lipoproteins
atherosclerosis and, 794, 795-796
cardiovascular assessment and, 720c, 721
coronary artery disease and, 850-851
metabolic syndrome and, 853t
High-dose rate implant radiation, 419, 420c
High-efficiency particulate air respirator
in severe acute respiratory syndrome, 666-667
in tuberculosis, 670, 672f
Higher intellectual function assessment, 938
High-flow oxygen delivery systems, 576-577, 577f, 577t, 578f
Highly active antiretroviral therapy, 375-379, 376-378c
High-output heart failure, 765
High-pitched rales, 563t
High-sensitivity C-reactive protein
in cardiovascular assessment, 721
in osteoarthritis, 325
in rheumatoid arthritis, 340
High-voltage electric shock in lightning injury, 151
Hilum, 556, 1527, 1527f
Hinge joint, 1142
Hip
fracture of, 1195-1197, 1196f
fat embolism syndrome and, 1182
long-term use of proton pump inhibitors and, 1248
osteoporosis-related, 1155
pain in, 1185
musculoskeletal assessment of, 1146
positioning for prevention of contracture, 544c
total hip arthroplasty and, 328-332, 330c, 330t, 332c, 332f
Hip spica cast, 1188t
Hip surgery, skin preparation for, 256f
Hirsutism, 473
in Cushing's disease, 1440
in endocrine problems, 1422
Hispanic Americans
beliefs regarding death, dying, and afterlife, 119t
coronary artery disease and, 850, 852
diabetes mellitus and, 1472
syphilis and, 1739
Histamine
allergic reaction and, 388, 389f
anaphylaxis and, 392
asthma and, 610
basophil production of, 311
Histamine cephalalgia, 954
Histamine$_2$-receptor antagonists
for acute pancreatitis, 1376
for gastritis, 1268
for gastroesophageal reflux disease, 1246c, 1247-1248
mechanical ventilation and, 696
for peptic ulcer disease, 1269c, 1274
preoperative, 261
Histocompatibility antigens, 307
Histoplasmosis, 371, 558-559
History
in acidosis, 206, 207c
in acquired immunodeficiency syndrome, 370
in acute coronary syndromes, 853
in acute glomerulonephritis, 1590-1591
in acute pancreatitis, 1373
in acute renal failure, 1603
in adrenal insufficiency, 1437
in allergic rhinitis, 389
in Alzheimer's disease, 970-971, 971t
in asthma, 612
in breast cancer, 1669-1670
in burn injury, 528, 529c
in cardiovascular assessment, 709-714
current health problems in, 712-714, 713t
family history and genetic risk in, 712
functional history in, 714, 714t
Gordon's Functional Health Patterns and, 711c
nutrition history in, 712
in cataract, 1092
in chronic glomerulonephritis, 1592
in chronic kidney disease, 1612
in chronic obstructive pulmonary disease, 624
in cirrhosis, 1347
in colorectal cancer, 1295
in Cushing's disease, 1440-1441
in cutaneous infection, 502
in dehydration, 178, 178c

History (*Continued*)
in diabetes mellitus, 1473
in endocrine assessment, 1419-1421, 1420*c*
in esophageal cancer, 1256
in fracture, 1183-1184
in gastroenteritis, 1320
in gastrointestinal assessment, 1219-1221, 1220*c*
in head and neck cancer, 598
in hearing assessment, 1111-1114, 1112*c*, 1113*c*, 1114*t*
in hearing loss, 1130-1131
in heart failure, 767-768
in hematologic assessment, 882*c*, 882-885, 883-884*t*
in hepatitis, 1358-1359
in hypertension, 798
in hyperthyroidism, 1450, 1450*f*
in hypothyroidism, 1457
in hypovolemic shock, 833
in infectious disease, 446-450
in intestinal obstruction, 1303-1304
intraoperative care and, 277
intraoperative medical record review and, 279
in irritable bowel syndrome, 1290
in leukemia, 903
in lung cancer, 642-643, 643*t*
in malnutrition, 1393
in multiple sclerosis, 1003
in musculoskeletal assessment, 1143-1145, 1144*c*
in neurologic assessment, 935-936, 937*c*
in obesity, 1403-1404
in osteoarthritis, 324
in osteomalacia, 1161-1162
in osteoporosis, 1155
in pain, 41
in pelvic inflammatory disease, 1748
in peptic ulcer disease, 1272-1273
before plastic surgery, 513
in pneumonia, 660-661
in polycystic kidney disease, 1583
postoperative care and, 286, 287*t*
preoperative, 244*c*, 244-245*t*, 244-247
in pressure ulcer, 488
in prostate cancer, 1720
in psoriasis, 506
in pulmonary embolism, 679
in pyelonephritis, 1587
rehabilitation and, 97
in renal assessment, 1533-1536, 1534*c*, 1535*t*
in renal cell carcinoma, 1595
in reproductive assessment, 1647-1649, 1648*c*, 1648*t*, 1649*c*
in respiratory assessment, 556-559, 558*c*, 558*t*, 560*t*
in septic shock, 841, 841*c*
in sickle cell disease, 895
in skin problems, 466*c*, 466-467
in spinal cord injury, 993
in stroke, 1032-1033
surgical risk and, 244*t*, 246
in traumatic brain injury, 1053, 1054*c*
in tuberculosis, 669
in ulcerative colitis, 1322-1323
in urinary incontinence, 1562, 1562*c*
in uterine leiomyoma, 1695
in vision assessment, 1075-1077, 1076*c*, 1076*t*
HIT; *See* Heparin-induced thrombocytopenia
HIV; *See* Human immunodeficiency virus infection
HIV protease, 379
HIV-associated dementia complex, 373
Hives, 150, 480
HIVID; *See* Zalcitabine
HLA; *See* Human leukocyte antigen
HMG-CoA reductase inhibitors, 796, 796*t*
HNP; *See* Herniated nucleus pulposus
HNPCC; *See* Hereditary nonpolyposis colorectal cancer
Hoarseness
in laryngitis, 658
radiation therapy-related, 599
in vocal cord nodule or polyp, 595
in vocal cord paralysis, 594
Hodgkin's lymphoma, 913*t*, 913-914
Holding area nurse, 265
Hole, retinal, 1101-1102, 1102*b*
HOLEP; *See* Holmium laser enucleation of prostate
Hollywood diet, 1405
Holmium laser enucleation of prostate, 1717
Home care management
in acquired immunodeficiency syndrome, 382, 383*c*
in acute coronary syndromes, 870, 870*c*, 871*c*
in acute pancreatitis, 1376
in Alzheimer's disease, 978, 978*c*
in back pain, 988
in bone cancer, 1171
in breast cancer, 1679, 1679*c*, 1680*c*
in burn, 545-546
in cataracts, 1094, 1095*c*
in chronic and disabling diseases, 108
in chronic kidney disease, 1633-1635, 1634*c*
in chronic obstructive pulmonary disease, 634
in cirrhosis, 1355
in colorectal cancer, 1300
in Crohn's disease, 1333
in Cushing's disease, 1445
in diabetes mellitus, 1516, 1516*c*
in diverticular disease, 1336
in dysrhythmias, 758
in endometrial cancer, 1701
in esophageal cancer, 1261
in fracture, 1194
in gastric cancer, 1286
in head and neck cancer, 605, 605*c*
in hearing loss, 1135
in heart failure, 776, 776*c*
in hospice, 121, 121*c*
in hypertension, 802-803
in hypoglycemia, 1508*c*
in hypothyroidism, 1459, 1460*c*
in infectious diseases, 453
in intestinal obstruction, 1306, 1306*c*
in leukemia, 911, 911*c*
in malnutrition, 1401
in multiple sclerosis, 1006
in myasthenia gravis, 1021
in oral cancer, 1238-1239
in osteoarthritis, 335-336
in oxygen therapy, 578-579, 579*f*
of pain, 58
in pancreatic cancer, 1384
in pelvic inflammatory disease, 1752
in peptic ulcer disease, 1278, 1279*c*
in pneumonia, 665, 665*c*
postoperative, 300
in pressure ulcer, 498
in prostate cancer, 1724
in pulmonary embolism, 683
in pyelonephritis, 1589
in renal transplantation, 1633-1635, 1634*c*
in rheumatoid arthritis, 346, 346*f*
in seizures, 960*c*
in septic shock, 844, 844*c*
in spinal cord injury, 999
in spinal tumor, 1002
in stroke, 1047-1048
in transsphenoidal hypophysectomy, 1432*c*
in traumatic brain injury, 1059
in tuberculosis, 670
in ulcerative colitis, 1328
in urinary incontinence, 1569
in uterine leiomyomas, 1697-1698, 1698*c*
in valvular heart disease, 783
Home oxygen therapy, 578-579, 579*f*
in chronic obstructive pulmonary disease, 634
in idiopathic pulmonary fibrosis, 639
Homeopathic medicine, 9
Homeostasis, 170-171, 171*f*
electrolytes and, 183
endocrine system and, 1412
glucose, 1467
negative feedback mechanism and, 1414
physiologic influences on, 171-174
diffusion in, 172*f*, 172-173
filtration in, 171*f*, 171-172, 172*f*
lymph and, 174
osmosis in, 173*f*, 173-174
renal disorders and, 1581, 1582*f*
skin and, 463*t*
Homocysteine
atherosclerosis and, 795
in cardiovascular assessment, 721
metabolic syndrome and, 853
Homograft for burn wound, 539
Homonymous hemianopsia, 1035, 1035*f*
Homozygous allele, 69
Hook and loop fastener straps, 103*t*
Hookworms, 1340
Hope, dying patient and, 120
Hordeolum, 1085-1087
Hormonal therapy
for breast cancer, 1677*t*, 1678
for cancer, 431*t*, 431-432
for dysfunctional uterine bleeding, 1699
for endometrial cancer, 1701
for fibrocystic breast condition, 1661
for prostate cancer, 1723
Hormone antagonists, 431*t*, 431-432
Hormone replacement therapy
in acute adrenal insufficiency, 1436*c*
breast cancer risk and, 1665*t*
in Cushing's disease, 1445*c*
in hypopituitarism, 1427-1428
in hypothyroidism, 1458
in menopause, 1689-1690, 1690*c*
for osteoporosis prevention, 1157, 1158*c*
Hormone(s), 1412-1413, 1413*f*, 1413*t*
adrenal, 1413*t*
anterior pituitary, 1413*t*, 1415*t*
glucose homeostasis and, 1467
posterior pituitary, 1413*t*, 1415, 1415*t*
regulation of fluid balance by, 175-176, 176*f*
renal, 1531*t*, 1531-1532
risk for infection and, 441*t*
thyroid, 1413*t*, 1417, 1417*t*
Horny layer of skin, 461, 461*f*
Hospice care, 113, 121, 121*c*
in amyotrophic lateral sclerosis, 1008
in lung cancer, 650
Hospital, infection control in, 443-444
Hospital emergency preparedness, 162-164, 163*t*, 164*t*
Hospital incident command system, 162-163, 163*t*
Hospital incident commander, 162-163, 163*t*
Hospital staff
emergency preparedness roles and responsibilities, 162-164, 163*t*, 164*t*
safety in emergency care, 128-130, 129*c*
Hospital-acquired infections
after thoracic aortic aneurysm repair, 813
health and hygiene of surgical team and, 270
pneumonia in, 659, 659*t*
Hot flash, 1644
LH-RH agonist-related, 1723
in menopause, 1689
House Ear Institute, 1127*t*
HSV; *See* Herpes simplex virus
Huber needle, 219
Huber Plus noncoring needle, 221*f*
Huffing, 91
Humalog, 1485*t*
Human B-type natruretic peptides, 772
Human immunodeficiency virus infection, 363-383
brain abscess in, 1066
chronic low self-esteem in, 381-382
diarrhea in, 380-381
disturbed thought processes in, 381
drug therapy for, 375-379, 376-378*c*
etiology and genetic risk in, 363*f*, 363-366, 364*f*, 365*t*
health care resources for, 383
health teaching in, 383, 384*c*
hemodialysis-related, 1626
home care management of, 382, 383*c*
impaired gas exchange in, 379
impaired skin integrity in, 381
incidence and prevalence of, 366*f*, 366-367, 367*f*
laboratory assessment in, 373-374
leukoplakia and, 1234
lung abscess in, 672
nursing diagnoses in, 374-375
nutritional status and, 380
pain in, 379-380
parenteral transmission of, 367-368
patient history and, 370
perinatal transmission of, 368
physical assessment in, 370-373, 371*c*, 372*t*
psychosocial assessment in, 373
risk for infection in, 375, 375*c*, 376*c*
sexual transmission of, 367, 368*c*
social isolation in, 382
testing for, 369-370, 370*c*
transmission and health care workers and, 368-369, 369*c*
Human leukocyte antigen, 307, 307*f*
in diabetes mellitus, 1471
renal transplantation and, 1631
in rheumatoid arthritis, 337, 339*c*
in Sjögren's syndrome, 396
Human lice, 504
Human lymphotropic virus, 408*t*
Human papillomavirus
cancers associated with, 408*t*
in cervical cancer, 1703
in genital warts, 1743-1743-1744, 1744*f*
Human papillomavirus test, 1652
Human papillomavirus vaccine, 1703, 1744
Human plasma for hypovolemic shock, 837
Human transplantation antigens, 307
Humeral shaft fracture, 1195
Humidification
during oxygen therapy, 573*f*, 573-574
in tracheostomy, 583
Humira; *See* Adalimumab
Humoral immunity, 309, 313-317, 314*f*, 315*f*
Humulin, 1485*t*
Huntington disease, 73, 75, 979-980
Hurricane Katrina, 160, 160*f*
Hyalgan; *See* Hyaluronate
Hyaluronate, 326-327
Hyaluronidase, 237
Hycamtin; *See* Topetecan
Hycort; *See* Hydrocortisone
Hydralazine, 348
Hydration
in chronic obstructive pulmonary disease, 632
in glucose-6-phosphate dehydrogenase deficiency, 898-899
in hyperparathyroidism, 1462
postoperative assessment of, 290
in sickle cell disease, 897
skin problems and, 467
Hydrea; *See* Hydroxyurea
Hydrocele, 731*f*, 1730-1731

Hydrocephalus
after brain tumor surgery, 1064
after stroke, 1044
after traumatic brain injury, 1052
in brain tumor, 1060
in meningitis, 963
Hydrochlorothiazide
for hypercalciuria, 1574
to reduce preload in heart failure, 772
Hydrocodone, 46
abuse of, 90t
equianalgesic dose of, 47t
Hydrocodone-acetaminophen, 46
Hydrocodone-ibuprofen, 46
Hydrocolloid dressing, 494-495t, 822
Hydrocortisone
for adrenal insufficiency, 1438, 1439c
for anaphylaxis, 393c
for septic shock, 843t
HydroDIURIL; *See* Hydrochlorothiazide
Hydrogel dressing, 494-495t
Hydrogen ions
overproduction of, 205-206
pH and, 199
Hydrogenation, 1403
Hydromorphone, 47
abuse of, 90t, 90-91, 91c
for burn pain, 536
for cholecystitis, 1369
epidural, 52
equianalgesic dose of, 47t
for pain in acquired immunodeficiency syndrome, 380
for postoperative pain, 297, 297c
preoperative, 261
for sickle cell disease pain, 896
Hydronephrosis, 1571, 1585f, 1585-1586
in benign prostatic hypertrophy, 1713
spinal cord injury-related, 998
Hydrophilic dressing, 493
Hydrophilic lotion, 480
Hydrophobic dressing, 493
Hydrops diet, 1128
Hydrostatic pressure, 171f, 171-172, 709
Hydrotherapy, 539
Hydrothorax, central venous catheter insertion-related, 231t
Hydroureter, 1570, 1585f, 1585-1586, 1713
Hydroxychloroquine, 396
for rheumatoid arthritis, 341c, 343
for systemic lupus erythematosus, 350
17-Hydroxycorticosteroids
in adrenal insufficiency, 1438
in Cushing's disease, 1442
Hydroxyurea, 422t
for polycythemia vera, 901
for sickle cell disease, 897
Hydroxyzine
for postoperative pain, 299
preoperative, 261
Hylan GF 20, 326-327
Hymenolepis nana, 1340
Hyoid bone, 553f, 554f
Hyoscyamine, 1558c
Hyperactive reflexes, 941, 941f
Hyperacusis, 1114
Hyperacute rejection, 319, 1633t
Hyperaldosteronism, 1445-1446
Hyperbaric oxygen therapy
for osteomyelitis, 1166
for pressure ulcer, 495
Hypercalcemia, 193-194, 194t
calcium supplementation-related, 1159
in cancer, 436
cardiovascular assessment and, 721-722
in chronic kidney disease, 1619
in hyperparathyroidism, 1461
in urolithiasis, 1571t
Hypercalciuria, 1574
Hypercapnia
central chemoreceptors and, 708
in hypokalemia, 189
Hypercarbia, 572
in acute respiratory failure, 686
in airway obstruction, 593
in chronic obstructive pulmonary disease, 626
oxygen-induced hypoventilation and, 573
in upper airway obstruction, 596
Hypercellularity in polycythemia vera, 901
Hypercortisolism, 1439-1445
acute adrenal insufficiency in, 1444
community-based care in, 1445, 1445c
excess fluid volume in, 1442-1443
history in, 1440-1441
imaging studies in, 1442
laboratory assessment in, 1441-1442
pathophysiology of, 1439-1440, 1440f, 1440t
physical assessment in, 1441, 1441c
psychosocial assessment in, 1441
risk for infection in, 1444
risk for injury in, 1443-1444
secondary hypertension in, 798
Hyperemia
in infection, 839
inflammation and, 312
Hyperesthesia in spinal cord injury, 993
Hyperextension injury of spinal cord, 990-991, 991f
Hyperflexion injury of spinal cord, 990, 991f
Hyperglycemia
after Whipple procedure, 1384
diabetes mellitus and, 1466, 1466t, 1475-1477
neuropathies and, 1470, 1470t
type 2, 1472
in hyperthyroidism, 1449
hypoglycemia *versus,* 1507t
insulin absence and, 1467
overproduction of growth hormone and, 1428
sulfonylurea-induced, 1483t
Hyperglycemic-hyperosmolar state
after pancreas transplantation, 1499
in diabetes mellitus, 1512c, 1512-1514, 1513f
diabetic ketoacidosis *versus,* 1510t
Hyperinsulinemia, 1495
Hyperkalemia, 190t, 190-191, 191c
in acute adrenal insufficiency, 1436c
in adrenal insufficiency, 1438
after pancreas transplantation, 1499-1500
burn-related, 524
in chronic kidney disease, 1610
in crush syndrome, 1182
in diabetes mellitus, 1467
enteral nutrition therapy and, 1400
in hypovolemic shock, 831
in polycythemia vera, 901
preoperative assessment of, 249
transfusion-related, 919
Hyperkinetic pulse, 716-717
Hyperleptinemia, 1402
Hyperlipidemia
atherosclerosis and, 794
in chronic kidney disease, 1611
diabetes mellitus and, 1466, 1468-1469
Hypermagnesemia, 196-197
Hypermenorrhea, 1695
Hypermetabolism, burn-related, 525
Hypermetropia, 1073, 1073f, 1102
Hypernatremia, 186t, 186-187, 1445, 1533
Hyperopia, 1073, 1073f, 1102
Hyperosmotic fluids, 174
Hyperoxaluria, 1571t, 1574
Hyperparathyroidism, 1461f, 1461t, 1461-1463, 1462c
Paget's disease of bone and, 1163
Hyperphosphatemia, 195
in chronic glomerulonephritis, 1592
in chronic kidney disease, 1610, 1610f
Hyperpigmentation, 1421-1422
in adrenal insufficiency, 1427f, 1427-1428
Hyperpituitarism, 1428f, 1428-1432, 1429f, 1430c, 1431f
Hyperplasia, 399, 400f
benign prostatic, 1646, 1712-1718
community-based care in, 1718
concept map for, 1716
drug therapy for, 1714-1715
laboratory assessment in, 1714
nursing diagnoses in, 1714
pathophysiology of, 1712-1713, 1713f
physical assessment in, 1713-1714, 1714c
surgical management of, 1715-1718, 1717f, 1718c
hyperparathyroidism and, 1454
Hyperplastic intestinal polyp, 1309
Hyperpnea
in acute respiratory distress syndrome, 687
in chronic kidney disease, 1613
Hyperresonance, 562t
Hyperresponsive airway in asthma, 610
Hypersensitivity, 387-398, 388t
autoimmunity and, 395-397, 396t
Goodpasture's syndrome in, 397
Sjögren's syndrome in, 396-397
suppressor T-cell and, 317
type I: rapid, 387-394
allergic rhinitis in, 388f, 388-391, 389f, 390c
anaphylaxis in, 391t, 391-394, 392c, 392f, 393c
latex allergy in, 394
type II: cytotoxic reactions, 394, 394f
type III: immune complex reactions, 394-395, 395f
type IV: delayed, 395
type V: stimulatory reactions, 395
Hypersensitivity vasculitis, 355
Hypertension, 796-804
in acute renal failure, 1603
after coronary artery bypass graft, 868
atherosclerosis and, 794
in black widow spider bite, 148
cardiovascular assessment and, 716
in chronic kidney disease, 1610-1611, 1618
concept map for, 800
coronary artery disease and, 852
diabetes mellitus and, 1468, 1472
in diabetic nephropathy, 1471
diagnostic tests for, 799
drug therapy for, 801t, 801-802
in Guillain-Barré syndrome, 1014
health teaching in, 803-804
heart failure and, 767
heath care resources for, 804
history in, 798
home care management in, 802-803
hypertensive crisis and, 802, 803c
ineffective therapeutic regimen management in, 802, 803c
lifestyle modifications in, 800-801
in nephrosclerosis, 1593
in nephrotic syndrome, 1593
nursing diagnoses in, 799
pathophysiology of, 796-798, 796-798t
peripheral arterial disease and, 807
in pheochromocytoma, 1446
physical assessment in, 798-799, 799f
in polycystic kidney disease, 1584-1585, 1585c
psychosocial assessment in, 799
in renovascular disease, 1593-1594
in scorpion sting, 149
in thyroid storm, 1455
vision changes in, 1075
Hypertensive crisis, 802, 803c
Hyperthermia
in infectious disease, 450, 451-452, 452c, 452t
malignant, 273, 275c
Hyperthyroidism, 1448-1455
drug therapy for, 1452-1454, 1453c
history in, 1450, 1450f
laboratory assessment in, 1451, 1451c
nursing diagnoses in, 1452
pathophysiology of, 1448-1450, 1449c
physical assessment in, 1450f, 1450-1451, 1451t
psychosocial assessment in, 1451
surgical management of, 1454-1455, 1455c
Hypertonia after stroke, 1034
Hypertonic fluids, 174
Hypertonic intravenous solutions, 214
Hypertonic saline
for hyponatremia, 186
for syndrome of inappropriate antidiuretic hormone secretion, 1435
Hypertriglyceridemia, 795
Hypertrophic cardiomyopathy, 787-790, 788t, 789f, 790c
Hypertrophic ungual labium, 1174t
Hypertrophy, 399, 400f
benign prostatic, 1646, 1712-1718
community-based care in, 1718
concept map for, 1716
drug therapy for, 1714-1715
laboratory assessment in, 1714
nursing diagnoses in, 1714
pathophysiology of, 1712-1713, 1713f
physical assessment in, 1713-1714, 1714c
prostate cancer and, 1720
surgical management of, 1715-1718, 1717f, 1718c
Hyperuricemia, 1571t
in gout, 353
Paget's disease of bone and, 1163
Hyperventilation
during electroencephalography, 947
in pulmonary embolism, 679
in respiratory regulation of acid-base balance, 203, 203f
in traumatic brain injury, 1056
Hypervolemia, 185
Hyphema, 1103
Hypnoanesthesia, 272t
Hypnosis
advantages and disadvantages of, 272t
for pain management, 57
Hypnotics
for general anesthesia, 272, 274t
preoperative, 261
Hypoactive reflexes, 941, 941f
Hypoalbuminemia, 1281
Hypocalcemia, 191-193, 192t, 193f
after parathyroidectomy, 1463
cardiovascular assessment and, 721
in chronic kidney disease, 1610, 1610f
in hyperparathyroidism, 1463
hypomagnesemia and, 196
plasmapheresis-related, 1014c
in thyroidectomy, 1454
Hypocapnia, 155
Hypodermoclysis, 237
Hypoesthesia, 993
Hypogammaglobulinemia, 385
Hypogastric artery, 804f
Hypoglossal nerve, 935t
Hypoglycemia
in adrenal gland hypofunction, 1436, 1436c
after Whipple procedure, 1384
in diabetes mellitus, 1506-1509, 1507t, 1508c
myocardial infarction and, 859
sulfonylurea-induced, 1483t
Hypogonadism, 1422
Hypokalemia, 187t, 187-189, 189c
after pancreas transplantation, 1499-1500
burn-related, 524
in diabetes mellitus, 1467

Hypokalemia *(Continued)*
in diabetic ketoacidosis, 1511
diuretic-induced, 772-773, 801
in hyperaldosteronism, 1445
plasmapheresis-related, 1014*c*
preoperative assessment of, 249
Hypokinetic pulse, 716
Hypomagnesemia, 196, 196*t*
cardiovascular assessment and, 722
in hyperparathyroidism, 1463
Hyponatremia, 185*t*, 185-186
burn-related, 524
in chronic kidney disease, 1609
enteral nutrition therapy and, 1400
in syndrome of inappropriate antidiuretic hormone secretion, 1435
Hypo-osmotic fluids, 174
Hypoparathyroidism, 1463
Hypoperfusion in diabetes mellitus, 1467
Hypophonia, 966*c*
Hypophosphatemia, 194-195, 195*c*, 195*t*
in chronic kidney disease, 1619
in hyperparathyroidism, 1461
in osteomalacia, 1162
Hypophysectomy, 58*f*, 1431*f*, 1431-1432, 1432*c*, 1443
Hypophysis, 930
Hypopigmentation, 1421-1422
Hypopituitarism, 1426-1428, 1427*c*
Hypoplasia, 902
Hypoproteinemia, 1392
Hyporeflexia, 188
Hypotension
after coronary artery bypass graft, 868
after esophageal surgery, 1260
in anaphylaxis, 392
in bee sting, 150
bromocriptine-related, 1431
dehydration and, 178
in heat stroke, 142
in hyperkalemia, 190
in hypermagnesemia, 196
in hypernatremia, 186
hyponatremia and, 185
in hypothermia, 153
in malignant hyperthermia, 273
in pit viper envenomation, 144
in pulmonary embolism, 679
in sepsis, 839
in septic shock, 843*t*
in spinal cord injury, 994
total hip arthroplasty and, 330*c*
in toxic shock syndrome, 1691, 1692*c*
in trauma patient, 136
in traumatic brain injury, 1054
Hypothalamic-hypophysial portal system, 1414
Hypothalamic-pituitary-thyroid gland axis feedback mechanism, 1417
Hypothalamus, 930, 931*f*, 1413*f*, 1414-1415, 1415*f*, 1415*t*
hormones of, 1413*t*
negative feedback mechanism and, 1414, 1414*f*
Hypothermia, 152-154
after coronary artery bypass graft, 868
after stroke, 1044
in drowning, 156
postoperative, 288, 299
in spinal cord injury, 994
in syndrome of inappropriate antidiuretic hormone secretion, 1435
trauma patient and, 138
Hypothyroidism, 1455-1460
decreased cardiac output in, 1458
decreased general metabolism *versus*, 1419*c*
disturbed thought processes in, 1458
history in, 1457
home care management in, 1459, 1460*c*
ineffective breathing pattern in, 1458
Hypothyroidism *(Continued)*
laboratory assessment in, 1457
myxedema coma and, 1459, 1459*c*
nursing diagnoses in, 1457-1458
pathophysiology of, 1455-1456, 1456*c*, 1456*f*
thyroiditis and, 1460
Hypotonia, 1034
Hypotonic fluids, 174
Hypotonic infusion, 187
Hypotonic intravenous solutions, 214
Hypoventilation
in combined ventilatory and oxygenation failure, 685
general anesthesia and, 275
intraoperative, 282
oxygen-induced, 573
in respiratory regulation of acid-base balance, 203, 203*f*
Hypovolemia
in acute pancreatitis, 1373
after abdominal aortic aneurysm resection, 812
in crush syndrome, 1182
in diabetes mellitus, 1467
in gastrointestinal bleeding, 1275-1276, 1276*c*
hyponatremia and, 185
isotonic dehydration and, 177
plasmapheresis-related, 1014*c*
thermal airway burn and, 530
Hypovolemic shock, 828, 828*t*, 830-838
in burn, 530, 534
causes of, 830*c*
community-based care in, 838
concept map for, 834
drug therapy for, 837*c*, 837-838
etiology of, 832
in fracture, 1182
history in, 833
incidence and prevalence of, 832
laboratory assessment in, 835, 836*c*
nursing diagnoses in, 835
oxygenation and tissue perfusion and, 826-827, 827*f*, 829*f*
pathophysiology of, 830-831, 831*t*
patient safety and, 836*c*
in peritonitis, 1317
physical assessment in, 833-835
in pit viper envenomation, 144
prevention of, 832-833, 833*c*
psychosocial assessment in, 835
risk factors in older adult, 841*c*
stages of, 831-832
surgical management of, 838
in traumatic brain injury, 1054
Hypoxemia
in asthma, 612
in chronic obstructive pulmonary disease, 623, 626
in high altitude pulmonary edema, 155
mechanical ventilation for, 689
oxygen therapy for, 571
in pneumonia, 663, 663*t*
postoperative, 287, 299, 300*c*
in pulmonary embolism, 678, 680-682, 680-682*c*
in sickle cell disease, 894
Hypoxia
dehydration and, 179
in diabetes mellitus, 1467
in drowning, 156
erythropoiesis and, 878
in high altitude-related illnesses, 154, 155
in hypokalemia, 189
in hypovolemic shock, 831, 835
in myocardial infarction, 849
oxygen therapy for, 571
in severe acute respiratory syndrome, 666
in severe sepsis, 840
in sickle cell disease, 894
tracheostomy patient and, 584
Hypoxia *(Continued)*
in traumatic brain injury, 1054
in upper airway obstruction, 596
Hypoxic ventilatory response, 155
Hysterectomy
in cervical cancer, 1704
in endometrial cancer, 1702
in ovarian cancer, 1706
in uterine leiomyomas, 1696-1697, 1697*c*, 1697*t*
in uterine prolapse, 1694
Hysterosalpingography, 1654-1655
Hysteroscopy, 1656-1657, 1688
Hytrin; *See* Terazosin

I

Iatrogenic hypoparathyroidism, 1463
Ibandronate, 1159*c*, 1160
IBS; *See* Irritable bowel syndrome
Ibuprofen, 46
after total hip arthroplasty, 331
for dysmenorrhea, 1685
for gout, 354
heart failure and, 767
for migraine headache, 952, 953*t*
nephrotoxicity of, 1506
for osteoarthritis, 326
for postoperative pain, 297-299, 298*c*
Ibutilde, 743*c*
ICD; *See* Implantable cardioverter-defibrillator
Ice application
in bee sting, 150
in black widow spider bite, 148
in brown recluse spider bite, 147
in scorpion sting, 149
Ice immersion in heat stroke, 142
ICF; *See* Intracellular fluid
ICG; *See* Impedance cardiography
Idamycin; *See* Idarubicin
Idarubicin, 421*t*
Idiopathic epilepsy, 956
Idiopathic hypoparathyroidism, 1463
Idiopathic osteoarthritis, 323
Idiopathic pulmonary fibrosis, 639
Idiopathic scoliosis, 1174
Idiopathic seizure, 956
Idiopathic thrombocytopenic purpura, 916
Idioventricular rhythm, 747
I/E ratio; *See* Inverse inspiration-expiration ratio
Ifex; *See* Ifosfamide
Ifosfamide, 422*t*
for testicular cancer, 1730
Ileal conduit, 1577*f*
Ileal reservoir, 1577*f*
Ileoanal anastomosis, 1326, 1327*f*
Ileoanal reservoir, 1327, 1327*f*
Ileostomy, 1325-1327, 1326*f*, 1327*f*, 1329*c*
Ileum, 1217*f*, 1219
Ilizarov technique, 1191-1192
Illness
cultural aspects of, 27-34
culture and cultural competence and, 27-38, 28*f*, 28*t*
health care disparities and, 28
Purnell's domains of culture and, 29*c*, 29*t*, 29-33, 30*c*, 31*t*, 32*f*, 33*f*
rehabilitation and, 94-110
constipation and, 106-107, 107*t*
coping issues in, 107-108
functional assessment and, 98-99
health care resources for, 109
health teaching and, 108-109
home care management and, 108
impaired physical mobility and, 99-101, 100*c*, 101*c*, 101*f*, 102*t*
impaired skin integrity and, 103-105, 104*c*
nursing diagnoses and, 99
patient history and, 97
Illness *(Continued)*
physical assessment and, 97*t*, 97-98
psychosocial assessment and, 99
rehabilitation team and, 95*f*, 95-97, 96*f*, 96*t*
self-care deficit and, 101-103, 103*t*
urinary elimination impairment and, 105*t*, 105-106
vocational assessment and, 99
terminal, 111-123
dyspnea management in, 117-118
euthanasia and, 121-122, 122*t*
hospice and palliative care in, 113
incidence of death and, 113
nausea and vomiting management in, 118
pain management in, 116-117
pathophysiology of dying and, 112
patient and family education in, 115*c*
perception of death and, 111-112, 112*t*
physical assessment and, 115*c*, 115-116
planning for death and, 113, 114*f*
postmortem care and, 121, 121*c*, 122*c*
psychosocial assessment and, 116, 116*c*
psychosocial management in, 119*t*, 119-121, 120*c*, 121*c*
refractory symptoms of distress and, 118
restlessness and agitation management in, 118
seizure management in, 118
weakness management in, 116
Ilotycin; *See* Erythromycin
Imagery, 9-10, 56
Imaging studies
in abdominal aortic aneurysm, 811-812
in acute coronary syndromes, 855
in acute pancreatitis, 1375
in acute renal failure, 1604
in adrenal insufficiency, 1438
in Alzheimer's disease, 973
in benign prostatic hypertrophy, 1714
in breast cancer, 1670-1671
in chronic kidney disease, 1614
in chronic obstructive pulmonary disease, 627
in cirrhosis, 1350
in colorectal cancer, 1296
in Cushing's disease, 1442
in endocrine problems, 1424
in fracture, 1185
in gastrointestinal problems, 1226
in head and neck cancer, 598
in hearing loss, 1116, 1131
in heart failure, 770
in hematologic assessment, 889
in infectious disease, 451
in intestinal obstruction, 1304
in leukemia, 904
in low back pain, 985
in meningitis, 963
in migraine headache, 951-952
in musculoskeletal disorders, 1148-1149, 1149*c*
in neurologic disorders, 943-946
cerebral angiography in, 943, 943*c*
computed tomography in, 943-945
magnetic resonance imaging in, 945-946
magnetoencephalography in, 946
patient preparation for, 944-945*t*
plain x-rays in, 943
positron emission tomography in, 946
single photon emission computed tomography in, 946
in osteoarthritis, 325
in osteoporosis, 1156-1157
in peptic ulcer disease, 1273-1274

Imaging studies *(Continued)*
in peripheral arterial disease, 805
in pneumonia, 663
preoperative, 249
in pulmonary embolism, 679
in pyelonephritis, 1588
in renal problems, 1543-1547
computed tomography in, 1545-1546
cystography and cystourethrography in, 1546
cystoscopy and cystourethroscopy in, 1546-1547
intravenous urography in, 1543-1545, 1545*c*
kidney, ureter, and bladder x-ray in, 1543
renal arteriography in, 1546
renography in, 1546
retrograde procedures in, 1547
ultrasonography in, 1546
in reproductive assessment, 1654-1655
in respiratory assessment, 564-566
in sickle cell disease, 896
in spinal cord injury, 994-995
in stroke, 1036
in traumatic brain injury, 1055
in urinary incontinence, 1563
in uterine leiomyoma, 1695
in vision assessment, 1079
Imatinib mesylate, 434, 435*t*, 905-906
Imbalanced nutrition: less than body requirements
in acquired immunodeficiency syndrome, 380
in acute pancreatitis, 1376
in burn injury, 543
in chronic kidney disease, 1615-1618, 1617*c*, 1617*t*
in chronic obstructive pulmonary disease, 632-633
in esophageal cancer, 1257
in fracture, 1194
in malnutrition, 1392-1402
community-based care in, 1401-1402
drug therapy for, 1395-1396
history in, 1393
intervention activities for, 1395*c*
laboratory assessment in, 1393-1394
nursing diagnoses in, 1394
nutrition management in, 1395
older adult and, 16, 1393*c*, 1395, 1396*c*
parenteral nutrition in, 1400-1401, 1401*c*
pathophysiology of, 1392
physical assessment in, 1393, 1394*t*
psychosocial assessment in, 1393
total enteral nutrition in, 1396-1400, 1397*f*, 1398*c*
Imdur; *See* Isosorbide
Imipramine
for pain, 54, 54*t*
for urinary incontinence, 1565*c*, 1567
Immediate memory, 938
Immobility
Guillain-Barré syndrome and, 1014-1015
pressure ulcer prevention and, 486
rehabilitation and, 99-101, 100*c*, 101*c*, 101*f*, 102*t*
Immobilization
for cast application in fracture, 1187*f*, 1187-1189, 1188*t*
in cervical spine injury, 995-996
in peripheral nerve trauma, 1023
in pit viper envenomation, 144
in thoracic and lumbosacral injuries, 996
Immune chromatography in gastritis, 1267
Immune complex reaction, 394-395, 395*f*
glomerulonephritis and, 1590, 1590*f*
Immune deficiencies, 362-386
Bruton's agammaglobulinemia in, 385
common variable immune deficiency in, 385
congenital, 385
human immunodeficiency virus infection in, 363-383
brain abscess in, 1066
chronic low self-esteem in, 381-382
diarrhea in, 380-381
disturbed thought processes in, 381
drug therapy for, 375-379, 376-378*c*
etiology and genetic risk in, 363*f*, 363-366, 364*f*, 365*t*
health care resources for, 383
health teaching in, 383, 384*c*
hemodialysis-related, 1626
home care management of, 382, 383*c*
impaired gas exchange in, 379
impaired skin integrity in, 381
incidence and prevalence of, 366*f*, 366-367, 367*f*
laboratory assessment in, 373-374
leukoplakia and, 1234
lung abscess in, 672
nursing diagnoses in, 374-375
nutritional status and, 380
pain in, 379-380
parenteral transmission of, 367-368
patient history and, 370
perinatal transmission of, 368
physical assessment in, 370-373, 371*c*, 372*t*
psychosocial assessment in, 373
risk for infection in, 375, 375*c*, 376*c*
sexual transmission of, 367, 368*c*
social isolation in, 382
testing for, 369-370, 370*c*
transmission and health care workers and, 368-369, 369*c*
leukemia and, 902
selective immunoglobulin A deficiency in, 385
therapy-induced, 384-385
Immune response, 306-321
antibody-mediated immunity and, 313-317, 314*f*, 315*f*
assessment in burn, 537, 538*t*
cell types involved in, 310*f*, 310-312, 311*t*, 312*f*
cell-mediated immunity and, 317-320, 318*f*, 318*t*
in heart failure, 767
immune system organization and, 308-309, 309*f*, 309*t*, 310*f*
infection and, 309-310
purpose of, 307, 309
self *versus* non-self and, 307*f*, 307-308, 308*c*, 308*f*
sequence of, 312-313
Immune serum globulin
for Bruton's agammaglobulinemia, 385
for Guillain-Barré syndrome, 1014
Immune system
autoimmunity and, 395-396, 396*t*
burn-related changes in, 525
cancer development and, 408-411, 409*c*, 409*t*, 410*t*
cirrhosis and, 1348*f*
Crohn's disease and, 1330
Cushing's disease and, 1441, 1441*c*
Guillain-Barré syndrome and, 1012
immunohemolytic anemia and, 899
organization of, 308-309, 309*f*, 309*t*, 310*f*
risk for infection and, 441
Immunity, 306
antibody-mediated, 313-317, 314*f*, 315*f*
host defense against infection and, 443
immune function changes related to aging and, 308*c*
Immunity *(Continued)*
macrophages and, 311
white blood cell and, 309*t*, 878, 878*t*
cancer and, 415
cell-mediated, 317-320, 318*f*, 318*t*
host defense against infection and, 443
immune function changes related to aging and, 308*c*
macrophages and, 311
tuberculosis and, 668
white blood cell and, 309*t*, 878, 878*t*
purpose of, 307
risk for infection and, 441
self *versus* non-self and, 307*f*, 307-308, 308*c*, 308*f*
Immunocompetent person, 306
Immunoglobulin A deficiency, 385
Immunoglobulin E
in allergic asthma, 612
rapid hypersensitivity reactions and, 387-388
Immunoglobulin G, 316
in cerebrospinal fluid, 948*t*
desensitization therapy and, 391
gastritis and, 1267
Immunoglobulin M, 316
gastritis and, 1267
Immunoglobulin(s), 316
Immunohemolytic anemia, 899
Immunologic interstitial and tubulointerstitial disorders, 1593
Immunologic renal disorders, 1589*t*, 1589-1593, 1590*f*
acute glomerulonephritis in, 1590*t*, 1590-1591
chronic glomerulonephritis in, 1592
nephrotic syndrome in, 1592-1593, 1593*c*
rapidly progressive glomerulonephritis in, 1591-1592
Immunometric assay, 1423
Immunomodulators
for asthma, 620-621
for ulcerative colitis, 1324
Immunosuppressed patient
lung abscess in, 672
methicillin-resistant *Staphylococcus aureus* and, 448
Immunosuppressive agents, 319-320
after transplantation
heart, 790
lung, 637
renal, 1633, 1634
for aplastic anemia, 900
for idiopathic pulmonary fibrosis, 639
for immunohemolytic anemia, 899
for multiple sclerosis, 1006
for myasthenia gravis, 1018-1019
for rheumatoid arthritis, 341*c*, 344
for scleroderma, 352
for Sjögren's syndrome, 396
Immunotherapy, 433*t*, 433-434
Imodium; *See* Loperamide
Impacted fracture, 1179*f*
Impaction of cerumen, 1122*f*, 1122-1123, 1123*c*
Impaired exchange impairment
in acquired immunodeficiency syndrome, 379
in burn, 535
in chronic obstructive pulmonary disease, 622, 628-630, 629*c*
in heart failure, 770, 771*c*
in pneumonia, 664, 664*c*
postoperative, 294, 295*c*
in spinal cord injury, 997
Impaired gas exchange
in acquired immunodeficiency syndrome, 379
in chronic obstructive pulmonary disease, 628-630, 629*c*
in heart failure, 770, 771*c*
Impaired gas exchange *(Continued)*
in pneumonia, 664, 664*c*
postoperative, 294, 295*c*
in spinal cord injury, 997
Impaired physical mobility, 99-101, 100*c*, 101*c*, 101*f*, 102*t*
in burn, 543-544, 544*c*, 544*f*
in fracture, 1193*f*, 1193-1194
in osteoarthritis, 335, 336*c*
in spinal cord injury, 997
in stroke, 1046
Impaired skin integrity
in acquired immunodeficiency syndrome, 381
in burn, 538-540, 539*t*
in chronic illness and disability, 103-105, 104*c*
postoperative, 294-296, 295*c*, 295*f*
in pressure ulcer, 491-496, 493*c*, 493-495*t*, 496*f*
Impaired urinary elimination
in chronic and disabling diseases, 105*t*, 105-106
in prostate cancer, 1721
in spinal cord injury, 997-998, 998*c*
Impaired verbal communication
in hearing loss, 1135, 1135*c*
in stroke, 1046, 1046*t*
Impairment, term, 95
Impedance, 708
Impedance cardiography, 728
Impedance plethysmography, 818
Impermeable membrane, 172-173
Implant
breast, 1662, 1675
cardiac, 758
cochlear, 1132
in high-dose rate implant radiation, 419, 420*c*
penile, 1726
Implantable cardioverter-defibrillator, 758
ejection fraction and, 765
health teaching in, 759, 761*c*
Implanted port, 218-219, 219*f*
Impotence; *See* Erectile dysfunction
Imuran; *See* Azathioprine
Incentive spirometry
in pneumonia, 664
preoperative patient education in, 255, 258*f*
Incision
in coronary artery bypass graft, 866
focused assessment after discharge from postanesthesia care unit and, 289*c*
splinting of, 257*c*
in total hip arthroplasty, 329
in tracheostomy, 580, 580*f*
Incision and drainage
in anorectal abscess, 1337
in Bartholin cyst, 1699
Incisional hernia, 1291-1293, 1292*f*
Incisional injury, 1183
Incomplete fracture, 1179
Incomplete spinal cord injury, 990
Incontinence, 1559-1570
after open radical prostatectomy, 1722
in Alzheimer's disease, 975
approaching death and, 115*c*
etiology of, 1561
functional, 1568-1569
health care resources for, 1569-1570
health teaching in, 1569, 1570*c*
history of, 1562, 1562*c*
home care management in, 1569
hospitalized older adult and, 23
imaging studies in, 1563
incidence and prevalence of, 1562
laboratory assessment in, 1563
nursing diagnoses in, 1563
older adult and, 1561, 1562*c*
physical assessment in, 1562-1563
pressure ulcer prevention and, 486
psychosocial preparation in, 1569

Incontinence (Continued)
reflex, 1568
in spinal tumor, 1001
stress, 1564c, 1564-1566, 1565c, 1565f, 1566t
in stroke, 1047
total or mixed, 1569
types of, 1560-1561t
urge, 1567-1568, 1568c
Increased intracranial pressure
in brain tumor, 1060, 1064
in encephalitis, 964
in meningitis, 962
in stroke, 1037c, 1037-1043
in traumatic brain injury, 1051, 1055-1057
Incretin agents, 1489
Incretin hormones
glucose homeostasis and, 1467
type 2 diabetes mellitus and, 1490
Incus, 1110, 1110f, 1111f
Independent living skills assessment before rehabilitation, 98-99
Independent nursing functions, 4
Inderal; *See* Propranolol
Indinavir, 377c, 379
Indirect contact transmission of infection, 442
Indirect Coombs' test, 886, 887c
Indirect inguinal hernia, 1291-1293, 1292f
Indirect traumatic brain injury, 1049
Indocin; *See* Indomethacin
Indocyanine green dye in burn assessment, 531
Indolent lymphoma, 914
Indomethacin, 354
Induction therapy in acute leukemia, 905
Induration in deep vein thrombosis, 817
Indwelling urinary catheter
for functional urinary incontinence, 1569
home care of, 1725c
postoperative monitoring of, 290
in spinal cord injury, 1000
in transurethral resection of prostate, 1715
urinary tract infection and, 1554
Ineffective airway clearance
in chronic obstructive pulmonary disease, 631-632, 632f, 633t
in pneumonia, 664
in spinal cord injury, 997
Ineffective breathing pattern
in burn injury, 535
in chronic obstructive pulmonary disease, 630-631, 631c
in hypothyroidism, 1458
in spinal cord injury, 997
Ineffective coping
in breast cancer, 1671-1672
in chronic and disabling diseases, 107-108
in coronary artery disease, 860-861, 861c
in osteoarthritis, 326
in spinal cord injury, 998
Ineffective therapeutic regimen management in hypertension, 802, 803c
Ineffective tissue perfusion
in acute coronary syndromes, 858-860, 859t
in burn, 533c, 533t, 533-535, 534f
in diabetes mellitus, 1506
in dysrhythmias, 750-751, 751c
in spinal cord injury, 995c, 995-997, 996f
in stroke, 1036-1037
Infarction
cerebral
in lightning strike, 151
in stroke, 1030
myocardial, 848-850, 849f
angina *versus*, 854c
Infarction (Continued)
chest pain in, 713t
in coronary artery disease, 847
in diabetes mellitus, 1468
emergency care in, 856-858, 857-858c
family history of, 936
heart failure and, 767
home care management after, 870, 870c, 871c
postmyocardial infarction heart failure and, 862, 862t
serum markers of myocardial damage in, 719-721
ventricular fibrillation and, 7u49
splenic, 784
Infection, 440-457
acute compartment syndrome-related, 1181
in acute sialadenitis, 1239-1240
of arteriovenous access, 1623, 1625t
bioterrorism and emerging infections and, 453-455, 454t, 455t
in brain abscess, 1065-1066
in burn patient, 538t, 540-543, 542-543c
catheter-related, 442
blood sampling and, 225
central venous catheter and, 234t
in epidural analgesia, 52
during chemotherapy, 425, 427c
in Cushing's disease patient, 1444
cutaneous, 499-503, 500c
anthrax in, 503-504
bacterial, 499, 501f
fungal, 501
pediculosis in, 504
prevention of, 501-502, 502c
scabies in, 504
viral, 499-501, 501f
in cystic fibrosis patient, 636
in cystitis, 1533, 1551-1559
community-based care in, 1558-1559
drug therapy for, 1555-1558, 1556-1558c
laboratory assessment in, 1554-1555
nursing diagnoses in, 1555
nutrition therapy for, 1558
pathophysiology of, 1551-1553, 1552t, 1553c
physical assessment in, 1553-1554, 1555c
prevention of, 1553, 1554c
of ear
in external otitis, 1121c, 1121f, 1121-1122
in furuncle, 1122
in labyrinthitis, 1127
in mastoiditis, 1125-1126
in otitis media, 1123-1125, 1124f, 1125c, 1125f
in perichondritis, 1122
prevention of, 1134c
in encephalitis, 963-965, 964c
of fracture, 1183, 1192-1193
fracture cast-related, 1189
in gastroenteritis, 1319t, 1319-1321, 1321c
Guillain-Barré syndrome and, 1012
health care resources for, 453
health promotion and maintenance and, 443c, 443-446, 444c, 445f
health teaching in, 453
helminthic, 1339-1340
hemodialysis-related, 1626
in hepatitis, 1356-1360, 1357t, 1358c, 1361c
history in, 446-450
home care management of, 453
human immunodeficiency virus, 363-383
brain abscess in, 1066
Infection (Continued)
chronic low self-esteem in, 381-382
diarrhea in, 380-381
disturbed thought processes in, 381
drug therapy for, 375-379, 376-378c
etiology and genetic risk in, 363f, 363-366, 364f, 365t
health care resources for, 383
health teaching in, 383, 384c
hemodialysis-related, 1626
home care management of, 382, 383c
impaired gas exchange in, 379
impaired skin integrity in, 381
incidence and prevalence of, 366f, 366-367, 367f
laboratory assessment in, 373-374
leukoplakia and, 1234
lung abscess in, 672
nursing diagnoses in, 374-375
nutritional status and, 380
pain in, 379-380
parenteral transmission of, 367-368
patient history and, 370
perinatal transmission of, 368
physical assessment in, 370-373, 371c, 372t
psychosocial assessment in, 373
risk for infection in, 375, 375c, 376c
sexual transmission of, 367, 368c
social isolation in, 382
testing for, 369-370, 370c
transmission and health care workers and, 368-369, 369c
humidifier-related, 574
hyperthermia in, 451-452, 452c, 452t
imaging assessment in, 451
immune status and, 441
inadequate antimicrobial therapy and, 449
infectious process and, 440-443, 441t, 442c
inflammation and immune response in, 306-321
antibody-mediated immunity and, 313-317, 314f, 315f
cell types involved in, 310f, 310-312, 311t, 312f
cell-mediated immunity and, 317-320, 318f, 318t
immune system organization and, 308-309, 309f, 309t, 310f
purpose of, 307, 309
self *versus* non-self and, 307f, 307-308, 308c, 308f
sequence of inflammatory response and, 312-313
intraoperative patient and, 281-282, 282f
laboratory assessment in, 450-451
in leukemia patient, 905c, 905-907, 912c
during mechanical ventilation, 696
in meningitis, 961t, 961-963, 962c, 962t, 963c
mental status change in older adult and, 935
nursing diagnoses in, 451
occupational exposure to, 449
ocular
in conjunctivitis, 1087-1088
corneal, 1089
drug therapy for, 1086c
in hordeolum, 1085-1087, 1087c
instillation of ophthalmic ointment for, 1085c
prevention of, 1074-1075
in trachoma, 1088
in osteomyelitis, 1164-1167, 1165f, 1166c
halo device-related, 996
intraosseous therapy-related, 239
lower extremity amputation-related, 1200
open fracture-related, 1183
Infection (Continued)
peritoneal dialysis-related, 1629-1630
in peritonitis, 1317c, 1317-1319
physical assessment in, 450
in pneumonia, 659-666
in acute pancreatitis, 1373
after brain tumor surgery, 1064
after open conventional esophageal surgery, 1254, 1254c
concept map for, 662
health care resources for, 666
health teaching in, 665-666
history in, 660-661
home care management in, 665, 665c
imaging assessment in, 663
impaired gas exchange in, 664, 664c
ineffective airway clearance in, 664
laboratory assessment in, 663, 663f
nursing diagnoses in, 663-664
pathophysiology of, 659, 659t
physical assessment in, 661, 663t
prevention of, 660, 660c
psychosocial assessment in, 661
risk in chronic obstructive pulmonary disease, 633
sepsis in, 664-665, 665t
ventilator-associated, 659, 660, 660c
postoperative
amputation-related, 1202
in brain tumor, 1064
in coronary artery bypass graft, 869
drug therapy for, 295-296
in esophageal cancer, 1260
laboratory assessment in, 490-491
in liver transplantation, 1363, 1364t
in lumbar spinal surgery, 987
in open esophageal surgery, 1260
in peripheral arterial disease, 809
in Whipple procedure, 1383t
pressure ulcer and, 496-498, 497c
in prostatitis, 1733-1734
psychosocial assessment in, 450
renal
in acute glomerulonephritis, 1590t, 1590-1591
in chronic glomerulonephritis, 1592
in chronic kidney disease, 1618
in nephritis, 347, 395, 1536
in pyelonephritis, 1586-1589, 1587c, 1587f
in rapidly progressive glomerulonephritis, 1591-1592
respiratory
in avian influenza, 667-668
in influenza, 658-659
in inhalation anthrax, 672-673, 673c
in laryngitis, 658
in lung abscess, 672
in peritonsillar abscess, 657
in pharyngitis, 655-657, 656c, 656t
in pulmonary empyema, 673-674
in rhinitis, 654
septic shock and, 838-839
in severe acute respiratory syndrome, 666-667
in sinusitis, 654-655, 655c
in tonsillitis, 657, 657c
sexually transmitted, 1737-1755, 1738t
chancroid in, 1753
chlamydia infection in, 1746-1747
complications caused by, 1738, 1739f
condom use and, 368c
focused assessment in, 1740c
genital herpes in, 1742c, 1742-1743
genital warts in, 1743-1744, 1744f
gonorrhea in, 1744-1746, 1745f
granuloma inguinale in, 1753-1754
Healthy People 2010 objectives in, 1739t
lymphogranuloma venereum in, 1753

Infection (*Continued*)
nursing diagnoses in, 1741*t*
oral antibiotic therapy for, 1752*c*
pelvic inflammatory disease in, 1747-1753, 1748*f*, 1749*t*, 1750-1751*c*
syphilis in, 1738-1742, 1740*f*
urethritis in, 1559
use of condoms and, 1743*c*
vaginal infections in, 1753
in sickle cell disease patient, 897
social isolation and, 452
in stomatitis, 1231-1234, 1233*c*, 1233*f*
in toxic shock syndrome, 1691, 1692*c*
tracheostomy-related, 584
tracheotomy-related, 581
transmission-based guidelines for, 446*t*, 446-449, 447*t*
in tuberculosis, 668-672
directly observed therapy in, 449
drug therapy for, 670, 671*c*
health care resources for, 672
health teaching in, 670-672
history in, 669
in HIV-infected patient, 372
home care management in, 670
laboratory assessment in, 669
lung abscess in, 672
nursing diagnoses in, 669
pathophysiology of, 668, 668*t*
physical assessment in, 669
in urethritis, 1559
bacterial prostatitis and, 1733
chlamydial, 1747
gonorrhea and, 1745*f*
in Reiter's syndrome, 355
sexually transmitted diseases and, 1739*t*
Infection control
after amputation, 1202
after bone marrow transplantation, 912*c*
health teaching in, 844*c*
in home care of HIV-infected patient, 384*c*
in inpatient health care setting, 443*c*, 443-444
methods of, 444*c*, 444-445, 445*f*
in pelvic inflammatory disease, 1749
in polycystic kidney disease, 1584*c*
in self-monitoring of blood glucose, 1490
skin and, 501-502, 502*c*
in total hip arthroplasty, 330*c*, 331
in urolithiasis, 1573-1574
Infection control nurse liaison, 445
Infectious arthritis, 356
Infectious process, 440-443, 441*t*, 442*c*
Infective endocarditis, 783-785, 784*c*
Inferior canaliculus, 1072*f*
Inferior myocardial infarction, 861-862
Inferior oblique muscle, 1073*f*, 1073*t*
Inferior punctum, 1072*f*
Inferior rectus muscle, 1073*f*, 1073*t*
Inferior turbinate, 553*f*
Inferior vena cava, 705*f*
renal system and, 1527*f*
right-sided heart catheterization and, 723*f*
Inferior vena cava interruption, 682, 820
Inferior wall myocardial infarction, 850
Infertility
fallopian tube cancer and, 1709
hypopituitarism and, 1426
sexually transmitted diseases and, 1739*t*
Infiltrating ductal carcinoma, 1663*f*, 1663-1664, 1664*f*
Infiltration in intravenous therapy, 226*t*
Inflammation, 306-321
in acute pancreatitis, 1371
in acute pericarditis, 785
in acute respiratory distress syndrome, 686
in acute sialadenitis, 1239
Inflammation (*Continued*)
antibody-mediated immunity and, 313-317, 314*f*, 315*f*
in arteriosclerosis, 794
in asthma, 610
in blepharitis, 1084
in burn injury, 525
cell types involved in, 310*f*, 310-312, 311*t*, 312*f*
cell-mediated immunity and, 317-320, 318*f*, 318*t*
in cerebral abscess, 1065
in cholecystitis, 1366
in conjunctivitis, 1087
in cystitis, 1551
in gastritis, 1265
in gout, 353
immune system organization and, 308-309, 309*f*, 309*t*, 310*f*
impaired wound healing and, 483*t*
infection and, 309-310
in laryngitis, 658
in patient with dark skin, 476, 476*c*
in pharyngitis, 655
in phlebitis, 817, 823
in pneumonia, 659
prevention of infection spread and, 443
in prostatitis, 1733-1734
purpose of, 307, 309
in pyelonephritis, 1586
in rapid hypersensitivity reactions, 387
in rheumatoid arthritis, 337
in rhinitis, 654
in scorpion sting, 148
self *versus* non-self and, 307*f*, 307-308, 308*c*, 308*f*
sequence of inflammatory response and, 312-313
in sinusitis, 654
in thyroiditis, 1460
in tonsillitis, 657
urethral, 1559
white blood cell and, 878, 878*t*
Inflammatory bowel disease, 1321-1334
Crohn's disease in, 1330*f*, 1330-1334, 1333*f*
complications of, 1322*t*
folic acid deficiency anemia in, 900
malabsorption in, 1311
pain management in, 1324*c*
ulcerative colitis *versus*, 1321*c*
ulcerative colitis in, 1321*c*, 1321-1330
diarrhea in, 1323-1325, 1324*c*
health care resources for, 1329*c*, 1329-1330
health teaching in, 1328-1329, 1329*c*
history in, 1322-1323
home care management in, 1328
laboratory assessment in, 1323
lower gastrointestinal bleeding in, 1290*f*, 1328
malabsorption in, 1311
nursing diagnoses in, 1323
pain in, 1327-1328, 1328*c*
pathophysiology of, 1321-1322, 1322*t*
physical assessment in, 1323
psychosocial assessment in, 1323
surgical management of, 1325-1327, 1326*f*, 1327*f*
Inflammatory breast cancer, 1663-1664, 1664*f*
Inflammatory cytokines, 317-318, 318*f*, 318*t*
as biological response modifiers, 433*t*, 433-434
heart failure and, 767
multiple myeloma and, 915
obesity and, 1402
osteoarthritis and, 323
septic shock and, 842
systemic inflammatory response and, 839
Inflammatory intestinal disorders, 1315-1343
anal fissure in, 1337-1338
anal fistula in, 1338
anorectal abscess in, 1337, 1337*c*
appendicitis in, 1316*f*, 1316-1317
Crohn's disease in, 1330*f*, 1330-1334, 1333*f*
diverticular disease in, 1334*f*, 1334-1337, 1335*c*
food poisoning in, 1340-1342, 1341*c*, 1341*t*
gastroenteritis in, 1319*t*, 1319-1321, 1321*c*
helminthic infestation in, 1339-1340
parasitic infection in, 1338-1339
peritonitis in, 1317*c*, 1317-1319
ulcerative colitis in, 1321-1330
diarrhea in, 1323-1325, 1324*c*
health care resources for, 1329*c*, 1329-1330
health teaching in, 1328-1329, 1329*c*
history in, 1322-1323
home care management in, 1328
laboratory assessment in, 1323
lower gastrointestinal bleeding in, 1328
nursing diagnoses in, 1323
pain in, 1327-1328, 1328*c*
pathophysiology of, 1321-1322, 1322*t*
physical assessment in, 1323
psychosocial assessment in, 1323
surgical management of, 1325-1327, 1326*f*, 1327*f*
Inflammatory phase of wound healing, 481*t*
Inflammatory skin disorders, 504-506, 505*c*
Infliximab
for ankylosing spondylitis, 355
for Crohn's disease, 1332
for rheumatoid arthritis, 342*c*, 343-344
for ulcerative colitis, 1324-1325
Inflow obstructions, 804, 804*f*, 805
Influenza, 658-659
avian, 667-668
pandemic, 160, 455
Informatics, 6, 6*f*
Informed consent, 252-254, 253*f*
Inframammary ridge, 1666
Infrapatellar notch, 324
Infratentorial tumor, 1060, 1061
Infusate, 214
Infusion catheter, 215
Infusion container, 219
Infusion Nurses Certification Corporation, 214
Infusion Nurses Society, 214, 234*t*
Infusion pressure, 224
Infusion systems, 219-222
add-on devices in, 220-221, 221*f*
administration sets in, 220, 220*c*
containers in, 219
rate-controlling devices in, 221-222
Infusion therapy, 213-240, 214*f*
alternative sites for, 236-239
arterial therapy in, 236
intraosseous therapy in, 238-239
intraperitoneal infusion in, 236-237
intraspinal infusion in, 237-238
subcutaneous infusion in, 237, 237*t*
blood sampling from catheter in, 225
central intravenous therapy in, 217-219, 218*f*, 219*f*
changing administration sets and needleless connectors in, 224
complications of, 225
central venous catheter insertion-related, 231-232*t*
during dwell of central venous catheter, 232-234*t*
local, 226-229*t*
systemic, 230*t*
Infusion therapy (*Continued*)
confirming tip location in, 222
controlling infusion pressure in, 224
documentation of, 225
flushing of catheter in, 224-225
health teaching in, 222
infusion systems in, 219-222
add-on devices in, 220-221, 221*f*
administration sets in, 220, 220*c*
containers in, 219
rate-controlling devices in, 221-222
nursing assessment in, 222-223
older adult and, 235-236, 236*f*
peripheral intravenous therapy in, 215*f*, 215-217, 216*c*, 216*f*, 216*t*
phlebitis scale for, 234*t*
prescribing of, 215
removal of catheter in, 225
securing and dressing of catheter in, 223*f*, 223-224, 224*f*
types of fluids in, 214-215
vascular access devices for, 215
Infusion therapy fluids, 214-215
Ingrown nail, 1174*t*
Inguinal area, 1646
Inguinal hernia, 1291-1293, 1292*f*
Inguinal ligament artery, 804*f*
INH; *See* Isoniazid
Inhalant abuse, 91
Inhalation anesthesia, 272*t*, 274*t*
Inhalation anthrax, 672-673, 673*c*
Inhalation burn injury, 524-525, 529, 529*t*
Inhaler, 618-619, 619*c*, 619*f*, 620*f*
Inheritance patterns, 71-74, 72*t*, 72-74*f*
Initial stage of shock, 831
Injection
of contrast agent, 943*c*
penile, 1726
periurethral, 1566*t*
safety practices in, 447
sites for insulin therapy, 1485, 1486*f*
Injection device in insulin therapy, 1487, 1487*f*
Injury
inflammation and immune response in, 306-321
antibody-mediated immunity and, 313-317, 314*f*, 315*f*
cell types involved in, 310*f*, 310-312, 311*t*, 312*f*
cell-mediated immunity and, 317-320, 318*f*, 318*t*
immune system organization and, 308-309, 309*f*, 309*t*, 310*f*
infection and, 309-310
purpose of, 307, 309
self *versus* non-self and, 307*f*, 307-308, 308*c*, 308*f*
sequence of inflammatory response and, 312-313
prevention of
bleeding precautions and, 428*c*
in emergency department, 129*c*
in hypocalcemia, 193
in Parkinson disease, 968
in patient receiving anticoagulants, 683*c*
in thrombocytopenia, 427*c*
risk for
in Alzheimer's disease, 976-977, 977*t*
in chronic kidney disease, 1618-1619
in Cushing's disease, 1443-1444
in diabetes mellitus, 1505
in hypercortisolism, 1443-1444
in leukemia, 910, 910*c*
Innate-native immunity, 316
Inner ear, 1110*f*, 1111
labyrinthitis of, 1127
tinnitus and, 1126, 1127*t*
Inner maxillary fixation in mandibular fracture, 593
Innohep; *See* Tinzaparin

InnoLet, 1488-1489
Inotropic agents
  to enhance contractility, 773-774
  for heart failure, 863-864c
  for hypertrophic cardiomyopathy, 788
  for hypovolemic shock, 837c, 838
Inpatient unit staff in emergency care, 128
INR; *See* International normalized ratio
Insect bites and stings, 146-150, 147f, 149f, 150c
Insensible water loss, 175
Insomnia, 1450
Inspection
  in abdominal assessment, 1222, 1222t
  in endocrine assessment, 1421-1422
  of eye, 1077
  of female genitalia, 1649
  of lungs and thorax, 560, 561f
  in musculoskeletal assessment, 1146
  of precordium, 717-718, 718f
  in skeletal assessment, 1145, 1145f
  of skin, 467-471, 468t, 469-471f, 471t
Inspra; *See* Eplerenone
Instillation
  of eardrops, 1121c
  of eyedrops, 1081c
  of ophthalmic ointment, 1085c
Institute for Healthcare Improvement, 3, 3t
Institute of Medicine
  core competencies of, 3-6
    collaboration with interdisciplinary health care team and, 5
    evidence-based practice and, 5-6, 6t
    informatics and, 6, 6f
    patient-centered care and, 3-5, 4c
    quality improvement and, 6
  initiative for end-of-life care, 112
  on lesbian health, 30
  National Patient Safety Goals and, 2
Instrumental activities of daily living, 98-99
Insufflation, 267
Insulase; *See* Chlorpropamide
Insulin
  anabolic effects of, 1418, 1418t
  bone and, 1142
  diabetes mellitus and
    absence in, 1467t, 1467-1468
    hypoglycemia and, 1509
    physiology of, 1466f, 1466-1467
  gene for, 63
  potassium transport and, 190-191
  refeeding syndrome and, 1399
  role in glucose diffusion across cell membrane, 173
  synthesis of, 70
Insulin pump, 1487, 1487f
Insulin resistance, 852-853, 853t, 1402, 1472
Insulin syringe, 1488, 1488c, 1489f
Insulin therapy, 1484-1489
  alternative methods of administration in, 1486-1489, 1487c, 1488b, 1489f
  complications of, 1486, 1487f
  factors influencing insulin absorption and, 1485-1486, 1486f, 1486t
  in hyperglycemic-hyperosmolar state, 1513-1514
  in intensive care unit, 1500
  preoperative, 254
  regimens in, 1484-1485
  types of insulin in, 1484, 1485t
  visually impaired patient and, 1505
Insulinoma, 1380
Insyte AutoGuard IV catheter, 215f
Intacs corneal ring placement, 1103
Intake and output monitoring
  in chronic kidney disease, 1618
  in Cushing's disease, 1443
  in fluid overload, 182
  in hyperparathyroidism, 1462
Intake and output monitoring *(Continued)*
  postoperative, 290
  in syndrome of inappropriate antidiuretic hormone secretion, 1435
Integrase, 363, 363f
Integrase inhibitors, 363-364, 378c, 379
Integrative medicine, 8
Integrilin; *See* Eptifibatide
Integumentary system, 460-478; *See also* Hair; Nails; Skin
  acidosis and, 207, 207c
  adrenal insufficiency and, 1437c
  age-related surgical risks and, 245c
  anemia and, 894c
  assessment of, 466-477
    biopsy in, 477
    diascopy in, 477
    hair and, 473
    inspection in, 467-471, 468t, 469-471f, 471t
    laboratory, 476-477
    nails and, 473-475, 474f, 474t, 475t
    palpation in, 471-472, 472t
    patient history in, 466c, 466-467
    in patient with dark skin, 475-476, 476c
    psychosocial, 476
    rehabilitation and, 97t, 98
    Wood's light examination in, 477
  changes associated with aging, 462-466, 463-464c, 465f, 466f
  chronic kidney disease and, 1613c, 1614
  diabetes insipidus and, 1433c
  immobility and, 102t
  leukemia and, 903c, 903-904
  nutrition screening assessment and, 1390c
  shock and, 829c
  structure and function of skin and, 461f, 461-462, 463t
Intensivist, 3
Intention tremor, 1004
Interbody cage fusion, 987
Intercostal nerve, 1022f
Interdisciplinary health care team collaboration, 5
  in emergency care, 127f, 127-128, 128f
Interferon therapy
  in multiple sclerosis, 1005
  in skin cancer, 512
Interferon(s), 433
Interleukin-1, 318t
  anakinra and, 344
  gastric cancer and, 1280
  osteoarthritis and, 323, 324
Interleukin(s), 318t
  as biological response modifiers, 433
  septic shock and, 842
Interlobar arteries, 1527f
Intermediate stage of shock, 832
Intermediate-acting insulin, 1484, 1485t
Intermittent claudication
  in Buerger's disease, 815
  cardiovascular assessment and, 714
  in peripheral arterial disease, 805
Intermittent peritoneal dialysis, 1628
Intermittent positive-pressure ventilation, 1008
Intermittent self-catheterization
  in chronic or disabling illness, 106
  for functional urinary incontinence, 1569
  for reflex urinary incontinence, 1568
Intermittent sequential pneumatic compression, 821
Internal auditory artery, 932f
Internal carotid artery, 932f
  brain circulation and, 931
  stroke and, 1033c
Internal derangement of knee, 1204-1205
Internal fixation, 1190-1192
Internal genitalia
  female, 1643, 1643f
  male, 1645f, 1645-1646
Internal hemorrhage in trauma patient, 136
Internal hemorrhoids, 1309, 1309f
Internal iliac artery, 804f
Internal mammary artery, 866, 867, 867f
Internal mammary nodes, 1644f
Internal os, 1643f
Internal radiation therapy, 419
  in bone cancer, 1169
  in breast cancer, 1676
  in endometrial cancer, 1700-1701, 1701c
  in oral cancer, 1237
  in prostate cancer, 1723
Internal urethral sphincter, 1532
International Medical Surgical Response Team, 162
International normalized ratio, 889
  in cardiovascular assessment, 721
  preoperative assessment of, 251c
  in warfarin therapy, 819
Internet, 6
Interphase of cell cycle, 67f
Interpreter, 29
Interrupted sutures, 282f
Interstitial brachytherapy, 1676
Interstitial cell tumor, 127, 1727t
Interstitial cystitis, 1551, 1553
Interstitial edema in traumatic brain injury, 1051
Interstitial fluid, 170, 183f
Interstitial laser coagulation, 1715
Interstitial pulmonary diseases, 638-641
Interstitial radiation therapy, 1237
Intertrochanteric hip fracture, 1196f
Intervention activities
  in acute coronary syndromes, 861c
  in adrenal insufficiency, 1439c
  for alcohol withdrawal, 84c
  in allergy management, 390c
  in Alzheimer's disease, 974c
  in bone cancer, 1171c
  in bone marrow transplantation, 911
  in caregiver support, 22c
  in chronic kidney disease, 1617c
  in chronic obstructive pulmonary disease, 629c
  in coronary artery disease, 861c
  in deficient fluid volume, 180c
  in diabetic neuropathy, 1502c
  in diabetic pain, 1505c
  in dysrhythmias, 751c
  in emergency care of burn patient, 533c
  for esophageal problems, 1258c
  in fever treatment, 452c
  in fracture-related peripheral neurovascular dysfunction, 1186c
  in Guillain-Barré syndrome, 1015c
  in heart failure, 771c
  in hypoglycemia, 1508c
  in hypokalemia, 189c
  in inflammatory bowel disease, 1324c
  for malnutrition, 1395c
  in metabolic acidosis, 209c
  in noninflammatory intestinal disorders, 1297c
  in osteoarthritis, 327c
  in oxygen therapy, 572, 572c
  for patient at risk for infection, 443c
  in peptic ulcer disease, 1276c
  for person at risk for genetic problem, 77c
  in pneumonia, 664c
  in polycystic kidney disease, 1584c
  for pressure ulcer, 493c
  in prevention of shock progression, 833c
  for problems of vocalization, 595c
  in pulmonary embolism, 680c
  for self-care assistance in rehabilitation, 103c
Intervention activities *(Continued)*
  in spinal cord injury, 995c
  in stroke, 1037c
  in urinary incontinence, 1567c
Interventional radiology
  in arteriovenous malformation, 1045
  in bone cancer, 1170
Intestinal disorders, 1289-1343
  inflammatory, 1315-1343
    anal fissure in, 1337-1338
    anal fistula in, 1338
    anorectal abscess in, 1337, 1337c
    appendicitis in, 1316f, 1316-1317
    Crohn's disease in, 1330f, 1330-1334, 1333f
    diverticular disease in, 1334f, 1334-1337, 1335c
    food poisoning in, 1340-1342, 1341c, 1341t
    gastroenteritis in, 1319t, 1319-1321, 1321c
    helminthic infestation in, 1339-1340
    parasitic infection in, 1338-1339
    peritonitis in, 1317c, 1317-1319
    ulcerative colitis in, 1321-1330; *See also* Ulcerative colitis
  noninflammatory, 1289-1314
    abdominal herniation in, 1291-1293, 1292f
    abdominal trauma in, 1307-1308
    colorectal cancer in, 1293-1302; *See also* Colorectal cancer
    hemorrhoids in, 1309f, 1309-1310
    intestinal obstruction in, 1302-1306, 1303f, 1304c, 1306c
    intestinal polyps in, 1308-1309, 1309f
    irritable bowel syndrome in, 1289-1291, 1290f
    malabsorption syndrome in, 1311-1312, 1312c
Intestinal obstruction, 1302-1306, 1303f, 1304c, 1306c
  in colorectal cancer, 1295
  in inflammatory bowel disease, 1322t
Intestinal peristalsis, 290
Intestinal polyp, 1290f, 1308-1309, 1309f
Intestinal preparation for surgery, 254
Intestinal villi, 1219
Intimate partner violence, 127
Intra-abdominal hypertension, 1308
Intra-abdominal pressure monitoring, 1308
Intra-arterial administration in chemotherapy, 423t
Intra-arterial catheter in hypovolemic shock, 838
Intra-arterial thrombolysis in stroke, 1037
Intracapsular hip fracture, 1196, 1196f
Intracavitary administration in chemotherapy, 423t
Intracavitary radiation in endometrial cancer, 1700-1701, 1701c
Intracellular fluid, 170
  electrolytes in, 183, 183f
  impermeability and, 173
  osmosis and, 174
  potassium in, 187
  sodium in, 184
Intracerebral hemorrhage
  after brain tumor surgery, 1064
  in lightning strike, 151
  in traumatic brain injury, 1051-1052, 1052f
Intracranial pressure
  brain tumor and, 1060, 1064
  encephalitis and, 964
  meningitis and, 962
  stroke and, 1037c, 1037-1043
  traumatic brain injury and, 1051, 1055-1057
Intractable pain, 52
Intradermal testing for allergy, 390

Intraductal papilloma, 1661*t*, 1662
Intradural spinal tumor, 1001
Intrahepatic obstructive jaundice, 1367
Intramedullary spinal tumor, 1000-1001
Intramural leiomyoma, 1694, 1695*f*
Intramuscular administration
  of opioid analgesics, 50*t*
  Z-track method of, 899*c*
Intranasal administration of opioid analgesics, 50*t*
Intraocular pressure, 1071-1072
  activities increasing, 1091*t*
  glaucoma and, 1095
  tonometry and, 1080, 1080*f*
Intraoperative autologous transfusion, 921
Intraoperative care, 264-284
  anesthesia and, 270-277
    advantages and disadvantages of various types of, 272*t*
    general, 272-275, 273*t*, 274*t*, 275*c*
    local or regional, 275-276, 276*f*, 276*t*, 277*f*
    moderate sedation and, 276-277
  history in, 277
  hypoventilation and, 282
  infection risk and, 281-282, 282*f*
  medical record review in, 278-279, 279*c*
  nursing diagnoses in, 279-280
  in pancreas transplantation, 1499
  preparation of surgical suite and, 267-270, 268*f*
  risk for perioperative positioning injury and, 280*f*, 280-281, 281*c*
  surgical team members and, 264-267, 266*f*, 267*f*
Intraoperative radiation therapy in breast cancer, 1677
Intraosseous therapy, 238-239
Intraperitoneal infusion, 236-237, 423*t*
Intrarenal azotemia, 1603-1604, 1604*c*
Intrarenal renal failure, 1601, 1602*t*
Intraspinal infusion, 237-238
Intrathecal contrast-enhanced computed tomography, 944*t*, 945
Intrathecal infusion, 237-238
  in chemotherapy, 423*t*
  of opioid analgesics, 51*t*, 52
  in spinal cord injury, 996
Intrauterine device for dysfunctional uterine bleeding, 1688
Intravaginal pessary, 1568-1569
Intravascular ultrasonography, 723
Intravenous access
  for blood sample, 888
  in hemodialysis, 1622-1623, 1623*t*, 1624*c*, 1624*f*
  patient preparation for, 255
  trauma patient and, 136-137
  vascular access devices for, 215
  veins for, 216*f*, 217
Intravenous administration
  in chemotherapy, 423, 423*t*
  of opioid analgesics, 50-51*t*, 536
Intravenous anesthesia, 272*t*, 274*t*
Intravenous immunoglobulin
  for Bruton's agammaglobulinemia, 385
  for Guillain-Barré syndrome, 1014
Intravenous pyelography, 1543-1545, 1544*t*, 1545*c*
Intravenous solutions, 180*t*, 214-215
Intravenous therapy
  for burn patient, 533, 533*c*, 533*t*
  central, 217-219, 218*f*, 219*f*
  complications of, 225
    central venous catheter insertion-related, 231-232*t*
    during dwell of central venous catheter, 232-234*t*
    local, 226-229*t*
    systemic, 230*t*
  documentation of, 225
  focused assessment after discharge from postanesthesia care unit, 289*c*
Intravenous therapy *(Continued)*
  in hypovolemic shock, 837
  in intestinal obstruction, 1305
  in intestinal parasitic infection, 1339
  peripheral, 215*f*, 215-217, 216*c*, 216*f*, 216*t*
  postoperative monitoring of, 290
  in pulmonary embolism, 682
  types of infusion fluids in, 180*t*, 214-215
Intravenous urography, 1543-1545, 1545*c*
  in bladder trauma, 1578
  in hydronephrosis and hydroureter and, 1586
  in pyelonephritis, 1588
  in renal trauma, 1598
  in urolithiasis, 1572
Intraventricular catheter
  for chemotherapy, 423*t*
  in traumatic brain injury, 1058, 1059*t*
Intravesical administration in chemotherapy, 423*t*
Intrinsic factor, 879, 880*f*, 900, 1218
Intrinsic renal failure, 1601, 1602*t*, 1603-1604, 1604*c*
Intropin; *See* Dopamine
Intubation
  endotracheal, 689-692, 690*f*, 691*c*
    in acute respiratory distress syndrome, 688
    in advanced cardiac life support, 756
    in drowning, 157
    postoperative evaluation of, 287
    problems in general anesthesia, 275
    in status epilepticus, 959
    in trauma patient, 136
    in upper airway obstruction, 596
  nasogastric, 1277*c*, 1397
    in abdominal trauma, 1308
    after esophageal surgery, 1254, 1260, 1260*c*
    in bariatric surgery, 1407
    calculation of drainage from, 291*t*
    decreased esophageal sphincter function and, 1244
    in diverticulitis, 1335
    in esophageal varices, 1354
    in gastrointestinal bleeding, 1276
    in ileostomy, 1327
    in intestinal obstruction, 1304-1305
    in laryngectomy, 602
    postoperative assessment of, 290-291
    preoperative preparation for, 255
    risk for aspiration and, 603-604
  nasotracheal
    securing of tube in, 691*c*
    in upper airway obstruction, 596
  orotracheal, 596
Intussusception, 1303, 1303*f*
Invasive breast cancer, 1663*f*, 1663-1664, 1664*f*
Invasive techniques for chronic pain, 57-58, 58*f*
Invasive temporary pacemaker system, 755
Inverse inspiration-expiration ratio, 693
Inverse square law of radiation exposure, 418, 419*f*
Inversion, 1146*f*
Invirase; *See* Saquinavir
Involuntary active euthanasia, 122*t*
Involuntary muscle, 1143
Iodine
  for hyperthyroidism, 1452, 1453*c*
  thyroid hormone production and, 1417
Ion, 183
Ionizing radiation
  breast cancer risk and, 1665*t*
  leukemia and, 902
  postirradiation sialadenitis and, 1240
Iontophoretic transdermal system, 48
IOP; *See* Intraocular pressure
IPD; *See* Intermittent peritoneal dialysis
IPPV; *See* Intermittent positive-pressure ventilation
Ipratropium
  for asthma, 616*c*, 620
  for dyspnea in dying patient, 117
Irbesartan, 771
Iressa; *See* Gefitinib
Irinotecan, 422*t*
  for colorectal cancer, 1297
  for esophageal cancer, 1258
Iris, 1071, 1071*f*, 1072*f*
  arcus senilis of, 465*f*, 1074, 1075*f*
  changes with aging, 1075*c*
Iritis
  in ankylosing spondylitis, 355
  in rheumatoid arthritis, 338
Iron
  hematologic assessment and, 887*c*
  supplementation in hookworm infection, 1340
  Z-track method of intramuscular administration, 899*c*
Iron deficiency anemia, 893*t*, 899, 899*c*, 1394*t*
Iron overload
  in myelodysplastic syndromes, 901
  in sickle cell disease, 897
  subcutaneous infusion therapy for, 237*t*
Irreducible abdominal hernia, 1292
Irregular bones, 1141
Irreversible stage of shock, 832
Irrigation
  for cerumen impaction, 113*c*, 1122, 1122*f*, 1123*c*
  of eye, 1104*c*
Irritability
  in hypernatremia, 186
  in premenstrual syndrome, 1685
Irritable bowel syndrome, 1289-1291, 1290*f*
Irritant-induced asthma, 640*c*
Ischemia
  in arteriovenous access for hemodialysis, 1623
  in Buerger's disease, 815
  in chronic stable angina pectoris, 848
  in compartment syndrome, 1181
  in coronary artery disease, 847
  in intestinal obstruction, 1303
  in myocardial infarction, 849
  in shock, 832
  signs and symptoms of, 810
  in strangulated hernia, 1292
Ischemic stroke, 1030-1031
Isentress; *See* Raltegravir
Ishihara chart, 1079, 1079*f*
Islet cell, 1466
Islet cell antibody, 1474
Islet cell transplantation, 1498-1499
Islets of Langerhans, 1418, 1418*f*
ISMO; *See* Isosorbide
Isocapneic hyperventilation, 629-630
Isoelectric line, 732
Isoenzymes of creatine kinase, 721
Isoflurane, 274*t*
Isolated systolic hypertension, 797
Isolation precautions
  for burn patient, 541
  in skin infection, 503
Isoleucine, 70*f*, 70*t*
Isometheptene combination, 953, 953*t*
Isoniazid, 670, 671*c*
Isoproterenol
  for anaphylaxis, 393*c*
  for cardiac arrest, 753*c*
Isoptin; *See* Verapamil
Isopto Carbachol; *See* Carbachol
Isopto Carpine; *See* Pilocarpine
Isosmotic fluids, 174
Isosorbide dinitrate, 857*c*
Isosorbide mononitrate, 857*c*
Isosthenuria, 1609
Isotonic dehydration, 177
Isotonic intravenous solutions, 214
Isotopes, 418
Isotretinoin, 515
Isuprel; *See* Isoproterenol
Itching, 480-481
  in bee sting, 150
  in brown recluse spider bite, 147
  in chronic cholecystitis, 1367
  dry skin and, 480
  epidural opioid-related, 53
  ocular drug effects and, 1076
  in pediculosis, 504
  in scabies, 504
  in skin problems, 467
  in tarantula bite, 148
  in uremia, 1536, 1614
  in vulvar cancer, 1707
  in vulvovaginitis, 1690
Itch-scratch-itch cycle, 480, 1691
ITP; *See* Idiopathic thrombocytopenic purpura
I.V. House, 224*f*
Ivermectin, 504

J

J point, 735*f*
J pouch, 1327, 1327*f*
Jackknife position, surgical, 280*f*
Jackson-Pratt drain, 292, 292*f*, 295
Jaeger card, 1078
Januvia; *See* Sitagliptin
Jarisch-Herxheimer reaction, 1741
Jaundice, 1221
  in acute pancreatitis, 1373
  in chronic cholecystitis, 1367
  in cirrhosis, 1345, 1345*t*
  in hepatitis, 1356, 1359
  in patient with dark skin, 476, 476*c*
  in sickle cell disease, 895
Jaw
  bisphosphonate-related osteonecrosis of, 1160
  fracture of, 593
Jejunostomy, 1397
  in laryngectomy, 602
  in pancreatic cancer, 1382
Jejunum, 1217*f*, 1219
JM-27 gene mutation, 1713
Job analysis, rehabilitation and, 99
Jock itch, 501
Joint capsule, 1142*f*
Joint cavity, 1142*f*
The Joint Commission, 2, 159
Joint effusion, 1146
  in osteoarthritis, 324
  in rheumatoid arthritis, 338
Joint(s), 1142*f*, 1142-1143
  complications related to intraoperative positioning, 281*c*
  dislocation of, 1208
  evidence-based instructions for protection of, 336*c*
  of hand, 1147*f*
  osteoarthritis and, 323-336
    chronic pain in, 326-328, 327*c*
    complementary and alternative therapies in, 327-328, 328*c*
    health care resources in, 336
    health promotion and maintenance in, 324
    health teaching in, 336, 336*c*
    home care management in, 335-336
    imaging assessment in, 325
    impaired physical mobility in, 335, 336*c*
    laboratory assessment in, 325
    nursing diagnoses in, 325-326
    pathophysiology of, 323*f*, 323-324
    patient history in, 324
    physical assessment in, 324-325, 325*t*
    psychosocial assessment in, 325
    total elbow arthroplasty in, 335

Joint(s) *(Continued)*
total hip arthroplasty in, 328-332, 330*c*, 330*t*, 332*c*, 332*f*
total knee arthroplasty in, 333*f*, 333-334, 334*c*
total shoulder arthroplasty in, 334-335
rheumatoid arthritis and, 337-347
body image and, 346
complementary and alternative therapies for, 345
diagnostic assessment in, 340
drug therapy for, 340-344, 341-342*c*
fatigue in, 346, 346*c*
gene therapy for, 345
health care resources in, 347
health teaching in, 347
home care management in, 346, 346*f*
laboratory assessment in, 339*c*, 339-340
nonpharmacologic interventions for, 344-345, 345*f*
pathophysiology of, 337, 337*c*
physical assessment in, 337-339, 338*f*
promotion of self-care in, 345-346
psychosocial assessment in, 339
subcutaneous infusion therapy in, 237*t*
scleroderma and, 351*f*, 351-353, 352*c*
Journaling, 9
Judaism, 119*t*
Jugular catheter in traumatic brain injury, 1058
Jugular vein, nontunneled percutaneous central catheter and, 218
Jugular venous distention
in acute renal failure, 1603
cardiovascular assessment and, 716
in coronary artery disease, 854
in dehydration, 178-179
in mitral regurgitation, 779*c*, 780
in pulmonary embolism, 679
in right-sided heart failure, 769
in status asthmaticus, 621
Junctional dysrhythmias, 747
Justice, 5
Juxtaglomerular complex, 1528, 1528*f*
Juxtamedullary nephron, 1527

K

Kadian; *See* Morphine
Kaletra; *See* Lopinavir-ritonavir
Kallidin, 1372
Kaposi's sarcoma, 372, 381, 1235
Karyotype, 67-68, 68*f*
Kava, 246*t*
Kayexalate; *See* Sodium polystyrene sulfonate
Kegel exercises
for urinary incontinence, 1564, 1564*c*
for uterine prolapse, 1693, 1693*c*
Kehr's sign, 1307
Keloid, 509, 509*f*
Keppra; *See* Levetiracetam
Keratin, 461
Keratinocyte, 461
Keratoconjunctivitis sicca, 1087
Keratoconus, 1089*f*, 1089-1091, 1090*f*, 1091*t*
Keratoplasty, 1090, 1090*f*
Keratosis, 597
Ketalar; *See* Ketamine
Ketamine, 274*t*
abuse of, 87-88
for burn pain, 536
for pain, 55
Ketoacids, 206
Ketoconazole
antacid interaction with, 1275
for cutaneous fungal infection, 503
for fungal infection in acquired immunodeficiency syndrome, 380
for prostate cancer, 1723
Ketogenesis, 1467
Ketone bodies, 1467, 1474-1475, 1539-1541
Ketoprofen, 46
Ketorolac, 45
after total hip arthroplasty, 331
for cholecystitis, 1369
for ocular inflammation, 1086*c*
for postoperative pain, 297, 298*c*
for urolithiasis, 1573
17-Ketosteroids, 1653*c*
Keyhole craniotomy, 1058
Keyhole surgery, 869-870
Kidney, 1526-1532
acid-base balance and, 204
acute renal failure and, 1601-1609
after liver transplantation, 1364*t*
chronic *versus*, 1601*t*
continuous renal replacement therapy for, 1608
dialysis therapies for, 1607*f*, 1607-1608
drug therapy for, 1605-1607, 1606*c*
health promotion and maintenance in, 1603
history in, 1603
imaging studies in, 1604
incidence and prevalence of, 1602-1603, 1603*t*
laboratory assessment in, 1604, 1605*c*
nursing diagnoses in, 1604
nutrition therapy for, 1607
phases of, 1602, 1602*t*
physical assessment in, 1603-1604, 1604*c*
posthospital care in, 1608
types of, 1601, 1602*t*
age-related changes in fluid balance and, 174*c*
antidiuretic hormone and, 175, 176*f*
blood pressure and, 708, 709
catecholamine receptors and, 1416*t*
changes associated with aging, 1533, 1534*c*
chronic kidney disease and, 1609*c*, 1609-1635
acute renal failure *versus*, 1601*t*
anxiety in, 1619-1620
cardiac changes in, 1610-1611, 1613, 1613*c*
concept map for, 1616
decreased cardiac output in, 1618
etiology and genetic risk in, 1611*t*, 1611-1612
excess fluid volume in, 1618
fatigue in, 1619
gastrointestinal changes in, 1611, 1613*c*, 1614
health care resources for, 1635
health promotion and maintenance in, 1612
health teaching in, 1635
hematologic changes in, 1611, 1613*c*, 1613-1614
hemodialysis in, 1620-1626; *See also* Hemodialysis
history in, 1612
home care management in, 1633-1635, 1634*c*
imaging studies in, 1614
imbalanced nutrition: less than body requirements in, 1615-1618, 1617*c*, 1617*t*
incidence and prevalence of, 1612, 1612*c*
integumentary manifestations in, 1613*c*, 1614
kidney changes in, 1609
laboratory assessment in, 1614
metabolic changes in, 1609-1610, 1610*f*
musculoskeletal manifestations in, 1613*c*, 1614
neurologic manifestations in, 1613*c*
Kidney *(Continued)*
nursing diagnoses in, 1615
osteomalacia and, 1161
peritoneal dialysis in, 1626-1630, 1627*t*, 1627-1629*f*, 1629*c*
physical assessment in, 1612-1614, 1613*c*
psychosocial assessment in, 1614
psychosocial preparation in, 1635
pulmonary edema in, 1620
renal transplantation in, 1630-1633, 1631*f*, 1632*f*, 1633*t*
reproductive manifestations in, 1613*c*
respiratory manifestations in, 1613, 1613*c*
risk for infection in, 1618
risk for injury in, 1618-1619
sickle cell disease and, 895-896
stages of, 1609, 1609*t*
cirrhosis and, 1348*f*
in control of potassium, 187
diabetes mellitus and, 1470-1471, 1506
disorders of, 1581-1599
acute glomerulonephritis in, 1590*t*, 1590-1591
chronic glomerulonephritis in, 1592
diabetic nephropathy in, 1594*t*, 1594-1595
hydronephrosis and hydroureter in, 1585*f*, 1585-1586
immunologic interstitial and tubulointerstitial disorders in, 1593
nephrosclerosis in, 1593
nephrotic syndrome in, 1592-1593, 1593*c*
polycystic kidney disease in, 1581-1585, 1582*f*, 1583*f*, 1583-1585*c*
pyelonephritis in, 1586-1589, 1587*c*, 1587*f*
rapidly progressive glomerulonephritis in, 1591-1592
renal cell carcinoma in, 1595*t*, 1595-1596
renal trauma in, 1596-1598, 1597*c*, 1597*t*
renovascular disease in, 1593-1594, 1594*c*
urethral stricture in, 1585*f*, 1585-1586
Goodpasture's syndrome and, 397
hepatitis A and, 1357*t*
hormonal functions of, 1531*t*, 1531-1532
hypovolemic shock and, 831
infusion therapy and, 235-236
leukemia and, 903*c*
microscopic anatomy of, 1527-1528, 1528*f*, 1529*f*
palpation of, 1536, 1537*f*
parathyroid hormone and, 1417, 1418*f*
physical assessment of, 1536-1537, 1537*f*
preoperative assessment of, 247-248
regulatory function of, 1528-1531, 1530*t*, 1531*f*
scleroderma and, 352
shock and, 829*c*
sickle cell disease and, 895-896
structure of, 1526-1527, 1527*f*
vasopressin and, 1415*t*
Kidney, ureter, and bladder x-ray, 1543, 1544*t*
in pyelonephritis, 1588
in reproductive assessment, 1654
in urolithiasis, 1572, 1572*f*
Kidney biopsy, 1547-1548
Kidney donor, 1631, 1631*f*
Kidney stones, 1570-1575
in gout, 353
in hyperparathyroidism, 1461
infection prevention in, 1573-1574
nutrition history in, 1535
Kidney stones *(Continued)*
Paget's disease of bone and, 1163
pathophysiology of, 1570-1571, 1571*t*
prevention of obstruction in, 1574*t*, 1574-1575, 1575*c*
spinal cord injury-related, 998
surgical management of, 1573
urinary tract infection and, 1551*t*
Kidney transplantation
in chronic kidney disease, 1630-1633, 1631*f*, 1632*f*, 1633*t*
in Goodpasture's syndrome, 394
Killer bee sting, 149-150
Killip classification of heart failure, 765, 862*t*
KinAir III bed, 104*f*
Kineret; *See* Anakinra
Kinins, 311
Kistner tracheostomy tube, 587
Klebsiella, 1753-1754
in pyelonephritis, 1587
in pyogenic liver abscess, 1361
in sepsis, 840
in urinary tract infection, 1552
Klinefelter syndrome, 68
Klonopin; *See* Clonazepam
Knee
below-the-knee amputation and, 1199
effusion in, 1146
patellar fracture of, 1197
sports-related injuries of, 1204-1206, 1205*c*, 1205*f*
total knee arthroplasty and, 333*f*, 333-334, 334*c*
Knee height caliper, 1389
Knee immobilizer, 1205*f*, 1205-1206
Knee to chest exercise, 986*c*
Knife wound, 1183
to head, 1050
Knock-knee deformity, 1146
Kock's pouch, 1326, 1326*f*, 1576, 1577, 1577*f*
Koebner's phenomenon, 511
KOH preparation, 477, 502
Koilonychia, 475*t*
Kosmix; *See* Zamifenacin
Kupffer cell, 1218
Kussmaul respiration
acidosis and, 207, 207*c*
in chronic kidney disease, 1610
in diabetes mellitus, 1467
in diabetic ketoacidosis, 1511
Kwashiorkor, 1392
Kwell; *See* Lindane
Kyphoplasty, 1160, 1198, 1198*c*
Kyphosis, 1145*f*
osteoporosis and, 1155, 1156*f*
in Paget's disease of bone, 1163
Kytril; *See* Granisetron

L

Labetalol, 802
Labia majora, 1642
Labia minora, 1642
Laboratory assessment
in acidosis, 208*c*, 208*f*, 208-209
in acquired immunodeficiency syndrome, 373-374
in acute coronary syndromes, 855
in acute glomerulonephritis, 1591
in acute pancreatitis, 1374*t*, 1374-1375
in acute renal failure, 1604, 1605*c*
in adrenal insufficiency, 1438, 1438*c*
in allergic rhinitis, 389
in Alzheimer's disease, 973
in asthma, 612
in atherosclerosis, 795
in benign prostatic hypertrophy, 1714
in breast cancer, 1670
in burn injury, 531-532, 532*c*
in cardiovascular assessment, 719-722, 720*c*

Laboratory assessment *(Continued)*
in chronic kidney disease, 1614
in chronic obstructive pulmonary disease, 626-627
in cirrhosis, 1349*t*, 1349-1350
in colorectal cancer, 1295-1296
in Crohn's disease, 1331
in Cushing's disease, 1441-1442
in cutaneous infection, 502
in cystitis, 1554-1555
in dehydration, 179
in diabetes mellitus, 1473*c*, 1473*t*, 1473-1475, 1474*c*, 1474*t*
in endocrine problems, 1423*c*, 1423-1424
in fracture, 1185
in gastritis, 1267
in gastrointestinal problems, 1223-1226, 1224-1225*c*
in head and neck cancer, 598
in heart failure, 769-770
in hematologic assessment, 886-889, 887*c*
in hepatitis, 1359-1360
in hyperkalemia, 190
in hyperthyroidism, 1451, 1451*c*
in hypothyroidism, 1457
in hypovolemic shock, 835, 836*c*
in infectious disease, 450-451
in intestinal obstruction, 1304
intraoperative medical record review and, 279
in leukemia, 904
in malnutrition, 1393-1394
in meningitis, 962, 962*t*
in multiple sclerosis, 1004
in musculoskeletal disorders, 1147-1148, 1148*c*
in neurologic evaluation, 943
in osteoarthritis, 325
in osteoporosis, 1156
in pelvic inflammatory disease, 1749
in peptic ulcer disease, 1273
in pneumonia, 663, 663*f*
postoperative, 293
preoperative, 248-249, 250-251*c*
in pressure ulcer, 490-491
in prostate cancer, 1720
in pulmonary embolism, 679
in pyelonephritis, 1588
in renal problems, 1537-1542, 1537-1543
blood tests in, 1537-1538, 1538*c*
urine tests in, 1538-1542, 1539*c*, 1540*t*
in reproductive problems, 1652-1654, 1653*c*
in respiratory disorders, 564, 565*c*
in rheumatoid arthritis, 339*c*, 339-340
in scleroderma, 352
in septic shock, 842*t*, 842-843
in sickle cell disease, 896
in skin problems, 476-477
in spinal cord injury, 994
in stroke, 1036
in systemic lupus erythematosus, 349-350
in testicular cancer, 1728
in traumatic brain injury, 1055
in tuberculosis, 669
in ulcerative colitis, 1323
in urinary incontinence, 1563
in uterine leiomyoma, 1695
in vision problems, 1079
Labyrinth, walking meditation and, 10
Labyrinthectomy, 1129
Labyrinthitis, 1127
Laceration
in closed head injury, 1050
ocular, 1104
renal, 1596-1598, 1597*f*
Lacrimal gland, 1072, 1072*f*
Lacrimal sac, 1072*f*
Lactase, 192, 1221
Lactase deficiency, 1311-1312, 1312*c*
Lactate, 202*c*
Lactate dehydrogenase
cerebrospinal fluid, 948*t*
in cholecystitis, 1369
in cirrhosis, 1349, 1349*t*
in musculoskeletal assessment, 1148*c*
in testicular cancer, 1728
Lactic acid
cerebrospinal fluid, 948*t*
in hypovolemic shock, 831, 836*c*
Lacto-ovo-vegetarian diet, 1387
Lactose intolerance, 192
cultural considerations in, 1221, 1387
osteomalacia and, 1161
testing for, 1311
Lacto-vegetarian diet, 1387
Laennec's cirrhosis, 1345
Lamellar keratoplasty, 1090
Lamictal; *See* Lamotrigine
Laminectomy
in back pain, 986-987
in spinal tumor, 1002
Lamivudine, 376*c*
Lamotrigine, 957*c*
Lamprene; *See* Clofazimine
Landouzy-Dejerine dystrophy, 1175*t*
Langerhans' cell, 460
Language area of brain, 930
Language assessment, 938
Language barriers, 29, 29*c*
Language Line Services, 29
Language Services Associates, 29
Lanoxin; *See* Digoxin
Lansoprazole
for gastroesophageal reflux disease, 1247*c*, 1248
for peptic ulcer disease, 1269*c*, 1274
for Zollinger-Ellison syndrome, 1279
Lantus, 1485*t*
Lanvis; *See* 6-Thioguanine
LAP; *See* Leukocyte alkaline phosphatase
Laparoscope, 269*f*
Laparoscopic adjustable-banded gastroplasty, 1406, 1406*f*
Laparoscopic cholecystectomy, 1369-1370
Laparoscopic Nissen fundoplication
in gastroesophageal reflux disease, 1248
in hiatal hernia, 1250-1253, 1253*c*
Laparoscopic radical prostatectomy, 1721
Laparoscopic surgery
in appendicitis, 1317
in pancreatic cancer, 1382
in reproductive assessment, 1656, 1656*f*
in uterine leiomyoma, 1695
Lapatinib, 435*t*
Large cell lung cancer, 641
Large intestine, 1219, 1220*c*
Large-bowel obstruction, 1302-1306, 1303*f*, 1304*c*, 1306*c*
Laryngeal edema
in anaphylaxis, 392
in bee sting, 150
Laryngeal nerve damage
in parathyroidectomy, 1463
in thyroidectomy, 1454
Laryngectomee, 602
Laryngectomy, 600, 600*t*, 605, 605*c*
Laryngectomy button, 601
Laryngectomy tube, 601, 601*f*
Laryngitis, 658
Laryngofissure, 600*t*
Laryngopharyngectomy, 599
Laryngopharynx, 553*f*, 554
Laryngospasm, 156
Larynx, 553*f*, 554, 554*f*
cancer of, 600, 600*t*
laryngitis and, 658
of older adult, 557*c*
physical assessment of, 559-560
trauma to, 596
vocal cord nodules and polyps and, 595, 595*c*, 595*f*
vocal cord paralysis and, 594-595
Lasan; *See* Anthralin
Laser, 266-267
Laser Doppler imaging in burn assessment, 531
Laser in-situ keratomileusis, 1103
Laser nurse coordinator, 266-267
Laser specialty nurse, 266-267
Laser surgery
in laryngeal cancer, 600*t*
in varicose veins, 823
Laser therapy
in cervical cancer, 1703-1704
in vaginal cancer, 1708
in vulvar cancer, 1707
Laser thermodiskectomy, 986
Laser trabeculoplasty, 1097
Laser-assisted angioplasty, 807
Laser-assisted laparoscopic lumbar diskectomy, 986
LASIK surgery, 1103
Lasix; *See* Furosemide
Latanoprost, 1099*c*
Late adulthood, 15-16
Late latent syphilis, 1740
Latency asthma, 640*c*
Latency period in cancer development, 403
Late-onset seizure in traumatic brain injury, 1057
Lateral corticospinal tract, 932*f*, 933
Lateral position
in acute respiratory distress syndrome, 688
surgical, 280*f*
Lateral rectus muscle, 1071*f*, 1073*f*, 1073*t*
Lateral wall myocardial infarction, 850
Lateralization, 1116
Latex allergy, 394, 445
Latrodectism, 148
Latrodectus facies, 148
Laundry, standard precautions and, 446*t*
Laurent Clerc National Dear Education Center, 1127*t*
Laxatives
in bowel training, 107
fluid balance disturbance and, 178
for irritable bowel syndrome, 1291
Layout of surgical suite, 267, 268*f*
LDH; *See* Lactate dehydrogenase
Le Fort fracture, 593
LEAD; *See* Lower extremity arterial disease
Lead axis, 732, 732*f*
Lead systems in electrocardiogram, 732, 733*t*
Leave-of-absence visit, 108
LEEPs; *See* Loop electrosurgical excision procedures
Lee-White clotting test, 904
Leflunomide, 342*c*, 343
Left anterior descending coronary artery, 706, 706*f*, 850
Left atrium, 706
Left bundle branch, 731, 731*f*
Left bundle branch block, 750
Left cerebral hemisphere stroke, 1034, 1034*c*
Left circumflex coronary artery, 706, 706*f*
Left lower quadrant, 1222*f*, 1222*t*
Left main coronary artery, 706, 706*f*
Left pulmonary artery, 705*f*
Left pulmonary vein, 705*f*
Left shift, 293, 311, 450
Left upper quadrant, 1222*f*, 1222*t*
Left ventricle, 705*f*, 706, 710*c*
Left ventricular end-diastolic pressure, 727
Left ventricular end-diastolic volume, 707-708
Left-sided heart catheterization, 722*t*, 722-724
Left-sided heart failure, 765, 766*f*
in aortic regurgitation, 780
in coronary artery disease, 862
history in, 767-768
in infective endocarditis, 784
physical assessment in, 768*c*, 768-769
Leg
deep vein thrombosis and, 816-821, 817*f*, 819*c*, 821*c*
low back pain and, 985
popliteal entrapment and, 816
positioning for prevention of contracture, 544*c*
restless legs syndrome and, 1024
ulceration in sickle cell disease, 895
Leg cast, 1187-1188, 1188*t*
Leg cylinder, 1188*t*
Leg exercises, 257*c*, 258
Leg surgery, skin preparation for, 256*f*
Legally competent person, 20
Leiomyoma
dysfunctional uterine bleeding and, 1688
uterine, 1694-1699, 1695*f*, 1697*c*, 1697*t*, 1698*c*
Lenalidomine, 915
Lens, 1071, 1071*f*, 1072*f*
cataract of, 1091*f*, 1091-1095, 1092*f*, 1092*t*, 1094*f*, 1095*c*
changes with aging, 1075*c*
Leonard catheter, 218
Lepirudin, 818
Leprosy, 516
Leptin, 1402, 1403
Leptin resistance, 1402
Lesbian health care, 30*c*, 30-31, 31*t*
Lesion, 467
classification of, 469-470*f*
configuration of, 471*t*
diagnostic assessment of, 476-477
in genital herpes, 1742
in lymphogranuloma venereum, 1753
Lethargy, 938
in acute renal failure, 1604
in hypovolemic shock, 835
in tuberculosis, 669
Leu-3 positive T-cell, 317
Leucovorin, 1297
Leukemia, 902-913
conditions associated with genetic predisposition for, 410*t*
fatigue in, 910-911, 911*c*
health care resources for, 912
health teaching in, 911-912, 912*c*
hematologic assessment in, 409*c*
hematopoietic stem cell transplantation in, 907*t*, 907-910, 909*f*
history in, 903
home care management in, 911, 911*c*
imaging studies in, 904
laboratory assessment in, 904
nursing diagnoses in, 904
pathophysiology of, 902-903
physical assessment in, 903*c*, 903-904
psychosocial assessment in, 904
psychosocial preparation in, 912
risk for infection in, 905*c*, 905-907, 912*c*
risk for injury in, 910, 910*c*
Leukeran; *See* Chlorambucil
Leukine; *See* Sargramostim
Leukocyte
cell-mediated immunity and, 317
cytokine receptors on, 318*f*
Fc receptors on, 314, 315*f*
functions of, 308, 309*t*, 878, 878*t*
inflammation and, 310*f*, 310-312, 311*t*, 312*f*, 313
Leukocyte alkaline phosphatase, 886
Leukocyte count
in cardiovascular assessment, 722
preoperative assessment of, 251*c*
in respiratory assessment, 565*c*

Leukocyte disorders, 902-916
Hodgkin's lymphoma in, 913*t*, 913-914
leukemia in, 902-913
conditions associated with genetic predisposition for, 410*t*
fatigue in, 910-911, 911*c*
health care resources for, 912
health teaching in, 911-912, 912*c*
hematologic assessment in, 409*c*
hematopoietic stem cell transplantation in, 907*t*, 907-910, 909*f*
history in, 903
home care management in, 911, 911*c*
imaging studies in, 904
laboratory assessment in, 904
nursing diagnoses in, 904
pathophysiology of, 902-903
physical assessment in, 903*c*, 903-904
psychosocial assessment in, 904
psychosocial preparation in, 912
risk for infection in, 905*c*, 905-907, 912*c*
risk for injury in, 910, 910*c*
multiple myeloma in, 915
non-Hodgkin's lymphoma in, 914-915
Leukocytosis
in acute pancreatitis, 1374*t*, 1375
in appendicitis, 1316
in Guillain-Barré syndrome, 1013
Leukoesterase, 1541
Leukopenia
in aplastic anemia, 900
in brown recluse spider bite, 147
in leukemia, 902
Leukoplakia, 1234
in head and neck cancer, 597
in vulvar cancer, 1707
Leukotriene antagonists
for allergic rhinitis, 391
for asthma, 618*c*, 620
Leukotriene(s)
asthma and, 610
basophil production of, 311
Leuprolide
for breast cancer, 1678
for endometriosis, 1687
for premenstrual syndrome, 1686
for prostate cancer, 1723
for uterine leiomyoma, 1696
Leustatin; *See* Cladribine
Levalbuterol, 618
Levaquin; *See* Levofloxacin
Level I trauma center, 135, 135*t*
Level II trauma center, 135, 135*t*
Level III trauma center, 135, 135*t*
Level IV trauma center, 135, 135*t*
Level of consciousness
in acute renal failure, 1604
after brain tumor surgery, 1064
after coronary artery bypass graft, 869
assessment of, 938
in brain abscess, 1066
in encephalitis, 964
in fat embolism syndrome, 1182
Glasgow Coma Scale and, 941, 941*f*
in hypovolemic shock, 835
seizure and, 955
in spinal cord injury, 993
in stroke, 1031*t*, 1033
in traumatic brain injury, 1053, 1055
in uncal herniation, 1052
Level of evidence rating scale, 6*t*
Levemir, 1485*t*
Levetiracetam, 957*c*
Levin tube, 291
Levitra; *See* Vardenafil
Levobetaxolol, 1099*c*
Levodopa-carbidopa
for Parkinson disease, 967
for restless legs syndrome, 1024
Levodopa-carbidopa-entacapone, 968
Levo-Dromoran; *See* Levorphanol
Levofloxacin
for chlamydial infection, 1747
for leprosy, 516
for ocular infection, 1086*c*
for urinary tract infection, 1556*c*
Levophed; *See* Norepinephrine
Levorphanol, 47*t*
Levosimendan, 774
Levothyroxine sodium, 1458
Lexapro; *See* Escitalopram oxalate
Lexiva; *See* Fosamprenavir
LH; *See* Luteinizing hormone
LH-RH agonists
for breast cancer, 1677*t*, 1678
for endometriosis, 1687
for premenstrual syndrome, 1686
for prostate cancer, 1723
for uterine leiomyoma, 1696
Libido, 1647
erectile dysfunction and, 1726
menopause and, 1689
premenstrual syndrome and, 1685
prostate cancer and, 1723
Librium; *See* Chlordiazepoxide
Licensed practical nurse, 4
Licensed vocational nurse, 4
Lichen planus, 516
Lichenification, 467, 470*f*, 480
Lichtenberg figures, 151
Licorice, 246*t*
LICOX Brain Tissue Oxygen Monitoring System, 1058
Lidocaine, 741*c*
Lidoderm patch, 55
Life review, dying patient and, 120
Lifestyle
after amputation, 1202-1203
coronary artery disease and, 871
culture and, 29-30
dysrhythmias and, 759, 759*c*
gastroesophageal reflux disease and, 1245*c*, 1245-1246
heart disease risk and, 710
heart transplant recipient and, 790
hypertension and, 800-801
musculoskeletal health and, 1144
myasthenia gravis and, 1021
osteoporosis and, 1157
practices to promote wellness, 16, 16*c*
pulmonary embolism risk and, 678
stroke prevention and, 1032
tension headache and, 955
Ligament, 1143
sprain of, 1208
Ligation in deep vein thrombosis, 820
Light palpation in abdominal assessment, 1223
Light reflex, 1110*f*, 1115
Light touch discrimination, 939
Lightheadedness, 1126-1127
after cardiac catheterization, 724
in aortic dissection, 814
in Lyme disease, 356
Lightning injuries, 150-152, 151*c*
Limb leads, 732, 733*t*
Limb salvage procedure, 1199
Limb-girdle dystrophy, 1175*t*
Limbic lobe, 931*t*
Limited scleroderma, 351
Lindane, 504
Linear scleroderma, 351
Linear skin lesion, 471*t*
Linezolid, 503*c*
Lingual tonsils, 553*f*
Lioresal; *See* Baclofen
Lip, 1217
squamous cell carcinoma of, 1234-1235
Lipid emulsions, 1400
Lipid(s)
atherosclerosis and, 794
cardiovascular assessment and, 720*c*, 721
coronary artery disease and, 850-851
Lipitor; *See* Atorvastatin
Lipoatrophy, insulin therapy-related, 1486
Lipohypertrophy, insulin therapy-related, 1486
Lipolysis, 1467
Lipolytic process in acute pancreatitis, 1372
Lipoprotein-a, 721
Liposuction, 514*t*, 1406
Lip-reading, 1135
Liquid formula diet, 1404
Liquid oxygen, 579, 579*f*
Liquifilm; *See* Fluorometholone
Lisfranc amputation, 1199*f*
Lithium carbonate, 1452, 1453*c*
Lithotomy position
for hysterosalpingography, 1655
surgical, 280*f*
Lithotripsy, 1573
Liver, 1218*f*, 1218-1219, 1344-1365
abscess of, 1361
as accessory organ of blood formation, 879
aging-related changes in, 1220*c*
anabolic effects of insulin on, 1418*t*
cancer of, 1362
catecholamine receptors and, 1416*t*
cirrhosis and, 1344-1356
complications of, 1345-1346, 1346*t*
concept map for, 1351
etiology of, 1346-1347, 1347*t*
excess fluid volume in, 1350-1353, 1352*c*, 1353*c*
health care resources for, 1356
health teaching in, 1355*c*, 1355-1356
hemorrhage in, 1353-1354
history in, 1347
home care management in, 1355
imaging studies in, 1350
laboratory assessment in, 1349*t*, 1349-1350
nursing diagnoses in, 1350
pathophysiology of, 1344-1345
physical assessment in, 1347-1349, 1348*f*, 1349*f*
portal-systemic encephalopathy in, 1354-1355
psychosocial assessment in, 1349
fatty, 1360-1361
glucose homeostasis and, 1467
hepatitis and, 1356-1360, 1357*t*, 1358*c*, 1361*c*
palpation of, 886
trauma to, 1361*c*, 1361-1362
Liver biopsy, 1360
Liver enzymes
in cirrhosis, 1349, 1349*t*
in gastrointestinal assessment, 1223, 1224*c*
Liver spots, 465*f*
Liver transplantation, 1357, 1362-1363, 1364*t*
Liver-spleen scan, 1229
Living related kidney donor, 1631
Living will, 113
LMWHs; *See* Low-molecular-weight heparins
LNF; *See* Laparoscopic Nissen fundoplication
Lobar bronchus, 554, 555*f*
Lobar pneumonia, 659
Lobectomy, 645, 646
Lobelia, 246*t*
Lobes
of brain, 931*f*, 931*t*
of lung, 555*f*, 556
Lobular carcinoma in situ, 1663
Lobule of ear, 1110*f*
Local anesthesia, 275-276, 276*f*, 276*t*, 277*f*
advantages and disadvantages of, 272*t*
for pain, 54*t*, 55
Local anesthesia infusion pump, 55
Local seizure, 956
Localized pain, 41
Lockout interval in patient-controlled analgesia, 52
Locus, 63, 66
Log rolling
after decompressive laminectomy, 997
after lumbar spinal surgery, 988
in spinal tumor, 1002
Lomanate; *See* Diphenoxylate hydrochloride with atropine sulfate
Lomefloxacin, 1556*c*
Lomine; *See* Dicyclomine
Lomotil; *See* Diphenoxylate hydrochloride with atropine sulfate
Lomustine, 422*t*
for brain tumor, 1062
for spinal tumor, 1002
Long bones, 1140
Long-acting beta$_2$ agonists, 616*c*, 620
Long-acting insulin, 1484, 1485*t*
Long-arm cast, 1188*t*
Long-handled reacher, 103*t*
Long-leg cast, 1188*t*
Long-leg cylinder, 1188*t*
Long-term memory, 938
Long-term non-progressors, 366
Loop diuretics
for fluid overload, 182
for high altitude cerebral edema, 156
for hypertension, 801
hyponatremia and, 186
to reduce preload, 772
Loop electrosurgical excision procedures, 1657, 1703, 1704*c*
Loop of Henle, 1528, 1528*f*, 1530*t*, 1531*f*
Looser's zone, 1162
Loperamide
for irritable bowel syndrome, 1291
for ulcerative colitis, 1324
Lopidine; *See* Apraclonidine
Lopinavir-ritonavir, 378*c*, 379
Lopressor; *See* Metoprolol
Lorazepam, 957*c*
for anxiety in head and neck cancer, 604
for bone marrow aspiration, 890
for chemotherapy-induced nausea and vomiting, 429*c*
for dying patient, 118
for pain, 55
preoperative, 261
for seizures after stroke, 1043
for status epilepticus, 959, 960
in symptom relief kit for home hospice, 121*c*
Lordosis, 1145*f*, 1146, 1174
Lortab; *See* Hydrocodone-acetaminophen
Losartan, 771
Losec; *See* Omeprazole
Loss, older adult and, 17-18, 18*c*
Loss of consciousness
in complex partial seizure, 956
in hypothermia, 153
in lightning strike, 151
in pulmonary embolism, 679
Lotion, 480
Lotronex; *See* Alosetron
Lou Gehrig's disease, 1007*c*, 1007-1008
Lovastatin, 796, 796*t*
Lovenox; *See* Enoxaparin
Lovett's scale for grading muscle strength, 1147*t*
Low back pain, 983-989
complementary and alternative therapies for, 986
diagnostic assessment in, 985
health care resources for, 989
health teaching in, 988*c*, 988-989
home care management in, 988
nonsurgical management of, 985-986, 986*c*
in osteoporosis, 1155-1156
pathophysiology of, 984
physical assessment in, 984-985

Low back pain *(Continued)*
prevention of, 984, 984*c*
surgical management of, 986-988, 987*c*
Low-carbohydrate diet, 1404-1405
Low-density lipoproteins
atherosclerosis and, 794, 795-796
cardiovascular assessment and, 720*c*, 721
coronary artery disease and, 850-851
Low-dose rate implant radiation, 419, 420*c*
Lower esophageal sphincter, 1217
achalasia and, 1255
gastroesophageal reflux disease and, 1243-1244
Lower extremity amputation, 1199*f*, 1199-1204, 1202*f*, 1203*f*, 1204*c*
Lower extremity arterial disease, 804
Lower extremity fracture, 1197-1198
care after cast removal, 1194*c*
casts used for, 1188*t*
deep vein thrombosis and, 1183
traction for, 1190*t*
Lower extremity ulcer, 806*c*
Lower gastrointestinal bleeding
common causes of, 1290*f*
in ulcerative colitis, 1290*f*, 1328
Lower gastrointestinal series, 1226
Lower leg surgery, skin preparation for, 256*f*
Lower motor neuron, 933
Lower motor neuron lesion, 994
Lower nephron nephrosis, 1601
Lower respiratory disorders, 609-652
asthma in, 610-621
drug therapy in, 615-621, 616-618*c*
exercise and activity in, 621
health teaching in, 613-615, 615*c*
history in, 612
laboratory assessment in, 612
oxygen therapy in, 621
pathophysiology of, 610-611, 611*f*
physical assessment in, 612, 614*f*
smoking cessation and, 614*c*
status asthmaticus and, 621
step system in, 613*c*
subcutaneous infusion therapy in, 237*t*
surgical risk and, 246
bronchiolitis obliterans organizing pneumonia in, 641
chronic obstructive pulmonary disease in, 621-635
activity intolerance in, 633
anxiety in, 633
health care resources in, 634, 634*c*
health teaching in, 634
history in, 624
home care management in, 634
imaging studies, 627
imbalanced nutrition: less than body requirements in, 632-633
impaired gas exchange in, 628-630, 629*c*
ineffective airway clearance in, 631-632, 632*f*, 633*t*
ineffective breathing pattern in, 630-631, 631*c*
laboratory assessment in, 626-627
nursing diagnoses in, 628
physical assessment in, 624*f*, 624-626, 626*f*
pneumonia and respiratory infection risks in, 633
prevention of, 624
psychosocial assessment in, 626
pulmonary function tests in, 627, 627*t*
cystic fibrosis in, 635-637
idiopathic pulmonary fibrosis in, 639
lung cancer in, 641-650
hematologic assessment in, 409*c*
history in, 642-643, 643*t*
nonsurgical management of, 644-645
Lower respiratory disorders *(Continued)*
palliation in, 650, 650*c*
pathophysiology of, 641-642
physical assessment in, 643-644
prevention of, 642
psychosocial assessment in, 644
sites of metastasis for, 405*t*
surgical management of, 645-649, 646*f*, 647*f*, 648*c*
occupational lung disease in, 639-641, 640*c*
pneumonia in, 659-666
in acute pancreatitis, 1373
after brain tumor surgery, 1064
after open conventional esophageal surgery, 1254, 1254*c*
concept map for, 662
health care resources for, 666
health teaching in, 665-666
history in, 660-661
home care management in, 665, 665*c*
imaging assessment in, 663
impaired gas exchange in, 664, 664*c*
ineffective airway clearance in, 664
laboratory assessment in, 663, 663*f*
nursing diagnoses in, 663-664
pathophysiology of, 659, 659*t*
physical assessment in, 661, 663*t*
prevention of, 660, 660*c*
psychosocial assessment in, 661
risk in chronic obstructive pulmonary disease, 633
sepsis in, 664-665, 665*t*
ventilator-associated, 659, 660, 660*c*
primary pulmonary hypertension in, 637-638, 638*t*
sarcoidosis in, 638-639
Lower respiratory tract, 554-556, 555*f*
Low-flow oxygen delivery systems, 574-576, 575*t*, 576*f*
Low-intensity pulse ultrasound, 1192
Low-molecular-weight heparins
for deep vein thrombosis, 819
total hip arthroplasty and, 329, 330-331
Low-pitched crackles, 563*t*
Low-profile gastrostomy device, 1397, 1397*f*
Loxoscelism, 147
LSD; *See* Lysergic acid diethylamide
Lucassin; *See* Terlipressin
Luer-Lok, 220, 224
Lufyllin; *See* Dyphylline
Lumbar peritoneal shunt, 1064
Lumbar plexus, 1022*f*
Lumbar puncture, 945*t*, 947-949, 948*t*
Lumbar spinal surgery, 986-988, 987*c*
Lumbar spine, 1146
Lumbar sympathectomy, 816
Lumbosacral back pain, 983-989
complementary and alternative therapies for, 986
diagnostic assessment in, 985
health care resources for, 989
health teaching in, 988*c*, 988-989
home care management in, 988
nonsurgical management of, 985-986, 986*c*
in osteoporosis, 1155-1156
pathophysiology of, 984
physical assessment in, 984-985
prevention of, 984, 984*c*
surgical management of, 986-988, 987*c*
Lumbosacral plexus, 1022*f*
Lumbosacral spine tumor, 1001*c*
Lumen, 1216
Lumen occlusion in central intravenous therapy, 233*t*
Lumigan; *See* Bimatoprost
Luminal; *See* Phenobarbital
Lumpectomy with lymph node dissection, 1673*f*
Lung, 555*f*, 555-556
abscess of, 672
burn-related changes in, 524-525
catecholamine receptors and, 1416*t*
cirrhosis and, 1348*f*
complications of mechanical ventilation and, 696
Goodpasture's syndrome and, 397
of older adult, 557*c*
physical assessment of, 560-564, 561*f*, 562*f*, 562*t*, 563*t*
scleroderma and, 352
shock and, 829*c*
Lung biopsy, 569
Lung cancer, 641-650
hematologic assessment in, 409*c*
history in, 642-643, 643*t*
nonsurgical management of, 644-645
palliation in, 650, 650*c*
pathophysiology of, 641-642
physical assessment in, 643-644
prevention of, 642
psychosocial assessment in, 644
sites of metastasis for, 405*t*
surgical management of, 645-649, 646*f*, 647*f*, 648*c*
Lung compliance
in acute respiratory distress syndrome, 686
in pulmonary sarcoidosis, 638
Lung diseases, 609-652
asthma in, 610-621
drug therapy in, 615-621, 616-618*c*
exercise and activity in, 621
health teaching in, 613-615, 615*c*
history in, 612
laboratory assessment in, 612
oxygen therapy in, 621
pathophysiology of, 610-611, 611*f*
physical assessment in, 612, 614*f*
smoking cessation and, 614*c*
status asthmaticus and, 621
step system in, 613*c*
subcutaneous infusion therapy in, 237*t*
surgical risk and, 246
bronchiolitis obliterans organizing pneumonia in, 641
chronic obstructive pulmonary disease in, 621-635
activity intolerance in, 633
anxiety in, 633
health care resources in, 634, 634*c*
health teaching in, 634
history in, 624
home care management in, 634
imaging studies, 627
imbalanced nutrition: less than body requirements in, 632-633
impaired gas exchange in, 628-630, 629*c*
ineffective airway clearance in, 631-632, 632*f*, 633*t*
ineffective breathing pattern in, 630-631, 631*c*
laboratory assessment in, 626-627
nursing diagnoses in, 628
physical assessment in, 624*f*, 624-626, 626*f*
pneumonia and respiratory infection risks in, 633
prevention of, 624
psychosocial assessment in, 626
pulmonary function tests in, 627, 627*t*
cystic fibrosis in, 635-637
idiopathic pulmonary fibrosis in, 639
lung cancer in, 641-650
hematologic assessment in, 409*c*
history in, 642-643, 643*t*
nonsurgical management of, 644-645
palliation in, 650, 650*c*
pathophysiology of, 641-642
physical assessment in, 643-644
Lung diseases *(Continued)*
prevention of, 642
psychosocial assessment in, 644
sites of metastasis for, 405*t*
surgical management of, 645-649, 646*f*, 647*f*, 648*c*
occupational, 639-641, 640*c*
oxygenation failure in, 685, 685*t*
pneumonia in, 659-666
concept map for, 662
health care resources for, 666
health teaching in, 665-666
history in, 660-661
home care management in, 665, 665*c*
imaging assessment in, 663
impaired gas exchange in, 664, 664*c*
ineffective airway clearance in, 664
laboratory assessment in, 663, 663*f*
nursing diagnoses in, 663-664
pathophysiology of, 659, 659*t*
physical assessment in, 661, 663*t*
prevention of, 660, 660*c*
psychosocial assessment in, 661
risk in chronic obstructive pulmonary disease, 633
sepsis in, 664-665, 665*t*
primary pulmonary hypertension in, 637-638, 638*t*
sarcoidosis in, 638-639
Lung transplantation
in chronic obstructive pulmonary disease, 630
in cystic fibrosis, 636-637
in idiopathic pulmonary fibrosis, 639
in primary pulmonary hypertension, 638
Lung volume
in acute respiratory distress syndrome, 686
in chronic obstructive pulmonary disease, 627
Lunula, 462, 462*f*
Lupron Depot; *See* Leuprolide
Lupus erythematosus, 347-350, 348*c*, 349*f*, 350*c*
Lupus Foundation, 350
Lupus nephritis, 347
Lurch, 1145
Lutein, 1101
Luteinizing hormone, 1415, 1415*t*, 1645
deficiency of, 1426, 1427*c*
erectile dysfunction and, 1726
menopause and, 1689*t*
overproduction of, 1430*c*
serum levels in reproductive assessment, 1653*c*
Luteinizing hormone-releasing hormone, 431*t*
LVED; *See* Left ventricular end-diastolic volume
LVEDP; *See* Left ventricular end-diastolic pressure
Lycopene, 1715, 1720
Lyme disease, 356, 356*c*
Lymph, 174
Lymph nodes, 174
cervical, 1235*f*
of female breast, 1644*f*
hematologic assessment and, 885
Lymphadenopathy
in infection, 450
in non-Hodgkin's lymphoma, 914
in pharyngitis, 656*c*
in serum sickness, 395
Lymphangitis, 148
Lymphangitis carcinomatosis, 117
Lymphatic spread of cancer cells, 405
Lymphedema, mastectomy and, 1680
Lymphoblastic leukemia, 902
Lymphocele, 1633
LymphoCide; *See* Epratuzumab
Lymphocyte, 315*f*

Lymphocyte count
in human immunodeficiency virus infection, 373
in respiratory assessment, 565*c*
Lymphocytic leukemia, 902
Lymphogranuloma venereum, 1753
Lymphokines, 317, 318
Lymphoma
in HIV-infected patient, 372
Hodgkin's, 913*t*, 913-914
non-Hodgkin's, 914-915
Lyphocin; *See* Vancomycin
Lyrica; *See* Pregabalin
Lysergic acid diethylamide, 87
Lysine, 70*f*, 70*t*
Lysis, 315
Lysodren; *See* Mitotane
Lysosome, 63*f*
Lysozyme, 443

M

M phase of cell cycle, 65*f*, 66, 67*f*, 401, 401*f*
Machine operator's lung, 640*c*
Macrobid; *See* Nitrofurantoin
Macrocyst in fibrocystic breast condition, 1661
Macrocytic anemia, 900
Macrodantin; *See* Nitrofurantoin
Macrophage, 311, 311*t*
antigen-antibody interactions and, 313
functions of, 309*t*, 878*t*
inflammation and, 312
Macrovascular complications in diabetes mellitus, 1468-1469
Macula, 1081*t*
Macula densa, 1528, 1528*f*
Macula lutea, 1071, 1071*f*
Macular degeneration, 1100-1101
Macular rash, 471-472
Macule, 469*f*
Mafenide acetate, 542*c*
MAG3 study 99m, 1544*t*
Magnesium, 195-197
in body fluids, 183*f*
hypermagnesemia and, 196-197
hypomagnesemia and, 196, 196*t*
imbalance after coronary artery bypass graft, 868
normal plasma values for older adult, 184*t*
serum, 184*t*
Magnesium ammonium phosphate stones, 1574*t*
Magnesium hydroxide
for gastritis, 1268, 1268*c*
for gastroesophageal reflux disease, 1246*c*, 1247
Magnesium sulfate
for dysrhythmias, 745*c*, 752
for hypomagnesemia, 196
Magnetic resonance angiography, 945*t*, 945-946
in renovascular disease, 1594
in stroke, 1035
Magnetic resonance cholangiopancreatography, 1371
Magnetic resonance imaging
in Alzheimer's disease, 973
in brain tumor, 1061
of breast, 1671
in cardiovascular assessment, 726
in chronic pancreatitis, 1378
in cirrhosis, 1350
in colorectal cancer, 1296
in deep vein thrombosis, 818
in ear assessment, 1116
in endocrine assessment, 1424
in gastrointestinal assessment, 1226
in Guillain-Barré syndrome, 1013
in head and neck cancer, 598
in infection assessment, 451
in lung cancer, 644
in musculoskeletal assessment, 1149, 1149*c*
Magnetic resonance imaging *(Continued)*
in neurologic assessment, 945*t*, 945-946
in ocular problems, 1079
in oral cancer, 1235
in prostate cancer, 1721
renal, 1544*t*
in reproductive assessment, 1655
in spinal cord injury, 994-995
in spinal tumor, 1001
in stroke, 1035
in testicular cancer, 1728
in traumatic brain injury, 1056
in uterine leiomyoma, 1695
Magnetic resonance spectroscopy, 945*t*, 945-946
Magnetic resonance-guided focused ultrasonography, 1696
Magnetoencephalography, 946
Mainstem bronchus, 554, 555*f*
Maintenance therapy
in acute leukemia, 905
in transplantation, 319-320
Major burn, 521*t*
Major calyx, 1527*f*
Major histocompatibility antigens, 307
Major histocompatibility complex, 307
Major surgery, 243*t*
Mal de ojo, 32
Malabsorption, 1311-1312, 1312*c*
in chronic pancreatitis, 1377
in Crohn's disease, 1331
in folic acid deficiency anemia, 900
in inflammatory bowel disease, 1322*t*
in ulcerative colitis, 1311
Malabsorption procedures, 1046*f*, 1406-1407
Malathion, 504
Male, 1712-1736
benign prostatic hypertrophy in, 1712-1718
community-based care in, 1718
concept map for, 1716
drug therapy for, 1714-1715
laboratory assessment in, 1714
nursing diagnoses in, 1714
pathophysiology of, 1712-1713, 1713*f*
physical assessment in, 1713-1714, 1714*c*
surgical management of, 1715-1718, 1717*f*, 1718*c*
breast cancer in, 1664
cancer incidence and death, 406*f*
epididymitis in, 1734
erectile dysfunction in, 1471, 1725-1726
gynecomastia in, 1662-1663, 1663*f*
androgen therapy-related, 1427
in cirrhosis, 1348-1349
hormonal manipulation in cancer and, 432
LH-RH agonist-related, 1723
in testicular cancer, 1727
hydrocele in, 731*f*, 1730-1731
orchitis in, 1734
penile cancer in, 1732
phimosis and paraphimosis in, 1732*f*, 1732-1733
priapism in, 1733
prostate cancer in, 1719-1725
complementary and alternative therapies in, 1723-1724
cryotherapy in, 1723
drug therapy, 1723
health promotion and maintenance in, 1719*c*, 1719-1720
health teaching in, 1724-1725, 1725*c*
heath care resources for, 1725
history in, 1720
home care management in, 1724
impaired urinary elimination in, 1721
laboratory assessment in, 1720
Male *(Continued)*
nursing diagnoses in, 1721
pathophysiology of, 1719, 1719*f*
physical assessment in, 1720
psychosocial assessment in, 1720
radiation therapy in, 1722-1723
surgical management of, 1721-1722, 1722*c*
prostatitis in, 1733-1734
reproductive system of
aging related changes in, 1646*c*
genitoreproductive history and, 1648, 1648*c*
physical assessment of, 1651
structure and function of, 1645*f*, 1645-1646
spermatocele in, 1731, 1731*f*
testicular cancer in, 1726*c*, 1726-1730, 1727*t*, 1728*c*, 1729*c*
urethritis in, 1559
bacterial prostatitis and, 1733
chlamydial, 1747
gonorrhea and, 1745*f*
in Reiter's syndrome, 355
sexually transmitted, 1739*t*
varicocele in, 1731*f*, 1731-1732
Malignancy; *See* Cancer
Malignant cell growth, 399
Malignant external otitis, 1121
Malignant fibrous histiocytoma, 1168
Malignant hypertension, 797
Malignant hyperthermia, 273, 274, 275*c*
Malignant lymphomas, 913*t*, 913-915
Malignant melanoma, 509, 510*f*, 510*t*
Malignant state in leukemia, 902
Malignant transformation, 403, 404*f*
Malignant tumor
classification by tissue of origin, 405*t*
grading of, 406*f*
Malleus, 1110, 1110*f*, 1111*f*
Malnutrition, 1392-1402
community-based care in, 1401-1402
in Crohn's disease, 1332
drug therapy for, 1395-1396
in Guillain-Barré syndrome, 1015
history in, 1393
intervention activities for, 1395*c*
laboratory assessment in, 1393-1394
mechanical ventilation and, 696
nursing diagnoses in, 1394
nutrition management in, 1395
older adult and, 16, 1393*c*, 1395, 1396*c*
parenteral nutrition in, 1400-1401, 1401*c*
pathophysiology of, 1392
physical assessment in, 1393, 1394*t*
psychosocial assessment in, 1393
total enteral nutrition in, 1396-1400, 1397*f*, 1398*c*
Malogen; *See* Testosterone propionate
Malpighian layers, 461, 461*f*
Malpositioned catheter, 232*t*
MALT; *See* Mucosa-associated lymphoid tissue lymphoma
Malunion, 1183
Mammary gland, 1643-1644, 1644*f*
pituitary hormones and, 1415*t*
Mammography, 1655, 1665-1666
Mammoplasty, 514*t*
MammoSite, 1677
Mandibular fracture, 593
Mandibulectomy, 1237-1238
Manipulative and body-based therapies, 9*t*, 11, 11*f*, 11*t*
Manning criteria for irritable bowel syndrome, 1290
Mannitol
for hyponatremia, 186
for traumatic brain injury, 1057
Manometry in gastroesophageal reflux disease, 1245
Mantoux test, 669
Manual resuscitation bag, 756
MAP; *See* Mean arterial pressure
Marasmic-kwashiorkor, 1392
Marasmus, 1392
Maraviroc, 378*c*, 379
Marcaine; *See* Bupivacaine
Marfan syndrome, 355-356, 814
Marie-Strüpell disease, 355
Marijuana, 88
Marshall-Marchetti-Krantz colposuspension, 1566*t*
Marsupialization in Bartholin cyst, 1699
Mask, standard precautions and, 446*t*
Masklike facies in Parkinson disease, 966, 966*f*
Mass
abdominal, 1222
breast, 1670*c*
reproductive assessment and, 1649, 1649*c*
Mass casualty event, 159
Mass casualty triage, 160-161, 161*t*
Mass spectrometry, 1423
Massage, 11, 11*f*, 11*t*
in end-of-life care, 117
for postoperative pain, 299
Massive hemothorax, 699
Mast cell, 610
Mast cell stabilizing drugs, 391
Mastectomy, 1672-1675, 1673*f*, 1675*c*
lymphedema and, 1680
prophylactic, 1669
Mastication, 1217
Mastoid, otitis media and, 1123
Mastoid process, 1109, 1110*f*, 1114
Mastoidectomy, 1125-1126
Mastoiditis, 1125-1126
Matrix of bone, 1141
Matulane; *See* Procarbazine
Maturation phase of wound healing, 481*t*
MAWDS mnemonic, 777
Maxair; *See* Pirbuterol
Maxidex; *See* Dexamethasone
Maxillary and nasoethmoid complex fracture, 593
Maxillary antral puncture and lavage, 655
Maxillary sinus, 553*f*
Maximum mandatory ventilation, 693
Maxitrol; *See* Neomycin sulfate-polymyxin B sulfate-dexamethasone
Maze procedure, 746
McBurney's point, 1316, 1316*f*
McDonald criteria for multiple sclerosis, 1004
McGill-Melzack Pain Questionnaire, 42*f*
MCH; *See* Mean corpuscular hemoglobin
MCHC; *See* Mean corpuscular hemoglobin concentration
McMurray test, 1205
MCP; *See* Metacarpophalangeal joint
MCV; *See* Mean corpuscular volume
MDI; *See* Metered dose inhaler
MDMA; *See* 3,4-Methylenedioxymethamphetamine
MDS; *See* Minimum Data Set
Meal planning strategies in diabetes mellitus, 1494, 1494*t*
Mean arterial pressure, 706
blood volume and, 829*t*
in continuous arteriovenous hemofiltration, 1608
hypovolemic shock and, 830-831, 831*t*, 833
oxygenation and tissue perfusion and, 827, 829*f*
Mean corpuscular hemoglobin
in hematologic assessment, 886, 887*c*
in malabsorption syndrome, 1311
Mean corpuscular hemoglobin concentration
in hematologic assessment, 886, 887*c*
in malabsorption syndrome, 1311
Mean corpuscular volume
in hematologic assessment, 886, 887*c*
in malabsorption syndrome, 1311

Meat, exchange system for, 1494*t*
Mebendazole
for enterobiasis, 1339
for hookworm infection, 1340
Mechanical débridement, 491, 539
Mechanical forces in pressure ulcer, 484-485, 485*f*
Mechanical nociceptor, 38
Mechanical obstruction, 1302
Mechanical patient lift, 100
Mechanical properties of heart, 707-708
Mechanical pump, 774, 774*f*
Mechanical traction, 1189
Mechanical ventilation, 692*c*, 692-697
in acute respiratory distress syndrome, 688
after brain tumor surgery, 1063
after coronary artery bypass graft, 869
for airway management in trauma patient, 136
in amyotrophic lateral sclerosis, 1008
in burn, 535
extubation in, 697
in flail chest, 698
in lung cancer, 649
managing ventilator system in, 695*t*, 695-696
modes of ventilation in, 693
monitoring in, 694-695
in myasthenia gravis, 1018
preventing complications in, 696
in respiratory acidosis, 209
in trauma patient, 136
in traumatic brain injury, 1056
types of ventilators in, 692-693, 693*f*
ventilator controls and settings in, 693-694
weaning from, 696-697, 697*t*
Mechlorethamine, 422*t*
Medial nerve, 281*c*
Medial nerve block, 276*f*
Medial rectus muscle, 1071*f*, 1073*f*, 1073*t*
Median cubital vein, 216*f*
Median nerve, 1022*f*, 1206-1207
Median vein, 216*f*
Mediastinal shift, 568
Mediastinitis
after coronary artery bypass graft, 869
after esophageal surgery, 1260
in inhalation anthrax, 673
Medical alert identification for laryngectomee, 606, 606*f*
Medical command physician, 163, 163*t*
Medical Emergency Team, 3
Medical errors, 2-7
core competencies and, 3-6
collaboration with interdisciplinary health care team and, 5
evidence-based practice and, 5-6, 6*t*
informatics and, 6, 6*f*
patient-centered care and, 3-5, 4*c*
quality improvement and, 6
in emergency department, 129*c*, 130
Institute for Healthcare Improvement and, 3, 3*t*
National Patient Safety Goals and, 2
Medical harm, 3
Medical language interpreter, 29
Medical nutritional supplements, 1395*c*
Medical record review, 278-279, 279*c*
Medical Reserve Corps, 162
Medical-surgical nursing, 2-7
core competencies and, 3-6
collaboration with interdisciplinary health care team and, 5
in emergency nursing, 130-131
evidence-based practice and, 5-6, 6*t*
informatics and, 6, 6*f*
patient-centered care and, 3-5, 4*c*
quality improvement and, 6
Institute for Healthcare Improvement and, 3, 3*t*
National Patient Safety Goals and, 2
Medicare hospice benefit, 113
Medication errors
intravenous drug therapy and, 215
older adult and, 19-20
patient-controlled analgesia and, 52
Medication event monitoring system, 1634
Medication history
in cardiovascular assessment, 711
in musculoskeletal trauma, 1184
in renal assessment, 1535-1536
in skin problems, 466*c*
in vision assessment, 1076, 1076*t*
Medication overuse headache with triptan use, 952
Medication(s); *See also* Drug therapy
causing hematologic system impairment, 883-884*t*
interference with warfarin, 821*c*
surgical risk and, 244*t*
Meditation, 10, 10*f*
Medroxyprogesterone acetate
for dysfunctional uterine bleeding, 1688
for endometrial cancer, 1701
Medulla, 930, 931*f*, 931*t*
Medullary cavity of bone, 1141*f*
Medullary pyramid, 1527*f*
Medullary thyroid carcinoma, 1460-1461
Mefoxin; *See* Cefoxitin
MEG; *See* Magnetoencephalography
Megace; *See* Megestrol acetate
Megaloblastic anemia, 900
Megestrol acetate
for endometrial cancer, 1701
to increase appetite, 1395-1396
Meglitinide analogues, 1479*c*, 1483
Melanin, 461-462
Melanocyte, 461
Melanocyte-stimulating hormone, 1415*t*
adrenal insufficiency and, 1427
adrenocorticotropic hormone hypersecretion and, 1428
Melanoma, 509, 510*f*, 510*t*
conditions associated with genetic predisposition for, 410*t*
ocular, 1104-1106
sites of metastasis in, 405*t*
Melatonin, 1678
Melena
in bleeding esophageal varices, 1345
in chronic kidney disease, 1614
in gastritis, 1267
in peptic ulcer disease, 1271-1272
in ulcerative colitis, 1328
Melphalan, 422*t*
Memantine, 976
Membranous urethra, 1645*f*
Memetasone, 620
Memory
Alzheimer's disease and, 971
assessment of, 938
older adult and, 935, 936*t*
traumatic brain injury and, 1058
Memory cell
antigen-antibody interactions and, 314, 316
functions of, 309*t*, 878*t*
Memory method of heart rate determination, 736
Memory training in Alzheimer's disease, 974, 974*c*
MEMS; *See* Medication event monitoring system
Menarche, 1644
primary dysmenorrhea and, 1684, 1685
Mended Hearts, Inc., 765, 872
Meniere's disease, 1127-1129
Meniett device, 1128
Meninges, 929
Meningioma, 410*t*, 1060-1061
Meningitis, 961*t*, 961-963, 962*c*, 962*t*, 963*c*
after brain tumor surgery, 1064
cerebral abscess and, 1065-1066
Meningitis *(Continued)*
gonorrhea-related, 1746
in inhalation anthrax, 672
labyrinthitis and, 1127
in Lyme disease, 356
Meningococcal meningitis, 961
Meningoencephalitis, 964
Meniscectomy, 1205
Meniscus injury, 1205*f*, 1205-1206
Menopause, 1644-1645, 1689*t*, 1689-1690, 1690*c*
Menorrhagia, 884-885
Menses, 1644
Menstrual cycle, 1644
dysfunctional uterine bleeding and, 1688-1689
endometriosis and, 1687*f*, 1687-1688
menopause and, 1689*t*, 1689-1690, 1690*c*
premenstrual syndrome and, 1685-1687, 1686*c*
primary dysmenorrhea and, 1684-1685
Menstruation, 1644
dysfunctional uterine bleeding and, 1688
toxic shock syndrome and, 1691, 1692*c*
Mental health
disaster workers in mental health interventions and, 165-166
older adult and, 20-22, 21*f*, 22*t*
Mental illness, emergency nursing and, 133
Mental status
after discharge from postanesthesia care unit, 289*c*
assessment of, 937*c*, 937-938
bee sting and, 150
coral snake envenomation and, 146
dehydration and, 179
fat embolism syndrome and, 1182
heat stroke and, 142
hypernatremia and, 186
hyponatremia and, 185
hypothermia and, 153
in hypovolemic shock, 835
infection in older adult and, 935
left-sided heart failure and, 769
pressure ulcer prevention and, 486
Meperidine, 48
abuse of, 90*t*, 90-91, 91*c*
for diverticulitis, 1335
equianalgesic dose of, 47*t*
for fracture pain, 1192
for moderate sedation, 276
for postoperative pain, 297, 298*c*
preoperative, 261
promethazine with, 54
Mephyton; *See* Vitamin K_1
Mepron; *See* Atovaquone
6-Mercaptopurine, 421*t*
Meridia; *See* Sibutramine
Mesalamine, 1324, 1325*t*
Mesna, 424*t*
MESNEX; *See* Mesna
Messenger ribonucleic acid, 70
Mestinon; *See* Pyridostigmine
Metabolic acidosis, 205-206, 209, 209*c*
causes of, 205*t*
in chronic obstructive pulmonary disease, 626-627
in diabetes mellitus, 1467
in intestinal obstruction, 1303
laboratory assessment of, 208, 208*c*, 208*f*
in septic shock, 842
Metabolic alkalosis, 208*c*, 210*t*, 210-211, 211*c*
in hyperaldosteronism, 1445
in intestinal obstruction, 1303
Metabolic bone diseases, 1153-1164
osteomalacia in, 1160-1162, 1161*t*
osteoporosis in, 1143, 1153-1160
Metabolic bone diseases *(Continued)*
community-based care for, 1160
drug therapy for, 1157-1160, 1158-1159*c*
exercise and, 1157
history in, 1155
hypocalcemia and, 193
imaging studies in, 1156-1157
laboratory assessment in, 1156
lifestyle changes in, 1157
nursing diagnoses in, 1157
nutrition therapy in, 1157
osteomalacia *versus*, 1161, 1161*t*
pathophysiology of, 1153*c*, 1153*t*, 1153-1155
physical assessment in, 1155-1156, 1156*f*
prevention of, 1155
psychosocial assessment in, 1156
surgery for, 1160
Paget's disease of bone in, 1162-1164, 1163*c*
Metabolic syndrome, 795, 852-853, 853*t*, 1472
Metabolism
body fluid chemistry and, 201-202
burn-related changes in, 525
changes in older adult, 1419*c*
chronic kidney disease and, 1609-1610, 1610*f*
hyperthyroidism and, 1449*c*
hypothyroidism and, 1456*c*
liver and pancreas role in, 1218
premenstrual syndrome and, 1686*c*
respiratory acid-base control mechanisms and, 202-204, 203*f*
thyroid hormones and, 1417, 1417*t*
Metacarpal fracture, 1195
Metacarpal joint arthroplasty, 335
Metacarpophalangeal joint
musculoskeletal assessment of, 1146, 1147*f*
positioning for prevention of contracture, 544*c*
rheumatoid arthritis of, 338, 338*f*
Metaglip; *See* Glipizide-metformin
Metamucil; *See* Psyllium hydrophilic mucilloid
Metaphase chromosome, 66, 67*f*
Metaphase of cell cycle, 67*f*, 68*f*
Metaprel; *See* Metaproterenol
Metaproterenol, 393*c*, 394
Metastasis, 404, 404*f*
in bone cancer, 1168
in brain tumor, 1060
in breast cancer, 405*t*, 1672
in cervical cancer, 1702, 1702*t*
in colorectal cancer, 405*t*, 1293, 1296
in esophageal cancer, 1255
in gallbladder cancer, 1371
in gastric cancer, 1280, 1281
in head and neck cancer, 597
in lung cancer, 641
in oral cancer, 1238
in pancreatic cancer, 1380
Metastatic calcifications in chronic kidney disease, 1610, 1610*f*
Metastatic tumor, 404
of brain, 1061
spinal, 1001
Metatarsal joint arthroplasty, 335
Metered dose inhaler, 618-619, 619*c*, 619*f*, 620*f*
Metformin, 1479-1480*c*, 1483-1484
Methadone
abuse of, 90*t*, 90-91, 91*c*
equianalgesic dose of, 47*t*
for pain, 48
Methamphetamines, 85-86, 86*f*, 86*t*
Methemoglobinemia, 568
Methicillin-resistant *Staphylococcus aureus*, 448
in cutaneous infection, 499, 502*c*
in infection in leukemia, 906

Methicillin-resistant *Staphylococcus aureus (Continued)*
in open fracture-related osteomyelitis, 1183
in osteomyelitis, 1165
Methimazole, 1452, 1453*c*
Methohexital sodium, 274*t*
Methotrexate
for ankylosing spondylitis, 355
for brain tumor, 1062
for cancer, 421*t*
for Crohn's disease, 1331
for idiopathic pulmonary fibrosis, 639
for multiple sclerosis, 1006
for psoriasis, 508
for rheumatoid arthritis, 340, 341*c*
for Sjögren's syndrome, 396
for systemic lupus erythematosus, 350
N-methyl-[e2]D[/e2]-aspartate antagonists, 55, 976
3,4-Methylenedioxymethamphetamine, 88
Methylprednisolone
for anaphylaxis, 393*c*
for multiple sclerosis, 1006
for spinal cord injury, 996
Methylxanthines
for anaphylaxis, 393*c*
for asthma, 617*c*, 620
Metipranolol, 1099*c*
Metoclopramide
for chemotherapy-induced nausea and vomiting, 429*c*
for gastroesophageal reflux disease, 1247*c*, 1248
preoperative, 261
Metolazone, 772
Metopirone; *See* Metyrapone
Metoprolol
for acute myocardial infarction, 859
for coronary artery disease, 857*c*
for heart failure, 774
Metronidazole
for brain abscess, 1066
for Crohn's disease, 1331
for diverticulitis, 1335
for intestinal parasitic infection, 1339
for pelvic inflammatory disease, 1751*c*
for peptic ulcer disease, 1269*c*
for portal-systemic encephalopathy, 1355
Metyrapone, 1442
Mevacor; *See* Lovastatin
Meval; *See* Diazepam
Mexate; *See* Methotrexate
Mexiletine, 55, 741*c*
Mexitil; *See* Mexiletine
MGUS; *See* Monoclonal gammopathy of undetermined significance
MHC; *See* Major histocompatibility complex
MI; *See* Myocardial infarction
Miacalcin; *See* Calcitonin
Microalbuminemia, 721
Microalbuminuria, 1541
in diabetic nephropathy, 1470, 1506
in heart failure, 769
Microaneurysm in diabetic retinopathy, 1469
Microcyst in fibrocystic breast condition, 1661
Microcytic red blood cell, 899
Microdiskectomy, 986
Microendoscopic diskectomy, 986
Micronase; *See* Glyburide
Microplating surgical system in facial fracture, 593
Microprocessor ventilator, 693
Microscopic observation drug susceptibility test, 669
Microthrombus formation
in hypovolemic shock, 832
in sepsis, 839, 839*f*
Microvascular bone transfer, 1167
Microvascular complications in diabetes mellitus, 1469, 1469*f*, 1470*t*
Microvascular decompression for trigeminal neuralgia, 1026
Micturition, 1533, 1535*t*
Midamor; *See* Amiloride
Midarm circumference, 1392
Midarm muscle mass, 1392
Midazolam, 274*t*
for bone marrow aspiration, 890
for moderate sedation, 276
preoperative, 261
Midbrain, 930, 931*f*, 931*t*
Mid-clavicular catheter, 217
Middle cerebral artery, 931, 932*f*
embolic stroke and, 1031, 1033*c*
Middle ear, 1110*f*, 1110-1111, 1111*f*
mastoiditis and, 1125-1126
otitis media, 1123-1125, 1124*f*, 1125*c*, 1125*f*
trauma to, 1126
tumor of, 1126
Middle turbinate, 553*f*
Mid-foot amputation, 1199*f*
Midline catheter, 217
in older adult, 235
removal of, 225
Midrin; *See* Isometheptene combination
Midurethral sling procedures, 1566*t*
MIE; *See* Minimally invasive esophagectomy
Miglitol, 1481*c*, 1484
Migraine headache, 951-954, 952*c*, 953*t*, 954*c*, 954*t*
Migration of central venous catheter, 232*t*
Migratory arthritis, 338
MIIHR; *See* Minimally invasive inguinal hernia repair
Miliary tuberculosis, 668
Milk hypothermia, 152-153
Miller Fisher variant of Guillain-Barré syndrome, 1013*t*
Milrinone
to enhance contractility, 773
for heart failure, 864*c*
for hypovolemic shock, 837*c*, 838
for pulmonary embolism, 682
Mind-body therapies, 9*t*, 9-11, 10*f*
Mineralocorticoids, 1415, 1416
Mini Nutritional Assessment, 1389, 1391*f*
Minimal bacteria diet, 906
Minimally invasive direct coronary artery bypass, 866, 868-870
Minimally invasive esophagectomy, 1259
Minimally invasive inguinal hernia repair, 1293
Minimally invasive surgery, 244*t*
bariatric, 1046*f*, 1406-1407
in brain tumor, 1062-1063
in cervical neck pain, 989
in colorectal cancer, 1299
in Crohn's disease, 1332
in diverticular disease, 1336
in gallstones, 1369-1370
in intestinal obstruction, 1306
in low back pain, 986
in pancreatic cancer, 1382
in peptic ulcer disease, 1278, 1278*f*
preparation of surgical suite for, 267-270, 271*f*
in prostate cancer, 1721
in shoulder arthroplasty, 334
in total hip arthroplasty, 329
in total knee arthroplasty, 333
in urolithiasis, 1573
in uterine leiomyoma, 1696
MiniMed Paradigm REAL-Time Insulin Pump, 1487*f*
Mini-Mental State Examination, 971, 972*f*
Minimum Data Set, 99
Minipress; *See* Prazosin
Minnesota Multiphasic Personality Inventory, 951
Minnesota tube, 1353
Minocin; *See* Minocycline
Minocycline
for leprosy, 516
for stomatitis, 1233
Minor burn, 521*t*
Minor calyx, 1527*f*
Minor head injury, 1049, 1056*c*
Minor skin irritations, 480*c*, 480-481
Minor surgery, 243*t*
Miosis, 174*f*, 1074
in cluster headache, 954
Miostat; *See* Carbachol
Mirapex; *See* Pramipexole
MIS; *See* Minimally invasive surgery
Misoprostol
added to nonsteroidal antiinflammatory drugs, 46
for peptic ulcer disease, 1269*c*, 1274
Mite infestation, 504
Mithracin; *See* Plicamycin
Mithramycin, 1462
Mitochondria, 63*f*, 898
Mitomycin, 421*t*, 1705
Mitosis, 65-66, 65-68*f*, 399, 400-401, 401*f*
Mitotane, 1442
Mitotic index of tumor, 407
Mitoxantrone, 421*t*, 1006
Mitral area, 718*t*
Mitral regurgitation, 779*c*, 779-780
Mitral stenosis, 779, 779*c*
Mitral valve, 705*f*, 706
Mitral valve annuloplasty, 782
Mitral valve prolapse, 779*c*, 780
Mitral valvuloplasty, 781
Mivacron; *See* Mivacurium
Mivacurium, 274*t*
Mixed aphasia, 1046, 1046*t*
Mixed conductive-sensorineural hearing loss, 1116, 1129, 1129*f*
Mixed connective tissue disease, 358
Mixed urinary incontinence, 1560*t*, 1561, 1569
Mixed venous oxygen saturation, 728
Mixing of insulins, 1486, 1486*t*
MMV; *See* Maximum mandatory ventilation
MNPI; *See* Myocardial nuclear perfusion imaging
Mobenol; *See* Tolbutamide
Mobility
after amputation, 1202, 1202*f*
Braden Scale for pressure ulcer risk and, 487*f*
burn injury and, 543-544, 544*c*, 544*f*
fracture and, 1193*f*, 1193-1194
Guillain-Barré syndrome and, 1014-1015
multiple sclerosis and, 1006
musculoskeletal assessment of, 1140-1151
anatomy and physiology review and, 1140-1143, 1141*f*, 1141*t*, 1142*f*
arthroscopy in, 1150*f*, 1150-1151
biopsy in, 1149-1150
electromyography in, 1150
of hand, 1146, 1147*f*
imaging studies in, 1148-1149, 1149*c*
laboratory assessment in, 1147-1148, 1148*c*
mobility and functional assessment in, 1145, 1146*f*
muscle strength in, 1147, 1147*t*
musculoskeletal changes associated with aging and, 1143, 1143*c*
neurovascular assessment in, 1147
patient history in, 1143-1145, 1144*c*
posture and gait evaluation in, 1145, 1145*f*
psychosocial assessment in, 1147
Mobility *(Continued)*
myasthenia gravis and, 1018
older adult and, 17, 17*f*
osteoarthritis and, 335, 336*c*
preoperative patient education, 258
pressure ulcer prevention and, 486
rehabilitation and, 99-101, 100*c*, 101*c*, 101*f*, 102*t*
spinal cord injury and, 999, 1000*c*
spinal tumor and, 1001
stroke and, 1046
Modafinil, 594
Moderate burn, 521*t*
Moderate hypothermia, 153
Moderate sedation, 276-277
Moderate traumatic brain injury, 1049
Modes of ventilation, 693
Modifiable risk factors
for cardiovascular disease, 709
for coronary artery disease, 850, 852
for osteoporosis, 1155
Modified Brooke formula, 533*t*
Modified Parkland formula, 533*t*
Modified radical mastectomy, 1673*f*, 1674
MODS; *See* Multiple organ dysfunction syndrome
Mohs' surgery, 512
Moist heat injury, 525
Moisture content of skin, 468-471, 472*t*
Braden Scale for pressure ulcer risk and, 487*f*
hematologic assessment in older adult and, 882*c*
Moisture-retentive dressing for wound débridement, 493*t*
Mole, 509
Moniliasis, oral, 1232, 1233*f*
Monitoring
in abdominal trauma, 1307-1308
after extubation, 697
in brain tumor surgery, 1063
in cardiac catheterization, 724
in cirrhosis, 1353*c*
electrocardiographic, 731-737, 732*f*
in burn, 530
in cardiovascular assessment, 724
complexes, segments, and intervals in, 733-736, 735*f*
continuous, 732-733, 734*f*
determination of heart rate in, 736, 736*f*
heart rhythm analysis in, 736-737
in hyperkalemia, 190
in hypocalcemia, 192
lead systems for, 732, 733*t*
in lightning strike, 152
in pit viper envenomation, 145
preoperative, 249
in stress test, 724-725
of epidural opioids, 53
in flail chest, 698
in fluid overload, 182
during fluid resuscitation in burn patient, 534
hemodynamic, 726-728, 727*c*, 727*f*
in hyperglycemic-hyperosmolar state, 1513
in hyperthyroidism, 1452
in hypokalemia, 189
in hypovolemic shock, 838
in mechanical ventilation, 694-695
in meningitis, 963
of oxygen therapy, 573
in pancreas transplantation, 1499
during peritoneal dialysis, 1630
in pulmonary embolism, 680
in renal cell carcinoma, 1596
self-monitoring of blood glucose, 1490-1492, 1491-1492*t*
in stroke, 1037*c*, 1037-1043
in transurethral resection of prostate, 1718
of wound, 496, 497*c*
Monk's pepper, 1686

Monoamine oxidase inhibitors, 968
Monoclonal antibodies
for colorectal cancer, 1297
for esophageal cancer, 1258
for non-Hodgkin's lymphoma, 914
for oral cancer, 1237
to prevent transplant rejection, 320
Monoclonal gammopathy of undetermined significance, 915
Monoclonal origin of abnormal cells, 915
Monocyte
count in respiratory assessment, 565*c*
functions of, 309*t*, 878*t*
Monodox; *See* Doxycycline
Monofilament sensation testing, 1501-1503, 1503*f*
Monokines, 318
Monopril; *See* Fosinopril
Monospot test, 657
Monosyllabic words, 1118
Mons pubis, 1642
Monteleukast, 610, 618*c*, 620
Montgomery straps, 294, 295*f*
Monurol; *See* Fosfomycin
Mood swings in hyperthyroidism, 1451
Moon face, 1440, 1440*f*, 1441
Moore prosthesis, 1196*f*
Morbid obesity, 1402
Morbidity, preoperative assessment of, 247
Morphine, 47
abuse of, 90*t*, 90-91, 91*c*
for acute myocardial infarction, 856, 858
after laryngectomy, 601
for burn pain, 536
for cholecystitis, 1369
controlled release, 47*t*
for diverticulitis, 1335
for dyspnea in dying patient, 117
in end-of-life care, 116
epidural, 52
equianalgesic dose of, 47*t*
for fracture pain, 1192
for moderate sedation, 276
for postoperative pain, 297, 297*c*
preoperative, 261
for pulmonary edema, 776, 1620
for sickle cell disease pain, 896
in symptom relief kit for home hospice, 121*c*
for traumatic brain injury, 1057
for urolithiasis, 1573
Morphine sulfate extended-release liposome, 53
Mortality, preoperative assessment of, 247
Morton's neuroma, 1173
Motherwort, 246*t*
Motility
Guillain-Barr[ac]e syndrome and, 1015
irritable bowel syndrome and, 1289
Motor aphasia, 1046, 1046*t*
Motor cortex, 929
Motor end plate, 1143
Motor function
assessment of, 939*f*, 939-940
in cancer, 416-417
changes with aging, 933-935
in hypothermia, 153
in Parkinson disease, 965, 966*c*
postoperative assessment of, 289-290
in spinal cord injury, 993-994, 994*c*
in stroke, 1034, 1034*c*
in transient ischemic attack, 1030*c*
in traumatic brain injury, 1055-1056
Motor neuron, 928
Motor vehicle accidents
older adult and, 18, 19*c*
spinal cord injury and, 990
traumatic brain injury and, 1052
Motrin; *See* Ibuprofen
Mottling in septic shock, 842
Mourning, 119
Mouth, 1217, 1217*f*, 1231-1242
acute sialadenitis and, 1239-1240
cancer of, 1234-1239, 1235*f*, 1236*c*, 1238*c*
chemotherapy-related mucositis and, 424, 428, 429*c*
hematologic assessment and, 885
maintenance of healthy oral cavity and, 1232*c*
oral tumors and, 1234
postirradiation sialadenitis and, 1240
premalignant lesions of, 1234
salivary gland tumor and, 1240
stomatitis and, 1231-1234, 1233*c*, 1233*f*
Movement
assessment in musculoskeletal trauma, 1184*c*
postoperative gas exchange impairment and, 294
pressure ulcer prevention and, 486
MRA; *See* Magnetic resonance angiography
MRB; *See* Manual resuscitation bag
MRCP; *See* Magnetic resonance cholangiopancreatography
MRI; *See* Magnetic resonance imaging
MRS; *See* Magnetic resonance spectroscopy
MRSA; *See* Methicillin-resistant *Staphylococcus aureus*
MS; *See* Multiple sclerosis
MS Contin; *See* Morphine, controlled release
MSH; *See* Melanocyte-stimulating hormone
MSRT; *See* International Medical Surgical Response Team
MTX; *See* Methotrexate
Mu opioids, 48
Mucolytic agents, 629
Mucomyst; *See* Acetylcysteine
Mucosa, gastrointestinal, 1216, 1217*f*
Mucosa-associated lymphoid tissue lymphoma, 914
Mucosal barrier fortifiers, 1269*c*, 1275
Mucosal edema, 392
Mucosal erythroplasia, 1234
Mucosal ischemia, tracheostomy-related, 583
Mucosil; *See* Acetylcysteine
Mucositis, chemotherapy-induced, 424, 428, 429*c*, 644
Mucous colon, 1289-1291, 1290*f*
Mucous fistula, 1299
Mucous membranes
asthma and, 610
chemotherapy-related mucositis and, 424, 428, 429*c*, 644
dehydration and, 179
drying during oxygen therapy, 573*f*, 573-574
erythroplakia and, 1234
fluid overload and, 182*c*
head and neck cancer and, 598
as indicator of respiratory adequacy, 564
leukoplakia and, 1234
Mucus production
in anaphylaxis, 392
in asthma, 612
in cystic fibrosis, 635
Multi-casualty event, 159
Multidisciplinary pain team, 35
Multidrug-resistant organism infections, 448
Multidrug-resistant tuberculosis, 670
Multigated blood pool scanning, 726
Multi-infarct dementia, 21
Multimodal analgesia, 52
Multimodal therapy in oral cancer, 1236
Multiple endocrine neoplasia type 1 syndrome
gastrinoma and, 1279
hyperpituitarism in, 1428
medullary thyroid carcinoma and, 1460
Multiple myeloma, 915
Multiple organ dysfunction syndrome
in abdominal trauma, 1308
in acute pancreatitis, 1373
death and, 112
hypovolemic shock and, 831, 832
septic shock and, 839*f*
in sickle cell disease, 897-898
Multiple sclerosis, 1002-1007, 1003*c*
Multisystem trauma in lightning strike, 152
Mumps orchitis, 1734
Murmur, 718, 719, 719*t*
in aortic regurgitation, 779*c*, 780
in aortic stenosis, 779*c*, 780
in infective endocarditis, 784
in leukemia, 903
in mitral regurgitation, 779*c*, 780
in mitral stenosis, 779, 779*c*
Muromonab-CD3, 320
Murphy's sign, 1368
Muscarinic receptor antagonists, 1291
Muscle, 1143
anabolic effects of insulin on, 1418*t*
cardiac, 706
complications of mechanical ventilation and, 696
innervation of, 933
Muscle atrophy
in carpal tunnel syndrome, 1207
in myasthenia gravis, 1017
in osteoarthritis, 324
in systemic lupus erythematosus, 348-349
Muscle biopsy, 949, 1149-1150
Muscle cramping in osteomalacia, 1162
Muscle enzymes, 1147-1148
Muscle flap, 1167
Muscle relaxants
for black widow spider bite, 148
for fibromyalgia, 358
for low back pain, 985
for spinal cord injury, 996
for tension headache, 955
for trigeminal neuralgia, 1025
Muscle rigidity
in black widow spider bite, 148
in malignant hyperthermia, 273
Muscle spasm
in black widow spider bite, 148
in multiple sclerosis, 1004
Muscle strain, 989, 1208
Muscle strength, 1147, 1147*t*
after bone cancer surgery, 1170
in hyponatremia, 185
older adult and, 557*c*
Muscle twitching
in amyotrophic lateral sclerosis, 1007*c*
in black widow spider bite, 148
in hyperkalemia, 190
in hypernatremia, 186
in myasthenia gravis, 1017, 1019*t*
in pit viper envenomation, 144
Muscle wasting in amyotrophic lateral sclerosis, 1007
Muscle weakness
in acute compartment syndrome, 1181
in amyotrophic lateral sclerosis, 1007
assessment before rehabilitation, 98
in black widow spider bite, 148
end-of-life care and, 116
in Guillain-Barré syndrome, 1012
in heat exhaustion, 142
in high altitude pulmonary edema, 155
in hyperaldosteronism, 1446
in hypercalcemia, 194
in hypernatremia, 186
in hyperthyroidism, 1450
in hypokalemia, 188
in hypomagnesemia, 196
in hyponatremia, 185
in hypophosphatemia, 195
in hypothermia, 153
in hypothyroidism, 1457
Muscle weakness *(Continued)*
in hypovolemic shock, 835
in influenza, 658
in leukemia, 903
musculoskeletal assessment and, 1144-1145
in myasthenia gravis, 1016
in osteomalacia, 1162
in pit viper envenomation, 144
in systemic lupus erythematosus, 349
Muscular dystrophy, 1174-1175, 1175*t*
Muscular system, 1143, 1147, 1147*t*
Muscularis, 1216
Musculocutaneous nerve, 1022*f*
Musculoskeletal assessment, 1140-1151
anatomy and physiology review and, 1140-1143, 1141*f*, 1141*t*, 1142*f*
arthroscopy in, 1150*f*, 1150-1151
biopsy in, 1149-1150
in bone cancer, 1168
in burn, 537
electromyography in, 1150
of hand, 1146, 1147*f*
in hematologic disorders, 885
imaging studies in, 1148-1149, 1149*c*
laboratory assessment in, 1147-1148, 1148*c*
mobility and functional assessment in, 1145, 1146*f*
muscle strength in, 1147, 1147*t*
musculoskeletal changes associated with aging and, 1143, 1143*c*
neurovascular assessment in, 1147
in Paget's disease of bone, 1163
patient history in, 1143-1145, 1144*c*
posture and gait evaluation in, 1145, 1145*f*
psychosocial assessment in, 1147
rehabilitation and, 97*t*, 98
Musculoskeletal disorders, 322-361, 1152-1177
ankylosing spondylitis in, 355
benign bone tumors in, 1167
bone cancer in, 1168-1172, 1171*c*
chronic fatigue syndrome in, 358
common foot problems in, 1173, 1174*t*
disease-associated arthritis in, 357, 357*t*
Dupuytren's contracture in, 1172
fibromyalgia in, 357*f*, 357-358
foot deformities in, 1172-1173, 1173*f*
ganglion in, 1172
gout in, 353-354, 354*f*
infectious arthritis in, 356
lupus erythematosus in, 347-350, 348*c*, 349*f*, 350*c*
Lyme disease in, 356, 356*c*
Marfan syndrome in, 355-356
mixed connective tissue disease in, 358
Morton's neuroma in, 1173
osteoarthritis in, 323-336
chronic pain in, 326-328, 327*c*
complementary and alternative therapies in, 327-328, 328*c*
health care resources in, 336
health promotion and maintenance in, 324
health teaching in, 336, 336*c*
home care management in, 335-336
imaging assessment in, 325
impaired physical mobility in, 335, 336*c*
laboratory assessment in, 325
nursing diagnoses in, 325-326
pathophysiology of, 323*f*, 323-324
patient history in, 324
physical assessment in, 324-325, 325*t*
psychosocial assessment in, 325
total elbow arthroplasty in, 335
total hip arthroplasty in, 328-332, 330*c*, 330*t*, 332*c*, 332*f*
total knee arthroplasty in, 333*f*, 333-334, 334*c*

Musculoskeletal disorders *(Continued)*
total shoulder arthroplasty in, 334-335
osteomalacia in, 1160-1162, 1161*t*
osteomyelitis in, 1164-1167, 1165*f*, 1166*c*
osteoporosis in, 1153-1160
community-based care for, 1160
drug therapy for, 1157-1160, 1158-1159*c*
exercise and, 1157
history in, 1155
imaging studies in, 1156-1157
laboratory assessment in, 1156
lifestyle changes in, 1157
nursing diagnoses in, 1157
nutrition therapy in, 1157
pathophysiology of, 1153*c*, 1153*t*, 1153-1155
physical assessment in, 1155-1156, 1156*f*
prevention of, 1155
psychosocial assessment in, 1156
surgery for, 1160
Paget's disease of bone in, 1162-1164, 1163*c*
plantar fasciitis in, 1173
polymyalgia rheumatica and temporal arteritis in, 355, 355*c*
polymyositis/dermatomyositis in, 354
progressive muscular dystrophies in, 1174-1175, 1175*t*
pseudogout in, 356
psoriatic arthritis in, 357
Reiter's syndrome in, 355
rheumatoid arthritis in, 337-347
body image and, 346
complementary and alternative therapies for, 345
diagnostic assessment in, 340
drug therapy for, 340-344, 341-342*c*
fatigue in, 346, 346*c*
gene therapy for, 345
health care resources in, 347
health teaching in, 347
home care management in, 346, 346*f*
laboratory assessment in, 339*c*, 339-340
nonpharmacologic interventions for, 344-345, 345*f*
pathophysiology of, 337, 337*c*
physical assessment in, 337-339, 338*f*
promotion of self-care in, 345-346
psychosocial assessment in, 339
scleroderma in, 351*f*, 351-353, 352*c*
scoliosis in, 1173-1174, 1174*f*
systemic necrotizing vasculitis in, 354-355
Musculoskeletal system
age-related changes in fluid balance and, 174*c*
age-related surgical risks and, 245*c*
alkalosis and, 210, 211*c*
chronic kidney disease and, 1613*c*, 1614
Cushing's disease and, 1441, 1441*c*
fluid overload and, 182*c*
hyperkalemia and, 190
hypermagnesemia and, 196
hypernatremia and, 186
hyperthyroidism and, 1449*c*
hypocalcemia and, 192, 193
hypokalemia and, 188
hypomagnesemia and, 196
hyponatremia and, 185
hypophosphatemia and, 195
hypothyroidism and, 1456*c*
immobility and, 102*t*
leukemia and, 903*c*
preoperative assessment of, 248
sickle cell disease and, 896
Musculoskeletal trauma, 1178-1213
amputations in, 1199*f*, 1199-1204, 1202*f*, 1203*f*, 1204*c*
carpal tunnel syndrome in, 1206-1207
Musculoskeletal trauma *(Continued)*
complex regional pain syndrome in, 1204
fractures in, 1179-1199
acute compartment syndrome and, 1180-1182, 1181*c*
acute pain in, 1192
cast application for, 1187*f*, 1187-1189, 1188*t*
chronic complications of, 1183
classification of, 1179*f*, 1179-1180
crush syndrome and, 1182
emergency care of, 1186, 1186*c*
fat embolism syndrome and, 1182*c*, 1182-1183
health care resources for, 1194
health teaching in, 1194, 1194*c*
hip, 1195-1197, 1196*f*
history in, 1183-1184
home care management in, 1194
hypovolemic shock and, 1182
imaging studies in, 1185
imbalanced nutrition: less than body requirements in, 1194
impaired physical mobility in, 1193*f*, 1193-1194
incidence and prevalence of, 1183
infection and, 1183, 1192-1193
laboratory assessment in, 1185
lower extremity, 1197-1198
nursing diagnoses in, 1185-1186
open reduction of, 1190-1192, 1191*f*
pelvic, 1198
peripheral neurovascular dysfunction and, 1186, 1186*c*
physical assessment in, 1184*c*, 1184-1185
prevention of, 1183
psychosocial assessment in, 1185
rib or sternum, 1198
skeletal pin site care in, 1191
stages of bone healing and, 1180, 1180*f*
traction for, 1189*f*, 1189-1190, 1190*t*
upper extremity, 1195
venous thromboembolism and, 1183
vertebral, 1198*c*, 1198-1199
rotator cuff injury in, 1208
sports-related injuries in, 1204-1206, 1205*c*, 1205*f*
strains and sprains in, 1208
tendon rupture and joint dislocation in, 1208
Muse; *See* Alprostadil
Music therapy
in end-of-life care, 117, 118
for pain management, 10
Mustargen; *See* Mechlorethamine
Mutamycin; *See* Mitomycin
Mutation, 70-71
in breast cancer, 73, 78, 1647, 1664, 1705
in Crohn's disease, 1330
in esophageal cancer, 1256
in gastric cancer, 1280
in pancreatic cancer, 1380
in prostate cancer, 1330
Myalgia
in acquired immunodeficiency syndrome, 380
in hepatitis, 1359
in hypothyroidism, 1457
in influenza, 658
in meningitis, 961
in pneumonia, 661
related to drug therapy in leukemia, 911
in severe acute respiratory syndrome, 666
in viral gastroenteritis, 1320
Myasthenia gravis, 1016-1022
community-based care in, 1021*t*, 1021-1022, 1022*c*
electromyography in, 1018
nonsurgical management of, 1018-1020, 1019*t*, 1020*c*
nursing diagnoses in, 1018
pathophysiology of, 1016
physical assessment in, 1-17*c*, 1016-1017
surgical management of, 1020-1021
Myasthenic crisis, 1017, 1019*t*
Mycobacterium avium complex, 371
Mycobacterium tuberculosis, 668
Mycophenolate mofetil, 319, 637
Mycostatin; *See* Nystatin
Mycotic aneurysm, 1031-1032
Mydriasis, 174*f*, 1074
Myelin, multiple sclerosis and, 1002-1003
Myelin sheath, 929
Myelocytic leukemia, 902
Myelodysplastic syndromes, 901-902
Myelogenous leukemia, 902
Myelography, 1148
Myelosuppression, irinotecan-related, 1297
Myelotomy, 58*f*
Myenteric nerve plexus, 1217*f*
Myfortic; *See* Mycophenolate
Mylotarg; *See* Gemtuzumab
Myoblast transfer therapy, 1175
Myocardial contractility, 708
Myocardial contraction, 706-707
Myocardial depressant factor, 832
Myocardial fibrosis, 352
Myocardial hypertrophy, 767
Myocardial infarction, 848-850, 849*f*
angina *versus*, 854*c*
chest pain in, 713*t*
in coronary artery disease, 847
in diabetes mellitus, 1468
emergency care in, 856-858, 857-858*c*
family history of, 936
heart failure and, 767
home care management after, 870, 870*c*, 871*c*
postmyocardial infarction heart failure and, 862, 862*t*
serum markers of myocardial damage in, 719-721
ventricular fibrillation and, 7u49
Myocardial nuclear perfusion imaging, 725-726
Myocarditis, 338
Myocardium, 704, 705*f*
areas for inspection and auscultation, 718*t*
blood flow to, 706, 706*f*
cardioversion and, 756
Myoclonic seizure, 956
Myocutaneous flap, 495-496, 496*f*
Myofibril sarcomere, 706
Myoglobin
burn and, 531
cardiovascular assessment and, 721
in myocardial infarction, 855
Myoglobinuria
in coral snake envenomation, 146
in malignant hyperthermia, 273
Myoglobinuric renal failure, 1181
Myomectomy
in dysfunctional uterine bleeding, 1689
in uterine leiomyoma, 1696
Myometrium, 1643*f*
dysmenorrhea and, 1685
Myopathy, 1145
Myopia, 1073, 1073*f*, 1102
Myositis, 349
Myosplint, 775
Myotonic dystrophy, 1175*t*
Myringoplasty, 1132, 1133*f*
Myringotomy, 1124-1125
Mysoline; *See* Primidone
Myxedema, 1455, 1456*f*
Myxedema coma, 1455-1456, 1459, 1459*c*

N

Nadir, 423, 910
Nadolol, 1353
Nafcillin, 1066
Nails, 462, 462*f*, 473-475
alterations in color of, 474*f*, 474*t*
changes related to aging, 464*c*, 466*f*
endocrine assessment and, 1422
hematologic assessment and, 882*c*
variations in shape of, 475*t*
Naldecon Senior EX; *See* Guaifenesin
Naloxone
for morphine reversal, 858
for opioid-induced respiratory depression, 49, 297
Naltrexone, 85
Namenda; *See* Memantine
Naprosyn; *See* Naproxen
Naproxen
for dysmenorrhea, 1685
for migraine headache, 952, 953*t*
nephrotoxicity of, 1506
for pain, 46
Narcan; *See* Naloxone
Narcolepsy, 594
Narcotics abuse, 90*t*, 90-91, 91*c*
Nares, 553*f*
Naropin; *See* Ropivacaine
Narrow-angle glaucoma, 1095*t*, 1095-1098, 1098*c*
NARTIs; *See* Nucleoside analog reverse transcriptase inhibitors
Nasal cannula, 574, 575*t*, 576*f*
Nasal continuous positive airway pressure, 578, 578*f*
Nasal drainage, 389
Nasal fracture, 590-591, 591*f*
Nasal packing
in nosebleed, 592
in rhinoplasty, 591, 591*f*
Nasal polyp, 592
Nasal prongs, 574, 575*t*, 576*f*
Nasal punctum block, 397
Nasalcrom; *See* Cromolyn sodium
NASH; *See* Nonalcoholic steatohepatitis
Nasoduodenal tube, 543, 1397, 1397*f*
Nasoenteric tube, 1397
Nasoethmoid complex fracture, 593
Nasogastric tube, 1277*c*, 1397
in abdominal trauma, 1308
after esophageal surgery, 1254, 1260, 1260*c*
in bariatric surgery, 1407
calculation of drainage from, 291*t*
decreased esophageal sphincter function and, 1244
in diverticulitis, 1335
in esophageal varices, 1354
in gastrointestinal bleeding, 1276
in ileostomy, 1327
in intestinal obstruction, 1304-1305
in laryngectomy, 602
postoperative assessment of, 290-291
preoperative preparation for, 255
risk for aspiration and, 603-604
Nasolacrimal duct, 1072*f*
Nasopharyngeal cancer, 592-593
Nasopharynx, 553*f*
Nasoseptoplasty, 591
Nasotracheal intubation
securing of tube in, 691*c*
in upper airway obstruction, 596
Natacyn; *See* Natamycin
Natalizumab, 1005
Natamycin, 1086*c*
Nateglinide, 1479*c*, 1483
National Amputation Foundation, 1203
National Brain Tumor Foundation, 1065
National Center for Complementary and Alternative Medicine, 8, 9*t*
National Cholesterol Education Program, 795
National Disaster Medical System, 162
National Guard, 162

National Medical Response Teams-Weapons of Mass Destruction, 162
National Multiple Sclerosis Society, 1007
National Nurse Response Team, 162
National Osteoporosis Foundation, 1160
National Patient Safety Goals, 2, 23
National Pharmacist Response Team, 162
National Scoliosis Foundation, 1174
National Spinal Cord Injury Association, 1000
Native Americans
  beliefs regarding death, dying, and afterlife, 119*t*
  breast cancer and, 1665*t*
  diabetes mellitus and, 1472
  musculoskeletal differences in, 1141*t*
Natrecor; *See* Nesiritide
Natriuresis, 772
Natriuretic hormones, 1531*t*
Natriuretic peptides, 175-176, 767
Natulan; *See* Procarbazine
Natural chemical débridement, 491
Natural immunity, 309, 316, 441*t*
Natural killer cell, 309*t*, 317, 878*t*
Natural menopause, 1689
Natural passive immunity, 316
Naturopathic medicine, 9
Nausea
  in acute glomerulonephritis, 1591
  in acute mountain sickness, 155
  in acute renal failure, 1603
  in bee sting, 149
  in black widow spider bite, 148
  in botulism, 1341-1342
  bromocriptine-related, 1431
  chemotherapy-related, 427-428, 429*c*
  in chronic kidney disease, 1611
  in coral snake envenomation, 146
  in diverticulitis, 1335
  end-of-life care and, 118
  epidural opioid-related, 53
  in food poisoning, 1341
  in heat exhaustion, 142
  in hypercalcemia, 194
  in hyperparathyroidism, 1461
  in hypokalemia, 188
  in hypomagnesemia, 196
  in irritable bowel syndrome, 1290
  in labyrinthitis, 1127
  in leukemia, 904
  in lung cancer, 644
  in meningitis, 961
  in migraine headache, 951
  opioid analgesic-related, 48, 49*t*
  in pit viper envenomation, 144
  postoperative
    in aortic dissection, 814
    assessment of, 290-291, 291*t*
    in cardiac catheterization, 724
    in gallstones, 1370
    in retinal detachment repair, 1102
  in tube feeding, 1399
  in tuberculosis, 669, 670
  in urolithiasis, 1571
  in vertigo, 1126
Navelbine; *See* Vinorelbine
Near point of vision, 1074
Near vision testing, 1078
Near-drowning, 156
Near-euglycemia blood glucose, 1469
Nearsightedness, 1073, 1073*f*, 1102
Near-syncope, 714
Nebulizer
  for chronic obstructive pulmonary disease, 629
  drying mucous membranes during oxygen therapy and, 574
Necator americanus, 1340
Neck
  cancer of, 597-606
    anxiety in, 604
    assessment in, 598*t*, 598-599
Neck *(Continued)*
    disturbed body image in, 604
    health care resources in, 606
    health teaching in, 605*c*, 605-606, 606*f*
    home care management in, 605, 605*c*
    nursing diagnoses in, 599
    pathophysiology of, 597-598
    psychosocial preparation for, 606
    respiratory obstruction in, 599-602, 600*t*, 601*f*, 603*f*
    risk for aspiration in, 603*c*, 603-604, 604*c*
    subcutaneous infusion therapy in, 237*t*
  hematologic assessment and, 885
  musculoskeletal assessment of, 1146
  positioning for prevention of contracture, 544*c*
  spinal tumor and, 1001*c*
  thyroid gland and, 1417, 1417*f*
  trauma to, 596-597
Neck dissection, 600
Neck pain, 989*f*, 989-990, 990*c*
Neck vein distention
  in acute renal failure, 1603
  cardiovascular assessment and, 716
  in dehydration, 178-179
  in mitral regurgitation, 779*c*, 780
  in pulmonary embolism, 679
  in right-sided heart failure, 769
  in status asthmaticus, 621
Necrosis
  in acute pancreatitis, 1372
  in myocardial infarction, 849
  in tarantula bite, 148
Necrotic arachnidism, 147
Necrotizing external otitis, 1121
Necrotizing hemorrhagic pancreatitis, 1372
Necrotizing vasculitis, 354-355
Nedocromil, 618*c*, 620
NEECHAM Confusion Scale, 21
Needle, standard precautions and, 446*t*
Needle biopsy of thyroid, 1424
Needle bladder neck suspension, 1566*t*
Needleless connection device, 221, 221*f*, 224
Needleless insulin injection device, 1487, 1487*f*
Needlestick injury, 368
Needlestick Safety and Prevention Act, 221
Negative deflection, 732, 732*f*
Negative feedback mechanism, 1413-1414, 1414*f*
Negative nitrogen balance, 1449
Neglect, elder, 22*c*, 22-23
Neglect syndrome after stroke, 1034-1035, 1047
Neisseria gonorrhoeae, 1654, 1744-1746, 1745*f*, 1748
Neisseria meningitidis, 961, 961*t*
Nelfinavir, 378*c*, 379
Nemasol; *See* Mebendazole
Nembutal; *See* Pentobarbital sodium
Neoadjuvant therapy in breast cancer, 1672-1673, 1676
Neobladder, 1576
Neomycin, 1354-1355
Neomycin sulfate-polymyxin B sulfate-dexamethasone, 1086*c*
Neoplasia, 400
Neoplasm; *See* Tumor
Neoral; *See* Cyclosporine
Neo-Synephrine; *See* Phenylephrine
Nephrectomy
  in pyelonephritis, 1588-1589
  in renal cell carcinoma, 1596
  in renal transplantation, 1631
  in renal trauma, 1598
Nephritis, 1536
  lupus, 347
  in serum sickness, 395
Nephrogenic diabetes insipidus, 1433
Nephrolithiasis, 1570-1575
  in gout, 353
  in hyperparathyroidism, 1461
  infection prevention in, 1573-1574
  nutrition history in, 1535
  Paget's disease of bone and, 1163
  pathophysiology of, 1570-1571, 1571*t*
  prevention of obstruction in, 1574*t*, 1574-1575, 1575*c*
  spinal cord injury-related, 998
  surgical management of, 1573
  urinary tract infection and, 1551*t*
Nephrolithotomy, 1573
Nephron, 1527-1528, 1527-1529*f*
Nephronex; *See* Nitrofurantoin
Nephropathy
  diabetic, 1468, 1470-1471, 1506, 1594*t*, 1594-1595
  glomerular disease and, 1590
Nephropathy, diabetic, 1468, 1470-1471, 1506, 1590, 1594*t*, 1594-1595
Nephrosclerosis, 1593
Nephrosis, 1536
Nephrostomy, 1586
Nephrotic syndrome, 1592-1593, 1593*c*
Nephrotomography, 1544*t*
Nephrotoxic substances, 1506, 1602-1603, 1603*t*7
Nephrotoxicity
  of acetaminophen, 46
  of antiviral drugs, 906
Nephrox; *See* Aluminum hydroxide gel
Nerve biopsy, 949
Nerve block, 275, 276*f*, 276*t*
Nerve conduction velocity testing, 1013
Nerve damage
  central venous catheter insertion-related, 232*t*
  intravenous therapy-related, 229*t*
Nerve graft, 1024
Nerve root pain, 985
  after lumbar spinal surgery, 987*c*
  in spinal tumor, 1001
Nervous colon, 1289-1291, 1290*f*
Nesiritide, 772
Nettle, 246*t*
Neulasta; *See* Pegfilgrastim
Neumega; *See* Oprelvekin
Neupogen; *See* Filgrastim
Neupro; *See* Rotigotine
Neuralgia, trigeminal, 1025*f*, 1025-1026
Neural-induced distributive shock, 828
Neuritic plaques, 970
Neuroaxial anesthesia, 329
Neuroendocrine pancreatic tumor, 1380
Neuroendocrine regulation, 1412
Neurofibrillary tangles, 970
Neurofibromatosis, 73
Neurogenic bladder, 994, 998
Neurogenic pulmonary edema, 1064
Neurogenic shock, 995
Neurogenic symptoms in hypoglycemia, 1507, 1507*t*
Neuroglial cell, 929
Neuroglycopenic symptoms in hypoglycemia, 1507, 1507*t*
Neurohypophysis, 1414
Neurokinin receptor antagonists, 429*c*
Neuroleptic drugs
  for Alzheimer's disease, 976
  for amyotrophic lateral sclerosis, 1008
  for Huntington disease, 980
Neurologic assessment, 928-949
  aging-related changes in neurologic system and, 933-935, 936*c*
  anatomy and physiology and, 928-933
    autonomic nervous system and, 933
    brain and, 929-931, 931*f*, 931*t*, 932*f*
    neuroglial cells and, 929
    neuron and, 928-929, 929*f*, 930*t*
    parasympathetic nervous system and, 933, 934*f*, 935*t*
    spinal cord and, 931-933, 932*f*
  cerebral angiography in, 943, 943*c*
Neurologic assessment *(Continued)*
  cerebral blood flow evaluation in, 946
  computed tomography in, 943-945
  electroencephalography in, 946-947, 947*c*
  electromyography in, 946
  evoked potentials in, 947
  in hematologic disorders, 886
  immediate postoperative, 289*t*
  laboratory assessment in, 943
  lumbar puncture in, 947-949, 948*t*
  magnetic resonance imaging in, 945-946
  magnetoencephalography in, 946
  muscle and nerve biopsies in, 949
  patient history in, 935-936, 937*c*
  patient preparation for, 944-945*t*
  physical assessment in, 936-942
    cerebellar function and, 940
    cranial nerve evaluation and, 938
    mental status and, 937*c*, 937-938
    motor function and, 939*f*, 939-940
    rapid neurologic assessment and, 941*f*, 941-942, 942*f*
    reflex activity and, 940*f*, 940-941, 941*f*
    sensory function and, 938-939
  plain x-rays in, 943
  positron emission tomography in, 946
  psychosocial assessment in, 942-943
  rehabilitation and, 97*t*, 98
  single photon emission computed tomography in, 946
  in stroke, 1033*c*, 1033-1034
  transcranial Doppler ultrasonography in, 949
  in traumatic brain injury, 1054-1055
Neurologic deficits
  in brain tumor, 1060
  hemodialysis-related, 1626
  in stroke, 1031, 1031*t*
Neurologic disorders, 927-1068
  Alzheimer's disease in, 21, 969-980
    caregiver role strain in, 978
    chronic confusion in, 974*c*, 974*t*, 974-976, 976*c*
    disturbed sleep pattern in, 977-978
    health care resources for, 979
    health promotion and maintenance in, 970
    health teaching in, 978-979
    history in, 970-971, 971*t*
    home care management of, 978, 978*c*
    imaging studies in, 973
    laboratory assessment in, 973
    nursing diagnoses in, 973-974
    pathophysiology of, 969-970
    physical assessment in, 971-973, 972*c*, 972*f*
    psychosocial assessment in, 973
    risk for injury in, 976-977, 977*t*
  amyotrophic lateral sclerosis in, 1007*c*, 1007-1008
  back pain in, 983-989
    complementary and alternative therapies for, 986
    diagnostic assessment in, 985
    health care resources for, 989
    health teaching in, 988*c*, 988-989
    home care management in, 988
    nonsurgical management of, 985-986, 986*c*
    pathophysiology of, 984
    physical assessment in, 984-985
    prevention of, 984, 984*c*
    surgical management of, 986-988, 987*c*
  cervical neck pain in, 989*f*, 989-990, 990*c*
  facial paralysis in, 1026
  Guillain-Barré syndrome in, 1011-1016, 1012*c*, 1012*t*, 1013*t*, 1014*c*, 1015*c*
  headaches in, 951-955

Neurologic disorders *(Continued)*
cluster headache in, 954-955
migraine in, 951-954, 952*c*, 953*t*, 954*c*, 954*t*
tension headache in, 955
Huntington disease in, 979-980
infections in, 961-965
encephalitis in, 963-965, 964*c*
meningitis in, 961*t*, 961-963, 962*c*, 962*t*, 963*c*
multiple sclerosis in, 1002-1007, 1003*c*
myasthenia gravis in, 1016-1022
community-based care in, 1021*t*, 1021-1022, 1022*c*
electromyography in, 1018
nonsurgical management of, 1018-1020, 1019*t*, 1020*c*
nursing diagnoses in, 1018
pathophysiology of, 1016
physical assessment in, 1-17*c*, 1016-1017
surgical management of, 1020-1021
Parkinson disease in, 965*t*, 965-969, 966*c*, 966*f*, 967*c*
peripheral nerve trauma in, 1022*f*, 1022-1024, 1023*f*
restless legs syndrome in, 1024
seizures and epilepsy in, 955-961
drug therapy for, 957-959, 957-959*c*
emergency care in, 959-961
management of, 959, 959*c*, 960*c*
nursing diagnoses in, 957
pathophysiology of, 955-956
surgical management of, 960-961
spinal cord injury in, 990-1000
etiology of, 992-993
extent of injury in, 991-992, 992*f*
health care resources for, 1000
health teaching in, 999*c*, 999-1000, 1000*c*
history in, 993
home care management in, 999
imaging studies in, 994-995
impaired adjustment in, 998
impaired elimination in, 997-998, 998*c*
impaired gas exchange in, 997
ineffective tissue perfusion in, 995*c*, 995-997, 996*f*
laboratory assessment in, 994
mechanisms of injury in, 990-991, 991*f*
nursing diagnoses in, 995
physical assessment in, 993-994, 994*c*
psychosocial assessment in, 994
self-care deficit in, 997
spinal cord tumor in, 1000-1002, 1001*c*
stroke in, 1030-1049
arteriovenous malformation and, 1044*f*, 1044-1045
atrial fibrillation and, 745-746
carotid artery angioplasty with stenting in, 1044
carotid endarterectomy in, 1045
community-based rehabilitation in, 1048
diastolic blood pressure and, 797
disturbed sensory perception in, 1047
drug therapy for, 1043-1044
etiology and genetic risk for, 1032, 1033*c*
extracranial-intracranial bypass in, 1045
family history of, 936
health care resources for, 1048-1049
health teaching in, 1048, 1048*f*
heat, 142-143, 143*c*
history in, 1032-1033
home care management in, 1047-1048
homocysteine and, 795
in idiopathic thrombocytopenic purpura, 916

Neurologic disorders *(Continued)*
imaging studies in, 1036
impaired physical mobility in, 1046
impaired swallowing in, 1045
impaired verbal communication in, 1046, 1046*t*
ineffective tissue perfusion in, 1036-1037
in infective endocarditis, 784
intracranial pressure monitoring in, 1037*c*, 1037-1043
laboratory assessment in, 1036
migraine headache and, 952
nursing care plan for, 1038-1043
nursing diagnoses in, 1036
pathophysiologic changes in brain and, 1030
physical assessment in, 1033*c*, 1033*f*, 1033-1035, 1034*c*
prevention of, 1032
psychosocial assessment in, 1035-1036
thrombolytic therapy for, 1037, 1037*c*
types of, 1030*f*, 1030-1032, 1031*t*
unilateral neglect in, 1047
urinary and bowel incontinence in, 1047
syndrome of inappropriate antidiuretic hormone secretion and, 1435*t*
traumatic brain injury in, 1049-1060
brain herniation in, 1052, 1053*f*
closed head injury in, 1050, 1050*f*
community-based care in, 1059-1060
drug therapy for, 1057
fluid and electrolyte management in, 1057
hemorrhage in, 1051-1052, 1052*f*
history in, 1053, 1054*c*
hydrocephalus after, 1052
imaging studies in, 1055
incidence and prevalence of, 1052
increased intracranial pressure in, 1051, 1055-1057
laboratory assessment in, 1055
minor head injury in, 1056*c*
nutrition management in, 1057-1058
in older adult, 1054*c*
open head injury in, 1049-1050
pathophysiology of, 1049, 1049*c*
physical assessment in, 1053-1055
prevention of, 1053
psychosocial assessment in, 1055
sensory, cognitive, and behavioral management in, 1058
surgical management in, 1058, 1059*t*
types of force in, 1050*f*, 1050-1051
trigeminal neuralgia in, 1025*f*, 1025-1026
Neurologic positioning in spinal cord injury, 995, 995*c*
Neurologic status
after coronary artery bypass graft, 869
after decompressive laminectomy, 997
in infective endocarditis, 784
in meningitis, 963
preoperative assessment of, 248
Neurologic system
age-related changes in fluid balance and, 174*c*
age-related surgical risks and, 245*c*
alkalosis and, 210, 211*c*
anemia and, 894*c*
chronic kidney disease and, 1612-1613, 1613*c*
cirrhosis and, 1348*f*
dehydration and, 179
diabetes insipidus and, 1433*c*
fluid overload and, 182*c*
hepatitis A and, 1357*t*
hypermagnesemia and, 196
hypernatremia and, 186

Neurologic system *(Continued)*
hyperthyroidism and, 1449*c*
hypocalcemia and, 192
hypokalemia and, 188
hypomagnesemia and, 196
hyponatremia and, 185
hypophosphatemia and, 195
hypothyroidism and, 1456*c*
immobility and, 102*t*
leukemia and, 903*c*, 904
nutrient deficiencies and, 1394*t*
postoperative complications of, 287*t*
premenstrual syndrome and, 1686*c*
sickle cell disease and, 896
systemic lupus erythematosus and, 349
Neurolysis, 57
Neuroma
acoustic, 1129
Morton's, 1173
upper extremity amputation-related, 1200
Neuromuscular blocking agents
for general anesthesia, 272, 274*t*
for traumatic brain injury, 1057
Neuromuscular changes
in acidosis, 207, 207*c*
in adrenal insufficiency, 1437*c*
in alkalosis, 210, 211*c*
in hypercalcemia, 194
in hyperkalemia, 190
in hypermagnesemia, 196
in hypocalcemia, 192
in hypomagnesemia, 196
in hyponatremia, 185
in shock, 829*c*
Neuromuscular scoliosis, 1174
Neuron, 928-929, 929*f*, 930*t*
Neurontin; *See* Gabapentin
Neuropathic pain, 38, 38*t*
Neuropathy, 1011-1028
cast-related, 1189
chemotherapy-related, 430-431, 431*c*
diabetic, 1468, 1469-1470, 1470*t*
chronic pain in, 1504-1505, 1505*c*
foot and, 1501-1503, 1502*c*, 1502*t*, 1503*c*, 1503*f*, 1504*c*
in facial paralysis, 1026
in Guillain-Barré syndrome, 1011-1016, 1012*c*, 1012*t*, 1013*t*, 1014*c*, 1015*c*
musculoskeletal assessment and, 1145
in myasthenia gravis, 1016-1022
community-based care in, 1021*t*, 1021-1022, 1022*c*
electromyography in, 1018
nonsurgical management of, 1018-1020, 1019*t*, 1020*c*
nursing diagnoses in, 1018
pathophysiology of, 1016
physical assessment in, 1-17*c*, 1016-1017
surgical management of, 1020-1021
in peripheral nerve trauma, 1022*f*, 1022-1024, 1023*f*
in restless legs syndrome, 1024
in trigeminal neuralgia, 1025*f*, 1025-1026
Neurotransmitters, 929, 930*t*
Alzheimer's disease and, 970
Neurovascular assessment
after coronary artery bypass graft, 869
after total hip arthroplasty, 331
after total knee arthroplasty, 334
after total shoulder arthroplasty, 335
in musculoskeletal disorders, 1147
in musculoskeletal trauma, 1184*c*
in osteomyelitis, 1167
in peripheral nerve trauma, 1024
Neutralization, antigen-antibody interaction and, 316
Neutropenia
chemotherapy-related, 426, 426*c*
in myelodysplastic syndromes, 901

Neutrophil
functions of, 309*t*, 878*t*
inflammation and, 310*f*, 310-311, 311*t*
Neutrophil count, 565*c*
Neutrophilia, 312
Nevirapine, 377*c*, 379
Nevus, 509
New memory, 938
New York Heart Association classification of cardiovascular disability, 714, 714*t*, 765
New-onset angina, 849
Nexavar; *See* Sorafenib
Nexium; *See* Esomeprazole
NFLD; *See* Nonalcoholic fatty liver disease
NHP; *See* Necrotizing hemorrhagic pancreatitis
Niacin
deficiency of, 1394*t*
to reduce cholesterol levels, 796
Niacin-lovastatin, 796
NIC intervention activities; *See* Intervention activities
Nicardipine, 802
NICHE project, 23
Niclocide; *See* Niclosamide
Niclosamide, 1340
Nicotine abuse, 84-85, 85*f*
Nicotine patch, 85
Nicotinic acid, 1128
Nifedipine
for achalasia, 1255
for primary pulmonary hypertension, 637
for Raynaud's phenomenon, 816
Night blindness, 1102
Night sweats
in menopause, 1689
in tuberculosis, 669
Nilandron; *See* Nilutamide
Nilutamide, 1723
Nimbex; *See* Cisatracurium
Ninth nerve neurectomy, 58*f*
Nipent; *See* Pentostatin
Nipple, 1669
Nipride; *See* Nitroprusside
Nitrates
for achalasia, 1255
for coronary artery disease, 857*c*
for heart failure, 863-864*c*
inhalation abuse of, 91
to reduce preload in heart failure, 773
in urine, 1541
Nitric acid, 930*t*
Nitrofurantoin
for pyelonephritis, 1588
for urinary tract infection, 1557*c*, 1558
Nitrofurazone, 542*c*
Nitroglycerin
for acute myocardial infarction, 856, 857*c*
for heart failure, 863*c*
for pulmonary edema, 775-776
Nitroglycerin patch, 857*c*
Nitrolingual translingual spray, 857*c*, 872
Nitropress; *See* Nitroprusside
Nitroprusside
for heart failure, 863*c*
for hypertensive crisis, 802
for hypovolemic shock, 837*c*, 838
for pulmonary embolism, 682
Nitrous oxide, 274*t*
Nizatidine
for gastritis, 1268
for gastroesophageal reflux disease, 1246*c*, 1247-1248
for gastrointestinal protection in Cushing's disease, 1444
for peptic ulcer disease, 1269*c*, 1274
Nizoral; *See* Ketoconazole
NMDA antagonists, 55
NNRT; *See* National Nurse Response Team

NNRTIs; *See* Non-nucleoside analog reverse transcriptase inhibitors
Nociceptive pain, 38, 38*t*
Nociceptor, 38
Nocturia, 1534*c*, 1535*t*, 1536
in benign prostatic hypertrophy, 1713
endocrine system and, 1421
hospitalized older adult and, 24
in hyperaldosteronism, 1446
in polycystic kidney disease, 1583
preoperative assessment of, 247
in prostate cancer, 1720
Nocturnal penile tumescence test, 1726
Nocturnal polyuria, 1533
Nodal osteoarthritis, 323
Node of Ranvier, 929, 929*f*
Nodule, 469*f*
in cirrhosis, 1345
vocal cord, 595, 595*c*, 595*f*
No-lift policy, 100
Nolvadex; *See* Tamoxifen citrate
Nonabsorbable sutures, 281-282, 282*f*
Nonalcoholic fatty liver disease, 1360-1361
Nonalcoholic steatohepatitis, 1360-1361
Noncardiogenic pulmonary edema, 686-689, 687*t*
Non-cardioselective beta blockers, 802
Noncompliance, infection control and, 449
Noncoring port access needle, 219
Non-English speaking patient, 29, 29*c*
preoperative informed consent and, 254
Non-germ cell tumor, 127, 1727*t*
Non-heart-beating kidney donor, 1631
Non-Hodgkin's lymphoma, 914-915
Noninfectious cystitis, 1552-1553
Noninfectious lower respiratory problems, 609-652
asthma in, 610-621
drug therapy in, 615-621, 616-618*c*
exercise and activity in, 621
health teaching in, 613-615, 615*c*
history in, 612
laboratory assessment in, 612
oxygen therapy in, 621
pathophysiology of, 610-611, 611*f*
physical assessment in, 612, 614*f*
smoking cessation and, 614*c*
status asthmaticus and, 621
step system in, 613*c*
subcutaneous infusion therapy in, 237*t*
surgical risk and, 246
bronchiolitis obliterans organizing pneumonia in, 641
chronic obstructive pulmonary disease in, 621-635
activity intolerance in, 633
anxiety in, 633
complications of, 623, 623*c*
health care resources in, 634, 634*c*
health teaching in, 634
history in, 624
home care management in, 634
imaging studies, 627
imbalanced nutrition: less than body requirements in, 632-633
impaired gas exchange in, 628-630, 629*c*
ineffective airway clearance in, 631-632, 632*f*, 633*t*
ineffective breathing pattern in, 630-631, 631*c*
laboratory assessment in, 626-627
nursing diagnoses in, 628
pathophysiology of, 621*f*, 621-623, 623*t*, 632*f*
physical assessment in, 624*f*, 624-626, 626*f*
pneumonia and respiratory infection risks in, 633
prevention of, 624
psychosocial assessment in, 626
Noninfectious lower respiratory problems *(Continued)*
pulmonary function tests in, 627, 627*t*
cystic fibrosis in, 635-637
idiopathic pulmonary fibrosis in, 639
lung cancer in, 641-650
history in, 642-643, 643*t*
nonsurgical management of, 644-645
palliation in, 650, 650*c*
pathophysiology of, 641-642
physical assessment in, 643-644
prevention of, 642
psychosocial assessment in, 644
surgical management of, 645-649, 646*f*, 647*f*, 648*c*
occupational pulmonary disease in, 639-641, 640*c*
primary pulmonary hypertension in, 637-638, 638*t*
sarcoidosis in, 638-639
Noninfectious upper respiratory problems, 590-608
epistaxis in, 591-592, 592*c*, 592*f*
facial trauma in, 593-594
head and neck cancer in, 597-606
anxiety in, 604
assessment in, 598*t*, 598-599
disturbed body image in, 604
health care resources in, 606
health teaching in, 605*c*, 605-606, 606*f*
home care management in, 605, 605*c*
nursing diagnoses in, 599
pathophysiology of, 597-598
psychosocial preparation for, 606
respiratory obstruction in, 599-602, 600*t*, 601*f*, 603*f*
risk for aspiration in, 603*c*, 603-604, 604*c*
laryngeal trauma in, 596
nasal fracture in, 590-591, 591*f*
nasal polyps in, 592
neck trauma in, 596-597
nose and sinus tumors in, 592-593
obstructive sleep apnea in, 594
upper airway obstruction in, 596, 597*f*
vocal cord nodules and polyps in, 595, 595*c*, 595*f*
vocal cord paralysis in, 591-595
Noninflammatory intestinal disorders, 1289-1314
abdominal herniation in, 1291-1293, 1292*f*
abdominal trauma in, 1307-1308
colorectal cancer in, 1293-1302
anticipatory grieving in, 1296, 1297*c*
drug therapy in, 1297
health care resources for, 1302
health promotion and maintenance in, 1294-1295, 1295*c*
health teaching in, 1300-1302, 1301*c*
history in, 1295
home management in, 1300
imaging studies in, 1296
laboratory assessment in, 1295-1296
metastasis in, 1296
nursing diagnoses in, 1296
pathophysiology of, 1293-1294, 1294*f*
physical assessment in, 1295
psychosocial assessment in, 1295
radiation therapy in, 1297
surgical management of, 1297*t*, 1297-1300, 1298*t*, 1299*f*, 1300*c*
hemorrhoids in, 1309*f*, 1309-1310
intestinal obstruction in, 1302-1306, 1303*f*, 1304*c*, 1306*c*
intestinal polyps in, 1308-1309, 1309*f*
irritable bowel syndrome in, 1289-1291, 1290*f*
malabsorption syndrome in, 1311-1312, 1312*c*
Noninvasive breast cancer, 1663
Noninvasive positive-pressure ventilation, 578, 578*f*
Noninvasive temporary pacing, 754-755
Nonmechanical obstruction, 1302
Nonmodifiable risk factors
for cardiovascular disease, 709
for coronary artery disease, 850
Non-nodal osteoarthritis, 323
Non-nucleoside analog reverse transcriptase inhibitors, 363, 377*c*, 379
Nonoccupational postexposure prophylaxis to HIV, 368*c*
Non-opioid analgesics, 45, 45*t*
Nonpharmacologic pain management, 55-57, 56*f*, 299*c*
Nonpitting edema, 472*t*
Nonpressure eye patch, 1088*c*
Nonprogressive stage of shock, 831-832
Nonproliferative diabetic retinopathy, 1469, 1469*t*
Non-rebreather mask, 575*t*, 575-576, 576*f*
Non-small cell lung cancer, 641
Nonspecific eczematous dermatitis, 505, 505*c*
Non-ST-elevation myocardial infarction, 855
Nonsteroidal antiinflammatory drugs
for acquired immunodeficiency syndrome, 380
acute gastritis risk and, 1266
for asthma, 618*c*, 620
for carpal tunnel syndrome, 1207
for dysmenorrhea, 1685
for endometriosis, 1687
for fibromyalgia, 358
gastrointestinal assessment and, 1219
heart failure and, 767
hematologic assessment and, 884
for low back pain, 985
for migraine headache, 952, 953*t*
nephrotoxic, 1603*t*
for ocular inflammation, 1086*c*
for osteoarthritis, 326
ototoxic, 1114*t*
for pain, 45-46
peptic ulcer disease risk and, 1272
for pericarditis, 786
for postoperative pain, 297-299
for rheumatoid arthritis, 341*c*, 343
for tension headache, 955
as trigger for asthma, 611
Nonsustained ventricular tachycardia, 747
Nontunneled percutaneous central catheter, 218, 225
Nonunion, 1183, 1192
Nonurgent triage category, 132, 132*t*
Nonverbal communication, 29
Non-weight-bearing pelvic fracture, 1198
Norcuron; *See* Vecuronium
Norepinephrine, 930*t*, 1416
Alzheimer's disease and, 970
for anaphylaxis, 393*c*
for cardiac arrest, 752, 753*c*
glucose homeostasis and, 1467
for hypovolemic shock, 837*c*, 838
Norfloxacin
for gastroenteritis, 1320
for urinary tract infection, 1556*c*
Normal adult blood pressure, 796, 796*t*
Normal flora, 440, 441*t*
Normal heart sounds, 718
Normal saline
for hypovolemic shock, 837
for trauma patient, 138
Normal sinus rhythm, 737, 737*f*
Normiflo; *See* Ardeparin
Normodyne; *See* Labetalol
Normotonic fluids, 174
Noroxin; *See* Norfloxacin
Norpace; *See* Disopyramide
North American pit vipers, 144-145, 145*f*
Nortriptyline
for diabetic neuropathy, 1504
for fibromyalgia, 358
for pain, 54, 54*t*
for urinary incontinence, 1565*c*
Norvir; *See* Ritonavir
Norwalk virus gastroenteritis, 1319*t*
Nose, 553*f*, 553-554
fracture of, 590-591, 591*f*
inspection of, 559
rhinitis and, 654
tumor of, 592-593
Nosebleed, 396, 591-592, 592*c*, 592*f*
Nosocomial infections, 444
after thoracic aortic aneurysm repair, 813
health and hygiene of surgical team and, 270
pneumonia in, 659, 659*t*
Nostril, 553*f*
Notification and activation of emergency preparedness plan, 161-162
Novantrone; *See* Mitoxantrone
Novelty diet, 1405
Novodigoxin; *See* Digoxin
Novo-Dipam; *See* Diazepam
Novo-Hydroxyzin; *See* Hydroxyzine
Novolin, 1485*t*
NovoLog, 1485*t*
Novo-Lorazem; *See* Lorazepam
Novomethacin; *See* Indomethacin
Novonidazole; *See* Metronidazole
Novopentobarb; *See* Pentobarbital sodium
Novopheniram; *See* Chlorpheniramine
Novo-Profen; *See* Ibuprofen
Novo-Propamide; *See* Chlorpropamide
Novosemide; *See* Furosemide
Novospiroton; *See* Spironolactone
NPO status, 254
NPRT; *See* National Pharmacist Response Team
NPSGs; *See* National Patient Safety Goals
NSAIDs; *See* Nonsteroidal antiinflammatory drugs
NSVT; *See* Nonsustained ventricular tachycardia
N-teleopeptide, 1156
NTP; *See* Noninvasive temporary pacing
NTX; *See* N-teleopeptide
N-type calcium channel blockers, 988
Nuchal rigidity
in meningitis, 962
in traumatic brain injury, 1056
Nuclear, biologic, and chemical threats, 160
Nuclear envelope, 63*f*
Nuclear scan, 1149
Nucleic acid amplification test
in chlamydial infection, 1747
in gonorrhea, 1745-1746
Nucleokinesis, 65*f*
Nucleolus, 63*f*
Nucleoside, 64, 64*f*
Nucleoside analog reverse transcriptase inhibitors, 363, 376-377*c*, 379
Nucleosome, 63*f*
Nucleotide, 63-64, 64*f*
Nucleus, 63, 63*f*
Nulliparity
breast cancer and, 1664, 1665*t*
fallopian tube cancer and, 1709
Numeric pain distress scale, 43, 43*f*
Numorphan, 48
Nurse
advocacy role of, 5
as caregiver, 4
in coordination of patient care, 5
in emergency and disaster, 163-164, 164*t*
in genetic counseling, 77-78
rehabilitation, 96, 96*t*
substance abuse and, 82

Nurses Improving Care for Health System Elders project, 23
Nursing, transcultural, 27
Nursing assistant on rehabilitation team, 96
Nursing care plan
for gastrectomy, 1282-1285
for open conventional esophageal surgery, 1250-1253
for stroke, 1038-1043
Nursing competencies, 3-6
collaboration with interdisciplinary health care team and, 5
evidence-based practice and, 5-6, 6*t*
informatics and, 6, 6*f*
patient-centered care and, 3-5, 4*c*
in peaceful death, 112*t*
quality improvement and, 6
Nursing diagnoses
in acidosis, 209
in acquired immunodeficiency syndrome, 374-375
in acute coronary syndromes, 855-856
in acute pancreatitis, 1375
in acute renal failure, 1604
in acute respiratory distress syndrome, 688
in Alzheimer's disease, 973-974
in benign prostatic hypertrophy, 1714
in bladder cancer, 1576
in bone cancer, 1169
in breast cancer, 1671
in burn
acute phase and, 537-538
emergent/resuscitation phase and, 532-533
in cardiac dysrhythmias, 750
in cataract, 1092-1093
in chronic kidney disease, 1615
in chronic obstructive pulmonary disease, 628
in cirrhosis, 1350
in colorectal cancer, 1296
in Cushing's disease, 1442
in cystitis, 1555
in deep vein thrombosis, 818
in dehydration, 179
in diabetes mellitus, 1475
in esophageal cancer, 1257
in fluid overload, 182
in fracture, 1185-1186
in gastritis, 1267
in gastroesophageal reflux disease, 1245
in Guillain-Barré syndrome, 1013
in head and neck cancer, 599
in hearing loss, 1131-1132
in heart failure, 770
in hypernatremia, 186
in hyperpituitarism, 1430
in hypertension, 799
in hyperthyroidism, 1452
in hypocalcemia, 193
in hypokalemia, 188
in hypothyroidism, 1457-1458
in hypovolemic shock, 835
in infectious disease, 451
in intraoperative care, 279-280
in leukemia, 904
in malnutrition, 1394
in mechanical ventilation, 689
in migraine headache, 952
in multiple sclerosis, 1004
in myasthenia gravis, 1018
in oral cancer, 1235-1236
in osteoarthritis, 325-326
in osteomyelitis, 1166
in osteoporosis, 1157
in oxygen therapy, 572
in Parkinson disease, 967
in pelvic inflammatory disease, 1749
in peptic ulcer disease, 1274
in pneumonia, 663-664
in polycystic kidney disease, 1584
in postoperative care, 293-294
Nursing diagnoses *(Continued)*
in preoperative care, 252
in pressure ulcer, 491
in prostate cancer, 1721
in psoriasis, 506-507
in pulmonary embolism, 679-680
in pyelonephritis, 1588
in rehabilitation, 99
in seizures and epilepsy, 957
in sexually transmitted diseases, 1741*t*
in sickle cell disease, 896
in spinal cord injury, 995
in stroke, 1036
in testicular cancer, 1728
in tracheostomy, 580
in tuberculosis, 669
in ulcerative colitis, 1323
in urinary incontinence, 1563
in uterine leiomyoma, 1695-1696
in valvular heart disease, 781
Nursing process, 4
Nursing research, 6
Nutrient deficiencies, 1394*t*
Nutrition, 1386-1410
after esophageal cancer, 1261
after ileostomy, 1329*c*
Braden Scale for pressure ulcer risk and, 487*f*
burn patient and, 543
culture and, 31
cystic fibrosis and, 636
health promotion and maintenance and, 1386-1387, 1387*t*, 1388*f*, 1389*f*
malabsorption syndrome and, 1311-1312
malnutrition and, 1392-1402
community-based care in, 1401-1402
drug therapy for, 1395-1396
history in, 1393
intervention activities for, 1395*c*
laboratory assessment in, 1393-1394
nursing diagnoses in, 1394
nutrition management in, 1395
older adult and, 1393*c*, 1395, 1396*c*
parenteral nutrition in, 1400-1401, 1401*c*
pathophysiology of, 1392
physical assessment in, 1393, 1394*t*
psychosocial assessment in, 1393
total enteral nutrition in, 1396-1400, 1397*f*, 1398*c*
myasthenia gravis and, 1020, 1020*c*
nutritional assessment and, 1387-1392
anthropometric measurements in, 1389-1392
initial nutritional screening and, 1389, 1390*c*, 1391*f*
nutritional status in, 1388-1389
obesity and, 1402-1408
behavioral management in, 1405-1406
community-based care in, 1408, 1408*c*
complementary and alternative therapies for, 1406
complications of, 1402-1403, 1403*t*
diet programs for, 1404-1405
drug therapy for, 1405
etiology and genetic risk for, 1403
exercise program for, 1405
heart disease risk and, 710-711
history in, 1403-1404
nutrition therapy for, 1405
pathophysiology of, 1402
prevention of, 1403, 1403*t*
psychosocial assessment in, 1404
surgical management of, 1406*f*, 1406-1407
older adult and, 16-17, 23
osteoporosis and, 1154
Parkinson disease and, 968
premenstrual syndrome and, 1686
Nutrition *(Continued)*
pressure ulcer prevention and, 485*c*
rehabilitation and, 104
risk for infection and, 441*t*
tracheostomy and, 586, 586*c*
traumatic brain injury and, 1057-1058
Nutrition history
in acidosis, 206
in cardiovascular assessment, 712
in dehydration, 178
in endocrine assessment, 1420-1421
in gastrointestinal assessment, 1219-1221
in musculoskeletal assessment, 1144
in obesity, 1404
in ocular problems, 1077
in renal assessment, 1535
in reproductive assessment, 1647
in skin problems, 467
Nutrition therapy
in acquired immunodeficiency syndrome, 380
in acute renal failure, 1607
in acute respiratory distress syndrome, 689
after abdominal surgery, 1318-1319
after laryngectomy, 602
in atherosclerosis, 795
in cancer, 415
in chronic kidney disease, 1615-1618, 1617*c*, 1617*t*
in chronic obstructive pulmonary disease, 633
in cirrhosis, 1352, 1354, 1355*c*
in Crohn's disease, 1332
in Cushing's disease, 1443
in cystitis, 1558
in diabetes mellitus, 1492-1495, 1494*t*, 1495*t*
in diverticulitis, 1335
in esophageal cancer, 1257, 1258*c*
in fluid overload, 182
in gastroesophageal reflux disease, 1245
in gout, 354
in heart failure, 778
in hypernatremia, 187
in hypocalcemia, 193
in hypoglycemia, 1508, 1508*c*
in hypokalemia, 189
in hyponatremia, 186
in hypophosphatemia, 195, 195*c*
in leukemia, 911
in obesity, 1405
in osteoporosis, 1157
in peptic ulcer disease, 1275
in portal-systemic encephalopathy, 1354
in pressure ulcer, 493
in pyelonephritis, 1588
to reduce preload, 772
in renal stones, 1574, 1574*t*
in rheumatoid arthritis, 345
in ulcerative colitis, 1325
in urge incontinence, 1567
in urinary incontinence, 1564
Nutritional assessment, 1387-1392
anthropometric measurements in, 1389-1392
initial nutritional screening and, 1389, 1390*c*, 1391*f*
nutritional status in, 1388-1389
rehabilitation and, 97*t*, 97-98
Nutritional screening, 1389, 1390*c*, 1391*f*
Nutritional status, 1388-1389
acquired immunodeficiency syndrome and, 380
aging and, 16-17
hematologic assessment and, 884
preoperative assessment of, 248
pressure ulcer prevention and, 486
respiratory assessment and, 559
socioeconomic status and, 1221
stomatitis and, 1233
Nutritional supplements for older adult, 1395*c*
Nutritionist on rehabilitation team, 96
Nutrition-metabolic pattern
in cardiovascular assessment, 711*c*
in dehydration, 178*c*
in endocrine assessment, 1420*c*
in gastrointestinal assessment, 1220*c*
in hematologic assessment, 882*c*
in renal assessment, 1534*c*
Nystagmus, 1078-1079
in labyrinthitis, 1127
in multiple sclerosis, 1004
vertigo and, 1126
Nystatin, 1233

O

OA; *See* Osteoarthritis
Obesity, 1402-1408
abdominal hernia and, 1292
behavioral management in, 1405-1406
breast cancer risk and, 1665*t*
community-based care in, 1408, 1408*c*
complementary and alternative therapies for, 1406
complications of, 1402-1403, 1403*t*
coronary artery disease and, 852, 854*c*
diet programs for, 1404-1405
drug therapy for, 1405
etiology and genetic risk for, 1403
exercise program for, 1405
gastroesophageal reflux disease and, 1246
heart disease risk and, 710-711
history in, 1403-1404
nutrition therapy for, 1405
osteoarthritis and, 323
pathophysiology of, 1402
preoperative assessment of, 248
prevention of, 1403, 1403*t*
psychosocial assessment in, 1404
surgical management of, 1406*f*, 1406-1407
type 2 diabetes mellitus and, 1472
Obligatory solute excretion, 1542
Obligatory urine output, 175
Oblique fracture, 1179*f*
Obstetric history, 1648
Obstipation, 1304
Obstruction
airway
after extubation, 697
in burn injury, 529, 529*t*, 535
in cancer, 417
in facial trauma, 593
in head and neck cancer, 599-602, 600*t*, 601*f*, 603*f*
respiratory acidosis and, 206
upper, 596, 597*f*
in vocal cord paralysis, 594
intestinal, 1302-1306, 1303*f*, 1304*c*, 1306*c*
in colorectal cancer, 1295
in inflammatory bowel disease, 1322*t*
in strangulated hernia, 1292
pyloric, 1272
of tracheostomy tube, 580
urinary
acute renal failure and, 1601
in hydronephrosis and hydroureter, 1585*f*, 1585-1586
in urinary tract infection, 1551*t*
in urolithiasis, 1574*t*, 1574-1575, 1575*c*
Obstructive jaundice, 1346*t*, 1367
Obstructive shock, 828*t*, 830
causes of, 830*c*
risk factors in older adult, 841*c*
Obstructive sleep apnea, 594, 1244
Occipital lobe, 931*t*
Occipital lymph nodes, 1235*f*
Occipital-to-posterior inferior cerebellar artery bypass, 1045

Occlusive dressing, 822
Occult blood test, 291
Occupational exposure to infection, 449
Occupational history
in cardiovascular assessment, 712
in musculoskeletal trauma, 1184
in respiratory assessment, 556
Occupational pulmonary disease, 639-641, 640*c*
Occupational Safety and Health Administration, 449
Occupational therapist, 96
Occupational therapy
after amputation, 1203
for pain management, 55
Occupational therapy assistant, 96
Octreotide
for acromegaly, 1431
for acute pancreatitis prevention, 1373
for chronic pancreatitis, 1378
for dumping syndrome, 1285
for esophageal varices, 1353
for gastrointestinal bleeding, 1277
for sulfonylurea-induced hypoglycemia, 1509
for Zollinger-Ellison syndrome, 1279
Ocu-Caine; *See* Proxymetacaine
Ocu-Carpine; *See* Pilocarpine
Ocufen; *See* Flurbiprofen
Ocuflox; *See* Ofloxacin
Ocular assessment, 1070-1083
anatomy and physiology review in, 1070-1074, 1071-1074*f*, 1073*t*
changes associated with aging and, 1074, 1075*c*, 1075*f*
corneal staining in, 1079-1080
electroretinography in, 1082
fluorescein angiography in, 1081*c*, 1081-1082
health promotion and maintenance and, 1074-1075, 1076*c*
imaging studies in, 1079
inspection in, 1077
laboratory assessment in, 1079
ophthalmoscopy in, 1080-1081, 1081*f*, 1081*t*
patient history in, 1075-1077, 1076*c*, 1076*t*
psychosocial assessment in, 1079
slit-lamp examination in, 1079, 1080*f*
tonometry in, 1080, 1080*f*
vision testing in, 1077-1079, 1078*f*, 1079*f*
Ocular compress, 1087*c*
Ocular irrigation, 1104*c*
Ocular melanoma, 1104-1106
Ocular muscles, 1072, 1073*f*, 1073*t*, 1075*c*
Ocular problems, 1084-1108
application of eye patch for, 1088*c*
application of ocular compress for, 1087*c*
blepharitis in, 1084-1085
cataracts in, 1091*f*, 1091-1095, 1092*f*, 1092*t*, 1094*f*, 1095*c*
chalazion in, 1087
conjunctival hemorrhage in, 1087
conjunctivitis in, 1087-1088
contusion of eye in, 1103
corneal abrasion, ulceration, and infection in, 1089
drug therapy for inflammation and infection of eye, 1086*c*
ectropion in, 1085
entropion in, 1085, 1085*c*, 1085*f*
foreign body in eye in, 1103-1104
glaucoma in, 1095*t*, 1095-1098, 1099-1100*c*
hordeolum in, 1085-1087
hyphema in, 1103
insertion and removal of ocular prosthesis, 1105*c*
instillation of ophthalmic ointment and, 1085*c*
irrigation of eye in, 1104*c*
Ocular problems *(Continued)*
keratoconjunctivitis sicca in, 1087
keratoconus and corneal opacities in, 1089*f*, 1089-1091, 1090*f*, 1091*t*
laceration of eye in, 1104
macular degeneration in, 1100-1101
ocular melanoma in, 1104-1106
penetrating injury of eye in, 1104
prevention of, 1074-1075
promotion of independent living in patient with impaired vision, 1098*c*
reduced vision in, 1106*c*, 1106-1107
refractive errors in, 1102-1103
retinal holes, tears, and detachments in, 1101-1102, 1102*f*
retinitis pigmentosa in, 1102
trachoma in, 1088
uveitis in, 1100
vitreous hemorrhage in, 1098-1100
Ocular prosthesis, 1105*c*
Oculomotor nerve, 935*t*, 1072
Ocupress; *See* Carteolol
Ocusert; *See* Pilocarpine
Odor of urine, 1539*t*
Odynophagia
in esophageal cancer, 1256
in gastroesophageal reflux disease, 1245
in pharyngitis, 655, 656*c*
Off-pump coronary artery bypass, 870
Ofloxacin
for chlamydial infection, 1747
for leprosy, 516
for ocular infection, 1086*c*
for urinary tract infection, 1556*c*
OGTT; *See* Oral glucose tolerance test
OKT3, 320
OKT4 positive T-cell, 317
Older adult, 15-26
acid-base imbalance in, 205*c*
acute pancreatitis in, 1373
alcohol-related problems and, 83
Alzheimer's disease in, 21, 969-980
caregiver role strain in, 978
chronic confusion in, 974*c*, 974*t*, 974-976, 976*c*
disturbed sleep pattern in, 977-978
health care resources for, 979
health promotion and maintenance in, 970
health teaching in, 978-979
history in, 970-971, 971*t*
home care management of, 978, 978*c*
imaging studies in, 973
laboratory assessment in, 973
nursing diagnoses in, 973-974
pathophysiology of, 969-970
physical assessment in, 971-973, 972*c*, 972*f*
psychosocial assessment in, 973
risk for injury in, 976-977, 977*t*
antiepileptic drugs and, 958
appendicitis in, 1316
asthma in, 612
benign prostatic hypertrophy in, 1717
body mass index of, 1390
bone healing in, 1180
bowel preparation in, 1543
burn injury and
cardiac output and, 534
complications of, 529*c*
cancer in
breast, 1668-1669
hematologic assessment in, 409, 409*c*
nausea and vomiting and, 428
oral, 1238*c*
cardiovascular changes in, 710*c*
cerumen impaction in, 1123*c*
changes in ear and hearing, 1111, 1112*c*
cholecystitis in, 1368
chronic respiratory disorder in, 610
Older adult *(Continued)*
complex partial seizure in, 956
coronary artery disease in
chest pain and, 854
coronary artery bypass graft surgery and, 871*c*
nursing focus on, 861*c*
silent myocardial ischemia and, 856
delirium in, 21-22, 22*t*
dementia in, 21
depression in, 20-21, 21*f*
diabetes mellitus in
diabetic retinopathy and, 1469
dietary considerations in, 1495
exercise and, 1497
hyperglycemic-hyperosmolar state and, 1512
hypoglycemia and, 1509
diverticulitis in, 1335
driving safety and, 18, 19*c*
drug use and misuse in, 18-20, 19*t*, 20*f*
dysrhythmias in, 760*c*
elder neglect and abuse and, 22*c*, 22-23
endocrine changes in, 1419*c*
end-stage kidney disease in, 1626
eye and vision changes in, 1075*c*
fall prevention and, 18, 129
fecal impaction in, 1306*c*
fluid and electrolyte imbalances in
body systems and, 174*c*
dehydration and, 177
normal plasma electrolyte values and, 184*t*
skin turgor and, 179, 179*f*
total body water and, 183
food pyramid for, 1387
gastrointestinal changes in, 1220*c*
health care issues in hospitals and, 23-25, 24*c*
health teaching and, 4*c*
heart failure in
cardiac drug selection and dosing considerations and, 773
diuretics for, 772
drug-induced, 767
Healthy People 2010 objectives and, 767, 768*t*
thyroid function tests in, 769
hematologic assessment in, 882*c*
herpes zoster in, 501
hip fracture in, 1195-1196
hypothyroidism in, 1457, 1458*c*
immune function of, 308*c*
impaired vision in, 1098*c*
infection in
Clostridium difficile, 455
human immunodeficiency virus, 366
methicillin-resistant *Staphylococcus aureus*, 448
pneumonia in, 661
risk for, 442*c*
urinary tract, 1553
infusion therapy for, 235-236, 236*f*
integumentary system of, 463-464*c*
iron deficiency anemia in, 899
lifestyles and practices to promote wellness in, 16, 16*c*
low back pain in, 984*c*
malnutrition in, 1392, 1393*c*, 1395, 1396*c*
mobility issues and, 17, 17*f*
musculoskeletal changes in, 1143*c*
neurologic changes in, 933-936, 936*c*
nutrition problems in, 16-17
oral candidiasis in, 1232
osteoarthritis in, 323
osteoporosis in, 1155
pain and, 39, 40*c*, 44
peritonitis in, 1335
pressure ulcer in, 25, 485
psychosocial preparation for illness and, 1681
rehabilitation and, 104*c*
Older adult *(Continued)*
renal changes in, 1534*c*
reproductive changes in, 1646*c*
respiratory system of, 557*c*
risk factors for shock, 841*c*
stress and loss and, 17-18, 18*c*
substance abuse in, 82
surgery and
intraoperative nursing interventions and, 279*c*
postoperative neurologic function and, 289
postoperative skin care and, 295*c*
preoperative assessment of fluid status and, 255
risks for surgical complications in, 245, 245*c*
total hip arthroplasty in, 330*c*
tracheostomy care and, 587
transfusion in, 919*c*
traumatic brain injury in, 1054*c*
urinary incontinence in, 1561, 1562*c*
ventilator dependence and, 697
wound healing and, 484
Olecranon fracture, 1195
Olfactory nerve, 935*t*
Oligomenorrhea, 1440
Oligospermia, 1728
Oliguria, 1535*t*
in acute renal failure, 1601, 1602*t*, 1603
after renal transplantation, 1632
preoperative assessment of, 247
in urolithiasis, 1572
Olsalazine, 1325*t*
Olympic tracheostomy button, 587
Omalizumab, 618*c*, 620-621
Omega-3 fatty acids
coronary artery disease and, 851
for osteoarthritis, 328
to reduce cholesterol levels, 796
for rheumatoid arthritis, 345
Omega-6 fatty acids, 328
Omentectomy, 1709
Omeprazole
for gastritis, 1268
for gastroesophageal reflux disease, 1247*c*, 1248
for gastrointestinal protection in Cushing's disease, 1444
for peptic ulcer disease, 1269*c*, 1274
for Zollinger-Ellison syndrome, 1279
Oncaspar; *See* Pegaspargase
Oncofetal antigens, 1223, 1224*c*
Oncogene, 402, 407
Oncogenesis, 403*t*, 403-405, 404*f*, 404*t*, 405*t*
Oncogenic osteomalacia, 1161
Oncologic emergencies, 434-437
hypercalcemia in, 436
sepsis and disseminated intravascular coagulation in, 435
spinal cord compression in, 436
superior vena cava syndrome in, 436*f*, 436-437
syndrome of inappropriate antidiuretic hormone secretion in, 435-436
tumor lysis syndrome in, 437, 437*f*
Oncology Nursing Society, 214
Oncovin; *See* Vincristine
Oncoviruses, 408, 408*t*
Ondansetron
for chemotherapy-induced nausea and vomiting, 429*c*
for postoperative nausea and vomiting, 290
100,000 Lives Campaign, 3, 3*t*
ON-Q local anesthesia infusion pump, 55
Onycholysis, 473
Oophorectomy, prophylactic, 1669
Oophoritis, 1748
Oozing skin, 470*f*
Opacity, corneal, 1089*f*, 1089-1091, 1090*f*, 1091*t*

Opana; *See* Numorphan
Open carpal tunnel release, 1207
Open commissurotomy, 782
Open conventional esophageal surgery, 1250-1253
Open fracture, 1179, 1179*f*
Open head injury, 1049-1050
Open lung biopsy, 569
Open magnetic resonance imaging, 946
Open radical prostatectomy, 1722, 1722*c*
Open reduction and internal fixation, 1190-1192, 1191*f*
in femoral fracture, 1197
in hip fracture, 1196*f*
Open retroperitoneal lymph node dissection, 1730
Open rhizotomy, 57
Open skull fracture, 1050
Open-chest cardiac massage, 758
Operating room preparation, 267-270, 268*f*
Operating room technician, 265
Ophthalmic artery, 1072
Ophthalmic ointment, 1085*c*
Ophthalmoscope, 1080
Ophthalmoscopy, 1080-1081, 1081*f*, 1081*t*
Ophthetic; *See* Proxymetacaine
Opioid analgesics, 45*t*, 46-51
abuse of, 81, 81*t*, 90*t*, 90-91, 91*c*
for black widow spider bite, 148
for burn pain, 536
for cholecystitis, 1369
emergency care of overdose of, 299*c*
in end-of-life care, 49, 116-117
equianalgesic chart for, 46, 47*t*
for frostbite, 154
for general anesthesia, 272, 274*t*
for osteoarthritis, 326
for pain in acquired immunodeficiency syndrome, 380
patient-controlled, 51*f*, 51-52
in pit viper envenomation, 145
for postoperative pain, 297-298*c*, 297-299
preoperative, 261
PRN range orders for, 51
routes of administration, 49-51, 50-51*t*
side effects of, 48-49, 49*t*
substance abuser and, 82
for traumatic brain injury, 1057
Opioid receptor, 48
Opium, 90, 90*t*
Opportunistic infections, 364, 370-372, 371*c*
Oprelvekin, 433*t*
Opsonins, 312
Optic blood vessels, 1072, 1081*t*
Optic disc, 1071, 1071*f*, 1081*t*
Optic fundus, 1071, 1071*f*, 1081*t*
Optic nerve, 1071*f*, 1072, 1072*f*
functions of, 935*t*
hyperthyroidism and, 1450
imaging in glaucoma, 1097
OptiPranolol; *See* Metipranolol
Oral administration
in chemotherapy, 423*t*
of opioid analgesics, 50*t*
Oral blood glucose-lowering agents, 1477-1483*c*
Oral cavity, 1217, 1231-1242
acute sialadenitis and, 1239-1240
cancer of, 1234-1239, 1235*f*, 1236*c*, 1238*c*
maintenance of healthy mouth and, 1232*c*
oral tumors and, 1234
postirradiation sialadenitis and, 1240
premalignant lesions of, 1234
salivary gland tumor and, 1240
stomatitis and, 1231-1234, 1233*c*, 1233*f*
Oral contraceptives
breast cancer risk and, 1665*t*
for premenstrual syndrome, 1686
secondary hypertension and, 798
Oral food challenge, 390
Oral glucose tolerance test, 1473*t*, 1474, 1474*c*
Oral hygiene
in acquired immunodeficiency syndrome, 380
after facial trauma, 593
chemotherapy-related mucositis and, 424, 428, 429*c*
dementia patient and, 1232
in mucositis, 645
in oral cancer, 1236
tracheostomy and, 585
Oral rehydration therapy
after ileostomy, 1327
in dehydration, 180
in heat exhaustion, 142
Oral transmucosal fentanyl citrate, 50*t*
Oral tumor, 1234
Oramorph; *See* Morphine, controlled release
Orbit, 1070
Orbital trauma, 1103-1104
Orbital-zygoma fracture, 593
Orchiectomy
in epididymitis, 1734
in prostate cancer, 1721
in testicular cancer, 1729
Orchitis, 1647, 1734
Orencia; *See* Abatacept
Orexins, 1402
Organ of Corti, 1110*f*
Organic brain syndrome, 21
Organic erectile dysfunction, 1725
Organidin; *See* Guaifenesin
Organs
in abdomen, 1222*t*
catecholamine receptors and, 1416*t*
Orientation
Alzheimer's disease and, 975
assessment of, 938
ORIF; *See* Open reduction and internal fixation
Orinase; *See* Tolbutamide
Orlistat, 1405
Oropharyngeal airway, 756
Oropharynx, 553*f*, 554
pharyngitis and, 655-657, 656*c*, 656*t*
squamous cell carcinoma of, 1234-1235
Orotracheal intubation, 596
ORT; *See* Oral rehydration therapy
Orthopnea
in acute respiratory failure, 686
in aortic regurgitation, 779*c*, 780
in aortic stenosis, 779*c*, 780
cardiovascular assessment and, 713
in chronic obstructive pulmonary disease, 624, 624*f*
in left-sided heart failure, 768
in lung cancer, 643
in mitral stenosis, 779, 779*c*
respiratory assessment and, 559
Orthosis, thoracolumbosacral, 1174, 1174*f*
Orthostatic hypotension, 799
alpha blocker-related, 1714-1715
bromocriptine-related, 1431
cardiovascular assessment and, 716
dehydration and, 178
in diabetic neuropathy, 1470
in hypernatremia, 186
in hyponatremia, 185
spinal cord injured patient and, 997
Orthotopic heart transplantation, 789, 789*f*
Orudis; *See* Ketoprofen
Oseltamivir
for avian influenza, 667
for influenza, 658
OSHA; *See* Occupational Safety and Health Administration
Osmitrol; *See* Mannitol
Osmolality, 173-174
Osmolarity, 173-174, 183*f*
Osmoreceptor, 174
Osmosis, 173*f*, 173-174
Ossicle, 1110, 1110*f*
ossiculoplasty and, 1134*f*
trauma to, 1126
Ossiculoplasty, 1134*f*
Osteitis deformans, 1162-1164, 1163*c*
Osteoarthritis, 323-336, 1143
cast-related, 1189
chronic pain in, 326-328, 327*c*
complementary and alternative therapies in, 327-328, 328*c*
health care resources in, 336
health promotion and maintenance in, 324
health teaching in, 336, 336*c*
home care management in, 335-336
imaging assessment in, 325
impaired physical mobility in, 335, 336*c*
laboratory assessment in, 325
nursing diagnoses in, 325-326
obesity and, 1402
pathophysiology of, 323*f*, 323-324
patient history in, 324
physical assessment in, 324-325
psychosocial assessment in, 325
rheumatoid arthritis *versus*, 325*t*
total elbow arthroplasty in, 335
total hip arthroplasty in, 328-332, 330*c*, 330*t*, 332*c*, 332*f*
total knee arthroplasty in, 333*f*, 333-334, 334*c*
total shoulder arthroplasty in, 334-335
Osteoblast, 1141
Osteoblastic activity, 1461
Osteocalcin, 1156
Osteochondroma, 1167
Osteoclast, 1141
Osteoclastic activity, 1461
Osteocyte, 1141, 1141*f*
Osteodystrophy in chronic kidney disease, 1614
Osteogenic sarcoma, 1163
Osteogenic tumor, 1167
Osteoid, 1141
Osteomalacia, 1160-1162, 1161*t*
Osteomyelitis, 1164-1167, 1165*f*, 1166*c*
halo device-related, 996
intraosseous therapy-related, 239
lower extremity amputation-related, 1200
open fracture-related, 1183
Osteonecrosis
bisphosphonate-related, 1160
in osteoarthritis, 328
in systemic lupus erythematosus, 348
Osteopenia, 1143, 1153
Osteophyte, 323
Osteoporosis, 1143, 1153-1160, 1644
cast-related, 1189
community-based care for, 1160
drug therapy for, 1157-1160, 1158-1159*c*
exercise and, 1157
growth hormone deficiency and, 1426
history in, 1155
hypocalcemia and, 193
imaging studies in, 1156-1157
inflammatory bowel disease and, 1322*t*
laboratory assessment in, 1156
lifestyle changes in, 1157
nursing diagnoses in, 1157
nutrition therapy in, 1157
osteomalacia *versus*, 1161, 1161*t*
pathophysiology of, 1153*c*, 1153*t*, 1153-1155
physical assessment in, 1155-1156, 1156*f*
prevention of, 1155
psychosocial assessment in, 1156
surgery for, 1160
Osteoporosis Society of Canada, 1160
Osteoprotegerin, 1154
Osteosarcoma, 1168
Osteotomy
in bunionectomy, 1172
in hammertoe, 1173
in osteoarthritis, 328
Ostomate, 1325
Ostomy
in colorectal cancer, 1298-1300, 1299*f*
health care resources for, 1302
home care of, 1301, 1301*c*
in total proctocolectomy with permanent ileostomy, 1325-1326, 1326*f*
Otitis media, 1123-1125, 1124*f*, 1125*c*, 1125*f*, 1131
Otorrhea, 961
Otosclerosis, 1126
Otoscope, 1115, 1115*f*
Otoscopic examination, 1115, 1115*f*
in external otitis, 1121
in hearing loss, 1131
in mastoiditis, 1125
in otitis media, 1123, 1124*f*
Ototoxic drugs, 906, 1113, 1114*t*
Outflow obstructions, 804, 804*f*, 805
Outpatient surgery, 244
Ova and parasites, 1225
Oval window, 1110
Ovarian cancer, 1705*t*, 1705-1707
BRCA1 and *BRCA2* gene mutations and, 1647
conditions associated with genetic predisposition for, 410*t*
Ovarian cyst, 1694
Ovary, 1413*f*, 1643, 1643*f*
anterior pituitary hormones and, 1415*t*
hormones of, 1413*t*
Overactive bladder, 1561
Overdose
of anesthesia, 275
of opioid analgesics, 299*c*
Overeaters Anonymous, 1406
Overflow incontinence, 1560*t*, 1561
in benign prostatic hypertrophy, 1713
in bladder infection, 1559
Overhead traction, 1190*t*
Overhydration, 181*f*, 181-183, 182*c*
Over-the-counter drugs
gastrointestinal assessment and, 1219
for migraine headache, 952
nephrotoxicity of, 1612
older adult and, 20
skin problems and, 466-467
Overweight, 710-711, 1402
Ovide; *See* Malathion
Oviduct, 1643*f*
Ovoid pupil, 1055
Ovulation, 1644
Oxaliplatin, 422*t*
for colorectal cancer, 1297
for esophageal cancer, 1257-1258
Oxazepam, 55
Oxcarbazepine, 957*c*, 985
Oxtriphylline, 620
Oxybutynin
for urinary incontinence, 1565*c*, 1567
for urolithiasis, 1573
Oxycocet; *See* Oxycodone-acetaminophen
Oxycodan; *See* Oxycodone-aspirin
Oxycodone, 46
abuse of, 90*t*, 90-91, 91*c*
equianalgesic dose of, 47*t*
Oxycodone-acetaminophen, 46
after total hip arthroplasty, 331
for postoperative pain, 297, 298*c*
Oxycodone-aspirin, 46, 297, 298*c*
OxyContin; *See* Oxycodone
Oxygen, 552
Oxygen concentrator, 579
Oxygen delivery systems, 574-578
high-flow, 576-577, 577*f*, 577*t*, 578*f*
low-flow, 574-576, 575*t*, 576*f*
Oxygen dissociation, 877

Oxygen partial pressure
in burn, 532c
normal range for adult, 202c
in respiratory assessment, 565c
uncompensated acid-base imbalances and, 208c
Oxygen saturation
in acute respiratory failure, 685
in septic shock, 841, 841t
Oxygen therapy, 571-579
in acute myocardial infarction, 858
in acute respiratory failure, 686
in airway management in trauma patient, 136
in anaphylaxis, 393
in asthma, 621
in avian influenza, 668
in bee sting, 150
in burn, 535
in chronic obstructive pulmonary disease, 628, 629c
in cluster headache, 955
in drowning, 157
in dyspnea in dying patient, 118
hazards and complications of, 572-574, 573f
in heat stroke, 142
in high altitude cerebral edema, 156
high-flow oxygen delivery systems in, 576-577, 577f, 577t, 578f
home-based, 578-579, 579f
in hypovolemic shock, 837
intervention activities in, 572c
low-flow oxygen delivery systems in, 574-576, 575t, 576f
in lung cancer, 649
noninvasive positive-pressure ventilation in, 578, 578f
nursing diagnoses in, 572
in pneumonia, 664, 664c
in postoperative hypoxemia, 299
in primary pulmonary hypertension, 638
in pulmonary edema, 775
in pulmonary embolism, 680
in respiratory acidosis, 209
in septic shock, 843
in sickle cell crisis, 897
transtracheal, 578
Oxygen toxicity, 573
Oxygenation
acute respiratory problems and, 677, 678f
cardiovascular system and, 704
chronic obstructive pulmonary disease and, 631-632, 632f, 633t
respiratory system role in, 552, 552f
shock and, 826-827, 827f, 829f
Oxygenation failure, 685, 685t
Oxygen-induced hypoventilation, 573
Oxymorphone, 47t
Oxytocin, 1415, 1415t

P

P wave, 731, 731f, 734, 735f
heart rhythm analysis and, 737
idioventricular rhythm and, 747
normal sinus rhythm and, 737, 737f
premature atrial complexes and, 740
sinus arrhythmia and, 738
supraventricular tachycardia and, 740
PAC; *See* Premature atrial complexes
PACE process, 5
Pacemaker
health teaching in, 759, 760c
invasive temporary pacemaker system, 755
permanent insertion of, 757
sinus node as, 739
Pacemaker cell, 730
Packed red blood cells
in hypovolemic shock, 837
indications for, 917t
Pack-years
cardiovascular disease and, 709
effect on lung function, 558
head and neck cancer and, 598
Paclitaxel, 421t
for breast cancer, 1678
for cervical cancer, 1705
for esophageal cancer, 1258
for fallopian tube cancer, 1709
for testicular cancer, 1730
PACU; *See* Postanesthesia care unit
PAD; *See* Peripheral arterial disease
Paget Disease Foundation, 1164
Paget's disease of bone, 1162-1164, 1163c
Pain, 35-61
in abdominal aortic aneurysm, 811
in achalasia, 1255
in acquired immunodeficiency syndrome, 379-380
acute, 36t, 36-38, 37t
in acute compartment syndrome, 1181
in acute coronary syndromes, 856c, 856-858, 857-858c
in acute pancreatitis, 1375-1377
addiction, pseudoaddiction, tolerance, and physical dependence and, 39-41
in ankylosing spondylitis, 355
in aortic dissection, 814
in appendicitis, 1316
assessment of, 41-44, 42f, 43f
attitudes and practices related to, 38-39
back, 983-989
complementary and alternative therapies for, 986
diagnostic assessment in, 985
in growth hormone overproduction, 1429
health care resources for, 989
health teaching in, 988c, 988-989
home care management in, 988
in large-breasted woman, 1662
nonsurgical management of, 985-986, 986c
in osteoporosis, 1155-1156
pathophysiology of, 984
physical assessment in, 984-985
prevention of, 984, 984c
in prostatitis, 1733
surgical management of, 986-988, 987c
in Bartholin cyst, 1699
in benign bone tumor, 1167
in black widow spider bite, 148
in bone cancer, 1169, 1172
in bone marrow aspiration, 890
in botulism, 1342
bromocriptine-related, 1431
in brown recluse spider bite, 147
in burn, 520, 521t, 535-536
in cancer, 416
categorization of, 36-38, 36-38t
chest
after cardiac catheterization, 724
in aortic stenosis, 779c, 780
assessment of, 712-713, 713t
in chronic stable angina pectoris, 848
in coronary artery disease, 853c, 853-855, 861c
in empyema, 674
in hypertrophic cardiomyopathy, 789
in inhalation anthrax, 673
in lung abscess, 672
in lung cancer, 643
management at home, 872c
in mitral valve prolapse, 779c, 780
in pneumonia, 661, 663t
in pulmonary embolism, 679, 679c
respiratory assessment and, 559
in tuberculosis, 669
in cholecystitis, 1368, 1369
chronic, 36t, 36-38, 37t
Pain (Continued)
in chronic pancreatitis, 1377
in complex regional pain syndrome, 1204
in connective tissue diseases, 323
in coral snake envenomation, 146
in coronary artery bypass graft, 869
in Crohn's disease, 1331
in deep vein thrombosis, 817
definitions of, 36
in diabetes mellitus, 1504-1505, 1505c
in diverticulitis, 1334-1335
in dysmenorrhea, 1684-1685
end-of-life care and, 116-117
in endometriosis, 1687
epidural infusion for, 53, 237
in *Escherichia coli* infection, 1341
in external otitis, 1121
in fibromyalgia, 357-358
in food poisoning, 1341
in fracture, 1192
in frostbite, 154
gastrointestinal assessment of, 1221
guided imagery for, 56
in Guillain-Barré syndrome, 1015
hand massage for, 11, 11t
headache, 951-955
in acute mountain sickness, 155
in cerebral aneurysm, 1033
in cluster headache, 954-955
in heat exhaustion, 142
in hyperaldosteronism, 1446
in hypopituitarism, 1426
in influenza, 658
in lightning strike, 151
in meningitis, 961
in migraine, 951-954, 952c, 953t, 954c, 954t
in pheochromocytoma, 1446
in pneumonia, 661
in severe acute respiratory syndrome, 666
in tension headache, 955
in toxic shock syndrome, 1691, 1692c
in viral gastroenteritis, 1320
health care resources for, 59
health teaching in, 58-59
in hemorrhoids, 1309, 1310
in hiatal hernia, 1249
home care management of, 58
in hookworm infection, 1340
hospitalized older adult and, 23
in hydrocele, 1731
in hypercalcemia, 194
in infective endocarditis, 784
in inflammatory bowel disease, 1327-1328, 1328c
in intestinal obstruction, 1304
intractable, 52
invasive techniques for, 57-58, 58f
in irritable bowel syndrome, 1290
in lung cancer, 650
musculoskeletal assessment and, 1144
in musculoskeletal trauma, 1184c, 1185
music therapy for, 10
neck, 989f, 989-990, 990c
nonpharmacologic therapy for, 55-57, 56f
in ocular foreign body, 1104
older adult and, 40
opioids abuse in, 82
in osteoarthritis, 324, 326-328, 327c
in osteomyelitis, 1165, 1166c
in otitis media, 1123
in Paget's disease of bone, 1162-1163
Pain Care Bill of Rights and, 35, 36t
in pancreatic cancer, 1380
in pancreatic pseudocyst, 1380
in pelvic inflammatory disease, 1748, 1751-1752
in peptic ulcer disease, 1273, 1274-1275
perception of, 39, 40c
Pain (Continued)
in pericarditis, 785
in peripheral arterial disease, 805
peritoneal dialysis-related, 1629
in peritonitis, 1317-1318
pharmacologic therapy for, 44-55, 45t
acetaminophen in, 46
adjuvant analgesics in, 54t, 54-55
epidural analgesia in, 52-54, 53f
non-opioid analgesics in, 45
nonsteroidal antiinflammatory drugs in, 45-46
opioid analgesics in, 46-51, 47t, 49-51t
patient-controlled analgesia in, 51f, 51-52
in pharyngitis, 655
in pheochromocytoma, 1446
in pit viper envenomation, 144
in plantar fasciitis, 1173
in polycystic kidney disease, 1584
postoperative, 38t, 297-299, 297-299c
in amputation, 1201
analgesics for, 52
in back surgery, 987
in bariatric surgery, 1407
in cardiac catheterization, 724
in cataract surgery, 1094
in laryngectomy, 601-602
in lung cancer, 649
in lung transplantation, 630
in oral cancer surgery, 1238
relationship with anxiety, 249
in renal cell carcinoma, 1596
in retinal detachment repair, 1102
in total hip arthroplasty, 331
in vulvectomy, 1708
in prostate cancer, 1720
in prostatitis, 1733
psychosocial assessment of, 44
in pyelonephritis, 1588-1598
referral in, 59
in reproductive system disorders, 1648, 1649c
in rotator cuff injury, 1208
in scleroderma, 351
scope of problem, 36, 36t
in scorpion sting, 148
sensation of, 939
in sickle cell disease, 895, 896-897, 897c
subcutaneous infusion therapy for, 237t
in sunburn, 480
in systemic lupus erythematosus, 349
in tarantula bite, 148
transmission of, 38, 39f
in trigeminal neuralgia, 1025
in ulcerative colitis, 1321, 1327-1328, 1328c
Pain Care Bill of Rights, 35, 36t
Pain relief visual analog scale, 43f
Pain scale, 43, 43f
Paint thinner abuse, 91
Palatine tonsils, 553f, 554
Palliative care, 113
Palliative surgery, 243t, 417
in bone cancer, 1169-1170
in esophageal cancer, 1258-1259
in lung cancer, 641, 650, 650c
Pallor, 468t
in coral snake envenomation, 146
in dark-skinned patient, 885
in hypovolemic shock, 835
in leukemia, 903
in peripheral arterial disease, 805
in septic shock, 842
in sickle cell disease, 895
in urolithiasis, 1571
Palm of hand, hand massage and, 11t
Palonosetron, 429c
Palpation
in abdominal assessment, 1223
of breast, 1667f
of lungs and thorax, 560-561

Palpation *(Continued)*
in musculoskeletal assessment, 1146
of scrotum, 1651
of skin, 471-472, 472*t*
of spleen, 885-886
of thyroid, 1422, 1422*f*
Palpitations, 738
in aortic regurgitation, 779*c*, 780
caffeine and, 747
cardiovascular assessment and, 713-714
in Lyme disease, 356
in mitral regurgitation, 779*c*, 780
in mitral stenosis, 779
in mitral valve prolapse, 779*c*, 780
in pheochromocytoma, 1446
Pamelor; *See* Nortriptyline
Pamidronate, 424*t*
for bone cancer, 1169
for osteoporosis prevention, 1160
for Paget's disease of bone, 1164
Panacinar emphysema, 611*f*
Pancreas, 1371-1384, 1413*f*, 1418, 1418*f*, 1418*t*
abscess of, 1379-1380
acute pancreatitis and, 1371-1377, 1372*f*, 1373*t*, 1374*t*
acute pain in, 1375-1376
community-based care in, 1376-1377
complications of, 1373, 1373*t*
history in, 1373-1374
laboratory assessment in, 1374*t*, 1374-1375
pancreatic abscess and, 1379-1380
pathophysiology of, 1371-1373, 1372*f*
physical assessment in, 1374
aging-related changes in, 1220*c*
anatomy and physiology of, 1217*f*, 1218, 1218*f*
cancer of, 1380-1384, 1381*c*, 1383*c*, 1383*t*
catecholamine receptors and, 1416*t*
chronic pancreatitis and, 1377-1379, 1378*c*, 1379*c*
diabetes mellitus and, 1465-1520
absence of insulin in, 1467*t*, 1467-1468
acute complications of, 1468
amputation and, 1200
atherosclerosis and, 794
blood glucose control in, 1505
blood glucose monitoring in, 1490-1492, 1491-1492*t*
chronic pain in, 1504-1505, 1505*c*
chronic pancreatitis and, 1377, 1379
classification of, 1466, 1466*t*
concept map for, 1476
coronary artery disease and, 852, 854*c*
cultural considerations in, 1472, 1473*t*
cystic fibrosis and, 636
diabetic ketoacidosis in, 1510-1512, 1512*c*
endocrine pancreas and, 1466
erectile dysfunction in, 1471
etiology and genetic risk in, 1471*t*, 1471-1472
evidence-based practice and, 1500
exercise therapy for, 1496-1497, 1497*c*
foot care in, 1501-1503, 1502*c*, 1502*t*, 1503*b*, 1503*f*, 1504*c*
glucose homeostasis and, 1467
health care resources for, 1516
health promotion and maintenance in, 1472
health teaching in, 1514-1515, 1516*c*, 1517*t*
heart disease and, 709
history in, 1473
home care management in, 1516, 1516*c*

Pancreas *(Continued)*
hyperglycemia in, 1475-1477
hyperglycemic-hyperosmolar state in, 1512*c*, 1512-1514, 1513*f*
hypoglycemia in, 1506-1509, 1507*t*, 1508*c*
incidence and prevalence of, 1472
ineffective renal tissue perfusion in, 1506
insulin physiology and, 1466*f*, 1466-1467
insulin therapy for, 1484-1489, 1485*t*, 1486*f*, 1486*t*, 1487*c*, 1487*f*, 1488*c*, 1489*f*
laboratory assessment in, 1473*c*, 1473*t*, 1473-1475, 1474*c*, 1474*t*
macrovascular complications in, 1468-1469
microvascular complications in, 1469, 1469*f*, 1470*t*
nephropathy in, 1470-1471
neuropathy in, 1469-1470, 1470*t*
newer drug therapies for, 1489-1490
nursing diagnoses in, 1475
nutrition therapy for, 1492-1495, 1494*t*, 1495*t*
oral drug therapy for, 1477-1483*c*, 1477-1484, 1483*t*
pancreatic transplantation for, 1498-1500
sensory alterations in, 1500-1501, 1501*f*
subcutaneous infusion therapy in, 237*t*
vision changes in, 1075
wound care in, 1503-1504
hormones of, 1413*t*
insulinoma of, 1380
pseudocyst of, 1380
tumor of, 1279
Pancreatic duct, 1218*f*
Pancreatic enzymes
for chronic pancreatitis, 1378, 1378*c*
malabsorption syndrome and, 1311
Pancreatic transplantation, 636-637, 1498-1500
Pancreaticoduodenectomy
in gastric cancer, 1281-1282
in pancreatic cancer, 1382
in Zollinger-Ellison syndrome, 1279
Pancreaticojejunostomy, 1382, 1383*f*
Pancreatitis
acute, 1371-1377
community-based care in, 1376-1377
complications of, 1373, 1373*t*
history in, 1373-1374
laboratory assessment in, 1374*t*, 1374-1375
pain in, 1375-1376
pancreatic abscess and, 1379-1380
pathophysiology of, 1371-1373, 1372*f*
physical assessment in, 1374
after pancreatic transplant, 1498
chronic, 1377-1379, 1378*c*, 1379*c*
Pancrelipase, 1378
Pancuronium, 274*t*
Pancytopenia
in aplastic anemia, 900
engraftment in bone marrow transplantation and, 909
in lupus erythematosus, 349-350
Pandemic infection, 160, 455
severe acute respiratory syndrome and, 666-667
Panendoscopy in head and neck cancer, 598-599
Panhypopituitarism, 1426
Panhysterectomy, 1697*t*
Panje Voice Button, 603*f*
Panlobular emphysema, 611*f*, 622
Panniculectomy, 1408

Panniculitis, 1404
Panniculus, 1404, 1408
Pannus, 337
Pantoprazole
for gastroesophageal reflux disease, 1247*c*, 1248
for peptic ulcer disease, 1269*c*, 1274
PAOP; *See* Pulmonary artery occlusive pressure
PAP; *See* Pulmonary artery pressure
Pap smear, 1652
in cervical cancer, 1703
in fallopian tube cancer, 1709
in genital herpes, 1744
in vulvar cancer, 1707
Papaverine, 1375
Paper correction fluid inhalation, 91
Papilla, 1217
duodenal, 1218*f*
renal, 1527, 1527*f*
Papillary thyroid carcinoma, 1460-1461
Papilledema
in brain tumor, 1061
in traumatic brain injury, 1055
Papilloma, intraductal, 1661*t*, 1662
Papillotomy, 1227
Papular rash, 472
Papule, 469*f*
in lichen planus, 516
in psoriasis vulgaris, 506, 507*f*
Paracentesis in cirrhosis, 1352, 1352*c*
Paradoxic chest movement, 698, 698*f*
Paradoxical blood pressure, 716
Paradoxical pulse, 786
Paradoxical splitting of heart sounds, 718
Paraesophageal hiatal hernia, 1249*f*, 1249-1254, 1253*c*, 1253*f*, 1254*c*
Paraffin dip, 56
Paralysis
after stroke, 1034
in amyotrophic lateral sclerosis, 1007
assessment before rehabilitation, 98
in botulism, 1341
in coral snake envenomation, 146
facial, 1026
in Guillain-Barré syndrome, 1012
in lightning strike, 151
in spinal tumor, 1001
vocal cord, 591-595
Paralysis agitans, 965
Paralytic drugs for mechanical ventilation in burn, 535
Paralytic ileus, 1302
after abdominal aortic aneurysm resection, 813
after lumbar spinal surgery, 987*c*
in botulism, 1341
burn-related, 531
hypokalemia and, 188
hypomagnesemia and, 196
in spinal cord injury, 994
Paramedic, 127
Parametritis, 1748
Paranasal sinuses, 553*f*, 553-554
Paraneoplastic syndromes
lung cancer and, 641, 642*t*
renal cell carcinoma and, 1595
Paraparesis, 993
Paraphimosis, 1732*f*, 1732-1733
Paraplatin; *See* Carboplatin
Paraplegia, 993
Paraseptal emphysema, 622
Parasitic infection
cutaneous, 504
gastrointestinal, 1338-1339
Parasympathetic nervous system, 928, 933, 934*f*, 935*t*
Parathormone, 1142
Parathyroid gland, 1413*f*, 1417, 1418*f*
hormones of, 1413*t*
hyperparathyroidism and, 1461*f*, 1461*t*, 1461-1463, 1462*c*
hypoparathyroidism and, 1463

Parathyroid hormone, 1417, 1418*f*
bone and, 1142
calcium and, 191
hyperparathyroidism and, 1461-1462
osteoporosis and, 1154, 1157-1159
physiologic actions of, 1461*f*
Parathyroidectomy, 1462-1463
Parenteral fluids, 214-215
Parenteral nutrition, 1400-1401, 1401*c*
during mechanical ventilation, 696
Parenteral transmission of acquired immunodeficiency syndrome, 367-368
Paresis assessment before rehabilitation, 98
Paresthesia
in black widow spider bite, 148
in carpal tunnel syndrome, 1206
in coral snake envenomation, 146
in Guillain-Barré syndrome, 1012
in hyperaldosteronism, 1446
in hyperkalemia, 190
in hypocalcemia, 192
in hypothyroidism, 1457
in low back pain, 985
in multiple sclerosis, 1006
plasmapheresis-related, 1014*c*
in rheumatoid arthritis, 338
in scorpion sting, 149
in vitamin B_{12} deficiency, 900
Parietal cell, 1218
Parietal lobe, 931*t*
Parietal pericardium, 705*f*
Parietal pleura, 556
Parkin 1 gene, 965
Parkinson disease, 965*t*, 965-969, 966*c*, 966*f*, 967*c*
Parkland formula, 533*t*
Parlodel; *See* Bromocriptine
Paromomycin, 1339
Paronychia, 474
Parotid gland, 1217*f*
Parotidectomy, 1240
Paroxetine
for Alzheimer's disease, 976
for pain, 54, 54*t*
for premenstrual dysphoric disorder, 1687
Paroxysmal nocturnal dyspnea
in aortic regurgitation, 779*c*, 780
cardiovascular assessment and, 713
in left-sided heart failure, 768
in mitral stenosis, 779, 779*c*
respiratory assessment and, 559
Paroxysmal supraventricular tachycardia, 740-741
Pars flaccida, 1110, 1110*f*
Pars tensa, 1110, 1110*f*
Partial corpus callosotomy, 961
Partial cystectomy, 1576
Partial laryngectomy, 600, 600*t*
Partial nephrectomy, 1598
Partial parenteral nutrition, 1400
Partial pneumonectomy, 646, 646*f*
Partial pressure of arterial carbon dioxide
in acute renal failure, 1605*c*
in acute respiratory failure, 685
in asthma, 612
in hypovolemic shock, 835, 836*c*
normal range for adult, 202*c*
oxygen-induced hypoventilation and, 573
in pulmonary embolism, 679
uncompensated acid-base imbalances and, 208*c*
Partial pressure of arterial oxygen
acidosis and, 209
in acute respiratory distress syndrome, 687
in acute respiratory failure, 685
in hypovolemic shock, 835, 836*c*
normal range for adult, 202*c*
oxygen-induced hypoventilation and, 573
uncompensated acid-base imbalances and, 208*c*

Partial rebreather mask, 575, 575*t*, 576*f*
Partial seizure, 956
Partial thromboplastin time, 889
in cardiovascular assessment, 721
in pulmonary embolism, 682*c*
Partial vaginectomy, 1709
Partial-thickness skin graft, 495-496
Partial-thickness wound
in burn injury, 522*f*, 522-523, 523*f*
healing of, 482-483, 484*f*
Particle concentration in body fluids, 173-174
Passive euthanasia, 121, 122*t*
Passive immunity, 316, 441
Passive range of motion, 1145, 1146*f*
Passive range-of-motion exercises, 102*t*
Passive smoke, heart disease and, 710
Patch, 469*f*, 506, 507*f*
Patch testing, 395
Patellar fracture, 1197
Patellar reflex, 940*f*
Patellar weight-bearing cast, 1188*t*
Patellofemoral pain syndrome, 1205
Pathogen, 440-441
Pathogenicity, 440
Pathologic fracture, 1179
in bone cancer, 1168
in chronic kidney disease, 1614
in Cushing's disease, 1444
in hyperparathyroidism, 1462
in Paget's disease of bone, 1163
Pathologic staging of cancer, 407
Patient, defined, 2
Patient and family education; *See* Health teaching
Patient autonomy, 5
Patient care assistant, 4
Patient care technician, 4
Patient disposition
in emergency care, 133
trauma nursing and, 138-139
Patient education; *See* Health teaching
Patient history; *See* History
Patient identification
in blood transfusion, 214
in emergency care, 129, 129*c*
intraoperative, 266*f*, 277
in mass casualty event, 161
preoperative, 260
Patient positioning
after abdominal surgery, 1318
after brain tumor surgery, 1063
after pancreatic cancer surgery, 1383
in burn
for impaired physical mobility, 543, 544*c*
for ventilatory support, 535
for hysterosalpingography, 1655
low back pain and, 985
perioperative positioning injury and, 280*f*, 280-281, 281*c*
postoperative gas exchange impairment and, 294
preventing pressure ulcers and, 485*c*
to promote circulation, 807
in spinal cord injury, 995, 995*c*
for thoracentesis, 568, 568*f*
in traumatic brain injury, 1056
Patient preparation
for allergy testing, 389
for arthroscopy, 1150
for bone marrow aspiration, 889-890
for bronchoscopy, 567-568
for cardiac catheterization, 722-723
for colonoscopy, 1228
for cystoscopy and cystourethroscopy, 1546
for endoscopic surgery, 267-269
for intubation, 690
for laparoscopy, 1656
for lung biopsy, 569
for magnetic resonance imaging, 1149*c*
for nephrostomy, 1586
for neurologic assessment, 944-945*t*
Patient preparation *(Continued)*
for Pap smear, 1652
preoperative, 260-261
for prosthesis in amputation, 1202, 1203*f*
for pulmonary function tests, 566
for skin biopsy, 477
for stress test, 724-725
for thoracentesis, 568, 568*f*
Patient safety, 2-7
after sinus surgery, 655*c*
in Alzheimer's disease, 976*c*, 977
in anticoagulant therapy, 819*c*
chest tube drainage systems and, 648*c*
core competencies and, 3-6
collaboration with interdisciplinary health care team and, 5
evidence-based practice and, 5-6, 6*t*
informatics and, 6, 6*f*
patient-centered care and, 3-5, 4*c*
quality improvement and, 6
in ear irrigation, 1123*c*
in electroencephalography, 947*c*
emergency nursing and, 128-130, 129*c*
in hypovolemic shock, 836*c*
infection control and, 443*c*, 443-444
in injection of contrast agent, 943*c*
Institute for Healthcare Improvement and, 3, 3*t*
in mechanical ventilation, 692*c*
in meningitis, 963*c*
nasogastric tube and, 1277*c*
national goals for, 2
older adult and
driving and, 18, 19*c*
fall prevention and, 24*c*
health teaching and, 4*c*
impaired vision and, 1098*c*
relocation stress and, 18*c*
using restraint alternatives and, 24*c*
in oxygen therapy, 574*c*
in Parkinson disease, 967*c*
in perineal wound care, 1300*c*
in pleurodesis, 650*c*
in preventing ventilator-associated pneumonia, 660*c*
in prevention of aspiration during swallowing, 603*c*
in procedures using contrast media, 1545*c*
reduced vision and, 1106
in sealed implants of radioactive sources, 1701*c*
in spinal cord injury, 999*c*
in thrombocytopenia, 910*c*
in tracheostomy care, 584*c*
in tracheostomy patient during swallowing, 586*c*
transfer techniques and, 100*c*
in transfusion therapy, 918*c*
T-tube care and, 1370*c*
in tube feeding, 1398*c*
in valvular heart disease, 783*c*
Patient selection
for hemodialysis, 1620
for peritoneal dialysis, 1626-1627
for renal transplantation, 1630
Patient Self-Determination Act of 1990, 113, 254
Patient transfer to surgical suite, 261
Patient transport, infection control and, 446
Patient-centered care, 3-5, 4*c*
Patient-controlled analgesia, 51*f*, 51-52
in back surgery, 987
for burn, 536
fentanyl in, 48
for fracture pain, 1192
in Guillain-Barré syndrome, 1015
in hip fracture, 1196
in laryngectomy, 601
postoperative, 297
for sickle cell disease pain, 896
Patient-controlled infusion pump, 51, 51*f*
Patterns of inheritance, 71-74, 72*t*, 72-74*f*
Pavabid; *See* Papaverine
Paverine injection, 1726
Pavulon; *See* Pancuronium
PAWP; *See* Pulmonary capillary wedge pressure
Paxil; *See* Paroxetine
PCA; *See* Patient-controlled analgesia
PCP; *See* Phencyclidine
PCWP; *See* Pulmonary capillary wedge pressure
PEA; *See* Pulseless electrical activity
Peak airway pressure, 693-694
Peak expiratory flow
in asthma, 612, 614-615
in chronic obstructive pulmonary disease, 627
Peak inspiratory pressure, 693-694
Peau d'orange skin in breast cancer, 1663, 1664*f*
Pedal edema, 1536
Pedicle flap, 496, 496*f*
Pedicle injury, 1596, 1597*f*
Pediculosis, 504
Pedigree, 71-72, 72*f*
Pedunculated polyp, 1309, 1309*f*
PEEP; *See* Positive end-expiratory pressure
PEF; *See* Peak expiratory flow
PEG; *See* Percutaneous endoscopic gastrostomy
Pegaspargase, 422*t*
Pegfilgrastim, 433*t*
PEG-Intron; *See* Pegylated interferon alpha-2b
Pegvisomant, 1431
Pegylated interferon alpha-2b, 1360
Pelvic belt, 1190*t*
Pelvic examination, 1650*f*, 1650-1651
in cervical cancer, 1703
in endometriosis, 1687
in ovarian cancer, 1706
in uterine prolapse, 1693
in vaginal cancer, 1708
Pelvic exenteration, 1704*f*, 1704-1705
Pelvic fracture, 1198
fat embolism syndrome and, 1182
pain in, 1185
traction for, 1190*t*
Pelvic inflammatory disease, 1747-1753
acute pain in, 1751-1752
anxiety in, 1752
community-based care in, 1752
drug therapy for, 1749-1751, 1750-1751*c*
fallopian tube cancer and, 1709
history in, 1748
infection control in, 1749
laboratory assessment in, 1749
Neisseria gonorrhoeae in, 1744
nursing diagnoses in, 1749
pathophysiology of, 1747-1748, 1748*f*
physical assessment in, 1748, 1749*t*
psychosocial assessment in, 1748-1749
Pelvic muscle exercises
for urinary incontinence, 1564, 1564*c*
for uterine prolapse, 1693, 1693*c*
Pelvic sling, 1190*t*
Pelvic tilt, 986*c*
Pelvis, bone cancer of, 1170-1171
Pemphigus vulgaris, 516
Pendra, 1492
Pendramine; *See* Penicillamine
Penectomy, 1732
Penetrance, 73
Penetrating keratoplasty, 1090
Penetrating trauma, 136
abdominal, 1307-1308
bladder, 1578
ocular, 1104
spinal, 991
Penicillamine, 1462
Penicillin
for brain abscess, 1066
serum sickness and, 395
for skin infection, 503
for syphilis, 1741
for urinary tract infection, 1556-1557*c*
Penile clamp, 1568-1569
Penile implant, 1726
Penile injection for erectile dysfunction, 1726
Penile urethra, 1645*f*
Penis, 1645, 1645*f*
cancer of, 1732
erectile dysfunction and, 1725-1726
after open radical prostatectomy, 1722
after prostatectomy, 1725
in diabetes mellitus, 1471
phimosis and paraphimosis and, 1732*f*, 1732-1733
priapism and, 1733
Penrose drain, 292, 292*f*, 295
Pentacarinat; *See* Pentamidine isethionate
Pentamidine isethionate, 379
Pentasa; *See* Mesalamine
Pentobarbital sodium
abuse of, 89
for burn pain, 536
Pentostatin, 421*t*
Pentothal; *See* Thiopental sodium
Pentoxifylline, 807
Pepcid; *See* Famotidine
Peppermint oil, 955
Peptic ulcer disease, 1270-1279
in chronic kidney disease, 1611
complementary and alternative therapies for, 1270*t*
complications of, 1271*c*, 1271*f*, 1271-1272
drug therapy for, 1268-1269*c*
etiology and genetic risk in, 1272
gastrointestinal bleeding in, 1275-1278, 1276*c*, 1277*c*, 1278*f*
health care resources for, 1279
health teaching in, 1278
history in, 1272-1273
home care management in, 1278, 1279*c*
imaging studies in, 1273-1274
laboratory assessment in, 1273
nursing diagnoses in, 1274
pain in, 1274-1275
pathophysiology of, 1270*f*, 1270-1271, 1271*f*
physical assessment in, 1273, 1273*t*
prevention of, 1272
psychosocial assessment in, 1273
Peptides, 930*t*
Pepto-Bismol; *See* Bismuth subsalicylate
Peptol; *See* Cimetidine
Percent relief scale, 43*f*
Percocet; *See* Oxycodone-acetaminophen
Percodan; *See* Oxycodone-aspirin
Percussion
in abdominal assessment, 1223
of chest, 561, 561*f*, 562*t*
of kidney, 1537
Percutaneous alcohol septal ablation, 789
Percutaneous cervical diskectomy, 989, 990*c*
Percutaneous electrical nerve stimulation, 55-56, 56*f*
Percutaneous endoscopic diskectomy, 986
Percutaneous endoscopic gastrostomy, 1397
Percutaneous liver biopsy, 1350
Percutaneous lumbar diskectomy, 986
Percutaneous lung biopsy, 569
Percutaneous renal biopsy, 1547-1548
Percutaneous stereotactic rhizotomy
for cluster headache, 955
for trigeminal neuralgia, 1025

Percutaneous transhepatic biliary drain
in gallstones, 1369
in pancreatic cancer, 1381
Percutaneous transhepatic cholangiography, 1226
Percutaneous transluminal coronary angioplasty, 807, 860, 865, 865*f*
Percutaneous ureterolithotomy, 1573
Pereyra procedure, 1566*t*
Perforation
in appendicitis, 1316
esophageal, 1262, 1262*c*
in peptic ulcer disease, 1272, 1277-1278
of tympanic membrane, 1124, 1124*f*
Perfusion
in acute coronary syndromes, 858-860, 859*t*
amputation and, 1201
burn injury and, 533*c*, 533*t*, 533-535, 534*f*
cardiovascular system and, 704
chronic obstructive pulmonary disease and, 631-632, 632*f*, 633*t*
diabetes mellitus and, 1467-1468, 1506
dysrhythmias and, 750-751, 751*c*
respiratory system role in, 552, 552*f*
shock and, 826-827, 827*f*, 829*f*
spinal cord injury and, 995*c*, 995-997, 996*f*
stroke and, 1036-1037
Pergolide, 1430
Periactin; *See* Cyproheptadine
Pericardial effusion, 786
Pericardial friction rub, 719, 785
Pericardial space, 705*f*
Pericardiectomy, 786
Pericardiocentesis, 786
Pericarditis, 785-786, 786*c*
chest pain in, 713*t*
in chronic kidney disease, 1611
in rheumatoid arthritis, 338
in systemic lupus erythematosus, 349
Pericardium, 704
Perichondritis, 1122
Perichondrium, 1122
Peridural analgesia, 52-54, 53*f*
Perilymph, 1110*f*
Perimenopause, 1689, 1689*t*
Perimetry, 1097
Perinatal transmission of acquired immunodeficiency syndrome, 368
Perineal comfort measures, 1337*c*
Perineal muscle electromyography, 1547
Perineum, 1642
Periodontal disease, 1235
Perioperative nursing staff, 265-267, 266*f*, 267*f*
Perioperative patient, 241-303
intraoperative care and, 264-284
advantages and disadvantages of anesthesia and, 272*t*
general anesthesia and, 272-275, 273*t*, 274*t*, 275*c*
history in, 277
hypoventilation and, 282
infection risk and, 281-282, 282*f*
local or regional anesthesia and, 275-276, 276*f*, 276*t*, 277*f*
medical record review in, 278-279, 279*c*
moderate sedation and, 276-277
nursing diagnoses in, 279-280
preparation of surgical suite and, 267-270, 268*f*
risk for perioperative positioning injury and, 280*f*, 280-281, 281*c*
surgical team members and, 264-267, 266*f*, 267*f*
postoperative care and, 285-303
acute pain and, 297-299, 297-299*c*
cardiovascular evaluation in, 287-289
fluid, electrolyte, and acid-base balance in, 290
Perioperative patient *(Continued)*
gastrointestinal assessment in, 290-291, 291*t*
hand-off report in, 286, 286*c*
health care resources and, 300-301
health teaching and, 300
history in, 286, 287*t*
home care management and, 300
hypoxemia and, 299, 300*c*
impaired gas exchange and, 294, 295*c*
impaired skin integrity and, 294-296, 295*c*, 295*f*
laboratory assessment in, 293
neurologic assessment in, 289*t*, 289-290
nursing diagnoses in, 293-294
pain assessment in, 292-293
postanesthesia care unit record and, 288*f*
psychosocial assessment in, 293
renal evaluation in, 290
respiratory evaluation in, 287, 289*c*
skin assessment in, 291*f*, 291-292, 292*f*
preoperative care and, 242-263
administering regularly scheduled drugs and, 254
categories and purposes of surgery and, 243-244*t*
dietary restrictions and, 254
focused assessment in, 251*c*
history in, 244*c*, 244-245*t*, 244-247
imaging and, 249
informed consent and, 252-254, 253*f*
intestinal preparation in, 254
laboratory assessment in, 248-249, 250-251*c*
nursing diagnoses and, 252
patient anxiety and, 258-260
patient self-determination and, 254
patient transfer to surgical suite, 261
physical assessment in, 247*c*, 247-248
preoperative chart review in, 260
preoperative drugs and, 261
preoperative patient preparation and, 260-261
preparation for tubes, drains, and vascular access in, 255
psychosocial assessment in, 248
skin preparation in, 255, 256*f*
surgical settings and, 244
teaching postoperative procedures and exercises and, 255-259, 256*c*, 257*c*, 258*f*, 259*f*
Perioperative positioning injury, 280*f*, 280-281, 281*c*
Periorbital ecchymosis, 1103
Periosteum, 1141*f*
Peripheral arterial disease, 804-810
acute peripheral arterial occlusion in, 810
community-based care in, 809*c*, 809-810, 810*c*
diagnostic tests for, 805-806
drug therapy for, 807
pathophysiology of, 804, 804*f*
physical assessment in, 805, 805*c*, 806*c*
surgical management of, 808*f*, 808-809
Peripheral artery aneurysm, 814
Peripheral blood smear, 886
Peripheral blood stem cell harvesting, 908
Peripheral chemoreceptor, 708
Peripheral cyanosis
in aortic stenosis, 780
cardiovascular assessment and, 715
Peripheral edema
cardiovascular assessment and, 715
in coronary artery disease, 854
Peripheral intravenous therapy, 215*f*, 215-217, 216*c*, 216*f*, 216*t*
Peripheral nerve trauma, 1022*f*, 1022-1024, 1023*f*
Peripheral nervous system, 933, 1022*f*
Peripheral neurectomy, 58*f*
Peripheral neuritis, 356
Peripheral neuropathy, 1011-1028
cast-related, 1189
chemotherapy-related, 430-431, 431*c*
in diabetes mellitus, 1501-1503, 1502*c*, 1502*t*, 1503*c*, 1503*f*, 1504*c*
in facial paralysis, 1026
fracture-related, 1186, 1186*c*
in Guillain-Barré syndrome, 1011-1016, 1012*c*, 1012*t*, 1013*t*, 1014*c*, 1015*c*
in myasthenia gravis, 1016-1022
community-based care in, 1021*t*, 1021-1022, 1022*c*
electromyography in, 1018
nonsurgical management of, 1018-1020, 1019*t*, 1020*c*
nursing diagnoses in, 1018
pathophysiology of, 1016
physical assessment in, 1-17*c*, 1016-1017
surgical management of, 1020-1021
in peripheral nerve trauma, 1022*f*, 1022-1024, 1023*f*
in restless legs syndrome, 1024
in trigeminal neuralgia, 1025*f*, 1025-1026
Peripheral oxygen saturation, 565*c*, 566
Peripheral parenteral nutrition, 1400
Peripheral pulses
in coronary artery disease, 854
in peripheral arterial disease, 805
premature ventricular complexes and, 748
Peripheral vascular assessment, 289
Peripheral vascular disease, 804-823
acute peripheral arterial occlusion in, 810
aneurysms of central arteries in, 810-814, 811*f*
aneurysms of peripheral arteries in, 814
aortic dissection in, 814
Buerger's disease in, 815
homocysteine and, 795
peripheral arterial disease in, 804-810
community-based care in, 809*c*, 809-810, 810*c*
diagnostic tests for, 805-806
drug therapy for, 807
pathophysiology of, 804, 804*f*
physical assessment in, 805, 805*c*, 806*c*
surgical management of, 808*f*, 808-809
peripheral venous disease in, 816-823
phlebitis in, 823
varicose veins in, 822-823
venous insufficiency in, 821-822, 822*c*
venous thromboembolism in, 816-821, 817*f*, 819*c*, 821*c*
popliteal entrapment in, 816
Raynaud's phenomenon in, 815-816, 816*f*
subclavian steal in, 815
thoracic outlet syndrome in, 815
vascular trauma and, 823
Peripheral vascular pressure, 708, 797
Peripheral venous access device for blood sampling, 888
Peripheral venous disease, 816-823
phlebitis in, 823
varicose veins in, 822-823
vascular trauma in, 823
venous insufficiency in, 821-822, 822*c*
venous thromboembolism in, 816-821, 817*f*, 819*c*, 821*c*
Peripheral-acting analgesics, 45
Peripherally inserted central catheter, 217-218
in older adult, 235
for parenteral nutrition, 1400
removal of, 225
Peristalsis
peritonitis and, 1317
postoperative assessment of, 290
Peritoneal cavity
intraperitoneal infusion and, 236-237
peritonitis and, 1317*c*, 1317-1319
Peritoneal dialysis
in acute renal failure, 1608
in chronic kidney disease, 1626-1630, 1627*t*, 1627-1629*f*, 1629*c*
dietary restrictions in, 1617*t*, 1618
health teaching in, 1635
hemodialysis *versus*, 1621*t*
Peritoneum
female, 1643*f*
male, 1645*f*
Peritonitis, 1317*c*, 1317-1319
after pancreatic cancer surgery, 1383
in cholecystitis, 1367
in diverticulitis, 1335
in peptic ulcer disease, 1272
peritoneal dialysis-related, 1629
Peritonsillar abscess, 657
Peritubular capillary, 1528, 1530*t*
Periungual lesions
in rheumatoid arthritis, 338
in scleroderma, 352
Periurethral injection of collagen, 1566*t*
Permanent pacemaker
health teaching in, 760*c*
insertion of, 757
Permax; *See* Pergolide
Permeable membrane, 171, 171*f*, 172*f*
Permethrin
for pediculosis, 504
for scabies, 504
Pernicious anemia, 900, 1266
Peroneal artery, 804*f*
Peroneal nerve, 281*c*
PERRLA mnemonic, 942
Persantine; *See* Dipyridamole
Persistent pain, 36*t*, 36-38, 37*t*
Personal emergency preparedness plan, 163
Personal protective equipment, 445, 445*f*, 446*t*, 666-667
Personal readiness supplies, 163, 164*t*
Person-to-person transmission of infection, 442
Pessary
for urinary incontinence, 1568-1569
for uterine prolapse, 1693*c*
PET; *See* Positron emission tomography
Pet visitation, 11
Petaling of cast, 1187
$PETCO_2$; *See* Pressure of end-tidal carbon dioxide
Petechiae, 471
in cirrhosis, 1347
in fat embolism syndrome, 1182
hematologic assessment and, 885
in idiopathic thrombocytopenic purpura, 916
in infective endocarditis, 784
in leukemia, 903-904
Peutz-Jeghers syndrome, 1309
Peyronie's disease, 1725
pH, 199
alkalosis and, 211
burn assessment and, 532*c*
effect on transmission of nerve impulse, 929
in hypovolemic shock, 835, 836*c*
of intravenous solutions, 214
normal adult range of, 202*c*
in respiratory assessment, 565*c*
uncompensated acid-base imbalances and, 208*c*
urine, 1538, 1539*t*

Phacoemulsification cataract extraction, 1094, 1094*f*
Phagocytosis, 311-312, 312*f*
macrophages and, 311
neutrophils and, 310
risk for infection and, 441*t*, 443
Phagosome formation, 312
Phalangeal joint arthroplasty, 335
Phalanx fracture, 1195
Phalen's maneuver, 1206-1207
Phantom limb pain, 1200, 1201
Phantom limb sensation, 1200
Pharmacogenomics, 423
Pharmacologic stress echocardiogram, 725
Pharmacologic therapy; *See* Drug therapy
Pharyngeal tonsils, 553*f*, 554
Pharyngitis, 655-657, 656*c*, 656*t*
Pharynx, 554
obstructive sleep apnea and, 594
of older adult, 557*c*
pharyngitis and, 655-657, 656*c*, 656*t*
physical assessment of, 559-560
Phenazo; *See* Phenazopyridine
Phenazopyridine, 1557*c*
Phencyclidine, 87
Phendimetrazine, 1405
Phenergan; *See* Promethazine
Phenobarbital, 957*c*
abuse of, 89
for dying patient, 118
Phenotype, 69
Phenoxybenzamine
for hypertension in pheochromocytoma, 1446-1447
for Raynaud's phenomenon, 816
Phentermine, 1405
Phentolamine, 1726
Phenylephrine
for cardiac arrest, 752-753
for hypovolemic shock, 837*c*
Phenytoin, 958*c*
antacid interaction with, 1275
for brain abscess, 1066
for cerebral edema, 1062
for pain in acquired immunodeficiency syndrome, 380
for status epilepticus, 959, 960
for stroke, 1043
for traumatic brain injury, 1057
Pheochromocytoma, 798, 1446-1447
Pheresis, 908
Philadelphia chromosome abnormality, 407, 903
Phimosis, 1651, 1732*f*, 1732-1733
Phlebitis, 817, 823
central venous catheter and, 233*t*
intravenous therapy-related, 227*t*
Phlebitis scale, 234*t*
Phlebostatic axis, 727*c*
Phlebothrombosis, 817
Phlebotomy, 901
Phonation
head and neck cancer and, 598
vocal cord paralysis and, 591-595
Phonophobia, 951
Phonophoresis, 985
Phosphate
in acid-base control, 202
retention in chronic kidney disease, 1610
serum
abnormal findings in, 1462*c*
in acute renal failure, 1605*c*
in musculoskeletal assessment, 1148*c*
Phosphate binders, 1606*c*
Phosphodiesterase inhibitor, 773
Phosphodiesterase-5 inhibitors, 1726
Phospholine Iodide; *See* Echothiophate
Phosphorus, 194-195
bone and, 1142
calcitonin and, 1417
chronic kidney disease and, 1610, 1617, 1617*t*
Phosphorus *(Continued)*
hyperphosphatemia and, 195
hypophosphatemia and, 194-195, 195*c*, 195*t*
normal plasma values for older adult, 184*t*
serum, 184*t*
Photic stimulation during electroencephalography, 947
Photocoagulation for retinal detachment, 1101
Photodynamic therapy
in cancer, 432*c*, 432-433
in esophageal cancer, 1258
in lung cancer, 645
in macular degeneration, 1101
Photophobia, 1076
in hyperthyroidism, 1450, 1455
in lightning strike, 151
in meningitis, 961
in migraine headache, 951
Photopsia, 1101
Photosensitizer used in photodynamic therapy, 1101
Phrenic nerve, 1022*f*
Physiatrist, 96
Physical abuse of older adult, 22*c*, 22-23
Physical activity
after hysterectomy, 1698*c*
after total hip arthroplasty, 331-332, 332*f*
asthma and, 621
Braden Scale for pressure ulcer risk and, 487*f*
coronary artery disease and, 852, 854*c*, 871, 871*c*
older adult and, 17, 17*f*
Physical assessment
in abdominal aortic aneurysm, 811
in acidosis, 207, 207*c*
in acquired immunodeficiency syndrome, 370-373, 371*c*, 372*t*
in acute coronary syndromes, 853*c*, 853-855
in acute glomerulonephritis, 1591
in acute pancreatitis, 1374
in acute renal failure, 1603-1604, 1604*c*
in acute respiratory distress syndrome, 687
in adrenal insufficiency, 1437*f*, 1437-1438
in allergic rhinitis, 389
in Alzheimer's disease, 971-973, 972*c*, 972*f*
in amputation, 1200
in asthma, 612, 614*f*
in atherosclerosis, 794-795
in back pain, 984-985
in benign prostatic hypertrophy, 1713-1714, 1714*c*
in bladder cancer, 1575
in brain abscess, 1065-1066
in breast cancer, 1670, 1670*c*
in burn
acute phase and, 537, 538*t*
emergent/resuscitation phase and, 529*t*, 529-531, 530*t*, 531*f*
cardiovascular, 714-719
blood pressure and, 716
extremities and, 715, 715*f*
general appearance and, 714
precordium and, 717-719, 718*f*, 719*t*
skin and, 715
venous and arterial pulses and, 716-717, 717*f*
in cataract, 1092
in cervical cancer, 1703
in cholecystitis, 1368*b*, 1368-1369
in chronic glomerulonephritis, 1592
in chronic kidney disease, 1612-1614, 1613*c*
in chronic obstructive pulmonary disease, 624*f*, 624-626, 626*f*
Physical assessment *(Continued)*
in cirrhosis, 1347-1349, 1348*f*, 1349*f*
in colorectal cancer, 1295
in Crohn's disease, 1331
in Cushing's disease, 1441, 1441*c*
in cutaneous infection, 500*c*, 502
in cystitis, 1553-1554, 1555*c*
in dehydration, 178-179, 179*f*
of ear and hearing, 1114-1115, 1115*f*
in endocrine problems, 1421-1422, 1422*f*
in end-of-life care, 115*c*, 115-116
in endometrial cancer, 1699-1700
in esophageal cancer, 1256, 1256*c*
in fracture, 1184*c*, 1184-1185
in gastritis, 1267, 1267*c*
in gastroesophageal reflux disease, 1244*c*, 1244-1245
in gastrointestinal problems, 1221-1223, 1222*f*, 1222*t*
in glaucoma, 1097
in hearing loss, 1131, 1131*c*
in heart failure, 768*c*, 768-769
in hematologic assessment, 885-886
in hepatitis, 1359
in hypertension, 798-799, 799*f*
in hyperthyroidism, 1450*f*, 1450-1451, 1451*t*
in hypothyroidism, 1457
in hypovolemic shock, 833-835
in infectious disease, 450
in intestinal obstruction, 1304, 1304*c*
intraoperative medical record review and, 279
in leukemia, 903*c*, 903-904
in lung cancer, 643-644
in malnutrition, 1393, 1394*t*
in meningitis, 962
in multiple sclerosis, 1003*c*, 1003-1004
in myasthenia gravis, 1016-1017, 1017*c*
neurologic, 936-942
cerebellar function and, 940
cranial nerve evaluation and, 938
mental status and, 937*c*, 937-938
motor function and, 939*f*, 939-940
rapid neurologic assessment and, 941*f*, 941-942, 942*f*
reflex activity and, 940*f*, 940-941, 941*f*
sensory function and, 938-939
in obesity, 1404
in osteoarthritis, 324-325, 325*t*
in osteoporosis, 1155-1156, 1156*f*
in Paget's disease of bone, 1162-1163
in pain, 41-44, 42*f*, 43*f*
in pelvic inflammatory disease, 1748, 1749*t*
in peptic ulcer disease, 1273, 1273*t*
in peripheral arterial disease, 805, 805*c*, 806*c*
in plastic surgery, 513
in pneumonia, 661, 663*t*
in polycystic kidney disease, 1583, 1583*c*
postoperative, 286-293, 288*f*
cardiovascular evaluation in, 287-289
fluid, electrolyte, and acid-base balance in, 290
gastrointestinal assessment in, 290-291, 291*t*
neurologic assessment in, 289*t*, 289-290
pain assessment in, 292-293
renal evaluation in, 290
respiratory evaluation in, 287, 289*c*
skin assessment in, 291*f*, 291-292, 292*f*
preoperative, 247*c*, 247-248
in pressure ulcer, 488
in prostate cancer, 1720
in psoriasis, 506, 507*f*
in pulmonary embolism, 679, 679*c*
in pyelonephritis, 1587, 1587*c*
Physical assessment *(Continued)*
rehabilitation and, 97*t*, 97-98
in renal cell carcinoma, 1595
in renal problems, 1536-1537, 1537*f*
in reproductive problems, 1649-1651, 1650*c*, 1650*f*
in respiratory disorders, 559-564, 561*f*, 562*f*, 562*t*, 563*t*
in rheumatoid arthritis, 337-339, 338*f*
in scleroderma, 351*f*, 351-352
in septic shock, 841*t*, 841-842
in sickle cell disease, 895-896
in spinal cord injury, 993-994, 994*c*
in spinal tumor, 1001
in stroke, 1033*c*, 1033*f*, 1033-1035, 1034*c*
in systemic lupus erythematosus, 348-349, 349*f*
in testicular cancer, 1726, 1728*c*
in traumatic brain injury, 1053-1055
in tuberculosis, 669
in ulcerative colitis, 1323
in urinary incontinence, 1562-1563
in uterine leiomyoma, 1695
in vision assessment, 1077-1079
Physical carcinogenesis, 408
Physical dependence, 39-40, 83
Physical measures for pain management, 55
Physical mobility
burn injury and, 543-544, 544*c*, 544*f*
fracture and, 1193*f*, 1193-1194
osteoarthritis and, 335, 336*c*
rehabilitation and, 99-101, 100*c*, 101*c*, 101*f*, 102*t*
spinal cord injury and, 997
stroke and, 1046
Physical restraints in Alzheimer's disease, 977
Physical therapist, 96
Physical therapy
after total hip arthroplasty, 329, 332
after total knee arthroplasty, 333*f*, 333-334, 334*c*
for pain management, 55
in pressure ulcer, 493
Physician
emergency medicine, 128
medical command, 163, 163*t*
Physician-assisted suicide, 122*t*
Pia mater, 929
PICC; *See* Peripherally inserted central catheter
PID; *See* Pelvic inflammatory disease
Piercings, 471
Piggyback set, 220
Piggybacking an intermittent drug, 220*c*
Pigmentation, 1421-1422
in adrenal insufficiency, 1427*f*, 1427-1428
of nails, 474*f*
Pill box, 19, 20*f*
Pilocarpine, 1099*c*
Pilonidal cyst, 508
Pin site care, 1191
Pink eye, 1087-1088
Pinna, 1109, 1110*f*
changes with aging, 1112*c*
inspection of, 1114
instillation of antibiotics and, 1121*f*
Pinworm infection, 1339
Pioglitazone, 1481*c*, 1484
Pioglitazone-metformin, 1483*c*
Pirbuterol, 618
Pit viper envenomation, 143*f*, 143-146, 144*c*, 144*f*, 145*t*, 146*t*
Pitressin; *See* Vasopressin
Pitting edema, 181, 181*f*, 472*t*
cardiovascular assessment and, 715
in mitral regurgitation, 779*c*, 780
in mitral stenosis, 779*c*
Pitting nails, 475*t*

Pituitary, 930, 1413*f*, 1414-1415, 1415*f*, 1415*t*
  diabetes insipidus and, 1432-1433, 1433*c*, 1434*c*
  dysfunction of
    after traumatic brain injury, 1057
    in brain tumor, 1060
  hyperpituitarism and, 1428*f*, 1428-1432, 1429*f*, 1430*c*, 1431*f*
  hypopituitarism and, 1426-1428, 1427*c*
  negative feedback mechanism and, 1414, 1414*f*
  syndrome of inappropriate antidiuretic hormone secretion and, 1433-1436, 1435*t*
  tumor of, 1061
Pituitary Cushing's disease, 1440
Pivot joint, 1143
Placebo, 40-41
Placebo effect, 40
Plague, 454*t*, 455
Plantar digital neuritis, 1173
Plantar fasciitis, 1173
Plaque
  atherosclerotic, 794, 794*f*, 848, 848*f*
  cutaneous, 469*f*, 506, 507*f*
Plaquenil; *See* Hydroxychloroquine
Plasma, 877
  composition of, 183*f*
  for hypovolemic shock, 837
Plasma cell
  antigen-antibody interactions and, 314
  functions of, 309*t*, 878*t*
  multiple myeloma and, 915
Plasma exchange
  in Goodpasture's syndrome, 397
  in rheumatoid arthritis, 345
  in type II hypersensitivity, 394
Plasma high-density lipoproteins, 720*c*, 721
Plasma low-density lipoproteins, 720*c*, 721
Plasma membrane, self *versus* non-self and, 307*f*, 307-308, 308*c*, 308*f*
Plasma thromboplastin antecedent, 881*t*
Plasma thromboplastin component, 881*t*
Plasma transfusion, 920
Plasma volume expanders, 1598
Plasmapheresis
  in acute glomerulonephritis, 1591
  in Goodpasture's syndrome, 397
  in Guillain-Barré syndrome, 1013-1014
  in myasthenia gravis, 1019
  in rheumatoid arthritis, 345
  in type II hypersensitivity, 394
Plasmin, 884
Plasminogen, 884
Plaster traction, 1189, 1190*t*
Plaster-of-Paris cast, 1187
Plastic infusion container, 219
Plastic surgery, 513-515, 514*t*, 545
Plate guard, 103*t*
Platelet aggregation, 878, 879, 889
Platelet count
  in acute myelogenic leukemia, 910
  in acute peripheral arterial occlusion, 810
  in cirrhosis, 1349-1350
  in hematologic assessment, 887*c*
  in idiopathic thrombocytopenic purpura, 916
Platelet disorders, 916
Platelet inhibitors, 884
Platelet transfusion, 920
  in idiopathic thrombocytopenic purpura, 916
  indications for, 917*t*
Platelet(s), 878-879, 879*f*
  drugs disrupting, 883-884*t*
  reduced function in leukemia, 903
Platinol; *See* Cisplatin
Platybasia, 1163
Plavix; *See* Clopidogrel
Pleiotropic cytokines, 318
Plethoric appearance in polycythemia vera, 901
Plethysmography
  in Buerger's disease, 815
  in peripheral arterial disease, 806
Pleura, 555*f*, 556
Pleural effusion, 561
  in acute pancreatitis, 1373
  in inhalation anthrax, 673
  in lung cancer, 650
Pleural friction rub, 563*t*
Pleural space
  empyema and, 673-674
  pneumothorax and, 698-699
Pleur-Evac drainage system, 647, 647*f*
Pleurisy, 338
Pleuritic pain
  in lung abscess, 672
  in pneumonia, 661, 663*t*
  in pulmonary embolism, 679, 679*c*
Pleurodesis, 650, 650*c*
Pleuropulmonary pain, 713*t*
Plexus, 933
Plicamycin, 421*t*, 1164
Ploidy, cancer and, 406*t*, 406-407, 407*t*
Pluripotency, 402
Pluripotent stem cell, 308
  aplastic anemia and, 900
PMDD; *See* Premenstrual dysphoric disorder
PMI; *See* Point of maximal impulse
PMS; *See* Premenstrual syndrome
PND; *See* Paroxysmal nocturnal dyspnea
Pneumatic compression devices, 258, 259*f*
Pneumococcus
  in peritonitis, 1317
  in tonsillitis, 657
Pneumoconiosis, 640*c*
Pneumocystis jiroveci pneumonia, 371, 379
Pneumonectomy
  care after, 649
  in lung cancer, 645, 646, 646*f*
Pneumonia, 659-666
  in acute pancreatitis, 1373
  after brain tumor surgery, 1064
  after open conventional esophageal surgery, 1254, 1254*c*
  concept map for, 662
  health care resources for, 666
  health teaching in, 665-666
  history in, 660-661
  home care management in, 665, 665*c*
  imaging assessment in, 663
  impaired gas exchange in, 664, 664*c*
  ineffective airway clearance in, 664
  laboratory assessment in, 663, 663*f*
  nursing diagnoses in, 663-664
  pathophysiology of, 659, 659*t*
  physical assessment in, 661, 663*t*
  prevention of, 660, 660*c*
  psychosocial assessment in, 661
  risk in chronic obstructive pulmonary disease, 633
  sepsis in, 664-665, 665*t*
  ventilator-associated, 659, 660, 660*c*
Pneumonitis, 338
Pneumothorax, 560, 698-699
  central venous catheter insertion-related, 231*t*
  clinical manifestations of, 569
  in status asthmaticus, 621
  tension, 699
  tracheotomy-related, 580
POCkit HSV-2 Rapid Test, 1742
Podagra, 353
Podofilox, 1744
Point mutation, 71
Point of maximal impulse, 717-718, 718*f*
Poisoning
  carbon monoxide, 529-530, 530*t*
  food, 1340-1342, 1341*c*, 1341*t*
Polyarteritis nodosa, 355
Polyarthralgia, 354
Polyarthritis
  in serum sickness, 395
  in systemic lupus erythematosus, 348
Polycystic kidney disease, 1581-1585, 1582*f*, 1583*f*, 1583-1585*c*
Polycythemia, 893
Polydipsia, 1467
Polyester-cotton knit cast, 1187
Polymerase chain reaction, 1742
Polymorphism, 71
Polymorphonuclear cell, 310
Polymyalgia rheumatica, 355, 355*c*
Polymyositis/dermatomyositis, 354
Polymyxin B, 543*c*
Polyp
  cervical, 1699
  of ear, 1120-1121
  intestinal, 1290*f*, 1308-1309, 1309*f*
  nasal, 592
  vocal cord, 595, 595*c*, 595*f*
Polypectomy, 592, 1309
Polyphagia, 1467
Polypharmacy, 19
Polyradiculoneuropathy, 1011-1016, 1012*c*, 1012*t*, 1013*t*, 1014*c*, 1015*c*
Polysomnography, 594
Polyuria, 1535*t*
  in chronic kidney disease, 1609
  in diabetes insipidus, 1432
  in diabetes mellitus, 1467
  in hyperaldosteronism, 1446
  nocturnal, 1533
Polyvinyl chloride infusion container, 219
Pons, 930, 931*f*, 931*t*
Pontine artery, 932*f*
Pontocaine; *See* Cocaine
Popliteal artery, 804*f*
Popliteal artery aneurysm, 814
Popliteal entrapment, 816
Popliteal pulse, 717*f*
Pores in capillary membrane, 172, 172*f*
Portable amplifier, 1132
Portable chest drainage system, 647*f*, 649
Port-A-Cath, 53
Portal hypertension, 1345
Portal hypertensive gastropathy, 1345
Portal of exit, 443
Portal-systemic encephalopathy, 1345-1346, 1346*t*, 1354-1355
Position-fixing device for obstructive sleep apnea, 594
Positioning
  in burn
    for impaired physical mobility, 543, 544*c*
    for ventilatory support, 535
  in chronic obstructive pulmonary disease, 632
  for hysterosalpingography, 1655
  low back pain and, 985
  for osteoarthritis pain relief, 327
  postoperative
    in abdominal surgery, 1318
    in brain tumor surgery, 1063
    gas exchange impairment and, 294
    in lung transplantation, 630
    for pain management, 299
    in pancreatic cancer surgery, 1383
  preventing pressure ulcers and, 485*c*
  to promote circulation, 807
  in rheumatoid arthritis, 344
  in spinal cord injury, 995, 995*c*
  for thoracentesis, 568, 568*f*
  in traumatic brain injury, 1056
Positioning injury, intraoperative, 280*f*, 280-281, 281*c*
Positive air-purifying respirator, 128
Positive deflection, 732, 732*f*
Positive end-expiratory pressure, 694
  in acute respiratory distress syndrome, 688
  in burn, 537
  obesity surgery and, 1407
Positive end-expiratory pressure (*Continued*)
  oxygen toxicity and, 573
  tracheostomy and, 583
Positive inotropic drugs
  to enhance contractility, 773
  for pulmonary embolism, 682
Positron emission tomography
  in Alzheimer's disease, 973
  in cardiovascular assessment, 726
  in head and neck cancer, 598
  in lung cancer, 644
  in neurologic assessment, 944*t*, 946
Postanesthesia care unit, 285-286
  hand-off report and, 286, 286*c*
  physical assessment in, 286-293, 288*f*
    cardiovascular evaluation in, 287-289
    fluid, electrolyte, and acid-base balance in, 290
    gastrointestinal assessment in, 290-291, 291*t*
    neurologic assessment in, 289*t*, 289-290
    pain assessment in, 292-293
    renal evaluation in, 290
    respiratory evaluation in, 287, 289*c*
    skin assessment in, 291*f*, 291-292, 292*f*
Postanesthesia care unit record, 288*f*
Postauricular lymph nodes, 1235*f*
Post-cholecystectomy syndrome, 1370-1371, 1371*t*
Post-concussion syndrome, 1049, 1059-1060
Post-dialysis care, 1625-1626, 1626*c*
Posterior cerebral artery, 931, 932*f*, 1033*c*
Posterior cervical lymph nodes, 1235*f*
Posterior chamber, 1071*f*, 1072*f*
Posterior colporrhaphy, 1694
Posterior communicating artery, 932*f*
Posterior cord lesion, 992
Posterior descending coronary artery, 706*f*
Posterior exenteration, 1704*f*, 1704-1705
Posterior fornix, 1643*f*
Posterior gray horn, 932*f*
Posterior inferior cerebellar artery, 932*f*
Posterior nasal bleeding, 591-592, 592*f*
Posterior pituitary, 1415*f*, 1432-1436
  diabetes insipidus and, 1432-1433, 1433*c*, 1434*c*
  hormones of, 1413*t*, 1415, 1415*t*
  syndrome of inappropriate antidiuretic hormone secretion and, 1433-1436, 1435*t*
Posterior rhizotomy, 58*f*
Posterior segment of eye, 1071*f*, 1072*f*
Posterior spinocerebellar tract, 932, 932*f*
Posterior thoracic landmarks, 561*f*
Posterior tibial artery, 804*f*
Posterior tibial pulse
  location of, 717*f*
  in peripheral arterial disease, 805
Posterior urethra, 1532*f*
Posterior uveitis, 1100
Posterior wall myocardial infarction, 850
Posterior white columns, 933
Posteroanterior chest x-ray, 564
Postexposure prophylaxis to HIV, 368*c*, 369*c*
Postherpetic neuralgia, 501
Postictal stage of seizure, 956
Post-infusion phlebitis, 227*t*
Postirradiation sialadenitis, 1240
Postmortem care, 121, 121*c*, 122*c*
Postmyocardial infarction heart failure, 862, 862*t*
Postnecrotic cirrhosis, 1345
Postoperative bleeding
  in bone marrow transplantation, 912*c*
  in coronary artery bypass graft, 868
  in renal biopsy, 1548
  in total hip arthroplasty, 330*c*, 331
  in transurethral resection of prostate, 1718

Postoperative blood salvage, 921
Postoperative care, 285-303
in abdominal aortic aneurysm resection, 812
in abdominal hernia, 1293
acute pain and, 297-299, 297-299*c*
in back surgery, 987*c*, 987-988
in bariatric surgery, 1407
in bladder cancer, 1576
in bone cancer, 1170
in brain tumor, 1063
in breast reconstruction, 1677*c*
in cataract surgery, 1094
in colorectal cancer, 1299
in corneal transplantation, 1090-1091, 1091*t*
in coronary artery bypass graft, 868-869
in diverticular disease, 1336
in esophageal cancer, 1260
in exploratory laparotomy, 1306
in external fixation, 1191
in gastric cancer, 1282-1285
hand-off report in, 286, 286*c*
in head and neck cancer, 600-602, 601*f*
health care resources and, 300-301
health teaching and, 300
in heart transplantation, 790
in hiatal hernia, 1253, 1253*c*, 1254*c*
history in, 286, 287*t*
home care management and, 300
in hypophysectomy, 1431-1432, 1432*c*
hypoxemia and, 299, 300*c*
in hysterectomy, 1697, 1697*c*
in ileostomy, 1327
impaired gas exchange and, 294, 295*c*
impaired skin integrity and, 294-296, 295*c*, 295*f*
laboratory assessment in, 293
in lung cancer, 646
in lung transplantation, 630, 637
in mastectomy, 1674-1675, 1675*c*
in myringotomy, 1125, 1125*c*
nursing diagnoses in, 293-294
in open radical prostatectomy, 1722, 1722*c*
in oral cancer, 1238, 1238*c*
in pancreas transplantation, 1499-1500
in pancreatic cancer, 1382-1383, 1383*t*
in peripheral arterial disease surgery, 809
physical assessment in, 286-293, 288*f*
cardiovascular evaluation in, 287-289
fluid, electrolyte, and acid-base balance in, 290
gastrointestinal assessment in, 290-291, 291*t*
neurologic assessment in, 289*t*, 289-290
pain assessment in, 292-293
renal evaluation in, 290
respiratory evaluation in, 287, 289*c*
skin assessment in, 291*f*, 291-292, 292*f*
in plastic surgery, 515
in pressure ulcer repair, 496
psychosocial assessment in, 293
in renal cell carcinoma, 1596
in renal transplantation, 1632
in retinal detachment, 1102
in sinus surgery, 655*c*
in stapedectomy, 1134
in testicular cancer, 1729
in thyroidectomy, 1454
in total hip arthroplasty, 329, 330*c*, 330*t*
in total knee arthroplasty, 333*f*, 333-334, 334*c*
in tracheostomy, 580
in transurethral resection of prostate, 1717*f*, 1717-1718, 1718*c*
in tympanoplasty, 1133
in urinary incontinence, 1566
Postoperative care *(Continued)*
in urolithiasis, 1573
in valve surgery, 782
in vulvectomy, 1707-1708
Postoperative complications, 287*t*
older adult and, 245, 245*c*
surgical risk factors and, 244*t*
Postoperative exercises, 255-258, 257*c*, 258*f*, 259*f*
Postoperative graft occlusion, 809
Postoperative infection
amputation-related, 1202
in brain tumor, 1064
in liver transplantation, 1363, 1364*t*
in lumbar spinal surgery, 987
in open esophageal surgery, 1260
Postoperative nausea
in aortic dissection, 814
assessment of, 290-291, 291*t*
in cardiac catheterization, 724
in gallstones, 1370
in retinal detachment repair, 1102
Postoperative pain, 38*t*, 297-299, 297-299*c*
analgesics for, 52
in back surgery, 987
in bariatric surgery, 1407
in cataract surgery, 1094
in laryngectomy, 601-602
in lung cancer, 649
in lung transplantation, 630
in oral cancer surgery, 1238
relationship with anxiety, 249
in renal cell carcinoma, 1596
in retinal detachment repair, 1102
in vulvectomy, 1708
Postpartum hemorrhage, 1426
Postpericardiotomy syndrome, 869
Post-pericardiotomy syndrome, 785
Postrenal azotemia, 1601, 1602*t*, 1604*c*
Posttraumatic stress disorder
after lightning strike, 151
after mass casualty event, 164*c*, 164-166
Postural drainage, 631, 632*f*
Postural hypotension, 799
alpha blocker-related, 1714-1715
bromocriptine-related, 1431
cardiovascular assessment and, 716
dehydration and, 178
in diabetic neuropathy, 1470
in hypernatremia, 186
in hyponatremia, 185
spinal cord injured patient and, 997
Posture
musculoskeletal assessment and, 1145, 1145*f*
Parkinson disease and, 966*c*, 968
Post-void residual, 105
Potassium, 187*t*, 187-189, 189*c*
adrenal gland assessment and, 1438*c*
aldosterone secretion and, 1416
in body fluids, 183*f*
burn-related changes in, 524, 532*c*
chronic kidney disease and, 1617, 1617*t*
depletion in diabetes mellitus, 1467
excessive diarrhea and, 1320
in gastrointestinal assessment, 1224*c*
hyperkalemia and, 190*t*, 190-191, 191*c*
in acute adrenal insufficiency, 1436*c*
in adrenal insufficiency, 1438
after pancreas transplantation, 1499-1500
burn-related, 524
in chronic kidney disease, 1610
in crush syndrome, 1182
in diabetes mellitus, 1467
enteral nutrition therapy and, 1400
in hypovolemic shock, 831
in polycythemia vera, 901
preoperative assessment of, 249
transfusion-related, 919
hypokalemia and, 187*t*, 187-189, 189*c*
Potassium *(Continued)*
after pancreas transplantation, 1499-1500
burn-related, 524
in diabetes mellitus, 1467
in diabetic ketoacidosis, 1511
diuretic-induced, 772-773, 801
in hyperaldosteronism, 1445
plasmapheresis-related, 1014*c*
preoperative assessment of, 249
hypovolemic shock and, 836*c*
imbalance after coronary artery bypass graft, 868
levels after pancreas transplantation, 1499-1500
normal plasma values for older adult, 184*t*
preoperative assessment of, 249, 250*c*
prevention of imbalance of, 759*c*
serum, 184*t*
tubular reabsorption of, 1530, 1531*f*
uncompensated acid-base imbalances and, 208, 208*c*
Potassium chloride, 188-189
Potassium hydroxide preparation, 477, 502
Potassium-sparing diuretics
for hyperkalemia, 190
for hypertension, 801
for hypokalemia, 189
Potency, erection and, 1647
Potentiators, 54
Pouch, colostomy, 1301
Pouch care, 1329*c*
PPE; *See* Personal protective equipment
PQRST mnemonic, 1221
PR interval, 731*f*, 734, 735*f*, 737, 738, 739*f*
PR segment, 731*f*, 734, 735*f*
Pramipexole
for Parkinson disease, 967
for restless legs syndrome, 1024
Pramlintide, 1489
Prandial insulin secretion, 1467
Prandin; *See* Repaglinide
Pravigard; *See* Aspirin-pravastatin
Prayer, 9
Praziquantel, 1340
Prazosin, 802
Preadmission testing, 248
Prealbumin
in malnutrition, 1393
nutritional status and, 486
Preauricular lymph nodes, 1235*f*
Precordial leads, 732, 733*t*
Precordium assessment, 717-719, 718*f*, 719*t*
Precose; *See* Acarbose
Precursor cell, 877, 877*f*
Predischarge assessment in rehabilitation, 108
Predisposition genetic testing, 75*t*
Prednisolone
after lung transplantation, 637
for ocular infection, 1086*c*
for transplant immunosuppression, 319
Prednisone
for adrenal insufficiency, 1439*c*
after lung transplantation, 637
for anaphylaxis, 393*c*
for aplastic anemia, 900
for asthma, 617*c*, 620
for dyspnea in dying patient, 117
for rheumatoid arthritis, 341*c*, 344
for transplant immunosuppression, 319
for ulcerative colitis, 1324
Predone; *See* Prednisone
Preemptive analgesia, 37
Pregabalin
for fibromyalgia, 358
for pain, 54, 54*t*
Pregnancy
genital herpes and, 1743
methotrexate contraindication in, 340
Pregnancy *(Continued)*
perinatal transmission of HIV and, 368
urinary tract infection during, 1558
Pregnanediol, 1653*c*
Prehospital care providers, 127*f*, 127-128, 128*f*
Prehypertension, 796, 796*t*
Preictal phase of seizure, 956
Pre-infarction angina, 849
Preload, 707-708, 772-773
Premalignant lesions of oral cavity, 1234
Premature atrial complexes, 740, 769
Premature complexes, 738-739
Premature ventricular complexes, 747-748, 748*f*
in digitalis toxicity, 773
in left-sided heart failure, 769
Premenstrual dysphoric disorder, 1685
Premenstrual syndrome, 1685-1687, 1686*c*
Preoperative autologous blood donation, 921
Preoperative care, 242-263
in abdominal aortic aneurysm resection, 812
in abdominal hernia, 1293
administering regularly scheduled drugs and, 254
assessment in, 244-249
in bariatric surgery, 1406
in bladder cancer, 1576
in bone cancer, 1170
in brain tumor, 1062
in cataract surgery, 1093
categories and purposes of surgery and, 243-244*t*
in colorectal cancer, 1298, 1298*t*
in corneal transplantation, 1090
in coronary artery bypass graft, 866
in Cushing's disease, 1443
dietary restrictions and, 254
in diverticular disease, 1336
in esophageal cancer, 1259
focused assessment in, 251*c*
in fracture, 1190
in gastric cancer, 1281
in head and neck cancer, 600
in heart transplantation, 789
in hiatal hernia, 1250
history in, 244*c*, 244-245*t*, 244-247
in hypophysectomy, 1431
imaging assessment in, 249
informed consent and, 252-254, 253*f*
in intestinal obstruction, 1305
intestinal preparation in, 254
laboratory assessment in, 248-249, 250-251*c*
in low back pain, 986
in lung cancer, 645-646
in lung transplantation, 630, 636-637
in mastectomy, 1674
in myringotomy, 1124-1125
nursing diagnoses and, 252
in oral cancer, 1237
in pancreas transplantation, 1499
in pancreatic cancer, 1382
patient anxiety and, 258-260
patient self-determination and, 254
patient transfer to surgical suite and, 261
in peripheral arterial disease surgery, 808
physical assessment in, 247*c*, 247-248
in plastic surgery, 515
preoperative chart review in, 260
preoperative drugs and, 261
preoperative patient preparation and, 260-261
preparation for tubes, drains, and vascular access in, 255
in pressure ulcer, 495
in prostate cancer, 1721
psychosocial assessment in, 248
in renal cell carcinoma, 1596

Preoperative care *(Continued)*
in renal transplantation, 1631
in retinal detachment, 1101
skin preparation in, 255, 256*f*
in stapedectomy, 1134, 1134*c*
surgical settings and, 244
teaching postoperative procedures and exercises and, 255-259, 256*c*, 257*c*, 258*f*, 259*f*
in testicular cancer, 1729
in thyroidectomy, 1454
in total hip arthroplasty, 328-329
in total knee arthroplasty, 333
in tracheostomy, 580
in transurethral resection of prostate, 1715
in tympanoplasty, 1132-1133
in ulcerative colitis, 1325
in urinary incontinence, 1566
in urolithiasis, 1573
in valve surgery, 782
in vulvar cancer, 1707
Preoperative chart review, 260
Preoperative drugs, 261
Preoperative teaching checklist, 252*t*
Prepuce, penile cancer and, 1732
Prerenal azotemia, 1601, 1602*t*, 1603, 1604*c*
Prerenal failure, 1601
Presbycusis, 1130
Presbyopia, 18, 1074, 1102, 1514
Prescribing of infusion therapy, 215
Presenile dementia, 969
Pressure dressings, 543-544, 544*f*
Pressure eye patch, 1088*c*
Pressure necrosis, cast-related infection and, 1189
Pressure of end-tidal carbon dioxide, 566
Pressure relief devices, 104, 104*f*, 486-488
Pressure support ventilation, 697*t*
Pressure ulcer, 484-499
assessment before rehabilitation, 98
concept map for, 492
dressings for, 491-493, 493-495*t*
drug therapy for, 493
in Guillain-Barré syndrome, 1015
health care resources for, 498, 499*c*
health teaching in, 498
history in, 488
home care management in, 498
identification of high-risk patient and, 486, 487*f*
intervention activities for, 493*c*
intraoperative development of, 296
laboratory assessment in, 490-491
new technologies for, 495
nursing diagnoses in, 491
nutrition therapy for, 493
older adult and, 25
pathophysiology of, 484-485, 485*f*
physical assessment in, 488
physical therapy for, 493
pressure-relieving and pressure-reducing techniques for, 486-488
prevention of, 485*c*, 485-486
psychosocial assessment in, 490
risk for infection and, 496-498, 497*c*
spinal cord injured patient and, 997
surgical management of, 495-496, 496*f*
wound assessment in, 488-490, 489*c*, 489*f*, 490*t*
Pressure-cycled ventilator, 692-693
Pressure-reducing techniques, 486-488
Presymptomatic genetic testing, 75*t*
Pretibial edema, 1536
Pretibial myxedema, 1449
Prevacid; *See* Lansoprazole
Prevention
of abdominal hernia, 1292
of acute coronary syndromes, 850-853, 853*t*, 854*c*
of acute renal failure, 1603
of acute respiratory distress syndrome, 687
Prevention *(Continued)*
of Alzheimer's disease, 970
of back pain, 984, 984*c*
of bradydysrhythmias, 759*c*
of burn, 527-528
of cancer, 411*t*, 411-412
of carpal tunnel syndrome, 1206
of cataract, 1091-1092
of chronic kidney disease, 1612
of chronic obstructive pulmonary disease, 624
of colorectal cancer, 1294-1295, 1295*c*
of coronary artery disease, 854*c*
of cystitis, 1553, 1554*c*
of diabetes mellitus, 1472
of diabetes mellitus-related amputation, 1201
of diabetic ketoacidosis, 1511-1512
of ear infection or trauma after ear surgery, 1134*c*
of fracture, 1183
of hearing loss, 1130
of hemorrhoids, 1309-1310
of hepatitis, 1358, 1358*c*
of hypoglycemia, 1509
of hypovolemic shock, 832-833, 833*c*
of lung cancer, 642
of migraine headache, 953, 954*c*
of obesity, 1403, 1403*t*
of osteoporosis, 1155
of ovarian cancer, 1706
of peptic ulcer disease, 1272
of pneumonia, 660, 660*c*
of pulmonary embolism, 678*c*
of sepsis, 840*t*, 840-841
of septic shock, 840*t*, 840-841
of severe acute respiratory syndrome, 666-667
of sickle cell crisis, 898*c*
of stroke, 1032
of syphilis, 1740
of traumatic brain injury, 1053
of vulvovaginitis, 1691*c*
Preventive therapy drugs for asthma, 615
Previous surgical procedures, surgical risk and, 246
Prezista; *See* Darunavir
Prialt; *See* Ziconitide
Priapism, 1733
in black widow spider bite, 148
in sickle cell disease, 895
Prick test, 389
Prilosec; *See* Omeprazole
Primacor; *See* Milrinone
Primary aldosteronism, 798
Primary arthroplasty, 328
Primary bone tumor, 1168
Primary brain injury, 1049*c*, 1049-1050, 1050*f*
Primary bronchus, 554, 555*f*
Primary diabetes insipidus, 1433
Primary dysmenorrhea, 1684-1685
Primary epilepsy, 956
Primary glomerular diseases and syndromes, 1589*t*
Primary gout, 353
Primary hypertension, 797-798, 798*t*; *See also* Hypertension
Primary immune deficiencies, 385
Primary open-angle glaucoma, 1095*t*, 1095-1098, 1098*c*
Primary osteoarthritis, 323
Primary osteoporosis, 1153, 1153*c*
Primary prevention of cancer, 411, 411*t*
Primary progressive multiple sclerosis, 1003
Primary pulmonary hypertension, 637-638, 638*t*
Primary sclerosing cholangitis, 1321-1322
Primary skin lesion, 467
Primary stomatitis, 1231
Primary survey, 126-138, 137*f*, 138*t*
Primary syphilis, 1739
Primary tumor, 404
Primidone, 958*c*
Principle of double effect, 122*t*
Prinzmetal's angina, 849
Prioderm; *See* Malathion
Priority setting in emergency nursing, 130
PRL; *See* Prolactin
Proaccelerin, 881*t*
Pro-Banthine; *See* Propantheline
Probenecid
for gout, 354
for pelvic inflammatory disease, 1751*c*
Procainamide, 741*c*
transient lupus-like syndrome and, 348
for valvular heart disease, 781
Procarbazine, 422*t*
for brain tumor, 1062
for spinal tumor, 1002
Procardia; *See* Nifedipine
Prochlorperazine, 121*c*
Procrit; *See* Epoetin alfa
Proctitis
gonorrhea and, 1745*f*
in lymphogranuloma venereum, 1753
Proctosigmoidoscopy, 1228
Procytox; *See* Cyclophosphamide
Profunda femoris artery, 804*f*
Progesterone, 1653*c*
Progestin, 431*t*
Proglycem; *See* Diazoxide
Prograf; *See* Tacrolimus
Progressive muscular dystrophies, 1174-1175, 1175*t*
Progressive stage of shock, 832
Progressive systemic sclerosis, 351*f*, 351-353, 352*c*
Progressive-relapsing multiple sclerosis, 1003
Proinflammatory cytokines, 318*t*
Proinsulin, 1466, 1466*f*
Projected pain, 41
Prokine; *See* Sargramostim
Prokinetic agents
for chemotherapy-related nausea and vomiting, 429*c*
for gastroesophageal reflux disease, 1247*c*, 1248
Prolactin, 1415*t*
overproduction of, 1428, 1429, 1430*c*
serum levels in reproductive assessment, 1653*c*
Prolactin-secreting tumor, 1428
Prolapse, uterine, 1691-1694, 1692*f*, 1693*c*, 1693*f*
Prolapsed hemorrhoids, 1309, 1309*f*
Proliferative diabetic retinopathy, 1469, 1469*t*
Prometaphase of cell cycle, 67*f*
Promethazine, 54
Promotors of cancer cell development, 403
Pronation, 1146*f*
Pronator drift, 939
Prone position
in acute respiratory distress syndrome, 688
surgical, 280*f*
Prone pushups, 986*c*
Pronestyl; *See* Procainamide
Propafenone, 742*c*
Propantheline
for urinary incontinence, 1565*c*, 1567
for urolithiasis, 1573
Proparacaine, 1086*c*
Prophase of cell cycle, 67*f*
Prophylactic mastectomy, 1669
Prophylactic oophorectomy, 1669
Prophylactic surgery in cancer, 417
Prophylaxis
in colorectal cancer surgery, 1298
in corneal laceration, 1104
for inhalation anthrax, 673*c*
in valve disease before invasive procedure, 781
Propine; *See* Dipivefrin hydrochloride
Propofol, 274*t*
Proportional pulse pressure, 769
Propoxyphene
abuse of, 90*t*
for rheumatoid arthritis, 344
Propranadol, 1452
Propranolol, 742*c*
for esophageal varices, 1353
for multiple sclerosis, 1006
Proprioception
after stroke, 1034, 1047
assessment of, 939, 940
Brown-Séquard syndrome and, 992
posterior spinocerebellar tract and, 932
Proprioceptive system, 1126
Propylthiouracil, 1452, 1453*c*
Proscar; *See* Finasteride
Prosopagnosia, 975
Prostadynia, 1733
Prostaglandin agonists, 1099*c*
Prostaglandin analogues, 1269*c*, 1274
Prostaglandin synthesis inhibitors, 194
Prostaglandin(s)
dysmenorrhea and, 1685
endometriosis and, 1687
migraine headache and, 951
renal production of, 1531*t*, 1532
Prostate, 1532*f*, 1645*f*, 1646
benign prostatic hypertrophy and, 1646, 1712-1718
community-based care in, 1718
concept map for, 1716
drug therapy for, 1714-1715
laboratory assessment in, 1714
nursing diagnoses in, 1714
pathophysiology of, 1712-1713, 1713*f*
physical assessment in, 1713-1714, 1714*c*
prostate cancer and, 1720
surgical management of, 1715-1718, 1717*f*, 1718*c*
examination of, 1651
needle biopsy of, 1658
prostatitis and, 1733-1734
Prostate cancer, 1719-1725
benign prostatic hypertrophy and, 1720
complementary and alternative therapies in, 1723-1724
conditions associated with genetic predisposition for, 410*t*
cryotherapy in, 1723
drug therapy, 1723
health promotion and maintenance in, 1719*c*, 1719-1720
health teaching in, 1724-1725, 1725*c*
heath care resources for, 1725
hematologic assessment in, 409*c*
history in, 1720
home care management in, 1724
impaired urinary elimination in, 1721
laboratory assessment in, 1720
nursing diagnoses in, 1721
pathophysiology of, 1719, 1719*f*
physical assessment in, 1720
psychosocial assessment in, 1720
radiation therapy in, 1722-1723
sites of metastasis for, 405*t*
surgical management of, 1721-1722, 1722*c*
Prostatectomy
in benign prostatic hypertrophy, 1717*f*
erectile dysfunction after, 1725
laparoscopic radical, 1721
open radical, 1722, 1722*c*
Prostate-specific antigen test, 1653*c*, 1654
in benign prostatic hypertrophy, 1714
in prostate cancer, 1720
Prostatic urethra, 1645*f*

Prostatitis, 1733-1734
benign prostatic hypertrophy *versus,* 1714
gonorrhea and, 1745*f*
Prosthesis
for hip fracture, 1196*f*
ocular, 1105*c*
penile, 1726
preoperative removal of, 260
in stapedectomy, 1134, 1134*f*
in total hip arthroplasty, 329
Prosthetic heart valves, 782
Protamine sulfate, 331, 680
Protease inhibitors, 279, 364, 377-378*c*
Protease(s), 621
Protective environment, 445
for burn patient, 536, 541
Protective gene, 71
Protein
in body fluids, 183*f*
in cerebrospinal fluid, 948*t*
hyperthyroidism and, 1449
intake in diabetes mellitus, 1493
metabolism of, 1218
restriction in chronic kidney disease, 1615, 1617*t*
restriction in diabetic nephropathy, 1506
self *versus* non-self and, 307, 307*f*
synthesis of, 70, 70*f*, 70*t*, 71*f*
thyroid hormone production and, 1417
in urine, 1539*t*, 1541, 1542*c*
Protein buffers, 202
Protein C, 882
Protein deficiency, 1394*t*
Protein S, 882
Protein-calorie malnutrition, 16, 1392
Protein-energy malnutrition, 16, 1392
Protein-sparing modified fast, 1404
Proteinuria, 1541
in diabetes mellitus, 1475
in diabetic nephropathy, 1594
in heart failure, 769
in nephrotic syndrome, 1593
in polycystic kidney disease, 1583
Proteolysis, 1372, 1467
Proteus
in brain abscess, 1065
in prostatitis, 1733
in pyelonephritis, 1587
in urinary tract infection, 1552
Prothrombin, 881*t*
Prothrombin time
in cardiovascular assessment, 721
in cirrhosis, 1349, 1349*t*
in deep vein thrombosis, 819
in hematologic assessment, 887*c*, 888
preoperative assessment of, 251*c*
in pulmonary embolism, 682*c*
Proton pump inhibitors
for acute pancreatitis, 1376
for gastritis, 1268
for gastroesophageal reflux disease, 1247*c*, 1248
mechanical ventilation and, 696
for peptic ulcer disease, 1269*c*, 1274
for Zollinger-Ellison syndrome, 1279
Protonix; *See* Pantoprazole
Protozoal infection, 371
Protraction, 1146*f*
Proventil; *See* Albuterol
Provigil; *See* Modafinil
Proximal convoluted tubule, 1528, 1528*f*, 1530*t*, 1531*f*
Proximal femoral fracture, 1196*f*
Proximal humeral fracture, 1195
Proximal interphalangeal joint
musculoskeletal assessment of, 1146, 1147*f*
positioning for prevention of contracture, 544*c*
rheumatoid arthritis of, 338, 338*f*
Proxymetacaine, 1086*c*

Pruritus, 480-481
in bee sting, 150
in brown recluse spider bite, 147
in chronic cholecystitis, 1367
dry skin and, 480
epidural opioid-related, 53
ocular drug effects and, 1076
in pediculosis, 504
in scabies, 504
in skin problems, 467
in tarantula bite, 148
in uremia, 1536, 1614
in vulvar cancer, 1707
in vulvovaginitis, 1690
PSE; *See* Portal-systemic encephalopathy
Pseudoaddiction, 39-40
Pseudoaneurysm, 1031
Pseudocyst, pancreatic, 1380
Pseudogout, 356
Pseudomonas aeruginosa
in conjunctivitis, 1087
in external otitis, 1121
in humidifier-related infection, 574
in osteomyelitis, 1165
in pyelonephritis, 1587
in sepsis, 840
Psoralen and ultraviolet light therapy, 507-508
Psoriasis, 506-508, 507*f*
Psoriatic arthritis, 357, 506
Psychiatric crisis nurse team, 127
Psychoactive drugs for chemical restraint, 25
Psychological dependence
cocaine and, 86
phencyclidine and, 87
Psychological factors in heart disease development, 711
Psychosocial assessment
in acidosis, 207-208
in acquired immunodeficiency syndrome, 373
in acute coronary syndromes, 855
in acute pancreatitis, 1374
in adrenal insufficiency, 1438
in Alzheimer's disease, 973
in amputation, 1200-1201
in bladder cancer, 1575-1576
in breast cancer, 1670
in cardiovascular assessment, 719
in cataract, 1092
in chronic kidney disease, 1614
in chronic obstructive pulmonary disease, 626
in cirrhosis, 1349
in colorectal cancer, 1295
in Crohn's disease, 1331
in Cushing's disease, 1441
in endocrine problems, 1422-1423
in end-of-life care, 116, 116*c*
in endometrial cancer, 1700
in esophageal cancer, 1256
in fracture, 1185
in gastrointestinal problems, 1223
in head and neck cancer, 598
in hearing loss, 1116, 1131
in heart failure, 769
in hematologic assessment, 886
in hepatitis, 1359
in hypertension, 799
in hyperthyroidism, 1451
in hypothyroidism, 1457
in hypovolemic shock, 835
in hysterectomy, 1696-1697
in infectious disease, 450
in leukemia, 904
in lung cancer, 644
in malnutrition, 1393
in multiple sclerosis, 1004
in musculoskeletal disorders, 1147
in neurologic assessment, 942-943
in obesity, 1404
in osteoarthritis, 325
in osteoporosis, 1156
in pain, 44

Psychosocial assessment *(Continued)*
in Parkinson disease, 966*c*
in pelvic inflammatory disease, 1748-1749
in peptic ulcer disease, 1273
in plastic surgery, 513
in pneumonia, 661
in polycystic kidney disease, 1583
postoperative, 293
preoperative, 248
in pressure ulcer, 490
in prostate cancer, 1720
in pulmonary embolism, 679
in pyelonephritis, 1587-1588
rehabilitation and, 99
in renal problems, 1537
in reproductive problems, 1651-1652
in respiratory disorders, 564
in rheumatoid arthritis, 339
in septic shock, 842
in sickle cell disease, 896
in skin problems, 476
in spinal cord injury, 994
in stroke, 1035-1036
in systemic lupus erythematosus, 349
in testicular cancer, 1728
in traumatic brain injury, 1055
in ulcerative colitis, 1323
in uterine leiomyoma, 1695
in vision assessment, 1079
Psychosocial management
in bone cancer, 1171*c*
in burn, 545
in end-of-life care, 119*t*, 119-121, 120*c*, 121*c*
Psychosocial preparation
in breast cancer, 1680-1681
in chronic kidney disease, 1635
in diabetes mellitus, 1515-1516
in head and neck cancer, 606
in leukemia, 912
in urinary incontinence, 1569
Psychosocial response
in acquired immunodeficiency syndrome, 383
in colorectal cancer, 1301
in hyperthyroidism, 1449*c*
in hypothyroidism, 1456*c*
in spinal cord injury, 998-999
survivor to mass casualty event and, 165-166
to valve surgery, 783
Psychosocial support
in labyrinthitis, 1127
in Parkinson disease, 969
in reduced vision, 1107
Psychotropic drugs
for Alzheimer's disease, 976
for Huntington disease, 980
Psyllium hydrophilic mucilloid, 107
PTC; *See* Percutaneous transhepatic cholangiography
PTCA; *See* Percutaneous transluminal coronary angioplasty
PTH; *See* Parathyroid hormone
Ptosis, 1077
in black widow spider bite, 148
in cluster headache, 954
in myasthenia gravis, 1016
in stroke, 1035
in uncal herniation, 1052
PTSD; *See* Posttraumatic stress disorder
PTT; *See* Partial thromboplastin time
PTU; *See* Propylthiouracil
Ptyalin, 1217
Pubic lice, 504
Public Health Department, disaster assistance and, 162
Pubovaginal sling procedures, 1566*t*
Pudendal plexus, 1022*f*
Pulley exercise, 1675*c*
Pulmicort; *See* Budesonide
Pulmonary arterial hypertension, 237*t*

Pulmonary artery
bronchioles and, 555*f*
right-sided heart catheterization and, 723*f*
Pulmonary artery catheter, 770
Pulmonary artery occlusive pressure, 726
Pulmonary artery pressure, 727, 770
Pulmonary artery wedge pressure, 864
Pulmonary autograft, 782
Pulmonary capillary wedge pressure, 727-728
in acute respiratory distress syndrome, 687
in heart failure, 770
nesiritide and, 772
Pulmonary circulation, 556
Pulmonary complications
after brain tumor surgery, 1064
in ascites, 1352
in chronic pancreatitis, 1377-1378
in peritonitis, 1317
in spinal cord injury, 994
in Whipple procedure, 1383*t*
Pulmonary contusion, 697-698
Pulmonary disorders, 609-652
acute respiratory distress syndrome in, 686-689, 687*t*
asthma in, 610-621
drug therapy for, 615-621, 616-618*c*
exercise and activity in, 621
health teaching in, 613-615, 615*c*
history in, 612
laboratory assessment in, 612
oxygen therapy in, 621
pathophysiology of, 610-611, 611*f*
physical assessment in, 612, 614*f*
smoking cessation and, 614*c*
status asthmaticus and, 621
step system in, 613*c*
subcutaneous infusion therapy in, 237*t*
surgical risk and, 246
avian influenza in, 667-668
bronchiolitis obliterans organizing pneumonia in, 641
chronic obstructive pulmonary disease in, 621-635
activity intolerance in, 633
anxiety in, 633
health care resources in, 634, 634*c*
health teaching in, 634
history in, 624
home care management in, 634
imaging studies, 627
imbalanced nutrition: less than body requirements in, 632-633
impaired gas exchange in, 628-630, 629*c*
ineffective airway clearance in, 631-632, 632*f*, 633*t*
ineffective breathing pattern in, 630-631, 631*c*
laboratory assessment in, 626-627
nursing diagnoses in, 628
physical assessment in, 624*f*, 624-626, 626*f*
pneumonia and respiratory infection risks in, 633
prevention of, 624
psychosocial assessment in, 626
pulmonary function tests in, 627, 627*t*
cystic fibrosis in, 635-637
endotracheal intubation in, 689-692, 690*f*, 691*c*
flail chest in, 698, 698*f*
hemothorax in, 699
idiopathic pulmonary fibrosis in, 639
influenza in, 658-659
inhalation anthrax in, 672-673, 673*c*
lung abscess in, 672
lung cancer in, 641-650
hematologic assessment in, 409*c*
history in, 642-643, 643*t*

Pulmonary disorders *(Continued)*
nonsurgical management of, 644-645
palliation in, 650, 650*c*
pathophysiology of, 641-642
physical assessment in, 643-644
prevention of, 642
psychosocial assessment in, 644
sites of metastasis for, 405*t*
surgical management of, 645-649, 646*f*, 647*f*, 648*c*
mechanical ventilation in, 692*c*, 692-697
extubation in, 697
managing ventilator system in, 695*t*, 695-696
modes of ventilation in, 693
monitoring in, 694-695
preventing complications in, 696
types of ventilators in, 692-693, 693*f*
ventilator controls and settings in, 693-694
weaning from, 696-697, 697*t*
occupational lung disease in, 639-641, 640*c*
pneumonia in, 659-666
concept map for, 662
health care resources for, 666
health teaching in, 665-666
history in, 660-661
home care management in, 665, 665*c*
imaging assessment in, 663
impaired gas exchange in, 664, 664*c*
ineffective airway clearance in, 664
laboratory assessment in, 663, 663*f*
nursing diagnoses in, 663-664
pathophysiology of, 659, 659*t*
physical assessment in, 661, 663*t*
prevention of, 660, 660*c*
psychosocial assessment in, 661
sepsis in, 664-665, 665*t*
pneumothorax in, 698-699
primary pulmonary hypertension in, 637-638, 638*t*
pulmonary contusion in, 697-698
pulmonary empyema in, 673-674
rib fracture in, 698
sarcoidosis in, 638-639
severe acute respiratory syndrome in, 666-667
syndrome of inappropriate antidiuretic hormone secretion and, 1435*t*
tension pneumothorax in, 699
tracheobronchial trauma in, 699
tuberculosis in, 668-672
directly observed therapy in, 449
drug therapy for, 670, 671*c*
health care resources for, 672
health teaching in, 670-672
history in, 669
in HIV-infected patient, 372
home care management in, 670
laboratory assessment in, 669
nursing diagnoses in, 669
pathophysiology of, 668, 668*t*
physical assessment in, 669
Pulmonary edema
after brain tumor surgery, 1064
in black widow spider bite, 148
in burn injury, 536
in chronic kidney disease, 1620
in coronary artery disease, 862
in Cushing's disease, 1442
fluid overload and, 182
in heart failure, 775*c*, 775-776
high-altitude, 154-156, 156*c*
in mitral stenosis, 779
in pit viper envenomation, 144
in scorpion sting, 149
in syndrome of inappropriate antidiuretic hormone secretion, 436, 1436
in thermal airway burn, 530
Pulmonary embolism, 677-684
anxiety and, 682-683
atrial fibrillation and, 745-746
decreased cardiac output in, 682
fat embolism syndrome *versus,* 1182*c*
fracture-related, 1183
health care resources for, 683-684, 684*c*
health promotion and maintenance and, 678, 678*c*
health teaching in, 683, 684*c*
history in, 679
home care management in, 683
hypoxemia in, 680-682, 680-682*c*
imaging assessment in, 679
laboratory assessment in, 679
nursing diagnoses in, 679-680
pathophysiology of, 677-678
physical assessment in, 679, 679*c*
potential for bleeding in, 683, 683*c*
psychosocial assessment in, 679
spinal cord injured patient and, 997
total hip arthroplasty and, 330-331
Pulmonary empyema, 673-674
Pulmonary fibrosis, 639, 689
Pulmonary function tests, 566-567, 567*t*
in asthma, 612
in chronic obstructive pulmonary disease, 627, 627*t*
in cystic fibrosis, 636
Pulmonary hygiene
after thymectomy, 1020
in Cushing's disease, 1444
infection in leukemia and, 906
in respiratory acidosis, 209
Pulmonary hypertension
in rheumatoid arthritis, 338
in scleroderma, 352
Pulmonary rehabilitation, 629, 634
Pulmonary sarcoidosis, 638-639
Pulmonary tuberculosis, 668-672
directly observed therapy in, 449
drug therapy for, 670, 671*c*
health care resources for, 672
health teaching in, 670-672
history in, 669
in HIV-infected patient, 372
home care management in, 670
laboratory assessment in, 669
nursing diagnoses in, 669
pathophysiology of, 668, 668*t*
physical assessment in, 669
Pulmonary vasculature, 557*c*
Pulmonary vein, 555*f*
Pulmonic area, 718*t*
Pulmonic valve, 705*f*, 706
Pulmozyme; *See* Dornase alfa
Pulse
after discharge from postanesthesia care unit, 289*c*
assessment in musculoskeletal trauma, 1184*c*
cardiovascular assessment and, 716-717, 717*f*
dehydration and, 178
hypernatremia and, 186
hypocalcemia and, 192
hypokalemia and, 188
hyponatremia and, 185
Pulse deficit, 289
Pulse oximetry, 566
in hypovolemic shock, 834-835
in pneumonia, 663
postoperative, 287
in pulmonary edema, 775
Pulse pressure
in aortic regurgitation, 780
in aortic stenosis, 780
cardiovascular assessment and, 716
hypovolemic shock and, 833-834
in left-sided heart failure, 769
postoperative assessment of, 287
Pulse therapy for rheumatoid arthritis, 344
Pulseless electrical activity, 747
Pulsus alternans, 717, 769
Pulsus paradoxus, 786
Pump
of infusion rate-controlling device, 222
insulin, 1487, 1487*f*
Punch biopsy, 477
Punctum, 1072, 1072*f*
Puncture wound
in pit viper envenomation, 144
in scorpion sting, 149
Pupil, 1071, 1071*f*
assessment of, 1077
changes with aging, 1075*c*
constriction and dilation of, 1073-1074
neurologic assessment and, 942
traumatic brain injury and, 1055
Pure motor Guillain-Barré syndrome, 1013*t*
Pure-tone air-conduction testing, 1117
Pure-tone audiometry, 1117
Pure-tone bone-conduction testing, 1117
Purified protein derivative, 395
Purines, 64, 64*f*
Purinethol; *See* 6-Mercaptopurine
Purkinje fiber, 731, 731*f*
Purnell's domains of culture, 29*t*, 29-33
biologic ecology in, 31
culture overview and communication in, 29, 29*c*
family and workplace issues in, 29-30
health care practices and practitioners in, 32*f*, 32-33, 33*f*
lesbian, gay, bisexual, and transgender health in, 30*c*, 30-31, 31*t*
nutrition in, 31
spirituality in, 31-32
Purpura, 1614
Purpuric lesion, 471
Pursed-lip breathing, 631*c*
Purulent exudate, 490*t*
Purulent otitis media, 1123-1125, 1124*f*, 1125*c*, 1125*f*
Pus
in pleural space, 673
wound infection and, 490, 490*t*
Pustule, 469*f*
PUVA therapy, 507-508
PVCs; *See* Premature ventricular complexes
PVD; *See* Peripheral vascular disease
PYD; *See* Pyridinium
Pyelolithotomy, 1588-1589
Pyelonephritis, 1586-1589, 1587*c*, 1587*f*
Pyloric obstruction, 1272, 1278
Pyloric sphincter, 1217
Pyloromyotomy, 1259
Pyloroplasty, 1278
Pylorus, 1217
Pyogenic liver abscess, 1361
Pyramid, 1527, 1527*f*
Pyramidal tract, 929, 933
Pyrantel pamoate
for enterobiasis, 1339
for hookworm infection, 1340
Pyrazinamide, 670, 671*c*
Pyridiate; *See* Phenazopyridine
Pyridimines, 64, 64*f*
Pyridinium, 1156
Pyridium; *See* Phenazopyridine
Pyridostigmine, 1019
Pyridoxine deficiency, 1394*t*
Pyuria
in cystitis, 1555
in urethritis, 1559
Pyuria-dysuria syndrome, 1559
PZA; *See* Pyrazinamide

Q

Q wave, 849, 849*f*, 855
Qi, 11
QRS complex, 731, 731*f*, 734, 735*f*
atrioventricular blocks and, 750
heart rhythm analysis and, 737
normal sinus rhythm and, 737, 737*f*
sinus bradycardia and, 739*f*
sinus tachycardia and, 739*f*
ventricular dysrhythmias and, 747
QRS duration, 734, 737, 738
QT interval, 731*f*, 735*f*, 735-736
Quad cough, 997
Quadrigeminy, 738
Quadriparesis, 993
Quadriplegia, 993
Quadripod cane, 101*f*
Quadruple gallop, 719
Qualitative ultrasound, 1156-1157
Quality improvement, 6
QuantiFERON-TB Gold test, 669
Quantitative computed tomography, 1156
Quantitative RNA assay, 374
Quinolones, 1556*c*
Quinsy, 657
Quixin; *See* Levofloxacin

R

R wave, 731*f*
Rabeprazole
for gastroesophageal reflux disease, 1247*c*, 1248
for peptic ulcer disease, 1269*c*, 1274
Race, 27-28
breast cancer and, 1664-1665
burn assessment and, 532
cancer development and, 410, 410*t*
chronic obstructive pulmonary disease and, 622
coronary artery disease and, 850, 852, 855
diabetes mellitus and, 1472, 1473*t*
lactose intolerance and, 1221
musculoskeletal differences in, 119*t*
Radial nerve, 281*c*, 1022*f*
Radial nerve block, 276*f*
Radial pulse, 717*f*
Radial vein, 216*f*
Radiating pain, 41
Radiation burn, 526-527, 527*c*
Radiation dose, 418
Radiation proctitis, 1723
Radiation therapy, 418*f*, 418-420, 419*f*, 420*c*
in bladder cancer, 1576
in bone cancer, 1169-1170
in brain tumor, 1062
in breast cancer, 1676-1678, 1677*t*
in cervical cancer, 1705
in colorectal cancer, 1297
in Cushing's disease, 1443
in endometrial cancer, 1700-1701, 1701*c*
in esophageal cancer, 1258
in gallbladder cancer, 1371
in gastric cancer, 1281
in head and neck cancer, 599
in lung cancer, 645, 650
in nasopharyngeal cancer, 593
in ocular melanoma, 1106
in oral cancer, 1237
in ovarian cancer, 1706
in pancreatic cancer, 1382
postirradiation sialadenitis and, 1240
in prostate cancer, 1722-1723
in skin cancer, 512
in spinal tumor, 1002
in testicular cancer, 1730
in thyroid cancer, 1461
in vaginal cancer, 1709
Radiation-induced immune deficiency, 384-385
Radical hysterectomy, 1697*t*, 1702
Radical nephrectomy, 1596
Radical pancreatectomy, 1382
Radical surgery, 244*t*

Radical vulvectomy, 1707, 1708*f*
Radicular pain, 1001
Radiculopathy, 985
after lumbar spinal surgery, 987*c*
in spinal tumor, 1001
Radioactive iodine therapy, 1452-1454
Radioallergosorbent test, 389
Radiofrequency ablation, 757
in atrial fibrillation, 746
in bone cancer, 1170
for chronic pain, 57
in renal cell carcinoma, 1595
Radiofrequency energy technique for varicose veins, 823
Radiography
in acute renal failure, 1604
in cirrhosis, 1350
in fracture, 1185
in gastrointestinal assessment, 1226
in infection assessment, 451
in intestinal obstruction, 1304
kidney, ureter, and bladder x-ray, 1543
in neurologic assessment, 943
in peritonitis, 1318
in pyelonephritis, 1588
in reproductive assessment, 1654
in respiratory assessment, 564-566
skull, 1424
in spinal tumor, 1001
in urolithiasis, 1572, 1572*f*
Radionuclide studies
in heart failure, 770
in hematologic assessment, 889
in musculoskeletal assessment, 1149
in ocular tumor, 1079
in Paget's disease of bone, 1163
Raloxifene, 1159*c*, 1160
Raltegravir, 378*c*, 379
Ramipril, 771
Ranexa; *See* Ranolazine
Range of motion
assessment before rehabilitation, 98
gait training and, 100-101
in mobility and functional assessment, 1145, 1146*f*
Range-of-motion exercises
after amputation, 1202
after bone cancer surgery, 1170
for burn patient, 543
types of, 102*t*
Ranitidine
for gastritis, 1268
for gastroesophageal reflux disease, 1246*c*, 1247-1248
for gastrointestinal protection in Cushing's disease, 1444
mechanical ventilation and, 696
for peptic ulcer disease, 1269*c*, 1274
preoperative, 261
RANKL; *See* Receptor activator of nuclear factor kappa-B ligand
Ranolazine, 860
Rapamune; *See* Sirolimus
Rapid hypersensitivity reactions, 387-394
allergic rhinitis in, 388*f*, 388-391, 389*f*, 390*c*
anaphylaxis in, 391*t*, 391-394, 392*c*, 392*f*, 393*c*
latex allergy in, 394
Rapid neurologic assessment, 941*f*, 941-942, 942*f*
Rapid plasma reagin test, 1652-1654, 1741
Rapid Response Team, 3
Rapid urease testing, 1267
Rapid-acting insulin, 1484, 1485*t*
Rapidly progressive glomerulonephritis, 1591-1592
Raptiva; *See* Efalizumab
RAS; *See* Reticular activating system
Rasagiline mesylate, 968
Rash, 471-472, 504-506, 505*c*
in pharyngitis, 656*c*
in serum sickness, 395
Rash *(Continued)*
in syphilis, 1739-1740, 1740*f*
in systemic lupus erythematosus, 348, 349*f*
in toxic shock syndrome, 1691, 1692*c*
RAST; *See* Radioallergosorbent test
Rate-controlling device in infusion system, 221-222
Rattlesnake envenomation, 144-145, 145*f*
Raynaud's disease, 815-816
Raynaud's phenomenon, 815-816, 816*f*
in polymyositis/dermatomyositis, 354
in scleroderma, 352
in systemic lupus erythematosus, 349
Reading comprehension, 938
Rebound headache with triptan use, 952
Recall memory, 938
Recent memory, 938
Receptive aphasia, 1046, 1046*t*
Receptor, 307*f*
Receptor activator of nuclear factor kappa-B ligand
osteoporosis and, 1154
Paget's disease of bone and, 1162
Reclast; *See* Zoledronic acid
Recombinant tissue plasminogen activator, 1037, 1037*c*
Reconstruction surgery, 513-515, 514*t*
in breast cancer, 1675, 1676*t*, 1677*c*
in burn, 545
in cancer, 417
in pelvic bone cancer, 1170-1171
of tendon, 1208
Recovery score rating, 286
Recreational therapist, 96
Rectal administration of opioid analgesics, 50*t*
Rectal bleeding
in colorectal cancer, 1295
in hemorrhoids, 1310
Rectal examination, 1650, 1651
in benign prostatic hypertrophy, 1714
in prostate cancer, 1719, 1719*c*, 1720
in urinary incontinence, 1563
Rectal pain, 1337
Rectal prolapse, 635
Rectocele, 1693, 1693*f*
Rectouterine pouch, 1643*f*
Rectovaginal examination, 1650
Rectovesical pouch, 1645*f*
Rectum, 1217*f*
colorectal cancer and, 1293-1302
anticipatory grieving in, 1296, 1297*c*
conditions associated with genetic predisposition for, 410*t*
drug therapy in, 1297
genetic testing for, 76
health care resources for, 1302
health promotion and maintenance in, 1294-1295, 1295*c*
health teaching in, 1300-1302, 1301*c*
hematologic assessment in, 409*c*
history in, 1295
home management in, 1300
imaging studies in, 1296
laboratory assessment in, 1295-1296
metastasis in, 1296
nursing diagnoses in, 1296
pathophysiology of, 1293-1294, 1294*f*
physical assessment in, 1295
psychosocial assessment in, 1295
radiation therapy in, 1297
sites of metastasis for, 405*t*
surgical management of, 1297*t*, 1297-1300, 1298*t*, 1299*f*, 1300*c*
female, 1643*f*
hemorrhoids and, 1309*f*, 1309-1310
male, 1645*f*
Recurrent laryngeal nerve damage, 1454
Red blood cell, 877-878, 878*f*
in urine, 1539*t*
Red blood cell count
in cardiovascular assessment, 722
in hematologic assessment, 887*c*
in respiratory disorders, 564, 565*c*
in rheumatoid arthritis, 340
Red blood cell disorders, 893-902
anemia in, 878, 893-898
after total hip arthroplasty, 331
aplastic, 900
bleeding gastrointestinal ulcer or polyp and, 886
chemotherapy-related, 424, 426
common causes of, 893*t*
community-based care in, 898, 898*c*
folic acid deficiency, 900
glucose-6-phosphate dehydrogenase deficiency, 898-899
hematologic assessment and, 885
immunohemolytic, 899
iron-deficiency, 899, 899*c*
sickle cell disease in, 894*f*, 894-898, 895*f*, 897*c*, 898*c*
systemic manifestations of, 894*c*
vitamin B_{12} deficiency, 900
myelodysplastic syndromes in, 901-902
polycythemia vera in, 901, 901*c*
Red blood cell transfusion, 919*t*, 919-920
in sickle cell disease, 897
Red reflex, 1081, 1081*t*
Redirection in Alzheimer's disease, 975
Reduced vision, 1106*c*, 1106-1107
Reducible abdominal hernia, 1292
Reduction mammoplasty, 514*t*, 1662
Reed-Sternberg cell, 913
Re-epithelialization, 482-483, 484*f*
ReFacto; *See* Factor VIII cryoprecipitate
Refeeding syndrome, 1399
Referral
burn center referral criteria and, 521*t*
in chronic pain, 59
Referred pain, 41
Reflex arc, 933, 934*f*
Reflex bladder, 105, 105*t*
Reflex sympathetic dystrophy, 1204
Reflex urinary incontinence, 1560*t*, 1568
Reflexes, 933, 934*f*
assessment of, 940*f*, 940-941, 941*f*
spinal cord injury and, 993-994
Refludan; *See* Lepirudin
Reflux
in alkaline reflux gastropathy, 1285
in esophageal diverticula, 1261
gastroesophageal, 1243-1248
in cystic fibrosis, 635
drug therapy for, 1246-1247*c*, 1246-1248
endoscopic therapies for, 1248, 1248*c*
laryngitis in, 658
nonpharmacologic interventions in, 1245*c*, 1245-1246
nursing diagnoses in, 1245
pathophysiology of, 1243-1244, 1244*t*
physical assessment in, 1244*c*, 1244-1245
surgical management of, 1248
in hiatal hernia, 1249
in pyelonephritis, 1586-1587
Reflux esophagitis, 1243
Refraction, 1073, 1102
Refractive errors, 1102-1103
Refractive structures and media of eye, 1071-1072, 1072*f*
Refractory stage of shock, 832
Refractory symptoms of distress, end-of-life care and, 118
Regeneration of peripheral nerve, 1023, 1023*f*
Regional anesthesia, 272*t*, 275-276, 276*f*, 276*t*, 277*f*
Regional osteoporosis, 1153
Registered nurse, 4
Reglan; *See* Metoclopramide
Regonol; *See* Pyridostigmine
Regurgitation, 706
aortic, 779*c*, 780
in esophageal diverticula, 1261
in gastroesophageal reflux disease, 1244
in hiatal hernia, 1249
mitral, 779*c*, 779-780
Rehabilitation, 94-110
after total hip arthroplasty, 332
after total knee arthroplasty, 334
in burn injury, 545-547, 546*t*
constipation and, 106-107, 107*t*
coping issues in, 107-108
functional assessment and, 98-99
health care resources for, 109
health teaching and, 108-109
home care management and, 108
impaired physical mobility and, 99-101, 100*c*, 101*c*, 101*f*, 102*t*
impaired skin integrity and, 103-105, 104*c*
nursing diagnoses and, 99
patient history and, 97
physical assessment and, 97*t*, 97-98
psychosocial assessment and, 99
rehabilitation team and, 95*f*, 95-97, 96*f*, 96*t*
self-care deficit and, 101-103, 103*t*
in stroke, 1048
urinary elimination impairment and, 105*t*, 105-106
vocational assessment and, 99
Rehabilitation assistant, 96
Rehabilitation case manager, 96
Rehabilitation nurse, 96, 96*t*
Rehabilitation team, 95*f*, 95-97, 96*f*, 96*t*
Rehabilitative surgery in cancer, 417
Rehydration
in frostbite, 154
in metabolic acidosis, 209
Reiki, 12
Reiter's syndrome, 355
Rejection of transplant, 319-320
corneal, 1091
heart, 790*c*
liver, 1363, 1364*t*
pancreatic, 1498
renal, 1632, 1633*t*
Relapsing-remitting multiple sclerosis, 1003
Relative acidosis, 205
Relative alkalosis, 210, 210*f*
Relative dehydration, 176
Relaxation techniques
for pain management, 56-57
for postoperative pain, 299
for urolithiasis, 1573
Relenza; *See* Zanamivir
Reliance insert, 1566
Religion
beliefs regarding death, dying, and afterlife, 119*t*
dying patient and, 120
ReliOn R, 1485*t*
Relocation stress syndrome, 18
Remicade; *See* Infliximab
Remifentanil, 274*t*
Reminiscence, dying patient and, 120
Reminiscence therapy in Alzheimer's disease, 975
Reminyl; *See* Galantamine
Remodeling of bone, 1153, 1180, 1180*f*
Remodulin; *See* Treprostinil
Remote memory, 938
Renal acid-base control mechanisms, 203*t*, 204
Renal angioplasty, 1594
Renal arteriography, 1546
Renal arteriole, 1527*f*
Renal artery, 1527*f*
Renal artery stenosis, 1594
after renal transplantation, 1633
secondary hypertension in, 798

Renal assessment, 1526-1549
anatomy and physiology review in, 1526-1533, 1527-1529*f*, 1530*t*, 1531*f*, 1531*t*, 1532*f*
bladder scan in, 1542-1543, 1543*f*
blood tests in, 1537-1538, 1538*c*
in burn, 530-531
computed tomography in, 1545-1546
cystography and cystourethrography in, 1546
cystoscopy and cystourethroscopy in, 1546-1547
in hematologic disorders, 885
intravenous urography in, 1543-1545, 1545*c*
kidney, ureter, and bladder x-ray in, 1543
patient history in, 1533-1536, 1534*c*, 1535*t*
physical assessment in, 1536-1537, 1537*f*
postoperative, 290
psychosocial assessment in, 1537
rehabilitation and, 97*t*, 98
renal arteriography in, 1546
renal biopsy in, 1547-1548
renal changes with aging and, 1533, 1534*c*
renography in, 1546
retrograde procedures in, 1547
in spinal cord injury, 994
ultrasonography in, 1546
urine tests in, 1538-1542, 1539*c*, 1540*t*
urodynamic studies in, 1547
Renal biopsy, 1547-1548
in acute glomerulonephritis, 1591
in acute renal failure, 1604
in chronic glomerulonephritis, 1592
Renal calculi, 1570-1575
in gout, 353
in hyperparathyroidism, 1461
infection prevention in, 1573-1574
nutrition history in, 1535
Paget's disease of bone and, 1163
pathophysiology of, 1570-1571, 1571*t*
prevention of obstruction in, 1574*t*, 1574-1575, 1575*c*
spinal cord injury-related, 998
surgical management of, 1573
urinary tract infection and, 1551*t*
Renal capsule, 1527, 1527*f*
Renal casts, 1539*t*, 1541
Renal cell carcinoma, 1595*t*, 1595-1596
Renal colic, 1536, 1571
Renal columns, 1527, 1527*f*
Renal compensation, 204
Renal cortex, 1527, 1527*f*, 1528*f*
Renal disorders, 1550-1599
acute glomerulonephritis in, 1590*t*, 1590-1591
acute renal failure in, 1601-1609
after liver transplantation, 1364*t*
chronic *versus*, 1601*t*
continuous renal replacement therapy for, 1608
dialysis therapies for, 1607*f*, 1607-1608
drug therapy for, 1605-1607, 1606*c*
health promotion and maintenance in, 1603
history in, 1603
imaging studies in, 1604
incidence and prevalence of, 1602-1603, 1603*t*
laboratory assessment in, 1604, 1605*c*
nursing diagnoses in, 1604
nutrition therapy for, 1607
phases of, 1602, 1602*t*
physical assessment in, 1603-1604, 1604*c*
posthospital care in, 1608
types of, 1601, 1602*t*
bladder cancer in, 1575-1578, 1577*f*
bladder trauma in, 1578
Renal disorders *(Continued)*
chronic glomerulonephritis in, 1592
chronic kidney disease in, 1609*c*, 1609-1635
acute renal failure *versus*, 1601*t*
anxiety in, 1619-1620
cardiac changes in, 1610-1611, 1613, 1613*c*
concept map for, 1616
decreased cardiac output in, 1618
etiology and genetic risk in, 1611*t*, 1611-1612
excess fluid volume in, 1618
fatigue in, 1619
gastrointestinal changes in, 1611, 1613*c*, 1614
health care resources for, 1635
health promotion and maintenance in, 1612
health teaching in, 1635
hematologic changes in, 1611, 1613*c*, 1613-1614
hemodialysis in, 1620-1626; *See also* Hemodialysis
history in, 1612
home care management in, 1633-1635, 1634*c*
imaging studies in, 1614
imbalanced nutrition: less than body requirements in, 1615-1618, 1617*c*, 1617*t*
incidence and prevalence of, 1612, 1612*c*
integumentary manifestations in, 1613*c*, 1614
kidney changes in, 1609
laboratory assessment in, 1614
metabolic changes in, 1609-1610, 1610*f*
musculoskeletal manifestations in, 1613*c*, 1614
neurologic manifestations in, 1613*c*
nursing diagnoses in, 1615
osteomalacia and, 1161
peritoneal dialysis in, 1626-1630, 1627*t*, 1627-1629*f*, 1629*c*
physical assessment in, 1612-1614, 1613*c*
psychosocial assessment in, 1614
psychosocial preparation in, 1635
pulmonary edema in, 1620
renal transplantation in, 1630-1633, 1631*f*, 1632*f*, 1633*t*
reproductive manifestations in, 1613*c*
respiratory manifestations in, 1613, 1613*c*
risk for infection in, 1618
risk for injury in, 1618-1619
sickle cell disease and, 895-896
stages of, 1609, 1609*t*
cystitis in, 1551-1559
community-based care in, 1558-1559
drug therapy for, 1555-1558, 1556-1558*c*
laboratory assessment in, 1554-1555
nursing diagnoses in, 1555
nutrition therapy for, 1558
pathophysiology of, 1551-1553, 1552*t*, 1553*c*
physical assessment in, 1553-1554, 1555*c*
prevention of, 1553, 1554*c*
diabetic nephropathy in, 1594*t*, 1594-1595
hydronephrosis and hydroureter in, 1585*f*, 1585-1586
immunologic interstitial and tubulointerstitial disorders in, 1593
nephrosclerosis in, 1593
nephrotic syndrome in, 1592-1593, 1593*c*
polycystic kidney disease in, 1581-1585, 1582*f*, 1583*f*, 1583-1585*c*
Renal disorders *(Continued)*
pyelonephritis in, 1586-1589, 1587*c*, 1587*f*
rapidly progressive glomerulonephritis in, 1591-1592
renal cell carcinoma in, 1595*t*, 1595-1596
renal trauma in, 1596-1598, 1597*c*, 1597*t*
renovascular disease in, 1593-1594, 1594*c*
secondary hypertension in, 798, 799
urethral stricture in, 1559, 1585-1586
urethritis in, 1559
urinary incontinence in, 1559-1570
etiology of, 1561
functional, 1568-1569
health care resources for, 1569-1570
health teaching in, 1569, 1570*c*
history of, 1562, 1562*c*
home care management in, 1569
imaging studies in, 1563
incidence and prevalence of, 1562
laboratory assessment in, 1563
nursing diagnoses in, 1563
older adult and, 1561, 1562*c*
physical assessment in, 1562-1563
psychosocial preparation in, 1569
reflex, 1568
stress, 1564*c*, 1564-1566, 1565*c*, 1565*f*, 1566*t*
total or mixed, 1569
types of, 1560-1561*t*
urge, 1567-1568, 1568*c*
urolithiasis in, 1570-1575
in gout, 353
in hyperparathyroidism, 1461
infection prevention in, 1573-1574
nutrition history in, 1535
Paget's disease of bone and, 1163
pathophysiology of, 1570-1571, 1571*t*
prevention of obstruction in, 1574*t*, 1574-1575, 1575*c*
spinal cord injury-related, 998
surgical management of, 1573
Renal failure, 1600-1639
acute, 1601-1609
after liver transplantation, 1364*t*
chronic *versus*, 1601*t*
continuous renal replacement therapy for, 1608
dialysis therapies for, 1607*f*, 1607-1608
drug therapy for, 1605-1607, 1606*c*
health promotion and maintenance in, 1603
history in, 1603
imaging studies in, 1604
incidence and prevalence of, 1602-1603, 1603*t*
laboratory assessment in, 1604, 1605*c*
nursing diagnoses in, 1604
nutrition therapy for, 1607
phases of, 1602, 1602*t*
physical assessment in, 1603-1604, 1604*c*
posthospital care in, 1608
types of, 1601, 1602*t*
acute compartment syndrome-related, 1181
after abdominal aortic aneurysm resection, 812
in brown recluse spider bite, 147
chronic, 1609*c*, 1609-1635
acute renal failure *versus*, 1601*t*
anxiety in, 1619-1620
cardiac changes in, 1610-1611, 1613, 1613*c*
concept map for, 1616
decreased cardiac output in, 1618
etiology and genetic risk in, 1611*t*, 1611-1612
excess fluid volume in, 1618
Renal failure *(Continued)*
fatigue in, 1619
gastrointestinal changes in, 1611, 1613*c*, 1614
health care resources for, 1635
health promotion and maintenance in, 1612
health teaching in, 1635
hematologic changes in, 1611, 1613*c*, 1613-1614
history in, 1612
home care management in, 1633-1635, 1634*c*
imaging studies in, 1614
imbalanced nutrition: less than body requirements in, 1615-1618, 1617*c*, 1617*t*
incidence and prevalence of, 1612, 1612*c*
integumentary manifestations in, 1613*c*, 1614
kidney changes in, 1609
laboratory assessment in, 1614
metabolic changes in, 1609-1610, 1610*f*
musculoskeletal manifestations in, 1613*c*, 1614
neurologic manifestations in, 1613*c*
nursing diagnoses in, 1615
osteomalacia and, 1161
peritoneal dialysis in, 1626-1630, 1627*t*, 1627-1629*f*, 1629*c*
physical assessment in, 1612-1614, 1613*c*
psychosocial assessment in, 1614
psychosocial preparation in, 1635
pulmonary edema in, 1620
renal transplantation in, 1630-1633, 1631*f*, 1632*f*, 1633*t*
reproductive manifestations in, 1613*c*
respiratory manifestations in, 1613, 1613*c*
risk for infection in, 1618
risk for injury in, 1618-1619
sickle cell disease and, 895-896
stages of, 1609, 1609*t*
in chronic glomerulonephritis, 1592
contrast-induced, 1543-1544
hemodialysis in, 1620-1626, 1621*t*
anticoagulation in, 1622
complications of, 1626
dialysis settings for, 1621
nursing care in, 1625, 1625*t*
patient selection for, 1620
post-dialysis care in, 1625-1626, 1626*c*
procedure of, 1621*f*, 1621-1622, 1622*f*
vascular access for, 1622-1625, 1623*t*, 1624*c*, 1625*f*
in lightning strike, 152
in pit viper envenomation, 144
in polycystic kidney disease, 1584-1585, 1585*c*
in pyelonephritis, 1589
spinal cord injury-related, 998
Renal medulla, 1527, 1527*f*, 1528*f*
Renal osteodystrophy, 1610, 1610*f*, 1614
Renal palpation, 1536, 1537*f*
Renal papilla, 1527, 1527*f*
Renal parenchyma, 1527, 1527*f*
Renal pelvis, 1527, 1527*f*
Renal pyramid, 1527, 1527*f*
Renal replacement therapies, 1620-1630
hemodialysis in, 1620-1626, 1621*t*
in acute renal failure, 1607*f*, 1607-1608
anticoagulation in, 1622
complications of, 1626
dialysis settings for, 1621
dietary restrictions in, 1617*t*
in hypothermia, 153
nursing care in, 1625, 1625*t*
patient selection for, 1620

Renal replacement therapies *(Continued)*
post-dialysis care in, 1625-1626, 1626*c*
procedure of, 1621*f*, 1621-1622, 1622*f*
vascular access for, 1622-1625, 1623*t*, 1624*c*, 1625*f*
peritoneal dialysis in
in acute renal failure, 1608
in chronic kidney disease, 1626-1630, 1627*t*, 1627-1629*f*, 1629*c*
dietary restrictions in, 1617*t*, 1618
health teaching in, 1635
hemodialysis *versus*, 1621*t*
Renal scan, 1544*t*
Renal system, 1526-1533
age-related changes in fluid balance and, 174*c*
age-related surgical risks and, 245*c*
changes associated with aging, 1533, 1534*c*
cirrhosis and, 1348*f*
diabetes insipidus and, 1433*c*
hepatitis A and, 1357*t*
immobility and, 102*t*
infusion therapy and, 235-236
kidney in, 1526-1532
hormonal functions of, 1531*t*, 1531-1532
microscopic anatomy of, 1527-1528, 1528*f*, 1529*f*
regulatory function of, 1528-1531, 1530*t*, 1531*f*
structure of, 1526-1527, 1527*f*
leukemia and, 903*c*
nutrition screening assessment and, 1390*c*
postoperative complications of, 287*t*
premenstrual syndrome and, 1686*c*
preoperative assessment of, 247-248
shock and, 829*c*
sickle cell disease and, 895-896
ureter in, 1532, 1532*f*
urethra in, 1533
urinary bladder in, 1532-1533
Renal threshold for glucose reabsorption, 1531
Renal transplantation
in chronic kidney disease, 1630-1633, 1631*f*, 1632*f*, 1633*t*
in Goodpasture's syndrome, 394
Renal ultrasonography, 1544*t*
in acute renal failure, 1604
in renal trauma, 1598
in urolithiasis, 1572
Renal vein, 1527*f*
Renal vein thrombosis, 1593
Renin, 1416, 1528, 1529*f*, 1531*t*, 1531-1532
hypertension and, 797
hypovolemic shock and, 831
Renin inhibitors, 802
Renin-angiotensin system
heart failure and, 766, 766*f*
hypertension and, 797
hypovolemic shock and, 831
Renography, 1546
Renovascular disease, 1593-1594, 1594*c*
ReoPro; *See* Abciximab
Repaglinide, 1479*c*, 1483
Repetitive stress injury, 1206
Replacement lens, 1094
Replication of deoxyribonucleic acid, 65*f*, 65-66, 66*f*
Reproductive assessment, 1642-1659
biopsy in, 1657*c*, 1657-1658
endoscopic studies in, 1656*f*, 1656-1657
imaging studies in, 1654-1655
laboratory assessment in, 1652-1654, 1653*c*
patient history in, 1647-1649, 1648*c*, 1648*t*, 1649*c*
physical assessment in, 1649-1651, 1650*c*, 1650*f*
Reproductive assessment *(Continued)*
psychosocial assessment in, 1651-1652
reproductive changes associated with aging and, 1646, 1646*c*
reproductive structure and function and, 1642-1646
female, 1642-1645, 1643*f*, 1644*f*
male, 1645*f*, 1645-1646
Reproductive problems, 1684-1736
female, 1684-1711
Bartholin cyst in, 1699
cervical cancer in, 1702*t*, 1702-1705, 1704*c*, 1704*f*
cervical polyp in, 1699
dysfunctional uterine bleeding in, 1688-1689
endometrial cancer in, 1699-1702, 1700*t*, 1701*c*
endometriosis in, 1687*f*, 1687-1688
fallopian tube cancer in, 1709
menopause in, 1689*t*, 1689-1690, 1690*c*
ovarian cancer in, 1705*t*, 1705-1707
ovarian cyst in, 1694
premenstrual syndrome in, 1685-1687, 1686*c*
primary dysmenorrhea in, 1684-1685
toxic shock syndrome in, 1691, 1692*c*
uterine leiomyoma in, 1694-1699, 1695*f*, 1697*c*, 1697*t*, 1698*c*
uterine prolapse in, 1691-1694, 1692*f*, 1693*c*, 1693*f*
vaginal cancer in, 1708-1709
vulvar cancer in, 1707-1708, 1708*f*
vulvovaginitis in, 1690-1691, 1691*c*
male, 1712-1736
benign prostatic hypertrophy in, 1712-1718, 1713*f*, 1714*c*, 1717*f*, 1718*c*
epididymitis in, 1734
erectile dysfunction in, 1725-1726
hydrocele in, 731*f*, 1730-1731
orchitis in, 1734
penile cancer in, 1732
phimosis and paraphimosis in, 1732*f*, 1732-1733
priapism in, 1733
prostate cancer in, 1719*c*, 1719*f*, 1719-1725, 1722*c*, 1725*c*
prostatitis in, 1733-1734
spermatocele in, 1731, 1731*f*
testicular cancer in, 1726*c*, 1726-1730, 1727*t*, 1728*c*, 1729*c*
varicocele in, 1731*f*, 1731-1732
sexually transmitted diseases and, 1737-1755, 1738*t*
chancroid in, 1753
chlamydia infection in, 1746-1747
complications caused by, 1738, 1739*f*
condom use and, 368*c*
focused assessment in, 1740*c*
genital herpes in, 1742*c*, 1742-1743
genital warts in, 1743-1744, 1744*f*
gonorrhea in, 1744-1746, 1745*f*
granuloma inguinale in, 1753-1754
Healthy People 2010 objectives in, 1739*t*
lymphogranuloma venereum in, 1753
nursing diagnoses in, 1741*t*
oral antibiotic therapy for, 1752*c*
pelvic inflammatory disease in, 1747-1753, 1748*f*, 1749*t*, 1750-1751*c*
syphilis in, 1738-1742, 1740*f*
urethritis in, 1559
use of condoms and, 1743*c*
vaginal infections in, 1753
Reproductive system
chronic kidney disease and, 1613*c*
female, 1642-1645, 1643*f*, 1644*f*
hyperthyroidism and, 1449*c*
hypothyroidism and, 1456*c*
male, 1645*f*, 1645-1646
Requip; *See* Ropinirole
Rescriptor; *See* Delavirdine
Rescue therapy
in acute rejection, 320
in asthma, 615
Rescula; *See* Unoprostone isopropyl
Research, 6
Resection
of abdominal aortic aneurysm, 812
in colorectal cancer, 1298
in esophageal cancer, 1259
in gastric cancer, 1281
in oral cancer, 1238
Reservoir, 441
Residual limb pain, 1201
Residual volume, 567*t*, 627
Residuals, 1397
Resistance gene, 71
Resistin, 1402
Resistive breathing, 630
Resistive range-of-motion exercises, 102*t*
Resonance, 562*t*
Respect, ethical principle of, 5
Respiratory acid-base control mechanisms, 202-204, 203*f*
Respiratory acidosis, 206
causes of, 205*t*
in chronic obstructive pulmonary disease, 626
laboratory assessment of, 208*c*, 208*f*, 208-209
Respiratory alkalosis, 208*c*, 210*f*, 210*t*, 210-211, 211*c*
acclimatization and, 155
in diabetes mellitus, 1467
in heart failure, 769-770
in high altitude pulmonary edema, 155
Respiratory anthrax, 672-673, 673*c*
Respiratory arrest
in lightning strike, 151
in status asthmaticus, 621
Respiratory assessment, 552*f*, 552-570
aging-related changes and, 556, 557*c*
anatomy and physiology in, 553-556, 553-556*f*
in burn, 529*t*, 529-530, 530*t*
capnometry and capnography in, 566
endoscopic examination in, 567-568
exercise testing in, 567
in heart transplant recipient, 790
in hematologic disorders, 885
imaging studies in, 564-566
indicators of respiratory adequacy and, 564
laboratory assessment in, 564, 565*c*
lung biopsy in, 569
lungs and thorax evaluation in, 560-564, 561*f*, 562*f*, 562*t*, 563*t*
nose and sinuses inspection in, 559
patient history in, 556-559, 558*c*, 558*t*, 560*t*
pharynx, trachea, and larynx assessment in, 559-560
psychosocial assessment in, 564
pulmonary function tests in, 566-567, 567*t*
pulse oximetry in, 566
rehabilitation and, 97, 97*t*
skin tests in, 567
in spinal cord injury, 994
thoracentesis in, 568-569, 569*f*
Respiratory bronchiole, 555, 555*f*
Respiratory compensation, 204
Respiratory depression
opioid analgesic-related, 48-49, 49*t*
postoperative assessment of, 287
respiratory acidosis and, 206
Respiratory distress
after parathyroidectomy, 1463
after thoracic aortic aneurysm repair, 813
in anaphylaxis, 392
in burn, 537
Respiratory distress *(Continued)*
in epistaxis, 592
in feeding tube misplacement and dislodgement, 1399
in inhalation anthrax, 673
in thyroidectomy, 1454
Respiratory failure, 685*t*, 685-686, 686*f*
in amyotrophic lateral sclerosis, 1007
in botulism, 1341
burn-related, 524
Respiratory hygiene/cough etiquette, 446*t*, 447, 658
Respiratory insufficiency
in ankylosing spondylitis, 355
in bee sting, 150
in black widow spider bite, 148
in coral snake envenomation, 146
in myasthenia gravis, 1018
in scorpion sting, 149
Respiratory problems, 609-701
acute respiratory distress syndrome in, 686-689, 687*t*
after brain tumor surgery, 1064
in ascites, 1352
asthma in, 610-621
drug therapy in, 615-621, 616-618*c*
exercise and activity in, 621
health teaching in, 613-615, 615*c*
history in, 612
laboratory assessment in, 612
oxygen therapy in, 621
pathophysiology of, 610-611, 611*f*
physical assessment in, 612, 614*f*
smoking cessation and, 614*c*
status asthmaticus and, 621
step system in, 613*c*
subcutaneous infusion therapy in, 237*t*
surgical risk and, 246
avian influenza in, 667-668
bronchiolitis obliterans organizing pneumonia in, 641
chronic obstructive pulmonary disease in, 621-635
activity intolerance in, 633
anxiety in, 633
health care resources in, 634, 634*c*
health teaching in, 634
history in, 624
home care management in, 634
imaging studies, 627
imbalanced nutrition: less than body requirements in, 632-633
impaired gas exchange in, 628-630, 629*c*
ineffective airway clearance in, 631-632, 632*f*, 633*t*
ineffective breathing pattern in, 630-631, 631*c*
laboratory assessment in, 626-627
nursing diagnoses in, 628
physical assessment in, 624*f*, 624-626, 626*f*
pneumonia and respiratory infection risks in, 633
prevention of, 624
psychosocial assessment in, 626
pulmonary function tests in, 627, 627*t*
in chronic pancreatitis, 1377-1378
cystic fibrosis in, 635-637
endotracheal intubation in, 689-692, 690*f*, 691*c*
epistaxis in, 591-592, 592*c*, 592*f*
facial trauma in, 593-594
flail chest in, 698, 698*f*
head and neck cancer in, 597-606
anxiety in, 604
assessment in, 598*t*, 598-599
disturbed body image in, 604
health care resources in, 606
health teaching in, 605*c*, 605-606, 606*f*
home care management in, 605, 605*c*

Respiratory problems *(Continued)*
nursing diagnoses in, 599
pathophysiology of, 597-598
psychosocial preparation for, 606
respiratory obstruction in, 599-602, 600*t*, 601*f*, 603*f*
risk for aspiration in, 603*c*, 603-604, 604*c*
subcutaneous infusion therapy in, 237*t*
hemothorax in, 699
idiopathic pulmonary fibrosis in, 639
influenza in, 658-659
inhalation anthrax in, 672-673, 673*c*
laryngeal trauma in, 596
laryngitis in, 658
lung abscess in, 672
lung cancer in, 641-650
hematologic assessment in, 409*c*
history in, 642-643, 643*t*
nonsurgical management of, 644-645
palliation in, 650, 650*c*
pathophysiology of, 641-642
physical assessment in, 643-644
prevention of, 642
psychosocial assessment in, 644
sites of metastasis for, 405*t*
surgical management of, 645-649, 646*f*, 647*f*, 648*c*
mechanical ventilation for, 692*c*, 692-697
extubation in, 697
managing ventilator system in, 695*t*, 695-696
modes of ventilation in, 693
monitoring in, 694-695
preventing complications in, 696
types of ventilators in, 692-693, 693*f*
ventilator controls and settings in, 693-694
weaning from, 696-697, 697*t*
nasal fracture in, 590-591, 591*f*
nasal polyps in, 592
neck trauma in, 596-597
nose and sinus tumors in, 592-593
obstructive sleep apnea in, 594
occupational lung disease in, 639-641, 640*c*
oxygen therapy for, 571-579
hazards and complications of, 572-574, 573*f*
high-flow oxygen delivery systems in, 576-577, 577*f*, 577*t*, 578*f*
home-based, 578-579, 579*f*
intervention activities in, 572*c*
low-flow oxygen delivery systems in, 574-576, 575*t*, 576*f*
noninvasive positive-pressure ventilation in, 578, 578*f*
nursing diagnoses in, 572
transtracheal, 578
in peritonitis, 1317
peritonsillar abscess in, 657
pharyngitis in, 655-657, 656*c*, 656*t*
pneumonia in, 659-666
concept map for, 662
health care resources for, 666
health teaching in, 665-666
history in, 660-661
home care management in, 665, 665*c*
imaging assessment in, 663
impaired gas exchange in, 664, 664*c*
ineffective airway clearance in, 664
laboratory assessment in, 663, 663*f*
nursing diagnoses in, 663-664
pathophysiology of, 659, 659*t*
physical assessment in, 661, 663*t*
prevention of, 660, 660*c*
psychosocial assessment in, 661
sepsis in, 664-665, 665*t*
pneumothorax in, 698-699
primary pulmonary hypertension in, 637-638, 638*t*

Respiratory problems *(Continued)*
pulmonary contusion in, 697-698
pulmonary embolism in, 677-684
anxiety and, 682-683
decreased cardiac output in, 682
health care resources for, 683-684, 684*c*
health promotion and maintenance and, 678, 678*c*
health teaching in, 683, 684*c*
history in, 679
home care management in, 683
hypoxemia in, 680-682, 680-682*c*
imaging assessment in, 679
laboratory assessment in, 679
nursing diagnoses in, 679-680
pathophysiology of, 677-678
physical assessment in, 679, 679*c*
potential for bleeding in, 683, 683*c*
psychosocial assessment in, 679
total hip arthroplasty and, 330-331
pulmonary empyema in, 673-674
rhinitis in, 654
rib fracture in, 698
sarcoidosis in, 638-639
severe acute respiratory syndrome in, 666-667
sinusitis in, 654-655, 655*c*
in spinal cord injury, 994
in syndrome of inappropriate antidiuretic hormone secretion, 1435*t*
tension pneumothorax in, 699
tonsillitis in, 657, 657*c*
tracheobronchial trauma in, 699
tracheostomy in, 580-587
air warming and humidification in, 583
body image and, 586
bronchial and oral hygiene in, 585
care of, 584-585, 585*c*, 585*f*
community-based care in, 587
complications of, 580-581, 581*t*
emotional care in, 586
nursing diagnoses in, 580
nutrition and, 586, 586*c*
prevention of tissue damage in, 583, 583*f*
speech and communication and, 586
suctioning in, 583-584, 584*c*
tubes in, 581-583, 582*f*
weaning from, 586-587
tuberculosis in, 668-672
directly observed therapy in, 449
drug therapy for, 670, 671*c*
health care resources for, 672
health teaching in, 670-672
history in, 669
in HIV-infected patient, 372
home care management in, 670
laboratory assessment in, 669
nursing diagnoses in, 669
pathophysiology of, 668, 668*t*
physical assessment in, 669
upper airway obstruction in, 596, 597*f*
vocal cord nodules and polyps in, 595, 595*c*, 595*f*
vocal cord paralysis in, 591-595
Respiratory rate
acclimatization and, 155
in acute respiratory failure, 686
in chronic obstructive pulmonary disease, 626
in coronary artery disease, 854
dehydration and, 179
in hypothermia, 153
in hypovolemic shock, 835
in pneumonia, 663*t*
postoperative, 287
in sepsis, 839, 840
Respiratory status
in acquired immunodeficiency syndrome, 379
in acute pancreatitis, 1376

Respiratory status *(Continued)*
after abdominal aortic aneurysm resection, 812-813
after lung cancer surgery, 649
in chronic obstructive pulmonary disease, 628
in Guillain-Barré syndrome, 1014, 1015*c*
preoperative assessment of, 247
Respiratory system
acidosis and, 207, 207*c*
age-related surgical risks and, 245*c*
alkalosis and, 211, 211*c*
anemia and, 894*c*
cancer effects on, 417
chronic kidney disease and, 1613, 1613*c*
cirrhosis and, 1348*f*
dehydration and, 179
fluid overload and, 182*c*
hyperthyroidism and, 1449*c*
hypokalemia and, 188
hypothyroidism and, 1456*c*
immobility and, 102*t*
leukemia and, 903, 903*c*
nutrition screening assessment and, 1390*c*
pathogen entry via, 441-442
postoperative complications of, 287*t*
esophageal surgery and, 1253-1254, 1254*c*, 1260
preventive procedures and exercises for, 255-258, 258*f*
premenstrual syndrome and, 1686*c*
role in oxygenation and tissue perfusion, 552, 552*f*
shock and, 829*c*
Respite care in Alzheimer's disease, 978
Responder cell, 318
Rest
in acquired immunodeficiency syndrome, 379
in acute pancreatitis, 1375
in deep vein thrombosis, 818
in hepatitis, 1360
in infective endocarditis, 785
in multiple sclerosis, 1007
in myasthenia gravis, 1020
for osteoarthritis pain relief, 327
in rheumatoid arthritis, 344
in ulcerative colitis, 1325
in valvular heart disease, 781
Rest pain in peripheral arterial disease, 805
Resting metabolic rate, 1405
Restless legs syndrome, 1024
Restlessness
in Alzheimer's disease, 976-977
approaching death and, 115*c*
end-of-life care and, 118
Restorative aide, 96
Restorative surgery, 243*t*, 1023-1024
Restraints
in Alzheimer's disease, 977
during intubation, 690
older adult and, 24*c*, 24-25
Restrictive cardiomyopathy, 787-790, 788*t*, 789*f*, 790*c*
Restrictive lung diseases, 638
Resurfacing of skin, 483
Resuscitation interventions, trauma nursing and, 138
Resuscitation/emergent phase of burn injury, 528*c*, 528-537
acute respiratory distress syndrome and, 537
history and, 528, 529*c*
ineffective breathing pattern and, 535
ineffective tissue perfusion and, 533*c*, 533*t*, 533-535, 534*f*
laboratory assessment in, 531-532, 532*c*
nursing diagnoses in, 532-533
pain and, 535-536
physical assessment in, 529*t*, 529-531, 530*t*, 531*f*
pulmonary edema and, 536

Retavase; *See* Recombinant tissue plasminogen activator
Rete pegs, 461, 461*f*
Retention bridge, 282*f*
Retention sutures, 282
Reteplase, 819-820
Reticular activating system, 930
Reticular formation, 931*f*
Reticulocyte count
in hematologic assessment, 886, 887*c*
in sickle cell disease, 896
Retina, 1071, 1071*f*
holes, tears, and detachments of, 151, 1101-1102, 1102*f*
hypertension and, 799
macular degeneration and, 1100-1101
Retinitis, 1100
Retinitis pigmentosa, 1102
Retinoic acid, 515
Retinopathy, diabetic, 1468, 1469
Retraction, 1146*f*
Retrograde ejaculation, 1718
Retrograde lymph node obstruction, 673
Retrograde procedures in renal assessment, 1547
Retrograde uteroscopy, 1573
Retroperitoneal hemorrhage, 811
Retropubic prostatectomy, 1717*f*
Retropubic suspension, 1566*t*
Retrovesical prostatectomy, 1717*f*
Retrovir; *See* Zidovudine
Retroviruses
highly active antiretroviral therapy and, 375-379, 376-378*c*
human immunodeficiency virus in, 363
Return of spontaneous circulation, 756
Reverse transcriptase, 363, 363*f*
Reversible ischemic neurologic deficit, 1030
Revia; *See* Naltrexone
Revimine; *See* Dopamine
Revision arthroplasty, 328
Revlimid; *See* Lenalidomine
Rewarming methods
after coronary artery bypass graft, 868
in frostbite, 154
in hypothermia, 153
Reyataz; *See* Atazanavir
Rh antigen system, 919-920
Rhabdomyolysis
in crush syndrome, 1182
in hypophosphatemia, 195
in lightning strike, 152
Rhegmatogenous detachment, 1101
Rheolytic thrombectomy, 866
Rheumatic aortic stenosis, 780
Rheumatic carditis, 787
Rheumatic diseases, 322-361
ankylosing spondylitis in, 355
chronic fatigue syndrome in, 358
disease-associated arthritis in, 357, 357*t*
fibromyalgia in, 357*f*, 357-358
gout in, 353-354, 354*f*
infectious arthritis in, 356
lupus erythematosus in, 347-350, 348*c*, 349*f*, 350*c*
Lyme disease in, 356, 356*c*
Marfan syndrome in, 355-356
mixed connective tissue disease in, 358
osteoarthritis in, 323-336
chronic pain in, 326-328, 327*c*
complementary and alternative therapies in, 327-328, 328*c*
health care resources in, 336
health promotion and maintenance in, 324
health teaching in, 336, 336*c*
home care management in, 335-336
imaging assessment in, 325
impaired physical mobility in, 335, 336*c*
laboratory assessment in, 325

Rheumatic diseases *(Continued)*
nursing diagnoses in, 325-326
pathophysiology of, 323*f*, 323-324
patient history in, 324
physical assessment in, 324-325, 325*t*
psychosocial assessment in, 325
total elbow arthroplasty in, 335
total hip arthroplasty in, 328-332, 330*c*, 330*t*, 332*c*, 332*f*
total knee arthroplasty in, 333*f*, 333-334, 334*c*
total shoulder arthroplasty in, 334-335
polymyalgia rheumatica and temporal arteritis in, 355, 355*c*
polymyositis/dermatomyositis in, 354
pseudogout in, 356
psoriatic arthritis in, 357
Reiter's syndrome in, 355
rheumatoid arthritis in, 337-347
body image and, 346
complementary and alternative therapies for, 345
diagnostic assessment in, 340
drug therapy for, 340-344, 341-342*c*
fatigue in, 346, 346*c*
gene therapy for, 345
health care resources in, 347
health teaching in, 347
home care management in, 346, 346*f*
laboratory assessment in, 339*c*, 339-340
nonpharmacologic interventions for, 344-345, 345*f*
pathophysiology of, 337, 337*c*
physical assessment in, 337-339, 338*f*
promotion of self-care in, 345-346
psychosocial assessment in, 339
scleroderma in, 351*f*, 351-353, 352*c*
systemic necrotizing vasculitis in, 354-355
Rheumatic endocarditis, 787
Rheumatic heart disease, 779
Rheumatoid arthritis, 337-347
body image and, 346
complementary and alternative therapies for, 345
diagnostic assessment in, 340
drug therapy for, 340-344, 341-342*c*
exercise in, 336*c*
fatigue in, 346, 346*c*
gene therapy for, 345
health care resources in, 347
health teaching in, 347
home care management in, 346, 346*f*
laboratory assessment in, 339*c*, 339-340
nonpharmacologic interventions for, 344-345, 345*f*
osteoarthritis *versus*, 325*t*
pathophysiology of, 337, 337*c*
physical assessment in, 337-339, 338*f*
promotion of self-care in, 345-346
psychosocial assessment in, 339
Sjögren's syndrome with, 396
subcutaneous infusion therapy in, 237*t*
systemic lupus erythematosus *versus*, 350, 350*c*
Rheumatoid factor, 337, 339, 339*c*
Rheumatoid spondylitis, 355
Rheumatology, 322
Rheumatrex; *See* Methotrexate
Rhinitis, 654
allergic, 388*f*, 388-391, 389*f*, 390*c*
Rhinoplasty, 514*t*, 515, 591, 591*f*
Rhinorrhea
in allergic rhinitis, 389
in anaphylaxis, 392
in cluster headache, 954
in influenza, 658
in meningitis, 961
Rhizotomy, 57, 58*f*
Rhonchus, 563*t*
Rhytidectomy, 514*t*, 515
Rib fracture, 698, 1183, 1198
Ribavirin, 658
Riboflavin deficiency, 1394*t*
Ribonucleic acid, 70, 70*t*, 71*f*
Ribosome, 63*f*
Rickets, 1161
Rifadin; *See* Rifampin
Rifampin
for inhalation anthrax, 673*c*
for leprosy, 516
for tuberculosis, 670, 671*c*
Right atrial pressure, 727
Right atrium, 704-706, 705*f*
Right bundle branch, 731, 731*f*
Right bundle branch block, 750
Right cerebral hemisphere stroke, 1034, 1034*c*
Right coronary artery, 706, 706*f*, 850
Right lower quadrant, 1222*f*, 1222*t*
Right marginal coronary artery, 706*f*
Right pulmonary artery, 705*f*
Right pulmonary vein, 705*f*
Right upper quadrant, 1222*f*, 1222*t*
Right ventricle, 705*f*, 706, 723*f*
Right ventricular area, 718*t*
Right-sided heart catheterization, 722*t*, 722-724, 723*f*
Right-sided heart failure, 765
in aortic stenosis, 780
history in, 768
in infective endocarditis, 784
mitral stenosis and, 779
in myocardial infarction, 864
in pericarditis, 785-786
physical assessment in, 768*c*, 769
Rigidity
in black widow spider bite, 148
in malignant hyperthermia, 273
in Parkinson disease, 966
Rilutek; *See* Riluzole
Riluzole, 1007
Rimantadine, 658
RIND; *See* Reversible ischemic neurologic deficit
Ringer's lactate
characteristics of, 180*t*
for hypovolemic shock, 837
for trauma patient, 136-137
Ringworm, 501
Rinne turning fork test, 1116
Risedronate
for osteoporosis prevention, 1159*c*, 1160
for Paget's disease of bone, 1164
Risk identification in preventing pressure ulcer, 486, 487*f*
Risser cast, 1188*t*
Ristocetin, 889
Ritonavir, 378*c*, 379
Rituals and customs surrounding food, 31
Rituxan; *See* Rituximab
Rituximab, 342*c*, 344, 434, 435*t*
Rivastigmine
for Alzheimer's disease, 976
for Parkinson disease, 968
RNA; *See* Ribonucleic acid
Robotic heart surgery, 870
Robotic technology, 269*f*, 269-270
Rods, 1071
Rohypnol; *See* Flunitrazepam
Role/relationship pattern, 711*c*
Rolling hiatal hernia, 1249*f*, 1249-1254, 1253*c*, 1253*f*, 1254*c*
ROM; *See* Range of motion
Romazicon; *See* Flumazenil
Romberg sign, 940
R-on-T phenomenon, 735
Rope turning exercise, 1675*c*
Ropinirole
for Parkinson disease, 967
for restless legs syndrome, 1024
Ropivacaine, 52
ROSC; *See* Return of spontaneous circulation
Rosenbaum Pocket Vision Screener, 1078
Rosiglitazone, 1481-1482*c*, 1484
Rosiglitazone-metformin, 1482*c*
Rotation, 1146*f*
Rotation injury of cervical spine, 991, 991*f*
Rotator cuff injury, 1208
Rotaviral gastroenteritis, 1319*t*
Rotigotine, 967
Rotter's nodes, 1644*f*
Roubac; *See* Trimethoprim-sulfamethoxazole
Rough endoplasmic reticulum, 63*f*
Round ligament, 1643*f*
Round window, 1110
Roundworms, 1339-1340
Roux-en-Y gastric bypass, 1406*f*, 1407
Rowasa; *See* Mesalamine
Roxanol; *See* Morphine
Roxicet; *See* Oxycodone-acetaminophen
Rubex; *See* Doxorubicin
Rubor
cardiovascular assessment and, 715
in peripheral arterial disease, 805
Rugae, 1266
Rule of nines, 531, 531*f*
Rumpel-Leede test, 888
Running traction, 1189
Rupture
of aneurysm, 811
of carotid artery, 601
of central venous catheter, 233*t*
of cerebral aneurysm, 1032
of tendon, 1208
Russell's traction, 1190*t*
RV; *See* Residual volume
Rythmol; *See* Propafenone

S

S_1 heart sound, 718
S_2 heart sound, 718
S_3 heart sound, 718-719, 854
S phase of cell cycle, 65, 65*f*, 401, 401*f*
Saccular aneurysm, 810
Sacral plexus, 1022*f*
Sacral spine, 1146
Safe injection practices, 447
Safe Return Program in Alzheimer's disease, 976
Safer sex practices, 367, 368*c*
Safety, 2-7
after sinus surgery, 655*c*
in Alzheimer's disease, 976*c*, 977
in anticoagulant therapy, 819*c*
chest tube drainage systems and, 648*c*
core competencies and, 3-6
collaboration with interdisciplinary health care team and, 5
evidence-based practice and, 5-6, 6*t*
informatics and, 6, 6*f*
patient-centered care and, 3-5, 4*c*
quality improvement and, 6
in ear irrigation, 1123*c*
in electroencephalography, 947*c*
emergency nursing and, 128-130, 129*c*
in hypovolemic shock, 836*c*
infection control and, 443*c*, 443-444
in injection of contrast agent, 943*c*
Institute for Healthcare Improvement and, 3, 3*t*
in magnetic resonance imaging, 1149*c*
in mechanical ventilation, 692*c*
in meningitis, 963*c*
nasogastric tube and, 1277*c*
National Patient Safety Goals and, 2
older adult and
driving and, 18, 19*c*
fall prevention and, 24*c*
health teaching and, 4*c*
impaired vision and, 1098*c*
Safety *(Continued)*
relocation stress and, 18*c*
using restraint alternatives and, 24*c*
in oxygen therapy, 574*c*
in paracentesis, 1352*c*
in Parkinson disease, 967*c*
in perineal wound care, 1300*c*
in pleurodesis, 650*c*
in preventing ventilator-associated pneumonia, 660*c*
in prevention of aspiration during swallowing, 603*c*
in procedures using contrast media, 1545*c*
reduced vision and, 1106
in sealed implants of radioactive sources, 1701*c*
spinal cord injured patient and, 999*c*
surgical suite preparation and, 267-270, 268*f*
in thrombocytopenia, 910*c*
tracheostomy patient and, 584*c*, 586*c*
transfer techniques and, 100*c*
in transfusion therapy, 918*c*
T-tube care and, 1370*c*
in tube feeding, 1398*c*
in valvular heart disease, 783*c*
in vascular access for hemodialysis, 1624*c*
St. John's wort, 12*t*
antihypertensives and, 802
potential postoperative effects of, 246*t*
Salem pump, 291
Salem sump tube, 1304-1305
Salicylates, 343
Saline breast implant, 1662
Saline solution
for heat stroke, 142-143
for hypovolemic shock, 837
properties of, 180*t*
for trauma patient, 138
Saliva, 1217
acute sialadenitis and, 1239
changes after oral cancer surgery, 1239
Salivary amylase, 1217
Salivary gland, 1217, 1217*f*
acute sialadenitis and, 1239-1240
postirradiation sialadenitis and, 1240
tumor of, 1240
Salmeterol, 616*c*, 620
Salmon calcitonin, 1160
Salmonella, 1340-1341
in osteomyelitis, 1165
in pyelonephritis, 1587
in pyogenic liver abscess, 1361
Salpingitis, 1647
gonorrhea and, 1745*f*
Neisseria gonorrhoeae in, 1744
pelvic inflammatory disease and, 1748
sexually transmitted diseases and, 1739*t*
Salpingoophorectomy, 1705
Salt substitutes, 778
Same-day admission, 244
Same-day surgery, 244
Sanctura; *See* Trospium
Sandimmune; *See* Cyclosporine
Sandostatin; *See* Octreotide
Sanguineous drainage, 291
Santyl; *See* Collagenase
Saphenous nerve, 1022*f*
Saphenous vein for coronary artery bypass graft, 867, 867*f*
Saquinavir, 378*c*, 379
Sarcoidosis, 638-639
Sarcoma
chondrosarcoma, 1168
Ewing's, 1168
Kaposi's, 372, 381
Sargramostim, 433*t*
SARS; *See* Severe acute respiratory syndrome
Saturated solution of potassium iodine, 1453*c*
Saw palmetto, 1715

Sawyer extractor, 145
SBAR process, 5
SBFT; *See* Small bowel follow-through
Scabies, 504
Scald injury, 525
Scales, 470*f*, 506, 507*f*
Scapular fracture, 1195
Scarring, 483-484
Scheduled toileting, 1567*c*, 1568
Schilling test, 1311
Schwartz-Bartter syndrome, 1435
Sciatic nerve, 1022*f*
Sclera, 1071, 1071*f*
  assessment of, 1077
  sickle cell disease and, 895
Scleral buckling procedure, 1102*f*
Scleritis, 338
Scleroderma, 351*f*, 351-353, 352*c*
Sclerotherapy
  for esophageal varices, 1354
  for lung cancer palliation, 650
  for varicose veins, 823
Scoliosis, 1145*f*, 1146, 1173-1174, 1174*f*
  in Marfan syndrome, 356
  in Paget's disease of bone, 1163
Scopolamine, 121*c*
Scorpion, 148-149, 149*f*
Scotoma, 1004
Scratch testing, 389
Screening
  for colorectal cancer, 1295*c*
  for diabetes mellitus, 1474
  nutritional, 1389, 1390*c*, 1391*f*
  for tuberculosis, 669
Scrotum, 1645, 1645*f*, 1651
Scrub, surgical, 270, 271*f*
Scrub nurse, 265, 267*f*
Sealed implant of radioactive sources, 420*c*
Sebaceous gland, 462, 462*f*
  burn-related skin changes and, 520, 522*f*
Seborrhea, 1084
Seborrheic keratoses, 508, 509*f*
Sebum, 462
Second heart sound, 718
Second intention healing, 481, 482*f*
Secondary administration set, 220, 220*c*
Secondary depression, 20
Secondary dysmenorrhea, 1685
Secondary epilepsy, 956
Secondary glaucoma, 1095*t*
Secondary glomerular diseases and syndromes, 1590*t*
Secondary gout, 353
Secondary hypertension, 798, 798*t*
Secondary injury in traumatic brain injury, 1051-1052, 1052*f*
Secondary osteoarthritis, 323, 324
Secondary osteoporosis, 1153, 1153*t*
Secondary prevention of cancer, 412
Secondary progressive multiple sclerosis, 1003
Secondary skin lesion, 467
Secondary stomatitis, 1231-1232
Secondary survey, 138
Secondary syphilis, 1739-1740
Secondary tuberculosis, 668
Secondary tumor, 404, 1001
Second-degree atrioventricular block, 750
Second-degree frostbite, 154
Second-generation sulfonylurea agents, 1478-1479*c*
Secondhand smoke, 84
  heart disease and, 710
  lung cancer and, 642
Second-look surgery in cancer, 417
Sectral; *See* Acebutolol
Secular aneurysm, 1031
Securement device, 223, 223*f*
Security guard in emergency room, 129
Sedation
  for bone marrow aspiration, 890
  for dyspnea in dying patient, 118
Sedation *(Continued)*
  opioid analgesic-related, 48-49, 49*t*
  preoperative, 261
Sedation scale, 49*t*
Sediment in urine, 1541
Segmental systolic blood pressure measurement, 805-806
Segmentectomy, 646
Segmented neutrophil, 310
Seizure, 955-961
  in acquired immunodeficiency syndrome, 381
  after stroke, 1043
  in alcohol withdrawal, 84
  in brain abscess, 1066
  in brain tumor, 1065
  in brown recluse spider bite, 147
  drug therapy for, 957-959, 957-959*c*
  emergency care in, 959-961
  end-of-life care and, 118
  in heat stroke, 142, 143
  in high altitude cerebral edema, 155
  in hypernatremia, 186
  in hypocalcemia, 193
  in hypophosphatemia, 195
  in lightning strike, 151
  management of, 959, 959*c*, 960*c*
  in meningitis, 962, 963
  nursing diagnoses in, 957
  pathophysiology of, 955-956
  in phencyclidine withdrawal, 87
  in pit viper envenomation, 144
  in sickle cell disease, 896
  surgical management of, 960-961
  in thyroid storm, 1455
Seizure precautions, 959
Selection advantage of tumor cell, 404
Selective estrogen receptor modulators
  for breast cancer, 1677*t*, 1678
  for osteoporosis prevention, 1160
Selective hypopituitarism, 1426
Selective immunoglobulin A deficiency, 385
Selective serotonin reuptake inhibitors
  for Alzheimer's disease, 976
  for depression in older adult, 21
  for fibromyalgia, 358
  for premenstrual dysphoric disorder, 1687
Selegiline, 968
Self *versus* non-self, 307*f*, 307-308, 308*c*, 308*f*, 319
Self-administration of drugs, 19-20, 20*f*
Self-determination, 5
Self-examination
  breast, 1666, 1667*f*
  skin, 510-511
  testicular, 1651, 1726, 1726*c*
  vulvar, 1650, 1650*c*
Self-management, 5
  after stroke, 1046
  after total hip arthroplasty, 332, 332*c*
  in Alzheimer's disease, 973, 975
  in genital herpes, 1742*c*
  in heart failure, 776-778, 777*t*, 778*c*
  in myasthenia gravis, 1019-1020
  in Parkinson disease, 968
  reduced vision and, 1098*c*, 1107
  rehabilitation and, 101-103, 103*c*, 103*t*
  in rheumatoid arthritis, 345-346
  in spinal cord injury, 997
Self-monitoring of blood glucose, 1490-1492, 1491-1492*t*
Self-perception/self-concept pattern, 1548*c*
Self-tolerance, 307
Sella turcica, 1414
Selzentry; *See* Maraviroc
Semicircular canal, 1110*f*, 1111
Semilunar valve, 705*f*, 706
Seminal vesicle, 1645*f*
Seminoma, 127, 1727*t*
Semirigid infusion container, 219
Semi-sit-ups, 986*c*
Sengstaken-Blakemore tube, 1353
Senile angioma, 466*f*
Senna, 246*t*
Sensation testing with monofilament, 1501-1503, 1503*f*
Sensorineural hearing loss, 1116, 1129-1130
  in acoustic neuroma, 1129
  anatomy of, 1129*f*
  conductive hearing loss *versus*, 1130*t*
  in Meniere's disease, 1127
Sensory aphasia, 1046, 1046*t*
Sensory deficits
  after peripheral nerve trauma, 1023
  after transient ischemic attack, 1030*c*
  after traumatic brain injury, 1058
  in cancer, 416-417
  in cataract, 1093
  in diabetes mellitus, 1500-1501, 1501*f*
  in Guillain-Barré syndrome, 1012
  in hearing loss, 1132, 1133*c*
  in spinal tumor, 1001
  in stroke, 1047
Sensory function
  assessment in musculoskeletal trauma, 1184*c*
  assessment of, 938-939
  Braden Scale for pressure ulcer risk and, 487*f*
  carpal tunnel syndrome and, 1206
  older adult and, 935
  postoperative assessment of, 289-290
  spinal cord injury and, 993
  stroke and, 1047
Sensory neuron, 928
Sensory problems
  in diabetes mellitus, 1500-1501, 1501*f*
  ear and hearing, 1120-1137
    acoustic neuroma in, 1129
    cerumen impaction in, 1122*f*, 1122-1123, 1123*c*
    ear trauma in, 1126
    external otitis in, 1121*c*, 1121*f*, 1121-1122
    furuncle in, 1122
    hearing loss in, 1129-1136; *See also* Hearing loss
    labyrinthitis in, 1127
    mastoiditis in, 1125-1126
    Meniere's disease in, 1127-1129
    middle ear neoplasm in, 1126
    otitis media in, 1123-1125, 1124*f*, 1125*c*, 1125*f*
    perichondritis in, 1122
    tinnitus in, 1126, 1127*t*
    vertigo and dizziness in, 1126-1127
  eye and vision, 1084-1108
    application of eye patch for, 1088*c*
    application of ocular compress for, 1087*c*
    blepharitis in, 1084-1085
    cataracts in, 1091*f*, 1091-1095, 1092*f*, 1092*t*, 1094*f*, 1095*c*
    chalazion in, 1087
    conjunctival hemorrhage in, 1087
    conjunctivitis in, 1087-1088
    contusion of eye in, 1103
    corneal abrasion, ulceration, and infection in, 1089
    drug therapy for inflammation and infection of eye, 1086*c*
    ectropion in, 1085
    entropion in, 1085, 1085*c*, 1085*f*
    foreign body in eye in, 1103-1104
    glaucoma in, 1095*t*, 1095-1098, 1099-1100*c*
    hordeolum in, 1085-1087
    hyphema in, 1103
    insertion and removal of ocular prosthesis, 1105*c*
    instillation of ophthalmic ointment and, 1085*c*
    irrigation of eye in, 1104*c*
    keratoconjunctivitis sicca in, 1087
Sensory problems *(Continued)*
    keratoconus and corneal opacities in, 1089*f*, 1089-1091, 1090*f*, 1091*t*
    laceration of eye in, 1104
    macular degeneration in, 1100-1101
    ocular melanoma in, 1104-1106
    penetrating injury of eye in, 1104
    promotion of independent living in patient with impaired vision, 1098*c*
    reduced vision in, 1106*c*, 1106-1107
    refractive errors in, 1102-1103
    retinal holes, tears, and detachments in, 1101-1102, 1102*f*
    retinitis pigmentosa in, 1102
    trachoma in, 1088
    uveitis in, 1100
    vitreous hemorrhage in, 1098-1100
Sensory receptor, 933
Sentinel lymph node biopsy, 1673-1674
Sepsis, 830
  after esophageal trauma, 1262
  burn wound, 537, 538*t*
  in cancer, 435
  infection and, 838-839
  in inhalation anthrax, 672
  in pelvic inflammatory disease, 1748
  in pneumonia, 664-665, 665*t*
  septic shock and, 839*f*, 839-840
  severe, 840
  in sickle cell disease, 897
Sepsis resuscitation bundles, 843, 843*t*
Sepsis-induced distributive shock, 449
September 11, 2001 disaster, 159-160
Septic clot, 678
Septic shock, 449, 828*t*, 830, 838-844
  drug therapy for, 843-844
  etiology and genetic risk in, 840
  health teaching in, 844, 844*c*
  history in, 841, 841*c*
  home care management in, 844, 844*c*
  incidence and prevalence of, 840
  infection and, 838-839
  in inhalation anthrax, 673
  laboratory assessment in, 842*t*, 842-843
  oncologic emergency and, 435
  physical assessment in, 841*t*, 841-842
  prevention of, 840*t*, 840-841
  progression of events in, 838, 838*f*
  psychosocial assessment in, 842
  resuscitation in, 843, 843*t*
  sepsis and, 839*f*, 839-840
Septicemia, 435
Septra; *See* Trimethoprim-sulfamethoxazole
Sequestosome 1, 1162
Sequestrectomy, 1167
Sequestrum, 1165, 1165*f*
Serax; *See* Oxazepam
Serevent; *See* Salmeterol
Serial-seven test, 938
SERMs; *See* Selective estrogen receptor modulators
Serologic testing, 451, 1742
Serosa, 1216, 1217*f*
Serosanguineous exudate, 490*t*
Serositis, 349
Serotonin, 930*t*
  Alzheimer's disease and, 970
  antidepressants and, 54
  basophil production of, 311
  lysergic acid diethylamide and, 87
  migraine headache and, 951
Serotonin antagonists, 429*c*
Serous drainage, 291
Serous otitis media, 1123-1125, 1124*f*, 1125*c*, 1125*f*
Serpiginous skin lesion, 471*t*
Sertraline
  for Alzheimer's disease, 976
  for fibromyalgia, 358
  for pain, 54, 54*t*
  for premenstrual dysphoric disorder, 1687

Serum albumin
  in cirrhosis, 1349, 1349*t*
  in gastrointestinal assessment, 1224*c*
  in malnutrition, 1393
  nutritional status and, 486
Serum alkaline phosphatase
  in gastrointestinal assessment, 1224*c*
  in Paget's disease of bone, 1163
Serum alpha-fetoprotein, 1362
Serum ammonia
  in cirrhosis, 1349, 1349*t*
  in gastrointestinal assessment, 1223, 1224*c*
Serum amylase
  in acute pancreatitis, 1374, 1374*t*
  in gastrointestinal assessment, 1223, 1224*c*
Serum bicarbonate, 1605*c*
Serum bilirubin
  in acute pancreatitis, 1374, 1374*t*
  in cirrhosis, 1349, 1349*t*
  in gastrointestinal assessment, 1224*c*
  in jaundice, 1346*t*
Serum calcium
  abnormal findings in, 1462*c*
  in acute pancreatitis, 1374*t*, 1375
  in acute renal failure, 1605*c*
  calcitonin secretion and, 1417
  in gastrointestinal assessment, 1224*c*
  in musculoskeletal assessment, 1148*c*
  parathyroid hormone and, 1417, 1418*f*
Serum cardiac enzymes, 720*c*
Serum cholesterol
  coronary artery disease and, 850-851
  in gastrointestinal assessment, 1225*c*
Serum complement, 339*c*, 340
Serum creatinine, 1537, 1538*c*, 1601, 1605*c*
Serum elastase, 1374, 1374*t*
Serum electrolyte concentrations and functions, 184*t*
Serum enzymes
  in cirrhosis, 1349, 1349*t*
  in gastrointestinal assessment, 1223, 1224*c*
Serum ferritin, 886, 887*c*
Serum globulin, 1349, 1349*t*
Serum glucose, 1374*t*, 1375
Serum immunoglobulin E, 389
Serum lactate, 841, 841*t*, 842
Serum lipase
  in acute pancreatitis, 1374, 1374*f*
  in gastrointestinal assessment, 1223, 1224*c*
Serum lipids
  cardiovascular assessment and, 720*c*, 721
  coronary artery disease and, 850-851
Serum magnesium
  in acute pancreatitis, 1374*t*, 1375
  in acute renal failure, 1605*c*
  in hyperparathyroidism, 1463
Serum markers of myocardial damage, 719-721, 720*c*
Serum muscle enzymes, 1148*c*
Serum parathyroid hormone, 1461-1462, 1462*c*
Serum phosphate
  abnormal findings in, 1462*c*
  in acute renal failure, 1605*c*
  in musculoskeletal assessment, 1148*c*
Serum potassium
  in acidosis, 208, 208*c*, 208*f*
  in acute renal failure, 1605*c*
  in gastrointestinal assessment, 1224*c*
Serum protein electrophoresis
  in myasthenia gravis, 1017
  in rheumatoid arthritis, 339*c*
Serum proteins, 1349, 1349*t*
Serum sickness, 145, 395
Serum sodium
  in acute renal failure, 1605*c*
  in syndrome of inappropriate antidiuretic hormone secretion, 1436
Serum testosterone, 1726
Serum tests
  in burn, 532*c*
  in cardiovascular assessment, 721-722
  in gastrointestinal assessment, 1224-1225*c*
  in reproductive assessment, 1653*c*
Serum thyroxine, 1451*c*
Serum transferrin, 886, 1393-1394
Serum triiodothyronine, 1451*c*
Serum trypsin, 1374, 1374*t*
Sesamoid bone, 1141
Sessile polyp, 1309, 1309*f*
Severe acute respiratory syndrome, 666-667
Severe head injury, 1049
Severe hypothermia, 153
Severe sepsis, 840
Sevoflurane, 274*t*
Sex chromosomes, 68, 68*f*
Sex hormones, 1416
Sex-linked recessive patterns of inheritance, 72*t*, 74, 74*f*
Sexual activity
  after hysterectomy, 1698*c*
  genital herpes and, 1743
  patient history of, 1647
  urinary tract infection and, 1551*t*, 1558-1559
  vaginal infection and, 1753
Sexual assault forensic nurse, 127
Sexual assault nurse examiner, 127
Sexual function
  after exenteration, 1705
  after spinal cord injury, 1000
  coronary artery disease and, 872
  intestinal ostomy and, 1302
  osteoporosis and, 1156
  in reproductive assessment, 1648
Sexual identity, 30-31, 31*t*
Sexual transmission of acquired immunodeficiency syndrome, 367, 368*c*
Sexuality
  after vulvectomy, 1708
  breast cancer and, 1670, 1681
  testicular cancer and, 1728-1729
Sexuality-reproductive pattern
  in cardiovascular assessment, 711*c*
  in endocrine assessment, 1420*c*
  in reproductive assessment, 1548*c*
Sexually transmitted diseases, 1737-1755, 1738*t*
  chancroid in, 1753
  chlamydia infection in, 1746-1747
  complications caused by, 1738, 1739*f*
  condom use and, 368*c*
  focused assessment in, 1740*c*
  genital herpes in, 1742*c*, 1742-1743
  genital warts in, 1743-1744, 1744*f*
  gonorrhea in, 1744-1746, 1745*f*
  granuloma inguinale in, 1753-1754
  Healthy People 2010 objectives in, 1739*t*
  lymphogranuloma venereum in, 1753
  nursing diagnoses in, 1741*t*
  oral antibiotic therapy for, 1752*c*
  pelvic inflammatory disease in, 1747-1753
    acute pain in, 1751-1752
    anxiety in, 1752
    community-based care in, 1752
    drug therapy for, 1749-1751, 1750-1751*c*
    history in, 1748
    infection control in, 1749
    laboratory assessment in, 1749
    nursing diagnoses in, 1749
    pathophysiology of, 1747-1748, 1748*f*
    physical assessment in, 1748, 1749*t*
    psychosocial assessment in, 1748-1749
  syphilis in, 1738-1742, 1740*f*
  urethritis in, 1559
  use of condoms and, 1743*c*
  vaginal infections in, 1753
Sharps, standard precautions and, 446*t*
Sharps injury, human immunodeficiency virus transmission and, 368
Shave biopsy, 477
Shaving, preoperative skin preparation and, 255, 256*f*
Shearing forces
  musculoskeletal trauma and, 1183
  pressure ulcer and, 485, 485*f*, 487*f*
Sheehan's syndrome, 1426
Shiatsu massage, 11
Shift to left, 450
Shiga toxin, 1341
Shiga toxin-producing *Escherichia coli*, 1341, 1341*c*
Shigellosis, 1319*t*, 1319-1321, 1321*c*
Shingles, 500*c*, 501, 501*f*
Shivering
  during cooling measures, 143
  in hypothermia, 153
  postoperative, 299
Shock, 826-846
  in acute pancreatitis, 1373, 1374
  in anaphylaxis, 392
  in black widow spider bite, 148
  cardiogenic, 862-863
  hypovolemic, 830-838
    in burn, 530, 534
    community-based care in, 838
    concept map for, 834
    drug therapy for, 837*c*, 837-838
    etiology of, 832
    history in, 833
    incidence and prevalence of, 832
    laboratory assessment in, 835, 836*c*
    nursing diagnoses in, 835
    pathophysiology of, 830-831, 831*t*
    patient safety and, 836*c*
    in peritonitis, 1317
    physical assessment in, 833-835
    in pit viper envenomation, 144
    prevention of, 832-833, 833*c*
    psychosocial assessment in, 835
    stages of, 831-832
    surgical management of, 838
  in myxedema coma, 1459
  oxygenation and perfusion and, 826-827, 827*f*, 829*f*
  septic, 449, 830, 838-844
    bundles for resuscitation in, 843, 843*t*
    drug therapy for, 843-844
    etiology and genetic risk in, 840
    health teaching in, 844, 844*c*
    history in, 841, 841*c*
    home care management in, 844, 844*c*
    incidence and prevalence of, 840
    infection and, 838-839
    in inhalation anthrax, 673
    laboratory assessment in, 842*t*, 842-843
    oncologic emergency and, 435
    physical assessment in, 841*t*, 841-842
    prevention of, 840*t*, 840-841
    progression of events in, 838, 838*f*
    psychosocial assessment in, 842
    sepsis and, 839*f*, 839-840
  systemic manifestations of, 829*c*
  types of, 828*t*, 828-830, 830*t*
Shock lung, 686-689, 687*t*
Shoes for diabetic patient, 1503
Short bones, 1140
Short peripheral catheter, 215*f*, 215-216, 216*c*, 216*t*, 225
Short-acting beta$_2$ agonists, 615-618, 616*c*
Short-acting insulin, 1484, 1485*t*
Short-arm cast, 1188*t*
Short-led cast, 1188*t*
Short-term fasting program, 1404
Shoulder
  complications related to intraoperative positioning, 281*c*
Shoulder *(Continued)*
  positioning for prevention of contracture, 544*c*
  rotator cuff injury of, 1208
  total shoulder arthroplasty and, 334-335
Shoulder spica cast, 1188*t*
Shunt
  arteriovenous, 1623*t*, 1624*c*
  transjugular intrahepatic portal-systemic
    in cirrhosis, 1353
    in esophageal varices, 1354
  ventriculoperitoneal, 1064
SIADH; *See* Syndrome of inappropriate antidiuretic hormone secretion
Sialadenitis, 1239-1240
Sialagogues, 1240
Sibutramine, 1405
Sicca syndrome, 396
Sick-day rules in diabetes mellitus, 1512*c*
Sickle cell crisis, 897, 897*c*, 898*c*
Sickle cell disease, 893*t*, 894*f*, 894-898, 895*f*, 897*c*, 898*c*, 1733
Sickle cell trait, 894, 895*f*
Sidearm traction, 1190*t*
Sigmoid colon, 1219
  cancer in, 1294*f*
  diverticular disease and, 1334
Sigmoid colostomy, 1299*f*
Sigmoidoscopy, 1228, 1296
Sigmoidostomy, 1577*f*
Sign language, 1135
Sildenafil, 1726
Silent myocardial ischemia, 856
Silent stroke, 1030
Silicone breast implant, 1662, 1675
Silicosis, 640*c*
Silvadene; *See* Silver sulfadiazine
Silver sulfadiazine, 542*c*
Simdax; *See* Levosimendan
Simon's foci, 668
Simple facemask, 575, 575*t*, 576*f*
Simple fracture, 1179, 1179*f*
Simple hemothorax, 699
Simple mastectomy, 1673*f*
Simple partial seizure, 956
Simple surgery, 244*t*
Simulect; *See* Basiliximab
SIMV; *See* Synchronized intermittent mandatory ventilation
Simvastatin, 796, 796*t*
Sinemet; *See* Levodopa-carbidopa
Single gene trait, 69, 69*f*
Single nucleotide polymorphisms, 71, 410
Single photon emission computed tomography
  in Alzheimer's disease, 973
  in head and neck cancer, 598
  in neurologic assessment, 944*t*, 946
  in stroke, 1035
Single-lumen cannula cuffed tracheostomy tube, 582*f*
Singulair; *See* Monteleukast
Sinoatrial node, 706, 731, 731*f*
Sinus arrhythmia, 737-738
Sinus bradycardia, 739*f*, 740
Sinus dysrhythmias, 739*f*, 739-740
Sinus surgery, 655, 655*c*
Sinus tachycardia, 273, 739, 739*f*
Sinus x-ray, 566
Sinuses, 553*f*, 553-554
  inspection of, 559
  sinusitis and, 654-655, 655*c*
  tumor of, 592-593
Sinusitis, 654-655, 655*c*
Sirdalud; *See* Tizanidine
Sirolimus, 320
SIRS; *See* Systemic inflammatory response
Sitagliptin, 1490
Site infection in intravenous therapy, 228*t*
Situational depression, 20

Sjögren's syndrome, 338, 340
Skeletal muscle, 1143
  hypovolemic shock and, 835
  movements of, 1146*f*
Skeletal muscle atrophy
  in osteoarthritis, 324
  in systemic lupus erythematosus, 348-349
Skeletal pin site care, 1191
Skeletal system, 1140-1143, 1141*f*, 1141*t*, 1142*f*
  assessment of, 1145, 1145*f*, 1146*f*
  chronic kidney disease and, 1613*c*, 1614
  malalignment in osteomalacia, 1162
Skeletal traction, 1189
Skelid; *See* Tiludronate
Skin, 460-518
  acidosis and, 207, 207*c*
  acne and, 515
  acquired immunodeficiency syndrome and, 381
  age-related changes in fluid balance and, 174*c*
  age-related surgical risks and, 245*c*
  AIDS wasting syndrome and, 373
  assessment of, 466-477
    after burn, 531, 531*f*
    biopsy in, 477
    in chronic and disabling diseases, 97*t*, 98
    diascopy in, 477
    hair and, 473
    inspection in, 467-471, 468*t*, 469-471*f*, 471*t*
    laboratory, 476-477
    nails and, 473-475, 474*f*, 474*t*, 475*t*
    palpation in, 471-472, 472*t*
    patient history in, 466*c*, 466-467
    in patient with dark skin, 475-476, 476*c*
    postoperative, 291*f*, 291-292, 292*f*
    psychosocial, 476
    Wood's light examination in, 477
  bacterial infection of, 499, 500*c*, 501*f*, 502*c*, 503*c*
  biological response modifiers and, 434
  burns and, 519-549
    acute respiratory distress syndrome and, 537
    compensatory responses to, 525, 526*f*
    disturbed body image and, 544-545
    etiology of, 525-527, 527*f*
    history in, 528, 529*c*
    imbalanced nutrition: less than body requirements in, 543
    impaired physical mobility in, 543-544, 544*c*, 544*f*
    incidence and prevalence of, 527
    ineffective breathing pattern in, 535
    ineffective tissue perfusion in, 533*c*, 533*t*, 533-535, 534*f*
    laboratory assessment in, 531-532, 532*c*
    in lightning strike, 151
    nursing diagnoses in, 532-533, 537-538
    pain in, 535-536
    pathophysiology of, 520*f*, 520-525, 521*t*, 522-524*f*
    physical assessment in, 529*t*, 529-531, 530*t*, 531*f*, 537, 538*t*
    prevention of, 527-528
    pulmonary edema in, 536
    rehabilitative phase of, 545-547, 546*t*
    risk for infection in, 540-543, 542-543*c*
    wound care management in, 538-540, 539*t*
  cardiovascular assessment and, 715
  catecholamine receptors and, 1416*t*
  changes associated with aging, 462-466, 463-464*c*, 465*f*, 466*f*
Skin (*Continued*)
  chronic kidney disease and, 1613*c*, 1614
  cirrhosis and, 1348*f*
  coronary artery disease and, 854
  Cushing's disease and, 1441, 1441*c*, 1443-1444
  cutaneous anthrax and, 503-504
  cyst and, 508
  dehydration and, 179
  dry, 480, 480*c*
  endocrine assessment and, 1421-1422
  estrogen changes in older adult and, 1419*c*
  fluid overload and, 182, 182*c*
  fungal infection of, 500*c*, 501
  hematologic assessment in older adult and, 882*c*
  hyperthyroidism and, 1449*c*, 1451
  hypothyroidism and, 1456*c*
  hypovolemic shock and, 835
  immobility and, 102*t*
  as indicator of respiratory adequacy, 564
  inflammatory conditions of, 504-506, 505*c*
  innervation of, 934*f*
  keloids and, 509, 509*f*
  leprosy and, 516
  leukemia and, 903*c*, 903-904
  lichen planus and, 516
  nevi and, 509
  nutrient deficiencies and, 1394*t*
  pediculosis and, 504
  pemphigus vulgaris and, 516
  plastic or reconstructive surgery and, 513-515, 514*t*
  postoperative complications of, 287*t*, 294-296, 295*c*, 295*f*
  premenstrual syndrome and, 1686*c*
  preoperative preparation of, 255, 256*f*
  pressure ulcer and, 484-499
    concept map for, 492
    dressings for, 491-493, 493-495*t*
    drug therapy for, 493
    health care resources for, 498, 499*c*
    health teaching in, 498
    history in, 488
    home care management in, 498
    identification of high-risk patient and, 486, 487*f*
    intervention activities for, 493*c*
    laboratory assessment in, 490-491
    new technologies for, 495
    nursing diagnoses in, 491
    nutrition therapy for, 493
    pathophysiology of, 484-485, 485*f*
    physical assessment in, 488
    physical therapy for, 493
    pressure-relieving and pressure-reducing techniques for, 486-488
    prevention of, 485*c*, 485-486
    psychosocial assessment in, 490
    risk for infection and, 496-498, 497*c*
    surgical management of, 495-496, 496*f*
    wound assessment in, 488-490, 489*c*, 489*f*, 490*t*
  prevention of infections of, 501-502, 502*c*
  pruritus and, 480-481
  psoriasis and, 506-508, 507*f*
  risk for infection and, 441*t*
  scabies and, 504
  scleroderma and, 351, 351*f*
  seborrheic keratoses and, 508, 509*f*
  septic shock and, 842
  shock and, 829*c*
  sickle cell disease and, 895
  Stevens-Johnson syndrome and, 516
  stimulation for pain management, 55
  structure and function of, 461*f*, 461-462, 463*t*
  sunburn and, 481
Skin (*Continued*)
  systemic lupus erythematosus and, 348, 348*c*, 350, 350*c*
  toxic epidermal necrolysis and, 516
  trauma to, 481*t*, 481-484, 482*f*, 483*t*, 484*f*
  urticaria and, 481
  viral infection of, 499-501, 500*c*, 501*f*
Skin appendages, 462, 462*f*
  burn-related skin changes and, 520, 522*f*
Skin barriers, 1333*f*
Skin biopsy, 477
  in discoid lupus erythematosus, 349
  in skin cancer, 512
Skin cancer, 509-512, 510*f*, 510*t*, 511*c*
  ABCD features in, 467
  conditions associated with genetic predisposition for, 410*t*
  hematologic assessment in, 409*c*
  ocular melanoma in, 1104-1106
  sites of metastasis for, 405*t*
Skin care
  in chronic and disabling diseases, 103-105, 104*c*
  in chronic diarrhea, 1312*c*
  in Crohn's disease, 1332, 1333*f*
  in cutaneous infection, 502-503
  in emergency care, 129-130
  in gastroenteritis, 1321
  hospitalized older adult and, 23-24, 24*c*
    infusion therapy and, 235
    postoperative interventions and, 295*c*
  in ileostomy, 1329*c*
  infection in leukemia and, 906
  in inflammatory bowel disease, 1328*c*
  in ostomy, 1325-1326
  in peripheral nerve trauma, 1024
  preventing pressure ulcers and, 485*c*
  in radiation therapy, 420, 420*c*
Skin color
  assessment of, 467, 468*t*
    hematologic assessment in older adult and, 882*c*
    in hypovolemic shock, 835
    in musculoskeletal trauma, 1184*c*
    in septic shock, 841, 842
  in classification of burn depth, 521*t*
  endocrine assessment and, 1421-1422
  in pancreatic cancer, 1380
Skin grafting
  in brown recluse spider bite, 147
  in burn, 539, 540
  for pressure ulcer repair, 495-496
Skin lesion, 467
  classification of, 469-470*f*
  configuration of, 471*t*
  diagnostic assessment of, 476-477
  in genital herpes, 1742
  in lymphogranuloma venereum, 1753
Skin rash, 471-472, 504-506, 505*c*
  in pharyngitis, 656*c*
  in serum sickness, 395
  in syphilis, 1739-1740, 1740*f*
  in systemic lupus erythematosus, 348, 349*f*
  in toxic shock syndrome, 1691, 1692*c*
Skin sheet, 98
Skin substitutes, 495
Skin testing
  for allergies, 389
  in respiratory assessment, 567
Skin traction, 1189, 1189*f*
Skin-fold measurements, 1392
Skinning vulvectomy, 1707, 1708*f*
Skull fracture, 1050
Skull radiography, 1424
Sleep, signs and symptoms of approaching death and, 115*c*
Sleep apnea, 594
Sleep disturbance
  in Alzheimer's disease, 977-978
  hospitalized older adult and, 23
Sleep-rest pattern
  in cardiovascular assessment, 711*c*
  in endocrine assessment, 1420*c*
Sliding board, 100, 100*c*
Sliding hiatal hernia, 1249*f*, 1249-1254, 1253*c*, 1253*f*, 1254*c*
Sling, pelvic, 1190*t*
Slip lock, 220
Slit-lamp examination, 1079, 1080*f*
Small bowel capsule endoscopy, 1227-1228
Small bowel follow-through, 1226
Small bowel radiographic series, 1226
Small cell lung cancer, 641
Small intestine, 1219
Small intestine biopsy, 1311
Small-bowel obstruction, 1302-1306, 1303*f*, 1304*c*, 1306*c*
Smallpox, 454*t*
Smart pump, 222
Smegma, 1651
Smoke poisoning, 530
Smoking, 84-85, 85*f*
  bladder cancer and, 1575
  Buerger's disease and, 815
  cancer development and, 408
  chronic obstructive pulmonary disease and, 622
  coronary artery disease and, 851-852, 854*c*
  esophageal cancer and, 1255
  head and neck cancer and, 598
  heart disease and, 709-710
  history in respiratory assessment, 558
  lung cancer and, 642
  occupational pulmonary disease and, 639
  osteoarthritis and, 323
  osteoporosis and, 1154
  peripheral arterial disease and, 807
  prostate cancer and, 1720
  surgical risk and, 246
Smoking cessation, 85
  after laryngectomy, 606
  in asthma, 614*c*
  in diabetes mellitus, 1506
Smooth endoplasmic reticulum, 63*f*
Smooth muscle, 1143
Snakebite, 143*f*, 143-146, 144*c*, 144*f*, 145*t*, 146*f*
Snellen chart, 1077-1078, 1078*f*
Snoring, postoperative assessment of, 287
SNPs; *See* Single nucleotide polymorphisms
Social history
  in cardiovascular assessment, 711-712
  in neurologic assessment, 937*c*
  in skin problems, 466*c*
Social isolation
  acquired immunodeficiency syndrome and, 382
  infection and, 452
  infectious disease and, 452
Social worker, 96
Sodium, 183-187
  adrenal gland assessment and, 1438*c*
  in body fluids, 183*f*
  burn-related changes in, 524, 532*c*
  chronic kidney disease and, 1609-1610
  hypernatremia and, 186*t*, 186-187
  hyponatremia and, 185*t*, 185-186
    burn-related, 524
    in chronic kidney disease, 1609
    enteral nutrition therapy and, 1400
    in syndrome of inappropriate antidiuretic hormone secretion, 1435
  normal plasma values for older adult, 184*t*
  preoperative assessment of, 250*c*
  serum, 184*t*
  tubular reabsorption of, 1530, 1531*f*
  twenty-four hour urine collection range and, 1542*c*

Sodium bicarbonate, 753, 753c
Sodium chloride, 187
Sodium nitroprusside
for heart failure, 863c
for hypertensive crisis, 802
for hypovolemic shock, 837c, 838
for pulmonary embolism, 682
Sodium polystyrene sulfonate, 190
Sodium pump, 173
Sodium restriction
in chronic kidney disease, 1617, 1617t
in cirrhosis, 1352
in fluid overload, 182
in heart failure, 778
in hypertension, 803
to reduce preload, 772
Sodium retention
in chronic kidney disease, 1610
in hyperaldosteronism, 1445
Sodium-potassium pump, 187
Soft contact lenses, 1103
Soft palate, 553f, 1217
Solenoid, 63f
Solubility, 174
Soluble beta protein precursor, 973
Solu-Cortef; *See* Hydrocortisone
Solu-Medrol; *See* Methylprednisolone
Solutes, 171, 1530
Solutions for intravenous therapy, 180t, 214-215
Solvent, 171
Solvents abuse, 91
Soma, 928, 929f
Somatic mutation, 70
Somatic pain, 38, 38t
Somatomedins, 1426
Somatosensory evoked potentials, 947
Somatostatin, 1373, 1418
Somavert; *See* Pegvisomant
Somogyi phenomenon, 1486, 1487f
Sonohysterography, 1688
Sonoran coral snake envenomation, 145-146, 146f
Sorafenib, 435t, 1595-1596
Sore throat, 655-657, 656c, 656t
Sotalol, 742c
Sound, 1115-1116
Spacer for inhaler, 619c, 619f
Spaces of Fontana, 1072f
Spandin; *See* Gusperimus
Sparfloxacin
for leprosy, 516
for urinary tract infection, 1556c
Spastic bladder, 105, 105t
Spastic colon, 1289-1291, 1290f
Spastic paralysis
after stroke, 1034, 1046
in spinal tumor, 1001
Spasticity
in amyotrophic lateral sclerosis, 1007
in multiple sclerosis, 1006
Special nursing team in emergency care, 127
Special populations, emergency nursing and, 127
Specialized nutrition support, 1396
Specialty bed, 104f, 104-105
Specialty nurse, 266-267
Specific gravity of urine, 1538, 1539t, 1604
SPECT; *See* Single photon emission computed tomography
Speech
after laryngectomy, 602
amyotrophic lateral sclerosis and, 1008
Guillain-Barr[ac]e syndrome and, 1015-1016
myasthenia gravis and, 1020
Parkinson disease and, 966c
stroke and, 1046, 1046t
tracheostomy and, 586
transient ischemic attack and, 1030c
Speech area of brain, 930
Speech audiometry, 1117-1118
Speech discrimination testing, 1117-1118
Speech reception threshold, 1117
Speech-language pathologist, 96
Speech-language pathology assistant, 96
Speed, 85
Speed shock in intravenous therapy, 230t
Sperm banking, 1729, 1729c
Spermatic cord, 1651
Spermatocele, 1731, 1731f
Spermatogenesis, 1645
Sphenoid sinus, 553f
Sphincter of Oddi, 1218f, 1219
Sphincterotomy, 1376
SPICES framework, 23
Spider angioma, 1347
Spider bite, 145-150, 147f, 149t, 150c
Spinal administration of opioid analgesics, 51t
Spinal anesthesia, 275, 276t, 277f, 329
Spinal cord, 983-1010
amyotrophic lateral sclerosis and, 1007c, 1007-1008
back pain and, 983-989
complementary and alternative therapies for, 986
diagnostic assessment in, 985
health care resources for, 989
health teaching in, 988c, 988-989
home care management in, 988
nonsurgical management of, 985-986, 986c
pathophysiology of, 984
physical assessment in, 984-985
prevention of, 984, 984c
surgical management of, 986-988, 987c
cancer-related compression of, 436
cervical neck pain and, 989f, 989-990, 990c
injury of, 990-1000
etiology of, 992-993
extent of injury in, 991-992, 992f
health care resources for, 1000
health teaching in, 999c, 999-1000, 1000c
history in, 993
home care management in, 999
imaging studies in, 994-995
impaired adjustment in, 998
impaired elimination in, 997-998, 998c
impaired gas exchange in, 997
ineffective tissue perfusion in, 995c, 995-997, 996f
laboratory assessment in, 994
in lightning strike, 151
mechanisms of injury in, 990-991, 991f
nursing diagnoses in, 995
physical assessment in, 993-994, 994c
psychosocial assessment in, 994
self-care deficit in, 997
multiple sclerosis and, 1002-1007, 1003c
pain transmission and, 38, 39f
structure and function of, 931-933, 932f
tumor of, 1000-1002, 1001c
Spinal cord stimulation for chronic pain, 57
Spinal deformity, 1145, 1145f
Spinal fusion, 986, 987
Spinal nerves, 933
Spinal shock, 993
Spinal stenosis, 984
Spinal tap, 944t, 947-949, 948t
Spine
ankylosing spondylitis and, 355
compression fracture of, 1198c, 1198-1199
fracture of, 1198c, 1198-1199
musculoskeletal assessment of, 1146
osteoarthritis of, 324-325
osteoporosis and, 1155-1156, 1156f
Paget's disease of bone and, 1163
scoliosis of, 1173-1174, 1174f
Spinocerebellar tract, 932
Spinothalamic tract, 932, 932f
Spiral fracture, 1179f
Spirituality, 31-32, 120
Spiriva; *See* Tiotropium
Spironolactone
for cirrhosis, 1352
for hyperaldosteronism, 1446
for hypokalemia, 189
to reduce preload in heart failure, 773
Spleen, 879, 885-886, 1218f
Splenectomy
in aplastic anemia, 900
in idiopathic thrombocytopenic purpura, 916
in immunohemolytic anemia, 899
in pancreatic cancer, 1382
Splenic infarction, 784
Splenomegaly, 1223, 1345, 1348
Splint
for carpal tunnel syndrome, 1207
for fracture, 1186, 1187, 1187f
Splinter hemorrhage, 784
Splinting
for reflex urinary incontinence, 1568
of surgical incision, 257c
Split-thickness skin graft, 495-496
Splitting of heart sounds, 718
Spondee, 1117
Spondylolisthesis, 984
Spondylolysis, 984
Spongy bone, 1141, 1141f, 1153
Spontaneous bacterial peritonitis, 1346, 1352
Spontaneous fracture, 1179
Spoon nails, 475t
Sporadic Paget's disease of bone, 1162
Spork, 103t
Sports-related injury, 1204-1206, 1205c, 1205f
Sprain, 989, 1208
Sprue, 1311
SPRYCEL; *See* Dasatinib
Sputum production
in pneumonia, 661, 663t
respiratory assessment and, 559
in tuberculosis, 669
Sputum specimen, 564
in acute respiratory distress syndrome, 687
in chronic obstructive pulmonary disease, 627
in pneumonia, 663, 663f
in tuberculosis, 669, 670
Squamous cell carcinoma, 509, 510f, 510t
esophageal, 1255
gallbladder, 1371
in head and neck cancer, 597
lung, 641
in oral cancer, 1234-1235
Squamous metaplasia, 597
SSRIs; *See* Selective serotonin reuptake inhibitors
ST segment, 731f, 734, 735f
myocardial infarction and, 849, 849f
variant angina and, 855
Stable plaque, 794
Staff safety
in emergency care, 128-130, 129c
surgical suite preparation and, 267-270, 268f
Staging of cancer, 406t, 406-407, 407t
bone, 1169
cervical, 1702t
Hodgkin's lymphoma, 913, 913t
lung, 642
multiple myeloma, 915
non-Hodgkin's lymphoma, 914
renal, 1595t
Staging of heart failure, 765
Stalevo; *See* Levodopa-carbidopa-entacapone
Stamey procedure, 1566t
Stance phase of gait, 1145f
Standard precautions, 446t, 447
in emergency care, 128
human immunodeficiency virus transmission and, 368, 369c
personal protective equipment and, 445
Standard wound dressing for burn, 539
Stapedectomy, 1133-1134, 1134c, 1134f
Stapes, 1110, 1110f, 1111f
Staphylococcus
in epididymitis, 1734
in external otitis, 1121
in food poisoning, 1341, 1341t
in furuncle of ear, 1122
in pelvic inflammatory disease, 1748
in peritonitis, 1317
in pyogenic liver abscess, 1361
in sepsis, 840
in urinary tract infection, 1552
Staphylococcus aureus
in acute sialadenitis, 1239-1240
in arteriovenous access infection, 1623
in Bartholin cyst, 1699
in conjunctivitis, 1087
in hordeolum, 1085
in infectious arthritis, 356
in infective endocarditis, 783-785, 784c
methicillin-resistant, 448, 499, 502c
in osteomyelitis, 1165
in pyelonephritis, 1587
in tonsillitis, 657
in toxic shock syndrome, 1691, 1692c
vancomycin-intermediate, 448-449
vancomycin-resistant, 448-449
Staples, 282f, 295
Starling's law, 766
Starlix; *See* Nateglinide
Start codon, 70t
Stasis dermatitis, 821
Stasis ulcer, 821
Statex; *See* Morphine
Statins, 796, 796t
Stationary chest tube drainage system, 646-647, 647f
Status asthmaticus, 621
Status epilepticus, 959-960
Stavudine, 376c
Stay sutures, 282, 282f
STDs; *See* Sexually transmitted diseases
Steal syndrome, 1623
Steam inhalation, 530
Steatorrhea, 1225
in cholecystitis, 1368
in chronic pancreatitis, 1378
in Crohn's disease, 1331
in cystic fibrosis, 635
in malabsorption syndrome, 1311
in Zollinger-Ellison syndrome, 1279
Steatosis, 1360-1361
Steinert dystrophy, 1175t
ST-elevation myocardial infarction, 855
Stem cell, 308, 309f, 877, 877f
Stem cell transplantation
in breast cancer, 1679
in leukemia, 907t, 907-910, 909f
in multiple myeloma, 915
platelet transfusion and, 920
in sickle cell disease, 897
Stenosis
aortic, 779c, 780
mitral, 779, 779c
renal artery, 798
Stent
in acute coronary syndromes, 865-866, 866f
carotid artery angioplasty with, 1044
in peripheral arterial disease, 807
in renovascular disease, 1594
in urolithiasis, 1573
Step system in asthma, 613c
Step voltage, 151
Stereotactic pallidotomy/thalamotomy, 969
Stereotactic radiosurgery, 1062, 1062f

Stereotyping, 28
Sterilization, 445
Sternal fracture, 1198
Sternal split approach in thymectomy, 1020
Steroids
  abuse of, 91-92
  for acute respiratory distress syndrome, 688
  after lung transplantation, 637
  for allergic rhinitis, 390
  for anaphylaxis, 393*c*
  for asthma, 617*c*, 620
  for bee sting, 150
  for bronchiolitis obliterans organizing pneumonia, 640*c*
  for chemotherapy-induced nausea and vomiting, 429*c*
  for Crohn's disease, 1331
  drug-induced immune deficiency and, 384
  for dyspnea in dying patient, 117
  for facial paralysis, 1026
  for immunohemolytic anemia, 899
  for inflammatory skin disease, 505
  for pain, 54*t*
  for psoriasis, 507
  for pulmonary sarcoidosis, 639
  for rheumatoid arthritis, 344
  for scleroderma, 352
  for septic shock, 843*t*
  for Sjögren's syndrome, 396
  for ulcerative colitis, 1324
Stevens-Johnson syndrome, 516
Stiffness
  in osteoarthritis, 324
  in scleroderma, 351
Stimulants
  abuse of, 81, 81*t*, 85-86, 86*f*, 86*t*
  for pain, 54*t*
Stimulation testing
  in endocrine assessment, 1423, 1423*c*
  in hypopituitarism, 1427
  thyroid, 1451*c*
Stimulatory reactions, 395
Sting
  bee and wasp, 149-150, 150*c*
  scorpion, 148-149, 149*f*
Stirrup, 1110, 1110*f*
Stoma
  in colostomy, 1298-1299, 1299*f*
  in ileostomy, 1325
  in laryngectomy, 601, 605
Stomach, 1217-1218, 1265-1288
  aging-related changes in, 1220*c*
  cancer of, 1279-1287
    assessment in, 1280*c*, 1280-1281
    chronic gastritis and, 1266
    community-based care in, 1286-1287
    nonsurgical management of, 1281
    pathophysiology of, 1279-1280
    postoperative afferent loop syndrome and, 1285-1286
    postoperative alkaline reflux gastropathy and, 1285
    postoperative dumping syndrome and, 1285, 1286*t*
    prevention of, 1280
    surgery for, 1281-1285, 1282*f*
    upper gastrointestinal bleeding in, 1271*f*
  gastritis and, 1265-1270, 1266-1269*c*, 1270*t*
  peptic ulcer disease and, 1270-1279
    complications of, 1271*c*, 1271*f*, 1271-1272
    etiology and genetic risk in, 1272
    gastrointestinal bleeding in, 1275-1278, 1276*c*, 1277*c*, 1278*f*
    health care resources for, 1279
    health teaching in, 1278
    history in, 1272-1273
    home care management in, 1278, 1279*c*
Stomach *(Continued)*
    imaging studies in, 1273-1274
    laboratory assessment in, 1273
    nursing diagnoses in, 1274
    pain in, 1274-1275
    pathophysiology of, 1270*f*, 1270-1271, 1271*f*
    physical assessment in, 1273, 1273*t*
    prevention of, 1272
    psychosocial assessment in, 1273
  Zollinger-Ellison syndrome and, 1279
Stomach lying exercise, 986*c*
Stomatitis, 1231-1234, 1233*c*, 1233*f*
  in chronic kidney disease, 1611
  in induction therapy in acute leukemia, 905
Stone disease, 1570-1575
  in gout, 353
  in hyperparathyroidism, 1461
  infection prevention in, 1573-1574
  nutrition history in, 1535
  Paget's disease of bone and, 1163
  pathophysiology of, 1570-1571, 1571*t*
  prevention of obstruction in, 1574*t*, 1574-1575, 1575*c*
  spinal cord injury-related, 998
  surgical management of, 1573
  urinary tract infection and, 1551*t*
Stool collection for fecal occult blood test, 1225
Stool softeners
  in bowel training, 107
  for hemorrhoids, 1310
  for prevention of increased intracranial pressure, 1044
Stool tests
  in gastritis, 1267
  in gastrointestinal assessment, 1225-1226
Stop codon, 70*t*
Straight cane, 101*f*
Strain, 1208
Strangulated abdominal hernia, 1292
Strangulated intestinal obstruction, 1303
Stratum corneum, 461, 461*f*
Stratum granulosum, 461, 461*f*
Streptococcus
  in acute sialadenitis, 1239-1240
  in brain abscess, 1065
  in external otitis, 1121
  in hordeolum, 1085-1087, 1087*c*
  in infective endocarditis, 783-785, 784*c*
  in pelvic inflammatory disease, 1748
  in peritonitis, 1317
  in peritonsillar abscess, 657
  in pharyngitis, 655
  in prostatitis, 1733
  in sepsis, 840
  in tonsillitis, 657
  in toxic shock syndrome, 1691, 1692*c*
Streptococcus pneumoniae
  in acute sialadenitis, 1239-1240
  in meningitis, 961, 961squeeze/combine
  in pneumonia, 665
  in sinusitis, 654
Streptozocin, 422*t*
Stress
  cardiac complications of hyperthyroidism and, 1452
  coronary artery disease and, 852
  multiple sclerosis and, 1007
  older adult and, 17-18, 18*c*
  substance abuse and, 81
  tension headache and, 955
  ulcerative colitis and, 1323
Stress debriefing, 164*c*, 164-165
Stress fracture, 1179-1180
Stress test
  in cardiovascular assessment, 724-725
  in coronary artery disease, 855
Stress ulcer, 1270-1279
  complementary and alternative therapies for, 1270*t*
  complications of, 1271*c*, 1271*f*, 1271-1272
Stress ulcer *(Continued)*
  drug therapy for, 1268-1269*c*
  etiology and genetic risk in, 1272
  gastrointestinal bleeding in, 1275-1278, 1276*c*, 1277*c*, 1278*f*
  health care resources for, 1279
  health teaching in, 1278
  history in, 1272-1273
  home care management in, 1278, 1279*c*
  imaging studies in, 1273-1274
  laboratory assessment in, 1273
  mechanical ventilation and, 696
  nursing diagnoses in, 1274
  pain in, 1274-1275
  pathophysiology of, 1270*f*, 1270-1271, 1271*f*
  physical assessment in, 1273, 1273*t*
  prevention of, 1272
  psychosocial assessment in, 1273
Stress urinary incontinence, 1560*t*, 1564*c*, 1564-1566, 1565*c*, 1565*f*
  surgical procedures for, 1566*t*
  in uterine prolapse, 1693
Stretch receptor, 709
Stretta procedure, 1248, 1248*c*
Striae, 1422
Striated muscle, 1143
Stricture
  esophageal, 1244, 1256
  intestinal, 1330
  urethral, 1559, 1585-1586
Stricturoplasty, 1332
Stridor
  after extubation, 697
  in anaphylaxis, 392
  in inhalation anthrax, 673
  postoperative assessment of, 287
  in thyroidectomy, 1454
Stroke, 1030-1049
  arteriovenous malformation and, 1044*f*, 1044-1045
  atrial fibrillation and, 745-746
  carotid artery angioplasty with stenting in, 1044
  carotid endarterectomy in, 1045
  community-based rehabilitation in, 1048
  in diabetes mellitus, 1469
  diastolic blood pressure and, 797
  disturbed sensory perception in, 1047
  drug therapy for, 1043-1044
  etiology and genetic risk for, 1032, 1033*c*
  extracranial-intracranial bypass in, 1045
  family history of, 936
  health care resources for, 1048-1049
  health teaching in, 1048, 1048*f*
  heat, 142-143, 143*c*
  history in, 1032-1033
  home care management in, 1047-1048
  homocysteine and, 795
  in idiopathic thrombocytopenic purpura, 916
  imaging studies in, 1036
  impaired physical mobility in, 1046
  impaired swallowing in, 1045
  impaired verbal communication in, 1046, 1046*t*
  ineffective tissue perfusion in, 1036-1037
  in infective endocarditis, 784
  intracranial pressure monitoring in, 1037*c*, 1037-1043
  laboratory assessment in, 1036
  migraine headache and, 952
  nursing care plan for, 1038-1043
  nursing diagnoses in, 1036
  pathophysiologic changes in brain and, 1030
  physical assessment in, 1033*c*, 1033*f*, 1033-1035, 1034*c*
Stroke *(Continued)*
  prevention of, 1032
  psychosocial assessment in, 1035-1036
  thrombolytic therapy for, 1037, 1037*c*
  types of, 1030*f*, 1030-1032, 1031*t*
  unilateral neglect in, 1047
  urinary and bowel incontinence in, 1047
Stroke volume, 707
  heart failure and, 766
  hypovolemic shock and, 833
  in septic shock, 841, 841*t*
Stromectol; *See* Ivermectin
Struvite stones, 1571*t*, 1574, 1574*t*
Stryker local anesthesia infusion pump, 55
Stuart-Prower factor, 881*t*
Stump, 1202-1203, 1203*f*
Stuporous patient, 938
Stye, 1085-1087
Subacute thyroiditis, 1460
Subarachnoid analgesia, 52
Subarachnoid screw or bolt, 1058, 1059*t*
Subarachnoid space, 237, 929
Subcapital hip fracture, 1196*f*
Subchondral bone plate, 1142*f*
Subclavian artery, 815
Subclavian dialysis catheter, 1607*f*, 1607-1608
Subclavian nodes, 1644*f*
Subclavian steal, 815
Subclavian vein
  for hemodialysis access, 1607*f*, 1607-1608
  nontunneled percutaneous central catheter and, 218
Subcutaneous administration of opioid analgesics, 50*t*
Subcutaneous device for hemodialysis access, 1623*t*, 1625, 1625*f*
Subcutaneous emphysema, 561
  dilation of lower esophageal sphincter and, 1255
  in laryngeal trauma, 596
  in musculoskeletal trauma, 1184
  pneumothorax and, 699
  tracheotomy-related, 581
Subcutaneous fat, 461, 461*f*, 462*f*
  burn and, 522*f*
  changes related to aging, 464*c*
  functions of, 463*t*
Subcutaneous infusion therapy, 237, 237*t*
Subcutaneous nodule, 338
Subdiaphragmatic nodes, 1644*f*
Subdural catheter, 1058, 1059*t*
Subdural hematoma, 1051-1052, 1052*f*, 1064
Subdural space, 929
Subendocardial myocardial infarction, 849
Sublimaze; *See* Fentanyl
Sublingual administration of opioid analgesics, 50*t*
Sublingual nitroglycerin, 1255
Subluxation, 1208
  in osteoarthritis, 323
  total hip arthroplasty and, 329-330, 330*c*
  total shoulder arthroplasty and, 334
Submaxillary lymph nodes, 1235*f*
Submental lymph nodes, 1235*f*
Submucosa, gastrointestinal, 1216, 1217*f*
Submucosal leiomyoma, 1694, 1695*f*
Submucous resection in nasal fracture, 591
Subscapular nodes, 1644*f*
Subscapular skin-fold measurement, 1392
Subserosal leiomyoma, 1694, 1695*f*
Substance abuse, 80-93
  alcohol and, 82-84, 83*t*, 84*c*, 84*t*
  barbiturates and, 89
  commonly abused substances, 81*t*
  depressants and, 88-89

Substance abuse (Continued)
hallucinogens and, 86-88
hospitalized patient and, 81-82
inhalants and, 91
nicotine and, 84-85, 85*f*
nurse and, 82
opioids and, 90*t*, 90-91, 91*c*
sickle cell disease and, 896
steroids and, 91-92
stimulants and, 85-86, 86*f*, 86*t*
stress and, 81
Substance abuser
hospitalized, 81-82
pain in, 40
surgical risks and, 245-246
Substance misuse, 80
Substance P, 930*t*
Substantia gelatinosa, 38, 39*f*
Substantia nigrans, 965
Subthalamic nucleus, 931*f*
Subtotal hysterectomy, 1697*t*
Subtotal thyroidectomy, 1454
Subtrochanteric hip fracture, 1196*f*
Succinylcholine, 274*t*
Sucralfate
for gastritis, 1268
mechanical ventilation and, 696
for peptic ulcer disease, 1269*c*, 1275
Suction lipectomy, 514*t*
Suctioning
in chronic obstructive pulmonary disease, 631-632
of laryngectomy tube, 601
postoperative gas exchange impairment and, 294
of tracheostomy tube, 583-584, 584*c*
Sufentanil, 52, 274*t*
Suffocation, 91
Suicide
lesbian and, 30
older adult and, 20
physician-assisted, 122*t*
Sulcrate; *See* Sucralfate
Sulfamylon; *See* Mafenide acetate
Sulfasalazine
for rheumatoid arthritis, 342*c*, 343
for ulcerative colitis, 1324, 1325*t*
Sulfisoxazole, 1086*c*
Sulfonamides, 1556*c*
Sulfonylureas, 1477-1479*c*, 1477-1483, 1483*t*
Sulfuric acid, 202
Summation gallop, 719
Sunburn, 481
Sundowning in Alzheimer's disease, 973
Superficial cervical lymph nodes, 1235*f*
Superficial dorsal vein, 216*f*
Superficial femoral artery, 804*f*
Superficial middle temporal artery-to-middle cerebral artery graft, 1045
Superficial partial-thickness burn, 521*t*, 522, 522*f*
Superficial peroneal nerve, 1022*f*
Superficial-thickness burn, 521*t*, 522*f*
Superinfection, 453
Superior canaliculus, 1072*f*
Superior cerebellar artery, 932*f*
Superior mesenteric artery syndrome, 1188
Superior oblique muscle, 1073*f*, 1073*t*
Superior punctum, 1072*f*
Superior rectus muscle, 1073*f*, 1073*t*
Superior turbinate, 553*f*
Superior vena cava, 705*f*
nontunneled percutaneous central catheter and, 218
peripherally inserted central catheter and, 217
right-sided heart catheterization and, 723*f*
Superior vena cava syndrome
in cancer, 436*f*, 436-437
dyspnea in dying patient and, 117
in lung cancer, 644
Supination, 1146*f*
Supine position, surgical, 280*f*
Supplies shortage after mass casualty incident, 164
Support staff in emergency care, 128
SUPPORT study, 112
Supportive therapy
in avian influenza, 667
in deep vein thrombosis, 818
in rhinitis, 654
Suppressed gene, 402
Suppression testing
in Cushing's disease, 1442
in endocrine assessment, 1423, 1423*c*
in hyperpituitarism, 1430
thyroid, 1451*c*
Suppressor T-cell, 317
Suppurant otitis media, 1123-1125, 1124*f*, 1125*c*, 1125*f*
Supraclavicular lymph nodes, 1235*f*
Supraglottic method of swallowing, 604*c*
Supraglottic partial laryngectomy, 600*t*
Suprane; *See* Desflurane
Suprapatellar area, 324
Supratentorial tumor, 1060, 1061
Supraventricular tachycardia, 740-741
Suprax; *See* Cefixime
Sural nerve, 1022*f*
Surfactant, 555
acute respiratory distress syndrome and, 686
drowning and, 156
Surgeon, 265
Surgery, 241-303
in abdominal aortic aneurysm, 812-813
in abdominal hernia, 1292-1293
in abdominal trauma, 1308
in acute pancreatitis, 1376
in appendicitis, 1316-1317
arthroplastic, 328-335
elbow, 335
hip, 328-332, 330*c*, 330*t*, 332*c*, 332*f*
indications and contraindications for, 328
knee, 333*f*, 333-334, 334*c*
shoulder, 334-335
in back pain, 986-988, 987*c*
in benign prostatic hypertrophy, 1715-1718, 1717*f*, 1718*c*
in burn
escharotomy and, 534*f*, 534-535
for infection, 541-543
to restore mobility, 544
tracheotomy and, 535
in cancer, 417-418
bladder, 1576
bone, 1170
breast, 1672-1675, 1673*f*, 1675*c*
cervical, 1703-1704
colorectal, 1297*t*, 1297-1300, 1298*t*, 1299*f*, 1300*c*
endometrial, 1700
esophageal, 1259*f*, 1259-1261, 1260*c*
gallbladder, 1371
head and neck, 599-600, 600*t*
lung, 645*f*, 645-649, 647*f*, 648*c*
oral cavity, 1237-1238, 1238*c*
ovarian, 1706
pancreatic, 1382
prostate, 1721-1722, 1722*c*
renal cell carcinoma, 1596
skin, 512
spinal tumor, 1001-1002
testicular, 1729
thyroid, 1461
in cardiomyopathy, 789
in carpal tunnel syndrome, 1207
cataract, 1093-1094, 1094*f*
categories and purposes of, 243-244*t*
for chronic pain, 57-58, 58*f*
in chronic pancreatitis, 1379
in chronic venous insufficiency, 822
in cirrhosis, 1353
coronary artery bypass graft, 866-870, 867*f*
Surgery (Continued)
in Cushing's disease, 1443
in cystic fibrosis, 636-637
in deep vein thrombosis, 820
in diabetes mellitus, 1498-1500
in dysfunctional uterine bleeding, 1688-1689
in endometriosis, 1688
in epilepsy, 960-961
in fracture, 1190-1192, 1191*f*
in gallstones, 1369-1371, 1370*c*, 1371*t*
in gastroesophageal reflux disease, 1248
in glaucoma, 1097-1098
for hearing loss, 1132-1133, 1133*f*, 1134*c*, 1134*f*
stapedectomy in, 1133-1134, 1134*c*, 1134*f*
tympanoplasty in, 1132-1133, 1133*f*, 1134*f*
in heart failure, 774*f*, 774-775
in hemorrhoids, 1310
in hiatal hernia, 1250-1254, 1253*c*, 1253*f*, 1254*c*
in hyperaldosteronism, 1446
in hyperparathyroidism, 1462-1463
in hyperpituitarism, 1431*f*, 1431-1432, 1432*c*
in hyperthyroidism, 1454-1455, 1455*c*
in hypovolemic shock, 838
in infective endocarditis, 785
in intestinal obstruction, 1305-1306
intraoperative care and, 264-284
general anesthesia and, 272-275, 273*t*, 274*t*, 275*c*
history in, 277
hypoventilation and, 282
infection risk and, 281-282, 282*f*
local or regional anesthesia and, 275-276, 276*f*, 276*t*, 277*f*
medical record review in, 278-279, 279*c*
moderate sedation and, 276-277
nursing diagnoses in, 279-280
preparation of surgical suite and, 267-270, 268*f*
risk for perioperative positioning injury and, 280*f*, 280-281, 281*c*
surgical team members and, 264-267, 266*f*, 267*f*
in mastoiditis, 1125-1126
in Meniere's disease, 1129
in myasthenia gravis, 1020-1021
in nasal fracture, 591, 591*f*
for obesity, 1406*f*, 1406-1407
in obstructive sleep apnea, 594
in osteomyelitis, 1167
in osteoporosis, 1160
in otitis media, 1124-1125
in Paget's disease of bone, 1164
in Parkinson disease, 969
in peptic ulcer disease, 1278, 1278*f*
in peripheral arterial disease, 808*f*, 808-809
in peritonitis, 1318
plastic, 513-515, 514*t*
postoperative care and, 285-303
acute pain and, 297-299, 297-299*c*
cardiovascular evaluation in, 287-289
fluid, electrolyte, and acid-base balance in, 290
gastrointestinal assessment in, 290-291, 291*t*
hand-off report in, 286, 286*c*
health care resources and, 300-301
health teaching and, 300
history in, 286, 287*t*
home care management and, 300
hypoxemia and, 299, 300*c*
impaired gas exchange and, 294, 295*c*
impaired skin integrity and, 294-296, 295*c*, 295*f*
laboratory assessment in, 293
Surgery (Continued)
neurologic assessment in, 289*t*, 289-290
nursing diagnoses in, 293-294
pain assessment in, 292-293
postanesthesia care unit record and, 288*f*
psychosocial assessment in, 293
renal evaluation in, 290
respiratory evaluation in, 287, 289*c*
skin assessment in, 291*f*, 291-292, 292*f*
preoperative care and, 242-263
administering regularly scheduled drugs and, 254
dietary restrictions and, 254
focused assessment in, 251*c*
history in, 244*c*, 244-245*t*, 244-247
imaging and, 249
informed consent and, 252-254, 253*f*
intestinal preparation in, 254
laboratory assessment in, 248-249, 250-251*c*
nursing diagnoses and, 252
patient anxiety and, 258-260
patient self-determination and, 254
patient transfer to surgical suite, 261
physical assessment in, 247*c*, 247-248
preoperative chart review in, 260
preoperative drugs and, 261
preoperative patient preparation and, 260-261
preparation for tubes, drains, and vascular access in, 255
psychosocial assessment in, 248
skin preparation in, 255, 256*f*
teaching postoperative procedures and exercises and, 255-259, 256*c*, 257*c*, 258*f*, 259*f*
in pressure ulcer, 495-496, 496*f*
in pyelonephritis, 1588-1589
risk for infection and, 441*t*
sinus, 655, 655*c*
in spinal cord injury, 996-997
in traumatic brain injury, 1058, 1059*t*
in trigeminal neuralgia, 1025-1026
in ulcerative colitis, 1325-1327, 1326*f*, 1327*f*
in urinary incontinence, 1566, 1566*t*
in urolithiasis, 1573
in uterine leiomyoma, 1696
in uterine prolapse, 1694
in valvular heart disease, 781-782, 782*c*
Surgical antimicrobial solution, 270
Surgical assistant, 265
Surgical attire, 270, 270*f*
Surgical consent form, 253*f*
Surgical débridement of pressure ulcer, 495-496, 496*f*
Surgical drain, 292, 292*f*
Surgical dressing, 282
Surgical excision of burn wound, 540
Surgical incision site, 289*c*
Surgical positions, 280*f*
Surgical risk factors, 244*t*
Surgical scrub, 270, 271*f*
Surgical settings, 244
Surgical staging of cancer, 407
Surgical suite preparation, 267-270, 268*f*
Surgical team, 264-267, 266*f*, 267*f*, 270, 270*f*
Surgical technologist, 265
Surgical wound infection, 281-282, 282*f*
Surveillance of infectious disease, 441
Survival skills information for diabetic patient, 1514-1515
Survivor guilt, 165-166
Susceptibility, 441, 557*c*
Susceptibility gene, 71
Suspensory ligament, 1645*f*
Sustained immunity, 316

Sustained maximal inspiration, 664
Sustiva; *See* Efavirenz
Sutures
intravenous catheter and, 223
postoperative care of, 295
risk for infection and, 281-282, 282*f*
SUX; *See* Succinylcholine
SVT; *See* Supraventricular tachycardia
Swallowing
approaching death and, 116
esophageal cancer and, 1256, 1257
esophageal diverticula and, 1261
myasthenia gravis and, 1017
nasal fracture and, 591
radiation therapy-related dysfunction of, 599
stomatitis and, 1233
stroke and, 1045
supraglottic method of, 604*c*
tracheostomy and, 586, 586*c*, 603*c*, 604
Swallowing therapy in esophageal cancer, 1257, 1258*c*
Sweat gland, 462, 462*f*
burn-related skin changes and, 520, 522*f*
Sweat gland duct, 461*f*
Sweating
in aortic dissection, 814
in black widow spider bite, 148
in hyperthyroidism, 1450
in inhalation anthrax, 673
insensible water loss and, 175
in pheochromocytoma, 1446
in urolithiasis, 1571
Swedish massage, 11
Sweeteners, 1493
Swelling; *See* Edema
Swimmer's ear, 1121*c*, 1121*f*, 1121-1122
Swing phase of gait, 1145*f*
Syme amputation, 1199*f*
Symlin; *See* Pramlintide
Symmetrel; *See* Amantadine
Sympathectomy, 58*f*, 1204
Sympathetic ganglionectomy, 816
Sympathetic nervous system, 933
compensatory responses in burn, 525, 526*f*
heart failure and, 765-766
Sympathetic tone of blood vessels, 827
Sympathomimetics
for anaphylaxis, 393*c*
for heart failure, 864*c*
Symptomatic genetic testing, 75*t*
Synapse, 929
Synaptic cleft, 929
Synaptic knob, 929
Synarthrodial joint, 1142
SynchroMed pump, 53, 53*f*
Synchronized intermittent mandatory ventilation, 693, 697*t*
Syncope
in aortic stenosis, 779*c*, 780
cardiovascular assessment and, 714
in complex partial seizure, 956
in diabetic neuropathy, 1470
in hypertrophic cardiomyopathy, 789
in mitral valve prolapse, 779*c*, 780
in pulmonary embolism, 679
Syndrome of inappropriate antidiuretic hormone secretion, 1433-1436, 1435*t*
after brain tumor surgery, 1064
after traumatic brain injury, 1057
in brain tumor, 1060
cancer-related, 435-436
Syndrome X, 852-853, 853*t*, 1472
Syngeneic transplant, 907, 907*t*
Synovectomy
in carpal tunnel syndrome, 1207
in rheumatoid arthritis, 340
Synovial joint, 1142*f*, 1142-1143
Synovial joint cartilage, 1143
Synovitis
in carpal tunnel syndrome, 1206
in osteoarthritis, 323
in rheumatoid arthritis, 338
Synovium, 1142*f*
Synthetic cast, 1187, 1187*f*
Synthetic dressing for burn wound, 540
Synthroid; *See* Levothyroxine sodium
Synvisc; *See* Hylan GF 20
Syphilis, 1738-1742, 1740*f*
Syringe, insulin, 1488, 1488*c*, 1489*f*
Syringe pump, 222
Systemic arterial pressure, 797
Systemic complications of intravenous therapy, 230*t*
Systemic inflammatory response, 839*f*, 839-840, 842*t*
Systemic lupus erythematosus, 347-350, 348*c*, 349*f*, 350*c*, 1590
Systemic necrotizing vasculitis, 354-355
Systemic sclerosis, 348*c*, 351*f*, 351-353, 352*c*
Systemic vascular resistance, 708
Systole, 706
Systolic blood pressure, 708
Systolic heart failure, 765
Systolic murmur, 719
Systolic ventricular dysfunction, 765

T

T wave, 734-735, 735*f*
acute cardiac tamponade and, 786
myocardial infarction and, 849, 849*f*
premature atrial complexes and, 740
supraventricular tachycardia and, 740
variant angina and, 855
T-ACE alcohol use assessment, 83, 83*t*
Tachycardia, 736
in acute renal failure, 1603
in cholecystitis, 1369
in chronic kidney disease, 1619
in heat stroke, 142
in high altitude pulmonary edema, 155
in hyperthyroidism, 1452
in hypothermia, 153
in malignant hyperthermia, 273
nonsustained ventricular, 747
in pneumonia, 661
in scorpion sting, 149
sinus, 739, 739*f*
supraventricular, 740-741
in syndrome of inappropriate antidiuretic hormone secretion, 1435
in thyroid storm, 1455
in traumatic brain injury, 1054
ventricular, 748, 749*f*
Tachydysrhythmias, 738, 738*c*
Tachypnea
in chronic kidney disease, 1613
in heat stroke, 142
in high altitude pulmonary edema, 155
in pneumonia, 661
Tacrolimus, 320, 1498
Tactile fremitus, 561, 661
Tadalafil, 1726
TAF; *See* Tumor angiogenesis factor
Tag system in mass casualty event, 161, 161*t*
Tagamet; *See* Cimetidine
Tai Chi, 11
Takayasu's arteritis, 355
Talcosis, 640*c*
Tambocor; *See* Flecainide
Tamiflu; *See* Oseltamivir
Tamofen; *See* Tamoxifen citrate
Tamoxifen citrate
for breast cancer, 1678
for endometrial cancer, 1701
Tampon, toxic shock syndrome and, 1692*c*
Tamsulosin, 1714
Tapazole; *See* Methimazole
Tape, 282*f*
Tapeworms, 1340
Tar preparations, 507
Taraceva; *See* Erlotinib
Tarantula, 148
Tarceva; *See* Erlotinib
Target tissues, 1412, 1413, 1415*t*
Targeted therapy, 434, 435*t*
in breast cancer, 1677*t*, 1678
in esophageal cancer, 1258
in lung cancer, 645
in pancreatic cancer, 1382
in renal cell carcinoma, 1595-1596
Taste changes after oral cancer surgery, 1239
Tattoo, 471
Taxanes
for breast cancer, 1677*t*
for ovarian cancer, 1706
Taxol; *See* Paclitaxel
Taxotere; *See* Docetaxel
Tazarotene, 507
Tazorac; *See* Tazarotene
TB; *See* Tuberculosis
TBPI; *See* Toe brachial pressure index
TC-cell, 317
T-cell lymphoma, 914
T-cell subsets, 317
TCER; *See* Transcervical endometrial resection
TCT; *See* Thyrocalcitonin
Tear, retinal, 1101-1102, 1102*b*
Tears, changes with aging, 1075*c*
Technetium scan
in cardiovascular assessment, 725
in heart failure, 770
Technology in patient care, 6, 6*f*
TEE; *See* Transesophageal echocardiography
Teeth, 1217
TEF; *See* Tracheoesophageal fistula
Tegretol; *See* Carbamazepine
Tekturna; *See* Aliskiren
Telemetry system, 733
Telephone amplifier, 1132
Teletherapy, 419
Telomere, 66-67, 67*f*
Telomeric deoxyribonucleic acid, 67*f*
Telophase of cell cycle, 67*f*
Temodar; *See* Temozolomide
Temozolomide, 422*t*, 1062
Temperature
assessment of sensation of, 939
body; *See* Body temperature
skin and, 463*t*, 472*t*
Temporal arteritis, 355, 355*c*
Temporal field blindness, 1066
Temporal herniation, 1053*f*
Temporal lobe, 931*t*
Temporal pulse, 717*f*
Temporary pacing, 754-755
Temporary vascular access in hemodialysis, 1623-1625, 1625*f*
Temporomandibular joint, rheumatoid arthritis of, 338
Temsirolimus, 435*t*, 1596
Tendon, 1142*f*, 1143
rupture of, 1208
Tenesmus
in intestinal parasitic infection, 1339
in ulcerative colitis, 1321
Tenofovir, 376*c*, 379
Tenofovir-emtricitabine, 377*c*
TENS; *See* Transcutaneous electrical nerve stimulation
Tensilon testing, 1017
Tension headache, 955
Tension pneumothorax, 699
Tentorium, 929
Tenuate; *See* Diethylpropion
Tequin; *See* Gatifloxacin
Teratogenic drugs
isotretinoin in, 515
tazoratene in, 507
Teratogenic effects, 1647
Teratoma, 127, 1727*t*
Terazosin
for benign prostatic hypertrophy, 1714
for hypertension, 802
Terbutaline, 618
Teriparatide, 1157-1159
Terlipressin, 1353
Terminal arteriole, 708
Terminal bronchiole, 554-555, 555*f*
Terminal illness, 111-123
dyspnea management in, 117-118
euthanasia and, 121-122, 122*t*
hospice and palliative care in, 113
incidence of death and, 113
nausea and vomiting management in, 118
pain management in, 116-117
pathophysiology of dying and, 112
patient and family education in, 115*c*
perception of death and, 111-112, 112*t*
physical assessment and, 115*c*, 115-116
planning for death and, 113, 114*f*
postmortem care and, 121, 121*c*, 122*c*
psychosocial assessment and, 116, 116*c*
psychosocial management in, 119*t*, 119-121, 120*c*, 121*c*
refractory symptoms of distress and, 118
restlessness and agitation management in, 118
seizure management in, 118
weakness management in, 116
Terminal knob, 929
Tertiary syphilis, 1740
Testex; *See* Testosterone propionate
Testis, 1413*f*, 1645*f*, 1646
anterior pituitary hormones and, 1415*t*
cancer of, 127, 1726*c*, 1726-1730, 1727*t*, 1728*c*, 1729*c*
hormones of, 1413*t*
hydrocele and, 1730-1731, 1731*f*
palpation of, 1422, 1651
self-examination of, 1651, 1726, 1726*c*
spermatocele and, 1731, 1731*f*
varicocele and, 1731*f*, 1731-1732
Testosterone, 1645
prostate cancer and, 1719
serum levels in reproductive assessment, 1653*c*
Testosterone propionate, 1160
Tetanus prophylaxis
in black widow spider bite, 148
in brown recluse spider bite, 147
burn patient and, 540
in lightning strike, 152
in pit viper envenomation, 145
in tarantula bite, 148
Tetany, 1454
Tetracaine, 1086*c*
Tetracycline
antacid interaction with, 1275
for peptic ulcer disease, 1269*c*, 1274
for stomatitis, 1233
for trachoma, 1088
Tetrahydrocannabinol, 88
Tetraplegia, 993
Texture of skin, 472*t*
Thalamotomy, 969
Thalamus, 930, 931*f*
Thalidomide, 433, 915
Thallium scan
in cardiovascular assessment, 725-726
in coronary artery disease, 855
in heart failure, 770
in musculoskeletal assessment, 1149
Thalomid; *See* Thalidomide
Theophylline
for anaphylaxis, 393
for asthma, 617*c*, 620
Therapeutic hypothermia, 756
Therapeutic Lifestyle Changes diet, 796
Therapeutic regimen noncompliance in hypertension, 802, 803*c*
Therapeutic touch
in end-of-life care, 117
in pain management, 12-13, 13*f*

y-induced immune deficiency, 384-385
Thermal ablation techniques in bone cancer, 1170
Thermal injury, 530
Thermazene; *See* Silver sulfadiazine
Thermodilution method of cardiac output, 728
Thermography in burn assessment, 531
Thermotherapy for benign prostatic hypertrophy, 1715
Thiazide diuretics
for hypercalciuria, 1574
for hypertension, 801
hyponatremia and, 186
to reduce preload in heart failure, 772
Thiazolidinediones, 1481-1482*c*, 1484
Thigh surgery, skin preparation for, 256*f*
ThinPrep Pap Test, 1652
6-Thioguanine, 421*t*
Thionamides, 1452, 1453*c*
Thiopental sodium, 274*t*
Thiopeta, 422*t*
Thioplex; *See* Thiopeta
Third intention healing, 481, 482*f*
Third spacing, 523-524, 524*f*, 1317
Third-degree atrioventricular block, 750
Third-degree frostbite, 154
Thirst
in diabetes insipidus, 1432
extracellular fluid osmolarity and, 174
fluid balance and, 175
Thoracentesis, 568-569, 569*f*
in lung cancer, 650
in pneumonia, 663
Thoracic aortic aneurysm, 811
Thoracic aortic aneurysm repair, 813
Thoracic chordotomy, 58*f*
Thoracic outlet syndrome, 815
Thoracic spine
musculoskeletal assessment of, 1146
tumor of, 1001*c*
Thoracoabdominal surgery, skin preparation for, 256*f*
Thoracolumbosacral orthosis, 1174, 1174*f*
Thoracoscopy, 644
Thoracostomy, 136
Thoracotomy
in empyema, 674
in hemothorax, 699
Thorax
barrel chest in asthma and, 612, 614*f*
physical assessment of, 560-564, 561*f*, 562*f*, 562*t*, 563*t*
Thorazine; *See* Chlorpromazine
Thorough skin self-examination, 510-511
Thought processes disturbance
in acquired immunodeficiency syndrome, 381
in hypothyroidism, 1458
3TC; *See* Lamivudine
Threshold of sound, 1117
Throat, 554
pharyngitis and, 655-657, 656*c*, 656*t*
physical assessment of, 559-560
Throat culture
in pharyngitis, 655-656
in tonsillitis, 657
Thrombectomy
in acute peripheral arterial occlusion, 810
in deep vein thrombosis, 820
emergency, 809
Thrombin, 880
Thromboangiitis obliterans, 815
Thrombocytopenia, 916
in aplastic anemia, 900
in brown recluse spider bite, 147
chemotherapy-induced, 424, 426-427, 427*c*, 644
heparin-induced, 818
in hypothermia, 153
in leukemia, 902
Thrombocytopenia *(Continued)*
low-molecular-weight heparins and, 331
in myelodysplastic syndromes, 901
patient safety in, 910*c*
Thrombolytic therapy
for acute myocardial infarction, 859
for acute peripheral arterial occlusion, 810
contraindications to, 859*t*
for deep vein thrombosis, 819-820
hematologic assessment and, 884
for postoperative graft occlusion, 809
for stroke, 1037, 1037*c*
Thrombophlebitis, 817
intravenous therapy-related, 227*t*
Thrombopoietin, 318*t*, 878
Thrombosis
in acute coronary syndromes, 848
after liver transplantation, 1364*t*
after renal transplantation, 1632-1633
after total hip arthroplasty, 329, 330*c*, 330-331
of arteriovenous access, 1623
central venous catheter and, 234*t*
intravenous therapy-related, 227*t*
ischemic stroke and, 1030
in venous thromboembolism, 816-817
Thrombotic stroke, 1030-1031, 1031*t*
Thrombotic thrombocytopenic purpura, 916
Thrush, 501
Thumb spica cast, 1188*t*
Thymectomy, 1020
Thymine, 64, 64*f*
Thymoma, 1016
Thyrocalcitonin, 191, 1417, 1417*t*
Thyrohyoid membrane, 554*f*
Thyroid, 1413*f*, 1417, 1417*f*, 1417*t*, 1448-1461
cancer of, 1460-1461
heart failure and, 769
hyperthyroidism and, 1448-1455
drug therapy for, 1452-1454, 1453*c*
history in, 1450, 1450*f*
laboratory assessment in, 1451, 1451*c*
nursing diagnoses in, 1452
pathophysiology of, 1448-1450, 1449*c*
physical assessment in, 1450*f*, 1450-1451, 1451*t*
psychosocial assessment in, 1451
surgical management of, 1454-1455, 1455*c*
hypothyroidism and, 1455-1460
decreased cardiac output in, 1458
decreased general metabolism *versus*, 1419*c*
disturbed thought processes in, 1458
history in, 1457
home care management in, 1459, 1460*c*
ineffective breathing pattern in, 1458
laboratory assessment in, 1457
myxedema coma in, 1459, 1459*c*
nursing diagnoses in, 1457-1458
pathophysiology of, 1455-1456, 1456*c*, 1456*f*
thyroiditis and, 1460
needle biopsy of, 1424
palpation of, 1422, 1422*f*
thyroiditis and, 1460
thyroid-stimulating hormone and, 1415*t*
Thyroid antibody, 1451*c*
Thyroid cartilage, 553*f*, 554, 554*f*, 1417*f*
Thyroid crisis, 1449-1450, 1454-1455, 1455*c*
Thyroid hormones, 1413*t*, 1417, 1417*t*
Thyroid notch, 554*f*
Thyroid scan, 1451-1452
Thyroid stimulation test, 1451*c*
Thyroid storm, 1449-1450, 1452, 1454-1455, 1455*c*
Thyroid suppression test, 1451*c*
Thyroidectomy, 1454, 1461
Thyroiditis, 1460
Thyroid-stimulating hormone, 1415*t*, 1417
deficiency of, 1426, 1427*c*
Graves' disease and, 1449
in hyperthyroidism, 1451, 1451*c*
in hypothyroidism, 1455, 1457
overproduction of, 1430*c*
Thyroid-stimulating hormone stimulation test, 1451*c*
Thyroid-stimulating immunoglobulins, 1449
Thyrotoxicosis, 1017, 1448
Thyrotropin, 1430*c*
Thyrotropin receptor antibody, 1451*c*
Thyrotropin-releasing hormone, 1417
Thyrotropin-releasing hormone stimulation test, 1451*c*
Thyroxine, 1417, 1417*t*
bone and, 1142
hyperthyroidism and, 1451, 1451*c*
hypothyroidism and, 1457
TIA; *See* Transient ischemic attack
Tiagabine, 958*c*
TIBC; *See* Total iron-binding capacity
Tibial fracture, 1191*f*, 1197
Tibial nerve, 281*c*, 1022*f*
Tic douloureux, 1025*f*, 1025-1026
Tidal volume, 693
Tidaling, 648
Tikosyn; *See* Dofetilide
Tilade; *See* Nedocromil
Tiludronate, 1164
Time-cycled ventilator, 693
Timolol, 1099*c*
Timoptic; *See* Timolol
Tinea, 501
Tinel's sign, 1207
Tinnitus, 1112, 1114
in acoustic neuroma, 1061, 1129
in labyrinthitis, 1127
in Meniere's disease, 1127
in vertigo, 1126
Tinzaparin, 330
Tiotropium
for asthma, 620
for chronic obstructive pulmonary disease, 629
TIPS; *See* Transjugular intrahepatic portal-systemic shunt
Tirofiban
for acute myocardial infarction, 859
for deep vein thrombosis, 819
for postoperative graft occlusion, 809
Tissue macrophage, 311, 311*t*
Tissue necrosis
in acute pancreatitis, 1372
in myocardial infarction, 849
in pit viper envenomation, 144
in tarantula bite, 148
Tissue perfusion
in acute coronary syndromes, 858-860, 859*t*
amputation and, 1201
burn injury and, 533*c*, 533*t*, 533-535, 534*f*
cardiovascular system and, 704
chronic obstructive pulmonary disease and, 631-632, 632*f*, 633*t*
diabetes mellitus and, 1467-1468, 1506
dysrhythmias and, 750-751, 751*c*
respiratory system role in, 552, 552*f*
shock and, 826-827, 827*f*, 829*f*
spinal cord injury and, 995*c*, 995-997, 996*f*
stroke and, 1036-1037
Tissue plasminogen activator
for acute peripheral arterial occlusion, 810
for deep vein thrombosis, 819
for postoperative graft occlusion, 809
Tissue plasminogen activator *(Continued)*
for pulmonary embolism, 681*c*
for stroke, 1037, 1037*c*
Tissue swelling; *See* Edema
Tissue thromboplastin, 881*t*
Tissue-specific membrane proteins, 307*f*
Tizanidine
for spinal cord injury, 996
for tension headache, 955
TJA; *See* Total joint arthroplasty
TLC, *See* Total lung capacity
T-lymphocyte
antigen-antibody interactions and, 313
cell-mediated immunity and, 317-320, 318*f*, 318*t*
delayed hypersensitivity reactions and, 395
functions of, 309*t*, 878*t*
TNF; *See* Tumor necrosis factor
TNM system, 407, 407*t*
Tobacco use, 84-85, 85*f*
bladder cancer and, 1575
Buerger's disease and, 815
cancer development and, 408
chronic obstructive pulmonary disease and, 622
coronary artery disease and, 851-852, 854*c*
esophageal cancer and, 1255
head and neck cancer and, 598
heart disease and, 709-710
history in respiratory assessment, 558
lung cancer and, 642
occupational pulmonary disease and, 639
osteoarthritis and, 323
osteoporosis and, 1154
peripheral arterial disease and, 807
prostate cancer and, 1720
surgical risk and, 246
TobraDex; *See* Tobramycin-dexamethasone
Tobramycin
for cystic fibrosis, 636
nephrotoxicity of, 1506
for ocular infection, 1086*c*
Tobramycin-dexamethasone, 1086*c*
Tobrex; *See* Tobramycin
Tocainide, 741*c*
Tocilizumab, 344
Toe
amputation of, 1199*f*
hallux valgus and, 1172-1173, 1173*f*
Morton's neuroma and, 1173
Toe brachial pressure index, 716
Toe surgery, skin preparation for, 256*f*
Tofranil; *See* Imipramine
Tolazamide, 1477-1478*c*
Tolbutamide, 1478*c*
Tolerance, 39-40
to alcohol, 83
opioid analgesics and, 90
Tolinase; *See* Tolazamide
Tolterodine
for benign prostatic hypertrophy, 1715
for prostate cancer, 1723
for urinary incontinence, 1565*c*, 1567
Tomography; *See* Computed tomography
Tongue, 553*f*, 1217
hematologic assessment and, 885
squamous cell carcinoma of, 1234-1235
Tonic seizure, 955-956
Tonic-clonic seizure, 955-956, 959*c*
Tonic-clonic status epilepticus, 960
Tonocard; *See* Tocainide
Tonometry, 1080, 1080*f*, 1097
Tono-Pen, 1080, 1080*f*
Tonsil
peritonsillar abscess and, 657
tonsillitis and, 657, 657*c*
Tonsillar lymph nodes, 1235*f*
Tonsillectomy, 657
Tonsillitis, 657, 657*c*

Topamax; *See* Topiramate
Topetecan, 422*t*
Tophi, 353, 354*f*
on pinna, 1114
Topical anesthetics
for hemorrhoids, 1310
for ocular infection, 1086*c*
for pain, 54*t*, 55
Topical antibiotics for external otitis, 1121
Topical antifungal agents, 503
Topical antivirals for ocular infection, 1086*c*
Topical capsaicin
after total knee arthroplasty, 333
for osteoarthritis, 327-328
Topical drugs
for burn infection prevention, 540-541
for osteoarthritis, 326
for psoriasis, 507
Topical enzyme preparations for wound débridement, 493*t*
Topical growth factors for pressure ulcer, 495
Topical opioid analgesics, 50*t*
Topical steroids
for external otitis, 1121
for ocular infection, 1086*c*
Topiramate, 958*c*
for migraine headache, 953, 953*t*
for pain, 54, 54*t*
for seizures after stroke, 1043
Topoisomerase inhibitors, 422, 422*t*
Toprol XL; *See* Metoprolol
Toradol; *See* Ketorolac
Torisel; *See* Temsirolimus
Tornalate; *See* Bitolterol
Torsades de pointes, 722
magnesium sulfate for, 752
prolonged QT interval in, 736
Torsemide, 772
Total abdominal hysterectomy, 1696-1697, 1697*c*, 1697*t*, 1706
Total ankle arthroplasty, 335
Total bilirubin, 896
Total body surface area in burn, 528, 531, 531*f*
Total body water
gender and, 175
older adult and, 183
Total catecholamines, 1542*c*
Total cerebrospinal fluid proteins, 948*t*
Total colectomy, 1299
with continent ileostomy, 1326, 1326*f*
with ileoanal anastomosis, 1326, 1327*f*
Total elbow arthroplasty, 335
Total enteral nutrition, 1396-1400, 1397*f*, 1398*c*
Total estrogens, 1653*c*
Total exenteration, 1704*f*, 1704-1705
Total gastrectomy, 1282*f*, 1282-1285
Total granulocyte count, 310
Total hemoglobin
preoperative assessment of, 251*c*
in respiratory assessment, 565*c*
Total hip arthroplasty, 328-332, 330*c*, 330*t*, 332*c*, 332*f*
Total hysterectomy, 1700
Total iron-binding capacity, 886, 887*c*, 888, 1393-1394
Total joint arthroplasty, 328
elbow, 335
hip, 328-332, 330*c*, 332*c*, 332*f*
knee, 333*f*, 333-334, 334*c*
prevention of complications in, 330*t*
shoulder, 334-335
Total laryngectomy, 600*t*, 600-602, 601*f*
Total lung capacity, 567*t*, 627
Total lymphocyte count, 1394
Total parenteral nutrition, 1400-1401, 1401*c*
in acute renal failure, 1607
after pancreas transplantation, 1500
in chronic pancreatitis, 1378
in Crohn's disease, 1332
in pancreatic cancer, 1382
Total penectomy, 1732
Total proctocolectomy with permanent ileostomy, 1325-1326, 1326*f*
Total prostate-specific antigen test, 1720
Total protein, 532*c*
Total serum cholesterol
atherosclerosis and, 795
coronary artery disease and, 850-851
Total serum lipids
cardiovascular assessment and, 720*c*
coronary artery disease and, 850-851
Total shoulder arthroplasty, 334-335
Total thyroidectomy
in hyperthyroidism, 1454
in thyroid cancer, 1461
Total urinary incontinence, 1569
Total vaginal hysterectomy, 1696-1697, 1697*t*
Total vaginectomy, 1709
Totect; *See* Dexrazoxane
Touch discrimination, 939
Toxic diffuse goiter, 1449
Toxic epidermal necrolysis, 516
Toxic hepatitis, 1356
Toxic megacolon, 1322*t*, 1324
Toxic multinodular goiter, 1449
Toxic shock syndrome, 1691, 1692*c*
Toxin, 441
Toxoplasma gondii, 1065
Toxoplasmosis encephalitis, 371
T-piece, 577, 577*t*, 578*f*, 697*t*
TPN; *See* Total parenteral nutrition
Trabecular bone, 1153
Trabeculation, 1555
Trachea, 554, 555*f*
endotracheal intubation and, 689-690, 690*f*
physical assessment of, 559-560
Trachea-innominate artery fistula, 581*t*
Tracheal stenosis, 581*t*
Tracheobronchial trauma, 699
Tracheobronchial tree, 554-555, 555*f*
Tracheoesophageal fistula
after laryngectomy, 602, 603*f*
tracheostomy-related, 581*t*
Tracheoesophageal prosthesis, 603*f*
Tracheomalacia, 581*t*
Tracheostomy, 580-587
air warming and humidification in, 583
body image and, 586
bronchial and oral hygiene in, 585
care of, 584-585, 585*c*, 585*f*
community-based care in, 587
complications of, 580-581, 581*t*
emotional care in, 586
in laryngeal cancer, 600
nursing diagnoses in, 580
nutrition and, 586, 586*c*
prevention of tissue damage in, 583, 583*f*
speech and communication and, 586
suctioning in, 583-584, 584*c*
tubes in, 581-583, 582*f*
weaning from, 586-587
Tracheostomy button, 587
Tracheostomy collar, 577, 577*t*
Tracheostomy tube, 581-583, 582*f*
mechanical ventilation and, 696
obstruction of, 580
suctioning of, 583-584, 584*c*
T-piece apparatus for, 577, 577*t*, 578*f*
Tracheotomy, 580
in burn, 535
complications of, 581
in facial trauma, 593
in head and neck cancer, 602
in upper airway obstruction, 596
Trachoma, 1088
Tracleer; *See* Bosentan
Tracrium; *See* Atracurium
Traction, 1189*f*, 1189-1190, 1190*t*
in cervical spine injury, 996, 996*f*
Traction retinal detachment, 1101
Traditional Chinese medicine, 9, 11
Traditional cholecystectomy, 1370
Tragus, 1110*f*
Trained medical interpreter, 29
Training in emergency nursing, 131, 131*t*
TRAM flap, 1675
Tramadol, 48
Trans fatty acids, 1403, 1493
Transabdominal ultrasonography, 1714
Transbronchial biopsy, 569
Transbronchial needle aspiration, 569
Transcellular fluids, 170-171
Transcervical approach in thymectomy, 1020
Transcervical endometrial resection, 1696
Transcranial Doppler ultrasonography, 949
Transcultural nursing, 27
Transcutaneous electrical nerve stimulation, 55-56, 56*f*
Transdermal administration of opioid analgesics, 50*t*
Transesophageal echocardiography
in cardiovascular assessment, 725
in pulmonary embolism, 679
in valvular heart disease, 780
Transfer of patient
after coronary artery bypass graft, 869
to surgical suite, 261
techniques for, 99-100, 100*c*
Transferrin, 888
Transformation zone of cervix, 1702
Transfusion reactions, 920-921
Transfusion therapy, 214, 917-921
in aplastic anemia, 900
autologous, 921
in burn, 524
filter in, 221
in hypovolemic shock, 837
indications for, 917*t*
in leukemia, 911
in myelodysplastic syndromes, 901
older adult and, 919*c*
pretransfusion responsibilities in, 917-919, 918*c*
reactions to, 920-921
in septic shock, 844
in sickle cell disease, 897
via peripherally inserted central catheter, 218
Transfusion-associated graft-*versus*-host disease, 921
Transfusion-related acute lung injury, 686
Transgender health care, 30*c*, 30-31, 31*t*
Transient ischemic attack, 784, 1030
Transillumination
scrotal, 1651
in sinusitis, 654
Transitional cell, 731
Transjugular intrahepatic portal-systemic shunt
in cirrhosis, 1353
in esophageal varices, 1354
Transmission
of nerve impulse, 929
of pain, 38, 39*f*
of specific trait, 71
Transmission-based guidelines, 446*t*, 446-449, 447*t*
Transmission-based precautions, 448
Transmural myocardial infarction, 849
Transmyocardial laser revascularization, 870
Transoral cordectomy, 600*t*
Transparent plastic surgical dressing, 294-295, 540
Transplantation
bone marrow
in leukemia, 907*t*, 907-910, 909*f*
in multiple myeloma, 915
fetal tissue, 969
heart
in cardiomyopathy, 789, 789*f*
in heart failure, 774
Transplantation *(Continued)*
liver, 1357, 1362-1363, 1364*t*
lung
in chronic obstructive pulmonary disease, 630
in cystic fibrosis, 636-637
in idiopathic pulmonary fibrosis, 639
in primary pulmonary hypertension, 638
pancreatic, 1498-1500
rejection of, 319-320
corneal, 1091
heart, 790*c*
liver, 1363, 1364*t*
pancreatic, 1498
renal, 1632, 1633*t*
renal
in chronic kidney disease, 1630-1633, 1631*f*, 1632*f*, 1633*t*
in Goodpasture's syndrome, 394
stem cell
in breast cancer, 1679
in leukemia, 907*t*, 907-910, 909*f*
in multiple myeloma, 915
platelet transfusion and, 920
in sickle cell disease, 897
tendon, 1208
Transport maximum for glucose reabsorption, 1531
Transrectal scan, 1655
Transrectal ultrasonography, 1714
Transsphenoidal hypophysectomy, 1431*f*, 1431-1432, 1432*c*
Transthoracic echocardiography
in infective endocarditis, 784
in valvular heart disease, 780
Transthoracic needle aspiration, 569
Transtracheal oxygen therapy, 578
Transurethral incision of prostate, 1715
Transurethral microwave therapy, 1715
Transurethral needle ablation, 1715
Transurethral resection of bladder tumor, 1576
Transurethral resection of prostate
in benign prostatic hypertrophy, 1715-1717, 1717*f*, 1718*c*
in prostate cancer, 1721
Transurethral suppository for erectile dysfunction, 1726
Transurethral ultrasound-guided laser incision of prostate, 1717
Transvaginal ultrasonography, 1655
in dysfunctional uterine bleeding, 1688
in endometrial cancer, 1700
in uterine leiomyoma, 1695
Transverse colon, 1219, 1294*f*
Transverse colostomy, 1298-1299, 1299*f*
Trastuzumab, 434, 435*t*
for breast cancer, 1678
for esophageal cancer, 1258
Trauma, 134-135
abdominal, 1307-1308
kidney injury in, 1596
liver injury in, 1361
pelvic fracture and, 1198
amputations in, 1199*f*, 1199-1204, 1202*f*, 1203*f*, 1204*c*
bladder, 1578
carpal tunnel syndrome in, 1206-1207
chest, 697-699
complex regional pain syndrome in, 1204
esophageal, 597, 1262, 1262*t*
facial, 593-594
fractures and, 1179-1199
acute compartment syndrome and, 1180-1182, 1181*c*
acute pain in, 1192
cast application for, 1187*f*, 1187-1189, 1188*t*
chronic complications of, 1183
classification of, 1179*f*, 1179-1180
crush syndrome and, 1182

Trauma *(Continued)*
emergency care of, 1186, 1186*c*
fat embolism syndrome and, 1182*c*, 1182-1183
health care resources for, 1194
health teaching in, 1194, 1194*c*
hip, 1195-1197, 1196*f*, 1248
history in, 1183-1184
home care management in, 1194
hypovolemic shock and, 1182
imaging studies in, 1185
imbalanced nutrition: less than body requirements in, 1194
impaired physical mobility in, 1193*f*, 1193-1194
incidence and prevalence of, 1183
infection and, 1183, 1192-1193
laboratory assessment in, 1185
lower extremity, 1197-1198
mandibular, 593
nasal, 590-591, 591*f*
nursing diagnoses in, 1185-1186
open reduction of, 1190-1192, 1191*f*
osteoporosis-related, 1155
pelvic, 1198
peripheral neurovascular dysfunction and, 1186, 1186*c*
physical assessment in, 1184*c*, 1184-1185
prevention of, 1183
psychosocial assessment in, 1185
rib, 698, 1198
skeletal pin site care in, 1191
skull, 1050
stages of bone healing and, 1180, 1180*f*
sternum, 1198
traction for, 1189*f*, 1189-1190, 1190*t*
upper extremity, 1195
venous thromboembolism and, 1183
vertebral, 1198*c*, 1198-1199
head, 1049-1060
brain herniation in, 1052, 1053*f*
closed head injury in, 1050, 1050*f*
community-based care in, 1059-1060
drug therapy for, 1057
fluid and electrolyte management in, 1057
hemorrhage in, 1051-1052, 1052*f*
history in, 1053, 1054*c*
hydrocephalus after, 1052
imaging studies in, 1055
incidence and prevalence of, 1052
increased intracranial pressure in, 1051, 1055-1057
laboratory assessment in, 1055
minor head injury in, 1056*c*
nutrition management in, 1057-1058
in older adult, 1054*c*
open head injury in, 1049-1050
pathophysiology of, 1049, 1049*c*
physical assessment in, 1053-1055
prevention of, 1053
psychosocial assessment in, 1055
sensory, cognitive, and behavioral management in, 1058
surgical management in, 1058, 1059*t*
types of force in, 1050*f*, 1050-1051
laryngeal, 596
liver, 1361*c*, 1361-1362
middle ear, 1126
neck, 596-597
ocular, 1092*c*
osteoarthritis related to, 323-324
peripheral nerve, 1022*f*, 1022-1024, 1023*f*
renal, 1596-1598, 1597*c*, 1597*t*
rotator cuff injury in, 1208
to skin, 481*t*, 481-484, 482*f*, 483*t*, 484*f*

Trauma *(Continued)*
spinal cord, 990-1000
etiology of, 992-993
extent of injury in, 991-992, 992*f*
health care resources for, 1000
health teaching in, 999*c*, 999-1000, 1000*c*
history in, 993
home care management in, 999
imaging studies in, 994-995
impaired adjustment in, 998
impaired elimination in, 997-998, 998*c*
impaired gas exchange in, 997
ineffective tissue perfusion in, 995*c*, 995-997, 996*f*
laboratory assessment in, 994
mechanisms of injury in, 990-991, 991*f*
nursing diagnoses in, 995
physical assessment in, 993-994, 994*c*
psychosocial assessment in, 994
self-care deficit in, 997
sports-related injuries in, 1204-1206, 1205*c*, 1205*f*
strains and sprains in, 1208
tendon rupture and joint dislocation in, 1208
tracheobronchial, 699
tympanic membrane, 1126
vascular, 823
Trauma activation criteria, 136
Trauma center, 135, 135*t*
Trauma nursing, 134-139
airway and cervical spine management in, 136, 137*f*
breathing interventions in, 137
circulation management in, 137-138
disability examination in, 138
disposition of patient and, 138-139
exposure assessment in, 138
mechanism of injury and, 136
secondary survey and resuscitation interventions in, 138
trauma center and, 135, 135*t*
trauma systems and, 136
Trauma systems, 136
Traumatic amputation, 1199
Traumatic aneurysm, 1031
Traumatic brain injury, 1049-1060
brain herniation in, 1052, 1053*f*
closed head injury in, 1050, 1050*f*
community-based care in, 1059-1060
drug therapy for, 1057
fluid and electrolyte management in, 1057
hemorrhage in, 1051-1052, 1052*f*
history in, 1053, 1054*c*
hydrocephalus after, 1052
imaging studies in, 1055
incidence and prevalence of, 1052
increased intracranial pressure in, 1051, 1055-1057
laboratory assessment in, 1055
minor head injury in, 1056*c*
nutrition management in, 1057-1058
in older adult, 1054*c*
open head injury in, 1049-1050
pathophysiology of, 1049, 1049*c*
physical assessment in, 1053-1055
prevention of, 1053
psychosocial assessment in, 1055
sensory, cognitive, and behavioral management in, 1058
surgical management in, 1058, 1059*t*
types of force in, 1050*f*, 1050-1051
Traumatic relocation syndrome, 973
Travatan; *See* Travoprost
Travel, diabetes mellitus and, 1417*c*
Travel history in respiratory assessment, 558-559
Traveler's diarrhea, 1319*t*, 1319-1321, 1321*c*
Travoprost, 1099*c*

Trazodone
for fibromyalgia, 358
for pain, 54, 54*t*
Trelstar; *See* Triptorelin
Tremor
assessment of, 939
in chronic glomerulonephritis, 1592
in multiple sclerosis, 1004
Trendelenburg position, 280*f*
Trental; *See* Pentoxifylline
Treponema pallidum, 1738-1742, 1740*f*
Treprostinil, 638
TRH; *See* Thyrotropin-releasing hormone
Triage
emergency nursing and, 131*t*, 131-132
mass casualty, 160-161, 161*t*
Triage nurse, 131
Triage officer, 163
Triamcinolone in benzocaine, 1233
Triamterene, 189
Triceps reflex, 940*f*
Triceps skin-fold measurement, 1392
Trichinosis, 1339-1340
Trichomoniasis, 1552, 1753
Tricuspid area, 718*t*
Tricuspid valve, 705*f*, 706
Tricyclic antidepressants
for diabetic neuropathy, 1504
for fibromyalgia, 358
for Guillain-Barré syndrome, 1015
for irritable bowel syndrome, 1291
for multiple sclerosis, 1006
for pain, 54, 54*t*, 54-55
for pain in acquired immunodeficiency syndrome, 380
for urinary incontinence, 1565*c*, 1567
Tridil; *See* Nitroglycerin
Trifluridine, 1086*c*
Trigeminal nerve
blink reflex and, 1072
divisions of, 1025*f*
functions of, 935*t*
Trigeminal neuralgia, 1025*f*, 1025-1026
Trigeminal rhizotomy, 58*f*
Trigeminy, 738
Trigger points, 357
Triggering techniques in bladder training, 105-106
Triglycerides
atherosclerosis and, 795
cardiovascular assessment and, 720*c*, 721
coronary artery disease and, 850-851
metabolic syndrome and, 853*t*
Trigone muscle, 1532, 1532*f*
Trigonitis syndrome, 1559
Triiodothyronine, 1417, 1417*t*
hyperthyroidism and, 1451, 1451*c*
hypothyroidism and, 1457
Triiodothyronine resin uptake, 1451, 1451*c*, 1452
Trileptal; *See* Oxcarbazepine
Trimethoprim-sulfamethoxazole
for diverticulitis, 1335
for gastroenteritis, 1320
for granuloma inguinale, 1754
for *Pneumocystis jiroveci* pneumonia, 379
for prostatitis, 1733-1734
for urinary tract infection, 1556*c*, 1558
Triptans, 952-953, 953*t*
Triptorelin, 1723
Trisenox; *See* Arsenic trioxide
Trivada; *See* Tenofovir-emtricitabine
Trivalent botulism antitoxin, 1342
Trizivir; *See* Zidovudine-lamivudine-abacavir
Trochlear nerve, 935*t*, 1072
Tropic hormones, 1414, 1415*t*
Tropical sprue, 1311
Troponins, 720, 720*c*, 855
Trospium, 1565*c*
Trousseau's sign
in hyperparathyroidism, 1463
in hypocalcemia, 192, 193*f*

True aneurysm, 810
Trunk, positioning for prevention of contracture, 544*c*
Truphylline; *See* Aminophylline
Trusopt; *See* Dorzolamide
Truss, 1292
Tryptophan, 70*f*, 70*t*
T-score in bone mineral density testing, 1153
TSH; *See* Thyroid-stimulating hormone
TSSE; *See* Thorough skin self-examination
TTP; *See* Thrombotic thrombocytopenic purpura
T-tube drain, 292, 292*f*, 1370, 1370*c*
Tubal abscess, 1748
Tube feeding, 1396-1400, 1397*f*, 1398*c*
in acute respiratory distress syndrome, 689
after laryngectomy, 602
burn patient and, 543
during mechanical ventilation, 696
Tube thoracostomy, 136
Tuberculin test, 669
Tuberculosis, 668-672
directly observed therapy in, 449
drug therapy for, 670, 671*c*
health care resources for, 672
health teaching in, 670-672
history in, 669
in HIV-infected patient, 372
home care management in, 670
laboratory assessment in, 669
lung abscess in, 672
nursing diagnoses in, 669
pathophysiology of, 668, 668*t*
physical assessment in, 669
Tubo-ovarian abscess, 1748
Tubular breath sounds, 562, 563*t*
Tubular infiltrate, 1529
Tubular reabsorption, 1529-1530
Tubular secretion, 1531
Tubulointerstitial disorders, 1593
TULIP; *See* Transurethral ultrasound-guided laser incision of prostate
Tumescence, erectile dysfunction and, 1726
Tumor
benign
acoustic neuroma, 1129
Bartholin cyst, 1699
of bone, 1167
of brain, 1060*t*, 1060-1061
cervical polyp, 1699
classification by tissue of origin, 405*t*
cutaneous, 508-509, 509*f*
of middle ear, 1126
ovarian, 1694
uterine leiomyoma, 1694-1699, 1695*f*, 1697*c*, 1697*t*, 1698*c*
bladder, 1575-1578, 1577*f*
bone, 1161
benign, 1167
malignant, 1168-1172, 1171*c*
osteomalacia and, 1161
brain, 1060*t*, 1060-1065, 1061*c*, 1062*f*, 1064*t*
colorectal, 1293-1302
anticipatory grieving in, 1296, 1297*c*
conditions associated with genetic predisposition for, 410*t*
drug therapy in, 1297
genetic testing for, 76
health care resources for, 1302
health promotion and maintenance in, 1294-1295, 1295*c*
health teaching in, 1300-1302, 1301*c*
hematologic assessment in, 409*c*
history in, 1295
home management in, 1300
imaging studies in, 1296
laboratory assessment in, 1295-1296

Tumor *(Continued)*
lower gastrointestinal bleeding in, 1290*f*
metastasis in, 1296
nursing diagnoses in, 1296
pathophysiology of, 1293-1294, 1294*f*
physical assessment in, 1295
psychosocial assessment in, 1295
radiation therapy in, 1297
sites of metastasis for, 405*t*
surgical management of, 1297*t*, 1297-1300, 1298*t*, 1299*f*, 1300*c*
development of, 399-413
carcinogenesis and oncogenesis and, 403*t*, 403-405, 404*f*, 404*t*, 405*t*
classification of, 405*t*, 405-406, 406*f*
external factors in, 407-408, 408*c*, 408*t*
grading, ploidy, and staging and, 406*t*, 406-407, 407*t*
pathophysiology and, 399-403, 400*f*
personal factors in, 408-411, 409*c*, 409*t*, 410*t*
prevention of, 411*t*, 411-412
esophageal, 1255-1261
community-based care in, 1261
history in, 1256
imbalanced nutrition: less than body requirements in, 1257
nonsurgical management of, 1257-1259, 1258*c*
nursing diagnoses in, 1257
pathophysiology of, 1255-1256
physical assessment in, 1256, 1256*c*
psychosocial assessment in, 1256
surgical management of, 1259*f*, 1259-1261, 1260*c*
gastrin-secreting, 1279
gynecologic, 1699-1709
cervical cancer in, 1702*t*, 1702-1705, 1704*c*, 1704*f*
endometrial cancer in, 1699-1702, 1700*t*, 1701*c*
fallopian tube cancer in, 1709
ovarian cancer in, 1705*t*, 1705-1707
vaginal cancer in, 1708-1709
vulvar cancer in, 1707-1708, 1708*f*
insulinoma, 1380
kidney, 1595*t*, 1595-1596
middle ear, 1126
nose and sinus, 592-593
oncologic emergencies and, 434-437
hypercalcemia in, 436
sepsis and disseminated intravascular coagulation in, 435
spinal cord compression in, 436
superior vena cava syndrome in, 436*f*, 436-437
syndrome of inappropriate antidiuretic hormone secretion in, 435-436
tumor lysis syndrome in, 437, 437*f*
oral cavity, 1234
pancreatic, 1380-1384, 1381*c*, 1383*f*, 1383*t*
pheochromocytoma, 1446-1447
pituitary, 1061
Cushing's disease and, 1440
hyperpituitarism and, 1428
hypopituitarism and, 1426
salivary gland, 1240
spinal cord, 1000-1002, 1001*c*
testicular, 1726*c*, 1726-1730, 1727*t*, 1728*c*, 1729*c*
in Zollinger-Ellison syndrome, 1279
Tumor, node, metastasis system, 407, 407*t*
Tumor angiogenesis factor, 404, 404*f*
Tumor doubling time, 407
Tumor lysis syndrome, 437, 437*f*
Tumor markers
in chemotherapy for breast cancer, 1678
in testicular cancer, 1728
Tumor necrosis factor, 318*t*, 343
Tumor-induced osteomalacia, 1161
Tuning fork tests, 1116, 1131
Tunnel infection, 1629-1630
Tunneled central catheter, 218, 218*f*
Turbidity
of infusion fluid, 219
of urine, 1538, 1539*t*
Turbinates, 553, 553*f*
Turgor, 472, 472*t*
dehydration and, 179, 179*f*
Turner syndrome, 68
Turner's sign
in abdominal trauma, 1307
in acute pancreatitis, 1374
TURP; *See* Transurethral resection of prostate
Twenty-four hour ambulatory esophageal pH monitoring, 1245
Twenty-four hour urinary hydroxyproline, 1163
Twenty-four hour urine collection, 1540*t*, 1542*c*
Twitching
in hyperkalemia, 190
in hypernatremia, 186
Two-point discrimination, 939
Tykerb; *See* Lapatinib
Tylenol; *See* Acetaminophen
Tylox; *See* Oxycodone-acetaminophen
Tympanic membrane, 1109, 1110, 1110*f*, 1111*f*
changes with aging, 1112*c*
instillation of antibiotics and, 1121
myringotomy and, 1125, 1125*f*
perforation of, 1124, 1124*f*, 1126
trauma to, 1126
Tympanic percussion sound, 1223
Tympanometry, 1118
Tympanoplasty, 1125-1126, 1132-1133, 1133*f*, 1134*f*
Tympany, percussion note, 562*t*
Type 1 diabetes mellitus, 1466*t*
dietary considerations in, 1495
etiology and genetic risk in, 1471, 1471*t*
exercise and, 1496
focused assessment in, 1516*c*
hypoglycemic unawareness in, 1507
subcutaneous infusion therapy in, 237*t*
Type 2 diabetes mellitus, 1466*t*, 1471*t*, 1472
complications of, 1468
concept map for, 1476
dietary considerations in, 1495
genetic risk for, 74
glucose homeostasis and, 1467
incretin and, 1490
major risk factors for, 1473*t*
oral drug therapy for, 1477-1483*c*, 1477-1484, 1483*t*
presbyopia in, 1514
Type A gastritis, 1266
Type B gastritis, 1266
Type I rapid hypersensitivity reactions, 387-394, 388*t*
allergic rhinitis in, 388*f*, 388-391, 389*f*, 390*c*
anaphylaxis in, 391*t*, 391-394, 392*c*, 392*f*, 393*c*
latex allergy in, 394
Type II cytotoxic reactions, 388*t*, 394, 394*f*
Type II pneumatocyte, 555, 686
Type III immune complex reactions, 388*t*, 394-395, 395*f*
Type IV delayed hypersensitivity reactions, 388*t*, 395
Type V stimulatory reactions, 388*t*, 395
Tyrosine, 70*f*, 70*t*
Tyrosine kinase inhibitors, 1382
Tysabri; *See* Natalizumab
Tzanck smear, 502

U

U wave, 735, 735*f*
Ulcer, 470*f*
in brown recluse spider bite, 146
corneal, 1089
in Crohn's disease, 1330
Curling's, 525
diabetic foot and, 1501
in intestinal parasitic infection, 1339
in osteomyelitis, 1165, 1166, 1166*c*
peptic, 1270-1279
complementary and alternative therapies for, 1270*t*
complications of, 1271*c*, 1271*f*, 1271-1272
drug therapy for, 1268-1269*c*
etiology and genetic risk in, 1272
gastrointestinal bleeding in, 1275-1278, 1276*c*, 1277*c*, 1278*f*
health care resources for, 1279
health teaching in, 1278
history in, 1272-1273
home care management in, 1278, 1279*c*
imaging studies in, 1273-1274
laboratory assessment in, 1273
nursing diagnoses in, 1274
pain in, 1274-1275
pathophysiology of, 1270*f*, 1270-1271, 1271*f*
physical assessment in, 1273, 1273*t*
prevention of, 1272
psychosocial assessment in, 1273
in peripheral arterial disease, 805, 806*c*
pressure, 484-499
assessment before rehabilitation, 98
concept map for, 492
dressings for, 491-493, 493-495*t*
drug therapy for, 493
in Guillain-Barré syndrome, 1015
health care resources for, 498, 499*c*
health teaching in, 498
history in, 488
home care management in, 498
identification of high-risk patient and, 486, 487*f*
intervention activities for, 493*c*
intraoperative development of, 296
laboratory assessment in, 490-491
new technologies for, 495
nursing diagnoses in, 491
nutrition therapy for, 493
older adult and, 25
pathophysiology of, 484-485, 485*f*
physical assessment in, 488
physical therapy for, 493
pressure-relieving and pressure-reducing techniques for, 486-488
prevention of, 485*c*, 485-486
psychosocial assessment in, 490
risk for infection and, 496-498, 497*c*
surgical management of, 495-496, 496*f*
wound assessment in, 488-490, 489*c*, 489*f*, 490*t*
in Raynaud's phenomenon, 816
in sickle cell disease, 895
in stomatitis, 1231-1234, 1233*c*, 1233*f*
in syphilis, 1738-1742, 1740*f*
in vulvovaginitis, 1691
in Zollinger-Ellison syndrome, 1279
Ulcerative colitis, 1321-1330
Crohn's disease *versus*, 1321*c*
diarrhea in, 1323-1325, 1324*c*
health care resources for, 1329*c*, 1329-1330
health teaching in, 1328-1329, 1329*c*
history in, 1322-1323
home care management in, 1328
laboratory assessment in, 1323
lower gastrointestinal bleeding in, 1290*f*, 1328
Ulcerative colitis *(Continued)*
malabsorption in, 1311
nursing diagnoses in, 1323
pain in, 1327-1328, 1328*c*
pathophysiology of, 1321-1322, 1322*t*
physical assessment in, 1323
psychosocial assessment in, 1323
surgical management of, 1325-1327, 1326*f*, 1327*f*
Ulnar fracture, 1195
Ulnar nerve, 281*c*, 1022*f*
Ulnar nerve block, 276*f*
Ulnar pulse, 717*f*
Ultane; *See* Sevoflurane
Ultiva; *See* Remifentanil
Ultram; *See* Tramadol
Ultrasonography
in abdominal trauma, 1307
BladderScan and, 105
of breast, 1670-1671
in cholecystitis, 1369
in chronic pancreatitis, 1378
in cirrhosis, 1350
in esophageal cancer, 1256-1257
in gallbladder cancer, 1371
in gastrointestinal assessment, 1229
in infection assessment, 451
in intravenous line placement, 216
in liver trauma, 1361
in musculoskeletal assessment, 1149
in ocular problems, 1079
in osteoporosis, 1156-1157
renal, 1544*t*, 1546
in acute renal failure, 1604
in renal trauma, 1598
in urolithiasis, 1572
in reproductive assessment, 1655
in testicular cancer, 1728
of thyroid gland, 1452
transcranial Doppler, 949
in uterine leiomyoma, 1695
Ultra-Stat epistaxis catheter, 592*f*
Ultraviolet light therapy, 507-508
Umbilical hernia, 1291-1293, 1292*f*
Umbo, 1110, 1110*f*
Uncal herniation, 1052, 1053*f*
Unclassified seizure, 956
Unconjugated bilirubin
in gastrointestinal assessment, 1224*c*
in jaundice, 1346*t*
Undermedication in postoperative pain, 297
Undermining in wound assessment, 490
Undernutrition, 1392-1402
community-based care in, 1401-1402
in Crohn's disease, 1332
drug therapy for, 1395-1396
in Guillain-Barré syndrome, 1015
history in, 1393
intervention activities for, 1395*c*
laboratory assessment in, 1393-1394
mechanical ventilation and, 696
nursing diagnoses in, 1394
nutrition management in, 1395
older adult and, 16, 1393*c*, 1395, 1396*c*
parenteral nutrition in, 1400-1401, 1401*c*
pathophysiology of, 1392
physical assessment in, 1393, 1394*t*
psychosocial assessment in, 1393
total enteral nutrition in, 1396-1400, 1397*f*, 1398*c*
Undescended testis, 1727
Unfractionated heparin, 818-819, 819*c*
Unilateral adrenalectomy
in Cushing's disease, 1443
in hyperaldosteronism, 1446
Unilateral neglect in stroke, 1047
Uninhibited bladder, 105, 105*t*
Uniphyl; *See* Theophylline
Unipolar chest leads, 732, 733*t*
Unipolar limb leads, 732, 733*t*
United Ostomy Association of America, Inc., 1302
Universal skin lesion, 471*t*

sed assistive personnel, 4
a boot, 822
noprostone isopropyl, 1099*c*
Unrelieved pain, 36*t*
Unroofing of skin lesion, 477
Unstable angina, 848, 849
Unstable bladder, 1561
Unstable plaque, 794
Upper airway obstruction, 596, 597*f*
Upper esophageal sphincter, 1217
  gastroesophageal reflux disease and, 1243
Upper extremity
  amputation of, 1199
  fracture of, 1195
    care after cast removal, 1194*c*
    casts used for, 1188*t*
    traction for, 1190*t*
  subclavian steal and, 815
  thoracic outlet syndrome and, 815
Upper gastrointestinal bleeding, 1271*c*, 1271*f*, 1271-1272
Upper gastrointestinal radiographic series, 1226
  in diverticulitis, 1335
  in peptic ulcer disease, 1273-1274
Upper motor neuron lesion, 994
Upper respiratory disorders, 590-608
  epistaxis in, 591-592, 592*c*, 592*f*
  facial trauma in, 593-594
  head and neck cancer in, 597-606
    anxiety in, 604
    assessment in, 598*t*, 598-599
    disturbed body image in, 604
    health care resources in, 606
    health teaching in, 605*c*, 605-606, 606*f*
    home care management in, 605, 605*c*
    nursing diagnoses in, 599
    pathophysiology of, 597-598
    psychosocial preparation for, 606
    respiratory obstruction in, 599-602, 600*t*, 601*f*, 603*f*
    risk for aspiration in, 603*c*, 603-604, 604*c*
    subcutaneous infusion therapy in, 237*t*
  laryngeal trauma in, 596
  nasal fracture in, 590-591, 591*f*
  nasal polyps in, 592
  neck trauma in, 596-597
  nose and sinus tumors in, 592-593
  obstructive sleep apnea in, 594
  upper airway obstruction in, 596, 597*f*
  vocal cord nodules and polyps in, 595, 595*c*, 595*f*
  vocal cord paralysis in, 591-595
Upper respiratory tract, 553*f*, 553-554, 554*f*
Upper trunk extension exercise, 986*c*
Uracil, 70
Urate stones, 1574*t*
Urea, chronic kidney disease and, 1609
Urea nitrogen
  in burn, 532*c*
  twenty-four hour urine collection range and, 1542*c*
Urecholine; *See* Bethanechol chloride
Uremia, 1535*t*, 1536
  in chronic kidney disease, 1609, 1609*c*
  pruritus in, 1614
Uremic colitis, 1611
Uremic frost, 1614
Uremic syndrome, 1609
Ureter, 1527*f*, 1532, 1532*f*
  hydronephrosis and hydroureter and, 1585*f*, 1585-1586
  physical assessment of, 1536-1537
Ureteral spasm, 1571
Ureteroiliosigmoidostomy, 1577*f*
Ureterolithiasis, 1570
Ureteropelvic junction, 1531
Ureteroplasty, 1589
Ureterosigmoidostomy, 1576, 1577*f*
Ureterostomy, 1577*f*
Ureterovesical junction, 1532, 1532*f*
Urethra, 1527*f*, 1532*f*, 1533, 1537
Urethral discharge, 1651, 1747
Urethral meatus, 1533
Urethral pressure profile, 1547
Urethral pressure profilometry, 1547, 1563
Urethral stricture, 1559, 1585-1586
Urethral syndrome, 1559
Urethritis, 1559
  bacterial prostatitis and, 1733
  chlamydial, 1747
  gonorrhea and, 1745*f*
  in Reiter's syndrome, 355
  sexually transmitted diseases and, 1739*t*
Urethroplasty, 1559
Urethroscopy, 1559
Urethrovaginal fistula, 1694
Urge urinary incontinence, 1560*t*, 1561, 1567-1568, 1568*c*
Urgency, 1535*t*
  in cystitis, 1553
Urgent surgery, 243*t*
Urgent triage category, 131-132, 132*t*
Uric acid, 1163
Uric acid stones, 1574*t*
Urinalysis, 1538-1541, 1539*t*
  in acute glomerulonephritis, 1591
  in benign prostatic hypertrophy, 1714
  in chronic glomerulonephritis, 1592
  in chronic kidney disease, 1614
  in cystitis, 1554-1555
  in heart failure, 769
  in hydronephrosis and hydroureter and, 1586
  in polycystic kidney disease, 1583
  postoperative, 293
  preoperative, 249
  in pyelonephritis, 1588
  in renal cell carcinoma, 1595
  in renal trauma, 1597-1598
  in urethritis, 1559
  in urinary incontinence, 1563
  in urolithiasis, 1572
Urinary antiseptics, 1557*c*
Urinary assessment, 1526-1549
  anatomy and physiology review in, 1526-1533, 1527-1529*f*, 1530*t*, 1531*f*, 1531*t*, 1532*f*
  bladder scan in, 1542-1543, 1543*f*
  blood tests in, 1537-1538, 1538*c*
  in burn, 530-531
  computed tomography in, 1545-1546
  cystography and cystourethrography in, 1546
  cystoscopy and cystourethroscopy in, 1546-1547
  in hematologic disorders, 885
  intravenous urography in, 1543-1545, 1545*c*
  kidney, ureter, and bladder x-ray in, 1543
  patient history in, 1533-1536, 1534*c*, 1535*t*
  physical assessment in, 1536-1537, 1537*f*
  postoperative, 290
  psychosocial assessment in, 1537
  rehabilitation and, 97*t*, 98
  renal arteriography in, 1546
  renal biopsy in, 1547-1548
  renal changes with aging and, 1533, 1534*c*
  renography in, 1546
  retrograde procedures in, 1547
  in spinal cord injury, 994
  ultrasonography in, 1546
  urine tests in, 1538-1542, 1539*c*, 1540*t*
  urodynamic studies in, 1547
Urinary bladder, 1527*f*, 1532-1533
  benign prostatic hypertrophy and, 1714
  cancer of, 1575-1578, 1577*f*
Urinary bladder *(Continued)*
  catecholamine receptors and, 1416*t*
  female, 1643*f*
  infection of, 1533, 1551-1559
    community-based care in, 1558-1559
    drug therapy for, 1555-1558, 1556-1558*c*
    laboratory assessment in, 1554-1555
    nursing diagnoses in, 1555
    nutrition therapy for, 1558
    pathophysiology of, 1551-1553, 1552*t*, 1553*c*
    physical assessment in, 1553-1554, 1555*c*
    prevention of, 1553, 1554*c*
  physical assessment of, 1536-1537
  trauma to, 1578
Urinary bladder training, 1567*c*, 1567-1568
Urinary catheter
  for functional urinary incontinence, 1569
  home care of, 1725*c*
  postoperative monitoring of, 290
  preoperative preparation for, 255
  in spinal cord injury, 1000
  in transurethral resection of prostate, 1715
  urinary tract infection and, 1554
Urinary conduit, 1577*f*
Urinary disorders, 1550-1580
  bladder cancer in, 1575-1578, 1577*f*
  bladder trauma in, 1578
  cystitis in, 1551-1559
    community-based care in, 1558-1559
    drug therapy for, 1555-1558, 1556-1558*c*
    laboratory assessment in, 1554-1555
    nursing diagnoses in, 1555
    nutrition therapy for, 1558
    pathophysiology of, 1551-1553, 1552*t*, 1553*c*
    physical assessment in, 1553-1554, 1555*c*
    prevention of, 1553, 1554*c*
  urethral strictures in, 1559
  urethritis in, 1559
  urinary incontinence in, 1559-1570
    etiology of, 1561
    functional, 1568-1569
    health care resources for, 1569-1570
    health teaching in, 1569, 1570*c*
    history of, 1562, 1562*c*
    home care management in, 1569
    imaging studies in, 1563
    incidence and prevalence of, 1562
    laboratory assessment in, 1563
    nursing diagnoses in, 1563
    older adult and, 1561, 1562*c*
    physical assessment in, 1562-1563
    psychosocial preparation in, 1569
    reflex, 1568
    stress, 1564*c*, 1564-1566, 1565*c*, 1565*f*, 1566*t*
    total or mixed, 1569
    types of, 1560-1561*t*
    urge, 1567-1568, 1568*c*
  urolithiasis in, 1570-1575
    in gout, 353
    in hyperparathyroidism, 1461
    infection prevention in, 1573-1574
    nutrition history in, 1535
    Paget's disease of bone and, 1163
    pathophysiology of, 1570-1571, 1571*t*
    prevention of obstruction in, 1574*t*, 1574-1575, 1575*c*
    spinal cord injury-related, 998
    surgical management of, 1573
Urinary elimination
  chronic and disabling diseases and, 105*t*, 105-106
  postoperative monitoring of, 290
Urinary elimination *(Continued)*
  prostate cancer and, 1721
  spinal cord injury and, 997-998, 998*c*
Urinary frequency, 1535*t*
  in benign prostatic hypertrophy, 1713
  in chlamydial infection, 1747
  in cystitis, 1553
  in prostate cancer, 1720
  in prostatitis, 1733
  in urolithiasis, 1571-1572
Urinary habit training, 1567*c*, 1568
Urinary hesitancy, 1535*t*
Urinary 17-hydroxycorticosteroids
  in adrenal insufficiency, 1438
  in Cushing's disease, 1442
Urinary incontinence, 1559-1570
  after open radical prostatectomy, 1722
  in Alzheimer's disease, 975
  approaching death and, 115*c*
  etiology of, 1561
  functional, 1568-1569
  health care resources for, 1569-1570
  health teaching in, 1569, 1570*c*
  history of, 1562, 1562*c*
  home care management in, 1569
  imaging studies in, 1563
  incidence and prevalence of, 1562
  laboratory assessment in, 1563
  nursing diagnoses in, 1563
  older adult and, 23, 1561, 1562*c*
  physical assessment in, 1562-1563
  pressure ulcer prevention and, 486
  psychosocial preparation in, 1569
  reflex, 1568
  in spinal tumor, 1001
  stress, 1564*c*, 1564-1566, 1565*c*, 1565*f*, 1566*t*
  in stroke, 1047
  total or mixed, 1569
  types of, 1560-1561*t*
  urge, 1567-1568, 1568*c*
Urinary retention
  after lumbar spinal surgery, 987*c*
  in botulism, 1341
  epidural opioid-related, 53
  in hydronephrosis and hydroureter and, 1586
  older adult and, 1534*c*
  postoperative monitoring of, 290
Urinary system, 1526-1533
  age-related changes in fluid balance and, 174*c*
  age-related surgical risks and, 245*c*
  changes associated with aging, 1533, 1534*c*
  cirrhosis and, 1348*f*
  diabetes insipidus and, 1433*c*
  hepatitis A and, 1357*t*
  immobility and, 102*t*
  infusion therapy and, 235-236
  kidney in, 1526-1532
    hormonal functions of, 1531*t*, 1531-1532
    microscopic anatomy of, 1527-1528, 1528*f*, 1529*f*
    regulatory function of, 1528-1531, 1530*t*, 1531*f*
    structure of, 1526-1527, 1527*f*
  leukemia and, 903*c*
  nutrition screening assessment and, 1390*c*
  pathogen entry via, 442
  postoperative complications of, 287*t*
  premenstrual syndrome and, 1686*c*
  shock and, 829*c*
  sickle cell disease and, 895-896
  ureter in, 1532, 1532*f*
  urethra in, 1533
  urinary bladder in, 1532-1533
Urinary tract infection, 442, 1550-1559
  cystitis in, 1533, 1551-1559
    community-based care in, 1558-1559
    drug therapy for, 1555-1558, 1556-1558*c*

Urinary tract infection *(Continued)*
laboratory assessment in, 1554-1555
nursing diagnoses in, 1555
nutrition therapy for, 1558
pathophysiology of, 1551-1553, 1552*t*, 1553*c*
physical assessment in, 1553-1554, 1555*c*
prevention of, 1553, 1554*c*
diabetic patient and, 1506
factors contributing to, 1551*t*
factors influencing outcome of, 1552*t*
pyelonephritis in, 1586-1589, 1587*c*, 1587*f*
spinal cord injury-related, 998
urethritis in, 1559
Urine bilirubin
in cirrhosis, 1349, 1349*t*
in jaundice, 1346*t*
Urine color, 1538, 1539*t*
Urine crystals, 1541
Urine culture and sensitivity, 1541
in benign prostatic hypertrophy, 1714
in cystitis, 1555
Urine electrolytes, 1541
Urine glucose testing, 1475
Urine osmolarity, 1542
Urine output
in acute renal failure, 1604-1605
after renal transplantation, 1632
after transurethral resection of prostate, 1718
in burn, 531
in chronic glomerulonephritis, 1592
in chronic kidney disease, 1614
in crush syndrome, 1182
dehydration and, 179
fluid balance and, 175
in hypovolemic shock, 833, 835
postoperative monitoring of, 290
in renal cell carcinoma, 1596
in renal trauma, 1598
in sepsis, 839
in septic shock, 842
in severe sepsis, 840
Urine pH, 1538, 1539*t*
Urine sediment, 1541
Urine sodium, 1604
Urine specimen collection, 1540*t*
Urine stream testing, 1547
Urine tests, 1538-1542, 1539*c*, 1540*t*
in acute renal failure, 1604
in Cushing's disease, 1442
in diabetes mellitus, 1474-1475
in endocrine assessment, 1423*c*, 1423-1424
in gastrointestinal assessment, 1225
in reproductive assessment, 1653*c*
Urine urobilinogen, 1225
Uripas; *See* Flavoxate
Uristat; *See* Phenazopyridine
Urobilinogen, 1539*t*
in cirrhosis, 1349, 1349*t*
in gastrointestinal assessment, 1225
in jaundice, 1346*t*
Urochrome pigment, 1538
Urodynamic studies, 1547, 1714
Urogenital diaphragm, 1645*f*
Urography, 1563
Urolithiasis, 1570-1575
in gout, 353
in hyperparathyroidism, 1461
infection prevention in, 1573-1574
nutrition history in, 1535
Paget's disease of bone and, 1163
pathophysiology of, 1570-1571, 1571*t*
prevention of obstruction in, 1574*t*, 1574-1575, 1575*c*
spinal cord injury-related, 998
surgical management of, 1573
urinary tract infection and, 1551*t*
Urosepsis, 1553
Urothelial cancer, 1575-1578, 1577*f*
Urothelium, 1532, 1532*f*
Urotoin; *See* Nitrofurantoin
Uroxatral; *See* Alfuzosin
Urozide; *See* Hydrochlorothiazide
Urticaria, 481
in bee sting, 150
spironolactone-related, 1446
Usher's syndrome, 1130
Uterine artery embolization, 1696
Uterine fibroid embolization, 1696
Uterine leiomyoma, 1688, 1694-1699, 1695*f*, 1697*c*, 1697*t*, 1698*c*
Uterine tube, 1643, 1643*f*
Utero-ovarian ligament, 1643*f*
Uterosacral ligament, 1643*f*
Uterus, 1643, 1643*f*
cancer of, 1699-1702, 1700*t*, 1701*c*
dysfunctional uterine bleeding and, 1688-1689
endometrial biopsy and aspiration of, 1657
endometriosis and, 1687*f*, 1687-1688
fibroids of, 1694-1699, 1695*f*, 1697*c*, 1697*t*, 1698*c*
hysteroscopy of, 1656-1657
oxytocin and, 1415*t*
prolapse of, 1691-1694, 1692*f*, 1693*c*, 1693*f*
UTI; *See* Urinary tract infection
Uvea, 1071, 1071*f*
Uveitis, 1100

V

Vaccination
hepatitis B, 1358
for human papillomavirus, 1703, 1744
for influenza, 658
for primary cancer prevention, 411
for tuberculosis, 669
Vacuum constriction device, 1726
Vacuum-assisted wound closure, 495
in Crohn's disease fistula, 1332
in open fracture, 1193
Vagal maneuvers, 753-754
Vagal nerve stimulation, 960
Vagal reflex, 754
Vagal stimulation
for supraventricular tachycardia, 754
tracheostomy-related, 584
Vagina, 1643, 1643*f*
cancer of, 1708-1709
dryness in menopause, 1690
fistula of, 1694
sexually transmitted infection of, 1753
vulvovaginitis and, 1690-1691, 1691*c*
Vaginal bleeding
in cervical cancer, 1703
in uterine leiomyoma, 1695
Vaginal cone therapy, 1564-1566, 1565*f*
Vaginal discharge
in cervical cancer, 1703
in chlamydial infection, 1747
in gonorrhea, 1745
in vaginal infection, 1753
in vulvovaginitis, 1690
Vaginal sponge, toxic shock syndrome and, 1692*c*
Vaginal ultrasound, 1688
Vaginectomy, 1709
Vagotomy, 1278, 1278*f*
Vagotomy syndrome, 1261
Vagus nerve, 707, 935*t*
Valacyclovir
for genital herpes, 1742
for viral skin infection, 503
Valdecoxib, 1685
Valerian root, 246*t*
Validation therapy, 975
Valium; *See* Diazepam
Valproate, 958*c*
Valproic acid, 957*c*
Valsalva maneuver
in bladder training, 105-106
increased blood pressure in, 1496
mechanical ventilation and, 696
Valsalva maneuver *(Continued)*
for reflex urinary incontinence, 1568
sinus bradycardia and, 740
Valsartan, 771
Valtrex; *See* Valacyclovir
Valvular heart disease, 779*c*, 779-783, 782*f*, 783*c*
Valvuloplasty, 781-782
Vancomycin
for brain abscess, 1066
for inhalation anthrax, 673*c*
for methicillin-resistant *Staphylococcus aureus*, 503*c*
Vancomycin-intermediate *Staphylococcus aureus*, 448-449
Vancomycin-resistant *Enterococcus*, 448
Vancomycin-resistant *Staphylococcus aureus*, 448-449
Vanillylmandelic acid, 1446
VAP; *See* Ventilator-associated pneumonia
Vaprisol; *See* Conivaptan
Vardenafil, 1726
Variant angina, 849, 855
Varicella-zoster virus infection, 372
Varices, esophageal, 1345
Varicocele, 1731*f*, 1731-1732
Varicocelectomy, 1731-1732
Varicose veins, 822-823
Variola virus, 454*t*
Vas deferens, 1645*f*, 1646
Vasa recta, 1528, 1530*t*
Vascular access
for blood sample, 888
for hemodialysis, 1622-1625, 1623*t*, 1624*c*, 1625*f*
patient preparation for, 255
trauma patient and, 136-137
vascular access devices for, 215
veins for, 216*f*, 217
Vascular access device, 215
Vascular autoregulation, 797
Vascular degeneration, 970
Vascular disease, 793-825
acute peripheral arterial occlusion in, 810
aneurysms in, 810-814
of central arteries, 810-814, 811*f*
of peripheral arteries, 814
aortic dissection in, 814
arteriosclerosis and atherosclerosis in, 793-796, 794*f*, 794*t*, 796*t*
Buerger's disease in, 815
hypertension in, 796-804
cardiovascular assessment and, 716
concept map for, 800
diagnostic tests for, 799
drug therapy for, 801*t*, 801-802
health teaching in, 803-804
heart failure and, 767
heath care resources for, 804
history in, 798
home care management in, 802-803
ineffective therapeutic regimen management in, 802, 803*c*
lifestyle modifications in, 800-801
nursing diagnoses in, 799
pathophysiology of, 796-798, 796-798*t*
physical assessment in, 798-799, 799*f*
psychosocial assessment in, 799
peripheral arterial disease in, 804-810
community-based care in, 809*c*, 809-810, 810*c*
diagnostic tests for, 805-806
drug therapy for, 807
pathophysiology of, 804, 804*f*
physical assessment in, 805, 805*c*, 806*c*
surgical management of, 808*f*, 808-809
peripheral venous disease in, 816-823
phlebitis in, 823
varicose veins in, 822-823
Vascular disease *(Continued)*
vascular trauma in, 823
venous insufficiency in, 821-822, 822*c*
venous thromboembolism in, 816-821, 817*f*, 819*c*, 821*c*
popliteal entrapment in, 816
Raynaud's phenomenon in, 815-816, 816*f*
subclavian steal in, 815
thoracic outlet syndrome in, 815
Vascular system, 708-709
burn-related changes of, 523-524, 524*f*
cardiovascular assessment and, 704-729
arterial system and, 708-709
blood pressure and, 716
cardiac catheterization in, 722*t*, 722-724, 723*f*
changes associated with aging and, 709, 710*c*
current health problems in, 712-714, 713*t*
echocardiography in, 725
electrocardiography in, 724
electronic-beam computed tomography scan in, 726
electrophysiologic studies in, 724
extremities and, 715, 715*f*
family history and genetic risk in, 712
functional history in, 714, 714*t*
general appearance and, 714
Gordon's Functional Health Patterns and, 711*c*
hemodynamic monitoring in, 726-728, 727*c*, 727*f*
laboratory assessment in, 719-722, 720*c*
magnetic resonance imaging in, 726
myocardial nuclear perfusion imaging in, 725-726
nutrition history in, 712
precordium and, 717-719, 718*f*, 719*t*
psychosocial assessment and, 719
skin and, 715
stress test in, 724-725
transesophageal echocardiography in, 725
venous and arterial pulses in, 716-717, 717*f*
venous system and, 709
Vascular trauma, 823
Vascularization, tumor cell and, 404*f*
Vasculitis
in lupus erythematosus, 347
necrotizing, 354-355
in rheumatoid arthritis, 337, 338
Vasoactive drugs, 1625*t*
for esophageal varices, 1353
Vasoconstriction
in acute coronary syndromes, 848
mean arterial pressure and, 827, 829*f*
in Raynaud's phenomenon, 816
sympathetic stimulation and, 766
Vasoconstrictors for hypovolemic shock, 837*c*, 838
Vasodilation
mean arterial pressure and, 827, 829*t*
in myocardial infarction, 849
peripheral arterial disease and, 807
in septic shock, 841
Vasodilators
for heart failure, 863-864*c*
to reduce preload in heart failure, 773
Vasogenic edema
in brain tumor, 1060
in traumatic brain injury, 1051
Vasogenic shock, 828*t*
Vasomotor symptoms in menopause, 1689

...ssin, 1415, 1415t, 1425, 1530, 1531t
in cardiac arrest, 753c
deficiency of, 1427c
diabetes insipidus and, 1432
fluid balance and, 175, 176f
syndrome of inappropriate antidiuretic hormone secretion and, 1433-1436, 1435t
Vasopressors
for anaphylaxis, 393c
for septic shock, 843t
Vasospasm
cerebral, 1032, 1043-1044
in Raynaud's phenomenon, 815-816, 816f
Vasotec; *See* Enalapril
Vatronol; *See* Ephedrine sulfate
Vaughn-Williams classification of antidysrhythmics, 751
VDRL; *See* Veneral Disease Research Laboratory test
Vecuronium, 274t
for mechanical ventilation in burn, 535
for traumatic brain injury, 1057
Vegan diet, 1387
Vegetarian food pyramid, 1387, 1389f
Vein inflammation, 817
Vein transilluminator, 216
Veinlite LED, 216
VeinViewer, 216
Velban; *See* Vinblastine
Velbe; *See* Vinblastine
Velcade; *See* Bortezomib
Velcro straps, 103t
Velsar; *See* Vinblastine
Veneral Disease Research Laboratory test, 1652-1654, 1741
Venipuncture, 235
Veno-occlusive disease, 910
Venous access
for blood sample, 888
in hemodialysis, 1622-1623, 1623t, 1624c, 1624f
patient preparation for, 255
trauma patient and, 136-137
vascular access devices for, 215
veins for, 216f, 217
Venous beading in diabetic retinopathy, 1469
Venous duplex ultrasonography, 817
Venous insufficiency, 821-822, 822c
Venous leg ulcer disease, 821
Venous port, 218-219, 219f
Venous pulses, 716-717
Venous spasm, 229t
Venous stasis, 258
Venous stasis ulcer, 821-822
Venous system, 709
Venous thromboembolism, 816-821, 817f, 819c, 821c
fracture and, 1183
homocysteine and, 795
in pancreatic cancer, 1380
total hip arthroplasty and, 329, 330c, 330-331
Venous ulcer, 805, 806c
Ventilation and perfusion scanning, 566
Ventilation-perfusion mismatch
in acute respiratory distress syndrome, 686
in oxygenation failure, 685, 685t
in ventilatory failure, 685
Ventilator, 692-694, 693f
Ventilator alarms, 695, 695t
Ventilator dependence, 696, 697
Ventilator-associated pneumonia, 659, 660, 660c, 696
Ventilatory failure, 685, 685t
Ventilatory support
after brain tumor surgery, 1063
in amyotrophic lateral sclerosis, 1008
in burn, 535
in head and neck cancer, 600-601
Ventilatory support *(Continued)*
in heart failure, 770, 771c
in respiratory acidosis, 209
in traumatic brain injury, 1056
Ventolin; *See* Albuterol
Ventral hernia, 1291-1293, 1292f
Ventricular aneurysm, 758
Ventricular assist device, 774, 774f
Ventricular asystole, 749f, 750
Ventricular dysrhythmias, 747-750, 748f, 749f, 849
Ventricular escape rhythm, 747
Ventricular failure, 765
Ventricular fibrillation, 748-750, 749f
in coronary artery disease, 850
in hypothermia, 153
in lightning strike, 151
Ventricular gallop, 718-719
Ventricular remodeling, 766, 849
Ventricular septal myectomy, 789
Ventricular standstill, 749f, 750
Ventricular tachycardia, 747, 748, 749f
Ventriculoatrial shunt, 1064
Ventriculomyomectomy, 789
Ventriculoperitoneal shunt, 1064
Ventriculostomy, 1064
Venturi mask, 576-577, 577f, 577t
Venule, 708, 709
VePesid; *See* Etoposide
Verapamil, 744c
Verbal communication, stroke and, 1046, 1046t
Verbal descriptive pain scale, 43
Vermiform appendix, 1219
Vermox; *See* Mebendazole
Versed; *See* Midazolam
Vertebrae
musculoskeletal assessment of, 1146
osteoporosis and, 1155-1156, 1156f
Paget's disease of bone and, 1163
scoliosis and, 1173-1174, 1174f
Vertebral artery, 932f
Vertebral fracture, 1198c, 1198-1199
Vertebrobasilar artery, 1033c
Vertebroplasty, 1160, 1198, 1198c
Verteporfin, 1101
Vertical compression injury of spine, 991, 991f
Vertical laryngectomy, 600t
Vertical-banded gastroplasty, 1406
Vertigo, 1112, 1114, 1117, 1126-1127
Very-low-calorie diet, 1404
Vesicants, extravasation of, 217, 423, 424c
Vesicle, 469f, 1742
Vesicoureteral reflux, 1551t
Vesicouterine pouch, 1643f
Vesicovaginal fistula, 1694
Vesicular breath sounds, 562, 563t
Vestibular system, 1126
Vestibule
of ear, 1110f, 1111
vaginal, 1642
Vestibulocochlear nerve, 1110f
acoustic neuroma of, 1129
functions of, 935t
Veterinary Medical Assistance Team, 162
Viagra; *See* Sildenafil
Vibramycin; *See* Doxycycline
Vicodin; *See* Hydrocodone-acetaminophen
Vicoprofen; *See* Hydrocodone-ibuprofen
Vidarabine, 1086c
Vidaza; *See* Azacitidine
Video angiography in burn assessment, 531
Video-assisted thoracoscopic surgery, 646
Videx; *See* Didanosine
Vinblastine, 421t, 1730
Vincristine, 422t
for brain tumor, 1062
for spinal tumor, 1002
Vinorelbine, 422t
Viokase; *See* Pancrelipase
Violin spider, 147, 147f
Vira-A; *See* Vidarabine
Viracept; *See* Nelfinavir
Viral burden testing, 374
Viral carcinogenesis, 408, 408t
Viral infection
in avian influenza, 667-668
cutaneous, 499-501, 500c, 501f
in encephalitis, 963-965, 964c
in gastroenteritis, 1319t, 1319-1321, 1321c
in genital herpes, 1742c, 1742-1743, 1743c
Guillain-Barré syndrome and, 1012
in hepatitis, 1356-1360, 1357t, 1358c, 1361c
human immunodeficiency virus, 363-383
chronic low self-esteem in, 381-382
diarrhea in, 380-381
disturbed thought processes in, 381
drug therapy for, 375-379, 376-378c
etiology and genetic risk in, 363f, 363-366, 364f, 365t
health care resources for, 383
health teaching in, 383, 384c
home care management of, 382, 383c
impaired gas exchange in, 379
impaired skin integrity in, 381
incidence and prevalence of, 366f, 366-367, 367f
laboratory assessment in, 373-374
nursing diagnoses in, 374-375
nutritional status and, 380
pain in, 379-380
parenteral transmission of, 367-368
patient history and, 370
perinatal transmission of, 368
physical assessment in, 370-373, 371c, 372t
psychosocial assessment in, 373
risk for infection in, 375, 375c, 376c
sexual transmission of, 367, 368c
social isolation in, 382
testing for, 369-370, 370c
transmission and health care workers and, 368-369, 369c
in influenza, 658-659
in leukemia, 906
in meningitis, 961-963, 962c, 962t, 963c
multiple sclerosis and, 1003
in osteomyelitis, 1164-1167, 1165f, 1166c
in pharyngitis, 655-657, 656c, 656t
in pneumonia, 659-666
concept map for, 662
health care resources for, 666
health teaching in, 665-666
history in, 660-661
home care management in, 665, 665c
imaging assessment in, 663
impaired gas exchange in, 664, 664c
ineffective airway clearance in, 664
laboratory assessment in, 663, 663f
nursing diagnoses in, 663-664
pathophysiology of, 659, 659t
physical assessment in, 661, 663t
prevention of, 660, 660c
psychosocial assessment in, 661
risk in chronic obstructive pulmonary disease, 633
sepsis in, 664-665, 665t
in rhinitis, 654
in severe acute respiratory syndrome, 666-667
skin culture in, 477
in stomatitis, 1231-1234, 1233c, 1233f
in tonsillitis, 657, 657c
Tzanck smear for, 502
Viral load testing, 374
Viramune; *See* Nevirapine
Virazole; *See* Ribavirin
Virchow's triad, 817
Viread; *See* Tenofovir
Viremia, 367
Virilization, 1427
Viroptic; *See* Trifluridine
Virtual colonoscopy, 1228
Virulence, 440
Visceral pain, 38, 38t
Visceral pericardium, 705f
Visceral pleura, 556
Visceral proteins, 1393
Vision assessment, 1070-1083
anatomy and physiology review in, 1070-1074, 1071-1074f, 1073t
changes associated with aging and, 1074, 1075c, 1075f
corneal staining in, 1079-1080
electroretinography in, 1082
fluorescein angiography in, 1081c, 1081-1082
health promotion and maintenance and, 1074-1075, 1076c
imaging studies in, 1079
inspection in, 1077
laboratory assessment in, 1079
ophthalmoscopy in, 1080-1081, 1081f, 1081t
patient history in, 1075-1077, 1076c, 1076t
psychosocial assessment in, 1079
slit-lamp examination in, 1079, 1080f
tonometry in, 1080, 1080f
vision testing in, 1077-1079, 1078f, 1079f
Vision Compensation Behaviors, 1106-1107
Vision problems, 1084-1108
after transient ischemic attack, 1030c
after traumatic brain injury, 1055
application of eye patch for, 1088c
application of ocular compress for, 1087c
blepharitis in, 1084-1085
cataracts in, 1091f, 1091-1095, 1092f, 1092t, 1094f, 1095c
chalazion in, 1087
conjunctival hemorrhage in, 1087
conjunctivitis in, 1087-1088
contusion of eye in, 1103
corneal abrasion, ulceration, and infection in, 1089
in diabetes mellitus, 1469, 1469f
drug therapy for inflammation and infection of eye, 1086c
ectropion in, 1085
entropion in, 1085, 1085c, 1085f
foreign body in eye in, 1103-1104
glaucoma in, 1095t, 1095-1098, 1099-1100c
hordeolum in, 1085-1087
in hyperthyroidism, 1450, 1450f, 1455
hyphema in, 1103
in hypopituitarism, 1426
insertion and removal of ocular prosthesis, 1105c
instillation of ophthalmic ointment and, 1085c
irrigation of eye in, 1104c
keratoconjunctivitis sicca in, 1087
keratoconus and corneal opacities in, 1089f, 1089-1091, 1090f, 1091t
laceration of eye in, 1104
macular degeneration in, 1100-1101
ocular melanoma in, 1104-1106
penetrating injury of eye in, 1104
promotion of independent living in patient with impaired vision, 1098c
reduced vision in, 1106c, 1106-1107
refractive errors in, 1102-1103
retinal holes, tears, and detachments in, 1101-1102, 1102f
retinitis pigmentosa in, 1102

- Vision problems *(Continued)*
  - trachoma in, 1088
  - uveitis in, 1100
  - vitreous hemorrhage in, 1098-1100
- Vision testing, 1077-1079, 1078*f*, 1079*f*
- Vision-like experiences, approaching death and, 116*c*
- Vistaril; *See* Hydroxyzine
- Visual acuity, 1077-1078, 1078*f*
  - cataract and, 1092
  - vitreous hemorrhage and, 1100
- Visual Analog Dyspnea Scale, 626, 626*f*
- Visual analog pain scale, 43, 43*f*
- Visual compensation behavior in cataract, 1093
- Visual evoked potentials, 947
- Visual field testing, 1078
- Vital signs
  - postoperative, 287-289
  - preoperative, 247
- Vitamin A deficiency, 1394*t*
- Vitamin B_{12}
  - deficiency of, 1394*t*
    - anemia in, 893*t*
    - neurologic manifestations of, 886
    - presbycusis and, 1130
  - supplementation in chronic gastritis, 1268
- Vitamin C deficiency, 1394*t*
- Vitamin D
  - bone and, 1142
  - chronic kidney disease and, 1610
  - deficiency of
    - in hyperparathyroidism, 1463
    - osteomalacia and, 1160-1162, 1161*t*
  - osteoporosis and, 1154
  - renal activation of, 1531*t*, 1532
  - skin and, 461, 463*t*, 520
  - steroid therapy and, 344
  - supplementation of
    - in hypophosphatemia, 195
    - in osteomalacia, 1162
    - for osteoporosis prevention, 1159-1160
- Vitamin K_1 for warfarin reversal, 680
- Vitamin supplementation
  - in acute renal failure, 1606*c*
  - in chronic kidney disease, 1617-1618
  - in cystic fibrosis, 635
  - in fibrocystic breast condition, 1661
  - in vitamin B_{12} deficiency, 900
- Vitiligo, 1113, 1422
- Vitrectomy, 1100
- Vitreous body, 1071, 1071*f*
- Vitreous hemorrhage, 1098-1100
- Vitreous humor, 1072*f*
- Vivol; *See* Diazepam
- VMA; *See* Vanillylmandelic acid
- VMAT; *See* Veterinary Medical Assistance Team
- Vocal cords, 553*f*
  - nodules and polyps of, 595, 595*c*, 595*f*
  - paralysis of, 591-595
- Vocal fremitus, 561
- Vocal resonance, 564
- Vocational assessment, rehabilitation and, 99
- Vocational counselor, 96
- Voice box, 553*f*, 554, 554*f*
- Voice sounds, 564
- Voice test for hearing, 1115
- Voided urine specimen, 1540*t*
- Voiding, 1533
- Voiding cystourethrography, 1544*t*
  - in bladder trauma, 1578
  - in urinary incontinence, 1563
- Volkmann's canal, 1141
- Volkmann's contracture, 1181
- Voltaren; *See* Diclofenac
- Volume expanders, 837
- Volume-cycled ventilator, 693, 693*f*
- Voluntary active euthanasia, 122*t*
- Volunteer assistance in disaster, 162
- Volutrauma, mechanical ventilation and, 696
- Volvulus, 1249, 1303, 1303*f*
- Vomiting
  - in acute glomerulonephritis, 1591
  - in acute mountain sickness, 155
  - in acute renal failure, 1603
  - in aortic dissection, 814
  - in bee sting, 149
  - in black widow spider bite, 148
  - in botulism, 1342
  - chemotherapy-related, 427-428, 429*c*
  - in chronic kidney disease, 1611
  - in coral snake envenomation, 146
  - in diverticulitis, 1335
  - end-of-life care and, 118
  - epidural opioid-related, 53
  - in *Escherichia coli* infection, 1341
  - in food poisoning, 1341
  - in gallstones, 1370
  - in heat exhaustion, 142
  - in hypercalcemia, 194
  - in hyperparathyroidism, 1461
  - in hypokalemia, 188
  - in hypomagnesemia, 196
  - in labyrinthitis, 1127
  - in lung cancer, 644
  - in malnutrition, 1392
  - in migraine headache, 951
  - opioid analgesic-related, 48, 49*t*
  - in peptic ulcer disease, 1273
  - in pit viper envenomation, 144
  - postoperative assessment of, 290-291, 291*t*
  - in tube feeding, 1399
  - in urolithiasis, 1571
  - in vertigo, 1126
- von Hippel-Lindau syndrome, 1595
- VP-16; *See* Etoposide
- VTE; *See* Venous thromboembolism
- Vulva, 1642
  - Bartholin cyst of, 1699
  - cancer of, 1705*t*, 1707-1708, 1708*f*
  - infection of, 1690-1691, 1691*c*
  - self-examination of, 1650, 1650*c*
- Vulvectomy, 1707, 1708*f*
- Vulvovaginitis, 1690-1691, 1691*c*
- Vytorin; *See* Ezetimibe-simvastatin

W

- Wada test, 961
- Waist circumference, 1402
- Waist-to-hip ratio, 1402
- Walker, 101*f*, 1193-1194
- Walker-assisted gait training, 101*c*
- Walking cast, 1188*t*
- Walking meditation, 10
- Walking wounded, mass casualty conditions and, 161
- Wandering in Alzheimer's disease, 976-977
- Warfarin
  - after stroke, 1043
  - after total hip arthroplasty, 330
  - for atrial fibrillation, 746
  - contraindication for phenytoin, 958
  - for deep vein thrombosis, 819
  - for primary pulmonary hypertension, 637
  - prothrombin time and, 888-889
  - for pulmonary embolism, 680, 681*c*
  - for valvular heart disease, 781
- Warfilone; *See* Warfarin
- Warm antibody anemia, 899
- Warm phase of peripheral nerve trauma, 1023
- Warming methods
  - in frostbite, 154
  - in hypothermia, 153
- Washed red blood cells, 917*t*
- Wasp sting, 149-150, 150*c*
- Watch test for hearing, 1115
- Water
  - diabetes insipidus and, 1432
  - fluid and electrolyte balance and, 171-174
    - diffusion and, 172*f*, 172-173
    - filtration and, 171*f*, 171-172, 172*f*
    - lymph and, 174
    - osmosis and, 173*f*, 173-174
  - homeostasis and, 170-171, 171*f*
  - insensible loss of, 175
  - tubular reabsorption of, 1530
- Water brash, 1245
- Water moccasin envenomation, 144-145, 145*f*
- Water retention
  - cardiovascular assessment and, 714
  - fluid overload and, 182-183
  - mechanical ventilation and, 696
  - in right-sided heart failure, 768
  - in syndrome of inappropriate antidiuretic hormone secretion, 1435
- Weakness
  - in acute compartment syndrome, 1181
  - in amyotrophic lateral sclerosis, 1007
  - assessment before rehabilitation, 98
  - in black widow spider bite, 148
  - end-of-life care and, 116
  - in Guillain-Barré syndrome, 1012
  - in heat exhaustion, 142
  - in high altitude pulmonary edema, 155
  - in hyperaldosteronism, 1446
  - in hypercalcemia, 194
  - in hypernatremia, 186
  - in hyperthyroidism, 1450
  - in hypokalemia, 188
  - in hypomagnesemia, 196
  - in hyponatremia, 185
  - in hypophosphatemia, 195
  - in hypothermia, 153
  - in hypothyroidism, 1457
  - in hypovolemic shock, 835
  - in influenza, 658
  - in leukemia, 903
  - musculoskeletal assessment and, 1144-1145
  - in myasthenia gravis, 1016
  - in osteomalacia, 1162
  - in pit viper envenomation, 144
  - in systemic lupus erythematosus, 349
- Weaning
  - from mechanical ventilation, 696-697, 697*t*
  - from tracheostomy, 586-587
- Weapons of mass destruction, 160
- Wearing off phenomenon in Parkinson disease, 967
- Weber tuning fork test, 1116
- Wedge resection in lung cancer, 646
- Weight
  - fluid overload and, 182-183
  - low back pain and, 986
  - nutritional assessment and, 1389-1390
  - obesity and, 1402
  - of older adult, 1390, 1419*c*
- Weight gain
  - in acute renal failure, 1603
  - cardiovascular assessment and, 714
  - in hypothyroidism, 1457
  - in patient undergoing rehabilitation, 100
- Weight loss
  - in burn patient, 537
  - in chronic obstructive pulmonary disease, 624
  - in chronic pancreatitis, 1377, 1378
  - in Crohn's disease, 1331
  - dehydration and, 178
  - in hyperparathyroidism, 1461
  - in leukemia, 904
  - in lung cancer, 644
  - in obstructive sleep apnea, 594
  - in pancreatic cancer, 1380
  - in rheumatoid arthritis, 338
  - in tuberculosis, 669
- Weight-bearing pelvic fracture, 1198
- Wellness promotion in older adult population, 16, 16*c*
- Wernicke's aphasia, 1046, 1046*t*
- Wernicke's area, 930
- West Nile virus, 964, 964*c*
- Western blot, 374
- Wet age-related macular degeneration, 1101
- Wet preparation, 1654, 1654*t*
- Wet-to-damp saline-moistened gauze for wound d[ac]ebridement, 493*t*
- Wheal, 470*f*
- Wheal-and-flare reaction, 149
- Wheelchair or chair to bed transfer, 100*c*
- Wheezing, 563*t*
  - in anaphylaxis, 392
  - in asthma, 612
  - in chronic obstructive pulmonary disease, 626
  - in left-sided heart failure, 769, 854
  - in pneumonia, 661
- Whipple procedure
  - in gastric cancer, 1281-1282
  - in pancreatic cancer, 1382-1384, 1383*f*, 1383*t*
  - in Zollinger-Ellison syndrome, 1279
- White blood cell
  - cell-mediated immunity and, 317
  - functions of, 308, 309*t*, 878, 878*t*
  - infection and, 838-839
  - inflammation and, 313
  - in urine, 1539*t*
- White blood cell count
  - in acute pancreatitis, 1374, 1374*t*
  - in allergic rhinitis, 389
  - in appendicitis, 1316
  - in brain abscess, 1066
  - in burn, 531-532
  - in cardiovascular assessment, 722
  - in cholecystitis, 1369
  - in cirrhosis, 1350
  - in cystitis, 1555
  - in diverticulitis, 1335
  - in hematologic assessment, 887*c*
  - in human immunodeficiency virus infection, 373
  - for infection assessment, 450
  - in intestinal obstruction, 1304
  - in meningitis, 962
  - in osteomyelitis, 1166
  - in peritonitis, 1318
  - preoperative assessment of, 251*c*
  - in respiratory assessment, 565*c*
  - in rheumatoid arthritis, 340
  - in sepsis, 841
  - in septic shock, 842
  - in severe sepsis, 840
  - in sickle cell disease, 896
- White blood cell disorders, 902-916
  - Hodgkin's lymphoma in, 913*t*, 913-914
  - leukemia in, 902-913
    - conditions associated with genetic predisposition for, 410*t*
    - fatigue in, 910-911, 911*c*
    - health care resources for, 912
    - health teaching in, 911-912, 912*c*
    - hematologic assessment in, 409*c*
    - hematopoietic stem cell transplantation in, 907*t*, 907-910, 909*f*
    - history in, 903
    - home care management in, 911, 911*c*
    - imaging studies in, 904
    - laboratory assessment in, 904
    - nursing diagnoses in, 904
    - pathophysiology of, 902-903
    - physical assessment in, 903*c*, 903-904
    - psychosocial assessment in, 904
    - psychosocial preparation in, 912
    - risk for infection in, 905*c*, 905-907, 912*c*
    - risk for injury in, 910, 910*c*
  - multiple myeloma in, 915
  - non-Hodgkin's lymphoma in, 914-915
- White blood cell transfusion, 917*t*, 920

…atter
…ain, 929
…pinal cord, 931, 932*f*
Whitehead, 515
Whole-pancreas transplantation, 1498
Wide excision in skin cancer, 512
Wig for cancer patient, 430
Williams position, 985
Windpipe, 554, 555*f*
Winpred; *See* Prednisone
Withdrawal behavior, approaching death and, 116*c*
Withdrawal syndrome, 80
  alcohol and, 84, 84*t*
  amphetamines and methamphetamines and, 86, 86*t*
  barbiturates and, 89
  cocaine and, 86
  nicotine and, 84-85
  opioid analgesics and, 90
  physical dependence and, 40
Withdrawing or withholding life-sustaining therapy, 121, 122*t*
Women's health
  autoimmune disorders and, 396
  blood cell counts and, 882
  breast cancer and, 1663-1681
    anxiety in, 1671-1672
    BRCA1 and *BRCA2* gene mutations and, 73, 78, 1647
    breast reconstruction in, 1675, 1676*t*, 1677*c*
    breast self-examination and, 1666, 1667*f*
    chemotherapy in, 1677*t*, 1677-1679
    clinical breast examination and, 1666-1668, 1667*f*
    complementary and alternative therapies in, 1672, 1672*t*
    conditions associated with genetic predisposition for, 410*t*
    cultural considerations in, 1664-1665
    etiology and genetic risk in, 1664, 1665*t*
    health care resources for, 1681
    health teaching in, 1679-1680
    history in, 1669-1670
    home care management in, 1679, 1679*c*, 1680*c*
    imaging studies in, 1670-1671
    incidence and prevalence of, 1664
    invasive, 1663*f*, 1663-1664, 1664*f*
    laboratory assessment in, 1670
    mammography and, 1665-1666
    metastasis in, 1672
    noninvasive, 1663
    nursing diagnoses in, 1671
    in older adult, 1668-1669
    options for high-risk women, 1669
    physical assessment in, 1670, 1670*c*
    psychosocial assessment in, 1670
    psychosocial preparation in, 1680-1681
    radiation therapy in, 1676-1678, 1677*t*
    sites of metastasis for, 405*t*
    stem cell transplantation in, 1679
    subtypes of, 1671

Women's health *(Continued)*
    surgical management of, 1672-1675, 1673*f*, 1675*c*
    in young women, 1664
  cancer incidence and death, 406*f*
  carpal tunnel syndrome and, 1206-1207
  chronic calcium loss and, 192
  coronary artery disease and, 709, 712
    age and, 850
    atypical angina in, 853
    family history and, 850
    health promotion behaviors and, 853
  gallstones and, 1368
  human immunodeficiency virus infection and, 366, 367*f*
  migraine headaches and, 951
  osteoporosis and, 1143, 1153-1160
    community-based care for, 1160
    drug therapy for, 1157-1160, 1158-1159*c*
    exercise and, 1157
    history in, 1155
    hypocalcemia and, 193
    imaging studies in, 1156-1157
    laboratory assessment in, 1156
    lifestyle changes in, 1157
    nursing diagnoses in, 1157
    nutrition therapy in, 1157
    pathophysiology of, 1153*c*, 1153*t*, 1153-1155
    physical assessment in, 1155-1156, 1156*f*
    prevention of, 1155
    psychosocial assessment in, 1156
    surgery for, 1160
  pelvic inflammatory disease and, 1747-1753
    acute pain in, 1751-1752
    anxiety in, 1752
    community-based care in, 1752
    drug therapy for, 1749-1751, 1750-1751*c*
    fallopian tube cancer and, 1709
    history in, 1748
    infection control in, 1749
    laboratory assessment in, 1749
    Neisseria gonorrhoeae in, 1744
    nursing diagnoses in, 1749
    pathophysiology of, 1747-1748, 1748*f*
    physical assessment in, 1748, 1749*t*
    psychosocial assessment in, 1748-1749
  sexually transmitted diseases and, 1738
  sickle cell disease and, 898
  smoking and, 556
  substance abuse and, 81
  total body water and, 175
  urinary tract infection during pregnancy, 1558
Wood's light examination, 477
Work history in respiratory assessment, 556
World Health Organization
  analgesic ladder of, 48
  classification of lymphoma, 914

World Health Organization analgesic ladder of, 48
Worm infestation, 1339-1340
Wound assessment
  postoperative, 291*f*, 291-292
  in pressure ulcer, 488-490, 489*c*, 489*f*, 490*t*
Wound contamination, 490
  preoperative skin preparation and, 255
Wound dehiscence, 291*f*, 291-292, 296
Wound evisceration, 291*f*, 291-292, 296, 296*c*
Wound exudate, 490, 490*t*
Wound healing, 481-484
  classification of burn depth and, 521*t*
  mechanisms of, 482-484, 484*f*
  older adult and, 484
  phases of, 481, 481*t*, 482*f*, 483*t*
  postoperative assessment of, 291*f*, 291-292
Wound infection
  in brain tumor, 1064
  in coronary artery bypass graft, 869
  drug therapy for, 295-296
  in esophageal cancer, 1260
  laboratory assessment in, 490-491
  in peripheral arterial disease, 809
  in Whipple procedure, 1383*t*
Wound management
  in burn, 538-540, 539*t*
  in diabetes mellitus, 1503-1504
  in frostbite, 154
  in open fracture, 1193
  postoperative, 294-296, 295*c*, 295*f*
    in colorectal cancer, 1300, 1300*c*
    in laryngectomy, 601
    in open esophageal surgery, 1260
    in pancreatic cancer, 1383*t*
    in vulvectomy, 1708
Wrapping of stump, 1203*f*
Wrinkles, 465*f*
Wrist
  arthroplasty of, 335
  carpal tunnel syndrome and, 1206-1207
  fracture of, 1183, 1195
  positioning for prevention of contracture, 544*c*
Wrist drop, 281*c*
Wrist splint, 1187*f*

X

X chromosome, 74
Xalatan; *See* Latanoprost
Xanax; *See* Alprazolam
Xeloda; *See* Capecitabine
Xenical; *See* Orlistat
Xenograft
  for burn wound, 539
  in valvular heart disease, 782, 782*f*
Xenon, 947
Xenon computed tomography, 944*t*, 945
Xeroradiography, 1148
Xerosis, 465*f*, 480, 480*c*
Xerostomia
  after oral cancer surgery, 1238
  in postirradiation sialadenitis, 1240
  radiation therapy-related, 420, 599
  in Sjögren's syndrome, 396
Xibrom; *See* Bromfenac
Xigris; *See* Drotrecogin
Xolair; *See* Omalizumab
Xopenex; *See* Levalbuterol
Xylocaine; *See* Lidocaine
Xylose absorption, 1224*c*

Y

Y chromosome, 74
Yeast infection, 501
Yersinia pestis, 454*t*

Z

Zafirlukast, 610
Zagam; *See* Sparfloxacin
Zalcitabine, 379
Zamifenacin, 1291
Zanaflex; *See* Tizanidine
Zanamivir
  for avian influenza, 667
  for influenza, 658
Zanosar; *See* Streptozocin
Zantac; *See* Ranitidine
Zapex; *See* Oxazepam
Zarontin; *See* Ethosuximide
Zaroxolyn; *See* Metolazone
Zeaxanthin, 1101
Zebeta; *See* Bisoprolol
Zenapax; *See* Daclizumab
Zenker's diverticula, 1261-1262
Zerit; *See* Stavudine
ZES; *See* Zollinger-Ellison syndrome
Zetia; *See* Ezetimibe
Ziagen; *See* Abacavir
Ziconitide, 988-989
Zidovudine, 377*c*, 379
Zidovudine-lamivudine, 376*c*
Zidovudine-lamivudine-abacavir, 377*c*
Zileuton
  for allergic rhinitis, 391
  for asthma, 610
Zinacef; *See* Cefuroxime
Zinc deficiency, 1394*t*
Zinecard; *See* Dexrazoxane
Zithromax; *See* Azithromycin
Zocor; *See* Simvastatin
Zofran; *See* Ondansetron
Zoladex; *See* Goserelin
Zoledronic acid
  for bone cancer, 1169
  for osteoporosis prevention, 1160
  for Paget's disease of bone, 1164
Zollinger-Ellison syndrome, 1279
Zoloft; *See* Sertraline
Zometa; *See* Zoledronic acid
Zonegran; *See* Zonisamide
Zonisamide, 958*c*
Zovirax; *See* Acyclovir
Z-track method of intramuscular administration, 899*c*
Zyflo; *See* Zileuton
Zyloprim; *See* Allopurinol
Zymar; *See* Gatifloxacin
Zyrtec; *See* Cetirizine
Zyvox; *See* Linezolid